GREENFIELD'S

SURGERY

SCIENTIFIC PRINCIPLES AND PRACTICE

FIFTH EDITION

Editors

Michael W. Mulholland, MD, PhD
Frederick A. Coller Distinguished Professor
Surgeon-in-Chief
Chairman, Department of Surgery
University of Michigan
Ann Arbor, Michigan

Keith D. Lillemoe, MD
Jay L. Grosfeld Professor and Chairman
Department of Surgery
Indiana University School of Medicine
Surgeon-in-Chief
Indiana University Hospital
Indianapolis, Indiana

Gerard M. Doherty, MD
N.W. Thompson Professor of Surgery
Head, Section of General Surgery
Chief, Division of Endocrine Surgery
University of Michigan
Ann Arbor, Michigan

Illustrations by Holly R. Fischer, MFA

Ronald V. Maier, MD
Jane and Donald D. Trunkey Professor and Vice Chair of Surgery
University of Washington
Surgeon-in-Chief
Department of Surgery
Harborview Medical Center
Seattle, Washington

Diane M. Simeone, MD
Lazar J. Greenfield Professor of Surgery and Molecular & Integrative Physiology
Chief, Division of Gastrointestinal Surgery
Associate Chair of Research
University of Michigan
Ann Arbor, Michigan

Gilbert R. Upchurch, Jr., MD
Professor of Surgery
Leland Ira Doan Research Professor of Vascular Surgery
Department of Surgery
University of Michigan
Ann Arbor, Michigan

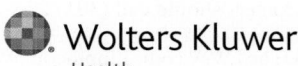

Wolters Kluwer | Lippincott Williams & Wilkins
Health
Philadelphia • Baltimore • New York • London
Buenos Aires • Hong Kong • Sydney • Tokyo

Acquisitions Editor: Brian Brown
Product Manager: Julia Seto
Production Manager: Bridgett Dougherty
Senior Manufacturing Manager: Benjamin Rivera
Marketing Manager: Lisa Lawrence
Design Coordinator: Stephen Druding
Production Service: Aptara, Inc.

Two Commerce Square
2001 Market Street
Philadelphia, PA 19103 USA
LWW.com

Printed in China

Library of Congress Cataloging-in-Publication Data

Greenfield's surgery : scientific principles and practice / editors, Michael W. Mulholland ... [et al.]; illustrations by Holly R. Fischer.—5th ed.
p. ; cm.
Other title: Surgery : scientific principles and practice
Includes bibliographical references and index.
Summary: "The Fifth Edition of Greenfield's Surgery has been thoroughly revised, updated, and refocused to conform to changes in surgical education and practice. Reflecting the increasingly clinical emphasis of residency programs, this edition features expanded coverage of clinical material and increased use of clinical algorithms. Key Points open each chapter, and icons in the text indicate where Key Points are fully discussed. Many of the black-and-white images from the previous edition have been replaced by full-color images"—Provided by publisher.
ISBN 978-1-60547-355-0 (hardback : alk. paper)
1. Surgery. 2. Medicine. I. Greenfield, Lazar J., 1934– II. Mulholland, Michael W. III. Title: Surgery : scientific principles and practice.
[DNLM: 1. General Surgery. 2. Surgical Procedures, Operative. WO 100 G812 2010]
RD31.S922 2010
617–dc22 2010024548

DISCLAIMER

Care has been taken to confirm the accuracy of the information presented and to describe generally accepted practices. However, the authors, editors, and publisher are not responsible for errors or omissions or for any consequences from application of the information in this book and make no warranty, expressed or implied, with respect to the currency, completeness, or accuracy of the contents of the publication. Application of the information in a particular situation remains the professional responsibility of the practitioner.

The authors, editors, and publisher have exerted every effort to ensure that drug selection and dosage set forth in this text are in accordance with current recommendations and practice at the time of publication. However, in view of ongoing research, changes in government regulations, and the constant flow of information relating to drug therapy and drug reactions, the reader is urged to check the package insert for each drug for any change in indications and dosage and for added warnings and precautions. This is particularly important when the recommended agent is a new or infrequently employed drug.

Some drugs and medical devices presented in the publication have Food and Drug Administration (FDA) clearance for limited use in restricted research settings. It is the responsibility of the health care provider to ascertain the FDA status of each drug or device planned for use in their clinical practice.

To purchase additional copies of this book, call our customer service department at (800) 638-3030 or fax orders to (301) 223-2320. International customers should call (301) 223-2300.

Visit Lippincott Williams & Wilkins on the Internet: at LWW.com. Lippincott Williams & Wilkins customer service representatives are available from 8:30 am to 6 pm, EST.

10 9 8 7 6 5 4 3 2 1

To my loving family.

—M.W.M.

To my wife, Cheryl, and our children, Chris, Shannon, Becky, and Heather for your love and support and to the surgical residents who have always stimulated me to stay "one step ahead."

—K.D.L.

To my wonderful family: Faith, Kevin, and Megan.

—G.M.D.

To Lauren, Michael, and Anna, for all you sacrifice for me.

—R.V.M.

Dedicated to the continual pursuit of Scientific knowledge to improve the lives of our patients.

—D.M.S.

To my family, Nancy, Rivers, Walker, Joe, and Antione, who remains supportive of my vocation as a surgeon

—G.R.U.

Keith D. Aaronson, MD
Associate Professor
Department of Internal Medicine
Division of Cardiovascular Medicine
University of Michigan
Ann Arbor, Michigan

N. Scott Adzick, MD
Surgeon in Chief
Department of Surgery
Children's Hospital of Philadelphia
Philadelphia, Pennsylvania

Sanjeev Aggarwal, MD
University Cardiothoracic Surgical
Louisville, Kentucky

Steven A. Ahrendt, MD
Associate Professor and Director
Section of Gastrointestinal Surgery
Department of Surgery and Pathology
University of Rochester
Rochester, New York

John J. Aiken, MD
Associate Professor of Pediatric Surgery
Medical College of Wisconsin
Milwaukee, Wisconsin

Gorav Ailawadi, MD
Assistant Professor
Department of Surgery
University of Virginia
Charlottesville, Virginia

Reginald Alouidor, MD
Assistant Professor of Surgery
Tufts University School of Medicine
Springfield, Massachusetts

Saman Arbabi, MD, MPH, FACS
Associate Professor
Department of Surgery
University of Michigan
Ann Arbor, Michigan

Subodh Arora, MD
Associate Professor of Surgery
George Washington University
Washington, DC

Ali Azizzadeh, MD
Assistant Professor
Cardiothoracic and Vascular Surgery
University of Texas at Houston Medical School
Medical Director, Vascular Laboratory, Staff Vascular Surgeon
Memorial Hermann Hospital
Houston, Texas

Ariel L. Barkan, MD
Professor of Medicine and Neurosurgery
University of Michigan
Ann Arbor, Michigan

Barbara L. Bass, MD
Professor
Department of Surgery
Weill Medical College of Cornell University
New York, New York;
Carolyn and John F. Bookout Chair
Department of Surgery
The Methodist Hospital
Houston, Texas

B. Timothy Baxter, MD
Professor
Department of Surgery
University of Nebraska Medical Center
Staff Surgeon
Department of Surgery
Nebraska Methodist Hospital
Omaha, Nebraska

Bradley D. Beasley, DPM, SWS
Private Practice
Restoration Foot and Ankle
Owasso, Oklahoma

Michael Belkin, MD
Associate Professor of Surgery
Harvard Medical School
Chief, Division of Vascular and Endovascular Surgery
Brigham and Women's Hospital
Boston, Massachusetts

Richard H. Bell, Jr., MD
Assistant Executive Director
The American Board of Surgery, Inc.
Philadelphia, Pennsylvania

Carlo Bellabarba, MD
Assistant Professor
Departments of Orthopaedics and Neurosurgery
University of Washington
Seattle, Washington

Christopher K. Bichakjian, MD
Assistant Professor
Department of Dermatology
University of Michigan
Ann Arbor, Michigan

Timothy R. Billiar, MD
The George Vance Foster Professor and Chair
Department of Surgery
Presbyterian University Hospital
University of Pittsburgh Medical Center
Pittsburgh, Pennsylvania

John D. Birkmeyer, MD
George D. Zuidema Professor of Surgery
Department of Surgery
University of Michigan
Director of Bariatric Surgery
Department of General Surgery
University Hospital
Ann Arbor, Michigan

C. Richard Boland, MD
Chief
Department of Internal Medicine, Division of Gastroenterology
Baylor University Medical Center
Dallas, Texas

Edward L. Bove, MD
Helen and Marvin Kirsch Professor
Professor and Section Head, Cardiac Surgery
C.S. Mott Children's Hospital
Ann Arbor, Michigan

Richard J. Bransford, MD
Assistant Professor
Department of Orthopaedics
University of Washington
Seattle, Washington

Robert S. Bresalier, MD
Professor of Medicine
Department of Gastrointestinal Medicine and Nutrition
University of Texas, MD Anderson Cancer Center
Houston, Texas

Jonathan R. Brody, PhD
Assistant Professor
Department of Surgery
Co-Director
Jefferson Pancreas, Biliary and Related Cancer Center
Thomas Jefferson University
Philadelphia, Pennsylvania

David L. Brown, MD, FACS
Associate Professor
Department of Surgery, Section of Plastic Surgery
University of Michigan
Ann Arbor, Michigan

Steven R. Buchman, MD
Professor, Plastic Surgery
Chief, Pediatric Plastic Surgery
Director, Craniofacial Anomalies Program
University of Michigan Health System
Ann Arbor, Michigan

Eileen M. Bulger, MD
Associate Professor
Department of Surgery
University of Washington School of Medicine
Associate Director
Emergency Surgical Services
Harborview Medical Center
Seattle, Washington

Andrew M. Cameron, MD, PhD
Assistant Professor
Department of Surgery
Johns Hopkins University School of Medicine
Director of Liver Transplant
Comprehensive Transplant Center
Johns Hopkins Hospital
Baltimore, MD

John L. Cameron, MD
Professor of Surgery
The Johns Hopkins University
Baltimore, Maryland

Darrell A. Campbell, Jr., MD
H. King Ransom Professor of Surgery
Department of Surgery
Chief of Staff
Office of Clinical Affairs
Division of Transplantation Surgery
University of Michigan
Ann Arbor, Michigan

Tony Capizzani, MD
Department of Surgery
University of Michigan Health System
Ann Arbor, Michigan

Marilia Cascalho, MD, PhD
Associate Professor of Surgery
Associate Professor of Microbiology and Immunology
Department of Transplant Biology
University of Michigan
Ann Arbor, Michigan

Darrell L. Cass, MD
Assistant Professor
Michael E. DeBakey Department of Surgery and Department of Pediatrics
Baylor College of Medicine
Co-Director, Texas Center for Fetal Surgery
Houston, Texas

Paul S. Cederna, MD
Associate Professor and Associate Chair
Department of Surgery
University of Michigan
Associate Chief of Staff
Office of Clinical Affairs
University of Michigan Health System
Ann Arbor, Michigan

Samuel Cemaj, MD
Assistant Professor
Department of Surgery
Creighton University Medical Center
Omaha, Nebraska

William F. Chandler, MD
Professor
Department of Neurosurgery
University of Michigan
Ann Arbor, Michigan

Andrew C. Chang, MD
Assistant Professor of Surgery
Section of Thoracic Surgery
University of Michigan
Ann Arbor, Michigan

Jens R. Chapman, MD
Professor of Orthopaedic Surgery and Sports Medicine
Joint Professor of Neurologic Surgery
Hans Joerg Wyss Endowed Chair
University of Washington School of Medicine
Harborview Medical Center
Seattle,Washington

Randall M. Chesnut, MD
Associate Professor, Neurosurgery
Director of Neurotrauma;
Chief, Neurosurgical Spine Service
University of Washington
Harborview Medical Center
Seattle, Washington

Kevin C. Chung, MD, MS
Assistant Dean for Faculty Affairs
University of Michigan Medical School
Professor of Surgery
Department of Surgery, Section of Plastic Surgery
University of Michigan Health System
Ann Arbor, Michigan

Robert E. Cilley, MD
Professor of Surgery and Pediatrics
Department of Surgery
Penn State University College of Medicine
Chief, Division of Pediatric Surgery
Department of Surgery
Milton S. Hershey Medical Center
Hershey, Pennsylvania

G. Patrick Clagett, MD
Professor and Chairman, Division of Vascular and Endovascular Surgery
Department of Surgery
University of Texas Southwestern Medical Center
Dallas, Texas

Bard C. Cosman, MD, MPH
Professor of Clinical Surgery
Department of Surgery
University of California, San Diego
Chief, Halasz General Surgery Section
Department of Surgical Service
VA San Diego Healthcare System
San Diego, California

Joseph Cuschieri, MD
Associate Professor
Department of Surgery
University of Washington School of Medicine
Harborview Medical Center
Seattle, Washington

Michael C. Dalsing, MD
Director of Vascular Surgery
Indiana University School of Medicine
Indianapolis, Indiana

Debra A. DaRosa, PhD
Professor of Surgery
Vice-Chair for Education
Department of Surgery
Northwestern University Feinberg School of Medicine
Chicago, Illinois

E. Patchen Dellinger, MD
Professor and Vice Chairman, Surgery
Associate Medical Director and Chief of General Surgery
University of Washington School of Medicine
Seattle, Washington

Eric J. DeMaria, MD
Director
Duke Health System Weight Loss Surgery Program
Durham, North Carolina

Eric J. Devaney, MD
Assistant Professor of Surgery
Section of Cardiac Surgery
University of Michigan
Ann Arbor, Michigan

Justin B. Dimick, MD, PhD
Assistant Professor
Department of Surgery
University of Michigan
Attending Surgeon
Department of Surgery
Ann Arbor VA Hospital
Ann Arbor, Michigan

Gerard M. Doherty, MD
N.W. Thompson Professor of Surgery
Head, Section of General Surgery
Chief, Division of Endocrine Surgery
University of Michigan
Ann Arbor, Michigan

Matthew O. Dolich, MD
Associate Clinical Professor
Department of Surgery
University of California Irvine
Irvine, California

Matthew J. Eagleton, MD
Assistant Professor
Department of Vascular Surgery
Cleveland Clinic Lerner College of Medicine of Case Western Reserve University
Staff, Vascular Surgery
The Cleveland Clinic Foundation
Cleveland, Ohio

Jonathan L. Eliason, MD
Assistant Professor
Department of Surgery
University of Michigan Health System
Ann Arbor, Michigan

Jean C. Emond, MD
Thomas S. Zimmer Professor
Department of Surgery
Director of Transplantation Services
Department of Surgery
New York Hospital—Columbia University Medical Center
New York, New York

Anthony L. Estrera, MD
Assistant Professor and Director, Cardiovascular Intensive Care Unit
Cardiothoracic and Vascular Surgery
University of Texas at Houston
Memorial Hermann Hospital
Houston, Texas

Mary E. Fallat, MD
Professor and Division Director of Pediatric Surgery
Department of Surgery
University of Louisville
Chief of Surgery and Trauma
Kosair Children's Hospital
Louisville, Kentucky

Emily Finlayson, MD
Assistant Professor
Division of General Surgery
University of California San Francisco
San Francisco, California

Robert J. Fitzgibbons, Jr., MD
Professor
Department of Surgery
Creighton University Medical Center
Omaha, Nebraska

Yuman Fong, MD
Murray F. Brennan Chair in Surgery
Chief, Gastric and Mixed Tumor Service
Department of Surgery
Memorial Sloan-Kettering Cancer Center
Professor of Surgery
Cornell University Medical College
New York, New York

Douglas L. Fraker, MD
Jonathan E. Rhoads Professor of Surgery
Department of Surgery
University of Pennsylvania
Philadelphia, Pennsylvania

David C. Frankenfield, MS, RD, CNSD
Chief Clinical Dietician
Penn State College of Medicine
M.S. Hershey Medical Center
Hershey, Pennsylvania

Chris E. Freise, MD
Associate Professor of Surgery
Transplant Division
University of California, San Francisco
San Francisco, California

Eric R. Frykberg, MD
Professor
Department of Surgery
University of Florida College of Medicine
Chief, Division of General Surgery
Shands Jacksonville Medical Center
Jacksonville, Florida

Joseph M. Galante, MD
Assistant Professor
Department of Surgery
University of California Davis Medical Center
Davis, California

Robert D. Galiano, MD
Assistant Professor
Department of Surgery
Northwestern University Feinberg School of Medicine
Attending Surgeon
Department of Surgery
Northwestern Memorial Hospital
Chicago, Illinois

Paul G. Gauger, MD
Professor
Department of Surgery, Division of Endocrine Surgery
University of Michigan
Ann Arbor, Michigan

Nicole S. Gibran, MD
Professor of Surgery
University of Washington
Director, University of Washington Burn Center
Harborview Medical Center
Seattle, Washington

A. Mark Gillinov, MD
Staff Surgeon, Judith Dion Pyle Chair in Heart Valve Surgery
Department of Thoracic and Cardiovascular Surgery
Cleveland Clinic
Cleveland, Ohio

Matthew A. Goettsch, MD
Department of Surgery
Creighton University Medical Center
Omaha, Nebraska

Jason S. Gold, MD
Assistant Professor of Surgery
Department of Surgery (Brigham and Women's Hospital)
Harvard Medical School
Boston, Massachusetts
Staff Surgeon
Department of Surgical Service
VA Boston Healthcare System
West Roxbury, Massachusetts

Joseph S. Gruss, MBBch, FRCSC
Professor
Department of Surgery
University of Washington
Marlys C. Larson Professor
Endowed Chair in Craniofacial Surgery
Seattle Childrens Hospital
Seattle, Washington

Ahmet Gurakar, MD
Medical Director, Liver Transplantation
The Johns Hopkins University School of Medicine
Baltimore, Maryland

Niraj J. Gusani, MD, MS, FACS
Assistant Professor
Department of Surgery, Division of Surgical Oncology
Penn State College of Medicine
Penn State Cancer Institue
Hershey, Pennsylvania

Jonathan W. Haft, MD
Assistant Professor
Department of Cardiac Surgery
University of Michigan
Ann Arbor, Michigan

Linnea S. Hauge, PhD
Assistant Professor of Surgery
Medical Education
Department of Surgery
University of Michigan
Ann Arbor, Michigan

Peter K. Henke, MD
Associate Professor of Surgery
Section of Vascular Surgery
University of Michigan
Ann Arbor, Michigan

Jennifer C. Hirsch, MD, MS
Assistant Professor
Department of Surgery and Pediatrics
University of Michigan
Ann Arbor, Michigan

Ronald B. Hirschl, MD
Arnold Coran Professor of Surgery
Head, Section of Pediatric Surgery
University of Michigan Health System
Ann Arbor, Michigan

Richard A. Hodin, MD
Professor
Department of Surgery
Harvard Medical School
Surgical Director, Crohn's and Colitis Center
Department of Surgery
Massachusetts General Hospital
Boston, Massachusetts

Richard A. Hopper, MD
Assistant Professor
Department of Plastic Surgery
University of Washington
Division Chief
Department of Pediatric Plastic Surgery
Seattle Children's Hospital
Seattle, Washington

Thomas J. Howard, MD
Willis D. Gatch Professor of Surgery
Department of Surgery
Indiana University School of Medicine
Indianapolis, Indiana
David B. Hoyt, MD
Executive Director
American College of Surgeons
Chicago, Illinois

David B. Hoyt, MD, FACS
John E. Connolly Professor of Surgery
Chairman, Department of Surgery
University of California, Irvine
Orange, California

Thomas S. Huber, MD, PhD
Professor and Chief
Division of Vascular Surgery
University of Florida College of Medicine
Attending Surgeon
Shands Hospital at the University of Florida
Gainesville, Florida

Tam T. Huynh, MD
Assistant Professor
Cardiothoracic and Vascular Surgery
University of Texas at Houston Medical School
Memorial Hermann Hospital
Houston, Texas

Ajay Jain, MD
Assistant Professor
Department of Surgery
University of Maryland
Chief, Section of Surgical Oncology
Department of Surgery
Baltimore VA Medical Center
Baltimore, MD

Craig M. Jarrett
Research Fellow
Department of Thoracic and Cardiovascular Surgery
Cleveland Clinic
Cleveland, Ohio

Timothy M. Johnson, MD
Professor of Dermatology, Otolaryngology, and Surgery
Chief, Cutaneous Surgery and Oncology Program
University of Michigan
Ann Arbor, Michigan

Gregory J. Jurkovich, MD
Professor
Department of Surgery
University of Washington
Chief, Trauma Service
Harborview Medical Center
Seattle, Washington

Jussuf T. Kaifi, MD, PhD
Assistant Professor
Department of Surgery, Division of Surgical Oncology
Pennsylvania State College of Medicine
Pennsylvania State Cancer Institute
Hershey, Pennsylvania

Larry R. Kaiser, MD
President
University of Texas Health Sciences Center
Alkek-Williams Chair
Cardiothoracic and Vascular Surgery
University of Texas Medical School at Houston
Houston, Texas

Eugene P. Kennedy, MD
Assistant Professor of Surgery
Thomas Jefferson University
Philadelphia, Pennsylvania

Sachin Kheterpal, MD, MBA
Assistant Professor
Department of Anesthesiology
University of Michigan Health System
Ann Arbor, Michigan

Lawrence T. Kim, MD
Professor
Department of Surgery
University of Arkansas for Medical Sciences
Chief
Department of Surgery
Central Arkansas Verterans Healthcare System
Little Rock, Arkansas

Eric T. Kimchi, MD, FACS
Assistant Professor
Department of Surgery, Division of Oncology
Penn State College of Medicine
Penn State Cancer Institute
Hershey, Pennsylvania

Tari A. King, MD
Associate Professor
Department of Surgery
Weill Medical College of Cornell
Associate Attending, Jeanne A Detrek Junior Faculty Chair
Memorial Sloan-Kettering Cancer Center
New York, New York

Andrew S. Klein, MD, MBA
Director, Comprehensive Transplant Center
Cedars-Sinai Medical Center
Los Angeles, California

Lauren Kosinski, MD
Assistant Professor
Department of Surgery
Medical College of Wisconsin
Froedtert Memorial Lutheran Hospital
Milwaukee, Wisconsin

Alexander S. Krupnick, MD
Instructor of Surgery
University of Washington School of Medicine
Seattle, Washington

John C. Kucharczuk, MD
Associate Professor of Surgery
University of Pennsylvania
Philadelphia, Pennsylvania

William M. Kuzon, Jr., MD, PhD
Professor and Section Head, Plastic Surgery
University of Michigan Health System
Ann Arbor, Michigan

Vibha Lama, MD
Assistant Professor
Department of Internal Medicine
University of Michigan Health System
Ann Arbor, Michigan

Wendy B. Landman, MD
Department of Radiology
Brigham and Women's Hospital
Boston, Massachusetts

Michael P. LaQuaglia, MD
Professor
Department of Surgery
Weill-Cornell Medical School
Chief
Department of Pediatric Surgerical Service
Memorial-Sloan Kettering Cancer Center
New York, New York

W. Anthony Lee, MD
Assistant Professor, Vascular Surgery
Department of Surgery
University of Florida College of Medicine
Gainesville, Florida

Steven K. Libutti, MD
Professor, Departments of Surgery and Genetics
Director
Montefiore-Einstein Center for Cancer Care
Montefiore Medical Center
Bronx, New York

Keith D. Lillemoe, MD
Jay L. Grosfeld Professor and Chairman
Department of Surgery
Indiana University School of Medicine
Surgeon-in-Chief
Indiana University Hospital
Indianapolis, Indiana

Jules Lin, MD
Assistant Professor
Section of Cardiothoracic Surgery
Department of Surgery
University of Michigan Health System
Ann Arbor, Michigan

Peter H. Lin
Professor of Surgery
Chief, Division of Vascular Surgery
Michael E. DeBakey Department of Surgery
Baylor College of Medicine
Houston, Texas

Virginia R. Little, MD
New York, New York

Ricardo V. Lloyd, MD, PhD
Professor of Pathology
Mayo Clinic College of Medicine
Consultant at Mayo Clinic
Rochester, Minnesota

G. Matthew Longo, MD
Assistant Professor, Department of Surgery
Section of General Surgery, Vascular Surgery
University of Nebraska Medical Center
Omaha, Nebraska

Kirk A. Ludwig, MD
The Vernon O. Underwood Professor
Department of Surgery
Medical College of Wisconsin
Chief of Colorectal surgery
Department of Surgery
Froedtert Memorial Lutheran Hospital
Milwaukee, Wisconsin

Robyn R. Macsata
Clinical Assistant Professor
Department of Surgery
Georgetown University Medical Center
Chief
Department of Vascular Surgery
VAMC
Washington, DC

Robert D. Madoff, MD
Professor
Department of Surgery
University of Minnesota
Minneapolis, Minnesota

David K. Magnuson, MD
Assistant Professor of Surgery and Pediatrics
Case Western Reserve University
Chief, Division of Pediatric Surgery
Rainbow Babies & Children's Hospital
Cleveland, Ohio

Raja S. Mahidhara, MD
Assistant Professor of Surgery
Section of Thoracic Surgery
University of Michigan Health System
Ann Arbor, Michigan

Ronald V. Maier, MD
Jane and Donald Trunkey Professor and Vice-Chairman of Surgery
University of Washington
Surgeon-in-Chief
Harborview Medical Center
Seattle, Washington

Michael R. Marvin, MD
Assistant Professor of Surgery
Department of Surgery, Divsion of Transplantation Surgery
University of Louisville
Chief
Department of Surgery, Divsion of Transplantation Surgery
Jewish Hospital
Louisville, Kentucky

Jeffrey B. Matthews, MD
Professor and Chairman
Dean for Clinical Affairs
Department of Surgery
University of Chicago
Surgeon-in-Chief
Department of Surgery
University of Chicago Hospital
Chicago, Illinois

Matthew T. Menard, MD
Co-Director of Endovascular Surgery
Division of Vascular and Endovascular Surgery
Brigham and Women's Hospital
Instructor in Surgery
Harvard Medical School
Boston, Massachusetts

Robert M. Merion, MD
Professor of Surgery
Department of Surgery
University of Michigan
Attending Transplant Surgeon
Department of Surgery
University of Michigan Health System
Ann Arbor, Michigan

Fabrizio Michelassi, MD
Lewis Atterbury Stimson Professor and Chairman
Department of Surgery
Weill Medical College of Cornell University
Surgeon-in-Chief
New York Presbyterian Hospital-Weill Cornell Medical Center
New York, New York

Tomislav Mihaljevic, MD
Staff
Department of Thoracic and Cardiovascular Surgery
Cleveland Clinic
Cleveland, Ohio

Dianna Milewicz, MD, PhD
Department of Internal Medicine
The University of Texas Health Science Center at Houston
Medical School
Houston, Texas

Barbara S. Miller, MD
Assistant Professor
Department of Surgery
Staff Physician
Division of Endocrine Surgery
University of Michigan

Mathew C. Miller, MD
Assistant Professor
Department of Otolaryngology
University of Rochester Medical Center
Rochester, New York

Charles C. Miller, III, PhD
Professor
Cardiothoracic and Vascular Surgery
Center for Clinical Research and Evidence-Based Medicine
Center for Biotechnology
University of Texas at Houston Medical School
Houston, Texas

Eugene Minevich, MD
Professor
Department of Surgery
Division of Pediatric Urology
Cincinnati Children's Hospital
Cincinnati, Ohio

Rebecca M. Minter, MD
Assistant Professor Surgery
Assistant Professor of Medical Education
Department of Surgery
University of Michigan Medical School
University of Michigan Health System
Ann Arbor, Michigan

Gregory L. Moneta, MD
Professor and Chief
Division of Vascular Surgery
Oregon Health & Science University
Portland, Oregon

Mark D. Morasch, MD
Associate Professor of Surgery
Division of Vascular Surgery
Northwestern University Feinberg School of Medicine
Attending Surgeon
Division of Vascular Surgery
Northwestern Memorial Hospital
Chicago, Illinois

Arden M. Morris, MD
Assistant Professor of Surgery
Section of General Surgery
Division of Colorectal Surgery
University of Michigan
Ann Arbor, Michigan

Monica Morrow, MD
Professor of Surgery
Weill Medical Collge of Cornell University
Chief, Breast Surgical Service
Department of Surgery
Memorial Sloan-Kettering Cancer Center
New York, New York

Jeffrey S. Moyer, MD, FACS
Assistant Professor
Department of Otolaryngology–Head and Neck Surgery
University of Michigan
Ann Arbor, Michigan

Michael W. Mulholland, MD, PhD
Professor and Chair
Department of Surgery
University of Michigan
Surgeon-in-Chief
Department of Surgery
University of Michigan Hospital
Ann Arbor, Michigan

Thomas A. Mustoe, MD
Chief of Plastic Surgery
Department of Surgery
Feinberg School of Medicine
Northwestern University
Chicago, Illinois

George B. Mychaliska, MD
Assistant Professor
Department of Pediatric Surgery
University of Michigan
Ann Arbor, Michigan

Christopher J. Myers, MD
Durham, North Carolina

Attila Nakeeb, MD
Associate Professor
Department of Surgery
Indiana University School of Medicine
Attending Surgeon
Indiana University Hospital
Indianapolis, Indiana

Avery B. Nathens, MD, PhD, MPH
Professor of Surgery
University of Toronto Faculty of Medicine
Toronto, Canada

Santhat Nivatvongs, MD
Professor of Surgery
Mayo Clinic College of Medicine
Rochester, Minnesota

Richard G. Ohye, MD
Assistant Professor, Departments of Surgery and Pediatrics and Communicable Diseases
Surgical Director, Pediatric Cardiac Transplantation
Director, Pediatric Cardiovascular Surgery Fellowship Program
University of Michigan
Ann Arbor, Michigan

Grant E. O'Keefe, MD
Professor of Surgery
Department of Surgery
University of Washington School of Medicine
Harborview Medical Center
Seattle, Washington

Keith T. Oldham, MD
Professor and Chief
Department of Surgery, Division of Pediatric Surgery
Medical College of Wisconsin
Surgeon-in-Chief
Department of Surgery
Children's Hospital of Wisconsin
Milwaukee, Wisconsin

John A. Olson, Jr., MD, PhD
Associate Professor
Department of Surgery
Duke University
Durham, North Carolina

Mary F. Otterson, MD
Professor
Department of Surgery
Medical College of Wisconsin
Physician
Department of Surgery
Froedtert Memorial
Milwaukee, Wisconsin

Francis D. Pagani, MD, PhD
Otto Gago, MD Professor in Cardiac Surgery
Director, Heart Transplant Program
Director, Center for Circulatory Support
Department of Surgery
University of Michigan
Ann Arbor, Michigan

Shawn J. Pelletier, MD
Assistant Professor
Department of Surgery
Division of Transplant Surgery
University of Michigan Health System
Ann Arbor, Michigan

Jeffrey H. Peters, MD
Professor and Chairman
Department of Surgery
University of Rochester School of Medicine and Dentistry
Surgeon-in-Chief
Strong Memorial Hospital
Rochester, New York

Rebecca P. Petersen, MD
Seattle, Washington

Allan Pickens, MD
Assistant Professor of Surgery
Section of Thoracic Surgery
University of Michigan Health System
Ann Arbor, Michigan

Richard N. Pierson, III, MD
Professor
Department of Surgery
University of Maryland
Director, Surgical Care
Baltimore VA Medical Center
Baltimore, Maryland

Henry A. Pitt, MD
Professor and Vice Chairman
Department of Surgery
Indiana University
Indianapolis, Indiana

Jeffrey L. Platt, MD
Professor Surgery
Professor of Microbiology and Immunology
Department of Transplantation Biology
University of Michigan
Ann Arbor, Michigan

Thomas H. Quinn, MD

Steven E. Raper, MD
Associate Professor
Department of Surgery
University of Pennsylvania
Attending Surgeon
Department of Surgery
Hospital of the University of Pennsylvania
Philadelphia, Pennsylvania

Philip A. Rascoe, MD
Department of Surgery
Hospital of the University of Pennsylvania
Philadelphia, Pennsylvania

John E. Rectenwald, MD, MS
Assistant Professor of Surgery
Section of Vascular Surgery
University of Michigan
Ann Arbor, Michigan

Daniel J. Reddy, MD
Professor
Department of Surgery
Wayne State University School of Medicine
Vascular Surgeon
Department of Surgery
John D. Dingell VA Medical Center
Detroit, Michigan

Rishindra M. Reddy, MD
Assistant Professor
Department of Surgery
University of Michigan
Ann Arbor, Michigan

Amy B. Reed, MD
Associate Professor of Surgery
Heart and Vascular Institute
Penn State College of Medicine
Chief
Department of Vascular Surgery
Milton S. Hershey Medical Center
Hershey, Pennsylvania

Taylor S. Riall, MD
Assistant Professor
Department of Surgery
University of Texas Medical Branch
Galveston, Texas

Barrie S. Rich, MD

William P. Robinson III, MD
Assistant Professor
Department of Surgery
University of Massachusetts Medical School
Worcestor, Massachusetts

Matthew R. Rosengart, MD
Assistant Professor
Department of Surgery
University of Pittsburgh School of Medicine
Pittsburgh, Pennsylvania

M. L. Chip Routt, Jr., MD
Professor
Department of Orthopaedic Surgery
University of Washington
Harborview Medical Center
Seattle, Washington

Grace S. Rozycki, MD
Professor and Vice Chair
Department of Surgery
Emory University School of Medicine
Director, Trauma/Surgical Critical Care
Grady Memorial Hospital
Atlanta, Georgia

Timothy W. Rutter, MD
Associate Professor
Department of Anesthesiology
University of Michigan
Ann Arbor, Michigan

Michael S. Sabel, MD
Assistant Professor of Surgery
Division of Surgical Oncology
University of Michigan
Ann Arbor, Michigan

Hazim J. Safi, MD
Professor and Chairman
Cardiothoracic and Vascular Surgery
University of Texas at Houston Medical School
UTH Medical Center
Houston, Texas

Ben Samstein, MD
Department of Surgery
New York-Presbyterian Hospital
New York, New York

George A. Sarosi, Jr., MD
Associate Professor
Department of Surgery
University of Florida College of Medicine
Staff Surgeon, Surgical Service
NF/SG VA Medical Center
Gainesville, Florida

Thomas T. Sato, MD
Associate Professor of Pediatric Surgery
Medical College of Wisconsin
Children's Hospital of Wisconsin
Milwaukee, Wisconsin

Willam P. Schecter, MD
Professor of Clinical Surgery
Department of Surgery
University of California, San Francisco
Staff Surgeon
Department of Surgery
San Francisco General Hospital
San Francisco, California

Randall P. Scheri, MD
Assistant Professor
Department of Surgery
Duke University
Durham, North Carolina

Richard D. Schulick, MD
Associate Professor of Surgery, Oncology, Gynecology and Obstetrics
Johns Hopkins Medical Institutions
Baltimore, Maryland

Federico G. Seifarth, MD
Department of Pediatric Surgery
Cleveland Clinic
Cleveland, Ohio

Curtis A. Sheldon, MD
Professor of Surgery
Department of Urology
University of Cincinnati
Director
Department of Pediatric Urology
Cincinnati Children's Hospital
Cincinnati, Ohio

Alexander D. Shepard, MD
Senior Staff Surgeon
Henry Ford Hospital
Detroit, Michigan

Anton N. Sidawy, MD, MPH
Chief, Surgical Service
VA Medical Center
Professor of Surgery
George Washington and Georgetown Universities
Washington, DC

Matthew J. Sideman, MD
Assistant Professor of Surgery
University of Texas Health Science Center San Antonio
San Antonio, Texas

Diane M. Simeone, MD
Lazar J. Greenfield Professor of Surgery and Molecular & Integrative Physiology
Chief, Division of Gastrointestinal Surgery
Associate Chair of Research
University of Michigan
Ann Arbor, Michigan

Niten Singh, MD, MS
Assistant Professor of Surgery
Uniformed Services University of the Health Sciences
Georgetown/Washington Hospital Center
Washington, DC

J. Stanley Smith, Jr., MD
Professor of Surgery
Department of Surgery
Pennsylvania State University College of Medicine
Breast Disease Team Leader
Breast Care Center
Penn State Hershey Medical Center
Hershey, Pennsylvania

Thomas G. Smith, III, MD
Assistant Professor
Division of Urology
Department of Surgery
The University of Texas Medical School at Houston
Houston, Texas

Christopher J. Sonnenday, MD, MHS
Assistant Professor
Department of Surgery
University of Michigan
Ann Arbor, Michigan

David I. Soybel, MD
Associate Professor of Surgery
Harvard Medical School
Staff Surgeon
Department of Surgery
Brigham & Women's Hospital
Boston, Massachusetts

Sunita D. Srivastava, MD
Assistant Professor
Section of Vascular Surgery, Department of Surgery
Cleveland Clinic Lerner College of Medicine of Case Western University
Staff, Department of Vascular Surgery
The Cleveland Clinic Foundation
Cleveland, Ohio

Benjamin W. Starnes, MD, FACS
Associate Professor and Chief
Department of Surgery, Division of Vascular Surgery
University of Washington
Harborview Medical Center
Seattle, Washington

Sharon L. Stein, MD
Assistant Professor of Surgery
Case Western Reserve University School of Medicine
Cleveland, Ohio

Peter Stock, MD
Professor
Surgical Director, Pediatric Renal Transplant Program
Surgical Director, Pancreas Transplant Program
Department of Surgery
San Francisco, California

Aurna Subramanian, MD
Assistant Professor of Medicine
Division of Infectious Diseases
Johns Hokins University School of Medicine
Baltimore, Maryland

Randall S. Sung, MD
Assistant Professor of Surgery
Department of General Surgery, Transplantation Division
University of Michigan
Ann Arbor, Michigan

Sandra A. Tan, MD, PhD
Assistant Professor
Department of Surgery
University of Florida
Gainesville, Florida

Kevin E. Taubman, MD
Assistant Professor
Department of Surgery
University of Oklahoma-Tulsa
Tulsa, Oklahoma

Theodoros N. Teknos, MD
Professor and David E. and Carole H. Schuller Chair in Head and Neck Oncologic Surgery
Director
Division of Head and Neck Surgery
Department of Otolaryngology
Ohio State University Medical School
Columbus, Ohio

Kevin K. Tremper, MD
Professor and Chair
Department of Anesthesiology
University of Michigan
Ann Arbor, Michigan

Richard H. Turnage, MD
Professor and Chair
Department of Surgery
University of Arkansas for Medical Sciences
Little Rock, Arkansas

Douglas J. Turner, MD
Assistant Professor
Department of Surgery
University of Maryland
Baltimore, Maryland

Gilbert R. Upchurch, Jr., MD
Professor of Surgery
Department of Surgery
Department of Surgery, Division of Vascular Surgery
University of Michigan
Ann Arbor, Michigan

Cosmas J.M. Vandeven, MD

Thomas K. Varghese, Jr., MD
Assistant Professor
Department of Surgery
Universtiy of Washington
Director of Thoracic Surgery
Department of Surgery
Harborview Medical Center
Seattle, Washington

Richard B. Wait, MD, PhD, FACS
Clinical Professor of Surgery
Department of Surgery
Tufts University School of Medicine
Boston, Massachusetts
Chairman of Surgery
Department of Surgery
Baystate Medical Center
Springfield, Massachusetts

Thomas W. Wakefield, MD
S. Martin Lindenauer Professor of Surgery
Department of Surgery, Section of Vascular Surgery
University of Michigan
Ann Arbor, Michigan

Thomas J. Watson, MD
Associate Professor
Department of Surgery
University of Rochester
Rochester, New York

Mitchell R. Weaver, MD
Department of Surgery
Henry Ford Hospital
Detroit, Michigan

Sharon M. Weber, MD
Professor
Department of Surgery
Chief, Surgical Oncology
University of Wisconsin Medical School
Madison, Wisconsin

Theordore H. Welling, MD
Assistant Professor
Department of Surgery
University of Michigan Health System
Ann Arbor, Michigan

Hunter Wessells, MD
Professor and Chair
Department of Urology
University of Washington
Attending Urologist
Harborview Medical Center
Seattle, Washington

Edward E. Whang, MD
Assistant Professor of Surgery
Department of Surgery
Brigham and Women's Hospital
Harvard Medical School
Boston, Massachusetts

Elizabeth C. Wick, MD
Assistant Professor
Department of Surgery
Johns Hopkins Medicine
Baltimore, Maryland

Edwin G. Wilkins, MD, MS
Associate Professor of Surgery
Section of Plastic Surgery
University of Michigan
Ann Arbor, Michigan

David H. Wisner, MD
Chair and Chief
Department of Surgery
University of California Davis
Sacramento, California

Sandra L. Wong, MD, MS
Assistant Professor
Department of Surgery
University of Michigan
Ann Arbor, Michigan

Amy D. Wyrzykowski, MD
Assistant Professor
Department of Surgery
Emory University
Associate Director
Surgical Intensive Care Unit
Grady Memorial Hospital
Atlanta, Georgia

Brett Yamane, MD
Department of Surgery
University of Wisconsin Hospital and Clinics
Madison, Wisconsin

Charles J. Yeo, MD
Samuel D. Gross Professor and Chairman
Department of Surgery
Thomas Jefferson University
Chief
Department of Surgery
Thomas Jefferson University Hospital
Philadelphia, Pennsylvania

Nicholas J. Zyromski, MD
Assistant Professor of Surgery
Indiana University School of Medicine
Indianapolis, Indiana

The editors are pleased to present the fifth edition of *Greenfield's Surgery: Scientific Principles and Practice*. The field of surgery has changed fundamentally in the years since the first edition of this text. Growth in the knowledge base of clinical surgery continues exponentially. Surgical practice has been transformed through advancements in physiologic and cellular investigation, integration of new techniques derived from imaging and robotics, from the concept of patient-centered care, and from the emerging field of biocomputation. The accelerating pace of scientific progress demands rapid adoption of new ideas into surgical therapy and a commitment to lifelong learning. Accordingly, the new edition of *Greenfield's Surgery* seeks to integrate new scientific knowledge with evolving changes in surgical care.

The fifth edition has been enhanced in every way, with changes to the book's editorial board, authorship, content, organization, and visual presentation. The fifth edition of Surgery: Scientific Principles and Practice reflects the founding principles and guidance of Lazar J. Greenfield, MD. His perceptive wisdom helped to create a truly unique book that balances scientific advance with clinical practice. With this new edition, we welcome a new editor—Diane M. Simeone, MD. Her expertise, energy, and vision have invigorated this volume.

We have solicited contributions from well over 200 authors, all chosen because of their scientific and clinical sophistication. Each contributor is currently an active practitioner in the field of surgery. Moreover, many have presented seminal articles and developed the new concepts in their disciplines that are featured in the text, for example, the new chapter "Policy Approaches to Improving Surgical Quality." Advances ranging from health services research to endovascular therapy mark the book as truly unique.

Organizationally, the book begins with topics of broad relevance to the practice of surgery, followed with chapters arranged by organ system. Trauma and transplantation are presented in the form of separate sections rather than subdivided chapters. The content within each has been presented as individual chapters in appreciation of the significance of each topic.

The book has been designed to create a text that not only looks better but also works better. The text is produced in a full range of colors, creating both visual impact and more opportunity to convey information quickly and with greater meaning. We continue our commitment to superb medical art in the form of line drawings—all created by a single artist. These illustrations have been enhanced to ensure a presentation that maximizes teaching effectiveness and clinical utility. Each chapter begins with a series of highlighted key teaching points, which are referenced within the text that follows. Individually numbered decision-making algorithms are featured throughout the book to provide diagnostic and management information in a simplified format. Tables carry classification bars, such as Diagnosis or Results, useful both when scanning the text for information and when accessing the book's contents digitally. The most important articles and chapters on the topic are highlighted in the reference list.

The fifth edition continues to be highly integrated with a new electronic format to provide supplemental educational material. These materials include review questions for reinforcement of concepts and for board examination preparation. Access to supplemental content produced by Lippincott Williams & Wilkins is an additional advantage of this electronic integration.

Today, *Greenfield's Surgery: Scientific Principles and Practice* has become the gold standard text in the field of Surgery. The editors continue their commitment to the education of contemporary surgeons, and to improved care of the patients that they serve. We believe that with the many improvements implemented in this fifth edition, it will continue be the text by which all other surgery texts are judged.

Michael W. Mulholland, MD, PhD

I express my appreciation for the efforts of the contributing authors, whose scholarship makes this work possible. We have been fortunate to maintain a happy working relationship with our publisher, Lippincott Williams & Wilkins, and I wish to specifically acknowledge the support of Brian Brown as acquisitions editor.

—M.W.M.

My gratitude to John Cameron, MD and the faculty and housestaff of the Johns Hopkins Hospital who both trained me and served as my role models for my career as an academic surgeon. Thanks also to the surgical faculty and housestaff at the Indiana University for providing a constant stimulus for greater achievement. It has been my honor and privilege to work with you over the last several years.

—K.D.L.

I appreciate the efforts of the faculties and residents at the University of Michigan, Washington University, and UCSF with whom I have had the privilege to work.

—G.M.D.

Thanks to the housestaff and students, whose dedication, inquisitiveness, and challenges provide the stimulus and rewards for this effort.

—R.V.M.

To my family: Ted, Samuel, and Amelia.

—D.M.S.

I am grateful to the residents and fellows at the University of Michigan. It has been a joy to train you and be trained by you.

—G.R.U.

CONTENTS

SECTION M: ARTERIAL SYSTEM

SECTION N: VENOUS SYSTEM

SECTION O: PEDIATRICS

SECTION P: GENITOURINARY SYSTEM

SECTION Q: SKIN AND SOFT TISSUE

LIST OF ALGORITHMS

PART ONE

SCIENTIFIC PRINCIPLES

CHAPTER 1 ■ READING EFFECTIVELY TO ATTAIN PROFICIENCY IN SURGERY

RICHARD H. BELL, Jr., LINNEA S. HAUGE, AND DEBRA A. DaROSA

SCIENTIFIC PRINCIPLES

KEY POINTS

1. During a residency in surgery, the successful surgeon-to-be advances from a novice, who must follow rules to achieve good outcomes, to becoming proficient, which means that accumulated knowledge and experience allows him/her to respond correctly to situations in a more automatic and effortless manner.
2. Real learning (more than just memorization for the short term) occurs when information becomes stored in long term memory. Learning with understanding occurs when the student or resident has accumulated sufficient knowledge in long-term memory that he/she recognizes familiar patterns in the new situations that are encountered.
3. Reading is a critical tool for acquiring surgical knowledge. Reading that leads to deep understanding can be facilitated by conscious strategies before, during, and after reading that increase the likelihood that information will be retained in long-term memory and be accessible when needed.
4. The student of surgery can and should develop conscious strategies for assessing the extent to which their reading results in deep comprehension of the educational material.

LEARNING, MEMORY, AND PROGRESSION TO EXPERTISE

If you are reading this book, the chances are high that you will be (or are or have been) a surgery resident on the first day of your first rotation of your first year. Imagine (or remember) the call to the emergency room to evaluate a new patient with a complex problem, perhaps a 70-year-old male with an upper gastrointestinal hemorrhage and known coronary artery disease. By that point in your education as a doctor, you will have learned enough basic rules about resuscitation to take a few steps—check the airway, start an intravenous line, send off blood for a type and cross match, perhaps place a Foley catheter. Soon, however, your knowledge, skills, and abilities are overwhelmed by the complexity of the situation. Perhaps the patient's blood pressure falls, or the electrocardiogram pattern changes. Chances are that you turn at that point to a senior or chief resident, who comes to your aid, seemingly cool in the face of chaos, and makes precise and rapid adjustments in the patient's treatment, develops a rapid differential diagnosis, and orders the appropriate diagnostic testing. Finally, the attending surgeon arrives with an air of confidence born of experience, seems to recognize the problems immediately, and, after an incisive set of questions, makes a decision to take the patient to the operating room. What has happened to allow the senior resident or senior surgeon to achieve that level of competence and confidence?

The beginning of a surgical residency marks the start of a new way of learning. Prior to that time, you may well have invested effort in accumulating knowledge of facts or understanding of concepts that you knew you were extremely unlikely to ever need beyond the next examination. Suddenly, however, as a resident you are placed in a situation where you need to rapidly acquire information that you can use to build a sophisticated understanding of diseases and operations. You have a huge amount to learn and don't have much time to waste on nonproductive educational activities. Much more than ever before, you need to retain the information you have encountered, store that information in ways that allow you to retrieve it in the future, and relate the information to other pieces of information you have acquired.

How can we describe the transition from the first-year resident with a limited repertoire to the respected senior surgeon? A model that is widely used is the Dreyfus model,[1] originally used to describe the performance progression of U.S. Air Force pilots. The Dreyfus system (Fig. 1.1) specifies five levels of accomplishment: novice, advanced beginner, competent, proficient, and expert.

1 A novice is capable of following rules, but not capable of changing the rules to adapt to new circumstances or knowing when the rules don't apply. For example, the novice is capable of generating a standard set of postoperative orders, but would not be able to significantly modify them for individual patients. When the novice sees a patient, he or she has had so little experience that he or she cannot call on mental images of a disease—the novice is forced to depend on analytic reasoning to try to tie the pathophysiology he or she has studied to symptoms and signs. The advanced beginner still functions largely on the basis of rules, but begins to develop some flexibility in applying them. The advanced beginner has had enough clinical experience to begin to recognize patterns in the patients he or she has encountered.

The competent surgeon begins to identify patterns in situations and has started to develop mental models of diseases and operations that guide his or her decision making. To a limited extent, the competent surgeon is able to apply knowledge of the known to new and unknown situations. At this stage, experience begins to supplant rules. The competent surgeon also begins to accept responsibility for the care of the patient and becomes more emotionally involved with patients.

The proficient surgeon is able to effortlessly recognize many situations, drawing on his or her extensive real-world experience and significant prior learning stored in memory. The proficient surgeon may appear to operate from instinct because of the fluidity of his or her decision making, but the "instinct" is derived from a store of experience that has created models that allow the surgeon to choose quickly among competing scenarios.

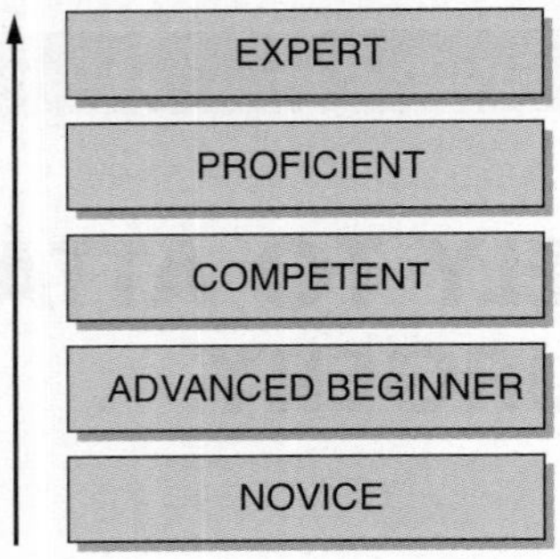

FIGURE 1.1. The Dreyfus model of performance (see also Carraccio C, Benson B, et al. From the educational bench to the clinical bedside: translating the Dreyfus developmental model to the learning of clinical skills. *Acad Med* 2008;83:761–767).

Finally, the expert seems to "always get it right." The expert routinely comes up with an optimal performance and appears to do it effortlessly. The expert's mental models of disease are so strong that he or she recognizes atypical features of cases that others miss. The expert may depend so much on "second nature" that he or she actually has difficulty describing his or her decision-making process. In general, the development of expertise in a given area takes 10 years or more. Most experts in surgery have focused on a particular area of surgery for decades.

The Science of Learning and Memory

The activities of your brain are conducted by cells, of which there are approximately 1 trillion. The number of brain cells does not increase during life; rather, the development of the brain results from increasing complex connections made between the brain's neurons, of which there are about 100 billion, the remainder of the brain cells being glial cells that organize and support the neurons. Neurons communicate with each other via dendrites and axons, the dendrites carrying impulses to the neuron and the axon carrying impulses from the neuron to the dendrites of surrounding neurons. Because an individual neuron can have thousands of dendrites, the number of possible interactions between cells becomes almost unlimited.

Learning occurs when the brain acquires new information; memory is the process through which that information is retained and stored for later retrieval.[2] When learning occurs, certain neurons start to function together. Repeated activation of those neurons makes subsequent activations faster and in some cases automatic, leading to the creation of memory. Storage of learning in memory in turn activates additional neuronal connections and associations.

Memory appears to be of three types: immediate memory, working memory, and long-term memory. Immediate memory allows you to recall enough information to quickly perform a task such as entering a patient's name into a computer and spelling it correctly. Working memory confers the ability to process information during the completion of tasks that take minutes to hours. Long-term memory refers to the storage of information for months or years. Storage of this type of information starts with the information being encoded by the hippocampus, which then exports it to long-term storage
2 areas. A very important goal in surgical education is to increase the likelihood that important information will be retained and stored in long-term memory. Two factors that have been shown to be important in ensuring retention are sense and relevance. Sense implies that the information fits in with the learner's previous experience. Relevance means that the information is much more likely to be retained if it has meaning for the learner and is related to the learner's real-life activities. Both of these principles are very important to keep in mind in the training of surgeons. As a resident, trying to read about endocrine surgery may not be very effective in promoting long-term memory if you are in the midst of a demanding vascular surgery rotation and have not had previous exposure to very many patients with endocrine problems.

Learning with Understanding

Learning with understanding occurs when the learner can make sense of new information in light of previous experience and can also see that the information is relevant to his or her learning needs. As one learns with understanding, pieces of information begin to relate to each other and eventually information is clustered in "mental models" or "scripts." Material that is learned with understanding can not only be recalled but can also be used when novel but related situations are encountered. Recent work suggests that it is the elaborateness and depth of these "illness scripts" that characterize the expert physician.[3] Learning with understanding is not easy. As noted previously, learning with understanding can be quite difficult if the learner is not sufficiently familiar with a subject to be well positioned to learn more. Sometimes the prior information that a learner possesses about a subject is incorrect and is difficult to eradicate. In surgery, learning with understanding is complicated when the learner is presented with conflicting information or misinformation from faculty or reading materials.

The remainder of this chapter deals with reading and how one can use a textbook in a way that is most likely to lead to learning with understanding and timely progress toward proficiency or expertise. Surgeons learn in many ways, and some are undoubtedly inclined to rely more on "doing" than reading. Reading is critical to learning to become a surgeon because it is a major way that experts transmit their accumulated understanding to those who are at lower stages in their comprehension. It is very hard to think of another way of learning that does this more efficiently. Having said this, reading is often not done well, not done efficiently, and not done at the right time and place. In the ensuing pages, we hope to offer practical advice about using this textbook and other printed materials to your maximal advantage in your surgical career.

READING FOR RETENTION AND TRANSFER—REMEMBERING FOLLOWS UNDERSTANDING

How do you read a chapter and more easily remember the material? What study strategies enable you to read efficiently, yet also permit you to retrieve the information from memory for use in patient care and on examinations? Why is it that sometimes you are asked a question on a topic about which you remember reading, but your recollection of the details is clouded? These are common concerns expressed by surgeons working to build and maintain a solid knowledge base in an era when the amount of knowledge is doubling every 18 months.[4] In this portion of the chapter, we will explain approaches individuals may take to learn new information and then describe reading and study activities that promote deep understanding and help translate new information into retrievable knowledge.

Surface Versus Deep Structured Learning Approaches

The retention of information in long-term memory is affected by a student's approach to learning. Individuals have tendencies to use either a surface or deep structured approach to reading and studying, although any given individual may change his or her approach at times. Readers who take a surface approach read "on autopilot," not processing or fully thinking about the information being read. These individuals may go through the motions of highlighting sections in the text, but they don't carefully choose key points. These learners tend to memorize facts indiscriminately, treat what is being read as unrelated bits of information, and find difficulty in later explaining what they read in their own words.[5] Surface readers glean satisfaction from the number of pages "covered," but then have difficulty remembering the content because the words were never translated into personally meaningful information. Surface-level readers search for facts that might appear on the test but not for the meaning of the text. A surface approach leads to temporary and superficial engagement with the educational material and does not promote long-term retention or understanding because little active thinking occurred during reading. A negative association has been reported between the surface study approach and exam performance. This approach is common in learners who are stressed, have performance anxiety, have little interest in the topic, possess limited time management skills and try to read too much in too little time, or lack the ability to discriminate between essential and less important concepts, thereby missing "the forest for the trees" and drowning in information overload.[6]

In contradistinction, deep structured learners are motivated by natural curiosity and a genuine need to know. Their purpose for reading is to acquire information that is considered relevant and personally meaningful. They take control of their own learning and seek to fully understand a topic. They recognize when they understand what is being read, and also recognize when they need more or different information to fully comprehend the material. These learners mentally engage with the information they read by questioning the material, asking themselves about key points, analyzing the material for relationships with what they already know through experience or prior knowledge, and identifying underlying principles to guide their thinking. A deep structured learning approach is an active, integrative process. It results in learners translating the words, charts, and other forms of information into an organized mental picture. This deep and structured approach leads to long-term retention.[7]

Study Considerations and Strategies

Some readers fall asleep while reading, or find themselves having to reread a paragraph several times. Others commit to studying for a block of time, only to start hours later because they found other things to do. Active reading requires a person's full attention. Even with the best of intentions, a reader's success can be compromised if concentration is lacking. It is important to minimize or eliminate visual or auditory distractions and to improve the study environment if there is poor lighting, clutter, or uncomfortable seating. Internal distractors (hunger, performance anxiety, sleepiness, etc.) require attention as well. In order to use study time well, keen and consistent concentration are needed.[8,9]

3 Table 1.1 demonstrates a three-step reading approach designed to promote deep structured learning.[10] In the first stage, learners prepare before reading by activating their prior knowledge and setting themselves up to read with a purpose. The second stage suggests ways to process the information while reading and make it personally meaningful. The last step reinforces the need to revisit and rehearse what was read to better transfer the information from short-term to long-term memory.

Before Reading: Activate Prior Knowledge

There is a well-established correlation between prior knowledge and reading comprehension.[11,12] Before reading new material, the learner should carefully reflect on what he or she already knows about the topic and how it relates to other subjects already studied. Prior knowledge is the foundation upon which new information is built. A person with a high level of prior knowledge on a given topic can comprehend what is being read in less time and with less effort than a person who has limited experience or knowledge about the subject. Prior knowledge helps learners construct concepts and make meaning out of what is being read.[13,14] By activating existing knowledge about a topic before reading more about it, the learner can identify knowledge gaps and then actively read with the clear aim to fill them. Several strategies exist for activating one's prior knowledge, including reflection and recording, interactive discussions, question and answer development, hypotheses development, and deciding what information about the subject matters the most.

Reflection and Recording. One of the simplest methods is to bring to mind the subject and note what you know about it. You can revisit existing knowledge by listing the chapter headings and subtitles and documenting what you already know. For example, assume that a chapter entitled "Shock" lists eight subtitles: pathophysiology, evaluation of shock, classification of hemorrhage, treatment of hemorrhagic shock, resuscitative fluids, special situations, experimental resuscitative fluids, and complications of shock. The process of briefly recording what

TABLE 1.1

STRATEGIES TO ACHIEVE DEEP STRUCTURED READING

■ BEFORE READING	■ DURING READING	■ AFTER READING
Activate prior knowledge: ■ Reflect and record ■ Discuss ■ Identify questions ■ Make predictions ■ Decide what matters most	Take notes: ■ Pictorial: Flow charts, maps, diagrams ■ Verbal: Cornell method ■ Combined: Virtual Web page design	Rehearse: ■ Periodic reviews ■ Self-assessment ■ Summarize

you already know about each of these areas stimulates memory, clarifies what is known, and highlights learning gaps or needs. This prepares you to read actively and selectively to fill knowledge voids while also efficiently verifying that your comprehension in areas where you have prior knowledge is sufficient.

Interactive Discussion with Others. Some people activate prior knowledge best through verbal exchange with others. Talking with a colleague about a specific topic can help highlight key points to be studied, highlight lessons learned through personal experiences, and clarify one's understanding about the topic. These discussions can also yield important questions about the topic that require attention as well as provide an organizational structure for thinking about the subject.

Question Development. Generating questions about a topic prior to reading helps you articulate what you think is important to know. It encourages you to think broadly about the subject and anticipate what information might be needed to take care of a patient with the given disease. You might anticipate a question posed by faculty or on an exam, or connect the topic with a patient care problem you've heard about, personally encountered, or anticipate being faced with in the future. When authoring questions on a topic, you should include questions related to word definitions, cause–effect relationships, and comparison–contrast information (how do the symptoms of appendicitis differ from other diseases causing abdominal pain?). The process of asking questions about a topic (I wonder why. . . .; what causes. . .?; how is X similar to Y. . .?; how is it different than Z. . .?; what if the patient is. . .?) requires you to think deeply about what you don't understand about the topic so reading can be focused to address identified learning needs. Noting questions before reading and then recording the answers while reading activates preknowledge, links the new information to forethought, and helps translate what is read to real-life situations, which makes the information all the more memorable.

Prediction or Hypothesis Development. Learners benefit from making predictions about various aspects of a topic by tapping into what they already know and predicting how it relates to the subject under study. For example, if reading about rectal cancer, the reader might predict that multimodality therapy is frequently employed, based on his or her preexisting knowledge of pelvic anatomy and lymphatic drainage and past experience with other gastrointestinal malignancies. By hypothesizing answers to key knowledge gaps, readers can test their assumptions through focused reading.

Deciding What Matters Most. Because time for study is limited, it is helpful to pause before reading about a topic to think about which aspects of it are critical, important, or useful to know. Focusing your reading can be done by any of the methods previously mentioned, as well as by simply listing personal learning objectives such as, "By the end of this study period concentrating on benign breast disease, I want to be able to do the following: (a). . .; (b). . . ." This process activates prior knowledge by determining what components of the topic are most important to you so you can then actively read the chapter with your objectives guiding your study.

During Reading: Taking Notes

If you don't possess a photographic memory or an expert's large store of prior knowledge on a subject so that material being read can be easily organized into long-term memory, note taking is needed or the material will be easily forgotten. It is inefficient to re-read each chapter or even review "highlighted" paragraphs. Interactive note taking leads to stronger memories and improved concentration while reading. According to Pauk and Owens,[15] note taking focuses attention on what is being read, which strengthens the original memory trace of the material. In addition, it results in a document available for later review and reinforcement. The aim is to create condensed notes driven by the identified learning needs from the "Before Reading" exercises described earlier, formatted for efficient future review and self-testing. Three note-taking methods are described in this section: visual notes, verbal notes, and combined visual/verbal notes.

Visual Notes. Visual notes help learners organize information because they show relationships and hierarchies of concepts. Types of graphic organizers include tables, pictures, flowcharts, mind maps, and diagrams.[16] Graphic organizers are often already published in the text and serve to highlight the importance of the information. Reading the published version, however, is less useful than constructing your own because creating your own version requires more information processing. Nevertheless, it can be useful to copy graphic organizers from a book to carry in a lab coat pocket to review during windows of available time or access when a clinical opportunity arises. Another strategy is to omit the data in parts of the published graph and later "fill in the blanks" to further reinforce understanding and retention.

Tables are useful for comparing and contrasting common types of details across variables. For example, a table would be helpful to learn about the various imaging techniques for pancreatic cancer. The column headings might include "Name of Test," "Cost," "Risks," "Sensitivity," "Specificity," and "Positive Predictive Value." This approach allows you to extract information from the book's narrative and place it in the correct location in the table format. The finished table enables you to compare and contrast the tests and create a "big picture" view of the multiple factors involved in choosing an optimal diagnostic tool.

A flowchart is a picture of the separate steps of a process in sequential order. Translating the material you read into a flowchart helps you think through "if–then" scenarios and can uncover your incorrect or unclear decision pathways. After reading a segment of a chapter on a particular disease entity, you can, for example, draw a scheme for working up a jaundiced patient or create an algorithm for the treatment of pulmonary embolus.

Mind maps, sometimes referred to as concept maps, relate facts or ideas to other facts or ideas. Relationships and patterns across information are easily seen in mind maps. A mind map is a structured graphic display of an individual's conceptual scheme within a well-circumscribed domain.[17,18] There are various approaches to developing mind maps, but most methods share similar steps. The first step, the brainstorming stage, occurs by drawing or writing the topic in the center of the page (Fig. 1.2). If the chapter under study is about gastroesophageal reflux disease (GERD), the reader would write the word "GERD" in the middle of a large sheet of blank paper. Lines are then drawn from the center topic outwardly to represent the main ideas or categories that are written or illustrated in the reading. Subheadings from the book could be used for these "spokes," or the reader can choose his or her own collection of key ideas. For example, one spoke might have printed on it "Diagnosis" and a second spoke may contain the word "Treatment." A third spoke might be "Epidemiology," and a fourth might read "Complications." Given that our minds don't think in a linear fashion, mind or concept maps enable readers to build branches and subbranches onto the main spokes or build more main spokes, depending on what they are thinking at the time. Any number of branches can be added to the major spoke lines. Learners continue to build their maps as their thoughts and "search and find" mental association powers are

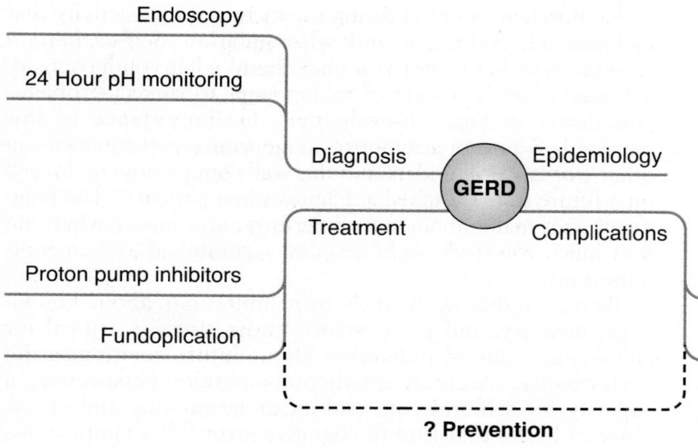

FIGURE 1.2. A basic "mind map" dealing with the topic of gastroesophageal reflux.

unleashed. Mapping allows for free-flow thinking and spontaneous thought and decreases the chances of premature closure about a topic or subtopic, which typically happens when using an outline approach.

Once the initial brainstorming map is completed, the "organizational stage" needs to occur. In this phase, readers redo their mind maps, sequencing the branches in sort of meaningful order. During this phase, readers may see hierarchies or new associations that can serve as a basis for organizing or modifying the map's branches or subbranches. Additional details on how to construct mind maps are published elsewhere.[19]

Other types of graphic organizers include diagrams or pictures. The latter can be helpful, for example, in summarizing a segment of a chapter that describes anatomy. Anatomic pictures can either be drawn or copied from the Internet or other printed source and used to note structures. Creating graphics helps readers activate background knowledge, strengthens metacognitive skills, strengthens their ability to construct meaning from the printed word, and reinforces understanding.

Verbal Notes. Research suggests that underlining (or highlighting) while reading leads to greater understanding than reading alone, but writing notes while reading is significantly better for retention than underlining. Creating summaries in your own words of the material you read is critical to converting learning into memory. If notes can't be done easily, then the information is not well enough understood to be incorporated for the long term. One note-making system worth considering is the Cornell method.[15] This method, pictured in Figure 1.3, provides a format for condensing and organizing notes. It makes use of paper with a 2.5-inch margin on the left and a 6-inch area on the right in which to write notes. While reading, you write cue words in the left margin and key phrases or points in the right. Later, when reviewing notes, you can view the cue word while simultaneously covering up the key phrases to discern whether you can extemporaneously come up with the key points. For example, while studying the principles of tumor biology, cue words in the left margin might read "how cancers develop," "role of the host," "clinical staging," etc. The bottom 2 inches of the page are used to write summary information or to note areas that need additional study. Templates for the Cornell method note formats and instructions about how to use them can be found on the Internet.

Combined Methods. There are many ways you can interact with the material you read, be it verbally or visually. With today's technology, you could set up a Web page for your reading notes. The Web page could include visual and verbal notes, all organized using a structure that makes sense to you.

After Reading: Rehearse

The importance of reviewing and rehearsing notes cannot be overemphasized in terms of its importance to long-term memory. Rehearsing material repeatedly helps it become "overlearned" and thus embedded in your memory. The passage of time can be detrimental to memory, but returning to review notes at the start of each study session can significantly increase retention. There is consistent evidence that the process of rehearsal and recitation transfers information from short-term memory into long-term memory.[20] Recitation or rehearsal can include reflecting on the topic, writing about it, answering the questions you posed at the prereading stage, and/or talking to yourself or others about it. It is best to write or talk aloud when rehearsing because it involves multiple senses, which increases the chances of remembering the material. Consider reviewing by offering to teach the topic to others—"to teach is to learn twice." When reviewing information, you will be more successful if your notes are

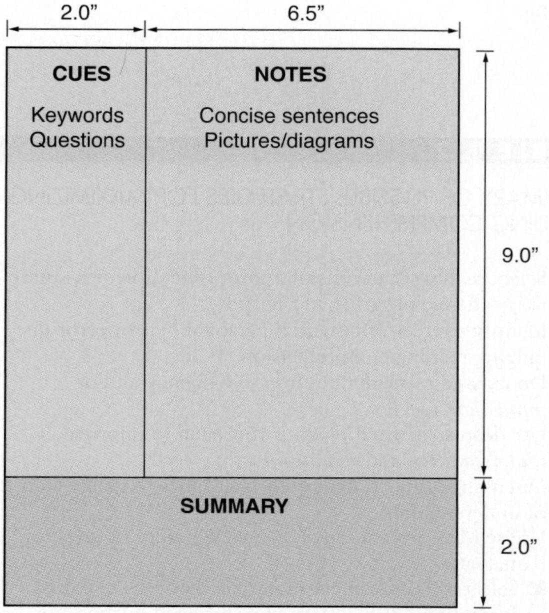

FIGURE 1.3. The Cornell method for note taking (see also Pauk W, Owens R. *How to Study in College*, 8th ed. Boston, MA: Houghton Mifflin Company Publishers; 2005).

SCIENTIFIC PRINCIPLES

organized in a manner that supports a systematic search, such as by hierarchies or categories. The rehearsal process requires processing the information by analyzing it, not merely reciting it.

Self-assessment is a helpful form of rehearsal. Multiple-choice practice exams are convenient, but open-ended questions allow for a richer interaction with the material and avoid some of the artifact in multiple-choice questions that is introduced by distractors. In summary, rehearsal is a critical part of learning. Periodic and consistent review will help you refresh and build your memory.

MONITORING YOUR LEVEL OF READING COMPREHENSION

Early in your education, your teachers helped you develop strategies to assess and improve reading comprehension. These strategies, known as *comprehension monitoring*, are likely so engrained in your reading process that now you give little thought to them.

4 Comprehension strategies are "specific, learned procedures that foster active, competent, self-regulated, and intentional reading."[21] The number and type of comprehension monitoring strategies that you use is predictive of retention.[22] Therefore, it is recommended that you do a personal inventory of your strategies before embarking on the difficult task of reading a surgery textbook to ensure that you are using your reading time as effectively as possible (Table 1.2).

Your goals for text comprehension should be related to your desired outcome. If you are reading to learn and remember the factual answers to questions you anticipate will be asked of you during an upcoming conference, your strategies may be confined to recitation or listing. If your goal is to understand how or why a patient responds to a particular drug, your need for deeper processing requires that you use more elaborate comprehension monitoring strategies such as schematic mapping or written summaries. Studying for a high-stakes examination, such as the American Board of Surgery Qualifying or Certifying Examination, requires more elaborate comprehension strategies aimed at deeper processing.

TABLE 1.2

SUMMARY OF POSSIBLE STRATEGIES FOR MAXIMIZING READING COMPREHENSION

- Select reading materials of appropriate difficulty, suitable for academic progress and purpose
- Identify sources of potential personal bias or error in judging reading comprehension
- Do massed re-reading to improve fluency and/or *immediate* recall
- Use deep structured reading approach to improve *understanding* and *retention*
- Discuss reading content with colleagues to gauge your level of understanding
- Use self-assessments such as review guides or question banks
  - Select self-assessment materials that are similar in format and difficulty to your targeted purpose for reading
  - During self-assessments, stop and reflect on justifications for answering questions

Comprehension monitoring is a metacognitive activity that includes self-evaluation and self-regulation. *Self-evaluation* refers to whether or not you understand what you have read. *Self-regulation* is the act of taking steps to correct problems you detect during self-evaluation. Of importance in this process is a sincere attempt to judge future performance—in other words, "do I understand this well enough now to do well on a future test? Or make a diagnosis in a patient?" The judgments you make about future performance impact what and how much you study, so honest and accurate self-assessment is important.

Being familiar with one's own limitations about knowledge, memory, and performance under stress is critical for enhancing accurate judgments about future comprehension performance. Accurate predictions require perspective, a capacity for self-criticism, and an understanding and acceptance of biases that lead to cognitive error.[23,24] Cognitive dispositions to respond (CDRs) to situations in predictable ways can lead to errors in critical thinking. An example of a CDR that can lead to cognitive error is "search satisfying," which occurs when a search is called off once something suitable is found. In diagnosing a source of pain, for example, a plausible explanation is encountered, causing you to cease the search for others. Awareness of these pitfalls and using a strategy for reducing cognitive error (continuing your search for other potential causes of pain) are known as cognitive forcing strategies. Getting perspective and reflecting on one's thinking process during reading, or in clinical situations, is an effective means for avoiding or minimizing potential errors in critical thinking.[23]

The judgments you make about reading comprehension are limited by the subjectivity inherent to self-evaluation.[25] The more familiar you are with a topic, the more likely you will overestimate your comprehension of it.[26] While we recommend that you read about topics related to your current rotation and patient encounters in order to take advantage of the retention effect of activating prior knowledge, be aware that when you are reading about a topic of immediate familiarity, you may overestimate your understanding of the material. Using a range of evaluation strategies to monitor your comprehension can help to avoid misinterpreting familiarity as understanding.

The more coherent or easier textual material is to process, the higher you will judge your comprehension to be.[26] Reading texts and review guides that provide abbreviated overviews of surgical topics may be an expeditious way to cover a topic. However, the easier-to-process text may give you the misimpression that you comprehend more than you actually do about the subject you are reading.

Massed re-reading, or reading text twice in a row, has been shown to improve memory of information in the text on free recall and also improve the accuracy of comprehension monitoring.[27] However, recent studies of massed re-reading compared to single reading demonstrate that massed re-reading is not an effective means of improving performance on multiple-choice tests.[28] Re-reading may be valuable when content is not familiar. However, the fluency gained during a re-read can be misunderstood as improved comprehension when, in fact, massed re-reading alone does not typically result in the deeper processing necessary for the level of comprehension that leads to retention.

Comprehension accuracy can be improved by reducing uncertainty about the context in which you will need to recall information.[26] Familiarizing yourself with the examination format and with the type of information that will be targeted in the test can improve your judgment about your readiness. Another recommendation for improving accuracy of judgments about comprehension involves using colleagues to anchor your judgments. Reducing the subjectivity inherent in self-evaluation can be accomplished by talking with others about the text after reading it.

Using your performance results from previous exams can serve as an effective guide for reading goals. A review book that mirrors the complexity of the questions you will face on an exam can also help reduce the uncertainty you may have about your future comprehension performance. Using a good review guide or question bank in conjunction with your textbook reading can both help you become familiar with test format and assess your retention. While taking practice tests, stop at intervals to review your answers (e.g., every 10 questions) and consider your justification for the responses you gave. This type of self-assessment has been shown to improve future test performance, a result attributed to the critical thinking or reasoning required by the process.[29] Rephrasing and justification about reasoning are also metacognitive strategies that can improve retention and future comprehension performance.

References

1. Carraccio C, Benson B, Nixon LJ, et al. From the educational bench to the clinical bedside: translating the Dreyfus developmental model to the learning of clinical skills. *Acad Med* 2008;83:761–767.
2. Sousa DA. *How the Gifted Brain Learns*. Thousand Oaks, CA: Corwin Press; 2003:22–25.
3. Schmidt H, Norman G, Boshuizen HP. A cognitive perspective on medical expertise: theory and implications. *Acad Med* 1990;65:611–621.
4. Mayberry J. Residency reform Halsted-style. *JACS* 2003;197:433–435.
5. Entwistle N. *Styles of Learning and Teaching: An Integrated Outline of Educational Psychology for Students, Teachers, and Lecturers*. New York: Wiley and Sons; 1981.
6. Ferguson E, James D, Madeley L. Factors associated with success in medical school: systematic review of the literature. *BMJ* 2002;324: 952– 957.
7. Reid W, Duvall E, Evans P. Relationship between assessment results and approaches to learning and studying in year two medical students. *Med Educ* 2007;41:754–762.
8. Furnham A, Bradley A. Music while you work: the differential distraction of background music on the cognitive test performance of introverts and extraverts. *Appl Cogn Psychol* 1999;11:445–455.
9. Furnham A, Gunter B, Peterson E. Television distraction and the performance of introverts and extraverts. *Appl Cogn Psychol* 2006;8:705–711.
10. Straker K, Kelman E. *Vital Skills: Study Strategies Every Nursing Student Must Know*. Houston, TX: Karista Press; 2007.
11. Maquire E, Frith C, Morris RG. The functional neuroanatomy of comprehension and memory: the importance of prior knowledge. *Brain* 1999;122: 1839–1850.
12. McNamara D, Kintsch W. Learning from texts: effects of prior knowledge and text coherence. *Discourse Process* 1996;22:247–288.
13. Spires H, Donley J. Prior knowledge activation: inducing engagement with information texts. *J Educ Psychol* 1998;90:249–260.
14. Kendou P, Van den Broek P. The effects of readers' misconceptions on comprehension of scientific text. *J Educ Psychol* 2005;97:235–245.
15. Pauk W, Owens R. *How to Study in College*, 8th ed. Boston, MA: Houghton Mifflin Company Publishers; 2005.
16. Kelman E, Straker K. *Study Without Stress: Mastering Medical Sciences*. Thousand Oaks, CA: Sage Publishers; 2000.
17. Allen D, Tanner K. Approaches to cell biology teaching: mapping the journey—concept maps as signposts of developing knowledge structures. *Cell Biol Educ* 2003;2:133–136.
18. Diwaker V, Ertmer P, Nour A. Helping students learn veterinary physiology through the use of concept maps. *J Vet Med Educ* 2007;34:652–657.
19. Buzan T, Buzan B. *The Mind Map Book*. London, UK: BBC Publishers; 2006.
20. Ericsson K, Kintsch W. Long-term memory. *Psychol Rev* 1995;102:211–245.
21. Trabasso T, Bouchard E. Teaching readers how to comprehend text strategically. In: Block CC, Pressley ME, eds. *Comprehension Instruction: Research-Based Best Practices*. New York: Guilford Press; 2002:176–200.
22. Ryan MP. Monitoring text comprehension: individual differences in epistemological standards. *J Educ Psychol* 1984;76:248–258.
23. Croskerry P. Cognitive forcing strategies in clinical decisionmaking. *Ann Emerg Med* 2003;41:110–120.
24. Croskerry P. The importance of cognitive errors in diagnosis and strategies to minimize them. *Acad Med* 2003;78:775–780.
25. Hacker DJ. Self-regulated comprehension during normal reading. In: Hacker DJ, Dunlosky J, Graesser AC, eds. *Metacognition in Educational Theory and Practice*. Mahwah, NJ: Erlbaum; 1998:165–191.
26. Zhao Q, Linderholm T. Adult metacomprehension: judgment processes and accuracy constraints. *Educ Psychol Rev* 2008;20:191–206.
27. Griffin TD, Wiley J, Thiede KW. Individual differences, rereading, and self-explanation: concurrent processing and cue validity as constraints on metacomprehension accuracy. *Mem Cognit* 2008;36:93–103.
28. Callender AA, McDaniel MA. The limited benefits of rereading educational texts. *Contemp Educ Psychol* 2009;34:30–41.
29. Austin Z, Gregory P, Chiu S. Use of reflection-in-action and self-assessment to promote critical thinking among pharmacy students. *Am J Pharm Educ* 2008;72:1–8.

CHAPTER 2 ■ SUBSTRATE METABOLISM IN SURGERY

STEVEN E. RAPER

KEY POINTS

1. Intermediary metabolism—as the metabolic manipulation and balancing of ingested carbohydrate, fat, and protein—ultimately can process all nutrients to acetyl coenzyme A (CoA) for energy production in the citric acid cycle.
2. Glucose must always be available for brain function; if not available directly from the diet, it can be mobilized for a brief period from glycogen stores and then derived from proteins in the liver and kidneys.
3. Free fatty acids are a direct source of energy catabolized by cardiac and skeletal muscle.
4. Hepatic protein synthesis, when excess amino acids are available, includes albumin, fibrinogen, and apolipoproteins and can reach 50 g per day.
5. The citric acid cycle includes a series of mitochondrial enzymes that transform acetyl CoA into water, carbon dioxide, and hydrogen-reducing equivalents; the hydrogen-reducing equivalents are then transformed into adenosine triphosphate (ATP) by the electron transport chain. Each molecule of acetyl CoA that enters the citric acid cycle yields 12 molecules of ATP.
6. Biotransformation of potentially toxic, often hydrophobic, compounds into hydrophilic, excretable compounds occurs mainly in the liver by the cytochromes P-450, the uridine diphosphate-glucuronyl (UDP-glucuronyl) transferases, the glutathione (GSH) S-transferases, and the sulfotransferases.

INTERMEDIARY METABOLISM: AN OVERVIEW

"[D]o You Have a More Exciting Word for 'Metabolism'?"*

Intermediary metabolism is the fate of dietary carbohydrate, fat, and protein after digestion and absorption. Although admittedly intricate, all surgeons should be familiar with the chemical reactions by which food is converted to energy. Understanding the major biochemical pathways is a prerequisite to making use of the rapid—and exciting—expansion of medical knowledge directed at improving health beginning at the cellular level. Some representative recent advances will be discussed at the end of the chapter.

The major intermediary metabolites are glucose, fatty acids, glycerol, and amino acids. Glucose is metabolized to pyruvate and lactate by glycolysis. Aerobic metabolism allows conver-
1 sion of pyruvate to acetyl coenzyme A (CoA). Acetyl CoA enters the citric acid cycle resulting in carbon dioxide, water, and reducing equivalents (a major source of adenosine triphosphate [ATP]). In the absence of oxygen, glycolysis ends in lactate. Glucose can be stored as or created from glycogen. Glucose can also enter the phosphogluconate pathway, where it is converted to reducing equivalents for fatty acid synthesis and ribose five-carbon sugars important in nucleotide formation. Glucose can be converted into glycerol for fat formation and pyruvate for amino acid synthesis. Gluconeogenesis allows synthesis of glucose from lactate, amino acids, and glycerol.

With regard to lipid metabolism, long-chain fatty acids arise from dietary fat or synthesis from acetyl CoA. Fatty acids can be oxidized to acetyl CoA by the process of β-oxidation or converted to acyl glycerols (fat) for storage as the main energy reserve. In addition to the fats noted previously, acetyl CoA can be used as a precursor to cholesterol and other steroids and in the liver can form the ketone bodies acetoacetate and 3-hydroxybutyrate, which are critical sources of energy during periods of starvation.

Proteins are degraded in two major ways: energy independent, usually in lysosomes, and energy requiring, usually through the ubiquitin pathway. Of amino acids generated in protein catabolism, about three fourths are reutilized for protein synthesis and one fourth are deaminated, with the resulting ammonia converted to urea. Amino acids may be divided into nutritionally essential and nonessential. Nonessential amino acids require fewer enzymatic reactions from amphibolic intermediates or essential amino acids. Each day, humans turn over 1% to 2% of total body protein.

CARBOHYDRATE METABOLISM

The products of intestinal carbohydrate digestion are glucose (80%) and fructose and galactose (20%). Fructose and galactose are rapidly converted to glucose, and the body uses glucose as the primary molecule for transport and uptake of carbohydrates by cells throughout the body. Blood glucose levels are tightly regulated by the liver despite wide fluctuations in dietary intake. About 90% of portal venous glucose is removed from the blood by liver cells through carrier-facilitated diffusion. Large numbers of carrier molecules on the sinusoidal domain of the hepatocyte are capable of binding glucose and transferring it to the cytoplasm. The rate of glucose transport is enhanced (up to 10-fold) by insulin. Given the critical role of glucose in survival, complex metabolic pathways have evolved for the storage of glucose in the fed state, the release of glucose from glycogen, and the synthesis of new glucose.

Blood glucose is stored, primarily in liver and muscle, as glycogen. Glycogen is a complex polymer of glucose with an average molecular weight of 5 million. The liver can convert up to 100 g of glucose into glycogen per day by glycogenesis. The liver can also release glucose into the blood by glycogenolysis, which is the breakdown of glycogen, or by gluconeogenesis, which is the formation of new glucose from substrates such as alanine, lactate, or glycerol. Hormones play a key role in the hepatic regulation of glycogen balance. Insulin, for example, stimulates glycogenesis and glycolysis; glucagon stimulates glycogenolysis and gluconeogenesis.[1]

Glycogenesis and Glycogenolysis

The first step in glycogen storage is the transport of glucose through the plasma membrane. Once in the hepatocyte, glucose and ATP are converted by the enzyme glucokinase to glucose-6-phosphate (G6P), the first intermediate in the synthesis of glycogen (Fig. 2.1). Because complete oxidation of one molecule of G6P generates 37 molecules of ATP, and storage uses only one molecule of ATP, the overall efficiency of glucose storage as glycogen is a remarkable 97%. Glycogenolysis does not occur by simple reversal of glycogenesis. Each succeeding glucose on a glycogen chain is released by glycogen phosphorylase (Fig. 2.2). Eventually, G6P is re-formed. G6P cannot exit from cells and must first be converted back to glucose. The conversion of G6P to glucose is catalyzed by glucose-6-phosphatase, which exists only in hepatocytes, kidney, and
2 intestinal epithelial cells. Neither brain nor muscle cells, which use glucose as a primary fuel source, contain the phosphatase enzyme. This lack of glucose-6-phosphatase ensures a ready supply of glucose for the energy needs of brain and muscle. Liver does not use glucose primarily for fuel but as a precursor for other molecules.

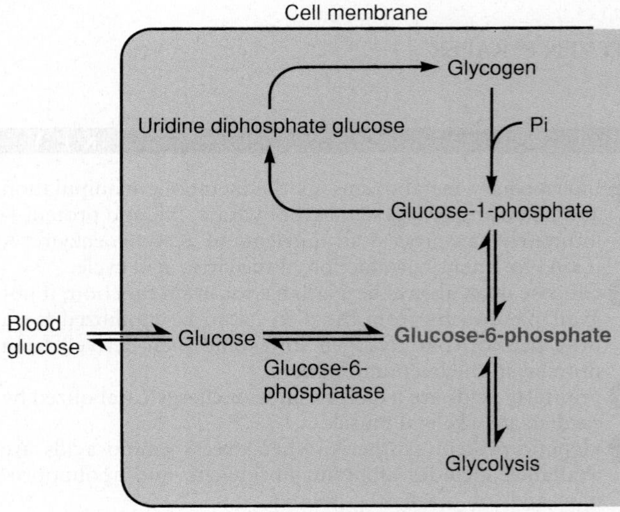

FIGURE 2.1. The chemical reactions of glycogenesis and glycogenolysis. Glucose-6-phosphatase allows hepatic glucose to be transported out of the hepatocyte for use in other tissues. Glucose-6-phosphate, in red, plays a central role in carbohydrate metabolism.

*Anonymous quote cited in Doenst T, Bugger H, Schwarzer M, et al. Three good reasons for heart surgeons to understand cardiac metabolism. *Eur J Cardiothoracic Surg* 2008;33:862–871.

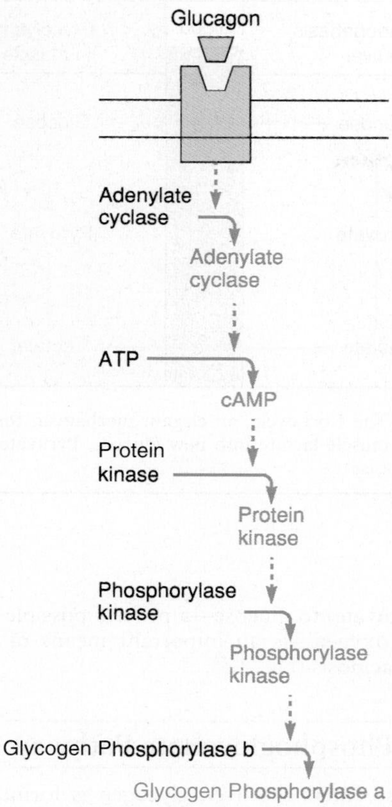

FIGURE 2.2. Glucagon-stimulated enzyme cascade, responsible for the control of glycogen metabolism. Inactive forms are shown in black, active forms in blue.

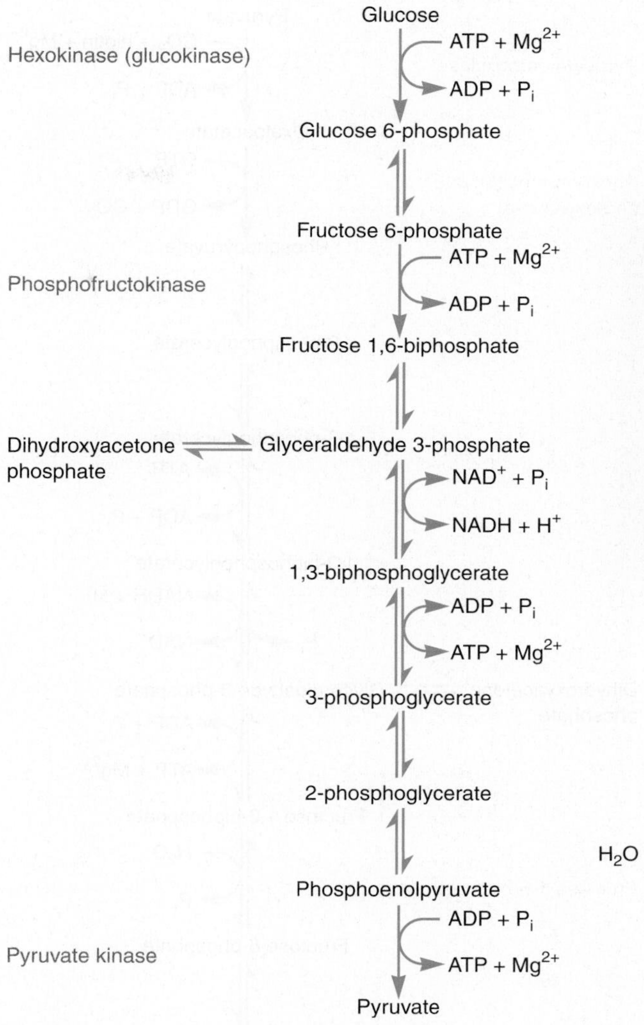

FIGURE 2.3. The glycolytic pathway. There is a net gain of two adenosine triphosphate molecules per glucose molecule. Phosphofructokinase is the key regulatory enzyme in this pathway; however, all the enzymes in red catalyze irreversible reactions. The pathway shown here is active only in the presence of aerobic conditions.

Glycolysis

Glycolysis is the pathway—in all mammalian cells—by which glucose is converted to pyruvate or lactate (Fig. 2.3). The glycolytic pathway is interesting in that glucose can be metabolized in the presence (aerobic) or absence (anaerobic) of oxygen. The aerobic conversion of glucose to pyruvate has three effects: (a) a net gain of two ATP molecules, (b) generation of two reducing equivalents of the nicotinamide adenine nucleotide (NADH + H^+), or (c) conversion of pyruvate to acetyl CoA with subsequent degradation of acetyl CoA in the citric acid cycle (see later). The conversion of glucose to pyruvate is regulated by three enzymes: hexokinase (glucokinase), phosphofructokinase, and pyruvate kinase, which are nonequilibrium reactions and as such, functionally irreversible.

Under anaerobic conditions, NADH + H^+ cannot be reoxidized by transfer of reducing equivalents through the electron transport chain to oxygen. Instead, pyruvate is reduced by the NADH + H^+ to lactate. Glycolysis takes place in the cytoplasm, in contrast to the citric acid cycle, which is a mitochondrial process. During times of glucose excess, as in the fed state, hepatic glycolysis can generate energy in the form of ATP, but the oxidation of ketoacids is a preferred hepatic energy source.

In erythrocytes, a unique variant of glycolysis enhances oxyhemoglobin dissociation. The first site in glycolysis for generation of ATP is bypassed, leading to the formation of 2,3-bisphosphoglycerate by an additional enzyme called bisphosphoglycerate mutase. Kinetics of the mutase present in erythrocytes allow the presence of high concentrations of 2,3-bisphosphoglycerate to build up. The 2,3-bisphosphoglycerate displaces oxygen from hemoglobin, allowing a shift of the oxyhemoglobin dissociation curve to the right.

Gluconeogenesis

There is an absolute minimum requirement for glucose in humans. Below a certain blood glucose concentration, brain dysfunction causes coma and death. When glucose becomes scarce, as in the fasting state, glycogenolysis occurs. Once glycogen stores have been depleted, the liver and kidneys are capable of synthesizing new glucose by the process of gluconeogenesis. Glucagon is produced in response to low blood sugar levels and stimulates gluconeogenesis. Gluconeogenesis is not a simple reversal of the glycolytic pathway. In glycolysis, as noted previously, the conversion of glucose to pyruvate is a one-way reaction. As a result, four separate, functionally irreversible enzyme reactions are required to convert pyruvate into glucose (Fig. 2.4). These enzymes are pyruvate carboxylase,

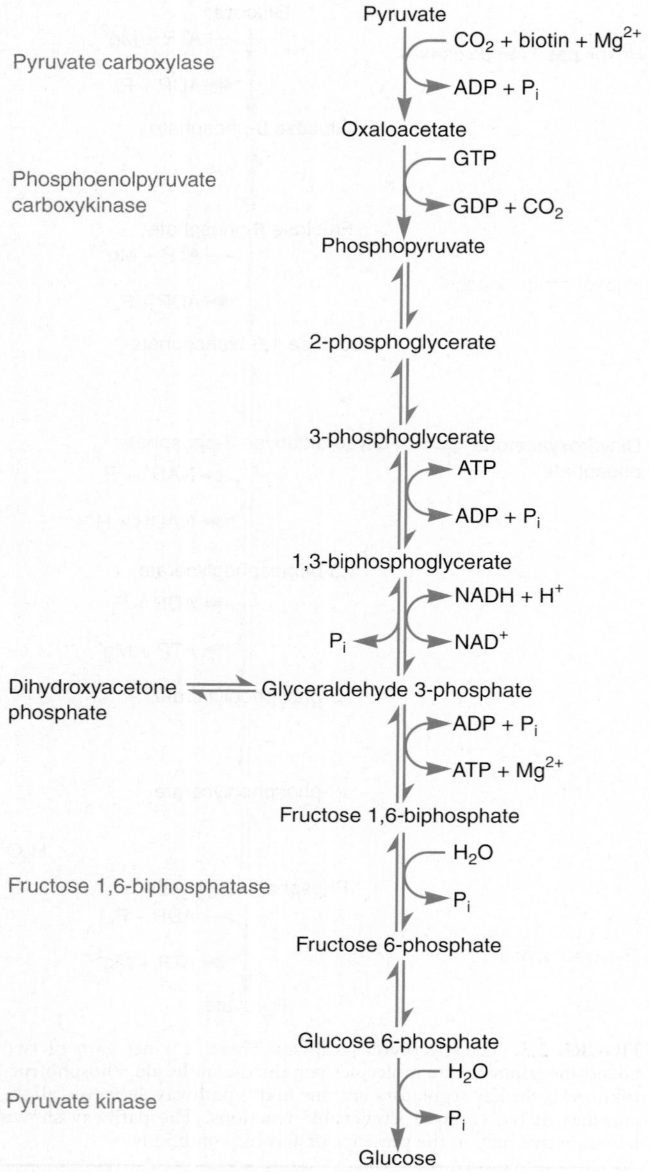

FIGURE 2.4. The gluconeogenesis pathway. The irreversible nature of the glycolytic pathway means that a different sequence of biosyntheses is required for glucose production. The enzymes in red catalyze irreversible reactions that are different from those in glycolysis. In mammals, glucose cannot be synthesized from acetyl coenzyme A, only from cytosolic pyruvate.

phosphoenolpyruvate carboxykinase, fructose-1,6-bisphosphatase, and glucose-6-phosphatase. Other enzymes are shared with the glycolytic pathway.

About 60% of the naturally occurring amino acids, glycerol, or lactate can also be used as substrates for glucose production. Alanine is the amino acid most easily converted into glucose. Simple deamination allows conversion to pyruvate, which is subsequently converted to glucose. Other amino acids can be converted into three-, four-, or five-carbon sugars and then enter the phosphogluconate pathway (see later). Gluconeogenesis is enhanced by fasting, critical illness, and periods of anaerobic metabolism. Active skeletal muscle and erythrocytes form large quantities of lactate. In patients with large wounds, lactate also accumulates. The conversion of lactate

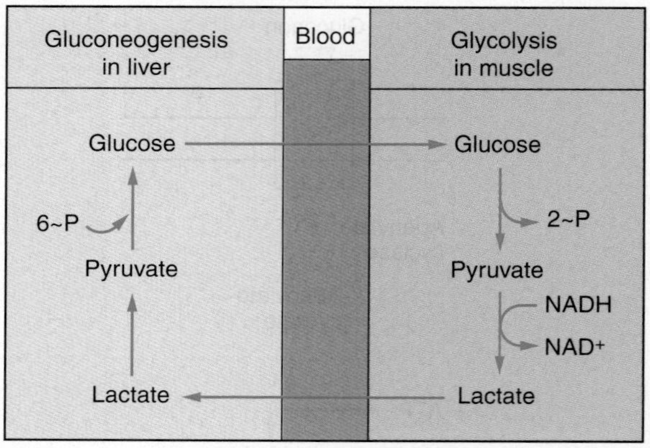

FIGURE 2.5. The Cori cycle, an elegant mechanism for the hepatic conversion of muscle lactate into new glucose. Pyruvate plays a key role in this process.

(through pyruvate) to glucose—a process possible only in the presence of oxygen—is an important means of preventing severe lactic acidosis (Fig. 2.5).

Phosphogluconate Pathway

When glucose enters the liver, glycogen is formed until the hepatic glycogen capacity is reached (about 100 g). If excess glucose is still available, the liver converts it to fat by the phosphogluconate pathway (also known as the pentose phosphate pathway) (Fig. 2.6). The cytosolic phosphogluconate pathway

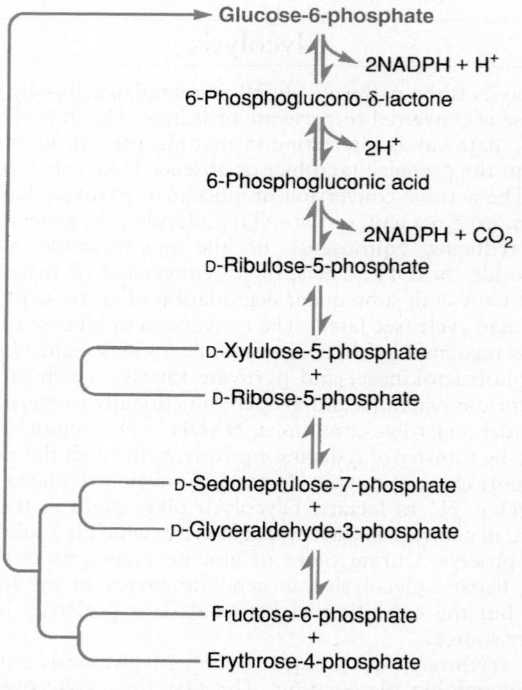

FIGURE 2.6. The phosphogluconate pathway. One of the major purposes of this pathway is to generate reduced nicotinamide adenine dinucleotide, which can serve as an electron donor and allow the liver to perform reductive biosynthesis.

can completely oxidize glucose, generating CO_2 and nicotinamide adenine dinucleotide phosphate (NADPH) through what is known as the oxidative phase. Hydrogen atoms released in the phosphogluconate pathway combine with oxidized nicotinamide adenine dinucleotide phosphate ($NADP^+$) to form reduced nicotinamide adenine dinucleotide phosphate ($NADPH + H^+$).[2] The oxidative phase is present only in tissues, such as the adrenal glands and gonads, that require reductive biosyntheses such as steroidogenesis or other forms of lipid synthesis. Essentially, all tissues contain the nonoxidative phase, which is reversible and produces ribose precursors for nucleotide synthesis. In erythrocytes, the phosphogluconate pathway provides reducing equivalents for the production of reduced glutathione by glutathione reductase. Reduced glutathione can remove hydrogen peroxide, which increases the conversion of oxyhemoglobin to methemoglobin and subsequent hemolysis.

LIPID METABOLISM

Lipid Transport

Lipid transport throughout the body is made complicated by the fact that lipids are insoluble in water. To overcome this physicochemical incompatibility, dietary triglycerides are first split into monoglycerides and fatty acids by the action of intestinal lipases. After absorption into the small intestinal cells, triacylglycerols are re-formed and aggregate into chylomicrons, which then enter the bloodstream by way of the lymph. Chylomicrons are removed from the blood by the liver and adipose tissue. The capillary surface of the liver contains large amounts of lipoprotein lipase, which hydrolyzes triglycerides into fatty acids and glycerol. The fatty acids freely diffuse into the hepatocytes for further metabolism. Similar to chylomicrons, very low-density lipoproteins (VLDLs) are synthesized by the liver and are the main vehicle for transport of triacylglycerols to extrahepatic tissues. The intestines and liver are the only two tissues capable of secreting lipid particles. In addition to chylomicrons and VLDLs, there are two other major groups of plasma lipoproteins: low-density lipoproteins (LDLs) and high-density lipoproteins (HDLs). LDLs and HDLs contain predominantly cholesterol and phospholipid.

The structure of all classes of lipoproteins is similar. There is a core of nonpolar lipids, either triacylglycerols or cholesteryl esters, depending on the particular lipoprotein. This nonpolar core is coated with a surface layer of amphipathic phospholipid or cholesterol oriented so that the polar ends are in contact with the plasma. A protein component is also present. The A apolipoproteins occur in chylomicrons and HDLs. The B apolipoproteins come in two forms: B-100 is the predominant apolipoprotein of LDLs, whereas the shorter B-48 is located in chylomicrons. The C apolipoproteins can transfer between VLDLs, LDLs, and HDLs. Apolipoprotein D and E also exist. Apolipoproteins have several functions in lipid transport and storage. Some, such as the B apolipoproteins, are an integral part of the lipoprotein structure. Other apolipoproteins are enzyme cofactors, such as C-II for lipoprotein lipase. Lastly, the apolipoproteins act as ligands for cell surface receptors. As an example, both B-100 and E serve as ligands for the LDL receptor.[3,4]

Fatty Acid Metabolism

Most human fatty acids in plasma are long-chain acids (C-16 to C-20). Because long-chain fatty acids are not readily absorbed by the intestinal mucosa, they must first be incorporated into chylomicrons. In contrast, short-chain and medium-chain fatty acids are absorbed directly into the portal circulation and are avidly taken up by the liver. Free fatty acids in the circulation are noncovalently bound to albumin and are transferred to the hepatocyte cytosol by way of fatty acid–binding proteins. Fatty acid CoA esters are synthesized in the cytosol after hepatic uptake of fatty acids. These fatty acid CoA esters can be converted into triglyceride, transported into mitochondria for the production of acetyl CoA and reducing equivalents, or stored in the liver as triglycerides. The rate-limiting step in the synthesis of triglyceride is the conversion of acetyl CoA to malonyl CoA. Malonyl CoA, in turn, inhibits the mitochondrial uptake of fatty acid CoA ester, favoring triglyceride synthesis. The liver also contains dehydrogenases that can unsaturate essential dietary fatty acids. Structural elements of all tissues contain significant amounts of unsaturated fats, and the liver is responsible for the production of these unsaturated fatty acids. As another example, dietary linoleic acid is elongated and dehydrogenated to the prostaglandin precursor arachidonic acid.

3 Under basal conditions, most free fatty acids are catabolized for energy by cardiac and skeletal muscle. Under conditions of adipocyte lipolysis, the liver can take up and metabolize fatty acids. Although fatty acid synthesis occurs in the cytosol, fatty acid oxidation occurs in the mitochondria. Fatty acid CoA esters bind carnitine, a carrier molecule, and in the absence of cytosolic malonyl CoA, they enter the mitochondria, where they undergo β-oxidation to acetyl CoA and reducing equivalents (Fig. 2.7). Acetyl CoA can then take one of the following routes: (a) enter the tricarboxylic acid cycle and be degraded to carbon dioxide, (b) be converted to citrate for fatty acid synthesis, or (c) be converted into 3-hydroxy-3-methylglutaryl CoA (HMG-CoA), a precursor of cholesterol and ketone bodies. The mitochondrial hydrolysis of fatty acids is a source of large quantities of ATP. The conversion of stearic acid to carbon dioxide and water, for instance, generates 136 molecules of ATP and demonstrates the highly efficient storage of energy as fat. By a process called β-oxidation, acetyl CoA molecules are cleaved from fatty acids. The acetyl CoA is then metabolized through the citric acid cycle under normal circumstances.

In times of unrestrained lipolysis, such as starvation, uncontrolled diabetes, or other conditions of triglyceride mobilization from adipocyte stores, ketone bodies—predominantly 3-hydroxybutyrate and acetoacetate—are formed in hepatic mitochondria from free fatty acids and are a source of energy for extrahepatic tissues. Ketogenesis is regulated predominantly by the rate of mobilization of free fatty acids. Once in the liver mitochondria, the relative proportion of acyl CoA destined to undergo β-oxidation is limited by the activity of an enzyme, carnitine palmitoyltransferase-1. Lastly, there are mechanisms that keep the levels of acetyl CoA entering the citric acid cycle constant, so that only at high mitochondrial levels will acetyl CoA be converted to ketone bodies. Even the brain, in times of starvation, can use ketone bodies for half of its energy requirements. At some point, however, the ability of liver to perform β-oxidation may be inadequate. Under such circumstances, hepatic storage of triglyceride or fatty infiltration of the liver can be significant, leading to the development of nonalcoholic steatohepatitis (NASH). Triglyceride storage by itself does not appear to be a cause of hepatic fibrosis, but fatty infiltration may be a marker for the derangement of normal processes by alcohol or drug toxicity, diabetes, or long-term total parenteral nutrition. A specific type of microvesicular fatty accumulation is also seen in a variety of diseases, such as Reye syndrome, morbid obesity, and acute fatty liver of pregnancy.

Cholesterol Metabolism

Cholesterol is an important regulator of membrane fluidity and is a substrate for bile acid and steroid hormone synthesis.

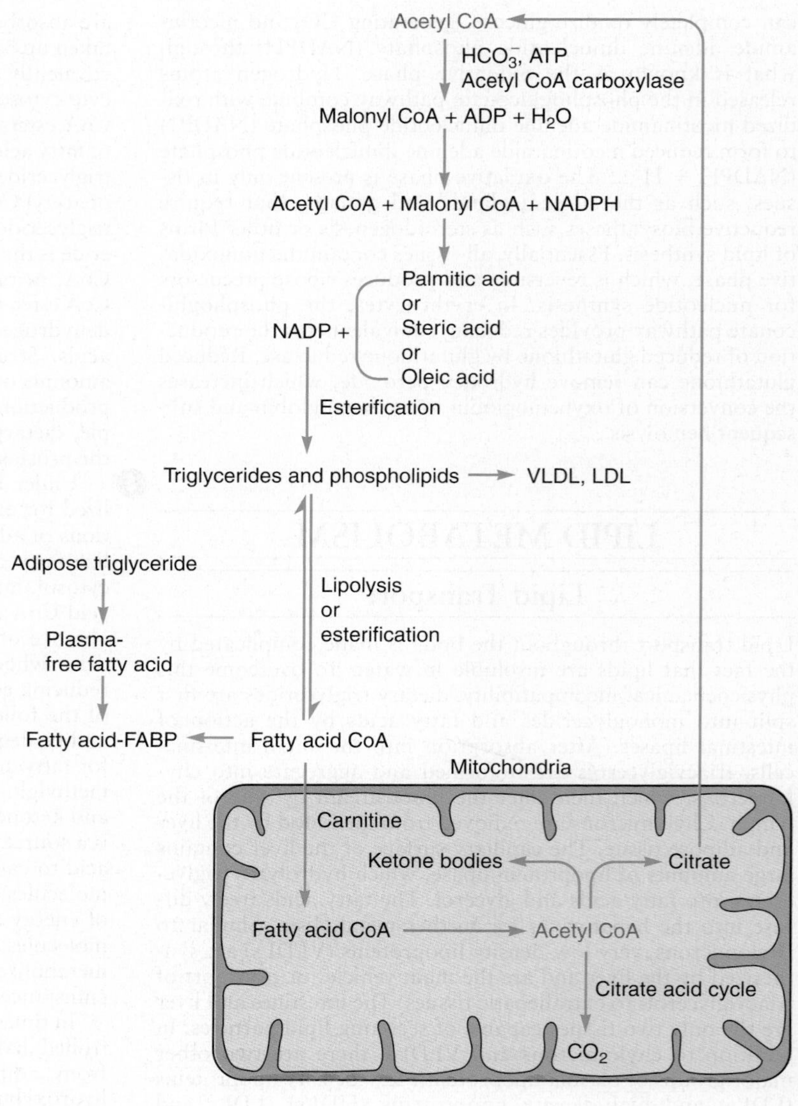

FIGURE 2.7. Diagram of hepatic fatty acid metabolism. Both dietary and newly synthesized fatty acids are esterified and subsequently degraded in the mitochondria for energy, first as reducing equivalents, then adenosine triphosphate via the electron transport chain.

Cholesterol may be available by dietary intake or by de novo synthesis. In mammals, most new cholesterol is synthesized in the liver from its precursor, acetyl CoA. Dietary cholesterol intake can suppress endogenous synthesis by inhibiting the rate-limiting enzyme in the cholesterol biosynthetic pathway, HMG-CoA reductase. A competitive antagonist, lovastatin, can also block HMG-CoA reductase and effectively lower plasma cholesterol by blocking cholesterol synthesis, stimulating LDL receptor synthesis, and allowing an increased hepatic uptake and metabolism of cholesterol-rich LDL lipoproteins. The structure of the LDL receptor is known and serves as a model for the structure and function of other cell membrane receptors (Fig. 2.8).

Cholesterol is lipophilic and hydrophobic, and most plasma cholesterol is in lipoproteins esterified with oleic or palmitic acid. The liver can process cholesterol esters from all classes of lipoproteins. Hepatocytes can also take up chylomicron remnants containing dietary cholesterol esters. Newly synthesized hepatic cholesterol is used primarily to synthesize bile acids for further intestinal absorption of dietary fats. A large proportion of the bile acids secreted by the liver into bile are returned to the liver via the enterohepatic circulation (Fig. 2.9). Abnormally elevated levels of cholesterol in VLDLs or LDLs are associated with atherosclerosis, whereas HDL levels are protective.

Phospholipids

The three major classes of phospholipids synthesized by the liver are lecithins, cephalins, and sphingomyelins. Although most cells in the body are capable of some phospholipid synthesis, the liver produces 90%. Phospholipid formation is controlled by the overall rate of fat metabolism and by the availability of choline and inositol. The main role of phospholipids of all types is to form plasma and organelle membranes. The amphiphilic nature of phospholipids makes them essential for reducing surface tension between membranes and surrounding fluids. Phosphatidylcholine, one of the lecithins, is the major biliary phospholipid and is important in promoting the secretion of free cholesterol into bile. Thromboplastin, one of the cephalins, is needed to initiate the clotting cascade. The sphingomyelins are necessary for the formation of the myelin nerve sheath.

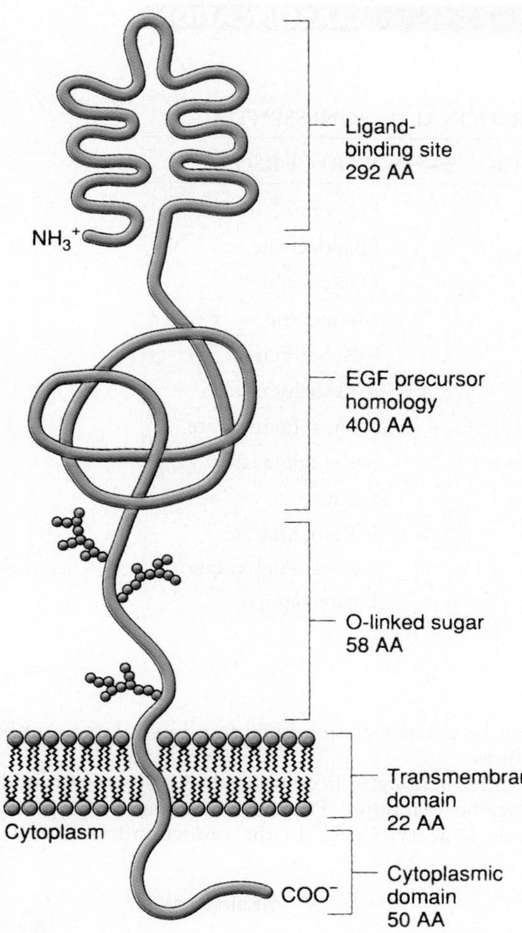

FIGURE 2.8. The low-density lipoprotein (LDL) receptor, an example of a transmembrane receptor that participates in receptor-mediated endocytosis. The LDL receptor specifically binds lipoproteins that contain apolipoprotein B-100 or E. Once internalized, the lipoproteins are degraded. AA, amino acids.

PROTEIN METABOLISM

Formation and Catabolism of Plasma Proteins

4 Essentially, all albumin, fibrinogen, and apolipoproteins are derived from the liver, which can add up to 50 g of protein to the plasma per day. Of the total hepatic protein synthesized, 75% is destined for export in plasma. Most newly synthesized proteins are not stored in the liver, and the rate of protein synthesis is primarily determined by the intracellular levels of amino acids. The tertiary structure of many proteins undergoes posttranslational modification after they have been synthesized in the liver's rough endoplasmic reticulum (ER). Glycosylation, or the addition of carbohydrate moieties, occurs in the smooth ER. Sialation, or the addition of sialic acid, occurs in the Golgi. Glycosylation is important in allowing some proteins to bind with specific receptors for subsequent hepatic uptake and processing. Removal of sialic acid residues, or desialation, from the terminal galactose molecules of glycoproteins allows them to bind to the asialoglycoprotein (ASGP) receptor in the liver and undergo degradation. Desialation, therefore, is important in the clearance of senescent proteins from the plasma.

Intracellular proteases hydrolyze proteins into peptides, and the peptides are in turn hydrolyzed by peptidases. Ultimately, free amino acids are generated. Unlike carbohydrate and lipids, excess amino acids are degraded if they are not immediately reincorporated into new proteins. Protein degradation occurs primarily by one of two routes. Asialoglycoproteins are internalized into lysosomes via receptor-mediated endocytosis. The lysosomal enzymes do not require ATP and are nonselective in their activities; more than 20 known hydrolytic enzymes are present in lysosomes. A second pathway involves the covalent attachment of ubiquitin, named for the fact that it exists in all mammalian cells, targeting proteins for destruction. This pathway is ATP dependent and generally is used for proteins with shorter half-lives.[5]

Amino Acid Synthesis

Essentially, all the end products of dietary protein digestion are amino acids, which are absorbed by the enterocytes into the portal circulation in an ionized state. Liver amino acid uptake occurs by one of several active transport mechanisms. Amino acids are not stored in the liver but are rapidly used in the production of plasma proteins, purines, heme proteins, and hormones. Under certain conditions, the amine group is removed from amino acids, and the carbon chain is used for carbohydrate, lipid, or nonessential amino acid synthesis.[6]

Ten nutritionally essential amino acids must be obtained from dietary intake (Table 2.1). However, human tissues contain transferases, which convert the α-keto acids of leucine, valine, and isoleucine so that the corresponding α-keto acids can be used as dietary supplements. The remaining nutritionally nonessential amino acids can be synthesized in one to three enzyme-catalyzed reactions. Hydroxyproline and hydroxylysine do not have a corresponding tRNA and arise by posttranslational modification of proline or lysine by mixed

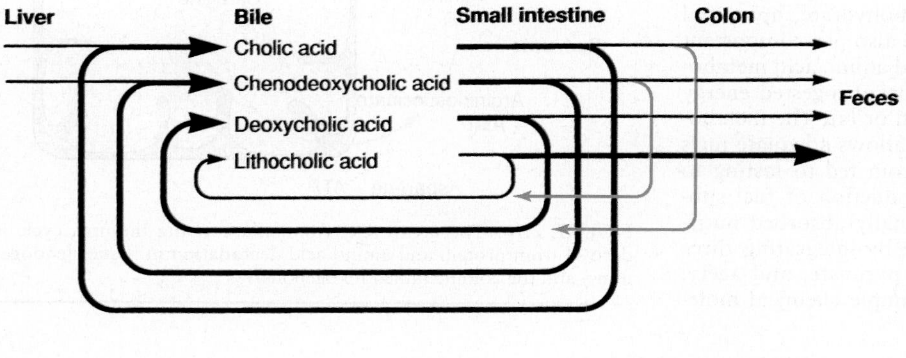

FIGURE 2.9. The enterohepatic circulation of bile acids. The primary bile acids, cholic acid and chenodeoxycholic acid, are synthesized in the liver from cholesterol. Deoxycholic acid and lithocholic acid are formed in the colon (*blue lines*) during bacterial degradation of the primary bile acids. All four bile acids are conjugated with glycine or taurine in the liver. Most of the lithocholic acid is also sulfated, which decreases reabsorption and increases fecal excretion. Bile acids are absorbed passively in the epithelium of the small and large intestine and actively in the distal ileum.

TABLE 2.1 **CLASSIFICATION**

AMINO ACIDS REQUIRED BY ADULT HUMANS

	NUTRITIONALLY NONESSENTIAL	
NUTRITIONALLY ESSENTIAL	AMINO ACID	PRECURSOR
Arginine	Alanine	Pyruvate
Histidine	Asparagine	Oxaloacetate
Isoleucine	Aspartate	Oxaloacetate
Leucine	Cysteine	Methionine
Lysine	Glutamate	α-Ketoglutarate
Methionine	Glutamine	α-Ketoglutarate
Phenylalanine	Glycine	3-Phosphoglycerate
Threonine	Hydroxyproline	α-Ketoglutarate
Tryptophan	Hydroxylysine	Lysine
Valine	Proline	α-Ketoglutarate
	Serine	3-Phosphoglycerate
	Tyrosine	Phenylalanine

function oxidases. Glutamate, glutamine, and proline are derived from the citric acid cycle intermediate α-ketoglutarate. Aspartate and asparagine are synthesized from oxaloacetate. Serine and glycine are synthesized from the glycolysis intermediate 3-phosphoglycerate. Cysteine and tyrosine are formed from essential amino acids (methionine and phenylalanine, respectively).[7]

Catabolism of Amino Acid Nitrogen

Ammonia, derived largely from the deamination of amino acids, is toxic to all mammalian cells. The ammonia formed as a result of the deamination of amino acids is detoxified by one of two routes.[8] The most important pathway involves the conversion of ammonia to urea by enzymes of the Krebs-Henseleit, or urea, cycle, which happens only in the liver (Fig. 2.10). A second route of ammonia metabolism involves synthesis of L-glutamine from ammonia and glutamate by renal glutamine synthetase.

THE CITRIC ACID CYCLE AND INTEGRATION OF METABOLIC PATHWAYS

The major function of the citric acid cycle is to act as a common pathway for the oxidation of carbohydrate, lipid, and protein. Conversely, the citric acid cycle also plays important roles in gluconeogenesis, lipogenesis, and amino acid metabolism. In the fed state, a large proportion of ingested energy from foodstuffs is converted to glycogen or fat. The metabolism of sugars, fats, and proteins, then, allows adequate fuels for all tissue types under conditions from fed to fasting to starvation. The body accomplishes production of fuel substrates for organs and regulates intestinally absorbed nutrients for tissue consumption or storage by integrating three key metabolites: glucose-6-phosphate, pyruvate, and acetyl CoA (Fig. 2.11). Each of these three simple chemical molecules can be extensively modified to allow a large number of metabolites.

5 The citric acid cycle is composed of a series of mitochondrial enzyme reactions. The substrate that drives the citric acid cycle is acetyl CoA.[9] In the mitochondria, acetyl CoA

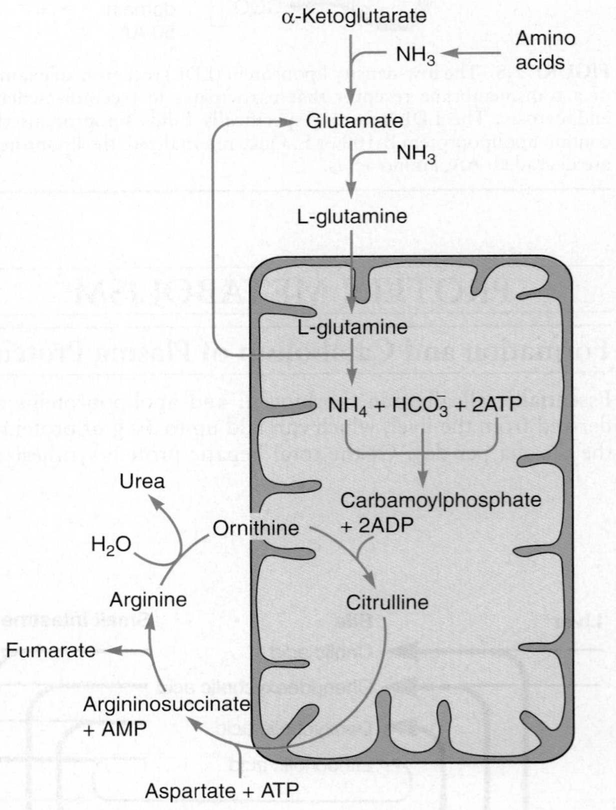

FIGURE 2.10. The urea cycle. Ammonia entering the urea cycle is derived from protein and amino acid degradation in tissues (endogenous) and the colonic lumen (exogenous).

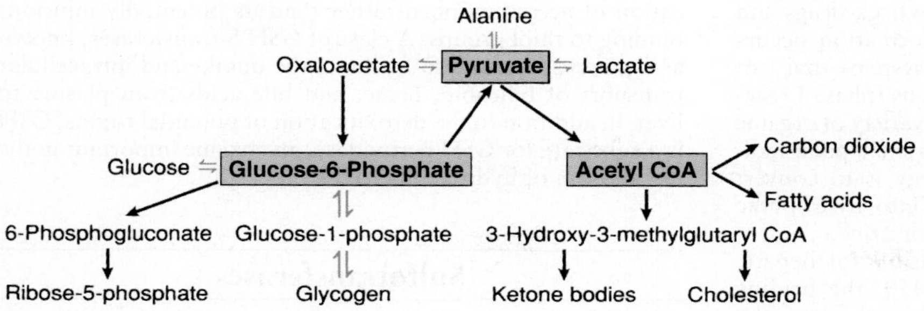

FIGURE 2.11. Summation of the key regulatory molecules used by the liver during diverse metabolic functions. Essentially, any compound found in the body can be synthesized in the liver from glucose-6-phosphate, acetyl coenzyme A, or pyruvate. As a consequence of the inability of mammalian liver to convert acetyl coenzyme A to pyruvate, fats cannot be converted to carbohydrates.

combines with oxaloacetate to form citrate. Through a series of enzymatic reactions involving both dehydrogenases and decarboxylases, citrate is catabolized to result in the generation of hydrogen-reducing equivalents and carbon dioxide (Fig. 2.12). Each molecule of acetyl CoA catabolized through the citric acid cycle yields three molecules of NADH + H^+ and one molecule of flavine adenine dinucleotide ($FADH_2$). These reducing equivalents are transported to the inner mitochondrial membrane and the electron transport chain to generate more ATP. Each molecule of NADH + H^+ is oxidized to yield three molecules of ATP, and each molecule of $FADH_2$ is oxidized to yield two molecules of ATP. One molecule of ATP is generated at the substrate level in the conversion of succinyl CoA to succinate; thus, the total molecules of ATP generated per molecule of acetyl CoA is 12.

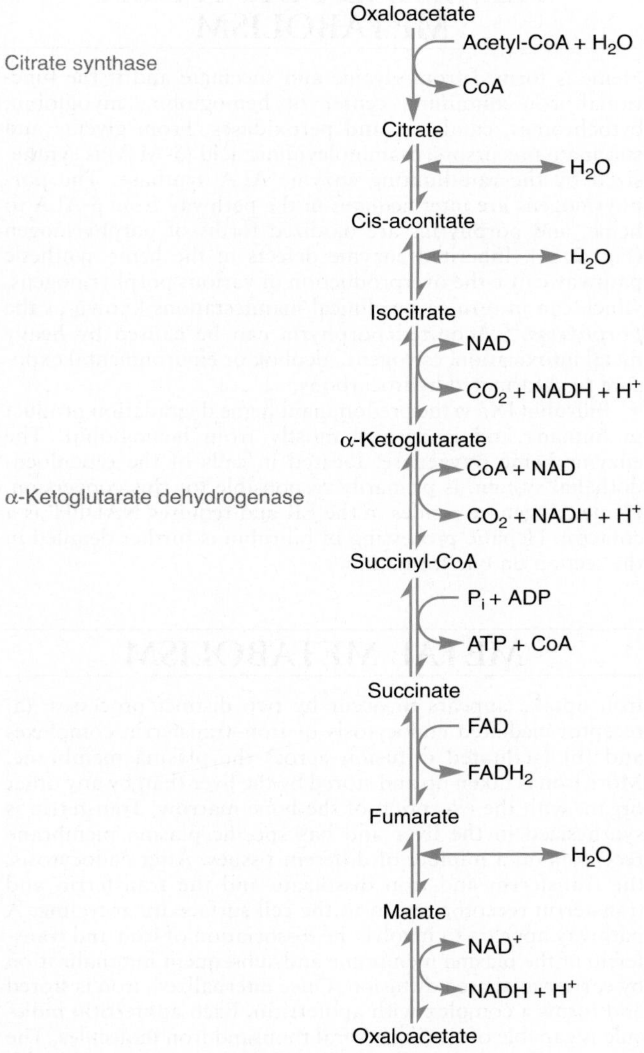

FIGURE 2.12. The citric acid cycle. Reduced nicotinamide adenine dinucleotide and reduced flavin adenine dinucleotide, formed in the citric acid cycle, are subsequently oxidized in mitochondria by means of the electron transport chain to generate adenosine triphosphate. Acetyl coenzyme A plays a key role.

G6P can be stored as glycogen or converted into glucose, pyruvate, or ribose-5-phosphate (a nucleotide precursor). Pyruvate can be converted into lactate, alanine (and other amino acids), and acetyl CoA, or it can enter the tricarboxylic acid cycle by conversion to oxaloacetate. Acetyl CoA is converted to HMG-CoA (a cholesterol and ketone body precursor) or citrate (for fatty acid and triglyceride synthesis), or it is degraded to carbon dioxide and water for energy. In humans, acetyl CoA cannot be converted into pyruvate due to the irreversible reaction of pyruvate dehydrogenase. Thus, lipids cannot be converted into either carbohydrates or glucogenic amino acids.

Regardless of the fed state of the human body, there is a requirement for glucose utilization. The nervous system and erythrocytes have an absolute requirement for glucose. Glucose is a source of glycerol-3-phosphate for adipose tissue, and most other tissues for integrity of the citric acid cycle. To maintain adequate glucose for survival, other fuels can be used depending on environmental conditions. Under conditions of carbohydrate shortage, ketone bodies and free fatty acids are utilized to spare oxidation of glucose in muscle. These alternate fuels increase intracellular citrate, which inhibits both phosphofructokinase and pyruvate dehydrogenase. In starvation, fatty acid oxidation results in the production of glycerol, which, along with gluconeogenesis from amino acids, is the only source of the required glucose. Ultimately, even the brain can substitute ketone bodies for about half of its energy requirements. The preferred energy substrates for liver are ketoacids derived from amino acid degradation even in well-fed states. This is designed to allow the consumption of glucose by obligate tissues. Glucose produced by the dephosphorylation of G6P rapidly diffuses out of the cell and is taken up by the brain, muscles, and other organs. Hepatic glycolysis is used primarily for the production of intermediates of metabolism and not for energy. Hepatic fatty acid degradation for energy is also inhibited under most circumstances and occurs only during adipocyte lipolysis.

BIOTRANSFORMATION

Biotransformation is defined as the intracellular metabolism of endogenous organic compounds (e.g., heme proteins and steroid hormones) and exogenous compounds (e.g., drugs and environmental compounds). Most biotransformation occurs chiefly in the liver, which contains enzyme systems that can expose functional groups, such as hydroxyl ions (phase I reactions), or alter the size and solubility of a wide variety of organic and inorganic compounds by conjugation with small polar molecules (phase II reactions). A general strategy is to convert hydrophobic, potentially toxic compounds into hydrophilic conjugates that can then be excreted into bile or urine.

6 The four general enzyme families responsible for hepatic biotransformation are the cytochromes P-450, the uridine diphosphate-glucuronyl (UDP-glucuronyl) transferases, the glutathione (GSH) S-transferases, and the sulfotransferases. Biotransforming enzymes are not distributed uniformly within the cells of the hepatic lobule. This heterogeneity may account for the ability of some drugs to cause damage preferentially in zone 3 hepatocytes (those nearest the central venule).

Cytochromes P-450

The cytochromes P-450 are named for their ability to absorb light maximally at 450 nm in the presence of carbon monoxide. These enzymes are bound to the ER and collectively catalyze reactions by using NADPH and oxygen. The P-450 isozymes present in mammalian liver catalyze reactions such as oxidation, hydroxylation, sulfoxide formation, oxidative deamination, dealkylation, and dehalogenation. Such reactions allow further phase II conjugation with polar groups such as glucuronate, GSH, and sulfate. The cytochromes P-450 can also create potentially toxic metabolites. Drugs such as acetaminophen, isoniazid, halothane, and the phenothiazines can be converted into reactive forms that cause cellular injury and death. The cytochromes also are responsible for the formation of organic free radicals, reactive metabolites that can directly attack and injure cellular components or act as haptens in the generation of an autoimmune response. Several of the most potent known carcinogens are aromatic hydrocarbons, which are modified by cytochromes P-450.

Uridine Diphosphate-glucuronyl Transferases

Glucuronidation is the conjugation of UDP-glucuronic acid to a wide variety of xenobiotics by either ester (acyl) or ether linkages. The transferases catalyzing these reactions reside in the ER. Many common compounds are metabolized in this way, including bilirubin, testosterone, aspirin, indomethacin, acetaminophen, chloramphenicol, and oxazepam. Clinically significant loss of activity can occur with acute ethanol exposure or acetaminophen overdose, when formation of UDP-glucuronic acid from UDP-glucose is outstripped by use. Some acyl linkages lead to the generation of electrophilic centers that can react with other proteins. The covalent linkage of conjugated bilirubin to albumin is believed to occur by this mechanism.

Glutathione S-transferases

The GSH transferases are more selective in the biotransformations they perform. GSH conjugation occurs only with compounds that have electrophilic and potentially reactive centers. The role of GSH conjugation catalyzed by the GSH S-transferases is demonstrated by acetaminophen. In metabolism of this drug, cytochromes P-450 create an electrophilic center that reacts with protein thiol groups or GSH.[10] The presence of GSH S-transferase allows the preferential detoxification of acetaminophen rather than its potentially injurious binding to thiol groups. A class of GSH S-transferases, known as *ligandins,* appears to facilitate the uptake and intracellular transport of bilirubin, heme, and bile acids from plasma to liver. In addition to the detoxification of potential toxins, GSH is a substrate for GSH peroxidase, an enzyme important in the metabolism of hydrogen peroxide.

Sulfotransferases

The sulfotransferases catalyze the transfer of sulfate groups from 3′-phosphoadenosine-5′-phosphosulfate (PAPS) to compounds such as thyroxine, bile acids, isoproterenol, α-methyldopa, and acetaminophen. They are located primarily in the cytosol. Although many P-450 derivatives can be further conjugated by either the sulfotransferases or the glucuronyl transferases, a limited ability of the liver to synthesize PAPS makes glucuronidation the predominant mechanism.

HEME AND PORPHYRIN METABOLISM

Heme is formed from glycine and succinate and is the functional iron-containing center of hemoglobin, myoglobin, cytochromes, catalases, and peroxidases. From glycine and succinate precursors, δ-aminolevulinic acid (δ-ALA) is synthesized by the rate-limiting enzyme ALA synthase. The porphyrinogens are intermediates in the pathway from δ-ALA to heme, and porphyrins are oxidized forms of porphyrinogen (Fig. 2.13). Inherited enzyme defects in the heme synthetic pathway cause the overproduction of various porphyrinogens, which can in turn cause clinical manifestations known as the *porphyrias.*[11] Acquired porphyria can be caused by heavy metal intoxication, estrogens, alcohol, or environmental exposure to chlorinated hydrocarbons.

Bilirubin IXa is the predominant heme degradation product in humans and is derived mostly from hemoglobin. The enzyme heme oxygenase, located in cells of the reticuloendothelial system, is primarily responsible for this conversion. Heme oxygenase resides in the ER and requires NADPH as a cofactor. Hepatic processing of bilirubin is further detailed in the section on bile formation.

METAL METABOLISM

Iron uptake appears to occur by two distinct processes: (a) receptor-mediated endocytosis of iron–transferrin complexes and (b) facilitated diffusion across the plasma membrane. More iron is taken up and stored by the liver than by any other organ, with the exception of the bone marrow. Transferrin is synthesized in the liver and has specific plasma membrane receptors on a number of different tissues. After endocytosis, the transferrin and iron dissociate and the transferrin and transferrin receptor return to the cell surface for recycling. A pathway appears to involve the dissociation of iron and transferrin at the plasma membrane and subsequent internalization by carrier-mediated diffusion. Once internalized, iron is stored and forms a complex with apoferritin. Each apoferritin molecule is capable of storing several thousand iron molecules. The iron–apoferritin complex, called *ferritin,* is responsible for iron storage under physiologic conditions. Iron storage in a protein-bound form is essential because free iron can catalyze free radical formation, leading to cell injury.[12]

Copper is transported to the liver bound to albumin or histidine and enters the hepatocytes by a process of facilitated

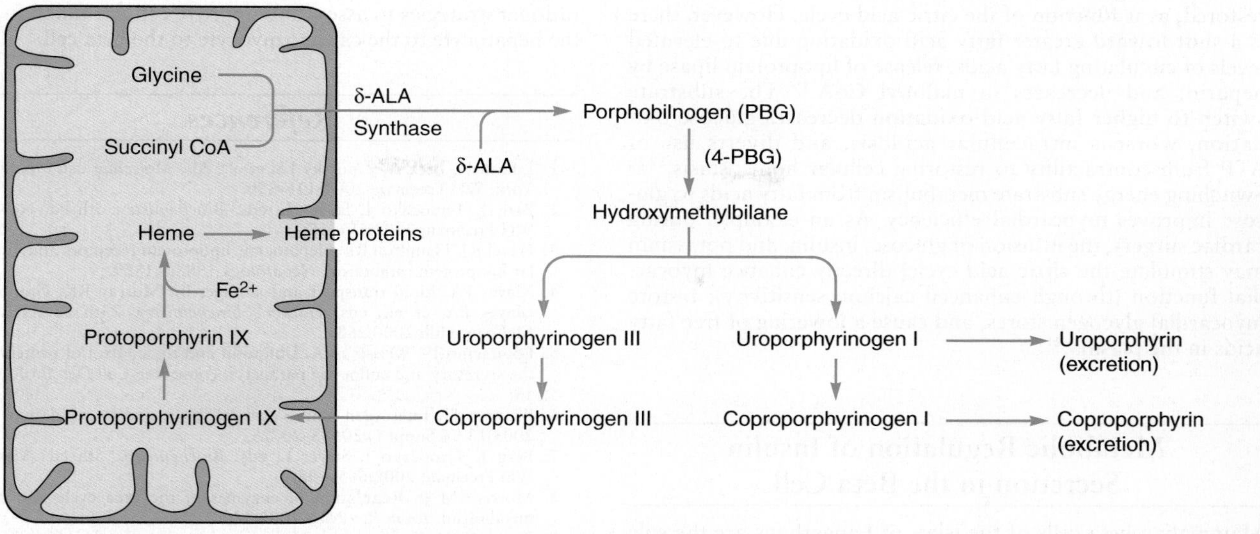

FIGURE 2.13. The heme biosynthetic pathway. Inherited defects of each of the heme biosynthetic enzymes except δ-aminolevulinic acid synthase have been described and lead to the clinical disorders known as the porphyrias.

diffusion. Once inside the cell, copper can bind to several intracellular proteins for storage or as a necessary enzyme cofactor. Copper-binding proteins include metallothionein, monoamine oxidase, cytochrome *c* oxidase, and superoxide dismutase. *Ceruloplasmin* is a liver-derived protein that binds hepatic copper for transport to other tissues. The low levels of ceruloplasmin seen in patients with Wilson disease suggest a pathogenetic defect.

Zinc is taken up by and competes for the same binding sites as copper. In hepatocytes, zinc binds predominantly to metallothionein and is excreted into bile, in which it enters the enterohepatic circulation. Other metals, usually found in trace amounts, are lead, cadmium, selenium, mercury, and nickel. These metals are usually bound to metallothionein or GSH, and intoxication is associated with free radical formation and liver injury.

INTERMEDIARY METABOLISM AND SPECIALIZED CELL FUNCTION

Once understood, the general principles of intermediary metabolism can be used to understand cell biology in specialized cell types. Several examples, not intended to be all-inclusive, are discussed to demonstrate how biochemical pathways influence cellular function.

Hepatocyte-specific Measures of Liver Reserve

To refine traditional estimates of liver reserve, such as the clinically based Childs-Pugh classification and cross-sectional imaging to quantitate liver volume, functional tests have been developed that measure the ability of an individual liver to carry out specific biochemical tasks and correlate this "functional capacity" with perioperative morbidity and mortality.[13] Although myriad functional studies have been described, several are known to be more predictive of liver function. None are widely used due to the lack of availability in clinical laboratories and the relatively small population of relevant patients.

Indocyanine green (ICG) is taken up by specific, ATP-independent carriers on the basolateral surface of the hepatocyte and excreted unmetabolized into bile through a mechanism that is dependent on hepatic ATP. ICG does not undergo enterohepatic recirculation. In the absence of adequate hepatocyte ATP stores, ICG builds up in and saturates hepatocytes, preventing otherwise available carriers from taking up more ICG. As a result, there is decreased clearance of ICG from serum, and clearance rates correlate with improved survival in major liver resections.[14] A limitation is the dependence of ICG clearance on hepatic blood flow, which can be significantly altered in cirrhosis.

Lidocaine is converted, by hepatocytes, into monoethylglycinexylidide (MEGX). The pathway includes oxidative N-dealkylation by the cytochromes P-450, and 97% of the conversion is done in the liver. There are data that show decreased complication rates when the MEGX test is used to predict the outcome of liver resection in cirrhotics.[15] The hippurate ratio is a measure of glycine conjugation of para-aminobenzoic acid to para-aminohippuric acid. These conjugations occur by non–P-450 phase II conjugation mechanisms.[16] The arterial ketone body ratio (AKBR) is also used to predict outcome. The AKBR is the fasting ratio of acetoacetic acid to β-hydroxybutyric acid and reflects mitochondrial oxidized nicotinamide adenine dinucleotide to reduced nicotinamide adenine dinucleotide.[13]

Cardiac Myocyte Substrate Utilization

Under normal conditions, the heart generates 70% of its ATP from fatty acid oxidation, 30% from glucose, and the rest from oxidation of lactate, amino acids, and ketone bodies.[17] In heart failure, the myocardium shifts away from fatty acid oxidation and toward glucose oxidation. This shift improves contractile function and slows the progression of pump failure.[18] In cardiac surgery, during reperfusion, oxygen levels are restored, as is function of the citric acid cycle. However, there is a shift toward greater fatty acid oxidation due to elevated levels of circulating fatty acids, release of lipoprotein lipase by heparin, and decreases in malonyl CoA.[19] The substrate switch to higher fatty acid oxidation decreases glucose oxidation, worsens intracellular acidosis, and diverts use of ATP from contractility to restoring cellular homeostasis.[17,20] Switching energy substrate metabolism from fatty acids to glucose improves myocardial efficiency. As an example, during cardiac surgery, the infusion of glucose, insulin, and potassium may stimulate the citric acid cycle; directly enhance myocardial function (through enhanced calcium sensitivity); restore myocardial glycogen stores; and cause a lowering of free fatty acids in the plasma.[21]

Metabolic Regulation of Insulin Secretion in the Beta Cell

Mammalian beta cells of the islets of Langerhans are the sole source of insulin. Insulin is secreted by a process known as stimulus-secretion coupling, which begins with glucose entering the beta cell via a specific glucose transporter known as GLUT-2. Intracellular glucose is metabolized beginning with phosphorylation by an equally unique hexokinase (glucokinase). The resulting glucose-6-phosphate is then metabolized by both glycolysis and the tricarboxylic acid cycle. The resulting ATP closes ATP-sensitive potassium channels, leading to cell membrane depolarization and opening of calcium channels. Free intracellular calcium then leads to insulin secretion.[22]

A distinguishing feature of beta cells compared to hepatocytes is that beta cells contain neither lactate transporters nor lactate dehydrogenase. As a result, neither lactate metabolism nor gluconeogenesis occurs in the beta cell.[23] Essentially, all glucose-derived carbon is funneled into the citric acid cycle, where 75% of the catabolic product is ATP, and the rest is used for protein synthesis. Pyruvate is forced into the citric acid cycle by a process called *anapleurosis*, or filling up. To overcome the unfavorable kinetics of driving pyruvate through the cycle, the beta cell contains seven times the usual level of pyruvate carboxylase.[24]

SUMMARY

The basics of intermediary metabolism have changed little over the past decade. Knowledge of the fundamental biochemical reactions by which substrates are metabolized, however, is being exploited at an ever-accelerating rate to support and perhaps enhance specialized cellular function. Variations on basic metabolic themes in individual cell types allow the development of rational strategies to assess and improve cellular function, from the hepatocyte to the cardiac myocyte to the beta cell.

References

1. Lodish H, Berk A, Zipursky LS, et al., eds. *Molecular cell biology*. New York: WH Freeman; 2004:301–350.
2. Berg J, Tymoczko J, Stryer L, eds. *Biochemistry*. 5th ed. New York: WH Freeman; 2002:551–576.
3. Havel RJ, Hamilton RL. Hepatocytic lipoprotein receptors and intracellular lipoprotein catabolism. *Hepatology* 1988;8:1869.
4. Mayes PA. Lipid transport and storage. In: Murray RK, Granner DK, Mayes PA, et al., eds. *Harper's biochemistry*. 25th ed. New York: McGraw-Hill; 2000:268.
5. Bonifacino JS, Weissman A. Ubiquitin and the control of protein fate in the secretory and endocytic pathways. *Annu Rev Cell Dev Biol* 1998;14:19.
6. Brosnan JT. Interorgan amino acid transport and its regulation. *J Nutr* 2003;133(6 Suppl 1):2068S–2072S.
7. Berg J, Tymoczko J, Stryer L, eds. *Biochemistry*. 5th ed. New York: WH Freeman; 2002:665–692.
8. Morris SM Jr. Regulation of enzymes of the urea cycle and arginine metabolism. *Annu Rev Nutr* 2002;22:87.
9. Kornberg H. Krebs and his trinity of cycles. *Nat Rev Mol Cell Biol* 2000;1:225.
10. Lee T, Li L, Ballatori N. Hepatic glutathione and glutathione S-conjugate transport mechanisms. *Yale J Biol Med* 1997;70:287–300.
11. Gross U, Hoffmann GF, Doss MO. Erythropoietic and hepatic porphyrias. *J Inherit Metab Dis* 2000;23:641.
12. Hentze MW, Muckenthaler MU, Andrews NC. Balancing acts: molecular control of mammalian iron metabolism. *Cell* 2004;117:285.
13. Mullin EJ, Metcalfe MS, Maddern GJ. How much liver resection is too much? *Am J Surg* 2005;190:87–97.
14. Minagawa M, Makuuchi M, Takayama T, et al. Selection criteria for repeat hepatectomy in patients with recurrent hepatocellular carcinoma. *Ann Surg* 2003;238:703–710.
15. Ercolani G, Grazi GL, Calliva R, et al. The lidocaine (MEGX) test as an index of hepatic function: its usefulness in liver surgery. *Surgery* 2000;127:464–471.
16. Lebel S, Nakamichi Y, Hemming A, et al. Glycine conjugation of para-aminobenzoic acid (PABA): a pilot study of a novel prognostic test in acute liver failure in children. *J Pediatr Gastroenterol Nutr* 2003;36:62–71.
17. Doenst T, Bugger H, Schwarzer M, et al. Three good reasons for heart surgeons to understand cardiac metabolism. *Eur J Cardiothoracic Surg* 2008;33:862–871.
18. Lopaschuk GD. Optimizing cardiac fatty acid and glucose metabolism as an approach to treating heart failure. *Semin Cardiothorac Vasc Anesth* 2006;10(3):228–230.
19. Wang W, Lopaschuk GD. Metabolic therapy for the treatment of ischemic heart disease: reality and expectations. *Expert Rev Cardiovasc Ther* 2007;5:1123–1134.
20. Liu Q, Docherty JC, Rendell JC, et al. High levels of fatty acids delay the recovery of intracellular pH and cardiac efficiency in post-ischemic hearts by inhibiting glucose oxidation. *J Am Coll Cardiol* 2002;39:718–725.
21. Taegtmeyer H. Clinical trials report. Metabolic modulation as a principle for myocardial protection. *Curr Hypertens Rep* 2003;5:443–444.
22. Leibiger IB, Leibiger B, Berggren P-O. Insulin signaling in the pancreatic beta cell. *Ann Rev Nutr* 2008;28:233–251.
23. Suckale J, Solimena M. Pancreas islets in metabolic signaling—focus on the beta cell. *Front Biosci* 2008;13:7156–7171.
24. Schuit F, De Vos A, Farfari S, et al. Metabolic fate of glucose in purified islet cells. Glucose-regulated anaplerosis in beta cells. *J Biol Chem* 1997;25;272(30):18572–18579.

SCIENTIFIC PRINCIPLES

CHAPTER 3 ■ NUTRITION AND METABOLISM

J. STANLEY SMITH, Jr. AND DAVID C. FRANKENFIELD

KEY POINTS

1. Recognize that the goal of perioperative or post-traumatic nutritional support is repletion or maintenance of protein and energy stores as a part of lean body mass to allow recovery from illness.
2. Starvation and systemic inflammatory response result in erosion of the fat-free mass and body weight (malnutrition) and are indicators for nutrition support if present.
3. Assess the patient's nutritional status by the subjective global assessment.
4. Identify nutritional requirements by estimating basal metabolic rate for age, gender, and body surface area and increase by 25% to 100% based on severity of stress.
5. Use enteral feedings whenever possible.
6. Remember the inflammatory response in metabolism is found in more disease states than trauma and sepsis.
7. Realize that inflammation increases energy utilization and alters the metabolism of glucose, protein, fat, and trace minerals.
8. Supply calories as glucose and fat with a calorie to nitrogen ratio of 150:1.
9. A strong relation between protein depletion and postoperative complications has been demonstrated in nonseptic, nonimmunocompromised patients undergoing elective major gastrointestinal surgery.
10. The maintenance of an intact brush border and intercellular tight junctions prevents the movement of toxic substances into the intestinal lymphatics and circulation; these functions may become altered in critically ill patients.
11. Re-assess the adequacy of nutritional support to determine further needs.
12. Cancer or AIDS cachexia cannot be cured, only managed, and so removing the stimulus for inflammation is not possible.
13. Excess glucose calories are converted to fat, are deposited in the liver, and result in hyperglycemia and glycosuria.

Nutrition support is indicated in surgical patients if they are significantly malnourished prior to surgery, if they are expected to remain NPO (non per os, "nothing by mouth") for more than 5 days postoperatively, or if they are critically ill.[1–4] The main feature of metabolism in the surgical patient is the presence of the inflammatory response. The inflammatory response is critical to survival from surgical or traumatic injury, yet it poses challenges in the nourishment of these patients. If the surgical injury is not sufficient to produce an inflammatory response, nutrition support in surgery is similar to that in simple starvation. Well-nourished patients with short-term undernutrition or mild inflammatory stress and limited weight loss do not have increased risk of complications during their surgical convalescence related to their nutritional status.[1–4] However, as America becomes more obese, good nutrition does not equate to a body weight above the ideal. In an Italian study, body mass index (BMI) and waist circumference were directly associated with systolic and diastolic blood pressure values. Processed meat, potatoes, and wine, typically consumed in the unhealthy American diet, were directly associated with increased blood pressure.[5]

1 The goal of nutrition support is to minimize protein loss and to provide key nutrients to maintain immune and other critical functions during and after surgical or traumatic injury. This chapter addresses the areas of nutritional assessment, metabolism, and therapy including the nutritional response to inflammation.

BASIC NUTRITIONAL METABOLIC PRINCIPLES

Body Composition

Total body mass is composed of aqueous and nonaqueous components. The nonaqueous portion is made up of bone mineral and the lipid portion of adipose tissue. The aqueous portion is divided between the body cell mass, which is made up of cellular components of skeletal muscle, organs, skin, blood, and adipose tissue, and the extracellular fluids and proteins, such as interstitial and intravascular volume, serum proteins, tendons, ligaments, and cartilage. The body cell mass is the metabolic engine of the body, while the extracellular contents form the supporting structure for the body cell mass. Total body water makes up about 55% to 60% of total body mass. In the prototypical 70-kg male, this is 40 liters, with about 22 liters intracellular, 14 liters interstitial, and 3.0 to 3.5 liters plasma. In obesity, there is generally expansion of both the body fat mass and the fat-free mass. Body composition also varies as a function of age and gender (Fig. 3.1)[6] and becomes further altered following injury or surgery.[7] In clinical practice, body composition is not measured but rather inferred by using the Quetelet index, more commonly known as body mass index (kg/m^2), which is most directly a measure of the total mass as a function of weight but which generally correlates with body fatness. A body mass index of 30 kg/m^2 or higher is indicative of obesity. However, there are people who are obese at lower levels of body mass index and others who are not obese despite a body mass index in excess of 30 kg/m^2.[8]

Body composition is altered following injury or surgery. The injury-induced changes are characterized by a rapid loss of lean body mass, a slower loss of body fat, and expansion of the extracellular fluid compartment, leading to a diminution of the metabolically active tissue even as total body weight increases.[9] The expansion of the extracellular water compartment is recognizable as edema, but the underlying changes in body cell mass and fat mass are difficult to recognize until late in the process, when they manifest as temporal or extremity wasting. Nonvisual assessment tools are limited. There is one report that midarm circumference correlates with outcomes in critically ill patients.[10] Bioelectrical impedance is another way

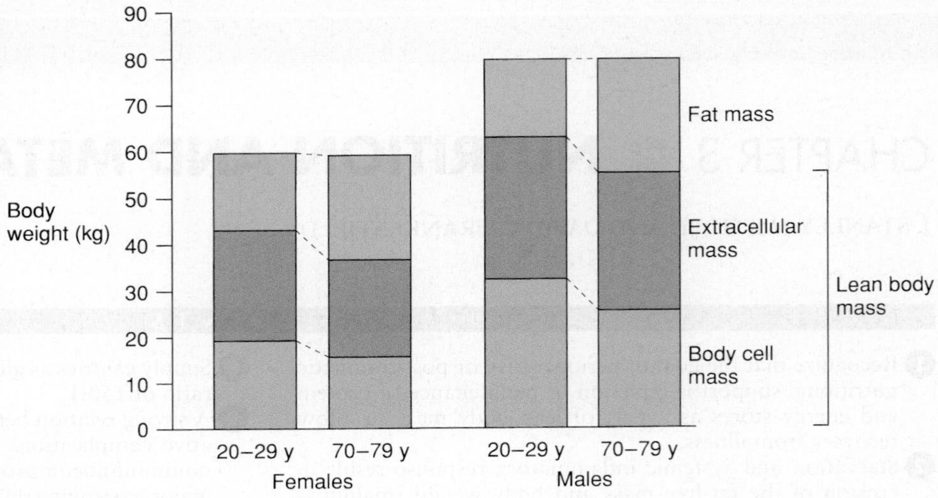

FIGURE 3.1. Body composition as a function of gender and age. (Data from Cohn SH, Vaartsky D, Yasumura S, et al. Compartmental body composition based on total-body nitrogen, potassium, and calcium. *Am J Physiol* 1980; 239:E524–E530.)

to measure the change in lean body mass, though its utility is still under investigation.

Bioelectrical impedance operates on the principle that electrical resistance is proportional to the fluid and electrolyte content of tissue. Since the lean body mass or body cell mass contains all of the fluid and electrolyte content, passage of an electrical current is a measure of the lean body or "fat-free" mass. This appears to work well in both healthy and critically ill patients and can give the practitioner a guide to accurately gauge nutritional and fluid support, especially in those patients with expanded extracellular water and increased body weight.[9]

Obese patients have an excess store of calories, but the body protein compartment is independent of the fat store. Obese people can be just as protein depleted as underweight people (i.e., it is possible to be overnourished and undernourished at the same time).

Energy and Substrate Metabolism

Conversion of Fuel to Work. From a simplistic mechanical standpoint, the human body is much like an engine. It uses oxygen to burn fuel (carbohydrate, fat, protein, ethanol) to generate energy used to perform work, and it exhausts or excretes the byproducts of this combustion (water, carbon dioxide, and heat) to the environment (Fig. 3.2). The human body does several kinds of work essential for life including mechanical work (e.g., locomotion, breathing), transport work (e.g., carrier-mediated uptake of nutrients into cells), and synthetic work (biosynthesis of proteins and other complex molecules). The energy used to do this work comes from the energy present in the chemical bonds of the nutrients we consume. Thus, the human body converts energy stored in the chemical bonds of nutrients into internal and external work. During starvation or following operative procedures when no nutrition is provided, the body oxidizes stored energy sources (i.e., body tissue) to generate this work. In humans, this process is relatively inefficient, since about half of this potential energy is lost as heat. Some of the heat generated during this process is used to help maintain body temperature via carefully controlled regulatory mechanisms in the hypothalamus. Excess heat is released primarily through the skin via evaporation, radiation, convection, and conduction. In surgical patients, these central regulatory mechanisms often become "reset," leading to the development of fever that under most circumstances is an appropriate response to injury and infection. An increase in body temperature, for example, results in an increase in enzymatic reactions that are necessary to support the inflammatory process.

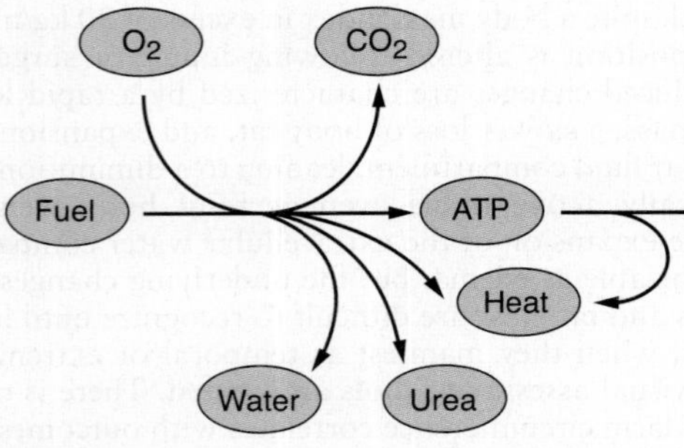

FIGURE 3.2. Fuel utilization in human metabolism.

The Calorie. Energy (heat) is measured in joules or calories. The joule is the SI unit of energy and is defined as the energy required to exert a force of 1 Newton for a distance of 1 meter. Unit of measure is $kg/m^2/s^{-2}$. The joule is intended to replace the calorie (technically referred to as the g-calorie) as the standard unit of energy on the basis that it is measured in metric terms. In the United States, the g-calorie or kg-calorie (kilocalorie) remains the most common way to express energy. A g-calorie is the amount of heat required to raise the temperature of 1 gram of water from 14.5°C to 15.5°C at a pressure of one standard atmosphere (and hence it can be argued that the calorie, like the joule, is a metric measurement). The kg-calorie is the amount of heat necessary to increase the temperature of 1 kg of water under the same circumstances. Joules and g-calories are small units of energy (1 joule is expended by a resting person every hundredth of a second) and so megajoules (MJ) and kilocalories are most often used in discussions of human nutrition. A megajoule is equivalent to 1,000,000 joules, while a kilocalorie is equivalent to 1,000 calories. The conversion of megajoules to kilocalories is 1 MJ = 239 kcal.

Respiration and Combustion. All work performed by the body is accompanied by oxidation of fuel via a series of decarboxylation/dehydrogenation reactions (glycolysis, tricarboxylic acid cycle). The fuel is derived from food or from body tissue. The energy released by these reactions is captured in adenosine triphosphate (ATP) via a series of redox reactions (electron transport system). In the final reduction reaction hydrogen is combined with oxygen to form water. The oxygen

TABLE 3.1 CLASSIFICATION

FUEL RESERVES OF A HEALTHY (70-kg) ADULT MALE

ENERGY SOURCE	kg	kcal VALUE
Fat	14	125,000
Protein		
Skeletal muscle	6	24,000
Other	6	24,000
Glycogen		
Muscle	0.15	600
Liver	0.075	300
Free glucose	0.02	80

present for that reduction and the carbon dioxide produced by decarboxylation are transported by the circulatory system and exchanged with the atmosphere by the lungs. Protein oxidation is a special case in which nitrogen is a byproduct besides carbon dioxide and water. The nitrogen is removed by the kidney after conversion to urea by the liver.

Body Fuels. Human metabolism is arranged such that the fuels consumed in the diet are preferentially utilized when they are present, with excess stored for the postprandial period. In the postprandial state, the body contains fuel reserves that it can mobilize in an orderly fashion as the time of fasting increases. These same fuel reserves are tapped during stress metabolism, though in a less orderly fashion (Table 3.1). By far the greatest energy component is calorically dense fat, providing 9 kcal/g. The body can store almost limitless amounts of fat. Body protein comprises the next largest source of potential energy, but amino acids yield only about 4 kcal/g, and the total reserve is smaller. Unlike fat reserves, body protein is a structural and functional component of the body. There is no storage form. Loss of body protein, if severe, has functional consequences. In undernourished and underfed states, proteolysis is mildly accelerated to generate amino acids to support gluconeogenesis and other key synthetic processes. In the long run, a chronic catabolic state can lead to erosion of body protein stores such that susceptibility to infection is increased, wound healing is impaired, and outcome is unfavorably impacted. Carbohydrate stores are minimal and exist as glucose or liver glycogen and can be depleted quickly unless replenished from exogenous sources. Though limited in stores, there is constant demand for carbohydrate in stress metabolism. Thus, carbohydrate and protein metabolism are linked because the body draws on endogenous protein to produce new glucose to meet the demand unmet by diet.

Carbohydrate

The basic unit of carbohydrate metabolism in humans is glucose. Nearly all dietary carbohydrate is converted to glucose, and glucose is the form of carbohydrate for oxidation. The human body has a constant need for glucose oxidation in the central nervous system and blood cells. A glucose supply of approximately 12 hours is available as liver glycogen, which is sufficient to cover glucose needs between meals. In periods of fasting extending beyond the glycogen supply, the body converts amino acids to glucose, recycles the available glucose, and eventually induces ketone production from fat, which can substitute for some but not all of the body's glucose need. Resumption of glucose intake completely reverses these metabolic adaptations. In surgical nutrition, the inflammatory response accelerates the rate of glucose production from amino acids, minimizes glucose recycling, and limits ketone production, leading to pronounced gluconeogenesis from amino acids. These metabolic adaptations are much less responsive to dextrose infusion after surgery or injury than in simple starvation.

Lipid

Lipids consist of a wide variety of hydrocarbon chains that can be classified several ways, including by chain length, degree of saturation, and location of the first double bond. Perhaps the most useful way to classify lipids for surgical nutrition is by chain length.

Short-chain fatty acids (two- to five-carbon chain length) are derived from the fermentation of dietary fiber in the colon. Much of this short-chain fatty acid is used by the commensal bacteria and is important in maintaining a healthy environment in the colon (i.e., optimal pH and bacterial populations). Some of the short-chain fatty acids are absorbed and are preferred fuels for the colonocytes. Short-chain fatty acid absorption is attended by absorption of water and sodium.

Medium-chain fatty acids (six- to nine-carbon chain length) are not typically found in the human diet but are used widely in enteral nutrition products (they are manufactured by fractionating the fatty acids of coconut oil). They are used because they are easier to digest and absorb than long-chain triglycerides. Being water soluble, medium-chain triglycerides do not require emulsification or micelle formation. Lipase is not required. The medium-chain triglycerides are absorbed directly into the portal circulation rather than via the lacteals into the lymphatic system. They yield 8.0 kcal/g on oxidation.

Long-chain fatty acids (greater than nine-carbon chain length) include the two fatty acids that are dietarily essential (linoleic and linolenic acid); are water insoluble; require bile salts for emulsification, lipase for digestion, and micelle and chylomicron formation for transport; and gain access to the bloodstream via the thoracic duct. In the cell, lipoprotein lipase is necessary for uptake, and carnitine is required to move the fatty acid from the cytosol into the mitochondria for oxidation. Long-chain triglycerides are the body's main form of energy storage. Some of the long-chain fatty acids are precursors for important inflammatory mediators (prostaglandins, leukotrienes, thromboxanes). The type of eicosanoid produced is partly influenced by the type of fatty acid available, and the type of fatty acid available is influenced by dietary fat intake.

Protein

Protein is a key nutrient in surgical nutrition and differs from carbohydrate and fat because it contains nitrogen. Twenty different amino acids are dietarily essential, and the quality of a food protein is determined by its content of these 20 amino acids. Proteins can be categorized structurally as amino acids, peptides, and proteins. The human gastrointestinal (GI) tract can absorb amino acids and small peptides, and must digest intact proteins into these smaller sizes for absorption. Protein is not stored by the body. All protein is functional.

Absorbed amino acids pass first through the liver, where portions are extracted for synthesis of circulating proteins. The branched-chain amino acids (leucine, isoleucine, and valine) are untouched by the liver and so are transported to and extracted by muscle. Dietary and endogenous amino acids eventually mix and distribute into intracellular and extracellular amino acid pools, where they are available upon demand for further metabolism. Excess amino acids are degraded and their carbon skeletons are oxidized to produce energy or are incorporated into glycogen or free fatty acids. In addition to

FIGURE 3.3. Whole body protein metabolism in a normal 70-kg man.

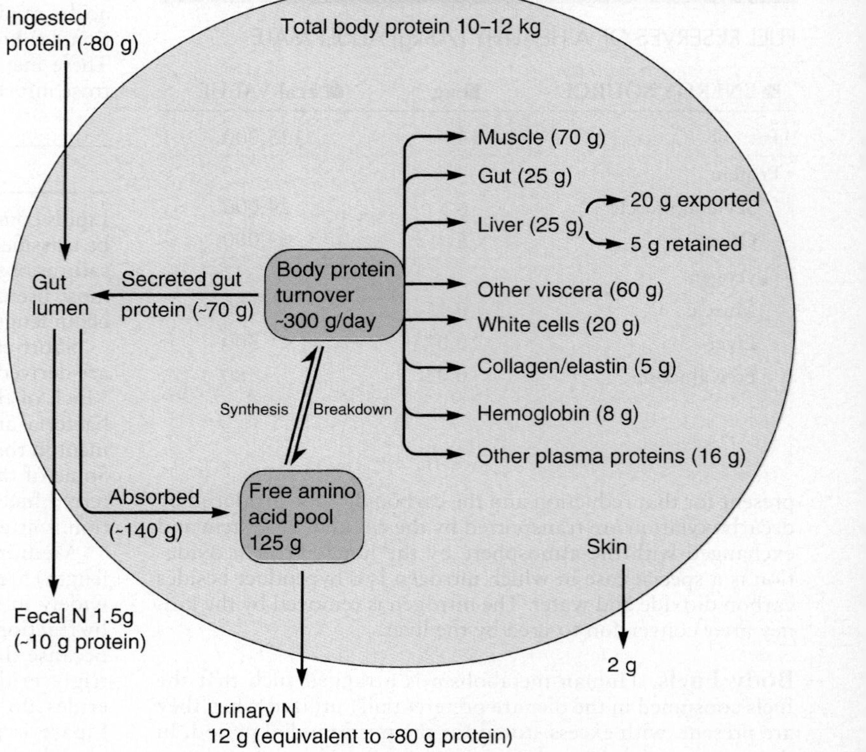

the metabolism of dietary amino acids, the existing proteins in the cell are continuously recycled, such that total protein turnover in the body is about 300 g/day (Fig. 3.3). Vertebrates cannot reutilize nitrogen with 100% efficiency; therefore, obligatory nitrogen losses occur, mainly in the urine. Most of the nitrogen lost in the urine is in the form of urea (85%), with lesser amounts excreted as creatinine and ammonia. Urinary nitrogen losses diminish in individuals fed a protein-free diet but never reach zero because of the body's inability to completely reutilize nitrogen. In stressed patients, this ability to adapt to starvation is compromised such that proteolysis of body proteins continues at a substantial rate (Fig. 3.4).

FIGURE 3.4. The response to starvation in normal, postoperative, and septic individuals. The normal person adapts to starvation by conserving body protein, which is manifested by a decrease in nitrogen excretion in the urine. Septic patients do not adapt to starvation by using ketones for energy and therefore urinary nitrogen losses are much greater.

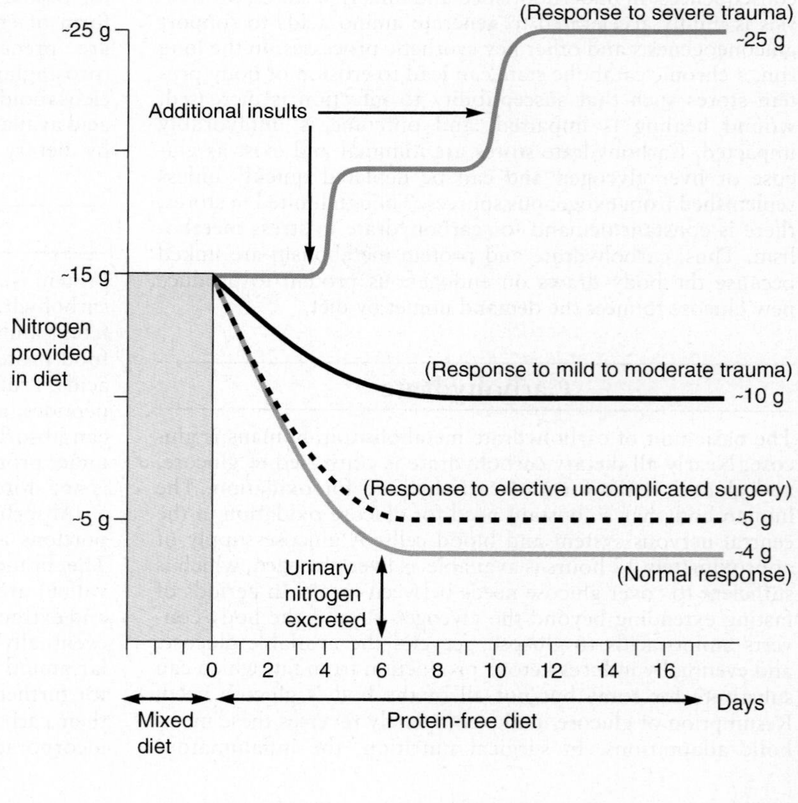

Although it is often assumed that skeletal muscle bears the brunt of this protein wasting, it is now apparent that net proteolysis also occurs in organs such as the gut and liver. If the ability to synthesize proteins is compromised by malnutrition or disease, function is generally correspondingly impacted. This may show clinically in patients as impaired wound healing, immunoincompetence, or breakdown of the gut mucosal barrier.

Metabolism of amino acids (from enteral or parenteral feedings) generates ammonia, which is one of the most toxic and reactive compounds in physiologic fluids. Yet, ammonia levels in blood are generally kept at nontoxic concentrations (20 to 40 μM); this is done primarily in the liver by converting ammonia to urea, a nontoxic soluble compound. A large portion of the ammonia used for urea synthesis arises from nitrogen catabolism in extrahepatic tissues. Excretory or transport amino acids, primarily glutamine and alanine, serve as vehicles for transporting ammonia in a nontoxic form from peripheral tissues to the visceral organs. In these organs, ammonia is reformed and then either excreted (via kidneys, where it acts as an important buffering system) or detoxified to urea (liver). From the intestinal tract, the large ammonia load delivered to the liver escapes the systemic circulation because of the biochemical pathways in the liver that detoxify it. Only the liver has all the enzymes of urea synthesis, and these enzymes are located only in periportal hepatocytes. Thus, diseases affecting the periportal areas lead to an increased ammonia load into the systemic circulation.

Nutrition Assessment

Metabolism is altered to varying degrees by surgical injury. In many cases, these alterations are adaptive, short-lived, and sustainable by a previously well-nourished person, even if they are denied food for a few days after surgery. However, in patients with preexisting malnutrition or with sufficiently severe metabolic insult in response to surgical injury or infection, early resumption of a nutrient supply is important in maximizing their recovery and minimizing their complication risk.[1–4] The aim of nutrition assessment is to identify the patient in need of early resumption of metabolic support and to determine the nutrient requirements to be fed to the patient.

2 Starvation versus Inflammation as the Cause of Malnutrition. Starvation and systemic inflammatory response result in erosion of the fat-free mass and body weight (malnutrition) and are indicators for nutrition support if present.[1–4] In starvation, the main features are reduced or absent nutrient intake with gradual loss of lean mass and body fat, preservation of serum protein levels, and reversal of the metabolic response upon feeding. The usual causes of starvation are functional (dysphagia, nausea, emesis, malabsorption) and psychosocial (food insecurity, social isolation, depression).

The main metabolic features of inflammatory response are elevated metabolic rate (hypermetabolism and hypercatabolism), an acute-phase protein response, and reduced sensitivity of the metabolic state to reversal by feeding. Impaired intake might also be present with an inflammatory response (i.e., the anorexia of illness). Inflammatory response is often the cause of malnutrition in patients with recent acute illness or chronic illness (e.g., cardiac cachexia, cancer cachexia).

3 Subjective Global Assessment. Subjective global assessment is a valid way to determine whether tissue erosion has occurred and whether the etiology is starvation or inflammation.[11,12] Subjective global assessment utilizes several types of information, including physical examination, weight history, recent nutrient intake, gastrointestinal symptoms, and history of disease. The patient is classified as class A (not malnourished), class C (definitely malnourished), or class B (all other cases that are moderate or indeterminant). A typical patient with class C malnutrition has a history of unintentional weight loss and physical signs of tissue erosion (temporal and/or extremity). The etiology (starvation vs. inflammation) is important to note, but it does not have a bearing on the classification of malnutrition severity.

Serum Proteins. Although still commonly used as markers of malnutrition, serum transport proteins usually do not decrease in response to starvation, even in advanced cases. When these proteins are decreased, it is usually a sign that the patient has had or continues to have an inflammatory response.[13] One of the features of inflammation is reprioritization of hepatic protein synthesis away from the transport proteins in favor of acute-phase reactants. C-reactive protein is an example of an acute-phase reactant that rises rapidly with inflammation and quickly falls back to normal when inflammation resolves.[13]

Nitrogen Balance. Nitrogen balance is an indicator of whether protein intake is keeping up with protein catabolism, and it may be the most important nutrition test in patients receiving nutrition support. Nitrogen balance is calculated from the amount of nitrogen consumed minus the amount excreted in a 24-hour period. Nitrogen intake is estimated from protein intake (g protein/6.25). The main route of nitrogen excretion is the urine (90% or more). Nitrogen is also lost through the skin and stool, but this loss is usually very small (<2 g/day), difficult to measure, and therefore usually accounted for with a constant of 2 in the balance equation. It is ideal to quantitate total urinary nitrogen (TUN), but many laboratories only measure urea nitrogen. If urea nitrogen (UUN) is measured, an additional 2 to 3 g should be added to the output side of the nitrogen balance equation to account for these unmeasured losses:

Nitrogen balance (g/d) = Protein intake/6.25 − (TUN + 2)
Nitrogen balance (g/d) = Protein intake/6.25 − (UUN + 2 + 3)

A nitrogen balance of –2 to +2 g/day indicates nitrogen equilibrium, and is the goal in surgical nutrition. Balances more negative than this should be managed by increasing the protein intake, and balances more positive than this are suggestive of error in the measurement (positive balance implies anabolism, but bedridden patients undergoing inflammatory response should not be anabolic). Limitations of the nitrogen balance technique include that it does not show when protein is being overfed, it takes several days for nitrogen to re-equilibrate in the body after protein intake has been changed, and renal dysfunction and GI bleeding may invalidate the study (renal dysfunction due to incomplete excretion of urea nitrogen, GI bleeding due to excess urea nitrogen production not associated with metabolism). Surgical critical care patients tend toward negative nitrogen balance unless large amounts of protein are administered,[14] and achievement of positive nitrogen balance has been linked to improved outcome, at least in one narrow segment of critically ill patients.[15]

Indirect Calorimetry. Resting energy expenditure can be measured at the bedside with indirect calorimetry. Patients must be either intubated or able to tolerate a hood placed over their face for collection of exhaled breath. Intubated patients must have a fraction of inspired oxygen less than 60%, while spontaneously breathing patients must be breathing room air only (no nasal cannulas, face masks, continuous positive airway pressure [CPAP] machines, etc.). No air leaks can be present. Protocols have been developed to measure resting energy expenditure with just a 5-minute test period (requiring a tight 5% coefficient of variation on the minute-to-minute measures of gas exchange), which saves time yet yields a reliable figure for 24-hour resting energy expenditure. If this 5% steady-state

TABLE 3.2 **CLASSIFICATION**

ACCURACY RATES OF METABOLIC RATE EQUATIONS IN HEALTHY INDIVIDUALS (PERCENTAGE OF INDIVIDUAL ESTIMATES FALLING WITHIN 10% OF MEASURED)

■ EQUATION	■ NONOBESE	■ OBESE
Harris-Benedict	69	64
Owen	73	51
WHO	69	57
Mifflin-St. Jeor	82	70

WHO, World Health Organization.
Data from Frankenfield DC, Rowe WA, Smith JS, et al. Validation of several established equations for resting metabolic rate in obese and non obese people. *J Am Diet Assoc* 2003;103:1152, plus supplemental data for a total of 200 subjects.

threshold is not met, a longer 30-minute measurement accepting a 10% coefficient of variation is accurate. These guidelines cover other aspects of measurement including environmental conditions, body posture, physical motion, feeding state, and interpretation of respiratory quotient.[16]

Estimation of Metabolic Rate. In most cases, energy expenditure is not measured, but estimated. Estimation of energy expenditure relies on the fact that all metabolic activity occurs within the fat-free mass. Fat-free mass is a function of body weight, height, age, and sex, and therefore, resting energy expenditure is likewise predictable from these variables. In obesity, these relationships are preserved, but the strength of the relationships is diminished. Several equations exist for predicting resting energy expenditure from these variables. For healthy people, the Mifflin-St. Jeor equation appears to be accurate more often than any of the other equations in existence (Table 3.2).[17] In non–intensive care unit (ICU) adult surgical patients without significant inflammatory response, this equation can probably be used without modification. In the more complex situation of critical illness, equations developed for this special population, taking into account the effect of inflammation on metabolic rate, improve the accuracy of calorie prediction and thus are better guides to calorie replacement (Table 3.3).[18,19] In general, energy needs increase with the presence of inflammatory response (Table 3.4).[20] Interestingly, the expenditure of kilocalories is only minimally increased after elective surgery. The largest increase in energy expenditure occurs in patients with severe multiple trauma or major thermal injury. However, the average-sized adult who sustains even a major burn rarely increases his or her energy expenditure to more than 3,000 kcal/day.

Overfeeding

While the provision of enough calories is beneficial, giving too many calories can "overfeed" the patient. Excess calories, especially in the form of sugars, lead to lipogenesis and hepatic steatosis interfering with hepatic function. To avoid overfeeding, critically ill patients may not fit the factors used to estimate their energy requirements and require indirect calorimetry to more accurately measure energy expenditure. There are two major consequences of overfeeding, hypophosphatemia and steatosis.

Nutrition Interventions

Elective Patients. Most patients undergoing elective operations are adequately nourished. Unless the patient has suffered significant preoperative malnutrition (subjective global assessment class C) or has a major intraoperative or postoperative complication, intravenous solutions containing 5% dextrose may be administered for 5 to 7 days before the return of feeding with no detrimental effect on outcome. Therefore, the increased cost of feedings and the potential complications associated with intravenous nutrition cannot be justified. On the other hand, malnourished patients should not be left unfed for more than a day or two after surgery. Assessment of nutritional status therefore should be completed early so that this information can be integrated into decision making and nutrition care planning. Enteral feeding is preferred to parenteral nutrition in patients who cannot resume an oral diet. Standard high-protein feeding formulas are adequate. Choice of product and volume of feeding are based on the results of the nutrition assessment. Most tube feedings today are manufactured with water-soluble dietary fiber, and the use of this nutrient should be standard in the feeding of surgical patients. If fluid intake must be limited, there are standard feeding formulas with a calorie concentration of 2.0/mL.

Critical Care. Timing and feeding route are primary considerations in nutrition intervention in the critically ill surgical

TABLE 3.3 **CLASSIFICATION**

ACCURACY RATES OF METABOLIC RATE EQUATIONS IN CRITICALLY ILL PATIENTS (PERCENTAGE OF INDIVIDUAL ESTIMATES FALLING WITHIN 10% OF MEASURED)

		■ YOUNG		■ ELDERLY	
■ EQUATION	■ ALL (n = 202)	■ NONOBESE (n = 52)	■ OBESE (n = 47)	■ NONOBESE (n = 52)	■ OBESE (n = 51)
Mifflin-St. Jeor	25	23	21	21	35
ACCP	35	44	34	50	12
Ireton-Jones	46	33	49	50	51
Swinamer	54	61	51	60	43
Faisy	53	65	72	37	39
Brandi	55	61	55	61	41
Penn State	67	69	70	77	53

ACCP, American College of Chest Physicians.
Data from Frankenfield DC, Smith JS, Cooney RN, et al. Relative association of fever and injury with hypermetabolism in critically ill patients. *Injury* 1997;28:617.

TABLE 3.4 **CLASSIFICATION**

METABOLIC RATES OF CRITICALLY ILL PATIENTS CATEGORIZED BY REASON FOR ADMISSION VS. FEVER STATUS (MEASURE OF RESTING ENERGY EXPENDITURE/HARRIS-BENEDICT ESTIMATE OF RESTING METABOLIC RATE)

■ REASON FOR ADMISSION	■ FEVER STATUS ■ T_{max} >38°C	■ T_{max} <38°C	■ REASON FOR ADMISSION MEANS
Trauma	145 + 22	123 + 14	134 + 23
Surgery	138 + 22	125 + 14	132 + 22
Medical	139 + 20	125 + 20	132 + 20
Fever status means	141 + 24	124 + 17	

No significant difference among the reasons for admission, the difference by fever status $p < 0.0001$, and no significant fever × reason for admission interaction.
Data from Frankenfield DC, Smith JS, Cooney RN, et al. Relative association of fever and injury with hypermetabolism in critically ill patients. *Injury* 1997;28:617.

patient. The best outcomes are achieved with enteral feeding started within 24 to 48 hours. Independent of nutritional status, any critically ill patient who is not expected to resume oral feeding within 5 days should be started on nutrition support within 48 hours.

Priorities of Care. Resuscitation, oxygenation, and arrest of hemorrhage are immediate priorities for survival. Wounds should then be repaired or stabilized as expeditiously as possible. Nutritional support is an essential part of the metabolic care of the critically ill trauma patient and should be instituted before significant weight loss occurs. Adequate nutrition supports normal responses that optimize wound healing and recovery.

At least four evidence-based guides to nutrition practice in 5 critical care exist.[1–4] There is general agreement among the guidelines that enteral nutrition is preferable to parenteral, that feeding should be started within 24 to 48 hours and should not be supplemented with parenteral nutrition as long as some tube feeding is tolerated, that blood glucose can be controlled to less than 140 mg/dL, that blue food dye should not be used for detection of aspiration, that the head of the bed should be elevated to 45 degrees to minimize aspiration risk, and that gastric feeding routes are as good as postpyloric routes unless the stomach is proven to be dysfunctional.

There is some divergence on whether immune or inflammation-modulating feeding formulas are indicated in some critically ill patients. There is at least one quality paper that has been published since the guidelines that supports the use of such feedings in patients with sepsis and risk for acute respiratory distress syndrome (ARDS) or acute lung injury.[21]

THE BODY'S RESPONSE WHEN STRESSED BY INJURY OR SURGERY

In the 1930s, Cuthbertson[22] described the time course for many of the posttraumatic responses and two distinct periods were identified. The early "ebb" or shock phase was usually brief in duration (12 to 24 hours) and occurred immediately following injury. Blood pressure, cardiac output, body temperature, and oxygen consumption were reduced. These events were often associated with hemorrhage and resulted in hypoperfusion and lactic acidosis. With restoration of blood volume, ebb phase alterations gave way to more accelerated responses. The flow phase was then characterized by hypermetabolism, increased cardiac output, increased urinary nitrogen losses, altered glucose metabolism, and accelerated tissue catabolism.

The "flow" phase responses to accidental injury are similar to those that occur following elective operation. The response to injury, however, is usually much more intensive and extends over a long period of time.

Characteristics of the Flow Phase of the Injury Response

Hypermetabolism. Hypermetabolism is defined as an increase in basal metabolic rate (BMR) above that predicted on the basis of age, sex, and body size in a healthy person. Metabolic rate is usually determined by measuring the exchange of respiratory gases and by calculating heat production from oxygen consumption and carbon dioxide production. The degree of hypermetabolism (increased oxygen consumption) is generally related to the severity of the inflammatory response to the injury, with temperature serving as a reasonable indicator of the higher metabolic rate.[16]

Altered Glucose Metabolism. Hyperglycemia commonly occurs following injury, and the elevation of fasting blood sugar levels generally parallels the severity of stress in the ebb phase. During the ebb phase, insulin levels are low and glucose production is only slightly elevated. Later, during the flow phase, insulin concentrations are normal or elevated; yet, hyperglycemia persists. This phenomenon suggests an alteration in the relationship between insulin sensitivity and glucose disposal, hence insulin resistance. Hepatic glucose production is increased and studies show that much of the new glucose generated by the liver arises from three-carbon precursors released from peripheral tissues.

Measurements of substrate exchange across injured and uninjured extremities of severely burned patients indicate that glucose is used in small amounts by the uninjured extremity. In contrast, the injured extremity extracts large amounts of glucose. The wound converts most of the glucose to lactate, which is recycled to the liver in the Cori cycle. Additional studies have shown that uninjured volunteers (controls) are able to dispose of an exogenous glucose load much more readily than injured patients. Moreover, the quantity of insulin elaborated by the injured was greater than in control subjects; nonetheless, these rising insulin concentrations failed to increase glucose clearance in these patients (insulin resistance). Other studies have demonstrated a failure to suppress hepatic glucose production in trauma patients during glucose loading or insulin infusion. Either of these perturbations usually inhibits hepatic glucose production in normal subjects. Thus, profound insulin resistance occurs in injured patients.

Alterations in Protein Metabolism. Extensive urinary nitrogen loss occurs following major injury. Like other responses, the loss of nitrogen following injury is related to the extent of the trauma. But it also depends on the previous nutritional status, as well as the age and gender of the patient, because these factors determine the size of the muscle mass. In unfed patients, protein breakdown rates exceed synthesis, and negative balance results. Providing exogenous calories and nitrogen increases protein synthesis, but, even with achievement of energy balance, the nitrogen loss is not attenuated.[23] Only providing enough nitrogen intake can balance the nitrogen loss.

Skeletal muscle is the major source of the nitrogen that is lost in the urine following extensive injury. Although it is now recognized that amino acids are released by muscle in increased quantities following injury, it has only recently been appreciated that the composition of amino acid efflux does not reflect the composition of muscle protein. The release is skewed toward glutamine and alanine, each of which comprise about one third of the total amino acids released by skeletal muscle, even though they make up only 5% of the protein mass of muscle. The kidney extracts glutamine, where it contributes ammonium groups for ammonia generation, a process that excretes acid loads. The gastrointestinal tract also takes up glutamine to serve as an oxidative fuel and substrate for RNA synthesis. The gut enterocytes convert glutamine primarily to ammonia and alanine, and these two substances are released into the portal venous blood. This ammonia is then removed by the liver and is converted to urea, and the alanine may be removed by the liver and serve as a gluconeogenic precursor. Following elective surgical stress, glutamine consumption by the bowel and the kidney is accelerated in a reaction that appears to be regulated by the increased elaboration of the glucocorticoids. Although skeletal muscle releases alanine at an accelerated rate, the gastrointestinal tract and kidney also release increased amounts of alanine. The alanine is then extracted by the liver to be used in the synthesis of glucose and acute-phase proteins. Hence, glutamine and alanine are important participants in the transfer of nitrogen from skeletal muscle to visceral organs; however, their metabolic pathways favor the production of urea and ammonia, both of which are terminal uses of nitrogen and must be excreted from the body.

Alterations in Fat Metabolism. To support the hypermetabolism, increased gluconeogenesis, and interorgan substrate flux, stored triglyceride is mobilized and oxidized at an accelerated rate. Glucose administration poorly attenuates this lipolysis, which may be the result of continuous stimulation of the sympathetic nervous system. Although mobilization and use of free fatty acids are accelerated in injured subjects, ketosis during brief starvation is blunted, and the accelerated protein catabolism remains unchecked. If unfed, severely injured patients rapidly deplete their fat and protein stores. Such malnutrition increases their susceptibility to added stresses of hemorrhage, surgery, and infection and may contribute to organ system failure, sepsis, and death.

Homeostatic Responses and Adjustments to Stress

Built into the body's defense mechanism is a complex and complicated set of orchestrated responses initiated within moments of injury or insult. These responses are essential for survival and are designed to maintain body homeostasis at a time when key physiologic processes are threatened. These responses are immediately set into motion by various components of the injury response such as volume loss, tissue damage, fear, and pain. Later factors reinitiating or perpetuating these responses include invasive infection and starvation. These events are generally related to the severity of injury; that is, the greater the insult is, the more pronounced the specific response. The synthesis of key hormones and peptides allows the body to respond to such insults with remarkable resilience. From an evolutionary standpoint, these biologic responses result from a process favoring survival of the fittest in the struggle to preserve the species. From a teleologic standpoint, these responses are designed to benefit the organism, enhance recovery, and ensure a relatively speedy return to health.

Whether the body is injured accidentally or within the carefully monitored confines of an operating room, the responses to such trauma are similar. However, such settings are also different in ways that influence the extent and magnitude of the stress response (Table 3.5). Accidental injury is unplanned and uncontrolled; tissues are torn, ripped, bruised, and contaminated. The associated volume loss may be substantial, leading to tissue hypoperfusion, which, if prolonged, results in cellular deterioration and death in tissues that were not initially traumatized. Pain, excitement, and fear are generally heightened and uncontrolled. As a consequence, the magnitude of the physiologic response to major accidental injury is considerable.

In contrast, the "elective" tissue trauma that is inflicted within the confines of an operating room is calculated, planned, and monitored. Although elective surgery causes pain, often interrupts food intake, and is generally associated with the removal of an organ or tissue, the perioperative management of elective surgical patients is often designed to attenuate such

TABLE 3.5

DIFFERENCES BETWEEN ELECTIVE SURGERY AND ACCIDENTAL INJURY

■ INSULT	■ ELECTIVE OPERATION	■ ACCIDENTAL INJURY (TRAUMA)
Tissue damage	Minimal; tissues are dissected with care and reapproximated	Can be substantial; tissues usually torn or ripped; debridement often necessary
Hypotension	Uncommon: preoperative hydration employed and fluid status is carefully monitored intraoperatively	Fluid resuscitation often not immediate; blood loss can be substantial leading to shock
Pain/fear/anxiety	Generally can be alleviated with preop medication	Generally present
Infectious complications	Uncommon; prophylactic antibiotics often administered	More common due to contamination, hypotension, and tissue devitalization
Overall stress response	Controlled and of lesser magnitude; starvation better tolerated	Uncontrolled; proportional to the magnitude of the injury; malnutrition poorly tolerated

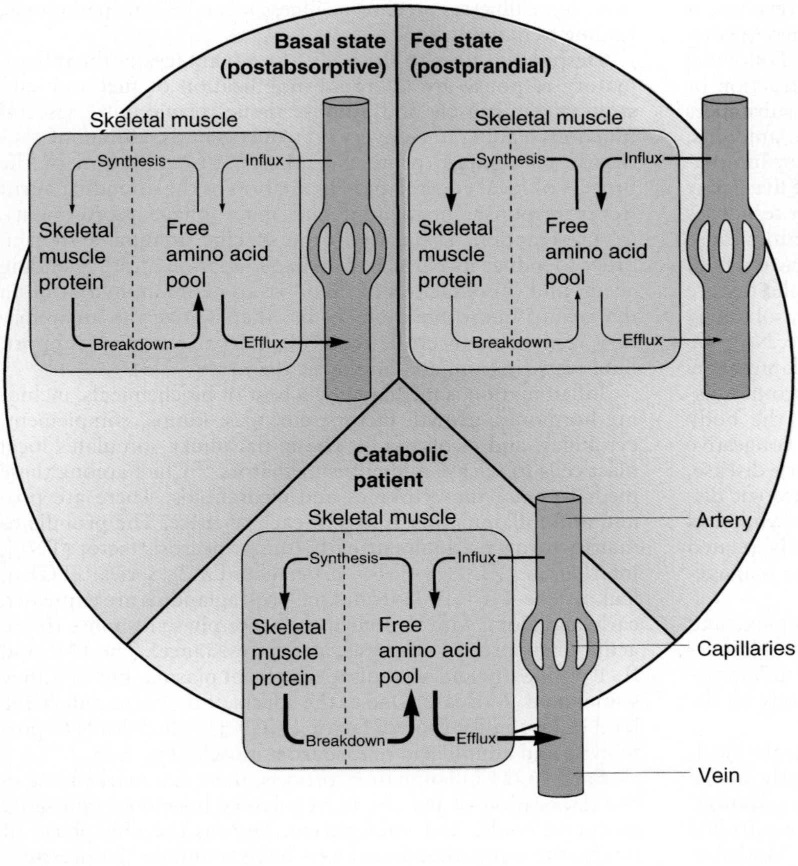

FIGURE 3.5. Relative rates of protein synthesis and breakdown in skeletal muscle in postabsorptive, postprandial, and catabolic states. After an overnight fast, muscle releases net amounts of amino acids to help maintain circulating pool. Breakdown exceeds synthesis, although this may not be measurable using standard techniques. Following a meal, muscle amino acid uptake is greater than release and protein synthesis is greater than catabolism. In the catabolic surgical patient, protein synthesis may be increased, but this rate is exceeded by the rate of breakdown. In the absence of nutritional support, profound muscle wasting can occur.

SCIENTIFIC PRINCIPLES

changes. Patients are assessed prior to surgery by anesthesiologists and surgeons to determine the need for preoperative nutritional support or additional medical consultation. Hydration prior to surgery is common, as is the administration of prophylactic antibiotics and drugs to relieve anxiety and fear. In the operating theater, the surgical site is "prepped" in a sterile fashion to minimize contamination, and numerous physiologic responses (i.e., blood pressure, pulse, urine output) are continually monitored. Blood and blood products are invariably available. During the operation, tissues are carefully dissected and incised to minimize tissue trauma; tissues are reapproximated with care when possible. Appropriately selected pharmacologic agents are used to block undesirable cardiovascular responses, and specific techniques such as epidural or local block anesthesia or patient-controlled analgesia are effective in minimizing postoperative pain. As a consequence, the physiologic responses to elective surgery are generally of a lesser magnitude than those following major accidental injury (Fig. 3.5). Improvements in surgical and anesthetic care now allow us to perform major elective operations with minimal morbidity and mortality. However, in the critically ill, an inflammatory cascade is launched, reaching beyond the limits of the beneficial response.

The Inflammatory Response. The response to operative stresses (elective injury) or accidental injury (trauma) is composed of two components: a neurohormonal arm and an inflammatory arm. These pathways work together to determine the magnitude of the response. The principal counterregulatory hormones involved are the catecholamines, the corticosteroids, and glucagon. The inflammatory component of injury involves the local elaboration of cytokines and the systemic activation of humoral cascades involving complement, eicosanoids, and platelet-activating factor (Fig. 3.6). These mediators promote wound healing by stimulating angiogenesis, white cell migration, and ingrowth of fibroblasts. During

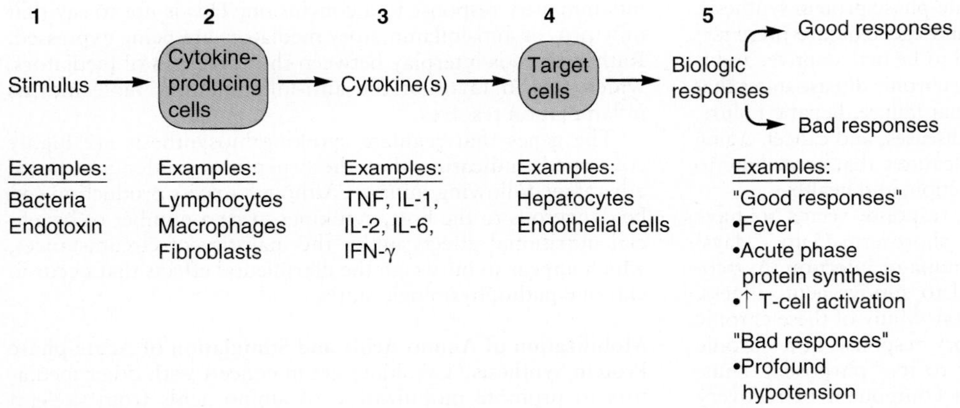

FIGURE 3.6. Cytokines can elicit both beneficial and deleterious responses.

elective surgical procedures, the local inflammatory response is confined to the wound and significant amounts of these mediators do not gain access to the systemic circulation. Following accidental injury where there is massive tissue destruction or prolonged hypotension leading to cell injury, these substances may be produced locally in the wound in excessive amounts, resulting in "spillover" into the systemic circulation. In addition, cells in other tissues (such as Kupffer cells in the liver) may become activated to produce these mediators. Such responses can lead to a systemic response in which these mediators cause detrimental effects such as hypotension and organ dysfunction.

6 The inflammatory response is the major metabolic feature of injury and infection, and is one of the main reasons why nutrition support in such patients can be a challenge. Now we are starting to appreciate the extent to which the inflammatory response underlies the nutritional issues of chronic diseases.[24,25] An inflammatory component exists in the body composition changes of such disparate diseases as congestive heart failure, cancer, chronic obstructive pulmonary disease, human immunodeficiency virus (HIV), and rheumatologic disorders.[26–29] Recognition that inflammation drives what has been traditionally thought of as purely nutritionally related effects of disease opens a whole new avenue for the management of the body wasting of disease (cachexia).

The inflammatory response is a primitive, complex, and indispensable part of the nonspecific immune system.[30] Importantly, the changes in body composition caused by inflammation are part of an orchestrated response by the body to the acute challenge to homeostasis.

Inflammation occurs at different levels. Small-scale localized inflammatory responses are occurring frequently in the body with no systemic consequences.[30] In fact, such responses may be an important mechanism for increasing the controlled exposure of the cellular immune system to antigen. Moderate inflammation is still localized, but its effects are more obvious. This would best be illustrated by the body's response to a piece of foreign material (e.g., a wood splinter), in which the classic signs of inflammation might be observed: rubor, tumor, calor, dolor, and functio laesa (redness, swelling, pain, heat, and loss of function).[30] Multiple traumatic/surgical injury produces a more exuberant inflammation, and systemic effects are more likely to be manifest (hypermetabolism, body protein catabolism, insulin resistance, fever, acute-phase protein response). However, dysregulation of this response causes the uncontrolled inflammation of septic multiple organ failure, in which widespread endothelial damage and organ dysfunction occur, along with deranged intermediary metabolism and, sometimes, cellular immune function collapse.[30,31] This type of inflammation-driven illness is a major cause of death in the ICU.[30] Severe loss of lean body mass is a feature of patients who survive this, but once convalescence is achieved, the inflammatory metabolism can normalize and the body can be repleted with proper nutrition and exercise.

7 The inflammatory response, for reasons not fully understood, can convert from an acute to a chronic condition, in which the systemic manifestations of altered acute-phase protein synthesis, impaired intermediary metabolism, and cachexia are present.[32] This form of inflammation is believed to be maladaptive, and is a common feature of many preexisting chronic disease states that occur in surgical patients, such as renal failure, hepatic failure, congestive heart failure, rheumatoid diseases, and cancer. Aging and obesity also have inflammatory features that contribute to the changes in body composition, function, and health.

Teleologically, the inflammatory response seems to have evolved as a defense mechanism for short-term (5 to 7 days) challenges to homeostasis, such as trauma or infection. As people began to live healthier lives and to survive acute illness, chronic illnesses became more common. Many of these chronic conditions stimulate the inflammatory response in a chronic manner, which is probably counter to its "purpose." Thus, while inflammation is an important component of recovery from acute illnesses, in chronic illness it can become pathologic, leading to malnutrition.

Despite the costs to the body, the advantages of the inflammatory response are (a) rapid mobilization of fuel and substrates from muscle and adipose tissue to maximize visceral functions leading to recovery (gluconeogenesis, glutamine synthesis, acute-phase protein synthesis), (b) initiation of the process of local control and elimination of the offending agent (fever response, neutrophil and macrophage recruitment), (c) presentation of signals to the specific immune system in order to induce its participation in elimination of the offending agent, and (d) reduction of fluid loss to maintain hydration in the face of interrupted intake. In other words, the inflammatory response is a crude form of internal nutrition support, fluid resuscitation, and antibiotic therapy.

Inflammation is mediated by a host of biochemicals, including hormones, growth factors, enzymes, kinins, complement, cytokines, and eicosanoids. The initial injury stimulates local mast cells to release numerous mediators.[33] Chief among these mediators are the cytokines and eicosanoids. There are pro- and anti-inflammatory forms of each of these. The proinflammatory forms predominate early (tumor necrosis factor [TNF], interleukin [IL]-1, IL-6, prostaglandin-2 series [PGE_2], leukotriene-4 [LT_4]). TNF and the prostaglandins are expressed early and along with IL-1 elicit the acute-phase response (fever, acute-phase protein synthesis, insulin resistance). The TNF and IL-1 peak early and then disappear from plasma, but first they stimulate IL-6 release. One of the effects of IL-6 is to reduce the level of insulinlike growth factor 1 (IGF-1), which leads to proteolysis and amino acid release from muscle (Fig. 3.6).

Early in the inflammatory process, there is a marked rise in the elaboration of the counterregulatory hormones glucagon, glucocorticoids, and epinephrine. During the ebb phase of injury, the sympathoadrenal axis helps maintain the pressure-flow relationships necessary for an intact cardiovascular system to maintain blood flow in a low-volume state. With the onset of hypermetabolism, a characteristic of the flow phase, these and other hormones exert a variety of metabolic effects. Glucagon along with insulin resistance has potent glycogenolytic and gluconeogenic effects on the liver, which signal the hepatocytes to produce glucose from hepatic glycogen stores and gluconeogenic precursors. Cortisol mobilizes amino acids from skeletal muscle and increases hepatic gluconeogenesis. The catecholamines stimulate hepatic glycolysis and gluconeogenesis and increase lactate production from peripheral tissues (skeletal muscle). Catecholamines also increase metabolic rate and stimulate lipolysis. The level of growth hormone is elevated, but there is resistance to its action (possibly because of suppressed levels of IGF-1), and thyroid hormone levels are reduced to low-normal concentrations.[33] Infusion of counterregulatory hormones into normal subjects reproduces many of the metabolic alterations that are characteristic of injury.[34]

As the inflammatory stimulus is controlled and eliminated, the anti-inflammatory cytokines (IL-4, IL-10, IL-13) and eicosanoids (PGE_3, LT_5) begin to predominate, and bring the inflammatory response to a conclusion. This is not to say that only pro- or anti-inflammatory mediators are being expressed. Rather, there is interplay between the two types of mediators, which tips in favor of the anti-inflammatory molecules as inflammation resolves.

The genes that regulate cytokine biosynthesis are highly conserved, indicating that these peptides confer a survival advantage following injury.[33] Although excess production can be dangerous to the host, cytokines exert a number of beneficial nutritional effects under the majority of circumstances, which appear to outweigh the detrimental effects that occur in extreme pathophysiologic states.

Mobilization of Amino Acids and Stimulation of Acute-phase Protein Synthesis. Cytokines act in concert with other mediators to promote mobilization of amino acids from skeletal muscle. This response provides key nutrients to support cellular metabolism at a time when food cannot be acquired. The primary metabolic component of the acute-phase response affected by IL-6 is a qualitative alteration in hepatic protein synthesis with a resulting alteration in plasma protein composition. Characteristically, proteins acting as serum transport and binding molecules (albumin, transferrin) are reduced in quantity, and acute-phase proteins (fibrinogen, C-reactive protein) are increased. Acute-phase proteins are elaborated, in part, for the purpose of reducing the systemic effects of tissue damage. While the true physiologic role of many of the acute-phase proteins remains unclear, many act as antiproteases, opsonins, or coagulation and wound-healing factors, and they likely inhibit the generalized tissue destruction that is associated with the local initiation of inflammation. For example, increases in fibrinogen enhance thrombus formation, while antiproteases reduce tissue damage caused by proteases released by dead or dying cells. C-reactive protein has been hypothesized to have a scavenger function and its serum level can be a measure of the inflammatory response. This acute-phase response normally confers a significant survival advantage following injury and infection.

Hypoferremia and Hypozincemia. Serum iron and zinc levels are reduced in septic patients, an event that is cytokine mediated. The decrease in serum iron is probably important in protecting the host against various bacteria. The reduction of iron can inhibit the growth rate of microorganisms that have a strict requirement for iron as a growth factor. Both TNF and IL-1 have been shown to mediate hypoferremia, hypozincemia, and other alterations in trace element metabolism.

In chronic disease states, the milieu of mediators remains predominantly proinflammatory, leading to prolonged tissue damage and systemic effects on immune function, body composition, and metabolism.

Induction of the inflammatory response requires a stimulus. Physical injury and invasion of antigen are the stimuli most often described (trauma, pancreatitis, infection). However, local areas of hypoxia can be an inflammatory stimulus, so that heart failure and chronic obstructive pulmonary disease (COPD) may be added to the list of conditions that might cause inflammation.[30,31] Conversion of self to non-self tissue (e.g., cancer) or faulty recognition of self versus nonself tissue (e.g., inflammatory bowel disease, rheumatologic conditions) can also elicit inflammation.[25]

SPECIFIC STIMULANTS OF THE STRESS RESPONSE

Volume Loss and Tissue Hypoperfusion

Following hemorrhage or plasma loss, the body immediately attempts to compensate in order to maintain adequate organ perfusion. Pressure receptors in the aortic arch and carotid artery and volume (stretch) receptors in the wall of the left atrium detect the fall in blood volume and immediately respond by signaling the brain. Heart rate and stroke volume increase. Afferent nerve signals are also initiated, which stimulate the release of both antidiuretic hormone (ADH) and aldosterone. ADH is produced by the posterior pituitary gland in response to hypotonicity and acts to increase water reabsorption in the kidney. Aldosterone is produced via the renin-angiotensin system when the juxtaglomerular apparatus in the kidney senses a fall in pulse pressure. Aldosterone increases renal sodium reabsorption to conserve intravascular water. These mechanisms are only partially effective and, in the absence of adequate resuscitation, severe hemorrhage often leads to a prolonged low-flow state (shock). Under these circumstances, oxygen delivery is inadequate to meet tissue demands and the cell is forced to switch to anaerobic metabolism, leading to lactic acidosis.

Tissue Damage

Injury of body tissues appears to be the most important factor setting the stress response into motion. Hypovolemia and starvation do not initiate a hypermetabolic/hypercatabolic response unless they result in infection or tissue injury. For example, prolonged underperfusion may lead to ischemia, cellular death, and the release of toxic products that can initiate the "stress" response. Afferent neural pathways from the wound signal the hypothalamus that injury has occurred; tissue destruction is generally sensed in the conscious patient as pain. Efferent pathways from the brain are immediately triggered and stimulate a number of responses designed to maintain homeostasis.

Pain and Fear

Pain and fear are established components of the stress response. Both lead to excessive production of the catecholamines preparing the body for the "fight or flight" response.

Lack of Nutrient Intake and the Consequences of Malnutrition

The metabolic response to injury and surgery demands increased energy expenditure. In many patients undergoing surgery, nutrient intake is inadequate for a period of time (1 to 5 days) following operation. If energy intake is minimal (e.g., 5% dextrose infusion), oxidation of body fat stores and erosion of lean body mass occur, with the resultant loss of weight. Body glycogen stores are limited and are depleted within 24 to 36 hours. Consequently, glucose, which is required by the central nervous system and white blood cells, must be synthesized de novo. Amino acids, released principally by skeletal muscle, are the major gluconeogenic precursors. Most injured patients can tolerate a loss of 15% of their preinjury weight without a significant increase in the risk of surgery. When weight loss exceeds 15% of body weight, the complications of undernutrition interact with the stress process and impair the body's ability to respond appropriately to the injury, and may impair responses to added complications such as infection.

8 The major goal of nutritional support, especially via the GI tract, in the surgical patient is to match the energy and nitrogen expenditure that occurs following injury in order to aid host defense.[35–37] In contrast to injured patients, the catabolic and hypermetabolic responses that occur after elective operations are of a lesser magnitude because there is less tissue destruction and the neurohormonal/inflammatory response is less intense. Consequently, well-nourished patients undergoing major operations do not require nutritional support after surgery unless it is anticipated that food intake will be precluded for more than 7 days.

Invasive Infection

The major complication observed in surgical patients is infection. Most patients, particularly those in intensive care units, are exposed to a variety of infectious agents in the hospital. Normal barrier defense mechanisms are disrupted by multiple indwelling pieces of plastic such as intravenous catheters and nasotracheal and nasogastric tubes. Breakdown of skin and mucous membranes allows portals of entry for bacteria.[38] Infection alone may initiate catabolic responses that are similar to those described following injury in noninfected patients. Both processes cause fever, hyperventilation, tachycardia, accelerated gluconeogenesis, increased proteolysis, and lipolysis, with fat utilized as the principal fuel source. Inflammatory cells release a variety of soluble mediators that aid host resistance and wound repair, but undernutrition may compromise the available host defense mechanisms and thereby increase the likelihood of invasive sepsis, multiple organ system failure, and death.

DETERMINANTS OF HOST RESPONSES TO SURGICAL STRESS

The pattern of physiologic changes elicited in response to surgical stress results from the specific interaction of an individual patient with the stressful stimulus. The host must be capable of transmitting and integrating injury signals, both neural and humoral, and then mounting an appropriate response that requires the interaction of a number of organ systems. The nature, intensity, and duration of the stress are fundamental determinants of both the host mediators activated and the physiologic changes observed. The responses that follow a minor elective operation are similar to those observed during a comparable, brief period of fasting and bed rest. On the other hand, major thermal injury results in a prolonged period of hypermetabolism and a severe drain on the body's energy and protein stores, resolving only with wound closure and resolution of the sepsis that may have developed. Thus, there are profound metabolic differences between the body's response to simple starvation and major stress (Table 3.6).

Body Composition

Body composition is a major determinant of the metabolic responses observed during surgical illness. Posttraumatic nitrogen excretion is directly related to the size of the body protein mass. The balance of nitrogen intake versus output from the body serves as a marker of protein metabolism. The net loss of a certain amount of nitrogen from the body implies the net breakdown of the corresponding amount of protein. In women, the size of the skeletal muscle mass is about one-half that of age-matched men; thus, it is the muscular young man in whom nitrogen losses are most marked after injury, and it is the elderly, sedentary woman in whom they are the least marked.[8]

Nutritional Status

9 A strong relation between protein depletion and postoperative complications has been demonstrated in nonseptic, nonimmunocompromised patients undergoing elective major gastrointestinal surgery.[23] Protein-depleted patients had significantly lower preoperative respiratory muscle strength and vital capacity, an increased incidence of postoperative pneumonia, and longer postoperative hospital stays. Impaired wound healing as well as decreased respiratory, hepatic, and muscle function in protein-depleted patients awaiting surgery have also been reported.

Age

Many of the changes in the metabolic responses to surgical illness that occur with aging can be attributed to alterations in body composition and to longstanding patterns of physical activity. Although weight remains more or less stable, fat mass tends to increase with age while muscle mass tends to decrease. The loss of strength that accompanies immobility, starvation, and acute surgical illness may have marked functional consequences. The capacity of muscle to serve as an energy source may be limited during prolonged illness in the elderly patient, and muscle strength may rapidly become inadequate for respiratory and other vital muscle function.

After the limited stress of elective operation, increases in energy expenditure are independent of age. Endocrine responses to elective operation and to trauma appear intact in older patients in terms of plasma cortisol levels and urinary excretion of adrenaline, noradrenaline, and 17-hydroxycorticosteroids.

The prevalence of cardiovascular and pulmonary diseases increases with age. Diminished arterial compliance, impaired vasoconstriction, altered autonomic function and sensitivity to catecholamines, and decreased baroreflex sensitivity may all impair the maintenance of cardiovascular homeostasis during acute surgical illness. Thus, the delivery of oxygen to the tissues may be impaired in the elderly and may be inadequate when oxygen demands are highest.

Gender

Observed differences between the metabolic responses of men and women in general reflect differences in body composition. Lean body mass, expressed as a proportion of body weight, is

TABLE 3.6

METABOLIC DIFFERENCES BETWEEN THE RESPONSE TO SIMPLE STARVATION AND TO INJURY

	SIMPLE STARVATION	SEVERE INJURY
Basal metabolic rate	−	++
Presence of mediators	−	+++
Major fuel oxidized	Fat	Mixed
Ketone body production	+++	±
Hepatic ureagenesis	+	+++
Negative nitrogen balance	+	+++
Gluconeogenesis	+	+++
Muscle proteolysis	+	+++
Hepatic protein synthesis	+	+++

lower in women than in men; this difference is thought to account for the lower net loss of nitrogen after major elective abdominal surgery in women.

The Gut Mucosal Barrier Dysfunction as a Mediator of the Stress Response

Under certain circumstances, the gut may become a source of sepsis and serve as the motor of the systemic inflammatory
10 response syndrome. The maintenance of an intact brush border and intercellular tight junctions prevents the movement of toxic substances into the intestinal lymphatics and circulation; these functions may become altered in critically ill patients. Maintenance of a gut mucosal barrier that effectively excludes luminal bacteria and toxins requires normal perfusion, an intact epithelium, and normal mucosal immune mechanisms.

Microbial translocation is the process by which microorganisms migrate across the mucosal barrier and invade the host.[37] Translocation can be promoted in three general ways: (a) altered permeability of the intestinal mucosa, (b) decreased host defense, and (c) an increased number of bacteria within the intestine. Hemorrhagic shock, hypoxemia, sepsis, distant injury, or administration of cell toxins leads to altered permeability. Glucocorticoid administration, immunosuppression, or protein depletion decreases host defense. Bacterial overgrowth in association with intestinal stasis may cause translocation. Even if actual migration of whole bacteria does not occur, the gut may absorb endotoxin into the portal venous system. A number of retrospective and epidemiologic studies have associated infection in specific patient populations with bacterial invasion from the gut. These studies have demonstrated an increase in mucosal permeability both in normal volunteers who received endotoxin and in infected burn patients. Because many of the factors that facilitate bacterial translocation occur simultaneously in surgical patients and their effects may be additive or cumulative, patients in an intensive care unit may be extremely vulnerable to the invasion of enteric bacteria or to the absorption of their toxins. Such patients do not generally receive enteral feedings and current parenteral therapy results in gut atrophy. Methods currently used to support critically ill patients neither facilitate repair of the intestinal mucosa nor maintain gut barrier function. Provision of early enteral feeds and glutamine do the most to prevent translocation.

Elective Operations and Physiologic Responses to Surgery

The physiologic responses to surgical stress are multiple and complex (Fig. 3.7). One of the earliest consequences of a surgical procedure is the rise in levels of circulating cortisol occurring in response to a sudden outpouring of adrenocorticotropic hormone (ACTH) from the anterior pituitary gland.

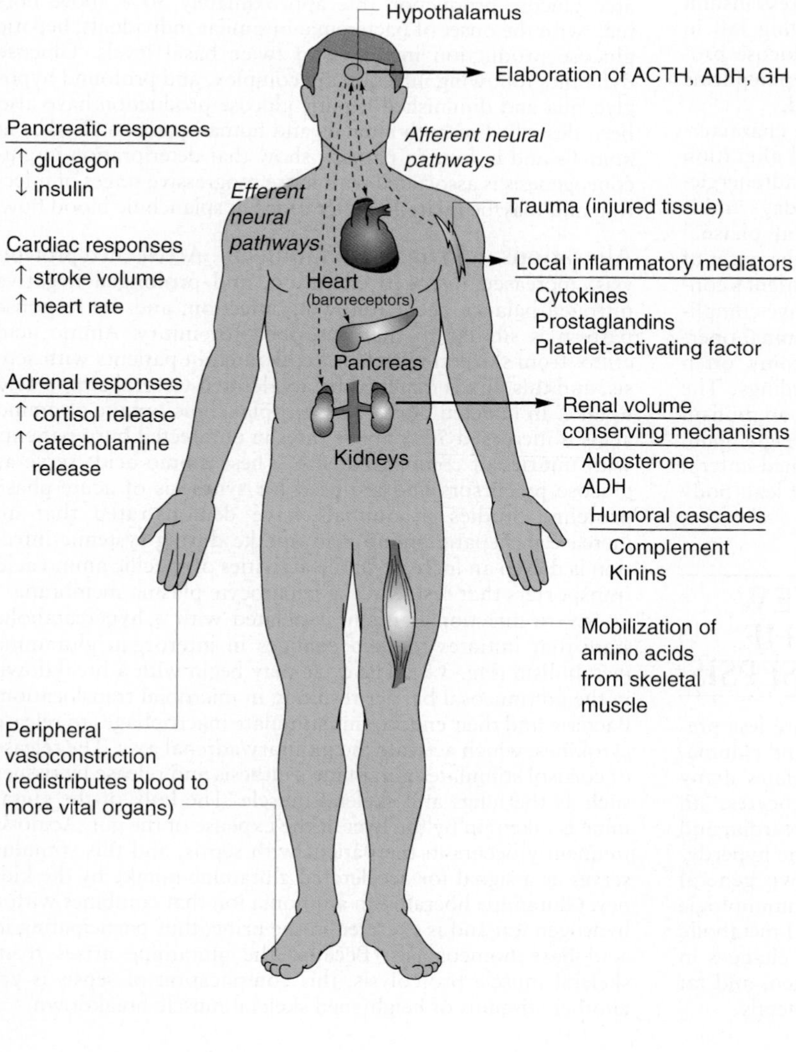

FIGURE 3.7. Homeostatic adjustments initiated after injury.

The rise in ACTH stimulates the adrenal cortex to elaborate cortisol, which remains elevated for 24 to 48 hours after operation. Cortisol has generalized effects on tissue catabolism and mobilizes amino acids from skeletal muscle that provide substrates for wound healing and serve as precursors for the hepatic synthesis of acute-phase proteins or new glucose. Associated with the activation of the adrenal cortex is stimulation of the adrenal medulla through the sympathetic nervous system, with elaboration of epinephrine and norepinephrine. These circulating neurotransmitters play an important role in circulatory adjustment, but may also elicit metabolic responses if the augmented secretion rate continues over a prolonged period of time.

The neuroendocrine responses to operation also modify the various mechanisms that regulate salt and water excretion. Alterations in serum osmolarity and tonicity of body fluids secondary to anesthesia and operative stress stimulate the secretion of aldosterone and ADH. Aldosterone is a potent stimulator of renal sodium retention, whereas ADH stimulates renal tubular water reabsorption. Thus, the ability to excrete a water load after elective surgical procedures is restricted and weight gain secondary to salt and water retention is usual following operation. Edema occurs to a varying extent in all surgical wounds, and this accumulation is proportional to the extent of tissue dissection and local trauma. This "third-spaced" fluid eventually returns to the circulation as the wound edema subsides and diuresis commences 2 to 4 days following the operation.

Alterations occur in the response of the endocrine pancreas following elective operation. In general, insulin elaboration is diminished, and glucagon concentrations rise. This response may be related to increased sympathetic activity or to the rise in levels of circulating epinephrine known to suppress insulin release. The rise in glucagon and the corresponding fall in insulin are a potent signal to accelerate hepatic glucose production, and, with the help of other hormones (epinephrine and glucocorticoids), gluconeogenesis is maintained.

The period of catabolism initiated by operation characterized by a combination of inadequate nutrition and alteration of the hormonal environment has been termed the "adrenergic-corticoid phase." This phase generally lasts 1 to 3 days and is followed by the "adrenergic-corticoid withdrawal phase," which lasts 1 to 3 days. This period is followed by the onset of anabolism, which occurs at a variable time in the patient's convalescence. In general, in the absence of postoperative complications, this phase starts 3 to 6 days after an abdominal operation of the magnitude of a colectomy or gastrectomy, often concomitant with the commencement of oral feedings. The patient then enters a prolonged period of early anabolism characterized by positive nitrogen balance and weight gain. Protein synthesis is increased as a result of sustained enteral feedings, and this change is related to the return of lean body mass and muscular strength.

SEPSIS: GENERAL OVERVIEW AND TIME COURSE OF THE METABOLIC RESPONSE TO SEPSIS

The response patterns following major infection are less predictable than those following elective operations and trauma. The invasion of the body by microorganisms initiates many host responses including mobilization of phagocytes, an inflammatory response at the local site, fever, tachycardia, and other systemic responses. Systemic events during the hyperdynamic phase of sepsis can be categorized into two general types of responses: (a) those related to the host's immunologic defenses and (b) those related to the body's general metabolic and circulatory adjustments to the infection. The changes in metabolism relate to alterations in glucose, nitrogen, and fat metabolism, as well as the redistribution of trace metals.

Systemic Metabolic Responses

Severe infection is characterized by fever, hypermetabolism, diminished protein economy, altered glucose dynamics, and accelerated lipolysis, much like the injured patient. Anorexia is commonly associated with systemic infection and contributes to the loss of lean body tissue. These effects are compounded in the patient with sepsis by multiorgan system failure, which includes the gastrointestinal tract, liver, heart, and lungs.

Hypermetabolism. Oxygen consumption is usually elevated in the infected patient. The extent of this increase is related to the severity of infection, with peak elevations reaching 50% to 60% above normal. Such responses often occur in the postoperative and postinjury periods secondary to severe pneumonia, intra-abdominal infection, or wound invasion. If the patient's metabolic rate is already elevated to a maximal extent because of severe injury, no further increase occurs. In patients with only slightly accelerated rates of oxygen consumption, the presence of infection causes a rise in metabolic rate that appears additive to the preexisting state. A portion of the increase in metabolism may be ascribed to the increase in reaction rate associated with fever (Q10 effect). Calculations suggest that the metabolic rate increases 10% to 13% for each elevation of 1°C in central temperature. On resolution of the infection, the metabolic rate returns to normal.

Altered Glucose Dynamics. The observation that glucose production is increased in infected patients appears to be additive to the augmented gluconeogenesis that occurs following injury. For example, uninfected burn patients have an accelerated glucose production rate approximately 50% above normal; with the onset of bacteremia in similar individuals, hepatic glucose production increases to twice basal levels. Glucose dynamics following infection are complex, and profound hypoglycemia and diminished hepatic glucose production have also been described in both animals and human patients. Studies in animals and in human patients show that deterioration in gluconeogenesis is associated with more progressive stages of infection and may be related to alterations in splanchnic blood flow.

Alterations in Protein Metabolism. Accelerated proteolysis, increased nitrogen excretion, and prolonged negative nitrogen balance occur following infection, and the response pattern is similar to that described for injury. Amino acid efflux from skeletal muscle is accelerated in patients with sepsis, and this flux is matched by accelerated visceral amino acid uptake. In infected burn patients, splanchnic uptake of amino acids is increased 50% above rates in uninfected burn patients with injuries of comparable size. These amino acids serve as glucose precursors and are used for synthesis of acute-phase proteins. Studies in animals have demonstrated that an increase in hepatic amino acid uptake during systemic infection is due to an increase in the activities of specific amino acid transporters that reside in the hepatocyte plasma membrane.

Severe infection is often associated with a hypercatabolic state that initiates marked changes in interorgan glutamine metabolism (Fig. 3.8). The cycle may begin with a breakdown in the gut mucosal barrier resulting in microbial translocation. Bacteria and their endotoxins stimulate macrophages to release cytokines, which activate the pituitary/adrenal axis. The release of cortisol stimulates glutamine synthesis and release by tissues such as the lungs and skeletal muscle. The bulk of the glutamine is taken up by the liver at the expense of the gut. Acidosis frequently occurs in the patient with sepsis, and this stimulus serves as a signal for accelerated glutamine uptake by the kidney. Glutamine liberates an ammonia ion that combines with a hydrogen ion and is excreted in the urine, thus participating in acid–base homeostasis. Because the glutamine arises from skeletal muscle proteolysis, this complication of sepsis is yet another stimulus of heightened skeletal muscle breakdown.

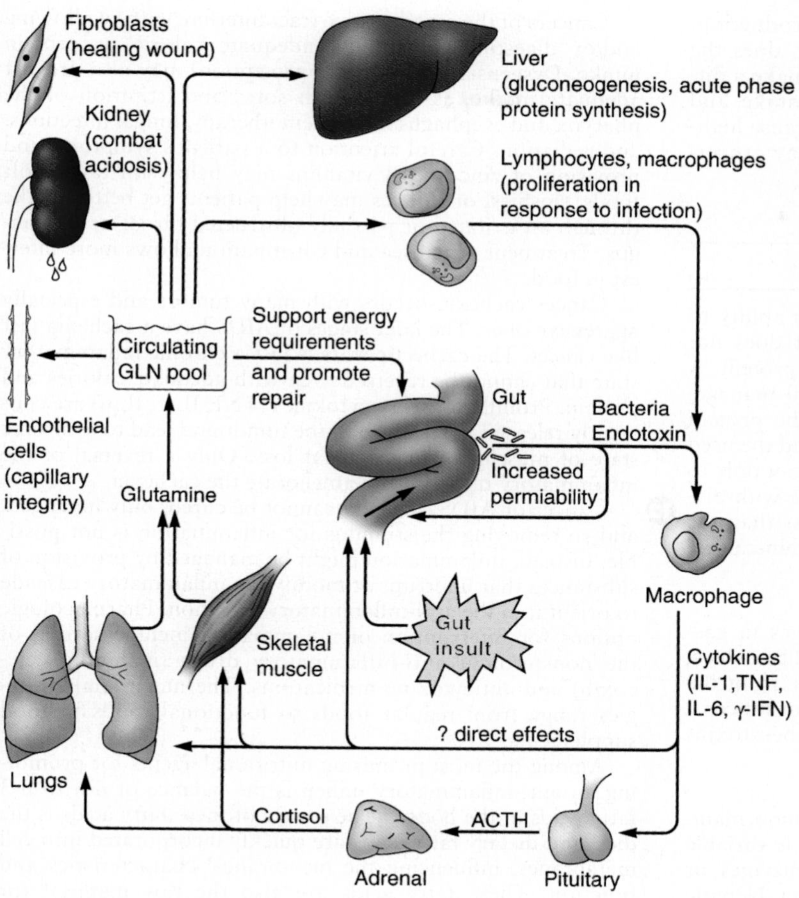

FIGURE 3.8. The interorgan glutamine cycle can be initiated by any local and/or systemic catabolic insult that redirects the flow of glutamine and results in glutamine depletion. In the case illustrated here, the patient develops a breakdown in the gut mucosal barrier, which causes an increase in bowel permeability and bacterial translocation. Bacteria and endotoxins stimulate macrophages to release cytokines (tumor necrosis factor [TNF], interleukin-1 [IL-1], IL-6), which exert direct effects on glutamine metabolism in various organs and also stimulate release of the counterregulatory hormones. These mediators work together to mobilize glutamine stores from muscle and to stimulate glutamine production by the lungs. A central goal is to support the increased glutamine requirements in other tissues. It is unclear why organs such as the gut should subserve other tissues, but it is apparent that if the cycle persists, or if the patient is unable to take oral feedings or remains glutamine deficient, a prolonged catabolic state develops.

Alterations in Fat Metabolism. Fat is a major fuel oxidized in infected patients, and the increased metabolism of lipids from peripheral fat stores is especially prominent during a period of inadequate nutritional support. Lipolysis is most probably mediated by the heightened sympathetic activity that is a potent stimulus for fat mobilization and accelerated oxidation. Serum triglyceride levels reflect the balance between rates of triglyceride production by the liver and use and storage by peripheral tissues. Marked hypertriglyceridemia has been associated with gram-negative infection on occasion, but plasma triglyceride concentrations are usually normal or low, indicating enhanced clearance by other organs. Infected patients cannot convert fatty acids to ketones efficiently in the liver, and hence do not adapt to starvation like fasted, unstressed individuals. It has been suggested that the low ketone levels of infection may be a consequence of the hyperinsulinemia associated with catabolic states.

Changes in Trace Mineral Metabolism. Changes in balance of magnesium, inorganic phosphate, zinc, and potassium generally follow alterations in nitrogen balance. Although the iron-binding capacity of transferrin is usually unchanged in early infection, iron disappears from the plasma, especially during severe pyrogenic infections; similar alterations are observed with serum zinc levels. These decreases cannot be totally accounted for by losses of the minerals from the body. Rather, both iron and zinc accumulate within the liver, and this accumulation appears to be another host defense mechanism. The administration of iron to the infected host, especially early in the disease, is contraindicated because increased serum iron concentrations may impair resistance. Unlike iron and zinc, copper levels generally rise, and the increased plasma concentrations can be ascribed almost entirely to the increase in ceruloplasmin produced by the liver.

Nutritional Requirements and Special Feeding Problems

As with all patients, the primary objectives of nutritional assessment are to evaluate the patient's present nutritional status and to determine energy, protein, and macro- and micronutrient requirements. Weight gain and anabolism are generally difficult to achieve during the septic process, but they do occur once the disease process has abated. Total energy requirements can be calculated using the stress equation; mild to moderate infections increase energy requirements 20% to 30%, and severe infection with fever increases caloric needs ~50% above basal levels. The most severe complication of sepsis is the multiple organ dysfunction syndrome, which may result in death. The current treatment of systemic infection consists of (a) removal or drainage of the septic source; (b) use of appropriate antibiotics; (c) supportive therapy of specific organ failure, whether cardiac, pulmonary, hepatic, renal, or gastrointestinal; and (d) vigorous support of the host through nutritional means.

Respiratory Insufficiency. A common problem associated with systemic infection is oxygenation and elimination of carbon dioxide in patients with a compromised pulmonary status. Patients often require intubation and vigorous ventilatory support, and hypermetabolism is a common feature of their illness. Hypermetabolism is accompanied by increased oxygen consumption, which drives carbon dioxide production as more substrate must be oxidized to support the hypermetabolic response. Within this model, composition of diet (carbohydrate vs. fat) is relatively unimportant in determining the carbon dioxide burden (carbohydrate at respiratory quotient [RQ] 1.0 releasing more CO_2 than fat at RQ 0.7). Avoidance of overfeeding is the primary concern in reducing the nutritional contribution to CO_2 production. Only in the most severely compromised patients does the change in CO_2 production from diet composition make a difference. The decision to reduce carbohydrate intake and increase lipid intake must be weighed carefully because high-fat diets, especially fats high in n-6 fatty acids, may exacerbate lung injury.

Renal Failure

Renal failure significantly compromises the body's ability to clear the byproducts of protein metabolism, but does not reduce the catabolic rate or the need for dietary protein. A nexus therefore exists between nutrition and renal management: should protein intake be determined by the protein needs of the patient or by a desire to limit uremia and the need for dialysis? Under such conditions, it is important not only to avoid overfeeding protein, but also to be aggressive with dialytic therapy so that protein is not restricted to less than the body's requirement. Careful assessment of protein-calorie needs is critical.

Gut Dysfunction. Sepsis causes marked changes in gastrointestinal function. The most common abnormality is ileus, which can result from intra-abdominal disease or from the effects of bacteria elsewhere. Breakdown of the gut mucosal barrier with translocation of luminal bacteria and their toxins can initiate a prolonged hypermetabolic state.

Hepatic Failure. Hepatic dysfunction is a common manifestation of septicemia. The degree of dysfunction is variable and may appear early as a slight elevation of liver enzymes, or it may cause severe jaundice and hyperbilirubinemia. Hepatic dysfunction generally resolves on resolution of the sepsis, but if the inflammatory process persists, adjustments in the feeding formulation are necessary. Balanced carbohydrate and fat intake are important with avoidance of overfeeding. The patient should be observed for the presence of encephalopathy; if this complication occurs and cannot be controlled by lactulose usage, then the protein load should also be reduced. Another indicator for limiting protein to less than 1.5 g/kg body weight is an elevated prothrombin time, as this indicates impairment of hepatic protein synthetic function. Of course, vitamin K and anticoagulants must be eliminated as causes of the change.

Cardiac Dysfunction. The myocardial dysfunction that occurs in sepsis may be secondary to the elaboration of cytokines such as TNF or IL-1, which have direct myocardial depressant activity. Alternatively, the heart failure may be secondary to pulmonary insufficiency with an increased pulmonary vascular resistance and right ventricular overload. Malnourished patients with sepsis may be sensitive to volume overload, and use of a concentrated enteral or parenteral feeding solution may be indicated to maximize calories and to minimize volume.

CANCER AND ACQUIRED IMMUNODEFICIENCY SYNDROME

11 Nutrition support of patients with cancer or acquired immunodeficiency syndrome (AIDS), whose inflammatory states are very similar, needs to be directed at two major areas: (a) providing nutrition when symptoms of the disease or side effects of treatment prevent adequate intake and (b) fighting the inflammatory state created by the disease.

Cancers of the aerodigestive tract interfere with swallowing and/or digestion, precluding adequate caloric or protein intake. Dysgeusia (altered taste perception) may also prevent adequate intake, as may mouth sores and irritation of the pharynx and esophagus from chemotherapy, fungal infections, and radiation. Careful attention to a patient's symptoms and provision of zinc and B vitamins may help with taste. Soft foods, slushies, or slurries may help patients get better intake through an irritated or partially obstructed throat or esophagus. Treatment of nausea and constipation allows more interest in food.

Cancer cachexia occurs with many tumors and especially aggressive ones. The later stages of AIDS have a cachexia just like cancer. The cachectic state is just a chronic inflammatory state that cannot be reversed even with adequate calories and protein. Proinflammatory cytokines (TNF, IL-1, IL-6) are constantly released in response to the tumor and lead to a chronic state of muscle wasting and fat loss. Only a reversal of the inflammatory response can ameliorate the cachexia.

12 Cancer or AIDS cachexia cannot be cured, only managed, and so removing the stimulus for inflammation is not possible. Instead, inflammation might be managed by provision of substances that interrupt or modify the inflammatory cascade to orient it in the anti-inflammatory direction. Pharmacologic options for interruption of inflammation include several of the nonsteroidal anti-inflammatory drugs (including celecoxib) and anticytokine medications. The nutritional strategies range from regular foods to functional foods to food supplements.

Among the most promising nutritional agents for promoting an anti-inflammatory milieu is the balance of n-6 to n-3 fatty acids in the body.[38] The source of these fatty acids is the diet, and dietary fatty acids are quickly incorporated into cell membranes, influencing the membranes' characteristics and function. These fatty acids are also the raw material for eicosanoid production.[39] The type of eicosanoid produced depends on the types of fatty acids contained in the cell membranes. The dietary and intravenous n-6 fatty acid is linoleic acid, which is incorporated into cell membranes as arachidonic acid, which gives rise to proinflammatory PG_2 and LT_4. The dietary n-3 fatty acids are α-linolenic, eicosapentaenoic, and docosahexaenoic acid and are incorporated into cell membranes as the more anti-inflammatory PG_3 and LT_5. These anti-inflammatory eicosanoids interrupt the release of IL-6, thus potentially allowing IGF-1 levels to normalize in the patient with cachexia.[40] The typical modern Western diet is high in the ratio of n-6 to n-3 fatty acids (about 15:1). A more therapeutic ratio would be 2:1 to 4:1. In managing cachexia, the nutritional recommendation is to increase calorie and protein intake by any means possible. This often means dairy foods and protein sources from cold-water fish, which tend to keep the n-3 level high.

In three studies, pancreatic cancer patients consumed 3 g of eicosapentaenoic acid (EPA), a marine source of n-3 fatty acid, in a calorie/protein liquid supplement.[41–43] By doing so, patients gained weight (as fat-free mass, an indicator of anabolism); increased their grip strength; reduced their levels of C-reactive protein, IL-6, and resting metabolic rate (markers of decreased inflammation); and improved their scores on quality-of-life and functional status questionnaires. In another randomized trial, daily supplementation of 18 g n-3 fatty acid improved survival time in malnourished patients with solid tumors.[44]

Another possible nutritional intervention in cachexia of chronic illness is amino acid supplementation, specifically arginine, glutamine, and/or branched chain amino acids (leucine, isoleucine, valine). It should be remembered that the metabolic pathways of all of these amino acids intersect in human metabolism, so supplementation with all of them may not be required. Be that as it may, two double-blind, randomized clinical trials of a commercially available amino acid supplement containing 14 g arginine, 14 g glutamine, and 3 g β-hydroxy-β-methylbutyrate (an analog of leucine) has shown that such supplementation can increase the fat-free mass of cachectic cancer patients (stage IV solid tumors) and patients with stage III AIDS.[45,46]

OTHER METHODS OF MODIFYING THE CATABOLIC RESPONSE TO SURGERY AND CRITICAL ILLNESS

Besides nutritional intervention, other methods to modify the physiologic and biochemical response to operation have been studied in an effort to reduce the magnitude of the stress response and to provide insight into possible mechanisms. Regional anesthetic techniques block afferent signals from the wound and interrupt sympathetic nervous efferent signals to the adrenal gland and possibly the liver, reducing the apparent magnitude of the stress response. Others have studied stress responses in sympathectomized animals by blocking the efferent limb of the neuroendocrine reflex response. These reports indicate that central nervous system blockade interrupts afferent signals stimulated by operative procedures.

More recent studies have documented the safety and efficacy of long-term exogenous recombinant growth hormone (GH) administration.[47] GH stimulates protein synthesis during hypocaloric feedings and increases retention of sodium and potassium by the kidney. The potential synergistic effects of specialized nutrition in combination with GH require further study. Cyclooxygenase inhibitors such as aspirin and ibuprofen attenuate the symptoms and endocrine responses that occur with critical illness without altering cytokine elaboration. It is anticipated that researchers may eventually be able to selectively block the deleterious effects of excessive cytokines yet preserve their beneficial effects.

Research Findings

One of the difficulties in applying the research on nutritional modulation of the inflammatory response is that research protocols target particular diseases, and so results are often not generalizable (i.e., a study that shows an improvement in body composition and quality of life in cancer patients cannot be generalized to patients with congestive heart failure).

Although novel approaches to the management of the inflammatory response are becoming clinical realities,[48] the current standard of supplemental macro- and micronutrients should not be ignored. Akner and Cederholm[23] reviewed the literature and found that in 60% of 36 randomized controlled trials, standard supplementation of nutrient intake improved function/morbidity, and in 80% of 41 randomized controlled trials, standard supplementation improved anthropometric variables. However, this leaves a large percentage of studies in which standard support of calorie, protein, and micronutrient intake did not have a positive effect. The intriguing question is whether in these negative studies a more targeted form of nutrition support would have had the desired effect.

CHOICE OF NUTRITION IN SURGICAL PATIENTS: ENTERAL OR PARENTERAL?

Although the physiologic advantage of enteral nutrition is apparent, preoperative nutritional repletion via the enteral route has not been as extensively studied as preoperative total parenteral nutrition (TPN). Although its use can be associated with the development of nausea, diarrhea, and distention, we recommend the use of enteral nutrition (via a feeding tube or as in-between-meal supplements) in malnourished patients if it is feasible. Candidates must have a functional GI tract and must be able to receive adequate amounts of calories and nitrogen. In many critically ill patients, enteral nutrition–related gastrointestinal complications are high and associated with decreased nutrient intake from the ordered levels.[49,50] Furthermore, forcing the enteral issue in patients who are intolerant of enteral nutrition is more detrimental than properly managed parenteral nutrition.

NUTRITION AS PRIMARY THERAPY

1. Patients with enterocutaneous fistulas (parenteral preferred but enteral could be used with a low-output fistula)

Patients with gastrointestinal-cutaneous fistulas represent the classic indication for TPN. In such patients, oral intake of food almost invariably results in increased fistula output, which can lead to metabolic disturbances, dehydration, and death. Several comprehensive reviews have concluded that total parenteral nutrition clearly impacts the treatment and course of disease for patients with GI fistulas. The following conclusions can be drawn from studies evaluating the use of TPN in patients with enterocutaneous fistulas: (a) TPN increases the spontaneous closure rate of enterocutaneous fistulas, but does not markedly decrease the mortality rate in patients with fistulas (improvements in mortality are mainly due to improved surgical and metabolic care); (b) if spontaneous closure of the fistula does not occur, patients are better prepared for operative intervention because of the nutritional support they received; and (c) certain fistulas (radiated bowel) are associated with a higher failure rate of closure than others and should be treated more aggressively surgically after a defined period of nutritional support (unless closure occurs).

2. Patients with short bowel syndrome (parenteral)

Prospective randomized trials designed specifically to examine the impact of TPN on patients with short bowel syndrome have not been initiated, mainly because such patients have no choice but to receive TPN. Most of these patients, who would have certainly died prior to the availability of TPN, now survive for long periods of time on home parenteral nutrition. In selected patients with residual small intestine (at least 18 inches), postresectional hyperplasia may develop with time such that they can tolerate enteral feedings. Studies by Wilmore and colleagues[39] have demonstrated that the requirement for TPN could be decreased or even eliminated in patients with short gut syndrome by providing a nutritional regimen consisting of supplemental glutamine, growth hormone, and a modified high-carbohydrate, low-fat diet. There was a marked improvement in the absorption of nutrients with this combination therapy and a decrease in stool output. In addition, TPN requirements were reduced by 50%, as were the costs associated with care of these individuals. Discontinuation of the growth hormone did not increase TPN needs in these patients once they had undergone successful gut rehabilitation.

3. Patients with hepatic failure (enteral preferred)

Individuals with liver disease may be malnourished because of excessive alcohol intake, diminished food intake, or an inflammatory state from viral infection. These individuals are protein depleted yet are intolerant of protein because of their tendency to become encephalopathic with a high nitrogen intake.

Because of liver damage and portasystemic shunting, these patients develop derangements in circulating levels of amino acids. The plasma aromatic–to–branched chain amino acid ratio is increased, favoring the transport of aromatic amino acids across the blood–brain barrier. These amino acids are precursors of false neurotransmitters that contribute to lethargy and encephalopathy. Treatment of individuals with liver failure with solutions enriched in branched chain amino acids and deficient in aromatic amino acids results in improved tolerance to the administered protein and clinical improvement in the encephalopathic state.

4. Patients with major thermal injury (enteral preferred if possible)

Aggressive nutritional support in patients with major burns seems to be associated with improved survival, particularly when increased amounts of dietary protein are provided.[51] Burned patients often require ventilatory support and/or suffer from ileus, which prevents using the GI tract for feeding. Even if the GI tract is usable, such patients are often unable to eat enough because of frequent trips to the operating room combined with the anorexia of severe injury. Most burn authorities believe that aggressive nutritional support in patients with major thermal injury has influenced outcome in a positive manner.

5. Patients with acute renal failure (enteral preferred if possible)

TPN with amino acids of high biologic value *may* decrease the mortality in patients with acute renal failure.[52] The use of solutions containing high-quality amino acids can improve nitrogen balance and diminish urea production. This translates into a decreased frequency of dialysis.

Total Parenteral Nutrition as Secondary Therapy

1. Prolonged ileus after operative procedure

Occasionally, patients develop a prolonged ileus after an abdominal procedure, which precludes the use of the intestinal tract as a route of feeding. Such an occurrence is generally unpredictable and the cause of the ileus is often not demonstrated. If the patient is unable to eat by the seventh postoperative day, TPN should be started. The ileus may persist for several weeks. Although provision of TPN does not influence the disease process per se, it is beneficial because it prevents further erosion of lean body mass.

2. Acute radiation and chemotherapy enteritis

Malnourished patients who receive abdominal or pelvic radiation or chemotherapy may develop mucositis and enterocolitis that precludes using the GI tract for prolonged periods of time. In such individuals, TPN should be provided until the enteritis resolves and oral feeding can be resumed.

3. Preoperative TPN in the perioperative setting

In general, one cannot justify the use of perioperative nutrition (particularly parenteral feedings) unless a clear benefit to the patient can be demonstrated. The results of prospective randomized trials evaluating the efficacy of preoperative TPN are conflicting because of the variations in the nutritional status of patients studied, the differences in types of diseases in these malnourished patients, the differences in the type and length of nutritional support administered, and the failure to accrue enough patients to avoid type II statistical error. The following questions are important to consider: Does preoperative nutritional support decrease the morbidity and mortality associated with major operative procedures? How long should nutritional support be administered? What type of nutritional repletion should be administered?

One of the best studies to date evaluating the efficacy of preoperative TPN was published by the Veterans Affairs Total Parenteral Nutrition Cooperative Study Group.[53] More than 3,500 patients requiring mainly elective abdominal surgery were entered into this prospective randomized trial. They were initially screened for evidence of malnutrition using subjective criteria and/or by determining their Nutritional Risk Index Score, which included objective criteria such as percentage of weight loss and serum albumin level. The patients were further divided into categories assigning them to one of four groups: well nourished, borderline malnourished, moderately malnourished, or severely malnourished. Patients in each malnourished category were randomized to receive at least 7 days of preoperative TPN or to proceed with surgery without preoperative TPN. Patients randomized to receive TPN received 1,000 kcal/day in excess of calculated caloric requirements. Lipid was provided on a daily basis. One criticism of this study was that patients were allowed to eat in addition to receiving parenteral feedings.

Analysis of the data from this study indicated that there was no difference in short-term or long-term complications between groups. Infectious complications including pneumonia, abscess, and line sepsis were statistically significantly higher for patients receiving TPN.[54] Noninfectious complications (impaired wound healing) were significantly lower only in those patients receiving TPN who were in the severely malnourished group (>15% weight loss and serum albumin <2.9 mg). This study strongly suggests that preoperative TPN should be provided only to severely malnourished patients who cannot be nourished by the enteral route. Contraindications to the use of preoperative TPN include patients requiring emergency operation and those who are only mildly or moderately malnourished. In such patients, TPN should be continued postoperatively only if the GI tract cannot be utilized for tube feedings. Nasojejunal or jejunostomy tubes should also be considered in patients undergoing major upper abdominal procedures in whom it is anticipated that oral feedings may not be resumed for 7 to 10 days after surgery.

Composition of Total Parenteral Nutrition Formulations

Total parenteral nutrition solutions are administered through a central venous catheter generally inserted into the subclavian vein (Fig. 3.9). The composition of a standard TPN solution is shown in Table 3.7. Because of the hyperosmolarity of such solutions, they must be delivered into a high-flow system to prevent venous sclerosis. Patients receiving TPN should be monitored regularly by measuring blood sugar, serum electrolytes, and liver function tests. Elevations in serum glucose are common in surgical patients receiving TPN, especially if the patient is stressed and is relatively glucose intolerant. Hyperglycemia can generally be controlled by adding insulin to the TPN formulation or by decreasing the amount of glucose in the solution. It has been shown that injured people can maximally oxidize about 4 to 5 mg of glucose/kg/min. For a 70-kg man, this is equal to approximately 400 to 500 g/day (1,600 to 13 2,000 kcal/day). Excess glucose calories are converted to fat, are deposited in the liver, and result in hyperglycemia and glycosuria. Glycosuria with its osmotic load leads to a water diuresis that leaves the patient with a hyperosmolar state that can progress to coma as the brain is depleted of water. The amounts of the various electrolytes provided to patients receiving TPN vary depending on factors such as previous nutritional and hydration status. Careful monitoring is critical because as new cell mass is built, potassium and phosphate can move into cells, leading to severe hypokalemia or hypophosphatemia. These electrolyte disturbances can develop rapidly and are much more life threatening than hyponatremia. Vitamin (Table 3.8) and trace mineral (Table 3.9) requirements must also be monitored.

TABLE 3.7

COMPOSITION OF A STANDARD CENTRAL VENOUS SOLUTION

Volume		
	10% Amino acid solution	500 mL
	50% Dextrose solution	500 mL
	Fat emulsion	—
	Electrolytes + vitamins + minerals	~50 mL
	Total volume	~1,050 mL
Composition		
	Amino acids	50 g
	Dextrose	250 g
	Total N	50/6.25 = 8 g
	Dextrose kcal	250 g × 3.4 kcal/g = 840 kcal
	mOsms/L	~2,000
Electrolytes Added to Total Parenteral Nutrition Solutions		
	Usual concentration	**Range of concentrations**
Sodium (mEq/L)	60	0–150
Potassium (mEq/L)	40	0–80
Acetate (mEq/L)	50	50–150
Chloride (mEq/L)	50	0–150
Phosphate (mEq/L)	15	0–30
Calcium (mEq/L)[a]	4.5	0–20
Magnesium (mEq/L)	5	5–15

[a]Generally added as calcium gluconate or calcium chloride: one ampule of calcium gluconate = 1 g of calcium = 4.5 mEq.

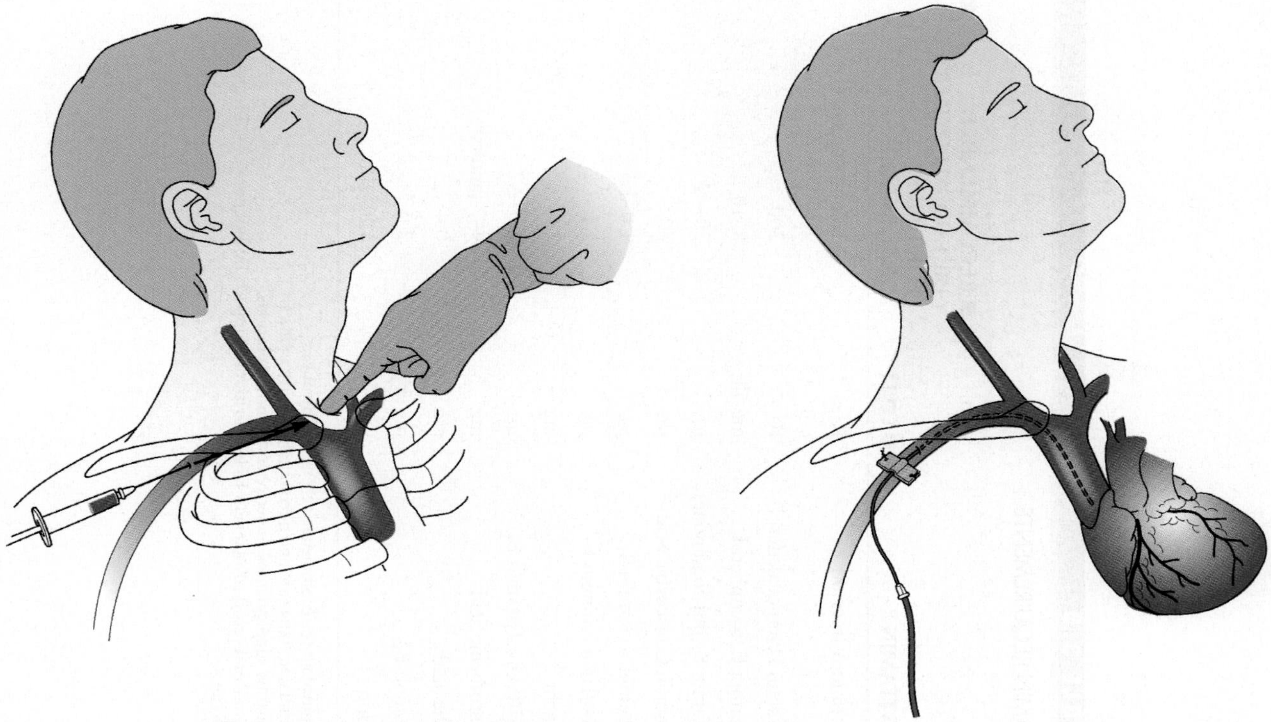

FIGURE 3.9. Technique for insertion of a subclavian catheter (see text for details).

TABLE 3.8

VITAMIN REQUIREMENTS

VITAMIN	UNIT	RECOMMENDED DIETARY ALLOWANCE FOR DAILY ORAL INTAKE	DAILY REQUIREMENT OF THE MODERATELY INJURED	DAILY REQUIREMENT OF THE SEVERELY INJURED	AMOUNT PROVIDED BY ONE VITAMIN PILL	DAILY AMOUNT PROVIDED BY STANDARD INTRAVENOUS PREPARATIONS
Vitamin A (retinol)	IU	1,760 (women)–3,300 (men)	5,000	5,000	10,000	3,300 (retinol)
Vitamin D (ergocalciferol)	IU	200	400	400	400	200
Vitamin E (tocopherol)	mg TE	8–10	Unknown	Unknown	15	10[a]
Vitamin K (phylloquinone)	μg	20–40[b]	20	20	0	0[c]
Vitamin C (ascorbic acid)	μg	60	75	300	100	100
Thiamine (vitamin B_1)	μg	1.0–1.5	2	10	10	3.0
Riboflavin (vitamin B_2)	μg	1.2–1.7	2	10	10	3.6
Niacin	mg	13–19	20	100	100	40
Pyridoxine (vitamin B_6)	μg	2.0–2.2	2	40	5	4.0
Pantothenic acid	mg	4–7 (adults)[b]	18	40	20	15
Folic acid	mg	0.4	1.5	2.5	0	0.4
Vitamin B_{12}	mg	3.0	2	4	5	5
Biotin	mg	100–200[b]	Unknown	Unknown	0	60

[a]Equivalent to recommended dietary allowance.
[b]Estimated to be safe and adequate in dietary intakes.
[c]Must be supplemented in peripheral venous solutions.
From Rombeau JL, Rolandelli RH. Nutritional support. In: Wilmore DW, Brennan MF, Harken RH, et al., eds. *Care of the Surgical Patient: II. Care in the ICU*. New York: Scientific American Medicine; 1989:6.

TABLE 3.9

MINERAL AND TRACE ELEMENT REQUIREMENTS

MINERAL	RECOMMENDED DIETARY ALLOWANCE FOR DAILY ORAL INTAKE (mg)	SUGGESTED DAILY INTRAVENOUS INTAKE (mg)	DAILY AMOUNT PROVIDED BY A COMMERCIALLY AVAILABLE MIXTURE (mg)
Zinc	15	2.5–5.0[a]	5.0
Copper	2–3[b]	0.5–1.5	1.0
Manganese	2.5–5.0[b]	0.15–0.8	0.5
Chromium	0.05–0.2[b]	0.01–0.015	0.1
Iron	8 (women)–10 (men)	3	0

[a]Burn patients require an additional 2 mg.
[b]Estimated to be safe and adequate in dietary intakes.
From Rombeau JL, Rolandelli RH. Nutritional support. In: Wilmore DW, Brennan MF, Harken RH, et al., eds. *Care of the Surgical Patient: II. Care in the ICU*. New York: Scientific American Medicine; 1989:6.

The use of lipids in TPN was developed to meet the requirement for essential fatty acids (linoleic acid) and the full caloric needs in hypermetabolic patients, recognizing the complications associated with infusing large amounts of dextrose. Intravenous fat emulsions are composed of soy or safflower oils (vegetable fat emulsions), which contain primarily long-chain triglycerides (LCTs) composed of fatty acids with 16- and 18-carbon chain lengths. The provision of fat provides essential linoleic acid, inhibits lipogenesis from carbohydrates, and lowers the RQ, which may benefit patients with respiratory compromise. However, the high content of n-6 polyunsaturated fatty acids (in particular, linoleic acid) in these emulsions may have harmful effects on pulmonary and immune function.[55] Standard intravenous fat emulsions may alter the cell membrane phospholipid composition of cells of the reticuloendothelial system, resulting in changes in membrane fluidity such that clearance of bacteria and toxins is impaired. In addition, n-6 polyunsaturated fatty acids may alter the local production of eicosanoids and cytokines such that chemotaxis is negatively impacted. Newer nutritional methods of modifying the catabolic response to injury and infection propose the use of the n-3 fatty acids, which may decrease eicosanoid biosynthesis and thereby diminish the vasoconstriction, platelet aggregation, and immunosuppression that may occur when n-6 derivatives are administered. Studies suggest that n-3 fatty acids may be of benefit to the critically ill patient. Omega-3 fatty acids have been added to enteral formulas, but are not in parenteral formulas available in the United States.

Fat is an important fuel source for critically ill patients. Septic and injured patients preferentially utilize endogenous fat as an energy source, which appears to be related in part to the effects of counterregulatory hormones on stimulating fat mobilization. These patients have a relative unresponsiveness to the administration of carbohydrates in that free fatty acid mobilization is only marginally decreased and free fatty acid oxidation is not suppressed, as in "pure starvation." Glucose infusion above energy expenditure in a hormonal milieu that favors fat mobilization and oxidation only leads to hepatic steatosis.

Potential Complications of Total Parenteral Nutrition

Advances in technology, monitoring, and catheter care have greatly reduced the incidence of complications associated with the use of TPN. The establishment of a nutrition support team (physician, dietician, nurse, pharmacist) and the recognition of such a team as an important part of overall patient care have also been key factors in reducing complications. Complications of TPN occur and can be divided into three types: mechanical, metabolic, and infectious (Table 3.10). The management of the patient who becomes septic while receiving TPN is shown in Algorithm 3.1.

The Effects of Total Parenteral Nutrition on the Gastrointestinal Tract

The majority of studies that have examined the effects of TPN on intestinal function and immunity have been done in animals. These studies clearly demonstrate that TPN has a downside, which is related to intestinal disuse. A unique feature of TPN is that subjects can remain on bowel rest for prolonged periods of time without concomitant malnutrition, thereby facilitating the study of intestinal disuse as an independent variable. In rats, TPN results in significant disruption of the intestinal microflora and bacterial translocation from the gut lumen to the mesenteric lymph nodes. In addition, when stresses such as burn injury, chemotherapy, or radiation are introduced in these models, animals on TPN have a much higher mortality. This body of literature suggests that TPN, under certain circumstances, may predispose patients to an increase in gut-derived infectious complications.[38]

A provocative study in human volunteers demonstrated that individuals receiving TPN had an accentuated systemic response to endotoxin challenge compared to enterally fed volunteers.[48] The study is consistent with an impairment in gut barrier function during parenteral feedings, which may promote the release of bacteria and/or cytokines, leading to pronounced systemic responses and possibly multiple organ failure.

Supporting the Gut in Critically Ill Patients

The intestinal tract has long been considered an organ of inactivity following operation or injury. Ileus is generally present, nasogastric decompression is often necessary, and the gut is usually dormant in the immediate postoperative period. In the past, digestion and absorption was thought to be the only physiologic role of the gut. Disuse of the GI tract, either via starvation or nutritional support by TPN, may lead to numerous physiologic derangements as well as changes in gut microflora, impaired gut immune function, and disruption of the integrity of the mucosal barrier. Thus, maintaining gut function in the perioperative period may be essential in order to minimize septic complications and organ failure.

Treatment strategies designed to support the gut during critical illness should be directed toward the provision of

TABLE 3.10

COMPLICATIONS ASSOCIATED WITH THE USE OF TPN

■ COMPLICATION	■ CAUSE	■ TREATMENT
MECHANICAL		
Pneumothorax	Puncture/laceration of lung pleura	Serial CXRs; chest tube if indicated
Subclavian artery injury	Penetration of subclavian artery during needle stick	CXR; serial monitoring of vital signs
Air embolism	Aspiration of air into the subclavian vein and right heart	Place patient in Trendelenburg and left lateral decubitus; aspirate air
Catheter embolization	Shearing off the tip when withdrawing catheter	Retrieve catheter transvenously under fluoroscopic guidance
Venous thrombosis	Clot formation in great vein secondary to catheter	Heparinization if clinically significant
Catheter malposition	Tip of catheter directed into IJ or opposite subclavian	Reposition under fluoroscopy
METABOLIC		
Hyperglycemia	Excessive glucose calories or glucose intolerance	Decrease glucose calories; administer insulin
Hypoglycemia	Sudden cessation of TPN	Bolus 50% glucose solution; monitor blood glucose
Carbon dioxide retention	Infusion of glucose calories in excess of energy needs	Decrease glucose calories and replace with fat
Hyperglycemic, hyperosmolar nonketotic coma (HHNC)	Dehydration from excessive diuresis	Discontinue TPN immediately; give insulin; monitor glucose/electrolytes
Hyperchloremic metabolic acidosis	Excessive chloride administration	Give Na and K as acetate salts
Azotemia	Excessive amino acid administration with inadequate calories	Decrease amino acids; increase glucose calories
Essential fatty acid deficiency	Inadequate essential fatty acid administration	Administer fat solution
Hypertriglyceridemia	Rapid fat infusion of decreased fat clearance	Slow rate of fat infusion
Hypophosphatemia	Inadequate administration of	Increase administration
Hypocalcemia	electrolyte in question	
Hypomagnesemia		
Hypokalemia		
Bleeding	Vitamin K deficiency	Administer Vitamin K
SEPTIC		
Line sepsis	Catheter tip infected	Remove catheter; antibiotics
Infection at skin site	Bacteria at site of catheter entry into skin	Remove catheter; local wound care

CXR, chest radiograph; IJ, internal jugular; TPN, total parenteral nutrition.

appropriate nutrition and maintenance of mucosal structure and function. Presumably, such efforts assist the gut in its role as a metabolic processing station and as a barrier.[56–58]

Nutrition Support: Enteral Feedings

Enteral feedings are probably the best single method of maintaining mucosal structure and function if the bowel is functional. The trophic effects of luminal nutrition are key and the beneficial effects are well documented even if relatively small amounts of nutrients are provided.[59]

Gut-specific Nutrients. It is now clear that the composition of the diet, as well as the route of delivery, plays an important role in maintaining gut structure and function. Several gut-specific nutrients have been studied, but glutamine has received the most attention. Glutamine has been classified as a nonessential or nutritionally dispensable amino acid. Since this categorization implies that glutamine can be synthesized in adequate quantities from other amino acids and precursors, it has not been considered necessary to include glutamine in nutritional formulas. It has been eliminated from TPN solutions because of its relative instability and short shelf life compared to other amino acids. With few exceptions, glutamine is present in oral and enteral diets only at the relatively low levels characteristic of its concentration in most animal and plant proteins (about 7% of total amino acids).

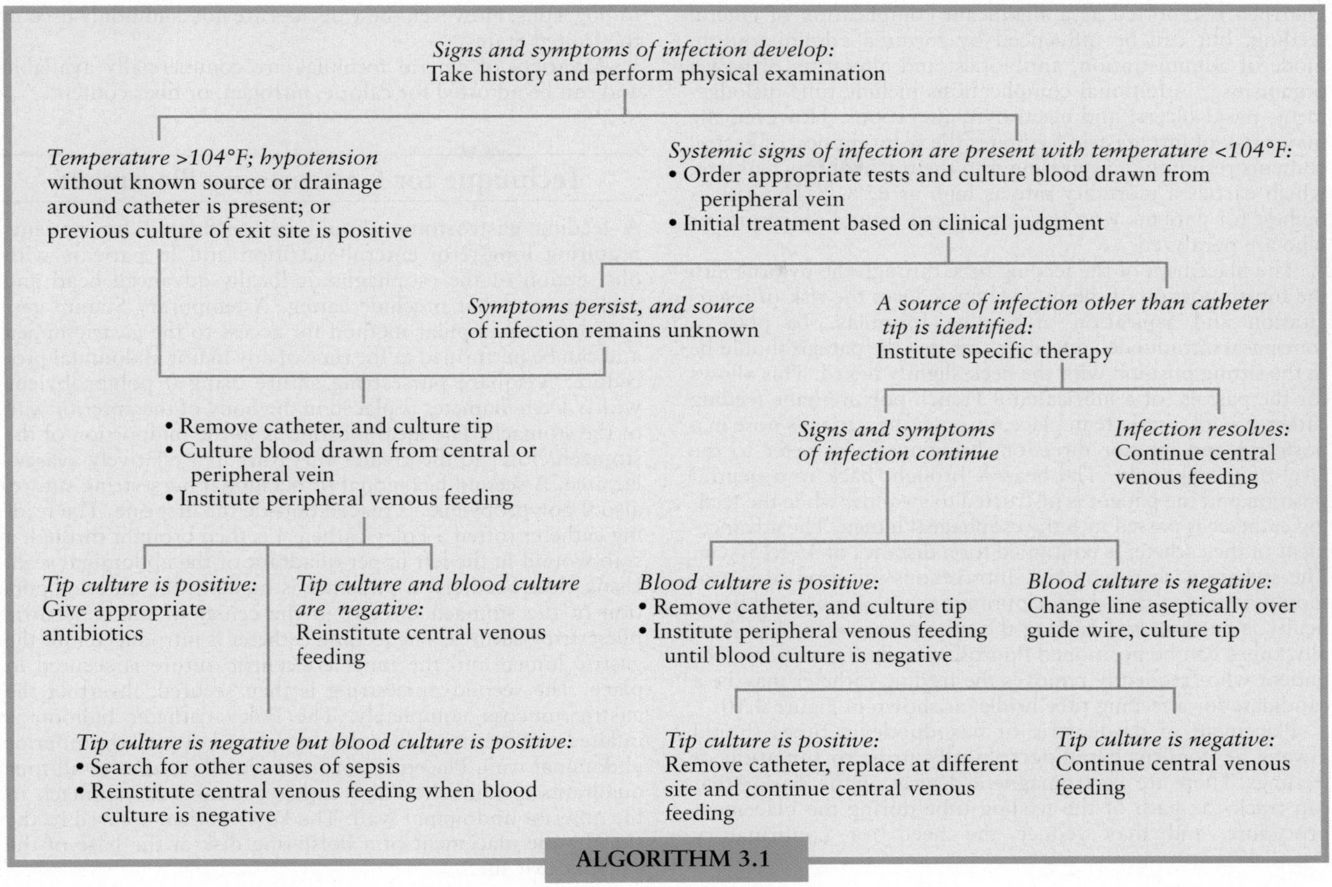
Signs and symptoms of infection develop:
Take history and perform physical examination
Temperature >104°F; hypotension without known source or drainage around catheter is present; or previous culture of exit site is positive
Systemic signs of infection are present with temperature <104°F:
• Order appropriate tests and culture blood drawn from peripheral vein
• Initial treatment based on clinical judgment
Symptoms persist, and source of infection remains unknown
A source of infection other than catheter tip is identified:
Institute specific therapy
• Remove catheter, and culture tip
• Culture blood drawn from central or peripheral vein
• Institute peripheral venous feeding
Signs and symptoms of infection continue
Infection resolves:
Continue central venous feeding
Tip culture is positive:
Give appropriate antibiotics
Tip culture and blood culture are negative:
Reinstitute central venous feeding
Blood culture is positive:
• Remove catheter, and culture tip
• Institute peripheral venous feeding until blood culture is negative
Blood culture is negative:
Change line aseptically over guide wire, culture tip
Tip culture is negative but blood culture is positive:
• Search for other causes of sepsis
• Reinstitute central venous feeding when blood culture is negative
Tip culture is positive:
Remove catheter, replace at different site and continue central venous feeding
Tip culture is negative:
Continue central venous feeding
ALGORITHM 3.1

ALGORITHM 3.1. Management of the total parenteral nutrition (TPN) patient who becomes septic.

Several recent studies have demonstrated that glutamine may be a conditionally essential amino acid during critical illness, particularly as it relates to supporting the metabolic requirements of the intestinal mucosa.[56–58] In general, these studies demonstrate that dietary glutamine is not required during states of health, but appears to be beneficial when glutamine depletion is severe and/or when the intestinal mucosa is damaged by insults such as chemotherapy and radiation therapy. Addition of glutamine to enteral diets reduces the incidence of gut translocation, but these improvements are dependent on the amount of supplemental glutamine and the type of insult studied. Glutamine-enriched TPN partially attenuates the villous atrophy that develops during parenteral nutrition. The use of intravenous glutamine in humans appears to be safe and effective and it has been shown to diminish complications and reduce hospital stay.

In contrast to glutamine, short-chain fatty acids (SCFAs) are the primary energy source for colonocytes. Diets enriched in SCFAs have been shown to increase colonic DNA content and mucosal morphometrics as well as strengthen colonic anastomoses in rats. From diet, SCFAs are obtained from consumption of dietary fiber and fermentation in the colon by bacteria.

Other Factors to Support the Gut Mucosa. Specific growth factors that may promote intestinal mucosal growth have been implicated in a number of physiologic processes including growth, tissue repair, and regeneration. Among these is epidermal growth factor (EGF), a polypeptide secreted by submaxillary glands and by Brunner glands of the small intestine. The most widespread effect of EGF on the gastrointestinal mucosa is the overall stimulation of DNA synthesis as evidenced by thymidine incorporation.

TECHNIQUES OF ENTERAL NUTRITIONAL SUPPORT

Enteral feeding causes the gut to release trophic factors, which improves intestinal mucosal integrity and reduces bacterial transmigration even if caloric goals are not met. It has also been associated with a decrease in postoperative infection rates and a significant increase in collagen deposition at anastomotic sites, increasing wound strength.[60,61] Therefore, it should always be considered first over parenteral feeding in the surgically ill patient.

Transnasal (Nasogastric and Nasoduodenal) Feeding Catheters

The use of transnasal feeding catheters for intragastric feeding or for duodenal intubation is a popular adjunct for providing nutritional support by the enteral route. The stomach is easily accessed by the passage of a soft flexible feeding tube. Intragastric feedings provide several advantages for the patient. The stomach has the capacity and reservoir for bolus feedings. Feeding into the stomach results in the stimulation of the biliary and pancreatic axis, which is probably trophic for the small bowel, and gastric secretions have a dilutional effect on the osmolarity of the feedings, reducing the risk of diarrhea.

Diarrhea is reported as a significant complication of enteral feeding, but can be influenced by formula administration, mode of administration, antibiotics, and alteration of bowel organisms.[62] Additional complications include tube dislodgement, nasal ulcers, and electrolyte alterations. However, the major risk of intragastric feeding is the regurgitation of gastric contents resulting in aspiration into the tracheobronchial tree, which carries a mortality rate as high as 62%.[62] This risk is highest for patients who have an altered mental sensorium or who are paralyzed.

The placement of the feeding tube through the pylorus into the fourth portion of the duodenum reduces the risk of regurgitation and aspiration of feeding formulas. To place a transnasal intraduodenal feeding catheter, the patient should be in the sitting position with the neck slightly flexed. This allows for the passage of a lubricated 8 French polyurethane feeding catheter, with a stylette in place, through the patient's nose in a posterior and inferior direction, bringing the catheter to the level of the pharynx. The head is brought back to a neutral position and the patient is instructed to swallow while the feeding catheter is passed into the esophageal lumen. The advancement of the catheter is continued for a distance of 45 to 50 cm. The stylette is then removed. Intravenous injection of a promotility agent, such as metoclopramide, can also be used if difficulty is encountered passing the tube postpyloric. Additionally, tubes can be positioned fluoroscopically if necessary. The patient who frequently removes the feeding catheter may be a candidate for a feeding tube bridle, as shown in Figure 3.10.

Placement of nasogastric or nasoduodenal tubes should always be confirmed radiographically prior to initiation of feedings. There are electromagnetic devices on the market that can track the path of the feeding tube during the placement procedure and may reduce the need for confirmatory radiographs. However, these devices are not commonly used in the United States.[63]

A variety of enteral formulas are commercially available and can be adjusted for calorie, nitrogen, or fiber content.

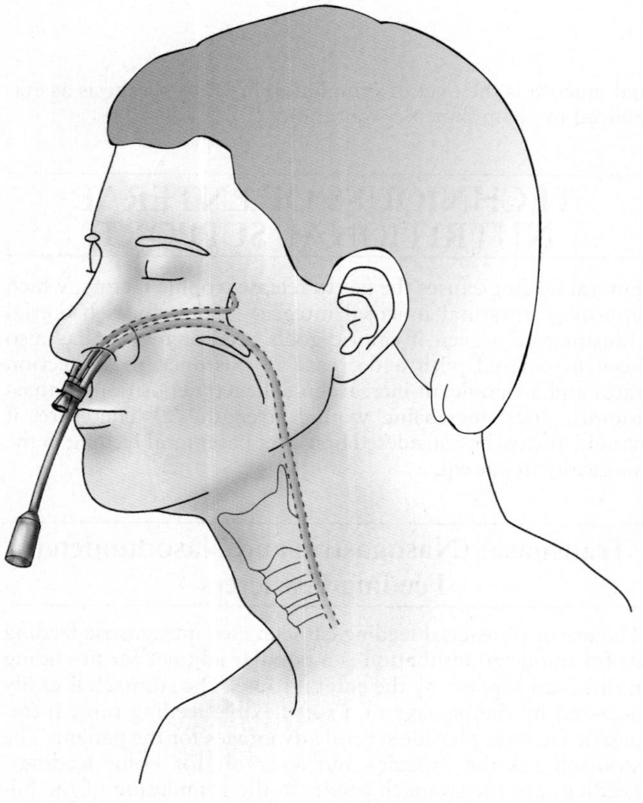

FIGURE 3.10. Use of a feeding tube bridle for patients who are prone to extubate the feeding catheter.

Technique for Gastrostomy Placement

A feeding gastrostomy should be considered for patients requiring long-term enteral nutrition and in patients with obstruction of the esophagus or locally advanced head and neck cancers that preclude eating. A temporary Stamm gastrostomy is a popular method for access to the gastric lumen and can be performed at the time of any major abdominal procedure. A square pursestring suture using 0 polypropylene with a 1-cm diameter is placed in the body of the anterior wall of the stomach. The ideal location is in the midportion of the stomach closer to the greater curvature in a relatively avascular area. A second hexagonal or octagonal pursestring suture, also 0 polypropylene, is placed outside the first one. The feeding catheter (often a Foley catheter) is then brought through a stab wound in the left upper quadrant of the abdominal wall. Using electrocautery, a puncture is made in the anterior portion of the stomach directly in the center of the concentric pursestring sutures. The feeding catheter is introduced into the gastric lumen and the inner concentric suture is secured in place. The second pursestring is then secured, inverting the gastric mucosa completely. The Foley catheter balloon is inflated and the stomach is drawn upward toward the anterior abdominal wall. Placement of Lembert silk sutures in all four quadrants around the Foley catheter secures the stomach to the anterior abdominal wall. The Foley is then secured to the skin by the placement of a bolstering disk at the base of the catheter exit site.

Technique of Percutaneous Endoscopic Gastrostomy

Percutaneous endoscopic gastrostomy (PEG) to provide access for gastric feedings can be performed without the need for a laparotomy or general anesthesia, and can be a useful modality for prolonged gastrointestinal decompression in patients with functional or mechanical obstruction.[64]

Using intravenous sedation and topical anesthetic, a gastroscope is passed through the mouth into the esophagus and stomach. The light from the gastroscope is then transilluminated through the anterior abdominal wall in the epigastrium or left subcostal area. The abdomen is prepped and draped and a wheal of local anesthetic is injected right at the area of transillumination. A 1-cm vertical incision is made and an Angiocath or needle is inserted through the abdominal wall into the stomach under the direct vision of the gastroscope. A wire loop is passed through the catheter into the stomach and grasped with a snare passed through the gastroscope. The scope and wire loop are withdrawn through the mouth and the wire is looped through a corresponding wire on the end of the PEG tube. By pulling the wire out through the abdominal wall, the PEG tube is pulled in through the mouth and out the anterior abdomen while followed through the esophagus by the scope. The scope then visualizes the inner part of the PEG tube to be sure it seats properly against the stomach wall. The tube protruding through the abdominal wall is then bolstered at the exit site to prevent accidental dislodgment. The PEG tube can later be removed with just a hard pull.

Disadvantages of PEG tube placement include PEG site metastasis in patients with head and neck cancers, although this is rare, with fewer than 30 cases reported in the literature.[64] A mini-laparoscopic technique has been developed for this reason and can also be used in patients where transillumination of the stomach is difficult or in patients who have had a subtotal gastrectomy with a small residual stomach.[65]

Feeding Catheter Jejunostomy Placement and Witzel Jejunostomy

A feeding catheter jejunostomy should be considered following any major upper abdominal procedure if prolonged enteral nutrition support is anticipated, in patients with gastroparesis, gastric outlet obstruction, or functional or structural defects, but with normal small bowel.[66]

The simplest method is a needle jejunostomy performed fairly quickly at the end of the definitive operation. A 14- or 16-gauge needle is used to create a tunnel subserosally approximately 30 to 40 cm distal to the ligament of Treitz and then the needle tip is introduced into the jejunal lumen. The feeding catheter is inserted through the needle and advanced 30 to 40 cm distally into the bowel lumen to the desired location, and the needle is withdrawn. The loop of jejunum is anchored to the parietal peritoneum with permanent sutures. The catheter is then secured to the skin with nylon sutures. A recent prospective study in major upper gastrointestinal surgery showed that feeding started earlier and progressed more easily with routine placement of a needle catheter jejunostomy.[59]

A feeding jejunostomy can also be performed by utilizing the Witzel technique. A loop of proximal jejunum 20 to 30 cm from the ligament of Treitz is delivered into the wound. A pursestring suture is placed on the antimesenteric border of the bowel and an incision is made with electrocautery in the intestinal wall in the center of the pursestring suture. A 14 French red rubber catheter is inserted into the lumen of the jejunum and advanced distally. The pursestring suture is then secured in place. A serosal tunnel is constructed with 000 silk sutures from the catheter's exit site extending 5 to 6 cm proximally. The catheter is then delivered through the abdominal wall through a separate stab incision. This loop of intestine is anchored to the peritoneum with two 000 silk sutures spread over 2 to 3 cm to prevent twisting of the loop and possible obstruction. The catheter is secured to the skin with a 3-0 nylon suture. Jejunal feeding catheters can be used immediately for feeding purposes following the operation.

Complications of feeding jejunostomies include small bowel perforations or volvulus, intraperitoneal leaks, cellulitis, occlusion, and dislodgement. Needle and Witzel jejunostomies are associated with a 2% and 10% complication rate, respectively.[67]

Jejunal tubes can also be placed endoscopically, usually via an extension tube through a gastrostomy. However, the extension tube can migrate proximally into the stomach and is prone to dysfunction. Direct insertion into the jejunum via endoscopy can provide a more stable access for feeding. The major advantage of this technique is tube patency, given that a 20 French tube can be inserted as opposed to the standard 9 French tube used with jejunal tube extensions.[66]

TECHNIQUES OF PARENTERAL NUTRITIONAL SUPPORT

Parenteral nutrition has several advantages over enteral nutrition. Delivery access is much simpler and reliable, nutrition does not have to be discontinued for further surgical procedures, and patients meet caloric goals consistently. However, intravenous feeding is not without serious complications and is associated with increased morbidity, including bacteremia, and prolonged ventilator dependency.[60] Even so, it still remains a valuable adjunct in caring for the critically ill patient.

Peripheral Intravenous Feedings

Peripheral intravenous nutrition delivered via a fine-bore midline catheter offers an alternative means of nutrition in patients who do not require central venous access, have adequate peripheral veins, and require only short-term nutritional support.[68,69] Indications for peripheral vein feeding include (a) as a supplement when enteral feedings can only be partially tolerated because of gastrointestinal dysfunction, (b) as a method of nutritional support when the gastrointestinal tract must be kept relatively empty for short periods during diagnostic workup, and (c) as preliminary feedings prior to subclavian catheter insertion in patients requiring TPN.

Peripheral intravenous feedings may be used for infusion of glucose, amino acid solutions, and fat emulsions. These solutions must be nearly isotonic to avoid peripheral vein sclerosis. Ten percent glucose solutions may be used to increase the efficacy of amino acid utilization. Fat emulsions can be administered simultaneously with glucose and amino acid solutions, because they provide an efficient fuel source and are isotonic. However, a disadvantage of peripherally administered solutions is limited caloric delivery to meet catabolic demands within tolerated fluid volumes.

The major complication of peripheral nutrition is peripheral vein thrombophlebitis (PVT), which necessitates routine daily catheter changes.[70] Several studies have shown that polyurethane cannulas develop fewer complications of thrombophlebitis and occlusion and can prolong feedings, compared to silicone cannulas.[68–70] Feed additives such as heparin and hydrocortisone can also extend the total period of feeding attainable and reduce the incidence of PVT.[9] In addition, long-chain triglycerides have been documented to prolong peripheral vein feeding by lessening the reaction of the venous endothelium to the nutritional infusate.[71]

Extravasation of infusion, occlusion of the catheter, and PVT are also influenced by the vein that is cannulated.[70] The cephalic vein is usually the vein of choice for standard intravenous insertion. However, the basilic vein is less narrow,[72] thus causing decreased inflammation between the catheter and the venous endothelium, making PVT less likely.[70]

A significant advantage of peripheral intravenous nutrition is avoiding central venous cannulation, which has considerable complications.

Central Venous Catheter Placement

The preferred method of access to the superior vena cava is by percutaneous cannulation of the subclavian vein. Alternate sites include the jugular approach, but with the catheter exiting in the neck region, this makes it more difficult to secure the dressing site and maintain sterility.

An individual who is experienced in the technique should perform the placement of a central venous catheter (CVC). The procedure is performed utilizing aseptic technique; the surgeon should wear a hat, mask, gown, and gloves. The procedure can take place in the operating room or in the patient's room if there is adequate lighting and assistance. An environment should be created to minimize patient anxiety, and informed consent must be obtained.

The following describes the standard Seldinger technique for insertion of a CVC via the subclavian vein; however, generally, the same approach is used when cannulating any central vein. The patient is placed in the Trendelenburg position with both arms at the sides and the head turned away from the site of insertion. The chest is shaved, prepped, and draped in a sterile fashion. Local anesthesia is infiltrated near the insertion site and the underlying tissues along the inferior border of the clavicle. The tip of the needle with the bevel pointed up is inserted into the skin and subcutaneous tissues at the midpoint of the clavicle aiming for the suprasternal notch. The needle is directed parallel to the patient's bed, insinuating beneath the clavicle and at all times with negative pressure applied to the syringe. The prompt inflow of blood into the syringe indicates entrance into the subclavian vein and the needle is advanced a few millimeters to ensure the entire bevel is within the lumen of the vessel. The needle is then rotated 90 degrees with the bevel pointed toward the foot of the bed to help direct advancement of the guide wire into the superior vena cava. The patient is instructed to perform a Valsalva maneuver to prevent an air embolism, the syringe is disconnected from the needle, and the guide wire is passed through the needle lumen. The needle is then withdrawn over the guide wire. The passage of the wire through the needle should be met with minimal resistance and the needle should be removed only after 15 cm of the wire has been passed into the vessel. A small incision is made at the guide wire exit site and a dilator is passed over the wire. The dilator is then removed over the wire and is replaced by the catheter, which is fully advanced. The wire is withdrawn and the catheter is flushed with sterile saline. The catheter is then sutured into position, the insertion site cleaned, and a sterile dressing placed. A portable chest radiograph (CXR) is done to confirm placement of the catheter tip, which should be located either in the proximal to middle superior vena cava or at the atriocaval junction, and to rule out pneumothorax.

Complications of central venous cannulation include pneumothorax, arterial puncture, neck or mediastinal hematoma (when using the jugular approach), and hemothorax.[73] To reduce the risk of bleeding complications in patients with a platelet count below 50,000, consideration should be given to transfuse fresh platelets prior to catheter insertion. There have been several studies, including the National Institute for Clinical Excellence guidelines formulated in September 2002, and revised in August 2005, that advocate the use of ultrasound (US) as the preferred method of CVC insertion, particularly through the jugular approach, and as a means to decrease the aforementioned complications from 10.5% to 4.6%.[73,74] US guidance in central venous cannulation also reduces time to insertion and may even decrease catheter-related sepsis.[75] If catheter sepsis is suspected, the CVC should be removed immediately and the tip cultured.

If a CVC is placed intraoperatively, the placement of the catheter is often not confirmed by CXR until several hours postoperatively. Incorrect CVC position, particularly in the right atrium, can be associated with adverse effects such as cardiac tamponade. Currently, studies are being conducted in the United States regarding electrocardiogram (ECG)-guided positioning for CVC placement. Using an ECG adapter connected to the central vein guide wire, an ECG monitor, and a right arm electrode, the CVC position in the right atrium would be confirmed by visualizing an elevated P wave on the monitor. The CVC could then be withdrawn until the P wave returned to normal configuration, indicating that the catheter was proximal to the atriocaval junction.[76] ECG-guided CVC positioning may decrease the frequency of CVC repositioning and repeated CXRs, and more importantly reduce cardiac complications.

An additional complication that is often overlooked is venous thrombosis. The clinical suspicion of subclavian vein thrombosis is only about 3%, whereas studies that use phlebography or radionuclide venography indicate that the incidence is as high as 35%.

Nutrition support of the surgical patient should strive to preserve body composition, provide needed nutrients, and minimize the inflammatory response to promote a decreased risk and better surgical outcome.

ACKNOWLEDGMENTS

We would like to thank Drs. Brian Cicuto and Melissa Boltz for their contributions to the Techniques section.

References

1. Kattelman KK, Hise M, Russell M, et al. Preliminary evidence for a medical nutrition therapy protocol: enteral feedings for critically ill patients. *J Amer Diet Assoc* 2006;106:1226–1241.
2. Kreyman KG, Berger MM, Deutz NEP, et al. ESPEN guidelines on enteral nutrition: intensive care. *Clin Nutr* 2006;25:210–223.
3. ASPEN Board of Directors and the Clinical Guidelines Taskforce. Guidelines for the use of parenteral and enteral nutrition in adult and pediatric patients. *JPEN J Parenter Enteral Nutr* 2002;26:(Suppl 1):1SA–138SA.
4. Heyland DK, Khaliwal R, Drover JW, et al. Canadian critical care clinical practice guidelines for nutrition support in mechanically ventilated, critically ill patients. *JPEN J Parenter Enteral Nutr* 2003;27:355–373.
5. Masala G, Bendinelli B, Versari D, et al. Anthropometric and dietary determinants of blood pressure in over 7000 Mediterranean women: the European Prospective Investigation into cancer and Nutrition–Florence cohort. *J Hypertens* 2008;26:2112–2120.
6. Cohn SH, Vaartsky D, Yasumura S, et al. Compartmental body composition based on total body nitrogen, potassium, and calcium. *Am J Physiol* 1980;239:E524–E530.
7. Frankenfield DC, Cooney RN, Smith JS, et al. Age-related differences in the metabolic response to injury. *J Trauma* 2000;48:49.
8. Frankenfield DC, Rowe WA, Cooney RN, et al. Limits of body mass index to detect obesity and predict body composition. *Nutrition* 2001;17:26.
9. Frankenfield DC, Cooney RN, Smith JS, et al. Bioelectrical impedance plethysmographic analysis of body composition in critically injured and healthy subjects. *Am J Clin Nutr* 1999;69:426.
10. Ravasco P, Camilo ME, Gouveia-Oliveira A, et al. A critical approach to nutritional assessment in critically ill patients. *Clin Nutr* 2002;21:73–77.
11. Baker JP, Detsky AS, Wesson DE, et al. Nutritional assessment. A comparison of clinical judgment and objective measures. *N Engl J Med* 1982;306: 969–972.
12. Lupo L, Pannarale O, Altomare D, et al. Reliability of clinical judgment in evaluation of the nutritional status of surgical patients. *Br J Surg* 1993;80: 1553–1556.
13. Povoa P. C-reactive protein: a valuable marker of sepsis. *Intensive Care Med* 2002;28:235–243.
14. Frankenfield DC, Smith JS, Cooney RN. Accelerated nitrogen loss after traumatic injury is not attenuated by achievement of energy balance. *JPEN J Parenter Enteral Nutr* 1997;21:324.
15. Scheinkestel CD, Kar L, Marshall K, et al. Prospective, randomized trial to assess caloric and protein needs of critically ill, anuric, ventilated patients requiring continuous renal replacement therapy. *Nutrition* 2003;19: 909–916.
16. Compher C, Frankenfield DC, Keim N, et al. Best practice methods to apply to measurement of resting metabolic rate in adults: a systematic review. *J Am Diet Assoc* 2006;106:881–903.
17. Frankenfield DC, Rowe WA, Smith JS, et al. Validation of several established equations for resting metabolic rate in obese and non obese people. *J Am Diet Assoc* 2003;103:1152.
18. Frankenfield D, Smith JS, Cooney RN. Validation of 2 approaches to predicting resting metabolic rate in critically ill patients. *JPEN J Parenter Enteral Nutr* 2004;28:259.
19. Frankenfield DC, Coleman A, Alam S, et al. Analysis of estimation methods for resting metabolic rate in critically ill adults. *JPEN J Parenter Enteral Nutr* 2009;33:27–36.
20. Frankenfield DC, Smith JS, Cooney RN, et al. Relative association of fever and injury with hypermetabolism in critically ill patients. *Injury* 1997;28: 617.
21. Pontes-Arruda A, Aragao AMA, Albuquerque JD. Effects of enteral feeding with eicosapentaenoic acid, gamma linolenic acid, and antioxidants in mechanically ventilated patients with severe sepsis and septic shock. *Crit Care Med* 2006;34:2323–2333.
22. Cuthbertson DP. *Q J Med* 1932;1:233.
23. Akner G, Cederholm T. Treatment of protein-energy malnutrition in chronic non-malignant disorders. *Am J Clin Nutr* 2001;74:6.
24. Kotler DP. Cachexia. *Ann Intern Med* 2000;133:622.
25. Kaysen G, Eisenrich JP. Characteristics and effects of inflammation in end-stage renal disease. *Semin Dial* 2003;16:438.
26. Espat NJ, Moldower LL, Copeland EM. Cytokine-mediated alterations in host metabolism prevent nutritional repletion in cachectic cancer patients. *J Surg Oncol* 1995;58:77.
27. Shulze PC, Gielen S, Adams V, et al. Muscular levels of proinflammatory cytokines correlate with a reduced expression of insulin like growth factor in chronic heart failure. *Basic Res Cardiol* 2003;98:367.
28. Debigaré R, Coté CH, Maltais F. Peripheral muscle wasting in chronic obstructive pulmonary disease. *Am J Respir Crit Care Med* 2001;164: 1712.
29. Chrousos GP. The hypothalamic-pituitary-adrenal axis and immune-mediated inflammation. *N Eng J Med* 1995;332:1351.
30. Steinborn W, Anker SD. Cardiac cachexia: pathophysiology and clinical implications. *Basic Appl Myol* 2003;13:191.
31. Anker SD, Coats AJS. Cardiac cachexia. A syndrome with impaired survival and immune and neuroendocrine activation. *Chest* 1999;115:836.
32. Fontana L, Weiss EP, Villareal DT, et al. Long-term effects of calorie or protein restriction on serum IGF-1 and IGFBP-3 concentration in humans. *Aging Cell* 2008;7:681–687.

33. Bessey PQ, Watters JM, Aoki TT, et al. Combined hormonal infusion simulates the metabolic response to injury. *Ann Surg* 1984;200:264.
34. Souba WW. Cytokines: key regulators of the nutritional/metabolic response to critical illness. *Curr Probl Surg* 1994;31:577.
35. Sena MJ, Utter GH, Cushieri J, et al. Early supplemental parenteral nutrition is associated with increased infectious complications in critically ill trauma patients. *J Am Coll Surg* 2008;207:459–467.
36. Dissanaike S, Pham T, Shalhub S, et al. Effect of immediate enteral feeding on trauma patients with an open abdomen: protection from nosocomial infection. *J Am Coll Surg* 2008;207:690–697.
37. Petrov MS, van Santvoort HC, Besselink MGH, et al. Enteral nutrition and the risk of mortality and infectious complications in patients with severe acute pancreatitis. *Arch Surg* 2008;143:1111–1117.
38. Bagga D, Wang L, Farius-Eisner R. Differential effects of prostaglandin derived from n-6 and n-3 polyunsaturated fatty acids on COX-2 and IL-6 secretion. *Proc Natl Acad Sci U S A* 2003;100:1751.
39. Scholz H. Prostaglandins. *Am J Physiol Regul Integr Comp Physiol* 2003; 285:R512.
40. Wigmore Sj, Fearon KC, Maingay JP, et al. Down-regulation of the acute-phase response in patients with pancreatic cancer cachexia receiving oral eicosapentaenoic acid is mediated via suppression of interleukin-6. *Clin Sci* 1997;92:215.
41. Barber MD, McMillan DC, Preston T, et al. The metabolic response to feeding in weight-losing pancreatic cancer patients and its modulation by a fish oil-enriched nutritional supplement. *Clin Sci* 2000;98:389.
42. Barber MD, Ross JA, Fearon KC, et al. Fish oil-enriched nutritional supplement attenuates progression of the acute phase response in weight-losing patients with advanced pancreatic cancer. *J Nutr* 1999;129:1120.
43. Barber MD, Ross JA, Fearon KC, et al. The effect of an oral nutritional supplement enriched with fish oil on weight loss in patients with pancreatic cancer. *Br J Cancer* 1999;81:80.
44. Gogos CA, Ginopoulis P, Salsa B, et al. Dietary omega-3 polyunsaturated fatty acids plus vitamin E restore immunodeficiency and prolong survival for severely ill patients with generalized malignancy. *Cancer* 1998;82:395.
45. May PE, Barber A, D'Olipio D, et al. Reversal of cancer-related wasting using oral supplementation with a combination of beta-hydroxy-beta-methylbutyrate, arginine, and glutamine. *Am J Surg* 2002;183: 471.
46. Clark RH, Feleke G, Din M, et al. Nutritional treatment for acquired immunodeficiency virus-associated wasting using beta-hydroxy-beta-methylbutyrate, glutamine, and arginine: a randomized, double-blind, placebo-controlled study. *JPEN J Parenter Enteral Nutr* 2000;24:133.
47. Jiang ZM, He GZ, Zhang SY, et al. Low-dose growth hormone and hypocaloric nutrition attenuates the protein-catabolic response after major operation. *Ann Surg* 1989;210:514.
48. Fong Y, Marano MA, Barber A, et al. Total parenteral nutrition and bowel rest modify the metabolic response to endotoxin in humans. *Ann Surg* 1989;210:449.
49. Ziegler TR, Young LS, Benfell K, et al. Clinical and metabolic efficacy of glutamine-enriched parenteral nutrition following bone marrow transplantation: a double-blind randomized controlled trial. *Ann Intern Med* 1992;116:821.
50. Byrne TA, Persinger RL, Young LS, et al. A new treatment for patients with the short bowel syndrome: growth hormone, glutamine, and a modified diet. *Ann Surg* 1995;222:243.
51. Alexander JW, MacMillan BG, Stinnert JD, et al. Beneficial effects of aggressive protein feeding in severely burned children. *Ann Surg* 1980;192: 505.
52. Abel RM, Beck CH, Abbott WM, et al. Improved survival from acute renal failure following treatment with intravenous essential L-amino acids and glucose: results of a prospective, double-blind study. *N Engl J Med* 1973; 288:695.
53. Buzby GP and The Veterans Affairs Total Parenteral Nutrition Cooperative Study Group. Perioperative total parenteral nutrition in surgical patients. *N Engl J Med* 1991;325:525.
54. Ishizuka M, Nagata H, Takagi K, et al. Total parenteral nutrition is a major risk factor for central venous catheter-related bloodstream infections in colorectal cancer patients receiving postoperative chemotherapy. *Eur Surg Res* 2008;41:341–345.
55. Batistella FD, Widergren JT, Anderson JT, et al. A prospective randomized trial of intravenous fat emulsion administration in trauma victims requiring total parenteral nutrition. *J Trauma* 1997;43:52.
56. van der Hulst RRWJ, van Kreel BK, von Meyenfeldt MF, et al. Glutamine and the preservation of gut integrity. *Lancet* 1993;341:1363.
57. Fukuda T, Seto Y, Yamada K, et al. Can immune-enhancing nutrients reduce postoperative complications in patients undergoing esophageal surgery? *Dis Esophagus* 2008;21:708–711.
58. Scheltinga MR, Young LS, Benfell K, et al. Glutamine-enriched intravenous feedings attenuate extracellular fluid expansion after standard stress. *Ann Surg* 1991;214:385.
59. Chin KF, Townsend S, Wong W, et al. A prospective cohort study of feeding needle catheter jejunostomy in an upper gastrointestinal surgical unit. *Clin Nutr* 2004;23:691.
60. Ochoa JB, Caba D. Advances in surgical nutrition. *Surg Clin North Am* 2006;86:1483–1493.
61. Kiyama T, Onda M, Tokunaga A, et al. Effect of early postoperative feeding on the healing of colonic anastomoses in the presence of intra-abdominal sepsis in rats. *Dis Colon Rectum* 2000;43:S54–S58.
62. Pancorbo-Hildalgo P, Garci-Fernandez C, Ramirez-Perez C, et al. Complications associated with enteral nutritional by nasogastric tube in an internal medicine unit. *J Clin Nurs* 2001;10:482–490.
63. Rao MM, Flindall I, Gatt M, et al. Use of Cortrak—an electromagnetic sensing device in placement of enteral feeding tubes. *Proc Nutr Soc* 2008;67: E109.
64. Sabnis A, Liu R, Chand B, et al. SLiC technique—a novel approach to percutaneous gastrostomy. *Surg Endosc* 2006;20:256–262.
65. Denzer U, Margener K, Kanzler S, et al. Mini-laparoscopically guided percutaneous gastrostomy and jejunostomy. *Gastrointest Endosc* 2003;58: 434–438.
66. Fan A, Baron T, Rumella A, et al. Comparison of direct percutaneous endoscopic jejunostomy and PEG with jejunal extension. *Am Soc Gastrointest Endosc* 2002;56:6.
67. Holmes J, Brundage S, Yuen P, et al. Complications of surgical feeding jejunostomy in trauma patients. *J Trauma* 1999;47:1009–1012.
68. Catton JA, Davies J, Dobbins BM, et al. The effect of heparin in peripheral intravenous nutrition via a fine-bore midline: a randomized double-blind controlled trial. *Clin Nutr* 2006;25:394–399.
69. Pluse SM, Horsman R, Kendall-Smith S. Fine-bore cannulas for peripheral intravenous nutrition: polyurethane or silicone? *Ann R Coll Surg Engl* 1998;80:154–156.
70. Everitt NJ, McMahon MJ. Influence of fine-bore catheter length on infusion thrombophlebitis in peripheral intravenous nutrition: a randomized controlled trial. *Ann R Coll Surg Engl* 1997;79:221–224.
71. Williams PL, Warwick R, Dyson M, et al. *Gray's Anatomy*, 37th ed. Edinburgh: Churchill Livingstone; 1989.
72. Smirniotis VK, Antoniou S, Kotsist E, et al. Incidence of vein thrombosis in peripheral intravenous nutrition: effect of fat emulsions. *Clin Nutr* 1999;18: 79–81.
73. Wigmore TJ, Smythe JF, Hacking RR, et al. Effect of the implementation of NICE guidelines for ultrasound guidance on the complication rates associated with central venous catheter placement in patients presenting for routine surgery in a tertiary referral centre. *Br J Anaesth* 2007;99:662–665.
74. Randolph AG, Cook DJ, Gonzales CA, et al. Ultrasound guidance for placement of central venous catheters. A meta-analysis of the literature. *Crit Care Med* 1996;24:2053–2058.
75. Slama M, Novara A, Safavian A, et al. Improvement of internal jugular vein cannulation using an ultrasound-guided technique. *Intensive Care Med* 1997;23:916–919.
76. Gebhard RE, Szmuk P, Pivalizza E, et al. The accuracy of electrocardiogram-controlled central line placement. *Anesth Analg* 2007;104:65–70.

CHAPTER 4 ■ WOUND HEALING

ROBERT D. GALIANO AND THOMAS A. MUSTOE

KEY POINTS

1. The inflammatory phase of acute wound healing begins immediately after injury. The initial response to the disruption of blood vessels is bleeding.
2. The proliferative phase of acute wound healing begins with the formation of a provisional matrix of fibrin and fibronectin as part of initial clot formation.
3. The transition from the proliferative phase to the remodeling phase of acute wound healing is defined by reaching collagen equilibrium.
4. Reconstruction of the epithelial barrier (epithelialization) begins within hours of the initial injury.
5. Visible scarring occurs only when the injury extends deeper than the superficial dermis.
6. A practical definition of a chronic wound is one that has failed to heal within 3 months. Although there are a variety of underlying causes, most chronic wounds can be categorized as pressure sores, diabetic foot ulcers, or leg ulcers.
7. Most chronic wounds occur in older patients, are associated with underlying ischemia or tissue hypoxia, and are contaminated by bacteria in the setting of a biofilm.
8. It takes at least 3 weeks for collagen to undergo sufficient remodeling and cross-linking to attain moderate strength.
9. The primary difference between a keloid and a hypertrophic scar is that a keloid extends beyond the boundary of the original tissue injury.
10. Stem cells hold great promise for achieving true tissue regeneration, as opposed to scar formation, following an injury.

Wound healing is a fundamental homeostatic event in response to injury. The process of wound healing brings into play an exquisitely controlled cascade of molecular and cellular responses that are evolutionarily conserved across multicellular organisms, as well as regulation of these processes once repair is complete. Our understanding of the intricate cross-talk present between cells in the wound and other cells throughout the body has led to an appreciation that the process of tissue repair involves a coordinated interplay between metabolic, nervous, inflammatory, immune, and vascular systems, all played out within the microcosm of the wound. Similarly, the realization that blood-borne progenitor cells participate to varying degrees in the healing wound has elevated our once-parochial view that wound healing is strictly a local phenomenon to the conceptialization of wound healing as a systemic process. Increased understanding of the cellular and molecular events involving growth factors and cytokines and the realistic prospects for pharmacologic manipulation have focused a great deal of research interest from a broad range of disciplines. The field of wound healing has expanded in complexity as well as scope: basic scientists as well as clinicians and allied health professionals all have contributed to advances in this fascinating field. Despite our greater understanding of the complexities involved, however, there remain a set of core principles that serve to direct and guide patient care. This chapter outlines a basic set of concepts regarding wound healing, with emphasis on the clinical principles of basic surgical techniques; the care of surgical incisions; and the management of both acute and chronic open wounds.

NORMAL WOUND HEALING

Wound healing is the body's response to injury. Injury can be acute or chronic and involve multiple tissues, but wound healing is most clearly illustrated by examining the response to full-thickness injury (e.g., a cut or an incision) to the epidermis and dermis. This injury sets in motion a sequence of interrelated reparative forces. Although the events overlap in time, it is helpful to consider the process as stages or phases of wound healing; these are presented as separate events. This provides for clear conceptualization of the individual events and conforms to standard conventions. These events, however, do not occur independently, and the degree of temporal overlap is significant (Fig. 4.1).[1]

Every tissue in the body undergoes reparative processes after injury. Bone has the unique ability to heal without scar. Liver has the potential to regenerate parenchyma and is the only organ that has maintained that ability in the adult human. With these exceptions, all other human tissues heal with scar. This chapter reviews the healing process of human skin with particular emphasis on surgical applications. Delineation of the individual mediators that participate in this process is still evolving, so the emphasis is on the underlying physiologic processes and the patterns of response.

Inflammatory Phase

1 The inflammatory phase of acute wound healing begins immediately after injury. The initial response to the disruption of blood vessels is bleeding. The homeostatic response to this is clot formation to stop hemorrhage. Platelet plug formation initiates the hemostatic process along with recruitment of clotting factors activated by collagen and basement membrane proteins exposed by the injury. Fibrin, converted from fibrinogen by the clotting cascade, binds the platelet plug and forms the provisional matrix for the cellular responses that follow. After injury, transient vasoconstriction is mediated by catecholamines, thromboxane, and prostaglandin F_{2a} (PGF_{2a}). Platelet degranulation, the emptying of the granules into the extracellular space, provides the contents of α granules and dense granules, most notably platelet-derived growth factor (PDGF) and transforming growth factor-β (TGF-β). These substances initiate chemotaxis and proliferation of inflammatory cells, beginning the inflammatory response that will ultimately heal the wound (Table 4.1). Transient vasoconstriction is necessary to decrease blood loss at the time of the initial

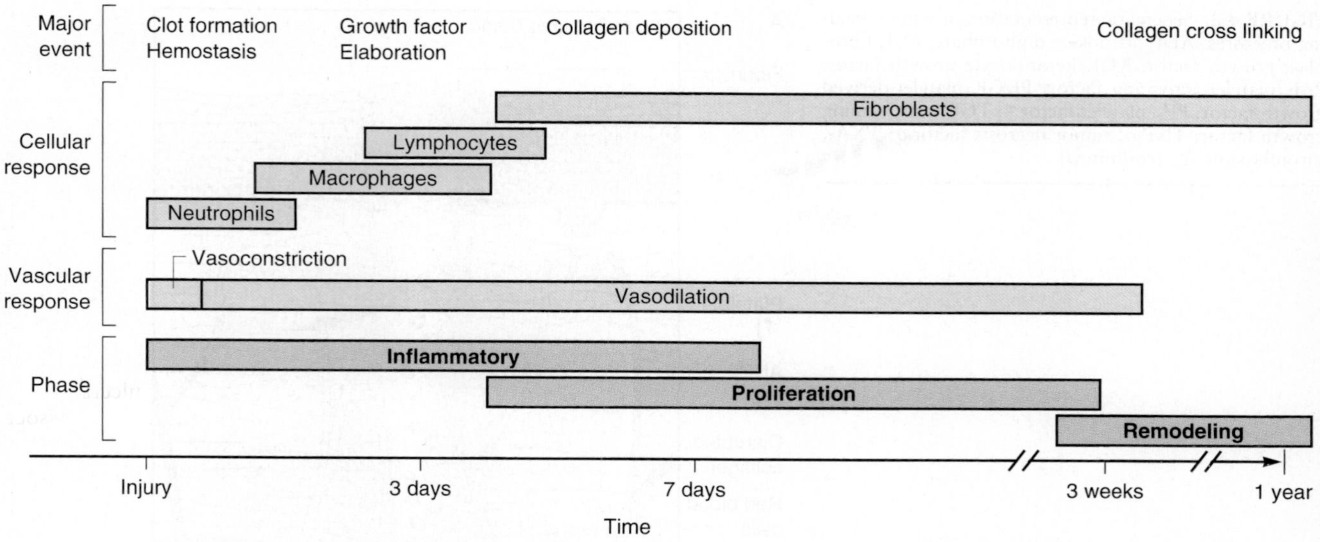

FIGURE 4.1. Timeline of phases of wound healing with dominant cell types and major physiologic events.

wounding and also to allow clot formation. Vasoconstriction lasts for 5 to 10 minutes. Once a clot has been formed and active bleeding has stopped, vasodilatation increases local blood flow to the wounded area, supplying cells and substrate necessary for further wound repair. The vascular endothelial cells also deform, increasing vascular permeability. The vasodilatation and increased endothelial permeability are mediated by histamine, PGE_2, and PGI_2 (prostacyclin), as well as vascular endothelial cell growth factor (VEGF). These vasodilatory substances are released by injured endothelial cells and mast cells and enhance the egress of cells and substrate into the wounded tissue (Fig. 4.2).

At this stage, the wound is full of debris from the initial injury. This material consists of a mixture of injured, devitalized tissue (fat, muscle, epithelium), clot (platelets, erythrocytes, fibrin), bacteria (from the skin surface and external environment), extravasated serum proteins (glycoproteins and mucopolysaccharides), and foreign material introduced at the time of injury (suture, dirt). During the next several days, the wound is cleared of bacteria, devitalized tissue, and foreign material by recruited and activated phagocytic cells. Polymorphonuclear leukocytes (PMNs) begin to arrive immediately, attaining large numbers within 24 hours. The process of clearing the wound of debris usually takes several days, but the time varies depending on the amount of material to be cleared. The PMNs are followed temporally by macrophages, which appear in wounds in significant numbers within 2 or 3 days. The macrophages are mononuclear phagocytic cells derived from circulating monocytes or resident tissue macrophages. They complete the process of removing all material not necessary for the ensuing steps of wound healing.

In the absence of significant bacterial contamination, macrophages promptly replace PMNs as the dominant cell type during the inflammatory phase. The role of the macrophages is not limited to phagocytosis.[2] In addition, macrophages are the sources of more than 30 different growth factors and cytokines. These growth factors induce fibroblast proliferation, endothelial cell proliferation (angiogenesis), and extracellular matrix production, and they recruit and activate additional macrophages. The result is the induction of a wound healing amplification cycle as growth factors recruit macrophages and elicit additional growth factor release. Specific antibodies that destroy PMNs or block certain aspects of amplification function (such as adhesion) have shown that experimental wounds heal normally in the absence of PMNs, but that healing is significantly impaired without functional macrophages (even in the absence of bacteria). These studies confirm the dominant role of the macrophage in the inflammatory phase of wound healing. The amplification process is so powerful that only scattered fibroblasts and endothelial cells are seen in a surgical incision or at the edge of an open wound at day 3, but by day 5 the wound is very cellular with active proliferation. By day 7, the incisional wound is strong enough to allow suture removal, and proliferating fibroblasts and angiogenesis give the wound an appearance similar in many respects to the stroma surrounding tumors.

Lymphocytes also appear in wounds in small numbers during the inflammatory phase. The role of lymphocytes in the wound healing process remains to be clarified but is thought to be related more to chronic inflammatory processes than to the initial response to wounding. Recently, it has become more appreciated that within this heterogeneous population of cells are several distinct subpopulations of blood-borne progenitor cells that likely contribute in varying degrees to tissue repair.

TABLE 4.1

PLATELET GRANULES AND MEDIATORS OF PLATELET AGGREGATION

PLATELET GRANULES
α Granules: Contain Platelet-specific Proteins
Platelet factor 4
β-Thromboglobulin
Platelet-derived growth factor
Transforming growth factor-β
Dense Granules
Adenosine diphosphate
Serotonin
Calcium
MEDIATORS OF PLATELET AGGREGATION
Thromboxane A_2
Thrombin
Platelet factor 4

FIGURE 4.2. Schematic representation of wound healing processes. ADP, adenosine diphosphate; FGF, fibroblast growth factor; KGF, keratinocyte growth factor; PAF, platelet-activating factor; PDGF, platelet-derived growth factor; PF_4, platelet factor 4; TGF, transforming growth factor; TNF-α, tumor necrosis factor-α; TXA_2, thromboxane A_2. (*continued*)

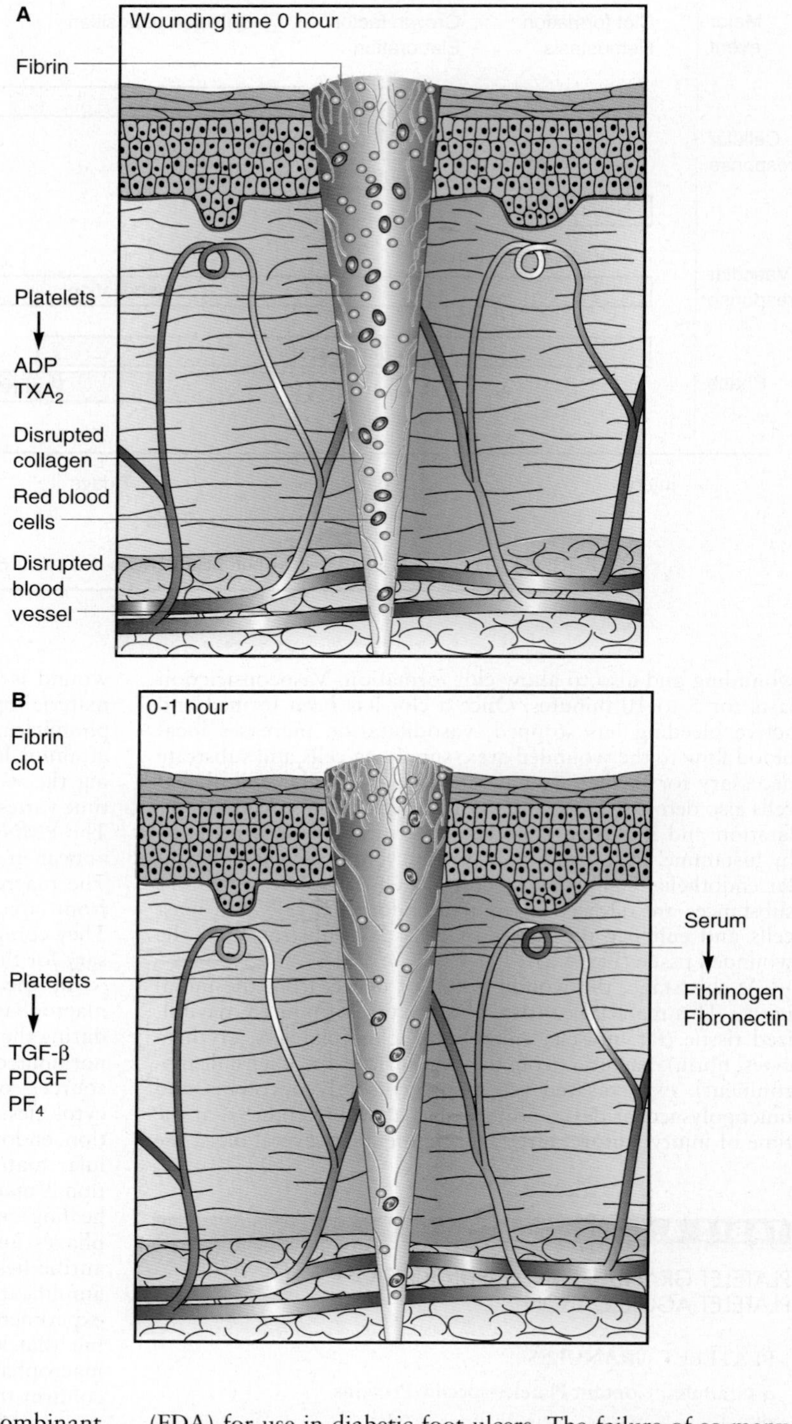

These will be discussed further later. Because recombinant growth factors are available in sufficient quantities for clinical use, the prospect of using growth factors as pharmacologic agents to stimulate wound healing (and potentially modulate abnormal scarring) has been the focus of much research. Dozens of growth factor studies have been performed in humans, based on animal studies that have demonstrated wound healing activity by about a dozen different growth factors (PDGF, TGF-β1, TGF-β2, TGF-β3, fibroblast growth factor 2 [FGF2], FGF7, keratinocyte growth factor [KGF], granulocyte-macrophage colony-stimulating factor [GMCSF], insulinlike growth factor 1 [IGF-1], IGF-1–binding protein [IGFBP1], and epidermal growth factor [EGF] represent a partial list). To date, only PDGF has been approved.[3] After a 7-year process involving 1,000 patients, PDGF (Regranex) was approved in 1997 by the U.S. Food and Drug Administration (FDA) for use in diabetic foot ulcers. The failure of so many clinical trials to demonstrate efficacy is a reflection of both the complexity and variability of human wounds, which make it difficult to demonstrate efficacy in all but the largest of studies and to demonstrate the multiple etiologic factors that result in chronic wounds.

Another product, an artificial skin equivalent made of a dermislike matrix covered with cultured epithelium from heterologous human foreskins (Apligraf), was approved by the FDA in 1998 for use in venous ulcers of more than 1 year's duration that had failed other therapies. This product's main effect is most likely due to the delivery of growth factors produced by the neonatal cells. Increased knowledge of the role of growth factors in wound healing has also provoked the evaluation of strategies using other pharmacologic agents to indirectly modulate growth factor levels in wounds.

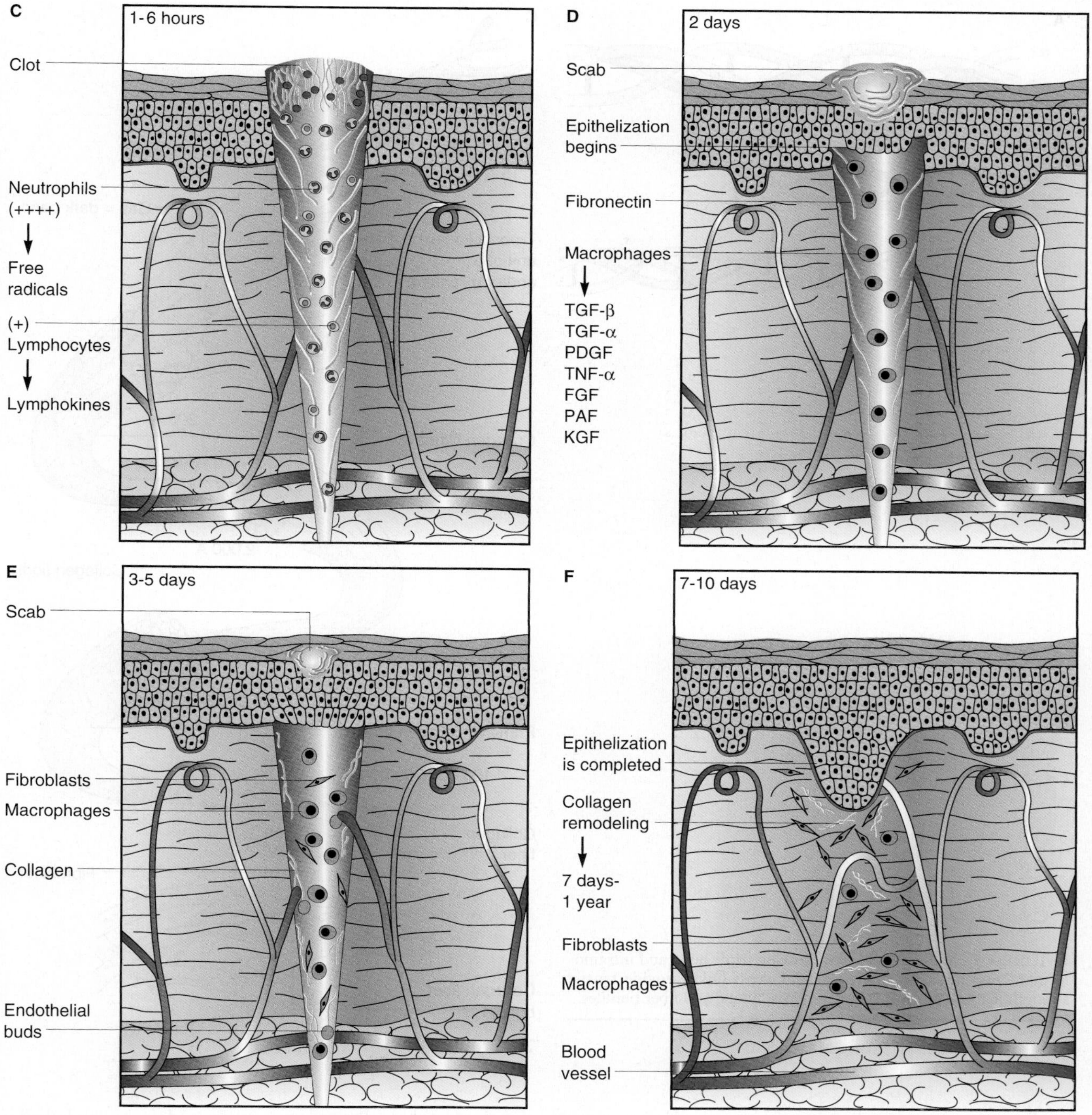

FIGURE 4.2. (*Continued*)

Proliferative Phase

2 The proliferative phase begins with the formation of a provisional matrix of fibrin and fibronectin as part of initial clot formation. Initially, the provisional matrix is populated by macrophages; however, by day 3, fibroblasts appear in the fibronectin–fibrin framework and initiate collagen synthesis. Fibroblasts proliferate in response to growth factors to become the dominant cell type during this phase. Growth factors produced by macrophages simultaneously induce angiogenesis, which induces the ingrowth and proliferation of endothelial cells, forming new capillaries. The process of neovascularization is driven in large part by the local tissue hypoxia present in the wound center, which in turn is orchestrated by the hypoxia-inducible factor-1 (HIF-1). This master transcription factor functions as the switch that turns on angiogenic processes, metabolic adaptations to hypoxia, an increase in iron transport, and erythropoiesis, functioning across local, regional, and systemic levels to restore blood flow to an injured area. Initially, the angiogenic cascade unleashed by HIF-1 results in a hypervascular network, which will be pruned later. This neovascularity is visible through the epithelium and gives the wound a pink or purple-red appearance. Capillary ingrowth provides the fibroblasts with oxygen and nutrients to sustain cell proliferation and support the production of the permanent wound matrix. This matrix is composed

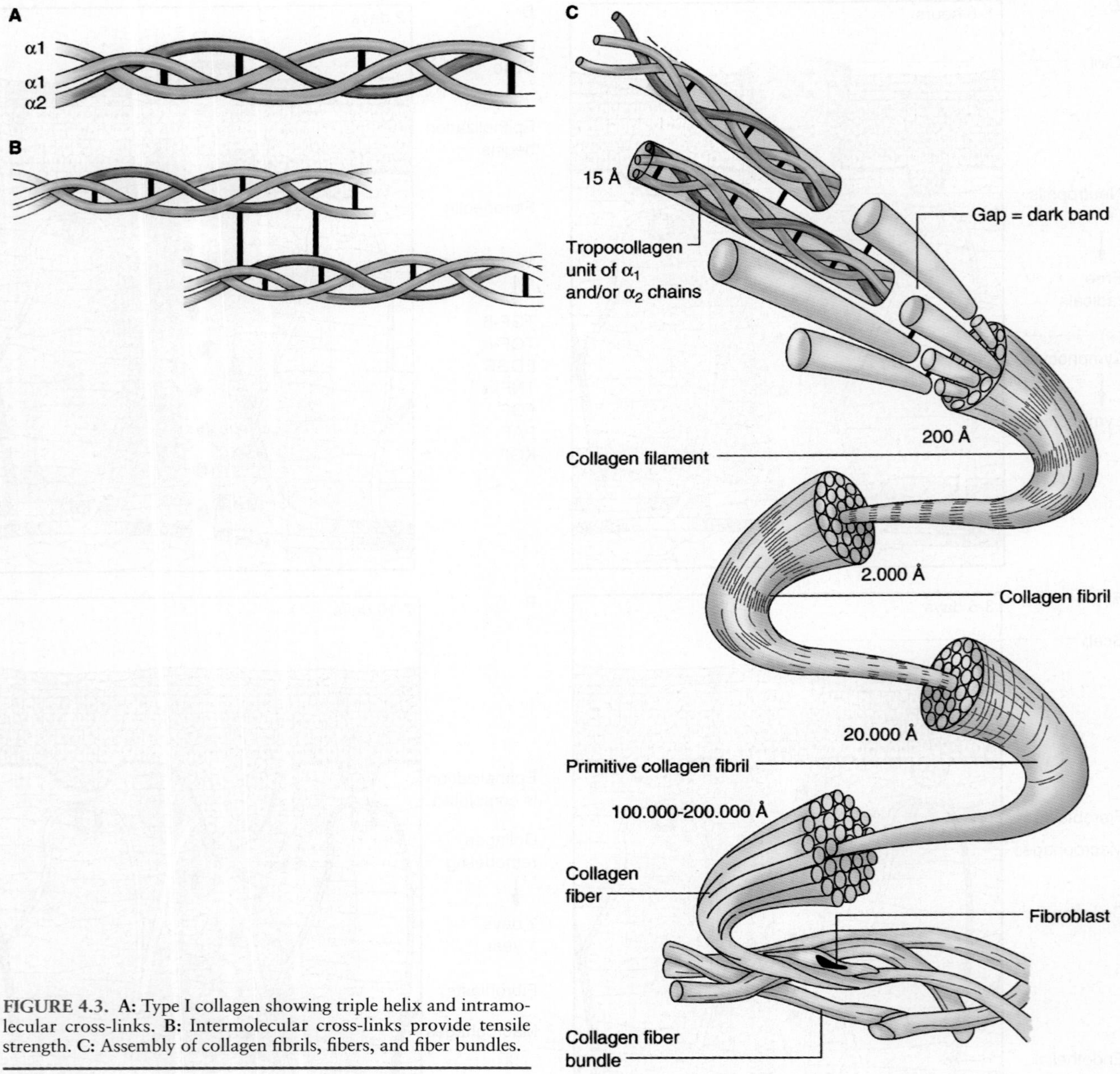

FIGURE 4.3. **A:** Type I collagen showing triple helix and intramolecular cross-links. **B:** Intermolecular cross-links provide tensile strength. **C:** Assembly of collagen fibrils, fibers, and fiber bundles.

of collagen and proteoglycans or ground substance and replaces the provisional fibronectin–fibrin matrix.

Collagen is the dominant structural molecule in the wound matrix and in the final scar. This is not surprising because collagen is the principal structural protein in skin, bone, and, indeed, all human tissues. Collagen is synthesized into an organized cablelike network in a multistep process with both intracellular and extracellular components (Fig. 4.3). The collagen molecule has abundant quantities of two unique amino acids, hydroxyproline and hydroxylysine. The hydroxylation process that forms these amino acids requires ascorbic acid (vitamin C) and is necessary for the subsequent stabilization and cross-linkage of collagen. Procollagen is formed within the fibroblasts as a long linear amino acid segment with regular repeats of hydroxyproline every third amino acid and with terminal extension peptides. Procollagen molecules aggregate in the case of type I collagen (the most common) as three α chains to form a triple-helical complex (Fig. 4.3A). The triple helix is maintained by intramolecular disulfide bonds between specific cystine residues. Procollagen is secreted in its triple-helical form; extracellular peptidases cleave the extension peptides at the amino and carboxy termini, leaving the central collagen molecule. Collagen cross-linking (Fig. 4.3B) then occurs in the extracellular space as the collagen molecules aggregate into larger structures. Lysyl oxidase catalyzes the conversion of lysine and hydroxylysine into aldehyde forms. These aldehydes form intermolecular bonds by undergoing spontaneous condensation. This produces stable, cross-linked collagen fibrils. These intramolecular and intermolecular bonds provide strength and stability. As the wound matures, fibrils cross-link to form large cables of collagen, providing increased tensile strength (Fig. 4.3C). The wound is then more appropriately considered a scar.

Although there are many types of collagen, type I predominates throughout the body. The principal collagen in scar is type I, with lesser amounts of type III collagen present. Other collagen types make important contributions to the basement membrane, cartilage, and other structures (Table 4.2).

TABLE 4.2

COLLAGEN TYPES

TYPE	PROPERTY OF AGGREGATE UNIT	TISSUE DISTRIBUTION
I	Rigid fibrils	All connective tissue except cartilage
II	Rigid fibrils	Cartilage and vitreous
III	Elastic fibrils	Elastic tissue (e.g., fetal skin, blood vessels, uterus)
IV	Sheet	Basement membrane
V	Fibril	Widespread
VI	Beaded filaments	Widespread
VII	Anchoring fibrils	Interface of basement membrane and underlying stroma
VIII	Sheet	Descemet membrane
IX	Fibril	Hyaline cartilage
X	Sheet	Hypertrophic cartilage
XI	Fibril	Hyaline cartilage
XII	Fibril	Similar to type I

Remodeling Phase: The Formation of Scars

3 The transition from the proliferative phase to the remodeling phase is defined by the achievement of collagen equilibrium. Collagen accumulation within the wound reaches a maximum within 2 to 3 weeks after wounding. Although supranormal rates of synthesis and degradation continue throughout remodeling, there is no further change in total collagen content.[4] Tensile strength gradually increases as random collagen fibrils are replaced by organized fibrils with more intermolecular bonds. During the initial phase of wound healing, there is a relative abundance of type III collagen in the wound. With remodeling, the normal adult ratio of 4:1 (type I to type III) collagen is restored. Under normal wound healing conditions, the capillary density gradually diminishes, and the number of fibroblasts is reduced. The wound loses its pink or purple vascular color and becomes progressively pale. The collagen undergoes constant remodeling. New collagen is formed, and collagen degradation by specific collagenases is ongoing. Collagenase activity is balanced against new production of collagen to produce a steady state. As equilibrium is achieved, the collagen fibrils align themselves in a longitudinal arrangement as dictated by stress placed on the wound. Scars never achieve the degree of order achieved by collagen in normal skin or tendons, but they do increase in strength for 6 months or longer, eventually reaching 70% of the strength of unwounded skin (Fig. 4.4).

The other important component of the extracellular matrix is the ground substance or proteoglycans. These substances are composed of a protein backbone with long hydrophilic carbohydrate side chains. The hydrophilic nature of these molecules accounts for much of the water content of scars. In the early immature wound, there is a disproportionately large amount of proteoglycans (particularly hyaluronic acid). During the maturation phase, the proteoglycan content returns to a level that closely approximates that of normal skin.

Until recently, the extracellular matrix (predominantly collagen and proteoglycans) was thought to be inert. It is becoming increasingly clear, however, that extracellular matrix signals certain cells through cell attachment receptors (integrins) and serves as a reservoir for growth factors. Via integrin receptors, the extracellular matrix influences intracellular signal transduction with an impact on cell motility and migration,

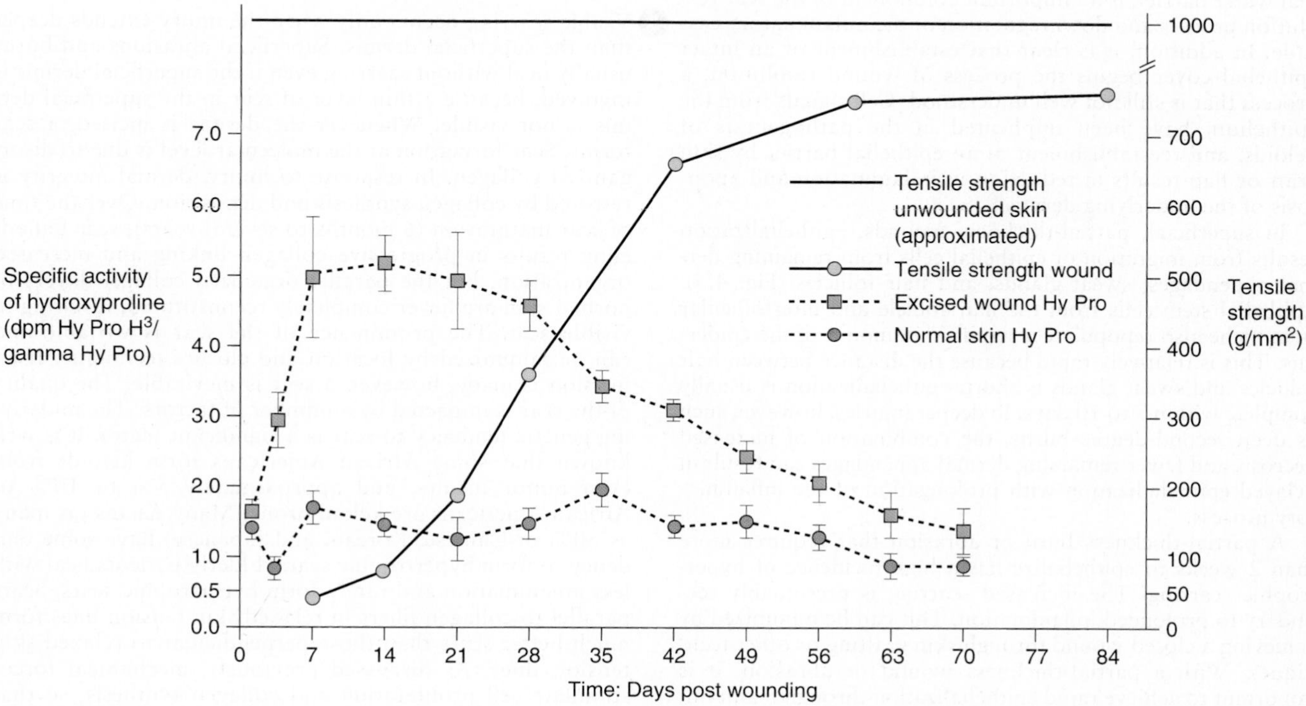

FIGURE 4.4. Relation of the rate of collagen synthesis to the gain of tensile strength of rat skin wounds. (Adapted from Madden JW, Peacock EE Jr. Studies on the biology of collagen during wound healing. 1. Rate of collagen synthesis and deposition in cutaneous wounds of the rat. *Surgery* 1968;64:288.)

cellular proliferation, and growth factor production. The role of proteoglycans as signaling molecules is just beginning to be understood. In addition, mechanical forces on tissue are transmitted from the matrix to the cells that are attached to the matrix, and increasing evidence indicates that mechanical forces result in signal transduction, which can result in cellular proliferation, apoptosis, and other signal transduction processes.[5]

Epithelialization

The skin is composed of two layers, the epidermis and the dermis. The outermost layer, the epidermis, is the protective barrier that forms the external interface between the body and the environment. The epidermis protects against water loss, allowing the other cells of the body to live in a liquid environment, as well as forming a barrier to bacteria and 4 other environmental factors. Reconstruction of the epithelial barrier (epithelialization) begins within hours of the initial injury. As an initial step, epithelial cells from the basal layer at the wound edge flatten and migrate across the wound, completing wound coverage within 18 to 24 hours in a coapted surgical wound. The cells along the margin are also dividing to re-form the characteristic basilar to apical differentiation of multilayered mature epithelium (see later). Epithelial cells exhibit contact inhibition; that is, they continue to migrate across an appropriate bed until a single continuous layer is formed. Epithelial cell migration occurs by a process in which the epithelial cells send out pseudopods, attaching to the underlying extracellular matrix by integrin receptors. Bacteria, large amounts of protein exudate from leaky capillaries, and necrotic tissue all compromise this process, delaying epithelialization. Delayed epithelialization results in a more profound and prolonged inflammatory process, thereby contributing to unsatisfactory or hypertrophic scarring. There is increasing evidence that reestablishment of a mature epithelium with a multilayered keratin layer (stratum corneum), which completely restores the normal water barrier, is an important component of the scar resolution process and downregulation of the inflammatory cascade. In addition, it is clear that establishment of an intact epithelial cover begins the process of wound resolution, a process that is still not well understood. Cell signals from the epithelium have been implicated in the pathogenesis of keloids, and reestablishment of an epithelial barrier by skin graft or flap results in reduction in inflammation and apoptosis of the underlying dermis.[6]

In superficial, partial-thickness wounds, epithelialization results from migration of epithelial cells from remaining dermal appendages, sweat glands, and hair follicles (Fig. 4.5). Epithelial stem cells from the hair follicle and interfollicular stem niche also repopulate a significant amount of the epidermis. This is relatively rapid because the distance between hair follicles and sweat glands is short; epithelialization is usually complete within 7 to 10 days. In deeper injuries, however, such as deep second-degree burns, the combination of increased necrosis and fewer remaining dermal appendages can result in delayed epithelialization with prolongation of the inflammatory process.

A partial-thickness burn or abrasion that requires more than 2 weeks to epithelialize has a high incidence of hypertrophic scarring. The increased scarring is presumably secondary to prolonged inflammation. This can be minimized by achieving a closed wound through skin grafting or other techniques. With a partial-thickness wound or abrasion, it is important to achieve rapid epithelialization through maintaining a moist environment and preventing bacterial proliferation by continually removing protein-containing exudates that provide a substrate for bacterial growth.

In full-thickness injury, the entire dermis is destroyed or removed. Epithelialization occurs only from the margins of the wound, at a maximal rate of 1 to 2 mm/d. In practice, adequate coverage of sizable wounds is rarely achieved. Thus, lower leg ulcers rarely heal faster than 1 cm/mo; that is, a 2-cm-diameter ulcer typically takes 2 months to heal under ideal conditions. In an open wound, the rate of epithelialization is critically dependent on the vascularity and health of the underlying granulation tissue (neodermis) across which it migrates. In addition, cellular migration is dependent on the condition of the matrix. Excess bacterial burden results in secondary PMN influx with protease degradation of the matrix and a hostile environment for cellular attachment and migration. Thus, although chronic wounds are manifested by a failure of epithelial migration, the cause is most often a problem in the underlying wound bed, such as local ischemia or excessive bacterial colonization.

The epithelial cells alone provide little strength when not anchored to dermis. They are therefore prone to injury. The basal epidermal cells are attached to the underlying dermis by hemidesmosomes. These structures attach to keratin filaments within the epithelial cells. The hemidesmosomes connect by a series of intermediate proteins to anchoring filaments, long proteins that intertwine with the collagen network of the dermis. Intact epithelium is resistant to sheer forces due to these strong dermal attachments. Without an adequate dermal base, however, epidermis provides unstable wound coverage and is characterized by chronic and recurrent wound breakdown; this is frequently noted in a heavily cicatrized bed.

After the first layer of cells restores the epithelial barrier, additional layers develop, restoring the basilar-to-apical order. As the cells mature, they resume keratin formation. This regenerates the stratum corneum of the epidermis, completes the restorative process of epithelialization, and provides stable coverage.

Scar

5 Visible scarring occurs only when the injury extends deeper than the superficial dermis. Superficial abrasions and burns usually heal without scarring even if the superficial dermis is involved, because a thin layer of scar in the superficial dermis is not visible. Whenever the dermis is incised, a scar forms. Scar formation at the molecular level is due to disorganized collagen. In response to injury, dermal integrity is restored by collagen synthesis and deposition. Over the time of scar maturation (6 months to several years), scar remodeling results in progressive collagen linking and increased organization, but the parallel organized collagen layers of normal skin are never completely reconstituted, resulting in visible scar. The prominence of the scar is variable and can be minimized by location and closure technique. If an incision is made, however, a scar is inevitable. The quality of the scar is impacted by a number of factors. The underlying genetic tendency to scar is a significant factor. It is well known that some African Americans form keloids from even minor insults, and approximately 5% to 10% of African Americans are keloid prone. Many Asians (as many as 50% of Chinese, Korean, and Japanese) have some tendency to form hypertrophic scars. Elderly patients heal with less inflammation and rarely form hypertrophic scars. Scars parallel to collagen fibers in relaxed skin tension lines form much better scars than those perpendicular to relaxed skin tension lines. As discussed previously, mechanical forces stimulate cell proliferation and collagen synthesis, so that scars closed under tension after skin excision or in locations subjected to tension such as the sternum or shoulder are prone to scar hypertrophy.[7]

FIGURE 4.5. Reepithelialization of a partial-thickness wound. (*continued*)

A

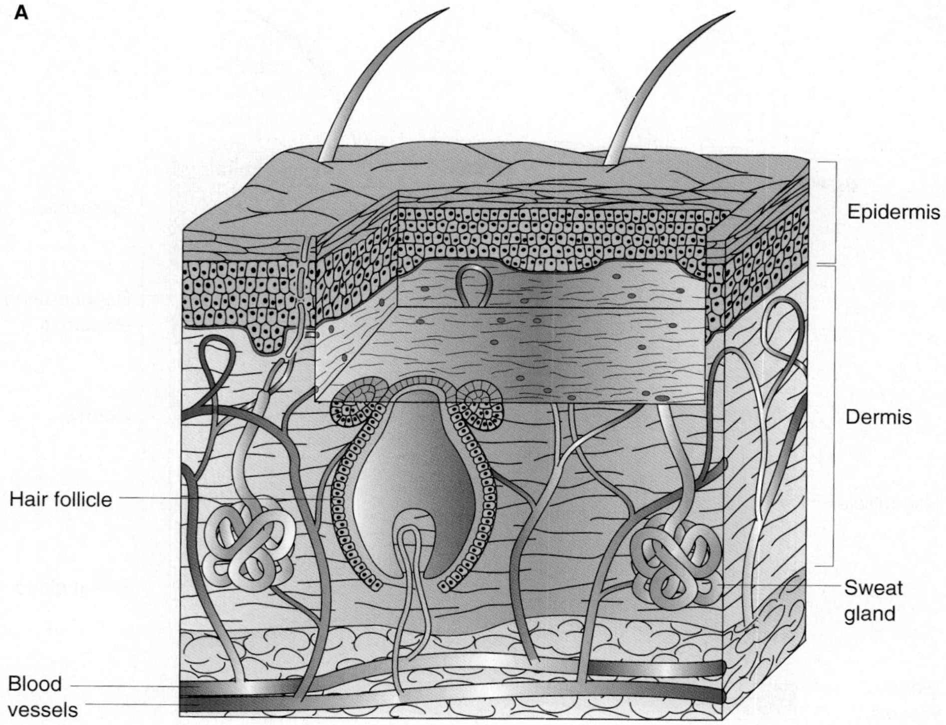

B

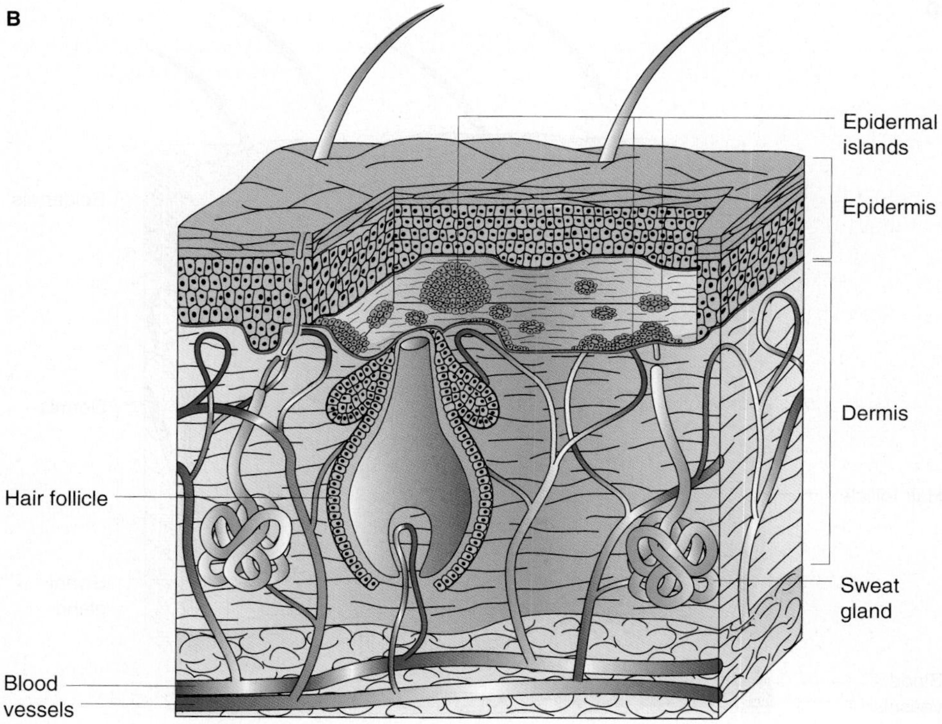

Stretch marks are a unique type of scar. Stretch marks occur when the collagen fibers in the dermis are stretched to the point of disruption, but the epidermis is not disrupted. This results in scar formation in the dermis that is visible through an intact, unscarred epidermis. There is no treatment for stretch marks other than excision of the skin (which of course results in scar from wound closure) or tissue destruction, which can in exceptional circumstances result in wound contraction and some shrinkage of the stretch marks (the rationale for treating stretch marks with laser).

Clinical Implications

Optimal Outcomes from Surgical Closure. This review of normal wound healing has numerous practical implications to the care of wounds and surgical incisions in order to ensure uncomplicated, expeditious healing as well as produce an optimal scar. Meticulous hemostasis reduces the inflammation and phagocytosis necessary to clear the wound of blood. The use of electrocautery should be judicious. Electrocautery results in a band of tissue necrosis that varies in thickness in relation to

FIGURE 4.5. (*Continued*)

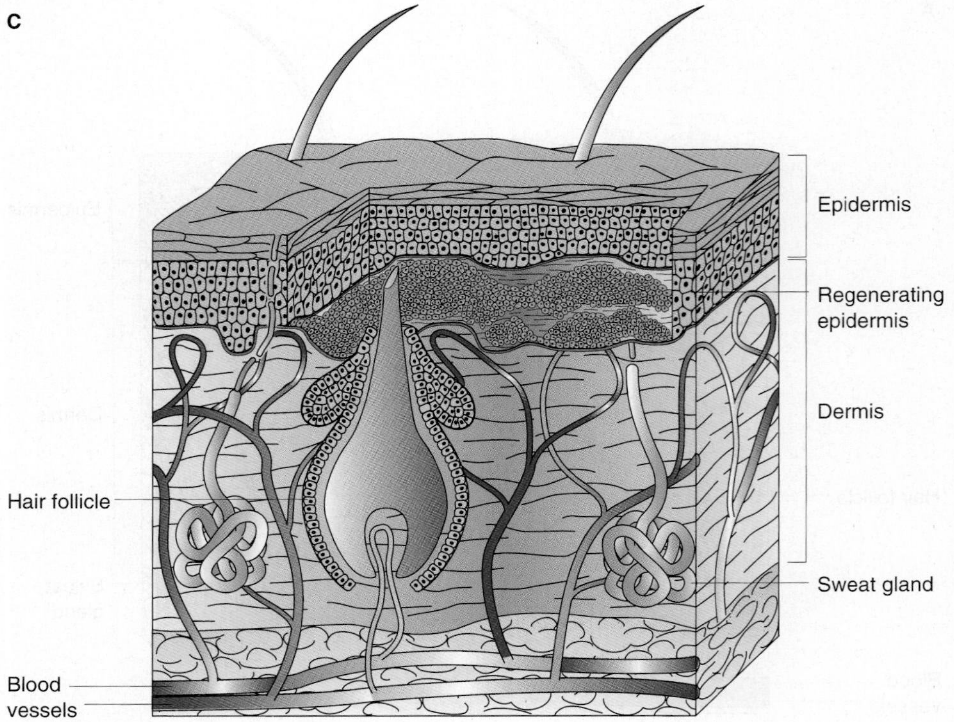

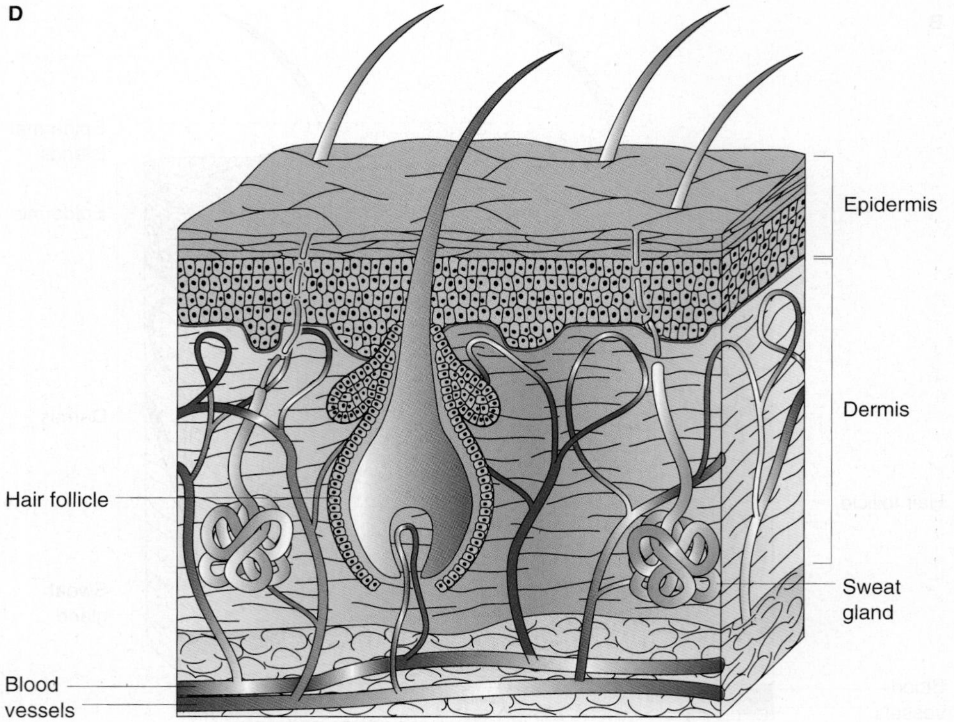

heat generated. The benefits in hemostasis from cautery must be balanced with the thermal injury that results, to minimize stimuli for inflammation. Atraumatic handling of tissue decreases the load of necrotic or nonviable cells at the wound margin. This is best achieved using fine forceps or skin hooks to retract and assist in coapting the dermis. Crush injury to the epidermis with forceps should be avoided. Deep sutures are best placed only into collagen-laden structures that can hold tension, that is, fascia and dermis. These tissues have the tensile strength to hold sutures under tension. Fat does not contain collagen and does not hold tension. Therefore, fatty tissue should not be sutured as a separate layer. Dead-space obliteration and fluid evacuation are best achieved by suction drainage rather than by adding additional foreign material to the wound in the form of suture material. Therefore, in closing a laparotomy incision, even in a morbidly obese patient with a large panniculus, the closure should be limited to the abdominal fascia, the skin, and rarely the Scarpa fascia. The choice and proper use of suture material is also important. Sutures should be chosen to provide the appropriate amount of strength to prevent dehiscence; this is balanced by the inflammation that results as a suture dissolves. In the skin, an absorbable intradermal suture that dissolves over a prolonged period will result in prolonged inflammation and a prominent scar. Well-placed sutures will also minimize the incidence of suture knot extrusion, which can also compromise the final appearance of the scar.

Under normal circumstances, epithelialization of an incision is complete within 24 to 48 hours, and there is no reason to protect the incision from water beyond this time. Allowing the patient to wash or shower 1 or 2 days after surgery has significant psychological benefit and gently débrides the incision and keeps it clean by rinsing away surface bacteria and debris. Blood and protein exudate are an excellent culture media for any skin surface bacteria. Showers reduce the chance of bacterial accumulation in surface crusts along the incision and on the sutures. This decreases inflammation and prevents breakdown of the fragile epithelial layer over the incision, improving the quality of the scar. Once the incision has epithelialized and the epidermis has matured, there is increasing acceptance of the concept that covering immature epidermis for a period of as long as 2 months with paper tape, silicone gel sheeting, or other materials improves scar outcome, most likely due to restoration of the water barrier function of mature stratum corneum.[7]

OPEN WOUNDS (ACUTE)

Open wounds, whether ulcers or open surgical incisions closing by secondary intention, heal with the same sequence of inflammation, matrix deposition, epithelialization, and scar maturation as previously described. However, there are some important differences. In the closed (sutured) incisional wound, the healing process progresses through an orderly temporal sequence. In an open wound, the healing events are spatially separated. In the healing wound, a bed of granulation tissue forms over the exposed subcutaneous tissue. Granulation tissue is composed of new capillaries; proliferating fibroblasts; and an immature matrix of collagen, proteoglycans, substrate adhesion molecules (including fibronectin, laminin, and tenascin), and acute and chronic inflammatory cells. In addition, there are variable amounts of bacteria and protein exudate, depending on the condition of the wound. At the advancing edge of epithelium, the process of acute inflammation is present. Behind the advancing edge, there is a proliferative area, and further behind, the scar is maturing and remodeling. An understanding of the biologic principles of wound healing has direct clinical implications in wound care, particularly in the case of chronic wounds (e.g., pressure sores, lower leg ulcers, diabetic foot ulcers).

The most important clinical factor in the healing of surgical incisions is the gain in tensile strength of the wound. This depends almost entirely on collagen deposition. The rate of collagen synthesis determines the initial wound strength; ultimate wound strength is determined by the degree of collagen organization and cross-linking. The healing of open wounds is defined primarily by epithelialization, and successful healing is related more to the maintenance of epithelial integrity than to the tensile strength of the scar. As discussed earlier, the rate of epithelialization in open wounds is limited by the rate of migration of the proliferating epithelial edge. Factors that regulate epithelial migration are an area of active research. There is clear evidence that the extracellular matrix (collagen, fibronectin, basement membrane proteins, and glycosaminoglycans) is composed of structural elements that are not inert. They function as an essential substrate, with adhesion molecules regulating intercellular communication. The cellular occupants of the matrix express specific receptors that recognize amino acid sequences on the matrix proteins. This allows for cellular attachment at specific sites, cell locomotion, and intracellular signal transduction. Rapid epithelialization is therefore dependent on an optimal matrix, synthesized by the underlying granulation tissue, as well as on optimal delivery of nutrients and oxygen by an adequate blood supply. The rate of epithelialization is also inversely related to the degree of bacterial presence in the wound, a variable that is directly related to the quality of the granulation tissue present.

Inflammatory cells in open wounds, especially the macrophages, release growth factors. Growth factors enhance migration and proliferation of fibroblasts and endothelial cells in wounds. In an open wound, this leads to the formation of granulation tissue, the cobblestonelike pink surface of healthy new tissue. The ability of an open wound to form granulation tissue is governed by the blood supply to the tissue and the relative absence of devitalized tissue and bacteria. Therefore, wounds that form granulation tissue should heal or be amenable to surgical closure with flaps or skin grafts. Wounds that do not form granulation tissue are very likely to be recalcitrant to all treatments except those directed at the underlying cause of the failure to form granulation tissue, that is, vascular bypass to restore adequate blood flow to an ischemic extremity wound or a vigorous surgical débridement to clear the wound of contaminating bacterial pathogens that impair the development of healthy granulation tissue and impede epidermal migration.

Débridement deserves mention, as it is frequently underutilized in clinical care. It is a simple technique that is unglamorous in comparison to other more complex surgical operations, yet is essentially critical to ensuring healing in a contaminated surgical wound. Débridement is a term that refers to clearance of tissue that is unnecessary and counterproductive to healing, and in practical terms usually refers to bacteria and necrotic, devitalized tissue. Débridement can take the form of nonsurgical techniques, such as autolytic, enzymatic, or biologic approaches, or alternatively a surgical technique can be used. The astute clinician will tailor the degree of débridement necessary to achieve the desired outcome while minimizing removal of healthy healing tissue. The importance of débridement is most clearly seen in chronic wounds, which will be more fully discussed later. The process of débridement removes bacteria and their products, which serve to propagate a counterproductive hyperinflammatory phase and which divert metabolic resources away from the healing wound. In a chronic wound, bacterial critical colonization often will result in a hyperinflammatory loop that is best short-circuited by a judicious débridement, allowing the wound to progress toward healing (Fig. 4.6).[8]

Wound Contraction

Wound contraction is an important event that contrasts the healing of open wounds with closed incisions. When open wounds contract, the surrounding skin is pulled over the wound to reduce its size. This can occur much faster than epithelialization. In addition to increasing the speed of wound closure, another advantage is that the open wound is resurfaced by the normal sensate skin surrounding the wound. Most animals are loose skinned, meaning that the skin (epithelium, dermis, subcutaneous fat) is only loosely attached to the underlying muscle fascia. Some animal wounds heal almost entirely by contraction; for example, a 2-cm ulcer heals to a

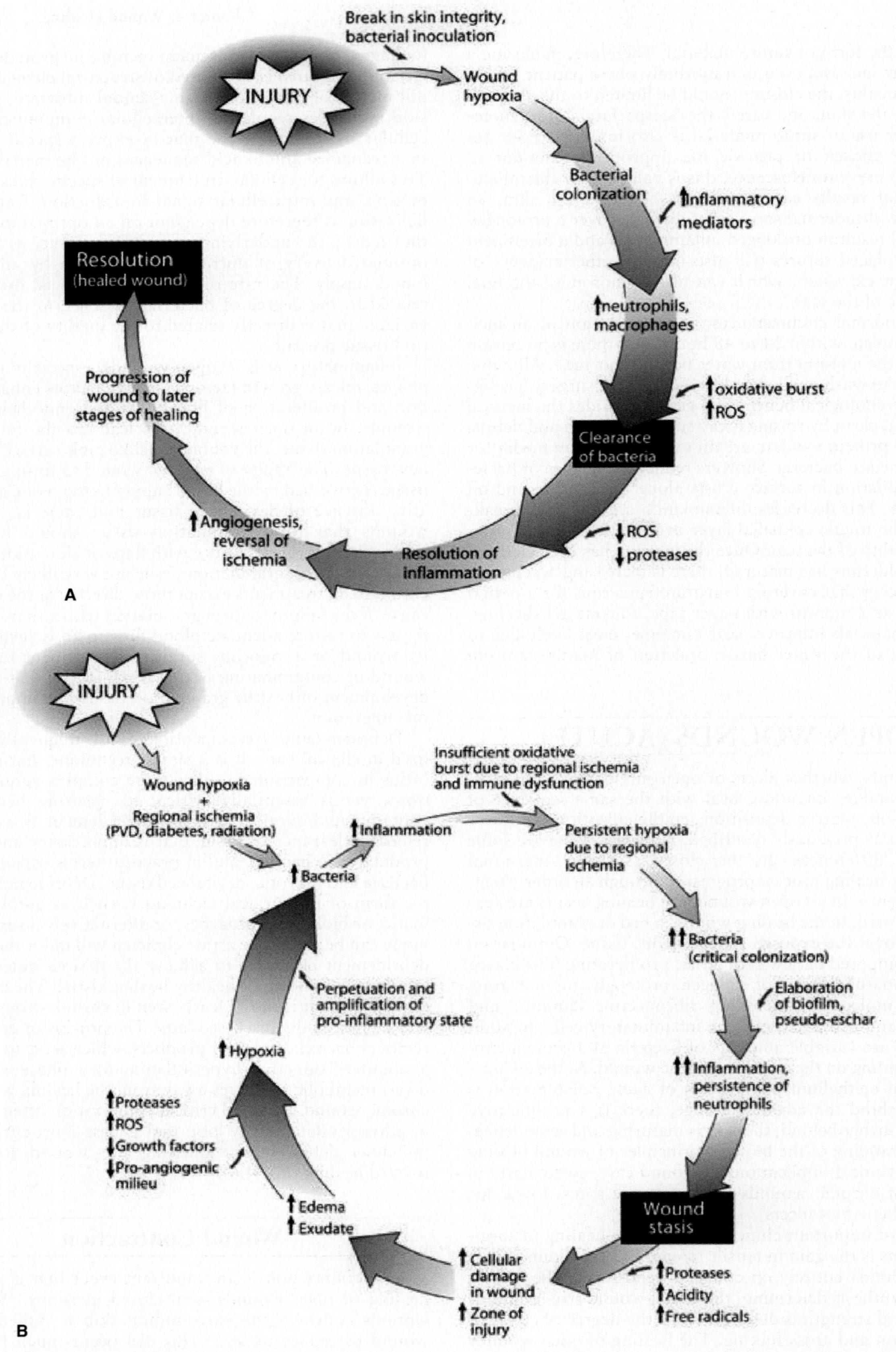

FIGURE 4.6. The inflammatory cascade in wound repair. A: In healthy patients with adequate tissue perfusion, the inflammatory burst is self-limited as reactive oxygen species (ROS) serve to clear bacteria from the wound bed to enable progression to the later phases of wound healing. Since the bacteria are cleared from the wound, the production of ROS and proteases is self-limited, minimizing bystander cellular damage. B: In a setting of regional hypoxia or other comorbidities, bacteria are not efficiently cleared, partly due to an ineffective oxidative burst, which requires oxygen. Bacteria will continue to accumulate in a biofilm state and a level of critical colonization or frank infection will result, leading to an amplified and/or prolonged inflammatory state with further tissue damage and persistent hypoxia as neovascularization is impaired. (Reproduced with permission from Thorne CM. *Grabb and Smith's Plastic Surgery,* 6th ed. Philadelphia, PA: Lippincott Williams & Wilkins; 2006, Figure 3.1.)

3-mm point in a matter of days in a loose-skinned animal. Humans, however, do not have this degree of skin mobility in most sites; the skin is tightly adherent and less elastic, particularly in the lower leg. Therefore, although contraction may account for 90% of the reduction in wound size on the perineum, it accounts for at most 30% to 40% of the healing of a lower leg ulcer. This is one important reason why leg ulcers are so slow to heal. All healing wounds generate a strong contractile force.[9] When this contractile force is exerted across a joint, such as the neck, axilla, or elbow, it may result in a scar contracture. A scar contracture is a scar that limits the functional range of motion of a joint.

At the cellular level, the forces that drive wound contraction come from the fibroblasts. Fibroblasts, like muscle cells, contain actin microfilaments. When these filaments increase in number, the cells take on the morphologic appearance of myofibroblasts. Myofibroblasts are seen in increased numbers in contracting wounds, but their role and derivation are unclear. It is unknown whether the fibroblasts that attach to the collagen fibrils by means of integrin receptors move collagen fibers together using a locomotor action or whether the contraction comes from intrinsic cellular contraction, but it is likely that contraction is due to a combination of the two. In addition, it is still unclear whether myofibroblasts are derived from tissue-resident fibroblasts that phenotypically assume the role of a myofibroblast in response to tissue strain and molecular mediators such as TGF-β1 or develop from blood-borne precursor cells such as fibrocytes that are recruited to an open wound. The forces of contraction continue as long as there is inflammation and collagen remodeling.

Unless created and dressed under sterile conditions, all open wounds are contaminated by the bacterial flora on the surrounding skin and from the environment. Even when dressed under sterile conditions, bacterial colonization will occur within about 48 hours from the surrounding skin. Bacterial *colonization* of the wound is routine and is not deleterious to normal healing. However, bacterial *infection,* defined as a bacterial presence that overwhelms the host response, is deleterious and can delay or prevent healing. Cellulitis or invasive bacterial infection of the surrounding skin is relatively easy to diagnose with experience. Treatment typically requires systemic antibiotic therapy. Distinguishing wound colonization from excess bacterial load resulting in excess inflammatory cells, protease degradation of matrix, and impaired healing, however, can be difficult. The burn wound experience has demonstrated that bacterial counts of more than 10^5 organisms per gram of tissue on quantitative analysis are associated with failure of surgical wound closure. This is an important technique, because clinical judgment is inadequate. The failure of wound closure in this circumstance is in part due to bacterial and phagocytic proteases that prevent healing. In a similar fashion, if the bacterial count is above this threshold in the wound granulation tissue, the endotoxins and excessive proteases, derived from both bacteria and PMNs, delay epithelialization. Several experimental systems have demonstrated that an excess of PMNs in a wound delays healing. Clinical experience with pilonidal wounds, with no other risk factors for impaired healing other than an increased bacterial burden, indicates that resolution of that one variable can result in rapid healing of wounds that have remained open for months or even years.

Any nonepithelialized wound leaks plasma. With more inflammation, capillary permeability is further increased. Increased microvascular permeability results from endothelial cell injury or dysfunction. This is mediated by many components of the inflammatory cascade, including histamine, kinins, complement, PGE_2, PGI_2, VEGF, and others. This exudate of serum proteins and inflammatory cells serves as a rich culture medium, which may continue the cycle of bacterial proliferation and leads to more exudate formation. The net result of this cycle is delayed or absent wound healing. In addition, the edema that results from capillary dysfunction increases the distance for diffusion from oxygen and nutrient sources to their metabolic targets.

Clinical Features

Basic principles of wound care should be tailored to assist the mechanisms elaborated earlier, leading to more rapid healing. Although many varieties of wound care are practiced, Winter and Scales[10] first recorded that epithelialization is more rapid under moist conditions than dry conditions. Without dressings, a superficial wound, or one with minimal devitalized tissue, forms a scab or crust. The scab forms when blood and serum coagulate, dry, and form a protective moisture barrier over the open wound (Fig. 4.7). Epithelialization occurs with controlled clot proteolysis and migration of the epithelium under the clot. If the wound is kept moist with an occlusive dressing, however, and the exudate does not become infected, then epithelial migration is optimized. A skin graft donor site, for example, epithelializes several days faster under an occlusive dressing than a dry dressing. In addition, the pain of an open wound or skin graft donor site is dramatically reduced under an occlusive dressing.

Moist healing can be achieved by occlusive dressings, ointments or creams, or continually moistened dressings. The traditional wet to dry dressing, however, if truly left to dry, simply produces desiccation and necrosis of the surface layer of the wound, delaying epithelialization. Although wet to dry dressings can be effective for débridement of wound exudate, they are generally less desirable than a moist healing environment combined with effective cleaning of the wound (i.e., water irrigation or a tailored surgical débridement).

Role of Oxygen

Oxygen is necessary for normal metabolic cellular function, but in wounds with actively proliferating and metabolically stimulated cells, it is even more critical. PMNs require ambient PO_2 levels of 25 mm Hg to produce superoxide radicals, which serve an essential role in bacterial killing. The enzyme system that generates superoxide and its derivative oxidant products functions optimally at PO_2 levels greater than 50 mm Hg. Collagen synthesis is also highly dependent on an adequate tissue oxygen tension. A fresh wound is initially avascular and is always hypoxic relative to the surrounding tissues. In the center of a new wound, the tissue PO_2 can drop to near zero. After angiogenesis and the delivery of oxygenated blood, the tissue PO_2 quickly rises. Generally, the tissue oxygen tension in a wound is lower than that of surrounding normal tissues. Atherosclerosis of major arteries, small vessel disease from other causes, impaired oxygen delivery, local scarring with fibrosis, and other events may reduce local tissue PO_2 levels from normal (about 40 mm Hg) to less than 25 mm Hg. If so, tissue hypoxia results in significantly impaired wound healing. In the postoperative patient, suboptimal skin perfusion due to even modest hypovolemia, smoking-related arteriopathy, or excess circulating epinephrine can result in a low tissue PO_2. Subcutaneous tissue oxygen levels have been correlated clinically with surgical complication rates. Supplemental oxygen, optimal fluid administration, pain control, and arterial reconstruction all have potential roles in the effort to enhance the tissue PO_2. Oxygen delivery to tissue is the primary determinant of healing; anemia alone is not specifically detrimental to wound healing.[11]

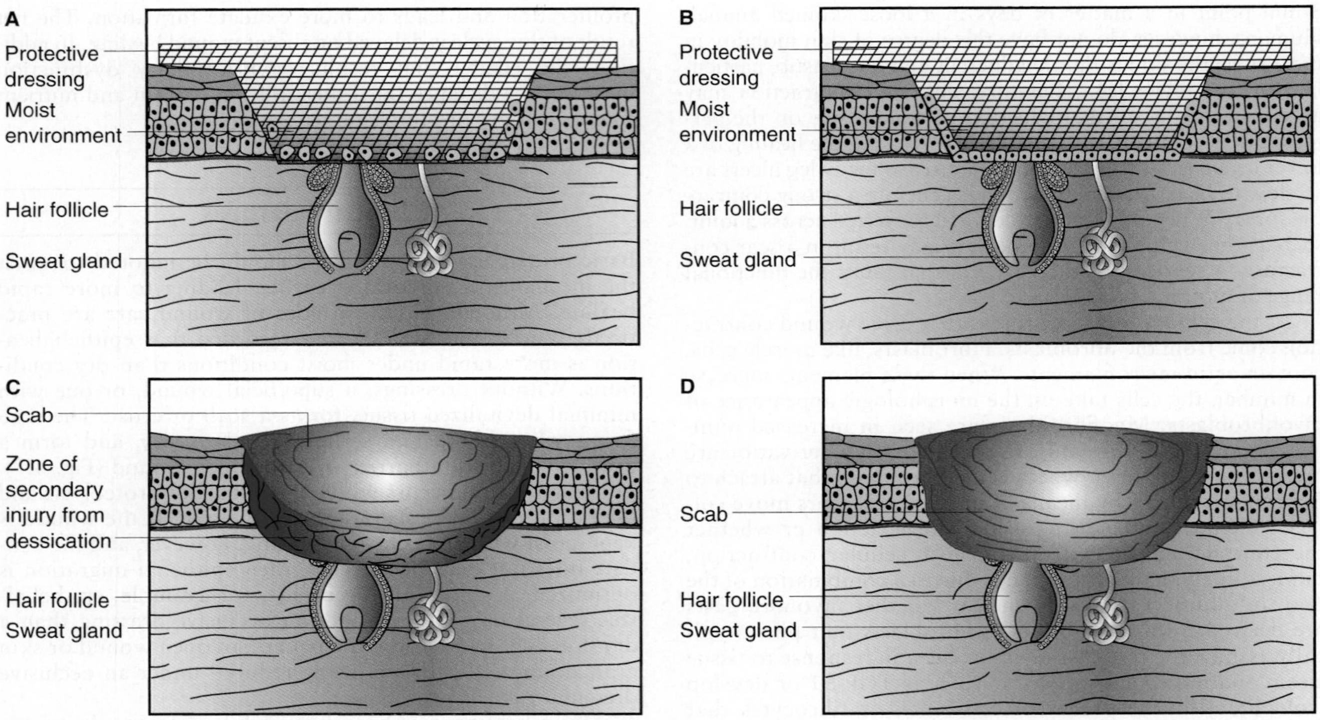

FIGURE 4.7. Rapid epithelialization occurs in a moist environment. Desiccation delays healing by causing tissue necrosis in the exposed wound. The scab ultimately forms a moisture barrier, and epithelialization occurs from the wound edge and any remaining dermal appendages.

Hyperbaric oxygen therapy (HBO) can achieve high oxygen levels in most wounds for the duration of the treatment, usually 1.5 hours at a time. The patient is placed in the hyperbaric chamber and is exposed to 2 to 2.5 atmospheres of pressure and 100% oxygen. Although oxygen is a necessary component in aerobic metabolism, it may also act as a signaling molecule for growth factor production. There is extensive clinical experience suggesting clinical efficacy of HBO, but conclusive prospective randomized trials have not been conducted. It is clear that HBO can raise the PO_2 in ischemic wounds, but the indications, length of treatment, and number of treatments are still empiric. Based on the success of a number of retrospective studies, the usage of HBO in recent years has become widespread, particularly with diabetic foot ulcers and wounds that have been irradiated.

The role of oxygen as a therapeutic agent has been in part stimulated by an increased understanding of the role of oxygen in intracellular signaling. Previously, oxygen was thought to play an essential role in oxidative metabolism, but oxygen sensors were thought to be limited to the kidney (erythropoietin synthesis), the carotid body, and other specialized organs. However, there has been a great deal of interest, in recent years, in the existence in every cell of signal transduction pathways in response to hypoxia. These pathways are mediated by the master transcription factor HIF-1 that is transported to the nucleus and binds to the promoter region to activate synthesis of many genes including growth factors and hormones such as VEGF, erythropoietin, and stromal cell–derived factor (SDF). Therefore, there is a plausible role for intermittent oxygen therapy to induce signal transduction and improve wound healing. The amount of oxygen necessary to result in a therapeutic effect is unknown, but in the acute surgical situation there are data indicating a beneficial effect from supplemental oxygen in the immediate postoperative period. For the treatment of chronic wounds, placing the wound in an enriched oxygen environment has had some anecdotal interest.[12] Another approach to increasing local tissue oxygenation is to increase blood flow. A number of studies have suggested that increasing local skin temperature has resulted in improved wound healing.

Role of Edema

In normal tissue, each cell is only a few cell diameters away from the nearest capillary and receives nutrients and oxygen by diffusion. However, with inflammation, venous insufficiency, or any other causes of edema formation, the sequestered extracellular and extravascular fluid increases the diffusion distance for oxygen and results in a lower tissue PO_2. In the case of lower extremity venous insufficiency, the chronic protein leak from the capillaries results in pericapillary deposition. This "cuffing" is a further barrier to oxygen and nutrient diffusion and possibly functions as a site of nonspecific binding of growth factors, making them less available to the wound environment. The importance of edema control is often underestimated. Even in extremities that are not noticeably swollen, elevation and other methods of edema control (elastic wraps, compression stockings, and sequential compression machines) can be of substantial benefit. The most important therapeutic maneuver in the healing of leg ulcers associated with venous insufficiency is edema control with leg elevation, compression stockings or compressive dressings, and, in severe cases, intermittent or sequential compression devices.

Role of Tissue Necrosis and Exudate

Open wounds often contain devitalized tissue as a result of injury and may be aggravated by infection or suboptimal tissue perfusion. If the amount of dead tissue is large, the impairment to healing is obvious, but it is often not fully appreciated that smaller amounts of necrotic tissue or fibrinous exudate also delay healing. In addition, any open wound constantly produces an exudate of serum proteins and dead inflammatory cells, which increases devitalized tissue, if present. The net result is increased exudate, higher bacterial counts, edema, more proteases and other inflammatory mediators, and a deleterious effect on healing. Therefore, devitalized tissue, especially dermis, generally requires surgical excision. If necrotic dermis is left in place, the underlying subcutaneous tissue (fat), which is less vascular, eventually becomes infected. Small amounts of devitalized tissue and exudate can be débrided or removed with dressings, enzyme application, whirlpools, water irrigation, or simple washing. However, the mechanical débriding action must be sufficient and frequent enough to remove the exudate and debris, producing a clean wound before healing is optimal. Because wounds are painful and the dressings or washings insufficient, the exudate is often not removed adequately. This results in delayed healing. The impact of water irrigation in cleaning a wound and reducing tissue bacterial counts has been underappreciated. Whirlpool can gently clean a wound and modestly reduce tissue bacteria counts, but water under pressure (pulse lavage, syringe irrigation with sufficient force, or even a shower stream or dental water pic) can reduce bacterial counts in tissue by several logs.

CHRONIC WOUNDS

6 A practical definition of a chronic wound is one that has failed to heal within 3 months. Although there are a variety of underlying causes, most chronic wounds can be categorized as pressure sores, diabetic foot ulcers, or leg ulcers. An important question is whether chronic wounds are intrinsically different than acute wounds. For instance, does local tissue senescence make healing a chronic wound impossible? Or do chronic wounds have the inherent potential to heal, but a combination of factors leads to delayed healing? Research in the past few years has begun to address the question of what is different
7 about the environment in a chronic wound. One important realization is that most chronic, nonhealing wounds are characterized by the presence of three variables: advanced age, local tissue ischemia with reperfusion injury, and excess bacterial load.[13]

Clinicians have long recognized that most chronic wounds do indeed have the potential to heal. Healing usually does not occur because of inadequate attention to the basic principles of open wound care—adequate cleansing, débridement, edema control, avoidance and treatment of ischemia, and achievement of a moist wound healing environment. However, the wound environment in many chronic wounds does differ in important ways from acute wounds. Studies have examined wound fluid and biopsies collected from chronic wounds. These reveal significant increases in tissue levels in proteases and collagenases, which are capable of degrading matrix proteins and growth factors. Degradation of growth factors inhibits their crucial functions of proliferation and chemotaxis. When wound fluid from a chronic wound is compared with fluid from an acute surgical wound, there is indeed a decreased level of growth factors. It is not clear what influence bacteria have in this process, although the direct release of bacterial proteases and the indirect effect of protease release from phagocytic cells are both relevant. It is unknown whether growth factor levels are depressed because of proteolysis, primary inhibition of release, or secondary phenotypic changes in the cells of the chronic wound.

Another important factor in the genesis of chronic wounds is the fact that their occurrence is generally in the aged, who have an impaired response to the stress factors of local tissue hypoxia, the increase in reactive oxygen species generated by inflammatory cells, and the existing bacterial burden. As mentioned previously, most chronic wounds are of three types: pressure sores, diabetic foot ulcers, and venous leg ulcers. In all three types, the inciting injury is an ischemia reperfusion injury. In the first two types, pressure exceeding tissue perfusion resulting in a period of ischemia is followed by reperfusion. Repeated cycles of ischemia and reperfusion are much more damaging than an ischemic insult by itself. Experimental evidence in animals supports the notion of an increase in tissue damage in response to an ischemia reperfusion injury.[13]

In chronic wounds, there is some evidence that cells in the periphery of the wound can become senescent after the prolonged stimulus of many months. This is likely a more problematic factor in the elderly and provides a theoretical basis for the efficacy of surgical débridement and excision of the "rind" or callus of a chronic wound, converting it to an acute wound and converting a nonhealing wound to a healing wound.

The final common denominator in the triad of factors that is present in most chronic wounds is excess bacterial presence. It has recently become appreciated that bacteria exist in wounds in the setting of a biofilm.[14] Biofilms represent a complex community of bacteria that are present within a secreted and assembled exopolysaccharide matrix. They interact with each other via the process of quorum sensing. The slime layer in which they encase themselves protects them from the inflammatory cells of the wound. In a wound that has reached critical colonization, the robust inflammatory process necessary for bacterial clearance actually becomes a deleterious process. The overproduction of free radicals and proteases serves to divert resources and nutrients away from the healing cells and results in significant bystander damage. This is of importance in a debilitated or elderly patient. As mentioned, the hostile wound environment and altered pH can degrade or inactivate growth factors to further impair healing. The presence of this leads to further tissue damage, eventually resulting in a vicious cycle of tissue injury, bacterial overgrowth, and further tissue injury in the form of bystander damage as the body's inflammatory cascade becomes unregulated (Fig. 4.6). Clearance of bacteria via a surgical débridement will break this cycle, reduce the inflammatory cascade, and allow progression of the wound through the appropriate stages of wound healing.

WOUND MANAGEMENT

Surgical Incisions

8 It takes at least 3 weeks for collagen to undergo sufficient remodeling and cross-linking to attain moderate strength. Figure 4.4 shows that at 1 to 2 weeks, the time when most sutures are removed, a wound has a small fraction of its eventual strength and may therefore disrupt with even modest stresses. Therefore, deep sutures are placed in collagen-containing structures to hold prolonged tension. Dermis, intestinal submucosa, muscular fascia, tendon, ligament, Scarpa fascia, and blood vessel wall represent a partial list of tissues with high collagen content. These deep sutures are often absorbable. The most common absorbable material, polyglactic acid (Vicryl, Dexon), retains tensile strength for about 3 weeks. Sutures used for tendon and abdominal fascia are usually permanent or, if absorbable, should ideally retain their tensile strength for close to 6 weeks. After 6 weeks, wounded tissue has gained about 50% of its eventual strength. To prevent hernia formation, heavy lifting is avoided after major abdominal surgery for 6 weeks. Tendon repairs are splinted and activity restricted to avoid full tension for a similar period.

As discussed in earlier sections, the fibroblasts in a wound respond to mechanical forces, and because skin has elastin fibers and tends to retract in response to injury, virtually all wounds are closed under some tension. If the tension forces are relatively large (in excisional wounds, for instance), sutures that effectively splint the wound, preventing the wound fibroblasts from experiencing large mechanical forces, will result in less collagen excess (scar hypertrophy) and less scar stretch. Most absorbable sutures retain their tensile strength for only 3 weeks or so. Studies in humans have demonstrated that this is insufficient to prevent scar widening and results in no better scars than those in which all sutures are removed at 7 days. Therefore, to achieve optimal scars in wounds closed under tension or in areas such as the shoulder, permanent sutures should be left in place for 6 months until collagen remodeling is essentially complete. A continuous intradermal Prolene suture or intradermal interrupted clear nylon sutures with buried knots will achieve that objective.

Open Wound Dressings

There are at least 150 dressing products commercially available at present. These include multiple topical antibiotics, irrigants, and débriding agents. Although PDGF (Regranex) and tissue engineered living cell constructs (Apligraf and Dermagraft) have been shown to decrease healing times in certain wounds, standard treatment, which adheres to the principles outlined earlier, may be successfully applied to the vast majority of wounds. There are many good alternative treatments, but to avoid confusion, they should be judged according to the following criteria:

1. How effectively is the wound cleaned or débrided?
2. Is moist wound healing achieved?
3. Is edema minimized in the periwound tissue?
4. Are new pressure (ischemia reperfusion) insults or wound soilage prevented?
5. Is tissue oxygenation (blood flow) adequate?

In some situations, reduction of tissue bacteria is also an important additional need; this is most often addressed by adequate cleaning and débridement. In the absence of large amounts of necrotic tissue, wound débridement does not need to be accomplished surgically. Proteinaceous exudate can be tenacious, however, and simple application of moist dressings may not be adequate to remove it. Water irrigation either in whirlpools or by water from a handheld shower spray or even from dental water cleaning devices can be gentle and yet generate enough power to effectively débride.[15] Frequent moist dressing changes can accomplish this as well, and in some cases, occlusive absorptive dressings can generate enough tissue proteases to effectively degrade proteins that the absorptive dressings remove (autolytic débridement). This deceptively simple principle is the most frequently overlooked in wound care. The typical open surgical wound often contains deep interstices that packing or other absorptive dressings may not effectively reach. The deeper portions of the wound may then accumulate exudate and bacteria. This is one example in which water irrigation may be particularly useful. Commonly used agents such as hydrogen peroxide are actually harmful to normal tissue and are weak oxidants and thus do a poor job of débriding. These are to be avoided. Enzymatic débriding agents can be effective when properly used.

As discussed, a desiccated wound undergoes delayed healing. Most wounds require an absorptive dressing to remove exudate. This can be gauze, which is inexpensive and effective but which requires frequent dressing changes and is not occlusive so that an ointment or cream must be added. Skin graft donor sites do well with an occlusive polyurethane film dressing. Most of the newer dressing products have been designed to be more absorptive and achieve moist healing without infection from excess exudate. An emphasis has been placed to decrease the frequency of dressing changes. It must be emphasized that although factors such as convenience, patient acceptance, and cost are good reasons for choosing a product, as long as moist healing is achieved, there is no evidence that one is better than another.

Edema is detrimental to wound healing and is often undertreated, in part because of difficulties in patient education. Edema can be a factor in virtually any ulcer of the lower extremity, although venous insufficiency is the most important. Because patients often have personal habits that are hard to modify, this can be a refractory problem. Patients often object to compression stockings, the most effective method for limiting edema. This leaves intermittent leg elevation, elastic wraps, and elevation of the foot of the bed as alternative measures. The critical factor is getting the patient to realize that leg swelling must be avoided, and so in the course of the day, each patient must modify behavior sufficiently to treat this problem.

Systemic Factors Affecting Wound Healing

Several important systemic factors or conditions influence wound healing. Interestingly, there are no known systemic conditions that lead to more rapid wound healing. The discussion that follows relates to factors that may retard or inhibit wound healing.

Nutrition. Wound healing requires energy and is an anabolic process. Patients who are severely malnourished or who are actively catabolic demonstrate impaired healing. Although there is no single measure of nutritional adequacy, the serum albumin level is the most readily available and clinically useful parameter. A serum albumin greater than 3.5 g/dL suggests adequate protein stores and positive nitrogen balance. However, albumin has a serum half-life of 19 days. Therefore, the serum albumin level does not drop early in a catabolic process and is slow to rise when protein stores are repleted and an anabolic state returns. Serum transferrin has a shorter half-life and, therefore, responds more promptly to nutritional fluctuations, but it is not part of a routine chemistry panel and has not gained widespread clinical usage. There is no consensus on nutritional parameters that accurately predict the development of surgical complications. In considering closure of a chronic wound such as a pressure sore, the ability to form granulation tissue and begin wound contraction are clinical indications of acceptable wound healing potential. The presence of a granulating, contracting wound argues strongly that the patient has adequate nutrition to undergo surgery. An albumin level of less than 3 mg/dL raises concern for potential wound healing problems. In clinical practice, the trajectory of prealbumin levels (i.e., an increased level measured weekly) may be more useful than a static level and suggests the restoration of adequate stores. Most surgeons avoid trying to close chronic wounds surgically until nutritional levels are considered acceptable, particularly in the elderly.

Vitamins play an important role in wound healing as well. Vitamin A is involved in the stimulation of fibroplasia, collagen cross-linking, and epithelialization. In animal studies, vitamin A reverses the inhibitory effects of glucocorticoids on the inflammatory phase of wound healing.[16] Although there is no conclusive evidence in humans, vitamin A may be useful clinically for steroid-dependent patients who have problematic wounds or who are undergoing an extensive surgical procedure. Vitamin A may be used either topically or systemically, but attention should be paid to the dosage and duration of therapy as vitamin A is fat soluble and has a well-defined toxicity state. An oral dose of 25,000 IU daily or topical application of 200,000 IU ointment three times a day should be sufficient.

Vitamin C is a necessary cofactor in the hydroxylation of lysine and proline in collagen synthesis and cross-linkage. The deficiency state, scurvy, is rarely seen in the Western world today. The utility of vitamin C supplementation in patients who are taking a normal diet is not established.

Vitamin E is applied to wounds and incisions by many patients. The evidence to support this practice is entirely anecdotal, and, in fact, large doses of vitamin E have been found to inhibit wound healing.[17] Only massage, pressure, and silicone sheeting have been shown to flatten and soften scars. Many people perceive a healing benefit from topical creams, but it is very difficult to exclude the two main variables in scar formation: (a) scars improve with passage of time and (b) there is natural variability in scar formation between different individuals and in the same individual in different locations and at different ages.

Essential fatty acids are required for all new cell synthesis. Essential fatty acid deficiency is first noted in areas of high cellular turnover, such as healing wounds, skin, and gastrointestinal mucosa. Early experience with total parenteral nutrition in which essential fatty acids were lacking showed that patients developed difficult wounds and dramatic skin changes. These were rapidly reversed with the addition of fat to the parenteral nutritional program.

Zinc and copper are also important cofactors for many enzyme systems that are important to wound healing. Deficiency states have been seen with parenteral nutrition but are rare and now readily recognized and treated with supplements.

Vitamin and mineral deficiency states clearly show the necessity of these agents for wound healing. However, these deficiency states are extremely rare in the absence of parenteral nutrition or other extreme dietary restrictions. There is no evidence to support the concept that supranormal provision of these factors enhances wound healing in normal patients. Significant complications, especially with excessive fat-soluble vitamin supplementation, are reported. However, malnutrition can be a significant problem in the elderly and debilitated patient. These patients require nutritional supplementation and should receive vitamin and mineral supplementation as part of their protein and caloric repletion.

Aging. There are important age-dependent aspects of wound healing. The elderly heal more slowly and with less scarring. There is gradual attenuation of the inflammatory response with age, and decreased wound healing is one of the consequences. In vitro studies have documented an age-dependent decrease in the proliferative potential of fibroblasts and epithelial cells. Clinically, these account for the formation of finer scars and improved cosmetic appearance in the elderly. Hypertrophic scars are rarely seen in the elderly. Sutures should be left in place longer to allow for the slower gain in tensile strength in the aged. This may be done without formation of suture marks as slower epithelialization occurs along the sutures. Although the aged usually heal from surgical incisions without complications, the combination of age and other adverse factors can result in severe healing deficits and high surgical complication rates (see the previous section on chronic wounds).

Pharmacologic Impairment to Wound Healing. Bone marrow suppression, a common consequence of chemotherapy, is detrimental to wound healing. Quantitative and qualitative lymphocyte and monocyte deficiency impairs cellular proliferation in the inflammatory phase of wound healing. Any chemotherapeutic agent that suppresses the bone marrow will impair healing. Fortunately, this is predictably reversible with cessation of chemotherapy. Glucocorticoids inhibit wound healing based on their anti-inflammatory and immunosuppressive effects. The anti-inflammatory effect of steroids is in part the result of inhibiting arachidonic acid metabolism, resulting in impaired macrophage migration and altered neutrophil function. Glucocorticoids also inhibit synthesis of procollagen by fibroblasts, delaying wound contraction. Steroid-dependent patients have a persistent decrease in wound tensile strength even after healing is complete. Patients who require chronic systemic steroids have attenuation of the dermis and are therefore susceptible to injury. Even minor shearing forces may produce tearing of the skin and full-thickness wounds due to the decreased tensile strength. The advent of antiangiogenic agents in the treatment of cancer unfortunately also contributes to impaired wound healing. Agents such as bevacizumab and sunitinib impair angiogenic growth factors such as VEGF. Since wound healing is an angiogenesis-dependent process, particularly recalcitrant wounds can result from use of these medications.

TABLE 4.3

FACTORS THAT CONTRIBUTE TO WOUND ISCHEMIA

Poor arterial inflow—atherosclerosis
Poor venous flow—venous stasis
Smoking
Radiation
Edema
Diabetes mellitus—accelerates atherosclerosis, microvascular dysfunction
Vasculitis
Fibrosis—chronic scarring
Pressure—pressure sores or decubitus ulcer

Ischemia. Adequate tissue oxygenation plays a critical role in wound healing.[18] Oxygen is needed for aerobic metabolism and also for proper neutrophil function, especially in bacterial killing. Oxygen is also a requirement for hydroxylation of proline and lysine to form stable collagen fibrils (Table 4.3).

Smoking. Smoking or nicotine patches inhibit oxygen delivery via sympathomimetic vasoconstriction. In addition, smoking elevates carboxyhemoglobin levels in the blood. This effect shifts the oxygen delivery curve to the left due to the high affinity of carboxyhemoglobin for oxygen, resulting in less available oxygen in the wound. Animal studies demonstrate that even moderate decreases in tissue oxygen tension result in severe impairment of wound healing with substantially increased infection rates. Smoking has been shown to increase wound complication rates when skin flaps are elevated with marginal distal blood supply.

Radiation. Radiation injury leads to arteriolar fibrosis and impaired oxygen delivery. In addition, there is progressive obliteration of blood vessels in the radiated area over time. Radiation also causes intranuclear and cytoplasmic damage to fibroblasts, and this change appears to limit their proliferative potential. It is important to realize that radiated tissues gradually and progressively deteriorate over time. Irradiated wounds will often require a flap (i.e., the introduction of healthy nonirradiated tissue) for successful closure.

Edema. Edema impairs local oxygen delivery. In addition, edema is often associated with increased venous pressure. This postcapillary obstruction decreases the perfusion pressure in the capillary bed, resulting in ischemia. Increased venous pressure also leads to protein extravasation and pericapillary cuffing. This effect acts as a diffusion barrier to oxygen, further impairing tissue oxygenation and wound healing.

Diabetes. Diabetes mellitus is often associated with decreased healing of open wounds and increased susceptibility to infection. Many factors contribute to poor healing in diabetic patients, and most of these reflect local wound ischemia. However, healing is not impaired in a normally perfused area in a patient with well-controlled diabetes in the absence of infection. This subject is discussed in detail later.

Neuropathy. There is considerable evidence that neuropeptides promote healing, and their decrease or absence in the setting of spinal cord injury is a factor in impaired wound healing and may be a factor in the neuropathy of diabetes. This is not currently a condition that can be treated effectively, although the neuropeptides that impact wound healing are a focus of active research.

Other Local Conditions. Peripheral arterial occlusive disease secondary to atherosclerosis can be a primary cause of impaired healing and may also be a cofactor with the other conditions discussed. In addition, conditions such as vasculitis, prolonged pressure, lower leg venous insufficiency, and tissue fibrosis affect wound healing through the mechanism of local tissue ischemia.

Chronic Wound Care

A chronic wound is commonly defined as an open wound that has failed to respond to standard care and remains open at 3 months. Typically, the wound size is static with an absence of a visible advancing epithelial edge. The etiology of a chronic wound is often multifactorial. One or more factors that impair wound healing, such as advanced age, ischemia, bacterial contamination, edema, and malnutrition or immunosuppression, are often present in patients with chronic wounds. A systematic approach is needed to identify the causative factor(s). Once all of the potentially applicable factors have been identified, those amenable to treatment should be addressed. Although age is fixed, some impact can be made on most other factors. Wounds should be débrided, and topical as well as systemic antibiotics may be indicated for true bacterial infection. Arterial revascularization can increase oxygenation in the wound, and elevation and compression dressings can decrease edema. Skin grafting or other surgical procedures are indicated as long as the underlying processes have been identified and appropriately treated. The underlying causes of some chronic wounds cannot be corrected in some patients, such as those with diabetes or venous insufficiency. Specific chronic wounds are discussed in the sections that follow.

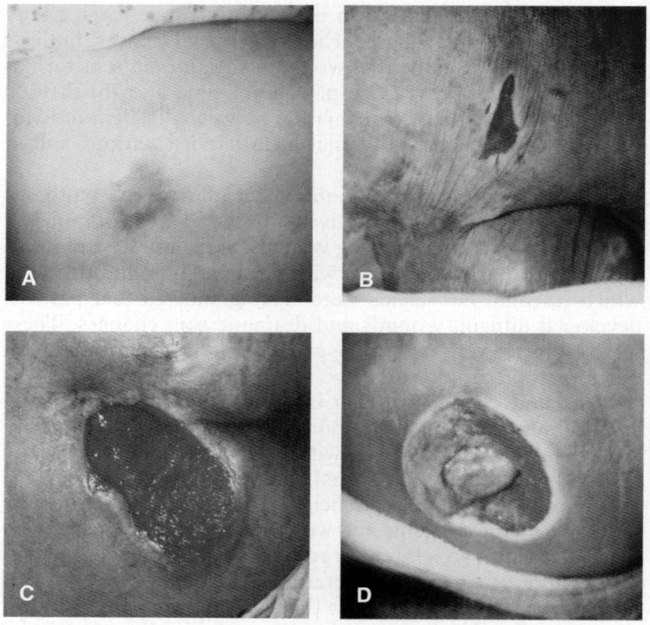

FIGURE 4.8. Pressure ulcer staging. **A:** Stage I—erythema. **B:** Stage II—breakdown of the dermis. **C:** Stage III—full-thickness skin breakdown. **D:** Stage IV—bone, muscle, and supporting tissue involved. (Reproduced with permission from Nettina SM. *The Lippincott Manual of Nursing Practice*, 7th ed. Philadelphia, PA: Lippincott Williams & Wilkins; 2001.)

Pressure Sores. Pressure sores are sometimes mistakenly referred to as bed sores or decubitus ulcers (Fig. 4.8). These sores do not always develop in bed or while lying flat in a decubitus position. All pressure sores, regardless of location, do involve prolonged pressure over a bony prominence followed by reperfusion, which produces much of the injury, particularly when there are repeated cycles. The ability of tissue to withstand pressure is defined by the duration of the pressure, the amount of pressure, and related sheer forces. The most frequent locations of pressure sores are overlying the ischium, sacrum, and trochanter. The heel, knee, ankle, and posterior scalp are less common locations.

Prolonged pressure produces ischemia in the tissue by occluding the microcirculation. This occurs when the tissue pressure exceeds the capillary filling pressure of 25 mm Hg. Pressure on the tissue overlying the sacrum can reach 80 mm Hg in a recumbent patient, so that tissue necrosis can occur within hours if not relieved by frequent changes in position.

Skin is more resistant to pressure than is the underlying subcutaneous fat (which has less blood supply) or muscle (which, although having an excellent blood supply, is very sensitive to ischemia). This sensitivity accounts for the common finding of a small skin ulceration overlying a large area of subcutaneous necrosis. Efforts to identify and control factors that contribute to impaired wound healing should be made. Nutrition is often a problem as is bacterial overgrowth. If the patient can avoid pressure on the involved area and other contributing factors are controlled, most pressure sores will heal. There is a higher incidence of recurrence if pressure sores are allowed to heal by secondary intention rather than by surgical closure. This difference is explained by the increased scarring that occurs with healing by secondary intention and the fact that this places the scar directly over the pressure point. Because scars are never as strong as intact skin, they are more prone to breakdown than intact skin that has been placed over these pressure points by surgical closure. Patients with significant life expectancy, such as young paraplegics who have a precipitating factor leading to development of a pressure sore, are best treated with surgical flap closure. The recurrence rate can be as high as 90% if chronic issues such as depression are not adequately treated (leading to neglect).

Leg Ulcers. Leg ulcers are perhaps the most common type of chronic ulcer. The underlying disease process is most often local tissue ischemia. The underlying cause of this local tissue ischemia should be identified and appropriate treatment initiated. About 90% of leg ulcers in the United States are secondary to venous insufficiency (valvular incompetence) (Fig. 4.9). Venous ulcers lead to local tissue ischemia by increased venous pressure, which lowers the transcapillary perfusion pressure, and by leg edema. Initial treatment should be directed to cleansing and débriding the wound of proteinaceous exudate and limiting the edema and protein loss with compression dressings and elevation. A common treatment has been the Unna boot, a paste bandage that is absorptive, limits edema, and can be changed weekly. This allows the physician to control treatment with weekly visits. If this dressing is made compressive by adding an elastic wrap, it is highly effective in reducing edema, absorbing exudate, and providing an occlusive wound environment. Its limitations are that it requires weekly visits and precludes normal showering or bathing. Another alternative that has become standard in many venous leg ulcer studies is the four-layered compression garment, in which multiple layers result in effective compression over many days. With effective compression, over 50% of venous ulcers can be healed within a 3- to 4-month period. Compression garments or elastic wraps with frequent dressing changes, thorough cleaning, and an occlusive dressing can be equally

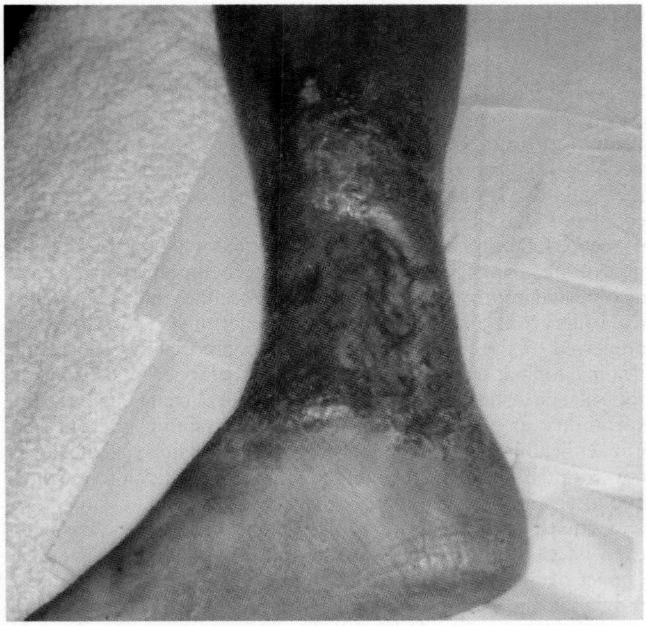

FIGURE 4.9. Venous ulcer. (Reproduced with permission from Nettina SM. *The Lippincott Manual of Nursing Practice,* 7th ed. Philadelphia, PA: Lippincott Williams & Wilkins; 2001.)

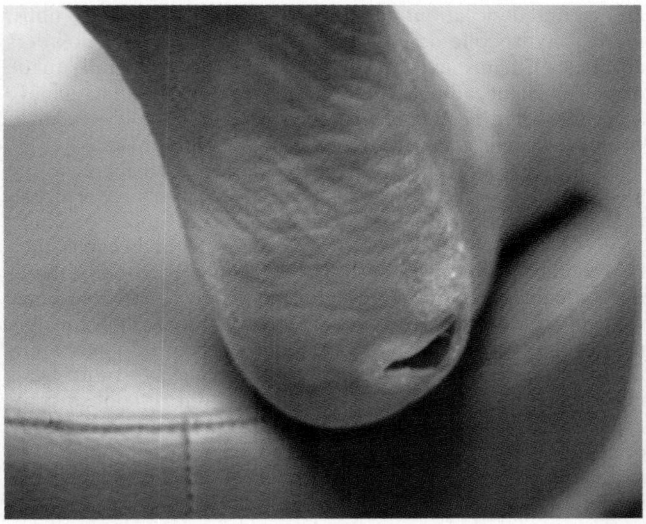

FIGURE 4.10. Diabetic ulcer of the heel. These lesions are noted at sites of pressure, such as the heel in this patient. (Reproduced with permission from Goodheart HP. *Goodheart's Photoguide of Common Skin Disorders,* 2nd ed. Philadelphia, PA: Lippincott Williams & Wilkins; 2003.)

effective. Surgical treatment of venous insufficiency is addressed elsewhere and is useful only in isolated instances in which an incompetent perforator can be identified proximal to an ulcer. Valve reconstruction has not achieved widespread acceptance in the United States.

Additional causes of leg ulcers include arterial insufficiency and other vasculitis syndromes. These are treated best by correcting the underlying disease and local wound care. If the underlying problem cannot be treated, there is little hope of securing a stable, healed wound. For example, vasculitic ulcers will often heal with the judicious use of steroids.

Diabetic Foot Ulcers. Diabetic foot ulcers are caused by pressure over bony prominences, usually the metatarsal heads or calcaneus, in the setting of neuropathy (Fig. 4.10). There is, however, no evidence to support the often-cited concept that these ulcers may result from small vessel disease. This theory originated with a nonblinded study of the microvasculature in amputation specimens by Goldenberg in 1959. Subsequent blinded studies have failed to reveal any architectural differences in small blood vessels of diabetic amputation specimens. However, there is evidence that there may be a *functional* microangiopathy in diabetic patients, with impairments in vasodilatation and angiogenesis after injury. The ischemia in diabetic foot ulcers is due to prolonged pressure on insensate toes and feet, with subsequent reperfusion. This pressure ischemia is enhanced by the increase in blood viscosity related to nondeforming erythrocytes, which develop because of nonenzymatic glycosylation of cell membrane proteins. These rigid red blood cells plug capillary beds and decrease microvascular flow. In addition, glycosylated hemoglobin has increased affinity for oxygen, thereby making less oxygen available to the tissues. Diabetic patients also have a predilection for infrapopliteal arterial occlusive disease and may therefore benefit from arterial reconstructive surgery. The requirements for successful treatment of diabetic ulcers include pressure relief with non–weight-bearing strategies and aggressive débridement of callus and marginally vascularized wound edges. Preventive measures with appropriate orthotic shoes are essential once healing is achieved. It should be remembered that it is in clean diabetic forefoot wounds that the clinical effectiveness of becaplermin gel has been demonstrated.

Diabetic foot ulcers are best treated in a multidisciplinary clinic with a combination of surgical and adjunctive measures. If vascular studies indicate significant underlying disease and reduced toe pressures, the leg should be revascularized if possible. Often, diabetics develop altered pressures on their metatarsals and midfoot secondary to neuropathy and loss of functioning intrinsic muscles in the foot. The Achilles tendon can also shorten due to the buildup of glycosylated end products within the matrix-rich tendon. In addition to orthotics, surgical procedures to partially correct the altered pressure patterns such as Achilles tendon lengthening can be beneficial. Aggressive surgical débridement to remove callus and convert the chronic wound to a well-vascularized acute wound can be therapeutic. Becaplermin gel has been most efficacious in the setting of aggressive serial débridements.

Agents to Optimize Wound Healing

Dressings. Becaplermin gel has been shown to speed healing in diabetic forefoot wounds and probably has a role in other chronic wounds for which there is a paucity of pharmacologic agents. The biologic dressings Apligraf and Dermagraft have been approved for use in venous ulcers and diabetic ulcers, respectively, and some clinicians feel they play a role in recalcitrant wounds. Many types of dressings are commercially available, and none have been demonstrated to be effective if standard care is ignored. Despite marketing claims, standard wound care, keeping wounds clean, moist, and as free of edema and bacteria as possible, are still the most important factors in ensuring wound healing.

The ideal dressing should be simple, inexpensive, highly absorptive, and nonadherent. It should achieve moist healing and have antibacterial properties. Other factors to be considered are less frequent dressing changes, an all-in-one dressing that does not require tape or an overlay, and a gentle adhesive that is effective but not injurious to the skin when removed.[19]

The simplest dressing is gauze and tape—it is inexpensive, is absorptive, and when used with an ointment, can achieve moist healing. The primary disadvantages are the necessity for frequent dressing changes and the potential for tape irritation and wound desiccation. Other products are classified into films, foams, hydrocolloids, hydrogels, and absorptive powders (Table 4.4). Films are semipermeable to water, generally made of polyurethane, and nonabsorptive. These are useful to achieve a moist wound healing environment over minimally exudative wounds, such as a split-thickness skin graft donor site.

Other dressing types have been designed to increase the absorptive capacity of the dressing. This requires fewer dressing changes and maintains an environment for moist healing.

The hydrocolloids deserve special mention because they have achieved widespread use. These contain hydrophilic materials, such as quar, karaya, gelatin, or carboxymethylcellulose, with an adhesive material and are covered by a semipermeable polyurethane film. The material adheres to the skin surrounding the wound, is highly absorptive, and achieves a moist healing environment. Adhesion is maintained until the absorptive capacity is exhausted, and then atraumatic removal is easily done. Similar materials have been extensively used for peristomal care. These are best used for open wounds that have only moderate exudate.

The increased absorptive capacity of these products allows infrequent, minimally traumatic dressing changes. This, along with ease of use and achievement of moist healing, are their principal advantages. Although the availability of these dressing products is accelerating at a dizzying pace, the overriding principle in the proper choice of a dressing is choosing one that will allow the optimal moisture balance within the wound. More exudative wounds will require a more absorptive dressing, whereas drier wounds (such as an arterial ulcer) will require a dressing regimen that gently hydrates the wound.

Antibiotics. The role of antibiotics in wound care is controversial. All open wounds are colonized with bacteria. Only when the surrounding tissue is invaded (cellulitis) are systemic antibiotics clearly indicated. Antibiotics may be useful in other situations, such as when the granulation tissue has a high bacterial count or in a case of reduced resistance to bacteria, such as in a diabetic foot ulcer, but these situations are not clearly defined. The routine use of systemic antibiotics for chronic wounds should be avoided to reduce the development of resistant bacterial strains within the wound.

Topical antibiotics are frequently used and can be useful. The ointment vehicle may help keep the wound moist, and the bacteria count in a wound may be lowered as a result. With most antibiotics, however, resistant organisms emerge quickly and development of allergic, hypersensitivity reactions are common. Most topical antibiotic ointments should be limited to 3 weeks of therapy to avoid developing a rash or other signs of inflammation as a result of the antibiotic ointment, not bacteria. The expense is substantial, and the benefits are not well demonstrated. Silver sulfadiazine, frequently used for burn care, is also useful for chronic wounds. Its broad spectrum of activity, the lack of relevant drug-resistant plasmids in bacteria, and its low cost make it a good choice.

In recent years, silver-impregnated dressings have become available and achieved widespread acceptance. They have the antibacterial activity of silver ions without the potential for allergy with sulfadiazine, combine a powerful broad-spectrum antibacterial activity without the problems of drug resistance, and have the absorptive activities of many dressings. However, although widely used, questions such as the concentration of silver needed for efficacy await better evidence before their routine use can be justified.

Débriding Agents. Collagenases have been used to débride wounds for 20 years and can be a highly effective adjunct in the treatment of chronic wounds with necrotic tissue. These agents may be used after surgical débridement to help clean a wound and to avoid a painful mechanical débridement. Currently, only one enzymatic agent is approved for reimbursement in the United States. Another method of wound débridement involves the use of medicinal maggots (biologic débridement). Maggots are effective débridement agents that selectively digest nonviable tissue and also secrete bioactive compounds in their secretions that likely impair bacterial growth.

Pharmacologic Agents. Growth factors found naturally in wounds have improved healing in both normal and complex animal wounds. The growth factors with the most evidence for efficacy are PDGF, TGF-β, epidermal growth factor, and members of the FGF family, although IGF-1, interleukin (IL)-1, IL-2, granulocyte-macrophage colony-stimulating factor, and VEGF have also shown improved rates of healing in animal models.[20,21] Clinical trials are in progress, and only becaplermin (PDGF) has been approved by the FDA. PDGF has shown efficacy in accelerating healing for patients with clean, well-vascularized diabetic forefoot ulcers. A limiting factor in these clinical trials has been the variability in patients in terms of both systemic factors that impact healing and the number of variables related specifically to the wounds. The clinical studies are therefore difficult to perform and interpret.

Growth hormone deserves brief mention because it has been used successfully in some situations to reverse the catabolic impact of many severe injuries. Wound healing is a fundamentally anabolic event (creating new tissue), and in the setting of a severe burn, growth hormone administration significantly accelerates donor site healing, presumably because of its effects in minimizing catabolism.

Negative-pressure Wound Therapy. In recent years, negative-pressure wound therapy (NPWT) such as the vacuum-assisted closure (VAC) device has gained increasing acceptance for a wide variety of difficult wounds. This treatment involves the application of a moderate vacuum to an occlusive dressing with a sponge or gauze to allow wicking of the exudates up into the dressing and out of the wound. On theoretical grounds, NPWT is an optimal wound therapy. The negative pressure results in reduction of wound edema and a resulting increase in local tissue perfusion. Continual removal of wound exudates removes the media for bacterial growth and results in removal of the bacteria as well, with a resulting reduction in bacterial burden, and the negative pressure accelerates wound contraction. At the cellular level, the microdeformation placed in cells in the wound bed is thought to upregulate the production of growth factors. NPWT has found uses in the treatment of chronic wounds and difficult acute wounds; for adherence of skin grafts; and, in recent years, in the treatment of open sternotomy wounds and exposed joint prostheses, as well as a variety of other applications. Often, use of NPWT has allowed secondary closure with a skin graft or straightforward secondary closure rather than a complex flap.[22,23]

EXCESSIVE SCARRING

Many factors are involved in the formation of an ideal scar. The most important of these are (a) accurate alignment of sharply incised tissue parallel to the natural lines of resting skin tension, (b) closure of the wound without tension on the epidermis and without underlying dead space, and (c) primary healing without complications such as infection or dehiscence. The patient's genetic makeup and the location of the wound on the body are also important factors. The more negative factors that are associated with a particular wound, the more likely it will form a scar that is less than ideal. In general terms, the three main factors associated with an adverse scar include genetic predisposition, tension, and inflammation. From an evolutionary viewpoint, wound healing has been programmed to be rapid and exuberant to minimize the problems of an open wound. As part of the aging process, the proliferative phase of wound healing becomes less exuberant, and although wound healing is slower, scars are improved (see the remodeling phase

TABLE 4.4

WOUND DRESSINGS

■ CLASSIFICATION	■ COMPOSITION	■ INDICATIONS	■ FUNCTIONS	■ EXAMPLES
Films	Semiocclusive (semipermeable)—polyurethane or copolyester	Acute partial- or full-thickness wounds with minimal exudate Nondraining primarily closed wounds	Mimics skin performance Is water vapor permeable Is water and bacterial impermeable Is retention dressing for gel Is retention dressing for tubes Provides moist environment	Op-site Bioclusive Tegaderm Blisterfilm Visulin
Hydrocolloids	Contain hydrophilic colloidal particles (quar, karaya, gelatin, carboxymethyl cellulose) in an adhesive mass (usually polysorbutylene)	Acute or chronic partial- or full-thickness wounds Stage I to IV decubitus ulcers	Absorbs fluid Débrides soft necrotic tissue by autolysis Protects wounds Provides good adhesiveness without adherence to wound Encourages granulation Promotes reepithelialization Protects wounds from trauma	Cutinova Hydro Duoderm Comfeel Restore Intrasite Ultec J&J ulcer dressing
Hydrogels	Contain 80%–99% water Cross-linked polymer such as polyethyleneoxide, polyvinyl pyrrolidone, or acrylamide	Acute or chronic partial-thickness wounds with minimal exudate	Creates moist environment Usually requires secondary dressing Has low absorbency Débrides minimally Decreases pain Does not adhere to wound	Vigilon Geliperm Elastogel Intrasite gel
Foams	Either hydrophilic or hydrophobic Nonocclusive Usually polyurethane or gel film coated High absorbency	Acute or chronic partial-thickness wounds that are highly secreting and require mechanical débriding	Débrides Has high absorbency Water vapor permeable	Cutinova Plus Lyofoam Allevyn
Impregnates	Fine-mesh gauze impregnated with moisturizing, antibacterial, or bactericidal compounds Nonadherent	Acute or chronic partial-thickness wounds with minimal or moderate exudate	Does not adhere to wound Promotes reepithelization	Aquaphor-Gauze Adaptic Biobrane
Absorptive powders and pastes	Consist of starch, copolymers, or collodial hydrophilic particles Can absorb up to 100 times their weight in fluid	Chronic full-thickness wounds with large amounts of exudate	Has high absorbancy Débrides necrotic and fibrous material from wound	Spand-Gel Geliperm Envisan paste Bard absorption Dressing Duoderm granules Hydrogran Hollister Exudate Absorber

Compiled by M.C. Crossland, RN, Wound Healing Center, Medical College of Virginia, Richmond, VA.

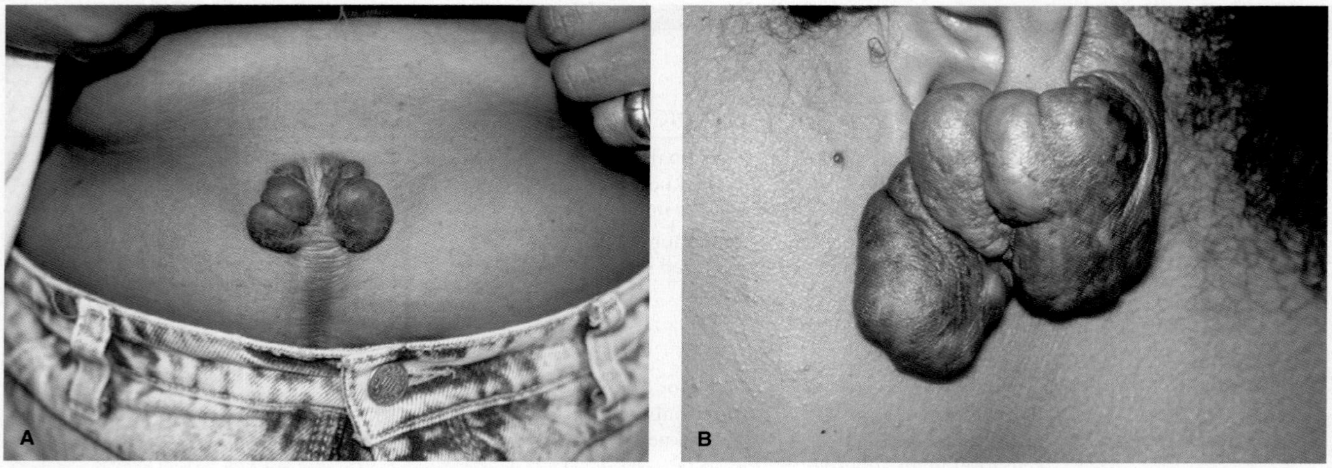

FIGURE 4.11. Keloids. A: This lesion is growing well beyond the border of cesarean section scar. B: The ear lobes are a common location. (Reproduced with permission from Goodheart HP. *Goodheart's Photoguide of Common Skin Disorders,* 2nd ed. Philadelphia, PA: Lippincott Williams & Wilkins; 2003.)

section). The distinctions between an unsightly scar, a hypertrophic scar, and a true keloid can be confusing. An accurate diagnosis of most scars can be made by clinical observation and the history of the lesion.

Keloids

True keloids are uncommon and occur predominantly in dark-skinned people with a genetic predisposition for keloid formation.[7] In most cases, the gene appears to be transmitted in an
9 autosomal dominant pattern. The primary difference between a keloid and a hypertrophic scar is that a keloid extends beyond the boundary of the original tissue injury. It behaves as a benign tumor and extends into or invades the normal surrounding tissue. This creates a scar that is larger than the original wound (Fig. 4.11).

Histologically, keloids contain an overabundance of collagen. The absolute number of fibroblasts is not increased, but the production of collagen continually outpaces the activity of collagenase, resulting in a scar of ever-increasing dimensions. The cause of keloid formation is unknown. Immunoglobulin G levels are increased, which suggests possible autoimmune stimulation resulting in a chronic inflammatory response with continued collagen deposition.

The treatment of keloids is difficult. The cause of keloids is unknown, and the underlying disorder is not resolved by any specific therapy. Some improvement is usually seen with excision followed by intralesional steroid injection.[24] In unresponsive cases, excision followed by a short course of radiotherapy has been successful, but the resulting scar is unpredictable and may potentially be worse. Keloids typically develop several months after injury and rarely, if ever, subside. Although many therapies have been tried, with anecdotal reports of success, none is ideal, and recurrence is frustratingly common.[25]

Hypertrophic Scars

Hypertrophic scars are histologically similar to keloids. They contain an overabundance of dermal collagen. Hypertrophic scars, however, respect the boundaries of the original injury and do not extend into normal unwounded tissue. They have less genetic predisposition, but hypertrophic scars also occur more frequently in Asian and African skin. They are often seen on the upper torso and across flexor surfaces. They usually develop within the first month after wounding and often subside gradually (Fig. 4.12).

Improvement of hypertrophic scars may be obtained with pressure garments, topical silicone gel sheeting applications, or reexcision and closure.[6,26] Reexcision and closure should be considered if conditions of the closure can be improved. This is especially true for wounds that originally healed by secondary intention or were complicated by infection: that is, wounds that were adversely affected by prolonged inflammation. Simple reexcision and closure is unlikely to improve a

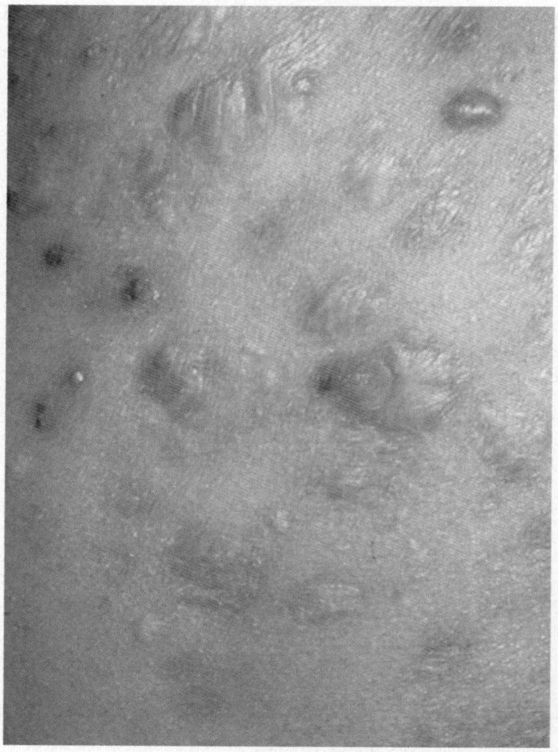

FIGURE 4.12. Hypertrophic scars. These lesions are characteristic of acne scars that occur on the trunk. (Reproduced with permission from Goodheart HP. *Goodheart's Photoguide of Common Skin Disorders,* 2nd ed. Philadelphia, PA: Lippincott Williams & Wilkins; 2003.)

scar that was closed with proper alignment and that healed primarily without complications.[27]

Unsightly Scars

A wound that is closed under tension or without adequate or accurate alignment, or a wound that runs across the lines of natural skin tension, is often unsightly. Surgical excision and closure with attention directed to correcting the underlying cause of the unsightly scar usually results in improvement. When reexcising either a hypertrophic scar or an unsightly scar from other causes, reclosure with attention to relieving mechanical tension by the use of semipermanent or permanent intradermal sutures and everting wound closure, followed by treatment with taping and/or silicone gel sheeting, and judicious use of injected intralesional steroids can result in substantial improvement in the quality of the scar in a high percentage of cases.

FETAL WOUND HEALING AND STEM CELLS: THE POTENTIAL FOR TISSUE REGENERATION

The ultimate and as yet unrealized goal of wound healing research is achieving tissue regeneration as opposed to scar formation. Much interest and research have focused on the process of fetal wound healing and the role of stem cells in tissue repair, as both hold significant potential for the directed manipulation of the healing wound to attain true tissue regeneration.

It has been demonstrated that humans and several other mammalian species undergo fetal skin healing with little or no scar if the injury occurs early enough during gestation.[28,29] The physiologic mechanisms involved in scarless fetal healing have been under active investigation. Adult wounds heal with a significant inflammatory response followed by abundant collagen deposition and remodeling into a mature scar. Numerous studies have shown that fetal wounds heal with little or no inflammation and no excess collagen formation. The fetal wound matrix is also higher in hyaluronic acid than the adult wound. This substance is seen only early in adult healing. Amniotic fluid is rich in hyaluronic acid and may provide the hyaluronic acid found in the fetal wound. Experiments that have exposed adult skin to amniotic fluid, however, demonstrate adult-type healing with scar formation. One important factor is that after the second trimester, fetal wounds begin to heal with scar, suggesting that the increased cell differentiation that occurs with maturation of the fetus is a critical factor in the scarless versus scarring phenotype.

Clearly, the fetal wound differs from the adult wound in several ways. The scarless healing appears multifactorial. Further research may identify factors (i.e., growth factors) that can be applied to wounds to diminish scar formation. This has potentially important application in virtually all of surgery but has proved to be elusive despite aggressive research interest.

Another promising and complementary approach for tissue regeneration has arisen from the realization that bone marrow–derived progenitor cells participate in the process of tissue repair. It is now appreciated that tissue hypoxia in a wound upregulates HIF-1, which in turn causes release of growth factors including VEGF and SDF-1. In addition to their well-recognized roles in angiogenesis and lymphocyte migration, respectively, both also serve to recruit marrow-derived progenitor cells such as endothelial progenitor cells and mesenchymal stem cells to the site of injury. The identification of other signals that mobilize and recruit stem cells to wounds is an area of active inquiry, as are the morphogenic pathways and cues that direct stem cells to develop into different tissue lineages. The role that such cells play in tissue repair is currently being elucidated, and the potential of these cells to augment healing in disease states such as diabetes, as well as in clinical states associated with impaired healing such as advanced age, holds tremendous promise for all fields of surgery.[30]

Tissue-derived stem cells also play a role in healing. It is likely that epithelial stem cells and dermis-resident cells have previously unappreciated functions in wound repair. The potential of other tissue-derived stem cells, such as adipose tissue–derived stem cells, in tissue repair is currently an area of intense research. 10 The directed manipulation of stem and progenitor cells will likely define future advances in regenerative medicine, which is a direct offshoot of wound healing science.

References

1. Singer AJ, Clark RA. Cutaneous wound healing. *N Engl J Med* 1999;341:738.
2. Leibovich SJ, Ross R. The role of the macrophage in wound repair: a study with hydrocortisone and antimacrophage serum. *Am J Pathol* 1975;78:71.
3. Cross KC, Mustoe TA. Growth factors in wound healing. *Surg Clin North Am* 2003;83:531–546.
4. Madden JW, Peacock EE. Studies on the biology of collagen during wound healing. I. Rate of collagen synthesis and deposition in cutaneous wounds of the rat. *Surgery* 1968;64:288.
5. Ruoslahti E. Stretching is good for a cell. *Science* 1997;276:1345–1346.
6. Mustoe TA. Editorial: treatment of scars and keloids. *BMJ* 2004;328:1329–1330.
7. Mustoe TA, Cooter R, Gold M, et al. International clinical guidelines for scar management. *Plast Reconstr Surg* 2002;110:560–572.
8. Galiano RD, Mustoe TA. Wound care. In: Thorne CH, ed. *Grabb and Smith's Plastic Surgery*, 6th ed. Philadelphia, PA: Lippincott Williams and Wilkins; 2006.
9. Peacock EE Jr. *Wound Repair*, 3rd ed. Philadelphia, PA: WB Saunders; 1984:23–32.
10. Winter GD, Scales JT. Effect of air drying and dressings on the surface of a wound. *Nature* 1963;197:91.
11. Jonsson K, Jensen JA, Goodson WH, et al. Tissue oxygenation, anemia, and perfusion in relation to wound healing in surgical patients. *Ann Surg* 1991;214:6.
12. Davidson JD, Mustoe TA. Commentary. Oxygen in wound healing: more than a nutrient. *Wound Repair Regen* 2001;9:175–177.
13. Mustoe TA. Understanding chronic wounds: a unifying hypothesis on their pathogenesis, and implications for therapy. *Am J Surg* 2004;187:S65–S70.
14. James GA, Swogger E, Wolcott R, et al. Biofilms in chronic wounds. *Wound Repair Regen* 2008;16:37.
15. Gross A, Cutright DE, Bhaskar SN. Effectiveness of pulsating water jet lavage in treatment of contaminated crushed wounds. *Am J Surg* 1972;124:373.
16. Seifter E, Rettura G, Padawer J, et al. Impaired wound healing in streptozotocin diabetes: prevention by supplemental vitamin A. *Ann Surg* 1981;194:42.
17. Ehrlich P, Tarver H, Hunt TK. Inhibitory effect of vitamin E on collagen synthesis and wound repair. *Ann Surg* 1972;175:235.
18. LaVan FB, Hunt TK. Oxygen and wound healing. *Clin Plast Surg* 1990;17:463.
19. Carver N, Leigh IM. Synthetic dressings. *Int J Dermatol* 1992;31:10.
20. Mustoe TA, Pierce GF, Thomason A, et al. Accelerated healing of incisional wounds in rats induced by transforming growth factor-β. *Science* 1987;237:1333.
21. Brown GL, Nanney LB, Griffen J, et al. Enhancement of wound healing by topical treatment with epidermal growth factor. *N Engl J Med* 1989;321:76.
22. Argenta LC, Morykwas MJ. Vacuum-assisted closure: a new method for wound control and treatment: clinical experience. *Ann Plast Surg* 1997;38:563–577.
23. Moues CM, Vos MC, van den Bemd GJ, et al. Bacterial load in relation to vacuum-assisted closure wound therapy: a prospective randomized trial. *Wound Repair Regen* 2004;12:11–17.
24. Griffith H. The treatment of keloids with triamcinolone acetonide. *Plast Reconstr Surg* 1966;38:202.
25. Lawrence WT. In search of the optimal treatment of keloids: report of a series and a review of the literature. *Ann Plast Surg* 1991;27:164.
26. Ahn ST, Monafo WW, Mustoe TA. Topical silicone gel: a new treatment for hypertrophic scars. *Surgery* 1989;106:781.
27. Khouri RK, Mustoe TA. Trends in the treatment of hypertrophic scars. *Adv Plast Reconstr Surg* 1991;8:129.
28. Mast BA, Diegelmann RF, Krummel TM, et al. Scarless wound healing in the mammalian fetus. *Surg Gynecol Obstet* 1992;174:441.
29. Siebert JW, Burd AR, McCarthy JG, et al. Fetal wound healing: a biochemical study of scarless healing. *Plast Reconstr Surg* 1990;85:503.
30. Gurtner GC, Werner S, Barrandon Y, et al. Wound repair and regeneration. *Nature* 2008;453:314.

CHAPTER 5 ■ HEMOSTASIS

PETER K. HENKE AND THOMAS W. WAKEFIELD

KEY POINTS

1. At the same time that thrombin forms, natural anticoagulant mechanisms oppose further thrombin formation and help to localize thrombin activity to areas of vascular injury. Just as thrombin generation is key to coagulation, antithrombin is the central anticoagulant protein.
2. The endothelial cell acts as a nonthrombogenic surface, and inflammation tips the balance to the procoagulant state.
3. Thrombosis and inflammation are closely linked, and may perpetuate each other. Leukocytes and chemokines are involved with normal deep venous thrombosis resolution.
4. Heparin agents are the primary anticoagulants for acute venous and arterial thrombosis, while a vitamin K antagonist is standard for long-term anticoagulation.
5. Factor VIII and IX deficiency states are involved in hemophilia A and B and von Willebrand disease.
6. Heparin-induced thrombocytopenia (HIT) occurs in 0.6% to 30% of patients in whom heparin is given; severe thrombocytopenia associated with thrombosis (HITTS) is much less frequent. Cessation of heparin is critical.

BASIC CONSIDERATIONS

Coagulation is an essential homeostatic mechanism for survival and involves tightly controlled processes to maintain vascular integrity including thrombosis localization, amplification, and neutralization. These coordinated steps occur at the vessel, cellular, and subcellular level. Understanding of pathologic thrombosis and its basic hemostatic processes is essential for surgeons. Thrombosis, directly or indirectly, is the underlying leading cause of death in the world.

Platelets form the initial hemostatic plug and are locally activated and aggregation induced (Fig. 5.1). Platelet aggregation is mediated by receptors that are part of the mammalian integrin family. This family includes the β_1 family, mediating platelet interaction with cells, collagen, fibronectin, and laminin; the β_2 family (LeuCAM), present on leukocytes mediating interactions between leukocytes and other cells important in inflammation; and the β_3 family (cytoadhesion), including the megakaryocyte-specific glycoprotein (Gp) IIb/IIIa receptor and the vitronectin receptor present on platelets and other cells.[1] Platelet aggregation is mediated by GpIIb/IIIa, which binds fibrinogen, von Willebrand factor (vWF), fibronectin, vitronectin, and thrombospondin to activated platelets. These high-density receptors are hidden on inactivated platelets and become exposed on the surface of activated platelets.

Once stimulated, activated platelets contract, with externalization of negatively charged procoagulant phospholipids, including phosphatidylserine and phosphatidylinositol (termed *platelet factor 3*).[2] This allows for the coagulation proteins to assemble on the surfaces of platelets, accelerating the coagulation reaction.[3,4] Platelet membranes contribute critical surfaces for coagulation complex assembly. During platelet activation, granules release their contents of calcium, serotonin, adenosine diphosphate (ADP), and adenosine triphosphate[3] and membranes are exposed that are rich in receptors for factors Va and VIIIa,[5,6] as well as fibrinogen, vWF, and ADP, a potent activator of other platelets. vWF is responsible for platelet adhesion through binding to GpIb,[7] whereas fibrinogen forms bridges between activated platelets by binding to GpIIb/IIIa on adjacent stimulated platelets.[8] The GpIIb/IIIa receptor contains a binding site for the tripeptide sequence arginine-glycine-aspartic acid (RGD), which is common to many of the receptor proteins. Unstimulated platelets can also attach to immobilized fibrinogen by the same receptor.[9] Platelet activation leads to the release of arachidonic acid metabolites such as thromboxane A_2, a powerful initiator of platelet aggregation.[10] Platelets also release microparticles (MPs), rich in tissue factor (TF) and other procoagulant products, that further accelerate the coagulation process.

Once the platelet plug has formed, the stage is set for coagulation protein assembly (Fig. 5.2). Initiating agents for coagulation include subendothelial collagen and TF, usually from vascular injury.[11] There is also growing evidence that blood-borne TF associated with leukocytes, or circulating in soluble form, is also involved with venous thrombogenesis.[12] Leukocyte adhesion to platelets may trigger leukocyte activation, causing recruitment of blood-borne TF onto the surface of leukocytes associated with thrombus or recruitment of TF-positive leukocytes onto the growing thrombus.[13] TF, both blood-borne and local, activates the extrinsic pathway of coagulation by complexing with activated factor VII (VIIa) and activating factors IX and X to factors IXa and Xa.[12] The enzyme responsible for the initial activation of factor VII is unknown. However, factors Xa and VIIa amplify activation of factor VII. Activated factor X, activated factor V (Va), ionized calcium, and factor II (prothrombin) form on the platelet phospholipid surface to initiate the prothrombinase complex, which catalyzes the formation of thrombin faster than can be achieved with factor Xa alone[3] (Fig. 5.3). When the amount of TF is limited, activation of factor IX rather than factor X is favored,[14] allowing for coagulation in situations of low TF concentration.

Thrombin is central to coagulation and acts to cleave fibrinopeptide A (FPA) from the α chain of fibrinogen and fibrinopeptide B (FPB) from the β chain. This leads to the release of fibrinopeptides and the formation of new fibrin monomers, which then cross-link, resulting in fibrin polymerization. Thrombin also activates factor XIII, which catalyzes the cross-linking of fibrin to make the clot firm, activates platelets, and activates factors V and VIII, two nonenzymatic cofactors, to Va and VIIIa.[3] This is important because only activated factors Va and VIIIa are involved in coagulation. Factor XIIIa also cross-links other plasma proteins, such as fibronectin and α_2-antitrypsin, resulting in their incorporation into clot.[15]

The intrinsic pathway of blood coagulation requires activation of factor XI to XIa. This may occur both by the contact activation system through activation of factor XII, plasma prekallikrein, and high-molecular-weight kininogen and, more

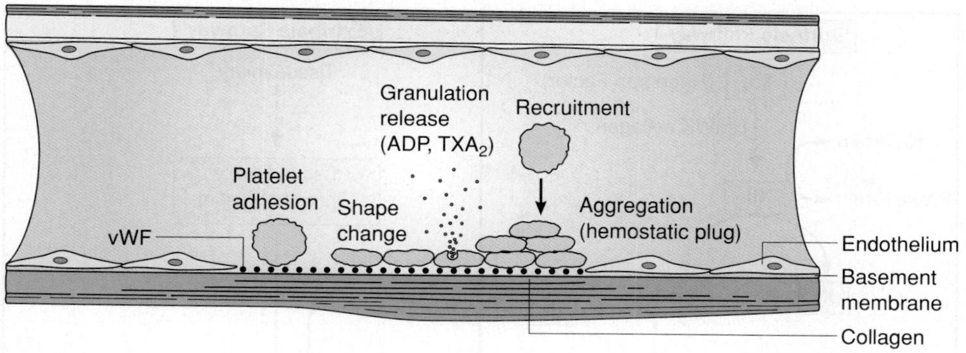

FIGURE 5.1. Primary hemostasis is achieved initially with a platelet aggregation as illustrated. Note that platelet adhesion, shape change, granule release followed by recruitment, and the hemostatic plug at the area of subendothelial collagen and collagen exposure are the initial events for thrombus formation.

important, through thrombin with negatively charged surfaces.[16] Factor XIa activates factor XI autocatalytically and also catalyzes the conversion of factor IX to IXa. After activation, factor VIIIa dissociates from vWF and assembles with factors IXa and X. Factor IXa, factor X, ionized calcium, and thrombin-activated factor VIII (VIIIa) then assemble on the platelet surface in a complex called the *Xase complex* to catalyze the activation of factor X to Xa[3] (Fig. 5.3). Factor Xa then shunts into the prothrombinase complex for further amplification of thrombin formation. The importance of a mechanism of factor XI activation independent of the contact activation system is apparent because patients deficient in those factors of the contact activation system, including factor XI, bleed, whereas patients deficient in factor XII, prekallikrein, and high-molecular-weight kininogen do not usually bleed.[15] The contact activation system is the most important coagulation process involved in extracorporeal bypass circuits, including cardiopulmonary bypass and extracorporeal membrane oxygenation (ECMO).

NATURAL ANTICOAGULANT MECHANISMS

1 At the same time that thrombin forms, natural anticoagulant mechanisms oppose further thrombin formation and help to localize thrombin activity to areas of vascular injury. Just as thrombin generation is key to coagulation, antithrombin (AT) is the central anticoagulant protein (Fig. 5.4). This glycoprotein of 70-kD molecular weight binds to thrombin, preventing the removal of FPA and FPB from fibrinogen; prevents the activation of factors V and VIII; and inhibits the activation and aggregation of platelets. In addition, AT directly inhibits factors IXa, Xa, and XIa.

A second natural anticoagulant is activated protein C (APC), which inactivates factors Va[17,18] and VIIIa, thus reducing the Xase and prothrombinase complex acceleration of the rate of thrombin formation. In the circulation, protein C is activated on endothelial cell surfaces by thrombin complexed with one of its receptors, thrombomodulin.[19–21] The formation of this thrombin–thrombomodulin (TM) complex accelerates the activation of protein C compared with thrombin alone. Thrombin, at the same time, by binding to TM, loses its platelet-activating activity[22] as well as its enzymatic activity for fibrinogen and factor V.[23] Protein S is a cofactor for APC.

Another innate anticoagulant is tissue factor pathway inhibitor (TFPI). This factor is bound to low-density lipoprotein (LDL) in plasma, and is also called lipoprotein-associated coagulation inhibitor. The protein binds to the TF–VIIa complex, inhibiting the activation of factor X to Xa and the formation of the prothrombinase complex.[15,24] A fourth natural anticoagulant is heparin cofactor II.[25] Its

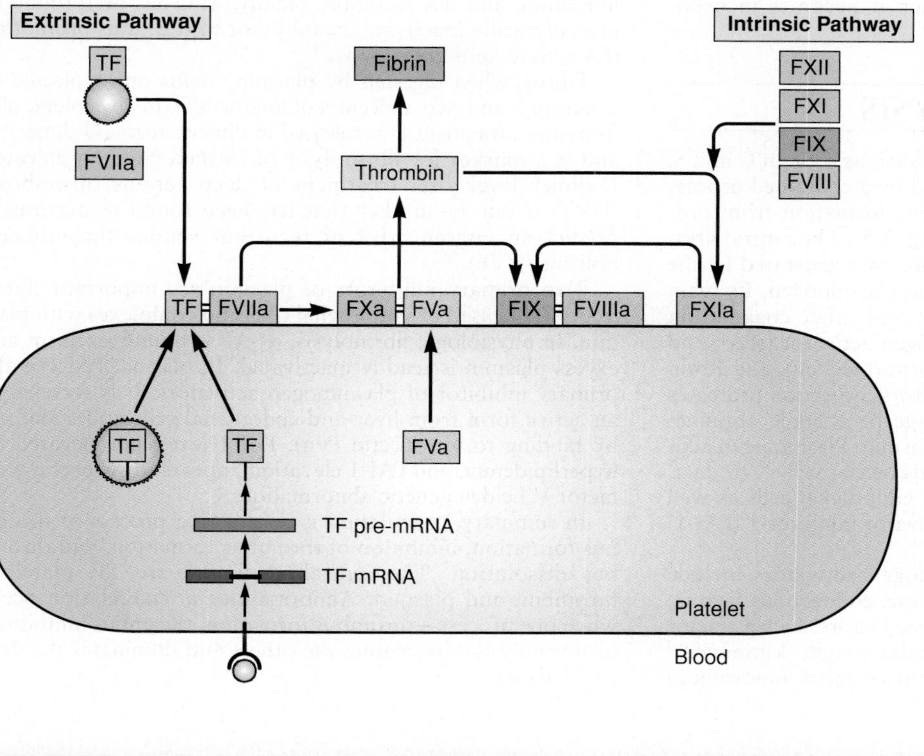

FIGURE 5.2. On the platelet surface, the clotting cascade involves both the intrinsic and extrinsic pathways. Tissue factor mRNA is transcribed and translated to active tissue factor, which activates factor VII to VIIa as a primary event.

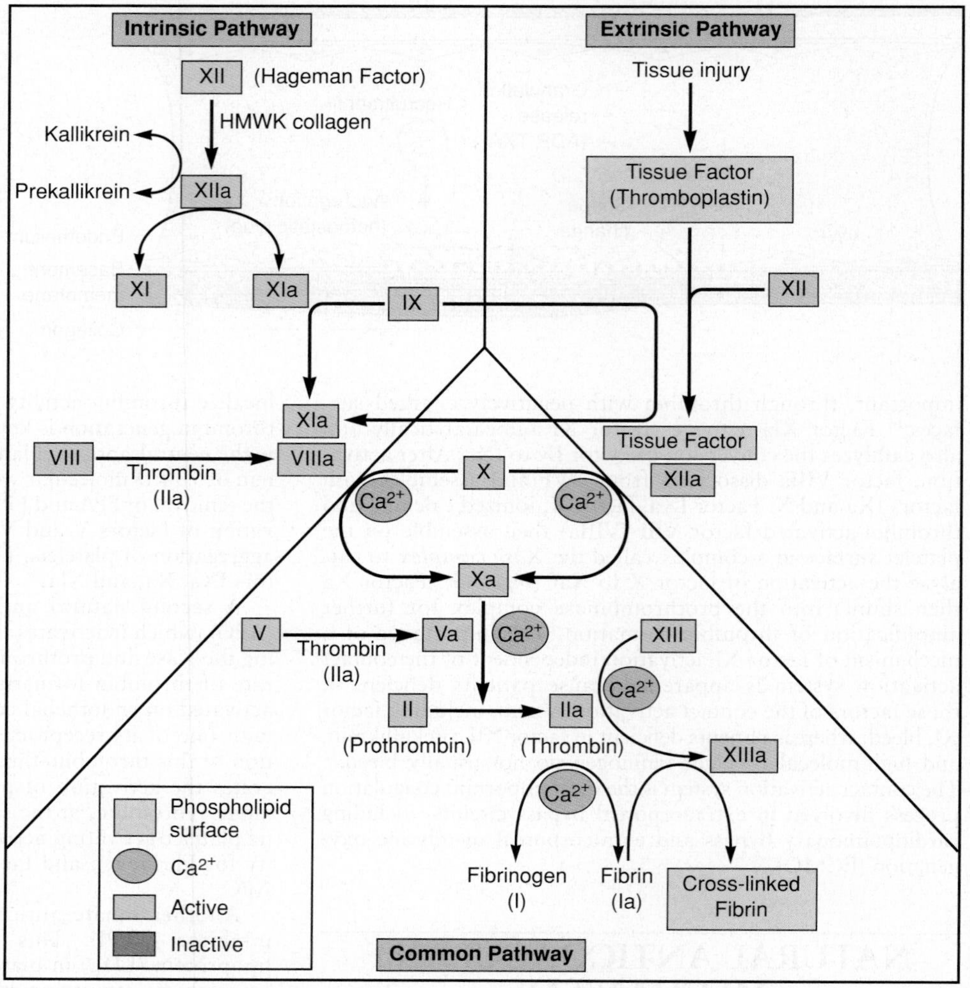

FIGURE 5.3. The classical pathway showing the interface between the intrinsic pathway, extrinsic pathway, and common pathway is illustrated with the ultimate production of thrombin. This catalyzes fibrin from fibrinogen and then cross-links the fibrin to form a stable clot.

concentration in plasma is estimated to be significantly less than that of AT, and its action is implicated primarily in the regulation of thrombin formation in extravascular tissues. Finally, thrombin is inactivated when it becomes incorporated into the clot.

FIBRINOLYSIS

In addition to natural anticoagulants such as protein C and S, physiologic clot formation is balanced by a contained process of clot lysis, which prevents thrombus formation from proceeding outside of the injured area (Fig. 5.5). The central fibrinolytic enzyme is plasmin, a serine protease generated by the proteolytic cleavage of the proenzyme plasminogen. Its main substrates include fibrin, fibrinogen, and other coagulation factors. Plasminogen, tissue plasminogen activator (tPA), and α_2-antiplasmin (α_2-AP) become incorporated into the fibrin clot as it forms.[3] Plasminogen activators are serine proteases that activate plasminogen, by cleavage of a single arginine-valine peptide bond, to the enzyme plasmin. Plasminogen activation provides localized proteolytic activity.[26–28] In fact, thrombin promotes tPA release from endothelial cells as well as the production of plasminogen activator inhibitor-1 (PAI-1) from endothelial cells.[29,30]

The major categories of plasminogen activators include exogenous factors, such as streptokinase; endogenous factors, such as tPA and urokinase; and intrinsic factors, such as factor XII, prekallikrein, and high-molecular-weight kininogen.[3] These later factors of the contact system are more important in clot lysis than thrombus formation. These enzymes may also liberate bradykinin from high-molecular-weight kininogen, resulting in an increase in vascular permeability, prostacyclin liberation, and tPA secretion. Finally, APC has been found to proteolytically inactivate the inhibitor to tPA, thus promoting tPA activity and fibrinolysis.[31]

Fibrin, when digested by plasmin, yields one molecule of fragment E and two molecules of fragment D. In physiologic clot formation, fragment D is released in dimeric form (D-dimer)[3,15] and is a marker for fibrinolysis of formed clot. An elevated D-dimer level after treatment of deep venous thrombosis (DVT) is one biomarker that has been found to accurately predict an ongoing risk of recurrent venous thromboembolisms (VTE).[32]

Two primary inhibitors of plasmin are important. First, α_2-AP is released by endothelial cells and complexes with plasmin. In physiologic fibrinolysis, α_2-AP is bound to fibrin and excess plasmin is readily inactivated. In plasma, PAI-1 is the primary inhibitor of plasminogen activators. It is secreted in an active form from liver and endothelial cells and stabilized by binding to vitronectin (Vn). PAI-1 levels are elevated by hyperlipidemia, and PAI-1 elevation appears to synergize with factor V Leiden genetic abnormalities.[33]

In summary, coagulation is an ongoing process of thrombus formation, inhibition of thrombus formation, and thrombus dissolution. The central mediators are TF, platelets, thrombin, and plasmin. Abnormalities in coagulation occur when one process—thrombus formation, thrombus inhibition, or fibrinolysis—overcomes the others and dominates the delicate balance.

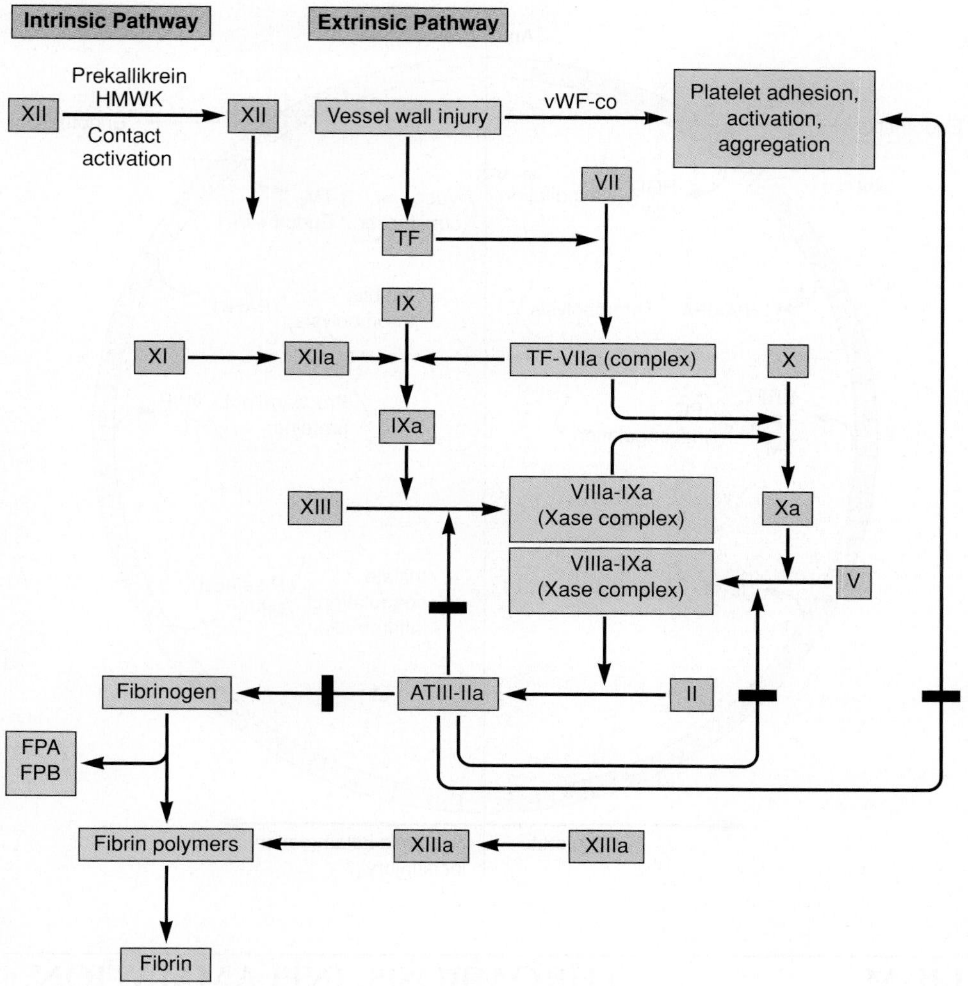

FIGURE 5.4. Antithrombin is a primary anticoagulant. Note that antithrombin complexes with IIa to inhibit fibrin polymerization, as well as factor Xa, and inactivates factor Va and VIIIa.

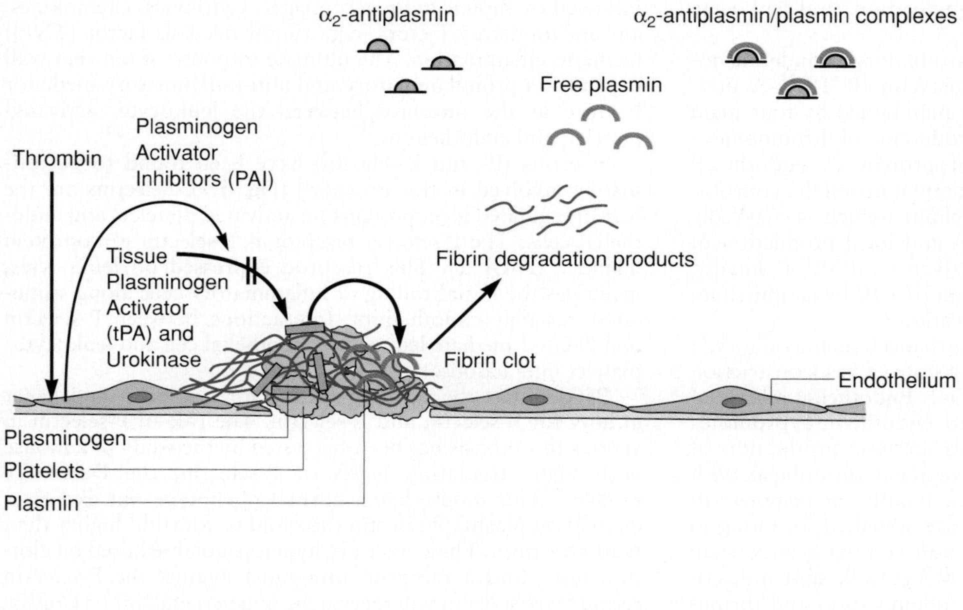

FIGURE 5.5. Hemostasis with thrombus production is a tight and intricate process that is tightly confined. Balancing thrombus production is tissue plasmin activator and urokinase plasminogen activator, which activate plasmin and cause thrombolysis. These are balanced by plasminogen activator inhibitor-1 and α_2-antiplasmin. Free plasmin is complexed rapidly. Fibrin degradation products, such as D-dimer, are produced.

SCIENTIFIC PRINCIPLES

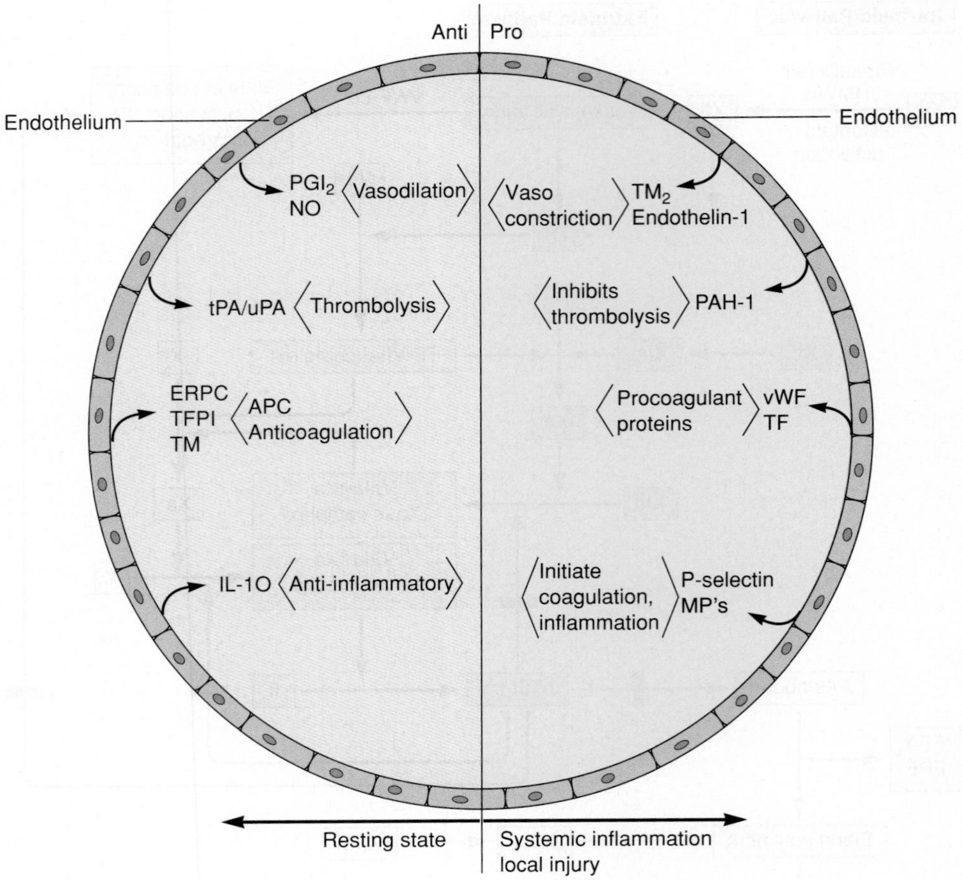

FIGURE 5.6. The endothelium is a primary interface allowing anticoagulant functions in the resting state, with prostacyclin, nitric oxide, plasminogen activators, and thrombomodulin. Procoagulant proteins are expressed on activated endothelium including selectins; procoagulant proteins, such as the von Willebrand factor; tissue factor; and plasminogen activator inhibitor-1.

ENDOTHELIUM AND HEMOSTASIS

Through its ability to express procoagulants and anticoagulant factors, vasoconstrictors and vasodilators, and key cell adhesion molecules and cytokines, the endothelial cell is a key regulator of hemostasis[34] (Fig. 5.6). Vascular endothelium maintains a vasodilatory and local fibrinolytic state in which coagulation, platelet adhesion and activation, and leukocyte activation are suppressed.

Endothelial products that are vasodilatory include adeno-
2 sine, nitric oxide (NO), and prostacyclin (PGI_2).[35] A nonthrombogenic endothelial surface is maintained by four main mechanisms including endothelial production of thrombomodulin and subsequent activation of protein C, endothelial expression of surface heparan- and dermatan-sulfate, constitutive expression of TFPI by endothelium (which is markedly accelerated in response to heparin), and local production of tPA and urokinase plasminogen activator (uPA).[34,36] Finally, the elaboration of NO and interleukin (IL)-10 by endothelium inhibits leukocyte adhesion and activation.[35]

During states of endothelial disturbances such as injury, a prothrombotic and proinflammatory state of vasoconstriction is supported by the endothelial surface. Endothelial release of platelet-activating factor (PAF) and endothelin-1 promotes vasoconstriction.[36] Endothelial cells increase production of vWF, TF, PAI-1, and factor V to augment thrombosis with exposure to prothrombotic stimuli. Finally, in response to endothelial injury, endothelial cells are activated, resulting in increased surface expression of cell adhesion molecules (such as P- or E-selectin), and promotes leukocyte adhesion and activation. This initiates and amplifies inflammation and thrombosis.

THROMBOSIS, INFLAMMATION, AND RESOLUTION

After venous thrombosis, an acute to chronic inflammatory response occurs in the vein wall and thrombus, leading to thrombus amplification and organization and vein recanalization (often at the expense of vein wall and vein valvular damage). Initially, there is an increase in neutrophils in the vein wall followed by monocytes/macrophages. Cytokines, chemokines, and inflammatory factors (e.g., tumor necrosis factor [TNF]) facilitate inflammation. The ultimate response of the vein wall depends on proinflammatory and anti-inflammatory mediator balance at the interface between the leukocyte, activated platelet, and endothelium.[37]

Selectins (P- and E-selectin) have been found to be intimately involved in this process[38] (Fig. 5.7). Selectins are the first upregulated glycoproteins on activated platelets and endothelial cells. The P-selectin receptor is P-selectin glycoprotein ligand-1 (PSGL-1). This receptor, expressed on leukocytes, facilitates the initial rolling of inflammatory cells along stimulated vascular endothelium. Interactions between P-selectin and PSGL-1 mediate leukocyte–endothelial cell and leukocyte–platelet interactions.

PSGL-1 has the greatest affinity for P-selectin and lesser affinity for E-selectin and L-selectin. The role of P-selectin in venous thrombosis has been suggested by the study of a mouse with high circulating levels of P-selectin, the Delta CT mouse.[39] This mouse has a normal phenotype but expresses circulating plasma P-selectin threefold to fourfold higher than wild-type mice. These mice are hypercoagulable based on clotting tests, and a receptor antagonist against the P-selectin receptor (rPSGL-Ig) will reverse the hypercoagulability. Consistently, wild-type mice administered soluble P-selectin become

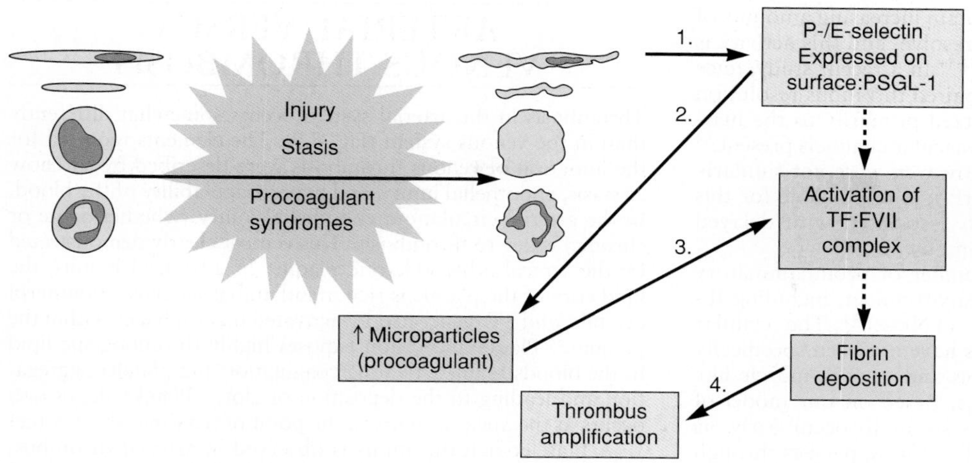

FIGURE 5.7. The interaction between stasis injury and procoagulant syndromes are represented by Virchow's triad. Endothelial and vascular injury causes leukocytes and platelets to express P- and E-selectin and the P-selectin glycoprotein ligand-1 (PSGL-1) receptor. Microparticles are released, which express tissue factor. This stimulates the coagulation pathway, fibrin production, and thrombus amplification.

hypercoagulable. In models of venous thrombosis, P-selectin inhibition given prophylactically decreases thrombosis in a dose-dependent fashion and can treat established venous thrombosis as effectively as heparin without anticoagulation.[40,41]

Microparticles (<1 micron fragments) may be central for P-selectin's effect. It is believed that with initial thrombosis, selectin upregulation leads to MP formation. These procoagulant MPs, which may express TF, are then recruited into the area of developing thrombosis, amplifying the process. Consistently, P-selectin and E-selectin gene deficiency results in less MP formation and less thrombosis.[42] In a mouse model of inferior vena cava (IVC) thrombosis, the Delta CT mouse has increased thrombosis, associated with elevated levels of MPs.[42] In a similar experimental study, the generation of procoagulant activity was shown to be dependent on P-selectin: PSGL-1 interactions related to MP formation.[43] The procoagulant nature of these MPs was demonstrated by their ability to normalize bleeding in factor VIII–deficient mice.

Inflammatory cells are important to the process of thrombus recanalization and organization[38] (Fig. 5.8). Thrombus DVT resolution resembles wound healing and involves profibrotic growth factors, collagen deposition, and matrix metalloproteinase (MMP) expression and activation. The fact that leukocytes invade the thrombus in a specific sequence suggests their importance in the normal thrombus resolution.[44]

❸

The first cell type in the thrombus is the neutrophil (polymorphonuclear leukocytes [PMNs]). Although PMNs may cause vein wall injury, they are essential for early thrombus resolution by promoting both fibrinolysis and collagenolysis.[45,46] In a rat model of stasis DVT, neutropenia was associated with larger thrombi at 2 and 7 days and was correlated with increased thrombus fibrosis and significantly lower thrombus levels of both uPA and MMP-9.[47] Neutropenic cancer patients are not protected from DVT, and multiple neutropenic episodes are associated with recurrent VTE in patients with malignant disease who required filter placement due to a failure of, or contraindication to, anticoagulation.[48]

The monocyte is likely the most important cell for later DVT resolution. Monocyte influx into the thrombus peaks at day 8 after thrombogenesis and correlates with elevated monocyte chemotactic protein-1 (MCP-1) levels,[49] which has been associated with DVT resolution.[50] Targeted deletion of the CC receptor-2 (CCR-2 KO) in the mouse model of stasis thrombosis was associated with late impairment of thrombus resolution, probably via impaired MMP-2 and MMP-9 activity. We also found that CCR-2 KO mice with stasis thrombosis supplemented with exogenous interferon-γ had full restoration of thrombus resolution, in part due to recovery of MMP-2 and MMP-9 activities, and without an increase in thrombus monocyte influx.[51]

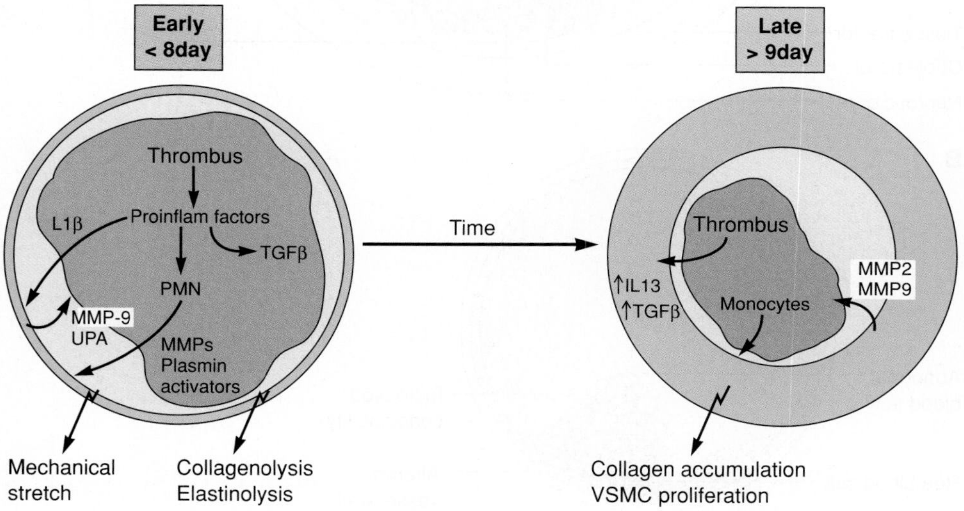

FIGURE 5.8. The proposed resolution mechanism involves both early thrombolysis with a large distending clot and then, over time, a fibrotic thrombus that resembles scar tissue as produced. Note that proinflammatory factors, as well as neutrophils and matrix metalloproteinases, are present early with subsequent vein wall injury related to collagenolysis and elastinolysis. Later, vascular smooth muscle cell proliferation appears to occur, with thrombus resolution and an increase in profibrotic growth factors such as interleukin-13 and transforming growth factor-β. This promotes collagen accumulation.

Thrombi have been found to contain increasing amounts of both tPA and uPA activity as they resolve, and this activity is expressed by invading monocytes.[52,53] In a recent study, mice genetically deleted for uPA had impaired thrombus resolution with reduced cell infiltration restricted primarily to the margins of the thrombus, with few neovascular channels present.[54] Mice genetically deleted for tPA, however, were not similarly affected, suggesting that uPA, not tPA, is responsible for this activity. Absence of uPA was also associated with delayed monocyte recruitment into the thrombus.

As the thrombus resolves, a number of proinflammatory factors are released into the local environment, including IL-1β and tumor necrosis factor-α (TNF-α).[44] The cellular sources of these different mediators have not been specifically defined but likely include leukocytes and smooth muscle like cells within the resolving thrombus. Based on our model of stasis DVT in the rat, elastinolysis seems to occur early, as measured by an increase in vein wall stiffness; persists through 14 days; and is accompanied by elevated MMP-2 and MMP-9 activities. However, early vein wall collagenolysis rather than deposition seems to occur within the first 7 days, representing an acute response to injury.[55]

Taken together, inflammation is important for thrombus organization and recanalization, with neutrophils setting the early stage for later monocyte activity.

ARTERIAL VERSUS VENOUS THROMBOSIS

Thrombosis in the arterial system occurs somewhat differently than in the venous system (Fig. 5.9). The elements required for the initiation of venous thrombosis were described by Virchow as stasis, endothelial injury, and hypercoagulability of the blood. In the arterial circulation, endothelial injury (whether acute or chronic) is key to thrombosis. This is most clearly demonstrated by the typical atherosclerotic plaque. In advanced lesions, the lipid core of the plaque is rich in inflammatory cells, cholesterol crystals, and TF (generated by activated macrophages within the plaque).[56] Plaque ulceration exposes highly thrombogenic lipid to the bloodstream, activating coagulation and platelet aggregation and leading to the deposition of clot.[57] Platelet deposition occurs at the apex of stenosis, the point of maximal shear force.

A platelet-rich thrombus is observed in arterial thrombus, while in contrast, venous blood stasis and changes in its composition (leading to hypercoagulability) incite the formation of thrombus from local procoagulant events, including small endothelial disruptions at venous confluences, saccules, and valve pockets. Hypercoagulable states have classically been highly associated with VTE, but do play a role in cardiovascular disease as well. For example, both factor V Leiden and

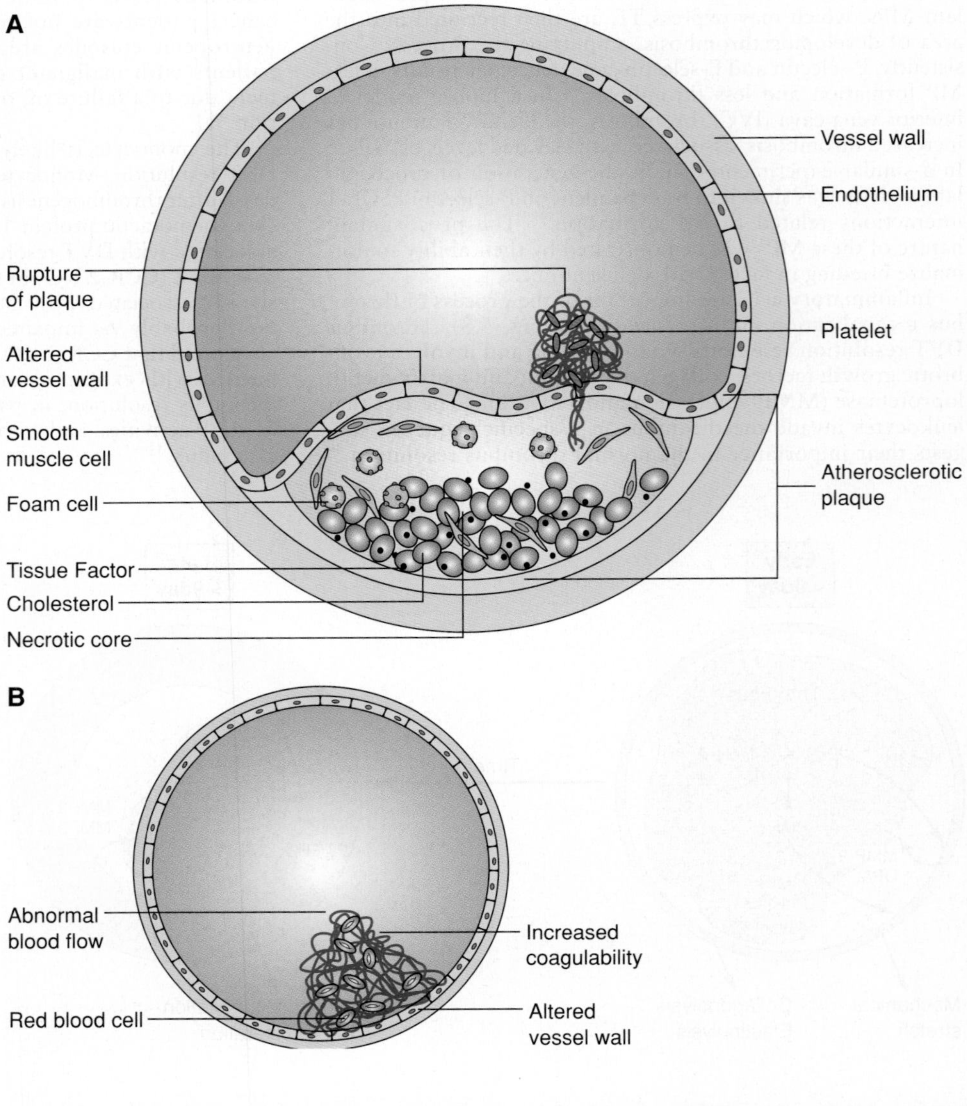

FIGURE 5.9. **A:** Depicted here is the typical atherosclerotic thrombotic nidus, which includes rupture of a plaque, composed of smooth muscle, foam cells, and leukocytes. Platelets are the primary intermediary in arterial thrombosis, as well as tissue factor. **B:** Increased coagulability, as well as vessel wall changes with procoagulant tissue factor expression, promotes thrombosis.

TABLE 5.1

FREQUENCY OF THROMBOSIS DUE TO HYPERCOAGULABLE STATES

HYPERCOAGULABLE STATE	FREQUENCY (%)
Factor V Leiden	20–60
Hyperhomocysteinemia	10
PT G20210A	4–6
Protein C deficiency	3–5
Protein S deficiency	2–3
Dysfibrinogenemia	1–3
Antithrombin	1–2
Dysplasminogenemia	<1

PT, prothrombin.

prothrombin 20210 A mutation are associated with coronary artery disease and stroke.[58]

PROCOAGULANT STATES

Refer to Tables 5.1 to 5.3 and Algorithm 5.1.

ACQUIRED PROCOAGULANT STATES

Most thrombotic clinical episodes have a proximate cause, although environmental risks and genetic predispositions to thrombosis may account for many of the VTE that manifest clinically. Risk factors for arterial thrombosis are primarily related to atherosclerosis, and are detailed elsewhere.

The most common risk factors for venous thrombosis are prior DVT, malignancy, immobility, intravenous catheters, increased age, major surgery, trauma, infections such as pneumonia and urinary tract infection, and certain cytotoxic chemotherapy regimens.[59–61] Certain medications such as oral contraceptives and hormonal replacement therapies also increase the risk of VTE.

Of primary importance to surgeons is how to best estimate perioperative VTE risk and apply appropriate prophylaxis. This can be done with a screening form, such as that devised by Caprini[62] (Fig. 5.10). Essentially, this is a focused assessment of VTE risks related to current illnesses and history that may not be fully covered in the routine history and physical examination. The recommendations are also well detailed in the routinely updated American College of Chest Physicians VTE evidence-based guidelines.[63] The higher the risk, the more intensive the prophylaxis is. For example, an outpatient hernia patient may require no prophylaxis outside of early ambulation, whereas an obese patient having a hip replacement would be best treated with anticoagulation as well as sequential compression devices for the lower extremities. However, all patients should be assessed for VTE risk. This is a quality and safety measure by U.S. governing bodies such as the Joint Commission and Centers for Medicare and Medicaid Services.

TABLE 5.2

SEVERITY OF VTE DUE TO HYPERCOAGULABLE STATES

High risk for thrombosis
- AT deficiency
- Protein C deficiency
- Protein S deficiency
- HIT/HITTS
- Antiphospholipid antibody syndrome

Lower risk for thrombosis
- Factor V Leiden
- Hyperhomocysteinemia
- PT G20210A
- Dysfibrinogenemia
- Dysplasminogenemia
- Elevated factors VIII, IX, and XI

AT, antithrombin; HIT, heparin-induced thrombocytopenia; HITTS, heparin-induced thrombocytopenia and thrombosis syndrome; PT, prothrombin; VTE, venous thromboembolism.

TABLE 5.3

ANATOMIC LOCATION OF VTE DUE TO HYPERCOAGULABLE STATES

Arterial
- Elevated fibrinogen
- Abnormal platelet aggregation
- Atherosclerosis
- Lipoprotein(a)

Both arterial and venous
- Hyperhomocysteinemia
- HITTS
- Antiphospholipid antibody
- Elevated PAI-1

Venous
- AT
- Protein C
- Protein S
- Factor V Leiden
- PT G20210A
- Dysfibrinogenemia
- Elevated factors XI, IX, and VIII

AT, antithrombin; HITTS, heparin-induced thrombocytopenia and thrombosis syndrome; PAI-1, plasminogen activator inhibitor; PT, prothrombin; VTE, venous thromboembolism.

Lupus Anticoagulant/Antiphospholipid Syndrome (Antiphospholipid Antibody)

This condition, despite its name, is a prothrombotic state and deserves expanded discussion. The antiphospholipid antibody syndrome consists of an elevated antiphospholipid antibody titer in association with thrombosis, recurrent fetal loss, thrombocytopenia, and livedo reticularis.[64,65] Strokes, myocardial infarction, visceral infarction, and extremity gangrene may also occur. Although the lupus anticoagulant has been noted often in patients with systemic lupus erythematosus (SLE), it does occur in patients without SLE. It may also be induced in patients by medications, cancer, and certain infections.[66]

This syndrome is associated with antiphospholipid antibodies that are most commonly immunoglobulin G (IgG). Antiphospholipid antibody syndrome is a particularly virulent hypercoagulable state that results in arterial and venous thrombosis at 5- to 16-fold greater risk.[66–68] A number of possible thrombotic mechanisms have been suggested, including inhibition of prostacyclin synthesis or release from endothelial cells,[69] inhibition of APC by thrombin/TM,[70] elevated PAI-1 levels,[67] platelet activation,[71] endothelial cell activation,[72] and interference with the endothelial cell–associated annexin V anticoagulant activity.[73] Increased

SCIENTIFIC PRINCIPLES

Patients with:
- Strong family history
- Young patients with thrombosis without obvious cause
- Multiple episodes of thrombosis without underlying anatomic abnormality
- Thrombosis in unusual locations

→ Procoagulant screen

Routine coagulation tests
Antithrombin III activity/antigen
Protein C activity/antigen
Protein S antigen
Mixing studies
APCR and factor V Leiden gene analysis
Prothrombin 20210 A gene analysis
Homocysteine
Anticardiolipin antibody
Functional plasminogen
Platelet aggregation testing
Fibrinogen

ALGORITHM 5.1

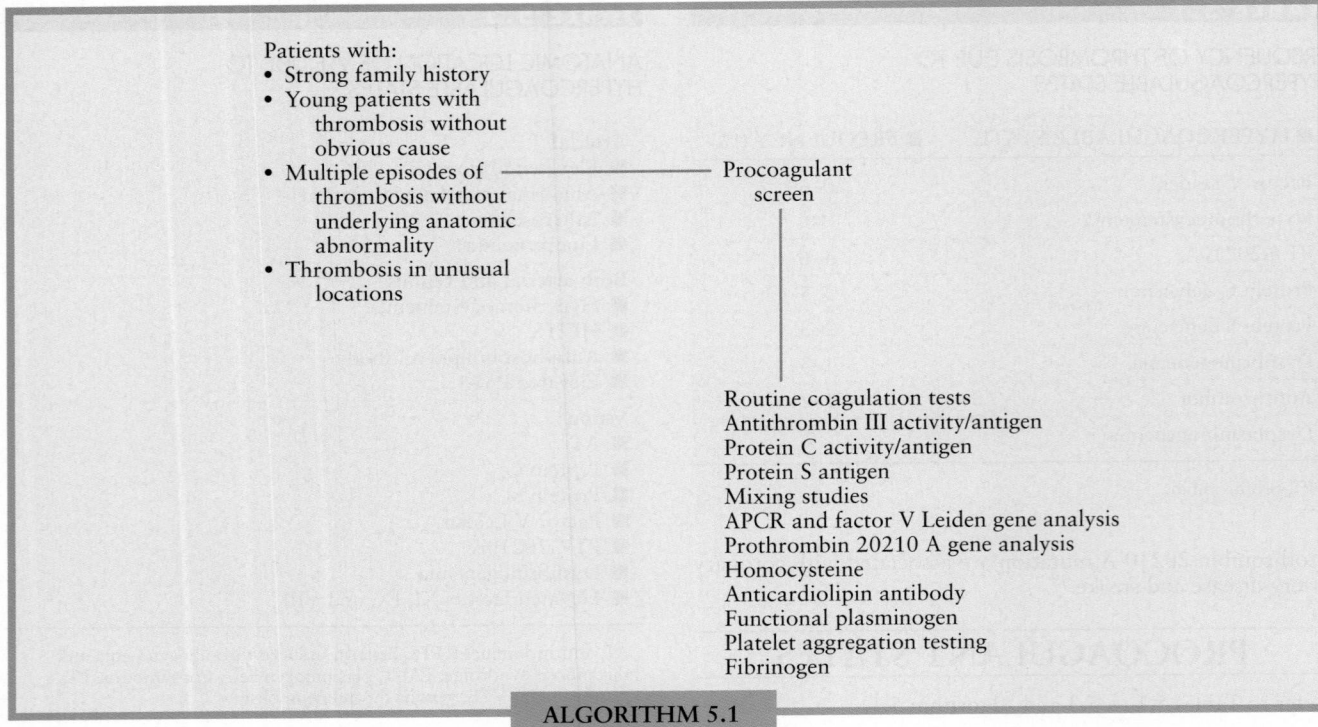

ALGORITHM 5.1. Coagulation analysis.

TF expression on monocytes and low free protein S plasma levels have also been found with the antiphospholipid syndrome and a history of thrombosis.[74]

At least one third of patients with lupus anticoagulants have a history of one or more thrombotic events, 70% or more being VTE.[75] Graft thrombosis has been observed in 27% to 50% of patients positive for antiphospholipid antibody.[76,77]

The diagnosis should be suspected in someone with a prolonged activated partial thromboplastin time (aPTT) with other standard coagulation tests normal, along with the presence of an increased antiphospholipid or anticardiolipin antibody titer and elevation of α_2-glycoprotein I.[3,78] The prolongation in the aPTT is strictly a laboratory phenomenon. The dilute Russell viper venom time confirms the presence of a lupus anticoagulant.

There is imperfect agreement between diagnostic tests for this abnormality. Approximately 80% of patients with a prolonged aPTT will have a positive antiphospholipid antibody, but only 10% to 50% of patients with a positive antiphospholipid antibody will have a prolonged aPTT.[79] Patients with both tests positive are reported to have the same thrombotic risk as those with either test alone.

Heparin followed by warfarin has been recommended for the treatment of the antiphospholipid syndrome.[66,75] For recurrent fetal loss, heparin or low-molecular-weight heparin (LMWH) use through pregnancy is recommended. In patients with lupus anticoagulants, heparin is monitored by antifactor Xa levels.

INHERITED PROCOAGULANT STATES

Defects with High Risk for Thrombosis

Antithrombin Deficiency. AT is a serine protease inhibitor (SERPIN) of thrombin, kallikrein, and factors Xa, IXa, VIIa, XIIa, and XIa. It is synthesized in the liver and has a half-life of 2.8 days. AT deficiency accounts for approximately 1% to 2% of episodes of VTE and may occur at unusual sites such as mesenteric or cerebral veins. Arterial and graft thrombosis have also been described in AT deficiency.[80,81] Most cases become apparent by 50 years of age.[82] Homozygous patients usually die in utero, whereas heterozygous patients usually demonstrate AT levels less than 70% of normal. Acquired AT deficiency results from liver disease, malignancy, sepsis, disseminated intravascular coagulation (DIC), malnutrition, and renal disease.[80]

The diagnosis of AT deficiency is suspected in a patient who cannot be adequately anticoagulated with heparin or who develops thrombosis while on heparin and is made by measuring AT antigen and activity levels. However, patients should not have been exposed to heparin or related compounds for at least 2 weeks to have accurate values. Heparin decreases AT levels 30%, and this effect can occur up to 10 days after stopping intravenous heparin therapy.[78] Conversely, warfarin increases AT levels.

For a patient with AT deficiency, anticoagulation with heparin requires the administration of fresh frozen plasma to provide AT, 2 units every 8 hours, decreasing to 1 unit every 12 hours, followed by oral anticoagulation. A reasonable alternative includes anticoagulation with direct thrombin inhibitors such as lepirudin, argatroban, or bivalirudin.[63] Aggressive prophylaxis against VTE is recommended during the perioperative period, and usually lifelong anticoagulation therapy is required after a first episode of significant VTE.[63,83]

Protein C and S Deficiencies. Protein C and its cofactor protein S are both vitamin K–dependent factors synthesized in the liver with half-lives of 4 to 6 hours and 12 to 14 hours, respectively. The majority of cases of protein C or protein S deficiency are inherited as autosomal dominant. Patients present with VTE, often between the ages of 15 and 30 years.[83,84] Protein C and S deficiency states are responsible for approximately

Venous Thromboembolism Risk Factor Assessment

Patient's Name ____________ Age: ___ Sex: ___ Wgt: ___ lbs Hgt: ___ inches

Choose All That Apply

Each Risk Factor Represents 1 Point

- ☐ Age 41-59 years
- ☐ Minor surgery planned
- ☐ History of prior major surgery
- ☐ Varicose veins
- ☐ History of inflammatory bowel disease
- ☐ Swollen legs (current)
- ☐ Obesity (BMI >30)
- ☐ Acute myocardial infarction (< l month)
- ☐ Congestive heart failure (< 1 month)
- ☐ Sepsis (< 1 month)
- ☐ Serious lung disease incl. pneumonia (< 1 month)
- ☐ Abnormal pulmonary function (COPD)
- ☐ Medical patient currently at bed rest
- ☐ Leg plaster cast or brace
- ☐ Central venous access
- ☐ Blood transfusion (<1 month)
- ☐ Other risk factor ____________

For Women Only (Each Represents 1 Point)

- ☐ Oral contraceptives or hormone replacement therapy
- ☐ Pregnancy or postpartum (<1 month)
- ☐ History of unexplained stillborn infant, recurrent spontaneous abortion (≥ 3), premature birth with toxemia or growth-restricted infant

Each Risk Factor Represents 2 Points

- ☐ Age 60-74 years
- ☐ Major surgery (> 60 minutes)*
- ☐ Arthroscopic surgery (> 60 minutes)*
- ☐ Laparoscopic surgery (> 60 minutes)*
- ☐ Previous malignancy
- ☐ Morbid obesity (BMI > 40)

Each Risk Factor Represents 3 Points

- ☐ Age 75 years or more
- ☐ Major surgery lasting 2-3 hours*
- ☐ BMI > 50 (venous stasis syndrome)
- ☐ History of SVT, DVT/PE
- ☐ Family history of DVT/PE
- ☐ Present cancer or chemotherapy
- ☐ Positive Factor V Leiden
- ☐ Positive Prothrombin 20210A
- ☐ Elevated serum homocysteine
- ☐ Positive Lupus anticoagulant
- ☐ Elevated anticardiolipin antibodies
- ☐ Heparininduced thrombocytopenia (HIT)
- ☐ Other thrombophilia
  Type ____________

Each Risk Factor Represents 5 Points

- ☐ Elective major lower extremity arthroplasty
- ☐ Hip, pelvis or leg fracture (< 1 month)
- ☐ Stroke (< 1 month)
- ☐ Multiple trauma (< 1 month)
- ☐ Acute spinal cord injury (paralysis) (< 1 month)
- ☐ Major surgery lasting over 3 hours*

Total Risk Factor Score ☐

*Select only one from the surgery category

Please see Following Page for Prophylaxis suggestions and Safety Considerations

A

FIGURE 5.10. A Caprini risk factor score sheet is shown here as an example of a preoperative risk factor scoring system. (*continued*)

2% to 5% of patients with VTE. However, cases of arterial thrombosis have also been reported.[85] If present as a homozygous state at birth, infants usually die from unrestricted clotting and fibrinolysis, a condition of extreme DIC termed *purpura fulminans*. Patients heterozygous for protein C deficiency usually have antigenic protein C levels less than 60% of normal.[78,86] Acquired protein C deficiency occurs with liver failure, DIC, and nephrotic syndrome.

Protein S is a cofactor to protein C and is regulated by complement C4b-binding protein. Free protein S is functionally active as an anticoagulant. The deficiency of protein S results in a clinical state identical to protein C deficiency. Nephrotic syndrome can lead to a reduction in free protein S,[87] whereas inflammatory states such as SLE can result in an elevation of C4b-binding protein, reducing free protein S.

The diagnosis of protein C or S deficiency is made by measuring plasma protein C and S levels.[3,88] For protein C, both antigen and activity are measured, whereas for protein S, only antigen is measured. A condition also exists in which there is an abnormality in the function of protein C itself, resulting in a decrease in protein C activity without a decline in antigenic protein C.[84]

Treatment consists of anticoagulation, initially with heparin, usually followed by lifelong oral anticoagulation after a first thrombotic event. However, not all patients with low levels develop VTE. Many heterozygous family members of homozygous protein C–deficient infants also are unaffected.[31] Thus, the institution of anticoagulation therapy in patients should occur only following an episode of thrombosis. However, aggressive anticoagulant prophylaxis during perioperative periods or high-risk environmental situations is necessary for asymptomatic heterozygote carriers.

With the initiation of oral anticoagulation, blood may become transiently hypercoagulable as the vitamin K–dependent factors with short half-lives are inhibited (factor VII, protein C) before the other vitamin K–dependent factors (factors II, IX, and X).[89] In someone already partially deficient in protein C or S, the levels of these anticoagulant factors will diminish even further with the initiation of warfarin. This results in temporary hypercoagulability, resulting in thrombosis in the microcirculation and warfarin-induced skin necrosis.[90] This leads to full-thickness skin loss, especially over fatty areas such as the breasts, buttocks, and abdomen. This complication can

VTE Risk and Suggested Prophylaxis For Surgical Patients

Total Risk Factor Score	Incidence of DVT	Risk Level	Prophylaxis Regimen
0-1	< 10%	Low Risk	No specific measures; early ambulation
2	10-20%	Moderate Risk	IPC, LDUH(5000 U BID) or LWMH (<3400 U)
3-4	20-40%	High Risk	IPC, LDUH (5000 U TID), or LMWH (>3400 U) or FXa I
5 or more	40-80% 1-5% mortality	Highest Risk	Pharmacological: LDUH, LMWH*, Warfarin* or FXa I* alone or in combination with IPC

Legend

IPC – Intermittent Pneumatic Compression
LDUH – Low Dose Unfractionated Heparin
LMWH – Low Molecular Weight Heparin
FXa I – Factor Xa Inhibitor

Prophylaxis Safety Considerations: Check box if answer is 'YES'

Anticoagulants: Factors Associated with Increased Bleeding

- ☐ Is patient experiencing any active bleeding?
- ☐ Does patient have (or has had history of) heparin-induced thrombocytopenia?
- ☐ Is patient's platelet count <100,000/mm^3?
- ☐ Is patient taking oral anticoagulants, platelet inhibitors (e.g., NSAIDS, Clopidogrel, Salicylates)?
- ☐ Is patient's creatinine clearance abnormal? If yes, please indicate value ________

If any of the above boxes are checked, the patient may not be a candidate for anticoagulant therapy and you should consider alternative prophylactic measures: IPC or Foot Pump.

Intermittent Pneumatic Compression (IPC)

- ☐ Does patient have severe peripheral arterial disease?
- ☐ Does patient have congestive heart failure?
- ☐ Does patient have an acute superficial/deep vein thrombosis?

If any of the above boxes are checked, then patient may not be a candidate for intermittent compression therapy and you should consider alternative prophylactic measures. (IVC filter?)

Examiner: ________________________ Date: __________

B

FIGURE 5.10. (*Continued*)

be prevented by initiating warfarin therapy under the protection of systemic heparin anticoagulation or a direct thrombin inhibitor.

Defects with Lower Risk for Thrombosis

Resistance to Activated Protein C (Factor V Leiden). Resistance to APC is reportedly present in 20% to 60% of cases of idiopathic VTE and is the most common underlying abnormality associated with VTE. This disorder is present in 1% to 2% of the general population.[91–93] It confers a relatively low risk for thrombosis, however, and is more common in whites than in nonwhite Americans.[91] As a result of the substitution of a single amino acid, glutamine for arginine, at position 506 in the protein for factor V, caused by a nucleotide substitution of guanine for adenine at 1691 in the factor V gene, hypercoagulability is conferred by resistance to inactivation of factor Va by APC.[94–96] Additionally, less VIIIa is interfered with, compounding the hypercoagulability.

Thrombotic manifestations are noted in those individuals both homozygous and heterozygous for this mutation. The relative risk for VTE in patients heterozygous for factor V Leiden is sevenfold, whereas the relative risk is 80-fold for those homozygous for factor V Leiden.[95] In contrast to factor deficiency states, persons homozygous for this mutation usually do not die in infancy. Additionally, thrombosis is potentiated in the presence of additional acquired risk factors.[95,97]

Combined defects with other hypercoagulable states, such as protein C and S deficiency or prothrombin G20210A, are not uncommon and increase the thrombotic risk.[98,99] In addition to cases of VTE, recurrent VTE is also more common in patients with this entity, with a relative risk 2.4-fold.[93] Although VTE predominates in patients with this syndrome, arterial thrombosis has also been reported.[100]

The diagnosis of APC resistance is made by a clot-based functional assay with the addition of APC (modified aPTT). Additionally, genetic analysis should be performed to confirm heterozygosity versus homozygosity, as treatment decisions may be different between the two states. If the patient has a known lupus anticoagulant syndrome, this entity may interfere with the clot-based APC resistance assay[101] and genetic analysis is more accurate.

Treatment options for APC resistance after VTE include anticoagulation, initially heparin or LMWH, followed by oral anticoagulation. The long-term use of warfarin is controversial. No data exist to suggest that long-term warfarin should be given after a first episode of VTE in a patient heterozygous for the mutation.[63] The fact that APC resistance is a relatively low risk for recurrent thrombosis (2.4-fold) suggests that not all patients after their first episode of VTE need long-term anticoagulant treatment. Patients must be evaluated in light of their overall risk for bleeding versus thrombosis.[83]

Prothrombin G20210A Polymorphism. Prothrombin (factor II), a vitamin K–dependent factor synthesized in the liver, becomes thrombin when activated. A genetic polymorphism in the distal 3′ untranslated region of the gene for prothrombin has been described in patients with VTE. This results in a normal prothrombin but at increased levels.[84,97,102] This polymorphism confers an increased risk for VTE by two- to sevenfold, and is associated with 4% to 6% of patients with VTE.[83,103,104] This thrombosis risk is increased in pregnant women,[105] in women with early myocardial infarctions,[106] and in synergy with factor V Leiden.[97] Most patients are heterozygous for this mutation, and whites are more often affected than those of Asian or African descent.[106] Genetic analysis is the marker for this abnormality.[107]

Patients who present with VTE should be treated according to current standards and akin to the treatment for heterozygous factor V Leiden. Individuals with prothrombin G20210A who have recurrent episodes of VTE should undergo lifelong anticoagulation, as should those patients with both prothrombin G20210A and factor V Leiden.[97]

Hyperhomocysteinemia. Hyperhomocysteinemia has been a known risk factor for atherosclerosis and vascular disease for more than 25 years, though a direct cause-and-effect relationship has not been established.[108–110] However, a recent meta-analysis suggests the risk of VTE to be 2.5-fold with elevated homocysteine levels.[111] Two enzyme deficiencies, N^5, N^{10}, methylene tetrahydrofolate reductase (MTHFR) or cystathionine β-synthase, are responsible for elevated homocysteine levels.[112] Deficiencies in vitamins B_6 and B_{12} and folate also contribute to elevations in homocysteine. Although mutations in these enzymes are not infrequent, the common polymorphism in MTHFR alone is not a factor in either the elevation of plasma homocysteine or thrombosis.[113]

Hyperhomocysteinemia also has been found to be a risk factor for VTE in those younger than 40 years,[114] in women,[108] and for recurrent venous thrombosis in patients between 20 and 70 years of age.[109] The combination of hyperhomocysteinemia and factor V Leiden results in an increased risk of venous and arterial thromboses.[115] Elevated plasma homocysteine results in abnormal endothelial function.[116–120] Fasting homocysteine levels are determined from serum, usually on two occasions. The test may also be performed after a methionine oral loading regimen.[121,122]

Homocysteine elevation is treated with folate supplements. Although the association between hyperhomocysteinemia and VTE has been established, treatment to lower homocysteine levels and the long-term effects of such treatment on procoagulant activity have yet to be validated.[108]

Other Disorders Associated with Thrombosis

Defective Fibrinolysis/Dysfibrinogenemia/Lipoprotein(a). Abnormal plasminogens (dysplasminogenemias), although rare (<1%), have been described in cases of spontaneous arterial or VTE.[123] Other defects in fibrinolysis may affect up to 10% of the normal population.[124] Abnormal fibrinogens may account for 1% to 3% of patients with venous thrombosis and those presenting with digital ischemia.[125] Numerous molecular defects have been classified. Defective thrombin binding or resistance to plasmin-mediated breakdown has been described.[126] Although not clearly documented, defects in plasminogen activators, tPA, or uPA may incite thrombotic events.[127] Moreover, elevated PAI-1 has been associated with DVT and myocardial infarction.[123] Although the relationship between VTE and abnormal fibrinolysis is debated, it is clear that in the postoperative period there is a connection between fibrinolysis and VTE.[123,128,129] Additionally, PAI-1 is upregulated by thrombin, endotoxin, and IL-1, explaining the elevated circulating levels of PAI-1 during infections.[130] Lipoprotein(a), associated with LDL, has both atherogenic and prothrombotic properties.[131–133] It prevents plasminogen from binding to cells or fibrin and inhibits fibrinolysis.[134] Elevated levels of lipoprotein(a) have been associated with VTE in childhood; it is a weak thrombotic risk factor in adults.[135]

When an individual with thrombosis presents with one of the previously mentioned abnormalities, standard anticoagulation is necessary.[136,137]

Abnormal Platelet Aggregation. It has been recognized for some time that there are patients who have thrombosis and may have hyperactive or hyperresponsive platelets, but this entity is poorly defined. Diabetes mellitus, which is known to be associated with hyperactive platelets and hyperlipidemic states, may be a contributing factor. Two clinical settings in which abnormal platelet aggregation has been associated with thrombosis include advanced malignancy of the lung and uterus and after carotid endarterectomy. Hyperactive platelets have also been noted during graft thrombosis in peripheral vascular reconstructions.[67] Although platelet aggregation assays may be helpful in making the diagnosis, these assays are not commonly performed or standardized and, thus, the incidence and importance of platelets to thrombosis are not well known. Bleeding time measurements are not specific and are not recommended for making this diagnosis.

Standard anticoagulant treatment is recommended for this condition. Aspirin and the thienopyridine derivatives such as clopidogrel may be useful, but their utility is unknown.[138]

Elevated Procoagulant Factors: VIII, IX, and XI

Elevated prothrombotic factors have only recently been associated with primary and recurrent VTE.[83,139] A dose-response effect has been observed, and elevated factor VIII has been best studied.[139–141] Factor VIII:C above the 90th percentile is associated with a five times increased risk of VTE.[141,142] Factor VIII:C elevation is also affected by blood type and race. Elevation of factor XI above the 90th percentile is associated with a twofold increase in VTE, independent of other hypercoagulability factors.[143] Similar increases in VTE risk have been observed with elevated factor IX.[144] Acquired and environmental factors precipitate VTE in patients with elevation of these factors, as opposed to inherited deficiencies of AT, protein C, and protein S that confer higher VTE risk.[145]

The diagnosis is made by the direct measurement of these factors with activity assays. If VTE occurs with one of these factors elevated, standard anticoagulant management should be undertaken.[137]

Disseminated Intravascular Coagulation

DIC is a primary form of acute thrombosis. Causes of DIC include abruptio placentae, gram-positive and gram-negative sepsis, endotoxemia, malignant tumors, pelvic operations, certain snake bites, hematologic malignancies, and hepatic failure.[3] Coagulation is activated by the release of TF into the circulation, which activates factor VII to VIIa, leading to massive thrombin production and fibrin generation. Fibrinolysis then becomes activated, leading to bleeding in the later stages of the syndrome because of the consumption of clotting factors, depletion of fibrinogen, and unchecked plasmin activity. Laboratory values in DIC reveal a decline in platelet count and fibrinogen level with a concomitant elevation in fibrin split products and the presence of a positive D-dimer test. A more chronic form of DIC has been reported, with the release of small amounts of TF into the circulation in conditions such as tumors of the prostate, diabetes mellitus, use of factor IX concentrates, total hip replacement, and abdominal aortic aneurysm.[3]

Testing for Hypercoagulable States

Patients with a strongly positive family history of thrombotic events, young patients with unprovoked arterial and venous thromboses, and patients with multiple episodes of thrombosis without an underlying anatomic abnormality should be investigated.[146] Whether unaffected relatives should be screened is controversial, and genetic counselors may be of assistance.

A hypercoagulable screen should include routine coagulation tests such as the aPTT and platelet count, AT activity and antigen assay, protein C antigen and activity levels, protein S antigen level, and mixing studies to identify a lupus anticoagulant (if indicated); APC resistance assay and factor V Leiden gene analysis; prothrombin G20210A genetic analysis; homocysteine level; an antiphospholipid antibody screen that includes anticardiolipin antibody; fibrinogen level; factor VIII, IX, and XI levels; and a functional plasminogen assay.

A confirmatory test for dysfibrinogenemia includes a fibrinogen clotting activity-to-antigen ratio. It may also be detected by a prolonged thrombin clotting time (TCT) or reptilase time.[147] Abnormal plasminogens are detected by the presence of reduced activity-to-antigen ratios. PAI-1 levels have to be measured directly by activity or antigen assay. Lipoprotein(a) levels are measured in serum.

BLEEDING DISORDERS

Although the surgeon deals more often with procoagulant states than bleeding disorders, it is important to recognize these disorders when they occur.

Coagulation Factor Deficiency

5 Coagulation factor deficiency states are important causes of bleeding, and the most common are factor VIII and IX deficiency states, termed hemophilia A and B, and type I von Willebrand disease (vWD).

Hemophilia A is inherited as a sex-linked recessive deficiency of factor VIII, with fewer cases secondary to spontaneous mutation. The incidence of this abnormality is approximately 1 in 10,000 births. Clinical findings range from bleeding into joints and muscles, epistaxis, hematuria, and bleeding after minor trauma, to prolonged postoperative bleeding, retroperitoneal bleeding, and intramural bowel hemorrhage. Laboratory screening tests usually reveal a prolongation of the aPTT along with decreased factor VIII levels; other test results are normal. The minimum level of factor VIII required for hemostasis is 30%, and spontaneous bleeding is uncommon with factor VIII levels greater than 5% to 10% of normal.[148] Levels less than 2% constitute severe, 2% to 5% moderate, and greater than 5% mild deficiency.[149] Severe deficiency with levels less than 1% poses the risk for spontaneous bleeding episodes. Although the half-life of factor VIII is 2.9 days in normal subjects, the half-life of factor VIII concentrates is only 9 to 18 hours.[3] Levels between 80% and 100% of normal should be attained for surgical bleeding or life-threatening hemorrhage. Acquired deficiency has been reported to occur with the development of antibodies to factor VIII after therapy. Inhibitor antibodies develop in approximately 10% to 15% of patients with hemophilia A, although the incidence of antibody formation may be much higher in previously untreated patients and in those with severe hemophilia A.

Recombinant factor VIII preparation has been developed and tested in children and infants. Despite the development of low levels of inhibitors in 20% of children at a mean 9 days after first administration, these inhibitors either disappeared or remained at low levels.[150] Because this recombinant preparation is virus free, the benefits outweigh the risks of low levels of inhibitor development for the treatment of hemophilia A.[151]

Factor IX deficiency (Christmas factor), known as hemophilia B, is transmitted as an X-linked recessive trait. It also may be acquired because of enhanced factor IX clearance in states such as the nephrotic syndrome, abnormal protein production in vitamin K deficiency, and acquired specific inhibitors to factor IX in various autoimmune diseases, such as SLE. It is clinically indistinguishable from hemophilia A, and laboratory screening tests reveal a prolonged aPTT, with other test results normal, although a greater proportion of patients have only mild or moderate deficiency.[152] Severe deficiency (approximately 30% of cases) is defined as a level of activity less than 4% of normal, whereas moderate deficiency is reported with activity levels between 20% and 40%.[3] Treatment consists of plasma or factor IX concentrates and vitamin K. It has been recommended that levels greater than 30% be achieved for hemostasis.[148]

vWF causes platelet adhesion to collagen, initiating platelet plug formation. It also forms a complex with factor VIII in the blood. Produced in endothelial cells and megakaryocytes (compared with the liver for factor VIII), it has a circulating half-life of 6 to 20 hours.[3] vWD, a deficiency of vWF, is the most common of the inherited coagulation disorders. A number of different subtypes have been identified for its deficiency state, and the syndrome is transmitted as both autosomal dominant (heterozygous) and autosomal recessive (homozygous) forms. Variants include types I and III (quantitative decreases in normal-appearing vWF) and type II (qualitative abnormalities in structure and function of vWF).[153] vWF deficiency is probably as common as hemophilia A, although the true incidence may surpass what is generally appreciated because many mild cases probably remain undiagnosed.

The classic syndrome is caused by a reduction of factor VIII activity (although not as great as in hemophilia A) and vWF (vWF–factor VIII complex). Clinical manifestations include easy bruisability, mild to moderate epistaxis, gingival bleeding, menorrhagia, rare joint or muscle bleeding, prolonged bleeding following surgery, and subcutaneous bleeding.[153] Spontaneous bleeding is not as common as in hemophilia A.

Abnormal laboratory tests include a prolonged bleeding time, a decreased level of factor VIII activity, decreased immunoreactive levels of the vWF, and an abnormal platelet aggregation response to ristocetin.[3] The most reliable source of vWF is cryoprecipitate, although many concentrates of factor VIII have vWF present and show promise. Desmopressin acetate (DDAVP) is available for the treatment of mild cases of type I and of type IIa and IIb vWD; serum levels of 25% to 50% are needed for hemostasis.[148] In other type II states and type III VWD, factor VIII concentrates are necessary. Recombinant factor VIII/vWF concentrates that avoid the infectious risks of transfusion are available.

Rare Factor Deficiencies

Other specific factor deficiencies are much less common and receive only a brief mention here. These include factors II, XI, V, VII, and X. These can be measured by serum assays, although this is not routinely available in many hospitals. The treatment is primarily fresh frozen plasma concentrates to give back the clotting factors.[3]

Deficiencies of fibrinogen can also lead to bleeding disorders. This is the only factor deficiency state in which the TCT is prolonged. It is generally believed that a fibrinogen level of 100 mg/mL should be achieved to stop bleeding related to fibrinogen abnormalities. Fibrinogen deficiency may also occur from consumption during DIC and from primary fibrinolytic states.

Platelet Disorders

Platelet disorders are another important cause of bleeding. Inherited defects of platelet receptors include defects of GpIIb/IIIa (Glanzmann thrombasthenia), characterized by impaired platelet binding to vWF, fibrinogen, and fibronectin. In patients with defects in GpIb (Bernard-Soulier syndrome), the absolute number of platelets is decreased, the platelets are larger, and platelet aggregation and adhesion are abnormal.[3] Acquired deficits occur in uremia; both GpIb and GpIIb/IIIa receptors are defective, resulting in impaired adhesion and aggregation. Acquired deficits also occur in patients who previously received platelet transfusions and then acquire immune-mediated antiplatelet antibodies.

Abnormalities in Fibrinolysis

Abnormalities in fibrinolysis may play a role in abnormal bleeding disorders. Genetic or acquired deficiencies in α_2-AP may be associated with bleeding, whereas deficiencies in factor XIII (fibrin stabilizing factor) may lead to highly lysable clot. α_2-AP deficiency is treated with e-aminocaproic acid or tranexamic acid. Homozygous patients with factor XIII deficiency and less than 1% of normal plasma activity often show bleeding from the umbilical cord at birth, bleeding after trauma or surgery, and delayed bleeding 24 to 36 hours later.[3] Intracranial bleeding also has been noted. Screening test results include a shortened euglobulin lysis time.[3] A specific assay for factor XIII activity exists. Treatment consists of fresh frozen plasma, cryoprecipitate, and factor XIII concentrates.

PHARMACOLOGIC AND NONPHARMACOLOGIC INTERVENTIONS

Heparin, Factor Xa, and Direct Thrombin Inhibitors

4 Heparin, discovered by Jay McLean in 1916, is a heterogeneous mixture of sulfated polysaccharide molecules of varying molecular weights, ranging from 2 to 40 kD. Heparin is obtained from beef lung or porcine intestine. Heparin accelerates the inhibition of thrombin and other serine proteases by AT. Heparin also directly binds and inhibits coagulation proteases and is important for the selective inhibitor of thrombin, heparin cofactor II.[154] After bolus injection, heparin's half-life is approximately 90 to 120 minutes, although the half-life depends on the amount injected—the more injected, the longer the half-life. Activated factor X and activated factor II are most sensitive to the heparin–AT complex. Heparin is cleared through the reticuloendothelial system and does not cross the placental barrier. Heparin is reversed with protamine sulfate by direct irreversible binding between the compounds.

Clinical use of heparin is for prophylaxis of, and treatment of, venous and arterial thrombosis.[155] In monitoring heparin, an aPTT 1.5 to 2.0 times control or a TCT two times control reflects adequate anticoagulation. Activated clotting times (ACTs) in a range of 150 to 200 seconds also suggest adequate anticoagulation. The use of low-dose unfractionated heparin (UFH) therapy is most commonly used for VTE prophylaxis.[63]

Because of the bleeding complications caused by UFH, LMWH for venous thrombosis prophylaxis and treatment is now primary.[63] Standard heparin is a mixture of polysaccharide molecules that vary in size from 2 to 40 kD. The anticoagulant effect is primarily centered over the lower end of the molecular-weight spectrum. Standard UFH is able to inhibit thrombin because it is large enough to make a ternary complex between itself, thrombin, and AT. LMWH is not large enough to make this complex because the minimum chain length necessary for formation of such a ternary complex is 18 saccharide units. LMWH demonstrates less AT activity, but for inhibition of factor Xa, such a ternary complex is not necessary. Thus, LMWH preparations are able to inhibit factor Xa. Each LMWH preparation has its own antifactor Xa–to–antifactor IIa (thrombin) ratio, depending on its size and molecular weight.[157] Most commercially available LMWH preparations have ratios between 4:1 and 2:1. Because the bleeding potential of heparin is related largely to its AT activity, LMWH has a lower bleeding potential. In addition, LMWH preparations have less antiplatelet activity and less risk for heparin-induced thrombocytopenia (HIT).

The LMWH preparations have other advantages over standard UFH. These include an improved pharmacokinetic profile due to reduced nonspecific binding to plasma proteins, less lipolysis, a half-life that is not dose dependent, more constant antifactor Xa inhibition, less interference with protein C activation, less complement activation and interference with appropriate platelet aggregation, less risk for osteoporosis, and a lower level of fibrin monomer production.[156] High and sustained plasma antifactor Xa levels exist for greater than 16 hours after LMWH administration in therapeutic doses, and its excretion is primarily renal. There is no available agent effective for complete LMWH reversal as measured by antifactor Xa levels,[157] although clinically the bleeding potential of LMWH can be reversed by protamine sulfate.

LMWH is the primary therapy for VTE. A number of level 1 evidence studies and meta-analyses have compared LMWH with UFH in the treatment of VTE.[158,159] Together, these studies demonstrate a lower risk of major bleeding, a lower risk of recurrent thromboembolic events, and a lower risk of death than with UFH. Even for nonmassive pulmonary embolism (PE), LMWH appears at least equivalent if not superior to UFH, but much more convenient.[160] It is not necessary to monitor LMWH with coagulation testing except in specific situations such as renal failure, pregnancy, or morbid obesity, and most dosage schemes use either fixed-dose or weight-adjusted dosing given subcutaneously. Because there is no need for coagulation testing, outpatient treatment has become a reality.

LMWH has also been studied in unstable angina[156] and has been found superior to placebo and equivalent or superior to UFH when evaluating the outcomes of death or myocardial infarction, without any increase in major bleeding.

The most common complication of heparin therapy is bleeding. The risk of hemorrhage is increased in the elderly; in postmenopausal women; and in patients with preexisting abnormalities of coagulation, thrombocytopenia, and uremia. Long-term therapy may be associated with alopecia and osteoporosis; osteoporosis has been found in patients receiving large doses of heparin for longer than 6 months.

Reversal of heparin anticoagulation with protamine sulfate may be associated with adverse hemodynamic and hematologic side effects, including hypotension, bradycardia, pulmonary artery hypertension or hypotension, declines in oxygen consumption, leukopenia, and thrombocytopenia.[161,162] Immunologic reactions may occur in patients with prior exposure to protamine, especially in diabetic patients taking NPH insulin that contains protamine or those previously exposed to protamine. Unfortunately, no other effective and safe agent for heparin neutralization exists, and in those situations when heparin must be reversed, such as at the completion of major aortic reconstructions and cardiopulmonary bypass, protamine must be given. Although it has been suggested that the rate of administration is the most crucial factor in protamine-related reactions, declines in hemodynamic parameters and oxygen consumption still occur with slow administration.[162]

The specific factor Xa inhibitor pentasaccharide fondaparinux (Arixtra, GlaxoSmithKline, Parsippany, NJ) potentiates approximately 300-fold factor Xa neutralization by AT. It has a half-life of 17 hours and does not bind to plasma proteins. It is primarily excreted through the kidneys. Large prospective randomized studies for both DVT and PE treatment have been conducted suggesting efficacy and safety similar to LMWH.[163] In orthopedic surgery, this agent is superior to the best currently available DVT prophylaxis using LMWH. In fact, in hip fracture and knee reconstruction surgery, this agent has decreased the incidence of DVT by greater than 50%. In a meta-analysis of more than 7,000 patients, fondaparinux significantly decreased the odds of VTE as compared to LMWH with no difference in critical bleeding, although major bleeding was slightly greater.[164–166] There is no good reversal drug for this agent, and this has been one of the factors that has prevented its wider adoption into the medical and surgical communities.

Oral Xa inhibitors are currently being developed. Rivaroxaban (BAY 59-7939), one such inhibitor, showed promising results in phase 2 trials when compared to enoxaparin for the prevention of VTE in those undergoing major orthopedic surgery.[167] Trials are currently under way in additional treatment applications.

Direct thrombin inhibitors have been developed for both oral and parental use, particularly in HIT. Unlike heparin, the direct thrombin inhibitors have the ability to inactivate fibrin-bound thrombin.[168] Direct thrombin inhibitors such as argatroban and lepirudin (hirudin analogue) have also been shown to be effective anticoagulants in patients with HIT and are dosed via the aPTT.[169] Argatroban has a relatively short half-life, is cleared by the liver, and is safe to use in those with renal insufficiency. Conversely, lepirudin is cleared renally, has a slightly longer half-life, and is the preferred anticoagulant in patients with hepatic insufficiency. A third parental thrombin inhibitor, bivalirudin is used in patients with unstable angina who are undergoing percutaneous cardiac intervention and cardiac surgery.

Although early trials with ximelagatran, a direct oral thrombin inhibitor, were not successful owing to the hepatic toxicity, a new agent in the same family, dabigatran, has promising data supporting its efficacy and safety. Results of a large phase 2 trial comparing dabigatran to enoxaparin for VTE prevention in those undergoing hip replacement demonstrated noninferiority to enoxaparin.[170]

Other new alternative agents are in various stages of development, such as oral heparins, oral factor IIa and Xa inhibitors, P-selectin inhibitors, factor VIIa inhibitors, TFPIs, and PAI-1 inhibitors.[170] These agents, available now and in the future, will likely revolutionize the whole field of thrombosis prophylaxis and treatment.

Heparin-induced Thrombocytopenia and Thrombosis Syndrome

6 A specific complication of heparin deserves detailed discussion. HIT occurs in 0.6% to 30% of patients in whom heparin is given, although severe thrombocytopenia associated with thrombosis (HITTS) occurs much less frequently.[171,172] Approximately one half of HIT patients have thrombosis that is noted clinically or by duplex imaging. In an analysis of 11 prospective studies, the incidence was reported to be 3%, with thrombosis in 0.9%.[173] Although earlier morbidity and mortality rates of 61% and 23% had been reported,[70] with early diagnosis and appropriate treatment, these rates have declined to 6% and 0%, respectively.[174] HIT is caused by a heparin-dependent IgG antibody that, when bound to platelet factor 4 (PF_4), induces platelet aggregation in part by inducing MP formation.[175,176] The antibody may not be heparin specific, as the degree of sulfonation of the heparinlike compound has been suggested to be critical for this aggregation.[177] Both porcine and bovine UFH as well as LMWH have been associated with HIT.[178] The syndrome usually begins 3 to 14 days after heparin is begun. Both arterial and venous thromboses have been reported, and even small exposures to heparin (heparin coating on catheters) can cause the syndrome.[171,179]

The diagnosis should be suspected when a patient experiences a 50% or greater decline in platelet count, when there is a fall in platelet count below 100,000/mL during heparin therapy, or in any patient who experiences thrombosis during heparin administration.[180] The syndrome may be difficult to diagnose as many hospitalized patients have multiple reasons for low platelet counts, and vigilance is important. A platelet count should be checked about every 2 days when on heparin therapy.

The laboratory diagnosis of HIT/HITTS is made by a number of assays. The serotonin release assay (SRA) was the "gold standard." An enzyme-linked immunosorbent assay (ELISA) test detecting the antiheparin antibody in the patient's plasma directed against the heparin–PF_4 complex is now commonly used.[171] This assay is less specific but easier to perform and interpret than the serotonin assay.

When the diagnosis is made (clinically), cessation of heparin is mandatory. This includes removing heparin from intravenous catheters and flushes.[179] Warfarin should not be administered until an adequate alternative anticoagulant has been started to prevent venous limb gangrene development.[181] LMWH preparations have high rates of cross-reactivity with the HIT antibody and therefore should not be merely substituted for UFH in patients with HIT.[182]

A number of anticoagulants are now available to substitute for patients with this diagnosis. The direct thrombin inhibitors hirudin (lepirudin/Refludan) and argatroban are the treatments of choice and are U.S. Food and Drug Administration approved for this indication.[180,183] These agents show no cross-reactivity to heparin antibodies.

Warfarin

Warfarin oral anticoagulant therapy remains the standard for long-term treatment of arterial and venous thromboembolism. Warfarin interferes with the vitamin K–dependent clotting factors II, VII, IX, and X and proteins C and S. In the liver, these factors are γ-carboxylated in a reaction catalyzed by the reduced form of vitamin K. During this reaction, 10 to 12 glutamic acid residues are converted to γ-carboxyglutamic acid residues. When these factors are released from the liver, they are secreted as active proteins.[3] The carboxyglutamic acid residues are responsible for these proteins binding to phospholipid membranes and the formation of the Xase and prothrombinase complexes on activated platelet surfaces. Warfarin prevents the reduction of vitamin K once it has functioned as a cofactor for the γ-carboxylation.

Because of variations in the thromboplastins used for the prothrombin time (PT) determinations in various countries, the international normalized ratio (INR) system, in which the sensitivity of thromboplastins has been standardized, was developed.[184] Using this system, the proper range for treatment of most thrombotic diseases by warfarin is an INR of 2 to 3.

Major complications of warfarin therapy include bleeding, recurrent thrombosis, and skin necrosis. Patients at highest risk for bleeding on warfarin include the elderly, patients with gynecologic or urologic disorders, women after childbirth, and patients given large warfarin loading doses. A specific complication of warfarin is skin necrosis, which occurs more frequently in patients with protein C deficiency. This usually involves full-thickness skin sloughing over fatty areas such as the breasts and buttocks but can also occur in other anatomic distributions such as the extremities and digits.

Warfarin should be continued for at least 3 months after an initial episode of DVT or arterial thromboembolism. Detailed guidelines for level of anticoagulation and duration are updated every 3 to 5 years.[63] Currently, 3 months of anticoagulant treatment is indicated for a provoked VTE event, while consideration of bleeding and thrombosis risk needs to be determined and a longer duration used if an unprovoked event occurred. Male gender, antiphospholipid syndrome, prior DVT, and thrombophilias all increase the risk of recurrence and support prolonged anticoagulation. Conversely, Asian race and a normal D-dimer at 1 month after ceasing anticoagulation support limited anticoagulation. Data that support prolonged therapy for unprovoked DVT include a recent multicenter trial comparing low-dose warfarin (INR 1.5 to 2.0) to placebo with 4-year follow-up.[185] Another study suggested that full-dose warfarin (INR 2.0 to 3.0) was superior to low-dose warfarin in these same patients without a difference in bleeding, suggesting that unprovoked DVT requires long-term oral anticoagulation of some still-to-be-defined duration.[186]

Antiplatelet Agents

Antiplatelet agents are used to prevent cardiovascular events such as coronary and peripheral arterial thrombosis. Platelet aggregation can be inhibited by several mechanisms, including (a) blocking cyclooxygenase, the first step in converting arachidonic acid to thromboxane and prostacyclin; (b) blocking thromboxane synthase, the enzyme leading to thromboxane A_2; (c) blocking the thromboxane A_2 receptor; (d) increasing intraplatelet levels of cyclic adenosine monophosphate (cAMP) or guanosine monophosphate (GMP), which inhibit the exposure of the platelet GpIIb/IIIa receptor; and (e) directly blocking the platelet receptor GpIIb/IIIa.

Aspirin inhibits cyclooxygenase, and thus both thromboxane and prostacyclin. In clinical situations, the use of lower doses of aspirin in an attempt to inhibit thromboxane generation but preserve prostacyclin generation is theoretical, and may have some efficacy. Dipyridamole (Persantine; Boehringer Ingelheim, Ridgefield, CT), inhibits the uptake of adenosine into platelets, endothelial cells, and red blood cells. This leads to increased platelet cAMP levels through a local increase in adenosine concentration, inhibiting platelet aggregation. Additionally, it also inhibits phosphodiesterase, the enzyme that normally degrades cAMP, leading to higher levels of cAMP, and augments the increase in cGMP produced by nitric oxide. Thienopyridines work by ADP receptor blockade, interfering with subsequent GIIb/IIIc fibrinogen binding.[187] In addition, monoclonal antibodies to GpIIb/IIIa itself or synthetic peptide blockers of this receptor containing the RGD sequence or the fibrinogen γ-chain carboxyl-terminal sequence directly inhibit the function of this receptor. Receptor blockage is the most specific way to inhibit aggregation, and when the GpIIb/IIIa receptor is blocked, even high concentrations of agonists cannot stimulate platelets.

Because of ticlopidine-associated neutropenia, an analogue of ticlopidine, clopidogrel, was developed. This thienopyridine compound is not associated with the same degree of neutropenia and has been shown to reduce the composite endpoints of stroke, myocardial infarction, and death in patients with vascular disease.[2] It is mandatory treatment for patients in whom a drug-eluting stent has been placed in the coronary arterial circulation and is used for periprocedural protection in those patients undergoing peripheral angioplasty and stenting.

Direct inhibitors of the GpIIb/IIIa receptor were first developed as murine-derived monoclonal antibodies. The compound C7E3Fab (ReoPro; Eli Lilly, Indianapolis, IN), a human chimeric monoclonal antibody directed at GpIIb/IIIa, is the first agent of this class to become clinically available.[2] Its receptor binding is nonspecific and it binds to other cell surface integrins. Other agents include RGD mimics that are competitive antagonists to the GpIIb/IIIa receptor, including the cyclic peptide eptifibatide (Integrilin; Key Pharmaceutical, Kenilworth, NJ) and the parenteral nonpeptide mimetics tirofiban (Aggrastet; Merck & Co., West Point, PA) and lamifiban.[188] All studies to date with these agents have involved coronary interventions.

Fibrinolytic Agents

Fibrinolytic agents are direct or indirect activators of plasminogen, the inactive proteolytic enzyme of plasma that binds to fibrin during the formation of thrombus. Fibrin-bound plasminogen is more susceptible to activation than is free plasminogen in plasma. Streptokinase isolated from group C β-hemolytic streptococci and acylated plasminogen–streptokinase (APSAC) act through a streptokinase–plasminogen complex; urokinase, single-chain urokinase-type plasminogen activator (SCU-PA), and recombinant tPA act directly on plasminogen without an intermediate drug–plasminogen complex[189] (Fig. 5.11). tPA (originally isolated from a melanoma cell line and now produced through recombinant DNA technology), APSAC, and SCU-PA are termed *fibrin selective* because of their high ratio of activity for fibrin-bound plasminogen compared with circulating plasminogen. For therapeutic uses, tPA or recombinant plasminogen activator (rPA) is primarily used, and the others are of historical significance only. tPA has a fibrin-binding site and a catalytic site that are widely separated from each other. This separation allows tPA to be activated to its fibrin target, thus establishing its fibrin-specific nature. Evidence-based recommendations for agent and indications are continually updated.[190,191]

Bleeding complications associated with fibrinolytic agents are related to the invasive procedures associated with drug delivery. Factors associated include hypofibrinogenemia and fibrin degradation products. The latter inhibit fibrin polymerization and, in combination with a decrease in the clotting factors V and VIII (from excess plasmin not neutralized by α_2-AP), inhibit the ability of blood to clot. Although coagulation tests in general do not correlate well with bleeding, a fibrinogen level less than 100 mg/dL is associated with an increased risk and severity of bleeding.

Platelets are both inhibited and stimulated by fibrinolytic agents. Because fibrinogen is a necessary cofactor for ADP-induced platelet aggregation, low fibrinogen levels aggravate a platelet defect. At the same time, plasminogen bound to platelets leads to impaired adhesion and a decrease in their ability to aggregate. Plasmin-induced cleavage of adhesive proteins, such as thrombospondin, fibronectin, and fibrin, also disrupts the bonds that hold platelet aggregates together.

Despite these mechanisms that decrease the clotting ability of blood during fibrinolytic therapy, it has been found that these agents promote reocclusion in up to 30% of cases early after thrombolysis through platelet activation, suggesting that platelet activation occurs early after lysis and platelet inhibition occurs later.[1] In addition, increased synthesis of endothelial cell PAI-1 has been demonstrated experimentally after treatment with tPA, another mechanism that could potentially contribute to early thrombotic reocclusion if the patients are not heparinized.[192]

Thrombolytic therapy for peripheral arterial applications is commonly used, especially when the agents are given via catheter infusion, and is a standard treatment for acute limb ischemia and peripheral bypass graft occlusion.[193] Several studies suggest its efficacy and safety for acute limb ischemia as comparable to surgery.[194,195] After thrombolytic therapy has reopened an occluded vessel or graft, however, radiologic or surgical correction of the lesion responsible for the thrombosis

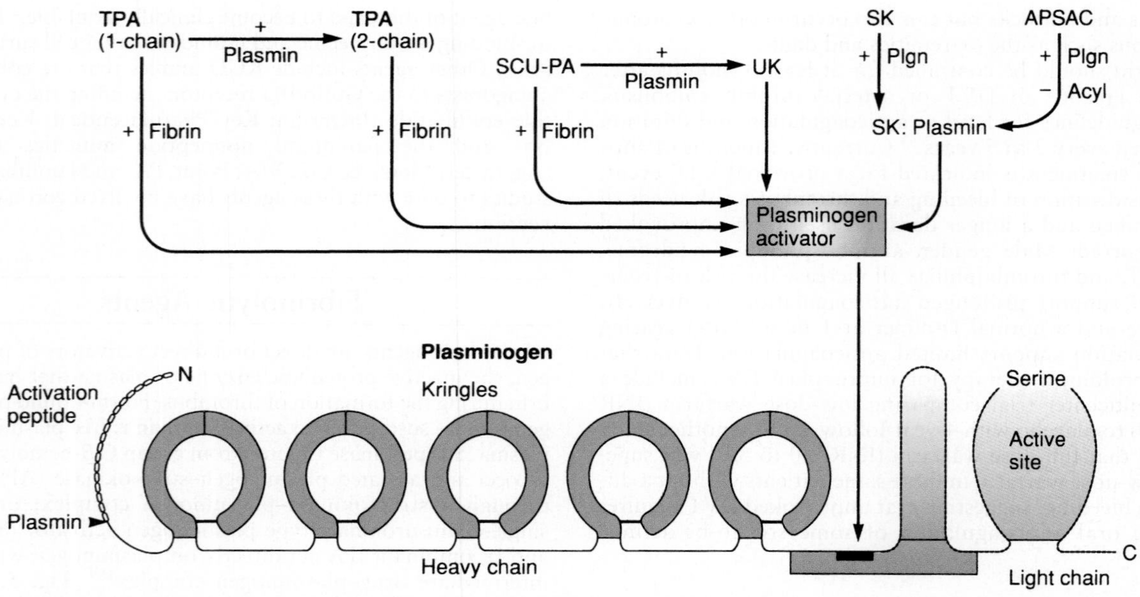

FIGURE 5.11. Sites of action of plasminogen activators on plasminogen. APSAC, acylated plasminogen–streptokinase; Plgn, plasminogen; SCU-PA, single-chain urokinase plasminogen activator; SK, streptokinase; TPA, tissue plasminogen activator; UK, urokinase.

must be addressed for long-term success.[196] The use of intraoperative thrombolytic therapy has been advocated for situations in which complete clot evacuation cannot be accomplished (as may occur in up to 40% of patients undergoing balloon embolectomy with an embolectomy catheter for acute arterial occlusion) or when the distal vasculature is occluded and precludes appropriate inflow patency.[197]

Complications associated with thrombolytic therapy for arterial thrombosis include bleeding, rethrombosis, embolization treated with further thrombolytic therapy, and sepsis from prolonged catheter placement. The most recent innovation in intra-arterial thrombolytic therapy involves lacing the entire length of the thrombus with high-dose tPA before continuous infusion and then using pulse-spray techniques, sometimes in conjunction with mechanical dissolution.[198]

Indications for DVT and PE thrombolytic therapy remain controversial.[197] Thirteen studies of thrombolytic therapy for acute DVT have been compiled from the literature.[199] In these studies, patients were assessed with venography. Of those patients treated with anticoagulants, only 4% had complete lysis and 14% revealed partial lysis. In contrast, 45% of patients treated with thrombolytic agents showed significant or complete clot lysis and an additional 18% revealed partial lysis. Importantly, catheter-directed thrombolysis for iliofemoral DVT is associated with significantly improved quality of life over time.[200] Thrombolytic therapy in PE has been extensively studied. Early studies evaluated the use of either urokinase or streptokinase. Although both agents rapidly lysed clot and improved pulmonary hemodynamics, there was no difference in patient mortality rate or recurrence rate of PE compared with heparin alone.[201,202] As a general guide, thrombolytic therapy for PE should be considered when there is angiographically documented lobar or greater PE causing acute pulmonary hypertension and right ventricular failure with hemodynamic compromise; lesser degrees of PE should be treated with standard heparin or LMWH anticoagulation.[63,203] Fibrinolytic therapy may also have a role and has been suggested for use in upper extremity effort thrombosis, catheter-induced venous thrombosis, and superior vena caval thrombosis. Contraindications to thrombolytic therapy, whether regional or systemic, are well defined (Table 5.4).

TABLE 5.4 INDICATIONS/CONTRAINDICATIONS

CONTRAINDICATIONS TO THROMBOLYTIC THERAPY

ABSOLUTE
- Neurosurgery within 3 mo
- Active internal bleeding
- Recent (<2 mo) cerebrovascular accident
- Intracranial disease
- Recent gastrointestinal bleeding

RELATIVE

Major
- Recent (<10 d) major surgery, obstetric delivery, or organ biopsy
- Left heart thrombus
- Active peptic ulcer or gastrointestinal abnormality
- Recent major trauma
- Uncontrolled hypertension (systolic >180 mm Hg; diastolic >110 mm Hg)
- Recent eye surgery

Minor
- Minor surgery or trauma
- Recent cardiopulmonary resuscitation
- Atrial fibrillation with mitral valve disease
- Bacterial endocarditis
- Hemostatic defects (i.e., renal or liver disease)
- Diabetic hemorrhagic retinopathy
- Pregnancy

CONTRAINDICATIONS TO STREPTOKINASE
- Known allergy
- Recent streptococcal infection
- Previous therapy within 6 mo

Table adapted from TASC II. *J Vasc Surg*. 2007;45:S45.

Dextran

Dextran is a high-molecular-weight polysaccharide produced from sucrose by *Leuconostoc mesenteroides*. Fractionation and hydrolysis produce a product with an average molecular weight of either 40 kD (dextran-40 [Rheomacrodex; Medisan, Parsippany, NJ]) or 70 kD (dextran-70). Dextran-40 has been studied in detail for its ability to augment patency of difficult lower extremity bypass grafts in the early postoperative period. Dextran-40 acts as a volume expander, causing hemodilution, decreasing blood viscosity, decreasing platelet adhesiveness, reducing factor VIII activity, and increasing the lysability of clots.[204] In addition, dextran has been found to coat endothelial cell surfaces, decreasing their electronegativity.

LABORATORY MONITORING OF COAGULATION AND ANTICOAGULATION

Tests of Platelet Function

Platelet tests include peripheral platelet counts, bleeding times, and platelet aggregation. Usually, a platelet count of 50,000/mL or more ensures adequate hemostasis, whereas counts less than 10,000/mL are dangerous and may lead to spontaneous bleeding. Thrombocytosis is considered to exist when the platelet count exceeds 500,000/mL, although in some cases (especially those involving myeloproliferative disorders or following splenectomy), counts may be greater than 1,000,000/mL.[3] Bleeding time assays assess the ability of platelets to form hemostatic plugs and are usually shorter than 8 minutes. A bleeding time between 8 and 15 minutes most often reflects a low plasma level of vWF, the use of antiplatelet drugs, the presence of lupuslike antibodies, or a factor XI deficiency.[3] A bleeding time greater than 15 minutes is clearly prolonged and indicates severe platelet functional impairment, very low levels of vWF, or a fibrinogenemia and severe factor V deficiency. Many of the platelet functions are best assessed with the platelet function analyzer (PFA-100; Dade Behring, Germany), available in most hospitals.[205]

Coagulation Tests

Coagulation tests include PT (intrinsic and extrinsic pathways and fibrinogen), aPTT (contact and intrinsic pathway), TCT (fibrinogen conversion to fibrin), and ACT (whole blood and platelets). The only abnormality that causes an isolated elevation in PT with all of the other test results normal is factor VII deficiency. In addition, the PT is sensitive to small decreases in factor V levels. The aPTT identifies abnormalities of the contact and intrinsic phases of coagulation. Conditions that cause a prolonged aPTT include the presence of heparin; deficiencies in factors VIII, IX, and XII; and the presence of lupuslike anticoagulants.[3] aPTT values have variably been shown to correlate with heparin dosages and serum heparin levels, and levels of 0.2 IU/mL or greater usually correlate with an aPTT of 1.5 times normal or greater.

The TCT is a measurement of the time it takes for exogenously added thrombin to turn plasma fibrinogen into fibrin clot. As such, it is extremely sensitive to levels of heparin and is an excellent means of measuring the level of heparin-induced anticoagulation. The beauty of the TCT is that it is not specific for any disease condition; thus, it may be used to differentiate factor deficiencies from the presence of heparin or to separate lupus anticoagulant from abnormalities in fibrinogen levels.[3]

The ACT is a measurement of the ability of whole blood to clot and as such is an available technique for monitoring intraoperative heparin levels. The ACT responds linearly to increasing heparin dosage and correlates well with observed clinical anticoagulation (thrombus-free surface on cardiopulmonary bypass devices).[206] Adequate anticoagulation for extracorporeal circulation is defined as an ACT of 480 seconds or more, but most cardiovascular surgeons would agree that any value between 300 and 600 seconds is acceptable. For peripheral vascular applications, values of 250 seconds or greater are considered appropriate levels, representative of full intraoperative anticoagulation. The ACT may be affected by hemodilution, cardioplegia solutions, hypothermia, platelet dysfunction, hypofibrinogenemia, and other coagulopathies, as well as by certain medications and excess protamine administration. Finally, factor Xa levels can be measured to accurately measure LMWH or direct Ia inhibitors. Clinically, this is useful in renal failure patients and morbidly obese patients.

Tests of Fibrinolysis

Tests of fibrinolysis are less well characterized. The euglobulin lysis test time is a crude screening test for problems with fibrinolysis.[3] Patients with accelerated fibrinolysis are often found to have a deficiency of α_2-AP (of which the total amount normally is only half of the total plasmin that can be generated) or the fibrin clot-stabilizing factor XIII.[3] A deficiency of PAI-1 also may lead to accelerated fibrinolysis. During normal clot formation and breakdown, the D-dimer fragment of fibrinogen is a marker for ongoing thrombosis and physiologic fibrinolysis, whereas for fibrinogenolysis, the two D fragments that are produced are not cross-linked into the D-dimer form.[3]

References

1. Coller BS. Platelets and thrombolytic therapy. *N Engl J Med* 1990;322(1):33–42.
2. Ferguson JJ, Waly HM, Wilson JM. Fundamentals of coagulation and glycoprotein IIb/IIIa receptor inhibition. *Eur Heart J* 1998;19(suppl D): D3–D9.
3. Hassouna HI. Laboratory evaluation of hemostatic disorders. *Hematol Oncol Clin North Am* 1993;7(6):1161–1249.
4. Monroe DM, Hoffman M. What does it take to make the perfect clot? *Arterioscler Thromb Vasc Biol* 2006;26(1):41–48.
5. Sims PJ, Faioni EM, Wiedmer T, et al. Complement proteins C5b-9 cause release of membrane vesicles from the platelet surface that are enriched in the membrane receptor for coagulation factor Va and express prothrombinase activity. *J Biol Chem* 1988;263(34):18205–18212.
6. Gilbert GE, Sims PJ, Wiedmer T, et al. Platelet-derived microparticles express high affinity receptors for factor VIII. *J Biol Chem* 1991;266(26):17261–17268.
7. Hickey MJ, Williams SA, Roth GJ. Human platelet glycoprotein IX: an adhesive prototype of leucine-rich glycoproteins with flank-center-flank structures. *Proc Natl Acad Sci U S A* 1989;86(17):6773–6777.
8. Bennett JS, Vilaire G, Cines DB. Identification of the fibrinogen receptor on human platelets by photoaffinity labeling. *J Biol Chem* 1982;257(14):8049–8054.
9. Savage B, Ruggeri ZM. Selective recognition of adhesive sites in surface-bound fibrinogen by glycoprotein IIb-IIIa on nonactivated platelets. *J Biol Chem* 1991;266(17):11227–11233.
10. Shapiro AD. Platelet function disorders. *Haemophilia* 2000;6(suppl 1):120–127.
11. Furie B, Furie BC. Mechanisms of thrombus formation. *N Engl J Med* 2008;359(9):938–949.
12. Mackman N, Tilley RE, Key NS. Role of the extrinsic pathway of blood coagulation in hemostasis and thrombosis. *Arterioscler Thromb Vasc Biol* 2007;27(8):1687–1693.
13. Himber J, Wohlgensinger C, Roux S, et al. Inhibition of tissue factor limits the growth of venous thrombus in the rabbit. *J Thromb Haemost* 2003;1(5):889–895.
14. Bauer KA, Kass BL, ten Cate H, et al. Factor IX is activated in vivo by the tissue factor mechanism. *Blood* 1990;76(4):731–736.
15. Davie EW, Fujikawa K, Kisiel W. The coagulation cascade: initiation, maintenance, and regulation. *Biochemistry* 1991;30(43):10363–10370.
16. Naito K, Fujikawa K. Activation of human blood coagulation factor XI independent of factor XII. Factor XI is activated by thrombin and factor XIa in the presence of negatively charged surfaces. *J Biol Chem* 1991;266(12):7353–7358.
17. Kisiel W, Canfield WM, Ericsson LH, et al. Anticoagulant properties of bovine plasma protein C following activation by thrombin. *Biochemistry* 1977;16(26):5824–5831.

18. Marlar RA, Kleiss AJ, Griffin JH. Mechanism of action of human activated protein C, a thrombin-dependent anticoagulant enzyme. *Blood* 1982;59(5):1067–1072.
19. Esmon CT, Owen WG. Identification of an endothelial cell cofactor for thrombin-catalyzed activation of protein C. *Proc Natl Acad Sci U S A* 1981;78(4):2249–2252.
20. Owen WG, Esmon CT. Functional properties of an endothelial cell cofactor for thrombin-catalyzed activation of protein C. *J Biol Chem* 1981;256(11):5532–5535.
21. Esmon NL, Owen WG, Esmon CT. Isolation of a membrane-bound cofactor for thrombin-catalyzed activation of protein C. *J Biol Chem* 1982;257(2):859–864.
22. Esmon NL, Carroll RC, Esmon CT. Thrombomodulin blocks the ability of thrombin to activate platelets. *J Biol Chem* 1983;258(20):12238–12242.
23. Esmon CT, Esmon NL, Harris KW. Complex formation between thrombin and thrombomodulin inhibits both thrombin-catalyzed fibrin formation and factor V activation. *J Biol Chem* 1982;257(14):7944–7947.
24. Mosnier LO, Bouma BN. Regulation of fibrinolysis by thrombin activatable fibrinolysis inhibitor, an unstable carboxypeptidase B that unites the pathways of coagulation and fibrinolysis. *Arterioscler Thromb Vasc Biol* 2006;26(11):2445–2453.
25. Tollefsen DM. Heparin cofactor II modulates the response to vascular injury. *Arterioscler Thromb Vasc Biol* 2007;27(3):454–460.
26. Dano K, Andreasen PA, Grondahl-Hansen J, et al. Plasminogen activators, tissue degradation, and cancer. *Adv Cancer Res* 1985;44:139–266.
27. Vassalli JD, Sappino AP, Belin D. The plasminogen activator/plasmin system. *J Clin Invest* 1991;88(4):1067–1072.
28. Kohler HP, Grant PJ. Plasminogen-activator inhibitor type 1 and coronary artery disease. *N Engl J Med* 2000;342(24):1792–1801.
29. Gelehrter TD, Sznycer-Laszuk R. Thrombin induction of plasminogen activator-inhibitor in cultured human endothelial cells. *J Clin Invest* 1986;77(1):165–169.
30. Dichek D, Quertermous T. Thrombin regulation of mRNA levels of tissue plasminogen activator and plasminogen activator inhibitor-1 in cultured human umbilical vein endothelial cells. *Blood* 1989;74(1):222–228.
31. Esmon CT. The regulation of natural anticoagulant pathways. *Science* 1987;235(4794):1348–1352.
32. Palareti G, Cosmi B, Legnani C, et al. D-dimer testing to determine the duration of anticoagulation therapy. *N Engl J Med* 2006;355(17):1780–1789.
33. Schulman S, Wiman B. The significance of hypofibrinolysis for the risk of recurrence of venous thromboembolism. Duration of Anticoagulation (DURAC) Trial Study Group. *Thromb Haemost* 1996;75(4):607–611.
34. Aird WC. Phenotypic heterogeneity of the endothelium: I. Structure, function, and mechanisms. *Circ Res* 2007;100(2):158–173.
35. Becker BF, Heindl B, Kupatt C, et al. Endothelial function and hemostasis. *Z Kardiol* 2000;89(3):160–167.
36. Gross PL, Aird WC. The endothelium and thrombosis. *Semin Thromb Hemost* 2000;26(5):463–478.
37. Wagner DD, Frenette PS. The vessel wall and its interactions. *Blood* 2008;111(11):5271–5281.
38. Wakefield TW, Myers DD, Henke PK. Mechanisms of venous thrombosis and resolution. *Arterioscler Thromb Vasc Biol* 2008;28(3):387–391.
39. Andre P, Hartwell D, Hrachovinova I, et al. Pro-coagulant state resulting from high levels of soluble P-selectin in blood. *Proc Natl Acad Sci U S A* 2000;97(25):13835–13840.
40. Myers DD Jr, Schaub R, Wrobleski SK, et al. P-selectin antagonism causes dose-dependent venous thrombosis inhibition. *Thromb Haemost* 2001;85(3):423–429.
41. Myers D, Wrobleski S, Londy F, et al. New and effective treatment of experimentally induced venous thrombosis with anti-inflammatory rPSGL-Ig. *Thromb Haemost* 2002;87(3):374–382.
42. Myers DD, Hawley AE, Farris DM, et al. P-selectin and leukocyte microparticles are associated with venous thrombogenesis. *J Vasc Surg* 2003;38(5):1075–1089.
43. Hrachovinova I, Cambien B, Hafezi-Moghadam A, et al. Interaction of P-selectin and PSGL-1 generates microparticles that correct hemostasis in a mouse model of hemophilia A. *Nat Med* 2003;9(8):1020–1025.
44. Wakefield TW, Strieter RM, Wilke CA, et al. Venous thrombosis-associated inflammation and attenuation with neutralizing antibodies to cytokines and adhesion molecules. *Arterioscler Thromb Vasc Biol* 1995;15(2):258–268.
45. Varma MR, Varga AJ, Knipp BS, et al. Neutropenia impairs venous thrombosis resolution in the rat. *J Vasc Surg* 2003;38:1090–1098.
46. Stewart GJ. Neutrophils and deep venous thrombosis. *Haemostasis* 1993;23(suppl 1):127–140.
47. Varma MR, Moaveni DM, Dewyer NA, et al. Deep vein thrombosis resolution is not accelerated with increased neovascularization. *J Vasc Surg* 2004;40(3):536–542.
48. Lin J, Proctor MC, Varma M, et al. Factors associated with recurrent venous thromboembolism in patients with malignant disease. *J Vasc Surg* 2003;37(5):976–983.
49. Hogaboam CM, Steinhauser ML, Chensue SW, et al. Novel roles for chemokines and fibroblasts in interstitial fibrosis. *Kidney Int* 1998;54(6):2152–2159.
50. Humphries J, McGuinness CL, Smith A, et al. Monocyte chemotactic protein-1 (MCP-1) accelerates the organization and resolution of venous thrombi. *J Vasc Surg* 1999;30(5):894–899.
51. Henke PK, Pearce CG, Moaveni DM, et al. Targeted deletion of CCR2 impairs deep vein thrombosis resolution in a mouse model. *J Immunol* 2006;177(5):3388–3397.
52. Northeast AD, Soo KS, Bobrow LG, et al. The tissue plasminogen activator and urokinase response in vivo during natural resolution of venous thrombus. *J Vasc Surg* 1995;22(5):573–579.
53. Soo KS, Northeast AD, Happerfield LC, et al. Tissue plasminogen activator production by monocytes in venous thrombolysis. *J Pathol* 1996;178(2):190–194.
54. Singh I, Burnand KG, Collins M, et al. Failure of thrombus to resolve in urokinase-type plasminogen activator gene-knockout mice: rescue by normal bone marrow-derived cells. *Circulation* 2003;107(6):869–875.
55. Henke PK, Varma MR, Moaveni DK, et al. Fibrotic injury after experimental deep vein thrombosis is determined by the mechanism of thrombogenesis. *Thromb Haemost* 2007;98(5):1045–1055.
56. Mackman N. Triggers, targets and treatments for thrombosis. *Nature* 2008;451(7181):914–918.
57. Ross R. Atherosclerosis—an inflammatory disease. *N Engl J Med* 1999;340(2):115–126.
58. Chan MY, Andreotti F, Becker RC. Hypercoagulable states in cardiovascular disease. *Circulation* 2008;118(22):2286–2297.
59. Gangireddy C, Rectenwald JR, Upchurch GR, et al. Risk factors and clinical impact of postoperative symptomatic venous thromboembolism. *J Vasc Surg* 2007;45(2):335–341; discussion 341–342.
60. Heit JA. The epidemiology of venous thromboembolism in the community. *Arterioscler Thromb Vasc Biol* 2008;28(3):370–372.
61. Heit JA, Silverstein MD, Mohr DN, et al. The epidemiology of venous thromboembolism in the community. *Thromb Haemost* 2001;86(1):452–463.
62. Caprini JA, Arcelus JI, Reyna JJ. Effective risk stratification of surgical and nonsurgical patients for venous thromboembolic disease. *Semin Hematol* 2001;38(2 suppl 5):12–19.
63. Geerts W. Antithrombotic and thrombolytic therapy, 8th ed: ACCP guidelines. *Chest* 2008;133:381s–451s.
64. Lockshin MD. Antiphospholipid antibody syndrome. *JAMA* 1992;268(11):1451–1453.
65. Lockshin MD. Antiphospholipid antibody. Babies, blood clots, biology. *JAMA* 1997;277(19):1549–1551.
66. Khamashta MA, Cuadrado MJ, Mujic F, et al. The management of thrombosis in the antiphospholipid-antibody syndrome. *N Engl J Med* 1995;332(15):993–997.
67. Eldrup-Jorgensen J, Flanigan DP, Brace L, et al. Hypercoagulable states and lower limb ischemia in young adults. *J Vasc Surg* 1989;9(2):334–341.
68. Galli M, Luciani D, Bertolini G, et al. Lupus anticoagulants are stronger risk factors for thrombosis than anticardiolipin antibodies in the antiphospholipid syndrome: a systematic review of the literature. *Blood* 2003;101(5):1827–1832.
69. Carreras LO, Defreyn G, Machin SJ, et al. Arterial thrombosis, intrauterine death and "lupus" anticoagulant: detection of immunoglobulin interfering with prostacyclin formation. *Lancet* 1981;1(8214):244–246.
70. Comp PC, DeBault LE, Esmon NL, et al. Human thrombomodulin is inhibited by IgG from two patients with non-specific anticoagulants (abstract). *Blood* 1983;62(suppl 1):244–246.
71. Vermylen J, Blockmans D, Spitz B, et al. Thrombosis and immune disorders. *Clin Haematol* 1986;15(2):393–412.
72. Ferro D, Pittoni V, Quintarelli C, et al. Coexistence of anti-phospholipid antibodies and endothelial perturbation in systemic lupus erythematosus patients with ongoing prothrombotic state. *Circulation* 1997;95(6):1425–1432.
73. Rand JH, Wu XX, Andree HA, et al. Pregnancy loss in the antiphospholipid-antibody syndrome—a possible thrombogenic mechanism. *N Engl J Med* 1997;337(3):154–160.
74. Reverter JC, Tassies D, Font J, et al. Hypercoagulable state in patients with antiphospholipid syndrome is related to high induced tissue factor expression on monocytes and to low free proteins. *Arterioscler Thromb Vasc Biol* 1996;16(11):1319–1326.
75. Greenfield LJ. Lupus-like anticoagulants and thrombosis. *J Vasc Surg* 1988;7(6):818–819.
76. Ahn SS, Kalunian K, Rosove M, et al. Postoperative thrombotic complications in patients with lupus anticoagulant: increased risk after vascular procedures. *J Vasc Surg* 1988;7(6):749–756.
77. Nielsen TG, Nordestgaard BG, von Jessen F, et al. Antibodies to cardiolipin may increase the risk of failure of peripheral vein bypasses. *Eur J Vasc Endovasc Surg* 1997;14(3):177–184.
78. de Moerloose P, Bounameaux HR, Mannucci PM. Screening test for thrombophilic patients: which tests, for which patient, by whom, when, and why? *Semin Thromb Hemost* 1998;24(4):321–327.
79. Lynch A, Marlar R, Murphy J, et al. Antiphospholipid antibodies in predicting adverse pregnancy outcome. A prospective study. *Ann Intern Med* 1994;120(6):470–475.
80. Flinn WR, McDaniel MD, Yao JS, et al. Antithrombin III deficiency as a reflection of dynamic protein metabolism in patients undergoing vascular reconstruction. *J Vasc Surg* 1984;1(6):888–895.
81. Towne JB, Bernhard VM, Hussey C, et al. Antithrombin deficiency—a cause of unexplained thrombosis in vascular surgery. *Surgery* 1981;89(6):735–742.
82. Pabinger I, Schneider B. Thrombotic risk of women with hereditary antithrombin III-, protein C- and protein S-deficiency taking oral contraceptive

medication. The GTH Study Group on Natural Inhibitors. *Thromb Haemost* 1994;71(5):548–552.
83. Seligsohn U, Lubetsky A. Genetic susceptibility to venous thrombosis. *N Engl J Med* 2001;344(16):1222–1231.
84. Bick RL. Prothrombin G20210A mutation, antithrombin, heparin cofactor II, protein C, and protein S defects. *Hematol Oncol Clin North Am* 2003; 17(1):9–36.
85. Donaldson MC, Belkin M, Whittemore AD, et al. Impact of activated protein C resistance on general vascular surgical patients. *J Vasc Surg* 1997; 25(6):1054–1060.
86. Franco RF, Reitsma PH. Genetic risk factors of venous thrombosis. *Hum Genet* 2001;109(4):369–384.
87. Siddiqi FA, Tepler J, Fantini GA. Acquired protein S and antithrombin III deficiency caused by nephrotic syndrome: an unusual cause of graft thrombosis. *J Vasc Surg* 1997;25(3):576–580.
88. Jennings I, Cooper P. Screening for thrombophilia: a laboratory perspective. *Br J Biomed Sci* 2003;60(1):39–51.
89. Dahlback B. Blood coagulation. *Lancet* 2000;355(9215):1627–1632.
90. Cole MS, Minifee PK, Wolma FJ. Coumarin necrosis—a review of the literature. *Surgery* 1988;103(3):271–277.
91. Ridker PM, Miletich JP, Hennekens CH, et al. Ethnic distribution of factor V Leiden in 4047 men and women. Implications for venous thromboembolism screening. *JAMA* 1997;277(16):1305–1307.
92. Rosendaal FR, Koster T, Vandenbroucke JP, et al. High risk of thrombosis in patients homozygous for factor V Leiden (activated protein C resistance). *Blood* 1995;85(6):1504–1508.
93. Svensson PJ, Dahlback B. Resistance to activated protein C as a basis for venous thrombosis. *N Engl J Med* 1994;330(8):517–522.
94. Kalafatis M, Mann KG. Factor V Leiden and thrombophilia. *Arterioscler Thromb Vasc Biol* 1997;17(4):620–627.
95. Mann KG, Kalafatis M. Factor V: a combination of Dr Jekyll and Mr Hyde. *Blood* 2003;101(1):20–30.
96. Simioni P, Prandoni P, Lensing AW, et al. The risk of recurrent venous thromboembolism in patients with an Arg506–>Gln mutation in the gene for factor V (factor V Leiden). *N Engl J Med* 1997;336(6):399–403.
97. De Stefano V, Martinelli I, Mannucci PM, et al. The risk of recurrent deep venous thrombosis among heterozygous carriers of both factor V Leiden and the G20210A prothrombin mutation. *N Engl J Med* 1999;341(11): 801–806.
98. Koeleman BP, Reitsma PH, Allaart CF, et al. Activated protein C resistance as an additional risk factor for thrombosis in protein C-deficient families. *Blood* 1994;84(4):1031–1035.
99. Koeleman BP, van Rumpt D, Hamulyak K, et al. Factor V Leiden: an additional risk factor for thrombosis in protein S deficient families? *Thromb Haemost* 1995;74(2):580–583.
100. Ouriel K, Green RM, DeWeese JA, et al. Activated protein C resistance: prevalence and implications in peripheral vascular disease. *J Vasc Surg* 1996;23(1):46–51, discussion 51–52.
101. Van Cott EM, Soderberg BL, Laposata M. Activated protein C resistance, the factor V Leiden mutation, and a laboratory testing algorithm. *Arch Pathol Lab Med* 2002;126(5):577–582.
102. Vicente V, Gonzalez-Conejero R, Rivera J, et al. The prothrombin gene variant 20210 A in venous and arterial thromboembolism. *Haematologica* 1999;84(4):356–362.
103. Cumming AM, Keeney S, Salden A, et al. The prothrombin gene G20210A variant: prevalence in a U. K. anticoagulant clinic population. *Br J Haematol* 1997;98(2):353–355.
104. Martinelli I, Sacchi E, Landi G, et al. High risk of cerebral-vein thrombosis in carriers of a prothrombin-gene mutation and in users of oral contraceptives. *N Engl J Med* 1998;338(25):1793–1797.
105. Gerhardt A, Scharf RE, Beckmann MW, et al. Prothrombin and factor V mutations in women with a history of thrombosis during pregnancy and the puerperium. *N Engl J Med* 2000;342(6):374–380.
106. Ridker PM, Hennekens CH, Miletich JP. G20210A mutation in prothrombin gene and risk of myocardial infarction, stroke, and venous thrombosis in a large cohort of US men. *Circulation* 1999;99(8):999–1004.
107. McGlennen RC, Key NS. Clinical and laboratory management of the prothrombin G20210A mutation. *Arch Pathol Lab Med* 2002;126(11): 1319–1325.
108. De Stefano V, Casorelli I, Rossi E, et al. Interaction between hyperhomocysteinemia and inherited thrombophilic factors in venous thromboembolism. *Semin Thromb Hemost* 2000;26(3):305–311.
109. den Heijer M, Blom HJ, Gerrits WB, et al. Is hyperhomocysteinaemia a risk factor for recurrent venous thrombosis? *Lancet* 1995;345(8954): 882–885.
110. den Heijer M, Koster T, Blom HJ, et al. Hyperhomocysteinemia as a risk factor for deep-vein thrombosis. *N Engl J Med* 1996;334(12):759–762.
111. den Heijer M, Keijzer MB. Hyperhomocysteinemia as a risk factor for venous thrombosis. *Clin Chem Lab Med* 2001;39(8):710–713.
112. Legnani C, Palareti G, Grauso F, et al. Hyperhomocyst(e)inemia and a common methylenetetrahydrofolate reductase mutation (Ala223Val MTHFR) in patients with inherited thrombophilic coagulation defects. *Arterioscler Thromb Vasc Biol* 1997;17(11):2924–2929.
113. Kottke-Marchant K. Genetic polymorphisms associated with venous and arterial thrombosis: an overview. *Arch Pathol Lab Med* 2002;126(3): 295–304.
114. Falcon CR, Cattaneo M, Panzeri D, et al. High prevalence of hyperhomocyst(e)inemia in patients with juvenile venous thrombosis. *Arterioscler Thromb* 1994;14(7):1080–1083.
115. Mandel H, Brenner B, Berant M, et al. Coexistence of hereditary homocystinuria and factor V Leiden—effect on thrombosis. *N Engl J Med* 1996;334(12):763–768.
116. Hayashi T, Honda G, Suzuki K. An atherogenic stimulus homocysteine inhibits cofactor activity of thrombomodulin and enhances thrombomodulin expression in human umbilical vein endothelial cells. *Blood* 1992; 79(11):2930–2936.
117. Loscalzo J. The oxidant stress of hyperhomocyst(e)inemia. *J Clin Invest* 1996;98(1):5–7.
118. Rodgers GM, Conn MT. Homocysteine, an atherogenic stimulus, reduces protein C activation by arterial and venous endothelial cells. *Blood* 1990; 75(4):895–901.
119. Tawakol A, Omland T, Gerhard M, et al. Hyperhomocyst(e)inemia is associated with impaired endothelium-dependent vasodilation in humans. *Circulation* 1997;95(5):1119–1121.
120. Upchurch GR, Welch GN, Randev V, et al. The effect of homocysteine on endothelial nitric oxide production. *FASEB J* 1995;9:A876.
121. George J, Alving BM, Ballem P. Platelets. In: McArthur JR, Benz EJ, eds. *Hemotology – 1994,* vol. 66. Washington, DC; 1994:1750.
122. Ueland PM, Refsum H, Brattstrom L. *Plasma Homocysteine and Cardiovascular Disease.* New York: Marcel Dekker; 1993.
123. Reiner AP, Siscovick DS, Rosendaal FR. Hemostatic risk factors and arterial thrombotic disease. *Thromb Haemost* 2001;85(4):584–595.
124. Towne JB, Bandyk DF, Hussey CV, et al. Abnormal plasminogen: a genetically determined cause of hypercoagulability. *J Vasc Surg* 1984;1(6): 896–902.
125. Kwaan HC, Levin M, Sakurai S, et al. Digital ischemia and gangrene due to red blood cell aggregation induced by acquired dysfibrinogenemia. *J Vasc Surg* 1997;26(6):1061–1068.
126. Roberts HR, Stinchcombe TE, Gabriel DA. The dysfibrinogenaemias. *Br J Haematol* 2001;114(2):249–257.
127. Nilsson IM, Ljungner H, Tengborn L. Two different mechanisms in patients with venous thrombosis and defective fibrinolysis: low concentration of plasminogen activator or increased concentration of plasminogen activator inhibitor. *Br Med J (Clin Res Ed)* 1985;290(6480):1453–1456.
128. Prins MH, Hirsh J. A critical review of the evidence supporting a relationship between impaired fibrinolytic activity and venous thromboembolism. *Arch Intern Med* 1991;151(9):1721–1731.
129. van Tilburg NH, Rosendaal FR, Bertina RM. Thrombin activatable fibrinolysis inhibitor and the risk for deep vein thrombosis. *Blood* 2000;95(9): 2855–2859.
130. Paramo JA, Perez JL, Serrano M, et al. Types 1 and 2 plasminogen activator inhibitor and tumor necrosis factor alpha in patients with sepsis. *Thromb Haemost* 1990;64(1):3–6.
131. Ishibashi S. Lipoprotein(a) and atherosclerosis. *Arterioscler Thromb Vasc Biol* 2001;21(1):1–2.
132. Liao JK, Shin WS, Lee WY, et al. Oxidized low-density lipoprotein decreases the expression of endothelial nitric oxide synthase. *J Biol Chem* 1995;270(1):319–324.
133. Valentine RJ, Kaplan HS, Green R, et al. Lipoprotein (a), homocysteine, and hypercoagulable states in young men with premature peripheral atherosclerosis: a prospective, controlled analysis. *J Vasc Surg* 1996;23(1): 53–61, discussion 61–63.
134. Griffin JH, Fernandez JA, Deguchi H. Plasma lipoproteins, hemostasis and thrombosis. *Thromb Haemost* 2001;86(1):386–394.
135. Nowak-Gottl U, Junker R, Hartmeier M, et al. Increased lipoprotein(a) is an important risk factor for venous thromboembolism in childhood. *Circulation* 1999;100(7):743–748.
136. Mosesson MW. Dysfibrinogenemia and thrombosis. *Semin Thromb Hemost* 1999;25(3):311–319.
137. Rosendaal FR. Venous thrombosis: a multicausal disease. *Lancet* 1999; 353(9159):1167–1173.
138. Harker LA. Platelets in thrombotic disorders: quantitative and qualitative platelet disorders predisposing to arterial thrombosis. *Semin Hematol* 1998;35(3):241–252.
139. Kamphuisen PW, Lensen R, Houwing-Duistermaat JJ, et al. Heritability of elevated factor VIII antigen levels in factor V Leiden families with thrombophilia. *Br J Haematol* 2000;109(3):519–522.
140. Koster T, Blann AD, Briet E, et al. Role of clotting factor VIII in effect of von Willebrand factor on occurrence of deep-vein thrombosis. *Lancet* 1995;345(8943):152–155.
141. O'Donnell J, Mumford AD, Manning RA, et al. Elevation of FVIII: C in venous thromboembolism is persistent and independent of the acute phase response. *Thromb Haemost* 2000;83(1):10–13.
142. Mansvelt EP, Laffan M, McVey JH, et al. Analysis of the F8 gene in individuals with high plasma factor VIII: C levels and associated venous thrombosis. *Thromb Haemost* 1998;80(4):561–565.
143. Meijers JC, Tekelenburg WL, Bouma BN, et al. High levels of coagulation factor XI as a risk factor for venous thrombosis. *N Engl J Med* 2000; 342(10):696–701.
144. van Hylckama Vlieg A, van der Linden IK, Bertina RM, et al. High levels of factor IX increase the risk of venous thrombosis. *Blood* 2000;95(12): 3678–3682.
145. Lane DA, Grant PJ. Role of hemostatic gene polymorphisms in venous and arterial thrombotic disease. *Blood* 2000;95(5):1517–1532.
146. Middeldorp S, Levi M. Thrombophilia: an update. *Semin Thromb Hemost* 2007;33(6):563–572.
147. Cunningham MT, Brandt JT, Laposata M, et al. Laboratory diagnosis of dysfibrinogenemia. *Arch Pathol Lab Med* 2002;126(4):499–505.

148. Collins JA. Blood transfusion and disorders of surgical bleeding. In: Sabiston DC, ed. *Textbook of Surgery*, 14th ed. Philadelphia: WB Saunders; 1991:85–102.
149. Lusher JM, Warrier I. Hemophilia. *Hematol Oncol Clin North Am* 1993; 7:1021.
150. Lusher JM, Arkin S, Abildgaard CF, et al. Recombinant factor VIII for the treatment of previously untreated patients with hemophilia A. Safety, efficacy, and development of inhibitors. Kogenate Previously Untreated Patient Study Group. *N Engl J Med* 1993;328(7):453–459.
151. Telfer JC. Clinical spectrum of viral infections in hemophilic patients. *Hematol Oncol Clin North Am* 1993;7:999.
152. Larson PJ, High KA. Biology of inherited coagulopathies: factor IX. *Hematol Oncol Clin North Am* 1993;7:999.
153. Ginsburg D. Biology of inherited coagulopathies: von Willebrand factor. *Hematol Oncol Clin North Am* 1993;7:1011.
154. Hirsh J, Raschke R, Warkentin TE, et al. Heparin: mechanism of action, pharmacokinetics, dosing considerations, monitoring, efficacy, and safety. *Chest* 1995;108(4 suppl):258S–275S.
155. Hirsh J. Heparin. *N Engl J Med* 1991;324(22):1565–1574.
156. Hirsh J. Low-molecular-weight heparin: a review of the results of recent studies of the treatment of venous thromboembolism and unstable angina. *Circulation* 1998;98(15):1575–1582.
157. Salzman EW. Low-molecular-weight heparin: is small beautiful? *N Engl J Med* 1986;315(15):957–959.
158. Leizorovicz A. Comparison of the efficacy and safety of low molecular weight heparins and unfractionated heparin in the initial treatment of deep venous thrombosis. An updated meta-analysis. *Drugs* 1996;52(suppl 7): 30–37.
159. Siragusa S, Cosmi B, Piovella F, et al. Low-molecular-weight heparins and unfractionated heparin in the treatment of patients with acute venous thromboembolism: results of a meta-analysis. *Am J Med* 1996;100(3): 269–277.
160. Simonneau G, Sors H, Charbonnier B, et al. A comparison of low-molecular-weight heparin with unfractionated heparin for acute pulmonary embolism. The THESEE Study Group. Tinzaparine ou Heparine Standard: Evaluations dans l'Embolie Pulmonaire. *N Engl J Med* 1997;337(10):663–669.
161. Horrow JC. Protamine: a review of its toxicity. *Anesth Analg* 1985;64(3): 348–361.
162. Wakefield TW, Ucros I, Kresowik TF, et al. Decreased oxygen consumption as a toxic manifestation of protamine sulfate reversal of heparin anticoagulation. *J Vasc Surg* 1989;9(6):772–777.
163. Buller HR, Davidson BL, Decousus H, et al. Subcutaneous fondaparinux versus intravenous unfractionated heparin in the initial treatment of pulmonary embolism. *N Engl J Med* 2003;349(18):1695–1702.
164. Eriksson BI, Bauer KA, Lassen MR, et al. Fondaparinux compared with enoxaparin for the prevention of venous thromboembolism after hip-fracture surgery. *N Engl J Med* 2001;345(18):1298–1304.
165. Bauer KA, Eriksson BI, Lassen MR, et al. Fondaparinux compared with enoxaparin for the prevention of venous thromboembolism after elective major knee surgery. *N Engl J Med* 2001;345(18):1305–1310.
166. Turpie AG, Bauer KA, Eriksson BI, et al. Fondaparinux vs enoxaparin for the prevention of venous thromboembolism in major orthopedic surgery: a meta-analysis of 4 randomized double-blind studies. *Arch Intern Med* 2002;162(16):1833–1840.
167. Eriksson BI, Borris LC, Friedman RJ, et al. Rivaroxaban versus enoxaparin for thromboprophylaxis after hip arthroplasty. *N Engl J Med* 2008; 358(26):2765–2775.
168. Di Nisio M, Middeldorp S, Buller HR. Direct thrombin inhibitors. *N Engl J Med* 2005;353(10):1028–1040.
169. Greinacher A, Volpel H, Janssens U, et al. Recombinant hirudin (lepirudin) provides safe and effective anticoagulation in patients with heparin-induced thrombocytopenia: a prospective study. *Circulation* 1999;99(1): 73–80.
170. Gross PL, Weitz JI. New anticoagulants for treatment of venous thromboembolism. *Arterioscler Thromb Vasc Biol* 2008;28(3):380–386.
171. Alving BM. How I treat heparin-induced thrombocytopenia and thrombosis. *Blood* 2003;101(1):31–37.
172. Ansell JE, Price JM, Shah S, et al. Heparin-induced thrombocytopenia. What is its real frequency? *Chest* 1985;88(6):878–882.
173. Cancio LC, Cohen DJ. Heparin-induced thrombocytopenia and thrombosis. *J Am Coll Surg* 1998;186(1):76–91.
174. Almeida JI, Coats R, Liem TK, et al. Reduced morbidity and mortality rates of the heparin-induced thrombocytopenia syndrome. *J Vasc Surg* 1998; 27(2):309–314; discussion 315–316.
175. Kelton JG, Smith JW, Warkentin TE, et al. Immunoglobulin G from patients with heparin-induced thrombocytopenia binds to a complex of heparin and platelet factor 4. *Blood* 1994;83(11):3232–3239.
176. Walenga JM, Jeske WP, Messmore HL. Mechanisms of venous and arterial thrombosis in heparin-induced thrombocytopenia. *J Thromb Thrombolysis* 2000;10(suppl 1):13–20.
177. Greinacher A, Michels I, Mueller-Eckhardt C. Heparin-associated thrombocytopenia: the antibody is not heparin specific. *Thromb Haemost* 1992; 67(5):545–549.
178. Warkentin TE, Levine MN, Hirsh J, et al. Heparin-induced thrombocytopenia in patients treated with low-molecular-weight heparin or unfractionated heparin. *N Engl J Med* 1995;332(20):1330–1335.
179. Laster J, Silver D. Heparin-coated catheters and heparin-induced thrombocytopenia. *J Vasc Surg* 1988;7(5):667–672.
180. Warkentin TE. Heparin-induced thrombocytopenia. *Dis Mon* 2005; 51(2–3):141–149.
181. Warkentin TE, Elavathil LJ, Hayward CP, et al. The pathogenesis of venous limb gangrene associated with heparin-induced thrombocytopenia. *Ann Intern Med* 1997;127(9):804–812.
182. Slocum MM, Adams JG Jr, Teel R, et al. Use of enoxaparin in patients with heparin-induced thrombocytopenia syndrome. *J Vasc Surg* 1996;23(5): 839–843.
183. Warkentin TE. Heparin-induced thrombocytopenia: a clinicopathologic syndrome. *Thromb Haemost* 1999;82(2):439–447.
184. Hirsh J. Oral anticoagulant drugs. *N Engl J Med* 1991;324(26):1865–1875.
185. Ridker PM, Goldhaber SZ, Danielson E, et al. Long-term, low-intensity warfarin therapy for the prevention of recurrent venous thromboembolism. *N Engl J Med* 2003;348(15):1425–1434.
186. Kearon C, Ginsberg JS, Kovacs MJ, et al. Comparison of low-intensity warfarin therapy with conventional-intensity warfarin therapy for long-term prevention of recurrent venous thromboembolism. *N Engl J Med* 2003;349(7):631–639.
187. Pettigrew LC. Antithrombotic drugs for secondary stroke prophylaxis. *Pharmacotherapy* 2001;21(4):452–463.
188. Madan M, Berkowitz SD, Tcheng JE. Glycoprotein IIb/IIIa integrin blockade. *Circulation* 1998;98(23):2629–2635.
189. Marder VJ, Sherry S. Thrombolytic therapy: current status (1). *N Engl J Med* 1988;318(23):1512–1520.
190. Hirsch AT, Haskal ZJ, Hertzer NR, et al. ACC/AHA 2005 guidelines for the management of patients with peripheral arterial disease (lower extremity, renal, mesenteric, and abdominal aortic): executive summary: a collaborative report from the American Association for Vascular Surgery/Society for Vascular Surgery, Society for Cardiovascular Angiography and Interventions, Society for Vascular Medicine and Biology, Society of Interventional Radiology, and the ACC/AHA Task Force on Practice Guidelines (Writing Committee to Develop Guidelines for the Management of Patients With Peripheral Arterial Disease) endorsed by the American Association of Cardiovascular and Pulmonary Rehabilitation; National Heart, Lung, and Blood Institute; Society for Vascular Nursing; TransAtlantic Inter-Society Consensus; and Vascular Disease Foundation. *J Am Coll Cardiol* 2006;47(6):1239–1312.
191. Norgren L, Hiatt WR, Dormandy JA, et al. Inter-Society Consensus for the Management of Peripheral Arterial Disease (TASC II). *J Vasc Surg* 2007; 45(suppl S):S5–S67.
192. Fujii S, Sawa H, Saffitz JE, et al. Induction of endothelial cell expression of the plasminogen activator inhibitor type 1 gene by thrombosis in vivo. *Circulation* 1992;86(6):2000–2010.
193. Henke PK, Stanley JC. The treatment of acute embolic lower limb ischemia. *Adv Surg* 2004;38:281–291.
194. Ouriel K, Veith FJ, Sasahara AA. A comparison of recombinant urokinase with vascular surgery as initial treatment for acute arterial occlusion of the legs. Thrombolysis or Peripheral Arterial Surgery (TOPAS) Investigators. *N Engl J Med* 1998;338(16):1105–1111.
195. Comerota AJ, Rao AK, Throm RC, et al. A prospective, randomized, blinded, and placebo-controlled trial of intraoperative intra-arterial urokinase infusion during lower extremity revascularization. Regional and systemic effects. *Ann Surg* 1993;218(4):534–541; discussion 541–543.
196. Gardiner GA Jr, Sullivan KL. Catheter directed thrombolysis for the failed lower extremity bypass graft. *Semin Vasc Surg* 1992;5:99.
197. Lee WK, Weaver FA. Thrombolytic agents. In: Cronenwett MD, Johnston W, eds. *Rutherford's Vascular Surgery*, 7th ed. Philadelphia: Elsevier; 2010:756.
198. Ouriel K. Endovascular techniques in the treatment of acute limb ischemia: thrombolytic agents, trials, and percutaneous mechanical thrombectomy techniques. *Semin Vasc Surg* 2003;16(4):270–279.
199. Comerota AJ, Aldridge SC. Thrombolytic therapy for deep venous thrombosis: a clinical review. *Can J Surg* 1993;36(4):359–364.
200. Comerota AJ, Throm RC, Mathias SD, et al. Catheter-directed thrombolysis for iliofemoral deep venous thrombosis improves health-related quality of life. *J Vasc Surg* 2000;32(1):130–137.
201. Urokinase pulmonary embolism trial. Phase 1 results: a cooperative study. *JAMA* 1970;214(12):2163–2172.
202. Urokinase-streptokinase embolism trial. Phase 2 results. A cooperative study. *JAMA* 1974;229(12):1606–1613.
203. Goldhaber SZ. Pulmonary embolism. *Lancet* 2004;363(9417):1295–1305.
204. Rutherford RB, Jones DN. The role of dextran-40 in preventing early graft thrombosis. In: Bergqvist D, Lindblad B, eds. *Pharmacological Intervention to Increase Patency After Arterial Reconstructions*. Malmo, Sweden; 1989:44.
205. Klouche M. Diagnostic methods for platelet function analysis. *Transfus Med Hemother* 2007;34:20–32.
206. Stenbjerg S, Berg E, Albrechtsen OK. Heparin levels and activated clotting time (ACT) during open heart surgery. *Scand J Haematol* 1981;26(4):281–284.

CHAPTER 6 ■ INFLAMMATION

MATTHEW R. ROSENGART AND TIMOTHY R. BILLIAR

KEY POINTS

1. Innate immunity, a system already poised to respond prior to any stimulus, provides the initial defense against microbes. Subsequent reinforcement is provided by the more specific adaptive immune system, which possesses exquisite specificity for subsequent exposure to individual microbes and the capacity to learn and modify subsequent responses to repeated exposures. Both are composed of cellular and humoral components.
2. Implicit with the capacity for pathogen elimination is the potential for destruction of host tissues. Numerous regulatory mechanisms provide temporal and spatial control of the inflammatory processes, including programmed cell death (i.e., apoptosis).
3. The T_H1 inflammatory response (i.e., cell-mediated immunity or delayed-type hypersensitivity) is induced by interleukin-12 (IL-12) derived from phagocytes and provides one major arm of the adaptive immune response; it is mediated by $CD4^+$ and $CD8^+$ lymphocytes and macrophages, which regulate production of opsonizing and complement fixing antibodies and are effectors of phagocyte-dependent responses.
4. The principal stimulus for T_H2 differentiation is IL-4, which is derived from T cells, mast cells, and basophils. As the cellular effectors of humoral immunity, they provide the other major arm of the adaptive immune response, which is mediated by T_H2 $CD4^+$ cells, B cells, plasma cells, and antibodies.
5. Over 30 randomized controlled clinical trials have been conducted to assess the efficacy of agents modulating inflammation, in particular systemic cytokine concentrations, in reducing mortality. Yet only one, activated protein C, has been approved by the U.S. Food and Drug Administration for use, and studies are ongoing to confirm its benefit.
6. The complement system is integral to both innate and adaptive immunity and has the capacity to independently eliminate organisms and facilitate host defense by marking foreign particles for phagocytosis through opsonization.
7. Additional systems, including the vascular (i.e., vasodilatation, adhesion receptors, kinin cascade) and neuroendocrine (i.e., adrenocorticotropic hormone, arginine vasopressin, corticotropin-releasing hormone), integrate with the immune system, sharing similar mediators and their receptors, to orchestrate an intense, coordinated response to any injurious/septic insult.
8. Our immune system differentiates pathogens and damaged cells from self using evolutionarily ancient sets of recognition molecules called pattern recognition receptors, which bind conserved molecular structures found in large groups of pathogens, termed pathogen-associated molecular patterns (PAMPs), an example being the Toll-like receptors (TLRs).
9. Danger-associated molecular patterns are the endogenous equivalent of PAMPS, represent danger signals or "alarmins," and share many characteristics similar to cytokines. They may be released following nonprogrammed cell death, such as necrosis, or secreted as mediators by immune cells, under which circumstance they may facilitate the inflammatory response.

The concept of inflammation has undergone considerable revision since the initial description of the four cardinal signs and symptoms by Celsus in the first century AD: "rubor et tumor cum calor et dolore," redness and swelling with heat and pain.[1] Centuries lapsed before John Hunter postulated that inflammation provides a survival mechanism to preserve the host. Ironically, he commented that an exuberant inflammatory response could be deleterious; the pathologic sequelae of excessive inflammation (i.e., acute respiratory distress syndrome [ARDS], multiple organ dysfunction syndrome [MODS]) are encountered more frequently as technology affords survival of the initial insult.[1] The 19th century witnessed milestone contributions to our understanding of this process. Rudolph Virchow detailed the cellular pathology of inflammation, Julius Cohnheim provided microscopic details of the acute phases of inflammation (vasodilatation, edema formation, and leukocyte emigration), and Elie Metchnikoff described the events of phagocytosis.[1–3] The evidence culminated into a cellular and humoral concept of inflammation, both of which were deemed critical in host defense against foreign pathogens.

In the 20th century, technologic advancements in molecular biology and biochemistry facilitated more detailed investigation and enabled the rapid expansion of knowledge of the many interwoven facets of the inflammation process. Evidence began to accumulate that the ramifications of these processes extended beyond the confines of the insult. Many humoral mediators, in addition to local effects, influenced distant targets as well, such as the liver and neurohormonal centers. Recently, it has become clear that the immune system, endocrine system, and nervous system comprise an integrated network sharing similar mediators and their receptors. Such an integrative view, introduced by J. Edwin Blalock, when combined with Hans Selye's concept of stress, led to the contemporary understanding of sickness behavior, defined by Robert Dantzer as a highly organized strategy of the organism to fight infections and to respond to other environmental stressors. Hence, what originated nearly two millennia ago as a simple concept founded on a constellation of signs and symptoms now is considered an intense, coordinated interplay of the nervous, vascular, endocrine, and immune systems to any injurious insult. It is the culmination of millions of years of evolution. Without it, life would be an arduous, painful, and brief existence, at best.

This chapter attempts to summarize this enormous quantity of information. An initial description of the elements involved in inflammation will provide the foundation upon which to discuss the sequence of events and interactions that comprise the inflammatory cascade.

INNATE VERSUS ADAPTIVE IMMUNITY

1 The initial security against microbes is the responsibility of our innate immunity, a system composed of both cellular and humoral components, already poised to respond prior to any stimulus.[4] Phylogenetically it is ancient and conserved, notably providing the primary mechanism of invertebrate host defense. The response it provides is uniform and consistent with each successive infection. Subsequent reinforcement is provided by the more specific and targeted efforts of the adaptive immune system. In contrast to innate immunity, subsequent exposure to the inciting agent during adaptive immunity elicits responses of increased magnitude and defensive capabilities.[4] This exquisite specificity for individual microbes, the capacity to "learn," "remember," and modify subsequent responses to repeated exposures, has provided the impetus for the name.

Both arms of immunity are composed of cellular and serum components. In the adaptive immune response this has been divided into humoral immunity, which is mediated primarily by antibodies, and cell-mediated immunity. These are not distinct systems and form an integrated system of host defense.

CELLULAR COMPONENTS

Neutrophils

Neutrophils are integral to both innate and humoral immunity, providing the initial defense against invading viral, bacterial, and parasitic pathogens. This importance is underscored by the fact that 55% to 60% of the hematopoietic output of bone marrow is dedicated to the production of neutrophils.[5] On exiting the marrow they circulate for 7 to 10 hours before taking up residence in the tissues for 1 to 2 days (Table 6.1).[6,7] They are uniquely sensitive to minute concentration gradients of microbial products and inflammatory mediators and rapidly accumulate at sites of infection, where they ingest and dispose of a wide array of pathogens with their vast microbicidal armamentarium. This pathogenicity, however, carries with it an implicit capacity for host injury and, accordingly, neutrophil function must be tightly regulated.

Recruitment. Neutrophil recruitment may be viewed as a sequence of events progressing from initial adhesion to activated endothelium, to subsequent extravasation and emigration toward inflammatory foci, to the ultimate elimination of foreign microorganisms through phagocytosis, to the generation of reactive oxygen species and the release of microbial substances.[4] These processes function in a similar context in other inflammatory cells that migrate to foci of infection or inflammation.

After injury, local and regional vasodilation induces hyperemia and facilitates the delivery of leukocytes. Extravasation of plasma creates edema, and in combination with the release of vasoactive substances leads to hemoconcentration, which promotes the peripheral margination of leukocytes.[8,9] Circulating neutrophils transiently interact with the endothelial cell surface molecules during "rolling," a process that involves a series of loose and reversible attachments (Fig. 6.1). These interactions are prerequisite for subsequent tighter interactions. The family of selectin receptors binds with their counterligands, the sialyl Lewis family, and other fucosylated and sulfated structures and mediate this process. E-selectin and P-selectin are present on endothelium and L-selectin is found on leukocytes.[4]

Consequent to stimulation with inflammatory mediators (thrombin, histamine, complement fragments, oxygen species, lipopolysaccharide [LPS], and cytokines such as interleukin-1 [IL-1], tumor necrosis factor-α [TNF-α], and interferon-γ [IFN-γ]), vascular endothelial cells express P- and E-selectin, which may engage the neutrophil surface glycoprotein P-selectin glycoprotein ligand 1 (PSGL-1) or sialyl Lewis. P-selectin is stored intracellularly and can be rapidly mobilized for expression within minutes of cellular activation. Endothelial cells also translocate ligands for neutrophil L-selectin and release mediators like platelet-activating factor (PAF) and IL-8. Cytokines such as TNF-α, granulocyte-macrophage colony-stimulating factor (GM-CSF), and granulocyte colony-stimulating factor (G-CSF) increase the affinity of leukocyte L-selectin for its counterreceptor. In addition to mechanical anchorage, these selectins induce signal transduction pathways that influence cellular function. P-selectin facilitates neutrophil degranulation and superoxide production, and cross-linking L-selectin primes the neutrophil for increased superoxide production.[10–12]

After rolling, L-selectin is rapidly shed in preparation for leukocyte diapedesis and emigration. Subsequent exposure to chemoattractant gradients results in conversion of the neutrophil to a state of tight stationary adhesion (Fig. 6.1). The receptors mediating this interaction are members of the β_2-integrin family, most importantly leukocyte function antigen 1 (LFA-1, CD11a/CD18) and Mac-1 (CD11b/CD18), and their expression is enhanced in response to selectin binding. Secretory vesicles are a major reservoir for these receptors. Both integrin receptors engage the intercellular adhesion molecules (ICAM)-1 and ICAM-2 in mediating adhesion; yet, each provides additional important functions. Leukocyte emigration is primarily an LFA-1–dependent process, as mice deficient in this receptor show reduced neutrophil attachment to ICAM-1 and endothelial cells. By contrast, mice lacking Mac-1 demonstrate impaired degranulation, superoxide production, and

TABLE 6.1

LEUKOCYTE SUBSETS

CELL	NEUTROPHIL	MONOCYTE	LYMPHOCYTE	EOSINOPHIL	BASOPHIL
Size (μm)	13	16–20	9–16	12–16	15
Differential (%)	40–75	2–6	20–45	1–6	<1
Life span	6 h to 7 d	1 d to years	Months to years	8 to 12 d	1 year
Activators	G-CSF, IL-8	M-CSF, GM-CSF, IFN-γ, TNF-α	IL-2, IL-12 (T_H1), IL-4 (T_H2)	G-CSF, IL-5	G-CSF, IL-3

G-CSF, granulocyte colony-stimulating factor; IL, interleukin, M-CSF, macrophage colony-stimulating factor; T_H, helper T cell; TNF, tumor necrosis factor.
Modified from Burkitt G, Young B, Heath JW, eds. *Wheater's Functional Histology: A Text and Colour Atlas,* 3rd ed. Edinburgh, New York: Churchill Livingstone; 1993.

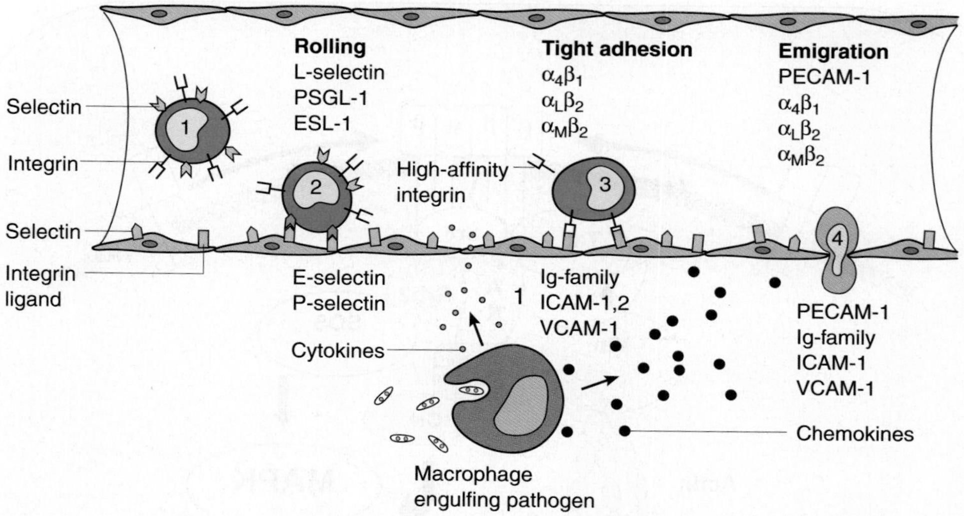

FIGURE 6.1. Leukocyte recruitment. *1.* Circulating leukocytes express integrins in a low-affinity conformation. *2.* Exposure to activated endothelium leads to rolling, which is mediated by L-selectin and P-selectin on the neutrophil and E-selectin on endothelium. *3.* Leukocyte exposure to cytokines released by macrophages phagocytosing pathogens induces a high-affinity integrin conformation integrins. Tight leukocyte–endothelial adhesion involves integrin engagement with counterligand expressed on the endothelium. *4.* Subsequent exposure to chemokines leads to diapedesis, which is further mediated by the family of β_1 and β_2 integrins. (Redrawn from Abbas AK, Lichtman AH. *Cellular and Molecular Immunology.* Philadelphia: Saunders; 2003.)

phagocytosis. Mac-1 also binds fibrinogen, heparin, and factor X and is implicated in neutrophil phagocytosis-induced apoptosis, a process essential for resolution of the inflammatory process (vide infra). The very late antigen 4 (VLA-4) binds vascular cellular adhesion molecule 1 (VCAM-1) and may provide an additional mechanism for tight adhesion. In addition to providing mechanical anchorage, these receptors interact with the cytoskeleton and other structural proteins and signaling cascades and are thought to represent a biochemical link between the external environment and intracellular signal transduction cascades that induce a cellular phenotype more appropriate for the current environment (Box A. Integrin signaling).[13–15]

Once tightly adhered, neutrophils must diapedese between endothelial cells and across the basement membrane to arrive at the focus of inflammation. Platelet/endothelial cell adhesion molecule 1 (PECAM-1) and integrin-associated protein are integral to transmigration (Fig. 6.1).[13,14,16,17] PECAM-1 is concentrated along the intercellular junctions of endothelial cells, and both leukocyte and endothelial PECAM-1 appear to be essential for neutrophil and monocyte diapedesis. Other candidate receptors include the β_1 integrins, or VLAs, which possess affinity for many constituents of the extracellular matrix, including laminin, fibronectin, and collagens, and the β_3 family of integrins including glycoprotein (Gp) IIβ/IIIα and the vitronectin receptor.[4] Further "directions" for migration to the focus of inflammation are delivered by the concentration gradients of chemotactic factors, including complement C5a, IL-8, leukotriene B_4 (LTB_4), and the bacterial product formylmethionyl-leucyl-phenylalanine (fMLP).[18–20]

The clinical significance of even minor derangements in any aspect of this process is evident in the disease leukocyte adhesion deficiency, characterized by complete absence of CD18, and therefore all β_2 integrins. Patients usually succumb to recurrent skin and mucosal infections within the initial 10 years of life.[4]

Phagocytosis. Microbial elimination commences when the neutrophil first encounters foreign pathogen. It is facilitated by opsonization, a process whereby microbes are coated by immune globulins and/or complement, which subsequently bind to their respective cell surface receptors, FcγRs and Mac-1.[21–23] Neutrophils constitutively express low-affinity immune globulin receptors FcγRII and FcγRIII and can be induced to express high-affinity FcγRI by incubation with IFN-γ or cross-linking β_2 integrins.[5,24] Complement-dependent phagocytosis is mediated by interactions between the leukocyte Mac-1 receptor and the complement opsonin iC3b.

Once engaged, FcγRs are phosphorylated on tyrosine residues within an immunoreceptor tyrosine activation motif (ITAM) by the Src family of kinases.[24] These phosphorylated sites serve as docking regions for a variety of proteins, in particular Syk. The importance of Syk is underscored by the observation that mice deficient in Syk are incapable of ingesting IgG-opsonized particles. A series of enzymes are subsequently activated including phosphoinositol 3-kinase, phospholipase C, and protein kinase C. Ultimately, the actin cytoskeleton undergoes rearrangement and the local plasmalemma is remodeled in the formation and sealing of the phagosome.[4,24]

This immature phagosome undergoes a series of maturation steps, whereby it acquires the machinery necessary for the killing and disposal of internalized microorganisms. Alterations in cytosolic calcium concentration induce the fusion of secretory vesicles and granules containing the microbicidal armamentarium with the immature phagosome.[24] Proteins effected by calcium concentration and that may govern phagosomal maturation include synaptogamins, actin, calmodulin, and the Src family of kinases.[24] The SNARE (soluble N-ethylmaleimide-sensitive-fusion-protein attachment protein receptor) proteins are thought to assist in fusion by engaging cognate receptors on the target membrane and approximating the two membranes. Antibodies to the SNARE 5, syntaxin 6 and SNAP-23, inhibited exocytosis of azurophilic and specific granules, respectively.[24]

Neutrophil Granules and Secretory Vesicles. There are two arms to the microbicidal capacity of the neutrophil: an oxygen-dependent pathway, or "respiratory burst," that generates toxic oxygen derivatives and an oxygen-independent

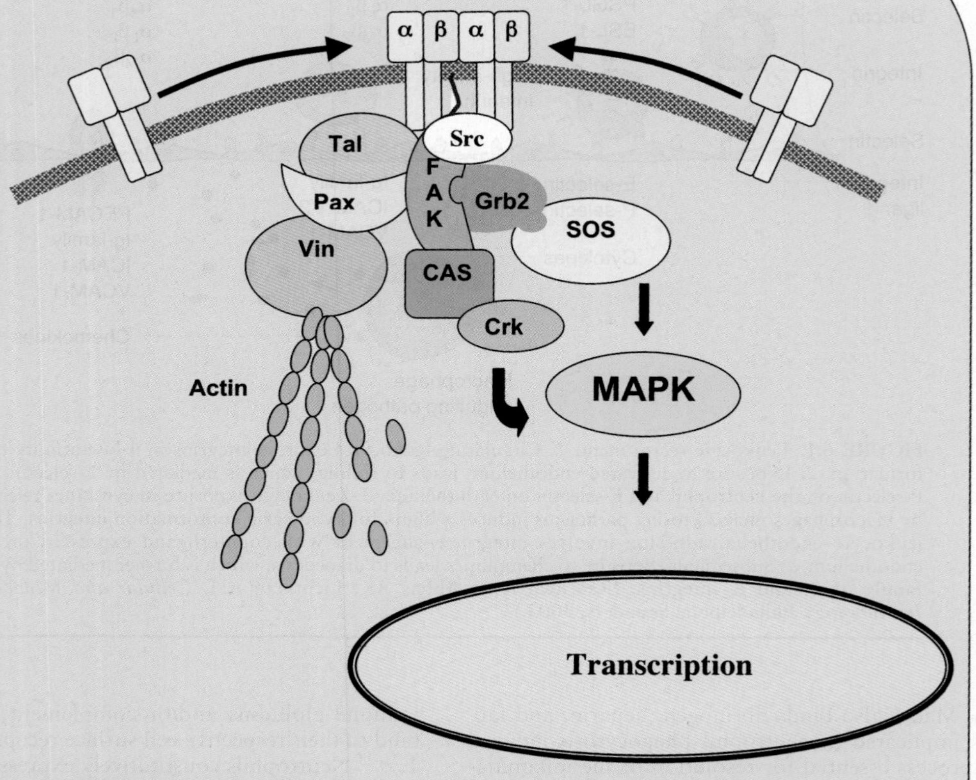

Integrin Signaling. Integrins comprise a large family of cell surface receptors that are composed of 2 subunits, α and β, and are activated by dimerization. The cytoplasmic tails are devoid of enzymatic activity, and hence, signal transduction is effected by adapter proteins that connect the receptor to the cytoskeleton, cytoplasmic kinases, and transmembrane growth factor receptors. As integrins bind the extracellular matrix they become clustered and associated with the cytoskeletal proteins talin, paxilin, and vinculin and signaling complexes. Actin stress fibers form, which increase integrin clustering. Ultimately, focal adhesion kinase (FAK) is recruited via interactions with talin and paxillin or with the β integrin subunit. Subsequent autophosphorlyation on tyrosine 397 provides a binding site for the Src homology 2 (SH2) domain of Src. The Src kinase phosphorylates a number of focal adhesion components including paxillin and tensin and p130CAS, a docking protein that recruits Crk, which can subsequently activate proximal elements in the JNK cascade of the MAPK family. FAK may also be phosphorylated by Src on tyrosine 925, creating a binding site for the complex of the adapter Grb2 and Ras guanosine 5'-triphosphate exchange factor mSOS. These interactions also lead to activation of MAPK cascades, and ultimately the induction of a variety of genes. *(Redrawn from Giancotti F & Ruoslahti E. Integrin Signaling. Science 1999: 1028-1032)*

BOX A

pathway that utilizes toxic proteinases.[25] These two components are compartmentalized into four distinct granules or vesicles that also contain adhesion molecules and important inflammatory mediators (Table 6.2).[26] They are mobilized in a hierarchical fashion in response to gradual elevations in the intracellular calcium level, which parallels their respective contents and the current needs of the cell.[27]

Primary, or azurophil (affinity for the dye azure A), granules target the destruction of phagocytosed organisms (Table 6.2). The myeloperoxidase (MPO) within these granules generates hypochlorous acid from products generated by nicotinamide adenine dinucleotide phosphate (NADPH) oxidase and also imparts the characteristic greenish color of pus.[9,27] Other major constituents include α-defensins, cytotoxic proteins that scaffold into transmembrane pores within the microbial cell wall and perturb the maintenance of vital transmembrane gradients, and bactericidal/permeability-increasing protein (BPI), which binds to gram-negative organisms and induces rearrangement of membrane lipids and inhibits growth.[27–30] Elastase cleaves constituents of the extracellular matrix, including proteoglycans, collagen (types I, III, IV), and fibronectin and, of course, elastin.[31] Azurocidin is chemotactic for monocytes and stimulates LPS-induced release of IL-6 and TNF-α from monocytes.[4,27]

The contents of specific granules, which are rich in antimicrobial substances, are released extracellularly (Table 6.2).[26]

TABLE 6.2

NEUTROPHIL GRANULES AND SECRETORY VESICLES

■ AZUROPHIL GRANULES	■ SPECIFIC GRANULES	■ GELATINASE GRANULES	■ SECRETORY VESICLES
MEMBRANE			
Myeloperoxidase (MPO)	Lysozyme	Gelatinase	Plasma proteins
Lysozyme	Phospholipase A_2	Lysozyme	
Cathepsins	Gelatinase	β_2-Microglobulin	
Elastase	Collagenase	Acetyltransferase	
Proteinase 3	Lactoferrin		
Azurocidin	TNF		
BPI	β_2-Microglobulin		
Defensins	Histaminase		
iNOS	Heparinase		
α_1-Antitrypsin	uPA		
α-Mannosidase			
Sialidase			
Acid mucopolysaccharide			
β-Glycerophosphatase			
Elastase			
CYTOSOL			
CD63	Mac-1	Mac-1	Mac-1
CD68	SNAP proteins	SNAP proteins	SNAP proteins
	CD15	Cytochrome b558	Cytochrome b558
	CD66	fMLP R	CR1
	CD67	DAG-deacylating enzyme	CD14
	Cytochrome b558	uPA R	CD45
	Fibronectin R		fMLP R
	Laminin R		uPA R
	Vitronectin R		C1q R
	Thrombospondin R		
	fMLP R		
	uPA R		

BPI, bactericidal/permeability-increasing protein; CD, cluster of differentiation; CR1, complement component C3b; DAG, diacylglycerol; fMLP, N-formylmethionyl-leucyl-phenylalanine; iNOS, inducible nitric oxide synthase; R, receptor; TNF, tumor necrosis factor; uPA, urokinase-type plasminogen activator. Modified from Faurschou M, Borregaard N. Neutrophil granules and secretory vesicles in inflammation. *Microbes Infect* 2003;5:1317–1327.

Lactoferrin, by sequestering iron, retards bacterial growth and can bind bacterial cell membranes and induce irreversible membrane damage and lysis.[27] Phospholipase A_2 (PLA_2) participates in the degradation of bacterial membrane phospholipids. Lysozyme, present in all granules, is a cationic antimicrobial peptide that cleaves peptidoglycan polymers of bacterial cell walls. Other extracellular matrix–degrading enzymes include gelatinase and collagenase.[27] These granules also possess receptors for a variety of extracellular matrix proteins and cell surface ligands, such as the β_2-integrin Mac-1 that mediates firm adhesion to the endothelium. In addition to the mechanical function of cellular anchorage, engagement of these receptors with their respective counterligands induces phenotypic alterations such as degranulation and enhanced reactive oxygen species production.[4,27]

Gelatinase granules contain an eclectic array of mediators that contribute to many aspects of inflammation (Table 6.2). They contain matrix metalloproteases, zymogens that upon proteolytic activation degrade the interstitial matrix including collagens, fibronectin, proteoglycans, and laminin; this may facilitate neutrophil extravasation and migration. They are a source of cell surface adhesion molecules.[4,27,30]

Secretory vesicles contain many of the cell surface adhesion molecules operant during and essential for leukocyte recruitment. Their membranes are dense with the β_2 integrins LFA and Mac-1, the complement receptor 1 (CR1), the LPS receptor CD14, and the FcγRIII. Through fusion with the plasmalemma, the cell surface is enriched with these receptors, which facilitates firm neutrophil-endothelial engagement and the capacity to respond to a variety of stimuli.[4,27] Not surprisingly, because of the essential nature of leukocyte recruitment, secretory vesicles possess the lowest threshold for release, followed by gelatinase, specific, and azurophil granules (Table 6.2).[27]

TABLE 6.3

MAJOR ROS AND THEIR METABOLISM

■ ROS MOLECULE	■ MAIN SOURCES	■ ENZYMATIC DEFENSE SYSTEMS	■ PRODUCTS
Superoxide ($O_2^{\bullet-}$)	Leakage from electron transport chain	Superoxide dismutase	$H_2O_2 + O_2$
	Activated phagocytes	Superoxide reductase	H_2O_2
	Xanthine oxidase		
	Flavoenzymes		
Hydrogen peroxide (H_2O_2)	From $O_2^{\bullet-}$ via superoxide dismutase	Glutathione peroxidase	H_2O + GSSG
	NADPH oxidase	Catalase	$H_2O + O_2$
	Glucose oxidase	Peroxiredoxins	H_2O
	Xanthine oxidase		
Hydroxyl radical ($O_2^{\bullet-}$)	From $O_2^{\bullet-}$ and H_2O_2 via transition metals		
Nitric oxide (NO)	Nitric oxide synthases	Glutathione/TrxR	GSNO

NADPH, nicotinamide adenine dinucleotide phosphate; ROS, reactive oxygen species; TrxR, thioredoxin.
Modifed from Nordberg J, Arner E. Reactive oxygen species, antioxidants, and the mammalian thioredoxin system. *Free Radic Biol Med* 2001;31: 1287–1312.

Oxidative Burst and Oxidant Metabolites. The generation of toxic oxygen metabolites or reactive oxygen species (ROS) is the cardinal characteristic of the neutrophil, but may also be produced by the monocyte/macrophage. Their essential antimicrobial properties are equally destructive to host tissues and implicated in the pathophysiology of many inflammatory disorders (Table 6.3). Counterintuitive to their role in cell destruction, recent evidence also supports a role of ROS in intracellular signal transduction.[32]

A free radical is any species possessing one or more unpaired electrons; the valence is irrelevant. They are categorized under the broader term ROS, which encompasses all molecules capable of radical formation. Despite a very brief existence (10^{-11} to 10^{-6} seconds), extensive damage may occur through the induction of free radical chain reactions. Species operant during both physiologic and pathophysiologic inflammation include the following: the superoxide anion ($O_2^{\bullet-}$), the hydroxyl radical (•OH), hydrogen peroxide (H_2O_2), and singlet oxygen, as well as the reactive nitrogen intermediates nitric oxide (NO) and peroxynitrite ($ONOO^-$) (Table 6.3). In addition to their antimicrobial properties, ROS may modulate the immune response by activating inflammatory cells and inducing proinflammatory cytokine secretion.[33,34]

2 Implicit with the capacity for pathogen elimination, however, is the potential for destruction of host tissues. Hence, numerous regulatory mechanisms provide temporal and spatial control of the ROS production. The NADPH oxidase complex itself exists in a disassembled state, and only upon cell activation and the need for ROS production are the subunits approximated and enzymatic function restored.[35] In addition, high plasma and tissue concentrations of proteinase inhibitors provide continuous surveillance and systemic control. However, such regulation is incomplete as evidenced by such diseases as rheumatoid arthritis, chronic obstructive pulmonary disease, and autoimmune vasculitis, which are the consequence of damage due to neutrophil-derived products.[35]

NADPH oxidase is a heteromeric complex composed of six subunits: flavocytochrome b558, the electron transporting apparatus, which is subdivided into Gp91(phox) and p22(phox); the cytosolic complex p40(phox), p47(phox), and p67(phox); and the oxidase factor rac-2 (Fig. 6.2).[35] Microorganisms or high concentrations of chemoattractants bind to cell surface receptors and initiate oxidase activation, heralded by phosphorylation of p47(phox). Cytochrome b558 (Gp91 and p22), which exists within the plasmalemma and the membranes of specific granules and secretory vesicles, is recruited by phagocytosis and granule fusion. Phosphorylation of p47(phox) induces a conformation change that enables its incorporation within the membrane, wherein it facilitates the translocation of rac2 and p67(phox), and stabilizes the association of this cytosolic complex with cytochrome b558, thereby rendering the complex functional.[35]

At the redox center of the oxidase, an electron is transferred from NADPH to oxygen, thereby generating superoxide[36]:

$$O_2 + e^- = O_2^{\bullet-}$$

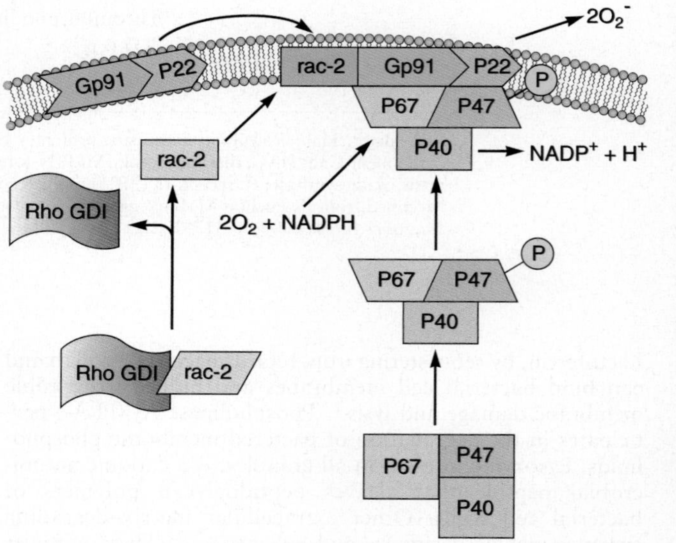

FIGURE 6.2. Reduced nicotinamide adenine dinucleotide phosphate (NADPH) oxidase assembly. In the resting neutrophil, the cytochrome subunits Gp91 and p22 are tightly bound in the membrane. p47(phox), p67(phox), and rac-s complex are in the cytosol. On activation, GDI releases rac-2, and p47(phox) becomes phosphorylated. This causes translocation of rac-2, p47(phox), and p67(phox) to the membrane and complex formation with the cytochrome components, thereby completing the assembly of the active oxidase. (Redrawn from Burg ND, Pillinger MH. *Clin Immunol* 2001;1:7–17.)

Other mechanisms of superoxide production include uncoupling of the xanthine dehydrogenase system, uncoupling of mitochondrial and endoplasmic reticulum electron transport chains, and nonenzymatic reactions such as autooxidation of hemoglobin.[37,38]

Superoxide is relatively weak and of low bactericidal potency. However, its membrane permeability and role as a reactant in reactions yielding highly toxic products confers upon it a high potential for cellular and tissue damage.[36]

Superoxide can spontaneously or enzymatically (superoxide dismutase) dismutate into hydrogen peroxide[35,36]:

$$2H^+ + O_2^{\bullet -} \Leftrightarrow H_2O_2 + O_2$$

It can also be converted to the more potent hydroxyl radical through the metal-catalyzed Haber-Weiss reaction[35,36]:

$$H_2O_2 + O_2^{\bullet -} + Fe^{3+} \Leftrightarrow O_2 + OH^- + {\bullet}OH + Fe^{2+}$$

or through the Fenton equation[35,36]:

$$H_2O_2 + Fe^{2+} \Leftrightarrow Fe^{3+} + OH^- + {\bullet}OH + Hb\text{-}Fe^{2+} + H_2O_2$$
$$\Leftrightarrow Hb\text{-}Fe^{3+} + OH^- + {\bullet}OH$$

Under physiologic conditions, lactoferrin found in neutrophil-specific granules provides the iron catalyst for the Haber-Weiss reaction. In the Fenton reaction, superoxide or other biologic reducing agents such as lactate or ascorbate donate electrons to generate the ferrous ions required to react with hydrogen peroxide to produce the hydroxyl radical.[35,36,39]

The hydroxyl anion is highly reactive and induces DNA strand breaks and base hydroxylations leading to adenosine triphosphate (ATP) depletion and gene mutations. It can attack lipid side chains of membrane phospholipids to form hydrogen peroxide and lipid hydroperoxides in a process called lipid peroxidation. These products can disrupt membrane function, serve as substrates for the production of cytotoxic aldehydes, or uncouple calcium-ATPase and increase cytosolic calcium concentration. Recent data also support a mechanism by which oxidation of critical sulfhydryl residues on the ryanodine receptors induce an "open" configuration and a leak of intracellular endoplasmic reticulum (ER) calcium into the cytosol.[40] This elevation of cytosolic calcium activates calcium-dependent proteases and phospholipases that propagate cellular damage.[39]

Superoxide can react with nitric oxide to produce peroxynitrite ($ONOO^-$) and hydroxyl radical[36,41]:

$$NO^{\bullet} + O_2^{\bullet -} \Leftrightarrow ONOO^- + H^+ \Leftrightarrow ONOOH \Leftrightarrow {\bullet}OH + NO_2^{\bullet}$$

The hemoprotein MPO yields the potently bactericidal hypochlorous acid (HOCl) from the reactants chloride and H_2O_2. HOCl oxidizes amino acids, nucleotides, and hemoproteins; can activate neutrophil collagenases and permit unabated elastase injury by inhibiting α_1-antitrypsin; and contributes to hydroxyl radical and singlet oxygen production.[33,39,42] Though short-lived, subsequent reactions with secondary amines generate secondary chloramines, which are equally toxic but much more stable. These metabolites can oxidize similar cellular components. They can combine with halide anions to generate toxic free halides or with taurine chloramines, which induces membrane attack complex (MAC) complement formation.[33,39,42]

In light of the pivotal role of MPO during inflammation and pathogen elimination, it is surprising that MPO deficiency is both common and relatively benign. Though MPO-deficient neutrophils show early depressed bacterial killing, bactericidal function normalizes within 60 minutes.[43] It is hypothesized that though bacterial killing is impaired, post-phagocytosis oxidase-dependent neutrophil apoptosis is normal, resulting in appropriate regulation of the inflammatory response.[43]

Singlet oxygen, a highly reactive and extremely short-lived species, is formed by an input of energy to O_2 that reverses the spin direction of one of the outermost unpaired electrons away from a parallel spin. It is produced during reactions of the MPO-H_2O_2-halide system and is a potential product of superoxide dismutation and the Haber-Weiss reaction. It is highly electrophilic, reacting with compounds containing electron-rich double bonds, and may react with membrane lipids to produce peroxides.[39]

The destructive potential of these ROS for both host and pathogen necessitates a mechanism of continuous tight spatial and temporal regulation. The oxidase complex itself exists spatially disaggregated; only upon cellular activation are its constituents assembled and enzymatic function restored (Fig. 6.2).[35,43] As elegant as is the mechanism by which to control ROS production, so too are the measures employed to eliminate these products when they are no longer needed. Superoxide, the proximal reactant necessary for many of the ROS-generating reactions, is removed by both spontaneous and enzymatic (superoxide dismutase) dismutation to H_2O_2 (Fig. 6.3). H_2O_2 is subsequently reduced to oxygen and water by catalase.[36,39] In the extracellular environment, this function is performed by glutathione (GSH) peroxidase, a selenium-dependent enzyme that reduces H_2O while oxidizing reduced GSH to its oxidized form. There is evidence that increasing GSH concentrations in monocytes and macrophages blocks ROS-mediated activation of nuclear factor (NF)-κB and subsequent proinflammatory cytokine production.[39] The utilization of N-acetylcysteine, a reducing agent that restores GSH, reduces hepatocellular injury in an animal model of warm liver ischemia/reperfusion.[32] It has also been shown to reduce contrast-induced nephropathy in patients undergoing imaging procedures requiring the use of iodinated contrast.[44] Mechanisms of preventing hydroxyl radical-induced tissue damage include the binding of transition metal ions by albumin, ceruloplasmin, haptoglobulin, lactoferrin, and transferrin.[33,36,39] Taurine is a scavenger for HOCl. Other antioxidants that may assist in controlling the reaction include vitamins E (tocopherol) and C. Vitamin C has many antioxidant properties, including the ability to regenerate α-tocopherol. It can prevent activation of neutrophil-derived collagenase and is a powerful scavenger of HOCl, superoxide, singlet oxygen, and hydroxyl radicals. Carotenoids have long double bonds to attract and sequester free radicals. Uric acid is a powerful scavenger of water-soluble radicals such as HOCl and singlet oxygen. It can

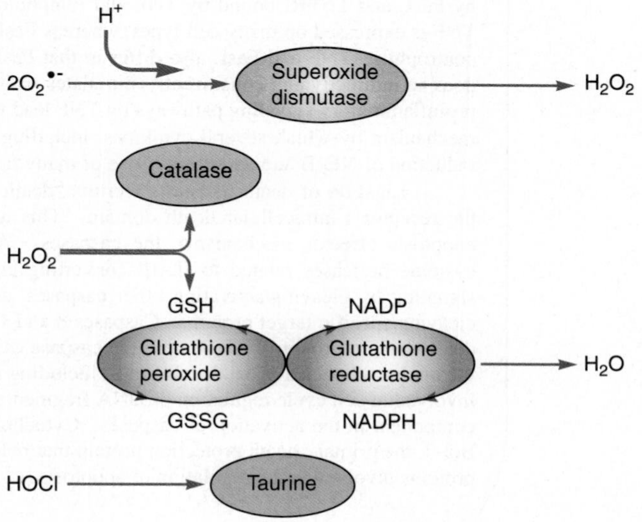

FIGURE 6.3. Scavengers of reactive oxygen species (ROS). (Redrawn from Klebanoff SJ. In: Gallin JI, Snyderman R, eds. *Inflammation: Basic Principles and Clinical Correlates,* 3rd ed. Philadelphia, PA: Lippincott Williams & Wilkins; 1999:723.)

also bind copper and iron ions to suppress hydroxyl radical formation. Stress proteins or heat-shock proteins are induced by oxygen radicals and ischemia and may play a role in defense. Furthermore, heme oxygenase-1 (HO-1) catalyzes the cleavage of heme to biliverdin, which is subsequently converted to bilirubin, an efficient free radical scavenger.[33,36,39]

All of the aforementioned participants of the NADPH oxidase are vital for health, as evidenced by those who suffer from chronic granulomatous disease.[35,43] These patients have deficient superoxide production and experience ineffective inflammatory reactions to infection. They commonly suffer from repeated bacterial infections (pneumonia, cutaneous abscesses and hepatic and perihepatic abscess, and osteomyelitis) by organisms that are catalase positive (*Staphylococcus aureus*). Organisms that produce large amounts of peroxide are less of a threat as the neutrophils can utilize bacterial peroxide to produce toxic metabolites. The use of prophylactic antibiotics and IFN-γ has reduced the frequency of serious infections in this patient population.[35,43]

Regulation of Inflammation. In addition to the previously described mechanisms for controlling the inflammatory response of neutrophils, there is substantial evidence supporting the role of apoptosis in resolving the inflammatory response (Box B).[45] Within 90 minutes of phagocytosis, over 250 genes are induced, of which more than 30 encode proteins integral to at least three distinct apoptotic pathways.[45] These observations suggest that the mechanism inducing apoptosis is

Apoptosis. Apoptosis is an integral component in the regulatory mechanisms that limit and resolve inflammation. Unlike cell necrosis, which is characterized by loss of membrane integrity, cellular edema and lysis, and release of intracellular products that incite an inflammatory reaction, apoptosis is a physiologic process of programmed cell death, characterized by DNA fragmentation and plasma membrane blebbing, with the compartmentalization of cytoplasmic and membrane particles into apoptotic bodies consisting of cytoplasmic and membrane fragments. Cytoplasmic contents are not released and consequently, an inflammatory response is not induced. Neutrophils are programmed to undergo apoptosis constitutively, and the signal transduction pathways culminating in apoptosis are activated early in acute inflammation. Subsequent neutrophil apoptotic particles are phagocytosed by resident macrophages. This is the preferred mechanisms for clearing neutrophils from inflammatory foci, and has also been implicated in the clearance of eosinophils, monocytes, and lymphocytes.

Apoptosis plays a prominent role in the immune system. Most developing T cells undergo apoptosis during the selection process in the thymus. Termination of the cellular immune response also involves cytokine-induced apoptosis. Apoptosis can be used by lymphocytes as a means of effecting death in other cells. CTL kill target cells by inducing apoptosis via a Fas-induced pathway and a perforin- and granzyme-mediated pathway. Increased apoptosis has been observed in lymphoid tissues of patients dying of sepsis, suggesting that excessive lymphocyte apoptosis may contribute to fatal sepsis.

Inducers of apoptosis include oxidant stress, radiation, viral infection, trauma, and cytokines. Many of the pathologic agents that induce apoptosis at low concentrations can cause necrosis at higher concentrations. Apoptogenic stimuli activate the apoptotic pathway through both receptor-dependent and independent pathways. The sphingomyelin breakdown product, ceramide, is implicated as a transducer of apoptosis. DNA damage secondary to radiation or oxygen radical formation results in the accumulation of the tumor suppressor gene p53. p53 promotes non-receptor-mediated modulation of apoptosis.

Receptor-mediated pathways involve the "death receptors" that belong to the TNF receptor superfamily. Ligands shown to induce apoptosis include FasL, TNF, TNF-related apoptosis-inducing ligand (TRAIL), nerve growth factor, and CD40L. The best-characterized death receptors are Fas bound by FasL and TNFRI bound by TNF and lymphotoxin α. Although primarily produced by macrophages, TNF is expressed on many cell types, whereas FasL is restricted to the surfaces of CTL, macrophages, and neutrophils. TNF and FasL also differ in that FasL directly activates a cell death pathway, whereas TNF does so indirectly and concurrently stimulates pathways that inhibit apoptosis. Independent and divergent proinflammatory signaling pathways by TNF lead to the induction of NFκB, an inhibitor of apoptosis. The mechanism by which several cytokines, including IL-1, IL-6, and GM-CSF, inhibit apoptosis is through induction of NFκB and apoptosis is one of many factors that ultimately determine the cell's fate.

Ligation of death receptors recruits "death domain" containing adaptor proteins that interact with the receptor's intracellular death domain. This interaction initiates the enzyme cascade responsible for apoptosis effector mechanisms, the caspases. All signaling pathways converge on the activation of cysteine proteases related to IL-1β converting enzyme called caspases. Caspases propagate apoptotic signaling by cleaving/activating other caspases, and eventually execute terminal events in apoptosis by cleaving specific target proteins. Caspases 8 and 10 activate apoptosis signaling by linking Fas-associated death domain protein (FADD) with the caspase cascades. Caspases 3 and 7 are the executor molecules in the nucleus that cleave death substrates, including nuclear structural proteins, protein kinases, and proteins involved in cell cycle regulation or DNA fragmentation. Cytochrome C release from mitochondria is a key component in the activation of caspases. Cytochrome C release, and therefore apoptosis, is inhibited by Bcl-2, the primary death protection protein that belongs to the Bel family of proapoptotic and antiapoptotic proteins involved in the regulation of apoptosis.

BOX B

initiated quite proximal in the inflammatory cascade, in fact, just subsequent to phagocytosis. The timely execution of a controlled cell death program in human PMNs is essential for preventing damage to healthy tissues and for the resolution of infection. Furthermore, evidence suggests that the phenotype of other immune cells, including monocytes and macrophages, is altered after encountering and phagocytosis of apoptotic neutrophils. During some processes such as infection or trauma, neutrophil apoptosis may be delayed, which might contribute to a failure to resolve inflammation.

The inflammatory capacity of neutrophils is also transcriptionally regulated. Genes encoding proinflammatory mediators or signal transduction molecules such as receptors for IL-8, IL-10, and IL-13 are downregulated early after activation and decrease rapidly after the initiation of apoptosis.[45] In addition, regulating oxidative stress and ROS achieve high priority as the genes involved in glutathione and thioredoxin metabolism and heme catabolism are upregulated as is the production of reduced glutathione.[45] Hence, activation-induced apoptosis in neutrophils stimulates self-directed regulation, an event that likely facilitates removal of neutrophils by macrophages. As aforementioned, removal of apoptotic neutrophils by activated macrophages also appears to serve a role in modifying their function and halting the inflammatory response.

Mononuclear Phagocytes

Monocytes circulate for about 1 to 2 days; thereafter, they constitutively hone to a particular tissue to differentiate into macrophages possessing a phenotype specific to the resident tissue (dendritic cells, Kupffer cells) (Table 6.1).[4,46,47] Resident macrophages are typically found at interfaces with blood (liver and spleen) and with lymph, where they can readily detect, ingest, and destroy invading organisms.[39] Mononuclear cells function as antigen-presenting cells in T-cell–mediated adaptive immune responses, presenting antigen in the appropriate context to effector T cells. They provide service integral to both innate and adaptive immune responses. Evidence also supports their role in providing an "alarm" both locally and systemically through the release of intracellular proteins (i.e., high-mobility group box 1 protein [HMGB1]) expressing damage-associated molecular patterns (DAMPs) that can function as a danger signal (see later).

Recruitment

Monocytes are recruited and emigrate to foci of inflammation utilizing similar mechanisms of adhesion and diapedesis as described for neutrophils (Fig. 6.1). PAF; C5a; the CC chemokines, regulated on activation, normally T-cell expressed and secreted (RANTES); macrophage inflammatory protein (MIP)-1α; and chemokines of the membrane cofactor protein (MCP) family are potent monocyte-macrophage chemotaxins.[48,49] The selectin family of adhesion receptors mediates the initial tethering of monocytes to endothelial cells.[18] Firm adhesion to the endothelium involves the interactions of β_1 and β_2 integrins on monocytes with the endothelial adhesion molecules ICAM-1 and VCAM-1.[18]

Phagocytosis. Phagocytosis involves both the IgG receptor (FcγR) and the receptor for the complement factor C3b. Terminal sugar patterns on microbial surfaces also allow recognition by macrophages for nonspecific phagocytosis.[22] However, phagosomal maturation differs from that which occurs in the neutrophil in that monocytes and macrophages have an endocytic pathway targeting the phagosome to a lysosome.[24] After endocytosis of a receptor–ligand complex, the contents of a vesicle are targeted to an early endosome, the ligand and receptor dissociate, and the receptor is recycled to the cell surface.[24] This early endosome undergoes a series of maturation steps in which it is acidified (pH 5.5 to 6.0). This acidification is requisite for optimal protease and hydrolase activity involved in pathogen killing. It may also be integral for phagosome maturation as titrating the acidity inhibits phagosome–lysosome fusion.[24] Ultimately, the endosome fuses with a lysosome, which is characterized by its extreme acidity (pH $<$5.0) and elevated concentration of proteases.[24] Lysosomes are the terminal destination of phagocytosed material to be degraded.

After fusion, MPO released into phagosomes can react with hydrogen and halides to yield toxic hypohalous acids, superoxide anion, hydrogen peroxide, and hydroxyl radical (Table 6.3). Macrophages may also use peroxidase generated by adjacent neutrophils, eosinophils, and monocytes and acquired through endocytosis to generate these ROS. In addition to supporting the inflammatory response, macrophages also play an important immunoregulatory role in inflammation by scavenging apoptotic neutrophils at sites of inflammation.[39]

Activation. IFN-γ derived primarily from T cells is the primary activator of macrophages.[4,47,50] Optimal macrophage activation requires both interferon IFN-γ and a sensitizing agent, both of which can be provided by activated T lymphocytes. CD40 ligand on T cells can bind CD40 on macrophages to sensitize the cell. Alternatively, membrane-associated TNF-α or lymphotoxin from lymphocytes can activate macrophage TNF-α synthesis and thereby sensitize the macrophage to IFN-γ.[39] IL-10 promotes monocyte maturation and macrophage differentiation.[51] Other activators include GM-CSF, TNF-α, IL-1, and LPS.

Activated monocytes and macrophages can produce approximately 100 different products, including GM-CSF, macrophage colony-stimulating factor (M-CSF), G-CSF, IL-1, TNF-α, and NO (Table 6.4).[39,52] Mononuclear phagocytes are important sources of chemoattractants such as IL-8, PAF, and LTB_4 that recruit other neutrophils and leukocytes. Their release of HMGB1 and other DAMP molecules serves as a danger signal to other immune cells in the local environment. However, systemic release of HMGB1 may be causally related to mortality in such inflammatory states as sepsis and trauma.[53,54] The respiratory burst and subsequent production of toxic ROS mirrors that of neutrophils.

Antigen Presentation. T cells recognize only those antigens associated with surface major histocompatability complex (MHC) molecules. MHC class I molecules are expressed on all nucleated cells, whereas MHC class II molecules are restricted to antigen-presenting cells (APCs). After phagocytosing pathogen, mononuclear cells process and display antigen to T cells, and in doing so, initiate the development of the adaptive response. There is evidence that the heat-shock protein receptor CD91 may also participate in this process (vide infra). This processed antigen is presented in the context of MHC molecules on the APC surface that are specifically recognized by T-cell receptors and essential for T-cell activation. $CD4^+$ T cells, or helper T cells (T_H), recognize antigen coexpressed with MCH class II molecules and induce B-cell differentiation into either memory or antigen-specific antibody-producing plasma cells. These T_H cells can also induce macrophage production of NO, ROS, and other inflammatory mediators. $CD8^+$ cytotoxic T lymphocytes (CTLs) recognize antigen in the context of MHC class I molecules and induce target cell lysis; they destroy host cells infected with intracellular pathogens or cells of malignant potential.[55] Activated mononuclear phagocytes release IL-12, a potent stimulus for T_H cells and the production of inflammatory cytokines, and elaborate IL-15, the function of which mirrors that of IL-2.[56,57]

The three professional APCs are dendritic cells (DCs), macrophages, and B cells. Dendritic cells are a specialized APC, which process and present antigen to naïve T cells.

TABLE 6.4

MONOCYTE/MACROPHAGE PRODUCTS

■ PRODUCT	■ FUNCTIONS
Enzymes	
Lysozyme	Antimicrobial
Urokinase	Plasminogen activation and fibrinolysis
Collagenase	Connective tissue degradation
ACE	Vasopressor
Cytokines	Multiple
IL-1	Multiple
TNF-α	Antiviral, immune modulation
Interferon α/β	Acute-phase response
IL-6	Anti-inflammatory
IL-10	Stimulate IFN-γ production
IL-12, IL-18	Neutrophil chemoattraction
IL-8	Fibroblast growth
FGF	Granulocyte, macrophage differentiation
GM-CSF	Chemoattractant
MIP-1α/β	Monocyte recruitment
MCP-1	Monocyte/T_H cell recruitment
RANTES	Opsonization, complement activation
Complement proteins	Coagulation
Coagulation factors	Localization, migration
Adhesion, matrix molecules	Iron transport
Fibronectin, proteoglycan	Vitamin transport
Transport proteins	Inflammation
Transferring	Inflammation
B_{12}-binding protein	Platelet activation
Bioactive lipids	Antimicrobial
Cyclooxygenase	Antimicrobial
Lipo-oxygenase	Antibacterial
PAF	
Reactive oxygen intermediates	
Superoxide, hydrogen peroxide oxygen singlet	
Reactive nitrogen intermediates	
NO, nitrates, nitrites	
Defensins	

ACE, angiotensin-converting enzyme; FGF, fibroblast growth factor; GM-CSF, granulocyte/macrophage colony-stimulating factor; IL, interleukin; MCP, membrane cofactor protein; MIP, macrophage inflammatory protein; NO, nitric oxide; PAF, platelet-activating factor; RANTES, regulated on activation, normally T-cell expressed and secreted; TNF, tumor necrosis factor.
Modified from Gordon S. Development and distribution of mononuclear phagocytes: relevance to inflammation. In: Gallin JL, Snyderman R, eds. *Inflammation: Basic Principles and Clinical Correlates,* 3rd ed. Philadelphia, PA: Lippincott Williams & Wilkins; 1999.

Monocytes stimulated with GM-CSF and IL-4 or IL-13 differentiate toward DCs. Maturation of the DC requires TNF-α or LPS stimulation.[39] Epidermal Langerhans cells, after encountering antigen, migrate through the lymphoid organs and differentiate into mature DCs and acquire the capacity to provide the costimulatory signal. DCs are particularly effective at presenting viral antigen. They present antigen in the context of both MHC I and MHC II and thereby induce both a T_H1 and T_H2 response, respectively. DCs can also present antigens derived from apoptotic cells in the context of MHC class I.[58–60]

Macrophages present antigenic peptides from ingested pathogens that persist in the phagosomes. These peptides, usually of bacterial origin, are expressed in conjunction with MHC class II molecules. B cells, by contrast, bind specific soluble molecules (insect toxins, venom, and allergens) via immunoglobulin. This is endocytosed, processed, and presented on surface MHC II.[39,60–62]

Lymphocytes

B, T, and natural killer (NK) cells comprise this lineage of inflammatory cells (Table 6.1). B and T cells are central to the adaptive immune response, whereas NK cells lack antigen specificity and primarily function during innate immune response. NK cells are the first line of defense against many viral infections; the loss of surface expression of MHC class I molecules on virus-infected cells serves as a target for NK cells.[39,63] Alternatively, NK cells bind cell-bound antibody and participate in antibody-dependent cell cytotoxicity. Cells targeted by either mechanism are induced to undergo cell death.

B Lymphocytes. B cells are of bone marrow origin, yet attain full maturation within extramedullary sites such as lymph nodes, the spleen, and the mucosal lymph nodules of the tonsils and Peyer patches. With activation, B cells differentiate into antibody-producing plasma cells, which through the elaboration of antibody, aid the neutralization of viruses and bacterial toxins and facilitate opsonization for phagocytosis and complement activation.[4] Activation requires antigen binding to cell surface receptors and stimulation by T_H cell–derived cytokines; they do not need the assistance of APCs. Polyclonal B-cell activation can occur in a T-cell–independent mechanism if the antigen has a large repeating polymeric sequence.[39,64]

T Lymphocytes. Development of T lymphocytes begins within the marrow and is completed in the thymus. The final population profile is determined by apoptotic processes of both positive and negative selection.[65] Any protein or antigen of host origin is presented by APCs, and thymocytes reactive to these self-proteins are deleted.[66] Alternatively, expansion of cell lines recognizing foreign, or rather non-self, antigen, occurs through positive selection. IL-7 provides the stimulation for proliferation and differentiation of developing T cells. Ultimately, two lines of mature cells, $CD4^+$ and $CD8^+$, will develop.[67]

Lymphocytes, the smallest of the leukocytes, constitute approximately 20% of circulating leukocytes.[4] Most circulating lymphocytes are T cells, and 60% of those are $CD4^+$, a marker of a T_H phenotype. The other 40% are $CD8^+$, called cytotoxic T cells, T_C. The normal ratio of $CD4^+$ to $CD8^+$ is 2:1.[4] Lymphocytes continuously recirculate through the lymph nodes, spleen, lymphatics, lymph nodules, and blood, providing continuous surveillance. Encounter with a particular antigen initiates activation toward an effector T cell. Activation of a T cell requires its specific antigen binding plus a costimulatory signal provided by the interaction between costimulatory molecules on the APC and their cognate receptors on the T cell.[39]

Naïve T cells circulate continuously between blood and lymphoid organs, making contact with many APCs and the epitopes of the antigens they express.[68] Initially, lymphocytes enter the cortical region of lymph nodes by migrating across the high endothelial venules, a process mediated by the selectin family of receptors. L-selectin, which is found constitutively on all lymphocytes, binds sialyl Lewis carbohydrate on the endothelium.[39] For example, L-selectin on lymphocytes binds GlyCAM-1 on the high endothelial venules in lymph nodes. In mucosal tissues, endothelial MAdCAM-1 guides L-selectin–mediated emigration. Migration across the endothelium requires integrins, in particular LFA-1.[69] Binding of LFA-1 to ICAM-1 and ICAM-2 on endothelial cells facilitates migration. Most lymphocytes are carried back to the blood by the efferent lymphatics. If a T lymphocyte recognizes its specific antigen on the surface of an APC, it remains for several days, then returns to the blood as an armed effector T cell.[39]

Adhesion molecules mediate many of the transient interactions between T cells and APCs required for the T cell to sample each antigen it encounters. Lymphocyte LFA-1 can bind the APC in a loose, reversible fashion by any of the ICAM molecules on APCs. If a match between T cell and antigen is found, conformational changes in LFA-1 greatly increase its affinity for ICAM-1 and ICAM-2 to stabilize the interaction. The T cell can then proliferate and differentiate into an effector cell. Effector T cells lose surface expression of L-selectin and no longer circulate through lymphoid tissue. Instead they express VLA-4, an integrin, which binds vascular endothelium at sites of infection. Effector T cells have increased LFA-1 and CD2 adhesion molecule expression that facilitate tight binding to the target cell.[70,71]

Antigen binding in the appropriate context provides the signal for clonal expansion and differentiation of T cells into effector and memory lymphocytes. The appropriate contact is composed of antigen complexed with MHC class II molecules on APCs, costimulators, and cytokines produced by the APCs and by the T cells themselves. This first encounter of naïve T cells with antigen is the primary immune response, which serves to induce the formation of effector and memory T cells. These activated T cells hone to peripheral tissues, where, upon reexposure to the antigen for which they are specific, they activate macrophages to eliminate phagocytosed microbes and induce B-cell differentiation and antigen-specific secretion. The $CD8^+$ CTLs kill infected host cells and tumor cells that display class I MHC–associated antigen. Naïve T cells require activation by dendritic cells, whereas effector T cells can respond to antigens presented by a wider variety of APCs, such as macrophages and B lymphocytes. Not surprisingly, differentiated effector and memory T cells possess lower thresholds for costimulation and require lower antigen concentration for activation than naïve T cells.

In general, antigen presented on MHC II molecules is the prototypical stimulus for $CD4^+$ T-cell activation and the subsequent production of a variety of cytokine mediators, including IL-2, which stimulate further expansion and activation. However, the circumstances under which this activation occurs may dictate disparate paths of differentiation, producing T-cell subsets with distinct cytokine profiles and effector functions. These differing phenotypes have been utilized to characterize two distinct subsets: T_H1 and T_H2.[56,57,72] IL-12 derived from phagocytes infected with intracellular pathogen provides the necessary signal for T_H1 differentiation.[39] IL-12 also stimulates production of IFN-γ, the principal macrophage activator, by NK cells and $CD4^+$ lymphocytes. Interferons stimulate T_H1 development by augmenting phagocytic IL-12 production and by maintaining IL-12 receptor expression on $CD4^+$ T cells. The principal effector action of T_H1 cells is the activation of macrophages through the production of IFN-γ, GM-CSF, TNF-α, CD40L, and FasL.[39,56,57,72] They regulate production of opsonizing and complement fixing antibodies and are effec-
3 tors of phagocyte-dependent responses. This inflammatory response is also referred to as cell-mediated immunity or delayed-type hypersensitivity, provides one major arm of the adaptive immune response, and is mediated by $CD4^+$ and $CD8^+$ lymphocytes and macrophages.

4 The principal stimulus for T_H2 differentiation is IL-4, which is derived from T cells, mast cells, and basophils.[56,57,72] These cells are the cellular effectors of humoral immunity and provide the other major arm of the adaptive immune response, which is mediated by T_H2 $CD4^+$ cells, B cells, plasma cells, and antibodies. They produce IL-4, IL-5, and CD40L, thereby inducing B-cell activation and antibody production and a host of other proinflammatory and anti-inflammatory cytokines.[39] Activation of mast cells and eosinophils by extracellular pathogens is associated with activation of T_H2 cells. T_H2 cells quell the inflammatory response by inhibiting macrophage functions and T_H1 responses; they are considered the anti-inflammatory arm of cell-mediated inflammation. Helper T cells that express both T_H1 and T_H2 patterns of cytokine expression have been called T_H0 cells, and further studies will certainly discern other subsets of T cells.[4,72]

T-cell activation, differentiation, and expansion are orchestrated by the T cell itself. The responding T cell, in an autocrine fashion, serves as both source and target of a variety of mediators stimulating growth. The principal autocrine growth factor is IL-2, which is induced by signaling regulated by the phosphatase calcineurin (see later).[73] IL-15 stimulates the proliferation of $CD8^+$ T cells, especially memory cells of the $CD8^+$ subset. After antigen exposure, the numbers of T cells specific for that antigen may increase to about 1 in 10 for $CD8^+$ and 1 in 1,000 to 10,000 for $CD4^+$ cells.[4]

After activation, some proliferating cells will differentiate into effector cells that eliminate antigens and may activate other immune cells. Mature $CD4^+$ cells induce the activation of mononuclear phagocytes and B cells. $CD8^+$ cells differentiate into CTLs that recognize viral and other intracellular pathogen antigens that are presented in the context of MHC class I molecules and induce target cell death by releasing the cytotoxins perforin and granzymes from cytoplasmic granules. Granzymes are serine proteases that trigger DNA fragmentation and apoptosis. Perforin stimulates cell membrane pore formation, which facilitates granzyme entrance into cells. Apoptosis can also be induced by the binding of Fas ligand on CTL to Fas on the target cell. CTLs also release the cytokines IFN-γ, TNF-α, and CC chemokines. IFN-γ and certain CC chemokines have antiviral properties, and both are potent activators of macrophage function. IL-2 produced by CTL and local helper $CD4^+$ lymphocytes expands the CTL, and IL-12 released by APC stimulates CTL activity. As with $CD4^+$ cells, early evidence suggests that the population of $CD8^+$ cells may be divided into T_C1 and T_C2 cells based on their cytokine profiles and effector functions.[39,55–57]

Other T cells will mature into long-lived functionally quiescent memory cells. A cell surface rich in adhesion molecules such as integrins and CD44 facilitates rapid and efficient migration to peripheral sites of infection and inflammation upon antigen reexposure.[4] These cells accumulate over time and in the adult human comprise more than half of the circulating T cells.

Mere antigen exposure is insufficient for activation of naïve T cells; proliferation and differentiation require costimulatory signals provided by molecules on APCs. The best-characterized costimulator pathway involves the T-cell surface molecule CD28 and its counterligand B7-1 and B7-2 expressed on activated APCs.[4,39] CD28 delivers signals that enhance T-cell survival by increasing expression of the antiapoptotic protein Bcl-X, the production of cytokines such as IL-2 and the IL-2 receptor, and the differentiation of immature T cells. In vitro, purified populations of $CD4^+$ cells challenged with antigen by APCs that express B7 proliferate and secrete cytokines, yet not if B7 is absent. The costimulatory signal must come from the same APC that provides the initial signal. DCs are the most potent APCs because they express both classes of MHC molecules and the B7 molecules. Macrophages and B cells must be activated to express the costimulatory molecules. This expression of costimulators is regulated so as to ensure that T-cell activation is temporally and spatially appropriate. For instance, during T-cell activation, engagement of CD40 ligand with

CD40 induces upregulation of B7 costimulators on the APCs. In addition, it increases the secretion of cytokines such as IL-12 that promote T-cell differentiation, and cytokines are secreted that promote T-cell differentiation and activation. A protein called CTLA-4 is homologous to CD28, binds B7-1 and B7-2, and is expressed on activated T cells. Unlike CD28, CTLA-4 functions to terminate T-cell responses and plays a role in self-tolerance. On the basis of many experimental studies of costimulators, antagonists against B7 molecules and CD40L are in clinical trials to prevent the rejection of organ allografts.[4,39]

The differentiation of naïve $CD8^+$ T cells to CTL requires a stronger costimulatory signal. This can be provided by either DCs, as they have the greatest intrinsic costimulatory activity, or by a $CD4^+$ helper T lymphocyte. Naïve helper T cells attached to the same APC as the $CD8^+$ T cell can be activated to elaborate IL-2. Attached effector T helper cells can stimulate the APC to express more costimulatory molecules. In the case of virulent viruses, cytotoxicity substitutes for CD28 costimulation, and so the typical costimulatory signal is not required for activation. For less virulent viruses, costimulation is necessary for CTL induction.[39,74] The absence of costimulation results in an unresponsive, or anergic, T cell. Recently this has been shown to be mediated by the serine/threonine kinase calcium/calmodulin-dependent protein kinase (CaMK) II (see later).[75] Anergic T cells do not produce IL-2 and therefore cannot proliferate and differentiate into effector cells even when presented with antigen at a later time.[39]

The affinity of most T-cell receptors (TCRs) for peptide–MHC complexes is low, with dissociation constants on the order of 10^{-5} to 10^{-7} and an estimated TCR–antigen interaction of less than 10 seconds. Furthermore, on any APC, fewer than 1,000 of the 10^5 available MHC molecules are likely to be displaying any one peptide at any particular time. Therefore, one APC can engage a small fraction of the 10^4 to 10^5 antigen receptors on a single T cell.[4] Activation of an individual T cell may require multiple sequential engagements of that cell's antigen receptors by peptide–MHC complexes on APCs. With engagement, there is clustering of membrane receptors, tyrosine phosphorylation of several proteins, and recruitment and activation of adaptor proteins. TCRs are devoid of enzymatic activity and must utilize other signal-transducing proteins.[4]

After TCR–MHC engagement, several membrane surface proteins and intracellular signaling proteins are rapidly recruited, including the TCR complex, CD4 or CD8, receptors for costimulators such as CD28, and enzymes and adaptor proteins.[4] After TCR clustering, activated tyrosine kinases that are associated with the cytoplasmic domains of CD3 phosphorylate tyrosine residues on both CD3 and TCR (Fig. 6.4). These phosphorylation sites provide docking sites for other tyrosine and protein kinases, such as Lck, an Src family of tyrosine kinase, and ZAP-70, a tyrosine kinase. These kinases become activated with phosphorylation. Activated ZAP-70 phosphorylates several adaptor proteins that subsequently induce a variety of signal transduction cascades. Adaptor proteins contain structural domains that bind other proteins and thereby facilitate the correct spatial orientation to promote the activation of signal transduction pathways. The ras pathway is also activated, which is an early step in the activation of the mitogen-activated protein kinases (MAPKs) that can activate a variety of transcription factors. Ras is a member of a family of guanine nucleotide–binding proteins (guanosine diphosphate [GDP]/guanosine triphosphate [GTP]) that are involved in diverse activation responses in different cell types. This pathway is an amplification process by which few upstream kinases lead to the activation of several downstream kinases. Ultimately, activation of the terminal extracellular regulated kinase (ERK 1/2) leads to the phosphorylation of the protein ELK, which stimulates the transcription of fos, a component of the activation protein 1 (AP-1) transcription factor (Box C). Concomitantly, c-Jun N-terminal kinase (JNK) is activated, which phosphorylates c-Jun, the second component of AP-1. The third member of the MAPK family, p38, is also activated. The activities of the MAPKs are terminated by specific protein tyrosine/threonine phosphatases that are regulated by the MAPKs themselves. Hence, the entire system is self-regulated by a negative feedback system.[4]

Activation of TCR also leads to the induction of phospholipase C (PLC), in particular PLCγ1 (Fig. 6.4). Phosphorylated PLCγ1 catalyzes the hydrolysis of phosphatidylinositol 4,5-bisphosphate (PIP_2) into inositol 1,4,5-triphosphate (IP_3) and diacylglycerol (DAG), and activates enzymes that generate

FIGURE 6.4. T-cell signaling and activation. (Redrawn from Abbas AK, Lichtman AH. *Cellular and Molecular Immunology.* Philadelphia: Saunders; 2003.)

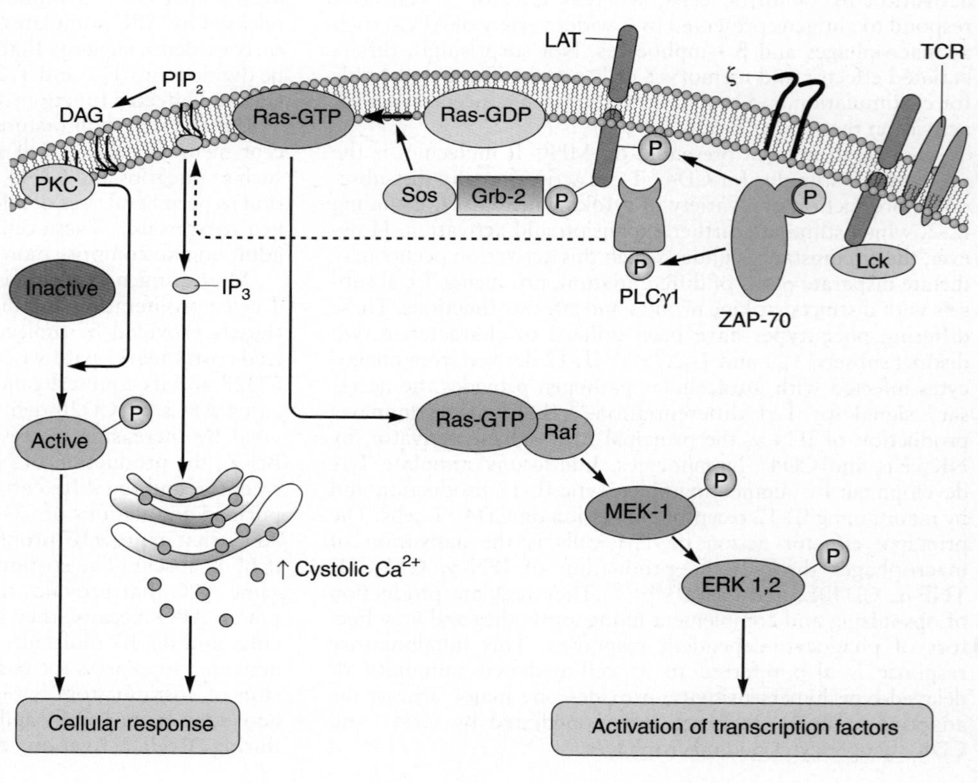

Transcription Factor	Stimuli	Effector Genes
AP-1	TNF, IL-1, UV light, H_2O_2, LPS, stress, ROS, hypoxia	TNF, IL-1, IL-2, IL-5, IFN-γ, ICAM-1, E-selectin, GM-CSF, MMPs, COX-2
NFκB	TNF-IL-1, UV light, H_2O_2, LPS, ROS	IL-1, IL-2, IL-6, IL-8, IL-12, TNF, E-selecting, VCAM-1, ICAM-1, MIP-1, MCP-1, RANTES, iNOS, eotaxin, PLA_2, G-CSF, GM-CSF, IFN-β
STAT	IFNs, CSFs, GFs, IL-1 to IL-15	FOS, E-selectin, Myc, ICAM-1, Fc γRI
NFAT	TCR, BCR, FcεR, FcγR, histamine and thrombin receptors	IL-2, IL-3, IL-4, IL-5, IL-8, IL-13, TNF, GM-CSF, IFN-γ, CD40L, FASL

Transcription Factors. AP, activator protein; CSF, colony-stimulating factor; COX, cyclooxygenase; GF, growth factor; ICAM, intercellular adhesion molecule; IFN, interferon; IL, interleukin; iNOS, inducible nitric oxide synthase; LPS, lipopolysaccharide; MMP, matrix metalloproteinase; MPO, myeloperoxidase; NFAT, nuclear factor of activated T cells; NFκB, nuclear factor kappa-B; PLA_2, phospholipase A_2; ROS, reactive oxygen species; STAT, signal transducer and activator or transcription; TNF, tumor necrosis factor; UV, ultraviolet; VCAM, vascular cell adhesion molecule. *(Modified from Gallin JI, Snyderman R, eds. Inflammation: basic principles and clinical correlates, 3rd ed. Philadelphia: Lippincott Williams & Wilkins, 1999)*

BOX C

additional active transcription factors. IP_3 increases cytosolic free calcium that leads to a large influx of both intracellular and extracellular calcium with subsequent activation of calcium- and calmodulin-dependent proteins. Calcineurin, a calcium/calmodulin-dependent phosphatase, is integral to T-cell activation via modulation of the activation of the transcription factors nuclear factor of activated T cells (NFAT) and NF-κB (Box C).[73,4] These transcription factors are essential for the induction of cytokine transcription, in particular IL-2 production. However, in the absence of costimulation, activation of the CaMK II opposes the actions of calcineurin as described earlier and produces an anergic cell.[75] DAG activates protein kinase C, which activates additional transcription factors. The role of PKC and calcium in T-cell function is made evident by studies in which pharmacologic activation of PKC and/or elevation of intracellular calcium concentration stimulates T-cell cytokine secretion and proliferation.[4] Regulation of those kinases operant in T-cell signaling involves protein tyrosine phosphatases. Through dephosphorylation, they modulate TCR signaling. Two phosphatases induced with TCR clustering are SHP-1 and SHP-2.

The ultimate goal of all these signaling transduction pathways is to activate transcription factors that bind to promoter regions and enhance transcription. Three transcription factors that are activated in T cells and appear critical for most T-cell responses are NFAT, AP-1, and NF-κB (Box C).

A third mechanism of T-cell activation involves lipid antigens such as cell wall protein from intracellular bacteria. These antigens bind CD1, an MHC-related cell surface molecule that presents these antigens to certain subtypes of T cells. A superantigen is an unprocessed bacterial or retroviral product that binds the MHC molecule and the T-cell receptor outside the usual antigen-binding sites. This engagement leads to a polyclonal and non-specific stimulation of a large proportion of the T-cell population. An overwhelming activation of all arms of the immune system ensues and underlies much of the pathophysiology of toxic shock syndrome. Intravenous immunoglobulin (IVIG), by binding this antigen, is thought to be of therapeutic benefit.

Eosinophils

Eosinophils are marrow-derived granulocytes that share some properties of neutrophils and are involved in the eradication of helminthic infections and allergen reaction (Table 6.1). IL-3, GM-CSF, and IL-5 promote eosinophil differentiation, the induction of effector functions, and survival by inhibiting apoptosis.[76] They emigrate through inflamed endothelium and upon exiting release inflammatory mediators and toxic agents from cytoplasmic granules. They generate superoxide anion and hydrogen peroxide, though less efficiently than neutrophils. Eosinophils act in conjunction with basophils and mast cells as primary effectors in allergy and inflammation. They express IgE receptors and stimulate histamine release from basophils and mast cells through major basic protein (MBP). They can also regulate basophil and mast cell function by releasing enzymes that inactivate histamine and slow-reacting substance of anaphylaxis (SRS-a). Upon exiting the marrow, their intravascular half-life is but a few hours; thereafter, they enter the mucosa of the lung, gastrointestinal, and genitourinary tracts.[39,76]

Recruitment and Activation. Eosinophils are primarily recruited to sites of parasitic infection and allergen challenge. Mast cells and macrophages responding to either allergen or parasite secrete cytokines (IL-5, PAF, LTB-4) that upregulate expression of endothelial adhesion molecules. Eosinophils

SCIENTIFIC PRINCIPLES

themselves are more responsive to CC chemokines (MIP-1α, RANTES, and MCP-3) and the cytokines produced with T_H2 activation. Engagement of the β_1-integrin VLA_4 of eosinophil with VCAM-1 and fibronectin on the endothelium initiates the process of emigration. IL-4 can activate both the binding and the upregulation of endothelial cell VCAM-1. Diapedesis and tissue infiltration also involve members of the β_2-integrin family (Mac-1 and LFA) similar to that employed during neutrophil recruitment.[39,77]

Eosinophils are activated by IL-3, GM-CSF, IL-5, PAF, CC chemokines, and C3a and C5a of complement. IL-5 is a potent activating agent and enhances the ability of eosinophils to release granule contents on FcR cross-linking. A positive feedback cycle ultimately is established, in which recruited eosinophils produce cytokines and chemokines that recruit more eosinophils and other leukocytes.

Granules. Eosinophils possess a compartmentalized armamentarium of toxic substances to assist in the elimination of organisms, in particular helminths. Their specific granules contain GM-CSF and MBP, the latter of which is cytotoxic to parasites and normal cells and is a stimulus for histamine release from mast cells and basophils.[78] The granule matrix contains eosinophil peroxidase (EPO), eosinophil-derived neurotoxin, lysosomal enzymes, catalase, TNF-α, transforming growth factor-β (TGF-β), and eosinophilic cationic proteins that stimulate formation of transmembrane pores to increase target cellular permeability.[79] EPO is released extracellularly on target cell surfaces where it generates hydrogen peroxide and hydrogen halides. Approximately 30% of oxygen consumed by stimulated eosinophils is utilized in the formation of halogenating species. Thiocyanate may be the major halide for the EPO-H_2O_2 system.[80] If ingested by a neighboring phagocyte, EPO can combine with H_2O_2 and halides to form hypohalous acids. EPO also stimulates neutrophil aggregation and adhesion to endothelial cells. Although they express Fc receptors for IgG, IgA, and IgE, they are relatively insensitive to activation by antigen-mediated cross-linking of these receptors. However, they can kill microorganisms by antibody-dependent cell-mediated cytotoxicity (ADCC).[4,39]

The primary targets of eosinophils are extracellular parasites. The size of these pathogens prohibits phagocytosis, and their integument is relatively resistant to the microbicidal products of neutrophils and macrophages; however, they can be killed by MBP, which is released after cross-linking of Fc-bound IgE coating the parasite. The T_H2 response to parasitic invasion produces IL-4, IL-5, and IL-13. IL-4 stimulates the production of specific IgE antibodies, which opsonize helminths. IL-5 activates eosinophils, which bind to the IgE-coated helminths via Fc receptors. Activated eosinophils then release their granule contents and generate reactive oxygen species and hypohalous acids. EPO also stimulates neutrophil aggregation and adhesion to endothelial cells. The sparse uncompartmental granules contain Charcot-Leyden crystals and have lysophospholipase activity. Finally, eosinophils produce and release lipid mediators such as PAF, prostaglandins, and leukotrienes, which probably contribute to the process of allergic diseases.[4,81,82]

Basophils and Mast Cells

Basophils and mast cells are central to the development of allergic inflammation and produce cytokines, lipid mediators, vasoactive amines, and proteases that participate in nonallergic inflammatory responses (Table 6.1). Both cells share a common progenitor cell, which diverges early during differentiation. The primary growth factors for basophil development are IL-3 and GM-CSF, whereas stem cell factor is the primary stimulus for mast cell maturation.[83] Although basophils and mast cells are distinct cell types, they are often grouped together because of their similarity in granule content, activating stimuli, and effector functions.[39]

Mature basophils constitute only 0.5% to 1% of the circulating leukocytes, and mast cells primarily reside fixed in connective tissue. Engagement of IgE-bound antigen with the high-affinity IgE antibody receptor, FcεR, provides the primary stimulus for basophil and mast cell activation and degranulation. In addition, diverse agents such as contrast media, opiates, anaphylatoxins, chemokines, and neuropeptides may serve as activators. Basophils and mast cells elaborate both preformed and newly synthesized inflammatory mediators. The main basophil proteoglycan is chondroitin sulfate A, whereas mast cells contain heparin, chondroitin sulfate, and chondroitin sulfate E and also store neutral proteases.[84] The lipid mediators LTB_4, LTC_4, and prostaglandin D_2 (PGD_2) are synthesized de novo in response to stimulation. The leukotrienes are powerful vasoconstrictors, bronchoconstrictors, and chemoattractants for neutrophils and eosinophils. PGD_2 inhibits platelet aggregation and is chemotactic for neutrophils. Both basophils and mast cells synthesize and secrete histamine. Histamine, or 2-(4-imidazolyl)-ethylamine, is formed by the carboxylation of histidine. It is stored in preformed granules at acid pH as a complex with proteins and proteoglycans. Mast cells carry greater quantities of histamine than do basophils. The classic vasoactive properties of arteriolar dilatation, increased vascular permeability, and bronchoconstriction are mediated by the H_1 receptors. H_2 receptors are involved in modulation of the immune response and stimulating gastric output and mucus secretion. H_3 receptors participate in neuroconduction.[39,84,85]

Platelets

Though classically considered in the context of hemostasis, platelets are integral to both normal and pathologic inflammation and link the processes of hemostasis, inflammation, and tissue repair. They are activated in a variety of inflammatory conditions, such as rheumatoid arthritis and inflammatory bowel disease, a testimony to their role in inflammation.[86] Upon activation, they release factors that enhance vascular permeability, chemokines, microbicidal proteins, and mitogens for endothelial cells, smooth muscle cells, and fibroblasts. They assist leukocytes in promoting the inflammatory reaction and killing microbes by providing an adhesive surface to facilitate emigration, by stimulating adhered leukocytes, and by further modulating chemokine synthesis (Table 6.5).[86,87]

Humans possess about 150 to 400 $\times 10^9$ platelets per liter of blood.[86] Thrombopoiesis is regulated by thrombopoietin (TPO) as well as a variety of other peptides (IL-3, IL-4, IL-6, IL-7, and IL-11). In fact, human IL-11 is clinically used to stimulate thrombopoiesis in patients undergoing chemotherapy.[88] After release from the marrow, they circulate with a half-life of approximately 12 days. Interferon-α is inhibitory for megakaryocyte growth, and the elevated levels induced with some viral and inflammatory conditions may explain the relative thrombocytopenia observed in these conditions.[86,89]

Recruitment and Activation. Platelets are activated and aggregate by exposure to thrombin or activated endothelium. Clot formation triggers the release of vasoactive agents (PGE_2, PGI_2, $PGF_{2\alpha}$, and platelet-derived growth factor [PDGF]) and inflammatory mediators. Serotonin, PGE_2, and PAF increase vascular permeability. The adhesion molecule PECAM-1 and the β_3 integrins mediate platelet plug formation, endothelial cell adhesion, and leukocyte emigration. The integrin IIb/IIIa and P-selectin facilitate platelet interactions with other inflammatory cells. The α granules are rich in membrane-bound P-selectin; upon fusion with the cell surface membrane they markedly enhance the cell surface density of this receptor. On stimulation, both receptors are expressed on the platelet surface in an activated state. IIb/IIIa binds various adhesive proteins containing the RGD sequence (i.e., fibrinogen), which serve as a mechanical

TABLE 6.5

PLATELET-DERIVED MEDIATORS

Chemoattractants	
	C5a
	12-HETE
	PAF
	α-Granule proteins
	PDGF
	PF-4
	RANTES
Growth Factors	
	Transforming growth factors-α and -β
	Fibroblast growth factor
	PDGF
Antimicrobial activity	
	Cationic bactericidal protein
	IgE-mediated oxidant production by platelets directed at schistosomes
Vascular Reactions	
	Prostaglandin E_2
	Prostaglandin I_2
	Prostaglandin $F_{2\alpha}$
	Serotonin
	PDGF
	Serotonin
	PAF
	Cationic proteins
	Vascular endothelial growth factor

HETE, hydroxyeicosatetraenoic acid; IgE, immunoglobulin E; PAF, platelet-activating factor; PDGF, platelet-derived growth factor; PF-4, platelet factor 4; RANTES, regulated on activation, normally T-cell expressed and secreted.
From Klinger MHF, Jelkmann W. Role of blood platelet in infection and inflammation. *J Interferon Cytokine Res* 2002;22:913–922.

link to other platelets, leukocytes, and the endothelium. Possibly the immobilization on the vessel wall of activated platelets with induced P-selectin biochemically and functionally promotes the adhesion of neutrophils to endothelial cells.[86,89]

Platelets are a primary source of chemoattractants for neutrophils. Neutral proteinases released from stimulated platelets cleave complement factor C5, liberating the chemoattractant C5a. PDGF binds strongly to the extracellular matrix, providing a long-acting source of chemoattractant. Platelet factor 4 (PF4) is a cationic protein that penetrates the vascular wall and is a chemoattractant. Activated platelets also bind monocytes via P-selectin and PSGL-1 and induce the expression and secretion of MCP-1 and IL-8. Thrombospondin released from activated platelets mediates monocyte binding to platelets. Together these substances promote leukocyte margination, activation, and recruitment to the sites of injury.[39]

Granules. The vasoactive substances and inflammatory mediators of platelets are either stored in cytoplasmic granules or synthesized de novo. A platelet contains about 35 α granules and five dense bodies. The dense granules contain adenosine diphosphate (ADP), ATP, serotonin, and calcium, mediators operant during the initial phase of inflammation. ADP is the principal platelet agonist during platelet aggregation and augments the oxidative burst of neutrophils. Serotonin increases vascular permeability and enhances the superoxide production by macrophages.[86]

The more abundant α granules contain fibrinogen, RANTES, MIP-1α, thrombospondin, P-selectin, PF4, PDGF, TGF-β, β-thromboglobulin, high-molecular-weight kininogen (HMWK), and many other biologically active proteins. PF4 and β-thromboglobulin initiate leukocyte recruitment and activation. PF4 induces neutrophil adherence to unstimulated endothelium and the release of secondary granules, whereas it inhibits monocyte apoptosis and promotes macrophage differentiation. PF4 can also stimulate histamine release from basophils. RANTES is deposited on the endothelium and recruits monocytes from the circulation. MIP-1α is chemotactic for $CD8^+$ T lymphocytes. PAF induces platelet aggregation, increases vascular permeability, and enhances phagocyte free radical formation and the adhesion of platelets to neutrophils. Platelet activation appears to occur in allergic asthma and may precede the delayed accumulation of eosinophils in the lung after allergen exposure. The α granules also carry several important growth factors, including vascular endothelial growth factor (VEGF), PDGF, and TGF-β. VEGF promotes extravasation and aids recruitment of leukocytes. PDGF is chemotactic for neutrophils and monocytes. TGF-β is chemotactic for and activates neutrophils and monocytes early during inflammation, but displays immunosuppressive effects during later stages of inflammation.[86]

Platelets are an important source of eicosanoids, including thromboxane and prostaglandins $F_{2\alpha}$ and E_2. Thromboxane synthetase in platelets is responsible for the production of thromboxane A_2 (TXA_2), a potent vasoconstrictor that also increases vascular permeability and stimulates platelet aggregation. Aspirin and other nonsteroidal anti-inflammatory drugs (NSAIDs) inhibit platelet function by inhibiting TXA_2 production. As this effect is irreversible, new platelets must be produced (7 to 10 days) to restore normal clot formation. $PGF_{2\alpha}$ causes vasoconstriction, whereas PGE_2 vasodilates and modulates pain.[90,91]

Platelets participate in transcellular lipoxygenase (LO) metabolism, which refers to the production of eicosanoids through interactions with neighboring inflammatory cells. Endothelial cells utilize platelet-derived endoperoxides to synthesize PGI_2. Platelets interact with neutrophils in several pathways, providing a direct link between thrombosis and inflammation. 12-Hydroxyeicosatetraenoic acid (HETE) released from activated platelets can be used by unstimulated neutrophils to produce the chemoattractant 12,20-HETE. 12-HETE and 5-HETE from activated platelets and neutrophils, respectively, can combine in either cell type to form 5,12-diHETE, an anti-inflammatory compound, which diverts production away from the proinflammatory leukotrienes. 12-LO from platelets and LTA_4 formed by neutrophils can produce the intermediate 5(6)-epoxytetraene. This intermediate produces lipoxins A_4 and B_4 that have primarily counterinflammatory functions.[39,87,90,92]

In addition to modulating inflammation, platelets possess some direct microbicidal activity. Platelets are activated and degranulate when exposed to certain bacteria. Electron microscopic studies have shown that activated platelets internalize bacteria and viruses. The α granules contain antibacterial proteins called thrombocidins (TCs) in humans that support the killing of adherent bacteria. The two antibacterial proteins isolated from human platelets (TC-1 and TC-2) are bactericidal for *Escherichia coli* and *S. aureus*.[86]

Noncellular Components

Cytokines. Cytokines are soluble protein mediators secreted by the cells of the innate and adaptive immunity in response to microbes and other antigens, including intra- and extracellular proteins, and mediate many of the functions of these cells (Table 6.6). They regulate and influence the host response to both pathogen-associated molecular patterns (PAMPs; i.e.,

TABLE 6.6

CYTOKINES

CYTOKINE	RECEPTOR	SIGNAL TRANSDUCTION	CELLULAR SOURCE	TARGETS	EFFECTS
INNATE/EARLY CYTOKINES					
TNF-α	TNF R	TRAFS Death domains	Mo/Mϕ, MC, Ba, Eo, NK, B, T, F, Ep	Endothelium PMN Many cells	↑ inflammation, coagulation, adhesion molecules ↑ activation ↑ apoptosis ↑ fever, APP, catabolism
IL-1	Ig family	IRAK	Mo/Mϕ, B, EC, Ep, F	Endothelium PMN Mo	↑ inflammation, coagulation, adhesion molecules ↑ activation and emigration ↑ activation and emigration ↑ shock, fever, APP production
Chemokines/IL-8	7 trans-membrane	G protein	Mo/Mϕ, T, PMN, F, EC, Ep	PMN T Mo/Mϕ EC Ba	↑ activation, adherence, and migration ↑ emigration ↑ emigration ↑ adhesion molecules ↑ histamine release
IL-12	Type I	JAK/STAT	Mϕ	T NK	T_H1 differentiation, interferon-γ synthesis, ↑ cytolytic activity
Interferons (Type I)	Type II	JAK/STAT	All	All	Antiviral, antitumor, increases MHC I activates T, Mϕ, NK cells
IL-10	Type II	JAK/STAT	Mo/Mϕ, T, B, MC	Mo/Mϕ T B, NK, MC	↓ IL-12, costimulators, MHC II ↓ T_H1 differentiation
IL-6	Type I	JAK/STAT	Mo/Mϕ, B, F, EC, Ep	T B Mo/Mϕ E	Differentiation ↑ antibody-producing cells APP synthesis
IL-15	Type I	JAK/STAT	Mϕ	NK T	Proliferation Proliferation
IL-18	Ig family	IRAK	Mϕ	T, NK	↑ interferon-γ
ADAPTIVE/LATE CYTOKINES					
IL-2	Type I	JAK/STAT	T	T B NK	T activation and proliferation, Fas apoptosis ↑ proliferation, antibody synthesis ↑ proliferation and activation Mo/Mϕ activation
IL-4	Type I	JAK/STAT	T, Ba, MC	T B Mo/Mϕ	T_H2 differentiation and proliferation, ↓ T_H1 Isotype switching to IgE ↓ interferon-γ-mediated function

(continued)

TABLE 6.6

CYTOKINES (*Continued*)

CYTOKINE	RECEPTOR	SIGNAL TRANSDUCTION	CELLULAR SOURCE	TARGETS	EFFECTS
IL-5	Type I	JAK/STAT			
Interferon-γ	Type II	JAK/STAT	T, NK	Mϕ T B	Mϕ activation T_H1 differentiation IgG secretion ↑ MHC I and II ↑ antiviral ↑ fever, anorexia, shock, capillary leak ↑ APP synthesis, inflammatory cytokine induction
TGF-β			All	T Mϕ B	↓ T proliferation and effector functions ↓ Mϕ function ↓ proliferation ↑ matrix protein synthesis
Lymphotoxin	TNF R	TRAFs Death domains	T	PMN	Recruitment and activation
IL-13	Type I	JAK/STAT	T	Mo/Mϕ B EC	↓ Mϕ function switching to isotype IgE ↑ adhesion molecules and CC chemokines

APP, acute-phase protein; B, B cell; Ba, basophil; EC, endothelial cell; Ep, epithelial cell; F, fibroblast; IL, interleukin; IRAK, IL-1R–associated kinase; JAK/STAT, Janus kinase/signal transducer and activator of transcription; MC, mast cell; MHC, major histocompatibility complex; Mo, monocyte; Mϕ, macrophage; NK, natural killer; PMN, polymorphonuclear leukocyte; T, T cell; TNF, tumor necrosis factor; TRAF, tumor necrosis factor receptor–associated factor.
Modified from Abbas AK, Lichtman AH. *Cellular and Molecular Immunology,* 5th ed. 2003:179, 181–182.

acute and chronic bacterial, viral, fungal, and parasitic infections) and DAMPs (i.e., trauma, burns, allograft rejection, ischemia/reperfusion injury, and autoimmune disease). They govern lymphocyte differentiation during adaptive immunity and activate effector cells of both arms of inflammation to eliminate microbes. Cytokines play important roles in tumor biology as well as angiogenesis. Though essential for a normal immune response, excessive cytokine release underlies a variety of pathophysiologic inflammatory states such as acute respiratory distress syndrome (ARDS) and multiple organ dysfunction syndrome (MODS).[93–96]

Cytokine secretion is brief, and as they typically are not stored preformed, necessitates transcription and de novo synthesis, which is also transient as the messenger RNA is unstable. Their functions are pleiotropic and redundant, which has been interpreted as a teleologic safety mechanism. However, such protective characteristics greatly limit the therapeutic 5 utility of either cytokine administration or blockade. In fact, over 30 randomized controlled clinical trials have been conducted to assess the efficacy of agents modulating inflammation, in particular systemic cytokine concentrations, in reducing mortality. Yet only one, activated protein C, has been approved by the U.S. Food and Drug Administration (FDA) for use, and studies are ongoing to confirm its benefit.[97] Cytokines often influence the synthesis and actions of other cytokines, such as IL-1–induced T-cell IL-2 production; this interaction may be synergistic (additive or multiplicative) or antagonistic. They may function in an autocrine, paracrine, or even endocrine function, although the inability to correlate plasma cytokine concentrations with the extent of tissue damage suggests that they are designed for local rather than systemic inflammation.[4,39,93]

Their actions are mediated by specific membrane receptors on target cells to which they bind with high affinity (kD α 10^{-10} to 10^{-12}); hence, only minute quantities are necessary to elicit a response. Such efficiency is accompanied by a narrow therapeutic index and potential for unwanted global effects (i.e., MODS) with even small systemic concentrations. The receptors and the cells expressing them are regulated by external stimuli, which provides some degree of specificity to the response even though the cytokines themselves are not antigen specific. Receptor binding alters cellular gene transcription (induction or suppression) that may result in proliferation, differentiation, and the acquisition of new or suppression/enhancement of preexisting functions.[4]

All cytokine receptors consist of at least one transmembrane protein with an extracellular portion for ligand binding and an intracellular domain mediating signal transduction. Current receptor classification is based on structural homologies among the extracellular cytokine-binding domains. Type I cytokine receptors contain a domain with two conserved pairs of cysteine residues and a membrane proximal sequence of tryptophan-serine-X-tryptophan-serine, where X is any amino acid (WSXWS). Type II receptors resemble type I receptors; however, the WSXWS motif is absent. The Ig superfamily consists of receptors with extracellular Ig domains. TNF receptors belong to a family of receptors with conserved cysteine-rich extracellular domains. Finally, seven-transmembrane α-helical receptors mediate the functions of cytokines called chemokines through GTP-binding (G) proteins.[4]

Translating ligand engagement to the signaling events that alter cellular phenotype involves a variety of signaling cascades dependent on the structure of the cytoplasmic tail of the particular receptor (Table 6.6). This is another method by which to classify cytokine receptors. These individual signaling cascades will be discussed in the context of the various cytokines and respective receptors employing them.

Early Cytokines/Innate Immunity

Tumor Necrosis Factor-*α*. TNF-*α* is the principal mediator in the initiation of the inflammatory response to gram-negative bacteria and other infectious pathogens. It is an important early mediator of inflammation and is essential for the normal initiation, maintenance, and repair of tissue injury. However, aberrant production may underlie the pathologic sequelae of many inflammatory and infectious states (i.e., MODS, rheumatoid arthritis, Crohn disease). Mononuclear phagocytes are the principal source of TNF-*α*, usually in response to the potent prototypical stimulus lipopolysaccharide.[98,99] LPS-induced TNF-*α* production may be augmented by concomitant stimulation with IFN-*γ*, IL-4, and IL-10, whereas corticosteroids are suppressive.[100] Secondary sources include mast cells, NK cells, and T and B lymphocytes, and stimuli include complement C5a, GM-CSF, hypoxia, IL-1, NO, ROS, and TNF-*α* itself.[39]

Shedding of extracellular domains of the two TNF-*α* receptors by metalloproteinases can further alter the biologic activity of TNF-*α* by decreasing the number of cell signaling sites on target tissues and increasing the amount of circulating inhibitors. Unlike other members of the TNF family that are primarily involved in regulation of cell proliferation, TNF-*α* has both proinflammatory and apoptosis-inducing properties.[93,101]

TNF-*α* is expressed on the cell membrane as a bioactive protein and is cleaved into its soluble form by a specific TNF-*α*–converting enzyme. There are two distinct TNF receptors present on virtually all cell types (Fig. 6.5).[102] Ligand binding to TNF-RII leads to recruitment of TNF receptor–associated factors (TRAFs) that ultimately activate the transcription factors NF-*κ*B and AP-1 and thereby influence gene expression and cellular phenotype.[4] Alternatively, binding to TNF-RI activates caspases and triggers apoptosis, in addition to signaling transcription factors. The manner by which either a proinflammatory or apoptotic path is chosen is unknown, although the net effect of TNF-*α* binding is probably the culmination of differential adaptor protein expression and downstream signal transduction cascades. TNF-RI appears to be more important in host defense as knockout TNF-RI mice show a greater degree of impairment in host defense than mice lacking TNF-RII.[4]

The principal function of TNF-*α* is to recruit neutrophils and monocytes to foci of infection and to activate these cells to eradicate microbes. TNF-*α* activates the endothelium to upregulate the expression of the adhesion molecules E- and P-selectin, ICAM-1, PECAM-1, and VCAM-1, and stimulates these cells and macrophages to secret chemokines (IL-8, MIP-1*α*, and Gro-*α*) that enhance the affinity of leukocyte integrins for their ligands and induce leukocyte chemotaxis and recruitment.[103] TNF-*α* also can induce HMGB1 release by activated macrophages, which generates a forward feedback mechanism, as HMGB1, by signaling through RAGE (see later), also induces TNF-*α* release.[104,105] TNF-*α* induces a state of hypercoagulability by stimulating the release of tissue factor, PAF, von Willebrand factor, and thromboplastin. By inhibiting tissue-type plasminogen activator and thrombomodulin, it suppresses fibrinolysis, decreases protein C and S activation, and increases thrombin formation. However, TNF-*α* also induces the release of a variety of anticoagulants (prostacyclin), fibrinolytics (urokinase-type plasminogen activator), and vasodilators (NO, PGE_2), which may balance the tendency toward a procoagulant state. Most likely, the ultimate effect of TNF-*α* depends on the location and quantity in which it is produced and the vascular bed with which it interacts.[4,93]

In severe infections, exuberant production and aberrant release of TNF-*α* enables it to function as an endocrine hormone

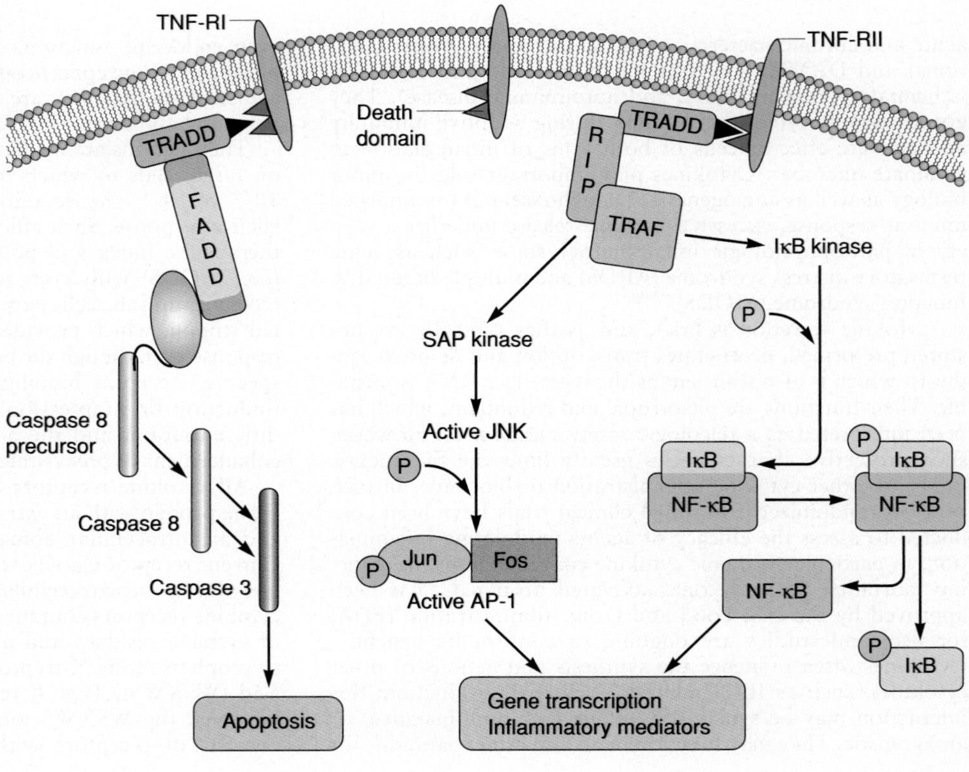

FIGURE 6.5. Tumor necrosis factor (TNF) receptor signaling pathway. (Redrawn from Abbas AK, Lichtman AH. *Cellular and Molecular Immunology.* Philadelphia: Saunders; 2003.)

and cause a plethora of pathologic sequelae. These systemic effects include fever (hence the name *endogenous pyrogen*) by stimulating the production of PGE_2 by the hypothalamus, acute-phase protein production by the liver, cachexia, inhibition of myocardial contractility and vascular tonus, and intravascular thrombosis due to loss of normal anticoagulant properties of the endothelium and the production of tissue factor. TNF-α is central to the pathogenesis of systemic inflammatory response syndrome (SIRS) and septic shock, and either state can be reproduced by administration of LPS or TNF-α.[106–108] The organ dysfunction characteristic of either state may result from the hypercoagulability and subsequent tissue ischemia induced by this cytokine. Antagonists of TNF-α can prevent mortality in experimental models, but clinical trials with anti–TNF-α antibodies or with soluble TNF-α receptors have been to no avail.[4,106]

Soluble TNF receptors formed by proteolytic processing of both types of receptors bind and neutralize TNF-α and serve as an endogenous regulator of cytokine activity.[39] Also, TNF-α directly induces the expression and release of TNF-α inhibitors, including IL-10, corticosteroids, and prostanoids, which in a negative feedback loop suppress TNF-α production and processing.[93] Hence, TNF-α serves as its own regulator.

Interleukin-1. Interleukin-1 functions similarly to TNF-α in mediating a proinflammatory host response to insult and is frequently released concomitantly with TNF-α (Table 6.6).[109] The major source of IL-1 is the mononuclear phagocyte. Synthesis and release are induced by LPS, cytokines (TNF-α, IL-2, TGF-β, all the interferons), antigen–antibody complexes, C5, and hypoxia.[93] IL-1 is also produced by neutrophils, B cells, helper T cells, epithelial cells, fibroblasts, renal mesangial cells, and endothelial cells.

There are two forms of IL-1: IL-1α and IL-1β. Both forms are active, bind to the same receptors, and mediate the same effects. Most IL-1 found in the circulation is IL-1β.[4]

The two IL-1 receptors (IL-1Rs) are members of the Ig superfamily. IL-1RI is universally expressed and transduces the majority of IL-1 responses.[110,111] IL-1RII expression is restricted to B cells, but may be induced on other cells. There is little evidence that this latter receptor serves any function, and in fact, it may serve as a decoy.[112] The cytoplasmic portion of IL-1RI is homologous to a domain of Toll-like receptors (TLRs), which mediate the cellular response to endotoxin (Fig. 6.6). Engagement of IL-1 with IL-1RI induces the activation of the IL-1 receptor–associated kinase (IRAK) and the subsequent induction of the transcription factors NF-κB and AP-1.[4,111]

The functions of IL-1 mirror those of TNF-α, and synergy between the two cytokines is evident.[109] IL-1 activates endothelial cells to increase cell surface expression of adhesion molecules and the production of prostaglandins, PAF, and a variety of colony-stimulating factors. In doing so, it facilitates the recruitment and activation of appropriate leukocyte populations for specific localized immune responses. IL-1 also induces a procoagulant state by suppressing fibrinolysis through enhanced plasminogen activator inhibitor-1 and decreased tissue-type plasminogen activator activity and increasing thrombosis by stimulating tissue factor–like procoagulant and thromboplastin

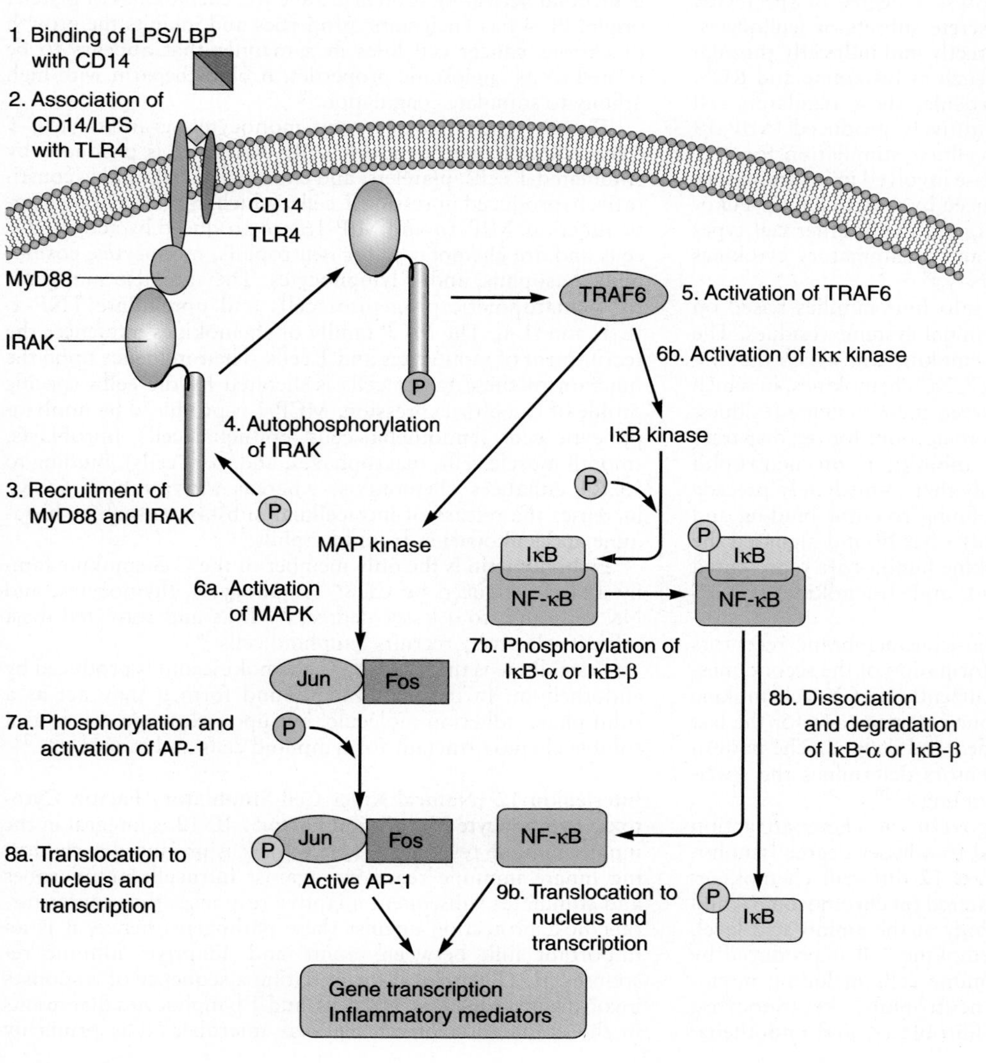

FIGURE 6.6. Toll-like receptor (TLR) signaling pathway. (Redrawn from Abbas AK, Lichtman AH. *Cellular and Molecular Immunology.* Philadelphia: Saunders; 2003.)

SCIENTIFIC PRINCIPLES

production and suppressing thrombomodulin release. It induces the synthesis of PAF, a potent vasoconstrictor and stimulus for platelet and leukocyte activation. However, similar to TNF-α, it also stimulates the production of prostacyclin and urokinase-type plasminogen activator, which promotes an antithrombotic state.[113] At larger concentrations, its effects become systemic, causing fever, the synthesis of acute-phase proteins, cachexia (inhibition of hunger and increased lipoprotein lipase activity), myalgia, somnolence, and hypotension. It stimulates arachidonic acid and prostaglandin metabolism and the release of pituitary stress hormones. It stimulates collagenase release and is a potent mitogen for neutrophils. Though similar in effect to TNF-α, probably by activating similar signaling cascades and transcription factors, IL-1 does not induce apoptosis, and even at high concentrations does not cause the physiologic derangements of septic shock.[39,109]

Mononuclear cells produce the natural inhibitor of IL-1, IL-1ra. This IL-1 structural homologue is an inactive competitive inhibitor and may function as an endogenous regulator of IL-1. As with TNF-α, attempts to inhibit IL-1 have not been of clinical benefit in human trials of sepsis.[39]

Chemokines. This is a large family of cytokines that primarily govern leukocyte chemotaxis, hence the name[114–118] (Table 6.6). Those bound on the endothelial surface induce leukocyte integrins to express a high-affinity state for their ligands, which is critical for tight leukocyte adherence and subsequent migration into the extravascular space. However, they are also constitutively produced and assist in orchestrating the migration of immune cells into lymphoid organs. Unlike other chemoattractants, members of this family possess a degree of specificity, influencing the recruitment of discrete subsets of leukocytes. They mediate their effects both directly and indirectly through the induction of other mediators such as histamine and ROS. Though some chemokines, in particular those regulating cell traffic through tissues, are constitutively produced (MIP-3β and RANTES), most necessitate cellular stimulation for synthesis and release, in particular, those involved in inflammatory reactions. They are typically produced by macrophages, leukocytes, endothelial cells, fibroblasts, and many other cell types stimulated by LPS, phagocytosis, and inflammatory cytokines such as IL-1, TNF-α, IL-6, and IFN-γ.[39]

Chemokines can be classified into four families based on the number and location of N-terminal cysteine residues. The two major families are the CC chemokines, in which the cysteine residues are adjacent, and the CXC chemokines, in which one amino acid is interposed between these cysteine residues. This amino acid sequence appears to account for the disparate influence, either promotion or inhibition, on neutrophil chemotaxis. The three amino acids that immediately precede the first cysteine are critical in defining receptor binding and neutrophil activation.[119,120] This area has been designated the ELR motif. The other two chemokine families are represented by lymphotactin (C chemokine) and fractalkine (CX3C chemokine).[39]

Chemokine receptors are seven-transmembrane receptors that signal by G proteins and the formation of the second messengers, IP_3 and DAG (Fig. 6.4). Currently six CXC chemokine receptors, 11 CC receptors, and one receptor each for the last two subfamilies have been identified and defined. The pattern of cellular expression of the receptors determines the specificity of the cellular response to binding.[4,120]

CXC chemokines primarily govern the chemoattraction and activation of neutrophils, and to a lesser degree lymphocytes, in particular T cells. At least 12 different chemokines have been identified. They are clustered on chromosome 4 and demonstrate 20% to 50% homology at the amino acid level. IL-8 is the prototypical CXC chemokine.[96] It is produced by an array of immune and nonimmune cells including monocytes, alveolar macrophages, neutrophils, keratinocytes, mesangial cells, epithelial cells, fibroblasts, and endothelial cells. TNF-α and IL-1 are key molecules for inducing IL-8. It is chemotactic for all granulocytes and influences nearly every aspect of neutrophil function. It stimulates neutrophil degranulation, phagocytosis, transendothelial migration, and shedding of L-selectin, upregulation of β_2 integrins, and augments superoxide production. It is also a potent angiogenic factor. It binds to both CXCR1 and CXCR2, receptors that also engage the chemokines GCP-2, GRO-α, and ENA-78. ENA-78 is a potent neutrophil chemotaxin produced by the endothelium in response to TNF-α or IL-1, neutrophils, or monocytes. Studies have demonstrated that ELR-containing CXC chemokines are angiogenic, whereas those lacking this motif are angiostatic.[39,93,119–121]

The interferon-influenced chemokines IP-10 and Mig do not target neutrophils, and the ELR motif is absent. They induce IFN-γ production and may play a more prominent role in mediating the inflammatory response to viral infections and autoimmune disorders. Mig is chemotactic for tumor-infiltrating lymphocytes, activated T cells, and monocytes and promotes CTL activity. IP-10 is chemotactic for monocytes, T cells, and NK cells and augments T-cell adhesion. Both chemokines bind the CXCR3 receptor found on IL-2–activated T cells. IFN-γ attenuates the expression of both IL-8 and ENA-78, and hence may serve as an important mechanism to the control and regulate inflammation.[39,93] Stromal cell–derived factor-1 (SDF-1) is the only known ligand for the CXCR4 receptor and in the presence of IL-7 stimulates proliferation of pre–B-cell clones and growth of bone marrow B progenitor cells. The receptor has gained much interest since it was identified as a coreceptor for human immunodeficiency virus type 1 (HIV-1). Platelet factor 4 and neutrophil-activating protein-2 are CXC chemokines of platelet origin. PL-4 has angiostatic properties and inhibits the growth of various cancer cell lines in a manner that appears to be related to its angiostatic properties. It binds heparin with high affinity to stimulate coagulation.[39]

The CC chemokines recruit monocytes, granulocytes, T cells, NK cells, and dendritic cells. RANTES is produced by stimulated T cells, platelets, and endothelial cells and is constitutively produced in resting T cells, which implies a homeostatic function. MIP-1α and MIP-1β are produced by activated T cells and are chemotactic for neutrophils, monocytes, eosinophils, basophils, and T lymphocytes. They are also mitogenic for hematopoietic progenitor cells and upregulate TNF-α, IL-1, and IL-6. The MCP family of chemokines influences the recruitment of monocytes and T cells. Their influence upon the function of these target cells is dictated by the cell's specific profile of receptor expression. MCP-1 is produced by nonlymphocytic cells (endothelial cells, epithelial cells, fibroblasts, smooth muscle cells, macrophages, and mast cells). Binding to CCR1 enhances chemotaxis, whereas activation of CCR2 increases the release of intracellular substances such as histamine and leukotrienes from basophils.[39]

Lymphotactin is the only member of the C chemokine family and is produced by $CD8^+$ lymphocytes, thymocytes, and NK cells and, to a lesser degree, by DCs and activated mast cells. It selectively recruits lymphoid cells.[39]

Fractalkine is the sole CX3C chemokine and is produced by endothelium. In its membrane-bound form it may act as a solid-phase adhesion molecule, but upon cleavage serves as a soluble chemoattractant for lymphoid cells and monocytes.[39]

Interleukin-12 (Natural Killer Cell Stimulatory Factor, Cytotoxic Lymphocyte Maturation Factor). IL-12 is integral in the innate immune response (Table 6.6). It is produced early during innate immune reactions against intracellular microbes and stimulates subsequent adaptive responses that confer further host protection against these pathogens; hence, it is an important link between innate and adaptive immune responses. IL-12 is critical for initiating a sequence of responses involving macrophages, NK cells, and T lymphocytes that results in the eradication of intracellular microbes. It is primarily derived from activated mononuclear phagocytes and dendritic cells, and most importantly stimulates IFN-γ from T cells and NK cells. There are two pathways leading to IL-12 production: a T-cell-dependent and a T-cell–independent pathway. During innate immunity, LPS, infection by intracellular bacteria, and viral infections may induce IL-12 production. In addition, interactions between CD40 ligand and CD40 on activated lymphocytes and antigen-presenting cells, respectively, induce the release of APC IL-12.[122,123] Thus, IL-12 is produced during the induction of and the effector phases of cell-mediated immune response when APCs present antigens to T cells.[4,39]

The IL-12 receptor is a heterodimer composed of β_1 and β_2 subunits, the latter of which is involved in signaling, although both are required for engaging ligand. The receptor signals through the Janus kinase (JAK)/signal transduction and activator of transcription (STAT) pathway (Fig. 6.7).[4] This signal transduction pathway is employed by numerous cytokines including IL-6, IL-12, IL-2, IL-7, IL-9, IL-4, and IL-10. A characteristic of this cytokine is the generation of a positive amplification loop, which heightens the inflammatory response. Expression of the IL-12 receptor is induced by IFN-γ. Activated NK cells and T_H1 cells produce IFN-γ that potentiates macrophage IL-12 production. IL-12 stimulates further production of IFN-γ by NK cells and T lymphocytes, which continues to fuel the reaction in a positive feedback mechanism. Ultimately, IFNγ activates macrophages to kill and degrade phagocytosed microbes. IL-12 potentiates bacterial LPS-induced macrophage TNF-α production. IL-12 antagonists reduce mortality in experimental models of LPS-induced septic shock; however, there is no evidence of their efficacy in human clinical trials.[4]

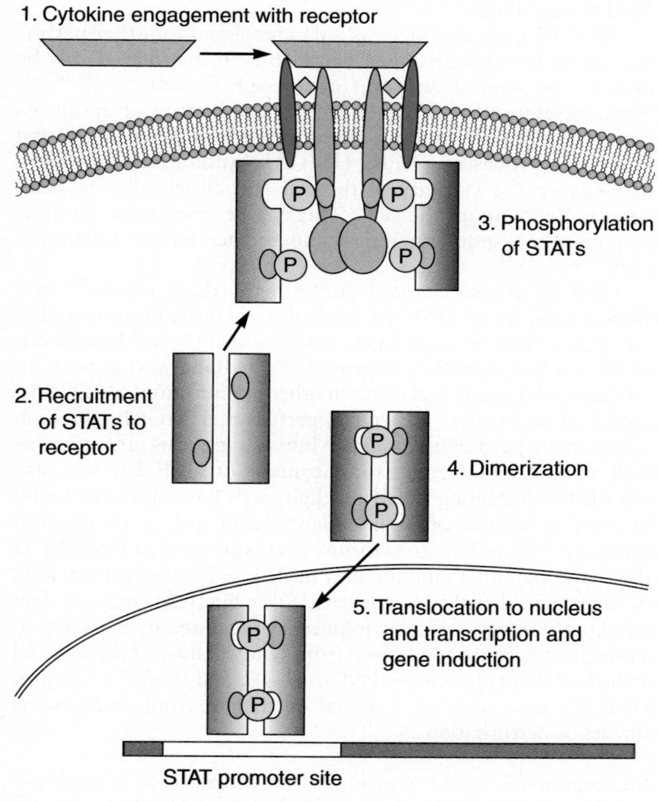

FIGURE 6.7. JAK/STAT signaling pathway. JAK (Janus kinase) components are associated in an inactive form with the cytoplasmic portion of cytokine receptors. Cytokine binding leads to receptor aggregation. Adjacent JAK proteins become activated and phosphorylate each other and tyrosine residues. Through the Src homology domain, STAT (signal transduction and activator of transcription) proteins bind phosphotyrosine residues on the cytoplasmic portion of cytokine receptors. Bound STAT proteins are phosphorylated by bound JAK proteins and subsequently dissociate. Phosphorylated STAT proteins dimerize and then move to the nucleus, where they induce transcription by binding to STAT-binding regions within the promoter. (Redrawn from Abbas AK, Lichtman AH. *Cellular and Molecular Immunology.* Philadelphia: Saunders; 2003.)

$CD4^+$ helper T lymphocytes, under the influence of IL-12, differentiate into T_H1 cells, which subsequently activate phagocytes in cell-mediated immunity. It enhances the cytolytic functions of activated NK cells and $CD8^+$ CTLs, and suppresses T_H2 cell differentiation and effector activity. The inhibition of T_H2 and IL-4 activity confers antiallergic properties to IL-12. IL-12 knockout mice demonstrate diminished IFN-γ production and defective T_H1 cell development and cell-mediated immunity against intracellular organisms.[4,39]

Interleukin-6. IL-6 regulates the acute-phase response to inflammation, characterized by altered thermoregulation (i.e., fever), perturbation in nitrogen balance (i.e., cachexia and catabolism), and the generation of the acute-phase reactants of innate immunity by the liver (Tables 6.6 and 6.7).[93,124] It functions in both innate and adaptive immunity to enable the host to recover. Despite in vitro data demonstrating that a variety of cells can produce IL-6, the most prominent in vivo sources of IL-6 are monocytes and macrophages stimulated with LPS or IL-1 or TNF-α–stimulated fibroblasts and endothelial cells.[125] Steroids inhibit the induction of IL-6. The receptor for IL-6 consists of cytokine-binding protein and a signal-transducing subunit, which belong to the type I cytokine receptor family. It signals through the JAK/STAT pathway (Fig. 6.7).[4]

In conjunction with IL-1 and TNF-α, IL-6 regulates the systemic manifestations of the acute-phase response.[124] It potentiates the immune response by inducing B-cell differentiation and activating T cells. It interacts with TNF-α to enhance T-cell proliferation and promotes neutrophil activation and accumulation. In adaptive immunity, IL-6 stimulates the growth of B

TABLE 6.7

ACUTE-PHASE PROTEINS

■ ACUTE-PHASE PROTEIN	■ FUNCTION
INCREASE	
C-reactive protein	Opsonin
Serum amyloid A	Apolipoprotein
α_1-Acid glycoprotein	Platelet inhibitor
Fibrinogen	Coagulation, tissue repair
α_2-Macroglobulin	Antiprotease
α_1-Protease inhibitor	Antiprotease
α_1-Antichymotrypsin	Antiprotease
Haptoglobulin	Antioxidant
Hemopexin	Antioxidant
Ceruloplasmin	Antioxidant
C3	Complement
Factor b	Complement
C1 inhibitor	Complement
C4b-binding protein	Complement
Mannose-binding lectin	Complement
DECREASE	
Albumin	Transport
Prealbumin	Transport
Transferrin	Transport

lymphocytes that have differentiated into antibody-producing plasma cells. IL-6 antagonizes LPS-induced TNF-α production and TNF-α–induced IL-1 production.[126,127]

High Mobility Group Box 1 Protein

HMGB1 was initially identified as an architectural chromatin-binding factor that bends DNA and directs protein assembly on specific DNA targets. It is abundant, ubiquitous, and evolutionarily conserved as evident by the 99% amino acid homology between rat and human proteins.[53] Thirty years after its original discovery, Tracey et al. demonstrated that HMGB1 acts as a late mediator of mortality in murine endotoxemia and sepsis. HMGB1 appeared 8 hours poststimulation and plateaued at 16 to 32 hours, very distinct from the acute rise and fall of early mediators (TNF-α, IL-1β) of severe sepsis and septic shock.[53] Recent studies show that systemic concentrations are elevated in those patients who die of sepsis.[128]

HMGB1 is the prototypical DAMP. When cells die by necrosis (i.e., nonprogrammed cell death), HMGB1 is released into the extracellular medium; in contrast, apoptotic cells modify their chromatin so that HMGB1 irreversibly binds, and thus is not released.[129,130] However, HMGB1 may also be released by activated macrophages and NK cells via an active process that necessitates shuttling the protein from nucleus to cytoplasm; this event does not require further synthesis.[129–131] Acetylation of HMGB1 appears essential for release; however, acetylation of histones, as occurs during apoptosis, strengthens its interaction with chromatin and inhibits release.[129,130] Interestingly, though apoptotic cells do not release HMGB1, macrophages engulfing apoptotic cells do. Recent studies have shown that nucleocytoplasmic shuttling of HMGB1 involves serine phosphorylation by CaMK IV that enables it to be translocated to the cytoplasm by 14-3-3 and CRM1 chaperones.[132,133] Subsequent release of cytoplasmic HMGB1 appears to involve active secretion through a secretory lysosomal pathway.[129,131]

HMGB1 has many of the intercellular signaling activities characteristic of cytokines and therefore is often classified as a proinflammatory cytokine and potent regulator of the inflammatory response. In light of the fact that it is released by macrophages responding to bacterial challenge or by injured cells, it may mediate inflammation consequent to sepsis or trauma. After release, signaling is thought to occur by binding to RAGE with subsequent activation of p21ras, MEK, the MAPKs, and NF-κB.[104,134] This receptor is expressed on mononuclear phagocytes, vascular smooth muscle cells, and neurons. Blocking antibodies to RAGE fail to completely prevent cellular activation, suggesting the presence of an alternate receptor. Recent studies suggest that both TLR2 and TLR4 may mediate HMGB1-induced activation of NF-κB in macrophages and neutrophils. This observation is very important as it demonstrates that a receptor classically considered specific for microbial danger signals may interact with an endogenous molecule.[53,104,134]

HMGB1–RAGE interactions induce numerous proinflammatory events. Endothelial cells increase the expression of adhesion molecules and also secrete TNF-α and IL-8.[135] In neutrophils, HMGB1 activates MAPKs and enhances the expression of proinflammatory cytokines in an NF-κB–dependent manner. In addition, it is chemotactic for neutrophils, monocytes, macrophages, and dendritic cells.[134] Intratracheal administration of HMGB1 to LPS-resistant mice stimulated lung neutrophil accumulation and the local production of proinflammatory cytokines.[134] HMGB1 has potent immunostimulatory actions and promotes the maturation of both myeloid and plasmacytoid dendritic cells. Systemic levels are markedly elevated in patients who die of sepsis, and animal studies suggest this association is causal.[128] Recombinant HMGB1 mimics the lethality of high-dose LPS and induces the release of TNF-α by macrophages. However, intravenous administration of HMGB1 does not cause shock like TNF-α. In a series of elegant studies, anti-HMGB1 antibodies conferred a dose-dependent protection in animal models of endotoxemia, even when the first dose of anti-HMGB1 antibodies was delayed for 2 hours.[54] This occurred without changes in TNF-α, IL-1β, or MIP-2 concentrations. Even more striking are the in vivo cecal ligation and perforation (CLP) models, in which anti-HMGB1 administration up to 24 hours after CLP significantly increased survival, 72% versus 28%.[54] This wider therapeutic window may enable the development of inhibitors of HMGB1 for treatment of sepsis.[134,136–138] More recent data call into question whether HMGB1 can promote directly the secretion of proinflammatory cytokines (TNF-α, IL-1α/β, IL-6, IL-8) and chemokines (MIP-1α/β) as initially reported. A direct proinflammatory activity of HMGB1 has not been reproduced consistently, raising some concern that this might be based on the formation of specific complexes with other molecules such as LPS. Recent studies show that highly purified recombinant HMGB1 has very weak direct proinflammatory activity.[139]

These observations have stimulated the search for other inhibitors of HMGB1. Ethyl pyruvate, a nontoxic food additive, dose dependently inhibits HMGB1 release and confers significant protection against the lethality of sepsis, even when the first dose is administered 24 hours after the onset of sepsis. In addition, it inhibits the translocation of NF-κB and p38 MAPK signaling.[134,136,140,141]

HMGB1 may also serve as a danger signal for other perturbations in homeostasis, as it can also be released passively by necrotic or injured cells but not apoptotic cells.[130,138,142,143] Hypoacetylation of chromatin on the induction of apoptosis enhances HMGB1 binding, thereby preventing release during apoptotic processes. Thus, HMGB1 binding to chromatin depends on the viability of the cell and clearly distinguishes necrotic from apoptotic cells. This enables the innate immune response to respond to injury and further induce inflammation.[130,138,142,143]

HMGB1 is also elevated during hemorrhage shock.[144] In a clinical case, serum HMGB1 levels increased significantly within 24 hours of hemorrhagic shock and returned toward basal levels as the clinical condition improved.[145] HMGB1 also appears to mediate cell damage and death in other noninfectious insults. In a model of warm liver ischemia/reperfusion, HMGB1 inhibition attenuates hepatocellular injury.[32] Interestingly, this protection, as well as reduced systemic concentrations of HMGB1, was also afforded by inhibiting CaMK.[32] High levels have also been found in other conditions of sterile inflammation such as rheumatoid arthritis.[146–148] In human arthritis, overexpression of HMGB1 at the site of joint inflammation may be detected in the synovial fluid of rheumatoid arthritis patients.[147,148] HMGB1 may in fact amplify the effect of local cytokines, as suggested by its ability to stimulate macrophages derived from synovial fluid of rheumatoid arthritis patients to release TNF-α, IL-1β, and IL-6.[146,149] Hence, HMGB1 may serve as a signal of danger from endogenous threats or perturbations.

Interleukin-15. IL-15 is produced by various cells in response to LPS and other stimuli, though the principal cellular source is mononuclear phagocytes (Table 6.6). It is structurally homologous to IL-2 as is its receptor and the IL-2R. IL-15 stimulates the proliferation of NK cells similarly to the manner by which IL-2 functions later in the adaptive immune response. It also acts as a T-cell growth and survival factor, especially for long-lived memory CD8$^+$ T cells.[4]

Interleukin-18. IL-18 is structurally homologous to IL-1 and utilizes a similar IRAK signaling pathway (Table 6.6). Macrophages responding to microbial challenge or exposure to LPS are the principal source. Its primary function is to stimulate the production of IFN-γ by NK cells and T cells, and in synergizing with IL-12, augments cell-mediated immunity. Knockout mice lacking IL-18 are deficient in IFN-γ production, and concomitant IL-12 deficiency eliminates all IFN-γ production and any T_H1 response.[4]

Interferons (Type I). Type I interferons possess potent antiviral and antitumor properties (Table 6.6). It is from this ability to interfere with viral infection that the name is derived. They are subcategorized into α and β interferons. Mononuclear phagocytes are the major source of interferon-α, whereas many cell types produce interferon-β. The most potent stimulus inducing the synthesis and release of either is viral infection, particularly double-stranded RNA produced during viral replication. Other inducers include IL-1, TNF-α, LPS, and antigen-activated T cells. Both groups bind to the same cell surface receptor and induce similar responses by signaling through the JAK/STAT pathway (Fig. 6.7).

These cytokines provide the first line of defense against viral infection and promote cell-mediated immunity against intracellular pathogen. They are secreted from virally infected cells to protect neighboring uninfected ones by inducing the synthesis of a number of enzymes that interfere with viral RNA or DNA transcription and viral replication. Through enhanced expression of class I MHC molecules, the type I interferons facilitate recognition of class I–associated viral antigens on infected cells by CTLs and increase the efficiency of CTL-mediated killing. Type I interferon stimulates the development of T_H1 cells by promoting these cells to express IL-12 receptor. They can also stimulate B-cell development, proliferation, and immunoglobulin heavy chain switching from IgM to IgG.[150–152] Knockout mice lacking the receptor for these cytokines are susceptible to viral infections. Interferons are currently in clinical use for hepatitis B and C infection, multiple sclerosis, chronic myelocytic leukemia (CML), and Kaposi sarcoma.[150–152]

Interleukin-10 (Cytokine Synthesis Inhibiting Factor). IL-10 inhibits activated macrophages and antigen-presenting cells and functions in a counterregulatory mechanism to suppress innate immune reactions (Table 6.6). It is produced mainly by macrophages, and hence functions by negative feedback. T lymphocytes, particularly the T_H2 subset, B cells, and some other nonlymphoid cells produce IL-10, in response to a variety of stimuli including LPS, TNF-α, IL-2, IL-4, and IL-13.

IL-10 binds to a type II (interferon) receptor. Though the manner by which it effects curtailment of the inflammatory response is unknown, its presence inhibits NK-κB activation and the generation of inflammatory mediators perhaps by inhibiting, in some manner, the activation of signal transduction cascades and gene activation in proinflammatory pathways.[4,153]

IL-10 terminates many of the functions of activated macrophages and participates in reestablishing homeostasis as the infection resolves. It downregulates proinflammatory cytokine (TNF-α, IL-1, IL-6, and IL-8) production, suppresses IL-12 production, and inhibits IFN-γ production and the innate and cell-mediated immune responses.[4,56,93] It represses the expression of costimulators and class II MHC molecules on antigen-presenting cells, thereby terminating T-cell activation and inhibiting cell-mediated immunity.[4] In neutrophils it inhibits cytokine release, superoxide generation, migration, and even survival.[154] In combination with IL-4, it inhibits IFN-γ release and IL-12 production to limit differentiation and function of T_H1 cells, favoring a T_H2 profile.[56]

IL-10 knockout mice develop inflammatory bowel disease, which is hypothesized to result from unregulated macrophage reaction to enteric microbes.[155] In observational studies of ARDS or MODS, serum IL-10 levels were often elevated, and those patients with the highest systemic concentrations died.[153] It is unclear whether this is actually a pathologic response or merely a marker of disease severity. Contemporary belief is that IL-10 is not a mediator of immunosuppression, but rather, important for immunoregulation.

Late Cytokines/Adaptive Immunity

Interleukin-2 (T-cell Growth Factor). Interleukin-2 stimulates the growth and proliferation of T lymphocytes and is responsible for T-cell clonal expansion after antigen recognition (Table 6.6).[156] IL-2 is produced by $CD4^+$, and to a lesser extent $CD8^+$ T cells. The receptor is heterotrimeric, consisting of three noncovalently associated proteins, α, β, and γ. The α and β chains are involved in cytokine binding, and the β and γ chains mediate signal transduction.[4] Antigen recognition enhances the expression of functional IL-2 receptors, which confers a degree of specificity, as those T cells recognizing antigen are preferentially induced to proliferate in response to IL-2. Though the α chain appears on T-cell activation and binds IL-2, signal generation necessitates the β and γ chains. Cells expressing the complete α, β, and γ complex bind IL-2 with higher affinity (kD of 10^{-11} M), and growth stimulation of such cells occurs at a low IL-2 concentration.[4] Upon antigen receptor–mediated T-cell activation, IL-2Rα is rapidly upregulated, which reduces the concentration of IL-2 needed to stimulate growth. Therefore, antigen-stimulated T cells are more responsive to IL-2 than naïve T cells. This receptor signals through numerous signal transduction pathways including the JAK/STAT and MAPK pathways (Figs. 6.4 and 6.7).

IL-2 functions in an autocrine and paracrine fashion to induce the proliferation of the antigen-specific cells. After exposure to IL-1, there is a rise in cyclins and activation of cyclin-dependent kinases that stimulate the progression from the G1 to the S phase of the cell cycle. A reduction in p27, an inhibitor of cyclin–kinase complexes, facilitates this progression, and the induction of Bcl-2, an antiapoptotic protein, facilitates survival. It also stimulates the production of other cytokines such as IFN-γ and IL-4.[4]

IL-2 promotes the proliferation and differentiation of many immune cells. NK cells are stimulated to grow and transform into lymphocyte-activated killer (LAK) cells. In combination with IFN-γ and IL-12, IL-2 can trigger a positive feedback cycle of NK activation. IL-2 stimulates B-cell growth and antibody synthesis. Repeated activation of $CD4^+$ T cells in the presence of IL-2 sensitizes these cells to apoptosis by Fas-Fas-ligand. IL-2 may also stimulate the development of regulatory T cells, and IL-2 knockout mice develop autoimmunity. Knockout mice lacking the γ chain develop X-linked severe combined immunodeficiency syndrome. This is probably due to an inability of immature T cells to respond to IL-7. IL-2 has been used in the management of cancer, in particular renal cell carcinoma.[157]

Interleukin-4. IL-4 is the major stimulus for the production of IgE antibodies and for the development of T_H2 cells from naïve $CD4^+$ T cells (Table 6.6). The principal cellular sources are $CD4^+$ T cells, mast cells, and basophils. The IL-4 receptor belongs to the type I cytokine receptor family and signals through the JAK/STAT pathway[158] (Fig. 6.7). IgE is integral in orchestrating the defense against parasitic infections. It stimulates IgE production and mast cell/eosinophil-mediated reactions, and induces B-cell Ig heavy chain class switching to the IgE isotype. However, IL-4 also serves a counterregulatory role by inducing T_H2 cell differentiation and growth. IL-4 antagonizes the macrophage-activating effects of IFN-γ and thus inhibits cell-mediated immunity.

Interleukin-5. IL-5 is produced by T_H2 cells and activated mast cells and activates eosinophils (Table 6.6). It signals through the type I cytokine receptor and the JAK/STAT pathway (Fig. 6.7). IL-5 is an inducer of eosinophil growth, differentiation, and activation, and also participates in the eradication of helminthic infection. IL-5 also stimulates the proliferation of B cells and the production of IgA antibodies.[4]

Interleukin-13. IL-13 is produced by T_H2 cells and some epithelial cells and is structurally homologous and functionally similar to IL-4 (Table 6.6). The receptor is found mainly on nonlymphoid cells and can be activated by either IL-13 or IL-4. IL-13 downregulates the expression of Fcγ on monocytes and macrophages, thereby decreasing antibody-dependent cellular cytotoxicity. It increases 15 S-HETE and lipoxin A_4, both of which antagonize proinflammatory leukotrienes. However, they can increase the expression of MHC class II and costimulatory molecules on monocytes and thereby serve an immunostimulatory function. The major action is to inhibit the activation of macrophages and to antagonize IFN-γ.[159]

Interferon-γ. IFN-γ is produced by NK cells, T_H1 cells, and $CD8^+$ cells, and as the principal stimulus for macrophage activation, provides necessary functions during both innate and adaptive immune responses (Table 6.6). It modulates cellular differentiation, cytotoxicity, cytokine production, cellular adhesion, and oxidative metabolism. During innate immunity, NK cells secrete it upon exposure to pathogen or IL-12. $CD8^+$ T cells and the T_H1 subset of $CD4^+$ T cells produce it in response to MHC-bound peptide antigen with a costimulatory signal. The IFN-γ receptor is composed of two homologous proteins belonging to the type II cytokine receptor family and functions through the JAK/STAT pathway (Fig. 6.7).[4]

The antiviral and antitumor properties of IFN-γ are redundant with those of type I interferons. In concert with TNF-α and IL-12, it forms one arm of a positive feedback loop fueling the activation of both NK cells and macrophages. Stimulated macrophages activate NK cells by releasing TNF-α and IL-12. These NK cells produce IFN-γ, which further stimulates macrophages to secrete more TNF-α and IL-12.[160,161]

IFN-γ induces the genes encoding the enzymatic machinery required for generating reactive oxygen species generation and provides the principal stimulus for macrophages to kill phagocytosed microbes. It regulates the expression of MHC class I and class II molecules and costimulators of APC, and induces the transcription of enzymes regulating antigen processing.[160,161]

IFN-γ synergizes with TNF-α to activate the endothelium and upregulate adhesion molecule expression; in doing so it facilitates lymphocyte recruitment and leukocyte recruitment. Interferon promotes the differentiation of naïve $CD4^+$ cells into T_H1 cells and inhibits the proliferation of T_H2 cells, in part by inducing IL-12, the major T_H1-inducing cytokine, from activated mononuclear phagocytes. It promotes B-cell switching to certain IgG subclasses, notably IgG2a, and inhibits the switching to IL-4–dependent isotypes such as IgE and IgG1. These IgG subclasses bind the Fcγ receptors on phagocytes and activate complement, thereby promoting phagocytosis of opsonized microbes. It activates PMNs and stimulates the cytolytic activity of NK cells. The net effect is to promote macrophage-rich inflammatory reactions while inhibiting IgE-dependent eosinophil-rich reactions. IL-10, by suppressing macrophage release of TNF-α and IL-12, negatively regulates IFN-γ production.

IFN-γ also demonstrates counterregulatory properties. It selectively inhibits LPS-induced expression of CXC chemokines. It upregulates macrophage production of IP-10, MIG, and ELR-negative chemokines that inhibit neutrophil chemotaxis and activation and decreases macrophage release of ELR-positive CXC chemokines (e.g., IL-8), which are chemotactic for neutrophils.[4]

Transforming Growth Factor-β. TGF-β is a homodimer synthesized and secreted by activated T cells, macrophages, and many other cells (Table 6.6). It is primarily immunosuppressive and inhibits the proliferation and activation of lymphocytes and other leukocytes. It promotes wound healing by increasing extracellular matrix protein synthesis and stimulating mononuclear cell and fibroblast influx.[162–164] Though the family consists of three closely related isoforms, most cells utilize TGF-β. Its effects are mediated through two high-affinity TGF receptors (type I and II) that signal through a serine/threonine kinase domain that phosphorylates transcription factors called SMADS.[4]

TGF-β inhibits the proliferation and differentiation of T cells and the activation of macrophages. It favors differentiation of $CD4^+$ cells to the T_H2 subset and inhibits MHC class II surface expression. By suppressing the expression of MHC class II antigen, it abrogates the adaptive immune response. Macrophages demonstrate diminished ROS production and TNF-α and NO release. It directly counteracts the influence of proinflammatory cytokines on PMNs and endothelial cells, and in combination with IL-4, IL-13, and IL-10 can antagonize the production or effects of these proinflammatory mediators. Knockout mice deficient in TGF-β develop uncontrolled inflammatory lesions.[4,39]

Cytokines That Stimulate Hematopoiesis. Cytokines are necessary for normal hematopoiesis. Several of the cytokines stimulated during both innate and adaptive immune responses are mitogenic for and induce differentiation of bone marrow progenitor cells.

CSFs are cytokines made by activated T cells, macrophages, endothelial cells, and bone marrow stromal cells that stimulate increased production of inflammatory leukocytes by bone marrow progenitors. Receptors for GM-CSF and G-CSF are of the class I family of cytokine receptors. GM-CSF is expressed by T and B cells, macrophages, mast cells, fibroblasts, and endothelium in response to stimuli such as IL-1, IL-2, LPS, and TNF-α. It stimulates neutrophils, monocytes, macrophages, and DCs and is a powerful inducer of hematopoiesis. It enhances cytokine release, degranulation, and phagocytosis of opsonized particles in neutrophils. In monocytes and macrophages it enhances cytotoxicity and cytokine release. It promotes the activity of APCs and the maturation of bone marrow cells into dendritic cells and monocytes.[165] G-CSF is produced by macrophages, endothelial cells, fibroblasts, and bone marrow stromal cells. It functions as an endocrine hormone to mobilize neutrophils and induces subsequent leukocyte proliferation and maturation. In 1991, the FDA approved G-CSF for use in patients with neutropenia.[166,167]

Stem cell factor or c-Kit ligand is synthesized by marrow stromal cells and binds to a cell surface tyrosine kinase receptor on pluripotent stem cells that is the protein product of the cellular proto-oncogene c-kit. Its effects appear permissive, as it is corequisite for stem cell responsiveness to other colony-stimulating factors, yet in isolation does not stimulate colony formation. It may also play a role in sustaining the viability and proliferative capacity of immature T cells in the thymus.[4]

IL-3 is a product of $CD4^+$ T cells that promotes the differentiation of immature marrow progenitors into all known mature cell types. It also promotes the growth and development of mast cells. Surprisingly, despite these important functions, murine knockouts do not manifest noticeable impairment of hematopoiesis.[4]

IL-7 is secreted by bone marrow stromal cells and promotes the growth and survival of immature precursors committed to the B- and T-lymphocyte lineages. Knockout mice, deficient in IL-7 or its receptor, are lymphopenic with diminished populations of B and T cells.[4]

The Complement System

6 The complement system is integral to both innate and adaptive immunity. It has the capacity to independently eliminate organisms and to facilitate host defense by marking foreign particles for phagocytosis through opsonization. Many pathophysiologic inflammatory diseases, immune complex diseases, ischemia/reperfusion injury, and ARDS are considered consequences of aberrant function of this system.[168–171]

The system consists of three pathways composed of approximately 30 serum and cell surface proteins that interact with one another and with other molecules of the immune system in a highly coordinated fashion. These cascades involve the sequential proteolytic activation of zymogens to generate enzymes with proteolytic activity. This mechanism for activation amplifies the response because each individual enzyme activated can cleave numerous zymogens in the next step and generate multiple activated enzyme molecules. Ultimately, the products of complement activation adhere to microbial cell surfaces or to antibody-bound microbes and other antigens to directly or indirectly eliminate these pathogens. Temporal and spatial regulation to the focus of infection is ensured both by the transience of activation of these enzymes in the absence of microbes or antigens and by several circulating proteins that provide surveillance.[168,170]

The complement cascade is divided into three distinct pathways: the classical pathway (humoral immunity), which is activated by antibody bound to antigen; the alternative pathway (innate immunity), in which complement is activated by components of microbial cell surfaces; and the mannose/lectin pathway (innate immunity), which is activated by a plasma lectin that binds to mannose residues on microbes. Despite differences in which the cascade is activated, all three complement pathways ultimately result in the cleavage of C3 and share the same subsequent late cascade.[168,170]

The alternative pathway functions in the absence of antibody and is phylogenetically the oldest pathway (Fig. 6.8). Bacteria, viruses, fungi, and parasites all function as stimuli. Initial activation begins with the cleavage of C3 and the stable attachment of its product C3b to the microbial surface. Bound C3b binds factor B, which is subsequently cleaved by a plasma serine protease called factor D to generate Bb. The C3bBb complex is called the alternative pathway C3 convertase and functions to cleave more C3. In doing so the convertase serves as an amplification step in both the classical and alternative pathways. Properdin prolongs the half-life of C3 convertase by delaying the release of Bb from C3bBb. C3b is the recognition component of the alternate pathway and is responsible for the opsonization of bacteria. C3a in conjunction with C5a and C4a induces acute inflammation by activating mast cells and neutrophils. These inflammatory mediators play a significant role in increasing blood vessel permeability, vasodilatation, edema formation, neutrophil adhesion and activation, chemotaxis, and the release of toxic oxygen species and lysosomal enzymes from phagocytic cells. The binding of another C3b to this complex generates the alternative pathway C5 convertase, C3bBb3b.[4,168,170]

Activation of the alternative pathway is restricted to the cell surface of microbes, as mammalian cells possess several regulatory proteins to rapidly degrade any C3bBb. Excessive amplification is regulated by β1H globulin factor H and factor I. H accelerates the decay and delays the formation of C3bBb. It also acts as a cofactor for I to degrade C3 into iC3b, which is unable to bind B to generate C3 convertase. Decay acceleration factor (DAF) hinders C3 convertase assembly and mediates its dissociation in all three pathways. Also, the protein properdin, which stabilizes this alternative pathway C3 convertase, has a higher affinity for microbial than mammalian cell surfaces.[4,168,170]

The classical pathway is the primary mediator of adaptive humoral immunity and is initiated by binding of the complement protein C1 to IgG or IgM molecules engaged with antigen (Fig. 6.8). Other substances such as lipid A in endotoxin and mitochondrial membranes may activate this pathway independent of antigen–antibody complexes in vitro.[168,172]

C1 is a calcium-dependent trimeric protein consisting of C1q, which recognizes and binds the Fc region of the immunoglobulin, and C1r and C1s, which are proteases. C1q engages the Fc portion of the immunoglobulin μ and γ heavy chains. Each Fc region has a single C1q binding site, yet for activation, each C1q molecule must bind to two Ig heavy chains. Hence, multiple antibodies must be approximated for activation, which restricts activation to foci of immunoglobin engagement. IgM exists as a pentamer enabling it to bind to two C1q molecules, and hence it is more efficient at complement activation.[4,168,172]

Interaction between C1q and the immunoglobin Fc region induces a conformational change in C1q that activates C1r, which subsequently cleaves and activates C1s. C1s cleaves C4 to generate C4b and C4a. The C4a anaphylatoxin possesses properties similar to those described for C3a. C4b localizes to immune complexes on the cell surface. C2, after complexing with C4b, is cleaved by C1s, thereby generating the classical C3 convertase C4b2a complex, which has the ability to cleave C3. The C3b generated can bind Bb, producing more C3 convertase and amplifying the signal. The key early steps of the alternative and classical pathways are analogous: C3 and factor B of the alternative pathway are homologous to C4 and C2 in the classical pathway. C3b can also combine with the classical C3 convertase to generate C4b2a3b, the classical C5 convertase.[4]

Numerous regulatory mechanisms exist to restrict activation to sites of inflammation. Excessive classical C3 convertase activity is prevented by the rapid decay of C2a from the complex, which renders the complex unstable. C1 inhibitor

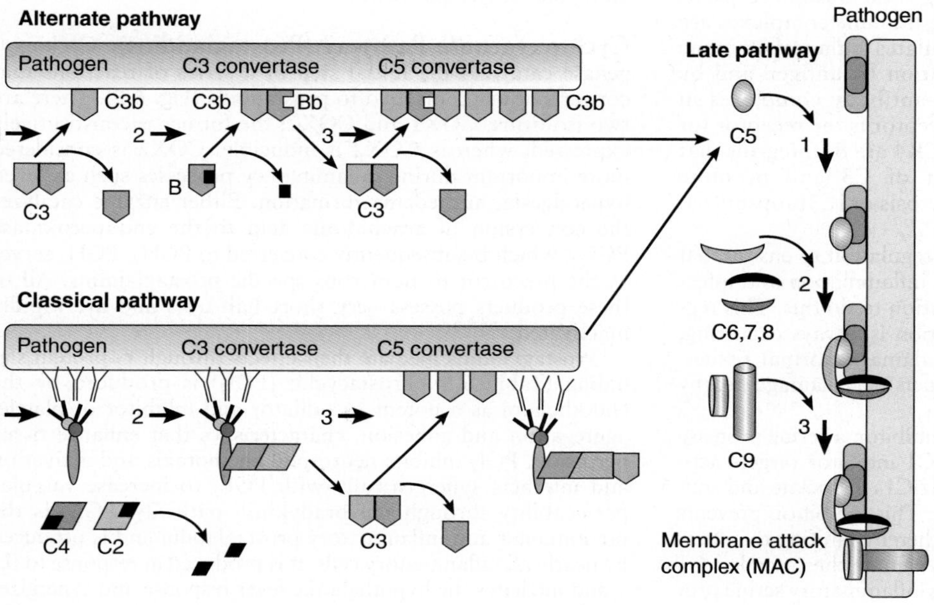

FIGURE 6.8. Complement pathways. **Alternate pathway:** *1.* C3 is cleaved to C3b. *2.* C3b binds and cleaves B to Bb to form C3 convertase (C3bBb). *3.* Another C3b binds C3 convertase to form C5 convertase (C3bBbC3b). **Classical pathway:** *1.* C1 binds immunoglobulin. *2.* C1 binds and cleaves C4 and C2 to C4b and C2a to form C3 convertase (C4b2a). *3.* C4b2a binds another C3b to generate C5 convertase (C4b2aC3b). **Late pathway:** *1.* C5 convertase cleaves C5 to form C5b, which integrates into the plasmalemma. *2.* C6–8 are recruited, forming the C5b–8 complex. *3.* C5b–8 recruits numerous C9 subunits, which form a pore in the pathogen cell wall. (Redrawn from Abbas AK, Lichtman AH. *Cellular and Molecular Immunology.* Philadelphia: Saunders; 2003.)

SCIENTIFIC PRINCIPLES

covalently binds C1s, reducing the half-life of activated C1 to only 13 seconds. C4-binding protein enhances spontaneous dissociation of C4b2a and also acts as a cofactor for C3b/C4b inactivator, which degrades C4b.[39]

The mannose-binding lectin (MBL) pathway is activated by the binding of microbial polysaccharides to circulating lectins; mannose-binding lectin serves as the recognition unit of the MBL pathway. This pathway recognizes polysaccharides with high mannose content and other oligosaccharides with characteristic linkages found exclusively on pathogens and not on normal host components. Binding is calcium dependent and results in the activation of mannose-binding lectin-associated serine proteases (MASP-1 and MASP-2). Activated MASP-2 cleaves and activates C4 and C2 in the same fashion as the classical complement pathway. Subsequent steps of complement activation of the MBL pathway mirror those of the classical complement pathway.[168,173,174]

The C5 convertases generated during either the classical or alternative pathway initiate a cascade of events that culminates in the formation of the cytocidal MAC. Specifically, C5 convertase cleaves C5, yielding C5a and C5b. C6 and C7 bind to generate the C5b67 complex. This hydrophobic moiety penetrates deeply into the lipid bilayer as a high-affinity receptor for C8. Binding of C8 forms the complex C5b–8 that recruits numerous C9 subunits, which polymerize to form pores in the plasma membrane. The pores structurally resemble the membrane pores formed by perforin, the cytolytic granule protein found in CTLs and NK cells. Their diameter may span 100 angstroms, which prevents the maintenance of vital ionic gradients and induces osmotic lysis and, ultimately, the death of target cells or pathogens. Patients with deficiencies in the terminal components of C5, C6, C7, and C8 are susceptible to meningococcal and gonococcal infections.[4,175] By contrast, recent studies suggest that aberrant induction of the complement system, specifically C5a, plays an integral role in inducing paralysis of the innate immunity and the development of ARDS and MODS.

The effects of complement are in part mediated through several complement receptors. Opsonization and phagocytosis are important mechanisms for pathogen destruction, and phagocytic cells express receptors for complement factor C3 components. Complement receptor type 1 (CR1), the C3b receptor for C3b and C4b, mediates engagement of and facilitates phagocytosis of complement-bound microbes and the clearance of immune complexes from the circulation. It is expressed on a variety of cells including RBCs, neutrophils, monocytes, eosinophils, and T and B cells. RBCs facilitate elimination by transporting these opsonized particles to the liver and spleen where the immune complexes are removed by phagocytes. CR2 stimulates humoral immune response by enhancing B-cell activation by antigen and by promoting the trapping of antigen–antibody complexes in germinal centers. In humans, this receptor is the receptor for Ebstein-Barr virus (EBV). CR3 and CR4 are β_2 integrins that bind the iC3b-processed fragment of C3 and promote macrophage and neutrophil phagocytosis of iC3b-opsonized antigen.[4,39]

This entire cascade is under strict regulation to ensure that any activation is restricted to sites of inflammation and infection. Several circulating proteins function to do this. This regulation is needed as low-level activation is always occurring, and if not quelled, would certainly damage normal tissues. Even when locally activated, byproducts may damage nearby cells and tissues.

C1r and C1s are inhibited by C1 inhibitor, a serine protease inhibitor that mimics C1r and C1s. C1 inhibitor targets activated C1qrs, and after attachment, C1r-C1s dissociate and activation of classical complement ceases. This inhibition prevents the accumulation of active C1r-C1s, thereby limiting the duration during which active C1r-C1s can initiate the cascade.[4] C1 inhibitor also inhibits other circulating inflammatory serine proteases including kallikrein and factor XII, both of which can activate the formation of bradykinin.[4] Hereditary angioneurotic edema is an inherited deficiency of C1 inhibitor and manifests as acute intermittent edema of the skin and mucosa causing abdominal pain, vomiting, diarrhea, and airway obstruction.

MCP, CR1, and DAF are regulatory proteins that bind to C3b and C4b deposited on cell surfaces and competitively inhibit the binding of other components of the C3 and C5 convertases, such as Bb and C2a, and thereby block further progression of the cascade. These proteins are only produced by mammalian cells. Deficiency of an enzyme required to form the linkages necessary to express DAF underlies paroxysmal nocturnal hemoglobinuria, a disease characterized by recurrent intravascular hemolysis due to unregulated complement activation on the surface of erythrocytes. Cell-associated C3b is proteolytically degraded by a plasma serine protease called factor I, which is active only in the presence of regulatory proteins such as MCP, factor H, C4BP, and CR1. MAC formation is inhibited by CD59, a membrane protein that incorporates itself into growing MACs and inhibits the incorporation of C9. It is not present in microbes. The function of these regulatory proteins may be overcome by increasing amounts of complement activation.[4]

Lipid Mediators

Eicosanoids. Eicosanoids are 20-carbon lipid inflammatory mediators derived from membrane arachidonic acid that are involved in numerous homeostatic processes and inflammation. These lipid mediators are not stored in tissues, but are synthesized de novo within seconds in response to a variety of stimuli, including mechanical trauma, or specific cytokines, growth factors, and other mediators (Fig. 6.9). Although most cells are capable of producing eicosanoids, neutrophils and macrophages are the predominant source during inflammation. They are rapidly degraded in the circulation, which limits their role primarily to that of autocrine and paracrine mediators of local inflammatory changes.[176–178]

The liberation of the precursor molecule, arachidonic acid, is the major rate-limiting step. The family of PLA_2, in particular type IV cytosolic PLA_2, is responsible for eicosanoid production; cells lacking type IV PLA_2 are devoid of eicosanoid synthesis.[179] Many PLA_2 are transcriptionally regulated by IL-1 and TNF-α, whereas others are regulated by the MAPK pathway and by calcium-dependent translocation to membranes. Once formed, arachidonic acid metabolism proceeds along one of two pathways.[176–178]

Cyclooxygenase Pathway (Prostaglandins). Cyclooxygenase catalyzes the initial step of a series of reactions that converts arachidonic acid to prostanoids (Fig. 6.9). There are two isoforms, COX1 and COX2; the former is constitutively expressed, whereas COX2 is inducible. COX2 is considered more important during inflammatory processes such as fever, hyperalgesia, and edema formation. Either enzyme catalyzes the conversion of arachidonic acid to the endoperoxidase PGG_2, which is subsequently converted to PGH_2. PGH_2 serves as the precursor to numerous specific prostaglandins. All of these products possess very short half-lives and are rapidly inactivated.[179,180]

Prostaglandins mediate their effects through G-protein signaling (Table 6.8). Prostacyclin (PGI_2) is produced by the endothelium as a potent vasodilator and inhibitor of platelet aggregation and adhesion, characteristics that enhance tissue perfusion. PGI_2 inhibits neutrophil chemotaxis and activation and interacts synergistically with PGE_2 to increase vascular permeability through the bradykinin pathway. PGE_2 is the predominant anti-inflammatory prostaglandin and is produced by nearly all inflammatory cells. It is produced in response to IL-1 and mediates the hypothalamic fever response and synergizes

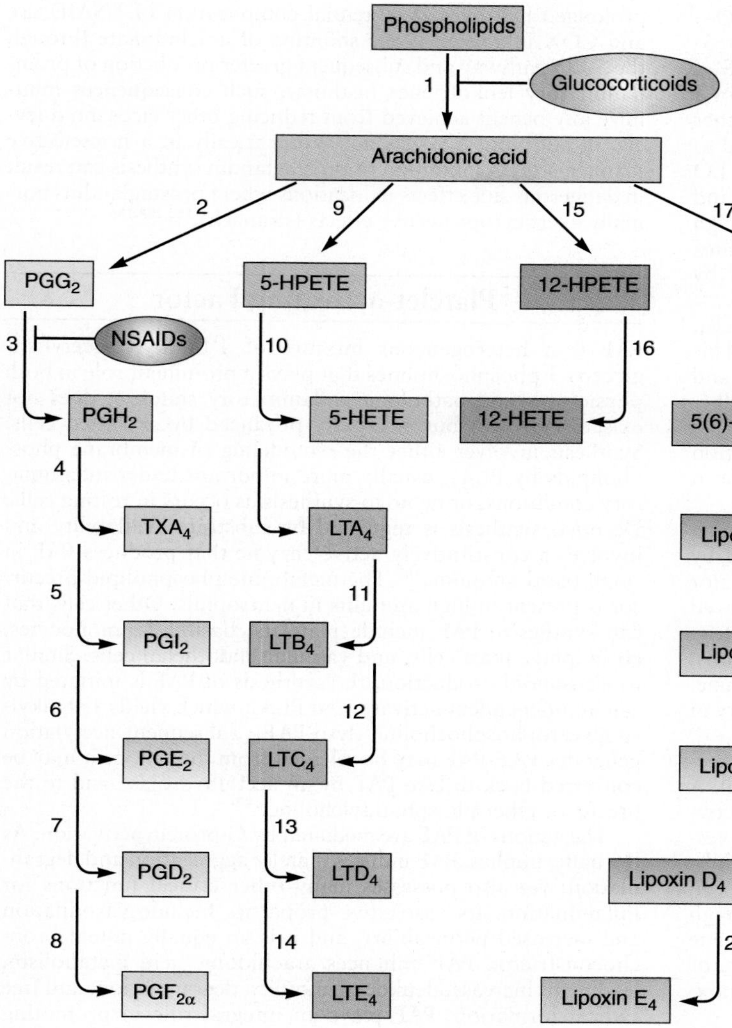

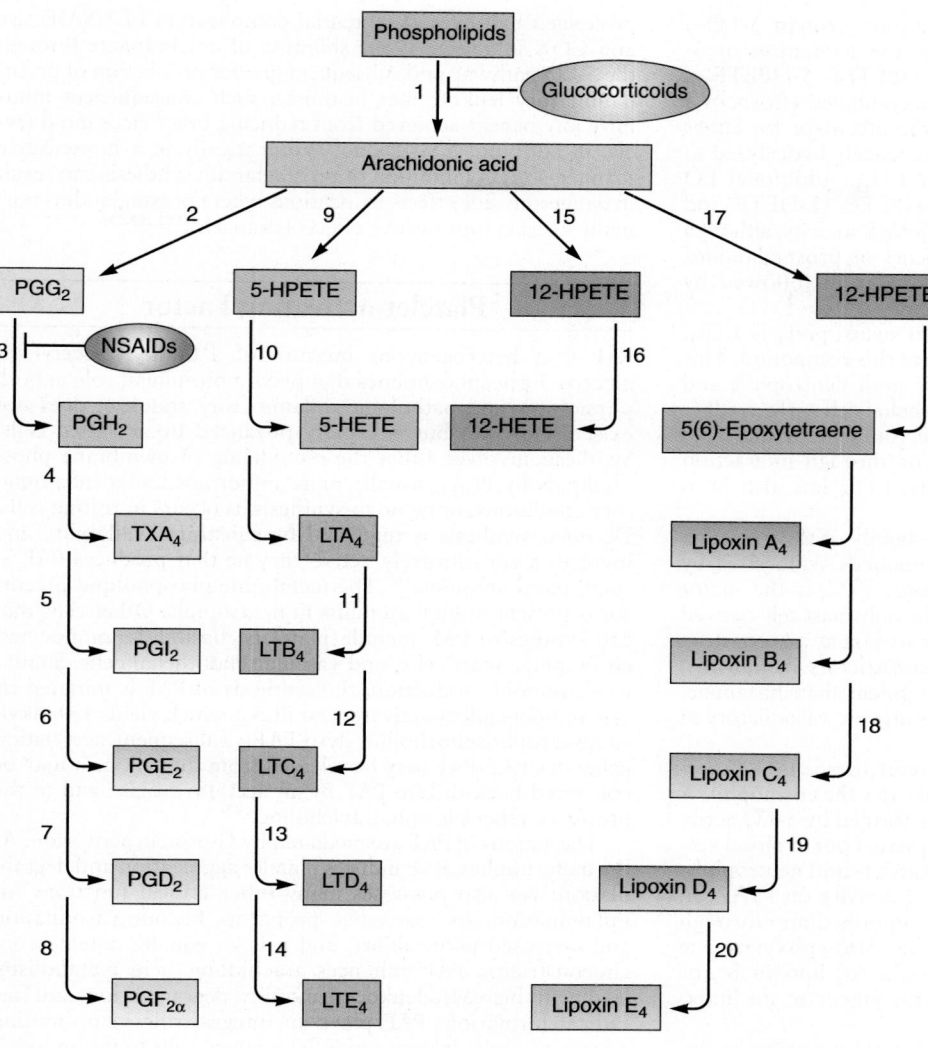

FIGURE 6.9. Eicosanoid production. *1.* Phospholipases. *2.* Cyclooxygenase. *3.* Hydroperoxidase. *4.* Thromboxane synthetase. *5.* Prostacyclin synthetase. *6.* E-isomerase. *7.* D-isomerase. *8.* F-reductase. *9.* 5-Lipoxygenase. *10.* Glutathione peroxidase. *11.* Hydrolase. *12.* Glutathione S-transferase. *13.* γ-Glutamyl transpeptidase. *14.* Cysteinyl glycanase. *15.* 12-Lipoxygenase. *16.* Peroxidase. *17.* 15-Lipoxygenase. *18.* GSH-cis-11-trans lipoxin A_4. *19.* α-Glutamyl transferase. *20.* Dipeptidase.

with bradykinin and histamine to mediate pain. It is a bronchodilator, inhibits both IL-1 production and T-cell responsiveness to IL-1, and at low concentrations suppresses TNF-α production. It also inhibits neutrophil chemotaxis and activation and T_H1 lymphocyte proliferation.[179,180] There is some suggestion from animal studies that PGE_2, PGE_1, and PGI_2 may be beneficial in response to sepsis through their endogenous counterregulatory properties. Administration of each of these has been shown to improve survival in several animal models of hypovolemic and traumatic shock, though clinical trials have failed to identify benefit.[180] PGD_2 is a potent bronchoconstrictor that inhibits neutrophil chemotaxis and activation. TXA_2, PGG_2, and PGH_2 oppose the actions of prostacyclin by promoting platelet aggregation and inducing bronchoconstriction. TXA_2 produced by platelets and macrophages is a powerful vasoconstrictor that induces neutrophil accumulation and increases vascular permeability.[176–178,181] There is substantial evidence that TXA_2 plays a significant role in early acute-phase organ injury.[180]

Lipoxygenase Pathway (Leukotrienes and Lipoxins). Leukotrienes and lipoxins are leukocyte-derived molecules synthesized by the oxidation of arachidonic acid by one of three LO enzymes: 5-LO, 12-LO, and 15-LO (Fig. 6.9). 5-LO

TABLE 6.8

PROSTANOID EFFECTS

	PGG_2	PGH_2	PGI_2	PGE_2	TXA_2
Chemotaxis	↑	↑	↓	↓	↑
Bronchial resistance	↑	↑	↓	↓	↑
Platelet aggregation	↑	↑	↓	↓	↑
Systemic vascular resistance			↓	↓	↑
Pulmonary vascular resistance	↑	↑	↓	↓	↑

PG, prostaglandin; TXA_2, thromboxane A_2.

associates with the perinuclear membrane protein 5-LO–activating protein (FLAP) to catalyze the formation of 5-hydroperoxyeicosatetraenoic acid (5-HPETE). 5-HPETE is subsequently converted to LTA_4 by the combined efforts of a dehydrase and 5-LO. LTA_4 serves as the precursor for either LTB_4 or LTC_4. LTC_4 can in turn be successively hydrolyzed to the dipeptide derivative LTD_4 and the LTE_4. Additional LO activity results in the production of 12-HPETE, 12-HETE, and 15-HPETE. These compounds exhibit biologic activity, although they are not as potent as the leukotrienes or prostaglandins. The leukotrienes are inactivated by oxidation followed by dehydration.[177–179,181,182]

The major lipoxygenase product of neutrophils is LTB_4, though macrophages may also synthesize this compound. This compound is potently chemotactic for both neutrophils and eosinophils, and by upregulating endothelial cell surface adhesion molecules promotes leukocyte recruitment. It increases vascular permeability, either directly or through interaction with neutrophils and endothelial cells. LTB_4 has also been shown to induce hyperalgesia.[92,179]

LTC_4, LTD_4, and LTE_4 comprise the family of slow-reacting substances of anaphylaxis (SRSA), compounds synthesized by mast cells during anaphylactic reactions. LTC_4 is the major eicosanoid product of eosinophils and the only mast cell–derived product of LO. These three leukotrienes are potent vasoconstrictors and the most powerful bronchoconstrictors in humans, being three orders of magnitude more potent than histamine. They also increase vascular permeability and are vasodilatory in skin.[43,179]

Lipoxins are biosynthesized by several routes in a tissue-specific manner. Current evidence implicates the eosinophil. A 5(6)-epoxytetraene intermediate can be formed by 5-LO activity on 15-HPETE. This reaction when carried out in blood vessels requires the interaction between platelets and neutrophils. On mucosal surfaces, 12-LO and 5-LO activity on LTA_4 can result in formation of this lipoxin intermediate through leukocyte–epithelial interactions. The 5(6)-epoxytetraene intermediate is then converted to lipoxin A_4, lipoxin B_4, or lipoxin C_4, the last of which serves as the precursor for lipoxins D_4 and E_4.[90,183,184]

Though many of the functions of lipoxins have yet to be elucidated, they appear to counterregulate the actions of leukotrienes. They inhibit leukotriene production by downregulating 5-LO as 15-LO is upregulated. The anti-inflammatory cytokines IL-4 and IL-13 further contribute to suppression of inflammatory responses by enhancing 15-LO activity. In addition to inhibiting synthesis, lipoxins inhibit the actions of LTB_4 and LTD_4. Lipoxins A_4 and B_4 are potent vasoactive compounds, though this effect is tissue specific for lipoxin B_4, as it induces vasoconstriction in some tissue beds. Lipoxins influence smooth muscle and vascular tonus by increasing NO and prostacyclin production, increasing arachidonate release, and reversing endothelin-induced vasoconstriction. Counterinflammatory functions of lipoxin A_4 include inhibition of leukotrienes, fMLP, and other chemoattractants. Lipoxin A_4 also downregulates LTB_4-mediated delayed-type hypersensitivity reactions.[90,183–185]

A large number of anti-inflammatory drugs, many of which are in clinical use, act by interfering with eicosanoid synthesis. The anti-inflammatory properties of corticosteroids are mediated at least in part by the inhibition of PLA_2 through the induction of lipocortin. They have been shown to selectively inhibit COX2 activation without affecting COX1. NSAIDs block the synthesis of both prostaglandins and thromboxanes by inhibiting COX activity. In contrast to the other NSAIDs, aspirin inhibits COX in an irreversible manner, and restoration of platelet function necessitates the administration of platelets. Recently aspirin, by either acetylating COX2 or by inducing the oxidation of arachidonic acid by cytochrome P450 or 5-LO, has been shown to stimulate the formation of 15R-HETE in endothelial or epithelial cells. These 15-epilipoxins exhibit higher potency in suppressing inflammation because of their prolonged half-lives. A potential complication of NSAID use and COX inhibition is the shunting of arachidonate through the 5-LO pathway and subsequent greater production of proinflammatory leukotrienes (asthma); such consequences minimize any benefit achieved from reducing other eicosanoid levels. In addition, NSAIDs act systematically in a nonselective manner, so that inhibition of prostaglandin synthesis can result in dangerous side effects in locations where prostaglandins normally exert cytoprotective effects (stomach).[180,184,186]

Platelet-activating Factor

PAF is a heterogeneous mixture of 1-0-alkyl-2-acetyl-sn-glycero-3-phosphocholines that plays a prominent role in both physiologic and pathologic inflammatory states. It does not exist preformed, but is rapidly produced by activated cells. Synthesis involves either the remodeling of membrane phospholipids by PLA_2, usually more important under inflammatory conditions, or de novo synthesis as occurs in resting cells. De novo synthesis is regulated by substrate availability and involves a constitutively active enzyme that produces PAF in small basal amounts.[187] The membrane phospholipid precursor is present in high amounts in neutrophils. Other cells that can synthesize PAF include platelets, basophils, monocytes, eosinophils, mast cells, and vascular endothelial cells. Similar to eicosanoid production, the synthesis of PAF is initiated by calcium-dependent activation of PLA_2, which yields 1-0-alkyl-sn-glycerophosphocholine (lyso-PAF); subsequent acetylation generates PAF. PAF may be released from the cell, or it may be converted back to lyso-PAF by an acetylhydrolase and to the precursor ether-phosphatidylcholine.[187]

The actions of PAF are mediated by G-protein activation. As the name implies, PAF induces platelet aggregation and degranulation, yet also possesses many other critical functions for inflammation. Its vasoactive properties include vasodilation and increased permeability, and it is an equally potent bronchoconstrictor. PAF enhances arachidonic acid metabolism, leading to increased leukocyte motility, degranulation, and free radical formation. PAF plays an integral role in promoting activation and adherence of inflammatory cells to the endothelium.[188] During the early inflammatory response, activated endothelial cells synthesize and express PAF on the cell surface. Leukocytes tethered by selectins to the endothelium are activated by endothelial PAF, which results in the induction of tight integrin-dependent adhesion and subsequent emigration and chemotaxis toward the inflammatory focus. Acyl-PAF, the major acetylated lipid from mast cells, basophils, and endothelial cells, is a less potent derivative of PAF that likely plays a similar role in the regulation of neutrophil recruitment. PAF also promotes platelet and neutrophil aggregation, thereby contributing to the prothrombotic state of acute inflammation. In circumstances of persistent pathologic stimuli, PAF may be liberated systemically, thereby causing the sequelae of an excessive inflammatory response. As a mediator of sepsis, PAF augments endotoxin-induced hypotension and neutrophil and platelet accumulation in the lungs. There is evidence that the NO-induced hypotension in experimental models of endotoxemia is mediated by PAF.[189] PAF infusion leads to a shock state that is similar to septic shock in that there is tissue hypoperfusion despite adequate fluid resuscitation. In animal studies, PAF has been shown to contribute many manifestations of sepsis including coronary vasoconstriction, reduced cardiac contractility, reduced preload, peripheral vasodilation, pulmonary vasoconstriction, increased microvascular permeability, gastrointestinal hemorrhage, and thrombocytopenia.[180] Two prospective randomized, placebo-controlled trials of PAF inhibition in sepsis have suggested a benefit.[180]

PAF acetylhydrolase, an enzyme regulated by dexamethasone, estrogen, and PAF itself, is the enzyme responsible for degradation of PAF.

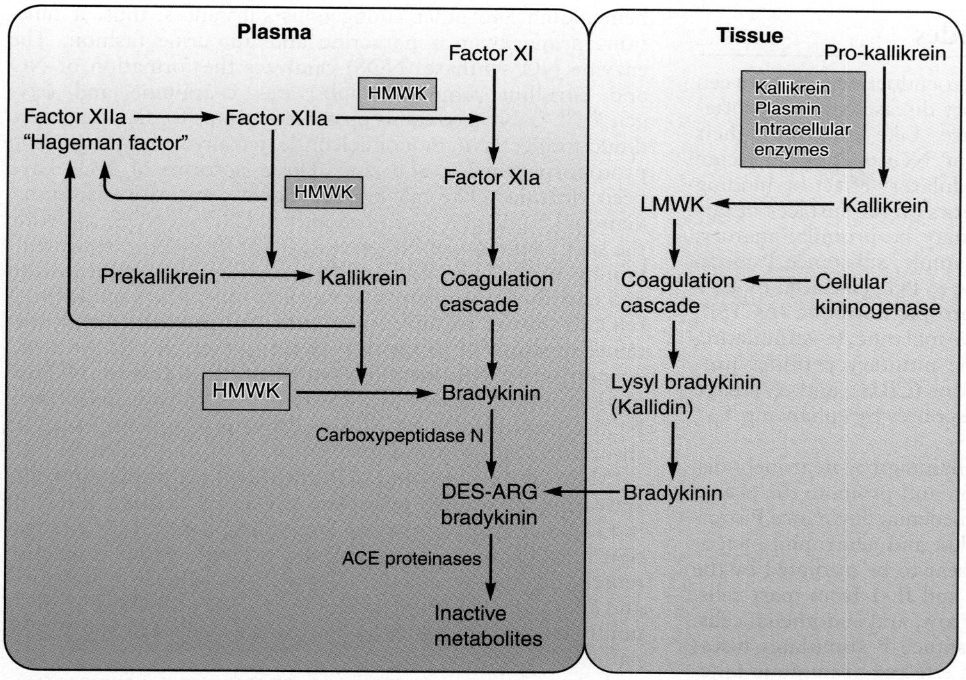

FIGURE 6.10. Kinin pathway. (Modified from Proud D, Kaplan AP. Kinin formation: mechanisms and role in inflammatory disorders. *Annu Rev Immun* 1988;6:49.)

Kinins

Kinins (i.e., bradykinin and lysyl bradykinin) are small vasoactive peptides generated during the inflammatory response (Fig. 6.10). Three mechanisms of kinin formation are operant during inflammation: (a) plasma proteins, (b) tissue proteins, and (c) cellular proteinases.[190–193]

Production of Bradykinin. Biosynthesis commences with the activation of Hageman factor (HF), or factor XII of the coagulation cascade (Fig. 6.10). HF is activated by exposure to anionic surfaces such as the basement membrane of injured endothelium, heparin, or lipid A of endotoxin. It can also be proteolytically cleaved and activated by kallikrein. Prekallikrein circulates complexed with HMWK, a nonenzymatic protein. Kininogen enhances the binding of prekallikrein to negatively charged surfaces. Activated HF converts prekallikrein to kallikrein, which in turn activates more HF in a positive feedback cycle. HFf, a cleavage product of activated HF, is also capable of activating prekallikrein. Kallikrein in plasma, tissues, and secretions specifically cleaves HMWK to release the nonapeptide bradykinin. In addition to bradykinin production, kallikrein participates in the activation of plasminogen and C1q of the complement system, yet another link between inflammation and the coagulation system. The only major plasma inhibitor of activated HF is C1 inhibitor. The primary inhibitors of kallikrein in plasma are C1 inhibitor and α_1-macroglobulin.[39,190]

Kinin Production in Tissue. Lysyl-bradykinin (kallidin) is the cleavage product of either HMWK or low-molecular-weight kininogen (LMWK) by tissue kallikreins, which are proteins distinct from their plasma counterparts. LMWK is present in higher concentrations intracellularly compared with HMWK. Whereas both HMWK and LMWK can be converted to lysyl-bradykinin by tissue kallikrein, only HMWK is cleaved by plasma kallikrein. Kallidin itself can be converted to bradykinin by a plasma aminopeptidase. Both kallidin and bradykinin use the same receptors and perform similar functions, but kallidin is approximately 85% as potent as bradykinin. Tissue kallikrein is synthesized from a preproenzyme and is converted intracellularly to tissue prokallikrein by enzymes that are not yet well characterized. The secreted prokallikrein is then converted to tissue kallikrein extracellularly by plasmin or plasma kallikrein. The only significant inhibitor of tissue kallikreins is α_1-proteinase inhibitor.[39,190]

Cellular Kininogenase Activity. Neutrophils, mast cells, and basophils are sources of kininogenase activity. Neutrophils produce leukokinins by way of cathepsin D. Their role in inflammation is unclear. Bradykinin is metabolized sequentially to the partially active eight-amino-acid peptide, des-Arg-bradykinin, by carboxypeptidase N, and then to inactive 5-amino-acid and three-amino-acid fragments by the angiotensin-converting enzyme (ACE). ACE is the predominant enzyme to inactivate bradykinin in the pulmonary vasculature. Arginine released as a byproduct of the carboxypeptidase N reaction may contribute further to the modulation of inflammation by acting as a substrate for the formation of NO.[39,190,194]

There are three kinin receptors, of which two are well characterized.[190,192] B1 receptors are expressed primarily on the vasculature under pathologic conditions such as tissue injury. They bind des-Arg-bradykinin and des-Arg-kallidin and may mediate the hypotension characteristic of sepsis as well as pain.[190,195] Both B1 and the more widely distributed B2 receptors are G-protein–coupled receptors. Activation of B2 receptors stimulates IP and phospholipase C (PLC), resulting in the accumulation of the second messengers IP_3, DAG, and calcium. The B2 receptors are more important in mediating the effects of inflammatory kinins, such as bradykinin and lysyl-bradykinin. These kinins induce arteriolar dilatation and mediate pain. Similar to histamine, bradykinin increases the gaps between postcapillary venule endothelial cells to increase vascular permeability. It is a potent constrictor of bronchial, uterine, and gastrointestinal smooth muscle, as well as the coronary and pulmonary vasculature.[192] Activation of endothelial B2 receptors stimulates production of NO to further enhance vasodilatation. Kinins have been implicated in mediating the antihypertensive and cardioprotective effects of ACE inhibitors.[196] ACE, in addition to catalyzing the formation of angiotensin II from angiotensin I, promotes the hydrolysis of bradykinin to inactive metabolites. In addition, bradykinin can modulate platelet function by stimulating endothelial cell secretion of PGI_2 and thromboxane through activation of PLA_2.[190]

Neuropeptides

Neuropeptides may provide the neuroendocrine link between psychological stress and inflammatory diseases such as psoriasis and inflammatory bowel disease. Like cytokines, their
7 actions are pleiotropic and redundant. Neuropeptides execute their inflammatory and immunomodulatory effect by binding to specific G-protein–coupled receptors on the surfaces of target cells, and the resultant effect may be proinflammatory, anti-inflammatory, or both. For example, substance P mediates the hypothalamic fever response to PGE_2 induced by IL-1 and TNF-α, whereas adrenocorticotropic hormone (ACTH), arginine vasopressin (AVP), and α-melanocyte–stimulating hormone (α-MSH) suppress it. The pituitary peptides prolactin, corticotropin-releasing hormone (CRH), and AVP have been shown to augment immune responses by enhancing T_H1 activity.[39,197,198]

Tachykinins are important proinflammatory neuropeptides that mediate pain and vasodilatation and promote the classic inflammatory signs of erythema and edema. Substance P stimulates monocyte and neutrophil influx and neutrophil phagocytosis. Its inflammatory effects appear to be mediated by the proinflammatory cytokines TNF-α and IL-1 from mast cells, monocytes, macrophages, bone marrow, and endothelial cells. During allergic inflammation, substance P stimulates histamine release from mast cells. As an effector of immune function, substance P promotes T-cell proliferation and antibody production. Substance P released locally by nerve terminals is important in mediating the perception of pain.[39,190]

CRH induces the release of IL-1, IL-6, and superoxide anion from macrophages and regulates its own proinflammatory effects through cortisol release. Cortisol downregulates production of proinflammatory cytokines such as IL-1, TNF-α, and IL-2; metalloproteinases; and inducible nitric oxide synthase (iNOS), and through this negative feedback loop, inhibits the production of CRH as well as ACTH and AVP. AVP, growth hormone, and prolactin are other important proinflammatory neuropeptides.[39,197,198]

Vasoactive intestinal peptide (VIP) and its homologues display both proinflammatory and anti-inflammatory effects. VIP is widely distributed throughout the central and peripheral nervous systems and serves as a chemoattractant for macrophages, neutrophils, and T cells, and may play an important role in granulomatous reactions. VIP stimulates the release of histamine, and IL-5 and is a potent vasodilator. It inhibits IL-6, TNF-α, and IL-12 release and iNOS expression in activated macrophages. VIP has also been shown to stimulate the production of the anti-inflammatory cytokine IL-10 by macrophages and inhibit T-lymphocyte proliferation and IL-2 and IFN-γ production.[199]

Somatostatin and α-MSH are primarily anti-inflammatory in action. Somatostatin, which colocalizes with substance P in sensory nerves, inhibits IgE formation and NK cell activity. α-MSH inhibits leukocyte chemotaxis and IFN-γ production and downregulates T_H1 activity. ACTH, calcitonin, and β-endorphin are other neuropeptides with predominantly anti-inflammatory properties.[39]

Calcitonin gene-related peptide (CGRP) is an immunomodulator that inhibits the activity of T cells and macrophages, in part through the induction of IL-10. It also is an inhibitor of antigen presentation. CGRP promotes vasodilatation and neutrophil influx and synergizes with bradykinin and histamine to promote edema formation.

Nitric Oxide. The endogenous synthesis of NO was first identified in 1987, and NO was the first gaseous molecule shown to be synthesized for the purpose of cell signaling.[200] NO is a weakly reactive radical that diffuses short distances from cell to cell independent of membrane channels or receptors. Its half-life is short because of its rapid inactivation by hemoglobin and other endogenous substances; thus, it functions primarily in a paracrine and autocrine fashion. The enzyme NO synthase (NOS) catalyzes the formation of NO and citrulline from the substrates L-arginine and oxygen.[50,201–203] NOS contains prosthetic groups for flavin-adenine dinucleotide, flavin mononucleotide, tetrahydrobiopterin, iron protoporphyrin IX, and zinc. Three isoforms of NOS have been identified. The calcium-dependent constitutive isoforms, neuronal NOS (nNOS) and endothelial NOS (eNOS), generate the small amounts of NO necessary for those processes maintaining physiologic homeostasis, such as neurotransmission and endothelial regulation of vascular tone. The expression of iNOS, however, requires stimulation and produces larger, sustained amounts of NO with both cytoprotective and cytotoxic properties. This distinction is not absolute, as certain cell populations express low basal levels of iNOS, and constitutive NOS transcripts can be enhanced by certain stimuli such as shear stress and hypoxia.[50,201–203]

Many of the physiologic effects of NO are mediated by the activation of soluble guanylate cyclase. Increased levels of intracellular cyclic guanosine monophosphate trigger a reduction in calcium concentration and promote vascular smooth muscle relaxation and the inhibition of platelet aggregation and adhesion. The cellular response to NO also likely involves multiple signal transduction mechanisms including the MAPK pathway.

Inflammation secondary to endotoxemia, hemorrhagic shock, and ischemia/reperfusion are associated with increased NO production by iNOS. iNOS, first described in macrophages, can be expressed in essentially any cell type in response to immunologic stimuli, and unlike nNOS and eNOS, does not depend on elevations in intracellular calcium levels for its activity.[50,201–203] Important activators of iNOS upregulation include LPS, IL-1, TNF-α, and IFN-γ. Expression is primarily transcriptionally regulated, although stabilization of iNOS mRNA also appears to play a role. IFN-γ stabilizes iNOS mRNA, whereas TGF-β can destabilize it. Transcription of the iNOS gene is controlled by NF-κB, IFN-γ–responsive element, and TNF-responsive element. Induction of iNOS can be inhibited by glucocorticoids, thrombin, macrophage deactivation factor, PDGF, IL-4, IL-8, IL-10, and IL-13.[50,201–203] Dexamethasone may inhibit iNOS induction by impairing the DNA-binding capacity of NF-κB and by increasing levels of I-κB.[204,205]

The endothelial dysfunction and vascular hyporeactivity characteristic of septic shock is mediated in part by iNOS production of NO.[206] NO has been shown to be the effective mediator of the negative myocardial inotropy of TNF-α, IL-6, and IL-2 and the TNF-α–induced vasodilatation in the systemic and microcirculations.[207] NO may indirectly increase prostaglandin production by increasing the catalytic activity of cyclooxygenase and decrease leukotriene production by inhibiting 5-lipoxygenase.[208] NO plays an autoregulatory role in the T_H1 subset of T_H cells by limiting their own proliferation.[209]

NO can mediate tissue injury in inflammation by modulating organ perfusion, mediating interactions with neutrophils, contributing to proinflammatory signaling, and regulating apoptosis.[210] Whereas eNOS primarily regulates perfusion during homeostasis, both eNOS and iNOS modulate organ flow in pathophysiologic states. Basal NO production from eNOS prevents the adherence of neutrophils to the endothelium and inhibits chemotaxis under physiologic conditions. Animal studies have demonstrated that pharmacologic inhibition of iNOS or genetic deletion of iNOS attenuates neutrophil accumulation in organs after ischemia/reperfusion injury.[211] Conversely, similar experiments in endotoxemia implicate an antiadhesive role for iNOS, suggesting that the effect of induced NO on neutrophil accumulation is insult specific.[210] Activated neutrophils can be stimulated by fMLP, PAF, and LTB_4 to produce NO. NO produced by neutrophils at sites of inflammation can combine with superoxide to form peroxynitrite as another means of effecting toxicity.[39,212]

The reaction of NO with superoxide is the only reaction that outcompetes the reaction of superoxide with superoxide dismutase. Although small amounts of peroxynitrite are produced under basal conditions from constitutively produced NO and superoxide from mitochondria and other cellular sources, endogenous antioxidants such as GSH, vitamins E and C, and superoxide dismutase likely limit its toxicity. A low concentration of peroxynitrite has been shown to inhibit neutrophil adhesion. Higher concentrations of peroxynitrite can initiate a wide range of toxic oxidative reactions through a peroxynitrous acid intermediate. These include the initiation of tyrosine nitration, lipid peroxidation, and direct inhibition of mitochondrial respiratory enzymes. The balance between superoxide and NO determines the reactivity of peroxynitrite; excess NO reduces the oxidation elicited by peroxynitrite. In addition, peroxynitrite may contribute to cytotoxicity by a more indirect pathway. Peroxynitrite-induced single-strand breaks in DNA activate the nuclear enzyme poly(ADP-ribose) synthetase, leading eventually to irreversible energy depletion of the cells and necrotic-type cell death.[39,41]

Inducible NOS plays a key role in host defense, with NO or peroxynitrite exhibiting potent antimicrobial activity against a number of pathogens including viruses, fungi, and bacteria. Although microbicidal susceptibility to NO-mediated killing can vary considerably between species, essential roles have been identified in tuberculosis and bacterial peritonitis.[213] Induced NO has been shown to be essential for the upregulation of the inflammatory response in hemorrhagic shock and is likely to be so in other inflammatory processes. NO produced by iNOS leads to the activation of NF-κB.[214] This is followed by the induction of proinflammatory cytokines and increased leukocyte recruitment and activation.

NO has demonstrated both proapoptotic and antiapoptotic effects depending on the circumstances. NO derived from eNOS may inhibit apoptosis.[215] Proapoptotic effects appear to be associated with pathophysiologic conditions in which iNOS is upregulated. Low concentrations of peroxynitrite have also been shown to induce apoptosis, whereas higher concentrations promote cell necrosis in vitro. The role of NO-mediated apoptosis in the regulation of the inflammatory response has yet to be more clearly defined.

In summary, NO mediates tissue injury both directly through the formation of peroxynitrite and indirectly through the amplification of the inflammatory process. Like many mediators, however, NO has dual regulatory functions and is therefore difficult to characterize as either proinflammatory or anti-inflammatory. In general, basal levels of NO produced by constitutive NOS may confer anti-inflammatory effects, whereas induced NO may tend to promote the upregulation of the inflammatory response. It is likely that an optimal level of NO is necessary in host defense; too little NO may be as harmful as too much.

Heme Oxygenase

Heme oxygenase catalyzes the breakdown of heme to iron, biliverdin, and carbon monoxide (CO).[216] Three isoforms of HO have been identified. HO-2 is constitutively expressed in many tissues, whereas HO-3 expression appears to be limited to the brain. HO-1 is not expressed constitutively in most tissues, but is rapidly upregulated by both heme and nonheme cellular stresses, including hypoxia, redox stress, and inflammation. Additionally, NO is a potent inducer of HO-1. HO-1 has profound antiapoptotic and anti-inflammatory effects. These cytoprotective effects have been attributed to the individual catalytic products of heme metabolism. Biliverdin is converted to bilirubin by biliverdin reductase, and bilirubin has been demonstrated to act as a potent intracellular antioxidant. Carbon monoxide alone can mimic many of the actions of HO-1 and has been shown to protect in models of sepsis, hemorrhagic shock, and ischemia/reperfusion when administered as an inhaled gas. The mechanisms of action of carbon monoxide have both similarities and dissimilarities with nitric oxide and are an area of active investigation.[216]

Hydrogen Sulfide

Hydrogen sulfide (H_2S) is a colorless, flammable gas, with the typical malodor of putrid eggs. It is highly lipophilic and freely penetrates the cell wall, which greatly facilitates its biologic activity.[217] Recent evidence highlights the widespread distribution of H_2S in the plasma, brain, and other tissues. H_2S is formed in mammalian cells largely by the activity of two pyridoxal phosphate-dependent enzymes, cystathione γ-lyase (CSE) and cystathionine β-synthetase (CBS), that utilize cysteine and homocysteine to form H_2S.[217] Large amounts of these enzymes occur in the brain (CBS), liver (CSE), kidney (CSE), and blood vessels (CSE). Interestingly, lipopolysaccharide exposure induces the expression of CSE, suggesting that H_2S may regulate inflammation.[218] Both pro- and anti-inflammatory actions have been described. H_2S levels and CSE expression are increased in animal models of endotoxemia, sepsis, and hemorrhagic shock.[218–220] It has been shown to increase leukocyte attachment and rolling in jejunal blood vessels and to increase ICAM-1 expression.[221] In human monocytes, H_2S donors induced the formation of proinflammatory cytokines and chemokines via a NF-κB mechanism.[222] Inhibitors of CSE reduced the inflammation in these animal models of sepsis and hemorrhage. By contrast, H_2S decreased LPS-induced upregulation of NF-κB in RAW 264.7 macrophages, and H_2S-releasing derivatives of diclofenac exhibited greater anti-inflammatory activity in endotoxic shock.[217,223,224]

RECOGNITION AND ACTIVATION PROCESSES

Exogenous and Endogenous Danger Recognition

Multicellular organisms have evolved an essential mechanism of
8 surveillance, defense, and repair of injured cells. Implicit with this system is the ability to differentiate pathogens and damaged cells from self. The initial response is orchestrated by the evolutionarily ancient and more universal innate immune system, which employs monoclonal sets of recognition molecules called pattern recognition receptors (PRRs).[225,226] PRRs bind conserved molecular structures found in large groups of pathogens, termed *PAMPs*. PAMPs are a diverse set of microbial molecules, which share a number of different recognizable biochemical features that alert the organism to intruding pathogens.[225–227] These PAMPs are recognized by cells of innate and acquired immunity, primarily through the Toll-like PRRs. Activation induces several signaling pathways, most notably NF-κB.[225,227] Consequent to this activation, an immune response is triggered to destroy the pathogen and/or pathogen-infected cells, and an adaptive response is initiated to select pathogen-specific T cells and antibodies for future occasions.

However, pathogens are not the only causative agents of tissue and cell damage. Cells, and thus tissues, can be injured by various noxious insults: heat, cold, chemicals, radiation, ischemia, or direct mechanical injuries. Evolution has enabled us to deal with these damages, which though not caused by pathogens, still necessitate repair. It is becoming apparent that specific receptors exist by which to recognize extrinsic threats (i.e., pathogen) and intrinsic altered self (cytokines, oxidized mitochondrial DNA, heat-shock proteins, and uric acid).[227]

Danger-associated Molecular Patterns

9 DAMPs, the endogenous equivalent of PAMPs, represent danger signals or "alarmins" and share many characteristics similar to cytokines.[227] DAMPs may be released following nonprogrammed cell death, such as necrosis, and under such circumstances tend to elicit inflammation. By contrast, programmed cell death (i.e., apoptosis) incorporates mechanisms such as acetylation to minimize the release of these mediators and any subsequent inflammatory response. Cells of the immune system also can be induced to secrete these mediators.[227] This secretion may occur by specialized secretion systems or by the classical ER-Golgi secretion pathway.[227] Under these circumstances, DAMPs may facilitate the inflammatory response by aiding the recruitment of innate immune cells, most notably dendritic cells. In doing so, they indirectly orchestrate the subsequent adaptive immune response and facilitate tissue repair.[227] The prototypical alarmin, HMGB1, has already been discussed. Here we briefly discus mediators recently added to this list.

S100 Proteins. The family of S100 proteins incorporates over 20 related calcium-binding proteins.[227] S100A8 and S100A9 form heterocomplexes in the cytosol of granulocytes, monocytes, and macrophages, whereas S100A12 exists as homodimers in the cytoplasm of granulocytes. S100 proteins are actively secreted at sites of inflammation via a nonclassical pathway. The receptors mediating their effects are still being defined, though it appears that S100A12 and S100B interact with RAGE, whereas S100A8/9 may interact with TLR receptors. S100 proteins have been shown to induce increased vascular permeability and a prothrombotic effect. Recent studies implicate S100 proteins in the pathogenesis of autoimmune arthritis and psoriasis.[227]

Uric Acid. Uric acid is released after cellular injury, and upon exposure to the extracellular environment, precipitates to form monosodium urate (MSU).[227] Uric acid stimulates dendritic maturation and, when coinjected with antigen in vivo, significantly enhances the generation of responses from $CD8^+$ T cells.[227] It has significant proinflammatory properties that are best evidenced in the disease gout, in which uric acid accumulates in tissues and induces inflammation-dependent arthritis. MSU crystals engage the inflammasome, resulting in the production of IL-1β and IL-18.[227] Macrophages from mice deficient in IL-1R or in various components of the inflammasome, such as caspase-1, ASC, and NaLP3, are defective in MSU-induced cytokine secretion and have reduced inflammation.[227] Extracellular uric acid is eliminated by uricase.[227]

Receptors for Danger Recognition. Innate immunity is not antigen specific, but rather programmed to respond to groups of evolutionarily conserved macromolecules that represent "patterns of danger" and signal a potential threat to the host. PRRs identify these PAMPS and include the Toll-like receptors and NOD-like receptors. Recent studies highlight the promiscuity of these PRRs in also recognizing and mediating DAMP-dependent signaling. In fact, multiple positive feedback loops between DAMPS and PAMPs and their overlapping receptors may represent the molecular basis for the observation that infections, as well as nonspecific stress factors, can trigger flares of autoimmune diseases (i.e., rheumatic).[147] Additional novel receptors have subsequently been identified and designated PRRs, including RAGE.[226,227]

CD14. The prototypical receptor identifying external infectious threats (i.e., gram-negative infections) is CD14. CD14 was identified as the LPS receptor when transfection of CD14-negative CHO cells with CD14 conferred responsiveness to LPS.[228] Its critical role in LPS recognition is underscored by the LPS-hyporesponsive phenotype of CD14-deficient mice. It has been identified on cells of the myeloid lineage, B cells, liver parenchymal cells, and fibroblasts. Differential expression is observed, ranging from high levels on peritoneal and pleural macrophages to lower levels on Kupffer cells, alveolar macrophages, monocytes, and PMNs. Expression may be modified as human PMNs express low levels of CD14 that is upregulated by TNF-α, G-CSF, GM-CSF, and fMLP. Prototypically, CD14 binds LPS bound to LPS-binding protein (LBP) in combination with MD-2 and presents it to TLR4.[228] MD-2 is required for cellular responsiveness to LPS, as demonstrated by both transfection studies and an analysis of a CHO cell line with a mutated MD-2 gene. Most of the available evidence indicates that a complex of TLR4/MD-2/CD14 directly binds LPS.[228] CD14 is also important in TLR2 signaling, whereby it presents bacterial products other than LPS.

Toll-like Receptors. CD14 is a glycosylphosphatidylinositol-linked receptor devoid of any transmembrane domain. This, in combination with the identification of a soluble form of CD14, necessitated identifying the manner by which LPS induced activation.[229] In 1996, the Toll protein in Drosophila was shown to be necessary for an effective immune response to the fungus *Aspergillus fumigatus*.[225] In 1998, Poltorak et al. discovered that the *lps* gene in LPS-hyporesponsive C3H/HEJ mice encoded a murine member of the TLR family. These data provided the initial evidence that mammalian TLRs function as PRRs.[230] Subsequent studies have confirmed that TLR4 is the "LPS receptor" and that it is essential for the defense against gram-negative microorganisms.[228]

Thirteen mammalian TLR receptors have been characterized. Each recognizes a specific set of conserved microbial molecules, and as a family, they can detect most microbes.[228] Interestingly, the subcellular localization of different TLRs correlates to some extent with the molecular patterns of their ligands and their function.[231] TLR1, TLR2, and TLR4 are located on the cell surface and are recruited to phagosomes after activation by their respective ligands. They are the receptors mediating the response to exogenous insults including bacterial infection and trauma. By contrast, TLR3, TLR7, and TLR9, all of which are involved in the recognition of nucleic acid–like structures (i.e., viral DNA), are expressed intracellularly.[225,232]

TLR4 is required for the innate response to gram-negative organisms and LPS, though other TLRs, such as TLR2, can also recognize and mediate this response.[226] TLR4 has been shown to trigger the response to additional ligands, including lipoteichoic acid (LTA) and peptidoglycans from gram-positive bacteria and the fusion protein of the respiratory syncytial virus.[233] Individuals with the D299G polymorphism in TLR4 demonstrate increased risk of gram-negative infections, and other studies have linked this with an increased incidence of SIRS.[234] In addition, this polymorphism has been associated with alterations in the susceptibility to other inflammatory and potentially infectious processes (carotid artery atherosclerosis, coronary artery disease).[234] Heat-shock protein 60 (HSP60) of chlamydial origin has been found in atherosclerotic plaques and can bind TLR4. Perhaps recognition of HSP60 by human TLR4 might exacerbate the inflammatory component of atherosclerosis, whereas people with the D299G polymorphism might be at least partly protected from this exacerbation.[234] TLR4 has been well characterized as a PRR for DAMPs, including heat-shock proteins (HSP60, HSP70, Gp96), hyaluronate, heparan sulfate, and other matrix proteins. Because of its ability to recognize endogenous proteins, TLR4 is implicated in a variety of diseases, including arthritis and atherosclerosis.[147,232]

TLR2 recognizes lipoproteins derived from the cell wall of bacteria such as *Treponema pallidum* and *Mycoplasma fermentans*, LTA from gram-positive bacteria, lipopeptides, LPS, and lipid A.[226,232,233] It also can recognize a host of DAMPs, including the heat-shock proteins, fibronectin, fibrinogen, heparan sulfate, and hyaluronate. Recent data suggest that TLR2 forms heterodimers with other TLRs, including TLR1 or TLR6, to recognize these DAMPs. A likely consequence of this cooperation is an increased repertoire of ligand specificities. The R753Q polymorphism in the TLR2 is associated with a decreased response to these bacteria and may increase susceptibility to staphylococcal infections or tuberculosis.[232,234]

Additional TLRs involved in inflammation include TLR9, which recognizes unmethylated CpG motifs present in bacterial DNA. By contrast, most of the host mammalian genome is methylated. TLR9-ligand engagement occurs intracellularly, in either endosomes or lysosomes, presumably following bacterial lysis. Recent evidence suggests that TLR9 can identify host DNA released by dead or dying cells, and hence may be involved in the autoimmune diseases such as systemic lupus erythematosus (SLE).[225] TLR5 recognizes flagellin of bacterial flagella.[232] TLR3 recognizes double-stranded RNA of both viral and endogenous sources. Because of the latter characteristic, TLR3 has been implicated in autoimmune arthritis.

TLRs induce signal transduction via their cytoplasmic Toll-interleukin-1 receptor (TIR) domains to promote the expression of a variety of host defense genes. These include inflammatory cytokines and chemokines, antimicrobial peptides, costimulatory molecules, MHC molecules, and other effectors. A considerable portion of the functional response is mediated by activating intracellular signaling pathways that culminate in the induction of the transcription factor NF-κB. Specifically, the CD14/MD-2/TLR4 complex, upon engagement with LPS-LBP, recruits the adapter protein MyD88, which subsequently engages the serine/threonine kinase IRAK. IRAK undergoes autophosphorylation and recruits TRAF6. Ultimately, activated I-κK phosphorylates and targets for degradation the NF-κB inhibitor I-κB, which enables the nuclear translocation of NF-κB and transcription of inflammatory genes. AP-1 and members of the MAPK transduction cascade are also activated by this mechanism. This pathway is critical to the production of IL-12, TNF-α, and IL-6. All TLRs signal through this conserved signaling cascade, and for some, MyD88 (TLRs 2, 6, 9) is their sole receptor-proximal adaptor. For instance, MyD88 is essential for clearance of *S. aureus*, a gram-positive bacteria, which would signal through TLRs 2, 6, 9.[225,226,233]

Subsequent studies utilizing MyD88-deficient mice suggested that alternate TLR pathways existed. These mice, in response to many TLR ligands, including peptidoglycan and unmethylated CpG motifs, did not activate NF-κB or MAPK. Surprisingly, however, LPS could still activate NF-κB and MAPK, though in a delayed fashion. Subsequently, a MyD88-independent pathway has been characterized that is utilized by TLR4 and utilizes a distinct adaptor protein called TIR domain–containing adapter protein (TIRAP) or Mal. A dominant negative mutant of TIRAP specifically impairs TLR4- and TLR2- but not IL-1R– or TLR9-induced NF-κB, indicating a specificity of TIRAP for the TLR4 pathway. A third TIR-containing adaptor molecule, TIR domain–containing adaptor inducing IFN-β (TRIF), also appears to mediate an MyD88-independent pathway.[225,226,233]

Most of this research has occurred in the realm of sepsis and provided insight into the manner by which organisms identify infectious threats and activate the inflammatory pathway to preserve the host. However, several circumstances of sterile inflammation suggest a role of the TLRs in mediating inflammation in response to endogenous danger signals (uric acid, mitochondrial DNA, HMGB1).[228] Hepatocellular injury consequent to ischemia/reperfusion (I/R) has been shown to be dependent on TLR4.[32]

RAGE. RAGE is an immunoglobulin superfamily molecule that belongs to the multiligand receptors that recognize families of ligands rather than a single polypeptide.[95,227,235,236] It has a single transmembrane spanning domain and a highly charged cytoplasmic tail that, though lacking known signaling motifs, is critical for cellular activation. Though RAGE knockout mice are viable and fertile, they display a wide range of defects. Most of these defects are subtler than expected, leading to the suggestion that other receptors with overlapping function might exist. Signaling appears to necessitate clustering into a particular orientation, which facilitates binding of cytosolic signaling complexes.[95,235] Its ligands include products of nonenzymatic glycosidation (e.g., advanced glycation end-products or AGEs), the amyloid-β precursor protein, the S100/calgranulin family of proinflammatory cytokinelike mediators, and HMGB1, and its expression is upregulated at sites of diverse pathologies including atherosclerosis and Alzheimer disease. In fact, RAGE-mediated cellular stimulation is thought to increase expression of the receptor itself, thereby generating a positive feedback mechanism and perpetuating the proinflammatory state.[95,235,236]

Recent studies demonstrate the activation of multiple signal transduction cascades subsequent to ligand binding, including the MAPK family (p38, ERK1/2, and JNK) and Rho GTPases (cdc42 and rac).[236] Like TLRs and IL-1R, RAGE engagement leads to NF-κB activation, suggesting that both receptor usage and signaling pathways evoke similar responses when cells are activated by PAMPs and DAMPs. It is currently hypothesized that RAGE–ligand interaction induces a new heightened basal state of activation. With a superimposed stimulus, cellular perturbation is magnified. Rather than returning to homeostasis, cellular signal transduction mechanisms favor augmented dysfunction.[95,235]

Studies have implicated RAGE to be an important receptor during various acute and chronic inflammatory processes as well as tumor biology. RAGE expression and function directly correlated with tumor growth in RAGE-transfected C6 glioma cells. In a murine tumor model, in mice treated with soluble RAGE, which functions as a decoy, there was a reduction in lung metastases, cellular invasion, and expression of matrix metalloproteinases.[236]

RAGE has also been identified as a receptor for S100A12, a member of the S100/calgranulin family of proinflammatory mediators. Endothelial cells cultured with S100A12 displayed RAGE-dependent expression of VCAM-1 and tissue factor. Mononuclear phagocytes displayed S100A12-RAGE chemotaxis, expression of tissue factor, and elaborated IL-1 and TNF-α. In vivo studies of delayed-type hypersensitivity demonstrated reduced inflammatory response when mice were treated with anti-RAGE F(ab′)2, anti-S100 F(ab′)2, or soluble RAGE. Treated animals also displayed reduced NF-κB activation and IL-1 and TNF-α expression.[236]

The angiopathy of diabetes is thought to be consequent to inflammatory processes generated by elevated glucose concentrations. Hyperglycemia has been demonstrated to activate numerous signaling cascades. One process that might mediate these effects is through the nonenzymatic formation of AGEs.[95,235,236] AGE–RAGE interactions on endothelium lead to the expression of procoagulant tissue factor and VCAM-1 and macrophage-released tissue factor. Animals treated with soluble RAGE showed decreases in atherosclerotic lesion area and number and a marked reduction in lesion complexity. Also, treated animals had reduced expression of adhesion molecules, tissue factor, MCP-1, and matrix metalloproteinases.[95,235,236]

CD91

The immunologic properties of HSPs were discovered by their ability to elicit antitumor immunity. It was later discovered that this antigenic specificity was determined by the peptides they chaperoned. APCs can bind and internalize HSP–peptide complexes derived from virus-infected cells or tumors and represent them on MHC class I molecules. In addition, APC engagement of HSP–peptide complexes induces maturation, the expression of costimulatory molecules, and the induction and release of cytokines (TNF-α, IL-1, IL-12, IL-6, GM-CSF, MIP-1, RANTES, and NO).[237,238]

CD91 had been identified as a receptor for the serum protein α_2-macroglobulin, a natural protease inhibitor that, like HSPs, is found across many species. In fact, α_2-macroglobulin is the evolutionary precursor of the C3 complement component. By binding pathogen proteases utilized during invasion and shuttling them for endocytosis, α_2-macroglobulin hinders pathogen invasion.[237,239]

However, such a method of host defense would be ineffective for intracellular pathogens that gain access by alternative means, such as mimicking host proteins and developing ligands for host receptors. Hence, another method of signaling danger is necessary. It is currently thought that upon cell death, HSPs contained within the cell transfer information regarding the infected intracellular environment to CD91. This large cell surface receptor, complexed with the HSPs, is internalized and delivers antigen into the classical MHC class I pathway. The MHCs bind and present them to $CD8^+$ T cells. On recognizing nonself, T cells are induced to proliferate and mediate killing. This mechanism could be generalized to implicate CD91 and HSP interactions in the recognition of all cellular stress that culminates in injury and death.[239]

CD91 was first identified by Binder et al. as the receptor for Gp96 and then by Basu et al. as a common receptor for other HSPs (HSP70, HSP90, and calreticulin).[240,241] This large multidomain 600-kD protein possesses multiple binding sites for at least 32 ligands. The binding of this receptor to many members of the HSP family has been corroborated by several independent functional and structural studies.[239]

Several in vivo studies suggest a physiologic relevance for HSP–CD91 interaction. Mice immunized with tumor-derived Gp96–peptide complexes reject a subsequent tumor challenge. If CD91 antiserum is mixed with the HSP-peptide inoculum, the mice fail to reject the tumors. Binder et al. noted that blocking of CD91 completely inhibits the phenomenon of re-presentation of peptides that are carried or chaperoned by HSPs, suggesting that not only is CD91 a receptor for HSPs, but it may also be the sole receptor involved in antigen re-presenting.[238,241]

HSPs have been shown to chaperone antigenic peptides (tumor, viral, minor histocompatibility antigens) from all cellular compartments. The HSPs thus appear to be a universal mechanism for antigen capture, and they permit a high-efficiency antigen uptake through a receptor-mediated mechanism.

Evidence that HSP–peptide–CD91 interactions serve to signal cellular stress is beginning to culminate. Basu et al. demonstrated that HSP70, HSP90, Gp96, and calreticulin are released from cells as a result of necrotic cell death, but not apoptotic cell death.[240] Similarly, Melcher et al. reported that tumor cells undergoing necrotic death are highly immunogenic as compared to those undergoing apoptotic death.[242] Actual necrosis may be unnecessary as stressed cells and cancer cells have been reported to express cell surface HSP molecules, which may activate APCs. Zheng et al. observed that physical contact of tumor cells artificially engineered to express cell surface HSPs with immature DCs elicits a powerful maturation of DCs.[243]

Other Heat Shock Protein Receptors. CD40 was reported as a receptor for HSP70 when anti-CD40 antibodies were observed to inhibit macrophage chemokine secretion in response to mycobacterial HSP70. Subsequently, Becker et al. noted the association of recombinant GST-tagged CD40 with murine HSP70.[244,245] They further demonstrated enhanced binding after the APCs were stimulated with LPS. As LPS induces expression of a number of cell surface molecules, the authors concluded that CD40 mediates recognition and binding of HSP70.[246]

CD36 has been implicated as a receptor for Gp96. Transfection of CD36 into CD36-negative cells has been shown to enhance Gp96 binding. In addition, $CD36^{-/-}$ macrophages have a 52% reduction in Gp96 binding compared with wild-type controls, suggesting some role for CD36 as an HSP receptor.[246]

LOX-1, a member of the same scavenger superfamily as CD91 and CD36, has been postulated to be an additional receptor for endocytic uptake of HSP70 and chaperoned peptides by human DCs. Anti–LOX-1 antibodies and LOX-1 ligand-acetylated albumin competed with HSP70 for binding to DCs.[113]

Both TLRs and CD14 have been implicated as receptors for HSPs, such as HSP70.[247] HSP70 stimulates macrophage IL-12p40 production that is partially abrogated by inhibiting downstream TLR signaling cascades. In addition, human HSP60 activated NF-κB and TNF-α production by 293 T cells transfected with either TLR-2 or TLR-4 and MD-2.[248] HSP60 also activated JNK and IKK signaling and TNF-α production by macrophages, an effect that was partially eliminated by knocking out MyD88 or TRAF6. Similar functional studies have proposed that CD14 might serve as an HSP70 receptor in APCs. All of these studies heavily suggest a role of TLRs or CD14 in HSP binding, although several investigators call into question the potential for contamination with LPS to be mediating much of these effects.[246]

The Stress Response

The stress response is the cellular reaction to any external perturbation or disruption in equilibrium and serves to restore homeostasis. It is often referred to as the heat-shock response after the identification in the 1960s of a group of genes expressed after exposure to heat, the heat-shock proteins (supra vide).[249] However, subsequent investigations delineated additional cellular proteins that were expressed in response to a wide variety of insults. Inducers of the stress response include physical stresses (burns, radiation, trauma), chemical agents and mediators (toxins, heavy metals, cytokines, ROS), infectious agents (bacteria, viruses, parasites), and allergens. Clinically, expression of HSP has been observed under conditions in which oxygen delivery is compromised, as in hemorrhage or ischemia.[250]

Activation of the stress response is characterized by both morphologic and metabolic cellular alterations. Morphologic alterations include the accumulation of unprocessed forms of mRNA in the nucleolus and increased numbers of actin microfilaments in the cytoplasm. Changes in cellular metabolism include a rapid reduction in intracellular ATP levels, most likely correlated with alterations in the integrity of mitochondria. The stress response is characterized by transient downregulation of most cellular products and by the upregulation of stress proteins.[251] It is the induction of stress proteins that confers the primary adaptive and protective effects of the stress response. After expression of stress genes, cells become resistant to subsequent stresses. Members of the stress protein family include heme oxygenase (supra vide); the multiple-drug resistance gene product or P-glycoprotein, ubiquitin, involved in targeting proteins for degradation; scavengers such as superoxide dismutase, ferritin, and metallothioneins; and the glycolytic enzymes enolase and glyceraldehyde 3-phosphate dehydrogenase. The most extensively characterized are the HSPs.[39]

Heat-shock proteins are molecular chaperones that may either be constitutively expressed or induced upon cellular stress.[252] Classification is based on their molecular mass and degree of homology. The most extensively studied is the HSP70 family, members of which possess a mean molecular mass of 70 kD and greater than 70% homology. Members of the HSP70 family bind ATP, and under conditions of energy depletion the stress response is induced. HSP70 is integral in cellular adaptation to and survival during environmental stresses. Both HSP72 and HSP73 are present in the cytosol and nucleus; the former is constitutively expressed, whereas expression of HSP72 is exclusively induced after stress. In most studies HSP72 is used as a marker of HSP induction.[39,250,253,254]

The HSP60 family members are also referred to as chaperones. The glucose-regulated protein group of HSP is induced with glucose starvation, inhibitors of N-glycosylation, and calcium ionophores. The decrease in glucose content may affect the pool of sugar donors during protein glycosylation. The low-molecular-weight HSPs (molecular masses of 20 to 30 kD) may be important regulatory components of the actin-based cytoskeleton.[250]

Transcription is mediated by the activation of heat-shock elements in the gene promoters. Two heat-shock transcriptional factors (HSFs) have been identified: HSF1 and HSF2. HSF1 activates transcription of the HSP72 gene in response to heat, heavy metals, and other inducers of the stress response. With stimulation, unbound HSF1 oligomerizes, translocates to the nucleus, and binds to the HSP promoter to activate the transcription of the gene. HSF2 is not activated by the classic inducers of heat-shock genes but may be important in controlling the activities of HSP gene expression in the normal or unstressed cell.[39,250,253,254]

HSP can play multiple roles in modulating the inflammatory response. A number of inflammatory states such as rheumatoid arthritis, ARDS, and asthma have been shown to benefit experimentally from increased HSP expression.[249–251,254] Functions of HSP during inflammation include enhancement of immune responses, thermotolerance, regulation of apoptosis, hemostasis, and cytoprotection against ROS and other inflammatory mediators. HSP–CD91 interaction is integral to the processing and representation of antigen by APCs. HSP may shift the balance between T_H1 and T_H2 toward an increase in more anti-inflammatory T_H2 cells. ROS, including H_2O_2, hydroxyl radical, and peroxynitrite, activate HSP synthesis. In the presence of iron, ROS also induce the oxidation-specific stress protein heme oxygenase or ferritin, proteins contributing protection against oxidative stress by binding iron and preventing it from participating in the Fenton reaction. Mechanisms of HSP-mediated cytoprotection from the toxic effects of ROS include the maintenance of cellular GSH levels (HSP27) and mitochondrial protection (HSP70). Hence, ROS induce a cytoprotective response that counteracts their own toxicity. Other inflammatory mediators such as NO have also been shown to induce expression of HSP.[39]

HSP may participate in intracellular signaling pathways that modulate the production or function of inflammatory mediators. For example, HSP90 has been shown to facilitate signaling that leads to NO formation by eNOS.[255] HSP70 has been reported to prevent apoptosis, which may promote propagation rather than resolution of inflammation. In addition, the body's immune response to bacterial and parasitic stress proteins likely protects the host from infection. The bacterial homologue of HSP60, GroEL, is a major target of the mammalian humoral response to bacterial infections. Many activators of HSF1 are potent inhibitors of the proinflammatory transcription factor NF-κB. Aspirin and other NSAIDs activate HSF while inhibiting NF-κB. Therefore, the anti-inflammatory effects associated with the stress response might be related more to the inhibition of NF-κB activation.[250,256]

The Acute-phase Response

The acute-phase response consequent to trauma or cellular injury is characterized by alterations in hepatic metabolism; activation of the central nervous system, leading to fever and adaptive behaviors; altered hematopoiesis; activation of complement and the fibrinolytic and coagulation cascades; and the release of neuropeptides, kinins, and hormones. It is a rapid, nonspecific response that accompanies both acute and chronic inflammatory disorders. Many of the processes induced during the acute-phase response are mediated by cytokines; IL-6, IL-1, and TNF-α play particularly central roles.[257,258] Though considered a defense mechanism promoting host survival, aberrant or unregulated production of many of these inflammatory mediators can be lethal.

Acute-phase Proteins. An acute-phase protein is defined as a protein whose concentration increases by at least 25% during inflammation (Table 6.7).[258,259] These changes are primarily due to altered hepatic synthesis, typically occur within approximately 6 hours of the inciting stimulus, and function to restore homeostasis. These functions include hemostatic functions (fibrinogen), microbicidal and phagocytic functions (complement components, C-reactive protein), antithrombotic properties (plasminogen, protein S), antioxidant properties (haptoglobin), and antiproteolytic actions (α_2-macroglobulin, α_1-protease, α_1-chymotrypsin). The negative acute-phase proteins albumin, prealbumin, transferrin, and retinol-binding protein decrease by at least 25%. Levels of the negative acute-phase proteins albumin and transferrin drop almost immediately after operation and remain depressed for several days. The rapid initial loss of these proteins is likely due to increased vascular permeability and loss to the extravascular space. The magnitude of the response is proportional to the severity of the stress and is specific to the genetic composition of the patient. Whereas trauma and burns lead to significant increases in acute-phase reactants, exercise and psychiatric illness induce more moderate responses.

The two major acute-phase proteins in humans are C-reactive protein (CRP) and serum amyloid A (SAA). CRP, named because of its reaction with pneumococcal C-polysaccharide, displays both proinflammatory and anti-inflammatory effects. It has been shown to activate complement, recognize foreign pathogens, bind phagocytic cells, and enhance activation of tissue factor, the main initiator of coagulation. CRP can also inhibit superoxide production by neutrophils and inhibit neutrophil adhesion by decreasing surface expression of L-selectin. Changes in plasma or serum CRP, although nonspecific, may reflect the magnitude of an inflammatory process and may aid the differentiation of inflammatory from noninflammatory conditions. Measurement of CRP is more precise than the erythrocyte sedimentation rate (ESR), which largely depends on plasma fibrinogen levels and is influenced by a variety of other, unrelated factors in the circulation. SAA may affect cholesterol metabolism and promote chemotaxis and adhesion of phagocytes during inflammation.[39]

C1 inhibitor is of special interest as an acute-phase protein because of its effects outside of the complement cascade. This antiprotease inhibits the activity of Hageman factor, limiting kinin production and factor XI production. Thus, enhanced expression of a complement inhibitor protein during the acute phase influences such diverse processes as the coagulation, fibrinolysis, and kinin pathways.

Systemic Manifestations of the Acute-phase Response. Systemic manifestations include neuroendocrine changes, shifts in the hematologic profile, and metabolic and chemical alterations. The classic neuroendocrine manifestation is fever. IL-1, IL-6, and TNF-α mediate the fever response by resetting the hypothalamic temperature set point through the synthesis of PGE_2. The secretion of neuropeptides such as CRH and AVP and of hormones such as glucagon, insulin, thyroxin, and aldosterone is also characteristic of the acute-phase response. CRH and AVP released by the hypothalamus increase ACTH and cortisol levels. The rise in plasma cortisol levels occurs rapidly and may function to inhibit the fever response and cytokine gene expression, thereby serving a potential regulatory function in the acute-phase response. Glucocorticoids also stimulate macrocortin synthesis, which by inhibiting synthesis of PLA_2, limits the availability of arachidonic acid for prostaglandin synthesis. Glucocorticoids increase the rate of synthesis of certain acute-phase proteins involved in connective tissue repair and clotting, as well as antioxidants and antiproteinases. They also may function to counteract the hypoglycemic response to insulin overproduction during infection or stress.

Other alterations include a prominent leukocytosis, thrombocytosis, and the "anemia of chronic disease." Metabolic changes include altered lipid metabolism and negative nitrogen balance. Changes in the chemical and enzymatic profile include increased hepatic production of metallothionein, iNOS, heme oxygenase, manganese superoxide dismutase, and GSH. Plasma levels of zinc and iron are noted to drop, whereas copper levels increase slightly. This persists for the duration of inflammation and is likely due to sequestration induced by IL-6, glucocorticoids, and catecholamines. Low levels of iron and zinc may confer protective antimicrobial effects because they are essential for microbial growth.[39]

Mediators of the Acute-phase Response. Bacterial products such as LPS are probably the most potent activators of tissue macrophages, the initiators of the acute-phase response. LPS, through its interactions with LPS-binding protein, CD14, and Toll-like receptors, induces macrophage synthesis of ROS, including NO; lipid derivatives such as PGE_2, thromboxane A_2, and PAF; and acute-phase cytokines. The primary signals inducing synthesis of acute-phase cytokines in the absence of bacterial infection may be free radicals, prostaglandins, or modified proteins acting like foreign materials.[39]

Acute-phase cytokines can be proinflammatory (IL-1, TNF-α, IFN-γ, IL-8) or anti-inflammatory (IL-10, IL-4, IL-13, TNF-β). However, it is IL-6– and IL-6–type cytokines that are most critical in the acute-phase response. IL-6 is the major inducer of acute-phase protein synthesis and, together with IL-1 and TNF-α, is responsible for the systemic features classically associated with the acute-phase response (fever, anorexia, leukocytosis, and hormonal changes).[39]

In addition to the aforementioned cytokines, IFN-γ is a potent inducer of complement components. The anti-inflammatory cytokine TGF-β stimulates synthesis of antiproteases, urokinase, and negative acute-phase proteins. IL-4 is inhibitory to some acute-phase proteins. Growth factors, including hepatocyte growth factor and TGF-β, are also able to modulate the synthesis of acute-phase proteins. Glucocorticoids augment the response to cytokines, and insulin attenuates the cytokine-induced rise in acute-phase proteins.[39]

Effects of the cytokines are influenced by cytokine receptors, receptor antagonists, and hormones. IL-1RA competes with IL-1 and attenuates the acute-phase response in vivo. Soluble receptors for IL-1 and TNF-α act as antagonists. In contrast, soluble receptors for IL-6 act as agonists.

Regulation of Acute-phase Cytokines and Proteins. Several major families of transcription factors participate in the upregulation of acute-phase cytokines and proteins, the most important being NF-IL-6, AP-1, and NF-κB.[260] NF-IL6 participates in the induced expression of the cytokines IL-1, TNF-α, IL-6, and IL-8, among others. Activation of cytokine gene expression by NF-κB is probably the most important pathway. The triggering of IL-6 in monocytes in vitro by IFN-γ involves a change in the amount of the phosphorylated transcription factor Sp1, together with the induction and activation of IFN-regulatory factor.

All known acute-phase proteins are regulated primarily at the transcriptional level. Activation of TNF-α and IL-1 receptors triggers signaling pathways that activate transcription factors AP-1 and NF-κB. Many type I acute-phase protein genes contain response elements for NF-κB, NF-IL-6, and AP-1. Acute-phase protein responses to IL-6 are mediated through the JAK/STAT signal transduction pathway. In addition, both IL-1 and IL-6 signal transduction mechanisms activate the MAPK pathway that activates transcription factor NF-IL-6, linking the IL-1 and IL-6 pathways.

Reperfusion Injury

Prolonged tissue ischemia produces irreversible injury and cell death. Timely restoration of perfusion may salvage some tissue, though paradoxically can induce injury as well. Reperfusion injury is the damage caused by the restoration of blood flow in previously ischemic tissue (i.e., myocardial ischemia, transplantation, vascular surgery). Injury is the direct consequence of activation of the inflammatory response, especially complement activation and neutrophil recruitment. Components of the complement cascade promote tissue damage through the generation of anaphylatoxins and by the formation of the MAC. Invading neutrophils injure tissue through the generation of ROS and the release of proteolytic enzymes. Recent evidence points to TLR4 as a sensor of tissue stress probably through the release of DAMPs from ischemic cells.[32] TLR4 stimulation leads to the activation of local and systemic inflammation in both warm and cold reperfusion. This inflammation contributes to tissue damage in this setting.

Alterations in the microvascular endothelium are central to the pathophysiologic process of reperfusion injury. Early loss of constitutive NO production facilitates neutrophil adherence and the upregulation of cell adhesion molecules such as P-selectin, and inhibits vasorelaxation and perfusion.[261] Low oxygen tension induces the conversion of xanthine dehydrogenase to xanthine oxidase. Reperfusion and reoxygenation yield the formation of superoxide anion and H_2O_2 and induce oxidant injury. Neutrophils and other cellular effectors are progressively recruited and activated, releasing ROS, cytokines, and NO, further contributing to increased vascular permeability and tissue injury. PAF released by neutrophils activates circulating platelets and promotes vascular plugging. Platelets also release factors that enhance platelet–neutrophil adhesion. Both cell types also release vasoconstricting agents that can further exacerbate no-reflow. Capillary plugging by neutrophils and platelets can impair local blood flow and cause the "no-reflow phenomenon."[39]

Neutrophils mediate direct toxicity to the surrounding tissue through the elaboration of ROS and granule contents. Peroxynitrite formed by the reaction of NO and superoxide can contribute directly to tissue injury during reperfusion. Neutrophil granule proteases such as elastase, collagenase, and gelatinase alter the vascular permeability and are highly destructive to local tissue. The significance of the neutrophil in mediating these effects is apparent in neutrophil depletion studies demonstrating attenuated tissue injury compared with subjects with normal numbers of neutrophils.[262] Animal studies using blocking monoclonal antibodies to selectins and β_2 integrins show improved organ function ischemia/reperfusion.[263]

The mechanism by which complement is activated with reperfusion is not completely understood. Ischemia may alter the cell's plasma membrane or through the exposure of basement membrane or subcellular organelle components, creating a complement-activating surface. Alternatively, binding of natural antibody may lead to induction of these cascades.[171] Complement activation has been shown to occur in the setting of therapeutic thrombolysis. The generation of plasmin-dependent fibrinolytic agents and plasmin after tissue plasminogen activator administration has been associated with complement activation.[264]

Anaphylatoxins are important effectors of complement-mediated injury. They alter vascular permeability and induce smooth muscle cell contraction and the release of histamine from mast cells and basophils. C3a and C5a are potent chemoattractants especially for neutrophils. C5 can be activated by oxygen free radicals, which are abundant. The subsequent generation of the MAC perturbs the maintenance of vital ion gradients, induces cell lysis, and facilitates neutrophil recruitment. In addition, it can induce the expression of numerous inflammatory mediators, including cytokines (TNF-α, IL-1, IL-8), ROS, prostaglandins, leukotrienes, and cell surface adhesion molecules.[265]

Systemic Inflammatory Response Syndrome

The inability of host defenses to control a localized inflammatory process or an unchecked inflammatory response can results in SIRS. A recent consensus conference defined SIRS as the presence of any two of the following physiologic parameters: (a) a temperature greater than 38°C or less than 36°C; (b) leukocytosis (>12,000), leukopenia (<4,000), or more than 10% bands; (c) pulse greater than 90 beats per minute; and (d) tachypnea (respiratory rate >20 or $PaCO_2$ <32 mmHg).[266] Infection underlies a significant minority of cases as a third of patients with SIRS will have a documented infection and meet the criteria for sepsis. There is a continuum from the development of SIRS to sepsis, severe sepsis, septic shock, and MODS.[267] The outcome depends on the balance between SIRS and host compensatory mechanisms. In one prospective study, 26% of patients with SIRS developed sepsis and 7% died.[268]

SIRS may be initiated by infectious or noninfectious causes, such as trauma, autoimmune reactions, or pancreatitis. Gram-negative organisms, rich in LPS, induce a potent inflammatory response mediated through the CD14/TLR4/MyD88 pathway previously described and account for the majority of infectious SIRS cases. Gram-positive organisms can generate a similarly impressive degree of inflammation either through TLR2 or alternative mechanisms; streptococcal superantigen may induce a global and nonspecific activation of T cells that culminates in massive systemic elaboration of cytokines and cardiovascular collapse termed *toxic shock syndrome*. Trauma, either through tissue injury (HMGB1–RAGE, HSP–CD91) or the ischemia/reperfusion consequent to hemorrhage, can culminate in inflammatory pathophysiology indistinguishable from that accompanying these other inflammatory states. As evidence continues to grow, we are replacing the former concept that these stimuli possess individual receptor-signaling mechanisms with one that emphasizes the similarities and integration. Though there are clearly mechanisms by which the host distinguishes normal self from endogenous (trauma) and exogenous (infection) dangers, there is considerable overlap in the receptors utilized and all stimuli appear to converge upon signaling mechanisms in attaining the goal of preserving the host.

The development of SIRS has been described as progressing through three stages: stage I, local cytokine production recruits inflammatory cells to the injured site; stage II, an acute-phase response is initiated and small quantities of cytokines are released into the circulation to enhance the local response; and stage III, homeostasis cannot be reestablished.[269] Enhanced levels of CRP, the major acute-phase protein in humans, occur in SIRS/sepsis, and clinical resolution is preceded by a drop in CRP levels.

The elaboration of proinflammatory cytokines (IL-1, TNF-α, and IL-6) is central to the pathogenesis of SIRS regardless of the initiating stimulus. Their elaboration triggers increased expression of adhesion molecules, leukocyte recruitment, and the production of secondary proinflammatory mediators, such as chemokines. Endotoxin, or LPS, is one of the most powerful triggers of SIRS. LPS activates the complement and coagulation cascades, induces endothelial cell activation, and increases TNF-α and IL-1 synthesis and the late release of HMGB1. However, noninfectious tissue injury induces a similar inflammatory response. LPS, TNF-α, and IL-1 also induce increased production of NO by iNOS in macrophages and other inflammatory cells. PGI_2, along with other metabolites or arachidonic acid, together with NO contributes to decreased systemic vascular resistance and hypotension. Autocrine and paracrine NO production also results in myocardial depression. Increased vascular permeability promotes extravasation of fluid and edema formation. Activated endothelial cells express tissue factor, PECAM, and TXA_2, which promote a procoagulant local environment that predisposes to microthrombi formation. Adherent leukocytes further exacerbate organ injury by mechanically impeding microvascular blood flow and by damaging the endothelial cells and surrounding connective tissue. The results are end-organ hypoperfusion, inadequate oxygen delivery, initiation of anaerobic metabolism, and end-organ failure. The metabolic and nutritional sequelae of this activated cytokine milieu includes fever, catabolism, cachexia, and altered fat, glucose, and trace mineral metabolism.

SIRS is counteracted by the concomitant induction of an anti-inflammatory response termed the *compensatory anti-inflammatory response syndrome* (CARS).[269] Many of the proinflammatory mediators that participate in SIRS modulate the immune function of lymphocytes and mononuclear cells. Proinflammatory mediators can inhibit their own synthesis or enhance the synthesis of natural antagonists by negative feedback mechanisms. Thus, at any given time, the clinical manifestation is SIRS, CARS, or an intermediate, mixed inflammatory response syndrome. The spectrum of features that characterize these syndromes has been termed *CHAOS* (cardiovascular shock, homeostasis, apoptosis, organ dysfunction, and immune suppression). Studies employing a variety of specific anticytokine agents have failed to observe an improvement in the outcome of patients with SIRS or sepsis. However, two studies of immunomodulation have noted significant effects in septic populations. The PROWESS study of activated protein C underscores the importance of the coagulation cascade during inflammation. This randomized controlled trial noted a 19.6% relative reduction and a 6.1% absolute reduction in mortality for those patients with severe sepsis who received activated protein C.[270] Another study used a combination of corticosteroid and mineralocorticoid replacement for those patients with sepsis who had relative adrenal insufficiency as defined by a less than 10 unit increase in cortisol after a Cortrosyn stimulation test. They documented a 33% related reduction and 10% absolute reduction in the risk of death for those patients who received steroids.[271]

Chronic Inflammation

There are no clear boundaries between an acute and a chronic inflammatory response. In general, if the source of an acute inflammatory process is incompletely eliminated, a state of chronic inflammation eventually ensues. Chronicity is usually not characterized by the signs classically associated with acute responses, such as swelling, heat, or redness. Pain is minimal if not absent. Microscopically, a mononuclear cell infiltrate predominates (lymphocytes, monocytes, plasma cells) with proliferation of fibroblasts and vascular elements.

Many agents can create a state of chronic inflammation, including persistent infectious agents, remnants of dead organisms, foreign bodies, and metabolic byproducts. Ultimately, chronicity of inflammation is a result of the immune response to a persistent antigen. Furthermore, a chronic inflammatory response can develop in the absence of a preceding acute response, such as infections with agents of low toxicity such as mycobacterium and treponema. $CD4^+$ T cells and macrophages are the primary cellular orchestrators of the chronic inflammatory response.[272] T_H1 cell-mediated immunity (CMI) responses are protective against most microbes and usually result in the elimination of the pathogen. If the microbe persists, the ongoing T_H1 response results in inflammatory tissue injury. Cytokines and growth factors released by T lymphocytes and macrophages stimulate proliferative responses. Neutrophils and eosinophils contribute to the release of proteolytic enzymes and oxygen derivatives. Eosinophilia occurs with chronic parasitic infections and hypersensitivity conditions. Fibroblasts are actively recruited by chemoattractants such as fibrin, collagens, and cytokines. Local IL-1 stimulates fibroblast proliferation and collagen production. Irreversible tissue damage can occur through the replacement of normal parenchyma with fibrous connective tissue. Fibroblasts can release metalloproteinases that degrade normal tissue, further contributing to tissue destruction. Mast cells are elevated in chronic conditions and may play a part in cell-mediated immune responses. Inflammatory cyst formation may occur as a result of epithelial hyperplasia.

References

1. Cotran RS. Inflammation: historical perspectives. In: Gallin J, Snyderman R, eds. *Inflammation: Basic Principles and Clinical Correlates*, 3rd ed. Philadelphia, PA: Lippincott Williams & Wilkins; 1999.
2. Heifets L. Centennial of Metchnikoff's discovery. *J Reticuloendothel Soc* 1982;31(5):381–391.
3. Cotran RS, Kumar V, Robbins T, eds. *Robbins Pathologic Basis of Disease*, 6th ed. Philadelphia: WB Sanders; 1999.
4. Abbas AK, Lichtman AH. *Cellular and Molecular Immunology*, 5th ed. Philadelphia, PA: Saunders; 2003.
5. Wheeler JG, Abramson JS. The neutrophil. Oxford, England: IRL Press at Oxford University Press; 1993.
6. Bainton D. The cells of inflammation: a general view. In: Weissmann G, ed. *The Cell Biology of Inflammation,* vol. 2. New York: Elsevier/North-Holland; 1980.
7. Dancey JT, Deubelbeiss KA, Harker LA, et al. Neutrophil kinetics in man. *J Clin Invest* 1976;58(3):705–715.
8. Omann GM, Hinshaw DB. Inflammation. In: Greenfield LJ, et al. eds. *Surgery: Scientific Principles and Practice*, 2nd ed. Philadelphia: Lippincott-Raven; 1997:130–159.
9. Trowbridge H, Emling R. In: Trowbridge HO, Emling RC, eds. *Inflammation: A Review of the Process*. Chicago, IL: Quintessence; 1997.
10. Dustin ML, Springer TA. Role of lymphocyte adhesion receptors in transient interactions and cell locomotion. *Annu Rev Immunol* 1991;9:27–66.
11. Kansas GS. Selectins and their ligands: current concepts and controversies. *Blood* 1996;88(9):3259–3287.
12. Tedder TF, Steeber DA, Chen A, et al. The selectins: vascular adhesion molecules. *FASEB J* 1995;9(10):866–873.
13. Frenette PS, Wagner DD. Adhesion molecules–part II: blood vessels and blood cells. *N Engl J Med* 1996;335(1):43–45.
14. Frenette PS, Wagner DD. Adhesion molecules–part 1. *N Engl J Med* 1996; 334(23):1526–1529.
15. Hynes RO. Integrins: versatility, modulation, and signaling in cell adhesion. *Cell* 1992;69(1):11–25.
16. Muller WA. Leukocyte-endothelial-cell interactions in leukocyte transmigration and the inflammatory response. *Trends Immunol* 2003;24(6): 327–334.
17. Vaporciyan AA, DeLisser HM, Yan HC, et al. Involvement of platelet-endothelial cell adhesion molecule-1 in neutrophil recruitment in vivo. *Science* 1993;262(5139):1580–1582.
18. Thornhill M, Haskard D. Leukocyte adhesion to endothelium. In: Horton M, ed. *Blood Cell Biochemistry. Macrophages and Related Cells,* vol. 5. New York: Plenum Press; 1993.
19. Rot A. The role of leukocyte chemotaxis in inflammation. In: Whicker J, Evans S, eds. *Biochemistry and Inflammation*. Boston, MA: Kluwer Academic; 1992.
20. Wagner JG, Roth RA. Neutrophil migration during endotoxemia. *J Leukoc Biol* 1999;66(1):10–24.
21. Indik ZK, Park JG, Hunter S, et al. Structure/function relationships of Fc gamma receptors in phagocytosis. *Semin Immunol* 1995;7(1):45–54.
22. Ezekowitz R. The mannose receptor and phagocytosis. In: Furth RV, ed. *Mononuclear Phagocytes: Biology of Monocytes and Macrophages*. Boston, MA: Kluwer Academic; 1992.
23. Ezekowitz RA, Sim RB, Hill M, et al. Local opsonization by secreted macrophage complement components. Role of receptors for complement in uptake of zymosan. *J Exp Med* 1984;159(1):244–260.
24. Lee WL, Harrison RE, Grinstein S. Phagocytosis by neutrophils. *Microbes Infect* 2003;5(14):1299–1306.
25. Zychlinsky A, Weinrauch Y, Weiss J. Introduction: forum in immunology on neutrophils. *Microbes Infect* 2003;5(14):1289–1291.
26. Borregaard N, Cowland JB. Granules of the human neutrophilic polymorphonuclear leukocyte. *Blood* 1997;89(10):3503–3521.
27. Faurschou M, Borregaard N. Neutrophil granules and secretory vesicles in inflammation. *Microbes Infect* 2003;5(14):1317–1327.
28. Lehrer RI, Ganz T, Selsted ME. Defensins: endogenous antibiotic peptides of animal cells. *Cell* 1991;64(2):229–230.
29. Elsbach P. The bactericidal/permeability-increasing protein (BPI) in antibacterial host defense. *J Leukoc Biol* 1998;64(1):14–18.
30. Beamer LJ, Carroll SF, Eisenberg D. The BPI/LBP family of proteins: a structural analysis of conserved regions. *Protein Sci* 1998;7(4):906–914.
31. Gabay JE, Scott RW, Campanelli D, et al. Antibiotic proteins of human polymorphonuclear leukocytes. *Proc Natl Acad Sci U S A* 1989;86(14): 5610–5614.
32. Tsung A, Klune JR, Zhang X, et al. HMGB1 release induced by liver ischemia involves Toll-like receptor 4 dependent reactive oxygen species production and calcium-mediated signaling. *J Exp Med* 2007;204(12): 2913–2923.
33. Chapple IL. Reactive oxygen species and antioxidants in inflammatory diseases. *J Clin Periodontol* 1997;24(5):287–296.
34. Kasahara Y, Iwai K, Yachie A, et al. Involvement of reactive oxygen intermediates in spontaneous and CD95 (Fas/APO-1)-mediated apoptosis of neutrophils. *Blood* 1997;89(5):1748–1753.
35. Roos D, van Bruggen R, Meischl C. Oxidative killing of microbes by neutrophils. *Microbes Infect* 2003;5(14):1307–1315.
36. Nordberg J, Arner ES. Reactive oxygen species, antioxidants, and the mammalian thioredoxin system. *Free Radic Biol Med* 2001;31(11): 1287–1312.
37. Winyard PG, Perret D, Harris G, et al. The role of toxic oxygen species in inflammation with special reference to DNA damage. In: Whicker JT, Evans SW, eds. *Biochemistry of Inflammation*. Boston, MA: Kluwer Academic; 1992.
38. Nohl H. Generation of superoxide radicals as byproduct of cellular respiration. *Ann Biol Clin (Paris)* 1994;52(3):199–204.
39. Schuchert RD, Billiar TR. Inflammation. In: Greenfield LJ, ed. *Surgery: Scientific Principles and Practice*, 3rd ed. Philadelphia, PA: Lippincott Williams & Wilkins; 2001.
40. Menshikova EV, Salama G. Cardiac ischemia oxidizes regulatory thiols on ryanodine receptors: captopril acts as a reducing agent to improve Ca2+ uptake by ischemic sarcoplasmic reticulum. *J Cardiovasc Pharmacol* 2000; 36(5):656–668.
41. Szabo C. The pathophysiological role of peroxynitrite in shock, inflammation, and ischemia-reperfusion injury. *Shock* 1996;6(2):79–88.
42. Warren J, Ward P, Johnson K. Oxygen radicals as mediators of inflammation. In: H PM, and M RC, eds. *Handbook of Inflammation*, vol. 6. New York: Elsevier Science Publishers BV; 1989.
43. Burg ND, Pillinger MH. The neutrophil: function and regulation in innate and humoral immunity. *Clin Immunol* 2001;99(1):7–17.
44. Marenzi G, Assanelli E, Marana I, et al. N-acetylcysteine and contrast-induced nephropathy in primary angioplasty. *N Engl J Med* 2006;354(26): 2773–2782.
45. Kobayashi SD, Voyich JM, DeLeo FR. Regulation of the neutrophil-mediated inflammatory response to infection. *Microbes Infect* 2003;5(14): 1337–1344.
46. Burkitt HG, Young B, Heath JW. In: Burkitt HG, Young B, Heath JW, eds. *Wheater's Functional Histology: A Text and Colour Atlas*, 3rd ed. Edinburgh, UK: 1993.
47. Ma J, Chen T, Mandelin J, et al. Regulation of macrophage activation. *Cell Mol Life Sci* 2003;60(11):2334–2346.
48. Ben-Baruch A, Michiel DF, Oppenheim JJ. Signals and receptors involved in recruitment of inflammatory cells. *J Biol Chem* 1995;270(20): 11703–11706.
49. Kuijpers T, Hakkert B, Knol E, et al. Membrane surface antigen expression on human monocytes: changes during purification, in vitro activation and transmigration across monolayers of endothelial cells. In: Furth RV, ed. *Mononuclear Phagocytes: Biology of Monocytes and Macrophages*. Boston, MA: Kluwer Academic; 1992.
50. Nathan C, Xie QW. Nitric oxide synthases: roles, tolls, and controls. *Cell* 1994;78(6):915–918.
51. de Waal Malefyt R, Yssel H, Roncarolo MG, et al. Interleukin-10. *Curr Opin Immunol* 1992;4(3):314–320.
52. MacMicking J, Xie QW, Nathan C. Nitric oxide and macrophage function. *Annu Rev Immunol* 1997;15:323–350.
53. Wang H, Yang H, Tracey KJ. Extracellular role of HMGB1 in inflammation and sepsis. *J Intern Med* 2004;255(3):320–331.
54. Wang H, Bloom O, Zhang M, et al. HMG-1 as a late mediator of endotoxin lethality in mice. *Science* 1999;285(5425):248–251.
55. Griffiths GM. The cell biology of CTL killing. *Curr Opin Immunol* 1995; 7(3):343–348.
56. Romagnani S. Understanding the role of Th1/Th2 cells in infection. *Trends Microbiol* 1996;4(12):470–473.
57. Mosmann TR, Coffman RL. TH1 and TH2 cells: different patterns of lymphokine secretion lead to different functional properties. *Annu Rev Immunol* 1989;7:145–173.
58. Lane PJ, Brocker T. Developmental regulation of dendritic cell function. *Curr Opin Immunol* 1999;11(3):308–313.
59. Banchereau J, Steinman RM. Dendritic cells and the control of immunity. *Nature* 1998;392(6673):245–252.
60. Braciale TJ, Morrison LA, Sweetser MT, et al. Antigen presentation pathways to class I and class II MHC-restricted T lymphocytes. *Immunol Rev* 1987;98:95–114.
61. Razi-Wolf Z, Freeman GJ, Galvin F, et al. Expression and function of the murine B7 antigen, the major costimulatory molecule expressed by peritoneal exudate cells. *Proc Natl Acad Sci U S A* 1992;89(9):4210–4214.
62. Lanzavecchia A. Receptor-mediated antigen uptake and its effect on antigen presentation to class II-restricted T lymphocytes. *Annu Rev Immunol* 1990;8:773–793.
63. Gumperz JE, Parham P. The enigma of the natural killer cell. *Nature* 1995;378(6554):245–248.
64. Janeway C, Travers P. Immunobiology: the immune system in health and disease. In: Janeway C, Travers P, eds. *Immunobiology: The Immune System in Health and Disease*, 3rd ed. 1997.
65. Surh CD, Sprent J. T-cell apoptosis detected in situ during positive and negative selection in the thymus. *Nature* 1994;372(6501):100–103.
66. von Schacky C. Mechanisms of tolerance induction in major histocompatibility complex class II-restricted T cells specific for a blood-borne self-antigen. *J Exp Med* 1994;180(6):2089–2099.
67. Zal T, Volkmann A, Stockinger B. Mechanisms of tolerance induction in major histocompatibility complex class II-restricted T cells specific for a blood-borne self-antigen. *J Exp Med* 1994;180(6):2089–2099.
68. Picker LJ. Control of lymphocyte homing. *Curr Opin Immunol* 1994;6(3): 394–406.

69. Dustin ML, Springer TA. T-cell receptor cross-linking transiently stimulates adhesiveness through LFA-1. *Nature* 1989;341(6243):619–624.
70. Springer TA. Traffic signals for lymphocyte recirculation and leukocyte emigration: the multistep paradigm. *Cell* 1994;76(2):301–314.
71. Janeway CA Jr, Bottomly K. Signals and signs for lymphocyte responses. *Cell* 1994;76(2):275–285.
72. Mosmann TR, Sad S. The expanding universe of T-cell subsets: Th1, Th2 and more. *Immunol Today* 1996;17(3):138–146.
73. Jain J, McCaffrey PG, Miner Z, et al. The T-cell transcription factor NFATp is a substrate for calcineurin and interacts with Fos and Jun. *Nature* 1993;365(6444):352–355.
74. Lee KP, Harlan DM, June CH. Role of co-stimulation in the host response to infection. In: Gallin JI, Snyderman R, eds. *Inflammation: Basic Principles and Clinical Correlates*, 3rd ed. Philadelphia, PA: Lippincott Williams & Wilkins; 1999.
75. Lin MY, Zal T, Ch'en IL, et al. A pivotal role for the multifunctional calcium/calmodulin-dependent protein kinase II in T cells: from activation to unresponsiveness. *J Immunol* 2005;174(9):5583–5592.
76. Broide DH, Hoffman H, Sriramarao P. Genes that regulate eosinophilic inflammation. *Am J Hum Genet* 1999;65(2):302–307.
77. Elsner J, Kapp A. Regulation and modulation of eosinophil effector functions. *Allergy* 1999;54(1):15–26.
78. Weller PF, Bach DS, Austen KF. Biochemical characterization of human eosinophil Charcot-Leyden crystal protein (lysophospholipase). *J Biol Chem* 1984;259(24):15100–15105.
79. Giembycz MA, Lindsay MA. Pharmacology of the eosinophil. *Pharmacol Rev* 1999;51(2):213–340.
80. Slungaard A, Mahoney JR Jr. Thiocyanate is the major substrate for eosinophil peroxidase in physiologic fluids. Implications for cytotoxicity. *J Biol Chem* 1991;266(8):4903–4910.
81. Wardlaw AJ, Moqbel R, Kay AB. Eosinophils: biology and role in disease. *Adv Immunol* 1995;60:151–266.
82. Wedi B, Raap U, Lewrick H, et al. Delayed eosinophil programmed cell death in vitro: a common feature of inhalant allergy and extrinsic and intrinsic atopic dermatitis. *J Allergy Clin Immunol* 1997;100(4):536–543.
83. Valent P, Schmidt G, Besemer J, et al. Interleukin-3 is a differentiation factor for human basophils. *Blood* 1989;73(7):1763–1769.
84. Nilsson G, Cost J, Metcalfke D. Mast cells and basophils. In: Gallin JI, Snyderman R, eds. *Inflammation: Basic Principles and Clinical Correlates*, 3rd ed. Philadelphia, PA: Lippincott Williams & Wilkins; 1999.
85. Metcalfe DD, Baram D, Mekori YA. Mast cells. *Physiol Rev* 1997;77(4):1033–1079.
86. Klinger MH, Jelkmann W. Role of blood platelets in infection and inflammation. *J Interferon Cytokine Res* 2002;22(9):913–922.
87. Marcus A. Platelets: their role in hemostasis, thrombosis, and inflammation. In: Gallin J, Synderman R, eds. *Inflammation: Basic Principles and Clinical Correlates*, 3rd ed. Philadelphia, PA: Lippincott Williams & Wilkins; 1999.
88. Du X, Williams DA. Interleukin-11: review of molecular, cell biology, and clinical use. *Blood* 1997;89(11):3897–3908.
89. Weyrich AS, Lindemann S, Zimmerman GA. The evolving role of platelets in inflammation. *J Thromb Haemost* 2003;1(9):1897–1905.
90. Serhan CN. Lipoxins and novel aspirin-triggered 15-epi-lipoxins (ATL): a jungle of cell-cell interactions or a therapeutic opportunity? *Prostaglandins* 1997;53(2):107–137.
91. Marcus AJ, Safier LB, Ullman HL, et al. Platelet-neutrophil interactions. (12S)-hydroxyeicosatetraen-1,20-dioic acid: a new eicosanoid synthesized by unstimulated neutrophils from (12S)-20-dihydroxyeicosatetraenoic acid. *J Biol Chem* 1988;263(5):2223–2229.
92. Serhan CN, Haeggstrom JZ, Leslie CC. Lipid mediator networks in cell signaling: update and impact of cytokines. *FASEB J* 1996;10(10):1147–1158.
93. Colletti LM, Cytokines. In: Greenfield LJ, ed. *Surgery: Scientific Principles and Practice*, 3rd ed. Philadelphia, PA: Lippincott Williams & Wilkins; 2001.
94. Thomson A. *The Cytokine Handbook*, 3rd ed. New York: Academic Press; 1998.
95. Schmidt AM, Yan SD, Yan SF, et al. The biology of the receptor for advanced glycation end products and its ligands. *Biochim Biophys Acta* 2000;1498(2–3):99–111.
96. Strieter RM, Lynch JP III, Basha MA, et al. Host responses in mediating sepsis and adult respiratory distress syndrome. *Semin Respir Infect* 1990; 5(3):233–247.
97. Opal SM, Patrozou E. Translational research in the development of novel sepsis therapeutics: logical deductive reasoning or mission impossible? *Crit Care Med* 2009;37(1 suppl):S10–S15.
98. Cerami A. Inflammatory cytokines. *Clin Immunol Immunopathol* 1992; 62(1 Pt 2):S3–S10.
99. Bauss F, Droge W, Mannel DN. Tumor necrosis factor mediates endotoxic effects in mice. *Infect Immun* 1987;55(7):1622–1625.
100. Philip R, Epstein LB. Tumour necrosis factor as immunomodulator and mediator of monocyte cytotoxicity induced by itself, gamma-interferon and interleukin-1. *Nature* 1986;323(6083):86–89.
101. Tartaglia LA, Ayres TM, Wong GH, et al. A novel domain within the 55 kd TNF receptor signals cell death. *Cell* 1993;74(5):845–853.
102. Adam-Klages S, Schwandner R, Adam D, et al. Distinct adapter proteins mediate acid versus neutral sphingomyelinase activation through the p55 receptor for tumor necrosis factor. *J Leukoc Biol* 1998;63(6):678–682.
103. Meager A. Cytokine regulation of cellular adhesion molecule expression in inflammation. *Cytokine Growth Factor Rev* 1999;10(1):27–39.
104. Chen G, Li J, Ochani M, et al. Bacterial endotoxin stimulates macrophages to release HMGB1 partly through CD14- and TNF-dependent mechanisms. *J Leukoc Biol* 2004;76(5):994–1001.
105. Kokkola R, Andersson A, Mullins G, et al. RAGE is the major receptor for the proinflammatory activity of HMGB1 in rodent macrophages. *Scand J Immunol* 2005;61(1):1–9.
106. Tracey KJ, Fong Y, Hesse DG, et al. Anti-cachectin/TNF monoclonal antibodies prevent septic shock during lethal bacteraemia. *Nature* 1987; 330(6149):662–664.
107. Tracey KJ, Lowry SF, Cerami A. Cachetin/TNF-alpha in septic shock and septic adult respiratory distress syndrome. *Am Rev Respir Dis* 1988; 138(6):1377–1379.
108. Tracey KJ, Lowry SF, Cerami A. Cachectin/TNF mediates the pathophysiological effects of bacterial endotoxin/lipopolysaccharide (LPS). *Prog Clin Biol Res* 1988;272:77–88.
109. Le J, Vilcek J. Tumor necrosis factor and interleukin 1: cytokines with multiple overlapping biological activities. *Lab Invest* 1987;56(3):234–248.
110. Sims JE, March CJ, Cosman D, et al. cDNA expression cloning of the IL-1 receptor, a member of the immunoglobulin superfamily. *Science* 1988; 241(4865):585–589.
111. Kuno K, Matsushima K. The IL-1 receptor signaling pathway. *J Leukoc Biol* 1994;56(5):542–547.
112. Colotta F, Dower SK, Sims JE, et al. The type II 'decoy' receptor: a novel regulatory pathway for interleukin 1. *Immunol Today* 1994;15(12):562–566.
113. Bevilacqua MP, Schleef RR, Gimbrone MA Jr, et al. Regulation of the fibrinolytic system of cultured human vascular endothelium by interleukin 1. *J Clin Invest* 1986;78(2):587–591.
114. Baggiolini M, Dewald B, Moser B. Human chemokines: an update. *Annu Rev Immunol* 1997;15:675–705.
115. Bacon K, Baggiolini M, Broxmeyer H, et al. Chemokine/chemokine receptor nomenclature. *J Interferon Cytokine Res* 2002;22(10):1067–1068.
116. Bacon KB, Greaves DR, Dairaghi DJ, et al. The expanding universe of C, CX3 C, and CC chemokines. In: Thomson A, ed. *The Cytokine Handbook*, 3rd ed. New York: Academic Press; 1998.
117. Rollins BJ, Chemokines. *Blood* 1997;90(3):909–928.
118. Schall TJ, Bacon KB. Chemokines, leukocyte trafficking, and inflammation. *Curr Opin Immunol* 1994;6(6):865–873.
119. Hebert CA, Vitangcol RV, Baker JB. Scanning mutagenesis of interleukin-8 identifies a cluster of residues required for receptor binding. *J Biol Chem* 1991;266(28):18989–18994.
120. Clark-Lewis I, Dewald B, Geiser T, et al. Platelet factor 4 binds to interleukin 8 receptors and activates neutrophils when its N terminus is modified with Glu-Leu-Arg. *Proc Natl Acad Sci U S A* 1993;90(8):3574–3577.
121. Clark-Lewis I, Kim KS, Rajarathnam K, et al. Structure-activity relationships of chemokines. *J Leukoc Biol* 1995;57(5):703–711.
122. D'Andrea A, Rengaraju M, Valiante NM, et al. Production of natural killer cell stimulatory factor (interleukin 12) by peripheral blood mononuclear cells. *J Exp Med* 1992;176(5):1387–1398.
123. Shu U, Kiniwa M, Wu CY, et al. Activated T cells induce interleukin-12 production by monocytes via CD40-CD40 ligand interaction. *Eur J Immunol* 1995;25(4):1125–1128.
124. Gauldie J, Richards C, Harnish D, et al. Interferon beta 2/B-cell stimulatory factor type 2 shares identity with monocyte-derived hepatocyte-stimulating factor and regulates the major acute phase protein response in liver cells. *Proc Natl Acad Sci U S A* 1987;84(20):7251–7255.
125. Van Snick J. Interleukin-6: an overview. *Annu Rev Immunol* 1990;8:253–278.
126. LeMay LG, Otterness IG, Vander AJ, et al. In vivo evidence that the rise in plasma IL 6 following injection of a fever-inducing dose of LPS is mediated by IL 1 beta. *Cytokine* 1990;2(3):199–204.
127. Tilg H, Trehu E, Atkins MB, et al. Interleukin-6 (IL-6) as an anti-inflammatory cytokine: induction of circulating IL-1 receptor antagonist and soluble tumor necrosis factor receptor p55. *Blood* 1994;83(1):113–118.
128. Sunden-Cullberg J, Norrby-Teglund A, Rouhiainen A, et al. Persistent elevation of high mobility group box-1 protein (HMGB1) in patients with severe sepsis and septic shock. *Crit Care Med* 2005;33(3):564–573.
129. Bonaldi T, Talamo F, Scaffidi P, et al. Monocytic cells hyperacetylate chromatin protein HMGB1 to redirect it towards secretion. *EMBO J* 2003; 22(20):5551–5560.
130. Scaffidi P, Misteli T, Bianchi ME. Release of chromatin protein HMGB1 by necrotic cells triggers inflammation. *Nature* 2002;418(6894):191–195.
131. Gardella S, Andrei C, Ferrera D, et al. The nuclear protein HMGB1 is secreted by monocytes via a non-classical, vesicle-mediated secretory pathway. *EMBO Rep* 2002;3(10):995–1001.
132. Tang D, Shi Y, Kang R, et al. Hydrogen peroxide stimulates macrophages and monocytes to actively release HMGB1. *J Leukoc Biol* 2007;81(3):741–747.
133. Zhang X, Wheeler D, Tang Y, et al. Calcium/calmodulin-dependent protein kinase (CaMK) IV mediates nucleocytoplasmic shuttling and release of HMGB1 during lipopolysaccharide stimulation of macrophages. *J Immunol* 2008;181(7):5015–5023.
134. Chen G, Ward MF, Sama AE, et al. Extracellular HMGB1 as a proinflammatory cytokine. *J Interferon Cytokine Res* 2004;24(6):329–333.
135. Fiuza C, Bustin M, Talwar S, et al. Inflammation-promoting activity of HMGB1 on human microvascular endothelial cells. *Blood* 2003;101(7):2652–2660.

136. Andersson U, Tracey KJ. HMGB1 in sepsis. *Scand J Infect Dis* 2003;35(9): 577–584.
137. Andersson U, Wang H, Palmblad K, et al. High mobility group 1 protein (HMG-1) stimulates proinflammatory cytokine synthesis in human monocytes. *J Exp Med* 2000;192(4):565–570.
138. Andersson UG, Tracey KJ. HMGB1, a pro-inflammatory cytokine of clinical interest: introduction. *J Intern Med* 2004;255(3):318–319.
139. Rouhiainen A, Tumova S, Valmu L, et al. Pivotal advance: analysis of proinflammatory activity of highly purified eukaryotic recombinant HMGB1 (amphoterin). *J Leukoc Biol* 2007;81(1):49–58.
140. Riedemann NC, Guo RF, Ward PA. Novel strategies for the treatment of sepsis. *Nat Med* 2003;9(5):517–524.
141. Sama AE, D'Amore J, Ward MF, et al. Bench to bedside: HMGB1-a novel proinflammatory cytokine and potential therapeutic target for septic patients in the emergency department. *Acad Emerg Med* 2004;11(8):867–873.
142. Erlandsson Harris H, Andersson U. Mini-review: the nuclear protein HMGB1 as a proinflammatory mediator. *Eur J Immunol* 2004;34(6): 1503–1512.
143. Rovere-Querini P, Capobianco A, Scaffidi P, et al. HMGB1 is an endogenous immune adjuvant released by necrotic cells. *EMBO Rep* 2004;5(8): 825–830.
144. Peltz ED, Moore EE, Eckels PC, et al. HMGB1 is markedly elevated within 6 hours of mechanical trauma in humans. *Shock* 2009;32:17–22.
145. Ombrellino M, Wang H, Ajemian MS, et al. Increased serum concentrations of high-mobility-group protein 1 in haemorrhagic shock. *Lancet* 1999;354(9188):1446–1447.
146. Jiang W, Pisetsky DS. Mechanisms of disease: the role of high-mobility group protein 1 in the pathogenesis of inflammatory arthritis. *Nat Clin Pract Rheumatol* 2007;3(1):52–58.
147. Rifkin IR, Leadbetter EA, Busconi L, et al. Toll-like receptors, endogenous ligands, and systemic autoimmune disease. *Immunol Rev* 2005;204:27–42.
148. Foell D, Wittkowski H, Roth J. Mechanisms of disease: a 'DAMP' view of inflammatory arthritis. *Nat Clin Pract Rheumatol* 2007;3(7):382–390.
149. Taniguchi N, Kawahara K, Yone K, et al. High mobility group box chromosomal protein 1 plays a role in the pathogenesis of rheumatoid arthritis as a novel cytokine. *Arthritis Rheum* 2003;48(4):971–981.
150. Bogdan C. The function of type I interferons in antimicrobial immunity. *Curr Opin Immunol* 2000;12(4):419–424.
151. De Maeyer E, De Maeyer-Guignard J. Type I interferons. *Int Rev Immunol* 1998;17(1–4):53–73.
152. Uze G, Lutfalla G, Mogensen KE. Alpha and beta interferons and their receptor and their friends and relations. *J Interferon Cytokine Res* 1995;15(1):3–26.
153. Selzman CH, Shames BD, Miller SA, et al. Therapeutic implications of interleukin-10 in surgical disease. *Shock* 1998;10(5):309–318.
154. Cassatella MA, Meda L, Bonora S, et al. Interleukin 10 (IL-10) inhibits the release of proinflammatory cytokines from human polymorphonuclear leukocytes. Evidence for an autocrine role of tumor necrosis factor and IL-1 beta in mediating the production of IL-8 triggered by lipopolysaccharide. *J Exp Med* 1993;178(6):2207–2211.
155. Neurath MF, Meyer zum Buschenfelde KH. Protective and pathogenic roles of cytokines in inflammatory bowel diseases. *J Investig Med* 1996; 44(9):516–521.
156. Smith KA. Interleukin-2: inception, impact, and implications. *Science* 1988;240(4856):1169–1176.
157. Smith KA. Lowest dose interleukin-2 immunotherapy. *Blood* 1993;81(6): 1414–1423.
158. Zurawski SM, Vega F Jr, Huyghe B, et al. Receptors for interleukin-13 and interleukin-4 are complex and share a novel component that functions in signal transduction. *EMBO J* 1993;12(7):2663–2670.
159. de Waal Malefyt R, Figdor CG, Huijbens R, et al. Effects of IL-13 on phenotype, cytokine production, and cytotoxic function of human monocytes. Comparison with IL-4 and modulation by IFN-gamma or IL-10. *J Immunol* 1993;151(11):6370–6381.
160. Billiau A, Heremans H, Vermeire K, et al. Immunomodulatory properties of interferon-gamma. An update. *Ann N Y Acad Sci* 1998;856:22–32.
161. Boehm U, Klamp T, Groot M, et al. Cellular responses to interferon-gamma. *Annu Rev Immunol* 1997;15:749–795.
162. Lawrence DA. Transforming growth factor-beta: an overview. *Kidney Int Suppl* 1995;49:S19–S23.
163. Lawrence DA. Transforming growth factor-beta: a general review. *Eur Cytokine Netw* 1996;7(3):363–374.
164. Wahl SM, Hunt DA, Wakefield LM, et al. Transforming growth factor type beta induces monocyte chemotaxis and growth factor production. *Proc Natl Acad Sci U S A* 1987;84(16):5788–5792.
165. Romani N, Gruner S, Brang D, et al. Proliferating dendritic cell progenitors in human blood. *J Exp Med* 1994;180(1):83–93.
166. Crawford J, Ozer H, Stoller R, et al. Reduction by granulocyte colony-stimulating factor of fever and neutropenia induced by chemotherapy in patients with small-cell lung cancer. *N Engl J Med* 1991;325(3):164–170.
167. Metcalf D, Nicola NA. Proliferative effects of purified granulocyte colony-stimulating factor (G-CSF) on normal mouse hemopoietic cells. *J Cell Physiol* 1983;116(2):198–206.
168. Cooper NR. Biology of the complement system. In: Gallin JI, Snyderman R, eds. *Inflammation: Basic Principles and Clinical Correlates*, 3rd ed. Philadelphia, PA: Lippincott Williams & Wilkins; 1999.
169. Frank MM, Fries LF. The role of complement in inflammation and phagocytosis. *Immunol Today* 1991;12(9):322–326.
170. Roitt I, Brostoff J, Male D. Complement. In: Roitt I, Brostoff J, Male D, eds. *Immunobiology*, 3rd ed. St. Louis, MO: Mosby; 1993.
171. Weiser MR, Williams JP, Moore FD Jr, et al. Reperfusion injury of ischemic skeletal muscle is mediated by natural antibody and complement. *J Exp Med* 1996;183(5):2343–2348.
172. Cooper NR. The classical complement pathway: activation and regulation of the first complement component. *Adv Immunol* 1985;37:151–216.
173. Matsushita M, Fujita T. Activation of the classical complement pathway by mannose-binding protein in association with a novel C1 s-like serine protease. *J Exp Med* 1992;176(6):1497–1502.
174. Sim RB, Malhotra R. Interactions of carbohydrates and lectins with complement. *Biochem Soc Trans* 1994;22(1):106–111.
175. Muller-Eberhard HJ. The membrane attack complex of complement. *Annu Rev Immunol* 1986;4:503–528.
176. Marnett LJ, Rowlinson SW, Goodwin DC, et al. Arachidonic acid oxygenation by COX-1 and COX-2. Mechanisms of catalysis and inhibition. *J Biol Chem* 1999;274(33):22903–22906.
177. Seeds MC, Bass DA. Regulation and metabolism of arachidonic acid. *Clin Rev Allergy Immunol* 1999;17(1–2):5–26.
178. Smith WL, Garavito RM, DeWitt DL. Prostaglandin endoperoxide H synthases (cyclooxygenases)-1 and -2. *J Biol Chem* 1996;271(52):33157–33160.
179. Funk CD. Prostaglandins and leukotrienes: advances in eicosanoid biology. *Science* 2001;294(5548):1871–1875.
180. Bulger EM, Maier RV. Lipid mediators in the pathophysiology of critical illness. *Crit Care Med* 2000;28(4 Suppl):N27–N36.
181. Gerritsen ME. Physiological and pathophysiological roles of eicosanoids in the microcirculation. *Cardiovasc Res* 1996;32(4):720–732.
182. Serhan CN. Inflammation. Signalling the fat controller. *Nature* 1996; 384(6604):23–24.
183. Leff JA. Leukotriene modifiers as novel therapeutics in asthma. *Clin Exp Allergy* 1998;28(suppl 5):147–153; discussion 171–173.
184. McMahon B, Godson C. Lipoxins: endogenous regulators of inflammation. *Am J Physiol Renal Physiol* 2004;286(2):F189–F201.
185. Marcus AJ. Transcellular metabolism of eicosanoids. *Prog Hemost Thromb* 1986;8:127–142.
186. De Caterina R, Sicari R, Giannessi D, et al. Macrophage-specific eicosanoid synthesis inhibition and lipocortin-1 induction by glucocorticoids. *J Appl Physiol* 1993;75(6):2368–2375.
187. Snyder F, Fitzgerald V, Blank ML. Biosynthesis of platelet-activating factor and enzyme inhibitors. *Adv Exp Med Biol* 1996;416:5–10.
188. Snyder F. Metabolic processing of PAF. *Clin Rev Allergy* 1994;12(4):309–327.
189. Noguchi K, Matsuzaki T, Shiroma N, et al. Involvement of nitric oxide and eicosanoids in platelet-activating factor-induced haemodynamic and haematological effects in dogs. *Br J Pharmacol* 1996;118(4):941–950.
190. Blais C Jr, Marceau F, Rouleau JL, et al. The kallikrein-kininogen-kinin system: lessons from the quantification of endogenous kinins. *Peptides* 2000;21(12):1903–1940.
191. Erdos EG. Kinins, the long march–a personal view. *Cardiovasc Res* 2002; 54(3):485–491.
192. Hall JM. Bradykinin receptors: pharmacological properties and biological roles. *Pharmacol Ther* 1992;56(2):131–190.
193. Schreiber AD. Plasma inhibitors of the Hageman factor dependent pathways. *Semin Thromb Hemost* 1976;3(1):32–51.
194. Volpe AR, Giardina B, Preziosi P, et al. Biosynthesis of endothelium-derived nitric oxide by bradykinin as endogenous precursor. *Immunopharmacology* 1996;33(1–3):287–290.
195. Dell'Italia LJ, Oparil S. Bradykinin in the heart: friend or foe? *Circulation* 1999;100(23):2305–2307.
196. Tschope C, Gohlke P, Zhu YZ, et al. Antihypertensive and cardioprotective effects after angiotensin-converting enzyme inhibition: role of kinins. *J Card Fail* 1997;3(2):133–148.
197. Chikanza IC, Grossman AB. Neuroendocrine immune responses to inflammation: the concept of the neuroendocrine immune loop. *Baillieres Clin Rheumatol* 1996;10(2):199–225.
198. Whicker JT, Evans SW. A role for neuropeptides in inflammation. In: Whicker JT, Evans SW, eds. *Biochemistry of Inflammation*. Boston, MA: Kluwer Academic; 1992.
199. Delgado M, Munoz-Elias EJ, Gomariz RP, et al. Vasoactive intestinal peptide and pituitary adenylate cyclase-activating polypeptide enhance IL-10 production by murine macrophages: in vitro and in vivo studies. *J Immunol* 1999;162(3):1707–1716.
200. Palmer RM, Ferrige AG, Moncada S. Nitric oxide release accounts for the biological activity of endothelium-derived relaxing factor. *Nature* 1987; 327(6122):524–526.
201. Moncada S, Palmer RM, Higgs EA. Nitric oxide: physiology, pathophysiology, and pharmacology. *Pharmacol Rev* 1991;43(2):109–142.
202. Alderton WK, Cooper CE, Knowles RG. Nitric oxide synthases: structure, function and inhibition. *Biochem J* 2001;357(Pt 3):593–615.
203. Geller DA, Billiar TR. Molecular biology of nitric oxide synthases. *Cancer Metastasis Rev* 1998;17(1):7–23.
204. De Vera ME, Taylor BS, Wang Q, et al. Dexamethasone suppresses iNOS gene expression by upregulating I-kappa B alpha and inhibiting NF-kappa B. *Am J Physiol* 1997;273(6 Pt 1):G1290–G1296.
205. Kleinert H, Euchenhofer C, Ihrig-Biedert I, et al. Glucocorticoids inhibit the induction of nitric oxide synthase II by down-regulating cytokine-induced activity of transcription factor nuclear factor-kappa B. *Mol Pharmacol* 1996;49(1):15–21.
206. Titheradge MA. Nitric oxide in septic shock. *Biochim Biophys Acta* 1999; 1411(2–3):437–455.
207. Finkel MS, Oddis CV, Jacob TD, et al. Negative inotropic effects of cytokines on the heart mediated by nitric oxide. *Science* 1992;257(5068):387–389.

208. Goodwin DC, Landino LM, Marnett LJ. Effects of nitric oxide and nitric oxide-derived species on prostaglandin endoperoxide synthase and prostaglandin biosynthesis. *FASEB J* 1999;13(10):1121–1136.
209. Allione A, Bernabei P, Bosticardo M, et al. Nitric oxide suppresses human T lymphocyte proliferation through IFN-gamma-dependent and IFN-gamma-independent induction of apoptosis. *J Immunol* 1999;163(8):4182–4191.
210. Ou J, Carlos TM, Watkins SC, et al. Differential effects of nonselective nitric oxide synthase (NOS) and selective inducible NOS inhibition on hepatic necrosis, apoptosis, ICAM-1 expression, and neutrophil accumulation during endotoxemia. *Nitric Oxide* 1997;1(5):404–416.
211. Isobe M, Katsuramaki T, Hirata K, et al. Beneficial effects of inducible nitric oxide synthase inhibitor on reperfusion injury in the pig liver. *Transplantation* 1999;68(6):803–813.
212. Xia Y, Zweier JL. Superoxide and peroxynitrite generation from inducible nitric oxide synthase in macrophages. *Proc Natl Acad Sci U S A* 1997;94(13):6954–6958.
213. Szabo C, Billiar TR. Novel roles of nitric oxide in hemorrhagic shock. *Shock* 1999;12(1):1–9.
214. Hierholzer C, Harbrecht B, Menezes JM, et al. Essential role of induced nitric oxide in the initiation of the inflammatory response after hemorrhagic shock. *J Exp Med* 1998;187(6):917–928.
215. Tzeng E, Kim YM, Pitt BR, et al. Adenoviral transfer of the inducible nitric oxide synthase gene blocks endothelial cell apoptosis. *Surgery* 1997;122(2):255–263.
216. Ryter SW, Alam J, Choi AM. Heme oxygenase-1/carbon monoxide: from basic science to therapeutic applications. *Physiol Rev* 2006;86(2):583–650.
217. Li L, Moore PK. Putative biological roles of hydrogen sulfide in health and disease: a breath of not so fresh air? *Trends Pharmacol Sci* 2008;29(2):84–90.
218. Li L, Bhatia M, Zhu YZ, et al. Hydrogen sulfide is a novel mediator of lipopolysaccharide-induced inflammation in the mouse. *FASEB J* 2005;19(9):1196–1198.
219. Mok YY, Atan MS, Ping CY, et al. Role of hydrogen sulphide in haemorrhagic shock in the rat: protective effect of inhibitors of hydrogen sulphide biosynthesis. *Br J Pharmacol* 2004;143(7):881–889.
220. Collin M, Anuar FB, Murch O, et al. Inhibition of endogenous hydrogen sulfide formation reduces the organ injury caused by endotoxemia. *Br J Pharmacol* 2005;146(4):498–505.
221. Zhang H, Zhi L, Moochhala SM, et al. Endogenous hydrogen sulfide regulates leukocyte trafficking in cecal ligation and puncture-induced sepsis. *J Leukoc Biol* 2007;82(4):894–905.
222. Zhi L, Ang AD, Zhang H, et al. Hydrogen sulfide induces the synthesis of proinflammatory cytokines in human monocyte cell line U937 via the ERK-NF-kappaB pathway. *J Leukoc Biol* 2007;81(5):1322–1332.
223. Oh GS, Pae HO, Lee BS, et al. Hydrogen sulfide inhibits nitric oxide production and nuclear factor-kappaB via heme oxygenase-1 expression in RAW264.7 macrophages stimulated with lipopolysaccharide. *Free Radic Biol Med* 2006;41(1):106–119.
224. Li L, Rossoni G, Sparatore A, et al. Anti-inflammatory and gastrointestinal effects of a novel diclofenac derivative. *Free Radic Biol Med* 2007;42(5):706–719.
225. Kimbrell DA, Beutler B. The evolution and genetics of innate immunity. *Nat Rev Genet* 2001;2(4):256–267.
226. Medzhitov R, Janeway C Jr. Innate immune recognition: mechanisms and pathways. *Immunol Rev* 2000;173:89–97.
227. Bianchi ME. DAMPs, PAMPs and alarmins: all we need to know about danger. *J Leukoc Biol* 2007;81(1):1–5.
228. Beutler B. Inferences, questions and possibilities in Toll-like receptor signalling. *Nature* 2004;430(6996):257–263.
229. Triantafilou M, Triantafilou K. Lipopolysaccharide recognition: CD14, TLRs and the LPS-activation cluster. *Trends Immunol* 2002;23(6):301–304.
230. Poltorak A, He X, Smirnova I, et al. Defective LPS signaling in C3 H/HeJ and C57BL/10ScCr mice: mutations in Tlr4 gene. *Science* 1998;282(5396):2085–2088.
231. Akira S, Takeda K. Toll-like receptor signalling. *Nat Rev Immunol* 2004;4(7):499–511.
232. Roach JC, Glusman G, Rowen L, et al. The evolution of vertebrate Toll-like receptors. *Proc Natl Acad Sci U S A* 2005;102(27):9577–9582.
233. Kopp E, Medzhitov R. Recognition of microbial infection by Toll-like receptors. *Curr Opin Immunol* 2003;15(4):396–401.
234. Cook DN, Pisetsky DS, Schwartz DA. Toll-like receptors in the pathogenesis of human disease. *Nat Immunol* 2004;5(10):975–979.
235. Schmidt AM, Yan SD, Yan SF, et al. The multiligand receptor RAGE as a progression factor amplifying immune and inflammatory responses. *J Clin Invest* 2001;108(7):949–955.
236. Stern D, Yan SD, Yan SF, et al. Receptor for advanced glycation endproducts: a multiligand receptor magnifying cell stress in diverse pathologic settings. *Adv Drug Deliv Rev* 2002;54(12):1615–1625.
237. Stebbing J, Bower M, Gazzard B, et al. The common heat shock protein receptor CD91 is up-regulated on monocytes of advanced melanoma slow progressors. *Clin Exp Immunol* 2004;138(2):312–316.
238. Binder RJ, Han DK, Srivastava PK. CD91: a receptor for heat shock protein gp96. *Nat Immunol* 2000;1(2):151–155.
239. Srivastava P. Interaction of heat shock proteins with peptides and antigen presenting cells: chaperoning of the innate and adaptive immune responses. *Annu Rev Immunol* 2002;20:395–425.
240. Basu S, Binder RJ, Suto R, et al. Necrotic but not apoptotic cell death releases heat shock proteins, which deliver a partial maturation signal to dendritic cells and activate the NF-kappa B pathway. *Int Immunol* 2000;12(11):1539–1546.
241. Binder RJ, Srivastava PK. Essential role of CD91 in re-presentation of gp96-chaperoned peptides. *Proc Natl Acad Sci U S A* 2004;101(16):6128–6133.
242. Melcher A, Todryk S, Hardwick N, et al. Tumor immunogenicity is determined by the mechanism of cell death via induction of heat shock protein expression. *Nat Med* 1998;4(5):581–587.
243. Zheng H, Dai J, Stoilova D, et al. Cell surface targeting of heat shock protein gp96 induces dendritic cell maturation and antitumor immunity. *J Immunol* 2001;167(12):6731–6735.
244. Heilmann HP, Doppelfeld E, Fernholz HJ, et al. Results of radiotherapy of bronchial carcinoma (author's transl). *Dtsch Med Wochenschr* 1976;101(43):1557–1562.
245. Becker T, Hartl FU, Wieland F. CD40, an extracellular receptor for binding and uptake of Hsp70-peptide complexes. *J Cell Biol* 2002;158(7):1277–1285.
246. Binder RJ, Vatner R, Srivastava P. The heat-shock protein receptors: some answers and more questions. *Tissue Antigens* 2004;64(4):442–451.
247. Asea A, Kraeft SK, Kurt-Jones EA, et al. HSP70 stimulates cytokine production through a CD14-dependant pathway, demonstrating its dual role as a chaperone and cytokine. *Nat Med* 2000;6(4):435–442.
248. Vabulas RM, Ahmad-Nejad P, da Costa C, et al. Endocytosed HSP60s use toll-like receptor 2 (TLR2) and TLR4 to activate the toll/interleukin-1 receptor signaling pathway in innate immune cells. *J Biol Chem* 2001;276(33):31332–31339.
249. Polla BS, Bachelet M, Dall'ava J, et al. Heat shock proteins in inflammation and asthma: Dr Jekyll or Mr Hyde? *Clin Exp Allergy* 1998;28(5):527–529.
250. Polla BS, Bachelet M, Elia G, et al. Stress proteins in inflammation. *Ann N Y Acad Sci* 1998;851:75–85.
251. Multhoff G, Botzler C. Heat-shock proteins and the immune response. *Ann N Y Acad Sci* 1998;851:86–93.
252. Perdrizet GA. Heat shock and tissue protection. *New Horiz* 1995;3(2):312–320.
253. Mathew A, Morimoto RI. Role of the heat-shock response in the life and death of proteins. *Ann N Y Acad Sci* 1998;851:99–111.
254. Ribeiro SP, Villar J, Slutsky AS. Induction of the stress response to prevent organ injury. *New Horiz* 1995;3(2):301–311.
255. Garcia-Cardena G, Fan R, Shah V, et al. Dynamic activation of endothelial nitric oxide synthase by Hsp90. *Nature* 1998;392(6678):821–824.
256. Wong HR, Ryan M, Wispe JR. Stress response decreases NF-kappaB nuclear translocation and increases I-kappaBalpha expression in A549 cells. *J Clin Invest* 1997;99(10):2423–2428.
257. Moshage H. Cytokines and the hepatic acute phase response. *J Pathol* 1997;181(3):257–266.
258. Pepys MB, ed. *Acute Phase Proteins in the Acute Phase Response.* New York: Springer-Verlag; 1989.
259. Gabay C, Kushner I. Acute-phase proteins and other systemic responses to inflammation. *N Engl J Med* 1999;340(6):448–454.
260. Koj A. Initiation of acute phase response and synthesis of cytokines. *Biochim Biophys Acta* 1996;1317(2):84–94.
261. Giraldez RR, Panda A, Xia Y, et al. Decreased nitric-oxide synthase activity causes impaired endothelium-dependent relaxation in the postischemic heart. *J Biol Chem* 1997;272(34):21420–21426.
262. Romson JL, Hook BG, Kunkel SL, et al. Reduction of the extent of ischemic myocardial injury by neutrophil depletion in the dog. *Circulation* 1983;67(5):1016–1023.
263. Vedder NB, Winn RK, Rice CL, et al. A monoclonal antibody to the adherence-promoting leukocyte glycoprotein, CD18, reduces organ injury and improves survival from hemorrhagic shock and resuscitation in rabbits. *J Clin Invest* 1988;81(3):939–944.
264. Agostoni A, Gardinali M, Frangi D, et al. Activation of complement and kinin systems after thrombolytic therapy in patients with acute myocardial infarction. A comparison between streptokinase and recombinant tissue-type plasminogen activator. *Circulation* 1994;90(6):2666–2670.
265. Morgan BP. Complement membrane attack on nucleated cells: resistance, recovery and non-lethal effects. *Biochem J* 1989;264(1):1–14.
266. Muckart DJ, Bhagwanjee S. American College of Chest Physicians/Society of Critical Care Medicine Consensus Conference definitions of the systemic inflammatory response syndrome and allied disorders in relation to critically injured patients. *Crit Care Med* 1997;25(11):1789–1795.
267. Bone RC. Sepsis, sepsis syndrome, and the systemic inflammatory response syndrome (SIRS). Gulliver in Laputa. *JAMA* 1995;273(2):155–156.
268. Rangel-Frausto MS, Pittet D, Costigan M, et al. The natural history of the systemic inflammatory response syndrome (SIRS). A prospective study. *JAMA* 1995;273(2):117–123.
269. Davies MG, Hagen PO. Systemic inflammatory response syndrome. *Br J Surg* 1997;84(7):920–935.
270. Bernard GR, Vincent JL, Laterre PF, et al. Efficacy and safety of recombinant human activated protein C for severe sepsis. *N Engl J Med* 2001;344(10):699–709.
271. Annane D, Sebille V, Charpentier C, et al. Effect of treatment with low doses of hydrocortisone and fludrocortisone on mortality in patients with septic shock. *JAMA* 2002;288(7):862–871.
272. Dvorak HF, Galli SJ, Dvorak AM. Cellular and vascular manifestations of cell-mediated immunity. *Hum Pathol* 1986;17(2):122–137.

CHAPTER 7 ■ SURGICAL INFECTIONS

E. PATCHEN DELLINGER

KEY POINTS

1. Surgical infections require surgical intervention, that is, "source control," which refers to a mechanical or anatomic procedure to drain an abscess, relieve an obstruction, repair a perforation, or resect dead, ischemic, or inflamed tissue or foreign body to promote resolution.
2. Source control is combined with empiric antibiotic therapy that is later modified based on microbiologic susceptibility patterns.
3. Empiric antibiotic therapy requires knowledge of the current patterns of pathogens involved and antibiotic susceptibility within the institution and, even, specific units, such as the intensive care unit.
4. Surgical site infections are dependent on numerous factors, including extent of contamination, hemostasis, tissue handling, length of operation, tissue hypoxia, patient temperature, and glucose control, in addition to minimizing comorbidities.
5. Antibiotic prophylaxis should be dosed to maintain adequate tissue concentrations during the period of potential contamination, starting approximately 1 hour or less prior to surgery; repeated after one to two half-lives during prolonged operations, with increased doses in large patients; and stopped within 24 hours postoperatively if not immediately at the end of the operation. Choose a first-generation cephalosporin if no anaerobes are expected and add metronidazole if anaerobic activity is likely. Consider vancomycin only if there is a history of methicillin-resistant *Staphylococcus aureus* (MRSA) colonization or infection, for a dialysis patient or a patient with recent hospitalization or antibiotic treatment, or if there is a high rate of MRSA surgical site infections in your institution.
6. With peritonitis, antibiotics active against aerobic gram-negative organisms prevent early mortality and those active against anaerobic organisms prevent abscesses. Thus, broad-spectrum antibiotics are needed.
7. Necrotizing soft tissue infections are hard to diagnose, present with external skin changes underrepresenting the extent of underlying disease, and have potential for major tissue loss and high morbidity and mortality.

1 Although there is no official definition of a surgical infection, it is commonly understood as an infection that will not resolve with antimicrobial therapy alone but also requires surgical intervention, sometimes called source control. The intervention may be as significant as a major laparotomy or thoracotomy or as simple as removing sutures from an infected surgical incision or draining a superficial abscess. It also includes interventions by radiologists or other specialists such as computed tomography (CT)-guided percutaneous drainage of an intra-abdominal abscess or placement of a stent through a biliary stricture in a patient with cholangitis. A unifying characteristic of all surgical infections is an anatomic manipulation, such as draining a closed space, closing a perforated viscus, or removing dead tissue or foreign body, that must be performed to achieve resolution of the infection. Many "medical" infections involve single pathogens that are able to establish themselves and grow through intrinsic pathogenic mechanisms despite intact skin or mucosa. Examples include pneumococcal pneumonia, streptococcal pharyngitis, meningococcal meningitis, and salmonella enteritis. Surgical infections typically occur after a mechanical breach of normal epithelial barriers and often involve multiple organisms, typically endogenous to the area of epithelial injury. Examples include peritonitis after perforated appendicitis or diverticulitis and surgical site infections (SSIs) caused by skin flora after clean operations. An exception to this principle for surgical infections is the occurrence of necrotizing soft tissue infections secondary to group A β-hemolytic streptococci (hemolytic streptococcal gangrene) or community-associated methicillin resistant *Staphylococcus aureus* (CA-MRSA), which can occur following trivial injuries or no known prior injury. In this chapter we also discuss nonsurgical infections that typically occur in hospitalized surgical patients. These include catheter-related bloodstream infections, pneumonia, and urinary tract infections (UTIs).

In approaching the topic of surgical infections, each area is approached in the following order: prevention, diagnosis, treatment. The first element of prevention is the natural host defense mechanisms of the patient. The most important of these for surgical infections is the epithelial covering that separates the sterile portions of the body from those with normal endogenous flora. Thus, the skin on the outside of the body and the gastrointestinal (GI) mucosa lining the alimentary tract are the sites of complex microbiologic flora and serve to bar those flora from the tissues in most cases. Once these mechanical barriers are breached, by trauma, medical or surgical procedures, neoplasm, inflammation, or ischemia, cellular and humoral defenses become important.

The array of host defenses is large and complex, and our understanding of these processes is continually advancing. Initial, nonspecific defenses begin with fixed tissue macrophages and circulating polymorphonuclear leukocytes (PNMs), which engulf and kill small numbers of invading microorganisms. The macrophages and dendritic cells also have the ability to ingest pathogens and to process their antigens for presentation to T lymphocytes for the subsequent development of specific antibodies by B lymphocytes. The first presentation of an antigen leads to the formation of IgM class antibodies that are produced over the next 1 to 2 weeks. Subsequent exposure to the same antigen leads to much more rapid production of IgG antibodies. Antibodies bound to microorganisms promote more efficient phagocytosis and killing and also serve to activate complement proteins, another element in the humoral defense system. The complement system exists in a quiescent form, which when activated leads to a cascade of activated complement proteins and fractions that enhance phagocytosis, increase vascular permeability, stimulate inflammation, and lead to direct lysis of some pathogens.

There are many interactions between the cellular and humoral aspects of host defense. Host defense cells manufacture the humoral components, and when activated, the humoral components stimulate the cells. In addition, there is extensive cross-talk among the cellular elements of host defenses involving a large number of cytokines including tumor necrosis factor (TNF) and many interleukins (ILs), signified by IL-*n*, with the number *n* increasing as new cytokines are discovered and characterized. The successful interaction of these elements is essential to normal host defenses, but when the mechanisms of control fail and cytokines spread beyond their intended local actions, these host defense mechanisms can turn against the host, resulting in a spectrum of conditions variously called the systemic inflammatory response syndrome (SIRS) and multiple organ dysfunction syndrome (MODS). Many attempts to modify this process through the development of specific antagonists to various elements of this system have so far failed to produce clinically useful products, although research continues.

When injury occurs and blood vessels are opened, the coagulation cascade, similar in some ways to the complement cascade, is also initiated. In recent years it has been recognized that a number of elements in the coagulation response and the inflammatory response are shared, and local thrombosis and fibrinogen deposition are prominent components of acute inflammation. Inflammation stimulates a procoagulant state and can also promote distant thromboembolic events. More recently, a clinical trial of activated protein C, a component of the coagulation cascade that has antithrombotic, anti-inflammatory, and profibrinolytic properties, has proved beneficial for some patients with combined SIRS, infection, and organ failure.[1]

PREVENTION

Despite the success of intrinsic host defenses, in many circumstances infections do occur, especially after surgical interventions, both elective and urgent. It is incumbent on the surgical team to understand and to apply what is known regarding elements of patient care and delivery of surgical procedures that reduce the risk of subsequent infection as much as possible. In general terms, these preventive measures can fall into three broad categories. The patient should come to an operative procedure with host defenses in the best possible condition. The procedure should be conducted in a manner that reduces to the minimum introduction of pathogens into the sterile compartments of the body. The perioperative management of the patient should be conducted in a manner that optimally supports and maintains the patient's host defenses. In actual practice, many items of patient care will relate to more than one of these goals. These items are discussed in more detail in the section dealing with SSIs.

DIAGNOSIS

Although details specific to the diagnosis of specific surgical infections and other infections in surgical patients are covered in those individual sections, some items of diagnosis are common to all. Some relatively straightforward infections such as superficial SSIs or subcutaneous abscesses are properly treated by simply opening the wound or draining the abscess without the use of antimicrobial agents and do not require routine culture. 2 However, most surgical infections require at least the initial use of antimicrobial agents that are most effective if active against the primary pathogens involved. If initial treatment is clearly successful, then knowledge of the specific pathogens and their susceptibilities is not critical for the treatment of that patient. However, when the patient does not respond as expected, then knowledge of the pathogens and their susceptibilities can be extremely useful, and this information will not be available unless the appropriate cultures were obtained prior to initiating antibiotic therapy.

Material sent to the microbiology laboratory from the operating room or the interventional radiology suite is preferable. Surface swabs taken from open or draining wounds or material from drains that have been in place for days have a high probability of returning information about contaminating or colonizing organisms that are not responsible for the infection needing treatment. Samples of tissue or fluid are always preferable to swabs from the operating room. Blood cultures are helpful when positive but are positive in less than one third of surgical infections in most reported series. An early source of information from such specimens is the Gram stain, which should be available to the physician in less than an hour after obtaining the specimen. The initial choice of antimicrobial agents for a serious infection will be quite different if the Gram stain shows gram-positive cocci than if the stain shows predominantly gram-negative rods. Microbial growth and preliminary identification will usually be available within 24 hours for most surgical pathogens, but susceptibility information will 3 not be reported for 1 or more additional days. Thus, knowledge of the susceptibility patterns in the hospital, or even more specifically, in a specific intensive care unit (ICU), can be invaluable in directing initial empiric antimicrobial choices for a critically ill patient.[2] This is another reason to culture severe infections. The body of information about pathogens and their susceptibilities locally helps to direct therapy for patients in the future, and these patterns can change over time. Thus, current culture information is always helpful. Although antimicrobial susceptibility data currently take 2 days or more in most cases, advances in the modern microbiology laboratory may someday provide this information more rapidly. Detection of specific nucleic acid sequences has the potential to identify certain common and well-characterized resistance genes such as the *mecA* gene that codes for methicillin resistance in *Staphylococcus aureus*. Other diagnostic advances that are making their way to the clinical microbiology laboratory include antigen and antibody detection systems and polymerase chain reaction (PCR) for amplifying small amounts of nucleic acids.

Diagnosis of infection always involves history and physical examination, but these are more efficiently discussed in relation to specific infections. Fever and leukocytosis are frequent accompaniments of infection but are not specific and are variously sensitive depending on the specific infection. They may drive further diagnostic efforts including physical and radiologic examination but are not sufficient reason to initiate antimicrobial treatment in isolation from other data. Radiologic examinations can be very helpful in some specific circumstances but should not substitute for or precede history and physical examination and clinical judgment.

TREATMENT

Treatment of surgical infections, as discussed initially in the definition of surgical infections, always involves a procedure and often involves the use of one or more antimicrobial agents. The generic term for a procedure directed at the resolution of a surgical infection is *source control*. Source control refers to the mechanical or anatomic procedure that is used to drain an abscess, relieve an obstruction, repair a perforation, or resect dead, ischemic, or inflamed tissue or a foreign body to promote the resolution of a surgical infection. In recent years there has been growing recognition that the literature regarding surgical infections is incomplete when it does not adequately describe and evaluate the effectiveness of source control.[3] This is particularly true for publications comparing different antimicrobial treatments of surgical infections. When the differences between two regimens are small, a difference in the delivery of source control to patients in the comparative regimens can skew the results.[4] The appropriate use of antimicrobial agents is also important in many situations and is addressed in the sections regarding specific infections.

Although the choice of specific agents, and to a lesser extent dosing, have been addressed, there are very little relevant data regarding the appropriate duration of antimicrobial treatment for most surgical infections. Trends in recent years have been to decrease this duration in many cases. Only in the area of prophylaxis are good data available.

SURGICAL SITE INFECTIONS

Infections that occur in a surgical incision were previously called wound infections. In recent years, a consensus conference involving surgical and medical societies and the Centers for Disease Control and Prevention (CDC) developed the concept of SSI.[5,6] This includes any infection that occurs in an operative site. An infection of the subcutaneous tissue only (the most common "wound infection") is termed a superficial SSI. One that involves the muscular and fascial layers and includes a partial or complete fascial dehiscence is a deep SSI. An infection that occurs within the organ or deep space of the wound such as peritonitis, an intra-abdominal abscess, an empyema, or a joint space infection is called an organ/space SSI. Data from the National Nosocomial Infection Surveillance (NNIS) system of the CDC shows that of all SSIs, 47% are superficial, 23% are deep, and 30% are organ/space.[7] Only 46% of these SSIs are diagnosed during the original hospitalization, whereas 16% are diagnosed after discharge as outpatients and 38% on readmission to the hospital. Although 58% of all organ/space SSIs are diagnosed during the original hospitalization, 59% of other SSIs are diagnosed only after discharge.[7]

Surgeons have traditionally divided wounds into the classes of clean, clean-contaminated, contaminated, and dirty (Table 7.1)[8] based on the probability that the wound would be contaminated by bacteria during the operative procedure. These classes roughly divide wounds into different risks for the development of SSI. More recently, examination of databases that include many thousands of wounds have led to the development of newer risk classification systems that provide a more accurate estimate of risk. The NNIS index[9] assigns up to one risk point for each of (a) contaminated or dirty wound, (b) American Society of Anesthesiologists (ASA) class 3 or higher, and (c) duration of operation exceeding the 75th percentile for that operation.[9] Thus, an operation may fall into one of four classes between 0 and 3. Table 7.2[9] demonstrates the increased precision of this system compared with the older system that refers only to wound class. This system can be used to roughly compare the performance of a hospital or surgical department against the NNIS database by comparing expected with observed infection rates.[10] Of course, much more precise risk data can be developed for single operative procedures through analysis of large databases in which the heterogeneity imposed by multiple different procedures is eliminated.[11,12]

Many other factors that influence the risk of SSI have been proposed, and a relatively complete summary of these factors is provided in a publication by the Hospital Infection Control Practices Advisory Committee (HICPAC) of the CDC.[6] Some of these are summarized in Table 7.3, which lists the category 1 recommendations that are readily influenced by the surgeon. It is likely that the majority of these are important in most operative procedures, although most have been generated through analysis of single procedures or limited classes of procedures and have not been reproduced in all cases. Many, such as the patient's weight and smoking status or the presence of an infection at a distant site, are modifiable prior to scheduled operation. Others, such as age or underlying immune disorders, cannot be improved. Some, such as diabetes, cannot be eliminated, but recent information suggests that tight control of perioperative glucose levels can greatly reduce the risk associated with this diagnosis.[13–15]

TABLE 7.1 CLASSIFICATION

WOUND CLASSIFICATION

■ CLASS	■ DEFINITION
Clean	An uninfected operative wound in which no inflammation is encountered and the respiratory, alimentary, genital, or infected urinary tract is not entered. In addition, clean wounds are closed primarily
Clean-contaminated	An operative wound in which the respiratory, alimentary, genital, or urinary tracts are entered under controlled conditions and without unusual contamination
Contaminated	Open, fresh, accidental wounds. Operations with major breaks in sterile technique or gross spillage from the gastrointestinal tract, and incisions in which acute, nonpurulent inflammation is encountered
Dirty	Old traumatic wounds with retained devitalized tissue and those that involve existing clinical infection or perforated viscera

TABLE 7.2 CLASSIFICATION

COMPARISON OF WOUND CLASSIFICATION AND NNIS SYSTEM FOR EVALUATING RISK OF SURGICAL SITE INFECTION

	■ NNIS RISK INDEX				
■ WOUND CLASS	■ 0	■ 1	■ 2	■ 3	■ ALL
Clean	1.0	2.3	5.4	—	2.1
Clean-contaminated	2.1	4.0	9.5	—	3.3
Contaminated	—	3.4	6.8	13.2	6.4
Dirty	—	3.1	8.1	12.8	7.1
All	1.5	2.9	6.8	13.0	2.8
Maximum ratio[a]	2.1	1.7	1.8	1.0	

NNIS, National Nosocomial Infection Surveillance System.
[a]Ratio of lowest to highest infection rate in wound class or in risk index.
Adapted from Dellinger EP, Ehrenkranz NJ, Jarvis WR, Surgical site infections. In: Jarvis WR, ed. *Bennett & Brachman's Hospital Infections*, 5th ed. Philadelphia, PA: Wolters Kluwer Health/Lippincott Williams & Wilkins; 2007:583–598.

Prevention

4 Preventing SSIs is clearly a prime responsibility of any operating surgeon. Although many surgeons think first of prophylactic antibiotics for prevention, and these are clearly important, antibiotics are most effective when they complement maximal efforts for prevention by other means. Two classic papers on surgical prophylaxis, each of which demonstrated the superiority of prophylactic antibiotics to placebo in randomized prospective trials, also demonstrated an increased infection

TABLE 7.3 TREATMENT

CATEGORY 1 RECOMMENDATIONS FROM THE HOSPITAL INFECTION CONTROL PRACTICES ADVISORY COMMITTEE FOR THE PREVENTION OF SURGICAL SITE INFECTIONS

- Do not operate on patients with active infections.
- Do not shave patient in advance.
- Control glucose in diabetic patients.
- Stop tobacco use in patient.
- Have patient shower with antiseptic soap.
- Prepare skin with appropriate agent.
- Surgeon's nails should be short.
- Surgeons scrub hands.
- Exclude infected surgeons.
- Give prophylactic antibiotics when indicated.
- Maintain prophylactic antibiotic levels during operation.
- Keep operating room doors closed.
- Use sterile instruments.
- Avoid flash sterilization.
- Wear a mask.[a]
- Cover all hair.[a]
- Wear sterile gloves.[a]
- Use gowns and drapes that resist fluid penetration.
- Handle tissue gently.
- Use closed suction drains (when used).
- Delay primary closure for heavily contaminated wounds.
- Use sterile dressing for 24–48 h.
- Use CDC definitions for SSI.
- Watch for SSI and give feedback to surgeons.

CDC, Centers for Disease Control and Prevention; SSI, surgical site infection.
[a]These items are required by Occupational Safety and Health Administration (OSHA) regulations and are not actually supported by class 1 data.
From Mangram AJ, Horan TC, Pearson ML, et al. Guideline for prevention of surgical site infection, 1999. Hospital Infection Control Practices Advisory Committee. *Infect Control Hosp Epidemiol.* 1999;20:250–278, with permission.

rate in the face of prophylaxis when hemostasis was not ideal[16] or when gross contamination was observed during the operative procedure.[17] Each patient should be brought to the operating room only after the correctable items noted in Table 7.3 have been corrected to the degree possible. In addition, in recent years several elements of the immediate perioperative management of surgical patients have been demonstrated to have a significant effect on the risk for SSI. Beyond these issues, most surgeons believe that the technical conduct of the operation, including the handling of tissues, number of ties and other foreign material and devitalized tissue, and length of operation, all influence the risk of SSI. Unfortunately, no validated method for assessing these issues exists. In addition, although data clearly demonstrate that the risk for SSI increases with increasing duration of operation and increasing transfusion, it is not clear that operations that take longer or require more transfusion are the same as shorter procedures that do not require transfusion. Thus, the precise role of these issues is not clear. Certainly, no surgeon should take longer than he or she thinks necessary for a procedure, nor should he or she transfuse a patient when it is not considered important.

Inspired Oxygen Tension. Multiple animal models of infection demonstrate that oxygen tension within the surgical wound correlates with risk for SSI. Low oxygen tensions increase risk, whereas higher tensions decrease it.[18] Another report examined the subcutaneous oxygen tension in 130 surgical patients in the postanesthesia recovery room.[19] The same inverse relationship was found between oxygen tension and risk for SSI. Recently, a prospective trial comparing inspired oxygen concentrations of 30% to 80% in patients having a colectomy demonstrated a significant decrease in infection rates in the high-inspired-oxygen group.[20] Subsequently, two papers from different groups of investigators have reported both contradictory and confirmatory results. One was a much smaller study of patients having mixed GI procedures and poorly balanced comparative groups with an opposite conclusion, a higher infection rate in the patients receiving 80% oxygen compared with 35%.[21] The other was a larger, well-done multicenter study that showed a clear reduction in SSI risk with 80% fraction of inspired oxygen (FiO_2) compared with 30%, but both groups had relatively higher infection rates than the first two studies.[22] Until more data are available, we must consider the ideal inspired oxygen concentration for reducing risk of SSI in surgical patients to be unsettled, although the preponderance of evidence leans toward a benefit to higher levels of FiO_2.[23]

Temperature Control. The temperature of a patient in the operating room is known to influence skin and subcutaneous blood flow and oxygen tension.[24] Animal models have demonstrated increased infection risk when body temperature is lowered. Recently, two prospective controlled trials have demonstrated a reduction in SSI in patients who were actively warmed. One trial in patients submitted to colectomy compared active warming in the operating room to no efforts at warming.[25] A threefold reduction in infection rate was found in the warmed patients. In another study of minor procedures (hernia repair, varicose vein operation, or breast procedure with incision >3 cm), active prewarming, either of the whole patient or of the operative site, also significantly reduced the incidence of SSI and of postoperative antibiotic use by physicians blind to the treatment group.[26] It is increasingly the standard to maintain normal body temperature for operative patients, but without specific protocols to achieve this in all patients, it frequently is not achieved.[27]

Glucose Control. It has long been known that diabetics have a higher risk for SSI than nondiabetic patients. It has been assumed that this is related to underlying defects in host defense associated with the diagnosis. Recently, analysis of a large series of patients, both diabetic and nondiabetic, having an open heart procedure demonstrated that the risk for SSI was most strongly correlated with the occurrence of hyperglycemia (glucose >200 mg/dL) during the first 48 hours after operation.[13] When this occurred, the risk for SSI was doubled regardless of whether the patient was diabetic or not. Forty-seven percent of the patients with hyperglycemia in this study were not diabetic. This relation has also been shown for a group of mixed GI and cardiovascular operations in diabetic patients.[28] Another cardiac surgery group has shown the same relationship between glucose levels and infection risk and has also demonstrated that improved perioperative glucose control with intravenous insulin infusions has reduced both the incidence of SSI and mortality in their diabetic patients.[14,29] Although the strongest evidence exists for diabetic cardiac surgical patients, it is likely that all hyperglycemic surgical patients will benefit from perioperative glucose control.[15]

Antibiotic Prophylaxis. Antibiotic prophylaxis for surgical procedures began shortly after the initial introduction of penicillin with the hope that antibiotics would reduce the risk of surgical wound infections. Prior to 1960, prophylactic antibiotics commonly were started after surgery, a technique that we now know is ineffective. Furthermore, antibiotics were given most often to patients at special risk of infection. Consequently, patients given antibiotics were more likely to develop infections than untreated patients.[30] Subsequent animal experiments and human trials demonstrated that giving antibiotics before wound contamination occurred (i.e., preoperatively)

TABLE 7.4 **RESULTS**

TYPICAL INFECTION RATES AND REDUCTION WITH PROPHYLAXIS

	PROPHYLAXIS (%)	PLACEBO (%)	NNT[a]
Colon	4–12	24–48	3–5
Other (mixed) GI	4–6	15–29	4–9
Vascular	1–4	7–17	10–17
Cardiac	3–9	44–49	2–3
Hysterectomy	1–16	18–38	3–6
Craniotomy	0.5–3	4–12	9–29
Total joint replacement	0.5–1	2–9	12–100
Breast and hernia operations	3.5	5.2	58

GI, gastrointestinal.
[a]Approximate number needed to treat (NNT) to avoid one surgical site infection.

significantly reduced SSI.[31] Subsequent study has shown that the ideal time for antibiotic administration is just before the incision because this regimen produces better tissue antibiotic concentrations at both the beginning and end of the operation than other administration times.[32–35]

Prophylactic antibiotics are indicated for all GI (including appendectomy), obstetric, gynecologic, oropharyngeal, vascular (abdominal and leg), and open heart procedures. Typical reductions in SSI rate in early placebo-controlled trials of prophylactic antibiotics are given in Table 7.4. The use of prophylactic antibiotics for clean operations remains controversial. Although prophylactic antibiotics reduce the infection rate even in clean procedures, the baseline infection rate is low in these cases.[36,37] Consequently, the number needed to treat for each infection prevented is so large that the reduction in infection risk may not justify the cost and complications associated with antibiotic administration. Nonetheless, prophylactic antibiotic treatment is used routinely for clean procedures such as open heart operations, joint replacement, vascular prostheses, and craniotomy, in which the consequences of SSI are especially severe.[38]

5 Antibiotics should be dosed to maintain adequate tissue concentrations throughout the period of potential contamination. For example, doses should be increased in larger patients.[39] Similarly, doses should be repeated after one or two half-lives have elapsed.[40,41] Numerous trials comparing shorter and longer durations of prophylactic antibiotics failed to show any benefit of extending antibiotic administration beyond the operating room.[42,43] Furthermore, prolonged prophylaxis is associated with recovery of resistant bacteria.[44] An expert panel assembled by the Center for Medicare and Medicaid Services (CMS) thus recommended that prophylactic antibiotics be initiated within the hour before starting an operation and stopped within 24 hours of completion.[45]

Naturally, the antibiotic(s) must be active against the relevant pathogens. This is most clearly illustrated by the requirement that the agent used have activity against enteric anaerobes for procedures involving the lower GI tract. Although yet to be studied in a systematic manner, there is general agreement that antibiotic agents used for prophylaxis should be different from agents usually chosen as first-line treatment of established infections. Thus, although imipenem/cilastatin or piperacillin/tazobactam would undoubtedly be efficacious as prophylactic agents for colon operations, they are not recommended for this purpose. Table 7.5 gives the spectrum of antibiotic recommendations that have been published by different professional societies and organizations. In general, one can choose a first-generation cephalosporin for operations not expected to encounter anaerobes and a second-generation cephalosporin with anaerobic activity for procedures in which anaerobic contamination is likely.

β-Lactam allergies are often cited as a problem for surgical antibiotic prophylaxis. However, many patients reported as allergic do not have true allergy and instead have experienced minor adverse reactions such as *Candida* overgrowth or GI upset. Before choosing an alternate prophylactic agent, one should confirm the nature of the previous reaction. Patients who have had immediate, anaphylactic-type reactions should not receive a cephalosporin, but most others can safely receive one or two doses in the perioperative period. For patients with true β-lactam allergies, vancomycin is the most common prophylactic choice when the primary risk of infection is from skin organisms, and clindamycin is another appropriate alternative. There are no controlled trials of prophylaxis in colon operations using agents appropriate for β-lactam–allergic patients. Logic suggests that the combination of clindamycin or metronidazole with either an aminoglycoside or a fluoroquinolone or the combination of clindamycin with aztreonam should be effective. Although vancomycin has been recommended for routine prophylactic use in hospitals with high rates of methicillin-resistant *Staphylococcus aureus* (MRSA), infection rates were not reduced in the only relevant prospective trial, and the number of infections due to sensitive staphylococci was increased in the vancomycin arm.[46] Vancomycin prophylaxis appears to be most appropriate in patients proved by preoperative nasal culture to be MRSA carriers.

Shaving. Removing hair at the operative site remains routine in many settings, although there is no evidence that it reduces infection rate. In contrast, studies show that avoiding hair removal or using depilatories rather than shaving reduces infection rates after clean operations.[47,48] For example, infection rates are reduced when hair is clipped rather than shaved, even when performed on the day of operation. It may be helpful to warn patients not to shave their operative sites before surgery as some do in an effort to be helpful. If hair removal at the incision site is considered necessary, it should be performed with clippers during the immediate preoperative period.

Delayed Primary Closure. A classic technique to avoid SSI has been to leave the wound open at the original procedure and then to attempt delayed primary closure a few days later or to leave the wound open for closure by secondary intention. This practice was widely used by the military during World War II, and although there have been many series recommending this practice, it has rarely been subject to controlled trial.

TABLE 7.5 **MANAGEMENT**

SUMMARY OF PUBLISHED GUIDELINES ON ANTIMICROBIAL PROPHYLAXIS FOR OPERATIONS TARGETED FOR SURVEILLANCE IN THE NATIONAL SURGICAL CARE IMPROVEMENT PROJECT (SCIP)

■ OPERATIONS	■ PROPHYLACTIC ANTIBIOTIC RECOMMENDATION	■ COMMENTS
Cardiothoracic surgery	Cefazolin Cefuroxime Vancomycin If β-lactam allergy: Vancomycin Clindamycin	Stop within 48 h of end of operation. The Society of Thoracic Surgeons (STS) Practice Guideline for Antibiotic Prophylaxis in Cardiac Surgery (2006) indicates that there is no reason to extend antibiotics beyond 48 h for cardiac surgery and very explicitly states that antibiotics should not be extended beyond 48 h even with tubes and drains in place for cardiac surgery.
Vascular surgery or hip or knee arthroplasty	Cefazolin Cefuroxime Vancomycin If β-lactam allergy: Vancomycin Clindamycin	Stop within 24 h of end of operation. Although not addressed in any of the published guidelines, the workgroup recommends that the prophylactic antimicrobial be completely infused prior to the inflation of a tourniquet.
Colon surgery	Parenteral: Cefoxitin or cefotetan or ampicillin-sulbactam or ertapenem OR Cefazolin plus metronidazole or cefuroxime plus metronidazole If β-lactam allergy: Clindamycin plus an aminoglycoside or a quinolone or aztreonam OR Metronidazole plus an aminoglycoside or a quinolone	Prophylaxis should stop within 24 h of end operation.
Vaginal or abdominal hysterectomy	Cefazolin Cefotetan Cefoxitin Cefuroxime Ampicillin-sulbactam If β-lactam allergy: Clindamycin plus an aminoglycoside or a quinolone or aztreonam OR Metronidazole plus an aminoglycoside or a quinolone OR Clindamycin monotherapy OR Metronidazole monotherapy	Prophylaxis should stop within 24 h of end operation.

Adapted from Bratzler DW, Houck PM. Antimicrobial prophylaxis for surgery: an advisory statement from the national surgical infection prevention project. *Clin Infect Dis* 2004;38:1706–1715, with permission. Available at: http://www.qualitynet.org/dcs/ContentServer?cid=1137346750659&pagename=Medqic%2FContent%2FParentShellTemplate&parentName=TopicCat&c=MQParents. Accessed December 1, 2008.

A recent prospective trial randomized patients undergoing an operative procedure with dirty wounds either to have primary closure of the incision or to have it left open with delayed primary closure.[49] Although the authors concluded that there were fewer SSIs in the group with wounds left open, it is instructive that there were very few differences in overall patient course, and more patients went home with open wounds requiring dressing changes when the wounds were left open than when they were closed primarily in the operating room. There were no differences in overall hospital stay or in charges.

Diagnosis of Surgical Site Infection

One can easily diagnose an SSI when the wound opens and discharges pus. However, it is preferable to make the diagnosis earlier and to initiate prompt intervention. Most SSIs are not clinically evident before the fourth or fifth postoperative day. The rare exceptions to this are infections caused by β-hemolytic streptococci and by histotoxic *Clostridium* sp. and, even more rarely, wound toxic shock. These can be evident within 1 day and, although rare, can be very severe. If a patient manifests severe systemic signs of infection during the first few days after an operation, the incision should be inspected for signs of infection (Algorithm 7.1). Streptococcal infections usually have local signs of inflammation with marked erythema and pain and wound fluid containing white blood cells (WBCs) and gram-positive cocci. Wounds infected by clostridia usually lack signs of inflammation but cause severe pain out of proportion to other findings and drain a thin, brackish wound fluid lacking leukocytes due to the action of the exotoxins on leukocytes inhibiting migration and causing lysis. In these cases, gram-positive rods without spores are evident on Gram smear. Wound blisters or desquamation of skin associated with SSI are late findings and predictive of significant morbidity.

Thirteen cases of wound toxic shock were confirmed by the CDC during an 18-month period, representing less than 1% of all cases of toxic shock reported during that period. More than half of these presented within 48 hours of an operation.[50] The earliest signs were fever, diarrhea, and vomiting. Erythroderma and hypotension were also present. Often, local signs of wound infection were initially absent. Drainage and irrigation of the wound in combination with a systemic antistaphylococcal antibiotic is recommended.

Although most wound infections are diagnosed within 2 weeks after the procedure, diagnosis may occasionally be considerably delayed. This is more likely when a significant amount of tissue covers the operative site such as abdominal incisions in morbidly obese patients. Because many patients have some fever in the first several days after a major operative procedure even without infection, fever is not a specific sign of postoperative infection (Fig. 7.1).[51] Many surgeons want to continue prophylactic antibiotics or to restart antibiotics in cases with early postoperative fever, but this is unlikely to be helpful. In addition, SSI cannot be treated without opening the incision. If antibiotics are given for an SSI without opening the wound, this can result in a delay in diagnosis and definitive treatment, additional morbidity, and additional complications such as wound dehiscence.

Therapy

The most important treatment for an SSI is to open the incision and evacuate the infected material. Antimicrobial agents are needed only when a patient exhibits a significant systemic response to the infection or when there is clinical evidence for

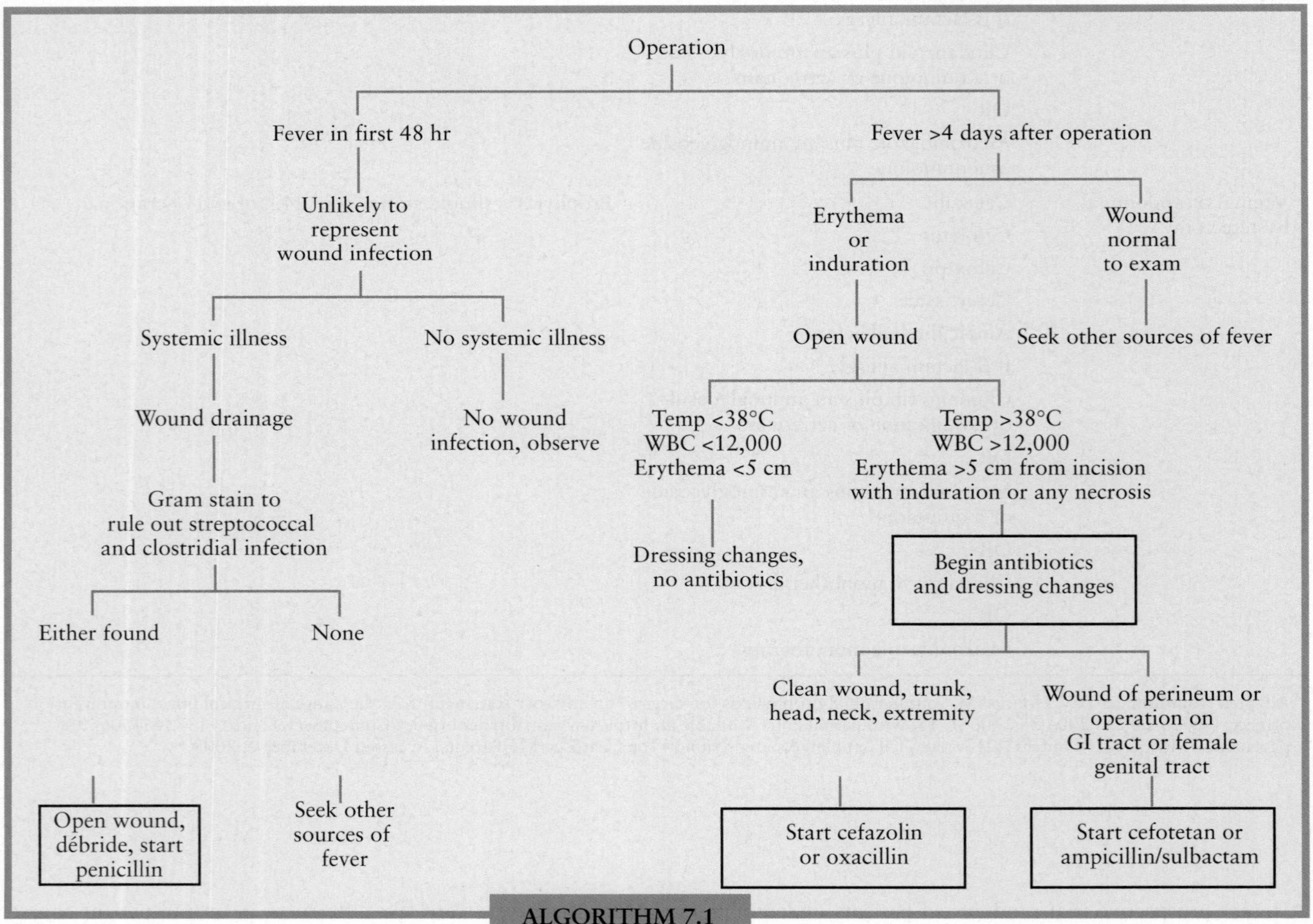

ALGORITHM 7.1

ALGORITHM 7.1. Managing potential surgical site infections. (Adapted from Dellinger EP. Post-operative wound infections. In: Schlossberg D, ed. *Clinical Infectious Disease*. New York: Cambridge University Press; 2008:769–773.)

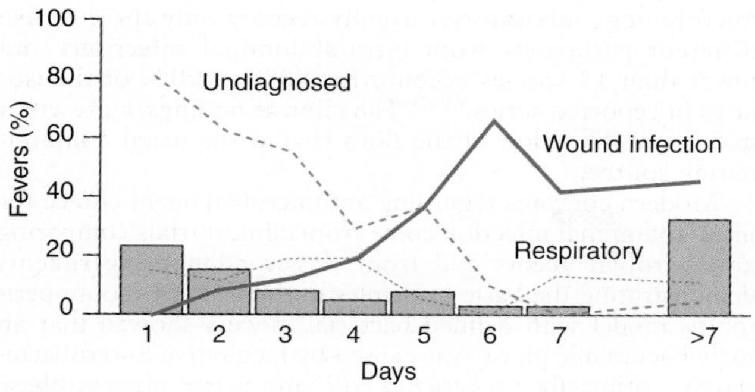

FIGURE 7.1. Percentage of all postoperative fevers occurring on the indicated day following an operative procedure. Lines indicate the percent of fevers occurring on each day attributable to the cause indicated. (After Dellinger EP. Approach to the patient with postoperative fever. In: Gorbach S, Bartlett J, Blacklow N, eds. *Infectious Diseases*. Philadelphia, PA: Lippincott Williams & Wilkins; 2004:817–823.)

invasive infection beyond the surgical wound. In most cases, the entire incision will be involved under the skin and will have to be opened. When an incision is first opened, it should be inspected by a surgeon who understands the procedure and the underlying anatomy. If the procedure was a laparotomy or a thoracotomy, the integrity of the closure of the abdominal or chest wall should be confirmed. In some cases, the incisional SSI is not the primary event but is a sign of more severe and more extensive infection at a deeper level, an organ/space SSI.

Antimicrobial agents should be started empirically at the time of diagnosis and opening of the wound only if there is a significant systemic reaction with temperature above 38°C, an elevated pulse rate, or an absolute WBC count above 12,000/mm^3 or if there is invasive infection in the subcutaneous space or at the fascial level. The agent chosen should be determined by Gram stain of the wound contents and by the prior procedure. SSIs after an operation that did not enter the alimentary tract and was not on the perineum or axilla are often caused by *S. aureus* or less commonly streptococcal species. If Gram stain confirms gram-positive cocci, one can use an initial dose of cefazolin or oxacillin. Antimicrobial treatment should be continued only as long as systemic signs of infection or local cellulitis continues to be present, usually 3 days or less.

For SSIs that follow operations in the axilla, gram-negative bacilli are found more often, and after operations on the perineum or involving the alimentary or genital tract, both facultative and obligate anaerobes are common. In these cases, if antimicrobial therapy is necessary, treatment can be started with cefazolin plus metronidazole or perhaps ertapenem. Patients allergic to penicillin and cephalosporins can receive ciprofloxacin or levofloxacin combined with metronidazole. Again, the treatment should usually be 3 days or less.

INTRA-ABDOMINAL INFECTIONS

Prevention

Most intra-abdominal infections are the result of spontaneous disease including such conditions as appendicitis, diverticulitis, obstructed or perforated carcinomas, or inflammatory bowel disease. Here, prevention depends on early diagnosis and treatment of the underlying condition. However, an increasing proportion of intra-abdominal infections from series published in the past few decades have been postoperative, reflecting the increasing number of operative procedures performed, the increasing risk status of the patients, and the complexity of the operations performed. In the case of postoperative intra-abdominal infections, there are few data available regarding prevention. It is safe to assume that factors that reduce risk of incisional SSI after abdominal operations are probably helpful in the case of organ/space or intra-abdominal infections as well. In addition, avoidance of unintended injury to bowel and optimal performance of GI anastomoses are critical. When contamination of the peritoneum does occur, either during operation or because of spontaneous disease, natural host defense mechanisms actually deal very successfully with small inocula by a combination of lymphatic clearance and phagocytosis by local macrophages. However, if contamination with a small inoculum is repeated, abscess formation is likely. And, if continued contamination occurs, local defenses are overwhelmed and peritonitis results.

Diagnosis

Intra-abdominal infections are usually divided into peritonitis, a poorly localized infection of the peritoneal space, or intra-abdominal abscess, a localized infection within the abdomen. Peritonitis can be relatively local within one quadrant or region of the abdomen, as in early gangrenous or perforated appendicitis, or diffuse in two or more abdominal quadrants. Diffuse peritonitis has a worse prognosis than peritonitis localized to one quadrant.[52] Abscesses may occur within the free peritoneal space in the subphrenic regions, lateral gutters, pelvis, or interloop within the intestinal folds, or they may occur in the retroperitoneum or within a solid organ (visceral) such as liver or spleen. Peritonitis has traditionally been divided into primary and secondary peritonitis, and in recent years the concept of tertiary peritonitis has been proposed. Primary peritonitis describes those patients with ascites due either to hepatic cirrhosis or to nephrotic syndrome who develop infected ascites presumably secondary to bacteremia and without evidence for perforation or underlying GI tract pathology. If the diagnosis of primary peritonitis can be made, these patients are best treated with antimicrobial agents alone and without operation. Because of their severe underlying disease, they are at high risk for poor outcome.

Secondary peritonitis refers to peritoneal infection that occurs secondary to another underlying disease such as bowel perforation. Tertiary peritonitis is a condition first recognized toward the end of the last century and describes patients who continue to have evidence of poorly localized intra-abdominal infection after initial operative and antimicrobial treatment of secondary infection. At subsequent interventions, these patients tend to have evidence of diffuse inflammation without bowel perforation, and cultures return a variety of bacteria that are not common pathogens in the peritoneum such as coagulase-negative staphylococci, *Candida* sp., enterococcus, and *Pseudomonas* sp.[53] The categorization of secondary intra-abdominal infection can also be divided into spontaneous infection, those cases arising from underlying disease, and postoperative infection, occurring after operative intervention or other procedures or trauma. Recent series show that approximately 66% of intra-abdominal infections are spontaneous and 34% are postoperative.[52]

The diagnosis of intra-abdominal infection is almost always first suggested by abdominal pain. This supplemented with a directed history and an exam demonstrating abdominal tenderness strengthens the case. Fever and elevated WBC count are often present, but early cases of appendicitis and diverticulitis will sometimes present with normal temperature and/or WBC count. In patients with diffuse peritonitis such as follows freely perforated bowel or ulcer, the diagnosis is usually made by clinical examination, and this can be followed by resuscitation and operative management without additional sophisticated studies. With abscess, however, the clinical picture is often less straightforward and the addition of cross-sectional imaging techniques, particularly CT scanning, can be very helpful, whereas radionuclide scans have limited usefulness in the diagnosis of intra-abdominal abscess.

Treatment: Source Control

The treatment of intra-abdominal infection always involves the combination of both source control and antimicrobial agents. Diffuse peritonitis involves inflammation and fluid production throughout the peritoneal surface, an area comparable to total body surface area. This is a major hemodynamic challenge and an inflammatory stress to the host organism and must be addressed by attention to circulating blood volume, respiratory status, and other systemic parameters just as in any other critical systemic illness. The fluid requirements of diffuse peritonitis approximate those of a 50% body surface area burn. These fluid shifts accompanied by the cytokine response to peritonitis can easily lead to respiratory and renal failure initially followed by MODS if not treated early and aggressively. Attention to airway, breathing, and circulation must occur simultaneously with antimicrobial management. The systemic disturbance associated with intra-abdominal infection is most readily measured by critical care scores such as the Acute Physiology and Chronic Health Evaluation (APACHE) II score, which has been demonstrated to correlate with mortality and inversely with successful initial treatment of intra-abdominal infection.[54]

Diffuse peritonitis essentially always implies an uncontrolled leak from the GI tract and always mandates operative exploration for source control. If intra-abdominal abscess is diagnosed or suspected, drainage is required, but this can often be accomplished by drains placed percutaneously using the radiologic guidance of fluoroscopy, CT, or ultrasound. Although no prospective trials have been performed comparing open drainage with percutaneous drainage, comparative series suggest that resolution of abscess and mortality are essentially equal between the techniques.[55] Open drainage of intra-abdominal abscess is usually reserved for those cases in which percutaneous access to the abscess is prevented by overlying viscera. Regardless of the approach to source control, review of multiple series suggests that in approximately one fourth of cases a second effort at source control will be necessary to resolve the infection. This may be another open operation, another percutaneous drain, or conversion from one approach to the other. A subsequent intervention is indicated when the patient fails to improve or worsens following the primary intervention. Ideally, the initial effort at source control should be successful. When the operating surgeon is asked to rate the initial source control procedure, outcome is greatly inferior when he or she is not satisfied with this procedure.[52,56,57] Regardless, current evidence suggests that second operations should only be pursued in the presence of clinical or radiographic evidence that the original infection has not resolved or that another infection has developed. Mandatory or scheduled relaparotomies are not helpful except to correct specific known defects such as retained packing after damage control or restoration of intestinal continuity that could not be completed at the original procedure.[58,59]

Treatment: Antimicrobial Therapy

6 The initial antimicrobial treatment of intra-abdominal infection is always empiric. The diagnosis is made clinically, and antimicrobial therapy is started when the diagnosis is made and while the patient is being prepared for the source control procedure. Cultures should be taken in the operating room or radiology suite, but bacterial identification will not be available for at least a day for aerobic and facultative species and for at least 2 days or more for anaerobes. Susceptibility data will not be available for an equivalent amount of time after that. Accordingly, the first 2 to 5 days of treatment are empiric and will be completed without specific susceptibility data. The potential bacterial flora of peritonitis is complex. At least 400 different bacterial species can be identified in the human colon.[60] Despite this, clinical microbiology laboratories usually recover only three to five different pathogens from intra-abdominal infections and fewer than 15 species account for 80% to 90% of the isolates in reported series.[61–64] The clinical findings represent a major simplification of the flora that is the usual contaminating source.

Modern concepts regarding antimicrobial agent choice for intra-abdominal infection come from clinical trials comparing antimicrobial agents and from classic animal experiments demonstrating the basic principles in this field. A mouse peritonitis model with defined bacterial inocula showed that an early bacteremic phase was caused by facultative Enterobacteriaceae, primarily *Escherichia coli,* and a late abscess phase was dependent on anaerobes, especially *Bacteroides fragilis.*[65,66] Antimicrobial agents active against Enterobacteriaceae prevented early mortality, and agents active against the anaerobes prevented late abscess formation. Clinical trials in humans have demonstrated that when antimicrobial regimens are compared, most demonstrate equivalence when both regimens have good activity against both anaerobes and Enterobacteriaceae. A smaller number of trials have demonstrated a clinically and statistically significant difference between antimicrobial regimens and have confirmed that in humans it is important to have coverage against Enterobacteriaceae and against anaerobes.

A number of observational studies have found a strong correlation between the presence of one or more organisms resistant to the antimicrobial agents being used and clinical failure.[63,67–69] One pathogen that has frequently been correlated with failure is *Enterococcus*, a common enteric organism.[70] However, no prospective trial has demonstrated a superior result for a regimen that has activity against enterococci when compared with one that does not. In addition, patients who have been hospitalized before the onset of intra-abdominal infection or who develop postoperative intra-abdominal infection have an increased risk of resistant organisms. Despite this, no prospective trial has demonstrated an advantage for a more comprehensive, or "broad spectrum," regimen for such patients.[67,71] For these reasons, a consensus has developed that an empiric antimicrobial regimen for the treatment of peritonitis should have broad activity against aerobic and facultative gram-negative bacilli and against enteric anaerobes. The regimen should not be completely inactive against *Staphylococcus* and *Streptococcus* sp. Single and combination antimicrobial regimens that have these characteristics and have been tested in prospective trials are listed in Table 7.6.[72,73] For some patients it may be helpful for the regimen to have activity against *Pseudomonas aeruginosa* and against *Enterococcus* sp., but accurate criteria for choosing such patients are lacking. A joint Surgical Infection Society and Infectious Diseases Society of America committee has concluded that it is reasonable, based on retrospective series and expert opinion, to provide agents with activity against *Enterococcus* and, in general, antibiotic combinations with broader spectra of activity for patients at high risk of failure due to the severity of physiologic disturbance at presentation and/or acquisition of the infection in a health care setting.[72–74]

NECROTIZING SOFT TISSUE INFECTIONS

Necrotizing soft tissue infection refers to a spectrum of surgical infections that involve tissue necrosis but are not localized or walled off as abscesses are. These include clostridial infections, which are rare, and nonclostridial infections. Historically, a great variety of labels have been applied to the nonclostridial infections, and in some cases attempts are made to distinguish one from another (Table 7.7).[75] However, these

TABLE 7.6 TREATMENT

ANTIMICROBIAL AGENTS FOR INTRA-ABDOMINAL INFECTION OF MILD TO MODERATE SEVERITY

Single agents
- Cefoxitin
- Ertapenem
- Moxifloxacin
- Tigecycline
- Ticarcillin/clavulanic acid

Combination regimens
- Cefazolin, cefuroxime, ceftriaxone, cefotaxime, ciprofloxacin, or levofloxacin plus metronidazole

Antimicrobial agents for intra-abdominal infection with severe physiologic disturbance, advanced age, or immunocompromised state

Single agents
- Imipenem/cilastatin
- Meropenem
- Doripenem
- Piperacillin/tazobactam

Combination regimens
- Cefepime, ceftazidime, ciprofloxacin, or levofloxacin plus metronidazole

conditions have more in common than the small differences recorded. All present with external signs at the skin level that are far less extensive than the underlying infection, and thus the potential for late diagnosis and treatment. Also, all possess the potential for major tissue loss, significant morbidity, and high mortality. Differences that have been stressed include the pathogen (β-hemolytic *Streptococcus* or CA-MRSA vs. mixed infection), the location (perineum vs. other location), and depth of involvement (involving only superficial tissues vs. muscle also involved). The most common term applied is necrotizing fasciitis, but in most cases the involvement is limited to skin and subcutaneous tissue, and the deeper muscular aponeurosis is not involved. Deeper tissues tend to be involved when the original injury (or operation) breached those areas (e.g., intramuscular hematoma). Necrotizing infection of the abdominal wall can occur after abdominal operations involving bowel entry or treatment of intra-abdominal infection, and the risk is increased when the patient is hemodynamically unstable or when the abdominal wall is closed under tension, causing ischemia in the wound.

TABLE 7.7 CLASSIFICATION

TERMS APPLIED TO SIMILAR NECROTIZING SOFT TISSUE INFECTIONS

- Gangrenous erysipelas
- Necrotizing erysipelas
- Hemolytic streptococcal gangrene
- Nonclostridial crepitant cellulitis
- Nonclostridial gas gangrene
- Synergistic necrotizing cellulitis
- Bacterial synergistic gangrene
- Necrotizing fasciitis
- Necrotizing cellulitis
- Fournier gangrene

Adapted from Dellinger EP. Necrotizing soft-tissue infections. In: Davis JM, Shires GT, eds. *Principles and Management of Surgical Infections*. Philadelphia, PA: J.B. Lippincott; 1991:23–39.

Histotoxic clostridial infections or myonecrosis, commonly called "gas gangrene," are less common than the nonclostridial infections, which are less likely to but still frequently contain gas due to microbial metabolism. Toxins, produced when clostridia grow in anaerobic conditions, kill muscle and inhibit neutrophil chemotaxis, thus facilitating the spread of infection and systemic toxicity.[76,77] The most common clostridial organism is *Clostridium perfringens*, followed by *Clostridium novyi*, *Clostridium septicum*, and *Clostridium sordelli*. Although nearly all cases of myonecrosis originate in a traumatic wound, *C. septicum* is capable of causing spontaneous myonecrosis if it gains access to the body through compromised bowel mucosa, which can occur with GI malignancies, such as colon cancer, or during chemotherapy for other malignancies.[78]

SCIENTIFIC PRINCIPLES

Diagnosis

The most important aspect for effective treatment of necrotizing soft tissue infections is early diagnosis. Delay in diagnosis affects outcome adversely. The following physical signs are strongly suggestive of necrotizing infection and merit exploration of the wound in the operating room: any skin necrosis, crepitus, gas in tissue detected by radiologic examination, bullae, or ecchymosis. Other suggestive criteria include marked, or "woody," edema beyond the area of inflammation or progression of the infection despite apparently appropriate antimicrobial therapy. Although necrotizing soft tissue infections have a reputation for progressing very rapidly, and many do, leading to potential early death, they can also be more indolent and simply persist until diagnosed and débrided.[79]

The diagnostic significance of infection-associated gas is worth an explanation. When aerobic and facultative bacteria are able to use oxidative metabolic pathways, they produce CO_2 as do mammals. CO_2 is highly soluble and is readily carried away by blood flow in perfused tissue. However, when facultative and anaerobic bacteria are forced to use nonoxidative metabolic pathways, they rely on fermentation, denitrification, or deamination. These processes produce nitrogen and hydrogen, which are relatively insoluble and accumulate in the surrounding tissue. Thus, the presence of gas in tissue with infection implies anaerobic metabolism, which is incompatible with living host tissue. This implies that the infection is in nonperfused, dead tissue and requires débridement or drainage.

The persistent difficulty of diagnosis using signs and symptoms has led clinicians to search for other aids to diagnosis. Multiple reports examining the role of ultrasound, CT scans, and magnetic resonance imaging suggest that these techniques have increased sensitivity for detecting abnormalities in affected tissues but are not specific and frequently are unhelpful in distinguishing between soft tissue infections that require operative intervention from those that do not.[79,80] In addition, biopsy and frozen section examination of affected tissues have been suggested.[81] However, if enough suspicion exists to do a biopsy, most experienced surgeons can recognize the extent of the process and need for débridement visually when the incision is made.[79]

Treatment

Operative management of these infections requires exposure of all affected tissue. This usually necessitates incision through uninvolved skin for a significant distance. Necrotic tissue should be débrided, and involved areas must be exposed, but this does not necessarily require excision of overlying tissues unless they are rendered ischemic by the incisions. Careful planning of incisions should be able to avoid this in most cases. On an extremity, amputation may be required for a clostridial infection, and, although this is uncommon for nonclostridial soft tissue infections, amputation may still be lifesaving and should not be delayed if indicated. Intraoperatively, lack of muscular contraction in response to electrical stimulation, using cautery, is frequently used to identify dying or dead muscle requiring more extensive débridement. All patients who require operative intervention for a necrotizing soft tissue infection should be scheduled for a second look in the operating room during the next 24 to 48 hours. Decisions regarding further operative intervention can be made at that time. Large wounds are common, and secondary closure or skin grafts may be required after the infection is completely resolved.

Antimicrobial treatment is initially empiric and must be directed against a presumed mixed flora or aerobic and anaerobic pathogens. The choice of agents is essentially the same as for intra-abdominal infection. Initially, high-dose penicillin, gentamicin, and clindamycin are frequently implemented. There is suggestive evidence from animal experiments that high-dose clindamycin, by binding to RNA in the bacteria, may reduce toxin formation by clostridial species and by toxin-producing streptococci and staphylococci.[82] As with other severe infections, patients with necrotizing soft tissue infections have a marked systemic response and require attention to fluid resuscitation, gas exchange, and renal function.

SEPSIS, SHOCK, AND MULTIPLE ORGAN DYSFUNCTION

A severe systemic response to infection including hemodynamic instability and progression to multiple organ dysfunction can occur after either medical or surgical infections. They can occur after either gram-positive or gram-negative infections but appear to be more common with gram-negative infections and are often triggered by a complex systemic host response to lipopolysaccharide (LPS). Within the context of surgical infections, the best outcome for a patient results from prompt diagnosis and treatment of infections to prevent the onset of sepsis. A number of studies show that early, aggressive correction of physiologic abnormalities seen in early sepsis[83] along with prompt aggressive treatment of the infection itself, both with antimicrobial agents and source control,[84,85] results in the best outcome. Currently, the only additional medical treatment with demonstrated benefit is the administration of activated protein C (drotrecogin alfa) to patients who fit the entry criteria for this trial with sepsis and concomitant organ dysfunction in more than one organ.[1] The risk of increased bleeding complications must be balanced against potential benefits, particularly following recent surgical procedures.

OTHER NOSOCOMIAL INFECTIONS IN SURGICAL PATIENTS

Surgical patients are also susceptible to a number of nonsurgical nosocomial infections during hospitalization. The appropriate care of these patients demands an understanding of the prevention and treatment of these infections.

Catheter-related Bloodstream Infections

Although both peripheral venous and arterial catheters and central venous catheters can be infected, diagnosis is often easier with peripheral catheters, and serious bloodstream infections are more common with central catheters. One of the first principles in preventing these infections is to restrict the use of catheters and to ask each day whether the patient actually needs the catheters that are in place. Another important element of prevention is the insertion technique, especially for central catheters. Although full barrier precautions with wide draping and use of glove, gown, hat, and mask by the inserting physician results in lower infection rates,[86] this is not always followed. An institutional education program to emphasize the importance of insertion technique has been shown to lower infection rates.[87] Skin preparation with a chlorhexidine solution results in lower infection rates than preparation with povidone-iodine solutions.[88] All intravascular devices are susceptible to infection, and the risk increases the longer the catheter is in place. However, changing central lines on a particular schedule does not decrease infection risk.[89,90] The final risk is related to the number of days that any catheter is in place. Subclavian central venous catheters have a lower risk of infection than internal jugular catheters. Recommendations for the use of antimicrobial-coated catheters are not well established because one must balance the risk of line infection against the risk of additional antimicrobial exposure to the patient and to the environment. When the local rate of infection is high, they are probably justified.[90] The single most impressive effort in reducing central line–associated infections has been a program that "bundles" all of these components together, uses a checklist, and empowers all members of the medical/surgical team to take responsibility for adherence to the bundle.[91]

The diagnosis of catheter-related bloodstream infection is made by isolating the same organism from the bloodstream and from a semiquantitative culture of the catheter tip. To make a diagnosis of catheter-related bloodstream infection without removing the catheter, draw simultaneous cultures through the line and from a different peripheral source. A line infection is indicated when the quantitative culture of the line is equal or greater than five times the peripheral quantity or when the line culture turns positive 2 hours or more before the peripheral culture. When the diagnosis is made, the catheter should be removed. Bacteremia should be treated by a specific antimicrobial agent and, for *S. aureus*, gram-negative rods, or fungi, should be continued for 10 to 14 days.[92] For coagulase-negative staphylococci, the most common pathogen, duration of treatment can be limited to the period of systemic response after removal of the catheter.

Pneumonia

Pneumonia is less common than SSI and UTI on surgical services but when it occurs is a major source of morbidity and mortality. Prevention of postoperative pneumonia is best accomplished by policies and procedures that emphasize the early extubation of ventilated patients, the use of noninvasive positive-pressure ventilation when feasible, and elevation of the head of the bed for ventilated patients. Diagnosis can be made by physical examination and chest radiograph in the spontaneously breathing postoperative patient. The diagnosis can be much more challenging in the ventilated ICU patient. These patients often have abnormal chest films and physical findings as well as fever and leukocytosis in the absence of pneumonia. In addition, all patients with an endotracheal tube for more than a few days are likely to have bacteria in tracheal aspirates independent of infection. Overtreatment of suspected infection is common, and restriction of treatment for patients without demonstrated pneumonia improves outcome.[93] On the other hand, delayed, specific treatment of true infection increases mortality.[94,95] For this reason, procedures that produce a more specific diagnosis of pneumonia and that help to rule out the diagnosis when pneumonia is not present, such as bronchoalveolar lavage and protected specimen brush cultures, have an important role in the care of ventilated ICU patients.[96–98] Cultures of expectorated sputum or of simple endotracheal aspirates are very nonspecific and of little use in diagnosing pneumonia. When pneumonia is diagnosed, treatment duration should be limited. Usually 7 to 8 days is sufficient.[99]

Urinary Tract Infection

The most common etiologic agent of UTI in hospitalized patients is the indwelling bladder catheter. Many surgical patients have urinary catheters placed in the operating room. A primary preventive measure for UTI is to use urinary catheters only when actually necessary due to the location of the operative procedure or the length and complexity of the operation. When a catheter is required it should be removed as soon as possible, often at the end of the operative procedure or on the first postoperative day. When a catheter must be left in place, a closed system should always be used. The risk of UTI doubles on any day when the integrity of a closed system is violated.

In a patient without a catheter, the diagnosis of UTI is traditionally made when a quantitative culture shows greater than 10^5 organisms per milliliter of urine. In patients with catheters, much lower colony counts may represent true infection. Attempts to clear bacteriuria when the catheter is in place usually fail. If the patient is symptomatic, specific antimicrobial treatment should be followed by a catheter change. If the patient is not symptomatic, specific antimicrobial treatment should be given after the catheter has been removed.

PATHOGENS

As noted in the beginning of this chapter, most surgical infections are caused by endogenous microorganisms that gain access to the body after violation of an epithelial barrier. Specific pathogens are identified through culture in the microbiology laboratory, but earlier information can be obtained through examination of a Gram-stained smear of material taken from the infected site. Gram-positive cocci are very commonly found in soft tissue infections and can represent *Staphylococcus* sp., either *S. aureus* or coagulase-negative staphylococci, or streptococcal species. Coagulase-negative staphylococci are the most common pathogens found in catheter-related bloodstream infections but cause serious infections in other locations rarely. *S. aureus* possess virulence characteristics that enable them to invade healthy tissues and form abscesses and are usually significant when recovered. Extensive use of β-lactam antibiotics has led to the emergence of MRSA in many areas, and recently some strains of vancomycin-intermediate *S. aureus* (VISA) and vancomycin-resistant *S. aureus* (VRSA) strains have emerged. In the first decade of the 21st century a new strain of MRSA has become common in the community in patients not recently exposed to the health care system. This is called community-acquired MRSA and is frequently characterized by a new virulence feature, the Panton-Valentin leucocidin that appears to stimulate more tissue necrosis. This organism has been associated with necrotizing soft tissue infections similar to those previously only associated with β-hemolytic streptococci.

β-Hemolytic streptococci, especially from group A, have significant virulence properties that allow them to invade uninjured or minimally injured tissues to cause severe soft tissue infections as previously discussed in the section on necrotizing soft tissue infections. They are uncommon surgical pathogens otherwise. Group D streptococci, or enterococci, are frequently recovered from intra-abdominal infections, but studies fail to demonstrate superior outcomes when antimicrobial regimens are directed toward enterococci. However, this species can clearly cause severe disease in immune-compromised patients, especially liver transplant patients. In this setting the occurrence of vancomycin-resistant enterococci (VRE) in recent years has presented a very difficult treatment challenge.

Facultative gram-negative rods, which can grow in either aerobic or anaerobic environments, are commonly associated with surgical infections, especially those arising from intra-abdominal sources. These include the familiar genera *Escherichia, Proteus, Klebsiella, Enterobacter, Morganella, Providencia,* and *Serratia.* These pathogens are most commonly treated with advanced-generation cephalosporins, expanded-spectrum penicillins, carbapenems, or fluoroquinolones. In recent years, a number of these pathogens have developed extended-spectrum β-lactam enzymes (ESBLs) capable of inactivating even third-generation cephalosporins. While these are more common outside of the United States, they are also found in the United States and have increased in recent years. Currently, carbapenem antibiotics are considered the antibiotic of choice for these organisms. An even newer resistance mechanism, *Klebsiella* pneumonia carbapenemase (KPC enzymes), has led to ESBL pathogens that are also resistant to the carbapenem antibiotics. In these cases only tigecycline; the old, relatively toxic antibiotics polymyxin B and E (colistin); and sometimes aminoglycosides have activity. Bacteria that are resistant to three of the following classes, β-lactams (including penicillins, cephalosporins, and monobactams), carbapenems, fluoroquinolones, and aminoglycosides, are termed multidrug-resistant (MDR) organisms.[100,101] Obligate aerobic gram-negative rods encountered in surgical patients include *Pseudomonas* sp. and *Acinetobacter* sp. These are most commonly found in the respiratory tract but can also occur in the abdomen. These pathogens often exhibit an even higher degree of antimicrobial resistance than the facultative gram-negative rods.

Anaerobic bacteria are the most common inhabitants of the GI tract in humans and cause significant disease in intra-abdominal infections, but they are not represented in infections proportional to their density in the bowel. The most common isolates are members of the *Bacteroides* genus, especially *B. fragilis* and *Bacteroides thetaiotaomicron.* The most effective antibiotics against these organisms are metronidazole, the carbapenems, and advanced-generation penicillins combined with a β-lactam inhibitor. Moxifloxacin and tigecycline also have activity against the common anaerobes. The anaerobic cocci are also susceptible to the same antibiotics. *Clostridium* sp., as noted in the section on necrotizing soft tissue infections, are most important in that setting. When anaerobes are recovered from a surgical infection or from the bloodstream, this means that bacteria are growing in the body in an anaerobic environment. These are always surgical infections and require source control in addition to antimicrobial treatment.

Fungi, most commonly *Candida* sp., are rarely primary causative agents in surgical infections. However, they are often secondary pathogens, overgrowing on skin and the gut under the influence of broad-spectrum antibacterial therapy. In this setting they become important opportunistic invaders. The most common strain found is *Candida albicans.* Most *Candida* infections are currently treated with fluconazole, but increasing use of this agent tends to provide pressure to increase the presence of resistant strains such as *Candida glabrata* or *Candida krusei.* In these cases, treatment with voriconazole, caspofungin, anidulafungin, micafungin, or amphotericin may be required.

Viruses do not cause surgical infections. Surgical patients are most susceptible to viral infection as a result of blood transfusion, which may transmit hepatitis B, hepatitis C, or the human immunodeficiency virus (HIV). Recent advances in nucleic acid detection technology have rendered the blood supply in the United States increasingly safe so that the current risk for transmission of any of these agents by transfusion is less than 1 in 2 million.[102] Transplant patients are susceptible to a number of viral infections due to their immune-compromised state, especially cytomegalovirus.

ANTIMICROBIAL AGENTS

Antimicrobial agents are used in combination with source control and other treatment modalities to prevent or resolve surgical infections. The goal should be to use these agents when they are required and to withhold them when they are not. Overuse of antimicrobial agents contributes to bacterial resistance and limits their effectiveness when they are needed. They should be used in a manner that ensures therapeutic levels at the site of infection for the appropriate duration. Pharmacodynamic principles of antibiotic use differ for different classes of drugs. The factors that go into an antibiotic's effectiveness include its minimal inhibitory concentration (MIC) for a particular pathogen, its half-life and mode of elimination from the body, and its mechanism of action.[103,104] β-Lactam antibiotics such as penicillins and cephalosporins bind to penicillin-binding proteins (PBPs) in the bacterial cell wall and inhibit bacterial cell wall synthesis. Once drug levels are achieved that are well above MIC, the rate of bacterial killing does not increase with higher drug levels. Their effectiveness depends on the percent of time during therapy that the drug levels exceed the MIC at the site of infection. Thus, a dose and time of administration that achieves levels above MIC for more than 50% of the time between doses will provide optimal therapy. This favors drugs with long half-lives or continuous administration of drugs with shorter half-lives. Time above MIC can also be prolonged with intermittent dosing if infusions are prolonged for 1 to 2 hours. Alternatively, aminoglycosides kill by inhibiting microbial protein synthesis, and higher levels of drug above the MIC kill bacteria more rapidly. In addition, these drugs exhibit a "postantibiotic effect" in which bacteria do not begin to grow again for a time after the drug levels have fallen below the MIC. This has led to the once-daily administration of aminoglycoside antibiotics, which achieve very high serum levels shortly after administration and take advantage of the postantibiotic effect after serum levels have fallen. In addition, renal toxicity of the drugs is equal or less with once-daily administration compared with three-times-daily administration, which was the former practice. For quinolones, the best results correlate with the ratio between the area under the curve (AUC) when time is graphed

TABLE 7.8 **CLASSIFICATION**

ANTIBIOTICS

Penicillin class	**Carbapenems**
The original	Imipenem/cilastatin
Penicillin G	Meropenem
Antistaphylococcal	Ertapenem
Methicillin	Doripenem
Nafcillin	**Fluoroquinolones**
Oxacillin	Ciprofloxacin
Limited gram-negative activity	Levofloxacin
Ampicillin	Gatifloxacin
Amoxicillin	Moxifloxacin
Broader gram-negative activity	**Aminoglycosides**
Carbenicillin	Gentamicin
Ticarcillin	Tobramycin
Piperacillin	Amikacin
β-Lactamase inhibitor combinations	Netilmicin
Ampicillin/sulbactam	**Various antianaerobic drugs**
Amoxicillin/clavulanate	Chloramphenicol
Ticarcillin/clavulanate	Clindamycin
Piperacillin/tazobactam	Metronidazole
Cephalosporin class	**Antimicrobials with activity against MRSA**
First generation	Vancomycin
Cephalothin	Quinupristin/dalfopristin
Cefazolin	Linezolid
Cephalexin	Daptomycin
Cephradine	Tigecycline
Second generation	**Antifungal drugs**
Cefuroxime	Amphotericin
Cefoxitin	Fluconazole
Cefmetazole	Voriconazole
Cefotetan	Caspofungin
Third generation	Anidulafungin
Cefotaxime	Micafungin
Ceftizoxime	
Ceftriaxone	
Cefoperazone	
Ceftazidime	
Cefepime	

MRSA, methicillin-resistant *Staphylococcus aureus*.

against serum concentration in mg/L. A ratio of AUC/MIC greater than 125 correlates with clinical success.

When antimicrobial agents are used to treat an infection, response to treatment should be evaluated in a regular and ongoing schedule. If improvement is not evident within 2 to 3 days of treatment, the situation should be assessed and an explanation sought. These questions should be asked: Was the original source control adequate? Has a complication of the source control procedure occurred? Has a superinfection developed? Is enough of the proper drug being given in an appropriate manner? The wrong antibiotic is not the most common cause of failure in treating a surgical infection.

Once the patient is improving, one needs to decide how long to continue antimicrobial agents. For most surgical infections, these agents can be stopped when the patient has demonstrated a return to normal temperature and WBC count with improvement in general condition as long as the source control was adequate. There is an absence of objective, prospective data demonstrating the necessary duration of drug treatment. Prolonged antimicrobial agent administration predisposes the patient to superinfections, to colonization with resistant bacteria, and to development of drug adverse reactions and organ damage.

This chapter does not provide a detailed discussion of each antimicrobial drug available. The list is very large and frequently changes. Detailed discussions of indications and doses for individual drugs are available in several reference or online sources, which are updated on a yearly basis. Common examples are the *Sanford Guide*, *The Medical Letter*, and the *Johns Hopkins Division of Infectious Diseases Antibiotic Guide* (http://hopkins-abxguide.org/). Table 7.8 lists the classes and individual drugs that are most commonly used by surgeons, grouped by class and antimicrobial activity.

References

1. Bernard GR, Vincent JL, Laterre PF, et al. Efficacy and safety of recombinant human activated protein C for severe sepsis. *N Engl J Med* 2001;344: 699–709.
2. Namias N, Harvill S, Ball S, et al. Empiric therapy of sepsis in the surgical intensive care unit with broad-spectrum antibiotics for 72 hours does not lead to the emergence of resistant bacteria. *J Trauma* 1998;45:887–891.
3. Marshall JC, Schein M. *Source Control: A Guide to the Management of Surgical Infections*. Berlin: Springer; 2002.
4. Solomkin JS, Yellin AE, Rotstein OD, et al. Ertapenem versus piperacillin/tazobactam in the treatment of complicated intraabdominal infections: results of a double-blind, randomized comparative phase III trial. *Ann Surg* 2003;237:235–245.
5. Horan TC, Gaynes RP, Martone WJ, et al. CDC definitions of nosocomial surgical site infections, 1992: a modification of CDC definitions of surgical wound infections. *Am J Infect Control* 1992;20:271–274.
6. Mangram AJ, Horan TC, Pearson ML, et al. Guideline for prevention of surgical site infection, 1999. Hospital Infection Control Practices Advisory Committee. *Infect Control Hosp Epidemiol* 1999;20:250–278; quiz 79–80.
7. Gaynes RP, Culver DH, Horan TC, et al. Surgical site infection (SSI) rates in the United States, 1992–1998: the National Nosocomial Infections Surveillance System basic SSI risk index. *Clin Infect Dis* 2001;33:S69–S77.
8. Howard JM, Barker WF, Culbertson W, et al. Postoperative wound infections: the influence of ultraviolet irradiation on the operating room and of various other factors. *Ann Surg* 1964;160:1–196.
9. Culver D, Horan T, Gaynes R. Comparing surgical site infection (SSI) rates using the NNIS SSI index and the standardized infection ratio. *Am J Infect Control* 1994;22:102.
10. Nosocomial infection rates for interhospital comparison: limitations and possible solutions. A Report from the National Nosocomial Infections Surveillance (NNIS) System. *Infect Control Hosp Epidemiol* 1991;12: 609–621.
11. Roy MC, Herwaldt LA, Embrey R, et al. Does the Centers for Disease Control's NNIS system risk index stratify patients undergoing cardiothoracic operations by their risk of surgical-site infection? *Infect Control Hosp Epidemiol* 2000;21:186–190.
12. Minnema B, Vearncombe M, Augustin A, et al. Risk factors for surgical-site infection following primary total knee arthroplasty. *Infect Control Hosp Epidemiol* 2004;25:477–480.
13. Latham R, Lancaster AD, Covington JF, et al. The association of diabetes and glucose control with surgical-site infections among cardiothoracic surgery patients. *Infect Control Hosp Epidemiol* 2001;22:607–612.
14. Furnary AP, Zerr KJ, Grunkemeier GL, et al. Continuous intravenous insulin infusion reduces the incidence of deep sternal wound infection in diabetic patients after cardiac surgical procedures [see comments]. *Ann Thorac Surg* 1999;67:352–360; discussion 60–62.
15. Ramos M, Khalpey Z, Lipsitz S, et al. Relationship of perioperative hyperglycemia and postoperative infections in patients who undergo general and vascular surgery. *Ann Surg* 2008;248:585–591.
16. Polk HC, Jr, Lopez-Mayor JF. Postoperative wound infection: a prospective study of determinant factors and prevention. *Surgery* 1969;66:97–103.
17. Hojer H, Wetterfors J. Systemic prophylaxis with doxycycline in surgery of the colon and rectum. *Ann Surg* 1978;187:362–368.
18. Hunt TK, Linsey M, Grislis H, et al. The effect of differing ambient oxygen tensions on wound infection. *Ann Surg* 1975;181:35–39.
19. Hopf HW, Hunt TK, West JM, et al. Wound tissue oxygen tension predicts the risk of wound infection in surgical patients. *Arch Surg* 1997;132: 997–1004; discussion 5.
20. Greif R, Akca O, Horn EP, et al. Supplemental perioperative oxygen to reduce the incidence of surgical-wound infection. Outcomes Research Group [see comments]. *N Engl J Med* 2000;342:161–167.
21. Pryor KO, Fahey TJ, 3rd, Lien CA, et al. Surgical site infection and the routine use of perioperative hyperoxia in a general surgical population: a randomized controlled trial. *JAMA* 2004;291:79–87.
22. Belda FJ, Aguilera L, Garcia de la Asuncion J, et al. Supplemental perioperative oxygen and the risk of surgical wound infection: a randomized controlled trial. *JAMA* 2005;294:2035–2042.
23. Dellinger EP. Increasing inspired oxygen to decrease surgical site infection: time to shift the quality improvement research paradigm. *JAMA* 2005; 294:2091–2092.
24. Rabkin JM, Hunt TK. Local heat increases blood flow and oxygen tension in wounds. *Arch Surg* 1987;122:221–225.
25. Kurz A, Sessler DI, Lenhardt R. Perioperative normothermia to reduce the incidence of surgical-wound infection and shorten hospitalization. Study of Wound Infection and Temperature Group [see comments]. *N Engl J Med* 1996;334:1209–1215.
26. Melling AC, Ali B, Scott EM, et al. Effects of preoperative warming on the incidence of wound infection after clean surgery: a randomised controlled trial. *Lancet* 2001;358:876–880.
27. Sessler DI. Perioperative heat balance. *Anesthesiology* 2000;92:578–596.
28. Pomposelli JJ, Baxter JK, 3rd, Babineau TJ, et al. Early postoperative glucose control predicts nosocomial infection rate in diabetic patients. *JPEN J Parenter Enteral Nutr* 1998;22:77–81.
29. Furnary AP, Gao G, Grunkemeier GL, et al. Continuous insulin infusion reduces mortality in patients with diabetes undergoing coronary artery bypass grafting. *J Thorac Cardiovasc Surg* 2003;125:1007–1021.
30. McKittrick LS, Wheelock FC, Jr. The routine use of antibiotics in elective abdominal surgery. *Surg Gynec Obstet* 1954;99:376–377.
31. Burke J. The effective period of preventive antibiotic action in experimental incisions and dermal lesions. *Surgery* 1961;50:161–168.
32. Classen DC, Evans RS, Pestotnik SL, et al. The timing of prophylactic administration of antibiotics and the risk of surgical-wound infection [see comments]. *N Engl J Med* 1992;326:281–286.
33. Dellinger EP. Prophylactic antibiotics: administration and timing before operation are more important than administration after operation. *Clin Infect Dis* 2007;44:928–930.
34. DiPiro JT, Vallner JJ, Bowden TA, et al. Intraoperative serum and tissue activity of cefazolin and cefoxitin. *Arch Surg* 1985;120:829–832.
35. van Kasteren ME, Mannien J, Ott A, et al. Antibiotic prophylaxis and the risk of surgical site infections following total hip arthroplasty: timely administration is the most important factor. *Clin Infect Dis* 2007;44: 921–927.
36. Platt R. Antibiotic prophylaxis in clean surgery: does it work? Should it be used if it does? *New Horiz* 1998;6:S53–S57.
37. Platt R, Zaleznik DF, Hopkins CC, et al. Perioperative antibiotic prophylaxis for herniorrhaphy and breast surgery. *N Engl J Med* 1990;322:153–160.
38. Dellinger EP, Gross PA, Barrett TL, et al. Quality standard for antimicrobial prophylaxis in surgical procedures. Infectious Diseases Society of America. *Clin Infect Dis* 1994;18:422–427.
39. Forse RA, Karam B, MacLean LD, et al. Antibiotic prophylaxis for surgery in morbidly obese patients. *Surgery* 1989;106:750–756.
40. Scher KS. Studies on the duration of antibiotic administration for surgical prophylaxis. *Am Surg* 1997;63:59–62.
41. Zanetti G, Giardina R, Platt R. Intraoperative redosing of cefazolin and risk for surgical site infection in cardiac surgery. *Emerg Infect Dis* 2001;7:828–831.
42. Kriaras I, Michalopoulos A, Turina M, Geroulanos S. Evolution of antimicrobial prophylaxis in cardiovascular surgery. *Eur J Cardiothorac Surg* 2000;18:440–446.
43. McDonald M, Grabsch E, Marshall C, et al. Single- versus multiple-dose antimicrobial prophylaxis for major surgery: a systematic review [see comments]. *Aust N Z J Surg* 1998;68:388–396.
44. Harbarth S, Samore MH, Lichtenberg D, et al. Prolonged antibiotic prophylaxis after cardiovascular surgery and its effect on surgical site infections and antimicrobial resistance. *Circulation* 2000;101:2916–2921.
45. Bratzler DW, Houck PM. Antimicrobial prophylaxis for surgery: an advisory statement from the national surgical infection prevention project. *Clin Infect Dis* 2004;38:1706–1715.
46. Finkelstein R, Rabino G, Mashiah T, et al. Vancomycin versus cefazolin prophylaxis for cardiac surgery in the setting of a high prevalence of methicillin-resistant staphylococcal infections. *J Thorac Cardiovasc Surg* 2002; 123:326–332.

47. Alexander JW, Fischer JE, Boyajian M, et al. The influence of hair-removal methods on wound infections. *Arch Surg* 1983;118:347–352.
48. Ko W, Lazenby WD, Zelano JA, et al. Effects of shaving methods and intraoperative irrigation on suppurative mediastinitis after bypass operations. *Ann Thorac Surg* 1992;53:301–305.
49. Cohn SM, Giannotti G, Ong AW, et al. Prospective randomized trial of two wound management strategies for dirty abdominal wounds. *Ann Surg* 2001;233:409–413.
50. Bartlett P, Reingold AL, Graham DR, et al. Toxic shock syndrome associated with surgical wound infections. *JAMA* 1982;247:1448–1450.
51. Dellinger EP. Approach to the patient with postoperative fever. In: Gorbach S, Bartlett J, Blacklow N, eds. Infectious Diseases, 3rd ed. Philadelphia: Lippincott Williams & Wilkins; 2004:817–823.
52. Seiler CA, Brugger L, Forssmann U, et al. Conservative surgical treatment of diffuse peritonitis. *Surgery* 2000;127:178–184.
53. Nathens AB, Rotstein OD, Marshall JC. Tertiary peritonitis: clinical features of a complex nosocomial infection. *World J Surg* 1998;22:158–163.
54. Christou NV, Barie PS, Dellinger EP, et al. Surgical Infection Society intra-abdominal infection study. Prospective evaluation of management techniques and outcome. *Arch Surg* 1993;128:193–198; discussion 8–9.
55. Levison MA. Percutaneous versus open operative drainage of intra-abdominal abscesses. *Infect Dis Clin Nort Am* 1992;6:525–544.
56. Ohmann C, Yang Q, Hau T, et al. Prognostic modelling in peritonitis. Peritonitis Study Group of the Surgical Infection Society Europe. *Eur J Surg* 1997;163:53–60.
57. Koperna T, Schulz F. Relaparotomy in peritonitis: prognosis and treatment of patients with persisting intraabdominal infection. *World J Surg* 2000; 24:32–37.
58. van Ruler O, Mahler CW, Boer KR, et al. Comparison of on-demand vs planned relaparotomy strategy in patients with severe peritonitis: a randomized trial. *JAMA* 2007;298:865–872.
59. Dellinger EP. Timing of reoperation for patients with severe peritonitis. *JAMA* 2007;298:923–924.
60. Finegold SM, Sutter VL, Mathisen GE. Normal indigenous intestinal flora. In: Hentges DJ, ed. *Human Intestinal Microflora in Health and Disease.* New York: Academic Press; 1983:3–31.
61. Solomkin JS, Dellinger EP, Christou NV, et al. Results of a multicenter trial comparing imipenem/cilastatin to tobramycin/clindamycin for intra-abdominal infections. *Ann Surg* 1990;212:581–591.
62. Barie PS, Vogel SB, Dellinger EP, et al. A randomized, double-blind clinical trial comparing cefepime plus metronidazole with imipenem-cilastatin in the treatment of complicated intra-abdominal infections. Cefepime Intra-abdominal Infection Study Group. *Arch Surg* 1997;132:1294–1302.
63. Mosdell DM, Morris DM, Voltura A, et al. Antibiotic treatment for surgical peritonitis. *Ann Surg* 1991;214:543–552.
64. Solomkin JS, Reinhart HH, Dellinger EP, et al. Results of a randomized trial comparing sequential intravenous/oral treatment with ciprofloxacin plus metronidazole to imipenem/cilastatin for intra-abdominal infections. The Intra-Abdominal Infection Study Group. *Ann Surg* 1996;223: 303–315.
65. Bartlett JG, Onderdonk AB, Louie T, et al. A review. Lessons from an animal model of intra-abdominal sepsis. *Arch Surg* 1978;113:853–857.
66. Weinstein WM, Onderdonk AB, Bartlett JG, et al. Antimicrobial therapy of experimental intraabdominal sepsis. *J Infect Dis* 1975;132:282–286.
67. Christou NV, Turgeon P, Wassef R, et al. Management of intra-abdominal infections. The case for intraoperative cultures and comprehensive broad-spectrum antibiotic coverage. The Canadian Intra-abdominal Infection Study Group. *Arch Surg* 1996;131:1193–1201.
68. Hopkins JA, Lee JC, Wilson SE. Susceptibility of intra-abdominal isolates at operation: a predictor of postoperative infection. *Am Surg* 1993;59: 791–796.
69. Montravers P, Gauzit R, Muller C, et al. Emergence of antibiotic-resistant bacteria in cases of peritonitis after intraabdominal surgery affects the efficacy of empirical antimicrobial therapy. *Clin Infect Dis* 1996;23:486–494.
70. Burnett RJ, Haverstock DC, Dellinger EP, et al. Definition of the role of enterococcus in intraabdominal infection: analysis of a prospective randomized trial. *Surgery* 1995;118:716–721.
71. Dupont H, Carbon C, Carlet J. Monotherapy with a broad-spectrum beta-lactam is as effective as its combination with an aminoglycoside in treatment of severe generalized peritonitis: a multicenter randomized controlled trial. The Severe Generalized Peritonitis Study Group. *Antimicrob Agents Chemother* 2000;44:2028–2033.
72. Mazuski JE, Sawyer RG, Nathens AB, et al. The Surgical Infection Society Guidelines on Antimicrobial Therapy for Intra-Abdominal Infections: An Executive Summary. *Surg Infect (Larchmt)* 2002;3:161–173.
73. Mazuski JE, Sawyer RG, Nathens AB, et al. The Surgical Infection Society Guidelines on Antimicrobial Therapy for Intra-Abdominal Infections: Evidence for the Recommendations. *Surg Infect (Larchmt)* 2002;3:175–233.
74. Solomkin JS, Mazuski JE, Baron EJ, et al. Guidelines for the selection of anti-infective agents for complicated intra-abdominal infections. *Clin Infect Dis* 2003;37:997–1005.
75. Anaya DA, Dellinger EP. Necrotizing soft-tissue infection: diagnosis and management. *Clin Infect Dis* 2007;44:705–710.
76. Stevens DL, Mitten J, Henry C. Effects of alpha and theta toxins from Clostridium perfringens on human polymorphonuclear leukocytes. *J Infect Dis* 1987;156:324–233.
77. Stevens DL, Tweten RK, Awad MM, et al. Clostridial gas gangrene: evidence that alpha and theta toxins differentially modulate the immune response and induce acute tissue necrosis. *J Infect Dis* 1997;176:189–195.
78. Dellinger EP. Necrotizing soft-tissue infections. In: Davis JM, Shires GT, eds. *Principles and Management of Surgical Infections*. Philadelphia: J. B. Lippincott; 1991:23–39.
79. Marshall JC, Maier RV, Jimenez M, et al. Source control in the management of severe sepsis and septic shock: An evidence-based review. *Crit Care Med* 2004;32:S513–S526.
80. Stevens DL, Bisno AL, Chambers HF, et al. Practice guidelines for the diagnosis and management of skin and soft-tissue infections. *Clin Infect Dis* 2005;41:1373–1406.
81. Stamenkovic I, Lew PD. Early recognition of potentially fatal necrotizing fasciitis. The use of frozen-section biopsy. *N Engl J Med* 1984;310: 1689–1693.
82. Stevens DL, Bryant AE, Hackett SP. Antibiotic effects on bacterial viability, toxin production, and host response. *Clin Infect Dis* 1995;2:S154–S157.
83. Rivers E, Nguyen B, Havstad S, et al. Early goal-directed therapy in the treatment of severe sepsis and septic shock. *N Engl J Med* 2001;345:1368–1377.
84. Kumar A, Roberts D, Wood KE, et al. Duration of hypotension before initiation of effective antimicrobial therapy is the critical determinant of survival in human septic shock. *Crit Care Med* 2006;34:1589–1596.
85. Kumar A, Wood K, Gurka D, et al. Outcome of septic shock correlates with duration of hypotension prior to source control implementation. In: *Interscience Conference on Antimicrobial Agents and Chemotherapy.* Washington, DC: American Society for Microbiology; 2004.
86. Raad II, Hohn DC, Gilbreath BJ, et al. Prevention of central venous catheter-related infections by using maximal sterile barrier precautions during insertion. *Infect Cont Hosp Epidemiol* 1994;15:231–238.
87. Sherertz RJ, Ely EW, Westbrook DM, et al. Education of physicians-in-training can decrease the risk for vascular catheter infection. *Ann Intern Med* 2000;132:641–648.
88. Maki DG, Ringer M, Alvarado CJ. Prospective randomised trial of povidone-iodine, alcohol, and chlorhexidine for prevention of infection associated with central venous and arterial catheters. *Lancet* 1991;338:339–343.
89. Cook D, Randolph A, Kernerman P, et al. Central venous catheter replacement strategies: a systematic review of the literature. *Crit Care Med* 1997; 25:1417–1424.
90. O'Grady NP, Alexander M, Dellinger EP, et al. Guidelines for the prevention of intravascular catheter-related infections. *MMWR Recomm Rep* 2002;51:1–29.
91. Pronovost P, Needham D, Berenholtz S, et al. An intervention to decrease catheter-related bloodstream infections in the ICU. *N Engl J Med* 2006; 355:2725–2732.
92. Mermel LA, Farr BM, Sherertz RJ, et al. Guidelines for the management of intravascular catheter-related infections. *Clin Infect Dis* 2001;32:1249–1272.
93. Singh N, Rogers P, Atwood CW, et al. Short-course empiric antibiotic therapy for patients with pulmonary infiltrates in the intensive care unit. A proposed solution for indiscriminate antibiotic prescription. *Am J Respir Crit Care Med* 2000;162:505–511.
94. Kollef MH, Sherman G, Ward S, et al. Inadequate antimicrobial treatment of infections: a risk factor for hospital mortality among critically ill patients. *Chest* 1999;115:462–474.
95. Mathevon T, Souweine B, Traore O, et al. ICU-acquired nosocomial infection: impact of delay of adequate antibiotic treatment. *Scand J Infect Dis* 2002;34:831–835.
96. Chastre J, Luyt CE, Combes A, et al. Use of quantitative cultures and reduced duration of antibiotic regimens for patients with ventilator-associated pneumonia to decrease resistance in the intensive care unit. *Clin Infect Dis* 2006;43(Suppl 2):S75–S81.
97. Croce MA, Fabian TC, Schurr MJ, et al. Using bronchoalveolar lavage to distinguish nosocomial pneumonia from systemic inflammatory response syndrome: a prospective analysis. *J Trauma* 1995;39:1134–1139; discussion 9–40.
98. Pereira Gomes JC, Pedreira WL Jr, Araujo EM, et al. Impact of BAL in the management of pneumonia with treatment failure: positivity of BAL culture under antibiotic therapy. *Chest* 2000;118:1739–1746.
99. Chastre J, Wolff M, Fagon JY, et al. Comparison of 8 vs 15 days of antibiotic therapy for ventilator-associated pneumonia in adults: a randomized trial. *JAMA* 2003;290:2588–2598.
100. Nicasio AM, Kuti JL, Nicolau DP. The current state of multidrug-resistant gram-negative bacilli in North America. *Pharmacotherapy* 2008;28: 235–249.
101. Boucher HW, Talbot GH, Bradley JS, et al. Bad bugs, no drugs: No ESKAPE! An update from the Infectious Diseases Society of America. *Clin Infect Dis* 2008;481–12.
102. Dodd RY, Notari EP, Stramer SL. Current prevalence and incidence of infectious disease markers and estimated window-period risk in the American Red Cross blood donor population. *Transfusion* 2002;42:975–979.
103. Ebert SC, Craig WA. Pharmacodynamic properties of antibiotics: application to drug monitoring and dosage regimen design. *Infect Control Hosp Epidemiol* 1990;11:319–326.
104. Leggett JE, Ebert S, Fantin B, et al. Comparative dose-effect relations at several dosing intervals for beta-lactam, aminoglycoside and quinolone antibiotics against gram-negative bacilli in murine thigh-infection and pneumonitis models. *Scand J Infect Dis Suppl* 1990;74:179–184.

CHAPTER 8 ■ SHOCK

JOSEPH CUSCHIERI

KEY POINTS

1. Shock is the clinical syndrome that results from inadequate tissue perfusion from numerous causes: hypovolemic, cardiogenic, extracardiac obstructive, and distributive.
2. Hypovolemic shock due to ongoing blood and/or plasma loss leads to progressive cardiovascular deterioration, ultimate hypotension, oliguria, confusion, irreversible cell injury, and death.
3. Cardiogenic shock results in decreased tissue perfusion due to intrinsic pump failure.
4. Extracardiac obstructive shock attenuates pump function due to external compression of inflow and outflow (tamponade, tension pneumothorax, etc.).
5. Septic and traumatic shock, forms of distributive shock, are systemic inflammatory responses to infection or tissue injury with cellular breakdown, producing severe hypotension requiring massive volume resuscitation and high risk of multiple organ failure and death.
6. Complications of an episode of shock include ischemia-reperfusion injury from oxidant stress; potential secondary immunosuppression with enhanced nosocomial infection risk; hypothermia and coagulopathy; and multiple organ failure syndrome, including abdominal compartment syndrome.
7. Treatment of shock involves aggressive volume resuscitation with control of the underlying etiology and careful monitoring of adequacy of end-organ perfusion to avoid under- and overresuscitation.

1 The current accepted concept of shock was first described in 1929 by Walter B. Cannon as inadequate blood flow that results in cellular hypoxia.[1] Persistence of this cellular hypoxia, in turn, results in cellular and organ dysfunction. Although this state can result from a number of causes, it was Blalock who first described hematogenic, neurogenic, cardiogenic, and vasogenic factors that were associated with shock.[2]

Prior to these concepts, the concept of shock was not understood since the nature and purpose of the heart and circulatory system were either unknown or misunderstood. Galen was the first to explore the purpose of the heart and circulatory system. He proposed that the arteries carried blood, not air, as previously thought, away from the heart. However, he incorrectly believed that arterial blood within the circulatory system subsequently dissolved in the body to release nutrients. Blood returning to the heart was not due to recirculation, but rather was rapidly remanufactured by the liver. Additionally, because much of his dissection work was carried out in frogs, he concluded falsely that the heart had only two chambers and blood passed from the right to left chamber through invisible pores in the septum.[3]

These conclusions remained unchallenged for nearly 1,500 years until Vesalius, in the 17th century, described dissection of the human body. He demonstrated that blood did not flow directly from the right to left ventricle. Although he provided elaborate drawings of the body's network of blood vessels, he did not anticipate that blood circulated through the body and was unable to discern the heart's purpose. Shortly thereafter, Harvey moved beyond anatomy and studied physiology; he discovered the closed nature of the circulation and concluded that the heart was the main pumping mechanism. Although the microscope had not yet been invented, he proposed the existence of capillaries that connect the arterial and venous system.[3]

In the following century, military surgeons such as Henri le Dran (1740) noted that injured soldiers left unattended for several hours suddenly deteriorated as if there had been a *secousse* (jolt) to the system, which probably led to use of the word "shock."[1] Surgeons began to notice that even when a wounded extremity was amputated, the physiologic effects of the injury often continued, and shock was increasingly recognized as a distinct systemic syndrome apart from the wound itself.[3]

Eventually, Cannon and then Blalock described our current concept of shock and its attributed systemic effects. In fact, Blalock was the first to recognize the third-space fluid loss that follows shock resuscitation that is greater than the quantity of initial blood loss.[4] As a result, therapy began to focus not only on restoring intravascular volume but also on replacing fluid lost to the interstitium with a balanced salt solution. Investigators then became increasingly intrigued by the fact that, at some point, shock becomes irreversible and is no longer responsive to further volume resuscitation. As stated more than 50 years ago by Wiggers, "at a certain stage an adequate circulation cannot be restored by merely filling the system, as one does an automobile radiator."[5] At some point the wound, infection, cardiac dysfunction, or other initiating event is no longer the primary threat. Other factors sustain the shock state, blood pressure cannot be restored, improvements are only transient, and death occurs shortly thereafter.

The current concept of shock has led to a reclassification into four distinct groups—hypovolemic, cardiogenic, extracardiac obstructive, and distributive—that may occur independent of each other, or more characteristically synergistic with each other.[6] Early recognition and prompt treatment are essential to modern treatment. If delayed, uncorrected hypovolemia and critical oxygen delivery deficits occur that lead to irreversible shock. However, it is believed that future therapies will move beyond simple recognition and fluid resuscitation, and indices of tissue oxygenation that target the internal machinery of the cell itself will be followed. Thus, investigators are increasingly looking to gain an understanding of the chain of events that occur that lead to organ damage and irreversibility. This chapter describes these events, discusses the therapeutic approaches utilized in current management, and offers a brief perspective on what may lie ahead in the future.

EVALUATION OF SHOCK

Shock is easily recognized by even the most inexperienced caregiver after the compensatory mechanisms have been overcome (Table 8.1). However, it is more difficult to recognize the

TABLE 8.1

SHOCK RECOGNITION

ORGAN SYSTEM	SIGN/SYMPTOM	CAUSE
CNS	Mental status changes (agitation/anxiety to coma)	Decreased cerebral perfusion
Circulatory		
Cardiac	Tachycardia	Adrenergic stimulation
	Atrial/ventricular dysrhythmias	Coronary ischemia
	Hypotension	Coronary ischemia, right heart failure
Systemic	Hypotension	Decreased SVR, decreased venous return
	Decreased CVP	Hypovolemia
	Increased CVP	Right heart failure
Respiratory	Tachypnea	Pulmonary edema, sepsis, compensation for metabolic acidosis
	Cyanosis	Hypoxia
Renal	Oliguria	Decreased perfusion, afferent arteriolar vasoconstriction
Skin	Cool, clammy	Vasoconstriction
	Warm, dry	Vasodilation

CNS, central nervous system; CVP, central venous pressure; SVR, systemic vascular resistance.

patient in compensated shock, who presents with vital signs that are almost normal. It is critically important to the patient's ultimate outcome that recognition and treatment of shock occur before decompensation. The clinical assessment must be guided by the knowledge that the severity of symptoms and signs of shock vary between patients and the degree of the type of shock present. The patient is evaluated based on clinical appearance, hemodynamic measurements, physiologic responses, and biochemical analyses.

Early during various shock states, vasoconstriction frequently causes the skin to be cool, with poor capillary refill. However, this must be contrasted to shock states induced by either neurogenic or septic states in which vasodilation is present causing the skin to be warm, with good capillary refill. Common to the various shock states is the presence of hyperventilation, a compensatory response due to progressive metabolic acidosis. As shock progresses, mental status changes occur, and decreased cerebral blood flow and increased catecholamine stimulation may lead to anxiety and restlessness. With continued shock, lethargy may result. True coma, however, seldom results due to shock alone, unless coincident complete cardiovascular collapse occurs, and is usually associated with other conditions such as direct brain injury or severe hypoxia.[7]

The hemodynamic assessment should include evaluation of the rate and character of the pulse, the blood pressure, and, in some cases, the central venous pressure (CVP) and pulmonary artery pressure.[8] Tachycardia is a normal response to volume loss but also to pain, anxiety, and fear, all of which are commonly present. Assessment of the pulse (full and strong or weak and thready) may be helpful in determining the proper diagnosis. Because of the body's ability to compensate for hypovolemia, changes in blood pressure do not occur reliably until 20% to 30% of blood volume has been lost. However, the pulse pressure usually narrows, even in compensated shock, because of the effects of vasoconstriction on the diastolic blood pressure. Importantly, the CVP reflects the adequacy of and not the true blood volume, and the state of the venous tone. Changes in CVP in response to treatment or from continuing hemorrhage are more revealing than a solitary measurement.

An indirect but extremely valuable measure of perfusion and volume status is urine output. A urinary catheter should be inserted in every patient being evaluated for shock. Hourly urine output should be 0.5 to 1 mL/kg for adult patients, at least 1 mL/kg for most pediatric patients, and 1 to 2 mL/kg for patients younger than 2 years of age. Lack of adequate appropriate urine output in the setting of previous normal kidney function should cause the caregiver to be highly concerned about the continued presence of inadequate perfusion and cellular hypoxia.

Although each of the physical examination components are important in the identification of shock, used alone these factors can lead to a potential underdiagnosis of compensated shock due to the robust ability of the human body to compensate to various degrees. As a result, biochemical markers have been added as a means to identify shock in its early stages. Biochemical analysis of shock is based on the shift from aerobic to anaerobic metabolism in underperfused tissues. Increased lactate production is associated with tissue hypoperfusion. In addition, lactate appears to be prognostic in several different shock states including hypovolemic, septic, and cardiogenic.[9] Resuscitation of shock results in a decrease in serum lactate levels, and the time required to normalize serum lactate levels appears to be an important prognostic factor for survival.[10,11]

Another biochemical marker of shock and resuscitation is the base deficit. This is defined as the amount of a fixed base (or acid) that must be added to an aliquot of blood to restore the pH to 7.40. Base deficit values have been categorized as normal (2 to –2), mild (–3 to –5), moderate (–6 to –9), and severe (>–10). Changes in base deficit toward normal with volume infusion can be used to judge the efficacy of resuscitation.[12–14] Further, base deficit has been shown to be superior to pH values in assessing the normalization of acidosis after shock resuscitation, and the time required for normalization of base deficit has perhaps even greater prognostic significance than that for lactate.[12,15]

These biochemical changes associated with the hypoperfusion of shock occur even with compensation. Because of the potential difficulties in diagnosing compensated shock, an arterial and/or venous blood gas analysis including base deficit and lactate should be obtained for every patient suspected of being in shock. Additionally, any patient with a lactate of ≥4 mmol/L or base deficit of ≥6 mEq/L should be considered to be in shock until proven otherwise.[13,16,17]

Although each of these factors can be used to characterize shock, no single measurement has been determined to be optimal or when used singly to be always accurate for identification and treatment of shock. Currently, other measurements are being investigated that demonstrate promise. These markers include measurements of central and mixed venous oxygen saturations, end-diastolic cardiac volume indices, and specific noninvasive end-organ tissue oxygen saturations.[18–23]

TYPES OF SHOCK

Although several different classifications for shock have been described, the most currently widely accepted classification of shock was proposed by Weil and Shubin in 1971.[6] This classification divides the shock syndrome into four distinct categories (Table 8.2). Despite this separation, however, there is considerable overlap between the categories, with some patients presenting with more than one factor at the same time. Given this overlap, it is helpful to evaluate the hemodynamic pattern in order to elucidate the etiology and manage the patient (Table 8.3).

Hypovolemic Shock

2 Hypovolemic shock is the form of shock most commonly encountered in surgical practice (Table 8.2). The essential feature is a reduction in intravascular volume to a level that prevents the heart from being able to pump sufficient blood to vital organ systems. Substantial blood (>20% circulating volume) or plasma (via soft tissue or enteric sequestration or gastrointestinal, urinary, or insensible losses) losses are required to produce this syndrome.

The signs and symptoms of shock vary with both the severity and duration of blood loss. A review of the Advanced Trauma Life Support classification system of the American College of Surgeons is useful to comprehend the manifestations and physiologic changes associated with hemorrhagic shock in adults.[24] Blood volume is estimated at 7% of ideal body weight, or approximately 4,900 mL in a 70-kg patient (Table 8.4).

Class I: Mild hemorrhage, up to 15% of total blood volume. This condition is exemplified by voluntary blood donation. In the supine position, there are no measurable changes in heart or respiratory rates, blood pressure, or pulse pressure. Capillary refill is normal. This degree of hemorrhage requires little or no treatment, and blood volume is restored within 24 hours by transcapillary refill and the other compensatory methods.

Class II: Loss of 15% to 30% of blood volume (800 to 1,500 mL). Clinical symptoms include tachycardia and tachypnea. The systolic blood pressure may be only slightly decreased, especially in the supine position, but the pulse pressure is narrowed (because of the diastolic increase from adrenergic discharge). Urine output is reduced only slightly (20 to 30 mL/h). Mental status changes (e.g., anxiety) are frequently present. Capillary refill is usually delayed. Patients with class II hemorrhage usually can be resuscitated with crystalloid solutions, but some may require blood transfusion.

Class III: Loss of 30% to 40% of blood volume (up to 2,000 mL). Patients with class III hemorrhage present with inadequate perfusion that is obvious; marked tachycardia and tachypnea; cool, clammy extremities with significantly delayed capillary refill; hypotension; and significant changes in mental status (e.g., confusion, combativeness). Class III hemorrhage represents the smallest volume of blood loss that consistently produces a decrease in systolic blood pressure. The resuscitation of these patients frequently requires blood transfusion in addition to administration of crystalloids.

Class IV: Loss of more than 40% of blood volume (more than 2,000 mL), representing life-threatening hemorrhage. Symptoms include marked tachycardia, a significantly depressed systolic blood pressure, and narrowed pulse pressure or unobtainable diastolic pressure. The mental status is depressed and the skin is cold and pale. Urine output is negligible. These patients require immediate transfusion for resuscitation and frequently require immediate surgical or other (e.g., angiographic embolization) intervention.

In practice, individual susceptibility to blood loss varies greatly and is affected by age, pregnancy, preexisting disease, prescription and nonprescription medications (e.g., beta-blockers), adequacy of compensatory mechanisms, and other factors that are poorly characterized. Presence of these factors should lead the caregiver to consider early use of invasive monitoring as an adjunct to appropriate fluid resuscitation.

Hypovolemia due to plasma losses may also lead to hypovolemic shock. The clinical findings of hemorrhagic shock are typically present, but significant differences do exist. Hemoconcentration, elevated blood urea nitrogen (BUN) and creatinine, and hypernatremia are typical of acute plasma and/or free water losses and are not necessarily present in other forms of shock. Appropriate evaluation of preload and urine output should be followed, with specific considerations for unique electrolyte abnormalities associated with specific plasma and fluid losses (e.g., gastric vs. colonic losses).

Cardiogenic Shock

3 The clinical definition of cardiogenic shock is decreased cardiac output with tissue hypoperfusion, despite presence of adequate intravascular volume. It is caused by a primary problem with the cardiac muscle, electrical conduction system, or valves. The most common cause is anterior wall myocardial infarction, although in surgical patients it is often precipitated by pulmonary embolus, myocardial contusion, or pulmonary hypertension.

Distinguishing cardiogenic shock from other shock etiologies is occasionally difficult. It is not uncommon to see combined cardiogenic and traumatic shock in the elderly patient, with one often being the precipitating event for the other. The hallmarks of the hemodynamic and neuroendocrine response to systemic hypoperfusion from other causes are also typical of cardiogenic shock. Eliciting a history of preexisting cardiac disease, and physical findings such as pulmonary rales, cardiac murmurs, an S3 gallop, and jugular venous distention may be helpful. An electrocardiogram may detect significant ischemia or other pathology. A chest radiograph may reveal bilateral pulmonary infiltrates typical of cardiogenic edema, and cardio-specific serum tests (troponin I, creatine phosphokinase [CPK]) may indicate myocardial damage.

Manifestations of cardiogenic shock develop as a consequence of failure of peripheral perfusion, the associated adrenergic response, and the inability of the heart to accommodate blood returning from the lungs and the periphery. In the absence of sepsis or tissue injury, however, there is not usually an associated increase in the metabolic needs of the peripheral tissues. Sympathetic-mediated constriction of the peripheral vasculature attempts to maintain central blood pressure and perfusion of cerebral and coronary circulations. The clinical

TABLE 8.2

CLASSIFICATION SYSTEM AND CAUSES OF SHOCK

■ CLASSIFICATION	■ ETIOLOGY	■ CAUSE
Hypovolemic	Hemorrhagic	Trauma
		Gastrointestinal
	Nonhemorrhagic	Absolute fluid loss (renal, gastrointestinal)
		Redistributive or "third spacing"
Cardiogenic	Myocardial	Ischemia
		Infarction
		Contusion
		Cardiomyopathy
		Myocarditis
		Pharmacologic/toxic (beta-blockers, calcium channel blockers, tricyclic antidepressants, anthracycline)
		Metabolic (hypophosphatemia, hypocalcemia, acidosis)
	Valve failure	Infection
		Injury
		Ruptured papillary muscle
		Stenosis
	Arrhythmias	Ischemia
		Pharmacologic/toxic
		Metabolic
Extracardiac obstructive	Extrinsic compression	Mediastinal tumors
	Increased intrathoracic pressure	Tension pneumothorax
		Positive-pressure ventilation
	Intrinsic vascular flow obstruction	Pulmonary embolism
		Air embolism
		Tumors (myxoma)
		Proximal aortic dissection
		Aortic coarctation
		Acute pulmonary hypertension
		Tamponade
		Pericarditis
Distributive	SIRS related	Trauma
		Sepsis
		Pancreatitis
		Burns
	Anaphylactic/anaphylactoid	Drugs
		Venoms
	Neurogenic	Spinal cord injury
	Toxic/pharmacologic	Vasodilators
		Benzodiazepines
	Endocrine	Adrenal insufficiency
		Thyroid
		Myxedema

SIRS, systemic inflammatory response syndrome.

TABLE 8.3

HEMODYNAMIC PATTERNS IN SHOCK

■ TYPE	■ CO	■ SVR	■ PAOP	■ CVP	■ SvO_2
Hypovolemic	↓	↑	↓	↓	↓
Cardiogenic					
Left ventricular MI	↓	↑	↑	N, ↑	↓
Right ventricular MI	↓	↑	N, ↓	↑	↓
Extracardiac obstructive					
Pericardial tamponade	↓	↑	↑	↑	↓
Pulmonary embolism	↓	↑	↑	↑	↓
Distributive					
Early	↑, N, ↓	↑, N, ↓	N	N, ↑	N, ↑
Early after fluid administration	↑	↓	N, ↑	N, ↑	↑, N, ↓
Late	↓	↑	N	N	↓

CO, cardiac output; CVP, central venous pressure; MI, myocardial infarction; N, normal; PAOP, pulmonary artery occlusion pressure; SvO_2, mixed venous oxygen saturation; SVR, systemic vascular resistance.

findings of cardiogenic shock may thus be similar to those of hypovolemic shock because both involve induction of the adrenosympathetic response.

Diminished or ineffective contractile activity of the right or left side of the heart allows blood to accumulate in the respective venous circulations. Shock from an acute left ventricular myocardial infarct occurs when more than 40% of the left ventricle is involved and may be present in approximately 20% of Q-wave infarcts.[25] Shock from an acute right ventricular myocardial infarct, on the other hand, is rare and only occurs in approximately 10% of all inferior wall infarcts.[26] Not only does the diagnosis of each infarct vary, but also the treatment and support vary significantly.

In any patient in shock, especially in those with compromised cardiac function, consideration should be given to the institution of mechanical ventilation. The work of breathing can be considerable, especially for the patient in a state of agitation or distress. Oxygen needs are decreased through intubation and mechanical ventilation. In this manner, the patient can be comfortably sedated with a secure airway; the work of breathing is undertaken by the ventilator, and gas exchange can be optimized. If there is a tenuous balance between myocardial oxygen needs and availability, the balance can thus be shifted in the patient's favor.

Like other forms of shock, cardiogenic shock tends to be self-perpetuating. Myocardial perfusion depends on the pressure gradient between the coronary artery and the left ventricle and the duration of diastole. Both are compromised by the hypotension and tachycardia that characterizes this condition. High-volume fluid resuscitation, sometimes necessary for treatment of other forms of shock, is poorly tolerated and likely to be detrimental to an individual with the compromised myocardial function of cardiogenic shock.

Extracardiac Obstructive Shock

4 A subset of patients with cardiogenic shock do not have intrinsic cardiac disease but have pump failure due to extrinsic compression that limits diastolic filling and cardiac output. Cardiac tamponade, tension pneumothorax, diaphragmatic herniation of abdominal viscera, mediastinal hematoma, and,

TABLE 8.4

CLASSIFICATION OF HEMORRHAGIC SHOCK

	■ CLASS I	■ CLASS II	■ CLASS III	■ CLASS IV
Blood loss (mL)	Up to 750	750–1,500	1,500–2,000	>2,000
Blood loss (%)	Up to 15	15–30	30–40	40
Heart rate	<100	>100	>120	>140
Blood pressure	Normal	Normal	Decreased	Decreased
Pulse pressure	Normal	Decreased	Decreased	Decreased
Respiratory rate	14–20	20–30	30–40	>35
Urine output (mL/h)	>30	20–30	5–15	Minimal
Mental status	Normal	Mildly anxious	Anxious and confused	Confused and lethargic
Fluid replacement	Crystalloid	Crystalloid	Crystalloid and blood	Crystalloid and blood

occasionally, positive-pressure mechanical ventilation may all precipitate cardiogenic shock by exerting constricting pressure on the myocardium. The key to diagnosis and appropriate therapy is the physical examination, supplemented by use of appropriate diagnostic modalities.

The classic physical findings of cardiac tamponade, Beck's triad, are hypotension, muffled heart sounds, and jugular venous distention. Unfortunately, these nonspecific clinical findings are seldom present together. Elevated jugular venous pressure, noted by either physical examination or measurement of CVP, although not specific for cardiac compression, is usually present. Pulsus paradoxus can be useful for the diagnosis of cardiac tamponade. Although it may be caused by other conditions, it is virtually always present in patients with tamponade.

Given the difficulty in evaluation of these patients, especially in combination with other shock states, early diagnostic evaluation, both invasive and noninvasive, of cardiac function is warranted. Recent guidelines suggest that any patient with concern for primary or secondary cardiac dysfunction should undergo early ultrasound evaluation. This early evaluation not only evaluates the primary cardiac function but also can lead to the early diagnosis and management of secondary causes of cardiac dysfunction including cardiac tamponade and pulmonary embolism.

Distributive Shock

Distributive shock occurs in a state of inappropriate oxygen utilization associated with the systemic inflammatory response syndrome (SIRS). Classically, SIRS is triggered by sepsis, but SIRS is associated with other immune processes including trauma, pancreatitis, and other types of tissue injuries. However, other types of distributive disturbances can occur unrelated to inflammation that may be directly due to loss of vascular tone from spinal cord injury, endocrine dysfunction, or anaphylaxis.

Septic Shock

5 Septic shock is defined as a SIRS response to infection in conjunction with arterial hypotension, despite adequate fluid resuscitation.[27] It occurs when bacterial products interact with cells of the immune system, leading to elaboration of mediators that cause circulatory disturbances and direct and indirect cell damage leading to the clinical manifestations of SIRS (Table 8.5).[28] Hemodynamic changes are defined as early (warm or hyperdynamic) or late (cold or hypodynamic). These stages are primarily characterized by the degree of ventricular contractility and peripheral vasomotor impairment present, but can be misclassified if not appropriately evaluated. Early septic shock is distinguished by peripheral vasodilation, flushed and warm extremities, and a compensatory elevation in cardiac output. Although an increase in venous capacitance diminishes venous return to the heart, cardiac output is maintained via tachycardia and the decrease in afterload due to systemic vasodilation.

Late septic shock is characterized by impaired myocardial contractility due to local and systemic release of cardiac depressants, worsening peripheral perfusion, vasoconstriction, extremity mottling, oliguria, and hypotension. Peripheral oxygen utilization may be severely impaired by bacterial toxins, such as lipopolysaccharide (LPS) and the inflammatory products of the host's own immune response, resulting in metabolic dysfunction and acidosis despite a high systemic oxygen delivery. This inappropriate oxygen utilization and systemic shunting lead not only to confusion regarding the adequacy of resuscitation, but also to progressive cell death. Together, both systemic hypoperfusion and the altered tissue metabolism create a vicious cycle that propagates the inflammatory response initiated in reaction to the initial infectious challenge leading to progressive cellular injury.

Due to both volume deficits and cardiovascular dysfunction, persistent perfusion deficits are common and contribute significantly to multiple organ failure and mortality. In fact, the fluid volume required for treatment may exceed that required for treatment of other forms of shock due to persistent microvascular endothelial capillary leak. As a result of this profound leak, interstitial and total body fluid balances become extreme, leading to the potential development of marked hypoxia and the abdominal compartment syndrome.

Although appropriate early resuscitation and cardiovascular support are essential to the treatment of septic shock, as important are early infection source control and appropriate administration of antimicrobials. In fact, numerous investigators have demonstrated that even a few hours' delay in initiation of antimicrobial therapy is associated with a significant increase in mortality.[29]

TABLE 8.5

SYSTEMIC INFLAMMATORY RESPONSE SYNDROME

Systemic inflammatory response syndrome: The systemic inflammatory response to a variety of severe clinical inflammatory factors is manifested by two or more of the following conditions:

- Temperature >38°C or <36°C
- Heart rate >90 bpm
- Respiratory rate >20 breaths/min or $PaCO_2$ <32 mm Hg
- WBC count >12,000 cells/mm^3, <4,000 cells/mm^3, or >10% immature (band) forms

bpm, beats per minute; $PaCO_2$, partial pressure of arterial carbon dioxide; WBC, white blood cell count.

Traumatic Shock

The major contributor to shock after injury is hypovolemia due to hemorrhage. Even when hemorrhage ceases or is controlled, patients can continue to suffer loss of plasma volume into the interstitium of injured tissues and develop progressive hypovolemic shock. In addition, tissue injury evokes a broader pathophysiologic immunoinflammatory response and a potentially more devastating degree of shock than that produced by hypovolemia alone.

The degree to which direct tissue injury and an inflammatory response participate in the development and progression of traumatic shock distinguishes it from purely hypovolemic shock. Thus, traumatic shock results from direct tissue or bony injury, resulting in not only hypovolemia caused by fluid and blood loss but also an immunologic and neuroendocrine response to tissue destruction and devitalization. This combined insult complicates what might otherwise be straightforward hemorrhagic shock by inducing a systemic response that utilizes many of the inflammatory mediators present in septic shock.[30] These mediators propagate and intensify the effects of the initial hypovolemia and make subsequent multiple organ failure far more likely than occurs with hypovolemic shock alone.

Although this condition can lead to increased fluid requirements, common problems associated with this condition such as rhabdomyolysis should be aggressively evaluated and treated with optimal resuscitation.[31] In addition, common patient characteristics are known to alter traumatic shock resuscitation, in particular, morbid obesity that can result in delayed correction of metabolic acidosis and increased risk for organ dysfunction.[32]

Thus, initial management of the seriously injured requires the assurance of an airway, breathing, and circulation; later management requires appropriate volume resuscitation and control of ongoing losses. Control of hemorrhage is a major concern and demands priority over attention to other injuries. After resuscitation and control of volume losses, efforts become necessary to minimize the potentially lethal postshock sequelae, including acute respiratory distress syndrome (ARDS) and multiple organ dysfunction syndrome (MODS).

Neurogenic Shock

Neurogenic shock is defined as failure of the nervous system to provide effective peripheral vascular resistance, resulting in inadequate end-organ perfusion. Warm, flushed, flaccid extremities; paraplegia; confusion; oliguria; and hypotension are the classic clinical findings. Injury to the proximal spinal cord, with interruption of the autonomic sympathetic vasomotor pathways, disrupts basal vasoconstrictor tone to peripheral veins and arterioles. Profound vasodilation of all microvascular beds below the level of cord injury diminishes venous return to the heart, reduces cardiac output, and precipitates hypotension. Injuries at or above the fourth thoracic vertebrae may disrupt sympathetic enervation to the heart, resulting in significant bradycardia and severe decompensation.

Similar to the initial therapy for shock resulting from hypovolemia, treatment of the relative hypovolemia due to vasodilation of neurogenic shock requires intravenous volume resuscitation. Restoration of the pathologically expanded intravascular space improves preload and cardiac output and may reverse hypotension. However, maintenance of adequate hemodynamics often requires vasopressor support in an effort to avoid the administration of excessive fluids. CVP monitoring to assess cardiac preload should be considered as a means of determining adequate and nonexcessive filling pressures, as loss of vasomotor capacity within the pulmonary circulation predisposes these patients to pulmonary edema. As spinal cord injury is often associated with other traumatic injuries, the diagnosis of isolated neurogenic shock must be a process of exclusion.

This condition should not be confused with spinal shock. Spinal shock is defined as a loss of sensation accompanied by motor paralysis with initial loss but gradual recovery of spinal reflexes following spinal cord injury. The reflexes caudal to the spinal cord injury are hyporeflexic or absent, while those rostral are unaffected. No circulatory compromise is associated with this condition; thus, it should not be considered a shock state.

Hypoadrenal Shock

The role of adrenocortical hormones in providing resistance to shock is well recognized. The reduction in effective blood volume and changes in blood chemistry that occur after adrenalectomy are similar to those of shock and hemorrhage. Adrenalectomized animals have markedly diminished tolerance to both trauma and hypovolemia. Adrenal cortical hormones also play a key role in maintaining normal capillary tone and permeability. In recent years, the concept of functional or relative adrenal insufficiency has received increasing attention as a cause of unrecognized shock and hypoperfusion. Most critically ill patients have elevated cortisol levels, but some have low concentrations in relation to the degree of stress imposed by their disease. Administration of physiologic doses of steroids to correct this insufficiency may result in stabilization of hemodynamics and possible survival benefits.[33] However, the concept of routine administration of physiologic doses of steroids has been questioned and thus routine and indiscriminate use is not recommended.[34]

Diagnosis of hypoadrenal shock is difficult, as classic signs of Addison disease are absent. The only clinical clues may be unexplained hypotension and refractory response to high-dose vasopressors. An isolated serum cortisol level is difficult to interpret because the range of values observed in critically ill patients varies considerably. A cortisol level below 15 μg/dL suggests a high likelihood of adrenal insufficiency, whereas a value above 35 μg/dL suggests an adequate renal function.[35] The adrenocorticotropic hormone (ACTH) stimulation test may be used to identify hypoadrenal patients when the diagnosis is unclear, but the utility of this test, particularly with an elevated baseline value, is of questionable utility.

The utility of the ACTH stimulation test is especially questionable in patients with persistent evidence of shock and elevated baseline levels of cortisol above 35 μg/dL. These patients actually demonstrate evidence of inadequate systemic cortisol utilization with a significant risk of morality, and thus may actually benefit from systemic administration of physiologic concentrations of corticosteroids.[35]

Although hypoadrenal shock may complicate various types of shock, there is conflicting evidence to support the use of supplemental corticosteroids in patients with septic shock if there is biochemical evidence of hypoadrenalism. Thus, supplemental corticosteroids should be used with extreme caution until further evidence is available.[27,36]

PHYSIOLOGIC RESPONSE TO HYPOVOLEMIA

Common to each shock state is usually an initial decrease in circulating intravascular volume. This reduction is due directly to fluid loss or secondarily to fluid redistribution. This reduction in circulating fluid volume initiates both a rapid and sustained compensatory response. Within minutes, a rapid compensatory response occurs primarily due to adrenergic output. Sustained responses, in contrast, occur slower and result in intravascular fluid reabsorption and renal conservation of water and electrolytes (Algorithm 8.1).

Rapid Response

Hypovolemia results in the initial secretion of epinephrine and norepinephrine from the adrenal gland due to decreased afferent impulses from arterial baroreceptors. Catecholamine release is acute, and limited to the first 24 hours following the onset of hypovolemia. This results in vasoconstriction, tachycardia, and increased myocardial contractility. Adrenergic-induced vasoconstriction of the systemic capacitance of small veins and venules shifts blood back to the central venous circulation, thus increasing right-sided filling pressures. Left-sided filling and pressure are augmented by pulmonary vasoconstriction. Concomitantly, vasoconstriction occurs in the skin, kidneys, and viscera, effectively shunting blood to the heart and brain. Adrenergic-induced vasoconstriction increases cardiac filling and causes increased contractility and reflex tachycardia, all of which combine to increase stroke volume and cardiac output.

Adrenergic-mediated vasoconstriction affects arterioles, pre- and postcapillary sphincters, and small veins and venules. Due to this specific vasoconstriction, decreased hydrostatic pressure distal to the precapillary sphincter occurs that leads to reabsorption of interstitial fluid [water, sodium (Na^+), and chloride (Cl^-)] into the vascular space. This functions to restore circulating blood volume and is known as transcapillary refill.[37]

Sustained Response

Sustained compensatory responses include the release of vasoactive hormones and fluid shifts from the interstitium and

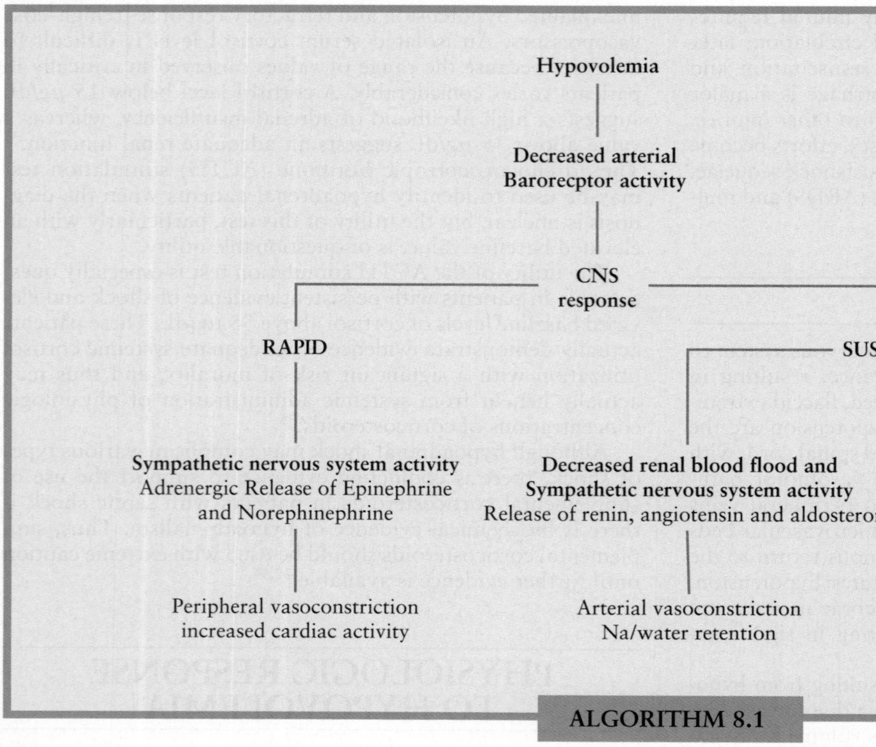

ALGORITHM 8.1. Neurohormonal response to hypovolemia.

the intracellular space to the intravascular compartment. Decreased renal blood flow, increased adrenergic activity, and compositional changes in tubular fluid lead to the secretion of renin from the juxtaglomerular complex. Renin results in increased formation and release of angiotensin I by the liver. Circulating angiotensin I is rapidly converted to angiotensin II by the lungs and is the most potent known arterial and arteriolar vasoconstrictor. Angiotensin II also stimulates the release of pituitary ACTH. Increased circulating levels of both angiotensin II and ACTH result in increased secretion of aldosterone. As a result, reabsorption of Na^+ in the distal renal tubules in exchange for potassium (K^+) and hydrogen ions occurs.

Additionally, due to hypovolemia and increased serum osmolarity, reduced stimulation of arterial baroreceptors occurs, leading to the release of arginine vasopressin (AVP), also known as antidiuretic hormone (ADH). This hormone not only functions as a potent vasoconstrictor but also causes increased reabsorption of water by increasing water permeability and passive Na^+ transport in the distal renal tubule. The overall net effect of aldosterone and AVP is to decrease glomerular filtration and increase salt and water tubular reabsorption in an effort to replace circulating intravascular volume deficits.

Finally, the increased release of the stress hormones (epinephrine, ACTH, cortisol, and glucagon) leads to glycogenolysis, lipolysis, and protein catabolism, causing a negative nitrogen balance and high extracellular concentration of glucose due to decreased insulin release and resistance. This leads to increased glucose utilization by insulin-independent tissues such as the brain and heart. In addition to glucose, products of anaerobic metabolism from hypoperfused cells accumulate in the extracellular compartment, inducing hyperosmolarity. This extracellular hyperosmolarity draws water from the intracellular space, increasing interstitial osmotic pressure, which in turn drives water, Na^+, and Cl^- across the capillary endothelium into the vascular space.

ORGAN-SPECIFIC COMPENSATORY RESPONSES TO SHOCK

Cardiac and Microvascular Response

Cardiovascular physiology is profoundly affected by shock (Table 8.3). Reduced stroke volume is caused by an absolute or relative loss of preload. Intrinsic neuroendocrine and renal compensatory responses, along with additional intravenous fluid, are needed to increase ventricular end-diastolic volume. Restoration of adequate preload alone is often sufficient to return cardiac output to levels required to overcome peripheral perfusion deficits. However, some cases are complicated by acquired myocardial contractility derangements. Contractile function under these conditions is less a function of preload and more related to intrinsic myocardial dysfunction.

A defining characteristic of shock is compromise of microvascular perfusion. Far from being a passive conduit, the microvasculature actively participates in the response to shock. Arteriolar vessels are innervated by sympathetic nerves, as are small veins and venules. The vasoconstriction of hypovolemic shock and the vasodilation of septic and neurogenic shock are a result of these autonomic responses. The majority of the circulating blood volume resides in the venous system, and normal physiologic compensation mechanisms rely on this venous blood pool as an autotransfusion reservoir. Collapse of underperfused veins passively propels blood toward the heart, while α-adrenergic venoconstriction actively mobilizes the venous pool. Profound peripheral vasoconstriction via α-adrenergic, vasopressin, angiotensin II, and endothelin-1 stimulation of arteriolar and precapillary smooth muscle sphincters selectively diminishes perfusion to dermal, renal, muscle, and, significantly, splanchnic vascular beds to preserve perfusion of critical central organs, primarily the central nervous system (CNS) and myocardium.[38]

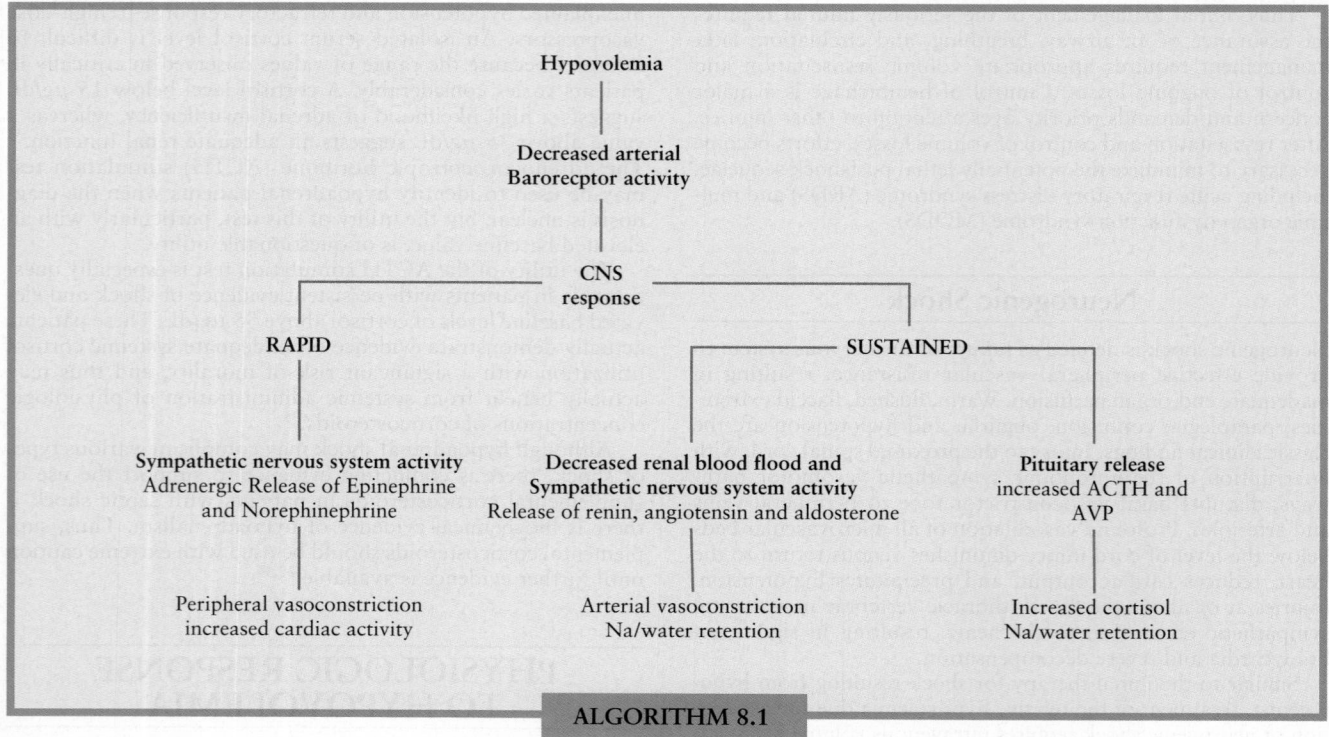

The capillary endothelial monolayer maintains a semipermeable barrier between the intra- and extraluminal spaces and is compromised by shock.[39] Circulating inflammatory mediators and byproducts of infection (LPS, thrombin, tumor necrosis factor alpha [TNF-α], interleukin [IL]-1, nitric oxide, and endothelin-1) generated in response to traumatic or septic shock have been shown to induce and sustain endothelial capillary leak. Although the exact mechanisms of endothelial monolayer dysfunction are unclear, the only available therapies to reverse microvascular decompensation are timely restoration of peripheral perfusion, rapid elimination of infectious and necrotic tissue, and pharmacologic and mechanical support of cardiopulmonary function.[40,41]

Neuroendocrine Response

The neuroendocrine reaction to shock consists of involuntary responses by the hypothalamus, autonomic nervous system, and secretory endocrine glands and is directed toward restoration of tissue perfusion and a redirected utilization of metabolic substrates. The autonomic response is initially triggered by hypoxia, hypotension, or hypovolemia detected by aortic and carotid baroreceptors and chemoreceptors (Algorithm 8.2). Subsequently, sympathetic vasoconstriction of specific vascular beds, induced by direct synaptic release of norepinephrine, results in redistribution of circulating blood volume from tissue of low metabolic activity to more metabolically demanding organs. Cardiac output, diminished by loss of preload, is augmented by inhibition of cardiac vagal activity and a resulting reflex tachycardia.

Circulating epinephrine and norepinephrine alter several aspects of glucose utilization, availability, and metabolism. The hyperglycemia of stress results from catecholamine-induced glycogenolysis, gluconeogenesis, and decreased pancreatic insulin release. Simultaneously, hypothalamic stimulation of the anterior pituitary induces release of ACTH, which in turn prompts cortisol and aldosterone release by the adrenal cortex. Elevated serum cortisol contributes to postinjury hyperglycemia by increasing gluconeogenesis, enhancing lipolysis, and diminishing peripheral utilization of glucose and amino acids. The pancreatic response is characterized by a decrease in insulin release and an increase in glucagon secretion, which further stimulates hepatic gluconeogenesis. The combined actions of catecholamines, cortisol, and glucagon are synergistic and create a shock-related hyperglycemia that is often refractory to insulin treatment.

Renal juxtaglomerular secretion of renin in response to adrenergic stimulation and renal hypoperfusion triggers the formation of angiotensin I in the liver, which is subsequently converted to angiotensin II by the lungs. Angiotensin II, a potent vasoconstrictor, augments shock-induced catecholamine-mediated peripheral and splanchnic vasoconstriction and stimulates aldosterone release from the adrenal cortex. Renal tubular reabsorption of sodium in response to elevated circulating aldosterone creates highly concentrated, low-volume urine. Vasopressin secretion by the posterior pituitary similarly contributes to compensatory restoration and maintenance of intravascular

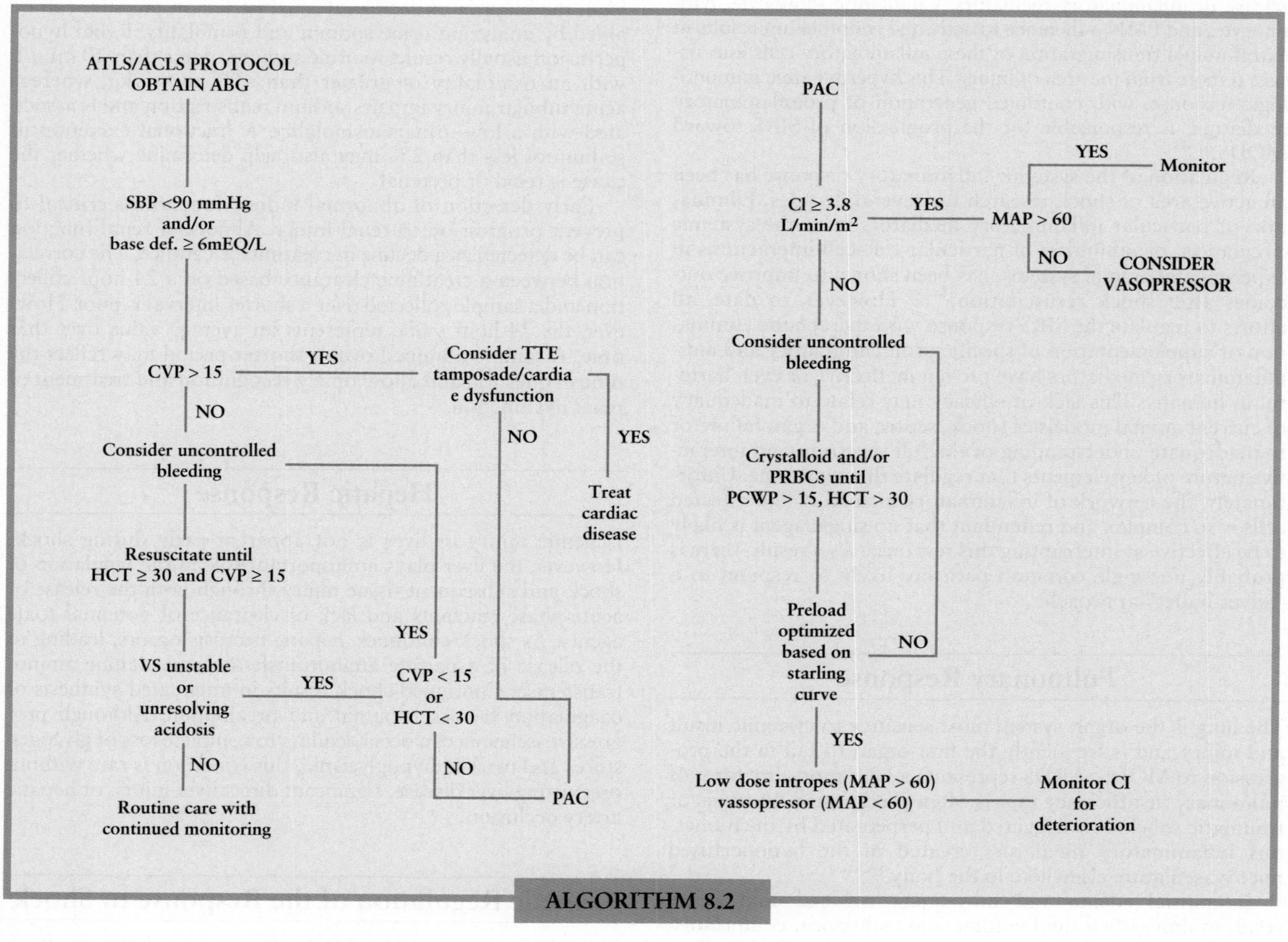

ALGORITHM 8.2. Shock resuscitation algorithm.

volume by promoting water reabsorption by the renal distal tubules and by causing peripheral and splanchnic vasoconstriction. A major result is a prolonged severe hypoperfusion of the splanchnic vascular bed, further augmenting the deleterious host response.

Immunoinflammatory Response

Many shock-inducing events, particularly those associated with septic or traumatic shock, simultaneously trigger a massive systemic inflammatory response. Although inflammatory mediators (TNF-α, ILs, chemokines, etc.) play an integral role in the recovery of local tissue to trauma and infection, an uncontrolled systemic inflammatory response contributes to organ failure. Immunologically active cells involved in the systemic inflammatory response include nucleated blood cells (monocytes, polymorphonuclear leukocytes [PMNs]) and platelets, microvascular endothelial cells, and tissue macrophages. These cells generate and secrete scores of signal-amplifying inflammatory mediators ranging in complexity from individual molecules (nitric oxide) to large multisubunit, extensively modified proteins (TNF-α, IL-1, etc.). Even transient systemic elevation of any of these mediators has profound physiologic consequences.

Local tissue destruction, microbial contamination, and infection similarly activate the coagulation cascade and induce platelet aggregation and release of numerous platelet-, endothelial-, and clot-derived vasoactive mediators. Persistent, profound, and recurring microvascular hypoperfusion of the splanchnic and other organs likewise causes local tissue ischemia, parenchymal cell injury, microvascular coagulation, activation of inflammatory cells, and release of inflammatory mediators. Circulating monocyte, lymphocyte, and PMN adherence to activated endothelium results in extraluminal transmigration of these inflammatory cells into tissues remote from the area of injury. This hyperdynamic immunologic response, with continued generation of proinflammatory mediators, is responsible for the progression of SIRS toward MODS.[42–45]

Regulation of the systemic inflammatory response has been an active area of shock research for several decades. Elimination of particular inflammatory mediators from the systemic circulation, or inhibition of particular cell–cell interactions in experimental animal systems, has been shown to improve outcomes after shock resuscitation.[46–48] However, to date, all efforts to regulate the SIRS response with therapeutic elimination or supplementation of specific proinflammatory and anti-inflammatory mediators have proven ineffective or even harmful in humans. This lack of efficacy may relate to inadequacy of current animal models of shock, sepsis, and organ failure or to inadequate understanding of the full spectrum and interactive nature of key elements that regulate this syndrome. Unfortunately, the network of inflammatory mediators and affected cells is so complex and redundant that no single agent is likely to be effective at interrupting this response. As a result, there is probably no single common pathway likely to respond to a "silver bullet" approach.

Pulmonary Response

The lung is the organ system most sensitive to systemic insult and injury and is frequently the first organ to fail in the progression to MODS. ARDS represents a high-mortality form of pulmonary insufficiency that is often precipitated by sepsis or traumatic shock. It is triggered and perpetuated by the numerous inflammatory mediators created in the hypoperfused microvasculature elsewhere in the body.[49–51]

Interstitial edema and subsequent reduced compliance result in diminished tidal volume and tachypnea, compromising gas exchange. Surfactant abnormalities contribute to alveolar collapse, resulting in loss of functional residual capacity (FRC) and the onset of pulmonary insufficiency. The pulmonary microvascular response mirrors the systemic response, with angiotensin and α-adrenergic–induced vasoconstriction creating significant elevations of pulmonary vascular resistance, further straining the heart. Pulmonary parenchymal injury may be propagated by excessive positive-pressure ventilation generated by alveolar overdistention in particular, further contributing to alveolar damage.

No specific measures are available to reverse the ARDS process; therefore, aggressive management of predisposing conditions is most appropriate. Once ARDS has become fully developed, treatment involves intensive supportive care while minimizing iatrogenic insults. As a result, early utilization of lung-protective strategies may diminish progressive ventilator-induced lung injury and improve outcome.[52]

Renal Response

Direct sympathetic-induced renal vasoconstriction increases afferent arteriole resistance in response to shock. This effect is reinforced by elevated circulating angiotensin II and catecholamines. The resulting decrease in renal blood flow and glomerular filtration rate (GFR), along with elevated circulating aldosterone and vasopressin (ADH), produce oliguria and prerenal azotemia. Acute tubular necrosis (ATN) may result from prolonged decreases in renal cortical blood flow, as well as from toxins generated during sepsis. Oliguric renal failure, like the pulmonary insufficiency of ARDS, is a common component of MODS.

Distinguishing low urine output due to oliguric renal failure from the oliguria of decreased renal perfusion pressure can be aided by analyzing urine sodium and osmolality. Renal hypoperfusion usually results in urine sodium of less than 20 mEq/L with an osmolality of greater than 400 mOsm/kg, whereas acute tubular injury impairs sodium reabsorption and is associated with a low urinary osmolality. A fractional excretion of sodium of less than 2% may also help determine whether the cause is renal or prerenal.

Early detection of abnormal kidney function is critical to prevent progression to renal injury. Abnormal renal function can be detected as a decline in creatinine clearance. The correlation between a creatinine clearance based on a 24-hour collection and a sample collected over a shorter interval is poor. However, the 24-hour value represents an average value over that time. A sample obtained over a shorter period may reflect the time in question and allow timely recognition and treatment of renal dysfunction.

Hepatic Response

Ischemic injury to liver is not apparent early during shock. However, the liver plays an important role in the regulation of shock and subsequent tissue injury through both the release of acute-phase reactants and lack of clearance of potential toxic agents. As shock continues, hepatic necrosis occurs, leading to the release of aspartate aminotransferase and alanine aminotransferase. Continued shock results in attenuated synthesis of coagulation factors, albumin and prealbumin. Although progressive ischemia can occur, leading to complete loss of glycogen stores and marked hypoglycemia, this condition is rare without preexisting liver disease, significant direct liver injury, or hepatic artery occlusion.

Genetic Regulation of the Response to Shock

Individuals vary considerably in their susceptibility to shock and in their ability to recover from its consequences. Recently, unique host-specific responses have been identified as important determinants of the outcome of sepsis and septic shock. Genetic predispositions in an individual's immunoinflammatory response may dictate whether infection is adequately or inadequately countered. These differences in response may be partially explained by single nucleotide polymorphisms (SNPs) in the genetic sequences for various inflammatory mediators. These subtle nucleotide variations may affect the transcription or translation of associated genes or the secretion or function of the corresponding proteins.

The recognition that genetic background may regulate the response to severe sepsis and septic shock has led to the identification of an array of genetic markers associated with enhanced risk of septic mortality. These SNPs are in genes encoding proteins involved in pathogen recognition (toll-like receptors 2, 4, and 5; CD14; and mannose-binding lectin), cytokine expression (TNF-α, IL-1, IL-6, and IL-10), and several other genes involved in mediating and controlling the innate immune response and the inflammatory cascade.[53,54]

Investigation into genetic polymorphisms should provide important insights into the pathophysiology of shock. SNP identification leading to early diagnosis of individuals at risk of developing or dying from the complications of shock may allow therapies to become more preemptive and effectively targeted.

LOSS OF COMPENSATORY RESPONSES TO SHOCK

If shock is prolonged, the arteriolar and precapillary sphincters become refractory and relax, while the postcapillary sphincter remains in spasm. Therefore, the capillary hydrostatic pressure increases, and Na^+, Cl^-, and water are moved into the interstitium, leading to depletion of intravascular volume.

Cellular membrane function is also impaired with prolonged shock. The normal negative membrane potential approaches neutrality, leading to increased permeability and interstitial flooding by K^+. This is caused, at least in part, by a decrease in the normal function of the adenosine triphosphate–dependent Na^+-K^+ membrane pump that is a result of cellular hypoxia. The loss of the membrane potential difference leads to cellular swelling due to an intracellular influx of Na^+ and fluid.

In addition to these cellular effects, severe and prolonged shock results in the development of progressive organ dysfunction. Although the mechanisms responsible are incompletely understood, it appears that the vital organs, in particular the lung early on, are limited in their ability to protect themselves during shock. As a result, direct endothelial injury occurs, resulting in leakage of various inflammatory mediators, which in turn results in accumulation of interstitial fluid and subsequent reduction in nutrient and gaseous diffusion. This condition, along with progressive microcirculatory thrombosis, is responsible for the late organ dysfunction characteristic of uncompensated shock.

COMPLICATIONS OF SHOCK

Ischemia-Reperfusion Injury

6 Inadequate microvasculature flow results in activation of leukocytes and converts local endothelial cells to a proinflammatory, prothrombotic phenotype. On reperfusion, the reintroduction of oxygen prompts these cells to generate superoxide anion, hydroxyl radicals, and hydrogen peroxide, further injuring local tissue. Microvascular endothelial adherence, monolayer transmigration, and local oxidative burst by activated neutrophils, along with the profound loss of endothelial monolayer integrity (i.e., microvascular capillary leak), contribute to massive interstitial edema after reperfusion. Although all tissues are sensitive to varying degrees, ischemia-reperfusion injury appears to be most detrimental to the pulmonary vasculature and the splanchnic circulations. Pulmonary interstitial edema and alveolar fluid accumulation are associated with the development of ARDS, whereas extensive visceral edema may contribute to development of abdominal compartment syndrome and mesenteric ischemia.

Second-hit Phenomena

Patients who have been successfully resuscitated from shock are at risk for what is referred to as the second-hit phenomenon. A single episode of severe or prolonged shock may precipitate organ failure, but, in addition, the initial insult may "prime" the inflammatory response, resulting in an augmented or prolonged response to a subsequent insult such as an infection, a second episode of blood loss, or major surgery.[55] For example, after the primary event, circulating neutrophils demonstrate enhanced superoxide anion production, increased endothelial cell adherence, augmented cytokine response, and increased cytotoxicity. Not only do circulating innate immune cells demonstrate this priming effect, but tissue-fixed cells, in particular the macrophage, demonstrate altered phagocytosis and augmented cytokine release.[56] This dysfunctional response leads to not only diminished microbial clearance and enhanced risk of nosocomial infection but also increased host tissue injury and subsequent development of MODS.

Multiple Organ Dysfunction Syndrome

Multiple organ dysfunction syndrome rarely develops as a result of isolated cardiogenic or neurogenic shock but is most often precipitated by septic and traumatic shock complicated by second-hit events such as repeated episodes of hypovolemia, subsequent infection, or repeated blood transfusions. Similarly, the presence of an unresolved inflammatory focus (such as devitalized necrotic tissue), undrained bodily fluids, or unresolved regional perfusion deficits can be the primary causes for the persistence of SIRS and the transition to MODS.

The effects of shock, resuscitation, and reperfusion and the subsequent development of MODS appear to depend on changes in the splanchnic and pulmonary microcirculations. These vascular beds appear to be major sites of the activation and subsequent immunoinflammatory mediator production that is responsible for the SIRS response. As splanchnic microcirculatory flow decreases in response to homeostatic vasoconstrictive responses during hypovolemia, excessive and prolonged hypoperfusion of the gut results in extensive microvascular injury and subsequent activation of endothelium, neutrophils, and macrophages. In addition, mucosal barrier disruption permits translocation of bacteria and bacterial toxins to circulate and reach the large tissue-fixed macrophage population in the liver. Extensive activation of the Kupffer cells in the liver results in the release of inflammatory mediators that cause distant organ injury through the systemic activation of other immune cells.

Not only is a proinflammatory phase of SIRS present, but there is also a compensatory anti-inflammatory phase of the SIRS response that is evolutionarily designed to counter the locally generated hyperimmune response and check systemic spread of proinflammatory mediators. If the compensatory anti-inflammatory response syndrome (CARS) results in excessive immunosuppression, it may contribute to susceptibility to primary and secondary infections that can then lead to organ failure.[57]

Numerous clinical trials utilizing proinflammatory and anti-inflammatory mediators as therapeutic interventions have been conducted. Unfortunately, few therapeutic agents designed to counter immune dysfunction have had significant impact on the prevention and treatment of MODS. In fact, with the exception of activated protein C, all attempts have failed to sufficiently and appropriately stimulate or suppress the SIRS response and improve outcomes.[58]

Abdominal Compartment Syndrome

Abdominal compartment syndrome is a highly morbid complication of reperfusion injury to the splanchnic viscera. This syndrome appears to be increasingly prominent due to aggressive resuscitation techniques that enable salvage of profoundly hypotensive and hypovolemic patients. Splanchnic ischemia and reperfusion result in extensive visceral capillary leak and interstitial edema of the bowel. Excessive volume resuscitation during this phase leads to grossly edematous viscera within the closed space of the abdomen, which dramatically increases intra-abdominal pressure, and compromises intra-abdominal organ function, increases renovascular resistance, limits diaphragmatic excursion, and may decrease cardiac output and elevate intracranial pressure. The clinical hallmarks of abdominal compartment syndrome are a distended and tense abdomen, diminished tidal volume, pulmonary edema, decreased cardiac output, oliguria, and elevated urinary bladder pressure. Presence of all or a major part of this syndrome should prompt consideration of an urgent operative laparotomy to decompress the abdomen and treat by leaving the abdomen open.

Hypothermia

Hypothermia (core temperature <35°C) is common during shock. In addition to immobilization, both prehospital and postadmission exposure can lead to conductive, convective, and evaporative heat loss, which should all be minimized. In addition, the administration of room temperature intravenous fluids and of cold-stored blood also contributes to hypothermia.[59] Hypothermia increases fluid requirements and independently increases acute mortality rates.[60]

As the core temperature decreases, the rate of oxygen consumption also decreases, to approximately 50% of normal at 28°C. The decrease in oxygen consumption is accompanied by increased production of acid metabolites. A leftward shift in the oxyhemoglobin dissociation curve also occurs with hypothermia but is partially compensated by the acidosis. Central nervous system effects progress from confusion and loss of manual dexterity to obtundation and frank coma as the core temperature decreases from 35°C to 26.5°C. The heart rate decreases to approximately half of baseline at 28°C, with a concomitant decrease in cardiac output. All cardiac electrical conduction intervals are prolonged, consistent with the changes in heart rate, and both atrioventricular dissociation and refractory ventricular fibrillation occur at 28°C. Other potential physiologic effects include ileus and pancreatitis (from cold enzyme activation) at temperatures lower than 35°C.

Compensatory responses to hypothermia include increased excretion of catecholamines, resulting in doubling of the basal metabolic rate, and increased production of thyroid hormones, further increasing the basal metabolic rate to five times baseline. Shivering can increase heat production as well, but it represents a significant energy expenditure, and has been shown to be inhibited during episodes of hypotension or hypoxemia.[61] Compensatory responses to hypothermia are lost at temperatures below 30°C or 31°C, and a state of complete poikilothermy is reached.

The treatment for hypothermia is rewarming. The core temperature should be obtained on admission of the trauma patient. Patients whose core temperatures are 33°C to 35°C can be treated with passive rewarming, warm blankets, and hot packs. Patients with core temperatures lower than 33°C require active rewarming. If the patient is unconscious, airway control should first be obtained. Because severe hypothermia causes vasoconstriction, noninvasive blood pressure measurements may not be feasible or accurate, and an arterial line should be placed for monitoring and blood gas sampling. The inspired gas through the ventilator should be heated to 41°C and fully saturated with water vapor to increase heat conductance in the lung. The intravenous fluids should also be warmed. Commercially available rapid infusion systems with countercurrent heating elements should be used. For extreme hypothermia, continuous mechanical arteriovenous rewarming can be performed for both circulatory support and rewarming. Recently developed microtechnology permits core rewarming by percutaneous placement of countercurrent warming coils directly in the inferior vena cava. Finally, other warming methods include lavage of heated saline through nasogastric and thoracostomy tubes as well as peritoneal lavage, but are not as effective.

Coagulopathy

Coagulopathy is a frequent problem complicating shock, especially in those patients who have received large volumes of crystalloid solution and blood for resuscitation. Although this problem is incompletely understood, it is clear that coagulation defects during shock are multifactorial. The presence of shock, the fluid volume required for resuscitation, the presence of hypothermia, and preexisting diseases all influence the likelihood and severity of coagulopathy.[62]

A major factor in coagulopathy is usually due to the dilutional thrombocytopenia that occurs after massive volume resuscitation. Although bleeding times can be prolonged with platelet counts less than 100,000 cells/mL, platelet counts of 50,000 cells/mL or greater are usually adequate for surgical hemostasis. Dilutional thrombocytopenia becomes more likely with infusions of more than one blood volume. Each unit of platelets administered increases the platelet count by 10,000 to 15,000 cells/mL. Control of surgically remediable hemorrhage is prudent before platelet transfusion to prevent the loss of the transfused platelets.

Dilution of other coagulation factors also plays a role in development of coagulopathy. Factors V and VIII are the most labile in banked blood, but levels of less than 10% of normal for factors VII, X, XI, XII, and XIII are all associated with abnormalities in hemostasis, as demonstrated by prolonged partial thromboplastin time and prothrombin time. Fresh frozen plasma can be administered as a source of all the soluble coagulation factors. The administration of cryoprecipitate may be necessary as a concentrated source of factor VIII and fibrinogen, particularly if adequate hemostasis is not obtained with the use of fresh frozen plasma.

Recent support has emerged for the use of recombinant activated factor VIIa. Although developed initially for use in hemophiliacs who developed inhibitors to factor VIII, anecdotal evidence has suggested that recombinant activated factor VIIa may serve to quickly reverse hemorrhage-induced coagulopathy.[63] However, currently no definitive data exist on which patients may benefit, and therefore further studies are required before routine use can be advocated.

Finally, evidence has suggested that coagulopathy and hemorrhage can be minimized following massive blood loss if early aggressive use of fresh frozen plasma is administered. Military data demonstrate that significant early coagulopathy is present after massive injury, even before blood component therapy is begun. Both civilian and military experience with a 1:1 ratio of packed red blood cells to fresh frozen plasma has been associated with reduced mortality.[64–66] However, this practice has been associated with an increase in the development of ARDS and organ dysfunction due to poorly defined mechanisms.[67] Thus, generalization of this data to all patients with hemorrhage other than the massively injured should be performed with caution until further prospective evidence is available.

TREATMENT

Fluid Therapy

Early investigators of hemorrhagic shock noted that decreased CVP and a reduction in total body oxygen delivery (DO_2) were key early findings. If the decrease in oxygen delivery was severe or prolonged, a reduction in total body oxygen consumption ensued. After adequate fluid resuscitation, oxygen delivery and consumption increased above the baseline value for several hours, as if the body was paying back an "oxygen debt." Failure of the patient to achieve this hyperdynamic response to resuscitation was almost always fatal. Because early death from shock appeared to be explained by the dynamics of oxygen delivery and utilization, therapy focused on restoring hemodynamics and oxygen transport with fluid and inotropes.

The provision of additional fluid beyond the amount of blood loss was associated with improved survival in both clinical and experimental studies of hemorrhagic shock, leading to widespread acceptance of aggressive fluid infusion. However, some researchers have recently described a significant increase in mortality associated with crystalloid overresuscitation and have postulated that excessive fluid administration increases the clinical risk of ARDS, MODS, increased intracranial pressure, and abdominal compartment syndrome.[68–70] Because massive volumes of fluid are only provided to patients with severe shock, it is unclear if it is the excessive fluid or the associated underlying shock that increases the risk of ARDS, organ failure, or death after massive fluid resuscitation.

7 A minimum of two large-bore (14- to 16-gauge) intravenous catheters should be established in adults. Isotonic fluid is then infused at the same time as blood is obtained for arterial blood gas analysis, screening, and typing. Fluid can be infused up to 200 mL/min through a 14-gauge catheter and up to 220 mL/min through a 7-French catheter. A fluid challenge of 10 to 25 mL/kg is administered to the hypotensive patient and the response is assessed (i.e., 2,000 mL or 40% of blood volume of a 70-kg man). This therapeutic challenge is an effective trial in determining the amount of preexisting or continuing volume loss. If the blood pressure returns to normal and is stabilized, the volume loss was relatively small, and the only treatment required may be infusion of isotonic fluid.

If the increase in blood pressure is transient after fluid bolus, then hemorrhage or continued fluid losses are severe and ongoing. Additional crystalloid is administered, and the need for blood transfusion is assessed. Patients who continue to require large amounts of fluid and blood to support perfusion usually have ongoing hemorrhage and require surgical intervention. No response or a minimal response to apparently adequate infusions of crystalloid solution and blood indicates exsanguinating hemorrhage and the need for urgent surgery.

Crystalloids. Balanced salt solutions are the most commonly used resuscitative fluids, and their use to restore extracellular volume significantly decreases the transfusion requirement after hemorrhagic shock. Lactated Ringer solution is isotonic, readily available, and inexpensive. It rapidly replaces the depleted interstitial fluid compartment and does not aggravate any preexisting electrolyte abnormalities. Previous investigations have shown that administration of lactated Ringer solution does not lead to aggravation of the lactic acidosis that is present in shock.[71] In fact, animal models have demonstrated that the use of blood plus lactated Ringer solution results in a more rapid return to normal lactate and pH than dose shed blood alone. As volume and perfusion are restored, lactate is mobilized and metabolized to bicarbonate in a single pass through the liver. In fact, mild metabolic alkalosis may occur 1 or 2 days after large-volume resuscitations with lactated Ringer solution. Normal saline solution is also effective for resuscitation of hypovolemic patients. Concerns about inducing hypernatremic, hyperchloremic metabolic acidosis with massive resuscitation volumes remain but appear of less relevance by further investigation with normal saline and the hypertonic saline solutions.

Recently several investigations have raised concerns about the proinflammatory effects of resuscitation with lactated Ringer solution. Some commercially available lactated Ringer solutions contain racemic lactate that is made of equal concentrations of D(−)- and L(+)-isomers of lactate. The D(−)-isomer has been demonstrated in vitro to result in enhanced production of reactive oxygen species by neutrophils and inflammatory gene expression by leukocytes.[72,73] In addition, increased apoptosis in both the small intestine and the liver was seen after resuscitation from hemorrhage with lactated Ringer solution, but not with hypertonic solutions or blood resuscitation.[74] These findings, however, are not consistent and do not appear dissimilar from saline resuscitation in other animal models.[75] Thus, further investigations are required to determine the overall inflammatory effect of crystalloid resuscitation and extent of D(−)-isomer use in current commercial fluids.

Colloids. Colloids have the theoretic advantages of increasing the colloid oncotic pressure and requiring smaller volumes for resuscitation than crystalloids.[76] Colloids commonly used for volume expansion in hypovolemia include albumin, dextran 70, dextran 40, and hydroxyethyl starch. Although each has unique individual characteristics, currently there is little justification for the routine addition of colloids to balanced salt solutions for volume replacement during shock.

Albumin solutions have been used during resuscitation to increase colloid oncotic pressure and, hypothetically, to protect the lung from interstitial edema; however, there is a relatively rapid flux of albumin across the pulmonary capillary membranes and relatively rapid clearance through the pulmonary lymphatics. In fact, colloid albumin infusion has been demonstrated to prolong the resuscitation phase and delay postresuscitation diuresis. Additionally, albumin may serve to depress circulating immunoglobulin levels and suppress albumin synthesis.

Dextran 40 and dextran 70 are polysaccharides with molecular weights of 40 and 70 kD, respectively. Dextran 40 (10%) is hyperoncotic and initially exerts a volume-expanding effect. However, because of its lower molecular weight, it is more rapidly excreted. Thus, dextran 40 is commonly used in cases of peripheral vascular disease and hyperviscosity syndromes. Dextran 70, conversely, is provided as a 6% solution and does not exert a hyperoncotic effect. The volume expansion is somewhat greater than the amount infused, and because of its large molecular size the effect is maintained for up to 48 hours. The dextran preparations, however, cause decreased platelet adhesiveness and decreased factor VIII activity. They also carry an incidence of allergic reaction of up to 5% and anaphylaxis of 0.6%.[76]

Hydroxyethyl starch is an amylopectin with volume-expanding effects for approximately 36 hours. It has side effects similar to those of dextran, but with less frequency. The incidence of anaphylaxis is 0.006%. A new hydroxyethyl starch, pentastarch, has a lower molecular weight and fewer hydroxyethyl groups than hydroxyethyl starch. Pentastarch has a shorter duration of action (2.5 hours) and has been reported to have even fewer side effects.[77,78]

The controversy regarding use of crystalloids versus colloids in resuscitation has not been resolved. Both types of solutions can restore circulating volume. The effects of the solutions on pulmonary function are at issue and are summarized as follows: (a) the use of crystalloid solutions decreases plasma oncotic pressure, thereby leading to lung edema at lower microvascular pressures; and (b) colloids given in the face of pulmonary injury can extravasate, promoting edema because of the reduced plasma interstitial oncotic gradient. In fact, a previous meta-analysis of colloid versus crystalloid resuscitation after hemorrhagic shock demonstrated a higher mortality rate among the colloid-resuscitated patients, partly because of pulmonary complications.[79] Therefore, since colloid infusion has not demonstrated a significant benefit over crystalloid resuscitation alone, it is not currently recommended in the management of hypovolemic shock.

Resuscitative Strategy. Aggressive fluid resuscitation is clearly a lifesaving modality, and a key strategy in the treatment of shock and prevention of secondary consequences (Algorithm 8.2). However, indiscriminate fluid loading causes problematic edema in the lungs, gut, brain, and other organs. The amount of fluid used for resuscitation should be titrated to carefully selected hemodynamic and oxygen transport endpoints. Solutions currently in development ("artificial blood") with oxygen transport capabilities may hold the potential of restoring oxygen transport while minimizing the need for large volumes.

Permissive Hypotension

Elevation of systemic arterial pressure in patients with disruption of the arterial system or major solid organ injury, especially after penetrating trauma, may cause acceleration of hemorrhage, disrupt natural clotting mechanisms, and cause dilution of clotting factors. Laboratory and clinical evidence support judicious use of intravenous fluids until hemorrhage is controlled by surgery, angiography, or direct pressure for penetrating trauma.[80] Fluid resuscitation for patients with multisystem blunt trauma, especially with concomitant traumatic brain injury, represents a more complicated decision process, as maintaining cerebral perfusion pressure is a competing priority. Avoidance of both excessive fluid administration and prolonged hypoperfusion is best achieved in all patients not by maintenance of a marginal blood pressure, but by rapid surgical or angiographic intervention to control bleeding.

Transfusion

Anemia prompts clinical concerns because it may signify blood loss or hematologic disease, but it rarely causes tissue ischemia. The hemoglobin level that causes concern should depend on the adequacy of other mechanisms involved in oxygen delivery such as arterial oxygen saturation and cardiac output, the specific clinical situation, and the organ systems most at risk, balanced against the risk of transfusion. Clinical evidence suggests that hemoglobin values above 7 mg/dL are adequate in most patients, including the critically ill, but this has not been explored during shock. In one prospective randomized trial in critically ill patients, it was clearly demonstrated that a reduction in complications and improvement in survival were noted when lower hemoglobin values were accepted.[81] However, this study excluded patients with hypovolemia, acute coronary syndrome, and sepsis. Thus, the role of transfusion during shock remains problematic.

Given this limitation, currently it is held that most patients with class I or II shock can be resuscitated with balanced salt solutions alone. Patients who lose more than 25% to 30% of total blood volume require blood for resuscitation, as do patients with persistent evidence of inadequate end-organ perfusion.[16] The decision about the extent of blood cross match prior to being transfused is determined in part by the urgency of the situation. Blood that has been fully typed and cross matched carries the least risk of transfusion reactions, but it also takes the most time to obtain. Other transfusion options include the use of type O or type-specific blood (Table 8.6).

Type O Blood. Type O (universal donor) blood is immediately available without a cross match. Because type O blood contains no AB cellular antigens, administration of packed red blood cells is relatively safe in patients of any blood type. Males should be transfused type O Rh-positive blood, while prepubescent females and females of childbearing age should be given type O Rh-negative blood to avoid sensitization that would complicate future pregnancies. The administration of more than 4 units of type O blood to a non–O-blood-type patient, however, theoretically can result in an admixture of blood type. A pretransfusion blood specimen should be sent to the blood bank when the patient is admitted, and type-specific blood should be transfused as soon as it is available.

Type-specific Blood. Type-specific blood is available from most blood banks within 5 to 10 minutes of receipt of the blood specimen, while the patient is being resuscitated with balanced salt solutions. Although not cross matched, this blood can be administered safely, as demonstrated in both military and civilian experiences.[82]

Autotransfusion. Autotransfusion involves collection of the shed blood and its reinfusion through a filter back into the patient. Autotransfusion can be as simple as aspiration of the blood into a citrate-containing collection chamber, followed by reinfusion through a 40-mm filter. A more elaborate system, the Haemonetics autotransfuser (Haemonetics Corp., Braintree, MA), centrifuges the collected blood and delivers washed, packed red blood cells for reinfusion. The advantages of autotransfusion include transfusion with warm, compatible blood without delays and with no risk of transmission of hepatitis, human immunodeficiency virus, or other blood-borne pathogens.

Autotransfused blood can produce disseminated intravascular coagulation and activation of fibrinolysis. In addition, collection of blood from the peritoneal cavity after hollow viscus injury, even with cell washing, may lead to bacterial contamination of the autotransfused blood.[83] Successful autotransfusion of contaminated blood has been demonstrated, but blood

TABLE 8.6

COMPARISON OF BLOOD AVAILABILITY

BLOOD	TYPING	ANTIBODY SCREEN	CROSS MATCH	TIME
Type O	No	No	No	Immediate
Type specific	Yes	No	No	<10 min
Type and screen	Yes	Yes	Yes	20–30 min
Type and cross match	Yes	Yes	Yes	45–60 min

obtained from enteric-contaminated cavities probably should not be used, except perhaps in extreme circumstances.[84] Despite the potential benefits, investigators have found that the autotransfuser was used in only 26% of the trauma patients for whom it was prepared.[85] Currently, no evidence exists that autotransfusion improves outcome compared to exclusive homologous blood transfusions in trauma patients.

Endpoints of Resuscitation

Endpoints of resuscitation can be categorized as either global or regional indicators of perfusion. Blood pressure and pulse are global measures and are relatively poor determinants of the adequacy of tissue oxygenation. They must also be interpreted in the context of patient age and preexisting medical conditions. Tachycardia is a component of SIRS and does not always resolve with increased preload. Arterial pressure is maintained by myriad compensatory mechanisms, even in the face of a significant volume deficit, and interpretation is complicated by highly variable baseline pressures, age, and preexisting medical conditions.

Base deficit and serum lactate are also global indicators of perfusion and may help in the detection of patients who are in otherwise compensated shock. Acidosis arising from regional tissues may not be apparent in peripheral blood samples, as is frequently the case in patients with intestinal ischemia, in whom systemic acidosis is a late finding. An elevated base deficit and lactate can be caused by electrolyte abnormalities, accelerated glycolysis or pyruvate production, and/or decreased clearance by the liver. They may also reflect dysfunction caused by a period of hypoperfusion that has already resolved and that does not need further treatment. A positive response toward correction, however, is indicative of appropriate resuscitation.

A pulmonary artery catheter (PAC) has obvious appeal as a monitor because ensuring adequate oxygen delivery is paramount in the treatment of shock (Algorithm 8.2). A progressive decline in systemic oxygen delivery (DO_2) results in an increase in the oxygen extraction ratio, evident as a reduction in pulmonary mixed venous oxygen saturation. When DO_2 is reduced below the level needed to maintain normal tissue metabolic activity, anaerobic metabolism occurs. This is evident as a decrease in total body oxygen consumption (VO_2). Adequate resuscitation requires eliminating any pathologic decrease in VO_2 by restoring oxygen delivery to an adequate level. In clinical practice, however, there is no precise level of VO_2 that can be used as an endpoint, as tissue oxygen needs vary according to the patient's condition, level of sedation, body temperature, and other factors, and are affected by endogenous and exogenously administered catecholamines.

Oxygen consumption may be especially difficult to interpret in patients with late-stage sepsis because acquired defects in mitochondrial respiration may prevent utilization of oxygen, resulting in decreased consumption and progressive acidosis despite normal or high DO_2.

The adequacy of resuscitation can also be assessed by measurement of end-organ function and perfusion, in addition to global measures. Blood flow to the most vital organs (brain and heart) is preserved during shock at the expense of flow to the skin, muscles, gut, and, ultimately, kidneys. Detection of ischemia in less vital organs could theoretically identify patients in compensated shock who have otherwise normal global indicators.

Low urine output ($<$0.5 to 1.0 mL/kg per hour) is an indicator of inadequate end-organ perfusion, but inappropriate urine output may initially be maintained by peripheral venoconstriction and maintenance of cardiac output due to tachycardia. The use of gastric tonometry to measure intramucosal pH has highlighted the uneven recovery from shock by visceral organs. Persistent visceral hypoperfusion, as demonstrated by intramucosal acidosis despite correction to normal hemodynamics, is associated with organ failure and poor outcomes. Unfortunately, direct measurement of visceral hypoperfusion, as well as hypoperfusion in other regional vascular beds, requires use of technically challenging, labor-intensive devices that often produce variable unreliable results and has not yet had widespread application. Presently, the goal of therapy is to restore tissue perfusion, both global and regional as measured by organ function, and to normalize cellular metabolism while avoiding excessive use of fluids and inotropes.

Recently, several biomarkers, in addition to base deficit and lactate, have demonstrated potential promise. Among the most promising is procalcitonin for the early recognition of sepsis. However, in addition to being significantly elevated during sepsis, procalcitonin has recently been demonstrated, similar to lactate and base deficit, to be prognostic of outcome from hypovolemia based on rate of clearance.[86] Thus, this biomarker along with potential others may lead to early recognition and treatment of shock.

MONITORS

Central Venous Pressure

CVP is determined by a number of factors, the most important of which are venous volume and venous compliance. Cardiac output and arterial dilation modulate CVP by affecting central venous volume, whereas sympathetic venoconstriction and thoracic and intra-abdominal pressure primarily affect central venous compliance. A variety of conditions can raise CVP despite a normal or even low cardiac preload. High ventilator pressures, expiratory airway obstruction, tension pneumothorax, cardiac tamponade, and obesity are additional non–volume-dependent causes of a relatively elevated CVP.

Circulating catecholamines cause vasoconstriction, with maintenance of venous pressure despite reduced circulating volume. In such cases, fluid therapy may reduce the intensity of vasoconstriction by reducing tone, with no net change in CVP. Following the change in CVP in response to a fluid challenge may be the only way to accurately estimate preload in some patients. Although an elevated CVP does not guarantee adequate preload, a low CVP is a reliable indicator of hypovolemia. Inspiratory stridor is the only condition that can falsely reduce CVP and mimic hypovolemia by significantly reducing intrapleural pressure.

Pulmonary Artery Catheter

Hemodynamic monitoring utilizing a flow-directed PAC has been a standard in the treatment of shock for decades and has been considered to be essential for optimal management of certain forms of shock. However, as a result of a multicenter study that reported that use of a PAC was associated with increased mortality, the indications for PAC use have recently been questioned.[87] PAC patients were retrospectively compared to matched control patients that were selected using a scoring system. This scoring system has not been validated, which raises the possibility that physicians inserted a PAC in the more critically ill patients.

Intensive care unit (ICU) staffing practices may have also been a factor explaining these surprising results. The study was conducted in "open" ICUs, where any physician on the medical staff could admit a patient to the unit and insert a PAC. Clinicians may not always interpret PAC data appropriately. In a multicenter study of physicians' knowledge and interpretation of PAC data, nearly half (47%) were unable to appropriately determine the wedge pressure from a clear tracing, and a similar percentage (44%) could not identify the determinants of oxygen delivery.[88] Studies have demonstrated improved outcome when patients are managed in ICUs staffed by specialists in critical care, despite their more frequent use of PACs.[89]

An additional consideration regarding the controversy over the utility of PACs is that currently used endpoints for PAC-guided resuscitation may be inappropriate. For example, efforts to augment systemic oxygen delivery have not demonstrated any benefits and, in fact, harm may be caused this approach, whereas treatments used to alter the variables ascertained with the catheter may themselves cause harm (fluid overload, excessive inotropes, blood transfusions). Finally, PACs are associated with specific complications, including the risk of central venous catheter insertion, endocarditis, and pulmonary artery injury, which may outweigh any potential benefits. As the safety and utility of the PAC have not yet been evaluated with prospective clinical trials in specific shock states, its usefulness in the management of shock remains to be determined.

Newer versions of the PAC have been developed that provide additional hemodynamic information, including continuous determination of cardiac output, ejection fraction, and calculated right ventricular end-diastolic volume. The pulmonary artery wedge pressure is a proxy for preload. However, the amount of precontractile stretch achieved with any given wedge or chamber pressure is modulated by the compliance of the ventricle. Therefore, cardiac chamber pressure may not be an accurate indicator of ventricular end-diastolic volume, just as end-diastolic volume may not be an accurate indicator of pulmonary wedge pressure and/or risk of pulmonary edema. The combination of both wedge pressure and end-diastolic volume may be optimal to maximize preload while avoiding excessive pulmonary capillary pressure.

A comparison of the pH and partial pressure of carbon dioxide (PCO_2) of mixed venous blood with a matched arterial blood sample can provide evidence of shock with tissue hypoxia. Hypoxic cells generate a hydrogen ion that is buffered by bicarbonate, resulting in increased production of H_2O and CO_2. An increase in venous PCO_2 results in an abnormal gap between mixed venous and arterial PCO_2 and pH and is a sign of anaerobic metabolism. With cessation of hydrogen ion production, this abnormal gap is quickly eliminated, whereas base deficit and hyperlactatemia may persist for several hours.

PHARMACEUTICAL SUPPORT

Therapeutic adjustments of preload and afterload form the basis of treatment strategies in all forms of shock. Optimal volume resuscitation should always precede measures to augment the contractile function of the heart. Inotropic augmentation of cardiac output may therefore be required when restoration of venous preload fails to provide sufficient cardiac output to satisfy tissue oxygen demands. The effect of inotropic agents depends on the specific adrenergic receptor affinity, chronotropic effects, and demands placed on myocardial oxygen consumption of the individual agents (Table 8.7). Vasodilators reduce demands on the myocardium and augment cardiac function via reduction in systemic vascular resistance (SVR) or afterload or by dilating the venous system and reducing cardiac preload. Afterload reduction may preserve stroke volume in the face of a failing myocardium, whereas

TABLE 8.7

PHARMACODYNAMICS OF INOTROPIC/VASOCONSTRICTOR AGENTS

		■ SITES OF ACTION				■ HEMODYNAMIC RESPONSE			
■ DRUG	■ METABOLISM	■ HEART β_1	■ HEART β_2	■ VESSELS α	■ VESSELS β_2	■ RENAL PERFUSION	■ CO	■ SVR	■ BP
Isoproterenol 1 mg/250 mL 1–2 μg/min initially	Renal	+++	+++	0	+++	+/–		–	+/–
Dobutamine 250 mg/250 mL 3 μg/kg/min initially	Hepatic	+++	0/+	0/+	0/+			–	0/+
Dopamine 200 mg/250 mL 2–5 μg/kg/min low dose 20–50 μg/kg/min high dose	Hepatic	+++	+	0	Low dose High dose	–	Low dose High dose	0/+ –	
Epinephrine 2 mg/250 mL 2 μg/min initially	Renal	+++	+++	+++	++	–		–	
Norepinephrine 4 mg/250 mL 4 μg/min initially	Renal	++	++	+++	0	–	+/–		
Phenylephrine	Renal	0	0	+++	0	–	–		

α (alpha), vasoconstrict peripheral arterioles; β_1 (beta-1) myocardial inotropy, chronotropy, enhance atrioventricular conduction; β_2 (beta-2) chronotropy, vasodilate mesenteric/skeletal bed, bronchodilation; dopaminergic, vasodilate mesenteric/renal bed.
BP, blood pressure; CO, cardiac output; SVR, systemic vascular resistance.

venodilation reduces pulmonary capillary wedge pressure and pressure-driven pulmonary edema. Agents that increase afterload may be needed when blood pressure falls below the autoregulatory range of the coronary, cerebral, and renal vascular beds.

Inotropes and Vasopressors

Dopamine. Dopamine is an endogenous sympathetic amine that is a biosynthetic precursor of epinephrine and functions as a central and peripheral neurotransmitter. The effects of dopamine vary from individual to individual, and are altered with increasing doses. The highest-affinity receptors are occupied at low serum concentrations (infusions <2 to 3 μg/kg per minute) and consist of dopaminergic receptors in the renal and splanchnic beds that serve to augment regional blood flow, increase urine output, and cause natriuresis. However, multiple studies, including prospective randomized trials, have failed to demonstrate that low-dose dopamine prevents acute renal failure or decreases the need for dialysis in critically ill patients. At modest concentrations (3 to 5 μg/kg per minute), dopamine occupies cardiac β_1-adrenergic receptors and increases myocardial contractility and heart rate. Higher doses (>5 μg/kg per minute) cause an increase in heart rate and blood pressure. α-Adrenergic receptors are stimulated at higher dose ranges (>10 μg/kg per minute), resulting in elevation of blood pressure and peripheral vascular resistance. Dopamine is therefore an effective agent for increasing blood pressure in hypotensive patients after appropriate fluid resuscitation. Because the relationship among a specific dose, receptor affinity, and clinical effect is unique to each patient, individual titration is required to achieve the desired effect.

Dobutamine. Dobutamine, a synthetic catecholamine, has a predominant affinity for β-adrenergic receptors. At clinically relevant doses (5 to 20 μg/kg per minute), dobutamine enhances myocardial contractility with mild to moderate changes in heart rate. It also induces peripheral vasodilation, which limits its utility in patients with hypotension. It is an appropriate agent when cardiac output augmentation, not blood pressure support, is required and when a drop in peripheral resistance and preload is clinically tolerable or beneficial. Treatment of cardiogenic shock following myocardial infarction or cardiac dysfunction following shock and reperfusion typically requires support of myocardial contractility and reduction of peripheral resistance, which makes dobutamine an excellent choice in this setting.

Epinephrine. Epinephrine, the endogenous adrenal catecholamine, is released physiologically in response to stress. It has a broad spectrum of systemic actions, including significant cardiovascular effects. When epinephrine is administered as a pharmacologic agent (0.01 to 0.05 μg/kg per minute), β_1-adrenergic effects predominate, causing increased stroke volume, heart rate, and contractility, along with modest β_2-receptor stimulation. At higher infusion rates, α-adrenergic receptors are stimulated, which overcome β_2-mediated peripheral vasodilation, resulting in an increase in blood pressure and SVR. Renal and splanchnic vasoconstriction, cardiac dysrhythmias, and increased myocardial oxygen demands limit the prolonged use of high-dose epinephrine. Transient increases in serum lactate have also been noted, possibly due to impaired regional blood flow. Epinephrine should be considered as a potential short-term agent for use in patients with impaired cardiac function not responsive to other agents such as dobutamine.

Norepinephrine. Norepinephrine, the sympathetic neurotransmitter, also has concentration-dependent cardiovascular effects. It should be considered as a drug with predominantly α-constrictor effects and less pronounced β-stimulation and is therefore appropriate for use in patients who remain hypotensive despite dopamine administration or as a dopamine alternative. Combined α- and β-stimulation typically results in an increase in afterload and renal glomerular perfusion pressure, with preservation of cardiac output. Despite the potential for renal vasoconstriction, as a result of its effects on mean arterial pressure, norepinephrine is associated with an increase in urine output and creatinine clearance in hypotensive, and particularly septic, patients. A primary concern is to ensure adequate volume resuscitation prior to utilization due to risk of severe tissue damage from excessive vasoconstriction on the hypovolemic patient.

Isoproterenol. Isoproterenol is a synthetic catecholamine with potent α-adrenergic effects. From a cardiovascular standpoint, both cardiac and peripheral effects are significant. Stimulation of cardiac α_1-receptors prompts an increase in contractility, heart rate, and conduction velocity. The chronotropic response, however, may predominate. These activities, in conjunction with peripheral vasodilation, generate significant increases in cardiac output and pulse pressure. Isoproterenol greatly increases myocardial oxygen demand and limits coronary filling due to tachycardia. As a result, indications for isoproterenol are limited to patients with hemodynamically significant bradyarrhythmias while preparations are made for electrical pacing.

Phenylephrine. Phenylephrine is a pure α-agonist and is an effective agent for increasing peripheral vascular resistance and arterial blood pressure. Although it has no direct effect on the myocardium, the increase in afterload increases left ventricular work and oxygen demand and may cause a decrease in stroke volume and cardiac output. It is often used as a first-line agent in patients with neurogenic shock, but its use is otherwise generally restricted to patients who remain hypotensive when the dosage of agents such as dopamine or norepinephrine cannot be increased due to excessive tachycardia.

Vasopressin. Vasopressin acts directly on V_1 receptors in vascular smooth muscle to cause vasoconstriction and increases the reactivity of vascular smooth muscle to catecholamines. Release of endogenous vasopressin is a normal physiologic response to shock. After septic or prolonged hemorrhagic shock, circulating vasopressin levels are decreased, possibly due to depletion of hypophyseal secretory stores. This relative deficiency may play a role in causing refractory hypotension. Vasopressin has minimal effects on normotensive patients, but in patients with septic shock it is effective in increasing SVR and mean arterial pressure. Vasopressin does not have inotropic properties but has potent splanchnic and coronary vasoconstrictors. It has been associated with decreased cardiac output due to myocardial ischemia and increased afterload and may worsen metabolic acidosis in patients in shock by causing splanchnic ischemia. As a result, early use of vasopressin at only physiologic concentrations to minimize associated other pressor use may be indicated.

Amrinone and Milrinone. Amrinone and milrinone are noncatecholamine inotropes with cardiovascular effects similar to dobutamine, but with minimal chronotropic activity. As steroidlike phosphodiesterase antagonists, they increase smooth muscle cyclic adenosine monophosphate (cAMP) and alter calcium metabolism. Cardiac contractility, stroke volume, heart rate, and cardiac output are increased, while a concomitant reduction in afterload offsets cardiac workload. The increase in cardiac performance with minimal demands on myocardial oxygen consumption offers some utility in the treatment of cardiogenic shock or as a potential alternative to dobutamine infusion. Both agents have a relatively long half-life of nearly 3 hours and should therefore be used with caution in patients at risk of developing hypotension, a major risk in the critically ill patient.

Vasodilators

Vasodilators are used as a means to augment cardiac function through optimization of preload and afterload, both of which reduce demands on the myocardium. The failing ventricle responds to afterload reduction with significant increases in stroke volume. The reason for this is that the compromised myocardium is working past the plateau and on the down slope of the Starling curve. As a result, afterload reduction with vasodilator agents may allow cardiac output to increase, resulting in improved oxygen delivery.

Nitroprusside. Nitroprusside is a balanced but potent arterial and venous smooth muscle vasodilator. It causes a reduction in afterload that increases cardiac output and has a less prominent venodilatory effect that reduces pulmonary venous pressure and preload. Hypotension may limit its use, particularly in the presence of contractility deficits or inadequate preload. Infusions (>3 μg/kg per minute) continued for greater than 48 hours require monitoring of serum thiocyanate levels and arterial pH to detect complications of cyanide toxicity.

Nitroglycerin. Nitroglycerin is primarily a venous smooth muscle vasodilator, with less significant arterial vasodilation effects than nitroprusside. Thus, although nitroprusside predominantly decreases afterload, nitroglycerin predominantly increases venous capacitance. It is an effective treatment for acute myocardial ischemia because it reduces excessive preload and ventricular end-diastolic pressure, thereby diminishing myocardial oxygen demand.

Miscellaneous Therapeutics

Corticosteroids. In septic shock, ACTH resistance may diminish the normal cortisol response. Also, peripheral tissue resistance to corticosteroids may develop through proinflammatory-induced downregulation of normal corticosteroid receptors. Initial clinical trials showed no reduction in mortality when short courses of high-dose corticosteroids were used as adjuncts in the treatment of septic shock. However, recent studies utilizing low or physiologic doses (<300 mg/day) of hydrocortisone for a longer duration (>5 days) of treatment have demonstrated a beneficial impact on mortality, particularly in septic patients.[33] Currently, routine use of ACTH stimulation tests is not advocated since they provide little more than prognostic information.[35] Given that hypoadrenal shock complicates various shock states, routine use is considered, but given the lack of proven benefit in other multicenter trials, use is currently not widely advocated without caution.[34]

Activated Protein C. Decades of cellular and humoral inflammation research have failed to produce an effective immunologic intervention in humans with septic shock and organ failure. However, coagulation pathway dysfunction, the mediators of which are also part of the innate host response to infection, has recently been shown to correlate with disease severity and mortality. Specifically, septic shock is associated with rapid depletion of protein C and blunted endogenous protein C activation. The protein C pathway serves to regulate thrombosis and may play a role in limiting the inflammatory response and diminishing endothelial cell injury in response to inflammatory cytokines.

In a large randomized phase III trial of recombinant activated protein C (APC) in severe sepsis, a 6.1% absolute reduction in 28-day mortality compared with placebo was demonstrated. The short- and long-term survival rates associated with APC were significantly better only in septic patients at high risk of death. However, treatment with APC was also associated with a slightly increased risk of serious bleeding compared with placebo, particularly during infusion (3.5% vs. 2.0%), and must be considered a major contraindication in the patient in the early postoperative period or with minimal organ dysfunction in sepsis.[90]

Metabolites and Electrolytes. Severe shock is frequently associated with hypocalcemia. Severe hypocalcemia that causes cardiac dysfunction or electrical instability should be rapidly treated. Calcium chloride rapidly corrects calcium deficits, whereas calcium gluconate must be degraded in the liver to release calcium ion, resulting in slower correction of deficits but less risk of tissue reaction. In the absence of evidence of cardiac dysfunction, attempts to restore plasma calcium to normal during shock are not warranted. Ischemia results in decreased cell membrane ATP and failure of the membrane calcium pump. Thus, reduced serum calcium levels during severe shock are probably due to movement of ionized calcium into the cells. Increased cytosolic calcium causes release of lysosomal enzymes and activation of phospholipases, protein kinases, and proteases that cause membrane damage and cytoskeletal destruction. Administration of exogenous calcium may merely worsen this uncontrolled intracellular calcium influx, whereas effective resuscitation will usually restore circulating calcium levels to normal.

Many shock resuscitation protocols emphasize correction of metabolic acidosis with fluids and inotropes until the pH begins to normalize. When interpreting an acid–base disorder, the presence of an anion gap is supportive evidence of lactic acidosis. However, a non–anion gap acidosis with worsening base deficit frequently occurs when normal saline is administered in large volumes. Efforts to correct a non–anion gap acidosis with additional fluids that may no longer be needed will only increase the risk of fluid overload.

Future Therapies

When initiating therapy for shock, the clinician does not know whether therapy has been started early, when salvage is still possible, or late, after irreversible changes have occurred within the cell and death is inevitable. Failure to respond to fluids, inotropes, and vasopressors with restoration of normal oxygen consumption and aerobic metabolism probably represents a defect in cellular and subcellular function in critical organ systems. There are many active areas of investigation that reflect the progression of our understanding of shock that have been outlined in this chapter and that have begun to move the field beyond the basics of fluid resuscitation and hemodynamic monitoring.

Efforts to control ischemia-reperfusion injury include controlled reperfusion with carbon monoxide or other compounds to reduce oxidative stress. Induced hypothermia may interrupt generation of harmful byproducts of ischemia and enable restoration of circulation and repair of structural injuries in a cellular environment where hypoxia is no longer critical. Additional biomarkers, such as procalcitonin, may allow earlier diagnosis and treatment of sepsis and shock.[86] New biosensors using near-infrared light may enable transcutaneous identification of critical limitations of blood flow and enable clinicians to more accurately target areas of regional hypoperfusion.[91] A search for agents that optimize circulation in the microvascular system by preventing activation of the endothelium may enable resuscitative efforts to restore oxygen to cells as needed to maintain normal respiration and provide critical nutrients. Ultimately, further understanding of functional genomics may enable clinicians to target transcription and translational events triggered by shock and thus alter outcome.

References

1. Cannon WB. Pharmacological injections and physiological inferences. *Science* 1929;70(1821):500–501.

2. Blalock A. Reminiscence: shock after thirty-four years. *Rev Surg* 1964;21:231–234.
3. Bogolioubov A, Keefe DL, Groeger JS. Circulatory shock. *Crit Care Clin* 2001;17(3):697–719.
4. Blalock A, Mason MF. Blood and blood substitutes in the treatment and prevention of shock: with particular reference to their uses in warfare. *Ann Surg* 1941;113(5):657–676.
5. Wiggers HC, Ingraham RC. Hemorrhagic shock: definition and criteria for its diagnosis. *J Clin Invest* 1946;25(1):30–36.
6. Weil MH, Shubin H. Proposed reclassification of shock states with special reference to distributive defects. *Adv Exp Med Biol* 1971;23(0):13–23.
7. Whittington LK, Roscelli JD, Parry WH. Hemorrhagic shock and encephalopathy: further description of a new syndrome. *J Pediatr* 1985;106(4):599–602.
8. Moore FA, McKinley BA, Moore EE, et al. Inflammation and the Host Response to Injury, a large-scale collaborative project: patient-oriented research core–standard operating procedures for clinical care. III. Guidelines for shock resuscitation. *J Trauma* 2006;61(1):82–89.
9. Vitek V, Cowley RA. Blood lactate in the prognosis of various forms of shock. *Ann Surg* 1971;173(2):308–313.
10. Abramson D, Scalea TM, Hitchcock R, et al. Lactate clearance and survival following injury. *J Trauma* 1993;35(4):584–588; discussion 588–589.
11. Nguyen HB, Rivers EP, Knoblich BP, et al. Early lactate clearance is associated with improved outcome in severe sepsis and septic shock. *Crit Care Med* 2004;32(8):1637–1642.
12. Davis JW, Kaups KL, Parks SN. Base deficit is superior to pH in evaluating clearance of acidosis after traumatic shock. *J Trauma* 1998;44(1):114–118.
13. Davis JW, Shackford SR, Holbrook TL. Base deficit as a sensitive indicator of compensated shock and tissue oxygen utilization. *Surg Gynecol Obstet* 1991;173(6):473–476.
14. Davis JW, Shackford SR, Mackersie RC, et al. Base deficit as a guide to volume resuscitation. *J Trauma* 1988;28(10):1464–1467.
15. Davis JW, Parks SN, Kaups KL, et al. Admission base deficit predicts transfusion requirements and risk of complications. *J Trauma* 1996;41(5):769–774.
16. Rivers E, Nguyen B, Havstad S, et al. Early goal-directed therapy in the treatment of severe sepsis and septic shock. *N Engl J Med* 2001;345(19):1368–1377.
17. Rivers EP, Kruse JA, Jacobsen G, et al. The influence of early hemodynamic optimization on biomarker patterns of severe sepsis and septic shock. *Crit Care Med* 2007;35(9):2016–2024.
18. Bouman CS, Oudemans-van Straaten HM, Schultz MJ, et al. Hemofiltration in sepsis and systemic inflammatory response syndrome: the role of dosing and timing. *J Crit Care* 2007;22(1):1–12.
19. Cui ZG, Kondo T, Matsumoto H. Enhancement of apoptosis by nitric oxide released from alpha-phenyl-tert-butyl nitrone under hyperthermic conditions. *J Cell Physiol* 2006;206(2):468–476.
20. Englehart MS, Schreiber MA. Measurement of acid-base resuscitation endpoints: lactate, base deficit, bicarbonate or what? *Curr Opin Crit Care* 2006;12(6):569–574.
21. Goodrich C. Endpoints of resuscitation: what should we be monitoring? *AACN Adv Crit Care* 2006;17(3):306–316.
22. Jones AE, Shapiro NI, Kilgannon JH, et al. Goal-directed hemodynamic optimization in the post-cardiac arrest syndrome: a systematic review. *Resuscitation* 2008;77(1):26–29.
23. Muehlschlegel S, Dunser MW, Gabrielli A, et al. Arginine vasopressin as a supplementary vasopressor in refractory hypertensive, hypervolemic, hemodilutional therapy in subarachnoid hemorrhage. *Neurocrit Care* 2007;6(1):3–10.
24. Cuschieri J, Umanskiy K, Solomkin J. PKC-zeta is essential for endotoxin-induced macrophage activation. *J Surg Res* 2004;121(1):76–83.
25. Goldberg RJ, Gore JM, Alpert JS, et al. Cardiogenic shock after acute myocardial infarction. Incidence and mortality from a community-wide perspective, 1975–1988. *N Engl J Med* 1991;325(16):1117–1122.
26. Roberts N, Harrison DG, Reimer KA, et al. Right ventricular infarction with shock but without significant left ventricular infarction: a new clinical syndrome. *Am Heart J* 1985;110(5):1047–1053.
27. Russel JA. The current management of septic shock. *Minerva Med* 2008;99(5):431–458.
28. Darville T, Giroir B, Jacobs R. The systemic inflammatory response syndrome (SIRS): immunology and potential immunotherapy. *Infection* 1993;21(5):279–290.
29. Kollef MH. Broad-spectrum antimicrobials and the treatment of serious bacterial infections: getting it right up front. *Clin Infect Dis* 2008;47(suppl 1):S3–S13.
30. Goris RJ. Pathophysiology of shock in trauma. *Eur J Surg* 2000;166(2):100–111.
31. Nespoli A, Corso V, Mattarel D, et al. The management of shock and local injury in traumatic rhabdomyolysis. *Minerva Anestesiol* 1999;65(5):256–262.
32. Mansfield ND, Forni LG. Recently published papers: treating sepsis, measuring troponin and managing the obese. *Crit Care* 2005;9(6):535–537.
33. Annane D, Sebille V, Charpentier C, et al. Effect of treatment with low doses of hydrocortisone and fludrocortisone on mortality in patients with septic shock. *JAMA* 2002;288(7):862–871.
34. Sprung CL, Annane D, Keh D, et al. Hydrocortisone therapy for patients with septic shock. *N Engl J Med* 2008;358(2):111–124.
35. Lipiner-Friedman D, Sprung CL, Laterre PF, et al. Adrenal function in sepsis: the retrospective Corticus cohort study. *Crit Care Med* 2007;35(4):1012–1018.
36. Groeneveld AB, Molenaar N, Beishuizen B. Should we abandon corticosteroids during septic shock? No. *Curr Opin Crit Care* 2008;14(4):384–389.
37. Gann DS, Carlson DE, Byrnes GJ, et al. Impaired restitution of blood volume after large hemorrhage. *J Trauma* 1981;21(8):598–603.
38. Parker MM. Pathophysiology of cardiovascular dysfunction in septic shock. *New Horiz* 1998;6(2):130–138.
39. Peters J, Mack GW, Lister G. The importance of the peripheral circulation in critical illnesses. *Intensive Care Med* 2001;27(9):1446–1458.
40. Cuschieri J, Gourlay D, Garcia I, et al. Modulation of endotoxin-induced endothelial function by calcium/calmodulin-dependent protein kinase. *Shock* 2003;20(2):176–182.
41. Cuschieri J, Gourlay D, Garcia I, et al. Modulation of endotoxin-induced endothelial activity by microtubule depolymerization. *J Trauma* 2003;54(1):104–112; discussion 112–113.
42. Barie PS, Hydo LJ. Epidemiology of multiple organ dysfunction syndrome in critical surgical illness. *Surg Infect (Larchmt)* 2000;1(3):173–185; discussion 185–186.
43. Baue AE. MOF, MODS, and SIRS: what is in a name or an acronym? *Shock* 2006;26(5):438–449.
44. Bhatia M, Moochhala S. Role of inflammatory mediators in the pathophysiology of acute respiratory distress syndrome. *J Pathol* 2004;202(2):145–156.
45. Matsuda N, Hattori Y. Systemic inflammatory response syndrome (SIRS): molecular pathophysiology and gene therapy. *J Pharmacol Sci* 2006;101(3):189–198.
46. Winn RK, Ramamoorthy C, Vedder NB, et al. Leukocyte-endothelial cell interactions in ischemia-reperfusion injury. *Ann N Y Acad Sci* 1997;832:311–321.
47. Winn RK, Sharar SR, Vedder NB, et al. Leukocyte and endothelial adhesion molecules in ischaemia/reperfusion injuries. *Ciba Found Symp* 1995;189:63–71; discussion 72–76, 77–78.
48. Winn RK, Vedder NB, Mihelcic D, et al. The role of adhesion molecules in reperfusion injury. *Agents Actions Suppl* 1993;41:113–126.
49. Costa EL, Schettino IA, Schettino GP. The lung in sepsis: guilty or innocent? *Endocr Metab Immune Disord Drug Targets* 2006;6(2):213–216.
50. Goodman ER, Kleinstein E, Fusco AM, et al. Role of interleukin 8 in the genesis of acute respiratory distress syndrome through an effect on neutrophil apoptosis. *Arch Surg* 1998;133(11):1234–1239.
51. Papadakos PJ. Cytokines, genes, and ARDS. *Chest* 2002;121(5):1391–1392.
52. Ventilation with lower tidal volumes as compared with traditional tidal volumes for acute lung injury and the acute respiratory distress syndrome. The Acute Respiratory Distress Syndrome Network. *N Engl J Med* 2000;342(18):1301–1308.
53. Imahara SD, O'Keefe GE. Genetic determinants of the inflammatory response. *Curr Opin Crit Care* 2004;10(5):318–324.
54. O'Keefe GE, Hybki DL, Munford RS. The G–>A single nucleotide polymorphism at the -308 position in the tumor necrosis factor-alpha promoter increases the risk for severe sepsis after trauma. *J Trauma* 2002;52(5):817–825; discussion 825–826.
55. Rotstein OD. Modeling the two-hit hypothesis for evaluating strategies to prevent organ injury after shock/resuscitation. *J Trauma* 2003;54(suppl 5):S203–S206.
56. Cuschieri J, Maier RV. Oxidative stress, lipid rafts, and macrophage reprogramming. *Antioxid Redox Signal* 2007;9(9):1485–1497.
57. Sharma S, Kumar A. Septic shock, multiple organ failure, and acute respiratory distress syndrome. *Curr Opin Pulm Med* 2003;9(3):199–209.
58. Bernard GR, Ely EW, Wright TJ, et al. Safety and dose relationship of recombinant human activated protein C for coagulopathy in severe sepsis. *Crit Care Med* 2001;29(11):2051–2059.
59. Gentilello LM. Advances in the management of hypothermia. *Surg Clin North Am* 1995;75(2):243–256.
60. Gentilello LM, Jurkovich GJ, Stark MS, et al. Is hypothermia in the victim of major trauma protective or harmful? A randomized, prospective study. *Ann Surg* 1997;226(4):439–447; discussion 447–449.
61. Stoner HB. Studies on the mechanism of shock. The impairment of thermoregulation by trauma. *Br J Exp Pathol* 1969;50(2):125–138.
62. Gubler KD, Gentilello LM, Hassantash SA, et al. The impact of hypothermia on dilutional coagulopathy. *J Trauma* 1994;36(6):847–851.
63. Dutton RP, McCunn M, Hyder M, et al. Factor VIIa for correction of traumatic coagulopathy. *J Trauma* 2004;57(4):709–719.
64. Gunter OL Jr, Au BK, Isbell JM, et al. Optimizing outcomes in damage control resuscitation: identifying blood product ratios associated with improved survival. *J Trauma* 2008;65(3):527–534.
65. Kashuk JL, Moore EE, Johnson JL, et al. Postinjury life threatening coagulopathy: is 1:1 fresh frozen plasma:packed red blood cells the answer? *J Trauma* 2008;65(2):261–270; discussion 270–271.
66. Spinella PC, Perkins JG, Grathwohl KW, et al. Effect of plasma and red blood cell transfusions on survival in patients with combat related traumatic injuries. *J Trauma* 2008;64(suppl 2):S69–S77; discussion S77–S78.
67. Sperry JL, Ochoa JB, Gunn SR, et al. An FFP:PRBC transfusion ratio >/ = 1:1.5 is associated with a lower risk of mortality after massive transfusion. *J Trauma* 2008;65(5):986–993.

68. Ball CG, Kirkpatrick AW, McBeth P. The secondary abdominal compartment syndrome: not just another post-traumatic complication. *Can J Surg* 2008;51(5):399–405.
69. Bream-Rouwenhorst HR, Beltz EA, Ross MB, et al. Recent developments in the management of acute respiratory distress syndrome in adults. *Am J Health Syst Pharm* 2008;65(1):29–36.
70. Vidal MG, Ruiz Weisser J, Gonzalez F, et al. Incidence and clinical effects of intra-abdominal hypertension in critically ill patients. *Crit Care Med* 2008;36(6):1823–1831.
71. Canizaro PC, Prager MD, Shires GT. The infusion of Ringer's lactate solution during shock. Changes in lactate, excess lactate, and pH. *Am J Surg* 1971;122(4):494–501.
72. Alam HB, Stanton K, Koustova E, et al. Effect of different resuscitation strategies on neutrophil activation in a swine model of hemorrhagic shock. *Resuscitation* 2004;60(1):91–99.
73. Koustova E, Stanton K, Gushchin V, et al. Effects of lactated Ringer's solutions on human leukocytes. *J Trauma* 2002;52(5):872–878.
74. Deb S, Martin B, Sun L, et al. Resuscitation with lactated Ringer's solution in rats with hemorrhagic shock induces immediate apoptosis. *J Trauma* 1999;46(4):582–588; discussion 588–589.
75. Corso CO, Okamoto S, Ruttinger D, et al. Hypertonic saline dextran attenuates leukocyte accumulation in the liver after hemorrhagic shock and resuscitation. *J Trauma* 1999;46(3):417–423.
76. Ross AD, Angaran DM. Colloids vs. crystalloids—a continuing controversy. *Drug Intell Clin Pharm* 1984;18(3):202–212.
77. Waxman K, Holness R, Tominaga G, et al. Hemodynamic and oxygen transport effects of pentastarch in burn resuscitation. *Ann Surg* 1989; 209(3):341–345.
78. London MJ, Ho JS, Triedman JK, et al. A randomized clinical trial of 10% pentastarch (low molecular weight hydroxyethyl starch) versus 5% albumin for plasma volume expansion after cardiac operations. *J Thorac Cardiovasc Surg* 1989;97(5):785–797.
79. Velanovich V. Crystalloid versus colloid fluid resuscitation: a meta-analysis of mortality. *Surgery* 1989;105(1):65–71.
80. Bickell WH, Wall MJ Jr, Pepe PE, et al. Immediate versus delayed fluid resuscitation for hypotensive patients with penetrating torso injuries. *N Engl J Med* 1994;331(17):1105–1109.
81. Hebert PC. Transfusion requirements in critical care (TRICC): a multicentre, randomized, controlled clinical study. Transfusion Requirements in Critical Care Investigators and the Canadian Critical Care Trials Group. *Br J Anaesth* 1998;81(suppl 1):25–33.
82. Gervin AS, Fischer RP. Resuscitation of trauma patients with type-specific uncrossmatched blood. *J Trauma* 1984;24(4):327–331.
83. Boudreaux JP, Bornside GH, Cohn I Jr. Emergency autotransfusion: partial cleansing of bacteria-laden blood by cell washing. *J Trauma* 1983;23(1): 31–35.
84. Glover JL, Smith R, Yaw PB, et al. Autotransfusion of blood contaminated by intestinal contents. *JACEP* 1978;7(4):142–144.
85. Jurkovich GJ, Moore EE, Medina G. Autotransfusion in trauma. A pragmatic analysis. *Am J Surg* 1984;148(6):782–785.
86. Seligman R, Meisner M, Lisboa TC, et al. Decreases in procalcitonin and C-reactive protein are strong predictors of survival in ventilator-associated pneumonia. *Crit Care* 2006;10(5):R125.
87. Connors AF Jr, Speroff T, Dawson NV, et al. The effectiveness of right heart catheterization in the initial care of critically ill patients. SUPPORT Investigators. *JAMA* 1996;276(11):889–897.
88. Iberti TJ, Fischer EP, Leibowitz AB, et al. A multicenter study of physicians' knowledge of the pulmonary artery catheter. Pulmonary Artery Catheter Study Group. *JAMA* 1990;264(22):2928–2932.
89. Reynolds HN, Haupt MT, Thill-Baharozian MC, et al. Impact of critical care physician staffing on patients with septic shock in a university hospital medical intensive care unit. *JAMA* 1988;260(23):3446–3450.
90. Dhainaut JF, Yan SB, Margolis BD, et al. Drotrecogin alfa (activated) (recombinant human activated protein C) reduces host coagulopathy response in patients with severe sepsis. *Thromb Haemost* 2003;90(4):642–653.
91. Hopf HW. Molecular diagnostics of injury and repair responses in critical illness: what is the future of "monitoring" in the intensive care unit? *Crit Care Med* 2003;31(suppl 8):S518–S523.

CHAPTER 9 ■ CRITICAL CARE

AVERY B. NATHENS AND RONALD V. MAIER

KEY POINTS

1. Critical care units provide monitoring to identify and guide intervention prior to life-threatening physiologic deterioration and utilize advanced technology to support failing organs until treatment and recovery can occur.
2. Oxygen delivery to tissues must match cellular metabolic needs. To prevent cellular failure, adequate tissue oxygenation relies on oxygen-carrying capacity of blood (hemoglobin), loading of oxygen (gas exchange), and cardiac output (heart function).
3. When oxygen delivery is inappropriate to meet demand, fluid administration is often used to increase cardiac output through an increase in stroke volume. Conventional static indices of assessing fluid responsiveness are inferior to dynamic indices.
4. Respiratory dysfunction involves inadequate gas exchange, ventilation, or both. Oxygenation requires matching pulmonary perfusion to alveolar ventilation, whereas CO_2 excretion relies primarily only on ventilation. Ventilator support should be tailored to individual needs, and the ventilatory strategy may have a significant impact on outcome.
5. Excessive transfusion (hematocrit >21) has been shown to correlate with increased complications and mortality.
6. Full nutritional support (enteral route preferred) based on estimated needs should be provided as soon as possible. Carbohydrates should match metabolic needs to protect against excess nitrogen losses from protein breakdown. Essential fatty acids, vitamins, and mineral intake should recognize excessive losses in the critically ill.
7. Acute renal failure rarely occurs as an isolated organ failure. Dialysis is indicated for fluid overload, acidosis, electrolyte abnormalities, or coagulopathy. The choice of renal replacement therapy should be based on patient and institutional factors.
8. Multiple scores of critical illness have been developed to produce both an objective prognosis in the critically ill and an assessment of outcome by quantifying the severity of multiple organ failure.

ORGANIZATIONAL STRUCTURE OF THE INTENSIVE CARE UNIT

A significant proportion of patients under the care of surgeons receive some form of critical care during their hospital stay. The exposure to the intensive care unit (ICU) may take one of several forms, ranging from routine postoperative monitoring in the high-risk surgical patient to the management of life-threatening postoperative complications. Additionally, many patients experience significant physiologic derangements due to their surgical illness (e.g., trauma, peritonitis) such that they require ICU care.

The ICU environment is conducive to the support of acute life-threatening organ dysfunction including the provision of mechanical ventilation, renal replacement therapy, and invasive cardiac monitoring. These services require specific equipment and nursing expertise not found in or available throughout the hospital setting. As a result of these requirements, the ICU is typically spatially separated from the acute care beds in most hospitals. This spatial separation leads to one of two possibilities for the provision of medical care by physicians. The surgeon responsible for the care of the patient's underlying disease may assume primary responsibility for the provision of critical care services. This approach is in keeping with the ethical standards of the American College of Surgeons under which surgeons are responsible for the postoperative care of their patients. In this context, the ICU is simply a location where advanced monitoring and organ support are available. The surgeon continues with clinical responsibilities outside the ICU while also caring for critically ill patients. This organizational approach is typically referred to as an "open" ICU.[1] Alternatively, the surgeon may relinquish care of the patient to an intensivist who ideally may be specifically trained in the care of the critically ill patient and certified by one of several medical specialty boards including internal medicine, anesthesiology, or surgery. In this context, the intensivist has no other responsibilities outside the ICU that would limit his or her immediate accessibility and is primarily available to the critically ill patient. This organizational approach is often referred to as a "closed" ICU or an intensivist-model ICU.[1]

The argument for maintaining the involvement of the operating surgeon as the primary physician responsible for the direction of critical care services is to ensure that there is continuity of care. Putatively, this continuity of care results in a well-defined, cohesive management plan that is necessary to ensure optimal outcomes. However, in a retrospective analysis of the effect of conversion from an open to a closed surgical ICU in a tertiary care academic center, complications and mortality were lower and the use of consultants was less frequent when patients were primarily cared for by surgeons or anesthesiologists who were board certified in critical care.[2] In another report in a similar surgical ICU setting, two different concurrent care models were compared. One group was managed exclusively by the critical care attending service and the other by the general surgery faculty and house staff. Despite increased severity of illness, the critical care cohort had a shorter ICU length of stay, fewer days of mechanical ventilation, fewer consultations, fewer complications, and lower hospital charges.[3] Last, in a large observational study, Pronovost et al.[4] evaluated outcomes following abdominal aortic surgery in the state of Maryland. This cohort of patients was well chosen because these individuals are at high risk of postoperative complications both related to the operative intervention and from significant comorbidity. These investigators demonstrated that daily rounds by a dedicated intensivist were associated with a significant reduction in the risk of postoperative complications and death.

Taken together, these data and a recent systematic review suggest that critically ill patients are best cared for by intensivists, but not at the total exclusion of the operating surgeon from decision making.[5] For surgical patients, this argues for the continued training and involvement of surgeons in the field for optimal critical care. In the absence of a surgical intensivist, the most recent recommendations from the American College of Critical Care Medicine are that the intensivist and the surgeon proactively collaborate closely in the ongoing care of the patients.[6]

PURPOSES OF THE INTENSIVE CARE UNIT

1 The ICU serves several purposes. First, the availability of both electronic physiologic monitors and a high nurse-to-patient ratio (typically 1:1 or 1:2) provides an opportunity for very early detection of a critical change in status of the patient. This change might relate to postoperative bleeding, the development of a neurologic deficit after craniotomy or spinal surgery (or injury to the brain or spinal cord), or changes in the patients' cardiorespiratory status. Common to all of these scenarios is a high likelihood of a need for urgent intervention. In this context, the ICU serves the purpose of monitoring to both identify and prevent adverse consequences in a patient at great risk.

The more familiar role of the ICU is an environment with all the resources available to support an acute deterioration of vital organ function. Approximately one third of all hospital costs are spent in the ICU environment, and with the exception of very specific clinical scenarios, most interventions studied appear to be cost-effective.[7,8] To ensure optimal outcomes and efficiency, it is critical that the physician understands the physiology of organ dysfunction, the tools he or she has available for their monitoring and support, their limitations, and who most likely will benefit. Without this understanding, the physicians with the extensive resources available in the ICU have the potential to inflict great harm. The most frequent challenges in the critical care environment are the support of the failing cardiovascular system, lungs, and kidneys. During this period of support, the patient must receive adequate nutritional support until the acute physiologic derangements have normalized. The focus of this chapter is on these aspects of critical care, followed by a discussion of prognostic scoring systems and ethics in the ICU.

ASSESSMENT AND MANAGEMENT OF THE FAILING CARDIOVASCULAR SYSTEM

2 Support of the failing cardiovascular system is geared toward achieving adequate tissue oxygen delivery, which amounts to ensuring tissue oxygen delivery meets demand. Under normal conditions, oxygen consumption ($\dot{V}O_2$) is normally 100 to 120 mL/m^2 per minute, or 200 mL/min for a typical adult. The critically ill surgical patient experiences a profound increase in $\dot{V}O_2$ induced by high circulating levels of catecholamines and inflammatory mediators. Inadequate levels of tissue oxygen delivery in the face of either normal or increased levels of $\dot{V}O_2$ result in anaerobic tissue metabolism and are reflected clinically as a state of shock (i.e., cellular dysfunction). Currently, we have little control over tissue oxygen consumption, save for avoiding or treating hyperthermia and pharmacologic paralysis.

Oxygen Delivery

Many interventions in the ICU focus on manipulating tissue oxygen delivery ($\dot{D}O_2$) to meet either normal or elevated levels of tissue $\dot{V}O_2$. The amount of O_2 that is delivered to peripheral tissues is the product of the O_2 content in arterial blood (CaO_2) and the cardiac output. Normally, CaO_2 is about 20 mL/dL and the normal cardiac index (CI) is 3.2 L/m^2 per minute, or 5 L/min for a typical adult. Therefore, the normal systemic delivery of O_2 ($\dot{D}O_2$) is 20 mL/dL $\times$ 50 dL/min, or 1,000 mL/min. Although the O_2 content is the most important measure of O_2 in blood, it is the partial pressure of oxygen (PO_2) and the oxyhemoglobin saturation that are more commonly measured in the ICU. Each gram of hemoglobin (Hgb) can bind 1.36 mL of O_2. If the Hgb level of the blood is normal (15 g/dL) and the Hgb is 98% saturated, the amount of O_2 bound to Hgb is 19.9 mL/dL. In addition, a small amount of O_2 is physically dissolved in the water that makes up plasma and red blood cells. The solubility coefficient for O_2 is 0.0031 mL/mm Hg per deciliter; therefore, the amount of O_2 dissolved in 1 dL of blood at a PaO_2 of 100 mm Hg is 0.3 mL, so that the O_2 content of normal arterial blood is 19.9 + 0.3 or 20.2 mL/dL, conveniently rounded off to 20 mL/dL. Through the same arithmetic, the O_2 content of venous blood (CvO_2), which is 80%

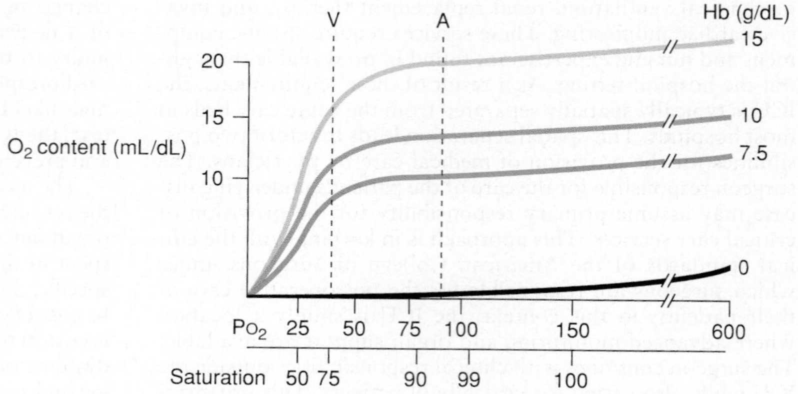

FIGURE 9.1. The relation of O_2 content, saturation, and PO_2. Typical normal levels in arterial and venous blood are defined at various levels of hemoglobin. (After Bartlett RH. *University of Michigan Critical Care Handbook*. Boston, MA: Little, Brown; 1996.)

saturated, is 16 mL/dL; hence, the normal arteriovenous difference in O_2 content (avO_2 difference) is 4 mL/dL. Expressed mathematically:

$$\dot{D}O_2 = CI \times CaO_2$$

where: $CaO_2 = 1.36 \times Hsb + 0.0031 \times PaO_2$ CI = stroke volume × heart rate and, therefore,

$$\dot{V}O_2 = CI \times (CaO_2 - CvO_2)$$

The relation among PO_2, saturation, and O_2 content for different concentrations of Hgb is shown in Figure 9.1. Note that the arterial partial pressure of oxygen (PaO_2) and saturations are the same as for normal arterial and venous blood due to an increase in CI, even though the O_2 content is severely decreased in anemia.

Relationship Between Oxygen Supply and Demand

Shock states are characterized by limitations in $\dot{D}O_2$ leading to a mismatch of oxygen supply and demand. For example, hemorrhagic shock leads to a reduction in preload (thus affecting stroke volume and CI) and a reduction in $\dot{D}O_2$, which is further decreased by the drop in CaO_2 due to loss of Hgb. The end result of this limitation in $\dot{D}O_2$ is tissue hypoxia, which is thought to play a causal role in the development of multiple organ failure. When $\dot{D}O_2$ falls below the level of $\dot{V}O_2$, $\dot{V}O_2$ becomes supply dependent and a state of anaerobic metabolism occurs.

The relation between $\dot{D}O_2$ and $\dot{V}O_2$ is reflected in the amount of O_2 in venous blood. Under normal conditions the amount of O_2 extracted is 20% of that delivered, with 80% of the O_2 still present in venous blood returning to the heart. This latter parameter, referred to as mixed venous oxygen saturation (SvO_2), is typically in the range of 70% to 80% and must be obtained from blood in either the right ventricle or pulmonary artery to allow mixing of superior vena caval, inferior vena caval, and coronary sinus blood as the relative rates of extraction in organs served by these circulations differ. In the critical care setting, SvO_2 is typically obtained from a pulmonary artery catheter (PAC) and can be monitored continuously using oximetric probes at the tip of the catheter. Reductions in SvO_2 are indicative of a mismatch between supply and demand. If $\dot{V}O_2$ increases with no further increase in delivery, then the percent of oxygen extraction must increase, resulting in a drop in SvO_2. More frequently, SvO_2 is affected by changes in $\dot{D}O_2$. Relatively small reductions in CI, arterial blood oxygen saturation (SaO_2), or Hgb concentrations can result in a significant drop in SvO_2. In the context of a very dynamic clinical situation with multiple perturbations occurring concurrently, continuous measurement of SvO_2 provides a good estimate of the net effect of any intervention on the balance between oxygen supply and demand.

In critically ill patients, $\dot{V}O_2$ is most frequently elevated compared to that seen during the normal state. $\dot{V}O_2$ is elevated in proportion to the degree of inflammation (either bacterial or sterile, as in burns and pancreatitis). A febrile patient with significant signs of sepsis typically has a $\dot{V}O_2$ that is 1.5 to 2 times normal. It is unusual for the $\dot{V}O_2$ of a critically ill patient to be more than twice normal. This occurs only in situations of severe muscular activity, as in seizures or tetany.

During this state of elevated tissue $\dot{V}O_2$, the normal response is a proportional increase in $\dot{D}O_2$; thus, it is normal for a hypermetabolic patient to have a high cardiac output and pulse rate, referred to as a hyperdynamic state. Not infrequently, patients cannot mount an increased $\dot{D}O_2$ in response to an increased $\dot{V}O_2$ because of any combination of hypoxia, anemia, and myocardial dysfunction. If this occurs, the amount of O_2 extracted from each deciliter of blood increases, reflected as a drop in SvO_2.

Hemodynamic Assessment

Given the importance of adequate oxygen delivery, it is evident that a tremendous amount of effort among intensivists is geared toward optimizing delivery. There are three important parameters that can be modified to affect systemic oxygen delivery: CI, Hgb, and hemoglobin saturation (SaO_2). While Hgb and SaO_2 are readily measured and manipulated, it is the monitoring (and subsequent manipulation) of CI that is most challenging. The cardiac output is a product of the stroke volume and heart rate. Most efforts at meeting tissue oxygen demands are directed toward increasing $\dot{D}O_2$ through an effect on stroke volume. Thus, the available tools in the critical care environment are geared toward understanding how stroke volume can best be manipulated to improve $\dot{D}O_2$.

3 The most common intervention to improve $\dot{D}O_2$ to reverse the shock state is through the administration of intravenous fluids. The sole reason for administering fluids is to increase the stroke volume. When fluids are administered, it is with the belief that the patient is on the steep part of the Starling curve and thus has preload-recruitable cardiac output (Fig. 9.2). In the ICU environment, there are two broad classifications of measures used to assess whether the administration of fluids will increase stroke volume (and thus cardiac output) (Table 9.1). While more frequently used, static indices of fluid responsiveness are generally less accurate than dynamic indices.

Static Indices of Fluid Responsiveness. Right atrial pressures as assessed through a central venous catheter are probably most frequently used as a measure of fluid responsiveness. It is generally believed that a low central venous pressure (CVP, reflecting a low right ventricular end-diastolic volume) reflects a low intravascular volume. It follows then that the administration of fluids in the context of a low CVP

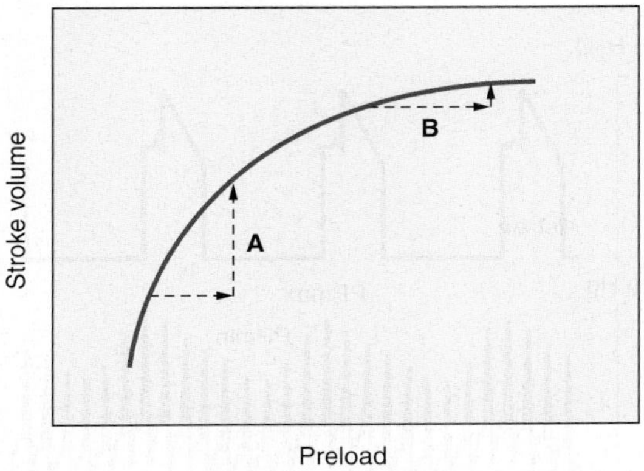

FIGURE 9.2. The concept of preload-recruitable stroke volume is demonstrated. If the ventricle is on the steep part of the Starling curve (**A**), then a given increase in preload will lead to a significant increase in stroke volume. By contrast, on the flatter part of the curve (**B**), the stroke volume increases marginally if at all with the same increase in preload. Dynamic indices of preload-recruitable stroke volume are more accurate than static indices in identifying where on this curve the patient is at any point in time.

should increase stroke volume. However, a number of studies have demonstrated that the CVP is a poor marker of fluid responsiveness.[9–11] In fact, it appears to be no more reliable than flipping a coin. Additionally, while many advocate that the change in CVP in response to a volume challenge might indicate fluid responsiveness, this index can also be unreliable. Thus, central venous catheters primarily serve the purpose of providing intravenous access. An oximetric central venous catheter has the additional advantage of providing the oxygen saturation level of blood in the superior vena cava. While this value overestimates mixed venous oxygen saturation, it might provide a useful parameter to evaluate the response to interventions as it trends well with the SvO_2.[12,13]

Other frequently measured static indices of fluid responsiveness are those measured through the use of the pulmonary artery catheter. The balloon-tip flow-directed pulmonary artery (or Swan-Ganz) catheter is inserted into the central venous system and is passed through the right heart and rests in the pulmonary artery where it provides continuous monitoring of pulmonary artery pressures. The catheter has more proximal ports such that central venous pressure is also monitored. Using the thermal dilution method, the catheter also provides information regarding CI. More recent modifications of the PAC have resulted in the capability of continuous measurement of cardiac output, SvO_2, and right ventricular end-diastolic volume. When the balloon is inflated, the catheter advances slightly and wedges into a small pulmonary artery branch. This pulmonary capillary wedge pressure (PCWP) provides an estimate of left ventricular end-diastolic pressure (LVEDP). The assumption is that a static, nonflowing column of blood that extends from the catheter's lumen to the pulmonary arterioles, capillaries, and veins of that lung segment provides a measure of the pressure downstream from the catheter tip ending in the left ventricle. Barring circumstances described later, LVEDP thus tracks left ventricular end-diastolic volume (LVEDV). LVEDV represents the volume of the left ventricle (i.e., myocardial stretch, or preload) that we aim to affect through increases in intravascular volume. If all assumptions are met, a patient with a low PCWP (and hence low LVEDV) should improve his or her stroke volume and thus his or her cardiac output with fluid administration. By contrast, if the PCWP is high, then cardiac output can only be improved through an increase in contractility or a reduction in afterload.

TABLE 9.1

INDICES TO EVALUATE FLUID RESPONSIVENESS IN MECHANICALLY VENTILATED PATIENTS

■ STATIC INDICES	■ DYNAMIC INDICES
Right atrial pressure (measured as central venous pressure)	Systolic pressure variation
Pulmonary capillary wedge pressure	Pulse pressure variation
Right ventricular end-diastolic volume index	Aortic blood velocity[a]

[a]Evaluable using Doppler echocardiography.

When the PCWP is used to guide administration of fluids, it is important to understand that several of the assumptions whereby PCWP tracks LVEDV might be violated. The ability to derive information regarding a volume (LVEDV) from a pressure (PCWP) first assumes that the myocardial compliance is normal. However, myocardial compliance is often affected by ischemia, massive volume resuscitation, high intra-abdominal or intrathoracic (e.g., high levels of positive end-expiratory pressure [PEEP]) pressures, or long-standing hypertension. Focusing on the PCWP to guide therapy in these circumstances will lead to an overestimate of preload. Mitral stenosis will also increase the PCWP, while LVEDV might be low. Not realizing the importance of these assumptions and how they might be violated often leads to incorrect treatment strategies.

Many have advocated the use of the right ventricular end-diastolic volume index (RVEDVI), a measure of right ventricular filling, as a better measure to assess for adequate preload and fluid responsiveness.[14] However, the relationship between volume responsiveness and either the PCWP or the RVEDVI is very complex, and many recent studies suggest these may not be optimal indices to guide fluid management.[9,10,15,16] Thus, the most reliable actionable information gleaned from the use of the PAC is limited to that assessed through measurement of the SvO_2 and from the CI.

The PAC is merely a monitoring device; thus, any benefit derived from its use will depend on the therapeutic strategies implemented following collection of various hemodynamic parameters. Despite the conceptual appeal of invasive hemodynamic monitoring and the information it provides, there are no data suggesting that the use of a PAC offers survival benefit.[17,18] In several studies, the PAC has been associated with harm, including increased resource utilization, mortality, higher rates of renal failure, thrombocytopenia, and thromboembolic events.[19,20] Given these data, it is important to realize that the PAC offers no clear significant benefit in the resuscitation of all critically ill patients. If there are specific subgroups that benefit, they have not yet been clearly identified in either retrospective or prospective studies. As a result of these findings, the use of the PAC by intensivists has dramatically declined.[21]

Dynamic Indices of Fluid Responsiveness. Dynamic assessments of fluid responsiveness are based on cyclical changes in systolic pressure, pulse pressure, and stroke volume in response to cardiorespiratory interactions.[22] The increase in pleural pressure during a positive-pressure breath during inspiration reduces right ventricular preload and leads to a reduction in right ventricular stroke volume. The reduction in right ventricular stroke volume leads to a decrease in left ventricular filling after two to three heartbeats, a reflection of the pulmonary transit time (Fig. 9.3). This reduction in left ventricular filling then manifests as a reduction in left ventricular stroke volume, which is at its minimum during expiration.

These changes in stroke volume are more pronounced in the presence of hypovolemia, and this finding has been used to advantage to identify patients who might be fluid responsive.

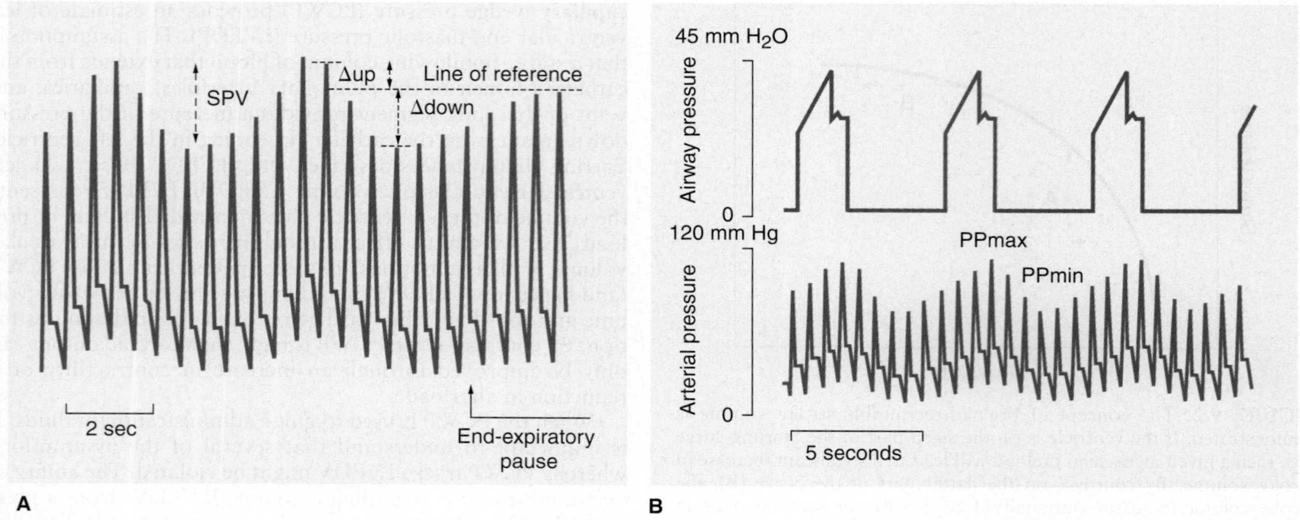

FIGURE 9.3. Demonstration of cyclic systolic (**A**) and pulse pressure variation (**B**) during the respiratory cycle of a mechanically ventilated patient. Systolic pressure variation (A) is demonstrated along with the reference line and end inspiration, from which Δdown can be determined. Pulse pressure variation is demonstrated in B. The pulse pressure is greatest at the end of the inspiratory period and at least several beats later (during the expiratory period). (From Michard F, Teboul JL. Using heart-lung interactions to assess fluid responsiveness during mechanical ventilation. *Crit Care* 2000;4:282–289, with permission.)

Systolic pressure variation (SPV) is the difference between maximal and minimal values of systolic blood pressure during one positive-pressure mechanical breath (Fig. 9.3). SPV is divided into two components: Δup and Δdown. ΔUp is the difference between the maximal value of systolic pressure over a single respiratory cycle and the reference systolic pressure. ΔDown is the difference between the reference systolic pressure and the minimal value of systolic pressure over a single respiratory cycle. In either case the reference systolic pressure is that pressure measured during an end-expiratory pause. SPV greater than 11% or Δdown greater than 5 mm Hg has been most strongly associated with fluid responsiveness.[23]

Pulse pressure variation has also been used as a dynamic index of fluid responsiveness and is directly proportional to left ventricular stroke volume (Fig. 9.3). Pulse pressure variation is measured as follows:

$$\Delta PP\ (\%) = 100 \times \frac{(PPmax - PPmin)}{(PPmax + PPmin)/2}$$

PPmax and PPmin are the maximal and minimal values of pulse pressure over a single respiratory cycle, respectively. Thus, ΔPP is simply the difference between PPmax and PPmin divided by the mean of the two values. A ΔPP (%) of greater than 13% is associated with fluid responsiveness and is believed to be more accurate than SPV.[9,15,22]

One additional means of evaluating fluid responsiveness using Doppler echocardiography has been described. Echocardiography can be used to estimate aortic blood velocity, which is a good measure of left ventricular stroke volume. Respiratory variation in aortic blood velocity has been shown to be an accurate measure of fluid responsiveness, yet is more invasive than other approaches due to the need for an esophageal Doppler probe.[24]

New Modalities for Cardiac Output Measurement

The difficulties in using the PAC along with the questions regarding their safety has been the impetus for the development of several less invasive means of monitoring cardiac output. Esophageal probes, placed in a similar fashion to a nasogastric tube, measure blood flow velocity in the descending aorta by means of a Doppler transducer. The measured parameter is the aortic velocity waveform, which is converted to stroke volume using a standardized algorithm. An accurate velocity measurement requires good alignment between the Doppler beam and blood flow. In general, the agreement between cardiac output obtained by means of the thermodilution technique and that obtained through measurement of the aortic velocity waveform appears to be acceptable, but challenging.[25]

Pulse contour analysis has also been investigated as a means to continuously monitor cardiac output. Pulse contour–derived cardiac output (PCCO) methods use the arterial pressure waveform as an input for a model of the systemic circulation to predict instantaneous flow. The pressure waveform is obtained from a peripheral arterial line (radial or femoral), which requires assumptions regarding the changes in pulse shape between these different locations. The values attributed to model parameters (e.g., arterial resistance and compliance) are initially estimated according to the patient's sex and age and from the pressure waveform. They are then refined following a calibration of mean cardiac output using an indicator technique (e.g., transpulmonary thermodilution or lithium chloride dilution). While there is good agreement between the cardiac output measured by thermodilution and that determined by pulse contour analysis, this technology has its limitations. PCCO appears to be inaccurate in the absence of sinus rhythm or in cases where the hemodynamic changes are occurring rapidly, as one might anticipate with hemorrhage or septic shock.[26–28] Presumably, alterations in vasomotor tone affect the pulse contour to the extent that the algorithms begin to fail.

SUPPORT OF THE FAILING RESPIRATORY SYSTEM

Impending or established respiratory failure is a common reason for admission of surgical patients to the ICU. However, it is important to recognize that not all patients requiring an airway (endotracheal or nasotracheal intubation) and mechanical ventilatory support have respiratory failure. There are a large proportion of patients who have airway instability requiring endotracheal intubation (postoperative patients, traumatic brain injury, intoxication) but whose need for mechanical ventilatory support is relatively limited. By contrast, patients with respiratory failure due to acute respiratory distress syndrome (ARDS), trauma, cardiogenic pulmonary edema, exacerbation of chronic obstructive pulmonary disease, or other less common etiologies require a mechanical ventilator to support gas exchange.

Pulmonary Gas Exchange

By gas exchange, we mean the process by which oxygen is taken up by the pulmonary capillaries from the alveolus and CO_2 ultimately excreted in each expired breath. These two processes—oxygen uptake and CO_2 excretion—are regulated by different mechanisms and have to be managed with these differences in mind.

Oxygen Uptake. Gas transfer in the lung and the causes of hypoxemia are demonstrated in Figure 9.4. Under normal conditions, red blood cells in the pulmonary capillaries become fully saturated and O_2 dissolves in the plasma; the result is a blood PO_2 of 100 mm Hg (when equilibrium is reached at the end of a resting expiration) and a saturation of 100% (alveolus *A* in Fig. 9.4). This equilibration may be disturbed by hypoventilation in relation to perfusion, or V/Q mismatch (alveolus *B* in Fig. 9.4); diffusion block caused by interstitial fibrosis or edema (alveolus C in Fig. 9.4); or perfusion of nonventilated alveoli (shunt), which is simply the extreme of hypoventilation (alveolus *D* in Fig. 9.4). Diffusion block and V/Q mismatch can usually be overcome by breathing 100% O_2; thus, persistent hypoxemia during exposure to high alveolar Po_2 is caused by total V/Q mismatch, called *transpulmonary shunting* or *venous admixture*. Under normal conditions, about 5% of the blood entering the left atrium has been shunted away from the pulmonary capillaries and oxygenation, either as a result of bronchial nutritive blood flow or through thebesian veins opening directly into the left side of the heart. This phenomenon, combined with the normal minor V/Q mismatch associated with shallow breathing at rest and positional effects on pulmonary blood flow, results in a normal arterial PO_2 of 90 to 100 mm Hg and a normal SaO_2 of 98%. The extent to which various degrees of transpulmonary shunting affect arterial oxygenation is shown in Figure 9.5. The shunt fraction is actually calculated by assuming that the blood in capillaries in those alveolar units that are functioning normally is fully saturated and oxygenated. In addition, it is assumed that the blood passing through areas of transpulmonary shunt is identical to venous blood. With these assumptions, the fraction of blood passing through the shunt can be calculated as the O_2 content of blood leaving the capillaries of normal alveoli minus the O_2 content of arterial blood divided by the O_2 content of blood leaving normal alveoli minus the O_2 content of venous blood.

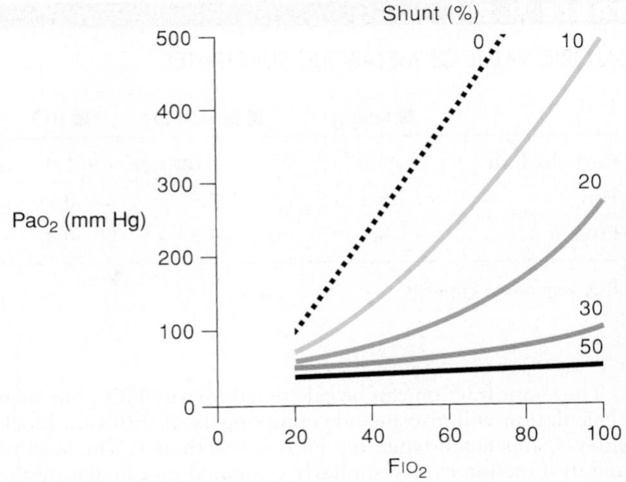

FIGURE 9.5. The PaO_2 values achieved at variable levels of FiO_2 and variable levels of shunt. These calculations assume normal hemoglobin and a venous saturation of 75%. (After Bartlett RH. *University of Michigan Critical Care Handbook*. Boston, MA: Little, Brown; 1996.)

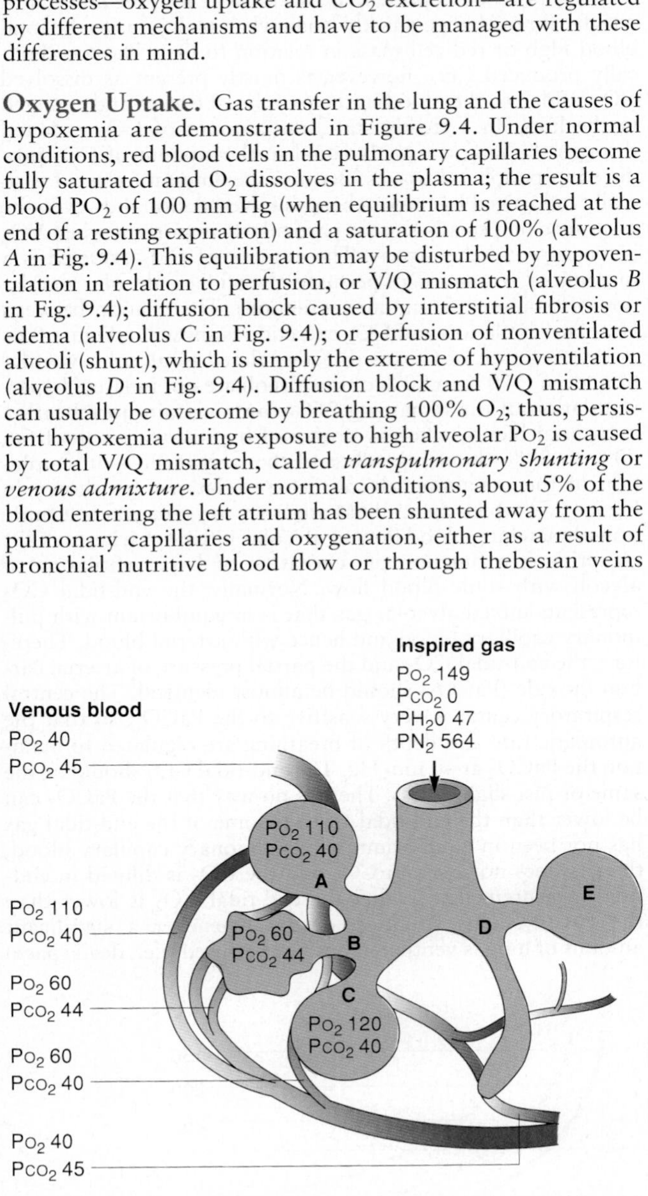

FIGURE 9.4. Variables affecting pulmonary gas exchange while air is breathed. In alveolus *A*, blood flow and ventilation are equal and normal. The values in the alveolus and the exiting blood represent the end of a normal resting exhalation. Alveolus *B* represents hypoventilation. Alveolus C represents diffusion block. Alveolus *D* represents collapse or transpulmonary shunt. Alveolus *E* is ventilated without blood flow. (After Bartlett RH. Posttraumatic pulmonary insufficiency. In: Cooper P, Nyhus L, eds. *Surgery Annual, 1971*. New York: Appleton-Century-Crofts; 1971.)

Obviously, the effect of the O_2 content of venous blood in the shunt calculation is considerable; when O_2 delivery is decreased because of low cardiac output or a low Hgb concentration, the venous saturation falls and the shunt fraction is increased. It is not generally appreciated that the reductions in mixed venous oxygen saturation as a result of inadequate cardiac output or severe anemia might lead to profound hypoxemia refractory to increases in the fraction of inspired oxygen (FiO_2). This effect occurs only in the presence of some degree of intrapulmonary shunting and is not evident in patients with normal lungs. For example, if one assumes there is some degree of shunt due to atelectasis, blood perfusing the atelectatic lung mixes with blood perfusing the more normal lung, so that overall pulmonary venous oxygen content is significantly lowered. Increasing the inspired O_2 to 100% may result in a large increase in PO_2 in the blood leaving the normal lung but little increase in arterial oxygen saturation because the pulmonary venous blood from normal alveoli was already maximally saturated. The large increase in PO_2 is associated with a small increase in O_2 *content* because the O_2 that raises the PO_2 (e.g., from 100 to 500 mm Hg) does increase the small amount dissolved in plasma. However, the oxygenation of the arterial blood is an average of the O_2 content of blood from the two areas of lung, not an average of the PO_2. Therefore, systemic hypoxia persists regardless of the FiO_2. This physiology should be kept in mind—at times improvements in arterial oxygen saturation may only be gained through increasing O_2 by improving CI or Hgb concentration, both of which would serve to increase the mixed venous oxygen saturation.

TABLE 9.2

CALORIC VALUE OF METABOLIC SUBSTRATES

	■ kcal/g	■ kcal/L O_2	■ RQ
Carbohydrate	4.0	5.0	1.0
Fat	9.5	4.7	0.7
Protein	4.8	4.5	0.8

RQ, respiratory quotient.

The shunt fraction can be calculated for any FiO_2, but such a calculation will also include components of diffusion block and V/Q mismatch when the FiO_2 is less than 1. The level of lung dysfunction can be similarly estimated by calculating the alveolar–arterial (Aa) gradient for O_2 or the PaO_2 divided by the FiO_2. The Aa gradient is calculated as follows:

$$AaO_2 \text{ gradient} = (P_B - P_{H_2O}) \times FiO_2 - PaCO_2/R - PaO_2$$

where P_B = barometric pressure (~60 mm Hg at sea level), P_{H_2O} = 47 mm Hg at 37°C, and R = respiratory quotient (usually 0.8), and the alveolar PCO_2 is identical to the arterial PCO_2.

With these assumptions, the normal Aa gradient is about 10 mm Hg, and an Aa gradient above 500 mm Hg corresponds to about 30% transpulmonary shunt. Dividing the PaO_2 by the FiO_2 is simply a shortened method to characterize the Aa gradient without all the calculations. The normal value is 500, and a value of 100 corresponds to a 30% shunt.

Finally, interruption of the blood flow to alveoli has no effect on oxygenation, except for the diversion of blood flow to all the other areas of lung (alveolus *E* in Fig. 9.4). If the remainder of the lung is basically normal, then occlusion of the pulmonary arteries should have no effect on oxygenation. Patients with pulmonary embolism can become hypoxic, however, because (a) blood flow must increase through areas of V/Q mismatch and shunting, (b) right atrial pressure increases to the point at which right-to-left shunting occurs through a patent foramen ovale, or (c) the residence time of red blood cells in pulmonary capillaries becomes so short that the time for oxygenation is inadequate. Of these causes, the latter can be largely corrected with supplemental O_2, which raises the gradient for O_2 diffusion in the pulmonary capillaries. Thus, response to supplemental O_2 can aid in discriminating an obstructive process (e.g., pulmonary embolism) from a diffuse injury and increased shunt (e.g., ARDS).

Excretion of CO_2. The rate of alveolar ventilation is the principal parameter affecting the excretion of CO_2. This differs from oxygen uptake because CO_2 is much more diffusible than O_2 and a large amount of CO_2 is excreted during a short period of hyperventilation.

The total amount of CO_2 produced by systemic metabolism is roughly equivalent to the amount of O_2 consumed (100 to 120 mL/m^2 per minute, or 200 mL per minute in a typical adult). The ratio between CO_2 produced and O_2 consumed is referred to as the *respiratory quotient* (RQ) and varies slightly depending on whether carbohydrate or fat is being metabolized, with a normal value being 0.8. An RQ of 1 or greater suggests that the principal nutrient being metabolized is carbohydrate, whereas an RQ of 0.7 indicates that primarily lipids are being utilized (Table 9.2).

The production of CO_2 is increased or decreased by each of the factors that cause an increase or decrease in $\dot{V}O_2$. Most of the CO_2 in blood is present as bicarbonate ion, the amount of which cannot change quickly (somewhat analogous to the total blood Hgb or red cell mass in relation to O_2). The metabolically produced CO_2, however, is mostly present as dissolved CO_2, added to the blood in the peripheral tissues and excreted in the lung. In a steady state, the amount of CO_2 excreted through the lung is exactly equal to the amount of CO_2 produced in peripheral tissues. Because the amount excreted is so easily influenced by minor changes in ventilation, however, the assurance of a steady state is particularly important when $\dot{V}O_2$ is measured at the airway. The amount of CO_2 excreted is a function of ventilation of perfused alveoli (i.e., alveolar ventilation per minute, or minute ventilation). The relation between alveolar ventilation and CO_2 excretion is shown in Figure 9.6.

As excretion of CO_2 is directly related to alveolar ventilation, even if 70% to 80% of the alveoli are not inflated, hyperventilation of the remaining 25% can maintain normocarbia in arterial blood, whereas profound hypoxemia results from 70% to 80% shunt regardless of the level of FiO_2 or ventilation of the remaining alveoli. These relations are shown in Figure 9.7, which again illustrates that oxygenation is a function of matching blood flow to alveolar inflation, whereas CO_2 excretion is a function of ventilation or hyperventilation of alveoli with some blood flow. Normally, the end-tidal CO_2 represents mixed alveolar gas that is in equilibrium with pulmonary capillary blood and hence with arterial blood. Therefore, the end-tidal CO_2 and the partial pressure of arterial carbon dioxide ($PaCO_2$) should be almost identical. The central respiratory center is very sensitive to the $PaCO_2$, so that the automatic rate and depth of breathing are regulated to maintain the $PaCO_2$ at 40 mm Hg. The end-tidal CO_2 should be the same or just slightly less. There is no way that the $PaCO_2$ can be lower than the end-tidal CO_2. If some of the end-tidal gas has not been in equilibrium with pulmonary capillary blood, the gas does not contain CO_2 and the CO_2 is diluted in end-tidal measurements, so that the end-tidal CO_2 is lower than the $PaCO_2$. This situation occurs whenever a significant amount of lung is ventilated but not perfused (i.e., dead space)

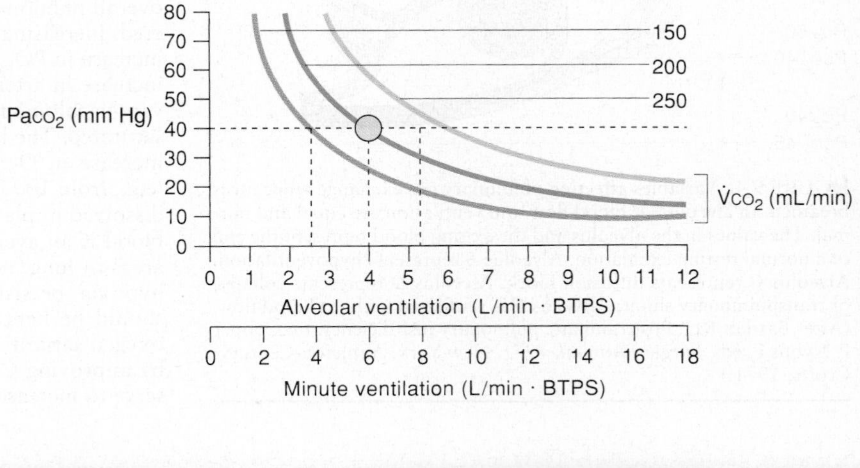

FIGURE 9.6. Alveolar ventilation required to excrete different levels of metabolically produced CO_2. (Adapted from Nunn JF. *Applied Respiratory Physiology.* London: Butterworth-Heineman; 1969;2:9.)

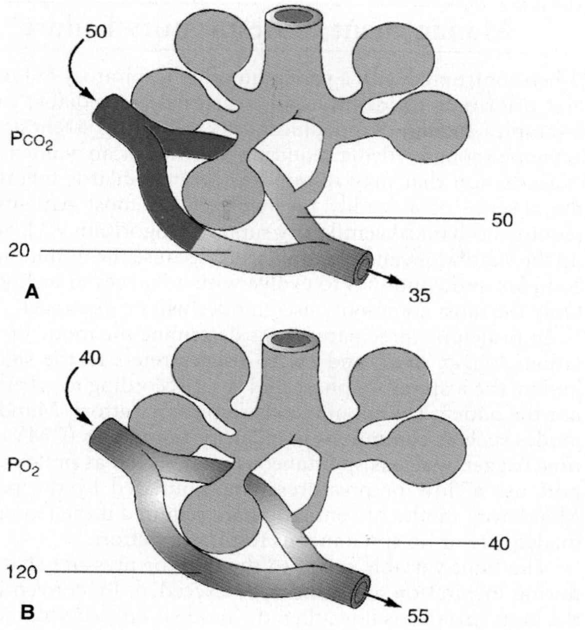

FIGURE 9.7. The effects of collapsed alveoli (transpulmonary shunt) on the exchange of O_2 and CO_2 in the lung. **A:** Exchange of CO_2 is limited by ventilation of perfused lung. **B:** Exchange of O_2 is limited by blood uptake of O_2 in ventilated lung. (After Bartlett RH. Pulmonary pathophysiology in surgical patients. *Surg Clin North Am* 1980;60:1323.)

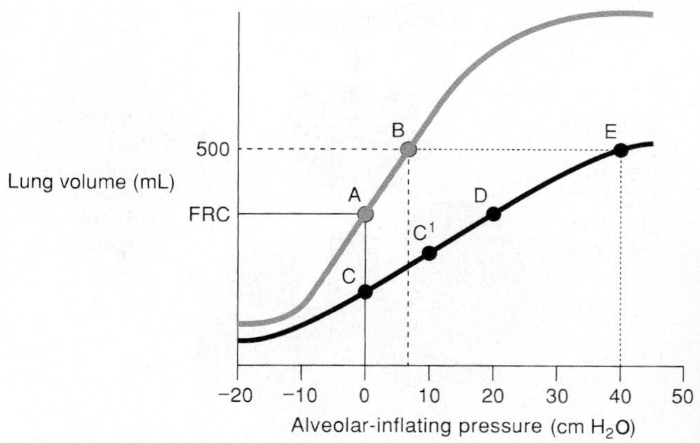

FIGURE 9.8. Volume–pressure (compliance) curves representing a normal lung (*A* and *B*) and an atelectatic or edematous lung (*C* through *E*). The functional reserve capacity is decreased (*A* to *C*), and more pressure is required for inflation (*C* to *E*). (After Bartlett RH. Use of mechanical ventilation. In: Holcroft J, ed. *Care of the Surgical Patient, Vol 1. Critical Care.* New York: Scientific American Medicine; 1989;2:9.)

or is overventilated and minimally perfused or when some of the end-tidal gas represents inflation gas that is simply compressed and released, never having reached the alveoli. The latter situation inevitably occurs under any positive-pressure ventilation circumstance but creates a significant end-tidal $PaCO_2$ gradient only when peak airway pressures are very high and when the compression volume is a significant component of each exhaled breath. However, the end-tidal CO_2 measurement becomes a useful continuous monitor of $PaCO_2$ when the lung is nearly normal, as in ventilator weaning. In addition, the gradient between end-tidal and arterial CO_2, when it is large, serves as an indirect measure of nonperfused alveoli (dead space) or compression volume, or both.

Pulmonary Mechanics

The interrelations of gas volumes and pressures in ventilation are referred to as *pulmonary mechanics*. How these volumes and pressures relate depend on pulmonary compliance. The standard compliance or volume–pressure curve, shown in Figure 9.8, is drawn by measuring volume and pressure at stages of lung *deflation* after total inflation. Volume–pressure curves for normal lungs in three different patients are shown in Figure 9.8. Notice that the curve for a normal 35-kg child is the same as that for an adult with major atelectasis. (It would be similar after pneumonectomy in an adult.) This emphasizes the point that the functional lung in acute respiratory failure is smaller, but not necessarily "stiffer." Computed tomographic studies of patients with ARDS support this concept. The lung injury in ARDS is heterogeneous such that, in the presence of normal tidal volumes, the relatively few alveoli that remain ventilated might very well be overdistended.[29] These findings have significant implications for iatrogenic injury and ventilatory strategies in these patients.

In the example shown in Figure 9.8, inflation of the normal lung with 500 mL of gas requires a pressure of 8 cm H_2O and moves the patient from point *A* to point *B*. When the pressure is released, exhalation occurs passively, and lung volume returns to point *A*. Periodic inflation to 25 or 30 cm H_2O would achieve near-total alveolar inflation without causing overdistention. In acute respiratory failure, the cause of decreased compliance is almost always associated with a decrease in the functional residual capacity (FRC) (Fig. 9.8). The decreased FRC represents lost alveoli, which are either collapsed or filled with fluid but still perfused with blood. Because the lung is smaller, the compliance curve is shifted to the right, and much higher pressures are required to achieve the same level of inflation. To inflate the lung to point *E*, for example, a pressure of 40 cm H_2O would be necessary. One way of managing ventilation in this circumstance is to maintain PEEP at 10 cm H_2O (C^1 in Fig. 9.8) and ventilate to point *D* with tidal breathing. The PEEP is set at this level to maintain the inflation of alveoli that might close at lower end-expiratory pressures. The elevated inspiratory pressures on top of the PEEP may also be helpful in recruiting closed alveoli. When that happens, the functional lung is bigger, and the entire compliance curve shifts back toward the left.

PEEP has beneficial effects on gas exchange and lung compliance; however, if used without understanding the potential downsides, it can cause harm. For example, high levels of PEEP in relatively compliant lungs might increase intrathoracic pressure sufficiently to inhibit venous flow and reduce preload and cardiac output. High intrathoracic pressures might also have dramatic effects on patients with elevated intracranial pressure due to increased impedance for cerebral venous return. Caution must also be exercised in patients with a unilateral lung process (e.g., aspiration, pulmonary contusion, alveolar hemorrhage), as the increased pressures might harm the uninjured normal lung through overdistention.

Several measurements must be taken to determine whether positive airway pressure is recruiting collapsed alveoli or simply distending normal alveoli (Fig. 9.9). As the most normal areas of lung have the best compliance, they are the most vulnerable to overdistention, and this vulnerability contributes to the steady progression of lung dysfunction in patients ventilated at either excessive pressures or tidal volumes. As collapsed alveoli are reinflated, compliance improves and oxygenation increases at the same ventilator settings as shunt decreases. These principles and measurements must be kept in mind during the treatment of the patient on a mechanical ventilator.

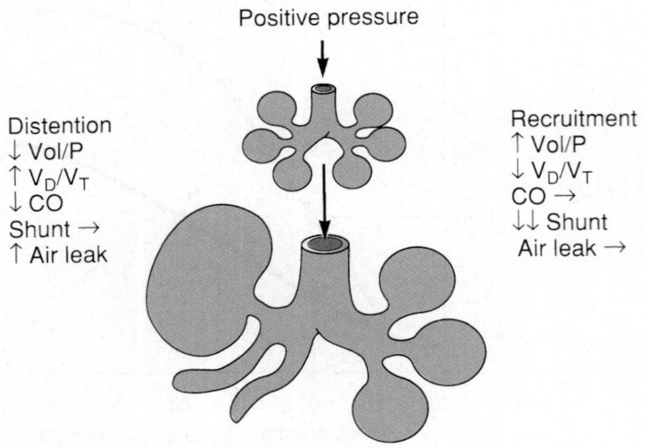

FIGURE 9.9. During mechanical ventilation, the gas volume may inflate alveoli equally (recruitment) or overdistend selected alveoli (distention). (After Bartlett RH. Pulmonary pathophysiology in surgical patients. *Surg Clin North Am* 1980;60:1323.)

Management of Respiratory Failure

When confronted with a patient in acute respiratory failure, the first priority is to identify and treat easily remediable causes. Examples include a pneumothorax requiring a chest tube, acute pulmonary edema requiring diuresis, or an acute asthma exacerbation that may respond to bronchodilator therapy. In the absence of a readily reversible cause, most patients will require mechanical ventilatory support (Algorithm 9.1). Setting up the ventilator can be intimidating because the terminology is complex and continues to evolve with advances in technology. Only the most commonly used modes will be discussed.

4 In principle, three parameters determine the mode of ventilation: *trigger, limit*, and *cycle*. Trigger refers to the signal to initiate the inspiratory phase and is set according to whether or not the patient has spontaneous respiratory effort. Mandatory modes such as continuous mandatory ventilation (CMV) use a time trigger, whereas spontaneous modes such as pressure support use a flow or pressure change initiated by the patient. Mandatory modes of ventilation are required if the patient has inadequate or no spontaneous respiratory effort.

The limit variable refers to the flow or pressure that is set during inspiration and cannot be exceeded. By convention, if the limit variable is flow, then the mode is labeled volume control (VC) ventilation (volume = flow × time). Alternatively, if

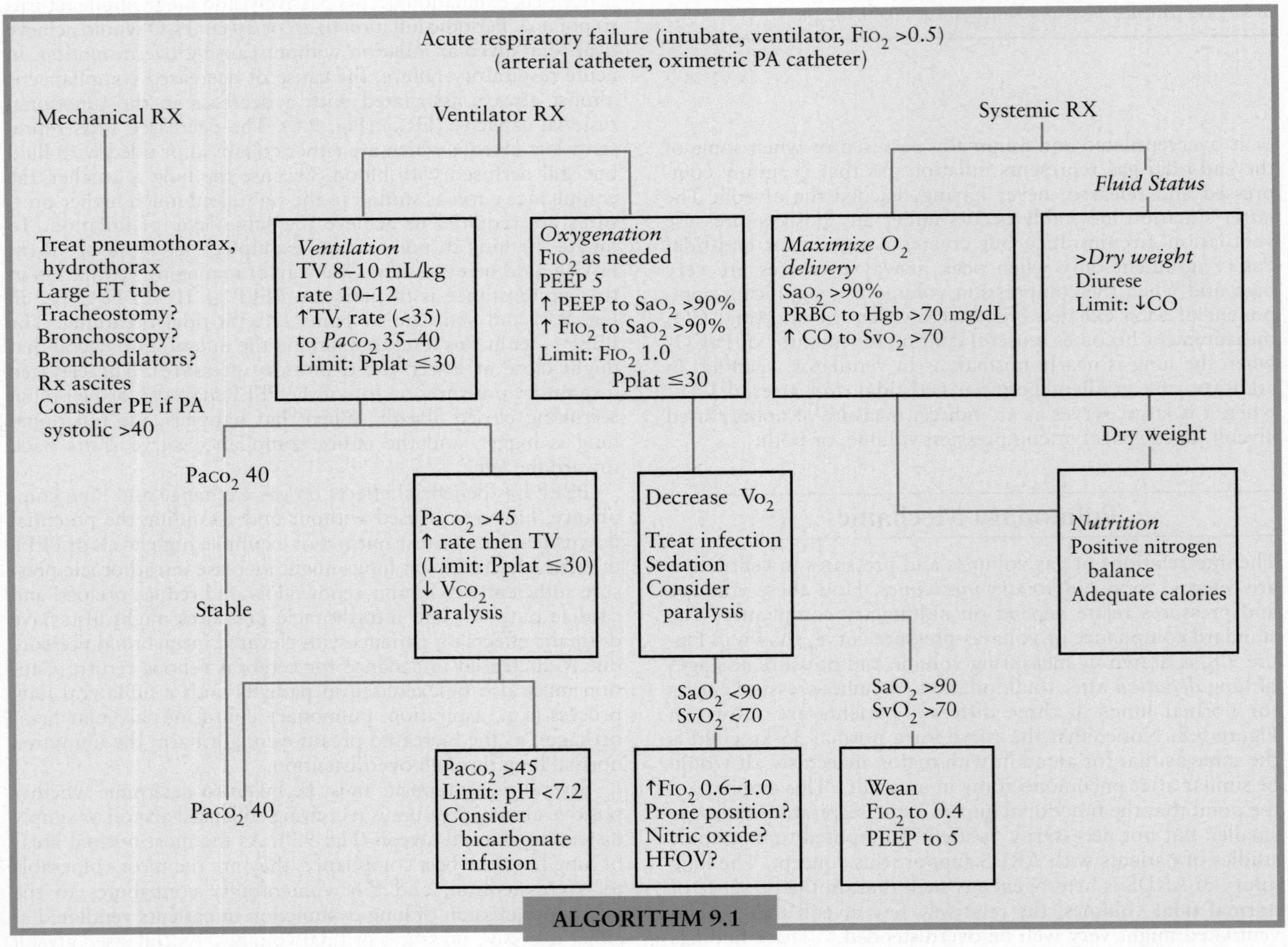

ALGORITHM 9.1. Management of respiratory failure. ET, endotracheal; PA, pulmonary artery; PCWP, pulmonary capillary wedge pressure; PE, pulmonary embolism; PEEP, positive end-expiratory pressure; PRBC, packed red blood cells; TV, tidal volume. (Modified from Bartlett RH. *University of Michigan Critical Care Handbook*. Boston, MA: Little, Brown; 1996.)

the limit variable is pressure, then the mode is termed pressure control (PC) or pressure support ventilation (PSV). Although both are pressure-limited modes, PSV requires spontaneous inspiratory effort, whereas PC can be used as either a mandatory or spontaneous mode.

Cycle is the variable that terminates the inspiratory cycle, which might be time, flow, pressure, or volume. In general, setting the cycle variable is equivalent to setting the inspiratory time and is manipulated based on pulmonary mechanics and the desired ratio of inspiratory to expiratory time. Intermittent mandatory ventilation (IMV) and assist control (A/C) modes both represent forms of volume control ventilation in which breaths are delivered at a set tidal volume with a set frequency. In A/C mode, if the patient initiates a breath, the tidal volume delivered will be the set volume, whereas in IMV mode, the tidal volume of spontaneous breaths is determined by the patient. However, when the ventilator is triggered (machine or patient), a fixed flow of gas is generated for a specific time providing a preset inspiratory volume (volume = flow × time). Volume-limited ventilation is generally easier to regulate but may be less comfortable for the awake patient as the flow curve is a square wave and markedly different from the normal inspiratory flow pattern in a nonventilated patient. The major advantage of volume-controlled modes of ventilation is the assurance that the patient will receive a guaranteed minimum minute ventilation.

PSV is the most frequently used form of pressure-limited ventilation. In this mode, the patient triggers a breath and a variable flow is delivered to meet a set pressure. Cycling in this mode is determined by the decrease in flow rate and causes the ventilator to stop the inspiratory phase. As the lung inflates, compliance decreases and flow decreases to maintain a constant inspiratory pressure. When flow reaches a percentage of the maximal flow rate (typically around 80% of maximum, depending on the ventilator model), inspiratory flow ceases, and the patient exhales passively. Tidal volumes will be determined by lung compliance—the more compliant the lung, the larger the tidal volume is at a set pressure. PSV is often used as a partial mode of ventilatory support in alert patients who may not tolerate more controlled forms of mechanical ventilation.

Pressure control ventilation (PCV) is related to pressure support in that the flow is descending in amplitude during the inspiratory cycle. In contrast to PSV, with PCV the inspiratory time is set by the ventilator, not the patient. PCV is generally used in the A/C, which allows full support of patient-initiated breaths in addition to those initiated by the ventilator (mandatory, or time triggered). The purported advantages of PCV relate to the decelerating flow curve, which is thought to allow more time for alveolar inflation and gas exchange. It is important to recognize that the tidal volume (and therefore minute ventilation) might change quite rapidly with changes in lung compliance. Thus, without continued reassessment of tidal volumes, there is a possibility that the patient might be significantly hypo- or hyperventilated. Pressure-regulated volume control (PRVC) is a mode similar to PCV in which the pressure is autoregulated (within a specified range) to ensure tidal volumes are maintained despite changes in lung compliance.

Ventilator Strategies. Endotracheal intubation and mechanical ventilation provide vital support yet are associated with disadvantages, including a greater risk of pneumonia and aggravation of alveolar injury, respectively. Additionally, there is increasing evidence that the manner by which patients are ventilated and weaned might have significant effects on outcome. For example, in a large randomized controlled trial, patients with ARDS or acute lung injury (a form of hypoxemic respiratory failure, Table 9.3[30]) ventilated with lower tidal volumes (6 mL/kg) had a significantly lower mortality than those ventilated at higher tidal volumes (12 mL/kg).[31] Clinical and experimental studies suggest that higher tidal volumes lead to ventilator-induced lung injury (by means of overdistending alveoli), which incites a secondary greater local and systemic inflammatory response. Patients ventilated with lower tidal volumes also had significantly lower ventilatory pressures (plateau pressures <30 cm H_2O); thus, it is unclear which offered benefit—the lower tidal volumes or the lower plateau pressures. Most centers have since adopted this lung-protective ventilatory strategy.

A frequent point of controversy in managing the hypoxemic patient is the relative merits of using high levels of PEEP and lower levels of FiO_2 or using lower levels of PEEP with a correspondingly higher FiO_2. By convention, many intensivists use higher levels of PEEP to maintain the FiO_2 less than 0.6, believing that higher levels of oxygen might induce hyperoxic lung injury. However, results from a randomized controlled trial comparing a high PEEP strategy with a high FiO_2 strategy demonstrated similar outcomes.[32] Given these data, the risks and benefits of using PEEP should be assessed for each patient depending on the nature of his or her underlying lung disease and associated conditions (e.g., low cardiac output state, high intracranial pressure, unilateral lung disease).

Refractory hypoxemia in the critically ill patient often presents a significant challenge. Two common approaches to assist in the management of these patients are prone positioning and high-frequency oscillatory ventilation (HFOV). Prone positioning requires that the patient be cared for in this position, typically for as few as 4 to as many as 24 hours a day for as long as 1 to 10 days, depending on the clinical response. This approach results in improved ventilation due to the triangular shape of the rib cage (wider posteriorly) and a reduction in atelectasis by reversing the compressive effects of the heart and

TABLE 9.3

RECOMMENDED CRITERIA FOR ACUTE LUNG INJURY AND ACUTE RESPIRATORY DISTRESS SYNDROME[a]

	TIMING	OXYGENATION	CHEST RADIOGRAPH	PULMONARY ARTERY WEDGE PRESSURE
Acute lung injury (ALI)	Acute onset	$PaO_2/FiO_2 \leq 300$ regardless of PEEP level	Bilateral infiltrates on frontal chest radiograph	≤18 when measured or no clinical evidence of left atrial hypertension
Acute respiratory distress syndrome (ARDS)	Acute onset	$PaO_2/FiO_2 \leq 200$ regardless of PEEP level	Bilateral infiltrates on frontal chest radiograph	≤18 when measured or no clinical evidence of left atrial hypertension

PEEP, positive end-expiratory pressure.
[a]In setting of known risk factors of either direct lung injury (aspiration, diffuse pulmonary infection, near drowning, toxic inhalation, pulmonary contusion) or indirect lung injury (sepsis, severe nonthoracic trauma, massive transfusion, cardiopulmonary bypass or ischemia/reperfusion insult).
Adapted from Bernard GR, Artigas A, Brigham KL, et al. The American-European Consensus Conference on ARDS. Definitions, mechanisms, relevant outcomes, and clinical trial coordination. *Am J Respir Crit Care Med* 1994;149:818–824.

diaphragm due to gravitational forces.[33] The prone position also improves the clearance of secretions. Persistence of improved perfusion to the posterior lung also improves perfusion/ventilation mismatch. In several clinical trials, prone positioning led to a 25% to 35% increase in the PaO_2/FiO_2 ratio, with sustained effects even beyond the period of proning.[34] Rates of pneumonia appear to be significantly lower due to a lesser risk of aspiration of secretions. While this approach appears to have significant merit, patient selection is important. Trauma patients in whom there are concerns regarding the stability of the spine are not appropriate, nor are patients at risk for cardiac arrest due to the challenges in performing cardiopulmonary resuscitation (CPR). In addition, to date, no overall benefit to survival has been demonstrated.

HFOV is a mode of ventilation using a piston pump oscillating at frequencies between 180 and 600 breaths/min (3 to 10 breaths/s). This piston pump moves air with very low tidal volumes (40 to 200 mL). Mean airway pressures are typically set just above the mean airway pressures used for conventional ventilation, yet the high frequency and lower tidal volumes lead to better lung recruitment and a higher end-expiratory lung volume as the alveoli do not have an opportunity to collapse. There is less cyclical recruitment-derecruitment of alveoli, leading to less alveolar shearing. At the same time, the lower tidal volumes prevent overdistention. Taken together, this mode of ventilation should reduce the potential for ventilator-induced lung injury, a finding demonstrated in small animal studies.[35] While large randomized controlled trials evaluating the efficacy of HFOV in patients with acute lung injury are under way, early studies suggest an improvement in PaO_2/FiO_2 ratios and a lower mortality rate.[36]

Weaning from Mechanical Ventilation. The process of weaning from the ventilator has changed significantly with evidence that the most rapid means of liberating a patient from the ventilator is through daily trials (30 to 90 minutes) of spontaneous breathing with low levels of continuous positive airway pressure (CPAP). This approach is superior to the gradual withdrawal of ventilation using pressure support or IMV.[37–39,40] If the patient tolerates the trial of spontaneous breathing, it is likely that he or she can be extubated with a low risk of requiring reintubation, providing he or she can protect the airway. Patients who fail a trial of spontaneous breathing should be rested for at least 24 hours using a stable, nonfatiguing form of ventilatory support. A partial support mode of ventilation (e.g., pressure support) probably offers benefit in terms of patient comfort while allowing a period of rest, as the patient can determine the respiratory rate, flow rate, inspiratory time, and tidal volume.

TRANSFUSION THERAPY IN THE INTENSIVE CARE UNIT

Virtually half of patients admitted to an ICU will receive a transfusion during the course of their ICU stay.[41] In those staying in the ICU for at least 1 week, 85% will require an average of 9 units over the course of their ICU stay.[42] The causes are multifactorial and include blood loss from the underlying disease(s), repeated blood draws for laboratory tests, and suppression of erythropoietin release and erythropoiesis. In the past, transfusions were provided liberally to maintain Hgb in the range of 10 g/dL with the belief that allogeneic transfusions were not harmful and would improve oxygen delivery to hasten recovery. However, many studies have demonstrated that tissue oxygen extraction is not improved following transfusion. This lack of enhanced tissue oxygenation is likely multifactorial and, in large part, related to the effects of storage on the erythrocyte. These effects result in increased hemoglobin oxygen affinity (due to loss of 2,3-diphosphoglycerate) and changes in membrane deformability leading to sludging in the microvascular circulation.[43–45] Additionally, a systematic review of cohort studies suggests that the transfusion of allogeneic red blood cells is associated with an increased risk of nosocomial infection, acute lung injury, and multiple organ failure.[46] It is noteworthy that these sequelae are not limited to allogeneic red blood cells, as they have also been strongly associated with the transfusion of fresh frozen plasma.[47,48]

5 A large clinical trial in which nonbleeding, euvolemic critically ill patients were randomized to either a liberal transfusion strategy (Hgb of 10 g/dL) or a restrictive strategy (Hgb of 7 g/dL) demonstrated that patients in the liberal group fared no better than those in the restrictive group who received far fewer transfusions.[49] In fact, younger patients (younger than 55 years of age) and those with Acute Physiology and Chronic Health Evaluation (APACHE) II scores of less than 20 had lower mortality and lower rates of organ dysfunction. In a subset of patients requiring prolonged ventilator support, the rate of liberation from mechanical ventilation was higher in patients randomized to the restrictive arm, suggesting there is no benefit to transfusing patients for the purposes of improving their ability to wean off the ventilator.[50] It appears that the risk of adverse outcomes related to a strict transfusion strategy is higher only in patients with unstable cardiovascular disease (unstable angina or acute myocardial infarction).[51]

Several approaches may be used to reduce transfusion requirements in the critically ill patient. Blood sampling should be reduced to only that which is required to alter patient care. Pulse oximetry should be used rather than arterial blood gases when there are changes in PEEP or FiO_2, and end-tidal CO_2 monitoring can guide changes in minute ventilation. Weekly recombinant human erythropoietin (rHuEPO) administration has been evaluated in patients with an anticipated prolonged ICU stay. In one randomized controlled trial, erythropoietin reduced transfusion requirements by approximately 20% and reduced the need for any transfusion by 17%, without affecting length of stay, rates of organ dysfunction, or mortality.[52] A subsequent meta-analysis of seven randomized controlled trials suggested a 0.4-unit reduction in red cells transfused and a 25% lower risk of receiving any transfusion.[53] Again, no effects on clinically relevant outcome were evident. Given these findings of limited benefit, erythropoietin receptor agonists are not recommended for use in critically ill patients. Further, the incremental cost-effectiveness with the use of these agonists is unacceptable. Estimates include almost $5 million to prevent one transfusion-related adverse event.[54]

METABOLISM AND NUTRITION

Metabolic and nutritional support are vital if the critically ill patient is to survive the ICU stay. Depletion of energy and protein reserves leads to an inability to wean off the ventilator, immunologic failure, and a high probability of death due to overwhelming infection. Thus, in the ICU a tremendous amount of effort is geared toward assessing and maintaining adequate nutritional support.

Energy Sources

The major sources of energy are carbohydrates (including ketones and alcohols) and fats. In addition, protein can be oxidized through gluconeogenesis and is often a significant source of energy in critically ill patients. The goal of nutritional support is to supply energy from sources other than protein, so that endogenous and exogenous protein can be used for anabolism rather than catabolism. In normal volunteers and surgical patients, the breakdown of protein is decreased by giving the subject exogenous fuel, typically in the form of carbohydrate or fat. This is referred to as the *protein-sparing effect.* Small amounts of glucose (400 cal/d) provide some degree of protein sparing, but full caloric support is required for maximal effect.

Carbohydrate is the major source of energy during the normal, nonstarving state. The brain and red cells are obligate users of glucose. They require glucose as the primary energy source under normal conditions. Other organs also use glucose preferentially as a source of energy. The brain and red blood cells can develop the capacity to use ketones as an energy source, a process called *starvation adaptation.* When fully oxidized, carbohydrate produces 4 cal of energy per gram of substrate metabolized, 5 cal of energy per liter of O_2 consumed, and one molecule of CO_2 for each molecule of O_2 consumed. The latter ratio is the RQ, discussed previously in the context of CO_2 production (see Table 9.2).

Fat is the most efficient source of energy. Fat produces 9 cal of energy per gram of substrate metabolized and 4.7 cal of energy per liter of O_2 consumed in this oxidation; its RQ is 0.7. Fat is stored as triglyceride, and for every three molecules of fatty acid oxidized to produce energy, one molecule of glycerol is also oxidized. Endogenous fat is the major source of energy during starvation. Glycogen stores are virtually depleted after a single day of fasting, following which fat becomes the major source of energy, with protein breakdown supplying glucose through the process of gluconeogenesis.

Metabolic Requirements

The typical expenditures of energy and protein in normal subjects and critically ill patients are shown in Figure 9.10. Protein and energy requirements are continuous. These are met by endogenous sources during fasting or through exogenous treatment (nutrition). Energy expenditure is referred to as the *basal metabolic rate,* or the *basal energy expenditure.* The term *basal metabolic rate* describes the energy required to maintain cell integrity in the resting state and at thermoneutrality. The latter term means an ambient temperature, usually close to 80°F (28°C), at which the heat loss and the need for increased heat production to maintain the body temperature are minimal. The basal energy expenditure (BEE) decreases with advancing age and varies with sex and body size. It is a function of cellular metabolism and hence of the body cell mass. The basal energy expenditure (in kilocalories)

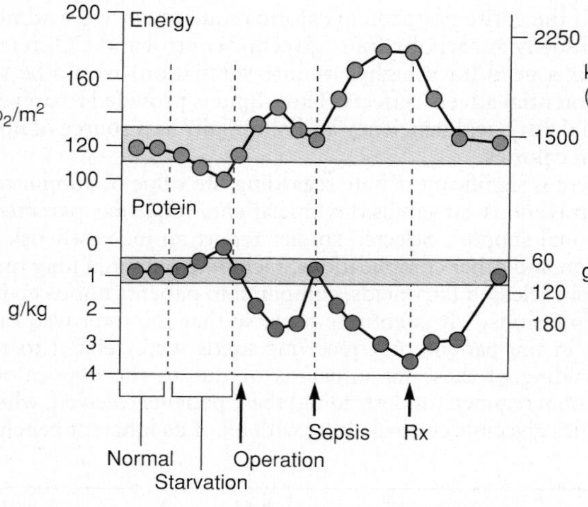

FIGURE 9.10. Energy and protein metabolism in normal, starving, operative, and septic states. (After Bartlett RH. Nutritional support. In: Dantzker DR, ed. *Cardiopulmonary Critical Care.* Orlando, FL: Grune & Stratton; 1986:263.)

is usually estimated from the Harris-Benedict equation, which incorporates age, sex, and body size:

Women:

$$\text{BEE} = 655 + (9.6 \times \text{weight in kilos}) + (1.8 \times \text{height in cm}) - (4.7 \times \text{age in years})$$

Men:

$$\text{BEE} = 66\ (13.7 \times \text{weight in kilos}) + (5 \times \text{height in cm}) - (6.8 \times \text{age in years})$$

Requirements are most often expressed as kcal/kg per day. Basal requirements in healthy adults are typically in the range of 25 kcal/kg per day.

Estimating and Measuring Energy Requirements

The actual metabolic rate of any given patient can be estimated by modifying the predicted basal rate according to the clinical condition. For example, the metabolic rate is decreased by 10% in a starving person and increased by 10% with minor activity. This further estimation of metabolic activity in the resting (as opposed to basal) state is referred to as the *resting energy expenditure.* Trauma, stress, sepsis, and surgical operations are all known to increase the metabolic rate. As a result, the BEE is usually multiplied by a stress factor to better approximate caloric requirements (Table 9.4). In general, to match utilization, the critically ill patient requires approximately 35 kcal/kg per day.

Although most of the studies on nutrition in critical illness have been based on estimated energy expenditure, actual measurement is much more accurate and is an important aspect of critical care. The most commonly used method of measurement is indirect calorimetry. In the ICU, indirect calorimetry is the only accurate and clinically feasible method of measuring energy expenditure. It is called indirect because the caloric burn rate is calculated from a measurement of oxygen uptake. Direct calorimetry implies a measurement of heat released by the body, which is technically difficult and clinically impractical. Indirect calorimetry relies on the fact that burning 1 kilocalorie requires approximately 200 mL of oxygen. Because of this very direct relationship between caloric burn and oxygen consumed, measurements of oxygen uptake (VO_2) and caloric burn rate are virtually interchangeable.

TABLE 9.4

PREDICTED INCREASE IN CALORIC REQUIREMENTS AS A FUNCTION OF STRESSOR

■ PHYSIOLOGIC STRESS	■ STRESS FACTOR
Operation	1.1
Peritonitis, major infection, or long bone fracture	1.25
Severe injury/infection or multiple organ failure	1.5
Thermal injury	
10% BSA	1.25
20%–30% BSA	1.5
40% BSA	1.75
>50% BSA	2.0

BSA, body surface area.

Indirect calorimetry can be carried out at the patient's bedside and requires the measurement of the differences in oxygen and carbon dioxide concentrations between a known volume of inspired and expired gas. Assuming the patient is in a steady state, oxygen consumption and carbon dioxide production can be quantitated. With measurement of O_2 consumption and CO_2 production, the RQ ($\dot{V}CO_2/\dot{V}O_2$) can be calculated, thus also providing an assessment of the relative oxidation of carbohydrates and fat (see Table 9.2). Thus, indirect calorimetry provides some indication of which substrates are being utilized to fulfill energy requirements. Normally the RQ is approximately 0.8; very infrequently the RQ might be in excess of 1 and as high as 2.5, indicative of lipogenesis (synthesis of fat from carbohydrates) and indicative of excess availability of carbohydrates.

Measurement of the RQ is helpful as an internal check on the accuracy of the calorimetry measurements and as a guideline to patient management. For example, if a patient has been receiving only 500 cal/d and has a metabolic rate of 2,500 cal/d, one would expect that the use of fat would be maximal, and the RQ should be 0.7 or less. If such a patient is treated with parenteral nutrition and glucose used as the major source of energy, the RQ should be 1 when the caloric replacement matches caloric losses. If the RQ exceeds 1, then some of the excess infused carbohydrate is being converted to fat and excess CO_2 is produced, which leads to a need for a higher minute ventilation. Thus, hypercaloric feeding with glucose can aggravate respiratory failure and the requirement for mechanical ventilation simply by increasing the load of CO_2.

Protein Metabolism

Estimating and Measuring Protein Requirements. In normal protein metabolism, a continuous excretion of nitrogen (mostly as urea) equivalent to about 50 g of protein each day is matched by a protein intake of 50 g/d. The rate of protein synthesis and breakdown is about 300 g/d, with most endogenous amino acids being recycled into new protein. In starvation, protein catabolism continues (although at a slower rate) without a corresponding protein intake, leaving the patient in a negative protein balance. This protein flux is most conveniently measured as nitrogen flux; consequently, the condition is commonly referred to as *negative nitrogen balance*. During critical illness, the rate of protein catabolism generally increases while intake stops, so that a significant negative nitrogen balance results. It is convenient to think of this protein breakdown as necessary to produce critically required glucose through gluconeogenesis when other carbohydrate stores have been exhausted.

Protein Sources. The fact that the nitrogen balance is negative does not mean that protein synthesis stops or slows down. On the contrary, the synthesis of new cells, inflammatory cells, collagen, coagulation factors, antibodies, and scores of other proteins occurs at an accelerated rate during critical illness. Amino acids derived from muscle tissue or other somatic and visceral proteins become the building blocks for protein in healing tissue and host defenses. Thus, the site of a traumatic or surgical wound or an area of acute inflammation diverts protein from other body tissues. Proteins that would otherwise strengthen the diaphragm or myocardium or participate in host defense processes are less available, thus significantly compromising the patient. A large part of the goal of nutritional management is to provide sources of energy so that endogenous proteins are not required for energy (i.e., protein sparing) and to supply exogenous proteins so that all the needs of protein synthesis can be met without a breakdown of endogenous sources. Although oversimplified, a convenient number to remember for the basal protein requirement is 0.8 g/kg per day. The average critically ill surgical patients might require 1.5 g/kg per day, whereas patients with severe thermal injury and head injuries might have requirements in excess of 2 g/kg per day.

Nitrogen Balance. Protein balance is most frequently determined through assessment of nitrogen balance. Nitrogen balance can be determined by measuring the amount of nitrogen excreted. This is most conveniently done by measuring the amount of urea excreted in the urine if one assumes that urea constitutes 85% of the total nitrogen excretion. Since each gram of nitrogen represents 6.25 g of protein, total protein intake can be compared with protein loss through an estimate of daily urea excretion. However, it is better to measure the total nitrogen in urine and other lost fluids because the percentage contained in urea can vary considerably.

Indirect assessments of protein reserves are based on the single measurement of body substances that are maintained at normal levels by rapid protein synthesis. A variety of visceral proteins that have relatively short half-lives have been assessed for their relationship to protein status. Prealbumin ($t_{1/2}$ = 2 days), retinol-binding protein ($t_{1/2}$ = 10 days), and transferrin ($t_{1/2}$ = 8 days) have all been used in the evaluation of nitrogen balance. Albumin has limited utility given its relatively long half-life ($t_{1/2}$ = 21 days). Some advocate insulinlike growth factor-1 as another short-lived serum visceral protein, with the major benefit being its relative independence of the inflammatory state of the patient. For example, prealbumin is a negative acute-phase reactant and serum levels will decrease in the presence of ongoing, acute inflammation. As a result, increasing levels of prealbumin might be consistent with the deposition of new protein or an abating inflammatory response, whereas a decrease might suggest a negative nitrogen balance or a new focus of inflammation or infection. For these reasons, these rapid-turnover visceral proteins should be used as only one measure of protein status.

Fat Metabolism

In a normal 80-kg man, about 1,000 cal are readily available as glycogen and other stored carbohydrates, 24,000 cal are available as protein, and approximately 140,000 cal are stored as fat. A 10,000-cal deficit accrued over 5 to 6 days of semistarvation in a critically ill patient is considered a severe, acute energy deficit. This seems paradoxical given the large amount of calories stored as fat. However, the problem of a 10,000-cal deficit is not the loss of a few kilograms of fat but rather the protein catabolism commonly associated with an energy deficit of this size.

With the exception of essential fatty acids, the critically ill patient has little need for the administration of exogenous lipid. If the entire nonprotein caloric requirement were administered solely as carbohydrate, glycemic control and CO_2 retention (or a need for a higher minute ventilation) would be the only potential adverse effects. Thus, lipid is provided to prevent essential fatty acid deficiency and minimally as a source of nonprotein calories.

There is significant debate regarding the value of administering intravenous fat emulsions in patients requiring parenteral nutritional support. Selected studies report an increased risk of infection and other complications, including potential lung toxicity from released fatty acids, compared to patients not receiving lipid emulsions.[55] It is entirely possible that the improved outcomes in the patients not receiving lipids were related to the withholding of these fat infusions or due to the hypocaloric nutritional regimen (underfeeding) these patients received, which simplifies glycemic control along with all of its inherent benefits.

Vitamins and Minerals

A hypermetabolic patient catabolizes vitamins more rapidly than normal and can reach a deficiency state sooner. Additionally, the oxidative stress associated with reperfusion injury and a systemic inflammatory response leads to depletion of endogenous antioxidants, including vitamins E and C. In this regard, there is evidence to suggest that high doses of vitamins E and C might improve outcome and lower the risk of multiple organ failure in critically ill surgical patients.[56] Adequate levels of other vitamins are readily available in commercially prepared formulations used for enteral or parenteral administration.

Mineral and trace metals must be managed more carefully than vitamins because a deficiency can occur more quickly and overdose can be deleterious. Calcium, phosphorus, and magnesium are lost continuously through the urine, stool, gastric juices, and other drainage. Although large body stores (particularly of calcium and phosphorous) are available, functional deficiency can develop rapidly. Enteral and parenteral feeding must include these elements and serum levels of calcium, phosphorus, and magnesium should be measured at regular intervals. In addition, zinc, copper, chromium, selenium, and manganese must be supplied to patients who are supported with enteral or parenteral feeding for more than 2 weeks.

Nutritional Support

6 Nutritional status should be assessed at the time of admission to the ICU with a view to determining whether the patient is malnourished and the likelihood of timing to return to normal oral intake. Patients who are malnourished at the time of admission should receive nutritional support as soon as possible, typically once the acute resuscitation phase is over. In a systematic review of randomized controlled trials, early enteral nutrition (initiation within 36 hours of admission) was associated with a significantly lower risk of infections and a shorter hospital length of stay.[57] A reasonable goal for nutritional support is to meet the caloric and protein requirements within 5 days of ICU admission in adequately nourished patients in whom a return to oral intake is not imminent (Algorithm 9.2).

The critically ill patient is best provided energy and protein using the gastrointestinal tract whenever possible. This route has fewer risks of complications and is less costly than the parenteral route. Enteral feeding can be accomplished through a tube passed directly into the duodenum or jejunum at surgery or through a soft, small-bore feeding tube passed into the stomach through the nose or mouth. It is generally possible to accomplish tube feeding with gastric infusion and there appears to be no specific benefit to postpyloric enteral feeding with respect to rates of pneumonia due to aspiration.[58] However, in the case of intolerance, postpyloric feeding should be considered. Intolerance of gastric feeding usually manifests as large volumes (>300 mL) of residual feeds in the stomach on aspiration from the feeding tube. In this scenario, the feeding

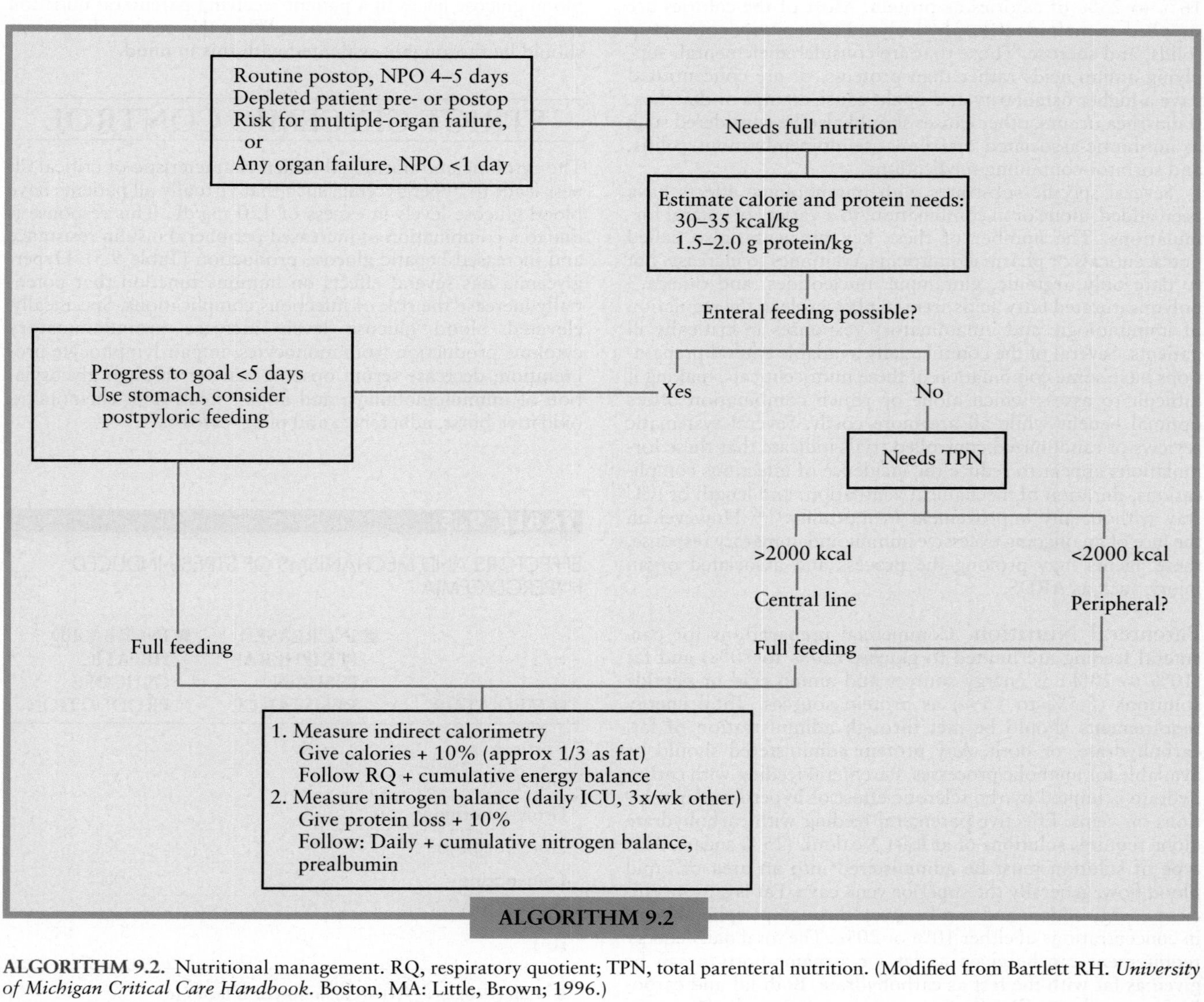

ALGORITHM 9.2. Nutritional management. RQ, respiratory quotient; TPN, total parenteral nutrition. (Modified from Bartlett RH. *University of Michigan Critical Care Handbook*. Boston, MA: Little, Brown; 1996.)

tube should be advanced beyond the pylorus using endoscopy or fluoroscopy. Alternatively, prokinetic agents like metoclopramide or erythromycin may be effective.

Feedings should be given by continuous infusion rather than as large boluses. The patient should be positioned in a semirecumbent or sitting position (at a minimum of a 30-degree angle) to prevent regurgitation and aspiration and to lower the risk of ventilator-associated pneumonia. Gastric residuals should be checked if the patient feels uncomfortable or appears distended, but it is not necessary to check the residual more than once a day under most circumstances. With continuous tube feeding, a residual of 200 to 300 mL is normal.

It is better to start with a small amount of full-strength formula rather than a large amount of diluted formula. The rate can be advanced and gradually increased until the desired volume is reached. Hypernatremia can occur in patients who receive high-protein formulas or concentrated formulas or in those patients with significant free water losses. Hypernatremia should be managed by administering free water via the feeding tube. A serious problem with tube feeding is complete cessation of feedings because of diarrhea or a large gastric residual. If the tube feeding needs to be curtailed for any reason, it should be reinstituted the next hour at a smaller volume and gradually increased until the prescribed caloric load is reached.

Enteral Formulations. Commercially available formulas for enteral feeding generally contain 1 to 2 cal/mL and include 16% to 25% of calories as protein. Most of the calories are supplied as maltodextrins, hydrolyzed corn syrup, corn syrup solids, and sucrose. Those that are considered elemental, supplying amino acids rather than proteins, or are concentrated have a higher osmolarity and might cause cramps or diarrhea. If diarrhea occurs, other causes should also be considered such as antibiotic-associated diarrhea, pseudomembranous colitis, and sorbitol-containing medications.

Several specific substrates with immunologic effects have been added, alone or in combination, to a variety of enteral formulations. The number of these key nutrients, also called nutraceuticals or pharmaconutrients, continues to increase, but to date only arginine, glutamine, nucleotides, and omega-3 polyunsaturated fatty acids seem to play a role in the regulation of immunologic and inflammatory responses in critically ill patients. Several of the commercially available enteral preparations have some combination of these nutraceuticals, making it difficult to assess which alone or which combination offers optimal benefit while all are more costly. Several systematic reviews of randomized controlled trials indicate that these formulations appear to reduce the incidence of infectious complications, duration of mechanical ventilation, and length of ICU stay without any improvement in mortality.[59,60] However, in the face of an ongoing excessive immunoinflammatory response, these agents may prolong the process and associated organ injury, such as ARDS.

Parenteral Nutrition. Commercial preparations for parenteral feeding are limited to glucose (20% to 70%) and fat (10% to 20%) as energy sources and amino acid or peptide solutions (5.5% to 15%) as protein sources. Total energy requirements should be met through administration of fat, carbohydrate, or both. Any protein administered should be available for anabolic processes. Parenteral feeding with carbohydrate is limited by the sclerotic effect of hyperosmolar solutions on veins. Effective parenteral feeding with carbohydrate alone requires solutions of at least 1 cal/mL (25% sugar). This type of solution must be administered into an area of rapid blood flow, generally the superior vena cava. Fat is a more efficient energy source and can be given through peripheral veins in concentrations of either 10% or 20%. The total daily energy requirement can be given as fat, or a major portion can be given as fat with the rest as carbohydrate. Both fat and carbohydrate are equally effective sources of energy. The ratio between fat and carbohydrate energy sources and the ratio between total energy sources and grams of protein vary depending on the clinical state. For example, a patient with cardiac failure may require a solution that is low in volume and low in sodium but high in calories and protein. A patient with multiple intestinal fistulas may require large volumes, which allow for fewer calories and grams of protein per milliliter. As a rule of thumb, half of the calories can be provided by carbohydrate, 30% as fat, and the remainder as protein.

The standard solution can be modified for individual patients by raising or lowering the concentration of glucose and amino acids and by varying the electrolyte and trace metal composition. Vitamins and trace minerals are added to the solution at regular intervals. The standard solution must be supplemented with intravenous fat to provide at least 100 g of fat emulsion each week to preclude fatty acid deficiency. Fat emulsion may be administered through a peripheral vein or through a central catheter at the same time as the hypertonic glucose solution.

The most common complication of total parenteral nutrition is infection on or around the intravascular catheter. Of course, infection can occur with any indwelling vascular catheter, but it is more likely in the presence of hypertonic glucose and protein solutions. If catheter infection is suspected, the catheter must be removed and a new location and catheter placed. Hyperglycemia is also common and should be aggressively managed with an insulin infusion. A sudden increase in blood glucose levels in a patient receiving parenteral nutrition is often an early sign of infection. When this occurs, the patient should be thoroughly evaluated with this in mind.

STRICT GLYCEMIC CONTROL

The cytokine and hormonal milieu characteristic of critical illness leads to hyperglycemia such that virtually all patients have blood glucose levels in excess of 120 mg/dL. This response is due to a combination of increased peripheral insulin resistance and increased hepatic glucose production (Table 9.5). Hyperglycemia has several effects on immune function that potentially increase the risk of infectious complications. Specifically, elevated blood glucose levels increase proinflammatory cytokine production from monocytes; impair lymphocyte proliferation; decrease serum opsonic activity through glycosylation of immunoglobulins; and impair neutrophil chemotaxis, oxidative burst, adherence, and phagocytosis.

TABLE 9.5

EFFECTORS AND MECHANISMS OF STRESS-INDUCED HYPERGLYCEMIA

MEDIATOR	INCREASED PERIPHERAL INSULIN RESISTANCE	INCREASED HEPATIC GLUCOSE PRODUCTION
Cortisol	X	
Glucagon		X
Growth hormone	X	
Norepinephrine		X
Epinephrine		X
TNF-α	X	
IL-1	X	

IL-1, interleukin 1; TNF-α, tumor necrosis factor-α.

TABLE 9.6

CLASSIFICATION OF ACUTE KIDNEY INJURY (RIFLE CLASSIFICATION)

■ RIFLE CATEGORY	■ GFR CRITERIA[a]	■ URINE OUTPUT CRITERIA	■ ICU MORTALITY
RISK	Increased serum creatinine × 1.5 or decrease of GFR >25%	Urine output <0.5 mL/kg/h for 6 h	5%
INJURY	Increased serum creatinine × 2 or decrease of GFR >50%	Urine output <0.5 mL/kg/h for 12 h	14.7
FAILURE	Increased serum creatinine × 3 or decrease of GFR >75% or serum creatinine ≥4 mg/dL	Urine output <0.3 mL/kg/h for 12 h or anuria for 12 h	36.5
LOSS	Complete loss of renal function for >4 wk	47.6	
END-STAGE KIDNEY DISEASE	Need for renal replacement therapy for >3 mo		

[a]Either GFR (glomerular filtration rate) or urine output criteria might be used to define the RIFLE classification.

Early evidence from randomized controlled trials suggested that strict glycemic control aiming for blood glucose in the range of 80 to 120 g/dL reduced mortality, principally due to a reduction in the risk of sepsis-induced organ failure.[61] More recent trials and meta-analyses suggest that the relationship between glycemic control and mortality is more complex.[62,63] It appears that there is no benefit and even a potential for harm in medical patients or mixed medical-surgical critical care units. By contrast, there appears to be a mortality benefit with a 40% lower risk of death in critically ill surgical and trauma patients.[62,63] The differential effects are not easily explained and might relate to the attributable mortality of sepsis in medical as compared to surgical populations. What is evident from many of these trials is that the rate of hypoglycemic episodes is over fivefold greater (as high as 20% of all patients) and the nursing workload associated with titration of a continuous insulin infusion is significant. To mitigate some of these concerns, evidence-based guidelines suggest a tightly controlled insulin protocol and a more moderate approach, with a blood glucose target under 140 mg/dL.

ACUTE RENAL FAILURE

Acute renal failure (ARF) complicates approximately 5% of ICU admissions. By definition, ARF is an abrupt decrease in kidney function that results in the accumulation of nitrogenous solutes. ARF may be oliguric (urine output <400 mL/d) or nonoliguric 7 (urine output is normal or increased while solute clearance is markedly decreased). It is now recognized that renal dysfunction occurs along a continuum, such that the term more appropriately used in the ICU is *acute kidney injury* (AKI), which is graded using the RIFLE (*r*isk, *i*njury, *f*ailure, *l*oss, *e*nd-stage kidney disease) classification (Table 9.6).[64,65] The mortality of ARF in the surgical ICU is high (50% to 90%) because ARF is usually just one component of severe multiple organ failure. The mortality from nonoliguric ARF is significantly less than that from oliguric ARF, although many patients progress to oliguria with its poor outcome. Regardless of urine output, the sequelae of ARF result from the retention of metabolic wastes indicated by a progressive rise in blood urea nitrogen (BUN) and serum creatinine concentrations. Hypervolemia and electrolyte imbalances further complicate the management of oliguric ARF.

Etiology of Acute Renal Failure

The pathogenesis of ARF is commonly classified as prerenal, postrenal, or intrinsic parenchymal disease (renal). In any patient with renal dysfunction, prerenal and postrenal (obstructive uropathy) causes should be excluded (Table 9.7). Obstructive etiologies can easily be excluded using ultrasonography to evaluate the kidneys, ureters, and bladder. Parenchymal disease is the most frequent cause of ARF in the ICU, with acute tubular necrosis (ATN) being the most common pathologic finding.

ATN is the death of tubular cells, which occurs due to either ischemia (ischemic ATN) or nephrotoxic agents (toxic ATN). Ischemic ATN is seen in the context of sepsis, hypovolemia, major surgery (likely related to changes in intravascular volume), or cardiogenic shock. Under conditions of diminishing renal blood flow, perfusion of the kidneys is first maintained by vasomotor responses, which dilate the afferent arteriole and constrict the efferent arteriole. As continued hypotension is detected by the juxtaglomerular apparatus, the renin-angiotensin system is activated in concert with the sympathetic release of other vasoactive hormones. These substances produce vasoconstriction systemically, including the afferent arteriole, and further exacerbate cortical hypoperfusion. Casts of cellular debris obstruct the lumen, and cellular edema occurs. As tubular cells become necrotic and slough off, the leakage of glomerular ultrafiltrate back across the proximal tubular membrane into the interstitium causes edema. Acute tubular necrosis consists of a spectrum of effects of cortical ischemia, ranging from polyuria with tubular dysfunction to temporary anuria to renal cortical necrosis with chronic anuria.

TABLE 9.7

STANDARD MEASUREMENTS IN THE DIAGNOSIS OF RENAL FAILURE

■ TEST	■ PRERENAL	■ PARENCHYMAL
Urine osmolarity (mOsm)	>500	250–350
U/P osmolality	>1.5	<1.1
U/P creatinine	>20	<10
Urine sodium	<20	>40
FE_{Na}	<1%	>3%

FE_{Na}, fraction of excreted sodium; U/P, urine-to-plasma ratio.

Toxic Acute Tubular Necrosis

Toxic ATN might occur as a result of pigments (myoglobin, hemoglobin), radiocontrast media, or drugs. Pigment nephropathy due to the effects of myoglobin following trauma, major burns, global ischemia, or operation is not uncommon in the surgical intensive care unit. Rarely, hemoglobinemia due to massive intravascular hemolysis might also give rise to pigment nephropathy. ARF due to circulating myoglobin occurs in almost half of patients with significant rhabdomyolysis. Rhabdomyolysis leads to ATN through three mechanisms: intrarenal vasoconstriction and ischemia, cast formation with tubular obstruction, and the direct toxic effects of myoglobin on the renal tubules. Although myoglobin is not a direct nephrotoxin, in the presence of aciduria, myoglobin is converted to ferrihemate, which is toxic to renal cells. Rhabdomyolysis should be suspected in patients with burns, trauma, seizures, alcohol or drug intoxication, prolonged ischemia in muscle groups, and extended coma.

The presence of myoglobin in the urine can be first suspected by the presence of dark, tea-colored urine and then confirmed with a positive urine dipstick, which reacts with the heme groups of both myoglobin and Hgb. The absence of red cells on microscopy confirms that the discolored urine is caused by myoglobin. High serum levels of creatinine phosphokinase (CPK) or myoglobin, in combination with evidence of urine myoglobin, confirm the diagnosis. One characteristic feature of early rhabdomyolysis-induced acute kidney injury that differs from other forms of ATN is the presence of a low fractional excretion of sodium (<1%), a potential manifestation of the importance of vasoconstriction and tubular occlusion in its pathogenesis.[66]

Patients with either CPK greater than 20,000 IU/L or serum myoglobin greater than 10,000 ng/mL are at highest risk for pigment nephropathy. Measures should be instituted to prevent pigment nephropathy and lower the likelihood of requiring renal replacement therapy (RRT). The most important measure is volume expansion with or without administration of diuretics to achieve a urine output of 150 to 200 mL/h. Mannitol is an ideal diuretic in this sense as it induces an osmotic diuresis and as an oxidant scavenger might reduce iron-mediated oxidative injury to the renal tubules. Many intensivists also attempt to alkalinize the urine (pH ≥7) through the administration of sodium bicarbonate solutions, although evidence supporting this approach is lacking. Forced diuresis should continue until the urine is clear of myoglobin.

Radiocontrast media is another frequent cause of toxic ATN in surgical patients and is the third most common cause of ARF in hospitalized patients. It is believed to be due to both renal vasoconstriction leading to medullary ischemia and oxidant injury. The incidence of contrast nephropathy is about 1% to 3% when defined as a 25% elevation in serum creatinine. Risk factors include mode of administration (intraarterial > intravenous), advanced age, preexisting renal dysfunction, diabetes, hypovolemia, nonsteroidal anti-inflammatory drug (NSAID) use, and type of radiocontrast agent.[67]

Contrast nephropathy is usually experienced as an asymptomatic, transient rise in creatinine but may progress to oliguric renal failure that requires hemodialysis (HD). Volume expansion with saline is probably the most effective means of preventing contrast nephropathy in high-risk patients. There are conflicting reports regarding the effectiveness of N-acetylcysteine and sodium bicarbonate in preventing acute kidney injury following radiocontrast media exposure. N-acetylcysteine may protect against the effects of free radicals, while sodium bicarbonate is believed to prevent their formation. Taken together, the evidence suggests that at a minimum, either of these adjunctive measures is not harmful and might be beneficial.[68]

Management of Acute Renal Failure

In surgical patients, ARF rarely occurs in isolation. Rather, ARF is only one component of a syndrome of multiple organ failure that is often accompanied by infection. The treatment of these patients, therefore, should be focused on managing the underlying disease processes. The development of ARF complicates the care of surgical patients by introducing difficulties in fluid, electrolyte, and nutritional management. The adverse effects of RRT further compound these problems. A favorable outcome can be achieved only through aggressive intervention. This includes surgical drainage of infectious foci, excision of necrotic tissue, early implementation of effective RRT, and full nutritional support (Algorithm 9.3).

General Care

With nonoliguric ARF, the treatment may differ little from that required for identical patients with normal renal function. The management of fluids, solutes, and nutrition is usually unaffected by nonoliguric ARF, although the BUN may be elevated. The extent of renal dysfunction is limited and almost always reversible. The use of renal replacement therapies (and their inherent complications) is rarely necessary.

Oliguria and anuria pose several management difficulties. In the absence of normal urine output, problems of fluid overload can lead to anasarca, pulmonary edema, and congestive heart failure. The pharmacokinetics of drugs becomes difficult to predict as a result of decreased elimination and increased volume of distribution. In light of these risks, the volume status of patients with ARF must be carefully monitored. Fluid intake and output must be precisely tabulated, and the body weight should be measured daily. Pulmonary artery catheterization may be necessary to monitor the fluid status of these patients more closely. Treatment options for hypervolemia consist of fluid restriction or fluid removal with some form of RRT. Fluid restriction, however, limits the administration of intravenous medications and may preclude adequate nutrition.

ARF can create severe derangements in electrolyte and acid–base physiology. Serum electrolytes should be measured at least daily. Of all the electrolyte abnormalities that can occur with ARF, hyperkalemia is the most serious. Under the conditions of hypercatabolism and tissue necrosis that characterize these patients, large amounts of potassium may be generated and accumulate during a short period of time. Acute hyperkalemia causes a decrease in cardiac excitability, which can ultimately result in asystole. The removal of potassium must be accomplished with RRT or ion exchange resins. Other electrolyte abnormalities, such as hyponatremia, hyperphosphatemia, hypocalcemia, and metabolic acidosis, are common in ARF and must be monitored closely. Treatment consists of appropriate additions or restrictions of intravenous solutions and effective use of RRT.

Platelet dysfunction and coagulopathy are often associated with ARF. A reproducible platelet defect can be demonstrated experimentally with a BUN of 100 mg/dL. This defect can be transiently reversed with administration of desmopressin (DDAVP). Platelet transfusion in this clinical setting will be ineffective because the transfused platelets will rapidly acquire the same dysfunction at the patient's platelets. Anemia also accompanies ARF in surgical patients. In addition to the loss of blood during hemorrhage or operation, the production of erythropoietin has been shown to decrease in direct proportion to the decrease in renal function.

Nutritional Support in Acute Renal Failure

The goal of nutritional support in ARF is to provide optimal amounts of calorie and protein substrates to minimize

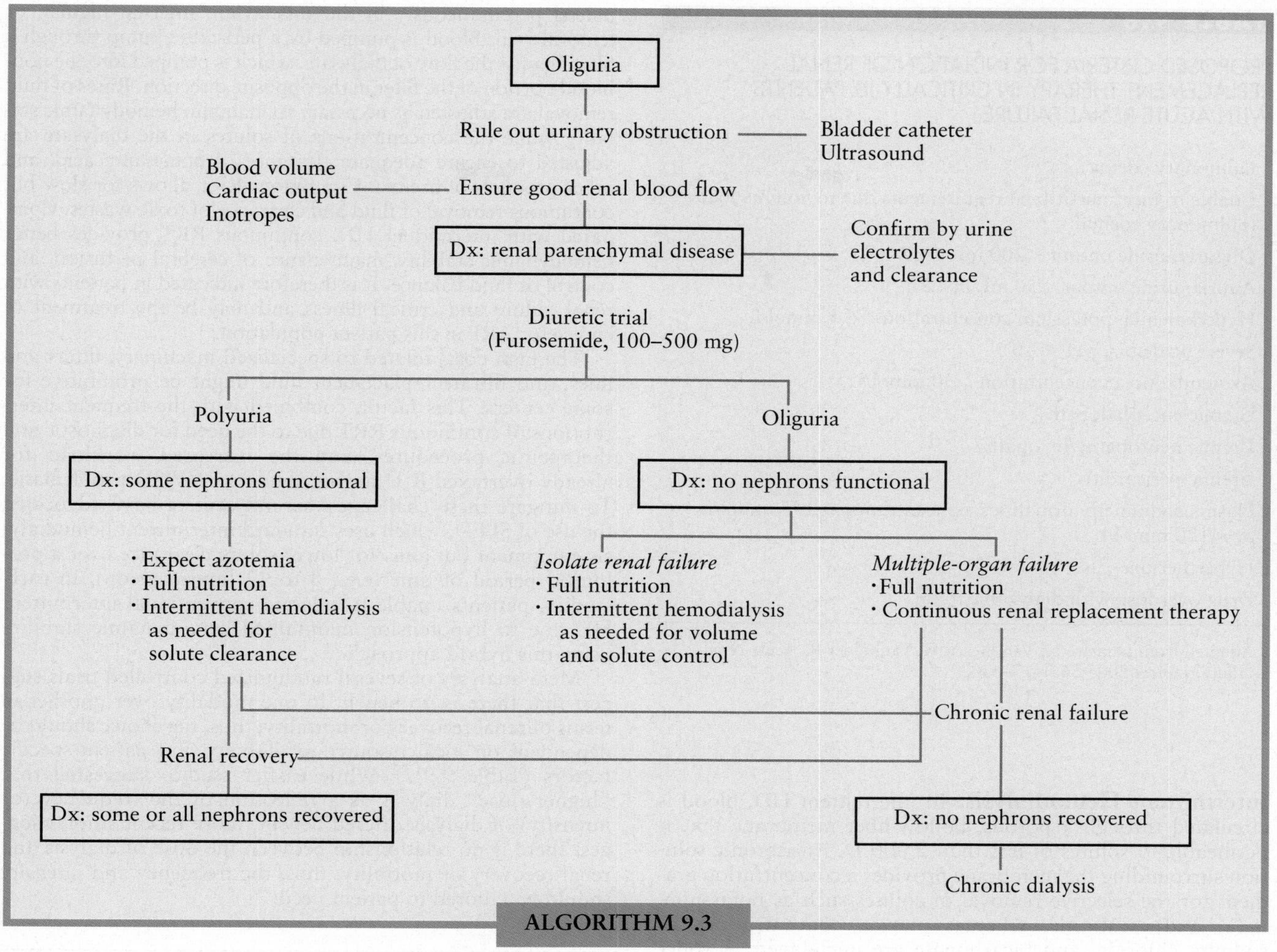

ALGORITHM 9.3. Management of acute renal failure. CAVH, continuous arteriovenous hemofiltration; CAVHD, continuous arteriovenous hemodialysis; PD, peritoneal dialysis.

autocatabolism and allow tissue anabolism, wound healing, and sustained immune function. In any discussion of nutrition and renal failure, it is necessary to point out the distinction between acute and chronic renal failure. Patients with chronic renal failure are generally healthy, and their energy requirements differ little from those of persons without chronic renal failure. Protein intake is required only for metabolic turnover and is restricted to minimize the generation of urea and other products of protein metabolism.

By contrast, the metabolic requirements of a patient with ARF are those of a critically ill, hospitalized patient. Actual measurement of resting energy expenditure has shown that the caloric requirements of patients with multiple organ failure and ARF are often 50% above those of normal, healthy subjects. Measured protein requirements may be increased to as much as 2.5 g/kg to provide for anabolic wound healing and sustained immune function. For these patients, protein restriction is counterproductive and potentially detrimental. Urea generation is best minimized by providing enough energy substrates (carbohydrates and lipids) to prevent the cannibalization of endogenous protein as an energy source.

A positive energy balance may also make the management of uremia and hyperkalemia less difficult. When a patient receives fewer calories than those expended, the difference must be made up from endogenous stores. In a well-nourished person, carbohydrate stores rarely exceed 2,500 kcal. After these stores have been depleted, lipid and protein stores are mobilized. In the diseased state, endogenous protein has been shown to be catabolized preferentially as an energy substrate in the absence of readily available glucose. With the catabolism of protein, urea is generated. In addition, catabolic wasting of tissues and cells liberates excess potassium. Maintaining a positive energy balance with glucose and lipids should reduce protein catabolism, urea generation, and hyperkalemia.

Renal Replacement Therapy

Indications for the use of RRT include fluid overload (pulmonary edema, congestive heart failure), hyperkalemia, metabolic acidosis, uremic encephalopathy, coagulopathy, and acute poisoning[69] (Table 9.8). The optimal timing of initiation of therapy has not been definitively established, but it is preferable to begin renal replacement before complications occur. In the only randomized controlled trial to date, there was no improvement in mortality or renal recovery in patients in whom RRT was initiated within 12 hours of developing ARF compared to initiation once conventional indications for dialysis were met.[70]

The three modalities of RRT frequently used in the critical care setting include intermittent HD, continuous RRT, and a recently introduced hybrid modality referred to as sustained low-efficiency dialysis (SLED).[71]

TABLE 9.8

PROPOSED CRITERIA FOR INITIATION OF RENAL REPLACEMENT THERAPY IN CRITICALLY ILL PATIENTS WITH ACUTE RENAL FAILURE

Pulmonary edema
Unable to meet nutritional requirements due to volume load (pulmonary edema)
Oliguria: urine output <200 mL in 12 h
Anuria: urine output <50 mL in 12 h
Hyperkalemia: potassium concentration >6.5 mmol/L
Severe acidemia: pH <7.0
Azotemia: urea concentration >30 mmol/L
Uremic encephalopathy
Uremic neuropathy/myopathy
Uremic pericarditis
Plasma sodium abnormalities: concentration >155 mmol/L or <120 mmol/L
Hyperthermia
Drug overdose with dialyzable toxin

Adapted from Lameire N, Van Biesen W, Vanholder R. Acute renal failure. *Lancet* 2005;365:417–430.

Intermittent Hemodialysis. In intermittent HD, blood is circulated through a porous, hollow-fiber membrane that is permeable to solutes of less than 2,000 D. An isotonic solution surrounding the membrane provides a concentration gradient for the selective removal of solutes such as potassium, urea, and creatinine, whereas plasma concentrations of sodium, chloride, and bicarbonate are unchanged. A roller pump is used to maintain an extracorporeal blood flow of about 300 mL/min through an arteriovenous shunt or a double-lumen venovenous access. The transmembrane pressure gradient created by the pump affects the desired amount of fluid removal. Full systemic anticoagulation is required for this procedure, although less heparin may be used in patients with a baseline coagulopathy. Solute and volume removal with HD is considered very efficient relative to removal with the other methods of renal replacement. This efficiency is reflected in the clearance of water-soluble drugs such as aminoglycosides, cephalosporins, and penicillins. Plasma concentrations may be decreased by as much as 50% per treatment; accordingly, these drugs should be administered after treatments with close monitoring of serum concentrations. HD is also the method of choice for the rapid removal of life-threatening toxins and poisons.

Although the incidence of complications of HD is insignificant in the treatment of patients with chronic renal failure, frequent and often profound complications may occur when it is used to treat critically ill patients with ARF. In the acute setting, HD has been shown to cause hypotension, hypoxemia, and hemolysis and to precipitate cardiac arrhythmia. These events limit the application of HD in patients who are hemodynamically unstable.

Continuous Renal Replacement Therapy. Continuous renal replacement techniques offer the advantage of improved hemodynamic stability with continuous clearance of toxic metabolites and fluid removal. Continuous venovenohemodialysis (CVVHD) is the most commonly used method in the ICU. In this technique, venous access is obtained by means of a temporary double-lumen central venous dialysis catheter, which is placed percutaneously in the subclavian, internal jugular, or femoral vein. Blood is pumped by a peristaltic pump through a filter against the flow of dialysate, which is pumped into the non-blood portion of the filter in the opposite direction. Rates of fluid removal are adjusted as necessary to maintain hemodynamic stability while the concentrations of solutes in the dialysate are adjusted to ensure adequate clearance of potassium, acid, and other products of uremia. Continuous RRT allows for slow but continuous removal of fluid and clearance of toxic wastes. Compared with intermittent HD, continuous RRT provides better hemodynamic stability, maintenance of cerebral perfusion, and control of fluid balance. It is therefore indicated in patients with renal failure and critical illness and may be the treatment of choice for ARF in this patient population.

The high costs related to specialized machinery, filters and lines, and filtrate replacement fluid might be prohibitive for some centers. This factor, combined with the frequent interruptions of continuous RRT due to the need for diagnostic and therapeutic procedures, and the increased workload for already overtaxed ICU nurses, renders CVVHD problematic. To mitigate these challenges, several centers have advocated the use of SLED, which uses standard intermittent hemodialysis equipment but aims for lower solute clearance over a prolonged period of time (e.g., 8 to 12 hours/session). In early studies, patients unable to tolerate conventional intermittent HD due to hypotension maintained hemodynamic stability using this hybrid approach.[71]

Meta-analyses of several randomized controlled trials suggest that there is no benefit to one modality over another in terms of renal recovery or mortality; thus, the choice should be dependent on local resource availability and patient-specific factors (Table 9.9).[72] While earlier studies suggested that "higher dose" dialysis as a reflection of the frequency (or intensity) of dialysis offered benefit, more recent studies suggest there is no relationship between the dose of dialysis and renal recovery or mortality; thus, the frequency and intensity should be tailored to patient need.[73]

Prognosis in Acute Renal Failure

The survival of patients with ARF depends on the successful treatment of the primary disease causing renal failure. The anephric patient supported with RRT survives until disease of some other organ system supervenes. The mortality among patients with multiple organ failure dependent on RRT ranges from 50% to 90%.

For patients who survive the acute phase of illness, the recovery of renal function after ARF depends on the type and extent of injury to the renal parenchyma. RRT may be required for several weeks until urine output and solute excretion return to acceptable levels. If renal function has not returned after 6 weeks, recovery is unlikely, and provisions should be made for long-term renal substitution therapy. In most studies, approximately 70% of survivors will require long-term renal replacement.

PROGNOSTICATION AND INTENSIVE CARE UNIT OUTCOME

8 The critical care environment is filled with an abundance of data. Data are collected at the time of admission and almost daily, allowing repeated assessment of physiologic status over time. This data-rich environment has led to the development of scoring systems that provide information regarding the likelihood of survival based on information available early during the course of the ICU stay. Many systems that have been developed focus not on prognosticating survival but rather on the

TABLE 9.9

ADVANTAGES OF INTERMITTENT HEMODIALYSIS AND CONTINUOUS RENAL REPLACEMENT THERAPY

■ INTERMITTENT HEMODIALYSIS	■ CONTINUOUS RENAL REPLACEMENT THERAPY
Advantages	
Lower risk of systemic bleeding	Better hemodynamic stability
Facilitates transport for other interventions	Fewer cardiac arrhythmias
More suitable for severe hyperkalemia	Improved nutritional support
Lower cost	Better pulmonary gas exchange
	Better fluid control
Disadvantages	
Availability of dialysis staff	Greater vascular access problems
More difficult hemodynamic control	Higher risk of systemic bleeding
Inadequate dialysis dose (frequency)	Long-term immobilization of patient
Inadequate fluid control	More filter problems (rupture, clotting)
Inadequate nutritional support	Greater cost
Not suitable for patients with intracranial hypertension	
No removal of cytokines (theoretical)	
Potential complement activation by nonbiocompatible membranes	

Adapted from Lameire N, Van Biesen W, Vanholder R. Acute renal failure. *Lancet* 2005;365:417–430.

assessment of potential outcome, typically in the degree of organ dysfunction. The differences in these two approaches are highlighted in Table 9.10.

Prognostic Scoring Systems

Prognostic scores were developed to maximize their predictive capacity. The APACHE, the simplified acute physiology score (SAPS II), and the mortality prediction model (MPM) systems constitute the three most widely used prognostic models.[74–76] Each model assumes that mortality will be influenced by extreme physiologic derangement that occurs early in the course of the illness and before optimal resuscitation. Each uses data that are available early in the ICU admission to construct a composite severity of illness measure.

The most frequently utilized prognostic score is the APACHE II system, consisting of data derived from 12 physiologic variables, age, and chronic health status, yielding a score of 0 to 71. Major limitations of this system include the fact that risk predictions are based on outcomes of treatment from 1979 to 1982; the system was not designed to predict

TABLE 9.10

SCORING SYSTEMS IN THE ICU

	■ PROGNOSTIC SCALES: SEVERITY OF ILLNESS	■ OUTCOME MEASURES: ORGAN DYSFUNCTION SCALES
Uses	Prognostication; risk stratification	Outcome prediction; evaluation of clinical course over time
Timing of ascertainment	Early during ICU stay	Following resuscitation; at any time during ICU stay
Selection of variables	Physiologic measures	Measures of physiology or therapeutic response
	Worst values	Stable, representative values
	Selected to maximize predictive capacity	Selected to reflect clinical construct
Calibration	Maximize prediction	Maximize description

ICU, intensive care unit.
From Marshall JC. Risk prediction and outcome description in critical surgical illness. In: Norton JA, Bollinger RR, eds. *Surgery Basic Science and Clinical Evidence*. New York: Springer Verlag; 2001:306.

TABLE 9.11

ORGAN DYSFUNCTION SCORING: THE MARSHALL MULTIPLE ORGAN DYSFUNCTION SCORE

ORGAN SYSTEM	0	1	2	3	4
Respiratory (PaO_2/FiO_2)	>300	226–300	151–225	76–150	≤75
Renal (serum creatinine, mg/dL)	≤1.1	1.2–2.3	2.4–3.9	4.0–5.6	>5.7
Hepatic (serum bilirubin, mg/dL)	≤1.1	1.2–3.5	3.6–7.1	7.2–14.1	>14.2
Cardiovascular (PAR[a])	≤10.0	10.1–15.0	15.1–20.0	20.1–30.0	>30.0
Hematologic (platelet count $\times 10^{-3}$)	>120	81–120	51–80	21–50	≤20
Neurologic (Glasgow Coma Scale score)	15	13–14	10–12	7–9	≤6

[a]Adapted from Marshall JC, Cook DJ, Christou NV, et al. Multiple organ dysfunction score: a reliable descriptor of a complex clinical outcome. *Crit Care Med* 1995;23:1638.

outcome for individual patients; and there is lead time bias—unless all admissions were entered at the same time in the course of the patient's illness, there will be errors in prediction. APACHE III is a more recent model and is derived from information on 17 variables.[77] APACHE III is proprietary and has not been widely adopted.

SAPS II is composed of 17 variables, which include 12 physiologic variables, age, type of admission (medical, surgical, scheduled surgical, unscheduled surgical), and variables that are related to specific underlying diseases. The MPM is less based on physiology than APACHE II or SAPS and was designed to measure mortality risk at 24 and 48 hours after ICU admission. This longer time interval provides a revised risk based on patient response to resuscitation and early treatment. There are minor differences across these prognostic measures in terms of their predictive capacity, but there are no data to support that one offers significant improvement over another. Pertinent to the discussion on futility, these severity of illness systems provide only estimates of mortality. For example, a mortality estimate of 75% means that approximately 75 of 100 patients with this probability would be expected to die, but it is not possible to ascertain whether any specific, individual patient will be 1 of the 75 patients that dies or 1 of the 25 that lives.

Outcome Measures

Organ failure is a relatively frequent occurrence in critically ill patients and has resulted in attempts to describe and quantify organ dysfunction. This is a difficult process because organ failure is dynamic and represents a broad spectrum of disease. Which organ systems to include and which measures one should use to quantitate organ dysfunction remain controversial. Most scores focus on six organ systems: respiratory, cardiovascular, hematologic, central nervous system, renal, and hepatic. These outcome measures have conceptual appeal for several reasons. First, they provide an estimate of baseline severity for entry into clinical trials, whereas serial evaluation might provide information on mortality risk. With these organ dysfunction measures, the burden of disease experienced by the patient throughout the course of ICU stay is captured. By contrast, with prognostic scoring systems there is but an early snapshot of the patient's physiologic status, whereas information regarding the remainder of the patient's course is lost.

The most commonly used outcome measures include the Sequential Organ Failure Assessment (SOFA) Score and the Multiple Organ Dysfunction (MOD) Score or Marshall Score, both of which capture data on the six aforementioned systems[78,79] (Table 9.11). A Marshall score of greater than or equal to 4 (≥6 in select studies) is used to indicate MOD. By contrast, posttraumatic multiple organ failure is often assessed using a discrete scoring system limited to only four organ systems (also known as the Denver Score).[80] Hematologic dysfunction and neurologic dysfunction are not captured, likely due to the frequency of coagulopathy and traumatic brain injury, which relate to the initial injury rather than the development of organ dysfunction. A Denver Score of greater than or equal to 4 is indicative of MOD. Like the prognostic scoring systems, no single measure of organ dysfunction is superior or predictive in the individual patient.

ETHICS IN THE INTENSIVE CARE UNIT

The availability of advanced technologies to prolong life in the ICU has resulted in a number of controversies centered on their appropriate use. The controversies have developed under the guise of the technologic imperative, implying that the availability of technology requires that this technology be used. To counter the technologic imperative, physicians have often invoked the concept of futility to limit its inappropriate use, resulting in confusion and, at times, conflict when caring for critically ill patients.

In the strictest sense, true medical futility occurs rarely and signifies interventions that simply should not be offered. For example, we do not offer ongoing medical care to a patient who meets criteria for brain death. The majority of interventions that physicians judge to be futile are not truly futile. They should more accurately be considered inadvisable or inappropriate because the chances of achieving the intended goal are exceedingly low, their benefits are controversial, or their costs are excessively great. Implicit in this definition is a clear understanding of the real or perceived therapeutic endpoint; that is, it is meaningless to say an intervention is futile without specifying the goal of the intended therapy. Conflicts arise when there are disagreements about the intended goal, whether the desired goal is appropriate, and whether the probability of success is sufficiently great. In this sense, there are both qualitative (value-driven) and quantitative (probabilistic) aspects to the understanding and application of futility in the ICU.

Quantitative futility describes a clinical situation in which the application of an intervention has a very low probability of producing a satisfactory outcome—usually survival. There have been a large number of prognostic scoring systems developed to compare outcomes in large groups of patients.

Although these scoring systems were not devised to predict outcome in individual patients, there has been some effort on the part of physicians to adapt these measures for this purpose. In effect, if the probability of survival is below a certain threshold, the intervention might be considered futile or inadvisable and not instituted. Physicians are not very capable at assigning an estimated probability of outcome for an individual patient. Further, this threshold varies across physicians and patients, making decisions based on quantitative futility difficult.

Qualitative futility describes the clinical situation in which the outcome is survival but with an unsatisfactory quality of life. Excellent examples of qualitative futility include patients in a persistent vegetative state or patients dependent on intensive medical care. Conflict arises when what is defined as unsatisfactory for one party might be acceptable for the other. For example, the family of a critically ill, severely debilitated elderly stroke patient might consider the maintenance of life of greatest importance, whereas the physicians believe that given the expected quality of life, further care would be futile.

Inappropriate declarations of futility are common; we rarely can predict with absolute certainty whether a patient will survive his or her ICU stay. In effect, we offer opinions colored by our own values, not objective data. The tendencies to frame value judgments as medical decisions based on such data are inappropriate. Therapeutic interventions should be directed not toward eliciting a desired physiologic effect but toward an agreed on goal that is consistent with the wishes of the patient while maintaining professional integrity. Failure to reach the prespecified goal renders the treatment futile. In one study of patients with an expected probability of death of greater than 95%, only 20% of patients had advance directives to guide care, leading to a lack of clarity of what the intended goal might be.[81] Further, 15% of families had unrealistic expectations regarding survival. In this latter group, rates of resource utilization (transfusion, advanced imaging modalities, dialysis, surgery) were significantly greater than patients whose families did not have unrealistic expectations. These data suggest that the families influenced the caregivers to use resources more extensively than would have been the case otherwise. In situations such as these, intensivists should consider the use of ethics consultations when the goals cannot be agreed on or when confusion exists. Consultation with an ethicist is not to decide the answer but to receive input from an impartial individual who often brings a fresh approach to a difficult situation. In one randomized controlled trial, the use of ethics consultations shortened the duration of ICU stay and reduced the use of life-sustaining treatments without altering overall mortality.[82] In this study, the majority of physicians, nurses, and patients/surrogates agreed that ethics consultations in the ICU were helpful in addressing treatment conflicts.

References

1. Brilli RJ, Spevetz A, Branson RD, et al. Critical care delivery in the intensive care unit: defining clinical roles and the best practice model. *Crit Care Med* 2001;29:2007–2019.
2. Ghorra S, Reinert SE, Cioffi W, et al. Analysis of the effect of conversion from open to closed surgical intensive care unit. *Ann Surg* 1999;229: 163–171.
3. Hanson CW III, Deutschman CS, Anderson HL III, et al. Effects of an organized critical care service on outcomes and resource utilization: a cohort study. *Crit Care Med* 1999;27:270–274.
4. Pronovost PJ, Jenckes MW, Dorman T, et al. Organizational characteristics of intensive care units related to outcomes of abdominal aortic surgery. *JAMA* 1999;281:1310–1317.
5. Pronovost PJ, Angus DC, Dorman T, et al. Physician staffing patterns and clinical outcomes in critically ill patients: a systematic review. *JAMA* 2002;288:2151–2162.
6. Haupt MT, Bekes CE, Brilli RJ, et al. Guidelines on critical care services and personnel: recommendations based on a system of categorization of three levels of care. *Crit Care Med* 2003;31:2677–2683.
7. Talmor D, Shapiro N, Greenberg D, et al. When is critical care medicine cost-effective? A systematic review of the cost-effectiveness literature. *Crit Care Med* 2006;34:2738–2747.
8. Halpern NA, Pastores SM, Greenstein RJ. Critical care medicine in the United States 1985–2000: an analysis of bed numbers, use, and costs. *Crit Care Med* 2004;32:1254–1259.
9. Bendjelid K, Romand JA. Fluid responsiveness in mechanically ventilated patients: a review of indices used in intensive care. *Intensive Care Med* 2003;29:352–360.
10. Coudray A, Romand JA, Treggiari M, et al. Fluid responsiveness in spontaneously breathing patients: a review of indexes used in intensive care. *Crit Care Med* 2005;33:2757–2762.
11. Marik PE, Baram M, Vahid B. Does central venous pressure predict fluid responsiveness? A systematic review of the literature and the tale of seven mares. *Chest* 2008;134:172–178.
12. Chawla LS, Zia H, Gutierrez G, et al. Lack of equivalence between central and mixed venous oxygen saturation. *Chest* 2004;126:1891–1896.
13. Dueck MH, Klimek M, Appenrodt S, et al. Trends but not individual values of central venous oxygen saturation agree with mixed venous oxygen saturation during varying hemodynamic conditions. *Anesthesiology* 2005; 103:249–257.
14. Cheatham ML, Nelson LD, Chang MC, et al. Right ventricular end-diastolic volume index as a predictor of preload status in patients on positive end-expiratory pressure. *Crit Care Med* 1998;26:1801–1806.
15. Huang CC, Fu JY, Hu HC, et al. Prediction of fluid responsiveness in acute respiratory distress syndrome patients ventilated with low tidal volume and high positive end-expiratory pressure. *Crit Care Med* 2008;36: 2810–2816.
16. Osman D, Ridel C, Ray P, et al. Cardiac filling pressures are not appropriate to predict hemodynamic response to volume challenge. *Crit Care Med* 2007;35:64–68.
17. Harvey S, Harrison DA, Singer M, et al. Assessment of the clinical effectiveness of pulmonary artery catheters in management of patients in intensive care (PAC-Man): a randomised controlled trial. *Lancet* 2005;366: 472–477.
18. Richard C, Warszawski J, Anguel N, et al. Early use of the pulmonary artery catheter and outcomes in patients with shock and acute respiratory distress syndrome: a randomized controlled trial. *JAMA* 2003;290: 2713–2720.
19. Connors AF, Speroff T, Dawson NV, et al. The effectiveness of right heart catheterization in the initial care of critically ill patients. *JAMA* 1996;276:889–897.
20. Rhodes A, Cusack RJ, Newman PJ, et al. A randomised, controlled trial of the pulmonary artery catheter in critically ill patients. *Intensive Care Med* 2002;28:256–264.
21. Wiener RS, Welch HG. Trends in the use of the pulmonary artery catheter in the United States, 1993–2004. *JAMA* 2007;298:423–429.
22. Michard F, Teboul JL. Using heart-lung interactions to assess fluid responsiveness during mechanical ventilation. *Crit Care* 2000;4:282–289.
23. Marik PE, Cavallazzi R, Vasu T, et al. Dynamic changes in arterial waveform derived variables and fluid responsiveness in mechanically ventilated patients: a systematic review of the literature. *Crit Care Med* 2009;37: 2642–2647.
24. Feissel M, Michard F, Mangin I, et al. Respiratory changes in aortic blood velocity as an indicator of fluid responsiveness in ventilated patients with septic shock. *Chest* 2001;2001:867–873.
25. Valtier B, Cholley BP, Belot JP, et al. Noninvasive monitoring of cardiac output in critically ill patients using transesophageal Doppler. *Am J Respir Crit Care Med* 1998;158:77–83.
26. Bein B, Meybohm P, Cavus E, et al. The reliability of pulse contour-derived cardiac output during hemorrhage and after vasopressor administration. *Anesth Analg* 2007;105:107–113.
27. Compton FD, Zukunft B, Hoffmann C, et al. Performance of a minimally invasive uncalibrated cardiac output monitoring system (Flotrac/Vigileo) in haemodynamically unstable patients. *Br J Anaesth* 2008;100:451–456.
28. Cooper ES, Muir WW. Continuous cardiac output monitoring via arterial pressure waveform analysis following severe hemorrhagic shock in dogs. *Crit Care Med* 2007;35:1724–1729.
29. Gattinoni L, Caironi P, Pelosi P, et al. What has computed tomography taught us about the acute respiratory distress syndrome? *Am J Respir Crit Care Med* 2001;164:1701–1711.
30. Bernard GR, Artigas A, Brigham KL, et al. The American-European consensus conference on ARDS. Definitions, mechanisms, relevant outcomes, and clinical trial coordination. *Am J Respir Crit Care Med* 1994;149: 818–824.
31. The Acute Respiratory Distress Syndrome Network. Ventilation with lower tidal volumes as compared with traditional tidal volumes for acute lung injury and the acute respiratory distress syndrome. *N Engl J Med* 2000; 342:1301–1308.
32. Brower RG, Lanken PN, MacIntyre N, et al. Higher versus lower positive end-expiratory pressures in patients with the acute respiratory distress syndrome. *N Engl J Med* 2004;351:327–336.
33. Albert RK, Hubmayr RD. The prone position eliminates compression of the lungs by the heart. *Am J Respir Crit Care Med* 2000;161:1660–1665.
34. Sud S, Sud M, Friedrich JO, et al. Effect of mechanical ventilation in the prone position on clinical outcomes in patients with acute hypoxemic respiratory failure: a systematic review and meta-analysis. *CMAJ* 2008;178: 1153–1161.
35. Chan KP, Stewart TE, Mehta S. High-frequency oscillatory ventilation for adult patients with ARDS. *Chest* 2007;131:1907–1916.

SCIENTIFIC PRINCIPLES

36. Derdak S, Mehta S, Stewart TE, et al. High-frequency oscillatory ventilation for acute respiratory distress syndrome in adults: a randomized, controlled trial. *Am J Resp Crit Care Med* 2002;166:801–808.
37. Ely EW, Baker AM, Dunagan DP, et al. Effect on the duration of mechanical ventilation of identifying patients capable of breathing spontaneously. *N Engl J Med* 1996;335:1864–1869.
38. Esteban A, Alia I, Tobin MJ, et al. Effect of spontaneous breathing trial duration on outcome of attempts to discontinue mechanical ventilation. Spanish Lung Failure Collaborative Group. *Am J Respir Crit Care Med* 1999;159:512–518.
39. Esteban A, Frutos F, Tobin MJ, et al. A comparison of four methods of weaning patients from mechanical ventilation. Spanish Lung Failure Collaborative Group. *N Engl J Med* 1995;332:345–350.
40. MacIntyre NR, Cook DJ, Ely EW Jr, et al. Evidence-based guidelines for weaning and discontinuing ventilatory support: a collective task force facilitated by the American College of Chest Physicians; the American Association for Respiratory Care; and the American College of Critical Care Medicine. *Chest* 2001;120:375S–395S.
41. Corwin HL, Gettinger A, Pearl RG, et al. The CRIT Study: anemia and blood transfusion in the critically ill—current clinical practice in the United States. *Crit Care Med* 2004;32:39–52.
42. Corwin HL, Parsonnet KC, Gettinger A. RBC transfusion in the ICU. Is there a reason? *Chest* 1995;108:767–771.
43. Silverman HJ, Tuma P. Gastric tonometry in patients with sepsis. Effects of dobutamine infusions and packed red blood cell transfusions. *Chest* 1992; 102:184–188.
44. Marik PE, Sibbald WJ. Effect of stored-blood transfusion on oxygen delivery in patients with sepsis. *JAMA* 1993;269:3024–3029.
45. Napolitano LM, Corwin HL. Efficacy of red blood cell transfusion in the critically ill. *Crit Care Clin* 2004;20:255–268.
46. Marik PE, Corwin HL. Efficacy of red blood cell transfusion in the critically ill: a systematic review of the literature. *Crit Care Med* 2008;36: 2667–2674.
47. Sarani B, Dunkman WJ, Dean L, et al. Transfusion of fresh frozen plasma in critically ill surgical patients is associated with an increased risk of infection. *Crit Care Med* 2008;36:1114–1118.
48. Gajic O, Dzik WH, Toy P. Fresh frozen plasma and platelet transfusion for nonbleeding patients in the intensive care unit: benefit or harm? *Crit Care Med* 2006;34:S170–S173.
49. Hebert PC, Wells G, Blajchman MA, et al. A multicenter, randomized controlled clinical trial of transfusion requirements in critical care. *N Engl J Med* 1999;340:409–417.
50. Hebert PC, Blajchman MA, Cook DJ, et al. Do blood transfusions improve outcomes related to mechanical ventilation? *Chest* 2001;119:1850–1857.
51. Hebert PC, Yetisir E, Martin C, et al. Is a low transfusion threshold safe in critically ill patients with cardiovascular diseases? *Crit Care Med* 2001;29: 227–234.
52. Corwin HL, Gettinger A, Pearl RG, et al. Efficacy of recombinant human erythropoietin in critically ill patients: a randomized controlled trial. *JAMA* 2002;288:2827–2835.
53. Zarychanski R, Turgeon AF, McIntyre L, et al. Erythropoietin-receptor agonists in critically ill patients: a meta-analysis of randomized controlled trials. *CMAJ* 2007;177:725–734.
54. Shermock KM, Horn E, Lipsett PA, et al. Number needed to treat and cost of recombinant human erythropoietin to avoid one transfusion-related adverse event in critically ill patients. *Crit Care Med* 2005;33:497–503.
55. Battistella FD, Widergren JT, Anderson JT, et al. A prospective, randomized trial of intravenous fat emulsion administration in trauma victims requiring total parenteral nutrition. *J Trauma* 1997;43:52–58.
56. Nathens AB, Neff MJ, Jurkovich GJ, et al. Randomized, prospective trial of antioxidant supplementation in critically ill surgical patients. *Ann Surg* 2002;236:814–822.
57. Marik PE, Zaloga GP. Early enteral nutrition in acutely ill patients: a systematic review. *Crit Care Med* 2001;29:2264–2270.
58. Montejo JC, Grau T, Acosta J, et al. Multicenter, prospective, randomized, single-blind study comparing the efficacy and gastrointestinal complications of early jejunal feeding with early gastric feeding in critically ill patients. *Crit Care Med* 2002;30:796–800.
59. Heyland DK, Novak F, Drover JW, et al. Should immunonutrition become routine in critically ill patients? A systematic review of the evidence. *JAMA* 2001;286:944–953.
60. Montejo JC, Zarazaga A, Lopez-Martinez J, et al. Immunonutrition in the intensive care unit. A systematic review and consensus statement. *Clin Nutr* 2003;22:221–233.
61. Van den Berghe G, Wouters P, Weekers F, et al. Intensive insulin therapy in the critically ill patients. *N Engl J Med* 2001;345:1359–1367.
62. Griesdale DE, de Souza RJ, van Dam RM, et al. Intensive insulin therapy and mortality among critically ill patients: a meta-analysis including NICE-SUGAR study data. *CMAJ* 2009;180:821–827.
63. Finfer S, Chittock DR, Su SY, et al. Intensive versus conventional glucose control in critically ill patients. *N Engl J Med* 2009;360:1283–1297.
64. Bellomo R, Ronco C, Kellum JA, et al. Acute renal failure – definition, outcome measures, animal models, fluid therapy and information technology needs: the Second International Consensus Conference of the Acute Dialysis Quality Initiative (ADQI) Group. *Crit Care* 2004;8:R204–R212.
65. Ostermann M, Chang RW. Acute kidney injury in the intensive care unit according to RIFLE. *Crit Care Med* 2007;35:1837–1843.
66. Bosch X, Poch E, Grau JM. Rhabdomyolysis and acute kidney injury. *N Engl J Med* 2009;361:62–72.
67. Pannu N, Wiebe N, Tonelli M. Prophylaxis strategies for contrast-induced nephropathy. *JAMA* 2006;295:2765–2779.
68. Hogan SE, L'Allier P, Chetcuti S, et al. Current role of sodium bicarbonate-based preprocedural hydration for the prevention of contrast-induced acute kidney injury: a meta-analysis. *Am Heart J* 2008;156:414–421.
69. Lameire N, Van Biesen W, Vanholder R. Acute renal failure. *Lancet* 2005; 365:417–430.
70. Bouman CS, Oudemans-Van Straaten HM, Tijssen JG, et al. Effects of early high-volume continuous venovenous hemofiltration on survival and recovery of renal function in intensive care patients with acute renal failure: a prospective, randomized trial. *Crit Care Med* 2002;30:2205–2211.
71. Marshall MR, Golper TA, Shaver MJ, et al. Sustained low-efficiency dialysis for critically ill patients requiring renal replacement therapy. *Kidney Int* 2001;60:777–785.
72. Rabindranath K, Adams J, Macleod AM, et al. Intermittent versus continuous renal replacement therapy for acute renal failure in adults. *Cochrane Database Syst Rev* 2007;(3)CD003773.
73. Palevsky PM, Zhang JH, O'Connor TZ, et al. Intensity of renal support in critically ill patients with acute kidney injury. *N Engl J Med* 2008;359: 7–20.
74. Knaus WA, Draper EA, Wagner DP, et al. APACHE II: a severity of disease classification system. *Crit Care Med* 1985;13:818–829.
75. Lemeshow S, Teres D, Klar J, et al. Mortality probability models (MPM II) based on an international cohort of intensive care unit patients. *JAMA* 1993;270:2478–2486.
76. Le G Jr, Lemeshow S, Saulnier F. A new Simplified Acute Physiology Score (SAPS II) based on a European/North American multicenter study. *JAMA* 1993;270:2957–2963.
77. Knaus WA, Wagner DP, Draper EA, et al. The APACHE III prognostic scoring system. *Chest* 1991;100:1619–1636.
78. Vincent JL, Moreno R, Takala J, et al. The SOFA (Sepsis-related Organ Failure Assessment) score to describe organ dysfunction/failure. On behalf of the Working Group on Sepsis-Related Problems of the European Society of Intensive Care Medicine. *Intensive Care Med* 1996;22:707–710.
79. Marshall JC, Cook DJ, Christou NV, et al. Multiple organ dysfunction score: a reliable descriptor of a complex clinical outcome. *Crit Care Med* 1995;23:1638–1652.
80. Sauaia A, Moore FA, Moore EE, et al. Early predictors of postinjury multiple organ failure. *Arch Surg* 1994;129:39–45.
81. Berge KH, Maiers DR, Schreiner DP, et al. Resource utilization and outcome in gravely ill intensive care unit patients with predicted in-hospital mortality rates of 95% or higher by APACHE III scores: the relationship with physician and family expectations. *Mayo Clin Proc* 2005;80: 166–173.
82. Schneiderman LJ, Gilmer T, Teetzel HD, et al. Effect of ethics consultations on nonbeneficial life-sustaining treatments in the intensive care setting: a randomized controlled trial. *JAMA* 2003;290:1166–1172.

CHAPTER 10 ■ FLUIDS, ELECTROLYTES, AND ACID–BASE BALANCE

RICHARD B. WAIT AND REGINALD ALOUIDOR

KEY POINTS

1. The human body is conceptualized as composed of at least four compartments: water, protein, fat, and bone ash.
2. Sodium (extracellular fluid [ECF]) and potassium (intracellular fluid [ICF]) are the dominant cations and, whereas composition varies between ECF and ICF, overall concentration of solutes in these fluids is identical.
3. Osmolality is kept constant by tight regulation of water balance by osmoreceptor-induced control of antidiuretic hormone and thirst.
4. Effective circulating volume is sensed by volume receptors (capacitance vessels, atria, hepatic, and central nervous system) and pressure receptors (aortic arch, carotid, and intrarenal) that alter sodium and water balance mediated by renin-angiotensin, aldosterone, atrial natriuretic peptide, dopamine, and renal prostaglandins.
5. Water losses involve both sensible (measurable) via urine, stool, and sweat and insensible (unmeasurable) via evaporative loss from both the skin and respiratory tract.
6. Goals of fluid therapy are to normalize hemodynamic parameters and body fluid electrolyte concentrations and can be achieved with crystalloids (preferable) or colloids, both correcting deficits and matching ongoing or expected losses.
7. The major cations (Na^+, K^+, Ca^{2+}, and Mg^{2+}) should be monitored and replaced, recognizing unique distributions and impact of various diseases.
8. Acid–base balance is carefully buffered within very narrow limits. Acid–base disturbance and compensation are frequently mixed, involving respiratory and metabolic-renal responses.

A thorough understanding of fluid and electrolyte composition and management is essential to the effective care of surgical and critically ill patients. Disease- and injury-related alterations in fluid volume and electrolyte physiology are complex and cannot be fully understood without first understanding normal physiologic mechanisms of fluid and electrolyte homeostasis, inclusive of acid–base balance considerations. In this chapter, these mechanisms are reviewed and used as a starting point for presentation of fluid and electrolyte pathophysiology and management of specific clinical situations.

BODY FLUIDS

Total Body Water and Body Fluid Compartments

1 Traditionally, most scientists used a two-compartment model of tissues within the body: the fat compartment and the fat-free or lean tissue compartment. Over the past 20 years, technology has added significantly to our knowledge of body composition, and more complex models have been developed, the simplest of which is the four-compartment model. In this model, the fat-free mass is actually composed of three separate compartments: water, protein, and bone ash. The remaining compartment is fat, which is considered to be triglycerides, because adipose tissue, a more general descriptor, also contains small amounts of water. *Total body water* (TBW) is defined as the total volume of water within the body. TBW has traditionally been measured using indicator dilution techniques in which radioactive tracers such as deuterium oxide (D_2O) were given to subjects and a steady state allowed to develop before measurements of the D_2O in the plasma were made. More recently, other techniques have added greatly to our ability to measure TBW content as well as the content of all of the elements within the body such as *neutron activation analysis,* in which the body is exposed to a source of thermal neutrons. These neutrons enter the atomic nuclei, resulting in the transformation of that nucleus to a more activated energy state. This activated state is transient and later returns to the baseline, resulting in energy release from the nucleus in the form of gamma radiation, which can then be measured using whole-body shielded gamma detectors.[1] In recent years multicomponent models of body composition based on dual-energy x-ray absorptiometry (DEXA), computed tomography (CT) scan, and magnetic resonance imaging (MRI) have been developed in order to provide estimates of the various components of the fat-free mass as well as the distribution of the adipose organ. These techniques can be useful when it is expected that the fat-free mass is altered and that the simple two-component model cannot be applied.[2] Using these techniques, total body oxygen, carbon, hydrogen, nitrogen, calcium, phosphorus, sulfur, potassium, sodium, and chlorine can be measured. These measurements, in turn, can be used to calculate steady-state body composition using standard formulas. For example, total body protein can be calculated as total body nitrogen $\times$ 0.625, because 99% of the body's nitrogen is found within protein. More complex mathematical models are needed when calculating the composition of components using elements that are distributed among more than one component of the body (e.g., TBW and fat).

The relationship between TBW and body weight varies according to percentage of body fat. Differences in percent TBW between individuals can generally be accounted for by differences in relative body fat content. Average TBW is 60% of body weight in adult men and 50% in adult women. In infants, water makes up approximately 80% of body weight. This figure decreases to approximately 65% by 1 year of age and continues to decrease slowly throughout life, primarily related to decreases in lean body mass. Estimates of TBW can be empirically adjusted for the obese and thin body habitus. In

TABLE 10.1

BODY FLUID COMPARTMENTS

	■ BODY WEIGHT (%)	■ TOTAL BODY WATER (%)
Total	60	100
Intracellular	40	67
Extracellular	20	33
Intravascular	5	8
Interstitial	15	25
Transcellular	2	4

obesity, estimates of TBW can be decreased by 10% to 20%. In very thin individuals, estimates can be increased by up to 10%.

TBW is distributed into specific compartments in dynamic equilibrium with one another. The principal of these are the intracellular and extracellular compartments (Table 10.1). Intracellular fluid (ICF) makes up approximately two thirds of the TBW, and the remaining one third is composed of extracellular fluid (ECF). The ECF compartment has traditionally been measured using *inulin*, which distributes itself primarily within the ECF. More recently, ECF estimates have been made by measuring the volume of distribution of either bromide or sulfate isotopes, both of which are distributed primarily within the ECF. Using these techniques, ECF volume estimates range from 30% to 33% of TBW, or approximately 20% of body weight.

ICF cannot be measured directly, however, because the majority of potassium within the body resides within the intracellular space; measurements of total body potassium (TBK) can be used to estimate intracellular water. This is accomplished using a technique similar to neutron activation analysis. Normally, potassium within the body exists in two states, nonradioactive ^{39}K and radioactive ^{40}K. Because ^{40}K represents a stable proportion of total K within the body (0.0118%), measurement of the gamma radiation of the ^{40}K radioisotope using the sensing equipment similar to that used in neutron activation analysis can be accomplished. The TBK can then be calculated as TBK (mmol) = $^{40}K/0.000118$.[3] If one knows the size of the ECF compartment and multiplies this by the known quantity of ^{40}K measured in a serum sample, the ICF can then be calculated by subtracting this total from the TBK.

The ECF compartment is subdivided into the intravascular and interstitial spaces. The intravascular space accounts for 25% of the ECF and contains the plasma volume, which is approximately 8% of the TBW or 5% of body weight. Interstitial water volume is calculated as ECF–intravascular space volume and constitutes approximately 25% of TBW, or 15% of body weight. The interstitial space extends from the blood vessels to the cells themselves and includes the complex ground substance making up the acellular tissue matrix. The water in this space exists in free and bound phases. The free phase contains water that is freely exchangeable with intravascular, lymphatic, and intracellular water and that is in a constant state of flux. The bound or *gel* phase is much less freely exchangeable and is composed of water that hydrates matrix materials such as glycosaminoglycans and mucopolysaccharides. The transcellular space, a third and smaller component of ECF, consists of water that is separated from other compartments by endothelial and epithelial barriers, including cerebrospinal, ocular, and synovial fluids, as well as fluid in the gastrointestinal (GI) tract. Under normal circumstances, fluid in the transcellular space is not easily exchangeable with that in other compartments.

Composition of Body Fluids

2 Sodium and potassium are the dominant cations in the body. Sodium is restricted primarily to the ECF and potassium to the ICF. Sodium content in the average adult is approximately 60 mEq/kg. Approximately 25% is confined to bone and is nonexchangeable. Of the exchangeable fraction, approximately 85% is in the ECF. Potassium, calcium, and magnesium make up the remainder of the cations present in the ECF. As mentioned, potassium is the dominant cation in the ICF. TBK is normally approximately 42 mEq/kg, and most of this potassium is intracellular and freely exchangeable. Magnesium and sodium ions also contribute to the cationic component of the ICF. These cations are balanced by phosphate and sulfate anions as well as bicarbonate and intracellular proteins (Table 10.2).

TABLE 10.2

ELECTROLYTE CONCENTRATIONS OF INTRACELLULAR AND EXTRACELLULAR FLUID COMPARTMENTS

	■ EXTRACELLULAR FLUID (mEq/L)		■ INTRACELLULAR FLUID (mEq/L)
	■ PLASMA	■ INTERSTITIAL	
Cations			
Na^+	140	146	12
K^+	4	4	150
Ca^{2+}	5	3	10^{-7}
Mg^{2+}	2	1	7
Anions			
Cl^-	103	114	3
HCO_3^-	24	27	10
SO_4^{2-}	1	1	—
HPO_4^{3-}	2	2	116
Protein	16	5	40
Organic anions	5	5	—

Similarly, ECF cations are in electrochemical balance with chloride, bicarbonate, phosphate, and sulfate anions, although chloride is the major contributor to this balance. In addition, anionic proteins contribute to ion balance in plasma but not in interstitial fluid, which is essentially an ultrafiltrate of plasma that normally contains little protein. As a result, the content of both cations and anions in interstitial fluid is slightly higher than in plasma (see Table 10.2).

The Donnan equilibrium describes the relationship between solutions of permeable and impermeable complex anions when these anions are unevenly distributed across a semipermeable membrane. This special type of equilibrium exists between the ICF and ECF because of the high concentration of protein and nondiffusible phosphates in the cell. Interstitial fluid, by comparison, contains little protein. These impermeable intracellular negative charges tend to favor diffusion of permeant anions into the ECF. The Donnan equilibrium also exists across the capillary endothelial membrane because the concentration of protein is higher on the blood side of the capillary than on the interstitial fluid side. Thus, the concentrations of diffusible ions are not necessarily equal across these membranes because of the presence of these complex anions.

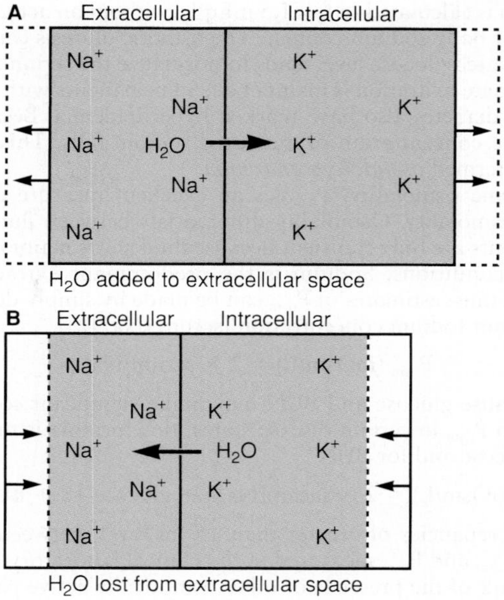

FIGURE 10.1. **A:** The equilibration of water from the extracellular to the intracellular space after the addition of free water to the extracellular fluid compartment. Osmolality transiently decreases in the extracellular compartment, causing water to move across the cell membranes into the intracellular space. **B:** Similar shifts after free water loss from the extracellular compartment. Water moves from the intracellular space to the extracellular space in response to the osmolal gradient that is established.

Concentration of Body Fluids

Despite the difference in composition between the ECF and ICF, the overall concentration of solutes in water in these fluids is identical. Transient concentration differences may develop; however, because water freely equilibrates between compartments, these quickly disappear. The concentration of solutes in the fluid compartments depends on the osmotic activity generated by the ion species contained in each compartment.

Osmotic Activity of Body Fluids

When two solutions are separated by a semipermeable membrane, water moves across the membrane to equalize the concentration of osmotically active particles to which the membrane is impermeable. The maintenance of osmotic equilibrium across a semipermeable membrane is based primarily on the number of solute particles rather than on the molar concentration of the solution on each side of the membrane. The correct measurement to reflect osmotic activity is made by multiplying the molar concentration of the substance by the number of particles into which it can freely dissociate in water. The unit of measurement of osmotically active particles is the osmole (Osm) or milliosmole (mOsm) rather than the conventional units of solute concentration such as milliequivalents per liter (mEq/L). When 1 mol of NaCl dissociates in water to Na^+ and Cl^-, it produces 2 Osm. The same relationship holds true of dissociating salts of multivalent ions such as calcium and magnesium. One mol of a nondissociating molecule, such as glucose, produces 1 Osm (1,000 mOsm). Osmolarity (mOsm/L) and osmolality (mOsm/kg water) define the osmotic activity of particles in solution. The measured osmolality of a solution may not equal the calculated osmolality if the ions do not totally dissociate. The osmotic coefficient of a solution describes the degree to which dissociation of the ions in solution occurs, and can be calculated as follows:

$$\text{Osmotic coefficient} = \text{observed (measured) osmolality/calculated osmolality}$$

Body fluids are aqueous solutions composed of water and various solutes within the different body fluid compartments. Because cells are bounded by a semipermeable membrane, adding free water to the fluid surrounding a cell causes water to move across the cell membrane to equalize the osmolality differential between the intracellular and extracellular compartments. On a larger scale, adding free water to the ECF of the body causes an immediate expansion of the extracellular space, followed by a redistribution of water into the intracellular compartment (Fig. 10.1A). Conversely, loss of free water from the extracellular space ultimately leads to a shift of water from the intracellular to the extracellular space (Fig. 10.1B). An osmotic gradient of just 1 mOsm generates a pressure gradient of 19.3 mm Hg.

Whereas *osmolality* defines the concentration of osmotically active particles in solution, *tonicity* refers to the effect of the particles on cell volume. Permeant solutes can freely cross cell membranes, whereas impermeant solutes cannot. Although permeant solutes contribute to the osmolality of a solution, they have no effect on tonicity because they contribute neither to oncotic gradients across cell membranes nor to alterations in cell volume. Sodium is an example of an impermeant solute that affects both osmolality and tonicity. Urea and ethanol are permeant solutes that contribute to osmolality but have little effect on tonicity because they distribute equally across membranes.

Both impermeant and permeant solutes can contribute to *hyperosmolar* and *hypo-osmolar* states. However, hypo-osmolar states are always accompanied by hypotonicity, whereas hyperosmolar states are not always associated with hypertonicity. There may be marked hyperosmolality without hypertonicity with elevation of blood urea nitrogen (BUN) levels because urea is a freely permeable molecule. In contrast, elevated levels of plasma glucose in diabetic patients are associated with hyperosmolarity and associated hypertonicity. Insulin increases the transport of glucose across cell membranes, rendering these osmoles *ineffective* and reducing hypertonicity. Plasma hyperglycemia is associated with the movement of intracellular water to the extracellular space. This causes expansion of ECF and plasma volume and a consequent decrease in the concentration of plasma sodium. For every 100 mg/dL elevation in blood glucose, measured serum

SCIENTIFIC PRINCIPLES

sodium is calculated to fall 1.5 mEq/L, without an actual alteration of body sodium content. The osmotic diuresis caused by the elevated glucose level tends to normalize the serum sodium if adequate hydration is maintained. Some patients with uncontrolled diabetes also have marked hyperlipidemia. Because of this, the concentration of measured sodium falls. This condition is termed *pseudohyponatremia*.

Plasma osmolality (P_{osm}) is an excellent measure of total body osmolality. Osmolality differentials between fluid compartments are only transient because fluid shifts maintain isosmotic conditions. Sodium is the predominant extracellular cation; thus, estimates of P_{osm} can be made by simply doubling the serum sodium concentration (serum $[Na^+]$):

$$P_{osm}\ (mOsm/L) = 2 \times serum[Na^+]$$

Because glucose and BUN may make significant contributions to P_{osm} in certain disease states, this formula is modified for glucose and for BUN:

$$P_{osm}\ (mOsm/L) = 2 \times serum[Na^+] + glucose/18 + BUN/2.8$$

Discrepancies of greater than 15 mOsm/L between calculated P_{osm} and P_{osm} measured in the clinical laboratory may be the result of the presence of other osmotically active particles, such as mannitol, ethanol, or ethylene glycol, or of a reduced fraction of plasma water secondary to high levels of myeloma proteins or hypertriglyceridemia.

Colloid Oncotic Pressure (Colloid Osmotic Pressure)

Plasma proteins are confined primarily to the intravascular space and contribute to the osmotic pressure developed between the plasma and the interstitial fluid. Normal plasma protein levels of 7 g/dL contribute approximately 0.8 mOsm/L. The van't Hoff equation is used to convert osmolality to osmotic pressure:

$$p = CRT$$

where p = osmotic pressure, C = osmolal solute concentration, R = gas constant, and T = absolute temperature. At body temperature, each milliosmole develops a 19.3-mm Hg pressure gradient; thus, normal plasma protein concentrations generate a colloid oncotic pressure of 15.4 mm Hg (19.3 mm Hg × 0.8 mOsm/L). When measured directly, plasma oncotic pressure equals approximately 24 mm Hg. The difference between the calculated and measured pressures is due to the shift in solute particles caused by the pressure of protein anions on one side of a semipermeable membrane as explained by the Donnan equilibrium.

Osmoregulation

3 Osmolality of body fluids stays fairly constant at approximately 285 to 295 mOsm/L as the result of tightly regulated water balance. Osmoreceptor cells in the paraventricular and supraoptic nuclei of the hypothalamus exert central control over the thirst mechanism and antidiuretic hormone (ADH) secretion from the posterior pituitary. In the presence of excess free water, ECF osmolality falls toward 280 mOsm/kg H_2O, thirst is inhibited, and ADH levels decline. In the absence of ADH, the permeability of renal collecting tubules to water is decreased, causing free water reabsorption to decrease and excretion to increase. Urine osmolality (U_{osm}) can decline to 100 mOsm/kg H_2O (Fig. 10.2). As excess free water is eliminated, P_{osm} begins to rise. Conversely, free water depletion causes an increase in P_{osm}. As P_{osm} approaches 295 mOsm/kg H_2O, thirst is stimulated as is ADH secretion. As ADH levels rise to approximately 5 pg/mL, the renal collecting tubules become maximally permeable to water. Water is reabsorbed from the collecting ducts in response to the concentration gradient developed in the renal medullary interstitium. Thus, the final concentration of urine depends on both the permeability of the collecting ducts (controlled by ADH secretion) and the concentration of the medullary interstitium. Maximal U_{osm} may approach 1,200 mOsm/kg H_2O. The net effect of these mechanisms is to promptly return high or low P_{osm} to normal. The high sensitivity of the osmoreceptors and the responsiveness of the ADH feedback system ensure that even small changes in P_{osm} result in marked alterations in urine concentration. This relation can be expressed as follows:

$$\text{Urine osmolality} = 95 \times \text{plasma osmolality}$$

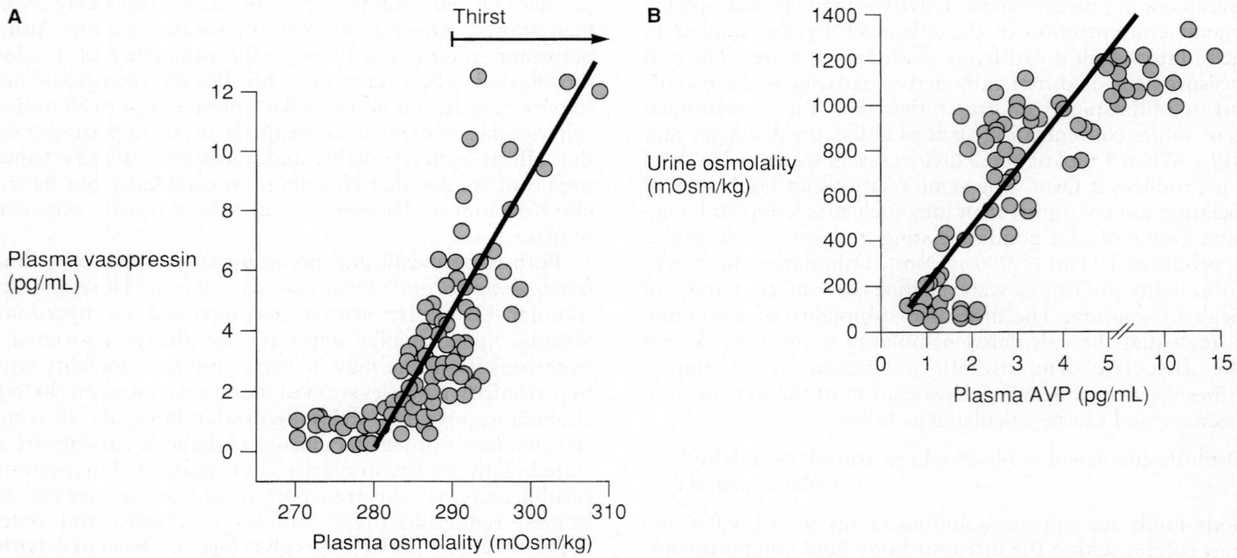

FIGURE 10.2. The relation of plasma antidiuretic hormone (arginine vasopressin, or AVP) secretion to plasma (A) and urine (B) osmolality in healthy adults in varying states of water balance. (Reproduced with permission from Robertson GL, Berl T. Water metabolism. In: Brenner BM, Rector FC Jr, eds. *The Kidney*. Philadelphia, PA: WB Saunders; 1986:392.)

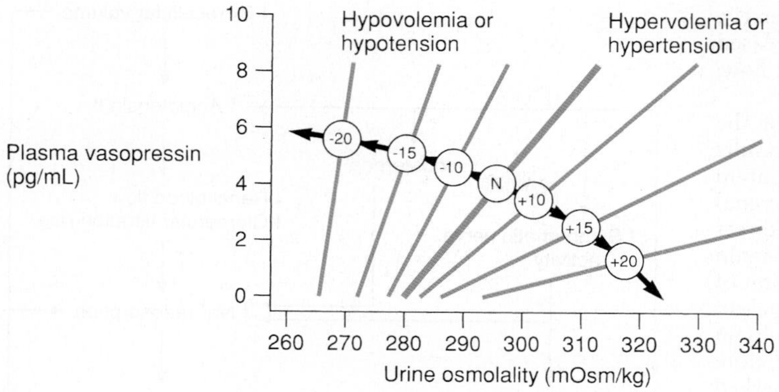

FIGURE 10.3. Effect of acute changes in blood volume or pressure on the osmoregulation of antidiuretic hormone (ADH; vasopressin). The heavy oblique line in the center represents the relation between plasma ADH and osmolality under normovolemic, normotensive conditions. The lines to the left and right show the shift in the relation when blood volume or blood pressure is acutely decreased or increased by the percentage indicated in the circles. (Reproduced with permission from Robertson GL. Physiology of ADH secretion. *Kidney Int* 1987;32(suppl 21):520.)

Thus, a 1-mOsm change in P_{osm} results in a 95-fold change in U_{osm}.

Angiotensin II and neural input from medullary baroreceptors can also influence ADH secretion and thirst, thus tying water balance to hemodynamic alterations. Relatively small changes in pressure have little effect on ADH secretion, but large decreases in pressure can cause tremendous increases in ADH release. Although changes in osmolality tend to have a much greater effect on ADH secretion than do hemodynamic changes, ADH responses to high or low P_{osm} can be profoundly affected by large changes in blood pressure (Fig. 10.3).

FLUID BALANCE

Sodium Concentration and Water Balance

Changes in TBW content are reflected by changes in the extracellular solute concentration. Because sodium is the primary extracellular cation and potassium is the predominant intracellular cation, the serum [Na^+] approximates the sum of the exchangeable total body sodium (Na_e^+) and exchangeable TBK (K_e^+) divided by TBW:

$$\text{Serum}[Na^+] = Na_e^+ + Na_e^+/TBW$$

Because total body solute content ($Na_e^+ + K_e^+$) remains relatively stable over time, changes in TBW content result in inversely proportional changes in serum Na^+ (Fig. 10.4). Thus,

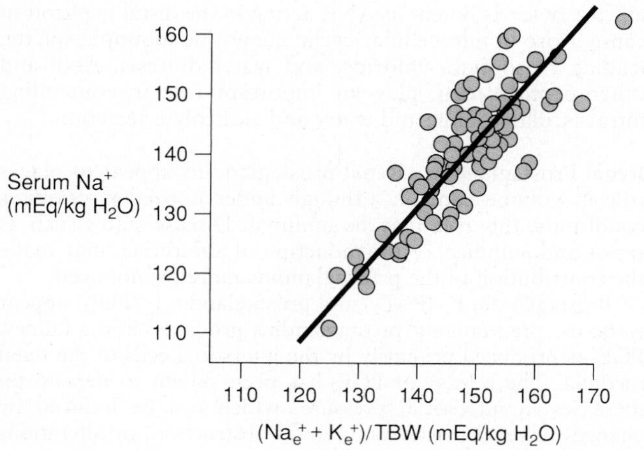

FIGURE 10.4. Relation between serum [Na^+] and the ratio of ($Na_e^+ + K_e^+$) to total body water (TBW). (Reproduced with permission from Edelman IS, Liebman J, O'Meara MP, et al. Interrelationships between serum sodium concentration, serum osmolarity and total exchangeable sodium, total exchangeable potassium and total body water. *J Clin Invest* 1958;37:1236.)

abnormalities in serum sodium are usually an indication of abnormal TBW content.

Volume Control

Changes in volume are detected both by osmoreceptors, which detect changes in P_{osm}, and baroreceptors, which are sensitive to changes in pressure. The osmoreceptors are responsible for the day-to-day fine-tuning of volume, whereas the baroreceptors contribute relatively little to the control of fluid balance under normal conditions.[4] As mentioned previously, large changes in circulating volume (10% to 20% blood volume loss) can modify the osmoregulation of ADH secretion. Cardiac atrial baroreceptors control volume by means of sympathetic and parasympathetic neural mechanisms, whereas atrial natriuretic peptide (ANP) released by atrial myocytes in response to atrial wall distention may influence sodium-linked volume control by inhibition of renal sodium reabsorption.

Baroreceptor Modulation of Volume Control. *Effective circulating volume* describes that portion of the extracellular volume that perfuses the organs of the body and affects the baroreceptors. The effective circulating volume normally corresponds to the intravascular volume. However, in disease states such as congestive heart failure and arteriovenous fistula, where a smaller percentage of intravascular volume than normal is available for organ perfusion, effective circulating volume is reduced.

4 Changes in the effective circulating volume are sensed by volume receptors in the intrathoracic capacitance vessels and atria, pressure receptors of the aortic arch and carotid arteries, intrarenal baroreceptors, and hepatic and cerebrospinal volume receptors. These stretch receptors respond to changes in pressure and circulating volume and, through a complex system of neural and hormonal actions, alter sodium and water balance in the kidneys. Hormonal effects are mediated by the renin-angiotensin system, aldosterone, ANP, dopamine, and the renal prostaglandins.

Baroreceptor Function. The low-pressure baroreceptors of the intrathoracic vena cava and atria are located in vessels that are distensible and not affected by sympathetic stimulation; thus, they are ideally situated to detect changes in venous volume.[5] These receptors send continuous signals through vagal afferent nerves to the cardiovascular control centers of the medulla and hypothalamus, which, in turn, send signals through parasympathetic and sympathetic fibers to the heart and kidneys. Changes in stretch of these vessels result in changes in the frequency of signal output from these receptors. Increases in atrial distention cause decreased nerve signal traffic, which ultimately causes increased sympathetic tone to the heart, which results in tachycardia and inhibition of sympathetic tone to the kidney. This leads to increased renal blood flow and decreased tubular sodium reabsorption. Conversely, low volume in the intrathoracic vessels results in increased sympathetic tone to the kidneys, decreased renal blood flow, and increased sodium reabsorption.

Experimental evidence indicates that stimulation of the sympathetic innervation of renal arterioles and tubules results in decreased renal blood flow and increased tubular sodium reabsorption. The effects of sympathetic activity on renal sodium reabsorption are probably mediated both by direct tubular innervation and by β-adrenergic stimulation of renin production. Whether this effect is crucial to fine regulation of sodium balance under normal physiologic conditions is unclear. Renal denervation in conscious, unstressed animals results in minimal alteration of either blood flow or sodium reabsorption. The effects of renal denervation become much more marked with anesthesia administration or hypotension, suggesting that sympathetic effects on renal function may be important during periods of physiologic stress.

Arterial baroreceptors are located in the aortic arch and carotid arteries. They respond to changes in heart rate, arterial pressure, and the rate of rise in the arterial pressure. Arterial baroreceptors are important during periods in which there are extremes in the changes in arterial pressure characteristics, as occur during hemorrhage. They are probably not involved in controlling subtle volume or pressure changes. In addition to large-vessel baroreceptors, there are arterial baroreceptors in the afferent arterioles of the kidneys. These baroreceptors modulate renin secretion. Increases in transmural pressure cause suppression of renin release, and decreases in transmural pressure stimulate renin release.

Hormonal Mediators of Volume Control

Renin-angiotensin System. Renin is a 40-kD proteolytic enzyme that is released from the juxtaglomerular cells of afferent arterioles in the kidney in response to several stimuli. These include changes in arterial pressure, changes in sodium delivery to the macula densa of the distal convoluted tubule, increases in β-adrenergic activity, and increases in cellular cyclic adenosine monophosphate.

Renin cleaves the decapeptide angiotensin I from circulating angiotensinogen, an α_2-globulin produced by the liver. Angiotensin I is cleaved to the octapeptide angiotensin II by angiotensin-converting enzyme (ACE), which is produced by vascular endothelial cells. One pass through the pulmonary microvasculature converts most angiotensin I to angiotensin II. Angiotensin II acts both locally and systemically to increase vascular tone. It also stimulates catecholamine release from the adrenal medulla, increases sympathetic tone through central effects, and stimulates catecholamine release from sympathetic nerve terminals. Angiotensin II affects sodium reabsorption by decreasing renal blood flow and glomerular filtration. This results in altered tubuloglomerular feedback, the mechanism by which changes in distal tubular NaCl delivery alter glomerular blood flow. Finally, angiotensin II increases sodium reabsorption by direct tubular action as well as by stimulation of aldosterone release from the adrenal cortex. The multiplicity of actions of angiotensin is depicted in Figure 10.5.

Aldosterone. Aldosterone is a mineralocorticoid produced in the zona glomerulosa of the adrenal cortex. Aldosterone increases renal tubular reabsorption of sodium. Aldosterone acts directly on the distal tubule cells by modifying gene expression and stabilizing the epithelial Na^+ channel in the open state and by increasing the number of channels in the apical membrane of these cells.[6] By increasing protein production in these tubular cells, aldosterone induces an influx of sodium, which causes an increase in cellular Na^+-K^+-adenosine triphosphatase activity. The net result is increased sodium reabsorption and increased potassium excretion. Although the primary regulator of aldosterone secretion is angiotensin II, aldosterone release is also stimulated by increased potassium levels, adrenocorticotropic hormone, endothelins, and prostaglandins.

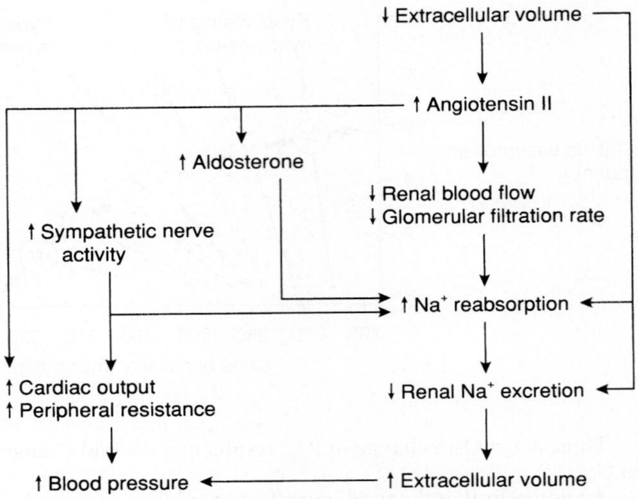

FIGURE 10.5. Multiple effects of increased angiotensin II release in response to the stimulus of decreased extracellular volume.

Atrial and Renal Natriuretic Peptides. ANP is synthesized and released by atrial myocytes in response to atrial wall distention. As mentioned previously, small changes in right atrial pressure produce large increases in plasma levels of ANP.[7,8] There is evidence that ANP has a direct inhibitory effect on renal sodium reabsorption, which is probably maximal at the level of the medullary collecting tubules. Although pharmacologic doses of ANP can cause changes in both renal blood flow and glomerular filtration rate, physiologic levels do not appear to have any major effect on these parameters. Other active fragments of the ANP prohormone have been found to have natriuretic activity. The best described is urodilatin, also known as *renal natriuretic* peptide. Urodilatin is a peptide with ANP-like activity that was first isolated from human urine. It is synthesized and luminally secreted by cortical collecting tubule cells. Like ANP, it is released in the kidney tubules in response to atrial distention and saline loading. It is at least twice as potent as ANP, acting in the distal nephron to cause a rise in intracellular cyclic guanosine monophosphate, leading to sodium, chloride, and water diuresis. ANP and other peptides may play an important role in controlling intravascular volume and water and electrolyte secretion.[9]

Renal Prostaglandins. Renal prostaglandins appear to play a role in volume control, although under normal physiologic conditions, this role may be minimal. Disease states such as sepsis and jaundice, or the induction of anesthesia, may make the contribution of the prostaglandins more pronounced.

Prostaglandin E_2 (PGE_2) and prostaglandin I_2 (PGI_2) appear to be the predominant prostaglandins produced in the kidney. PGE_2 is produced primarily by the interstitial cells of the renal medulla. The release of PGE_2 has been shown to depend on increases in interstitial pressure, which can be induced by changes in renal perfusion, ureteral obstruction, or alterations in oncotic pressure. Under these conditions, PGE_2 increases sodium excretion in the absence of changes in glomerular filtration rate. PGE_2 antagonizes the action of vasopressin (ADH) and inhibits ADH-induced sodium reabsorption along the medullary collecting duct and thick ascending limb. PGI_2 is produced by the glomeruli and endothelial cells of the kidney and is present in the greatest concentrations in the renal cortex. PGI_2 is a vasodilator, and its effects on renal vascular resistance increase both renal blood flow and glomerular filtration rate. PGI_2 production is augmented by increases in angiotensin, catecholamines, and sympathetic tone and may act to counterbalance their vasoconstricting effects. Although under normal physiologic conditions inhibition of prostaglandin production has little effect on renal function, administration of nonsteroidal anti-inflammatory agents, which inhibit cyclooxygenase, to patients with conditions known to cause renal dysfunction (e.g., cirrhosis) can precipitate renal failure, presumably because of loss of the protective effects of the renal prostaglandins.[10]

Endothelins. Endothelins are peptide vasoconstrictors that are involved in volume and pressure regulation. Endothelin is produced and released by endothelial and other cells act on adjacent smooth muscle cells. In addition to increasing peripheral resistance, endothelin infusion has a direct inotropic effect on the myocardium. In contrast to its vasoconstrictive effects, endothelin stimulates the release of other vasoactive mediators, particularly endogenous vasodilators like nitric oxide, which act to limit its intense vasoconstrictor effect.

Endothelin exerts a complex influence on sodium and water exchange through varied interactions with many other hormones that govern fluid and electrolyte balance. One net effect of endothelin is a decrease in the filtered load of sodium in the kidney. This results in inhibition of water reabsorption and decreased sodium excretion. Endothelin increases ANP secretion, activates ACE, and inhibits renin release by the juxtaglomerular apparatus. At low doses, endothelin-1 produces a dose-dependent natriuresis and diuresis. Endothelin also modulates the biosynthesis of aldosterone, thereby inhibiting water reabsorption through aldosterone-controlled mechanisms. Vasopressin-mediated water reabsorption is also inhibited. Endothelin appears to have complex interactions with other regulators of renal perfusion and handling of water and electrolytes, which has stimulated research to evaluate the contribution of endothelin to the pathophysiology of various renal diseases.[11]

Nitric Oxide. Nitric oxide is a short-lived free radical produced from L-arginine by nitric oxide synthases. Although this substance has numerous biologic functions that are beyond the scope of this chapter, including regulation of vascular tone and tissue blood flow,[12] its effects in the kidney as they relate to fluid and electrolyte homeostasis deserve mention. Nitric oxide is produced in renal smooth muscle cells, mesangial cells, tubules, and endothelial cells and participates in the regulation of renal hemodynamics and renal handling of water and electrolytes. Nitric oxide and PGI_2 each independently cause renal vasodilation in response to a variety of stimuli. Nitric oxide is important in the regulation of medullary (vasa recta) blood flow. Pressure-dependent sodium excretion is ablated by inhibitors like L-NG-monomethyl-arginine and restored with L-arginine. Nitric oxide also contributes to tubuloglomerular feedback, which modulates the delivery and reabsorption of sodium and chloride in the renal tubules. Nitric oxide synthase in macula densa cells is activated by tubular solute reabsorption to release nitric oxide as a vasodilating component of the tubuloglomerular feedback response. Nitric oxide also participates in regulating renin release by the juxtaglomerular apparatus. Finally, nitric oxide produced in the proximal tubule may mediate the effects of angiotensin on tubular reabsorption.[12]

Normal Water and Electrolyte Exchange

The body's normal homeostatic mechanisms control both the volume and composition of the fluid compartments such that a remarkably stable internal milieu is maintained. Surgical patients are prone to fluid and electrolyte abnormalities, not only because of disease but also because perioperative fluid replacement may sidestep some of these homeostatic mechanisms. Although it is important to recognize and correct disease, trauma, and stress-related abnormalities, it is equally important to understand normal fluid and electrolyte balance and to avoid iatrogenic perturbations of these systems.

TABLE 10.3

WATER LOSSES IN A 60- TO 80-kg MAN

	■ AVERAGE DAILY VOLUME (mL)	■ MINIMAL DAILY VOLUME (mL)
Sensible losses		
Urinary	800–1,500	300
Intestinal	0–250	0
Sweat	0	0
Insensible losses		
Lungs and skin	600–900	600–900

Adapted from Shires GT, Canizaro PC. Fluid and electrolyte management of the surgical patient. In: Sabiston DC, ed. *Textbook of Surgery.* Philadelphia, PA: WB Saunders; 1986:77, with permission.

5 **Normal Water Exchange.** Water losses are both sensible (measurable) and insensible (unmeasurable). Sensible losses include losses through urine, stool, and sweat. Table 10.3 summarizes the normal sensible and insensible losses encountered in a 24-hour period. The volumes of these losses may vary considerably. Urinary loss usually varies in proportion to intake plus other losses. The minimal amount of water needed to excrete normal metabolic waste products is approximately 300 mL/d.

Water loss in stool is usually small, on the order of 150 mL/d, but may increase markedly in disease conditions. The GI tract has a net secretory action down to the level of the jejunum, and the reabsorptive capacity of the remainder of the small and large intestines keeps water loss by this route to a minimum. Bowel obstruction, severe diarrhea, and enterocutaneous fistulas are examples of conditions that may increase GI losses of water and electrolytes.

Sweat does not usually account for much of the daily water loss. Sweating is an active process involving the secretion of a hypotonic mixture of electrolytes and water, and it should be differentiated from the insensible water loss of evaporation from the skin.

Insensible water loss is the evaporatory loss of water from both the skin and the respiratory tract (see Table 10.3). Evaporatory skin losses are determined by the body surface area and temperature of the patient, as well as by the relative humidity of the environment. Evaporation through the skin functions as a mechanism for heat loss and is proportional to calories expended. Approximately 30 mL of water is lost for every 100 kcal expended. Respiratory exchange depends on the ambient temperature and the relative humidity as well as on the rate of air exchange. Respiratory water loss is also energy dependent; thus, at normal respiratory rates, 13 mL of water is lost for every 100 kcal expended. Overall, normal insensible water losses average approximately 8 to 12 mL/kg per day. Insensible water loss increases 10% for each degree of body temperature above 37.2°C (99°F). In addition, patients with tracheostomies who breathe unhumidified air lose additional free water. Conversely, patients who are on respirators or who breathe air that is 100% humidified have no respiratory losses and may gain free water.

A person normally consumes approximately 2,000 mL/d of water, although this quantity is highly variable. Approximately one third of this amount comes from water bound to food, and the remainder originates from free water intake. In addition, water may be gained when carbohydrates and proteins, which are kept in solution by water in the cell, are metabolized. Although this gain is usually minimal, catabolic states may increase the amount of oxidative free water gain to approximately 500 mL/d. To maintain proper fluid volumes, intake and excretion are well balanced through thirst mechanisms and the changes in renal excretion described earlier.

Normal Salt Exchange. In industrialized nations, daily sodium intake averages 100 to 250 mEq/d. This intake is balanced by losses through sweat, stool, and urine. Fine control of sodium balance is achieved by renal sodium excretion. In cases of hyponatremia, the kidney is capable of reducing urinary losses of sodium to less than 1 mEq/d. Conversely, urinary excretion can be increased to rates up to 5,000 mEq/d if necessary to achieve sodium balance. The normal sodium requirement is in the range of 1 to 2 mEq/kg per day.

Potassium balance in the body is also finely controlled. Because most potassium remains in the intracellular compartment, potassium homeostasis is maintained by a balance between intake and GI and renal losses and by a balance between extracellular and intracellular potassium. With a normal diet, approximately 40 to 120 mEq of potassium is ingested daily. Of this potassium, 10% to 15% is excreted in the feces, and the remainder is excreted in the urine. Normal daily potassium requirements are approximately 0.5 to 1 mEq/kg per day. Abnormal renal function markedly changes this figure; consequently, potassium intake must be minimized in patients with renal failure.

FLUID AND ELECTROLYTE THERAPY

Parenteral Solutions

Crystalloids. Solutions of electrolytes and water are collectively referred to as *crystalloids* and are the most widely used fluids for parenteral administration. Crystalloids are inexpensive, are highly effective for fluid maintenance and replacement, and have outstanding safety profiles. Crystalloid-induced hypercoagulability has been reported.[13–15] Its causes are multifactorial and poorly understood. It can possibly be corrected with addition of fibrinogene[16] and/or antithrombin III, but this does not often represent a significant clinical problem.

A number of electrolyte solutions are available for parenteral administration (Table 10.4). Selection of the appropriate fluid requires assessment of the patient's maintenance fluid requirements, existing fluid deficits, and anticipated ongoing fluid losses. When a single solution does not accurately replace the electrolyte components of the losses or deficits, more than one type of solution may be administered. Ions such as potassium, magnesium, or calcium may be necessary and can be added to parenteral solutions to suit the patient's requirements.

Lactated Ringer solution is commonly used to replace losses of fluid with the ionic composition of plasma, such as blood loss, edema fluid, and small-bowel losses. It is ideal for the replacement of existing fluid deficits when serum electrolyte concentrations are normal. Although sodium content (130 mEq/L) is low compared with plasma, normal renal function usually ensures that the extra free water in this solution (150 mL/L) is excreted. Hyponatremia can occur with extended use of lactated Ringer solution or with use in patients who have impaired renal function, especially dilutional abnormalities such as those secondary to increased ADH secretion. Because the lactate anions in lactated Ringer solution are readily metabolized to bicarbonate in the liver, this solution does not appear to contribute to acidosis if tissue perfusion has been maintained or restored. Recent work comparing the DL racemic mixture of lactate in lactated Ringer solution with its L-isomer have implicated the D-isomer in leukocyte activation, although at present there are no compelling data to suggest that resuscitation with this solution increases the inflammatory response.[17] Utilization of only the L-isomer in resuscitation solutions eliminates this theoretical problem.

Isotonic saline (0.9% or normal saline) contains 154 mEq of both sodium and chloride. Although this solution can be useful in patients with hyponatremia or hypochloremia, the excess of both sodium and chloride can lead to electrolyte and acid–base disturbances. Infusion of large volumes of 0.9% saline can lead to total body sodium overload and hyperchloremia. The added chloride load can result in a hyperchloremic metabolic acidosis or can aggravate preexisting acidosis. In addition, the pH of this solution and of the related solutions (0.45%, 0.33%, and 0.2% saline) is 4.0 to 5.0.

Following correction of deficits, less concentrated saline solutions are more appropriate to replace ongoing fluid losses (i.e., nasogastric tube losses) and for maintenance fluid therapy. Although the practical differences between 0.45%, 0.33%, and 0.2% saline solutions are not large, the specific fluid product selection is best determined by calculated requirements. These fluids are hypoosmotic and hypotonic with respect to plasma. In theory, rapid infusion of very hypotonic solutions can result in red blood cell lysis. For this reason, 5% dextrose (50 g of dextrose per liter) is added to these solutions to increase tonicity. In addition, 5% dextrose represents 200 kcal in each liter of solution.

TABLE 10.4

ELECTROLYTE CONTENT OF COMMONLY USED INTRAVENOUS CRYSTALLOID SOLUTIONS

	ELECTROLYTE (mEq/L)					
SOLUTION	Na^+	K^+	Ca^{2+}	Mg^{2+}	Cl^-	...
0.9% NaCl	154	—	—	—	154	—
0.45% NaCl	77	—	—	—	77	—
0.33% NaCl	56	—	—	—	56	—
0.2% NaCl	34	—	—	—	34	—
Lactated Ringer	130	4	4	—	109	28
3.0% NaCl	513	—	—	—	513	—
5.0% NaCl	855	—	—	—	855	—

Hypertonic saline solutions (HTSs) (3% NaCl and 5% NaCl) are generally used to replace sodium deficits in patients with symptomatic hyponatremia. However, these and even more concentrated (7.5% NaCl) solutions have also been used for resuscitation of hemorrhagic shock, head trauma, and burn patients.[18,19] Hypertonic saline appears to increase intravascular volume in these patients more quickly than isotonic solutions, and the total resuscitation volume requirement may be decreased. When HTS is used for resuscitation of patients with severe sepsis, it has been shown to result in improvements in oxygen transport, cardiac output, and pulmonary capillary wedge pressure.[18] The systemic and mesenteric oxygen extraction coefficient improves without worsening of other markers of perfusion. This is achieved by rapid mobilization of fluids from the intracellular compartment to the extracellular compartment. The osmotic gradient produced by HTS redistributes fluids from the perivascular and intracellular spaces to the intravascular space with consequent plasma volume expansion (up to fourfold). These cardiovascular and hemodynamic effects are short-lived, in general lasting from 60 to 120 minutes. The addition of colloids such as dextran or hetastarch can prolong the effect.

The osmotic effect of hypertonic saline may benefit patients with acute severe brain injury.[20] By reducing the water content of the brain, HTS can help to control intracerebral pressure after injury. In addition, HTS has immunomodulatory effects, which are well documented.[21] HTS reduces the systemic inflammatory response syndrome (SIRS) and may attenuate multiple organ dysfunction syndrome (MODS).[21] HTSs are not without adverse effects, however. Patients are at risk for electrolyte abnormalities such as hypernatremia. Extravasation into the soft tissues can produce significant soft tissue edema and even necrosis. Further clinical trials will be needed to determine the indications and efficacy of hypertonic solutions.

Colloids. Colloid plasma volume expander solutions offer the potential benefits of promoting retention of fluid in the intravascular space and of reducing excess interstitial fluid (edema). Worldwide, albumin and artificial colloids are relied on to varying degrees in fluid management of the surgical patient. In the United States, concerns regarding the effectiveness, cost, and potential complications of colloid administration have limited their use to specific clinical situations.

Albumin. Albumin (69 kD), derived from human plasma and heat-treated to reduce infection risk, is available in 5% and 25% solutions. These act by increasing plasma oncotic pressures and theoretically retarding or even reversing movement of water into the interstitial space. However, many of the conditions associated with edema are also associated with abnormalities in microvascular permeability. Examples include the pulmonary circulation in the adult respiratory distress syndrome, regional circulatory beds in burns or infections, and the systemic circulation in sepsis. Exogenously administered protein in colloid solutions can extravasate into the interstitial space and intensify, rather than decrease interstitial edema. The debate continues as recent large studies have added to the question of the benefits and disadvantages of resuscitation with colloids versus crystalloids.[22] The SOAP trial (Sepsis Occurrence in Acutely Ill Patients) demonstrated increased mortality in intensive care unit patients treated with colloids, whereas the SAFE trial (Saline vs. Albumin Fluid Evaluation) found no overall difference in organ dysfunction or survival.[24]

Hetastarch. Hydroxyethyl starches (HESs) are synthetic plasma expanders derived from hydrolyzed amylopectin, with variable degrees of substitution (DS) of hydroxyl groups for carbon groups on glucose molecules. HES is available commercially in the United States as a 6% solution of high-molecular-weight (450,000), highly hydroxyethyl substituted (DS 0.7) HES (hetastarch) in 0.9% saline. Hetastarch has been used as a resuscitative solution in a variety of clinical settings with variable results. Coagulopathy and bleeding complications have been widely reported after administration of highly substituted, high-molecular-weight HES.[25,26] This appears to be associated with reduced factor VIII and von Willebrand factor levels, a prolonged partial thromboplastin time, and impaired platelet function.[27] Because of its long half-life, coagulopathy does not quickly reverse after cessation of HES administration. Reports of renal insufficiency or renal failure after HES 450/0.7, HES 250/0.45 (Pentaspan), and HES 200/0.62 administration add to the concerns regarding overuse of these volume expanders, particularly in patients with preexisting renal impairment.

Hextend, a balanced 6% hetastarch (molecular weight [MW] 720,000) in lactated Ringer solution, has been forwarded as a much-improved alternate resuscitation product as compared to 6% hetastarch in saline. In a phase III trial of Hextend and 6% hetastarch in saline, Hextend was found to be as effective for resuscitation but without adversely affecting the coagulation profile.[28] Although the safety profile of this alternative colloid resuscitative fluid appears to be better than that of 6% hetastarch in saline, the data regarding its safety in situations of massive resuscitation are not clear. In a recent study using an experimental model of traumatic brain injury, Hextend was found to reduce fluid requirements, eliminate the need for mannitol, and improve neurologic outcome as compared to crystalloid and mannitol resuscitation. Furthermore, it had no adverse effect on coagulation.[29] In another recent experimental report, Hextend was found to have no significant platelet-inhibitory effects.[30]

Low-molecular-weight, low-substituted (MW 130 kD; DS 0.4) HES (Voluven) has recently been introduced and demonstrated to have a far smaller effect on coagulation than other HES solutions.[31] In addition, there is evidence that renal impairment does not occur after administration of HES 130/0.4, in contrast to the high-molecular-weight, highly substituted HES solutions.[32] Although numerous reports now suggest that this type of alternative HES is a very good option when plasma volume expansion is indicated, the safety of wide use of large-volume Voluven administration remains to be demonstrated.

Dextrans. Dextrans are glucose polymers synthesized by *Leuconostoc mesenteroides* bacteria grown on sucrose media. These are available as synthetic plasma expanders in 40,000-MW (dextran 40; Rheomacrodex) and 70,000-MW (dextran 70; Macrodex) solutions. Although neither is used frequently for volume expansion, dextran 70 has been preferred because of its significantly longer half-life and better retention in plasma. The most accepted current use of dextran solutions is to lower blood viscosity. Both should be avoided in patients with known renal dysfunction, but dextran 40 has been shown to represent a particular risk for renal injury.[33] Anaphylactoid reactions can occur with either dextran 40 or 70.

Gelatins. Gelatin solutions produced from bovine collagen are effective as plasma volume expanders and are available outside the United States in urea-linked (Gelofusin) and succinate-linked (Haemaccel) formulations. Gelofusin has been used in similar clinical settings to HES, with similar clinical results, although one randomized trial comparing the two colloids in trauma patients suggested that HES (MW 250; DS 4.5) was more effective in reducing capillary leak.[34] Coagulopathy does not appear to be an issue with gelatins, although renal impairment has been reported with these colloids as well. Allergic reactions ranging in severity from pruritus to anaphylaxis can occur with both gelatin formulations.[35]

Artificial Oxygen Carriers. Although the subject of transfusion is beyond the scope of this chapter, new developments in the area of oxygen-carrying synthetic volume expanders deserve brief mention. Early difficulties with perfluorocarbon-based solutions have increased the intensity of investigation to develop hemoglobin-based oxygen-carrying (HBOC) solutions, and the results of recent clinical trials with these substances have been encouraging.[36] In the future, these solutions may prove beneficial when volume expansion in conjunction with increased oxygen-carrying capacity is required and will avoid the immunologic consequences of allogenic blood transfusions.

Goals of Fluid and Electrolyte Therapy

6 The goals of fluid therapy are to normalize hemodynamic parameters and body fluid and electrolyte concentrations. This is accomplished by correction of both volume and electrolyte abnormalities, as well as by replacement of both normal daily losses and additional ongoing losses associated with disease states and surgical treatments.

CORRECTION OF VOLUME ABNORMALITIES

Volume Deficits

Hypovolemia is common among surgical and trauma patients. Its occurrence may be related to direct loss of blood or other fluids but frequently occurs in the absence of external fluid loss. In critically ill patients, this can be due to vasodilation or diffuse capillary leak. Large volumes of fluid can be sequestered in extravascular spaces (third-space losses) as a consequence of inflammation, sepsis, or shock-related endothelial injury and increased endothelial permeability.[37] This situation is characterized by a movement of proteins and fluid from the intravascular to the interstitial compartment. Examples of disorders that cause third-space losses include bowel obstruction with edema of the bowel wall and transudation of fluid into the bowel lumen and pancreatitis with often massive retroperitoneal fluid extravasation. Third-space fluid in the interstitial space is poorly exchangeable with the intravascular compartment while the disease process persists. With the resolution of pathologic conditions and normalization of microvascular permeability, these fluid losses stop and sequestered fluid is returned to the intravascular space at variable rates.

Volume deficits can be either acute or chronic. Chronic volume deficits may manifest as decreased skin turgor, weight loss, sunken eyes, hypothermia, oliguria, orthostatic hypotension, and tachycardia. In addition, serum BUN and creatinine may be elevated, with a high BUN/creatinine ratio (above 15:1), and the hematocrit may be elevated as well. Assuming no change in red cell mass, the hematocrit can be expected to increase 6 to 8 percentage points for each liter deficit in intravascular volume. In this situation, urine concentration is usually high, and urine sodium excretion is low (<20 mEq/L Na^+). Unlike urine sodium levels, plasma sodium is not an indicator of intravascular volume. Plasma sodium concentration remains normal when fluid loss is isotonic, despite the volume of fluid lost.

Acute volume losses are usually manifested by changes in vital signs. If organ perfusion is compromised, urine output may be low. Attempts to quantify volume deficits are usually of little value. The volume of fluid required to restore blood pressure, heart rate, and urine output is the best estimate of what the volume deficit has been. Fluid resuscitation for hypovolemia is initiated with an isotonic solution such as lactated Ringer solution. Urine flow in critically ill patients is monitored with an indwelling Foley catheter with a goal of at least 0.5 mL/kg per hour output. After fluid resuscitation has been initiated, a thorough history and physical examination may help to determine the origins of the volume deficits, and the underlying causes can be appropriately addressed. Invasive monitoring with a central venous or pulmonary artery catheter should be considered early in the resuscitation of elderly patients or patients with certain disease states such as severe cardiac disease or renal failure.

Volume Excess

Clinical manifestations of volume excess may occur with excessive parenteral volume administration, particularly in at-risk patients such as the elderly and those with cardiac disease. Volume overload can occur if appropriate adjustments to fluid therapy are not made. Possible manifestations of volume overload are weight gain, elevated central venous pressure (CVP), pulmonary congestion or edema, and peripheral edema. Intravascular volume excess is treated by volume restriction and use of loop diuretics.

MAINTENANCE FLUID THERAPY

Calculation of maintenance fluid replacement does not include replacement of either preexisting deficits or ongoing additional losses. Basal requirements for water and electrolytes are determined by sensible and insensible losses. Insensible water loss averages 8 to 12 mL/kg per day and increases 10% for every degree of body temperature above 37.2°C. Urinary and fecal losses must be added to this figure. Maintenance fluid volume requirements can be calculated based on body weight taking into account a larger per kilogram volume requirement of smaller body weight individuals (Table 10.5). A 10-kg child requires 100 mL/kg per day or 1,000 mL/d. A 70-kg man requires 1,000 mL/d for the first 10 kg (100 mL/kg × 10 kg), plus 500 mL/d for the second 10 kg (50 mL/kg × 10 kg), plus 1,000 mL/d for the last 50 kg (20 mL/kg × 50 kg), for a total daily water requirement of 2,500 mL/d. In patients who may be intolerant of hypervolemia (i.e., cardiac disease, elderly patients), the requirement per kilogram over 20 kg is decreased to 15 mL/kg per day.

For maintenance therapy, 1 to 2 mEq/kg per day of sodium is required, with any administered excess managed by urinary sodium excretion. Potassium requirements are approximately 0.5 to 1 mEq/kg per day. If sodium is replaced at 2 mEq/kg per day and potassium is replaced at 1 mEq/kg per day, a 70-kg patient requires 2,500 mL of water containing 140 mEq of sodium and 70 mEq of potassium. Each liter of parenteral solution would contain 56 mEq of sodium and 28 mEq of potassium. The solution that best fits this patient's daily maintenance requirements is 0.33% saline solution (56 mEq/L Na^+). Potassium chloride can be added to each liter of solution (20 to 30 mEq/L), with appropriate adjustments for the patient's electrolyte and renal functional status.

7 Short-term maintenance therapy generally does not require addition of calcium, phosphate, or magnesium. However, in

TABLE 10.5

CALCULATION OF MAINTENANCE FLUID REQUIREMENTS

BODY WEIGHT	FLUID REQUIREMENT[a]	
For 0–10 kg	Give 100 mL/kg/d	A
For the next 10–20 kg	Give an additional 50 mL/kg/d	B
For weight >20 kg[b]	Give 20 mL/kg/d	C

[a]Maintenance fluid requirements = sum of A + B + C.
[b]For elderly patients or patients with cardiac disease, this amount should be reduced to 15 mL/kg/d.

TABLE 10.6

ELECTROLYTE CONCENTRATIONS IN GASTROINTESTINAL SECRETIONS

	ELECTROLYTE (mEq/L)					
SECRETION	Na^+	K^+	Cl^-	. . .	H^+	RATE (mL/d)
Salivary	50	20	40	30	—	100–1,000
Gastric						
Basal	100	10	140	—	30	1,000
Stimulated	30	10	140	—	100	4,200
Bile	140	5	100	—	—	500–1,000
Pancreatic	140	5	75	—	—	1,000
Duodenum	140	5	80	—	—	100–2,000
Ileum	140	5	70	—	—	100–2,000
Colon	60	70	15	—	—	—

patients with chronic disorders, patients who experience significant volume shifts, or patients who require long-term parenteral fluid therapy, these electrolytes should be measured and corrected by the most practical route. If the enteral route is unavailable, these are administered in parenteral nutrition solutions along with trace elements, vitamins, and appropriate caloric sources.

REPLACEMENT OF ONGOING FLUID LOSSES

Once volume deficits have been replaced and maintenance fluids have been calculated and given, the overall fluid balance of the patient can be maintained by replacement of fluid losses beyond those considered to be maintenance. Ongoing losses from nasogastric tubes, stomas, fistulas, and other measurable sources are recorded during the course of care and can be replaced in fairly straightforward fashion. The electrolyte contents of these fluids can be estimated or measured and used to guide the choice of replacement fluid type (Table 10.6).

Intraoperative Fluid Therapy

Anesthesia interrupts normal baroreceptor reflexes, so the patient with volume depletion that was compensated preoperatively by increased vascular resistance and heart rate may become acutely hypotensive on induction of anesthesia. For this reason, adequate resuscitation before surgery is mandatory. During operative procedures fluid losses result from blood loss, third-space sequestration, and evaporative losses from open wounds. Operative blood loss can often be measured. Evaporative losses and shifts of intravascular fluid to the extravascular space (third space) cannot be measured but should be anticipated. Intraoperative replacement with isotonic solutions is usually accomplished at rates of 500 to 1,000 mL/h. Close monitoring of blood pressure and urine output, as well as judicious use of invasive monitoring techniques, aids the surgeon and anesthesiologist in avoiding problems associated with intraoperative volume depletion.

Postoperative Fluid Therapy and Monitoring

Fluid therapy during the postoperative period is adjusted to the patient's volume status at the completion of the operative procedure, as well as to anticipated ongoing fluid losses. Isotonic solutions should be used for volume resuscitation during the early postoperative period. It is best not to give potassium supplements during this period, unless they are specifically required as indicated by serum electrolyte measurements, until adequate renal function is confirmed.

Routine monitoring of postoperative fluid status consists of serial vital signs and urine output measurements. Fluid intake and output data are recorded in the patient's medical record and used to plan ongoing fluid therapy. Weight should also be recorded daily. In the postsurgical patient, rapid fluctuations in weight are generally related to changes in TBW. Adequate fluid is given to maintain a urine output of greater than 0.5 mL/kg per hour. Urine specific gravity can also be measured and serves as an indicator of both volume status and renal ability to concentrate and dilute the urine. Urine specific gravity of greater than 1.010 to 1.012 indicates that the urine is being concentrated (relative to plasma), and a urine specific gravity of less than 1.010 indicates that dilute urine is being produced. Both volume depletion and cardiac failure are accompanied by increased urine concentration and low urine outputs. Urine specific gravity in the range of plasma (1.010 to 1.012) may indicate either adequate hydration or the inability of the kidneys either to dilute or concentrate the urine.

Renal failure in the postoperative period may be accompanied by low urine volumes (oliguric renal failure, <500 mL/d) or normal or high urine volumes (nonoliguric or high-output renal failure). Measurement of urine electrolytes and creatinine clearance can help clarify questions regarding volume status and renal function. CVP measurement can be used to more accurately assess volume status and guide fluid administration. Normal CVP may range from 5 to 12 mm Hg. Higher pressures usually indicate volume overload or cardiac failure, whereas pressures below this range indicate intravascular volume depletion. There are significant limitations to CVP measurement as a reflection of circulating volume, particularly in critically ill patients. Abnormalities of cardiac performance and vascular tone may confound interpretation of CVP measurements, and pulmonary artery catheterization may be required to resolve volume status questions.

ELECTROLYTES

Concentration Changes in Body Fluids

Volume excess or deficits are often isotonic but may be accompanied by changes in extracellular sodium concentration and osmolality. The mechanisms controlling normal osmoregulation

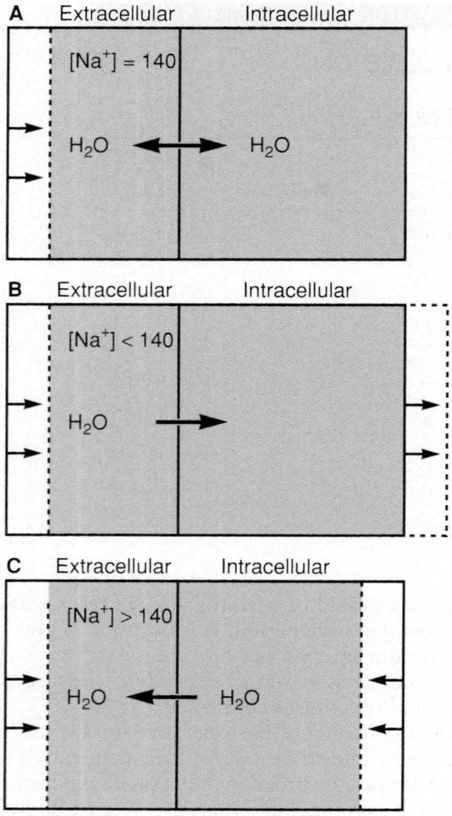

FIGURE 10.6. A: Isotonic dehydration. Extracellular fluid is lost, but sodium concentration and osmolality remain unchanged. There is no change in intracellular volume. **B:** Hypotonic dehydration caused by an extracellular fluid deficit with hyponatremia. Water moves into the intracellular space, causing further extracellular depletion and intracellular fluid (ICF) expansion. **C:** Hypertonic dehydration caused by loss of extracellular free water, resulting in hypernatremia. Water from the ICF shifts to the extracellular space, resulting in contraction of both ICF and extracellular fluid compartments.

may be affected by the same processes responsible for controlling volume. Volume depletion is the most common disorder of volume status encountered in surgical and trauma patients. These patients usually present with isotonic dehydration (Fig. 10.6A). In this condition, the volume lost is isotonic with plasma. Examples of isotonic volume deficits include blood loss, third-space losses, and GI losses. Volume depletion may also be accompanied by hypo-osmolar conditions (hypotonic dehydration; see Fig. 10.6B) and is often iatrogenic and the result of incomplete volume resuscitation with hypotonic solutions. Dehydration associated with hyperosmolar states (hypertonic dehydration; see Fig. 10.6C) is infrequent and usually indicates impaired consciousness and thirst mechanisms or a patient's inability to drink or obtain water. As mentioned previously, volume excesses often occur some time after hospitalization rather than at presentation. The most frequent concentration defect associated with volume excess is hyponatremia.

Hyponatremia

Causes. Hyponatremia may result from direct sodium loss or from dilution of sodium by excessive free water under hypovolemic, euvolemic, or hypervolemic conditions. Hyponatremia is frequently seen in the postoperative or postinjury period when ADH is elevated as a component of the normal stress response to injury. Inflammatory and stress cytokines such as C-reactive protein, interleukin-6, interleukin-1, and tumor necrosis factor all increase ADH levels. Volume expansion due to increased ADH-stimulated free water reabsorption may stimulate natriuresis and exacerbate hyponatremia. Because volume expansion and hyponatremia diminish the effects of ADH on the collecting tubules, hyponatremia is usually self-limited under these circumstances, with serum sodium concentration rarely falling below 130 mEq/L unless exacerbated by exogenous free water administration.

TABLE 10.7

CAUSES OF THE SYNDROME OF INAPPROPRIATE ADH SECRETION

Tumor hypersecretion of ADH	Lung
	Pancreas
	Bladder
	Prostate
CNS disorders	Head trauma
	Neurosurgical interventions
	Brain tumors
	Alcohol withdrawal
	Stroke
Other	Infection
	Medication induced

ADH, antidiuretic hormone; CNS, central nervous system.

The *syndrome of inappropriate ADH secretion* (SIADH) occurs as the result of ADH release under circumstances that are inappropriate to the patient's volume status. The diagnosis can be made when hyponatremia occurs in the presence of euvolemia (or hypervolemia) and normal renal and adrenal function. SIADH can be encountered in a wide range of clinical problems (Table 10.7). The diagnosis requires that the patient have a low plasma osmolality with a high urine osmolality secondary to high urinary sodium excretion in a low volume of urine. Treatment of hyponatremia in the setting of SIADH depends on the presence of symptoms, the severity of the hyponatremia, and its duration. In the acute setting most patients will respond to fluid restriction. Fluids are restricted to 50% to 75% of daily maintenance (700 to 1,000 mL/m^2 per day) and electrolytes should be measured every 6 to 8 hours. Patients who are symptomatic require aggressive treatment with hypertonic saline solutions such as 3% NaCl. Patients with chronic hyponatremia may not respond to water restriction and can benefit from drugs. Medication options include vasopressin receptor antagonists (VRAs) and osmotic loop diuretics. Demeclocycline, a tetracycline antibiotic, can be used to block vasopressin. A new class of peptide and nonpeptide VRA are in development. Currently, conivaptan (Vaprisol), a nonselective VRA, is the only drug of this class approved in the United States. Oral formulations such as relcovaptan, SSR-149,415, and V2 selective drugs (lixivaptan, mozvaptan, stavaptan, and tolvaptan[38]) await approval by the Food and Drug Administration for use in the United States.

Hyponatremia can also be associated with low effective circulating volume. This most commonly occurs in edematous states or cirrhosis with ascites, but it can also result from dehydration with concomitant volume replacement with hypotonic solutions. Because of the low intravascular volume, renal plasma flow and glomerular filtration rate are low, resulting in increased sodium reabsorption by the kidneys. This renal compensation may not be sufficient to correct the abnormality.

Although hyponatremia most often results from excess free water, it can occur in the presence of excess solute, as previously

TABLE 10.8

SYMPTOMS OF HYPONATREMIA

Central nervous system	Headaches Confusion Delirium Coma Seizures
Gastrointestinal	Anorexia Nausea Vomiting
Musculoskeletal	Weakness Fatigue Muscle cramps

described, with increased P_{osm} in hyperglycemic conditions (pseudohyponatremia). Other types of solute may contribute to hyperosmolality and water shifts from the intracellular to the extracellular space, with consequent hyponatremia. These include exogenously administered or ingested mannitol, ethanol, methanol, or ethylene glycol. In addition to shifts in water, cellular exchange of potassium for sodium as a compensatory mechanism for potassium loss may result in hyponatremia. In both hyperosmolar and hypokalemic conditions, total body sodium remains normal.

Finally, hyperproteinemia and hyperlipidemia can cause falsely low sodium values. This pattern of *pseudohyponatremia* is due to an anomaly of laboratory measurement of sodium and is not accompanied by any symptoms attributable to hyponatremia.

Clinical Features. Chronic hyponatremia is often asymptomatic until serum $[Na^+]$ falls below 110 to 120 mEq/L. A more acute drop in serum $[Na^+]$ to the 120 to 130 mEq/L range may result in central nervous system (CNS), musculoskeletal, or GI symptoms (Table 10.8). Symptoms related to the CNS result largely from cellular water intoxication, and permanent CNS injury can occur if hyponatremia is left untreated.

Diagnosis. Differentiating the causes of hyponatremia may be difficult. Once hyperosmolar hyponatremia (caused by hyperglycemia, mannitol administration, or radiologic contrast medium) has been excluded and pseudohyponatremia has been eliminated from the differential diagnosis, the clinician must determine whether the effective circulating volume is low (hyponatremic dehydration) or normal.

Hyponatremic dehydration may be caused by renal or extrarenal sodium losses. Renal sodium losses are usually the result of diuretic use, chronic renal failure, adrenal insufficiency, or a defect in aldosterone secretion. The hallmark of these disorders is a urine sodium level above 20 mEq/L in the face of hyponatremia. This is in contradistinction to extrarenal sodium loss such as that caused by vomiting; diarrhea; or fluid loss through nasogastric tubes, fistulas, or drains. The dehydration resulting from these conditions causes increased renal sodium reabsorption and urine sodium levels below 20 mEq/L. Normal or high effective circulating volume in combination with hyponatremia is almost always caused by SIADH or by increased sensitivity of the renal collecting tubules to the action of normal levels of ADH.

Treatment. Hypovolemic patients with hyponatremia can frequently be treated by rehydration with isotonic saline or lactated Ringer solution because symptoms in this situation are often caused by dehydration rather than hyponatremia. Overly rapid normalization of volume may lead to hypernatremia, and serum $[Na^+]$ must be serially monitored during volume replacement. Most surgical patients with hyponatremia are euvolemic or hypervolemic. Asymptomatic patients in this category are best treated by free water restriction.

Patients who have significant symptoms require aggressive treatment with a clear recognition that overzealous therapy may lead to CNS injury. Rapid infusion of hypertonic saline may result in central pontine myelinolysis and the quadriplegia, dysarthria, and dysphasia of the "locked in" syndrome. This risk is greatest in patients who have been hyponatremic for longer than 48 hours. In these patients, 3% or 5% saline solution is given relatively slowly to increase serum $[Na^+]$ at a rate not exceeding 0.5 mEq/L per hour. The amount of sodium needed to increase the serum $[Na^+]$ to a desired level can be calculated as follows:

$$Na^+ \text{ required(in mEq)} = (\text{desired}[Na^+]_s - \text{actual}[Na^+]_s) \times \text{TBW}$$

where $[Na^+]_s$ = serum sodium concentration. For example, a 70-kg patient has been hyponatremic for more than 48 hours and has a serum sodium level of 120 mEq. Correction of hyponatremia during the first 24 hours is limited to 0.5 mEq/L per hour × 24 hours = 12 mEq/L. Assuming TBW 60% of body weight:

$$Na^+ \text{ required} = (132 - 120) \times (0.6[70]) = 504 \text{ mEq}$$

Because 5% saline contains 850 mEq/L of sodium, the volume of 5% saline required to provide 504 mEq of sodium in the first 24 hours of treatment is as follows:

$$504 \text{ mEq}/850 \text{ mEq} = 0.593 \text{ L } 5\% \text{ saline}$$

For more acute symptomatic hyponatremia (<48 hours' duration), more rapid treatment may be used. Five percent or 3% hypertonic saline may be administered at a rate of 1 to 2 mEq/L per hour. Hyperacute hyponatremia, which may result from inadvertent infusion of large volumes of water or from dialysis accidents, can be treated at rates of 5 mEq/L per hour. The treatment goal is to achieve a serum sodium level above 125 mEq/L or to achieve resolution of symptoms.

Hypernatremia.

Hypernatremia is a less common problem in surgical patients than hyponatremia but can occur due to a number of causes (Table 10.9). Although hypernatremia is

TABLE 10.9

CAUSES OF HYPERNATREMIA

■ VOLUME STATUS	■ CAUSE
Low	Free water loss Insensible—skin, respiratory Gastrointestinal loss Excessive hyperosmotic peritoneal dialysis Renal Diuretics, diabetes insipidus, nonoliguric renal failure
Normal	Same as "Low" volume status but with improper correction
High	Free water loss Increased mineralocorticoids—hyperaldosteronism, hypercortisolism Iatrogenic Excessive sodium administration

usually the result of excessive free water loss associated with hypovolemia, it can also occur in euvolemic and hypervolemic states. Euvolemic hypernatremia tends to occur for the same reasons as in hypovolemic situations, with the added factor of improper correction of free water loss (i.e., with sodium-containing fluids). Water loss may be due to nonrenal or renal causes. Nonrenal free water losses can be characterized as insensible as in respiratory losses in patients with tracheostomies who breathe unhumidified air or skin losses in patients with high fevers. Large volumes of free water can also be lost when hypertonic glucose solutions are used for peritoneal dialysis. *Diabetes insipidus,* seen most frequently in head trauma or neurosurgical patients, is due to depressed secretion of ADH. The free water diuresis in this condition can at times be massive.

Hypernatremia can also be caused by increased total body content of sodium, which is usually related to exogenous administration of sodium. Infusion of excessive amounts of sodium bicarbonate during acute resuscitation from cardiopulmonary arrest is frequently associated with subsequent hypernatremia. Administration of solutions containing large amounts of sodium for replacement of free water deficits may also lead to hypernatremia.

Clinical Features. Moderate degrees of hypernatremia are tolerated well, and symptoms rarely develop unless serum $[Na^+]$ levels exceed 160 mEq/L or serum osmolality exceeds 320 to 330 mOsm/kg. Rapid onset of hypernatremia is associated with earlier onset of symptoms. The symptoms of hypernatremia are related to the hyperosmolar state. Cellular dehydration occurs as water passes into the extracellular space. CNS effects predominate. The most common symptoms are restlessness, irritability, ataxia, fever, tonic spasms, and seizures. Subarachnoid hemorrhage may also occur.

Treatment. Once hypernatremia becomes symptomatic, it is associated with significant morbidity and mortality if prompt treatment is not instituted. Rapid correction carries a significant risk of cerebral edema and brainstem herniation. In chronic hypernatremia, the cells in the brain gradually adapt by increasing intracellular osmotic solute content, thereby regaining cellular volume. These cellular changes are not readily reversed. A sudden decrease in extracellular sodium concentration, and therefore osmolality, results in cell swelling. Because chronic hypernatremia is relatively well tolerated, there are few advantages to correcting the free water deficit rapidly. Free water is administered to correct serum $[Na^+]$ at a rate not exceeding 0.7 mEq/L per hour. The amount of water required to correct a hypernatremic state depends on the free water deficit, the insensible free water losses, and the urinary free water excretion rate. The water requirement to replace the free water deficit can be calculated using the following formula:

$$\text{water requirement} = \frac{\text{desired change in } [Na^+]_s \times \text{TBW}}{\text{desired } [Na^+]_s}$$

For example, a 70-kg patient with a TBW of 42 L (TBW 60% of body weight) has a serum sodium of 170 mEq/L. The maximum desired change in serum sodium over 1 day would be approximately 16 mEq (0.7 mEq/L per hour). Therefore, water requirement = 16 × 42/154 = 4.3 L.

The desired level of serum sodium would not be achieved unless insensible losses (approximately 8 mL/kg per day) and urinary free water losses were also replaced. Urinary losses of free water can be determined by calculating free water clearance:

$$CH_2O = V - C_{osm}\,V - \frac{U_{osm} \times V}{P_{osm}}$$

where CH_2O = free water clearance rate, C_{osm} = osmolar clearance rate, V = urine flow rate, and U_{osm} and P_{osm} = urine and plasma osmolalities, respectively.

The U_{osm} and P_{osm} can be estimated by the total sodium and potassium concentrations. Therefore,

$$CH_2O = V - \frac{(U_{Na} + U_k) \times V}{[Na^+]_s}$$

where U_{Na} and U_K = urinary sodium and potassium concentrations, respectively. A positive number signifies net free water loss and adds to the water requirement, whereas a negative number indicates free water absorption and is subtracted from the water requirement. Thus, the total water requirement to achieve the desired decrease in serum $[Na^+]$ is the sum of the calculated water deficit plus the calculated insensible water loss plus the urinary free water clearance.

Compositional Changes in Body Fluids

Potassium. Potassium is the major intracellular cation and is the major determinant of intracellular osmolality. Normally, intracellular potassium concentration is approximately 150 mEq/L, whereas extracellular potassium levels range from 3.5 to 5 mEq/L. Because of the large difference between intracellular and extracellular potassium concentrations, a transmembrane potential is generated. Alterations in the potassium concentration gradient have profound effects on transmembrane potential and consequently on cellular function. This is especially true for cardiac, skeletal, and smooth muscle. The membrane potential (E_m) developed in cells is described by the Nernst equation:

$$E_m = -\log 60\ [K_I]/[K_E]$$

where $[K_I]$ and $[K_E]$ = intracellular and extracellular potassium concentrations, respectively.

Normally, the membrane potential of cells is approximately −90 mV as produced by a $[K_I]/[K_E]$ ratio of 30:1. Intracellular potassium levels are relatively stable, but extracellular potassium levels are often altered in pathologic situations. Overall potassium balance is determined by potassium intake and by renal and extrarenal excretion.

Approximately 90% of ingested potassium is excreted in the urine, and the remainder (5 to 10 mEq/d) primarily in feces. Most potassium filtered by the glomerulus is reabsorbed in the proximal tubule, so that net excretion is determined by the amount of potassium secreted by the distal tubule and collecting duct of the nephron. In these nephron segments, movement of potassium into the tubular lumen is determined by the difference between intracellular and luminal fluid K^+ concentrations, the permeability of the luminal cell membranes to K^+, and the electrical potential gradient across the luminal cell membrane. Potassium secretion is stimulated by increased urine flow in the distal nephron segments, increased sodium delivery to these segments, high plasma potassium concentrations, and alkalosis. In addition, humoral factors, including aldosterone, vasopressin, and β-adrenergic agonists, stimulate renal excretion of K^+. Because of the central role of the kidneys in potassium excretion, renal failure can lead to hyperkalemia. Nonrenal losses may increase greatly in hyperkalemic states or in renal failure.

Extracellular potassium levels can be greatly influenced by the acute shifts of potassium into or out of the cells. Insulin causes potassium to move into the cell, inducing a change in membrane potential and stimulating glycolysis. Alkalosis causes K^+ to shift into cells in exchange for H^+. Conversely, acidemia induces the cellular exchange of intracellular K^+ for extracellular H^+. A redistribution of K^+ into the ECF can also occur in hyperosmolar conditions because the movement of water into the extracellular compartment causes "solvent drag," which may increase the flux of potassium.

Hyperkalemia

Causes. Hyperkalemia rarely develops from excessive potassium intake given the high capacity for renal potassium excretion. In the surgical patient, diminished renal function is probably the most common problem leading to hyperkalemia. Both chronic and acute renal failure result in a defect in potassium excretion. Nonoliguric renal failure may lead to hyperkalemia despite apparently adequate urine output. Serum potassium levels may increase by 0.3 to 0.5 mEq/L per day in noncatabolic patients with acute renal failure, but this level can increase to 0.7 mEq/L per day or more in catabolic patients or those with other sources of potassium intake. Hospitalized patients may also receive excess potassium in intravenous fluids and total parenteral nutrition formulas. Less obvious sources include medications that are bound to potassium (i.e., β-lactam antibiotics).

In patients with chronic renal disease, potassium balance is normalized by increased colonic potassium excretion, as well as increased potassium excretion per functional nephron. Infusion of cationic amino acid solutions, such as arginine and lysine, can be associated with hyperkalemia because these amino acids are taken up by cells in exchange for potassium. Patients with impaired renal function or diabetes are also at risk for developing hyperkalemia when given ACE inhibitors and/or angiotensin or aldosterone receptor inhibitors.[39]

Cellular disruption with release of potassium may result in hyperkalemia. The classic example of this is hyperkalemia associated with crush injuries. Reperfusion of ischemic limbs can lead to substantial elevations in potassium when reflow of blood washes out the byproducts of ischemia-induced cell lysis. Hyperkalemia may also occur when potassium is released from lysed erythrocytes in large hematomas or after massive blood transfusion. Similarly, potassium release from tumor lysis may result in increased serum potassium. Hyperkalemia can also be associated with the depolarizing muscle relaxants (e.g., succinylcholine). Although unusual, hyperkalemia can also result from absorption of potassium after the use of solutions containing high potassium levels, such as cardioplegia solutions or organ preservation solutions.

Clinical Features. The clinical manifestations of hyperkalemia are primarily related to membrane depolarization caused by a decrease in the $[K_I]/[K_E]$ ratio. The most life-threatening manifestations are related to the cardiac effects of membrane depolarization. Mild hyperkalemia results in peaked T waves on the electrocardiogram (ECG) and can cause paresthesias and/or weakness. More severe forms of hyperkalemia cause flattened P waves, prolongation of the QRS complex, and deep S waves on the ECG. Ventricular fibrillation and cardiac arrest can follow. Neuromuscular manifestations of severe hyperkalemia include weakness progressing to flaccid paralysis.

Treatment. The treatment of hyperkalemia is dictated by the serum level and by ECG changes or symptoms. Severe hyperkalemia with ECG abnormalities requires urgent treatment. The effects of hyperkalemia on membrane potentials can be reduced by increasing calcium levels. Rapid infusion of 10% to 20% calcium gluconate may be lifesaving. The effects are transient and usually last approximately 30 minutes. Administration of sodium bicarbonate is another temporary measure. The increase in serum sodium antagonizes the effects of hyperkalemia on the membrane potential, whereas the increase in extracellular pH shifts potassium into the cells. Movement of potassium into the intracellular compartment can also be achieved by giving 10 to 20 units of regular insulin. To avoid insulin-induced hypoglycemia, 25 to 50 g of glucose (50 to 100 mL of 50% glucose solution) is administered concurrently.

Definitive therapy of hyperkalemia requires increasing potassium excretion. This may be accomplished by the administration of K^+/Na^+ exchange resins such as sodium polystyrene sulfonate (Kayexalate). The usual oral dose is 40 g dissolved in 20 to 100 mL of sorbitol. Each gram removes approximately 1 mEq of potassium. Kayexalate can also be given as a retention enema in a dose of 50 to 100 g in 200 mL of water. Retention of the enema may be facilitated by inflating the balloon of a Foley catheter in the rectum. Each gram removes approximately 0.5 mEq of potassium. Peritoneal dialysis or hemodialysis is indicated for severe hyperkalemia and for patients with renal failure.

Hypokalemia

Causes. Hypokalemia can be caused by TBK depletion secondary to decreased potassium intake, increased extrarenal potassium losses, or increased renal potassium losses. Normally, hypokalemia is not secondary to diminished potassium intake, although intravenous fluid replacement with potassium-free solutions for prolonged periods can result in hypokalemia, especially in patients with ongoing potassium losses.

Decreased serum potassium levels may also be caused by redistribution of potassium into the intracellular space. Acute increases in blood pH secondary to bicarbonate administration during resuscitation can cause acute hypokalemia, as can administration of insulin to hyperglycemic diabetic patients. Causes of hypokalemia are listed in Table 10.10.

Clinical Features. Symptoms of hypokalemia, like those of hyperkalemia, are manifestations of disturbances in the $[K_I]/[K_E]$ ratio with resultant alterations in membrane potentials. As potassium levels fall below 2.5 mEq/L, muscle weakness is common. Severe hypokalemia can cause paralysis involving the muscles of respiration. Intestinal peristalsis can be impaired and result in intestinal ileus. Cardiac muscle abnormalities are reflected by the predisposition to digitalis intoxication; the development of cardiac arrhythmias, including ventricular fibrillation; and sensitization to epinephrine. ECG abnormalities include flattened T waves, depressed ST segments, prominent U waves, and prolongation of the QT interval. Renal changes include decreased renal blood flow and glomerular filtration rate. These effects may be relatively minor, and they may be accompanied by polyuria, polydipsia, metabolic alkalosis, and sodium retention. Decreased peripheral vascular resistance with ensuing hypotension may be due to a decrease in vascular sensitivity to angiotensin II.

Treatment. The primary treatment of hypokalemia is potassium replacement, although the patient's acid–base balance should be considered before initiating therapy. The route and rate of potassium replacement depends on the presence and severity of symptoms. Since potassium is primarily an intracellular ion,

TABLE 10.10

CAUSES OF HYPOKALEMIA

- Shift of potassium to the intracellular space
- Acute alkalosis
- Administration of glucose and insulin
- Catecholamines
- Increased gastrointestinal loss
- Diarrhea
- Mucus-secreting colon tumors (villous adenoma)
- Excessive renal loss
- Metabolic alkalosis
- Magnesium deficiency
- Hyperaldosteronism (adrenal adenoma or hyperplasia)

potassium deficits cannot be directly calculated but they can be estimated. On average, a reduction in serum potassium of 1 mEq/L represents a TBK deficiency of approximately 100 to 200 mEq. Potassium should be given orally if possible. Oral formulations include potassium salts such as potassium chloride, potassium phosphate, and potassium bicarbonate. Potassium should be administered intravenously if the symptoms are severe, if the serum concentration is below 2 mEq/L, or if the patient is unable to take oral potassium. Intravenous potassium is highly irritating to peripheral veins and should not be administered at a rate greater than 20 mEq/h and ideally should be administered at 10 mEq/h or less. Under close cardiac supervision and continuous monitoring in emergent circumstances, as much as 40 mEq/h can be administered via a central line.

Calcium. Calcium is a divalent cation found in abundance in the human body. Approximately 99% of total body calcium is located in bone in the form of hydroxyapatite crystals. Although the bulk of this calcium is not readily exchangeable, the calcium on the surface of bones can be exchanged and serves as the major store of calcium for maintenance of calcium balance. Calcium homeostasis depends on exchange of calcium between bone and ECF, renal excretion, and intestinal absorption. These three processes are controlled to a great extent by parathyroid hormone (PTH).

The total plasma calcium concentration is approximately 10 mg/dL. In ECF, calcium exists in three forms: ionized, nonionized, and protein bound. Ionized calcium, which makes up approximately 45% of total calcium, is responsible for most physiologic actions of calcium in the body, and its level is tightly controlled by regulatory mechanisms. Normal serum concentration of ionized calcium is approximately 4.5 mg/dL. Some nonionized calcium is complexed with nonprotein anions, including phosphate and citrate, and does not easily dissociate. These molecular forms make up only 15% of the total calcium present in plasma. Approximately 40% of extracellular nonionized calcium is bound to proteins. Most is bound to albumin, with the remainder bound to α- and β-globulins.

Changes in either plasma protein levels or pH can alter the proportion of calcium in the ionized state. The protein binding of calcium is pH dependent because of competition by H^+ for protein-binding sites. Prompt correction of changes in ionized calcium by various homeostatic mechanisms usually prevents symptoms from occurring, but rapid changes in pH can result in symptoms. The change in ionized calcium can be predicted if the changes in pH and protein concentrations are known. A 0.1 change in pH alters protein-bound calcium by 0.17 mg/dL in the same direction as the pH change. Thus, acidosis decreases protein-bound calcium levels and increases ionized calcium levels. Similarly, a change in albumin concentration of 1 g/dL changes protein-bound calcium by 0.8 mg/dL in the same direction. Because little of the calcium is bound to globulins, changes in globulin concentration of 1 g/dL change protein-bound calcium by only 0.16 mg/dL.

Despite a 10,000-fold concentration gradient with the ECF, intracellular calcium concentration is normally maintained at extremely low levels, 10^{-7} mol/L. This is accomplished by active transport of calcium out of the cell and by sequestration of calcium in mitochondria and the endoplasmic reticulum. Calcium influx occurs through calcium channels, and cytosolic calcium is often bound to specific calcium-binding proteins such as calmodulin. These control mechanisms are key to the central role of calcium as a second messenger in multiple cellular functions such as neural transmission, muscle contraction, and enzyme regulation.

Calcium Homeostasis. Calcium homeostasis is maintained through a balance of bone exchange, renal excretion, and intestinal absorption. All of these functions are controlled to a great degree by PTH. Of these three homeostatic mechanisms, calcium exchange with bone is the most important. Decreased levels of ionized calcium lead to increases in PTH and increases in 1,25-dihydroxyvitamin D_3, both of which stimulate bone absorption by increasing osteoclastic activity. Increased levels of ionized calcium result in decreased PTH and 1,25-dihydroxyvitamin D_3, which decreases bone absorption. In addition, an elevated ionized calcium concentration results in increased calcitonin and 24,25-dihydroxyvitamin D, which increases osteoblastic activity.

Intestinal absorption of calcium depends primarily on 1,25-dihydroxyvitamin D_3, which stimulates calcium absorption from all parts of the small intestine. Renal excretion of calcium is regulated by PTH and vitamin D, which increase distal tubular reabsorption of calcium, and by calcitonin, which inhibits calcium reabsorption. Both metabolic and respiratory alkalosis can increase calcium excretion. Acidosis has the opposite effect. The fundamentals of the regulation of calcium homeostasis are depicted in Figure 10.7.

Hypercalcemia

Causes. The most common causes of hypercalcemia are hyperparathyroidism and malignancy. Hyperparathyroidism is termed *primary* when one or more parathyroid glands produce inappropriately elevated amounts of PTH in relation to the serum calcium level. This is the result of a parathyroid adenoma in approximately 80% to 90% of cases. Chief cell hyperplasia accounts for an additional 15% of cases, whereas parathyroid cancer is responsible for less than 1% of cases. In secondary hyperparathyroidism, elevated PTH secretion occurs because of an abnormality of an organ system other than the parathyroid glands. Usually this is the result of renal failure, although Paget disease, osteogenesis imperfecta, and multiple myeloma are other known etiologies. Renal failure can contribute to hypocalcemia in several ways: (a) poor renal excretion of phosphate produces rises in serum phosphate levels that result in decreased serum calcium levels, (b) gut absorption of calcium is decreased because of a deficiency in renal vitamin D metabolism, and (c) diseased kidneys are not capable of clearing the breakdown products of PTH. Tertiary hyperparathyroidism is the development of parathyroid hyperplasia with autonomous PTH production. As a result, up to 30% of patients with prerenal transplantation hyperparathyroidism have persistent elevations in the PTH and calcium after renal transplantation despite the fact that renal function has returned toward normal.

Hypercalcemia can be caused by malignant disease, either because of bony destruction from metastases, or from autonomous tumor secretion of PTH-like substances that alter calcium homeostasis. Common causes of hypercalcemia associated with bone destruction include multiple myeloma, lymphoma, or metastatic breast carcinoma. Interleukin-1, colony-stimulating factor, and tumor necrosis factor have been implicated as local mediators of the osteolytic activity associated with tumor metastases. Tumors that elaborate humoral factors resulting in hypercalcemia are primarily squamous cell carcinomas of the head and neck, esophagus, lung, kidney, and genitourinary tract. Secretion of PTH-like peptides, prostaglandins, transforming growth factor, and vitamin D metabolites has been reported. Humorally mediated hypercalcemia may also occur with metastatic tumors, especially breast carcinoma.

Other causes of hypercalcemia include the use of thiazide diuretics, acute adrenal insufficiency, granulomatous disease, milk-alkali syndrome, hyperthyroidism, and prolonged immobilization in otherwise young and healthy patients.

Clinical Features. The clinical manifestations of hypercalcemia depend on both the severity and duration of the abnormality. Neuromuscular effects may be the earliest manifestations and include muscle fatigue, weakness, personality disorders, psychoses, confusion, depression, and coma. Cardiovascular effects are less prominent, with hypertension being the most frequent problem encountered. ECG changes include shortening

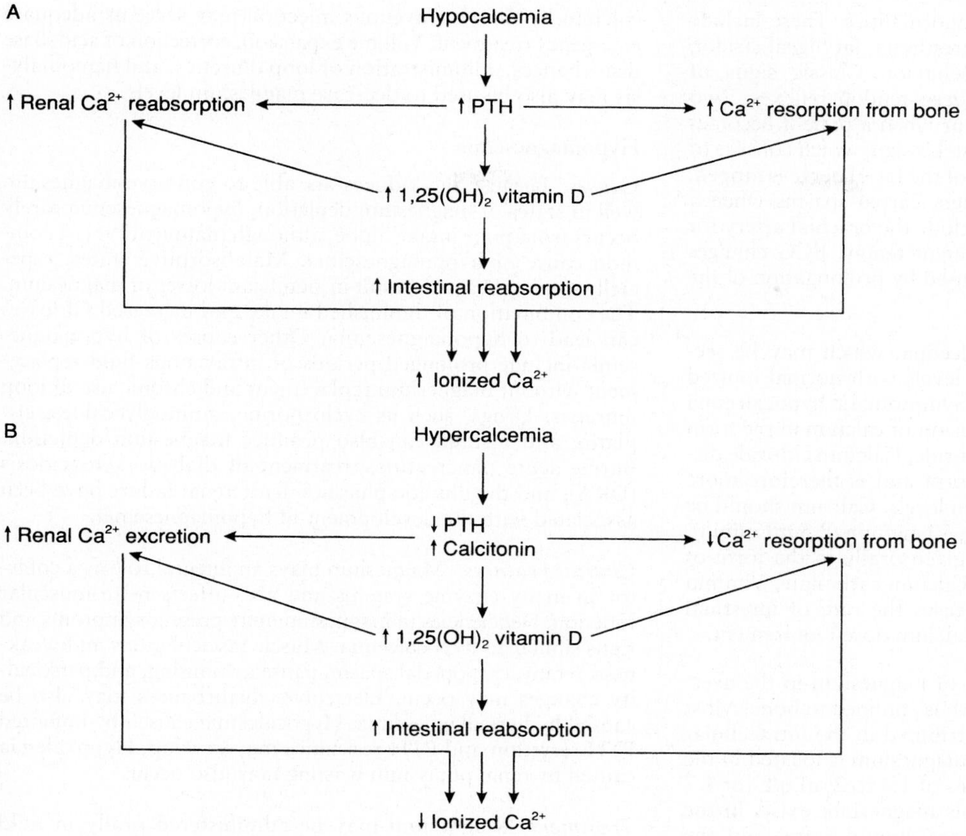

FIGURE 10.7. Effects of hypocalcemia (A) and hypercalcemia (B) on the mediators of calcium homeostasis. PTH, parathyroid hormone.

of the QT interval. GI side effects, such as nausea, vomiting, and abdominal pain, are not uncommon. Pancreatitis and increased gastric acid secretion with ulcer formation have also been reported.

The renal side effects of chronic hypercalcemia are numerous and can be severe. The combination of increased renal calcium excretion and decreased intestinal calcium reabsorption in response to hypercalcemia results in a new state of equilibrium at a higher serum concentration of calcium. A decrease in glomerular filtration rate, which may be a direct effect of hypercalcemia or secondary to dehydration from vomiting, can exacerbate the hypercalcemia by increasing calcium reabsorption by the kidney. In addition, nephrocalcinosis can occur, ultimately leading to chronic renal failure. Nephrolithiasis, interstitial nephropathy, renal tubular acidosis (RTA), and nephrogenic diabetes insipidus may also accompany prolonged hypercalcemia.

Treatment. Elevation of serum calcium concentrations to greater than 14 mg/dL requires prompt treatment to prevent potentially lethal complications of hypercalcemia. This is even more urgent for hypercalcemia associated with hyperphosphatemia because of the risk of metastatic calcification. Immediate measures are directed toward maximizing renal excretion of calcium. Because these patients are often dehydrated, 0.9% or 0.45% saline solution with 20 to 30 mEq/L of potassium is administered intravenously. Hydration should proceed at rates of 200 to 300 mL/h to promote diuresis. Once adequate hydration is achieved, furosemide may be given at a rate of 20 to 80 mg every 1 to 2 hours. To enhance calcium excretion, the patient should remain in positive fluid balance. Replacement of potassium and magnesium may also be needed.

Long-term treatment depends on the underlying cause of the hypercalcemia. Primary hyperparathyroidism is treated by parathyroidectomy. Secondary or tertiary hyperparathyroidism may be treated by either subtotal parathyroidectomy or total parathyroidectomy with autonomous parathyroid transplantation. Hypercalcemia secondary to tumor secretion of hormonal mediators may be controlled by extirpation of the tumor. In the presence of metastatic bone disease, inhibition of bone resorption with mithramycin or calcitonin may yield good results. In addition, hypercalcemia due to metastatic breast carcinoma or hematologic malignancies may respond to steroid therapy. Intravenous administration of bisphosphonates has been shown to be extremely effective and safe for treatment of patients with hypercalcemia associated with cancer.[40] Patients with renal failure benefit from dialysis using a low-calcium dialysate.

Hypocalcemia

Causes. Hypocalcemia secondary to hypoparathyroidism can complicate thyroid or parathyroid surgery by either inadvertent total parathyroidectomy or loss of parathyroid function due to devascularization. This has been reported to occur in as many as 2% to 3% of patients undergoing total thyroidectomy, although this figure appears to be declining. After resection of a parathyroid adenoma, hypocalcemia can occur because of atrophy of the remaining glands. Calcium replacement therapy may be required until the remaining glands resume normal function.

Hypocalcemia can also complicate acute pancreatitis owing to calcium precipitation into the peripancreatic tissues. In addition, pancreatic and small-bowel fistulas may result in loss of calcium-rich fluid. Longstanding vitamin D deficiency secondary to malnutrition, malabsorption, or lack of exposure to sunlight can lead to hypocalcemia. Renal failure can lead to a deficiency in 1,25-dihydroxyvitamin D_3 and result in diminished intestinal absorption of calcium. Severe magnesium deficiency can also lead to hypocalcemia because of suppression of PTH levels.

Clinical Features. Serum calcium levels below 8 mg/dL may be associated with symptoms and signs that are primarily manifestations of neuromuscular abnormalities. These include muscle cramps, perioral tingling, paresthesia, laryngeal stridor, tetany, seizures, and psychotic behavior. Classic signs of hypocalcemia include hyperactive deep tendon reflexes. Two well-described physical findings occur when a patient becomes hypocalcemic. One of these is Chvostek's sign, which consists of facial muscle spasm when the trunk of the facial nerve is tapped. The other finding is Trousseau's sign, carpal spasms when a blood pressure cuff is inflated to occlude the brachial artery for 3 minutes. This finding indicates latent tetany. ECG changes include a prolonged QT interval caused by prolongation of the ST segment.

Treatment. Asymptomatic hypocalcemia, which may be secondary to low protein or albumin levels with normal ionized calcium levels, need not be treated. Symptomatic hypocalcemia is best treated with intravenous infusion of calcium in the form of calcium gluconate or calcium chloride. Calcium chloride dissociates primarily to the ionized form and is therefore more efficacious in raising ionized calcium levels. Calcium should be administered at a rate not exceeding 50 mg/min (2.5 mEq/min). Prolonged calcium replacement is given orally in the form of calcium lactate, calcium citrate, or calcium carbonate. Vitamin D_3, also known as calcitriol, increases the rate of intestinal absorption and decreases the oral calcium dose requirement.

Magnesium. Total body content of magnesium in the average adult is 2,000 mEq, half of which is confined to bone. Most of the remaining magnesium is distributed in the intracellular space. Less than 1% of total body magnesium is located in the extracellular space, at concentrations of 1.4 to 2 mEq/L (or 1.7 to 2.3 mg/dL). Sixty percent of this magnesium exists in the ionized form, 25% is in the protein-bound state, and the remainder is complexed with nonprotein anionic species.

Approximately 25 mEq/d of magnesium is consumed in the diet, a variable amount of which is absorbed by the small intestine. Magnesium absorption may be influenced by the levels of 1,25-dihydroxyvitamin D_3. Bone stores constitute the other major source of available magnesium, although regulation of magnesium exchange with bone is poorly understood.

Magnesium is excreted primarily by the kidneys. Approximately 40% of the filtered magnesium is reabsorbed in the proximal tubule, predominantly in the ascending limb of Henle. Thus, loop diuretics cause a marked increase in magnesium excretion. Magnesium excretion is also increased by hypermagnesemia, hypercalcemia, metabolic acidosis, and phosphate depletion. Conversely, magnesium excretion is decreased by metabolic alkalosis.

Hypermagnesemia

Causes. Because of the ability of the kidneys to excrete large magnesium loads, hypermagnesemia rarely occurs if renal function is normal. In chronic or acute renal failure, administration of magnesium-containing antacids or laxatives is frequently the cause of hypermagnesemia. Severe burns, crush injuries, and other causes of rhabdomyolysis may lead to high magnesium levels due to the release of magnesium from injured tissues. Severe metabolic acidosis, extracellular volume depletion, and renal insufficiency with creatinine clearances below 30 mL/min may also cause hypermagnesemia.

Clinical Features. Neuromuscular function is depressed by hypermagnesemia because of the inhibition of synaptic acetylcholine release. Loss of deep tendon reflexes can occur with magnesium levels above 8 mg/dL. Paralysis and eventually coma can develop if levels exceed 12 to 18 mg/dL. Hypotension or even cardiac arrest can occur if levels exceed 18 mg/dL.

Treatment. Magnesium-containing medications must be avoided in patients with hypermagnesemia. Calcium antagonizes the effects of magnesium, and infusion of 5 to 10 mEq of calcium by slow intravenous injection may serve as adequate emergency treatment. Volume expansion, correction of acid–base disturbances, administration of loop diuretics, and hemodialysis may also be used to decrease magnesium levels.

Hypomagnesemia

Causes. Because the kidneys are able to conserve magnesium well in states of magnesium depletion, hypomagnesemia rarely occurs from poor intake alone, although malnutrition is a common cause of hypomagnesemia. Malabsorptive states, especially steatorrhea, can result in significant losses of magnesium. The combination of diminished intake and increased GI losses can lead to hypomagnesemia. Other causes of hypomagnesemia include prolonged periods of intravenous fluid replacement without magnesium replacement and chronic use of loop diuretics. Drugs, such as cyclosporine, aminoglycosides, cisplatin, and insulin, can also produce magnesium depletion. Burns, acute pancreatitis, treatment of diabetic ketoacidosis (DKA), and the diuretic phase of acute renal failure have been associated with the development of hypomagnesemia.

Clinical Features. Magnesium plays an integral role as a cofactor in many enzyme systems and also affects neuromuscular function. Deficiencies in magnesium may present symptoms and signs similar to hypocalcemia. Muscle fasciculations and weakness, tetany, carpopedal spasm, nausea, vomiting, and personality changes may occur. Electrolyte disturbances may also be caused by hypomagnesemia. Hypocalcemia caused by impaired PTH secretion and PTH resistance may develop. Hypokalemia caused by renal potassium wasting may also occur.

Treatment. Magnesium may be administered orally in mild cases of hypomagnesemia, but large oral doses frequently lead to diarrhea. Correction of major deficits is therefore managed by intravenous administration of magnesium sulfate at a dose of 50 to 100 mEq/d. Treatment of patients who have severe symptoms with up to 3 g of magnesium sulfate may be accomplished by bolus intravenous injection followed by an infusion of 1 to 2 mEq/kg per day.

ACID–BASE BALANCE

Definitions

An acid is defined as a chemical that can donate a hydrogen ion (H^+), for example, HCl and H_2CO_3, and a base is a chemical that can accept a H^+, for example, OH^- and HCO_3^-. Ampholytes are both acids and bases; an example is $H_2PO_4^-$, which can donate a H^+ to become HPO_4^{2-} but can also accept H^+ to become H_3PO_4. Because HCl is a strong acid that almost completely dissociates, Cl^- is not considered a base. Bases are commonly anions, but neutral substances can also function as bases (e.g., ammonia and creatinine). Some chemicals do not fit the classic definition of an acid, although they retain acidic properties when dissociated in water. For example, when $CaCl_2$ is dissolved in water, the Ca^{2+} accepts OH^- to form $Ca(OH)_2$. Because $[H^+] \times [OH^-]$ in water remains constant at 10 to 14, the consumption of OH^- by Ca^{2+} results in increased dissociation of water. Consequently, the concentration of hydrogen ions increases, and $CaCl_2$ dissolved in water is an acidic solution.

The concentration of hydrogen ions $[H^+]$ determines the acidity of a solution. The pH is the negative logarithm of $[H^+]$ expressed in moles per liter (mol/L). The concentration of H^+ in biologic systems is in the range of nanomoles (10^{-9} mol) per liter (nmol/L). When

$$[H^+] = 40 \text{ nmol/L} = 4 \times 10^{-10} \text{ mol/L}$$

then

$$\text{pH} = -\log[H^+] = -(-7.4) = 7.4$$

When

$$[H^+] = 80 \text{ nmol/L} = 8 \times 10^{-10} \text{ mol/L}$$

then

$$pH = -\log[H^+] = -(-7.1) = 7.1$$

The degree to which an acid dissociates determines its strength. If an acid, HA, dissociates to H^+ and A^-, then

$$[H^+] \times [A^-]/[HA] = K$$

where K = dissociation constant. The greater the value of K, the greater the ability to dissociate and therefore the greater the strength of the acid. Because most acids have a K value considerably below 1.0,

$$pK = -\log K$$

Rearranging,

$$[H^+] = K \times [HA]/[A^-]$$
$$-\log[H^+] = -\log K \times -\log[HA]/[A^-]$$
$$pH = pK \times \log[A^-]/[HA]$$

This is the derivation for the Henderson-Hasselbalch equation.

Buffer Systems

Buffers are chemicals in solution that tend to minimize changes in pH that would otherwise occur after the addition of acid or alkali. If a strong acid is added to the salt of a weak acid and a strong base, the reaction produces another salt and a weak acid:

$$HCl + NaHCO_3 \rightarrow NaCl + H_2CO_3$$

Thus, the decrease in pH that would have occurred in the absence of $NaHCO_3$ is minimized. Conversely, if a strong base is added to a weak acid, the base is neutralized:

$$NaOH + H_2CO_3 \rightarrow NaHCO_3 + H_2O$$

The elevation in pH after the addition of NaOH is prevented.

One type of buffer is a mixture of a weak acid and its salt, which forms an amount of weak acid or base equivalent to the amount of strong acid or base added to the system. The presence of such buffer systems in the body is crucial in minimizing changes in pH secondary to the daily production of the 70 mEq of acid generated from dietary precursors. There is a relatively narrow range of pH for optimal function of the chemical reactions necessary for cell function.

The principal intracellular buffers are organic phosphates, bicarbonate, and peptides. In addition, hemoglobin functions as a significant buffer in red blood cells. The major extracellular buffer is bicarbonate. An approximation of the total body buffer capacity is 15 mEq/kg. More than half of the total body alkaline buffer content is located outside the ECF and may in large part reside in bone.[41] The buffer pair carbonic acid/bicarbonate (H_2CO_3/HCO_3^-) is the focus of the ensuing discussion because it is the primary buffer system of the body and the components of this buffer system are easily measured. Because all body buffer systems are in equilibrium, the state of the H_2CO_3/HCO_3^- system essentially reflects the state of all the body buffers.

From a chemical point of view, the ideal buffer should have a pK that approximates the pH to be preserved. The H_2CO_3/HCO_3^- buffer system has a pK of only 6.1, but this buffer system is efficient because of the presence of large amounts of bicarbonate, the conversion of its acid H_2CO_3 to CO_2 that is rapidly excreted through the lungs, and an inexhaustible supply of CO_2, although at low concentrations.

The H_2CO_3/HCO_3^- buffer system is defined by the Henderson-Hasselbalch equation:

$$pH = pK + \log[HCO_3^-]/[H_2CO_3]$$

In the clinical use of this equation, $[H_2CO_3]$ is replaced by $[CO_2]$ because measurement of the low concentrations of $[H_2CO_3]$ present in body fluids is difficult, whereas $[CO_2]$, which is in equilibrium with $[H_2CO_3]$ in a fixed ratio, can be readily measured. Making this substitution, the equation becomes

$$pH = pK + \log[HCO_3^-]/[CO_2]$$

Because the pK for this buffer system is 6.1,

$$pH = 6.1 + \log[HCO_3^-]/[CO_2]$$

Using normal values for $[HCO_3^-]$ (24 mEq/L) and $[CO_2]$ (1.2 mmol/L),

$$pH = 6.1 + \log 24/1.2$$
$$= 6.1 + \log 20 = 7.4$$

A pH of 7.4 is maintained as long as the ratio of $[HCO_3^-]$ to $[CO_2]$ remains 20:1. The amount of $[CO_2]$ in solution is estimated from partial pressure of carbon dioxide (PCO_2) and its solubility coefficient (0.03 in plasma). Making these substitutions,

$$pH = 6.1 + \log[HCO_3^-]/(PCO_2 \times 0.03)$$

Anion Gap

The anion gap is defined as follows:

$$\text{Anion gap} = [Na^+] - ([Cl^-] + [HCO_3])$$

Normally, the difference between the serum $[Na^+]$ and the sum of the chloride and bicarbonate anion concentrations is a reflection of the sum of the serum proteins, sulfate anions, inorganic phosphates, and organic acids present in low concentrations. The anion gap is usually 12 ± 2 mEq/L. Variances from the normal may be caused by a change in unmeasured anions or cations. Calculation of the anion gap may help define both simple and mixed forms of acid–base disturbances. Acidosis associated with a high anion gap is usually secondary to increases in endogenously produced acids (e.g., lactic acidosis or ketoacidosis), decreases in renal excretion of acid, or ingestion of toxins.

Acid–Base Disturbances

8 There are four primary acid–base disturbances, each of which are related to changes in either $[HCO_3^-]$ or PCO_2. Metabolic acidosis is a decrease in pH as a result of a primary decrease in $[HCO_3^-]$, whereas metabolic alkalosis is an increase in pH caused by a primary increase in $[HCO_3^-]$. Respiratory acidosis is a decrease in pH secondary to a primary increase in PCO_2, and respiratory alkalosis is an increase in pH caused by a primary decrease in PCO_2. In each of these disorders, compensatory changes occur to minimize changes in the relative ratio of $[HCO_3^-]$ to PCO_2 and thereby blunt the effect of the primary disturbance on pH (Table 10.11).

Metabolic Acidosis. Three mechanisms result in a decrease in extracellular bicarbonate concentration and metabolic acidosis:

1. Dilutional acidosis. Rapid infusion of an alkali-free solution results in dilution of the bicarbonate concentration.
2. Cellular retention of K^+ in exchange for Na^+ and H^+. Buffering of the H^+ may result in a transient decrease in extracellular bicarbonate concentration.
3. Decreased body bicarbonate content. This occurs when net loss of bicarbonate exceeds bicarbonate generation.

TABLE 10.11

HCO_3^- AND PCO_2 DERANGEMENTS IN PRIMARY AND SECONDARY ACID–BASE DISTURBANCES

		PRIMARY		SECONDARY	
DISORDER	pH	HCO_3^-	PCO_2	HCO_3^-	PCO_2
Metabolic acidosis	↓	↓			↓
Metabolic alkalosis	↑	↑			↑
Respiratory acidosis	↓		↑	↑	
Respiratory alkalosis	↑		↓	↓	

The first two mechanisms are relatively infrequent and usually produce only mild, self-limiting metabolic acidosis; however, aggressive "overresuscitation" of surgical or trauma patients with normal saline solution may result in a dilutional acidosis. Most clinically significant metabolic acidosis is related to net loss of bicarbonate, which occurs when consumption due to either loss or titration is greater than bicarbonate generation. Under normal circumstances of ingestion of the average amount of protein in the American diet, approximately 70 mEq of acid is generated daily. The major source of acid production is sulfuric acid from the metabolism of sulfur-containing amino acids. In addition, normal physiologic processes result in the generation of organic acids, the titration of which consumes bicarbonate. Although the resulting organic anions are further metabolized with regeneration of bicarbonate, urinary excretion of some organic anions occurs and results in net loss of bicarbonate.

These sources of acid gain are partially offset by net GI absorption of metabolizable anions, such as citrate, which are metabolized to yield bicarbonate. The remainder of the excess acid is balanced by renal excretion of acid with simultaneous generation of bicarbonate. A decrease in body bicarbonate content may therefore be the result of a primary increase in net acid generation, termed *extrarenal acidosis,* or a primary reduction in renal acid excretion, termed *renal acidosis.*

In extrarenal acidosis, the normal compensatory mechanism is increased renal excretion of acid, usually as ammonia, with generation of bicarbonate. This mechanism is sensitive to decreases in bicarbonate concentration and has the capacity to generate large amounts of bicarbonate.

In contrast, renal acidosis is not as readily compensated because the renal abnormality is the primary mechanism. The level to which serum bicarbonate concentration decreases depends on several factors, including the magnitude of the disparity in acid production and acid excretion as well as its duration. In general, the development of renal acidosis is slow but progressive, whereas the development of extrarenal acidosis is rapid but usually self-limiting. Despite persistent net loss of bicarbonate, extracellular bicarbonate concentration may stabilize at a subnormal level rather than continue to decrease. This may be due to bone buffering, which has the capacity to buffer as much as 28 to 37 mEq/d of acid.

Mechanisms Resulting in Decreased Body Bicarbonate Content

Increased Production of Organic Acids. Increased protein intake and tissue catabolism resulting in greater metabolism of sulfur-containing amino acids can lead to generation of increased amounts of sulfuric acid. With normal kidney function, any decline in serum bicarbonate concentration stimulates renal acid excretion, which can compensate nearly completely for the increase in acid production.

Administration of Exogenous Acid. Ingestion of a sufficient quantity of exogenous acid can exceed renal compensatory capacity and result in metabolic acidosis. Examples of acids that may be ingested include ammonium chloride, calcium chloride, nitric acid, sulfuric acid, and hydrochloric acid.

Nonrenal Loss of Bicarbonate. Diarrhea, intestinal or pancreatic fistulas, and burns can cause metabolic acidosis secondary to loss of bicarbonate. Urinary diversion with segments of GI tract (ureterosigmoidostomy and ureteroileostomy) can result in loss of bicarbonate with reabsorption of NH_4Cl from the urine. The potential for fistulas to result in metabolic acidosis depends on the concentration of bicarbonate in the fluid and the rate of external drainage. Thus, metabolic acidosis is less common with biliary fistulas than pancreatic fistulas because bicarbonate concentration in bile is usually less than 50 to 60 mEq/L, and the amount of drainage tends to be modest. Bicarbonate concentration in pancreatic juice approaches 150 mEq/L, and the drainage can be profuse.

Organic Acidosis. Organic acidosis describes conditions of acidosis brought about by abnormal endogenous production of specific acid compounds. The two most common types of organic acidosis are *ketoacidosis* and *lactic acidosis.*

Ketoacidosis. Normally, free fatty acids generated from breakdown of triglycerides in adipose tissue are either used as an energy source by tissues such as muscle or carried to the liver, where they are reesterified to triglycerides. Ketoacids are produced by mitochondrial metabolism of free fatty acids to acetyl CoA, with subsequent formation of acetoacetate and b-hydroxybutyrate (redox forms of the same compound). Under normal conditions, a small amount of ketoacidosis is produced. During prolonged starvation, production of ketoacids increases to modest levels, providing an important source of energy to nonhepatic tissues, particularly the brain.

In DKA, the ketoacid production is excessive because of insulin deficiency, which drives ketoacid production by increasing free fatty acid release from adipose tissue, increasing transport of free fatty acids into hepatic mitochondria, promoting conversion of acetyl CoA to ketoacids, and impairing extrahepatic use of ketoacids.[42] Insulin deficiency also contributes to hyperglycemia by decreasing the metabolism of glucose by extrahepatic tissues and increasing hepatic production of glucose. The resulting osmotic glucose diuresis causes increased renal excretion of sodium and water. Additional losses of sodium and potassium occur as the result of renal excretion of the excess ketoacid anions. Potassium excretion is further enhanced by hyperaldosteronism due to the increased delivery of sodium to the distal tubule that occurs in association with the osmotic diuresis. Despite TBK depletion, serum potassium concentration is often increased in DKA secondary to metabolic acidosis, renal insufficiency, insulin deficiency, and hyperosmolality. These pathophysiologic changes result in the typical clinical presentation, which includes dehydration, polyuria, polydipsia, hyperglycemia, hyperventilation, and metabolic acidosis with an increased anion gap. Spontaneous decarboxylation of acetoacetate to acetone occurs with excretion of acetone through the lungs, resulting in the characteristic odor described in DKA. Patients may demonstrate impaired mental status or coma in severe cases.

In hyperosmolar, hyperglycemic, and nonketotic coma, moderate acidosis may be observed. The mechanism of the acidosis is not clear. In contrast to the moderate hyperglycemia, averaging 600 mg/dL, seen in DKA, the marked hyperglycemia, averaging 1,200 mg/dL, that occurs in hyperosmolar nonketotic hyperglycemia is not associated with ketoacidosis.

Lactic Acidosis. Lactic acidosis can be characterized as type A (caused by tissue hypoxia) or type B (other causes). Hypoxia impairs the mitochondrial oxidation of the reduced form of nicotinamide adenine dinucleotide (NADH) to NAD, which is necessary for glycolysis. Under these conditions, NADH is oxidized by the reduction of pyruvate, the end product of glucose metabolism in the Embden-Meyerhof pathway, to lactic acid. Thus, generation of lactic acid is the final step of anaerobic glycolysis. Lactic acid is normally produced by muscle, blood elements, intestine, and skin and is used by the liver and kidney. Normal serum lactate concentration is below 2 mEq/L. Lactic acidosis secondary to hypoxia is usually due to increased production of lactate as well as decreased use, and serum lactate concentration is greater than 6 mEq/L.

The most common cause of type B lactic acidosis is ethanol intoxication. Lactic acidosis is caused by increased generation of NADH by the metabolism of alcohol, which interferes with hepatic gluconeogenesis and, therefore, lactate use.

In lactic acidosis, the L-isomer is usually elevated because of the specificity of mammalian lactate dehydrogenase. Various bacteria found in colonic flora are capable of generating large amounts of D-lactic acid. D-Lactic acidosis has been reported in humans only in the presence of short-gut syndrome because the small bowel normally absorbs the dietary substrate for bacterial D-lactic acid production. In addition, the colon must be selectively colonized by bacteria that possess D-lactate dehydrogenase. Typically, the patient has short-gut syndrome, and the acidosis is preceded by food ingestion and is accompanied by characteristic neurologic findings, including mental confusion, slurred speech, staggering gait, and nystagmus. These neurologic manifestations are secondary to bacterial neurotoxins. The acidosis is accompanied by an increased anion gap, but L-lactate and ketone levels are normal. Treatment includes oral antibiotics, recolonization of the colon with non–D-lactate dehydrogenase–forming bacteria, and a low-carbohydrate diet.

Metabolic Acidosis Caused by Drugs and Toxins. Acetylsalicylic acid (aspirin) is rapidly metabolized to salicylic acid and then more slowly to other metabolites that are excreted by the kidney. Ingestion of more than 4 to 6 g/d results in salicylate intoxication with an anion gap metabolic acidosis, as well as renal excretion of unmetabolized salicylic acid. Acidosis increases the toxicity of salicylate by increasing the concentration of its nonionized form, which can achieve high intracellular concentrations. A respiratory alkalosis occurs due to direct stimulation of the respiratory center. Manifestations of salicylate overdose include tinnitus, asterixis, noncardiogenic pulmonary edema, hypotension, vascular collapse, vomiting, seizures, and coma. Treatment consists of alkalinization of the urine to prevent reabsorption of salicylate and hemodialysis in patients with severe neurologic symptoms.

Ethylene glycol, the principal component of antifreeze, is converted by alcohol dehydrogenase to glycoaldehyde, then to glycolic acid with production of one NADH at each step. The acidosis produced by ingestion of ethylene glycol is secondary to accumulation of glycolic acid, although lactate also accumulates because of the production of NADH. Bicarbonate is not regenerated when the glycolate is further metabolized, so exogenous alkali is required to replace what was titrated. In addition, 3% to 10% of ethylene glycol is converted to oxalic acid, which may result in hypocalcemia and contribute to acute renal failure. Three stages of toxicity are described. CNS dysfunction characterizes the first stage. This is followed by cardiopulmonary failure and finally by oliguric acute renal failure. Treatment includes the administration of ethanol, which has greater affinity for alcohol dehydrogenase and delays the metabolism of ethylene glycol to its toxic metabolites. Treatment also includes hemodialysis or peritoneal dialysis to remove ethylene glycol and glycolate.

Metabolism of methanol by alcohol dehydrogenase results in the formation of formaldehyde and formic acid, both of which are severely toxic. The acidosis is associated with an increase in anion gap secondary to the accumulation of formate. The clinical presentation includes blurred vision or blindness associated with the funduscopic findings of hyperemic discs and retinal edema, malaise, headache, abdominal pain, vomiting, convulsions, and coma. Treatment includes ethanol infusion to delay the metabolism of methanol by alcohol dehydrogenase, hemodialysis, bicarbonate administration, and intravenous folate to enhance metabolism of formate.

Renal Acidosis: Decreased Net Acid Excretion. The impaired ability of the kidney to excrete acid may be secondary to a decrease in the number of functioning nephrons and is termed *uremic acidosis* or *renal tubular acidosis.* Uremic acidosis, which can occur in both acute and chronic renal failure, is primarily caused by a reduction in ammonia excretion secondary to a reduction in the number of functioning proximal tubular cells. In addition, decreased proximal tubular bicarbonate reabsorption contributes to the development of acidosis. Although the onset of uremic acidosis may be related to declining renal function, its appearance can also be influenced by diet-dependent protein and organic anion ingestion, use of diuretic therapy that stimulates acid excretion, and the extent of tubular versus glomerular injury.

RTA can be classified as distal (type I) or proximal (type II), depending on the primary site of the renal tubular defect leading to acidosis. Distal RTA is characterized by a defect in urinary acidification. It is associated with either hypokalemia or hyperkalemia, depending on the underlying pathophysiologic mechanisms. Proposed mechanisms of distal RTA with hypokalemia include reduced H^+ pump activity and increased tubular permeability with back-leak of secreted H^+ into the tubular cell. In RTA with hyperkalemia, the mechanism is decreased luminal negativity secondary to impaired sodium reabsorption. The major defect in proximal RTA is proximal tubular dysfunction resulting in diminished reabsorption of filtered bicarbonate. Urinary excretion greater than 15% of the filtered load of bicarbonate at normal serum bicarbonate levels is pathognomonic for proximal RTA. Other indicators of proximal tubular dysfunction include glycosuria, aminoaciduria, uricosuria, and phosphaturia.

Clinical Features of Acute Metabolic Acidosis. The major cardiovascular effects of acute metabolic acidosis are peripheral arteriolar dilatation, decreased cardiac contractility, and central venous constriction. These can lead to cardiovascular collapse and pulmonary edema. Catecholamine secretion is stimulated by metabolic acidosis, and in mild cases (pH >7.1), heart rate may be increased. In more severe metabolic acidosis (pH <7.1), the direct effects of acidosis override the catecholamine effects and result in bradycardia and decreased contractility. These depressive effects are magnified by beta-blockers. In addition to these cardiovascular effects, metabolic acidosis can increase oxygen delivery by shifting the oxygen–hemoglobin dissociation curve to the right. In more prolonged metabolic acidosis, this may be partially offset by decreased production of 2,3-diphosphoglycerate in red blood cells because of a slower rate of glycolysis. Metabolic acidosis can also cause gastric distention, abdominal pain, nausea, and vomiting.

Compensatory Mechanisms

Renal Compensation. The kidney is extremely sensitive to changes in serum bicarbonate concentration and responds by increasing net acid excretion primarily by increasing ammonia excretion. Maximal renal compensation requires 2 to 4 days. In addition, the maximal amount of ammonia excreted during acidosis depends on factors that include the rate of glutamine delivery, effects on glomerular filtration rate by associated conditions such as dehydration, and the type of anion that accompanies the acid because renal acid secretion is stimulated to varying degrees by different anions. Although renal compensation is effective in achieving normal net acid excretion with extrarenal causes of metabolic acid, variable results are seen with renal acidosis. Compensation at times is complete for proximal RTA, whereas compensation usually is incomplete for distal RTA.

Respiratory Compensation. Delay in achieving maximal renal response to an increased acid load causes blood pH to decline, which stimulates hyperventilation. Although effective in promptly raising blood pH, early ventilatory compensation is only partial. Full respiratory compensation can occur in 12 to 24 hours. The magnitude of the decrease in PCO_2 in response to a given degree of metabolic acidosis can be used to determine whether the metabolic acidosis is complicated by coexisting respiratory acidosis or respiratory alkalosis. Although a number of sophisticated mathematic models relating PCO_2 to serum bicarbonate, serum hydrogen ion, and pH have been described, the following is a simple equation that is readily applicable to the clinical situation:

$$dPCO_2 = 1.2 \times d[HCO_3^-] \pm 2.0$$

where $dPCO_2$ = expected decrease in PCO_2 given the measured decrease in serum bicarbonate concentration. For example, if serum bicarbonate is 18, $d[HCO_3^-]$ is 6 (24 – 18). The expected $dPCO_2$ is 7.2 ± 2, or PCO_2 = 32.8 (40 – 7.2) ± 2 mm Hg. This equation is applicable in mild to moderate metabolic acidosis because pulmonary edema complicating severe metabolic acidosis interferes with maximal ventilatory compensation.

Treatment

Acute Metabolic Acidosis. In surgical and trauma patients, metabolic acidosis is often the result of inadequate tissue perfusion and consequent lactic acidosis. Volume resuscitation alone may be enough to correct this acidosis. Attempts to correct acidosis with exogenous bicarbonate without addressing inadequate tissue perfusion will be unsuccessful. Bicarbonate is best reserved for patients with metabolic acidosis that is either not easily reversible or is so severe that the patient is in danger of cardiovascular collapse. Older patients and those with cardiovascular disease have decreased tolerance for acidosis, and it may be appropriate to administer bicarbonate in these groups before the pH has fallen to critically low levels. The amount of bicarbonate required to increase its serum concentration to any given level cannot be calculated. The goal is to increase the pH to 7.2 to 7.3 by administering one or two ampules of bicarbonate (44.5 to 50 mEq/amp) initially, basing the need for additional bicarbonate on repeated arterial blood gas results. Rapid correction to achieve normal serum bicarbonate concentration may be harmful because organic anions are precursors of bicarbonate, and their eventual metabolism combined with administered bicarbonate may result in metabolic alkalosis. This may be further complicated by persistent hyperventilation in the face of rapidly normalized serum bicarbonate concentration, resulting in the superimposition of a respiratory alkalosis. In addition, rapid correction of serum bicarbonate concentration may not allow reversal of 2,3-diphosphoglycerate depletion in red blood cells. The resulting leftward shift of the oxygen–hemoglobin dissociation curve may result in tissue hypoxia.

Chronic Acidosis. Distal RTA may be treated with daily doses of alkali to correct acidosis and prevent nephrocalcinosis and nephrolithiasis, and potassium supplementation if hypokalemia is also present. Mild proximal RTA in adults does not require specific therapy. Severe cases ($[HCO_3^-]$ <18) are treated with thiazide diuretics and a low-salt diet aimed to achieve modest volume depletion, which reduces bicarbonate requirement. Children are particularly susceptible to the growth-retarding effects of even mild acidosis, and the threshold for treatment should be low.

Diabetic Ketoacidosis. The correction of both acidosis and hyperglycemia is best achieved by administration of insulin. Metabolism of the anions of the ketoacids begins promptly with insulin therapy and results in the generation of bicarbonate. In addition, insulin inhibits ketone formation and gluconeogenesis and stimulates peripheral uptake of ketones and glucose. An intravenous (IV) dose of 20 IU of regular insulin may be given to initiate therapy, followed by a continuous intravenous infusion of 5 to 10 IU/h. Insulin administration should continue until acidosis resolves. Volume resuscitation requirements in DKA averages 4 to 5 L in the first 24 hours. By alternating liters of normal and half-normal saline, risk of cerebral edema is minimized. Potassium should be administered even in the face of normal or high serum potassium, because hypokalemia develops as acidosis and hyperglycemia are corrected. Unrecognized hypokalemia is a major cause of death from DKA.

Hyperosmolar Nonketotic Acidosis. The key to successful treatment is to seek, recognize, and treat any underlying cause for the hyperosmolar nonketotic hyperglycemia, such as gram-negative sepsis. Hyperglycemia is corrected by the administration of insulin, as described previously. Volume depletion can be more severe than that seen with DKA. Potassium supplementation must be given as well.

Metabolic Alkalosis

Causes. Sustained metabolic alkalosis occurs only if extracellular bicarbonate concentration is increased and renal excretion of excess bicarbonate is inhibited. Extracellular bicarbonate concentration increases can occur through several mechanisms. In surgical patients, loss of HCl is a frequent cause of metabolic alkalosis, most commonly due to vomiting or nasogastric drainage in the face of gastric outlet obstruction. External loss of gastric acid results in a net gain in bicarbonate (generated by equimolar gastric secretion of HCl), which causes the alkalosis. Although the kidney can excrete excess bicarbonate, this must be accompanied by excretion of sodium. Renal excretion of sodium is limited in the face of the volume depletion that also occurs with external losses of gastric secretion. As volume depletion progresses, sodium is conserved in exchange for hydrogen, and urine will become acidic, even in the presence of severe metabolic alkalosis. This phenomenon is referred to as *paradoxic aciduria.*

Increased extracellular bicarbonate concentration can occur with administration of either bicarbonate or precursors of bicarbonate, such as lactate, citrate, or calcium carbonate, or as a result of increased renal production of bicarbonate. Conditions in which acid excretion exceeds endogenous acid production and in which the renal threshold for bicarbonate reabsorption is increased can result in metabolic alkalosis.

Such conditions include moderate potassium depletion, excess mineralocorticoids, and high PCO_2.

Hypokalemia and cellular exchange of potassium for hydrogen can also lead to metabolic alkalosis. Hypokalemia results in enhanced proximal tubular bicarbonate reabsorption and distal tubular acid excretion. When potassium leaves the cell, it is exchanged for either sodium or hydrogen to maintain electrical neutrality. Loss of potassium from the body then results in a net gain in bicarbonate in the ECF.

Maintenance of elevated extracellular bicarbonate concentration can occur by a number of mechanisms. Volume contraction leads to decreases in renal blood flow and glomerular filtration rate that reduce the filtered load of bicarbonate. This, in addition to increased proximal tubular reabsorption of bicarbonate, maintains high extracellular concentrations of bicarbonate. High PCO_2 causes an increase in renal threshold for bicarbonate secondary to decreased intracellular pH of the renal tubular cell. The net result is increased bicarbonate reabsorption.

Hypercalcemia and low PTH levels both result in increased proximal tubular reabsorption of bicarbonate, which may be enhanced by a decrease in glomerular filtration rate. Renal failure also leads to an inability of the kidney to excrete excess bicarbonate. Diuretics can cause or exacerbate metabolic alkalosis by both causing rapid contraction of intravascular volume and increasing renal excretion of acid. Chloride deficiency is another common factor that maintains an alkalotic state. In some instances of metabolic alkalosis, urinary excretion of chloride is markedly reduced. Reversal of metabolic alkalosis in these cases can be readily achieved by administration of chloride-containing solutions. Although chloride deficiency per se can result in an increased renal threshold for bicarbonate and in increased renal reabsorption of bicarbonate, this apparent association may also be related to volume contraction. Metabolic alkalosis can be divided into chloride-responsive and chloride-resistant types.

Respiratory Compensation. The major compensatory mechanism in metabolic alkalosis is respiratory because the presence of the metabolic alkalosis implicates renal dysfunction in either generating or failing to excrete increased amounts of bicarbonate. Hypoventilation is limited by the development of hypoxemia, which stimulates ventilation, and PCO_2 rarely exceeds 60 mm Hg (Table 10.12). Among the four major types of acid–base disorders, this compensatory mechanism is the least effective. For a given degree of metabolic alkalosis, the following equation can be used to predict the compensatory increase in PCO_2:

$$dPCO_2 = 0.7 \times d[HCO_3^-] \pm 5$$

where $dPCO_2$ = expected increase in PCO_2 given the measured increase in serum bicarbonate concentration.

Clinical Features. Clinical signs of metabolic alkalosis may not be prominent because the condition usually develops relatively slowly. If acute, CNS manifestations of confusion, obtundation, stupor, and coma may be present as well as tetany and neuromuscular irritability.

Treatment. Correction of the underlying cause is the mainstay of treatment in this disorder. In general, correction of potassium depletion and volume depletion corrects the metabolic alkalosis. Renal excretion of bicarbonate cannot occur in the face of persistent volume depletion. Volume depletion should be corrected with chloride-containing solutions. In patients without intravascular volume deficits, renal excretion of bicarbonate can be enhanced by administration of the carbonic acid anhydrase inhibitor diuretic acetazolamide. If renal excretion of bicarbonate cannot be increased because of underlying renal insufficiency or if the metabolic alkalosis is severe, acid may be administered to titrate directly the excess extracellular bicarbonate. Acids that can be used include ammonium chloride, arginine hydrochloride, lysine hydrochloride, or dilute hydrochloric acid (0.1 N). Partial correction of the alkalosis is the initial goal. A general guide is that 2.2 mEq/kg of acid decreases serum bicarbonate by approximately 5 mEq/L. In the face of renal failure, dialysis may be necessary to remove excess bicarbonate.

Respiratory Alkalosis.

Respiratory alkalosis is defined as increased extracellular pH secondary to decreased PCO_2 with hyperventilation. Hyperventilation and the ensuing fall in PCO_2 may be secondary to hypoxia, reflex stimulation from decreased pulmonary compliance, drugs, mechanical ventilation, and other causes.

Hypoxia stimulates ventilation through peripheral chemoreceptors in the carotid and aortic body. Decrease in arterial partial pressure of oxygen (PO_2), rather than in oxygen content, is the main stimulus. Acute drops in arterial PO_2 result in sustained hyperventilation only when the PCO_2 decreases below 60 mm Hg. Although hyperventilation occurs with even slight degrees of hypoxia, the resulting increase in brain pH suppresses the stimulus for hyperventilation unless severe hypoxia is present. In contrast, chronic hypoxia results in hyperventilation even with mildly decreased PCO_2 because brain pH is lowered by metabolic compensation. The two most common causes of hypoxia resulting in respiratory alkalosis are pulmonary disease and exposure to high altitudes.

Compensatory Mechanisms. Tissue buffering is the initial response to a decrease in PCO_2. Red blood cells provide one third of the buffering. Consumption of bicarbonate results from cellular liberation of H^+. Although immediate, the

TABLE 10.12

CALCULATIONS FOR ESTIMATING THE COMPENSATORY RESPONSES TO PRIMARY ACID–BASE DISTURBANCES

TYPE OF DISORDER	COMPENSATION REQUIREMENT	TIME
Metabolic acidosis	$dPCO_2 = d[HCO_3^-] \times 1.2 \pm 2$	12–24 h
Metabolic alkalosis	$dPCO_2 = d[HCO_3^-] \times 0.7 \pm 5$	12–24 h
Acute respiratory acidosis	$d[HCO_3^-] = dPCO_2 \times 0.07 \pm 1.5$	Minutes
Chronic respiratory acidosis	$d[HCO_3^-] = dPCO_2 \times 0.4 \pm 3$	3–5 d
Acute respiratory alkalosis	$d[HCO_3^-] = dPCO_2 \times 0.2 \pm 2.5$	Minutes
Chronic respiratory alkalosis	$d[HCO_3^-] = dPCO_2 \times 0.5 \pm 2.5$	2–3 d

magnitude of tissue buffering is slight and can be predicted by the following formula:

$$d[HCO_3^-] = dPCO_2 \times 0.2 \pm 2.5$$

Renal compensation is achieved not by increasing excretion of bicarbonate but by decreasing net acid excretion, primarily through reductions in ammonia excretion and increases in organic anion excretion. These organic anions are excreted as sodium and potassium salts. As a result, potassium excretion is increased, resulting in hypokalemia. Complete renal compensation requires 2 or 3 days.

Clinical Features. Chronic respiratory alkalosis is usually asymptomatic because compensatory mechanisms are successful in maintaining pH close to normal. Acute respiratory alkalosis may cause sensations of breathlessness, dizziness, and nervousness and can result in circumoral and extremity paresthesias, altered levels of consciousness, and tetany. These signs are related to decreased cerebral blood flow secondary to the decreased PCO_2 and decreased ionized calcium concentration secondary to the increased blood pH.

Treatment. The underlying stimulus for the hyperventilation should be addressed. The cause of hypoxemia should be determined and corrected. In acute symptomatic respiratory alkalosis, rebreathing or breathing 5% CO_2 temporarily relieves the symptoms. If the condition is secondary to mechanical ventilation, adjustment of tidal volume or respiratory rate should result in resolution of the respiratory alkalosis.

Respiratory Acidosis.

Respiratory acidosis, the decrease in extracellular pH from a primary increase in PCO_2, is due to inadequate ventilation. Causes of hypoventilation include the various causes of CNS depression, as well as impaired thoracic ventilatory mechanics, airway obstruction, and chronic obstructive pulmonary disease. In addition, inappropriate ventilator settings may result in respiratory acidosis in patients on mechanical ventilation.

Compensatory Mechanisms. Increased PCO_2 results in increased H_2CO_3, which dissociates into H^+ and HCO_3^-. Cellular exchange of Na^+ and K^+ for H^+ allows the reaction to continue in this direction with increased extracellular bicarbonate. This tissue buffering is accomplished within minutes. Persistently elevated PCO_2 also stimulates increased renal acid excretion, primarily the chloride salt of ammonia, and results in increased renal generation of HCO_3^-. Full renal compensation occurs over 3 to 5 days. The following formula describes chronic respiratory acidosis:

$$d[HCO_3^-] = dPCO_2 \times 0.4 \pm 3$$

Clinical Features. The magnitude of clinical manifestations depends on the chronicity and rate of development of respiratory acidosis. Acute increases in PCO_2 result in cerebral acidosis, manifested by drowsiness, restlessness, and tremor, as well as stupor or coma in more severe cases. Cerebral vasculature dilation occurs in response to acidosis, resulting in increased cerebral blood flow. This may, in turn, result in increased intracranial blood pressure, headache, and papilledema. Systemic acidosis results in peripheral vasodilatation, depressed cardiac contractility, and insensitivity to catecholamines.

Treatment. Treatment should be directed to the underlying cause of hypoventilation. Endotracheal intubation to achieve adequate ventilation is key to the treatment of acute respiratory acidosis of any cause. The treatment of chronic, compensated respiratory acidosis may be complicated by the accompanying hypoxemia. In chronic hypercapnia, the central chemoreceptors may be insensitive, and the accompanying hypoxemia may supply the main respiratory drive through stimulation of peripheral chemoreceptors. In such patients, complete correction of the hypoxemia may further suppress respiration and worsen the respiratory acidosis. In addition, PCO_2 should not be normalized rapidly. Reequilibration of cerebral bicarbonate concentration lags behind systemic changes. Thus, even if PCO_2 is normal, cellular and cerebral metabolic alkalosis may develop.

Mixed Acid–Base Disorders.

Combinations of two or more of the four primary acid–base disorders may occur and should be suspected when blood pH approaches normal despite abnormal PCO_2 and $[HCO_3^-]$, or when compensatory changes appear to be either excessive or inadequate (Fig. 10.8).

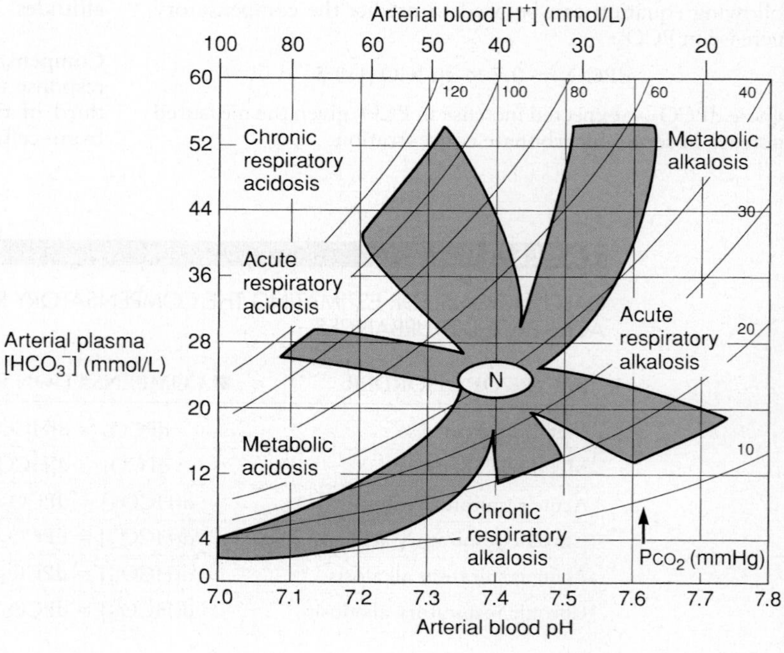

FIGURE 10.8. Acid–base nomogram. Shown are the 95% confidence limits of the normal respiratory and metabolic compensations for primary acid–base disturbances. (Reproduced with permission from Cogan MG, Rector FC Jr. Acid–base disturbances. In: Brenner BM, Rector FC Jr, eds. *The Kidney*. Philadelphia, PA: WB Saunders; 1986:473.)

Familiarity with the acid–base disorders associated with various clinical situations and the expectation of mixed abnormalities allows appropriate interpretation of arterial blood gases and serum electrolyte determinations. A summary of the calculations for estimating the compensatory responses and timing of these responses is presented in Table 10.12.[43]

References

1. Kehayias JJ, Valtuena S. Neutron activation analysis determination of body composition. *Curr Opin Clin Nutr Metab Care* 1999;2:453–463.
2. Forbes G. Body Composition: overview. *J Nutr* 1999;129(1):270S–272S.
3. Pietrobeloi A, Wang Z, Heymsfield SB. Techniques used in measuring human body composition. *Curr Opin Clin Nutr Metab Care* 1998;1:439–448.
4. Briggs JP, Sawaya BE, Schnerman J. Disorders of salt balance. In: Kokko JP, Tannen RL, eds. *Fluid and Electrolytes.* Philadelphia, PA: WB Saunders; 1990:70.
5. Thompson CA, Tatro DL, Ludwig DA, et al. Baroreflex responses to acute changes in blood volume in humans. *Am J Physiol* 1990;259:R792–R798.
6. Stockand JD. New ideas about aldosterone signaling in epithelia. *Am J Physiol Renal Physiol* 2002;51:F559–F576.
7. Boland DG, Abraham WT. Natriuretic peptides in heart failure. *Congest Heart Fail* 1998;4:23–33.
8. Falcao LM, Fausto P, Luciano R, et al. BNP and ANP as diagnostic and predictive markers in heart failure with left ventricular systolic dysfunction. *J Renin Angiotensin Aldosterone Sys* 2004;5:121–129.
9. Schrier R, Abraham W. Mechanisms of disease: hormones and hemodynamics in heart failure. *N Engl J Med* 1999;341:577–585.
10. Wait RB, Kahng KU. Renal failure complicating obstructive jaundice. *Am J Surg* 1989;157:256–263.
11. Naicker S, Bhoola KD. Endothelins: vasoactive modulators of renal function in health and disease. *Pharmacol Ther* 2001;90(1):61–68.
12. Roland CB, Aihua D, Mark L, et al. The complex role of nitric oxide in the regulation of glomerular filtration. *Kidney Int* 2002;61:782–785.
13. Ruttmann TG, James MFM, Lombard EM. Haemodilution induced enhancement of coagulation is attenuated in vitro by restoring antithrombin III to predilution concentrations. *Anaesth Intensive Care* 2001;29:489–493.
14. Ng KFJ, Lam CCK, Chan LC. In vivo effect of haemodilution with saline on coagulation: a randomized controlled trial. *Br J Anaesth* 2002;88:475–480.
15. Ruttmann TG, James MFM, Finlayson J. Effects on coagulation of intravenous crystalloid or colloid in patients undergoing peripheral vascular surgery. *Br J Anaesth* 2002;89:226–230.
16. De Lorenzo C, Calatzis A, Welsch U, et al. Fibrinogen concentrate reverses dilutional coagulopathy induced in vitro by saline but not by hydroxyethyl starch 6%. *Anesth Analg* 2006;102:1194–2000.
17. Koustova E, Standon K, Gushchin V, et al. Effects of lactated Ringer's solution on human leukocytes. *J Trauma* 2002;53:872–878.
18. Hanneman L, Reinhart K, Korrel R, et al. Hypertonic saline in stabilized hyperdynamic sepsis. *Shock* 1996;5:130–134.
19. Wade CE, Kramer GC, Grady JJ, et al. Efficacy of 7.5% saline and 6% dextran-70 in treating trauma. A meta-analysis of controlled clinical studies. *Surgery* 1997;122:609–616.
20. Doyle J, Davis D, Hoyt D. The use of hypertonic saline in the treatment of traumatic brain injury. *J Trauma* 2001;50:367–383.
21. Rizoli SB, Rhind SG, Shek PN, et al. The immunomodulatory effects of hypertonic saline resuscitation in patients sustaining traumatic hemorrhagic shock. *Ann Surg* 2006:243:47–57.
22. Finfer S, Bellomo R, Boyce N, et al. A comparison of albumin and saline for fluid resuscitation in the intensive care unit. *N Engl J Med* 2004;350:2247–2256.
23. Vincent JL, Sakr Y, Reinhart K, et al. Is albumin administration in the acutely ill associated with increased mortality? Results of the SOAP study. *Crit Care* 2005;9:R745–R754.
24. Greg M. Conflicting clinical trial data: a lesson from albumin. *Crit Care* 2005;9:649–650.
25. Alexey AS, Raili S, Anne HK, et al. Rapidly degradable hydroxyethyl starch solutions impair blood coagulation after cardiac surgery: a prospective randomized trial. *Anesth Analg* 2009;108:30–36.
26. Martin G, Bennett-Guerrero E, Wakeling H, et al. A prospective, randomized comparison of thrombelastographic coagulation profile in patients receiving lactated Ringer's solution, 6% hetastarch in a balanced-saline vehicle, or 6% hydroxyethyl starch in saline during major surgery. *J Cardiothorac Vasc Anesth* 2002;16:441–446.
27. Omar MN, Shouk TA, Khaleq MA. Activity of blood coagulation and fibrinolysis during and after hydroxyethyl starch (HES) colloidal volume replacement. *Clin Biochem* 1999;32:269–274.
28. Gan TJ, Bennett-Guerrero E, Phillips-Bute B, et al. Hextend, a physiologically balanced plasma expander for large volume use in major surgery: a randomized phase III clinical trial. Hextend Study Group. *Anesth Analg* 1999;88:992–998.
29. King DR, Cohn SM, Proctor KG. Changes in intracranial pressure, coagulation, and neurologic outcome after resuscitation from experimental traumatic brain injury with hetastarch. *Surgery* 2004;136:355– 363.
30. Deusch E, Thaler U, Kozek-Langenecker SA. The effects of high molecular weight hydroxyethyl starch solutions on platelets. *Anesth Analg* 2004;99:665–668.
31. Franz A, Bräunlich P, Gamsjäger T, et al. The effects of hydroxyethyl starches of varying molecular weights on platelet function. *Anesth Analg* 2001;92:1402–1407.
32. Jungheinrich C, Scharpf R, Wargenau M, et al. The pharmacokinetics and tolerability of an intravenous infusion of the new hydroxyethyl starch 130/0.4 (6%, 500 mL) in mild-to-severe renal impairment. *Anesth Analg* 2002;95:544–551.
33. Biesenbach G, Kaiser W, Zazgornik J. Incidence of acute oligoanuric renal failure in dextran 40 treated patients with acute ischemic stroke stage III or IV. *Ren Fail* 1997;19:69–75.
34. Allison KP, Gosling P, Jones S, et al. Randomized trial of hydroxyethyl starch versus gelatine for trauma resuscitation. *J Trauma* 1999;47:1114–1121.
35. Russell WJ, Fenwick DG. Anaphylaxis to Haemaccel and cross reactivity to Gelofusin. *Anaesth Intensive Care* 2002;30:481–483.
36. Moore EE, Moore FA, Fabian TC, et al. Human polymerized hemoglobin for the treatment of hemorrhagic shock when blood is unavailable: the USA Multicenter Trial. *J Am Coll Surg* 2009;208:1–13.
37. Fleck A, Raines G, Hawker F, et al. Increased vascular permeability: a major cause of hypoalbuminaemia in disease and injury. *Lancet* 1985;1:781–784.
38. Schrier RW, Gross P, Gheorghiade M, et al. Tolvaptan, a selective oral vasopressin V2-receptor antagonist, for hyponatremia. *N Engl J Med* 2006;355(20):2099–2112.
39. Palmer BF. Managing hyperkalemia caused by inhibitors of the renin-angiotensin-aldosterone system. *N Engl J Med* 2004;351:585–592.
40. Stewart AF. Hypercalcemia associated with cancer. *N Engl J Med* 2005;352:373–379.
41. Lemann J Jr, Lennon EJ. Role of diet, gastrointestinal tract, and bone in acid–base homeostasis. *Kidney Int* 1972;1:275–279.
42. Hood VL, Tannen RL. Mechanisms of disease: protection of acid-base balance by pH regulation of acid production. *N Engl J Med* 1998;339:819–826.
43. Carroll HJ, Oh MS. *Water, Electrolyte and Acid–base Metabolism.* Philadelphia, PA: J.B. Lippincott; 1989:206.

CHAPTER 11 ■ BURNS

NICOLE GIBRAN

KEY POINTS

1. Burns should be triaged to a burn center with a multidisciplinary care team according to American Burn Association criteria.
2. Burn depth evolves over 72 hours, making early surgical decisions difficult.
3. Inhalation injury constitutes three types of injury—upper airway thermal burns, chemical pneumonitis, and carbon monoxide toxicity—and with a thermal injury is associated with increased mortality.
4. Fluid resuscitation during the first 24 to 48 hours after injury must be titrated to urine output (30 mL/h for adults; 1 to 1.5 mL/kg per hour for children <20 kg) and mean arterial blood pressure (≥60 mm Hg).
5. Prophylactic systemic antibiotics other than tetanus prophylaxis are contraindicated.
6. Of all interventions in the care of patients with thermal injuries, early excision and grafting has had the most significant impact on burn patient survival.
7. Patients should be treated for background pain, breakthrough pain, and procedural pain as well as for anxiety.
8. Rehabilitation should start at admission with active range of motion if possible and passive range of motion with splinting if the patient is not able to participate.
9. Toxic epidermal necrosis is best treated at a burn center with biological dressing to allow the underlying skin to heal; systemic steroids are associated with worse mortality rates.
10. Necrotizing fasciitis should be highly suspected if a patient has signs of sepsis together with marked induration and edema with skin blistering/sloughing and a white blood cell count greater than 20,000 and hyponatremia (Na <135).

Comprehensive care of the patient with thermal injuries involves sophisticated surgical decision making, critical care management, rehabilitation, and psychosocial interventions. With early excision and grafting and better critical care management, survival rates have improved markedly since the mid-1970s. Therefore, in the 21st century, clinical goals must focus on optimizing outcomes and returning patients to their premorbid level of function. This chapter presents a management philosophy that correlates increasing understanding of burn pathophysiology with optimal clinical management of patients with thermal injuries and promotes a systematic multidisciplinary approach.

MANAGEMENT PHILOSOPHY

Whereas the coordinated care provided by a burn center may primarily benefit patients with complicated life-threatening large burn injuries, excellent multidisciplinary management of smaller burns bears long-term beneficial impact on patient outcome—both aesthetic and functional. The focused systematic approach of an organized burn center allows for early surgical excision and closure of burn wounds, critical care support, patient and family psychosocial support, patient and family education, continuous long-term rehabilitation, reentry into society, and reconstructive surgical needs.[1] Therefore, patients with burns that meet American Burn Association criteria (Table 11.1) for transfer to a burn center soon after initial assessment are likely to benefit from a multidisciplinary specialized burn care plan. (Guidelines for the Operations of Burn Centers [pp. 79–86], Resources for Optimal Care of the Injured Patient: 2006, Committee on Trauma, American College of Surgeons.)

With modern burn care, survival with an excellent quality of life should be expected for most patients with severe burns. Predicting mortality is difficult in burned patients. There remain no reliable formulas for predicting burn survival in spite of the easily remembered "Age + % total body surface area burn = mortality" formula.[2] In one statistical evaluation, age over 60 years, full-thickness burn size over 40% total body surface area (TBSA), and the presence of inhalation injury were found to be important prognostic factors.[3] One retrospective study of patients with burns over 65% TBSA suggested that the nontangible presence of family and friends at the bedside was more common in survivors than in patients who died.[4] Experienced burn surgeons report that they may limit resuscitation based on burn size, availability of donor sites, patient age, comorbidity, and inhalation injury; however, this approach to providing comfort care for devastating injuries must be carefully and thoroughly discussed by knowledgeable burn care providers with consideration for patient values and interests (unpublished data).

Successful burn patient outcomes require a well-organized care plan. The national trend to include family members in all aspects of patient treatment including access to trauma and intensive care unit (ICU) rooms[5,6] is a natural extension from the multidisciplinary care teams supported by the burn community.[7] Deciding whether outpatient management is appropriate for a patient with small burns (1% to 5% TBSA) that do not involve joints or vital structures or when to discharge a patient with a large burn requires clear communication with the patient and family.

Outpatient management often fails because insufficient teaching in a busy emergency room leads to inadequate pain control, wound infection, and limited movement. Indications for burn patient hospitalization include wound care needs, physical therapy, and pain management. In spite of major issues regarding access to care and hospital overcrowding, even patients with minor burns benefit from a short hospital stay immediately after the injury and before swelling, infection, or functional limitations hinder long-term recovery. A burn specialty therapist can educate the patient about expected range-of-motion exercises and activity programs; early understanding of importance of exercise can prevent range-of-motion limitation and subsequent swelling that often leads to infection and uncontrollable pain. Pain, including background pain (pain experienced with ordinary daily activities), breakthrough pain (the pain that occurs in spite of scheduled pain medicines), and procedural pain (pain experienced during wound care or intensive therapy sessions), and anxiety should be carefully

TABLE 11.1

AMERICAN BURN ASSOCIATION CRITERIA FOR PATIENT TRANSFER TO A BURN CENTER

Burn injuries that should be referred to a burn center include the following:

1. Partial-thickness burns >10% total body surface area (TBSA)
2. Burns that involve the face, hands, feet, genitalia, perineum, or major joints
3. Third-degree burns in any age group
4. Electrical burns, including lightning injury
5. Chemical burns
6. Inhalation injury
7. Burn injury in patients with preexisting medical disorders that could complicate management, prolong recovery, or affect mortality
8. Patients with burns and concomitant trauma (such as fractures) in which the burn injury poses the greatest risk of morbidity or mortality.
   If the trauma poses the greater immediate risk, the patient may be initially stabilized in a trauma center before being transferred to a burn center.
   Physician judgment will be necessary in such situations and should be in concert with the regional medical control plan and triage protocols.
9. Burned children in hospitals without qualified personnel or equipment for the care of children
10. Burn injury in patients who will require special social, emotional, or long-term rehabilitative intervention

assessed. Analgesic and anxiolytic medication should be titrated to individual levels. Inadequate pain management frequently leads to hospital readmission. Pain levels may increase as epithelial buds emerge in a healing partial-thickness burn and new-onset stinging pain may indicate a superficial wound infection. Change in symptoms indicates that the burn should be evaluated for signs of infection, including wound erythema or breakdown of a previously healed wound.

Simple wound care is a key to successful transition to outpatient management. For all but major burns greater than 40% TBSA, once-daily dressing changes are adequate. Burns are effectively washed during a daily shower or bath with tap water and nonperfumed soap. Using a soapy washcloth to wipe the topical ointment bacteria that have accumulated over the past day from the wound provides adequate wound care; there is no need to scrub the wound to débride superficial exudates. Intact blisters provide a useful protective biologic wound dressing unless they limit mobility, in which case blisters should be incised, débrided, and covered with a topical antimicrobial dressing that allows full range of motion.

A common misconception is that joint immobilization promotes burn wound healing. In reality, extremity immobilization leads to swelling, which worsens tissue injury, exacerbates pain, and increases the risk of wound infection. Patients with hand burns must learn exercises to maintain range of motion and patients with foot burns must ambulate without assistive devices, so that muscle contraction facilitates lymphatic drainage of the extremity. Patients must elevate burned extremities when they are not actively exercising to reduce swelling. Many burn patients underestimate the time and commitment they must dedicate to physical therapy for optimal functional recovery.

EPIDEMIOLOGY

Because burns are an unreported disease, the annual incidence of thermal injuries is unknown. However, extrapolation from

TABLE 11.2

RISK FACTORS FOR BURN INJURIES

Alcohol and drugs
Age (very young/very old)
Smoking
Socioeconomic status
Occupation
Violence
Epilepsy

2003 Centers for Disease Control and Prevention (CDC) data (http://www.cdc.gov/ncipc/) on fire-related injuries suggests that approximately 1 million burn injuries occur annually in the United States. Fire-related deaths in the United States in 2003 are estimated to be 3,700 (1.3 deaths per 100,000); this compares to 322,000 (5.2 deaths per 100,000) worldwide deaths (http://www.who.int/violence_injury_prevention).

In general, burn injuries affect vulnerable populations (Table 11.2): the very young and old, the impaired, and those in lower socioeconomic groups. Workplace injuries comprise a significant component of burn injuries among young adults. Structural fires historically were associated with large numbers of patients with large burns. However, introduction of smoke detectors has dramatically reduced the numbers of these burns except in cases where the alarms are tampered with or when the inhabitants are cognitively or physically impaired. As with other trauma, alcohol and drugs are often implicated in the epidemiology of burn injuries. Suggestion of a nonaccidental injury or potential neglect mandates admission for full evaluation of the home situation; if the history and the burn distribution are consistent with abuse, the patient must be referred to protective services. Likewise, suggestion of a self-induced burn injury should trigger admission for psychological evaluation; the presence of multiple small cigarette burns in various phases of healing is an absolute indication for admission to the hospital for psychological evaluation, even though the burns themselves may be easily cared for at home with bandages. Patients with language barriers may also benefit from a brief hospital admission to be sure they understand the treatment plan. Underinsured and homeless patients may not have the resources to care for a wound outside the hospital and should be admitted for initial wound care and comprehensive discharge planning.

In spite of regulations established after mass burn casualties such as the Cocoanut Grove Fire in Boston in 1942, the risk of burn mass casualties in public places continues to be a public concern as evidenced in the 2002 Rhode Island nightclub fire that killed 100 people and injured approximately 200 others. Extensive legislative efforts and public outreach programs have decreased the incidence of many nonaccidental burn injuries. Examples including state mandates that hot water heaters in multidwelling facilities be set at 120°F have led to a decreased incidence of nonaccidental hot water injuries.[8] Inconsistent application of these laws across states remains a problem. Smoke detectors and annual drives to change the batteries have decreased serious injuries in house fires. Federal requirements that children's sleepwear be fire retardant, implemented in 1972, represented a transiently successful national burn prevention program that died in 1996 when Congress reversed regulations. Abuse and neglect continue to impact pediatric patients and require ongoing public awareness campaigns.[9] One recent national legislative lobbying effort has been the implementation of laws requiring that cigarettes have reduced propensity to ignite furniture or mattresses by using less-dense tobacco, less-porous paper, a smaller diameter, a filter tip, and no added citrates to the paper.[10] As of December

2008, 37 states and the District of Columbia have passed legislation requiring that cigarettes sold in those states meet fire-safe requirements (www.firesafecigarettes.org).

BIOLOGY OF SKIN

Two distinct layers, the epidermis and the dermis, comprise the skin. The outer epidermis acts as the barrier against the environment and protects against infection, toxin absorption, ultraviolet light exposure, fluid evaporation, and thermal regulation. It has five progressively differentiated layers of keratinocytes, leading to the outermost nonviable and relatively impermeable stratum corneum, which provides the barrier mechanism that protects the underlying tissues. In contrast, the dermis is a complicated cellular and extracellular layer that contributes cutaneous durability and elasticity. The fibroblast, the principal cell of the dermis, synthesizes and degrades mesenchymal proteins. Since there is no single fibroblast marker, it is not entirely clear that the spindle-shaped cells that populate the dermis constitute a single cell type. The epidermis and dermis both harbor bone marrow–derived inflammatory cells that contribute to cutaneous inflammatory responses. Dermal connective tissue projections known as dermal papillae interdigitate with epidermal projections known as rete ridges to create the dermal-epidermal junction. Here, the basement membrane, a complex extracellular matrix layer made up of structural proteins that anchor the basal keratinocytes to the papillary dermis, separates the two cutaneous layers.

BURN PATHOPHYSIOLOGY

Jackson's 1953 classification of burn wound depth remains a basis for our understanding of the pathophysiology of cutaneous thermal injury.[11] He described three zones of tissue injury following burn injury (Fig. 11.1A, B). The central, most severely damaged area is the zone of coagulation because the tissue is coagulated or necrotic and irreparably injured; this region represents a full-thickness burn (third degree) (Fig. 11.1C) that will not heal and must be débrided and grafted. Surrounding the zone of coagulation is a zone of stasis, characterized by vasoconstriction and ischemia. With careful wound management, this partial-thickness burn (second degree) (Fig. 11.1D) can convert to a shallower wound; however, edema, infection, or poor perfusion increases the risk that the injured tissue will convert to a deeper burn that will require excision and grafting. The outermost area of a burn is the zone of hyperemia or superficial partial-thickness burn (Fig. 11.1D), which usually heals quickly without scarring. Superficial burns such as sunburns are often referred to as first-degree burns and are not included in burn size calculations.

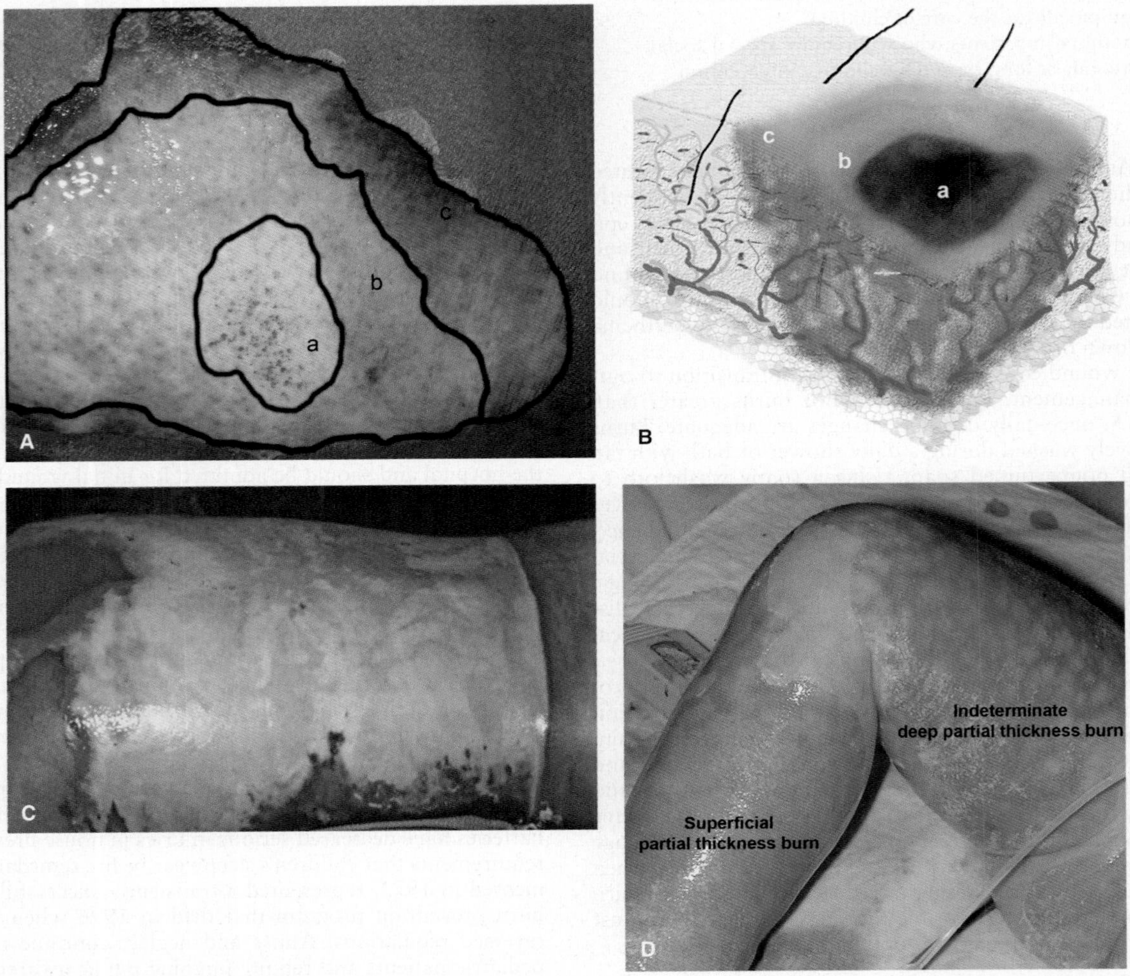

FIGURE 11.1. Zone of injury correlates with burn depth. **A, B:** The central zone of coagulation (*a*) represents a full-thickness burn (as shown in **C**); the surrounding zone of stasis (*b*) represents a partial-thickness burn (as shown in **D**) that may extend into the reticular dermis (deep partial thickness) or the papillary dermis (superficial partial thickness). The peripheral zone of hyperemia (*c*) correlates with a superficial or first-degree burn and might be similar to a sunburn.

Tissue repair represents a continuum that begins immediately following injury. An initial hemostatic response involves coagulation and microvasculature constriction. The extrinsic and intrinsic coagulation pathways also provide provisional matrix scaffolding for subsequent cellular migration into the wound bed. Tissue factor activation of the coagulation cascade leads to cleavage of fibrinogen to fibrin, which serves as both clot matrix and wound bed matrix. Wound inflammatory cells generate plasmid for clot resolution, a process tightly regulated by plasminogen activator inhibitors to ensure that the clot does not resolve too rapidly. Interestingly, animal studies suggest that exogenous tissue plasminogen activator promotes conversion of the zone of stasis in an acute burn wound to a zone of hyperemia.[12]

The well-recognized vasodilatation and capillary leak associated with the resuscitative phase of a burn injury follow the early transient vascular constriction. Vascular permeability contributes to inflammatory cell migration into the wound bed but also causes extravascular leak, which complicates overall patient outcome by causing pulmonary edema, compartment syndrome, and conversion of burns to a deeper injury. Many inflammatory cytokines contribute to this response. In addition to the many interleukins and prostaglandins, sensory nerve–derived neuropeptides induce histamine release by mast cells,[13] cytokine and adhesion molecule upregulation by keratinocytes and endothelial cells, inflammatory cell chemotaxis, and fibroblast proliferation.[14] Serotonin, histamine, bradykinin, and the arachidonic acid metabolites prolong vasodilatation and capillary permeability.[15]

Resident cutaneous cells may be the most important contributors to cutaneous inflammation. *Skin-associated lymphoid tissue* includes bone marrow–derived cells, such as Langerhans cells and dermal dendrocytes, and keratinocytes and microvascular endothelial cells.[16] Keratinocytes and dermal microvascular cells synthesize cytokines, including interleukins,[17–21] monocyte chemoattractant protein-1,[22] and tumor necrosis factor.[23,24] Before margination into the wound bed, neutrophils adhere to endothelial cell adhesion molecules and plug the capillaries, thereby inducing further cytokine release and potential tissue ischemia. In burn wounds, the zone of stasis represents ischemic tissue that may convert to a zone of coagulation with neutrophil-mediated reperfusion injury. Whereas inhibition of the neutrophil-endothelial adherence in deep dermal rabbit contact burns speeds healing,[25] these studies have not been verified in human burn patients.

Granulation tissue, with its capillary arcades, is well-recognized clinical evidence that a wound is healthy and is ready for closure. However, normal excisional wound closure occurs with angioinhibition,[26,27] suggesting that secondary wound repair may not require angiogenesis. Skin grafts and tissue flaps do require angiogenesis for engraftment. Whereas delivery of oxygen and nutrients to a skin graft by imbibition—or diffusion—suffices for a few days, skin graft take requires neovascularization, which occurs by inosculation, the linkage between existent capillaries in the graft and in the wound bed. Excessive wound granulation actually hinders burn wound healing as it prevents migration of the epithelial tongue; many burn surgeons débride the granulation tissue in a healing burn before applying a skin graft to maximize graft take because of the associated bacterial contamination and exuberant inflammatory response. Excessive granulation tissue has been associated with increased hypertrophic scar formation in the healed wound.[28,29]

An epithelialized burn equals a healed burn. Full-thickness wounds heal from the wound edges (Fig. 11.2A), but an advancing epithelial tongue can migrate for approximately 1 cm before it stops migrating and heaps up at the wound edge. In contrast, partial-thickness wounds heal from epidermal

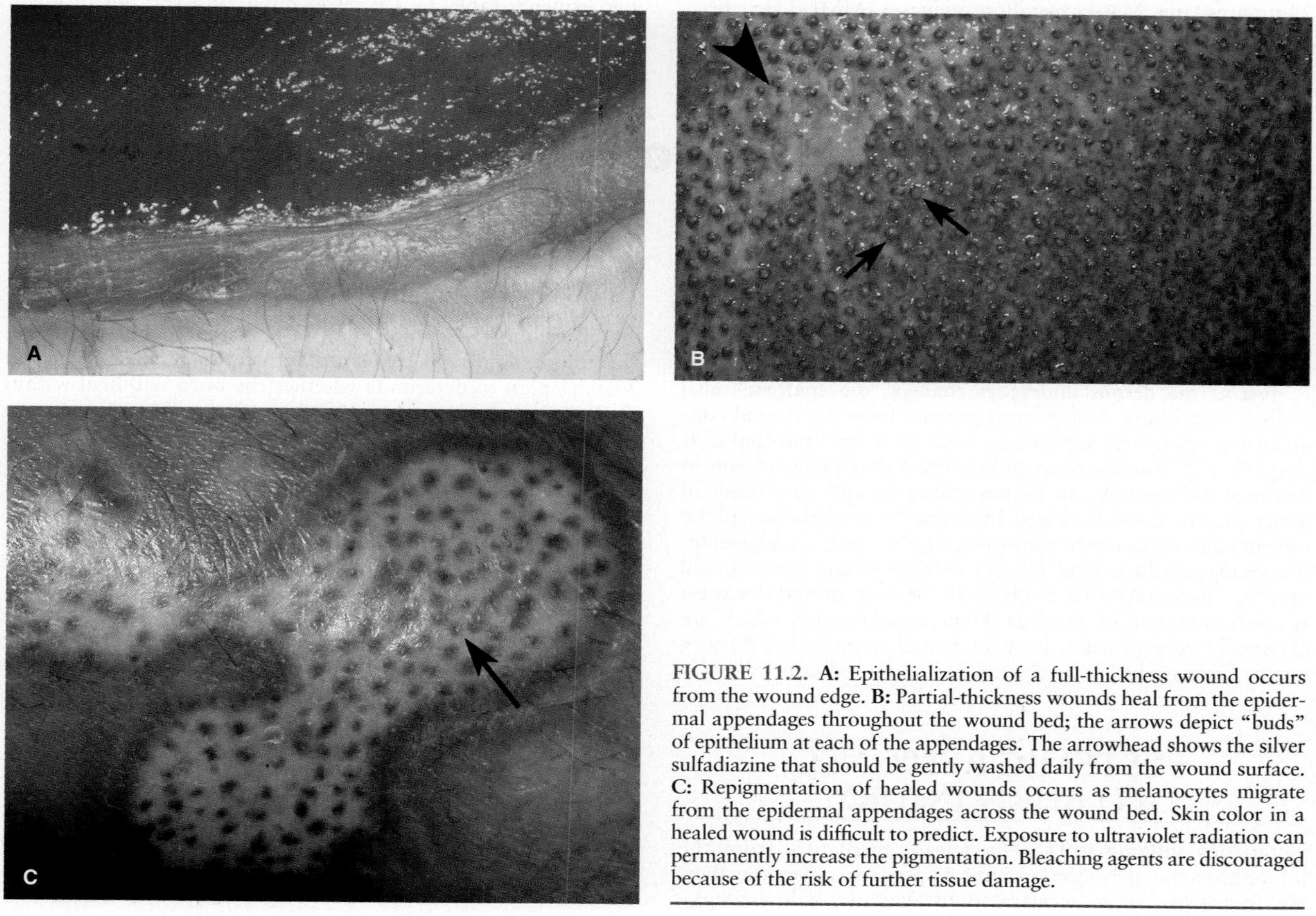

FIGURE 11.2. **A:** Epithelialization of a full-thickness wound occurs from the wound edge. **B:** Partial-thickness wounds heal from the epidermal appendages throughout the wound bed; the arrows depict "buds" of epithelium at each of the appendages. The arrowhead shows the silver sulfadiazine that should be gently washed daily from the wound surface. **C:** Repigmentation of healed wounds occurs as melanocytes migrate from the epidermal appendages across the wound bed. Skin color in a healed wound is difficult to predict. Exposure to ultraviolet radiation can permanently increase the pigmentation. Bleaching agents are discouraged because of the risk of further tissue damage.

appendages (i.e., hair follicles, sweat glands, and sebaceous glands) in the wound bed (Fig. 11.2B). Whereas completion of this process by no means represents the end of burn wound healing, epithelialization restores the three protective barrier functions of the outer layer of the skin: fluid maintenance, temperature regulation, and prevention of microbial or toxin invasion. Epithelialization may also represent an essential transition in the wound inflammatory state. Growing evidence suggests that epidermal–dermal interactions regulate cutaneous morphogenetic processes such as fetal skin development and wound repair.[30] Just as the epidermis responds to mesenchyme-derived mediators,[31] activated keratinocytes in the advancing epidermal tongue may secrete cytokines and growth factors to promote dermal inflammation.[32,33] Once cell–cell contact is achieved with complete wound epithelialization, release of the inflammatory mediators may stop. Evidence for epidermal influence on dermal inflammatory responses includes clinical observations that partial-thickness wound coverage with viable allograft eliminates granulation tissue formation and promotes healing.[34] Because it takes time for a mature basement membrane to develop, epithelialized wounds undergo epidermolysis (blistering) until the anchoring structures mature.

Whereas clinicians consider an epithelialized wound to be "healed," long-term dermal and subcutaneous fibrogenesis may be the most critical determinants of long-term wound appearance and cutaneous tensile strength. Deposition of fibrin, thrombin, fibronectin, and vitronectin into the site of injury promotes cellular migration and proliferation for angiogenesis and fibrogenesis. As fibroblasts migrate into the wound from the margins, they synthesize collagen. The result is deposition of collagen III and subsequently collagen I in a dense mat that is characteristic of dermal scar. As collagen I fibrils are cross-linked into cables, dermal breaking strength increases but never meets that of uninjured skin. Matrix remodeling begins with fibrin clot dissolution and ends with a mature wound 12 to 24 months later. Matrix metalloproteinases (MMPs) have been implicated in keratinocyte migration,[35] angiogenesis,[36] and dermal matrix remodeling.[37,38] Expression levels of MMPs appear to be decreased in hypertrophic scars.[39]

Contraction, resulting from centrifugal forces in the center of the wound, constitutes an important wound closure mechanism. Myofibroblasts, specialized fibroblasts characterized by intracellular smooth muscle actin filaments,[29] may contribute to this means of closure. A pathologic extension of wound contraction over joints is a contracture—a debilitating scarring process that compromises return to function in many patients with large burns. Constant attention to stretching, exercising, and splinting can minimize contracture development, but surgical release of the tight bands may be necessary to restore normal function of the extremities, neck, or mouth.

Just as the dermis undergoes changes, the epidermis also evolves after injury. Melanocytes migrate from the wound edge and from epidermal appendages soon after the epithelial cells (Fig. 11.2C). Patients must be informed that pigmentation in healed burn wounds can be unpredictable and may result in either increased or decreased melanin. Most clinicians advise patients that exposure to ultraviolet rays exacerbates pigmentation changes in the wound. Use of topical bleaching agents should also be discouraged. Patients with healing partial-thickness wounds complain of pruritus. Hypertrophic scars, which are classically very pruritic, have increased numbers of sensory nerves compared to normal scars and uninjured skin.[40,41]

SYSTEMIC RESPONSE TO BURN INJURY

Cutaneous inflammatory cells release mediators from the injured tissue to drive the systemic response to cutaneous thermal injury, leading to accelerated intravascular volume depletion, inadequate tissue perfusion, and, ultimately, risk of multiorgan dysfunction. Therefore, patients with large burns require continuous intravenous replacement to compensate for the capillary leak. The leak associated with a burn larger than 30% TBSA (or smaller if there is concomitant inhalation injury) can cause clinically significant interstitial edema in soft tissues including muscle compartments, the lungs, and the abdomen. The potential morbidity from the edema includes compartment syndrome in injured and noninjured extremities, abdominal compartment syndrome, and pulmonary edema leading to development of adult respiratory distress syndrome. Careful attention to fluid status of the acutely injured burn patient can avoid resuscitation failures including inadequate and excessive resuscitation.

INITIAL EVALUATION

A burn patient is a trauma patient and should be addressed with the same organized approach to serious injuries that begins with the primary survey to assess airway, breathing, and circulation. A systematic early comprehensive secondary survey is mandatory, especially for burn patients with associated trauma such as seen in motor vehicle collisions. Evidence suggests that even a small burn injury significantly worsens prognosis in patients with multiple injuries and high injury severity scores.[42] Therefore, close coordination between the trauma and burn teams is indicated, especially during the resuscitative phase of response to injury.

Since workup of a trauma patient is covered extensively in Chapter 17, this section focuses on elements of the workup relevant to evaluation of the burn component of the injuries. Expeditious transfer of a critically burned patient to a burn ICU is essential to avoid hypothermia and resuscitation complications; this mandates rapid evaluation in the emergency department. Table 11.3 is an example of a transfer protocol that outlines initial management of the burn patient prior to transfer to a burn center.

A crucial part of the initial evaluation of the extent of burn injury is estimation of the size and depth of the burn. This is the basis for subsequent fluid resuscitation and care plans. Because
2 the zones of injury in a burn wound evolve for up to 72 hours (see earlier discussion on the zones of injury), burn depth determination at the initial examination can be erroneous. Although numerous burn depth indicators have been investigated, including laser Doppler flow meters, intravenous fluorescein, burn wound biopsy, thermography, light reflectance, magnetic resonance imaging, and intravenous dyes,[43–45] no technology has been more accurate than an experienced burn surgeon. Therefore, many indeterminate burns must be in a "wait and watch" plan to determine whether the burn will heal within 3 weeks or whether excision and grafting will be necessary to close the wound.

Two simple formulas exist to estimate burn size. The rule of nines (Fig. 11.3) provides an anatomic estimate in which each arm is considered to be 9% TBSA, each leg 18%, the anterior trunk 18%, the posterior trunk 18%, and the head 9%; this method underestimates head size in children. Another easy method involves using the patient's full palm, including digits, to represent 1% TBSA. First-degree burns should not be included in the calculation of burned areas. Soot should be gently cleaned from the patient since it often misleads an unfamiliar evaluator and erroneously increases the estimated burn size.

Initial assessment of the burn patient requires few laboratory or radiologic studies. Patients with a history of exposure to noxious fumes should have partial pressure of arterial oxygen (PaO_2), partial pressure of arterial carbon dioxide ($PaCO_2$), pH, and carboxyhemoglobin (CO) percentage determined. Patients with isolated burns without other injuries rarely need blood products during the resuscitative phase of

TABLE 11.3

UNIVERSITY OF WASHINGTON BURN CENTER TRANSFER STABILIZATION PROTOCOL

1. Remove source of heat.
   - Remove clothing that is burned, covered with chemicals, or constrictive.
2. Intubate patients for:
   - Loss of consciousness, increasing stridor or hoarseness, evidence of posterior pharyngeal burns, or burns exceeding 60% total body surface area (TBSA).
3. Initiate fluid resuscitation.
   - Estimate the burn size based on the rule of nines or based on patient palm size (1% TBSA) to calculate the resuscitation fluid volume (Fig. 11.3).
   - Administer lactated Ringer solution at 3 mL/kg/% TBSA burn.
   - For children who weigh <20 kg, also administer D_5 ½NS at maintenance IV rate.
     a. Except for maintenance fluids in children, dextrose solutions cause osmotic diuresis and confuse assessment of resuscitation.
   - Unless mean arterial blood pressure is <60 mm Hg, IV fluid boluses are not necessary for burn resuscitation.
4. Insert nasogastric tube in intubated patients and patients with burns ≥20% TBSA.
   - Enteral tube feedings should be started if the patient will not be transported to a burn center within 12 h.
   - If feeding is contraindicated, a proton pump inhibitor should be started.
5. Insert Foley catheter in patients with burns >20% TBSA to assess urine output as a measure of resuscitation.
   - Adequate urine output is 30 mL/h in adults and 1.5 mL/kg/h in a child weighing <20 kg.
   - Observe urine for burgundy color (seen with massive injuries or electrical burns). The high incidence of renal failure associated with myoglobinemia from these injuries warrants prompt and aggressive intervention.
   - If the urine is red or brown, consult burn center staff for fluid management.
6. Escharotomy
   - If transfer will occur within 12 h of injury, escharotomies are rarely needed.
   - Burned extremities should be elevated.
7. Medications
   - A tetanus shot should be given on admission to the emergency department.
   - Antibiotics are NOT indicated for acute burn management.
   - Short-acting pain and anxiety medication may be titrated in small doses.
8. Wound care
   - Débridement and application of topical antimicrobials are usually unnecessary.
   - Transport patient in dry sheets and blankets, keeping patient warm.
   - Avoid hypothermia.
9. Special considerations for chemical burns
   - Remove ALL clothing.
   - Brush powered chemicals off wound: flush burns for a minimum of 30 min with running water. Be careful to protect yourself.
   - Irrigate burned eyes with a gentle stream of saline. Follow with an ophthalmology consult if transport is not imminent.
10. Special considerations for electrical injuries
    - Elevate burned extremities above the level of the heart on pillows.
    - Monitor distal pulses and neurologic examination.
    - Maintain urine output >100 mL/h if myoglobinuria present

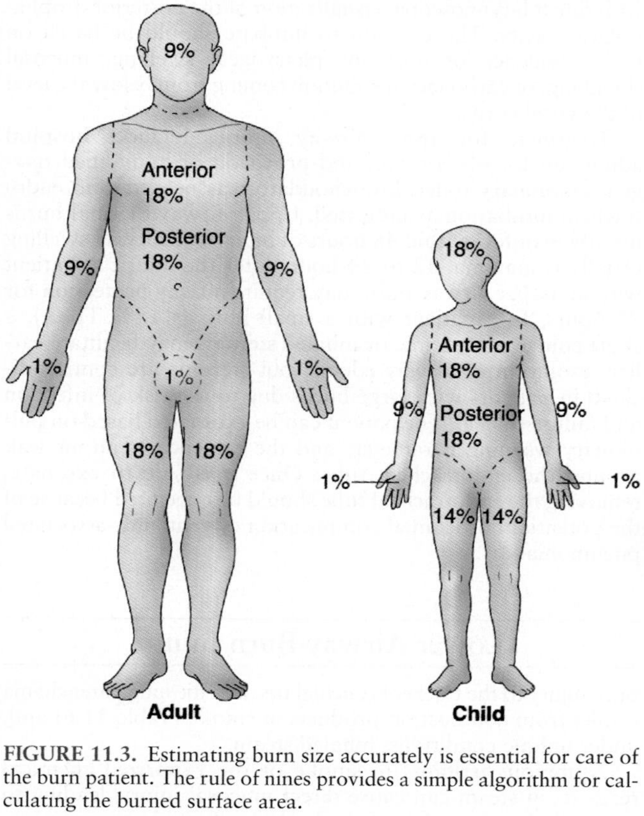

FIGURE 11.3. Estimating burn size accurately is essential for care of the burn patient. The rule of nines provides a simple algorithm for calculating the burned surface area.

their care but a routine blood sample can be sent to the blood bank as a type and screen. Routine hematology and chemistry profiles have limited use, but baseline electrolyte levels and renal function (blood urea nitrogen [BUN], creatinine), hematocrit, white blood cell count, and platelet count should be established. The efficacy of following laboratory values such as base deficits and lactic acid levels has not been established in burn patients. Urinalysis may be helpful to diagnose myoglobinuria in patients with electrical injuries or deep thermal burns, but if the urine appears clear, treatment is not warranted. Need for radiographic assessments must be based on mechanism of injury, but a baseline chest radiograph is sufficient for an isolated burn without other evidence of trauma.

AIRWAY ASSESSMENT AND MANAGEMENT

3 Airway assessment and management in the burn patient must include diagnosis of an inhalation injury since this significantly increases morbidity and mortality of patients with thermal injuries. Diagnosis of an inhalation injury should be considered for any patient involved in a closed space fire, but inhalation injury may also occur in a patient who is injured outdoors; a patient who throws gasoline onto a bonfire can inhale the petroleum fumes or liquid and sustain a significant chemical pneumonitis. Clues in the physical examination include singed nasal hairs and facial burns, but these do not in themselves indicate the presence of an inhalation injury. The decision to intubate should be based on respiratory and mental status;

TABLE 11.4

CARBOXYHEMOGLOBIN LEVEL CORRELATIONS WITH PATIENT SYMPTOMS

■ CARBOXYHEMOGLOBIN LEVEL (%)	■ SYMPTOMS
<10	None
15–25	Nausea, headache
30–40	Confusion, stupor, weakness
40–60	Coma
>60	Death

hoarseness, wheezing, or stridor suggests pharyngeal swelling and indicates intubation. In patients with these signs and symptoms, direct laryngoscopy should be performed to confirm posterior pharyngeal mucosal sloughing or carbonaceous sputum coming up through the vocal cords. Patients with large burns who will receive massive intravenous resuscitation volumes should be intubated for airway protection as swelling progresses. With swelling or with face burns, securing the endotracheal tube can be a challenge and requires that an umbilical tie be used rather than tape; arch bars allow the tube to be wired in place, which facilitates wound care and minimizes pressure points. Nasotracheal intubation should be avoided if possible because of the risks of sinusitis and erosion of the nasal columella, especially if the nose is burned. Intubated patients with inhalation injuries should have the head of their bed elevated to 45 degrees to reduce swelling and to prevent aspiration and ventilator-associated pneumonia.

Inhalation Injury

Inhalation injury complicates approximately one third of all major burns. Whereas isolated inhalation injuries do not result in high mortality, they significantly increase mortality in patients with cutaneous burns.[46–51] Presumably, the combined injuries lead to recurrent or persistent bacteremia from the burn wound that potentiates the pulmonary injury. Unfortunately, no reliable long-term outcome data exist about late sequelae related to inhalation injury.

Carbon Monoxide Poisoning. Carbon monoxide (CO) toxicity is the most commonly diagnosed form of inhalation injury since clinical signs and symptoms correlate with arterial carboxyhemoglobin levels (Table 11.4).

CO toxicity is easily treated with 100% inhaled oxygen, which rapidly accelerates CO dissociation from hemoglobin (Table 11.5). Hyperbaric oxygen treatment has been proposed as an expeditious way to reduce carboxyhemoglobin levels, but data are controversial.[52–54] Hyperbaric treatment may be appropriate in the patient who has isolated CO toxicity with impaired neurologic status and a markedly elevated carboxyhemoglobin level (≥25%).

However, the risks for a burn patient (≥10% TBSA) undergoing resuscitation in an isolated hyperbaric chamber may be too significant. Reported life-threatening complications in burn patients undergoing hyperbaric therapy include aspirations, inadequate resuscitation with hypovolemia and metabolic acidosis, inadequate ventilation with respiratory acidosis, electrolyte abnormalities with associated cardiac dysrhythmias, hypothermia, and barotraumas.[55] Inhalation injury complicated by cardiac arrest is uniformly fatal regardless of aggressive therapy, including hyperbaric oxygen.[52] Hydrogen cyanide toxicity, which may occur in structural fires, disrupts cellular oxidation and causes lactic acidosis, which resolves with ventilation in most patients without the need for sodium thiosulfate treatment.[56] Data are beginning to emerge on the safety of hydroxocobalamin administration for cyanide toxicity, but benefits of this early intervention have not been adequately verified to warrant this as a standard of care.[57]

TABLE 11.5

CARBON MONOXIDE–HEMOGLOBIN HALF-LIFE WITH OXYGEN TREATMENT

■ CARBOXYHEMOGLOBIN HALF-LIFE	■ TREATMENT MODALITY
4 h	Room air
45–60 min	100% oxygen
20 min	100% oxygen at 2 atm (hyperbaric oxygen [HBO])

Upper Airway Thermal Injury

Upper airway burns occur due to hot air or chemical toxins and can be diagnosed by direct visualization of the posterior pharynx at the time of intubation. The heat absorptive capacity of the oropharynx is sufficiently efficient that thermal burns to the lower airway are rare; steam can cause a lower airway thermal burn.

Direct thermal damage tends to occur in the upper airway because the oropharynx has a substantial capacity to absorb heat. Upper airway thermal injury constitutes an important indication for intubation, because it is mandatory to control the airway before airway edema develops during resuscitation.

The diagnosis of upper airway thermal injury is achieved with direct laryngoscopic visualization of the posterior oropharyngeal cavity. The decision to intubate should be based on visual evidence of posterior pharyngeal swelling, mucosal sloughing, or carbonaceous sputum coming from below the level of the vocal cords.

Treatment for upper airway injuries includes hospital admission for observation and provision of humidified oxygen, pulmonary toilet, bronchodilators as needed, and endotracheal intubation as indicated. Upper airway thermal burns usually manifest within 48 hours of injury and airway swelling usually is maximal 12 to 24 hours after the injury. A patient with an upper airway burn may require airway protection for 72 hours. In a patient with a small burn (<15% TBSA), a short course of systemic or inhaled steroids may facilitate earlier resolution of airway edema, but steroids are contraindicated in patients with large burns due to the risk of infection and failure to heal. The patient can be extubated based on pulmonary weaning parameters and the presence of an air leak around the endotracheal tube. Once it is safe to extubate, removing the endotracheal tube should be expedited because of the potential nosocomial complication of ventilator-associated pneumonia.

Lower Airway Burn Injury

Burn injury to the tracheobronchial tree and the lung parenchyma results from combustion products in smoke (Table 11.6) and, under unique conditions, inhaled steam.

Numerous irritants in smoke or the vaporized chemical reagents in steam can cause direct mucosal injury, leading to mucosal slough and bronchial edema, bronchoconstriction,

TABLE 11.6

PRODUCTS OF COMBUSTION THAT CAN BE PREDICTED TO CAUSE SIGNIFICANT PULMONARY PARENCHYMAL INJURY

■ SOURCE	■ PRODUCT OF COMBUSTION
Organic matter	Carbon monoxide Carbon dioxide
Petroleum products (gasoline, kerosene, propane, plastics)	Carbon monoxide, nitrogen oxide, benzene
Wood, paper, anhydrous ammonia	Nitrogen oxides (NO, NO_2)
Polyvinyl chloride (plastics)	Hydrogen chlorine
Wool, silk, polyurethane (nylon)	Hydrogen cyanide
Wood, cotton, paper	Aldehydes
Polyurethane (nylon)	Ammonia

and bronchial obstruction. Tracheobronchial mucosal damage and loss of ciliary clearance of the debris induce parenchymal inflammation, which leads to exudate formation and microvascular permeability, and ultimately[50] may progress to pulmonary edema, pneumonia, or acute respiratory distress syndrome (ARDS). Significant inhalation of aerosolized toxins can reduce myocardial contractility and cause resuscitation failure. Whereas diagnosis of lower airway inhalation injury can be confirmed by bronchoscopy, a scoring system to correlate degree of pulmonary injury and outcome has yet to be developed. Xenon[133] ventilation-perfusion scan[58] has also been used for diagnosis but often underdiagnoses the extent of injury and does not change the clinical outcome.[59] Therefore, these technologies may help with documentation of a clinical diagnosis but they are not crucial to subsequent management. Given the high rate (up to 50%) of pneumonia[46] in patients with lower airway inhalation injuries, successful treatment requires aggressive pulmonary toilet and frequent chest physiotherapy.

Acute Respiratory Distress Syndrome

ARDS is an independent risk factor for death in burn patients.[60,61] Understanding of ARDS pathophysiology and management has improved since its initial description in the late 1960s,[62] but 40% to 70% of patients with ARDS still die.

ARDS is defined by the clinical findings of pulmonary edema, hypoxemia, diffuse pulmonary infiltrates, and reduced lung compliance; radiographic findings may be nonspecific. Histologically, ARDS has diffuse alveolar epithelial damage, microvascular permeability, and subsequent inflammatory cell infiltration into the lung parenchyma; interstitial and alveolar edema; hyaline membrane formation; and, ultimately, fibrosis.

The development of ARDS is often presaged by high fluid resuscitation requirements reflecting increased microvascular permeability and leading to increased pulmonary edema. ARDS commonly develops within 7 days after injury. Burn patients with inhalation injury have as much as a 73% incidence of respiratory failure (defined by hypoxemia, pulmonary infections, or prolonged ventilator support) and a 20% incidence of ARDS compared to burn patients without inhalation injury, who have a 5% incidence of respiratory failure and a 2% incidence of ARDS.[63] Advanced age may also be a risk factor for development of ARDS.[64] Acute lung injury rarely develops in patients with inhalation injury but without cutaneous burns.[51,65]

FLUID RESUSCITATION

Most patients undergo resuscitation without difficulty. However, approximately 15% of patients with thermal injuries fail resuscitation[66] in spite of significant attention to improving fluid management of the burn patient.[67] Vascular access should be obtained early during the evaluation before swelling obscures venous markings. Two large-bore peripheral intravenous (IV) lines should provide adequate prehospital venous access; since the early burn is not contaminated with bacteria, these IV lines can be placed through eschar, but care should be taken to secure them well. For children, intraosseous cannulae can provide temporary lifesaving resuscitation, but intravenous access should be obtained as soon as possible.

Multiorgan failure due to inadequate resuscitation and decreased tissue perfusion was a common cause of death in burn patients before formulas were developed to estimate fluid needs.[68] Several proposed fluid resuscitation formulas estimate fluid requirements in the patient with large burns, suggesting that no one formula satisfactorily estimates fluid requirements for all patients. It is essential to remember that each of these formulas estimates fluid needs. However, fluid volumes should be constantly adjusted based on patient physiologic responses during resuscitation (urine output, alert sensorium, and blood pressure). Patients may require more or less fluid depending on the size and depth of burn (deeper burns often are associated with a greater inflammatory response and higher fluid needs), presence of inhalation injury, associated injuries, or comorbidities. Other clinical indicators of higher volume requirements include mechanical ventilation and high base deficit.[69]

One of the commonly used resuscitation formulas has been the Baxter (or Parkland) formula, which calls for 3 to 4 mL of crystalloid per percentage TBSA burned over 24 hours. Half of this volume is delivered during the first 8 hours after injury; the other half is delivered over the subsequent 16 hours. If a patient receives all of the 24-hour estimated volume during the first 2 hours after injury, that fluid will likely leak into the interstitial extracellular tissues and the patient still must receive the estimated hourly crystalloid volumes to maintain intravascular volumes. The reliability of the Parkland formula directly depends on an accurate initial assessment of burn depth and size as described earlier. The trend since Baxter originally proposed this formula has been to administer more fluid than patients require. Some studies report volumes approaching 8 mL/kg per percent TBSA burn,[70] but whether this impacts long-term outcome is difficult to demonstrate.[71]

4 Reliable clinical resuscitation endpoints include maintaining a mean arterial blood pressure greater than 60 mm Hg and urine output of 30 mL/h for adults. Pediatric fluid requirements often exceed formula estimates[72] likely due to less-well-developed renal concentrating abilities. Therefore, the urinary output goal for infants and very young children (<20 kg) should be 1.5 mL/kg per hour. Large-volume crystalloid boluses should be restricted to hypotensive episodes and should be accompanied by an increase in the hourly volume by 10%. Decreased urine output for 1 to 2 hours does not require a large-volume crystalloid bolus and should be managed by increasing the hourly resuscitation fluid rate by 10%. Stabilization of the flux of mediators and closure of capillary leaks occur gradually 12 to 48 hours after the burn injury. As capillary leak resolves, the amount of fluids needed to maintain these endpoints should progressively decrease and the IV rate generally can be slowly weaned by 10% per hour. Most burn patients do not require pulmonary arterial pressure monitoring

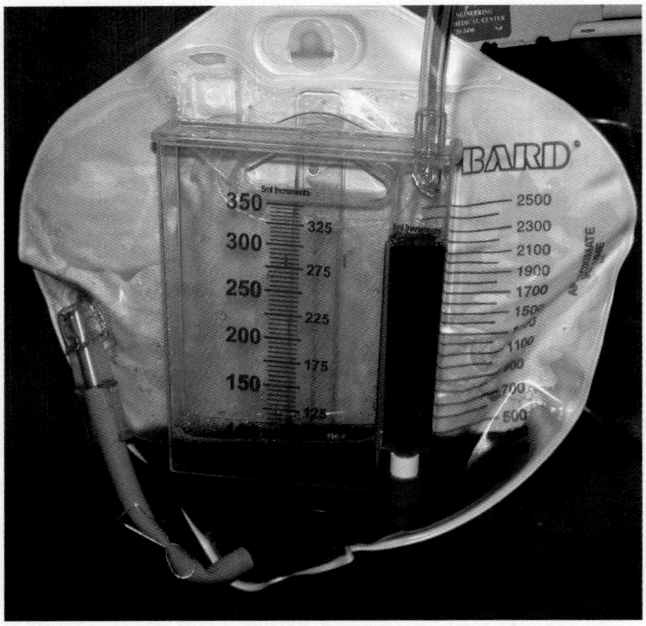

FIGURE 11.4. Myoglobinuria with dark pigment in the urine.

during resuscitation and will be overresuscitated if IV fluid administration is based on pulmonary artery wedge pressures. A pulmonary artery catheter may be useful in patients with underlying cardiac comorbidity at risk for cardiac shock and congestive heart failure.

Patients with extremely deep burns, electrical burns, or compartment syndrome may develop rhabdomyolysis with myoglobinuria (Fig. 11.4) and subsequent acute tubular necrosis. In these patients, a brisk urine output of 100 mL/h should be maintained. Alkalinization of the urine with intravenous sodium bicarbonate (0.12 to 0.5 mEq/kg per hour) theoretically increases myoglobin solubility and decreases precipitation in the renal tubules but requires careful serum pH monitoring and lacks clinical verification. Rarely, osmotic diuresis with mannitol is required to maintain urine output, but this treatment should be carefully considered since osmotic diuresis reduces urine output reliability as an endpoint for determining intravascular volume status.

Colloid administration (albumin or fresh frozen plasma) after the capillary leak has closed (12 to 72 hours postinjury) may restore intravascular volume in patients with persistent low urine output and hypotension despite adequate crystalloid administration. In such cases, 5% albumin (0.3 to 0.5 mL/kg per percent TBSA burn) can be administered over 24 hours. Plasmapheresis also reduces intravenous fluid requirements in patients who do not respond to standard crystalloid resuscitation. Indications for plasmapheresis include a sustained mean arterial pressure of less than 60 mm Hg and urine output less than 30 mL/h in a patient whose ongoing fluid needs are more than twice fluid volume estimates. Early plasmapheresis (12 to 24 hours postinjury) appears to decrease the incidence of complications from administration of excessive fluid such as extremity compartment syndromes, abdominal compartment syndrome, and pulmonary edema. The mechanism by which plasmapheresis works is unknown, but theoretically the plasma exchange removes circulating cytokines that cause vasodilatation and capillary leak and drive the systemic inflammatory response.

Once resuscitation is complete (24 to 48 hours postinjury), insensible losses and hyperthermia associated with a hyperdynamic state may require ongoing maintenance intravenous or enteral fluid administration. Reliable daily weights are often useful for determining insensible fluid losses or fluid retention.

Fluid Resuscitation Complications

Overresuscitation[70,73] causes complications such as poor tissue perfusion, abdominal or extremity compartment syndrome, pulmonary edema, and pleural effusions. Increased abdominal pressure decreases lung compliance and impedes lung expansion, resulting in elevated airway pressures and hypoventilation.

Because of the risk for compartment syndrome in patients undergoing large-volume resuscitation, burned extremities should be elevated and hourly neurovascular examinations should be performed; tight bands of eschar are often evident before vascular inflow is compromised and indicate the need for escharotomies. Decreased chest compliance with circumferential burns can also improve with thoracic escharotomies, especially in children. An effective thoracic escharotomy must extend along each anterior axillary line and connect at the infraclavicular and subcostal lines (Fig. 11.5A). Extremity escharotomies should extend through the skin only and should not violate the fascia; the arm must be in anatomic position when medial and lateral incisions are made (Fig. 11.5B). Eschar on the dorsal hand must often be released to restore signals in the palmar arch (Fig. 11.5C); there is no benefit to digital escharotomies and risk of injury to the digital arteries and nerves is significant.

Abdominal compartment syndrome also classically decreases venous return, causes oliguria, and increases intra-abdominal pressures exceeding 25 mm Hg.[74] Bedside decompressive laparotomy through burn wounds, if necessary (Fig. 11.6), can alleviate abdominal compartment syndrome[75] in patients with hemodynamic instability, hypoventilation, and elevated abdominal pressures. In addition, pulmonary edema increases risk of ARDS.

Recently, orbital compartment syndrome has been reported as one more complication related to high-volume resuscitation. Patients with massive fluid resuscitation with or without facial burns develop intraocular pressures as high as 90 mm Hg, which returns to a normal range with lateral canthotomy.[76]

Composition of the resuscitation fluid is important to prevent electrolyte imbalance and acidosis. Typically, lactated Ringer solution is the primary resuscitative fluid because of the risk for metabolic hyperchloremic acidosis and hypernatremia in patients who receive large volumes of 0.9% normal saline solution. The resuscitative fluid solution should not contain glucose because hyperglycemia and osmotic diuresis may confound resuscitation. Pediatric patients who weigh less than 20 kg do not have large glycogen stores in their liver and should receive 0.45% saline with 5% dextrose at a maintenance rate (3 to 4 mL/kg per hour).

WOUND MANAGEMENT

Topical Antimicrobials

5 It is worth emphasizing that prophylactic systemic antibiotics do not have a role in the management of the patient with acute burn injuries.[77] Because eschar is devitalized and avascular, systemic antibiotics cannot reach the eschar surface where the bacterial colonization occurs. Topical antimicrobial agents delay wound colonization and infection, but they themselves have not changed mortality in the way that early excision and grafting did. All agents commonly used in the United States have benefits and side effects (Table 11.7).

Silver sulfadiazine is the most commonly used antimicrobial agent for burns because it has a broad spectrum of antimicrobial activity, is soothing, and has no significant metabolic or electrolyte implications. Because silver sulfadiazine does not penetrate eschar, it is ineffective against already established burn wound infections. Silver sulfadiazine has been associated with

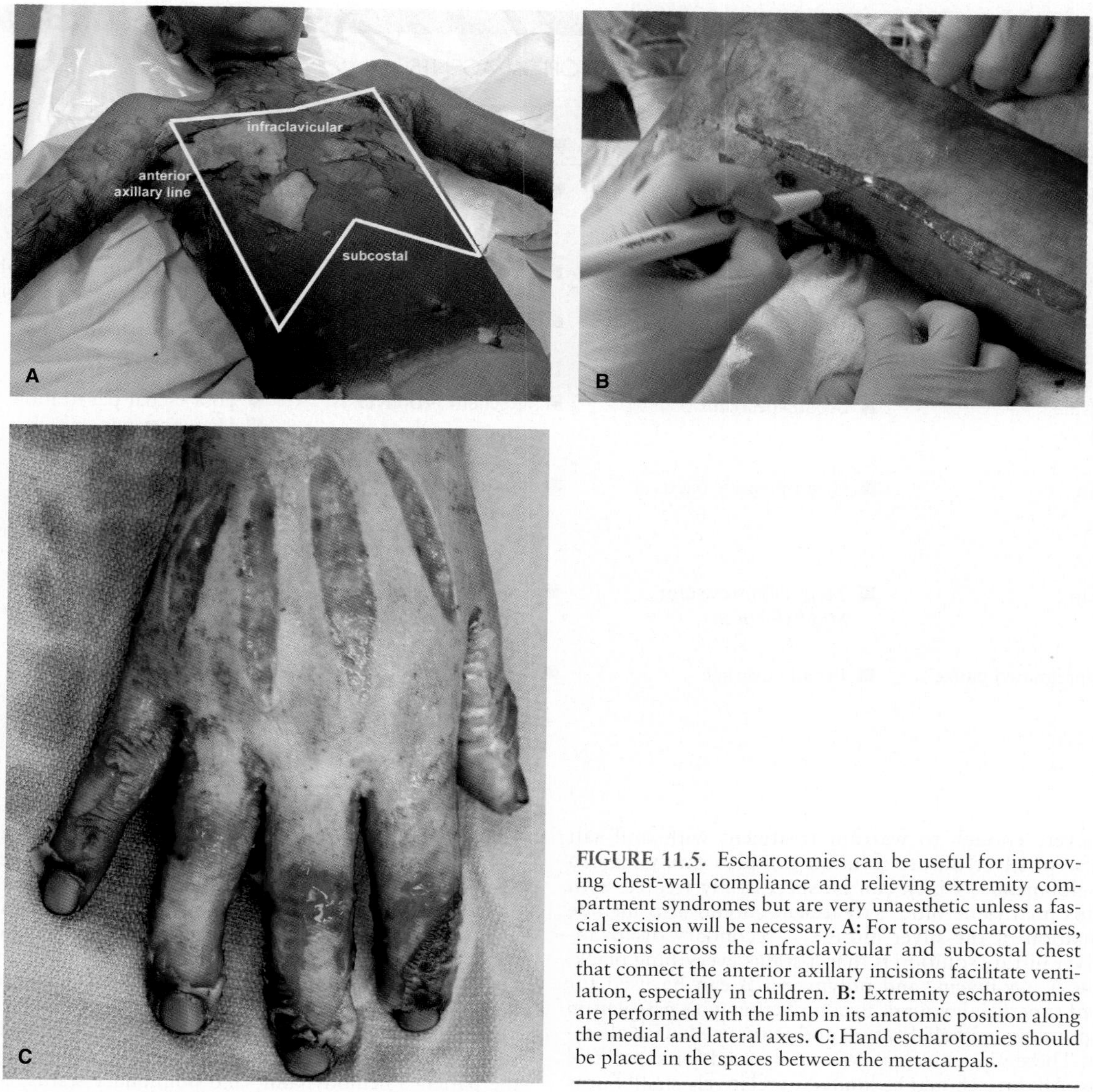

FIGURE 11.5. Escharotomies can be useful for improving chest-wall compliance and relieving extremity compartment syndromes but are very unaesthetic unless a fascial excision will be necessary. A: For torso escharotomies, incisions across the infraclavicular and subcostal chest that connect the anterior axillary incisions facilitate ventilation, especially in children. B: Extremity escharotomies are performed with the limb in its anatomic position along the medial and lateral axes. C: Hand escharotomies should be placed in the spaces between the metacarpals.

early postburn neutropenia, but this is more likely related margination of neutrophils due to the overall inflammatory response to injury rather than to the topical agent. The neutropenia is typically self-limited and rarely requires a change in antimicrobial therapy. Patients with sulfa allergies typically do not have adverse

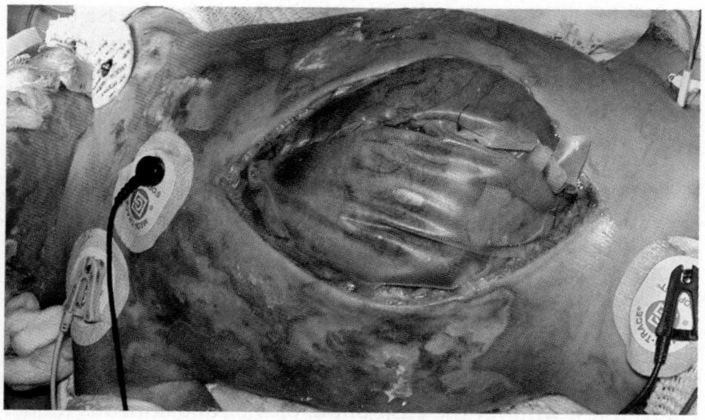

FIGURE 11.6. Decompressive laparotomy can be safely performed through a burn but significantly increases morbidity and should be avoided by closely monitoring fluid resuscitation.

reactions to silver sulfadiazine; a test patch in a small area of the burn will cause pain or a rash in the unusual case of an allergy.

Mafenide acetate is unique because it penetrates eschar, making it effective in both treating and preventing burn wound infections. This attribute has led to its frequent use on the ears to protect against suppurative chondritis; however, silver sulfadiazine appears to be equally effective.[78] Mafenide provides excellent coverage against gram-negative organisms. Mafenide is available as either a cream or a solution, which is a useful topical agent for skin grafts when the wound bed is considered likely to benefit from postoperative antimicrobial treatment. The major disadvantage is that mafenide inhibits carbonic anhydrase and causes metabolic acidosis that may complicate ventilator management. Topical mafenide can be painful, especially on application to partial-thickness burns.

Silver nitrate provides broad-spectrum antimicrobial coverage, including good activity against staphylococci and gram-negative organisms, but it does not penetrate eschar well. Dressings must be irrigated with the aqueous 0.5% solution every 4 hours to keep the dressing moist and prevent precipitation of the silver nitrate onto the wound surface. Since concentrated silver nitrate causes a chemical burn, the bacteriostatic solution used for burn wounds is very hypotonic (it is reconstituted in water rather than saline to avoid silver chloride precipitation) and causes osmotic dilution in the tissues, leading to hyponatremia and hypochloremia. These can

TABLE 11.7

ADVANTAGES AND DISADVANTAGES OF ANTIMICROBIAL TOPICAL AGENTS

■ ANTIMICROBIAL AGENT	■ COVERAGE	■ ADVANTAGES	■ DISADVANTAGES
Silver sulfadiazine	■ Broad spectrum, especially *Pseudomonas*	■ Soothing	■ Poor eschar penetration ■ May impede epithelial cell migration
Mafenide acetate	■ Broad spectrum, including *clostridium*	■ Good eschar penetration ■ Excellent for both treatment and prophylaxis	■ Carbonic anhydrase inhibition with 2° metabolic acidosis ■ Painful
Silver nitrate	■ Broad spectrum	■ Excellent prophylaxis	■ Poor eschar penetration ■ Hyponatremia ■ Methemoglobinemia
Bacitracin	■ Gram-positive bacteria	■ Good for shallow facial burns	■ Expensive ■ Often delivered in combination with neomycin and polymyxin B, which are nephrotoxic
Mupirocin	■ Methicillin-resistant *Staphylococcus*	■ Excellent for methicillin-resistant *Staphylococcus*	■ Very expensive
Silver-impregnated gauze	■ Broad coverage	■ Good for shallow burns, grafts, and donor sites	■ Hides wound ■ Can cause discomfort when dried ■ Nonadhesive and slips from wound

become severe enough to warrant treatment with oral salt tablets. Use of silver nitrate solution can also rarely lead to methemoglobinemia, which can be successfully treated with intravenous methylene blue[79]; treatment should also include discontinuation of the silver nitrate. A secondary disadvantage of silver nitrate solution is that it stains everything black.

Bacitracin, neomycin, and polymyxin B can be used for coverage of superficial wounds in conjunction with petrolatum gauze to promote epithelialization and minimize bacterial colonization. These ointments are commonly used for superficial face burns. All three should be limited to relatively small burns because of potential nephrotoxicity. Mupirocin has the advantage of being effective against methicillin-resistant *Staphylococcus aureus* (MRSA) and its use should be restricted for this indication.

Several recently introduced dressings are impregnated with silver, which has unique antimicrobial properties and works by disrupting bacterial cellular respiration. These dressings can be used for superficial partial-thickness burns, donor sites, and meshed skin grafts. An advantage of these dressings is a reduced need for dressing changes since they can stay in place until a shallow burn or donor site heals. The reduced frequency of dressing changes simplifies burn care but can hinder evaluation of evolving partial-thickness burns, so its use should be limited to wounds that are likely to heal or do not need frequent evaluations. Since the silver-impregnated dressings are nonadherent, an adhesive tape such as Hypafix (Smith & Nephew) must be placed along the edge of the dressing to secure the dressing to the wound bed. After 10 to 14 days, the tape can be removed and the dressings can be washed and towel-dried daily until they peel off the epithelialized wound.

Burn Excision and Grafting

6 The beneficial impact of early excision and grafting on outcomes following thermal injuries has been remarkable. Because of this change in therapy from a nonoperative to an operative approach,[80–83] mortality in burn patients has dramatically dropped and functional outcomes have improved over the past 30 years. Other advantages include shortened length of hospital stay,[84] lower costs,[85] and fewer reconstructive surgeries.[86] The timing for initial excision of deep burn wounds should occur as soon after the resuscitative phase of recovery as feasible. Excising large burns during the first 24 hours complicates fluid resuscitation with the risk of hypothermia and bleeding and is not recommended. By 3 to 4 days after injury, burn excision and wound coverage should be a safe option depending on the patient's hemodynamic and pulmonary status, comorbidities, and associated injuries. A patient with large, deep, partial-thickness or full-thickness burns should undergo the initial excision within 7 days of injury. Staged excisions can be performed every 2 to 3 days until the entire burn wound is excised. However, many burns are not homogeneous with both shallow and deep areas. Such indeterminate-depth burns can be safely treated with topical antimicrobial ointment for 7 to 10 days until the deeper portion that requires grafting becomes evident; this situation is common in patients with scald or grease burns. By 72 hours after injury, an experienced burn care provider can often differentiate burns that will heal with topical antimicrobial treatment within 3 weeks from deeper injuries that will require excision.

Surgical excision of the burn wound involves one of two technical approaches: fascial excision or tangential excision. Fascial excision involves excising the burned tissue and the underlying subcutaneous tissue down to the muscle fascia using electrocautery, which limits surgical bleeding (Fig. 11.7A). Advantages of a fascial excision include an easily defined, well-vascularized plane that can readily accept a graft. A major disadvantage to this approach is the inevitable removal of healthy, viable subcutaneous tissue, which leads to unaesthetic contour deformities; without the cushioning of the subcutaneous tissue, the grafts on the fascia are often fragile for years after the injury.

Tangential excision involves sequential excision of eschar until the wound bed displays diffuse punctate bleeding[87] indicative of viable tissue that can support a skin graft (Fig. 11.7B).

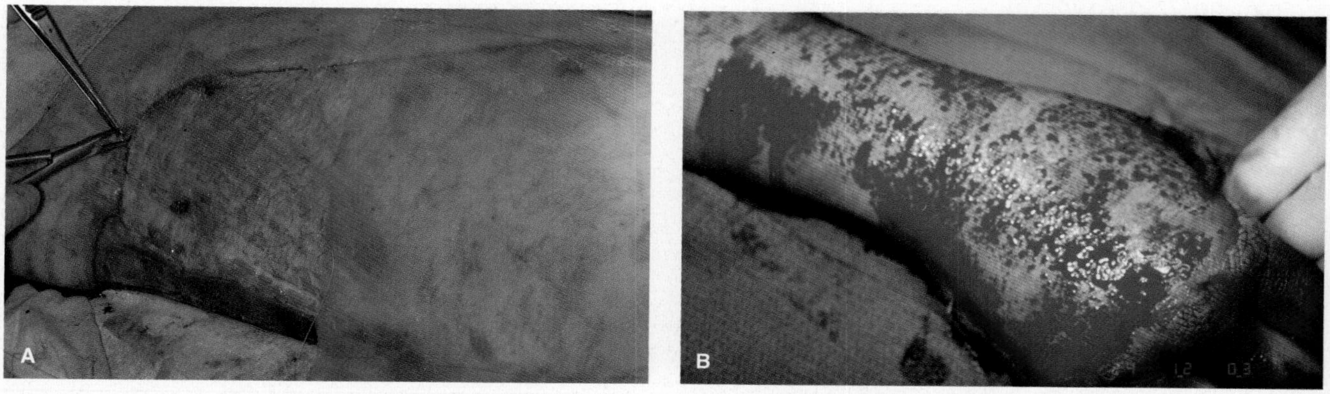

FIGURE 11.7. **A:** Fascial excision limits bleeding but results in suboptimal aesthetic outcomes and should be avoided if possible. If necessary because of burn depth, care can be taken to tack down the edges to minimize the ledge that interferes with function. **B:** Tangential excision requires serial tissue removal until the wound bed has diffuse punctate bleeding; ideally this allows a thin pearly white dermal layer to remain in the wound bed.

Tangential excision can be performed with a handheld knife (Weck or Watson) adjusting the guard to control depth of excision. A disadvantage of tangential excision includes diffuse bleeding from the wound bed. As surgeons have become more comfortable with early excision and grafting, they have developed strategies to minimize surgical blood loss. Topical epinephrine solution (1:10,000), electrocautery, and compression were recognized early on to minimize blood loss. With experience, other methods evolved including using pneumatic tourniquets for extremity burns and using subeschar injection of dilute epinephrine solution to vasoconstrict the capillaries before excision. Both of these techniques require substantial experience to assess tissue viability since there will be no diffuse bleeding in the wound bed. A commercially available fibrinogen and thrombin spray system (Artiss Fibrin Sealant; Baxter, Deerfield, IL) improves hemostasis and promotes graft adherence to the wound bed with fewer and smaller underlying postoperative fluid collections.[88,89]

Wound Closure Alternatives

Once the eschar is excised to viable tissue, the wound should be closed as soon as possible, ideally with immediate autografting. Whereas the best cutaneous replacement would be full-thickness skin grafts, this is not possible for most patients, especially those with large burns and limited donor sites. Traditionally, wounds that could not be autografted immediately were covered with a biologic dressing while donor sites healed. Human allograft is one temporary biologic dressing that is meshed 1:1 and applied to excised wound beds to allow wound drainage. Allograft vascularizes and engrafts and provides physiologic wound closure for 2 to 4 weeks, at which point it typically is rejected and must be replaced with either new allograft or preferably autograft from reharvested donor sites. Porcine xenograft can also be used as a cheaper alternative, but it will not vascularize and will not engraft. When widely meshed skin grafts are necessary, overlayed sheets of allograft can be used on top of the autografts to protect the wound bed as the meshed interstices epithelialize.[90] This minimizes wound bed desiccation and reduces pain. The disadvantage of this technique is the long time until definitive wound closure, the need to recrop donor sites, and the potential for significant hypertrophic scar formation in the interstices of the widely meshed grafts (Fig. 11.8A) and in the reharvested donor sites.

Alternative approaches using skin substitutes have improved patient long-term functional and aesthetic outcomes. Two types of skin substitutes exist: epidermal and dermal. Both technologies have advantages and disadvantages (Table 11.8).

Epidermal skin substitutes consisting of cultured autologous keratinocytes with or without a subjacent layer of autologous fibroblasts suggested great promise for scarless wound closure in the late 1980s.[91] Whereas future advances in burn wound management will depend on improvements in cultured epithelial cell technology,[92,93] current available products have not significantly evolved burn wound management. Dermal substitutes have been more successful in early clinical use.[94,95] Integra dermal template (Integra Lifesciences, Plainsboro, NJ) is one commercially available product, designed to be combined with ultra-thin autograft[96] or cultured epithelium. Its advantage is that it is a bilaminate product composed of a temporary outer silastic layer and an inner matrix layer of type 1 collagen and chondroitin sulfate.[97,98] The silastic layer provides early wound closure following eschar excision and the inner layer serves as a template that autologous fibroblasts, endothelial cells, and other mesenchymal cells populate. Once the product is vascularized (2 to 3 weeks), an ultra-thin autograft can be placed on the neodermis.[96] Histologic evaluation suggests that the Integra neodermis architecture is more comparable to uninjured dermis than regular scar (Fig. 11.9A). Integra use has been reported to have improved long-term aesthetic and functional results (Fig. 11.9B) but requires

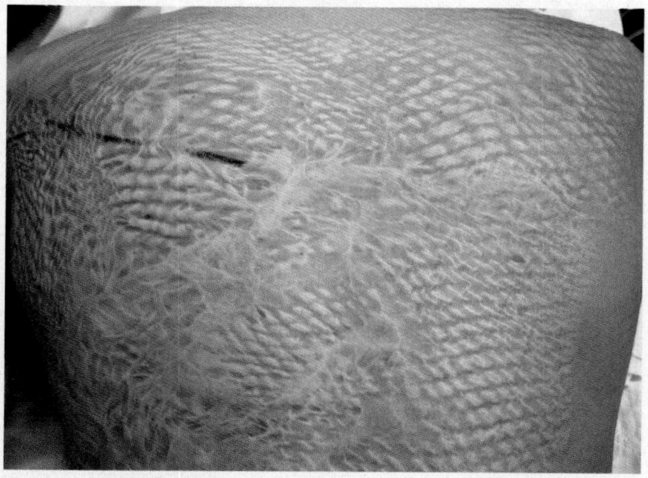

FIGURE 11.8. Traditional widely meshed skin grafts leave hypertrophic interstices long after the wounds are mature.

TABLE 11.8

ADVANTAGES AND DISADVANTAGES OF SKIN SUBSTITUTES

	■ DERMAL SUBSTITUTES	■ EPIDERMAL SUBSTITUTE
Pros	■ Useful with limited donor sites ■ Replaces mesenchyme ■ Thin donor sites ■ Decreases scar formation	■ Useful with limited donor sites ■ Replaces epidermis ■ Fewer donor sites
Cons	■ Expensive ■ Prone to infection ■ Requires completely viable wound bed ■ Requires fastidious postoperative wound care	■ Expensive ■ Prone to infection ■ Prone to sheering ■ Prolonged immobilization with delayed rehabilitation ■ Prolonged length of stay

meticulous surgical excision and postoperative care to minimize infection.[99] A topical antimicrobial agent is usually necessary postoperatively; if neodermal quantitative cultures demonstrate more than 10^6 colony-forming units, directed systemic antibiotics might also be indicated. A significant advantage is the rapid healing and minimal scarring in ultra-thin donor sites (Fig. 11.9C).

Another promising dermal substitute is AlloDerm (LifeCell, Woodlands, TX), a cryopreserved human dermal allograft.[100] The advantage of this product is the native mesenchymal structure without the allogenic cellular components that cause allograft rejection. This dermal substitute requires immediate autografting since there is no outer barrier.

METABOLIC AND NUTRITIONAL SUPPORT

Patients with major thermal injury develop a hypermetabolic state characterized by increased basal metabolic rate, increased oxygen consumption, negative nitrogen balance, and weight loss. Subsequently, these patients have increased caloric requirements[101] to prevent delayed wound healing, decreased immune competence, and cellular dysfunction.

Protein catabolism in a 60-kg patient with a large burn may result in loss of 150 to 200 g of nitrogen per day. Nitrogen excreted in the urine can be measured, but large amounts of nitrogen lost from wounds are insensible. Therefore, measured

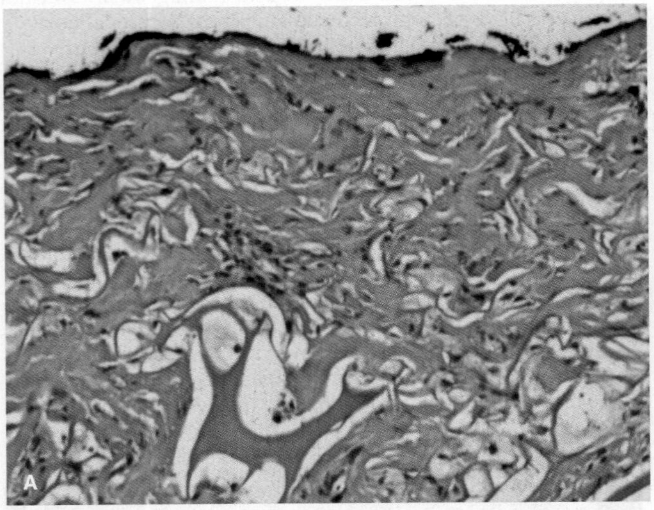

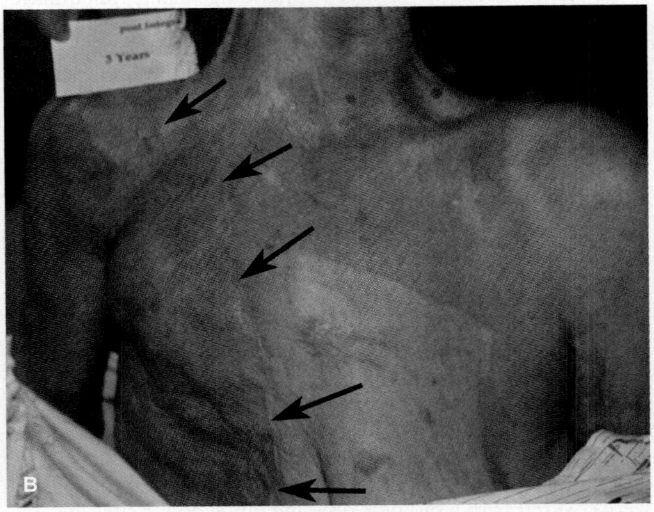

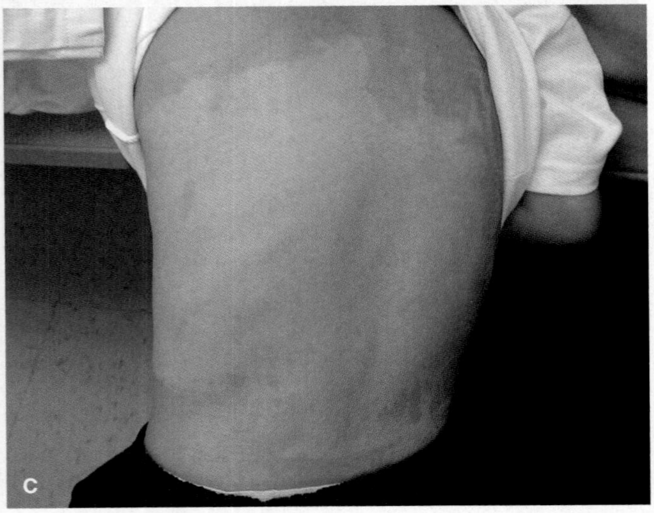

FIGURE 11.9. **A:** Histology of Integra neodermis appears more like uninjured dermis than regular scar. **B:** Integra covered with ultra-thin skin grafts (*arrows*) is softer and more elastic than the traditional wide meshed graphs. **C:** Donor sites for the ultra-thin grafts heal quickly without the long-term scars typical of standard-depth donor sites.

TABLE 11.9

NUTRITIONAL ASSESSMENT OF BURN PATIENTS

	WOUND SIZE (% TBSA)	NITROGEN LOSS FROM WOUNDS (g/kg/d)	PROTEIN LOSS FROM WOUNDS IN A 60-kg ADULT (g/d)	NUTRITIONAL NEEDS
Small burn	<10	0.02	~8	Oral intake only
Moderate burn	11–30	0.05	~19	Supplemental enteral feeding if oral intake is insufficient
Large burn	>31	0.12	~45	Enteral feeding to meet nutritional goals with oral intake as tolerated

24-hour total urea nitrogen levels underestimate nitrogen losses in burn patients (Table 11.9).[102]

The catabolic state continues until the wounds are closed. Once a patient becomes anabolic, preburn muscle takes three times as long to regain as it did to lose.[103,104] Several equations can be used to estimate calorie needs. The Harris-Benedict equation estimates basal energy expenditure according to gender, age, height, and weight; the basal energy expenditure is multiplied by an activity factor that reflects the severity of injury or the degree of illness. For burns, this multiplier is 2, the maximal factor for this formula. The Harris-Benedict equation overestimates caloric needs for patients with a moderate burn size. The Curreri formula[105] based on patient weight and burn size overestimates caloric needs for patients with large burns and is best used for patients with small or moderate-sized burns (<40% TBSA).[106,107]

Infection, ARDS, or creation of donor sites increases catabolism and alters caloric needs.[108] Healing and skin grafting close wounds and decrease the catabolic state. Hence, repeated evaluation of the metabolic state of a burn patient is necessary to account for changes in wound size and clinical condition. As discussed earlier, 24-hour total urea nitrogen levels in the urine must be augmented to estimate nitrogen losses from the wound. Serum albumin levels are not sensitive markers of adequate nutrition; they are typically low in patients with burns larger than 20% TBSA.[109] Transthyretin or prealbumin levels correlate more closely with catabolic status and a trend over several weeks may correlate with patient caloric needs.[110] C-reactive protein levels provide an indication of the patient's general inflammatory state and may correlate with catabolic status.[111] Indirect calorimetry may be useful for measuring caloric needs in intubated burn[112] patients by quantifying oxygen consumption and carbon dioxide expiration and calculating nutritional requirements based on the formula: kcal/day = $(3.9 \times VO_2 + 1.1 \times VCO_2) \times 1.44$. Pulmonary artery catheters can also indirectly provide this information by using the Fick equation: kcal/day = cardiac output $\times$ (arterial pO_2 − venous pO_2) $\times 10 \times 6.96$. Recent reports suggest that in children, respiratory quotients may not accurately estimate feeding needs.[113]

Enteral Nutrition

Prolonged ileus and stress ulcers in burn patients have been largely eliminated by early feeding.[114] Multiple studies have shown that patients with major thermal injury can receive adequate calories soon after injury. At the University of Washington Burn Center, tube feeding is started a median of 5 hours after admission (unpublished quality improvement data).

Benefits of gastric feeding versus duodenal feeding continue to be debated. Although feeding distal to the pylorus theoretically should cause less aspiration risk, enteral formulas can be found in pulmonary secretions of 7% of patients receiving gastric feeds compared with 13% of patients receiving transpyloric feeding.[115] Hence, for burn patients with high caloric needs, the delay in feeding for confirmation of tube placement may not be worth the effort.

Continuation of tube feeds during surgery in intubated burn patients who require multiple operations maximizes caloric intake and decreases wound infection.[116] However, intraoperative repositioning may necessitate stopping feeds preoperatively, especially if the patient will be prone. Critically ill burn patients who have undergone decompressive laparotomy for abdominal compartment syndrome also tolerate continuous tube feedings.[117]

Glucose Management

Hyperglycemia negatively impacts wound healing and increases morbidity and mortality in critically ill patients, even those without underlying diabetes mellitus.[118] Increased risk of infection, reduced skin graft take, and higher mortality[119] underscore the importance of maintaining blood sugars between 80 to 120 mg/dL.[118] In spite of the initial excitement about the beneficial effect of tight glucose control on outcomes of critically injured patients, increasing data suggest that very tight control does not improve outcomes in trauma patients[120] and should be studied prospectively in burn patients.[121]

Albumin

Hypoalbuminemia typically persists in burn patients until the wounds are healed. Patients with large burns typically have serum albumin levels of 1.7 g/dL and rarely exceed 2.5 g/dL.[109] Administration of exogenous albumin to attain serum levels above 1.5 g/dL does not appear to impact length of stay, complication rate, or mortality.[122]

Nutritional Supplementation

Studies to determine benefits of specialized nutritional supplements such as arginine, glutamine, and omega-3 fatty acids in burn patients are contradictory.[123–125] However, there are reports that anabolism can be promoted in burn patients with metabolically active agents such as insulin, recombinant human growth factor, the anabolic steroid oxandrolone, and propranolol.[126] Oxandrolone in particular has been reported to improve weight gain and functional recovery in burn survivors.[127] Propranolol has now been fairly well characterized as having a beneficial effect in pediatric patients[128] and should be investigated in a multicenter trial for adults. Early administration of the antioxidants α-tocopherol and ascorbic acid reduces the incidence of organ failure and shortens ICU length of stay in critically ill trauma patients.[77] Whereas a multicenter study will be necessary to demonstrate similar results in burn patients, the potential benefit and the low cost make antioxidant supplementation an attractive low-risk intervention for burn patients at risk for multiorgan dysfunction.

INFECTION

We have determined that as many as 80% of patients with large burns developed an infection from one or more sources during the hospital stay (unpublished data). Judicious antibiotic use must be employed to limit development of opportunistic infections in patients and to establish responsible epidemiologic infection control in the burn unit. Therefore, targeted systemic antibiotics should be used for diagnosed infections based on clinical judgment and supportive laboratory and radiologic findings. Prophylaxis against gram-positive organisms leads to development of gram-negative bacterial infections or fungal and mold infections and are therefore contraindicated in patients with burns.[129] Fungal wound infection has been reported to be independently associated with mortality in burn patients regardless of burn size, age, or presence of inhalation injury.[130] Tetanus prophylaxis continues to be recommended since the disease is so devastating and vaccination has few theoretical risks. However, current medical literature has few reports of tetanus developing in patients who have been immunized during childhood.[131]

DEEP VEIN THROMBOSIS

The incidence of deep vein thrombosis (DVT) has been reported to be as high as 25% in hospitalized burn patients.[132] It has also been reported to be responsible for only 0.14% of deaths in burn patients; hence, a standard of care for DVT prophylaxis in burn patients has never been defined.[133] One study has suggested that age and burn size have a synergistic effect on DVT/pulmonary embolism risk, with the sum of age and TBSA burn having the strongest independent effect ($p < 0.001$).[134] At the University of Washington Regional Burn Center, patients with burns larger than 20% TBSA developed clinically evident thromboembolic disease in 9% of those who received prophylaxis with unfractionated heparin and in 18% of those who received low-molecular-weight heparin (unpublished quality improvement data). On the basis of these data, patients with burns larger than 20% TBSA receive prophylaxis with subcutaneous unfractionated heparin, 5,000 U three times per day. A dropping platelet count suggests heparin-induced thrombocytopenia, which causes generalized microvascular thrombosis and can be associated with thromboembolic disease.

ANEMIA

Acute blood loss soon after injury is uncommon in a patient with an isolated burn injury; therefore, a dropping hematocrit during resuscitation may be a sign that a patient has associated injuries or a bleeding diathesis. Procedures such as central venous line placement or escharotomies should not be associated with significant blood loss.

Patient age, overall condition, and comorbidity should contribute to the determination for the need for a transfusion. The risks of viral transmission, transfusion reaction, and cost must also be considered. For a healthy patient who does not need surgery, a hematocrit as low as 20% may be well tolerated. However, inhalation injury, infection, or multiorgan failure may require a higher hematocrit to maximize oxygen-carrying capacity. Patients with large burns and anticipated blood loss should receive iron supplements. Erythropoietin is an expensive recombinant supplement that has not been shown to prevent anemia or decrease transfusion requirements in acutely burned patients.[135]

PAIN MANAGEMENT

Pain management for patients with burn injuries works best with simple pharmaceutical approaches. Use of several narcotics with varying half-lives will confuse health care providers, 7 the patient, and the family. However, burn patients experience three different classes of pain, background, breakthrough, and procedural pain, which require different approaches.

Burn patients experience background pain 24 hours per day until their wounds are healed; long-acting pain relievers are well suited for this type of discomfort. A hospitalized patient with large burns can be easily treated with methadone or controlled-release morphine sulfate. An outpatient with a small burn often does well with a nonsteroidal anti-inflammatory drug; ideally these should be stopped at least 7 days before surgery.

Breakthrough pain occurs when exercise or other activities of daily living exacerbate background burn wound discomfort. Short-acting narcotics or acetaminophen can alleviate occasional breakthrough pain. Persistent breakthrough pain suggests that the long-acting medication dosage should be increased.

Procedural pain occurs during wound care and dressing changes and usually requires treatment with a short-acting narcotic. For inpatients with larger burns, oral narcotics or transmucosal fentanyl citrate[136,137] works well for wound care; IV morphine or fentanyl can be used for uncontrolled pain. For outpatients, oxycodone (5 to 15 mg) usually suffices for daily wound care. Anxiety about wound care or therapy is often misconstrued as pain, especially in children, and is likely undertreated.[138] Therefore, patients with large burns requiring daily wound care should be evaluated for potential benefit from a short-acting anxiolytic agent for procedures. Complications of excessive narcotic use, such as prolonged sedation, delirium, and, more urgently, loss of airway control, must be avoided in young children and elderly patients, who may have decreased narcotic tolerance.[139]

Nonpharmacologic approaches can augment pain management in burn patients. Hypnosis can be administered either by trained health care providers or by patients themselves to reduce narcotic use in burn patients.[140] Virtual reality has also shown promise as a distraction modality to enhance patient comfort during wound care and intense therapy.[141]

Discomfort in the healed wound due to paresthesias and itching may persist for months after injury but generally does not respond to narcotics; exercise and deep massage are effective modalities that patients should be encouraged to use. Diphenhydramine, cyproheptadine, or cetirizine may relieve itching. Use of doxepin ointment may also abrogate itching in healed wounds. Keeping the wound moist with a topical salve or lotion may be as effective as other pharmacologic approaches.

SPECIALIZED BURN AREAS

Burns of the Face, Ocular Adnexa, and Ears

The structures in the midface can be difficult to excise and reconstruct. Therefore, the face is commonly treated nonoperatively with topical antimicrobial agents for 10 days.[142,143]

Areas that remain unhealed at that time should be excised and grafted with thick sheet autograft. The nasal tip and alar rims are especially difficult to reconstruct and excision should be sparing. Periocular burns can lead to acute and late sequelae. Early after injury, edema can cause conjunctival desiccation with eventual keratitis and corneal ulceration. Lubrication with ophthalmologic antibiotics is mandatory but tarsorrhaphy may be necessary. If the lid burns are deep, earlier excision and full-thickness skin grafting may be indicated. Ear burns can lead to suppurative chondritis if infection develops. Many texts suggest that all ear burns must be treated with mafenide cream,[144] but studies have verified that silver sulfadiazine has comparable results.[78] More importantly, pressure on the burned auricle from objects such as pillows and tight dressings or ties should be avoided by using a foam egg crate for a pillow and very loose dressings.

Burns of the Hands and Feet

Optimal functional outcome of hand burns is facilitated by an organized, multidisciplinary approach to the injuries with emphasis on the therapist. The initial evaluation of the burned hand must include evaluation of capillary refill, temperature, and Doppler signals in the palmar arch. It is not enough simply to demonstrate that there is blood flow in the radial or ulnar arteries. If the arm or upper arm is circumferentially burned, escharotomies of the proximal upper extremity and dorsal hand may be indicated (Fig. 11.5B, C). Digital escharotomies are never indicated because the potential injury to the digital vessels and nerves outweighs the benefits. For high-voltage electrical injury or deep fourth- or fifth-degree thermal burns, fasciotomy may be required for forearm compartment syndrome or progressive neurovascular impairment. In equivocal cases, it is most prudent to proceed to decompression promptly rather than wait until ischemia has advanced.

Extremity elevation benefits hand burns by limiting edema and subsequently allowing range of motion and limiting risk
8 of infection. Active range of motion should be the goal for all hand burns; this will decrease edema and maintain manual function. If the patient is unable to cooperate, passive range of motion should be performed at least twice per day. Splinting the hand in a functional position, with the metacarpophalangeal joints at 70 to 90 degrees, the interphalangeal joints in extension, the thumb in neutral position with the first web space open, and the wrist in 20 to 30 degrees of extension, may be indicated for a critically injured patient. Deep partial-thickness and full-thickness burns should be excised and sheet grafted as soon as practical (Fig. 11.10). Hands are immobilized in a functional position for 5 days after surgery to prevent shearing of the graft before range-of-motion exercises are resumed. Deeper hand burns that involve the extensor mechanisms, joint capsules, or bone are difficult clinical problems. They also often require temporary or long-term axial Kirschner wire fixation of open and unstable interphalangeal or metacarpophalangeal joints. These burns may require groin or abdominal flap coverage[145] to achieve a tissue bed that can be grafted. With these approaches patients with deep hand burns should be able to function independently.

Palm burns are especially common in the toddler age group as they begin to explore and touch hot surfaces such as ovens or gas-fireplace glass. Since palmar skin is thick, many burns do not require resurfacing. Therefore, a nonoperative approach facilitates preservation of the specialized attachment of the palmar skin to the underlying fascia and regeneration of the unique Pacinian mechanoreceptors in the palmar skin. If necessary, full-thickness injuries that do not heal in 3 to 4 weeks or show signs of healing by contraction should be grafted with full-thickness or thick split-thickness sheet grafts and splinted in extension to maintain the palm in an open position. Likewise, burns of the plantar surface of the feet should be grafted with full-thickness or thick split-thickness sheet grafts if they fail to heal within 3 weeks.

Genital Burns

Genital burns should be investigated for suggestion of abuse or neglect. A burned foreskin must be reduced to a normal

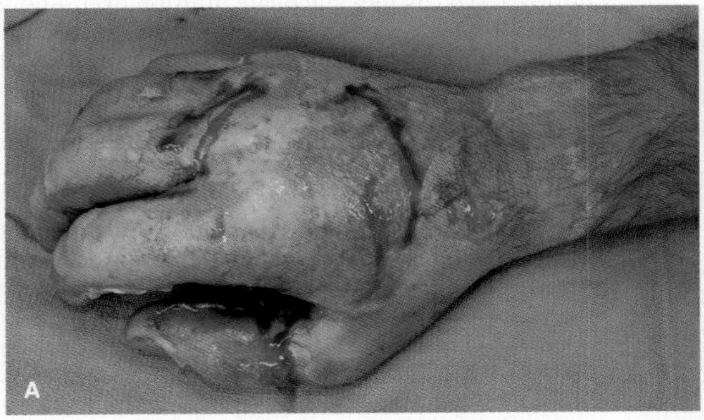

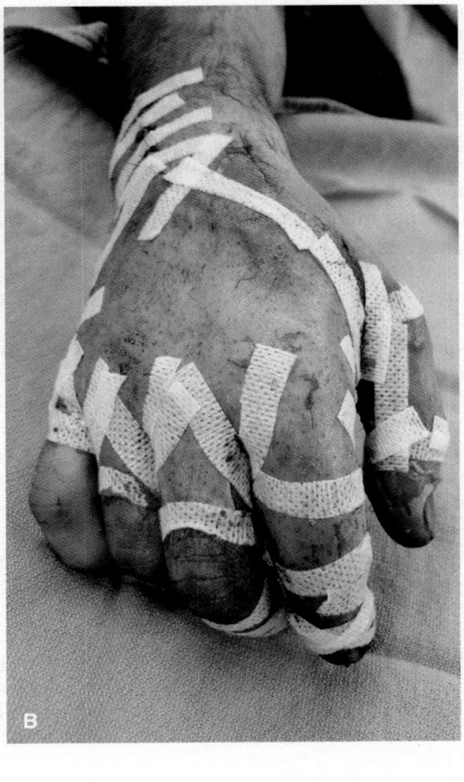

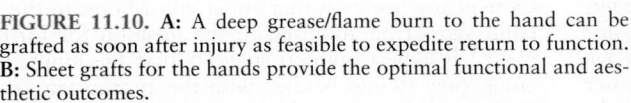

FIGURE 11.10. A: A deep grease/flame burn to the hand can be grafted as soon after injury as feasible to expedite return to function. **B:** Sheet grafts for the hands provide the optimal functional and aesthetic outcomes.

position so edema does not cause paraphimosis. Penile and scrotal burns often heal well without excision and grafting. Urethral stenting and bladder catheter drainage are not required for genital burn management and increase the risk of urinary tract infection. Bladder catheters should be removed when close monitoring of the urine output is no longer required. Likewise, diversion of the intestinal tract is not required in the management of perineal burns.

MISCELLANEOUS BURN INJURIES

Electrical Injuries

As with many areas of burn care management, electrical burns have little level 1 evidence to support treatment algorithms.[146] Electrical injuries can be grouped into three categories: high voltage, involving contact with more than 1,000 volts; low voltage, caused by contact with less than 1,000 volts; and those caused by lightning. Electrical flash burns occur when a high-voltage current arcing (jumping) from a high-tension wire toward a human being generates heat and produces a flash skin burn; this does not involve electrical current and should not be confused with an electrical injury. Low-voltage injuries may cause locally destructive injuries but rarely cause systemic sequelae. High-voltage injuries can cause local destruction at the contact wounds, a deep-tissue injury secondary to the passage of current, deep wounds where the current arcs across joints, flash burns or deep flame burns if clothing ignites, axial spine fractures due to tetanic contraction of paravertebral muscles, and other blunt injuries related to a fall. Hence, patients with high-voltage electrical burns require a complete trauma evaluation including radiographic skeletal series, cardiac monitoring, bladder catheterization to evaluate the urine for presence of myoglobinuria, and serial neurovascular exams in extremities at risk for compartment syndrome; because many electrical injuries involve the hand, carpal tunnel syndrome and impaired median nerve function deserve special immediate attention. Increased compartment pressures due to edema of the injured muscle leads to additional ischemic injury and rhabdomyolysis and warrant immediate fasciotomy; likewise, progressive loss of median nerve function suggests that a carpal tunnel release may be indicated. Surveys of trauma and burn surgeons suggest that practices vary with regard to cardiac monitoring and musculoskeletal workup; given a paucity of evidence-based data on outcomes following electrical injuries, establishing standards of care for treating this injury is challenging.

A low-voltage electrical injury especially unique to children occurs when a child puts an electrical extension cord connector into his or her mouth to pull the two plugs apart. The classic finding is a full-thickness tissue injury to the lateral mouth (Fig. 11.11) with delayed bleeding from the labial branch of the facial artery when the eschar falls off. Maintaining the oral opening is essential to prevent contracture.

Late sequelae of high-voltage electrical injuries include progressive sensory and/or motor neurologic loss and early cataract formation; these can develop within weeks to months of the injury. All patients admitted for evaluation and treatment of a high-voltage electrical injury should undergo a comprehensive neurologic and ophthalmologic examination to establish baseline status.

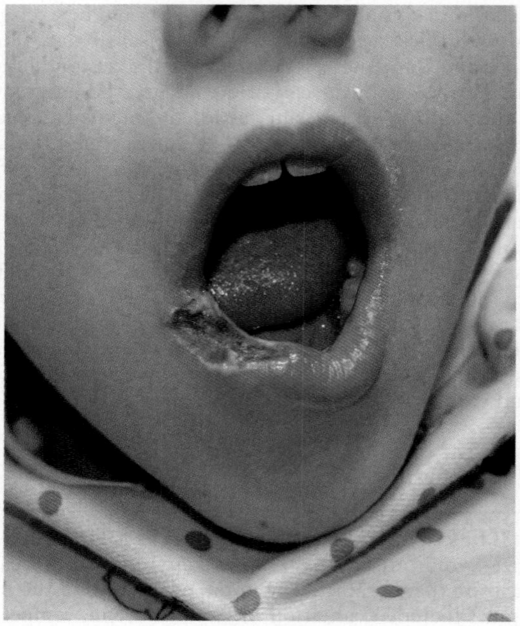

FIGURE 11.11. Full-thickness tissue destruction due to an electrical burn to the commissure of the mouth in young children can lead to oral contractures. The importance of range-of-motion exercises must be emphasized to the parents.

Chemical Injuries

Regardless of whether a chemical burn is alkali or acid, the initial treatment should be copious irrigation with tap water for 30 minutes. Cement and concrete powder or powdered lye should be brushed dry from the patient since contact with water activates the aluminum hydroxide. For eye burns, topical ophthalmic anesthetics can facilitate relief of the conjunctivitis and blepharospasm that limits affective irrigation; ophthalmologic antibiotics should be used if a fluorescent examination confirms presence of a corneal abrasion.

Hydrofluoric acid is one chemical that does have a specific antidote since exposure can induce life-threatening hypocalcemia as the fluoride binds calcium in the tissue.[147] In addition to irrigation with water, topical calcium gluconate gel can be soothing[148] but is inefficient. These burns are often located on the hands of manual workers and can be treated with slow intra-arterial calcium gluconate infusion over 4 hours.[149] This approach requires cardiac monitoring in an ICU. If the burn involves a large area and hypocalcemia persists, emergency burn wound excision may be indicated.

Tar Injuries

Tar is often heated to more than 300°F and commonly causes a deep burn, especially if the source is the "mother pot." Adherent tar can be initially cooled by tap water irrigation to limit the progression of the injury. It can be easily removed from the skin (Fig. 11.12) with a lipophilic solvent such as Medi-Sol (The Orange-sol Group of Companies, Gilbert, AZ). Once the wound is exposed, it can be treated like other thermal injuries with topical antimicrobial ointments until the need for surgery is determined.

NONACCIDENTAL BURN INJURIES

Neglect and abuse affect enough children that providers should consider these diagnoses in any child that has burns. If there is any question that either contributes to the injury, the child should be admitted to the hospital for further assessment.[9] If expert opinion suggests that the injuries are suspicious, they should be filed with the appropriate local agency. Radiographic evaluation of the head, ribs, and long bones

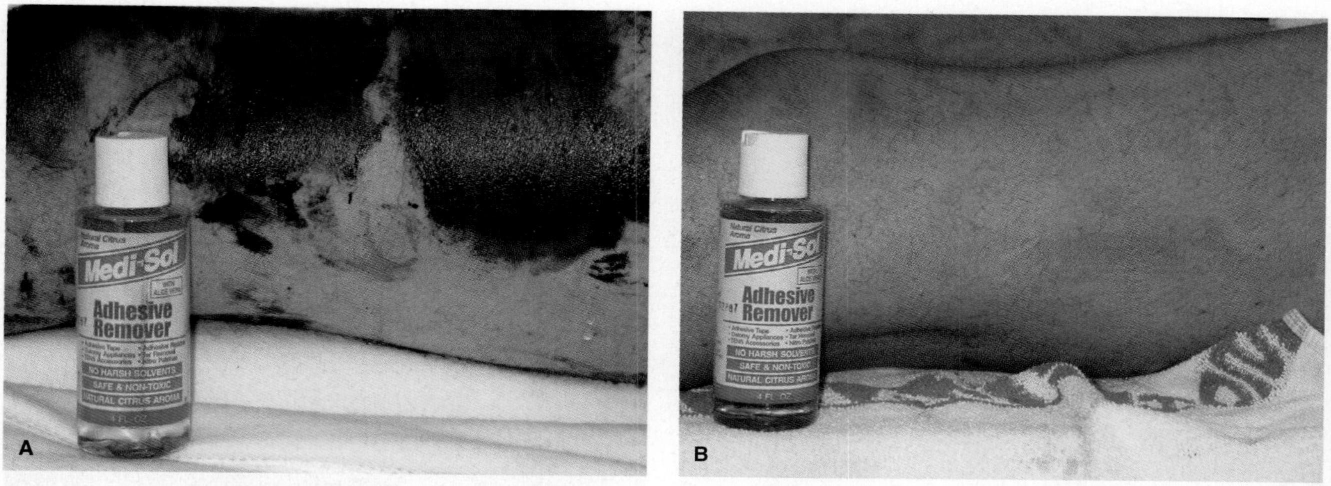

FIGURE 11.12. **A:** Congealed tar should be removed with a lipophilic solvent to determine whether there is a burn underneath. **B:** Cleaning wounds thoroughly with Medi-Sol is safe and essential for correctly determining an accurate burn size.

should be obtained for further documentation of other types of abuse; ophthalmologic evaluation should also be performed to rule out retinal detachment, often a sign of shaken baby syndrome. Too often abuse in other vulnerable populations is overlooked; learning disabled and the elderly[150] are at-risk groups and suspicious injuries should be reported to adult protective services.[151] Finally, self-mutilation should be treated cautiously. Even patients with multiple small burns such as cigarette burns should be admitted for psychological evaluation.[152]

NONBURN CONDITIONS COMMONLY CARED FOR IN BURN CENTERS

Wound care and critical care services in burn centers[153,154] lend themselves to management of other conditions with large cutaneous deficits such as purpura fulminans, toxic epidermal necrolysis, staphylococcal scalded skin syndrome, or major soft tissue avulsions.

9 Toxic epidermal necrolysis (TEN) (Fig. 11.13A), scalded skin syndrome (Fig. 11.13B), and graft versus host disease (Fig. 11.13C) are similar blistering disorders with vastly different etiologies. TEN, a variant of erythema multiforme major, involves epidermal slough at the dermal-epidermal junction. Common associations include sulfa drugs, anticonvulsants, and nonsteroidal anti-inflammatory agents, but nonspecific viral syndromes may be the only prodromic event leading to the skin loss. This condition is characterized by sloughing of all stratified squamous epithelial cell surfaces including the oral mucosa and anus. Typically, the skin between the blisters can be sheared with minimal digital pressure in a test known as a Nikolsky sign. Treatment depends on extent of skin slough. Small, scattered areas can be treated with silver-impregnated dressing or greasy gauze. When epidermal sloughing involves more than 25% TBSA, gentle débridement of the confluent areas of sloughed skin and placement of a biologic dressing such as xenograft[155] is indicated to prevent skin desiccation and superinfection (Fig. 11.13D); this approach has been associated with a 19% mortality rate,[156] which is lower than national reports of mortality after TEN. Systemic steroid treatment is associated with poorer prognosis, as are topical treatment with silver nitrate solution and total peripheral nutrition.[157] Recent suggestions that the process can be effectively limited with intravenous immunoglobulin (IVIG) treatment[158] have not been definitively demonstrated in clinical trials. Prophylactic antibiotics are associated with increased mortality. Patients with severe oropharyngeal involvement may require intubation for airway protection and early enteral tube feeding while the oral lesions heal. Daily ophthalmologic evaluation is essential to prevent synechiae forming. Likewise, daily separation of the external genitalia and vaginal lubrication are indicated to prevent painful mucosal scarring.

Differentiation between TEN and staphylococcal scalded skin syndrome can be difficult on clinical grounds, and if there is a question, a skin biopsy for histologic confirmation is warranted. Patients with scalded skin syndrome typically do not present with positive blood cultures since the staphylococcal exotoxin is responsible for the epidermal separation at the granular layer. These wounds are more superficial than TEN and usually heal quickly. Mucous membrane and conjunctiva involvement are not typical and may provide a useful differentiation between staphylococcal scalded skin syndrome and toxic epidermal necrolysis.

Empiric antistaphylococcal antibiotics should be administered, but a detailed physical examination should be performed to identify a source of infection.

Purpura fulminans is typically a complication of meningococcal or streptococcal sepsis.[159] Many patients with this condition have multiorgan failure due to the underlying septic shock coupled with the significant vasopressive agents required for cardiovascular support; ischemia affects end organs including patchy cutaneous necrosis (Fig. 11.14A), especially the digits (Fig. 11.14B). Treatment of the wounds is supportive until the patient is stable enough to undergo excision and grafting; excision or amputation may be indicated earlier if the necrotic wounds become superinfected. Amputations are common in survivors.

Necrotizing Soft Tissue Infection

10 Necrotizing fasciitis should be considered in any patient with cellulitis and a history of IV drug abuse, diabetes, obesity, vascular insufficiency, or immunosuppression. Signs and symptoms that differentiate a necrotizing infection (Fig. 11.15A) from uncomplicated cellulitis reflect the severity of illness and are summarized in Table 11.10. Delayed diagnosis and surgical treatment are associated with significantly increased mortality. If a necrotizing soft tissue infection is suspected, wider surgical débridement should be performed emergently (Fig. 11.15B). A central venous catheter should be placed for fluid

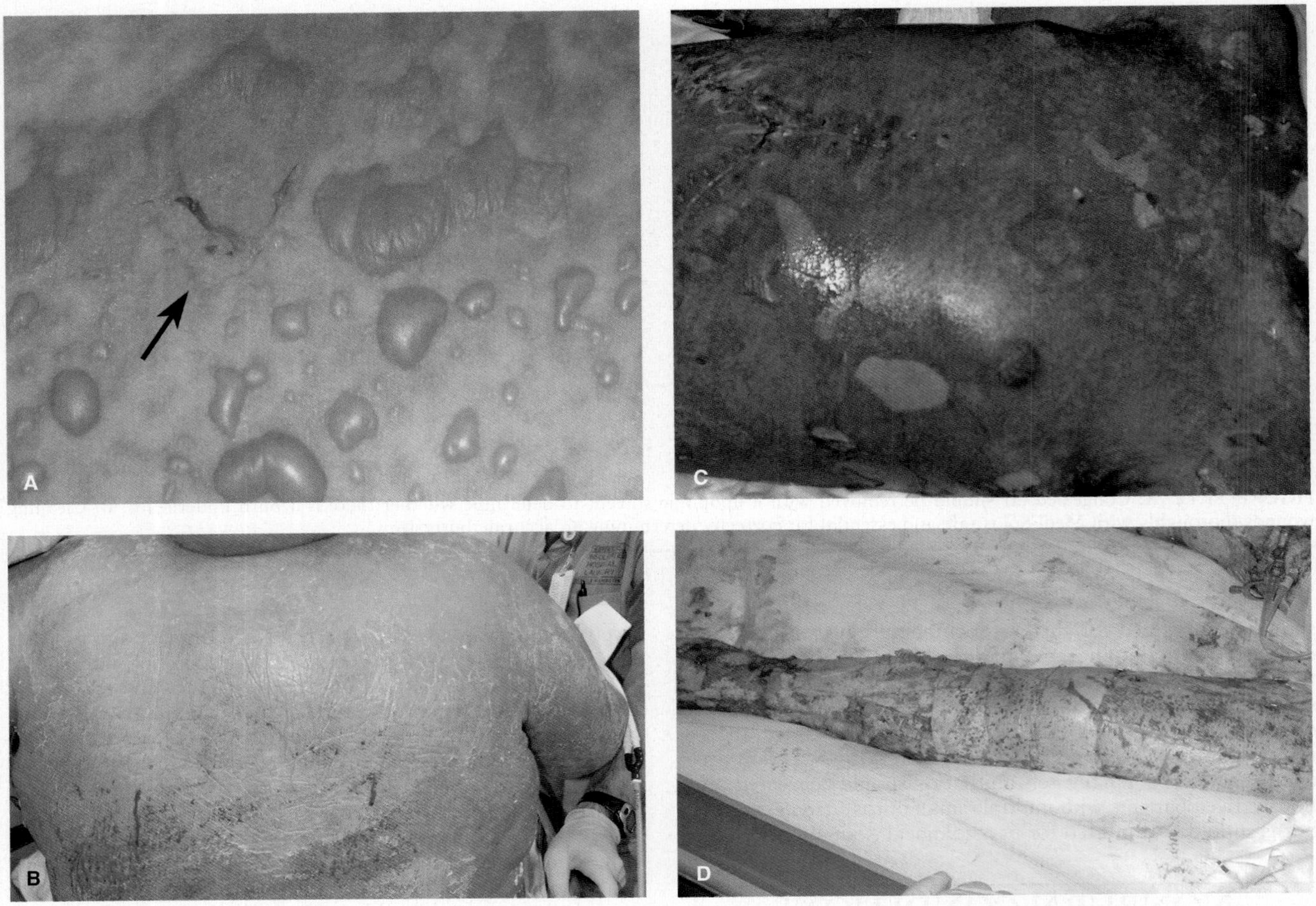

FIGURE 11.13. A: Toxic epidermal necrolysis (TEN), a severe variant of erythema multiforme major, causes distinct blisters and a characteristic Nikolsky sign (*arrow*) of normal-appearing skin sloughing between the bullae. B: Scalded skin with diffuse erythema appears more diffuse and when the skin sloughs, the underlying epidermis is often healed. C: Graft versus host disease can be confused in appearance with TEN, but history of a recent transplant (solid or hematologic) is pathognomonic. D: Removal of the sloughed skin and protection of the underlying viable wound bed by applying a biologic dressing such as xenograft improves survival in patients with TEN.

resuscitation and preoperative antibiotics penicillin (4 million units), gentamicin (7 mg/kg), and clindamycin (1,200 to 1,600 mg) should be administered. During wide débridement of necrotic tissue, an immediate Gram stain and culture swab should be obtained and reviewed. One should assume clostridia infection if there are gram-positive rods with a paucity of white blood cells and assume β-hemolytic streptococcal infection if there are abundant gram-positive cocci. Plans should be made to reexplore the wound within 24 hours of the original operation; this may be sooner if the patient undergoes clinical deterioration or if the white blood cell count increases. Broad-spectrum antibiotics should be continued

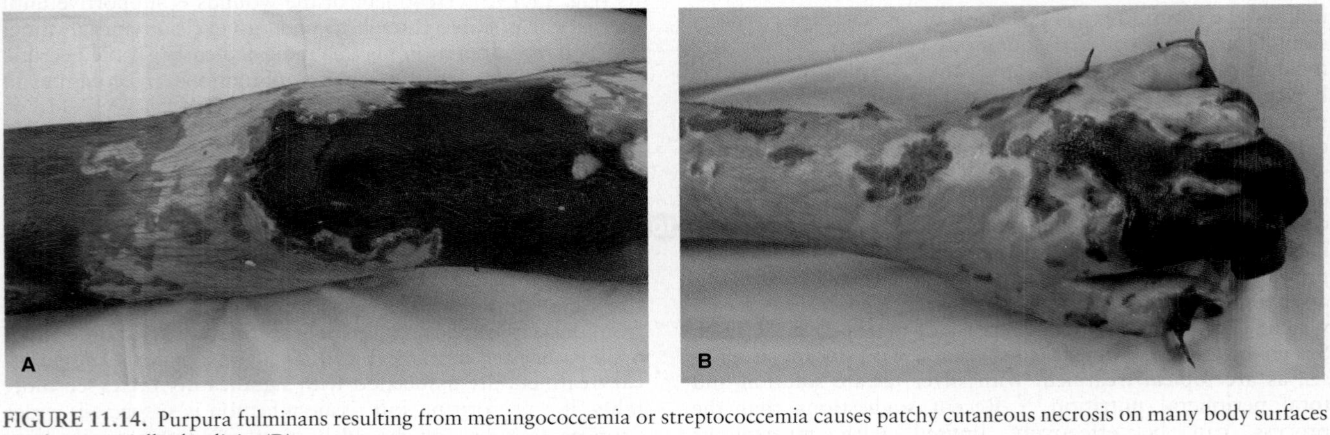

FIGURE 11.14. Purpura fulminans resulting from meningococcemia or streptococcemia causes patchy cutaneous necrosis on many body surfaces (A), but especially the digits (B).

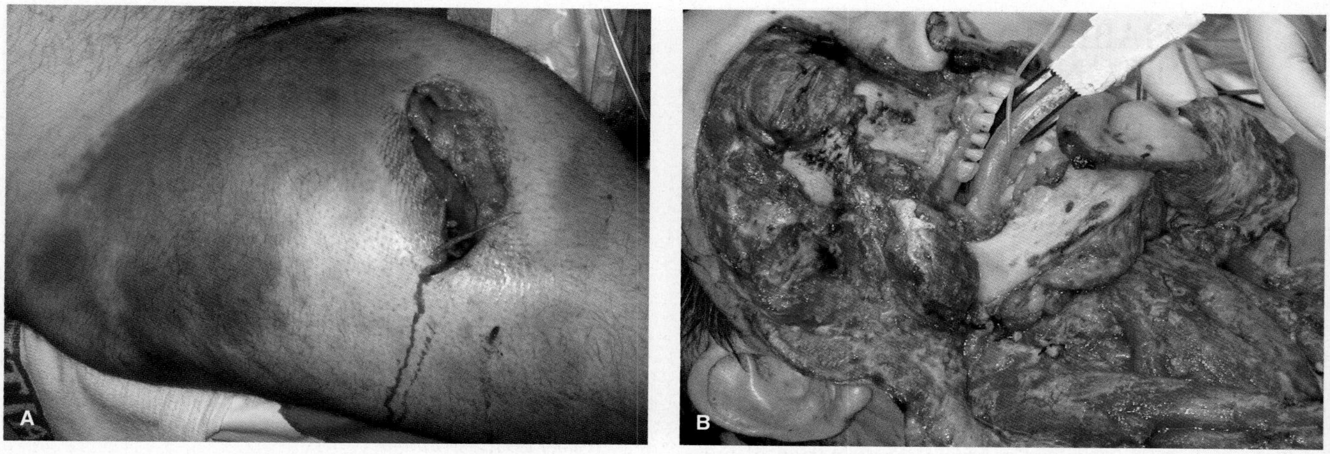

FIGURE 11.15. A: Necrotizing soft tissue infections must be differentiated from cellulitis based on systemic physiology. B: Wide surgical débridement of all involved tissues is the mainstay of treatment for this life-threatening tissue infection, even if it exposes vital structures.

until the microbiology results are final. For patients in septic shock, perioperative IVIG may be indicated to bind the toxin. Anecdotal evidence also indicates that plasmapheresis might improve outcome in septic patients.

HYPERTROPHIC SCARRING AND RECONSTRUCTIVE SURGERY

Hypertrophic scar formation is a devastating complication of burns and partial-thickness wounds (Fig. 11.16). The scars are raised, hyperemic, warm, and very pruritic, reflecting the histologic findings of increased microvessels[28] and nerves.[40,41] We know from clinical experience that hypertrophic scars form in wounds that take longer to heal, suggesting that wound depth is important. We also know that they occur in anatomic locations such as the presternal chest and central face more frequently than sites such as the forehead, scalp, and palms or soles. Hypertrophic scars are more prevalent in patients with pigmented skin, especially Asians and Hispanics. The decreased incidence in elderly patients with atrophic skin and senescent cellular responses suggests that high cellular activity may contribute to scar formation. Despite the misery associated with hypertrophic scar formation, our understanding of the pathophysiology is very limited; this basic lack of knowledge is aggravated by the absence of an animal model of scar hypertrophy. However, recent studies suggest that the female red Duroc pig generates a fibroproliferative scar[160] that parallels many clinical, histologic, and biochemical findings in human hypertrophic scar tissues.

The ability to regulate development of hypertrophic scars is limited, as is treatment for the symptoms. Custom-fit compression garments are worn within 2 weeks of wound healing and often continue until the wounds mature at 1 or 2 years after injury. Topical silicone anecdotally improves hypertrophic scar size and symptoms, but the mechanism is not clear and skin irritation and rashes can accompany use. Intradermal steroid injection has also been described but is very painful and unreliable in the management of hypertrophic scarring; furthermore, the wound size that can be treated is limited by the risk of systemic steroid effects. Patients with persistent symptomatic hypertrophic scarring that limit function or activities of daily living often require excision and primary wound closure or wound closure with sheet autografts or tissue flaps. Patients who have survived large burns may require several sequential reconstructive procedures during the first few years after injury to attain optimal cosmetic and functional results.

TABLE 11.10

SIGNS AND SYMPTOMS OF NECROTIZING SOFT TISSUE INFECTION

White blood cell count >20,000
Thin, gray drainage
Marked induration
Edema of entire limb
Hyponatremia (Na <135 mEq/L)
Skin blistering/sloughing
Skin necrosis
Crepitus/soft tissue gas on radiography
Pain out of proportion to skin findings
Sepsis (tachycardia, hypotension, high fluid requirements)

If patient meets any of these criteria, consider early surgical consultation.

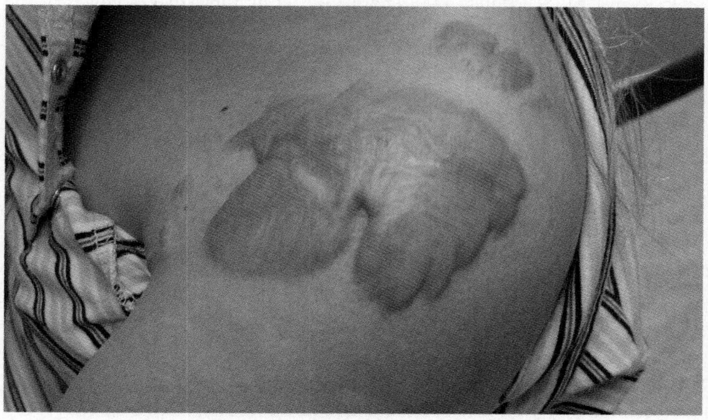

FIGURE 11.16. Hypertrophic scars in healed deep partial-thickness burns cause considerable patient discomfort and misery due to the itching, warmth, raised appearance, and often functional limitations.

REHABILITATION AND RECONSTRUCTION

As survival following major burns has improved, more emphasis has been placed on functional recovery, societal reintegration, and return to school or work. In the early 1990s, the National Institute of Disability and Rehabilitation Research (NIDRR; http://www.ed.gov/offices/osers/nidrr), whose mission is to generate, disseminate, and promote new knowledge to improve independent living options for disabled persons, recognized that burn survivors would likely benefit from organized rehabilitation model systems that had been established for survivors of traumatic brain injuries. Since then, the NIDRR has continuously funded projects to advance knowledge in burn rehabilitation by providing multicenter grants to four centers of excellence.

Physical function requires continual participation of burn occupational and physical therapists from the time of the acute injury until long after discharge from the hospital. Initially, therapists are involved with twice-daily passive or active range-of-motion exercises of all joints and positioning and splinting of the hands, extremities, or neck. In patients with small burns or in those with almost healed large injuries, therapy involves strengthening, ambulation, active and passive range of motion, performance of activities of daily living, and, in older adolescents and adults, development of work-related skills and, if necessary, development of adaptive skills with modified utensils or prosthetic devices. Therapists often provide the essential human bridge between inpatient and outpatient care.

Posttraumatic stress, anxiety, or depression frequently manifests after severe burns. Whereas burns that involve the hands or face can be anticipated to induce these symptoms, they cannot be otherwise predicted based on burn size or location. Preinjury psychiatric conditions, family dysfunction, or substance abuse further complicate psychosocial recovery. The major impact that psychological recovery has on the burn patient's ability to recover functionally underscores the need for coordinated participation of burn psychologists and social workers in the multidisciplinary care of burn patients. These staff members typically interact with the patient, family, and local outpatient support services throughout hospitalization and assist with coordinating discharge plans.

References

1. Gibran NS, Klein MB, Engrav LH, et al. UW Burn Center A model for regional delivery of burn care. *Burns* 2005;31(suppl 1):S36–S39.
2. Baux S, Mimoun M, Saade H, et al. Burns in the elderly. *Burns* 1989;15:239–240.
3. Ryan CM, Schoenfeld DA, Thorpe WP, et al. Objective estimates of the probability of death from burn injuries. *N Engl J Med* 1998;338:362–366.
4. Muangman P, Sullivan SR, Wiechman S, et al. Social support correlates with survival in patients with massive burn injury. *J Burn Care Rehabil* 2005;26:352–356.
5. Wall RJ, Engelberg RA, Downey L, et al. Refinement, scoring, and validation of the Family Satisfaction in the Intensive Care Unit (FS-ICU) survey. *Crit Care Med* 2007;35:271–279.
6. Gooding TD, Newcomb L, Mertens K. Patient-centered measurement at an academic medical center. *Jt Comm J Qual Improv* 1999;25:343–351.
7. Warden GD, Brinkerhoff C, Castellani D, et al. Multidisciplinary team approach to the pediatric burn patient. *QRB Qual Rev Bull* 1988;14:219–226.
8. Erdmann TC, Feldman KW, Rivara FP, et al. Tap water burn prevention: the effect of legislation [see comments]. *Pediatrics* 1991;88:572–577.
9. Bennett B, Gamelli R. Profile of an abused burned child. *J Burn Care Rehabil* 1998;19:88–94; discussion 87.
10. Barillo DJ, Brigham PA, Kayden DA, et al. The fire-safe cigarette: a burn prevention tool. *J Burn Care Rehabil* 2000;21:162–164; discussion 164–170.
11. Jackson D. The diagnosis of the depth of burning. *Br J Surg* 1953;40:588–596.
12. Isik S, Sahin U, Ilgan S, et al. Saving the zone of stasis in burns with recombinant tissue-type plasminogen activator (r-tPA): an experimental study in rats. *Burns* 1998;24:217–223.
13. Payan D, Levine J, Goetzl E. Modulation of immunity and hypersensitivity by sensory neuropeptides. *J Immunol* 1984;132:1601–1604.
14. Ansel JC, Kaynard AH, Armstrong CA, et al. Skin-nervous system interactions. *J Invest Dermatol* 1996;106:198–204.
15. Arturson G. Pathophysiology of the burn wound. *Ann Chir Gynaecol* 1980;69:178–190.
16. Streilein J, Tigelaar R. SALT: skin-associated lymphoid tissue. In: Daynes R, Spikes J, eds. *Experimental and Clinical Photoimmunology*. Boca Raton, FL: CRC Press; 1983:151–172.
17. Kupper TS, Deitch EA, Baker CC, et al. The human burn wound as a primary source of interleukin-1 activity. *Surgery* 1986;100:409–415.
18. Nijsten MW, Hack CE, Helle M, et al. Interleukin-6 and its relation to the humoral immune response and clinical parameters in burned patients. *Surgery* 1991;109:761–767.
19. Rennekampff HO, Hansbrough JF, Kiessig V, et al. Bioactive interleukin-8 is expressed in wounds and enhances wound healing. *J Surg Res* 2000;93:41–54.
20. Sehgal PB. Interleukin-6: molecular pathophysiology. *J Invest Dermatol* 1990;94:2S–6S.
21. Nickoloff BJ, Karabin GD, Barker JN, et al. Cellular localization of interleukin-8 and its inducer, tumor necrosis factor-alpha in psoriasis. *Am J Pathol* 1991;138:129–140.
22. Gibran NS, Ferguson M, Heimbach DM, et al. Monocyte chemoattractant protein-1 mRNA expression in the human burn wound. *J Surg Res* 1997;70:1–6.
23. Kock A, Schwarz T, Kirnbauer R, et al. Human keratinocytes are a source for tumor necrosis factor alpha: evidence for synthesis and release upon stimulation with endotoxin or ultraviolet light. *J Exp Med* 1990;172:1609–1614.
24. Rodriguez JL, Miller CG, Garner WL, et al. Correlation of the local and systemic cytokine response with clinical outcome following thermal injury. *J Trauma* 1993;34:684–694.
25. Bucky LP, Vedder NB, Hong HZ, et al. Reduction of burn injury by inhibiting CD18-mediated leukocyte adherence in rabbits. *Plast Reconstr Surg* 1994;93:1473–1480.
26. Jang YC, Arumugam S, Gibran NS, et al. Role of alpha(v) integrins and angiogenesis during wound repair. *Wound Repair Regen* 1999;7:375–380.
27. Bloch W, Huggel K, Sasaki T, et al. The angiogenesis inhibitor endostatin impairs blood vessel maturation during wound healing. *FASEB J* 2000;14:2373–2376.
28. Kischer CW, Pindur J, Krasovitch P, et al. Characteristics of granulation tissue which promote hypertrophic scarring. *Scanning Microsc* 1990;4:877–887.
29. Gabbiani G. The cellular derivation and the life span of the myofibroblast. *Pathol Res Pract* 1996;192:708–711.
30. Wu L, Pierce GF, Galiano RD, et al. Keratinocyte growth factor induces granulation tissue in ischemic dermal wounds. Importance of epithelial-mesenchymal cell interactions. *Arch Surg* 1996;131:660–666.
31. Kaplan ED, Holbrook KA. Dynamic expression patterns of tenascin, proteoglycans, and cell adhesion molecules during human hair follicle morphogenesis. *Dev Dyn* 1994;199:141–155.
32. Bohnert A, Hornung J, Mackenzie IC, et al. Epithelial-mesenchymal interactions control basement membrane production and differentiation in cultured and transplanted mouse keratinocytes. *Cell Tissue Res* 1986;244:413–429.
33. Garner WL. Epidermal regulation of dermal fibroblast activity. *Plast Reconstr Surg* 1998;102:135–139.
34. Kirsner RS, Falanga V, Eaglstein WH. The biology of skin grafts. Skin grafts as pharmacologic agents [see comments]. *Arch Dermatol* 1993;129:481–483.
35. Ashcroft GS, Horan MA, Herrick SE, et al. Age-related differences in the temporal and spatial regulation of matrix metalloproteinases (MMPs) in normal skin and acute cutaneous wounds of healthy humans. *Cell Tissue Res* 1997;290:581–591.
36. Raza SL, Cornelius LA. Matrix metalloproteinases: pro- and anti-angiogenic activities. *J Investig Dermatol Symp Proc* 2000;5:47–54.
37. Stricklin GP, Li L, Jancic V, et al. Localization of mRNAs representing collagenase and TIMP in sections of healing human burn wounds. *Am J Pathol* 1993;143:1657–1666.
38. Hembry RM, Ehrlich HP. Immunolocalization of collagenase and tissue inhibitor of metalloproteinases (TIMP) in hypertrophic scar tissue. *Br J Dermatol* 1986;115:409–420.
39. Dasu MR, Hawkins HK, Barrow RE, et al. Gene expression profiles from hypertrophic scar fibroblasts before and after IL-6 stimulation. *J Pathol* 2004;202:476–485.
40. Crowe R, Parkhouse N, McGrouther D, et al. Neuropeptide-containing nerves in painful hypertrophic human scar tissue. *Br J Dermatol* 1994;130:444–452.
41. Liang Z, Engrav LH, Muangman P, et al. Nerve quantification in female red Duroc pig (FRDP) scar compared to human hypertrophic scar. *Burns* 2004;30:57–64.
42. Santaniello JM, Luchette FA, Esposito TJ, et al. Ten year experience of burn, trauma, and combined burn/trauma injuries comparing outcomes. *J Trauma* 2004;57:696–700; discussion 700–701.
43. Afromowitz MA, Callis JB, Heimbach DM, et al. Multispectral imaging of burn wounds: a new clinical instrument for evaluating burn depth. *IEEE Trans Biomed Eng* 1988;35:842–850.
44. Heimbach D, Engrav L, Grube B, et al. Burn depth: a review. *World J Surg* 1992;16:10–15.

45. Atiles L, Mileski W, Purdue G, et al. Laser Doppler flowmetry in burn wounds. *J Burn Care Rehabil* 1995;16:388–393.
46. Rue LW III, Cioffi WG, Mason AD, et al. Improved survival of burned patients with inhalation injury. *Arch Surg* 1993;128:772–778; discussion 778–780.
47. Stassen NA, Lukan JK, Mizuguchi NN, et al. Thermal injury in the elderly: when is comfort care the right choice? *Am Surg* 2001;67:704–708.
48. Muller MJ, Pegg SP, Rule MR. Determinants of death following burn injury. *Br J Surg* 2001;88:583–587.
49. Jurkovich GJ, Moylan JA. Inhalation injury–a major burn complication. *Physician Assist* 1983;7:59–62, 65–68.
50. Heimbach DM, Waeckerle JF. Inhalation injuries. *Ann Emerg Med* 1988; 17:1316–1320.
51. Hantson P, Butera R, Clemessy JL, et al. Early complications and value of initial clinical and paraclinical observations in victims of smoke inhalation without burns. *Chest* 1997;111:671–675.
52. Hampson NB, Zmaeff JL. Outcome of patients experiencing cardiac arrest with carbon monoxide poisoning treated with hyperbaric oxygen. *Ann Emerg Med* 2001;38:36–41.
53. Hampson NB, Mathieu D, Piantadosi CA, et al. Carbon monoxide poisoning: interpretation of randomized clinical trials and unresolved treatment issues. *Undersea Hyperb Med* 2001;28:157–164.
54. Juurlink DN, Stanbrook MB, McGuigan MA. Hyperbaric oxygen for carbon monoxide poisoning. *Cochrane Database Syst Rev* 2000;(1): CD002041.
55. Grube BJ, Marvin JA, Heimbach DM. Therapeutic hyperbaric oxygen: help or hindrance in burn patients with carbon monoxide poisoning? *J Burn Care Rehabil* 1988;9:249–252.
56. Barillo DJ, Goode R, Esch V. Cyanide poisoning in victims of fire: analysis of 364 cases and review of the literature. *J Burn Care Rehabil* 1994;15: 46–57.
57. Borron SW, Baud FJ, Barriot P, et al. Prospective study of hydroxocobalamin for acute cyanide poisoning in smoke inhalation. *Ann Emerg Med* 2007;49:794–801, e1–e2.
58. Schall GL, McDonald HD, Carr LB, et al. Xenon ventilation-perfusion lung scans. The early diagnosis of inhalation injury. *JAMA* 1978;240: 2441–2445.
59. Bingham HG, Gallagher TJ, Powell MD. Early bronchoscopy as a predictor of ventilatory support for burned patients. *J Trauma* 1987;27: 1286–1288.
60. Darling GE, Keresteci MA, Ibanez D, et al. Pulmonary complications in inhalation injuries with associated cutaneous burn. *J Trauma* 1996;40: 83–89.
61. Bulger EM, Jurkovich GJ, Gentilello LM, et al. Current clinical options for the treatment and management of acute respiratory distress syndrome. *J Trauma* 2000;48:562–572.
62. Ashbaugh DG, Bigelow DB, Petty TL, et al. Acute respiratory distress in adults. *Lancet* 1967;2:319–323.
63. Hollingsed TC, Saffle JR, Barton RG, et al. Etiology and consequences of respiratory failure in thermally injured patients. *Am J Surg* 1993;166: 592–596; discussion 596–597.
64. Dancey DR, Hayes J, Gomez M, et al. ARDS in patients with thermal injury. *Intensive Care Med* 1999;25:1231–1236.
65. Tasaki O, Goodwin CW, Saitoh D, et al. Effects of burns on inhalation injury. *J Trauma* 1997;43:603–607.
66. Cancio LC, Reifenberg L, Barillo DJ, et al. Standard variables fail to identify patients who will not respond to fluid resuscitation following thermal injury: brief report. *Burns* 2005;31:358–365.
67. Pham TN, Cancio LC, Gibran NS. American Burn Association practice guidelines burn shock resuscitation. *J Burn Care Res* 2008;29:257–266.
68. Sharar SR, Heimbach DM, Green M, et al. Effects of body surface thermal injury on apparent renal and cutaneous blood flow in goats. *J Burn Care Rehabil* 1988;9:26–30.
69. Cancio LC, Chavez S, Alvarado-Ortega M, et al. Predicting increased fluid requirements during the resuscitation of thermally injured patients. *J Trauma* 2004;56:404–413; discussion 413–414.
70. Friedrich JB, Sullivan SR, Engrav LH, et al. Is supra-Baxter resuscitation in burn patients a new phenomenon? *Burns* 2004;30:464–466.
71. Klein MB, Hayden D, Elson C, et al. The association between fluid administration and outcome following major burn: a multicenter study. *Ann Surg* 2007;245:622–628.
72. Graves TA, Cioffi WG, McManus WF, et al. Fluid resuscitation of infants and children with massive thermal injury. *J Trauma* 1988;28:1656–1659.
73. Pruitt BA Jr. Protection from excessive resuscitation: "pushing the pendulum back." *J Trauma* 2000;49:567–568.
74. Greenhalgh DG, Warden GD. The importance of intra-abdominal pressure measurements in burned children. *J Trauma* 1994;36:685–690.
75. Hobson KG, Young KM, Ciraulo A, et al. Release of abdominal compartment syndrome improves survival in patients with burn injury. *J Trauma* 2002;53:1129–1133; discussion 1133–1134.
76. Sullivan SR, Ahmadi AJ, Singh CN, et al. Elevated orbital pressure: another untoward effect of massive resuscitation after burn injury. *J Trauma* 2006;60:72–76.
77. Durtschi MB, Orgain C, Counts GW, et al. A prospective study of prophylactic penicillin in acutely burned hospitalized patients. *J Trauma* 1982;22: 11–14.
78. Engrav LH, Richey KJ, Walkinshaw MD, et al. Chondritis of the burned ear: a preventable complication if. *Ann Plast Surg* 1989;23:1–2.
79. Chou TD, Gibran NS, Urdahl K, et al. Methemoglobinemia secondary to topical silver nitrate therapy–a case report. *Burns* 1999;25:549–552.
80. Jackson D, Stone P. Tangential excision and grafting of burns: the method and a report of 50 consecutive cases. *Br J Plast Surg* 1972;25:416–426.
81. Burke JF, Quinby WC, Bondoc CC. Early excision and prompt wound closure supplemented with immunosuppression. *Surg Clin North Am* 1978; 58:1141–1150.
82. Gray DT, Pine RW, Harnar TJ, et al. Early surgical excision versus conventional therapy in patients with 20 to 40 percent burns. A comparative study. *Am J Surg* 1982;144:76–80.
83. Janzekovic Z. A new concept in the early excision and immediate grafting of burns. *J Trauma* 1970;10:1103–1108.
84. Herndon DN, Barrow RE, Rutan RL, et al. A comparison of conservative versus early excision. Therapies in severely burned patients. *Ann Surg* 1989;209:547–552; discussion 552–553.
85. Merrell SW, Saffle JR, Sullivan JJ, et al. Increased survival after major thermal injury. A nine year review. *Am J Surg* 1987;154:623–627.
86. Engrav L, Heimbach D, Reus J, et al. Early excision and grafting vs. nonoperative treatment of burns of indeterminant depth: a randomized prospective study. *J Trauma* 1983;23:1001–1004.
87. Monafo W, Aulenbacher C, Pappalardo C. Early tangential excision of the eschars of major burns. *Arch Surg* 1972;104:503.
88. Gibran N, Luterman A, Herndon D, et al. Comparison of fibrin sealant and staples for attaching split-thickness autologous sheet grafts in patients with deep partial- or full-thickness burn wounds: a phase 1/2 clinical study. *J Burn Care Res* 2007;28(3):401–408.
89. Foster K, Greenhalgh D, Gamelli RL, et al. Efficacy and safety of a fibrin sealant for adherence of autologous skin grafts to burn wounds: results of a phase 3 clinical study. *J Burn Care Res* 2008;29:293–303.
90. Alexander J, MacMillan B, Law E, et al. Treatment of severe burns with widely meshed skin autograft and meshed skin allograft overlay. *J Trauma* 1981;21:433.
91. Compton CC, Gill JM, Bradford DA, et al. Skin regenerated from cultured epithelial autografts on full-thickness burn wounds from 6 days to 5 years after grafting. A light, electron microscopic and immunohistochemical study. *Lab Invest* 1989;60:600–612.
92. Boyce ST, Kagan RJ, Yakuboff KP, et al. Cultured skin substitutes reduce donor skin harvesting for closure of excised, full-thickness burns. *Ann Surg* 2002;235:269–279.
93. Boyce ST, Warden GD. Principles and practices for treatment of cutaneous wounds with cultured skin substitutes. *Am J Surg* 2002;183:445–456.
94. Heimbach D, Luterman A, Burke J, et al. Artificial dermis for major burns. A multi-center randomized clinical trial. *Ann Surg* 1988;208:313–320.
95. Heimbach DM, Warden GD, Luterman A, et al. Multicenter postapproval clinical trial of Integra dermal regeneration template for burn treatment. *J Burn Care Rehabil* 2003;24:42–48.
96. Fang P, Engrav LH, Gibran NS, et al. Dermatome setting for autografts to cover INTEGRA. *J Burn Care Rehabil* 2002;23:327–332.
97. Yannas IV, Burke JF, Orgill DP, et al. Wound tissue can utilize a polymeric template to synthesize a functional extension of skin. *Science* 1982;215: 174–176.
98. Burke JF, Yannas IV, Quinby WC Jr, et al. Successful use of a physiologically acceptable artificial skin in the treatment of extensive burn injury. *Ann Surg* 1981;194:413–428.
99. Muangman P, Deubner H, Honari S, et al. Correlation of clinical outcome of Integra application with microbiologic and pathological biopsies. *J Trauma* 2006;61:1212–1217.
100. Sheridan R, Choucair R, Donelan M, et al. Acellular allodermis in burns surgery: 1-year results of a pilot trial. *J Burn Care Rehabil* 1998;19:528–530.
101. Curreri PW, Luterman A. Nutritional support of the burned patient. *Surg Clin North Am* 1978;58:1151–1156.
102. Waxman K, Rebello T, Pinderski L, et al. Protein loss across burn wounds. *J Trauma* 1987;27:136–140.
103. Demling RH, Orgill DP. The anticatabolic and wound healing effects of the testosterone analog oxandrolone after severe burn injury. *J Crit Care* 2000;15:12–17.
104. Hart DW, Wolf SE, Mlcak R, et al. Persistence of muscle catabolism after severe burn. *Surgery* 2000;128:312–319.
105. Curreri PW, Richmond D, Marvin J, et al. Dietary requirements of patients with major burns. *J Am Diet Assoc* 1974;65:415–417.
106. Schane J, Goede M, Silverstein P. Comparison of energy expenditure measurement techniques in severely burned patients. *J Burn Care Rehabil* 1987;8:366–370.
107. Gore DC, Rutan RL, Hildreth M, et al. Comparison of resting energy expenditures and caloric intake in children with severe burns. *J Burn Care Rehabil* 1990;11:400–404.
108. Khorram-Sefat R, Behrendt W, Heiden A, et al. Long-term measurements of energy expenditure in severe burn injury. *World J Surg* 1999;23: 115–122.
109. Sheridan RL, Prelack K, Cunningham JJ. Physiologic hypoalbuminemia is well tolerated by severely burned children. *J Trauma* 1997;43: 448–452.
110. Rettmer RL, Williamson JC, Labb'e RF, et al. Laboratory monitoring of nutritional status in burn patients [see comments]. *Clin Chem* 1992;38: 334–337.
111. Manelli JC, Badetti C, Botti G, et al. A reference standard for plasma proteins is required for nutritional assessment of adult burn patients. *Burns* 1998;24:337–345.

112. Saffle JR, Larson CM, Sullivan J. A randomized trial of indirect calorimetry-based feedings in thermal injury. *J Trauma* 1990;30:776–782; discussion 782–783.
113. Liusuwan Manotok RA, Palmieri TL, Greenhalgh DG. The respiratory quotient has little value in evaluating the state of feeding in burn patients. *J Burn Care Res* 2008;29:655–659.
114. Raff T, Hartmann B, Germann G. Early intragastric feeding of seriously burned and long-term ventilated patients: a review of 55 patients. *Burns* 1997;23:19–25.
115. Esparza J, Boivin MA, Hartshorne MF, et al. Equal aspiration rates in gastrically and transpylorically fed critically ill patients. *Intensive Care Med* 2001;27:660–664.
116. Jenkins ME, Gottschlich MM, Warden GD. Enteral feeding during operative procedures in thermal injuries. *J Burn Care Rehabil* 1994;15:199–205.
117. Mayes T, Gottschlich MM, Warden GD. Nutrition intervention in pediatric patients with thermal injuries who require laparotomy. *J Burn Care Rehabil* 2000;21:451–456; discussion 450–451.
118. Van Den Berghe G, Wouters PJ, Bouillon R, et al. Outcome benefit of intensive insulin therapy in the critically ill: insulin dose versus glycemic control. *Crit Care Med* 2003;31:359–366.
119. Gore DC, Chinkes D, Heggers J, et al. Association of hyperglycemia with increased mortality after severe burn injury. *J Trauma* 2001;51:540–544.
120. Shin S, Britt RC, Reed SF, et al. Early glucose normalization does not improve outcome in the critically ill trauma population. *Am Surg* 2007;73:769–772; discussion 772.
121. Cochran A, Davis L, Morris SE, et al. Safety and efficacy of an intensive insulin protocol in a burn-trauma intensive care unit. *J Burn Care Res* 2008;29:187–191.
122. Greenhalgh DG, Housinger TA, Kagan RJ, et al. Maintenance of serum albumin levels in pediatric burn patients: a prospective, randomized trial. *J Trauma* 1995;39:67–73; discussion 73–74.
123. Saffle J, Wiebke G, Jennings K, et al. Randomized trial of immune-enhancing enteral nutrition in burn patients. *J Trauma* 1997;42:793–800; discussion 800–802.
124. Garrel D, Patenaude J, Nedelec B, et al. Decreased mortality and infectious morbidity in adult burn patients given enteral glutamine supplements: a prospective, controlled, randomized clinical trial. *Crit Care Med* 2003;31:2444–2449.
125. Herndon DN. Nutritional and pharmacological support of the metabolic response to injury. *Minerva Anestesiol* 2003;69:264–274.
126. Demling RH, DeSanti L. Oxandrolone induced lean mass gain during recovery from severe burns is maintained after discontinuation of the anabolic steroid. *Burns* 2003;29:793–797.
127. Nathens AB, Neff MJ, Jurkovich GJ, et al. Randomized, prospective trial of antioxidant supplementation in critically ill surgical patients. *Ann Surg* 2002;236:814–822.
128. Jeschke MG, Norbury WB, Finnerty CC, et al. Propranolol does not increase inflammation, sepsis, or infectious episodes in severely burned children. *J Trauma* 2007;62:676–681.
129. Karyoute SM, Badran IZ. Tetanus following a burn injury. *Burns Incl Therm Inj* 1988;14:241–243.
130. Horvath EE, Murray CK, Vaughan GM, et al. Fungal wound infection (not colonization) is independently associated with mortality in burn patients. *Ann Surg* 2007;245:978–985.
131. Wahl WL, Brandt MM, Ahrns KS, et al. Venous thrombosis incidence in burn patients: preliminary results of a prospective study. *J Burn Care Rehabil* 2002;23:97–102.
132. Rue LW 3rd, Cioffi WG Jr, Rush R, et al. Thromboembolic complications in thermally injured patients. *World J Surg* 1992;16:1151–1154; discussion 1155.
133. Still JM Jr, Belcher K, Law EJ, et al. A double-blinded prospective evaluation of recombinant human erythropoietin in acutely burned patients. *J Trauma* 1995;38:233–236.
134. Harrington DT, Mozingo DW, Cancio L, et al. Thermally injured patients are at significant risk for thromboembolic complications. *J Trauma* 2001;50:495–499.
135. Sharar SR, Carrougher GJ, Selzer K, et al. A comparison of oral transmucosal fentanyl citrate and oral oxycodone for pediatric outpatient wound care. *J Burn Care Rehabil* 2002;23:27–31.
136. Honari S, Patterson DR, Gibbons J, et al. Comparison of pain control medication in three age groups of elderly patients. *J Burn Care Rehabil* 1997;18:500–504.
137. Martin-Herz SP, Patterson DR, Honari S, et al. Pediatric pain control practices of North American burn centers. *J Burn Care Rehabil* 2003;24:26–36.
138. Carrougher GJ, Ptacek JT, Honari S, et al. Self-reports of anxiety in burn-injured hospitalized adults during routine wound care. *J Burn Care Res* 2006;27:676–681.
139. Ohrbach R, Patterson DR, Carrougher G, et al. Hypnosis after an adverse response to opioids in an ICU burn patient. *Clin J Pain* 1998;14:167–175.
140. Groene D, Martus P, Heyer G. Doxepin affects acetylcholine induced cutaneous reactions in atopic eczema. *Exp Dermatol* 2001;10:110–117.
141. Hoffman HG, Patterson DR, Seibel E, et al. Virtual reality pain control during burn wound debridement in the hydrotank. *Clin J Pain* 2008;24:299–304.
142. Klein MB, Moore ML, Costa B, et al. Primer on the management of face burns at the University of Washington. *J Burn Care Rehabil* 2005;26:2–6.
143. Cole JK, Engrav LH, Heimbach DM, et al. Early excision and grafting of face and neck burns in patients over 20 years. *Plast Reconstr Surg* 2002;109:1266–1273.
144. Mills DCd, Roberts LW, Mason ADJ, et al. Suppurative chondritis: its incidence, prevention, and treatment in burn patients. *Plast Reconstr Surg* 1988;82:267–276.
145. Matsumura H, Engrav LH, Nakamura DY, et al. The use of the Millard "crane" flap for deep hand burns with exposed tendons and joints. *J Burn Care Rehabil* 1999;20:316–319.
146. Arnoldo B, Klein M, Gibran NS. Practice guidelines for the management of electrical injuries. *J Burn Care Res* 2006;27:439–447.
147. Caravati EM. Acute hydrofluoric acid exposure. *Am J Emerg Med* 1988;6:143–150.
148. Chick LR, Borah G. Calcium carbonate gel therapy for hydrofluoric acid burns of the hand. *Plast Reconstr Surg* 1990;86:935–940.
149. Vance MV, Curry SC, Kunkel DB, et al. Digital hydrofluoric acid burns: treatment with intraarterial calcium infusion. *Ann Emerg Med* 1986;15:890–896.
150. Bird PE, Harrington DT, Barillo DJ, et al. Elder abuse: a call to action. *J Burn Care Rehabil* 1998;19:522–527.
151. Bowden ML, Grant ST, Vogel B, et al. The elderly, disabled and handicapped adult burned through abuse and neglect. *Burns Incl Therm Inj* 1988;14:447–450.
152. Assin WD. Multiple cigarette burn wounds in a chronic paranoid schizophrenic. *S Afr Med J* 1996;86:1437.
153. Barillo DJ, Hallock GG, Mastropieri CJ, et al. Utilization of the burn unit for nonburn patients: the "wound intensive care unit." *Ann Plast Surg* 1989;23:426–429.
154. Barillo DJ, McManus AT, Cancio LC, et al. Burn center management of necrotizing fasciitis. *J Burn Care Rehabil* 2003;24:127–132.
155. Marvin JA, Heimbach DM, Engrav LH, et al. Improved treatment of the Stevens-Johnson syndrome. *Arch Surg* 1984;119:601–605.
156. Imahara SD, Holmes JHT, Heimbach DM, et al. SCORTEN overestimates mortality in the setting of a standardized treatment protocol. *J Burn Care Res* 2006;27:270–275.
157. Palmieri TL, Greenhalgh DG, Saffle JR, et al. A multicenter review of toxic epidermal necrolysis treated in U.S. burn centers at the end of the twentieth century. *J Burn Care Rehabil* 2002;23:87–96.
158. Viard I, Wehrli P, Bullani R, et al. Inhibition of toxic epidermal necrolysis by blockade of CD95 with human intravenous immunoglobulin. *Science* 1998;282:490–493.
159. Warner PM, Kagan RJ, Yakuboff KP, et al. Current management of purpura fulminans: a multicenter study. *J Burn Care Rehabil* 2003;24: 119–126.
160. Zhu KQ, Engrav LH, Gibran NS, et al. The female, red Duroc pig as an animal model of hypertrophic scarring and the potential role of the cones of skin. *Burns* 2003;29:649–664.

CHAPTER 12 ■ ANESTHESIOLOGY AND PAIN MANAGEMENT

SACHIN KHETERPAL, TIMOTHY W. RUTTER, AND KEVIN K. TREMPER

SCIENTIFIC PRINCIPLES

KEY POINTS

1. Anesthetics are generalized depressants of consciousness, pain, cardiopulmonary function, motor function, and recall.
2. To prevent movement and to facilitate the surgical exposure, neuromuscular blocking agents are generally used. These drugs are competitive or noncompetitive inhibitors of the neurotransmitter acetylcholine at the neuromuscular junction.
3. Opioids produce profound analgesia and respiratory depression. They have no amnesic properties, minimal direct myocardial depressive effects, and no muscle-relaxant properties.
4. Propofol is unique because it is rapidly cleared through hepatic metabolism to inactive metabolites in a way that the patient becomes alert soon after cessation of the infusion. However, as the duration and dose of the maintenance infusion is increased, the time to return of consciousness is also significantly increased.
5. Peripheral nerve blockade can be used in lieu of general anesthesia to provide surgical anesthesia or as a postoperative pain management technique. Use of long-acting local anesthetics or placement of an indwelling continuous catheter provides long-term (16 hours to several days) pain relief.
6. The concept of airway management should be focused on not just endotracheal intubation, but also mask ventilation. Until the airway can be secured via intubation, the patient must be supported through mask ventilation. The key elements of an airway examination are an assessment of obesity, mouth opening, neck flexion and extension, Mallampati oropharyngeal classification, presence of beard, and mandibular protrusion ability.
7. Hypertension is the most common preexisting medical disease in patients presenting for surgery and is a major risk factor for renal, cerebrovascular, peripheral vascular, and coronary artery diseases as well as for congestive heart failure.
8. The appropriate duration to defer elective surgery after coronary stenting remains controversial, but recent guidelines from the American College of Cardiology/American Heart Association recommend 12 months for drug-eluting stents and 6 weeks for bare-metal stents. The role for antiplatelet therapy remains a major question, but data suggest that cessation of recommended antiplatelet therapy in the perioperative period may have significant coronary thrombotic risks without major improvement in bleeding adverse events.
9. The three goals of the preoperative evaluation are (a) to develop an anesthetic plan that considers the patient's medical condition, the requirements of the surgical procedure, and the patient's preferences; (b) to ensure that the patient's chronic disease is under appropriate medical therapy before an elective procedure; and (c) to gain rapport with and the confidence of the patient, answer any questions, and allay fears.
10. Patients receiving chronic pain or opioid addiction therapy with buprenorphine (Subutex, Suboxone) can be particularly challenging to manage in the postoperative period and should be immediately referred to their primary care physician and an anesthesiologist to create a pain management plan prior to the day of surgery. Buprenorphine is mixed opioid agonist/antagonist that tightly binds at the μ receptor and has a long and varied half-life (24 to 60 hours). It can inhibit the analgesic benefits of traditional opioids in the postoperative period, resulting in uncontrolled pain, decreased patient satisfaction, and the potential for adverse events due to the need for very high doses of opioids.
11. As positive-pressure ventilation impedes venous return within a closed thorax, decreases in systolic pressure associated with a respiratory pattern can be detected. In patients with sinus rhythm with stable cardiac contractility, the degree of systolic pressure variation (SPV) reflects the intravascular volume status of the patient. The normal range of SPV is 5 to 10 mm Hg.
12. Postoperative acute pain management may require a multimodal approach that incorporates opioids, peripheral nerve blockade, and nonopioid analgesics. Chronic pain patients can be particularly difficult to manage and may require preoperative optimization by an anesthesiologist.

The "state of general anesthesia" is a combination of hypnosis, amnesia, analgesia, and muscle relaxation. This state can be achieved by administration of single or multiple anesthetic agents via inhalational or intravenous routes. Historically, anesthesia was achieved by inhaling volatile anesthetic vapors that produced each of these conditions in proportion to the concentration achieved in the central nervous system. Anesthesia can also be achieved by using a balance of multiple pharmacologic agents, each targeted to produce a specific effect. These are the hypnotic/sedatives, analgesics, and neuromuscular blocking agents. As the concentration of hypnotic/sedative and analgesic agents increases, cardiovascular and respiratory functions may be progressively blunted. For this reason, modern anesthetics usually require titration of these agents to optimize conditions for the surgery while maintaining cardiovascular stability.

The goals of modern anesthesia are (a) to create a reversible anesthetic state quickly and safely by choosing the appropriate techniques and agents considering the patient's medical condition, (b) to maintain this state throughout the surgical procedure while compensating for the effects of varying degrees of painful stimuli and fluid loss, and (c) to reverse the muscle relaxation and hypnosis, bringing the patient back to a homeostatic state while maintaining sufficient analgesia to minimize postoperative pain. This process is accomplished with a high degree of safety 30 to 40 million times a year in the United States, despite the serious potential complications of technical or judgment errors. The high degree of success of both surgical and anesthetic outcomes is due to the efforts of thousands of surgeons and anesthesiologists who have advanced the art and science of their field.[1] Although modern surgical techniques, regional or neuraxial blockade procedures, and systemic analgesics have made it possible to ameliorate perioperative pain, significant challenges in postoperative pain management remain. Pain not only is unpleasant, but it also has significant adverse physiologic effects and physicians should encourage patients to alert health care personnel when pain is felt.

ANESTHETIC AGENTS AND THEIR PHYSIOLOGIC EFFECTS

Inhalation Agents

1 Anesthetics are generalized depressants of consciousness, pain, cardiopulmonary function, motor function, and recall. The potent inhalation agents (e.g., isoflurane, sevoflurane, desflurane) produce these effects in a dose-dependent fashion. The measurement used to compare the potency of inhalation agents is the minimum alveolar concentration (MAC), an empirically derived number defined as the expired percent concentration required to prevent movement on painful stimulation (incision) in half of experimental subjects. There is significant patient-to-patient variability independent of underlying comorbidities. Compounding this variability are the effects of age, weight, preexisting heart disease, liver disease, and medications other than the inhalational anesthetic. Table 12.1 lists the commonly used inhalation agents and their MACs and side effects. In general, all agents depress blood pressure by myocardial depression and vasodilation, resulting in system hypotension. There is a generalized depression of cerebral function and cerebral metabolic rate of oxygen consumption, although cerebral blood flow may increase because of cerebrovascular dilatation and a loss of coupling. Renal blood flow and glomerular filtration rate are reduced by 20% to 50%. The body's normally tight regulation of core body temperature is lost, resulting in a redistribution of heat from the core to the periphery. The combination of these effects, the cold environment of the operating room, and open body cavities make the patient extremely vulnerable to hypothermia (core body temperature <36°C).

Intravenous Sedatives/Hypnotics

Several commonly used intravenous sedative/hypnotic medications can also be used in lieu of an inhalational anesthetic to achieve the hypnotic component of the state of anesthesia. A constant intravenous infusion of these medications is used to achieve and maintain a blood concentration that results in the loss of consciousness and prevents recall. Unlike the inhalational agents, there currently is no ability to measure the patient's expired or blood concentration of these intravenous agents. As a result, the infusion rate is titrated to effect by observing patient movement (if muscle relaxants are not used concurrently) and hemodynamic responses to procedural stimuli. Of note, the sedative/hypnotic intravenous agents do not possess clinically useful muscle relaxant or analgesic properties and must be combined with other agents to deliver a "balanced" anesthetic. The most commonly used intravenous agent for maintenance of anesthesia is propofol, a lipid-soluble substituted isopropyl phenol that produces hypnosis and sedation through interactions with γ-aminobutyric acid (GABA), the

TABLE 12.1

COMMON INHALATION AGENTS: MINIMUM ALVEOLAR CONCENTRATIONS AND EFFECTS

AGENT	MINIMUM ALVEOLAR CONCENTRATION (%)	STRENGTHS	WEAKNESSES
Nitrous oxide	105	Analgesia Rapid uptake and elimination Little cardiac or respiratory depression	Sympathetic stimulation Expansion of closed air spaces Interference with vitamin B_{12} metabolism Limitation of FiO_2
Isoflurane	1.15	Good muscle relaxation Stable cardiac rate and rhythm Usability in neurosurgery	Pungent odor
Desflurane	6	Rapid induction and emergence	Pungent odor Causes coughing High vapor pressure (Boiling point 23.5°C) Requires special pressurized vaporizer High cost
Sevoflurane	1.71	Rapid induction and emergence Less pungent Good for mask induction	Moderate cost Metabolized in liver and produces increased plasma fluoride Canister fires with Baralyme

FiO_2, fraction of inspired oxygen.
Adapted from Miller FL, Marshall BE. The inhaled anesthetics. In: Longnecker DE, Murphy FL, eds. *Introduction to Anesthesia,* 8th ed. Philadelphia, PA: WB Saunders; 1992:77.

primary inhibitory neurotransmitter of the central nervous system. When administered as a continuous infusion, propofol can achieve minimal levels of sedation, deep sedation, or general anesthesia. Additional details regarding the use and side effects of propofol are discussed later. Other classic agents such as benzodiazepines can also be used as maintenance infusions, but do not enable the rapid return to consciousness that propofol offers. A novel, highly specific α_2-receptor agonist, dexmedetomidine, has recently demonstrated an exciting role as an intravenous sedative/hypnotic that also has analgesic effects. In the perioperative setting, it is currently limited to use as an adjunct to propofol and inhalational anesthetics.

Muscle Relaxants

2 To prevent movement and to facilitate the surgical exposure, neuromuscular blocking agents are generally used. These drugs are competitive or noncompetitive inhibitors of the neurotransmitter acetylcholine at the neuromuscular junction. The only noncompetitive inhibitor used clinically is succinylcholine. This drug rapidly binds to the nicotinic receptors and produces depolarization at the neuromuscular junction, clinically obvious as fine muscle fasciculations occurring about 60 seconds after injection. Succinylcholine cannot be reversed, but has a short duration of action (<10 minutes) because it is quickly hydrolyzed in the plasma by cholinesterase. Because of rapid onset, succinylcholine is frequently used to facilitate endotracheal intubation when it must be accomplished quickly.

All other clinically useful muscle relaxants are termed *competitive inhibitors* and do not cause depolarization when they attach at the neuromuscular junction. Because these agents compete with acetylcholine, the block produced is in direct proportion to the concentration of the agent relative to the concentration of acetylcholine. If the concentration ratio is low enough, competitive relaxants can be reversed if the concentration of acetylcholine is artificially elevated. Acetylcholine concentration can be increased by giving a drug that blocks its metabolism, an anticholinesterase (e.g., neostigmine). The neuromuscular blocking agent is still present, but motor function returns if the acetylcholine concentration is high enough to overwhelm the blocking agent. There is a ceiling to which anticholinesterase drugs can safely elevate circulating acetylcholine; therefore, high levels of nondepolarizing relaxants cannot be reversed. Reversing neuromuscular relaxants is not analogous to using naloxone to reverse the effects of opioids. The reversal agent neostigmine does not compete or combine with the relaxant.

Unfortunately, there are systemic consequences to increasing the plasma concentration of acetylcholine. Acetylcholine is the predominant neurotransmitter in the preganglionic sympathetic and parasympathetic nervous systems and in the postganglionic parasympathetic nervous system. For this reason, an anticholinergic drug (atropine or glycopyrrolate) must be given with the anticholinesterase to prevent the undesirable effects of a generalized acetylcholine overdose. The common neuromuscular blocking drugs and their doses, durations, and side effects are listed in Table 12.2; common regimens of reversal agents are shown in Table 12.3.

A novel class of compounds, known as *selective relaxant binding agents,* is currently under phase III clinical trials. They are able to rapidly reverse the effects of profound levels of muscle relaxation created by steroidal muscle relaxant agents such as rocuronium, vecuronium, or pancuronium. Rather than attempting to increase the concentration of acetylcholine, these agents actually bind free muscle relaxant molecules within its cyclodextrin ring structure. This decreases the concentration of free muscle relaxant and allows acetylcholine to function normally at the neuromuscular junction. The cyclodextrin–muscle relaxant combination is then eliminated via the kidney. The first cyclodextrin used for this purpose, known as sugammadex, is being reviewed by the U.S. Food

TABLE 12.2

COMMON NEUROMUSCULAR BLOCKING DRUGS AND REVERSAL AGENTS

MUSCLE RELAXANT	INTUBATING DOSE (mg/kg)	INFUSION DOSE (mg/kg/min)	STRENGTHS	WEAKNESSES
DEPOLARIZING				
Succinylcholine	1.0	100[a]	Fastest onset (30 to 60 s) Short duration[b] (5 min)	Associated with malignant hyperthermia, dysrhythmias, bradycardia, and hyperkalemia, especially in patients with burns or neurologic injury
NONDEPOLARIZING				
Long acting (>1 h)				
Pancuronium	0.1	0.3	No histamine release	Tachycardia Slow onset Long duration
Intermediate acting (≈1 h)				
Cisatracurium	0.2	0.1	Spontaneous degradation, not affected by renal or liver disease	Moderate cost
Vecuronium	0.1	1	No cardiovascular effects	
Rocuronium	0.8	10	Fast onset, no cardiovascular effects	

[a]This should not be used for longer than 1 h.
[b]Duration is dramatically increased in patients with abnormal plasma pseudocholinesterase.

TABLE 12.3

DRUGS FOR ANTAGONIZING NONDEPOLARIZING NEUROMUSCULAR BLOCKADE[a]

■ DOSE	■ TIME TO PEAK EFFECT (min)	■ DOSE	■ USE WITH	■ COMMENTS
ANTICHOLINESTERASES				
Edrophonium	1–2	0.5–1.0 mg/kg	—	Very fast onset, not commonly used
Neostigmine	3–5	0.04–0.07 mg/kg	—	Most commonly used
Pyridostigmine	10–12	0.2–0.3 mg/kg	—	Not used clinically for neuromuscular reversal
ANTICHOLINERGICS				
Glycopyrrolate	—	0.008 mg/kg (0.5–0.6 mg/70 kg)	Neostigmine Pyridostigmine	Not commonly used in adults
Atropine	—	0.007–0.02 mg/kg (0.05–1.5 mg/70 kg)	Edrophonium	CNS effects because it crosses the blood–brain barrier

CNS, central nervous system.
[a]For reliable results in reversing the effects of nondepolarizing muscle relaxants, administration of anticholinesterases is delayed until spontaneous recovery permits three of four responses to a train-of-four stimulus. For patients with more profound blockade, larger amounts of anticholinesterases may be required, but doses of neostigmine higher than 0.14 mg/kg are unlikely to produce additional improvement.
Adapted from Watling SM, Dasta JF. Prolonged paralysis in intensive care unit patients after the use of neuromuscular blocking agents: a review of the literature. *Crit Care Med* 1994;22:884.

and Drug Administration (FDA) and European Union for clinical use.[2] These drugs could revolutionalize the practice of anesthesiology by enabling the rapid (<3 minutes) reversal of profound muscle relaxation as surgical conditions warrant.

Nondepolarizing relaxants are occasionally used in critically ill patients who are difficult to manage. For example, neuromuscular blockade can facilitate ventilation of patients with adult respiratory distress syndrome who require complex modes of ventilation. It is imperative that these drugs be given in conjunction with analgesics and amnesic agents. Neuromuscular blocking agents have no analgesic or amnesic properties and only prevent motion of voluntary muscles. Patients can be totally aware and in pain but unable to communicate. When prolonged muscle relaxation is required, it is best to administer the relaxant by continuous infusion and then monitor the effect with a nerve stimulator. For these settings, relaxants should be administered only to achieve the degree of relaxation necessary and in a dose that allows reversal at any time. Table 12.2 includes the recommended ranges of infusion rates. In recent years, there have been reports of patients who have prolonged residual motor weakness after the muscle relaxant is cleared.[3] These problems have been primarily noted with the drug pancuronium, especially when the patients are also being treated with steroids.

All muscles in the body are not equally sensitive to muscle relaxants. The diaphragm is most resistant to neuromuscular blockade, whereas the neck and pharyngeal muscles that support the airway are most sensitive. It is possible for an intubated patient to spontaneously ventilate and even to produce a large negative inspiratory effort and yet develop complete airway obstruction when extubated because of the effects of residual muscle relaxant on the upper airway muscles. The definitive clinical test for complete reversal of neuromuscular blockage is the patient's ability to sustain a head lift from the bed for 5 seconds.

Opioids (Narcotics) and Other Intravenous Analgesics

Narcotics and synthetic analogues belong to the class of drugs called *opioids*. The most commonly used drugs in this family are morphine, fentanyl, and codeine. Since the mid-1980s, a series of synthetic opioids have been developed with fentanyl as the prototype. More recently developed synthetics (sufentanil, alfentanil, and remifentanil) are more potent and of 3 varying duration (Table 12.4). Opioids produce profound analgesia and respiratory depression. They have no amnesic properties, minimal direct myocardial depressive effects, and no muscle-relaxant properties. Opioids can produce significant hemodynamic effects indirectly by releasing histamine or blunting the patient's sympathetic vascular tone because of analgesic properties. The latter effect depends on the degree of sympathetic tone that is present at baseline. Acutely injured patients may be hypovolemic and in pain, with high sympathetic tone and peripheral vascular resistance. Patients in this condition can experience dramatic drops in systemic blood pressure with minimal doses of opioids. For this reason, it is important to titrate narcotics in small incremental doses. Because of the lack of direct myocardial depression and the absence of histamine release with the synthetic opioids, they are frequently used as the primary anesthetic in combination with an amnesic agent and a muscle relaxant in patients with significant myocardial dysfunction.

When opioids are titrated intravenously, patients first become apneic because of the respiratory depressive effect (shifting the CO_2 response curve), but they still breathe on command. As the dose increases, patients become apneic and unresponsive. An unusual side effect of high-dose intravenous (IV) opioids is chest-wall muscle rigidity, which can make it extremely difficult to ventilate a patient without the assistance of a muscle relaxant.

Opioids are primarily analgesic and not amnesic. Patients can be totally aware and have substantial recall of conversations despite appearing completely anesthetized. All opioids can be reversed with naloxone. The duration of action of naloxone can be shorter than that of the opioid, and patients must be observed carefully after they have been treated with naloxone. Naloxone reversal of opioids can be dangerous because the agent acutely reverses not only the analgesic effects of the opioid but also the analgesic effects of native endorphins. Naloxone treatment has been associated with acute pulmonary edema and myocardial ischemia and should not be used electively to reverse the effects of a narcotic. It is

TABLE 12.4

ANALGESICS

	POTENCY	SEDATION DOSE	DURATION	INFUSION DOSE
OPIOIDS				
Morphine	1	0.02–0.1 mg/kg IV	2–7 h	—
Fentanyl	100	0.5–1 mg/kg IV	30–60 min	—
Sufentanil	1,000	Not recommended		
Alfentanil	25	10–20 mg/kg IV	10–15 min	
Remifentanil[b]	—	Not recommended	10 min	0.1–0.2 mg/kg/min
OTHER ANALGESICS AND ANESTHETICS				
Propofol		0.1–0.5 mg/kg IV[a,c]		25–50 mg/kg/min =
Ketamine		0.1–0.5 mg/kg IV[a] 1.0–2.0 mg/kg IM		80 mg/kg/min

IM, intramuscular; IV, intravenous.
[a]May produce apnea.
[b]Will produce apnea.
[c]Produces pain on injection that can be reduced by treatment with 20 mg of lidocaine IV.

appropriately used in an emergency situation when the airway is poorly controlled and the patient is not ventilating because of an opioid overdose.

Propofol

Propofol is a lipid-soluble substituted isopropyl phenol that produces a rapid induction of anesthesia in 30 seconds followed by awakening in 4 to 8 minutes after a single bolus. Intravenous propofol can effectively produce total anesthesia (for less stimulating procedures), including amnesia, some
4 analgesia, and some degree of muscle relaxation. Propofol is unique because it is rapidly cleared through hepatic metabolism to inactive metabolites in a way that the patient becomes alert soon after cessation of the infusion. However, as the duration and dose of the maintenance infusion is increased, the time to return of consciousness is also significantly increased. This context-sensitive half-life of propofol must be incorporated into expectations of a "quick wake-up." Propofol has direct antiemetic properties and is a valid alternative to inhalational anesthetics in patients who have demonstrated a history of prolonged, refractory postoperative nausea and vomiting. It has an important role in intensive care units when used as a continuous infusion sedative at dosages of 25 to 50 μg/kg/min. However, prolonged infusions have been associated with a lethal metabolic derangement known as propofol infusion syndrome, characterized by a profound metabolic acidosis and cardiovascular compromise.[4] Propofol can produce significant hypotension when IV induction doses are administered. It also produces significant pain on injection in peripheral veins. Pain can be diminished or eliminated by pretreatment with IV lidocaine via the vein to be used for propofol administration. Propofol is insoluble in aqueous solution and therefore comes dissolved in a lipid emulsion that has the associated risk of bacterial contamination. Once a vial of propofol is opened, it is not recommended that it be used after 6 hours.

Ketamine

Ketamine is a phencyclidine derivative that produces anesthesia characterized by dissociation between the thalamus and limbic systems. Induction of anesthesia is achieved within 60 seconds after IV injection of 1 to 2 mg/kg or within 2 to 4 minutes of intramuscular (IM) injection of 5 to 10 mg/kg. Patients appear to be in a cataleptic state in which their eyes remain open with a slow nystagmic gaze. The drug produces intense amnesia and analgesia but has been associated with unpleasant visual and auditory hallucinations that can progress to delirium. The incidence of these problems can be significantly reduced if benzodiazepines are also administered with the drug. At low doses (0.1 to 0.2 mg/kg IV or 2 mg/kg IM), patients continue to spontaneously ventilate but cannot be expected to protect the airway should vomiting occur. At higher doses, ketamine acts as a respiratory depressant and produces complete apnea. Ketamine also has direct and indirect sympathetic nervous system stimulatory effects, which can be useful in hypovolemic patients. These effects are diminished or absent in patients who are catecholamine depleted. The sympathetic stimulatory effect increases myocardial oxygen consumption and intracranial pressure, and ketamine is relatively contraindicated in patients with ischemic heart disease or space-occupying intracerebral lesions. Ketamine is frequently used as an IV analgesic during debridement procedures, at doses listed in Table 12.4. Intramural ketamine (1.0 to 2.0 mg/kg) is also very useful for sedating patients who are difficult to manage (e.g., combative adult or mentally retarded patient) so IV access can be obtained.

Amnesics and Anxiolytics

Benzodiazepines are the primary class of agents used as amnesics and anxiolytics. The prototype drug, diazepam, has been more recently replaced by its water-soluble analogue of shorter duration, midazolam. Lorazepam also belongs in this family of agents, but because it has a very long duration of action, it is not routinely used intraoperatively. Lorazepam has intensive care unit applications (Table 12.5). Benzodiazepines produce anxiolysis and some degree of amnesia but have no analgesic properties. Intraoperatively, midazolam is always used in conjunction with an opioid or inhalation agent. Midazolam can be used in combination with the short-acting opioid fentanyl to produce conscious sedation for minor procedures. Benzodiazepines can produce apnea and have synergistic adverse effects with narcotics. Very small doses of midazolam

TABLE 12.5

ANXIOLYTICS AND AMNESICS (BENZODIAZEPINES)

■ NAME	■ DOSE (mg/kg)	■ DURATION (h)	■ STRENGTHS	■ WEAKNESSES
Midazolam (Versed)	0.05 (infusion dose 0.25 mg/kg/min)	0.5	Water soluble Short duration Good for sedation for short procedures	Acute respiratory depression
Diazepam (Valium)	0.1	1	Intermediate duration	Irritation on IV injection Phlebitis Acute respiratory depression after IV overdose
Lorazepam (Ativan)	0.02–0.08	6–8	Long duration	—
BENZODIAZEPINE REVERSAL				
Flumazenil (Romazicon)	4–20 (0.2 mg repeated every 2 to 10 min until reversal is achieved) Maximum dose 1 mg	45–90 min	—	May produce seizures, panic, arrhythmias

IV, intravenous.

and fentanyl can quickly produce an unconscious apneic patient. As with all anesthetics, benzodiazepines used as IV agents for sedation should be given in small incremental doses to achieve the desired effect. A reversal agent is also available for benzodiazepines (flumazenil). The recommended dosages of these drugs and the reversal agents appear in Table 12.5.

Local Anesthetics

Local anesthetics constitute a class of drugs that temporarily block nerve conduction by binding to neuronal sodium channels. As the concentration of the local anesthetic increases around the nerve, autonomic transmission will be blocked first, followed by sensory transmission, and then motor nerve transmission. These drugs can be injected locally into tissue to produce a field block, around peripheral nerves to produce a specific dermatomal block, around nerve plexuses to produce a major conductive block, or into the subarachnoid or epidural space to produce extensive neuroaxial blockade. All the methods have been used to assist in the provision of an alternative form of balanced anesthesia by supplementing analgesia and muscle relaxation.

Adverse consequences associated with the use of local anesthetics fall into three categories: acute central nervous system toxicity due to excessive plasma concentration, hemodynamic and respiratory consequences due to excessive conduction block of the sympathetic or motor nerves, and allergic reactions. Whenever a local anesthetic is injected, there can be inadvertent intravascular injection or an overdose of the drug because of rapid uptake from the tissues. All can produce seizures. Complications can be minimized by withdrawing before injection to avoid an intravascular injection and limiting dosages to the safe range (Table 12.6).

When local anesthetics are administered for a spinal or epidural block, they produce a progressive blockade of the sympathetic nervous system, which produces systemic vasodilation. Sympathetic nerves travel along the thoracolumbar region with the first four thoracic branches, including the cardiac sympathetic accelerators. A sympathetic blockade of this entire region produces profound systemic vasodilatation and bradycardia. This condition is referred to as *total sympathectomy,* and the hypotension that ensues is usually below the minimal cerebral perfusion pressure required to maintain consciousness. Affected patients are bradycardic, hypotensive, unconscious, and usually apneic. This disastrous situation is easily remedied if treated quickly with a vasopressor (phenyl ephrine or ephedrine) and atropine. If not treated promptly, the situation proceeds to cardiac arrest. In this emergency situation, the treatment of high doses of epinephrine is 10 to 40 μ/kg, or 1 to 4 mg for an adult. The doses of epinephrine are higher than in a usual cardiac arrest because of the total sympathectomy.[5] Because the level of sympathetic block is two to six dermatomal levels higher than the sensory block, it is often difficult to obtain a high spinal sensory level without approaching a total sympathectomy.

Local anesthetics are chemically divided into two groups, esters and amides. The esters (2-chloroprocaine and tetracaine) produce metabolites that are related to *p*-aminobenzoic acid and have been associated with allergic reactions. Amides (lidocaine and bupivacaine) are rarely associated with allergic reactions. If an allergic reaction does occur, it is most likely due to the preservative (methyl paraben) used in multidose vials of lidocaine.

NEURAXIAL AND PERIPHERAL NERVE BLOCKADE

Although general anesthesia is employed for millions of surgical procedures each year in the United States, many operations can be performed safely using neuraxial or peripheral nerve blockade. The two primary neuraxial techniques, a "single-shot" spinal and continuous epidural catheter, can be used for lower extremity and lower abdominal procedures. In both techniques, a small dose of local anesthetic is administered near spinal nerve roots in order to temporarily ablate sensory input from the peripheral somatic and visceral structures. In the case of a spinal anesthetic—also known as a subarachnoid block—the intrathecal sac surrounding the cauda equina at vertebral interspace L2-3 or below is located using a sterile, small-caliber

TABLE 12.6

LOCAL ANESTHETICS

	■ MAXIMUM SINGLE DOSE (mg)	■ DURATION (h)	■ COMMENTS
AMIDES			
Lidocaine	500	1[a]	Fast onset
Ropivacaine	200	4–12[a]	Less cardiac toxicity than bupivacaine
Bupivacaine	200	4–12[a]	Exaggerated cardiotoxicity with IV injection Slow onset Long duration
ESTERS[b]			
2-Chloroprocaine	1,000	0.5–1[a]	Fast onset Lowest toxicity
Tetracaine	80	0.5–1	Slow onset

IV, intravenous.
[a]Addition of 100 μg of epinephrine (0.1 mL of 1:1,000) lowers the toxicity and increases the duration of the local anesthetic.
[b]Metabolism to paraaminobenzoic acid may cause allergic reactions.

needle (25 gauge typically). Once cerebrospinal fluid is observed in the hub of a needle, 1 to 2 mL of local anesthetic (typically bupivacaine or lidocaine) is injected into the intrathecal space. The needle is then completely withdrawn. This local anesthetic serves to directly inactivate efferent and afferent transmission at the nerve roots it comes in contact with. Because local anesthetics are not specific to specific nerve fiber types, blockade of sensory, motor, and sympathetic nerves occurs. The spread of local anesthetic within the subarachnoid space is primarily determined by three factors: (a) the vertebral interspace accessed, (b) the density of the local anesthetic in relation to the density of cerebrospinal fluid (a concept known as *baricity*), and (c) the position of the patient during injection and immediately thereafter. In order to eliminate the risk of needle puncture of the spinal cord, subarachnoid blocks are only performed below L2-3 in adults and L3-4 in children. The local anesthetic solution may be combined with vasoconstrictors such as epinephrine or opioids such as fentanyl or morphine in order to increase the density or duration of the sensory blockade. Surgical anesthesia ranging from 1 to 2 hours can be achieved using a subarachnoid block. Because of concerns regarding permanent nerve damage, intrathecal catheters are typically not used.[6,7] As a result, most subarachnoid blocks are "single-shot" techniques that cannot be redosed.

In the case of epidural techniques, the nerve roots are blocked outside the thecal sac in potential space between the ligamentum flavum and dura mater. This space is accessed sterilely using a 19-gauge introducer needle and a loss of resistance technique. Once the space is identified, a 21-gauge catheter is inserted into the space via the introducer needle and the needle is removed. After testing to reduce the likelihood of inadvertent intravascular or intrathecal placement of the catheter, the epidural catheter can be taped in place. Because the epidural catheter can be left in place for several days, redosing is possible. Dilute local anesthetics combined with vasoconstrictors or opioids are the mainstay of epidural therapy. Epidural neuraxial techniques can be used for surgical anesthesia, as an adjunct to general anesthesia, or for postoperative pain relief. Epidural catheters can be placed in the thoracic or lumbar regions because the intrathecal sac is not being accessed; associated dermatomal spread and analgesia is observed. Epidural techniques often fail to result in a dense sacral nerve root blockade, so this may be a poor choice for surgical anesthesia at or below the knee.

Peripheral nerve blockade (PNB) has been used for surgical anesthesia of the extremities since the days of intravenous regional anesthesia described by Bier in 1908. Peripheral nerve blockade differs from neuraxial techniques in that it targets peripheral nerves after they have formed from the combinations of nerve roots. Upper extremity, lower extremity, and visceral peripheral nerves are targets of these peripheral nerve blocks. Historically, anatomic landmark-based identification of peripheral nerves was complemented by use of electrical stimulator needles with the hope of eliciting specific motor responses confirming correct needle placement. However, current anesthesia techniques now employ real-time ultrasound guidance of a PNB needle under direct visualization. Vascular structures and nerves are visualized in relation to a PNB needle in order to decrease the likelihood of intravascular or intraneural injection
5 and increase the likelihood of an efficacious block. Peripheral nerve blockade can be used in lieu of general anesthesia to provide surgical anesthesia or as a postoperative pain management technique. Use of long-acting local anesthetics or placement of an indwelling continuous catheter provides long-term (16 hours to several days) pain relief.

SEDATION ANALGESIA FOR MINOR SURGICAL PROCEDURES

There are a variety of minor surgical procedures that can be accomplished safely and comfortably with anesthesia provided by infiltration of local anesthetics (most commonly 1% lidocaine) and mild sedation/anxiolysis provided by IV agents. All IV benzodiazepines, narcotics, and other IV anesthetics produce apnea if given in a high enough dose. Because there is a substantial patient-to-patient variability in response to a given dose,

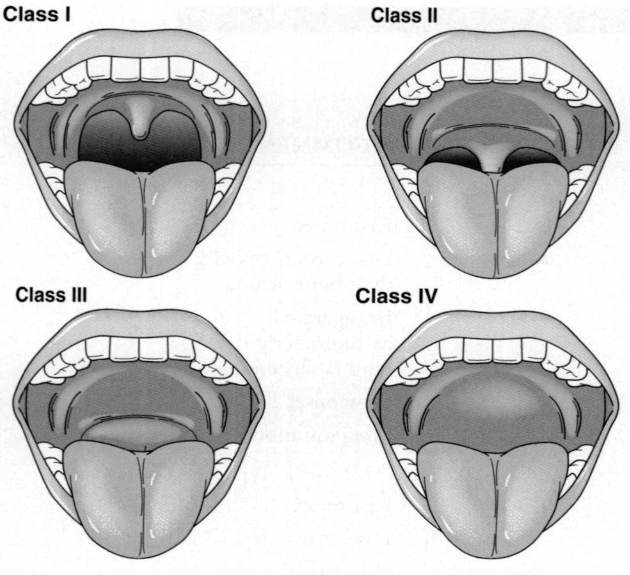

FIGURE 12.1. Classification of the patient's upper airway based on the size of the tongue and the pharyngeal structures visible on mouth opening. Class I, soft palate and anterior/posterior tonsillar pillars, and uvula visible; Class II, tonsillar pillars and part of uvula hidden by base of tongue; Class III, soft and hard palate visible; Class IV, soft palate not visible, only hard palate visible. (Reproduced with permission from Stoelting RK, Miller RD. *Basics of Anesthesia,* 5th ed. New York: Churchill Livingston; 2007:146.)

it is important that IV anxiolytics be given in small incremental doses slowly to achieve a safe sedated state. Another important factor to remember is that the anesthesia is provided by infiltration of the local anesthetic and not by the IV sedative. IV agents including narcotics cannot overcome the pain associated with a surgical incision. If large doses of narcotics are given for this purpose, once the surgical stimulus ends, the patient may quickly become apneic. The duration of the respiratory depression for even short-acting narcotics is much longer than the painful stimulus of the incision. Because of the potentially serious consequences of an apneic episode, the Joint Commission has required that all patients receiving sedation for minor surgical or medical procedures undergo the following[8]:

1. A preprocedure evaluation including an airway examination (Fig. 12.1)
2. Appropriate monitoring: pulse oximetry as a minimum
3. Documentation of the patient's vital signs and arterial saturation as well as the dose and timing of sedatives provided during the procedure
4. Documentation of a recovery period and a return to a safe recovered state

TABLE 12.7

SEDATION SCALE

■ SEDATION SCALE	■ DESCRIPTION
1	Awake and alert
2	Awake and sedated
3	Asleep but arousable to touch or verbal stimuli
4	Asleep but arousable to painful stimulus
5	Asleep and not arousable to painful stimulus

The preprocedure evaluation should include current medications, coexisting disease, and a brief physical examination including an evaluation of the airway. The most common drug used to provide sedation is midazolam. This is a fast-onset, relatively short-acting benzodiazepine that can be easily titrated to produce a sedated yet cooperative arousable state. It is usually given to adults in incremental doses of 1 mg (0.01 mg/kg in children). Narcotics such as fentanyl even in small doses act synergistically with benzodiazepines to cause a more sedated state with a much higher incidence of apnea. To assess the effect of the drug, a validated sedation scale can be of value. The scale used at the University of Michigan is presented in Table 12.7.[9]

AIRWAY EVALUATION FOR THE NONANESTHESIOLOGIST

An essential skill for all clinicians is the assessment of a patient airway. It is important to determine how difficult it may be to obtain control of the airway if a patient should require airway
6 or ventilatory support. The concept of airway management should be focused on not just endotracheal intubation, but also mask ventilation. Until the airway can be secured via intubation, the patient must be supported through mask ventilation.[10] The key elements of an airway examination are an assessment of obesity, mouth opening, neck flexion and extension, Mallampati oropharyngeal classification, presence of beard, and mandibular protrusion ability (Table 12.8).[11]

TABLE 12.8

STANDARD AIRWAY EXAMINATION FOR NONANESTHESIOLOGISTS

■ EXAM ELEMENT	■ CONCERNING FINDINGS
Body mass index (kg/m^2)	Body mass index ≥31
Mouth opening	Interincisor or intergingival distance >3 cm
Mallampati classification	Class III or IV (see Fig. 12.1)
Mandibular protrusion	Inability to protrude lower incisors to meet or extend past upper incisors
Neck anatomy	Radiation changes, or thick obese neck
Cervical spine mobility	Limited extension or possibly unstable cervical spine
Beard	Presence of full beard

Despite decades of research, there is no perfect combination of clinical tests to predict difficult intubation. However, the presence of abnormalities in three or more of the aforementioned elements increases the likelihood of a difficult mask ventilation and/or difficult intubation by more than eight times.[11] In patients with multiple (three or more) airway abnormalities, the presence of a beard is an easily corrected characteristic: the patient should be asked to shave the beard in order to improve the ability to manage the airway. Assessment of oropharyngeal classification is performed by having patients open their mouth and maximally protrude the tongue without phonation. This Mallampati oropharyngeal assessment can be classified depending on whether the uvula can be completely seen (class 1), only partly seen (class 2), or not seen, with only the hard and soft palate visible (class 3), or only the hard palate visible (class 4; see Fig. 12.1).[12]

RISKS ASSOCIATED WITH ANESTHESIA

7 Because the anesthetic agents effectively obtund or completely block nearly all physiologic protective mechanisms, there is an associated risk even without a surgical procedure. Fortunately, with the advent of newer agents and monitoring techniques, it is estimated that the mortality rate due to anesthesia alone has decreased from about 1 in 10,000 patients in the 1950s to as low as 1 in 200,000 or less for healthy patients today.[13] Although a 1 in 200,000 risk of death or serious neurologic impairment may appear small, when dire consequences occur in a young patient undergoing a purely elective procedure, the consequences are devastating for everyone involved. When patients are placed in a condition in which they cannot breathe, there is always the possibility of a technical or judgmental error resulting in hypoxia and brain damage or death. It has been estimated that between 50% and 75% of anesthetic-related deaths are due to human error and are preventable. Because the consequences of an anesthetic mishap are usually severe, the emotional and financial costs are high.

The most common problems associated with adverse outcomes are related to the airway and include inadequate ventilation, unrecognized esophageal intubation, unrecognized extubation, and unrecognized disconnection from the ventilator. The incidence of these problems has been significantly reduced by including capnometry and pulse oximetry in addition to other noninvasive monitors, although a cause-and-effect relation has been difficult to prove. Efforts to improve outcome can be approached at three levels: (a) reduction of the incidence of rare but catastrophic anesthetic-related problems, (b) improvement of the care and experience of every patient undergoing anesthesia and surgery, and (c) improvement of the preparation and management of patients with preexisting medical conditions who have higher morbidity and mortality rates. The first goal has been addressed in part with improved monitoring techniques and anesthesia training. Others have been advanced by the addition of comprehensive pain management, as discussed later in this chapter. Issues of preexisting medical disease and how they affect the anesthetic plan are also briefly discussed later in this chapter.

Cardiovascular Diseases

Hypertension. Hypertension is the most common preexisting medical disease in patients presenting for surgery and is a major risk factor for renal, cerebrovascular, peripheral vascular, and coronary artery diseases, as well as congestive heart failure (CHF). It is particularly associated with lipid disorders, diabetes, and obesity. It is these associated comorbidities that are most likely to lead to morbidity and mortality in the perioperative period, and therefore, the presence of hypertension should prompt the surgeon to review the history and physical examination for them. Hypertensive patients should be treated medically to render them normotensive before elective surgery. In general, antihypertension medications should be continued throughout the perioperative period. Recently this strategy has been questioned for patients treated with angiotensin receptor blockers (ARBs), such as valsartan, candesartan, losartan, or angiotensin-converting enzyme inhibitors (ACE-Is), such as lisinopril, captopril, or ramipril. Patients treated with these medications have experienced substantial intraoperative hypotension, which is unresponsive to standard vasopressors. This ACE-I/ARB hypotension has been treated successfully with terlipressin, vasopressin, and methylene blue.[14–16] Some now recommend withholding ACE-Is/ARBs the morning of surgery, and data among general surgery patients indicate that withholding the medications for at least 10 hours prior to induction of anesthesia may be appropriate.[17,18] Patients on concomitant diuretic therapy are at greatest risk for intraoperative hypotension requiring treatment.[19,20]

The incidence of hypotension and myocardial ischemia intraoperatively is higher in untreated hypertensive patients than in adequately treated hypertensive patients if the preoperative diastolic pressure is 110 mm Hg or higher.[21] Inadequately treated hypertensive patients undergoing carotid endarterectomies have an increased incidence of neurologic deficits, and those with a history of prior myocardial infarctions have an increased incidence of reinfarction. Patients commonly have an elevated blood pressure on admission to the hospital. Hypertensive patients can have exaggerated responses to painful stimuli and have a higher incidence of perioperative ischemia.

Coronary Artery Disease. Much of the anesthetic preoperative evaluation has historically been focused on the detection and treatment of coronary artery disease. Coronary artery disease is present in about 25% of patients who undergo surgery each year.[21] It is the leading cause of death in the United States and continues to be a major cause of postoperative morbidity and mortality.[22] The goal of the preoperative cardiac evaluation is to identify patients who are at increased risk of perioperative cardiac morbidity and ensure that their chronic conditions are optimized. Although perioperative cardiac events are the leading cause of death following anesthesia and surgery, it has been difficult to define patient characteristics that accurately predict a high risk of adverse outcome.[23] It has been even more difficult to modify that risk effectively.[24] Preoperative CHF is clearly a significant risk factor, as is recent myocardial infarction or unstable angina (Table 12.9). Diabetes mellitus, atherosclerotic vascular disease, and hypertension also appear to confer risk, although less than with CHF or unstable angina. Perioperative risk in patients with valvular heart disease varies with the severity of the disease as represented by CHF, pulmonary hypertension, and dysrhythmias. Dysrhythmias are also a concern in the presence of coronary artery disease. Age and stable angina remain controversial as predictors of perioperative risk, with equal numbers of supporting and refuting studies. The value of revascularization remains controversial as well. In patients without significant pulmonary disease, the ability to climb two flights of stairs without stopping or experiencing symptoms of angina or shortness of breath is considered a good practical test of cardiac reserve. Unfortunately, many patients with ischemic heart disease have concomitant pulmonary disease or other medical problems that limit their activity. A history of myocardial infarction is important information. Large retrospective studies have found that the incidence of reinfarction is related to the time elapsed since the previous myocardial infarction.[25–27] The incidence of reinfarction appears to stabilize at about 6%

TABLE 12.9

CLINICAL PREDICTORS OF INCREASED PERIOPERATIVE CARDIOVASCULAR RISK (MYOCARDIAL INFARCTION, HEART FAILURE, DEATH)

MAJOR
Unstable coronary syndromes
Acute or recent MI[a] with evidence of important ischemic risk by clinical symptoms or noninvasive study
Unstable or severe[b] angina (Canadian class III or IV)[c]
Decompensated heart failure
Significant arrhythmias
High-grade atrioventricular block
Symptomatic ventricular arrhythmias in the presence of underlying heart disease
Supraventricular arrhythmias with uncontrolled ventricular rate
Severe valvular disease
Intermediate
Mild angina pectoris (Canadian class I or II)
Previous MI by history or pathologic Q waves
Compensated or prior heart failure
Diabetes mellitus (particularly insulin dependent)
Renal insufficiency
MINOR
Advanced age
Abnormal ECG (left ventricular hypertrophy, left bundle-branch block, ST-T abnormalities)
Rhythm other than sinus (e.g., atrial fibrillation)
Low functional capacity (e.g., inability to climb one flight of stairs with a bag of groceries)
History of stroke
Uncontrolled systemic hypertension

ECG, electrocardiogram; MI, myocardial infarction.
[a]The American College of Cardiology National Database Library defines recent MI as >7 d but ≤1 mo (30 d); acute MI is within 7 d.
[b]May include "stable" angina in patients who are unusually sedentary.
[c]Campeau L. Grading of angina pectoris. *Circulation* 1976;54:522.

TABLE 12.10

CARDIAC RISK[a] STRATIFICATION FOR NONCARDIAC SURGICAL PROCEDURES

High (reported cardiac risk often >5%)
Emergent major operations, particularly in the elderly
Aortic and other major vascular surgery
Peripheral vascular surgery
Anticipated prolonged surgical procedures associated with large fluid shifts and/or blood loss
Intermediate (reported cardiac risk generally <5%)
Carotid endarterectomy
Head and neck surgery
Intraperitoneal and intrathoracic surgery
Orthopedic surgery
Prostate surgery
Low[b] (reported cardiac risk generally <1%)
Endoscopic procedures
Superficial procedures
Cataract surgery
Breast surgery

[a]Combined incidence of cardiac death and nonfatal myocardial infarction.
[b]Do not generally require further preoperative cardiac testing.

after 6 months. The highest rate of reinfarction occurs in the 0- to 3-month period. Mortality from reinfarction, for patients undergoing noncardiac surgery (Table 12.10), has been reported to be between 20% and 50% and usually occurs within the first 48 hours after surgery.

Perioperative cardiac adverse event risk reduction has undergone significant changes over the past decade. Previous retrospective studies demonstrating value to coronary revascularization spurred aggressive preoperative coronary artery disease identification and management. However, recent data have questioned the value of coronary revascularization among asymptomatic patients in not only the perioperative period, but also in the general medical population.[28,29] The most recent American College of Cardiology (ACC)/American Heart Association (AHA) guidelines reserve preoperative coronary revascularization for patients demonstrating asymptomatic left main coronary artery disease, three-vessel disease, reduced ejection fraction, unstable angina, or acute myocardial infarction.[30] Furthermore, large retrospective and prospective studies have demonstrated that the institution perioperative beta blockade also bears significant risks that must be weighed against possible benefits.[31,32] As a result, the most recent ACC/AHA guidelines reserve the institution of beta-blocker therapy for only high-risk procedures or high-risk patients.[30] Patients already on beta-blocker therapy should be continued on the therapy throughout the perioperative period.[33] The widespread use of 3-hydroxy-3-methylglutaryl coenzyme A (HMG-CoA) reductase inhibitors, commonly known as statins, for cardiovascular disease and hyperlipidemia has introduced another medication into the surgical preoperative evaluation. Although prospective data establishing the value of instituting preoperative statin therapy are limited, there is general consensus that these medications should not be withdrawn during the perioperative period.[34]

All patients in high-risk groups or with a history of ischemic heart disease must be evaluated and properly treated before elective surgery. All elective surgery should be delayed for 6 months after myocardial infarction. If this is not feasible, invasive monitoring should be considered in the perioperative period and intensive postoperative observation should continue for at least 48 hours. The intrusiveness of the surgical procedure also plays a part in the overall risk and need for preoperative workup of heart disease. The AHA has produced and updated an algorithm for the recommended preoperative workup (Algorithm 12.1).[33]

Percutaneous Coronary Intervention with Stenting. The widespread use of percutaneous intervention for coronary artery disease via angioplasty with or without stenting has introduced a new level of clinical complexity. In-stent thrombosis is a feared complication with profound morbidity and mortality. Given the known proinflammatory and prothrombotic physiologic state induced by acute illness, surgery, and anesthesia, coronary stents may be at elevated risk for thrombosis during the perioperative period. Large retrospective studies have demonstrated that the risk of perioperative in-stent thrombosis is increased if noncardiac surgery is performed soon after percutaneous coronary intervention.[35,36]

8 The appropriate duration to defer elective surgery after

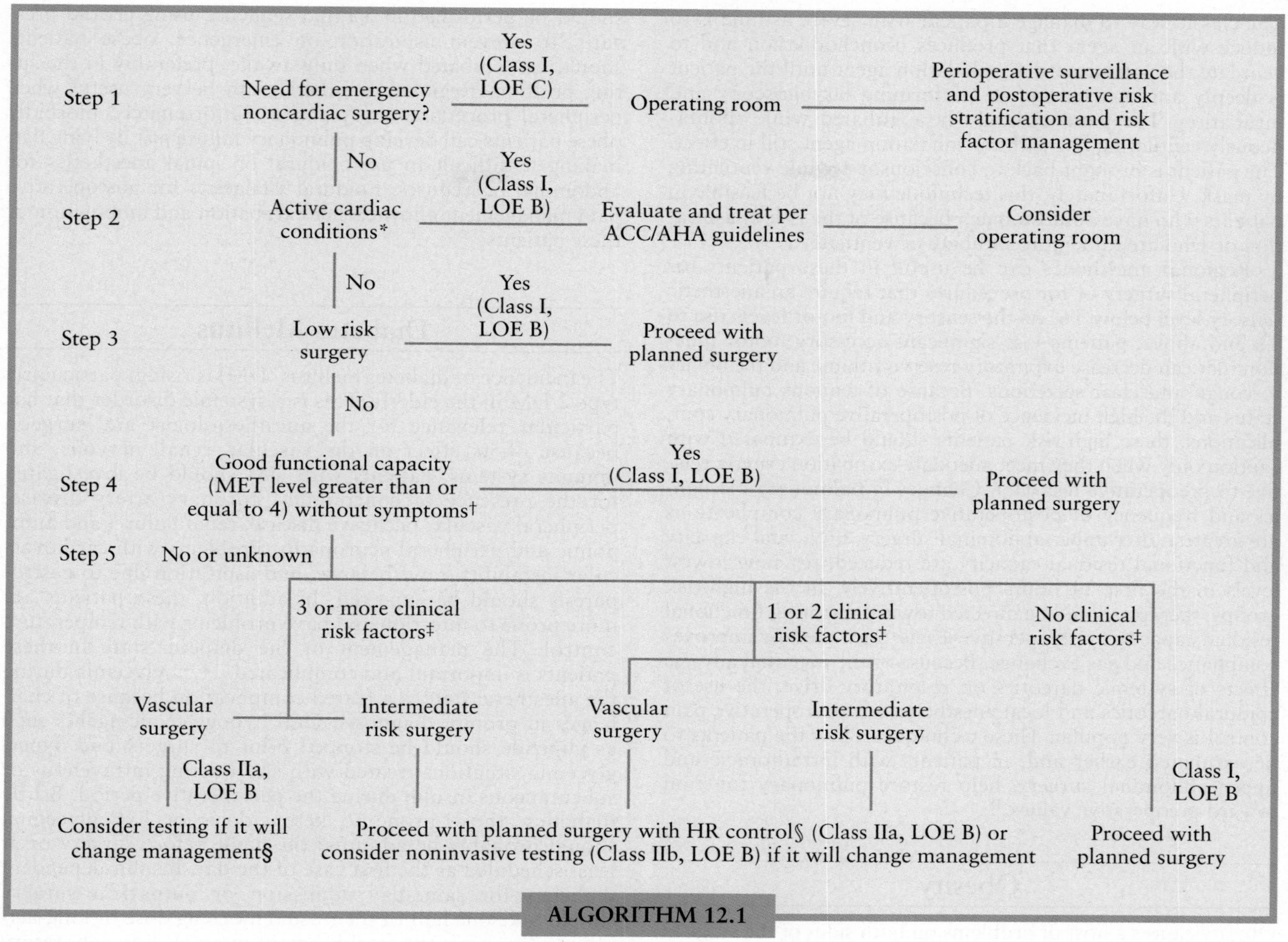

ALGORITHM 12.1. Decision aid for preoperative cardiac evaluation prior to noncardiac surgery. This decision tree for preoperative evaluation takes into account not only the patient's physical status but also the severity of the surgical procedure. ACC, American College of Cardiology; AHA, American Heart Association; LOE, level of evidence.

coronary stenting remains controversial, but recent ACC/AHA guidelines recommend 12 months for drug-eluting stents and 6 weeks for bare-metal stents.[30] The role for antiplatelet therapy remains a major question, but data suggest that cessation of recommended antiplatelet therapy in the perioperative period may have significant coronary thrombotic risks without major improvement in bleeding adverse events.[35,36] The decision to stop antiplatelet therapy within 1 year of a drug-eluting stent or 6 weeks of a bare-metal stent placement should be made with caution. The continuation of aspirin therapy in patients with coronary stents was previously thought to increase the risk of bleeding. However, recent data and recommendations suggest that the continuation of single antiplatelet therapy with aspirin throughout the perioperative period even 1 year after stenting may be appropriate.[30]

Congestive Heart Failure. CHF has been described as the single most important factor predicting postoperative cardiac morbidity.[37] All elective surgical procedures should be deferred until congestive failure is medically optimized. If surgery cannot be deferred, aggressive perioperative management is warranted with a goal of optimizing cardiac output. In contrast to isolated ischemic heart disease, CHF is more easily diagnosed by history, physical examination, and basic preoperative laboratory workup, including electrocardiography (ECG) and chest radiography. Because patients with left, right, or both left and right ventricular dysfunction are less tolerant of the fluid shifts associated with surgery and the myocardial depression associated with the anesthetic, they constitute the highest-risk group for postoperative cardiac complications.

Pulmonary Disease

Pulmonary disease is classically divided into acute and chronic restrictive and obstructive disease. Restrictive disease is defined by processes that reduce lung volumes, and obstructive disease is characterized by reduced flow rates on pulmonary function tests.

Obstructive diseases are present in patients with forced expiratory volume in 1 second (FEV_1)/forced vital capacity (FVC) ratios of less than 50%. Obstructive pulmonary disease can be either chronic or acute (asthma). In either case, the reversible component of obstruction should be reversed before elective surgery. Patients are maintained on bronchodilator medications, and those with chronic secretions are appropriately hydrated and receive therapy to mobilize secretions. In patients with reactive airway disease, the endotracheal tube can induce severe bronchospasm. Even in patients who are well treated preoperatively, reactive bronchospasm can complicate anesthetic induction and the emergence from anesthesia. The principal method used to prevent or diminish this "foreign body"–induced bronchospasm is intubation of the patient at a deep level of anesthesia when reflexes are blunted.

The classic way to manage a patient with severe asthma is to induce with an agent that produces bronchodilation and to ventilate the patient with an inhalation agent until the patient is deeply anesthetized before performing laryngoscopy and intubation. The patient should be extubated while spontaneously ventilating but with the inhalation agent still in effect. The patient is brought back to consciousness while ventilating by mask. Unfortunately, this technique may not be feasible in patients who have a full stomach because of the risk of aspiration or who are difficult to intubate or ventilate.

Regional anesthetics can be useful in these patients for peripheral surgery or for procedures that require an anesthetic sensory level below T6. As the sensory and motor levels rise to T6 and above, patients lose significant accessory motor function that can decrease expiratory reserve volume and the ability to cough and clear secretions. Because of tenuous pulmonary status and the high incidence of postoperative pulmonary complications, these high-risk patients should be extubated with caution only when they meet adequate extubation criteria relative to preoperative test data. Changes in pulmonary mechanics and frequency of postoperative pulmonary complications are greatest after upper abdominal surgery. Both vital capacity and functional residual capacity are reduced, reaching lowest levels in the first 24 hours postoperatively. In the high-risk groups, therapy should be directed toward restoring functional residual capacity to preoperative levels. Such therapy improves compliance and gas exchange. Because of the potential adverse effects of systemic narcotics on respiratory drive, the use of epidural narcotics and local anesthetics for postoperative pain control is very popular. These techniques allow the patients to be extubated earlier and, in patients with intrathoracic and upper abdominal surgery, help restore pulmonary function toward preoperative values.[38]

Obesity

Obesity causes a host of problems on both sides of the surgical drapes. Obesity is defined as a body mass index greater than or equal to 30 kg/m^2. Body mass index (BMI) can be easily calculated by dividing the patient's weight in kilograms by the square of his or her height in meters. The pathophysiologic changes associated with morbid obesity (BMI $\geq$40 kg/m^2) affect the respiratory, cardiovascular, and gastrointestinal systems. Patients have an external restrictive disease that reduces functional residual capacity and worsens with the supine position. Breathing effort increases and ventilation becomes diaphragmatic and position dependent. Obese patients frequently desaturate at night and have a high incidence of sleep apnea. Because of increased blood volume and frequent desaturations, obese patients can develop pulmonary hypertension and right-sided heart failure. Obese individuals have a high incidence of coronary artery disease. Because of size alone, they have increased cardiovascular demands with limited cardiac reserve and exercise tolerance. Obese patients have a high incidence of hiatal hernia and gastroesophageal reflux, increasing the risk for aspiration on induction and emergence from anesthesia. Issues as mundane as venous access can cause significant problems in this patient group.

A significant concern of the anesthesiologist is gaining adequate control of the airway. The combined problems of aspiration risk, rapid desaturation caused by reduced functional residual capacity and increased oxygen demand, and technical difficulties associated with intubation due to anatomic fat deposits make intubation a high-risk procedure. If problems occur, there can be significant technical difficulties in obtaining a rapid cricothyrotomy. For these reasons, a nasal or oral awake intubation can be useful. Patients should receive prophylactic administration of H_2-receptor antagonists and a nonparticulate antacid to improve the pH of gastric contents. If intubations are to be done after induction of anesthesia, they should be performed in a rapid sequence using cricoid pressure. To prevent aspiration on emergence, obese patients should be extubated when fully awake, preferably in the sitting position. Regional anesthetics can be very useful when peripheral procedures are planned. Unfortunately, morbidly obese patients can develop pulmonary failure just by lying flat, making it difficult to use epidural or spinal anesthetics for abdominal procedures. Epidural analgesics for postoperative pain management allow earlier extubation and ambulation of these patients.[38]

Diabetes Mellitus

The incidence of diabetes mellitus (DM) is rising, particularly type 2 DM in the elderly. This is a systemic disorder that has particular relevance for the anesthesiologist and surgeon because of its effect on the vascular, renal, nervous, and immune systems. Patients with DM should be investigated for the presence of concomitant coronary artery disease, peripheral vascular occlusive disease, renal failure, and autonomic and peripheral neuropathy. Problems with cardiovascular instability, fluid balance, and aspiration due to gastroparesis should be expected. In addition, these patients are more prone to infection and have problems with temperature control. The management of the diabetic state in these patients is important and complicated. Hypoglycemia during the anesthetic state is a feared complication because of challenges in prompt diagnosis. Oral hypoglycemic agents such as glipizide should be stopped prior to surgery and hyperglycemic situations treated with short-acting intravenous or subcutaneous insulin during the perioperative period. Brittle diabetics, those prone to ketoacidosis or hypoglycemia, should probably be admitted the night before surgery or at least scheduled as the first case of the day. Insulin-dependent diabetics for same-day admission or outpatient surgery should take one half of their usual morning dose of long-acting insulin. After the establishment of an IV line, laboratory blood samples are drawn and infusion of dextrose is started. Additional insulin is then given according to the results of frequent (every 1 to 2 hours) blood sugar monitoring. Alternatively, simultaneous IV infusion of dextrose and insulin may be used to keep the blood sugar in the range of 120 to 180 mg/dL. Again, these patients, whenever possible, should be done as the first case of the day to interfere as little as possible with the diabetic regimen.

Renal Insufficiency and Failure

Because the kidneys play a vital role in metabolic, synthetic, and fluid management homeostasis, renal failure is associated with many effects on the cardiovascular, pulmonary, hematologic, gastrointestinal, and immune system. Preexisting renal insufficiency is a known risk factor for postoperative myocardial infarction and renal failure.[39,40] Optimizing the fluid and metabolic status of a patient in end-stage renal disease is of vital importance. Elective surgery should be delayed until such optimization is performed. In emergent situations, the urgent need for hemodialysis should be considered intraoperatively or postoperatively to avoid life-threatening electrolyte and fluid derangements. Although postoperative renal failure has historically been the focus of cardiac surgery researchers, national data suggest that 1% of patients undergoing general surgery procedures will also experience postoperative acute kidney injury, with a sixfold rise in 30-day mortality. Risk factors for postoperative acute kidney injury in patients undergoing general surgery are listed in Table 12.11. These data should be considered during the patient consent process.

TABLE 12.11

PREDICTORS OF POSTOPERATIVE ACUTE KIDNEY INJURY AFTER GENERAL SURGERY PROCEDURES

Age ≥56 y
Male sex
Emergency surgery
Intraperitoneal procedures
Preoperative renal insufficiency (serum creatinine >1.2 mg/dL)
Ascites
Active congestive heart failure
Diabetes mellitus requiring oral hypoglycemic or insulin therapy
Hypertension requiring chronic medication

From Kheterpal S, Tremper K, Heung M, et al. Development and validation of an acute kidney injury risk index for patients undergoing general surgery. *Anesthesiology.* 2009;110:505–515.

RISKS ASSOCIATED WITH REGIONAL TECHNIQUES IN PATIENTS BEING TREATED WITH LOW-MOLECULAR-WEIGHT HEPARIN

Low-molecular-weight heparin (LMWH) has become a routine method of prophylactically treating patients who are at risk for deep venous thrombosis. It has several advantages over traditional heparin and has therefore been adopted in Europe and the United States over the past few years. Unfortunately, there has been an increased number of reported cases of epidural hematoma formation when regional anesthetics are provided in patients who are being treated with LMWH.[41] For that reason, the Society of Regional Anesthesia has published the following guidelines for central conduction block (spinal and epidural anesthesia) to try to minimize the incidence of this devastating complication:

1. The presence of blood during needle and catheter placement will require a delay of 24 hours, postoperatively, before initiation of LMWH therapy.
2. For patients on LMWH (once a day dosing), needle placement should occur at least 12 hours after the last LMWH dose. For patients receiving higher dosing (e.g., enoxaparin 1 mg/kg twice a day), placement should occur at least 24 hours after the last LMWH dose.
3. It is recommended that patients who have an indwelling epidural catheter will receive LMWH only when there is an extreme risk of deep vein thrombosis (DVT) and there is frequent monitoring of the patient's neurologic status (every hour); the catheter should not be removed within 12 hours of the last dose.
4. Following removal of an epidural catheter, LMWH dosing should not occur for at least 2 hours.[41]

PREOPERATIVE EVALUATION

9 The three goals of the preoperative evaluation are (a) to develop an anesthetic plan that considers the patient's medical condition, the requirements of the surgical procedure, and the patient's preferences; (b) to ensure that the patient's chronic disease is under appropriate medical therapy before an elective procedure; and (c) to gain rapport with and the confidence of the patient, answer any questions, and allay fears.

Optimally, to complete this task, an anesthesiologist would meet every patient before the planned surgical procedure to review the medical history, complete a physical examination, discuss the options and associated anesthetic risks, and develop an anesthetic plan. In the past, this was accomplished when the anesthesiologist visited the patient in the hospital the night before surgery. Currently, it is rare to have patients admitted the night before surgery even before the most comprehensive and complex surgical procedures. The evaluation must still be accomplished, but it must be done on an ambulatory basis, which creates associated logistical problems.

A patient's medical conditions should be optimized before an elective surgical procedure. This optimization is best performed by the primary care physician, with medical specialty consultation if necessary. If the procedure is deemed a surgical emergency, the anesthesiologist is responsible for assessing the patient quickly, developing the appropriate anesthetic plan, and proceeding to the operating room as soon as possible. In an emergency situation, the anesthesiologist is not obligated to seek medical consultation to evaluate chronic medical problems because time is essential. The following questions must be answered when evaluating a patient undergoing an elective surgical procedure (Table 12.12). What must be included in

TABLE 12.12 RESULTS

HOSPITAL MORTALITY RATES IN RELATION TO AGE, PREOPERATIVE DISEASE, AND SURGERY

PREOPERATIVE DISEASE AND SURGERY	<50[a]	AGE (y) 50–69[a]	>70[a]
Chronic heart failure	0.1%/0.5%	0.4%/2%	0.8%/4%
Renal failure	0.2%/1%	0.9%/2%	2%/9%
Abdominal surgery	0.3%/2%	1%/6%	3%/12%
Chronic heart failure and renal failure	0.7%/3%	3%/13%	6%/24%
Chronic heart failure and abdominal surgery	0.9%/4%	4%/17%	7%/30%
Renal failure and abdominal surgery	2%/8%	2%/32%	16%/50%
Chronic heart failure, renal failure, and abdominal surgery	6%/26%	22%/60%	37%/76%

[a]Figures are for elective surgery (first number) and emergency surgery (second number).
From Pedersen T, Eliasen K, Henriksen E. A prospective study of mortality associated with anesthesia and surgery: risk indicators of mortality in hospitals. *Acta Anaesthesiol Scand* 1990;34:176, with permission.

the preoperative evaluation? Second, who is involved in this process? When and where are all the steps in this process to be conducted? How should all the information be coordinated so that it is available to the appropriate personnel at the appropriate time?

The following steps must be completed before moving the patient into the operating room:

1. A comorbidity-focused history and physical examination
2. Appropriate laboratory studies and medical consultations
3. An anesthesiologist preoperative evaluation with assignment of an American Society of Anesthesiologists (ASA) physical status
4. Discussion with the patient of the options and risks
5. Development and communication of the anesthetic plan to the patient and surgeon
6. Acute optimization of any pertinent medical conditions

The history and physical examination have repeatedly been shown to be the most valuable parts of the preoperative assessment. It is primarily the surgeon's responsibility to obtain a basic history that includes current medical conditions, current medication, and previous surgical and anesthetic history. Questions that are of unique interest to the anesthesiologist are those that involve previous anesthetic problems experienced by the patient or blood relatives and the patient's exercise tolerance. This evaluation not only determines the laboratory tests that may be required but also allows for the assignment of ASA physical status (PS) (Table 12.13). The classification serves as a general measure of the patient's state of well-being, taking into account all problems the patient brings to the operating room, including systemic disturbances caused by the surgical illness. Although studies of anesthetic mortality show a correlation with the physical status classification, this categorization does not describe the risk directly. The risk of any operation is determined not only by patient-related factors but also by procedure-specific ones. For patients with complex medical problems, it is frequently helpful to supplement the surgical history and physical examination with a recent assessment by the patient's primary physician.

The value of preoperative laboratory studies has undergone substantial reevaluation since the mid-1980s. In the past, a surgical procedure was an opportunity to obtain a battery of baseline laboratory tests, even for ASA PS-1 patients. The current thinking is that a laboratory test should not be ordered unless a change in the surgical or anesthetic plan is anticipated. The only preoperative screening test required at the University of Michigan, for instance, is an ECG within a year of the planned surgical procedure for men older than 40 and women older than 50 years of age. Pregnancy tests should be obtained only for women who state that they could be pregnant. For procedures with significant anticipated blood loss, a type and cross match is ordered, and a preoperative hematocrit is also required. All other tests should have an indication based on history and physical examination. A current strategy for selecting tests indicated by patient history is presented in Table 12.14. Electronic patient questionnaires have also been developed, allowing the appropriate laboratories to be selected based on the patient's response to questions.[42]

Discussions of the options of anesthetic techniques and anesthetic risks are best performed by the anesthesiologist who will provide the anesthetic. If the surgeon prefers a specific anesthetic technique, this is best communicated directly to the anesthesiologist rather than recommended to the patient. The development of the anesthetic plan must be determined by the anesthesiologist.

The history, physical examination, and laboratory studies should be performed by the surgeon as soon as the surgical procedure is scheduled. The results of the laboratory studies must be evaluated well in advance of the day of surgery so that positive findings can be attended to in a timely manner. For healthy patients (ASA PS-1 and PS-2), the preoperative anesthetic assessment can be conducted by the anesthesiologist on the day of the procedure. If the patients have complex medical problems (ASA PS-3 or greater) or have significant concerns they want to discuss with an anesthesiologist, they should be evaluated before the day of surgery. Because of the logistical problems of scheduling, most institutions have developed preoperative anesthesia clinics where this process can take place. When specialty medical consultation is considered, the following questions should be answered. Does this patient have ischemic heart disease that requires further medical management

TABLE 12.13 **CLASSIFICATION**

PHYSICAL STATUS CLASSIFICATION OF THE AMERICAN SOCIETY OF ANESTHESIOLOGISTS

PHYSICAL STATUS CLASSIFICATION	DESCRIPTION
PS-1	A normal, healthy patient
PS-2	A patient with mild systemic disease that results in no functional limitation *Examples:* Hypertension, diabetes mellitus, chronic bronchitis, morbid obesity, extremes of age
PS-3	A patient with severe systemic disease that results in functional limitation *Examples:* Poorly controlled hypertension, diabetes mellitus with vascular complications, angina pectoris, prior myocardial infarction, pulmonary disease that limits activity
PS-4	A patient with severe systemic disease that is a constant threat to life *Examples:* Congestive heart failure, unstable angina pectoris, advanced pulmonary, renal, or hepatic dysfunction
PS-5	A moribund patient who is not expected to survive without the operation *Examples:* Ruptured abdominal aneurysm, pulmonary embolus, head injury with increased intracranial pressure
PS-6	A declared brain-dead patient whose organs are being removed for donor purposes
Emergency operation (E)	Any patient in whom an emergency operation is required *Example:* An otherwise healthy 30-year-old woman who requires dilation and curettage for moderate but persistent vaginal bleeding (PS-1E)

TABLE 12.14

SIMPLIFIED STRATEGY FOR PREOPERATIVE TESTING

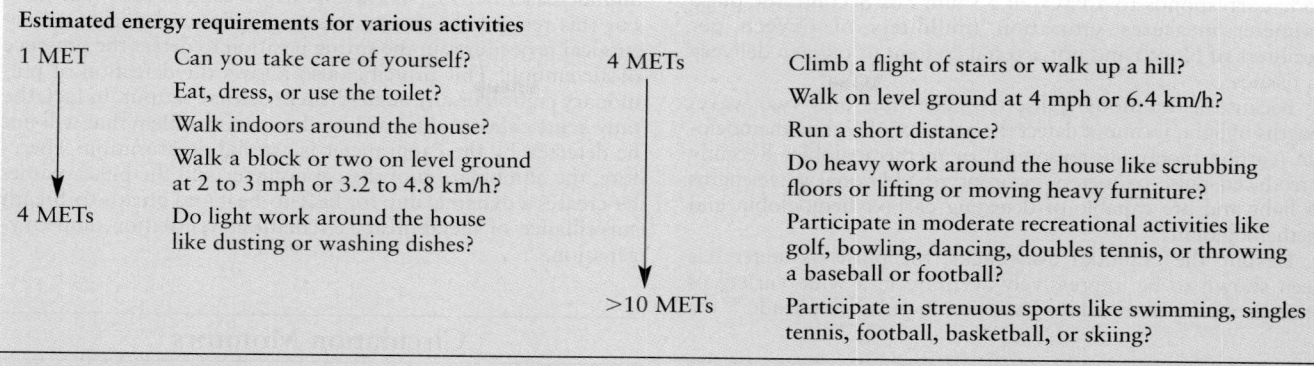

Estimated energy requirements for various activities

1 MET	Can you take care of yourself?	4 METs	Climb a flight of stairs or walk up a hill?
↓	Eat, dress, or use the toilet?	↓	Walk on level ground at 4 mph or 6.4 km/h?
	Walk indoors around the house?		Run a short distance?
	Walk a block or two on level ground at 2 to 3 mph or 3.2 to 4.8 km/h?		Do heavy work around the house like scrubbing floors or lifting or moving heavy furniture?
4 METs	Do light work around the house like dusting or washing dishes?		Participate in moderate recreational activities like golf, bowling, dancing, doubles tennis, or throwing a baseball or football?
		>10 METs	Participate in strenuous sports like swimming, singles tennis, football, basketball, or skiing?

MET, metabolic equivalent.

or workup? Is medical treatment of these problems optimized? If not, what needs to be done and how long will it take?

In addition, the patient's medication regimen should be reviewed to ensure that appropriate medications are continued or discontinued in the days and hours leading up to an elective procedure. In general, diuretics and ACE-I/ARB medications should not be taken the day of surgery. Several important classes of medications should be continued per the patient's normal regimen: chronic pain therapy (including opioids), beta-blockers, statins, and proton pump inhibitors. The decision regarding anticoagulant therapy is a complex one that must take into account the indication for therapy, the likelihood and impact of surgical bleeding, and the risk of perioperative thrombosis. Insulin and oral hypoglycemic agents should be continued at a reduced dose given the fasting state of
10 the surgical patient. Patients receiving chronic pain or opioid addiction therapy with buprenorphine (Subutex, Suboxone) can be particularly challenging to manage in the postoperative period and should be immediately referred to their primary care physician and an anesthesiologist to create a pain management plan prior to the day of surgery. Buprenorphine is mixed opioid agonist/antagonist that tightly binds at the μ receptor and has a long and varied half-life (24 to 60 hours). It can inhibit the analgesic benefits of traditional opioids in the postoperative period, resulting in uncontrolled pain, decreased patient satisfaction, and the potential for adverse events due to the need for very high doses of opioids.[43] A management protocol used at the University of Michigan is demonstrated in Algorithm 12.2.

An obvious problem that concerns anesthesiologists is the potential of a difficult intubation. This can be assessed as discussed earlier (see Fig. 12.1 and Table 12.8). Even if a patient has no medical problem, the possibility of a difficult airway warrants that the patient be seen preoperatively and evaluated. These patients can always be approached by an awake fiberoptic technique, but this takes planning and can cause a significant delay if there is no prior warning.

MONITORING THE SURGICAL PATIENT

One of the more obvious changes in anesthesia care has been the routine use of an array of electronic monitoring devices to provide continuous surveillance of physiologic status. Because the art and science of anesthesiology involves titrating pharmacologic agents to produce desired physiologic effects, there must be a measured parameter to which drug dosages are titrated. Depending on the severity of preexisting disease and the extent and duration of the surgical procedure, invasive techniques can be used to provide comprehensive continuous data to guide the titration of fluid therapy and cardiovascular agents.

Monitors of Oxygenation

Pulse oximetry has been called the most significant advance in patient monitoring to date. This device continuously, noninvasively, and inexpensively provides arterial hemoglobin saturation (SaO_2) and peripheral pulse by measuring light absorption in a manner similar to that of a laboratory cooximeter. A laboratory cooximeter shines light through a cuvette filled with a blood sample. Each hemoglobin species absorbs light in direct proportion to its concentration (Beer-Lambert law). A cooximeter requires one wavelength of light for each hemoglobin species to be measured, that is, one wavelength for oxyhemoglobin and one for reduced hemoglobin. To measure other hemoglobins, such as carboxyhemoglobin or methemoglobin, the device requires four wavelengths of light.

The traditional pulse oximeter uses two wavelengths of light, one red and one infrared, that shine through a tissue bed, usually a finger. Opposite the light sources is a photodiode that measures the transmitted light intensity. A large proportion of the light absorbed as it passes through the tissues is not associated with arterial blood but with other components of the tissue, such as skin, muscle, bone, and venous blood. Therefore, the device analyzes only the pulsatile component of absorption and assumes that anything that pulses within the tissue bed is arterial blood, hence the name *pulse oximeter.* Actually, the pulse oximeter measures the ratio of the pulsatile component of red light absorbed to the pulsatile component of the infrared light absorbed. This ratio changes with SaO_2. The exact relation between this ratio and SaO_2 has been empirically determined from volunteer studies and is programmed into the electronics of the oximeter. If any artifacts occur in a pulsatile nature, they may be erroneously integrated into the equation, causing erroneous SaO_2 estimates.

Several things should be remembered when interpreting a pulse oximeter's output. First, the device measures SaO_2 and not arterial oxygen tension (PaO_2). The PaO_2 must drop below 80 mm Hg before any significant change in SaO_2 occurs. As the PaO_2 drops below 60 mm Hg, the SaO_2 rapidly falls as the inflection point of the sigmoidal oxyhemoglobin dissociation curve is approached. As a rough rule of thumb, as SaO_2 drops below 90%, the PaO_2 can be estimated by subtracting 30 points from the SaO_2. For example, a SaO_2 of 85% corresponds to a PaO_2 of 55 mm Hg. Second, the pulse oximeter measures saturation (milliliters of oxygen per deciliters of blood) and not arterial content or oxygen delivery to tissues.

Because a traditional pulse oximeter uses only two wavelengths of light, it cannot detect the presence of carboxyhemoglobin (carbon monoxide poisoning) or methemoglobin. Recently introduced pulse oximeters incorporate additional wavelengths of light and are capable of detecting carboxyhemoglobin and methemoglobin.[44]

Despite the potential drawbacks, the pulse oximeter has been shown to be impressively accurate in a wide variety of patients with a tremendous variation in pulse amplitude.[45]

Ventilation Monitors

By definition, a patient is appropriately ventilated when arterial carbon dioxide tension ($PaCO_2$) is 40 mm Hg. Measuring the respiratory rate can document only the presence of ventilation, not its adequacy. Capnography, or end-tidal CO_2 monitoring, is the visual display of the CO_2 concentration at the airway. To understand the utility of capnography, one must understand dead-space components and how they affect CO_2 removal from the body.[46] Dead space (DS) is defined as the portion of the tidal volume (VT) that does not participate in gas exchange.

$$VT = DS + VA$$

The alveolar volume (VA) is the volume of the inspired gas that reaches well-perfused alveoli. The remainder of the VT, which equals the DS, can be divided into three subcomponents: apparatus dead space (DS_{ap}), anatomic dead space (DS_{an}), and alveolar dead space (DS_{al}). At the end of inspiration, the respiratory apparatus (e.g., endotracheal tube) is filled with inspired gas that should not contain CO_2. Similarly, all the anatomic airways (trachea, bronchi, and all conducting airways down to the alveoli) should be filled with inspired gas and should therefore contain no CO_2. In this model, there are two types of alveoli: those that are well perfused and those that are not perfused. The alveolar gas should completely equilibrate with the arterial blood and contain CO_2 at the same tension as the arterial blood; ideally, $PaCO_2$ should equal 40 mm Hg. As the patient expires, the CO_2 detected at the patient's mouth first reflects the DS_{ap} gas having no CO_2; followed by the DS_{an} gas, again with no CO_2; and finally the alveolar gases, containing both dead-space and well-perfused alveolar gas. When mixed alveolar gas reaches the airway, it produces a rapid rise in the CO_2 concentration to a level somewhere between the concentration in the alveolar gas (40 mm Hg) and the DS_{al} (0 mm Hg), depending on each component's proportion of volume. For example, if half of the alveoli are DS_{al} and $PaCO_2$ equals 40 mm Hg, then the plateau value of the capnogram should be 20 mm Hg, implying that half of the alveoli are not being perfused. With inspiration, the CO_2 value again drops to 0 until another expiration, and a square wave appears again as the alveolar gas is detected at the mouth. With each breath, there should be a square wave, whose height approaches the $PaCO_2$ value as the amount of the DS_{al} gas approaches 0.

In a healthy young adult, there is no significant DS_{al} gas, and the end-tidal CO_2 value equals the $PaCO_2$. Therefore, the difference between these values indicates the proportion of DS_{al} in the patient. The presence of a capnogram itself implies that there is metabolism (the production of CO_2), circulation (blood flow to the lungs), and ventilation (respiratory rate and an intact ventilator circuit).

Providing this information on a breath-to-breath basis, the continuous capnogram is extremely useful in many critical situations. It can be used as a surveillance monitor of both the respiratory circuit and the cardiovascular system. Any acute decrease in cardiac output will decrease blood flow to the lungs and increase the DS_{al}, causing an acute drop in end-tidal CO_2. For this reason, the device was originally used during neurosurgical procedures in the sitting position to detect the presence of air emboli. This principle also allows the detection of pulmonary emboli or any acute drop in cardiac output. In fact, the only acute catastrophic cardiopulmonary problem that will not be detected by the capnometer is arterial desaturation. Therefore, the combination of the capnometer and the pulse oximeter creates a dynamic duo for beat-to-beat and breath-to-breath surveillance of metabolism, circulation, ventilation, and oxygenation.

Circulation Monitors

Hemodynamic stability can be monitored by a variety of methods, the most basic of which is systemic arterial blood pressure. Intermittent, noninvasive measurement of systemic blood pressure with an oscillometric blood pressure cuff is the standard in the operating room, and its accuracy equals that of clinical measurements by auscultation. Blood pressure cuffs can be cycled as quickly as once per minute, but when used for an extended duration, they should be cycled no more than once every 3 to 5 minutes. When tighter control or observation is required in patients with significant comorbidities or large swings in hemodynamics due to surgical circumstances, invasive arterial monitoring is used. Although pressure measurements provided by invasive techniques are different from those of noninvasive techniques, they usually coincide closely. A continuous invasive arterial tracing can also be used to assess the adequacy of fluid resuscitation by following the systolic pressure variation (SPV) with positive-
11 pressure ventilation. As positive-pressure ventilation impedes venous return within a closed thorax, decreases in systolic pressure associated with a respiratory pattern can be detected. In patients with sinus rhythm with stable cardiac contractility, the degree of SPV reflects the intravascular volume status of the patient. The normal range of SPV is 5 to 10 mm Hg. A systolic pressure decrease of greater than 10 mm Hg during positive-pressure ventilation implies inadequate preload and the need for more aggressive fluid resuscitation.[47]

In this context, central venous access may be reserved for patients and procedures with the potential for large, rapid volume resuscitation requirements. Transesophageal echocardiography (TEE) is now commonly used to assess cardiac function. This technique is easily used in the anesthetized, intubated patient and can quickly assess systolic and diastolic function as well as valvular dysfunction. Increasing familiarity in the use of TEE by noncardiac anesthesiologists may result in the pulmonary artery catheter being reserved for very specific patients demonstrating the need for pulmonary artery pressure monitoring or continuous cardiac output trending.

"Awareness" and Level of Consciousness Monitors

When delivering a general anesthetic, one of the major imperatives is to achieve and maintain a loss of consciousness. Normally, this is achieved through careful observation of vital signs (heart rate, blood pressure), physical examination signs (movement in a patient without neuromuscular blockade), and delivery of inhalational or intravenous agents at doses consistent with a loss of consciousness. However, this "science" is inexact and must account for patient age, comorbidities, chronic medications, surgical stimulus, and patient-to-patient variability. As a result, patients may rarely experience "awareness under anesthesia"—a state characterized not only by consciousness but also by recall of intraoperative events. The laypress and public have increased their scrutiny of this perioperative event.

First, appropriate expectations and effective communication of the anesthetic are required. Recent literature has demonstrated that patients undergoing regional anesthesia are as likely to report unpleasant "awareness" as patients undergoing a general anesthetic.[48] This is despite the reality that loss of consciousness is only a goal of general anesthesia. Clearly, anesthesiologists must communicate the anesthetic plan and expectations more accurately.

Second, several level of consciousness monitors have been developed in hopes of providing the anesthesiologist with additional objective data to guide their assessment and actions. The current generation of monitors generally uses electroencephalographic (EEG) analysis to provide the clinician with an assessment of the relative "depth" of anesthesia achieved. Several commercially available monitors such as the bispectral index (BIS) from Aspect Medical Systems and Entropy from General Electric Healthcare are in common clinical use. Data evaluating the value of these EEG-based monitors in reducing awareness are conflicting, with several large trials producing varying results.[49,50] As a result, the ASA has not adopted awareness monitors as a standard of care and leaves the decision to use such monitoring technology to each provider, patient, and situation.[51] Further large, randomized studies comparing EEG-based monitoring techniques to routine clinical care in a typical general surgery population are currently under way and may provide valuable data.

COMMON PROBLEMS IN THE POSTOPERATIVE PERIOD

Postanesthesia care units are required in any setting where surgical procedures are conducted. The increased scope of surgery and the invasive technology used to monitor sicker patients has increased the service at and training required to operate these facilities. In 1994, the ASA revised the 1988 Standards for Postanesthesia Care (Table 12.15).

The scoring systems used to assess the postoperative patient direct attention to the primary areas of concern. The postanesthesia recovery score is an attempt to evaluate postanesthesia patient status[52] (Table 12.16). This basic information should be incorporated in a record that provides clear documentation of postoperative events. Documentation should also include details of postoperative outpatient care, with a note indicating postoperative telephone contact made to elucidate problems. Problems should receive appropriate follow-up, and written postoperative discharge instructions should be provided for the patient.

Investigators have reported that 24% of patients experience a postanesthesia care unit complication. Nausea, vomiting, and the need for airway support constitute 70% of these complications[53] (Fig. 12.2). The need to maintain airway support was by far the most common respiratory complication. The duration of the procedure as well as ASA classification and type of procedure had a significant bearing on the incidence of complications in this study. Hypothermia was also a common problem that prolonged postoperative postanesthesia care unit stay (Fig. 12.3). Hypothermia has the deleterious effects of altering drug metabolism and delaying recovery. Furthermore, it causes shivering, which increases the metabolic demand for oxygen.

Among cardiovascular complications in the postoperative period, none is more important or more difficult to diagnose than myocardial ischemia. The association of perioperative myocardial ischemia with cardiac morbidity has been clearly documented.[25] In a series of high-risk patients undergoing noncardiac surgery, researchers noted that "early postoperative myocardial ischemia is an important correlate of adverse cardiac outcomes."[25] Diagnosis is complicated by the fact that only 10% to 30% of patients suffering documented myocardial infarction have pain and that postoperative ECG T-wave changes are often nonspecific.[54] Instead, one must seek secondary indications of ongoing ischemia or "angina equivalents," such as hypotension, arrhythmias, elevated filling pressures, or postoperative oliguria. Arrhythmias are common and are significant primarily because of the association with myocardial ischemia or hypoxemia.

Nausea and vomiting are rarely unifactorial and cause considerable discomfort to patients. Opioids are responsible for stimulating the emesis center in a significant cohort of patients. These patients may provide a clear history of opioid sensitivity and anesthetic and analgesic regimens may be tailored to limit the exposure of these patients to these drugs. In general, however, there is little evidence to favor one anesthetic or anesthetic technique over another, although propofol appears to have an antiemetic effect. Nitrous oxide, often considered causative, does not appear to increase the incidence of nausea according to well-documented studies. It is not unusual for an antiemetic agent to be included preoperatively or as part of the anesthetic technique, especially in patients with a positive history or those deemed to be at risk, such as menstruating young women undergoing laparoscopy. Standard usage includes phenothiazines, butyrophenones, $5HT_3$ antagonists, and steroids. A multimodal approach that avoids redosing of a given medication class has been demonstrated to be most beneficial.[55] Despite decades of research, classic medications such as droperidol remain a mainstay of therapy. The FDA recently added a black-box warning to droperidol due to concerns of QT prolongation, but such concerns have not been validated when compared to other perioperative medications; as a result, many institutions continue to use droperidol for postoperative nausea and vomiting prophylaxis.[56,57]

The most common cause of delayed emergence is the residual effects of anesthesia. The differential diagnosis of delayed emergence is best approached by ruling out physiologic, pharmacologic, and neurologic cases, in this order (Table 12.17). There should be little confusion about the implication of muscle relaxants because physical indications of ventilatory distress, combined with the readings of the blockade monitor, should clearly indicate the role of these drugs. Where appropriate, opioids can be reversed using titrated doses of naloxone. Flumazenil can be used for reversal of benzodiazepines.

POSTOPERATIVE ACUTE PAIN MANAGEMENT

Postoperative pain is an inevitable consequence of surgery. Its severity is site dependent (Table 12.18), but the magnitude of the pain experienced by individual patients after similar surgical procedures is influenced by a multitude of factors. Variation in patient experience has been clearly demonstrated by several authors and is reflected in deficiencies in postoperative pain control.[58] The recognition of this clinical problem has prompted interest in underlying pain mechanisms and in innovative ways to alleviate postoperative suffering.

In 1965, the crucial role of nociceptive C fiber feedback behavior and its modulation by cells in the substantia gelatinosa of the dorsal horn was recognized.[59] Repetitive stimulation of these fibers by cellular mediators, such as kinins and catecholamines, promotes neural excitation, prolongs repetitive firing, and lowers the threshold to further excitation. As a

TABLE 12.15

STANDARDS FOR POSTANESTHESIA CARE

■ STANDARDS		■ CRITERIA TO BE FULFILLED
Standard I[a]	All patients who have received general, regional, or monitored anesthesia care shall receive appropriate postanesthesia management.	1. A PACU or an area that provides equivalent postanesthesia care shall be available to receive patients after anesthesia care. All patients who receive anesthesia care shall be admitted to the PACU or its equivalent *except* by specific order of the anesthesiologist responsible for the patient's care. 2. The medical aspects of care in the PACU shall be governed by policies and procedures that have been reviewed and approved by the department of anesthesiology. 3. The design, equipment, and staffing of the PACU shall meet requirements of the facility's accrediting and licensing bodies.
Standard II	A patient transported to the PACU shall be accompanied by a member of the anesthesia care team who is knowledgeable about the patient's condition. The patient shall be continually evaluated and treated during transport with monitoring and support appropriate to the patient's condition.	
Standard III	On arrival in the PACU, the patient shall be reevaluated and a verbal report provided to the responsible PACU nurse by the member of the anesthesia care team who accompanies the patient.	1. The patient's status on arrival in the PACU shall be documented. 2. Information concerning the preoperative condition and the surgical/anesthetic course shall be transmitted to the PACU nurse. 3. The member of the anesthesia care team shall remain in the PACU until the PACU nurse accepts responsibility for the nursing care of the patient.
Standard IV	The patient's condition shall be evaluated continually in the PACU.	1. The patient shall be observed and monitored by the methods appropriate to the patient's medical condition. Particular attention shall be given to monitoring oxygenation, ventilation, circulation, and temperature. During recovery from all anesthetics, a quantitative method of assessing oxygenation such as pulse oximetry shall be employed in the initial phase of recovery. This is not intended for application during the recovery of the obstetric patient in whom regional anesthesia was used for labor and vaginal delivery. 2. An accurate written report of the PACU period shall be maintained. Use of an appropriate PACU scoring system is encouraged for each patient on admission, at appropriate intervals prior to discharge, and at the time of discharge. 3. General medical supervision and coordination of patient care in the PACU should be the responsibility of an anesthesiologist. 4. There shall be a policy to ensure the availability in the facility of a physician capable of managing complications and providing cardiopulmonary resuscitation for patients in the PACU.
Standard V	A physician is responsible for discharging the patient from the PACU.	1. When discharge criteria are used, they must be approved by the department of anesthesiology and the medical staff. They may vary depending on whether the patient is discharged to a hospital room, tothe ICU, to a short stay unit, or home. 2. In the absence of the physician responsible for the discharge, the PACU nurse shall determine that the patient meets the discharge criteria. The name of the physician accepting responsibility for discharge shall be noted on the record.

ICU, intensive care unit; PACU, postanesthesia care unit.
[a]For nursing care issues, refer to Standards of Postanesthesia Nursing Practice, published by the American Society of Postanesthesia Nurses.
Based on the American Society of Anesthesiologists (ASA)'s Standards for Postanesthesia Care. A copy of the full text can be obtained from ASA, 520 N. Northwest Highway, Park Ridge, IL 60068-2573.

TABLE 12.16

POSTANESTHESIA RECOVERY SCORE[a]

■ PARAMETER	■ SCORE
ACTIVITY	
Voluntary movement of all limbs to command	2
Voluntary movement of two extremities to command	1
Unable to move	0
RESPIRATION	
Breathes deeply and coughs	2
Dyspnea, hypoventilation	1
Apneic	0
CIRCULATION	
Blood pressure equals 80% of preanesthetic level	2
Blood pressure equals 50%–80% of preanesthetic level	1
Blood pressure equals <50% of preanesthetic level	0
CONSCIOUSNESS	
Fully awake	2
Arousable	1
Unresponsive	0
COLOR	
Pink	2
Pale, blotchy	1
Cyanotic	0

[a]Patients should score at least 7 before discharge from the postanesthesia care unit.

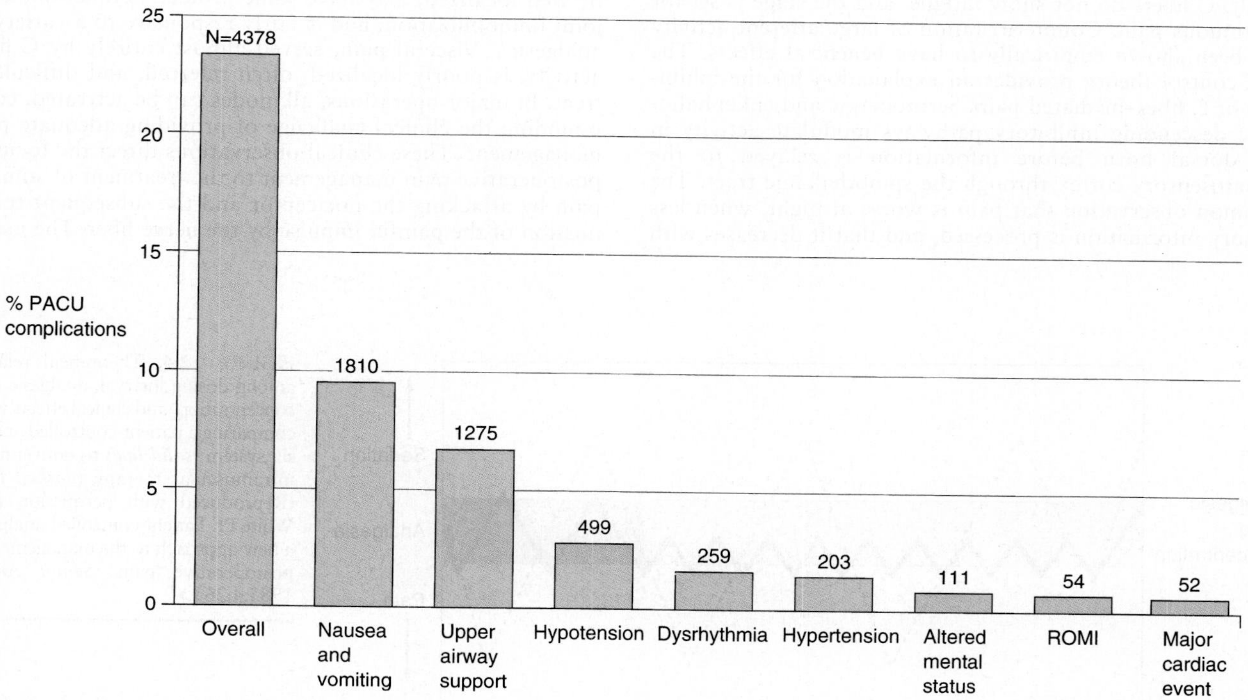

FIGURE 12.2. Major postanesthesia care unit complications by percentage of occurrence and number of patients experiencing each complication. Nausea and vomiting were the most frequently observed complications. ROMI, rule out myocardial infarction. (Reproduced with permission from Hines R, Barash PG, Watrous G, et al. Complications occurring in the postanesthesia care unit: a survey. *Anesth Analg* 1992;74:505.)

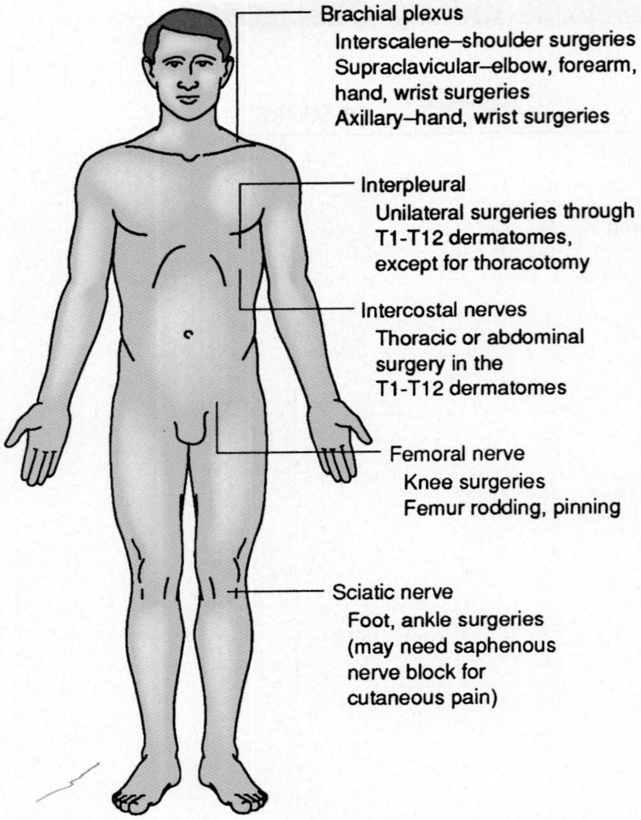

FIGURE 12.3. Surgical procedures in which peripheral nerve blockade can provide postoperative pain relief.

TABLE 12.17

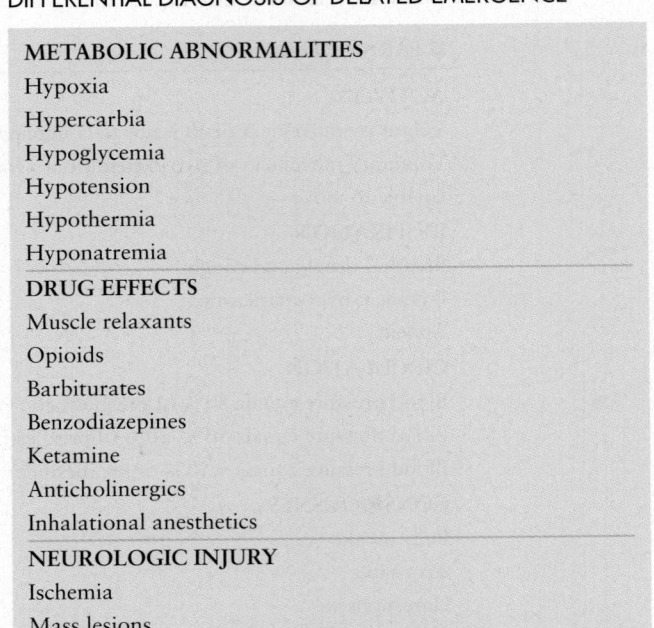

DIFFERENTIAL DIAGNOSIS OF DELAYED EMERGENCE

METABOLIC ABNORMALITIES
Hypoxia
Hypercarbia
Hypoglycemia
Hypotension
Hypothermia
Hyponatremia
DRUG EFFECTS
Muscle relaxants
Opioids
Barbiturates
Benzodiazepines
Ketamine
Anticholinergics
Inhalational anesthetics
NEUROLOGIC INJURY
Ischemia
Mass lesions
Seizure disorders

result, C fibers do not show fatigue, and the stage is set for continuous pain. Counterirritation of large afferent activity has been shown empirically to have beneficial effects. The gate-control theory provides an explanation for the inhibition of C fiber–mediated pain. Serotonergic and enkephalinergic descending inhibitory pathways modulate activity in the dorsal horn before information is relayed to the somatosensory cortex through the spinothalamic tract. The common observation that pain is worse at night, when less sensory information is processed, and that it decreases with daytime activity is an example of how this complex neural system functions.

Superficial somatic pain is well localized and has a protective function. Superficial somatic pain is readily treated by common analgesic techniques. Deep somatic pain may not be well localized; may have some protective function, as in joint immobilization; and is fairly responsive to a variety of analgesics. Visceral pain, served almost entirely by C fiber activity, is poorly localized, often referred, and difficult to treat. In major operations, all modes can be activated, compounding the clinical challenge of providing adequate pain management. These clinical observations direct the focus of postoperative pain management to the treatment of somatic pain by attacking the nociceptor and the subsequent transmission of the painful impulse by the nerve fiber. The use of

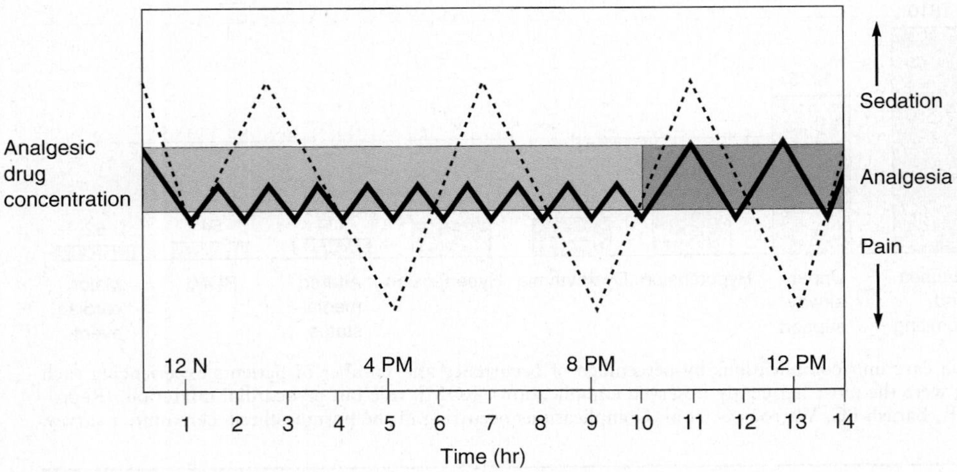

FIGURE 12.4. Theoretical relation among dosing interval, analgesic drug concentration, and clinical effects when comparing a patient-controlled analgesia system (*solid line*) to conventional intramuscular therapy (*dashed line*). (Reproduced with permission from White PF. Patient-controlled analgesia: a new approach to the management of postoperative pain. *Semin Anesth* 1985;4:261.)

TABLE 12.18

PERCENTAGE OF PATIENTS WHO REQUIRE ANALGESIC INJECTIONS

OPERATION	NO ANALGESIC NEEDED (%)	THREE OR MORE ANALGESIC INJECTIONS (%)
Minor chest wall	82	0
Inguinal hernia	52	0
Appendectomy	25	10
Lower abdominal surgery	18	40
Upper abdominal surgery	10	45–65

TABLE 12.19

PROBLEMS THAT CAN OCCUR DURING PATIENT-CONTROLLED ANALGESIA (PCA) THERAPY

OPERATOR ERRORS
Misprogramming PCA device
Failure to clamp or unclamp tubing
Improperly loading syringe or cartridge
Inability to respond to safety alarms
Misplacing PCA pump key
PATIENT ERRORS
Failure to understand PCA therapy
Misunderstanding PCA pump device
Intentional analgesic abuse
MECHANICAL ERRORS
Failure to deliver on demand
Defective one-way valve at Y-connector
Faulty alarm system
Device malfunctions

nonsteroidal anti-inflammatory drugs with or without the injection of local anesthetics into the wound is very effective. If done preemptively at the time of surgery, this approach can significantly benefit the patient's postoperative experience.[60] Examples of nerve blocks for various procedures are shown in Figure 12.4.

Including potent opioids in the treatment of deep pain, both somatic and visceral, has been routine. However, the responses to standard regimens have been notoriously unreliable, from inadequate pain relief to narcosis, with complications at both ends of the scale. It was not until the 1980s that variations in response were linked to variable serum concentrations of analgesic drugs. Interpatient variation in serum levels to any standard dose can be fivefold, and interpatient therapeutic concentrations can vary on a similar scale. When factored together, there is the potential for a 25-fold variation in patient response to a standard drug prescription. Each patient has an individual therapeutic window. The clinical implications are enormous.

In 1968, investigators demonstrated the virtue of small IV doses given on demand.[60] As a result, the patient experienced greater pain relief, yet used the same or less total narcotic. Although there was significant patient variation, the demand from any individual patient, though cyclic, was constant. Patient-controlled analgesia (PCA) and the technologic and administrative systems to provide it have developed to a point of some sophistication, requiring servicing and a support structure with its own set of problems (Table 12.19). PCA administration requires a receptive environment, education of all personnel, and adequate patient instruction. PCA has received widespread acceptance by patients, nursing staff, and physicians because it provides more prompt and painless analgesia that more closely matches the patient's need over time. PCA is as safe as conventional IM medication. Morphine and meperidine are commonly used drugs, and an example of orders is shown in Table 12.20.

Transdermal narcotic delivery is receiving attention and may become available for postoperative pain. The method is both practical and inexpensive and aims to maintain continuous delivery and constant blood levels. Fentanyl has been the drug of choice and has been well received by patients. The method appears to be safe, but there is a significant lag time between application and the attainment of therapeutic blood levels.

The discovery of endorphins in the 1970s and recognition of their importance in modulating pain at spinal sites led to the supposition that it would be possible to selectively apply opioids directly to receptors. This led to the development of epidural opiate analgesia, in which opioids are applied directly to the receptors at spinal sites. The goal of epidural analgesia is to obtain maximal analgesia while minimizing systemic side effects. For severe acute postoperative pain caused by major surgery, epidural analgesia has proved to be a superior modality

TABLE 12.20

EXAMPLE OF ORDERS FOR PATIENT-CONTROLLED ANALGESIA (PCA)

1. Patient is to be initiated on PCA with standard monitoring protocol.		
2. Drug selection	Morphine 1 mg/mL	Hydromorphone 0.2 mg/mL
3. Loading initial dose (start PRN for pain)	2–5 mg	0.2–0.5 mg
Maximum total loading dose	10 mg	1 mg
4. Pump setting PCA dose	1–2 mg	0.1–0.2 mg
Lockout interval	6–10 min	6–10 min
4-Hour limit	30–45 mg	4–5 mg

University of Michigan Hospitals online order form Acute Pain Service, Patient Controlled Analgesia Standard Orders.

SCIENTIFIC PRINCIPLES

TABLE 12.21

OPIOID PROTOCOLS IN EPIDURAL OPIATE ANALGESIA

	MORPHINE[a]	FENTANYL[b]
Length of onset	Longer (30–60 min)	Shorter (15–30 min)
Duration	Longer (6–24 h for single bolus)	Shorter (1–2 h for single bolus)
Cephalad spread and side effects	More prone	Less prone
Indication	Favored for lumbar administration after abdominal surgery	Favored for thoracic administration after chest surgery
Dose	Typically 3–5 mg, q6–8h	Typically 50–75 mg/h (±dilute bupivacaine)

[a]Hydrophilic: slow in, slow out.
[b]Lipophilic: fast in, fast out.

for pain control. In high-risk cases, there is evidence that it has an overall beneficial effect on morbidity.[38]

The effective use of this sophisticated modality requires education and the establishment of protocols with rigorous attention to detail. The potential for respiratory depression demands adherence to monitoring standards. Morphine and fentanyl, often in combination with a dilute local anesthetic solution, are most often prescribed. A typical order form with monitored parameters is shown in Table 12.21.

A comprehensive postoperative pain management service demands resources and must use the physical and pharmacologic modalities available while recognizing the significant subjective component of any individual's pain problem. The ability to recognize the impact of acute pain or an underlying chronic pain disorder requires that experience be brought to bear on difficult problems. The active involvement of nursing staff and surgeons is essential for the patient to achieve maximal benefit. It is incumbent on the pain-management service to render efficient, continuous, and cost-effective care.

12 Postoperative acute pain management may require a multimodal approach that incorporates opioids, peripheral nerve blockade, and nonopioid analgesics. Chronic pain patients can be particularly difficult to manage and may require preoperative optimization by an anesthesiologist. These patients require very large doses of IV analgesics and need to be maintained orally. The best way to evaluate an appropriate starting dose is to convert the preoperative opioid regimen to an IV morphine equivalent then add what would be required to treat

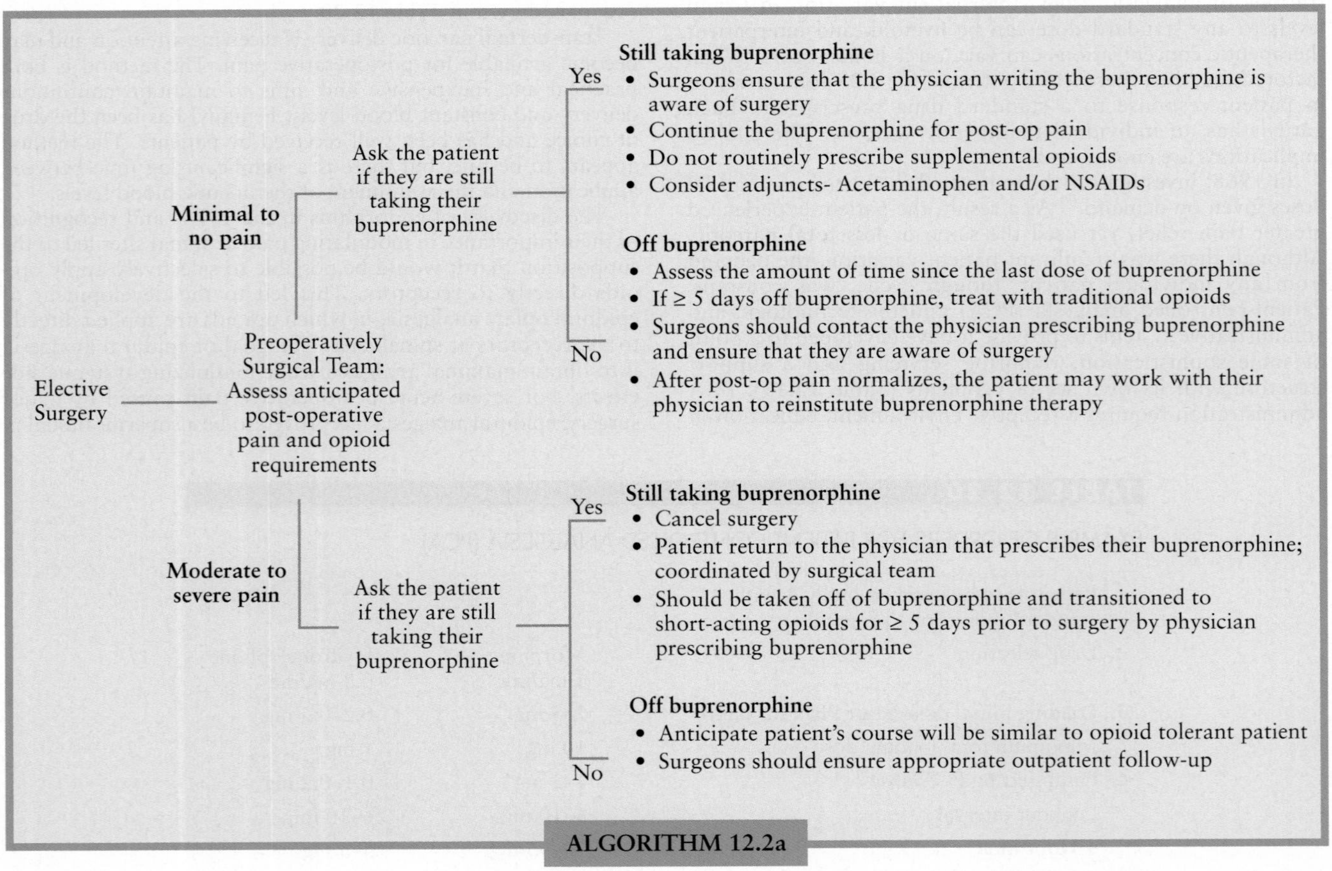
Elective Surgery
Preoperatively Surgical Team: Assess anticipated post-operative pain and opioid requirements
Minimal to no pain
Ask the patient if they are still taking their buprenorphine
Yes
Still taking buprenorphine
• Surgeons ensure that the physician writing the buprenorphine is aware of surgery
• Continue the buprenorphine for post-op pain
• Do not routinely prescribe supplemental opioids
• Consider adjuncts- Acetaminophen and/or NSAIDs
No
Off buprenorphine
• Assess the amount of time since the last dose of buprenorphine
• If ≥ 5 days off buprenorphine, treat with traditional opioids
• Surgeons should contact the physician prescribing buprenorphine and ensure that they are aware of surgery
• After post-op pain normalizes, the patient may work with their physician to reinstitute buprenorphine therapy
Moderate to severe pain
Ask the patient if they are still taking their buprenorphine
Yes
Still taking buprenorphine
• Cancel surgery
• Patient return to the physician that prescribes their buprenorphine; coordinated by surgical team
• Should be taken off of buprenorphine and transitioned to short-acting opioids for ≥ 5 days prior to surgery by physician prescribing buprenorphine
No
Off buprenorphine
• Anticipate patient's course will be similar to opioid tolerant patient
• Surgeons should ensure appropriate outpatient follow-up
ALGORITHM 12.2a

ALGORITHM 12.2. Algorithm for managing a patient on chronic buprenorphine therapy. APS, acute pain service; ICU, intensive care unit; PCA, patient-controlled anesthesia; NSAIDs, nonsteroidal anti-inflammatory drugs. (*continued*)

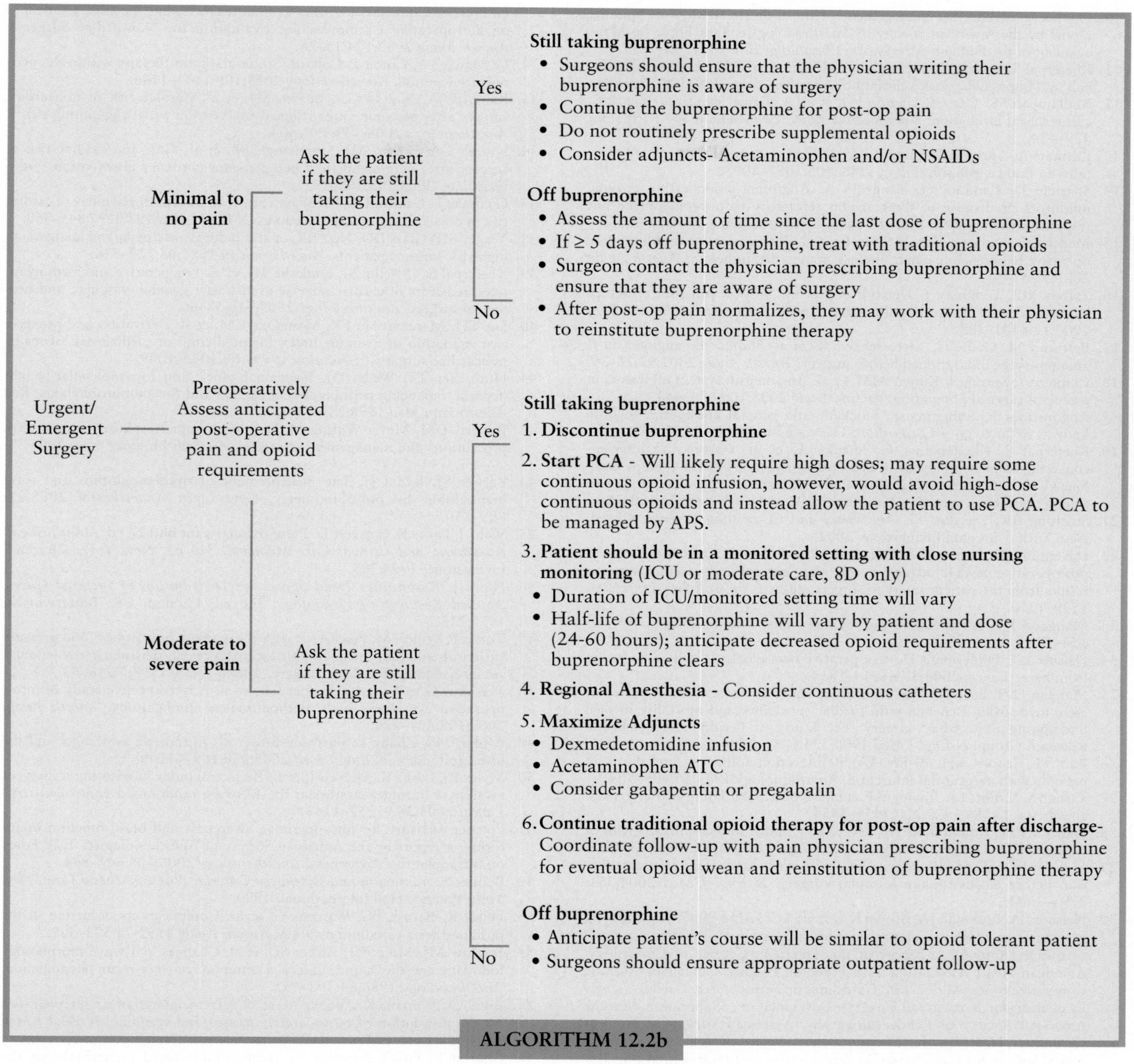
Urgent/ Emergent Surgery
Preoperatively Assess anticipated post-operative pain and opioid requirements
Minimal to no pain
Ask the patient if they are still taking their buprenorphine
Yes
Still taking buprenorphine
• Surgeons should ensure that the physician writing their buprenorphine is aware of surgery
• Continue the buprenorphine for post-op pain
• Do not routinely prescribe supplemental opioids
• Consider adjuncts- Acetaminophen and/or NSAIDs
No
Off buprenorphine
• Assess the amount of time since the last dose of buprenorphine
• If ≥ 5 days off buprenorphine, treat with traditional opioids
• Surgeon contact the physician prescribing buprenorphine and ensure that they are aware of surgery
• After post-op pain normalizes, they may work with their physician to reinstitute buprenorphine therapy
Moderate to severe pain
Ask the patient if they are still taking their buprenorphine
Yes
Still taking buprenorphine
1. Discontinue buprenorphine
2. Start PCA - Will likely require high doses; may require some continuous opioid infusion, however, would avoid high-dose continuous opioids and instead allow the patient to use PCA. PCA to be managed by APS.
3. Patient should be in a monitored setting with close nursing monitoring (ICU or moderate care, 8D only)
• Duration of ICU/monitored setting time will vary
• Half-life of buprenorphine will vary by patient and dose (24-60 hours); anticipate decreased opioid requirements after buprenorphine clears
4. Regional Anesthesia - Consider continuous catheters
5. Maximize Adjuncts
• Dexmedetomidine infusion
• Acetaminophen ATC
• Consider gabapentin or pregabalin
6. Continue traditional opioid therapy for post-op pain after discharge- Coordinate follow-up with pain physician prescribing buprenorphine for eventual opioid wean and reinstitution of buprenorphine therapy
No
Off buprenorphine
• Anticipate patient's course will be similar to opioid tolerant patient
• Surgeons should ensure appropriate outpatient follow-up
ALGORITHM 12.2b

ALGORITHM 12.2. (*Continued*)

the acute surgical pain (see Table 12.4). The use of nonopioid and nonpharmacologic treatments is essential in the management of acute postoperative pain in this patient population. Peripheral nerve blockade, aggressive use of acetaminophen and nonsteroidal anti-inflammatory agents, and novel agents such as dexmedetomidine may be necessary to minimize the adverse effects associated with uncontrolled postoperative pain. As mentioned earlier, these patients may need to be evaluated by an anesthesiologist prior to the day of surgery. This should be an institutional requirement for patients on chronic buprenorphine therapy, as demonstrated in Algorithm 12.2.

References

1. Calverly R. Anesthesia as a specialty: past, present and future. In: Barash P, Cullen B, Stoelting R, eds. *Clinical Anesthesia* Philadelphia, PA: JB Lippincott, 1992.
2. Plaud B, Meretoja O, Hofmockel R, et al. Reversal of rocuronium-induced neuromuscular blockade with sugammadex in pediatric and adult surgical patients. *Anesthesiology* 2009;110:284–294.
3. Watling SM, Dasta JF. Prolonged paralysis in intensive care unit patients after the use of neuromuscular blocking agents: a review of the literature. *Crit Care Med* 1994;22:884–893.
4. Kam PC, Cardone D. Propofol infusion syndrome. *Anaesthesia* 2007;62: 690–701.
5. Rosenberg JM, Wahr JA, Sung CH, et al. Coronary perfusion pressure during cardiopulmonary resuscitation after spinal anesthesia in dogs. *Anesth Analg* 1996;82:84–87.
6. Drasner K, Smiley R. Continuous spinal analgesia for labor and delivery: a born-again technique? *Anesthesiology* 2008;108:184–186.
7. Standl TG. Catheter tip position and baricity of the local anesthetic have an impact on maldistribution in microcatheter CSA. *Anesthesiology* 1999; 90:1227–1229.
8. The Joint Commission on Accreditation of Healthcare Organizations (JCAHO). *Comprehensive Accreditation Manual for Hospitals: The Official Handbook: Conscious Sedations*. Oakbrook Terrace, IL: JCAHO; 1999:73–77.
9. Naughton N. *Sedation Analgesia for Diagnostic and Therapeutic Procedures.* New Jersey: Human Press; 2003.

10. Practice guidelines for management of the difficult airway: an updated report by the American Society of Anesthesiologists Task Force on Management of the Difficult Airway. *Anesthesiology* 2003;98:1269–1277.
11. Kheterpal S, Han R, Tremper KK, et al. Incidence and predictors of difficult and impossible mask ventilation. *Anesthesiology* 2006;105:885–891.
12. Mallampati SR, Gatt SP, Gugino LD, et al. A clinical sign to predict difficult tracheal intubation: a prospective study. *Can Anaesth Soc J* 1985;32: 429–434.
13. Lienhart A, Auroy Y, Pequignot F, et al. Survey of anesthesia-related mortality in France. *Anesthesiology* 2006;105:1087–1097.
14. Sparicio D, Landoni G, Zangrillo A. Angiotensin-converting enzyme inhibitors predispose to hypotension refractory to norepinephrine but responsive to methylene blue. *J Thorac Cardiovasc Surg* 2004;127:608.
15. Medel J, Boccara G, Van de Steen E, et al. Terlipressin for treating intraoperative hypotension: can it unmask myocardial ischemia? *Anesth Analg* 2001;93:53–55.
16. Talbot MP, Tremblay I, Denault AY, et al. Vasopressin for refractory hypotension during cardiopulmonary bypass. *J Thorac Cardiovasc Surg* 2000;120:401–402.
17. Bertrand M, Godet G, Meersschaert K, et al. Should the angiotensin II antagonists be discontinued before surgery? *Anesth Analg* 2001;92:26–30.
18. Comfere T, Sprung J, Kumar MM, et al. Angiotensin system inhibitors in a general surgical population. *Anesth Analg* 2005;100:636–644.
19. Augoustides JG. Angiotensin blockade and general anesthesia: so little known, so far to go. *J Cardiothorac Vasc Anesth* 2008;22:177–179.
20. Kheterpal S, Khodaparast O, Shanks A, et al. Chronic angiotensin-converting enzyme inhibitor or angiotensin receptor blocker therapy combined with diuretic therapy is associated with increased episodes of hypotension in noncardiac surgery. *J Cardiothorac Vasc Anesth* 2008;22:180–186.
21. Stoelting RK, Dierdorf SF. *Anesthesia and Co-existing Disease*, 4th ed. New York: Churchill Livingstone; 2002.
22. Davenport DL, Ferraris VA, Hosokawa P, et al. Multivariable predictors of postoperative cardiac adverse events after general and vascular surgery: results from the patient safety in surgery study. *J Am Coll Surg* 2007;204: 1199–1210.
23. Mangano DT. Perioperative cardiac morbidity. *Anesthesiology* 1990;72: 153–184.
24. Fleisher LA, Poldermans D. Perioperative beta blockade: where do we go from here? *Lancet* 2008;371:1813–1814.
25. Mangano DT, Browner WS, Hollenberg M, et al. Association of perioperative myocardial ischemia with cardiac morbidity and mortality in men undergoing noncardiac surgery. The Study of Perioperative Ischemia Research Group. *N Engl J Med* 1990;323:1781–1788.
26. Rao TL, Jacobs KH, El-Etr AA. Reinfarction following anesthesia in patients with myocardial infarction. *Anesthesiology* 1983;59:499–505.
27. Tarhan S, Moffitt EA, Taylor WF, et al. Myocardial infarction after general anesthesia. *JAMA* 1972;220:1451–1454.
28. Boden WE, O'Rourke RA, Teo KK, et al. Optimal medical therapy with or without PCI for stable coronary disease. *N Engl J Med* 2007;356:1503–1516.
29. McFalls EO, Ward HB, Moritz TE, et al. Coronary-artery revascularization before elective major vascular surgery. *N Engl J Med* 2004;351: 2795–2804.
30. Fleisher LA, Beckman JA, Brown KA, et al. ACC/AHA 2007 Guidelines on perioperative cardiovascular evaluation and care for noncardiac surgery: executive summary: a report of the American College of Cardiology/ American Heart Association Task Force on Practice Guidelines (Writing Committee to Revise the 2002 Guidelines on Perioperative Cardiovascular Evaluation for Noncardiac Surgery): Developed in collaboration with the American Society of Echocardiography, American Society of Nuclear Cardiology, Heart Rhythm Society, Society of Cardiovascular Anesthesiologists, Society for Cardiovascular Angiography and Interventions, Society for Vascular Medicine and Biology, and Society for Vascular Surgery. *Circulation* 2007;116:1971–1996.
31. Devereaux PJ, Yang H, Yusuf S, et al. Effects of extended-release metoprolol succinate in patients undergoing non-cardiac surgery (POISE trial): a randomised controlled trial. *Lancet* 2008;371:1839–1847.
32. Lindenauer PK, Pekow P, Wang K, et al. Perioperative beta-blocker therapy and mortality after major noncardiac surgery. *N Engl J Med* 2005; 353:349–361.
33. Fleisher LA, Beckman JA, Brown KA, et al. ACC/AHA 2006 guideline update on perioperative cardiovascular evaluation for noncardiac surgery: focused update on perioperative beta-blocker therapy—a report of the American College of Cardiology/American Heart Association Task Force on Practice Guidelines (Writing Committee to Update the 2002 Guidelines on Perioperative Cardiovascular Evaluation for Noncardiac Surgery). *Anesth Analg* 2007;104:15–26.
34. Le Manach Y, Coriat P, Collard CD, et al. Statin therapy within the perioperative period. *Anesthesiology* 2008;108:1141–1146.
35. Rabbitts JA, Nuttall GA, Brown MJ, et al. Cardiac risk of noncardiac surgery after percutaneous coronary intervention with drug-eluting stents. *Anesthesiology* 2008;109:596–604.
36. Nuttall GA, Brown MJ, Stombaugh JW, et al. Time and cardiac risk of surgery after bare-metal stent percutaneous coronary intervention. *Anesthesiology* 2008;109:588–595.
37. Goldman L, Caldera DL, Nussbaum SR, et al. Multifactorial index of cardiac risk in noncardiac surgical procedures. *N Engl J Med* 1977;297:845–850.
38. Yeager MP, Glass DD, Neff RK, et al. Epidural anesthesia and analgesia in high-risk surgical patients. *Anesthesiology* 1987;66:729–736.
39. Kheterpal S, O'Reilly M, Englesbe MJ, et al. Preoperative and intraoperative predictors of cardiac adverse events after general, vascular, and urological surgery. *Anesthesiology* 2009;110:58–66.
40. Lee TH, Marcantonio ER, Mangione CM, et al. Derivation and prospective validation of a simple index for prediction of cardiac risk of major noncardiac surgery. *Circulation* 1999;100:1043–1049.
41. Horlocker TT, Wedel DJ. Neuraxial block and low-molecular-weight heparin: balancing perioperative analgesia and thromboprophylaxis. *Reg Anesth Pain Med* 1998;23:164–177.
43. Roberts DM, Meyer-Witting M. High-dose buprenorphine: perioperative precautions and management strategies. *Anaesth Intensive Care* 2005;33: 17–25.
44. Barker SJ, Badal JJ. The measurement of dyshemoglobins and total hemoglobin by pulse oximetry. *Curr Opin Anaesthesiol* 2008;21: 805–810.
45. Wahr J, Parks R, Boisvert D. Pulse oximetry. In: Blitt H, ed. *Monitoring in Anesthesia and Critical Care Medicine,* 3rd ed. New York: Churchill Livingstone; 1994:385.
46. Nunn J. *Respiratory Dead Space and Distribution of Inspired Gases, Applied Respiratory Physiology,* 2nd ed. London, UK: Butterworths; 1977:213.
47. Coriat P, Vrillon M, Perel A, et al. A comparison of systolic blood pressure variations and echocardiographic estimates of end-diastolic left ventricular size in patients after aortic surgery. *Anesth Analg* 1994;78:46–53.
48. Mashour GA, Wang LY, Turner CR, et al. A retrospective study of intraoperative awareness with methodological implications. *Anesth Analg* 2009;108:521–526.
49. Avidan MS, Zhang L, Burnside BA, et al. Anesthesia awareness and the bispectral index. *N Engl J Med* 2008;358:1097–1108.
50. Myles PS, Leslie K, McNeil J, et al. Bispectral index monitoring to prevent awareness during anaesthesia: the B-Aware randomised controlled trial. *Lancet* 2004;363:1757–1763.
51. Practice advisory for intraoperative awareness and brain function monitoring: a report by the American Society of Anesthesiologists Task Force on Intraoperative Awareness. *Anesthesiology* 2006;104:847–864.
52. Bonner S. *Admission and Discharge Criteria. Post Anesthesia Care.* New York: Prentice Hall International; 1990.
53. Hines R, Barash PG, Watrous G, et al. Complications occurring in the postanesthesia care unit: a survey. *Anesth Analg* 1992;74:503–509.
54. Breslow MJ, Miller CF, Parker SD, et al. Changes in T-wave morphology following anesthesia and surgery: a common recovery-room phenomenon. *Anesthesiology* 1986;64:398–402.
55. Apfel CC, Korttila K, Abdalla M, et al. A factorial trial of six interventions for the prevention of postoperative nausea and vomiting. *N Engl J Med* 2004;350:2441–2451.
56. Charbit B, Funck-Brentano C. Droperidol-induced proarrhythmia: the beginning of an answer? *Anesthesiology* 2007;107:524–526.
57. Nuttall GA, Eckerman KM, Jacob KA, et al. Does low-dose droperidol administration increase the risk of drug-induced QT prolongation and torsade de pointes in the general surgical population? *Anesthesiology* 2007; 107:531–536.
58. Marks RM, Sachar EJ. Undertreatment of medical inpatients with narcotic analgesics. *Ann Intern Med* 1973;78:173–181.
59. Melzack R, Wall PD. Pain mechanisms: a new theory. *Science* 1965;150: 971–979.
60. Tverskoy M, Cozacov C, Ayache M, et al. Postoperative pain after inguinal herniorrhaphy with different types of anesthesia. *Anesth Analg* 1990;70:29–35.

CHAPTER 13 ■ CANCER

STEVEN K. LIBUTTI

KEY POINTS

1. There are six important capabilities that a cell or a group of cells must acquire to be capable of growing, invading, and metastasizing and thus becoming a cancer: (a) self-sufficiency in growth signals, (b) insensitivity to antigrowth signals, (c) evading apoptosis, (d) limitless replicative potential, (e) sustained angiogenesis, and (f) tissue invasion and metastases.
2. The ability of a cell to become self-sufficient in its growth and no longer rely on the normal temporal sequences of programmed cell growth is often the result of mutations in the genes involved in growth regulation and control.
3. Transformation from the normal phenotype to invasive malignancy appears to involve a loss of normal tumor suppressive and growth inhibitory responses as well as the acquisition of inappropriate proliferative signals.
4. Angiogenesis is necessary for tumor growth and progression and is a potential site for targeted molecular therapy.
5. Gene therapy and immunotherapy for cancer are areas of active investigation that have not yet reached standard practice.
6. Operative resection or regional therapy of metastatic disease can be helpful for patients.

Few medical diagnoses carry with them the fear and dread that a diagnosis of cancer brings to the patient. Historically, Hippocrates is credited with first distinguishing between benign and malignant tumors. Hippocrates described invasive carcinoma using the Greek term for crab, *karkinos,* based on the similarities between the invasive tongue of solid tumors and the claws of the crab. *Karkinos* forms the root for the term *carcinoma.* The word *cancer* is derived from the Latin, *cancrum,* for crab.

The term has come to represent a constellation of malignant processes involving a host of tissue types, each with differing potentials for invasion and metastases. Each pathologic type of cancer has different approaches for its diagnosis and management. However, there are certain basic characteristics that define the transition from normal cell division and proliferation into abnormal, unregulated growth and invasion, which is the hallmark of cancer. The breadth and depth of information regarding the processes involved in the development, diagnosis, and treatment of cancer are complex; this chapter gives an overview to provide a basis for further investigation and discovery.

EPIDEMIOLOGY

The earliest recorded writings related to cancer were made in the Edwin Smith Papyrus in Egypt around 1600 BC. Since that time and throughout recorded history, references are made to various malignancies of the bone and soft tissue that were attributed to sources as varied as vital humors and parasites. Cancer affects approximately 9.6 million Americans, and a total of 1.4 million new cancer diagnoses and 570,000 cancer-related deaths are expected in the United States in the year 2008. For persons younger than the age of 85, cancer is the leading cause of death in the United States and has been since 1999. Although overall mortality rates from cancer have declined in both men and women, the rate of decline in deaths due to heart disease has been much more rapid (Fig. 13.1).

Between 1995 and 2004, the cancer incidence rates in men stabilized, while the incidence rates in women have stabilized between 1999 and 2004. The overall death rate due to cancer has continued to decease in men since 1990 and in woman since 1991. Cancers differ in men and women by both type and incidence. The most common cancers in men by incidence are prostate (25%), lung and bronchus (15%), and colon and rectum (10%). In women, the most common cancers by incidence are breast (26%), lung and bronchus (14%), and colon and rectum (10%). In both men and women, lung and bronchial cancers continue to account for the largest number of cancer-related deaths (31% men; 26% women). This is followed by prostate cancer in men (10%) and breast cancer in women (15%) accounting for the second most common histologies resulting in death. Colon and rectal cancer remains the third most common cause of cancer-related deaths in both men (8%) and women (9%) (Table 13.1). Although the overall incidence of cancer, as well as mortality due to cancer, decreased between 1994 and 2008, for several tumor types there has been either an increase in incidence or relatively little change over that time. For example, melanoma of the skin increased in incidence among men from 3% to 5% and among women from 3% to 4% between 1994 and 2008. The incidence of thyroid cancer increased from 2% to 4% between 1994 and 2008 for women, in whom thyroid cancer occurs more frequently than in men (3:1). Despite the decline in incidence and associated death among common cancer types in both men and women, cancer continues to pose a significant cost to the United States in both human and financial terms.

In 2003, cancer cost the United States an estimated $189.5 billion. Roughly one third of these costs were due to direct medical costs, and more than two thirds were related to nonmedical costs, including lost productivity and lost workdays. The Centers for Disease Control and Prevention (CDC) has estimated that cancer screening and early detection could reduce colorectal cancer deaths by 30%, breast cancer deaths by 16%, and cervical cancer deaths by 60%. Further, it is estimated that in the year 2003, more than 180,000 cancer deaths were due to the consequences of tobacco use. Although the connection between cigarette smoking and lung cancer is an obvious and well-established one, smoking plays a role in approximately 30% of all other cancer deaths (e.g., kidney, oral, bladder). As newer and more effective adjuvant therapies, most notably, biologic agents, are developed and validated, these costs will undoubtedly increase.

Major efforts are under way in cancer prevention. Some causative agents, such as tobacco, are obvious. Other factors that influence the development of cancer include genetic predisposition, diet and exercise, and environmental factors. For

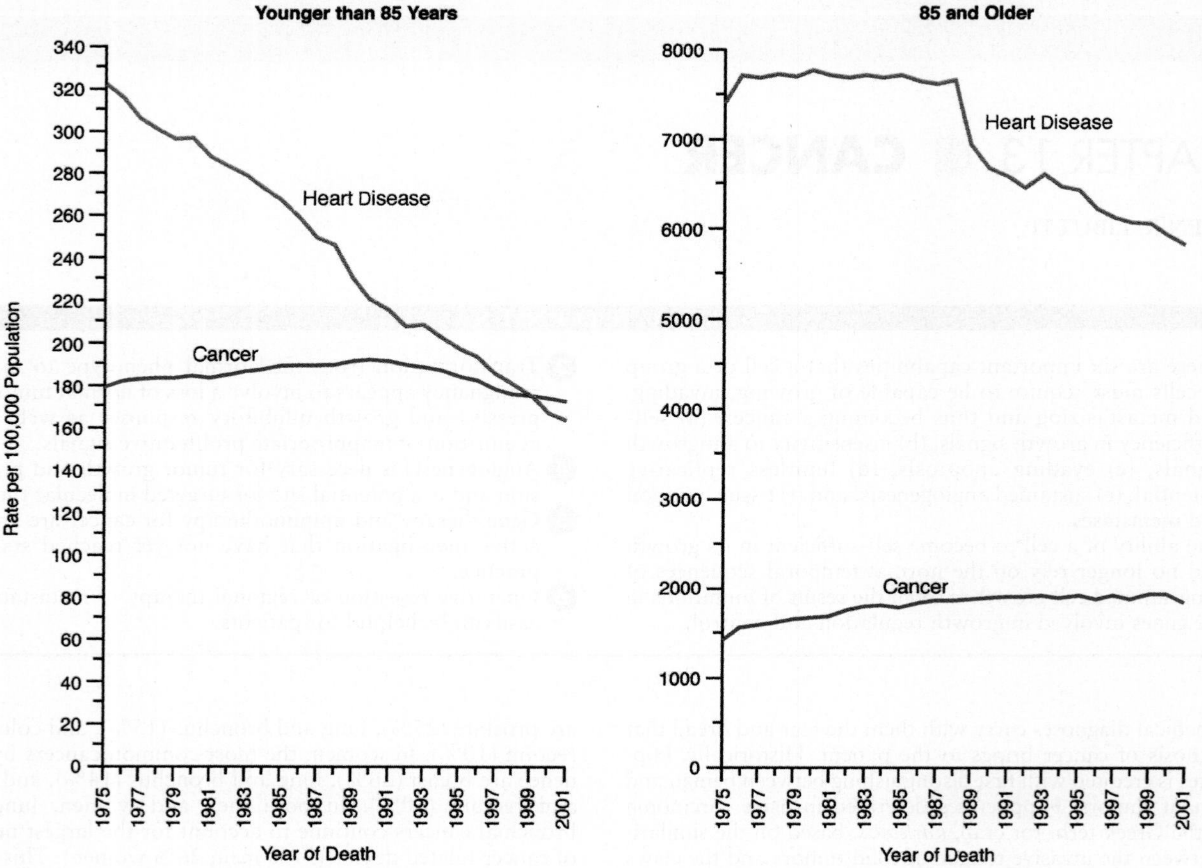

FIGURE 13.1. Age-adjusted death rates from cancer and heart disease. (Jemal A, et al. *CA Cancer J Clin* 2008;58:71–96.)

several cancer types, environmental influences have a complex interaction with other known and unknown factors leading to the development of the disease. For example, chronic hepatitis (both hepatitis B and hepatitis C) increases the incidence of hepatocellular carcinoma, but not all patients with hepatocellular carcinoma have chronic hepatitis, and not all patients with chronic hepatitis develop hepatocellular carcinoma. The relationship of cervical cancer to human papillomavirus (HPV) infection is well established. Estimates for the impact of screening demonstrate that reducing the transmission of HPV could have a significant impact on reducing the incidence of cervical cancer. Recently, a new vaccine for HPV was developed at the National Cancer Institute (NCI) and approved for use in women. A program of early vaccination for at-risk individuals will hopefully lead to a decreased incidence of cervical cancer. Sun exposure (or artificial ultraviolet [UV] light exposure) influences the incidence of melanoma skin cancer; however, melanoma can develop in patients without a significant history of sun or UV exposure. Although some genetic factors, such as mutations in the *BRCA1* or *BRCA2* genes, significantly increase the risk of developing breast cancer, the majority of patients with breast cancer have no such germline mutations. More work is needed to understand the complex interactions of genetics and environment on the cell to better identify avoidable risk factors. This may help to prevent the development of cancer.

ETIOLOGY

At its most basic, cancer can be defined as abnormal cell growth. Often described as a foreign invader in the body, it is more accurate to think of cancer as the body's own cellular growth machinery gone wrong. Throughout history, a variety of theories emerged in an attempt to explain the findings of abnormal tissue growth and invasion. Hippocrates ascribed the formation of cancer to an excess of black bile (one of the four humors or body fluids) collecting in various body sites. This theory was unchallenged through the Middle Ages. In the 18th century, John Hunter was a proponent of the concept that cancer derived from the lymph system. The notion was that tumors arose from lymph, which is constantly expressed by the blood.

In the 19th century, Yohans Mueller dispelled the lymph theory by demonstrating that cancer was made up of cells. However, Mueller did not believe that cancer arose from normal cells but rather from "budding elements" (blastema) that arose between normal tissues. This theory was later rejected by Mueller's student Rudolph Virchow, who demonstrated that all cells, including cancer cells, had their origin from other cells. Virchow proposed that chronic irritation led to the formation of cancer and that cancers could spread through tissues like a fluid. The idea that cancer resulted from irritation and trauma persisted into the 20th century.

Modern thinking recognizes a series of important events that are required for a cell to become cancerous and to grow, 1 invade, and metastasize. Hanahan and Weinberg described six important capabilities that a cell or a group of cells must acquire to be capable of growing, invading, and metastasizing and thus becoming a cancer. These six properties are as follows (Fig. 13.2):

1. Self-sufficiency in growth signals
2. Insensitivity to antigrowth signals
3. Evading apoptosis
4. Limitless replicative potential
5. Sustained angiogenesis
6. Tissue invasion and metastases

TABLE 13.1

THE 10 LEADING CANCER TYPES FOR THE ESTIMATED NEW CANCER CASES AND DEATHS, BY GENDER, FOR THE UNITED STATES IN 2008

MALES			FEMALES		
CANCER	INCIDENCE		CANCER	INCIDENCE	
ESTIMATED NEW CASES[a]					
Prostate	186,320	(25%)	Breast	182,460	(26%)
Lung and bronchus	114,690	(15%)	Lung and bronchus	100,330	(14%)
Colon and rectum	77,250	(10%)	Colon and rectum	71,560	(10%)
Urinary bladder	51,230	(7%)	Uterine corpus	40,100	(6%)
Non-Hodgkin lymphoma	35,450	(5%)	Non-Hodgkin lymphoma	30,670	(4%)
Melanoma of the skin	34,950	(5%)	Thyroid	28,410	(4%)
Kidney and renal pelvis	33,130	(4%)	Melanoma of the skin	27,530	(4%)
Oral cavity and pharynx	25,310	(3%)	Ovary	21,650	(3%)
Leukemia	25,180	(3%)	Kidney and renal pelvis	21,260	(3%)
Pancreas	18,770	(3%)	Leukemia	19,090	(3%)
All sites	**745,180**	**100%**	**All sites**	**692,000**	**100%**
ESTIMATED DEATHS					
Lung and bronchus	90,810	(31%)	Lung and bronchus	71,030	(26%)
Prostate	28,660	(10%)	Breast	40,480	(15%)
Colon and rectum	24,260	(8%)	Colon and rectum	25,700	(9%)
Pancreas	17,500	(6%)	Pancreas	16,790	(6%)
Liver and intrahepatic bile duct	12,570	(4%)	Ovary	15,520	(6%)
Leukemia	12,460	(4%)	Non-Hodgkin lymphoma	9,370	(3%)
Esophagus	11,250	(4%)	Leukemia	9,250	(3%)
Urinary bladder	9,950	(3%)	Uterine corpus	7,470	(3%)
Non-Hodgkin lymphoma	9,790	(3%)	Liver and intrahepatic bile duct	5,840	(2%)
Kidney and renal pelvis	8,100	(3%)	Brain and other nervous system	5,650	(2%)
All sites	**294,120**	**100%**	**All sites**	**271,530**	**100%**

[a]Excludes basal and squamous cell skin cancers and in situ carcinoma except urinary bladder. Estimates are rounded to nearest 10.
Adapted from Jemal A, et al. *CA Cancer J Clin* 2008;58:71–96.

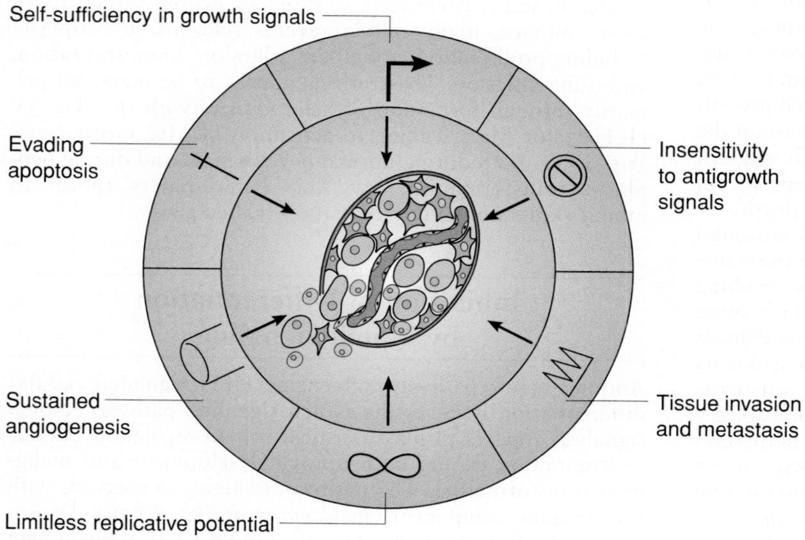

FIGURE 13.2. Acquired capabilities of cancer. (Adapted from Hanahan D, Weinberg R. The hallmarks of cancer. *Cell* 2000;100:57.)

SCIENTIFIC PRINCIPLES

Each of these capabilities is placed in the perspective of current research efforts in the sections that follow.

CANCER BIOLOGY

The basic unit of tissues and organs is the cell. The control of cell growth and differentiation is the focal point in understanding the processes involved in malignant transformation. Cells normally grow, divide, perform necessary functions to maintain homeostasis, and die in a programmed fashion throughout most tissues and organs. A cancer cell is one that has alterations in this carefully controlled program that lead to the phenotype of cancer. Hanahan and Weinberg's model describes four of the six functional capabilities, which directly relate to changes within the cell itself. These are the acquired ability for self-sufficient growth, insensitivity to antigrowth signals, ability to evade apoptosis, and limitless replicative potential. The other two functional capabilities—sustained angiogenesis and tissue invasion and metastases—involve changes not only within the individual cancer cell but also in the interaction and relationship with other host elements.

Oncogenes and Tumor Suppressor Genes

❷ The ability of a cell to become self-sufficient in its growth and no longer rely on the normal temporal sequences of programmed cell growth is often the result of mutations in the genes involved in growth regulation and control. Activating mutations of proto-oncogenes create oncogenes. For example, a point mutation of a single nucleotide in the *ras* gene can result in cell-transforming activity. Approximately one half of human colon cancers have a mutation in the *ras* oncogene.

The three Ras proteins (h-, k-, and n-ras) are members of a large superfamily of Ras-related proteins that share significant structural homology as well as guanosine triphosphatase (GTPase) activity. All known *ras* genes include an identical nine-amino-acid domain in the N-terminal half of the protein. This undergoes a conformational shift when Ras binds to GTP. These Ras-related proteins function as molecular switches, involved in the control of a variety of cellular functions including growth, organization, and transport. The biologic activity of Ras is controlled by a number of factors known as guanine nucleotide exchange factors that promote the formation of the active GTP-bound state (e.g., SOS), and the GTPase-activating proteins (e.g., NF1-GAP) that promote formation of the inactive guanosine diphosphate (GDP)-bound state. Structural mutations involving codons 12, 13, and 61 result in mutant Ras proteins that lack this GTPase activity. These oncogenic Ras proteins are locked in the active GTP-bound conformation, leading to constitutive activation of downstream targets. This can be thought of as an "on-off" switch for cell growth that is locked in the "on" position due to the mutation in the *ras* oncogene. In addition to stimulating growth signals, mutant Ras proteins can also facilitate survival signals within the cell, allowing the cell to evade programmed cell death.

Oncogenes can also be activated through chromosomal rearrangements known as translocations that involve the transfer of one segment of a chromosome to another. The resulting shift in position of genes can change the way in which those genes are regulated. An example of this is the Philadelphia chromosome that appears in chronic myelogenous leukemia (CML). This chromosomal rearrangement results when the small c-*abl* proto-oncogene is translocated from chromosome 9 to the small *bcr* locus on chromosome 22. The result of this creates the small *bcr/abl* oncogene. This oncogene leads to an increase in tyrosine kinase activity and therefore downstream signaling in the cell, leading to uncontrolled cell growth.

Oncogenes also affect the development of familial endocrine tumors. An activating mutation of the RET proto-oncogene on chromosome 10 causes the development of medullary thyroid cancer in patients suffering from multiple endocrine neoplasia (MEN) 2a and MEN 2b. Patients with MEN 2 uniformly develop medullary thyroid cancer, and many also develop other tumors (such as adrenal pheochromocytomas) due to the constitutive activation of this gene.

Another class of genetic change that predisposes to cancer, both sporadically and within inherited cancer syndrome families, is inactivating mutations of tumor suppressor genes. Tumor suppressor genes typically code for proteins that play an important role in cellular growth control. When these genes are mutated, growth dysregulation can occur. In the familial setting, these mutations inactivate one allele of a growth control gene in the germline. An inactivating mutation of the second allele of the gene in a susceptible cell causes loss of the growth control function in that cell, contributing to the development of the characteristic tumor. Tumors that develop sporadically due to mutations of tumor suppressor genes require accumulation of inactivating changes in both copies of the gene within a single cell. This explanation of tumor suppressor genes is known as the Knudsen hypothesis. Examples of this include mutations of the *BRCA1* or *BRCA2* genes, which together account for 75% of familial breast cancer cases. *BRCA1* acts as a tumor suppressor gene in that mutation of one copy followed by inactivation of the second copy of the gene in a cell results in malignant transformation. Another example of a tumor suppressor gene is the *MEN1* gene that is inactivated in MEN type 1, the *vHL* gene inactivated in von Hippel-Lindau syndrome, and the adenomatous polyposis coli (*APC*) gene locus that can lead to the development of colorectal cancers when mutated.

Myc Regulation of Cellular Differentiation

In human neoplasia, many components of the dedifferentiated phenotype appear to involve regulation by helix-loop-helix motif (HLH) proteins. At least three major pathways have been identified that impact on HLH-regulated cellular differentiation. These include amplification/overexpression of the c-*myc* proto-oncogene, overexpression of Id transcriptional repressors, and activation of Notch signaling. With respect to Myc, the c-*myc* proto-oncogene is amplified in many human tumors, including lung cancer, breast cancer, cervical cancer, and ovarian cancer. In addition, increased expression of c-*myc* is noted in up to one third of breast and colon carcinomas. c-*myc* appears to represent a central switch through which a number of oncogenic pathways including BCR-ABL, b-catenin, and c-*src* converge to stimulate neoplasia (Fig. 13.3). c-*myc* impacts many cellular events relevant to neoplasia including proliferation, apoptosis, adhesion, immortalization, and differentiation. These effects appear to be mediated primarily through formation of heterodimers with the class IV HLH factor Max, leading to activation of Myc target genes (Fig. 13.4). Both during normal development and during neoplastic transformation, Myc/Max heterodimers appear to inhibit expression of differentiation-related genes.

Inhibition of Differentiation by Notch Signaling

Another major pathway influencing HLH-regulated cellular differentiation involves the Notch signaling pathway. Notch signaling appears to play a critical role in regulating cellular differentiation during both normal development and malignant transformation. The pathway is highly conserved, with homologous components in *Caenorhabditis elegans, Drosophila*, zebrafish, mice, and humans (Table 13.2). Four human Notch family members have been identified. Notch proteins

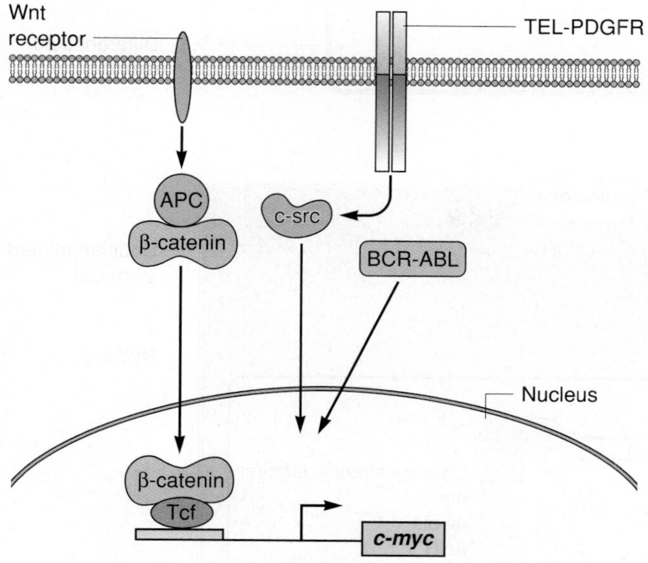

FIGURE 13.3. The *c-myc* gene is a central oncogenic switch for oncogenes and the tumor suppressor adenomatous polyposis coli (APC). The APC tumor suppressor protein mediates the degradation of β-catenin. The Wnt oncoprotein is shown activating its receptor, which results in the stabilization of free β-catenin, which sustains activating mutations in human cancers; β-catenin is a cofactor for the transcription factor Tef. Tef activates *c-myc* expression through specific DNA binding sites. The oncogenic fusion protein TEL-PDGFR hypothetically activates *c-src*, as does native PDGFR, resulting in the activation of *c-myc*. The BRC-ABL oncoprotein likewise requires *c-myc* for its activity. (Adapted from Dang CV. *c-Myc* target genes involved in cell growth, apoptosis, and metabolism. *Mol Cell Biol* 1999;19:1.)

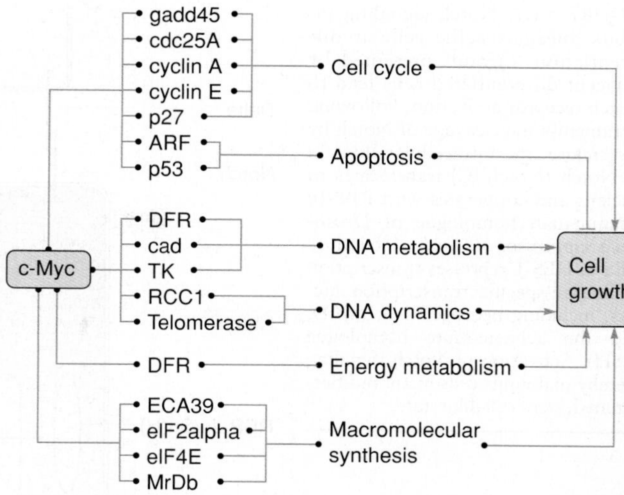

FIGURE 13.4. Links between c-Myc, selected putative target genes, cellular functions, and cell growth. The diagram illustrates the complexity of the connections between c-Myc and its putative target genes, which are shown clustered according to their functions. The various cellular functions cooperate to promote cell growth. It should be noted that this diagram does not reflect the controversies over the authentication of the various target genes. (Adapted from Dang CV. c-Myc target genes involved in cell growth, apoptosis, and metabolism. *Mol Cell Biol* 1999;19:1.)

TABLE 13.2

CONSERVED COMPONENTS OF THE NOTCH SIGNALING PATHWAY

	■ *CAENORHABDITIS ELEGANS*	■ *DROSOPHILA*	■ MAMMALS
Notch receptors	Lin-12	Notch	Notch1 Notch3
	Glp-1		Notch2 Notch4
Extracellular ligands (DSL proteins)	Lag-2	Delta	Delta-1
	Apx-1		Delta-1
			Delta-like 1 (Dll-1)
			Delta-like 3 (Dll-3)
		Serrate	Jagged1 (Serrate1)
			Jagged2 (Serrate2)
Intracellular effectors	Lag-1	Suppressor of hairless [Su(H)]	CBF-1/RBP-Jκ
		Deltex	Deltex
			NFκB
Target genes		Enhancer of split [E(spl)]	HES (Hairy/enhancer of split)
		bHLH	bHLH
		Groucho	TLE
Processing molecules	SUP-17	Kuzbanian	Kuzbanian
Modifiers		Fringe	Lunatic fringe
			Manic fringe
			Radical fringe
		Numb	Numb
			Numb-like
		Disheveled	Disheveled 1,2,3

SCIENTIFIC PRINCIPLES

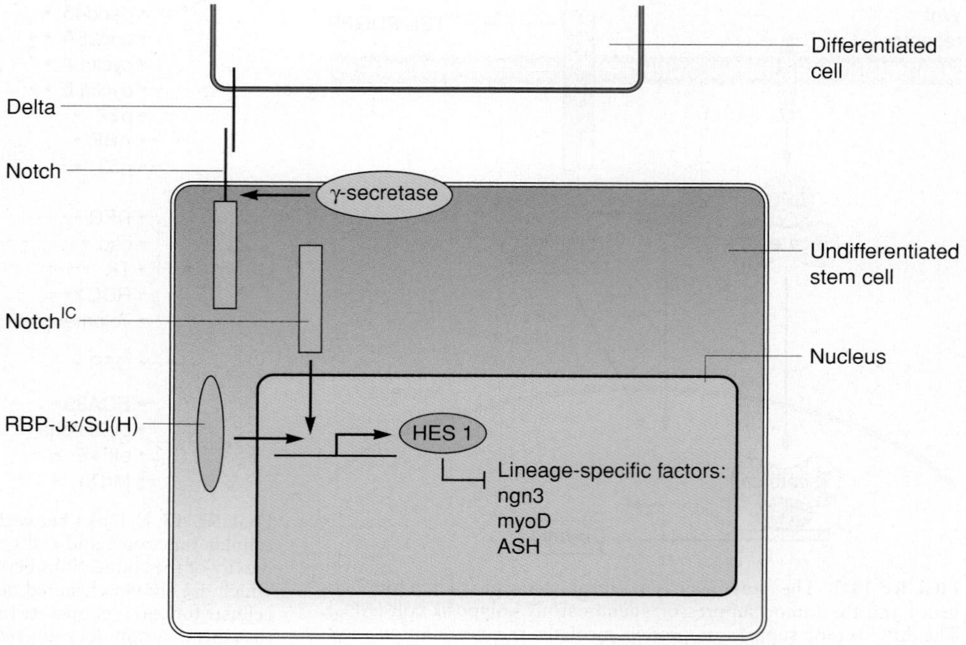

FIGURE 13.5. Notch signaling inhibits lineage-specific cellular differentiation. Ligands presented by adjacent differentiated cells lead to Notch receptor activation. Following intramembrane cleavage of Notch by γ-secretase, the intracellular domain of Notch (Notch-IC) translocates to nucleus and cooperates with RBP-Jκ (mammalian homologue of *Drosophila Suppressor of Hairless*) to induce HES-1. HES-1 represses transcription of lineage-specific transcription factors, including neurogenin 3, myoD, and the achaete-scute homologue (ASH). Activation of Notch signaling thereby maintains cells in an undifferentiated, stem cell–like state.

are transmembrane receptors containing extracellular tandem epidermal growth factor (EGF)-like repeats as well as three Lin/Notch repeats that function in ligand binding and Notch activation. As transmembrane receptors, Notch proteins are unique in apparently lacking any enzymatic activity. Instead, Notch proteins undergo proteolytic cleavage on activation by binding to DSL ligands (e.g., Delta, Serrate, Lag-2). Recent data suggest that proteolytic cleavage of Notch may be accomplished by γ-secretase, an enzyme also responsible for proteolytic production of β-amyloid from amyloid precursor protein. Following proteolytic cleavage, the Notch intracellular domain (Notch-IC) is released to interact with a number of cytoplasmic and nuclear proteins, including CSL proteins such as *Drosophila Suppressor of Hairless* and mammalian CBF-1. Interactions between Notch-IC and CSL proteins result in transcriptional activation of Hairy/Enhancer of Split (HES) class VI HLH protein. Once bound to DNA, HES proteins recruit a corepressor known as Groucho, thereby preventing expression of a number of cell lineage–specific class II bHLH proteins, including MyoD, neurogenin 3, and achaete-scute homologues (Fig. 13.5).

Notch signaling therefore represents a mechanism to prevent lineage-specific cellular differentiation. During development, this function plays a critical role in lateral inhibition as well as in boundary formation. Notch signaling is also implicated in various forms of neoplasia. Notch-IC is capable of transforming rat kidney cells in cooperation with adenoviral E1A and substitutes for activated ras in this assay. Notch receptors and ligands are upregulated in human cervical cancer, and activating translocations involving Notch family members have been identified in acute T-cell leukemia. Notch also appears to be required for immortalization of B lymphocytes by Epstein-Barr virus and represents a site for activating integration by the mouse mammary tumor virus. Additional studies have identified an important role of the Notch target gene HES-1 in regulating differentiation status in non–small cell lung cancer.

Telomerase and Cell Immortalization/Senescence

Senescence is the process during which a normal cell ages and dies. This process is controlled, in part, by specialized heterochromatic structures at the ends of eukaryotic chromosomes called telomeres that function to stabilize and protect the chromosome. During normal somatic cell replication, telomeres become progressively shorter with each cell division, resulting in chromosome instability. It has been postulated that the shortening of telomeres represents a checkpoint mechanism by which cellular senescence is signaled in normal replicating cell populations.

Telomerase is an RNA-dependent DNA polymerase that stabilizes telomeres by synthesizing the six oligonucleotide repeat TTAGGG. This stabilization can allow indefinite replication and thus "cell immortalization." Although inactive in most somatic cells, telomerase remains activated in germ cells and lymphocytes. A unique characteristic of the cancer cell is immortality with the ability to divide repeatedly without undergoing normal cellular senescence. A correlation between telomerase and cancer has recently been documented by the detection of telomerase activity in a high percentage of primary human malignancies including cancer of the lung, colon, breast, and prostate. By remaining in the activated state, telomerase may contribute to the uncontrolled replicative capacity of the cancer cell. This finding has stimulated much discussion of the potential diagnostic, prognostic, and therapeutic implications of telomerase in the management of cancer.

Cell Survival/Programmed Cell Death

Virtually all cell populations are controlled through a balance of cell survival and cell death. Under certain conditions, such as terminal differentiation, growth factor deprivation, or DNA damage, survival signals to the cell are overtaken by death signals. Cell death can occur in a variety of forms, but the most common forms of cell death are necrosis and apoptosis. Necrotic cell death takes place primarily from noxious stimuli to the cell due to chemical or heat exposure, ischemia, or other insults. In contrast, apoptosis, or programmed cell death, occurs via a complex, genetically determined process. Apoptosis is a continual process in many normal as well as altered cell populations. For instance, during embryogenesis, organ formation occurs through a series of remolding events that include apoptosis. Apoptosis is also an active process in many disease states. Following myocardial infarction, induction of apoptosis can occur in the damaged cardiac muscle cells.

The process of apoptosis is described as a cascade of events, each mediated by intracellular proteins, ultimately leading to apoptotic cell death. After receiving a cell death stimulus, induction of genes that promote apoptosis occurs, thereby shifting the intercellular balance toward proteins with proapoptotic activity. Two of the best-studied apoptotic genes are *Bcl-2* and *Bax*. Normally, the levels of antiapoptotic *Bcl-2* allow for continued cell survival. During the apoptotic state, *Bcl-2* levels are downregulated, shifting the balance toward proapoptotic proteins such as *Bax*. Downstream regulators of the apoptotic cascade are recruited including endonucleases, which cleave chromatin, resulting in nuclear fragmentation. This results in the formation of apoptotic bodies and other morphologic characteristics of apoptosis such as cell shrinkage and loss of contact with adjacent cells. In contrast, necrotic cell death is characterized by cellular swelling and ultimate rupture of the cell membrane. Just as apoptosis is active in embryogenesis and the molding of organ structure and function, it is also important in disease states such as cancer. In general, cancer cells that are resistant to cell death have altered their balance of apoptotic regulators. For instance, cancer cells that are resistant to conventional therapies such as radiation and chemotherapy often have increased levels of antiapoptotic proteins such as Bcl-2. To change the balance toward apoptotic cell death, some newer therapies attempt to upregulate proapoptotic proteins such as Bax or, conversely, downregulate antiapoptotic proteins such as Bcl-2.

In addition to the induction of apoptosis by these proteins, programmed cell death can also occur via recognition events of the immune system. Specifically, the Fas antigen (CD-95, APO-1) is a cell surface protein of the tumor necrosis factor (TNF) family. When stimulated by its ligand (FasL) under certain conditions, Fas-bearing cells can undergo apoptotic cell death. This is a possible mechanism of cytotoxic T-cell– and natural killer cell–mediated death as well as other autoimmune responses.

Abnormal Growth Regulation in Cancer

3 Transformation from the normal phenotype to invasive malignancy appears to involve a loss of normal tumor suppressive and growth inhibitory responses as well as the acquisition of inappropriate proliferative signals. The presence of inappropriate proliferative signals has been well documented in most malignancies and includes overexpression of peptide growth factors (transforming growth factor β [TGF-β], amphiregulin, heparin-binding EGF) and of growth factor receptors (e.g., HER2/neu). Alternatively, there may be mutational activation of the signal transduction pathways for the growth factors (e.g., *ras* and *src* oncogenes), activation of oncogenes that are directly involved in stimulating progression of the cell cycle regulation (*myc, cyclin D1,* etc.), or inactivation of genes that provide checkpoint control on cell cycle progression (e.g., the retinoblastoma gene *p53*).

Cell Cycle Regulation in Cancer

The cell cycle involves cellular events controlling replication of chromosomal DNA during the S phase and the separation of replicated chromosomes during cell division (mitosis or meiosis, M phase). The cell cycle is an indispensable process for survival of an organism and is highly conserved throughout evolution. The S phase and M phase are separated by gap periods, or G phases. The G1 phase precedes the S phase and the G2 phase precedes the M phase (Fig. 13.6). G0 describes cells that are in a nonreplicating, quiescent state. G0 cells are often differentiated cells that may be metabolically active, but are not involved in the process of cellular replication. The cell has mechanisms for responding to extracellular signals to recruit G0 cells into the cell cycle.

The process of cell cycle progression is tightly regulated. The factors responsible for advancing cell cycle progression were initially described in yeast and in amphibian eggs. Cyclins were discovered as proteins that oscillated during specific periods of the cell cycle. Subsequent work led to the identification of the catalytic partners of the cyclins, called cyclin-dependent kinases (CDKs). Specific sets of cyclins with their partner CDKs drive progression through specific periods of the cell cycle (Fig. 13.7). Mistakes in DNA replication or in chromosomal segregation are detected and prevented from propagation. This function, termed *cell cycle checkpoint control,* involves regulation of the levels and activities of the cyclins and CDKs and also involves the regulation of programmed cell death (apoptosis).

Quiescent cells may be recruited to the cell cycle by mitogenic stimulation (e.g., growth factor exposure). Normal cells depend on exogenous mitogenic stimulation only during the first two thirds of the G1 phase. At this two-thirds point, also called the restriction (R) point, the cell may commit itself to advance into the S phase and subsequent phases of the cell cycle (Fig. 13.8). The retinoblastoma protein (pRB) is the molecular switch that controls passage through the R point. Unphosphorylated or hypophosphorylated pRB blocks R point transition, whereas phosphorylation of pRB prevents it from blocking cell cycle progression.

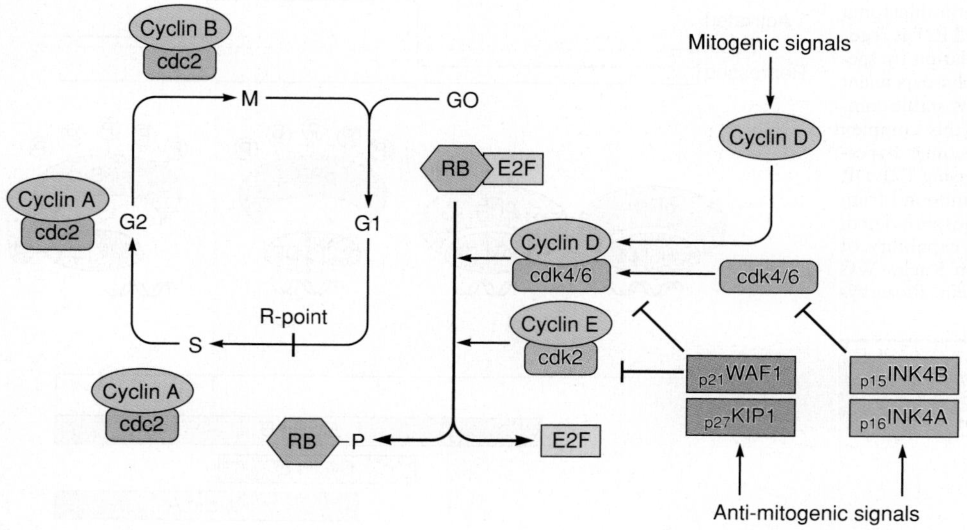

FIGURE 13.6. The cell cycle clock machinery. G0, M, G1, S, and G2 refer to the quiescence, mitosis, first gap, DNA synthesis, and second gap phases of the cell cycle, respectively. The restriction point (R-point) is shown preceding S-phase entry. RB and RB-p represent unphosphorylated and hyperphosphorylated forms of the retinoblastoma protein. (Adapted from Lundberg AS, Weinberg RA. Control of the cell cycle and apoptosis. *Eur J Cancer* 1999;35:531.)

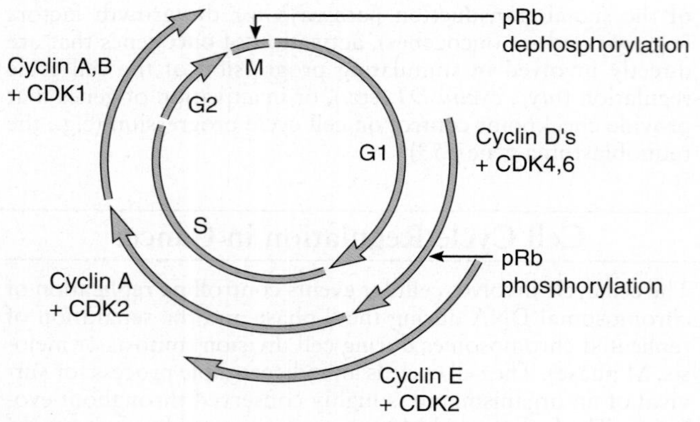

FIGURE 13.7. The cell cycle clock. This version of the cell cycle shows where the retinoblastoma protein (pRB) is either phosphorylated or dephosphorylated to regulate cell cycle transit.

Expression of a specific subset of the cyclins called D-type cyclins (D1, D2, and D3) is increased in early to mid-G1 in response to mitogenic signals. The D-type cyclins assemble with their catalytic partners, CDK4 and CDK6, and the cyclin D–CDK complex enters the cell nucleus where it becomes phosphorylated by a CDK-activating kinase (CAK). A critical function of the cyclin D–dependent kinases is the phosphorylation of the Rb protein. Growth factor activation of Ras signaling and the MAPK cascade induces transcription of the cyclin D1 gene, decreases the turnover of the cyclin D1 protein, and regulates cyclin D–CDK assembly. Expression of the D-type cyclins is dependent on continuous mitogenic stimulation. Progression through the mid- to late G1 phase of the mammalian cell cycle is dependent on the cyclin D–dependent protein kinases.

Cyclin D–dependent kinases initiate the phosphorylation of Rb in mid-G1, and then subsequent activation of the cyclin E–CDK2 complex leads to further phosphorylation of Rb on additional sites. Cyclin A–dependent CDK (CDK2) becomes activated during the S phase and cyclin B–dependent CDK (CDC2) becomes activated during G2 and M. These cyclin-dependent kinases help to maintain Rb in a hyperphosphorylated state until mitosis has been completed and Rb is returned to its hypophosphorylated state at the beginning of G1. Hypophosphorylated Rb inhibits the transcriptional activity of E2F protein family members. Hyperphosphorylation of Rb in late G1 phase disrupts its association with E2F family members, thereby enabling them to express their activity as transcription factors. The activation of the E2F transcription factor complex is required for the expression of a set of genes whose activities are required for S-phase progression. These include gene products that regulate nucleotide metabolism and DNA synthesis, as well as cyclins E and A.

The activities of CDKs are governed by other proteins called CDK inhibitors (CKIs). There are two families of CKIs based on structure and their CDK targets. One class includes the INK4 proteins (inhibitors of CDK4), which specifically bind and inhibit the activities of CDK4 and CDK6. This family is composed of four such proteins ($p16^{INK4a}$, $p15^{INK4b}$, $p18^{INK4c}$, and $p19^{INK4d}$). The Cip/Kip family comprises the other family of CKIs. This family includes the proteins $p21^{Cip1}$, $p27^{Kip1}$, and $p57^{Kip2}$. The CKIs of the Cip/Kip family were originally thought to interfere with the activities of cyclin D–, cyclin E–, and cyclin A–dependent kinases. This view has now evolved with further data confirming that the Cip/Kip proteins are potent inhibitors of cyclin E– and cyclin A–dependent CDK2 activity; however, this family of CKIs appears to act as positive regulators of cyclin D–dependent kinases. Increased levels of cyclin D/CDK4 during the G1 phase results in sequestration of the Cip/Kip CKIs, thereby preventing them from associating with and inhibiting cyclin E– and cyclin A–dependent CDK2. Activated CDK2 catalyzes hyperphosphorylation of Rb and also triggers the proteolytic destruction of $p27^{Kip1}$.

In addition to transcriptional activation and induction of cyclin gene expression, proteolysis is a critical function in the regulation of the cell cycle. As mentioned previously, proteolytic destruction of $p27^{Kip1}$ is triggered during the S phase. Once the S phase has been initiated, the cell is no longer reliant on mitogenic signals or the D-dependent cyclins for progression through the remainder of the cell cycle. Cyclin E is degraded as cells progress through the S phase, cyclin A is degraded during G2, and cyclin B is degraded by the completion of the M phase to reset the system and thereby reestablish a period of mitogen dependence in the next G1 phase (Fig. 13.9).

Disruption of the growth suppressive function of Rb is a common event in cancer. This may occur as the result of mutational inactivation of Rb itself or because of the disruption of p16 function. Increased expression and activation of cyclin D and CDK4 (via amplification or transcriptional activation) are also common events in human cancer and result in the same type of inactivation of growth inhibitory function of Rb. Interestingly, complete loss of Cip/Kip function has not been

FIGURE 13.8. Interactions of the retinoblastoma protein (pRB). The interaction of pRB and E2F is regulated by cell cycle–dependent phosphorylation by specific cyclins acting with their partner cyclin-dependent kinases. Underphosphorylated pRB forms stable complexes with E2F/DP heterodimers and this complex actively represses transcription. pRB becomes hyperphosphorylated in late G1, thereby releasing E2F/DP, which is transcriptionally active when unbound from pRB. Late in the S phase, DP becomes phosphorylated, thereby neutralizing the DNA-binding capability of the E2F/DP heterodimer. (Adapted from Kaelin WG Jr. Functions of the retinoblastoma protein. *Bioessays* 1999;21:950.)

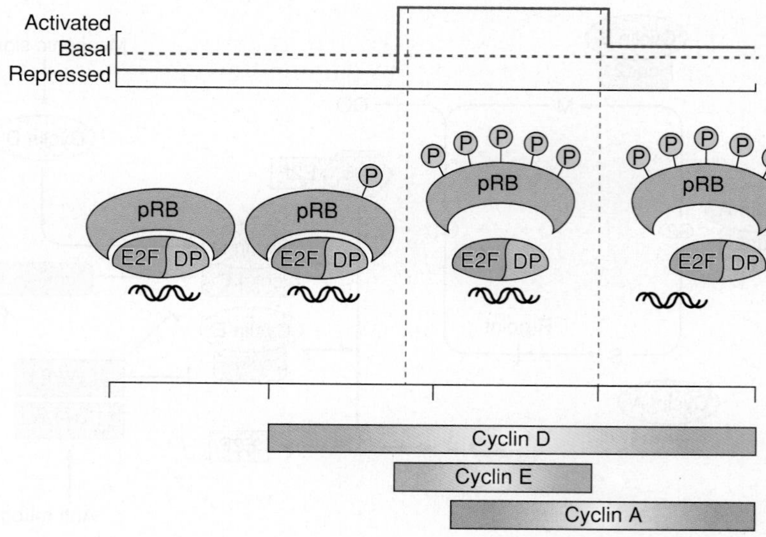

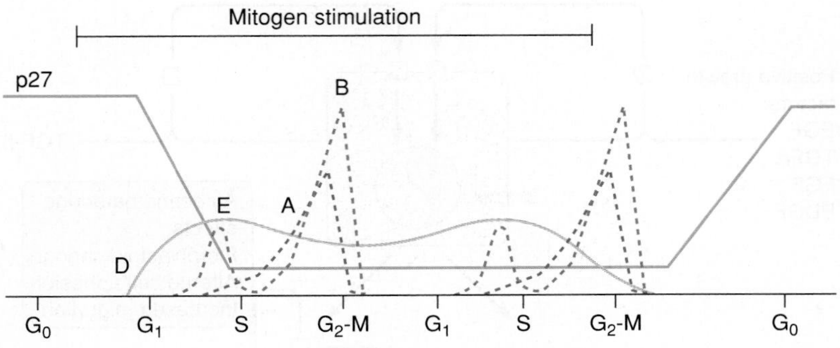

FIGURE 13.9. Fluctuations of cyclins and cyclin kinase inhibitors during the cell cycle. Cyclins E, A, and B undergo periodic oscillation during each cell cycle. In contrast, the D-type cyclins tend to remain elevated in cycling cells under the influence of growth stimuli. Levels of the inhibitor $p27^{Kip1}$ tend to remain high in quiescent cells but are decreased in proliferating cells. (Adapted from Sherr CJ. Cancer cell cycles. *Science* 1996;274: 1672.)

observed in cancer nor have cyclin E gene amplification or mutations resulted in increased cyclin E–dependent CDK activity.

The CKIs appear to function as checkpoint controls to ensure that cell cycle progression occurs under the proper environmental conditions and that the proper intracellular signaling has been completed prior to the initiation of DNA synthesis. Further checkpoints are the DNA damage and replication controls that block mitosis when DNA is damaged or DNA replication is incomplete. These checkpoint controls are essential for maintaining genomic stability, the failure of which allows cells to divide when DNA is damaged or DNA synthesis is incomplete or in the presence of faulty chromosomal segregation.

All cancer cells have abnormalities in one or more of the components of cell cycle control involved in G1- to S-phase transition. In some cases, loss of Rb function itself is the event that releases the cells from extracellular signaling constraints. Mutational loss of Rb function occurs in the vast majority of retinoblastomas and less frequently in other tumor types such as lung cancers and soft tissue sarcomas. In the absence of functional Rb protein, E2F is active and there is no requirement for activation of cyclin D/CDK4 to initiate DNA synthesis. Amplification of the cyclin D1 gene is common in several types of human tumors such as breast, head and neck, esophageal, and hepatic malignancies. Increased expression of cyclin D1 without gene amplification is common in colorectal cancer. Deletion of the $p16^{INK4a}$ gene is also common in human cancers, particularly in melanomas and in a subset of pancreatic cancers. Hereditary loss of $p16^{INK4a}$ function is associated with increased risk for melanoma and pancreatic cancer. All of the previous defects in cell cycle regulators result in loss of the same G1/S checkpoint control. It is rare for more than one of the previously mentioned defects to be identified in the same tumor.

Genomic Instability in Cancer

Genomic instability, with a high frequency of chromosomal loss and gain, genome doubling, and subtler genetic mutations, is a common characteristic of cancer cells. Genomic instability increases the chance of specific gene mutations that are ultimately responsible for the various phenotypes of cancer cells. Cancer cells acquire defects in the checkpoints that control normal mitosis, with its equal distribution of chromosomes into daughter cells and cytokinesis. Failure of this checkpoint may result in unequal distribution of chromosomes or failure to undergo cytokinesis, and either polyploidy (4N, 8N, etc.) or aneuploidy.

The tumor suppressor protein p53 plays a critical role in maintaining genomic stability. p53 function is required to initiate checkpoint-activated cell cycle arrest and programmed cell death in response to DNA damage. This function of p53 is necessary to ensure the integrity of the cellular genome by protecting it from the adverse effects of DNA damage. The p53 protein functions as an important transcription factor mediating expression of a variety of genes whose products may directly regulate growth arrest or apoptosis. Growth arrest induced by p53 may enable a cell to repair DNA that has been damaged. Alternatively, p53 also functions to induce apoptosis to prevent propagation of a cell lineage containing mutated DNA sequences.

Expression of p53 may be induced by either DNA damage or by inappropriate mitogenic signaling. An example of an important p53-responsive gene product involved in cell cycle arrest is the cyclin kinase inhibitor protein $p21^{Cip1}$. Several p53-responsive gene products appear to be involved in the apoptotic response. These include Bax, Fas/Apo, Killer/Dr5, and the redox regulator gene products known as PIGs (p53-induced genes). The expression of Mdm2 is also induced on activation of the p53 gene. Mdm2 is a negative feedback regulator of p53 whose function is to target p53 for rapid degradation. Interestingly, one of the two products of the *INK4a/ARF* locus, $p14^{ARF}$ inhibits the function of Mdm2, thereby stabilizing and activating p53 and promoting cell cycle arrest and apoptosis in response to inappropriate mitogenic signals. The other product of the *INK4a/ARF* locus is $p16^{Ink4a}$, the important inhibitor of CDKs 4 and 6, and a mediator of G1 cell cycle.

The protein product of the *Myc* proto-oncogene also regulates both cell proliferation and apoptosis in cell culture systems. *Myc* expression is capable of preventing cells from exiting the cell cycle and of promoting continuous cell cycle progression. Expression of *Myc* also inhibits differentiation in certain cell types. Similar to the situation in which inappropriately increased E2F triggers apoptosis, inappropriate *Myc* expression can also trigger apoptosis. Both increased E2F and *Myc* increase the expression of the ARF protein (p14 and p19), and as described previously, increased expression of ARF stabilizes p53, leading to both growth arrest and apoptosis.

There is a growing list of additional proteins that are involved in sensing and repairing DNA damage, or in ensuring correct chromosomal segregation during mitosis. Loss of function of these important genomic "caretaker" systems appears to be common in cancer cells, and this loss facilitates genomic instability with the accumulation of additional genetic lesions. The cumulative genetic mutations lead to tumor cells with selective advantages for aggressive biologic behavior including invasiveness and metastatic capacity, resistance to immunosurveillance, resistance to apoptosis, and the ability to resist cancer therapeutic interventions.

Loss of Growth Inhibitory Effects of Transforming Growth Factor β in Cancer

TGF-β regulation of epithelial cell proliferation is altered by transformation. Loss of responsiveness to the growth inhibitory effects of TGF-β occurs in many cancer cell types, including pancreatic, breast, and colorectal carcinoma cells. Thus, loss of growth inhibitory responses to TGF-β appears to

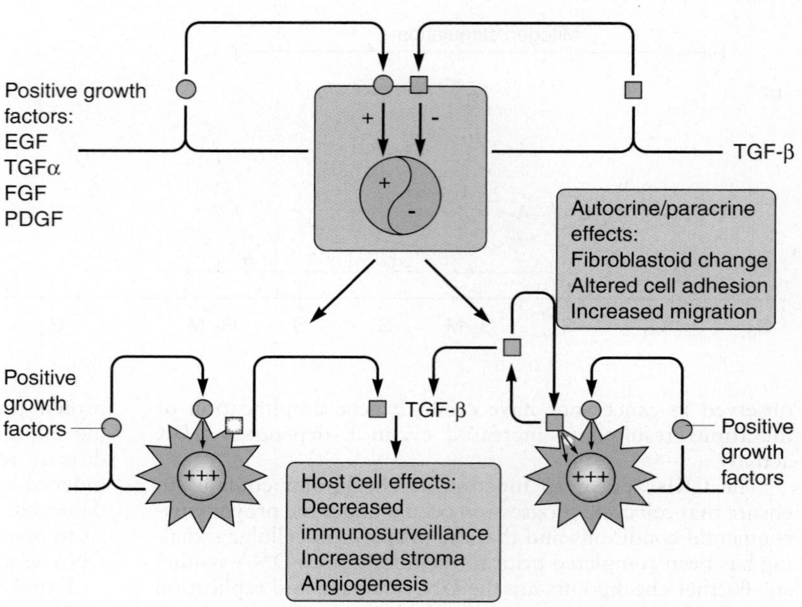

FIGURE 13.10. The effect of the transforming growth factor β (TGF-β) signaling pathway on cells is context dependent. Normal cells respond to TGF-β with growth inhibition and TGF-β appears to function as a tumor suppressor under normal conditions. Although complete loss of the TGF-β receptors is expected to eliminate all autocrine (but not paracrine) effects of tumor-derived TGF-β, postreceptor mutations should not. Tumor cells often lose the ability to undergo growth arrest in response to TGF-β. Despite this loss of growth inhibitory effect, TGF-β autocrine effects on cell morphologic change and cell adhesion and cell migration (all likely to be advantageous for tumor cells) appear to be retained along with the paracrine effects.

be a common and important event that attends malignant transformation of epithelial cells (Fig. 13.10).

Transforming Growth Factor β Signaling Abnormalities in Cancer

The association of colorectal cancers, pancreatic carcinomas, and breast cancers with genetic lesions in the TGF-β signal transduction pathway underscores the importance of TGF-β in maintaining homeostasis in the digestive tract and in the breast. One of the mechanisms by which tumor cells become resistant to the growth inhibitory actions of TGF-β is through downregulation or mutation of TGF-β type II receptor (TβRII). Loss of TGF-β receptor function causes cellular loss of negative growth regulation by TGF-β. Several studies have suggested that a decrease in expression or inactivation of TβRII is a key step for the neoplastic transformation of epithelial cells in both the breast and the colon. Activation of Ras protein, which occurs frequently in colorectal cancer, results in a decreased expression of the TβRII.

TβRII inactivation has been detected in a subgroup of colorectal carcinomas associated with the microsatellite instability or RER (replication error) phenotype identified in approximately 13% of all colorectal cancers. Recent studies have also confirmed the presence of TβRII mutations in an additional 15% of microsatellite stable (MSS) colon cancers and TGF-β signaling abnormalities distal to TβRII in an additional 55% of these MSS colon cancers. It is of interest and seemingly paradoxical that the subset of colorectal cancers that exhibit microsatellite instability (and TβRII mutations) tend to be proximal colon cancers and have a better prognosis (stage for stage) than the majority of sporadic colorectal cancers that do not share these genetic defects.

Mutational loss of function of TGF-β signal transduction proteins has been identified in human colorectal cancer. Madr2 (Smad2) mutation was observed in 4%, and DPC4 (Smad4) mutation has been reported in up to 30% of human colorectal cancers. Also, loss of heterozygosity (LOH) of Smad3 has been detected in 2 (one sporadic and one HNPCC) of 17 cancers examined. These types of mutations may have a significantly different phenotypic outcome as compared with that resulting from loss of the TβRII. Smad4 mutation has also been identified in familial juvenile polyposis, a syndrome characterized by a predisposition to hamartomatous polyps and gastrointestinal cancer. These studies suggest that disruption of Smad signaling may be involved in either the initiation or progression of certain cancers.

Transforming Growth Factor β as a Tumor-promoting Factor

There are several lines of evidence that TGF-β may actually promote malignant transformation and tumor progression for several different cell types and under selected circumstances. TGF-β expression tends to be increased in a wide variety of cancers (including colon cancer) relative to adjacent normal tissues. Transformation of cells with dominant oncogenes (e.g., Ha-*ras* or v-*src*) activates transcription of the TGF-β1gene. Studies of human colorectal cancers have demonstrated that high-level expression of TGF-β in the primary tumor is associated with advanced stages and is an independent predictor of risk for recurrence and decreased survival.

There are several potential mechanisms for this tumor-promoting effect. For example, TGF-β may suppress tumor immunosurveillance. TGF-β exhibits growth inhibitory effects on moderate to well-differentiated primary colon carcinomas but stimulates the proliferation and invasion of poorly differentiated and metastatic colonic carcinomas. Treatment with TGF-β can induce estrogen-independent tumorigenicity of human breast cancer cells. TGF-β treatment can also substitute for wounding as a promoter of fibrosarcomas in chickens infected with the Rous sarcoma virus.

Transformation of preinvasive epithelial neoplasm to the invasive phenotype with metastatic potential is characterized by several profound changes in gene expression and in cellular and tissue morphology. The changes in cellular morphology and tissue architecture can be observed histologically and are accompanied by dramatic changes in the behavior of the transformed cells. The metastatic phenotype is associated with the acquisition of fibroblastoid features and the ability of the cells to invade stroma and blood vessels. There is mounting evidence that autocrine TGF-β expression by tumor cells can play a major role in the epithelial to fibroblastoid conversion that accompanies malignant transformation in mammary cells and in keratinocytes. TGF-β1 overexpression enhanced progression of carcinogen-induced skin cancers toward the malignant spindle cell phenotype in transgenic mice expressing high levels of TGF-β in the skin. The TGF-β–induced epithelial to mesenchymal transition in Ha-*ras*–transformed mammary epithelial cells involves disrupted cell–cell adhesion and the loss of epithelial cell polarity in addition to causing the cells to become more spindle shaped and invasive. The loss of cell polarity in response to TGF-β appears to be the result of a disruption of ZO-1 and F-actin proteins comprising the tight junctions in mammary epithelial cells.

There also is an important regulatory interaction between the TGF-β and cyclooxygenase-2 (COX-2) pathways. Forced overexpression of COX-2 in the nontransformed RIE-1 cells results in downregulation of the TβRII, and forced overexpression of COX-2 in a human colon cancer cell line results in increased secretion of TGF-β1 from those cells. TGF-β synergistically enhances the expression of COX-2 in conditionally Ha-*ras*–transformed RIE-1 cells, and the increase in COX-2 expression by TGF-β in the context of *ras* transformation occurs primarily through a marked increase in the stability of the COX-2 mRNA.

The predominant effect of TGF-β appears to be dependent on the context of the responding cell. Thus, the divergent effects of TGF-β in carcinogenesis may depend on the proliferative capacity and state of differentiation of the epithelial cell, both of which may be altered during the process of neoplastic transformation. Clearly, TGF-β signaling has an important tumor suppressive role; however, after transformation has occurred, TGF-β effects may be detrimental and may actually promote tumor cell survival, invasion, and metastasis. Recent work suggests that these effects may involve TGF-β regulation of COX-2 and other pathways that may contribute to tumor cell aggressiveness.

TUMOR HOST INTERACTIONS

There are many complex pathways within the tumor cell that allow it to express a phenotype different from that of normal replicating cells. There are important interactions between the tumor cell and surrounding normal cells that enhance the attributes normally ascribed to cancer. In the Hanahan and Weinberg six capability model, the two capabilities most involved in these tumor interactions are sustained angiogenesis and tissue invasion and metastasis. Both of these processes involve a carefully coordinated interplay between a variety of cell types, each influencing the other's growth and development.

Tumor Angiogenesis

4 The observation that tumors require the establishment of a vasculature to grow larger than several millimeters is one that was clearly elucidated by Judah Folkman in 1971. Since that time there has been a growing realization that tumors must develop a network of vessels to grow, invade, and metastasize. A variety of signals allow tumor cells to stimulate vessel ingrowth. One of the more commonly studied cytokines is vascular endothelial growth factor (VEGF). Many studies have linked the ability of a tumor to produce VEGF with its malignant potential. This has been shown in breast cancer, colon cancer, and kidney cancer, as well as others. VEGF is actually a family of cytokines, which act on the endothelial cell through a variety of surface receptors. The most common VEGF isotypes (A, B, and C) act on predominantly three endothelial cell receptors (VEGF-R 1, 2, and 3). VEGF receptors 1 and 2 bind VEGF and act predominantly to modulate endothelial cell proliferation and maturation in blood vessels. VEGF-C, working through VEGF receptor 3, exerts its effects predominantly on the endothelial cells of the lymphoid system.

Several lines of evidence have demonstrated the importance of VEGF as a tumor-derived factor for stimulating and recruiting a blood supply. Models have been developed that demonstrate the importance of VEGF in tumorigenesis. Using a transgenic mouse model of pancreatic islet carcinoma (RIP1-Tag2), Hanahan et al. demonstrated that five VEGF lineage genes are expressed in normal islets and throughout islet tumorigenesis. When this group produced an islet beta cell–specific knockout of VEGF-A, the resulting islets in these animals had reduced vascularity but retained their normal physiology. In RIP1-Tag2 mice in which most of the oncogene expressing cells had deleted the VEGF-A gene, both angiogenic switching and tumor growth were disrupted, as was the degree of neovessel formation. This elegant work demonstrates the crucial role of VEGF in angiogenesis. Although such experimental work is compelling, clinical data support this notion further.

A humanized mouse monoclonal antibody against VEGF (bevacizumab, Avastin, Genentec, Inc.) has recently completed phase III clinical trials and has received Food and Drug Administration (FDA) approval based on its activity in patients with colon cancer. In a prospective randomized phase III trial in renal cancer, James Yang et al. demonstrated that systemic administration of anti-VEGF antibody to patients with metastatic renal cell carcinoma resulted in a significant prolongation in the time to disease progression when compared with patients receiving a placebo. Herb Hurwitz et al. combined anti-VEGF antibody with a three-drug chemotherapy regimen consisting of 5-fluorouracil (5FU), leucovorin, and irinotecan for patients with metastatic colorectal carcinoma and compared this combination with the three-drug chemotherapy regimen alone. The addition of the anti-VEGF antibody to the standard chemotherapy regimen resulted in an improved response rate and an improved disease-free and overall survival. This clear relationship between blockade of factors known to induce tumor vasculature leading to antitumor effects seen clinically in patients underscores the importance of the angiogenic process in human tumors.

To gain a better understanding of the complex relationships between tumor cells and the surrounding stromal cells, including the endothelium, a basic understanding of the molecular processes involved in endothelial cell growth and differentiation is important. Indeed, regulation of vessel growth and proliferation is an important component of normal homeostatic mechanisms. Following embryogenesis and tissue formation, the growth of new blood vessels in normal tissues is carefully controlled and regulated. In addition to VEGF, there are a number of other regulatory cytokines, both initiators of vessel formation and inhibitors, that are regulated in a careful balance. An understanding of this balance may allow a more informed selection of targets for future cancer therapies. In addition to VEGF, other stimulatory cytokines have been shown to play an important role in a tumor's ability to recruit a vasculature. Among these, acidic fibroblast growth factor (aFGF) and basic fibroblast growth factor (bFGF) as well as placental-derived growth factors play important roles.

In addition to a careful balance of cytokines, integrin signaling plays an important role in regulating angiogenesis. When quiescent blood vessels are compared to activated or actively proliferating blood vessels, the panel of expressed integrins differs. Integrins such as $\alpha v\beta 3$, which plays an important role in endothelial cell adhesion to vitronectin (a component of the extracellular matrix), is differentially expressed in the vasculature of certain tumors when compared to other histologies and to normal tissues. Endothelial cells differ in their expression of various surface proteins depending on the tissue in which they reside. Work by investigators such as Pasqualini and Arap has demonstrated the diversity of endothelial cells and underscores the important observation that not all endothelial cells are the same.

In landmark studies using phage display techniques, Pasqualini and Arap have demonstrated that endothelial cells have unique surface markers that define their differences based on their tissue of origin. These so-called endothelial cell zip

SCIENTIFIC PRINCIPLES

TABLE 13.3

ENDOGENOUS NATURALLY OCCURRING ANGIOGENESIS INHIBITORS

Angiostatin/other plasminogen kringles	IP-10
Antithrombin (cleaved)	METH-1 and -2
Endostatin	MIG
Fibronectin fragments	p16
PEX	p53
16-kD Prolactin	Canstatin
Prothrombin kringle-2	PEDF
Maspin	Platelet factor-4
Restin	Proliferin-related protein
Vasostatin	PSA
IL-1, -4, -10, -12, -18	Protamine
Arresten	Retinoic acid
IFNs	Soluble FGF receptor
TIMPs	TGF-β1
1,25-$(OH)_2$-vitamin D	TNF-α
2-Methoxyestradiol	Troponin I
Angiopoietin-2	TSP-1 and -2
EMAP-II	
gro-β	

EMAP, endothelial monocyte octivating polypeptide; FGF, fibroblast growth factor; IFNs, interferons; IL, interleukin; PSA, prostate-specific antigen; TGF, transforming growth factor; TIMPs, tissue inhibitor of metalloproteinases; TNF, tumor necrosis factor; TSP, thrombospondin.

codes may provide a unique target for delivering endothelial cell–directed therapies. This diversity may also explain, in part, the differences in response rates of various tumors to different angiogenesis inhibitors.

A series of elegant experiments performed by Kalluri et al. focused on the relationship of endothelial cell surface integrin expression to the response of those endothelial cells to the effects of various angiogenesis inhibitors. Kalluri showed that endothelial cells expressing $\alpha v\beta 3$ responded to the collagen IV derivative tumstatin and not to endostatin. Conversely, endothelial cells expressing the integrin $\alpha 5\beta 1$ responded to endostatin rather than tumstatin. This was confirmed in animals bearing tumors. This specificity for certain integrin profiles is a critical observation in choosing the appropriate angiogenesis inhibitor and may explain, in part, the early clinical results with this class of agents.

A host of counterregulatory angiogenesis inhibitors have also been elucidated. These include thrombospondin 1, angiostatin, endostatin, and a series of collagen IV derivatives known as canstatin, arresten, and tumstatin. Table 13.3 lists some of these angiogenesis inhibitors; however, the field is rapidly growing and evolving and therefore any list must be considered representative rather than all-inclusive. The balance between proangiogenic factors and angiogenesis inhibitors was termed the "angiogenic switch" by Hanahan and Folkman. Tumors can activate this switch by changing the relative balance between inducers and inhibitors. How this balance is altered is the subject of ongoing study.

An intriguing possibility is that naturally occurring angiogenesis inhibitors play a gatekeeper function by inhibiting the progression of premalignant lesions by preventing their ability to recruit a blood supply. Thrombospondin 1 (TSP-1) has been implicated as a putative regulator of such a process. Preclinical mouse models as well as studies of clinical samples have shown an inverse relationship between the level of TSP-1 expressed and the invasive potential of the tumor. This relationship has also been identified in cervical cancer specimens.

Both endostatin and tumstatin have also been implicated in such a gatekeeping role. A curious clinical observation is that patients suffering from Down syndrome have a distinctly lower incidence of the common solid tumors than the general population. As Down syndrome patients have lived longer, they have a much lower rate of lung, breast, and colon cancers. Down syndrome is caused by trisomy of chromosome 21, which is the location of the gene coding for collagen XVIII, the precursor of endostatin. Down syndrome patients have higher circulating levels of endostatin than the normal population, perhaps due to the extra copy of the collagen XVIII gene on the additional chromosome 21. Kalluri has postulated that these elevated levels of circulating endogenous angiogenesis inhibitors may function as endothelium-specific tumor suppressors. An attractive future strategy for tumor prevention might involve exogenous administration of these inhibitors or, alternatively, administration of small molecules that raise the circulating levels of endogenous inhibitors, thus decreasing the ability of noninvasive lesions from developing an invasive phenotype.

Tissue Invasion and Metastasis

Although the primary tumor can cause significant morbidity and even death, by far the majority of deaths due to cancer result from metastatic disease. Metastatic disease remains the most difficult component of cancer to treat, and therefore a thorough understanding of the processes that lead to the ability of cancer cells to spread to and grow in distant sites is critical. In the past, much work focused on the complex process of metastasis was observational; however, new tools now make it possible to study the pathways involved at a molecular level.

For tumor cells to invade into surrounding tissue and gain access to the lymphatics and blood vessels, a number of changes must take place. The normal cell surface proteins, which mediate contact inhibition and allow for normal anchoring to the extracellular matrix (ECM), must be perturbed. Two classes of such proteins are the cell–cell adhesion molecules (CAMs) and the integrins.

One example of an important CAM is E-cadherin, a member of the calcium-dependent cadherin family. E-cadherin is expressed on epithelial cells and helps to mediate antigrowth signals between cells. E-cadherin forms bridges between cells and transmits antigrowth signals via contact with β-catenin in the cytoplasm and downstream signaling via Lef/Tcf transcription factor. Mutations in E-cadherin or β-catenin can result in the loss of antigrowth signals and contact inhibition, leading to epithelial carcinomas.

A member of the immunoglobulin super family, N-CAM, is another example of a CAM that plays a pivotal role in preventing invasion and metastasis. Mutations in N-CAM can result in a change in isoform from an adhesive to a poorly adhesive phenotype. These mutations have been identified in small cell lung cancer and Wilms tumor.

Integrins play a critical role in anchoring cells to the ECM. Different cell types rely on different integrins to perform this function. Successful interaction between an integrin and the ECM can suppress growth signals. Integrins are often made up of an α and a β subunit. The switching between these subunits can result in differing phenotypes with respect to cell growth and invasion.

Beyond contact inhibition and anchorage dependence, cells must also shift in their ability to produce enzymes, which allow for the degradation of the basement membrane and ECM to allow invasion and migration. Differential expression of proteases can allow for tissue invasion and access to lymphatics and vessels, which can provide a conduit to distant organ sites.

Once a tumor cell loses contact inhibition and expresses proteases, there is no guarantee that it will be able to grow in a distant organ such as the lung or liver. In addition to surviving the trip to the distant site, it must be able to take up residence in the organ and grow. Not every tumor cell that successfully reaches a distant site will be able to multiply and grow successfully. Some organs do not readily allow for the growth of cells of certain histologies (e.g., colon cancer does not commonly metastasize to the kidney). In some very elegant experiments, Fidler has studied this "seed and soil" phenomenon.

Fidler et al. looked at the ability of orthotopically placed colon cancer cells implanted in the cecum of mice to effectively metastasize to other organs. When these cells were implanted in the cecum and normal mesenteric vascular anatomy drained the site through the mesenteric vein to the portal vein and into the liver, liver metastases were seen to develop in these animals. However, when Fidler rerouted the venous drainage from the colon by reimplanting the mesenteric vein into the renal vein, metastases did not develop in the kidney. Clearly, some growth factors were present in the target organ or cell surface interactions between the tumor cell and the cells of the target organ that allowed colon cancer to grow in the liver but not in the kidney. Such organ predilection for tumor metastases has also been observed clinically.

Ocular melanoma, melanoma that develops from the pigmented cells within the eye, can metastasize systemically. The most common site of metastases for ocular melanoma is the liver. In fact, the majority of patients with metastatic ocular melanoma present initially with isolated liver metastasis. There is no clear-cut anatomic drainage pattern from the eye to the liver. In fact, when liver metastases are successfully treated, ocular melanoma can grow in other sites, such as the lungs and subcutaneous tissues. However, the liver as a first site for the spread of ocular melanoma clearly indicates some "seed and soil" relationship that promotes the ability of these cells to grow in a specific site.

Other examples of specific sites for metastatic disease are more easily understood based on venous drainage. Colon cancers arising above the peritoneal reflection often metastasize to the liver consistent with the mesenteric venous drainage via the portal system. Rectal cancers below the peritoneal reflection, which are drained by the pudendal veins into the caval system, often metastasize first to the lungs.

Although much of the focus of understanding tumor invasion and metastasis has focused on the tumor cells themselves, there is increasing evidence that the host may play a facilitative role in the ability of cells to invade and metastasize. Kent Hunter and his group at the NCI have investigated the role of host genetics and tumor metastasis. Hunter's group observed that, although a typical tumor can shed millions of cells into the bloodstream daily, very few clinically relevant metastases are ultimately formed. Using transgenic mouse models, Hunter has demonstrated that tumor cells carrying mutations in key metastasis-associated genes may demonstrate the ability to metastasize in certain strains of mice while they are unable to metastasize in other strains despite their ability to form tumor nodules. Expression of genes that are important for the ability of tumor cells to metastasize has also been shown to be altered in the host tissues themselves. The hypothesis that particular genetic mutations or polymorphisms in the host may make one patient more prone to metastatic disease than another is an intriguing one that warrants further investigation. If such markers could be identified, then patients at higher risk for metastases could be treated with more aggressive adjuvant therapies following surgical resection. By contrast, those patients without such a predisposition may do well with surgical resection of the primary lesion alone.

THE FUTURE OF CANCER THERAPY

Throughout the 20th century, the standard approaches for the treatment of cancer included surgical resection, radiation therapy, and chemotherapy. Although advances in specific technical applications and in combinations of therapies were made, these three broad modalities remained the foundation of therapeutic approaches. This section focuses on novel strategies for treating cancer that may serve to complement and in some cases replace the traditional paradigm of surgery, radiation, and chemotherapy.

Targeted Molecular Therapies

The explosion in information and the increase in our understanding of the basic pathways involved in the transformation of normal cells into invasive cancers have ushered in a new field of oncologic research. The concept behind molecular therapeutics is that a more thorough understanding of the alterations in specific pathways that result in the cancer phenotype may allow for the development of agents that either block a precancer phenotype or replace factors that inhibit the transformation to cancer. It could be argued that many standard chemotherapies work in this manner. Alkylating agents as well as antimetabolites indeed target specific structures such as DNA, which are critical for tumor cells to divide and proliferate. However, these agents for the most part do not distinguish between normal cells and tumor cells. The promise of molecular therapy is the ability to make such a distinction. The importance of this is obvious. By distinguishing normal cells from neoplastic cells, toxicity may be reduced and efficacy increased.

One example of this strategy is the development, application, and subsequent FDA approval of the agent imatinib (Gleevec). Imatinib is an inhibitor of the Bcr-Abl kinase and was initially developed as a treatment for Bcr-Abl–positive leukemias. Imatinib was also found to inhibit other receptors, which signaled through kinases such as PDGF-receptor as well as c-Kit. This observation led to the application of imatinib to tumors beyond leukemias such as gastrointestinal stromal tumors (GISTs). The understanding of the importance of receptor signaling in the transformation of neoplastic cells allowed for the development of an agent that targeted these receptor kinases, thus blocking their activity.

Additional receptor kinase inhibitors have been developed against other receptors that have been shown to play an important role in cancer invasion and metastasis. EGF-R has been shown to play an important role in head and neck cancers, non–small cell lung cancers, and pancreatic cancers. Several agents have been developed that block the activity of this receptor. The small molecule tyrosine kinase inhibitor gefitinib (Iressa) has received FDA approval for the treatment of non–small cell lung carcinoma. Cetuximab (Erbitux) has been used for head and neck cancers as well as colon cancer. Table 13.4 gives a representative list of a number of targets and the agents that have been developed to inhibit them. The VEGF receptors also signal through kinases and can be blocked by a variety of agents still in clinical trials. These agents have been utilized alone and in combination with more conventional cytotoxic chemotherapies.

The expression of HER2 (neu) in breast cancer has been shown to influence the aggressiveness of these tumors. For those patients with breast cancer that expresses HER2, the agent trastuzumab (Herceptin), a humanized monoclonal antibody, has been used with success to block HER2 signaling.

SCIENTIFIC PRINCIPLES

TABLE 13.4

MOLECULAR TARGETS AND THE AGENTS DEVELOPED TO MODULATE THEM

■ TARGET	■ AGENT	■ MANUFACTURER
Bcr-abl	Gleevec	Novartis
HER2 (neu)	Herceptin	Genentech
Ras	R11577	Johnson & Johnson
VEGF	Avastin	Genentech
VEGF	VEGF Trap	Regeneron
EGFR	Iressa	AstraZeneca
EGF	ABX-EGF	Abgenix
Cyclin-dependent kinase	Flavopiridol	Aventis
Protein linase C	Affinitak	Isis Pharmaceuticals

EGF, endothelial growth factor; EGFR, epidermal growth factor receptor; VEGF, vascular endothelial growth factor.
Adapted from Becker J. Signal transduction inhibitors: a work in progress. *Nature Biotechnol* 2004;22:15.

Herceptin in combination with chemotherapy for patients with tumors expressing HER2 has been shown to be superior to chemotherapy alone.

These targeted agents represent an important new strategy, and the number of new agents in the study is likely to increase as new targets are identified. In many cases, the evaluation of these agents will require the development of novel monitoring techniques that can reveal if the targeted pathway is being effectively modulated. One example of this is the use of fluorodeoxyglucose (FDG) positron emission tomography (PET) scans and imatinib in the monitoring and treatment of patients with GISTs.

Another area of active investigation is the development of agents that modulate the methylation status of DNA. DNA methylation is an epigenetic event, which commonly occurs in the cell and allows for the control of gene expression. Methyl groups added to specific sequences (known as CpG islands) generally in the region of promoters result in the silencing of gene expression.

Hypermethylation often occurs in cancer. Most often, the genes that are susceptible to hypermethylation are those involved in cell cycle regulation, DNA repair, apoptosis, drug resistance, differentiation, angiogenesis, and metastasis. Hypermethylation can result in the inactivation of normally reactive tumor suppressors, which would otherwise prevent malignant transformation. Agents that result in DNA demethylation are undergoing active study as anticancer therapies. Agents such as decitabine reverse methylation in a number of tumor lines and have been shown to act on solid tumors as well in clinical trials. Other strategies involve targeting histone-deacetylase (HDAC). HDAC is an important enzyme that is activated by DNA methylation to repress gene expression. HDAC inhibitors have been shown to increase gene expression from methylated genes.

Although the majority of cancers demonstrate hypermethylation, there are some that have evidence of hypomethylation, such as breast, cervical, and brain tumors. Hypomethylation is thought to activate tumorigenesis by turning on oncogenes such as c-*myc* and H-ras. Clearly, agents that result in demethylation will not be universally applicable to all cancers, and site-specific methylating agents may also be needed.

Another exciting field of investigation is in the ability to silence specific gene transcripts. If a tumor is known to overexpress K-ras, having the ability to turn off this expression would be advantageous. Small interfering RNA (siRNA) is a type of RNA designed to bind to messenger RNA, resulting in the degradation and removal of the message. RNA interference can be incorporated into a strategy to decrease the available message for subsequent translation. These siRNA can be generated as short oligonucleotide DNA fragments or delivered in a plasmid form for expression within a cell. In vitro and in vivo experiments have demonstrated the efficiency of this strategy of gene silencing and efforts are under way to develop methods for delivering siRNA in a clinical setting.

Gene Therapy

5 Despite the controversy surrounding human clinical trials using gene therapy, this strategy remains a promising approach for the treatment of patients with cancer. Gene therapy involves the delivery of a cDNA coding sequence for a particular gene of interest via a vector to a host organism with subsequent expression of that gene and production of the gene product. The gene product can provide a missing protein whose function in the case of cancer results in the suppression of the neoplastic phenotype or the protein can result in the lysis or destruction of the tumor or the tumor's associated vasculature. Many genes have been considered as likely candidates for gene delivery strategies to treat tumors. There are also several different vector systems that can be utilized to deliver these genes.

Vectors. The choice of a vector, which is a term used to describe the carrier for the gene sequence that is being delivered, depends to a certain degree on the route of administration, the target tissue, the amount of gene product one hopes to produce, and finally the duration of expression of the gene that is necessary to effect a response. Vectors tend to be categorized into two major classes. Nonviral vectors including plasmid DNA, liposomes, nanoparticles, and other synthetic carriers are attractive in that there is generally little to no immune response from the host and no endogenous viral proteins produced. In addition, these vector systems tend to be transient in their expression and, unless otherwise engineered, do not integrate into the host genome. The downside of nonviral vectors is that both the level of gene product expression and the duration of expression tend to be less than with viral vector systems. Viral vectors have the advantage of efficient transfection or transduction of host cells and sustained elevated levels of gene expression. The disadvantage is their potential immunogenicity, which may render multiple administrations less successful as well as increase the potential for host tissue toxicity.

Both nonviral and viral vector systems can be engineered to target specific tissue beds or tissue types and be delivered in a nontargeted way to host organs such as the liver. The choice between a targeted or nontargeted vector generally depends on the particular gene to be expressed and the ultimate goals of the therapy. This strategy has been illustrated by the application of antiangiogenic gene therapy to the treatment of cancer.

The goal of antiangiogenic gene therapy is to deliver an angiogenesis inhibitor in such a way that the body produces the protein of interest, thus eliminating the difficulties in recombinant production and the need for repeat administration of these proteins. Two strategies have been employed to deliver antiangiogenic agents via gene therapy (Fig. 13.11). The first is to engineer the vector system to target the gene of interest to the tumor cell or the tumor-associated vasculature. The advantage here is that relative tissue levels of the agent of interest can be significantly higher than those that are achieved through systemic production. In addition, genes that produce

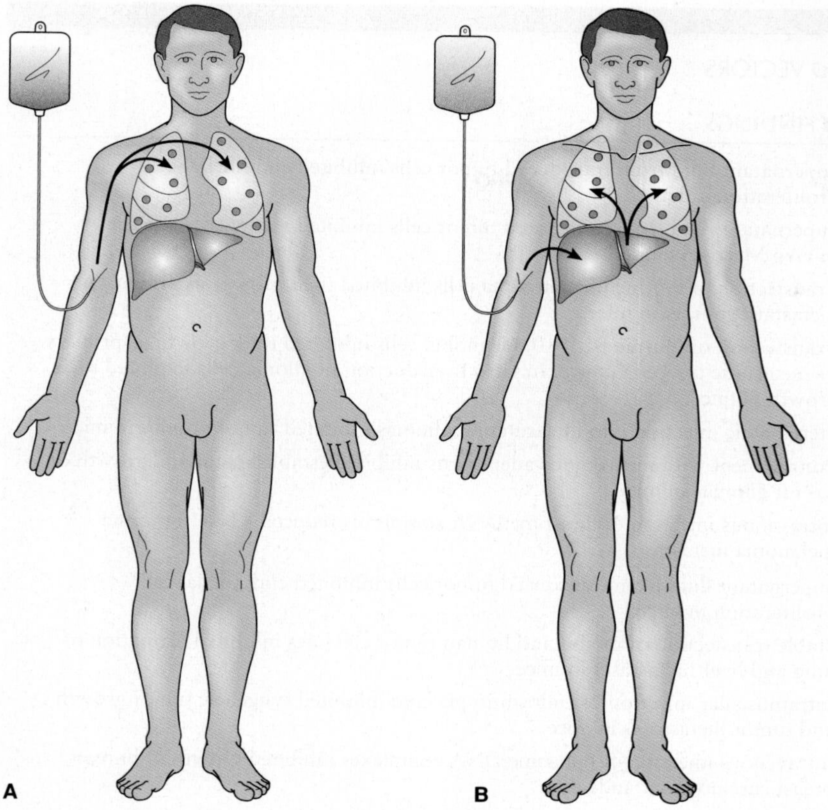

FIGURE 13.11. Strategies for antiangiogenic gene therapy. **A:** Tumor-directed antiangiogenic gene therapy facilitates paracrine activity and avoids systemic toxicity. **B:** Systemic antiangiogenic gene therapy utilizes normal host tissue such as the liver as a "factory" to elevate systemic levels of the gene product. (Adapted from Feldman AL, Libutti SK. Progress in antiangiogenic gene therapy of cancer. *Cancer* 2000;89;1181.)

a product with direct cytotoxicity to the cancer cell or the tumor's associated vasculature can be administered in a targeted way so as to reduce potential toxicity to normal tissues.

An alternative strategy is to deliver a vector to an organ such as the liver resulting in efficient transfection of hepatocytes with the gene for the angiogenesis inhibitor. The goal in this strategy is to harness the liver as a "factory" to produce circulating levels of the angiogenesis inhibitor to prevent the further growth and spread of micrometastatic disease throughout the body. Viral vectors such as adenovirus or adeno-associated virus with their native predilection for liver infection owing to CAR receptor uptake have been the vectors of choice for this approach. However, nonviral vectors such as liposomes tend to be taken up by the reticular endothelial system in the liver as well, and they also result in sustained gene expression and circulating levels of the protein. Table 13.5 lists various genes coding for angiogenesis inhibitors as well as the vectors used for their delivery that have been studied.

In addition to gene therapy strategies that employ the replacement of a gene such as p53 or the delivery of a cytotoxic gene such as thymidine kinase and ganciclovir therapy, the use of cytotoxic vectors alone has shown some promise. Vaccinia virus is a cytoplasmic virus that is related to the virus causing smallpox. Vaccinia virus delivery results in the infection and subsequent lysis of the cells infected. Studies utilizing vaccinia targeted to tumors have demonstrated the potential for this strategy in inhibiting the growth and spread of tumors.

Several clinical trials have been conducted utilizing gene therapy for cancer. Adenovirus carrying p53 has been studied in both direct arterial infusion into the liver as well as the treatment of glioma, lung cancer, ovarian cancer, and breast cancer. Recurrent head and neck cancer has also been studied. So-called suicide gene therapy utilizing the herpes simplex virus thymidine kinase gene and the prodrug ganciclovir has been studied in the clinic. Patients with mesothelioma have been studied in a phase I trial using this strategy, as have patients with prostate adenocarcinoma using direct injection of an adenovirus expressing hsv-tk followed by ganciclovir exposure. These studies have demonstrated the safety of this strategy, although studies to evaluate efficacy are still under way.

The future of gene therapy for cancer is dependent on several important lines of investigation. Improved vectors are needed that minimize toxicity, allow for specific targeting, decrease the host's immune response or prevent a host immune response, and can be produced efficiently for clinical use. The judicious selection of the appropriate genes to deliver in such a strategy is dependent on further investigation into the molecular pathways that are important to the malignant phenotype.

Immunotherapy

Harnessing the body's immune system to attack cancer is an attractive strategy and area of investigation. Tumors express antigens that are often different from the antigens expressed by the normal cells. There are two main approaches for the use of immunotherapy to treat patients with cancer. The first involves the use of vaccine therapy to stimulate the body's native immune system, mainly antigen-presenting cells and lymphocytes, to react specifically against the tumor antigens resulting in tumor regression. The second is the transfer of lymphocytes isolated from the patient's tumor tissue (tumor infiltrating lymphocytes [TILs]) that have been selected for their immunoreactivity against the patient's tumor.

Vaccine therapy may utilize peptides derived from the protein sequence of the cancer antigen, gene therapy with vectors carrying a coding sequence for the peptide or antigen, or, alternatively, the delivery of whole tumor lysate providing a variety of antigenic stimuli. Once vaccinated, the protein or peptide is processed by antigen-presenting cells in the context of the patient's class I major histocompatibility complex (MHC) molecule, thus stimulating a lymphocyte response to the tumor.

TABLE 13.5

ANTIANGIOGENIC GENE THERAPY: GENES AND VECTORS

■ GENE	■ DELIVERY VECTOR	■ FINDINGS
Angiostatin	Adeno-associated virus	Supernatant fluid from transduced tumor cells inhibited endothelial cell proliferation in vitro.
	Cationic liposome: DNA complex	Supernatant fluid from transfected tumor cells inhibited angiogenesis in the in vivo Matrigel model.
	In vitro transfection	Transfection of murine fibrosarcoma cells inhibited their growth as primary or metastatic tumors in mice.
	In vitro transfection Retrovirus	Transfection of murine B16F10 melanoma cells inhibited their growth as primary or metastatic tumors in mice. In vitro transduction of glioma cells inhibited their growth in mice.
	Adenovirus	Stereotactic injection into intracerebral gliomas inhibited tumor growth in mice.
	Adenovirus	Pretreatment with intravenous adenovirus inhibited establishment and growth of C6 rat gliomas in mice.
	Cationic liposome:DNA complex	Intravenous injection of liposome:DNA complexes reduced B16F10 murine melanoma metastasis.
Endostatin	Adeno-associated virus	Supernatant fluid from transduced tumor cells inhibited endothelial cell proliferation in vitro.
	In vitro transfection	Stable transfection of mouse and human tumor cell lines inhibited formation of lung and liver metastases in mice.
	Polymerized plasmid DNA	Intramuscular injection of endostatin plasmid inhibited syngeneic tumor growth and tumor metastases in mice.
	Cationic liposome:DNA complex	Intravenous injection of liposome:DNA complexes inhibited growth of human breast carcinoma in nude mice.
	Adenovirus	Intravenous injection of recombinant adenovirus inhibited growth of subcutaneous tumors in nude mice.
	Adenovirus	Intravenous injection of recombinant adenovirus inhibited subcutaneous tumor growth and prevented lung metastases in nude mice.
IL-4	Retroviral packaging cells	Stereotactic injection inhibited angiogenesis and growth of intracerebral rat gliomas and was immunostimulatory.
IL-10	In vitro transfection	Transfection of human melanoma cells inhibited angiogenesis, tumor growth, and establishment of metastases.
	In vitro transfection	Transfection of human prostate cancer cells inhibited their growth in nude mice
IL-12	Semliki Forest virus	Intratumoral injection inhibited B16 melanoma angiogenesis and growth in mice independent of immune response.
IFN-a TIMP-1	In vitro retroviral transduction Adenovirus	Transduction of human prostate carcinoma cells inhibited their ability to form tumors and lymph node metastases in nude mice. Adenoviral infection of endothelial cells inhibited their migration in vitro.
TIMP-2	In vitro transfection	Transfection of B16F10 murine melanoma cells inhibited angiogenesis, tumor growth, and metastases in mice.
TSP-1	Liposome:DNA complex	Intravenous injection of DNA complexes encoding a TSP-1 fragment inhibited human breast carcinoma growth in mice.
p16	Adenovirus	Pretreatment with virus inhibited the ability of glioma cells to induce angiogenesis in a dorsal air sac model in nude mice.
p53	Liposome:DNA complex	Intravenous injection inhibited human breast carcinoma growth associated with decreased blood vessel density in nude mice.
	Liposome:DNA complex	Intravenous injection reduced angiogenesis and inhibited establishment of B16F10 lung metastases in C57BL/6 mice.
PF-4	Adenovirus	Coinjection of adenovirus with glioma cells under renal capsule of nude mice inhibited tumor growth and vascularity.
EMAP-II	Vaccinia	Intravenous injection of vaccinia enhanced tumor sensitivity to TNF associated with endothelial cell TNF receptor upregulation.

From Feldman AL, Libutti SK. Progress in antiangiogenic gene therapy of cancer. *Cancer* 2000;89:1181.

Cancer vaccines have been utilized in clinical trials studying a variety of human tumors. Patients with melanoma, breast cancer, colon cancer, head and neck cancer, and renal cancers have been studied. Although several studies have demonstrated successful immunization of patients to tumor antigens, to date, there have been no successful trials demonstrating significant cancer regression to vaccine therapy alone.

Cell transfer therapy has demonstrated antitumor activity in patients. To date, the most effective immunotherapy that has been utilized for patients with melanoma and renal cell cancer has been the infusion of interleukin-2 (IL-2). IL-2 is a lymphocyte-stimulating cytokine that has a variety of effects on T cells. Response rates to the systemic administration of IL-2 for patients with both melanoma and kidney cancer are 15% to 20%, with complete responses being approximately 9%. Complete responses are often durable with a majority of patients enjoying a long-term disease-free survival beyond 10 years. Therefore, any new immunotherapy strategy must improve on these IL-2 results.

TILs can be grown successfully from melanoma. These lymphocytes can then be tested for their reactivity against the melanoma using cell lysis assays. The advantage of cell transfer approaches is the ability to administer extremely large numbers of highly selective cells that have demonstrated avidity for the tumor antigens as well as the ability to affect tumor cell lyses. In studies at the NCI, Rosenberg et al. have demonstrated the ability to effect regression of metastatic melanoma refractory to standard treatment in patients receiving a nonmyeloablative preparative chemotherapy regimen followed by the administration of selected TILs and IL-2. Response rates of 40% have been achieved with such an approach. A new strategy involving the introduction of specific and reactive T-cell receptors into peripheral blood mononuclear cells may obviate the need for harvesting tumor-infiltrating lymphocytes and open the possibility of using this strategy to treat solid tumors other than melanoma.

Clearly, there is a role for immunotherapy in the treatment of cancer. The future involves a better understanding of the complex interactions that lead to the immune response so as to better harness this knowledge for the development for more effective therapies. Such an understanding of the molecules that suppress or activate the immune response has led to the identification of lymphocyte surface molecules such as CTLA-4. CTLA-4 is an important regulator of T-lymphocyte proliferation and function. When active, CTLA-4 suppresses lymphocyte activation. Antibodies against CTLA-4 have been utilized in clinical trials demonstrating that inhibition of this suppression can result in an immune response against tumors.

ROLE OF THE SURGEON IN CANCER TREATMENT

Modern cancer therapy involves a multidisciplinary approach consisting of a variety of specialists with diverse talents. These individuals can be physicians, nurses, physical therapists, pain and palliative care specialists, dietitians, and clergy. The cancer patient often presents with a complex series of medical and nonmedical issues that require a coordinated approach for the optimal delivery of care. The surgeon's role in this coordinated effort is critical. For many patients, their first experience with the health care team is with a surgeon for the management of their primary tumor. This requires that the surgeon have a good understanding of the roles of the other members of the team and an ability to coordinate their interactions to provide the patient with the best possible outcome.

Typically, surgeons are associated with the management of early-stage disease and are usually called on only to manage the complications of stage IV disease, such as bowel obstruction or bleeding. This paradigm is changing as it has become increasingly evident that aggressive surgical approaches may be of benefit to patients with advanced-stage tumors. Throughout this text are descriptions of the role of surgeons for the management of early-stage disease. Therefore, this section focuses on surgeons' impact in the management and care of cancer patients with metastatic tumors.

6 Surgical resection of metastatic disease has been practiced for decades. For certain tumor types, most notably, colorectal cancer and sarcoma, surgical resection of metastases in the lung or liver has been associated with improved survival. This approach relies on the fact that metastatic disease is well localized to one or two organs and that resection of those sites can be done safely and completely.

In 2008, it is estimated that there will be approximately 150,000 new cases of colorectal cancer. Of these patients, 20% to 40% will develop liver metastases as the sole or dominant site of their disease progression. Approximately 10% to 20% of patients with liver metastases will have disease that can be resected and patients may potentially benefit from the intervention. For patients with metastatic colorectal cancer confined to the liver, the options for therapy include resection for those with resectable disease with or without the addition of the adjuvant therapy, and systemic therapies for those with unresectable disease relying on combinations of irinotecan, 5FU, leucovorin, oxaliplatin, and, most recently, bevacizumab (Avastin). Bevacizumab is an antiangiogenic agent that blocks VEGF. It was recently approved by the FDA for the treatment of advanced colon cancer. Regional therapies involving hepatic artery infusion or isolated hepatic perfusion are also options for patients with unresectable disease, as are radiofrequency ablation and cryotherapy.

For patients with resectable metastatic colon cancer involving the liver (similar results exist for isolated disease involving the lung), resection of disease is followed by 5-year survival in a significant fraction. A variety of studies evaluating the outcome and operative mortality for patients undergoing complete resection of isolated colorectal cancer metastasis to the liver demonstrate 5-year survival ranging from 26% to 40%. There is at present no systemic chemotherapy regimen that significantly improves on the 10% 5-year survival observed in the earliest 5FU and leucovorin studies. Therefore, it is important to identify those patients with metastatic colorectal cancer isolated to the liver who would be candidates for surgical resection and therefore potentially a cure.

It is important to properly stratify patients to determine which ones will likely derive the greatest benefit from resection. In a 1999 study, Fong et al. at Memorial Sloan-Kettering Cancer Center reported on the results of an analysis of more than 1,000 patients treated by surgical resection for stage IV colon cancer isolated to the liver. They analyzed prognostic factors using univariate and multivariate statistics and determined the factors that predicted a positive outcome for their patients. Among the influential factors were disease-free interval between resection of the primary tumor and first sign of liver metastasis, number of tumors in the liver, carcinoembryonic antigen (CEA) value, size of the largest liver lesion, and the nodal status of the primary tumor. Depending on the number of these factors, a prediction of the 5-year survival and median overall survival in months could be determined (Table 13.6).

This type of information is critical in deciding which patients would most likely benefit from an aggressive surgical resection for their liver lesions. These outcomes are improved by the ability to accurately stage patients preoperatively with modalities such as high-resolution computed tomography (CT), magnetic resonance imaging (MRI), and PET using FDG. Intraoperative ultrasound is also critical to the careful intraoperative staging of these patients not only for the detection of additional liver lesions but also for the accurate determination of anatomic relationships to choose the appropriate resection to perform. Improved operative techniques such as segmental resections, use of stapling devices and coagulation

TABLE 13.6

PREDICTORS OF MORTALITY AND SURVIVAL FOLLOWING RESECTION OF HEPATIC COLORECTAL METASTASES

PROGNOSTIC FACTOR	*p* VALUE	RR DEATH
Disease-free interval <12 mo	0.002	1.56
Tumor number >1	0.01	1.56
CEA >200 μg/L	0.05	1.45
Size >5 cm	0.01	1.46
Node positive primary	0.05	1.34

SURVIVAL BASED ON NUMBER OF FACTORS

NUMBER OF FACTORS	5-y SURVIVAL (%)	MEDIAN OS
0	57	74
1	57	73
2	47	50
3	16	30
4	8	15

CEA, carcinoembryonic antigen; OS, overall survival; RR, relative risk. Adapted from Fong Y, Fortner J, Sun RL, et al. Clinical score for predicting recurrence after hepatic resection for metastatic colorectal cancer: analysis of 1,001 consecutive cases. *Ann Surg* 1999;230:309.

devices, minimization of blood loss by extrahepatic ligation of the hepatic vein prior to dissection, and intermittent inflow occlusion of the porta hepatis have led to a significant reduction in morbidity and mortality. However, despite these advances, many patients are not candidates for surgical resection. The surgeon can still play a role in the aggressive management of these patients.

Regional therapies for cancer have been the subject of study for more than 50 years. A variety of regional therapies are presently available to treat isolated hepatic metastases that might not otherwise be amenable to surgical resection due to the number of lesions, underlying liver disease, or other comorbid medical conditions. These techniques include cryoablation, radiofrequency ablation, intra-arterial hepatic infusion chemotherapy, chemoembolization of tumors, intralesional injection of chemotherapy or alcohol, and regional perfusion through operative or percutaneous techniques. Isolated operative hepatic perfusion and percutaneous hepatic perfusion are two promising strategies for the treatment of patients with isolated hepatic colorectal cancer metastasis.

Isolated hepatic perfusion (IHP) is a complex surgical procedure that was first reported in the early 1960s. It involves the complete isolation of the vascular inflow and outflow of the liver to deliver, via the hepatic arterial circulation, high doses of chemotherapy or cytokines to treat lesions within the liver but to spare the rest of the body from potential toxicity. The liver is ideally suited to such an approach because the majority of liver tumors (approaching 100%) derive their blood supply from the hepatic arterial vessels, whereas the normal liver receives 75% of its blood flow from the portal system. This

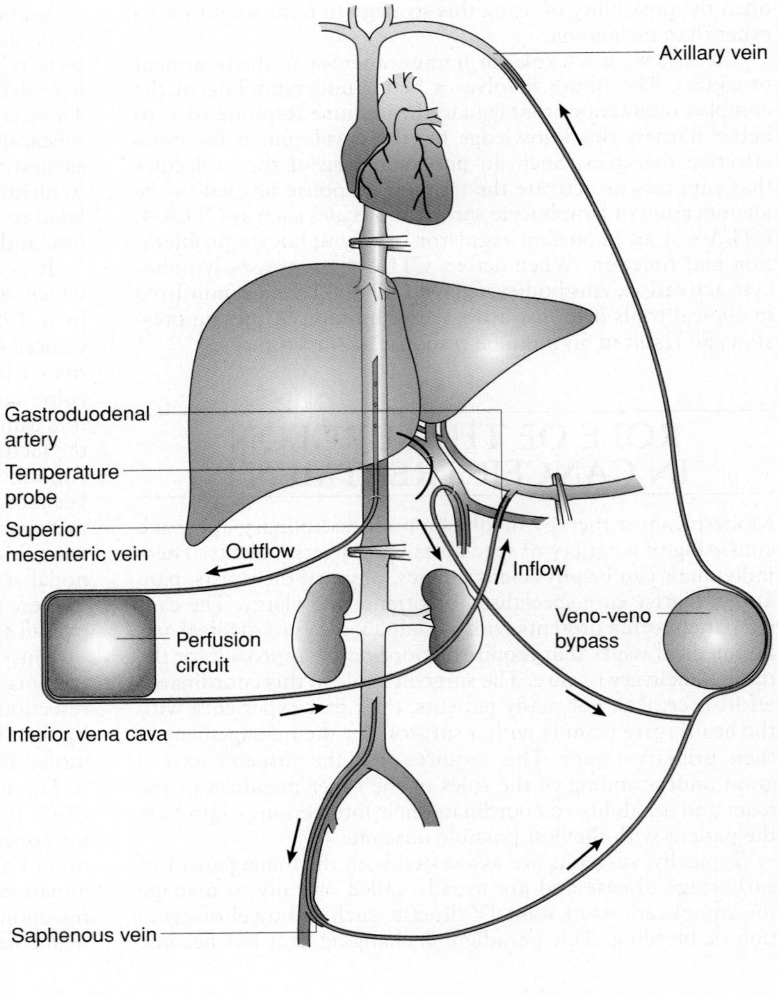

FIGURE 13.12. Schematic diagram of the perfusion and veno-veno bypass circuits used during an isolated hepatic perfusion. For the perfusion circuit, blood is collected from the hepatic veins via an isolated segment of retrohepatic vena cava that has been carefully prepared by ligating dividing venous tributaries and the adrenal vein. This blood is returned to a heat oxygenator and is perfused back into the liver via the common hepatic artery (through a catheter in the gastroduodenal artery). The perfusate consists of packed red blood cells and chemotherapy in a crystalloid solution. Infrahepatic blood and portal blood is shunted via an extracorporeal bypass circuit to the axillary vein to maintain venous return to the heart.

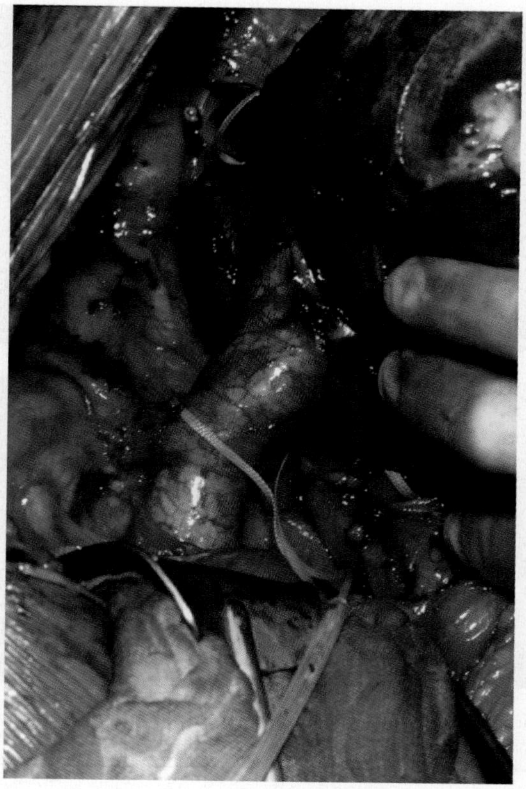

FIGURE 13.13. A view of the retrohepatic vena cava following dissection for an isolated hepatic perfusion.

allows the differential delivery of chemotherapy to the liver tumor by infusing the agent directly into the hepatic arterial circulation. The venous effluent from the hepatic veins is collected in an isolated segment of retrohepatic vena cava and this blood is recirculated back through a perfusion circuit that maintains a constant perfusion of oxygenated blood carrying chemotherapy and cytokines to the liver.

Extrahepatic circulation is maintained by shunting the infrahepatic caval blood as well as the portal circulation through a pump to the axillary vein to maintain systemic blood pressure (Fig. 13.12). Careful dissection of the liver with special attention to the retrohepatic vena cava is required to divide collaterals and prevent systemic exposure to the perfusion agent (Fig. 13.13). The portal structures must also be completely dissected to isolate the portal vein and hepatic vessels for cannulation (Fig. 13.14). The advantages of such an approach are the complete separation of the regional and systemic circulation eliminating or significantly reducing systemic toxicity. Dose escalation of the chemotherapeutic agents is now limited only by the liver's tolerance to these agents as opposed to bone marrow or other systemic sites. The liver generally has a much greater reserve and ability to recover than the bone marrow. This technique also allows the utilization of hyperthermia via this closed circulatory system that can be heated and oxygenated by an extracorporeal heart lung machine.

A number of centers both in the United States and in Europe have explored this technique; the largest experience has been in the Surgery Branch of the NCI. Alexander et al. have reported results for 51 patients with unresectable colorectal cancer metastases treated with an IHP using the chemotherapy melphalan (with or without TNF) with or without follow-up hepatic arterial infusion (HAI) with FUDR/LV. Results included a response rate of approximately 75% with a median survival of 16 months for those patients not receiving follow-up HAI therapy and 27 months for those receiving HAI therapy following their IHP. These results demonstrate that significant responses and an acceptable duration of response can be achieved for an aggressive surgical approach for patients with significant liver disease (Fig. 13.15).

The application of IHP to unresectable liver metastases demonstrates the potential role for the surgeon in the management of patients with metastatic cancer. Clearly, however, such an intervention requires significant resources and skill, which may not be available at every major medical center. Therefore, a need to adapt this strategy to a therapy that can be more safely and easily administered and that allows repeated administrations (IHP can only be performed once) would be desirable. Investigators are therefore evaluating whether or not a percutaneous approach to hepatic isolation can be utilized.

This technique relies on the use of balloons placed via a catheter percutaneously introduced into the vena cava through the femoral vein. The balloons can occlude above the hepatic veins and above the renal veins to isolate a segment of the vena cava. The catheter isolates hepatic venous effluent to allow for extracorporeal filtration of chemotherapy delivered to the liver through a separate catheter introduced into the hepatic artery

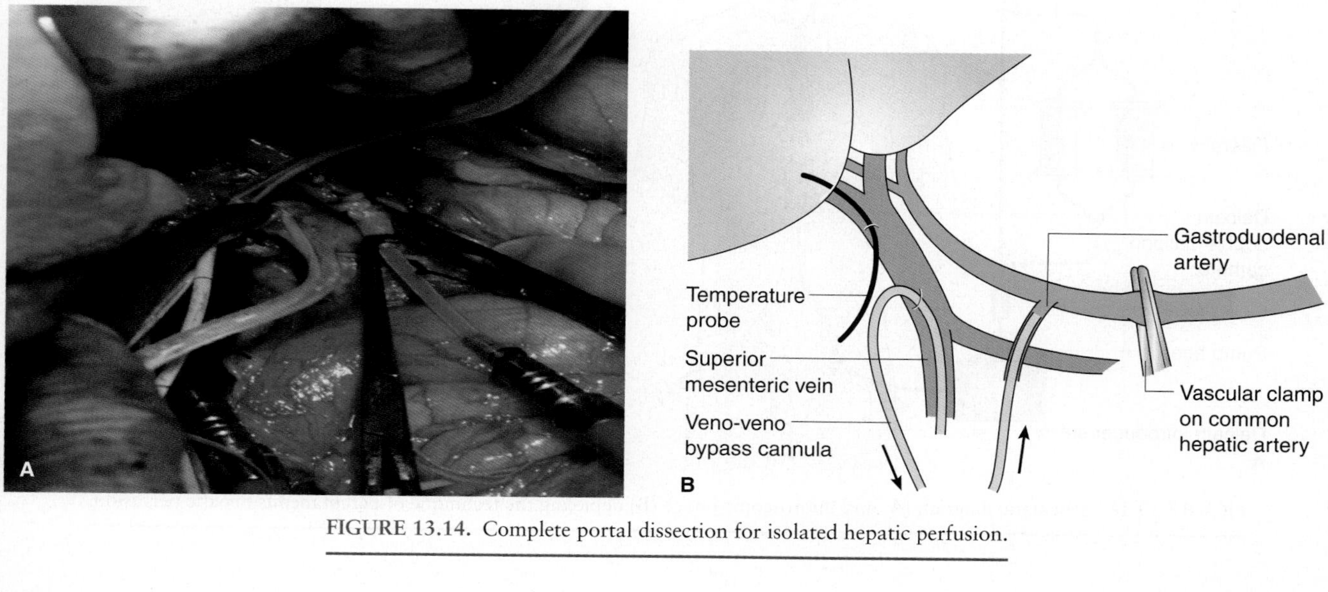

FIGURE 13.14. Complete portal dissection for isolated hepatic perfusion.

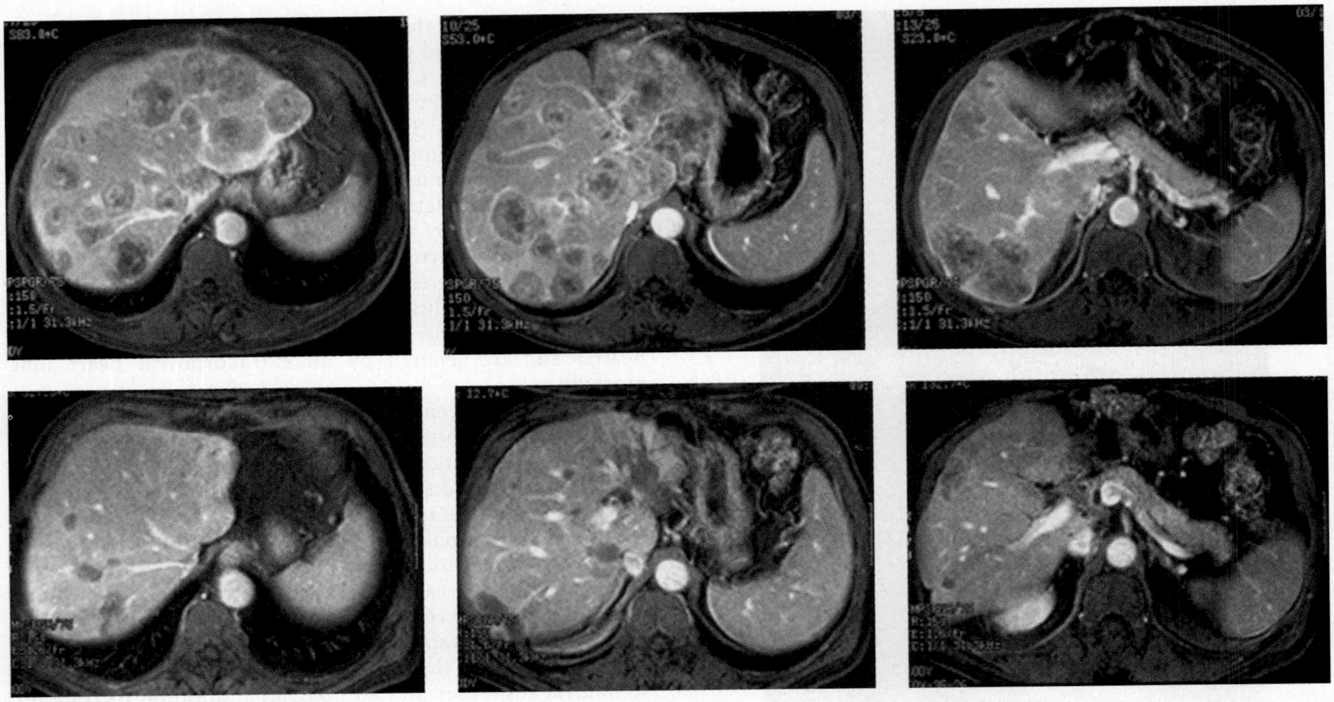

FIGURE 13.15. Magnetic resonance imaging of the liver for a patient with colorectal cancer metastatic to the liver before (*top*) and after (*bottom*) an isolated hepatic perfusion (IHP).

(Fig. 13.16). The filtered blood is then returned via the internal jugular vein to maintain venous return. A phase I trial was recently completed at the NCI demonstrating a safe dose of melphalan that can be delivered in this fashion. A multicenter phase III trial is now under way to evaluate the utility of this approach for metastatic melanoma (cutaneous and ocular) to the liver compared to best standard therapy.

Regional therapy can be applied to other locations in the body such as the limb (isolated limb perfusion for melanoma or sarcoma) and the peritoneal cavity. Peritoneal carcinomatosis secondary to a number of histologies including colorectal cancer, gastric cancer, pancreatic cancer, and malignant mesothelioma can be addressed. Traditionally, surgeons have played a role in managing the complications of this entity such as ascites and obstruction. However, techniques such as surgical debulking and intraperitoneal chemotherapy are gaining prominence as a viable management strategy for treating patients with peritoneal carcinomatosis. Surgeons have a unique role to play and can make a significant impact in treating this condition.

Malignant peritoneal mesothelioma can result in significant abdominal pain and distention accompanied by anorexia and

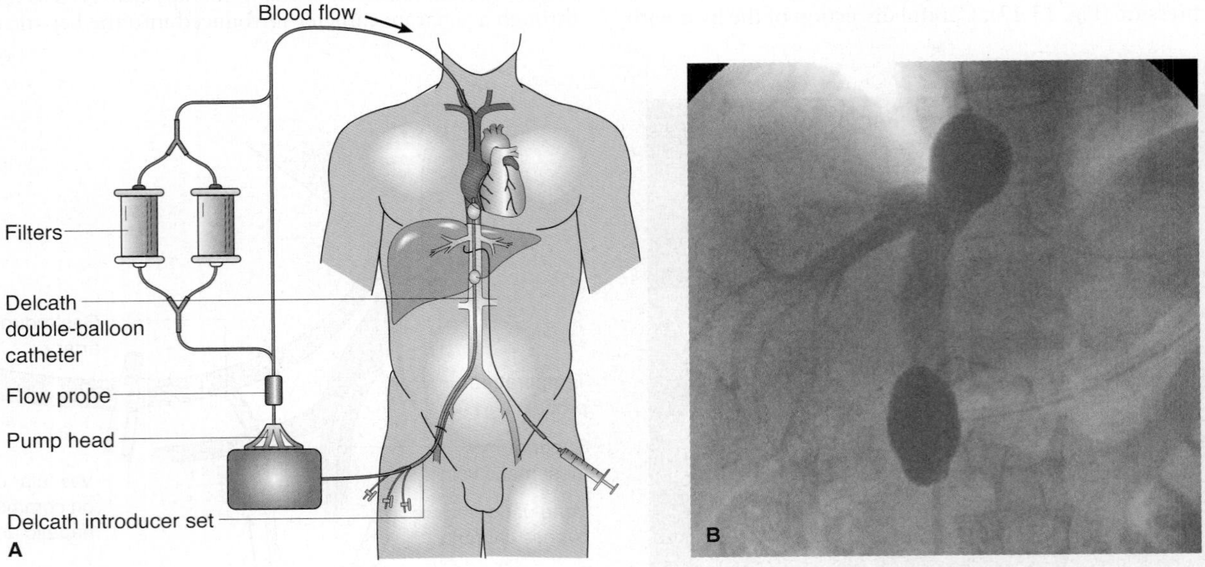

FIGURE 13.16. Schematic diagram (**A**) and fluoroscopic image (**B**) depicting the technique of percutaneous hepatic perfusion.

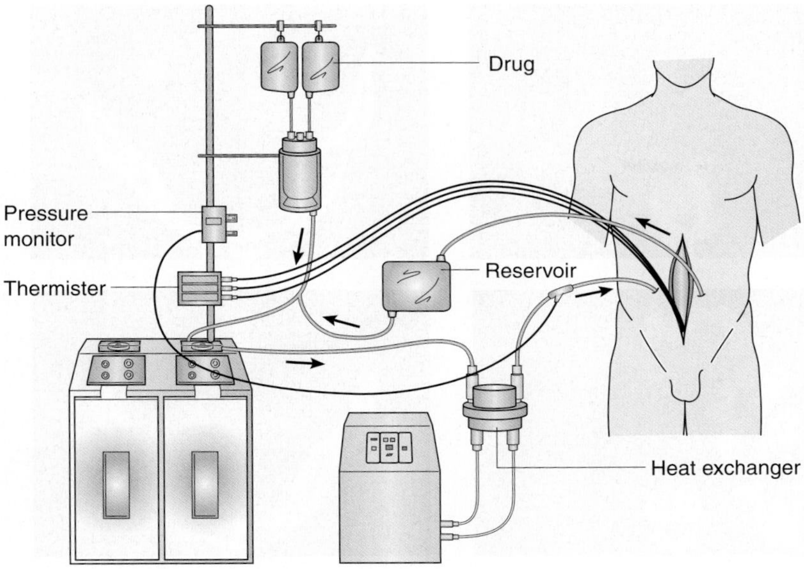

FIGURE 13.17. Diagram of the setup for continuous hyperthermic peritoneal perfusion.

weight loss, ascites, and bowel obstruction. These complications can lead to death and there are no effective systemic treatment options. Although agents such as cisplatin and carboplatin as well as paclitaxel (Taxol) and doxorubicin (Adriamycin) have been used to treat this condition, response rates are low (<20%) and survival is poor. The technique of continuous hyperthermic peritoneal perfusion (CHPP) involves an exploratory laparotomy with lysis of adhesions, tumor resection, omentectomy, and peritonectomy of involved peritoneal surfaces (Fig. 13.17). Organs such as the spleen, if significantly involved with tumor, are also resected. At the completion of resection, the abdomen is closed after the insertion of inflow and outflow catheters and temperature probes. Carcinomatosis can involve the surfaces of the mesentery, which can be very difficult to resect (Fig. 13.18). Best efforts are made to strip the peritoneal surface over the mesentery and to fulgurate small lesions with ball electrocautery.

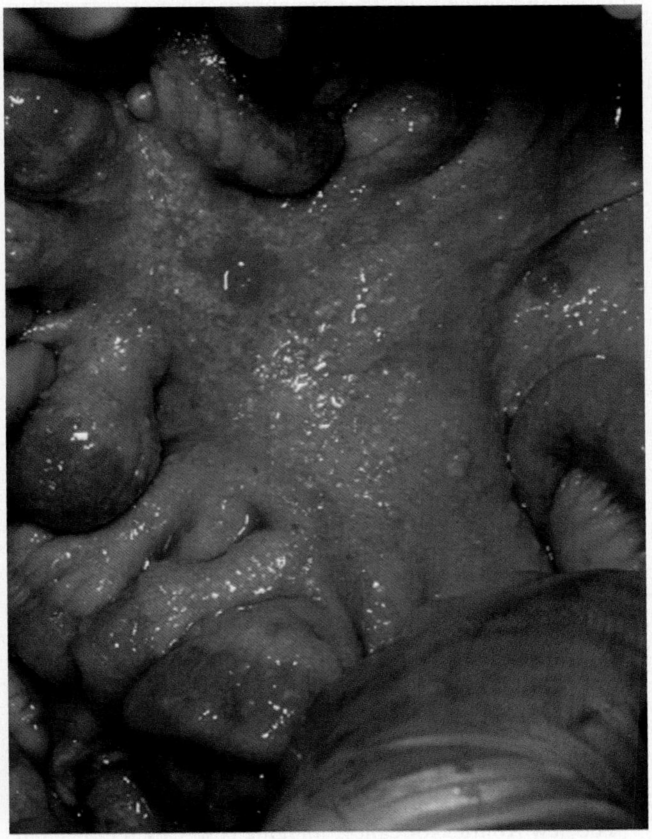

FIGURE 13.18. Intraoperative photo demonstrating significant carcinomatosis involving the mesentery of the small bowel.

These catheters are connected to a perfusion circuit with a roller pump and heat exchange coil to circulate hyperthermic intraperitoneal chemotherapy agents. At the completion of the perfusion the abdomen is irrigated, and a peritoneal dialysis catheter can be inserted for postoperative dwell therapy with additional regional chemotherapy.

In a study of CHPP for intraperitoneal mesothelioma, Park et al. summarized the results of 18 patients with peritoneal mesothelioma treated with CHPP from 1993 through 1998. Of these 18 patients, 13 had clinically significant ascites. Patients were treated with operative debulking and CHPP with cisplatin. After a median follow-up of 19 months, there were no operative or treatment-related mortalities, and the overall operative morbidity was 24%. Morbidity included wound infection, atrial fibrillation, pancreatitis, ileus, and line sepsis.

Nine of 13 patients with ascites had complete resolution of their ascites following a single procedure. Three other patients had resolution of their ascites after a second CHPP. The median progression-free survival was 26 months, and the overall 2-year survival was 80%. Although this study did not prospectively compare CHPP to systemic cisplatin, trials of intravenous cisplatin report survival data that are similar to untreated patients. The results of CHPP can be dramatic for patients suffering with the very morbid condition of abdominal ascites (Fig. 13.19).

Thus, the surgeon can play an important role in the management of not only patients with primary tumors but also patients with stage IV disease. Surgeons must familiarize themselves with the other available nonoperative options for their patients with cancer so the correct therapy can be selected for the appropriate patient. Further study is needed to identify therapies that will benefit patients with advanced disease.

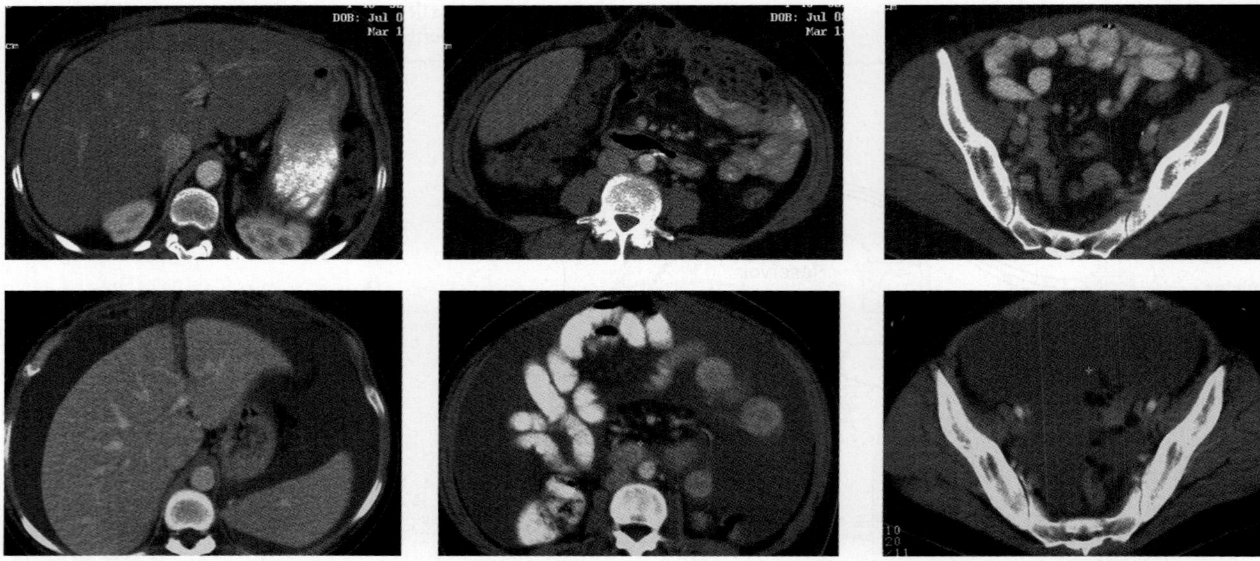

FIGURE 13.19. Computed tomography scan of a patient with ascites from peritoneal mesothelioma before (*top*) and after (*bottom*) a tumor debulking and continuous hyperthermic peritoneal perfusion.

CANCER DETECTION AND BIOMARKERS

Methods to enable more accurate early detection of cancer are an active area of investigation. Some of these methods are amenable to cancer screening, allowing assessment of large populations of at-risk patients to detect disease at its earliest possible time. Other methods are best applied to patients who have already been treated for their cancer and are being followed for signs of recurrence. This section highlights three areas that illustrate the possibilities for early cancer detection.

Imaging

Standard imaging techniques such as CT, MRI, and ultrasound have been applied to patients as a means of both screening and follow-up. Standard plain radiographs have also been used in this setting. As CT scans and MRIs have become more advanced with higher resolution and shorter scanning times, the sensitivity for lesion detection has been dramatically improved. One example has been the development of both CT and magnetic resonance (MR) colonography.

Colonography has been proposed as a means to screen patients for colon polyps and tumors in an effort to avoid the need for an optical endoscopic colonoscopy. Virtual colonoscopy using CT scanning was evaluated as a screening procedure for colorectal neoplasia in asymptomatic adults at the National Naval Medical Center in Bethesda, Maryland. A total of 1,233 asymptomatic adults (mean age 58 years) underwent a same-day CT colonography as well as an optical colonoscopy. The radiologist used a three-dimensional endoluminal display for the detection of polyps on the virtual colonoscopy. The physicians performing the optical colonoscopy did not know the results of the virtual colonoscopy for the initial examination. The sensitivity and specificity of virtual colonoscopy compared to optical colonoscopy were then compared to the findings of a final unblinded optical colonoscopy, which was used as the reference standard.

Sensitivity of the virtual colonoscopy for adenomatous polyps was 94% for polyps greater than 8 mm in diameter and 89% for polyps that measured at least 6 mm in diameter. The sensitivity of optical colonoscopy for adenomatous polyps was 88% to 92% for polyps greater than 8 mm in diameter and 92% for polyps measuring at least 6 mm in diameter. Of the patients screened, two polyps were found to be malignant and both of them were detected by virtual colonoscopy. With sensitivities and specificities that are approaching or better than those of optical colonoscopy, virtual colonoscopy using CT may become a screening procedure of choice. When lesions are detected, a follow-up optical colonoscopy can be performed to biopsy the lesion.

Noninvasive imaging can also be utilized in patients following the treatment of a cancer to detect early recurrence. In a study at the NCI, standard imaging techniques such as CT, MRI, and ultrasound were compared to PET using FDG, anti-CEA antibody immunoscintigraphy, and a blind second-look laparotomy for patients with a rising serum CEA following definitive management of colorectal cancer. In this study FDG-PET and blind second-look laparotomy were found to be the most sensitive methods for detection of recurrent disease. As a noninvasive screening method, FDG-PET was both sensitive and specific for the detection of recurrent disease in patients with a rising serum CEA and therefore is now recommended as an appropriate screening modality prior to any planned surgical management (Fig. 13.20). FDG-PET is also useful in the metastatic workup of patients with malignant melanoma, primary lung carcinoma, and esophageal cancers.

Dynamic enhanced MRI (DEMRI) has become a useful noninvasive imaging modality for the evaluation of the functional status of a tumor. Tumor blood flow and blood volume can be calculated from DEMRI images and thus, this noninvasive imaging method can be used to follow the response of a tumor to a variety of therapies. DEMRI has been successfully utilized for imaging primary breast cancers as well as for imaging metastatic sites from a variety of histologies. Images obtained from DEMRI can be utilized to determine residual areas of tumor activity following therapies to more accurately guide biopsies and further regional treatment.

The new frontier for cancer imaging is so-called molecular imaging. Although this term can encompass a variety of imaging approaches and methods, it is most commonly used to categorize techniques that rely on imaging a tissue based

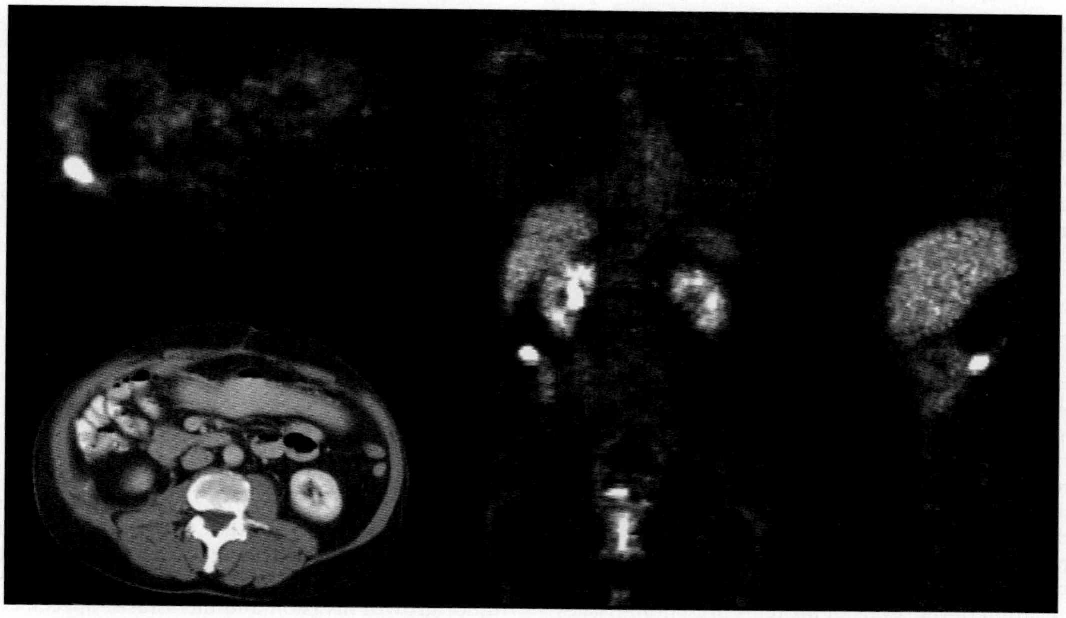

FIGURE 13.20. Fluorodeoxyglucose positron emission tomography scan demonstrates a recurrent colon cancer in the bed of a previous right hemicolectomy that was not detected on computed tomography scan in a patient with a rising serum carcinoembryonic antigen.

on specific expression of receptors or pathways. In combination with molecular therapies, such imaging methods may allow for noninvasive monitoring of the activity of targeted agents.

A number of preclinical models have been developed to test molecular imaging strategies. Weissleder et al. have designed a number of noninvasive methods for imaging the activity of enzymes and pathways to predict the efficacy of molecular agents. One example is their use of iron oxide nanoparticles cross-linked to Cy-3 and Cy-5 fluorescent dyes. Using cathepsin-B cleavable linking peptides, activity can be measured via cleavage and determination of the ratio of the various fluorophores. By using fluorophores as well as iron particles, both fluorescent imaging and MRI of the tissue in question can be performed.

Specific tissue receptors can also be imaged noninvasively. Tumor vasculature is known to have an increased expression of integrins such as $\alpha v\beta 3$. Using RGD cyclic pentapeptides labeled with PET positron emitters, tissues with enhanced $\alpha v\beta 3$ expression can be imaged. Such techniques can be used to locate areas of increased tumor neovascular density and can also be utilized to follow the targeting or activity of $\alpha v\beta 3$-specific agents.

Gene Expression Profiling

With the completion of the sequencing of the human genome, a wealth of information is now available regarding the roughly 30,000 genes that code for various proteins involved in normal cellular homeostasis. The dysregulation of these genes that occurs in neoplastic tissue can now be studied using microarray-based technologies.

Microarrays for the study of gene expression can utilize a variety of platforms, the most common of which are cDNA and oligonucleotide sequences. Nucleic acid sequences can be spotted on glass slides or on proprietary chips, allowing 20,000 or more coding sequences to be placed on a single slide (chip). These techniques allow high-throughput screening of these genes from a variety of sources capable of yielding substrate RNA. Using linear RNA amplification techniques, even the smallest samples of RNA from fine-needle aspirates (FNAs) or microdissected tissues can be utilized for profiling. Gene expression profiling can be used to answer a variety of questions including the differences in gene expression pathways between malignant and normal tissues. Expression profiles can also be determined in tissues prior to and following therapies to better understand mechanism of action of a treatment. Recently, genomics approaches have been validated for the stratification of women with breast cancer for treatment with adjuvant therapy. Such approaches are useful in determining which patients may benefit from adjuvant chemotherapy or hormonal therapy and which patients will not, thereby avoiding unnecessary toxicity in patients unlikely to benefit from the therapy.

Complex bioinformatics software programs have been developed to allow a more thorough analysis of the data sets obtained through these studies. The National Institutes of Health (NIH) Center for Information Technology and the NCI have posted a series of bioinformatics tools to allow investigators to better study and understand the results of their microarray experiments. This Web site can be found at http://nciarray.nci.nih.gov/.

One example of the utility of microarray approaches for the diagnosis of cancer is the differentiation of benign versus malignant thyroid lesions. Approximately 10 million new thyroid lesions are diagnosed each year in the United States. Only 5% of these lesions are malignant. Although fine-needle aspiration has been utilized in an attempt to identify those patients with a thyroid cancer who require further management, straightforward cytologic examination of FNA samples often leads to indeterminate or nondiagnostic studies. A molecular method for distinguishing benign from malignant thyroid lesions would be helpful in identifying those patients who would most benefit from a surgical intervention.

Utilizing cDNA microarray, our group compared expression profiles of thyroid cancers (papillary thyroid cancers and follicular variant papillary thyroid cancers) to benign thyroid lesions. Cluster analysis developed a model to predict the malignant potential of the tissue. Using this strategy, we identified 10 genes capable of differentiating a benign lesion from a malignant lesion. By using this technique, the diagnosis of thyroid cancer from FNA may be improved.

Microarray approaches have also been used to grade lymphoma as well as predict potential response to therapies. Childhood sarcomas have also been subclassified using a similar molecular approach. As these technologies improve, more widespread use of these molecular-based diagnostics will be feasible.

Proteomics

Genes mainly code for proteins that perform the various structural and functional roles in the cell. Proteins undergo a series of modifications to perform these jobs, most importantly glycosylation and phosphorylation. Although cDNA and oligonucleotide microarrays can determine levels of gene expression, they cannot elucidate the modifications that take place at the protein level.

Proteomics, or the direct study of proteins, allows for not only a quantification of the levels of proteins present in tissues but also a determination of the phosphorylation status of these proteins. Serum proteomics is an exciting new technology, which holds promise for the diagnosis of cancer from a sample of blood. Such an approach is now being applied to clinical samples.

Based on the assumption that patients harboring a malignancy have circulating proteins in their serum that are not present in unaffected patients, serum proteomics endeavors to distinguish a "biosignature" profile of human cancer. By taking samples from a population of patients with cancer and comparing the proteomic profile of their serum to that of a population of people without cancer, a pattern can be elucidated that identifies the at-risk population. The novelty of this approach is that, unlike investigating single specific biomarkers such as CEA for colon cancer or CA 19–9 for pancreas cancer, a serum proteomic approach requires no hypotheses about which proteins will be important to identify. In fact, thousands of proteins can be queried and utilized to form the biosignature. The most informative of these can be determined using various bioinformatics strategies to reduce the number to a manageable assay.

Applying this approach to patients with ovarian cancer, high-resolution spectral data have been obtained that demonstrated a specific pattern capable of distinguishing patients with stage I ovarian cancer from patients with more advanced ovarian cancer, as well as from normal healthy controls. As these techniques improve, they will no doubt be applied to other tumor histologies and will add to the armamentarium of diagnostic tests available to the clinician.

CLINICAL TRIALS

As knowledge increases regarding the pathways involved in tumorigenesis, novel agents will be identified that show promise in treating cancer. Although much can be learned about these agents in preclinical models, the ultimate evaluation of a new cancer therapeutic requires carefully conducted clinical trials.

Clinical trials involve the participation of patient volunteers. These volunteers agree to participate in studies that pose specific scientific questions to find improved strategies to prevent, diagnose, screen for, or treat a particular disease process. There are a number of types of clinical trials.

Prevention trials are designed to evaluate strategies or therapies aimed at preventing the development of cancer. These studies are most often conducted with healthy patient volunteers who have not yet developed cancer but may or may not have a predisposition to develop cancer. Screening trials are aimed at finding improved ways to determine which patients or populations of patients are most at risk for developing cancer and therefore detect cancers in these patients at the earliest time point to be more effective in treating their disease.

Diagnostic trials are geared toward the study of procedures or tests that can identify cancer at its earliest possible stage. The testing of new diagnostics is often performed on patients who are already known to have cancer based on standard diagnostic tests. Supportive care (quality of life) trials are designed to investigate ways to improve the quality of life of patients in whom further therapies may not be available. These trials are of critical importance as they can often determine where new therapies may have a dramatic improvement in the symptoms of cancer and therefore decrease the suffering due to cancer in those patients.

Genetic studies can be standalone trials or a part of another trial. These studies may rely on the analyses of germline mutations in patients (e.g., studies of patients with familial cancer syndromes) or may rely on studies of somatic mutations in the tumor tissues themselves to understand pathways involved in tumor growth invasion and metastasis. Special considerations must be made when performing genetic studies that involve germline analysis as the findings of such studies may have far-reaching implications for the patient. Appropriate genetic counseling must be a part of the informed consent process for these studies.

The most common and familiar types of clinical trial are treatment trials, which are designed to evaluate new cancer therapies. Treatment trials are divided into different phases of evaluation for new anticancer agents. Phase I trials are performed to evaluate the safety and toxicity profile of a compound and are generally conducted in a dose escalation format. Patients receive progressively higher doses of the agent to determine the maximum tolerated dose and any dose-related toxicities. This allows for determination of the safe dose for evaluation in the next phase. Pharmacokinetics and pharmacodynamics can also be studied. These studies generally enroll 20 to 30 patients in cohorts of three patients per study dose level.

Phase II trials are focused on determining the efficacy of a given agent at its maximum tolerated dose (MTD). These trials generally focus on a given histology (or small number of histologies) to define the response rate and duration of response for the test compound. Responses are generally scored by measuring changes in the size of measurable lesions, typically using imaging studies or physical measurements of accessible tumors. Responses can also utilize changes in circulating biomarkers or other functional measures of tumor activity.

Most current treatment trials rely on the response evaluation criteria in solid tumors (RECIST) criteria for determining the activity of the test agent. When objective tumor response is the primary endpoint of the trial, only patients with measurable disease at baseline are generally included. Measurable disease is defined as the presence of at least one measurable lesion. Measurable lesions must allow for the accurate measurement in at least one dimension with the longest diameter greater than 20 mm using conventional techniques or 10 mm or larger utilizing spiral CT scan.

Nonmeasurable lesions are defined as all other lesions including smaller lesions, bone lesions, leptomeningeal disease, ascites, effusions, and so forth. Lesions can be measured utilizing best available methods such as CT and MRI or, in the case of accessible lesions such as cutaneous lesions, by direct caliper measurements. The RECIST criteria do not allow for the measurement of tumor markers alone to assess response.

The RECIST criteria call for the documentation of both target and nontarget lesions. The target lesions are defined as all measurable lesions up to a maximum of five lesions per organ

TABLE 13.7

BEST OVERALL RESPONSE CALCULATIONS BASED ON RECIST CRITERIA

TARGET LESIONS	NONTARGET LESIONS	NEW LESIONS	OVERALL RESPONSE
CR	CR	No	CR
CR	Incomplete response/SD	No	PR
PR	Non-PD	No	PR
SD	Non-PD	No	SD
PD	Any	Yes or no	PD
Any	PD	Yes or no	PD
Any	Any	Yes	PD

CR, complete response; PD, progressive disease; PR, partial response; RECIST, response evaluation criteria in solid tumors; SD, stable disease.

and 10 organs in total that are representative of all involved organs. These should be measured at baseline. The criteria define, for the purpose of measurements, the total size of target lesions. This is defined as a sum of the longest diameter (LD) for all target lesions, which is calculated and reported as the baseline sum LD. This baseline sum LD is what is used as the point of reference to characterize all subsequent measurements and therefore objective responses. All other lesions that are not designated target lesions are defined as nontarget lesions and are scored only based on presence or absence rather than directed measurements.

Based on changes from the sum LD, the following response criteria are defined. For the evaluation of target lesions, a complete response (CR) is defined as the disappearance of all target lesions. A partial response (PR) is defined as at least a 30% decrease in the sum of the LD of target lesions when compared to the reference baseline sum LD. Progressive disease (PD) is defined as at least a 20% increase in the sum of the LD of target lesions or the appearance of one or more new lesions. Stable disease (SD) is defined as neither a sufficient shrinkage to qualify for PR nor a sufficient increase to qualify for PD.

With respect to the evaluation of nontarget lesions, a CR is defined as the disappearance of all target lesions and normalization of a tumor marker if measured. An incomplete response or stable disease is defined as persistence of one or more nontarget lesions and/or maintenance of tumor marker levels above the normal limits. Progressive disease is defined as one or more new lesions or the unequivocal progression of existing nontarget lesions.

The evaluation of response is generally recorded as the best overall response. Table 13.7 defines how best overall response is calculated based on both target and nontarget lesions. Once an overall response is calculated, the duration of this response is measured from the time that measurement criteria are met for CR or PR until the first date that recurrence or PD is objectively documented.

Strict approaches to the definition of response are critically important in evaluating the efficacy of agents in phase II trials. Notions such as "marginal response," although potentially descriptive, are not rigorously supported and therefore not interpretable with respect to the activity of an agent. Adherence to the strict definitions allows for a more critical evaluation and therefore more useful decision making with respect to the development of a new cancer therapy. Once a response rate and duration of response are determined for an agent, a decision is made on whether or not to take that agent to further clinical evaluations.

Phase III clinical trials are conducted once the maximum tolerated dose of an agent has been tested in the phase II trial in a variety of histologies and has demonstrated reasonable response and duration of response data. Although phase I and phase II trials can often be conducted with fewer than 30 patients, phase III trials generally require hundreds or thousands of patients to have the appropriate statistical power and a sufficient variety of patient types to demonstrate definitive activity.

Phase III trials are typically designed to compare the test agent to standard therapy. The strongest design is a prospective randomized trial, in some cases blinding of the investigators and/or the patient to the receipt of the experimental therapy. Although phase III trials are the definitive studies to demonstrate the superiority of a new therapy over the previous standard, the majority of new cancer agents approved by the FDA are approved after successful phase II studies.

Recently, the concept of phase 0 trials has been introduced. These studies are usually conducted either prior to a phase I or between a phase I and phase II study. The purpose of a phase 0 trial is to evaluate the effects of an agent using novel biomarkers or other surrogates in a small number of patients at a dose that is predicted to be nontoxic. Such trials are especially useful in the evaluation of novel biologic or targeted therapies.

In addition to understanding the basic mechanics and nomenclature for clinical trials, research with human subjects must be conducted according to strict scientific and ethical principles. All federally supported clinical trials and trials evaluating new drugs or devices that are subject to FDA regulation are required to be reviewed and approved by an institutional review board (IRB). Most institutions require that all clinical trials and all human subjects research, regardless of funding, be reviewed and approved by their IRB.

The IRB is typically made up of physicians, nonphysician health professionals, laypersons, and statisticians who have the capacity to critically evaluate research studies or protocols to determine relative risk benefit for the patient volunteers. The IRB has the power to stop or hold clinical trials secondary to questions regarding patient safety. It is important that the IRB consider, in its evaluation of the risks and benefits of a particular protocol, the scientific design and questions being asked to determine if they are likely to be answered with the patient population under study. It is also important for the IRB to determine whether any conflicts of interest may exist with regard to the investigator conducting the trial and the agents being tested. If such conflicts exist, they should be clearly delineated in the protocol and consent document so that potential patient volunteers are given a complete disclosure of any potential conflicting motivations for the investigators conducting the study.

As newer agents are identified and new classes of agents defined (biologic agents, molecularly targeted agents, antiangiogenic agents, etc.), modifications and adaptations of the traditional clinical trial phases may be implemented. As agents are identified that impact on a particular pathway, methods for measuring the activity of that pathway may need to be incorporated into the response criteria. Classic stopping rules for traditional chemotherapeutic agents, such as evidence of progressive disease, may need to be adjusted for agents that have a slow onset of activity and require prolonged administration to have an antitumor effect. Issues such as these are under constant evaluation by the FDA and the NIH, and updated information is constantly evaluated. For up-to-date changes in clinical trial strategies as well as access to searches for available clinical trials, the Web site http://www.cancer.gov is a useful online reference.

Bibliography

Anisimov VN. Aging and cancer in transgenic and mutant mice. *Front Biosci* 2003;8:s883–s902.

Anisimov VN. The relationship between aging and carcinogenesis: a critical appraisal. *Crit Rev Oncol Hematol* 2003;45:277–304.

Artavanis-Tsakonas S, Rand MD, Lake RJ. Notch signaling: cell fate control and signal integration in development. *Science* 1999;284:770–776.

Bartlett DL, Libutti SK, Figg WD, et al. Isolated hepatic perfusion for unresectable hepatic metastases from colorectal cancer. *Surgery* 2001;129: 176–187.

Blagosklonny MV. How cancer could be cured by 2015. *Cell Cycle* 2005;4(2): 269–278.

Boguski MS, McCormick F. Proteins regulating Ras and its relatives. *Nature* 1993;366:643–654.

Costouros NG, Diehn FE, Libutti SK. Molecular imaging of tumor angiogenesis. *J Cell Biochem Suppl* 2002;39:72–78.

Dang CV. c-Myc target genes involved in cell growth, apoptosis, and metabolism. *Mol Cell Biol* 1999;19:1–11.

Diamandopoulos GT. Cancer: an historical perspective. *Anticancer Res* 1996; 16:1595–1602.

Feldman AL, Libutti SK. Progress in antiangiogenic gene therapy of cancer. *Cancer* 2000;89:1181–1194.

Fidler IJ. The pathogenesis of cancer metastasis: the – 'seed and soil' hypothesis revisited. *Nat Rev Cancer* 2003;3:453–458.

Finkelstein SE, Heimann DM, Klebanoff CA, et al. Bedside to bench and back again: how animal models are guiding the development of new immunotherapies for cancer. *J Leukoc Biol* 2004;76:333–337.

Folkman J, Kalluri R. Cancer without disease. *Nature* 2004;427:787.

Fong Y, Fortner J, Sun RL, et al. Clinical score for predicting recurrence after hepatic resection for metastatic colorectal cancer: analysis of 1001 consecutive cases. *Ann Surg.* 1999;230:309–321; discussion 318.

Forman MR, Hursting SD, Umar A, et al. Nutrition and cancer prevention: a multidisciplinary perspective on human trials. *Annu Rev Nutr* 2004;24: 223–254.

Frijhoff AF, Conti CJ, Senderowicz AM. Advances in molecular carcinogenesis: current and future use of mouse models to screen and validate molecularly targeted anticancer drugs. *Mol Carcinog* 2004;39:183–194.

Hackel PO, Zwick E, Prenzel N, et al. Epidermal growth factor receptors: critical mediators of multiple receptor pathways. *Curr Opin Cell Biol* 1999;11: 184–189.

Hanahan D, Weinberg RA. The hallmarks of cancer. *Cell* 2000;100:57–70.

Hunter KW. Host genetics and tumour metastasis. *Br J Cancer* 2004;90:752–755.

Jemal A, Murray T, Ward E, et al. Cancer statistics, 2005. *CA Cancer J Clin* 2005; 55:10–30.

Kurdziel KA, Figg WD, Carrasquillo JA, et al. Using positron emission tomography 2-deoxy-2-[18F]fluoro-D-glucose, 11CO, and 15-O-water for monitoring androgen independent prostate cancer. *Mol Imaging Biol* 2003;5: 86–93.

Libutti SK, Alexander HR Jr, Choyke P, et al. A prospective study of 2-[18F] fluoro-2-deoxy-D-glucose/positron emission tomography scan, 99mTc-labeled arcitumomab (CEA-scan), and blind second-look laparotomy for detecting colon cancer recurrence in patients with increasing carcinoembryonic antigen levels. *Ann Surg Oncol* 2001;8:779–786.

Libutti SK, Barlett DL, Fraker DL, et al. Technique and results of hyperthermic isolated hepatic perfusion with tumor necrosis factor and melphalan for the treatment of unresectable hepatic malignancies. *J Am Coll Surg* 2000;191: 519–530.

Libutti SK, Choyke P, Carrasquillo JA, et al. Monitoring responses to antiangiogenic agents using noninvasive imaging tests. *Cancer J Sci Am* 1999;5: 252–256.

Mazzanti C, Zeiger MA, Costouros NG, et al. Using gene expression profiling to differentiate benign versus malignant thyroid tumors. *Cancer Res* 2004; 64:2898–2903.

Park BJ, Alexander HR, Libutti SK, et al. Treatment of primary peritoneal mesothelioma by continuous hyperthermic peritoneal perfusion (CHPP). *Ann Surg Oncol* 1999;6:582–590.

Park JW, Kerbel RS, Kelloff GJ, et al. Rationale for biomarkers and surrogate end points in mechanism-driven oncology drug development. *Clin Cancer Res* 2004;10:3885–3896.

Petricoin E, Wulfkuhle J, Espina V, et al. Clinical proteomics: revolutionizing disease detection and patient tailoring therapy. *J Proteome Res* 2004;3: 209–217.

Preston RJ. Quantitation of molecular endpoints for the dose-response component of cancer risk assessment. *Toxicol Pathol* 2002;30:112–116.

Rosenberg SA. Shedding light on immunotherapy for cancer. *N Engl J Med* 2004; 350:1461–1463.

Rosenberg SA, Yang JC, Restifo NP. Cancer immunotherapy: moving beyond current vaccines. *Nat Med* 2004;10:909–915.

Rosenblatt KP, Bryant-Greenwood P, Killian JK, et al. Serum proteomics in cancer diagnosis and management. *Annu Rev Med* 2004;55:97–112.

Rye PD, Stigbrand T. Interfering with cancer: a brief outline of advances in RNA interference in oncology. *Tumour Biol* 2004;25:329–336.

Sekiguchi M, Sakumi K. Roles of DNA repair methyltransferase in mutagenesis and carcinogenesis. *Jpn J Hum Genet* 1997;42:389–399.

Selkirk SM. Gene therapy in clinical medicine. *Postgrad Med J.* 2004;80: 560–570.

Sudhakar A, Sugimoto H, Yang C, et al. Human tumstatin and human endostatin exhibit distinct antiangiogenic activities mediated by alpha v beta 3 and alpha 5 beta 1 integrins. *Proc Natl Acad Sci U S A* 2003;100:4766–4771.

Sund M, Hamano Y, Sugimoto H, et al. Function of endogenous inhibitors of angiogenesis as endothelium-specific tumor suppressors. *Proc Natl Acad Sci U S A* 2005;102:2934–2936.

Tandle A, Blazer DG 3rd, Libutti SK. Antiangiogenic gene therapy of cancer: recent developments. *J Transl Med* 2004;2:22.

Thomas DM, Fleming NI, Holloway AJ, et al. Molecular medicine: a clinician's primer on microarrays. *Intern Med J* 2004;34:565–569.

Widschwendter M, Jones PA. DNA methylation and breast carcinogenesis. *Oncogene* 2002;21:5462–5482.

Zurita AJ, Arap W, Pasqualini R. Mapping tumor vascular diversity by screening phage display libraries. *J Control Release* 2003;91:183–186.

Zwick E, Hackel PO, Prenzel N, et al. The EGF receptor as central transducer of heterologous signalling systems. *Trends Pharmacol Sci* 1999;20: 408–412.

CHAPTER 14 ■ POLICY APPROACHES TO IMPROVING SURGICAL QUALITY

JOHN D. BIRKMEYER AND JUSTIN B. DIMICK

KEY POINTS

1. Commonly used quality indicators, including both volume- and risk-adjusted outcomes, readily identify groups of hospitals and surgeons with superior outcomes. They are not reliable in profiling performance for individual providers, however.
2. In surgery, the most familiar process compliance strategy is the pay-for-performance program of the Surgical Care Improvement Project, which aims to increase adoption of evidence-based practices related to perioperative care.
3. Current process measures do not reliably identify hospitals or surgeons with better outcomes. Higher leverage measures, including those that reflect important aspects of surgical decision making or operative performance, are needed.
4. Although prophylactic strategies aimed at avoiding complications in the first place are obviously important, "rescuing" patients once a complication has occurred may be even more critical in reducing current variations in hospital mortality rates.
5. Outcomes measurement and feedback may provide early benefits by capitalizing on the surgical "Hawthorne effect," but they do not inform hospitals or surgeons about how best to improve.
6. The optimal strategy for improving surgical quality may depend on political realities, the clinical context, and which outcomes stakeholders hope to improve.

Improving the quality of surgical care is a public health imperative. Based on our extrapolations from national Medicare data, approximately 50,000 patients die every year undergoing surgery in the United States; perhaps 10 times that number experience serious complications. A growing body of literature suggests that a large proportion of surgical morbidity and mortality may be avoidable. Almost 10 years ago, the Institute of Medicine estimated that between 44,000 and 98,000 Americans die every year as a result of medical errors, at least half of whom are surgical patients.[1,2] Evidence that morbidity and mortality vary widely across hospitals and surgeons further suggests opportunities for improvement. In addition to variation among individual providers,[3–5] surgical outcomes differ according to a number of provider attributes, including procedure volume, surgeon subspecialty training, and other factors.[6–8]

In response, payers, policy makers, and professional organizations have implemented a variety of different strategies aimed at improving surgical quality.[9] Some of these efforts, including payers' Centers of Excellence programs, aim to direct surgical patients to hospitals or surgeons with the best results (selective referral). Others, instead, strive to "raise the tide," focusing on improving outcomes at all hospitals, particularly those with subpar results. Among broad-based quality improvement efforts currently under way, pay-for-performance programs are incentivizing hospital and surgeon compliance with specific process measures, most related to perioperative care (process compliance model). For example, the Surgical Care Improvement Project aims to improve practices related to prophylaxis against surgical site infection, venous thromboembolism, and ventilator-acquired pneumonia. In contrast, professional organizations, including the American College of Surgeons (ACS) and its National Surgical Quality Improvement Program (NSQIP), are focusing on outcomes measurement and feedback to hospitals (outcomes measurement model).[10,11] These efforts are less prescriptive with regard to clinical practice and instead assume that hospitals and surgeons can figure out themselves how best to improve at the local level.

Although some might use different labels, selective referral, process compliance, and outcomes measurement represent the three dominant strategies for surgical quality improvement currently being employed in the United States. In this chapter, we review the relative strengths and weaknesses of each approach (Table 14.1). We also consider the optimal strategy for different clinical contexts and procedures, and how each strategy could be improved in the future.

SELECTIVE REFERRAL

With this approach, payers (usually) identify hospitals with the best results with selected procedures and direct care to these facilities. To achieve this end, they can employ selective contracting or tiered health plans and benefits packages that give patients financial incentives (lower copays or monthly premiums) to select higher-quality providers. Although also intended to enhance accountability and motivate quality improvement at the local level, public reporting of hospital performance is another obvious tool for effecting selective referral.

Among current examples of selective referral, the Leapfrog Group, a large coalition of public and private employers and purchasers, is promoting "evidence-based hospital referral" for selected procedures (coronary artery bypass graft surgery, aortic valve replacement, abdominal aortic aneurysm repair, bariatric surgery, esophagectomy, and pancreatic resection) based on both procedure volume criteria and hospital mortality rates.[12] Cardiac surgery, bariatric surgery, and breast cancer care are becoming increasingly popular targets for payers' Centers of Excellence programs.

Such strategies reflect the natural response of payers (and many patients) to data indicating variation in provider performance with surgery. Among their advantages, selective referral can often be implemented expediently and inexpensively, particularly when based on simple structural measures of quality (e.g., 1 procedure volume). For many procedures, commonly used quality indicators can reliably identify groups of hospitals and

TABLE 14.1

CHARACTERISTICS OF THREE DIFFERENT MODELS FOR REDUCING VARIATION AND IMPROVING SURGICAL MORTALITY

	SELECTIVE REFERRAL	PROCESS COMPLIANCE	OUTCOMES MEASUREMENT
Goal/mechanism	Steer patients to best hospitals or surgeons	Improve care in all settings by increasing hospital compliance with evidence-based processes of perioperative care	Improve care in all settings by providing feedback on surgical outcomes; hospitals and surgeons implement improvement efforts at the local level
Examples	Leapfrog Group evidence-based hospital referral program Payers' Centers of Excellence programs in cardiac and bariatric surgery	Surgical Care Improvement Project (SCIP), other pay-for-performance programs focusing on practices related to reducing surgical site infection (SSI) and venous thromboembolism	Society of Thoracic Surgery database for cardiothoracic surgery American College of Surgeons' National Surgical Quality Improvement Program
Advantages	Inexpensive, expedient Traction with patients and payers	Likely to achieve rapid improvements in aspects of perioperative care	Measurement alone may be effective in improving outcomes ("Hawthorne effect")
Disadvantages	Highly polarizing (for providers) Hard to identify best providers (at individual level)	Improving processes related to secondary outcomes (e.g., SSI) may not reduce variation in mortality	Lack of insights about how best to improve; may limit ultimate extent of improvement Expensive

surgeons with superior outcomes. For example, data readily obtained from administrative data, including procedure volume and hospital mortality, not only describe past performance, but also forecast future performance with many procedures.[13]

Unfortunately, such measures are considerably less useful in discriminating performance among individuals, in part because provider-specific outcomes are statistically unstable. For example, Krumholz et al. used clinical data from the Cooperative Cardiovascular Project to assess the usefulness of the HealthGrades hospital ratings for acute myocardial infarction (based primarily on risk-adjusted mortality rates from Medicare data).[14] Relative to one-star (worst) hospitals, five-star (best) hospitals had significantly lower mortality (16% vs. 22%, $p < 0.001$) after risk adjustment with clinical data. However, the HealthGrades ratings poorly discriminated among any two individual hospitals. In only 3% of head-to-head comparisons did five-star hospitals have statistically lower mortality rates than one-star hospitals.

Selective referral strategies have other downsides. Strategies that displace patients from their usual site of care and regular physicians may interfere with coordination of care. They tend to be highly polarizing, dividing hospitals and surgeons into winners and losers. In alienating the latter, a price of selective referral may be lost opportunities for engaging physicians in other types of quality improvement efforts. And finally, selective referral improves outcomes exclusively to the extent that it steers care away from poor performers. It provides no mechanism for helping other hospitals and surgeons improve their outcomes.

PROCESS COMPLIANCE

2 Another approach to improving surgical outcomes is to encourage hospitals and surgeons to increase their compliance with processes of care associated with better outcomes. This model is best represented by ongoing pay-for-performance programs of both public and private payers. For example, payers are linking hospital reimbursement to satisfactory adherence to evidence-based practices related to perioperative care, as defined by the Surgical Care Improvement Project (SCIP), a joint effort of the Centers for Medicare and Medicaid Service (CMS) and the Centers for Disease Control and Prevention.[15] At the present time, these include specific processes aimed at reducing rates of surgical site infection, postoperative cardiac events, venous thromboembolism, and ventilator-associated pneumonia.

Efforts aimed at improving compliance with specific processes of care are considerably less polarizing than selective referral. In theory, anyone can "win." To the extent that surgeons can "play to the quiz," process-based pay-for-performance programs have the potential to achieve rapid and significant improvements in many aspects of perioperative care. At the University of Michigan Hospital, for example, the proportion of colorectal surgery patients receiving an appropriate antibiotic within 60 minutes prior to incision increased virtually overnight, from 70% to over 95%, following implementation of a pay-for-performance program by one of its major private payers. Studies in primary care suggest that pay-for-performance programs may be particularly effective in improving process compliance among poor performers and thus reducing overall variation.[16,17]

Nonetheless, the extent to which process compliance will 3 improve surgical outcomes remains uncertain. Studies to date have generally failed to demonstrate a strong relationship between provider performance and specific process measures and patient outcomes. For example, based on data suggesting that patients in whom more nodes are detected seem to have a more favorable prognosis after cancer surgery, many pay-for-performance programs recently began rewarding hospitals for examining at least 12 lymph nodes from the surgical specimens of patients undergoing colectomy for colon cancer. In a recent study, hospitals varied widely in their success in achieving the 12-node minimum.[18] However, hospitals scoring well on this process measure had virtually identical 5-year survival rates as those scoring poorly. In another study by Hawn et al.,[19] hospitals' compliance with SCIP-1 (proportion of patients receiving appropriate antibiotics within 60 minutes of surgical incision) had little relation to their rates of surgical site infection. Such studies highlight the complexity of surgical care and the limitations of focusing on a small number of discrete steps.

Even if current process compliance strategies were successful in reducing rates of specific complications, it is not certain that they would also reduce mortality, arguably the most important end result of many major procedures. To explore this issue empirically, we recently assessed hospital compliance with several process measures targeted by the Surgical Care

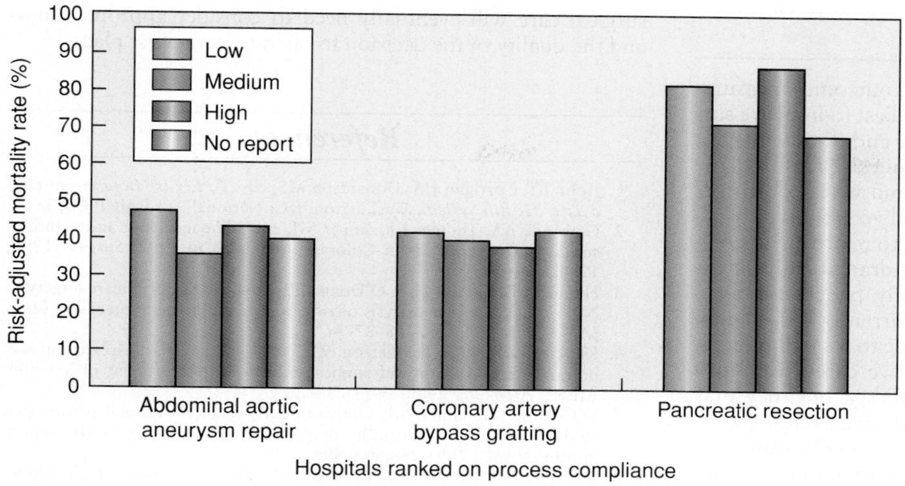

FIGURE 14.1. Association between overall hospital compliance with Surgical Care Improvement Project (SCIP) measures (from the Centers for Medicare and Medicaid Service's Hospital Compare Program) and risk-adjusted mortality rates with several high-risk procedures, based on 2005–2006 national Medicare data.

Improvement Project, as compiled by CMS's Hospital Compare Program. Process compliance varied widely across hospitals (56% in the lowest vs. 91% in the highest hospital tercile). However, hospital compliance with SCIP process measures had no significant relationship with perioperative mortality for high-risk surgery (Fig. 14.1).

4 Although prophylactic strategies aimed at avoiding complications in the first place have obvious appeal, "rescuing" patients once a complication has occurred may be even more critical in reducing mortality. In a large study of Medicare patients by Silber et al., hospital mortality with specific procedures seemed to be primarily related to failure to rescue (the likelihood of mortality given a complication), and only weakly correlated with complication rates.[20] We conducted a similar analysis based on data from the American College of Surgeons National Surgical Quality Improvement Program. Participating hospitals were ranked and sorted according to their risk-adjusted mortality rates. Hospitals in the best quintile had mortality rates of only 2.2%, versus 7.2% in the highest-mortality quintile. As seen in Figure 14.2, high-mortality hospitals had only slightly higher overall complication rates (odds ratio 1.2, $p < 0.001$) than low-mortality hospitals. However, their failure-to-rescue rates were markedly higher (odds ratio 3.2, $p < 0.001$).

OUTCOMES MEASUREMENT

In contrast to payers and regulators, professional organizations in surgery are focusing primarily on disseminating

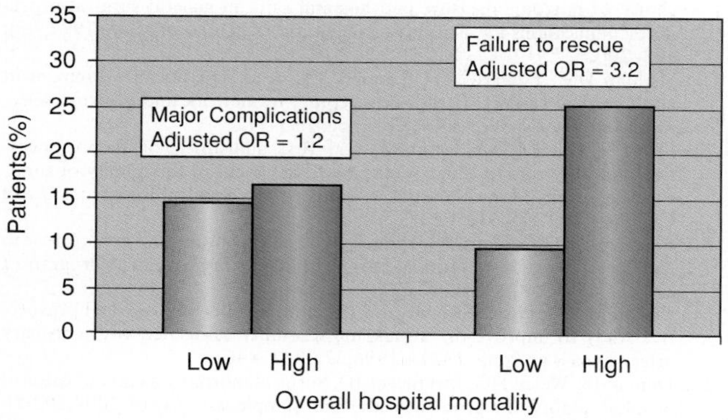

FIGURE 14.2. Major complication rates and failure-to-rescue rates at hospitals in the lowest and highest quintiles of overall risk-adjusted mortality, based on 2005–2006 data from the American College of Surgeons' National Surgical Quality Improvement Program (NSQIP). OR, odds ratio.

nationwide systems for tracking surgical outcomes. Their goal is to provide hospitals and surgeons with rigorous feedback about their outcomes relative to those of their peers, in the hopes that they will identify opportunities for improvement and respond accordingly. This model is less prescriptive than the process compliance approach and assumes that hospitals and surgeons can decide best how to improve care at the local level.

The Society of Thoracic Surgeons was among the first to embrace this model and now a large majority of U.S. hospitals involved in cardiac surgery contribute to its national outcomes database.[21] First developed by the Department of Veterans Affairs, the NSQIP has been adapted for use in the private sector by the ACS and has become the most recognized outcomes measurement platform for noncardiac surgery.[10,22] Although the ACS's NSQIP has traditionally assessed morbidity and mortality for random samples of patients undergoing any major procedures, the program will soon begin procedure-specific data collection and outcomes reporting.[23]

This model of centralized quality measurement but local quality improvement has particular appeal among surgeons. They view good outcomes as the best criterion of surgical quality, but do not like directives about how to achieve them. There is strong evidence that this model can be very effective in reducing both overall mortality and variation across providers. In northern New England, for example, mortality with coronary artery bypass grafting fell by more than 25% almost immediately following feedback of mortality data to hospitals and surgeons; variation in mortality rates across hospitals fell even more dramatically.[24] This surgical "Hawthorne effect" has been similarly observed in Veterans Affairs hospitals nationwide after implementation of the NSQIP.[4] Although what actually changed about clinical practice to effect this improvement has never been fully characterized, overall morbidity rates fell by over 40%.

Among their disadvantages, outcomes measurement programs often involve extensive data collection (mainly to ensure adequate risk adjustment) and thus can be expensive. Annual costs for hospitals participating in the ACS's NSQIP exceed $100,000. Outcomes measures, particularly when assessed at the level of specific procedures, are often hindered by small sample sizes and too "noisy" to inform hospitals and surgeons of their true performance.[25] Type I and type II errors can lead to oversteering and understeering, respectively, in targeting
5 quality improvement efforts. Finally, outcomes measurement provides no insights about best practices and how individual providers or the profession as a whole can improve. Outcomes feedback alone may also be insufficient for addressing specific types of quality problems, including surgeon inexperience, technical proficiency, and judgment.

SUMMARY

Selective referral, process compliance, and outcomes measurement reflect different philosophies on how best to improve surgical quality and have distinct advantages and disadvantages. The optimal strategy may depend on political realities, the clinical context (e.g., which procedure), and which outcomes stakeholders hope to improve.[9] As currently configured, selective referral strategies may be best applied to relatively uncommon procedures for which outcomes vary dramatically across hospitals and surgeons (e.g., esophagectomy, pancreatic resection). Process compliance strategies are currently focusing on "low-hanging fruit"—improving adherence to a small number of evidence-based practices in perioperative care. They may not be effective in reducing surgical mortality, but they may ultimately prove successful to reducing adverse events important to patients (e.g., surgical site infection). Finally, outcomes measurement efforts—the major thrust of professional organizations—are likely to improve outcomes to the extent that they can capitalize on the surgical Hawthorne effect. In addition to spurring quality improvement at the local level, these efforts may ultimately provide a platform for public reporting and provider accountability in surgery.

Each of the three strategies would benefit from advances in quality measurement and improvement. Selective referral could be improved by measures that more reliably capture performance for individual hospitals and surgeons. Optimal measures would not only describe past performance, but also forecast future outcomes for patients and payers trying to identify the best hospitals and surgeons for specific procedures. As described elsewhere, individual measures of structure (including procedure volume), process of care, and outcomes have major limitations in reflecting provider-specific quality.[26] Composite quality measures, which empirically combine information from several quality domains, appear very promising and may soon become the standard in selective referral.[27,28] Simple composites combining procedure volume and operative mortality have already been adopted by the Leapfrog Group.

Effective process compliance strategies await higher-leverage processes of care on which to base them. A better understanding of mechanisms underlying variation in surgical mortality and other important outcomes is essential for identifying such practices. For example, which types of clinical events and complications account for differences in mortality across hospitals? Which specific processes of care and organizational factors explain different rates of these clinical events? Previous research provides only preliminary answers to these basic questions. High-leverage processes of care may ultimately prove harder to codify than the perioperative processes that SCIP and payers are now focusing upon, and may involve those related to preoperative decision making (e.g., which patients to operate on in the first place) and surgeon proficiency in the operating room.

To fully realize their potential, outcomes measurement strategies need a more potent "effecter arm." Performance feedback may be the essential first step, but hospitals and surgeons need more guidance on what they can do to improve. As described earlier, a better understanding of mechanisms underlying variation and suboptimal outcomes will be crucial in this regard. In the meantime, professional organizations should develop better systems for developing and disseminating practice guidelines, providing expert-based consultative services to underperforming providers, and educating surgeons about the principles of continuous quality improvement.

Regardless of the underlying improvement strategy, payers and professional organizations should ensure that surgical quality is not defined too narrowly. At the present time, each is focusing almost exclusively on measures of technical quality around the surgical episode. However, a large body of evidence suggests that the use of surgery varies even more widely across providers than do the outcomes of surgery. Despite the practical and methodologic challenges involved, policy approaches to improving surgical care will eventually need to consider appropriateness and the quality of the decision to operate in the first place.

References

1. Kohn LT, Corrigan JM, Donaldson MS, eds. *To Err Is Human: Building a Safer Health System.* Washington, DC: National Academy Press; 1999.
2. Gawande AA, Thomas EJ, Zinner MJ, et al. The incidence and nature of surgical adverse events in Colorado and Utah in 1992. *Surgery* 1999;126(1):66–75.
3. Hannan EL, Kilburn H Jr, O'Donnell JF, et al. Adult open heart surgery in New York State. An analysis of risk factors and hospital mortality rates. *JAMA* 1990;264(21):2768–2774.
4. Khuri SF, Daley J, Henderson WG. The comparative assessment and improvement of quality of surgical care in the Department of Veterans Affairs. *Arch Surg* 2002;137(1):20–27.
5. O'Connor GT, Plume SK, Olmstead EM, et al. A regional prospective study of in-hospital mortality associated with coronary artery bypass grafting. *JAMA* 1991;266:803–809.
6. Dudley RA, Johansen KL, Brand R, et al. Selective referral to high volume hospitals: estimating potentially avoidable deaths. *JAMA* 2000;283:1159–1166.
7. Halm EA, Lee C, Chassin MR. Is volume related to outcome in health care? A systematic review and methodologic critique of the literature. *Ann Intern Med* 2002;137:511–520.
8. Houghton A. Variation in outcome of surgical procedures. *Br J Surg* 1994;81:653–660.
9. Birkmeyer NJ, Birkmeyer JD. Strategies for improving surgical quality—should payers reward excellence or effort? *N Engl J Med* 2006;354(8):864–870.
10. Fink A, Campbell DJ, Mentzer RJ, et al. The National Surgical Quality Improvement Program in non-Veterans Administration hospitals: initial demonstration of feasibility. *Ann Surg* 2002;236:344–353.
11. Rowell KS, Turrentine FE, Hutter MM, et al. Use of national surgical quality improvement program data as a catalyst for quality improvement. *J Am Coll Surg* 2007;204:1293–1300.
12. The Leapfrog Group. The Leapfrog Group fact sheet. Available at: http://www.leapfroggroup.org/about_us/leapfrog-factsheet. Accessed December 1, 2008.
13. Birkmeyer JD, Dimick JB, Staiger DO. Operative mortality and procedure volume as predictors of future hospital performance. *Ann Surg* 2006;243:411–417.
14. Krumholz HM, Rathore SS, Chen J, et al. Evaluation of a consumer-oriented internet health care report card: the risk of quality ratings based on mortality data. *JAMA* 2002;287(10):1277–1287.
15. Gold JA, Gold JA. The surgical care improvement project. *Wis Med J* 2005;104(1):73–74.
16. Rosenthal MB, Dudley RA. Pay-for-performance: will the latest payment trend improve care? *JAMA* 2007;297(7):740–744.
17. Rosenthal MB, Frank RG, Li Z, et al. Early experience with pay-for-performance: from concept to practice [see comment]. *JAMA* 2005;294(14):1788–1793.
18. Wong SL, Ji H, Hollenbeck BK, et al. Hospital lymph node examination rates and survival after resection for colon cancer [see comment]. *JAMA* 2007;298(18):2149–2154.
19. Hawn MT, Itani KM, Gray SH, et al. Association of timely administration of prophylactic antibiotics for major surgical procedures and surgical site infection. *J Am Coll Surg* 2008;206(5):814–819; discussion 9–21.
20. Silber JH, Rosenbaum PR, Williams SV, et al. The relationship between choice of outcome measure and hospital rank in general surgical procedures: implications for quality assessment. *Int J Qual Health Care* 1997;9(3):193–200.
21. Shahian DM, Edwards FH, Ferraris VA, et al. Quality measurement in adult cardiac surgery: part 1—conceptual framework and measure selection. *Ann Thorac Surg* 2007;83(suppl 4):S3–S12.
22. Khuri SF, Daley J, Henderson W, et al. Risk adjustment of the postoperative mortality rate for the comparative assessment of the quality of surgical care: results of the National Veterans Affairs Surgical Risk Study. *J Am Coll Surg* 1997;185:315–327.
23. Birkmeyer JD, Shahian DM, Dimick JB, et al. Blueprint for a new American College of Surgeons: National Surgical Quality Improvement Program. *J Am Coll Surg* 2008;207:777–782.
24. O'Connor GT, Plume SK, Morton JR, et al. Results of a regional prospective study to improve the in-hospital mortality associated with coronary artery bypass grafting. *JAMA* 1996;275:841–846.
25. Dimick JB, Welch HG, Birkmeyer JD. Surgical mortality as an indicator of hospital quality: the problem with small sample size. *JAMA* 2004;292(7):847–851.
26. Birkmeyer JD, Birkmeyer NJ, Dimick JB. Measuring the quality of surgical care: structure, process, or outcomes? *J Am Coll Surg* 2004;198:626–632.
27. O'Brien SM, Shahian DM, DeLong ER, et al. Quality measurement in adult cardiac surgery: part 2—statistical considerations in composite measure scoring and provider rating. *Ann Thorac Surg* 2007;83:S13–S26.
28. Staiger DO, Dimick JB, Baser O, et al. Empirically derived composite measures of surgical performance. *Med Care* 2009;47:226–233.

CHAPTER 15 ■ MEASURING THE QUALITY OF SURGICAL CARE

JUSTIN B. DIMICK AND JOHN D. BIRKMEYER

KEY POINTS

1. The National Quality Forum (NQF) has recently emerged as the leading organization endorsing quality measures. Many other organizations, including the Joint Commission and the Centers for Medicare and Medicaid Services (CMS), rely on endorsement by the NQF before applying a measure to practice.
2. Quality measures fall into three categories: structure, process, and outcomes. Health care structure refers to fixed attributes of the system in which patients receive care. Process of care measures are the clinical details of care provided to patients. Outcome measures reflect the end result of care, from a clinical perspective or as judged by the patient.
3. Composite measures, created by combining multiple individual quality indicators, are becoming increasingly used in the assessment of surgical quality. Most existing pay-for-performance efforts, including the CMS pilot, use composite measures to assess the quality of medical and surgical diagnoses.
4. No quality measure is perfect. Clinical leaders, patient advocates, payers, and policy makers will have to make decisions about when imperfect measures are good enough to act upon. A measure should be implemented only with the expectation that acting on it will result in a net improvement in health quality.
5. It is important to ensure a good match between the performance measure and the primary goal of measurement. The right measure depends on whether the underlying goal is (a) quality improvement or (b) selective referral—directing patients to higher-quality hospitals and/or providers.
6. For quality improvement purposes, a good performance measure must be actionable. Measurable improvements in the given process should translate to clinically meaningful improvements in patient outcomes.
7. With selective referral, a good measure will steer patients to better hospitals or physicians. As one basic litmus test, a measure based on prior performance should reliably identify providers likely to have superior performance now and in the future.
8. One of the biggest limitations of surgical quality measurement is the statistical "noise" from the small sample sizes at most hospitals. This problem makes it difficult to isolate the quality signal from the background statistical noise. An emerging technique, reliability adjustment, directly addresses this problem. This technique, based on hierarchical modeling, quantifies and subtracts statistical noise from the measurement process.
9. Another significant limitation of existing approaches to surgical quality assessment is a lack of good measures of global quality. As payers and purchasers of health care move forward with value-based purchasing, there is a growing need for better composite scores. In this chapter, we discuss an emerging technique for creating empirically weighted composite measures of surgical performance.
10. An emerging technique for creating empirically weighted composite measures of surgical performance is improving the quality and efficiency of surgical care. Quality measures are only useful if they inform improvement efforts. Future refinements in measurement should therefore aim to meet the diverse needs of the improvement efforts of patients, payers, and providers.

With growing recognition that the quality of surgical care varies widely, good measures of performance are in high demand. Patients and their families need accurate information to help them choose the safest hospitals for surgery.[1] Employers and payers need reliable measures for their value-based purchasing programs.[2] Motivated in part by these external pressures, clinical leaders need better measures to guide their quality improvement efforts.[3]

Despite a broadening array of measures, there remains considerable uncertainty about which measures are most useful.[4,5] Current measures are remarkably heterogeneous, encompassing different elements of health care structure, process, and outcomes. With the proliferation of value-based purchasing, which requires a global assessment of quality, there has been a rapid growth in the use of composite measures.[6] Although each of these types of performance measures has strengths, each is also associated with conceptual, methodologic, and/or practical problems (Table 15.1).

This chapter provides an overview of existing quality indicators followed by a review of the main strengths and limitations of each type of measure: structure, process, outcomes, and composites. The chapter then closes with recommendations for selecting the right measure and a description of emerging techniques that address some of the limitations of existing quality measures.

OVERVIEW OF CURRENT MEASURES

An ever-broadening array of performance measures has been
1 developed for assessing surgical quality. Over the past few years, the National Quality Forum (NQF) has emerged as the leading organization endorsing quality measures. Table 15.2 includes surgical quality measures endorsed by the NQF. Many other organizations, including the Joint Commission and the Centers for Medicare and Medicaid Services (CMS), rely on endorsement by the NQF before applying a measure to practice. The number of measures relevant to surgery endorsed by the NQF has grown rapidly. Many of these new measures are part of CMS's Surgical Care Improvement Program (SCIP), which includes process measures related to prevention of

TABLE 15.1

EXAMPLES, STRENGTHS, AND LIMITATIONS OF DIFFERENT APPROACHES TO MEASURING SURGICAL PERFORMANCE

	■ EXAMPLE	■ STRENGTHS	■ LIMITATIONS
Structure	Hospital or surgeon volume Surgeon specialty training	Inexpensive and readily available Strong relationship to important outcomes	Not actionable for quality improvement Not good at discriminating individual provider performance
Process	Appropriate selection, timing, and duration of antibiotic prophylaxis Use of internal mammary artery for coronary artery bypass grafting	Actionable as targets for improvement Everybody can achieve 100% compliance	Most known processes relate to secondary outcomes High-leverage processes are unknown for most procedures
Outcome	Risk-adjusted mortality Risk-adjusted morbidity	Seen as the bottom line of patient care Buy-in from providers	Sample sizes too small at individual hospitals
Composite	The Leapfrog Group's Survival Predictor STS Composite score for coronary artery bypass grafting	Addresses problems with small sample size Makes sense of multiple conflicting measures	Too broad to identify specific areas that need improvement

STS, Society of Thoracic Surgeons.

TABLE 15.2

OVERVIEW OF CLINICAL PERFORMANCE MEASURES RELEVANT TO SURGERY THAT HAVE BEEN ENDORSED BY THE NATIONAL QUALITY FORUM (NQF) AS OF AUGUST 2007

■ DIAGNOSIS OR PROCEDURE	■ PERFORMANCE MEASURE
Coronary artery bypass	Use of internal mammary artery Preoperative beta-blocker Deep sternal wound infection rate Prolonged intubation Renal insufficiency Surgical re-exploration Hospital volume
Aortic valve replacement	Risk-adjusted mortality rate Hospital volume
Mitral valve replacement	Risk-adjusted mortality rate Hospital volume
Any cardiac surgery	Antiplatelet, antilipid, and beta-blockers on discharge Participation in a cardiac surgery registry Preoperative beta-blocker Renal insufficiency Prolonged intubation Stroke
Surgery for breast cancer	Radiation therapy after breast conservation surgery
Surgery for colon cancer	Adjuvant chemotherapy for appropriate candidates At least 12 lymph nodes identified in surgical specimen
Surgery for rectal cancer	Adjuvant radiation therapy for patients with rectal cancer
Any surgical procedure	Venous thrombosis prophylaxis Appropriate timing, selection, and discontinuation of prophylactic antibiotics
Any hospitalized patient, including all after surgery	Central venous catheter infection rate Urinary catheter-associated infection rate Ventilator-associated pneumonia rate

TABLE 15.3

OVERVIEW OF PERFORMANCE MEASURES CURRENTLY USED FOR SURGERY

DIAGNOSIS OR PROCEDURE	PERFORMANCE MEASURE	DEVELOPER/ ENDORSER
Critically ill patients	Board-certified intensivist staffing	LF
Abdominal aneurysm repair	Hospital volume	AHRQ, LF
	Risk-adjusted mortality rates	AHRQ
	Prophylactic beta-blocker use	LF
Carotid endarterectomy	Hospital volume	AHRQ
Esophageal resection for cancer	Hospital volume	AHRQ
Pancreatic resection	Hospital volume	AHRQ, LF
	Risk-adjusted mortality rates	AHRQ
Pediatric heart surgery	Hospital volume	AHRQ
	Risk-adjusted mortality rates	AHRQ
Hip replacement	Risk-adjusted mortality rates	AHRQ
Craniotomy	Risk-adjusted mortality rates	AHRQ
Cholecystectomy	Laparoscopic approach	AHRQ
Appendectomy	Avoidance of incidental appendectomy	AHRQ

AHRQ, Agency for Healthcare Research and Quality; LF, Leapfrog Group.

surgical site infections, postoperative cardiac events, venous thromboembolism, and respiratory complications.

While the NQF is the central organization for evaluating candidate measures, many other organizations continue to create their own quality indicators (Table 15.3). The Agency for Healthcare Research and Quality (AHRQ) has focused on quality measures that can be used with administrative data. For example, the AHRQ maintains and distributes state and national administrative data as part of their Healthcare Cost and Utilization Project (HCUP). Processes of care are generally not available in these datasets, so the AHRQ measures focus mainly on structure (e.g., hospital volume) and outcomes (e.g., mortality rates).

The Leapfrog Group, a coalition of large employers and health care purchasers, has issued perhaps the most visible set of surgical quality indicators for its value-based purchasing initiative. Although originally focused exclusively on structural measures, including volume standards, their current standards also include selected processes and risk-adjusted outcomes. In the future, the Leapfrog Group will use a composite of operative mortality and hospital volume as the primary measure for their evidence-based hospital referral initiative.[7] We will discuss composite measures in detail later in this chapter.

INDIVIDUAL QUALITY MEASURES

❷ Quality measures fall into three categories: structure, process, and outcomes.

Structure

Health care structure refers to fixed attributes of the system in which patients receive care. Many structural measures describe hospital-level attributes, such as the resources or staff coordination and organization (e.g., nurse-to-patient ratios, hospital teaching status). Other structural measures reflect attributes of individual physicians (e.g., subspecialty board certification, procedure volume).

Strengths. Structural measures of quality have several attractive features. First, they are strongly related to patient outcomes. For example, with esophagectomy and pancreatic resection, operative mortality rates at high-volume hospitals are often 10% lower, in absolute terms, than low-volume centers.[8,9] In some instances, structural measures such as procedure volume are more predictive of subsequent hospital performance than any known processes of care or even direct mortality measures (Fig. 15.1).

Perhaps the most important advantage of structural variables is the ease with which they can be assessed. Many can be determined using readily available administrative data. Although some structural measures require surveying hospitals or providers, such data are much less expensive to collect than measures requiring detailed patient-level information.

Limitations. Perhaps the greatest limitation of this approach is that structural measures are not readily actionable. For example, a small hospital cannot readily make itself a high-volume center. Thus, while selected structural measures may be useful for selective referral initiatives, they have limited value for quality improvement purposes. Structural measures are also limited in their ability to discriminate the performance of individual providers. For example, in aggregate, high-volume hospitals have much lower mortality rates than lower-volume centers for pancreatic resection.[8,9] However, some individual high-volume hospitals may have high mortality rates, and some low-volume hospitals may have low mortality rates.[10] Although the true performance of individual hospitals is difficult to confirm empirically (for sample size reasons), this lack of discrimination is one reason structural measures are often viewed as "unfair" by many providers.

Process of Care

Process of care measures are the clinical details of care provided to patients. Although long the predominant quality indicators for medical care, their popularity in surgery is growing rapidly. Perhaps the best example of the trend toward using

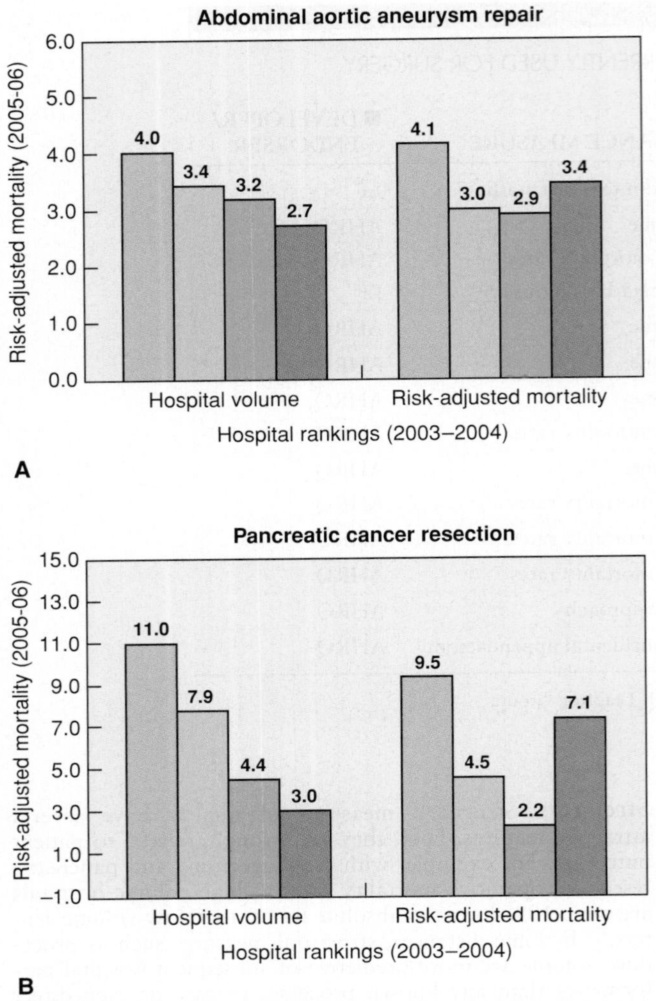

FIGURE 15.1. Ability of hospital rankings based on 2003–2004 mortality rates and hospital volume to predict risk-adjusted mortality in 2005–2006. Data shown for abdominal aortic aneurysm repair (**A**) and pancreatic cancer resection (**B**). Source: National Medicare data.

process measures is the CMS's SCIP. As previously mentioned, this quality measurement initiative focuses exclusively on processes related to prevention of surgical site infections, postoperative cardiac events, venous thromboembolism, and respiratory complications.

Strengths. Since processes of care reflect the care actually delivered by physicians, they have face validity and enjoy greater buy-in from providers. They are also directly actionable and provide good substrate for quality improvement activities. Although risk adjustment may be important for outcomes, it is not required for many process measures. For example, the appropriate prophylaxis against postoperative venous thromboembolism is a widely used process measure. Since virtually all patients undergoing open abdominal surgery should be offered some form of prophylaxis, there is little need to collect detailed clinical data for risk adjustment.

Limitations. The biggest limitation of process measures is the lack of correlation between processes of care and important outcomes.[4] There is a growing body of empirical data showing very little correlation between processes of care and important outcomes.[11–13] Most data come from literature on medical diagnoses, such as acute myocardial infarction. For example, the Joint Commission and CMS process measures for acute myocardial infarction explained only 6% of the observed variation in risk-adjusted mortality for acute myocardial infarction.[12]

Although few analogous studies have been done in surgery, there are some reasons to believe that existing process measures explain very little of the variation in important surgical outcomes. First, most process measures currently used in surgery relate to secondary outcomes. While none would dismiss the value of prophylactic antibiotics in reducing risks of superficial wound infection, this process is not related to the most important adverse events of major surgery, including death.

Second, process measures in surgery often relate to complications that are very rare. For example, there is consensus that venous thromboembolism prophylaxis is necessary and important. The SCIP measures, endorsed by the NQF, include the use of appropriate venous thrombosis prophylaxis. However, pulmonary embolism is very uncommon, and improving adherence to these processes will therefore not avert many deaths. Until we understand which processes of care account for those adverse events leading to death, process measures will have limited usefulness in surgical quality measurement.[4,11–13]

Outcomes

Outcome measures reflect the end result of care, from a clinical perspective or as judged by the patient. Although mortality is by far the most commonly used measure in surgery, other outcomes that could be used as quality indicators include complications, hospital readmission, and a variety of patient-centered measures of quality of life or satisfaction. The best example of this type of measurement is found in the National Surgical Quality Improvement Program (NSQIP).[14] The NSQIP is a surgeon-led clinical registry for feeding back risk-adjusted morbidity and mortality rates to participating hospitals. After its successful implementation in Veterans Affairs (VA) hospitals, it was introduced into the private sector with good results.[15] Under the guidance of the American College of Surgeons, hospital participation in the NSQIP continues to grow, with more than 200 hospitals currently participating. Several changes to the NSQIP measurement platform, which were discussed in the previous chapter, will help make the program less expensive and more useful.[3]

Strengths. There are at least two key advantages of outcomes measures. First, outcome measures have obvious face validity, and thus are likely to get the greatest "buy-in" from hospitals and surgeons. Surgeon enthusiasm for the NSQIP and the continued dissemination of the program clearly underline this point. Second, the act of simply measuring outcomes may lead to better performance—the so-called Hawthorne effect. For example, surgical morbidity and mortality rates in VA hospitals have fallen dramatically since implementation of the NSQIP two decades ago.[14] No doubt many surgical leaders at individual hospitals made specific organizational or process improvements after they began receiving feedback on their hospitals' performance. However, it is very unlikely that even a full inventory of these specific changes would explain such broad-based and substantial improvements in morbidity and mortality rates.

Limitations. Hospital- or surgeon-specific outcome measures are severely constrained by small sample sizes. For the large majority of surgical procedures, very few hospitals (or surgeons) have sufficient adverse events (numerators) and cases (denominators) for meaningful, procedure-specific measures of morbidity or mortality. For example, Dimick et al. used data from the Nationwide Inpatient Sample to study seven procedures for which mortality rates have been advocated as quality indicators by the AHRQ.[16] For six of the seven procedures, a very small proportion of US hospitals had adequate caseloads to rule out a mortality rate twice the national average (Fig. 15.2). Although

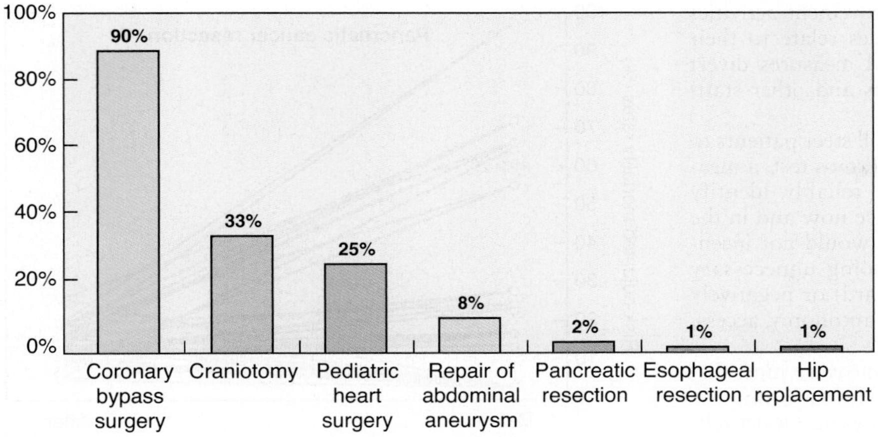

FIGURE 15.2. Big problems with small samples: the proportion of hospitals in the United States with sufficient caseloads (sample size) to reliably use mortality rates to measure quality.

identifying poor-quality outliers is an important function of outcomes measurement, focusing on this goal alone significantly underestimates problems with small sample sizes. Discriminating among individual hospitals with intermediate levels of performance is even more difficult.

Another significant limitation of outcomes assessment is the expense of data collection. Reporting outcomes requires the costly collection of detailed clinical data for risk adjustment. For example, it costs over $100,000 annually for a private sector hospital to participate in the NSQIP. Because of the expense of data collection, the American College of Surgeons' (ACS's) NSQIP currently collects data on only a sample of patients undergoing surgery at each hospital. Although this sampling strategy decreases the cost of data collection, it exacerbates the problem of small sample size with individual procedures. As discussed in the next chapter, changes in the next iteration of the NSQIP are aimed at reducing the expense of data collection without compromising the risk adjustment.

COMPOSITE MEASURES

3 Composite measures, created by combining multiple individual quality indicators, are becoming increasingly used in the assessment of surgical quality.[6,7,17] Most existing pay-for-performance efforts, including the CMS pilot, use composite measures to assess the quality of medical and surgical diagnoses. The Society of Thoracic Surgeons (STS) Measurement Taskforce has created a new composite score that combines elements of outcomes and processes of care into a single measure.[17] With growing enthusiasm for this approach, the AHRQ recently published a technical review of composite measures.[18]

Strengths

Composite measures have two main advantages over individual quality indicators. First, pooling multiple measures overcomes the problem with small sample sizes described earlier. Second, this approach deals with the problem of multiple conflicting measures, and simplifies quality measurement by providing a single, summary measure of performance. For example, the STS measure for cardiac surgery combines several measures of process and outcomes to create a single score with three categories: one star, two stars, and three stars.[17]

Limitations

Composite measures have both technical and practical limitations. Perhaps the biggest technical challenge is weighting the input measures. Most existing composite measures are created using equal weighting, expert opinion, or the "all or none" approach. For example, the STS cardiac surgery composite score calculates a domain-specific score for morbidity, mortality, process of care, and perioperative medications, and then places equal weight on each domain.[17] Unfortunately, these simplistic weighting schemes do not take into account the simple fact that some measures are more important than others. Ideally, input measures would be weighted empirically, based on how strongly they are related to important outcomes.[18] An emerging technique for creating such empirically weighted composite measures of surgical performance will be discussed at the end of the chapter.[19]

Composite measures also have a practical limitation. By design, composite measures reflect global performance with a procedure or specialty. It is hard to know exactly where improvement is needed with this global assessment. Thus, it is important to deconstruct the composite measures into the individual process and outcome measures. Actionable targets for improvement (e.g., high complication rates or failure to adhere to specific processes) can then be addressed.

CHOOSING THE RIGHT MEASURE

4 No quality measure is perfect. Clinical leaders, patient advocates, payers, and policy makers will have to make decisions about when imperfect measures are good enough to act upon. A measure should be implemented only with the expectation that acting on it will result in a net improvement in health quality. Thus, the direct benefits of implementing a particular measure cannot be outweighed by the indirect harms. Unfortunately, these benefits and harms are often difficult to measure and heavily influenced by the specific context and who—patients, payers, or providers—is doing the accounting. For this reason, there is no simple answer for where to "set the bar."

5 It is important to ensure a good match between the performance measure and the primary goal of measurement. The right measure depends on whether the underlying goal is (a) quality improvement or (b) selective referral—directing patients to higher-quality hospitals and/or providers. Although many pay-for-performance initiatives have both goals, one often predominates. For example, the ultimate objective of the CMS's pay-for-performance initiative with prophylactic antibiotics is improving quality at all hospitals (quality improvement). Conversely, the Leapfrog Group's efforts in surgery are primarily aimed at getting patients to hospitals likely to have the best outcomes (selective referral).

6 For quality improvement purposes, a good performance measure must be actionable. Measurable improvements in the given process should translate to clinically meaningful improvements

in patient outcomes. Although quality improvement activities are rarely "harmful," their major downsides relate to their opportunity cost. Initiatives hinged on bad measures divert resources (e.g., time and focus of physicians and other staff) away from more productive activities.

7 With selective referral, a good measure will steer patients to better hospitals or physicians. As one basic litmus test, a measure based on prior performance should reliably identify providers likely to have superior performance now and in the future. At the same time, an ideal measure would not incentivize perverse behaviors (e.g., surgeons doing unnecessary procedures to meet a specific volume standard) or negatively affect other domains of quality (e.g., patient autonomy, access, and satisfaction).

Many believe that a good performance measure must discriminate performance at the individual level. From the provider perspective in particular, a "fair" measure must reliably reflect the performance of individual hospitals or physicians. Unfortunately, as described earlier, small caseloads (and sometimes case mix variation) conspire against this objective for most procedures. Patients, however, should value information that improves their odds of good outcomes on average. Many measures meet this latter interest while failing on the former (e.g., hospital volume standards). There may be no simple solution to resolving the basic tension implied by performance measures that are unfair to providers yet informative for patients. However, it underscores the importance of being clear about both the primary purpose (quality improvement or selective referral) and whose interests are receiving top priority (provider or patient).

DEVELOPING BETTER MEASURES

Although great progress has been made, the science of quality measurement is in its infancy. In fact, there are solutions on the
8 horizon for many of the limitations discussed earlier. One of the biggest limitations of surgical quality measurement is the statistical "noise" from the small sample sizes at most hospitals. This problem makes it difficult to isolate the quality signal from the background statistical noise. In other words, it is often hard to know whether hospitals or surgeons have poor performance because they provide low-quality care or because they were unlucky. For obvious reasons, labeling surgeons and hospitals correctly is extremely important.

An emerging technique, reliability adjustment, directly addresses the problem of statistical noise.[20] This technique, based on hierarchical modeling, quantifies and subtracts statistical noise from the measurement process. Essentially, it "shrinks" providers' performance back toward average unless they deviate to such an extreme that it is safe to assume they are truly different. In this way, it gives providers the benefit of the doubt. Figure 15.3 shows the risk-adjusted mortality rates for pancreatic resection in Medicare patients before and after reliability adjustment. Prior to reliability adjustment, the mortality rates varied from 0% to 100%. After reliability adjustment, the mortality rates only vary from 2% to 22%, yielding a range of performance that is clinically more realistic. Reliability adjustment is gaining popularity outside surgery (e.g., ambulatory care) and is becoming widely recognized as a valid tool for improving the accuracy of quality measurement.[20,21]

Despite wide use in other fields, reliability adjustment is only beginning to find application in surgery. Perhaps the most prominent example is the Massachusetts state cardiac surgery report card, which publishes "smoothed" mortality rates for each hospital.[22] These are obtained with reliability adjustment using hierarchical modeling techniques, as described earlier. This approach will also soon be applied to the morbidity and mortality rates in the ACS's NSQIP, as described with other changes in a recent "Blueprint" for a new ACS NSQIP.[3] As the

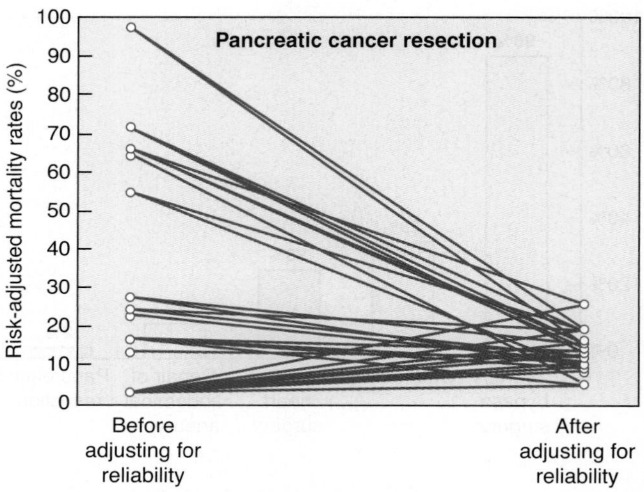

FIGURE 15.3. Variation in hospital mortality rates before and after adjusting for reliability. Twenty randomly sampled hospitals are shown. Source: National Medicare data, 2005–2006.

advantages of this technique become more widely known, there is no doubt it will become the standard technique for reporting risk-adjusted outcomes.

9 Another significant limitation of existing approaches to surgical quality assessment is a lack of good measures of global quality. As payers and purchasers of health care move forward with value-based purchasing, there is a growing need for better composite scores. Unfortunately, as discussed earlier, most approaches are not thoughtful about how they weight input measures. However, there is an emerging technique for creating empirically weighted composite measures of surgical performance.[19] To create these measures, a "gold standard" quality measure is first identified (e.g., risk-adjusted mortality). The relationships between all input measures and this "gold standard" measure are then determined. A composite is then created that weights the input measures based on how reliable they are (a measure of precision) and how closely they are related to the "gold standard" outcome. Staiger et al. recently published the methods for creating these measures using aortic valve replacement.[19] They found that a composite measure of risk-adjusted mortality and hospital volume with aortic valve replacement combined with risk-adjusted mortality for other cardiac procedures explained 70% of the hospital-level variation in mortality and was better at predicting future performance than any individual measure (Fig. 15.4).

Although both of these emerging techniques will enhance our ability to profile hospitals on technical quality, we also need to develop better measures of surgical decision making. Wide geographic variations in the use of surgical procedures imply substantial underuse, misuse, and overuse. Escalating health care costs are at least in part due to overuse and misuse of surgical interventions. Measures of appropriateness or utilization will need to become part of our armamentarium if meaningful attempts at reducing these variations are to be made. Although appropriateness criteria have been extensively studied, there is growing consensus that they are impractical on a large scale.[23] The task of tabulating all of the potential scenarios in which a procedure is "appropriate" or "inappropriate" is daunting. Even when these exhaustive lists are created, reasonable clinicians may still disagree in a large proportion of cases.[23] Appropriateness criteria should be limited to "low-hanging fruit," those procedures with a few, well-agreed-upon indications for operation.

For the majority of procedures, however, another approach is needed. One promising approach is the measurement of

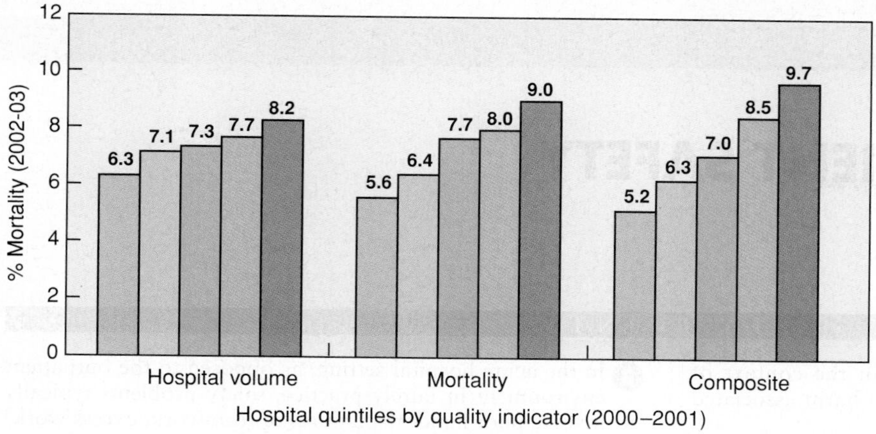

FIGURE 15.4. Ability of various historical (2000–2001) quality indicators to forecast subsequent (2002–2003) risk-adjusted mortality with aortic valve replacement (AVR). Hospitals sorted into quintiles according to hospital volume alone, risk-adjusted mortality alone, and composite measure based on AVR mortality, AVR hospital volume, and mortality and volume with other cardiac procedures.

utilization at the level of the Physician-Hospital Network (PHN). The PHN is a virtual organization for physicians and the hospital with which they are affiliated.[24,25] PHNs are felt by some health policy experts to be the right level of accountability for measuring the quality of the extended health care system. Rates of surgery for each PHN could be used for public reporting, value-based purchasing, or tiered health plans. This approach would allow patients to choose hospitals based on how "aggressive" they are. Public disclosure of surgery rates would also put downward pressure on hospitals with high rates of surgery, potentially discouraging expanding capacity when it may not be necessary.

The near future will no doubt bring other major advances in the science of quality measurement. The accelerating pace of technology will surely play a role. As electronic medical records become more widely adopted, clinical data will be more easily abstracted from the patient record. Such improvements in technology will provide cost-efficient risk adjustment and more practicable approaches for assessing the adherence to important processes of care. While improvements in technology and infrastructure are of great benefit, involvement of surgeons in health services research will also be important. Studies using tools of clinical epidemiology are needed to generate evidence linking high-leverage processes of care to important outcomes. These processes of care could then be applied to existing quality measurement platforms. Surgeon-scientists with scholarship in quality improvement will be instrumental in providing these insights and leading this high-impact academic field forward.

10 When measuring quality, it is important to keep in mind the ultimate goal: improving the quality and efficiency of surgical care. Quality measures are only useful if they inform improvement efforts. Future refinements in measurement should therefore aim to meet the diverse needs of the improvement efforts of patients, payers, and providers. In the previous chapter, the three dominant approaches for improving surgical quality were discussed: selective referral, process compliance, and outcomes measurement. These three policy approaches roughly mirror the three types of quality measures (structure, process, and outcomes), providing real-world examples of how various stakeholders weigh the pros and cons of quality indicators, and ultimately choose an assessment approach by matching the measure to the purpose.

References

1. Lee TH, Meyer GS, Brennan TA. A middle ground on public accountability. *N Engl J Med* 2004;350:2409–2412.
2. Galvin R, Milstein A. Large employers' new strategies in health care. *N Engl J Med* 2002;347:939–942.
3. Birkmeyer JD, Shahian DM, Dimick JB, et al. Blueprint for a new American College of Surgeons: National Surgical Quality Improvement Program. *J Am Coll Surg* 2008;207:777–782.
4. Birkmeyer JD, Dimick JB, Birkmeyer NJ. Measuring the quality of surgical care: structure, process, or outcomes? *J Am Coll Surg* 2004;198:626–632.
5. Landon BE, Normand SL, Blumenthal D, et al. Physician clinical performance assessment: prospects and barriers. *JAMA* 2003;290(9):1183–1189.
6. O'Brien SM, DeLong ER, Dokholyan RS, et al. Exploring the behavior of hospital composite performance measures: an example from coronary artery bypass surgery. *Circulation* 2007;116:2969–2975.
7. Dimick JB, Staiger DO, Baser O, et al. Composite measures for predicting surgical mortality in the hospital. *Health Aff* 2009;28:1189–1198.
8. Halm EA, Lee C, Chassin MR. Is volume related to outcome in health care? A systematic review and methodologic critique of the literature. *Ann Intern Med* 2002;137:511–520.
9. Dudley RA, Johansen KL, Brand R, et al. Selective referral to high volume hospitals: estimating potentially avoidable deaths. *JAMA* 2000;283:1159–1166.
10. Rathore SS, Epstein AJ, Volpp KG, et al. Hospital coronary artery bypass graft surgery volume and patient mortality, 1998–2000. *Ann Surg* 2004;239:110–117.
11. Fonarow GC, Abraham WT, Albert NM, et al. Association between performance measures and clinical outcomes for patients hospitalized with heart failure. *JAMA* 2007;297:61–70.
12. Bradley EH, Herrin J, Elbel B, et al. Hospital quality for acute myocardial infarction: correlation among process measures and relationship with short-term mortality. *JAMA* 2006;296:72–78.
13. Hawn MT, Itani KM, Gray SH, et al. Association of timely administration of prophylactic antibiotics for major surgical procedures and surgical site infection. *J Am Coll Surg* 2008;206:814–819.
14. Khuri SF, Daley J, Henderson W, et al. The Department of Veterans Affairs' NSQIP: the first national, validated, outcome-based, risk-adjusted, and peer-controlled program for the measurement and enhancement of the quality of surgical care. National VA Surgical Quality Improvement Program. *Ann Surg* 1998;228:491–507.
15. Fink AS, Campbell DA Jr, Mentzer RM Jr, et al. The National Surgical Quality Improvement Program in non-Veterans Administration hospitals: initial demonstration of feasibility. *Ann Surg* 2002;236:344–353.
16. Dimick JB, Welch HG, Birkmeyer JD. Surgical mortality as an indicator of hospital quality: the problem with small sample size. *JAMA* 2004;292:847–851.
17. O'Brien SM, Shahian DM, DeLong ER, et al. Quality measurement in adult cardiac surgery: part 2—statistical considerations in composite measure scoring and provider rating. *Ann Thorac Surg* 2007;83(suppl 4):S13–S26.
18. AHRQ Inpatient Quality Indicators Composite Measure. Draft technical report. Available at: http://qualityindicators.ahrq.gov/news/AHRQ_IQI_Composite_Draft.pdf. Accessed June 27, 2007.
19. Staiger DO, Dimick JB, Baser O, et al. Empirically derived composite measures of surgical performance. *Med Care* 2009;47(2):226–233.
20. Hofer TP, Hayward RA, Greenfield S, et al. The unreliability of individual physician "report cards" for assessing the costs and quality of care of a chronic disease. *JAMA* 1999;281:2098–2105.
21. Zaslavsky AM, Beaulieu ND, Landon BE, et al. Dimensions of consumer-assessed quality of Medicare managed-care health plans. *Med Care* 2000;38:162–174.
22. Adult Coronary Artery Bypass Graft Surgery in the Commonwealth of Massachusetts. Fiscal Year 2006 Report, October 1, 2005–September 30, 2006. Available at: http://www.massdac.org/reports/CS%20FY2006.pdf. Accessed June 17, 2010.
23. Casparie AF. The ambiguous relationship between practice variation and appropriateness of care: an agenda for further research. *Health Policy* 1996;35:247–265.
24. Bynum JP, Bernal-Delgado E, Gottlieb D, et al. Assigning ambulatory patients and their physicians to hospitals: a method for obtaining population-based provider performance measurements. *Health Serv Res* 2007;42:45–62.
25. Fisher ES, Staiger DO, Bynum JP, et al. Creating accountable care organizations: the extended hospital medical staff. *Health Aff (Millwood)* 2007;26:w44–w57.

CHAPTER 16 ■ PATIENT SAFETY

DARRELL A. CAMPBELL, Jr.

KEY POINTS

1. Safety means "freedom from harm"; in the context of patient care, safety means freedom from harm associated with any medical action or treatment.
2. Even though the system should be constructed to back up human fallibilities, it is instructive to recognize these fallibilities. This subject is hard to quantify, but a good list, developed in a family practice environment, reads as follows: hurry, distraction, lack of knowledge, premature closure of the diagnostic process, and inadequate aggressiveness in patient management.
3. In the acute hospital setting, as opposed to the outpatient environment in family practice, safety problems typically involve poor handoffs, failures of teamwork, excess workload, and fatigue.
4. Another approach to the implementation of safe practices is to educate and train physicians and nurses within the context of a team.
5. The future of the patient safety movement depends on the development of an effective safety reporting mechanism.

IMPORTANT DEFINITIONS: SAFETY VERSUS QUALITY

The terms *quality* and *safety* have important bearings on any discussion of patient care. These are related subjects but have different meanings, and these differences should be underscored before any dialogue about patient safety begins. 1 Safety means "freedom from harm"; in the context of patient care, safety means freedom from harm associated with any medical action or treatment. Quality is a more global term referring to a "degree of excellence." It is theoretically possible for a hospital to be safe but for quality to be average or poor. It is not possible for a hospital to be of high quality and unsafe. In this chapter we focus primarily on the subject of patient safety, but admit that some aspects of the subject drift into the area of quality as well.

THE PROBLEM

By now, all are familiar with the report issued by the Institute of Medicine (IOM) in 2000 entitled *To Err Is Human.*[1] The report was an exhaustive review of the status of safety in our nation's hospitals. The bottom line—which served as a "burning platform" for the patient safety movement—was the astonishing calculation that between 44,000 and 98,000 Americans died annually in hospitals as the result of preventable medical error. The report produced a flurry of outrage from consumer groups and denials and refutations from medical groups, but when the dust settled, what was left was the recognition, by all groups, that something was seriously wrong in our medical care delivery system.

Comparisons are often made between the safety of airline travel and medical care. One airline disaster every 2 or 3 years produces calls for new regulation, better airports, more frequent mechanical checks, and earlier retirement for pilots. But consider medical care. If even the lower number of preventable deaths extrapolated by the IOM report (44,000 annually) were seen as accurate, and one accepted that an average of 350 passengers were on board every major commercial aircraft flight, deaths from medical error would be equivalent of 63 separate midair collisions per year in the airline industry, or five per month. Imagine the public outcry this would produce, the laws that would be quickly passed, and the boon to train travel that would result. But this is not what has happened in medicine. The government response has been weak at best, and the medical community has been slow to acknowledge, and even slower to respond, to the safety imperative.

CULTURE

Culture is defined as "how we do things around here." That is, there is a certain level of acceptance for what goes on in a given hospital. That acceptance is based on two precepts, which in the past have not been challenged. One precept is that medical errors exist because "humans will always make mistakes." While superficially true, this statement fails to acknowledge that modern human factors engineering strategies can militate against commonly encountered errors. A concrete example of how human factors engineering can be brought into play involves something as simple as a connector for medical tubing. If the connector is designed such that it is not possible to connect an O_2 line to a CO_2 valve, a potentially catastrophic mistake becomes impossible. More globally, work hour restrictions for medical trainees, which reduce fatigue, could be expected to result in fewer errors by exhausted and stressed doctors. To date, human factors engineering has not been brought into the delivery of medical care effectively. While humans will always be capable of making mistakes, the number of mistakes will be reduced if design is targeted to what we know about human fallibilities.

The second precept accounting for complacency is the notion that a medical error is the result of poor individual performance rather than an imperfect system of care. If an individual made the error, in isolation, the only thing to do about it would be to fire the hapless caregiver, or immerse him or her in intensive remedial education. The problem with this approach is that it doesn't apply to the next hapless caregiver faced with the same situation. And so, since there is a high turnover in most medical environments, mistakes continue to happen, caregivers continue to be fired, and nothing really changes. This sequence has been ingrained in the medical culture, and is why the medical community has been slow to respond to the safety crisis.

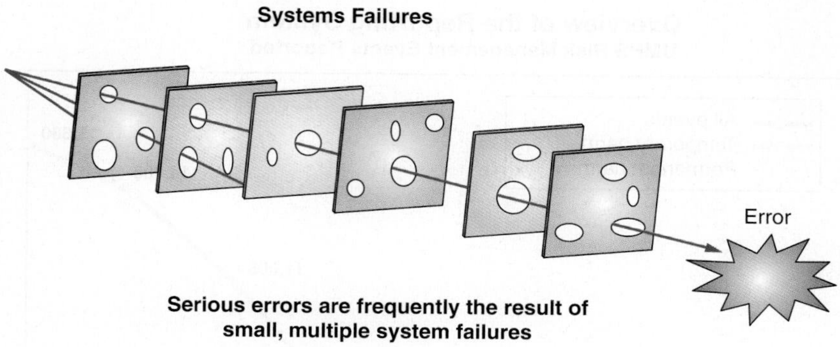

Systems Failures
Error
Serious errors are frequently the result of small, multiple system failures

FIGURE 16.1. Systems failures.

SWISS CHEESE AND MEDICAL ERRORS

A popular paradigm in the medical safety area is the "Swiss cheese" model, introduced by James Reason[2] (Fig. 16.1). This model is a visual representation of the multiple system layers that could prevent a medical error from occurring. A beam of light, representing a latent error, passes through a hole in the cheese, which represents a system vulnerability. The latent error passing through the system via vulnerability will result in a medical error. If enough systems are set up with vulnerabilities, but in different locations, it becomes progressively harder for the latent error to become manifest clinically. The point here is that, while we recognize that both humans and systems of care have vulnerabilities, the prevention of error lies at the door of hospital leadership. Positive results come from the establishment of effectively redundant systems of error prevention. This concept is a major paradigm shift in the patient safety movement.

2 Even though the system should be constructed to back up human fallibilities, it is instructive to recognize these fallibilities. This subject is hard to quantify, but a good list, developed in a family practice environment, reads as follows: hurry, distraction, lack of knowledge, premature closure of the diagnostic process, and inadequate aggressiveness in patient management.[3] The first three issues are probably obvious, but premature closure of the diagnostic process is a problem needing emphasis. Humans often fall into this trap. We see issues as black and white in an attempt to make sense out of complex circumstances. Hurry, distraction, and lack of knowledge contribute. Relevant pieces of Swiss cheese, which could counteract this tendency, include electronic diagnosis and decision-making aids; an institutional policy fostering physician interactions, teamwork, and second opinions; and setting and adhering to reasonable workload standards.

3 Depending on the environment, other fallibilities are exposed. In the acute hospital setting, as opposed to the outpatient environment in family practice, safety problems typically involve poor handoffs, failures of teamwork, excess workload, and fatigue.[4]

But what about the concept of individual responsibility? One cannot show up for work with a careless attitude, engage in irresponsible actions, and expect to be held unaccountable from poor performance because of the emphasis on systems. This is a delicate balance for any health care system. The underlying principle here is that most employees of a hospital wake up each morning wanting to do a good job, and to avoid mistakes, and hence (with exceptions) the general philosophy should be that a major improvement in safety will be at the level of system engineering rather than individual fallibility. When the onus of individual fallibility is lessened (not removed entirely), there then emerges a new sense of system responsibility, with increased willingness to identify system errors and to participate in safety enhancement as a group. This collaborative participation does not occur when one is worried about punitive consequences for reporting and the possibility of job loss.

LEADERSHIP AND POLICY

How does one change a culture? This is not done easily. There are two crucial elements, which, if effective, can change the culture direction positively. The first element is set by the example of hospital leadership. When the rank and file sees that the hospital CEO places patient safety at the top of the list and backs this priority up with funding, a lot of good things happen. When the CEO emphasizes a change in hospital policy, with an emphasis on safety, the change is reinforced. We introduced two policies that serve as examples to make this point. The first, the "full disclosure" policy, stipulated that employees were obligated (not just encouraged) to disclose fully to patients important errors made in rendering their care. Remarkably, this policy resulted in fewer malpractice claims against the system, but more important, it underscored for employees the institutional emphasis on openness and honesty.[5] The second policy change implemented was the "speak up with safety concerns" policy, which stipulated that no caregiver could be punished for voicing a concern involving patient safety, regardless of feelings hurt or hierarchy violated. Again, this written policy clearly articulated a health system goal—that patient safety trumped all other considerations.

One manifestation of an improved safety culture is an increased error reporting rate. Clearly, the error reporting rate will not go up if there exists widespread fear of retribution for reporting. What is desired is an increased rate of error reporting, but a decreasing rate of events resulting in temporary or permanent harm. This pattern suggests that caregivers are vigilant, care about safety, and are reporting on "near misses." The data from "near misses" represent a treasure chest of information that can be used to prevent actual mistakes. We have seen increased reporting in association with the purchase of a new electronic reporting format. Whether a change in culture or a change in reporting format is responsible for the increased level of reports is hard to say, but we believe that it is some combination of both (Fig. 16.2).

ASSESSING THE CULTURE

If one places priority on "improving" a safety culture, it is necessary that the "culture" can be measured. Validated culture surveys exist, which, if applied periodically in a hospital environment, give important insight into the success of safety culture initiatives. We use the Agency for Healthcare Research and Quality (AHRQ) safety culture instrument primarily and survey all caregivers at approximately 2-year intervals. We use the resulting information in three ways. First, we use the aggregate response to answer the question, "Are we improving the safety culture?" and, if not, "What are the areas that need to be addressed institutionally?" On our last survey, a clear sore point at our institution was difficulty with "handoffs," that is, the transfer of information between caregivers and teams. We then developed a taskforce focused on fixing the problem, over

FIGURE 16.2. Overview of the reporting system.

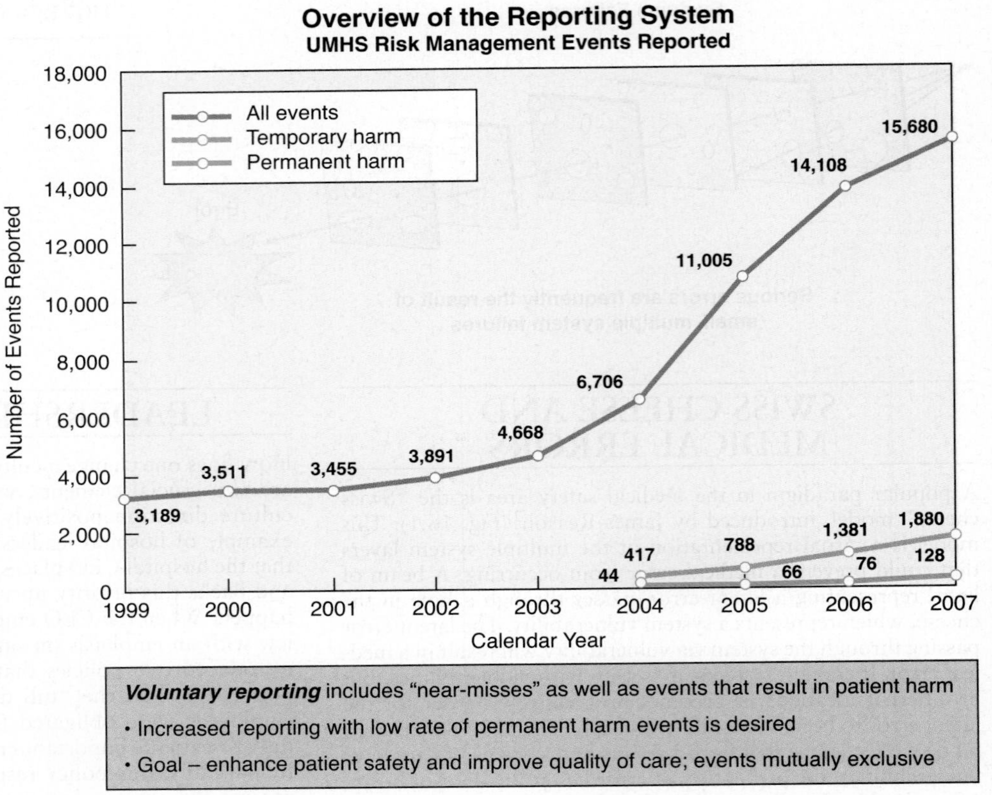

both the short and long term. The long-term solution is an electronic one; the short-term solution is a paper-based handoff tool. This effort was a direct result of information gained from the safety culture survey.

A second way we use the safety culture survey data is to identify specific hospital units that are struggling with a dispirited or complacent attitude toward the safety effort. Such problems often result from poor nurse leadership, disruptive physicians, or a lack of perceived resources. Armed with information about the safety culture (or lack of it), the institution can implement a focused strategy customized to the problem. Figure 16.3 shows results from our survey arranged by individual nursing unit, demonstrating certain units in need of help with error reporting and, conversely, units where the culture is good and institutional resources are not needed. A third source of information derived from the survey comes from narrative comments entered by individual caregivers. This is a very rich source of information and, since it is anonymous, often draws a fine line under issues that are hard to talk about in any other forum. Issues of suspected physician impairment, abusive behavior, or lack of leadership skills are sometimes identified.

Two important questions regarding safety culture and our efforts to improve it remain. First, using the AHRQ tool, have we seen an aggregate improvement over the past two survey intervals? Many safety initiatives have been instituted over this period of time, and yet the aggregate culture data haven't shown much change. We interpret this information to mean that much more work needs to be done, and that changing a culture is a hard thing to do, akin to changing direction of an aircraft carrier. Also, over the period of time we have been studying our culture, our institutional activity has gone up dramatically, the complexity of our patients has increased, and nursing turnover has been high. Under these circumstances, no change in the safety culture data might be viewed more optimistically.

A second question is, Are there individual strategies we have used that influence the safety culture positively? If so, we could use these strategies more broadly. The answer to this question is yes. Patient safety rounds have been an important strategy that has improved the safety culture. Over the course of the past several years, we have made safety rounds on over 125 occasions, at 2-week intervals. Safety rounds are carried out by leadership (chief of staff, chief of nursing, CEO, etc.) and a pointed 45-minute discussion ensues with the unit caregivers, including nurses, aides, clerks, and transporters. The culture effects of this endeavor are profound. When caregivers believe that leadership is willing to listen, takes safety very seriously, and will put resources behind the articulated concerns, an overall feeling of confidence and support of the safety effort follows. Figure 16.4 demonstrates that caregivers having participated in patient safety rounds viewed the patient safety environment much more positively than those who had not.

But is a positive safety culture actually associated with improved safety? The assumption is yes, but data were hard to come by until recently. In Michigan, a multihospital collaborative was initiated (the Keystone Project), the object of which was to implement evidence-based practices known to decrease the incidence of bloodstream infections (BSIs).[6] One hundred and seven hospitals were involved, and caregivers responded to the Safety Attitudes Questionnaire (SAQ), similar to the AHRQ tool described previously. Results (incidence of BSIs) were correlated with answers to the SAQ. The results are seen in Figure 16.5. There was an important association noted between the best results (percent reduction in BSIs) and the most positive answers to SAQ questions. This is only an association (and subject to the usual caveats about associations vs. cause and effect), but important nonetheless. These results support the underlying hypothesis that when leadership prioritizes safety and implements actions to support safety, caregivers reflect this in their answers to the SAQ and this is associated with improved patient safety.

THE EVIDENCE BASE FOR PATIENT SAFETY

As important as it is to lay a strong foundation in safety culture, the energy and enthusiasm of caregivers to provide safe

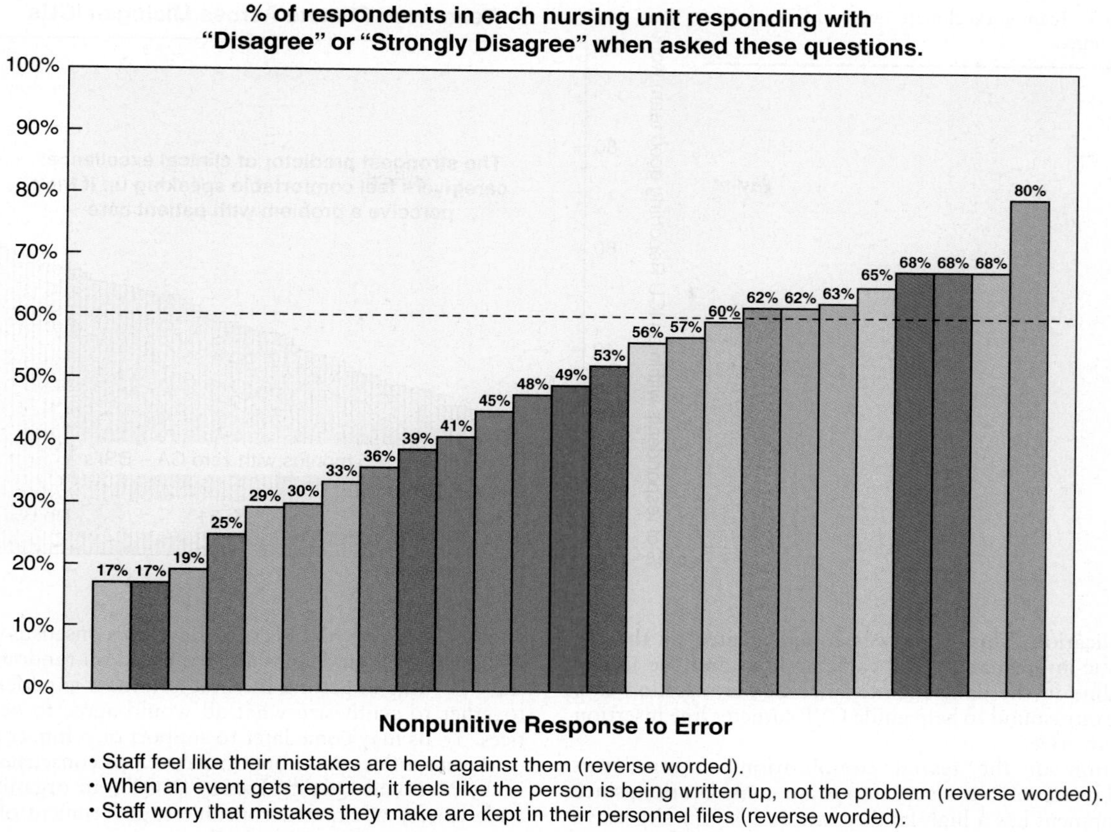

FIGURE 16.3. Nonpunitive response to error.

patient care must be rooted in activities that have been found to be effective. Unfortunately, there does not exist at this point a large base of evidence in patient safety, largely because the field is relatively young. Recently, the World Health Organization (WHO) convened a group to carefully analyze existing studies and highlight effective strategies with an evidence base.[7] These are listed in Table 16.1. Comments about specific evidence-based actions follow.

With regard to the administration of perioperative beta-blockers to prevent postoperative myocardial ischemia, it is very clear that patients already on such medications must be given them postoperatively. However, an initial interest in beta-blocker administration for patients never having received them previously evaporated as the result of the POISE trial.[8] This was an international randomized controlled trial focusing on this specific issue, and the result, after analyzing many thousands of patients, was that giving beta-blockers perioperatively to naïve patients caused more harm than good. Specifically, treated patients developed more troublesome bradycardia and hypotension than controls, and this resulted in a higher incidence of stroke, obviating the potential benefit of the drug in preventing myocardial ischemia.

Using maximum sterile barriers for central venous pressure (CVP) catheter insertion to prevent bloodstream infection may seem obvious, and the implementation of this protocol has resulted, in many studies, in a dramatic fall in the incidence of

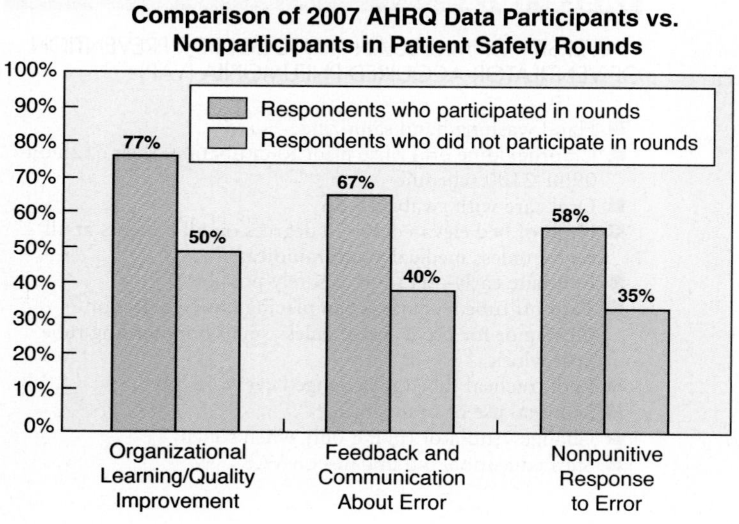

FIGURE 16.4. Comparison of 2007 Agency for Healthcare Research and Quality (AHRQ) data participants versus nonparticipants in patient safety rounds.

SCIENTIFIC PRINCIPLES

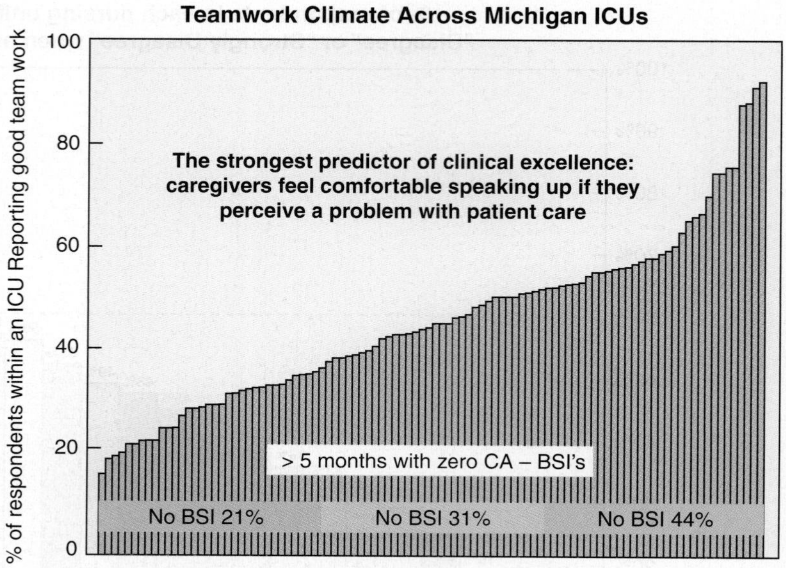

FIGURE 16.5. Teamwork climate across Michigan intensive care units.

this complication. This strategy is complemented by the use of antibiotic-impregnated CVP catheter lines and the use of chlorhexidine in the daily maintenance of the insertion site. The use of ultrasound to help guide CVP catheter line insertion is clearly effective.

Prevention of the feared complication of ventilator-associated pneumonia is a very important consideration, since this development has a high fatality rate and is very expensive to treat. There is some evidence that the continuous aspiration of subglottic secretions is important. Our institution has been successful in decreasing the ventilator-acquired pneumonia rate dramatically (Fig. 16.6) using the multipronged strategy described in Table 16.2.

DEVELOPING CONSENSUS

Given the paucity of real evidence to achieve what we think of as safe patient care, and because there is an urgent need to act, another strategy has been to develop consensus guidelines. Although such guidelines are not based on randomized trials, there is value in getting the best and most experienced minds together to synthesize what all would agree to be best practices. Trials may come later to support or refute consensus.

A very influential group that develops consensus guidelines is the National Quality Forum (NQF), an organization of a wide variety of experts, consumers, government officials, and corporate directors. The NQF several years ago published its list of "30 Safe Practices" recommended for implementation. Because this chapter is oriented toward surgery, Table 16.3 lists a selection of the 30 Safe Practices germane to the inpatient setting.

Consensus and Accreditation

The NQF works closely with the Joint Commission. When the NQF has reached consensus on a specific safety practice, this is often translated into a Joint Commission requirement for hospital accreditation, in this setting recognized as Joint Commission "patient safety goals." These goals are more specific than consensus guidelines and have more "bite" to them, in that all hospitals need to fulfill these requirements in order to be

TABLE 16.1

EVIDENCE-BASED INTERVENTIONS FOR SAFE PATIENT CARE

- Appropriate use of prophylaxis to prevent venous thromboembolism
- Use of perioperative beta-blockers in appropriate patients to prevent perioperative morbidity and mortality
- Use of maximum sterile barriers while placing central intravenous catheters to prevent infections
- Asking that patients recall and restate what they have been told during the informed consent process
- Continuous aspiration of subglottic secretions to prevent ventilator-associated pneumonia
- Use of pressure-relieving bedding materials to prevent pressure ulcers
- Use of real-time ultrasound guidance during central line insertion to prevent complications
- Patient self-management for warfarin to achieve appropriate outpatient anticoagulation and prevent complications
- Appropriate provision of nutrition, with a particular emphasis on early enteral nutrition in critically ill and surgical patients
- Use of antibiotic-impregnated central venous catheters to prevent catheter-related infections

TABLE 16.2

UNIVERSITY OF MICHIGAN PROTOCOL FOR PREVENTION OF VENTILATOR-ACQUIRED PNEUMONIA (VAP)

- Hand washing/hand sanitizing
- Chlorhexidine oral rinse prior to intubation, then q12h on 0900–2100 schedule
- Oral care with swabs q2–3h
- Head of bed elevated 30–45 degrees on all patients at all times, unless medically contraindicated
- Extubate early—as soon as safely possible
- Turn off tube feedings when placing patients flat for turning or for procedures, unless small-bore feeding tube postpyloric
- Endotracheal tube tape changed every 48 h
- Minimal use of saline lavage
- Change ventilator tubing only when soiled
- Staff education and updates on VAP

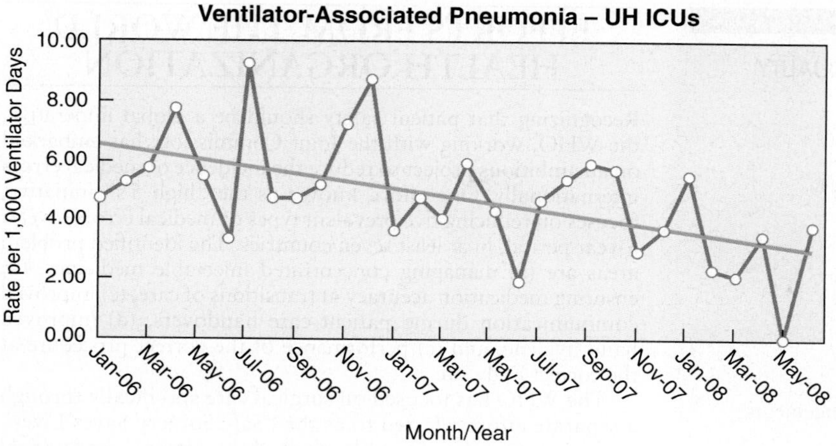

FIGURE 16.6. Ventilator-associated pneumonia—University Hospital intensive care units.

accredited. For example, goal 7, "Reduce the risk of health care associated infections," stipulates, among other things, that hospitals have specific strategies in place to prevent surgical site infections (SSIs); that they provide regular feedback about SSI rates to caregivers, with follow-up for 30 days; that they discontinue the use of shaving as a method of preoperative hair removal; and so on. Goal 8, "Reduce the risk of patient harm resulting from falls," stipulates that each hospital implement a specific falls reduction program.

Consensus, Accreditation, and Payment

The Centers for Medicare and Medicaid Services (CMS) has a lot to say about implementation of safety practices in that they pay a large fraction of the nation's health care bill. As it regards safety in surgery and hospital care, CMS has embarked on two important strategies. The first is the Surgical Care Improvement Project (SCIP), whose stated goal is to reduce the incidence of selected surgical complications 25% by the year 2010. To do this, CMS produced several specific process measures that are required to be met by hospitals before receiving full payment for services. Private insurers soon followed suit. SCIP measures are listed in Table 16.4. In contrast to the more broadly defined consensus guidelines, SCIP measures have a strong evidence base. Whether this effort will be translated into national improvement in results remains to be determined. The Joint Commission has also integrated certain SCIP measures into its evaluation requirements.

Another important strategy embarked upon by the CMS is known as "nonpayment for hospital-acquired conditions," otherwise referred to as the "never event" policy. In this strategy the CMS has determined that it will not reimburse for flagrant medical errors, such as wrong patient, wrong side, or wrong site surgery. Administrators and surgeons don't object to this policy as far as it goes. But great concern has been raised about other conditions on the "never event" list, such as venous thromboembolism (VTE) or patient falls. The controversy arises because in these cases there does not exist an evidence base that would allow a hospital to eliminate these events entirely. Perfectly appropriate VTE prophylaxis, for example, only reduces the incidence of postoperative VTE by 50%. This situation seems unfair, and the list of "never event" conditions is progressively growing longer. Whether this strategy will really improve quality and make patients safer remains to be proven.

TABLE 16.3

NATIONAL QUALITY FORUM SAFE PRACTICES

- Create a culture of safety.
- Obtain explicit informed consent.
- ICU patients managed by critical care certified providers.
- Implement computerized physician order entry.
- Implement protocol for wrong side/site prevention.
- Evaluate for venous thromboembolism/implement prophylactic protocols.
- Develop facility-wide anticoagulation services.
- Adhere to effective measures for preventing bloodstream infections.
- Implement appropriate methods (antibiotic administration) for the prevention of surgical site infection.
- Evaluate each patient at admission for the risk of malnutrition.
- Develop effective hand sanitizing policies.

ICU, intensive care unit.

TABLE 16.4

SURGICAL CARE IMPROVEMENT PROGRAM (SCIP) PROCESS AND OUTCOME MEASURES

Infection (INF)

- SCIP INF 1: Prophylactic antibiotic received within 1 h prior to surgical incision
- SCIP INF 2: Prophylactic antibiotic selection for surgical patients
- SCIP INF 3: Prophylactic antibiotics discontinued within 24 h after surgery end time (48 h for cardiac patients)
- SCIP INF 4: Cardiac surgery patients with controlled 6 a.m. postoperative blood glucose
- SCIP INF 6: Surgery patients with appropriate hair removal.
- SCIP INF 7: Colorectal surgery patients with immediate postoperative normothermia

Venous Thromboembolism (VTE)

- SCIP VTE 1: Surgery patients with recommended venous thromboembolism prophylaxis ordered
- SCIP VTE 2: Surgery patients who received appropriate venous thromboembolism prophylaxis without 24 h prior to surgery to 24 h after surgery

TABLE 16.5

AGENCY FOR HEALTHCARE RESEARCH AND QUALITY PATIENT SAFETY INDICATORS

1. Hospital-level patient safety indicators

- Complications of anesthesia
- Death in low-mortality DRGs
- Decubitus ulcer
- Failure to rescue
- Foreign body left in during procedure
- Iatrogenic pneumothorax
- Selected infections due to medical care
- Postoperative hip fracture
- Postoperative hemorrhage or hematoma
- Postoperative physiologic and metabolic derangements
- Postoperative respiratory failure
- Postoperative pulmonary embolism or deep vein thrombosis
- Postoperative sepsis
- Postoperative wound dehiscence in abdominopelvic surgical patients
- Accidental puncture and laceration
- Transfusion reaction
- Birth trauma—injury to neonate
- Obstetric trauma—vaginal delivery with instrument
- Obstetric trauma—vaginal delivery without instrument
- Obstetric trauma—cesarean delivery

2. Area-level patient safety indicators

- Foreign body left in during procedure
- Iatrogenic pneumothorax
- Selected infections due to medical care
- Postoperative wound dehiscence in abdominopelvic surgical patients
- Accidental puncture and laceration
- Transfusion reaction
- Postoperative hemorrhage or hematoma

DRGs, diagnosis-related groups.

PATIENT SAFETY INDICATORS

The AHRQ is another national group, funded by the National Institutes of Health. Several years ago the AHRQ developed 21 patient safety indicators (PSIs), which are thought to reflect on an institution's safety. These indicators are captured from a hospital's coding system, using International Classification of Diseases-9 (ICD-9) codes after patient discharge. The PSIs are listed in Table 16.5. While useful information can be obtained from this system, a disadvantage is that the data are obtained from medical billing coders, and may not accurately reflect whether a complication was actually preventable. An example might be the PSI labeled "accidental puncture and laceration." An enterotomy made during the course of a difficult dissection in an irradiated and multiply operated abdomen would fit into this category and be interpreted by nonsurgeons as an "accident." The surgeon who was carefully dissecting under these circumstances would definitely not agree. Despite such limitations, the AHRQ PSIs will be publicly reported as a safety indicator by the government next year, and already form the basis of certain proprietary safety indices, such as those put forth by HealthGrades.com or the University Health System Consortium.

EFFORTS FROM THE WORLD HEALTH ORGANIZATION

Recognizing that patient safety should be a global imperative, the WHO, working with the Joint Commission, has embarked on an ambitious project to reduce the incidence of medical errors internationally. One effort, known as the "high 5's" initiative, focuses on reducing five prevalent types of medical errors, over a 5-year period, in at least seven countries. The identified problem areas are (a) managing concentrated injectable medicines, (b) ensuring medication accuracy at transitions of care, (c) improved communication during patient care handovers, (d) improved hand hygiene, and (e) performance of the correct procedure at the correct body site.

The WHO has focused on surgical care specifically through a separate effort referred to as the "Safe Surgery Saves Lives" campaign. One very tangible result of this effort is the Surgical Safety Checklist, shown in Table 16.6.[9] Now being tested in eight countries, the vision is that a standardized forum for intraoperative communication will be adopted internationally, much in the same way that the international aviation community has endorsed standardized flight checklists.

IMPLEMENTATION STRATEGIES

Establishing a safe culture is important, and emphasizing an evidence base and consensus guidelines is important, but ensuring implementation of what is known to be safe practice is critical and may be the most difficult of all safety strategies to accomplish. Several strategies have been helpful in our environment.

Adding Pharmacists to Rounds

Our medical center is a tertiary care referral center; the complexity of cases is high and always going higher. Transplants, complex oncologic problems, extracorporeal membrane oxygenation (ECMO) patients, and others with multisystem organ failure fill a large portion of our beds. The pharmacologic aspects of these cases are complex. Adding to the difficulty of managing such patients is the educational aspect of our enterprise, which guarantees a constant supply of new faces on rounds. To address these issues and to prevent errors, we have implemented a policy of adding a clinical pharmacist to each of our high-complexity services. The role of this individual is to suggest appropriate drugs, screen for allergies and incompatibilities, and monitor for important side effects. The program has been invaluable in improving patient safety at our institution and at others.[10]

Rapid Response Team

Mortality rates for in-hospital cardiac arrest have been high for decades, despite advances in cardiopulmonary resuscitation (CPR) techniques and cardiotropic medications. This is true particularly for "floor arrests," those cases of arrest occurring outside of the intensive care unit (ICU). In our center, and in many others, analysis of CPR cases has led to frustration that insufficient attention had been paid to the patient's condition in the hours prior to the arrest, at a time when interventions could conceivably have been very helpful.

One approach to this problem has been to develop a rapid response team (RRT), which is activated when certain physiologic parameters fall outside a specified range. Such parameters identified at our center are heart rate ($<$40 or $>$140 with new symptoms), respiratory rate ($<$8 or $>$36), blood pressure (systolic $<$80 or $>$220, diastolic $>$110 with symptoms), and unexplained change in cognition or neurologic status of adult inpatients. A key feature of the RRT activation is that it is seen as

TABLE 16.6

WORLD HEALTH ORGANIZATION SURGICAL SAFETY CHECKLIST

■ BEFORE INDUCTION OF ANESTHESIA	■ BEFORE SKIN INCISION	■ BEFORE PATIENT LEAVE OPERATING ROOM
■ SIGN IN	■ TIME OUT	■ SIGN OUT
■ Patient has confirmed: ■ Identity ■ Site ■ Procedure ■ Consent ■ Site marked/not applicable ■ Anesthesia safety check completed ■ Pulse oximeter on patient and functioning ■ Does patient have: ■ A known allergy? ■ No ■ Yes ■ Difficult airway/aspiration risk? ■ No ■ Yes ■ Risk of >500 mL blood loss (7 mL/kg in children)? ■ No ■ Yes, and adequate intravenous access and fluids planned	■ Confirm all team members have introduced themselves by name and role ■ Surgeon, anesthesia professional, and nurse verbally confirm ■ Patient ■ Site ■ Procedure ■ Anticipated critical events ■ Surgeon reviews: What are the critical or unexpected steps, operative duration, anticipated blood loss? ■ Anesthesia team reviews: Are there any patient-specific concerns? ■ Nursing team reviews: Has sterility (including indicator results) been confirmed? Are there equipment issues or any concerns? ■ Has antibiotic prophylaxis been given within the last 60 min? ■ Yes ■ Not applicable ■ Is essential imaging displayed? ■ Yes ■ Not applicable	■ Nurse verbally confirms with the team: ■ The name of the procedure recorded ■ That instrument, sponge, and needle counts are correct (or not applicable) ■ How the specimen is labeled (including patient name) ■ Whether there are any equipment problems to be addressed ■ Surgeon, anesthesia professional, and nurse review the key concerns for recovery and management of this patient

mandatory for nursing; no judgment is required. If the parameters are exceeded, the RRT is activated. This relieves some of the anxieties experienced by nurses in the past about communication with physicians, particularly at odd hours. In our center, activation of the RRT results in the timely arrival of an experienced surgical intensive care unit nurse and a respiratory therapist. If the conditions are found to warrant it, a hospitalist is called. This occurs in 15% of cases. There is controversy in the literature as to whether the RRT effort actually is effective.[11] However, the concept has so much face validity that most hospitals have accepted it as an important strategy to improve a safety culture.

An interesting, and entirely unexpected, offshoot of the RRT has been the process, by the RRT team, of visiting nursing floors on a shift-by-shift basis prior to any RRT activation. This process lets the team become more familiar with patients who might subsequently warrant RRT activation. Visits often foster a discussion among caregivers and family as to whether any intervention is appropriate or warranted.

Crew Resource Management

4 Another approach to the implementation of safe practices is to educate and train physicians and nurses within the context of a team. The team is defined, goals are set, and individual responsibilities are assigned. The completion of tasks (or omission) is apparent to members of the team, which provides a fail-safe structure. There has been considerable interest in crew resource management in the area of medicine since it has been conclusively shown to add value to aviation cockpit training. Crew resource management is probably best applied in small, well-defined areas, with relatively consistent staffing patterns, such as an operating room. In one report, a perioperative crew resource management training program consisted of an e-learning module, the development of laminated checklists and pocket-sized cards, briefing scripts, a communication whiteboard, and a hands-on training program facilitated by experienced personnel. Even with focused effort at crew resource management, perioperative safety practice implementation was found to be less than perfect,[12] but the field, at least in medicine, is in its infancy, and it will probably be an important part of safety strategies in years to come.

Developing Collaborative Groups of Hospitals

Under conditions where motivated hospitals get together to discuss safety, the result is often a more consistent implementation of safety practices and better results. The development of a collaborative group directed at safety and/or quality allows for comparative evaluation of quality and safety, and often results in a spirit of friendly competition, which improves the aggregate level of safety.

A prominent example of such collaboration was mentioned previously, the Michigan Hospital Association–sponsored Keystone Initiative. Here, evidence-based practice for the care of patients in the ICU was monitored and found to be low across the state. A protocol was adopted for over 100 ICU groups, which included elevation of the head of the bed 30 degrees, ulcer prophylaxis, regular respiratory weaning trials, and a central line insertion protocol, with line maintenance involving chlorhexidine patches. When the latter protocol was implemented, a profound drop in the incidence of bloodstream infections across the state was seen, and the estimated cost savings exceeded $160 million.[6]

In a different example, 34 Michigan hospitals formed the Michigan Surgical Quality Collaborative. These hospitals, using the American College of Surgeons' National Surgical Quality Improvement Project (ACS NSQIP) as a quality reporting infrastructure, convene at 3-month intervals and share information about surgical results. Hospitals with the fewest complications in a specific area discuss why they feel they have been successful. "Best practices" are then distributed in a network including through the Internet, a hardcopy newsletter, and YouTube. Each hospital implements strategies it feels are appropriate for its situation. The result has been a sharp drop in the incidence of surgical complications. The results suggest that a collaborative quality organization, with regular and intensive sharing of data and best practices, is an essential vehicle for quality improvement.

PATIENT AND FAMILY INVOLVEMENT

One element of the patient safety movement that will become more important in the future is the involvement of the patient in various hospital safety strategies. A valuable source of information, and an important feedback mechanism, is lost when the patient, or family, is not a part of the care process. Two examples of the value of patient involvement involve hand washing and urgent care.

For hand washing, an effective hospital strategy prompts patients to ask physicians, "Have you washed your hands?" when they come into the patient's room. Physicians frequently wear buttons in this effort, which say, "Ask me if I've washed my hands." While it may seem trivial and somewhat demeaning to the physicians, the fact remains that the percentage of physicians and nurses washing their hands prior to patient contact remains far below 100%, and the prevalence of patient infection with *Clostridium difficile*, vancomycin-resistant *Enterococcus*, and other hospital-acquired infections remains high. In this context, patient involvement could be seen as a very important piece of Swiss cheese.

Another example of patient and family involvement in the care process is the concept of "family activation" of the rapid response team. Family members are often more aware of changes in a patient's condition than nurses or doctors, for the obvious reason that they know the personality and traits of the patient in detail. "He wouldn't complain about this unless it was really bad" is an important source of information from a wife. In the past, this clue to an evolving situation was sometimes lost on caregivers more focused on vital signs and urine output. In "family activation" of the rapid response team, family members are allowed to call a phone number activating the rapid response team if they feel that more attention is needed to a given situation. While it might seem that this would let loose a flood of such calls, in actuality, this has not been the case.

DEVELOPING A TAXONOMY FOR PATIENT SAFETY

Ultimately, comparative data on the safety of patient care in this country will be available to the public, much in the same way that the safety of retail products, medications, and automobiles is currently reported. For any reporting system to be valuable and fair, the definitions of safety events need to be refined and agreed upon. It is not possible to compare the safety of different hospitals if definitions used are not standardized. Many national organizations are working on this topic. The WHO has recently developed an "International Classification for Patient Safety" designed to "define, harmonize and group patient safety concepts into an internationally agreed upon classification in a way that is conducive to learning and improve patient safety across systems." This work, while difficult, is essential for the patient safety movement.[9]

PUBLIC REPORTING OF SAFETY DATA

We live in an age of transparency. The public wants—and deserves—information about the safety record of a given hos-
5 pital. And yet such information is hard to find. The future of the patient safety movement depends on the development of an effective safety reporting mechanism. This is because, in the absence of a large-scale database, information is not disseminated effectively, and one hospital may easily make the same mistake as its sister hospital down the street. One major impediment to the development of a national safety database is the lack of a standardized taxonomy of patient safety events. This problem is being addressed, as was just described.

Public reporting has been initiated using both voluntary and mandatory designs. Two examples of successful voluntary reporting systems are the National Nosocomial Infection Survey, a branch of the Centers for Disease Control and Prevention, and the MEDMARX program of the U.S. Pharmacopeia. Mandatory safety reporting systems are often state initiated and provide various sanctions for hospitals known to be engaged in unsafe practices. This penalty provides a disincentive to report, however. Only a few states have successful mandatory reporting systems.

One very successful example of a voluntary reporting system, albeit in the field of aviation, is the Aviation Safety Reporting System. This system analyzes 30,000 reports annually. Its success has depended on these factors: the system is simple, it is safe (for the reporting pilots), and it provides value.[13] The patient safety movement would do well to emulate this system. When it does, and the taxonomy is standardized, doctors, nurses, and administrators will be considerably more willing to make safety data available to the public.

References

1. Kohn LT, Corrigan JM, Donaldson M, eds., Committee on Quality of Health Care in America IoM. *To Err Is Human: Building a Safer Health System*. Washington, DC: National Academy Press; 2000.
2. Reason J. Education and debate. Human errors: models and management. *BMJ* 2000;320:768–770.
3. Ely JW, Levinson W, Elder NC, et al. Perceived causes of family physicians' errors. *J Fam Pract* 1995;40:337–344.
4. Singh H, Thomas E, Petersen L, et al. Medical errors involving trainees: a study of closed malpractice claims from 5 insurers. *Arch Intern Med* 2007; 167(19):2030–2036.
5. Boothman RC, Blackwell AC, Campbell DA Jr, et al. A better approach to medical malpractice claims? The University of Michigan Experience. *J Health Life Sci Law* 2009;2(2):125–159.
6. Pronovost P, Needham D, Berenholtz S, et al. An intervention to decrease catheter-related bloodstream infections in the ICU. *N Engl J Med* 2007; 356(25):2660.
7. Ovretveit J. *Which interventions are effective for improving patient safety? A synthesis of research and policy issues.* WHO HEN Copenhagen and MMC. Stockholm, Sweden: Karolinska. http://homepage.mac.com.
8. POISE Study Group. Effects of extended-release metoprolol succinate in patients undergoing non-cardiac surgery (POISE trial): a randomized controlled trial. *Lancet* 2008;371:1839–1847.
9. *World Alliance for Patient Safety Progress Report 2006–2007*. Geneva, Switzerland: World Health Organization; 2008.
10. Kucukarslan SN, Peters MP, Mlynarek M, et al. Pharmacists on rounding teams reduce preventable adverse drug events in hospital general medicine units. *Arch Intern Med* 2003;163:2014–2018.
11. Hillman K, Chen J, Cretikos M, et al., MERIT Study Investigators. Introduction of the medical emergency team (MET) system: a cluster-randomised controlled trial. *Lancet* 2005;365:2091–2097.
12. France D, Leming L, Jackson T. An observational analysis of surgical team compliance with perioperative safety practices after crew resource management training. *Am J Surg* 2008;195:546–553.
13. Leape L. Reporting of adverse events. *N Engl J Med* 2002;347(20): 1633–1638.

PART TWO

SURGICAL PRACTICE

CHAPTER 17 ■ TRAUMA AND TRAUMA CARE: GENERAL CONSIDERATIONS

RONALD V. MAIER

KEY POINTS

1. Injury is an epidemic in America, killing 150,000 and hospitalizing 3.0+ million while costing more than $250 billion per year. Trauma is the leading cause of death to age 45 years, the fourth leading cause of death overall, and the leading contributor to years of potential life lost before age 65 overall. The major causes of injury-related death, in decreasing order, are motor vehicle crashes, penetrating trauma, falls, and burns.
2. Trauma deaths occur at three time periods following injury, each having a unique pattern and etiology: 50% at the scene, 30% within the "golden hour" or acute resuscitation phase, and 20% delayed from several days to several weeks after injury.
3. Modern trauma care is derived from the care of wounds and casualty management developed during major wars, and trauma systems are based on military experiences of improved survival in injured personnel produced by rapid transport to definitive care.
4. Trauma systems require a lead agency with designating authority, a formal verification process utilizing American College of Surgeons or similar standards, a limit on the number of centers based on patient needs, and triage criteria to deliver the right patient to the right hospital at the right time. The impediments of distance, discovery, training, and maintenance of expertise make rural trauma care a remaining major challenge.
5. Scoring systems allow objective quantification of the injury to assess impact on outcome and to track differences in outcome, both serially within an institution and between institutions and regional systems.
6. Traumatic injury results in deformation and structural damage of tissue dependent on the kinetic energy transferred to the host, which, in turn, is dependent on the mass and, to a much greater extent, the velocity of the injuring force. Varying mechanisms of injury produce predictable patterns of damage.
7. The interdisciplinary science of injury control requires a team approach that involves surgical and medical specialists, epidemiologists, statisticians, biomechanical engineers, public health practitioners, and economists.

EPIDEMIOLOGY

Injury has been a frequent cause of death in the United States since accurate statistics were first collected in the middle of the 19th century. With decreases in infectious diseases and the industrialization of society, injury has become a leading public health concern, which shows little sign of abating (Table 17.1).
1 In the United States, more than 3 million people are hospitalized annually as a result of unintentional injury, and approximately 35 to 40 million emergency department visits occur for the evaluation and treatment of injuries.[1] According to the most recent Centers for Disease Control and Prevention National Center for Injury Prevention and Control (CDC-NCIPC) statistics, 163,750 deaths resulted from injury in the United States in 2006 (Fig. 17.1).[2] Unintentional injuries account for about three fourths of these deaths (121,599 in 2006), and nearly one half of these were caused by motor vehicle crashes (MVCs), including occupant, pedestrian, and motorcyclist. Falls, occurring primarily among the elderly, are the second major cause of death from unintentional injuries. In 2002, there were 3,482 unintentional drownings and 14,050 burn injuries, with 2,670 deaths. Intentional injuries are responsible for just over 40,000 deaths per year, of which 66% are suicides and 34% homicides. Firearms account for 60% of all suicides and 72% of all homicides.[3] Injury causes not only mortality but also significant morbidity. Each year, 37 million people are treated in emergency departments for injury and approximately 10% will require hospitalization.[2] It is estimated that the direct costs associated with fatal and nonfatal injuries total over $60 billion per year.[3] However, the overall impact of injury on society exceeds $250 billion per year due to years of lost productivity and chronic impairments. Of the 16 million people living with impairments in the United States, 44% cite injury as the cause of their disability.[4] More than one half of all hospitalized trauma patients have fractures, dislocations, or ligamentous injuries. Orthopedic injuries are particularly problematic for the elderly.

Perhaps the single most responsible factor for the increase in the incidence of trauma has been the motor vehicle. Deaths from MVCs skyrocketed during the 1910s through 1920s, rising from an infrequent occurrence to a peak of 30 deaths per 100,000 per year during the 1930s and 1940s. During this time, trauma achieved its current status as the leading cause of death and disability among young Americans. Of these patients, more than 40% are between the ages of 25 and 44 years, and 20% are between 15 and 24 years. People under the age of 45 sustain almost 80% of all injuries and account for 75% of the total lifetime medical costs. Young males are the highest-risk group, not because of physiologic distinctions, but because of the propensity to engage in high-risk activities. According to data provided by the NCIPC, reported in 2001, considering all injury-related deaths (total of 157,070), 56.6% occurred in the age group of 15 to 49 years, predominantly in the male population.[5] Overall, the risk of dying following injury for the male population is seven times higher than that for the female population.[5] Trauma (intentional and unintentional injury) is currently the leading cause of death up to the age of 44 years and the fourth leading cause of death overall (after heart disease, cancer, and stroke).

Although morbidity and mortality figures are important, another important variable related to injury costs for society is measured in years of potential life lost (YPLL) before age 65. In the United States, these are the most productive for society[6]

TABLE 17.1

SIGNIFICANT HISTORICAL DEVELOPMENTS RELATED TO TRAUMA CARE

■ PERIOD OR PERSON	■ CONTRIBUTION
Greek medicine	Wound care and fracture management
Roman Empire	Realization that laudable pus was undesirable Healing by second intention
16th century, Paré	Use of dressing and ligature in wound management
French and Indian War, John Hunter	Differentiation between primary and secondary wound healing
Early 1800s, Dominique Jean Larrey	Developed the principle of the ambulance and the concept of triage
Crimean War, 1853–1856	Demonstrated value of nursing care (Florence Nightingale)
Samuel Gross, 1862	Described shock as "the rude unhinging of the machinery of life"
Civil War	Rediscovery of importance of field ambulance, nonsuppurative wound care Initial use of antiseptics Further development of nursing care by Clara Barton, American Red Cross founder
World War I	Principle of débridement and delayed closure for wounds more than 8 h old Established primary closure for wounds <8 h old only Field ambulance mechanized with automobile availability Recognition that shock was due to blood or fluid loss and use of seawater to replace blood volume
World War II	Débridement and delayed closure practiced Diverting colostomies standard care for colon injuries Blood transfusion, rapid evacuation, specialized surgical units close to the front
Korean War	Development of Mobile Army Surgical Headquarters (MASH) units, use of helicopters, development of vascular surgery, field research leading to better understanding of posttraumatic renal failure
Vietnam War	Development of an airbase regional emergency medical system with transport from injury to intervention in 1 h or less Better fluid resuscitation to prevent renal failure Recognition of acute respiratory distress syndrome
Operation Enduring Freedom (OEF, Afghanistan) and Operation Iraqi Freedom (OIF)	More damage control operations, flying critical care air transport (CCAT) Optimal utilization of blood components: ratio of red blood cells to fresh frozen plasma to cryoprecipitate

and reflect the potential productivity that is lost as a result of premature death. As a result of its effect on younger age groups, traumatic deaths are the leading contributor to YPLL when compared with deaths associated with either cancer or cardiovascular diseases. In 1996, the age-adjusted YPLL before age 65 (per 100,000 population) was 1,919, 1,554, and 1,223 for injury, cancer, and heart diseases, respectively.[1] On average, for each traumatic death, there are 36 YPLL, compared with 16 for cancer and 12 for cardiovascular diseases.[6]

The leading causes of injury in decreasing rank include MVCs, firearms, falls, those related to cutting or piercing instruments, and burns. Fatalities after injury are mainly caused by MVCs (32%), gunshot wounds (22%), and falls (9%).[7] Recently, in the rapidly growing elderly population, deaths due to falls eclipsed those due to MVCs.

Several important differences are found among the various ethnic groups in the United States in terms of the epidemiology of injury. The three leading causes of traumatic death for persons younger than 35 years are the same overall: MVCs, homicide, and suicide. However, in the African American population, the leading cause of death in this age group is homicide, whereas the mortality rate from MVCs is about 42 of 100,000 among Native Americans, 20 per 100,000 among the white population, and 11 per 100,000 in the Asian population.[6] Similarly, suicide rates are higher for American Indians than for any other group.[1]

The impact of injury in children younger than 15 is also significant. The leading causes of injury in this group are MVCs, burns, drowning, falls, and poisoning. Injury in this age group leads to a significant number of deaths, disabilities, days of missed school, medical costs, and missed workdays for parents. Adolescents are also at increased risk for injury. In fact, more adolescents die from injuries than from all other diseases combined (Fig. 17.1).[8] Of all deaths in this age group, 40% are caused by intentional injuries, such as homicide and suicide.[9] Considering only adolescents 15 to 19 years of age, one fourth of the deaths are caused by firearms.[10]

Alcohol ingestion is a major cause of fatal vehicular crashes. Although significant progress has been made in the prevention of drinking and driving, 32% of all traffic fatalities in 2007 were still alcohol related.[11] More importantly, 60% of the time that a child passenger dies in a car crash, the driver was intoxicated.[11] In addition, other commonly abused drugs, such as marijuana and cocaine, have been implicated in 18% of MVC-related fatalities.[12] Thus, those who participate in injury research and prevention must take into account both the unique characteristics of the specific target population and other important epidemiologic factors such as alcohol and drug use.

Although its position as the leading killer of young people has not changed, the overall mortality rate of trauma has gradually decreased during the past two decades. Prevention efforts

10 Leading Causes of Death, United States
2006, All Races, Both Sexes

Rank	Age Groups										
	<1	1-4	5-9	10-14	15-24	25-34	35-44	45-54	55-64	65+	All Ages
1	Congental Anomalies 5,819	Unintentional Injury 1,610	Unintentional Injury 1,044	Unintentional Injury 1,214	Unintentional Injury 16,229	Unintentional Injury 14,954	Unintentional Injury 17,534	Malignant Neoplasms 50,334	Malignant Neoplasms 101,454	Heart Disease 510,542	Heart Disease 631,636
2	Short Gestation 4,841	Congenital Anomalies 515	Malignant Neoplasms 459	Malignant Neoplasms 448	Homicide 5,717	Suicide 4,985	Malignant Neoplasms 13,917	Heart Disease 38,095	Heart Disease 65,477	Malignant Neoplasms 387,515	Malignant Neoplasms 559,888
3	SIDS 2,323	Malignant Neoplasms 377	Congenital Anomlies 182	Homicide 241	Suicide 4,189	Homicide 4,725	Heart Disease 12,339	Unintentional Injury 19,675	Chronic Low. Respiratory Disease 12,375	Cerebro-vascular 117,010	Cerebro-vascular 137,119
4	Maternal Pregnancy Comp. 1,683	Homicide 366	Homicide 149	Suicide 216	Malignant Neoplasms 1,644	Malignant Neoplasms 3,656	Suicide 6,591	Liver Disease 7,712	Unintentional Injury 11,446	Chronic Low. Respiratory Disease 106,845	Chronic Low. Respiratory Disease 124,583
5	Unintentional Injury 1,147	Heart Disease 161	Heart Disease 90	Heart Disease 163	Heart Disease 1,076	Heart Disease 3,307	HIV 4,010	Suicide 7,426	Diabetes Mellitus 11,432	Alzheimer's Disease 71,660	Unintentional Injury 121,599
6	Placenta Cord Membranes 1,140	Influenza & Pneumonia 125	Chronic Low. Respiratory Disease 52	Congenital Anomlies 162	Congenital Anomlies 460	HIV 1,182	Homicide 3,020	Cerebro-vascular 6,341	Cerebro-vascular 10,518	Diabetes Mellitus 52,351	Diabetes Mellitus 72,449
7	Respiratory Distress 825	Septicemia 88	Cerebro-vascular 45	Chronic Low. Respiratory Disease 63	Cerebro-vascular 210	Diabetes Mellitus 673	Liver Disease 2,551	Diabetes Mellitus 5,692	Liver Disease 7,217	Influenza & Pneumonia 49,346	Alzheimer's Disease 72,432
8	Bacterial Sepsis 807	Perinatal Period 65	Influenza & Pneumonia 40	Cerebro-vascular 50	HIV 206	Cerebro-vascular 527	Cerebro-vascular 2,221	HIV 4,377	Suicide 4,583	Nephritis 37,377	Influenza & Pneumonia 56,326
9	Neonatal Hemorrhage 618	Benign Neoplasms 60	Septicemia 40	Septicemia 44	Influenza & Pneumonia 184	Congenital Anomlies 437	Diabetes Mellitus 2,094	Chronic Low. Respiratory Disease 3,924	Nephritis 4,368	Unintentional Injury 36,689	Nephritis 45,344
10	Circulatory System Disease 543	Cerebro-vascular 54	Benign Neoplasms 38	Benign Neoplasms 38	Complicated Pregnancy 179	Influenza & Pneumonia 335	Septicemia 870	Viral Hepatitis 2,911	Septicemia 4,032	Septicemia 26,201	Septicemia 34,234

FIGURE 17.1. Ten leading causes of death, United States, 2006, all races, both sexes. (Data from the National Center for Injury Prevention and Control Department within the Centers for Disease Control and Prevention. 10 Leading Causes of Death, United States, 2006, All Races, Both Sexes. http://webapp.cdc.gov/sasweb/ncipc/leadcaus10.html.)

have been especially notable in the field of transportation safety. Fatal crashes decreased by 3.6% from 2006 to 2007, and the fatality rate dropped to 1.36 fatalities per 100 million vehicle miles of travel in 2006, the lowest since records began in the 1920s.[13] Improved safety standards for vehicles, better roads, and a moderate decrease in alcohol-related crashes are the dominant contributing factors to this decline. However, some of the success in combating motor vehicle–related trauma has been offset by increases in death from intentional injury, principally that related to firearms. Deaths from firearms now outnumber those from traffic injuries in several states.[14]

MORTALITY PEAKS AFTER TRAUMA INJURY

2 Trauma deaths occur at three traditionally recognized times after injury (Fig. 17.2). Approximately half of all trauma-related deaths occur within seconds or minutes of injury and are related to lacerations of the aorta, heart, brainstem, brain, and spinal cord. Few of these patients are saved by health care systems, regardless of efficacy. In general, the only effective interventions for this primary peak in injury-induced mortality are aggressive prevention strategies, either devices, such as automobile restraints and bicycle helmets, that prevent or lessen injury, or laws, such as drinking and driving penalties and motorcycle helmet laws, that limit certain risk-enhancing behavior patterns.[15]

The second mortality peak occurs within hours of injury and accounts for approximately 30% of deaths, about half of which result from hemorrhage and half from central nervous system (CNS) injuries. Important reductions in mortality rates during this period ("the golden hour") have resulted from the development of trauma and emergency medical services (EMS) with rapid transport systems. Overall, preventable trauma mortality rates, as defined by expert panels, have been reduced from approximately 25% to 30% to 2% to 3% where well-organized trauma care systems exist.[16,17] Currently, an estimated 85% of U.S. residents have potential access to level 1/2 trauma centers within 60 minutes,[18] but for 28% this is by helicopter only. The nearly 50 million Americans who do not have access to organized trauma care within an hour live mostly in rural areas. Further development of trauma systems and evidence-based care protocols and expansion of these systems to rural areas will undoubtedly result in further reductions in mortality rates during this early postinjury period.

The third mortality peak includes deaths that occur from day 1 to 2 after trauma resuscitation and acute care to weeks

FIGURE 17.2. Three periods of peak mortality after injury.

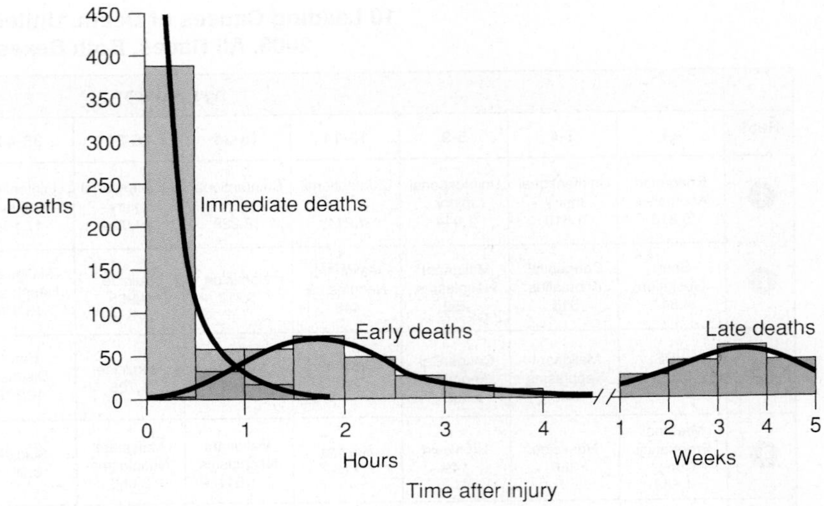

later. This late mortality generally is attributed to infection and multiple organ failure (MOF).[19] Of all trauma deaths, 10% to 20% occur during this period. The development of efficient evidence-based trauma care, however, is changing the epidemiology of these deaths. During the first week after trauma, refractory intracranial hypertension complicating severe traumatic brain injury (TBI) now accounts for a significant number of these deaths. The incidence of sepsis and MOF-related deaths following trauma has continued to diminish as a result of aggressive early resuscitation with improved goal-directed endpoints along with advanced organ support and ongoing critical care. Sepsis and MOF now account for approximately 5% of overall mortality and only 30% of later mortality where organized trauma systems and sophisticated intensive care unit (ICU) care exist. In addition to severe TBI, fatal pulmonary embolism also now accounts for a significant number of these late deaths.[20] Lastly, the aging of America has created an ever-increasing population of fragile elders with significant comorbidities, decreased organ reserve, and minimal ability to recover from the primary trauma insult. As a result, increasing challenges are the ethics of end-of-life and palliative care decision making. In the severely injured very elderly patient, just because "it can be done" does not necessarily justify that "it should be done." From both unnecessary patient suffering and consumption of limited critical resources viewpoints, thoughtful, ethical, and appropriate intervention or lack of intervention must be applied.

Optimal efforts to reduce the morbidity and mortality of trauma must include specific programs for each of the three separate mortality peaks. Early deaths can best be reduced with injury prevention programs and educational outreach or legislated use of protective devices and control of dangerous behavior. Focus on the regional planning and fiscal support of trauma system development will affect the number of avoidable deaths during the second "golden hour" mortality peak. Finally, late deaths will be diminished as research generates better understanding of the extensive physiologic processes and cell biology related to inflammation, immune dysfunction, sepsis, coagulopathy, multiple organ failure, and CNS injury and development of proven evidence-based care.[21,22]

TRAUMA CARE AND TRAUMA SYSTEMS

Trauma care providers have an important role in combating the injury epidemic in the United States. Few areas exist in which public health interests so closely overlap those of direct delivery of care. The most significant advances in the care of the injured patient that have occurred in the past 50 years are in surgery, anesthesia, imaging technology, and a better understanding of the basic cellular and genomic responses to shock and inflammation. But, in addition and unique to trauma care has been the coordinated societal effort at developing a trauma *system* of care, one that spans the continuum from injury occurrence, notification, and transportation to emergency and surgical interventions, critical care, rehabilitation, and eventual community reincorporation. These advances are highlighted both in the treatment of individual patients and in the establishment of effective systems of prehospital, hospital, and rehabilitative care. Trauma systems have become the paradigm for regionalized health care in the 21st century.[22]

Over time, these trauma systems have become more inclusive, attempting to recruit all appropriate institutions and covering all levels of resources, to optimize access to care for all injured patients. The ideal system, however, must still be "selective" to avoid expensive duplication of resources resulting from excessive designation of frequently competing institutions that then exceeds the needs of the injured patient population. An approach of matching resources to patient population needs produces efficient utilization of expensive resources along with generation of high patient volumes and clinical experience, leading to improved patient outcomes while still being able to respond to the needs of each injured member of society. Such a functional system requires a lead authority, usually located in the state department of health, which is empowered to not only designate the appropriate number of institutions that meet the various levels of standards but also hold those institutions to appropriate standards. A triage plan is required that optimizes delivery of "the right patient to the right institution at the right time," as dictated by the patient's injuries. Further transfer guidelines allows near-seamless movement or transfer from hospital to hospital as dictated by patient need and availability of appropriate resources. Ongoing quality assurance (QA) or improvement (QI) derived from evidence-based medicine (EBM) assesses appropriate implementation of what is acknowledged as the correct approach in providing care to increase survival and decrease morbidity and long-term disability. While access to the system should be universal and is universally advocated, this has been a great, unresolved challenge, particularly in the vast rural areas of America and for an increasing number of underinsured and uninsured Americans everywhere. The development of this regionalization paradigm has been politically charged due to perceived loss of patients and potential revenue through triage and bypass of institutions to optimize patient care. And, most recently, the shortage of general surgeons and appropriate surgical specialists has created an enormous threat to maintenance of the system and patient access to care. Only with persistence and increasing societal, legislative, and financial support can these hurdles be overcome. Both active resistance and cultural inertia have led to significant delays in the full deployment of the trauma system. However, the quality of care, improvement in outcome, and recognized decrease in morbidity and disability strongly support and stimulate the need for ongoing system development so more and more states and regions have fully integrated trauma systems, accessible to every injured patient.[23]

MILITARY HERITAGE AND DEVELOPMENT OF TRAUMA SYSTEMS

3 Our approach to modern trauma has grown primarily out of the care of wounds and casualty management resulting from war and recent increases in global terrorist attacks. Advances in rapid transport, volume resuscitation, wound management (both débridement and infection control), blood banking and appropriate utilization, enteric injury management, damage control concepts, vascular surgery, and surgical critical care and the need for early nutritional management have all come from or been significantly enhanced by military experiences. Salient historical events are shown in Table 17.1. Although by no means complete, this table provides examples of the many and significant contributions derived from extensive military experiences treating casualties with multiple injuries.

Care of the trauma patient poses several challenges not encountered in other aspects of surgical care. First, injury frequently occurs at a site remote from medical care. This problem couples with the importance of a time-critical injury requiring means for identifying and transporting critically injured patients quickly. Additionally, the polytrauma patient often requires complex surgical care that crosses specialty lines, requiring that an interdisciplinary team be available with little advanced planning or notification. The primacy of time renders an *ad hoc approach* to the delivery of trauma care unacceptable and is the principal impetus for the development of organized systems of trauma care.

It was the American experience in the Korean War that laid the earliest foundation for the current system of trauma care in the United States. The terrain made it difficult to evacuate the wounded along the traditional chain from the front lines to definitive care, as occurred during World War I and World War II.[24] Simultaneously, helicopters had evolved and were used to rapidly move the wounded from combat zones to mobile army surgical hospitals (MASHs). Additional experience with rapid evacuation to definitive surgical care was obtained during the Vietnam War, such that mean transport times dropped from 4 hours to 1.25 hours to 27 minutes in World War II, the Korean War, and the Vietnam War, respectively. Over these three conflicts, there was a concomitant reduction in mortality rates from 4.5% in World War II to 1.9% in the Vietnam War. It is likely that several factors contributed to the reduction in mortality over this interval; first among them was the military control of airspace that permitted the rapidity with which the injured soldier reached definitive medical care.[24] Most recently, the addition of flying critical care air transport for large numbers of critically ill casualties in B17 transports during Iraqi Enduring Freedom (IEF) has allowed transport to definitive optimal care facilities out of the war zone.

In Vietnam, the importance of rapid transport and a prepared receiving facility was well recognized. The distribution of trained personnel, equipment, and medical care was designed such that no soldier in Vietnam was more than 35 minutes away from a medical facility capable of giving definitive, resuscitative lifesaving treatment.[24] This model of prehospital care became the framework and expectation for prehospital civilian care in the United States over the next several decades.

In 1966, coincident with the observations made in Vietnam, the National Academy of Science/National Research Council report on trauma explicitly stated that the quality of civilian trauma care in the United States was below the standard achieved in Vietnam, such that "Expert consultants returning from both Korea and Vietnam have publicly asserted that if seriously wounded, the chances of survival would be better in the zone of combat than on the average city street."[25] In response to this report and in an attempt to improve trauma care delivery, the American College of Surgeons and its Committee on Trauma developed criteria for the designation of trauma centers and the establishment of regional trauma systems in 1976.[26]

Civilian progress in trauma care, in general, has followed the evolution of military medical systems. In 1922, the importance of orthopedic trauma was first recognized in the United States with the establishment of the Committee on the Treatment of Fractures. This evolved into the Committee on Trauma of the American College of Surgeons in 1949. Increased awareness of traffic injuries and fatalities during the 1950s and 1960s began to raise surgical awareness and public concern leading to the opening of a dedicated trauma entity in 1961 at the University of Maryland, and the concept of the "golden hour" was established. In 1966, the National Academy of Sciences and the National Research Council's important white paper, entitled *Accidental Death and Disability: The Neglected Disease of Modern Society*, increased public awareness and led to a federal agenda for the general improvement in trauma care.[25] Coupled with leadership from key academic centers and often by surgeons with recent military experience, the spread of advanced military concepts in trauma systems began. The Maryland Institute of Emergency Medicine became the first organized, statewide, regionalized system in 1973, while Harborview Medical Center in Seattle created the first fire department–based prehospital medical care delivery system for both acute cardiac and trauma events in 1969.[22] Prehospital provider programs grew from these early attempts and were formalized, as emergency medical technicians (EMTs) and other paramedical personnel were identified, and training programs were established. In 1973, the Emergency Medical Service (EMS) Act became federal law, providing specific endorsement and financial assistance for the development of comprehensive prehospital emergency medical service systems. In addition to federal efforts, state and local legislatures began to organize strategies to care for injured patients by using prehospital care systems to stabilize and deliver patients to major hospitals where appropriate care could be given.

Two other factors influenced the development of regionalized systems of trauma care in the late 1970s. First, major teaching hospitals in large cities had become regional trauma centers by default because of their experience and involvement in the trauma care of indigent patients. While the original country hospital system proved nonviable fiscally in the 1960s in most major cities, with strong academic leadership, these centers were taken over as major training centers and were able to develop as models for regionalization of trauma care. Second, and of at least equal importance, the American College of Surgeons Committee on Trauma developed a task force to publish *Optimal Hospital Resources for the Care of the Seriously Injured* in 1976, thus establishing a standard for evaluation of care. The most current version was published in 2006 and is the most comprehensive to date.[26] It establishes criteria for prehospital and trauma care and emphasizes the importance of ongoing QA and QI to confirm optimal outcomes. In addition, the American College of Surgeons Committee on Trauma

TABLE 17.2

TRAUMA CENTER DESIGNATION LEVELS IN THE UNITED STATES

■ TRAUMA CENTER LEVELS	■ DESCRIPTION	■ ESTIMATED NUMBER
1	Typically located in large urban environments, major cities. Provides full spectrum of trauma care 24 h/d with 24-h availability of in-house surgeon. Acts as a community leader in trauma research, education, and prevention. Expected to admit >1,200 trauma, >20% of whom are severely injured.	190
2	In population-dense areas, supplements the resources of the level 1 center, whereas in more rural environments, may play the lead role in the community. Provides full spectrum of trauma care, 24 h/d. Surgeons must be rapidly available on short notice. Should coordinate outreach programs to incorporate smaller centers within the region.	263
3	Must have the capability to manage the initial care of most injured patients. General surgeon must be promptly available for major resuscitation. Will have transfer agreements in place to rapidly transfer patients to higher levels of care. Will have educational programs for physicians, nurses, and allied health care workers.	251
4/5	Provides initial evaluation and assessment of injured patients in rural and urban environments. Requires 24-h coverage by a physician (level 4 only). No specific requirement for surgeon or availability of specialists. Most injured patients will require transfer to larger facilities. Will have transfer agreements in place to rapidly transfer patients to higher levels of care as appropriate.	450

Data from U.S. Department of Health and Human Services. *A 2002 National Assessment of State Trauma System Development*. Washington, DC: Emergency Medical Services Resources and Disaster Readiness for Mass Casualty Events; 2003. Table from Nathens AB, Brunet FP, Maier RV. Development of trauma systems and effect on outcomes after injury. *Lancet* 2004;363:1794–1801, with permission from Elsevier.

developed the Advanced Trauma Life Support course in 1980, which has contributed greatly to uniformity in the initial evidence-based care of the injured and the development of a common language for diverse care providers.[27]

TRAUMA SYSTEM COMPONENTS

Trauma centers are the core or "hub" of an organized system of trauma care. As originally conceived, the trauma center was an institution with all the resources necessary for immediate and definitive care of the critically injured patient. These centers, with their interested and committed staff, also served as the primary teaching sites for those interested in furthering their education in the care of the injured and performing the research to advance the evidence-based care of the injured. This description remains as the most consistent with a level 1 trauma center as an institution that takes a lead role for the provision of trauma care within a region. However, with an increasing understanding that it is neither desirable nor efficient that every injured patient must be transported to a center with all necessary resources available, a classification scheme for the designation of various levels of centers has evolved to allow a broad range of institutions to participate while still ensuring that standards are met to provide the appropriate level of care for the severity of injury (Table 17.2). This tiered approach improves the efficiency of trauma care by allowing higher-resource-level centers to focus on the more severely injured patient and reduces the likelihood that patients with minor injuries will be transported outside their community when they might best be cared for closer to home. Currently, more than 1,000 designated trauma centers exist in the United States, with just under half designated as level 1 or 2.[28]

The trauma center represents the core of the trauma system; however, the system is much broader in scope. Specifically, mechanisms must be in place to ensure that severely injured patients are triaged and ultimately transported to a center where they can receive definitive care. If a patient is injured at a site remote from a level 1 center, agreements must be in place to facilitate interfacility transfer from outlying centers. A QA program, both at the hospital level and at the system level, is critical to ensure optimal patient outcomes. Within a center, these QA programs allow for the evolution of evidence-based care protocols, whereas at the system level, they ensure adequate triage and the integrity of the triage and interfacility transfer process. These and other critical trauma system components were identified by West et al.[29] and then expanded by Bazzoli et al.[30] (Table 17.3)[30] Many have advocated that both injury prevention and postacute hospital care (e.g., rehabilitation) be included under the conceptual umbrella of the trauma system to better reflect the entire continuum needed for optimal trauma care.[31]

TABLE 17.3

ESSENTIAL TRAUMA SYSTEM COMPONENTS

- Presence of a lead agency with legal authority to designate trauma centers
- Use of a formal process for trauma center designation
- Use of American College of Surgeons (or similar) standards for trauma center verification
- Use of an out-of-area survey team for trauma center designation
- A mechanism to limit the number of designated trauma centers in a community based on community need
- Written triage criteria that form the basis for bypassing nondesignated centers
- Presence of ongoing monitoring systems for quality assurance (e.g., trauma registry)
- Statewide availability of trauma centers

From Nathens AB, Brunet FP, Maier RV. Development of trauma systems and effect on outcomes after injury. *Lancet* 2004;363: 1794–1801, with permission from Elsevier.

The process of trauma center designation begins with a health regulatory agency–directed on-site verification of resources and commitment by either state health authorities or surveyors from the American College of Surgeons Committee on Trauma (ACSCOT) Verification Review Committee. Hospitals undergo verification at fixed intervals, consistent with either ACSCOT or regional regulatory requirements.

4 A lead agency with the legal authority to designate trauma centers is critical to the development of an organized system of trauma care. In many regions, the state or regional department of health holds this authority. This authority usually extends beyond the designation of trauma centers to encompass the development of criteria for the triage of patients and oversight of prehospital EMS care provided. Legal authority is critical because with the instatement of triage criteria, the potentially nearer, nondesignated centers are bypassed by EMS personnel in deference to a regional trauma center. In addition, the number, location, and level of centers must be based on population demographics (i.e., number of patients) and geography, rather than mere institutional interest, not only to ensure that the needs of the patients are met but also, importantly, to prevent unnecessary competitive duplication of expensive resources and optimize volume and experience in the trauma center. This process is apt to bring with it the fears of monopolistic business practices and resistance from the nondesignated centers. The identification of trauma centers in a region is perceived as a loss of market competition among the hospitals within that region, which might result in the loss of income for the nondesignated centers. Ensuring the system is backed by legislation helps to mitigate, but does not eliminate, these issues.

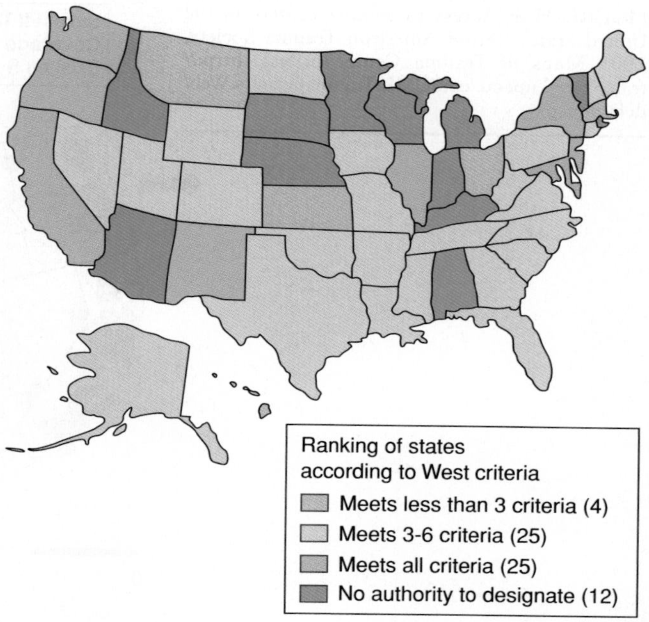

FIGURE 17.3. Regional trauma system in the United States as of 2002. States are ranked by the number of trauma system components implemented in their region. (From U.S. Department of Health and Human Services. *A 2002 National Assessment of State Trauma System Development, Emergency Medical Services Resources, and Disaster Readiness for Mass Casualty Events*. 2003. From ftp://ftp.hrsa.gov/hrsa/trauma/nationalassessment.pdf. Accessed November 2004.)

TRAUMA SYSTEM IMPLEMENTATION AND EFFECTIVENESS IN THE UNITED STATES

Progress in the implementation of organized systems of care in the United States has been difficult and is still limited in many areas. A major ongoing restraint is that the funding required to support the design, implementation, and maintenance of a well-integrated, coordinated regional system of trauma care is lacking. This is paradoxical in the face of the enhanced awareness and threat of terrorism, which virtually always involves mass casualties requiring the resources of the trauma care system. However, despite this chronic relatively limited funding, progress has been made; 38 states have implemented, or are in the process of implementing, organized systems of trauma care (Fig. 17.3).[32]

Several lines of evidence suggest that an organized system of trauma care reduces mortality from injury. West and Trunkey[33] evaluated the preventable death rate caused by trauma in San Francisco County, California, where a single institution was responsible for all major trauma care, with the death rate in Orange County, California, where more than 40 centers managed trauma patients. In San Francisco County, only 1% of deaths were considered preventable, whereas almost three quarters of all deaths in Orange Country were potentially salvageable. Subsequently, Orange County implemented a trauma system and demonstrated an eightfold reduction in the rate of preventable death as patients were triaged and cared for at designated trauma centers.[34] Population-based studies have also been used to evaluate the benefits of regional trauma centers. For example, Rutledge et al.[35] demonstrated that counties with designated trauma centers in North Carolina had a 20% reduction in per capita trauma deaths compared with counties without trauma centers, whereas Nathens et al.[36] demonstrated that states with an organized system of trauma care reduced MVC-related mortality by 10%. These results have been confirmed by MacKenzie et al. in the only prospective study analyzing injured patients cared for in level 1 trauma centers versus community hospitals where a 25% reduction in mortality was shown.[23] However, these benefits are not achieved instantaneously, taking as long as a decade following enacting legislation to become manifest.[37,38] It is likely that, after formal legislative implementation of the trauma system, a gradual change in care delivery and the process of quality improvement leads to better outcomes. Presumably, prehospital protocols improve such that the patients are more appropriately triaged to centers with adequate resources, whereas the trauma centers themselves evolve as they begin to commit an appropriate proportion of their resources to trauma and become more experienced due to increased volumes and thus capable of providing more optimal care.[39–41]

RURAL TRAUMA SYSTEMS

Rural trauma care has been considered one of the great challenges in trauma system development.[42] Approximately one third of the U.S. population resides in rural areas and account for those outside the "golden hour" for transport to a level 1 or 2 trauma facility, yet over half of all deaths caused by MVCs occur in the rural environment. To put this in greater perspective, the rate of death from MVCs is 600 times greater in rural Texas than in New York City.[43] Several factors play into this excess mortality. With a lower population density, discovery times, of necessity, are longer. Further, both EMS response times and transport times are longer; together, these factors increase the risk of prehospital death by as much as sevenfold.[44] In addition, prehospital personnel in rural environments are often volunteers with limited training. For example, in the rural state of Vermont, only 2% of all EMS providers are trained as paramedics capable of providing advanced life support (ALS).[42] Many EMS providers in rural areas attend to fewer than 10 severely injured patients annually, making it virtually impossible for providers to maintain

TRAUMA

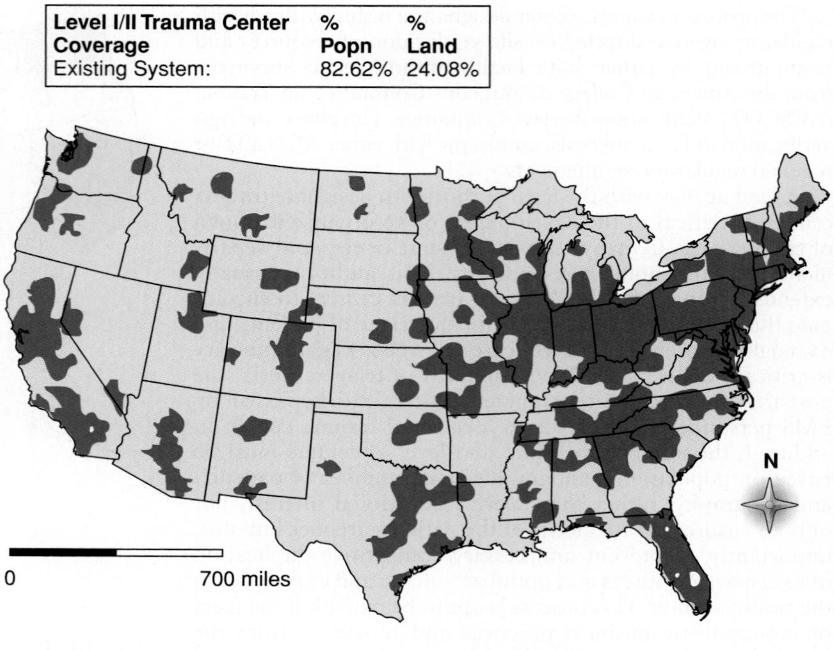

FIGURE 17.4. Access to trauma centers in the United States. (From American Trauma Society. 2009 Maps of Trauma Center Access. http://tramah.cml.upenn. edu/CML.TraumaCenters.Web/default.aspx.)

an adequate level of experience despite adequate training. Similarly, physicians working in rural environments have limited exposure to the major trauma patient. Together, these data support the premise that enhanced training (with subsequent maintenance of skills), combined with mandatory time in the field, provides the best opportunity for optimal outcomes.

Given these impediments to providing adequate and timely trauma care, some rural states have implemented *inclusive trauma systems* such that virtually all hospitals are required to participate as designated trauma centers to the extent that their resources allow.[45] This approach is in contrast to *exclusive systems,* where most injured patients are transported to relatively few centers, which may be at great distance. Each region must decide the appropriate balances of patient needs and resources available. At a minimum, the structure of an inclusive system must ensure that the initial receiving hospital will have a plan as well as appropriate human material resources in place to provide initial, emergent management of the severely injured patient. In addition, once patients are assessed by the receiving center, they must be transferred as indicated to higher-level trauma centers for definitive care.

To facilitate this process, many hospitals (designated as level 3, 4, or 5 trauma centers) have interfacility transfer protocols and agreements with level 1 or level 2 centers to expedite the transfer process. In the rural settings, these lower-level trauma centers play a critical role in initial stabilization and triage.[46] Although conceptually sound, the efficacy of this approach is unproved. For example, when rural centers were designated in Oregon, evidence showed clearly that the distribution of trauma patients within the system changed; however, no significant measurable improvements in overall outcome were evident in this limited population of the most severely injured patients.[47,48]

SUMMARY

There is clear evidence that trauma system implementation reduces injury-related mortality.[23,34–36] However, despite increasing trauma system implementation across the United States, approximately one third of major trauma victims are not cared for at regional trauma centers.[49] The reasons for this are multifactorial; however, it is likely that access is not uniformly consistent across states and within regions. For example, the availability of trauma centers varies greatly across states, ranging from 0.9 to 6.6 centers per million population, and 25% of the land mass of America is not within 1 hour of a level 1 or 2 trauma center (Fig. 17.4).[28,48] In addition, many of the states have not fulfilled many of the key components of trauma system design to ensure that populations within more sparsely populated regions have access to high-level trauma care (Fig. 17.3); thus, rural access to trauma care remains a major challenge in trauma system design.

SCORING SYSTEMS AND INJURY AND OUTCOME ASSESSMENTS

5 Many scoring systems have been developed in an effort to match injuries and trauma patients to allow comparison within and among institutions. Although all provide considerable help, none is perfect. The impetus for injury severity scoring systems is provided by the need to identify and classify severely injured patients in the prehospital phase, predict mortality, assess outcome results, and improve communication. Outcome analyses based on these parameters are a major objective of these types of scoring systems.[50] These systems also permit tracking of patient outcomes within an institution over time.

One simple way to classify trauma patients is to place them into three groups according to severity of injury: (a) those patients with injuries that are rapidly fatal, (b) those with injuries that are potentially fatal, and (c) those with injuries that are not fatal. The first group includes patients who have exsanguinating injuries, massive head injuries, high cervical spinal cord transection, or major airway disruption producing death in less than 10 minutes. Of traumatic injuries, 5% and half of all injury-related deaths fall within this category. The third group, which accounts for 80% of trauma patients, includes patients with injuries that are minor or confined to soft tissue and isolated extremity fractures. Significant risk to life is seldom seen in this group and urgent treatment is not essential. These patients survive without significant disability even if prolonged delays occur before definitive therapy. The real impact of improved prehospital care and organized trauma systems is on the second category of patients (15% to

TABLE 17.4

REVISED TRAUMA SCORE COMPONENTS

GLASGOW COMA SCALE	SYSTOLIC BLOOD PRESSURE (mm Hg)	RESPIRATORY RATE (Breaths/Min)	CODED VALUE
13–15	>89	10–29	4
9–12	76–89	>29	3
6–8	50–75	6–9	2
4–5	1–49	1–5	1
3	0	0	0

20% of the total): those who can be saved and morbidity minimized if effective medical care is provided quickly. It is for this group that trauma systems and scoring have been developed.[41]

Revised Trauma Score and Triage

The revised trauma score (RTS) developed by Champion and Sacco[50] in 1981 was for years the most widely applied scoring system for the initial evaluation of trauma victims. It mathematically combines the physiologic parameters of blood pressure, respiratory rate, and Glasgow Coma Scale Score to assess injury severity and predict which patients need the most timely and sophisticated medical care. Table 17.4 shows the components of the RTS.

While this mathematical model is uncommonly used today, the physiologic parameters included are still critical factors used to estimate injury severity and need for triage. In addition to physiologic scores, specific anatomic aspects of injury are also correlated with poor injury outcomes. Penetrating injuries to the head, neck, torso, and proximal extremities; multiple broken ribs and flail chest; two or more proximal long-bone fractures; pelvic fractures; limb paralysis; and amputation proximal to the wrist have all been identified as anatomic indicators of severe injury. Finally, the mechanism of injury is used to identify patients who are at high risk for significant injuries and are best evaluated at a trauma center. These data have been integrated with factors of age and comorbid disease into a triage decision scheme that is recommended by the American College of Surgeons and Centers for Disease Control and Prevention (Algorithm 17.1).

The major criticism of this triage scheme is that it leads to the frequent triage of patients to trauma centers that may not be necessary (i.e., overtriage). On the other hand, it diminishes the number of patients with severe injury who are overlooked and left potentially undertreated (undertriage). Overtriage is the inherent and necessary cost of a sufficiently sensitive scoring system. The exception to this approach is during disaster and mass casualty events when overtriage can consume limited resources and adversely impact overall patient outcomes and thus must be severely restricted.

Abbreviated Injury Scale

The Abbreviated Injury Scale (AIS)[51] was developed in 1971 for use in blunt trauma and has subsequently been updated on a periodic basis. The 1990 revision of the AIS includes descriptors for penetrating trauma. Injury severity is determined in six different body areas on a scale of 0 to 6, where 0 indicates no injury, 5 indicates critical injury, and 6 indicates a nonsurvivable injury. The AIS evaluates individual injuries but does not account for multiple injuries. Thus, it is an injury-specific anatomic index.[52] Table 17.5 shows an example of the AIS for abdominal injuries. The shortcoming of the AIS is that it evaluates each injury independently and recognizes only the most severe injury in each body area. Thus, AIS scores fail to account for multiple serious injuries within the same body compartment, thereby underscoring the true severity of the injury.

Injury Severity Score

In 1974, Baker et al.[52] developed the Injury Severity Score (ISS), which is calculated by assigning AIS values to the most severe injury in each of six body areas: head and neck (score = 1), face (= 2), chest (= 3), abdomen and pelvic contents (= 4), extremities and pelvis (= 5), and general and cutaneous (= 6). To derive the ISS, the scores for the three most severely injured areas are squared and added. ISS values vary from 0 to 75. If the value of the AIS is 6 (i.e., nonsurvivable injury) in any body area, the ISS is automatically 75.

The result is that substantial quadratic correlation between injury severity based on the ISS and death can be developed. The ISS is extremely helpful and has been widely used. However, it does not adjust for patient age or patient-related comorbid risk factors, such as chronic disease. Further, the severity of a head injury is disproportionately underscored in that combinations of injuries in other areas can result in a higher ISS score than a fatal head injury. Despite these drawbacks, the ISS is an excellent tool for the study of groups of patients with multiple injuries from blunt trauma and allows comparison of outcomes and quality assurance. To address the concern of ignoring the impact of multiple injuries in one body region, a modified new ISS, or NISS, has been developed that includes the three most severe injuries, regardless of body region. Intuitively, this approach has advantages in patients with penetrating trauma where injuries are often concentrated in a single body region. In either blunt or penetrating trauma, this modification improves predictability and appears to better reflect and weight significant injuries than the ISS alone.[53]

TABLE 17.5

ABBREVIATED INJURY SCALE SCORING SYSTEM FOR ABDOMINAL INJURIES

SCORE	INJURY EXAMPLES
1	Abdominal wall abrasion
2	Liver, stomach, colon, mesentery contusion
3	Minor liver or spleen laceration Bowel laceration without perforation
4	Major liver or spleen laceration Bowel laceration with perforation
5	Major liver or spleen laceration with tissue loss Bowel laceration with tissue loss

TRAUMA

FIELD TRIAGE DECISION SCHEME: THE NATIONAL TRAUMA TRIAGE PROTOCOL

1

Measure vital signs and level of consciousness

Glasgow Coma Scale	< 14 or
Systolic blood pressure	< 90 or
Respiratory rate	< 10 or > 29 (< 20 in infant < one year)

Yes: **Take to a trauma center.** Steps 1 and 2 attempt to identify the most seriously injured patients. These patients should be transported preferentially to the highest level of care within the trauma system.

No: Assess anatomy of injury

2

- All penetrating injuries to head, neck, torso, and extremities proximal to elbow and knee
- Flail chest
- Two or more proximal long-bone fractures
- Crushed, degloved, or mangled extremity
- Amputation proximal to wrist and ankle
- Pelvic fractures
- Open or depressed skull fracture
- Paralysis

Yes: **Take to a trauma center.** Steps 1 and 2 attempt to identify the most seriously injured patients. These patients should be transported preferentially to the highest level of care within the trauma system.

No: Assess mechanism of injury and evidence of high-energy impact

3

Falls

- Adults: > 20 ft. (one story is equal to 10 ft.)
- Children: > 10 ft. or 2-3 times the height of the child

High-Risk Auto Crash

- Intrusion: > 12 in. occupant site; > 18 in. any site
- Ejection (partial or complete) from automobile
- Death in same passenger compartment
- Vehicle telemetry data consistent with high risk of injury

Auto v. Pedestrian/Bicyclist Thrown, Run Over, or with Significant (> 20 MPH) Impact
Motorcycle Crash > 20 MPH

Yes: **Transport to closest appropriate trauma center,** which depending on the trauma system, need not be the highest level trauma center.

No: Assess special patient or system considerations

4

Age

- Older Adults: Risk of injury death increases after age 55
- Children: Should be triaged preferentially to pediatric-capable trauma centers

Anticoagulation and Bleeding Disorders
Burns

- Without other trauma mechanism: Triage to burn facility
- With trauma mechanism: Triage to trauma center

Time Sensitive Extremity Injury
End-Stage Renal Disease Requiring Dialysis
Pregnancy > 20 Weeks
EMS Provider Judgment

Yes: Contact medical control and consider transport to a trauma center or a specific resource hospital.

No: Transport according to protocol

ALGORITHM 17.1

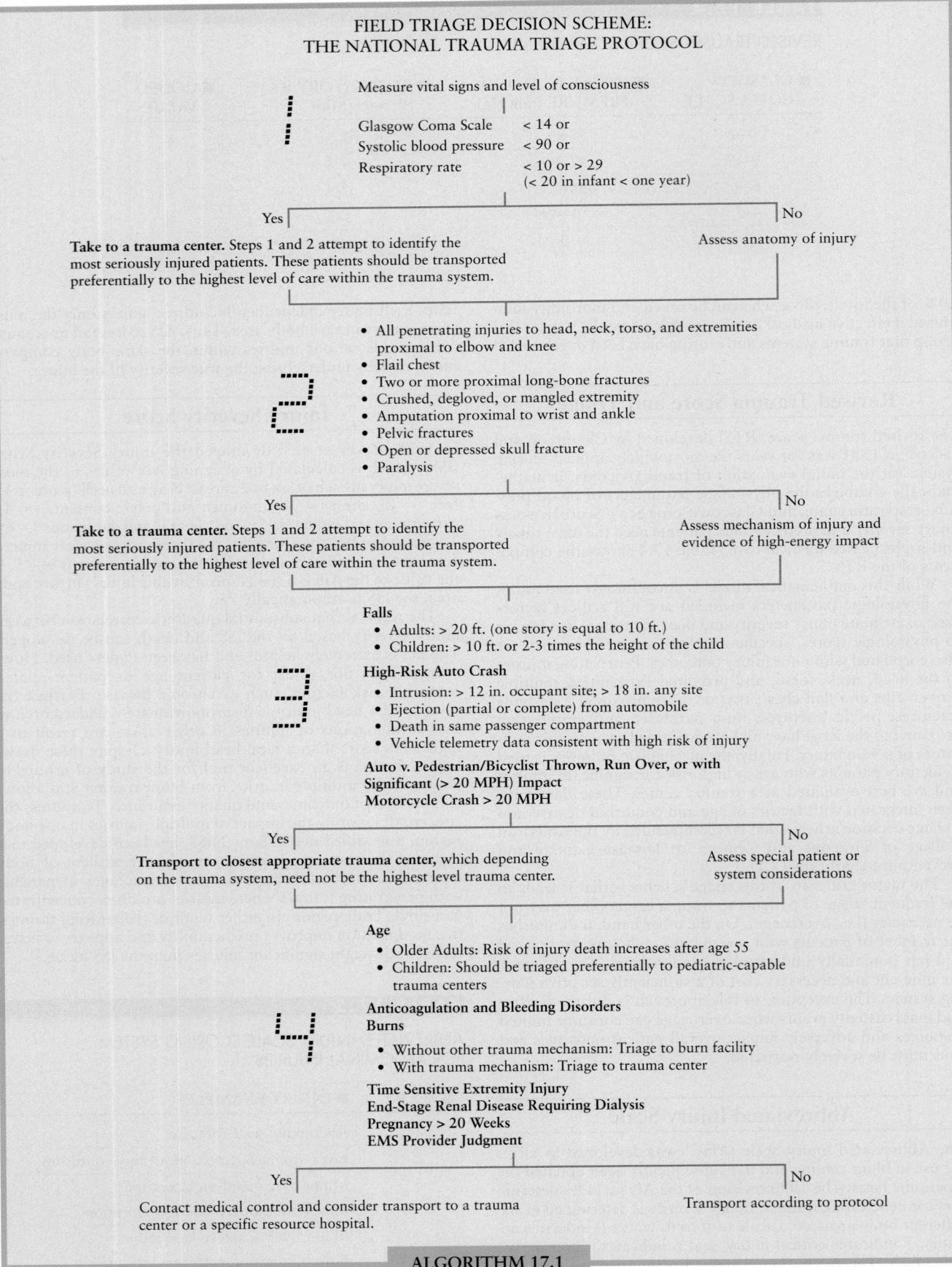

ALGORITHM 17.1.

Trauma and Injury Severity Score

The Trauma and Injury Severity Score (TRISS) methodology[54] is of importance because it attempts to combine the trauma score, or physiologic component of injury, and the ISS, or anatomic component of injury. It also incorporates the patient's age.

The TRISS method yields a specific probability of survival. Adjustments are made for age and mechanism of injury sustained (blunt or penetrating). The methodology allows patient groups to be compared. Individuals with an unexpected outcome, either survival or death, can be specifically identified and investigated. TRISS can be used for QI evaluations both within and between institutions. Typically, a cutoff point (e.g., predictability of survival, Ps = 50%) is chosen, and records of the deaths of patients with a probability of survival greater than the cutoff value are submitted for peer review. TRISS also can be used to examine cases in which the survivors exceeded the cutoff value to help, in part, identify specific system components that improve outcome. In addition, TRISS can be used to compare trauma outcomes between different institutions or regions.

BIOMECHANICS OF INJURY

6 All traumatic injury occurs as a result of deformation of tissues beyond a threshold that results in structural damage. In general, injury is categorized as either penetrating or nonpenetrating (blunt) trauma or thermal injury. Blunt trauma injury is produced as the tissues are either compressed (crushed) or as deceleration (shear) occurs. In penetrating trauma, the injury is produced by crushing and separation of tissues along the path of the penetrating object.

Energy Transfer

The severity of any injury is directly proportional to the amount of kinetic energy transferred to the tissues, whether by a projectile or by blunt impact. Kinetic energy (KE) is a function of the mass (M) of an object and its velocity (V):

$$KE = (M \times V)/2$$

Changes in velocity alter the kinetic energy transfer more significantly than changes in mass. This fact becomes critical when assessing the extent of damage from high-velocity and low-velocity gunshot wounds. Likewise, a small child and a large adult, though significantly different in size and weight, are subjected to similar levels of energy transfer in a high-speed vehicular collision, the primary determinant being velocity rather than mass.

Cavitation

Cavitation occurs as tissue impacted by a moving body recoils from the point of impact, away from the object. The resulting transient tissue cavity can be caused by rapid acceleration or deceleration. Extreme strain occurs at points of anatomic fixation during the formation of these temporary cavities. Forces can be produced both along the longitudinal axis (tensile or compression strain) and across the transverse axis (shear strain). These types of forces cause deformity, tearing, and soft tissue failure or fracture. With penetrating trauma, transfer of kinetic energy from the projectile causes transient cavitation. A permanent cavity is produced by tissue displacement and destruction. Cavitation is the cause of tissue damage and loss beyond the immediate course of the projectile.

Biomechanics of Blunt Trauma

Blunt trauma results in two types of forces during impact. First, changes in speed (acceleration or deceleration) create shear strain, and second, deformity changes (stretch or compression) create tensile strain. For example, shear stress to the head secondary to deceleration leads to brainstem stretching, and injury to the spinal cord occurs from shear stress at points of attachment. Contrecoup brain injuries include stretch forces placed on bridging veins, which may lead to hemorrhage and a subdural hematoma.

Differential acceleration in the thorax makes the aorta the most common site of life-threatening shear injuries, the most frequent point of injury being the ligamentum arteriosum. Here, the descending aorta is tightly fixed to the thoracic spine, whereas more proximally it is relatively mobile. Shear stress in this area allows the proximal aorta to move forward in relation to the fixed distal aorta and, therefore, to tear. Abdominal injuries can result as a consequence of acceleration of the viscera at a rate out of proportion to movement of the points of attachment, in particular, vascular attachments. The kidneys, small intestine, large intestine, liver, and spleen are all vulnerable to this type of shear injury and vascular disruption. Similarly, with deceleration, the liver may continue to travel relative to the ligamentum teres, generating shear forces that transect or lacerate the hepatic parenchyma. An inappropriately applied, high-riding lap seatbelt, particularly in a small child, can also produce a shear plane across the edge of the belt, causing severe intestinal injury during crash-induced deceleration. Rapid deceleration can also place sudden flexion and extension forces on the spine with a seatbelt placed inappropriately high across the lower thoracic and upper lumbar spines, causing fractures, subluxation, or ligamentous injury (Chance fracture dislocation).

Tensile strain creates injury by directly compressing (crushing) or stretching the tissue. For the head, tensile strain results in fractures of the skull, which in turn may cause intracranial bleeding or contusions of the underlying brain parenchyma. In the thorax, external chest compression can lead to cardiac contusion, pulmonary contusion, pneumothorax, and fractured ribs or a flail chest. In the abdomen, the pancreas, liver, spleen, and occasionally kidneys are subject to tensile strain injuries, particularly following a frontal (or, for the kidney, flank) impact. In addition, direct compression of the abdomen may increase intra-abdominal pressure, rupturing the diaphragm. Similarly, external compression of the pelvis is associated with bladder rupture and other pelvic injuries.

MOTOR VEHICLE COLLISIONS

Specific patterns of injury are recognized for various types of motor vehicle collisions. These include (a) head-on or frontal impact, (b) rear impact, (c) lateral or side impact, (d) rotational impact, and (e) rollover. Some estimates of injury pattern are possible by analysis of damage to the vehicle, but the presumption should usually be that any or all of these forces may have been involved. In general, a vehicle's occupant receives a kinetic energy transfer similar to that of the vehicle itself. As an automobile collides with an object, passengers collide with the interior of the automobile, and the internal organs collide with the body wall or are sheared from anatomic attachments.

It has been shown that better automotive design has greatly improved the outcome for occupants when the safety features of the vehicle are in use at the time of the crash. Active safety restraint systems include shoulder and lap seatbelts, air bags (frontal and lateral), and door locks; passive restraint systems include front and rear energy-absorbing collapsible chassis, lateral bars, and improved lateral wall design.

FIGURE 17.5. Down-and-under (A) and up-and-over (B) mechanisms of injury after frontal deceleration impact.

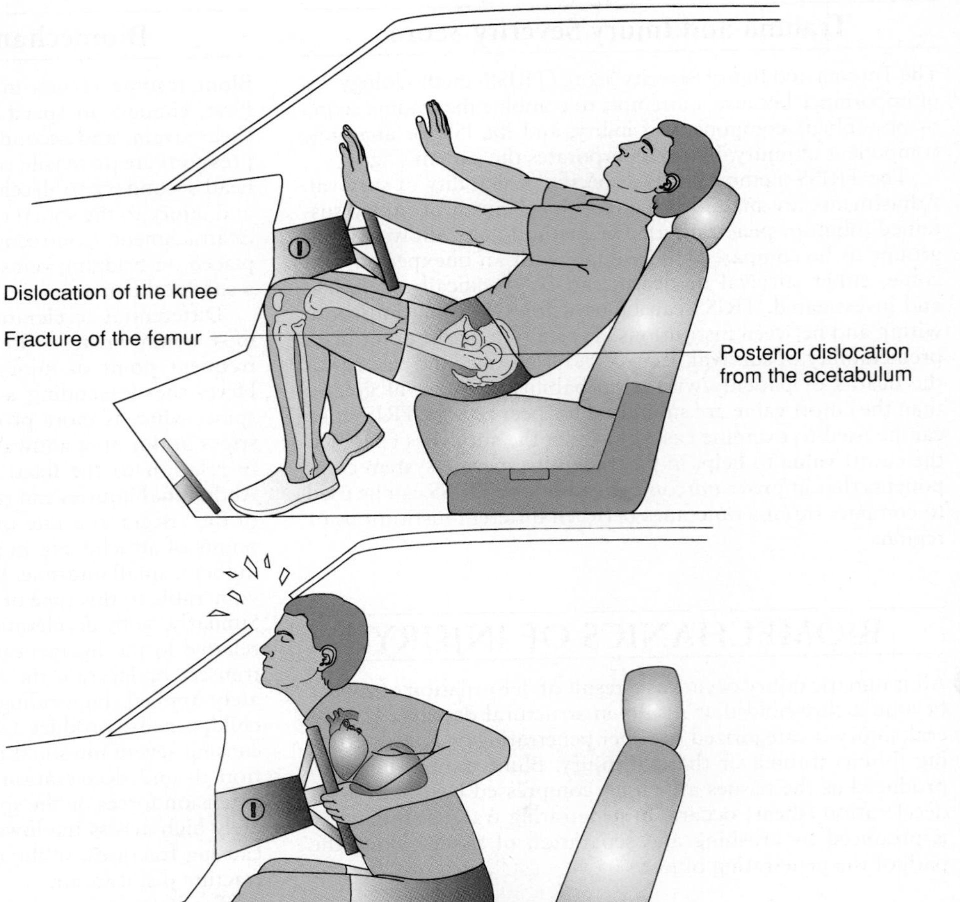

Frontal and Rear Impact

With a frontal impact, the vehicle stops abruptly, and unrestrained front-seat occupants move in one of two predictable pathways: down and under the dashboard or up and over the dash or steering wheel (Fig. 17.5). With the former movement, the knees strike the dashboard and the upper legs absorb the primary energy transfer. Dislocated knees, fractured femurs, and posterior fracture dislocations of the hips are expected. With an up-and-over impact, the upper body flexes forward, moving up and over the steering wheel. The chest or abdomen impacts the steering wheel and the head impacts the windshield. The head stops the forward momentum of the torso and the cervical spine absorbs the kinetic energy. Predictable injury patterns resulting from the up-and-over component of a frontal impact are given in Table 17.6.

Rear-impact collisions occur when stationary objects or slow-moving vehicles are struck from behind. The amount of kinetic energy generated depends on the difference between the velocities of the two vehicles, rather than the sum, in forward collisions. After a rear impact, the vehicle and its occupants accelerate forward, during which time cervical spine hyperextension with possible injury may occur. If the vehicle slows to a stop spontaneously, often the occupants are not severely

TABLE 17.6

PREDICTABLE INJURY PATTERNS RESULTING FROM THE UP-AND-OVER COMPONENT OF FRONTAL IMPACT

- Rib fractures, pulmonary contusion, flail chest, and myocardial contusion from anterior chest-wall compression against the steering wheel
- Hollow abdominal viscera and solid organ compression, resulting in intestinal perforation and lacerations of the mesentery and solid organs, with accompanying hemorrhage
- After the anterior chest stops intrathoracic organs continue to move, resulting in shear injuries such as lacerations of the aorta or liver
- Shear injuries to the kidneys and other solid viscera
- Injury to the brain from direct compression with scalp lacerations, skull fractures, and cerebral contusions, or from deceleration and shear stress, which cause diffuse axonal injury and cerebral contusion or subdural hematoma
- Acute neck flexion, hyperextension, or both, causing a cervical spine injury

injured. If the car strikes another object, the occupants are thrown forward, with injury potential similar to that seen with a frontal impact. Thus, rear-impact collision can potentially cause two types of injury: those from the primary rear impact and those resulting from the secondary frontal impact.

Lateral and Rotational Impact and Rollover

Two patterns of injury result from lateral impact, depending on whether energy is transferred to the vehicle directly or imparts motion to the vehicle. If the target vehicle remains in place or there is significant passenger compartment intrusion, typical injuries include lateral crushing compression injuries to the torso, pelvis, and spine. Energy delivered to the chest with lateral compression can cause a flail chest, pulmonary contusion, and ruptured liver or spleen. Depending on the location of the occupant's arm, humeral and clavicular fractures may occur. The pelvis and femur are often impacted by the door, forcing the femoral head medially and causing an acetabular impaction fracture. Head injuries range from simple lacerations to cerebral contusions with intracranial hemorrhage.

When the vehicle does not move away from the point of lateral impact, an occupant who is restrained remains fixed in place and is more vulnerable to the intruding vehicle. More commonly, the force of the impact moves the vehicle, and passenger restraints markedly reduce injury. In this case, the occupant begins motion with the car and is pulled away from the impact point by the restraint. As the torso is pushed/pulled medially into the car, the head stays in its original position, producing lateral flexion and rotation to the cervical spine, which may lead to fractures and ligamentous injury. Passengers sustaining lateral impact also should be considered for injuries resulting from secondary collisions with other passengers and objects within the vehicle.

Rotational impact injuries occur when a car strikes a moving vehicle laterally. The moving vehicle rotates around the point of impact, resulting in a combination of the injuries seen in head-on and lateral impacts.

During rollover crashes, the automobile may impact many times from many different angles, and as a result, the occupant may have virtually any type of injury. All potential injury mechanisms should be considered. Rollover crashes with passenger ejection are associated with a profound increase in fatality rates (up to 10-fold), in part because the repeated second impacts can cause injuries that compound or exceed those resulting from the initial impact. Rollover crashes with passenger ejection are considered to have the greatest injury potential.

Restraint Device Injury

Theoretically, three-point passenger restraints, when used properly, allow the kinetic energy transferred by the impact to be absorbed by the bony pelvis and chest. If improperly positioned, however, lap belts may rise above the pelvis, delivering the compression force to the soft tissues of the abdominal cavity or retroperitoneum, and shoulder harnesses can enhance flexion and rotational stress on the cervical spine. The number of injuries related to restraint devices is increasing, reflecting the broader general use of these systems and increasing rate of high-speed collisions. While there is no question of the overall efficacy of these devices, the clinician must recognize possible specific restraint-related injuries.

Injuries caused by lap belts incorrectly strapped above the anterior iliac crest occur most frequently in small children. These include shear injury to intestines most commonly, compression injuries of the intra-abdominal organs (liver, pancreas, spleen, small bowel, large bowel), increased intra-abdominal pressure with diaphragmatic rupture, and anterior flexion compression and posterior distraction injury of the lumbar spine. For these reasons and others, children shorter than 4 feet 9 inches tall, under 80 pounds, and younger than 8 years old should be placed in booster seats to allow appropriate positioning of seat belts. In addition, diagonal shoulder straps should be worn in combination with lap belts to prevent the forward motion of the trunk and excessive spine flexion. Diagonal shoulder straps should not be worn alone because this can be associated with chest and neck injuries if the pelvis is not also secured by the lap belt. Injuries associated with sliding underneath shoulder straps include carotid artery contusion, with or without thrombosis and disruption, and clavicle and rib fractures.

Air bags have enormous potential for injury prevention because they prevent the initial collision of passenger and automobile interior that occurs with frontal or lateral impacts. To be effective, air bags must be used in combination with seatbelts because they deflate immediately and therefore do not prevent secondary collisions. Lateral air bags are also increasingly incorporated in vehicles. Injuries such as lateral collisions of the head with the middle column and lateral compression of the chest wall and pelvis are in part prevented by these devices. Air bags are not effective in rear-impact collisions. However, given the predominance of frontal impact collisions, public health considerations by far favor that air bags should be strongly emphasized.

MOTORCYCLES

Motorcycle injuries involve four types of impacts: frontal, angular, ejection, and rear-end collision. In a frontal impact, the center of gravity is above and behind the front axle as the motorcycle tips forward and the rider travels over the handlebars. Injuries to the head, chest, or abdomen occur, depending on which part of the anatomy strikes the handlebars. If the rider's feet are placed on the pegs, the upper leg strikes the handlebars on forward motion, causing bilateral midshaft femur fractures. Angular or lateral impact from another vehicle or the ground when "laying the bike down" to avoid a collision generally results in crush injuries of the lower extremities. With ejection, the rider is thrown into the air until the head, chest, or extremities strike another object. Injury occurs at the point of impact, and, just as with the occupant ejected from the automobile, the potential for severe injury is high. This mechanism of injury is frequent and contributes importantly to the extraordinary injury potential for motorcycle riders.

In rear-end collisions, the motorcycle is usually at a stop when it is hit by a second vehicle from behind. The injury pattern is that of rapid acceleration with hyperextension and subsequent crush injuries on sudden stop.

PEDESTRIANS

Two general patterns are seen in motor vehicle versus pedestrian impacts, depending on whether the pedestrian is an adult or a child. In adults, the initial impact is often by the car bumper, producing fractures to the tibia and fibula. As the victim falls over the moving vehicle, the pelvis and upper femur are struck by the front of the vehicle's hood, and the abdomen and thorax continue onto the top of the hood. The secondary strike can result in fractures of the femur or pelvis and produce serious intra-abdominal or intrathoracic injury. Injury to the head depends on whether the patient's head strikes the car hood or is protected with the arms. A third impact occurs as the victim falls away, striking the ground. This impact commonly leads to head injury as well.

In children, the initial impact is predictably higher and may produce injury to the pelvis or upper femur. The second impact occurs when the front of the hood strikes the thorax. The final impact may not occur on top of the hood but rather as the

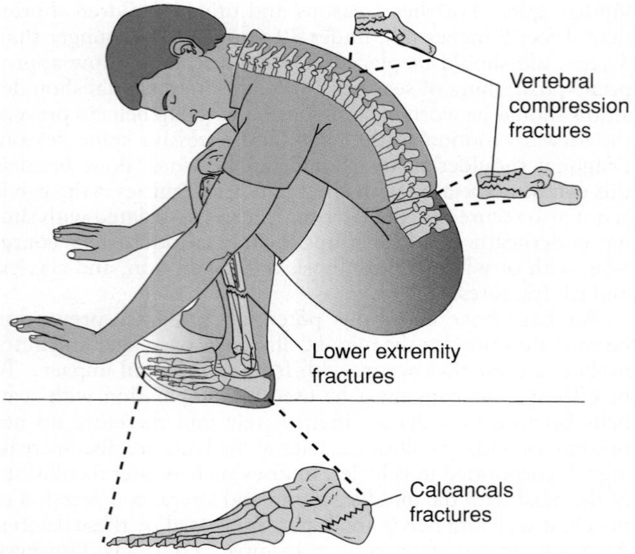

FIGURE 17.6. Hyperflexion and axial loading injury after a fall.

TABLE 17.7

PATTERNS OF INJURY TO THE HEAD, NECK, TRUNK, AND EXTREMITIES ASSOCIATED WITH ORTHOPEDIC INJURIES

■ DIAGNOSED INJURY	■ ASSOCIATED INJURY
Fracture—temporal, parietal bone	Epidural hematoma
Maxillofacial fracture	Cervical spine fracture
Sternal fracture	Cardiac contusion
First and second rib fracture	Descending thoracic aorta, intra-abdominal bleeding
Fractured scapula	Pulmonary contusion
Fractured ribs 8–12, right	Lacerated liver
Fractured ribs 8–12, left	Lacerated spleen
Fractured pelvis	Ruptured bladder, urethral transection
Fractured humerus	Radial nerve injury
Supracondylar humerus fracture	Brachial artery injury
Distal radius fracture	Median nerve compression
Supracondylar femur fracture	Popliteal artery thrombosis
Anterior dislocation shoulder	Axillary nerve injury
Posterior dislocation of hip	Sciatic nerve injury
Posterior dislocation of knee	Popliteal artery thrombosis

child is dragged underneath the vehicle. As the child falls backward, multiple impacts with the ground, underside of the vehicle, and wheels are possible, so virtually any type of injury may occur. Because of the potential for forceful impact and the direct blow to the middle torso, any child struck by a vehicle must be considered to have potentially severe crush injuries.

FALLS

Falls result in multiple impacts. Energy transfer is a result of the velocity that develops during the fall, so the height of the fall usually determines the magnitude of injury. Falls from more than three times the height of the victim, or from more than 20 feet, are considered severe. The surface on which the victim lands and its degree of compressibility (e.g., water vs. concrete) also have an effect on the energy transfer and the types of shear and tensile strain that occur. A typical injury pattern after falls in which the victim lands on his or her feet is transaxial and includes bilateral calcaneal fractures, lower extremity fractures, and multiple compression fractures of the thoracic and lumbar spine (Fig. 17.6). Of increasing importance are low-level falls (ground level falls [GLFs]) in the very elderly where the presence of significant comorbidities and medications (such as Coumadin) greatly enhance the risks of complications and mortality, even with relatively minor injuries.

GENERAL ANATOMIC CONSIDERATIONS IN BLUNT INJURY

The first and second ribs, sternum, scapula, and femur are considered to be some of the strongest and least vulnerable bones in the body. Therefore, fractures of these bones are indicators of severe trauma. Clear association exists between first and second rib fractures and injuries to the head, chest, and abdomen. Similarly, fractures to the sternum, though unusual, have a relatively high frequency of associated myocardial contusion. Fractures to the scapula indicate significant thoracic trauma. A femur fracture in a frontal impact injury should raise the concern of acetabular fractures or dislocation of the knee. An inventory of specific orthopedic injuries and their commonly associated findings is provided in Table 17.7. These associations should be routinely considered during the initial evaluation following major blunt trauma.

The anatomic orientation of certain structures also leads to predictable injury patterns. For example, the right ventricle is the most anterior portion of the heart and therefore is the most commonly contused area. The association of splenic injury with rib fractures on the lower left side and liver injuries with rib fractures on the lower right side is also frequently seen after blunt trauma.

BIOMECHANICS OF PENETRATING INJURIES

Penetrating trauma involves the transfer of energy to a relatively small tissue area. The velocity of a gunshot wound is exceedingly high compared with any type of blunt trauma. The kinetic energy [KE = (M × V)/2] of a bullet disrupts and fragments cells and tissues, moving them away from the path of the bullet. The actual size of the area of impact is determined by three factors: profile, tumble (spin and yaw), and fragmentation.

The profile, or frontal area, of a knife, screwdriver, or smooth bullet is that of a pointed missile. If the missile is crushed or deformed as a result of impact, the frontal area changes shape and disperses the impact over a wider tissue area, producing more rapid and greater energy exchange to the tissue and therefore greater injury. A knife or jacketed bullet does not

TABLE 17.8

MUZZLE VELOCITY, KINETIC WEIGHT OF PROJECTILE, AND APPROXIMATE MAXIMUM KINETIC ENERGY OF FREQUENTLY USED FIREARMS

DESCRIPTION (CALIBER)	PROJECTILE WEIGHT (g)	MUZZLE VELOCITY (ft/s)	KINETIC ENERGY (ft/lb)
Pistols			
.22 Short	29	1,000	72
.38 Special	158	870	263
9-mm Luger	125	1,150	440
.45	250	860	410
.357 Magnum	158	1,430	695
.44 Magnum	240	1,470	1,150
Rifles			
.22 Long	40	1,150	150
.56-mm M-16	55	3,200	1,248
.30-30 Winchester	170	2,200	1,830

deform significantly during impact, whereas a hollow-point bullet flattens, spreads, and fragments on impact.

Tumble results when the center of gravity of a bullet is eccentric, usually because it is located near the base rather than the apex of the bullet. Spin and axial movements (yaw) are bullet movements that occur after a gun is fired. At impact, spin and yaw continue to carry the base of the bullet forward, resulting in end-over-end motion or tumble. This increases the area and, thus, the amount of energy exchange and results in greater tissue damage. Multiple gunshot wounds are an example of the effect of fragmentation injury. The frontal impact damage can be estimated by classifying penetrating injuries into low-, medium-, and high-energy capacities.

Low-Energy Stab Wounds

Low-energy missiles include knives and other objects that produce damage by their sharp cutting edges. Cavitation is minimal and injury can be predicted simply by tracing the pathway of the weapon within the body. Knowledge of the type of weapon is sometimes helpful. Remember that the attacker may stab and move the knife or weapon inside the body, which can lead to more injury than that perceived from the cutaneous wound. Importantly, the ability to estimate the potential scope of injury by examination of the entrance wound is not reliable for stab or gunshot wounds.

Low- and Medium-Energy Gunshot Wounds

Low-energy gunshot wounds are defined as those with an initial muzzle velocity of less than 1,200 ft/s. Medium-velocity projectiles have muzzle velocities between 1,200 and 2,000 ft/s. Most handguns and some rifles are low- or medium-energy weapons. Table 17.8 provides a comparison of bullets and initial muzzle velocities for firearms frequently associated with penetrating civilian trauma. The primary point is that these weapons both damage the tissue directly in the path of the missile and produce cavitation injury to tissues in close proximity to the path. The size of the cavitation injury is directly proportional to the velocity of the bullet. However, the extent of tumble, fragmentation, and profile change in the projectile also influence the amount of injury.

High-Energy Weapons

The essential difference between high-energy weapon wounds and the typical civilian gunshot wounds is that their projectiles produce a much larger cavity or pressure cone than low- and medium-velocity missiles. The temporary cavity extends well beyond the actual bullet tract, producing a wider injury. The vacuum created by the cavitation pulls clothing, bacteria, and other debris from the surrounding areas into the wound, creating the additional risk of contamination. The proliferation of semiautomatic weapons also has resulted in an increased number of wounds a victim may experience. Instead of a single gunshot wound, the surgeon may be faced with multiple wounds in multiple body locations.

Shotgun Injuries

Blast injuries caused by close-range shotgun fire (10 to 15 ft.) constitute devastating injuries composed of extensive tissue destruction. Besides specific organ injury, blast injuries due to wadding from the shell and extensive foreign body contamination have the highest potential for secondary infection. These injuries, in general, should be surgically explored, devitalized tissue should be extensively débrided, and the wounds should be left open and packed with sterile dressing that should be changed; the wounds should be reviewed serially for additional débridement in the operating room.[57]

GENERAL ANATOMIC CONSIDERATIONS OF PENETRATING INJURIES

Evaluation of each entrance and exit wound helps to assess but does not confirm the number of projectiles, their courses, and which organs are at risk of injury. Close-range entrance wounds for bullets typically cause tattooing, burning, and abrasion as a result of the spin. Depending on the range, there may be direct burning of skin. Tattooing occurs if the muzzle is within 12 inches of the skin at the time of firing. The range from which a gun is fired is also significant in that the air resistance that slows bullet velocity and reduces kinetic energy is proportional to the distance traveled.

Once a missile penetrates tissue, the energy is distributed predictably within a closed space, and, depending on the organs impacted and the types of tissue traversed, certain injuries can be anticipated. For example, a bullet penetrating the skull may have insufficient residual energy to traverse and exit the opposite side of the skull. Instead, it may follow the curvature of the interior of the skull, generating a more severe brain injury than would result from a simple linear passage.

In the thorax, lung parenchyma has low mass and, therefore, sustains less damage from penetrating injury than any other thoracic tissue. Similarly, blood vessels that are not fixed may be pushed aside without significant damage. However, injury to adjacent blood vessels in proximity can result in intimal damage with subsequent thrombosis even if the vessel as a whole remains intact. Large fixed vessels such as the aorta and

FIGURE 17.7. Axial traverse (A) and transdiaphragmatic (B) wounding mechanisms with associated injury potential for combined thoracic and abdominal injuries.

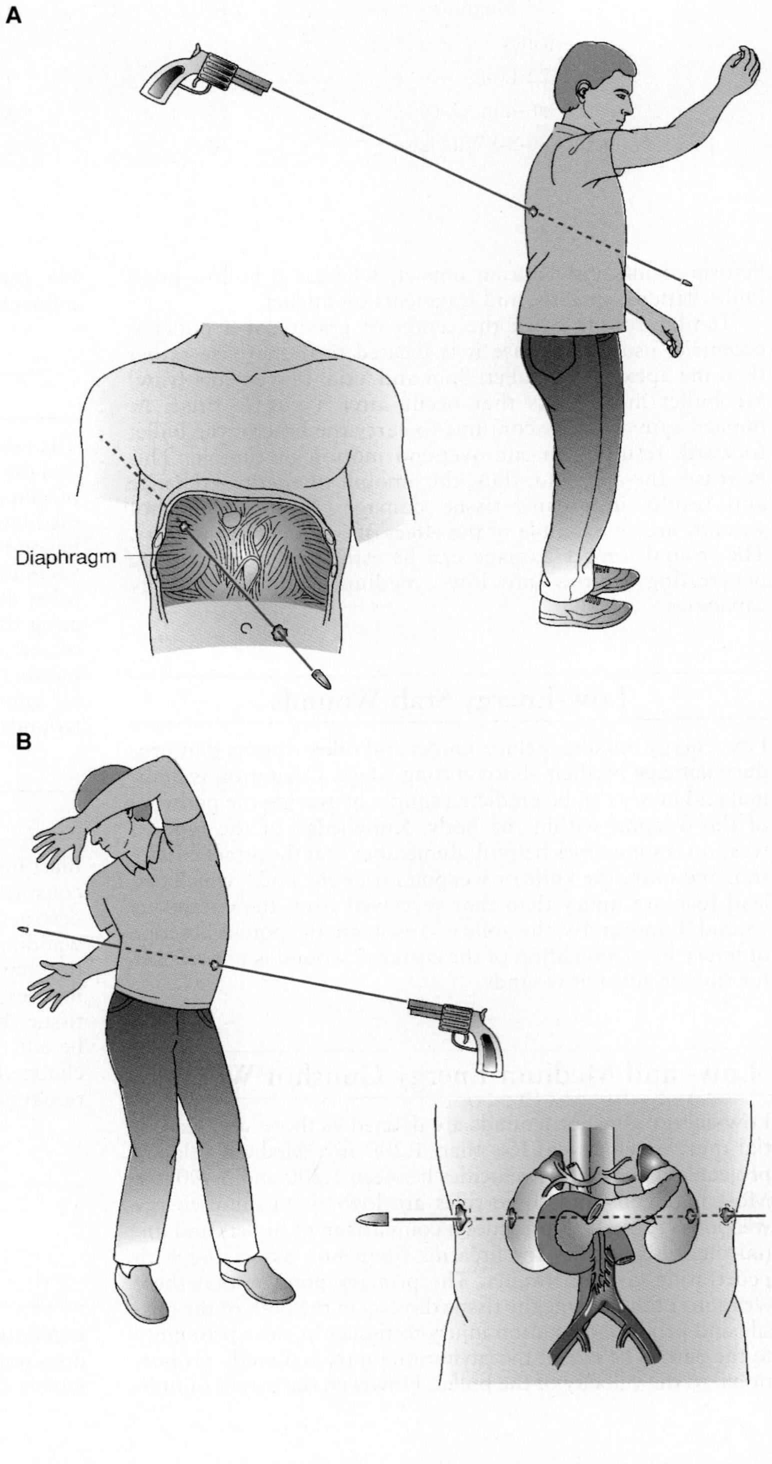

TABLE 17.9

INJURIES ASSOCIATED WITH SPECIFIC VASCULAR TRAUMA

- Superior mesenteric artery or superior mesenteric vein injury with pancreas and liver
- Renal artery injury with liver, kidney, and colon
- Inferior vena cava injury with liver, small bowel, colon, pancreas, and duodenum
- Axillary artery injury with brachial plexus trauma

vena cava are particularly susceptible to fatal injury. If bones are penetrated, bone fragments may become secondary missiles and can lacerate the surrounding tissues, including vascular structures. Muscles may expand out of the path of a missile, but this can result in vascular stretching and hemorrhage. Lower-velocity bullets may not follow a straight path but rather ricochet through the body cavity or track along fascial planes, injuring other organs.

Penetrating injuries should also be evaluated with regard to topography for potential anatomically associated proximity injuries. For example, penetrating wounds of the neck are commonly associated with injury to the jugular veins, trachea, pharynx, and carotid artery. Injuries to the trachea are commonly associated with injuries to the esophagus, and injuries to the carotid artery are commonly associated with internal jugular vein injury. In penetrating wounds to the thorax, possibilities of injury to the heart, lung, and diaphragm should be considered (Fig. 17.7A). The anterior location of the right ventricle makes it particularly vulnerable to penetrating trauma. All penetrating wounds below the nipple line or inframammary groove must be considered for potential intra-abdominal injury due to elevation of the diaphragm during expiration. Similarly, wounds that cross the midline, so-called transaxial wounds, are important to recognize (Fig. 17.7B). In the thorax, this indicates that every mediastinal structure is at risk, and in the abdomen, the possibility of major vascular injury, particularly to the aorta and vena cava, should be considered. Associated abdominal injuries often include hepatic and splenic injuries, as well as diaphragmatic, pulmonary, and gastric injuries. Duodenal and pancreatic injuries are commonly seen with injuries to the liver, inferior vena cava, stomach, and colon. Examples of injuries associated with specific vascular trauma are listed in Table 17.9. In all, gunshot wound penetration of the abdomen has associated injuries requiring surgical repair in 60% to 80% of patients.

THE ONGOING CHALLENGE OF TRAUMA

Spurred by two sentinel publications by the National Academy of Sciences and the National Research Council (NAS/NRC), injury has become recognized as a public health problem that has a greater impact on the United States than cancer or cardiovascular disease. In 1966, the NAS/NRC published a white paper entitled *Accidental Death and Disability: The Neglected Disease of Modern Society.*[25] Many have identified this publication as the inaugural event of what has become a sustained effort sponsored by the U.S. government to control unintentional injury and the injury epidemic. A 20-year follow-up study, entitled *Injury in America: A Continuing Public Health Problem,* appeared in 1985, outlining further efforts that would be needed to address the persistent problem of injury and the injury epidemic. The most recent contribution of the NRC Institute of Medicine (IOM) is the three-part series by the Committee on the Future of Emergency Care in the United States, including (a) *Hospital-Based Emergency Care: At the Breaking Point,* which describes the changing role of the hospital emergency department and the epidemic of overcrowding, uncompensated care, lack of availability of surgical specialists, liability exposure, lack of hospital disaster preparedness, and insufficient support for trauma research[58]; (b) *Emergency Medical Services at the Crossroads,* which describes the fragmented EMS system, inadequate communication systems, lack of coordinated regional patient flow, insufficient reimbursement, lack of national training standards, lack of integration into disaster preparedness, and absence of clinical evidence to support care protocols[59]; and (c) *Emergency Care for Children: Growing Pains,* which explains the 20 years of progress of EMS for Children (EMS-C) and the impacts of EMS magnified on EMS-C including training, readiness, medication issues, disaster preparedness, and research.[60] These excellent reviews identify the multiple ongoing stresses that have kept emergency and trauma care from achieving the goals necessary to optimally impact the epidemic of injury in America. Over the past four decades and especially since the development of the NCIPC at the Centers for Disease Control and Prevention, the health care community has been encouraged to assume, and has assumed, an enlarged role in injury control. Medical and surgical specialists, epidemiologists, statisticians, biomechanical engineers, public health practitioners, and economists are continuing to create the collaborations necessary to develop and implement the required sophisticated interdisciplinary approaches necessary for optimal injury control.

7

References

1. Bonnie R, Fulco CE, Liverman CT. Magnitude and costs. In: Bonnie R, Fulco CE, Liverman CT, eds. *Reducing the Burden of Injury, Advancing Prevention, and Treatment.* Washington, DC: National Academy Press; 1999:41–59.
2. National Center for Health Statistics National Vital Statistics System. *10 Leading Causes of Death, United States.* Atlanta: Office of Statistics and Programming, National Center for Injury Prevention and Control, Centers for Disease Control and Prevention; 2006.
3. Centers for Disease Control and Prevention. *Injury Topics and Fact Sheets.* Atlanta: Centers for Disease Control and Prevention; 2007.
4. LaPlante MP, Carlson D, National Institute on Disability and Rehabilitation Research. *Disability in the United States: Prevalence and Causes, 1992.* Washington, DC: U.S. Department of Education Office of Special Education and Rehabilitative Services, U.S. Government Printing Office; 1996.
5. National Center for Injury and Prevention Control. *Overall Injury and Adverse-event-related Deaths and Rate per 100,000.* Atlanta: National Center for Injury and Prevention Control, Centers for Disease Control and Prevention; 2005.
6. Baker SP. *The Injury Fact Book,* 2nd ed. New York: Oxford University Press; 1992.
7. Rice DP, Mackenzie EJ, Centers for Disease Control, Johns Hopkins University, School of Hygiene and Public Health, Injury Prevention Center. *Cost of Injury in the United States: A Report to Congress, 1989.* San Francisco, CA; Baltimore, MD: Institute for Health & Aging, University of California Injury Prevention Center, School of Hygiene and Public Health, Johns Hopkins University; 1989.
8. Centers for Disease Control and Prevention. *Injury Mortality: National Summary of Injury Mortality Data 1984–1990.* Atlanta, GA: Centers for Disease Control and Prevention; 1993.
9. Runyan CW, Gerken EA. Epidemiology and prevention of adolescent injury. A review and research agenda. *JAMA* 1989;262:2273–2279.
10. Fingerhut LA, National Center for Health Statistics. *Firearm Mortality Among Children, Youth, and Young Adults 1–34 Years of Age, Trends and Current Status: United States, 1985–90.* Hyattsville, MD: U.S. Department of Health and Human Services, Public Health Service, Centers for Disease Control and Prevention, National Center for Health Statistics; 1993.
11. National Highway Traffic Safety Administration (NHTSA). *Traffic Safety Facts 2007: Alcohol.* Washington, DC: NHTSA; 2008.
12. National Highway Traffic Safety Administration (NHTSA). *The Incidence and Role of Drugs in Fatally Injured Drivers.* Washington, DC: NHTSA; 1993.

13. National Highway Traffic Safety Administration (NHTSA). *Traffic Safety Facts 2007*. Washington, DC: NHTSA; 2008.
14. Rosengart M, Cummings P, Nathens A, et al. An evaluation of state firearm regulations and homicide and suicide death rates. *Inj Prev* 2005; 11:77–83.
15. Kraus JF, Peek C, McArthur DL, et al. The effect of the 1992 California motorcycle helmet use law on motorcycle crash fatalities and injuries. *JAMA* 1994;272:1506–1511.
16. Lowe DK, Gately HL, Goss JR, et al. Patterns of death, complication, and error in the management of motor vehicle accident victims: implications for a regional system of trauma care. *J Trauma* 1983;23:503–509.
17. Shackford SR, Hollingworth-Fridlund P, Cooper GF, et al. The effect of regionalization upon the quality of trauma care as assessed by concurrent audit before and after institution of a trauma system: a preliminary report. *J Trauma* 1986;26:812–820.
18. Branas CC, MacKenzie EJ, Williams JC, et al. Access to trauma centers in the United States. *JAMA* 2005;293:2626–2633.
19. Baker CC, Oppenheimer L, Stephens B, et al. Epidemiology of trauma deaths. *Am J Surg* 1980;140:144–150.
20. Shackford SR, Mackersie RC, Holbrook TL, et al. The epidemiology of traumatic death. A population-based analysis. *Arch Surg* 1993;128: 571–575.
21. National Research Council, Committee on Trauma Research, National Academies Press. *Injury in America: A Continuing Public Health Problem*. Washington, DC: National Academy Press; 1985.
22. Maier RV. Trauma: the paradigm for medical care in the 21st century. *J Trauma* 2003;54:803–813.
23. MacKenzie EJ, Rivara FP, Jurkovich GJ, et al. A national evaluation of the effect of trauma-center care on mortality. *N Engl J Med* 2006;354: 366–378.
24. Neel S. Army aeromedical evacuation procedures in Vietnam: implications for rural America. *JAMA* 1968;204:309–313.
25. National Committee of Trauma and Committee of Shock. *Accidental Death and Disability: The Neglected Disease of Modern Society*. Washington, DC: National Academy of Sciences/National Research Council; 1966.
26. American College of Surgeons Committee on Trauma. *Resources for Optimal Care of the Injured Patient 2006*. Chicago, IL: American College of Surgeons; 2006.
27. American College of Surgeons Committee on Trauma. *ATLS Student Course Manual,* 8th ed. Chicago, IL: American College of Surgeons; 2008.
28. MacKenzie EJ, Hoyt DB, Sacra JC, et al. National inventory of hospital trauma centers. *JAMA* 2003;289:1515–1522.
29. West JG, Williams MJ, Trunkey DD, et al. Trauma systems. Current status–future challenges. *JAMA* 1988;259:3597–3600.
30. Bazzoli GJ, Madura KJ, Cooper GF, et al. Progress in the development of trauma systems in the United States. Results of a national survey. *JAMA* 1995;273:395–401.
31. American Trauma Society. *Trauma Systems: Agenda for the Future*. U.S. Department of Transportation, National Highway Traffic Safety Administration; 2003.
32. U.S. Department of Health and Human Services. *A 2002 National Assessment of State Trauma System Development, Emergency Medical Services Resources and Disaster Readiness for Mass Casualty Events*. Washington, DC: US Department of Health and Human Services; 2003.
33. West JG, Trunkey DD, Lim RC. Systems of trauma care. A study of two counties. *Arch Surg* 1979;114:455–460.
34. West JG, Cales RH, Gazzaniga AB. Impact of regionalization. The Orange County experience. *Arch Surg* 1983;118:740–744.
35. Rutledge R, Fakhry SM, Meyer A, et al. An analysis of the association of trauma centers with per capita hospitalizations and death rates from injury. *Ann Surg* 1993;218:512–521; discussion 521–524.
36. Nathens AB, Jurkovich GJ, Rivara FP, et al. Effectiveness of state trauma systems in reducing injury-related mortality: a national evaluation. *J Trauma* 2000;48:25–30; discussion 30–31.
37. Mullins RJ, Mann NC, Hedges JR, et al. Preferential benefit of implementation of a statewide trauma system in one of two adjacent states. *J Trauma* 1998;44:609–616; discussion 617.
38. Nathens AB, Jurkovich GJ, Cummings P, et al. The effect of organized systems of trauma care on motor vehicle crash mortality. *JAMA* 2000;283: 1990–1994.
39. O'Keefe GE, Jurkovich GJ, Copass M, et al. Ten-year trend in survival and resource utilization at a level I trauma center. *Ann Surg* 1999;229: 409–415.
40. Peitzman AB, Courcoulas AP, Stinson C, et al. Trauma center maturation: quantification of process and outcome. *Ann Surg* 1999;230:87–94.
41. Gruen RL, Jurkovich GJ, McIntyre LK, et al. Patterns of errors contributing to trauma mortality: lessons learned from 2594 deaths. Ann Surg 2006; 244(3):371–380.
42. Rogers FB, Shackford SR, Osler TM, et al. Rural trauma: the challenge for the next decade. *J Trauma* 1999;47:802–821.
43. Baker SP, Whitfield RA, O'Neill B. Geographic variations in mortality from motor vehicle crashes. *N Engl J Med* 1987;316:1384–1387.
44. Grossman DC, Kim A, Macdonald SC, et al. Urban-rural differences in prehospital care of major trauma. *J Trauma* 1997;42:723–729.
45. Narad RA, Becker JL, Frecceri C. A decentralized trauma system design for a rural area. *Prehosp Disaster Med* 1996;11:134–139; discussion 139–140.
46. Grossman DC, Hart LG, Rivara FP, et al. From roadside to bedside: the regionalization of trauma care in a remote rural county. *J Trauma* 1995; 38:14–21.
47. Mann NC, Hedges JR, Mullins RJ, et al. Rural hospital transfer patterns before and after implementation of a statewide trauma system. OHSU Rural Trauma Research Group. *Acad Emerg Med* 1997;4: 764–771.
48. Clay Mann N, Mullins RJ, Hedges JR, et al. Mortality among seriously injured patients treated in remote rural trauma centers before and after implementation of a statewide trauma system. *Med Care* 2001;39: 643–653.
49. Nathens AB, Jurkovich GJ, MacKenzie EJ, et al. A resource-based assessment of trauma care in the United States. *J Trauma* 2004;56:173–178; discussion 178.
50. Champion HR, Sacco WJ, Carnazzo AJ, et al. Trauma score. *Crit Care Med* 1981;9:672–676.
51. American Association for Automotive Medicine. *The Abbreviated Injury Scale (AIS)*, rev. ed. Des Plaines, IL: American Association for Automotive Medicine; 1990.
52. Baker SP, O'Neill B, Haddon W Jr, et al. The injury severity score: a method for describing patients with multiple injuries and evaluating emergency care. *J Trauma* 1974;14:187–196.
53. Osler T, Baker SP, Long W. A modification of the injury severity score that both improves accuracy and simplifies scoring. *J Trauma* 1997;43: 922–925; discussion 925–926.
54. Boyd CR, Tolson MA, Copes WS. Evaluating trauma care: the TRISS method. Trauma Score and the Injury Severity Score. *J Trauma* 1987;27: 370–378.
55. Hoyt DB, Hollingsworth-Fridlund P, Winchell RJ, et al. Analysis of recurrent process errors leading to provider-related complications on an organized trauma service: directions for care improvement. *J Trauma* 1994;36: 377–384.
56. U.S. Department of Health and Human Services (DHHS). *Model Trauma Care System Plan*. Washington, DC: DHHS; 1992.
57. Hoekstra SM, Bender JS, Levison MA. The management of large soft-tissue defects following close-range shotgun injury. *J Trauma* 1990;30: 1489–1493.
58. Committee on the Future of Emergency Care in the United States Health System. *Hospital-Based Emergency Care at the Breaking Point*. Washington, DC: Institute of Medicine of the National Academies; 2007.
59. Committee on the Future of Emergency Care in the United States Health System. *Emergency Medical Services at the Crossroads*. Washington, DC: Institute of Medicine of the National Academies; 2007.
60. Committee on the Future of Emergency Care in the United States Health System. *Emergency Care for Children Growing Pains*. Washington, DC: Institute of Medicine of the National Academies; 2007.

CHAPTER 18 ■ PREHOSPITAL AND RESUSCITATION CARE

EILEEN M. BULGER

KEY POINTS

1. Emergency medical service systems provide a rapid, tiered response to the injured, beginning with an Emergency Medical Technician-Basic (first responder) and followed by an Emergency Medical Technician-Paramedic, as needed.
2. Duration at the scene should be individualized to the patient's injuries and physiologic status. "Scoop and run" versus "stay and play" approaches cannot be generalized.
3. Airway control is paramount and, if required, should be achieved using an orotracheal approach with neck immobilization and neuromuscular blockade, if needed.
4. A multidisciplinary team of specialists, led by the "captain of the ship," usually a trauma surgeon, is available in level 1 and 2 trauma centers to provide coordinated optimal care for any and all injuries.
5. Trauma assessment and care are provided in a logical, consistent manner. The primary survey identifies and simultaneously treats life-threatening injuries, including airway loss, inadequate ventilation, ongoing hemorrhage, and central nervous system damage. The secondary survey identifies all other injuries, including those with potential long-term disability.

Care of the injured patient begins in the prehospital setting with a tightly integrated multidisciplinary emergency medical service (EMS) system. The goal of the EMS system is to provide immediate access to lifesaving medical care. This care usually entails the use of a first-response team, such as the fire department or other public safety personnel with the capability of providing basic life support (BLS) within minutes of an injury. When available, a rapid transport team capable of providing advanced life support (ALS) moves the injured patient to a trauma center where a multidisciplinary team meets the patient to continue resuscitation, identify injuries, and provide expeditious therapy, with the aim of completing all of these processes within 1 hour (called the *golden hour*). The goal of the EMS system is to assess for life-threatening injuries, initiate emergency care, and transport the injured patient as expeditiously and safely as possible to the nearest appropriate trauma center.

PREHOSPITAL CARE

Personnel

1 The initial goal of any EMS system is to provide a rapid response by personnel trained in BLS skills to the scene of the injured patient. In most cases, this function is performed by an Emergency Medical Technician-Basic (EMT-B). The EMT-B's responsibility is to assess rapidly the patient's airway, breathing, and circulation and look for evidence of obvious external hemorrhage. The EMT-B's skills include extrication, spinal protection, immobilization, splinting, and control of external hemorrhage. In most EMS systems, BLS is followed by ALS. ALS personnel are usually Emergency Medical Technician-Paramedic (EMT-P) or specially trained nurses or physicians and may have air or ground transportation capabilities. ALS personnel are trained in a variety of advanced skills including endotracheal intubation, intravenous (IV) access and drug administration, needle and/or surgical cricothyrotomy, and needle thoracentesis. However, significant variability exists among different ALS systems regarding the procedures permitted and medications allowed for use by an EMT-P.[1,2]

2 An area of frequent controversy in the literature involves the philosophy of rapid transport ("scoop and run") versus field stabilization ("stay and play") for the injured patient.[3] The choice of approach for the individual patient often requires complex judgments. Decisions made by experienced on-scene EMTs, communicating online with trauma center control that will receive the patient, provide the best patient outcome.[4,5] The procedures performed and the time invested depend on factors such as the patient's hemodynamic stability, level of consciousness, complexity of extrication, distance from the receiving trauma center, and experience of the prehospital personnel. Injured patients who are at risk for progressive deterioration from continued hemorrhage are better served with stabilization procedures done en route rather than at the scene.[4]

Nationally standardized training programs for EMTs, both BLS and ALS, have become popular. These programs, Basic Trauma Life Support (BTLS) and Prehospital Trauma Life Support (PHTLS), provide EMS personnel a curriculum to assist in making these complex decisions.

Assessment and Management Priorities

3 **Airway Assessment.** Because the most immediately life-threatening problem to the injured patient is loss of airway patency, this is the first priority of the first-response team on arrival at the injury site. Patients who are awake, alert, and talking obviously have a patent airway, but those who are unconscious or have evidence of respiratory insufficiency require immediate attention. Typical BTLS skills, such as suctioning, chin lift or jaw thrust, the placement of oropharyngeal airways, and the use of bag mask devices, are usually sufficient, at least temporarily, to restore oxygenation. On arrival of ALS personnel, a more definitive airway can be secured by endotracheal intubation. Endotracheal intubation is the best procedure for airway control for patients who are in shock, have abnormal breathing patterns, or are unable to protect the

airway because they are unconscious. Endotracheal intubation is a skill that requires proper training and regular use of the technique. In addition, ongoing quality assurance and continuing education are needed to maintain skills over time.

Training of paramedical personnel almost always includes endotracheal intubation, but the indications for intubation vary. The indications for intubation are often dependent on whether ALS providers are allowed to use neuromuscular blocking agents (NMBAs), such as succinylcholine, to facilitate intubation. In systems that do not have clearance to use NMBAs, intubation is limited to severely injured patients without airway reflexes. The use of NMBAs has been associated with increased success at achieving prehospital intubation with minimal complication rates.[6–12] However, the absolute benefit of prehospital intubation for patients with traumatic brain injury remains controversial. Concerns have been raised that transient hypoxia associated with intubation or inadvertent hyperventilation after intubation could worsen outcome for these patients.[13,14] In contrast, early intubation reduces the risk of gastric aspiration, which can be exacerbated by positive-pressure ventilatory assistance by bag valve mask and cause gastric distention.

Common indications for endotracheal intubation in the field include respiratory distress, unconsciousness, hypovolemic shock, significant head injury, severe chest injury, and facial burns. More liberal indications for endotracheal intubation include all patients with significant mechanism of injury and unstable vital signs or altered mental status. Intubation in an uncontrolled environment such as the prehospital setting can be difficult. Patients with head injuries are at high risk for cervical spine injuries, so in-line mobilization techniques are necessary. In patients in whom intubation is not successful, the use of a pharyngeal lumen airway or Combitube may be an option.[15] Nasotracheal intubation is an effective technique if practiced frequently, but requires patient-initiated airflow to open the glottis; most paramedical personnel lack training in this technique, and patients with potential basilar skull fracture are not candidates for this approach. In some cases, needle or surgical cricothyroidotomy in the field may be the only way to establish an airway. Reasonable results have been obtained in the prehospital setting using cricothyroidotomy, but as with endotracheal intubation, mastering this skill requires ongoing training.[16,17]

A recent expert panel, convened by the Brain Trauma Foundation, emphasized the importance of several system factors in the implementation of a prehospital Rapid Sequence Intubation (RSI) program.[18] These include strong medical direction and oversight, protocol development, an implementation plan that includes both cognitive and technical training, appropriate prehospital triage, skill maintenance, and performance improvement. Furthermore, they note that "competent" performance of RSI is not limited to successful tube placement but also includes avoiding desaturations during RSI as well as subsequent hyperventilation, both of which have been associated with impaired outcome for patients with severe traumatic brain injury.

Breathing. After establishment of a patent and controlled airway, the next priority is to ensure that air exchange is taking place. Immediately life-threatening injuries that preclude air exchange include tension pneumothorax, massive open chest wounds, sucking chest wounds, and tracheal disruption. There are no maneuvers likely to correct tracheal disruption in the field. Both open chest wounds and sucking chest wounds respond to endotracheal intubation and positive-pressure ventilation. Tension pneumothorax occasionally requires field decompression. Field techniques to deal with tension pneumothorax include needle thoracostomy and chest tube thoracostomy in the midclavicular line of the second intercostal space. A recent review of prehospital needle thoracostomy suggested this was a relatively safe procedure but should be reserved for patients with physiologic signs consistent with tension pneumothorax.[19] Some trauma systems allow paramedical personnel to place chest tubes in the field or en route under medical control.[20] Chest tube placement probably is not necessary in urban trauma systems with short response times but may be of value in rural areas.

In addition to addressing mechanical factors that impair ventilation, such as tension pneumothorax, recent evidence has also suggested that we need to pay greater attention to the ventilation rate we provide the patient once the airway has been established.[21,22] This is particularly important for a patient who may have a traumatic brain injury (TBI). Historically, hyperventilation was used routinely in the management of patients with severe TBI as a means to decrease intracranial pressure; however, this was abandoned once the effects on cerebral blood flow were evident. In 1991, a randomized controlled trial of prolonged hyperventilation versus conventional ventilation of severe TBI patients in the intensive care unit demonstrated significantly impaired neurologic outcome 3 and 6 months after injury in the hyperventilation group.[23] This led to the recommendation that routine hyperventilation be avoided in severe TBI.[24,25] However, inadvertent hyperventilation early after injury remains a common problem and the impact of this transient period of hyperventilation on outcome has only recently been explored.

The cerebral arterial vasculature is extremely sensitive to changes in arterial carbon dioxide tension. Upon the induction of hypocapnia there is an immediate vasoconstriction of the cerebral arterioles, reducing cerebral blood volume (CBV), intracranial pressure (ICP), and, more important, cerebral oxygen delivery.[26] This leads to a shift in cerebral metabolism to an anaerobic state reflected by an immediate drop in jugular venous oxygen saturation and an increase in cerebral lactic acid production.[27–29] While hypocapnia results in the favorable drop in intracranial pressure, the subsequent cerebral ischemia causes secondary injury to the traumatized brain (Fig. 18.1).

Positive-pressure ventilation may cause additional secondary insults by increasing intrathoracic pressure, thus decreasing venous return to the heart. This decrease in preload, especially in the patient with concomitant hemorrhagic volume loss, may manifest as systemic hypotension, further exacerbating secondary brain injury. This decrease in venous return may paradoxically cause increased ICP by causing venous congestion in the jugular venous system.[30,31] Animal models of low blood flow states, such as hemorrhagic shock or cardiac arrest, have demonstrated significant impairment of hemodynamics associated with hyperventilation.[32–35] Recently, results of an animal

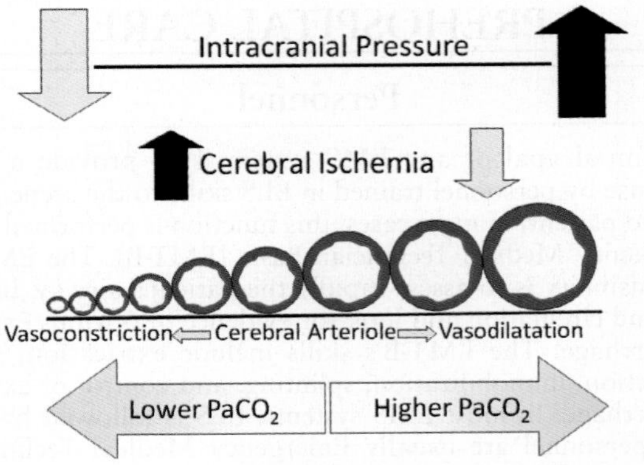

FIGURE 18.1. Physiology of the cerebrovascular response to changes in arterial carbon dioxide tension ($PaCO_2$). As $PaCO_2$ increases, there is cerebral vasodilatation, which may increase cerebral blood flow but at the expense of increased intracranial pressure. As $PaCO_2$ decreases, vasoconstriction leads to decreased intracranial pressure but at the expense of impaired cerebral blood flow.

study assessing cerebral perfusion during hemorrhagic shock and varying ventilation rates reported significant compromise of cerebral perfusion and oxygenation at a rate of 12 breaths per minute that was not evident at 6 breaths per minute.[36]

Most prehospital providers ventilate patients with bag valve devices with 100% oxygen connected to either a facemask or directly to an endotracheal tube or other supraglottic airway. Many of these bags have a volume in excess of 1,200 mL. Uncontrolled bag ventilation can easily lead to inadvertent hyperventilation early after injury. Davis et al. have reported that three quarters of recorded end-tidal CO_2 values for intubated TBI patients were <30 mm Hg in the prehospital setting.[37] Likewise, Thomas et al. have reported end-tidal CO_2 readings of <25 mm Hg in one third of patients and <30 mm Hg in two thirds of patients transported by prehospital air transport.[38] There is some variability among prehospital systems, however, as in Seattle we observed that only 18% of intubated trauma patients arrived with an arterial carbon dioxide tension ($PaCO_2$) <30 mm Hg.[22]

A recent study suggests that intubated trauma patients arriving to the emergency room have improved outcome if the arrival $PaCO_2$ is within the range of 30 to 35 mm Hg.[22] In a subsequent study, patients who were able to achieve a target ventilation range as reflected by a $PaCO_2$ of 30 to 39 mm Hg while in the emergency department (ED) had a significantly better outcome than those not able to achieve this range even after exclusion of patients who were severely hypercapnic ($PaCO_2$ >50 mm Hg).[21] For patients with a severe TBI as defined by a Head Abbreviated Injury Scale (AIS) score of 4 to 5, patients in the target range had a significant survival advantage (mortality odds ratio [OR] 0.33, 95% confidence interval [CI] 0.15–0.75). Furthermore, patients who arrived, based on their prehospital ventilation, outside the target range appeared to benefit from correction to the target range while in the ED. These studies emphasize the importance of tracking serial arterial blood gas results during ED ventilation of intubated TBI patients.

In light of these data, some authors have advocated the use of end-tidal CO_2 monitoring in the prehospital environment to minimize inadvertent hyperventilation.[39,40] While assessment of end-tidal CO_2 is important to confirm endotracheal tube placement[41,42] and monitor for tube dislodgement, it is less reliable as a marker of ventilation status. Impaired perfusion secondary to hypovolemic shock or impaired pulmonary gas exchange due to thoracic injuries can have significant effects on the end-tidal CO_2 values. In a recently completed study, the correlation between $PaCO_2$ and end-tidal CO_2 was very poor (R^2 0.277 for a cohort of intubated trauma patients managed in the ED).[43]

Circulation. The most common cause of death during the first hour after injury is hemorrhage. Therefore, after establishment of a patent airway and adequate air exchange, the next priority is support of the circulation. Direct pressure usually controls obvious external hemorrhage. There are a number of new topical agents designed to promote clot formation, which can be used in conjunction with direct pressure.[44,45] Studies are ongoing to determine the optimal product. For extremity injuries where direct pressure is not adequate to control the hemorrhage, recent data from the military experience in Iraq support that tourniquets should be considered as a lifesaving maneuver.[44,46] To initiate resuscitation, one or two large-bore IV lines may be placed in the upper extremities en route to the trauma center. However, placement of lines must not delay transport unless the patient is undergoing a complex extrication or is more than 30 minutes from a trauma center.[47] The standard of care in the prehospital setting for hypotensive patients is volume replacement and rapid transport to a trauma center. Historically, the pneumatic antishock garment was also used in this setting but has been largely abandoned based on data demonstrating increased mortality particularly in patients with thoracic trauma.[48] However, the pneumatic antishock garment is still occasionally used as a splint for combined pelvic and lower extremity injuries.

The appropriate volume and type of fluid used for initial resuscitation of the hypotensive trauma patient remains controversial. Recent experimental and clinical evidence raises the possibility that internal hemorrhage from major vascular injuries should not be treated with IV fluid infusion until the bleeding can be controlled in the operating room.[49] In the hypotensive state, major vascular injuries have a chance to clot and temporarily stop hemorrhaging; however, if IV volume restores normal blood pressure, the clot can dislodge and the rate of bleeding can increase significantly. However, the clinical data supporting this approach are based on a single trial that focused on patients with penetrating torso trauma and with a short transport time to the trauma center.[49] The role of limited volume resuscitation in blunt trauma is unknown and could be particularly harmful to patients with TBI. Currently the standard resuscitation fluid for trauma patients is a crystalloid solution of either lactated Ringer solution or normal saline. Several recent studies have suggested that hypertonic saline solutions may be even more beneficial as the initial resuscitation fluid for hypotensive trauma patients and those with TBI; clinical trials are ongoing.[50–52]

The controversy between the scoop-and-run philosophy and the field-resuscitation philosophy in seriously injured patients is best resolved by common sense. Patients who are a short distance from a trauma center should be expeditiously transported to the trauma center with attempts made during transport to obtain IV access. This strategy facilitates initiation of resuscitation on arrival at the trauma center. Alternatively, patients who are a long distance from a trauma center or who require long extrication times most likely will benefit from the administration of IV fluids. Similarly, the goal is an acceptable blood pressure (~90 to 100 mm Hg), not necessarily normal and obviously not hypertensive. Current standardized training programs (BTLS, PHTLS) for EMS personnel suggest that, at minimum, a trauma patient who does not require extrication should be assessed, treated, and packaged for transportation in less than 8 to 10 minutes.

TRIAGE

Another key decision that needs to be made in the prehospital environment is to select the appropriate facility to receive the patient. The Centers for Disease Control and Prevention recently convened an expert panel to revise the Field Triage Decision Scheme for transport to a designated trauma center (Fig. 18.2).[53] This decision tree is based on four steps in the evaluation process. Step 1 involves an initial evaluation of physiologic status and level of consciousness including Glasgow Coma Scale (GCS) score, systolic blood pressure, and respiratory rate. Step 2 focuses on specific injury patterns likely to require trauma center care. Step 3 addresses the mechanism of injury, and Step 4 considers the extremes of age and other mitigating comorbidities. If at any point in the algorithm the patient meets the suggested criteria, then transport to a designated trauma center is recommended. This algorithm has been endorsed by the American College of Surgeons Committee on Trauma.

RESUSCITATION PHASE

Development of trauma centers and trauma systems has produced documented improvement in survival of multiply injured patients in numerous reports.[54–58] Trauma centers are hospitals committed to the total care of the trauma patient, 24 hours a day. Multidisciplinary trauma teams consist of

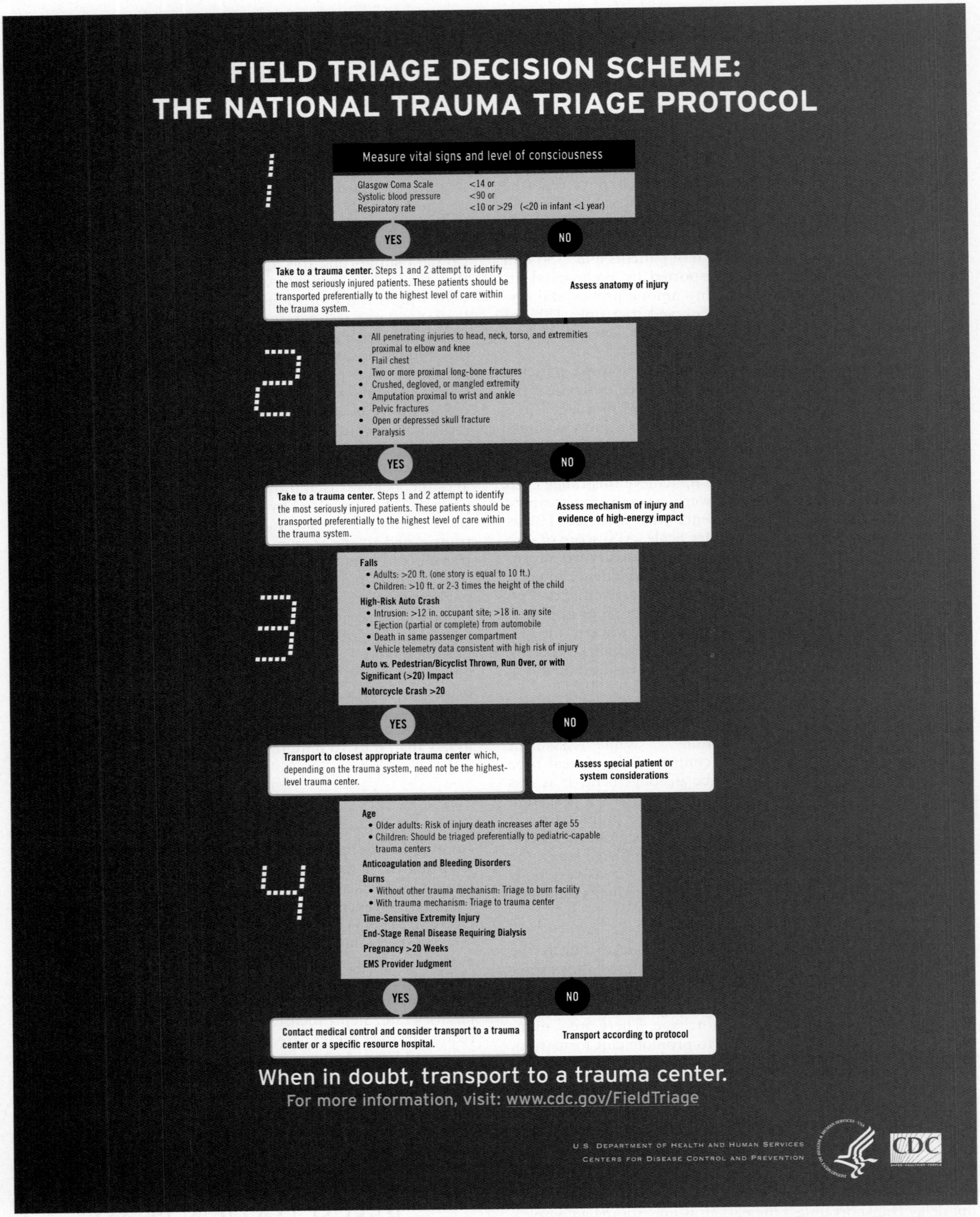

FIGURE 18.2. Field triage decision scheme. (Reprinted with permission from American College of Surgeons Committee on Trauma. *Resources for the Optimal Care of the Injured Patient*. Chicago, IL: American College of Surgeons; 2006:22).

emergency physicians, general and orthopedic surgeons and neurosurgeons, critical care nurses, and diagnostic technicians. After notification of a major injury from the scene, the trauma team assembles in a specially equipped resuscitation room prior to the patient's arrival. On arrival, care is immediately transferred to the trauma team, and the resuscitation phase is initiated without a delay. If feasible, seriously injured patients should bypass hospitals without these resources and be taken to the nearest trauma center.

Many patients have relatively minor injuries that do not require mobilization of this expensive team and resources. Therefore, an important function of a trauma system is to allow communication between prehospital personnel and the trauma center to identify those patients who will benefit from trauma center care. A written prehospital report describing the mechanism and extent of injury, vital signs, GCS score, and treatment started by the prehospital personnel should also be provided. These details alert the trauma center team to look for specific injury patterns based on mechanism of injury and guide further workup. Assessment and treatment then follow a logical sequence based on nationally standardized protocols using the Advanced Trauma Life Support (ATLS) format.[59]

Trauma Team Composition

4 The trauma team consists of members from different disciplines, each of whom sees the patient from a particular point of view. Of necessity, the team must have a single "captain of the ship" whose responsibility it is to organize and prioritize treatment efforts. In a well-orchestrated team, the team leader integrates and coordinates several tasks simultaneously. In most level 1 and 2 trauma centers, the team captain is a general surgeon trained in trauma care. In the ideal situation, the trauma surgeon should be present when the patient arrives. In many rural and nonacademic level 3 trauma centers, the initial team captain is an emergency physician, with a general surgeon assuming the role on arrival. Academic institutions with both emergency medicine and surgical residency programs have the obligation of training both specialties to assume the role of trauma team leadership.

Although responsibilities vary between institutions, anyone involved in the resuscitation of trauma patients must master several procedures: all types of airway management, including cricothyroidotomy; establishment of vascular access through both percutaneous and open approaches; decompression of the pleural space using needle or tube thoracostomy; and decompression of the pericardial space by pericardiocentesis, subxiphoid window, or emergency thoracotomy.

Primary Survey: Initial Assessment

5 The first priority of the trauma team is to repeat the assessment of the airway, breathing, circulation, and level of consciousness of the patient. This assessment is referred to as the *primary survey*. Although in reality the primary survey is performed in a simultaneous fashion, it is described here in its individual components and their appropriate priorities.

The first priority is reassessment of the airway. Airway obstruction often responds to simple maneuvers such as suctioning, chin lift, jaw thrust, or placement of an oropharyngeal airway. Protection of the cervical spine with in-line immobilization is imperative during these maneuvers. Persistence of respiratory insufficiency requires endotracheal intubation. Unsuccessful intubation necessitates emergent cricothyroidotomy. Occasionally, the anatomy does not allow cricothyroidotomy, as can occur with laryngeal fracture. In these cases, a formal tracheotomy must be performed. After an airway is established, a physician auscultates the chest to confirm air exchange, confirms return of carbon dioxide via the endotracheal tube, and obtains a chest radiograph to ensure proper tube position with the tip proximal to the carina. Appropriate placement of endotracheal tubes inserted in the prehospital setting should also be confirmed at this time.

The next priority is to ensure adequate ventilatory exchange by rapid auscultation of both lung fields and assessment for mechanical factors that may interfere with breathing. These factors include compression of the lung from hemothorax, pneumothorax, or visceral herniation; loss of chest-wall stability from flail chest; lung damage from pulmonary contusion; and airway obstruction from aspiration. A dramatic presentation with cyanosis, intense respiratory effort without air movement, distended neck veins, and lack of breath sounds on chest auscultation indicates that a tension pneumothorax is present. Clinical diagnosis of tension pneumothorax requires immediate needle thoracostomy followed by chest tube thoracostomy. Sucking chest wounds should be sealed with an occlusive dressing secured on three sides to function as a flap valve. Most other problems become evident on the initial chest radiograph and are relieved by chest tube insertion, suctioning, or repositioning of the endotracheal tube. The optimal position for chest tube insertion is the midaxillary line at the fifth or sixth interspace, avoiding the axilla, the large muscles of the back and chest, and the breast. Insertion of a finger into the chest before chest tube placement ensures entry into the pleural space and provides the opportunity to search digitally for defects in the diaphragm.

After establishment of an airway, ventilation, and appropriate pleural drainage, the next priority is assessment of the patient's circulatory status. Blood pressure, pulse, skin perfusion, temperature, capillary refill, mental status, presence of breath sounds, and neck vein distention are all useful clinical indicators of hemodynamic status. The first issue is to establish whether the patient is in hypovolemic shock and, if so, to determine the source of hemorrhage. Circulatory collapse in the injured patient is almost always caused by hypovolemia secondary to hemorrhage. Occasionally, concurrent heart disease, spinal cord injury, or cardiac tamponade may contribute. The mainstay of treatment for hypotension in the injured patient, regardless of cause, is volume resuscitation with crystalloid solution and, if hypotension is persistent, packed red blood cells (RBCs). A lack of response to IV infusion of 2 L of lactated Ringer solution indicates significant, ongoing hemorrhage and necessitates immediate blood transfusion.

Effective resuscitation from hemorrhagic shock requires both restoration of intravascular volume and control of hemorrhage. Most hypotensive patients are already compensating maximally on arrival in the ED and many have ongoing hemorrhage. The less responsive a patient is to initial volume resuscitation, the more urgent is the need for hemorrhage control. One need not wait for a response to resuscitation before taking the patient to the operating room. Another situation that requires vigilance is the cool, pale patient with relatively normal vital signs. These patients are compensating maximally and have a normal blood pressure because of intensive peripheral vasoconstriction. However, this compensatory mechanism is of only limited duration, and such patients require immediate rapid volume infusion, blood transfusion, and operative control of bleeding. A similar trap exists for patients with the mangled extremity syndrome or multiple open fractures. Patients may have lost significant blood volume at the injury scene. Before resuscitation, there may be relatively little hemorrhage from the open wounds; however, initiation of IV fluids may increase blood pressure and cause vasodilation, resulting in increased hemorrhage. These patients require immediate volume resuscitation and operative control of their wounds.

The final priority in the primary survey is a brief neurologic evaluation to assess the components of the GCS (Table 18.1). The GCS is scored by assessing eye opening, verbal responses, and motor responses with a maximal (normal) score of 15. In addition, pupillary size, reactivity and equality of the two, and

TABLE 18.1 **DIAGNOSIS**

GLASGOW COMA SCALE (GCS)

EYE OPENING	
Spontaneous	4
To voice	3
To pain	2
None	1
VERBAL RESPONSE	
Oriented	5
Confused	4
Inappropriate words	3
Incomprehensible sounds	2
None	1
MOTOR RESPONSE	
Obeys commands	6
Purposeful movement (pain)	5
Withdraw (pain)	4
Flexion (pain)	3
Extension (pain)	2
None	1
GCS SUBTOTAL	3–15

the presence of other lateralizing signs are assessed. Mental status may improve in response to volume resuscitation; however, a patient with a GCS score of 8 or less is assumed to have a significant brain injury. In this case, aggressive resuscitation, including appropriate adequate ventilation (see discussion under prehospital care, breathing), restoration of circulating volume, and the provision of adequate oxygenation, is an important consideration.

ED resuscitative thoracotomy is an aggressive, desperate attempt to save a dying patient. The dramatic return to full consciousness of a clinically dead patient after release of a pericardial tamponade from a stab wound to the heart provides complete justification for ED thoracotomy to those who have witnessed it. However, the widespread use of the technique in all patients arriving without vital signs has resulted in an extremely low survival rate at a very high cost. At first glance, the cost of an unsuccessful ED thoracotomy would seem to be nothing more than that of sterilizing the instruments and the physician's time. Many times, however, vital signs are temporarily restored, and the patient dies in the operating room or in the intensive care unit after massive blood transfusion and the use of considerable resources. Even worse is the rare patient who survives in a permanent vegetative state. The cost of the care for these patients must be included in any cost–benefit analysis. In addition, the risk of injury to a caregiver with viral contaminated blood or other infectious agents is unnecessary.

Boyd et al.[60] performed a meta-analysis of 24 reports concerning the outcome of ED thoracotomy. They found that the overall survival rate after ED thoracotomy was 11% (264 of 2,294 patients). There were no survivors among patients with no signs of life at the trauma scene. Signs of life were defined as supraventricular electrical activity, pupillary reaction, and agonal respirations. In addition, there were no neurologically intact survivors among blunt trauma patients who were without signs of life on arrival in the ED. Considering these findings, the researchers proposed an algorithm that would indicate ED thoracotomy for penetrating trauma only if the patient had signs of life at the scene and had lost signs of life less than 5 minutes before arrival in the ED. Blunt trauma patients would be allowed ED thoracotomy only if the patient had signs of life on arrival in the ED. For patients who meet these criteria and lose cardiac function, airway placement and fluid resuscitation are initiated simultaneously with, or are immediately followed by, left anterior thoracotomy, pericardiotomy, and internal cardiac massage (Algorithm 18.1).

Secondary Survey

The secondary survey is directed at specific identification of suspected and unsuspected injuries. It consists of a thorough physical examination that includes observation and palpation of the entire body for evidence and characterization of injury. However, performance of the secondary survey depends on the results of the primary survey and the patient's response to initial resuscitative efforts. The secondary survey for a patient in hemorrhagic shock unresponsive to initial resuscitative efforts during the primary survey consists only of rapid identification of the bleeding site and rapid transport to the operating room for definitive control of hemorrhage. At the other end of the spectrum, a completely stable patient with relatively minor injuries undergoes a complete physical examination with confirmatory laboratory and radiographic tests before initiation of the treatment phase. The secondary survey can be interrupted at any time if a patient's status deteriorates. Adjuvants to the secondary survey include radiographic examinations and laboratory testing. For the purposes of description, the secondary survey is discussed by its individual components.

Head and Face. The head-to-toe examination usually begins with palpation of the skull and the head to identify hematomas, lacerations, and fractures. Scalp lacerations can cause significant blood loss and should be closed with a full-thickness running suture to provide hemostasis. Potential ocular injuries are assessed by testing visual acuity, pupillary function, and ocular range of motion. A funduscopic examination is important to identify increased intracranial pressure, vitreal hemorrhage, or retinal detachment. The findings of ecchymosis over the mastoid process, hemotympanum, otorrhea, rhinorrhea, or periorbital ecchymosis often indicate basilar skull fracture. Thorough palpation and attempts to displace facial bones identify step-offs or instability associated with facial fractures. Reassessment of the airway and a careful bimanual examination of the oral cavity identify loose teeth as well as mandibular and maxillary fractures. Bleeding from nasal fractures may require posterior and anterior packing for hemostasis; transnasal posteriorly placed Foley catheter balloons often work well to stanch bleeding.

Neck. Examination of the cervical region is conducted while axial immobilization of the cervical spine is maintained. The cervical collar is removed and the neck is examined for tracheal deviation, subcutaneous emphysema, hematomas, lacerations, or distended jugular veins. The posterior cervical spine is palpated to elicit tenderness or other signs of obvious fracture. Evidence of laryngeal fracture includes subcutaneous emphysema, tenderness, "step-off" (distortion of the thyroid and cricoid cartilage), and voice change. The presence of a fractured larynx is a relative contraindication to endotracheal intubation because of the possibility of extending the injury or creating a false passage leading to loss of the airway. Patients with suspected laryngeal fractures should be taken to the operating room immediately for formal tracheotomy. Carotid pulses are assessed, and bruits or expanding hematomas that may be suggestive of carotid artery injury are identified.

Penetrating injuries should not be probed, cannulated, or explored past the platysma because uncontrollable hemorrhage may ensue if a clot is dislodged from a major vascular injury. Wounds that have penetrated the platysma are evaluated either by formal operative exploration of the neck or by

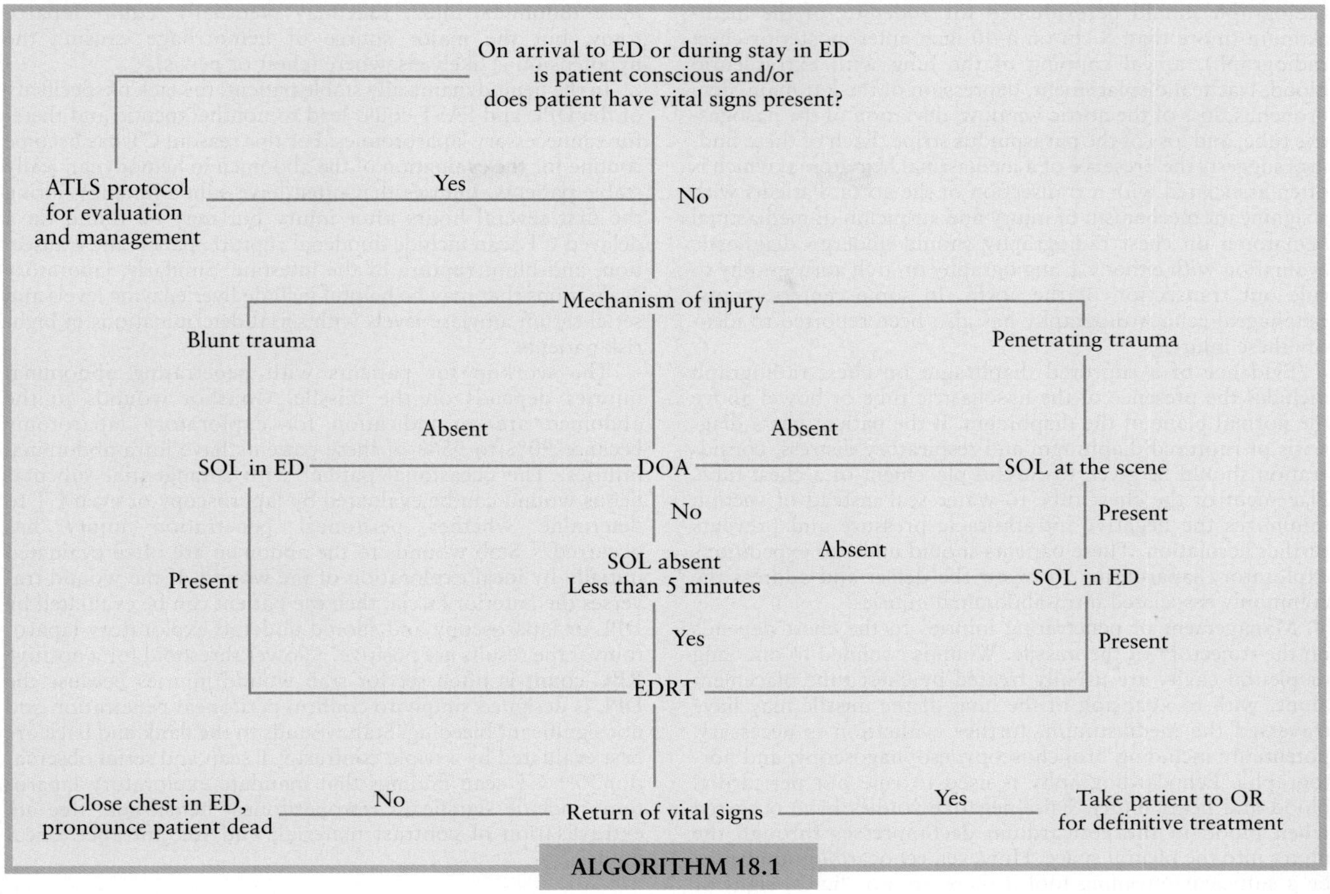

ALGORITHM 18.1. Emergency thoracotomy for penetrating trauma. ED, emergency department; ATLS, Advanced Trauma Life Support; SOL, signs of life; DOA, dead on arrival; EDRT, emergency department resuscitative thoracotomy; OR, operating room. (Adapted from Boyd M, Vanek VW, Bourguet CC. Emergency room resuscitative thoracotomy: when is it indicated? *J Trauma* 1992;33:714–721.)

some combination of angiography, triple endoscopy (pharyngoscopy, laryngoscopy, and esophagoscopy), radiographic contrast study, computed tomography (CT) scan, and observation.[61] Injuries encompassing the area from the cricoid cartilage to the angle of the mandible are usually explored. Angiography is mandatory for injuries between the cricoid cartilage and the clavicle and for injuries between the angle of the mandible and the base of the skull. Radiographic evaluation of the cervical spine should include anteroposterior, lateral, and odontoid views. A CT scan is often used to evaluate suspected bony injuries, and careful flexion and extension films may be necessary to rule out potentially unstable ligamentous injuries of the cervical spine.

Chest. The chest wall is inspected for evidence of instability and for lacerations, including sucking chest wounds, abrasions, and contusions. Auscultation is performed to identify hemothorax or pneumothorax, and palpation is used to elicit tenderness that may be associated with rib fractures. As has been mentioned, tension pneumothorax can be identified by cyanosis, tracheal deviation, distended neck veins, lack of breath sounds, and inability to move air. Tension pneumothorax causing cardiopulmonary collapse is a clinical (not radiologic) diagnosis that requires immediate treatment by needle thoracostomy followed by chest tube insertion.

Virtually all other life-threatening and potentially life-threatening chest injuries are diagnosed or suspected on chest radiography. Hemothorax is identified by opacification of a hemithorax and is treated by chest tube thoracostomy. Most pulmonary parenchymal bleeding stops with reexpansion of the lung and complete evacuation of the pleural space. Additional chest tubes should be placed, if necessary, to completely evacuate the thorax. However, thoracotomy is indicated if the initial blood loss exceeds 1,500 mL or if the rate of ongoing blood loss shortly following injury exceeds 200 to 300 mL/h in an adult.[62] Pulmonary contusion is identified by radiographic findings of an irregular interstitial pattern or frank consolidation in the lung parenchyma. The clinical manifestations of pulmonary contusion vary from mild dyspnea to overt pulmonary failure with development of acute respiratory distress syndrome. The magnitude of the injury is rarely appreciated during the initial evaluation, and it is important to follow up with serial blood gas determinations and a repeat chest radiograph at 6 hours.

All patients with chest trauma should have an electrocardiographic (ECG) evaluation and continuous monitoring during the first hour in the ED. If the ECG is normal, the patient may be discharged, if otherwise appropriate. Patients with ECG changes during the initial hour may have a blunt cardiac injury and should be monitored for at least 24 hours. If there is any sign of myocardial failure, the patient should undergo echocardiography. Most blunt cardiac injuries are self-limited and require only monitoring and treatment of significant dysrhythmias during the first 24 to 48 hours. Rarely, patients have manifestations of overt myocardial failure and require full support, including an intra-aortic balloon pump.

Patients with rapid deceleration blunt injuries to the chest may sustain a transection of the thoracic aorta. The chest radiograph should be evaluated for widening of the mediastinum (more than 8 cm on a 40-inch anteroposterior chest radiograph), apical capping of the lung with extrapleural blood, tracheal displacement, depression of the left main-stem bronchus, loss of the aortic window, deviation of the nasogastric tube, and loss of the paraspinous stripe. Each of these findings suggests the presence of a mediastinal hematoma, which is often associated with a transection of the aorta. Patients with a significant mechanism of injury and suspicion of mediastinal hematoma on chest radiography should undergo diagnostic evaluation with either CT angiography or arch aortography to rule out transection of the aorta. In some centers, transesophageal echocardiography has also been reported to identify these injuries.

Evidence of a ruptured diaphragm on chest radiograph includes the presence of the nasogastric tube or bowel above the normal plane of the diaphragm. If the patient has a diagnosis of ruptured diaphragm and respiratory distress, consideration should be given to careful placement of a chest tube. Placement of the chest tube to water seal instead of suction minimizes the negative intrathoracic pressure and prevents further herniation. These patients should undergo expeditious exploratory laparotomy to repair the defect and address the commonly associated intra-abdominal injuries.

Management of penetrating injuries to the chest depends on the trajectory of the missile. Wounds confined to one lung or pleural cavity are usually treated by chest tube placement alone, with reexpansion of the lung. If the missile may have traversed the mediastinum, further evaluation is necessary, potentially including bronchoscopy, esophagoscopy, and aortography. Echocardiography is used to rule out pericardial blood and heart injury. False-negative studies have occurred when blood in the pericardium decompresses through the injury into the pleural space. However, echocardiography may be a sufficient screening tool if there are no clinical signs or symptoms of cardiac injury and no hemothorax. Gunshot wounds below the nipple line, the upper limit of diaphragm excursion, place the abdominal cavity at risk and thus require abdominal exploration as well.

Abdomen. The abdominal examination should attempt to determine whether there is a significant injury requiring surgical intervention. Although physical examination is often accurate and reliable, it can be misleading in 20% to 30% of patients.[63] This inaccuracy is particularly true in patients who are obtunded from head injury, alcohol, drug use, or shock. If patients are hemodynamically unstable, it is important to determine rapidly whether free intraperitoneal hemorrhage is responsible for the hypotension. Diagnostic peritoneal lavage (DPL) or the focused abdominal sonogram for trauma (FAST) accomplishes this goal rapidly and safely. Both are reported to be extremely reliable in the hemodynamically unstable patient.[64,65] Both studies are operator dependent, however, and the choice of the best approach may depend on local hospital resources. DPL has the advantage of also being very sensitive for hollow viscus injury and thus is often preferred in the setting of a seatbelt sign with increased concern for bowel perforation.

DPL is considered grossly positive if more than 10 mL of blood is freely aspirated after catheter insertion. If less than 10 mL of blood or no blood is aspirated, 1 L of warmed crystalloid solution is infused into the peritoneum and then drained. A sample of the drained fluid is sent to the laboratory for RBC and leukocyte count, amylase and bilirubin level, and Gram stain for the presence of bacteria. DPL is considered microscopically positive if the RBC count is higher than 100,000/mL. If the goal is to find the source of hemorrhage in a hypotensive patient, then a grossly positive DPL pinpoints the abdomen as at least one source, and the patient should undergo immediate laparotomy. In contrast, a microscopically positive DPL indicates intra-abdominal injury that may eventually require laparotomy, but the major source of hemorrhage causing the hypotension is likely elsewhere (chest or pelvis).[66]

In the hemodynamically stable patient, the lack of specificity of the DPL and FAST could lead to nontherapeutic and therefore unnecessary laparotomies. For this reason, CT has become routine for the evaluation of the abdomen in hemodynamically stable patients. Injuries that often have subtle findings during the first several hours after injury but may be found on a delayed CT scan include duodenal rupture, pancreatic transection, and blunt rupture of the intestine. Similarly, laboratory evaluations that may be helpful include liver enzyme levels and serial serum amylase levels with serial determinations in high-risk patients.

The workup for patients with penetrating abdominal injuries depends on the missile. Gunshot wounds to the abdomen are an indication for exploratory laparotomy because 90% to 95% of these patients have intra-abdominal injuries. The occasional patient with a tangential subcutaneous wound can be evaluated by laparoscopy or even CT to determine whether peritoneal penetration injury has occurred.[67] Stab wounds to the abdomen are often evaluated initially by local exploration of the wound. If the wound traverses the anterior fascia, then the patient can be evaluated by DPL or laparoscopy and should undergo exploratory laparotomy if the results are positive. A lower threshold for a positive RBC count is often set for stab wound injuries because the DPL is designed simply to confirm peritoneal penetration and not significant bleeding. Stab wounds to the flank and back are best evaluated by a triple-contrast CT scan and serial observation.[68,69] CT scan findings that mandate exploratory laparotomy include significant retroperitoneal hematoma, free air, extravasation of contrast material, and free intraperitoneal fluid.

Pelvis. After evaluation of the abdomen, the pelvis is assessed by physical examination. The bones of the pelvis are palpated gently to elicit tenderness that could indicate fracture. Evidence of instability of the pelvic ring warrants placement of a sheet around the pelvis to reduce the pelvic volume and minimize venous bleeding in the retroperitoneum. This procedure can be performed in the field or on arrival in the ED. In some systems the pneumatic antishock garment is used for this purpose, but better reduction can often be achieved with a simple bed sheet tied around the iliac crests. The genitalia should be inspected for scrotal hematoma or blood at the urethral meatus, which indicates probable urethral transection. A bimanual pelvic examination in women identifies evidence of vaginal laceration, indicating an open pelvic fracture. A rectal examination is performed to identify blood indicative of bowel injury and, occasionally, a mobile, "floating" prostate, which indicates urethral transection. Evidence of a free-floating prostate, blood at the urethra, or scrotal hematoma should prompt a retrograde urethrogram before placement of a bladder catheter is attempted. All patients sustaining significant blunt torso trauma should undergo plain radiography of the pelvis to diagnose potential pelvic fracture.

If the patient is hemodynamically unstable, the pelvic fracture must be considered a potential source of hemorrhage. This consideration is important because pelvic fracture bleeding is retroperitoneal and rarely controllable at exploratory laparotomy. Venous bleeding is treated by reducing the volume of the pelvis, and arterial bleeding should be evaluated and treated by early angiography and embolization. Some authors have reported success with operative preperitoneal packing when angiography is not immediately available and the patient is rapidly exsanguinating.[70–72] If the patient is hemodynamically stable, the pelvic fracture should be evaluated further with additional plain radiographs and CT scans (Algorithm 18.2).

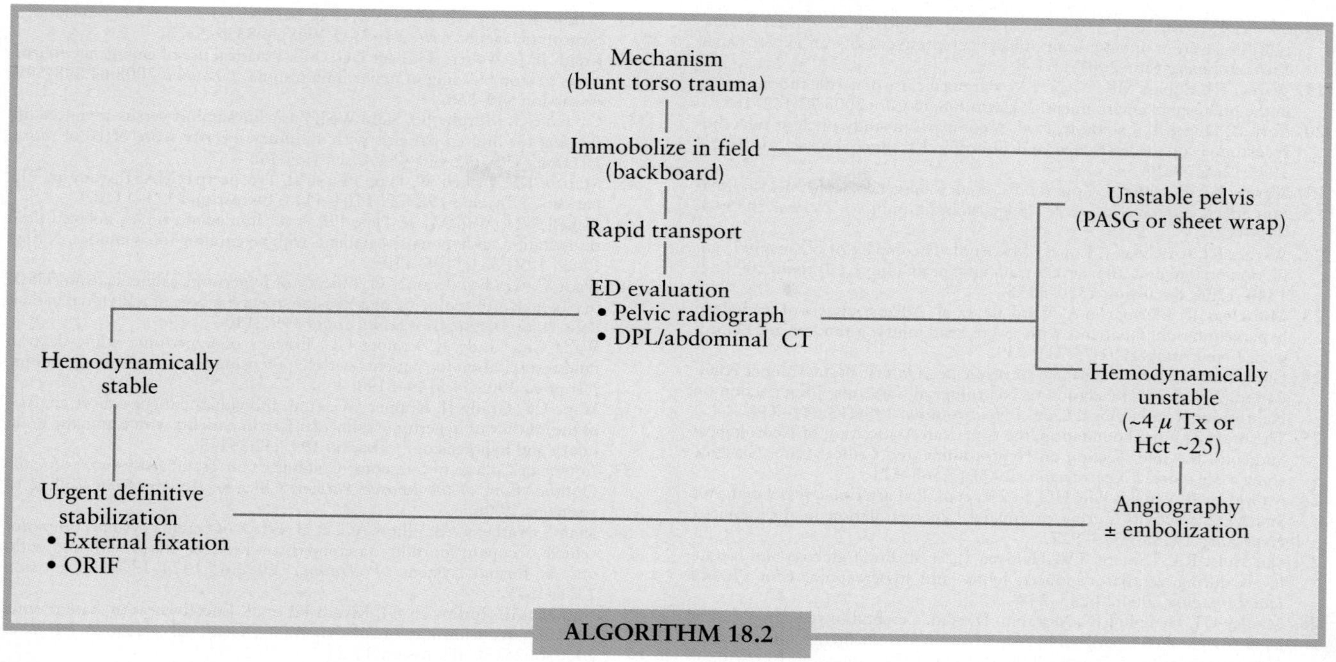

ALGORITHM 18.2. Emergency management of pelvic fractures. PASG, pneumatic antishock garment; ED, emergency department; DPL, diagnostic peritoneal lavage; CT, computed tomography; Tx, transfusion; Hct, hematocrit; ORIF, open reduction internal fixation.

Extremities. Finally, the extremities are evaluated for open wounds with potential sources of hemorrhage or occult open fractures. Evaluation of pulses may indicate vascular injury. Palpation and passive range-of-motion tests diagnose potential long-bone fractures, dislocations, and ligamentous injuries. Dislocations require prompt reduction, especially if there is any evidence of neurovascular compromise. Penetrating wounds to the extremities necessitate evaluation for potential vascular injury by palpation of pulses, auscultation for bruits, and recognition of expanding hematomas. Proximity wounds can be evaluated by duplex ultrasound scan or arteriography. With any injury, development of a compartment syndrome due to bleeding or associated edema should also be considered.

SUMMARY

The ideal trauma system consists of a prehospital care team that quickly and safely transports an injured patient to a trauma center where a multidisciplinary trauma team immediately begins resuscitation of the patient. Treatment of immediately life-threatening injuries begins during transport and continues after arrival at the trauma center. Rapid initial evaluation, followed by a more detailed secondary survey, allows identification of injuries while therapy is simultaneously begun. The primary survey focuses on identification and simultaneous treatment of life-threatening injuries, including airway obstruction, mechanical factors in the chest that impair ventilation, and control of hemorrhage. The next priority is assessment and intervention for neurologic injuries including traumatic brain injury and spinal cord injury. Once these issues have been addressed, the secondary survey is performed to identify all other injuries. The secondary survey is interrupted as necessary to treat life-threatening and limb-threatening injuries as they are identified. If interruption becomes necessary, the secondary survey is completed at a later time.

References

1. Lavery RF, Dora J, Tortella BJ, et al. A survey of advanced life support practices in the United States. *Prehospital Disaster Med* 1992;7:144–150.
2. McDonald CC, Bailey B. Out-of-hospital use of neuromuscular-blocking agents in the United States. *Prehosp Emerg Care* 1998;2:29–32.
3. Liberman M, Mulder D, Sampalis J. Advanced or basic life support for trauma: meta-analysis and critical review of the literature. *J Trauma* 2000;49:584–599.
4. Pepe PE, Maio RF. Evolving challenges in prehospital trauma services. Current issues and suggested evaluation tools. *Prehospital Disaster Med* 1993;8:25–34.
5. Sampalis JS, Lavoie A, Williams JI, et al. Impact of on-site care, prehospital time, and level of in-hospital care on survival in severely injured patients. *J Trauma* 1993;34:252–261.
6. Bulger EM, Copass MK, Maier RV, et al. An analysis of advanced prehospital airway management. *J Emerg Med* 2002;23:183–189.
7. Hedges JR, Dronen SC, Feero S, et al. Succinylcholine-assisted intubations in prehospital care. *Ann Emerg Med* 1988;17:469–472.
8. Wayne MA, Friedland E. Prehospital use of succinylcholine: a 20-year review [see comments]. *Prehosp Emerg Care* 1999;3:107–109.
9. Ochs M, Davis D, Hoyt D, et al. Paramedic-performed rapid sequence intubation of patients with severe head injuries. *Ann Emerg Med* 2002;40:159–167.
10. Sloane C, Vilke GM, Chan TC, et al. Rapid sequence intubation in the field versus hospital in trauma patients. *J Emerg Med* 2000;19:259–264.
11. Davis DP, Ochs M, Hoyt DB, et al. Paramedic-administered neuromuscular blockade improves prehospital intubation success in severely head-injured patients. *J Trauma* 2003;55:713–719.
12. Ma OJ, Atchley RB, Hatley T, et al. Intubation success rates improve for an air medical program after implementing the use of neuromuscular blocking agents. *Am J Emerg Med* 1998;16:125–127.
13. Davis DP, Hoyt DB, Ochs M, et al. The effect of paramedic rapid sequence intubation on outcome in patients with severe traumatic brain injury. *J Trauma* 2003;54:444–453.
14. Davis DP, Dunford JV, Poste JC, et al. The impact of hypoxia and hyperventilation on outcome after paramedic rapid sequence intubation of severely head-injured patients. *J Trauma* 2004;57:1–8; discussion 8–10.
15. Davis DP, Valentine C, Ochs M, et al. The Combitube as a salvage airway device for paramedic rapid sequence intubation. *Ann Emerg Med* 2003;42:697–704.
16. Salvino CK, Dries D, Gamelli R, et al. Emergency cricothyroidotomy in trauma victims. *J Trauma* 1993;34:503–505.
17. Boyle MF, Hatton D, Sheets C. Surgical cricothyrotomy performed by air ambulance flight nurses: a 5-year experience [see comments]. *J Emerg Med* 1993;11:41–45.

18. Davis DP, Fakhry SM, Wang HE, et al. Paramedic rapid sequence intubation for severe traumatic brain injury: perspectives from an expert panel. *Prehosp Emerg Care* 2007;11:1–8.
19. Warner KJ, Copass MK, Bulger EM. Paramedic use of needle thoracostomy in the prehospital environment. *Prehosp Emerg Care* 2008;12:162–168.
20. York D, Dudek L, Larson R, et al. A comparison study of chest tube thoracostomy: air medical crew and in-hospital trauma service. *Air Med J* 1993;12:227–229.
21. Warner KJ, Cuschieri J, Copass MK, et al. Emergency department ventilation effects outcome in severe traumatic brain injury. *J Trauma* 2008;64: 341–347.
22. Warner KJ, Cuschieri J, Copass MK, et al. The impact of prehospital ventilation on outcome after severe traumatic brain injury. *J Trauma* 2007;62: 1330–1336; discussion 1336–1338.
23. Muizelaar JP, Marmarou A, Ward JD, et al. Adverse effects of prolonged hyperventilation in patients with severe head injury: a randomized clinical trial. *J Neurosurg* 1991;75:731–739.
24. Guidelines for the management of severe head injury. Brain Trauma Foundation, American Association of Neurological Surgeons, Joint Section on Neurotrauma and Critical Care. *J Neurotrauma* 1996;13:641–734.
25. The Brain Trauma Foundation, the American Association of Neurological Surgeons, the Joint Section on Neurotrauma and Critical Care. Glasgow coma scale score. *J Neurotrauma* 2000;17:563–571.
26. Muizelaar JP, van der Poel HG, Li ZC, et al. Pial arteriolar vessel diameter and CO2 reactivity during prolonged hyperventilation in the rabbit. *J Neurosurg* 1988;69:923–927.
27. van Hulst RA, Lameris TW, Haitsma JJ, et al. Brain glucose and lactate levels during ventilator-induced hypo- and hypercapnia. *Clin Physiol Funct Imaging* 2004;24:243–248.
28. Manley GT, Hemphill JC, Morabito D, et al. Cerebral oxygenation during hemorrhagic shock: perils of hyperventilation and the therapeutic potential of hypoventilation. *J Trauma* 2000;48:1025–1032; discussion 1032–1033.
29. Sheinberg M, Kanter MJ, Robertson CS, et al. Continuous monitoring of jugular venous oxygen saturation in head-injured patients. *J Neurosurg* 1992;76:212–217.
30. Citerio G, Vascotto E, Villa F, et al. Induced abdominal compartment syndrome increases intracranial pressure in neurotrauma patients: a prospective study. *Crit Care Med* 2001;29:1466–1471.
31. Bloomfield GL, Ridings PC, Blocher CR, et al. A proposed relationship between increased intra-abdominal, intrathoracic, and intracranial pressure. *Crit Care Med* 1997;25:496–503.
32. Pepe PE, Lurie KG, Wigginton JG, et al. Detrimental hemodynamic effects of assisted ventilation in hemorrhagic states. *Crit Care Med* 2004;32: S414–S420.
33. Pepe PE, Roppolo LP, Fowler RL. The detrimental effects of ventilation during low-blood-flow states. *Curr Opin Crit Care* 2005;11:212–218.
34. Idris AH, Staples ED, O'Brien DJ, et al. Effect of ventilation on acid-base balance and oxygenation in low blood-flow states. *Crit Care Med* 1994; 22:1827–1834.
35. Yannopoulos D, Aufderheide TP, Gabrielli A, et al. Clinical and hemodynamic comparison of 15:2 and 30:2 compression-to-ventilation ratios for cardiopulmonary resuscitation. *Crit Care Med* 2006;34:1444–1449.
36. Davis DP. Early ventilation in traumatic brain injury. *Resuscitation* 2007;76(3):333–340.
37. Davis D, Buono C, Serrano JA, et al. The impact of hyper and hypoventilation on outcome in traumatic brain injury (abstract). *Acad Emerg Med* 2005;12(suppl 5):138–139.
38. Thomas SH, Orf J, Wedel SK, et al. Hyperventilation in traumatic brain injury patients: inconsistency between consensus guidelines and clinical practice. *J Trauma* 2002;52:47–52; discussion 52–53.
39. Davis DP, Dunford JV, Ochs M, et al. The use of quantitative end-tidal capnometry to avoid inadvertent severe hyperventilation in patients with head injury after paramedic rapid sequence intubation. *J Trauma* 2004;56:808–814.
40. Helm M, Schuster R, Hauke J, et al. Tight control of prehospital ventilation by capnography in major trauma victims. *Br J Anaesth* 2003;90:327–332.
41. Grmec S, Mally S. Prehospital determination of tracheal tube placement in severe head injury. *Emerg Med J* 2004;21:518–520.
42. Silvestri S, Ralls GA, Krauss B, et al. The effectiveness of out-of-hospital use of continuous end-tidal carbon dioxide monitoring on the rate of unrecognized misplaced intubation within a regional emergency medical services system. *Ann Emerg Med* 2005;45:497–503.
43. Warner KJ, Cuschieri J, Garland B, et al. The utility of early end-tidal capnography in monitoring ventilation status following severe injury. *J Trauma* 2009;66(1):26–31.
44. Mabry R, McManus JG. Prehospital advances in the management of severe penetrating trauma. *Crit Care Med* 2008;36:S258–S266.
45. Perkins JG, Cap AP, Weiss BM, et al. Massive transfusion and nonsurgical hemostatic agents. *Crit Care Med* 2008;36:S325–S339.
46. Kragh JF Jr, Walters TJ, Baer DG, et al. Practical use of emergency tourniquets to stop bleeding in major limb trauma. *J Trauma* 2008;64:S38–S49; discussion S49–S50.
47. Cayten CG, Murphy JG, Stahl WM. Basic life support versus advanced life support for injured patients with an injury severity score of 10 or more. *J Trauma* 1993;35:460–466; discussion 466–467.
48. Mattox KL, Bickell W, Pepe PE, et al. Prospective MAST study in 911 patients. *J Trauma* 1989;29:1104–1111; discussion 1111–1112.
49. Bickell WH, Wall MJ Jr, Pepe PE, et al. Immediate versus delayed fluid resuscitation for hypotensive patients with penetrating torso injuries. *N Engl J Med* 1994;331:1105–1109.
50. Wade C, Grady J, Kramer G. Efficacy of hypertonic saline dextran (HSD) in patients with traumatic hypotension: meta-analysis of individual patient data. *Acta Anaesthesiol Scand Suppl* 1997;110:77–79.
51. Wade CE, Grady JJ, Kramer GC. Efficacy of hypertonic saline dextran fluid resuscitation for patients with hypotension from penetrating trauma. *J Trauma* 2003;54:S144–S148.
52. Wade CE, Grady JJ, Kramer GC, et al. Individual patient cohort analysis of the efficacy of hypertonic saline/dextran in patients with traumatic brain injury and hypotension. *J Trauma* 1997;42:S61–S65.
53. American College of Surgeons, Committee on Trauma. *Resources for the Optimal Care of the Injured Patient*. Chicago, IL: American College of Surgeons; 2006.
54. Shafi S, Nathens AB, Elliott AC, et al. Effect of trauma systems on motor vehicle occupant mortality: a comparison between states with and without a formal system. *J Trauma* 2006;61:1374–1378; discussion 1378–1379.
55. Nathens AB, Jurkovich GJ, Rivara FP, et al. Effectiveness of state trauma systems in reducing injury-related mortality: a national evaluation. *J Trauma* 2000;48:25–30; discussion 30–31.
56. Nathens AB, Brunet FP, Maier RV. Development of trauma systems and effect on outcomes after injury. *Lancet* 2004;363:1794–1801.
57. Nathens AB, Jurkovich GJ, Cummings P, et al. The effect of organized systems of trauma care on motor vehicle crash mortality. *JAMA* 2000;283: 1990–1994.
58. MacKenzie EJ, Rivara FP, Jurkovich GJ, et al. A national evaluation of the effect of trauma-center care on mortality. *N Engl J Med* 2006;354: 366–378.
59. American College of Surgeons, Committee on Trauma. *Advanced Life Support for Doctors*. Chicago, IL: American College of Surgeons; 2008.
60. Boyd M, Vanek VW, Bourguet CC. Emergency room resuscitative thoracotomy: when is it indicated? *J Trauma* 1992;33:714–721.
61. Jurkovich GJ, Zingarelli W, Wallace J, et al. Penetrating neck trauma: diagnostic studies in the asymptomatic patient. *J Trauma* 1985;25: 819–822.
62. Karmy-Jones R, Jurkovich GJ, Nathens AB, et al. Timing of urgent thoracotomy for hemorrhage after trauma: a multicenter study. *Arch Surg* 2001; 136:513–518.
63. Miller FB, Cryer HM, Chilikuri S, et al. Negative findings on laparotomy for trauma. *South Med J* 1989;82:1231–1234.
64. Nagy KK, Roberts RR, Joseph KT, et al. Experience with over 2500 diagnostic peritoneal lavages. *Injury* 2000;31:479–482.
65. Rozycki GS, Ballard RB, Feliciano DV, et al. Surgeon-performed ultrasound for the assessment of truncal injuries: lessons learned from 1540 patients. *Ann Surg* 1998;228:557–567.
66. Evers BM, Cryer HM, Miller FB. Pelvic fracture hemorrhage. Priorities in management. *Arch Surg* 1989;124:422–424.
67. Fabian TC, Croce MA, Stewart RM, et al. A prospective analysis of diagnostic laparoscopy in trauma. *Ann Surg* 1993;217:557–564; discussion 564–565.
68. Pham T, Heinberg E, Cuschieri J, et al. The evolution of the diagnostic workup for stab wounds to the back and flank. *Injury* 2009;40(1): 48–53.
69. Boyle EM Jr, Maier RV, Salazar JD, et al. Diagnosis of injuries after stab wounds to the back and flank. *J Trauma* 1997;42:260–265.
70. Cothren CC, Osborn PM, Moore EE, et al. Preperitoneal pelvic packing for hemodynamically unstable pelvic fractures: a paradigm shift. *J Trauma* 2007;62:834–839; discussion 839–842.
71. Totterman A, Madsen JE, Skaga NO, et al. Extraperitoneal pelvic packing: a salvage procedure to control massive traumatic pelvic hemorrhage. *J Trauma* 2007;62:843–852.
72. Bach A, Bendix J, Hougaard K, et al. Retroperitoneal packing as part of damage control surgery in a Danish trauma centre—fast, effective, and cost-effective. *Scand J Trauma Resusc Emerg Med* 2008;16:4.

CHAPTER 19 ■ HEAD TRAUMA

RANDALL M. CHESNUT

KEY POINTS

1. Traumatic brain injury (TBI) results from both primary (impact disruption of brain and vascular tissue) and secondary (hypoxia, hypotension, pyrexia, effects of elevated intracranial pressure [ICP] and biochemical processes) insults.
2. Secondary insults are often the determining factor in outcome and, unlike primary injury, are amenable to medical intervention and, thus, are generally the focus of care.
3. Increases in ICP are deleterious because of herniation or ischemia (due to decreased cerebral blood flow), and the first-order attempt to avoid ischemia should be maintaining the cerebral perfusion pressure at greater than 60 mm Hg.
4. Assessment of the head-injured patient requires evaluation of (a) level of consciousness (using the Glasgow Coma Scale); (b) pupil asymmetry, dilation, or loss of light reflex; and (c) best motor response to painful stimulus.
5. Computed tomography is the diagnostic test of preference and should be used serially in settings of increased risk of progression of TBI.
6. Initial increases in ICP are treated by removal of mass lesions (blood collections or edematous injured brain), cerebrospinal fluid drainage, mild hyperventilation ($PaCO_2$ 30 to 35 mm Hg), or hyperosmolar therapy using mannitol or hypertonic saline to decrease edema. Hyperventilation should be avoided early ($PaCO_2$ 35 to 38 mm Hg) and used cautiously ($PaCO_2$ 30 to 35 mm Hg) later to treat unresponsive elevated ICP.
7. Refractory ICP elevation may be treated medically with more aggressive hyperventilation ($PaCO_2$ <30 mm Hg), barbiturates, or hypothermia, generally guided by aggressive, multimodality monitoring. Decompressive craniectomy constitutes an effective surgical treatment for refractory intracranial hypertension.

EPIDEMIOLOGY

In the field of trauma, other than for exsanguinating injuries, brain trauma is the injury most commonly responsible for mortality, accounting for about half of deaths at the scene. The injuries are generally blunt, occurring most frequently in motor vehicle crashes (MVCs). As many as two thirds of all MVC victims sustain some degree of brain injury. Complications from closed head injuries are the single largest cause of morbidity and mortality in patients who reach the hospital alive. Of patients who require long-term rehabilitation, head trauma is usually the primary injury.

These data are generally applicable to children as well. Although the mechanisms vary, head injuries are the major cause of morbidity and mortality in childhood trauma victims, accounting for an annual mortality rate of 1 per 1,000 in this age group.

Recently, with the aging of the population, a new spectrum of brain injury is blossoming, consisting of persons aged 60 years or older whose primary mechanism of injury is a fall. These patients have less inherent neurologic plasticity, limiting their recovery potential. As well, they often have significant comorbidities and may be on one or more anticoagulants. Management of these patients often takes a course differing from that optimal for the younger population.

In the mid-1990s, gunshot wounds surpassed other mechanisms as the most common cause of brain injuries.[1] Because of a case mortality ratio of approximately 94%, however, they continue to represent only a fraction of the brain injuries that come to definitive hospital care. In addition, because civilian gunshot wounds to the head are frequently isolated injuries, their spectrum of care varies more toward individual neurosurgical management.

PATHOPHYSIOLOGY

1 Traumatic injury to the brain involves a primary brain injury that occurs at impact and leads to disruption of brain substance and blood vessels. In addition, secondary brain injury may result from hypoxia, hypotension, pyrexia, the effects of increased intracranial pressure (ICP), and altered cellular biochemical processes that are often ongoing long after the primary insult.

Primary Injury

Energy transfer to the head causes direct disruption of neurons, glia cells, and microvasculature localized at the area of impact. As the brain rebounds within the skull, it is also vulnerable to impact with the opposite inner table. Therefore, countercoup injury to the contralateral brain is relatively common, in some cases being the more severe site of damage.

Particularly when the mechanism includes rotational forces, head trauma can result in widespread disruption of white matter axons throughout the brain, producing the condition termed *diffuse axonal injury* (DAI). Such injuries often damage a large number of widely distributed neurologic systems. When such injuries involve ascending pathways in both hemispheres or in the brainstem, the result is a depressed level of consciousness. The brain is also subject to torsion injury resulting from rotation around the fixed brainstem. This type of injury can damage the reticular activating system, producing unconsciousness.

Intracranial hemorrhage can take many forms. Direct laceration of epidural arteries from impact fractures or bleeding from fracture lines produces epidural hematomas, which damage the brain by compression. Disruption of bridging subdural veins and bleeding from cortical tissue damage produces a subdural hematoma, which is generally associated with disruption of underlying brain tissue. Intracerebral contusions, lacerations, and hematomas are caused by direct tissue disruption with associated vascular injury, producing neuronal damage and intraparenchymal bleeding.

Penetrating injury damages the brain through tissue injury caused directly by the projectile and, in the case of projectiles with relatively high velocity, result in disruption of neural tissue at a greater distance from the track via cavitation injury. In survivors, the extent and degree of the cavitation injury (related linearly to the mass and in a squared fashion to the velocity of the projectile) are often the primary determinant of outcome. Another source of morbidity is vascular injury, producing aneurysms, pseudoaneurysms, and other vascular anomalies that may present immediately or be delayed.

Whether a projectile or direct impact causes contusion, subdural hematoma, epidural hematoma, or diffuse axonal injury, little can be done therapeutically to change the magnitude or location of the primary injury once it has occurred. As such, most of our present care focus is on secondary injuries.

Secondary Injury

Secondary brain injuries result from events occurring after the primary insult, either from the direct consequences of the process initiated by the primary injury or from deleterious
2 exogenous influences. The occurrence and magnitude of secondary insults are often the determining factor in outcome from brain injury. In contrast to primary injuries, secondary insults are amenable to medical management and even prevention; they are the focus toward which the medical treatment of brain injury is primarily directed.

Primary tissue injury initiates a variety of biochemical processes, including free radical–mediated lipid peroxidation, excitotoxic "super-activation" of glutamate-aspartate neurotransmitter systems, and alterations in membrane receptor and ionic channel characteristics, among others. A variety of genomic processes are also activated, including apoptotic cell death, which is a focus of much current research. These processes can proceed for significant periods of time following primary injury and often are self-sustaining. The goal of the numerous clinical trials involving treatment of patients with brain trauma with various pharmacologic agents is to determine the means by which these processes may be attenuated or reversed. Unfortunately, to date, no clinically useful tools have been obtained from such research.

The primary external secondary injury processes occurring following brain injury are hypotension and hypoxia. Hypotension is the number one treatable determinant of severe head injury. A single episode of systolic blood pressure less than 90 mm Hg occurring during the period from injury through resuscitation doubles the mortality and significantly increases the morbidity of any given brain injury.[2] Furthermore, an early hypotensive episode strongly increases the probability of later intracranial hypertension. For these reasons, rapid and complete restoration of blood pressure is the most important goal in the resuscitation of the brain-injured patient. The old saw of "keeping the brain injury patient dry" by restricting fluids has been found to be completely erroneous and has been abandoned. Also for this reason, the somewhat unconventional suggestion of using pressors as temporizing agents during volume resuscitation has been incorporated into brain injury care.[2]

Hypoxia (apnea or cyanosis in the field or a partial pressure of arterial oxygen [PaO_2] <60 mm Hg) is also an independent predictor of poor outcome.[2,3] The frequency and magnitude of hypoxia have been notably decreased by modern airway management techniques, particularly early endotracheal intubation and assisted ventilation, in addition to ensuring adequate oxygen-carrying capacity through the avoidance of anemia.

Another important source of secondary injury is pyrexia. Fever is correlated with poorer outcome both by degree and duration.[3] Although the precise mechanism of this effect remains unclear, increased metabolism and the resultant metabolic recruitment of additional blood flow (and blood volume) is presumed to play a role.

Intracranial Pressure. ICP is a function of the aggregate volumes of brain, cerebrospinal fluid (CSF), and blood within the fixed intracranial compartment. Mild or slow expansion of one or two of these compartments can be buffered by compensatory decreases in either the CSF or blood compartments (into the spinal subarachnoid space or the venous sinuses, respectively). When this buffering capacity is exceeded, the compliance of the brain is compromised and small additional increases in any intracranial compartmental volume will produce marked elevations in ICP.

3 Intracranial hypertension is considered deleterious via two somewhat separable mechanisms: herniation and ischemia. Herniation occurs when a pressure gradient exists across an incomplete barrier, such as the tentorium, falx cerebri, or foramen magnum. It is deleterious because of the tissue damage that occurs and direct compression of adjacent vessels. Transtentorial herniation, the most recognized form, is manifest by anisocoria, motor posturing, autonomic disturbances, and death. The specter of herniation is the major determinant of the absolute threshold of ICP management, which is generally accepted as 20 to 25 mm Hg (although this range has not been well determined empirically). A major unanswered question is how ICP should be managed when separated from perfusion, both in terms of measuring the probability of herniation and in determining whether there are detrimental effects of elevated pressure per se. It is hoped that ongoing research in the area of cerebral compliance will produce clinically useful information regarding these issues.

The second deleterious aspect of intracranial hypertension is elevated resistance to cerebral blood flow (CBF), resulting in or exacerbating ischemia. This resistance can be very roughly approximated by cerebral perfusion pressure (CPP), which is defined as the difference between mean arterial blood pressure and ICP:

$$\text{CPP} = \text{mean arterial pressure} - \text{ICP}$$

Under normal circumstances, cerebral pressure autoregulation maintains CBF stable over a wide range of CPP (approximately 50 to 150 mm Hg) (Fig. 19.1). Following injury to the brain, this autoregulation is generally disrupted. This disruption can be complete, resulting in a pressure-passive system.[4] More frequently, the disruption is incomplete, characterized by a normal sigmoid shape but with abnormal elevation of the lower breakpoint above the normal value of 50 mm Hg (sigmoid dashed line). A probable consequence of this disruption is that a CPP that is satisfactory for uninjured patients may be associated with a lower CBF following head trauma (range of hypoperfusion).

In a pressure-passive system, cerebral blood volume (CBV) will increase in proportion to CPP. In such an instance, the goal is to keep the CPP just above the level of cerebral ischemia, thereby minimizing iatrogenic intracranial hypertension driven by increased CBV. In the situation of incomplete disruption, the goal is to keep CPP within the range of autoregulation, because this not only avoids ischemia but also may decrease ICP if autoregulatory vasoconstriction in response to increased CPP serves to decrease CBV.

Confounding this situation are reports that CBF may be disproportionately depressed during the early postinjury period. It is particularly critical, therefore, that CPP be supported assiduously from the first point of patient contact. Because hyperventilation causes vasoconstriction, thereby decreasing CBF, the use of hyperventilation during this early period is somewhat more hazardous than after the first 24 to 48 hours.

The preceding physiologic reasoning supported the increase in use of cerebral perfusion pressure therapy, wherein CPP was elevated to 70 mm Hg or higher throughout the course of intracranial hypertension. The efficacy of CPP therapy has been suggested by studies without internal controls reporting decreased morbidity and mortality associated with CPP therapy

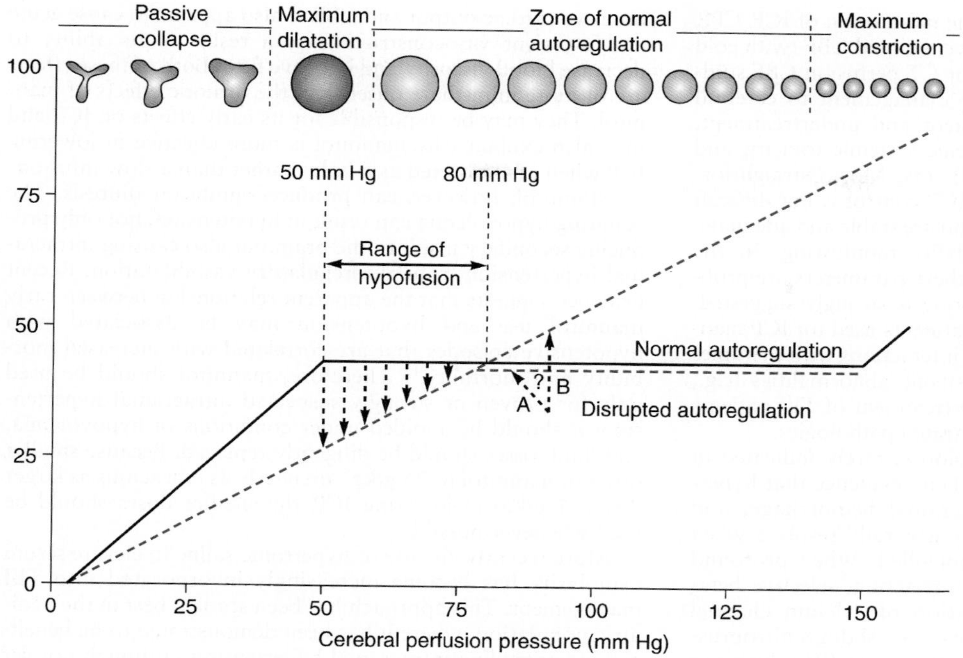

FIGURE 19.1. Cerebral pressure autoregulation. The normal relationship is indicated by the *solid line* with autoregulatory breakpoints at 50 and 150 mm Hg. Two disrupted states are also diagrammed. Complete loss of autoregulation (*straight dashed line B*) results in a pressure-passive system wherein cerebral blood flow (CBF) (and cerebral blood volume [CBV]) increases linearly with cerebral profusion pressure (CPP). The more common form of disruption is indicated by the sigmoid (*dashed line A*) where the major alteration is a right shift in the lower breakpoint. The *circles* at the top of the figure represent the diameters of the resistance vessels in the normal situation. The area of the circles represents CBV. Shifting this relationship to the right by 30 mm Hg would represent the partially disrupted state. (© R.M. Chesnut, MD., reproduced with permission.)

as compared to historical controls that practiced more conventional ICP-based therapy. The result of such reports was that CPP-based therapy at significantly elevated values became widely accepted as standard practice.

Subsequent reports, however, suggested that such acceptance might have been premature. Potential errors in selecting the historical control groups against which CPP-based therapy results were compared have prevented differentiating the effects of artificially increasing CPP from those of simply avoiding in-hospital hypotensive episodes. When control groups are selected to address this deficiency, it becomes apparent that CPP-based therapy may simply be a proxy for avoidance of transient ischemia.[5] Such a possibility is further supported by analysis of data from the National Institutes of Health (NIH)-funded North American Brain Injury Study on Hypothermia, which suggested that dips of CPP below 60 mm Hg are much more highly correlated with outcome than the efficacy of maintaining CPP above 70 mm Hg.[6] In addition, it appears that elevating CPP may increase the duration of intracranial hypertension.[7,8] This might be caused by the elevation of hydrostatic forces favoring the formation of vasogenic edema, thereby iatrogenically prolonging brain swelling and ICP elevation. Finally, the results of a prospective randomized investigation of CPP-based versus ICP-based management suggest that there is no overall difference in outcome between the two strategies, with the major effect of CPP-based therapy being the alteration in the mode of exitus from early, ICP-related deaths to delayed mortality from systemic complications (especially acute respiratory distress syndrome [ARDS]).[9] Such considerations imply that, although attention to CPP (and, thus, cerebral perfusion) is important, the proper method of managing CPP remains to be determined. It is clear, however, that routinely elevating CPP to values above 70 mm Hg is not associated with improved outcome.[10] This is reflected in the most recent revision of the Guidelines for the Management of Severe Brain Injury wherein the recommended CPP threshold has been decreased to 60 mm Hg based on an updated evidence review.[11]

Ultimately, the goal of managing blood pressure and CBF is to maintain a level of perfusion that meets the metabolic demands of the cell. The major problem with managing traumatic brain injury (TBI) based on pressure measurements is that alterations in cerebral metabolism will be missed. This may be of significant importance because the usual course of cerebral metabolism is to decrease following injury, slowly returning toward normal in patients who improve. One implication of such a metabolic course is that CBF values that would be dangerous under normal metabolic conditions might be satisfactory when cerebral metabolism is depressed. Indeed, because metabolic flow autoregulation is generally preserved following TBI, low values of CBF might often reflect flow:metabolism matching. One result of such a course of metabolic change might be that CPP elevation is reasonable during the early (i.e., first 12 to 24 hours) posttraumatic period when metabolism is near normal and ischemia is both probable and extremely devastating. Subsequently, when metabolism falls, CPP elevation may not be necessary and, indeed, may be counterproductive.

Absolute metabolic information is not readily available in the clinical situation. The relative balance between metabolic needs and substrate delivery, however, can often be usefully estimated by monitoring the oxygen saturation in the internal jugular vein ($JVSO_2$) or the tissue oxygen tension in the brain (P_bO_2). Although limited by problems of averaging, incomplete sampling of the total cerebral tissue volume, and technical issues of accuracy, the monitoring of $JVSO_2$ is a clinically useful method of detecting some otherwise occult episodes of ischemia as well as tailoring therapy to individual patient needs as they evolve.[12] By adding measurement of the arteriojugular lactate difference (AVDL), some occult areas of ischemia or anaerobic metabolism can also be detected that would not be apparent if only $JVSO_2$ were measured.

More recently, it has become possible to measure brain tissue oxygen tension ($PtiO_2$) using implantable Clark electrodes. This makes it possible to follow the balance between oxygen consumption and delivery, thereby providing the potential of detecting actual ischemia. These electrodes are easily implanted, either in a tunneled fashion or through a threaded bolt. Although absolute thresholds have not been rigorously determined, values above 15 to 20 mm Hg are generally considered adequate and values below 5 mm Hg are associated with increasingly poor outcome in a duration-dependent fashion.[13,14] The major limitations of this system are the extremely focal nature of this monitoring and technical issues with reliability. Although there is theoretical attractiveness to monitoring at the border of focal injuries (the "penumbra"), most monitoring is performed within normal brain.

We have found that combining the monitoring of ICP, CPP, $JVSO_2$, AVDL, $PtiO_2$, and quantitative regional CBF (with cold xenon computed tomography [CT] or CT perfusion CBF studies) has allowed us to safely tailor management to cerebral needs, thereby avoiding overtreatment and undertreatment, minimizing the likelihood of iatrogenic systemic toxicity, and shortening intensive care unit (ICU) stay. Most "straightforward" cases of brain injury, where ICP control is not difficult and systemic determinants of perfusion are stable and adequate, do not require invasive multimodality monitoring. In the approximately 10% of cases where these parameters are problematic, however, expanded monitoring is strongly suggested. Given the toxicity of many of the treatments used for ICP management and their often unfavorable interactions with therapies that may be indicated for other systemic abnormalities (e.g., ARDS), it is important to avoid overtreatment of TBI patients by targeting interventions at demonstrated pathologies.

Treatment of systemic hypertension is rarely indicated in the patient with head injury. There is no evidence that hypertension promotes continued intracranial hemorrhage, and hypertension related to brain injury generally resolves when the intracranial hypertension is controlled. When profound hypertension requires treatment, short-acting, selective beta-blockers or intravenous (IV) titration of calcium channel blockers should be used. Vasodilators (e.g., sodium nitroprusside) should be avoided because they increase CBV, which can exacerbate ICP.

As noted, metabolic autoregulation is the other and somewhat more fundamental type of intrinsic CBF control. Vasoconstriction is nonlinearly proportional to pH and, therefore, subject to manipulation of partial pressure of arterial carbon dioxide ($PaCO_2$). As a result, hyperventilation-induced alkalosis produces vasoconstriction, resulting in a decrease of both CBF and CBV. Although the latter is beneficial in controlling ICP, the former is potentially deleterious and mandates caution when using hyperventilation. For reasons outlined earlier, hyperventilation is best avoided whenever possible during the early postinjury course when the risk of ischemia is extremely high. Also, because of rapid compensatory buffering of iatrogenic hypocapnic alkalosis, the beneficial effects of hyperventilation tend to be relatively short-lived.

Cerebral Edema and Osmolar Therapy

Cerebral edema during the early postinjury period is generally cytotoxic (intracellular). Later, vasogenic (extracellular) edema may also play a role in brain swelling. Although resulting from different mechanisms (cellular membrane dysfunction and blood–brain barrier breakdown), our present treatment for cerebral edema in trauma is limited to the administration of osmotic agents, most classically mannitol. Generalizing the documented efficacy of corticosteroids to decrease tumor-related cerebral edema to the setting of trauma-induced edema has proven to be ineffective and actually harmful and is now considered contraindicated.[11,15]

Hyperosmolar agents increase the osmotic gradient, drawing fluid from the interstitial compartment into plasma, thereby reducing brain volume. In regions where the blood–brain barrier has been disrupted, however, such agents are minimally effective and can actually leak into tissues.[16] Fortunately, the area of blood–brain barrier breakdown is generally much smaller than the area of edema that it creates so that hyperosmolar therapy is generally effective in lowering ICP. Nevertheless, caution should be exercised when there are large areas of suspected blood–brain barrier breakdown (such as in regions of infarction) where large-scale parenchymal sequestration of osmotic agents might exacerbate edema formation and increase local mass effect.

Mannitol also has other mechanisms of action. It creates an acute increase in intravascular volume, which may transiently improve cardiac output and CBF. It also appears to cause acute and transient vasoconstriction as a result of its ability to decrease blood viscosity and improve flow. Both of these effects are of more immediate onset than the osmotic effects of mannitol. They may be responsible for its early effects on ICP and may also explain why mannitol is more effective in lowering ICP when administered as a bolus rather than a slow infusion.

Mannitol, however, can produce significant diuresis. The resulting hypovolemia can result in hypotension, not only producing secondary insult to the brain but also causing intracranial hypertension from autoregulatory vasodilatation. Recent evidence suggests that the apparent relationship between early mannitol use and hypotension may be associated with hypotensive episodes that are correlated with increased morbidity and mortality.[17] Therefore, mannitol should be used only for proven or strongly suspected intracranial hypertension; it should be avoided under conditions of hypovolemia, and fluid losses should be diligently replaced. Because smaller doses of mannitol (0.25 g/kg) are nearly as efficacious as larger doses (1 g/kg) in lowering ICP, the smaller doses should be used whenever possible.

More recently, the use of hypertonic saline to elevate serum osmolarity has become increasingly incorporated into TBI management. This approach has been studied best in the pediatric population, where it has been demonstrated to be beneficial in controlling intracranial hypertension (although not yet rigorously shown to improve clinical outcome). In those studies, 3% sodium chloride solution has generally been used, infused at 0.5 to 1.0 mL/kg per hour. As a result of such publications, the Guidelines for the Management of Severe Pediatric Brain Injury contained recommendations placing the use of hypertonic saline–based osmotherapy at the same level as the use of mannitol, leaving the choice to the physician.[18]

In the treatment of adult TBI, hypertonic saline has been widely incorporated into routine therapy, with concentrations ranging from 3% to 23% being used for continuous infusion or "bolus" injection. Unfortunately, at present, there is little solid evidence available to help clarify the optimal usage of hypertonic saline in TBI. In bolus form, it appears effective in acutely lowering ICP, but comparison data on its relative efficacy and duration with respect to mannitol are lacking. Also, rapid infusion of higher concentrations of hypertonic saline through a central line can produce temporary asystole. When used for continuous infusion, hypertonic saline is effective in raising serum osmolarity while maintaining vascular volume and has widely replaced scheduled dosing of mannitol.

Regardless of whether mannitol or hypertonic saline is the agent used to raise the serum osmolarity, when withdrawing therapy, the serum sodium and osmolarity should be allowed to return to within normal limits prior to removing the ICP monitor. The risk of rebound intracranial hypertension associated with the administration of hypotonic solutions such as half-normal saline or lactated Ringer solution can thereby be minimized.

CLINICAL ASSESSMENT

The objectives during early clinical assessment of the patient with head injury are multiple and must be accomplished simultaneously. These include establishing adequate oxygenation, ventilation, and circulatory stability and evaluating the extent of brain injury while treating ICP elevations. Although some evidence indicates that systemic hypotension may infrequently be the result of a head injury, always initially presume that hypotension in a trauma patient is the result of hypovolemia. It is a significant error to withhold volume resuscitation in a misdirected effort to control cerebral edema.

During initial assessment, mental status changes cannot be presumed to be the result of drugs or alcohol, although routine toxicology screening is appropriate. It should be presumed

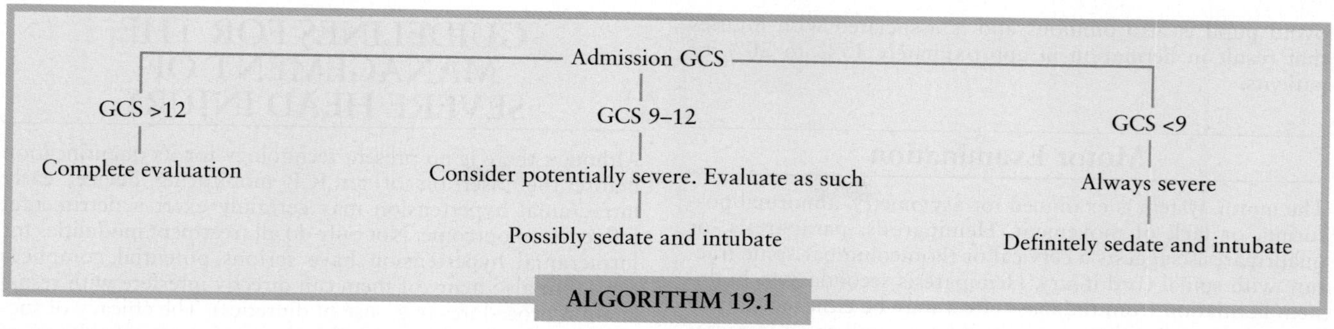

ALGORITHM 19.1. Glasgow Coma Scale (GCS) triage guide for initial evaluation of head injury. For the motor scale, the best response for any limb is recorded.

that any change in mental status or the neurologic examination in general, or any evidence of herniation (e.g., anisocoria), suggests an expanding intracranial mass lesion. Under such circumstances, therapeutic ICP reduction becomes the first priority and diagnostic imaging or surgical decompression must be accomplished emergently.

Do not assume that apparent neurologic unresponsiveness represents a lack of sensitivity to pain. Noxious stimuli, such as placement of urinary drainage catheters, nasogastric tubes, or IV catheters, can precipitate ICP peaks during resuscitation. These procedures should be done quickly and efficiently, optimally after sedation. Endotracheal intubation is particularly likely to induce herniation in borderline cases. Whenever practical, consider premedication with analgesics, sedatives, or IV or endotracheal lidocaine before airway instrumentation.

With regard to the brain injury, several critical assessments are necessary and should be precisely recorded because trends 4 are at least as important as any single observation. The three key parameters are level of consciousness, pupillary reflexes and size, and the motor examination.

Glasgow Coma Scale

The single most important assessment for a patient with head injury is to evaluate the level of consciousness. In this regard, the Glasgow Coma Scale (GCS) has become an international standard that is easily, rapidly, and reliably obtained (Algorithm 19.1). Components of the GCS include assessment of eye opening, verbal response, and motor response. It is not, and was never intended to be, a neurologic examination and should not be substituted for such information.

It has been suggested that early estimations of GCS, done in the field by emergency personnel, are often inaccurate.[19] In some areas, alternate, simpler systems (e.g., the AVPU scale) are accepted for this reason. The Guidelines for the Prehospital Care of Severe Brain Injury, however, support the continued use of the GCS for all prehospital care providers.[20] Special training has been developed by the Brain Trauma Foundation to optimize its accuracy (http://www.braintrauma.org/). The routine use of GCS provides a useful measure of initial injury severity and allows stratification for initial therapy as well as for outcome analysis.

For triage purposes, patients can be stratified using their GCS scores into those with severe injuries (GCS score <8), moderate injuries (GCS score 8 to 12), or mild injuries (GCS score >12; see Algorithm 19.1). Patients with severe head injuries require immediate endotracheal intubation, mechanical ventilation, and complete resuscitation; any clinical evidence of intracranial hypertension (e.g., signs of herniation) mandates maximal therapy to decrease ICP.

Many significant injuries occur in patients with GCS scores between 8 and 12. Although this is defined as the moderate injury group, all these patients require maximal brain resuscitation until a definitive diagnosis can be made. A patient with a GCS score of 12 or more tends to be confused but responsive to verbal stimulation. These patients need serial neurologic evaluations because they are in the group that can "talk and die" because of missed or delayed intracranial pathology. In general, for any brain injury, however, and whenever expedient, attention to other major injuries can take relative priority over cerebral imaging or management, whenever necessary.

Pupils

Pupillary asymmetry, dilation, or loss of light reflex in an unconscious patient usually reflects herniation because of the mass effect from intracranial hemorrhage ipsilateral to the dilated pupil. The probability of an intracranial mass lesion can be roughly approximated given the degree of anisocoria (≥1 mm or ≥3 mm), the mechanism of injury (± motor vehicle crash), and age (Fig. 19.2).[21] Occasionally, pupillary signs may indicate direct second or third nerve injury or trauma to the globe, but this must always be a diagnosis of exclusion. An unequal and nonreactive pupil is the cardinal sign that herniation is occurring, and rapid lowering of ICP is essential. An

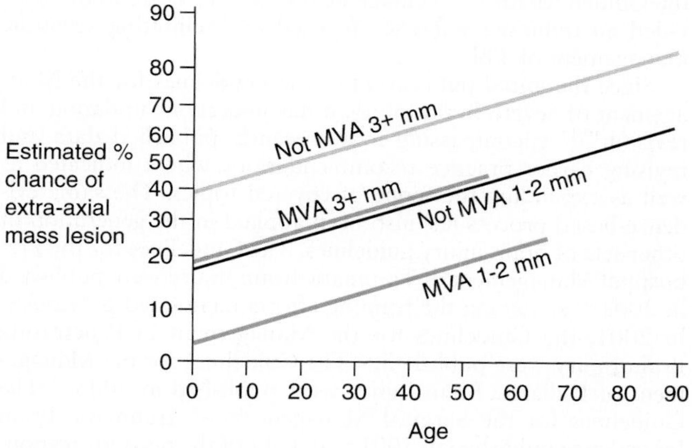

FIGURE 19.2. Estimated percentage chance of an extra-axial intracranial mass lesion greater than 25 mL as a function of degree of anisocoria, age, and mechanism of injury. Mechanism of injury was defined as motor vehicle accident (MVA) or other mechanism (not MVA). (Reproduced with permission from Chesnut RM, Gautille T, Blunt BA, et al. The localizing value of asymmetry in pupillary size in severe head injury: relation to lesion type and location. *Neurosurgery* 1994;34:840–845.)

ovoid pupil is also ominous and is associated with injuries that result in herniation in approximately 15% to 20% of patients.

Motor Examination

The motor system is examined for asymmetry, abnormal posturing, or lack of movement. Hemiparesis, paraparesis, or quadriparesis suggests a cervical or thoracolumbar spine fracture with spinal cord injury. Hemiparesis secondary to brainstem herniation from the mass effect may be either ipsilateral or contralateral to the side of the dilated pupil or an intracranial mass lesion.[21] Hemiparesis may also result from significant brain contusion. In the unconscious patient, a painful stimulus should be used to evaluate motor function. All four extremities should be examined and the results noted, because only the response of the best limb will be reflected in the GCS score.

INITIAL TREATMENT

Evidence-based Medicine and the Management of Traumatic Brain Injury

The publication of the first edition of the Guidelines for the Management of Severe Brain Injury in 1996 represented a significant step in standardizing the management of TBI based on published, peer-reviewed literature.[22] This document represents the application of a strict evidence-based process to 14 topics relevant to TBI care. Following an exhaustive, explicitly defined literature search covering each topic, the recovered literature was carefully classified along a three-point continuum of scientific rigor. As such, each article was ranked as class I, class II, or class III and the analysis of the scientific basis of each topic was predicated on the most scientifically rigorous (highest literature class) reports available. This process produced a set of standards, guidelines, and options for treatment where **standards** (based on class I evidence) represent principles with a high degree of clinical certainty, **guidelines** (based on class II evidence) reflect principles with a moderate degree of clinical certainty, and **options** (based on class III evidence) reflect principles for which unclear clinical certainty exists. By specifically defining the scientific foundation on TBI management issues, the Guidelines for the Management of Severe Brain Injury provided an unbiased reference focused on facilitating scientific management of TBI.

Since the initial publication of the Guidelines for the Management of Severe Brain Injury, it has undergone updating and revision[10,11] encompassing more recently published data and revising earlier practice recommendations where indicated as well as expanding the scope of covered topics. The same evidence-based process has also been applied in the generation of other sets of brain injury guidelines. The Guidelines for the Prehospital Management of Traumatic Brain Injury were published in 2002,[20] spawning the training efforts mentioned previously. In 2001, the Guidelines for the Management of Penetrating Brain Injury were published.[23] The Guidelines for the Management of Pediatric Brain Injury were published in 2003.[18] The Guidelines for the Surgical Management of Traumatic Brain Injury were published in 2001.[24] In light of the need for responsiveness of all evidence-based reports to the publication of new literature, the Brain Trauma Foundation has established a process to ensure that all of these reports are regularly updated and expanded through the Neurosurgical Evidence-based Medicine Center at the University of Washington.

Wherever applicable, the findings contained in these guidelines have been incorporated into this text. For details, the reader is referred to the source documents.

GUIDELINES FOR THE MANAGEMENT OF SEVERE HEAD INJURY

Although there is no present technology for its quantification before the insertion of an ICP monitoring device, early intracranial hypertension may certainly exert a detrimental influence on outcome. Not only do all treatment modalities for intracranial hypertension have serious potential complications, but also many of them can directly interfere with resuscitation procedures (e.g., use of diuretics). The efficacy of successful systemic resuscitation in improving the likelihood of survival from trauma in general is well accepted. In addition, the acknowledged negative influence of secondary insults (e.g., hypotension and hypoxia) on outcome from severe head injury renders systemic resuscitation a *condicio sine qua non*, which provides a vital infrastructure on which treatment of intracranial hypertension must be based. Therefore, all treatment must be consistent with optimal systemic resuscitation. When definite signs of transtentorial herniation occur, they should be interpreted as definitive evidence of intracranial hypertension and prompt, rapid, and definitive treatment specifically focused toward lowering ICP should be implemented consistent with continued physiologic resuscitation.

The composition and volume of the IV fluids used to resuscitate patients with head injuries should be selected with the purpose of restoring intravascular blood volume. Although the widely disseminated but scientifically unsupported adage of "keeping TBI patients dry" has now been discarded, the concept of restricting free water remains desirable. As such, isotonic crystalloid solution in the form of 0.9% normal saline (NS) is preferable to lactated Ringer solution as a resuscitation fluid for TBI. For some time, a growing body of indirect scientific support appeared to support the use of 250 mL of 7.5% NS as the first resuscitation fluid in TBI victims.[25–27] However, a recent randomized controlled trial from Australia has suggested that this may not be of benefit under optimal resuscitation conditions.[28] The branch of the ongoing Resuscitation Outcomes Consortium (ROC) Hypertonic Saline Trials focusing on prehospital treatment of TBI patients is currently attempting to readdress this problem.

The endpoints of resuscitation do not change depending on the presence or absence of a head injury. Blood volume should be normal, with an appropriate blood pressure and central venous pressure, adequate urine output and peripheral perfusion, and progressive improvement of any base deficit. The systolic blood pressure should never be allowed to drop below 90 mm Hg. Some evidence indicates an advantage to targeting a mean arterial pressure of 80 to 90 mm Hg during resuscitation until ICP monitoring can be initiated. Once ICP is available, a minimal CPP of 60 mm Hg should initially be the goal.

Resuscitation in the Absence of Clinical Signs of Herniation

Algorithm 19.2 is based on the Guidelines for the Management of Severe Brain Injury[10,11,22] and the Guidelines for the Prehospital Management of Severe Brain Injury[20] for use by prehospital and initial at-hospital care providers and emergency physicians to guide decision making in resuscitating TBI victims and determining the necessity of ICP-lowering therapy. "Signs of increased ICP" implies pupillary abnormalities, motor posturing, or neurologic deterioration not related to medications. When these signs are not present, mannitol is not given and the goal of ventilation is eucapnia. When such signs are present, the patient is hyperventilated to a $PaCO_2$ of 30 to 35 mm Hg and mannitol may be given if the patient's volume status is normal.

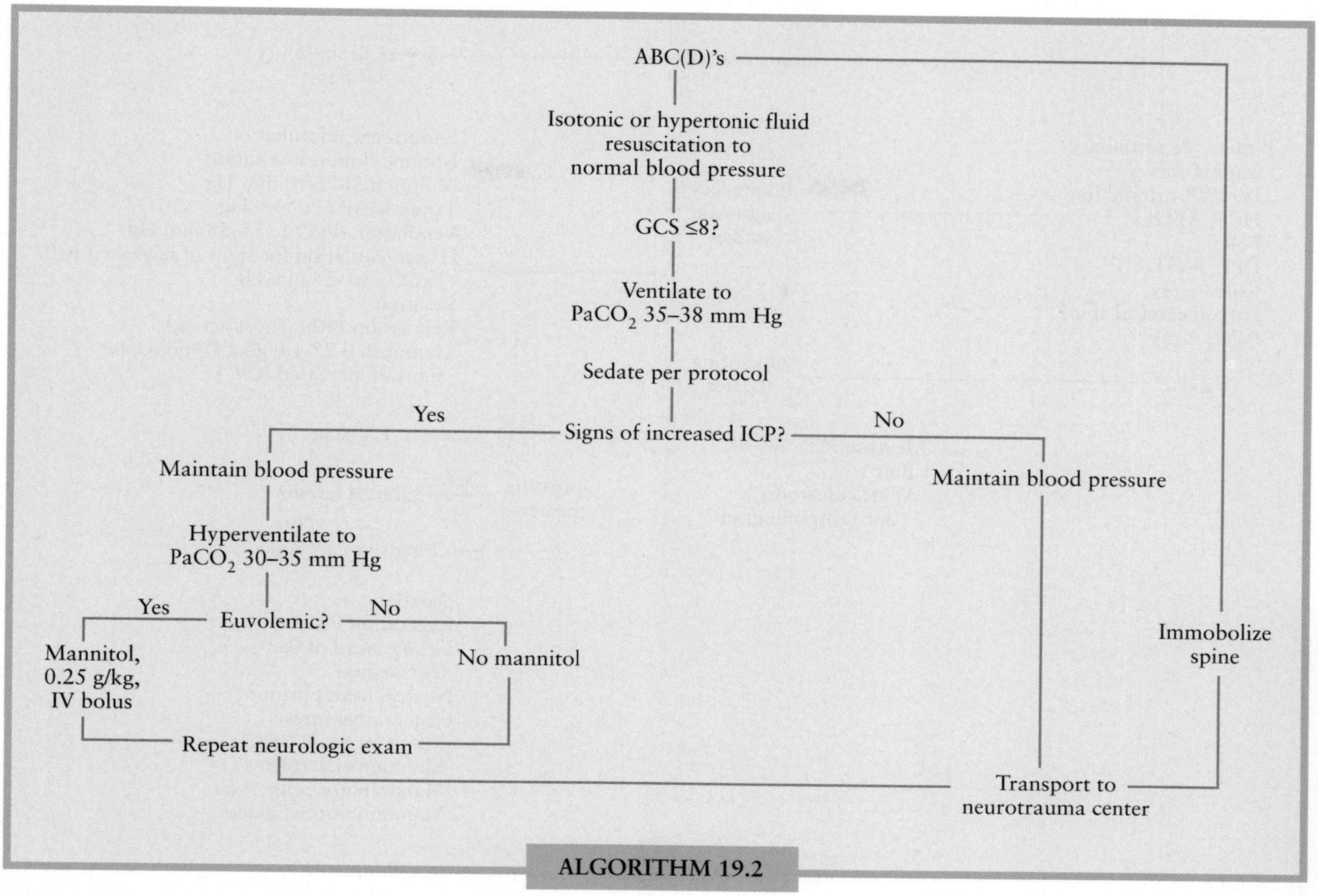

ALGORITHM 19.2. Prehospital evaluation and treatment of a patient with severe traumatic brain injury. "Signs of increased ICP" is the decision point for determining the necessity of intracranial pressure (ICP)-lowering therapy. These signs include pupillary abnormalities, motor posturing, or neurologic deterioration not related to medications. The order of steps is determined by the risk-benefit ratio for individual treatment maneuvers. This algorithm should be viewed as "expert opinion" and used as a framework, which may be useful in guiding an approach to field management of such patients. (© R.M. Chesnut, MD., FCCM, reproduced with permission.)

Algorithm 19.3 is based on the Guidelines for the Management of Severe Brain Injury[10,11,22] for evaluation and treatment of the severe TBI patient from arrival at the trauma center prior to the placement of an ICP monitor. As with any trauma patient, the first step is Advanced Trauma Life Support (ATLS) resuscitation. When appropriate, brain-specific therapies are incorporated into the treatment course. Brain-friendly initial ICU management should lead directly to monitoring of ICP.

Elevating the head of the bed (reverse Trendelenburg position in the absence of clearance of the axial skeleton) has been shown to generally lower the CPP in the absence of adequate volume resuscitation.[29] Because this may elevate the ICP per se, it is not advised until complete resuscitation has been accomplished.

The confusion and agitation often attendant to head injury often can drive intracranial hypertension and renders sedation desirable. Therefore, patients with suspected head injury should generally receive sedatives and analgesics whenever possible. Particularly in the TBI patient, the difference between sedation and analgesia should be kept in mind and the two agents titrated specific to their respective indications. Short-acting agents are preferable in the interest of following the neurologic examination.

In addition to eliminating any possibility of spontaneous ventilation and mandating complete ventilatory control, pharmacologic relaxation has the undesirable effect of limiting the neurologic examination to the pupils and the CT scan. Its use in the absence of evidence of herniation, therefore, should be limited to situations where sedation and analgesia alone are not sufficient to optimize safe and efficient patient transport and resuscitation.

The "prophylactic" administration of mannitol is not suggested, because of its volume-depleting diuretic effect. In addition, although it is desirable to approximate the lower end of the normal range of $PaCO_2$ during transport of a patient suspected of having brain injury, the risk of exacerbating early ischemia by vigorous hyperventilation outweighs the questionable benefit in the patient without evidence of herniation. Therefore, ventilation parameters consistent with optimal oxygenation and "normal" ventilation are recommended. The minute ventilation should be targeted at 100 mL/kg per minute until quantitative measurement of end-tidal carbon dioxide ($EtCO_2$) or $PaCO_2$ is available. The Guidelines for the Prehospital Management of Severe Brain Injury suggest the use of $EtCO_2$ monitoring during prehospital resuscitation and transport whenever possible. In the absence of signs of intracranial hypertension, ventilation should be adjusted to accomplish a $PaCO_2$ of 35 mm Hg when arterial gas values become available.

Resuscitation in the Presence of Clinical Signs of Herniation

Signs of intracranial hypertension consist of evidence of transtentorial herniation (pupillary dilation or loss of reactivity

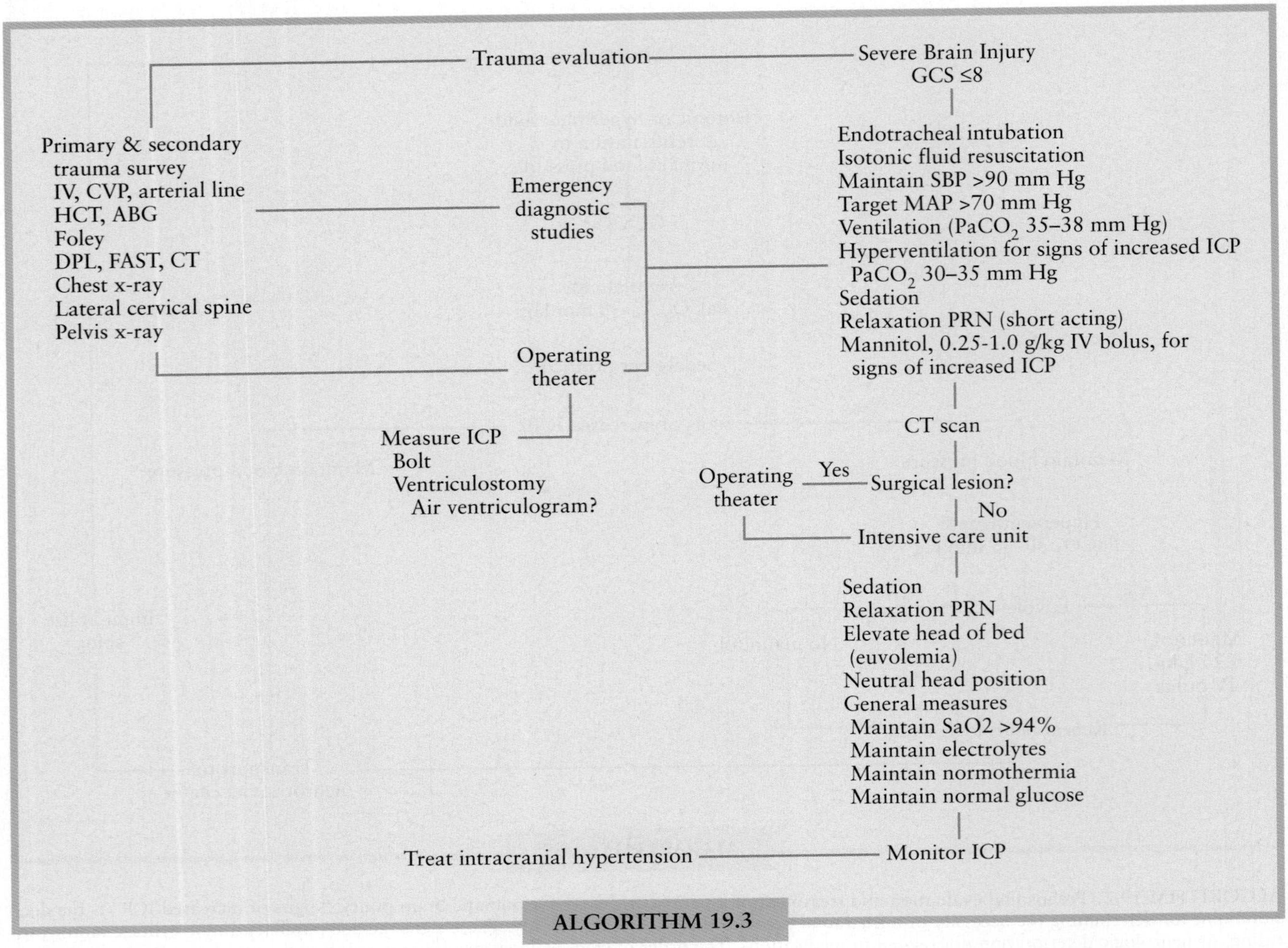

ALGORITHM 19.3. Evaluation and treatment of the patient with severe traumatic brain injury on arrival at the trauma center. The order of steps is determined by the risk-benefit ratio for individual treatment maneuvers. This algorithm should be viewed as "expert opinion" and used as a framework, which may be useful in guiding an approach to initial hospital management of such patients prior to the initiation of ICP monitoring. (© R.M. Chesnut, MD., reproduced with permission.)

or motor posturing or flaccidity) or progressive neurologic deterioration not attributable to other causes (e.g., sedation). When such signs occur, aggressive treatment of suspected intracranial hypertension is indicated. Hyperventilation to a $PaCO_2$ target of approximately 30 mm Hg should be accomplished by increasing the minute ventilation to approximately 120 to 140 mL/kg per minute or as directed by quantitative CO_2 monitoring. Because hypotension can produce both neurologic deterioration and intracranial hypertension, the use of mannitol is less desirable unless adequate volume resuscitation has been accomplished. If such is the case, however, mannitol should be administered by bolus infusion. Under such circumstances, it is critical that the diagnosis and treatment of the neurologic injury be accomplished with utmost haste. These patients must be transported to a trauma center with neurosurgical coverage.

Radiographic Priorities

Neurosurgical evaluation and assessment are initiated as soon
5 as the potential for significant head injury is realized. Prompt radiographic evaluation is essential and CT scanning is the imaging modality of choice for virtually all acute neurologic conditions. Patients with mild head injuries can usually be observed with sequential examinations and radiographic evaluation may be unnecessary unless the results determine whether the patient can be discharged from the hospital. In contrast, however, a cogent argument can be made for the liberal application of CT scanning to even patients with minimal evidence of TBI as a method of making safe, efficient, and economic triage decisions.[30] In any instance, evidence of neurologic deterioration or the occurrence of a situation wherein the neurologic examination cannot be followed (e.g., the need for general anesthesia) mandates CT scanning, intraoperative ICP monitoring, or both. General indications for neurologic imaging (generally, CT scanning) are listed in Table 19.1.

Patients with moderate or severe injuries require prompt neurosurgical consultation and rapid radiographic evaluation using the CT scanner. Hemodynamically stable patients with significant neurologic deterioration should go to the CT scanner immediately following ATLS resuscitation. In hemodynamically unstable patients who require immediate surgical intervention to sustain intravascular volume, lifesaving exploratory thoracotomy or laparotomy must take precedence. In such cases, it is a mistake to delay further investigation of the intracranial compartment pending the end of the case and transport to the CT scanner. A number of methods can be employed to evaluate the intracranial compartment during such lifesaving, extracranial surgery, including insertion of an

TABLE 19.1 DIAGNOSIS

INDICATIONS FOR NEUROLOGIC IMAGING

- Suspected skull penetration by a foreign body
- Discharge of cerebrospinal fluid (CSF), blood, or both from the nose
- Hemotympanum or discharge of blood or CSF from the ear
- Protracted unconsciousness
- Altered state of consciousness at the time of examination
- Focal neurologic signs or symptoms
- Any situation precluding proper surveillance
- Head injury plus additional trauma
- Possible head injury in the presence of additional pathologic findings, such as stroke
- Head injury with alcohol or drug intoxication

ICP monitor or ventriculostomy (with air ventriculography, if deemed necessary), transcranial Doppler evaluation, or even placement of exploratory burr holes in the instance of herniation. For this reason, neurosurgical consultation should be initiated on arrival in theater rather than at the finish of the case.

At the other end of the spectrum, in cases where there is an obvious surgical brain injury, the choice and timing of diagnostic systemic maneuvers should be subject to modification. Such patients should be transported directly to theater and examinations such as focused assessment with sonography in trauma (FAST) or diagnostic peritoneal lavage performed as the patient is being prepped for craniotomy. In such instances, obviously, early communication between the trauma surgery and neurosurgery departments is critical.

The spine should be cleared radiographically or immobilized and protected in every patient with a severe head injury. Although only 13% of patients with severe head injuries have spinal cord injuries, the potentially devastating consequences of an overlooked spine injury require constant vigilance.

Plain Skull Radiographs. With the routine availability of 24-hour CT scanning capabilities, plain skull radiography has largely become obsolete in TBI. The likelihood of a surgical intracranial hematoma is strongly correlated with the presence or absence of a skull fracture if the neurologic examination is factored in.[31] Nevertheless, the superiority of CT imaging in all aspects of evaluating TBI has relegated the use of skull films to unusual circumstances.

Computed Tomography. The CT finding that correlates most highly with intracranial hypertension is compression or obliteration of the basilar cisterns (Fig. 19.3). Not only does this finding portend a stormy ICP course, but also the primary predictor of outcome in patients with this CT picture is the peak level of intracranial hypertension occurring during the first 72 hours.[32,33] When cisternal compression is paired with a midline shift of more than 5 mm, the prognosis is even more ominous. ICP monitoring should be immediately initiated in any patient with cisternal compression and intracranial hypertension should be vigorously treated. Such patients, particularly those with minimal evidence of contusions, die primarily from secondary brain insults, which implies that they are potentially salvageable.

Acute epidural hematomas correlate well with skull fractures. The most common association is a linear, nondisplaced fracture in the temporoparietal region, crossing the middle meningeal artery. The classic clinical course involves a lucid interval following a brief loss of consciousness with subsequent neurologic deterioration. However, such a course occurs in less than 50% of epidural hematoma cases, so clinical suspicion must remain high. The typical CT appearance is a high- or mixed-density concave extra-axial hematoma with smooth borders (Fig. 19.4).

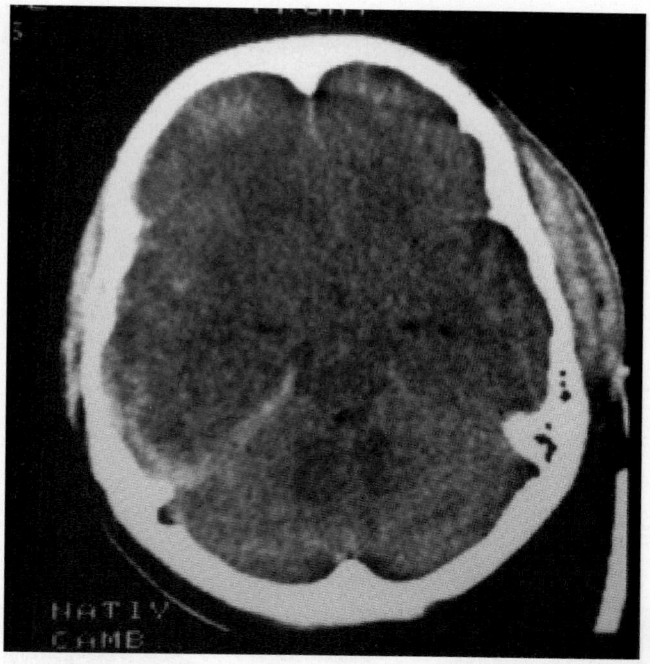

FIGURE 19.3. A computed tomography scan that is highly predictive of intracranial hypertension. The basilar cisterns are obliterated and the sulci are flattened.

Acute subdural hematomas occur over the convexity of the brain. The hematoma may evolve from rupture of bridging cortical veins or bleeding from the underlying parenchymal

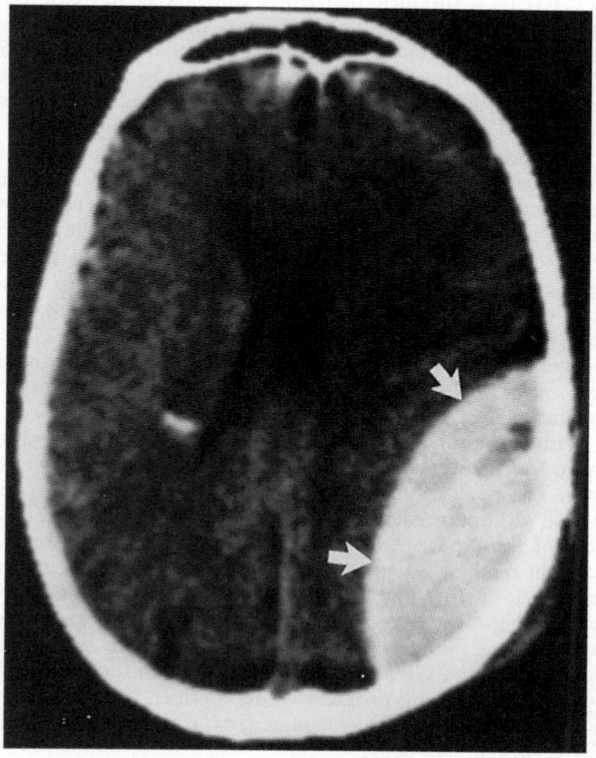

FIGURE 19.4. Typical computed tomography scan appearance of mixed-density, lens-shaped, acute epidural hematoma with mass effect.

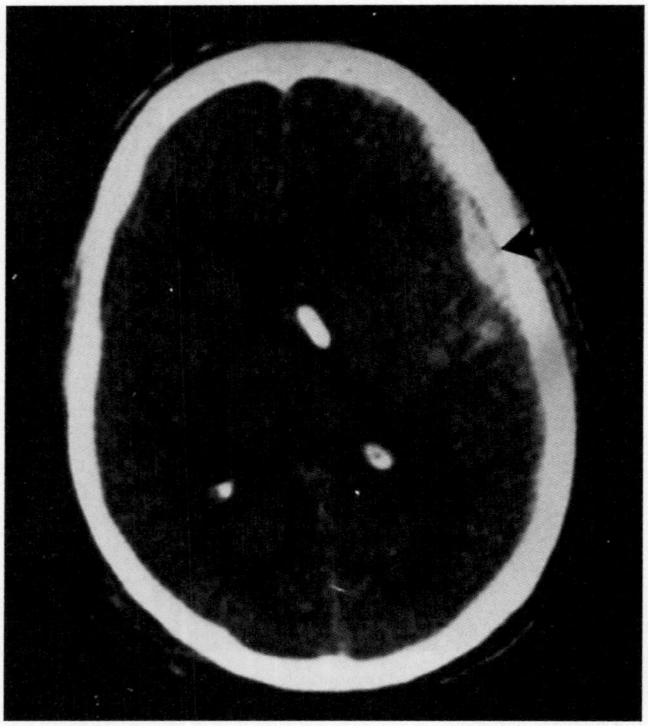

FIGURE 19.5. Usual computed tomography scan appearance of a crescent-shaped, high-density blood collection conforming to the contour of the cerebral hemisphere in a subdural hematoma.

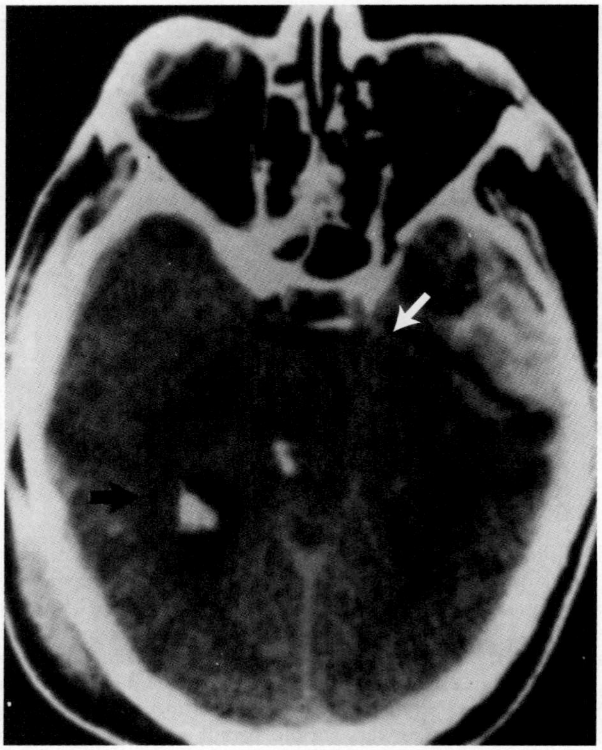

FIGURE 19.6. Contusion and associated intracerebral hematoma in the frontotemporal area.

injury, the latter being a common source. It is this subjacent tissue damage that generally determines the neurologic outcome of patients not succumbing to intracranial hypertension. On CT scan, a subdural hematoma appears as an extra-axial high- or mixed-density crescentic mass that spreads out over the hemisphere, following the cortical irregularities (Fig. 19.5). The midline shift may be out of proportion to the size of the hematoma because of the contributing mass effect from an underlying brain contusion or hemispheric swelling.

Intracerebral hemorrhage and cerebral contusion are common after trauma and are readily visualized with CT scanning. Brain contusion appears as a focal, heterogeneous density with hemorrhage interspersed with injured tissue (Fig. 19.6). Intracerebral hematomas are generally more homogenous in their high-density appearance. Both of these lesions tend to "blossom" over time because of some continued hemorrhage and the development of edema. It is important, therefore, to closely observe and monitor the ICP of such patients because significant and hazardous mass effect may evolve, requiring surgical extirpation.

With temporal or deep frontal contusions, late deterioration may occur, generally because of progressive edema development. The peak of such deterioration appears to be around 1 week, although cases have occurred as late as 10 to 14 days. Most of these patients will complain of severe or increasing headache or their CT images will show progressive edema formation. As such, a high index of suspicion must be accompanied by liberal use of follow-up CT imaging and, in particular, not dropping the level of surveillance until both the clinical situation and the CT appearance are stable. In the instance of such lesions showing progressive mass effect, the insertion of an ICP monitor may be considered, even in a patient with a relatively high GCS score.

The typical CT appearance of subarachnoid hemorrhage is a layer of blood over the cerebral cortex, layering over the tentorium and commonly filling the basal cisterns. Cerebral edema appears as areas of decreased density, which may be either focal or diffuse. Posttraumatic edema formation generally takes hours to days to develop unless compounded by hypoxia or hypotension. The "swollen brain" commonly seen in the setting of trauma may be caused by edema or increased CBV (unclotted, intravascular blood is low density). Diffuse axonal injury, typical of acute acceleration-deceleration injury, appears on CT scan as small areas of focal hemorrhage in the brainstem, thalamus or deep nuclear region, corpus callosum, and hemispheric white matter and may be accompanied by cerebral swelling. Finally, gunshot wounds or other penetrating injuries can be evaluated with CT scanning to allow accurate preoperative assessment of the anatomic injury for prognostic and therapeutic planning purposes.

One significant issue of recent origin is the "blossoming" or appearance of new lesions subsequent to CT images obtained at very short intervals following injury. Most of the "classic" TBI studies presented initial CT data from studies done hours following trauma. With improved prehospital transport and the ready availability of CT imaging, many initial studies are now performed 15 to 30 minutes after injury. As a result of such ultra-early CT scanning, there is now a risk of missing significant intracranial lesions by obtaining imaging before their appearance or during an early phase of their evolution. For this reason, in any patient with intracranial pathology or intracranial hypertension, we routinely obtain an early follow-up CT image at 4 to 6 hours after admission. Although such repeat imaging only uncommonly reveals new surgical pathology, documented lack of evolution may allow liberalization of the patient's care plan (e.g., transfer out of ICU or allowance of nonemergent extracranial surgery). Alternatively, any evidence of progression on follow-up CT imaging mandates that no decrease in surveillance should occur until further imaging establishes stability. At the time of follow-up brain imaging, a CT scan of the cervical spine can also be done in an effort to facilitate its clearance.

Ancillary Imaging. As noted earlier, there is a significant association between TBI and injury to the axial skeleton, particularly to the cervical spine. In addition, particularly when associated with basilar skull fractures or facial fractures, TBI suggests the possibility of damage to the major arteries of the neck. As such, particular attention should be given to careful radiographic clearance of the spine and consideration of studies such as CT angiography of the great vessels rostral to the aortic arch.

DEFINITIVE MANAGEMENT

Surgical Decompression and Outcome

Skull Fracture (Including Basal Skull Fractures). Depressed skull fractures are easily seen on plain frontal or lateral skull films and on CT. The mechanism of injury is usually a direct blow to the skull by a blunt object. Closed depressed skull fractures that are comminuted and those with a fragmented outer margin displaced beneath the inner table have characteristically been treated surgically, although growing evidence indicates that many may be treated nonoperatively if there is no neurologic dysfunction or CT evidence of underlying tissue injury. Open fractures are also generally treated surgically, although, again, growing evidence indicates that fresh, noncomminuted fractures without neurologic deficit, CSF or brain extrusion, gross contamination, or underlying tissue injury can be closed and treated with prophylactic antibiotics. When surgery is indicated, the goals are to débride the injury, accomplish secure CSF containment, restore cosmetic contours, and close the wound in a manner to ensure healing.

Basilar skull fractures are usually diagnosed with CT imaging or on clinical evidence, as they are poorly visualized on plain films. Clinical signs include otorrhea or rhinorrhea, subcutaneous ecchymoses overlying the mastoid region (Battle sign), bilateral periorbital ecchymoses (raccoon eyes), or hemotympanum. A basilar skull fracture may involve the paranasal sinuses, piriform sinus, petrous bone, sphenoid sinus, or sella turcica. Injuries to adjacent structures, such as the seventh or eighth cranial nerves, brainstem, and carotid or basilar arteries, are not uncommon. These are generally visualized with CT scanning, although special protocols may be required. If vascular injury is suggested (such as by fracture lines involving the carotid canal), CT or catheter angiography should be considered. In the acute CSF leak, no specific therapy is indicated. The leak should not be tamponaded unless it is brisk. Antibiotics should not be administered solely for prophylaxis of meningitis. Most CSF leaks stop spontaneously with minimal treatment (e.g., elevating the head of the bed). Leaks that continue more than 72 hours generally require temporary CSF diversion (e.g., via lumbar drainage or ventriculostomy). CSF drainage that does not respond to diversion will require surgery. Although most instances of rhinorrhea cease without surgery, the most common operation for persistent CSF leaks is exploration of the floor of the frontal fossa. The goal of such surgery is to identify the dural defect (often associated with herniation of a small tongue of brain tissue) and either close it primarily, patch it, or otherwise isolate the subarachnoid compartment from the skull base.

Mass Lesions. The possibility of a mass lesion must be entertained in any patient who develops evidence of herniation (see Fig. 19.2). Under optimal circumstances, this herniation can be reversed medically (with hyperventilation and hyperosmolar agents), allowing an emergent CT scan, which will demonstrate the location and size of any intracranial mass lesions and any herniation caused by nonsurgical processes.

When CT scanning is not immediately available or herniation is refractory to medical management, emergency trephination is a useful and lifesaving option. The first burr hole is placed in the ipsilateral temporal region and the dura is opened if an epidural hematoma is not in evidence (Fig. 19.7). If this exploration is negative, a second hole is placed in the opposite temporal region. If this is unrewarding, serial trephines are performed in the region of the parietal boss and the frontal convexity, first on the ipsilateral side, then contralaterally. A burr hole exploration is not negative until six holes have been drilled. A positive trephine is turned into a craniotomy, and the hematoma is thoroughly evacuated.

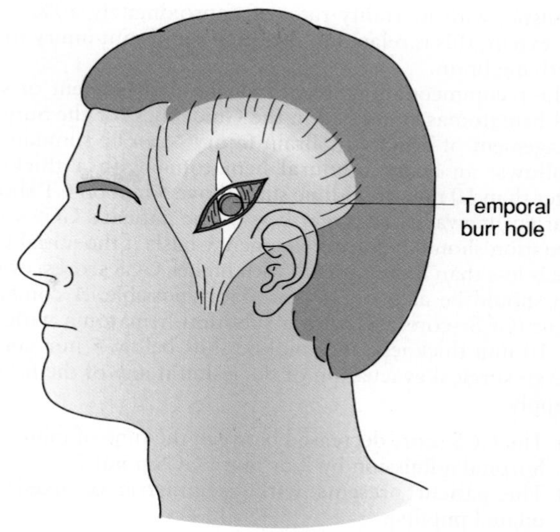

FIGURE 19.7. Location for placement of initial exploratory burr hole in the temporal region for emergency diagnosis and decompression.

Epidural Hematomas. Epidural hematomas are frequently of arterial origin and have a tendency to expand. Prognosis varies directly with level of consciousness at time of surgery, ranging from 0% mortality for patients conscious throughout, to 27% with the classic lucid interval, to over 50% if the patient never regains consciousness. Aggressive surgical management has resulted in an overall mortality of about 9%.[33]

The recommendations regarding the management of epidural hematomas contained in the Guidelines for the Surgical Management of Traumatic Brain Injury[24] can be summarized as follows: an epidural hematoma larger than 30 mL, clot thickness greater than 15 mm, or midline shift over 5 mm should be surgically evacuated regardless of the patient's GCS score. In patients with a GCS score of 8 or less, evacuation should be emergent. If the GCS score is higher than 8, evacuation should be done as soon as possible but must not interfere with other resuscitative efforts unless there is evidence of progressive deterioration. It is strongly recommended that patients with any acute epidural hematoma with anisocoria undergo surgical evacuation as soon as possible. Epidural hematomas of less than 30 mL, clot thickness below 15 mm, and midline shift less than 5 mm should be considered for evacuation because the risk of evacuation appears less than the dangers of enlargement and neurologic injury. Epidural hematomas of this size in patients with GCS scores above 8 may be considered for nonoperative management, including frequent neurologic monitoring in an ICU setting and serial CT imaging. Although the mean time for enlargement of such lesions is approximately 8 hours after trauma, they may occur at intervals up to 36 hours.

Subdural Hematomas. Subdural hematomas are the more common extra-axial mass lesion, particularly in non–motor-vehicle trauma. For subdural hematomas, the prognosis is less optimistic, with mortality rates of approximately 50%. To a great extent, this is related to the often significant injury to the underlying brain.

The recommendations regarding the management of subdural hematomas contained in the Guidelines for the Surgical Management of Traumatic Brain Injury[24] can be summarized as follows: an acute subdural hematoma with a thickness greater than 10 mm or midline shift above 5 mm on CT should be surgically evacuated, regardless of the patient's GCS score. Evacuation should be on an emergency basis if the initial GCS score is less than 8. In patients with higher GCS scores, evacuation should be as soon as reasonably possible. A comatose patient (GCS score ≤8) with a subdural hematoma with less than 10 mm thickness and midline shift below 5 mm should undergo surgical evacuation of the lesion if any of the following apply:

- The GCS score decreased between the time of injury and hospital admission by 2 or more GCS points.
- The patient presents with asymmetric or fixed and dilated pupil(s).
- The ICP exceeds 20 mm Hg.

Patients with subdural hematomas of less than 10 mm thickness and midline shift below 5 mm and GCS scores greater than 8 can be treated nonoperatively.

It appears that outcome from subdural hematomas is proportional to the timing of evacuation. When surgery is planned, it should be performed within 4 hours whenever possible.[34] If surgical evacuation of an acute subdural hematoma in a comatose patient (GCS score ≤8) is indicated, it should be done using a full craniotomy with or without bone flap removal and duraplasty.

All patients with acute subdural hematoma and coma (GCS score <9) should undergo ICP monitoring, including in the initial stages following evacuation.

Frequently, consideration is given to leaving off the bone flap and performing a duraplasty following the evacuation of acute subdural hematomas, particularly when the surgeon feels that there is evidence of brain swelling. Unfortunately, there is a relative dearth of information on this group of patients. An "in press" study of 155 such patients at Harborview Medical Center reveals that it appears to be effective in patients younger than 50 years of age and should be considered when the preoperative CT reveals intraparenchymal lesions or significant subarachnoid hemorrhage (Marcelo Vilela, unpublished data). In that group, the most powerful predictors of outcome in terms of variables amenable to clinical manipulation were postoperative intracranial hypertension (>35 mm Hg), CPP less than 60 mm Hg, or intraoperative hypotension (<90 mm Hg).

Parenchymal Lesions. Surgery for intraparenchymal mass lesions remains controversial. Arguments against surgery include the risks of the operation itself as well as damage to tissue that may otherwise go on to recover. Arguments for surgery focus on preventing the hazards of intracranial hypertension caused by the lesion itself or progressive edema formation as the lesion matures. Much of the difficulty in determining the applicability of surgery in individual situations arises from our inability to consistently predict which patients will rapidly deteriorate (e.g., proceed on to herniation) or fail nonoperative therapy by developing intracranial hypertension refractory to medical therapy. Unfortunately, this controversy has not been adequately addressed by well-done clinical investigations, so recommendations remain based on class III evidence. One thing that does appear consistent is that lesions of the anterior temporal lobe or the deep basilar frontal lobe are particularly dangerous because of the risk of precipitous herniation without impressive ICP elevation.

The recommendations regarding the management of traumatic parenchymal lesions contained in the Guidelines for the Surgical Management of Traumatic Brain Injury[24] can be summarized as follows: in general, patients with any lesion greater than 50 mL in volume should be treated operatively. Additionally, patients who have parenchymal mass lesions and signs of progressive neurologic deterioration referable to the lesion, medically refractory intracranial hypertension, or signs of mass effect on CT scan should be considered for surgery.

Patients with GCS scores of 6 to 8 should be treated operatively if they have frontal or temporal contusions greater than 20 mL in volume with either midline shift over 5 mm or cisternal compression on CT scan.

Patients with parenchymal mass lesions may be managed nonoperatively if they do not show evidence for neurologic compromise, have controlled ICP, and have no significant signs of mass effect on CT scan. Such patients should be managed with intensive monitoring and serial imaging. Surgery should be readdressed if difficulties with control of intracranial hypertension lead to consideration of "second tier" therapies (e.g., hypothermia or barbiturate coma) so as to avoid the secondary complications of such therapy. In all nonoperatively treated patients with parenchymal mass lesions, surgery should be considered before reaching the medical "point of failure."

Surgical management may involve decompression to "make room" for the lesion-induced swelling, evacuation and débridement of the offending lesions, or a combination. Because evacuation of such lesions does not always eliminate the development of intracranial hypertension, extensive craniotomy with expansible duraplasty and without replacing the bone flap should be considered at the time of operation.

Diffuse Injury. The mortality rate of diffuse brain injury is directly related to the significance of the associated intracranial hypertension. As such, the mortality rate of diffuse injury with open basilar cisterns is approximately 13%, whereas compression or absence of cisterns has an associated mortality rate of about 38%. Diffuse injuries are not amenable to surgical therapy unless decompressive craniectomy is indicated for control of intractable intracranial hypertension.

Diffuse axonal injury is a reasonably distinct subset of diffuse brain injury. It is characterized on CT scan as small areas of focal hemorrhage in the brainstem, thalamus or deep nuclear region, corpus callosum, and hemispheric white matter, which may be associated with cerebral swelling. Intracranial hypertension is an inconsistent part of this syndrome. When ICP is elevated, however, successful management improves outcome. These patients tend to recover to varying extents; many of them will significantly improve in their level of consciousness but will generally be left with diffuse neurologic deficits (e.g., spasticity, cognitive impairments). Although a favorable prognosis seems to be correlated with fewer lesions on imaging studies and early improvement in level of consciousness, prognostication is difficult in individual cases of diffuse axonal injury.

Posterior Fossa Lesions. Posterior fossa lesions are particularly dangerous because the progression from a benign lesion to a critical lesion is so precipitous and deadly. Patients may rapidly deteriorate from awake and alert to comatose, with signs of herniation ("upward" [caused by uncompensated swelling in the posterior fossa] or "downward" [from hydrocephalus]). Because of difficulties with the technology and uncertainty as to what pressures might be critical, monitoring of posterior fossa intracranial pressure is rarely performed. Vigilant clinical observation, tempered with a high degree of preemptive concern, therefore, represents the only form of monitoring currently applicable.

The recommendations regarding the management of traumatic posterior fossa lesions contained in the Guidelines for the Surgical Management of Traumatic Brain Injury[24] can be summarized as follows: rapid suboccipital craniectomy for evacuation of acute traumatic posterior fossa mass lesions is recommended in patients with neurologic dysfunction or deterioration referable to the lesion or mass effect on CT scan. Mass effect on CT scan appears as distortion, dislocation, or obliteration of the fourth ventricle; compression or loss of visualization of the basal cisterns; or presence of obstructive hydrocephalus.

In general, surgery is recommended for any clot larger than 3 cm in diameter, whereas conservative management may be considered with clots smaller than 3 cm when not associated with acute subdural or epidural hematomas. Because of the potential for rapid, unheralded deterioration, evacuation should be performed as soon as possible in patients with indications for surgical intervention.

Depressed Skull Fractures. Skull fractures are a common result of head trauma and, when closed and not displaced, rarely require treatment per se. When displaced (generally defined as beyond the inner table of the skull), surgical intervention should be considered for the management of underlying intracranial pathology or cosmesis. The best available evidence does not support elevation for the prevention or treatment of epilepsy. As such, nonoperative management of closed (simple) depressed skull fractures is a routine treatment option.

The recommendations regarding the management of traumatic open (compound) depressed skull fractures contained in the Guidelines for the Surgical Management of Traumatic Brain Injury[24] can be summarized as follows: treatment of open, depressed fractures is focused primarily on avoidance of infection. Cosmesis is a secondary consideration. In general, patients with open (compound) skull fractures depressed greater than the level of the skull inner table should undergo operative intervention to prevent infection. Indications for nonoperative management are given in Table 19.2.

When surgery is indicated, early operation is recommended to reduce the incidence of infection. Elevation and débridement is recommended as the surgical method of choice. Primary bone fragment replacement is a surgical option in the absence of wound infection at the time of surgery.

All management strategies for open (compound), depressed fractures should include antibiotics regardless of whether surgery is undertaken. The exact nature of the antibiotics used and the duration of treatment remain inadequately delineated in the existing literature. The general tendency is the use of broad-spectrum antibiotics (vs. gram-positive and gram-negative aerobic and anaerobic bacteria) for 1 to 2 weeks.

Penetrating Injuries. Penetrating injuries to the brain present several unique management problems, including the prophylaxis and treatment of intracranial infection, the possibility of epilepsy, and the risk of occult vascular injuries. The recommendations regarding the management of penetrating brain trauma contained in the Guidelines for the Management of Penetrating Brain Injury[23] can be summarized as follows: Although plain radiographs may be useful in determining intracranial trajectory, CT scanning of the head is the modality of choice in penetrating brain injury (PBI). In addition to the standard axial views with bone and soft tissue windows, coronal sections may be helpful in patients with skull base or high convexity involvement.

Angiography or CT angiography should be considered in patients with PBI. It is strongly recommended in cases in which the wound's trajectory passes through or near the Sylvian fissure, supraclinoid carotid, cavernous sinus, or a major venous sinus because of the increased risk of traumatic aneurysm or arteriovenous malformation. Sentinel signs of vascular abnormalities are large initial hematomas or the delayed development of substantial and otherwise unexplained subarachnoid hemorrhage or hematoma. When discovered, such vascular lesions should be definitively managed.

A major complication of penetrating injury is infection, both meningitis and abscess. Most infections occur within 3 weeks (55%) to 6 weeks (90%). The major risk factors appear to be CSF leaks, air sinus wounds, or wound dehiscence. The incidence of infection with the use of broad-spectrum antibiotic treatment ranges from 1% to 11%. Although the main causative agent appears to be *Staphylococcus*, gram-negative bacteria are also frequent and *Clostridium* or other anaerobic organisms may be found with appropriate culture techniques. As such, antibiotic prophylaxis is indicated in all penetrating injuries. The choice of antibiotics and the proper duration for their administration have not been formally investigated. Broad-spectrum regimens, including anaerobic coverage, lasting for 7 to 14 days appear to be a reasonable approach.

Seizures are much more frequent following PBI than nonpenetrating injury in general. Between 30% and 50% of patients with PBI develop seizures; 4% to 10% of those have their first seizure within the first week after injury and 80% during the first 2 years. About 18% may not have their first seizure until 5 or more years after injury. The risk decreases markedly with time. When followed for 15 years after a PBI, nearly 50% of patients with epilepsy eventually stop having seizures. Of patients with PBI, 95% remain seizure-free if they have no seizures during the first 3 years after injury.

Although there is a distinct lack of rigorous study, the increased incidence of early seizures has led to the recommendation that antiseizure medications (e.g., phenytoin, carbamazepine, valproate, phenobarbital) should be used during the first week after PBI. Prophylactic treatment with anticonvulsants beyond the first week after PBI has not been shown to prevent the development of new seizures and is not recommended.

The surgical management of penetrating wounds to the brain has undergone significant evolution over the past two decades. In the more distant past (and until recently, in terms of U.S. military policy), it was routine to fully explore penetrating injury tracts to completely remove all foreign substances. Reoperation was common for this purpose. Based on class III evidence from military actions of other countries (most from the Middle East), however, it is now recognized that outcomes are not measurably worse in patients who do not undergo aggressive débridement. At present, surgical débridement of the missile tract in the brain is not recommended in the absence of significant mass effect. As well, routine surgical removal of fragments lodged distant from the entry site or reoperation solely to remove retained bone or missile fragments is not recommended.

Treatment of small bullet entrance wounds to the head in patients whose scalp is not devitalized and have no significant intracranial pathology should consist of local wound care and closure. In more extensive wounds with nonviable scalp, bone, or dura, surgical management with more extensive débridement

TABLE 19.2 INDICATIONS/CONTRAINDICATIONS

INDICATIONS FOR NONOPERATIVE MANAGEMENT OF COMPOUND DEPRESSED SKULL FRACTURES

No clinical or radiographic evidence of:

- Gross wound contamination
- Significant intracranial hematoma
- Gross cosmetic deformity
- Frontal sinus involvement
- Dural penetration
- Depression >1 cm
- Wound infection
- Pneumocephalus

TRAUMA

followed by primary closure or grafting to secure a watertight wound is recommended. Closure of the dura and prevention of CSF leakage are extremely important goals in managing penetrating wounds. In patients with significant fragmentation of the skull, débridement of the cranial wound with either craniectomy or craniotomy is recommended.

Mass lesions should be surgically managed to prevent intracranial hypertension. As such, débridement of necrotic brain tissue and safely accessible bone fragments is recommended when they produce significant mass effect. As well, evacuation of intracranial hematomas is recommended if they produce significant mass effect as defined by the production of midline shift of over 5 mm or intracranial hypertension. This is one of the reasons that monitoring of ICP in penetrating injuries is an important adjunct to surgical decision making.

Repair of an open-air sinus injury with watertight closure of the dura is recommended.

Decompressive Craniectomy for Control of Intracranial Hypertension

Craniectomies done in conjunction with hematoma evacuation (usually on admission) must be separated from craniectomies done only for brain edema treatment (ICP/CPP management). The former consist of "leaving the bone out" and not closing the dura after surgery, which is done to evacuate extra-axial or intracranial mass lesions. Such surgery, per se, is not done simply to increase the size and compliance of the cranial compartment to allow for brain swelling. This procedure was discussed earlier in the section on subdural hematomas.

Craniectomies done solely to treat brain swelling involve intentionally removing very large bone flaps, leaving them out, and performing duraplasties to prevent the dura from constraining the bulging brain. The most common scenario is that of diffuse swelling wherein bilateral frontotemporoparietal flaps are removed. When edema is localized primarily to one hemisphere (producing intracranial hypertension with midline shift), unilateral craniectomy is usually performed. In both cases, the bone flaps are as large as possible and particular attention is paid to removing the temporal squame forming the lateral wall of the middle cranial fossa.

Other surgical approaches to managing the swollen brain include subtemporal decompression and temporal lobectomy. In subtemporal decompression, the procedure is focused entirely on removing the lateral wall of the middle cranial fossa to decompress the temporal lobe. Temporal lobectomy involves removing a portion of the temporal lobe to "make room." The right temporal lobe is generally chosen because of its less elegant nature. By definition, the operation involves removing undamaged or only partially damaged brain, which certainly decreases its attractiveness when alternatives exist. In addition, it is generally realized that the amount of room made by such operation is rapidly filled by swollen brain such that intracranial hypertension often soon returns. In the author's practice, this operation has been completely replaced by decompressive craniectomy.

The goal of decompressive craniectomy is to completely obviate further ICP treatment, whenever possible. To this end, extensive bone removal and duraplasty are recommended.

Although it has not been rigorously studied in well-controlled prospective fashion, the present evidence base definitely supports decompressive craniotomy within 48 hours of injury as a treatment option for patients with diffuse, medically refractory posttraumatic cerebral edema and resultant intracranial hypertension. One of the difficulties in determining the proper timing for such a procedure is the issue of when intracranial hypertension becomes medically refractory. The point of failure of second-tier treatments is a clear but quite delayed threshold point. In general, decompressive craniectomy should be considered as an option to instituting such second-tier treatment. In the interest of performing decompression before damage occurs from ICP elevation or cerebral ischemia, many support its use prophylactically as soon as a high degree of suspicion arises that medical management will fail before ICP control is attained. Examples of such decision points are patients with diffuse parenchymal injury with clinical and radiographic evidence for impending transtentorial herniation (e.g., obscuration of the basal cisterns or midline shift >5 mm) where the initial ICP is very high or where early management requires rapid escalation in the intensity of treatment.

Intracranial Pressure Monitoring. All patients with severe brain injuries and a significant percentage of those with moderate injuries require continuous ICP monitoring. The most recent revision of the Guidelines for the Management of Severe Brain Injury indicates that class II evidence supports monitoring of all patients with a postresuscitation GCS score equal to or less than 8 who have any CT evidence of intracranial pathology.[11] Class III level evidence supports monitoring in patients with severe TBI and a normal CT scan if they have two or three of the following: (a) age older than 40 years, (b) any history of hypotension, or (c) abnormal motor posturing. ICP monitoring in other patients is left to the discretion of the physician. ICP monitoring should be considered in any patient with a GCS score of 12 or less who cannot be closely monitored clinically or whose CT scan demonstrates evidence of intracranial hypertension (i.e., mass lesion, obscured or absent basal cisterns, or midline shift).

Although many techniques are available, the most common involve small fiberoptic or strain gauge catheter tip pressure sensors placed several millimeters into the brain or fluid-coupled catheters placed into the lateral ventricles. The minimally invasive catheters are reliable and have a very low complication rate, making them an ideal choice in instances where a minimum-risk ICP monitoring technique is desired (e.g., in a moderate head injury that needs general anesthetic). They are also useful when the ventricles are too small to cannulate or there is an uncorrected coagulopathy. Ventriculostomy catheters have the added capability of allowing CSF drainage for ICP control. They are technically more difficult to place, however, and the complication rate is somewhat higher. In any case, safe and effective monitoring technology is available for any instance in which ICP monitoring is desired.

Monitoring ICP not only provides early warning of herniation but also, by allowing calculation of CPP, opens up the possibility of more precisely optimizing CBF and preventing ischemic secondary brain injury. Because all methods of lowering ICP or raising CPP have potentially harmful side effects, using such agents to treat suspected intracranial hypertension without monitoring ICP is not recommended.

Monitoring of Cerebral Ischemia. One of the major influences of ICP on outcome is its interference with cerebral perfusion. It is concern for this aspect that has prompted the widespread incorporation of CPP management into TBI treatment as a rough estimate of cerebral vascular resistance. Much research has been done on cerebral perfusion after TBI but, given the variability of the cerebral metabolic rate following TBI, due to both injury- and treatment-related factors, it is much more valuable to monitor for cerebral ischemia. As noted previously, there are currently several methods that are readily clinically available for ICU measurement of the adequacy of cerebral oxygen delivery. Placing a catheter into the jugular bulb via a retrograde venous route allows sampling of the saturation of oxygen in the blood leaving the brain. Jugular venous oxygen saturation values below 50% are associated with cerebral ischemia and worsened recovery, whereas saturations above approximately 85% suggest hyperemic flow. Unfortunately, this method averages a large volume of the brain and does not include blood from all of the supratentorial parenchyma so that it cannot completely rule out ischemia. Looking for increased cerebral lactate production has been offered as a method of detecting cerebral ischemia that might be masked by the mixing of blood from ischemic and nonischemic areas, but the sensitivity of this measurement appears limited.

An alternative monitoring method is the insertion of an oxygen-sensing (Clark) electrode into the brain parenchyma to measure P_bO_2. P_bO_2 values of less than 20 mm Hg are suggestive of ischemia. There is a growing body of evidence supporting the utility of this method, although definitive studies remain to be done. This technique samples only a very small, focal volume of tissue, so its placement is a matter of some discussion. At present, it is generally placed into normal brain, although some argue that trying to place it into the penumbra of an injury site would be preferable.

Cerebral microdialysis constitutes a third method of monitoring for evidence of cerebral ischemia by allowing the measurement of tissue lactate and pyruvate and calculating the lactate/pyruvate ratio. Like P_bO_2 monitoring, this newer technique also samples a very focal region. At present, although cerebral microdialysis is very sensitive and is being used with growing frequency, it is primarily considered as a research tool.

Of note, these monitors are not mutually exclusive. They may be used to supplement each other or to verify findings from one technique that are suspect. Such a consideration becomes particularly important when significant prolongation or escalation of therapy is being considered based on an abnormal value from one monitoring system.

MEDICAL MANAGEMENT

General Measures

Aggressive restoration of intravascular volume, maintenance of adequate cerebral perfusion pressure, and avoidance of hypoxia are *conditiones sine quibus non* of medical treatment for intracranial hypertension. Volume resuscitation should be vigorous and thorough, with a target of euvolemia. The poorly founded, dangerous, and outmoded practice of restricting fluid volume should be abandoned. Restrict free water by using isotonic fluids, which makes normal saline preferable to lactated Ringer solution. Optimally, continuous monitoring of central venous and arterial pressures should be instituted early.

Control of pain and the response to noxious stimulation is necessary to avoid iatrogenic elevation of ICP. It should not be assumed that the comatose patient has a blunted pain response. Analgesia should be combined with sedation, using short-acting agents whenever possible to facilitate repeated neurologic examination. It is preferable to use sedatives that concomitantly decrease cerebral metabolism to increase the margin for hypoperfusion tolerance. Propofol and dexmedetomidine hydrochloride are good choices in adults for this reason.

The Guidelines for the Management of Severe Brain Injury do not support the early administration of antiepileptic medication for the prophylaxis of late seizures.[11] With respect to the prevention of early seizures (e.g., occurring within 10 to 14 days), prophylaxis does decrease their frequency but without proved benefit to outcome. As such, administration of antiepileptic agents for the first 2 weeks is at the discretion of the physician. One reasonable approach is to treat only in cases where seizures could compromise tenuous ICP control or when seizures are likely not to be detected (e.g., during neuromuscular blockade).

Fever will elevate ICP and is independently correlated with decreased recovery in severe TBI.[3] Local measures (e.g., cooling blankets, fans) should be used in conjunction with acetaminophen to keep temperatures below 37.5°C to 38°C when ICP requires treatment. Scheduled indomethacin may prove effective in cases where acetaminophen is not.

Venous drainage of the brain should be facilitated by avoiding constriction of the jugular system in the neck and elevating the head of the bed in euvolemic patients. In addition, attention should be paid to intrathoracic pressures, particularly when considering the use of positive end-expiratory pressure (PEEP) or continuous positive airway pressure (CPAP). Increased intra-abdominal pressure can also embarrass jugular drainage and elevate ICP.

Finally, meticulous general critical care is important, because the protracted ICU stay and the necessity for intubation, mechanical ventilation, and other artificial support systems significantly increase the risk of nosocomial and iatrogenic complications.

Recent investigations in the trauma population in general have demonstrated an increased risk of complications, such as the acute respiratory distress syndrome and the systemic inflammatory response syndrome, in patients who undergo transfusion. This has led to a reticence to transfuse and a strong tendency toward accepting hematocrit levels in the low 20s. On the other hand, evidence indicates that the injured brain is exquisitely sensitive to secondary insults such as ischemia. Unfortunately, there is little evidence that the damage caused by such events can be treated or reversed so that the general neurosurgical recommendation is to maintain an oxygen-carrying capacity that is higher than that afforded by such low hemoglobin levels, more commonly striving to values of approximately 30. As such, when the question of cerebral oxygenation arises in the setting of a hematocrit between approximately 21 and 30, monitoring the adequacy of cerebral oxygen delivery (e.g., by following jugular venous saturation or brain tissue oxygen tension) should be considered. In the absence of definitive studies, the choice of a general, empirical threshold for transfusion remains nebulous.

Control of Established Intracranial Hypertension. All of the previously discussed "pre-ICP monitoring" steps may be used in direct response to intracranial hypertension, their application and intensity tapered to achieve ICP control. These interventions should be considered the basic steps in this respect and should be optimized prior to adding further treatments.

6 Cerebrospinal fluid drainage, hyperventilation, mannitol, barbiturates, and so on are the mainstays of therapy to control documented intracranial hypertension. Each, however, has significant potential complications, which can obviate their beneficial effects. Therefore, they should not be employed unless intracranial hypertension is established by monitoring, and caution and vigilance must attend their usage. Although the treatment of intracranial hypertension is not the primary focus of this chapter, some brief comments will be useful.

As noted, the treatment of intracranial hypertension should be initiated on a base of adequate sedation and analgesia, control of fever, and optimization of systemic physiologic conditions that might exacerbate ICP elevation (e.g., intrathoracic pressure). Neuromuscular blockade may be added to sedation and analgesia if further ICP control is desired. It does not always work, so a trial is often considered. Blockade to the level of one to two twitches out of a train-of-four is a reasonable target in this population.

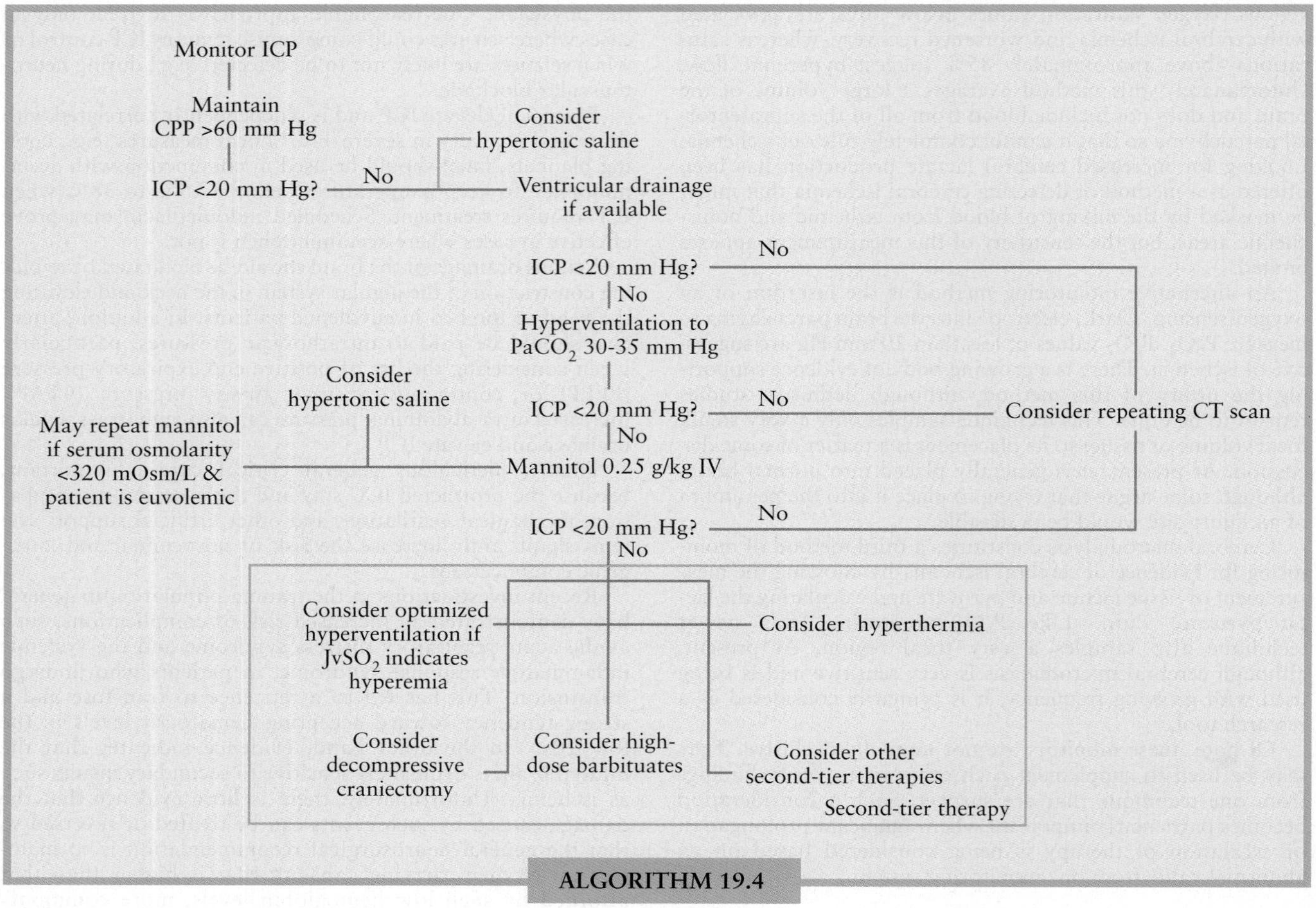

ALGORITHM 19.4. Treatment of established intracranial hypertension, based on the Guidelines for the Management of Severe Brain Injury. The order of steps is determined by the risk-benefit ratio for individual treatment maneuvers. This algorithm should be viewed as "expert opinion" and used as a framework, which may be useful in guiding an approach to elevated ICP.

Treatment for intracranial hypertension in adults from the original edition of the Guidelines for the Management of Severe Brain Injury is outlined in Algorithm 19.4. When consulting this algorithm, remember that it represents a consensus opinion (class III evidence) and that, for this reason, a treatment algorithm was not included in the 2008 revision (being left to subsequent, currently ongoing construction by a consensus development team). When this algorithm was developed, the role of hypertonic saline was not addressed.

When available via ventriculostomy, CSF drainage should be the first method of managing intracranial hypertension. There is no consensus on what pattern of drainage is most efficacious. It must be noted that ICP measurement cannot be performed when the ventricular catheter is open to drain. For this reason, we generally drain against approximately 10 cm H_2O for 2-minute intervals, then reclamp the catheter and measure the ICP. Requiring such cycling more than five times in 1 hour constitutes a need for consideration of therapeutic escalation.

As discussed, mannitol is useful for treating intracranial hypertension. There are no specific physiologic indications for the use of mannitol over other agents. Mannitol should be avoided under conditions of hypovolemia or increased serum osmolarity (i.e., >320 mOsm/L). When administered, mannitol should be given as a bolus. It appears that lower doses (e.g., 0.25 g/kg) may be equally as effective in lowering ICP as larger doses (e.g., 1 g/kg).[11] No adequate evidence exists to guide the choice between mannitol and hypertonic saline when osmolar treatment is being considered.

Hypertonic saline is becoming an increasingly common tool in the management of traumatic brain injury. Its efficacy in reversing intracranial hypertension has been best demonstrated in children, where administration of 3% NaCl to osmolarity thresholds of up to 360 mOsm/L and serum sodium levels of up to 160 mEq/L are tolerated. Because of a lack of outcome-based studies, however, the independent ability of such treatment to improve outcome remains unclear.

There has been a strong tendency to extrapolate such use of hypertonic saline to the treatment of intracranial hypertension in adults where it has been less well studied. For continuous intravenous infusion, doses are generally in the 0.5- to 1.0-mEq/kg per hour range and concentrations of 3% to 5% are commonly used. For "bolus" injection in response to an episode of intracranial hypertension, concentrations ranging from 3% to 23% are being used with the caveat (noted earlier) that the rate of injection of the higher concentrations into central lines should be limited in view of transient adverse effects on myocardial conductivity.

The tolerable limits for serum osmolarity and sodium levels have not been well defined in adults, but the levels used in children appear to be reasonably tolerated. A risk of rebound cerebral edema appears to exist when levels are allowed to drop too quickly after the administration of 3% saline is stopped. Our present practice is to not consider the patient "out of the woods" for such rebound until the serum sodium has returned to within normal limits. As such, we generally leave the ICP monitor in place and caution against major, nonemergent surgical cases.

Hyperventilation is generally effective in lowering ICP. As noted, however, it works on the arterial side, via vasoconstriction-induced decreases in CBV, which allows the possibility of inducing ischemia by embarrassing CBF. At present, no clinically applicable method exists for measuring CBV, and it is unclear how often elevated CBV per se is a primary physiologic abnormality in intracranial hypertension. Therefore, lowering CBV to treat intracranial hypertension includes risks that need be minimized.

In keeping with the Guidelines for the Management of Severe Brain Injury, hyperventilation ($PaCO_2$ <35 mm Hg) should be avoided during the first 24 hours following TBI.[11] Thereafter, if intracranial hypertension continues, hyperventilation to $PaCO_2$ values between 30 and 35 mm Hg may be considered. Whenever hyperventilation is used, and certainly when $PaCO_2$ values of less than 30 mm Hg are targeted, methods of monitoring the effects on CBF or flow-perfusion matching should be considered, such as quantitative CBF measurement, jugular venous saturation monitoring, or following cerebral tissue oxygen saturation.

7 When ICP control does not respond to these management steps, second-tier therapies should be considered. These include barbiturate therapy, hypothermia, decompressive craniectomy, and optimized hyperventilation (among other approaches). The details of the choice between second-tier agents are beyond the scope of this chapter. In general, the choice should be based on and directed using as much multimodality monitoring as is available, because the risk-benefit ratio of most of these treatments is very narrow.

References

1. Centers for Disease Control. Surveillance data on traumatic brain injury. *MMWR Morb Mortal Wkly Rep* 1997;46:8–11.
2. Chesnut RM, Marshall LF, Klauber MR, et al. The role of secondary brain injury in determining outcome from severe head injury. *J Trauma* 1993;34:216–222.
3. Jones PA, Andrews PJ, Midgley S, et al. Measuring the burden of secondary insults in head-injured patients during intensive care. *J Neurosurg Anesthesiol* 1994;6:4–14.
4. Lang EW, Chesnut RM. A bedside method for investigating the integrity and critical thresholds of cerebral pressure autoregulation in severe traumatic brain injury patients. *Br J Neurosurg* 2000;14:117–126.
5. Chesnut RM. Avoidance of hypotension: conditio sine qua non of successful severe head-injury management. *J Trauma* 1997;42:S4–S9.
6. Clifton GL, Miller ER, Choi SC, et al. Fluid thresholds and outcome from severe brain injury. *Crit Care Med* 2002;30:739–745.
7. Chesnut RM. Hyperventilation versus cerebral perfusion pressure management: time to change the question. *Crit Care Med* 1998;26:210–212.
8. Cruz J. The first decade of continuous monitoring of jugular bulb oxyhemoglobin saturation: management strategies and clinical outcome. *Crit Care Med* 1998;26:344–351.
9. Robertson CS, Valadka AB, Hannay HJ, et al. Prevention of secondary ischemic insults after severe head injury. *Crit Care Med* 1999;27:2086–2095.
10. Bullock R, Chesnut RM, Clifton G, et al. Guidelines for the management of severe head injury—revision. *J Neurotrauma* 2000;17:457–627.
11. Bratton S, Bullock R, Carney N, et al. Guidelines for the management of severe brain injury: 2007 revision. *J Neurotrauma* 2007;24(suppl 1):S1–S106.
12. Robertson CS, Cormio M. Cerebral metabolic management. *New Horiz* 1995;3:410–422.
13. Kiening K, Unterberg A, Bardt T, et al. Monitoring of cerebral oxygenation in patients with severe head injuries: brain tissue PO_2 versus jugular vein oxygen saturation. *J Neurosurg* 1996;85:751–757.
14. van Santbrink H, Maas AI, Avezaat CJ. Continuous monitoring of partial pressure of brain tissue oxygen in patients with severe head injury. *Neurosurgery* 1996;38:21–31.
15. Edwards P, Arango M, Balica L, et al. Final results of MRC CRASH, a randomised placebo-controlled trial of intravenous corticosteroid in adults with head injury—outcomes at 6 months. *Lancet* 2005;365:1957–1959.
16. Kaufmann AM, Cardoso ER. Aggravation of vasogenic cerebral edema by multiple-dose mannitol. *J Neurosurg* 1992;77:584–589.
17. Chesnut RM, Gautille T, Blunt BA, et al. Neurogenic hypotension in patients with severe head injuries. *J Trauma* 1998;44:958–963; discussion 963–964.
18. Adelson PD, Bratton SL, Carney NA, et al. Guidelines for the acute medical management of severe traumatic brain injury in infants, children, and adolescents. *Pediatr Crit Care Med* 2003;4:S1–S71.
19. Marion DW, Carlier PM. Problems with initial Glasgow Coma Scale assessment caused by prehospital treatment of patients with head injuries: results of a national survey. *J Trauma* 1994;36:89–95.
20. Gabriel EJ, Ghajar J, Jagoda A, et al. Guidelines for prehospital management of traumatic brain injury. *J Neurotrauma* 2002;19:111–174.
21. Chesnut RM, Gautille T, Blunt BA, et al. The localizing value of asymmetry in pupillary size in severe head injury: relation to lesion type and location. *Neurosurgery* 1994;34:840–845; discussion 845–846.
22. Bullock R, Chesnut R, Clifton G, et al. Guidelines for the management of severe head injury. *J Neurotrauma* 1996;13:639–734.
23. Aarabi B, Alden TD, Chesnut RM, et al. Guidelines for the management of penetrating brain injury. *J Trauma* 2001;51:S1–S86.
24. Bullock MR, Chesnut RM, Ghajar J, et al. Guidelines for the surgical management of traumatic brain injury. *Neurosurgery* 2006;58:1–191.
25. Vassar MJ, Fischer RP, O'Brien PE, et al. A multicenter trial for resuscitation of injured patients with 7.5% sodium chloride. The effect of added dextran 70. The Multicenter Group for the Study of Hypertonic Saline in Trauma Patients. *Arch Surg* 1993;128:1003–1011; discussion 1011–1013.
26. Vassar MJ, Perry CA, Gannaway WL, et al. 7.5% sodium chloride/dextran for resuscitation of trauma patients undergoing helicopter transport. *Arch Surg* 1991;126:1065–1072.
27. Vassar MJ, Perry CA, Holcroft JW. Prehospital resuscitation of hypotensive trauma patients with 7.5% NaCl versus 7.5% NaCl with added dextran: a controlled trial. *J Trauma* 1993;34:622–632; discussion 632–633.
28. Cooper DJ, Myles PS, McDermott FT, et al. Prehospital hypertonic saline resuscitation of patients with hypotension and severe traumatic brain injury: a randomized controlled trial. *JAMA* 2004;291:1350–1357.
29. Rosner MJ, Coley IB. Cerebral perfusion pressure, intracranial pressure, and head elevation. *J Neurosurg* 1986;65:636–641.
30. Stein SC, Ross SE. Mild head injury: a plea for routine early CT scanning. *J Trauma* 1992;33:11–13.
31. Mendelow AD, Teasdale G, Jennett B, et al. Risks of intracranial haematoma in head injured adults. *Br Med J Clin Res Ed* 1983;287:1173–1176.
32. Marmarou A, Anderson RL, Ward JD, et al. Impact of ICP instability and hypotension on outcome in patients with severe head trauma. *J Neurosurg* 1991;75:S159–S166.
33. Marshall LF, Gautille T, Klauber MR, et al. The outcome of severe head injury. *J Neurosurg* 1991;75:S28–S36.
34. Seelig JM, Becker DP, Miller JD, et al. Traumatic acute subdural hematoma: major mortality reduction in comatose patients treated within four hours. *N Engl J Med* 1981;304:1511–1518.

CHAPTER 20 ■ MAXILLOFACIAL TRAUMA

RICHARD A. HOPPER AND JOSEPH S. GRUSS

KEY POINTS

1. Maxillofacial trauma is directly related to social structure, geography, and economics. Facial injury patterns vary according to age, risk taking, and daily activities.
2. Facial trauma is common (up to one third of all multisystem trauma patients), is frequently associated with life-threatening injuries, and should provide a warning of potential concomitant airway, central nervous system, and orthopedic injuries.
3. Initial management of maxillofacial trauma follows Advanced Trauma Life Support (ATLS) principles and involves airway management, control of hemorrhage, and rapid identification of injuries with significant morbidity, ocular injury, cerebrospinal fluid leakage, neurologic damage, and malocclusion.
4. Structured history and physical examination and computed tomography scan–guided diagnosis with reconstruction of major facial buttress damage using open reduction and internal fixation in a timely fashion are critical to optimize final functional and esthetic outcome.

Facial trauma often accompanies life-threatening injuries and is a warning of concomitant airway, central nervous system, visceral, and orthopedic injuries.[1] Although it is the associated life-threatening injuries that demand immediate attention, it is the severity of facial trauma that has a direct correlation with the ability of patients to return to preinjury work.[2] Because of the significant role that facial appearance serves in our ability to function daily, and the density of functional units within the craniofacial skeleton, injuries in this region can cause lifelong debility that precludes functioning in society.

The current management of complex facial trauma aims to restore and maintain the normal anatomy of the craniofacial skeleton. Comprehensive clinical examination and computed tomography are used to establish the severity and extent of facial fractures and to identify injuries that require urgent treatment. Definitive operative treatment is performed as soon as the patient is stable in order to minimize the secondary problems of massive edema, bony collapse, and soft tissue shrinkage. Craniofacial surgical techniques are employed to expose the facial skeleton through limited incisions, to achieve anatomic reduction of the fractures, to restore occlusion and orbital volume, and then to use rigid internal fixation for stabilization of the reconstructed skeletal framework for uncomplicated fracture healing. Since the long-term results of timely treatment far exceed those of delayed treatment, it is essential that the definitive care phase of a trauma victim include the early detection, evaluation, acute management, and appropriate referral of maxillofacial injuries.

EPIDEMIOLOGY

Maxillofacial trauma includes soft tissue injuries, dentoalveolar damage, facial bone fractures, and combinations of these. (1) The epidemiology of these injuries is directly related to social structure, geography, and economics, all of which influence the activities of a population. There is consequently significant regional and national variability in the etiology and incidence of maxillofacial trauma patterns.[1–3] Despite this epidemiologic variation, maxillofacial injuries are relatively common in all societies, and are present in up to one third of seriously injured patients with multisystem trauma.[4]

The incidence of facial trauma as a whole peaks in the first decade of life and slowly degrades over the remaining decades of life.[1–3,5] The incidence of facial bone fractures, on the other hand, peaks in the third decade of life. Counter to the trend of increasing incidence of facial bone fractures in the first three decades of life, the actual relative risk per accident of facial bone fractures increases with increasing age (4.4% per year of life) due to the associated decrease in bone density.[1] Most injuries in the first decade of life are isolated soft tissue lacerations and/or dentoalveolar trauma (tooth impaction, alveolar process fractures, crown fractures, etc.) as opposed to the facial bone fractures seen in the adult population.

The etiology of facial trauma includes motor vehicle collisions (automobile, motorcycle, bicycle, and pedestrian), interpersonal violence, falls, industrial mishaps, sports-related injuries, and ballistic injuries. In the United States and Japan, motor vehicle collisions and interpersonal violence continue to be the major causes of facial bone fractures,[2,5] whereas in European studies, sports and activities of daily life incidents are predominant.[1] There is also a relationship between mechanism of injury and age. Over all age groups, motor vehicle collisions are the predominant mechanism of injury for inpatient facial fractures. In infants and toddlers (age 0 to 4 years), falls are the second most common mechanism; in the early school years (age 5 to 14 years), pedestrian and bicycle collisions are the second most common mechanism. After age 14, violence and assault become more common.[6]

(2) Approximately 20% of all facial soft tissue, dentoalveolar, and facial fracture trauma patients have associated injury to additional organ systems.[1] Motor vehicle collision victims with facial injuries have a relatively high associated rate of neurologic (32%), orthopedic (31%), visceral (24%), and ophthalmologic (14%) injuries. Personal assault has a lower association with neurologic (11%) and ophthalmologic (4%) injuries.[3] When facial fractures are present in patients suffering an occupational injury, there is an average of four associated injuries for every facial fracture present, and 2.4 associated injuries for every facial fracture present in a patient suffering a motorcycle crash.

INITIAL EVALUATION

(3) Although maxillofacial injuries can be visually distracting to the trauma team members, they must not cause deviation from

the established Advanced Trauma Life Support (ATLS) protocols. Rarely is facial trauma itself directly life threatening; however, as mentioned earlier, it should be viewed as a strong indicator of a significant mechanism of injury with associated injuries. Within the ATLS algorithms, there are considerations specific to maxillofacial injuries.

Airway Management

Airway compromise in maxillofacial injuries can result from direct laryngeal injury, foreign bodies (including aspirated teeth and bone fragments), or active bleeding from an upper airway source. Treatment of the compromised airway is complicated by the likelihood that 10% of facial trauma patients have cervical spine injuries.[7] As initial treatment, any blood clots should be suctioned from the oropharynx, and a finger sweep used to remove foreign material from the oral airway. Comminuted fractures of the mandible can lead to loss of support of the hyomandibular complex and consequent ptosis and retroposition of the tongue. Manual anterior traction on the mandible symphysis will often temporarily resolve this obstruction until definitive control of the airway can be achieved.

For definitive control of the airway, an artificial oral or nasal airway is often possible, but the use of blind nasal intubation should be carried out with caution. Nasal intubations can exacerbate bleeding from the nasal and nasopharyngeal regions, and the tube may be inadvertently placed into the cranial fossa in the obtunded patient with a comminuted skull base fracture. In the case of severe maxillofacial injuries such as a gunshot wound to the face, intubation is often easier than expected, since the missing or pathologically mobile jaws allow an unprecedented view of the glottis. As with all facial trauma patients, those with significant maxillofacial injury should have a secured airway early in the trauma assessment. The secondary swelling that occurs over the first few hours following the trauma can impede, or in some cases prevent, oral intubation.

Emergent tracheotomy is rarely indicated except in the unusual circumstance of laryngeal fracture or the inability to intubate orally due to massive bleeding or swelling. Semielective tracheostomy in the operating room is reserved for those cases with expected prolonged intubation due to massive soft tissue and bony injuries or impaired consciousness.

Massive Hemorrhage

The elaborate vascularity of the head and neck can result in rapid significant blood loss. Fortunately, the location of the injuries allows sufficient access for direct pressure to control the hemorrhage. Efforts should be made when possible to expose and visualize the source of bleeding prior to suture ligature or cautery in order to avoid collateral damage to adjacent structures, primarily neural structures.

Nasopharyngeal bleeding is common in maxillofacial injuries. The blood supply to the nose arises from both the internal and external carotid systems. The external carotid artery supplies the internal maxillary artery, whose sphenopalatine branch supplies the posterior nasal septum and lateral nasal walls, and the facial artery, whose superior labial branch supplies the anterior inferior nasal cavity. The internal carotid artery gives off the ophthalmic artery, which in turn supplies the anterior and posterior ethmoidal arteries that perfuse the superior and anterior nasal septum. The most common site of epistaxis is at the Kiesselbach plexus at the confluence of the anterior ethmoidal and superior labial arteries. Anterior bleeding is best controlled by formal anterior nasal packing of half-inch gauze coated with antibiotic ointment. The tail of the gauze is left exposed, and with the aid of a nasal speculum, good lighting, and bayonet forceps, the gauze is carefully layered and packed back and forth along the nasal floor until the roof is reached. The direction of packing is directly posterior, then inferior. Prefabricated nasal packing is also available.

Posterior nasal bleeding, such as from the sphenopalatine artery, requires posterior packing. A 16- or 18-French Foley catheter is inserted into the nasopharynx through the nostril. The balloon is then inflated and pulled anteriorly against the vomer and posterior soft palate. The catheter is secured in this position with a clamp at the nostril. A rolled gauze is used to protect the columella from pressure necrosis. Posterior packing will stop the posterior bleeding from draining into the airway, but will divert the flow of blood anteriorly out the nose. The posterior packing must therefore be augmented with anterior packing.

Surgical ligation of the external carotid artery will not control bleeding from its injured branches due to the robust collateralization present. Selective ligation, such as of the ethmoidal vessels through a radix incision or of the internal maxillary artery through a Caldwell-Luc incision, is possible but rarely feasible in the emergency department. If the patient is stable enough to undergo a general anesthetic, the most effective way to address bleeding that is not controlled by packing is through reduction and rigid fixation of the fractures.

Recalcitrant bleeding is treated by angiographic embolization. The source vessels are identified angiographically and then occluded with embolization material such as Gelfoam. At Harborview Regional Medical Center in Seattle, from 1985 to 2000, of the 62,366 trauma cases, 7,147 had craniofacial trauma. During this same period, of the 3,529 cases of radiographic embolization, only 4 were performed on patients with craniofacial trauma. This emphasizes that although radiographic embolization is a component of the treatment algorithm of maxillofacial bleeding, the vast majority of cases can be treated with other means.[8]

Ocular Injury

Direct injury to the eyeball should be suspected in all patients with orbital fractures or lacerations to the periorbital region. One prospective study reported a 29% incidence of ocular injury in 49 patients with orbital fractures.[9] Pain, decreased vision, and the appearance of spots before the eyes are all highly suggestive of globe damage. During the neurologic phase of trauma assessment, a brief clinical ophthalmologic examination should be performed. This would include visual acuity, pupillary response to light and accommodation, extraocular range of motion, globe position, and turgor. If there are any abnormal findings on the examination, an immediate ophthalmologic consult should be obtained for examination of the retina and ocular pressures. Injuries that may require immediate ophthalmologic treatment or result in permanent sequelae include corneoscleral lacerations, lens dislocation, major hyphema, acute glaucoma, and retinal detachment.

Blindness at the time of presentation is fortunately rare, but is an extremely poor prognostic factor for future sight. Patients with light perception at the time of presentation but who then demonstrate progressive loss of vision during the trauma assessment must be treated aggressively. The most common etiology of this presentation is traumatic optic neuropathy secondary to optic nerve compression from a retrobulbar hematoma, a bone fragment, or edema. The management of progressive vision loss remains controversial, for it is unclear which patients benefit from emergent optic nerve decompression. If the eyeball is tense, then immediate lateral canthotomy is indicated to release the confining force of the lids. If there is a clear source of compression visualized on computed tomography (CT), immediate operative decompression is indicated.[10] All other patients are treated with high-dose steroids.[11]

Cerebrospinal Fluid Rhinorrhea

Cerebrospinal fluid (CSF) leaks should be actively searched for in patients with craniofacial or high maxillary fractures. Clear or serosanguineous nasal discharge, anosmia, or a salty taste in the mouth is highly suggestive. A CSF leak into the nasal cavity implies a defect in the pia-arachnoid and an abnormal communication between the subarachnoid space and the external environment. The thin bone in the anterior skull base and the close adherence of the dura to the anterior fossa and cribriform plate predispose to penetration of fracture fragments into the subarachnoid space. Common associated fracture patterns that are detailed later in the chapter include LeFort II and III midface fractures, naso-orbital ethmoid (NOE) patterns, orbital roof fractures, and displaced fractures of the posterior table of the frontal sinus. CSF is differentiated from serum on laboratory examination by its low protein concentration and from normal nasal secretions by the presence of glucose but no mucin.

Most CSF fistulas close spontaneously. Morgan et al.[12] reported a 35% incidence of CSF rhinorrhea in 300 patients with severe facial fractures, of which 66% resolved spontaneously by the fifth postinjury day, and 87% by the 10th day. Fistulas that do not close spontaneously can be visualized on a metrizamide contrast CT scan, followed by surgical exploration and obliteration of the fistula using a dural patch.

Occlusion

Occlusion is the contact of the posterior masticating (chewing) and anterior incising (cutting) surfaces of the maxillary and mandibular teeth. Malocclusion is an indicator of orthognathic fracture and/or dental injury. The maxillary teeth should overlap the mandible teeth in normal occlusion in three ways: (a) overjet describes the horizontal projection of the upper front teeth in front of the lower teeth, (b) overbite describes the vertical overlap of the upper front teeth over the lower teeth, and (c) the posterior maxillary arch should be wider than the mandible arch on both sides by the space of one cusp. Typical malocclusion patterns seen following fractures include an anterior open bite (gap between the upper and lower front teeth), that indicates the fractured maxilla is impacted upward or that both condyles of the mandible have collapsed; a posterior open bite (gap between the upper and lower back teeth) often associated with a unilateral condylar fracture; or a posterior cross-bite (back teeth lateral or medial to the normal arch form) that indicates either a mandible fracture or a comminuted fracture of the maxilla and palate. These malocclusion patterns indicate that surgical intervention is indicated.

Missing or fractured teeth should be documented. If a tooth is missing, the oral cavity and airway should be carefully checked for the foreign body. Securing the tooth to an adjacent one with a wire can often salvage a loose or dislocated tooth. If a tooth is fractured with unstable fragments, the fragments should be removed to prevent entrance into the airway.

Neurologic Injury

Injury to the muscles of facial expression or the seventh cranial nerve can be particularly debilitating, due to their importance in interpersonal interactions. The most common cause of facial nerve injury is fracture of the temporal bone in the intraosseous canal.[13] Penetrating injury to the facial branches of the seventh nerve requires exploration and repair, whereas nonpenetrating injury is observed for recovery over a period of 3 to 6 months. Injury to the middle branches of the nerve distal to the parotid (zygomatic and buccal) can be masked by cross-innervation with other branches. The marginal mandibular (lower lip depressors) and temporal (brow elevation) branches have the least degree of cross-innervation, and therefore more commonly result in functional problems.

COMPUTED TOMOGRAPHY DIAGNOSIS OF MAXILLOFACIAL FRACTURES: THE FACIAL BUTTRESSES

The functional units of the face are held together and stabilized by several vertical and horizontal skeletal buttresses (Fig. 20.1). These buttresses represent regions of relatively dense bone that serve to support the functional units of the face in an optimal relation and define the form of the face by projecting the overlying soft tissue envelope.[14] Additionally, the facial buttresses stabilize the face to the cranial base and determine the proper relationship between these two important structural units. Conceptualizing and describing maxillofacial fractures according to the involved buttresses is useful because they are directly related to the definitive surgical treatment. Each buttress can be visualized on the craniofacial CT scan. There are four transverse and four paired vertical buttresses. Due to the reliance of facial form and function on these buttresses, as well as the mechanical force exerted on them, the craniofacial trauma surgeon typically treats any significant buttress displacement using anatomic reduction and rigid internal fixation.

4

As structural units that support the face, the buttresses must either directly or indirectly interface with the skull base or cranium as a stable reference. From superior to inferior, the **transverse facial buttresses** are as follows:

1. *Upper transverse maxillary buttress* runs from the temporal bone across the zygomatic arch and inferior orbital rim, superiorly to the frontal bone via the frontal process of the maxilla, and then across to the contralateral temporal bone via a similar path. This buttress crosses the zygomaticotemporal, the zygomaticomaxillary, and the nasofrontal sutures,

FIGURE 20.1. Illustration of adult skull demonstrating the four paired vertical and four transverse buttresses, all existing in areas of relative increased bone thickness.

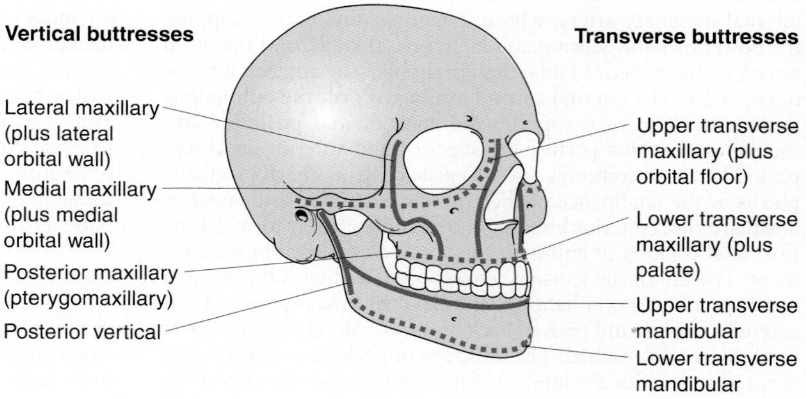

which are commonly involved in fracture patterns. The sagittal extensions of this buttress are the orbital floors.

2. *Lower transverse maxillary buttress.* From the pterygoid projection of the skull base, it extends along the bone of the maxillary alveolar arch to the contralateral pterygoids. The sagittal extension of this buttress is the hard palate.
3. *Upper transverse mandibular buttress* is at the level of the mandible's alveolar arch.
4. *Lower transverse mandibular buttress* is at the inferior border of the mandible.

The **paired vertical buttresses** from lateral to medial are as follows:

1. *Posterior vertical mandibular buttress.* Composed of the ascending ramus and condyle of the mandible, this buttress links the transverse mandibular buttresses with the skull base.
2. *Lateral maxillary buttress* is composed of the column of bone from the alveolar bone of the posterior maxillary molars across the zygomaticomaxillary suture and body of the zygoma, extending superiorly to the lateral orbital rim and across the zygomaticofrontal suture. The sagittal projection of this buttress includes the lateral orbital wall as it joins the sphenoid bone of the skull base.
3. *Medial maxillary buttress* is composed of the column of bone from the alveolar bone of the anterior maxillary dentition, extending superiorly along the rim of the piriform aperture and frontal process of the maxilla, then across the nasofrontal junction to frontal bone. The sagittal projection of this buttress includes the medial orbital wall.
4. *Posterior maxillary buttress* is composed of the column of bone at the pterygomaxillary junction where the pterygoid plates of the sphenoid join the posterior maxilla. These last three vertical buttresses support the transverse buttress of the maxillary occlusion.

Although other anatomic buttresses of the face can be conceptualized, the ones listed here meet the following critical criteria: (a) they are all linked either directly or through another buttress to the cranium or cranial base as a stable reference point, (b) they have sufficient bone thickness to accommodate metal screw fixation, and (c) with the exception of the posterior maxillary buttress, they are surgically accessible through standard limited surgical incisions. Accurate reduction and fixation of these facial buttresses restores projection, width, and height of the facial skeleton relative to the cranial base and, more important, establishes a functional support for the teeth and globes.

PATTERNS OF INJURY

Naso-orbito-ethmoid Fractures

NOE fractures involve the central upper midface between the eyes, disrupting the confluence of the medial maxillary buttress with the upper transverse maxillary buttress. Fractures of the NOE complex can be one of the most difficult fracture patterns to accurately repair. Failure to restore the sagittal projection of this region and correct the rotation of the frontal process of the maxilla (superior portion of the medial maxillary buttress) will result in a lack of upper nasal projection and telecanthus (increased distance between the inner corner of the eyes), both of which are difficult to correct as a secondary operation. The eyelids insert around the lacrimal fossa through the medial canthal tendon. If the tendon insertion is not returned to its correct position, the patient loses the normal shadow definition on either side of the nose, the medial corner of the palpebral fissure drifts laterally, and the eyes appear too far apart. If the distance between the medial canthi is greater than 30 mm, a NOE pattern should be suspected.

By definition, NOE fractures include damage to the ethmoid sinus and walls. If there is bilateral comminution and displacement in this region, the nasofrontal ducts that drain the frontal sinus are also likely disrupted. In this situation, the surgeon obliterates the frontal sinus by removing all of the sinus mucosa and filling the sinus with bone, fat, or some other tissue. Failure to diagnose disruption of the nasofrontal ducts and obliterate the sinus increases the risk of developing a frontal sinus mucocele postoperatively.

Zygoma and Orbital Fractures

Following nasal fractures, zygomatic fractures are the most common injury resulting from blunt trauma. The zygoma has two attachments to the cranium and two to the maxilla and forms a large portion of the orbital floor and lateral wall. These paired "cornerstone" bones are therefore surgically important in establishing orbital volume and in serving as a reference for maxilla reduction in LeFort-type maxillary fractures. The two major buttresses of the zygoma are the upper transverse maxillary (across the zygomaticotemporal and zygomaticomaxillary sutures) and the lateral vertical maxillary (across the zygomaticomaxillary and frontozygomatic sutures). Fractures typically occur across these three buttress-related sutures, leading to the term *tripod fracture.* This term fails to recognize the posterior relationship of the zygoma with the sphenoid bone of the skull base. A displaced orbitozygomatic fracture is really a quadripod fracture. If the two buttresses of the zygoma are reduced and fixated, it is still possible to have a rotational deformity of the zygoma about the zygomaticosphenoid suture. The surgeon pays particular attention to the alignment of the zygoma and sphenoid at the lateral orbital wall, since angulation here after fixation of the remaining buttresses reflects a residual rotational deformity and an associated increased orbital volume.

If the zygomatic arch component of the transverse buttress is comminuted and is needed as a reference to establish facial projection following a panfacial injury, the only way to access this region is via the coronal scalp degloving approach, which carries with it an associated increased blood loss, operating time, and risk for potential complications.

Orbital floor fractures can occur in isolation but are also commonly associated with zygoma fractures through posterior propagation of the fracture from the upper transverse maxillary buttress at the inferior orbital rim. The size and displacement of the orbital floor fragment must be known preoperatively to decide what treatment, if any, is required. The width of the defect of the floor can be estimated from the coronal reformat images, and the depth by counting the number of coronal cuts containing the fracture. Multiplying these two gives an estimate of the area of the defect. Attention to the shape and position of the inferior rectus muscle on the coronal CT scan can provide information regarding the damage to the fascial sling of the globe. If the rectus remains flattened on cross section and in the correct position, the surgeon will likely encounter minimal entrapped periorbital tissue. If, however, the inferior rectus is round and inferiorly displaced, the fascial sling is disrupted and the periorbita and muscle have prolapsed into the orbital floor defect (Fig. 20.2A). Entrapment of the inferior rectus in children can be easily missed because the flexible bone can spring back in place like a trapdoor, looking normal on CT scan except for the entrapped muscle beneath it (Fig. 20.2B). This trapdoor fracture requires urgent treatment within 24 to 72 hours to minimize the chance of motility problems.[15]

Maxillary Fractures

With the exception of alveolar and palate fractures, maxillary fractures are commonly described according to the classification described by Rene LeFort in 1901[16] (Fig. 20.3). LeFort fractures involve a separation of all or a portion of the maxilla

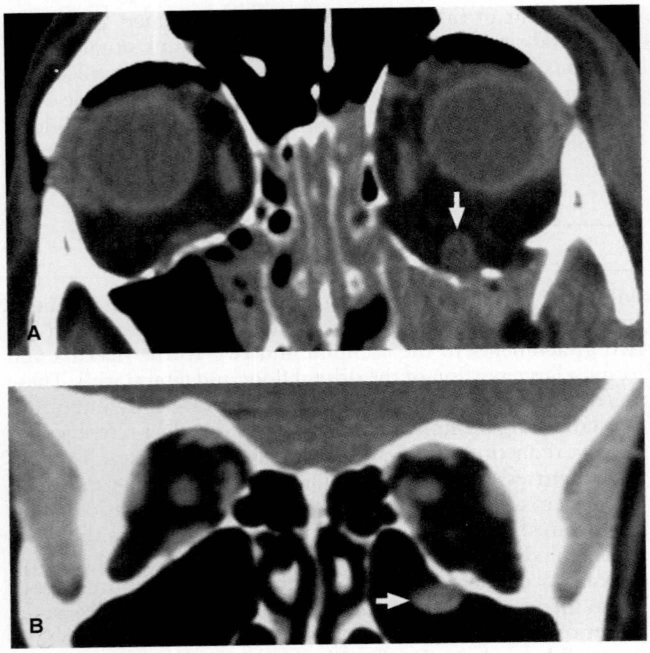

FIGURE 20.2. Computed tomography coronal plane noncontrast images demonstrating two patterns of orbital floor blowout fractures. **A:** A left orbital floor fracture with evidence of entrapment of the inferior rectus muscle. The inferior rectus (*arrow*) is displaced inferiorly into the maxillary sinus. Note how the muscle cross section has changed from ovoid to circular. The fascial support has been disrupted and the muscle is entrapped. **B:** A pediatric trapdoor left orbital floor blowout fracture. The orbital floor was disrupted by the impact, but then sprung back in place, trapping the inferior rectus muscle (*arrow*) within the maxillary sinus. Since the bone has returned to its anatomic location, this diagnosis can easily be missed unless attention is paid to the location of the extraocular muscles. Trapdoor fractures require emergent treatment to optimize the chance of recovery.

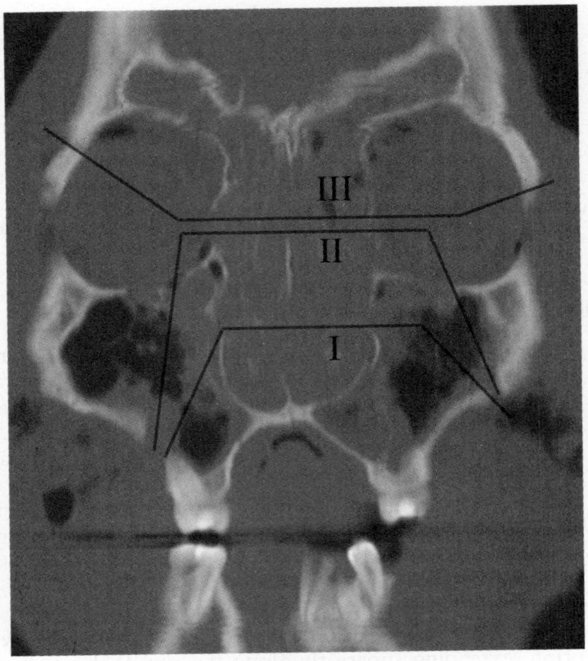

FIGURE 20.3. Computed tomography coronal plane noncontrast image demonstrating bilateral LeFort I, II, and III fractures in the same patient. The LeFort I pattern has fractures through the inferior portions of the medial and lateral maxillary buttresses, the LeFort II pattern is through the zygomaticomaxillary and frontomaxillary sutures, and the LeFort III pattern is complete craniofacial dissociation. To confirm the diagnosis, pterygomaxillary disjunction and fractures of the zygomatic arches would need to be observed on axial plane images.

from the skull base. For this to occur, the posterior vertical maxillary buttress at the junction of the posterior maxillary sinus with the pterygoid plates of the sphenoid must be disrupted. This can either be through the posterior walls of the sinus or through the plates themselves as seen on axial CT images. Once a pterygomaxillary disjunction has been diagnosed, the remaining facial buttresses are inspected to determine the class of LeFort fracture. If the inferior portions of both the lateral and medial maxillary buttresses are fractured, a LeFort I fracture has occurred, and the maxillary arch (lower transverse maxillary buttress) will move in relation to the rest of the face and skull. If the inferior lateral maxillary buttress (zygomaticomaxillary suture) and the superior medial maxillary buttresses (frontomaxillary sutures) are fractured, then the entire maxilla will move in relation to the skull base as a LeFort II fragment. If the upper transverse (zygomatic arch), superior lateral (frontozygomatic), and superior medial (maxillofrontal) maxillary buttresses are fractured, then craniofacial separation has occurred as a LeFort III pattern, with the entire face moving in relation to the skull base.

For all LeFort fractures, the maxillary dental arch is mobile; therefore, the patient must be placed in maxillomandibular fixation prior to plating of the fractures. All buttresses can be plated with the exception of the buttress common to all LeFort patterns—the pterygomaxillary posterior vertical buttress. Similar to zygomatic fractures, if there is severe comminution of a buttress, bone grafting may be required.

Mandible Fractures

Unlike the rest of the facial buttresses, isolated mandible fractures are typically diagnosed with plain radiograph series. In a trauma patient with multiple injuries, however, the diagnosis is often made on CT scan imaging as a disruption of the mandible arch. Fractures can occur at any point on the mandible including, in decreasing order of frequency, the body, angle, condylar neck, symphysis and parasymphysis, ramus, and alveolar ridge. The condyles are best visualized on coronal images. Many condylar fractures are not directly fixated because of the difficulty accessing this region surgically as a result of the proximity of the facial nerve, as well as the risk of iatrogenic temporomandibular joint (TMJ) dysfunction. If there are bilateral condylar neck fractures associated with a severely comminuted LeFort fracture, one condyle is typically exposed, reduced, and plated in order to reestablish a stable vertical buttress for reestablishing facial height. Intracapsular condylar injuries have a high risk of ankylosis and are treated conservatively with early range of motion if occlusion can be established.

TIMING OF DEFINITIVE REPAIR

There are two windows for optimum treatment of maxillofacial injuries. The first is in the first 6 to 12 hours following injury, before the onset of edema. With the exception of emergencies such as optic nerve compression, uncontrollable facial bleeding, or pediatric trapdoor orbital fractures, this phase is not feasible in a multisystem trauma victim due to the priority of other injuries. The most common timing for maxillofacial injuries is after the initial postinjury edema has subsided and the patient is cleared for the operating room. This is typically 3 to 7 days postinjury. Although facial fractures can be reduced up to 3 weeks postinjury, the soft tissue fibrosis and the early fracture callus make the procedure progressively more difficult starting 10 days after the injury. Mandible fractures have been traditionally treated as open fractures, with definitive treatment within 24 hours.

SUMMARY

Maxillofacial injuries in a trauma victim should be considered an indicator of associated severe injuries. The initial evaluation within the ATLS protocol includes special considerations of airway management, ocular assessment, control of bleeding, identification of CSF leaks, and neurologic injury. The definitive treatment of maxillofacial injuries, following a structured history and physical examination, includes identification of damage to the facial buttresses on CT imaging. Displaced buttress fractures require open reduction and internal fixation in a timely fashion to minimize secondary soft tissue contracture and optimize the final functional and esthetic outcome.

References

1. Gassner R, Tuli T, Hachl O, et al. Cranio-maxillofacial trauma: a 10 year review of 9,543 cases with 21,067 injuries. *J Craniomaxillofac Surg* 2003; 31(1):51–61.
2. Girotto JA, MacKenzie E, Fowler C, et al. Long-term physical impairment and functional outcomes after complex facial fractures. *Plast Reconstr Surg* 2001;108(2):312–327.
3. Haug RH, Prather J, Indresano AT. An epidemiologic survey of facial fractures and concomitant injuries. *J Oral Maxillofac Surg* 1990;48(9): 926–932.
4. Sastry SM, Sastry CM, Paul BK, et al. Leading causes of facial trauma in the major trauma outcome study. *Plast Reconstr Surg* 1995;95(1): 196–197.
5. Iida S, Kogo M, Sugiura T, et al. Retrospective analysis of 1,502 patients with facial fractures. *Int J Oral Maxillofac Surg* 2001;30(4):286–290.
6. Imahara SD, Hopper RA, Wang J, et al. Patterns and outcomes of pediatric facial fractures in the United States: a survey of the National Trauma Data Bank. *J Am Coll Surg* 2008;207(5):710–716.
7. Sinclair D, Schwartz M, Gruss J, et al. A retrospective review of the relationship between facial fractures, head injuries, and cervical spine injuries. *J Emerg Med* 1988;6(2):109–112.
8. Ho K, Hutter JJ, Eskridge J, et al. The management of life-threatening haemorrhage following blunt facial trauma. *J Plast Reconstr Aesthet Surg* 2006;59(12):1257–1262.
9. Jabaley ME, Lerman M, Sanders HJ. Ocular injuries in orbital fractures. A review of 119 cases. *Plast Reconstr Surg* 1975;56(4):410–418.
10. Stanley RB Jr, Sires BS, Funk GF, et al. Management of displaced lateral orbital wall fractures associated with visual and ocular motility disturbances. *Plast Reconstr Surg* 1998;102(4):972–979.
11. Li KK, Teknos TN, Lai A, et al. Traumatic optic neuropathy: result in 45 consecutive surgically treated patients. *Otolaryngol Head Neck Surg* 1999;120(1):5–11.
12. Morgan BD, Madan DK, Bergerot JP. Fractures of the middle third of the face—a review of 300 cases. *Br J Plast Surg* 1972;25(2):147–151.
13. Coker NJ. Management of traumatic injuries to the facial nerve. *Otolaryngol Clin North Am* 1991;24(1):215–227.
14. Gruss JS, Mackinnon SE. Complex maxillary fractures: role of buttress reconstruction and immediate bone grafts. *Plast Reconstr Surg* 1986; 78(1):9–22.
15. Grant JH III, Patrinely JR, Weiss AH, et al. Trapdoor fracture of the orbit in a pediatric population. *Plast Reconstr Surg* 2002;109(2):482–489; discussion 490–495.
16. LeFort R. Etude experimentale sur les fractures do la machoire siperieuve. *Riv Chir de Paris* 1901;23:208.

CHAPTER 21 ■ NECK INJURIES

SAMAN ARBABI

KEY POINTS

1. The numerous vital structures in the neck are concentrated in a small anatomic area at risk of injury, unprotected by bone or dense muscular covering.
2. Anatomically, in addition to large bilateral anterior and posterior triangles, the anterior neck is divided into three zones: zone I, extending from the sternal notch to the cricoid cartilage; zone II, from the cricoid cartilage to the angle of the mandible; and zone III, from the angle of the mandible to the base of the skull.
3. Mechanism and anatomic location of trauma are frequently predictive of pattern and number of vital structures injured.
4. Mandatory versus selective exploration of a penetrating neck injury is determined by anatomic and physical findings in addition to local resources and physician capabilities.
5. Patterns of fractures of the face, skull, and neck, along with significant soft tissue trauma and subcutaneous emphysema, predict the likelihood of airway or vascular injury, with computed tomography angiography being the most appropriate screening diagnostic test.

(1) The numerous vital structures of the neck are concentrated in a small anatomic area, generally unprotected by bone or dense muscular covering. Yet, because of its relatively small size, only 5% to 10% of traumatic injuries involve the neck. Although neck injuries occur infrequently, they often require prompt surgical management. Disruption of the airway or carotid circulation is an immediate, life-threatening problem, and esophageal or peripheral nerve injury can cause chronic morbidity. Penetrating injuries are most common and most severe, with fatality rates ranging from 1% to 2% for stab wounds, from 5% to 12% for gunshot wounds, and up to 50% for rifle or shotgun blasts.[1–3] Up to 50% of these deaths are preventable with appropriate early care. Significant blunt neck trauma is less common but can be particularly difficult to manage because it often involves the airway. Carotid or vertebral artery injury can also occur as a consequence of acute cervical spine hyperextension, even in the absence of bony injury. The initial diagnosis of these injuries can be difficult, yet the consequences of missing an injury are severe.

As a general guideline, all patients with penetrating neck wounds that traverse the platysma muscle should be admitted to the hospital for evaluation, observation, and treatment. Likewise, all patients with blunt traumatic injuries of the neck should be admitted. This section of the text focuses on the

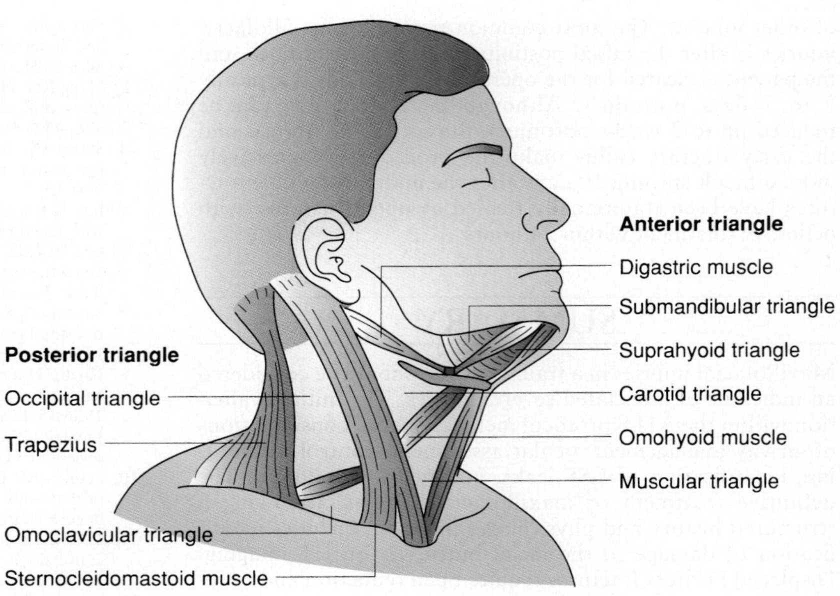

FIGURE 21.1. Anatomic triangles of the neck. The posterior triangle is composed of the smaller occipital and omoclavicular triangles. The anterior triangle has as smaller divisions the carotid, muscular, submandibular, and suprahyoid triangles.

available and preferred diagnostic and treatment options for patients with blunt or penetrating neck trauma.

ANATOMY

The neck is classically divided into a number of anatomic triangles (Fig. 21.1). The two large anterior and posterior triangles are particularly important in neck trauma. Wounds to the posterior triangle rarely involve the esophagus, airway, or major vascular structures, although if the blow is directed inferiorly, intrathoracic injury can occur. In contrast, penetrating wounds that enter through either the sternocleidomastoid muscle or the anterior triangle carry a high likelihood of vascular, airway, or esophageal injury (Fig. 21.2).

The anterior neck is further divided into three zones defined by horizontal planes. Zone I represents the base of the neck and is variably defined. In the Roon and Christensen classifi-

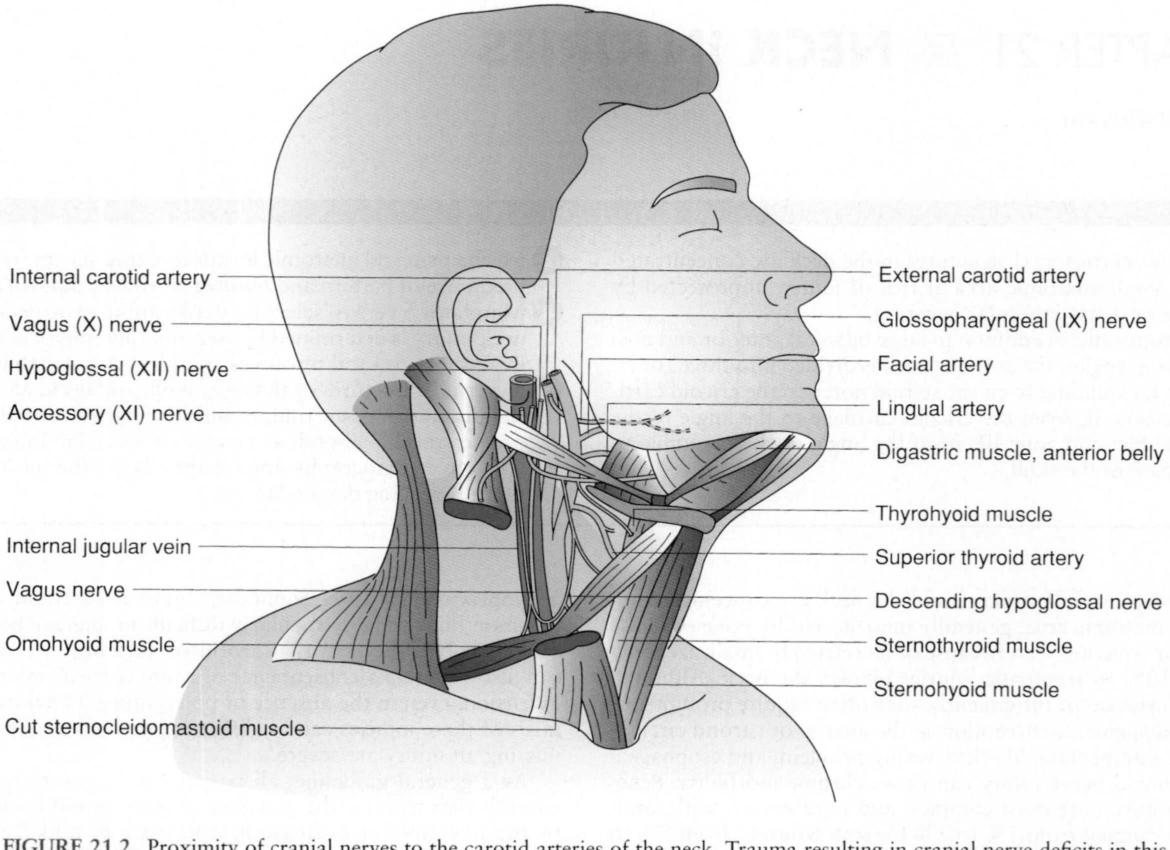

FIGURE 21.2. Proximity of cranial nerves to the carotid arteries of the neck. Trauma resulting in cranial nerve deficits in this region is often associated with vascular injury.

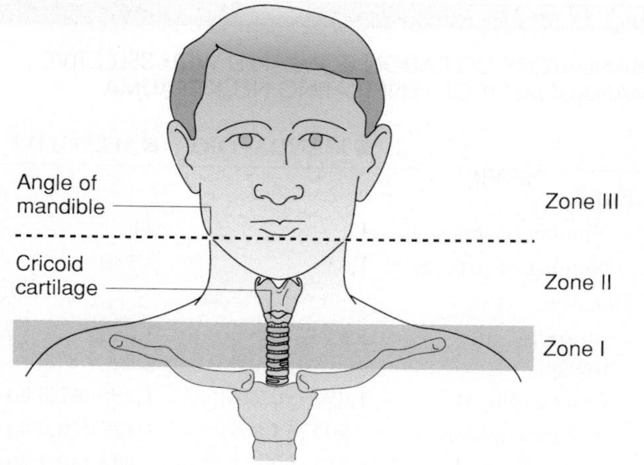

FIGURE 21.3. Zones of the neck. The junction of zones I and II is variously described as being at the cricoid cartilage or at the top of the clavicles. The important implication of a zone I injury is the greater potential for intrathoracic great vessel injury.

cation,[4] zone I is defined as extending from the sternal notch to the lower border of the cricoid cartilage (Fig. 21.3). Injuries here carry the highest mortality rate because of the risk of major vascular and intrathoracic injury. Zone II is the central and largest portion of the neck. It extends from the top of zone I to the angle of the mandible. Zone II injuries are most common but carry a lower mortality rate than either zone I or III injuries, because injury is usually apparent and exposure of vital structures is readily accomplished. Zone III is that part of the neck above the angle of the mandible. The risk of injury to the distal carotid artery, salivary glands, and pharynx is greatest in this zone. Exposure in this region can be particularly difficult.

The other major anatomic landmark in the neck is the platysma muscle. This thin, broad muscle lies just beneath the skin and covers the entire anterior triangle and anteroinferior aspect of the posterior triangle. Wounds that fail to penetrate the platysma are considered superficial and do not warrant extensive evaluation. Wounds that penetrate the platysma must be considered a serious surgical problem that mandates hospital admission and further evaluation.

INITIAL MANAGEMENT

The same priorities for initial care of the multiply injured patient apply to the management of isolated neck trauma. Airway control remains the primary tenet of initial trauma care, and it takes precedence over all other aspects of the evaluation and resuscitation. If injury involves the airway itself or surrounding structures, this management task takes on special significance. Rapid inspection for air movement, crepitus, hoarseness, and subcutaneous emphysema is the first step. Supplemental oxygen should always be administered, and adequate lighting and suction are essential. If spontaneous ventilation appears adequate, close observation and pulse oximetry monitoring are suggested, because acute decompensation can occur with little warning. If spontaneous respirations are inadequate, if blood or other material obstructs the airway, or if progressive cervical swelling from hemorrhage threatens to occlude the airway, emergency intubation is necessary. Procrastination converts a simple intubation into a difficult and bloody emergency tracheostomy. Direct visualization of the vocal cords and oral endotracheal intubation are usually preferred. If cervical spine injury has not been excluded, hyperextension of the neck must be avoided. Two-man intubation with in-line cervical traction is the preferred alternative to nasotracheal intubation.

A massive pharyngeal or neck hematoma can totally occlude the airway, making direct intubation impossible. Attempts at blind nasotracheal intubation can further aggravate mucosal or laryngeal injury, and an emergency surgical airway (cricothyroidotomy or tracheostomy) is required. Occasionally, blunt laryngeal trauma is so severe as to disrupt and occlude the airway. The preferred method of controlling the airway in this setting is controversial, but provisions for a surgical airway must be at hand. Options include primary tracheostomy or a single attempt at endoscopically assisted endotracheal intubation. Temporization with transtracheal needle-jet insufflation can be a valuable adjunct in these settings, and mandatory in the young child.

Concurrent with airway control is awareness of potential cervical spine injury, particularly in unconscious patients who have sustained blunt head and neck trauma. The head and neck should be supported in the neutral position until this possibility is excluded radiographically and by physical examination. In the emergency room, support of the head and neck during manipulation or procedures is best accomplished by a strong, steady assistant rather than by collars, sandbags, or tape. The lateral cervical spine film is an essential component of the initial evaluation of patients with either blunt or penetrating neck trauma, both to assess the bony cervical spine and to evaluate soft tissues for edema or malplaced air.

The initial management subsequent to control of the airway follows the ABC guidelines of trauma care advocated by the Advanced Trauma Life Support course of the American College of Surgeons, with particular attention directed at adequacy of ventilation, treatment of shock, and baseline neurologic examination. Patients with blunt neck trauma often have concomitant thoracic injuries, and penetrating neck wounds may follow a caudal trajectory, injuring lung or intrathoracic great vessels, particularly if the entrance is in zone I.[5] Rapid physical examination of the thorax is therefore part of the initial evaluation of neck trauma patients and should include inspection, palpation, and auscultation. Pneumothorax must be treated rapidly by needle decompression or tube thoracostomy, or both, and treatment should not necessarily be delayed for radiographic confirmation, particularly in the unstable patient. Major neck hemorrhage is treated with direct pressure. Blind clamping of vessels is discouraged to avoid inadvertent injury to adjacent nerves or esophagus. Adequate peripheral intravenous access is required in all patients with neck trauma and usually requires at least two peripheral intravenous catheter lines of 16 gauge or larger contralateral to the side of greatest neck injury. Blood is drawn for typing and cross matching and routine laboratory evaluations, and fluid resuscitation is initiated based on the degree of shock and anticipated hemorrhage. A rapid yet thorough neurologic examination is also part of the initial management, with particular attention to the patient's level of consciousness and the status of cranial and brachial plexus nerves. Changes in the results of neurologic examination are key indicators of progressive injury.

3 After the initial resuscitation, a complete physical examination is performed to detect associated injuries and to better define the extent of neck trauma. Close visual inspection of the neck alerts the physician to the possibility of underlying injuries and the mechanism of injury. For example, an oblique 4- to 6-cm bruise on the neck of a restrained passenger in a motor vehicle accident should alert the physician to the possibility of blunt cervical vascular trauma from a seat belt injury. Neck wounds should not be probed for fear of dislodging a clot and reinstituting hemorrhage. The neck should be palpated with attention to normal anatomic landmarks and areas of tenderness. Crepitus or subcutaneous emphysema indicates

TABLE 21.1 **DIAGNOSIS**

CLINICAL SIGNS OF SIGNIFICANT INJURY IN PENETRATING NECK TRAUMA

■ VASCULAR	■ DIGESTIVE TRACT
Shock	Hemoptysis
Active bleeding	Dysphagia or odynophagia
Large or expanding hematoma	Hematemesis
Pulse deficit	Subcutaneous emphysema
■ AIRWAY	**■ NEUROLOGIC**
Dyspnea Stridor	Focal or lateralized neurologic deficit
Hoarseness	
Dysphonia or voice change	
Subcutaneous emphysema	

TABLE 21.2

MANDATORY OPERATION COMPARED WITH SELECTIVE MANAGEMENT OF PENETRATING NECK TRAUMA

	■ MANDATORY	■ SELECTIVE
Patients		
Number of series	11	24
Number of patients	1,653	2,540
Outcome		
Mortality rate (range)	5.85% (0.3%–11.0%)	3.75% (0%–9.8%)
Cases explored	1,492 (90.2%)	1,596 (62.8%)
Positive explorations	803 (53.8%)	1,117 (70.0%)
Cases observed	161 (9.8%)	944 (37.2%)
Delayed exploration	3 (1.9%)	20 (2.1%)
System injured		
Arterial injuries	213 (12.9%)	303 (11.9%)
Venous injuries	310 (18.8%)	459 (18.0%)
Esophagus or pharynx	163 (9.9%)	191 (7.5%)
Larynx or trachea	150 (9.1%)	181 (7.1%)

Modified from Asensio J, Valenziano C, Falcone R, et al. Management of penetrating neck injuries: the controversy surrounding zone III injuries. *Surg Clin North Am* 1991;71:267.

injury to the trachea, esophagus, or lung until proven otherwise. Never assume that a penetrating skin wound itself is responsible for subcutaneous air. If the patient is able to talk, determine the presence of hoarseness, dysphagia, or dysphonia. Hemoptysis and hematemesis are also signs of tracheal or esophageal injury. Table 21.1 lists the clinical signs of significant injury that usually mandate neck exploration to exclude or treat vascular, airway, esophageal, or nerve injuries.

All patients with blunt or penetrating neck trauma should have a chest radiograph to rule out thoracic trauma. Stable patients should have soft tissue neck films to look for retropharyngeal hematoma, tracheal narrowing or deviation, retained missile fragments and pathways, and subcutaneous or retropharyngeal air. Computed tomography (CT) of the neck is particularly helpful in blunt trauma to evaluate laryngeal structures to look for laryngeal fractures. Patients with blunt neck trauma whose neurologic examination is inconsistent with findings on head CT should undergo studies to evaluate for cervical vascular injury.

SELECTIVE VERSUS MANDATORY EXPLORATION

There is uniform agreement that all unstable patients and all patients with clinical signs of significant neck injury require prompt exploration. All other patients with wounds that penetrate the platysma should at least be admitted to the hospital and observed. Controversy exists, however, in the management of asymptomatic, stable patients with penetrating neck
4 injury. Two distinct schools of thought exist, one advocating mandatory surgical exploration of all wounds that penetrate the platysma[2,6,7] and the other favoring a more selective approach.[8–12] A comprehensive review of selective versus mandatory operative management published in 1991 documents similar rates for injury incidence, overall mortality, and delayed complications, as well as similar hospital costs, but with a significant reduction of negative neck explorations in the selective management group[13] (Table 21.2). Most recent studies have advocated some type of selective management in a clinical setting with explicit guidelines and expertise in the appropriate use of various diagnostic modalities.[14–17]

Advocates of a mandatory exploration policy cite the low morbidity and negligible mortality rate after negative neck exploration as justification for the high rate of negative findings (40% to 60%). The disastrous complications of missed injuries further support this stance. A 67% mortality rate is reported after delayed operations for neck vascular injuries, and a 44% mortality rate for delayed operations for esophageal injuries.[3] A 1986 literature review reported an overall mortality rate of 16.7% for patients initially observed after penetrating neck trauma who subsequently required surgical exploration.[18] In addition, a few reports have documented major structural injury in a small percentage of patients who undergo exploration despite a clinically silent physical examination; in one report, 5.5% of patients with wounds that appeared innocuous but were nevertheless explored had significant injuries.[7] Transcervical gunshot injuries represent a special category of neck wounds, with one report documenting the high likelihood of injuries to cervical structures (83%) and supporting aggressive surgical exploration in all cases.[19]

Supporters of a more selective approach berate the high incidence of negative explorations, the cost of a surgical exploration, and the fact that some injuries are missed in spite of a surgical exploration. They also argue that the original data supporting mandatory neck exploration are based on World War II and Vietnam War experience with large-caliber, high-velocity projectiles, unlike the typical knife or hand gun injury observed in civilian trauma. The wide availability and diagnostic accuracy of angiography, endoscopy, and esophagography further support a selective management plan. Merion et al.,[12] as part of a review of the cost of managing penetrating neck trauma, analyzed 27 reported series in which the clinical courses of more than 4,000 patients with penetrating neck trauma were documented. Of patients treated by surgeons advocating selective exploration, 52% underwent immediate operation, compared with almost 90% of patients treated by those advocating mandatory exploration. Reexamination of these series revealed that mortality rate was no different in the two groups, and only 2.4% of initially observed patients required subsequent operation.[18]

No uniform policy has been adopted for selective management of penetrating neck injury patients in the absence of positive clinical findings. There is general agreement that zone I and III injuries require diagnostic studies such as helical CT angiography, angiography, endoscopy, and esophageal contrast studies.[20] The management of zone II injury, however, is variable and subject to the experience and preference of individual surgeons and trauma centers.[14–17] The disagreement concerns whether patients should routinely undergo surgical neck exploration, undergo extensive diagnostic evaluation similar to zone I and III injuries, or simply be observed. With the evolution of helical CT angiography (CTA), however, most recent studies support some kind of selective management of stable patients with penetrating neck injuries. A single-center study, evaluating stable penetrating neck trauma patients during a 16-month period, demonstrated helical CTA to have 100% sensitivity and 93.5% specificity in detecting all vascular and aerodigestive injuries sustained.[21] In some trauma centers, CTA has replaced conventional angiography in the initial assessment of stable penetrating trauma patients, since CTA is less costly and faster, does not require assembly of an angiographic team, and has fewer potential complications.[22] Angiography still remains the "gold standard" and is performed in patients who have inadequate studies, streak artifacts due to foreign bodies, or inconclusive CTA results. Performing diagnostic tests, such as endoscopy and esophageal contrast studies, in addition to CTA, is controversial. The accuracy of helical CT scan in detecting esophageal injury has not been studied extensively. In one study, two (50%) of four esophageal injuries in patients with penetrating trauma were missed by CT. It is important to note that esophagography missed the same two esophageal injuries as well.[23] The conclusion is that CT scan is no better or worse than esophagography in screening for esophageal injury. Further support for use of helical CT in penetrating trauma is the identification of the trajectory track. Such findings may increase suspicion of injury to the aerodigestive tract, thus delineating the need for observation, esophagoscopy, or operative exploration. Because a number of clinical reviews demonstrate similar patient outcomes, each institution or surgeon should adopt a management plan most consistent with local resources and experience.

At Harborview Medical Center in Seattle, all patients with neck wounds who are in hypovolemic shock or who have evolving stroke are immediately explored for vascular control. Most of those with neck wounds that penetrate the platysma in zone II undergo exploration, as do all patients with clinical signs of tracheal, esophageal, or major vascular injury. The track of the offending agent is followed throughout its course to exclude any possible vascular, tracheal, esophageal, or neurologic injury. Endoscopy is usually performed intraoperatively if pharyngeal, esophageal, or tracheal injury is suspected but cannot readily be identified. Some asymptomatic, stable patients with penetrating zone II neck injury are evaluated initially with CTA. Zone I and III penetrating injuries are selectively managed, based on clinical presentation and the results of diagnostic studies. Hemodynamically unstable patients undergo immediate exploration, with operative incision based on the most likely source of vascular injury. Zone I injuries are managed like mediastinal traversing wounds.[19,24] CTA is performed in hemodynamically stable patients with penetrating wounds to zone I to identify potential injuries to the thoracic outlet vessels or to better plan the operative approach. Depending on the penetrating wound trajectory seen on CTA, esophagography is performed to detect esophageal injury. Endoscopy is considered a complementary procedure to the esophagography, and should follow if there is any question of an abnormality.[25] CTA is also performed for zone III injuries, because of the possible inaccessibility of internal carotid artery lesions or to demonstrate a need for systemic anticoagulation. Angiography is performed in patients with inadequate or inconclusive CTA. In addition, most of the vascular lesions identified at the base of the skull are best managed by interventional angiography techniques.

Evolution in Diagnostic Modalities

Hemodynamically stable patients who sustain trauma with potential injury to the neck may be candidates for nonoperative management. Most of these patients lack the "hard" signs of injury such as expanding hematoma, active bleeding, significant air leak, or airway compromise.[26] These patients may be observed with assistance of diagnostic modalities when indicated. Traditionally, the most common studies are radiographic survey of the cervical spine, four-vessel angiography, esophagoscopy and/or esophagography, and bronchoscopy. Performing these studies, however, may be expensive and time consuming. In addition, four-vessel angiography is an invasive test with potential for complications. Therefore, a more selective approach to screen for cerebrovascular injuries is warranted and has been practiced.[27] Recently, with improvement of less invasive diagnostic methods such as helical CTA or magnetic resonance angiography (MRA), there has been an effort to substitute such modalities in place of routine angiography.[28,29]

5 CTA offers definitive advantages and has emerged as the primary diagnostic screening modality.[26] In fact, high-resolution CTA has replaced angiography in evaluation of selected patients with potential for cerebrovascular injuries in some trauma centers. The allure for helical CT is that it is a relatively fast, noninvasive test that can evaluate cervical spine, trachea, soft tissue, and vascular structures at the same time. Earlier data demonstrated CTA to be inadequate for screening of patients with blunt neck injury.[30] The diagnostic accuracy of high-resolution helical CTA, however, has improved with advances in image technology and increasing experience and expertise in evaluating these studies in trauma patients. Helical CT technology is rapidly changing, and the single-detector row is being replaced with multidetector row configuration, generating 1-mm-thick sections that are reconstructed at 0.5-mm intervals.[31] The recent data from the radiologic literature are favorable, reporting a sensitivity and specificity of 90% and 100%, respectively, in diagnosis of carotid and vertebral artery injuries in selected patients with penetrating neck injury.[31–33] Four major published studies have concluded that 16-channel detectors can be used to accurately screen at-risk patients for blunt cervical vascular injuries.[34–37] Eastman et al. compared digital subtraction angiography to CTA in a prospective study and identified 46 blunt cervical vascular injuries among 43 patients.[35] The overall sensitivity, specificity, positive predictive value, negative predictive value, and accuracy of CTA for the diagnosis of blunt cervical vascular injuries were 97.7%, 100%, 100%, 99.3%, and 99.3%, respectively.[35] The accuracy of helical CT in detecting blunt cervical vascular injuries remains controversial, however. A recent prospective comparative study of 16-channel detector CTA and angiography for detection of blunt cervical vascular injuries in at-risk trauma patients demonstrated the sensitivity, specificity, positive predictive value, and negative predictive value of CTA to be 74%, 86%, 65%, and 90%, respectively.[38] In addition, although CTA is less invasive than traditional angiography, the volume of contrast material used for helical CTA may be higher.[33] This is especially true when a focused study of the unilateral carotid or vertebral artery is desired rather than four-vessel angiography. Therefore, a digital subtraction angiography may be preferred in patients with high risk for contrast-induced nephrotoxicity.[33] Further studies of helical CTA in evaluation of trauma patients are warranted before uniform acceptance of this diagnostic modality; however, with the arrival of 64-detector scanners and increased

experience with the technology, CTA is likely to replace angiography in screening for cervical vascular injuries.

There is encouraging evidence regarding the use of duplex ultrasound and MRA as screening diagnostic tools.[39,40] In a multicenter study, duplex ultrasound demonstrated 86% (12 of 14) of the arterial injuries but was unable to discern dissection of the internal carotid artery at the base of the skull in two patients; proximal flow characteristics were also normal in both of these patients.[39,41] Use of MRA in screening of trauma patients has been limited due to practical problems such as monitoring the patient in the magnetic resonance imaging suite and lack of around-the-clock access. Most data regarding evaluation of cerebrovascular structures by MRA are in nontrauma patients.[42–44] In these studies MRA demonstrated a high accuracy in detecting vascular disease but remained less reliable than the "gold standard" digital subtraction angiography. The sensitivity of MRA in detecting cerebrovascular injuries in 143 blunt trauma patients was only 50%.[30] This study, however, utilized a 0.2 Tesla open magnet, and current studies utilize 1.5 Tesla magnets with significantly better image quality. Improving image quality and increasing experience in interpreting the findings may improve the accuracy of MRA in detecting cerebrovascular injury.

In the past, CT was frequently utilized to evaluate the cervical spine after incomplete or inadequate plain films. However, evaluation of the cervical spine for identification of fractures following blunt trauma has been changing from the traditional three-view plain film to helical CT scan with sagittal reconstruction. This is especially true in patients who require a CT scan of the head. Obtaining a helical CT scan of the cervical spine as the initial study has expedited time, as the initial study has expedited time to spine clearance,[45] increased sensitivity,[46] and decreased costs.[47]

The combination of the aforementioned findings makes helical CT scan an ideal screening tool for neck injuries. One advantage of helical CTA is that it can be incorporated in the workup of a blunt trauma patient who is having a head CT scan to evaluate intracranial structures because of concomitant head injury. Ideally, the cervical spine, soft tissue, and vascular structures are evaluated, without extra trips to the plain radiology or angiography suite. Other modalities such as MRA do not have the versatility of the helical CT scan, require the presence of around-the-clock expertise, still lack sufficient evidence to demonstrate their accuracy, and may possess high costs, all of which may make them impractical to use as mass screening tools for trauma patients.

OPERATIVE EXPLORATION

Of patients with penetrating neck trauma (depending on mechanism), 25% to 50% present with obvious signs of injury requiring prompt operation. An additional 10% to 20% of patients without clinical signs of injury are discovered to have significant vascular, esophageal, or airway injury on further diagnostic testing. A physician treating patients with neck trauma must be capable of performing a complete neck exploration and repair of vascular and aerodigestive injuries. Neck exploration should be performed in the operating room under general endotracheal anesthesia. In the hemodynamically stable patient with a patent airway, intubation can be deferred until laryngoscopy and bronchoscopy have been performed. A nasogastric tube is usually passed to ensure an empty stomach. Preparation and draping of the patient before induction of anesthesia allows control of hemorrhage if the patient starts to gag at the time of placement of the endotracheal tube. The chest is also auscultated before surgery, and a chest radiograph is routinely performed, because penetrating injuries may follow a downward path with pleural penetration. A pneumo-thorax may not develop until positive-pressure ventilation is applied, and it may initially present as unexplained hypotension during anesthesia.

The incision is planned to allow full exposure of the tract of the injury (Fig. 21.4). The oblique incision along the anterior border of the sternocleidomastoid muscle is preferred for unilateral and high (zone III) injuries, whereas the transverse collar incision is preferable for bilateral or neck-traversing wounds. Extension of either neck incision into a median sternotomy affords excellent exposure of the thoracic great vessels. Proximal and distal control of the major vessels potentially involved must also be considered in the length and position of the incision, and the patient is always surgically prepared for a possible median sternotomy. The tract of the injury is followed to its depth, systematically examining each structure in or near the tract.

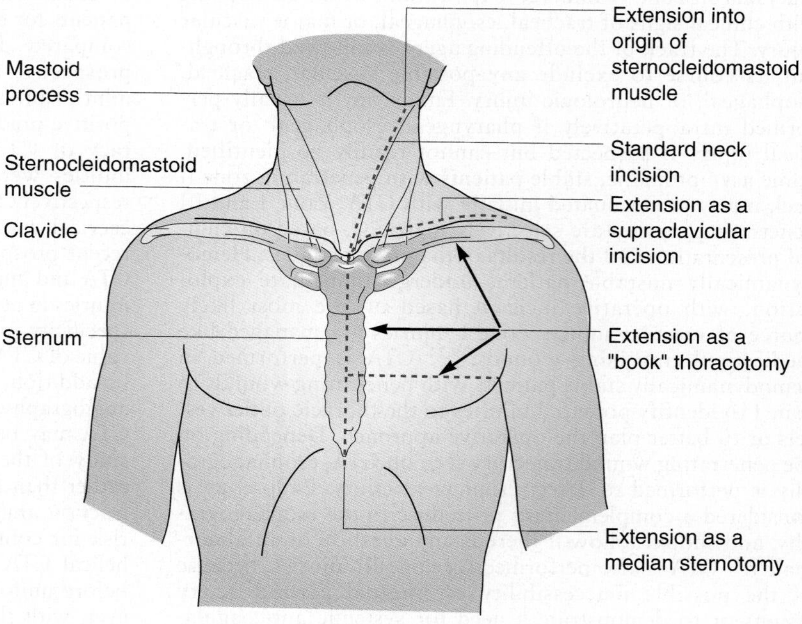

FIGURE 21.4. Neck exploration incisions. Extension of oblique or collar incision into a median sternotomy affords excellent exposure of the great vessels.

MANAGEMENT OF SPECIFIC INJURIES

Blood Vessels

Blood vessels are the most commonly injured structures in the neck. Major arterial and venous injuries occur in 18% and 26% of penetrating neck wounds, respectively.[48] There has been an increase in reported blunt carotid injuries, most likely due to better recognition.[49–51] Most recent studies report an incidence rate of 1% to 2% for blunt cervical vascular injuries. The initial diagnosis, however, remains a difficult one and must always be suspected with an appropriate mechanism of injury.

Carotid Artery

In one of the largest series reported in English literature, 85 blunt carotid injuries were recognized in 67 patients over 11 years in a level I trauma center.[51] Motor vehicle crashes were the most common injury mechanism (82%), followed by motorcycle crashes (7%) and assaults (6%). All but two of the patients had associated injuries, and combinations of blunt carotid injury with closed head and cervical spine injuries occurred in 48% and 6% of patients, respectively. The initial physical examination demonstrated neurologic examination that was not compatible with brain CT in 34% and soft tissue injury in the anterior neck in 14% of the patients. A neurologic deficit developed subsequent to hospital admission in 43% of the patients. The average interval from injury to definitive diagnosis was 53 hours, highlighting the point that, although its recognition is often delayed, blunt carotid trauma must be suspected in patients who develop focal neurologic signs or symptoms after a latent interval. In a multicenter review, 29% of patients developed significant neurologic deficits more than 12 hours after admission.[41] Other physical findings—expanding hematoma, audible bruit, pulsatile neck mass, palpable thrill, Horner syndrome, or any neurologic symptom not explained by other injuries—may be absent at the initial examination. Cervical vascular injury should be suspected in trauma patients with neurologic deficit not explained by head CT. Because some evidence suggested improved outcome with early diagnosis,[41,50,51] a high index of suspicion must exist if the mechanism of injury involves a direct blow to or compression of the neck, basilar skull fracture, cervical hyperextension and rotation, or blunt bilateral perioral fractures. Table 21.3 lists screening criteria for blunt cerebrovascular injury in asymptomatic trauma patients.[27,30]

The mortality rate remains high with blunt carotid injury, ranging from 20% to 40%, with permanent neurologic impairment in 25% to 80% of survivors.[41,50–52] There is a reasonably good neurologic outcome, better than 55%, for an uncomplicated arterial dissection and a uniformly poor outcome, with close to 100% mortality, for complete arterial disruption or bilateral arterial occlusion.[41,50,51] Treatment is highly variable and the efficacy has not been proven in a prospective study.[50,51,53] Therapy depends on the type and location of the vascular lesion, concomitant injuries, availability of the interventional techniques, and preference of the treating surgeon. Arterial dissections can be best managed by systemic anticoagulation.[51] For patients with contraindication to full anticoagulation, aspirin and antiplatelet therapy have been suggested.[50] Anticoagulation is to prevent propagation, embolization, and thrombosis. Stenting and primary surgical therapy, in anatomically favorable locations, have also been used in the management of arterial dissection in small studies.[41,50,51,54] If it is anatomically feasible, pseudoaneurysms are resected. Larger inaccessible pseudoaneurysms are a difficult management challenge; the treatment includes anticoagulation, balloon occlusion, stenting, ligation, or extracranial-intracranial bypass.[53,55,56] Patients with carotid-cavernous fistulas have been treated with balloon occlusion with variable results.[41,51] The outcome of an arterial injury with complete vascular thrombosis depends more on the neurologic status than on any treatment regimen. Nonsurgical management seems appropriate for most of these patients.[52] The rare and fortunate patient with complete carotid thrombosis without neurologic deficits can best be treated with anticoagulation to prevent further or contralateral damage.

Patients with penetrating carotid artery injury most commonly present with exsanguinating hemorrhage. The principles of operative repair of vascular structures in the neck are the same as those for other major vessels. What makes neck vascular trauma unique is the intolerance of the perfused end organ (brain) to even short periods of ischemia. The indication for repair versus ligation of a carotid injury in part depends on the neurologic presentation. Patients without a neurologic deficit should have restoration of vascular continuity, with a good neurologic outcome anticipated. Patients with all grades of neurologic deficits short of coma should also have primary vascular repair.[57] Although the experience with revascularization of patients suffering acute stroke from arteriosclerotic occlusive disease suggests that hemorrhagic infarction and death can result from revascularization, several reviews of acute revascularization in the trauma patient note that the combined morbidity and mortality rate is significantly lower in patients undergoing primary repair (15%) compared with those treated with arterial ligation (50%).[58–60] In comatose patients, neither repair nor ligation appears to influence what is a uniformly poor prognosis. Ligation of the carotid artery is indicated in the comatose patient with no prograde flow, in the presence of uncontrollable hemorrhage, or if technical reasons prohibit repair. There currently is little experience or evidence to favor extracranial-intracranial bypass in the patient requiring carotid artery ligation for trauma, although it has been used selectively in patients requiring selective carotid occlusion.[61,62]

TABLE 21.3 **DIAGNOSIS**

SCREENING CRITERIA FOR SUSPECTED BLUNT CEREBROVASCULAR INJURY IN ASYMPTOMATIC PATIENTS

- Cervical spine fracture in proximity to internal carotid or vertebral artery
- Skull base fracture extending into the carotid canal
- Le Fort II or III facial fracture
- Extensive soft tissue neck injury such as seat belt injury or hanging
- Diffuse axonal injury
- Mechanism associated with severe cervical hyperextension or hyperflexion
- Significant cervical soft tissue injury

Vertebral Artery

Traumatic injury to the vertebral artery, once only rarely diagnosed, is now more commonly identified because of the liberal application of neck angiography after both penetrating and blunt neck injuries. Blunt vertebral artery injuries occur more commonly than blunt carotid injuries, probably because of the close association of bony and ligamentous structures. Mechanisms reported to cause vertebral artery injury are remarkably diverse, including hyperextension and rotation, direct blows, chiropractic manipulation, yoga exercises, volleyball, and even "head banging" to heavy metal rock music.[63,64] Unilateral vertebral artery occlusion seldom results in a neurologic deficit, despite a 15% incidence of congenital unilateral hypoplastic vertebral arteries.[65] Treatment of blunt vertebral artery injury with thrombosis usually is nonoperative: systemic anticoagulation (if possible) is recommended to avoid further propagation

FIGURE 21.5. Normal anatomy of the vertebral artery, showing its division into four parts.

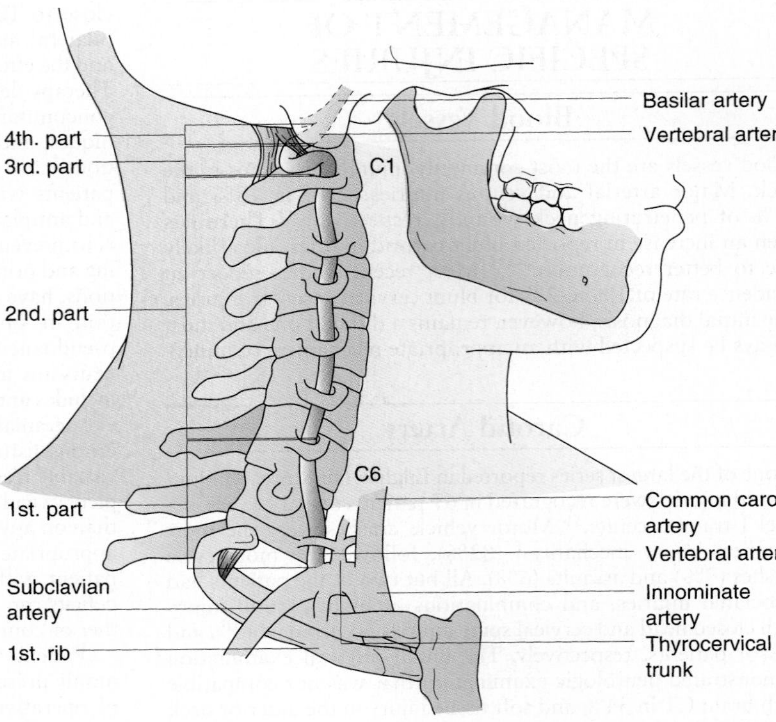

of existing thrombus. More often with penetrating wounds, acute hemorrhage, pseudoaneurysm, and formation of an arteriovenous fistula are reasons for surgically addressing a known vertebral artery injury. Operative exposure and exploration can be difficult. The extraosseous first portion of the vertebral artery can be exposed by a supraclavicular incision with transection of the sternal head of the sternocleidomastoid muscle (Fig. 21.5). More distal exposure (second or third portion) is best obtained by an anterior approach.[66,67] An incision is made along the anterior border of the sternocleidomastoid muscle, and the carotid sheath is identified and retracted either anterosuperiorly or posteroinferiorly to expose the prevertebral space (Fig. 21.6). Hemoclips are blindly applied where the vertebral artery is free of the osseous vertebral canal between the transverse processes, behind the longus cervicis (colli) muscle. High ligation of the vertebral artery at the C1-2 level (fourth portion) is a satisfactory method of obtaining distal control without unroofing the bony canal of the vertebral artery.[1,65] Percutaneous embolization both distal and proximal to the site of arterial injury simplifies the management, but it requires a skilled and experienced interventional angiographer to cross the site of injury without causing further, uncorrectable damage. Contralateral vertebral angiography is recommended to accurately determine the extent of injury or the adequacy of embolization.

Trachea and Larynx

Blunt laryngeal trauma typically results from an anterior impact force (e.g., dashboard, steering wheel) that drives the larynx posteriorly against the rigid cervical spine. The impact can produce a simple or comminuted fracture of laryngeal cartilage, disruption of the mucosa of the endolarynx, or perforation and tears of the hypopharynx. Figure 21.7 depicts the critical laryngeal anatomy and the most common blunt injury pattern. These injuries are frequently occult and are often initially overlooked as attention is directed to injuries of the head, face, and thorax. Delayed recognition of blunt laryngeal trauma is the single greatest contributor to mortality, followed by aspiration of blood, missed esophageal injury, and overlooked concomitant intra-abdominal injury. Subtle clinical signs and symptoms of laryngeal injury cannot be ignored. One report identifies hoarseness as the most common symptom, followed by shortness of breath, inability to tolerate the supine position, pain, dysphagia, and aphonia. Tenderness was identified as the most common clinical sign, followed by subcutaneous emphysema, neck contusion, tracheal deviation, and hemoptysis.[68] Liberal use of neck CT and fiberoptic endoscopy aids in the diagnosis.[69]

Unlike blunt laryngeal trauma, penetrating injuries to the trachea and larynx are usually readily apparent and dramatic in their clinical presentation. Subcutaneous emphysema (occasionally massive), pain, hoarseness, and respiratory distress are hallmarks of tracheal injury. However, rapid endotracheal intubation by field paramedics can mask a high tracheal injury. Concomitant esophageal, vascular, and thoracic injuries are frequent. A 20-year review of 106 tracheobronchial injuries documented a 22% incidence of concomitant esophageal injuries, a 16% incidence of major vessel injury, and a 40% incidence of hemopneumothorax.[70]

As with any trauma victim, the first treatment priority for those with laryngotracheal injuries is to secure an adequate airway. With a laryngeal injury, this usually straightforward task can be extremely challenging. If an emergency airway is required, direct endotracheal intubation can be attempted initially if the laryngeal structures are well visualized and the endotracheal tube is passed over a flexible endoscope. However, this risks further damage to the trachea even in the most experienced hands. Equipment and preparation for emergency tracheostomy should always be at hand, and tracheostomy is usually recommended if an emergency airway is required, even though it also carries some risk of further injury.[71] Pulse oximetry monitoring is essential, and care must be taken to prevent episodes of hypoxia while alternative airway access techniques are attempted. Transtracheal needle-jet insufflation can temporize a critical situation and allow a more controlled tracheostomy.

Operative repair is usually not required for patients with simple laryngeal edema, hematomas without mucosal disruption, small lacerations of the endolarynx not involving the anterior commissure or the free margin of the vocal fold, and

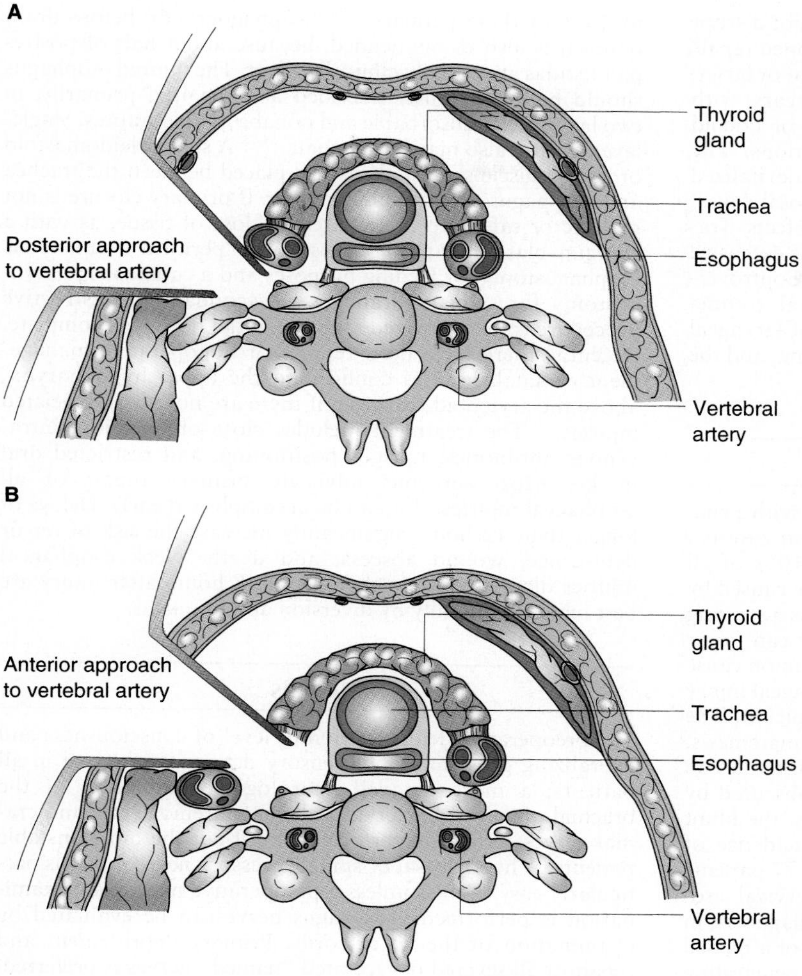

FIGURE 21.6. Operative approach to the vertebral artery. **A:** Carotid artery and sheath retracted anteriorly. **B:** Carotid artery and sheath retracted posteriorly.

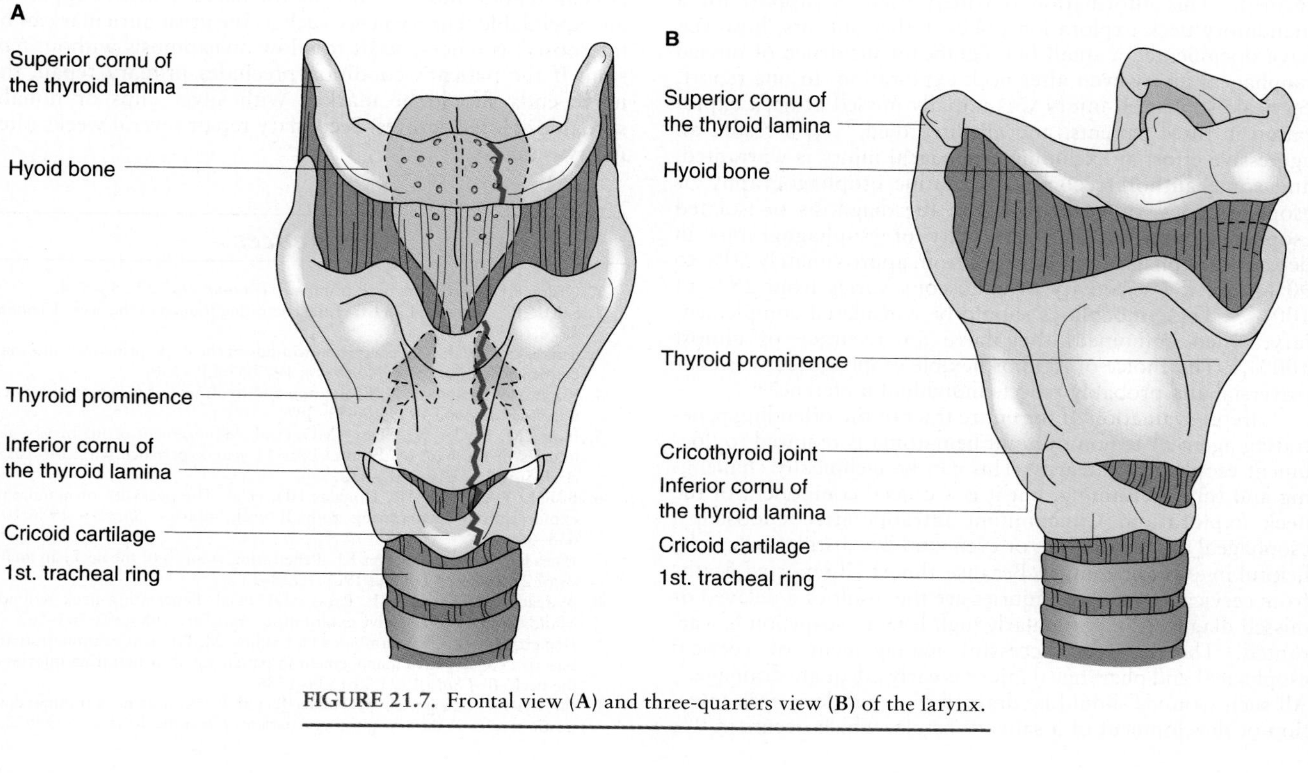

FIGURE 21.7. Frontal view (**A**) and three-quarters view (**B**) of the larynx.

small lacerations of the supraglottic larynx that do not disrupt the integrity of this site.[71] Indications for primary open repair of the larynx include virtually all penetrating tracheal or laryngeal wounds, vocal cord disruption, mucosal tears with exposed cartilage, thyrohyoid separation, thyroid or cricoid cartilage fractures, and hypopharyngeal perforations. The basic tenets of operative care are débridement of devitalized cartilage, reduction of cartilaginous fractures, mucosal coverage of exposed cartilage, and closure of tracheal defects. Tracheostomy is not always required, but it is useful if extensive edema or prolonged airway control is anticipated. Controversial areas in the surgical care of laryngotracheal trauma patients include the timing of operation, the role of laryngeal stints, the use of steroids, indications for skin grafting, and the techniques of operative exposure of the larynx.[72]

Pharynx and Esophagus

Esophageal injuries occur in only 5% of patients with penetrating neck wounds. Esophageal perforation from external blunt trauma is rare and accounts for less than 10% of all esophageal perforations.[73,74] Most blunt injuries are caused by a direct blow to the neck with a hard object, such as a steering wheel in high-speed motor vehicle crashes, but it can occur from minor trauma. Esophageal injury is an uncommon cause of pneumomediastinum. The diagnosis of an esophageal injury can be difficult and requires a high index of suspicion. The clinical signs of esophageal injury, such as hematemesis, odynophagia, neck pain, crepitus, and air in the soft tissues on chest and neck radiographs, are often absent or obscured by concomitant laryngotracheal injury.[75] In one study, the blunt cervicothoracic esophageal injury had a 56% incidence of associated tracheolaryngeal injury.[74] In a review of 77 patients with penetrating esophageal injuries, 45 had cervical esophageal wounds.[76] Overall, physical findings were diagnostic in only 26% of patients. Furthermore, the morbidity of a missed esophageal injury is catastrophic. One review of penetrating neck wounds contained 109 cases of esophageal injuries; the mortality rate was 2% if operation was immediately performed but increased to 44% if operation was delayed because of an initially missed injury and to 100% if no operation was performed.[3] This information is widely used as support for a mandatory neck exploration policy. Other authors, however, have documented a small but significant incidence of missed esophageal injury even after neck exploration. In one report, cervical esophageal injury was initially missed at neck exploration in three patients, and all three died.[76] As a result, an aggressive effort at excluding esophageal injury is warranted, and some authors recommend routine esophagography or esophagoscopy, or both, to aid in the diagnosis of isolated esophageal injuries. The sensitivity of esophagography in detecting esophageal injury varies from approximately 50% to 90%, and the sensitivity of endoscopy varies from 29% to 100%.[18] These modalities should be considered complementary; when combined, they have an accuracy of almost 100%.[25] The choice of rigid or flexible esophagoscopy is controversial and probably reflects individual preferences.

Careful evaluation of the entire tract of the offending penetrating agent or region of blunt hematoma is required to document esophageal integrity. This can be technically challenging and time consuming, but it is a crucial component of the neck exploration. Concomitant intraoperative endoscopy, esophageal air insufflation, or even vital dye instillation can be helpful in excluding injury. Because almost all reported deaths from cervical esophageal injuries are the result of a delayed or missed diagnosis, a particularly high level of suspicion is warranted. The key to successful management of cervical esophageal and pharyngeal injury is early adequate drainage.[77] All such wounds should be drained to avoid deep neck infection or development of a salivary fistula, which occurs in 9% to 18% of these patients.[75,78] Esophagography before drain removal is also recommended, because about half of postrepair fistulas are initially clinically silent. The injured esophagus should be meticulously débrided and repaired primarily, in two layers, with absorbable and nonabsorbable sutures. Single-layer closure also may be adequate.[75,78] A sternocleidomastoid or strap muscle should always be placed between the trachea and esophagus in a combined repair. If primary closure is not realistic or safe, due to an extensive loss of tissue, as with a shotgun blast, it may be necessary to perform a cutaneous esophagostomy for feeding purposes and a cutaneous pharyngostomy for salivary drainage. A secondary reconstructive procedure is then required after the initial healing is complete. Recently, there have been reports of nonoperative management of small injuries confined to the upper hypopharynx, above the arytenoid cartilage, if there are no other associated injuries.[77] The treatment includes close observation, intravenous antibiotics, upright positioning, and restricted oral intake. Most surgeons advocate primary repair of all esophageal injuries, if it can be accomplished early. Delays of longer than 12 hours significantly increase the risk of repair dehiscence, wound abscess, and death. Neck esophageal injuries diagnosed more than 24 to 48 hours after injury are best managed initially by diversion and drainage.

Nerves

The preoperative determination of level of consciousness and lateralizing gross motor or sensory deficits is required in all patients; a more detailed neurologic examination of the brachial plexus, deep cervical plexus, phrenic nerve, and cranial nerves should be performed in all but the most unstable patients. A hypoglossal or spinal accessory nerve injury is particularly easy to miss unless a preoperative neurologic examination is performed. The vagus nerve can be evaluated by examination of the vocal cords. Primary débridement and repair of all severed or lacerated "named" nerves is preferred, with the use of fine interrupted nonabsorbable sutures on the perineurium. Repair of a *single* recurrent nerve injury is controversial. An avulsed recurrent laryngeal nerve (blunt laryngotracheal disruption) should be implanted into the posterior cricoarytenoid muscle.[79] If a motor nerve deficit is apparent, an expendable sensory nerve such as the great auricular can be interposed as a nerve graft to allow anastomosis without tension. If the patient's condition precludes primary repair, the nerve ends should be marked with silver clips or nonabsorbable colored sutures. Secondary repair several weeks after injury is advised.

References

1. Ordog GJ. Penetrating neck trauma. *J Trauma* 1987;27:543–554.
2. Saletta JD, Lowe RJ, Lim LT, et al. Penetrating trauma of the neck. *J Trauma* 1976;16:579–587.
3. Sankaran S, Walt AJ. Penetrating wounds of the neck: principles and some controversies. *Surg Clin North Am* 1977;57:139–150.
4. Roon AJ, Christensen N. Evaluation and treatment of penetrating cervical injuries. *J Trauma* 1979;19:391–397.
5. Flint LM, Snyder WH, Perry MO, et al. Management of major vascular injuries in the base of the neck. An 11-year experience with 146 cases. *Arch Surg* 1973;106:407–413.
6. Bishara RA, Pasch AR, Douglas DD, et al. The necessity of mandatory exploration of penetrating zone II neck injuries. *Surgery* 1986;100: 655–660.
7. Jones RF, Terrell JC, Salyer KE. Penetrating wounds of the neck: an analysis of 274 cases. *J Trauma* 1967;7:228–237.
8. Ayuyao AM, Kaledzi YL, Parsa MH, et al. Penetrating neck wounds. Mandatory versus selective exploration. *Ann Surg* 1985;202:563–567.
9. Demetriades D, Charalambides D, Lakhoo M. Physical examination and selective conservative management in patients with penetrating injuries of the neck. *Br J Surg* 1993;80:1534–1536.
10. Jurkovich GJ, Zingarelli W, Wallace J, et al. Penetrating neck trauma: diagnostic studies in the asymptomatic patient. *J Trauma* 1985;25:819–822.

11. Mansour MA, Moore EE, Moore FA, et al. Validating the selective management of penetrating neck wounds. *Am J Surg* 1991;162:517–520; discussion 520–521.
12. Merion RM, Harness JK, Ramsburgh SR, et al. Selective management of penetrating neck trauma. Cost implications. *Arch Surg* 1981;116:691–696.
13. Asensio JA, Valenziano CP, Falcone RE, et al. Management of penetrating neck injuries. The controversy surrounding zone II injuries. *Surg Clin North Am* 1991;71:267–296.
14. Biffl WL, Moore EE, Rehse DH, et al. Selective management of penetrating neck trauma based on cervical level of injury. *Am J Surg* 1997;174: 678–682.
15. Irish JC, Hekkenberg R, Gullane PJ, et al. Penetrating and blunt neck trauma: 10-year review of a Canadian experience. *Can J Surg* 1997;40: 33–38.
16. Klyachkin ML, Rohmiller M, Charash WE, et al. Penetrating injuries of the neck: selective management evolving. *Am Surg* 1997;63:189–194.
17. Sofianos C, Degiannis E, Van den Aardweg MS, et al. Selective surgical management of zone II gunshot injuries of the neck: a prospective study. *Surgery* 1996;120:785–788.
18. Carducci B, Lowe RA, Dalsey W. Penetrating neck trauma: consensus and controversies. *Ann Emerg Med* 1986;15:208–215.
19. Hirshberg A, Wall MJ, Johnston RH Jr, et al. Transcervical gunshot injuries. *Am J Surg* 1994;167:309–312.
20. Sclafani SJ, Cavaliere G, Atweh N, et al. The role of angiography in penetrating neck trauma. *J Trauma* 1991;31:557–562; discussion 562–563.
21. Inaba K, Munera F, McKenney M, et al. Prospective evaluation of screening multislice helical computed tomographic angiography in the initial evaluation of penetrating neck injuries. *J Trauma* 2006;61:144–149.
22. Munera F, Cohn S, Rivas LA. Penetrating injuries of the neck: use of helical computed tomographic angiography. *J Trauma* 2005;58:413–418.
23. Gonzalez RP, Falimirski M, Holevar MR, et al. Penetrating zone II neck injury: does dynamic computed tomographic scan contribute to the diagnostic sensitivity of physical examination for surgically significant injury? A prospective blinded study. *J Trauma* 2003;54:61–64; discussion 64–65.
24. Richardson JD, Flint LM, Snow NJ, et al. Management of transmediastinal gunshot wounds. *Surgery* 1981;90:671–676.
25. Weigelt JA, Thal ER, Snyder WH 3rd, et al. Diagnosis of penetrating cervical esophageal injuries. *Am J Surg* 1987;154:619–622.
26. Gracias VH, Reilly PM, Philpott J, et al. Computed tomography in the evaluation of penetrating neck trauma: a preliminary study. *Arch Surg* 2001;136:1231–1235.
27. Biffl WL, Moore EE, Offner PJ, et al. Optimizing screening for blunt cerebrovascular injuries. *Am J Surg* 1999;178:517–522.
28. Rogers FB, Baker EF, Osler TM, et al. Computed tomographic angiography as a screening modality for blunt cervical arterial injuries: preliminary results. *J Trauma* 1999;46:380–385.
29. LeBlang SD, Nunez DB Jr. Helical CT of cervical spine and soft tissue injuries of the neck. *Radiol Clin North Am* 1999;37:515–532, v–vi.
30. Miller PR, Fabian TC, Croce MA, et al. Prospective screening for blunt cerebrovascular injuries: analysis of diagnostic modalities and outcomes. *Ann Surg* 2002;236:386–393; discussion 393–395.
31. Nunez DB Jr, Torres-Leon M, Munera F. Vascular injuries of the neck and thoracic inlet: helical CT-angiographic correlation. *Radiographics* 2004; 24:1087–1098; discussion 1099–1100.
32. Munera F, Soto JA, Nunez D. Penetrating injuries of the neck and the increasing role of CTA. *Emerg Radiol* 2004;10:303–309.
33. Munera F, Soto JA, Palacio DM, et al. Penetrating neck injuries: helical CT angiography for initial evaluation. *Radiology* 2002;224:366–372.
34. Biffl WL, Egglin T, Benedetto B, et al. Sixteen-slice computed tomographic angiography is a reliable noninvasive screening test for clinically significant blunt cerebrovascular injuries. *J Trauma* 2006;60:745–751; discussion 751–752.
35. Eastman AL, Chason DP, Perez CL, et al. Computed tomographic angiography for the diagnosis of blunt cervical vascular injury: is it ready for primetime? *J Trauma* 2006;60:925–929; discussion 929.
36. Utter GH, Hollingworth W, Hallam DK, et al. Sixteen-slice CT angiography in patients with suspected blunt carotid and vertebral artery injuries. *J Am Coll Surg* 2006;203:838–848.
37. Berne JD, Reuland KS, Villarreal DH, et al. Sixteen-slice multi-detector computed tomographic angiography improves the accuracy of screening for blunt cerebrovascular injury. *J Trauma* 2006;60:1204–1209; discussion 1209–1210.
38. Malhotra AK, Camacho M, Ivatury RR, et al. Computed tomographic angiography for the diagnosis of blunt carotid/vertebral artery injury: a note of caution. *Ann Surg* 2007;246:632–642; discussion 642–643.
39. Davis JW, Holbrook TL, Hoyt DB, et al. Blunt carotid artery dissection: incidence, associated injuries, screening, and treatment. *J Trauma* 1990; 30:1514–1517.
40. Mascalchi M, Bianchi MC, Mangiafico S, et al. MRI and MR angiography of vertebral artery dissection. *Neuroradiology* 1997;39:329–340.
41. Cogbill TH, Moore EE, Meissner M, et al. The spectrum of blunt injury to the carotid artery: a multicenter perspective. *J Trauma* 1994;37:473–479.
42. U-King-IM JM, Trivedi RA, Graves MJ, et al. Contrast-enhanced MR angiography for carotid disease: diagnostic and potential clinical impact. *Neurology* 2004;62:1282–1290.
43. Ho KY. MR angiography of carotid arteries. *JBR-BTR* 2004;87:29–32.
44. Hathout GM, Duh MJ, El-Saden SM. Accuracy of contrast-enhanced MR angiography in predicting angiographic stenosis of the internal carotid artery: linear regression analysis. *AJNR Am J Neuroradiol* 2003;24: 1747–1756.
45. Daffner RH. Cervical radiography for trauma patients: a time-effective technique? *AJR Am J Roentgenol* 2000;175:1309–1311.
46. Hanson JA, Blackmore CC, Mann FA, et al. Cervical spine injury: a clinical decision rule to identify high-risk patients for helical CT screening. *AJR Am J Roentgenol* 2000;174:713–717.
47. Grogan EL, Morris JA Jr, Dittus RS, et al. Cervical spine evaluation in urban trauma centers: lowering institutional costs and complications through helical CT scan. *J Am Coll Surg* 2005;200:160–165.
48. Beitsch P, Weigelt JA, Flynn E, et al. Physical examination and arteriography in patients with penetrating zone II neck wounds. *Arch Surg* 1994; 129:577–581.
49. Welling RE, Saul TG, Tew JM Jr, et al. Management of blunt injury to the internal carotid artery. *J Trauma* 1987;27:1221–1226.
50. Eachempati SR, Vaslef SN, Sebastian MW, et al. Blunt vascular injuries of the head and neck: is heparinization necessary? *J Trauma* 1998;45: 997–1004.
51. Fabian TC, Patton JH Jr, Croce MA, et al. Blunt carotid injury. Importance of early diagnosis and anticoagulant therapy. *Ann Surg* 1996;223: 513–522; discussion 522–525.
52. Fakhry SM, Jaques PF, Proctor HJ. Cervical vessel injury after blunt trauma. *J Vasc Surg* 1988;8:501–508.
53. Pretre R, Reverdin A, Kalonji T, et al. Blunt carotid artery injury: difficult therapeutic approaches for an underrecognized entity. *Surgery* 1994;115: 375–381.
54. Okada Y, Shima T, Nishida M, et al. Traumatic dissection of the common carotid artery after blunt injury to the neck. *Surg Neurol* 1999;51: 513–519; discussion 519–520.
55. Gewertz BL, Samson DS, Ditmore QM, et al. Management of penetrating injuries of the internal carotid artery at the base of the skull utilizing extracranial-intracranial bypass. *J Trauma* 1980;20:365–369.
56. Sundt TM Jr, Pearson BW, Piepgras DG, et al. Surgical management of aneurysms of the distal extracranial internal carotid artery. *J Neurosurg* 1986;64:169–182.
57. Brown MF, Graham JM, Feliciano DV, et al. Carotid artery injuries. *Am J Surg* 1982;144:748–753.
58. Liekweg WG Jr, Greenfield LJ. Management of penetrating carotid arterial injury. *Ann Surg* 1978;188:587–592.
59. Unger SW, Tucker WS Jr, Mrdeza MA, et al. Carotid arterial trauma. *Surgery* 1980;87:477–487.
60. Weaver FA, Yellin AE, Wagner WH, et al. The role of arterial reconstruction in penetrating carotid injuries. *Arch Surg* 1988;123:1106–1111.
61. Martin WS, Gussack GS. Pediatric penetrating head and neck trauma. *Laryngoscope* 1990;100:1288–1291.
62. Vazquez Anon V, Aymard A, Gobin YP, et al. Balloon occlusion of the internal carotid artery in 40 cases of giant intracavernous aneurysm: technical aspects, cerebral monitoring, and results. *Neuroradiology* 1992;34: 245–251.
63. DeBehnke DJ, Brady W. Vertebral artery dissection due to minor neck trauma. *J Emerg Med* 1994;12:27–31.
64. Egnor MR, Page LK, David C. Vertebral artery aneurysm–a unique hazard of head banging by heavy metal rockers. Case report. *Pediatr Neurosurg* 1991;17:135–138.
65. Golueke P, Sclafani S, Phillips T, et al. Vertebral artery injury–diagnosis and management. *J Trauma* 1987;27:856–865.
66. Hatzitheofilou C, Strahlendorf C, Kakoyiannis S, et al. Penetrating external injuries of the oesophagus and pharynx. *Br J Surg* 1993;80: 1147–1149.
67. Meier DE, Brink BE, Fry WJ. Vertebral artery trauma: acute recognition and treatment. *Arch Surg* 1981;116:236–239.
68. Myers EM, Iko BO. The management of acute laryngeal trauma. *J Trauma* 1987;27:448–452.
69. Fuhrman GM, Stieg FH III, Buerk CA. Blunt laryngeal trauma: classification and management protocol. *J Trauma* 1990;30:87–92.
70. Kelly JP, Webb WR, Moulder PV, et al. Management of airway trauma. I: tracheobronchial injuries. *Ann Thorac Surg* 1985;40:551–555.
71. Schaefer SD. The acute management of external laryngeal trauma. A 27-year experience. *Arch Otolaryngol Head Neck Surg* 1992;118:598–604.
72. Gussack GS, Jurkovich GJ. Treatment dilemmas in laryngotracheal trauma. *J Trauma* 1988;28:1439–1444.
73. Beal SL, Pottmeyer EW, Spisso JM. Esophageal perforation following external blunt trauma. *J Trauma* 1988;28:1425–1432.
74. Jacobs I, Niknejad G, Kelly K, et al. Hypopharyngeal perforation after blunt neck trauma: case report and review of the literature. *J Trauma* 1999;46:957–958.
75. Glatterer MS Jr, Toon RS, Ellestad C, et al. Management of blunt and penetrating external esophageal trauma. *J Trauma* 1985;25:784–792.
76. Defore WW Jr, Mattox KL, Hansen HA, et al. Surgical management of penetrating injuries of the esophagus. *Am J Surg* 1977;134:734–738.
77. Stanley RB Jr, Armstrong WB, Fetterman BL, et al. Management of external penetrating injuries into the hypopharyngeal-cervical esophageal funnel. *J Trauma* 1997;42:675–679.
78. Winter RP, Weigelt JA. Cervical esophageal trauma. Incidence and cause of esophageal fistulas. *Arch Surg* 1990;125:849–851; discussion 851–852.
79. Snow JB Jr. Diagnosis and therapy for acute laryngeal and tracheal trauma. *Otolaryngol Clin North Am* 1984;17:101–106.

CHAPTER 22 ■ CHEST TRAUMA

THOMAS K. VARGHESE Jr.

KEY POINTS

1. Thoracic injuries are a significant source of morbidity and mortality.
2. Injuries identified during the primary survey should be corrected as soon as they are identified.
3. Immediate life-threatening injuries identified during the secondary survey are not obvious on physical examination. A high degree of suspicion is needed along with appropriate use of diagnostic studies.
4. Several manifestations of thoracic trauma are indicative of a greater risk of associated injuries. Subcutaneous emphysema is associated with airway or lung injury. Injuries to the upper ribs (1 through 3), scapula, and sternum are associated with significant mechanisms of injury.
5. In situations where a significant mechanism of force has occurred, underlying head, spine, and thoracic injuries should be suspected.

1 Thoracic injuries account for 25% of immediate trauma-related deaths, second only to head and spinal cord injuries.[1] For those who survive the initial trauma, an additional 25% will die within the first year from complications.[2] Initial assessment and treatment of patients with thoracic trauma consists of the primary survey and intervention, resuscitation of vital functions, detailed secondary survey, and definitive care.

Major thoracic injuries can be grouped together as the
2 "fatal 14" (Table 22.1). The lethal six (airway obstruction, tension pneumothorax, open pneumothorax, flail chest with pulmonary contusion, massive hemothorax, and cardiac tamponade) are immediate life-threatening injuries that should be corrected as they are being identified during the primary
3 survey. The hidden eight (simple pneumothorax, hemothorax, pulmonary contusion, tracheobronchial tree injury, blunt cardiac injury, traumatic aortic disruption, traumatic diaphragmatic tear, and esophageal rupture) are potentially life-threatening injuries that should be detected during the secondary survey with subsequent definitive treatment.

TREATMENT OF INJURIES DURING THE PRIMARY SURVEY

Airway Assessment

The first priority in treating trauma patients is airway management. Trauma personnel rarely see acute airway injuries presenting to the emergency department (ED), which is likely the result of the high fatality rate at the scene secondary to aspiration of blood, secretions, and debris causing an acute airway obstruction. Acute management of the airway should follow the guidelines proposed and updated regularly by the American College of Surgeons Committee on Trauma for Advanced Trauma Life Support (ATLS). The cornerstones of airway management are adequate oxygenation, ventilation, and protection from aspiration. Airway patency and air exchange should be assessed by listening for air movement at the patient's nose, mouth, and lung fields; inspecting the oropharynx for airway obstruction; and observing for intercostal and supraclavicular muscle retractions. Orotracheal intubation with appropriate cervical spine immobilization and direct laryngoscopy is the most common important first step in establishing a secure airway. However, extreme caution is needed in the face of significant maxillofacial trauma and suspicion of laryngeal trauma. The flexible bronchoscope can serve as an important aid in the diagnosis and management of the injured airway. However, this may take some time to perform even in the most experienced hands. The status of the larynx may be assessed with a bronchoscope and a decision can be made to continue with orotracheal tube insertion over the bronchoscope versus proceeding with placement of a surgical airway.

A cricothyrotomy may play a lifesaving role when orotracheal intubation is not possible and should not be delayed by excessive attempts at orotracheal intubation. It is contraindicated in the presence of a rare laryngeal or cricoid cartilage injury. It may also be difficult to perform in the face of an expanding neck hematoma or significant subcutaneous emphysema. And, while a tracheostomy in the acute setting is difficult to perform, it is indicated in the face of severe laryngeal trauma, as well as in the setting of a disrupted cervical trachea, where the endotracheal tube can be placed directly through the injured area (Fig. 22.1).

Posterior dislocation of the clavicular head also can cause upper airway obstruction after injury to the upper chest. The injury should be suspected when there is presence of a palpable defect in the sternoclavicular joint associated with stridor or change in voice quality. Closed reduction of the dislocation can be achieved either by extension of the shoulders or by direct grasping of the clavicle with a towel clip to manually reduce the dislocation.

BREATHING

Complete exposure of the patient's chest and neck allows for assessment of breathing and the neck veins. Signs of chest injury or hypoxia include increased respiratory rate or change in breathing pattern.

Tension Pneumothorax

4 Tension pneumothorax develops secondary to a bronchopleural fistula (BPF) acting as a one-way valve, allowing for air entry into the pleural space from a defect in the lung

TABLE 22.1

CLASSIFICATION OF MAJOR THORACIC INJURIES ("FATAL 14")

A. Injuries identified during the primary survey ("lethal six")
   - i. Airway obstruction
   - ii. Tension pneumothorax
   - iii. Open pneumothorax
   - iv. Flail chest with pulmonary contusion
   - v. Massive hemothorax
   - vi. Cardiac tamponade

B. Injuries identified during the secondary survey ("hidden eight")
   - i. Simple pneumothorax
   - ii. Hemothorax
   - iii. Pulmonary contusion
   - iv. Tracheobronchial tree injury
   - v. Blunt cardiac injury
   - vi. Traumatic aortic disruption
   - vii. Traumatic diaphragmatic tear
   - viii. Esophageal rupture

parenchyma or airway (Fig. 22.2). The one-way valve effect can also occur through a defect in the chest wall. As a result of the sudden increase of air in the pleural space, the ipsilateral lung collapses, and the mediastinum shifts to the opposite side. This interferes with expansion of the contralateral lung and causes accompanying compromise of venous return to the heart. The associated hypotension is due to impaired filling pressures of the myocardium.

The most common cause of tension pneumothorax is positive-pressure mechanical ventilation in patients with visceral pleural injury. It can also occur as a complication of a simple pneumothorax after penetrating or blunt chest trauma when the lung parenchyma fails to seal. Traumatic defects in the chest wall may also cause a tension pneumothorax if the defect itself acts as a one-way flap valve or if the defect is incorrectly covered with an occlusive dressing without chest tube placement.

A tension pneumothorax is a clinical diagnosis reflecting air under pressure in the pleural space. In the setting of clinical suspicion and physical signs, treatment should be immediate and not be delayed for a chest radiograph. Signs and symptoms of tension pneumothorax include chest pain, respiratory distress, tachycardia, hypotension, tracheal deviation, unilateral absence of breath sounds, and neck vein distention. As these signs are similar to cardiac tamponade, differentiation should be made by hyperresonance on percussion and absence of breath sounds on the affected side. Both tension pneumothorax and massive hemothorax are associated with decreased breath sounds on auscultation. Differentiation on physical examination is made by percussion; hyperresonance confirms a pneumothorax, whereas dullness is present with a massive hemothorax. The possibility of an occult acute tension pneumothorax should also be entertained in the setting of a critically ill patient being mechanically ventilated who has a high peak airway pressure (>30 cm H_2O), requires high positive end-expiratory pressure (PEEP; >15 cm), has a history of thoracic trauma or chronic obstructive pulmonary disease, or decompensates immediately after an intervention (e.g., central line placement, bronchoscopy, deep endotracheal suctioning). Immediate treatment includes emergency needle decompression and aspiration, followed by chest tube placement. A standard large-bore intravenous catheter is inserted into the second intercostal space in the midclavicular line of the affected hemithorax. This maneuver converts the injury to a simple pneumothorax. Definitive therapy soon follows in the form of insertion of a chest tube, usually in the fifth intercostal space just anterior to the midaxillary line.

Open Pneumothorax

Chest wall defects that are significantly large can remain open and result in an open pneumothorax. Such wounds usually

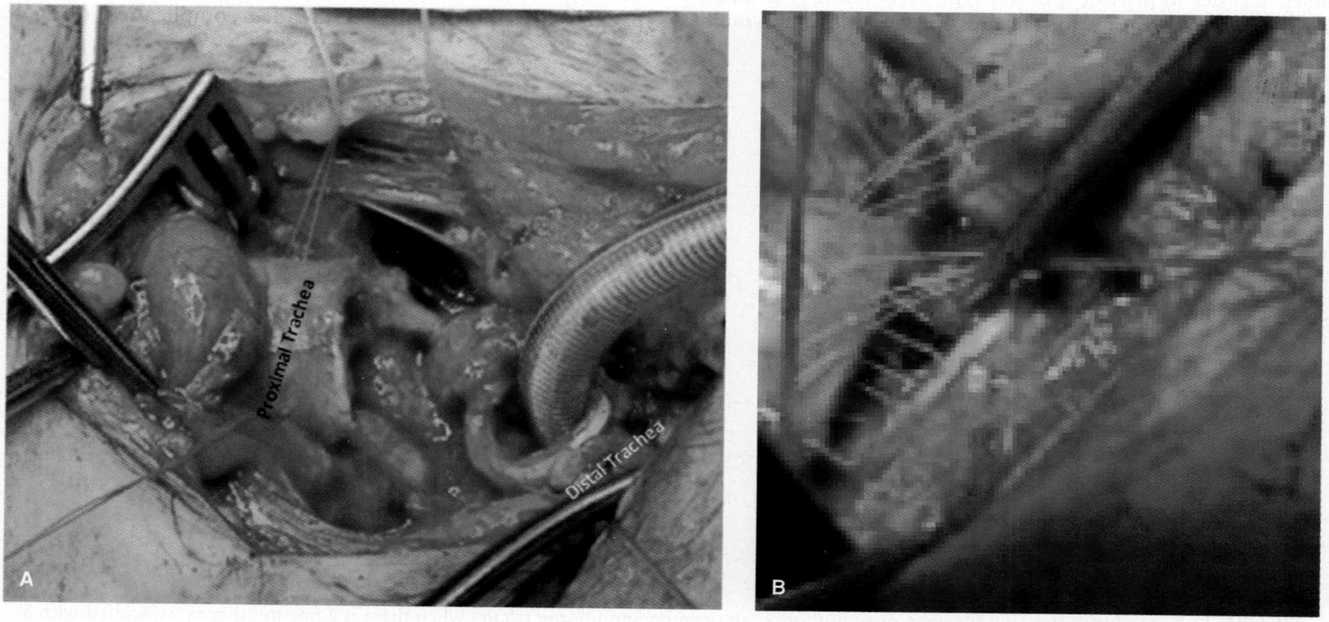

FIGURE 22.1. A 27-year-old patient with history of a 200-lb bag of fertilizer falling onto the back of the neck with subsequent hyperextension and disruption of the cervical trachea. **A:** Patient's airway is stabilized with an endotracheal tube placed into the distal trachea. **B:** Primary repair of the cervical trachea is performed with interrupted 4–0 Vicryl sutures.

TRAUMA

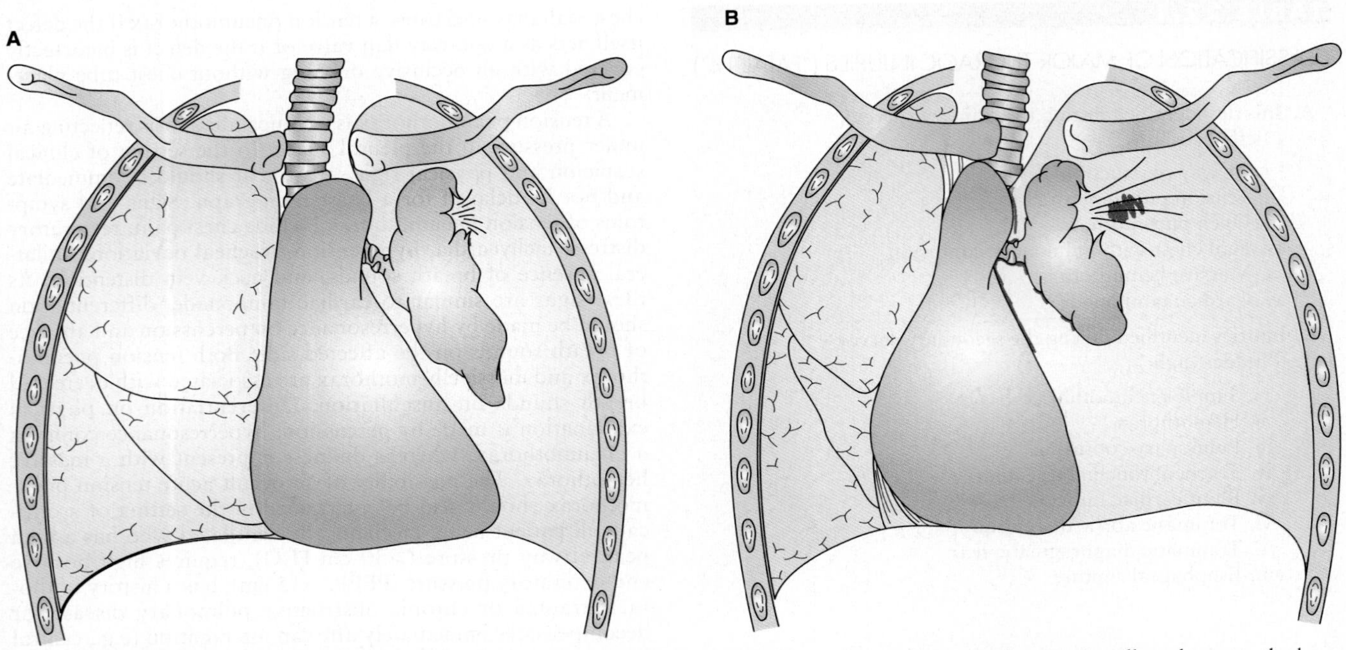

FIGURE 22.2. A: Simple pneumothorax: air collects between the lung and chest wall. B: Tension pneumothorax: air collects between the lung and chest wall, with associated mediastinal shift. This leads to compression of venous structures and subsequent decreased venous return to the heart.

occur from high-velocity missiles or shotguns fired at close range. The large opening leads to immediate equilibration between the atmospheric pressure and intrathoracic pressure. If the opening of the chest wall is at least two-thirds the circumference of the trachea, air passes preferentially through the chest wound with each breath rather than down the tracheobronchial tree. Ventilation is thus compromised leading to significant hypoxia and hypercarbia. The airway is controlled with early intubation and mechanical ventilation. The defect is promptly closed with a sterile occlusive dressing, large enough to overlap the wound's edges and taped securely only on three sides in order to provide a flutter-type valve effect (Fig. 22.3). As the patient breathes in, the dressing occludes the wound, preventing air entry through the chest wall. When the patient exhales, the open end of the dressing allows air to escape from the pleural space. A chest tube is placed remotely from the wound.

The next priority is to address any underlying intrathoracic injuries. If definitive surgical intervention is needed, an attempt is made to make the thoracotomy in such a fashion to preserve blood supply and muscle mass of the chest wall adjacent to the defect. After repair of intrathoracic injuries and débridement of devitalized tissue, the next step is to plan the definitive closure of the wound. In the interim, aggressive wound débridement, drainage of pneumothorax and/or hemothorax, and simple packing are appropriate.[3] A dreaded complication of chest

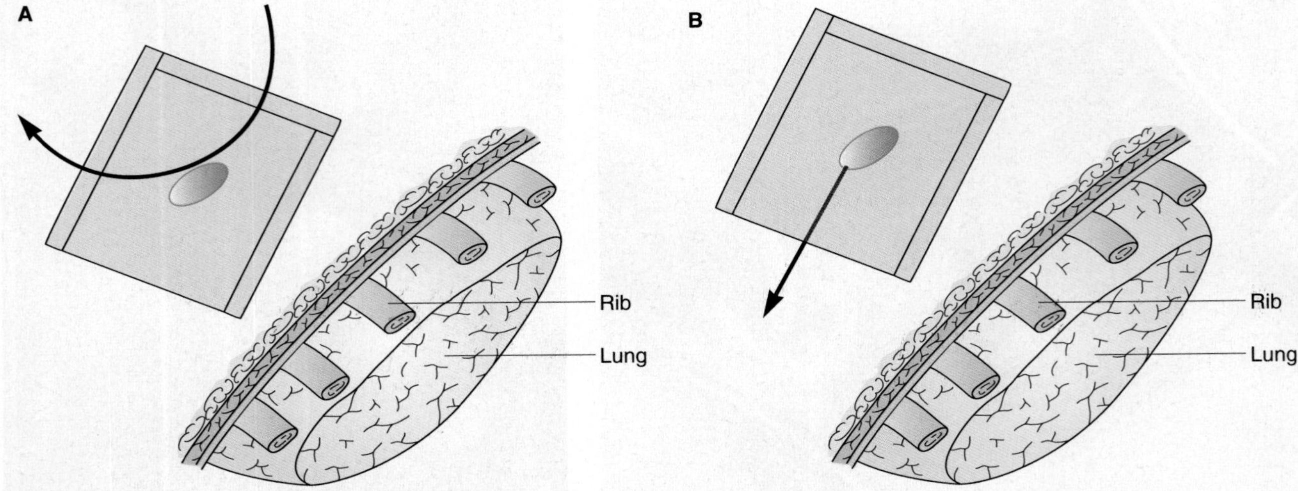

FIGURE 22.3. Occlusive dressing for open pneumothorax: an open pneumothorax occurs when there is a pneumothorax associated with a chest wall defect such that the pneumothorax communicates with the exterior. Treatment entails placing an occlusive dressing as well as an intercostal drain (chest tube). The occlusive dressing is airtight on three sides. A: Inspiration: the occlusive dressing prevents air entry into the chest. B: Expiration: air escapes from the wound and exits at the inferior aspect of the dressing.

wounds is necrotizing infection.[4] These infectious complications need wide local débridement and reconstruction. Most chest wall defects can be closed with viable autogenous tissue, usually through rotation of local flaps of the pectoral muscle, latissimus dorsi, or rectus abdominus. Collaboration between trauma surgeons, plastic surgeons, and thoracic surgeons is often helpful in these complex cases. Extensive injuries may dictate the need for mesh reconstruction with either Gore-Tex or methyl methacrylate.

Flail Chest with Pulmonary Contusion

Flail chest requires complete dissociation of a portion of the chest wall by segmental fractures of two or more adjacent ribs (Fig. 22.4). It may also arise from either disruption of the ribs from the sternum at the costochondral cartilage or a fracture
5 in the ribs (sternal flail; Fig. 22.5). In addition to the disarray in chest wall mechanics, the force needed to cause the injury often leads to significant underlying intrathoracic, primarily pulmonary parenchyma, injury. Although chest wall instability leads to paradoxical motion of the chest wall during inspiration and expiration, the major difficulty in flail chest is the injury to the lung (pulmonary contusion). Additional restriction in chest wall movement from the associated pain further exacerbates hypoxia.

There has been intense debate about the role of surgical intervention for flail chest. In the preventilator era, intervention centered on external fixation techniques such as external strapping, the placement of sandbags, or even external fixation combined with traction.[5] The significant rate of complications, prolonged bed rest needed for fracture union, and high failure rates led to early ventures in internal fixation. However, the use of positive-pressure mechanical ventilation (internal splinting) led to the observation of adequate stabilization in most patients, and hence the enthusiasm for surgical intervention waned. Only select patients who had persistent flail despite mechanical ventilation had a variety of attempted rib fracture repairs done with plates, wires, and intramedullary techniques. Recently, two randomized trials suggested that patients may

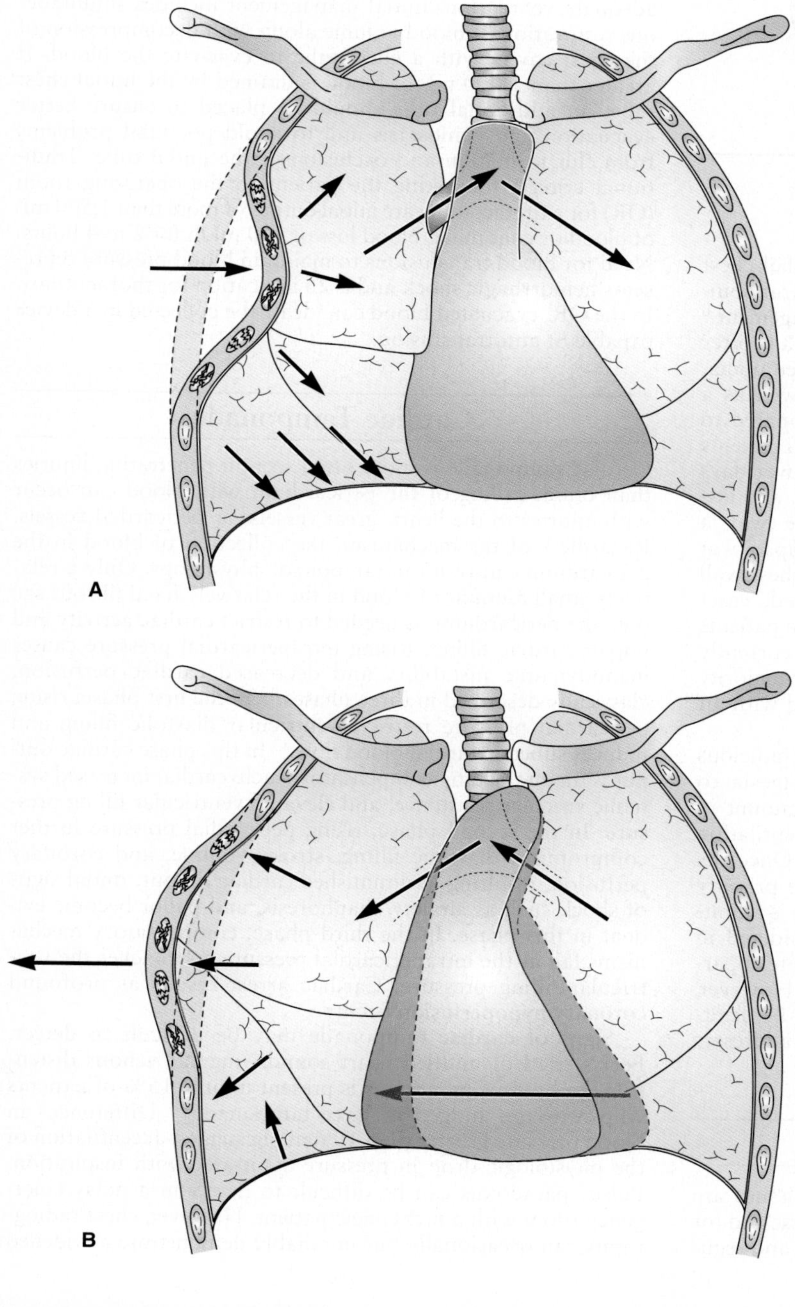

FIGURE 22.4. Pathophysiology of flail chest. **A:** Inspiratory phase: chest wall collapses inward, causing air to move out of the bronchus of the involved lung into the trachea and bronchus of the uninvolved lung, causing a shift of mediastinum to the uninvolved side. **B:** Expiratory phase: chest wall balloons outward so that air is expelled from the lung on the uninvolved side and enters the lung on the involved side with an associated shift of mediastinum to the involved side.

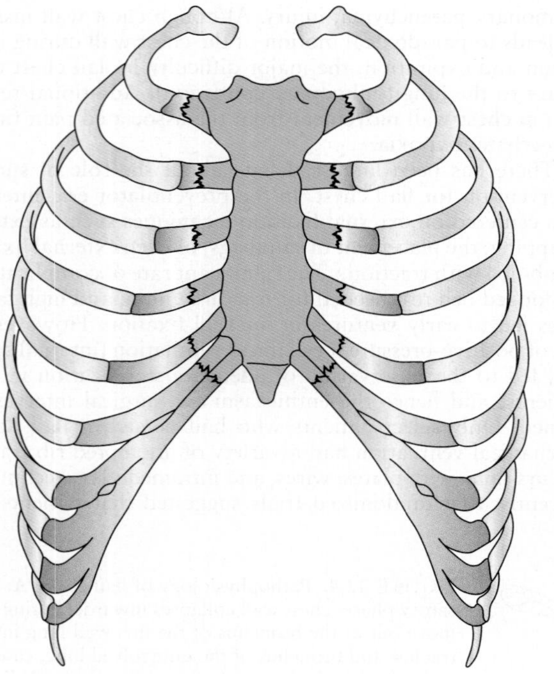

FIGURE 22.5. Sternal flail.

benefit from early operative repair. In one trial, 37 flail chest patients who required mechanical ventilation were randomized to surgical stabilization or nonoperative management.[6] The surgical group had fewer days on the ventilator, a shorter intensive care unit (ICU) stay, a lower incidence of pneumonia, and a better pulmonary function at 1 month, as well as a higher return to work percentage at 6 months, compared to the nonoperative group. A second trial randomized 40 patients in similar fashion.[7] The surgical group again had fewer days on the ventilator, decreased ICU and inpatient stays, and less pneumonia than the nonoperative cohort. There was a reported higher forced vital capacity and total lung capacity at 2 months, as well as decreased incidence of visual chest wall deformity or persistent flail. Other nonrandomized, case-control studies have supported these findings in those patients without major pulmonary contusions.[8–11] However, currently most trauma centers maintain the belief that the vast majority of patients with flail chest are satisfactorily managed without surgical intervention.

Initial treatment of flail chest entails oxygenation, judicious fluid administration, and providing adequate analgesia to improve ventilation. Prevention of hypoxia is paramount in these patients, and thus a period of intubation and ventilation may be necessary until all injuries are delineated. Once the ventilation status is stabilized, the remainder of the primary and secondary survey are completed, and the patient is admitted to the ICU. Surgical intervention may be considered in those patients who remain ventilator dependent despite apparent resolution of underlying pulmonary contusions. However, the definitive role for surgical intervention may not be determined until a randomized multicenter clinical trial addresses this issue.

CIRCULATION

After acute life-threatening airway and breathing issues are addressed during the primary survey, the patient is assessed for hypovolemia. The pulse is noted for its quality, rate, and regularity. Neck veins should be noted for distention. Cardiac contusions can lead to arrhythmias, which can be exacerbated with hypoxia and acidosis. Major thoracic injuries that affect circulation should be addressed during the primary survey, such as massive hemothorax and cardiac tamponade.

Massive Hemothorax

Massive hemothorax results from the collection of more than 1,500 mL of blood (30% to 40% of total blood volume) rapidly in the chest. This occurs most often with a penetrating wound with a systemic or hilar vessel injury, though it can also occur with blunt trauma. Penetrating anterior chest wounds medial to the nipple line and posterior wounds medial to the scapula should alert to the likelihood of an injury to the great vessels, hilar structures, and the heart. A massive hemothorax is suspected when shock accompanies absence of breath sounds and dullness to percussion on one side of the chest. Blood loss is complicated by hypoxia, as the significant rapid accumulation of blood in the chest compromises respiratory efforts by mechanically compressing the lung and preventing adequate ventilation. Initial management includes simultaneous restoration of blood volume along with decompression of the chest cavity with a chest tube to evacuate the blood. If greater than 1,000 mL of blood is drained by the initial chest tube, an additional tube should be placed to ensure better evacuation and hemostasis and to avoid potential problems from clot formation and occlusion of the initial tube. Traditional criteria for taking the patient to the operating room (OR) for a thoracotomy are initial output of more than 1,500 mL of blood or continuing blood loss of 200 mL/h for 2 to 4 hours. Need for blood transfusions to maintain blood pressure represents hemorrhagic shock and is an indication for thoracotomy. In the OR, evacuated blood can ideally be collected in a device capable of autotransfusion.

Cardiac Tamponade

Cardiac tamponade is more often seen in penetrating injuries than blunt. Filling of the pericardium with blood can occur with injuries to the heart, great vessels, or pericardial vessels. Regardless of the mechanism, the collection of blood in the pericardium can result in tamponade physiology. Only a relatively small amount of blood in the relatively fixed fibrous sac (i.e., the pericardium) is needed to restrict cardiac activity and impair cardiac filling. Rising intrapericardial pressure causes hemodynamic instability and decreased cardiac perfusion, classically described in three phases.[12] In the first phase, rising pericardial pressure restricts ventricular diastolic filling and reduces subendocardial blood flow.[13] In this phase cardiac output is maintained by compensatory tachycardia, increased systemic vascular resistance, and elevated ventricular filling pressure. In the second phase, rising pericardial pressure further compromises diastolic filling, stroke volume, and coronary perfusion, resulting in diminished cardiac output. Initial signs of shock such as anxiety, diaphoresis, and pallor become evident in this phase. In the third phase, compensatory mechanisms fail as the intrapericardial pressure approaches the ventricular filling pressure. Cardiac arrest results as profound coronary hypoperfusion occurs.

Signs of cardiac tamponade may be difficult to detect. Beck's triad of muffled heart sounds, jugular venous distention, and pulsus paradoxus is present in only 15% of patients who are later judged to have tamponade.[14] Differences in blood pressure greater than 10 mm Hg suggest accentuation of the physiologic drop in pressure associated with inspiration. Pulsus paradoxus can be difficult to detect in a noisy emergency room with a tachypneic patient. However, chest radiography can occasionally but unreliably demonstrate a widened cardiac shadow. Central venous pressure (CVP) reflecting elevated pressures can lead to the diagnosis, but may be absent due to hypovolemia. Elevated CVP and pulseless electrical activity (PEA) are nonspecific signs. Prompt diagnosis and evacuation of pericardial blood are indicated for patients who do not respond to the usual measures of resuscitation for hemorrhagic shock and have the potential for cardiac tamponade. Methods that are rapid and accurate in assessing cardiac injuries include focused sonogram in trauma (FAST) and echocardiography.[15] The presence of a pericardial effusion is diagnostic. However, its absence does not necessarily rule out injury.[16] Specifically, echocardiography cannot reliably rule out cardiac injury in the setting of an associated left pleural effusion. This occurs due to the effusion obscuring the pericardium or the effusion occurring as a result of a pericardial tear and escape of blood from the pericardium into the pleural space. In this circumstance, the pericardial sac may be empty.

In the first two phases of cardiac tamponade, patients may be aggressively managed with definitive airway control and volume resuscitation, and may be temporized with an attempted pericardiocentesis. However, definitive intervention requires taking the patient to the OR for a pericardial window or immediate median sternotomy. A pericardial window is typically performed through the subxiphoid approach, although there is a role for thoracoscopy in the stable patient with an associated hemothorax or if the abdominal route is to be avoided in the case of intra-abdominal contamination.[17] When the diagnosis is highly likely due to pattern or injury, hemodynamic responses, and/or ultrasound (FAST) results, a primary median sternotomy may be indicated prior to further physiologic deterioration for both definitive diagnosis and treatment. In the third phase of tamponade, patients have profound hypotension and should undergo ED thoracotomy (EDT) for evacuation of pericardial blood. Following the release of tamponade, the source of bleeding is directly controlled.

Emergency Department Thoracotomy. With the advent of regionalized trauma systems, the number of patients who, rather than dying in the field, arrive in extremis has increased. Closed heart massage for cardiac arrest or PEA is ineffective in patients with hypovolemia. Patients with penetrating thoracic injuries who arrive pulseless but with signs of life (reactive pupils, spontaneous movements, or organized electrocardiographic [ECG] activity) are candidates for immediate resuscitative thoracotomy. The other set of patients who may benefit from EDT are those patients with either blunt or penetrating thoracic injuries who lose their vitals in the trauma bay. EDT refers to the use of a resuscitative thoracotomy in the ED for those patients in extremis. A left anterolateral thoracotomy incision is preferred for EDT (Fig. 22.6). This enables the procedure to be performed in the supine position and allows for ongoing cardiac massage, and extension into the right hemithorax can be achieved with a clamshell thoracotomy and subsequent exposure of both pleural spaces, as well as mediastinal structures. EDT is performed to correct the cause of cardiovascular collapse from mechanical sources or extreme hypovolemia. The objectives of EDT are to (a) release pericardial tamponade, (b) control cardiac hemorrhage, (c) control intrathoracic bleeding, (d) evacuate massive air embolism, (e) perform open cardiac massage, and (f) temporarily occlude the descending thoracic aorta.[18] The highest survival rate following EDT is in patients with penetrating cardiac wounds, especially with pericardial tamponade.[19] The rationale for temporary thoracic aortic clamping with massive hemorrhage is twofold. First, aortic clamping redistributes the patient's limited blood volume to the myocardium and brain. Second, there may be decreased ongoing subdiaphragmatic blood loss in those patients with significant intra-abdominal injuries. However, once the patient's blood volume has been restored after repair of the injury, the aortic cross-clamp should be removed expeditiously. Persistent clamping in this situation can result in increased myocardial demand, increasing acidosis from malperfusion, and risk of paraplegia.

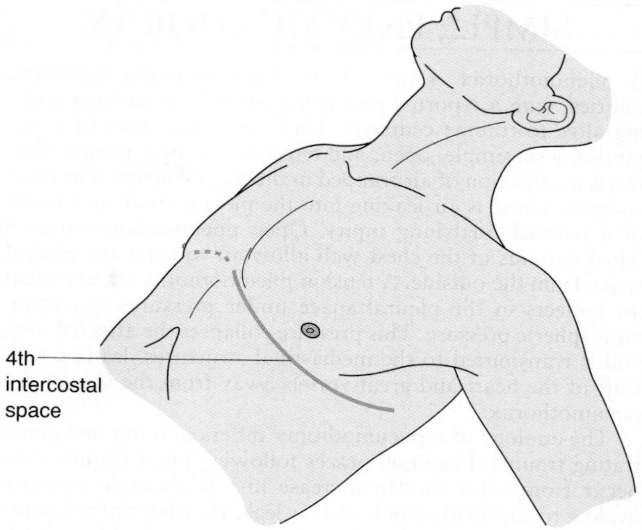

FIGURE 22.6. Left anterolateral thoracotomy incision.

In a patient with a penetrating chest injury who develops profound hypotension and cardiac arrest following endotracheal intubation and positive-pressure ventilation, a bronchovenous air embolism should be suspected. The traumatic alveolar-venous communication leads to migration of the air embolism to the coronary circulation, with resultant myocardial ischemia and shock. The associated low pulmonary venous pressure from intrathoracic blood loss and high bronchoalveolar pressure from positive-pressure ventilation increase the gradient for air transfer across the bronchovenous channels.[20] Immediate thoracotomy with pulmonary hilar cross-clamping prevents further pulmonary venous embolism. The pericardium is opened, and with the patient in Trendelenburg position, air trapped in the ventricles is removed by aspiration. Cardiac massage may also dissolve air present in the coronary arteries. Aspiration of the aortic root is also done to remove any additional accumulated air.

Analysis of the literature on EDT indicates that the success rates approach 35% in the patient arriving in shock with penetrating cardiac wounds and 15% for all penetrating wounds.[18] In contrast, the results of EDT are poor in the setting of blunt trauma, with a survival of only 1% to 2%. Patients undergoing cardiopulmonary resuscitation (CPR) prior to arrival in the ED should be stratified based on the type of injury and transport time to assess the potential utility of EDT.

TREATMENT OF INJURIES DURING THE SECONDARY SURVEY

The secondary survey includes detailed physical examination, a chest radiograph (ideally upright, injuries permitting), arterial blood gas measurements, pulse oximetry, and ECG monitoring. The chest radiograph is examined for adequate lung expansion, presence of fluid, widening of the mediastinum, mediastinal shift, and loss of anatomic detail. Multiple rib fractures and fractures of the first and second ribs are indicative of a severe force delivered to the chest. Unlike the previously described immediate life-threatening conditions, injuries detected during the secondary survey are not obvious on physical examination. A high degree of suspicion is needed, along with appropriate studies.

SIMPLE PNEUMOTHORAX

A pneumothorax is one of the most common traumatic injuries, with a reported prevalence of 20% in patients arriving alive to trauma centers.[21] There are three types of pneumothoraces: simple, open, and tension. A simple pneumothorax is a collection of air trapped in the pleural space. The most common cause is air leaking into the pleural space as a result of a parenchymal lung injury. Open pneumothorax occurs when wounds of the chest wall allow air to enter the pleural space from the outside. A tension pneumothorax occurs when air collects in the pleural space under pressures exceeding atmospheric pressure. This pressure collapses the affected lung and is transmitted to the mediastinal structures, leading to a shift of the heart and great vessels away from the side of the pneumothorax.

The etiology of a pneumothorax differs in blunt and penetrating trauma. Pneumothoraces following blunt trauma may occur from (a) a sudden increase in intrathoracic pressure leading to ruptured alveoli and air leak, (b) rib fractures lacerating the lung, (c) deceleration injuries tearing the lung, or (d) blunt forces directly crushing and disrupting alveoli. In penetrating trauma, the etiology is the direct laceration of lung parenchyma.

A definitive diagnosis is made on chest radiography (Fig. 22.7). Associated findings include subcutaneous emphysema, decreased breath sounds, and overlying chest wounds. With the increased use of computed tomography (CT) in the evaluation of the trauma patient, it is apparent that pneumothoraces can be missed on supine anteroposterior (AP) chest radiography. This rate of missed pneumothorax has been estimated to be as high as 20% to 35%. The patient's symptoms and physiologic response to the pneumothorax is significantly more important than the apparent size and should dictate the urgency of treatment.

There is debate regarding the management of patients whose pneumothorax is visible only on CT and not on a chest radiography. The reported incidence of these occult pneumothoraces is between 2% and 8% of all blunt trauma patients.[22,23] In one retrospective study, the size of the occult pneumothorax was correlated with the need for a chest tube, and recommendation was made for chest tube placement in all pneumothoraces greater than 5 × 80 mm in size.[24] These authors also suggested a chest tube be placed for those with two or more rib fractures. In another prospective study,[25] 8 out of 15 patients on positive-pressure ventilation required chest tubes, with three of these patients having developed tension pneumothoraces. The authors thus recommended chest tubes to be placed for all patients with occult pneumothoraces and requiring positive-pressure ventilation. In contrast, Brasel et al. in a prospective study of 44 patients found that neither size nor positive-pressure ventilation correlated with the development of clinically significant pneumothorax that needed a chest tube.[26] Thus, the treatment of an occult pneumothorax should be done in the context of the whole patient. In the stable patient an occult pneumothorax may be observed, but in those with multiple injuries, it would be wiser to place a chest tube. Serial examinations in those patients observed include repeat chest radiographs at 6 and 24 hours.

Currently, the standard treatment for a traumatic pneumothorax found on the screening AP chest radiograph is placement of a chest tube to allow for reexpansion of the lung and apposition of visceral and parietal pleurae. Supplemental oxygen may be tried to enhance reabsorption of the pneumothorax, but it is unlikely that high inspired oxygen tensions (>60%) will provide any more benefit than O_2 given by nasal prongs.[27]

HEMOTHORAX

Hemothorax is the collection of blood within the pleural space. This can occur as a result of pulmonary parenchymal lacerations, intercostal artery or vein laceration, or disruption of major pulmonary or bronchial vessels. Because parenchymal tears result in low-pressure pulmonary vessel injury, they usually stop bleeding with chest tube intervention and full expansion of the lung. The presence of retained blood in the chest can lead to complications such as empyema and restrictive fibrothorax. Early evacuation of hemothorax is thus ideal. The vast majority of hemothoraces can be drained with chest tube placement alone. Chest tubes fail to completely evacuate a hemothorax in approximately 5% of cases.[28] Conditions that can increase the chance of complications in retained fluid collections include prolonged ventilation, pleural disruption, the development of pneumonia, and other distant sites of

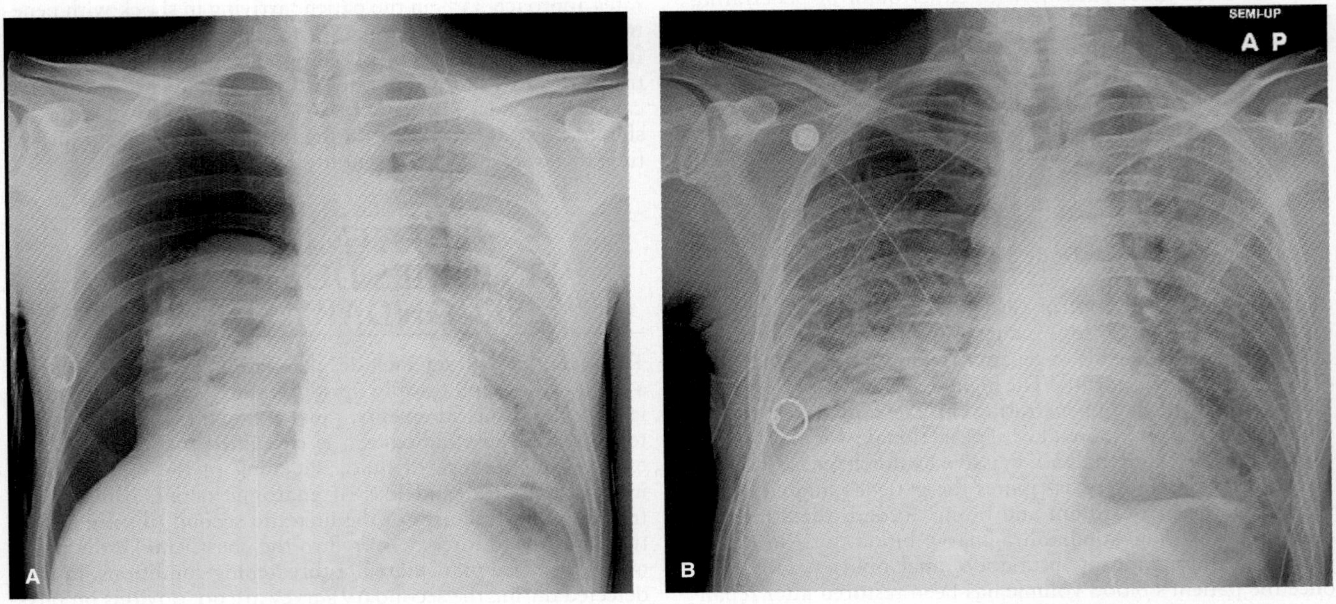

FIGURE 22.7. **A:** Chest radiograph demonstrating simple pneumothorax. **B:** Resolution of pneumothorax after chest tube placement.

infection. This is in contrast to the stable, nonventilated patient with small effusions (less than one fourth of the hemithorax) following blunt trauma with no obvious pleural disruption, who may be observed without intervention.[29]

Recognizing the true extent of a hemothorax can be challenging. Plain chest radiographs, especially done with portable equipment, can be misleading and typically underestimate the true extent of the fluid collection. Chest CT is much more accurate in quantification of total amount of blood, as well as assessment for loculations, entrapped lung, and parenchymal damage.[30] Moderate effusions in the ventilated patient or effusions in those patients with other risk factors for complications should be drained. However, it may be difficult to drain hemothoraces in patients where recognition occurs more than 24 hours after injury due to clot formation and early loculation. In these patients, chest tube placement may lead to inadequate drainage while increasing the pain, splinting, and risk of pneumonia. One option is the instillation of a thrombolytic agent via the chest tube. Intrapleural streptokinase (250,000 IU) or urokinase (40,000 IU) has been reported to have an efficacy ranging from 65% to 90%.[31] Although the risk of rebleeding is negligible, disadvantages to their use include associated fever, severe pain, several days for full effect, and ultimate inability to break down some loculations.

Video-assisted thoracoscopic surgery (VATS) is an effective minimally invasive means of definitively addressing significant hemothoraces persisting after failed chest tube drainage or a delayed diagnosis. The VATS approach is well suited for the treatment of hemothorax, breaking down areas of loculation, and completely evacuating gelatinous exudates and clots from the pleural space. Early fibrinous peels can usually be removed from the visceral pleural surface to free any lung entrapment. At the conclusion of the procedure, strategically placed chest tubes lead to full expansion of the lung and resolution of the process. In one prospective study, patients undergoing VATS early after trauma had decreased length of time requiring chest tube drainage, decreased hospital length of stay (2.7 days less), and subsequent decreased hospital cost ($6,000 less) compared to patients treated with a second chest tube.[32] There were no failures or complications, and no patients required conversion to a full thoracotomy with early VATS. In contrast, placement of a second chest tube failed to completely evacuate the retained hemothorax, requiring operative intervention in over 40% of patients.

VATS should be considered carefully to identify patients in whom it may not be feasible. Possible contraindications include (a) compromised pleural cavity due to previous granulomatous infections, empyema, or thoracotomy; (b) inability to tolerate single-lung ventilation secondary to contralateral pulmonary resection, acute or chronic respiratory insufficiency, high levels of required oxygen on mechanical ventilation, or hemodynamic instability; and (c) bleeding diathesis.[33] In these situations, a formal thoracotomy should be considered. Decortication of a mature visceral pleural peel requires an open approach, as do those situations where dense adhesions are anticipated. If a patient presents late (>3 months following the injury), a fibrothorax typically forms. This rare group of patients should initially be managed nonoperatively, if there is no evidence of infection, as there may be remodeling and adaptation at 6 to 9 months. If surgical intervention is needed, there is no added difficulty in performing the procedure at this later date.

PULMONARY CONTUSION AND PARENCHYMAL INJURIES

A pulmonary contusion is a serious injury to the lung parenchyma and is the most common potentially life-threatening chest injury. Most reviews report a mortality of 5% to 30%, and contusion is the direct cause of death in 25% to 50% of fatalities. Transmission of force (with or without rib fractures) leads to interstitial hemorrhage with resulting alveolar collapse, atelectasis, and consolidation of the uninjured areas of lung.[34] As edema forms around the area of initial injury, compliance decreases and work of ventilation increases. Resulting hypoxia occurs due to increased shunting of blood through unventilated lung.[35] The hypoxia and respiratory embarrassment typically are maximal within the first 24 to 48 hours and are exacerbated by the extent of injury and the associated need for volume replacement.[36] Chest radiographs usually appear normal at the time of initial presentation but then progress to show patchy infiltrates or nonsegmental areas of opacification within the first 4 to 6 hours after injury, usually in areas that underlie rib, clavicle, or sternal fractures. There is a direct correlation between the extent of abnormalities seen on chest radiography and the severity of the injury, and any abnormalities seen on the admission trauma series portend a severe pulmonary contusion. The degree of injury severity can be better assessed by chest CT, where pulmonary contusion appears as an ill-defined area of consolidation. However, routine assessment by CT does not significantly alter therapy or improve outcomes.[37]

TABLE 22.2

SIGNS OF PULMONARY CONTUSION

- Hypoxemia (PaO_2 <60 mm Hg) on room air
- Hypercarbia
- Increased work of breathing
- Hemoptysis
- Loss of lung compliance
- Elevated intrapulmonary shunting
- Ventilation/perfusion mismatch

The full assessment of pulmonary contusions is made through the correlation of clinical signs with radiographic findings and laboratory values (Table 22.2).[38] Any patient who has suffered a high-impact blunt impact to the chest should be suspected of having a pulmonary contusion. Arterial blood gases demonstrate an arterial hypoxemia on room air and hypercarbia. The degree of clinical lung injury can be assessed using a ratio of partial pressure of arterial oxygen (PaO_2) to the fraction of inspired oxygen (FiO_2)[39]:

- PaO_2/FiO_2 ratio less than 300 = acute lung injury
- PaO_2/FiO_2 ratio less than 200 = acute respiratory distress syndrome

A study by Tyburski et al.[40] demonstrated that quantifying the extent of pulmonary contusions on chest radiography and serial PaO_2/FiO_2 ratios in the first 24 hours after injury can aid in predicting the need for ventilatory support and patient outcome. An initial PaO_2/FiO_2 ratio less than 300 that continues to remain less than 300 at 24 hours after injury was the most significant factor correlating with the need for mechanical ventilation.

Management of pulmonary contusions is supportive initially, with goals of adequate oxygenation and decreased work of breathing. Early measures include supplemental oxygen to prevent hypoxemia, chest expansion through the use of incentive spirometry, Acapella flutter valve therapy to promote deep breathing and coughing, control of pain, and increased activity and mobilization to promote perfusion in all areas of the lung. Fluid volume should be restricted as much as possible, as obligatory capillary leaks lead to worsening pulmonary edema. Control of pain is critical in patients with limited chest excursion as a result of pain from rib fractures, chest wall contusion, and other injuries. Inadequate pain relief can lead to hypoventilation, promotion of atelectasis, and worsening hypoxemia. Epidural analgesia or patient-controlled analgesia using opioids and fentanyl patch should be considered, especially in the setting of rib fractures.[35]

Adequate oxygenation should be maintained to achieve a PaO_2 of 60 mm Hg and an oxygen saturation of 90%. Early intubation in this patient population is controversial at present. Intubation should be reserved for the classical indications, although the need for intubation and mechanical ventilation can lead to a 44% incidence of pneumonia. There is no role for routine antibiotic prophylaxis in this patient population. Hemodynamic monitoring with a central mixed venous oxygen saturation catheter can help in monitoring severe pulmonary injuries. A decrease in venous oxygen saturation (60% to 70%) is indicative of inadequate oxygenation and perfusion.

It has been estimated that 20% to 30% of patients who undergo thoracotomy following trauma will require some form of lung resection. Most patients who present with penetrating injuries have peripheral injuries that are simple to manage, whereas extensive blast or blunt trauma often results in combinations of diffuse contusion and lung maceration that is extremely difficult to salvage. The most common procedures required are simple suture repair or wedge resection. Tractotomy is used to either define and, in particular, control bleeding to the tracheobronchial tree in deep injuries or to manage peripheral injuries that pass through the parenchyma. Mortality rates as high as 3% to 50% following lobectomy and 70% to 100% following pneumonectomy reflect the severity of lung and overall injury in patients requiring extensive resection. The use of nonanatomic and stapling techniques has been advocated as a method of both damage control and rapid definitive resection with reduced operative time and blood loss and increased parenchymal salvage.[41]

TRACHEOBRONCHIAL TREE INJURY

Disruption or injury to a major bronchus or trachea is a rare potentially fatal condition that is often overlooked on initial assessment. It has been reported to occur in 1% to 3% of motor vehicle collisions, and more than 80% die in the field.[42,43] Those who reach the hospital alive have a high mortality rate from associated injuries. The injury, alone or in combination, is in the distal trachea within 2 cm of the carina in 76% of cases and in the right main stem within 2 cm of the carina in 43%. Approximately 50% of the injuries are circumferential.[44] In contrast, penetrating injuries involve the cervical trachea in greater than 80% of cases.

A high degree of suspicion is needed to detect these injuries in a timely manner. Clinical signs include subcutaneous emphysema, continuous large air leaks seen in chest tubes, and hemoptysis.[45] Although a chest radiograph is nonspecific, a pneumothorax, cervical emphysema, or pneumomediastinum may be present. A chest CT scan is more sensitive for detecting pneumomediastinum, and occasionally a "fallen lung sign" may be present, where the lung is seen to fall away from the hilum.[46] A persistent pneumothorax, despite a well-placed chest tube, and a continuous air leak throughout the entire respiratory cycle are also signs of a possible tracheobronchial disruption.

The first priority is airway control. Orotracheal intubation with appropriate cervical spine precautions and direct laryngoscopy is typically an appropriate first step in securing the airway. Caution should be used in the setting of maxillofacial trauma or suspicion of laryngeal trauma. Flexible bronchoscopy plays a role in the diagnosis and management of the injured airway. It can be used even in the most difficult airway while maintaining cervical spine immobilization. It allows for the accurate placement of distal tubes in the airway that can act as a stent for the disrupted trachea or mainstem bronchi. The status of the larynx can be assessed and a decision made to continue with the tube insertion over the bronchoscope versus aborting intubation and proceeding with a definite surgical airway. Tracheostomy is preferred over a cricothyroidotomy, as the latter can lead to complete airway separation and loss of ability to intubate in this setting. A smooth-end endotracheal tube such as an Armoured wired endotracheal tube of at least 8.0 French should be used. Adequate suctioning and bronchoscopy are possible with the 8.0 size, and the smooth-end reinforced tube reduces the risk of aggravating the airway tear, is easier to place, can be passed across the injury site, and can be manipulated during surgery. On occasion, the distal airway must be intubated through the operative field to allow for adequate exposure.

A patient who deteriorates after intubation, ventilation, and appropriate chest tube placement and subsequently develops a massive air leak should have immediate bronchoscopy. The timing and type of definitive repair depend on the site, extent, and association with other injuries. The proximal two thirds of the trachea is best approached via a low collar incision. This also allows access to the esophagus and cervical vessels in case of associated injury. The collar incision can be extended down into the manubrium with an upper sternal split ("T incision") for greater exposure of the middle third of the trachea, as well as facilitate control of the proximal innominate artery and vein. If there is any suspicion of injury to a great vessel, the ascending aorta, or the heart, median sternotomy should be employed.[43] The distal one third of the trachea and right mainstem bronchus is best approached by a right posterolateral thoracotomy via the fourth or fifth intercostal space. A left posterolateral thoracotomy through the fourth or fifth intercostal space gives one access to the left mainstem bronchus and the proximal left subclavian artery, descending thoracic aorta, and lower esophagus. However, the very proximal left mainstem is difficult to expose and requires mobilization of the arch by dividing the ligamentum arteriosum.[47]

Repair of simple lacerations of the trachea and bronchi are repaired primarily using interrupted sutures of 3–0 polyglactin 910 (Vicryl) to reestablish mucosal-to-mucosal continuity. Débridement of devitalized tissues should be performed with caution to leave the greatest amount of trachea available for repair. Suture lines performed through the chest are reinforced with pedicled flaps of pleura or pericardium wrapped around the anastomosis. Alternatively, intercostal muscle can be used. Repairs made through the neck are reinforced using mobilized strap muscles. In the case of more complex injuries involving complete transection of the trachea, the trachea can be mobilized anteriorly and around the hila to allow for structures to shift superiorly. Care is taken to avoid lateral dissection as much as possible, as the vascular supply enters on the sides. Interrupted 3–0 Vicryl sutures are placed after careful débridement. Pericartilaginous sutures are placed on the rigid portion of the trachea, and simple interrupted sutures are placed on the membranous portion (Fig. 22.1). At the end of the procedure, the patient's chin may be sutured to the anterior chest to prevent the patient from extending the neck and stressing the suture line ("guardian stitch"). This stitch is left in for 1 week and removed after confirmation of integrity of the suture line is done by flexible bronchoscopy. Distal airway injuries associated with lobar destruction can be managed by lobectomy.[45] Stricture and dehiscence occur in 3% of patients following tracheobronchial reconstruction, with stricture often presenting as new-onset wheezing. If the stricture is limited, dilation and temporary stenting can allow remodeling and thus provide a permanently patent and functioning airway.

BLUNT CARDIAC INJURY

Blunt cardiac injury (BCI) encompasses a spectrum of pathology ranging from clinically silent transient dysrhythmia to deadly free wall rupture. BCI occurs most often from motor vehicle crashes[48] where rapid deceleration occurs. An alternative mechanism is a direct blow to the precordium. Any patient involved in a motor vehicle crash with sudden deceleration or who sustains significant chest trauma is thus at risk. Several forces may be involved in

BCI, including shearing from rapid deceleration, compression of the heart between the spine and sternum, abrupt pressure fluctuations in the chest and abdomen, and blast injury.[49,50] The right heart is most commonly injured, likely related to its close proximity to the anterior chest wall and sternum.

The clinical features of BCI can vary widely. Most patients with severe BCI, such as uncontained myocardial rupture, do not reach the emergency department alive.[51,52] Of those who do, hypotension may reduce pressure on the injured myocardium, which may rupture as fluid resuscitation restores blood pressure. Atrial rupture occurs far less often than ventricular rupture, most likely due to anatomy and lower compliance. Septal injury and isolated valvular injury are extremely rare. Of the valves, the aortic valve is most often injured, followed by the mitral and tricuspid valve. Depending on the valve involved and the degree of injury, the clinical presentation falls between acute valvular insufficiency with right- or left-sided heart failure, a widened pulse pressure, and a new cardiac murmur. Treatment of septal or valvular injury is surgical.

The most common and controversial form of BCI is cardiac contusion. The absence of a clear definition and accepted "gold standard" of diagnosis makes assessment of cardiac contusion difficult. The exact incidence is thus unknown, and can be difficult to determine in the multiply injured trauma patient with many reasons for hypotension. BCI often presents with other injuries. In one autopsy series, sternal fractures were found in 76% of cases involving cardiac injury.[53] However, a sternal fracture does not necessarily imply an associated BCI and lack of fracture does not rule out BCI.

Commotio cordis, a rare type of BCI in which low-impact trauma causes sudden cardiac arrest, usually occurs from being struck by a projectile during sports. The cardiac arrest is theorized to occur from the timing of the blow during a period of electrical susceptibility.

While BCI is often associated with thoracic trauma, it can occur in any patient with multisystem trauma. The ECG is the single most important screening test for hemodynamically stable patients with potential BCI. An ECG consistent with BCI may reveal persistent sinus tachycardia, another dysrhythmia, a new bundle branch block, or ST depressions or elevation. A screening ECG is obtained in all blunt trauma patients with chest pain or tenderness, history suggestive of heart disease, and active signs or symptoms consistent with heart disease. These may include signs of heart failure or abnormal heart sounds.

Patients with unexplained tachycardia that persists over several hours despite adequate fluid resuscitation and pain control, a new bundle branch block, or significant dysrhythmia are admitted for cardiac monitoring and echocardiography. Echocardiography can provide important information in a patient with BCI, but is not as important in the hemodynamically stable patient without dysrhythmia.[49,54,55] In the rare case of blunt thoracic trauma with evidence of myocardial infarction on ECG, serial biomarkers should be measured (troponin I, creatine kinase [CK]-MB), and consultation done with both cardiology and cardiac surgery. In other patients without history of findings of severe cardiac injury but in whom concern persists, a brief course of ED observation over 6 hours can be done with a minimum of two ECGs obtained during the observation. Floor telemetry is appropriate for the patient with minor abnormalities (e.g., intermittent premature ventricular or atrial contractions), no significant concomitant injuries, and normal hemodynamics. All other patients should be admitted to the ICU for close monitoring, with associated cardiology consultation.

TRAUMATIC AORTIC DISRUPTION

Patients involved in high-energy blunt trauma involving rapid deceleration (such as a motor vehicle crash at speeds over 40 miles per hour or a fall from a height of 10 feet) are at significant risk for blunt aortic injury (BAI). BAIs cause immediate death from aortic transection in 80%. In a minority of patients, the adventitia and mediastinal structures contain the rupture, allowing the patient to survive the ambulance transport to the ED. In patients who survive to reach the hospital, the most common site of disruption is just distal to the origin of the left subclavian artery at the ligamentum arteriosum. This site is the juncture of the mobile aortic arch and immobile descending thoracic aorta, additionally tethered by the intercostal arteries. In a sudden deceleration, the descending aorta stops with the rest of the body, while the heart and aortic arch continue to move forward. Shear force develops at the juncture of these two segments of aorta, creating a tear.[56]

TABLE 22.3

CHEST RADIOGRAPHY FINDINGS ASSOCIATED WITH A MAJOR VASCULAR INJURY IN THE CHEST

- Widened mediastinum
- Obliteration of the aortic knob
- Deviation of the trachea to the right
- Depression of the left mainstem bronchus
- Elevation of the right mainstem bronchus
- Obliteration of the aortopulmonary window (space between the aorta and pulmonary artery)
- Deviation of the nasogastric tube (esophagus) to the right
- Widened paratracheal stripe
- Widened paraspinal interfaces
- Presence of a pleural or apical cap
- Left hemothorax
- Fractures of the first rib, second rib, or scapula

Specific signs and symptoms of traumatic aortic disruption are frequently absent. A high index of suspicion prompted by noting the mechanism of injury (rapid deceleration) and findings on chest radiography should be maintained, and the patient appropriately assessed. Findings on chest radiography that indicate a likelihood of major vascular injury in the chest are shown in Table 22.3. Any abnormality on chest radiography should be followed by a CT scan of the chest. A normal CT scan essentially rules out BAI.[57–59] An equivocal CT scan should be followed by angiography to exclude aortic injury in those where suspicion of injury remains.[60] Transesophageal echocardiography (TEE) can be used in those patients too unstable for chest CT. TEE has a high sensitivity and specificity for BAI and can be performed either in the ED or in the OR. It also has utility in assessing valvular incompetence and pericardial effusions.

When BAI is diagnosed, the goal of management is to prevent propagation of adventitial dissection and subsequent free rupture by controlling the shearing forces exerted on the aorta. This is accomplished by lowering the heart rate with a beta-blocker and decreasing the blood pressure with intravenous nitroprusside or nitroglycerin in those cases where the beta-blocker alone is not sufficient. Intravenous esmolol, due to its rapid action and short half-life, is an ideal beta-blocker to use as an initial agent. Beta blockade should be initiated prior to any other blood pressure–reducing medications, as other drugs may result in a compensatory elevation in heart rate and thereby increase the shearing force. In patients in whom beta-blockers are contraindicated, a calcium channel blocker such as diltiazem can be used. The goal is to maintain a heart rate below 100 and a systolic blood pressure around 100 mm Hg.[61]

Surgical options include thoracotomy with open repair or interposition graft, and endovascular stenting. Surgery should not be delayed if clinical or radiographic signs of impending rupture are present such as reaccumulating hemothorax, rapid enlargement of a pseudoaneurysm, or contrast extravasation. Surgery should also ideally be done early in those patients who are hemodynamically stable without other major injuries, as the risk of rupture is high if left untreated. There are, however, reports of patients who safely undergo delayed repair of BAI after diagnosis and careful management of wall stress.[62–64] After controlling for comorbidities, these patients were found to have outcomes similar to those undergoing immediate repair. Many of these patients had other associated injuries that led to the delay in repair.

Paralysis is the dreaded complication of aortic reconstruction. Risk factors include preoperative hypotension, cross-clamp time (>30 minutes), and not using mechanical circulatory support.[65,66] High mortality and paraplegia rates associated with open surgical intervention limit its utility. This led to the use of endovascular stents in BAI. The efficacy of stenting versus surgery in the emergent setting was specifically addressed in a nonrandomized study of 60 consecutive patients with acute rupture of the thoracic aorta; 28 patients were treated surgically and 32 were treated with an endovascular stent graft.[67] Findings of the study included a significantly lower perioperative mortality rate (3.1% vs. 17.8%). At a mean follow-up of 36 months, four additional deaths occurred in stented patients, three of which were attributed to late procedural complications (one aneurysm, one dissection, and one traumatic transection). No additional procedure-related deaths occurred in the surgical patients. Reintervention rates were similar in the two groups. All of the surgical reinterventions were early reexplorations for bleeding. In the patients treated with stents, one required early drainage of an empyema and two required late interventions for endovascular leaks (one repeat stent, complicated by paraplegia; one surgical repair with stent removal). Ongoing studies are awaited to assess the long-term durability of endovascular grafts.

TRAUMATIC DIAPHRAGMATIC INJURY

The true incidence of diaphragmatic injuries is hard to estimate because of missed and delayed diagnosis. A query of the National Trauma Data Bank (NTDB) of 952,242 patients from 565 trauma centers during the years 2000 to 2004 revealed an overall incidence of 0.63% (n = 6,038). Thirty-five percent occurred from blunt trauma and 65% from penetrating diaphragmatic injuries.[68] The frequency, however, may be even higher, as one prospective study where all patients admitted with left-sided penetrating thoracoabdominal trauma were evaluated with laparoscopy demonstrated 26 out of 110 (24%) patients with a diaphragmatic injury.[69]

There are several possible mechanisms for diaphragm rupture: increased abdominal pressure from forceful impact that causes stretching with avulsion or, more commonly, lacerations; or fractured ribs that can perforate the muscle.[70] Tears tend to be in a radial orientation along the posterolateral aspect of the diaphragm. Diagnosis is easiest on the left when herniated bowel enters into the chest. Severe associated injuries occur in greater than 50% of cases. The liver and spleen are the most commonly associated injury. Diaphragmatic injury may be associated with epigastric and abdominal pain, referred shoulder pain, shortness of breath, or shock. However, some patients are asymptomatic, and initial chest radiography may be nondiagnostic, particularly if the patient is on positive-pressure ventilation. CT allows for the production of sagittal and coronal reformatting, which appears to improve accuracy. In one large series, the sensitivity for CT in diagnosing left-sided diaphragmatic tears was 78% and for right-sided tears was 50%, with 100% specificity.[71] Accuracy is poor in the absence of visceral herniation. Right-sided injuries are more difficult to diagnose because the liver and diaphragm have a similar appearance on CT (Fig. 22.8). Coexisting injuries, atelectasis, and aspiration can also obscure the diaphragm and decrease sensitivity.

Often diaphragmatic injuries are found incidentally during laparotomy or thoracotomy to treat coexistent injuries. Treatment is by direct repair whenever the injury is diagnosed; an "airtight" closure is not necessary, and excess tension and ischemia are to be avoided to prevent disastrous tissue loss in the difficult to mobilize diaphragm.

ESOPHAGEAL RUPTURE

Diagnosis, management, and outcome for traumatic esophageal perforations are affected by etiology, location, and duration between event and intervention. In trauma, there is a tendency for the diagnosis to be delayed.[72] Esophageal injury lacks specific symptoms and generally occurs in multiple trauma, making it difficult to diagnose. Historically, injuries diagnosed greater than 24 hours after injury were treated with diversion. In recent times, the trend has changed to intervention based on the clinical stability of the patient, underlying esophageal pathology, and quality of the mediastinal tissues. There is now an emphasis on primary repair when possible, with some form of tissue reinforcement.

Traumatic injuries, which tend to involve the cervical esophagus in younger patients, have a mortality rate ranging from 9% to 19%.[72] The most common traumatic injury occurs following penetrating neck injury, accounting for more than 80% of all traumatic perforations. Only 0.5% to 5% of penetrating neck injuries, however, are associated with esophageal involvement. Blunt trauma patients rarely sustain esophageal rupture; when they do occur, it is mostly in the cervical area, typically caused by a sudden blow to the anterior hyperextended neck. Virtually all thoracic traumatic perforations are a consequence of penetrating trauma. Transmediastinal gunshot wounds involving "low-velocity" missiles that course close to the spine can result in through-and-through injuries.

Signs of injury may include blood in the nasogastric aspirate, subcutaneous cervical air, and neck hematoma, but none is sensitive.[72,73] Initial symptoms of cervical perforations may be simply hoarseness, spitting up blood, subcutaneous air, or anterior tracheal deviation. Untreated, fever, erythema, swelling, increasing crepitus, airway distress, and, finally, frank abscess formation occur. Infection often spreads along the precervical plane to involve upper mediastinal structures, leading to signs and symptoms of mediastinitis. Patients who present with zone II injuries that are associated with penetration of the platysma should be considered at risk for esophageal injury. Thoracic perforations typically have a subtle initial presentation but can quickly progress to mediastinitis, empyema, and septic shock.

Plain radiography may reveal pneumomediastinum, pleural effusion, mediastinal contour changes (which progress with inflammation), or gas bubbles in the nasogastric tube or esophagus, if a tracheoesophageal communication exists. CT scans may show subtle air leaks at the site of perforation, although the sensitivity of such findings is unclear. Pneumomediastinum without a clear cause is an indication for further assessment by a contrast study. Diagnosis is primarily made by contrast study. Although many radiologists favor Gastrografin studies, 15% of perforations can be missed with this type of study alone. Dilute or thin barium studies are thus preferred as the initial diagnostic study. A contrast study confirms the location of the leak and the side toward which the leak is going, and also demonstrates other pathology such as strictures that may need to be addressed.

Esophagoscopy and contrast studies are complementary in the trauma setting. Esophagoscopy can miss 15% to 40% of traumatic injuries, but when combined with contrast studies the sensitivity approaches 90% to 100%. Ideally, flexible esophagoscopy should be performed in the OR, as definitive intervention can be done when an injury is found.

The principles of surgical intervention include control of the leak, débridement of all devitalized tissues, wide drainage, and nutritional support. Broad-spectrum antibiotic coverage is essential.[79] Ideally, primary repair should be done whenever possible. Additional reinforcement with tissues such as pleura,

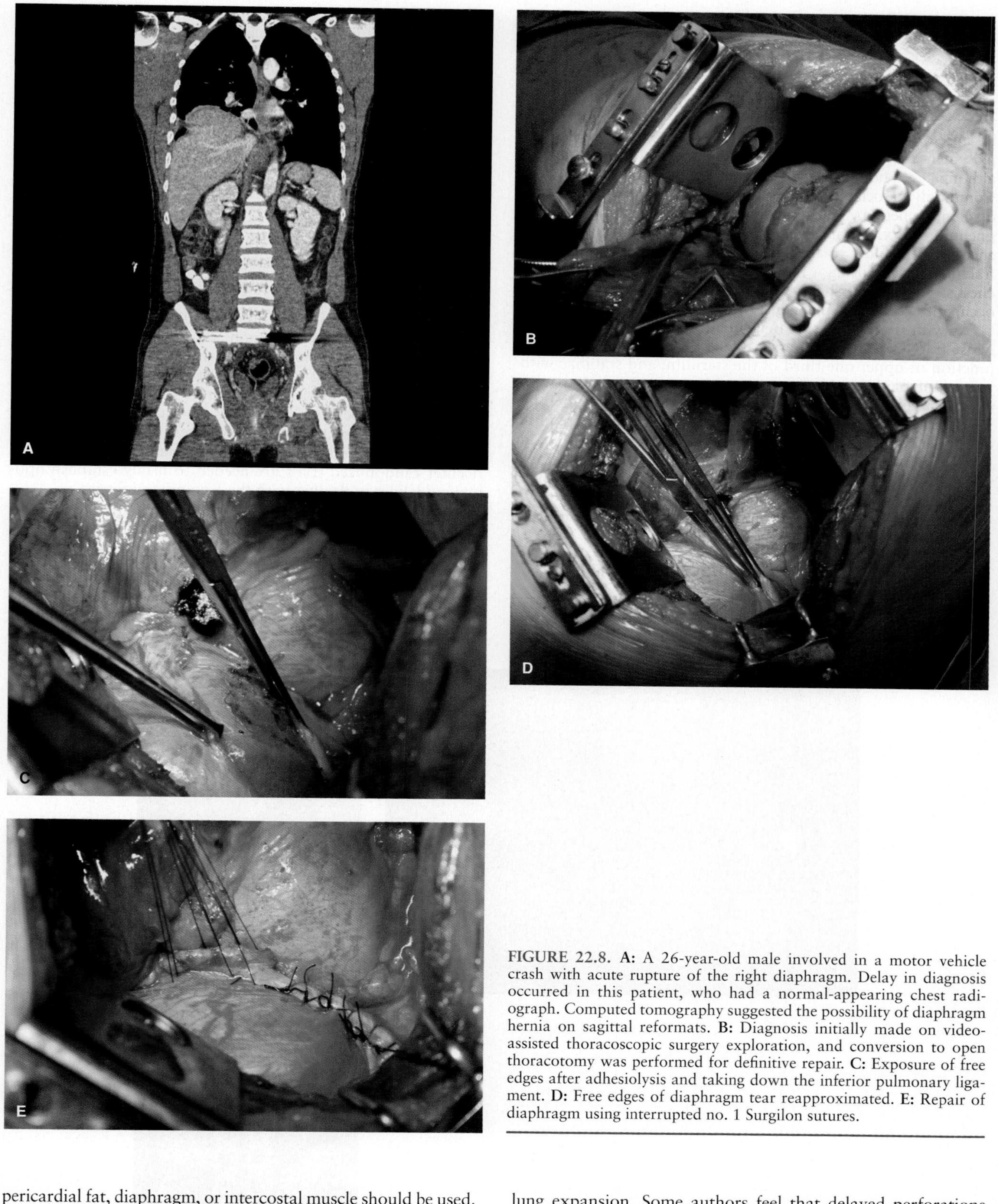

FIGURE 22.8. **A:** A 26-year-old male involved in a motor vehicle crash with acute rupture of the right diaphragm. Delay in diagnosis occurred in this patient, who had a normal-appearing chest radiograph. Computed tomography suggested the possibility of diaphragm hernia on sagittal reformats. **B:** Diagnosis initially made on video-assisted thoracoscopic surgery exploration, and conversion to open thoracotomy was performed for definitive repair. **C:** Exposure of free edges after adhesiolysis and taking down the inferior pulmonary ligament. **D:** Free edges of diaphragm tear reapproximated. **E:** Repair of diaphragm using interrupted no. 1 Surgilon sutures.

pericardial fat, diaphragm, or intercostal muscle should be used. In the cervical area, the sternocleidomastoid or other strap muscles can be mobilized as an onlay patch. When there is underlying preexisting esophageal pathology, the long-term results with primary repair are often poor, and hence esophageal resection may be needed in these cases. The presence of significant inflammation of tissues and/or degree of shock may mandate other approaches. In the setting of a delayed perforation, it is imperative that a thorough decortication is done to allow for adequate lung expansion. Some authors feel that delayed perforations should be treated with diversions (cervical fistula or drainage with a T-tube). When the tear or perforation is very large, resection can be performed expeditiously. A long cervical esophagostomy can be brought out onto the anterior chest wall below the clavicle. This allows for better securement of an ostomy collection device over the stoma. This procedure has the advantages of being more comfortable for the patient and maximizing the length of residual esophagus for later reconstruction.

SPECIAL THORACIC TRAUMA ISSUES

Sternal Fractures

5 Because of the force required, the degree of sternal fracture displacement correlates with the risk for associated thoracic injury, although even nondisplaced fractures carry a significant risk.[74,75] Commonly associated injuries include rib fractures, blunt cardiac injury, hemopericardium, spinal fracture, hemothorax, and pneumothorax. Sternal fractures usually result from a high-energy direct blow to the anterior chest wall. Typically these fractures occur during a motor vehicle crash when the driver's chest strikes the steering column or rapid deceleration causes an occupant's chest to slam against the cross-shoulder seatbelt.

As with rib fractures, management is primarily supportive. Most fractures are transverse, involve the sternal manubrial junction or upper one third of the sternum, and stabilize with pain control. Unstable fractures, fractures associated with chronic pain, or those associated with infection (indicated by new sternal click in the setting of fever or erythema) require operative intervention. Options include wires in figure-of-eight fashion, plates, or both (Fig. 22.9). Longitudinal fractures may require closure similar to that for closing a sternotomy incision. Sternal fractures complicated by mediastinal abscess may require serial widespread débridement and irrigation, followed by eventual closure with muscle or omental flaps.[76]

Rib Fractures

Rib fractures represent the most frequent chest injury. Patients with three or more rib fractures, especially elderly patients, are at significant risk for complications, such as pulmonary contusion and pneumonia, even in the absence of other injuries. In a multivariate analysis of 17,308 patients with rib fractures, age and Injury Severity Score were independent risk factors for development of pneumonia and mortality, with the incidence of pneumonia in this study being 6%, with an overall mortality of 4%.[80] These findings support the concept of aggressive pain management for patients with rib fractures to prevent atelectasis and to improve functional residual and vital capacity and the ability to clear secretions. Although the initial therapy for rib fractures has been supportive, the outcome of a strictly nonoperative approach may at times not be ideal. Rib fracture repair has had waxing and waning enthusiasm among select centers for over 50 years, but the operative indications have not yet been clearly established. Potential indications for rib fracture repair include flail chest; painful, movable rib fractures refractory to conventional pain management; chest wall deformity/defect; rib fracture nonunion; and during thoracotomy for other traumatic indication.[5] Rib fracture repair can at times be technically challenging secondary to the human rib's relatively thin cortex and its tendency to fracture obliquely. Many techniques of rib fracture repair have been described, including using wire sutures, intramedullary wires, staples, and various plates made of metal or absorbable materials (Fig. 22.10). Multicenter randomized trials are needed to firmly establish optimal guidelines in dealing with these common injuries.

Empyema

Posttraumatic empyema is likely to require surgical intervention because the blood and infection create a vigorous inflammatory reaction and early aggressive management of retained or contaminated hemothorax may reduce morbidity.[77,78]

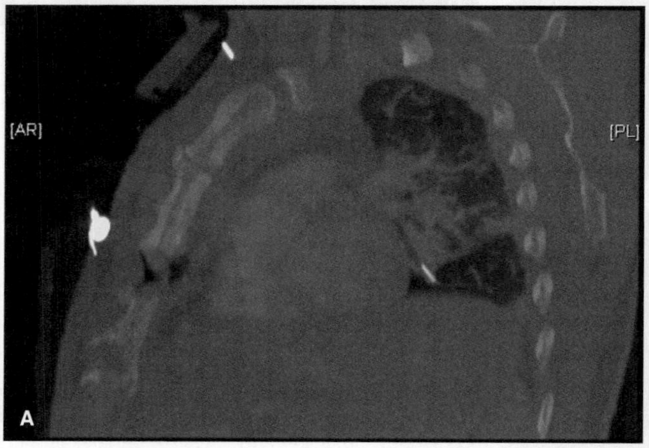

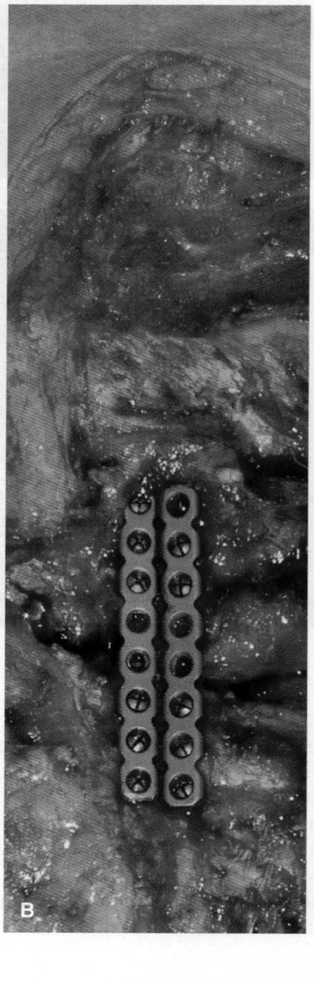

FIGURE 22.9. **A:** Computed tomography scan demonstrating transverse sternal fracture. **B:** Sternal plating performed using the titanium locking plates (Sternal Fixation System—Synthes CMF, West Chester, Pennsylvania).

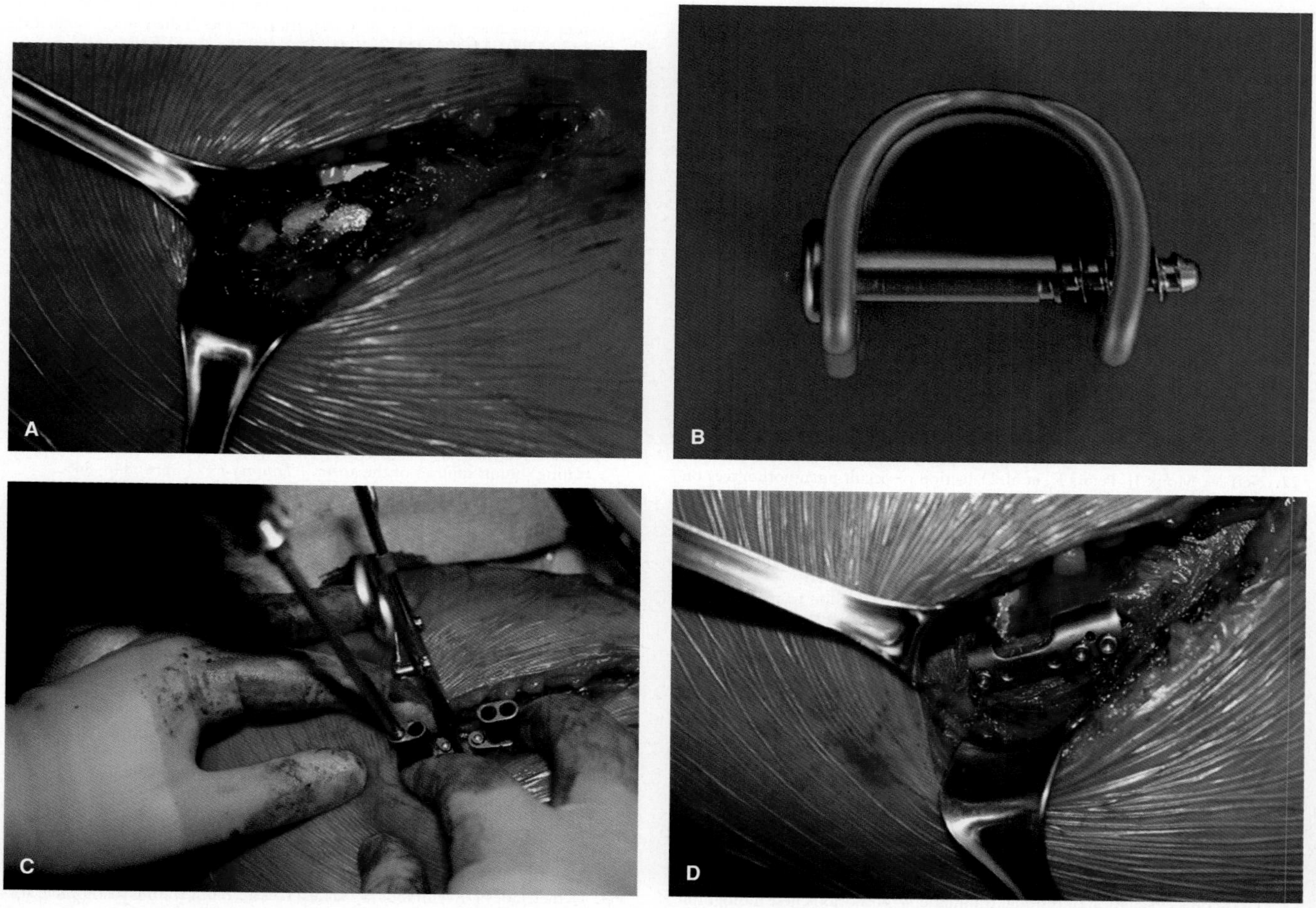

FIGURE 22.10. **A:** Exposure of rib fracture via cutdown technique. **B:** U-plate theoretically overcomes the inherent softness of the human rib by grasping the rib over its superior margin and by securing the plate with anterior-to-posterior locking screws that do not rely on screw purchase in bone (Acute Innovations Rib-Loc Plating System, Portland, Oregon). **C:** Securing the U-plate in place over the fractured rib. **D:** Final position of U-plate on fixed rib.

Patients with hemothoraces after chest tube placement with opacification of more than one-third hemithorax on chest radiography should be considered for drainage. Other risk factors include mechanical ventilation, splinting secondary to pain, hollow viscus injury, and chest tube placed in the emergency room. The primary reason that simple drainage or even thoracoscopic approaches may fail in treating empyema in the trauma population is the presence of a dense visceral peel preventing parenchymal reexpansion. Early and aggressive approaches including thoracotomy and formal pleurodesis are thus warranted in the trauma population.

SUMMARY

Thoracic trauma is common in the multiply injured patient and is a significant source of morbidity and mortality. The ability to recognize injuries in a timely manner can be lifesaving. The primary survey includes management of airway obstruction, tension pneumothorax, open pneumothorax, flail chest and pulmonary contusion, massive hemothorax, and cardiac tamponade. The secondary survey includes identification and initial treatment of potentially life-threatening injuries such as simple pneumothorax, hemothorax, pulmonary contusion, tracheobronchial tree injury, blunt cardiac injury, traumatic aortic disruption, traumatic diaphragmatic injury, and blunt esophageal injury. A deliberate and systematic approach in this patient population is essential in delivering effective care.

References

1. LoCicero J III, Mattox KL. Epidemiology of chest trauma. *Surg Clin North Am* 1989;69(1):15–19.
2. Kemmerer WT, Eckert WJ, Gathwright JB, et al. Patterns of thoracic injuries in fatal traffic accidents. *J Trauma* 1961;1:595.
3. White C, Isik F. Reconstruction of complex chest wall defects. In: Karmy-Jones R, Nathens A, Stern E, eds. *Thoracic Trauma and Critical Care.* Boston, MA: Kluwer Academic Publishers; 2002:247–251.
4. Losanoff JE, Metzler MH, Richman BW, et al. Necrotizing chest wall infection after blunt trauma: case report and review of the literature. *J Trauma* 2002;53:787–789.
5. Nirula R, Diaz JJ Jr, Trunkey DD, et al. Rib fracture repair: indications, technical issues and future directions. *World J Surg* 2009;33:14–22
6. Tanaka H, Yukioka T, Yamaguti Y, et al. Surgical stabilization of internal pneumatic stabilization? A prospective randomized study of management of severe flail chest patients. *J Trauma* 2002;52:727–732.
7. Granetzny A, Abd El-Aal M, Emam E, et al. Surgical versus conservative treatment of flail chest: evaluation of the pulmonary status. *Interact Cardiovasc Thorac Surg* 2005;4:583–587.
8. Ahmed Z, Mohyuddin Z. Management of flail chest injury: internal fixation versus endotracheal intubation and ventilation. *J Thorac Cardiovasc Surg* 1995;110:1676–1680.
9. Voggenreiter G, Neudeck F, Aufmkolk M, et al. Operative chest wall stabilization in flail chest: outcomes of patients with or without pulmonary contusion. *J Am Coll Surg* 1998;187:130–138.
10. EAST Practice Management Workgroup for Pulmonary Contusions. *Flail chest.* 2006. Available at: http://www.east.org/tpg.asp. Accessed December 1, 2008.
11. Nirula R, Allen B, Layman R, et al. Rib fracture stabilization in patients sustaining blunt chest injury. *Am Surg* 2006;72:307–309.
12. Shoemaker WC, Carey JS, Yao ST, et al. Hemodynamic alterations in acute cardiac tamponade after penetrating injuries to the heart. *Surgery* 1970;67:754.

13. Wechsler AS, Auerbach BJ, Graham TC, et al. Distribution of intramyocardial blood flow during pericardial tamponade. *J Thorac Cardiovasc Surg* 1974;68:847.
14. Knott-Craig CJ, Dalton RP, Rossouw GJ, et al. Penetrating cardiac trauma: management strategy based on 129 surgical emergencies over 2 years. *Ann Thorac Surg* 1992;53:1006–1009.
15. Kirkpatrick AW, Brown DR, Crickmer S, et al. Hand-held portable sonography for the on-mountain exclusion of a pneumothorax. *Wilderness Environ Med* 2001;12:270–272.
16. Aaland MO, Bryan FC III, Sherman R. Two-dimensional echocardiogram in hemodynamically stable victims of penetrating precordial trauma. *Am Surg* 1994;60:412–415.
17. Villavicencio RT, Aucar JA, Wall MJ Jr. Analysis of thoracoscopy in trauma. *Surg Endosc* 1999;13:3–9.
18. Cothren CC, Moore EE. Emergency department thoracotomy. In: Feliciano DV, Mattox KL, Moore EE, eds. *Chapter in Trauma*, 6th ed. New York: McGraw-Hill; 2008:245–260.
19. Beall AC Jr, Dietrich EB, Crawford HW, et al. Surgical management of cardiac injuries. *Am J Surg* 1996;112:686.
20. Graham JM, Beall AC Jr, Mattox KL, et al. Systemic air embolism following penetrating trauma to the lung. *Chest* 1977;72:449.
21. Di Bartolomeo S, Sanson G, Nardi G, et al. A population-based study on pneumothorax in severely traumatized patients. *J Trauma* 2001;51:677.
22. Neff M, Monk JJ, Peters K, et al. Detection of occult pneumothoraces on abdominal computed tomographic scans in trauma patients. *J Trauma* 2000;49:281.
23. Rhea J, Novelline R, Lawrason J, et al. The frequency and significance of thoracic injuries detected on abdominal CT scans of multiple trauma patients. *J Trauma* 1989;29:502.
24. Garramone RJ, Jacobs L, Sahdev P. An objective method to measure and manage occult pneumothorax. *Surg Gynecol Obstet* 1991;173:257.
25. Enderson BL, Abdalla R, Frame SB, et al. Tube thoracostomy for occult pneumothorax: a prospective randomized study of its use. *J Trauma* 1993; 35:726.
26. Brasel K, Satfford R, Weigelt J, et al. Treatment of occult pneumothorax from blunt trauma. *J Trauma* 1999;46:987.
27. England G, Hill R, Timberlake G, et al. Resolution of experimental pneumothorax in rabbits by graded oxygen therapy. *J Trauma* 1998;45:333.
28. Eddy AC, Luna GK, Copass M. Empyema thoracis in patients undergoing emergent closed tube thoracostomy for thoracic trauma. *Am J Surg* 1989; 157:494–497.
29. Coselli JS, Mattox KL, Beall AC Jr. Reevaluation of early evacuation of clotted hemothorax. *Am J Surg* 1984;148:786–790.
30. Velmahos GC, Demetriades D, Chan L, et al. Predicting the need for thoracoscopic evacuation of residual traumatic hemothorax: chest radiograph is insufficient. *J Trauma* 1999;46:65–70.
31. Inci I, Ozcelik C, Ulku R, et al. Intrapleural fibrinolytic treatment of traumatic clotted hemothorax. *Chest* 1998;114:160–165.
32. Meyer DM, Jessen ME, Wait MA, et al. Early evacuation of traumatic retained hemothoraces using thoracoscopy: a prospective, randomized trial. *Ann Thorac Surg* 1997;64:1396–1400; discussion 1400–1401.
33. Carrillo EH, Heniford BT, Etoch SW, et al. Video-assisted thoracic surgery in trauma patients. *J Am Coll Surg* 1997;184(3):316–324.
34. Cohn SM. Pulmonary contusion: review of the clinical entity. *J Trauma* 1997;42:973–979.
35. Richardson JD, Spain DA. Injury to the lung and pleura. In: Mattox KL, Feliciano DV, Moore EE, eds. *Trauma*, 4th ed. New York: McGraw-Hill Publishers; 2000:523–543.
36. Tranbaugh RF, Elings VB, Christensen J, et al. Determinants of pulmonary interstitial fluid accumulation after trauma. *J Trauma* 1982;22:820–826.
37. Guerrero-Lopez F, Vazquez-Mata G, Alcazar-Romero PP, et al. Evaluation of the utility of computed tomography in the initial assessment of the critical care patient with chest trauma. *Crit Care Med* 2000;28: 1370–1375.
38. Keough V, Pudelek B. Blunt chest trauma: review of selected pulmonary injuries focusing on pulmonary contusion. *AACN Clin Issues* 2001;12(2): 270–281.
39. Ware LB, Mathay MA. Medical progress: the acute respiratory distress syndrome. *N Engl J Med* 2000;342(18):1344–1349.
40. Tyburski JG, Collinge JD, Wilson RF, et al. Pulmonary contusions: quantifying the lesions on chest x-ray films and the factors affecting prognosis. *J Trauma* 1999;46:833–838.
41. Cothren C, Moore EE, Biffl WL, et al. Lung-sparing techniques are associated with improved outcome compared with anatomic resection for severe lung injuries. *J Trauma* 2002;53:483–487.
42. Kirsh MM, Orringer MB, Behrendt DM, et al. Management of tracheobronchial disruption secondary to nonpenetrating trauma. *Ann Thorac Surg* 1976;22:93–101.
43. Kiser AC, O'Brien SM, Detterbeck FC. Blunt tracheobronchial injuries: treatment and outcomes. *Ann Thorac Surg* 2001;71:2059–2065.
44. Velly JF, Martigne C, Moreau JM, et al. Post traumatic tracheobronchial lesions. A follow-up study of 47 cases. *Eur J Cardiothorac Surg* 1991;5: 352–355.
45. Jones WS, Mavroudis C, Richardson JD, et al. Management of tracheobronchial disruption resulting from blunt trauma. *Surgery* 1984;95:319–323.
46. Wintermark M, Schnyder P, Wicky S. Blunt traumatic rupture of a mainstem bronchus: spiral CT demonstration of the "fallen lung" sign. *Eur Radiol* 2001;11:409–411.
47. Wood D. Tracheobronchial trauma. In: Karmy-Jones R, Nathens A, Stern E, eds. *Thoracic Trauma and Critical Care*. Boston, MA: Kluwer Academic Publishers; 2002:109–122.
48. Fulda G, Brathwaite C, Rodriguez A, et al. Blunt traumatic rupture of the heart and pericardium: a ten-year experience (1979–1989). *J Trauma* 1991;31(2):167–173.
49. Schultz J, Trunkey D. Blunt cardiac injury. *Crit Care Clin* 2004;20(1):57–70.
50. Elle M. Blunt cardiac injury. *Mt Sinai J Med* 2006;73(2):542–552.
51. Leavitt B, Meyer J, Morton J, et al. Survival following nonpenetrating traumatic rupture of cardiac chambers. *Ann Thorac Surg* 1987;44(5):532–535.
52. Mandavia D, Hoffner R, Mahaney K, et al. Bedside echocardiography by emergency physicians. *Ann Emerg Med* 2001;38(4): 377–382.
53. Turk E, Tsokos M. Bunt cardiac trauma caused by fatal falls from height: an autopsy-based assessment of injury pattern. *J Tauma* 2004;57(2):301–304.
54. Hossack K, Morenao C, Vanway C, et al. Frequency of cardiac contusion in nonpenetrating chest injury. *Am J Cardiol* 1988;61(4):391–394.
55. Nagy K, Krosner S, Roberts R, et al. Determining which patients require evaluation for blunt cardiac injury following blunt chest trauma. *World J Surg* 2001;25(1):108–111.
56. Feczko J, Lynch L, Pless J, et al. An autopsy case review of 142 nonpenetrating (blunt) injuries of the aorta. *J Trauma* 1992;33(6):846–849.
57. Kram H, Appel P, Wohlmuth D, et al. Diagnosis of traumatic thoracic aortic rupture: a 10-year retrospective analysis. *Ann Thorac Surg* 1989;47(2): 282–286.
58. Mirvis S, Shanmuganathan K, Buell J, et al. Use of spiral computed tomography for the assessment of blunt trauma patients with potential aortic injury. *J Trauma* 1998;45(5):922–930.
59. Woodring J, Dillon M. Radiographic manifestations of mediastinal hemorrhage from blunt chest trauma. *Ann Thorac Surg* 1984;37(2):171–178.
60. Dyer D, Moore E, Ilke D, et al. Thoracic aortic injury: how predictive is mechanism and is chest computed tomography a reliable screening tool? A prospective study of 1,561 patients. *J Trauma* 2000;48(4):673–683.
61. Fabian T, Davis K, Gavant M, et al. Prospective study of blunt aortic injury: helical CT is diagnostic and antihypertensive therapy reduces rupture. *Ann Surg* 1998;227(5):666–677.
62. Maggisano R, Nathens A, Alexandrova N, et al. Traumatic rupture of the thoracic aorta: should one always operate immediately? *Ann Vasc Surg* 1995;9(1):44–52.
63. Pacini D, Angeli E, Fattori R, et al. Traumatic rupture of the thoracic aorta: ten years of delayed management. *J Thorac Cardiovasc Surg* 2005; 129(4):880–884.
64. Demetriades D, Velmahos G, Scalea T, et al. Blunt traumatic thoracic aortic injuries: early or delayed repair—results of an American Association for the Surgery of Trauma prospective study. *J Trauma* 2009;66(4):967–973.
65. Karmy-Jones R, Carter YM, Nathens A, et al. Impact of presenting physiology and associated injuries on outcome following traumatic rupture of the thoracic aorta. *Am Surg* 2001;67:61–66.
66. Fabian TC, Richardson JD, Croce MA, et al. Prospective study of blunt aortic injury: multicenter trial of the American Association for the Surgery of Trauma. *J Trauma* 1997;42:374–380; discussion 380–383.
67. Doss M, Wood J, Balzer J, et al. Emergency endovascular interventions for acute thoracic aortic rupture: four-year follow-up. *J Thorac Cardiovasc Surg* 2005;129(3):645–651.
68. Davis JW, Eghbalieh B. Injury to the diaphragm. In: Feliciano D, Mattox K, Moore E, eds. *Trauma*, 6th ed. New York: McGraw Hill; 623–635.
69. Murray JA, Demetriades D, Asesnio JA, et al. Occult injuries to the diaphragm: prospective evaluation of laparoscopy in penetrating injuries to the lower left chest. *J Am Coll Surg* 1998;187:626.
70. Mirvis ME. Imaging of acute thoracic injury: the advent of MDCT screening. *Semin Ultrasound CT MR* 2005;26(5):305–331.
71. Kileen K, Mirvis S, Shanmuganathan K. Helical CT of diaphragmatic rupture caused by blunt trauma. *AJR Am J Roentgenol* 1999;173(6):1611–1616.
72. Asensio JA, Chahwan S, Forno W, et al. Penetrating esophageal injuries: multicenter study of the American Association for the Surgery of Trauma. *J Trauma* 2001;50:289–296.
73. Gill S, Dierking J, Nguyen K, et al. Seatbelt injury causing perforation of the cervical esophagus: a case report and review of the literature. *Am Surg* 2004;70(1):32–34.
74. von Garrel T, Ince A, Junge A, et al. The sternal fracture: radiographic analysis of 200 fractures with special reference to concomitant injuries. *J Trauma* 2004;57(4):837–844.
75. Peek G, Firmin R. Isolated sternal fracture: an audit of 10 years' experience. *Injury* 1995;26(6):385–388.
76. Cuschieri J, Kralovich KA, Patton JH, et al. Anterior mediastinal abscess after closed sternal fracture. *J Trauma* 1999;47:551–554.
77. Richardson JD, Carrillo E. Thoracic infection after trauma. *Chest Surg Clin N Am* 1997;7:401–427.
78. Weissberg D, Refaely Y. Pleural empyema: 24-year experience. *Ann Thorac Surg* 1996;62:1026–1029.
79. Glatterer M, Toon R, Ellestad C, et al. Management of blunt and penetrating external esophageal trauma. *J Trauma* 1985;25(8):784–792.
80. Brasel K, Guse C, Layde P, et al. Rib fractures: relationship with pneumonia and mortality. *Crit Care Med* 2006;34:1642–1646.

CHAPTER 23 ■ ABDOMINAL TRAUMA

DAVID H. WISNER, JOSEPH M. GALANTE, MATTHEW O. DOLICH, AND DAVID B. HOYT

KEY POINTS

1. To aid in the evaluation for injury, the abdomen can be divided into four areas: intrathoracic abdomen (diaphragm, liver, spleen, stomach), true abdomen (small and large intestines, distended bladder, gravid uterus), pelvic abdomen (rectum, bladder, urethra, small intestine, female reproductive organs), and retroperitoneal abdomen (kidneys, ureters, pancreas, second and third duodenum, aorta, vena cava). With the exception of the true abdomen, all of these areas are difficult to assess by physical examination alone.
2. The top three patterns of injury are liver, intestines, and spleen caused by blunt (usually vehicular crashes, vehicle vs. pedestrian, and falls) and penetrating (gunshot and shotgun) trauma.
3. Adjunctive assessment is critical using hematocrit; white blood cell count; biochemical markers (amylase, lipase, creatinine, bilirubin, liver function tests); imaging, including ultrasound (focused abdominal sonography for trauma [FAST]), computed tomography (CT), and angiography; and diagnostic peritoneal lavage (DPL), as indicated by mechanism, pattern, and risk.
4. The objective is to determine who needs an operation—not what organ is injured. The primary effect of solid organ injury is bleeding (monitored by hematocrit and FAST, DPL, or CT), and visceral injury, peritonitis (diagnosed by physical examination, laboratory, DPL, and, increasingly, CT).
5. Operative treatment of specific injuries is dictated by pattern, extent, and overall stability of the patient and associated injuries. Blunt and penetrating injuries are, in large part, treated by similar principles. Grossly unstable patients require a "damage control" approach and return on a later day, when stable.
6. Specific pattern of injury (e.g., lower abdominal lap belt bruising along with lumbar spine fracture) may indicate need for operative intervention for intestinal injury and should be recognized early to minimize morbidity.
7. Approach to retroperitoneal hematoma depends on cause, location, and other injuries. The retroperitoneum is divided into zones to aid decision making: central (zone 1) is associated with pancreaticoduodenal injuries or major vascular injury and must be explored; flank (zone 2) is associated with perinephric bleeding and injuries are explored if enlarging, pulsatile, or caused by penetrating trauma; and pelvic (zone 3) is associated with pelvic fractures, entered at great risk, and best left alone.

Within the broad scope of trauma care, the knowledge to comprehensively manage abdominal trauma is the sine qua non of the trauma surgeon. Most civilian abdominal injuries are caused by blunt trauma secondary to high-speed automobile crashes, although penetrating injuries are common in urban environments. The inability to appropriately manage abdominal injuries accounts for most of the preventable deaths that follow multiple trauma. Failure to recognize occult abdominal hemorrhage and to control bleeding from intra-abdominal organs leads to significant morbidity, and such injuries account for approximately 10% of the traumatic deaths that occur annually in the United States.

ANATOMIC CONSIDERATIONS

The abdomen is defined by the diaphragm at its superior aspect and by the infragluteal fold at its caudal aspect; it includes the entire circumference of the torso. Abdominal injury is often accompanied by trauma to other sites, such as the central nervous system, the chest, and the musculoskeletal system. The pattern of extra-abdominal injury can often predict the abdominal organs at risk of injury. To simplify the initial trauma evaluation, the abdomen can be divided into four areas: intrathoracic abdomen, true abdomen, pelvic abdomen, and retroperitoneal abdomen (Fig. 23.1). With the exception of the true abdomen, all of these areas are difficult to assess by physical examination alone.

1 (key point marker)

The intrathoracic abdomen is the portion of the upper abdomen that lies beneath the rib cage (Fig. 23.1A). Bony and cartilaginous structures make this area essentially inaccessible to palpation. Its contents include the diaphragm, liver, spleen, and stomach. Each of these organs can be injured when blunt or penetrating impact is delivered to the rib cage.

The pelvic abdomen is defined by the bony pelvis (Fig. 23.1B). Its contents include the rectum, bladder, urethra, small intestine, and, in female patients, the uterus, fallopian tubes, and ovaries. Trauma to the pelvis, particularly pelvic fractures, can damage the organs within, while penetrating injuries of the buttocks can injure any or all of the pelvic organs. Injury to these structures may be extraperitoneal and, therefore, difficult to diagnose. For this reason, suspected injuries may require adjunctive procedures such as bladder catheterization, urethrocystography, and sigmoidoscopy for diagnosis.

The retroperitoneal abdomen contains the kidneys, ureters, pancreas, second and third portions of the duodenum, great vessels, aorta, and vena cava (Fig. 23.1C). Injury to these structures can occur secondary to penetrating or blunt trauma. The kidneys can be damaged by injury to the lower ribs posteriorly, and any of these structures can be damaged by crushing injuries to the front or side of the torso. Again, injury to these structures may result in few physical findings, and physical examination and diagnostic peritoneal lavage (DPL) are of little use. Accurate evaluation of the retroperitoneal abdomen usually relies on computed tomography (CT), angiography, and ultrasound.

The true abdomen contains the small and large intestines, the bladder when distended, and the uterus when gravid. Perforation of these organs is usually manifested by pain from peritonitis and is associated with significant abdominal physical

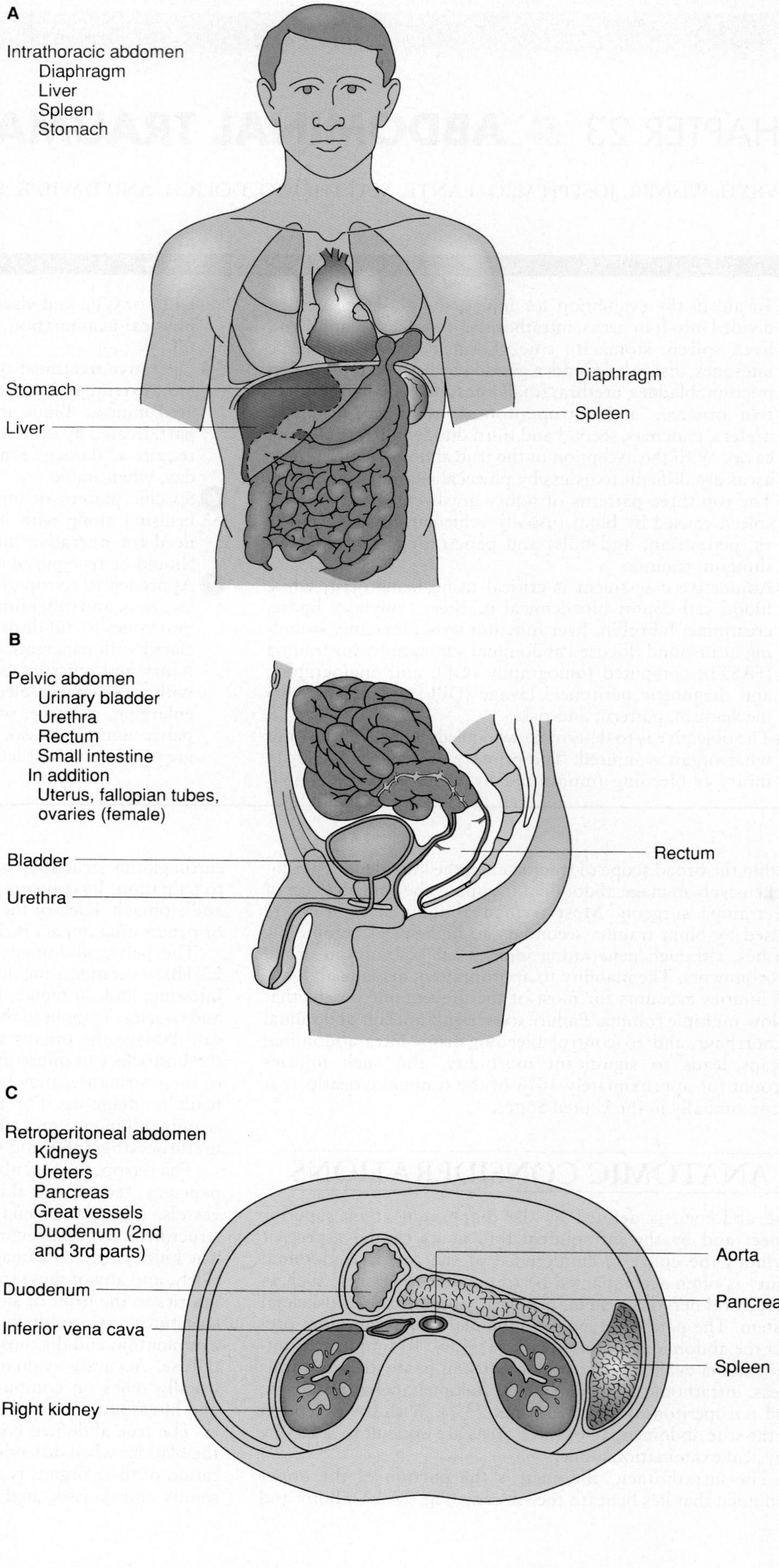

FIGURE 23.1. Four traditional anatomic divisions of the abdomen. **A:** Intrathoracic abdomen. Contents of this area are subdiaphragmatic but cephalad to the costal margin. With respiration, the diaphragm is presumed to ascend to the level of the nipples (fourth intercostal space anteriorly). A ruptured left hemidiaphragm is illustrated with herniation of the stomach and distal transverse colon into the left hemithorax. **B:** Similarly, the contents of the pelvic abdomen are within the bony pelvis. **C:** The structures in the retroperitoneal abdomen. The true (intraperitoneal) abdomen contains the remainder of the viscera, and the inventory of its contents is dynamic, depending on body position and respiration (not shown).

findings. While CT will usually provide substantial evidence when a solid organ injury is present, DPL can be a useful adjunct if intestinal injury is suspected.

The unique anatomy of the pediatric abdomen can substantially influence the pattern of injury. The high costal margin and low pelvic brim increase the amount of unprotected abdominal organs relative to the rest of the body. The thin abdominal musculature, diminished fat pad, and pliable ribs all contribute to vulnerability of the abdominal organs to trauma.

PENETRATING INJURY

2 While stab wounds are more common, handguns are more likely to cause serious penetrating injury to the abdomen. Significant intra-abdominal injury occurs in approximately 80% to 90% of patients who sustain abdominal gunshot wounds but in only 20% to 30% of patients with stab wounds. The difference in injury potential between gunshot wounds and stab wounds is a function of both depth of penetration and the higher kinetic energy associated with gunshot wounds. Selective management may be the best method for treating stab wounds. The frequency of organ injury after penetrating abdominal trauma is shown in Table 23.1.

Injuries to both thoracic and abdominal cavities occur in 25% of patients with penetrating wounds of the abdomen. Patients with penetrating wounds of the thorax also may have significant intra-abdominal injury because a bullet or knife can readily traverse the diaphragm. Patients with gunshot wounds to the abdomen and lower chest may routinely undergo laparotomy because the probability of intra-abdominal injury is high. Nonetheless, in patients where the trajectory may be tangential to the peritoneum or may have only traversed the liver, CT may be considered to allow the option of nonoperative management.

BLUNT TRAUMA

Automobile crashes are the cause of at least 60% of all traumatic injuries. Table 23.2 shows the frequency with which specific organs are injured by blunt abdominal trauma. Some series list the liver rather than the spleen as the most commonly injured intra-abdominal organ; this difference probably reflects the means of diagnosis. Small liver injuries are often detected in patients who undergo CT scan of the abdomen, whereas splenic injuries in adults are more likely to be clinically significant and to require surgical intervention.

Solid organs are most frequently injured from blunt trauma. The sudden application of pressure to the abdomen is more likely to rupture a solid organ than a hollow viscus. The more elastic tissues of young people tolerate trauma better than those of older people, and this accounts in part for the differences in incidence and pattern of injuries between children and adults with blunt abdominal trauma.

TABLE 23.1

FREQUENCY OF ORGAN INJURY IN PENETRATING ABDOMINAL TRAUMA

■ ORGAN	■ OCCURRENCE (%)
Liver	37
Small bowel	26
Stomach	19
Colon	17
Major vascular	13
Retroperitoneal	10
Mesentery and omentum	10
Spleen	7
Diaphragm	5
Kidney	4
Pancreas	4
Duodenum	2
Biliary system	1
Other	1

TABLE 23.2

FREQUENCY OF ORGAN INJURY IN BLUNT ABDOMINAL TRAUMA IN ADULTS

■ ORGAN	■ OCCURRENCE (%)
Liver	30
Spleen	25
Retroperitoneal hematoma	13
Kidney	7
Urinary bladder	6
Intestine	5
Mesentery	5
Pancreas	3
Diaphragm	2
Urethra	2
Vascular	2

PREHOSPITAL CARE

Little can be done outside a hospital for patients with abdominal injuries. For penetrating wounds, sterile dressings should be applied and the patient should be carefully monitored. Foreign bodies embedded in the trunk should not be removed because major bleeding can follow. Evisceration is best left undisturbed except for application of a moist sterile dressing and protection of the eviscerated organ from further injury. General principles of stabilization and evaluation should be followed, including ensuring an adequately functioning airway, inserting intravenous lines (preferably in the upper extremity), beginning fluid resuscitation, and providing rapid transport to a trauma center. Recent controversy surrounding the issue of the value of fluid resuscitation in the early posttraumatic period has arisen. In blunt trauma, aggressive volume resuscitation to return toward normal vital signs and level of consciousness is generally indicated, though a preoccupation with fluid resuscitation at the scene should not delay rapid transport to a trauma center. In penetrating abdominal trauma, smaller resuscitation volumes to achieve a systolic blood pressure only greater than 70 to 80 mm Hg may improve outcomes and diminish total blood loss.[1] The prehospital application of the pneumatic antishock garment in the treatment of abdominal trauma is rarely indicated and may lead to increased blood loss from injury manipulation and delay in transfer and impair pulmonary and cardiac function due to upward pressure on the diaphragm and increase in afterload.

HOSPITAL RESUSCITATION AND DIAGNOSIS

Diagnosis and treatment should proceed concurrently according to established protocols. A functioning airway must be established, particularly in the comatose patient, before evaluation of the abdomen occurs. If necessary, an endotracheal tube is placed and assisted ventilation is begun. Upper extremity, large-bore intravenous catheters are initiated, and resuscitation is begun with a balanced salt solution (e.g., lactated Ringer or normal saline). Early crystalloid resuscitation is mandatory, especially in the presence of a head injury, despite theoretic considerations that instillation of intravenous fluids increases bleeding and causes a dilutional coagulopathy.[2] When operative intervention is indicated, however, it should not be delayed by overzealous and prolonged attempts at fluid resuscitation.

HISTORY AND PATTERN OF INJURY

Penetrating injuries present little diagnostic challenge other than the question of whether to explore the abdomen operatively. An attempt should be made to establish details of the trauma event and the weapon used. The blunt trauma assessment can be aided considerably by an accurate history. If the patient was involved in an automobile crash in which he or she struck the steering wheel or if no seatbelt was used, specific thoracic and epigastric abdominal trauma should be suspected. If the patient was restrained, it can be helpful to determine whether the restraint was a two-point lap belt or a three-point shoulder belt. The patient who sustains rib fractures involving the lower left chest has a 15% chance of associated splenic injury; the patient with rib fractures on the right has a 10% chance of liver injury. A compression fracture of the lumbosacral region carries a 20% risk of significant renal parenchymal injury.

PHYSICAL EXAMINATION

The objective of the physical examination in abdominal trauma is to rapidly identify the patient who needs laparotomy. Precise definition of specific organ injury is unnecessary. In addition, the specificity and sensitivity of physical examination alone, however, are not adequate to make these determinations. Associated injuries often cause tenderness and spasm in the abdominal wall and make diagnosis difficult. Lower rib fractures, pelvic fractures, or abdominal wall contusions can mimic the signs of peritonitis.

In patients with gunshot wounds, no presumptions should be made about entrance and exit wounds. Unfounded presumptions can lead to inaccurate estimations about the number of times a patient was shot and the course of the bullets. If time permits, radiographs should be obtained to determine the location of any bullets or bullet fragments that remain in the patient. Penetrating wounds should be marked with radiopaque clips to allow radiographic delineation of the injury tract.

Because the primary manifestation of blunt solid organ injury is hemorrhage, the patient should be monitored closely during the initial assessment, and continuing or refractory shock is presumed to result from continuing or massive hemorrhage. The patient should be examined from head to toe for signs of blunt trauma and for penetrating wounds. Small abrasions or areas of ecchymosis suggest significant local intra-abdominal injury. The abdominal wall and back should be carefully inspected, and posterior ecchymosis should raise the possibility of retroperitoneal injury. The absence of bowel sounds is consistent with an ileus, but it is a nonspecific finding and, in the context of a busy emergency department, it is insensitive for discriminating between patients who do and do not need laparotomy.

Palpation can reveal localized tenderness, spasm, or rigidity of the abdominal wall. These findings and the finding of rebound tenderness are consistent with peritonitis and perforation of hollow viscera. Exploratory laparotomy is required for this presumed diagnosis. Suprapubic tenderness and pelvic lateral wall tenderness, which can indicate a pelvic fracture, are assessed in the conscious patient. Inspection of the perineum and urethral meatus for blood is routine to look for signs of pelvic fracture and possible urethral injury.

As assessment continues, rectal examination is performed and sphincter tone is evaluated. The integrity of the rectal wall and the position and excess mobility of the prostate associated with urethral injury are evaluated. The stool should be tested for the presence of gross or occult blood. A urinary catheter is placed, and a urine sample is sent for analysis for microscopic hematuria. If injury to the urethra is suspected, retrograde urethrography (RUG) should be performed before attempted catheterization and possible aggravation of injury and a suprapubic catheter placed if necessary.

The physical findings for injuries to these different structures are sometimes a function of the time between injury and examination. Hollow viscus perforations may require several hours before peritonitis becomes apparent. Colonic or gastric perforations produce peritonitis more rapidly, small bowel perforations less so. Hematomas and bruising from retroperitoneal or pelvic fracture bleeding may not be apparent initially. Frequent reevaluation is an essential strategy in the nonoperative treatment of patients with blunt abdominal trauma.

LABORATORY STUDIES

3 The hematocrit is the primary blood study of value in the initial evaluation of a patient with abdominal trauma. Leukocyte counts, serum creatinine, glucose, serum amylase/lipase, and serum electrolyte determinations are often obtained for reference but usually have little value in the immediate management period, but are critical for serial assessments and trending the results.

The diagnosis of massive hemorrhage is usually obvious from hemodynamic parameters, and the hematocrit merely confirms the diagnosis. Iatrogenic dilutional anemia is common and, in the presence of hemodynamic stability, is well tolerated. In the less severely injured, serial hematocrits showing a persistent downward trend identify ongoing bleeding requiring operative or angiographic intervention. Urinalysis confirms the presence of microscopic hematuria. For blunt trauma, radiographic evaluation (usually by CT) of the kidneys and bladder should be initiated if the patient has gross hematuria or microscopic hematuria and shock (systolic blood pressure <90 mm Hg in an adult) at any point during the prehospital or emergency department course.

The serum amylase is insensitive and nonspecific as a marker for major pancreatic or enteric injury. Injuries to the head and face commonly cause increased plasma amylase concentrations. Serum lipase levels are not elevated by facial trauma and are possibly more specific than amylase levels. Sensitivity and specificity of lipase levels, however, especially in the early postinjury period, are still relatively low. Sensitivity and specificity of both the amylase and lipase improve with serial testing. Persistent or increasing elevations of the amylase or lipase should, therefore, raise concern of significant intra-abdominal injury and are an indication for aggressive radiographic or surgical investigation.

RADIOGRAPHIC EVALUATION

Radiologic studies of potential value in the evaluation of abdominal trauma include a chest radiograph, retrograde urethrography and cystography, CT scans, ultrasound, and angiography. In addition, all injuries from penetrating trauma should be evaluated with a plain radiograph with the use of radiodense markers on the wound sites to allow evaluation of the missile trajectory. With blunt trauma, an anteroposterior film of the pelvis can delineate pelvic fractures not detectable on physical examination. The initial pelvic film or chest radiograph can also demonstrate fractures of the thoracic or lumbar spine. A transverse fracture of the vertebral bodies, or Chance fracture, should increase the search for serious blunt intestinal injury. The value of plain abdominal films after blunt trauma is extremely limited and they should not be routinely obtained.

4 Of greater value are CT scans, ultrasound, and angiography. CT has real value in the accurate assessment of solid organ injuries, particularly of the liver, kidney, and spleen; contrast-enhanced CT has great accuracy in the delineation of intra-abdominal bleeding. The accuracy of CT scan in evaluation of hollow viscus injury is somewhat more limited, but improvements in CT technology have led to increasing sensitivity of CT in the detection of the more subtle signs of injury to the intestine.[3,4] CT is also highly specific in the evaluation of retroperitoneal injuries and is the single most useful and informative diagnostic study for patients with abdominal trauma.

CT scanning can also be used on occasion for penetrating injuries when it is uncertain whether the track of the knife or bullet violated the retroperitoneum or the peritoneal cavity. Such an approach is most useful in patients with back and flank wounds but is also occasionally helpful in patients with anterior wounds if it is likely that the knife did not reach the peritoneal cavity or the bullet traversed a tangential path. Patients with any signs of peritonitis or hemodynamic instability after penetrating trauma are obviously not candidates for diagnostic CT scanning, nor is any trauma patient displaying hemodynamic instability.

Angiography is reserved for specific situations, such as suspected aortic or renal arterial injuries, or ongoing hemorrhage from pelvic, hepatic, or splenic injuries. It is not considered an initial screening investigation.

Laparoscopy has been used for both diagnosis and treatment of trauma patients.[5] Although limited to evaluation of the diaphragm in blunt trauma, after penetrating trauma laparoscopy is helpful when it is unclear whether the peritoneum has been penetrated. In patients in whom peritoneal penetration is seen, the use of laparoscopy to further explore the peritoneal cavity and repair injuries is more controversial. The adequacy of abdominal exploration, particularly examination of the bowel and retroperitoneum, has been questioned, and repair of large injuries through the laparoscope can be tedious. In patients with a lower chest wound, however, laparoscopy can identify both peritoneal penetration and diaphragmatic injury. An isolated diaphragmatic injury or associated nonbleeding liver laceration is one area in which repair of the diaphragm through the laparoscope has proved feasible. Of note, when laparoscopy is used in patients with potential diaphragmatic injury, the positive pressure in the peritoneal cavity can lead to tension pneumothorax if the chest is not adequately vented.

DIAGNOSTIC PERITONEAL LAVAGE AND ABDOMINAL ULTRASOUND

Diagnostic peritoneal lavage and focused abdominal sonography for trauma (FAST) are standard techniques to detect significant intra-abdominal hemorrhage after blunt trauma. FAST is less useful after penetrating trauma for potential intestinal injury.

The specific indications for DPL or FAST in blunt trauma include the following:

- Unconscious patient with question of potential abdominal injury
- Patient with a high-energy injury, suspected intra-abdominal injury, and equivocal physical findings
- Patient with multiple injuries and unexplained shock
- Patient with major noncontiguous or thoracoabdominal injuries
- Patient with spinal cord injury
- Intoxicated patient in whom abdominal injury is suspected
- Patient who has a suspected intra-abdominal injury with equivocal diagnostic findings and who will be undergoing prolonged general anesthesia for another injury, making continued reevaluation impossible

Relative contraindications to DPL but not to FAST are previous abdominal operations, pregnancy, and morbid obesity. Obvious peritonitis is a contraindication to either study. If the patient is hemodynamically stable, CT scan is prudent, and if the patient is unstable, immediate exploratory laparotomy, rapid abdominal tap, or FAST to confirm gross hemoperitoneum is indicated.

Diagnostic peritoneal lavage is not generally useful for patients with abdominal gunshot wounds, most of whom require laparotomy.[6] If local exploration of a stab wound suggests penetration of the fascia or peritoneum, DPL can help distinguish significant and insignificant injuries. It is most sensitive in the diagnosis of hemoperitoneum, but significant hemoperitoneum does not necessarily accompany hollow viscus lacerations. In blunt trauma, DPL is considered positive if 10 mL of grossly bloody aspirate is obtained before instillation of lavage fluid or (of much less importance) if the siphoned lavage fluid has more than 100,000 red blood cells (RBCs) per milliliter (equal to 20 mL of blood). Evaluation of lavage fluid in stab wounds should be based on a more sensitive protocol. In general, more than 1,000 RBCs/mL is considered a positive DPL, and laparotomy should follow. In both cases, presence of bile, amylase, bacteria, or particulate matter should indicate visceral injury and need for laparotomy.

Diagnostic peritoneal lavage and CT scan are both satisfactory tests for the diagnosis of visceral injury after blunt abdominal trauma. DPL has some advantages, including rapidity, higher sensitivity, lower cost, and immediate interpretation (Table 23.3). The major disadvantages are a 1% to 3% risk of iatrogenic intraperitoneal injury and the high sensitivity of the test. The high sensitivity can lead to nontherapeutic laparotomies (i.e., when there are no injuries requiring repair). False-positive DPL findings may result from traversing a pelvic hematoma that has dissected into the anterior infraumbilical abdominal wall if an infraumbilical approach is used in a patient with a pelvic fracture. A pelvic radiograph should be obtained before DPL, and if a pelvic fracture is present, the incision is placed cephalad to the umbilicus.

Before DPL, the bladder should be emptied with a Foley catheter. The abdomen is prepared with povidone-iodine solution and draped with sterile towels. The infraumbilical midline is infiltrated using lidocaine with epinephrine, and a 3-cm incision is carried down to the linea alba. This is opened, and a peritoneal

TABLE 23.3 DIAGNOSIS

COMPARISON OF DIAGNOSTIC PERITONEAL LAVAGE AND COMPUTED TOMOGRAPHY IN THE DIAGNOSIS OF VISCERAL INJURY AFTER BLUNT ABDOMINAL TRAUMA

	DIAGNOSTIC PERITONEAL LAVAGE	COMPUTED TOMOGRAPHY
False-negative result	<1%	5%–20%
False-positive result	5%–12%	5%
Time to complete	5 min	55 min
Cost	$125	$900

dialysis catheter is placed through the peritoneum under direct vision. After peritoneal entry, the catheter is directed at a 45-degree angle into the pelvis and aspirated. If the aspirate returns 10 mL of bloody fluid, the study is considered positive and is terminated. If little or no blood is aspirated, 1,000 mL of warm normal saline (or 10 mL/kg in a child) is rapidly infused into the peritoneal cavity. After the infusion is complete, the empty intravenous bottle is placed on the floor, allowing the intraperitoneal fluid to be siphoned into the bottle for analysis.

Ultrasound (FAST) has become increasingly popular in the initial diagnostic management of abdominal trauma and, when available, can be used in the circumstances outlined earlier for DPL.[7] FAST has been used as a screening modality for all patients with blunt trauma to determine which stable patients should undergo further diagnostic imaging with CT scanning.[8–10] It has also been used in hemodynamically unstable patients to rapidly determine the presence of intraperitoneal fluid and the need for immediate surgery analogous to the use of gross blood on DPL.[11]

In FAST, the ultrasound probe is used to interrogate serially the subhepatic space, the pericolic gutters, the left upper quadrant, the pericystic area in the pelvis, and the pericardial space. A small amount of physiologic fluid is occasionally seen in the pelvis, but anything more should be considered abnormal and should prompt either operative exploration or further investigation.

There is a steep learning curve for the use of FAST in the emergency department, but in the hands of experienced personnel it is effective in determining the presence or absence of intraperitoneal blood. Emergency department ultrasound is not very sensitive for the identification of specific organ injuries and is insensitive for the diagnosis of bowel injuries. It has proved much better for the evaluation of blunt trauma than for penetrating trauma, although interrogation of the pericardial space with an ultrasound probe placed in the subxiphoid position is sensitive for the presence of pericardial blood in patients with potential penetrating cardiac injuries.

The general approaches to the diagnosis of blunt and penetrating trauma are outlined in Algorithms 23.1 and 23.2.

INDICATIONS FOR SURGERY

It is the job of the general surgeon directing a trauma team to integrate the various specialties involved in the care of the multiply injured patient. Judgments about specialized procedures for problems that are not life threatening need to be made with an overall view of the patient's physiologic status. Indications for laparotomy include signs of peritonitis, evisceration, clinical deterioration during observation, and, in the presence of

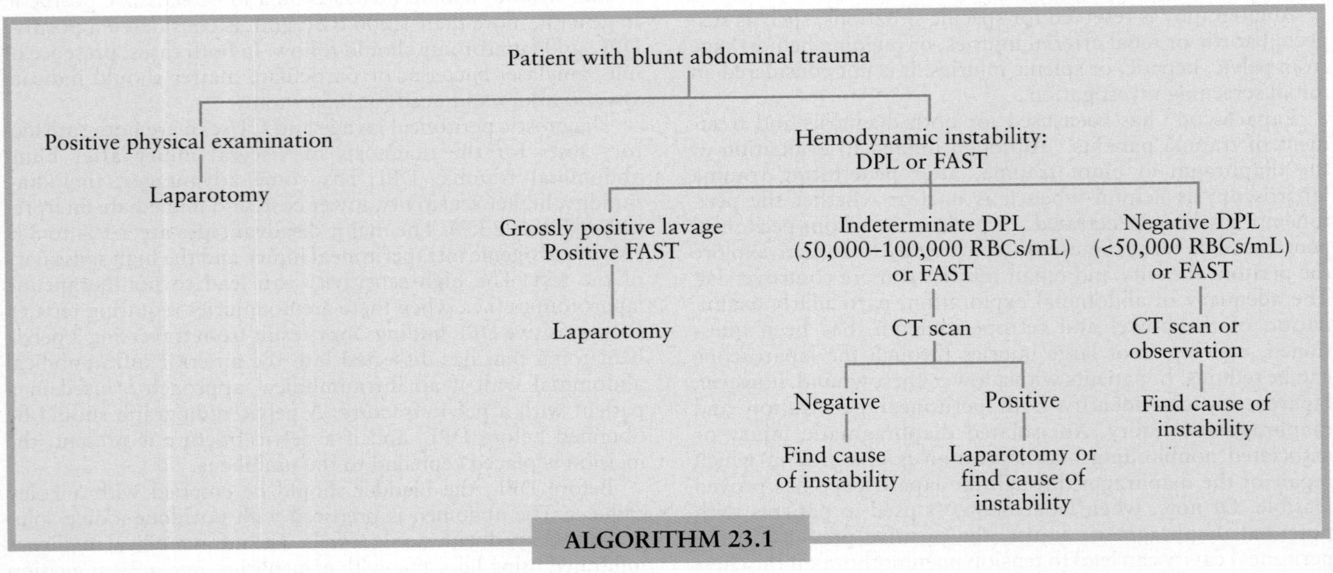

ALGORITHM 23.1. Diagnosis of blunt abdominal trauma.

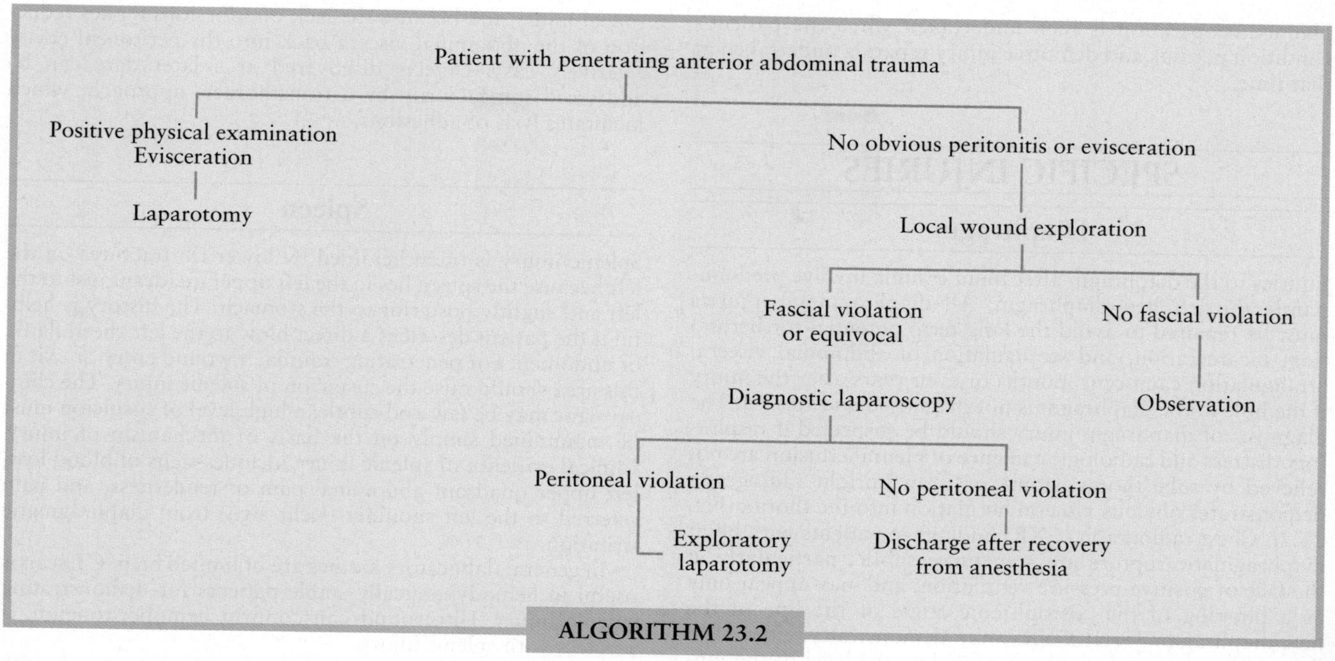

ALGORITHM 23.2. Diagnosis of low-velocity penetrating abdominal trauma.

hemodynamic instability, a DPL or FAST examination consistent with hemoperitoneum.

Broad-spectrum antibiotics are given as soon as the decision to perform a laparotomy is made. The spectrum of coverage should include anaerobic, in addition to aerobic, including gram-positive cocci, organisms. Good evidence suggests that antibiotics do not need to be continued for longer than 24 hours postoperatively, even if contamination from an injured hollow viscus has occurred.[12,13] Tetanus prophylaxis should be administered. If fully immunized as a child, a patient is adequately treated with a booster immunization. If adequate childhood immunization is absent, unlikely, or unknown, then passive immunization should be provided with hyperimmune globulin.

OPERATIVE APPROACH

The patient should be placed supine on the operating room table and the entire anterior torso from the sternal notch to the middle thighs should be prepared and draped to allow for maximum exposure and harvesting of the saphenous vein, if necessary for vascular repair. A midline incision is preferred and there are few reasons to deviate from this choice. This incision also allows extension into a median sternotomy in the event that more proximal control of the vena cava is needed or if the patient is found to have a cardiac injury.

After the abdomen is opened, obvious blood and clot are removed, and packing of the four quadrants is accomplished as indicated by ongoing bleeding. If the peritoneal cavity is full of blood, the location of clot is often a clue to the site of bleeding. Inflow occlusion can be accomplished, if needed, by clamping the aorta at the diaphragmatic hiatus adjacent to the esophagus. Obvious hollow viscus wounds should be rapidly controlled by sutures, clamps, or staples. This initial closure does not need to be definitive and is done primarily to minimize contamination during the course of the operation. Retroperitoneal bleeding may be the source of exsanguinating hemorrhage if rupture into the free peritoneal cavity has occurred. If not, these hematomas can be left for investigation at a later time, depending on their location. Hematomas of the pelvis that are associated with pelvic fractures should not be disturbed. Stable hematomas in the perinephric space lateral to the midline are also best left undisturbed. Central hematomas that can involve injury to the major vascular structures, pancreas, or duodenum are noted and explored after control of injuries within the peritoneal cavity.

After packing has controlled hemorrhage and ongoing contamination has been stopped, time is taken to allow resuscitation of the patient's circulating blood volume. Warming is necessary if massive blood loss has occurred and all fluids must be infused through warming devices, such as the level I. Sustained periods of hypotension should be avoided at all costs, which usually can be accomplished with packing. A complete and thorough exploratory laparotomy is performed methodically to investigate the entire contents of the abdomen for occult injuries.

5 In some patients, a temporizing approach to intra-abdominal injuries, or "damage control," is appropriate.[14] Minimizing operative time is emphasized and the definitive management of all injuries is not necessary. Appropriate candidates for damage control laparotomy are patients with profound coagulopathy, severe acidosis, hypothermia, massive intra-abdominal injuries, or severe associated nonabdominal injuries. Hollow viscus injuries should be temporarily controlled to prevent ongoing contamination, but restoration of gastrointestinal continuity is not performed. The abdominal wall is routinely left open either because of excessive tension and/or need to reoperate for definitive repair, and resuscitative efforts are continued with particular emphasis on correcting coagulopathy, acidosis, and hypothermia. A variety of techniques are available to temporarily avoid abdominal wall closure and still adequately cover and protect the abdominal viscera. Temporary vacuum dressing of the abdominal wall with plastic sheets, dressings, suction drains, and Ioban drapes or similar commercial devices has shown promise as a means of protecting the viscera while maintaining the pliability of the abdominal wall to allow for later fascial closure.[15] A

planned reoperation is then undertaken when the patient's condition permits and definitive injury repair is undertaken at that time.

SPECIFIC INJURIES

Diaphragm

Injuries to the diaphragm after blunt trauma involve predominantly the left hemidiaphragm. All diaphragmatic injuries must be repaired to avoid the long-term potential for herniation, incarceration, and strangulation of abdominal viscera. Strangulation can occur months or even years after the injury if the hole in the diaphragm is not diagnosed and treated. The diagnosis of diaphragm injury should be suspected if respiratory distress and radiologic evidence of pleural effusion are not relieved by tube thoracostomy or if an upright radiograph demonstrates obvious visceral herniation into the thorax (Fig. 23.2). Chest radiograph (CXR) findings in patients with blunt diaphragmatic rupture are sometimes subtle, particularly in the face of positive-pressure ventilation, and may appear only as a blurring of the costophrenic angle or the line of the hemidiaphragm. Serial CXRs may demonstrate evidence of delayed herniation. Low-thoracic (below the level of the nipples) penetrating injuries should be presumed to have traversed the diaphragm. During exploratory laparotomy, the entire diaphragmatic surface should be exposed and directly visualized. Linear lacerations can be repaired with a simple running suture or interrupted horizontal mattress sutures, whereas larger lacerations and tissue deficits occasionally require repair with prosthetic material or resuspension of the diaphragm to higher ribs. Exploration of acute traumatic diaphragmatic rupture is usually accomplished through the abdomen because of the high risk for associated intraperitoneal injury and because the lack of adhesions makes reduction of the abdominal viscera back into the peritoneal cavity relatively easy. Defects discovered at a later date can be addressed satisfactorily by a transthoracic approach, which facilitates lysis of adhesions.

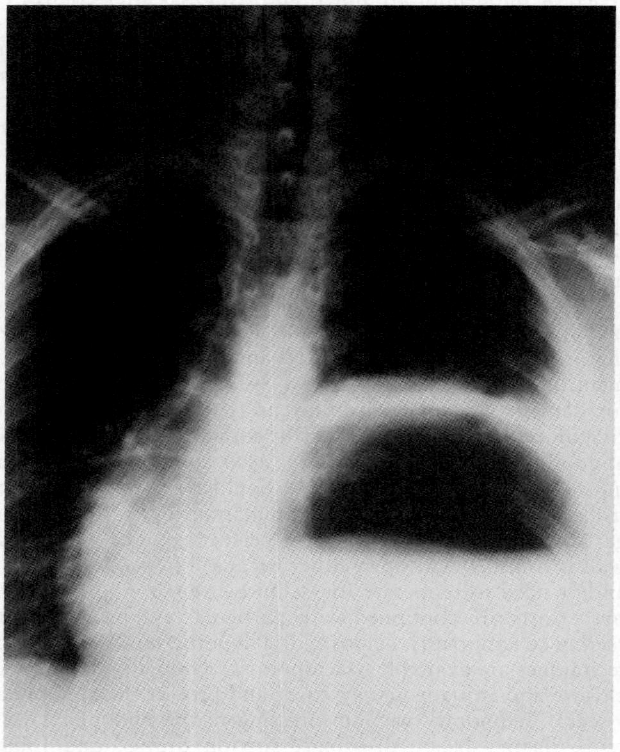

FIGURE 23.2. Chest radiograph showing gastric bubble in the left chest consistent with a rupture of the left hemidiaphragm.

Spleen

Splenic injury is often heralded by lower rib fractures on the left because the spleen lies in the left upper quadrant just to the left and slightly posterior to the stomach. The history is helpful if the patient describes a direct blow to the left chest, flank, or abdomen. For penetrating trauma, a wound entry or exit in this area should raise the suspicion of splenic injury. The clinical signs may be few and subtle; a high level of suspicion must be maintained simply on the basis of mechanism of injury. Clinical evidence of splenic injury includes signs of blood loss, left upper quadrant abdominal pain or tenderness, and pain referred to the left shoulder (Kehr sign) from diaphragmatic irritation.

In general, laboratory studies are of limited help. CT scan is useful in hemodynamically stable patients for demonstrating splenic injury. Ultrasound can confirm hemoperitoneum, if present, with splenic injury.

Historically, splenic injury was routinely treated with splenectomy. During the last few decades, several factors have contributed to a change in this management strategy. Postsplenectomy sepsis, with its high attendant mortality rate, has been characterized, particularly in the treatment of children. In addition, the relative success rates for splenic salvage techniques and nonoperative management have been well established. Nonoperative approaches focus on the clinical presentation of the patient rather than the CT scan appearance, although the presence of a "blush" on the CT scan is indicative of potential ongoing bleeding and an increased likelihood of need for operative intervention[16] (Fig. 23.3). The presence of a "blush" has also been used as a trigger for angiographic embolization in hemodynamically stable patients to prevent ongoing or recurrent bleeding. Care should be exercised to not confuse a nonbleeding pseudoaneurysm with a "true blush" of ongoing bleeding. Although increasingly practiced, nonoperative management is not without dangers and limitations. Potential disadvantages include a more prolonged hospitalization and possibly more exposure to transfused blood, but the

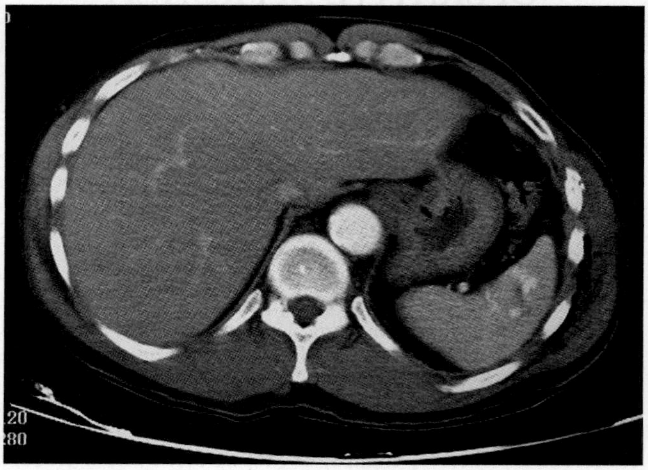

FIGURE 23.3. A cut from a computed tomography scan through the upper abdomen of a patient with a splenic injury. The spleen has evidence of several areas of contrast "blush."

principal risks are ongoing hemorrhage and missed associated intra-abdominal injuries, particularly to the pancreas or bowel.

The spleen is evaluated for hemorrhage during the course of laparotomy. If hemorrhage is noted, a decision must be made regarding splenic salvage. This assessment requires complete mobilization of the spleen from its lateral and posterior attachments, and care must be taken to prevent further injury. The spleen and tail of the pancreas must be mobilized together to evaluate adequately the extent of splenic injury. Ongoing bleeding is controlled during mobilization by manual compression. Topical hemostatic agents usually control capsular tears of the spleen. Lacerations of the splenic substance can be controlled with interlocking absorbable sutures. Major lacerations of the splenic substance can be treated with segmental splenic resection or wrapped in absorbable mesh. Splenic salvage should not be attempted if the patient has protracted hypotension or other severe injuries or if undue delays are encountered in the attempt to repair the spleen. With penetrating injury, damage to adjacent structures, such as the stomach, pancreas, colon, and diaphragm, must be anticipated and investigated.

The nonoperative management of splenic trauma is most attractive if the diagnosis has been made with an abdominal CT scan, the patient is hemodynamically stable, and no other signs of abdominal injury are present. Nonoperative management is successful in such circumstances approximately 90% of the time in adults, and even more often in children. Follow-up CT scans are routinely obtained by some surgeons, but they are probably not necessary if the patient is doing well clinically.[17] In general, nonoperative management should be carried out for the initial 24 to 48 hours in an intensive care unit, and patients should remain hospitalized until the hematocrit remains stable postmobilization. The maximum risk of continued or recurrent bleeding is within the first 48 hours after injury, but there is a decreasing risk of delayed bleeding within the first week postinjury and cases of delayed bleeding even months after injury have been reported.[18]

Complications after splenectomy include early transient thrombocytosis, which usually resolves spontaneously within 2 or 3 months. Anticoagulation is neither necessary nor helpful. Delayed hemorrhage, pancreatitis, pancreatic leak, and subphrenic abscess also may occur. Subphrenic abscess is primarily related to associated hollow viscus injuries and is uncommon. Routine "prophylactic" drainage of the subphrenic space should not be done; it is associated with an increased incidence of abscess.

Postsplenectomy Sepsis. Fatal pneumococcal septicemia after splenectomy was first noted in the mid-1950s in children. Postsplenectomy sepsis syndrome is caused by failure to clear one of several encapsulated bacteria in the absence of the spleen. The incidence is inversely related to age and is higher with underlying hematologic disorders such as lymphoma or thalassemia. The incidence of life-threatening sepsis in adult trauma patients is low (<1% to 2%) and the overall clinical significance is not easily defined. Concern about the possibility of postsplenectomy sepsis should not obscure the fact that the initial priority is to arrest hemorrhage and deal with the patient's immediate life-threatening injuries.

If splenectomy is performed, postoperative follow-up is important.[19] Immunization with the polyvalent pneumococcal vaccine has become the standard of care, and booster immunization is recommended every 3 years. Immunization for *Haemophilus influenzae*, meningococcus, and annually for influenza virus is also recommended. In addition, prophylactic antibiotics, usually oral penicillin, should be given any time the patient is to undergo instrumentation, such as during dental repair or surgery. Postsplenectomy patients should be advised of their increased potential for postsplenectomy sepsis and should carry an identification card to alert health care workers of this possibility if they develop an infection. Also recommended is that they should be given a several-day supply or prescription for oral antibiotics to be taken at the first sign of infection. All infections should be considered emergencies and treated aggressively with intravenous antibiotics in the hospital.

Liver

The liver, the largest organ in the abdominal cavity, is commonly damaged in blunt and penetrating abdominal trauma as well as in thoracoabdominal injuries. Some series have found that the incidence of liver injuries exceeds that of injuries to the spleen. In any case, the two together account for approximately 75% of all blunt intra-abdominal injuries. Trauma sufficient to lacerate the liver is often associated with injuries to other organs. Spontaneous hemostatic mechanisms are sufficiently effective that approximately 85% or more of patients with liver injuries can be managed nonoperatively.

Patients with significant liver injuries usually have a history of major blunt energy transfer to the right thorax or upper abdomen. Physical findings may be minimal because early bleeding may not cause peritoneal irritation or abdominal distention. Any patient with unexplained persistent or recurrent hypotension after blunt abdominal trauma must be considered at risk for a severe liver injury. DPL or FAST is most helpful in quickly establishing the diagnosis of hemoperitoneum, and if the results are positive, laparotomy is appropriate. In hemodynamically stable patients or patients who respond well to resuscitation, the presence of a liver injury may be suspected based on physical examination or ultrasound. A CT scan with intravenous contrast is indicated to illustrate the magnitude of injury and the presence of associated injuries. The injury should be graded according to the American Association for the Surgery of Trauma (AAST) Liver Trauma Scale. The grade of liver injury, the presence of active extravasation (or "blush"), and a rough estimate of the amount of free fluid pres-ent should be noted. However, the decision to proceed to laparotomy is not determined by the grade of injury but should be based on the patient's clinical response to resuscitation and the presence of other injuries, real or suspected. While earlier recommendations considered a severity grade (AAST grade IV or V) to be an indication for laparotomy, the relatively high mortality of operation and the proven success of nonoperative management do not support this approach.

Liver injuries seen on CT scan in hemodynamically stable patients can be treated nonoperatively as long as the patient is followed closely and the possibility of associated hollow viscus or pancreatic injury is borne in mind.[20] Penetrating injuries isolated to the liver can be managed in a similar manner as blunt injuries.[21] If active contrast extravasation is demonstrated, angiographic embolization should be considered along with the need for operative intervention, although it is not proven whether embolization improves outcomes. However, since active extravasation has been identified in patients without a "blush" on CT, embolization may be considered in all patients with significant bleeding.[22] Overall reported success of nonoperative management is greater than 90% in most series. When broken down by grade of injury, the success rate of nonoperative management for injuries grades I through III approaches 95%. In stable patients with ongoing bleeding, angiographic embolization as an adjuvant to a protocol of nonoperative management may lower the number of blood transfusions and the number of operations.

Patients with grades III through V liver injuries are generally admitted to the intensive care unit for monitoring of vital signs and serial hematocrit determinations. Patients with grades I and II injuries may be appropriate for a ward bed with appropriate laboratory and physical examinations. When no evidence of further bleeding is seen, patients can be mobilized and started on a diet. There is no mandated period of bed rest that has been shown to improve success rates of nonoperative management. A repeat CT scan before discharge is not required and normal physical activity is traditionally resumed 3 months postinjury. Liver injuries that do require definitive surgical care present a complex and life-threatening series of problems.

Operative Management. Patients with real or suspected liver injuries who illustrate persistent or recurrent shock require surgical intervention. Injuries vary from simple capsular tears and nonbleeding lacerations, to complex fractures with lobar destruction and extensive parenchymal disruption, to bile duct disruption, to hepatic artery and central venous injuries. The principles of operative management of liver injury are the same regardless of the severity of injury. They involve control of bleeding, removal of devitalized tissue, and establishment of adequate drainage.

Simple lacerations that have stopped bleeding at the time of surgery do not require drainage unless they are deep into the parenchyma, in which case they have an increased probability of postoperative biliary leakage. Subcapsular hematomas are preferably left intact if there is no associated parenchymal injury. Lacerations that continue to bleed despite attempts at local control, including packing, require exploration of the liver wound, and specific vessels and biliary radicals are individually ligated. In the event that bleeding continues, the structures of the porta hepatis should be compressed as a diagnostic maneuver (Pringle maneuver; Fig. 23.4). If the bleeding stops, it is presumed to originate from the portal veins or the hepatic artery. If the bleeding continues, it is presumed to arise principally from the main hepatic veins or inferior vena cava, although this distinction is seldom clear-cut in the operating room. The portal triad can be intermittently occluded to allow improved visualization during placement of sutures as parenchymal vessels are ligated. When selective parenchymal ligation fails, ligation of the hepatic artery is an alternative if the trial Pringle occlusion has had a salutary effect. This is rarely necessary but can occasionally produce dramatic hemostasis. The vessel is occluded as close to the liver injury as possible and after initial efforts at hemostasis have failed.

An alternative for deep lacerations with persistent bleeding is resectional débridement of the involved segment of the liver. This is accomplished by the finger fracture technique, removing devitalized liver or the appropriate portion of the liver. This is required in approximately 5% to 8% of all patients with liver injuries. Subsegmental resection is usually adequate; if segmentectomy or lobectomy is required, a knowledge of the anatomy is imperative so as not to compromise inflow or outflow of the remaining segments. This decision should be made early in the exploration, the blood bank notified, adequate help procured, and exposure obtained.[23] Exposure is best accomplished by complete division of the capsular attachments of the liver. This alternative is associated with operative mortality rates as high as 30% and as such should be avoided unless absolutely necessary.

An additional technique uses an absorbable mesh individually wrapping each lobe of the liver and attaching the mesh to the falciform ligament. This technique is useful, with or without packing, when there are multiple superficial lacerations of the liver with active bleeding and can be used as an alternative to parenchymal débridement.

If blood loss is significant and the patient remains difficult to resuscitate, is hypothermic or acidotic, and has a coagulopathy from massive transfusion, however, an early decision to pack the injury and perform further resuscitation after the abdomen is closed is most appropriate. Packing is done to significantly compress the injured liver with laparotomy pads placed above and below the liver. An absorbable mesh can be

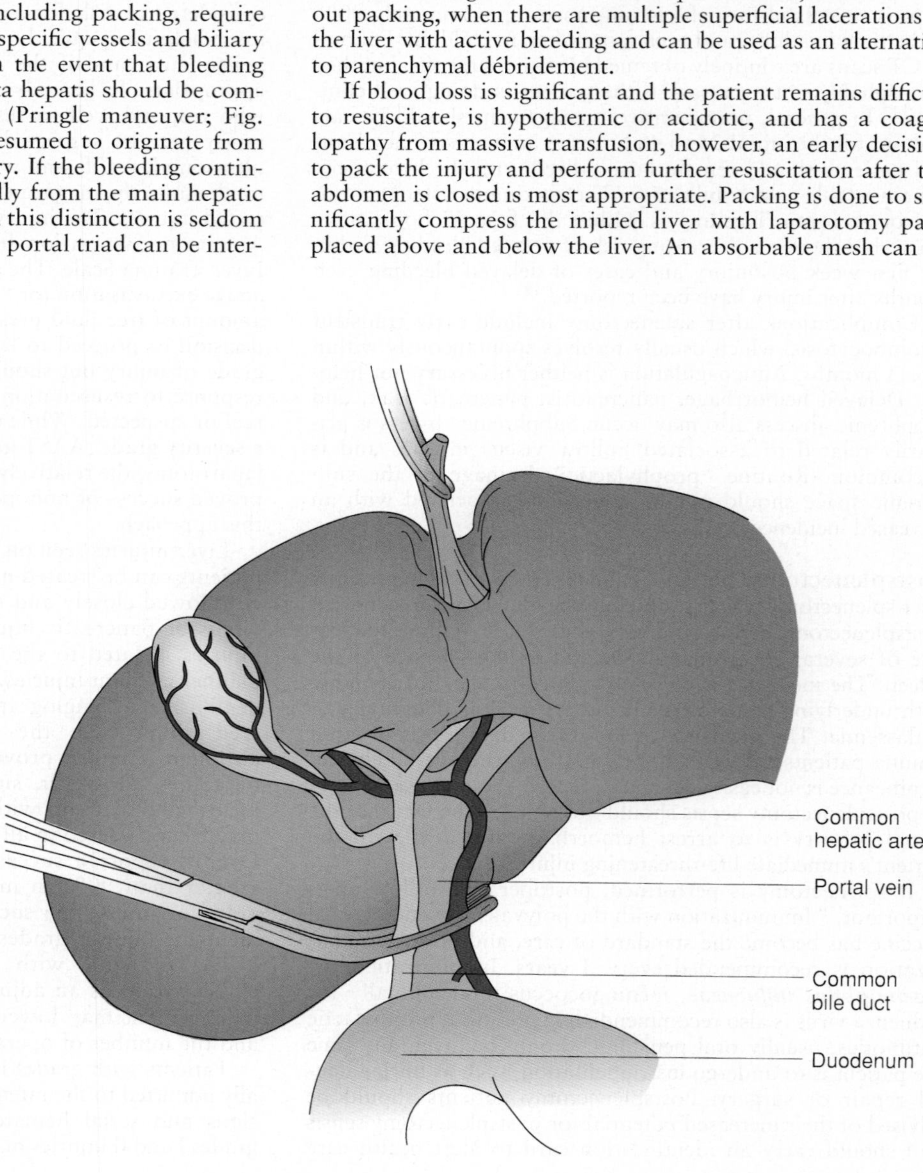

FIGURE 23.4. Pringle maneuver compression of the portal triad structures with a noncrushing vascular clamp for hepatic inflow control. If possible, clamp times should be limited to 15- to 20-minute intervals.

placed over the raw surface and left in place to preserve hemostasis when the packs are removed. For packing to be successful, it should be used early, before coagulopathy has become too severe. A system to evacuate fluid in a closed system should be constructed, or, more commonly, a commercial device is applied (wound vac). Subsequent operative removal of the packs 24 to 72 hours later can be accompanied occasionally by resection and suture ligation as needed. After hemostasis has been achieved, the area may be drained, although this may not diminish the incidence of biloma.

Inability to control bleeding by any of the previously described techniques suggests significant retrohepatic vena caval or adjacent hepatic vein bleeding. Early consideration should be given to complete vascular isolation or the placement of an intracaval shunt. This approach is rarely necessary and should be undertaken only if packing has not controlled hemorrhage from the liver and appropriate expertise is available (Fig. 23.5). To accomplish this, the midline laparotomy incision is extended into the chest, either by a right anterior thoracotomy or, preferably, by a median sternotomy. Infrahepatic (cephalad to the renal veins) and suprahepatic (usually intrapericardial) control of the vena cava is obtained. A shunt or other large conduit (chest tube or endotracheal tube) is then inserted through a right atrial pursestring suture into the vena cava, and vascular occlusion around the conduit at these sites is obtained. The resultant vascular isolation is always imperfect but may allow better visualization of hepatic vein and vena caval lacerations for direct suture ligation or repair. Total venous occlusion may be equally effective and serves the same general purpose but requires adequate volume loading prior to clamping to preserve cardiac function. The risk of hypotension is significant with either approach, in the former because of significant blood loss during atrial cannulation, and with the latter owing to diminished venous return to the right atrium. Last, in select institutions the availability of venous bypass may be an alternative.

The major complications after liver injury include hemorrhage, respiratory insufficiency, coagulopathy, hypoglycemia, biliary fistula or other bile duct injury, hemobilia, and subdiaphragmatic or intraparenchymal abscess formation. The coagulopathy after liver resection is usually the result of hypothermia and inadequate replacement of blood components. In cases of major liver hemorrhage, it is imperative to work with anesthesia to confirm that adequate fresh frozen plasma is being given along with blood cell replacement. In addition to aggressive component replacement, addition of

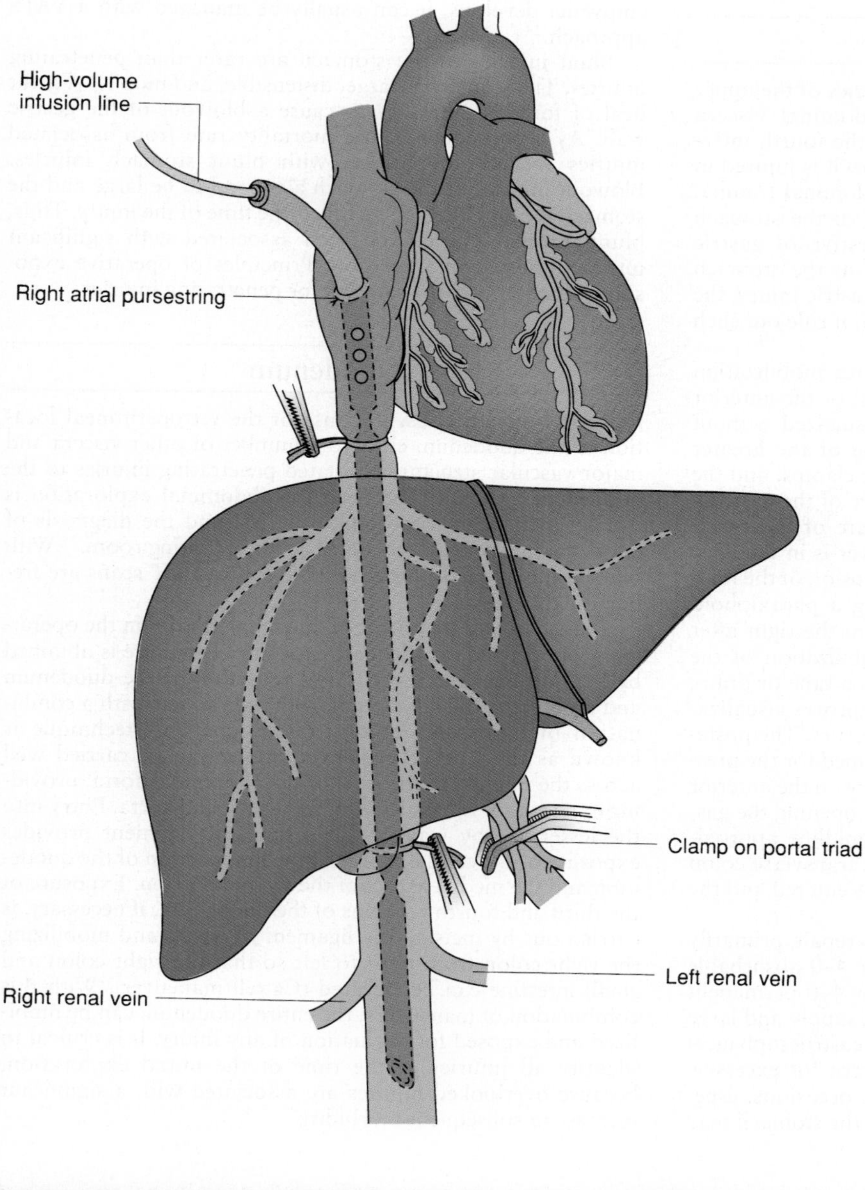

FIGURE 23.5. Intracaval shunt used for retrohepatic venous injuries, combined with a Pringle maneuver for isolation of the retrohepatic vena cava for operative repair.

activated factor VII (FVIIa) has anecdotally been lifesaving in select cases. Patients undergoing major hepatic resection or liver destruction need continuous glucose infusion, often 10% dextrose, during the early postoperative period. Hypoalbuminemia is common but does not usually require albumin administration and should be treated simply with aggressive nutritional support. Hyperbilirubinemia is transient and usually peaks in 2 to 3 weeks after major resection. Intrahepatic and subphrenic abscesses can develop, particularly if significant débridement has been necessary. They are diagnosed by clinical evidence of sepsis combined with ultrasound or CT scan and often can be treated with percutaneous drainage. When percutaneous drainage is unsuccessful, drainage can be effected surgically either transperitoneally or posteriorly through the bed of the 12th rib. Biliary fistulas or bilomas usually resolve spontaneously, and major extrahepatic ductal injuries are rare. For the rare biliary leak or fistula that does not close spontaneously, placement of a temporary intrabiliary stent either at the site of injury or, preferably, via the sphincter of Oddi (to decrease intrabiliary pressure) is recommended. A T-tube placed in an otherwise normal common bile duct is inappropriate unless the extrahepatic biliary tree is injured. Hemobilia is a rare complication, occurring with intrahepatic bleeding into the bile ducts, and is best diagnosed with angiography or endoscopy. Angiographic embolization is the treatment of choice.

Stomach

The stomach is vulnerable to penetrating injuries of the upper abdomen and lower chest. The upper abdominal viscera underlie the lower ribs to a level as high as the fourth intercostal space during full expiration. The stomach is injured in 5% to 10% of patients with penetrating abdominal trauma. Hematemesis or blood found on aspiration of the stomach with a nasogastric tube is a finding suggestive of gastric injury. Although many patients with blood in the stomach after penetrating abdominal trauma have a gastric injury, the absence of blood in the gastric aspirate does not rule out such an injury.

At laparotomy, adequate exposure requires mobilization and visualization of the entire stomach. Most of the anterior surface of the stomach can be adequately visualized without extensive mobilization by grasping the edge of the greater curve of the stomach with fingers or Babcock clamps, and the stomach is pulled down and spread. Exposure of the gastroesophageal junction can be difficult if the flare of the costal margin is narrow or if the left lobe of the liver is in the way. Improved exposure is accomplished with extension of the midline incision as high as possible by creating a paraxiphoid extension. The left hepatic lobe is retracted to the right after division of the left triangular ligament. Mobilization of the gastroesophageal junction, encirclement with a tape or drain, and caudal traction into the operative field improves visualization and the performance of any necessary repairs. The posterior wall of the stomach should also be examined for the presence of injuries, particularly if there is an injury on the anterior surface. The posterior stomach is exposed by opening the gastrocolic ligament bluntly to the left of the midline approximately halfway between the stomach and the transverse colon in a relatively avascular area. The lesser sac is entered and the posterior wall of the stomach examined.

Injuries to the stomach are usually easy to repair, primarily in two layers, with an inner layer of 3–0 or 4–0 absorbable sutures followed by an outer layer of 3–0 or 4–0 permanent Lembert sutures. Because of the ample blood supply and large lumen of the stomach in all areas except the gastroesophageal junction and pylorus, there is minimal concern for excessive inversion and luminal compromise. On rare occasions, especially after shotgun wounds, large injuries of the stomach may require resection. Injuries to the pylorus are rare. If viable tissue is present, it should be closed with a Heineke-Mikulicz pyloroplasty; a concomitant vagotomy is not necessary.

Because of the stomach's position high in the abdomen, penetrating injuries to the stomach are frequently associated with lacerations of the diaphragm. During spontaneous ventilation, there is negative pressure in the pleural cavity and positive pressure in the abdomen, and the resultant pressure gradient causes movement of gastric fluid and particulate matter from the abdomen into the chest. The degree of contamination can be deceptive in the operating room because most occurs before the institution of positive-pressure ventilation and laparotomy. Because even small amounts of contamination can result in an empyema, combined injuries to the stomach and diaphragm require the pleural cavity to be lavaged before closure of the diaphragm. The diaphragmatic laceration should be enlarged enough to allow lavage from the abdomen. The course of the phrenic nerve in the diaphragm should be borne in mind, and enlargement of the diaphragmatic laceration should be done either radially or as peripherally as possible. Occasionally, adequate lavage is difficult because of the amount of pleural contamination or if enlargement of the diaphragmatic laceration cannot be done without risk of de-nervation. In such instances, the patient should be closely followed postoperatively for evidence of the development of an empyema or undergo "prophylactic" video-assisted thora-scopic surgery (VATS) to lavage the chest. If empyema develops, it can usually be managed with a VATS approach.[24]

Blunt injuries to the stomach are rarer than penetrating injuries. The stomach is large, distensible, and mobile. A great deal of force is necessary to cause a blowout of the gastric wall. As a consequence, the mortality rate from associated injuries is high in patients with blunt stomach injuries. Blowout injuries of the stomach also tend to be large and the stomach is more likely to be full at the time of the injury. Thus, blunt trauma injuries are often associated with significant intraperitoneal contamination. Principles of operative exposure and repair are the same as for penetrating injuries.

Duodenum

Penetrating Injuries. Because of the retroperitoneal location of the duodenum close to a number of other viscera and major vascular structures, isolated penetrating injuries to the duodenum are rare. The need for abdominal exploration is usually dictated by associated injuries, and the diagnosis of duodenal injury is usually made in the operating room.[25] With blunt trauma, gastrointestinal (GI) contrast CT scans are frequently diagnostic.

Diagnosis and treatment of duodenal injuries in the operating room depend on adequate exposure. Exposure is obtained by incising the lateral peritoneal reflection of the duodenum and mobilizing the duodenum from right to left with a combination of blunt and cautery dissection. This technique is known as the Kocher maneuver, and it can be carried well across the midline to the level of the abdominal aorta, providing exposure of the underlying vena cava and aorta. Entry into the lesser sac by way of the gastrocolic ligament provides exposure of the caudal aspect of the first portion of the duodenum and the medial aspect of the second portion. Exposure of the third and fourth portions of the duodenum, if necessary, is carried out by incising the ligament of Treitz and mobilizing the right colon from right to left so that the right colon and small intestine can be elevated (Cattell maneuver). With this combination of maneuvers, the entire duodenum can be mobilized and exposed for evaluation of any injury. It is critical to identify all injuries at the time of the initial exploration, because overlooked injuries are associated with a significant increase in subsequent morbidity.

TABLE 23.4 **DIAGNOSIS**

IMPORTANT ASPECTS TO NOTE FOR DUODENAL INJURIES

Anatomic relation to the ampulla of Vater
Character of the injury (e.g., a simple laceration vs. destruction of the duodenal wall)
Involved circumference of the duodenum
Associated injuries to the biliary tract, pancreas, or major vascular structures

Grading systems have been devised to characterize duodenal injuries. Although useful for research purposes, the specifics of the grading systems are less important than several simple aspects of the duodenal injury (Table 23.4). Most penetrating injuries to the duodenum are simple lacerations that can be repaired primarily. Such repairs should be done in two layers, with an inner absorbable layer of 3–0 or 4–0 sutures followed by an outer layer of 3–0 or 4–0 permanent Lembert sutures. The closure should be oriented transversely, if possible, to avoid luminal compromise, but transverse orientation is not as critical in the duodenum as it is in the rest of the small intestine. The biliary tract does not require drainage in such cases unless an associated biliary tract injury is present, and the duodenum does not require tube decompression, although both of these maneuvers have been advocated in the past. The periduodenal area should be drained with closed suction drainage.

Injuries that encompass as much as 40% or 50% of the duodenal wall can be successfully closed primarily. Primary repair of injuries larger than this, however, can lead to luminal compromise. If the duodenum has been transected or almost transected, the edges should be débrided and a two-layer primary anastomosis done without tension after mobilization of the duodenum, provided that the transection is not close to the ampulla of Vater. Large injuries of the duodenum can be reinforced with a jejunal patch by bringing up a loop of jejunum and laying it onto the area of injury so that the serosa of the jejunum buttresses the duodenal repair (Fig. 23.6). Alternatively, a Roux-en-Y duodenojejunostomy can drain a large defect internally. If there are severe associated injuries to the pancreas or biliary tract, pancreaticoduodenectomy may be necessary. The morbidity associated with pancreaticoduodenectomy is substantial, and this operation is indicated only if the extent of injury is so great that the necessary resection has, in essence, been done by the injury.

Some duodenal repairs are tenuous. This is a particular problem if there is associated pancreatic injury, raising concern about the digestive action of activated pancreatic enzymes on the repair. Pyloric exclusion defunctionalizes the duodenum and protects the repair from activated pancreatic enzymes until it has had time to heal. A gastrotomy along the greater curvature of the stomach provides access to the pylorus, which is closed with a large running nonabsorbable suture or, alternatively, the pylorus is stapled shut. GI continuity is restored by a gastrojejunostomy (Fig. 23.7). Tube decompression of the duodenum may be performed in extreme duodenal injuries, but the biliary tract does not require decompression except in cases of an associated biliary tract injury. As with all duodenal injuries, the periduodenal area should be externally drained to control postoperative leak as a controlled fistula. With creation of a gastrojejunal anastomosis and no concomitant procedure to decrease gastric acid production, H_2 blockers or proton pump inhibitors should be given in the postoperative period to prevent marginal ulceration. After a number of weeks, the vast majority of patients have reconstituted normal GI continuity. The closure of the pylorus breaks down, regardless of whether the pylorus was closed with absorbable or nonabsorbable suture. As the pylorus reopens, the inherently ulcerogenic gastrojejunostomy gradually closes of its own accord and, thus, does not require a concomitant vagotomy.

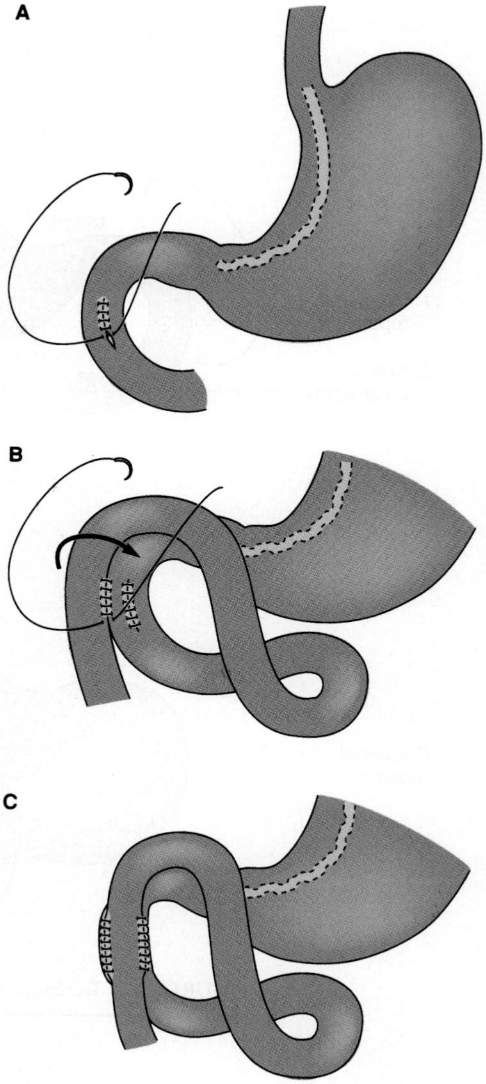

FIGURE 23.6. A jejunoileal patch can be used to reinforce repairs of the duodenum. **A:** The duodenum is first repaired. **B:** The retrocolic loop of jejunum is brought up to the area of repair. **C:** The serosa is sewn over the repair.

Blunt Injuries. Blunt injuries to the duodenum are less common and more difficult to diagnose than penetrating injuries. They can occur in isolation or with pancreatic injury. The need for immediate abdominal exploration is frequently not obvious. Because the duodenum is located in the retroperitoneum, findings on physical examination of the abdomen may be subtle except in cases of associated intra-abdominal injuries. Nonetheless, the physical examination is still one of the best methods for determining the presence of a duodenal injury. This is particularly true if the admission examination is indeterminate, emphasizing the need for serial abdominal examinations.

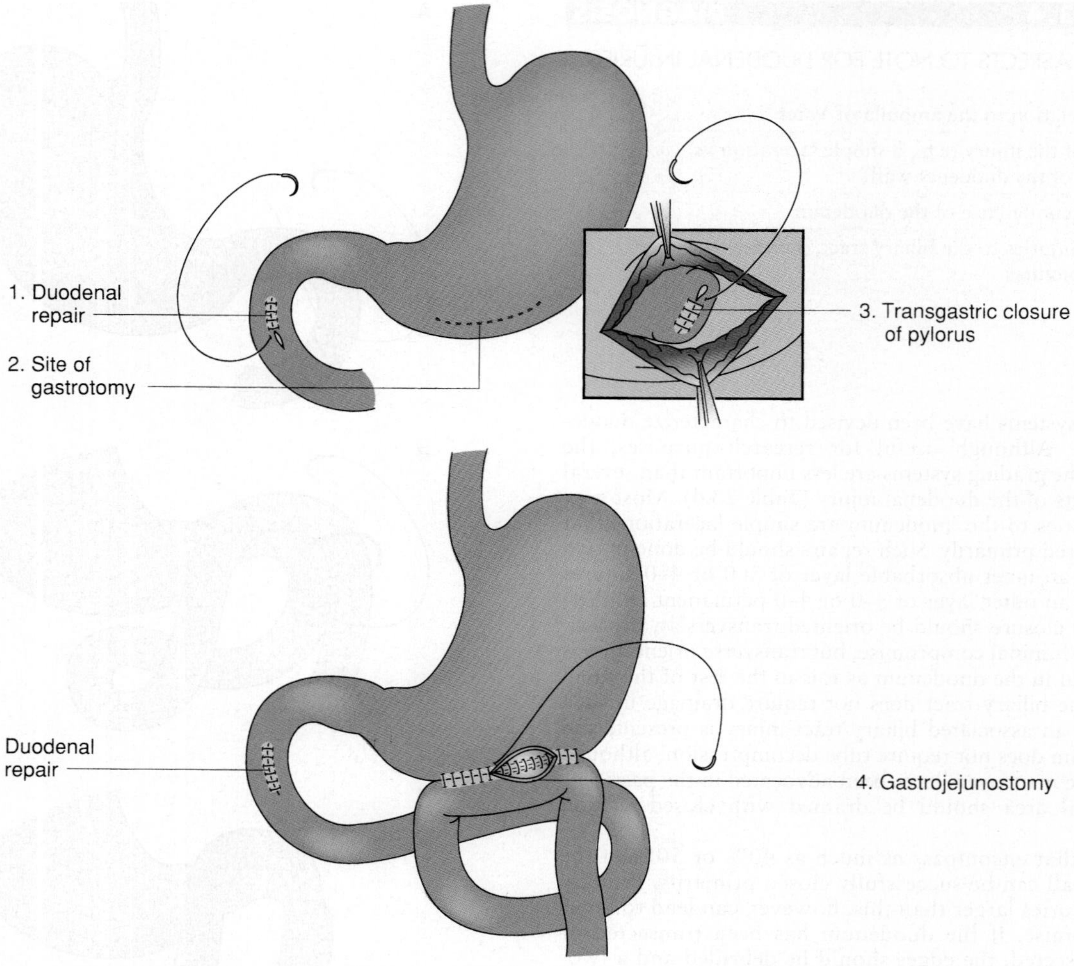

FIGURE 23.7. Technique of pyloric exclusion for complex duodenal injury.

The serum amylase concentration is helpful in the diagnosis of blunt duodenal injuries; however, the test lacks sensitivity. The duodenum is retroperitoneal, the concentration of amylase in the fluid that leaks is variable, and amylase concentrations often take hours, even days, to increase after injury. Serial determinations of serum amylase are better than a single, isolated determination on admission, but sensitivity is still not good and delays are inherent in serial determinations.

Upper GI series and CT scans with GI contrast are reasonably sensitive for the presence of duodenal injury after blunt trauma. Performance of these tests requires a stable patient without any other obvious indications for abdominal exploration. An advantage of CT over upper GI series is that the rest of the retroperitoneum and peritoneal viscera are also visualized. With either study, extravasation of contrast material from the duodenum constitutes an absolute indication for surgical intervention and repair.

Operative exposure and repair of the duodenum after blunt trauma are the same as for penetrating injuries. Crush injuries are more common after blunt trauma and occasionally require extensive resection, but the injuries can be treated frequently by simple techniques of repair if they are diagnosed in a timely fashion.

Intramural hematoma of the duodenum is a rare injury specific to patients with blunt trauma. It is most common in children after isolated localized force to the upper abdomen (e.g., bicycle handlebar ends). Intramural hematomas occur when the duodenum is crushed and bleeding occurs in the submucosal or subserosal layers of the duodenum. The duodenum is not perforated. Such hematomas can lead to obstruction of the lumen. If the diagnosis is not made at the time of the initial injury, the obstruction usually takes several days to develop, presumably because of increased accumulation of intramural water as the hemoglobin in the hematoma begins to break down and osmotic forces increase absorption of water. If exploration takes place shortly after injury, intramural hematomas of the duodenum are seen as periduodenal hematomas. All hematomas in the area of the duodenum should be explored to rule out the possibility of perforation. Such exploration includes a Kocher maneuver and mobilization of the duodenum, which in most instances successfully drains subserosal hematomas. Submucosal hematomas, if large and potentially obstructing, may require drainage with a deeper, separate myotomy-type incision. If surgery does not occur shortly after injury, obstructive symptoms become manifest after a number of days. An upper GI series or CT scan should be performed to demonstrate obstruction. The obstruction is usually in the second portion of the duodenum and, in the classic picture, demonstrates a coiled-spring appearance. Debate surrounds the treatment of intramural hematomas of the duodenum if the diagnosis is delayed, but the weight of opinion argues for initial nonoperative treatment. This strategy is usually successful because the hematoma gradually resolves and the obstructive symptoms subside without long-term residual sequelae. If obstructive symptoms persist beyond 10 to 14 days from the time of diagnosis, abdominal exploration should be undertaken to drain the hematoma, relieve the obstruction, and rule out a missed injury.

Complications. The duodenum is particularly susceptible to leak of repairs because of the presence of intraluminal digestive enzymes. Adequate drainage of the periduodenal area helps to ensure that such leaks are controlled and do not result in an intra-abdominal abscess. Placement of a decompressive duodenal tube to protect duodenal repairs is not necessary. If a duodenal repair breaks down and the duodenum is adequately drained, a duodenal fistula results. In the absence of distal obstruction, foreign body, or persistent infection (the chances of which are minimized by adequate drainage), most of these controlled fistulas ultimately close. They may be slow to resolve, and a wait of several months is advised to allow them to resolve spontaneously. Support with total parenteral nutrition increases the rate of spontaneous closure. If a fistula fails to close after an appropriate waiting period, further surgical intervention is warranted. It consists of reexploration of the abdomen and construction of a defunctionalized Roux-en-Y duodenojejunostomy as a form of internal drainage.

Pancreas

Penetrating Injuries. Penetrating injuries to the pancreas are usually diagnosed in the operating room.[26] The pancreas is located in the retroperitoneum, surrounded by a number of other viscera and major vascular structures. As a result, an isolated injury to the pancreas is unusual, and patients with penetrating pancreatic trauma usually have obvious indications for abdominal exploration. Preoperative serum amylase and lipase concentrations are not helpful; they are elevated only in a few patients with penetrating pancreatic injuries.

On abdominal exploration, signs of pancreatic injury include a projectile path that passes near the pancreas, a central hematoma in the upper abdomen, and injuries to the duodenum, vena cava, suprarenal aorta, or mesenteric vessels. In all these instances, the pancreas should be thoroughly explored.

The anterior surface of the pancreas is visualized by entry into the lesser sac of the peritoneal cavity. This is done in the same fashion as outlined previously for exposure of the posterior aspect of the stomach, with division of the gastrocolic ligament in a relatively avascular area to the left of the midline. A thin layer of peritoneum overlies the anterior surface of the pancreas at this point, and complete visualization of the surface sometimes requires incision of this layer.

The tail of the pancreas can be more fully visualized, especially in its posterior aspect, by mobilization of the spleen and the tail of the pancreas as a unit. This is accomplished by incision of any lateral attachments of the spleen to the abdominal wall and mobilization of the spleen with blunt dissection laterally to medially by development of the plane between the anterior surface of the left kidney and the posterior aspect of the spleen. This brings the spleen into the abdominal wound and elevates the posterior aspect of the pancreatic tail for inspection. The posterior aspect of the body of the pancreas is visualized by opening the avascular area at the inferior margin of the body and tail of the pancreas with a combination of sharp and blunt dissection. The pancreas can then be mobilized inferiorly to superiorly. This maneuver is also important to mobilize the pancreas in preparation for distal pancreatic resection.

The posterior aspect of the head of the pancreas can be exposed by an extensive Kocher maneuver. In combination with entry into the lesser sac, this also allows for bimanual palpation of the pancreatic head, with one hand placed on the anterior surface of the pancreas through the hole in the lesser sac and the other hand placed behind the pancreas in the plane developed by the Kocher maneuver.

In the evaluation of penetrating pancreatic injuries, an important key to operative management is whether a ductal injury is present. Transduodenal intraoperative pancreatography has been recommended. The advantage of this maneuver is that it allows for more definitive determination of the type of operative intervention that should be undertaken. The major disadvantage is that it necessitates entry into the duodenum when there is no associated duodenal injury, which turns simple pancreatic injuries into combined pancreaticoduodenal injuries, with an attendant significant increase in potential postoperative morbidity. A further argument against intraoperative pancreatography is that most injuries to the pancreas can be adequately evaluated and decisions made about appropriate operative treatment without radiographic examination of ductal anatomy. In rare circumstances in which the patient's condition permits and the necessary equipment and expertise are available, the use of intraoperative endoscopic retrograde cholangiopancreatography (ERCP) provides an excellent option.

The operative management of penetrating pancreatic injuries depends on both the location and severity of the injury.[27] With respect to location, injuries can be subdivided into those of the head, body, and tail of the pancreas. With respect to severity, injuries can be classified by the degree of parenchymal disruption and the presence or absence of ductal injury.

Contusions of the pancreas, regardless of location, should be either simply observed or drained. The optimal type of drainage is a matter of some debate, and a variety of different drainage methods have been espoused. The type of drain used after pancreatic injury is probably not as important as ensuring that adequate drainage has been effected. If drains are used, they should be left in place for at least 5 to 7 days to ensure that a drain tract develops. Pancreatic fistulas can develop on a delayed basis 3 to 7 days after injury, and if the drains are removed before that time, drainage may be inadequate. The morbidity rate for patients with undrained pancreatic secretions is much greater than for those with drained pancreatic secretions.

The timing of drain removal should be based on both the amount and character of the pancreatic drainage. Drain outputs in excess of 150 to 200 mL/d are suggestive of pancreatic fistulas. Determinations of drain amylase concentration are helpful, but amylase concentrations within a few days of injury, even if very high levels (>50,000 IU/L), do not correlate with the development of a pancreatic fistula or other complications. Determinations at 7 days after injury correlate with the persistence of a pancreatic fistula or other pancreatic complication only if the level is higher than 100,000 IU/L, whereas the negative predictive value of a concentration below 100,000 IU/L is poor and does not rule out the presence or subsequent development of a pancreatic complication.

Treatment of major parenchymal disruptions depends on location and the presence of ductal injury. Injuries to the body or tail of the pancreas should be evaluated for possible ductal disruption. It can be difficult to determine definitively whether an injury has occurred to the duct by inspection of the parenchymal injury. If a ductal injury is obvious or likely, the distal pancreas should be resected and the proximal pancreas and pancreatic duct oversewn. Distal resection can include up to 80% of the gland, if necessary. Subsequent endocrine or exocrine insufficiency is rare if the pancreas is normal. If a ductal injury is not present or is unlikely, the pancreas should be drained. Major parenchymal disruptions of the head of the pancreas should be drained, regardless of the presence of ductal disruption, because the morbidity of pancreaticoduodenectomy or attempts at internal drainage is greater than the morbidity of simply draining the area of injury. If a pancreatic fistula develops, drains can control it. If the fistula does not resolve with time, the pancreas can be drained internally or resected at a later date.

For massive injuries to the duodenum and head of the pancreas, pancreaticoduodenectomy with reconstruction should be reserved for cases in which débridement of devitalized tissue results in a de facto removal of the duodenum and head of the pancreas. Penetrating injuries to the ampulla of Vater also may require formal pancreaticoduodenectomy.

Internal drainage of the pancreas has been suggested as a means of treating ductal injuries without the need for resection of viable and functional pancreatic tissue. Although in theory this approach preserves pancreatic function and minimizes the risk of postoperative pancreatic insufficiency, it has major risks. The pancreaticojejunal anastomosis is susceptible to break down and leak, especially if suboptimal conditions of associated injury and hemodynamic instability exist. The construction of a Roux-en-Y jejunal limb requires the opening of the intestine and the creation of a small bowel anastomosis. If the intestine has not been injured, this procedure increases the amount of contamination associated with the injury as well as the likelihood of postoperative morbidity. For these reasons, most major trauma centers rarely carry out internal drainage procedures in the early postinjury period, relying instead on either resection or drainage. Internal drainage is usually reserved for cases in which persistent pancreatic fistulas or pseudocysts develop late[28] and is done on a delayed basis.

Distal pancreatectomy for traumatic injuries should be performed only after the pancreas has been thoroughly mobilized and exposed. In some cases, the pancreas has already been transected, and the site of resection has therefore already been determined for the surgeon. If this is not the case, the pancreas should be transected just proximal to the site of known or presumed ductal injury. If associated splenectomy is planned, elaborate dissection is unnecessary. The splenic artery can be identified near the superior margin of the pancreas and ligated. The splenic vein also can be individually ligated at this point. Commonly, the splenic vein lies behind the body and tail of the pancreas, and its isolation requires more dissection. As an alternative to extensive dissection to isolate the splenic vein behind the pancreas, the vein can be transected along with the pancreatic parenchyma. Individual ligation of the splenic vein stump can be done after the distal pancreas and spleen have been removed. It is helpful first to mobilize the spleen and tail of the pancreas.

The pancreas should be mobilized at the site of transection and can be encircled with a rubber drain. Mobilization and encirclement are best done by an approach to the pancreas along its inferior margin and mobilization inferiorly to superiorly. The pancreas can be divided either distal to a bowel clamp or with a stapler. There are some indications that a sutured closure is less likely to break down and lead to fistula formation than a stapled closure. If a bowel clamp is used, the pancreatic stump should be oversewn with a nonabsorbable running suture. It is recommended that an individual figure-of-eight suture be placed in the cut end of the pancreatic duct. This proves exceedingly difficult in patients with normal pancreatic ductal systems because the duct is small and not easily identified in the cut edge of the pancreatic stump. A pancreatic duct that can be seen easily may indicate preexisting proximal ductal obstruction. In this case, the duct should be individually ligated. If the cut end of the duct is not immediately apparent, time and effort should not be taken to locate and individually ligate it.

It is possible to perform a distal pancreatectomy without a concomitant splenectomy. Splenic salvage involves individual ligation and division of the branches of the splenic artery and vein that supply the body and tail of the pancreas. This adds to operative time and can increase the risk of bleeding, particularly if there is an associated injury to the spleen treated with splenorrhaphy. Splenic salvage should be attempted, therefore, only in hemodynamically stable patients with minimal or no associated intra-abdominal or extra-abdominal injuries.

Pancreatic injuries can lead to a number of complications, including pancreatic fistulas, pseudocysts, bleeding in the area of the pancreatic bed, and pancreatitis. Pancreatic fistulas after trauma are characterized by persistent drainage of pancreatic enzymes and secretions from the pancreatic injury for a number of weeks after injury. Most of these fistulas close spontaneously, especially if there is no proximal obstruction of the pancreatic ductal system. A trial of total parenteral nutrition may improve the rate and incidence of spontaneous closure. Experience with the use of somatostatin in patients with posttraumatic pancreatic fistulas is limited. Somatostatin given to patients with pancreatic fistulas after elective pancreatic resections seems to decrease the amount of fistula drainage but has not consistently decreased the time to fistula closure and may impact pancreatic healing.

Pseudocysts that develop after pancreatic trauma often resolve on their own or with percutaneous aspiration or drainage. If, after 4 to 6 weeks of observation with serial ultrasound or CT scans, the pseudocyst does not show signs of resolution, it should be drained internally, into either the stomach or a defunctionalized limb of jejunum, depending on its location.

Bleeding in the area of the pancreatic bed is usually an early complication caused by inadequate drainage with resultant autodigestion of the pancreas and surrounding tissue. Bleeding can be avoided by identifying all injuries at the time of exploration and ensuring adequate drainage. If massive bleeding does occur, it should be dealt with through angiographic or operative intervention.

Pancreatitis is another complication of pancreatic injury and is worsened by inadequate drainage of pancreatic secretions. Treatment consists of provision of adequate drainage and supportive care. If the pancreatitis is localized to the distal pancreas and a trial of conservative management fails, distal pancreatectomy should be considered.

Blunt Injuries. The major difference between penetrating and blunt injuries of the pancreas concerns diagnosis. Penetrating injuries are usually discovered on abdominal exploration for associated injuries, but blunt injuries can occur in isolation and the preoperative diagnosis can be difficult. Blunt pancreatic injuries are relatively rare, which increases the difficulty of diagnosis. In one series of pancreatic injuries, delays in diagnosis of blunt injuries ranged up to several days. Making the diagnosis as quickly as possible is important because delays in diagnosis are associated with significantly increased morbidity and mortality.

The body of the pancreas lies directly anterior to the vertebral column and is vulnerable to crush injuries when the anterior abdominal wall is forcibly compressed, as can occur from a seatbelt, steering wheel, or sharp blow to the epigastrium. In such instances, the pancreas may be the only intra-abdominal organ injured.

Physical examination of the abdomen is useful, but because of the retroperitoneal location of the pancreas, the results can be misleadingly benign until a number of hours to days after injury. This emphasizes the importance of serial examinations. In most cases, the abdomen becomes progressively more tender to palpation during the first 24 to 48 hours after injury and the need for abdominal exploration becomes more obvious. The physical examination of the abdomen is much less reliable in young children and in patients with head injuries.

Serum amylase and lipase concentrations drawn on admission have low positive and negative predictive values but are helpful in providing an initial value of these enzymes for comparison with subsequent serial determinations. Serial amylase and lipase concentrations are helpful in monitoring the courses of patients with normal or only mildly elevated admission values, but overreliance on these methods can result in dangerous delays in diagnosis.

Computed tomography scan of the abdomen allows for visualization of the retroperitoneum, including the pancreas. In the case of isolated injury to the pancreas, the sensitivity of the CT scan is at its lowest shortly after injury. Although CT diagnosis of pancreatic injury improves greatly after a number of hours have passed, immediate CT scan of the abdomen sometimes misses pancreatic injuries, particularly if expert interpretation is not available. Serial CT scans, with GI contrast to evaluate the duodenum, should be performed if pancreatic injury is of concern.

Endoscopic retrograde cholangiopancreatography is an attractive diagnostic method for pancreatic injury because it is less invasive than abdominal exploration and also provides information about the status of the ductal system, but there are several practical disadvantages to the technique. Most successful studies using ERCP have involved stable patients studied hours to days after injury at a referral center specifically because of suspicion of a pancreatic injury. These patients are a select group, different from patients who are recently injured. In addition, ERCP is not universally available and, even in large centers, is often unavailable at the odd hours necessary for early diagnosis in acutely injured patients. Many endoscopists are also fearful of inducing an exacerbation of pancreatitis in patients with mild pancreatic injuries lacking ductal involvement. Magnetic resonance cholangiopancreatography (MRCP) is a newer possibility for diagnosis of pancreatic ductal injury in patients with blunt trauma and has also been used as an alternative to ERCP for the investigation of possible postinjury or postoperative complications.[29] Experience to date with MRCP is limited, but it has the advantage of being noninvasive and does not cause pancreatitis. Further experience will be necessary to determine whether the false-negative and false-positive rates of MRCP are acceptable in the diagnosis of pancreatic injury.

Basic principles of exposure and operative management of blunt injuries of the pancreas are the same as for penetrating injuries. In many instances of severe injury, the pancreas already has been transected by the trauma, making the pancreatic resection somewhat simpler to carry out. Isolated injuries of the pancreas from blunt trauma also lend themselves to distal pancreatectomy with splenic preservation. As in penetrating injury, splenic salvage should be attempted only in stable patients without associated splenic rupture or severe associated intra-abdominal or extra-abdominal injuries. Complications of blunt pancreatic injury are similar to those outlined for penetrating injuries.

Small Intestine

Penetrating Injuries. Because the small intestine occupies more volume in the peritoneal cavity than any other organ, it is the intra-abdominal viscus most frequently injured by penetrating abdominal trauma. The severity of injury ranges from trivial rents in the bowel serosa or mesentery to massive perforation or devascularization injuries requiring extensive resection.

Diagnosis of small-bowel injury can be made by a number of methods. Physical examination of the abdomen reveals peritoneal signs in many patients with penetrating small-bowel injuries. Patients with gunshot wounds routinely undergo laparotomy. Recently, some have advocated that all patients with penetrating abdominal trauma, including gunshot wounds, who do not exhibit signs of peritonitis or hemodynamic instability should undergo abdominal CT.[30] If CT is performed, free air or stranding is an indication for early laparotomy due to the likelihood of bowel injury. However, for abdominal gunshot wounds, most trauma surgeons continue to limit this approach to only very limited tangential or right upper quadrant trajectories.

In stable patients with abdominal stab wounds, local wound exploration may be able to identify a subset of patients without fascial violation who may be discharged from the emergency department. Patients with multiple stab wounds, tangential stab wounds, or indeterminate results of exploration will require further evaluation to identify intraperitoneal injury. Laparotomy for other anterior abdominal stab wounds that violate the abdominal wall fascia should be selective. One method is to use serial abdominal examinations, hematocrits, and leukocyte counts. If the patient shows increasing signs of intraperitoneal injury, abdominal exploration is performed. Another approach is DPL, with a variety of criteria for positivity in patients with anterior abdominal wounds, ranging from 1,000 RBCs/mL of lavage fluid up to the conventional 100,000 RBCs/mL used in patients with blunt trauma. Lastly, CT has been used to determine the track of the wound and potential peritoneal penetration with or without evidence of intestinal or other visceral injury.

Regardless of the approach taken for the preoperative diagnosis of penetrating injuries of the small intestine, the operative approach is the same. The abdomen should be explored through a standard midline incision, and initial attention should be directed toward bleeding from associated injuries or from the small bowel mesentery. Bleeding from the mesentery usually can be controlled with suture ligation or with a rapid running closure of the mesenteric rent. This closure does not need to constitute definitive repair, but, if indicated, it temporarily controls bleeding until definitive treatment is delineated. Care should be taken not to compromise the vascular integrity of the bowel by overzealous suturing of the mesentery.

After bleeding has been controlled, steps to prevent ongoing leakage of intestinal contents from the injured small bowel should be taken. This is done by rapid examination of the small intestine and by application of Babcock or Allis clamps, a temporizing running single-layer closure, or stapled control of the injured areas. Definitive repair or resection should not be done until the entire length of the intestine has been carefully examined because knowledge of the extent of injury is necessary for a logical and rational approach to operative management. It makes no sense, for example, to repair a segment of small intestine only to determine after further exploration that injuries to adjacent segments of the bowel dictate resection of an entire larger segment.

The entire length of the small intestine should be carefully examined, starting at the ligament of Treitz and moving sequentially, proximally to distally, to each successive loop. This should be done in a systematic manner and should include inspection of the small-bowel mesentery by fanning out the mesentery and examining each new loop. When a suspect area is seen along the mesenteric border of the intestine, the mesentery should be cleared away to allow adequate visualization. The small intestine has a good blood supply and easily tolerates this maneuver. Any blood or other debris found on the serosa of the bowel should be wiped away. Sometimes, such debris overlies an otherwise unsuspected area of injury. Compression of the intestine in areas of suspected injury may also demonstrate a leak that would otherwise be missed.

In theory, the number of holes found in the small intestine should add up to an even number because the number of entrance and exit wounds should be identical. This rule is sometimes violated in practice, however, because the intestine is extensively coiled in the peritoneal cavity and tangential wounds of the bowel are common. Rather than focusing on the number of holes in the bowel, attention should be directed to a close inspection of the entire length of the intestine. After all areas of injury have been identified, a decision about repair or resection is made. Areas of massive destruction of the bowel or the mesentery, with associated ischemia, should be treated with resection. If after débridement more than 40% to 50% of the circumference of the wall of the small intestine is missing, that segment also should be resected. Caution should be exercised in using stapled anastomoses in trauma patients if extensive bowel wall edema is present. With normal intestinal wall thickness, however, stapled anastomoses are particularly useful when time is of the essence and should be constructed in a side-to-side, functional end-to-end fashion.

Knife wounds to the small intestine are usually easy to manage and rarely require extensive débridement or resection. On rare occasions, a large rent in the small bowel mesentery results in enough devascularization to require resection of a segment of intestine.

Minor mesenteric lacerations should be treated with suture ligation of bleeding points and closure of the rent. Major lacerations with devascularization should be treated with resection and primary anastomosis. Small-bowel anastomoses, when properly done and after adequate débridement of devitalized tissue, have an excellent rate of healing even with severe associated injuries, shock, and peritonitis.

Shotgun wounds to the abdomen from close range are often associated with massive tissue destruction, which should be débrided and anastomosis completed as appropriate. Medium- or longer-range shotgun wounds sometimes result in a diffuse pattern of shot injury, creating multiple small perforations of the small intestine. In such instances, the general principles outlined should be followed and obvious areas of injury repaired. It is sometimes impossible to ensure closure of all the numerous areas of perforation, and planned repeat laparotomy may be required to rule out occult injuries.

On rare occasions, injuries to the small intestine occur in patients who are hemodynamically unstable as a result of associated injuries. In such instances, the small intestine can be treated most expeditiously by application of the gastrointestinal anastomosis stapler as necessary to remove the injured areas of bowel as a "damage control" technique. A second operation is planned and definitive anastomosis is deferred with the stapled ends of the intestine returned to the abdomen until the second procedure is performed.

6 **Blunt Injuries.** Blunt injuries to the small intestine are much less common than penetrating injuries. As with other blunt intra-abdominal injuries, they are more difficult to diagnose because the need for urgent intra-abdominal intervention is not always obvious. Blunt perforations and devascularizations of the small intestine often occur in isolation, either as the only injury or as the only intra-abdominal injury present. This makes early diagnosis even more difficult.[31]

Seatbelts, in particular high-riding lap belts in children, have been implicated in the pathogenesis of blunt injuries of the small intestine. The intestine or mesentery is sheared across the seatbelt to the point of rupture or disruption of its mesentery, resulting in either perforation or devascularization. Because of the severe degree of force necessary to produce a blunt intestinal injury, there is a frequent association with transverse fractures of a lumbar vertebral body (Chance fracture), caused by flexion or distraction over the seatbelt.

Abdominal examination is usually positive shortly after injury, but initial findings in some cases can be subtle, resulting in delays in diagnosis. The presence of a Chance fracture and a lower abdominal lap belt transverse contusion warrants a high index of suspicion and a thorough search for intestinal injury. If head injury or intoxication makes physical examination of the abdomen unreliable, the initial CT scan should be closely scrutinized for clues of intestinal injury. CT, particularly if done early after injury, is not completely reliable in ruling out blunt intestinal injury. The injury itself may not be obvious, and it is important to look for findings that may indicate blunt abdominal injury. This includes free fluid without solid organ injury, focal bowel wall thickening, free air, or extravasation of oral contrast (if used). Small amounts of intraperitoneal fluid should not be ignored. If the CT is scrutinized for all of these findings, then the sensitivity of CT is actually quite high. If these findings are present, the CT may be repeated in 4 to 6 hours to evaluate for progression of the injury.[32] A follow-up DPL can also be valuable if there are concerns about radiation or contrast. If the patient is fully evaluable and does not have any signs or symptoms of injury, these studies may be obviated for careful serial exams. If abdominal pain or tenderness is present, a follow-up study is prudent. Optimally, the intestinal injury should be identified within 6 to 8 hours. Intervention greater than 12 to 24 hours will have a substantial increase in morbidity and mortality. Blunt injuries to the small intestine are most common in either the proximal jejunum or the distal ileum, probably because the intestine is fixed at these two points and more vulnerable to shear and stretch injuries. Multiple injuries to the small intestine from blunt trauma occur in approximately 25% of cases. Second or even third areas of injury should be carefully sought if a blunt intestinal injury is discovered on abdominal exploration.

After the suspicion of blunt intestinal or other intra-abdominal injury has been raised and the decision to explore the abdomen has been made, the basic principles of abdominal exploration and operative management of blunt small-bowel injuries are the same as for penetrating injuries. Because of the nature of the mechanism of injury, the perforations are usually amenable to primary repair. Mesenteric rents that cause devascularization and require resection are relatively more common after blunt injury than after penetrating injury. The radiologic and physical findings associated with these types of injuries are initially more subtle, but become obvious after the devascularized bowel perforates. This may lead to a delay in laparotomy and definitive control.

Colon and Rectum

Most injuries to the colon and rectum are the result of penetrating or perforating trauma. Blunt trauma accounts for only approximately 5% of colonic injuries. Rectal injuries can occur in association with pelvic fractures and the possibility of rectal injury must be considered in any patient with a significant pelvic fracture, in addition to evaluation of other pelvic viscera such as the bladder, distal ureters, uterus, and vagina.

Signs and symptoms of peritonitis result from injury to the colon and rectum but are not specific. Injury to the extraperitoneal rectum is particularly difficult to recognize because peritonitis does not result. Conventional laboratory studies usually are not helpful. Plain radiographs may show free air in the peritoneal cavity, but this finding is relatively uncommon; when it is not present, the patient cannot be assumed to be free of bowel perforation. DPL may be of value if intraperitoneal colonic injury is present, yielding lavage fluid with blood, bacteria, or fecal material. If the injury is confined to the extraperitoneal colon and rectum, however, DPL is of no value. Extraperitoneal colonic or rectal injury is extremely difficult to diagnose. The possibility of rectal injury must be considered in any patient with penetrating trauma to the lower abdomen or buttocks. CT scan may be useful in delineating the trajectory of a bullet, and further workup can be selectively applied based on the proximity of the trajectory to the extraperitoneal rectum.[33] Digital rectal examination is essential. The presence of blood on examination is strong evidence for colon or rectal injury, and proctoscopic and sigmoidoscopic examinations should be performed. As blood may be the only finding indicating an injury, it is essential that the operating surgeon perform the sigmoidoscopy first so that less experienced endoscopists do not contaminate the field with procedure-induced blood. Water-soluble contrast studies also may be useful, but direct bowel examination usually is preferable. Approximately 95% of colon injuries are caused by gunshot, shotgun, or stab wounds, and, whenever the possibility of colonic injury is entertained, broad-spectrum intravenous

TABLE 23.5 MANAGEMENT

PRINCIPLES OF OPERATIVE MANAGEMENT OF COLON AND RECTAL INJURIES

Placement of the patient in the lithotomy position to provide simultaneous exposure of both the perineum and abdomen
Wide débridement of all dead and devitalized tissue
A totally defunctioning colostomy (simple loop colostomy may be inadequate)
Rectal wall closure, if the injury is easily accessible
Retrorectal drainage, primarily in severe injuries
Distal rectal stump washout if easily feasible
Broad-spectrum intravenous antibiotics, nutritional support, and serial débridement

prophylactic antibiotics should be started immediately and continued postoperatively using a standard protocol limiting their use to no more than 2 to 3 days.

The longstanding controversy between primary repair of low-risk colonic injuries and repair or resection with exteriorization has been largely resolved.[34] Primary repair is preferred after additional risk factors that increase the incidence of complications have been excluded, such as preoperative hypotension, intraperitoneal hemorrhage exceeding 1 L, more than two additional injured organs (hepatic, pancreatic, and splenic injuries have the highest morbidity rates), gross fecal spillage, or an elapsed time since injury of more than 6 hours. Many patients with penetrating colon injuries, however, can be treated with primary closure even in the presence of these risk factors. Resection and colostomy are an overly conservative approach, and recent series indicate that primary repair may be safe even in the presence of some risk factors.[35] Exteriorization of the repaired segment has also been advocated, but the success of this technique is low and has little benefit over diverting colostomy alone. Overall primary repair is indicated for most colon wounds, but each surgeon must decide in the context of the individual patient's risks. Postoperative complications include abscess formation, anastomotic leak, peristomal hernia, and the morbidity and mortality associated with colostomy closure.

The morbidity and mortality from rectal injuries is primarily a result of inadequate initial therapy and the complications associated with delayed sepsis. Rectal injury must be suspected in any penetrating injury that enters the buttocks or tracks into the true pelvis, or if a pelvic fracture produces a ring disruption or large displaced bone fragments. Sigmoidoscopic examination is essential. The principles of operative management of colon and rectal injuries are outlined in Table 23.5.

Complete rectal destruction is a rare injury for which primary abdominoperineal resection with packing may be necessary. If done, the packing should be removed operatively in approximately 48 hours. Complications of rectal injuries include pelvic abscesses, urinary or rectal fistulas, rectal incontinence and stricture, urinary incontinence, and loss of sexual function.

Retroperitoneal Hematoma

The optimal management of retroperitoneal hematoma depends on a number of factors, including its cause, its location, and the presence of associated injuries. The retroperitoneum can be divided into anatomic zones for purposes of decision making (Fig. 23.8 and Table 23.6). Retroperitoneal

7

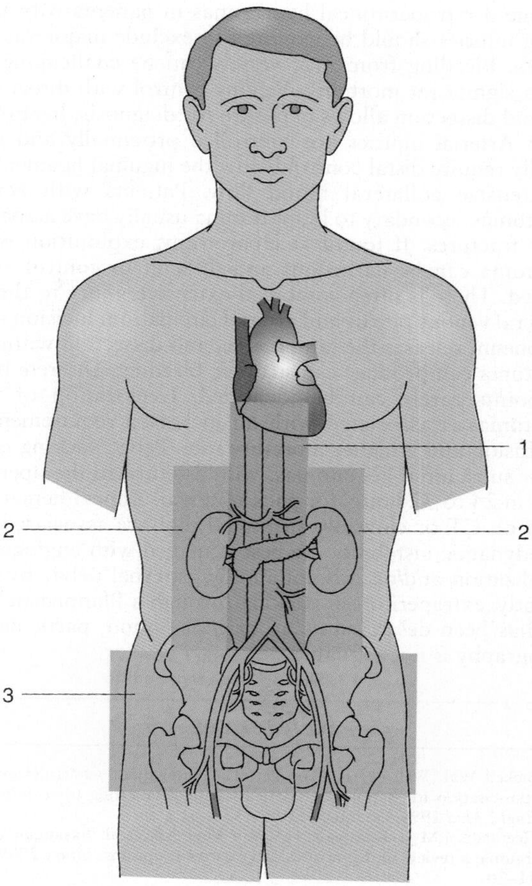

FIGURE 23.8. Zones of the retroperitoneum.

hematomas in zone 1, regardless of cause or size, are formally explored with inspection of each of the relevant structures. This is required because of the high incidence of associated major vascular, pancreatic, or duodenal injuries and the high morbidity and mortality rates if these are overlooked.

Zone 2 hematomas caused by penetrating injuries are routinely explored if encountered in the operating room. Whether proximal control of the renal pedicle should be obtained before exploration of a perinephric hematoma is controversial. In cases of severe ongoing hemorrhage, time should not be taken to obtain proximal control, and the kidney should be mobilized directly. If time and the degree of hemorrhage permit, however, it is acceptable to obtain vascular control before mobilization of the kidney. Zone 2 hematomas caused by blunt trauma can be left alone if they are not expanding.

TABLE 23.6

ZONES OF THE PERITONEUM

ZONE	LOCATION	ASSOCIATED INJURIES
1	Central retroperitoneum	Pancreaticoduodenal injuries or major abdominal vascular injury
2	Flank or perinephric area	Injuries to the genitourinary tract or to the colon (i.e., with penetrating trauma)
3	Pelvis	Pelvic fractures

TRAUMA

Zone 3 retroperitoneal hematomas in patients with penetrating injuries should be explored to exclude major vascular injuries. Bleeding from iliac vessels can be challenging and have a significant mortality. Venous control with direct pressure and dissection allows exposure for diagnosis, ligation, or repair. Arterial injuries are controlled proximally and occasionally require distal control below the inguinal ligament due to extensive collateral blood flow. Patients with zone 3 hematomas secondary to blunt trauma usually have associated pelvic fractures. If found at laparotomy, exploration of the hematoma can be hazardous and difficult to control and is avoided. There is often combined extensive injury to the rich presacral venous plexus and arterial circulation. Incision of the peritoneum releases the tamponade, and dissection within the hematoma can produce catastrophic bleeding. Discrete bleeding points rarely can be identified. Exploration of these hematomas is associated with an increased requirement for transfusion and a higher mortality rate. Pelvic packing is useful for substantial hematomas, with a return to the operating room in 24 to 72 hours for pack removal. Zone 3 hematomas found on CT or clinically suspected that are associated with hemodynamic instability are best managed with angiographic embolization and/or, less commonly, external pelvic fixation. Recently, extraperitoneal packing through a Pfannenstiel incision has been described as an exigent option, particularly if angiography is not available.[36]

References

1. Bickell WH, Wall MJ Jr, Pepe PE, et al. Immediate versus delayed fluid resuscitation for hypotensive patients with penetrating torso injuries. *N Engl J Med* 1994;331:1105–1109.
2. Geeraedts LM Jr, Kaasjager HA, van Vugt AB, et al. Exsanguination in trauma: a review of diagnostics and treatment options. *Injury* 2009;40(1): 11–20.
3. Malhotra AK, Fabian TC, Katsis SB, et al. Blunt bowel and mesenteric injuries: the role of screening computer tomography. *J Trauma* 2000;48: 991–1000.
4. Killeen KL, Shanmuganathan K, Poletti PA, et al. Helical computed tomography of bowel and mesenteric injuries. *J Trauma* 2001;51:26–36.
5. Villavicencio RT, Aucar JA. Analysis of laparoscopy in trauma. *J Am Coll Surg* 1999;189:11–20.
6. Moore E, Moore J, Van Duzer-Moore S, et al. Mandatory laparotomy for gunshot wounds penetrating the abdomen. *Am J Surg* 1980;140:847–851.
7. Rozycki GS, Ballard RB, Feliciano DV, et al. Surgeon-performed ultrasound for the assessment of truncal injuries: lessons learned from 1,540 patients. *Ann Surg* 1998;228:557–567.
8. McKenny MG, Martin L, Lentz K, et al. 1,000 Consecutive ultrasounds for blunt abdominal trauma. *J Trauma* 1996;40:607–612.
9. Branney SW, Moore EE, Cantrill SV, et al. Ultrasound based key clinical pathway reduces the use of hospital resources for the evaluation of blunt abdominal trauma. *J Trauma* 1997;42:1086–1090.
10. Shackford SR, Rogers FB, Osler TM, et al. Focused abdominal sonogram for trauma: the learning curve of nonradiologist clinicians in detecting hemoperitoneum. *J Trauma* 1999;46:553–564.
11. Wherrett LJ, Boulanger BR, McLellan BA, et al. Hypotension after blunt abdominal trauma: the role of emergent abdominal sonography in surgical triage. *J Trauma* 1996;41:815–820.
12. Luchette FA, Borzotta AP, Croce MA, et al. Practice management guidelines for prophylactic antibiotic use in penetrating abdominal trauma: the EAST Practice Management Guidelines Work Group. *J Trauma* 2000;48: 508–518.
13. Kirton OC, O'Neill PA, Kestner M, et al. Perioperative antibiotic use in high-risk penetrating hollow viscus injury: a prospective randomized, double-blind, placebo-control trial of 24 hours versus 5 days. *J Trauma* 2000;49: 822–832.
14. Rotondo MF, Schwab CW, McGonigal MD, et al. "Damage control": an approach for improved survival in exsanguinating penetrating abdominal injury. *J Trauma* 1993;35:375–382.
15. Suliburk JW, Ware DN, Balogh Z, et al. Vacuum-assisted wound closure achieves early fascial closure of open abdomens after severe trauma. *J Trauma* 2003;55:1155–1160.
16. Schurr MJ, Fabian TC, Gavant M, et al. Management of blunt splenic trauma: computed tomographic contrast blush predicts failure of nonoperative management. *J Trauma* 1995;39:507–512.
17. Thaemert BC, Cogbill TH, Lambert PJ. Nonoperative management of splenic injury: are follow-up computed tomographic scans of any value? *J Trauma* 1997;43:748–751.
18. Peitzman AB, Heil B, Rivera L, et al. Blunt splenic injury in adults: multi-institutional study of the Eastern Association for the Surgery of Trauma. *J Trauma* 2000;49:177–189.
19. Davidson RN, Wall RA. Prevention and management of infections in patients without a spleen. *Clin Microbiol Infect* 2001;7:657–660.
20. Croce MA, Fabian TC, Menke PG, et al. Nonoperative management of blunt hepatic trauma is the treatment of choice for hemodynamically stable patients: results of a prospective trial. *Ann Surg* 1995;221:744–753.
21. Demetriades D, Hadjizacharia P, Constantinou C, et al. Selective nonoperative management of penetrating abdominal solid organ injuries. *Ann Surg* 2006;244(4):620–628.
22. Brown CV, Kasotakis G, Wilcox A, et al. Does pelvic hematoma on admission computed tomography predict active bleeding at angiography for pelvic fracture? *Am Surg* 2005;71(9):759–762.
23. Polanco P, Leon S, Pineda J, et al. Hepatic resection in the management of complex injury to the liver. *J Trauma* 2008;65(6):1264–1269.
24. Scherer LA, Battistella FD, Owings JT, et al. Video-assisted thoracic surgery in the treatment of posttraumatic empyema. *Arch Surg* 1998;133: 637–642.
25. Levison MA, Peterson SR, Sheldon GF, et al. Duodenal trauma: experience of a trauma center. *J Trauma* 1984;24:475–480.
26. Wisner DH, Wold RL, Frey CF. Diagnosis and treatment of pancreatic injuries: an analysis of management principles. *Arch Surg* 1990;125: 1109–1113.
27. Patton JH, Lyden SP, Croce MA, et al. Pancreatic trauma: a simplified management guideline. *J Trauma* 1997;43:234–240.
28. Lucas CE. Diagnosis and treatment of pancreatic and duodenal injury. *Surg Clin North Am* 1977;57:49–65.
29. Fulcher AS, Turner, MA, Yelon JA, et al. Magnetic resonance cholangiopancreatography (MRCP) in the assessment of pancreatic duct trauma and its sequelae: preliminary findings. *J Trauma* 2000;48:1001–1007.
30. Shanmuganathan K, Mirvis SE, Chiu WC, et al. Penetrating torso trauma: triple-contrast helical CT in peritoneal violation and organ injury—a prospective study in 200 patients. *Radiology* 2004;231(3):775–784.
31. Wisner DH, Chun Y, Blaisdell FW. Blunt intestinal injury: keys to diagnosis and management. *Arch Surg* 1990;125:1319–1322.
32. Ekeh AP, Saxe J, Walusimbi M, et al. Diagnosis of blunt intestinal and mesenteric injury in the era of multidetector CT technology—are results better? *J Trauma* 2008;65(2):354–359.
33. Velmahos GC, Constantinou C, Tillou A, et al. Abdominal computed tomographic scan for patients with gunshot wounds to the abdomen selected for nonoperative management. *J Trauma* 2005;59(5):1155–1160.
34. Stone HH, Fabian TC. Management of perforating colon trauma: randomization between primary closure and exteriorization. *Ann Surg* 1979; 190:430–436.
35. Demetriades D, Murray JA, Chan L, et al.; Committee on Multicenter Clinical Trials. American Association for the Surgery of Trauma. Penetrating colon injuries requiring resection: diversion or primary anastomosis? An AAST prospective multicenter study. *J Trauma* 2001;50(5): 765–775.
36. Osborn PM, Smith WR, Moore EE, et al. Direct retroperitoneal pelvic packing versus pelvic angiography: a comparison of two management protocols for haemodynamically unstable pelvic fractures. *Injury* 2009;40(1): 54–60.

CHAPTER 24 ■ GENITOURINARY TRAUMA

THOMAS G. SMITH III AND HUNTER WESSELLS

KEY POINTS

1. Upper urinary tract injury is an infrequent result of trauma, and the majority of injuries result from blunt mechanisms.
2. Risk of renal injury requiring further evaluation is indicated by gross hematuria or microscopic hematuria with an episode of hypotension in adults or significant microscopic hematuria in children.
3. Most renal injuries are managed nonoperatively, with indications for exploration being symptomatic renal hemorrhage causing hypotension, expanding or pulsatile retroperitoneal hematoma at laparotomy, and grade V injury.
4. Ureteral injuries due to external violence are rare and require a heightened index of suspicion due to lack of consistent physical findings.
5. Injuries to the bladder require prompt diagnosis, with intraperitoneal injuries necessitating surgical repair.
6. Initial management of urethral injuries varies based on location (anterior vs. posterior) and severity, the most severe requiring urinary diversion with a suprapubic tube.
7. Primary open reconstruction of posterior urethral injuries secondary to pelvic fracture is discouraged, and primary endoscopic realignment should be undertaken only by a surgeon experienced with this technique.

The incidence of trauma is rising, and the World Health Organization estimates that without change or intervention, road traffic injuries will be the sixth leading cause of death by the year 2020 worldwide. Internal injuries were the fifth leading nonfatal injury noted, while pelvic fracture was the 12th, accounting for 6.3% and 2.6%, respectively, of all traffic injuries worldwide.[1] In the United States, abdominal organ injuries resulted in 6.3% of total injuries, while pelvic injuries resulted in 4.5%.[2] Based on current U.S. population data, approximately 15,000 persons will sustain renal injuries requiring hospital evaluation annually. Urethral and bladder injuries occur in approximately 10% to 15% of pelvic fractures, and the number of pelvic fractures in 2007 was greater than 67,000. Thus, in the United States, the number of bladder and urethral injuries sustained in 2007 can be estimated between 5,000 and 10,000 persons. While injuries to the genitourinary system as a whole are rarely life-threatening, the potential morbidity is quite high and the resultant effects on quality of life marked. Although few prospective randomized studies examining genitourinary trauma management exist, genitourinary injuries have reproducible clinical presentations, and imaging modalities have improved our ability to identify and treat these injuries. We review the fundamental principles guiding the evaluation and treatment of genitourinary trauma including the American Association for the Surgery of Trauma (AAST) organ injury scale (Table 24.1) and the Société Internationale D'Urologie (SIU) guidelines for management.

UPPER URINARY TRACT INJURY

Kidney

1 Injury to the upper urinary tract (kidney, ureter) is rare following trauma, with an incidence of renal injury of 4.89 per 100,000 persons.[3] Injury occurs in 1.14% to 3.25% of trauma patients, predominantly males aged 20 to 30 years.[4,5] Injuries are categorized as either blunt (81% to 95%) or penetrating (5% to 19%) trauma.[6] The majority of blunt traumatic injury is the result of motor vehicle collision (47% to 66%), with fall second (13% to 16%) and motor vehicle–pedestrian collision third (4% to 7%) in two large population-based studies.[3,7] Penetrating injury predominantly is due to firearms (15% to 18%) and stab wounds (6% to 10%).[8]

Anatomically, the kidneys lie in the retroperitoneum, protected by the ribcage, retroperitoneal fat, perirenal fat within Gerota capsule, and overlying viscera (right: liver, colon, duodenum, adrenal; left: spleen, colon, adrenal, pancreas). The collecting system begins within the kidney, forms the renal pelvis, and concentrically narrows at the ureteropelvic junction (UPJ) to become the ureter. The ureter then traverses the retroperitoneum inferiorly, protected by retroperitoneal fat and the psoas muscle. After crossing over the common iliac vessels, the ureter descends into the pelvis, coursing caudad to the base of the bladder and entering the trigone obliquely at the ureterovesical junction (UVJ).

Recognizing the factors that predispose to upper urinary tract injury facilitates early diagnosis and management, which is associated with improved outcomes (Algorithm 24.1). Hematuria is the most sensitive clinical sign of *renal* injury, yet
2 the degree does not predict injury severity. Our Harborview Medical Center guidelines for imaging of suspected blunt renal injury are consistent with the recent SIU Consensus Panel: in adults, gross hematuria or microhematuria (greater than 3 red blood cells [RBC]/high-powered field [hpf]) with a period of hypotension (systolic blood pressure [SBP] <90 mm Hg), and in children (younger than 15 years), greater than 50 RBC/hpf.[6] Contrast-enhanced computed tomography (CT) is the preferred imaging modality in stable patients, and the widespread use of CT provides accurate staging of upper urinary tract injuries using the AAST scale (Fig. 24.1).[6,9] The scan consists of early venous phase contrast-enhanced images detecting vascular blush, parenchymal integrity, retroperitoneal hematoma, and renal parenchymal perfusion. Delayed (10 minutes) imaging is essential for identifying collecting system injury (urinary extravasation, hydronephrosis) and ureteral continuity to the bladder. Conventional intravenous urography (IVU) with tomography, though inferior to CT, can be used for staging when CT is not available.[10,11] The ability of a single-shot urography to stage injuries is limited to an operative setting and should not be used for clinical staging. Focused abdominal ultrasound for trauma (FAST) remains investigational for

TABLE 24.1 **CLASSIFICATION**

AMERICAN ASSOCIATION FOR THE SURGERY OF TRAUMA (AAST) ORGAN INJURY SCALES FOR URINARY TRACT

INJURED STRUCTURE	AAST GRADE	CHARACTERISTICS OF INJURY
Kidney[a]	I	Contusion with microscopic or gross hematuria, urologic studies normal; nonexpanding subcapsular hematoma without parenchymal laceration
	II	Nonexpanding perirenal hematoma confined to renal retroperitoneum; laceration <1.0 cm parenchymal depth of renal cortex without urinary extravasation
	III	Laceration >1.0 cm parenchymal depth of renal cortex without collecting system rupture or urinary extravasation
	IV	Parenchymal laceration extending through renal cortex, medulla, and collecting system with urinary extravasation; injury to main renal artery or vein with contained hemorrhage
	V	Completely shattered kidney; avulsion of renal hilum that devascularizes kidney
Ureter[a]	I	Contusion or hematoma without devascularization
	II	<50% transection
	III	50% transection
	IV	Complete transection with <2 cm devascularization
	V	Avulsion with >2 cm devascularization
Bladder[b]	I	Contusion, intramural hematoma; partial-thickness laceration
	II	Extraperitoneal bladder wall laceration <2 cm
	III	Extraperitoneal bladder wall laceration >2 cm or intraperitoneal bladder wall laceration <2 cm
	IV	Intraperitoneal bladder wall laceration >2 cm
	V	Intraperitoneal or extraperitoneal bladder wall laceration extending into bladder neck or ureteral orifice (trigone)
Urethra	I	Contusion with blood at urethral meatus and normal urethrography
	II	Stretch injury with elongation of urethra, but without extravasation of urethrography contrast material
	III	Partial disruption with extravasation of urethrography contrast material at injury site with visualization in the bladder
	IV	Complete disruption with <2 cm urethral separation and extravasation of urethrography contrast material at injury site, without visualization in the bladder
	V	Complete transection with 2 cm urethral separation or extension into the prostate or vagina

[a]Advance one grade for bilateral injuries, up to grade III.
[b]Advance one grade for multiple injuries, up to grade III.
Adapted from Wessells H. Injuries to the urogenital tract. In Souba WW, Fink MP, Jurkovich GJ, et al., eds. *ACS Surgery*, 6th ed. New York: WebMD; 2002;10:3.

detecting urologic injury and is inferior to CT.[12,13] Renal arterial angiography is rarely used diagnostically but therapeutically is indicated to treat isolated, symptomatic (early or late) renal bleeding, arteriovenous fistula, or pseudoaneurysm using embolization.[14]

3 Most injuries can be managed nonoperatively.[3,15] Grade I and II injuries often require no further management. The bulk of blunt grade III and nonvascular grade IV injuries can be managed expectantly. Select penetrating injuries in hemodynamically stable patients can be managed on observation protocols as well.[16] The absolute indications for renal exploration include hemodynamic instability secondary to renal hemorrhage, expanding or pulsatile retroperitoneal hematoma at laparotomy, and pedicle avulsion. Furthermore, in patients undergoing laparotomy for concomitant intraperitoneal injuries, exploration should be considered for deep grade III or IV lacerations, with or without devitalized kidney fragments, because the incidence of complications from nonoperative management can potentially be reduced.[10,17] If renal exploration is contemplated or necessary, demonstration of contralateral renal function is important in the event ipsilateral nephrectomy is performed. In patients in whom immediate laparotomy is performed without preoperative imaging, an intraoperative single-shot urogram (kidneys, ureter, bladder [KUB] 10 minutes following intravenous injection of 2 mL/kg contrast) can provide this limited information.[11,18] Failure to demonstrate contrast excretion from the contralateral kidney may indicate a solitary kidney, hilar injury, hypoperfusion, or global renal insufficiency secondary to chronic renal disease. Exploration of a solitary kidney should be performed only when absolute indications exist.

The kidney and upper urinary tract are accessed through a midline abdominal incision. Using the inferior mesenteric vein (IMV) as a landmark, a posterior peritoneal window is created medial to the IMV overlying the aorta, which allows access, dissection, and control of the proximal renal vasculature.[19,20] Alternatively, mobilization of the right or left colon provides access to the renal hilum and direct rapid mobilization of the kidney.[21] If this method is employed, manual compression of the renal pedicle followed by vascular clamping may be required. Cooling is not routinely employed due to time constraints and potential for worsening hypothermia. After obtaining control of the renal artery and vein with vessel loops, the retroperitoneum is entered by mobilizing the colon (if not previously performed) and exposing the Gerota fascia, which is then opened, allowing one to dissect away the perinephric fat.

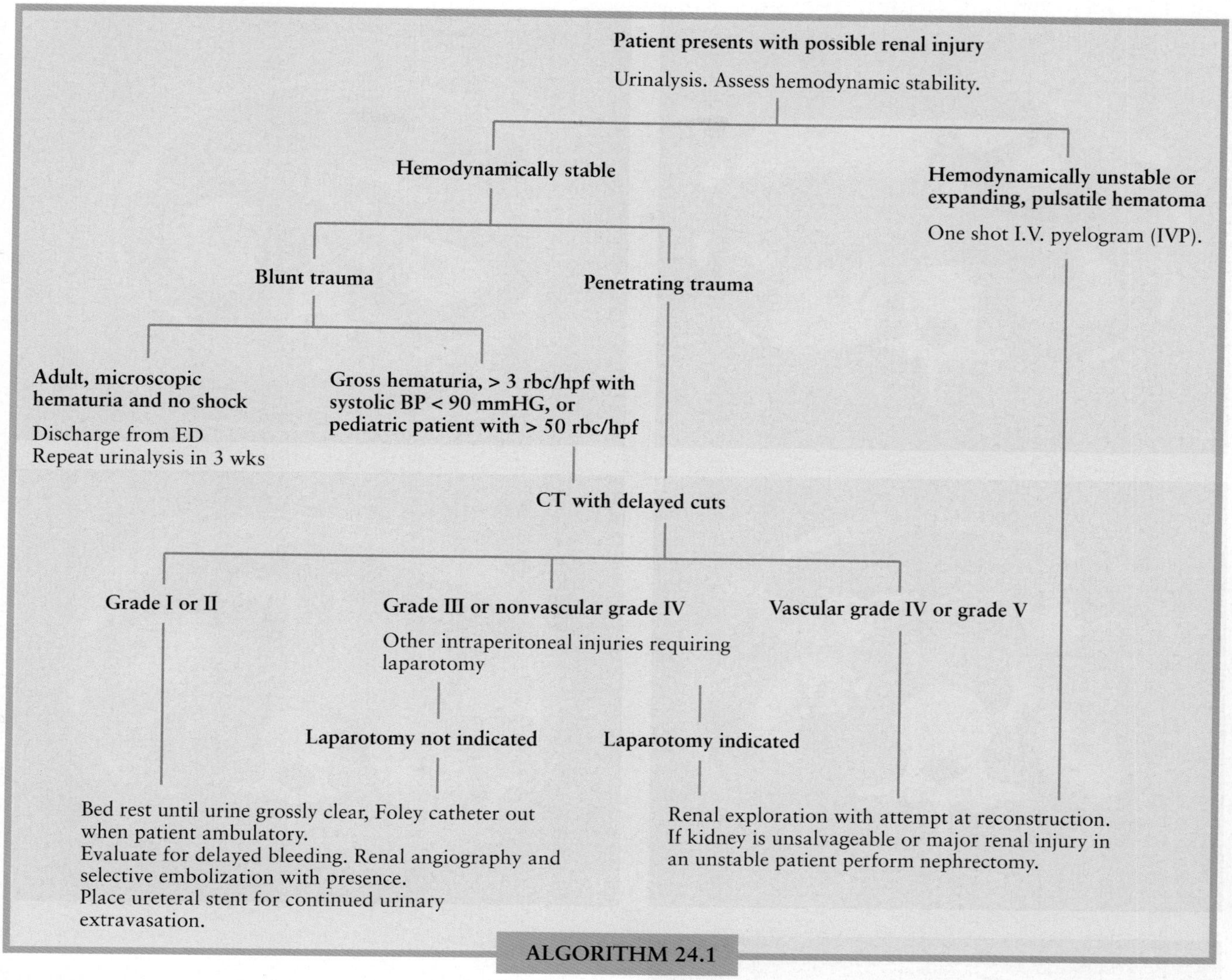
Patient presents with possible renal injury
Urinalysis. Assess hemodynamic stability.
Hemodynamically stable
Hemodynamically unstable or expanding, pulsatile hematoma
One shot I.V. pyelogram (IVP).
Blunt trauma
Penetrating trauma
Adult, microscopic hematuria and no shock
Discharge from ED
Repeat urinalysis in 3 wks
Gross hematuria, > 3 rbc/hpf with systolic BP < 90 mmHG, or pediatric patient with > 50 rbc/hpf
CT with delayed cuts
Grade I or II
Grade III or nonvascular grade IV
Other intraperitoneal injuries requiring laparotomy
Vascular grade IV or grade V
Laparotomy not indicated
Laparotomy indicated
Bed rest until urine grossly clear, Foley catheter out when patient ambulatory.
Evaluate for delayed bleeding. Renal angiography and selective embolization with presence.
Place ureteral stent for continued urinary extravasation.
Renal exploration with attempt at reconstruction.
If kidney is unsalvageable or major renal injury in an unstable patient perform nephrectomy.
ALGORITHM 24.1

ALGORITHM 24.1. Evaluation and management of suspected kidney injury.

The capsule of the kidney is routinely left intact for closure following renal reconstruction. During renal exploration, sharp débridement, hemostasis, collecting system repair, and pledgeted, bolstered closure of the renal capsule using absorbable suture is performed. A perinephric suction drain is placed away from the repair in the retroperitoneum and removed when drainage subsides, usually less than 50 mL/d. If concern exists regarding the nature of the drainage, an aliquot of fluid can be sent for creatinine concentration to evaluate for the presence of urine.

In the case of renal artery thrombosis, surgical revascularization is rarely helpful because of the time delay from injury to revascularization. Intervention is commonly limited to patients with solitary kidney or bilateral injuries.[22,23] An emerging therapy is vascular stent placement through the injury or thrombus; however, most series are limited and results mixed.[24] Venous injuries often result in massive bleeding and may require nephrectomy. Isolated proximal left renal vein injuries can potentially be managed by controlling and oversewing the caval stump because left renal vein collateral drainage is present via the gonadal, adrenal, and lumbar veins. Right renal venous injury requires repair, if feasible, or nephrectomy due to lack of collateral circulation.

Frequent clinical monitoring for ongoing bleeding is essential.[6] Postoperative complications of ileus, urinoma, atelectasis, and infection can occur. Secondary bleeding of nonoperatively managed and explored kidneys should be managed angiographically, because nephrectomy is likely with exploration. Late complications are uncommon and include renin-mediated hypertension from chronic renal ischemia, arteriovenous malformations, and segmental arteriolar pseudoaneurysm.

Ureter

4 Ureteral injuries are rare (1%), with fewer than 10 (due to external causes) presenting annually in busy trauma centers.[25] As these injuries often present without clear signs or symptoms, many are missed at the initial assessment and delayed diagnosis is common (Algorithm 24.2).[26] The most common source of injury to the ureter is iatrogenic during hysterectomy. These injuries occur with ligation of the infundibulopelvic ligament where the ureter crosses the uterine artery.[27] In the adult population, penetrating injuries, gunshot wounds followed distantly by stab wounds, are the most frequent source of injury associated with external violence.[28,29] A high degree of suspicion should accompany the evaluation of penetrating wounds and injury should be suspected when organs anatomically related to the ureter sustain injury: iliac vessels, bladder, sigmoid colon, and lumbar spine or transverse processes. Significant deceleration and hyperextension mechanisms can result in blunt avulsion as well. In children, the

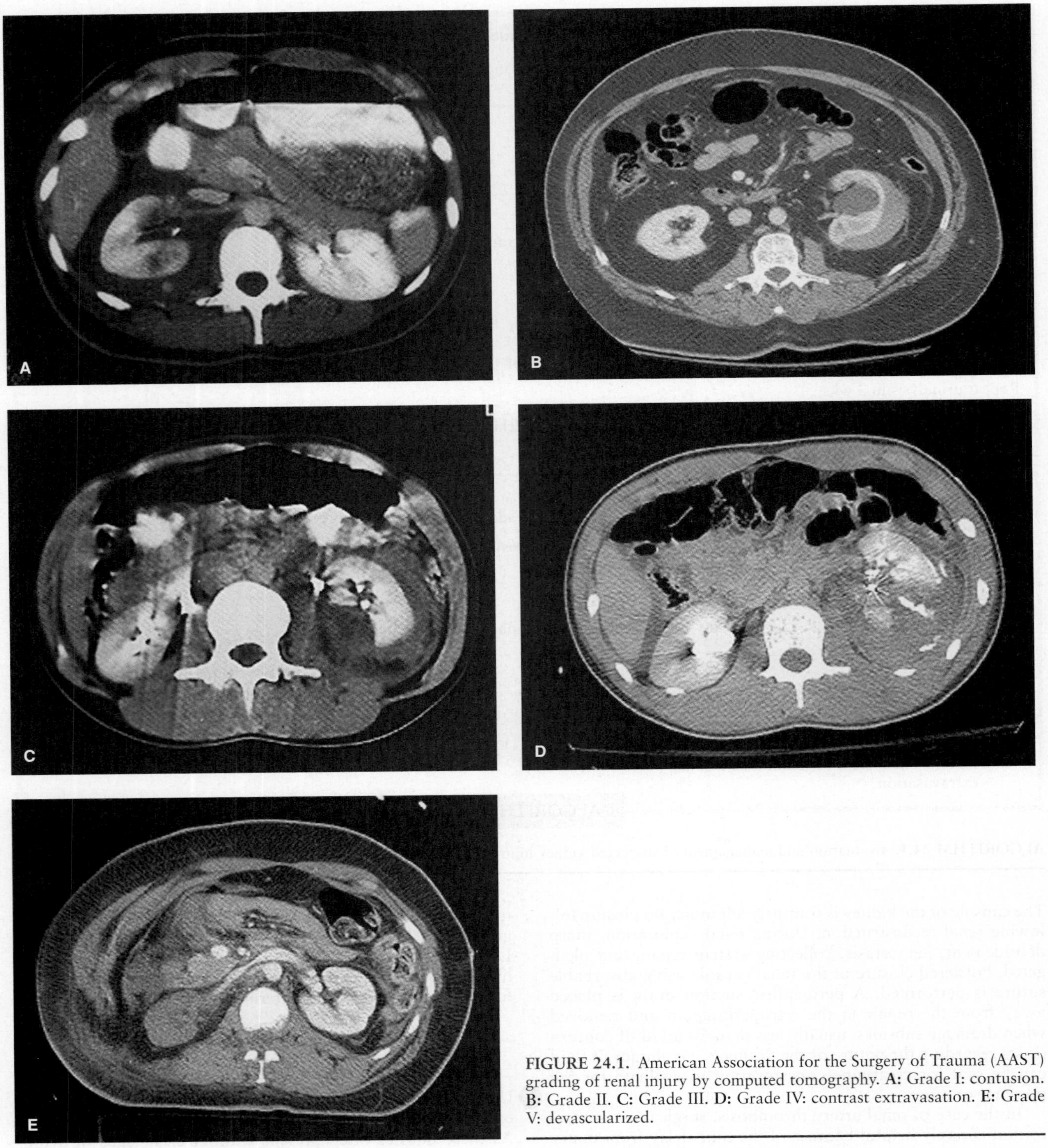

FIGURE 24.1. American Association for the Surgery of Trauma (AAST) grading of renal injury by computed tomography. **A:** Grade I: contusion. **B:** Grade II. **C:** Grade III. **D:** Grade IV: contrast extravasation. **E:** Grade V: devascularized.

injury occurs at the UPJ, resulting in avulsion of the ureter due to increased hyperextensibility of the spine.

Anatomically, the ureters begin posterior to the renal hilum at the UPJ. Subsequently, they course inferiorly through the retroperitoneum, along the anterior aspect of the psoas muscle. Upon entering the pelvis, the gonadal vessels run over the ureters, which subsequently traverse over the iliac vessels. Finally, the ureters continue caudally and enter the inferior aspect of the bladder obliquely. The blood supply is segmental and arises from the adjacent anatomic structures within the retroperitoneum and pelvis (proximal-lateral, mid-/true pelvis–medial, and inferior-posterolateral).

Often, patients with penetrating ureteral injuries undergo surgical exploration for associated injuries, allowing the ureter to be inspected directly.[30,31] Definitive reconstruction should be performed only if the patient is stable. When the defect is too long for primary repair or patients are hemodynamically unstable, damage control techniques for urinary diversion include débridement, drainage of the bladder and retroperitoneum, cutaneous ureterostomy diversion with a feeding tube, or ligation of the ureter with percutaneous nephrostomy tube placement. Complete débridement precedes ureter reconstruction, and the level and length of ureter dictate the type of repair (Fig. 24.2). UPJ disruptions require formal reconstruction by reanastomosis

Patient presents with possible ureteral injury

High index of suspicion: few physical signs and delayed presentation
Urinalysis. Assess hemodynamic stability

Patient is stable

CT w/ delayed cuts

Patient is unstable

One shot I.V. pyelogram (IVP) at laparotomy
Evaluate for periureteral hematoma.

Normal Studies

Observation

Abnormal Studies

Perform laparotomy

Delayed recognition, abscess or urinoma:
Percutaneous nephrostomy and abscess drainage
Ureteral stent if possible

Explore entire ureter and renal pelvis for location and type of injury
Repair injury over stent unless damage control

Percutaneous drains for post-op urinoma or abscess

ALGORITHM 24.2

ALGORITHM 24.2. Evaluation and management of suspected ureteral injury.

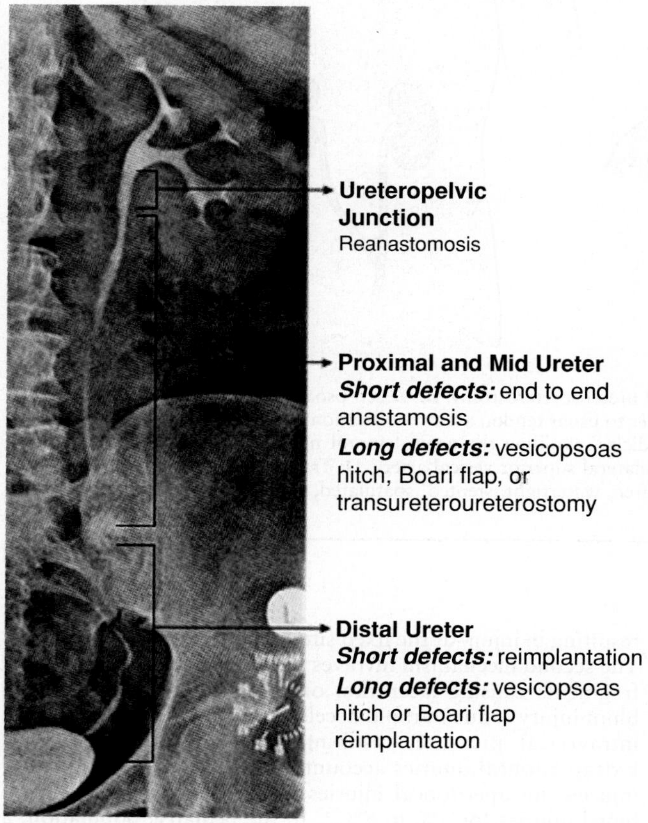

FIGURE 24.2. Ureteral reconstruction by location of injury.

or ureteropyelostomy. For ureteral injuries occurring in the proximal to midureter without associated renal injury, simple mobilization of the colon without hilar control can be used to gain access to the ureters. Short midureteric injuries are repaired by spatulated end-to-end anastomosis and low pelvic ureteric injuries are repaired by ureteroneocystostomy (Fig. 24.3). A nonrefluxing anastomosis is preferred in children, while a refluxing implant is acceptable in adults.

Patients presenting with a delay in diagnosis have symptoms of fever, flank pain, fullness, tenderness, atelectasis, or oliguria as a result of urinoma, hematoma, or abscess.[32] Operative intervention at the time of delayed diagnosis can result in nephrectomy. Therefore, management includes nephrostomy tube placement, percutaneous urinoma drainage, and Foley catheter insertion. Stent placement across an injury is delayed for 1 to 2 weeks and reconstruction is planned at 3 to 6 months to allow for resolution of periureteral inflammation. Long-term complications of unrecognized ureteral injury include fistula, fluid collections, ureteral stricture, and obstructive uropathy.

All individuals who have sustained injury to the upper urinary tract require follow-up, consisting of imaging in the form of radionuclide scanning or IVU at 3 and 12 months to evaluate for hydronephrosis and document parenchymal function.[33] Interval ultrasound to evaluate for urinoma or abscess is an acceptable imaging modality and limits radiation exposure.

LOWER URINARY TRACT INJURY

Bladder

5 Injury to the bladder is rare, occurring in 1% to 2% of trauma patients most commonly secondary to blunt trauma.[34]

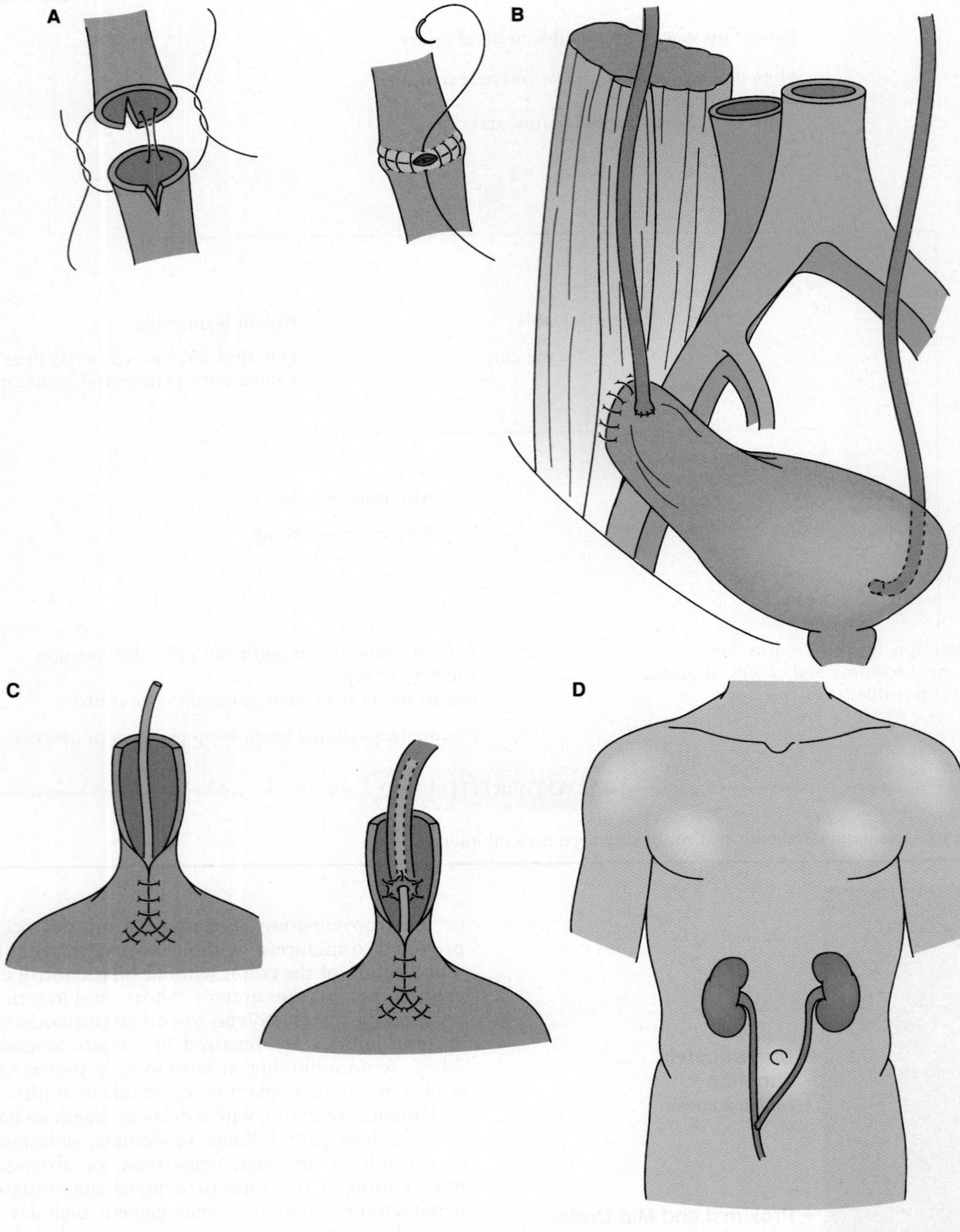

FIGURE 24.3. Techniques of ureteral repair. A: End-to-end ureteroureterostomy. B: Vesico-psoas hitch reconstruction with reimplantation performed by suturing of the bladder to psoas tendon after mobilization of both obliterated umbilical, plus or minus contralateral superior vesical, pedicles, avoiding the genitofemoral nerve. C: Boari flap performed using a tubularized bladder flap based on the ipsilateral superior vesical artery. D: Transureteroureterostomy (TUU). For all repairs the principles include tension-free, watertight, stented, spatulated, mucosa-to-mucosa anastomosis using absorbable suture with drain placement.

Penetrating trauma accounts for 0% to 45% of bladder trauma and blunt trauma accounts for the remainder.[35] Pelvic fractures are frequently associated with lower urinary tract injuries. An associated pelvic fracture is present in nearly 90% of cases, though only 5% to 10% of pelvic fractures result in bladder injury.[36] In pelvic fracture two mechanisms predominate as causes of bladder injury, usually resulting in extraperitoneal rupture. The first involves shearing forces at deceleration resulting in injury at the fixed sites of pelvic fascial attachment. The second mechanism involves direct injury from pelvic bone fragments causing laceration of the bladder. Intraperitoneal blunt injury is due to rapid deceleration creating a rapid rise in intravesical pressure, resulting in a "burst"-type injury. Extraperitoneal injuries account for 54% to 55% of bladder injuries, intraperitoneal injuries for 38% to 40%, and combined injuries for 5% to 8%.[37] In the pediatric population, a larger proportion of injuries are intraperitoneal because of the relative intra-abdominal location of the bladder. However, the overall incidence is lower. The incidence of pelvic fracture is also lower in children, but, in contradistinction to adults, bladder neck injuries are more common in boys with a pelvic crush injury rather than urethral injuries as seen in adults.[38]

Gross hematuria is a reliable sign of bladder injury, occurring in 95% of patients, and in the setting of blunt or penetrating trauma should prompt evaluation using cystography, urethrography, or both.[39,40] Acutely, patients presenting with bladder injury may complain of inability to void or suprapubic pain, though these symptoms may be masked by pain from more significant injuries.[35] With delayed presentation, frequent symptoms are abdominal distention, ileus, fever, or urinary ascites as a result of persistent leakage, pelvic urinoma, or abscess formation. If concomitant bladder neck injury occurs, voiding dysfunction may be present as well. Laboratory analysis demonstrates acidosis, hyperkalemia, hyperchloremia, hypernatremia, and uremia with intraperitoneal bladder injuries because of the frequency of these injuries with pelvic fracture. Particular attention is paid to thorough evaluation of the lower urinary tract for concurrent injury. Penetrating and iatrogenic trauma to the pelvis or perineum generally results in associated visceral, urethral, or genital injuries, but without bony disruption.[41]

Imaging of the bladder, if indicated, consists of cystography, and is performed in the clinically stable patient. Harborview Medical Center criteria for bladder imaging after blunt trauma include pelvic ring fracture with greater than 30 RBC/hpf or gross hematuria; an additional indication is the presence of a free intraperitoneal low-density fluid collection within the first 24 hours postinjury. Isolated acetabular fractures without pelvic ring involvement do not need cystography without other indications. CT cystography is used more liberally because of the central role of CT scanning in trauma assessment.[42] For CT cystography, the bladder is filled retrograde with contrast and the scan is performed after 300 to 400 mL of contrast is instilled. Static cystography (consisting of a scout pelvic image and a second image with 300 to 400 mL of contrast instilled in the bladder) remains an acceptable means of assessing for bladder rupture. Postdrainage films are essential for static cystography, and oblique images may identify posterior defects.[37] Extraperitoneal contrast extravasation is confined to the pelvis on CT and appears as a "flame-shaped" opacity on static cystography (Fig. 24.4). Characteristic patterns of intraperitoneal contrast extravasation include pooling

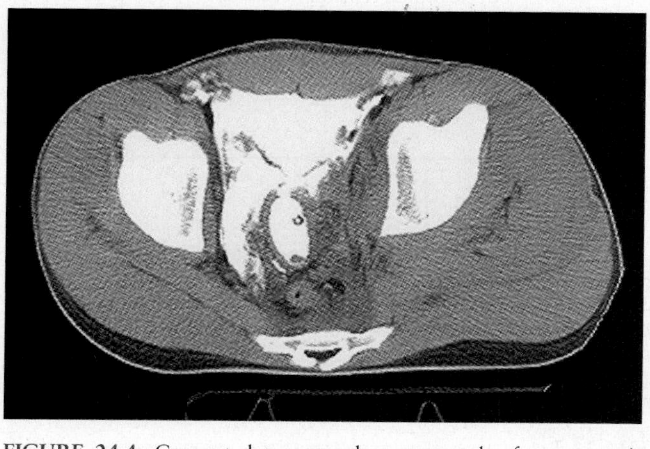

FIGURE 24.4. Computed tomography cystography for extraperitoneal bladder injury.

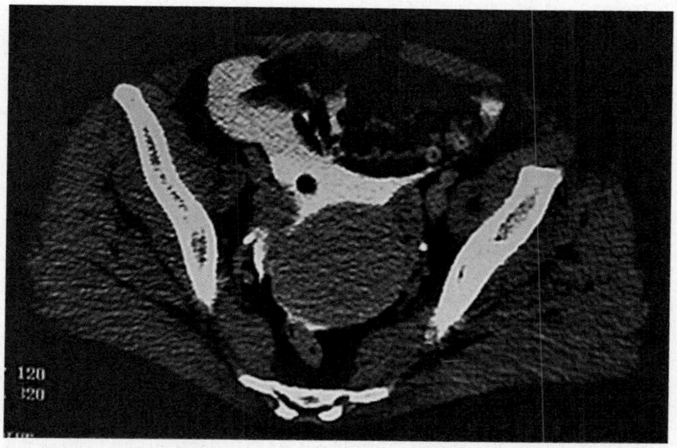

FIGURE 24.5. Computed tomography cystography for intraperitoneal bladder injury.

in the cul-de-sac, paracolic gutter, or retrohepatic space on CT or outlining of bowel loops on static cystography (Fig. 24.5).

Most extraperitoneal bladder injuries can be managed conservatively with catheter drainage. Indications for repair of bladder injury are intraperitoneal bladder injury; exploratory laparotomy for concomitant injuries; penetrating bladder trauma; extraperitoneal bladder injuries with concomitant vaginal, rectal, bladder neck injury, foreign body, or bony spicules protruding into the bladder lumen; and open reduction internal fixation (ORIF) for pelvic fractures (in an effort to reduce secondary contamination of orthopedic hardware). Delayed exploration, reconstruction, or drainage may be required to remedy problems that fail to resolve with conservative measures or are diagnosed in a delayed fashion. During exploration and repair, when possible, avoid disruption of a pelvic hematoma, which may cause significant hemorrhage. The ureteral orifices and bladder wall are inspected through an anterior cystotomy or the laceration/injury itself. Sites of injury within the bladder lumen are repaired with 3–0 interrupted full-thickness synthetic absorbable suture, while the cystotomy, external injuries, or perforations are closed with a two-layer running fashion using 2–0 synthetic absorbable suture. Foley drainage alone is adequate in most cases. Suprapubic catheter diversion using a Malecot catheter (22 to 24 French) is used when irrigation for heavy bleeding is required.[43] Closed suction drains are placed away from the site of repair and can be removed in 48 hours unless the drainage fluid demonstrates a creatinine level higher than serum. The urethral Foley catheter is usually left in place for 7 to 10 days and removed following cystogram demonstrating a healed, watertight repair.

Urethra

The anatomy of the urethra varies throughout its course and is divided for practical purposes into the anterior and posterior segments (Fig. 24.6). The mechanism of injury varies depending on the segment, but most commonly is due to blunt mechanisms. Anterior urethral injuries are the result of straddle-type falls or blows to the perineum. Posterior urethral injuries are often associated with pelvic fracture and involve varying degrees of prostatomembranous distraction.[44] Female urethral injuries are uncommon, 0% to 6%, and are usually associated with pelvic fracture and resultant laceration by bony fragments.[45] Gross blood at the urethral meatus in males is the most reliable sign and warrants evaluation for injury. Females

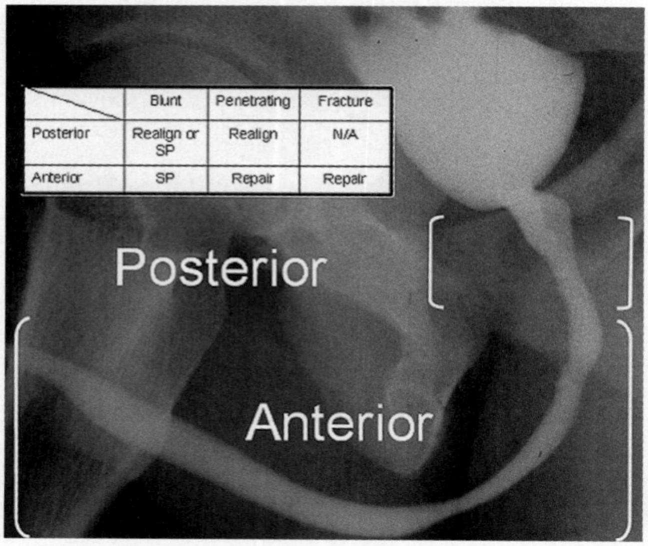

Blunt
Penetrating
Fracture
Posterior
Realign or SP
Realign
N/A
Anterior
SP
Repair
Repair
Posterior
Anterior

FIGURE 24.6. Normal retrograde urethrogram and management by segment and mechanism of injury.

with vaginal bleeding and pelvic fracture should be evaluated for gynecologic as well as urethral injuries. Further examination includes digital rectal examination evaluating for hematoma, bony spicules, Hemoccult blood, or a "high-riding prostate." These findings on examination and the presence of perineal ecchymosis or scrotal hematoma suggest anterior pelvic disruption and urethral injury (Algorithm 24.3).

When gross blood is present at the urethral meatus, retrograde urethrography (RUG) is indicated before catheterization.[46,47] RUG is readily performed using portable fluoroscopy in the emergency department or operating room. The fossa navicularis is occluded with the partially filled (2- to 3-mL) balloon tip of the catheter, the penis is stretched, and contrast is gently injected, opacifying the urethra. Oblique images are taken, when possible, to establish the absence of or the presence and location of extravasation, which is indicative of injury. If no extravasation is present, the catheter is advanced into the bladder. Failure to recognize these types of injuries can result in conversion of a partial injury to a complete injury if 6 blind catheter placement is performed.[36] Early management of most posterior urethral injuries involves urinary diversion with a suprapubic catheter. Grades I and II urethral injuries can be managed without a catheter provided the patient can void. Partial anterior injuries are managed with a urethral catheter alone, and a pericatheter urethrogram is done at 7 to 10 days to confirm healing before its removal. Whereas primary débridement and closure with diversion are advocated

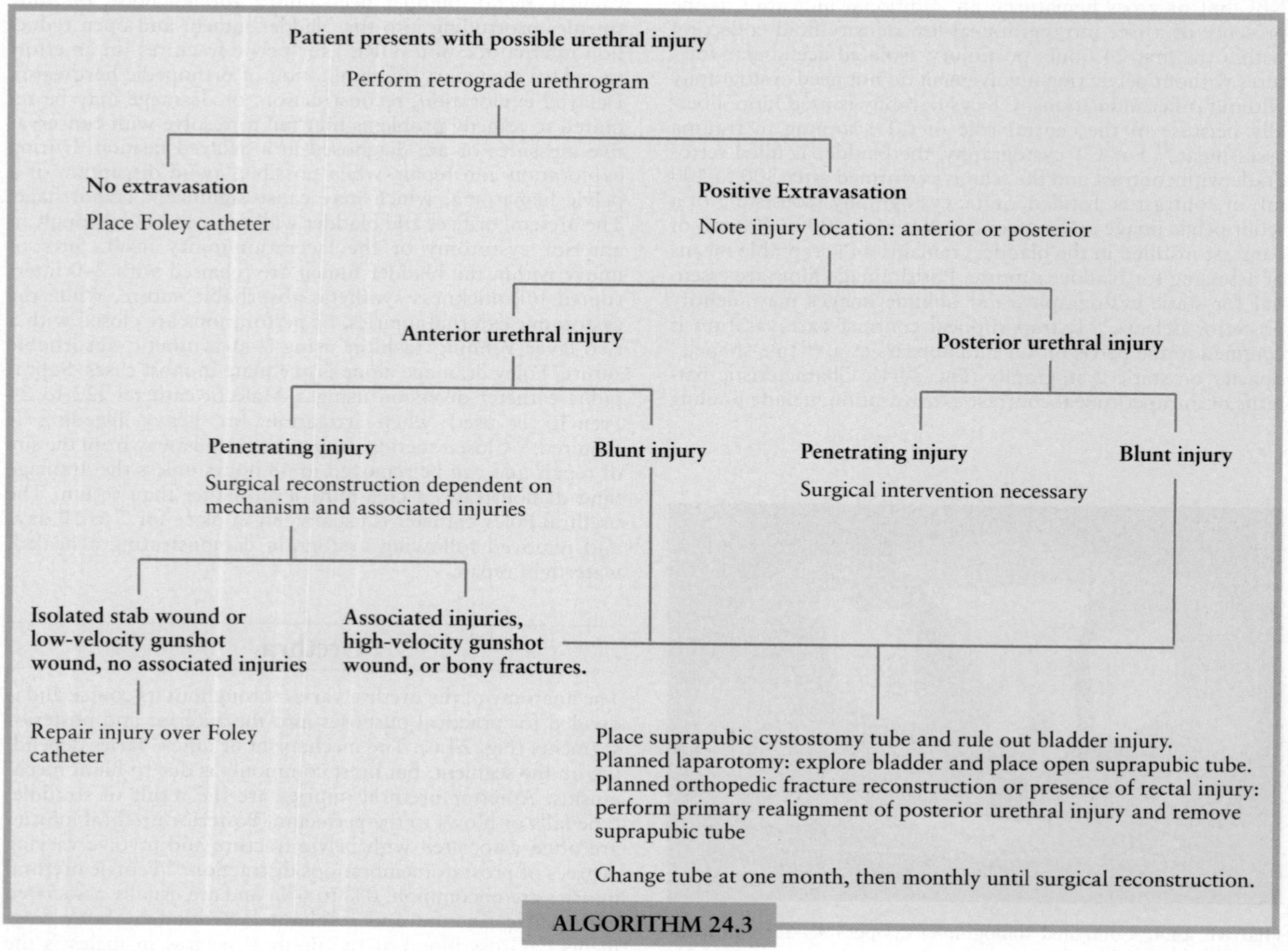

Planned laparotomy: explore bladder and place open suprapubic tube.

Change tube at one month, then monthly until surgical reconstruction.

ALGORITHM 24.3. Evaluation and management of suspected urethral injury.

for anterior stab wounds or low-velocity gunshot wounds, high-velocity injuries should be managed with a suprapubic catheter and delayed reconstruction.[48] Most posterior injuries can be managed with urinary diversion and delayed (3 to 6 months) reconstruction following resorption of the pelvic
7 hematoma. Aggressive early operative reconstruction is discouraged, although endoscopic techniques of primary realignment show promise in potentially decreasing rates of stricture formation while providing equivalent results with regard to continence and erectile dysfunction.[49] Early realignment is achieved employing endoscopes and fluoroscopy, then placing a catheter, by Seldinger technique, over a guidewire.[50] This has become a more commonplace method of initial urethral repair at high-volume trauma centers. Whether a patient receives a suprapubic cystostomy tube or a urethral Foley catheter as drainage, an appropriate plan of follow-up for tube changes, removals, and definitive reconstructive efforts is imperative, due to potential morbidities including infection, encrustation, hematuria, and obstructive uropathy. When definitive reconstruction is planned, antegrade voiding cystourethrography and retrograde urethrography are performed.

References

1. Peden M, Scurfield R, Sleet D, et al. *World Report on Road Traffic Injury Prevention.* Geneva, Switzerland: World Health Organization; 2004.
2. Clarke DE, Fantus RJ, eds. *National Trauma Data Bank Annual Report.* Chicago: American College of Surgeons; 2007.
3. Wessells H, Suh D, Porter JR, et al. Renal injury and operative management in the United States: results of a population-based study. *J Trauma* 2003;54(3):423–430.
4. Krieger JN, et al. Urological trauma in the Pacific Northwest: etiology, distribution, management and outcome. *J Urol* 1984;132(1):70–73.
5. Baverstock R, Simons R, McLoughlin M. Severe blunt renal trauma: a 7-year retrospective review from a provincial trauma centre. *Can J Urol* 2001;8(5):1372–1376.
6. Santucci RA, et al. Evaluation and management of renal injuries: consensus statement of the renal trauma subcommittee. *BJU Int* 2004;93(7):937–954.
7. Wright JL, et al. Renal and extrarenal predictors of nephrectomy from the National Trauma Data Bank. *J Urol* 2006;175(3 Pt 1):970–975; discussion 975.
8. Shariat SF, et al. Evidence-based validation of the predictive value of the American Association for the Surgery of Trauma kidney injury scale. *J Trauma* 2007;62(4):933–939.
9. McAndrew JD, Corriere JN Jr. Radiographic evaluation of renal trauma: evaluation of 1103 consecutive patients. *Br J Urol* 1994;73(4):352–354.
10. Corriere JN Jr, McAndrew JD, Benson GS. Intraoperative decision-making in renal trauma surgery. *J Trauma* 1991;31(10):1390–1392.
11. Morey AF, et al. Single shot intraoperative excretory urography for the immediate evaluation of renal trauma. *J Urol* 1999;161(4):1088–1092.
12. McGahan JP, et al. Use of ultrasonography in the patient with acute renal trauma. *J Ultrasound Med* 1999;18(3):207–213; quiz 215–216.
13. Perry MJ, Porte ME, Urwin GH. Limitations of ultrasound evaluation in acute closed renal trauma. *J R Coll Surg Edinb* 1997;42(6):420–422.
14. Hagiwara A, et al. The role of interventional radiology in the management of blunt renal injury: a practical protocol. *J Trauma* 2001;51(3):526–531.
15. Hammer CC, Santucci RA. Effect of an institutional policy of nonoperative treatment of grades I to IV renal injuries. *J Urol* 2003;169(5):1751–1753.
16. Wessells H, et al. Criteria for nonoperative treatment of significant penetrating renal lacerations. *J Urol* 1997;157(1):24–27.
17. Husmann DA, et al. Major renal lacerations with a devitalized fragment following blunt abdominal trauma: a comparison between nonoperative (expectant) versus surgical management. *J Urol* 1993;150(6):1774–1777.
18. Stevenson J, Battistella FD. The 'one-shot' intravenous pyelogram: is it indicated in unstable trauma patients before celiotomy? *J Trauma* 1994;36(6):828–833; discussion 833–834.
19. Carroll PR, Klosterman P, McAninch JW. Early vascular control for renal trauma: a critical review. *J Urol* 1989;141(4):826–829.
20. McAninch JW, Carroll PR. Renal trauma: kidney preservation through improved vascular control-a refined approach. *J Trauma* 1982;22(4):285–290.
21. Gonzalez RP, et al. Surgical management of renal trauma: is vascular control necessary? *J Trauma* 1999;47(6):1039–1042; discussion 1042–1044.
22. Haas CA, et al. Traumatic renal artery occlusion: a 15-year review. *J Trauma* 1998;45(3):557–561.
23. Carroll PR, et al. Renovascular trauma: risk assessment, surgical management, and outcome. *J Trauma* 1990;30(5):547–552; discussion 553–554.
24. Breyer BN, et al. Endovascular management of trauma related renal artery thrombosis. *J Trauma* 2008;64(4):1123–1125.
25. Brandes S, et al. Diagnosis and management of ureteric injury: an evidence-based analysis. *BJU Int* 2004;94(3):277–289.
26. Boone TB, Gilling PJ, Husmann DA. Ureteropelvic junction disruption following blunt abdominal trauma. *J Urol* 1993;150(1):33–36.
27. St Lezin MA, Stoller ML. Surgical ureteral injuries. *Urology* 1991;38(6):497–506.
28. Elliott SP, McAninch JW. Ureteral injuries from external violence: the 25-year experience at San Francisco General Hospital. *J Urol* 2003;170(4 Pt 1):1213–1216.
29. Perez-Brayfield MR, et al. Gunshot wounds to the ureter: a 40-year experience at Grady Memorial Hospital. *J Urol* 2001;166(1):119–121.
30. Palmer LS, et al. Penetrating ureteral trauma at an urban trauma center: 10-year experience. *Urology* 1999;54(1):34–36.
31. Velmahos GC, Degiannis E. The management of urinary tract injuries after gunshot wounds of the anterior and posterior abdomen. *Injury* 1997;28(8):535–538.
32. Ghali AM, et al. Ureteric injuries: diagnosis, management, and outcome. *J Trauma* 1999;46(1):150–158.
33. Knudson MM, et al. Outcome after major renovascular injuries: a Western trauma association multicenter report. *J Trauma* 2000;49(6):1116–1122.
34. Corriere JN Jr, Sandler CM. Management of the ruptured bladder: seven years of experience with 111 cases. *J Trauma* 1986;26(9):830–833.
35. Gomez RG, et al. Consensus statement on bladder injuries. *BJU Int* 2004;94(1):27–32.
36. Brandes S, Borrelli J Jr. Pelvic fracture and associated urologic injuries. *World J Surg* 2001;25(12):1578–1587.
37. Corriere JN Jr, Sandler CM. Diagnosis and management of bladder injuries. *Urol Clin North Am* 2006;33(1):67–71.
38. Tarman GJ, et al. Lower genitourinary injury and pelvic fractures in pediatric patients. *Urology* 2002;59(1):123–126; discussion 126.
39. Morey AF, et al. Bladder rupture after blunt trauma: guidelines for diagnostic imaging. *J Trauma* 2001;51(4):683–686.
40. Iverson AJ, Morey AF. Radiographic evaluation of suspected bladder rupture following blunt trauma: critical review. *World J Surg* 2001;25(12):1588–1591.
41. Franko ER, Ivatury RR, Schwalb DM. Combined penetrating rectal and genitourinary injuries: a challenge in management. *J Trauma* 1993;34(3):347–353.
42. Deck AJ, et al. Computerized tomography cystography for the diagnosis of traumatic bladder rupture. *J Urol* 2000;164(1):43–46.
43. Parry NG, et al. Traumatic rupture of the urinary bladder: is the suprapubic tube necessary? *J Trauma* 2003;54(3):431–436.
44. Basta AM, Blackmore CC, Wessells H. Predicting urethral injury from pelvic fracture patterns in male patients with blunt trauma. *J Urol* 2007;177(2):571–575.
45. Black PC, et al. Urethral and bladder neck injury associated with pelvic fracture in 25 female patients. *J Urol* 2006;175(6):2140–2144; discussion 2144.
46. Chapple C, et al. Consensus statement on urethral trauma. *BJU Int* 2004;93(9):1195–1202.
47. Palmer JK, Benson GS, Corriere JN Jr. Diagnosis and initial management of urological injuries associated with 200 consecutive pelvic fractures. *J Urol* 1983;130(4):712–714.
48. Husmann DA, Boone TB, Wilson WT. Management of low velocity gunshot wounds to the anterior urethra: the role of primary repair versus urinary diversion alone. *J Urol* 1993;150(1):70–72.
49. Mouraviev VB, Coburn M, Santucci RA. The treatment of posterior urethral disruption associated with pelvic fractures: comparative experience of early realignment versus delayed urethroplasty. *J Urol* 2005;173(3):873–876.
50. Brandes S. Initial management of anterior and posterior urethral injuries. *Urol Clin North Am* 2006;33(1):87–95.

CHAPTER 25 ■ VASCULAR TRAUMA

BENJAMIN W. STARNES

KEY POINTS

1. The overwhelming majority of vascular injuries can be diagnosed with a thorough history and physical examination and a high clinical index of suspicion.
2. Contrast arteriography is the traditional "gold standard" for diagnosing vascular injury, whereas computed tomography angiography can be rapidly obtained, provides more information about other injuries, and is less invasive with fewer complications.
3. Threat to life or limb from active hemorrhage is self-evident.
4. The management of injured extremities is superseded by the management of the overall patient: "life over limb." Limb salvage is a treatment modality not to be taken lightly or as a mandatory preference.
5. The guiding principle for the management of vascular injuries is proximal and distal control of the injured vessel.
6. The ascending aorta and innominate and right subclavian arteries are best approached by median sternotomy. The proximal left subclavian artery and descending thoracic aorta are best approached via left thoracotomy.
7. Left colon mobilization is useful for exposure of the paravisceral aorta, left renal artery, infrarenal aorta, and left iliac artery. Similarly, the inferior vena cava, right renal artery, infrarenal aorta, and right iliac artery can be approached by an extensive Kocher maneuver and mobilization of the right colon.
8. Endovascular repair of traumatic thoracic aortic disruption is associated with lower mortality and lower rates of paraplegia than traditional open repair.

A large body of literature currently exists regarding the management of traumatic vascular injuries with traditional open surgical techniques. Likewise, there is an evolving literature on the management of vascular trauma with endovascular techniques. Over the past several decades, catheter-based and endovascular techniques have been used with increasing frequency for the management of trauma. This is particularly true for the management of solid organ injury and vascular injuries resulting from pelvic fracture. The endovascular management of vascular trauma seems particularly appealing in the management of blunt truncal injuries, especially in the setting of severe concomitant brain and lung injury. Extremity and neck injuries are currently best handled by traditional methods of surgical proximal and distal control, the exception to this being base-of-skull injuries where there is no ability for distal vessel control and "watershed" areas between the trunk and extremities where surgical management for the unfamiliar surgeon can be quite difficult. This chapter reviews current literature with regard to broad principles of both open and endovascular management of traumatic vascular injuries with regions being broadly defined as neck, trunk, and extremity.

EPIDEMIOLOGY OF VASCULAR INJURY: DISTRIBUTION OF INJURIES

Trauma is the leading cause of death in persons under the age of 45 and consumes an enormous amount of health care dollars in terms of acute and long-term care. Vascular injury in particular is highly morbid and can lead to rapid exsanguination under certain circumstances. In a review of 5,760 cardiovascular injuries sustained by 4,459 patients, Mattox et al. described the predominantly young male population presenting with a majority (90%) of penetrating injury.[1] Truncal (including neck) vascular injuries predominated at 66%, with lower extremity regions representing only 19% of all vascular injuries. The mechanism of vascular injury varies, with most being caused by high- or low-velocity weapons (70% to 80%) (Fig. 25.1). This is followed by stab wounds (10% to 15%) and blunt trauma (5% to 10%).[1]

PHYSIOLOGIC CONSEQUENCE OF VASCULAR INJURY

The principal physiologic consequence of vascular injury results from either profound hemorrhage with associated metabolic consequences of total body ischemia or end-organ ischemia of the vascular bed fed by the injured vessel. Factors affecting ischemic tolerance include the nature of injury (complete vs. incomplete disruption), adequacy of collateral blood flow, underlying metabolic state, associated injuries, sensitivity of the end organ to ischemia, and the time required to repair the injury. The brain is the most sensitive tissue to ischemia due to the high basal energy requirements and the absence of robust glycogen stores. Warm brain ischemia lasting longer than 6 minutes results in irreversible injury. Other than bone, skeletal muscle is probably most resistant to ischemia. Peripheral nerves and muscle can tolerate up to 6 hours of ischemia without permanent damage.

Tissue ischemia causes anoxic cell death. Restoration of oxygen-rich blood flow after ischemic injury produces a reperfusion injury mediated by oxygen-free radicals.[2] These oxygen-free radicals initiate multiple proinflammatory processes, including lipid peroxidation, which causes diffuse injury to the microvasculature resulting in increased permeability, edema formation, and an increase in interstitial pressure. This overall process ultimately leads to stasis within the microvasculature, worsening ischemia, and cell lysis, including rhabdomyolysis. The resultant tissue destruction causes hyperkalemia, metabolic acidosis, and myoglobin-induced renal failure and may ultimately prove fatal.

DIAGNOSIS OF VASCULAR INJURY

1 The overwhelming majority of vascular injuries can be diagnosed with a thorough history and physical examination and

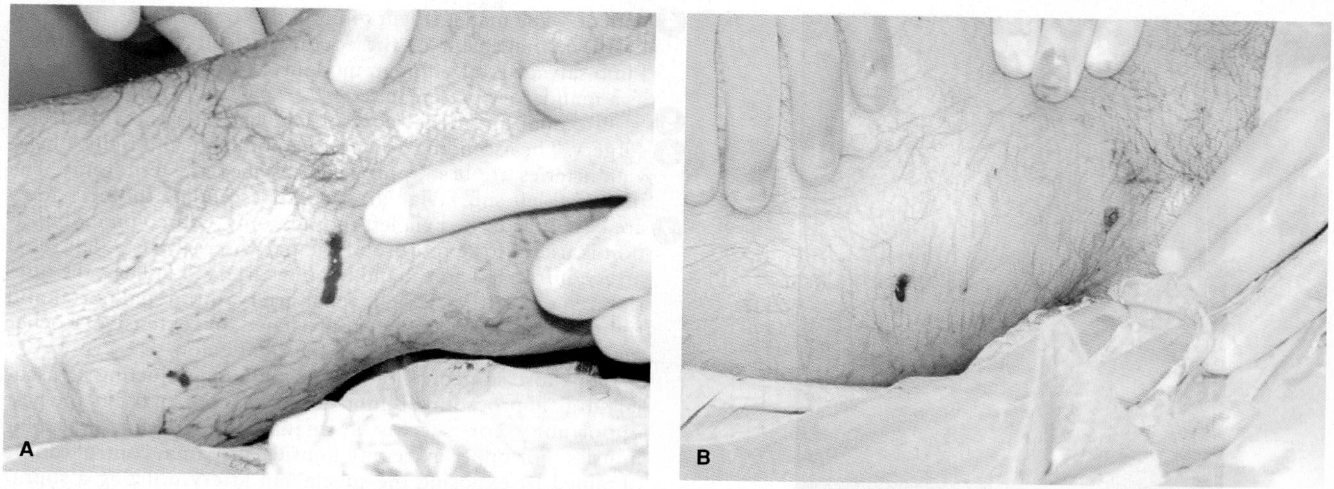

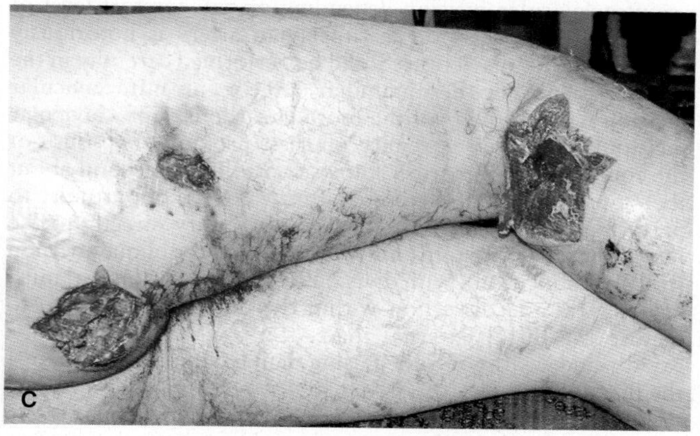

FIGURE 25.1. Three high-velocity gunshot wounds to the right lower extremity emphasizing a remarkable level of tissue destruction. **A:** Single entrance wound below knee. **B:** Two entrance wounds in proximal thigh. **C:** Notice the stellate appearance of the exit wounds.

high clinical index of suspicion. A history of pulsatile bleeding or, alternatively, a description of a large amount of blood at the scene of injury should elicit suspicion for vascular injury. Victims of a high-speed motor vehicle crash or those who fall from extreme heights must be assumed to have significant vascular injury until proven otherwise.

Physical examination findings are extremely variable but should be categorized according to "hard" and "soft" signs for vascular injury. Hard signs suggesting a vascular injury include pulsatile bleeding, expanding hematoma, palpable thrill, audible bruit, and evidence of ischemia as dictated by the six "P's": pulselessness, pain, pallor, paresthesia, paralysis, and poikilothermia. Soft signs of vascular injury include a history of moderate hemorrhage, injury in proximity to a named vessel, decreased but present pulse, nonexpanding hematoma, and associated peripheral neurologic deficit.[3] The presence of distal pulses can be deceiving and are intact in up to 20% of cases of major proximal vascular injury.

Intracavitary vascular injuries should be suspected in those patients presenting with hypotension and evidence of penetrating injury to the torso. A history of rapid deceleration or high transfer of kinetic energy, as occurs with a high-speed motor vehicle crash, should also elicit suspicion for a truncal vascular injury. Common findings associated with thoracic aortic injury include first rib fracture, thoracic spine fracture, flail chest, and sternal fracture. A widened upper mediastinum on anteroposterior chest radiography, loss of normal aortic contour, or thoracic outlet hematoma may suggest significant aortic injury.

The proper measurement of the ankle-brachial index (ABI) is essential for diagnosing more occult vascular injuries. The ABI is measured by obtaining the highest arterial occlusion pressure utilizing a manual blood pressure cuff at the ankle and a 9-MHz continuous wave Doppler probe placed over both the dorsalis pedis and posterior tibial arteries. This pressure value is then divided by the highest brachial systolic blood pressure, thereby providing the corresponding index. A normal index is greater than 1.0, and any index below 0.9 in an otherwise healthy patient is an indication for more definitive diagnostic tests to include duplex ultrasonography and/or arteriography.[4,5] Hypovolemic patients may have values as low as 0.75 and thus should undergo repeat measurement after resuscitation or further workup if not equally low in both extremities. Repeat physical examinations, coupled with repeat ABI measurements after therapeutic intervention, to include realignment of long bone fractures, are of paramount importance.

Arteriography remains the "gold standard" for diagnosing vascular injuries and providing a road map to guide surgical repair (Fig. 25.2). Standard arteriography is not always feasible or even practical in the multiply injured patient and is certainly not always indicated for single-level injury with associated hard signs of vascular trauma.[6] However, it can prove invaluable in the management of patients presenting with multiple levels of penetrating injury. Arteriography has traditionally been considered mandatory for patients presenting with complex knee injuries and/or posterior knee dislocations, although more recently, selective duplex examination has been used in patients with an otherwise normal vascular examination. Contrast arteriography has traditionally been the "gold standard" for diagnosing vascular injury, whereas computed tomographic angiography (CTA) is highly sensitive and specific, can be rapidly obtained, provides more information about other injuries, and is less invasive with fewer complications.[7,8]

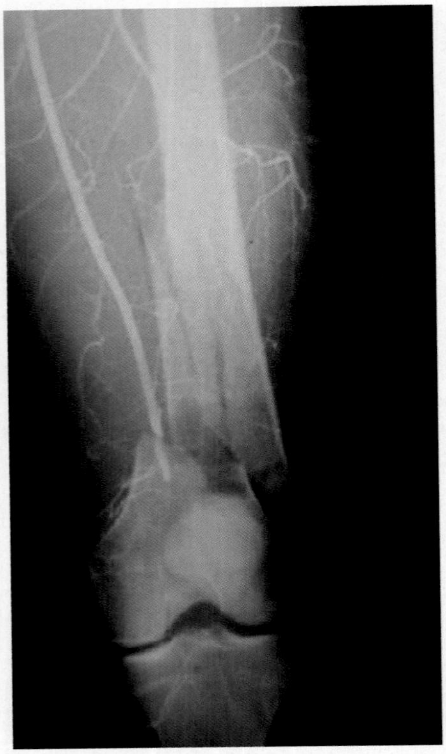

FIGURE 25.2. Arteriogram demonstrating vascular injury to the proximal popliteal artery as a result of distal left femur fracture.

PRINCIPLES OF MANAGEMENT

As stated previously, time is of the essence with patients presenting with vascular injury, and different vascular beds have different tolerance to ischemia. Preoperative antibiotics should be administered to all of these patients and every effort should be made to avoid vascular reconstruction in the setting of heavy contamination or simultaneous pancreatic injury. Patients with suspected vascular injuries should be prepared for operation with standard surgical approaches in mind and with additional preparations allowing for access of more proximal vascular control. In addition, preparation should be made for recovery of an adequate vein from an uninvolved extremity to be used as a reconstructive conduit. Hence, patients with suspected vascular injuries in the neck or upper extremity should have the entire chest prepped into the field to allow for rapid performance of median sternotomy or thoracotomy, as well as preparation of one or both of the lower extremities to allow for recovery of the greater saphenous vein for conduit. Patients with suspected abdominal vascular injuries should have the chest, abdomen, and both groins prepped. Patients with suspected lower extremity vascular injuries should have the abdomen and both lower extremities circumferentially prepped into the field. When managing a vascular injury in a lower extremity, the greater saphenous conduit should be obtained from the uninjured extremity.

The phrase "damage control" implies a rescue situation in which prevention of further injury is achieved. When applied to vascular injuries, damage control is defined as control of exsanguinating hemorrhage, rapid restoration of blood flow to an ischemic vascular bed, and prevention of further injury
3 such as extremity compartment syndrome. Danger from active hemorrhage is self-evident. When dealing with the multiply injured patient, limb salvage may be a secondary priority or not a priority at all depending on the physiologic status of the
4 patient.[9] The management of injured extremities is superseded by the management of the overall patient: "life over limb." Limb salvage is a treatment modality not to be taken lightly or as a mandatory preference.

5 Proximal and distal control is a basic tenant of vascular
6 surgery. The ascending aorta and innominate and right subclavian arteries are best approached by median sternotomy. The proximal left subclavian artery and descending thoracic aorta
7 are best approached via left thoracotomy. Left colon mobilization is useful for exposure of the paravisceral aorta, left renal artery, infrarenal aorta, and left iliac artery. Similarly, the inferior vena cava (IVC), right renal artery, infrarenal aorta, and right iliac artery can be approached by extensive Kocher maneuver and mobilization of the right colon.

For those surgeons not accustomed to conducting a vascular surgical procedure, remote proximal control offers the best opportunity for success in managing extremity vascular injuries. For upper extremity injuries, proximal control can be obtained by exposing the subclavian artery utilizing a supra- or infraclavicular incision depending on the comfort level of the operating surgeon. The subclavian artery is notoriously fragile and thus dissection should be performed carefully in the stable patient. For the unfamiliar surgeon, an infraclavicular incision is preferred over the more hazardous supraclavicular incision. For lower extremity injuries, proximal exposure of the common femoral artery allows controlled dissection about the more distal injured vessel and provides the opportunity to perform arteriography. The challenging injury directly to the femoral triangle requires a lower abdominal oblique incision (transplant incision), with division of all three abdominal muscular layers and dissection within the preperitoneal space to expose the distal external iliac artery, which can then be rapidly and easily controlled using digital compression against the iliac fossa.

As a rule, longitudinal incisions over named vascular structures allow for the widest exposure and best control. Curvilinear and "lazy S"-type incisions should be made across joints to include the antecubital and popliteal fossa. The posterior approach to the traumatic popliteal artery injury is rarely used in any setting. Exposure can often be demanding, particularly in the setting of debris, dirt, bone dust, and bone fragments in a wound. This presentation demands the time-honored tradition of adequate and aggressive débridement of devitalized tissue.

Systemic heparinization (50 to 75 U/kg intravenously) should be initiated in stable patients in whom vascular control of the injury has been quickly established, estimated prehospital blood loss is relatively low, and ongoing bleeding sources are minimal. Unstable patients with diffuse hemorrhage from bone fragments, torn muscle, and additional injuries and patients who are already hypothermic and coagulopathic should not get systemic anticoagulation during repair of a vascular injury. Alternatively, local administration of heparinized saline solution directly into the injured vessel prior to repair may aid in preventing thrombotic complications. The decision to anticoagulate is left to the discretion of the operating surgeon, who must be in close contact with the anesthesia providers in order to fully understand the patient's clinical status.

As with all vascular operations, there are several important elements for success. Key among these is careful handling of tissue, use of magnification loupes, adequate lighting, and use of fine instruments with fine, monofilament suture. After exposure, injured vessels should be carefully débrided back to normal- and healthy-appearing tissue. Inflow and back-bleeding should then be assessed. If there is no back-bleeding, gentle thrombectomy with appropriate-sized Fogarty embolectomy catheters should be performed. The use of a standard pulmonary artery catheter may be useful in this scenario if no standard embolectomy catheters are available.[10] Minimal manipulation of intima is imperative to prevent

TABLE 25.1 TREATMENT

TREATMENT OF VASCULAR INJURY

■ TYPE OF REPAIR	■ USES AND INDICATIONS
Lateral repair	When vessel not compromised >25% circumference
Patch angioplasty	When vessel not compromised >50% circumference
Primary end-to-end anastomosis	<2 cm defect, mobilize ends, spatulate
Interposition graft	>2 cm defect, reversed vein > polytetrafluoroethylene, most common repair
Extra-anatomic bypass	Extensive defect, multiple-level injury, contamination
Suture ligation	Strongly consider prophylactic fasciotomy, distal embolectomy, and anticoagulation

vessel thrombosis in the early postoperative setting. After adequate débridement, the vessels should be flushed with a heparinized saline solution both proximally and distally. A tension-free repair should then ensue. Options for repair are many and are listed in Table 25.1. As a general rule, the most often utilized vascular procedures are ligation and interposition bypass graft. With combined injuries, arterial repair should precede venous repair except when venous repair requires little effort. This is to minimize ischemic burden from an already severely injured vascular bed.

The temptation to reconstruct, repair, or even ligate an arterial injury in the setting of a highly contaminated wound should be thoroughly resisted. Recent studies have shown that a high failure rate ensues due to infection and subsequent thrombosis.[11] In a contaminated wound, every effort should be made to perform adequate débridement and then reassess for adequate collateral macroperfusion with every means available. If ligation of a major artery is required, distal embolectomy should be routinely performed followed by distal infusion or systemic administration of heparin to preserve collateral circulation.[12] If feasible, patients should undergo abdominal decompression, prophylactic fasciotomy, observation, and then definitive revascularization once control of wound sepsis has been accomplished. Alternatively, routing of bypass grafts through uncontaminated fields offers the best chance for success in the management of these challenging injuries.

Key to the success of vascular repair is appropriate use of available conduit for reconstruction. It is widely held that the best alternative conduit for reconstruction is autologous saphenous vein. The saphenous vein is the workhorse for vascular surgeons and can be used in multiple locations. It is important to remember the concept of directional flow within veins and thus reverse or turn around the saphenous vein prior to using it as a conduit for revascularization. The saphenous vein may also be used as patch material or refashioned in the form of a panel or spiral graft for reconstruction of larger vessels. The saphenous vein should always be recovered from the uninvolved extremity. This is done to provide maximal venous drainage from the injured extremity should the deep system be involved or the patient develop deep vein thrombosis in the postoperative period. Proximal saphenous vein can still be utilized in the rare patient presenting with upper extremity vascular injury and bilateral major traumatic below-knee injuries.

The repair of extremity venous injuries has been controversial. Data from Dr. Norman Rich and the Vietnam Vascular Registry supports an effort at repair of most major venous injuries if possible.[13,14] The decision to repair versus ligate a major extremity venous injury depends on the available resources, existing comorbidities, coexistent injuries in the same patient, and, of course, the hemodynamic stability of the patient. Rich retrospectively demonstrated a lower incidence of chronic venous insufficiency and postphlebitic syndrome in those patients undergoing venous repair as opposed to ligation in the lower extremity.[13] However, the same general principles do not hold true for venous injuries in the upper extremity, where ligation is better tolerated with minimal chronic morbidity.

OPERATIVE MANAGEMENT OF SPECIFIC REGIONS

Management of Vascular Injury in the Neck

Injuries to the neck have been notoriously difficult to manage. A clear anatomic division of the neck into zones has allowed a selective approach to penetrating neck trauma. Zone I lies below the cricoid cartilage, and zone III lies above the angle of the mandible. Zone II, which is between I and III, has classically been managed with immediate exploration and direct evaluation of the aerodigestive tract and the carotid and jugular vessels. The most commonly injured structures in the neck are the blood vessels, with the incidence of major vascular trauma following penetrating neck trauma being 20%.[15] Physical examination and determination of hard signs predict those patients with significant injuries who might benefit from immediate exploration.[16] Direct surgical repair remains the "gold standard" for injuries in all zones, but endovascular approaches are appealing in that some of these injuries can be remotely approached from within the thoracic inlet and base of the skull, thus avoiding the morbidity of the required extensive surgical exposure. Unique advantages for an endovascular approach to the extracranial cerebrovascular system include avoidance of general anesthetic and the ability to monitor neurologic status during the intervention.

Penetrating zone I and III injuries that require immediate operative intervention are not candidates for a purely endovascular approach. However, endovascular techniques may be utilized in a "hybrid" fashion to support the standard open repair of these injuries. Zone I injuries with hard signs of vascular injury may have an enlarging hematoma at the thoracic inlet, high chest tube output, or shock. These injuries notoriously involve the great vessels. Immediate control involves a high anterior thoracotomy, sternotomy, or clavicular resection to obtain adequate proximal control. Once the patient is prepared in the operating room, an occlusion balloon can be rapidly utilized from the groin to provide endoluminal proximal control of the great vessels, allowing conduct of a surgical exposure in a more controlled fashion and possibly avoiding sternotomy for proximal exposure. With an occlusion balloon in place, an arteriogram will help locate the injury and allow for operative planning. After the injury is exposed, a vascular clamp replaces the occlusion balloon, or, alternatively, if proximal vessel length is not adequate, the occlusion balloon remains in place for repair.

In patients with soft signs of a cervical vascular injury and hemodynamic stability, there is ample time for further evaluation. Arteriography may identify an intimal flap, dissection, pseudoaneurysm, complete or partial transection, or thrombosis. Operative repair of these lesions has been shown to reduce overall mortality and stroke rates for both penetrating and blunt trauma as compared to observation or ligation.[17] However, several centers have found that early anticoagulation alone also improves overall neurologic status and mortality in a cohort of patients with high internal carotid artery trauma who did not undergo operative repair and were able to tolerate anticoagulation with heparin.[18–20]

Vertebral artery injury is a rare occurrence, but the identification of vertebral artery injuries has actually increased owing to the liberal use of screening tests (ultrasound or CTA) during workup. When encountered, vertebral artery injuries can be difficult to expose and control. The first portion of the vertebral artery is fairly accessible, but once the vessel enters the bony foramen of the cervical canal, blind clipping or packing with bone wax carries the risk of cervical nerve root damage. Transcatheter embolization has been utilized for vertebral artery transections, pseudoaneurysms, and arteriovenous fistulas with a combination of embolization techniques including wire-guided crossing of a transected vessel to gain occlusive control of the distal bleeding vessel.[21–24]

Management of Vascular Injury in the Trunk

Truncal vascular trauma is a highly lethal event. The majority of patients experiencing blunt or penetrating injury to the aorta in either the chest or abdomen do not routinely survive to reach a higher level of care and often die in the field. A blunt mechanism of injury associated with rapid deceleration also causes predictable injury patterns within the thoracic and abdominal aorta and iliac, renal, and visceral arteries. Associated severe brain and lung injury directly and indirectly increase the perioperative risk associated with general anesthesia and a traditional open surgical approach.

Management of Vascular Injury in the Chest

Blunt aortic injury (BAI) is a highly lethal event, with 80% to 85% of patients expiring at the scene of injury. Of those presenting to a trauma center, 40% to 50% die within 24 hours of injury.[25] Conventional treatment involves thoracotomy for open repair, with associated mortality rates ranging from 15% to 28% and paraplegia rates as high as 19%.[26] In patients experiencing traumatic thoracic aortic injury, thoracotomy may worsen potential associated lung injuries and increase mortality risk.[27] The past decade has seen significant advances in the endovascular management of BAI with resultant dramatic decreases in morbidity and mortality. U.S. Food and Drug Administration (FDA)-approved devices are now commercially available in the United States for the endovascular repair of thoracic aortic pathology. During the evaluation and early care prior to surgery for these injuries, control of the shear forces on the disrupted aorta using beta-blockers is mandatory. Systolic blood pressures should be maintained at about 100 mm Hg.

In March 1997, Fabian et al. published a landmark prospective study of BAI inclusive of 50 trauma centers across North America now referred to as the American Association for the Surgery of Trauma 1 (AAST-1) trial.[28] There were 274 cases of blunt aortic injury studied over 2.5 years with average time from injury to repair of 16.5 hours. Overall mortality was 31%, with 63% of deaths attributable to aortic rupture. Of patients presenting in extremis or who sustained rupture while waiting for surgery, the mortality was 100%. Postoperative paraplegia occurred in 8.7% of patients. Ninety-three percent of injuries occurred at the proximal descending aorta in the region of the aortic isthmus.[28] Two months after this landmark publication, Semba et al. reported their initial experience using endoluminal grafts to repair a multitude of aortic pathology.[29] In their series of 95 patients, one patient underwent endoluminal repair for blunt aortic injury and survived. Since then, the use of endovascular techniques to manage this devastating injury has increased. An endovascular approach for repair of blunt thoracic aortic injury decreases the morbidity associated with posterolateral thoracotomy and single-lung ventilation in patients who often have multiple associated injuries, including rib fractures, flail chest, or pulmonary injury (Fig. 25.3).

Recently, the AAST Multi-institutional Thoracic Aortic Injury Study Group published the results of the AAST-2 trial. Over a period of 26 months, 193 patients with BAI from 18 centers were studied. Over 65% of the injuries were managed with endovascular repair with a resultant decrease in mortality from 22% to 13% and a reduction in paraplegia rates from 8.7% to 1.6%.[30] 8 Endovascular repair of traumatic thoracic disruption is associated with lower mortality and lower rates of paraplegia than traditional open repair. These findings are extremely compelling and should elicit a dramatic shift in the primary management of BAI by surgeons caring for this patient population.

A majority of patients experiencing BAI are young and hence have small aortic anatomy. Most commercially available grafts are designed for the treatment of aneurysmal disease and not meant for young aortas. The smallest commercially available grafts specifically designed for the thoracic aorta are 22 mm (Talent; Medtronic/AVE, Santa Rosa, CA) and 26 mm (TAG; W.L. Gore, Flagstaff, Arizona). Most experts would recommend an oversizing of 10% to 15% based on the aortic diameters defined in the landing zones for BAI. Aggressive oversizing has led to stent graft failures and "infolding" of the grafts with resultant endoleak and collapse.[31,32] A variety of different infrarenal "cuffs" and limb extensions have been used by some authors to avoid these problems in small aortas.[33]

Not all patients presenting with blunt aortic injury should be considered for endovascular repair. Some authors have

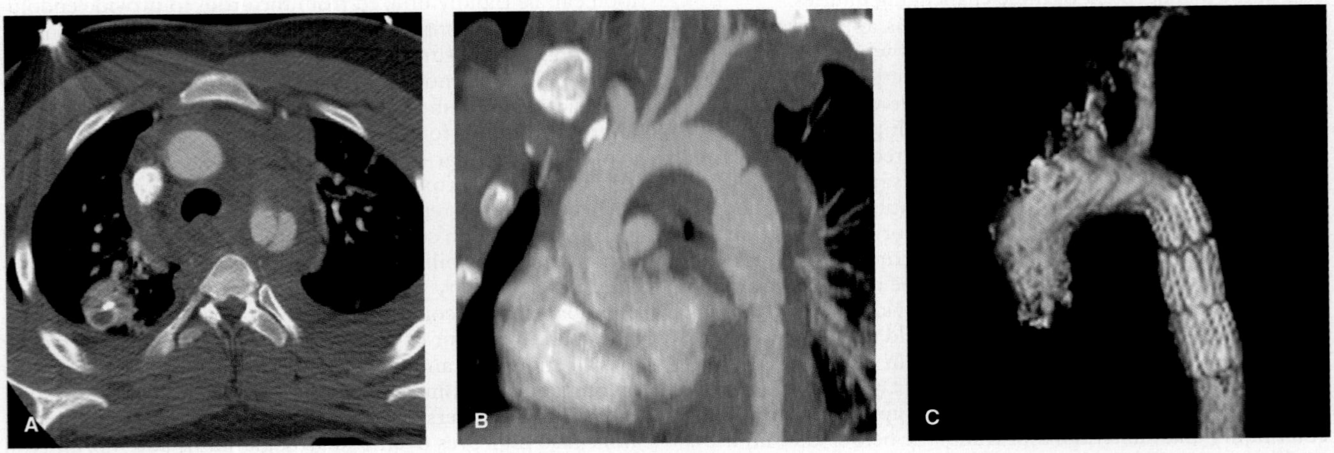

FIGURE 25.3. A: Axial computed tomography angiography (CTA) image of blunt aortic injury. B: Oblique sagittal CTA image of the same injury. C: Follow-up CTA reconstruction after successful stent graft repair.

advocated using the Injury Severity Score (ISS) to guide therapy.[27] A predicted mortality based on an ISS of greater than 100% should elicit an approach to simply supporting the patient with conservative measures, including long-term control of blood pressure with beta-blocking agents and other antihypertensive agents as required in the resistant patient.

Management of Vascular Injury in the Abdomen

The management of abdominal vascular trauma is a formidable challenge faced by many trauma surgeons. In a review of 5,760 vascular injuries in 4,539 patients, Mattox et al. described abdominal vascular injuries accounting for 33.7% of all vascular injuries.[1] Abdominal vascular injuries remain the most common cause of death following penetrating abdominal trauma. Many patients experiencing abdominal vascular injury, whether penetrating or blunt, have simultaneous hollow viscus injury, which makes operative management difficult when considering the need for prosthetic graft placement in a potentially contaminated field.

The so-called "seat belt aorta" is defined as injury to the aorta after direct compression against the bony structures of the spine. The most common site of this injury is directly below the inferior mesenteric artery. Atherosclerotic aortic plaques are also thought to be a contributing factor because less force is required to damage the aortic intima with an existing rigid plaque within the lumen.[34] It has been strongly suggested that an initial attempt at endovascular repair be made for blunt abdominal aortic injury. This approach is less invasive, avoids a retroperitoneal dissection and application of an aortic cross-clamp, and may be performed immediately after closure of a laparotomy for grossly contaminated injuries.[35]

Blunt trauma is the most common method of injuring a renal artery. There are only a few isolated reports in the literature describing renal artery stenting for traumatic injury with either balloon-expandable or self-expanding stents.[36–38] Potential benefits to this approach include the rapidity with which repair can be accomplished following the diagnosis by conventional or CTA. Unfortunately, in a majority of these injuries, the diagnosis is often delayed, which significantly impacts outcome for the affected kidney. While nonoperative complication rates, even with close and careful observation, have been reported to be as high as 82%,[39] treatment remains controversial when the end organ is not threatened. Most groups recommend treatment within 6 to 12 hours as the most critical factor in preserving renal function.[40]

Injuries to the celiac or superior mesenteric artery are best managed with traditional open surgical exposure and ligation and/or repair. Endovascular management of acute traumatic injury to these arteries has not been described as yet. Reasons for this probably stem from a requirement for assessment of bowel viability in conjunction with definitive arterial repair. The combination of endovascular and laparoscopic techniques in approaching these injuries may prove worthwhile in the future.

Iliac artery injuries are among the most challenging for trauma surgeons. Morbidity and mortality rates from these types of injuries approach 15% and 40%, respectively.[41,42] Proximal and distal control can be exceedingly difficult, while the utility of angiographic embolization of bleeding pelvic vessels in association with severe blunt pelvic trauma is well documented. As with the thoracic and abdominal aorta, blunt trauma is an infrequent cause of iliac vascular injury. However, morbidity and mortality associated with such injuries are profound. Like the abdominal aorta, the presence of atherosclerotic plaque within the iliac vessels has been associated with an increased susceptibility to intimal disruption.[43] Lyden et al. reported on the successful management of common iliac artery dissection with self-expanding stents after blunt abdominal trauma.[44] Long-term follow-up is not available for iliac stenting in the setting of injury from blunt arterial trauma; however, one would surmise that long-term patency rates are not too dissimilar and perhaps better than those from standard iliac artery angioplasty and stenting.

Injury to the vena cava is a rare event, occurring in 0.5% to 5% of penetrating injuries and 0.6% to 1% of blunt abdominal injuries.[45] Despite their rarity, injuries to the vena cava represent 30% to 40% of all abdominal vascular injuries and are commonly associated with a mortality as high as 50%.[46]

Management of Vascular Injury in Watershed Regions

Managing injuries to the thoracic outlet often requires incisions that are potentially profoundly morbid. Many injuries in this location are fortunately contained hematomas that allow for definitive preoperative diagnosis. This may allow for a window of opportunity to use endovascular techniques to manage supra-aortic truncal injuries to the innominate, carotid, or subclavian arteries while avoiding a thoracotomy.[47,48] Likewise, ileofemoral injuries are also difficult to control. A multicenter trial evaluated the use of Wallgraft Endoprostheses (Boston Scientific, Natick, Massachusetts) for the management of 62 patients with iliac, subclavian, or femoral arterial injuries.[49] While the majority (78%) of these injuries were iatrogenic in nature and not representative of a purely primary vascular injury series, the data provide compelling support for endovascular management.[49] In this study, the majority of injuries treated were in the iliac arteries (53.2%), while the remainder were located in the subclavian (29%) or femoral (17.7%) arteries. Eighty-five percent of patients avoided surgery entirely within the first year after placement of the stent graft.

In addition, operative complications for emergent procedures with the stent graft were significantly reduced compared with those of surgical repair (21% vs. 57%), and late complications for emergent procedures were not different from the rate for surgical repair (6% vs. 12.5%). Similarly, postprocedure mortality associated with emergent stent graft procedures was significantly reduced compared with that of emergent surgical repair (9% vs. 27%), and late all-cause mortality was significantly reduced compared with emergent surgical repair (15% vs. 34%).

These data should be interpreted with caution as the numbers are small and the comparison between iatrogenic injuries and standard traumatic vascular injuries is probably incomparable. Despite these differences, endovascular therapy has become an essential tool for the trauma or vascular surgeon managing these difficult injuries.

Management of Vascular Injury in the Extremity

The Mangled Extremity Severity Score (MESS) was created as objective criteria to predict amputation after lower extremity trauma. The four criteria include (a) skeletal/soft tissue injury, (b) limb ischemia, (c) shock, and (d) patient age. An MESS score greater than or equal to 7 in the original series predicted amputation with 100% accuracy.[50] Many such scores have been developed to attempt to predict the need for urgent amputation, but this accuracy has not been reproducible. The high specificity of these multiple scoring systems confirm that limb salvage can be predicted. However, the converse is not true; low variable sensitivities fail to support their validity as a predictor of amputation and should not be used for this purpose in the individual patient.[51]

The overwhelming majority of injured extremities requiring vascular repair for limb salvage will involve the common femoral, superficial femoral, popliteal, axillary, or brachial arteries. Isolated injuries to the ulnar, radial, and tibial arteries can be managed with arterial ligation in a majority of cases, as long as at least one vessel is patent to perfuse the extremity. In general, incisions of election should be made as a preference over incisions of opportunity provided by an existing wound. This is not always possible as the wound may provide adequate exposure for definitive control of the vascular injury.

The use of a tourniquet has long been a controversial topic. Inappropriately applied tourniquets actually cause an increase in bleeding from an extremity wound. This paradoxical effect results from occlusion of the lower-pressure venous outflow and inadequate occlusion of the higher-pressure arterial inflow. As a result, an increase in the bleeding from the wound can lead to early exsanguination. A properly applied tourniquet causes a significant amount of pain, which should be managed with intravenous or intramuscular pain medication. The temptation to remove a properly placed tourniquet due to patient discomfort should be resisted until operative control has been achieved. Tourniquets are often applied to hypotensive patients prior to resuscitation, and hence less pressure is required to arrest arterial hemorrhage. Once resuscitation is initiated and more normal systolic pressures are achieved, patients may bleed through their tourniquet. Thus, tourniquets should be monitored and tightened for effectiveness. In the emergency department, pneumatic tourniquets can be used as a proximal clamp for temporizing measures in the multiply injured patient with ongoing workup and those with massive soft tissue destruction and mangled extremities.

Temporary intraluminal shunts allow for rapid restoration of blood flow to an ischemic limb or vascular bed while other procedures to include wound débridement, external fixation of fractures, or more lifesaving procedures such as trauma laparotomy or thoracotomy can be accomplished.[52–54] Shunts may be easily and rapidly placed after proximal vascular control with either a pneumatic tourniquet or vascular clamp and secured in place with Rummel tourniquets or simple silk ties to prevent dislodgement. After placement, patency should be confirmed with intraoperative continuous wave Doppler of the shunt. The specific use of Sundt shunts minimizes risk of dislodgement due to their design when appropriately inserted. The Sundt shunt (Integra Lifesciences Corp., Plainsboro, New Jersey) is lined with an inner coil to prevent kinking or collapse (Fig. 25.4), except for one small area within the shunt of discontinuous coils, which should be used for clamping if needed. Clamping the shunt in any other location will crush the coil and occlude the shunt.

One of the most important factors in managing the acutely injured extremity is the liberal use of fasciotomy to avoid or treat compartment syndrome.[55] A thorough understanding of the technique of fasciotomy for both the upper and lower extremities as well as the feet and hands is mandatory (Fig. 25.5). A key principle for performance of a standard four-compartment fasciotomy in the lower extremity includes two long skin incisions, each at least 15 cm, on both the medial and lateral aspects of each affected extremity. Indications for fasciotomy are listed in Table 25.2.

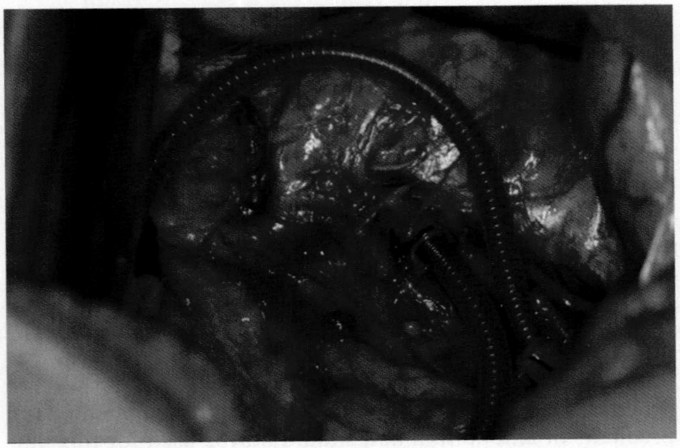

FIGURE 25.4. Temporary intraluminal shunt prior to definitive repair of an arterial injury.

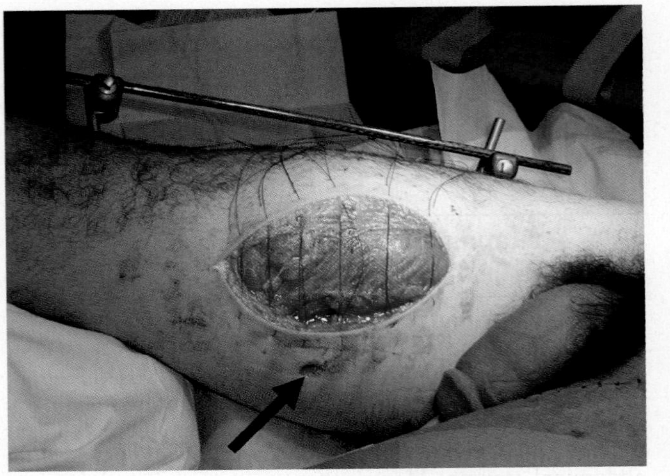

FIGURE 25.5. Thigh fasciotomy in a patient with penetrating injury to the right lower extremity causing vascular and skeletal injury.

Repair of traumatic lesions using endovascular techniques has had limited application in the extremities. The acutely injured patient with hard signs of a peripheral vascular injury can usually be controlled with direct tamponade or, rarely, a tourniquet. While time is of the essence in a patient with significant ischemia or neurologic deficit, peripheral vascular beds are fairly resistant to temporary ischemic times of 4 to 6 hours,[56] and this allows the surgeon time for catheter access and endoluminal examination of the injury in the operating room. While open repair may be required for complete vessel transection, endovascular treatment or proximal control can be advantageous for a high brachial artery injury or common femoral artery injury that is associated with an extensive hematoma. This would avoid an extensive dissection near the brachial plexus and, in the groin, would avoid a suprainguinal dissection into the pelvis.

Pseudoaneurysms and arteriovenous fistulas of the peripheral vascular system occur infrequently aside from iatrogenic injuries. Iatrogenic injuries secondary to femoral access sites account for the majority of pseudoaneurysms and arteriovenous fistulas that are managed with endovascular techniques.

TABLE 25.2 INDICATIONS/CONTRAINDICATIONS

INDICATIONS FOR FASCIOTOMY

>4–6 h evacuation delay to revascularization
Combined arterial and venous injuries
Crush injuries
High-kinetic-energy mechanism
Vascular repair
Arterial or venous ligation
Comatose, closed head injury, or epidural analgesia
Tense compartments
Prophylactic

After ultrasound-directed pressure and thrombin injection have failed to thrombose pseudoaneurysms,[57,58] covered stents can be successfully used to exclude pseudoaneurysms from the circulation.[59] Iatrogenic vascular injuries secondary to orthopedic procedures have also been successfully managed with endovascular principles.[60]

Traumatic pseudoaneurysms and arteriovenous fistulas are significantly higher in the military population as a result of fragmentation wounds[61] and are only rarely encountered in civilian trauma. These injuries may not be readily apparent at the time of injury and can present several years later.[62,63] While intimal flaps or segmental narrowing appears to resolve spontaneously, pseudoaneurysms and arteriovenous fistulas tend to enlarge, embolize, or thrombose.[64] When identified, endovascular treatment has ranged from transcatheter embolization with coils or balloons, and occasionally Gelfoam packing is required as an adjunct.[65–68] Remote endoluminal occlusion in these patients either avoids an exploration in an acute grossly infected cavitary wound or avoids an incision through a scar that would have potential healing complications.

POSTOPERATIVE MANAGEMENT

Patients who have undergone repair of vascular injuries from trauma should be monitored in the intensive care unit for at least the first 24 hours after surgery. This should include electrocardiographic monitoring and pulse oximetry, particularly because hemorrhagic shock and reperfusion of an ischemic limb may result in systemic physiologic derangements such as hypoxia, hyperkalemia, and acidosis. Acidosis, anemia, and hypothermia should be aggressively corrected. For isolated extremity vascular injuries, mild coagulopathy may be tolerated after revascularization as long as continued bleeding is minimal. Patients may have substantial hypothermia, tissue edema, and vasospasm in the injured limb, making palpation of pulses difficult. Hypothermia should therefore be aggressively corrected and evaluation of vascular status should rely on Doppler evaluation with ABIs rather than palpable pulses. During this early postoperative period, palpation for distal pulses and search for Doppler signals should occur hourly. Any change at the completion of the surgical repair in pulse or particularly Doppler signals from the baseline examination warrants an investigation, either by rechecking ABIs and/or performing an arteriogram. Patients who had heavily contaminated wounds on initial presentation should have a planned return trip to the operating room within 24 hours for repeat irrigation and débridement of wounds.

MILITARY-SPECIFIC APPLICATIONS

The modern battlefield has a staunch reputation of being unclean, noisy, and lacking valuable resources.[69] In addition, high-kinetic-energy injuries such as those resulting from high explosives, munitions, and high-velocity missiles often cause soft tissue destruction that is not routinely seen in civilian settings. Extremity injuries predominate, representing 50% to 70% of all injuries treated during Operation Iraqi Freedom, and exsanguination from extremity wounds is the leading preventable cause of death on the modern battlefield.[70] Recent advances in military medicine have translated into a greater percentage of wounded soldiers surviving during Operations Enduring and Iraqi Freedom than in any other previous American conflict.[70] Despite the relative lack of proper angiographic equipment on the modern battlefield, some surgeons are challenging this standard and attempting to perform "damage control" endovascular procedures in the field. This technology cannot be ignored for future military conflicts.

Major extremity vascular injury in armed conflict represents one of the most formidable challenges for the trauma surgeon. These injuries are often present in patients with concomitant multisystem injury from fragmentation munitions. Arterial injuries are frequently associated with venous, peripheral nerve, extensive soft tissue, and skeletal injury. Combined arterial and venous vascular injuries are not uncommon and often may preclude limb salvage if not addressed. Patients with these injuries often arrive in hemorrhagic shock, and treatment of these injuries usually requires staged and multidisciplinary approaches.[71]

OUTCOMES

Outcomes after vascular injury are time dependent, necessitating a sense of urgency in overall management. The results of expeditiously treated vascular injuries are encouraging. Mortality rates are highest when associated with truncal vascular injuries and mostly involve the aorta or its primary branches. Most often, however, the mortality is related to other associated injuries.

The ultimate outcome measure for lower extremity vascular trauma is the functional limb preservation rate. Amputation rates after peripheral vascular trauma continue to decrease, with several modern series reporting rates of less than 2%. This decrease in amputation rate probably relates to a shortening of the duration of ischemia by improvements in evacuation, rapid diagnosis and treatment, and the use of intraluminal shunts. Early amputation is more likely if a delay in diagnosis occurs or there has been a significant blunt component (crush) to the injury. Late amputation is not well documented but is typically done for intractable pain, complex wound issues, disability, or chronic infection, which frequently includes osteomyelitis. Long-term functional outcome is not dependent on the durability of the vascular repair but, alternatively, on the integrity of the neuromuscular and skeletal elements.[72]

CONCLUSIONS

The application of endovascular technology to the management of penetrating and blunt traumatic vascular injuries represents an exciting and significant advance in modern trauma centers. Utilization of these techniques to stabilize a patient in extremis or to serve as a "bridge" to future elective procedures represents an attractive alternative with potentially lower morbidity and mortality rates than conventional open surgical management. It is of the utmost importance that these procedures be carried out by experienced providers in a committed trauma center environment conducive to such repair. A wide variety of imaging equipment as well as endovascular inventory must be readily available for the successful management of these injuries.

Surgeons should emphasize the use of endovascular surgery as a modern "damage control" technique.[73] Likewise, training paradigms for the credentialing of qualified trauma surgeons should include exposure to basic endovascular techniques. It is likely that in one or two decades, all endovascular procedures relating to trauma will be performed by trauma specialists.

References

1. Mattox KL, Feliciano DV, Burch J, et al. Five thousand seven hundred sixty cardiovascular injuries in 4459 patients. Epidemiologic evolution 1958 to 1987. *Ann Surg* 1989;209(6):698–705.
2. Odeh M. The role of reperfusion-induced injury in the pathogenesis of the crush syndrome. *N Engl J Med* 1991;324(20):1417–1422.
3. Moore W. *Vascular Surgery: A Comprehensive Review,* 6th ed. Philadelphia: WB Saunders & Co. 2002:677–696.
4. Schwartz M, Weaver F, Yellin A, et al. The utility of color flow Doppler examination in penetrating extremity arterial trauma. *Am Surg* 1993; 59(6):375–378.
5. Schwartz MR, Weaver FA, Bauer M, et al. Refining the indications for arteriography in penetrating extremity trauma: a prospective analysis. *J Vasc Surg* 1993;17(1):116–122.

6. Nanobashvili J, Kopadze T, Tvaladze M, et al. War injuries of major extremity arteries. *World J Surg* 2003;27(2):134–139.
7. Eastman AL, Chason DP, Perez CL, et al. Computed tomographic angiography for the diagnosis of blunt cervical vascular injury: is it ready for primetime? *J Trauma* 2006;60(5):925–929.
8. Methodius-Ngwodo WC, Fortson JK, Stephenson E Jr. Craniofacial necrotizing fasciitis of the eyelids, and nasal region after traumatic assault to the face: successful outcome with early intervention. *Am Surg* 2008;74(8): 777–778.
9. Beekley AC, Watts DM. Combat trauma experience with the United States Army 102nd Forward Surgical Team in Afghanistan. *Am J Surg* 2004;187(5): 652–654.
10. Starnes BW, Bruce JM. Popliteal artery trauma in a forward deployed Mobile Army Surgical Hospital: lessons learned from the war in Kosovo. *J Trauma* 2000;48(6):1144–1147.
11. Fox CJ, Gillespie DL, O'Donnell SD, et al. Contemporary management of wartime vascular trauma. *J Vasc Surg* 2005;41(4):638–644.
12. Levin PM, Rich NM, Hutton JE Jr. Collateral circulation in arterial injuries. *Arch Surg* 1971;102(4):392–399.
13. Rich NM. Management of venous trauma. *Surg Clin North Am* 1988; 68(4):809–821.
14. Rich NM, Leppaniemi A. Vascular trauma: a 40-year experience with extremity vascular emphasis. *Scand J Surg* 2002;91(1):109–126.
15. Beitsch P, Weigelt JA, Flynn E, et al. Physical examination and arteriography in patients with penetrating zone II neck wounds. *Arch Surg* 1994; 129(6):577–581.
16. Demetriades D, Charalambides D, Lakhoo M. Physical examination and selective conservative management in patients with penetrating injuries of the neck. *Br J Surg* 1993;80(12):1534–1536.
17. Ramadan F, Rutledge R, Oller D, et al. Carotid artery trauma: a review of contemporary trauma center experiences. *J Vasc Surg* 1995;21(1):46–55.
18. Fabian TC, Patton JH Jr, Croce MA, et al. Blunt carotid injury. Importance of early diagnosis and anticoagulant therapy. *Ann Surg* 1996;223(5):513–522.
19. Mokri B. Traumatic and spontaneous extracranial internal carotid artery dissections. *J Neurol* 1990;237(6):356–361.
20. Biffl WL, Moore EE, Ryu RK, et al. The unrecognized epidemic of blunt carotid arterial injuries: early diagnosis improves neurologic outcome. *Ann Surg* 1998;228(4):462–470.
21. Beaujeux RL, Reizine DC, Casasco A, et al. Endovascular treatment of vertebral arteriovenous fistula. *Radiology* 1992;183(2):361–367.
22. Cohen JE, Rajz G, Itshayek E, et al. Endovascular management of exsanguinating vertebral artery transection. *Surg Neurol* 2005;64(4):331–334.
23. Mwipatayi BP, Jeffery P, Beningfield SJ, et al. Management of extra-cranial vertebral artery injuries. *Eur J Vasc Endovasc Surg* 2004;27(2):157–162.
24. Yee LF, Olcott EW, Knudson MM, et al. Extraluminal, transluminal, and observational treatment for vertebral artery injuries. *J Trauma* 1995;39(3): 480–484.
25. Jamieson WR, Janusz MT, Gudas VM, et al. Traumatic rupture of the thoracic aorta: third decade of experience. *Am J Surg* 2002;183(5):571–575.
26. Von Oppell UO, Dunne TT, De Groot MK, et al. Traumatic aortic rupture: twenty-year metaanalysis of mortality and risk of paraplegia. *Ann Thorac Surg* 1994;58(2):585–593.
27. Kasirajan K, Heffernan D, Langsfeld M. Acute thoracic aortic trauma: a comparison of endoluminal stent grafts with open repair and nonoperative management. *Ann Vasc Surg* 2003;17(6):589–595.
28. Fabian TC, Richardson JD, Croce MA, et al. Prospective study of blunt aortic injury: multicenter trial of the American Association for the Surgery of Trauma. *J Trauma* 1997;42(3):374–380.
29. Semba CP, Kato N, Kee ST, et al. Acute rupture of the descending thoracic aorta: repair with use of endovascular stent-grafts. *J Vasc Interv Radiol* 1997;8(3):337–342.
30. Demetriades D, Velmahos GC, Scalea TM, et al. Diagnosis and treatment of blunt thoracic aortic injuries: changing perspectives. *J Trauma* 2008; 64(6):1415–1418.
31. Steinbauer MG, Stehr A, Pfister K, et al. Endovascular repair of proximal endograft collapse after treatment for thoracic aortic disease. *J Vasc Surg* 2006;43(3):609–612.
32. Fang TD, Peterson DA, Kirilcuk NN, et al. Endovascular management of a gunshot wound to the thoracic aorta. *J Trauma* 2006;60(1):204–208.
33. Karmy-Jones R, Hoffer E, Meissner MH, et al. Endovascular stent grafts and aortic rupture: a case series. *J Trauma* 2003;55(5):805–810.
34. Brunsting LA, Ouriel K. Traumatic fracture of the abdominal aorta. Rupture of a calcified abdominal aorta with minimal trauma. *J Vasc Surg* 1988;8(2): 184–186.
35. Berthet JP, Marty-Ane CH, Veerapen R, et al. Dissection of the abdominal aorta in blunt trauma: endovascular or conventional surgical management? *J Vasc Surg* 2003;38(5):997–1003.
36. Villas PA, Cohen G, Putnam SG III, et al. Wallstent placement in a renal artery after blunt abdominal trauma. *J Trauma* 1999;46(6):1137–1139.
37. Whigham CJ Jr, Bodenhamer JR, Miller JK. Use of the Palmaz stent in primary treatment of renal artery intimal injury secondary to blunt trauma. *J Vasc Interv Radiol* 1995;6(2):175–178.
38. Lee JT, White RA. Endovascular management of blunt traumatic renal artery dissection. *J Endovasc Ther* 2002;9(3):354–358.
39. Carrillo EH, Bergamini TM, Miller FB, et al. Abdominal vascular injuries. *J Trauma* 1997;43(1):164–171.
40. Carroll PR, McAninch JW, Klosterman P, et al. Renovascular trauma: risk assessment, surgical management, and outcome. *J Trauma* 1990;30(5): 547–552.
41. Carrillo EH, Spain DA, Wilson MA, et al. Alternatives in the management of penetrating injuries to the iliac vessels. *J Trauma* 1998;44(6): 1024–1029.
42. Burch JM, Richardson RJ, Martin RR, et al. Penetrating iliac vascular injuries: recent experience with 233 consecutive patients. *J Trauma* 1990; 30(12):1450–1459.
43. Tsai FC, Wang CC, Fang JF, et al. Isolated common iliac artery occlusion secondary to atherosclerotic plaque rupture from blunt abdominal trauma: case report and review of the literature. *J Trauma* 1997;42(1):133–136.
44. Lyden SP, Srivastava SD, Waldman DL, et al. Common iliac artery dissection after blunt trauma: case report of endovascular repair and literature review. *J Trauma* 2001;50(2):339–342.
45. Burch JM, Feliciano DV, Mattox KL, et al. Injuries of the inferior vena cava. *Am J Surg* 1988;156(6):548–552.
46. Kuehne J, Frankhouse J, Modrall G, et al. Determinants of survival after inferior vena cava trauma. *Am Surg* 1999;65(10):976–981.
47. Patel AV, Marin ML, Veith FJ, et al. Endovascular graft repair of penetrating subclavian artery injuries. *J Endovasc Surg* 1996;3(4):382–388.
48. Becker GJ, Benenati JF, Zemel G, et al. Percutaneous placement of a balloon-expandable intraluminal graft for life-threatening subclavian arterial hemorrhage. *J Vasc Interv Radiol* 1991;2(2):225–229.
49. White R, Krajcer Z, Johnson M, et al. Results of a multicenter trial for the treatment of traumatic vascular injury with a covered stent. *J Trauma* 2006;60(6):1189–1195.
50. Johansen K, Daines M, Howey T, et al. Objective criteria accurately predict amputation following lower extremity trauma. *J Trauma* 1990;30(5): 568–572.
51. Bosse MJ, MacKenzie EJ, Kellam JF, et al. A prospective evaluation of the clinical utility of the lower-extremity injury-severity scores. *J Bone Joint Surg Am* 2001;83-A(1):3–14.
52. Johansen K, Bandyk D, Thiele B, et al. Temporary intraluminal shunts: resolution of a management dilemma in complex vascular injuries. *J Trauma* 1982;22(5):395–402.
53. Granchi T, Schmittling Z, Vasquez J, et al. Prolonged use of intraluminal arterial shunts without systemic anticoagulation. *Am J Surg* 2000;180(6): 493–496.
54. Eger M, Golcman L, Goldstein A, et al. The use of a temporary shunt in the management of arterial vascular injuries. *Surg Gynecol Obstet* 1971; 132(1):67–70.
55. Jacob JE. Compartment syndrome. A potential cause of amputation in battlefield vascular injuries. *Int Surg* 1974;59(10):542–548.
56. Wolma FJ, Larrieu AJ, Alsop GC. Arterial injuries of the legs associated with fractures and dislocations. *Am J Surg* 1980;140(6):806–809.
57. Lonn L, Olmarker A, Geterud K, et al. Treatment of femoral pseudoaneurysms. Percutaneous US-guided thrombin injection versus US-guided compression. *Acta Radiol* 2002;43(4):396–400.
58. Lonn L, Olmarker A, Geterud K, et al. Prospective randomized study comparing ultrasound-guided thrombin injection to compression in the treatment of femoral pseudoaneurysms. *J Endovasc Ther* 2004;11(5):570–576.
59. Waigand J, Uhlich F, Gross CM, et al. Percutaneous treatment of pseudoaneurysms and arteriovenous fistulas after invasive vascular procedures. *Catheter Cardiovasc Interv* 1999;47(2):157–164.
60. Wilson JS, Miranda A, Johnson BL, et al. Vascular injuries associated with elective orthopedic procedures. *Ann Vasc Surg* 2003;17(6):641–644.
61. Rich NM, Hobson RW, Collins GJ Jr. Traumatic arteriovenous fistulas and false aneurysms: a review of 558 lesions. *Surgery* 1975;78(6):817–828.
62. Jackson MR, Brengman ML, Rich NM. Delayed presentation of 50 years after a World War II vascular injury with intraoperative localization by duplex ultrasound of a traumatic false aneurysm. *J Trauma* 1997;43(1): 159–161.
63. Yilmaz AT, Arslan M, Demirkilic U, et al. Missed arterial injuries in military patients. *Am J Surg* 1997;173(2):110–114.
64. Frykberg ER, Vines FS, Alexander RH. The natural history of clinically occult arterial injuries: a prospective evaluation. *J Trauma* 1989;29(5): 577–583.
65. Edwards H, Martin E, Nowygrod R. Nonoperative management of a traumatic peroneal artery false aneurysm. *J Trauma* 1982;22(4):323–326.
66. Parodi JC. Endovascular repair of aortic aneurysms, arteriovenous fistulas, and false aneurysms. *World J Surg* 1996;20(6):655–663.
67. Rosa P, O'Donnell SD, Goff JM, et al. Endovascular management of a peroneal artery injury due to a military fragment wound. *Ann Vasc Surg* 2003;17(6):678–681.
68. Toyota N, Kimura F, Yoshida S, et al. Peroneal artery aneurysm treated by transcatheter coil embolization and temporary balloon occlusion in Behçet's disease. *Cardiovasc Intervent Radiol* 1999;22(3):257–259.
69. Champion HR, Bellamy RF, Roberts CP, et al. A profile of combat injury. *J Trauma* 2003;54(suppl 5):S13–S19.
70. Gawande A. Casualties of war–military care for the wounded from Iraq and Afghanistan. *N Engl J Med* 2004;351(24):2471–2475.
71. Martin RR, Mattox KL, Burch JM, et al. Advances in treatment of vascular injuries from blunt and penetrating limb trauma. *World J Surg* 1992; 16(5):930–937.
72. Bosse MJ, MacKenzie EJ, Kellam JF, et al. An analysis of outcomes of reconstruction or amputation after leg-threatening injuries. *N Engl J Med* 2002;347(24):1924–1931.
73. Starnes BW, Beekley AC, Sebesta JA, et al. Extremity vascular injuries on the battlefield: tips for surgeons deploying to war. *J Trauma* 2006;60(2): 432–442.

CHAPTER 26 ■ ORTHOPAEDIC TRAUMA

JENS R. CHAPMAN, RICHARD J. BRANSFORD, AND CARLO BELLABARBA

KEY POINTS

1. Orthopaedic injuries occur in 70% of multiply injured patients and, of missed injuries, 75% are orthopaedic, which mandates systematic, thorough secondary and tertiary surveys. Delayed recognition leads to potential ongoing blood loss and associated secondary insults contributing to complications, such as pulmonary failure.
2. Life-threatening blood loss can occur secondary to long bone fractures, which are treated by realignment, splinting, and compression wrapping; pelvic ring disruption, treated by sheet wrapping to decrease pelvic volume and stabilize fractures; and spine fracture dislocations, treated with immobilization, realignment, and airway and vascular support. Open, bleeding wounds require direct intervention, including potential amputation or completion amputation.
3. Making the decision to amputate is difficult but preferable to saving a disabling, nonfunctional, or painful extremity. Loss of significant tissue, prolonged ischemia, and disruption of nerves plus scores, such as the Mangled Extremity Severity Score (MESS), aid in this decision.
4. Compartment syndromes are defined as inadequate tissue perfusion to meet oxygen requirements resulting from increased pressure in a confined anatomic space. The earliest reliable sign is excessive pain to passive or active movement of muscles in the compartment. Pressure monitoring with pressure differences between the compartment and diastolic pressure of less than 30 mm Hg require urgent operative decompression.
5. Major joint dislocations such as of the hip, femoral neck fracture, open fractures with contamination, talar neck fracture with dislocation, and thoracic fracture dislocations are common injuries with potential for long-term disability that require aggressive early intervention.
6. Spinal cord injuries are leading causes of long-term morbidity and mortality. Aggressive prevention programs, adequate recognition and resuscitation to optimize perfusion, and timely decompression and stabilization are required to optimize recovery. The use of steroids in the management of spinal cord injuries is no longer the standard of care.

The initial resuscitation phase of an acutely traumatized patient aims to identify and treat the immediately life-threatening conditions with priorities placed on maintaining or restoring airway, breathing, and circulation. Injuries to the head, chest, and abdomen receive undisputed priority in rationale-based trauma assessment and treatment algorithms. 1 Musculoskeletal injuries, which have more than a 70% incidence in multiply injured patients and a high potential for considerable long-term morbidity, if not addressed properly, play an important role in successful trauma management.[1] Systematic and effective incorporation of musculoskeletal treatment algorithms in trauma assessment and care can play a crucial role in improving long-term patient outcomes and decreasing mortality. On a conceptual basis, orthopaedic injuries can be differentiated into the three general impact categories: (a) life-threatening injuries, (b) limb-threatening injuries, and (c) injuries with adverse long-term functional implications.

To minimize the effects of musculoskeletal injuries on the care of trauma patients, implementation of a protocolized approach to diagnosis is helpful. Since approximately 75% of missed injuries are orthopaedic in nature, a systematic musculoskeletal systems evaluation is recommended.[2–5] Inadequate visualization of the region of injury or failure to perform a formal secondary or tertiary trauma survey are the most common causes of delay in diagnosis.

Initial musculoskeletal assessment of an acutely injured patient ideally is performed concurrently with the other components of the trauma patient evaluation, including serial documentation of vital signs and mental status and an anteroposterior radiograph of the pelvis, a lateral radiograph of the cervical spine, and an anteroposterior roentgenogram of the chest. Preferably, formal musculoskeletal systems assessment and initial care take place during the exposure of the patient, with palpation of the trunk and all extremities, manual realignment of deformed limbs, palpation of pulses, and detailed neurologic examination.[6] While maintaining full spine precautions using the multiperson team technique, a formal "log-roll" turn remains a standard procedure for full clinical trauma assessment at the earliest feasible time with full palpation of the axial spine from the occiput through the coccyx and denotation of direct or indirect injury signs. Open injuries and penetrating wounds are evaluated for their impact on the patient's vital functions and limb viability and then are dressed sterilely and splinted until definitive care is rendered. Appropriate antibiotic management for open fractures and tetanus immunization should be administered in the emergency setting. A systematic neurologic examination and documentation are preferably performed consistent with the published standards recommended by the American Spinal Cord Injury Association, including perianal and rectal examination for presence of blood, voluntary contraction, sensation, tone, and reflexes.[7] For all trauma patients a protocol for secondary and tertiary evaluation should be in place to minimize the occurrence and impact of delayed injury recognition. This is particularly important for patients with cognitive impairment and patients who have been removed from the normal trauma care evaluation algorithm because of exigent circumstances.

LIFE-THREATENING INJURIES

Musculoskeletal trauma may directly or indirectly lead to 2 patient demise on an acute, subacute, or delayed basis. Acutely life-threatening conditions may arise from large-scale blood loss seen with major arterial injuries in conjunction with long bone fractures, pelvic ring disruption, or spine fracture dislocations. Subacute life-threatening circumstances may result from occult blood loss with delayed recognition and response.[8] Delayed patient loss of life may occur as either a direct or indirect result of musculoskeletal injuries. Secondary pulmonary deterioration and sepsis after multiple fractures are leading causes of such delayed patient loss of life. Although the exact cause of posttraumatic sepsis and pulmonary deterioration remains incompletely understood and is likely multifactorial, the timing and technique of resuscitation and musculoskeletal injury treatment, including factors such as the duration of recumbence and immobility, undoubtedly play a considerable role in the onset and prevention of these serious events.[9–11]

Injuries to the musculoskeletal system may be of sufficient severity to cause acutely life-threatening hemodynamic instability because of hypovolemia or neurologic alterations. Injuries with disruption of vascular structures leading to acute or subacute hypovolemia include pelvic ring disruptions, multiple long bone fractures, traumatic forequarter or hindquarter amputations, scapulothoracic dissociations, and upper- to midthoracic-level fracture dislocations, as well as any form of distractive spinal column injury.[12–15] The blood loss in each of these injuries may be occult if the injury is closed. The source of bleeding may be of arterial, venous, or combined origin, which can dissect along soft tissue planes even at low pressures into larger recesses such as the retroperitoneal pelvis, thigh, chest, or lumbodorsal fascia plane. Thus, constant suspicion of this "third-spacing" phenomenon in conjunction with severe musculoskeletal injuries remains a major differential diagnosis of hypovolemia. Diagnostic modalities such as computed tomography (CT) scans or even plain radiographs can assist in identifying such abnormal fluid collections. Aggressive countermeasures in this setting may include simple bedside measures such as temporary pressure dressings, pelvic sheet application, and limb realignment and splinting.[16]

A major factor affecting mortality in musculoskeletal injury has arisen with the increasing care challenges for injuries to the elderly. The adverse relationship between survival beyond 1 year following trauma for patients 80 years or older in the presence of numerous comorbidities and certain injuries, such as hip fractures, type 2 odontoid fractures, and fractures in ankylosing spinal conditions, has become an increasingly well-documented public health concern. Large-scale outcome studies continue to define the role of early aggressive multidisciplinary management versus more palliatively directed management options for this increasingly aged segment of the population.[17–20]

However, currently for these two large populations—the multiply injured secondary to high kinetic forces and the very elderly with low-velocity mechanisms, multiple comorbidities, and relatively trivial orthopaedic injuries—improved survival outcomes appear to be primarily attributable to multispecialty care approaches. In turn, communication between the different specialties was found to be a critical contributor to improved patient survival in comparisons of level I trauma centers to community care centers in studies comparing results from fracture care in general and for thoracolumbar fractures specifically.[20,21]

A number of common injuries that potentially pose an immediate threat to patient survival are reviewed here.

Pelvic Ring Disruption

Open-book pelvic injuries, which characteristically consist of an anterior-posterior distractive separation of the anterior pelvic ring and external rotation of the pelvic wings, can be associated with massive diffuse venous plexus bleeding into the traumatically expanded lower abdominal cavity. Because of the typically venous nature of the associated substantial blood volume loss, attempts at stopping the hemorrhage with interventional angiographic embolization may frequently be futile. Emergent reduction and compression of this traumatically expanded space may, however, be an effective emergent management strategy. This procedure can be achieved with a number of percutaneous surgical intervention measures, such as external fixation or a pelvic clamp, which can be placed in an emergency room setting. More recently, simple application of a "pelvic sheet" has been introduced as a similarly effective noninvasive volume reduction strategy to reduce lower abdominal and pelvic volumes. This simple technique consists of wrapping a folded linen sheet around the affected patient's pelvic ring from posterior to anterior and then clamping it tightly in front (Fig. 26.1).[16] The realignment of the injured pelvis is assessed with an anteroposterior radiograph. Definitive surgical stabilization with one or more definitive management options, ranging from minimally invasive to open instrumentation techniques, can be deferred to a later time when resuscitation is completed.

Major Limb Injuries

Major blood loss may occur from proximal limb trauma such as open fractures; traumatic amputations such as forequarter

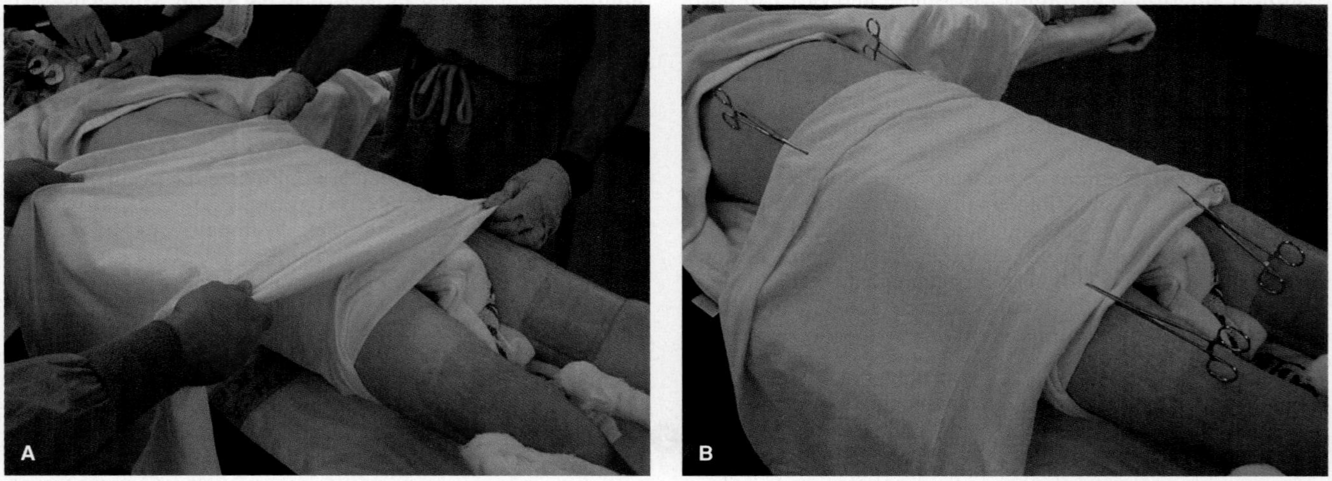

FIGURE 26.1. **A:** Application of pelvic sheet to provide external stability and reduce pelvic volume. **B:** Pelvic sheet in place swaddling patient's pelvis with application of pressure over both iliac wings and trochanteric area. The clamps are applied as cephalad, caudal, and lateral as possible to prevent obfuscation of subsequent imaging. Should groin access be necessary, the sheet may be fenestrated without significant compromise of the pelvic binding ability.

amputations; and closed disruptive injuries such as scapulothoracic dissociation.[21] Because bleeding commonly comes from arterial sources, emergent embolization following attempts at closed injury reduction and application of nonconstrictive compression dressings will frequently significantly reduce further blood loss. However, emergent operative intervention to control bleeding may have to be considered, especially in the presence of proximal limb or forequarter amputations.[14] Scapulothoracic dissociation injuries can be commonly identified on chest radiographs but may elude casual observation due to postinjury reduction. A combination of arterial injuries with venous bleeding in addition to brachial plexus disruption may pose a significant source of hemorrhage. If technically feasible, application of a chest–arm compressive spica dressing may limit fluid extravasation into the soft tissue planes of the torso. Should these measures prove unsuccessful, interventional angiography can prevent ongoing arterial bleeding. Surgical exploration of the injured shoulder girdle in a patient with known scapulothoracic dissociation is prone to significant hemorrhage in the acute setting and is not advisable.[12,13]

Spine Injuries

Life-threatening conditions may arise from several types of spinal column injuries. Upper cervical spinal cord or brainstem injury may be caused by bony or ligamentous disruption from the craniocervical junction through the C4 level. Patients with craniocervical injuries in particular are at risk for anoxia due to loss of respiratory drive secondary to concurrent brainstem or upper cervical cord injury. A particular worry in dealing with all spinal injuries is the potential for "occult" or underdiagnosed extent of spinal trauma, with potential for devastating consequences due to the delay in diagnosis. There are several potential spinal conditions typically overlooked. Spinal dislocations or ligamentous injuries may not be recognized on initial imaging tests because of a partial "rebounding mechanism" leading to a spontaneous, yet inherently unstable, skeletal reduction. Distractive spine injuries are especially worrisome due to their highly unstable nature and high propensity for associated neurovascular injury.[22] Other patients affected by critical but often occult or underappreciated spinal injuries are individuals whose spinal column has been subject to autofusion from a variety of conditions. Patients with ankylosing spondylitis, diffuse idiopathic skeletal hyperostosis (DISH), or high-grade spondylosis challenge clinicians due to their propensity to sustain subtle yet highly unstable injuries in the setting of their underlying complex anatomy. Due to the underlying disease processes, spinal injuries in this setting are more prone to increased bleeding and secondary displacement imposed by cantileverage of the fused spinal column above and below the injury zone.[18] In addition to delayed or secondary spinal cord injury, there have been reports of esophageal disruption or aortic injury as causes of delayed death or major morbidity in patients affected by ankylosing spinal disorders. Any form of distractive spinal injury or fracture in an ankylosing spinal disorder should result in expedient and aggressive immobilization to protect the spinal cord and column. Such temporizing measures can include placement of sandbags around the head and immobilizing the head with tape to provisional application of a halo ring and vest, unless contraindicated. For patients with the more common flexion-type cervical spine injuries, leading to jumped or perched facets or significant malalignment on lateral cervical radiographs, strong consideration should be given to urgent closed skeletal reduction under controlled circumstances. Acute reduction of cervical spine fracture dislocations in an emergency room setting prior to getting a magnetic resonance imaging (MRI) scan has been shown to be a safe and effective intervention for patients with spinal cord injury and may decrease the incidence and severity of secondary pulmonary insufficiency, acute respiratory distress syndrome (ARDS). Cervical traction to accomplish reduction of cervical fractures is the most commonly performed approach. Application of Gardner-Wells head tongs and sequential increase in weight along with intermittent neurologic evaluation is performed in a controlled environment that includes fluoroscopy and automated vital sign monitoring.[22] Contraindications to application of Gardner-Wells tongs include the presence of a skull fracture in the area of intended pin application and the presence of distractive-type neck injuries.

Spinal injury with secondary neurogenic shock should also be considered in the differential diagnosis of patients affected by sustained severe hypotension. This condition can result from fracture dislocations of the subaxial cervical spine or the upper thoracic spine with spinal cord injury and direct disruption of sympathetic nerve input (Fig. 26.2). Neurogenic shock

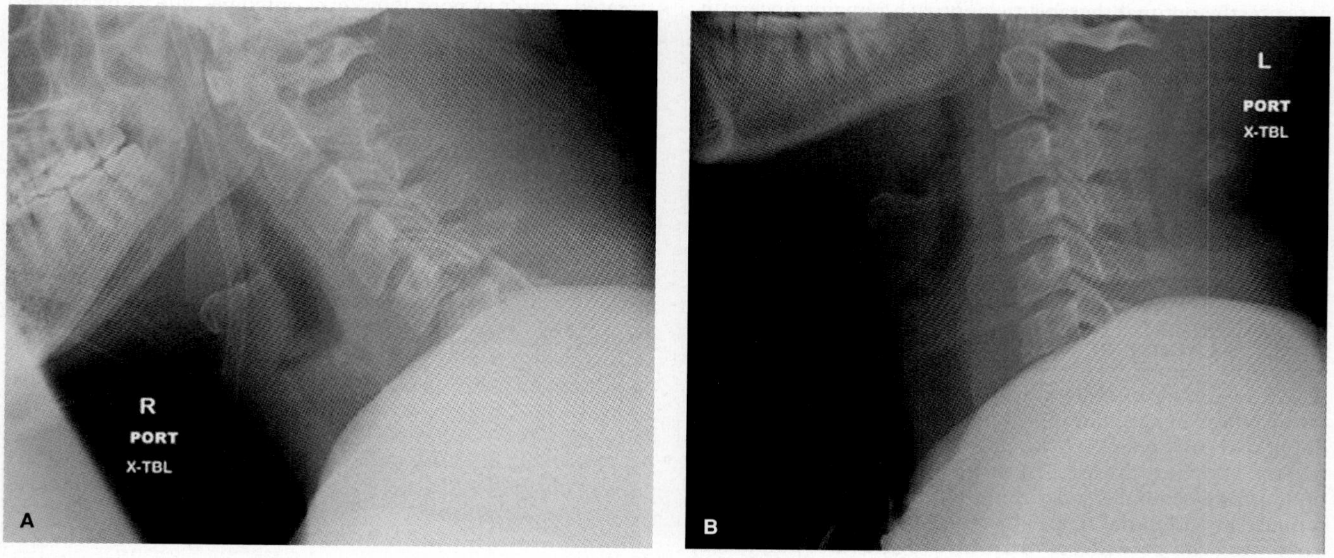

FIGURE 26.2. **A:** Initial lateral cervical radiograph of a young man after a motorcycle crash. He presented with paraplegia and neurogenic shock. Once the shock was under control, the next phase in care was rapid closed reduction of the cervical spine. **B:** Postreduction radiograph. Patient went on to definitive surgical stabilization at 48 hours after resuscitation and stabilization.

TABLE 26.1

COMPARISON OF NEUROGENIC AND HEMORRHAGIC SHOCK

■ PARAMETER	■ HEMORRHAGIC SHOCK	■ NEUROGENIC SHOCK
Blood pressure	⇓	⇓
Heart rate	⇑	⇓
Urine output	⇓	⇔
Skin	Pale, clammy	Warm, pink
Mental status	Anxious	Normal
Central venous pressure	⇓	⇓

is typically manifested by systemic hypotension with loss of peripheral vascular resistance, normal to increased urine output, a relative bradycardia, and warm, well-perfused extremities (Table 26.1). Protracted efforts at treating this condition with excessive intravascular fluid administration are usually unsuccessful and may lead to fluid overload and cardiopulmonary deterioration. Neurogenic hypotension or shock is preferably treated with intravenous pressors in addition to the judicious fluid resuscitation used to fill primarily dilated venous capacitance vessels. Correcting neurogenic hypotension permits the remainder of the workup to be completed safely, and perfusion and oxygenation of a damaged spinal cord are enhanced. Optimizing perfusion through appropriate resuscitation reduces the potential for enlarging the zone of primary spinal cord injury while enhancing any potential neurologic recovery.[23]

Respiratory dysfunction and failure as a result of prolonged supine bed rest in cervical traction or delayed mobilization due to spine trauma in general has been described repeatedly.[24–26] In addition, emergent surgery for spinal injury is commonly recommended for patients with neural compromise in association with highly unstable injury patterns that are unreducible by closed means.

While type 2 odontoid fractures constitute the most common type of spinal fracture requiring hospitalization in elderly patients, the optimal therapeutic approach remains uncertain. These fractures are frequently unstable and are associated with high mortality rates both in the acute and in the subacute phase of care, apparently irrespective of treatment choice. Similar to femoral neck fractures in the elderly, technical advances in fracture care have seemingly not improved survival rates or functional outcomes at 1 year after injury. Current treatment options range from an all-out aggressive multispecialty effort in patients deemed capable of returning to meaningful function to palliative care in those with poor outcome potential.[19,27]

Timing of Surgical Intervention

A lack of consensus remains as to the ideal timing of fracture stabilization in the multiply injured patient.[9] There is little doubt that early definitive skeletal stabilization can reduce secondary "fracture disease," such as pulmonary decompensation, thromboembolism, decubitus ulcers, and soft tissue compromise in an injured limb. However, untimely and extensive early surgical procedures may also aggravate pulmonary injury and dysfunction if the invasiveness of fracture stabilization surgery incurs hypovolemia and necessitates major fluid resuscitation.[21] Any secondary perioperative hypotension may also aggravate central nervous system and spinal cord injury as a major "second hit" phenomenon. In general, however, every reasonable attempt should be made to provide surgical débridement and some form of stabilization to high-grade open long bone and joint injuries.[28–30] Temporary stabilization of the pelvic ring—as outlined earlier in this chapter—can be a major resuscitation aid in an "open-book-type" pelvic ring injury.[16] And, specifically, stabilization of femoral shaft fractures within 24 hours specifically has been shown to reduce the rate of ARDS.[31]

The success of treatment of open fractures is closely related to the severity of soft tissue injury and the amount of primary bone loss. Limiting the timing to surgical débridement to within 8 hours has been proposed as a key variable to reduce the risk of osteomyelitis and delayed fracture union in tibial fractures in the past. However, the evolving current opinion is that the quality of the débridement is likely of far greater importance than compliance to a specific time frame for débridement.[32] Similarly, timing of thoracolumbar surgery for stabilization of acute fractures with or without spinal cord injury has been the subject of long-standing divergent opinions, with the definition of "early" still being subject to debate. While undeniably, respiratory distress and pneumonia remain the leading cause of death in spinal cord injury, there is some modest evidence suggesting that early surgery may enhance chances for spinal cord injury recovery or protect the patient from secondary neural injury. Additionally, the ability to mobilize a patient into an upright position early following injury may play an important role in reducing the risk of pulmonary decompensation and nosocomial pneumonia.[24–26]

In general, early surgical intervention for musculoskeletal trauma should be expedient and effective in stabilization while minimizing extent of surgical exposure, dissection-related blood loss, and anesthetic duration. There is a well-accepted advantage of integrating musculoskeletal trauma care into general trauma care efforts, with optimal communication between services necessary to best suit the care of an individual patient to his or her specific needs.[20]

LIMB-THREATENING INJURIES

Although the majority of orthopaedic injuries in trauma patients are not life-threatening, they may be a significant source of morbidity.[33] This is particularly true when the injury may directly lead to loss of limb or, if unrecognized or undertreated, result in poor long-term outcomes due to diminished function or chronic pain.[34] Injuries in which survival of the limb is immediately threatened include disruption of the major arterial blood supply, due to open fractures, from high-energy or penetrating trauma (Figs. 26.3 and 26.4). Furthermore, any

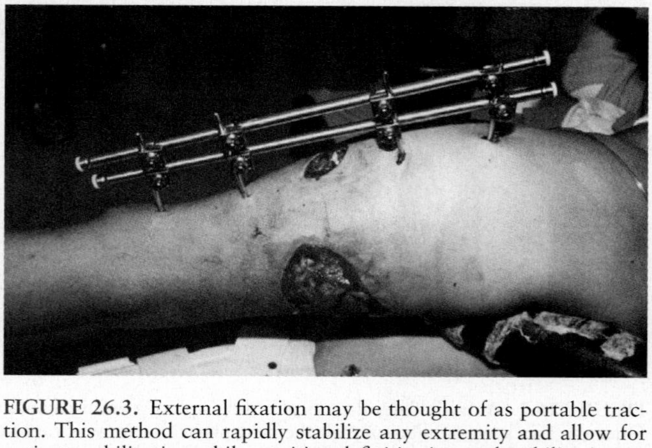

FIGURE 26.3. External fixation may be thought of as portable traction. This method can rapidly stabilize any extremity and allow for patient mobilization while awaiting definitive internal stabilization.

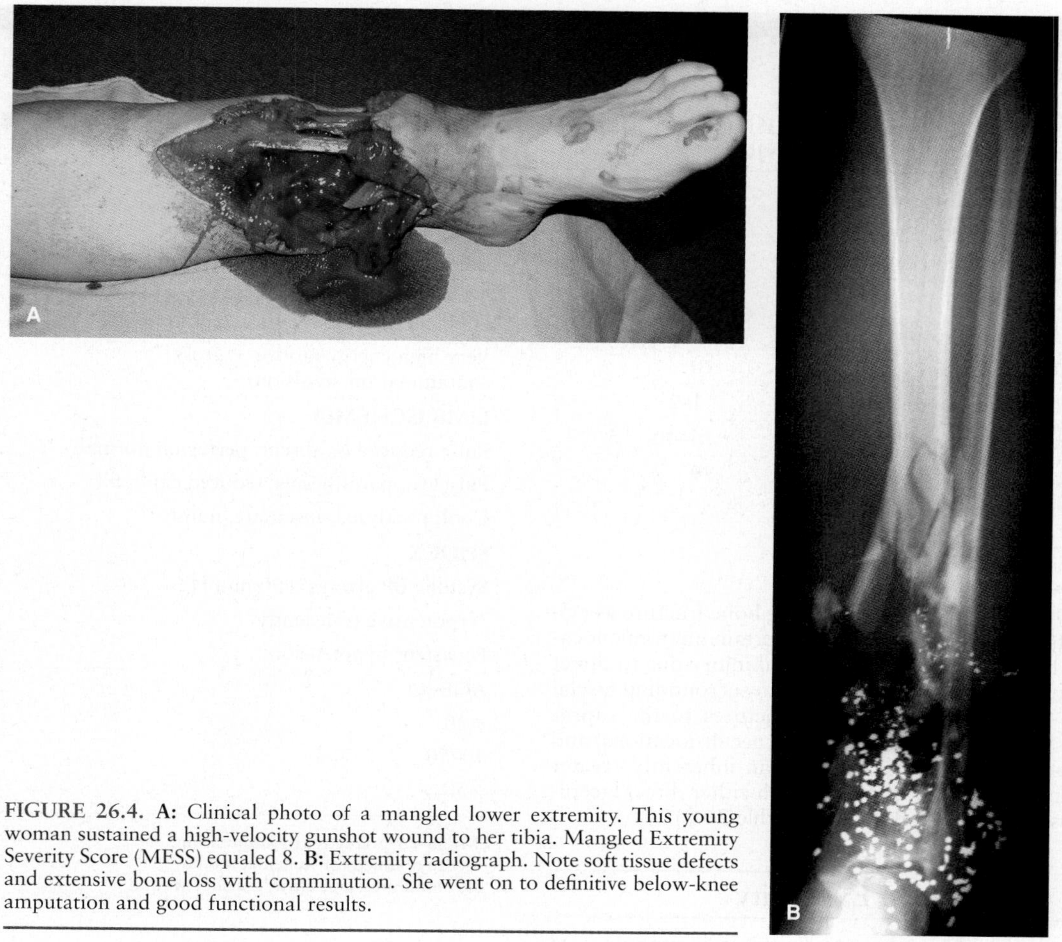

FIGURE 26.4. **A:** Clinical photo of a mangled lower extremity. This young woman sustained a high-velocity gunshot wound to her tibia. Mangled Extremity Severity Score (MESS) equaled 8. **B:** Extremity radiograph. Note soft tissue defects and extensive bone loss with comminution. She went on to definitive below-knee amputation and good functional results.

crushing or mangling-type limb injury may result in loss of blood supply on a delayed basis even in the absence of direct arterial injury due to diffuse intimal damage or through subsequent evolution of a compartment syndrome.

Efforts at identifying limb-threatening conditions early with appropriate clinical and radiographic evaluation allows for integration of expedient care for the threatened extremity within the larger treatment needs of the multiply injured patient. Timing of injury care in limb-threatening situations is highly time sensitive, with ischemic limb injuries usually requiring revascularization within 6 to 8 hours and release of symptomatic elevated fascial compartment pressures within a similar time frame.[35,36] However, distraction prompted by other injuries or impaired cognitive function by the patient may cause considerable delay in caring for a limb at risk. The most effective strategy is implementation of a formal secondary and tertiary trauma survey protocol in all high-risk patients.

Typical clinical signs of limb ischemia consist of disproportionate symptoms of pain and/or tenderness. Important clinical findings, which also require documentation during the initial evaluation, include findings of lacerations, bruising, swelling, and skin discoloration, along with any crepitus or excess tension of the soft tissue envelope on palpation. Finally, functional testing of joints, including range of motion and stability to stress, allows for a more integrated understanding of limb function. When possible, active range of motion with testing of manual resistance motor strength is obtained in nonobtunded patients. Clinical testing of perfusion of a traumatized limb ranges from simple palpation of pulses and assessment of skin color, temperature, capillary refill, and spontaneous blanching to more objective testing such as determining systolic ankle-brachial indices (ABIs), Doppler duplex evaluation of blood flow, and angiographic contrast studies.[35–37]

Although limb preservation is generally a preferred treatment goal by far, a timely and well-performed amputation may decrease the injury burden to critically injured patients, decrease acute multiple organ dysfunction, and improve long-term functional outcome. With present medical advances, limb salvage has become increasingly possible technically but at the cost of more surgeries and prolonged invalidity with very doubtful long-term functional gains. In contrast, excellent functional results can be obtained, especially in lower extremity amputations, with state-of-the-art amputee care. Therefore, amputation should not constitute a treatment failure but rather be considered a prudent treatment choice. This decision process is in drastic contrast to loss of limb resulting from an avoidable delay of diagnosis and/or failure to institute timely treatment.[38]

Vascular Injuries

After realignment of deformed limbs in a trauma patient, any potentially injured limb should have its vascular and neurologic status evaluated. Diagnosis of clinically significant vascular injury may be made by using the systolic ABI and/or confirming such by angiography if indicated. An ABI of greater than 0.9 is considered low risk for arterial injury, and immediate arteriography is not indicated.[35] In contrast, delay in the diagnosis of vascular injury following limb trauma with a warm ischemia time of 6 hours or more leads to a markedly increased rate of amputation.[37] Extremity trauma typical for an increased risk of vascular injury includes any penetrating

TABLE 26.2

RISK OF VASCULAR INJURY

LOCATION AND TYPE OF INJURY	RISK OF VASCULAR INJURY (%)
Proximal humerus fracture (open or closed, high energy)	<1
Femur shaft fracture (closed)	<1
Femur shaft fracture (open)	1.9
Tibia/fibula fracture (closed)	1
Tibia/fibula fracture (open)	10
Supracondylar femur fracture	1–2
Knee dislocation	16–40
Floating knee (ipsilateral femur and tibia fractures)	29

injury, open fracture, or high-energy long bone fracture as evidenced by history or fracture pattern. Certain anatomic locations have a higher prevalence for arterial injury due to direct proximity of bone or vascular tethering to surrounding fascial structures.[37] For instance, displaced fractures to the supracondylar femur and proximal humerus, knee dislocations, and scapulothoracic dissociations are all at an inherently greater risk of concurrent vascular injury through either direct laceration or by distractive intimal damage (Table 26.2).

Mangled Extremity

3 The descriptive term "mangled extremity" is commonly used to describe a limb injury with combined major soft tissue and high-grade osseous damage, with or without vascular injury, of such magnitude that limb survival is questionable even under the best of circumstances. The diagnosis of a mangled extremity is usually readily made by the dramatic nature of its clinical presentation. Feasibility of functional limb salvage, however, is far more difficult to ascertain in the acute setting and requires the ability to make difficult decisive treatment decisions with limited information. To aid in the decision-making process, several scoring systems have been proposed to help clinicians systematically review factors that play an important role in predicting outcomes. The most widely used of these scoring systems is the Mangled Extremity Severity Score (MESS; Tables 26.3 and 26.4).[39]

When the MESS is calculated to be greater than 7, consideration for primary amputation has been recommended. Attempts to salvage limbs with prolonged warm ischemia time, massive soft tissue contamination, neurologic injury, and skeletal instability may lead to not only increased morbidity but also overwhelming sepsis and death. Even if limb salvage has been successfully accomplished, long-term quality of life and functional outcomes scores have called into question the benefit to the patient of reconstructing highly traumatized limbs.[38]

Additional critical factors to consider before embarking on the reconstruction of a severely injured lower extremity are age, injury load on the patient, presence of comorbidities, severity of soft tissue injury and type of contamination, time to débridement, warm ischemia time, and integrity of neurologic function. In the lower extremity, the presence of severe ipsilateral foot trauma has been associated with extremely unsatisfactory functional outcomes and thus should sway the treating surgeon toward primary amputation.[40] Similarly, disruption of lower extremity nerves below the knee level with loss of protective sensation, primarily on the foot, usually indicates a poor outlook for most patients, regardless of reconstruction method.[41]

TABLE 26.3

MANGLED EXTREMITY SEVERITY SCORE (MESS)

PARAMETER	POINTS[a]
SKELETAL/SOFT TISSUE INJURY	
Low energy (stab, simple fracture, civilian GSW)	1
Medium energy (open/multiple fractures, dislocations)	2
High energy (crush injury, military GSW)	3
Very high energy (above + gross contamination, avulsion)	4
LIMB ISCHEMIA	
Pulse reduced or absent, perfusion normal	1*
Pulseless, paresthesias, reduced cap refill	2*
Cool, paralyzed, insensate, numb	3*
SHOCK	
Systolic BP always >90 mm Hg	0
Hypotensive transiently	1
Persistent hypotension	2
AGE (y)	
<30	0
30–50	1
>50	2

[a]MESS ≥7 predictive of amputation.
*Score doubled for ischemia >6 h.
BP, blood pressure; GSW, gunshot wound.

Diagnosis of neurologic injury in the extremity is often difficult in a multiply injured patient, and it may elude even the most thorough physical examination if the patient has an impaired cognitive status. Unfortunately, even advanced imaging studies such as MRI or electrophysiologic studies rarely provide accurate diagnostic data in the acute trauma setting. Specifically, electromyography would not be expected to show signs of neurologic injury until 3 weeks after injury. Therefore, a thorough clinical evaluation and/or direct surgical exploration of neural elements in case of surgical exposure of an affected nerve can be all the decision-making help that a treating physician may have. In contrast to the upper extremity,

TABLE 26.4

MANGLED EXTREMITY SCORING SYSTEMS

AUTHOR, YEAR	SCORING SYSTEM
Johansen et al., 1990 (MESS)	Mangled Extremity Severity Score
Howe et al., 1987	Predictive Salvage Index (PSI)
Russell et al., 1991	Limb Salvage Index (LSI)
McNamara et al., 1994	Nerve Injury, Ischemia, Soft Tissue Injury, Skeletal Injury, Shock, and Age Score (NISSA)
Tscherne et al., 1982 (HFS-97)	Hannover Fracture Scale-97

where repair of transected or avulsed neural elements has a reasonable chance of recovery, in the lower extremity this has been associated with significantly less-satisfactory rates of neurologic recovery and is rarely indicated. Therefore, in general, the boundaries of replantation or limb salvage attempts have a higher propensity toward the acceptable outcome in upper extremity trauma in contrast to severe injury in the lower extremities.

Compartment Syndrome

4 Compartment syndromes are defined as a mismatch between tissue perfusion and tissue oxygen requirements secondary to elevation of interstitial tissue perfusion pressure in an anatomically confined space. The most common site for compartment syndromes is the lower leg, with the posterior superficial and anterior compartments being most commonly affected. Other locations include the thigh, foot, and forearm. On occasion a compartment syndrome can also arise in the gluteal and psoas compartments. Pain medication, multiple injuries, impaired cognitive function, and bulky splints hinder accurate physical examination and thus prevent or delay detection of this condition. The earliest and most relevant warning sign of an evolving compartmental syndrome is pain out of proportion to that which is expected with passive stretch maneuvers of the muscles of the fascial compartment.[42] Other signs such as tension and local tenderness of the fascial compartment are variable and clinically not apparent in the thigh and gluteal region. Pallor, pulselessness, or neurologic signs such as paresthesia or weakness are ominous late signs of compartment syndrome and indicate prolonged ischemia in most circumstances. In patients for whom compliance with physical examination is diminished, a high degree of suspicion and vigilant monitoring is required. Invasive monitoring of intracompartmental pressures may provide information critical to surgical decision making if clinical examination is unobtainable, unreliable, or equivocal. The perfusion gradient (diastolic blood pressure minus compartmental pressure) in the monitored compartment should be greater than 30 mm Hg. If the perfusion gradient falls below 30 mm Hg, then the compartment is at a considerably elevated risk for ischemia and fasciotomy should be considered. The definitive treatment of pathologically elevated compartment pressure consists of a decompressive fasciotomy performed in a timely fashion. Presently, there are no fixed time guidelines regarding decompression of an evolving compartment syndrome. Depending on the affected anatomic region and a number of other variables, decompression within 6 hours from the time of insult is recommended for preservation of tissue.[43,44] Routine fasciotomies should also be considered after revascularization of a specific extremity or following other reperfusion conditions after a prolonged period of hypotension.[26–28]

Infection

There are multiple causes for posttraumatic infection. Aside from primary inoculation at the site of injury, the most common cause of infection in a trauma situation is presence of devitalized tissue. Adequate resuscitation efforts with maintenance of oxygenation and tissue perfusion pressures and judicious surgical débridement are important key steps in preventing musculoskeletal infection. Aside from host factors, effective early skeletal stabilization in combination with meaningful surgical débridement and supplemental antibiotic prophylaxis can decrease the likelihood of musculoskeletal infection. From an orthopaedic perspective, the expedient initial skeletal stabilization in an acutely injured patient is the most important adjuvant to decreasing the injury burden of a multiply injured patient. Specifically, intramedullary nails and temporary external fixation can expedite stabilization to permit improved mobility and care of patients with serious extremity trauma. Similar to the injured abdomen, the role of damage control surgery in orthopaedics, with limitation to only the most critical injuries and in an expedited approach, has become a popular concept and appears to be life and organ sparing in many cases; however, it remains subject to further validation.

INJURIES ASSOCIATED WITH LONG-TERM MORBIDITY

Certain injuries of the musculoskeletal system are associated with increased long-term morbidity if not treated expeditiously. Though not life threatening or limb threatening, these injuries may represent a considerable source of long-term daily disability for the traumatized patient after many of the most
5 severe injuries have healed. Major joint dislocations such as of the hip, femoral neck fractures, open fractures with contamination, talar neck fractures with displacement or dislocation, and thoracic fracture dislocations are examples of injuries with potential significant long-term disability and negative illness impact.

Hip dislocations can be identified on the initial anteroposterior pelvic trauma screening radiograph recommended by the Advanced Trauma Life Support (ATLS) protocol. For dislocations of the hip or fractures surrounding the femoral head and neck, early reduction and stabilization are desirable. Hip dislocations specifically should be viewed with urgency. Earliest feasible closed reduction followed by CT scan is a widely accepted standard of care. Vascular supply to the femoral head is tenuous and is derived largely from the vessels that reach the head after branching from the medial femoral circumflex artery. These vessels then travel through the posterior lateral aspect of the hip joint capsule as the posterior superior retinacular arteries. Prolonged dislocation of the femoral head leads to disruption of these retinacular arteries and may give rise to avascular necrosis (AVN) of the femoral head.[45,46] Anterior hip dislocations, though much less common, may lead to occlusion of the femoral artery with prolonged pressure from the displaced femoral head. Delay in reduction of this major joint dislocation also makes reduction progressively harder because of spasm-induced muscular contractions. CT of the pelvis following closed reduction of the hip is required to assess for articular debris. Presence of debris within the weight-bearing portion of the hip may lead to accelerated cartilage wear and arthrosis and should prompt consideration for early joint débridement through a suitable arthrotomy. Larger acetabular fragments may require stabilization through internal fixation to ensure congruent joint alignment.

Femoral neck fractures compromise perfusion of the femoral head by virtue of disruption of both vascular supply and outflow.[45,46] Early stable internal fixation with anatomic reduction and release of an intracapsular hematoma is associated with decreased incidence of AVN or nonunion of femoral neck fractures. Particularly in younger patients, few satisfactory reconstructive surgery options exist for either scenario. While for elderly patients primary hemiarthroplasty or immediate total hip arthroplasty has become the standard of care, posttraumatic hip arthroplasty in younger patients rarely provides a lasting treatment option.[45–47]

In general, any open fracture, regardless of contamination, requires formal débridement and irrigation. Removal of all foreign material and devitalized tissue at the earliest possible time has been shown to decrease the overall infection rate, both for acute wound infection and chronic osteomyelitis.[28–30] If the patient is too ill to have adequate débridement in an operating room environment, it should be done as thoroughly as possible in the resuscitation or intensive care arena. Internal fixation of fractures can then be safely performed after appropriate soft tissue management has occurred, which can also ultimately aid soft tissue healing.[29,30]

Displaced fractures of the talar neck with or without dislocation of the talar body are associated with a poor prognosis. Urgent reduction of the fracture or dislocation should be undertaken as soon as the diagnosis is made. If skin viability is compromised by underlying bone fragments and is not improved by closed reduction, immediate open reduction and fixation should occur. Although the presence of a talar neck fracture has been considered an indication for urgent operative reduction and stabilization in the past due to the potential for AVN, more recent studies have indicated that emergent surgical intervention may not affect the incidence of AVN. Operative débridement of open wounds and internal fixation of these injuries should be performed at the earliest reasonable time.[48–50] Delay of reduction of peritalar fractures or dislocations can be expected to lead to soft tissue breakdown, greatly increasing subsequent reconstruction challenges. Neglect of these fractures is associated with a higher incidence of AVN of the talus, subsequent severe arthrosis, and long-term disability.

Neurologic Injury

The presence of a neurologic deficit can be a major source of poor outcomes. Annually, there are approximately 11,000 new spinal cord injuries in the United States. While life expectancy of patients following thoracolumbar spinal cord injury and even higher levels of quadriplegia approximates that of their respective age cohorts, this injury entity still lacks an evidence-based proven treatment of choice. On the whole, no other condition affects patient outcome as profoundly as
6 spinal cord injury. At present, spinal cord injury therapeutic protocols follow four basic philosophies: (a) minimize the occurrence of preventable spinal cord injuries through education of the population at large and high-risk target groups specifically; (b) avoid secondary spinal cord injury or progression of injury through minimizing the occurrence of missed spinal column injuries; (c) optimize chances for spinal cord recovery through a number of measures including adequate resuscitation, timely decompression and stabilization of the spine, and pharmacologic measures aimed at reduction of swelling of neural membranes; and (d) implement a formal spinal cord rehabilitation program at the earliest possible time.[51] Highly publicized reports on breakthrough successes of treatment, including systemic hypothermia or stem cell therapies, are currently based more on opportunistic media reporting rather than objective medical evidence.[52]

Recovery from spinal cord injury is a highly variable and somewhat unpredictable occurrence. Injury mechanism, age, and health of the patient are major factors influencing the outcomes of spinal cord injury. To date there are no reproducible methods to achieve spinal cord regeneration. Pharmacologic treatment with methylprednisolone had been a widely followed practice in North America after several prominent studies. However, its ongoing routine use has become increasingly controversial due to questions about the study methodology and potential for serious adverse effects of treatment.[53,54] More than a decade after its widespread implementation, it has become apparent that the recommended high-dose intravenous application of 30 mg/kg methylprednisolone bolus given over 1 hour followed by a drip of 5.4 mg/kg per hour over 23 hours has not produced the anticipated dramatic change in the fate of most spinal cord injury patients. The administration of intravenous methylprednisolone has become a treatment option rather than a standard of care.[54] Unfortunately, for the foreseeable future there are no medical or cellular treatment regimens for spinal cord injury available outside of controlled clinical trials.

SUMMARY

The diagnosis and management of musculoskeletal injuries in the multiply injured patient population are often complex. Early recognition of injuries leads to diminished morbidity (both early and long term), earlier stabilization of patient hemodynamics, decreased length of stay in the intensive care setting, decreased rates of transfusion, earlier patient mobilization, and decreased mortality.[55] Improved understanding of how each organ injury complex of multisystem trauma impacts overall patient well-being will improve patient outcomes through enhanced, appropriate collaborative care and communication by the many specialists needed for an optimal outcome. While orthopaedic consultation may be readily available at major level I trauma centers, this is an increasing challenge in the greater community. Similarly, there is a significant trend toward improved survival in multiply injured patients and patients with concurrent thoracolumbar injuries when care is provided at level I centers. Overall, the orthopaedist treating multisystem trauma must understand the basics of general surgery trauma care, and the trauma surgeon needs to recognize, stabilize, and involve the orthopaedic surgeon early in the case of musculoskeletal trauma to optimize appropriate management and minimize morbidity and mortality.

References

1. Court-Brown CM. Care of accident victims. *Br Med J* 1989;298:115.
2. Davis JW, et al. The etiology of missed cervical spine injuries. *J Trauma* 1993;34:342.
3. Hanson DA, et al. Cervical spine injury: a clinical decision rule to identify high-risk patients for helical CT screening. *Am J Roentgenol* 2000;174:713.
4. Soundappand SV, et al. Role of an extended tertiary survey in detecting missed injuries in children. *J Trauma* 2004;57:114.
5. Brooks A, et al. Missed injury in major trauma patients. *Injury* 2004;35:407.
6. Stephen DJG, et al. Early detection of arterial bleeding in acute pelvic trauma. *J Trauma* 1999;47:638.
7. American Spinal Injury Association. *Standards of ASIA Standards for Neurological and Functional Classification of Spinal Cord Injury, Revised 1992*. Chicago, IL: American Spinal Injury Association; 1992.
8. Evers BM, et al. Pelvic fracture hemorrhage: priorities in management. *Arch Surg* 1989;124:422.
9. Pape HC, et al. The timing of fracture treatment in polytrauma patients: relevance of damage control orthopedic surgery. *Am J Surg* 2002;183:622.
10. Hildebrand F, et al. Damage control: extremities. *Injury* 2004;35:678.
11. Olson SA. Pulmonary aspects of treatment of long bone fractures in the polytrauma patient. *Clin Orthop* 2004;422:66.
12. Johansen K, et al. Traumatic scapulothoracic dissociation: a case report. *J Trauma* 1991;31:147.
13. Ebraheim NA, et al. Scapulothoracic dissociation (closed avulsion of the scapula, subclavian artery, and brachial plexus): a newly recognized variant, a new classification, and a review of the literature and treatment options. *J Orthop Trauma* 1987;1:18.
14. Hovius SE, et al. Acute management of traumatic forequarter amputations: case reports. *J Trauma* 1991;31:1415.
15. Dendrinos G, et al. Traumatic hemipelvectomy: a case report and comments on associated injuries. *Acta Orthop Trauma Surg* 1992;111:293.
16. Routt ML, et al. Circumferential pelvic anti-shock sheeting: a temporary resuscitation aid. *J Orthop Trauma* 2002;16:45.
17. Empara JP, Dargent-Molina P, Bréart G. Effect of hip fracture on mortality in elderly women: the EPIDOS prospective study. *J Am Geriatr Soc* 2004; 52(5):685–690.
18. Chapman JR, Bransford R. Geriatric spine fractures – an emerging health care crisis. *J Trauma* 2007;62(suppl 6):S61–S62.
19. Smith HE, Kerr SM, Maltenfort M, et al. Early complications of surgical versus conservative treatment of isolated type II odontoid fractures in octogenarians: a retrospective cohort study. *J Spinal Disord Tech* 2008; 21(8):535–539.
20. Haas B, Jurkovich GJ, Wang J, et al. Survival advantage in trauma centers: expeditious intervention or experience? *J Am Coll Surg* 2009;208:28–36.
21. Vale FL, et al. Combined medical and surgical treatment after acute spinal cord injury: results of a prospective pilot study to assess the merits of aggressive medical resuscitation and blood pressure management. *J Neurosurg* 1997;87:239.
22. Grant GA, et al. Risk of early closed reduction in cervical spine subluxation injuries. *J Neurosurg* 1999;90(suppl 1):13.
23. Hawryluk GW, Rowland J, Kwon BK, et al. Protection and repair of the injured spinal cord: a review of completed, ongoing, and planned clinical trials for acute spinal cord injury. *Neurosurg Focus* 2008;25(5):E14.

24. Krengel WF, et al. Early stabilization and decompression for incomplete paraplegia due to thoracic-level spinal cord injury. *Spine* 1993;18:2080.
25. McHenry TP, Mirza SK, Wang JJ, et al. Risk factors for respiratory failure following operative stabilization of thoracic and lumbar spine fractures. *J Bone Joint Surg Am* 2006;88(5):997–1005.
26. Chipman JG, Deuser WE, Beilman GJ. Early surgery for thoracolumbar trauma decreases complications. *J Trauma* 2004;56:52–57.
27. Frangen TM, Zilkens C, Muhr G, et al. Odontoid fractures in the elderly: dorsal C1/C2 fusion is superior to halo-vest immobilization. *J Trauma* 2007;63(1):83–89.
28. Gosselin RA, et al. Antibiotics for preventing infection in open limb fractures. *Cochrane Database Syst Rev* 2004;(1):CD003764.
29. Verhelle N, et al. How to deal with bone exposure and osteomyelitis: an overview. *Acta Orthop Belg* 2003;69:481–494.
30. Gustilo RB, et al. The management of open fractures. *J Bone Joint Surg Am* 1990;72:299.
31. Bone LB, et al. Early versus delayed stabilization of femoral fractures: a prospective randomized study, 1989. *Clin Orthop Relat Res* 2004;422: 11–16.
32. Al-Arabi YB, Nader M, Hamidian-Jahromi AR, et al. The effect of timing of antibiotics and surgical treatment on infection rates in open long bone fractures: a 9 year prospective study from a general hospital. *Injury* 2007; 38(8):900–905.
33. Myerson MS, et al. Morbidity after crush injuries to the foot. *J Orthop Trauma* 1994;8:343.
34. Bondurant FJ, et al. The medical and economic impact of severely injured lower extremities. *J Trauma* 1988;28:1270.
35. Mills WJ, et al. The value of the ankle-brachial index for diagnosing arterial injury after knee dislocation: a prospective study. *J Trauma* 2004;56: 1261.
36. Klineberg EO, et al. The role of arteriography in assessing popliteal artery injury in knee dislocations. *J Trauma* 2004;56:786.
37. Subasi M, et al. Popliteal artery injuries associated with fractures and dislocations about the knee. *Acta Orthop Belg* 2001;67:259.
38. MacKenzie EJ, et al. Functional outcomes following trauma-related lower-extremity amputation. *J Bone Joint Surg Am* 2004;86-A(8):1636–1645. Erratum in: *J Bone Joint Surg Am* 2004;86-A(11):2503.
39. Johansen K, et al. Objective criteria accurately predict amputation following lower extremity trauma. *J Trauma* 1990;30:568.
40. Hansen ST Jr. Salvage or amputation after complex foot and ankle trauma. *Orthop Clin North Am* 2001;32(1):181–186.
41. Grant GA, et al. Evaluation and surgical management of peripheral nerve problems. *Neurosurgery* 1999;44:825–839; discussion 839–840.
42. McQueen M, et al. Compartment monitoring in tibial fractures. The pressure threshold for decompression. *J Bone Joint Surg Br* 1996;78:99.
43. Heckman MM, et al. Compartment pressure in association with closed tibial fractures. The relationship between tissue pressure, compartment, and the distance from the site of the fracture. *J Bone Joint Surg Am* 1994;76:1285.
44. Brostrom LA, et al. Acute compartment syndrome in forearm fractures. *Acta Orthop Scand* 1990;61:50.
45. Tornetta P 3rd. Hip dislocation: current treatment regimens. *J Am Acad Orthop Surg* 1997;5(1):27–36.
46. Kregor PJ. The effect of femoral neck fractures on femoral head blood flow. *Orthopedics* 1996(Dec);19:1031–1036.
47. Bhandari M, Devereaux PJ, Swiontkowski MF, et al. Internal fixation compared with arthroplasty for displaced fractures of the femoral neck. A meta-analysis. *J Bone Joint Surg Am* 2003;85-A:1673–1681.
48. Vallier HA, et al. Talar neck fractures: results and outcomes. *J Bone Joint Surg Am* 2004;86:1616.
49. Canale ST, et al. Fractures of the neck of the talus. Long-term evaluation of seventy-one cases. *J Bone Joint Surg Am* 1978;60:143.
50. Hawkins LG. Fractures of the neck of the talus. *J Bone Joint Surg Am* 1970; 52:991.
51. McLain RF. Functional outcomes after surgery for spinal fractures: return to work and activity. *Spine* 2004;29(4):470–477; discussion Z6.
52. Kwon BK, Mann C, Sohn HM, et al. Hypothermia for spinal cord injury. *Spine J* 2008;8(6):859–874.
53. Bracken MB. Methylprednisolone and acute spinal cord injury: an update of the randomized evidence. *Spine* 2001;26(suppl 24):S47–S54.
54. Coleman WP, et al. A critical appraisal of the reporting of the National Acute Spinal Cord Injury Studies (II and III) of methylprednisolone in acute spinal cord injury. *J Spinal Disord* 2000;13(3):185–199.
55. Meek RN. Delaying emergency fracture surgery – fact or fad. *J Orthop Trauma* 2006;20(5):337–340.

CHAPTER 27 ■ PEDIATRIC TRAUMA

MARY E. FALLAT

KEY POINTS

1. Injury is the leading cause of death in children under 14 years of age and prevention, utilizing a public health model, is the most effective method to reduce deaths in children.
2. Community hospitals that stabilize injured children prior to transport to trauma centers commonly obtain unnecessary computed tomography imaging first and many of these children later require duplicate scans of the same anatomic region for various reasons, exposing the child to additional inappropriate risk and cost.
3. The injured child requires a patient- and family-centered approach to care. Increasingly, family members should be permitted during all phases of resuscitation and care.
4. The upper cervical spine is at increased risk for injury in the child because of a larger relative head mass and underdeveloped ligaments, and diagnosis is more challenging due to normal anatomic variants.
5. Plasticity of the thorax and transmission of kinetic energy to the lung make parenchymal injury such as pulmonary contusion more common and bony injury such as rib fractures less common.
6. Abdominal solid organ injury is unlikely to require surgery.
7. Hollow viscus injury is difficult to diagnose and requires a high index of suspicion, serial abdominal examinations, and select diagnostic studies, particularly with patterns of injury such as a "lap belt" contusion.
8. Children with unusual patterns of injury including retinal hemorrhages, multiple subdural hematomas without skull fracture, genital or perianal injury, burns in unusual places, and multiple new and old fractures mandate evaluation for inflicted trauma.
9. Although the child may have a higher survival rate following traumatic brain injury (TBI), the long-term negative impact of a minor TBI on learning and personal quality of life is much greater.
10. Children are emotionally vulnerable and follow-up should provide support to recognize and care for posttraumatic stress disorder in this population.
11. The Emergency Medical Services for Children (EMSC) program emphasizes a step-by-step approach to injury prevention by establishing goals and objectives with measurable outcomes.

EPIDEMIOLOGY

1 Unintentional injury is the leading cause of death among children ages 14 years and under in the United States and remains the greatest public health problem affecting young people.[1] Despite the fact that death and disability resulting from trauma surpass all major diseases in young Americans, far more federal funding is spent each year to reduce the incidence

of cancer, stroke, heart disease, and acquired immunodeficiency syndrome (AIDS) than injury.

Injury prevention is the most effective method of reducing death in children and adolescents.[2] The science of injury prevention is complex and involves societal decisions that trade safety for other benefits. For example, individual states have chosen both to raise the speed limit past 55 miles per hour to reduce travel time and to rescind motorcycle helmet laws to preserve individual freedom, rather than to protect the populace from increased death and disability due to vehicular crashes.[2] Health care workers can ultimately play a pivotal role in injury prevention by carefully documenting and collecting data regarding how injuries occur, which will serve dual roles of identifying populations at risk and providing compelling evidence to lawmakers in support of effective injury prevention legislation.

Trauma registries are one way to show trends or patterns of specific injuries and to use cumulative data to build a case for legislation. The National Pediatric Trauma Registry (NPTR)[3] and the National Trauma Registry of the American College of Surgeons (NTRACS)[4] are examples of national registries that have identified and can elucidate areas to target for prevention initiatives. The predominant mechanism of injury varies by age, with inflicted injuries most common in infants, falls more common in young children, pedestrian injuries in toddlers and elementary school-age children, and motor vehicle trauma in adolescents. Disparities in clinical and functional outcome have also been identified using registry data, providing opportunities for targeted initiatives. For example, worse outcome at discharge has been documented in black children after traumatic brain injury (TBI) compared with equivalently injured white children.[5,6]

Other disparities in pediatric trauma care deserve mention. Mortality rates for all types of trauma are greater in rural parts of the country than in cities and suburbs. The reasons for this are protean and include longer times from injury to definitive care,[7] in-hospital delays to definitive treatment,[8] less time for injury prevention education in schools and primary care offices, and socioeconomic and ethnic factors. Other associations have been identified that increase susceptibility to trauma. Children with behavioral disorders such as attention-deficit hyperactivity disorder (ADHD) have one and one-half times the odds of sustaining a variety of injuries from multiple causes than those without behavioral disorders, even after controlling for known demographic correlates.[9] Sometimes age works in favor of youth, with less morbidity after high-level falls in those 14 years of age and younger.[10]

The "trimodal" mortality curve described in adults is not seen in children. Children who die from injury do so either at the scene or within a few hours of hospital admission. Late deaths due to sepsis or organ failure are rare.[11] After injury control, prompt recognition and emergent treatment of life-threatening injuries are the most important ways to decrease death and disability caused by pediatric trauma. Whether or not outcome for a pediatric trauma victim is affected if care is rendered at a children's versus adult trauma center remains a somewhat controversial and unanswered question.[12]

PREHOSPITAL CARE

Pediatric runs represent approximately 10% of all prehospital emergency calls in the United States. Although educational courses such as Pediatric Education for the Prehospital Professional (PEPP)[13] and Pediatric Advanced Life Support (PALS)[14] have augmented the knowledge base of some prehospital providers, the recommended amount of pediatric training included in the U.S. Department of Transportation National Highway Traffic Safety Administration Emergency Medical Technician-Paramedic National Standard Curriculum is temporally limited and basic. The adequacy of prehospital airway management and the ability to obtain venous access in children by individual providers are associated with proper training, experience, skill maintenance, and online and offline medical oversight for prehospital care services.[15,16]

A goal of pediatric prehospital care is to prevent secondary brain injury associated with hypoxia or hypotension by controlling the airway and striving for normocapnia and normotension with appropriate fluid resuscitation. All ambulances must be equipped with pediatric equipment in various sizes, including blood pressure cuffs, masks, endotracheal tubes, and intravenous (IV) access devices.[17] Prehospital care of injured pediatric patients for short transports may be limited to maintaining spinal precautions, assurance of an adequate airway, administration of oxygen, and rapid transport to definitive care. Placement of a definitive airway and establishment of IV or intraosseous (IO) access is recommended for longer transport times.

An inclusive trauma system must provide for the needs of injured children as well as adults, with triage by the prehospital provider to the closest appropriate facility with the capabilities of caring for major trauma. This may be a free-standing pediatric trauma center or a regional trauma center with a verified pediatric component.[18] The receiving center must have the necessary personnel and equipment to care for the injured child, as outlined in *Resources for Optimal Care of the Injured Patient: 2006* by the American College of Surgeons Committee on Trauma.[19] Despite evidence for improved outcomes of severely injured children admitted to high-level trauma centers, almost one third of children with severe TBI fail to receive care in such centers and regionalization efforts in many parts of the country are still in their infancy.[20]

INITIAL RESUSCITATION AND EVALUATION

Preparation is the key to a successful pediatric trauma resuscitation. In institutions using a team approach, interventions may be done simultaneously (i.e., for airway and circulation).

The best protection for the airway in the child who is breathing spontaneously is maintenance of a superior and anterior position of the midface (sniffing position), while keeping the cervical spine immobilized. If the airway is inadequate, it can be opened with a gentle jaw thrust. The mouth is cleared of blood and foreign material and supplemental oxygen is used. In a young child, respiratory compromise can result from gastric dilatation or from compression of the diaphragm by intra-abdominal blood or air, necessitating the use of a gastric tube. The tube should be inserted orally if there is concern for a basilar skull or midface fracture.

Children with obvious respiratory distress, those with a Glasgow Coma Scale (GCS) score of less than or equal to 8, or those who arrive in shock must have immediate tracheal intubation. The proper-size endotracheal tube can be estimated by choosing one that corresponds to the diameter of the child's small finger or the external nares or using an appropriate reference as a guide. An excellent approach is the use of color-coded drawers containing all of the equipment necessary for a certain-size child and using a length-based pediatric resuscitation tape to estimate the child's weight.[21] In children younger than 8 years, nasotracheal intubation is avoided because of the more anterior and cephalad positioned airway, relatively large adenoids and tonsils, a soft short trachea, and the potentially serious complications associated with blind nasal passage. After preoxygenation, a pharmacologically assisted intubation using a neuromuscular blocker and a sedative is performed, unless the child has a GCS of 3 or has arrested. A chest radiograph should be obtained to confirm proper position of the endotracheal tube. If the airway cannot be secured by the most senior person in the resuscitation room, a temporizing needle cricothyrotomy is placed and jet insufflation initiated until an

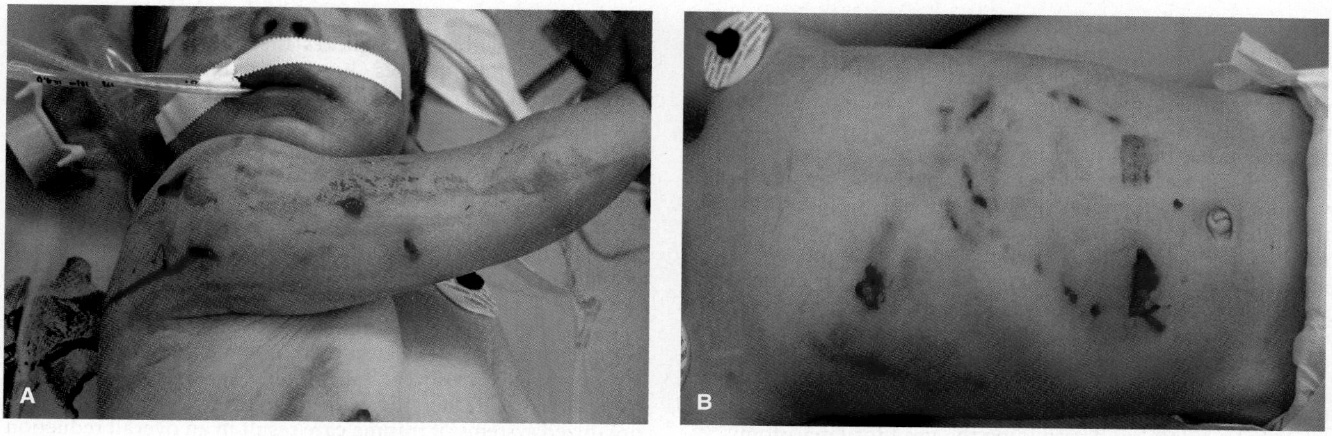

FIGURE 27.1. Child with multiple dog bites on face, extremities, and torso.

airway can be established in the operating room. Tracheostomy in young children is reserved for experienced surgeons under operating room conditions only.

Because of small blood volumes in children, shock can occur rapidly from blood loss from external wounds (Fig. 27.1). Bleeding should be controlled with pressure bandages. Preferred sites for percutaneous IV access in the child are the back of the hand, the antecubital fossa, and the saphenous vein at the ankle. If a child is in shock, and no IV line can be established after two attempts, an IO needle is placed in an uninjured proximal tibia. Alternatively, a percutaneous femoral venous line can be placed by an experienced physician. It is important to follow a protocol so that time is not wasted with too many attempts at percutaneous IV access before resuscitation can begin. Baseline laboratory work can be drawn concurrent with establishing IV access, including a complete blood count (CBC), serum aspartate aminotransferase, and amylase. A urinalysis is done if there is occult blood in a urine dip for blood. A clot to hold or type and cross match is sent to the blood bank as indicated by the physiologic status of the child. An arterial blood gas is sent if the child required tracheal intubation. A prothrombin time (PT) and partial thromboplastin time (PTT) are indicated for a GCS below 13, low systolic blood pressure, open/multiple bony fractures, and major soft tissue wounds.[22] There are no routine laboratory tests that have utility as good screening tools for pediatric abdominal trauma.[23]

A child's systolic blood pressure should be at least 70 mm Hg plus twice the age in years.[14] In general, a blood pressure of less than 70 mm Hg systolic is considered shock in a child, with the exception of small infants. Hypotension is a late sign of shock because of increased physiologic reserve in children compared with adults. The initial signs of shock can be subtle in a child and manifested only by tachycardia or lethargy. Once hypotension has developed, a child has already lost approximately 40% of the circulating blood volume and traumatic arrest is imminent if treatment is delayed.

Fluid resuscitation begins with 20 mL/kg of warmed isotonic crystalloid given by rapid IV/IO push. This is approximately one fourth of the blood volume of a child. This fluid bolus can be repeated twice, but if the child remains in shock, the source of bleeding should be quickly identified and addressed. Transfusion of O-negative packed red blood cells may be needed at an initial volume of 10 mL/kg. A Foley catheter should be inserted, assuming no blood at the urethral meatus or an unstable pelvic fracture. In addition to reestablishing normotension, a proper response to resuscitation includes slowing of the heart rate, return of extremity skin color and warmth, clearing of the sensorium, and a sustained urine output of 1 to 2 mL/kg per hour.

Small children are especially prone to hypothermia, which may render the child unresponsive to resuscitation efforts. Use of convective air blankets, warm IV fluids, and warm blankets is indicated as soon as feasible.

During the resuscitation, radiographic studies of the chest and pelvis are performed and cervical spine protection is maintained until age-appropriate views can be obtained (anteroposterior, lateral, and odontoid). It is difficult to obtain an open-mouth odontoid view in an infant or young child.[24] Clearing of the cervical spine is relatively elective; time should not be wasted on these films if other injuries take priority. In the hemodynamically unstable child, a quick sonographic evaluation of the pericardium and the peritoneum (the focused sonographic assessment for trauma [FAST] examination) for blood can be helpful in establishing the priorities of treatment. Blood in the pericardial or peritoneal cavity in the persistently unstable child demands surgical intervention. In the physiologically normal child, a computed tomography (CT) scan of the abdomen and pelvis with IV contrast is indicated in certain sit-
2 uations (Table 27.1). In this era of increasingly fast and sensitive radiographic testing, the multidetector-row CT has gained popularity, as has the total-body CT. There are three arguments against the routine use of total-body CT in children: (a) the medical radiation burden and increased cancer induction risk, (b) cost-effectiveness, and (c) the risk of pseudodisease with overinterpretation of clinically unimportant findings.[25] Community hospitals that stabilize injured children prior to transport to trauma centers commonly obtain CT imaging first. Many of these children later require duplicate scans of the same anatomic region for various reasons (scan inadequate or not sent with the patient, computer software incompatible, hard copies sent with inadequate tissue window images to allow assessment), exposing the child to additional risk and cost.[26]

TABLE 27.1 INDICATIONS/CONTRAINDICATIONS

INDICATIONS FOR COMPUTED TOMOGRAPHY OF THE ABDOMEN AND PELVIS

- History of shock but now stable
- Unexplained drop in hematocrit
- Positive FAST examination
- Presence of hematuria
- Presence of lower rib or pelvic fractures
- Unreliable abdominal examination because of head injury
- Presence of abdominal pain/ecchymosis
- Uncorrected base deficit

FAST, focused sonographic assessment for trauma.

Although ultrasound is reasonably sensitive in detecting the presence of fluid in the abdomen, its accuracy is highly dependent on the operator. Some data suggest that hospital resources are conserved when the FAST examination is incorporated into the algorithm in the evaluation of the pediatric abdomen after blunt trauma.[27] Ultrasound, however, may not detect the presence of intraparenchymal solid organ injuries without free blood, may miss small amounts of blood early in the resuscitation, cannot be used to grade the degree of injury to a solid organ, and cannot exclude pancreatic or bowel injury. In addition, the finding of blood in the peritoneum in a stable child does not dictate laparotomy. For all of these reasons, the role of FAST in pediatric trauma patients remains controversial. Neither ultrasound nor CT reliably detects the presence of a bowel injury. Serial abdominal examinations are indicated, and a diagnostic peritoneal lavage (DPL) may occasionally be helpful in determining the need for laparotomy.

Throughout this critical period of resuscitation and evaluation, there are a few additional focused needs of children to consider. One is the management of pain, which is often overlooked, even when pain scale charts or prompts are used.[28] Another is the emotional needs of the child. A frightened child is emotionally labile and may regress to infantile behavior. A calm and reassuring approach with attempted explanation of procedures gains the most cooperation. There is evidence that the psychological effects surrounding a traumatic event are long lasting, even if the trauma is relatively minor. The needs of the "injured" family must be met by providing a continual flow of information to the distressed parents or guardian during the resuscitation. A chaplain or member of the family support services staff can admirably serve this vital role on a pediatric trauma team. There is now a body of literature providing advice on "breaking bad news."[29–32]

3 In addition, with the shift in medical training from disease-centered to patient-centered and family-centered care, there has been increasing interest in and allowance of family presence during invasive procedures and cardiopulmonary resuscitation.[33,34] Although this concept has had limited exposure in the emergency pediatric trauma setting, family members often desire to be present and are more accepting of death and more satisfied with the level of care that their loved one received if they witness the events of the resuscitation.[35] Pediatric health care workers who have more frequent contact with seriously ill children are more likely to accept parental presence.[34]

MANAGEMENT OF SPECIFIC INJURIES

Neurologic and Extracranial Head Trauma

Traumatic brain injury is the leading cause of traumatic death and disability in children. The annual clinical burden remains high, with 50,658 TBI-associated hospitalizations in 2000 and a corresponding financial burden of $1 billion.[36] Unfortunately, the majority of the proinflammatory response caused by TBI occurs within 6 hours of injury, making early treatment initiatives challenging. Multiple pathways contribute to the endpoint of hypoxic ischemic injury, and a host of clinical trials evaluating single-modality translational treatment strategies have yielded uniformly disappointing results with no intervention resulting in improved outcome.[37] The National Institutes of Health (NIH) is currently promoting prospectively designed studies that will employ multiple therapeutic agents in combination. Emerging strategies that may be considered include hypertonic saline resuscitation, hypothermia, and cellular therapeutics (bone marrow progenitor cell therapy).[38] Each has its own inherent benefits, risks, and complications, and hypertonic saline and hypothermia ideally need to be started very soon after injury. Most treatments for TBI are designed to mitigate the secondary effects of the initial injury. Progenitor cell therapy explores the potential of reparative treatments and involves harvesting bone marrow from patients with severe TBI within a few days of injury, separating the cells, and reinfusing progenitor cells.

Treatment guidelines for the acute prehospital and the acute medical management of severe TBI in infants, children, and adolescents have been published, with the goal of assimilating the data that exist and presenting them within an evidence-based framework.[39,40] The methodology revealed a significant dependence on information derived from the adult population or personal experience due to a paucity of high-quality clinical trials in brain-injured children, thus limiting the strength of the recommendations. However, there is some evidence that pediatric patients with severe TBI should be treated in a pediatric trauma center rather than an adult trauma center and that organized systems of trauma care result in an overall reduction in the mortality rate for individuals with severe TBI.[12] The following represent reasonable initiatives or strategies based on the clinical evidence that exists.

Primary treatment of a child with a TBI preferably begins at the scene of the injury with correction of hypoxemia and shock by restoring oxygenation, ventilation, and perfusion. Supplemental oxygen should be administered. There is no evidence to support an advantage of endotracheal intubation (ETI) over bag valve mask (BVM) ventilation for the prehospital management of the airway in children with TBI who have short transport times to the hospital.[41] If prehospital ETI is instituted for pediatric TBI patients, specialized training and use of end-tidal CO_2 detectors is considered necessary. The airway should be secured in patients who have severe head injury (GCS <9), the inability to maintain an adequate airway, or hypoxemia not corrected by supplemental oxygen. Hypocarbia (partial pressure of arterial carbon dioxide [$PaCO_2$] <30 to 35), due to excessive ventilation in an emergent situation from large manual tidal volumes and rates, correlates directly with decreased functional outcomes from TBI and must be avoided. Hypotension should be identified and corrected as rapidly as possible with fluid resuscitation. Hypotension is defined as systolic blood pressure below the fifth percentile for age or by clinical signs of shock. The lower limit of systolic blood pressure (fifth percentile) for age may be estimated by the following formula: 70 mm Hg + (2 × age in years).[14] A retrospective study evaluating the temporal relationship of hypotension to severe TBI found that a poor discharge Glasgow Outcome Score was predicted by hypotension occurring during the first 6 hours after injury.[42]

A thorough neurologic examination is performed and documented, including the GCS score. The verbal portion of the score has several adaptations for application in infants and toddlers (Table 27.2), but it is the motor score that correlates

TABLE 27.2 CLASSIFICATION

PEDIATRIC VERBAL SCORE

VERBAL RESPONSE	VERBAL SCORE
Appropriate words or social smile, fixes and follows	5
Cries but consolable	4
Persistently irritable	3
Restless, agitated	2
None	1

Adapted from American College of Surgeons Committee on Trauma. *Advanced Trauma Life Support Course for Doctors: Student Course Manual*, 7th ed. Chicago, IL: American College of Surgeons; 2004:257.

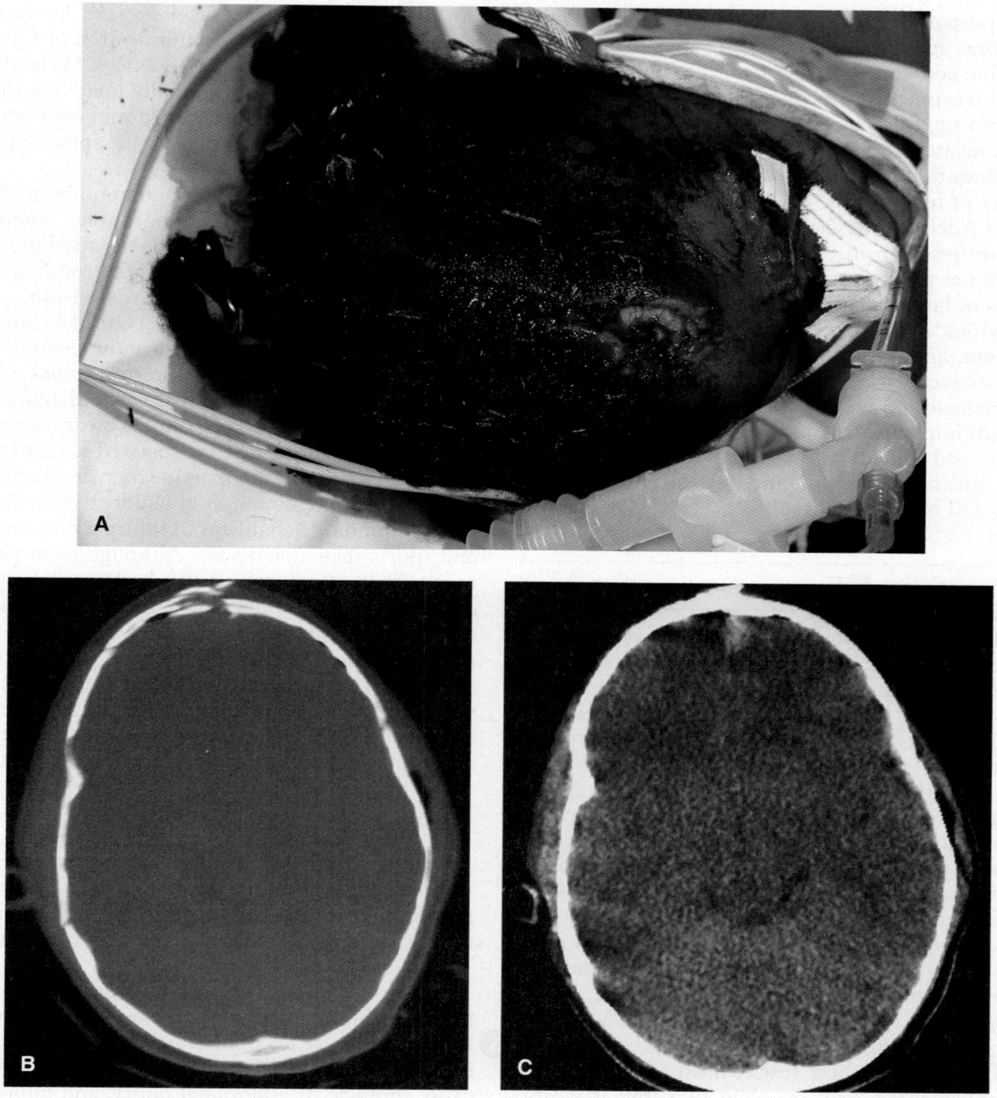

FIGURE 27.2. **A:** Scalp wound with underlying open frontal skull fracture. **B:** Bone window computed tomography image showing comminuted frontal skull fracture, pneumocephaly, and multiple additional skull fractures. **C:** A small frontal contusion is seen beneath the skull fracture.

best with outcome. Except for the most minor cases, a head CT scan is performed in all children with evidence of neurologic injury (Fig. 27.2). For those with severe TBI, serial scans ordered for increased ICP and neurologic deterioration best correlate with the need for operative intervention.[43]

Secondary measures to treat TBI in children include evacuation of an intracranial space-occupying hematoma, normalization of intracranial pressure (ICP), maintenance of tissue oxygenation, external ventricular drainage, and decompressive craniectomy in rare cases of conservative treatment failure.[44,45] Although mass lesions from hemorrhage requiring surgical intervention are relatively uncommon in children, cerebral edema is common and deserves treatment. Children with a GCS score of 8 or less and those with evidence of cerebral edema on CT scan are best managed with sedation, paralysis, endotracheal intubation, and mechanical ventilation to keep the $PaCO_2$ at approximately 35 mm Hg. Prophylactic hyperventilation has the potential to reduce cerebral blood flow to damaged or marginal brain tissue to ischemic levels. In a retrospective cohort analysis of significant pediatric TBI done after publication of the 2003 acute TBI medical management guidelines, the incidence of severe hypocarbia decreased but remained relatively high and predicted mortality.[46]

Evidence exists showing poorer outcomes with sustained ICP greater than 20 mm Hg, making ICP-guided therapy potentially beneficial.[47] For example, an ICP transducer (or ventriculostomy catheter) can be placed (with the exception of young infants with open cranial sutures) and therapy targeted to maintain ICP less than 20 mm Hg and a cerebral perfusion pressure of at least 40 to 65 mm Hg. Hyperosmolar therapy with either mannitol or hypertonic saline is an effective first-line option for controlling ICP. However, mannitol leads to a significant diuresis and potential subsequent volume requirement. Brain metabolism is minimized by treating fever and avoiding seizures. The use of anticonvulsants early may be associated with reduced mortality.[48] The occurrence of posttraumatic seizures and epilepsy increases with injury severity, younger age, and longer follow-up duration, and both are associated with adverse outcome.[49] Despite aggressive treatment, the overall mortality rate from severe head injury in pediatric patients is approximately 8%, and the coexistence of extracranial injury significantly reduces recovery potential.[50]

The significant reported variation in the use of paralytic agents, seizure medications, induced hypothermia, and intracranial pressure monitoring across pediatric critical care units suggests that standardized treatment protocols should be implemented so that more meaningful data can be accrued.[48,51] Other authors have enunciated the importance of establishing age-dependent guidelines that cover the spectrum of TBI management and recovery of function.[52]

Jankowitz and Adelson[53] describe five key areas for prioritization and future research in pediatric TBI: (a) prevention, including educational programs in combination with mandatory interventions or laws that are directed at sports programs, recreational activities, and vehicular modifications; (b) development, assessment, and implementation of a standard initial assessment tool to accurately define the severity of TBI and facilitate management; (c) use of multimodality, monitor-guided therapy; (d) implementation of an algorithm that standardizes anatomic and functional imaging at designated intervals to provide meaningful data; and (e) development of pediatric-specific TBI outcome measures.

Spinal Trauma

The incidence of pediatric spine injuries has been reported as 2% to 5% of all spine injuries.[54,55] Spinal trauma is frequently associated with concomitant system injuries including head, abdominal, and thoracic injuries and long bone fractures.[56] Head injury is the most common injury associated with spinal trauma. Any patient suspected of having a spinal injury must be immobilized until the entire vertebral column and spinal cord have been assessed. Spine injuries after minor trauma in children are less common than in adults because of the greater mobility and elasticity of the pediatric spine and a smaller body mass. However, the ligamentous laxity and increased mobility in the immature spine may predispose to lethal distraction injuries during forceful trauma.[57] Spinal trauma may occur with or without spinal cord injury (SCI). The mechanisms of SCI can be broadly classified as axial loading, dislocation, lateral bending, rotation, and hyperflexion/hyperextension. Severe injuries often result from a combination of these.[58] The CT scan is the best test to evaluate persistent symptoms or abnormalities seen on plain film, but it is not required as often as it is performed and poses a radiation risk. A CT "topogram" or scout film may be helpful to localize areas that need to be scanned.[24] The use of an algorithm to determine which patients need plain films and which patients need more thorough evaluation may be helpful.[59,60] Magnetic resonance imaging (MRI) should be performed to evaluate for clinical signs or symptoms of SCI.[58]

4 Certain anatomic features predispose younger children (age younger than 8 years) to injury of the upper cervical spine, from the occiput to C3.[61] These include a proportionately heavier head and weaker ligaments that permit greater mobility of C1 on C2 compared with the lower spine; horizontally inclined articulating facets and immature vertebral joints that facilitate sliding; growth centers that are susceptible to shear forces during rapid deceleration or hyperflexion-extension; and a higher fulcrum of flexion.[61] The fulcrum of cervical movement is located higher in young children (C2-3) compared to adolescents and adults (C5-6). In children older than 8 years, cervical spine fractures are primarily seen caudal to C4.[61] As a result of the anatomic and biomechanical differences between the immature pediatric spine and the mature adult spine, 60% to 80% of all pediatric vertebral injuries occur in the cervical region.[58]

Some normal anatomic variables make interpretation of cervical spine films in children challenging and misdiagnosis or misinterpretation common.[61,62] Pseudosubluxation occurs normally in approximately 19% to 40% of children and is most commonly seen as anterior displacement of C2 on C3 but can also be seen at the C3-4 level.[61] An increased distance between the dens and the anterior arch of C1 may also occur without any pathologic consequences. Skeletal growth centers may resemble fractures, especially involving the odontoid and the spinous processes. If there is doubt over whether an abnormality exists, it is wise to protect the spine until expert consultation can be arranged.

An abnormality seen more commonly in children is spinal cord injury without radiographic abnormality (SCIWORA).[61,63] This phenomenon is attributed to the elastic nature of the child's spine and may result from longitudinal distraction, hyperflexion, hyperextension, or spinal cord ischemia. The five specific SCI clinical syndromes that have been described in SCIWORA are the central cord syndrome, Brown-Sequard syndrome, anterior spinal artery syndrome, partial SCI, and complete SCI.[58] The diagnosis is established by MRI, and prognosis for recovery after a complete SCI may be poorer than after a SCI associated with a fracture.[57]

Thoracic and lumbar spine injuries including multilevel injuries are more common in children older than 9 years. The most common mechanisms of injury are motor vehicle crashes and sports-related activities. Although most patients with thoracolumbar spinal trauma can be treated conservatively, indications for surgery include persistent instability, significant compression fracture of the vertebral body, spinal kyphotic deformity of more than 20 degrees, vertebral dislocation, and spinal cord compression associated with progressive neurologic symptoms.[56] Some pediatric patients with devastating spinal cord injuries can recover substantial neurologic function. High-dose steroid therapy for spinal cord injury is controversial.[64–66]

Thoracic Trauma

Thoracic trauma is seen in 4% to 6% of children presenting to pediatric trauma centers and rarely occurs in isolation.[67] Mortality risk is increased due to associated injuries, particularly TBI.

There are important anatomic and physiologic differences between children and adults who present with thoracic injury.
5 Rib fractures are uncommon in children because the chest wall is more compliant. Displaced rib fractures can occasionally cause thoracic or abdominal injury, and multiple rib fractures are associated with increased morbidity and mortality. Posterior rib fractures in infants have a high association with inflicted trauma. Aortic and great vessel injuries are uncommon because of greater vessel elasticity and mobility of mediastinal structures. Enhanced pulmonary vasoconstriction results in less bleeding.

The most common injuries in children are pulmonary contusion, hemothorax, and pneumothorax. Pulmonary parenchymal injury following blunt trauma may result from direct compression, shearing forces, contrecoup compression, or laceration from fractured ribs. Chest radiography is the primary screening modality for thoracic injury, both to identify life-threatening injuries and to locate tubes and catheters (Fig. 27.3). Pulmonary contusion is characterized by areas of alveolar and interstitial hemorrhage and edema that appear as ill-defined opacities that do not follow anatomic boundaries.[68] Secondary edema from disruption of the alveolar-capillary interface peaks at 24 to 36 hours following injury, and the radiographic appearance of the lungs may worsen over the first several days. Pneumothorax and pneumomediastinum most commonly occur following alveolar or small airway rupture. Air dissects medially along peribronchial tissues toward the mediastinum or pleural space. If the air dissection is extensive, increased air pressure shifts the flexible mediastinum, compressing the contralateral lung and twisting the great vessels (tension pneumothorax).[68] If this condition is not emergently corrected, venous return to the heart is decreased and shock or cardiac arrest may ensue.

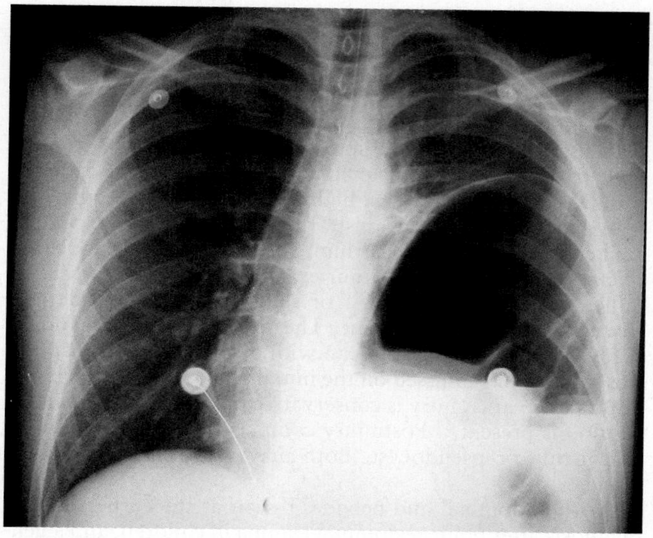

FIGURE 27.3. Anteroposterior chest radiograph showing an air–fluid level in the left chest and diaphragm elevation indicative of a traumatic diaphragmatic hernia. The cardiac silhouette is deviated into the right chest.

Pulmonary contusion may not be obvious on the initial chest radiograph but may be seen on CT scan. Hemothoraces and pneumothoraces are managed as in adults. Tracheobronchial disruption should be suspected in a child with a tension pneumothorax, massive subcutaneous emphysema, and/or a continuing air leak or persistent collapse of the lung despite a functioning chest tube. The diagnosis is confirmed by bronchoscopy, although multidetector CT (MDCT) scan has the perceived ability to provide detection and detail of pleural, parenchymal, mediastinal, and chest-wall injury, and also seems to have some utility for esophageal, tracheal, and mainstem bronchial disruption and cardiac injury.[69]

Blunt cardiac injuries can occur in children and range from mild to lethal.[70] The primary mechanisms of injury associated with this diagnosis are motor vehicle and pedestrian-related trauma. It is extremely rare for a hemodynamically normal patient with a normal sinus rhythm to develop a subsequent cardiac dysrhythmia or cardiac failure.[70] Significant cardiac injuries rarely occur in isolation, and most of these children die at the scene.[71] A few survive and are transported to trauma centers. Use of the FAST examination of the pericardium is a good tool to rapidly identify pericardial fluid in these children and allow for prompt treatment.

Thoracic aortic rupture is a rare injury in children but is highly lethal if undiagnosed. A report from the NPTR described 28 patients (from a total of 25,301) with traumatic aortic disruptions and a mortality rate of 57%.[72] Multisystem trauma from motor vehicle crashes or pedestrian collisions are the most common mechanisms. An appropriate mechanism of injury in conjunction with a chest radiograph demonstrating a wide mediastinum should raise suspicion and prompt investigation. Dynamic spiral CT angiography has become a definitive method of diagnosis. Good outcomes can be expected from early diagnosis, temporizing antihypertensive therapy, and definitive operative management including increasing use of endovascular stenting, although there are now reports of successful nonoperative management of both thoracic and abdominal aortic injuries in children.[73]

Abdominal Trauma

Twenty-five percent of children who sustain trauma have abdominal injuries. Unstable patients should undergo a FAST examination in the trauma room, and those with positive findings in the setting of continued hemodynamic abnormality despite fluid resuscitation should be taken to the operating room. The FAST examination will miss solid organ intraparenchymal injuries without free fluid, and stable pediatric trauma patients with major injury mechanisms or abdominal tenderness are evaluated with an abdominal and pelvic CT scan using IV contrast and then serial physical examinations during inpatient observation.[74–76] Six findings have been independently associated with intra-abdominal injury, including systolic blood pressure below normal for age, abdominal tenderness, associated femur fracture, serum aspartate aminotransferase concentration greater than 200 IU/L or serum alanine aminotransferase concentration greater than 125 IU/L, urinalysis showing more than 5 RBCs per high power field, and an initial hematocrit of less than 30%.[77]

6 The approach to solid organ injuries (liver, spleen, kidney) discovered on CT scan is primarily nonoperative, as most (more than 90%) of these injuries will heal with conservative management. The kidney is relatively large and anterior, and a significant abdominal blow often manifests with hematuria. However, hematuria is more often associated with a liver or spleen injury than with a radiographically significant renal injury. The indications for operation in children with solid organ injury include evidence of ongoing bleeding, uncorrected base deficit, persistent hemodynamic abnormality, the development of peritoneal signs or other signs and symptoms of an associated gastrointestinal (GI) injury, or major urinary extravasation with a renal injury.[78] Although most pediatric

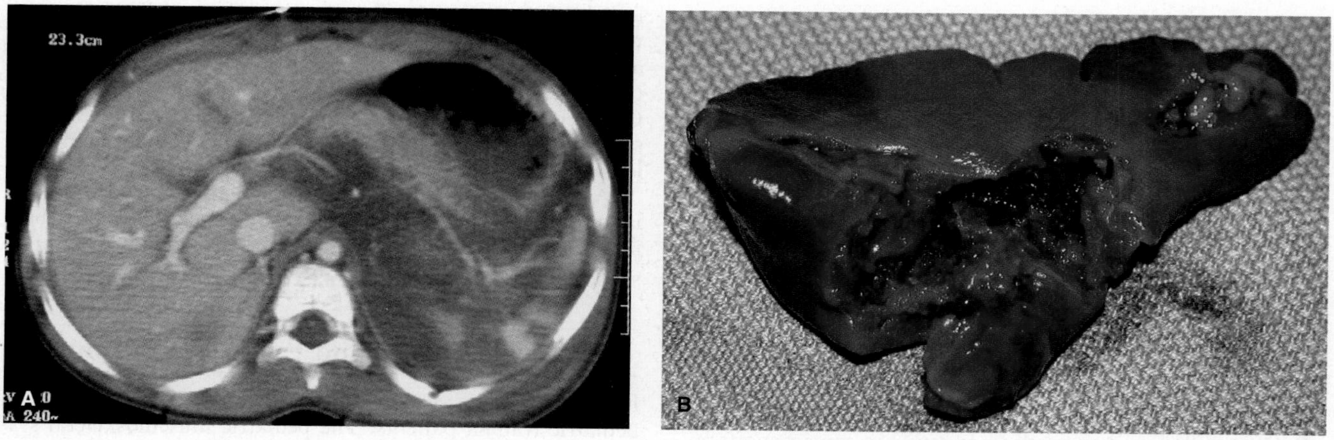

FIGURE 27.4. A: Abdominal computed tomography image showing grade V splenic rupture with extravasation of contrast. B: Ruptured spleen.

TABLE 27.3 **GRADING**

EVIDENCE-BASED STANDARDS FOR RESOURCE UTILIZATION IN CHILDREN WITH ISOLATED BLUNT SPLEEN AND LIVER INJURIES

	CT GRADE			
	I	II	III	IV
ICU stay	None	None	None	1 d
Hospital stay	2 d	3 d	4 d	5 d
Predischarge imaging	None	None	None	None
Postdischarge imaging	None	None	None	None
Activity restriction	3 wk	4 wk	5 wk	6 wk

CT, computed tomography; ICU, intensive care unit.
Reprinted with permission from Stylianos S. Evidence-based guidelines for resource utilization in children with isolated spleen or liver injury. APSA Trauma Committee. *J Pediatr Surg* 2000;35:164–169.

patients with blunt abdominal trauma do not require operation, the need for surgical judgment in determining which children fail nonoperative therapy is critical (Fig. 27.4).

There is now general consensus on the indications for intensive care and transfusion and the need for and timing of follow-up imaging procedures, along with the activities allowed after discharge of a child with a liver or spleen injury.[79,80] A prospective study by the American Pediatric Surgical Association of stable patients with traumatic grades I through IV liver and spleen injuries revealed a very low incidence of nonoperative failures (zero in some centers), a general agreement that transfusions were not required unless the hemoglobin fell below 7 g/dL, and that only children with grade IV injuries needed initial observation in an intensive care unit (ICU).[81] Children may be allowed out of bed when the hematocrit stabilizes, abdominal pain resolves, and hematuria is no longer present (renal injuries). Routine follow-up imaging is unnecessary in the absence of recurrent signs or symptoms of an abdominal complication. Recommendations on activity level after discharge have also been tested prospectively with a very low failure rate (Table 27.3). A reasonable approach to the stable child with a solid organ injury is outlined in Table 27.4. There is evidence that children with splenic injuries treated at trauma centers versus nontrauma centers more often undergo splenectomy, suggesting that dissemination of these guidelines may be both educational and reduce the numbers of children having operations following splenic trauma.[82] A recent study reported that children with high-grade (IV and V) liver injuries have a longer recovery, more complications, and greater use of resources than children with similar injuries to the spleen.[83]

TABLE 27.4 **TREATMENT**

APPROACH TO THE STABLE CHILD WITH A SOLID ORGAN INJURY

- Documentation of the degree of injury by computed tomography scan
- A brief hospital stay based on physiologic status
- Allow ambulation when pain and tenderness resolve
- Allow oral intake when pain and tenderness resolve
- Discharge when eating, ambulating without pain, and stable hematocrit
- Selectively repeat computed tomography scan for those with recurrent signs or symptoms following initial resolution
- Office follow-up before release to return to contact sports and physical education at school

Pancreatic injuries occur in a low percentage of pediatric trauma patients but carry a high morbidity and mortality risk if overlooked. The mechanism of injury is usually a circumscribed blow to the epigastrium, such as with the handlebars of a bicycle. Pancreatic injuries also may be the result of inflicted trauma, either a fist or shoe. Abdominal tenderness frequently is initially absent. The most sensitive diagnostic study is an abdominal CT scan with oral and IV contrast, but this injury can be missed on the initial scan. The approach to a blunt pancreatic injury is conservative unless major ductal disruption is present.[84] Postinjury complications include pancreatic fistula or pseudocyst. Both may resolve with drainage alone.

With abdominal and pelvic CT scan as the cornerstone of diagnosis after blunt abdominal trauma in children, and a general nonoperative approach to solid organ injuries, much attention has been directed toward the diagnosis of small-intestinal injuries in these patients.[85–87] Blunt intestinal injuries occur in 1% to 5% of pediatric patients with abdominal trauma. 7 Hollow viscus injury is difficult to diagnose and requires a high index of suspicion, serial abdominal examination, and select diagnostic studies. Mechanisms of injury involve intrusion-type blows and can include restrained or unrestrained motor vehicle passengers involved in crashes, pedestrians struck by motor vehicles, inflicted trauma, bike handlebar injuries, and direct blows to the abdomen or back (Fig. 27.5). The initial findings on physical examination may be subtle. Findings on CT scan may be equally subtle and include extravasation of oral contrast material, free intra-abdominal air, localized bowel wall thickening or dilatation, and signs of a mesenteric hematoma.[86] The presence of free pelvic fluid that is not associated with a solid organ injury is especially concerning for an intestinal injury. The presence of a small-intestinal injury also should be suspected when there is abdominal wall ecchymosis associated with spinal (Chance) fractures caused by the inappropriate high-riding use of a lap belt above the iliac crests without a shoulder harness (lap belt complex).[88] Occasionally, a blunt injury to the abdomen results in a hematoma that causes obstruction but not a transmural bowel wall ischemic injury. This is most common in the duodenum and usually resolves with conservative treatment.[85] In the presence of clear evidence of a hollow viscus injury, some pediatric surgeons are advocating initial diagnostic and possible therapeutic laparoscopy rather than laparotomy.[89] At least one study in children who had a missed or delayed diagnosis of GI tract injury showed no significant differences in ICU stay, total length of stay, associated injuries, and mortality compared with children who had a timely diagnosis. However, there was a significant increase in complications including abscess, fistula, wound infection, and delayed intestinal obstruction. Children whose injuries are initially missed exhibit evolving signs of peritonitis including fever, increasing abdominal pain, leukocytosis, and tachycardia (Fig. 27.6).[87]

Associated injuries to the abdominal aorta can also be seen in restrained children who are in high-speed crashes. These injuries are rare and may be diagnosed using CT angiography or aortography, and some can be managed nonoperatively.[73]

Pelvic Fractures and Extremity Trauma

Fractures are the second most common injury occurring in pediatric trauma patients. The pediatric musculoskeletal system differs greatly from the adult, presenting unique injury patterns and challenges in diagnosis and treatment.[90] Pediatric

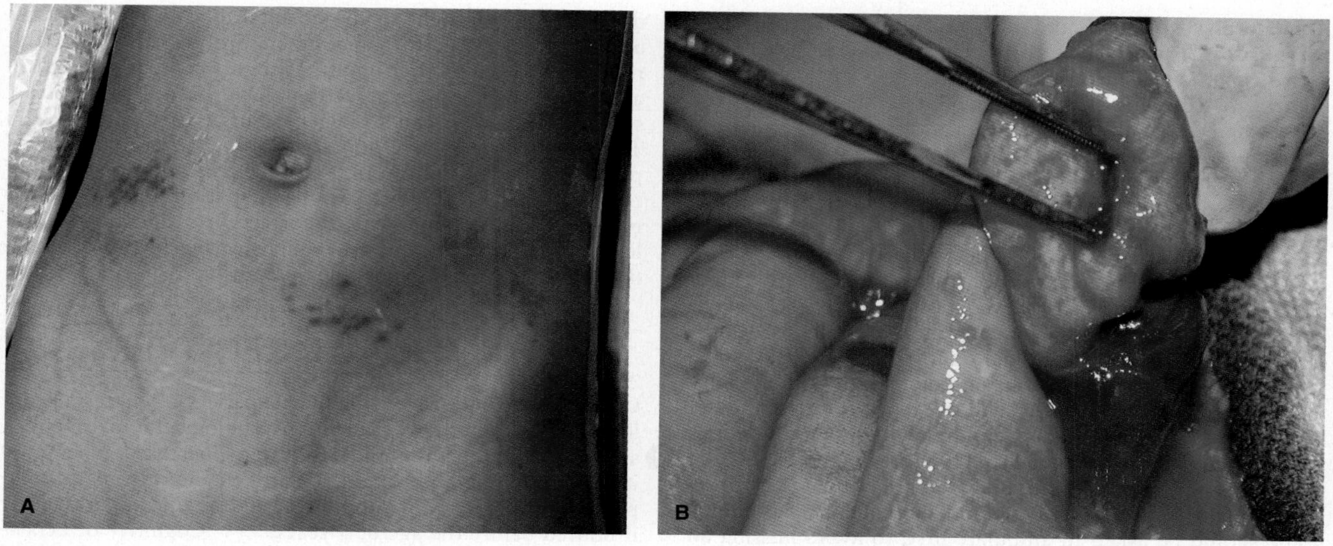

FIGURE 27.5. A: Ecchymosis of the abdominal wall resulting from improperly positioned seatbelt on the torso of a small child. B: Deserosalized segment of jejunum containing enterotomy.

bone contains more collagen leading to reduced tensile strength, reduced propagation of fractures, and improved resilience, but this quality makes radiographic evaluation more challenging. The periosteum is more metabolically active in children, leading to rapid callus formation and union of fractures and a higher potential for remodeling. The growth and change that occur at growth plates facilitate fracture remodeling and rapid healing, but physeal damage can also lead to deformity due to asymmetric limb growth.

Some fractures are unique to children. Greenstick fractures occur when the bone bends before it breaks, and the periosteal sleeve maintains apposition, creating a "hinge effect" without complete fracture of the bone.[90] Supracondylar fractures are the most common pediatric elbow fracture. Most (95%) are extension fractures due to a fall on an outstretched hand with the elbow hyperextended. Fracture reduction needs to proceed urgently in some cases. The physical examination should focus on the degree of swelling and neurovascular status. Excessive elbow swelling and ecchymosis together with increasing pain or pain with passive finger extension are concerning for ischemia. This injury is also predisposed to development of a compartment syndrome, although all injured extremities must be monitored carefully with frequent neurovascular examinations for this reason.

Injuries to peripheral nerves are common in all forms of pediatric upper extremity trauma, making early neurologic examination essential. In children who are unconscious, electrodiagnostic studies may be helpful if a neurologic deficit is detected later. Nerve exploration should be considered for open fractures, fractures that require open reduction, or nerve palsies that develop after fracture reduction. For closed fractures associated with nerve palsy at initial evaluation, observation is recommended with exploration reserved for lack of recovery on examination or electrodiagnostic testing after 4 months.[91]

Depending on age, location, and type of fracture, options for stabilization and alignment include casting, traction followed by casting, various methods of internal fixation including flexible rods and plates, and external fixation.[92] External fixation is particularly well suited for open complex fractures, fractures complicated by extensive soft tissue injury, open fractures complicated by a vascular injury, or fractures in multiple trauma victims who will require prolonged rehabilitation.

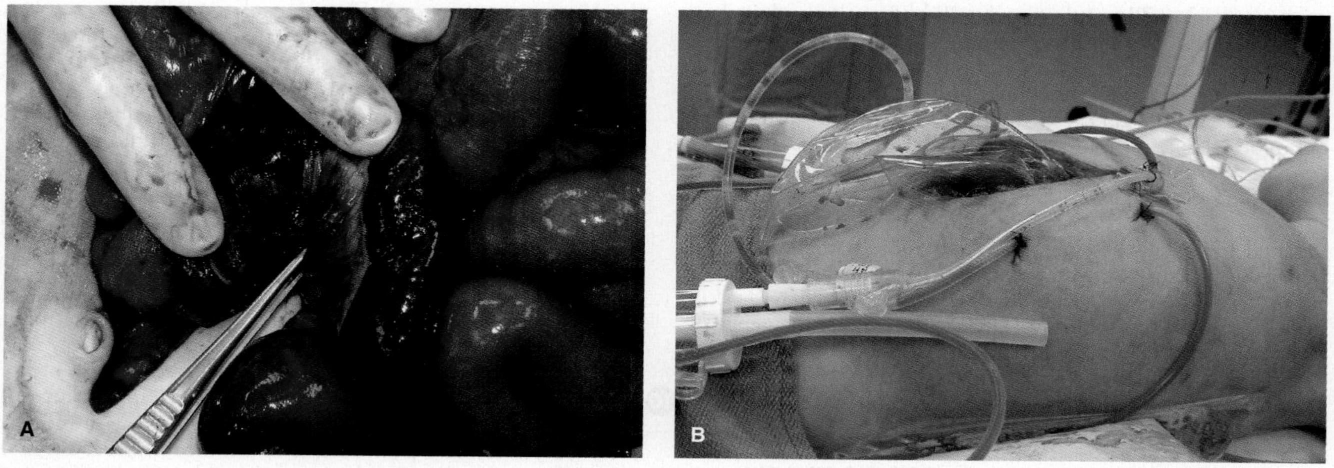

FIGURE 27.6. A: Jejunal hematoma and perforation at the ligament of Treitz resulting from child maltreatment. This child presented in hypovolemic shock and had a damage-control laparotomy. B: The abdomen was treated open for several days using a conventional, commercially available pediatric silo.

Angiography (diagnostic and/or therapeutic) may be needed in patients with suspected limb ischemia or pelvic bleeding.[93] There is some evidence that arterial trauma in ischemic but nonthreatened limbs of very young children (<2.5 years old) can be managed with systemic heparinization.[94]

Blood loss associated with bony injuries, especially in the pelvis, is proportionately greater in the child than in the adult, and this must be considered during volume resuscitation. At significant risk for hemorrhage are patients with bilateral anterior and posterior pelvic fractures.[95] The presence of multiple pelvic fractures also predicts the presence of associated genitourinary and abdominal injuries.[92] However, most pelvic injuries in children are not serious and are treated nonsurgically, with protected weight bearing and gradual return to activity.

Delay in diagnosis of fractures is common in both the minimally and the multiply injured child. A representative study of 149 multiply injured Canadian children with 494 total injuries reported a 6% incidence of delayed fracture diagnosis (46% of the 13 missed injuries).[96] Children who are evaluated in emergency departments after trauma and subsequently discharged home should be asked to ambulate first, to avoid missing an occult fracture.

Fractures can be associated with prolonged immobility, particularly when combined with a TBI. Adults are commonly treated prophylactically to prevent venous thromboembolism. At least one report indicates that pediatric inpatients with the diagnosis of trauma are not at increased risk to develop deep venous thrombosis of the lower extremities.[97] Nevertheless, adolescent patients who will have prolonged immobility from multiple fractures, pelvic fractures, or spinal trauma may be candidates for prophylactic therapy.

INFLICTED TRAUMA

All physicians caring for injured children have an ethical and legal responsibility to recognize and report the possibility of child maltreatment/abuse or inflicted injuries. The Centers for Disease Control and Prevention estimates that abuse and neglect is responsible for 4.5 of every 10,000 deaths in children 4 years of age and younger. Sadly, most children who die or sustain serious injury from inflicted trauma have a history of previous injury. Deaths or additional injuries are potentially preventable if the abusive behavior is recognized and remediated or the child is removed to foster care.[98] Inconsistency between the history and the anatomic injury or discrepancies in injury mechanism reported by involved adults should alert the medical provider to suspect maltreatment. Frequently, the child has been taken to several different emergency departments to avoid
8 raising suspicion. Physical signs of inflicted trauma include laceration or tear of the upper frenulum, retinal hemorrhages, multiple subdural hematomas without an acute skull fracture, genital or perianal injuries, burns in unusual areas (including burns caused by cigarettes), multiple torso bruises, and radiographic evidence of multiple old or healed fractures. The spectrum of injuries is variable, but head injuries are the most common injury reported in addition to being the most common cause of death. There is some evidence that children with inflicted TBI have worse outcomes than those with noninflicted injuries as measured with standardized functional and outcome status tools.[99] Visceral trauma is often associated with skin bruising and may also be associated with a higher incidence of thoracic trauma.[100] If maltreatment is suspected, hospital admission is mandatory and a formal report to the appropriate social agency is required by law in most states.

PERFORMANCE INDICATORS

The pediatric trauma system requires constant reevaluation. Because death after trauma is relatively less common in children who are brought to the hospital alive (compared with adults), pediatric performance filters are primarily aimed at reducing morbidity after injury. There are currently few pediatric performance indicators that have been systematically studied. The American College of Surgeons Committee on Trauma *Resources for Optimal Care of the Injured Patient*[19] provides a list of indicators used for verification of pediatric trauma centers (Table 27.5). Participation in systemwide reviews and a commitment to correction of identified problems are required of all professionals caring for injured children to ensure the best possible outcomes.

FUNCTIONAL RECOVERY

Children who survive trauma may experience long-term problems related to both physical and psychological impairment. A
9 subset of children with mild TBI display increased hyperactivity or inattention and conduct disorders, and/or somatic complaints of headaches, photophobia, and dizziness, particularly if injured before the age of 5 years.[101,102] Cognitive or behavioral changes may be evident as well as problems with school performance or sleep disorders. There are longitudinal studies indicating that depression is a significant problem among adults with pediatric-onset SCI, contributing to poorer outcomes and lower quality of life.[103] Many children with persistent disability noted at the time of hospital discharge do not receive appropriate rehabilitation services (physical therapy, occupational therapy, and speech services) because of lack of availability, insurance coverage, or parental perception of need.[104] When availability of rehabilitative resources for injured children is lacking, full recovery from injury is limited.[105] One recommendation is to involve the child's pediatrician or primary care physician in the follow-up care, regardless of the postacute services that the child may be receiving.[106]

Many published studies describe acute and long-term impairments in behavior, attention, memory, education, and adaptive function following TBI in school-aged children and adolescents.[107] Studies in preschool children indicate long-term impairment in educational performance and daily skills. For children with long-term disabilities resulting from TBI, there is a major impact on both their personal quality of life and that of their family.[108] In addition, many families caring for children after severe TBI are socially disadvantaged, with a large proportion of single, working, minority mothers.[109,110]

Within the first month after a traumatic event, individuals may display reexperiencing, avoidance, hyperarousal symptoms, and dissociation (feelings of unreality or emotional numbing).[111] Brief education is appropriate to explain that these symptoms are normal reactions that are likely to resolve. Symptoms that persist for more than a month or are particularly distressing in their intensity may be indicative of posttraumatic stress disorder (PTSD). Symptoms of this disorder in young children include sleep disturbances and nightmares, separation anxiety, difficulties in concentration, intrusive thoughts, difficulties in talking with parents and friends, mood disturbance, deterioration in academic performance, specific fears, and accident-related play. PTSD was reported in 35% of children involved in motor vehicle crashes compared with only 3% of children injured while playing sports.[112] Interventional programs that are aimed at both recognition and treatment of PTSD symptoms have the potential to improve functional recovery after injury in children.

A few studies have looked at health-related quality of life
10 (HRQOL) following various injuries. Multiple dimensions of HRQOL are negatively affected among children with moderate or severe TBI and do not improve significantly over the first year after injury.[113] Children requiring hospitalization for extremity fractures suffer dramatic declines in physical and psychosocial well-being during the first 3 months after injury, although children with upper extremity fractures do better

TABLE 27.5

EXAMPLES OF PEDIATRIC PROCESS AND OUTCOMES MEASURES: COMPLICATIONS/PERFORMANCE INDICATORS

■ MEASURE	■ DEFINITION	■ PURPOSE
Missed intubation	More than one attempt to place endotracheal tube appropriately	Efficiency of airway care is the defining variable in outcome for severely injured children. Who, when, what, and how many attempts were required for successful control of the airway are objective measures of system performance.
Unplanned extubation	Unintentional extubation by patient or provider	Failure to maintain the airway can be life threatening. This indicator reflects adequacy of pediatric critical care nursing care.
Extubation within 24 h of rapid-sequence intubation (excluding operative procedures)	Patient can be extubated <24 h after drug-assisted intubation, excluding operative procedure	This measure is the objective monitor of appropriateness of using rapid-sequence intubation, an intrinsically dangerous process. Patients who can be extubated within 24 h may not have required chemical paralysis and intubation in the first place.
Hypocapnia or hypercapnia	Overventilation or underventilation, especially in the first 12 h after injury	These measures are a reflection of efficacy and precision of care in the critical first 12 h after initial stabilization.
Resuscitation volumes	Infusion of more than 50 mL/kg during the first 2 h in child with normal initial vital signs	Judicious fluid management requires careful titration of filling pressures with oxygen-carrying capacity. Inordinate volumes of crystalloid, especially in the absence of clinical findings of hypoperfusion, will potentially exacerbate fluid sequestration in the brain and/or lung. This indicator reflects appropriate attention to clinical detail and accurate recording.
Vascular access problems	Any acquisition of vascular access that takes longer than 5 min to accomplish, especially if intraosseous infusion is not used	This indicator is an objective measure of preparation and facility in accomplishment of a critical, size-related component of pediatric resuscitation.
Unplanned operation following nonoperative management	Any operation for control of hemorrhage in a patient being managed nonoperatively	This indicator is an objective measure of the appropriateness of nonoperative management.
Unplanned hypothermia	Core temperature <35°C for >2 h	Although mild hypothermia has been associated with improved outcomes following brain injury, moderate to severe hypothermia causes a variety of hematologic and metabolic derangements and must be avoided in children.
Nosocomial pneumonia	Pneumonia, defined by NTDS[a]	Pneumonia is a major cause of avoidable morbidity and cost. Recognition of pneumonia is especially important in children without evidence of pulmonary injury or aspiration.
Missed injury	Any injury related to the initial traumatic event diagnosed >24 h after admission	This indicator is an objective measure of the specificity and accuracy of the initial assessment.

[a]From

than those with lower extremity fractures. Many children with tibia and/or fibula fractures still report poorer physical functioning 1 year postinjury.[114]

INJURY PREVENTION

Public health experts recommend that injury prevention efforts focus on injuries that are common, severe, and readily preventable. Examples include mechanisms likely to result in head or spinal cord injuries, where there is a high mortality or hospitalization rate and a long-term disability rate and effec- 11 tive countermeasures exist. The Emergency Medical Services for Children (EMSC) program emphasizes a step-by-step approach to injury prevention by establishing goals and objectives with measurable outcomes (Table 27.6).[115]

Physicians have been cited as the parent's first choice for information on injury control and child safety, but most physicians know little about injury prevention.[116] Major educational programs must be aimed at all caregivers to have a significant impact on pediatric trauma mortality rates.

Methods aimed at reducing childhood injury can be described as active or passive. The most successful prevention strategies are those that work automatically (i.e., are passive). Making roadways and vehicles safer has done more to decrease injuries from motor vehicle crashes than asking drivers to adhere to the speed limit or refrain from drinking alcohol before driving. Active intervention requires a behavioral change to be effective, such as securing a child in a safety seat. Recent studies emphasize specific patterns of injury in pediatric car crash victims, advocate continued public education for positioning children in the back seat of cars, and advocate

TABLE 27.6 **PREVENTION**

NATIONAL EMSC PROGRAM APPROACH TO INJURY PREVENTION

1. **Conduct a community assessment.** Bring individuals and groups who represent the community at large together to assess regional accomplishments and determine available resources.
2. **Define the injury problem.** Based on the community assessment and any available data, define a problem in specific, quantifiable terms.
3. **Set goals and objectives.** Make your goal a broad, general statement about the long-term changes the prevention initiatives are designed to make and the objective(s) specific, time limited, and quantifiable, in terms of either a *process* or an *outcome*.
4. **Plan and test interventions.** Interventions are the actions that you take to accomplish your goals and objectives. Use the E's of prevention to design options:
   - *Engineering* of products and environments
   - *Enactment* of legislation to promote safety
   - *Education* of children, caregivers, healthcare professionals, and legislators
   - *Evaluation* of the efficacy of specific interventions
5. **Implement and evaluate interventions.** Quantitate your results to determine whether your goals and objectives have been met.

After EMS for Children. Preventing childhood emergencies: a guide to developing effective injury prevention initiatives. Available at: http://www.childrensnational.org/EMSC/PublicRes/DownloadDocs.aspx. Accessed Feb 14, 2010.

for use of appropriate restraint systems (and appropriate use of restraint systems) for young children.[117–120]

Successful injury prevention programs have resulted in a significant reduction in the number of burn injuries in children, specifically with the development of fire-retardant sleepwear and working smoke detectors. There has been less success in reducing injuries to pediatric pedestrians: risk factors for pedestrian injuries in children include an age of 5 to 9 years, male sex, poverty, household crowding, inadequate parental supervision, family stress, and minority race or ethnic group.[1] Environmental contributions include living on streets with high traffic, lack of pedestrian-control devices, absence of alternatives to the street for play, and a high density of curbside parking. Successful environmental modifications, termed *traffic calming,* have been pioneered in Europe and include diversion of high-speed traffic away from the core of the city and residential areas and decreasing the speed limit to 10 to 20 mph. These changes reduce the risk of injury for all pedestrians, but especially for children. Bicycle helmets are effective in reducing the risk of head injuries by 85% and the risk of brain injuries by 88%, and legislation mandating their use coupled with public awareness translates into a decrease in injury rate.[121] There is evidence that educating pediatricians improves the use of car seats for children. Although the rate of use of car seats for newborns and infants is approximately 75%, their use in toddlers is estimated at only 29%, and more than half of car seats for children are not used correctly. In the child over 4 years or 40 pounds, there is ample evidence that booster seats should be used rather than adult-type restraints. More states now have legislation aimed at this high-risk population.

In the United States, all-terrain vehicle (ATV) crashes account for a rising number of neurologic injuries and deaths in all ages, including children. The injury and death rate substantially increased beginning in 1998 when the 1988 Consent Decrees between the Consumer Product Safety Commission and the ATV industry expired. This agreement included regulations that restricted operators younger than 16 years, halted the sale of three-wheeled vehicles, and included a mandatory educational safety training module and safety warnings.[122] Although helmets may reduce the risk of head injuries, many states do not have helmet laws, and juvenile passengers not only frequently drive ATVs but also do not wear helmets.[123] At least one study of pediatric ATV injuries found no advantage to wearing a helmet.[124]

A substantial proportion of motor vehicle crashes are alcohol related, and alcohol-related crashes are a serious problem even for the youngest drivers. Drivers under 21 years are more likely than older drivers to be involved in fatal crashes, and their added risk for fatal crash involvement increases more sharply at all levels of alcohol use.[125] This group has been the target of several interventions to reduce alcohol-impaired driving. These interventions include "zero tolerance" blood alcohol concentration (BAC) standards for drivers under the legal drinking age; graduated driver licensing programs that require new drivers to progress through stages and allow them increased driving privileges as they gain experience; and the 1984 Uniform Drinking Age Act, which required states to adopt a minimum legal drinking age of 21 years. Collectively, these and other targeted interventions have contributed to a decrease in alcohol-related fatal crashes across all age groups during 1982 to 2001, with the largest decrease among drivers under 21 years.[125,126]

Preventing penetrating trauma is more complicated but still can be done effectively. Laws that make gun owners responsible for storing firearms in a manner that makes them inaccessible to children have resulted in a 23% reduction in unintentional shooting deaths among children where they are in effect.[127] An injury prevention program in Harlem that included improving environmental safety, supporting community development, providing safe and supervised activities for children and adolescents, and providing effective health education resulted in a 50% reduction in assault and gun injuries in the intervention community, compared with increased injuries in a neighboring community.[128] Thus, there is hope for curbing the epidemic of pediatric injuries, but it will require a combination of legislative efforts, education of all child care providers, enforcement of existing safety laws, and use of widespread, community-based prevention programs using methods that have proved effective. Comprehensive injury data will allow us to direct our efforts into programs that target serious, common injuries with practical interventions.

References

1. Mendelson K, Fallat M. Pediatric injuries: prevention to resolution. *Surg Clin North Am* 2007;87:207–228.
2. Brussoni M, Towner E, Hayes M. Evidence into practice: combining the art and science of injury prevention. *Inj Prev* 2006;12:373–377.
3. Tepas JJ 3rd. The national pediatric trauma registry: a legacy of commitment to control of childhood injury. *Semin Pediatr Surg* 2004;13:126–132.
4. National Trauma Registry of the American College of Surgeons (NTRACS). www.dicorp.com. Accessed Feb 14, 2010.
5. Haider A, Efron D, Haut E, et al. Black children experience worse clinical and functional outcomes after traumatic brain injury: an analysis of the National Pediatric Trauma Registry. *J Trauma* 2007;62:1259–1263.
6. Martin C, Falcone R Jr. Pediatric traumatic brain injury: an update of research to understand and improve outcomes. *Curr Opin Pediatr* 2008; 20:294–299.
7. Svenson JE, Spurlock C, Nypaver M. Factors associated with the higher traumatic death rate among rural children. *Ann Emerg Med* 1996;27:625–632.
8. Esposito TJ, Sanddal ND, Dean JM, et al. Analysis of preventable pediatric trauma deaths and inappropriate trauma care in Montana. *J Trauma* 1999;47:243–253.
9. Brehaut JC, Miller A, Raina P, et al. Childhood behavior disorders and injuries among children and youth: a population based study. *Pediatrics* 2003;111(2):262–269.
10. Demetriades D, Murray J, Brown C, et al. High-level falls: type and severity of injuries and survival outcome according to age. *J Trauma* 2005;58: 342–345.

11. Calkins C, Bensard DD, Moore EE, et al. The injured child is resistant to multiple organ failure: a different inflammatory response? *J Trauma* 2002;53(6):1058–1063.
12. Ochoa C, Choski N, Upperman J, et al. Prior studies comparing outcomes from trauma care at children's hospitals versus adult hospitals. *J Trauma* 2007;63:S87–S91.
13. American Academy of Pediatrics. Pediatric Education for the Prehospital Professionals, 2nd ed. Sudbury, MA: Jones and Bartlett.
14. American Heart Association. Pediatric Advanced Life Support. Provider Manual. 2006.
15. Nicholl J, Hughes S, Dixon S, et al. The costs and benefits of paramedic skills in pre-hospital trauma care. *Health Tech Assess* 1998;2:1–73.
16. Paul TR, Marias M, Pons PT, et al. Adult versus pediatric prehospital trauma care: is there a difference? *J Trauma* 1999;47:455–459.
17. American College of Surgeons Committee on Trauma, American College of Emergency Physicians, National Association of EMS Physicians, Pediatric Equipment Guidelines Committee EMSC Partnership for Children Stakeholder Group, American Academy of Pediatrics. Equipment for ambulances. *Bull Am Coll Surg* 2009;94:23–29.
18. Potoka DA, Schall LC, Gardner MJ, et al. Impact of pediatric trauma centers on mortality in a statewide system. *J Trauma* 2000;49:237–245.
19. American College of Surgeons, eds. *Resources for Optimal Care of the Injured Patient*. Chicago, IL: American College of Surgeons; 2006.
20. Hartman M, Watson R, Linde-Zwirble W, et al. Pediatric traumatic brain injury is inconsistently regionalized in the United States. *Pediatrics* 2008; 122:e172–e180.
21. Luten R, Wears RL, Broselow J, et al. Managing the unique size-related issues of pediatric resuscitation: reducing cognitive load with resuscitation aids. *Acad Emerg Med* 2002;9(8):840–847.
22. Holmes JF, Goodwin HC, Land C, et al. Coagulation testing in pediatric blunt trauma patients. *Ped Emerg Care* 2001;17(5):324–328.
23. Capraro A, Mooney D, Waltzman M. The use of routine laboratory studies as screening tools in pediatric abdominal trauma. *Ped Emerg Care* 2006;22:480–484.
24. Swischuk L. Emergency pediatric imaging: changes over the years (part 1). *Emerg Radiol* 2005;11:193–198.
25. Westra S, Wallace E. Imaging evaluation of pediatric chest trauma. *Radiol Clin North Am* 2005;43:267–281.
26. Chwals WJ, Robinson AV, Sivit CJ, et al. Computed tomography before transfer to a level I pediatric trauma center risks duplication with associated increased radiation exposure. *J Ped Surg* 2008;43:2268–2272.
27. Partrick DA, Bensard DD, Moore EE, et al. Ultrasound is an effective triage tool to evaluate blunt abdominal trauma in the pediatric population. *J Trauma* 1998;45:57–63.
28. Rogovik AL, Rostami M, Hussain S, et al. Physician pain reminder as an intervention to enhance analgesia for extremity and clavicle injuries in pediatric emergency. *J Pain* 2007;8:26–32.
29. Oliver RC, Fallat ME. Traumatic childhood death: how well do parents cope? *J Trauma* 1995;39:303–307.
30. Oliver RC, Sturtevant JP, Scheetz JP, et al. Beneficial effects of a hospital bereavement intervention program following traumatic childhood death. *J Trauma* 2001;50(3):440–448.
31. Jurkovich GJ, Pierce B, Pananen L, et al. Giving bad news: the family perspective. *J Trauma* 2000;48:865–873.
32. Kirshblum S, Fichtenbaum J. Breaking the news in spinal cord injury. *J Spinal Cord Med* 2008;31:7–12.
33. Meyers TA, Eichhorn DJ, Guzzetta C, et al. Family presence during invasive procedures and resuscitation. *Am J Nurs* 2000;100:32–41.
34. O'Brien MM, Creamer KM, Hill EE, et al. Tolerance of family presence during pediatric cardiopulmonary resuscitation: a snapshot of military and civilian pediatricians, nurses, and residents. *Ped Emerg Care* 2002;18(6): 409–413.
35. Hanson C, Strawser D. Family presence during cardiopulmonary resuscitation: Foote Hospital emergency department's nine-year perspective. *J Emerg Nurs* 2002;18:104–106.
36. Schneier A, Shields B, Hostetler S, et al. Incidence of pediatric traumatic brain injury and associated hospital resource utilization in the United States. *Pediatrics* 2006;118:483–492.
37. Hutchison J, Ward R, Lacroix J, et al. Hypothermia therapy after traumatic brain injury in children. *N Engl J Med* 2008;358:2447–2456.
38. Walker P, Harting M, Baumgartner J, et al. Modern approaches to pediatric brain injury therapy. *J Trauma* 2009;67:S120–S127.
39. Adelson PD, Bratton SL, Carney NA, et al. Guidelines for the acute medical management of severe traumatic brain injury in infants, children and adolescents. *Pediatr Crit Care Med* 2003;4(3)(suppl):S1–S18.
40. Badjatia N, Carney N, Crocco TJ, et al. Guidelines for prehospital management of traumatic brain injury 2nd edition. *Prehosp Emerg Care* 2007; 12:S1–52.
41. Gausche M, Lewis R, Stratton S, et al. Effect of out-of-hospital pediatric endotracheal intubation on survival and neurological outcome: a controlled clinical trial. *JAMA* 2000;283:783–790.
42. Samant U IV, Mack C, Koepsell T, et al. Time of hypotension and discharge outcome in children with severe traumatic brain injury. *J Neurotrauma* 2008;25:495–502.
43. Figg R, Stouffer C, Vander Kolk W, et al. Clinical efficacy of serial computed tomographic scanning in pediatric severe traumatic brain injury. *Pediatr Surg Int* 2006;22:215–218.
44. Meier U, Zeilinger FS, Henzka O. The use of decompressive craniectomy for the management of severe head injuries. *Acta Neurochir* 2000;76: 475–478.
45. Rutigliano D, Egnor M, Priebe C, et al. Decompressive craniectomy in pediatric patients with traumatic brain injury with intractable elevated intracranial pressure. *J Ped Surg* 2006;41:83–87.
46. Curry R, Hollingworth W, Ellenbogen R, et al. Incidence of hypo- and hypercarbia in severe traumatic brain injury before and after 2003 pediatric guidelines. *Pediatr Crit Care Med* 2008;9:141–146.
47. Jagannathan J, Okonkwo DO, Yeoh HK, et al. Long-term outcomes and prognostic factors in pediatric patients with severe traumatic brain injury and elevated intracranial pressure. *J Neurosurg Pediatr* 2008;2: 240–249.
48. Tilford JM, Simpson PM, Yeh TS, et al. Variation in therapy and outcome for pediatric head trauma patients. *Crit Care Med* 2001;29(5):1056–1061.
49. Statler K. Pediatric posttraumatic seizures: epidemiology, putative mechanisms of epileptogenesis and promising investigational progress. *Dev Neurosci* 2006;28:354–363.
50. Tepas JJ III, DiScala C, Ramenofsky MLO, et al. Mortality and head injury: the pediatric perspective. *J Pediatr Surg* 1990;25:92–96.
51. White JRM, Farukhi Z, Bull C, et al. Predictors of outcome in severely head-injured children. *Crit Care Med* 2001;29(3):534–540.
52. Giza C, Mink R, Madikians A. Pediatric traumatic brain injury: not just little adults. *Curr Opin Crit Care* 2007;13:143–152.
53. Jankowitz BT, Adelson PD. Pediatric traumatic brain injury: past, present and future. *Dev Neurosci* 2006;28:264–275.
54. Parisini P, DiSilvestre M, Greggi T. Treatment of spinal fractures in children and adolescents: long-term results in 44 patients. *Spine* 2002;27(18): 1989–1994.
55. Slotkin J, Lu Y, Wood K. Thoracolumbar spinal trauma in children. *Neurosurg Clin N Am* 2007;18:621–630.
56. Dogan S, Safavi-Abbassi S, Theodore N, et al. Thoracolumbar and sacral spinal injuries in children and adolescents: a review of 89 cases. *J Neurosurg* 2007;106:426–433.
57. Carreon L, Glassman S, Campbell M. Pediatric spine fractures—a review of 137 hospital admissions. *J Spinal Disord Tech* 2004;17:477–482.
58. Jagannathan J, Dumont A, Prevedello D, et al. Cervical spine injuries in pediatric athletes: mechanisms and management. *Neurosurg Focus* 2006; 21:1–5.
59. Eubanks J, Gilmore A, Bess S, et al. Clearing the pediatric cervical spine following injury. *J Am Acad Orthop Surg* 2006;14:552–564.
60. Khanna G, El-Khoury G. Imaging of cervical spine injuries of childhood. *Skeletal Radiol* 2007;36:477–494.
61. Orenstein JB, Klein BL, Gotschall CS, et al. Age and outcome in pediatric cervical spine injury: 11-year experience. *Pediatr Emerg Care* 1994;10: 132–137.
62. Givens TG, Polley KA, Smieth GR, et al. Pediatric cervical spine injury: a three-year experience. *J Trauma* 1996;41:310–314.
63. Kriss VM, Kriss TC. SCIWORA (spinal cord injury without radiographic abnormality) in infants and children. *Clin Pediatr* 1996;35:119–124.
64. Bracken MB, Collins WF, Freeman DF, et al. Efficacy of methylprednisolone in acute spinal cord injury. *JAMA* 1984;251:45–52.
65. Bracken MB, Shephard MJ, Collins WF, et al. A randomized, controlled trial of methylprednisolone or naloxone in the treatment of acute spinal-cord injury: results of the Second National Acute Spinal Cord Injury Study. *N Engl J Med* 1990;322:1405–1411.
66. Tsutsumi S, Ueta T, Shiba K, et al. Effects of the second national acute spinal cord injury study of high-dose methylprednisolone therapy on acute cervical spinal cord injury-results in spinal injuries center. *Spine* 2006;31: 2992–2996.
67. Woosley CR, Mayes TC. The pediatric patient and thoracic trauma. *Thorac Cardiovasc Surg* 2008;20:58–63.
68. Sivit C. Pediatric thoracic trauma: imaging considerations. *Emerg Radiol* 2002;9:21–25.
69. Mirvis SE. Imaging of acute thoracic injury: the advent of MDCT screening. *Semin Ultrasound CT MRI* 2005;26:305–331.
70. Dowd MD, Krug S. Pediatric blunt cardiac injury: epidemiology, clinical features, and diagnosis. *J Trauma* 1996;40:61–67.
71. Scorpio RJ, Wesson DE, Smith CR, et al. Blunt cardiac injuries in children: a postmortem study. *J Trauma* 1996;41:306–309.
72. Cooper A, Barlow B, DiScala C, et al. Mortality and truncal injury: the pediatric perspective. *J Pediatr Surg* 1994;29:33–38.
73. Anderson S, Day M, Chen M, et al. Traumatic aortic injuries in the pediatric population. *J Ped Surg* 2008;43:1077–1081.
74. Murphy R, Ghosh A, Mackway-Jones K. Ultrasound or computed tomography in paediatric blunt abdominal trauma. *Emerg Med J* 2002;19: 554–556.
75. Baka AG, Delgado CA, Simon HK. Current use and perceived utility of ultrasound for evaluation of pediatric compared with adult trauma patients. *Pediatr Emerg Care* 2002;18(3):163–167.
76. Taylor GA, Fallat ME, Potter BA, et al. The role of computed tomography in blunt abdominal trauma in children. *J Trauma* 1988;28:1660–1664.
77. Holmes JF, Sokolove PE, Brant WE, et al. Identification of children with intra-abdominal injuries after blunt trauma. *Ann Emerg Med* 2002;39(5): 500–509.
78. Henderson C, Sedberry-Ross S, Pickard R, et al. Management of high grade renal trauma: 20-year experience at a pediatric Level I trauma center. *J Urol* 2007;178:246–250.
79. Fallat ME, Casale AJ. Practice patterns of pediatric surgeons caring for stable patients with traumatic solid organ injury. *J Trauma* 1997;43: 820–824.

80. Stylianos S, APSA Trauma Committee. Evidence-based guidelines for resource utilization in children with isolated spleen or liver injury. *J Pediatr Surg* 2000;35:164–169.
81. Stylianos S, APSA Liver/Spleen Trauma Study Group. Compliance with evidence-based guidelines in children with isolated spleen or liver injury. *J Pediatr Surg* 2002;37:453–456.
82. Stylianos S, Egorova N, Guice K, et al. Variation in treatment of pediatric spleen injury at trauma centers versus nontrauma centers: a call for dissemination of American Pediatric Surgical Association benchmarks and guidelines. *J Am Coll Surg* 2006;202:247–251.
83. Yang JC, Sharp SW, Ostlie DJ, et al. Natural history of nonoperative management for grade 4 and 5 liver and spleen injuries in children. *J Pediatr Surg* 2008;43:2264–2267.
84. Keller MS, Stafford PW, Vane DW. Conservative management of pancreatic trauma in children. *J Trauma* 1997;42:1097–1100.
85. Grosfeld JL, Rescorla FJ, West KW, et al. Gastrointestinal injuries in childhood: analysis of 53 patients. *J Pediatr Surg* 1989;24(6):580–583.
86. Jamieson DH, Babyn PS, Pearl R. Imaging gastrointestinal perforation in pediatric blunt trauma. *Pediatr Radiol* 1996;26:188–194.
87. Canty TG, Canty TC Jr, Brown C. Injuries of the gastrointestinal tract from blunt trauma in children: a 12-year experience at a designated pediatric trauma center. *J Trauma* 1999;46:234–240.
88. Newman KD, Bowman LM, Eichelberger MR, et al. The lap belt complex: intestinal and lumbar spine injury in children. *J Trauma* 1990;30:1133–1140.
89. Feliz A, Shultz B, McKenna C, et al. Diagnostic and therapeutic laparoscopy in pediatric abdominal trauma. *J Pediatr Surg* 2006;41:72–77.
90. Carson S, Woolridge DP, Colletti J, et al. Pediatric upper extremity injuries. *Pediatr Clin North Am* 2006;53:41–67.
91. Hosalkar HS, Matzon JL, Chang B. Nerve palsies related to pediatric upper extremity fractures. *Hand Clin* 2006;22:87–98.
92. Norman D, Peskin B, Ehrenraich A, et al. The use of external fixators in the immobilization of pediatric fractures. *Arch Orthop Trauma Surg* 2002;122:379–382.
93. Puapong D, Brown C, Katz M, et al. Angiography and the pediatric trauma patient: a 10-year review. *J Pediatr Surg* 2006;41:1859–1863.
94. Lazarides M, Georgiadis G, Papas T, et al. Operative and nonoperative management of children aged 13 years or younger with arterial trauma of the extremities. *J Vasc Surg* 2006;43:72–76.
95. McIntyre RC, Bensard DD, Moore EE, et al. Pelvic fracture geometry predicts risk of life-threatening hemorrhage in children. *J Trauma* 1993;35:423–429.
96. Letts M, Davidson D, Lapner P. Multiple trauma in children: predicting outcome and long- term results. *Can J Surg* 2002;45(2):126–131.
97. Vu L, Nobuhara K, Lee H, et al. Determination of risk factors for deep venous thrombosis in hospitalized children. *J Pediatr Surg* 2008;43:1095–1099.
98. Hudson M, Kaplan R. Clinical response to child abuse. *Pediatr Clin North Am* 2006;53:27–39.
99. Keenan HT, Bratton SL. Epidemiology and outcomes of pediatric traumatic brain injury. *Dev Neurosci* 2006;28:256–263.
100. Roaten J, Partrick D, Bensard D, et al. Visceral injuries in nonaccidental trauma: spectrum of injury and outcomes. *Am J Surg* 2005;190:827–830.
101. McKinlay A, Dalrymple-Alford JC, Horwood LJ, et al. Long term psychosocial outcomes after mild head injury in early childhood. *J Neurol Neurosurg Psychiatry* 2002;73(3):281–288.
102. Lee L. Controversies in the sequelae of pediatric mild traumatic brain injury. *Pediatr Emerg Care* 2007;23:580–583.
103. Anderson C, Vogel L, Chlan K, et al. Depression in adults who sustained spinal cord injuries as children or adolescents. *J Spinal Cord Med* 2007;30:S76–S82.
104. Nakayama DK, Gardner MJ, Rogers KD. Disability from bicycle-related injuries in children. *J Trauma* 1990;30:1390–1394.
105. Wesson DE, Scorpio RJ, Spence LJ, et al. The physical, psychological, and socioeconomic costs of pediatric trauma. *J Trauma* 1992;33:252–257.
106. Slomine B, McCarthy M, Ding R, et al. Health care utilization and needs after pediatric traumatic brain injury. *Pediatrics* 2006;117:e663–e674.
107. Catroppa C, Anderson VA, Morse SA, et al. Outcome and predictors of functional recovery 5 years following pediatric traumatic brain injury (TBI). *J Pediatr Psychol* 2008;33:707–718.
108. Montgomery V, Oliver R, Reisner A, et al. The effect of severe traumatic brain injury on the family. *J Trauma* 2002;52(6):1121–1124.
109. Keenan H, Runyan D, Nocera M. Child outcomes and family characteristics 1 year after severe inflicted or noninflicted traumatic brain injury. *Pediatrics* 2006;117:317–324.
110. Keenan H, Runyan D, Nocera M. Longitudinal follow-up of families and young children with traumatic brain injury. *Pediatrics* 2006;117:1291–1297.
111. Winston FK, Kassam-Adams N, Vivarelli-O'Neill C, et al. Acute stress disorder symptoms in children and their parents after pediatric traffic injury. *Pediatrics* 2002;109(6):e90.
112. Stallard P, Velleman R, Baldwin S. Prospective study of post-traumatic stress disorder in children involved in road traffic accidents. *BMJ* 1998;317:1619–1623.
113. McCarthy M, MacKenzie E, Durbin D, et al. Health-related quality of life during the first year after traumatic brain injury. *Arch Pediatr Adolesc Med* 2006;160:252–260.
114. Ding R, McCarthy M, Houseknecht E, et al. The health-related quality of life of children with an extremity fracture. *J Pediatr Orthop* 2006;26:157–163.
115. EMS for Children. Preventing childhood emergencies: a guide to developing effective injury prevention initiatives. Available at: www.childrensnational.org/EMSC/PubRes/DownloadDocs.aspx. Accessed Feb 14, 2010.
116. Eichelberger MR, Gotschall CS, Feely HB, et al. Parental attitudes and knowledge of child safety: a national survey. *Am J Dis Child* 1990;144:714–720.
117. Brown J, Jing Y, Wang S, et al. Patterns of severe injury in pediatric car crash victims: Crash Injury Research Engineering Network database. *J Pediatr Surg* 2006;41:362–367.
118. Quinones-Hinojosa A, Jun P, Manley G, et al. Airbag deployment and improperly restrained children: a lethal combination. *J Trauma* 2005;59:729–733.
119. Zuckerbraun B, Morrison K, Gaines B, et al. Effect of age on cervical spine injuries in children after motor vehicle collisions: effectiveness of restraint devices. *J Pediatr Surg* 2004;39:483–486.
120. Jermakian JS, Locey CM, Haughey LJ. Lower extremity injuries in children seated in forward facing child restraint systems. *Traffic Inj Prev* 2007;8:171–179.
121. Pardi L, King B, Salemi G, et al. The effect of bicycle helmet legislation on pediatric injury. *J Trauma Nurs* 2007;14:84–87.
122. Kute B, Nyland J, Roberts C, et al. Recreational all-terrain vehicle injuries among children. *J Pediatr Orthop* 2007;27:851–855.
123. Carr A, Bailes J, Helmkamp J, et al. Neurological injury and death in all-terrain vehicle crashes in West Virginia: a 10-year retrospective review. *Neurosurgery* 2004;54:861–867.
124. Gittelman M, Pomerantz W, Groner J, et al. Pediatric all-terrain vehicle-related injuries in Ohio from 1995 to 2001: using the Injury Severity Score to determine whether helmets are a solution. *Pediatrics* 2006;117:2190–2195.
125. Elder RW, Shults RA. Involvement by young drivers in fatal alcohol-related motor-vehicle crashes—United States, 1982–2001. *MMWR Morb Mortal Wkly Rep* 2002;51(48):1089–1091.
126. Hedlund JH, Ulmer RG, Preusser DF. *Determine Why There Are Fewer Young Alcohol-Impaired Drivers* (publication no. DOT-HS-809–348). Washington, DC: National Highway Traffic Safety Administration; 2001.
127. Cummings P, Grossman DC, Rivara FP, et al. State gun safe storage laws and child mortality due to firearms. *JAMA* 1997;278:1084–1086.
128. Durkin MS, Kuhn L, Davidson LL, et al. Epidemiology and prevention of severe assault and gun injuries to children in an urban community. *J Trauma* 1996;41:667–673.

CHAPTER 28 ■ GERIATRIC TRAUMA AND END-OF-LIFE DECISIONS

WILLIAM P. SCHECTER

KEY POINTS

1. Age older than 65 years significantly increases the risk of death after injury.
2. The Injury Severity Score is the most significant variable increasing the risk of death in the elderly.
3. Elderly patients taking warfarin have a significantly increased risk of death after head injury.
4. The most common cause of injury in the elderly is a fall.
5. Elderly trauma victims are often undertriaged despite the increased risk of death and disability associated with advanced age.
6. Long-term survival after cardiopulmonary resuscitation in the elderly is unusual.
7. Withholding or withdrawing life support is the most common event preceding death in the intensive care unit.
8. Decisions to limit critical care must be made in the best interests of the individual patient.

The elderly represent the most rapidly growing sector of our population.[1] Twenty percent of the population of the United States will be 65 years of age or older by the year 2030. Forty percent of all trauma patients will be 65 years or older by the year 2050 if current estimates are correct.[2] Unintentional injury is the ninth leading cause of death for the population aged 65 and older.[1] Both the dramatic demographic shift in favor of the elderly and the importance of injury as a cause of morbidity and mortality mandate a careful consideration of geriatric trauma, intensive care, and end-of-life decisions.

DEFINITION OF GERIATRIC TRAUMA

Geriatric trauma is usually defined as injury to individuals aged 65 years and older. However, the mortality rate from moderate injury (Injury Severity Score [ISS] 9 to 24) is already increased at age 45.[3]

PREDICTORS OF MORBIDITY AND MORTALITY

Age, the presence of comorbidities, mortality after injury, and injury severity all affect the risk of morbidity. Older patients are more likely on chronic drug treatment prior to injury and to have chronic medical conditions limiting physiologic reserve. Although elderly patients tend to sustain more severe injuries,[4] they have almost twice the mortality rate compared with younger patients when stratified for ISS and preexisting med-
1 ical conditions.[5] Trauma patients older than age 65 are 4.6 times more likely to die than younger patients ($p < 0.001$) after controlling for ISS and preexisting medical conditions.[6] The risk of death after injury in the presence of both cardiovascular disease and diabetes is greater in patients over age 65 compared with younger patients with the same diseases.[6] Functional recovery is also impaired. Elderly survivors of trauma are more likely to lose the ability to walk and transfer independently. The risk is even greater for patients older than age 80.[7]

Comorbidities

Comorbidities are more common in the elderly population and are associated with an increased risk of death following injury. Eighty percent of patients over age 65 have at least one comorbidity and 5% have at least two.[1] The increased relative risk of death with cirrhosis is 4.5, coagulopathy 3.2, chronic heart disease 1.8, chronic obstructive pulmonary disease 1.8, and diabetes 1.2.[8] In addition, renal disease and malignancy increase the risk of death following injury.[9,10]

Injury Severity

The average ISS of patients over age 75 is 18, compared with an average ISS of 11 to 12 in younger patients.[4] Forty-eight percent of patients with an ISS greater than 25 died in a study
2 of 852 trauma patients older than 65. The ISS was the most significant variable correlated with the risk of death. Other variables associated with a mortality rate greater than 80% were hypoventilation, hypotension, and a Glasgow Coma Scale Score (GCS) of 3.[11]

REASONS FOR INCREASED MORBIDITY AND MORTALITY IN GERIATRIC PATIENTS

Decreased Physiologic Reserve

The cardiac index decreases 1% per year and systemic vascular resistance increases 1% per year. Both the response to adrenergic stimulation and the maximal heart rate are reduced with age.[12] As a result, trauma patients over age 65 have a significantly lower cardiac index, oxygen delivery, and oxygen consumption than younger patients.[13] Hypoperfusion causing prolonged acidosis leads to a higher mortality rate in trauma patients over age 55 compared with younger patients.[14]

TRAUMA

Effect of Beta-Blockers

Twenty percent of elderly patients with coronary artery disease and 10% with hypertension take beta-blockers,[15] which inhibit their ability to respond to hypovolemia with tachycardia. Geriatric trauma patients often may not fulfill hemodynamic criteria for trauma team activation despite significant injury.[16] Preinjury beta blockade is associated with an increased risk of death.[17]

Effect of Anticoagulation

Warfarin is an important drug in the management of a number of chronic medical conditions common in geriatric patients including atrial fibrillation, deep vein thrombosis, and the presence of a prosthetic heart valve. The risk of spontaneous intracranial hemorrhage for patients taking oral anticoagulation is 1%.[18]

3 All elderly patients on warfarin require careful evaluation after injury. A retrospective study of 144 geriatric patients on warfarin with a history of mild head trauma demonstrated clinically significant intracranial injury in 7% of the patients.[19]

The mortality rate for 25 elderly head injury patients on warfarin with an average international normalized ratio (INR) of 3.2 ± 0.1 was 48%.[20] Patients on warfarin with a supratherapeutic INR (6.5) and severe brain injury (GCS <8) had an even worse outcome, with a mortality rate of 87.8%. Even patients with "minor" brain injury (GCS 13 to 15) who present with an elevated INR (4.4) have a mortality rate of 80.6% caused by continued intracranial hemorrhage after presentation to the hospital.[21]

Rapid correction of an elevated INR is essential after trauma. Correction of an elevated INR with fresh frozen plasma (FFP) and vitamin K within 2 hours reduced the mortality rate from 48% to 10% in patients on warfarin with intracranial hemorrhage and a GCS less than or equal to 14.[22,23] However, if rapid correction of the INR is required in an emergency, prothrombin complex concentrates (PCCs) are recommended.[24] Factor VIIa is also effective in reversing the anticoagulation effects of warfarin in patients with intracranial hemorrhage.[25]

Elderly patients taking aspirin or clopidogrel appear to be at increased risk for death after head injury. Although one study showed no difference in the frequency of intracranial hemorrhage in patients with or without low-dose aspirin,[26] two other studies showed a significantly increased mortality rate for patients taking antiplatelet drugs compared to controls.[20,27] The effect of platelet transfusions on the mortality rate is unclear.[27,28]

MECHANISM OF INJURY

4 The most common mechanism of injury in the elderly is falls,[29] followed by motor vehicle collisions and pedestrian/vehicle accidents. These injuries result in significant morbidity, mortality, and cost.[30,31] The mortality rate for elderly patients after pedestrian/vehicle accidents is higher than in any other age group.[31]

INJURY PREVENTION IN THE GERIATRIC POPULATION

The known physiologic, anatomic, metabolic, and neurologic changes associated with aging offer opportunities for intervention to reduce the risk of injury. Primary care providers and family members have an important role in identifying and modifying risk factors associated with injury. Patients taking multiple medications, particularly sedatives and hypnotics, are at increased risk for falls.[32] A careful review and appropriate reduction of unnecessary polypharmacy can reduce the risk of hemodynamic and neurologic side effects that predispose to injury. Periodic screening of geriatric patients for postural hypotension,[33] gait and station abnormalities,[34,35] visual acuity,[36] and cognitive deficits[37] can identify patients prone to fall.

Interventions such as medication change, external compression stockings, and education of caregivers can reduce the risk of postural hypotension.[38] An organized program of strengthening and coordination exercises can improve strength and balance.[39] Modification of environmental factors such as improved lighting; removing obtrusive furniture, slippery floors, and floor coverings; and provision of grab rails and raised toilet seats in washrooms and other high-risk areas are potential interventions that can reduce the risk of falling.[40] Other important injury prevention measures include automobile seat belts, bicycle helmets, smoke detectors, and hot water heaters limited to less than 48.8°C (120°F).[32]

AGE AS A CRITERION FOR TRAUMA CENTER TRIAGE

5 Age is an important criterion for trauma center triage for all of the reasons cited previously. Yet, available evidence indicates that elderly trauma victims are undertriaged.[41] Significantly fewer elderly compared with younger patients with appropriate triage criteria were transported to trauma centers in a study of trauma victims in Maryland.[42]

The reasons for undertriage of geriatric trauma patients are not known. One possible cause is late presentation of physical findings associated with hypovolemia.[16] Undertriage of geriatric trauma patients is a serious problem because treatment of these patients in a trauma center results in a significantly lower mortality rate.[43]

Head Injury

The initial presentation of intracranial hemorrhage in geriatric patients may be subtle if preexisting cerebral atrophy or impaired intellectual function is present.[29] Subdural hematoma is relatively common because of the fragile bridging veins and increased distance between the dura and brain. Epidural hematoma is less common because of increased dural adherence to the cranium with advancing age.[29]

The mortality rate and functional recovery after head injury are much worse in geriatric as compared to younger patients.[44] The effect of age as an independent predictor of death begins at age 45.[44] The odds of death, persistent vegetative state, or other severe disability increase by 50% with each decade increase in age.[45] Geriatric trauma patients who present with a GCS less than 8 and an intracranial space-occupying lesion have such a high mortality rate and such a low functional recovery rate[46,47] that some investigators have suggested withdrawal of aggressive support after 72 hours in the absence of significant improvement.[12] The adverse effect of chronic anticoagulation therapy on outcome after head injury was discussed earlier.

Splenic Injury

Although nonoperative management of hemodynamically stable patients with splenic injury is now standard care,[48] this approach must be used with caution in geriatric patients because of decreased physiologic reserve in the event of sudden hemorrhage. The success rate of nonoperative management of splenic injury (approximately 80%) appears to be the same in patients younger and older than age 55.[49–53] However, the mortality rate was significantly higher in patients older than age 55 for both successful (8% vs. 4%, $p < 0.05$) and unsuccessful (29% vs. 12%, $p = 0.54$) nonoperative management. Nonoperative management of splenic injury was overall less successful for elderly patients with higher-grade splenic injuries compared with younger patients.[54]

Skeletal Injury

Rib Fractures. Rib fractures are serious injuries in elderly patients and are associated with significant morbidity and mortality rates. The risk of pneumonia after isolated thoracic trauma in geriatric patients is three times the risk in younger patients.[55,56] The mortality rate associated with one to two rib fractures is 12% but is approximately 40% if more than six rib fractures are present.[57]

Chest-wall analgesia and pulmonary toilet are important in the management of rib fractures.[58] Parenteral opiates should be used with caution because of the risk of respiratory depression. Intercostal nerve blockade with local anesthetics effectively controls chest-wall pain, but unfortunately the duration of anesthesia is limited.[59] Epidural analgesia is probably the most effective method of pain control after rib fracture[60] and may be associated with a reduction in mortality rate.[56] Elderly patients with rib fractures should be admitted to the hospital, be monitored carefully, and receive chest-wall analgesia.

Hip Fractures. Hip fractures are common in elderly osteoporotic women. Patients with periarticular fractures often require primary prosthetic replacement to avoid the risks of delayed union or nonunion, loss of fixation, and osteonecrosis.[61] Timely surgical intervention is critical. The risk of death doubles if surgical treatment of hip fracture is delayed for more than 2 days.[62] However, elderly hip fracture patients should receive careful evaluation and optimization of acute and chronic medical conditions during the first 24 hours after injury prior to surgery.[63]

Other Extremity Fractures. Geriatric patients are at increased risk for poor functional outcome regardless of the type of extremity fracture.[61] The timing of orthopaedic surgery depends on the nature and severity of associated injuries and the physiologic status of the patient. As a general principle, surgical correction of unstable extremity fractures should occur as soon as possible after resuscitation, treatment of life-threatening injuries, and optimization of comorbid conditions.

Pelvic Fracture. Pelvic fracture is the most serious skeletal injury in the elderly, with a mortality rate approaching 81% for open pelvic fractures. Pelvic fracture patients older than 55 are three times more likely to require blood transfusions and more likely to require angioembolization than younger patients.[64] The overall mortality rate for geriatric patients (12.3% to 21%) is significantly higher than for younger patients (2.3% to 6%).[64,65]

INTENSIVE CARE IN GERIATRIC TRAUMA

A recent study of intensive care unit (ICU) resource utilization indicated that elderly trauma patients had a lower ICU admission rate (36.7%) compared to younger patients (45.5%). The lower ICU admission may be due to the death of more geriatric trauma patients prior to ICU admission. Once admitted, geriatric trauma patients have a longer period of ICU stay compared to younger patients.[5] The risk of death increases with the number of complications,[66] many of which are preventable.[67]

Thirty-nine percent of geriatric trauma patients develop nosocomial infections compared with 17% of younger patients ($p < 0.005$). Nosocomial infections are associated with a mortality rate of 28% for patients older than age 65. Patients with preexisting chronic obstructive pulmonary disease are at particular risk for nosocomial pneumonia.[68] Aggressive measures to prevent, diagnose, and treat nosocomial infections are essential to improve the outcome of geriatric intensive care patients.[12]

The most appropriate method of hemodynamic monitoring is unknown. Although pulmonary artery catheter (PAC) monitoring has been recommended for critically ill geriatric trauma patients,[12] the PAC is associated with an increased risk of death[69] and pulmonary embolism,[70] as well as complications related to insertion and nosocomial infection.[71]

Transthoracic echocardiography (TTE) and transesophageal echocardiography (TEE) permit minimally invasive assessment of cardiac anatomy, ventricular filling, wall motion, and ejection fraction. Unfortunately, TTE and TEE require extensive training for both the technical performance and interpretation of the examination and require multiple examinations at different points in time.[72–74] Anticipated improvements in technology offer the hope of efficacious noninvasive hemodynamic monitoring.

OUTCOME FROM CARDIOPULMONARY RESUSCITATION IN THE ELDERLY

6 Long-term survival following cardiopulmonary resuscitation (CPR) in the elderly is unusual.[75–77] Asystole[78] and failure to restore cardiac activity after 5 minutes of CPR[79] are variables associated with particularly poor outcome. Advance directives from patients help guide therapeutic discussions for geriatric patients after serious illness or injury.

ADVANCE DIRECTIVES AND HEALTH CARE PROXIES

Advance directives may be executed via a living will or health care proxy.[80] A living will is a legal document in which a competent person expresses preferences for care in the event of serious illness or injury precluding participation in therapeutic decisions.[81] Unfortunately, a living will can neither predict all potential health care scenarios nor predict a change in patient preferences due to changing circumstances. Trauma surgeons, who have usually not met the patient prior to injury, must at times be guided by a document written years previously without the benefit of a discussion with the patient.

A health care proxy is an individual appointed by a competent person to make proxy decisions in the event of incompetence due to serious illness or injury. Patients and the general public desire advance directives.[82,83] Lack of physician initiative in discussing advance directives with patients is the major impediment to advance directives.[82]

WITHHOLDING AND WITHDRAWING SUPPORT IN GERIATRIC TRAUMA PATIENTS

7 Withholding or withdrawing life support is now the most common event preceding death in the ICU.[84] Reasons cited by health care providers for limiting ICU care include brain

death, futility, patient suffering, and anticipated poor quality of life.[85]

The concept of brain death was introduced by Beecher in 1968 to respond to the challenges of the emerging fields of organ transplantation and intensive care.[86] Current diagnostic criteria include the presence of all of the following signs: (a) irreversible coma, (b) absent brainstem reflexes, and (c) apnea. These findings must be confirmed by serial examinations separated by 6 hours in adults over age 18. Confirmatory tests demonstrating absence of cerebral blood flow must be done if the diagnosis is in doubt.[87]

Futility is a word denoting continued intensive care without hope of survival. Unfortunately, uncertainty and disagreement regarding the futility of continued intensive care in an individual patient are common. Opinions regarding futility are influenced by the skill, experience, and professional background of the clinician as well as personal and cultural values.[88] While perceived patient suffering is a challenge for the ICU staff, withdrawal of support based solely on patient suffering is not indicated.

Data on the quality of life of geriatric trauma survivors are sparse. The use of anticipated poor quality of life as a criterion to withdraw support is dangerous. Clinicians may substitute their own concept of acceptable quality of life for the patient's. All trauma patients may struggle with the psychological, cosmetic, and functional sequelae of injury.[89,90] However, withholding or withdrawing support based solely on anticipated poor quality of life is not indicated.

Competition for the limited number of ICU beds is a daily occurrence. The appropriate allocation of this limited resource is a challenge for trauma surgeons.[91] Although social justice is a basic principle of medical ethics,[92] in the absence of a mass casualty event[93] the best interests of the individual patient must guide the clinician's decisions. The medical profession must provide transparent outcome data to inform open public debate regarding appropriate resource allocation. The body politic must set the rules. The medical profession must provide the best possible care given the rules.

Withholding and withdrawing intensive care for hopelessly ill geriatric trauma patients is a necessary part of clinical practice. Unfortunately, advance directives or health care proxies are often absent. The challenge is to identify the patients who
8 are hopelessly ill. Decisions to limit critical care should be made in the best interests of the patient based on the following principles[94]:

1. Diagnostic precision: All patients deserve a precise diagnosis and a search for treatable disease. All patients will be "hopelessly ill" if clinicians fail to diagnose a missed injury, drain pus under pressure, or resect dead tissue.
2. Recognition of an uncertain prognosis: Clinicians must recognize the uncertainty of their prognosis. All patients should be given every chance to improve before withdrawal of support if the prognosis is uncertain.
3. A risk-benefit analysis: The primary responsibility is to the individual patient and the family. The patient's interests are paramount. All decisions must be made in the patient's best interest.
4. Patient autonomy: The autonomy of all patients must be respected, both the competent and incompetent. Clinicians must not substitute their own concepts of quality of life for the patient's.
5. Due deliberation prior to decision: Clinicians should not rush to judgment. A careful consideration of all the issues is essential prior to making these critical decisions.
6. Communication with the patient, family, and professional colleagues: Close communication with the patient, family, and friends is important. Communication utilizes a critical resource for busy clinicians—time. However, failure to spend a small amount of time each day with the patient and professional colleagues will result in the expenditure of huge amounts of time later on coping with the inevitable conflict and psychological distress caused by lack of communication.
7. Cultural sensitivity: Framing the discussion in the cultural context of the patient and family is extremely helpful. If the clinician is unfamiliar with the culture, assistance from colleagues with the appropriate cultural and linguistic skills can be very helpful in improving the quality of communication.
8. Consensus prior to the final decision: Consensus is absolutely essential prior to withdrawal of support. Dogmatism and unilateral action lead to hostility and legal action. Agreement among all parties can almost always be achieved with daily meetings. Allowing another few days to pass to achieve respectful consensus is a wise course. If consensus cannot be achieved, involvement of the hospital ethics committee may help resolve the conflict. If concerted efforts are made to achieve meaningful communication, failure to reach consensus should be a rare event.

SUMMARY

An increasing number of geriatric patients will require care as a result of injury. Physiologic changes due to aging and multiple comorbidities both increase the geriatric patient's susceptibility and adversely affect the physiologic response to injury. Public and professional injury prevention education efforts have the potential to reduce the risk of injury in the elderly. Aggressive evaluation and treatment of the geriatric trauma patient are essential to minimize potentially preventable death and complications. In spite of all efforts, many desperately ill geriatric trauma patients require prolonged intensive care, presenting medical, rehabilitation, and ethical challenges to the trauma team.

References

1. He W, Sengupta M, Velkoff VA, et al. *65+ in the United States*. Washington, DC: US. Government Printing Office; 2005.
2. MacKenzie EJ, Morris JA Jr, Smith GS, et al. Acute hospital costs of trauma in the United States: implications for regionalized systems of care. *J Trauma* 1990;30:1096–1101; discussion 1101–1103.
3. Morris JA Jr, MacKenzie EJ, Damiano AM, et al. Mortality in trauma patients: the interaction between host factors and severity. *J Trauma* 1990; 30:1476–1482.
4. Shabot MM, Johnson CL. Outcome from critical care in the "oldest old" trauma patients. *J Trauma* 1995;39:254–259; discussion 259–260.
5. Taylor MD, Tracy JK, Meyer W. Trauma in the elderly: intensive care unit resource use and outcome. *J Trauma* 2002;53:407–414.
6. Perdue PW, Watts DD, Kaufmann CR, et al. Differences in mortality between elderly and younger adult trauma patients: geriatric status increases risk of delayed death. *J Trauma* 1998;45:805–810.
7. Grossman M, Scaff DW, Miller D, et al. Functional outcomes in octogenarian trauma. *J Trauma* 2003;55:26–32.
8. Morris JA Jr, MacKenzie EJ, Edelstein SL. The effect of preexisting conditions on mortality in trauma patients. *JAMA* 1990;263:1942–1946.
9. Grossman MD, Miller D, Scaff DW, et al. When is an elder old? Effect of preexisting conditions on mortality in geriatric trauma. *J Trauma* 2002;52: 242–246.
10. Milzman DP, Boulanger BR, Rodriguez A, et al. Pre-existing disease in trauma patients: a predictor of fate independent of age and injury severity score. *J Trauma* 1992;32:236–243; discussion 243–244.
11. Knudson MM, Lieberman J, Morris JA Jr, et al. Mortality factors in geriatric blunt trauma patients. *Arch Surg* 1994;129:448–453.
12. Jacobs DG, Plaisier BR, Barie PS, et al. Practice management guidelines for geriatric trauma: the EAST Practice Management Guidelines Work Group. *J Trauma* 2003;54:391–416.
13. Epstein CD, Peerless J, Martin J, et al. Oxygen transport and organ dysfunction in the older trauma patient. *Heart Lung* 2002;31:315–326.
14. Shulman AM, Claridge JA, Young JS. Young versus old: factors affecting mortality after blunt traumatic injury. *Am Surg* 2002;68:942–947; discussion 947–948.
15. Fishkind D, Paris BE, Aronow WS. Use of digoxin, diuretics, beta blockers, angiotensin-converting enzyme inhibitors, and calcium channel blockers in older patients in an academic hospital-based geriatrics practice. *J Am Geriatr Soc* 1997;45:809–812.

16. Demetriades D, Sava J, Alo K, et al. Old age as a criterion for trauma team activation. *J Trauma* 2001;51:754–756; discussion 756–757.
17. Neideen T, Lam M, Brasel K. Pre-injury beta blockers are associated with increased mortality in geriatric trauma patients. *J Trauma* 2008;65(5): 1016–1020.
18. Hart RG, Boop BS, Anderson DC. Oral anticoagulants and intracranial hemorrhage. Facts and hypotheses. *Stroke* 1995;26:1471–1477.
19. Li J, Brown J, Levine M. Mild head injury, anticoagulants, and risk of intracranial injury. *Lancet* 2001;357:771–772.
20. Mina AA, Knipfer JF, Park DY, et al. Intracranial complications of preinjury anticoagulation in trauma patients with head injury. *J Trauma* 2002; 53:668–672.
21. Cohen DB, Rinker C, Wilberger JE. Traumatic brain injury in anticoagulated patients. *J Trauma* 2006;60:353–357.
22. Mina AA, Bair HA, Howells GA, et al. Complications of preinjury warfarin use in the trauma patient. *J Trauma* 2003;54:842–847.
23. Ivascu FA, Howells GA, Junn FS, et al. Rapid warfarin reversal in anticoagulated patients with traumatic intracranial hemorrhage reduces hemorrhage progression and mortality. *J Trauma* 2005;59(5):1131–1137; discussion 1137–1139.
24. Levy JH, Tanaka KA, Dietrich W. Perioperative hemostatic management of patients treated with vitamin K antagonists. *Anesthesiology* 2008;109(5): 918–926.
25. Lin J, Hanigan WC, Tarantino M, et al. The use of recombinant activated factor VII to reverse warfarin-induced anticoagulation in patients with hemorrhages in the central nervous system: preliminary findings. *J Neurosurg* 2003;98:737–740.
26. Spektor S, Agus S, Merkin V, et al. Low-dose aspiring prophylaxis and risk of intracranial hemorrhage in patients older than 60 years of age with mild or moderate head injury: a prospective study. *J Neurosurg* 2003;99: 661–665.
27. Ohm C, Mina AA, Howells GA, et al. Effects of antiplatelet agents on outcomes for elderly patients with traumatic intracranial hemorrhage. *J Trauma* 2005;58:518–522.
28. Ivascu FA, Howells GA, Junn FS, et al. Predictors of mortality in trauma patients with intracranial hemorrhage on preinjury aspiring or clopidogrel. *J Trauma* 2008;65(4):785–788.
29. Mandavia D, Newton K. Geriatric trauma. *Emerg Med Clin North Am* 1998;16:257–274.
30. Roudsari BS, Ebel BE, Corso PS, et al. The acute medical care costs of fall-related injuries among the US older adults. *Injury* 2005;36:1316–1322.
31. Kong LB, Lekawa M, Navarro RA, et al. Pedestrian-motor vehicle trauma: an analysis of injury profiles by age. *J Am Coll Surg* 1996;182:17–23.
32. Miller KE, Zylstra RG, Standridge JB. The geriatric patient: a systemic approach to maintaining health. *Am Fam Physician* 2000;61(4): 1089–1094.
33. Tinetti ME, Baker DI, Mcavay G, et al. A multifactorial intervention to reduce the risk of falling among elderly people living in the community. *N Engl J Med* 1994;331(13):821–827.
34. Vellas BJ, Wayne SJ, Romero L, et al. One-leg balance is an important predictor of injurious falls in older persons. *J Am Geriatr Soc* 1997;45(6): 735–738.
35. Mathias S, Nayak US, Isaacs B. Balance in elderly patients: the "get-up and go" test. *Arch Phys Med Rehabil* 1986;67(6):387–389.
36. Sach TH, Foss AJ, Gregson RM, et al. Falls and health status in elderly women following first eye cataract surgery: an economic evaluation conducted alongside a randomised controlled trial. *Br J Ophthalmol* 2007; 91(12):1675–1679.
37. Fuller GF. Falls in the elderly. *Am Fam Physician* 2000;61(7):2159–2168.
38. Jensen J, Lundin-Olsson L, Nyberg L, et al. Fall and injury prevention in older people living in residential care facilities. A cluster randomized trial. *Ann Intern Med* 2002;36(10):733–741.
39. Mian OS, Baltzopoulos V, Minetti AE, et al. The impact of physical training on locomotor function in older people. *Sports Med* 2007;37(8): 683–701.
40. Hui-Chi H. A checklist for assessing the risk of falls among the elderly. *J Nurs Res* 2004;12(2):131–142.
41. Zimmer-Gembeck MD, Southard PA, Hedges JR, et al. Triage in an established trauma system. *J Trauma* 1995;39:922–928.
42. Ma MH, MacKenzie EJ, Alcorta R, et al. Compliance with prehospital triage protocols for major trauma patients. *J Trauma* 1999;46:168–175.
43. Meldon SW, Reilly M, Drew BL, et al. Trauma in the very elderly: a community-based study of outcomes at trauma and nontrauma centers. *J Trauma* 2002;52:79–84.
44. Vollmer DG, Torner JC, Jane JA, et al. Age and outcome following traumatic coma: why do older patients fare worse? *J Neurosurg* 1991;75: S37–S49.
45. Hukkelhoven CW, Steyerberg EW, Rampen AJ, et al. Patient age and outcome following severe traumatic brain injury: an analysis of 5600 patients. *J Neurosurg* 2003;99:666–673.
46. Kotwica Z, Jakubowski JK. Acute head injuries in the elderly. An analysis of 136 consecutive patients. *Acta Neurochir (Wien)* 1992;118:98–102.
47. Kilaru S, Garb J, Emhoff T, et al. Long-term functional status and mortality of elderly patients with severe closed head injuries. *J Trauma* 1996;41: 957–963.
48. Knudson MM, Maull KI. Nonoperative management of solid organ injuries. Past, present, and future. *Surg Clin North Am* 1999;79: 1357–1371.
49. Barone JE, Burns G, Svehlak SA, et al. Management of blunt splenic trauma in patients older than 55 years. Southern Connecticut Regional Trauma Quality Assurance Committee. *J Trauma* 1999;46:87–90.
50. Cocanour CS, Moore FA, Ware DN, et al. Age should not be a consideration for non-operative management of blunt splenic injury. *J Trauma* 2000; 48:606–610.
51. Falimirski ME, Provost D. Nonsurgical management of solid abdominal organ injury in patients over 55 years of age. *Am Surg* 2000;66:631–635.
52. Krause KR, Howells GA, Bair HA, et al. Nonoperative management of blunt splenic injury in adults 55 years and older: a twenty-year experience. *Am Surg* 2000;66:636–640.
53. Meyers JG, Dent DL, Stewart RM, et al. Blunt splenic injuries: dedicated trauma surgeons can achieve a high rate of nonoperative success in patients of all ages. *J Trauma* 2000;48:801–805; discussion 805–861.
54. Harbrecht BG, Peitzman AB, Rivera L, et al. Contribution of age and gender to outcome of blunt splenic injury in adults: multicenter study of the eastern association for the surgery of trauma. *J Trauma* 2001;51:887–895.
55. Bergeron E, Lavoie A, Clas D, et al. Elderly trauma patients with rib fractures are at greater risk of death and pneumonia. *J Trauma* 2003;54: 478–485.
56. Bulger EM, Arneson MA, Mock CN, et al. Rib fractures in the elderly. *J Trauma* 2000;48:1040–1046.
57. Stawicki SP, Grossman MD, Hoey BA, et al. Rib fractures in the elderly: a marker of injury severity. *J Am Geriatr Soc* 2004;52:805–808.
58. Easter A. Management of patients with multiple rib fractures. *Am J Crit Care* 2001;10(5):320–327.
59. Karmakar MK, Ho AM. Acute pain management of patients with multiple fractured ribs. *J Trauma* 2003;54(3):615–626.
60. Parris R. Towards evidence based emergency medicine: best BETs from the Manchester Royal Infirmary. Epidural analgesia/anaesthesia versus systemic intravenous opioid analgesia in the management of blunt thoracic trauma. *Emerg Med J* 2007;24(12):848–849.
61. Chang TT, Schecter WP. Injury in the elderly and end-of-life decisions. *Surg Clin North Am* 2007;87:229–245.
62. Zukerman JD, Sakales SR, Fabian DR, et al. Hip fractures in geriatric patients. Results of an interdisciplinary hospital care program. *Clin Orthop Relat Res* 1992;27:213–225.
63. Sexson SB, Lehner JT. Factors affecting hip fracture mortality. *J Orthop Trauma* 1987;1:298–305.
64. Henry SM, Pollak AN, Jones AL, et al. Pelvic fracture in geriatric patients: a distinct clinical entity. *J Trauma* 2002;53:15–20.
65. O'Brien DP, Luchette FA, Pereira SJ, et al. Pelvic fracture in the elderly is associated with increased mortality. *Surgery* 2002;132:710–714; discussion 714–715.
66. Smith DP, Enderson BL, Maull KI. Trauma in the elderly: determinants of outcome. *South Med J* 1990;83:171–177.
67. Pellicane JV, Byrne K, DeMaria EJ. Preventable complications and death from multiple organ failure among geriatric trauma victims. *J Trauma* 1992;33:440–444.
68. Bochicchio GV, Joshi M, Knorr KM, et al. Impact of nosocomial infections in trauma: does age make a difference? *J Trauma* 2001;50:612–617; discussion 617–619.
69. Connors AF Jr, Speroff T, Dawson NV, et al. The effectiveness of right heart catheterization in the initial care of critically ill patients. SUPPORT Investigators. *JAMA* 1996;276:889–897.
70. Sandham JD, Hull RD, Brant RF, et al. A randomized, controlled trial of the use of pulmonary-artery catheters in high-risk surgical patients. *N Engl J Med* 2003;348:5–14.
71. Webster CS, Merry AF, Emmens DJ, et al. A prospective clinical audit of central venous catheter use and complications in 1000 consecutive patients. *Anaesth Intensive Care* 2008;31(1):80–86.
72. Manasia AR, Nagaraj HM, Kodali RB, et al. Feasibility and potential clinical utility of goal-directed transthoracic echocardiography performed by noncardiologist intensivists using a small hand-carried device (SonoHeart) in critically-ill patients. *J Cardiothorac Vasc Anesth* 2005;19:155–159.
73. Jensen MB, Sloth E, Larsen KM, et al. Transthoracic echocardiography for cardiopulmonary monitoring in intensive care. *Eur J Anaesthesiol* 2004; 21:700–707.
74. Khoury AF, Afridi I, Quinones MA, et al. Transesophageal echocardiography in critically ill patients: feasibility, safety, and impact on management. *Am Heart J* 1994;127:1363–1371.
75. Applebaum GE, King JE, Finucane TE. The outcome of CPR initiated in nursing homes. *J Am Geriatr Soc* 1990;38:197–200.
76. Gordon M, Cheung M. Poor outcome of on-site CPR in a multilevel geriatric facility: three and a half years experience at the Baycrest Centre for Geriatric Care. *J Am Geriatr Soc* 1993;41:163.
77. Taffet GE, Teasdale JA, Luchi RJ. In-hospital cardiopulmonary resuscitation. *JAMA* 1988;260:2069.
78. Tresch DD. CPR in the elderly: When should it be performed? *Geriatrics* 1991;46(47):54.
79. Kinsella JD, Singer PA, Siegler M. Legalized active euthanasia: an Aesculapian tragedy. *Bull Am Coll Surg* 1989;74:6.
80. McCarthy EP, Pencina MJ, Kelley-Hayes M, et al. Advance care planning and health care preferences of community-dwelling elders: the Framingham Heart Study. *J Gerontol A Biol Sci Med Sci* 2008;63(9):951–959.
81. Silverman HJ, Vinicky JK, Gasner MR. Advance directives: implications for critical care. *Crit Care Med* 1992;20(7):1027–1031.
82. Emanuel LL, Barry MJ, Stoeckle JD, et al. Advance directives for medical care–a case for greater use. *N Engl J Med* 1991;324:889–895.

83. Shmerling RH, Bedell SE, Lilienfeld A, et al. Discussing cardiopulmonary resuscitation: a study of elderly outpatients. *J Gen Intern Med* 1988;3: 317–321.
84. Turner JS, Michell WL, Morgan CJ, et al. Limitation of life support: frequency and practice in a London and a Cape Town intensive care unit. *Intensive Care Med* 1996;22(10):1020–1025.
85. Smedira NG, Evans BH, Grais LS, et al. Withholding and withdrawal of life support from the critically ill. *N Engl J Med* 1990;322:309–315.
86. Beecher HK. A definition of irreversible coma. Report of the Ad Hoc Committee of the Harvard Medical School to Examine the Definition of Brain Death. *JAMA* 1968;205:337–340.
87. Morenski JD, Oro JJ, Tobias JD, et al. Determination of death by neurological criteria. *J Intensive Care Med* 2003;18:211–221.
88. Youngner SJ. Who defines futility? *JAMA* 1988;260:2094–2095.
89. Sluys K, Haggmark T, Iselius L. Outcome and quality of life 5 years after major trauma. *J Trauma* 2005;59:223–232.
90. Pande I, Scott DL, O'Neill TW, et al. Quality of life, morbidity and mortality after low trauma hip fracture in men. *Ann Rheum Dis* 2006;65: 87–92.
91. Abrams FR. The doctor with two heads. The patient versus the costs. *N Engl J Med* 1993;328:975–976.
92. Gillon R. Medical ethics: four principles plus attention to scope. *BMJ* 1995;310(6974):261–262.
93. Staudenmayer K, Schecter WP. Civilian hospital response to mass casualty events: basic principles. *Bull Am Coll Surg* 2007;92(8):16–20.
94. Schecter WP. Withdrawing and withholding life support in geriatric surgical patients. Ethical considerations. *Surg Clin North Am* 1994;74(2): 245–259.

CHAPTER 29 ■ TRAUMA IN PREGNANCY

AMY D. WYRZYKOWSKI AND GRACE S. ROZYCKI

KEY POINTS

1. Care of the injured pregnant patient brings the challenge of treating two patients, both with unique physiologic responses to the trauma.
2. Anatomic and physiologic changes of pregnancy can alter the maternal response to injury. Knowledge of these changes should be kept in mind as the evaluation and resuscitation of the pregnant trauma patient proceeds.
3. Priorities for the resuscitation of the injured pregnant patient are the same as for any other trauma patient. Patient care, however, is altered to accommodate the unique anatomic and physiologic characteristics of the gravid woman.
4. Following injury, the fetus is highly susceptible to hypoxia and decreased perfusion. Hypoxia, hypovolemia, and acidosis must be promptly treated and aggressively normalized.
5. If fundal height is at the umbilicus, the fetus should be presumed viable.
6. A Kleihauer-Betke test should be performed in all Rh-negative pregnant women to determine if fetomaternal transfusion has occurred.
7. Fetal evaluation includes fundal height measurement and recording heart tones, heart rate, and movement. Focused abdominal sonogram for trauma is an excellent noninvasive, radiation-free method of evaluating the mother, uterus, and fetus.
8. Trauma may require urgent transfusion, which should be type O, Rh-negative blood.
9. Liberal but judicious use of radiographic studies is advised for the evaluation of the pregnant trauma patient. An imaging study deemed necessary should not be withheld for fear of potential hazard to the fetus.
10. Although the myometrium is relatively elastic, the placenta is not, predisposing it to shear forces at the uteroplacental interface, which may lead to abruptio placentae. Abruptio placentae is the most common cause of fetal demise following trauma and may present as an occult process.

(1) Although injured pregnant patients make up only approximately 1% of all trauma admissions,[1–6] the magnitude of the problem is much greater because two patients are being cared for simultaneously. Studies have found that trauma is responsible for up to 46.3% of deaths in pregnant women.[7,8] In fact, the problem may be underestimated because gravid status may not be routinely recorded on death certificates.[9]

In several series, the rate of fetal death parallels the extent of maternal injury.[3,8,10] In others, fetal death rates have been reported to be three to four times greater than the maternal death rate, implying that the survival of the mother is not always sufficient to ensure fetal well-being.[1,2,5,11] Although most trauma involving pregnant patients occurs during the second or third trimester, some reports of domestic abuse show that this occurs most frequently before 18 weeks' gestation and then diminishes between 20 and 30 weeks' gestation.[1,9,11–13] Motor vehicle crashes occur with equal frequency throughout the gestational period and are the leading cause of fetal death secondary to maternal trauma.[13–15] An understanding of the anatomic and physiologic changes unique to pregnancy as well as of the principles of resuscitation and treatment after trauma are important to provide the best care for both the injured mother and her unborn child.

ANATOMY AND PHYSIOLOGY UNIQUE TO THE GRAVID PATIENT

(2) Anatomic and physiologic changes of pregnancy can alter the maternal response to injury (Table 29.1). Knowledge of these changes should be kept in mind as the evaluation and resuscitation of the pregnant trauma patient proceed.

Anatomic Changes

By the 12th week of gestation, the gravid uterus is considered an intra-abdominal organ. Important marks for estimating gestational age include the umbilicus (20 weeks' gestation) and the costal margins (34 to 36 weeks' gestation). During the final 2 weeks of normal gestation, the fetal head descends into the pelvis, placing the fetus at risk for skull fractures or traumatic brain injuries with maternal pelvic fractures. With increasing gestational age, the uterus becomes relatively thin (1.5 cm at term) and the amount of amniotic fluid decreases.[16] As a result, with advancing gestational age, the fetus is more

TABLE 29.1

PHYSIOLOGIC ALTERATIONS IN PREGNANCY

■ SYSTEM	■ CHANGE	■ IMPLICATION
Neurologic	Eclampsia may mimic traumatic brain injury (headache, seizures, hypertension)	Exclude traumatic brain injury (head computed tomography scan)
		May mask shock
Cardiovascular	Cardiac output increased by 1.0–1.5 L/min	Delayed signs of shock
	Heart rate ↑ 10–15 bpm	Supine hypotension syndrome
	Blood pressure ↓ 5–15 mm Hg in second trimester but returns to normal in third trimester	
	Plasma volume increase by 50%	
	Vena cava compression	
Respiratory	Residual lung volume decreased	Decreased buffering capacity
	Chronic respiratory alkalosis	
Gastrointestinal	Decreased gastrointestinal motility	Increased propensity toward aspiration and vomiting
Genitourinary	Dilatation of renal system	Physiologic hydronephrosis and urinary stasis
Laboratory values	Increased white blood cell count Decreased hematocrit	Difficulty interpreting clinical picture regarding hemorrhage
	Increased fibrinogen and factors VII, VIII, X, and XII	Hypercoagulable stage

vulnerable to injury, especially when the mother receives a direct blow to the abdomen. Although the myometrium is relatively elastic, the placenta is not, predisposing it to shear forces at the uteroplacental interface, which may lead to abruptio placentae (Fig. 29.1).

Cardiovascular

Maternal blood volume (plasma and erythrocytes) begins to increase during the first trimester but expands most rapidly

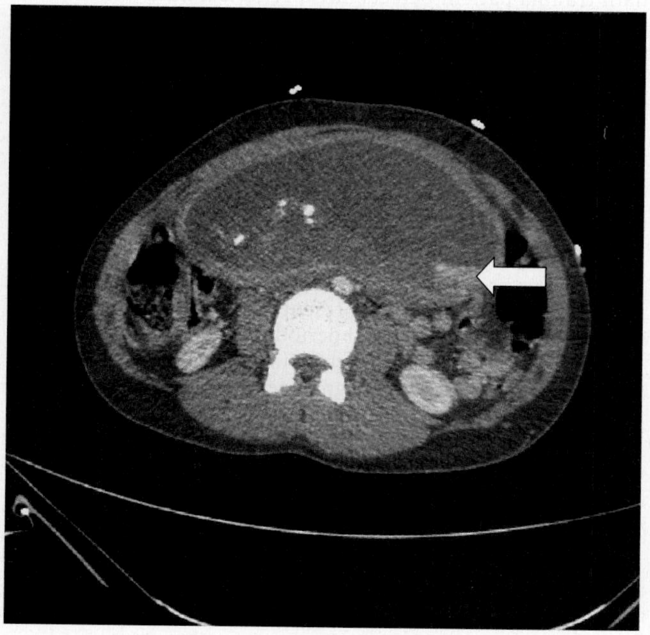

FIGURE 29.1. Placental abruption. Computed tomography scan demonstrating placental abruption. The arrow points to an area of active extravasation of contrast consistent with ongoing hemorrhage. (Reprinted with permission from Jeffrey M. Nicholas, MD, FACS.)

during the second trimester, reaching approximately 45% (6.5 to 8 L) above nonpregnant levels.[17–19] The increase in plasma volume is proportionally greater than the enlarged erythrocyte volume and results in the physiologic anemia of pregnancy. Near term, the plasma volume continues to expand, but the red cell mass begins to increase, resulting in a near-normal hematocrit. Pregnancy-induced hypervolemia supplies the extraordinary demands of the enlarged uterus, allows for fewer red blood cells to be lost during parturition, minimizes the loss of oxygen-carrying capacity associated with hemoglobin, and protects the mother from the hypotensive effects of impaired venous return.[20] This physiologic hypervolemia masks volume loss after trauma and may give the clinician an unfounded sense of security about the patient's hemodynamic stability. Almost 35% of the mother's blood volume may be lost before maternal signs of shock are noted.[21] Placental vasculature is dilated at baseline, but exquisitely sensitive to catecholamines. Maternal hypovolemia and the presence of circulating catecholamines may result in increased uterine vascular resistance, diminished placental blood flow, and diminished fetal oxygenation even with normal maternal vital signs.[22] In fact, fetal distress may be the first manifestation of maternal hypovolemia.[23]

As pregnancy progresses, cardiac output increases up to 50% above normal until the 24th week of gestation, after which it plateaus. This increase in cardiac output is a result of a modest rise in heart rate and stroke volume related to the expanded blood volume and the direct inotropic effect of estrogen.[24]

If the pregnant patient is in the supine position, the inferior vena cava is partially obstructed by the gravid uterus. This decreases venous blood return to the heart, lowers cardiac output, and results in supine hypotension. Turning the pregnant patient onto her left side improves venous return and increases cardiac output by approximately 30%.[25]

Overall, cardiac work is increased with pregnancy because of the volume load and estrogen effect, despite a decrease in systemic vascular resistance mediated by prostaglandin, progestin, intracellular calcium flux, and endothelial-derived factors.[26] Early in pregnancy, the blood pressure, especially the diastolic level, decreases but then slowly returns to normal by term. Mean normal values for the first trimester are 105 mm Hg systolic and 60 mm Hg diastolic; for the second trimester, 102 and 55 mm Hg, respectively; and for the third trimester, 108 and 67 mm Hg, respectively. Significant elevation above these levels may indicate pregnancy-induced hypertension.[27]

Finally, the enlarged uterus causes the heart to be displaced upward and to the left. This change, along with the common development of a serous pericardial effusion,[28] results in an enlarged cardiac silhouette and increased pulmonary vascular markings on the chest radiograph.[29]

Pulmonary

The thoracic cavity undergoes significant reconfiguration during pregnancy. The subcostal angle increases and the chest circumference expands 5 to 7 cm. As the uterus enlarges, the level of the diaphragm rises approximately 4 cm. The rise of the diaphragm decreases the volume of the lungs at rest, reducing both total lung capacity and functional residual capacity. At the same time, there is a 5% to 10% increase in inspiratory capacity. The net result of these changes is that pregnancy is a state of chronic hyperventilation with a 30% to 40% increase in minute ventilation inducing a chronic respiratory alkalosis. The maternal alkalosis facilitates the transfer of fetal CO_2 to the maternal circulation. Acidosis in the pregnant patient significantly compromises fetal–maternal gas exchange and must be avoided.[30]

Gastrointestinal

As pregnancy progresses, the enlarged uterus stretches the abdominal wall and compresses the viscera. This results in a diminished response to peritoneal irritation and altered or referred pain perception, diminishing the accuracy of the clinical exam. Progesterone diminishes the tone of the lower esophageal sphincter and decreases both gastric tone and motility. As a result, the pregnant patient is at significant risk for aspiration.

Renal

Throughout pregnancy, the renal collecting system enlarges to meet the demands of the increased blood volume and urine formation. The renal pelvis and ureter dilate early in the first trimester, resulting in a mild hydronephrosis and hydroureter.[31] Urinary stasis in the collecting system predisposes the pregnant woman to pyelonephritis. In the first trimester, the renal blood flow and the glomerular filtration rate increase by up to 50%; consequently, the levels of creatinine and blood urea nitrogen (BUN) decrease.[32] The clinical significance is that normal or slightly elevated levels of creatinine or BUN may signify renal dysfunction.

Musculoskeletal

The relaxation of the interosseous ligaments during pregnancy causes increased mobility of the sacroiliac and sacrococcygeal joints and widening of the symphysis pubis. These changes, coupled with an enlarged uterus, result in lordosis, disrupt the maternal center of gravity, and increase the risk for falls.

Laboratory Values

The peripheral blood leukocyte count increases to approximately 12,000 cells/mL during gestation and may be as high as 25,000 cells/mL during labor.[33] The platelet count may appear falsely low because of dilution from increases in plasma volume. Fibrinogen (factor I) and factors VII, VIII, IX, and X are increased considerably during pregnancy, but prothrombin (factor II) is increased only slightly. Although there is a slight decrease in the protein S level and its activity,[34] levels of antithrombin III and protein C show no significant change during pregnancy. The level of plasminogen (profibrinolysin) in plasma increases significantly, most likely induced by estrogen.

INITIAL ASSESSMENT AND MANAGEMENT

3 Priorities for the resuscitation of the injured pregnant patient are the same as for any other trauma patient. Patient care, however, is altered to accommodate the unique anatomic and physiologic characteristics of the gravid woman.[35]

The best therapy for the unborn child is expedient maternal resuscitation. An adequate airway with supplemental
4 oxygenation is essential to prevent fetal hypoxemia. Because fetal blood functions on a different oxyhemoglobin dissociation curve, small positive increments in maternal oxygen concentration improve oxygen content and physiologic reserve for the fetus, even if maternal arterial oxygen content does not change appreciably. Maternal hemorrhagic shock, with its resultant release of catecholamines, causes uterine artery vasoconstriction, reducing uterine perfusion and compromising fetal viability. Hence, vigorous crystalloid resuscitation is encouraged, even for patients who appear normotensive. In late pregnancy, compromised cardiac output and blood pressure secondary to vena cava compression can be relieved by placing the patient in the left lateral decubitus or right hip-flexed position. A nasogastric tube should be inserted because of the pregnant patient's increased propensity toward vomiting and aspiration. Urinary volume per hour should be monitored to provide some indication of perfusion status. A focused abdominal ultrasound examination should be performed to look for intraperitoneal hemorrhage in the mother. Goodwin et al. found that ultrasound in the pregnant trauma patient detects intraperitoneal fluid with a sensitivity, specificity, and accuracy similar to that of nonpregnant patients.[36]

History and Physical Examination

The secondary survey consists of a thorough history (including obstetric history), physical examination, and fetal monitoring if indicated by gestational age.[37] Maternal prenatal history is crucial and may alter management decisions if medical problems such as preeclampsia, diabetes, essential hypertension, or congenital heart disease are present. Obstetric history includes the date of the last menstrual period, the expected date of confinement, the perception of fetal movement, and the status of the current and previous pregnancies. If the mother is unable to provide the gestational age, it can be estimated from the
5 fundal height. Fundal height at the umbilicus represents approximately 20 weeks' gestation and the fetus should be considered viable unless an obstetrician determines otherwise. Pelvic and rectal examinations are performed with special attention to vaginal discharge (amniotic fluid or blood), effacement, dilation, and fetal station.[38] Vaginal bleeding is always abnormal and may be a sign of labor, placental abruption, placenta previa, or uterine rupture.[39,40]

6 Fetomaternal hemorrhage occurs in 20% of injured pregnant patients. The Kleihauer-Betke (KB) test detects fetal cells in the maternal circulation, indicating fetomaternal hemorrhage, and should be obtained in all Rh-negative pregnant women. If an Rh-negative woman has a positive KB test, she

should receive Rh immunoglobin. The initial dose is 300 μg followed by an additional 300 μg for each 30 mL of estimated fetomaternal transfusion.[41,42]

Fetal Assessment and Monitoring

7 Fetal evaluation consists of uterine assessment, fundal height measurement, and recording of heart tones, heart rate, and movement. Uterine tenderness and contraction may be related to abruptio placentae, which can occur in the absence of vaginal bleeding. Continuous fetal monitoring is the best predictor of a healthy or distressed fetus. Normal fetal heart rate is 120 to 160 beats per minute; both fetal tachycardia and bradycardia may indicate fetal distress. There is still no consensus on the indications for fetal monitoring in trauma patients. A guideline for patients with major injuries, including shock, is to provide continuous fetal monitoring for at least 24 hours.[43]

DIAGNOSTIC MODALITIES

After patient stabilization, several diagnostic modalities are used to define the extent and type of injury for the mother and
8 fetus. Initially, laboratory studies are obtained. If blood is urgently needed, type O, Rh-negative blood is chosen. Evaluation of the abdomen may be performed by ultrasound, computed tomography (CT) scan, or diagnostic peritoneal lavage.[44] Reliance on ultrasound to evaluate both the mother and the fetus obviates the need to perform a CT scan in some cases and can provide valuable information on fetal motion, heart tones, location, and placement. If diagnostic peritoneal lavage is elected, the open, supraumbilical technique is recommended.

9 Liberal but judicious use of radiographic studies is advised for the evaluation of the pregnant trauma patient. An imaging study deemed necessary should not be withheld for fear of potential hazard to the fetus. Factors contributing to the sequelae of prenatal exposure to ionizing radiation are the stage of development, the exposure time, the dose delivered, and the dose absorbed. The absorbed radiation dose varies according to many factors, including instrument model, desired image quality, and distance from the radioactive source. The roentgen (R) is the unit of exposure, and the centigray (cGy) or rad is the unit of absorbed dose. Approximate absorbed fetal doses for radiographic tests are presented in Table 29.2. There is no medical justification for terminating pregnancy in women exposed to 5 cGy or less.[45] A 0.1% increase in the rate of spontaneous abortion during the first 2 weeks of development follows a dose of 10 cGy, and there is a 1% increase in congenital abnormalities at the same dose.[46] Another concern is the potential for late neoplasia development. The risks for radiation-induced cancer after in utero exposure during the second and third trimesters are estimated to be 1 in 15,000 children if exposed to 1 mGy x-radiation.[47] If the fetus receives 50 mGy, the risk is increased to 1 in approximately 300 children. Prudent judgment and foresight by the physician should ensure that specific radiographic studies are ordered and accurately performed to avoid repetition.

TABLE 29.2 **DIAGNOSIS**

APPROXIMATE FETAL DOSES FROM COMMON DIAGNOSTIC PROCEDURES

■ EXAMINATION	■ MEAN EXPOSURE (mGy)	■ MAXIMUM DOSE (mGy)
CONVENTIONAL X-RAY EXAMINATIONS		
Abdomen	1.4	4.2
Chest	<0.01	<0.01
Intravenous pyelogram	1.7	10
Lumbar spine	1.7	10
Pelvis	1.1	4
Skull	<0.01	<0.01
Thoracic spine	<0.01	<0.01
FLUOROSCOPIC EXAMINATIONS		
Upper gastrointestinal	1.1	5.8
Barium enema	6.8	24
COMPUTED TOMOGRAPHY		
Abdomen	8.0	49
Chest	0.06	0.96
Head	<0.005	<0.005
Lumbar spine	2.4	8.6
Pelvis	25	79

Adapted from Sharp C, Shrimpton JA, Bury RF. *Diagnostic Medical Exposures*. London: National Radiology Board; 1998.

BLUNT TRAUMA

Motor vehicle crashes remain the chief cause of blunt trauma in the pregnant patient. As pregnancy progresses, the uterus becomes more vulnerable, rising out of the protective bony pelvis, and it absorbs most of the impact of blunt abdominal trauma. These factors often result in direct fetal injury, usually skull fracture or intracerebral hemorrhage. Pelvic fractures in the gravid patient may cause extensive maternal retroperitoneal hemorrhage as a result of engorged pelvic veins.

Uterine rupture is a catastrophic and fortunately rare complication of blunt abdominal trauma. The incidence is approximately 0.6%.[39] Fetal mortality approaches 100% and associated maternal mortality is 10%.[22]

10 *Abruptio placentae* is the most common cause of fetal death after maternal injury. This carries a 30% to 70% rate of fetal death and a 1% maternal mortality rate. Over 50% placental separation invariably results in fetal demise.[48] Abruptio placentae can occur in the absence of obvious abdominal injury, because maternal shock is a far greater stimulus for abruption than are the mechanical forces of trauma disrupting the placenta.[38] Abruptio placentae is more common in the presence of hypertension, diabetes mellitus, advanced age, multiparity, and maternal use of tobacco or cocaine. Abruptio placentae presents with vaginal bleeding (in 80% of cases), abdominal pain, disseminated intravascular coagulation due to thromboplastin release, and inexplicable maternal hypovolemia. It invariably occurs within 48 hours after trauma, and pregnant patients who are at risk should be monitored accordingly.

The pregnant patient with minor injury should be observed for several hours. Most patients with insignificant trauma do not require admission unless specific signs and symptoms, such as vaginal bleeding, abdominal cramps, or leakage of amniotic fluid, are present. In one series, only 1 of 11 patients had symptoms after minor trauma, and pregnancy outcome was successful.[6] Occult abruptio placentae has been reported after motor vehicle accidents in which the patient displayed only subtle clinical signs and symptoms. Because placental separation can occur with rapid deceleration injuries, a three-point restraint system appropriately applied is recommended for pregnant automobile passengers.[49–51] The mechanism of injury may provide invaluable information regarding potential injuries in even a healthy-appearing patient. At a minimum, a prompt and thorough maternal assessment, fetal assessment, and comprehensive search for injuries are necessary for evaluating the pregnant patient with minor trauma.

PENETRATING TRAUMA

The perinatal mortality rate from penetrating injury to the mother has been reported to range from 47% to 71%.[52] In general, pregnant women with gunshot wounds to the abdomen should undergo celiotomy. For those who sustain stab wounds to the abdomen, management is based on the likelihood of intra-abdominal injury. The abdominal examination may be unreliable because of a diminished response to peritoneal irritation and altered or referred pain perception. If the clinical presentation is unclear (e.g., absence of peritonitis or evisceration), then a diagnostic peritoneal lavage performed with the open technique in the supraumbilical area may be diagnostic.

OPERATIVE MANAGEMENT

General anesthesia is preferred for the gravid patient with multisystem injury. The risks of anesthesia are related to the physiologic changes that accompany pregnancy. For example, because aspiration is more likely, rapid-sequence induction with cricoid pressure is preferred. Both thiopental and etomidate are good induction agents in pregnancy. As a general rule, ketamine should be avoided as it increases uterine tone and may decrease placental perfusion. Both depolarizing and nondepolarizing neuromuscular blocking agents cross the placenta. This must be remembered because if delivery is required, the infant will be hypotonic and apneic. Volatile agents should be used, if tolerated, as they relax the uterine smooth muscle and blunt the maternal catecholamine response, both of which improve uterine perfusion.[53]

The standard vertical midline incision is used for maternal celiotomy. Adequate visualization of viscera is mandatory, and the pregnant uterus should not interfere with abdominal exploration or repair of an injury. If labor ensues, vaginal delivery is almost always encouraged. Even early in the postoperative period, vaginal delivery is still preferred and does not appear harmful to the mother or the neonate. Cesarean section prolongs the operative time and increases blood loss, generally by approximately 1 L. Indications for cesarean section during celiotomy for trauma are listed in Table 29.3.

If fetal delivery is cesarean, the uterus is incised longitudinally. After the amniotic membranes are ruptured, the fetus is delivered, and the placenta is removed. The uterus is closed in a running-locking fashion using large, absorbable suture. Once the uterus is evacuated, postpartum hemostasis begins. In cases of uterine atony, bimanual compression of the uterus and the intravenous administration of oxytocin are begun. In addition, the surgeon should examine the uterus and cervix for any lacerations and ensure that the uterus is thoroughly evacuated. Other measures to control severe hemorrhage include intravenous methyl ergonovine, or intramyometrial injection of 15-methyl prostaglandin F_{2a}. For the most part, massive hemorrhage associated with emergent cesarean section in the injured women is associated with a pelvic fracture. Packing of the pelvis or embolization of the internal iliac arteries may be needed as well.

Successful outcome of a postmortem cesarean section depends on the duration of the gestation and the time interval between maternal death and delivery. Under optimal conditions, at 26 to 28 weeks' gestation, the estimated fetal survival rate is approximately 50%. Therefore, postmortem cesarean section is justified if the estimated gestational age is at least approximately 26 to 28 weeks. If the time between maternal death and delivery is less than 5 minutes, the fetal prognosis is considered excellent. If the time since maternal death is prolonged to approximately 20 minutes, fetal prognosis is poor. Uncertainty about maternal death time is not a contraindication for this procedure.[54]

TABLE 29.3 **TREATMENT**

INDICATIONS FOR CESAREAN SECTION DURING CELIOTOMY FOR TRAUMA

- Maternal shock, pregnancy near term
- Threat to life from exsanguination (injury or disseminated intravascular coagulation)
- Mechanical limitation of maternal treatment
- Risk of fetal distress exceeding risk of prematurity
- Unstable thoracolumbar spinal injury

CRITICAL CARE MANAGEMENT

Critical care management of the traumatized pregnant patient covers a wide range of topics. The basic principles of hemodynamic monitoring, adequate ventilatory support, nutrition, and careful assessment of volume status apply to the injured pregnant patient and are covered in more detail in other chapters. Knowledge of the disease processes that can arise in the pregnant patient within the first 24 hours after injury allows the physician to render high-quality critical care to the traumatized patient and her unborn child.[55]

When administrating medication to the gravid patient, potential risk versus therapeutic benefit must be considered especially carefully. Prophylactic tetanus immunization should be given appropriately, with anti-D globulin for patients who are Rh negative and at risk for isoimmunization. Prophylactic antibiotics are administered if needed, but tetracycline and most sulfa drugs should be avoided.

CARDIOPULMONARY RESUSCITATION

The enlarged uterus compresses the vena cava, resulting in a 25% decrease in cardiac output as a result of decreased venous return. To improve the effects of cardiopulmonary resuscitation (CPR), patients before 24 weeks' gestation can be maintained in the supine position but with manual displacement of the uterus laterally. After 24 weeks' gestation, a procedure table with a 30-degree left lateral tilt is helpful, although CPR is only 80% effective when performed with the patient in this position. Emergent cesarean section may be needed if the patient does not respond to CPR within approximately 5 minutes.[56,57] Morris et al. found that if the fetus is viable (presence of fetal heart tones) and is at least 26 weeks' gestation, emergent cesarean section is justified; they found that infants who met these criteria had a survival rate of 75%.[58]

TOXEMIA OF PREGNANCY OR PREECLAMPSIA (PREGNANCY-INDUCED HYPERTENSION)

Any traumatized pregnant patient presenting with seizures or coma should have head injury excluded. Toxemia of pregnancy should also be included in the differential diagnosis. In the severe state, eclampsia is manifested by hypertension, pulmonary edema, elevated liver function enzymes, proteinuria (i.e., HELLP syndrome), and seizure activity. The pathophysiologic cause is vasospasm, which affects hepatic, renal, cerebral, and placental blood flow. Despite the presence of pulmonary edema, intravascular volume depletion is often present, and a fluid challenge may be appropriate. Rapid control of the hypertension is achieved with hydralazine.[59] However, elevated maternal oxygen consumption disrupts uterine vascular oxygen supply and maternal equilibrium, resulting in fetal distress. Smoother control of reduction in blood pressure and myocardial oxygen consumption is accomplished by achieving volume expansion before vasodilation. Inotropic support, in combination with vasodilator treatment, maximizes oxygen delivery and affects afterload reduction. Magnesium sulfate has a slight hypotensive effect but does not decrease systemic vascular resistance.

THROMBOEMBOLISM

Pregnant patients are at increased risk of thromboembolism from all three components of the Virchow triad: stasis, intimal damage, and hypercoaguability. Increased venous capacitance, vena cava compression, and weight gain promote venous stasis. Labor and trauma cause intimal damage, and hypercoaguability results from elevated levels of fibrinogen and intrinsic coagulation factors with the gravid state. Advanced age and multiparity further increase these risks. No method of prophylaxis has been demonstrated to be both safe and universally effective in preventing thromboembolism, either in the patient with multiple injuries or in the pregnant patient. In general, warfarin is avoided because it is associated with congenital anomalies if given to the mother in the first trimester and has been shown to cause serious fetal bleeding when administered during the second and third trimesters.[60,61] If chemical venous thromboembolism prophylaxis is indicated in the pregnant patient, the American College of Chest Physicians currently recommends the use of low-molecular-weight heparin over unfractionated heparin.[62]

AMNIOTIC FLUID EMBOLISM

Amniotic fluid embolism after trauma in pregnancy or parturition is characterized by hypotension, hypoxemia, and coagulopathy. The diagnosis is often difficult, and an 80% mortality rate has been reported. Amniotic fluid debris enters the maternal venous circulation, causing sudden dyspnea and hypotension. A mixed metabolic acidosis and respiratory alkalosis ensue. The chest radiograph shows characteristic pulmonary edema or an acute respiratory distress syndrome (ARDS) pattern. Hemodynamically, the patient has an elevated pulmonary capillary wedge pressure and a low systemic vascular resistance. Disseminated intravascular coagulation develops in approximately 30% of these patients. Although most cases of amniotic fluid embolism occur during labor, it has been reported to occur after abdominal trauma[63] and abruptio placentae. This diagnosis is established on clinical findings, and the treatment consists of supportive care (i.e., oxygenation, maximization of hemodynamic parameters, and correction of coagulopathy).

INTERPERSONAL VIOLENCE

Although motor vehicle crashes and falls are the most common causes of trauma during pregnancy, reports indicate that 4% to 17% of pregnant women are victims of interpersonal violence.[2–4] In fact, this number may be underestimated because population-based prevalence estimates are often unavailable, pregnancy is not consistently recorded on death certificates,[9] and, as with many abuse crimes, it is not frequently reported.

Poole et al. reported that 64 (31.5%) of 203 injured pregnant patients experienced interpersonal violence.[11] Of the eight fetal deaths in this series, three occurred 7 days after injury and five occurred in women with an Injury Severity Score of zero. These findings indicate that severe trauma to the fetus may occur without obvious injury to the mother, emphasizing the need for the physician to question the patient directly about abuse. Furthermore, physicians should be encouraged to take measures for early intervention, such as establishing a link with agencies that deal with battered women, so that physical protection, emotional support, and information about legal rights are readily available.

SUMMARY

The pregnant trauma victim presents a unique challenge to the resuscitating physician. Two patients are being treated, and a high degree of expertise is needed to treat both. Initially, evaluation should involve the cooperative efforts of the emergency physician, trauma surgeon, obstetrician, and obstetric nurse. If the pregnancy is near term or delivery is anticipated, a pediatrician and pediatric surgeon should be consulted. The pregnancy should not distract the surgeon from initiating basic resuscitation. Equally important, the injury should not confound the obstetrician. The expertise of the obstetric nurse is useful in coordinating the overall care plan for the mother and her unborn child. Expedient, accurate resuscitation of the mother takes priority because the best chance for fetal survival is maternal survival.

References

1. Rogers FB, Rozycki GS, Osler TM, et al. A multi-institutional study of factors associated with fetal death in injured pregnant patients. *Arch Surg* 1999;134:1274–1277.
2. Kissinger DP, Rozycki GS, Morris JA, et al. Trauma in pregnancy: predicting pregnancy outcome. *Arch Surg* 1991;126:1079–1086.
3. Drost TF, Rosemurgy AS, Sherman HF, et al. Major trauma in pregnant women: maternal/fetal outcome. *J Trauma* 1990;30:574–578.
4. Hoff WS, D'Amelio LF, Tinkoff GH, et al. Maternal predictors of fetal demise in trauma during pregnancy. *Surg Gynecol Obstet* 1991;172:175–180.
5. Esposito TJ, Gens DR, Smith LG, et al. Trauma during pregnancy: a review of 79 cases. *Arch Surg* 1991;126:1073–1078.
6. Pearlman MD, Tintinalli JE, Lorenz RP. A prospective controlled study of outcome after trauma during pregnancy. *Am J Obstet Gynecol* 1990;162:1502–1510.
7. Fildes J, Reed L, Jones N, et al. Trauma: the leading cause of maternal death. *J Trauma* 1992;32:643–645.
8. Shah KH, Simons RK, Holbrook T, et al. Trauma in pregnancy: maternal and fetal outcomes. *J Trauma* 1998;45(1):83–96.
9. Dietz P, Rochat R, Goldner T, et al. Pregnancy status poorly reported on death certificates. In: Osewe PL, ed. *Georgia Epidemiology Report* (Report #11–16). Atlanta, GA: Department of Human Resources; 1995:1–4.
10. Scorpio RJ, Esposito TJ, Smith LG, et al. Blunt trauma during pregnancy: factors affecting fetal outcome. *J Trauma* 1992;32:213–216.
11. Poole GV, Martin JN Jr, Perry KG Jr, et al. Trauma in pregnancy: the role of interpersonal violence. *Am J Obstet Gynecol* 1996;174:1873–1878.
12. Biester EM, Tomich PG, Esposito TJ, et al. Trauma in pregnancy: normal revised trauma score in relation to other markers of maternofetal status—a preliminary study. *Am J Obstet Gynecol* 1997;176:1206–1212.
13. Connolly A, Katz VL, Bash KL, et al. Trauma and pregnancy. *Am J Perinatol* 1997;14:331–336.
14. Weiss HB, Songer TJ, Fabio A. Fetal deaths related to maternal injury. *JAMA* 2001;286:1863–1868.
15. Weiss HB, Lawrence B, Miller T. Prevalence and risk of hospitalized pregnant occupants in car crashes. In: *Annual Proceedings/Association for the Advancement of Automotive Medicine* 2002;46:355–366.
16. Cunningham FG, MacDonald PC, Gant NF, et al., eds. In: *Williams Obstetrics,* 20th ed. Norwalk, CT: Appleton & Lange; 1997:191–225.
17. Pritchard JA. Changes in blood during pregnancy and delivery. *Anesthesiology* 1965;26:393.
18. Whittaker PG, MacPhail S, Lind T. Serial hematologic changes and pregnancy outcome. *Obstet Gynecol* 1996;88:33.
19. Scott DE. Anemia during pregnancy. *Obstet Gynecol Ann* 1972;48:638.

20. Smith CV, Phelan JP. Trauma in pregnancy. In: Clark SL, Cotton DB, Hankins GDV, et al., eds. *Critical Care Obstetrics,* 2nd ed. Boston, MA: Blackwell; 1991:498.
21. Brinkman CRI, Mofid M, Assali NS. Circulatory shock in pregnant sheep: effects of hemorrhage on uteroplacental and fetal circulation and oxygenation. *Am J Obstet Gynecol* 1974;118:77–90.
22. Weintraub AY, Leron E, Mazor M. The pathophysiology of trauma in pregnancy: a review. *J Matern Fetal Neonatal Med* 2006;19(10):601–605.
23. Tsuei BJ. Assessment of the pregnant trauma patient. *Injury* 2006;37(5): 367–373.
24. Gonick B. Intensive care monitoring of the critically ill pregnant patient. In: Creasy RK, Resnick R, eds. *Maternal-fetal Medicine: Principles and Practice*, 2nd ed. Philadelphia, PA: WB Saunders; 1989:845.
25. Bieniarz J, Branda LA, Maqueda E. Aortocaval compression by the uterus in late pregnancy: III. Unreliability of the sphygmomanometric method in estimating uterine artery pressure. *Am J Obstet Gynecol* 1968;102: 1106.
26. Greiss FC, Anderson SG. Effect of ovarian hormones on the uterine vascular bed. *Am J Obstet Gynecol* 1970;107:829.
27. Clark SL, Cotton DB, Lee W. Central hemodynamic assessment of normal term pregnancy. *Am J Obstet Gynecol* 1989;161:1439.
28. Enein M, Zina AAA, Kassem M, et al. Echocardiography of the pericardium in pregnancy. *Obstet Gynecol* 1987;69:851.
29. Lee W, Cotton DB. Cardiorespiratory changes during pregnancy. In: Clark SL, Cotton DB, Hankins GDV, et al., eds. *Critical Care Obstetrics*, 2nd ed. Boston, MA: Blackwell; 1991:2.
30. Gordon MC. Maternal physiology in pregnancy. In: Gabbe SG, Niebyl JR, Simpson JL, eds. *Obstetrics: Normal and Problem Pregnancies*, 4th ed. Philadelphia, PA: Churchill Livingstone; 2002:63–91.
31. Bailey RR, Rollerston GL. Kidney length and ureteric dilatation in the puerperium. *Br J Obstet Gynaecol* 1971;78:55.
32. Chesley LC. Renal function during pregnancy. In: Carey HM, ed. *Modern Trends in Human Reproductive Physiology*, Vol 1. London: Butterworths; 1963:205–214.
33. Taylor DJ, Phillips P, Lind T. Puerperal hematological indices. *Br J Obstet Gynaecol* 1981;88:601.
34. Bremme K, Ostlund E, Almqvist I, et al. Enhanced thrombin generation and fibrinolytic activity in normal pregnancy and the puerperium. *Obstet Gynecol* 1992;80:132.
35. Advanced Trauma Life Support. American College of Surgeons Committee on Trauma. *Trauma in Women,* 6th ed. Chicago, IL: American College of Surgeons; 1997:313–324.
36. Goodwin H, Holmes JF, Wisner DH. Abdominal ultrasound examination in pregnant blunt trauma patients. *J Trauma* 2001;50(4):689–694.
37. Higgins SD. Perinatal protocol: trauma in pregnancy. *J Perinatol* 1988;8: 288–292.
38. Neufeld JDG, Moore EE, Marx JA, et al. Trauma in pregnancy. *Emerg Med Clin North Am* 1987;5:623–640.
39. Mattox KL, Goetzl L. Trauma in pregnancy. *Crit Care Med* 2005; 33(10)(suppl):S385–S389.
40. Muench MV, Canterino JC. Trauma in pregnancy. *Obstet Gynecol Clin North Am* 2007;34(3):555–583.
41. Kleihauer E, Braun H, Betke K. Demonstration von fetalem hamoglobin in den erythrocyten eines blutausstrichs. *Klin Wochenschr* 1957;35:637.
42. Dhanraj D, Lambers D. The incidences of positive Kleihaour-Betke test in low-risk pregnancies and maternal trauma patients. *Am J Obstet Gynecol* 2004;190:1461–1463.
43. Depp R. Clinical evaluation of fetal status. In: Scott JR, DiSaia PJ, Hammond CB, et al., eds. *Danforth's Obstetrics and Gynecology,* 6th ed. Philadelphia, PA: JB Lippincott; 1990:315–334.
44. Reed KL. Ultrasound in obstetrics. In: Scott JR, DiSaia PJ, Hammond CB, et al., eds. *Danforth's Obstetrics and Gynecology*, 6th ed. Philadelphia, PA: JB Lippincott; 1990:297–314.
45. Brent RL. The effect of embryonic and fetal exposure to x-ray, microwaves, and ultrasound: counseling the pregnant and nonpregnant patient about these risks. *Semin Oncol* 1989;16:347–368.
46. Bushong SC. *Radiologic Science for Technologists*. Washington, DC: Mosby; 1983:550.
47. Stovall M, Blackwell CR, Novada DH, et al. Fetal dose from radiotherapy with photon beams: report of AAPM Radiation Therapy Committee Task Group No. 36. *Med Phys* 1995;22:63–82.
48. Higgins SD, Garite TJ. Late abruptio placentae in trauma patients: implications for monitoring. *Obstet Gynecol* 1984;63(3)(suppl):10S–12S.
49. Crosby WM. Automobile trauma in pregnancy: prevention and treatment. *Prim Care Update Ob/Gyn* 1996;3:6.
50. Crosby WM, Costiloe J. Safety of lap-belt restraint for pregnant victims of automobile collisions. *N Engl J Med* 1971;284:632.
51. Pearlman MD, Viano D. Automobile crash simulation with the first pregnant crash test dummy. *Am J Obstet Gynecol* 1996;175:977–981.
52. Franger AL, Buchsbaum HJ, Peaceman AM. Abdominal gunshot wounds in pregnancy. *Am J Obstet Gynecol* 1989;160:1124–1128.
53. Hull SB, Bennett S. The pregnant trauma patient: assessment and anesthetic management. *Int Anesthesiol Clin* 2007;45(3):1–18.
54. Rothenberger D, Quattlebaum FW, Perry JF. Blunt maternal trauma: a review of 103 cases. *J Trauma* 1978;18:173.
55. Naylor DF Jr, Olson MM. Critical care obstetrics and gynecology. *Crit Care Clin* 2003;19:127–149.
56. Marx GF. Cardiopulmonary resuscitation of late-pregnant women. *Anesthesiology* 1982;56:156.
57. Oates S, Williams GL, Rees GA. Cardiopulmonary resuscitation in late pregnancy. *BMJ* 1988;297:40.
58. Morris JA, Rosenbower TJ, Jurkovich GJ, et al. Infant survival after cesarean section for trauma. *Ann Surg* 1996;223:481–449.
59. Common complications of pregnancy: hypertensive disorders in pregnancy. In: Cunningham FG, MacDonald PC, Gant NF, et al., eds. *Williams Obstetrics*, 20th ed. Norwalk, CT: Appleton & Lange; 1997: 693–744.
60. Ginsberg JS, Hirsch J. Use of antithrombotic agents during pregnancy. *Chest* 1998;114:524S–530S.
61. Easterling TR, Otto C. Heart disease. In: Gabbe SG, Niebyl JR, Simpson JL, eds. *Obstetrics: Normal and Problem Pregnancies*. Philadelphia, PA: Churchill Livingstone; 2002:29,1016.
62. Bates SM, Greer IA, Pabinger I, et al. Venous thromboembolism, thrombophilia, antithrombotic therapy, and pregnancy: American College of Chest Physicians evidence-based clinical practice guidelines 8th edition. *Chest* 2008;133(suppl):8445–8465.
63. Judich A, Kuriansky J, Engelberg I, et al. Amniotic fluid embolism following blunt abdominal trauma in pregnancy. *Injury* 1998;29:475–477.

CHAPTER 30 ■ CRITICAL CARE AND POSTINJURY MANAGEMENT

GRANT E. O'KEEFE

KEY POINTS

1. Adequate resuscitation is critical to avoid ongoing occult hypoperfusion and subsequent complications by using a protocol for physiologic endpoints, including central venous pressure.
2. Hypothermia occurs due to ongoing heat loss and metabolic failure requiring large amounts of energy production and thus oxygen consumption. There is no proven benefit for hypothermia in traumatic brain injury (TBI) outcomes.
3. Coagulopathy is common and due to both dilution and consumption while being aggravated by hypothermia. Early empiric replacement of coagulation components reduces mortality.
4. TBI is a major cause of injury-related death, with care directed at avoiding secondary brain injury, control of elevated intracranial pressure, and early recognition of treatable mass lesions.
5. Elevated intra-abdominal pressure (abdominal compartment syndrome) causes a tense distended abdomen, hypoxia, oliguria despite adequate volume, and impaired cardiac output, requiring decompression and an open abdomen in severe cases.
6. Acute lung injury and acute respiratory distress syndrome require adequate, frequently higher levels of positive end-expiratory pressure; low tidal volumes; and moderate

levels of fraction of inspired oxygen to optimize recovery.

7 Venous thromboembolism remains an important and potentially preventable cause of morbidity and mortality. Prophylactic anticoagulation in high-risk patients must often be balanced with increased risk of hemorrhage.

8 Nosocomial infections are the most common complication requiring aggressive prevention, diagnosis, and preemptive empiric antibiotic therapy with subsequent de-escalation for ventilator-associated pneumonia, urinary tract infections, catheter-related bloodstream infections, and surgical site infections.

Most deaths occurring in trauma patients who survive to reach a trauma center occur in the intensive care unit (ICU). Furthermore, the most costly complications occur in and require treatment in the ICU.[1,2] Most of these deaths and complications are the consequence of severe hemorrhage and traumatic brain injury, and others are related to injury-induced alterations in coagulation and inflammatory and innate immune responses. Understanding their biology, epidemiology, and clinical features will help focus our resuscitative and definitive care efforts in these patients.[3,4]

Trauma patients experience shared physiologic changes and complications with noninjured critically ill patients. They also experience others that, if not unique to, are particularly relevant to trauma patients. The sections that follow are organized temporally in an effort to reflect when specific situations are most likely to be encountered in the postinjury period. The time periods that follow provide a framework in which to think about the challenges these patients face as they arrive in the ICU from the operating room, emergency department, and elsewhere.

STABILIZATION AND SECONDARY SURVEY (INITIAL 24 HOURS POSTINJURY)

This phase is often a continuation of emergency department or operating room stabilization of vital functions and the ongoing diagnosis and management of life-threatening injuries. In other circumstances, resuscitation is complete, but secondary or "tertiary" surveys to search for occult injuries are undertaken, optimal support of vital organ function is continued, and careful monitoring for deterioration is required.

Hemodynamic Resuscitation: Monitoring and Targets

Tissue injury, local and global ischemia, and hypoxia are well-known contributors to subsequent multiple organ dysfunction syndrome (MODS), nosocomial infection, and other complications after severe injury.[5,6] The duration and degree of shock both increase the risk for subsequent organ dysfunction and severe nosocomial infection after various types of trauma
1 (blunt, penetrating, and burn injury).[6,7] Therefore, rapid and adequate resuscitation is a critical component of the initial ICU care of trauma patients. However, there are no definitive markers of adequate resuscitation. Arterial base deficit and arterial lactate concentration are good indicators of the severity of injury and are a function of the degree and duration of shock. However, they correlate poorly with other "real-time" measures of tissue perfusion. Excessive attempts to normalize these values may lead to overresuscitation. Serum lactate concentrations and base deficit often remain elevated for hours after perfusion is appropriately restored, in part because they reflect adrenergic stimulation of Na^+-K^+/ATPase, which increases lactate production unrelated to tissue hypoxemia.[8,9] In addition, other biochemical or physiologic markers may only be obtained by invasive means, which are not warranted in most cases.

Therefore, and in recognition of the limitations of these physiologic endpoints, this early phase should initially be guided by the objectives of normalizing heart rate and blood pressure, achieving adequate urine output (0.5 mL/kg per hour in adults and 1.0 mL/kg per hour in children), and approximating an appropriate central venous pressure (CVP; 10 to 15 mm Hg), measurements that can be obtained simply from an indwelling bladder catheter, an arterial line, and a central venous line. Measuring CVP is important in the critically injured to guide resuscitation and may help distinguish hypovolemia from other less common causes of shock, such as pump failure from myocardial contusion or tamponade.[10] Overly aggressive crystalloid resuscitation or, conversely, inappropriate early use of vasopressor agents prior to adequate resuscitation have each been associated with poor outcomes after trauma.[11] Taken together, this information mandates careful attention to resuscitation strategies, collection of appropriate data, and judicious use of crystalloid and vasoactive agents.[12,13]

Clinical trials have shown that routine pulmonary artery catheter (PAC) use does not improve outcome in critically ill patients.[14] Furthermore, observational studies in trauma patients also do not demonstrate an overall survival advantage.[11] However, there are circumstances where additional information is needed to guide resuscitation. Invasive monitoring may be indicated when the patient remains hypotensive despite seemingly adequate intravascular volume, based on an adequate CVP, or when shock is accompanied by severe hypoxemia and additional fluid resuscitation may, in fact, worsen oxygenation. In patients who arrive in the ICU with unstable parameters after receiving large-volume resuscitations in the operating room or emergency department, invasive monitoring may be helpful in clarifying the patient's intravascular volume status and help determine whether additional volume, vasoactive medication, or both are necessary. When a PAC is used, recommended targets are a cardiac index of ~3.5 to 4.0 L/min per m^2 and an oxygen delivery index ~500 mL/min per m^2.

In addition, there are a number of potential alternatives to invasive monitoring with a PAC. These include continuous measurement of central venous oxyhemoglobin saturation ($ScvO_2$) (rather than mixed venous oxyhemoglobin saturation [$SmvO_2$] with a PAC), which has been shown to improve survival when used early in the management of patients with sepsis.[15] Transthoracic echocardiography and transesophageal Doppler have been studied as possible alternatives to invasive PAC monitoring. Limited transthoracic echocardiography can be used to assess preload and cardiac index. However, there are often physical impediments to its use (particularly subcutaneous air), its correlation with concurrent measurements from a PAC is modest, and it has not been shown to predictably influence patient management or outcome.[16] Transesophageal Doppler monitoring of cardiac function is a more promising technique. When used to guide resuscitation in the initial 12 hours after admission to the ICU, it influences volume resuscitation choices and may improve outcomes in critically ill trauma patients.[17] A summary of resuscitation targets is included in Table 30.1.

Hypothermia

2 Hypothermia (core temperature ≤34.5°C) is less common in trauma patients arriving in the ICU than it was in the past. This is likely due to more aggressive prevention in the emergency department, radiology suite, and operating room. However, it remains a preventable and treatable situation that contributes

TABLE 30.1

HEMODYNAMIC RESUSCITATION PARAMETERS DURING INITIAL 24 HOURS AFTER INJURY

Urine output: 30 mL/kg/h
Hemoglobin: 12–15 g/dL
Heart rate: ≤100/min
Arterial blood pressure: ≥120 mm Hg
Central venous pressure: 10–15 mm Hg
Cardiac index: 3.5–4.0 L/min/m^2
Oxygen delivery: 500–550 mL O_2/min/m^2
Mixed venous oxyhemoglobin saturation: ≥65%
Central venous oxyhemoglobin saturation: ≥70%

to complications and death. Thermoregulation is compromised in severely injured patients by shock and failure of cellular metabolism. Hypothermia from metabolic failure is often exacerbated by external heat loss through the four general mechanisms of energy transfer: (a) radiation, (b) convection, (c) evaporation, and (d) conduction.[18] Minimizing heat loss through careful attention to the patient's environment is central to preventing hypothermia and its consequences. In theory, the prevention of hypothermia simply requires the elimination or minimization of heat loss by these four mechanisms. This primarily involves keeping the patient covered and dry. Warm air contains little heat (specific heat = 0.25 kcal/kg per °C) and is of little help in warming a cold patient. However, a warm air environment or warm air circulating blanket is an excellent way to prevent heat loss.

A considerable amount of energy and, therefore, oxygen is required to warm a hypothermic patient.[18,19] The amount of energy required to warm a hypothermic patient by 3°C (34°C to 37°C, for example) is substantial and can be a significant metabolic stress. Based on the following formula, where specific heat of the human body is 0.83 kcal/kg per °C:

$$Q\text{ (heat)} = \text{mass (in kg)} \times 0.83\text{ kcal/kg/°C} \times [\text{Temp}_1 - \text{Temp}_2\ (\Delta\text{Temp})]$$

$$Q\text{ (heat)} = 70\text{ kg} \times 0.83\text{ kcal/kg/°C} \times [37°\text{C} - 34°\text{C}] = \underline{\mathbf{181\ kcal}}$$

It will take 181 kcal of energy to return the patient to 37°C. A patient would have to double his or her oxygen consumption for 3 hours (or increase it by 50% for 6 hours) in order to generate this amount of heat. Patients in shock or recovering from shock are unable to meet such a high metabolic demand and should be actively warmed, rather than having to rely on their own metabolism (termed *passive warming*). A number of techniques for actively rewarming patients are available. These include overhead radiant heat warmers, whose effectiveness requires that they be placed relatively close to the patient (within 70 cm) and that the patient be fully exposed to the radiant heat, rather than covered by a blanket, in which case the blanket is warmed. Not surprisingly, risk of thermal injury is significant. Body cavity lavage (pleural or peritoneal) can potentially transfer large amounts of energy, but may not be practical in the multiply injured patient or due to the significant logistic challenges. Airway warming with heated, humidified oxygen transfers relatively little energy, similar to increasing ambient temperature in general, and should not be relied upon for treatment of hypothermia. The most effective method for rewarming is full cardiopulmonary bypass, which has been used successfully in severely hypothermic trauma victims. Although a heparin-bonded system avoids the need for systemic anticoagulation, limited availability and overall implementation technical challenges hamper its usefulness.[20,21] Other forms of extracorporeal rewarming of blood have been used and tested in hypothermic trauma patients. These include arteriovenous and venovenous bypass systems. Each uses a countercurrent exchange warmer; the advantage of the venovenous system is that it does not rely on the patient's blood pressure to maintain adequate flow, but it does require a more complex system than an arteriovenous system.[22,23] Given the consequences of moderate to severe hypothermia, active rewarming should be used in any critically injured patient with a temperature of 34.5°C or below. Extracorporeal rewarming is the most effective option and radiant heat warmers are a secondary alternative. Although induced hypothermia increases survival after nontraumatic cardiac arrest, it should not be used in critically ill trauma patients.[24] Furthermore, induction of hypothermia has not been proven beneficial in the treatment of traumatic brain injury in either adults or children. Therefore, there are currently no circumstances where allowing a critically ill trauma patient to remain hypothermic is beneficial.

3 **Hemostatic Abnormalities.** Coagulopathies are common in critically injured trauma patients and their cause is multifactorial (Table 30.2). It is evident that hemorrhage accompanied by crystalloid and red blood cell transfusion results in dilution of coagulation factors, yet the implications of this dilution are not clear. Correlation between the amount of blood transfused and specific factor levels or the global measures of coagulation (activated partial thromboplastin time [aPTT], prothrombin time [PT]) are relatively low, and coagulopathy after non–trauma-related blood loss alone seems to generally occur after rather large transfusions (10 to 12 units of packed red blood cells).[25,26] The effect of pure dilution on platelet counts is even less clear, with wide variations in the incidence of thrombocytopenia being reported. Basing coagulation factor replacement and platelet transfusion needs on predictive formulas is generally inaccurate.[27]

A number of other factors have been linked to hemostatic abnormalities after trauma. Tissue trauma leads to platelet aggregation and activation of coagulation. Variable induction of these processes depending on the nature and severity of the trauma likely explain the lack of correlation of measured hemostatic deficits with blood loss, resuscitation, and blood transfusion volumes. For example, traumatic brain injury can result in coagulopathy that is independent of blood loss and transfusion volumes.[28] The exact mechanism is uncertain and likely more complicated than release of brain tissue thromboplastins, as has been previously theorized. Marked reductions in circulating fibrinogen concentrations (<50 mg/dL) are often seen, suggesting that hyperfibrinolysis plays an important role. Extremity injuries, including fractures and extensive soft tissue trauma, expose circulating coagulation factors and platelets to subendothelial collagen and tissue factor. However, clinically significant coagulopathies are unlikely to occur solely as the result of tissue trauma and require additional contributing factors. The effect of hypothermia on hemostasis is significant

TABLE 30.2

FACTORS CONTRIBUTING TO COAGULOPATHY IN TRAUMA

Dilution of coagulation factors
Hypothermia (impaired enzyme activity, platelet dysfunction, enhanced fibrinolysis)
Acidosis
Tissue trauma (brain injury, fractures, soft tissue injuries)
Preexisting hemostatic defects (von Willebrand disease, hemophilia, chronic liver disease)
Medications (warfarin, antiplatelet agents)

and generally multifactorial, and is effectively reversed only by achieving normothermia and not with blood components.

In the event of severe hemorrhage and clinical evidence of coagulopathic bleeding, treatment must not wait for laboratory confirmation or for precise characterization of the defect(s). The development of diffuse hemorrhage intraoperatively, abnormal bleeding from intravenous sites, and marked bloody drain (thoracostomy, other surgically placed drains, etc.) output are obvious but late signs of a coagulopathy.

Review of the likely contributing factors will help direct appropriate blood component therapy while waiting for definitive laboratory diagnosis of the specific abnormalities. Laboratory characterization and treatment can be based on four tests: the platelet count, PT, aPTT, and fibrinogen levels. In most circumstances, a combination of platelet, plasma, and cryoprecipitate transfusions are required and are sufficient to treat hemostatic abnormalities after trauma. There are no definitive platelet count, aPTT, or PT thresholds that require treatment, but general recommendations follow. Isolated increases in the aPTT (normal PT) should not be treated with blood products as they are not due to deficiencies in the common pathway factors (X, V, II, and I). The results may be spurious (blood drawn through heparinized tube) or due to a lupus anticoagulant or hemophilia. In the initial postinjury period, platelet counts should be maintained above 50,000/μL in all cases, and above 100,000/μL in the presence of an injury with major hemorrhage (severe liver injury requiring packing, pelvis fracture with large hematoma, etc.) or when the consequence of ongoing bleeding is devastating, such as in the case of an intracranial hemorrhage, cerebral contusion, and possibly spinal fractures. Combined moderate abnormalities in the aPTT and PT (1.5 to 3.0 times the upper limit of normal) should be treated with 2 to 4 units of plasma. Marked elevations in PT and aPTT may reflect very low fibrinogen levels. In this case or when measured fibrinogen is less than or equal to 100 mg/dL, cryoprecipitate should also be given. A normal aPTT should be the target in patients with injuries that have resulted in major hemorrhage as indicated. In the presence of a traumatic intracranial bleed (epidural, subdural, or intracerebral hematoma), the risk for hemorrhage progression has been associated with the aPTT, but as there is no particular threshold where bleeding clearly increases, the treatment goal should be to maintain the aPTT within the normal range.[29]

Recombinant factor VIIa has been used recently in severely coagulopathic trauma patients. Factor VIIa binds to tissue factor exposed at the site of injury and rapidly stimulates coagulation. Small studies have reported its usefulness in coagulopathic trauma patients who continue to bleed despite treatment with platelets, plasma, and cryoprecipitate.[30–32] Factor VIIa also may be indicated in bleeding trauma patients who have been receiving warfarin and for the rare trauma patient with hemophilia A who also has factor VIII inhibitors.

Management of Traumatic Brain Injury and Intracranial Hypertension

Severely injured patients, particularly those who have sustained their injuries by a blunt mechanism, often have a traumatic brain injury (TBI) in addition to torso and extremity injuries. 4 The three principal challenges in the management of TBI are (a) avoiding secondary brain injury, (b) control of elevated intracranial pressure (ICP), and (c) early identification of any progression of mass lesions that would require surgical decompression. These issues are discussed in detail in the section devoted to trauma to the central nervous system. Management of patients with traumatic brain injuries requires the use of various monitoring and therapeutic strategies based on clinical course, computed tomography (CT) scan findings, and response to treatment. Significant deterioration in clinical course, physical examination, or ICP should be considered an absolute indication for repeat CT scan. This is the only practical method for the prompt identification of patients in whom surgically correctable mass lesions develop during the initial phase of care.

Important additional and avoidable causes of secondary brain injury include hypotension, hyperthermia, seizure activity, hyperglycemia, and hypoxemia. Taken together, these contribute to deterioration in the severity of brain function and are often preventable. Hypotension at any point (even brief time periods) approximately doubles the likelihood of death from a given brain injury and must be avoided.[33,34] Posttraumatic seizures increase cerebral metabolic rate, may increase ICP, and may cause important secondary brain injury. Prevention with intravenous phenytoin for the first 7 days after injury is indicated and effective.[35] Normocapnia (partial pressure of arterial carbon dioxide [$PaCO_2$] 35 to 40 mm Hg) should be maintained to avoid cerebral vasoconstriction and concomitant hyperfusion. However, brief, but not excessive, hyperventilation (keep $PaCO_2$ >25 mm Hg) as a temporizing measure to treat sudden increases in ICP or herniation may be necessary while preparing for definitive treatment (craniotomy, ventriculostomy for cerebrospinal fluid drainage, etc.).

Mechanical Ventilation

This will be discussed in more detail elsewhere, but there are a number of important considerations in the delivery of mechanical ventilation during this resuscitative and diagnostic phase. First, abnormal gas exchange, leading to hypoxemia, commonly exists in patients who are being resuscitated from hemorrhagic shock. Pulmonary edema may arise more as a consequence of overly aggressive crystalloid resuscitation than the transiently increased endothelial permeability consequent to shock. Transient hypoxemic respiratory failure is observed in trauma patients and may reflect a somewhat different pathophysiologic process than that which exists in the more prolonged hypoxemic respiratory failure seen with subsequent acute lung injury (ALI) and acute respiratory distress syndrome (ARDS).[36] However, the goals of support at this point are primarily to ensure adequate resuscitation from shock, support oxygen delivery, and prevent any ongoing oxygen insufficiency. Therefore, it is important to distinguish the approach to mechanical ventilation in these first hours from the approach used once the patient has been successfully resuscitated and may have developed moderate to severe ALI. Initial ventilator settings aim to achieve adequate ventilation and oxygenation. This typically requires a minute ventilation of greater than or equal to 12 L/min and employs a fairly traditional approach. This includes volume-controlled ventilation, with a tidal volume of 8 to 10 mL/kg, a rate of 18 to 22 breaths/min, positive end-expiratory pressure (PEEP) of at least 5 to 10 cm H_2O, and a fraction of inspired oxygen (FiO_2) greater than or equal to 50%. Contrary to limits imposed for treatment of ALI or ARDS, it is appropriate to accept end-inspiratory static (Pst) pressures up to 40 cm H_2O and not aggressively limit tidal volume to 6 mL/kg and static pressures to less than 30 cm H_2O during this initial phase.

Rarely, circumstances occur in the severely injured patient that require unconventional ventilation strategies. These patients may be profoundly hypoxemic despite high FiO_2 concentrations and elevated PEEP and/or may have a massive air leak due to severe parenchymal or airway injury. These patients have typically received a massive volume of fluid during the acute resuscitation, have sustained severe thoracic trauma, and/or often both. There are no established proven best approaches to managing these patients. However, some principles can apply. First, large air leaks require treatment at this stage only if they are significantly affecting patient oxygenation due to diversion of the inspired gas away from gas-exchanging alveoli. Bronchoscopy should be considered to identify proximal airway injuries, but patient instability may preclude both bronchoscopy and definitive operative management. Therefore, regardless of the anatomy of the injury, in these severely hypoxemic patients, initial treatment options are often nonsurgical. Approaches include maneuvers to minimize air leak, such as high-frequency oscillatory ventilation (HFOV) and single-lung isolation (double-lumen endotracheal tube or bronchial blockers) to support effective gas exchange.

Abdominal Compartment Syndrome

5 Elevated intra-abdominal pressure (intra-abdominal hypertension) leading to pulmonary, renal, or cardiac dysfunction is termed the *abdominal compartment syndrome* (ACS). According to most studies, death is almost certain if greatly excessive pressure is not relieved.[37] Intra-abdominal hypertension can be defined as an intra-abdominal pressure of greater than or equal to 20 cm H_2O.[38] Experimental data indicate that hepatic arterial, portal venous, and hepatic microcirculatory blood flow are markedly reduced when intra-abdominal pressure is increased to greater than or equal to 20 cm H_2O.[39] Typically, it is observed after severe abdominal trauma that requires celiotomy and control of intra-abdominal hemorrhage.[40,41] It has also been described in the setting of intra-abdominal injuries that were initially managed nonoperatively (e.g., severe liver or kidney injuries).[42] In addition, excessive large-volume resuscitations, even in the absence of any direct abdominal trauma, can also lead to ACS.[12,43,44]

The diagnosis often begins with a triad of clinical findings: (a) tense, distended abdomen; (b) increased end-inspiration airway pressures; and (c) oliguria despite appropriate volume resuscitation. Additional clinical measurements, particularly those that reflect poor cardiac performance, may be helpful in making the diagnosis. Signs consistent with ACS are a reduced cardiac output, elevated systemic vascular resistance, and elevated pulmonary capillary wedge pressure with simultaneous low or normal calculated estimates of end-diastolic volumes. The addition of corroborative findings from invasive hemodynamic monitoring may help clarify the diagnosis and direct the appropriate treatment.

Bladder pressure is the most widely used surrogate for intra-abdominal pressure. It is measured with the patient supine, by distending the bladder with 100 mL of sterile saline. The drainage tubing is then occluded, and an 18-gauge needle inserted sterilely and connected to the pressure transducer through the aspiration port on the catheter tubing. An adequate pressure "tracing" is indicated by visible respiratory variation, which is usually less than 5 to 10 mm Hg.[45] The mean pressure should be used as an estimate of the intra-abdominal pressure, although this aspect of the procedure is not well characterized. A simpler method (although not validated) involves filling the bladder with 100 mL of sterile saline and elevating the clear tubing vertically above the pubic symphysis. The height of the fluid column is measured and converted to mm Hg (1.3 cm H_2O = 1 mm Hg).

Established ACS with associated organ dysfunction is treated with surgical decompression of the abdomen.[38] In contrast, elevated intra-abdominal pressures, regardless of the actual measured value, in the absence of physiologic derangement is not an indication for decompressive celiotomy. Similarly, high intrathoracic pressures and marked FiO_2 and PEEP requirements are not necessarily sufficient to warrant decompression. Progressive renal dysfunction (oliguria, rising creatinine) despite adequate preload and ongoing resuscitation should warrant abdominal decompression. Persistent shock, particularly when vasopressor agents are needed to supplement fluid resuscitation, also warrants decompressive celiotomy. There are no absolute thresholds for airway pressure, urine output, or arterial blood lactate that indicate or contraindicate decompressive celiotomy. Of note, ACS can occur in patients whose fascia has not been definitively closed, but where some other technique of temporary abdominal closure has been performed and is sufficient to generate excessive intra-abdominal pressures. One causal factor that seems common to all cases of ACS is the use of very aggressive crystalloid resuscitation, including attempts to reach elevated O_2 delivery to reverse a perceived oxygen debt. Therefore, attempts to achieve "supranormal" endpoints (cardiac index of $\geq$4 L/min per m^2 or oxygen delivery index of $\geq$600 mL/min per m^2), which often require the excessive resuscitation volumes that contribute to ACS, should be avoided.[11]

ORGAN SYSTEM SUPPORT AND DEFINITIVE CARE (1 TO 7 DAYS POSTINJURY)

Coordinating Multidisciplinary Care and the Timing of Operative Interventions

Decisions made during this phase will significantly influence patient outcome, and this period should not simply be considered a period of observation and general support. During and following resuscitation, patients require careful reevaluation as part of a tertiary survey to establish subsequent priorities in care. Communicating with other specialties to determine the timing of additional diagnostic tests and operative procedures is crucial during the first week after injury. It is typically the role of the general surgeon or surgical intensivist to oversee and coordinate the timing of subsequent surgical care. The definitive care of fractures and non–life-threatening torso injuries should be delayed when patients are hemodynamically unstable, acidotic, hypothermic, or coagulopathic or have intracranial hypertension.[46] Once these are addressed and corrected (typically within 48 hours), definitive repair can be undertaken. Generally, the more delayed operative stabilization of fractures, such as femoral, spine, and pelvic, is associated with an increased risk of respiratory complications.[47,48] On the other hand, it is important not to risk worsening organ function, particularly respiratory failure and TBI, by exposing patients to prolonged operative procedures and concomitant blood loss and potential hypotension at a time when they are least able to tolerate an additional physiologic challenge. Rather than the absolute timing of definitive procedures, it appears that the duration of the operation and the associated physiologic stress are the most important factors in determining how well the patient tolerates the intervention.[46,49] It is important, therefore, to discuss the details and expected course of each operative procedure with the consultant surgeon.

Mechanical Ventilation and Acute Respiratory Failure

Within 24 to 48 hours, many severely injured patients can be rapidly liberated from mechanical ventilation, are able to adequately protect their airway, and can be extubated. Prompt recognition of when the patient is ready to be liberated from mechanical ventilation can be best accomplished by performing a trial of spontaneous breathing rather than relying on any single measure (or even a combination of measures) of respiratory muscle strength or endurance.[50,51] Many patients require more prolonged mechanical ventilation, either for respiratory failure or often because they are unable to protect their airway, particularly in cases of TBI. In some cases, mechanical ventilation is supportive, gas exchange is not particularly impaired, and the lung fields on chest radiography are relatively normal. In these circumstances, mandatory volume-controlled (also termed "assist-control") ventilation aimed to maintain the partial pressure of arterial oxygen (PaO_2) at 80 to 100 mm Hg and the $PaCO_2$ at 35 to 45 mm Hg is appropriate. This can be accomplished using tidal volumes of 8 to 10 mL/kg of predicted body weight, positive end-inspiratory pressure of 5 to 10 cm H_2O, an FiO_2 of 40% to 60%, and a respiratory rate of 12 to 24 breaths/min. Slight adjustments above or below any of these thresholds are acceptable to achieve these targets. There is no proven advantage to using any other mode or technique of delivering positive-pressure ventilation.

6 Severe ALI and ARDS develop in a substantial fraction of critically ill trauma patients and contribute to prolonged and costly ICU care.[4,52] ALI is defined by the following set of clinical criteria: (a) diffuse patchy pulmonary infiltrates on chest radiograph, (b) PaO_2/FiO_2 less than or equal to 300, and (c) cardiac failure excluded as a cause for pulmonary edema; ARDS is defined by the same criteria except for a PaO_2/FiO_2 less than or equal to 200. While the pathophysiology is not entirely clear, an intense alveolar inflammatory response that correlates with the severity of the initial insult exists in these patients that may be influenced by positive-pressure ventilation, based on the following[53–55]: first, alveolar edema can be reduced by preventing end-expiratory collapse with sufficient PEEP.[56] Second, a marked inflammatory response can be induced in otherwise normal lungs in experimental animals exposed to positive-pressure ventilation, particularly when alveoli are allowed to repeatedly collapse (0 cm H_2O PEEP) and repeatedly overexpand with each inspiratory cycle.[57] Third, a similar inflammatory response is seen in patients with ARDS, and this inflammatory response can be reduced by a strategy that reduces end-expiratory collapse and end-inspiratory distention.[55] In clinical trials, mortality was reduced when patients were treated with protocols designed to limit alveolar stretch using a tidal volume of 6 mL/kg compared to subjects ventilated with higher tidal volumes (~12 mL/kg).[58,59] These trials included patients with ALI and ARDS due to many different risk factors, including trauma and massive transfusion. This approach is therefore applicable and considered the standard of care for trauma patients with ALI and ARDS. Judicious use of PEEP to maintain moderate FiO_2 levels ($\leq$60%) should typically be employed. An acceptable approach is based on PEEP and FiO_2 combinations used by the ARDS Network.[58] There is no benefit to using relatively higher or lower levels of PEEP or FiO_2 to achieve levels of PaO_2 greater than 80 to 90 in these patients.[60]

Nutritional and Metabolic Support

Nutritional and metabolic support is an important but often neglected component of caring for critically injured patients. Once resuscitation from shock is complete, a hypermetabolic and hyperdynamic cardiovascular response ensues, which has features characteristic of the more general acute-phase response, frequently referred to as systemic inflammatory response syndrome (SIRS). Important changes include increased energy expenditure and protein breakdown with a shift in metabolic priorities to favor the production of proteins characterized as acute-phase reactants, produced primarily by the liver.[61] Although the initial injury and subsequent complications are the prime drivers, the type and timing of nutritional and metabolic support are important modifiers of this response and can help reduce the loss of nitrogen derived from structural protein catabolism.

The route of administration, timing, amount, and nutrient composition of nutritional support are of particular relevance to critically injured patients. When compared to total parenteral nutrition (TPN), enteral nutrition (EN) is associated with greater constitutive protein concentrations (prealbumin and albumin) and lower acute-phase reactant proteins (such as C-reactive protein) in the initial days after trauma. These effects may be due to a direct effect of the route of nutrient delivery or to an associated reduction in infectious complications seen with EN.[62] Therefore, nutritional support should be delivered enterally when possible. Small randomized clinical trials and subsequent meta-analyses have shown that enteral nutrition results in fewer nosocomial infections than parenteral nutrition. The evidence is more complete in patients with severe torso trauma, but can be generalized to those with severe extremity injuries.[63,64]

Starting EN within the first 48 hours of injury appears beneficial. However, it is first important to ensure that the patient has been fully resuscitated, as intestinal ischemia may be the result of feeding a patient with splanchnic hypoperfusion due to ongoing hypovolemia. This may also lead to intolerance, gastroparesis, and aspiration. There is no proven definitive advantage of a very aggressive approach to feeding (6 to 12 hours after injury) when compared to EN delayed until 48 to 72 hours after injury. Nevertheless, it has been demonstrated that starting EN within 12 hours of being resuscitated from shock is safe and tolerated by approximately 80% of patients when a defined protocol for EN is used.[65]

The amount and composition of nutritional support, whether delivered enterally or parenterally, can be estimated or directly measured and the metabolic response to this support should be monitored. Caloric requirement estimates are derived from the Harris-Benedict equation in which basal energy expenditure (BEE) and, thus, caloric needs are calculated from an equation based on the patient's age, height, weight, and gender. The equations are as follows:

$$\text{Females: BEE} = 655 + 9.7\ (\text{wt in kg}) + 1.8\ (\text{ht in cm}) - 4.7\ (\text{age})$$

$$\text{Males: BEE} = 66 + 13.75\ (\text{wt in kg}) + 5\ (\text{ht in cm}) - 6.8\ (\text{age})$$

Depending on the severity of injury, the BEE expenditure is multiplied by a "stress" factor that estimates the energy expenditure above basal requirements. On average, this factor is approximately 1.4. Caloric needs according to this formula are approximately 25 to 30 kcal/kg per day. Head-injured patients typically have higher energy expenditure than other trauma patients (140% BEE), whereas spinal cord–injured patients often have lower metabolic demands (94% BEE). It is reasonable to estimate the initial caloric requirements using the Harris-Benedict equation, but when critical illness is prolonged beyond 7 to 10 days, direct measurements should be used to determine energy expenditure and refine nutritional support. Metabolism consumes oxygen and produces carbon dioxide. Therefore, oxygen consumption (VO_2) and carbon dioxide production (VCO_2) can be used to calculate caloric needs using the abbreviated de Weir equation: $EE = 1.44 \times [(3.9 \times VO_2) + (1.1 \times VCO_2)]$. Measuring VCO_2 requires a metabolic cart and is often inaccurate when FiO_2 requirements are high.

Although protein calories are included in the estimated caloric requirements, it is hoped that delivered protein is not broken down as an energy source, but rather used as a source of amino acids. Protein or nitrogen requirements are generally estimated relative to caloric goals. A kilocalorie/nitrogen (mg) ratio of 100:1 is considered appropriate for critically injured, catabolic patients. Elemental formulas may be better tolerated in patients who have been without EN for more than a few days, although there is no definitive advantage over nonelemental ones. The use of "immune-enhancing" formulas, in which additional amino acids such as arginine, omega-3 fatty acids, and various antioxidants are added, is controversial. The anti-inflammatory effects of omega-3 fatty acids are the most promising, and these nutrients seem beneficial in critically ill patients.[66] Similarly, the addition of antioxidants (selenium, vitamin C, and vitamin E) delivered enterally or intravenously and started early in the postinjury phase may reduce postinjury organ failure.[67]

Prevention of Gastric Stress Ulcer Hemorrhage

The incidence of clinically relevant stress ulceration or gastritis has substantially dropped. Whether this is a function of overall better general supportive care, particularly adequate resuscitation, or due to specific preventative measures is uncertain. Nevertheless, trauma patients in the ICU receiving mechanical ventilation for over 48 to 72 hours constitute a high-risk group in whom the risk for upper gastrointestinal hemorrhage is reported to be from 4% to 12%.[68,69] Histamine-2–receptor antagonists may be the most effective agent for preventing upper gastrointestinal hemorrhage in the ICU, and many practitioners choose them for prophylaxis.[70,71] However, nosocomial pneumonia and, in trauma patients, other nosocomial infections as well are increased in patients receiving histamine-2 antagonists when compared to those given sucralfate.[72,73] The use of sucralfate avoids gastric acid neutralization and the potential systemic effects of histamine-2–receptor antagonists. Proton pump inhibitors markedly suppress gastric acid secretion but are no more effective than other agents in reducing clinically relevant hemorrhage from stress gastritis. Once enteral nutrition via the stomach has been initiated and shown to be tolerated, there is no proven benefit to continuing any of the gastric-protective interventions.

Pain Relief

Approaches to pain relief and sedation assume great importance in this phase of care of the critically ill trauma patient. In particular, adequate pharmacologic relief of thoracic pain due to multiple rib fractures may be critical to avoiding intubation and to hastening liberation from mechanical ventilation and extubation. It appears that, when possible, thoracic epidural analgesia results in fewer cases of nosocomial pneumonia and fewer days of mechanical ventilation than systemically administered opioid analgesia.[74] Given the multiple painful stimuli experienced by trauma patients in the ICU (fractures, surgical incisions, lacerations, contusions, etc.), it is reasonable to consider regional analgesia not just for those with multiple rib fractures. However, contraindications to the use of epidural analgesia are commonly encountered and include severe traumatic brain injury, spinal fracture, coagulopathy, or any injury that would preclude appropriate positioning for accessing the epidural space. While sedation is critical to optimize patient rest and recovery, overdosing and deposition of active byproducts can lead to prolonged oversedation and inability to extubate in a timely fashion. All patients receiving sedation should undergo a "sedation holiday" every 24 hours, allowing the patient to return to baseline mentation and permit serial daily monitoring of overall neurologic status.

Venous Thromboembolic Disease

7 Venous thromboembolic disease (VTE), which can manifest as deep venous thrombosis (DVT) or pulmonary embolism (PE), is common after trauma and can have serious or fatal consequences. Pulmonary embolism is the most devastating manifestation and an important cause of posttraumatic death. Both can occur at any time after injury, and many occur as early as the initial 48 hours.[75] In particular, spinal cord injuries and lower extremity and severe pelvic fractures are strong risk factors for VTE.[76] However, patients without these injuries are also at risk for thromboembolic complications. Other important risk factors include increasing age, immobility, and the need for blood transfusions.[76,77] That most trauma patients are at risk and that both DVT and PE can occur early pose difficult practical problems to apply effective prevention strategies due to the high risk for ongoing or secondary bleeding and associated complications.

Low-molecular-weight heparin is more effective than unfractionated heparin for prophylaxis and should be used in patients in high-risk groups. One large randomized trial demonstrated that proximal DVT risk was approximately 30% lower in patients receiving low-molecular-weight heparin (30 mg twice daily) than in those receiving unfractionated heparin (5000 IU twice daily).[76,78] However, the risk of bleeding may be higher when patients are given low-molecular-weight heparin, and it is not recommended for use in those with intracranial hemorrhage or ongoing extracranial bleeding. Alternative prophylactic methods exist to address the risk of DVT in patients who cannot receive prophylactic or therapeutic heparin. Intermittent pneumatic compression devices can be used in patients with contraindications to heparin prophylaxis. Although once thought that these devices increased local and regional fibrinolysis by increasing tissue factor pathway inhibitor and decreasing plasminogen activator inhibitor activities, recent evidence suggests that this is not the case. Any benefit from pneumatic compression is likely due to improved venous blood flow.[79,80] In addition, prophylactic placement of a vena cava filter (VCF) is appropriate for patients at high risk for VTE who cannot receive prophylactic anticoagulation.[81] This has become an increasingly acceptable alternative with the development of retrievable filters.[82] Alternatively, sonographic screening, followed by VCF placement in only those with documented DVT, can be used in patients with a contraindication to prophylactic and therapeutic anticoagulation.[83] VTE prophylaxis is considered standard trauma care and should be approached with a specific protocol to ensure that all patients receive appropriate management.[84]

MANAGEMENT OF INFECTIOUS COMPLICATIONS (8 DAYS AND BEYOND)

Infectious complications can occur earlier in the postinjury period, but they assume heightened importance as patients remain in the ICU beyond the first week. At this point, prevention, surveillance, rapid diagnosis, and effective treatment become an important focus of the critical care team.

Nosocomial Pneumonia

8 Pneumonia is the most common pulmonary complication and the most common infection in trauma victims. It most often occurs in association with tracheal intubation, and when associated with mechanical ventilation is referred to as ventilator-associated pneumonia (VAP). Posttraumatic VAP occurs due to a combination of factors including alterations in host defense mechanisms and concomitant colonization with pathogenic bacteria. Taken together, recumbent positioning and translaryngeal intubation facilitate microaspiration of secretions that have pooled in the hypopharynx. Although gastric bacterial colonization may lead to oropharyngeal and tracheal colonization, oropharyngeal colonization frequently precedes both gastric and tracheal colonization.[69] Alterations in host innate immune mechanisms likely contribute to the risk for pneumonia by impairing cellular immune responses to aspirated bacteria. Examples of alterations in host innate immune mechanisms that exist in critically ill patients include reductions in immune cell expression of bacterial antigen receptors (Toll-like receptors 2 and 4) and alterations in intracellular signalling (decreased nuclear factor-κB heterodimer formation) leading to reduced cytokine responses.[85,86]

Posttraumatic nosocomial pneumonia is caused by a range of gram-negative and gram-positive organisms. *Pseudomonas* species and *Staphylococcus aureus* are the two most common pathogens and together are responsible for up to 40% of cases.[87,88] Multidrug-resistant bacteria are becoming a greater challenge. Both gram-negative organisms, such as *Acinetobacter* species, and gram-positive organisms, such as methicillin and vancomycin-resistant staphylococci and enterococci, have emerged as important pathogens.

Prevention strategies reduce the incidence of VAP. For example, elevating the head of the bed to 45 degrees effectively reduces VAP, presumably by minimizing gastroesophageal reflux and pooling in the hypopharynx with microaspiration.[89] This is the single most important preventative strategy, but may not be possible in certain circumstances. It may be contraindicated in patients with vertebral, spinal cord, or pelvic injuries. Various strategies to eradicate potential pathogens from the patient's gastrointestinal tract have also been tested. While aimed at reducing all types of infectious complications, their effect on nosocomial pneumonia may be most pronounced because this is the most common infection. These strategies have been typically referred to as selective digestive decontamination (SDD) or selective oropharyngeal decontamination (SOD), when applied in a more limited manner.[90] Despite being the subject of many clinical trials and meta-analyses, the effectiveness of SDD is controversial and it has not gained widespread use.[91] However, a large clinical trial has demonstrated a reduction in mortality when SDD was applied to critically ill patients expected to have a high risk of mortality.[92] In trauma patients, SDD appears to reduce the number of infections but not fatality rates.[93]

The diagnosis and treatment of VAP is ideally based on direct sampling and quantitative cultures of distal pulmonary secretions, typically with bronchoscopic guidance. Bronchoscopy is most useful in patients with specific clinical factors suggesting they have pneumonia. These factors are leukocytosis, fever, purulent tracheal secretions, and persistent or progressive pulmonary infiltrates on chest radiography. While not sufficient to diagnose VAP, these criteria should prompt bronchoscopic sampling for quantitative cultures, which can be obtained from bronchoalveolar lavage (BAL) or with a protected specimen brush (PSB). The threshold for diagnosis of pneumonia is greater than or equal to 10^4 colony-forming units/mL based on BAL samples and greater than or equal to 10^3 colony-forming units/mL based on PSB samples. A clinical approach using bronchoscopically obtained specimens leads to more appropriate use of antibiotics, shorter ICU stays, and lower mortality in patients with pneumonia, including trauma patients.[94]

Treatment initially is empiric and must be started immediately to minimize mortality; antibiotic choice depends on initial Gram stain identification of predominant organisms and the knowledge of prevailing antibiotic sensitivities of organisms specific to the unit or hospital. Once the organism and specific antibiotic sensitivities are identified, treatment should be modified accordingly ("de-escalation") using the most appropriate antibiotic or combination for the specific organisms. The duration of antibiotic therapy is controversial. An inadequate duration of treatment may increase the risk for recurrent VAP with resistant organisms, whereas excessive treatment is costly, may result in the selection of other resistant organisms, and does not seem to improve outcome. Generally, antibiotic treatment for 8 days, assuming adequate initial treatment, is as effective as a 15-day course of treatment. However, for VAP caused by non–lactose-fermenting gram-negative rods (e.g., *Acinetobacter* and *Pseudomonas*), a 15-day course results in lower recurrence.[88] Treatment failure with these organisms is common and associated with higher mortality. The two most important factors associated with treatment failure and poor outcomes are delayed or inadequate initial antibiotic therapy,[95] both of which may occur in up to 34% of cases.[96] This can be prevented by following the approach indicated earlier. However, even in the presence of timely and appropriate antibiotic therapy, treatment failure occurs and is correlated with the initial severity of illness based on Acute Physiology and Chronic Health Evaluation (APACHE) II scores and comorbidities.[96]

Vascular Catheter–related Infections

Intravascular catheters are an important source of nosocomial infections. These infections can be classified as primary bloodstream infections, catheter-related bloodstream infections (in which cultures of the blood and of the catheter reveal the same pathogen), and exit site infections (in which there is local catheter site evidence of infection without positive blood or catheter cultures).[97] Approximately 10% of critically ill patients will develop a vascular catheter–related infection during their ICU stay, and this translates into approximately 9 infections per 1,000 patient-days.[97] In the absence of infection at the site of insertion, the diagnosis of catheter-related infections is difficult. Options for diagnosing catheter-related infections include culture of a catheter segment or of blood drawn through the catheter alone or simultaneously with blood drawn from a peripheral vein. These specimens can be quantitatively, semiquantitatively, or qualitatively cultured. In general, quantitative catheter segment cultures are the most accurate (highest combined sensitivity and specificity) for the diagnosis of infection. Unpaired quantitative culture of blood (drawn via the vascular catheter alone, without paired peripheral samples) is slightly less accurate.[98] Therefore, when infection is suspected but the insertion site is not inflamed or draining, the catheter should be removed for intratissue catheter segmental culture or blood should be drawn from the catheter for quantitative culture.[98]

Preventative strategies can lower the incidence of catheter-related infections in the ICU. Full sterile barriers are appropriate for insertion of central venous catheters and reduce subsequent infection rates, but they may not be required for the insertion of peripheral arterial catheters.[99,100] Chlorhexidine gluconate results in fewer bloodstream infections in comparison to povidone-iodine when used for insertion site preparation.[101] Using a silver-impregnated antimicrobial subcutaneous cuff attached to central venous catheters or antibiotic-impregnated catheters decreases the incidence of catheter infections. However, while impregnating catheters with antimicrobials (rifampin-minocycline) may reduce the risk of catheter-related infections, antibiotic resistance can develop.

Hyperglycemia does not seem to be an important risk factor for catheter-related infections. However, TPN administration is a risk factor for catheter-related and other bloodstream infections. Avoiding unneeded TPN use and preventing even short periods of excessive caloric intake will help reduce the incidence of these infections.[102,103]

Other Infections

Other infections are less common in trauma patients but are still of considerable importance and reflect the spectrum of infections seen in other cohorts of critically ill patients. Wound and urinary tract infections, intra-abdominal abscesses, and less commonly considered complications such as *Clostridium difficile* colitis and acalculous cholecystitis must be considered in the days to weeks after injury. Any patient developing diarrhea or a rapidly rising white blood cell count, particularly following or during a course of antibiotic therapy, should have a stool specimen sent for *C. difficile* toxin and, in the critically ill, metronidazole begun empirically.

Fungal infections are uncommon but are serious complications in critically ill trauma victims. They typically develop after a prolonged ICU course in patients who have received multiple antibiotics for nosocomial bacterial infections. They are responsible for 5% to 17% of bloodstream infections in critically ill patients and various *Candida* species are responsible for the majority of these infections.[104–106] Candidemia refers to the growth of *Candida* from blood cultures, and systemic candidiasis refers to the situation in which microabscesses are present in multiple organs and tissues and are extremely difficult to eradicate.

The single most relevant risk factor for the development of candidemia in nonneutropenic trauma patients is the use of broad-spectrum antibiotics. Colonization with *Candida* organisms is another important risk factor that can be useful in identifying the highest-risk patients.[105,107] Fungal infections acquired in the ICU are an important risk factor for death in critically ill patients in general as well as in trauma patients.[104] Although antifungal prophylaxis with fluconazole seems safe and may reduce the incidence of invasive fungal infections in high-risk surgical patients, it is typically not indicated in trauma patients.[107] The diagnosis of candidemia is challenging, and the clinical presentation is neither sensitive nor specific for fungal infection. However, invasive *Candida* infections can occur without cultures being positive. Therefore, treatment is often empiric, based on a high clinical suspicion, typically in a patient colonized by *Candida* with sepsis who is not responding to antibiotic therapy. Treatment is generally with fluconazole or another azole antifungal agent. *Candida glabrata* and *Candida krusei* should be considered resistant to fluconazole, and resistance to amphotericin has been documented to occur.[108] Therefore, if these organisms are suspected or determined to be responsible for infection, amphotericin or one of the agents in the echinocandin class should be used as initial therapy. Voriconazole is a newer azole antifungal that is effective against azole-resistant *Candida* species. It is an acceptable alternative to amphotericin and the echinicadins.[109,110]

References

1. Sauaia A, Moore FA, Moore EE, et al. Epidemiology of trauma deaths: a reassessment. *J Trauma* 1995;38(2):185–193.
2. O'Keefe GE, Jurkovich GJ, Copass M, et al. Ten-year trend in survival and resource utilization at a level I trauma center. *Ann Surg* 1999;229(3): 409–415.
3. Acosta JA, Yang JC, Winchell RJ, et al. Lethal injuries and time to death in a level I trauma center. *J Am Coll Surg* 1998;186(5):528–533.
4. O'Keefe GE, Maier RV, Diehr P, et al. The complications of trauma and their associated costs in a level I trauma center. *Arch Surg* 1997;132(8): 920–924.
5. Sauaia A, Moore FA, Moore EE, et al. Early predictors of postinjury multiple organ failure. *Arch Surg* 1994;129(1):39–45.
6. Fitzwater J, Purdue GF, Hunt JL, et al. The risk factors and time course of sepsis and organ dysfunction after burn trauma. *J Trauma* 2003;54(5): 959–966.
7. Moore FA, Moore EE, Sauaia A. Blood transfusion. An independent risk factor for postinjury multiple organ failure. *Arch Surg* 1997;132(6): 620–624.
8. Luchette FA, Jenkins WA, Friend LA, et al. Hypoxia is not the sole cause of lactate production during shock. *J Trauma* 2002;52(3):415–419.
9. James JH, Luchette FA, McCarter FD, et al. Lactate is an unreliable indicator of tissue hypoxia in injury or sepsis. *Lancet* 1999;354(9177): 505–508.
10. Moore FA, McKinley BA, Moore EE, et al. Inflammation and the Host Response to Injury, a large-scale collaborative project: patient-oriented research core–standard operating procedures for clinical care. III. Guidelines for shock resuscitation. *J Trauma* 2006;61(1):82–89.
11. Sperry JL, Minei JP, Frankel HL, et al. Early use of vasopressors after injury: caution before constriction. *J Trauma* 2008;64(1):9–14.
12. McKinley BA, Kozar RA, Cocanour CS, et al. Normal versus supranormal oxygen delivery goals in shock resuscitation: the response is the same. *J Trauma* 2002;53(5):825–832.
13. Balogh Z, McKinley BA, Cocanour CS, et al. Secondary abdominal compartment syndrome is an elusive early complication of traumatic shock resuscitation. *Am J Surg* 2002;184(6):538–543.
14. Sandham JD, Hull RD, Brant RF, et al. A randomized, controlled trial of the use of pulmonary-artery catheters in high-risk surgical patients. *N Engl J Med* 2003;348(1):5–14.
15. Rivers E, Nguyen B, Havstad S, et al. Early goal-directed therapy in the treatment of severe sepsis and septic shock. *N Engl J Med* 2001;345(19): 1368–1377.
16. Gunst M, Ghaemmaghami V, Sperry J, et al. Accuracy of cardiac function and volume status estimates using the bedside echocardiographic assessment in trauma/critical care. *J Trauma* 2008;65(3):509–516.
17. Chytra I, Pradl R, Bosman R, et al. Esophageal Doppler-guided fluid management decreases blood lactate levels in multiple-trauma patients: a randomized controlled trial. *Crit Care* 2007;11(1):R24.
18. Gentilello LM. Advances in the management of hypothermia. *Surg Clin North Am* 1995;75(2):243–256.
19. Gentilello LM, Moujaes S. Treatment of hypothermia in trauma victims: thermodynamic considerations. *J Intensive Care Med* 1995;10(1): 5–14.
20. Chughtai TS, Gilardino MS, Fleiszer DM, et al. An expanding role for cardiopulmonary bypass in trauma. *Can J Surg* 2002;45(2):95–103.
21. Perchinsky MJ, Long WB, Hill JG, et al. Extracorporeal cardiopulmonary life support with heparin-bonded circuitry in the resuscitation of massively injured trauma patients. *Am J Surg* 1995;169(5):488–491.
22. Gentilello LM, Jurkovich GJ, Stark MS, et al. Is hypothermia in the victim of major trauma protective or harmful? A randomized, prospective study. *Ann Surg* 1997;226(4):439–447.
23. Knight DA, Manifold CA, Blue J, et al. A randomized, controlled trial comparing arteriovenous to venovenous rewarming of severe hypothermia in a porcine model. *J Trauma* 2003;55(4):741–746.
24. Hypothermia after Cardiac Arrest Study Group. Mild therapeutic hypothermia to improve the neurologic outcome after cardiac arrest. *N Engl J Med* 2002;346(8):549–556.
25. Harvey MP, Greenfield TP, Sugrue ME, et al. Massive blood transfusion in a tertiary referral hospital. Clinical outcomes and haemostatic complications. *Med J Aust* 1995;163(7):356–359.
26. Counts RB, Haisch C, Simon TL, et al. Hemostasis in massively transfused trauma patients. *Ann Surg* 1979;190(1):91–99.
27. Ciavarella D, Reed RL, Counts RB, et al. Clotting factor levels and the risk of diffuse microvascular bleeding in the massively transfused patient. *Br J Haematol* 1987;67(3):365–368.
28. Hulka F, Mullins RJ, Frank EH. Blunt brain injury activates the coagulation process. *Arch Surg* 1996;131(9):923–927.
29. Oertel M, Kelly DF, McArthur D, et al. Progressive hemorrhage after head trauma: predictors and consequences of the evolving injury. *J Neurosurg* 2002;96(1):109–116.
30. Dutton RP, McCunn M, Hyder M, et al. Factor VIIa for correction of traumatic coagulopathy. *J Trauma* 2004;57(4):709–719.
31. Grounds M. Recombinant factor VIIa (rFVIIa) and its use in severe bleeding in surgery and trauma: a review. *Blood Rev* 2003;17(suppl 1):S11–S21.
32. Hedner U, Erhardtsen E. Potential role for rFVIIa in transfusion medicine. *Transfusion* 2002;42(1):114–124.
33. Winchell RJ, Simons RK, Hoyt DB. Transient systolic hypotension. A serious problem in the management of head injury. *Arch Surg* 1996;131(5): 533–539.
34. Manley G, Knudson MM, Morabito D, et al. Hypotension, hypoxia, and head injury: frequency, duration, and consequences. *Arch Surg* 2001; 136(10):1118–1123.
35. Temkin NR, Dikmen SS, Wilensky AJ, et al. A randomized, double-blind study of phenytoin for the prevention of post-traumatic seizures. *N Engl J Med* 1990;323(8):497–502.
36. Dicker RA, Morabito DJ, Pittet JF, et al. Acute respiratory distress syndrome criteria in trauma patients: why the definitions do not work. *J Trauma* 2004;57(3):522–526.
37. Ivatury RR, Porter JM, Simon RJ, et al. Intra-abdominal hypertension after life-threatening penetrating abdominal trauma: prophylaxis, incidence, and clinical relevance to gastric mucosal pH and abdominal compartment syndrome. *J Trauma* 1998;44(6):1016–1021.
38. Hong JJ, Cohn SM, Perez JM, et al. Prospective study of the incidence and outcome of intra-abdominal hypertension and the abdominal compartment syndrome. *Br J Surg* 2002;89(5):591–596.
39. Diebel LN, Wilson RF, Dulchavsky SA, et al. Effect of increased intra-abdominal pressure on hepatic arterial, portal venous, and hepatic microcirculatory blood flow. *J Trauma* 1992;33(2):279–282.
40. Morris JA Jr, Eddy VA, Blinman TA, et al. The staged celiotomy for trauma. Issues in unpacking and reconstruction. *Ann Surg* 1993;217(5): 576–584.
41. Chen RJ, Fang JF, Chen MF. Intra-abdominal pressure monitoring as a guideline in the nonoperative management of blunt hepatic trauma. *J Trauma* 2001;51(1):44–50.
42. Yang EY, Marder SR, Hastings G, et al. The abdominal compartment syndrome complicating nonoperative management of major blunt liver injuries: recognition and treatment using multimodality therapy. *J Trauma* 2002;52(5):982–986.
43. Hobson KG, Young KM, Ciraulo A, et al. Release of abdominal compartment syndrome improves survival in patients with burn injury. *J Trauma* 2002;53(6):1129–1133.
44. Biffl WL, Moore EE, Burch JM, et al. Secondary abdominal compartment syndrome is a highly lethal event. *Am J Surg* 2001;182(6):645–648.
45. Kron IL, Harman PK, Nolan SP. The measurement of intra-abdominal pressure as a criterion for abdominal re-exploration. *Ann Surg* 1984; 199(1):28–30.
46. Pape HC. Effects of changing strategies of fracture fixation on immunologic changes and systemic complications after multiple trauma: damage control orthopedic surgery. *J Orthop Res* 2008;26(11):1478–1484.
47. McHenry TP, Mirza SK, Wang J, et al. Risk factors for respiratory failure following operative stabilization of thoracic and lumbar spine fractures. *J Bone Joint Surg Am* 2006;88(5):997–1005.
48. Brundage SI, McGhan R, Jurkovich GJ, et al. Timing of femur fracture fixation: effect on outcome in patients with thoracic and head injuries. *J Trauma* 2002;52(2):299–307.
49. Probst C, Probst T, Gaensslen A, et al. Timing and duration of the initial pelvic stabilization after multiple trauma in patients from the German trauma registry: is there an influence on outcome? *J Trauma* 2007;62(2): 370–377.
50. Ely EW, Baker AM, Dunagan DP, et al. Effect on the duration of mechanical ventilation of identifying patients capable of breathing spontaneously. *N Engl J Med* 1996;335(25):1864–1869.
51. O'Keefe GE, Hawkins K, Boynton J, et al. Indicators of fatigue and of prolonged weaning from mechanical ventilation in surgical patients. *World J Surg* 2001;25(1):98–103.

52. Treggiari MM, Hudson LD, Martin DP, et al. Effect of acute lung injury and acute respiratory distress syndrome on outcome in critically ill trauma patients. *Crit Care Med* 2004;32(2):327–331.
53. Pugin J, Ricou B, Steinberg KP, et al. Proinflammatory activity in bronchoalveolar lavage fluids from patients with ARDS, a prominent role for interleukin-1. *Am J Respir Crit Care Med* 1996;153(6 Pt 1):1850–1856.
54. Pugin J, Verghese G, Widmer MC, et al. The alveolar space is the site of intense inflammatory and profibrotic reactions in the early phase of acute respiratory distress syndrome. *Crit Care Med* 1999;27(2):304–312.
55. Ranieri VM, Suter PM, Tortorella C, et al. Effect of mechanical ventilation on inflammatory mediators in patients with acute respiratory distress syndrome: a randomized controlled trial. *JAMA* 1999;282(1):54–61.
56. Dreyfuss D, Soler P, Basset G, et al. High inflation pressure pulmonary edema. Respective effects of high airway pressure, high tidal volume, and positive end-expiratory pressure. *Am Rev Respir Dis* 1988;137(5):1159–1164.
57. Chu EK, Whitehead T, Slutsky AS. Effects of cyclic opening and closing at low- and high-volume ventilation on bronchoalveolar lavage cytokines. *Crit Care Med* 2004;32(1):168–174.
58. ARDS Network. Ventilation with lower tidal volumes as compared with traditional tidal volumes for acute lung injury and the acute respiratory distress syndrome. *N Engl J Med* 2000;342:1301–1308.
59. Amato MB, Barbas CS, Medeiros DM, et al. Effect of a protective-ventilation strategy on mortality in the acute respiratory distress syndrome. *N Engl J Med* 1998;338(6):347–354.
60. Brower RG, Lanken PN, MacIntyre N, et al. Higher versus lower positive end-expiratory pressures in patients with the acute respiratory distress syndrome. *N Engl J Med* 2004;351(4):327–336.
61. Gabay C, Kushner I. Acute-phase proteins and other systemic responses to inflammation. *N Engl J Med* 1999;340(6):448–454.
62. Kudsk KA, Minard G, Wojtysiak SL, et al. Visceral protein response to enteral versus parenteral nutrition and sepsis in patients with trauma. *Surgery* 1994;116(3):516–523.
63. Moore FA, Feliciano DV, Andrassy RJ, et al. Early enteral feeding, compared with parenteral, reduces postoperative septic complications. The results of a meta-analysis. *Ann Surg* 1992;216(2):172–183.
64. Kudsk KA, Croce MA, Fabian TC, et al. Enteral versus parenteral feeding. Effects on septic morbidity after blunt and penetrating abdominal trauma. *Ann Surg* 1992;215(5):503–511.
65. Kozar RA, McQuiggan MM, Moore EE, et al. Postinjury enteral tolerance is reliably achieved by a standardized protocol. *J Surg Res* 2002;104(1):70–75.
66. Marik PE, Zaloga GP. Immunonutrition in critically ill patients: a systematic review and analysis of the literature. *Intensive Care Med* 2008;34(11):1980–1990.
67. Nathens AB, Neff MJ, Jurkovich GJ, et al. Randomized, prospective trial of antioxidant supplementation in critically ill surgical patients. *Ann Surg* 2002;236(6):814–822.
68. Cook DJ, Fuller HD, Guyatt GH, et al. Risk factors for gastrointestinal bleeding in critically ill patients. Canadian Critical Care Trials Group. *N Engl J Med* 1994;330(6):377–381.
69. Maier RV, Mitchell D, Gentilello L. Optimal therapy for stress gastritis. *Ann Surg* 1994;220(3):353–360.
70. Cook D, Guyatt G, Marshall J, et al. A comparison of sucralfate and ranitidine for the prevention of upper gastrointestinal bleeding in patients requiring mechanical ventilation. Canadian Critical Care Trials Group. *N Engl J Med* 1998;338(12):791–797.
71. Daley RJ, Rebuck JA, Welage LS, et al. Prevention of stress ulceration: current trends in critical care. *Crit Care Med* 2004;32(10):2008–2013.
72. Cook DJ, Reeve BK, Guyatt GH, et al. Stress ulcer prophylaxis in critically ill patients. Resolving discordant meta-analyses. *JAMA* 1996;275(4):308–314.
73. O'Keefe GE, Gentilello LM, Maier RV. Incidence of infectious complications associated with the use of histamine2-receptor antagonists in critically ill trauma patients. *Ann Surg* 1998;227(1):120–125.
74. Bulger EM, Edwards T, Klotz P, et al. Epidural analgesia improves outcome after multiple rib fractures. *Surgery* 2004;136(2):426–430.
75. Owings JT, Kraut E, Battistella F, et al. Timing of the occurrence of pulmonary embolism in trauma patients. *Arch Surg* 1997;132(8):862–866.
76. Geerts WH, Code KI, Jay RM, et al. A prospective study of venous thromboembolism after major trauma. *N Engl J Med* 1994;331(24):1601–1606.
77. Montgomery KD, Geerts WH, Potter HG, et al. Practical management of venous thromboembolism following pelvic fractures. *Orthop Clin North Am* 1997;28(3):397–404.
78. Geerts WH, Jay RM, Code KI, et al. A comparison of low-dose heparin with low-molecular-weight heparin as prophylaxis against venous thromboembolism after major trauma. *N Engl J Med* 1996;335(10):701–707.
79. Macaulay W, Westrich G, Sharrock N, et al. Effect of pneumatic compression on fibrinolysis after total hip arthroplasty. *Clin Orthop* 2002;(399):168–176.
80. Killewich LA, Cahan MA, Hanna DJ, et al. The effect of external pneumatic compression on regional fibrinolysis in a prospective randomized trial. *J Vasc Surg* 2002;36(5):953–958.
81. Rogers FB, Shackford SR, Ricci MA, et al. Routine prophylactic vena cava filter insertion in severely injured trauma patients decreases the incidence of pulmonary embolism. *J Am Coll Surg* 1995;180(6):641–647.
82. Ashley DW, Gamblin TC, McCampbell BL, et al. Bedside insertion of vena cava filters in the intensive care unit using intravascular ultrasound to locate renal veins. *J Trauma* 2004;57(1):26–31.
83. Knudson MM, Ikossi DG. Venous thromboembolism after trauma. *Curr Opin Crit Care* 2004;10(6):539–548.
84. Cuschieri J, Freeman B, O'Keefe G, et al. Inflammation and the host response to injury a large-scale collaborative project: patient-oriented research core standard operating procedure for clinical care X. Guidelines for venous thromboembolism prophylaxis in the trauma patient. *J Trauma* 2008;65(4):944–950.
85. Ikushima H, Nishida T, Takeda K, et al. Expression of Toll-like receptors 2 and 4 is downregulated after operation. *Surgery* 2004;135(4):376–385.
86. Adib-Conquy M, Adrie C, Moine P, et al. NF-kappaB expression in mononuclear cells of patients with sepsis resembles that observed in lipopolysaccharide tolerance. *Am J Respir Crit Care Med* 2000;162(5):1877–1883.
87. Singh N, Rogers P, Atwood CW, et al. Short-course empiric antibiotic therapy for patients with pulmonary infiltrates in the intensive care unit. A proposed solution for indiscriminate antibiotic prescription. *Am J Respir Crit Care Med* 2000;162(2 Pt 1):505–511.
88. Chastre J, Wolff M, Fagon JY, et al. Comparison of 8 vs 15 days of antibiotic therapy for ventilator-associated pneumonia in adults: a randomized trial. *JAMA* 2003;290(19):2588–2598.
89. Drakulovic MB, Torres A, Bauer TT, et al. Supine body position as a risk factor for nosocomial pneumonia in mechanically ventilated patients: a randomised trial. *Lancet* 1999;354(9193):1851–1858.
90. Nathens AB, Marshall JC. Selective decontamination of the digestive tract in surgical patients: a systematic review of the evidence. *Arch Surg* 1999;134(2):170–176.
91. Bastin AJ, Ryanna KB. Use of selective decontamination of the digestive tract in United Kingdom intensive care units. *Anaesthesia* 2009;64(1):46–49.
92. de Smet AM, Kluytmans JA, Cooper BS, et al. Decontamination of the digestive tract and oropharynx in ICU patients. *N Engl J Med* 2009;360(1):20–31.
93. Stoutenbeek CP, van Saene HK, Little RA, et al. The effect of selective decontamination of the digestive tract on mortality in multiple trauma patients: a multicenter randomized controlled trial. *Intensive Care Med* 2007;33(2):261–270.
94. Fagon JY, Chastre J. Diagnosis and treatment of nosocomial pneumonia in ALI/ARDS patients. *Eur Respir J Suppl* 2003;42:S77–S83.
95. Clec'h C, Timsit JF, De Lassence A, et al. Efficacy of adequate early antibiotic therapy in ventilator-associated pneumonia: influence of disease severity. *Intensive Care Med* 2004;30(7):1327–1333.
96. Gursel G, Aydogdu M, Ozyilmaz E, et al. Risk factors for treatment failure in patients with ventilator-associated pneumonia receiving appropriate antibiotic therapy. *J Crit Care* 2008;23(1):34–40.
97. Eggimann P, Harbarth S, Constantin MN, et al. Impact of a prevention strategy targeted at vascular-access care on incidence of infections acquired in intensive care. *Lancet* 2000;355(9218):1864–1868.
98. Siegman-Igra Y, Anglim AM, Shapiro DE, et al. Diagnosis of vascular catheter-related bloodstream infection: a meta-analysis. *J Clin Microbiol* 1997;35(4):928–936.
99. Rijnders BJ, Van Wijngaerden E, Wilmer A, et al. Use of full sterile barrier precautions during insertion of arterial catheters: a randomized trial. *Clin Infect Dis* 2003;36(6):743–748.
100. Raad II, Hohn DC, Gilbreath BJ, et al. Prevention of central venous catheter-related infections by using maximal sterile barrier precautions during insertion. *Infect Control Hosp Epidemiol* 1994;15(4 Pt 1):231–238.
101. Chaiyakunapruk N, Veenstra DL, Lipsky BA, et al. Chlorhexidine compared with povidone-iodine solution for vascular catheter-site care: a meta-analysis. *Ann Intern Med* 2002;136(11):792–801.
102. Dissanaike S, Shelton M, Warner K, et al. The risk for bloodstream infections is associated with increased parenteral caloric intake in patients receiving parenteral nutrition. *Crit Care* 2007;11(5):R114.
103. Sena MJ, Utter GH, Cuschieri J, et al. Early supplemental parenteral nutrition is associated with increased infectious complications in critically ill trauma patients. *J Am Coll Surg* 2008;207(4):459–467.
104. Laupland KB, Kirkpatrick AW, Church DL, et al. Intensive-care-unit-acquired bloodstream infections in a regional critically ill population. *J Hosp Infect* 2004;58(2):137–145.
105. Vincent JL, Anaissie E, Bruining H, et al. Epidemiology, diagnosis and treatment of systemic Candida infection in surgical patients under intensive care. *Intensive Care Med* 1998;24(3):206–216.
106. Dissanaike S, Pham T, Shalhub S, et al. Effect of immediate enteral feeding on trauma patients with an open abdomen: protection from nosocomial infections. *J Am Coll Surg* 2008;207(5):690–697.
107. Pelz RK, Hendrix CW, Swoboda SM, et al. Double-blind placebo-controlled trial of fluconazole to prevent candidal infections in critically ill surgical patients. *Ann Surg* 2001;233(4):542–548.
108. Pappas PG, Rex JH, Sobel JD, et al. Guidelines for treatment of candidiasis. *Clin Infect Dis* 2004;38(2):161–189.
109. Johnson E, Espinel-Ingroff A, Szekely A, et al. Activity of voriconazole, itraconazole, fluconazole and amphotericin B in vitro against 1763 yeasts from 472 patients in the voriconazole phase III clinical studies. *Int J Antimicrob Agents* 2008;32(6):511–514.
110. Pfaller MA, Diekema DJ, Rinaldi MG, et al. Results from the ARTEMIS DISK Global Antifungal Surveillance Study: a 6.5-year analysis of susceptibilities of Candida and other yeast species to fluconazole and voriconazole by standardized disk diffusion testing. *J Clin Microbiol* 2005;43(12):5848–5859.

CHAPTER 31 ■ ENVIRONMENTAL INJURIES

GREGORY J. JURKOVICH

KEY POINTS

1. Of 3,000 species of snakes worldwide, only 375 are venomous, with approximately 20 deaths per year in the United States caused by snakebites compared with 100,000 species of Hymenoptera that cause approximately 40 deaths per year, mostly as a result of severe anaphylactic reactions.
2. Snakebite morbidity is a result of venom composition, time of year, size of snake, and depth and amount of envenomation. Venoms consist of numerous (up to 30 or more) proteins that disrupt endothelial cells and blood flow, produce neuromuscular blockade, or generate a coagulopathy via procoagulants. Coral snake venom also has direct neurotoxins and cardiotoxins.
3. Snakebites induce immediate pain, edema, and erythema at the site, and spread at greater than 30 cm/h indicates severe envenomation. Initial incision and suction provides little benefit, as does a proximal tourniquet, which may cause harm. Use of purified ovine antivenin is effective and has replaced equine antivenin with its associated risk of serum sickness.
4. Spider bites produce toxicity by local tissue necrosis (brown recluse and hobo spiders) and painful muscle contractions (black widow spider) in the United States. Deaths may be caused by stinging Hymenoptera, including bees (particularly aggressive Africanized bees), fire ants, and scorpions.
5. Hypothermia risk is high in the severely injured patient as a result of exposure, loss of normal protective metabolism (i.e., shivering), rapid massive infusion of cold fluids/blood, and open thoracic and abdominal cavities.
6. Loss of protective responses to hypothermia occurs between 33°C and 30°C with an initial intensive sympathetic-type reaction with tremulousness, profound vasoconstriction, tremendous increases in oxygen consumption, and accelerated heart rate and minute ventilation.
7. Hypothermia affects both blood gases and coagulation parameters with increased PAO_2 and decreased PCO_2, whereas coagulopathy is aggravated as a result of platelet dysfunction and impaired enzyme activity. However, both blood gases and coagulation parameters should be assessed at 37°C because if the arterial blood gas value is normal at 37°C, it will be acceptable at lower temperatures, whereas coagulopathy at 37°C requires blood component therapy separate from warming to correct the cold-induced coagulopathy.
8. Hypothermia increases risk of mortality at every level of injury. And, although hypothermia delays mortality in experimental shock models, there is no improvement in outcome when applied to severe traumatic brain injury, and patients rapidly rewarmed require less resuscitation volume and have improved survival.
9. Hypothermia is treated either passively by preventing further losses and allowing endogenous rewarming or actively either externally by use of warm blankets, heating pads, or lights and immersion in warm water or internally by core rewarming, which includes heated intravenous fluids; heated peritoneal, thoracic, gastric, bladder, or colonic lavage; heated moist inhaled air; extracorporeal circulatory rewarming (continuous arteriovenous rewarming), or closed circuit intravascular countercurrent heat exchange devises.
10. Frostbite involves ice crystal formation and unpredictable loss of tissue. Early definitive rewarming (avoiding refreezing) by submersion in 40°C to 42°C water is preferable with subsequent meticulous care, possible early thrombolytic therapy, and awaiting demarcation and avoidance of early débridement to optimize outcomes and tissue salvage.

ENVENOMATION

Snakes and Snakebites

1 There are more than 3,000 species of snakes worldwide, of which approximately 375 are venomous. Although estimates vary greatly, possibly 300,000 venomous bites each year are responsible for 30,000 deaths annually worldwide. In the United States, an estimated 45,000 snakebites occur annually, of which 7,000 are from venomous snakes, resulting in 14 to 20 deaths each year.[1–4] The American Association of Poison Control Centers provides an annual report of snakebites that are reported to poison centers in the United States; this information can be accessed at http://www.aapcc.org/. It is likely that many snakebites go unreported. For example, in 2007 only three deaths due to bites and stings from all sources were reported. A recent review of all human rattlesnake bites from 1993 to 2007 published in the Annual Reports of the American Association of Poison Control Centers revealed that while the incidence of severe (reported) bites is decreasing by 2% per year, annual rates of fatalities showed no significant change from 1983 through 2007.[4a]

From 2001 through 2005 there were 23,676 human exposures (average = 4,735/year) to native venomous snakes in the United States reported to U.S. poison centers in all states except Hawaii: 98% were to viper (Crotalidae) snakes and 2% to elapids. Overall, 77% of victims were male, 70% were adults older than 20 years, 12% were aged younger than 10 years, and interestingly, 65 cases involved pregnant women. The overall hospital admission rate was 53%. Outcomes were generally more severe with rattlesnake and copperhead envenomations and in children younger than 6 years of age. The fatality rate of reported cases was 0.06%.[4b]

The five main families of poisonous snakes found worldwide are the Colubridae, Elapidae, Hydrophiidae, Viperidae, and Crotalidae. The Colubridae family consists primarily of the boomslang and the bird snake, which are mainly found in Africa. The Elapidae family includes the cobras, the coral snakes, and the adders, which are found throughout Asia, Africa, the Americas,

TABLE 31.1

SNAKES OF THE FAMILY CROTALIDAE

GENUS	COMMON NAME	CHARACTERISTICS	RANGE
Agkistrodon	Water moccasin and copperhead	No rattles; large plates on crown	North America, southeastern Europe, Asia
Bothrops	New World pit vipers	No rattles; small scales on crown; large scales on ventral tail	Mexico to South America
Crotalus	Rattlesnakes	Rattles; small scales on crown	North, Central, and South America
Lachesis	Bushmaster	No rattles; small scales on crown; small scales on ventral tail	Central and South America
Sistrurus	Massasaugas and pygmy	Rattles; large plates on crown	North America
Trimeresurus	Rattlesnakes	No rattles; small scales on crown	Asia

and Australia. The Hydrophiidae family consists of the sea snakes, which are found throughout the Pacific and along the west coast of South America. The Viperidae family consists of Old World vipers, which are found throughout Africa, Europe, and the Middle East, and are noted by their lack of a heat-sensing pit. The Crotalidae are the true pit vipers and are found worldwide. Some classification systems note the pit vipers as a subfamily of the Viperidae.[5]

The native venomous snakes of North America are members of the phylum Chordata, class Reptilia, order Squamata, suborder Serpentes, and the two families Crotalidae and Elapidae (Table 31.1).

Rattlesnakes are members of the family Crotalidae and the genus *Crotalus* or *Sistrurus*. Water moccasins (or cottonmouths) and copperheads are also members of the Crotalidae family, but of the genus *Agkistrodon*. The coral snake is the major representative of the Elapidae family and of the genus *Micrurus* or *Micruroides*. Other well-known members of the Elapidae family that are not indigenous to North America are the cobras and mambas. The distribution of venomous snakes in the United States is extensive, with at least one native species found in every state except Maine, Alaska, and Hawaii. Rattlesnakes are particularly widely distributed, whereas the water moccasin is found in the southeastern United States, Mississippi Valley, Illinois, and Indiana. The copperhead's range is primarily from central Massachusetts to northern Florida and west to Illinois and Texas.

The Crotalidae, or pit vipers, have a number of characteristics that help distinguish them from benign snakes (Fig. 31.1). Their unique and characteristic thermoreceptor "pit" is an infrared sensor located between the nostril and the eye that helps the snake localize its prey. Pit vipers also have a vertical elliptical pupil, a triangular head, and retractable fangs. Venomous snakes have a single row of plates distal to the anal plate on their ventral surface, whereas harmless snakes have a double row of caudal plates.

Coloration is so variable that it is nearly useless as a distinguishing characteristic. An exception is the coloration of the Elapidae coral snake, which can be identified by the simple rhyme, "Red on yellow kill a fellow; red on black venom lack." Coral snakes have circular bands of colors with red adjacent to yellow, whereas the nonvenomous but similar-looking king snake has red on black bands that do not completely encircle it. The eastern coral snake has a completely black nose, whereas the king snake usually does not.

Most snakebites in the United States occur in the Sunbelt region between April and October, with the peak incidence occurring in the summer months of July and August. Prehibernation and posthibernation snakes appear to be more aggressive. The victims of snakebites are typically men between 18 and 50 years of age. Up to 60% of snakebite victims are deliberately handling snakes,[6] and alcohol consumption in snakebite victims is common.[7]

Not every poisonous snakebite results in envenomation, and even the presence of fang marks does not necessarily correlate with envenomation. Venom is produced in Duvernoy glands, which are located on the dorsal sides of the head and correspond to the parotid glands. The location of this large gland gives the head its characteristic triangular shape. During the bite, the venom is forced through the hollow fangs by the palatine muscles and extruded out the orifices, which are located just proximal to the tip. Therefore, clothing, gloves, and shoes may significantly diminish the depth of penetration and limit the amount of envenomation.

2 The severity of envenomation is related to the amount of venom injected, the concentration of the venom, and the size of the snake. Direct intravenous envenomation is unusual but particularly severe.[8] Snakebites with a distance between the fangs of more than 15 mm are representative of a large snake and therefore suggest a potentially more significant envenomation. Hibernation also seems to play a role in severity. After hibernation, snakes are relatively dehydrated because they have been in a prolonged fasting state, and therefore they produce a more potent, concentrated venom. The degree of envenomation also varies because 10% to 25% of bites have no significant envenomation, even when fang marks are noted on the victim. With each strike, the snake may discharge between 25% and 75% of its venom, so that successive or repetitive strikes tend to diminish the amount of venom available. Snakes that are angered or fearful may discharge greater amounts of venom. Table 31.2 lists the grading scale for pit viper bites.[24–28]

Snake Venom. The function of venom is to kill or immobilize prey and to aid in digestion. Venom consists of a complex array of proteins and enzymes that have historically been characterized as neurotoxins, hemotoxins, and cardiotoxins.[9] The components of pit viper venom, however, affect almost every organ system; thus, labeling snake venom as a specific organ toxin is probably inaccurate.[5] More than 26 different proteins and nonenzymatic peptides have been isolated from various venoms.[2,5] The Crotalidae venom consists of approximately 90% water, 5 to 15 enzymes, 3 to 12 nonenzymatic proteins and peptides, and more than 6 other unidentified substances. A partial list of these enzymes is shown in Table 31.3 and includes several proteolytic enzymes, phospholipase, nucleotidase, acetylcholinesterase, and amino acid oxidase.

These low-molecular-weight peptides and polypeptides (6 to 100 kD) appear to act by damaging vascular endothelial cells. Electron microscopic analysis of tissue from human snakebite victims has demonstrated disruption of the vascular endothelium and other plasma membranes. Microangiopathic vascular injury leads to increased permeability, peripheral

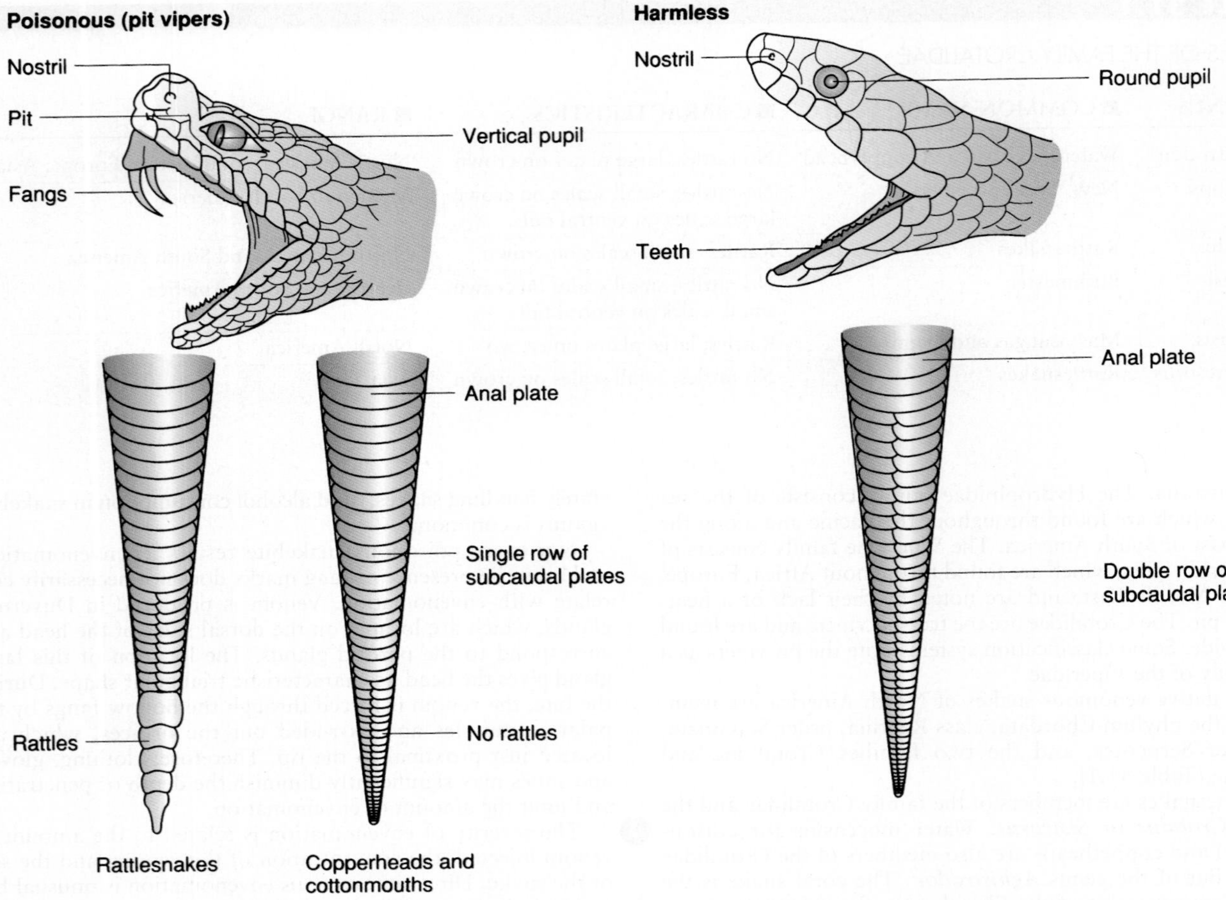

FIGURE 31.1. Characteristics of snakes that differentiate poisonous pit vipers from harmless snakes.

TABLE 31.2 CLASSIFICATION

GRADING OF PIT VIPER BITES

■ GRADE	■ DESCRIPTION OF BITE
0	Visible bite but no envenomation; swelling/erythema around the fang mark <2.5 cm; minimal pain and tenderness; no systemic symptoms
I	History of immediate pain with bite; swelling and erythema 5–15 cm from fang marks; no systemic signs or symptoms
II	Moderate pain; erythema and edema of 15–40 cm; mild systemic signs such as weakness and emesis; may have abnormal laboratory findings
III	Severe pain; erythema and edema >40 cm, with petechiae and bullae; systemic signs and symptoms such as vertigo, DIC, or coagulopathy; abnormal laboratory values
IV	Lethal envenomation with widespread edema, shock, seizures, coma, renal failure, bleeding, DIC, paralysis

DIC, disseminated intravascular coagulation.

TABLE 31.3

ENZYMES OF SNAKE VENOMS

Proteolytic enzymes
Arginine ester hydrolase
Thrombinlike enzyme
Collagenase
Hyaluronidase
Phospholipase A_2 (A)
Phospholipase C
Lactate dehydrogenase
Phosphomonoesterase
Phosphodiesterase
Acetylcholinesterase
RNase
DNase
5′-Nucleotidase
L-Amino acid oxidase

edema, pulmonary edema and hemorrhage, significant interstitial fluid sequestration, and hypotension. Other venom proteins appear to induce a neuromuscular blockade or coagulopathy. Procoagulant venom factors seem to dominate, primarily exerting their effect late in the clotting cascade by activating factor X or prothrombin or by directly converting fibrinogen to fibrin.[10] Tissue destruction is aided by several different proteins. L-Amino acid oxidase causes extensive tissue destruction and splits fibrinogen, leading to platelet trapping and unstable clot formation, thus contributing to the genesis of disseminated intravascular coagulation (DIC). Phospholipase A_2 causes hydrolysis of lecithin at the C-2 position, resulting in the formation of lysolecithin. This event alters the permeability of erythrocyte membranes and muscle cell plasma membranes, leading to hemolysis and tissue edema. Hyaluronidase induces the lysis of ground substance and thereby aids in the distribution of the venom throughout body tissues.

The Elapidae snake venom also contains specific and unique neurotoxins and cardiotoxins, which have a more direct effect on the neuroactivity of the prey. Coral snake venom directly blocks action of acetylcholine receptor sites that do not appear to be responsive to neostigmine. This blockade results in ptosis, dysphagia, and slurred speech and can lead to seizures, coma, and death within 8 to 72 hours. While coral venom is extremely toxic, there has been only one confirmed death in the United States from a coral snake bite in the past 40 years, the victim delaying medical attention; alcohol was involved.[10a]

Signs and Symptoms of Envenomation by Snakebite. 3 The important signs and symptoms of snakebites include both local and systemic effects. Immediate pain and progressive edema and erythema at the site of the bite are the norm. Local signs and symptoms progressing at a rate of greater than 30 cm/h, in addition to microscopic hematuria and bleeding from the puncture sites, indicate significant envenomation.[11] Delayed toxicity has been observed on occasion, and rarely severe toxicity has followed resolution of initial local symptoms.[12] Occasionally, a bite by a nonpoisonous garter snake (*Thamnophis* species) can be confused at an early stage with the bite of a poisonous snake of the Crotalidae family. Edema and erythema can be produced by toxic salivary secretions of a parotidlike gland (Duvernoy glands) if the skin has been broken.[13] Systemic signs fail to develop, however, and the local signs resolve spontaneously within a few days.

Myonecrosis at or near the bite site is affected by both the direct toxic effects of the venom and the added ischemia of edema and increased compartment pressures. The development of a frank compartment syndrome after a snakebite of the extremity can occur but is unusual, occurring in only 1 of 272 Eastern diamondback and water moccasin bites in one report.[14] Studies using purified venom injected into the anterolateral leg compartment of mongrel dogs determined that only intramuscular injection leads to an increase in compartmental pressure.[15] Compartment syndromes are unusual because most snakebites do not penetrate through the superficial fascia; the principal cause of myonecrosis is probably direct toxicity of the venom rather than ischemia from elevated compartment pressure. Nonetheless, in one report of 36 rattlesnake bites, three definitive diagnoses of compartment syndrome were made on the basis of elevated compartment pressures.[16] The indication for fasciotomy remains controversial, with some authors recommending fasciotomy in nearly all cases,[17] but others believing that aggressive use of antivenin precludes the need for fasciotomy in most instances.

Shock is a common finding with significant systemic envenomation, resulting from increased microvascular permeability and the loss of plasma volume. Bradycardia and arrhythmia result from the cardiotoxins. Renal failure may occur from hypoperfusion and shock, from DIC with renal tubular necrosis, or as a direct toxic effect of the venom. Sheehan syndrome of pituitary necrosis has been reported after a Russell viper bite, likely a result of the procoagulant activity of the viper's venom.[18]

The hematologic effects of venom cause both local and systemic problems. Venom appears to activate factor X as well as factors V and IX or directly converts fibrinogen to fibrin, leading to activation of the coagulation cascade and a consumptive coagulopathy.[18] The prothrombin time (PT) and partial thromboplastin time (PTT) are commonly increased, which may result in persistent bleeding, ecchymosis, or petechiae at the puncture site or affected extremity. Microscopic hematuria and bleeding from any preexisting condition, such as peptic ulcer or menstrual bleeding, may aggravate the situation. Venom also causes a mild defibrinogenation state, with unstable clot formation consuming fibrinogen but sparing platelets. This state may contribute to DIC.

Venom also appears to cause myriad neurologic effects, especially the venom from the Elapidae family. The venom of coral snakes, cobras, and sea snakes contains an acetylcholinesterase receptor antagonist that causes ptosis, slurred speech, and impaired swallowing leading to hypersalivation. This venom also has central nervous system activity that results in progressive weakness, paresthesia, and eventually respiratory muscle failure and respiratory arrest. Seizures and psychotic behavior may develop that can lead to coma or death in 8 to 72 hours. The toxins responsible include neurotoxin A, which appears to act on the central nervous system, and neurotoxin B, which acts at the myoneural junction.

Clinical Evaluation of Snakebites. Victims of snakebites require the same aggressive supportive and resuscitative care as any trauma patient. Attention to airway and breathing are the first priority, followed by cardiovascular assessment and resuscitation. A detailed history is often helpful in determining the type and size of snake, the circumstances of the bite, and timing. Key points should include snake description, first-aid measures applied, known allergies and comorbidities, and history of snakebites or use of antivenin. A complete and detailed physical examination should specifically look for fang marks (usually a single pair, rarely more than one strike), distance between fang marks (indicates size of the snake), and measurement of the zone of erythema and edema initially surrounding the fang marks and subsequently over time. Signs of toxicity to be searched for include petechiae, bruises, bullae, or blisters. Measurements at the same site should be repeated every 15 minutes until edema and erythema progression has ceased. Frequent clinical examinations should focus on neurologic, hematologic, and hemodynamic profiles.

Initial laboratory testing should include electrolytes, complete blood count with platelet count, PT, PTT, fibrinogen level, blood urea nitrogen, and serum creatine plus urinalysis. Depending on the patient's age and comorbidities, an electrocardiogram and chest radiograph should be included. Type and cross-matching for blood is advised, particularly if the patient presents with a more severe grade of injury. Tetanus immunization status should be queried and brought up to date if needed. Enzyme-linked immunosorbent assays (ELISAs) have been developed to directly measure serum venom antigens in patients and to help identify the species of snake.[18] ELISA is sensitive to 5 mg/L of venom and can assess serum, urine, blister fluid, or aspiration fluid. This test is helpful when attempting to determine the specific snake to direct monovalent antivenin therapy. Radioimmunoassay is extremely sensitive, with some venoms being detected to levels of 0.4 mg/L. The applicability of this assay is limited because of its expense and the fact that it may take 24 hours to produce a definitive result.[19] In the United States, however, there is only one Crotalidae antivenin and only one coral snake antivenin; therefore, this more detailed identification is usually unnecessary.

Treatment of Snakebite Envenomation. First aid is simply immobilization and splinting of the injected part at the level of the heart or at a slightly dependent position, much as a fracture of the extremity would be treated. The utility of incision and suction at the puncture site has been debated for years, and probably should not be advised. In dogs, up to half of the venom can be removed if incision and suction are begun within 3 minutes of the bite,[19] and in rabbits, a suction device (the Sawyer extractor pump) has been shown to remove up to 37% of radiolabeled venom in rabbits when applied 3 minutes after envenomation[34]; however, these results have not been verified in humans. Russell[2] has indicated that if immediate incision and suction is started and continued for 1 hour, at best 11% of the venom may be removed.[20] Most authorities do not recommend incision and suction therapy.[1,20,20a,21]

The use of a proximal tourniquet should also be discouraged because it may lead to venous congestion and increased edema and ischemia without demonstrated benefit. Cryotherapy (ice pack) is discouraged universally because it increases tissue ischemia. The effects of cryotherapy and steroids were studied in envenomated mongrel dogs, and it was found that no added benefit could be demonstrated by using corticosteroids or cryotherapy as adjuvants to antivenin alone.[22]

Tetanus prophylaxis and the prevention of secondary infections are important objectives of snakebite treatment. Species of the gram-negative bacteria *Aerobacter, Proteus,* and *Pseudomonas* are particularly common causes of bacterial infection, and appropriate systemic antibiotics are given routinely. Cholinergic agonists may be of benefit after an Elapidae bite because this venom has a significant effect on acetylcholine receptors. Calcium gluconate may also be of benefit after an Elapidae bite to control the onset of seizures. Some snake venoms have been shown to contain metallopeptides, and for this reason, ethylenediaminetetraacetic acid (EDTA) has been tried experimentally in animals as a chelator to inactivate these proteins. The use of this agent is to be discouraged, however, because it appears to hasten death in laboratory animals for unknown reasons.[16] Systemic steroids have no effect in the initial treatment of snakebites, but they play a significant role in treatment of serum sickness that often follows antivenin therapy.[23]

Antivenin is the mainstay of treatment of significant envenomation throughout the world.[1] While more than 100 antivenin* products are available worldwide, prior to 2007 there were two antivenins available in the United States for Crotalinae bites and one for Elapidae bites. In 2007, the manufacturer of Crotalidae equine polyvalent antivenin (Wyeth-Ayerst, St. David's, Pennsylvania) stopped distribution of this antivenin in the United States, although unexpired stock may still exist. The Crotalidae equine antivenin by Wyeth-Ayerst was a polyvalent, hyperimmune equine serum produced by horse envenomation with the eastern diamondback, western diamondback, tropical rattlesnake, and fer-de-lance. The high rate of hypersensitivity and serum sickness reactions was the primary reason for halting its use. Anaphylaxis is reported in 3% to 54% of patients treated with equine antivenin, but only 14% of those treated with ovine CroFab.[5,25] The anaphylaxis is a type I immunoglobulin E–mediated reaction to the horse serum, which results in massive mast cell degranulation.

The other available antivenin for Elapidae bites is the eastern coral snake antivenin, also manufactured by Wyeth-Ayerst.

Since 2000, the sheep (ovine)-produced antivenin, polyvalent Crotalidae ovine immune Fab (CroFab, Protherics) (referred to as "FabAV"), has been the standard of treatment for most North American snakebites. FabAV contains only the venom-binding portion of immunoglobulin G. CroFab (Crotalidae Polyvalent Immune Fab [Ovine]; Fougera, Melville, New York) is a sterile, nonpyrogenic, purified, lyophilized preparation of ovine Fab (monovalent) immunoglobulin fragments obtained from the blood of healthy sheep immunized with one of the following North American snake venoms: *Crotalus atrox* (western diamondback rattlesnake), *Crotalus adamanteus* (eastern diamondback rattlesnake), *Crotalus scutulatus* (Mojave rattlesnake), and *Agkistrodon piscivorus* (cottonmouth or water moccasin). To obtain the final antivenin product, the four different monospecific antivenins are mixed. Each monospecific antivenin is prepared by fractionating the immunoglobulin from the ovine serum, digesting it with papain, and isolating the venom-specific Fab fragments on ion exchange and affinity chromatography columns.[33]

CroFab is standardized by its ability to neutralize the lethal action of each of the four venom immunogens following intravenous injection in mice. The potency of the product varies with each batch; however, a minimum number of mouse LD50 neutralizing units against each of the four venoms is included in every vial of final product. A schema for using CroFab to treat snakebites is given in Algorithm 31.1. This product is roughly five times more potent than the older equine Crotalidae polyvalent antivenin; it has rapidly replaced the equine antivenin once widely used against all North American crotalids, primarily because of fewer allergic reactions.[5,29,30] Recurrence of the effects of venom after an initial response to antivenin has been well recognized, hence the subsequent smaller doses 6, 12, and 18 hours following an effective initial response. As the algorithm illustrates, however, the equine antivenin may still have a role in the patient who is a nonresponder to CroFab, and an equine antivenin remains the most effective antivenin for coral snake bites.

The occurrence of anaphylaxis during or after administration of any antivenin mandates immediate cessation of therapy and countermeasures, including antihistamines (oral diphenhydramine), epinephrine infusion, and/or corticosteroids. The adequacy of the airway and volume status must be ensured. The risk of continuing antivenin must be weighed against the potentially fatal consequences of severe envenomation. Concomitant administration of intravenous antihistamine and epinephrine in small, titrated microdrip doses to prevent the most severe manifestations of systemic anaphylaxis has been described in an allergic patient in whom antivenin therapy was deemed essential. This technique requires close physician observation because there are risks from both anaphylaxis and the treatment itself.

The other major complication of any antivenin therapy is serum sickness. Serum sickness occurs in approximately 50% to 75% of all patients treated with an equine-based antivenin but only 16% with the ovine source of antivenin.[5,24] Serum sickness is a type III hypersensitivity reaction in which soluble antigen–antibody complexes are deposited diffusely in the presence of antigen access. In 26 patients who were treated with a total of 507 vials of Crotalidae antivenin, there was a 23% incidence of immediate hypersensitivity reaction and a 50% incidence of serum sickness.[24] Of patients who received more than eight vials of antivenin, 83% experienced serum sickness compared with 38% of patients who received fewer than eight vials. Serum sickness symptoms of urticaria, itching, nephritis, and arthralgia can occur at any time up to 3 weeks after antivenin therapy. The exact number of vials of antivenin required to induce serum sickness is unknown, but it appears that increasing amounts of antivenin lead to a higher incidence of serum sickness, with almost universal occurrence after the administration of 7 to 10 vials of antivenin. The treatment for serum sickness is systemic corticosteroids in decreasing doses over a 7- to 14-day period.

Treatment of snakebites with antivenin has changed with the more widespread use of the ovine polyvalent CroFab. As illustrated in Algorithm 31.1, patients with a suspected or

*Regarding the terminology for envenomation, the term *venom* describes the poisonous fluid produced by snakes, spiders, scorpions, etc., and the term *venin* describes any poisonous substance found in venom; *antivenin* is the term used by both *Stedman's Medical Dictionary* and *Webster's English Dictionary* to describe an antitoxin or antiserum against an animal or insect venom.

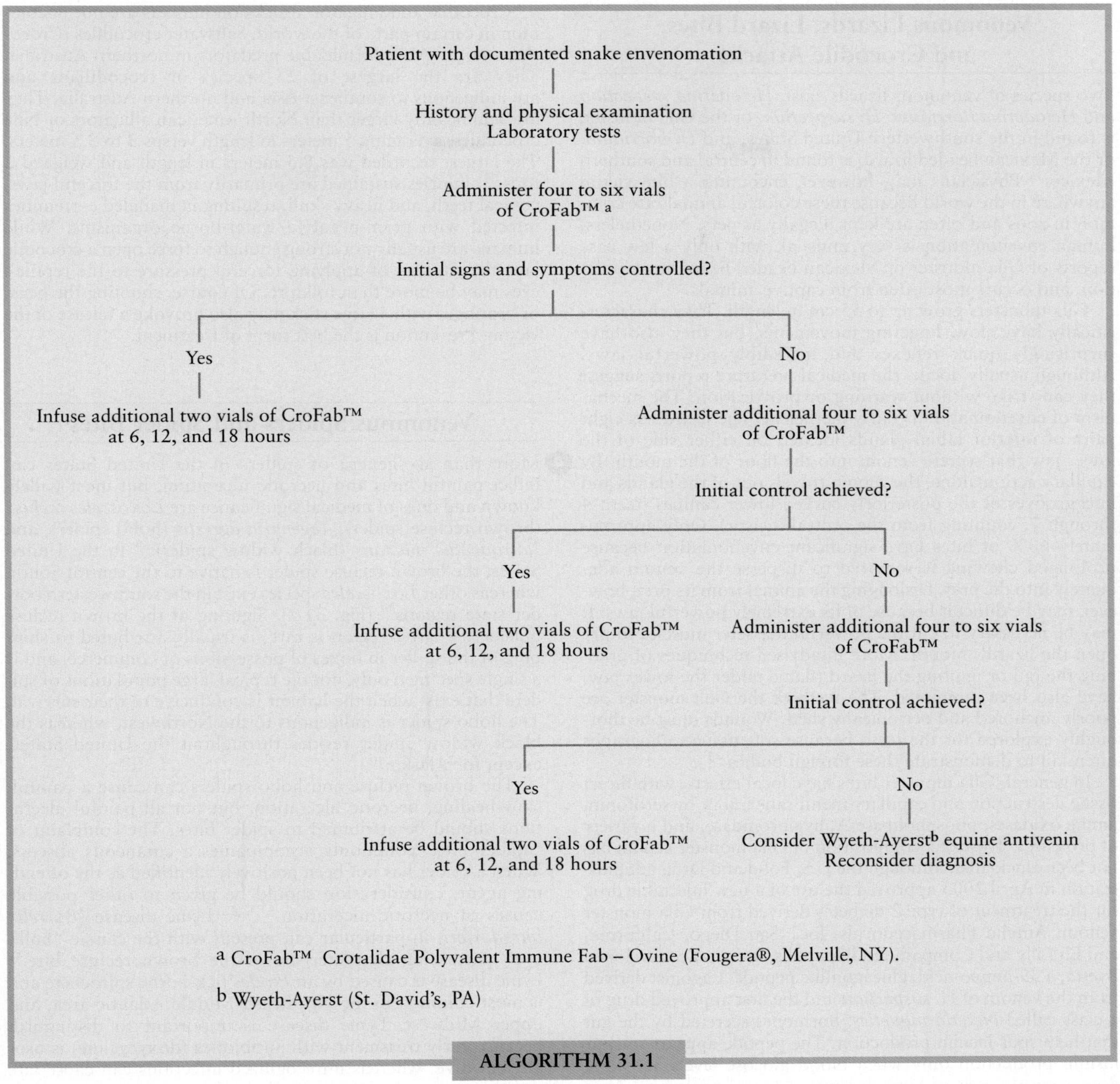
Patient with documented snake envenomation
History and physical examination
Laboratory tests
Administer four to six vials of CroFab™ a
Initial signs and symptoms controlled?
Yes
No
Infuse additional two vials of CroFab™ at 6, 12, and 18 hours
Administer additional four to six vials of CroFab™
Initial control achieved?
Yes
No
Infuse additional two vials of CroFab™ at 6, 12, and 18 hours
Administer additional four to six vials of CroFab™
Initial control achieved?
Yes
No
Infuse additional two vials of CroFab™ at 6, 12, and 18 hours
Consider Wyeth-Ayerst b equine antivenin
Reconsider diagnosis
a CroFab™ Crotalidae Polyvalent Immune Fab – Ovine (Fougera®, Melville, NY).
b Wyeth-Ayerst (St. David's, PA)
ALGORITHM 31.1

ALGORITHM 31.1. Treatment of snakebite envenomation with antivenin. (Adapted from Gold BS, Dart RC, Barish RA. Bites of venomous snakes. *N Engl J Med* 2002;347:347–356; and Cribari C. *Management of Poisonous Snakebites*. Chicago, IL: American College of Surgeons Committee on Trauma Poster; 2004.)

confirmed envenomation are recommended to receive an initial four to six vials of CroFab. If signs and symptoms of envenomation are controlled, additional vials are administered in a delayed fashion to prevent recurrence of symptoms. However, if the initial treatment fails to control envenomation, an additional four to six vials of CroFab are repeated twice, and then consideration should be given to using the "older" Wyeth-Ayerst polyvalent equine antivenin. The estimated initial amount of Crotalidae antivenin needed should correlate with the presenting clinical grade of envenomation. The package insert for Wyeth-Ayerst Crotalidae Antivenin Polyvalent provides detailed instructions for preparing, administering, and dosing this agent.

Although early surgical excision of the bite wound has been advocated by some, most authorities regard antivenin as the primary therapy and reserve surgery for the occasional compartment syndrome or débridement of necrotic tissue at the site of the bite several days after envenomation. Unless deep intramuscular envenomation has occurred and antivenin therapy has been delayed, fasciotomy is rarely required. Because the musculature and deep compartments of the hand are relatively superficial, however, intramuscular penetration may occur at these sites. Myonecrosis and interstitial edema may cause enough compartmental hypertension in these sites that linear finger fasciotomy and digital release are helpful. Fasciotomy may help reduce the ischemic tissue damage caused by increased pressure but does not alleviate the myonecrosis caused by the direct toxic effect of the venom.[31,32] Noninvasive arterial studies may help select patients who require special surgical intervention for ischemia.[33]

Venomous Lizards, Lizard Bites, and Crocodile Attacks

Two species of venomous lizards exist, *Heloderma suspectum* and *Heloderma horridum*. *H. suspectum*, or the Gila monster, is found in the southwestern United States, and *H. horridum*, or the Mexican beaded lizard, is found in central and southern Mexico.[35] Physicians may, however, encounter a bite victim anywhere in the world because these colorful animals are common in zoos and often are kept illegally as pets. Nonetheless, human envenomation is very unusual, with only a few case reports of Gila monster or Mexican beaded lizard envenomation, and occurs most often from captive animals.[35,36]

Gila monsters grow up to 55 cm in length. They characteristically have slow, lingering movements, but they also have surprisingly quick reflexes and incredibly powerful jaws. Although usually docile, the medical literature reports suggest they can strike without warning or provocation. The mechanism of envenomation is fairly inefficient. The lizard has eight pairs of inferior labial glands located on either side of the lower jaw that secrete venom into the floor of the mouth. By capillary action alone, the venom travels out of the glands and into grooves of the posteriorly curved lower canines (teeth 4 through 7, counting from the central incisor). Only approximately 60% of bites have significant envenomation because prolonged chewing is required to disperse the venom adequately into the prey. Dislodging the animal from its prey, however, may be difficult because of its extremely powerful jaws. It may be necessary to cut the powerful masseter muscles to pry open the lizard's mouth. More ill-advised techniques of grabbing the tail or igniting the lizard (flame under the lower jaw) have also been attempted. The teeth of the Gila monster are poorly anchored and periodically shed. Wounds must be thoroughly explored for the teeth because soft tissue radiographs often fail to demonstrate these foreign bodies.[35]

In general, Gila monster bites have local effects, with direct tissue destruction and capillary membrane injury by serotonin, amine oxidases, phospholipase A, hyaluronidase, and a variety of proteases. The exact composition of Gila monster venom has not been elucidated, although the U.S. Food and Drug administration in April 2005 approved the use of a new injectable drug for the treatment of type 2 diabetes derived from Gila monster venom. Amylin Pharmaceuticals, Inc. (San Diego, California) and Eli Lilly and Company (Indianapolis, Indiana) codeveloped Byetta, a 39-amino-acid, glucagonlike peptide-1 agonist derived from the venom of *H. suspectum* and the first approved drug of a class called *incretin mimetics*, hormones secreted by the gut that help spur insulin production. The peptide appears to spur insulin production only when blood glucose levels are high, decreasing the risk of hypoglycemia. Clinical trials have been initiated comparing this drug alone and in combination with metformin and sulfonylureas.[37]

The most common clinical symptom of a Gila monster bite is pain, usually subsiding in 8 to 10 hours, although it may persist for several days. Generalized weakness, dizziness, perspiration, and anxiety are other common symptoms. Hypotension is a common clinical finding with envenomation, usually responding to fluid resuscitation alone. There has been one reported case of significant systemic hypotension and myocardial infarction in a 23-year-old man after a Gila monster bite.[38] Other common signs include erythema, edema, and even lymphangitis, probably from pathogens injected at the time of the bite because injection of sterile venom produces none of these clinical signs. Rather severe nausea and vomiting can also be seen. Laboratory abnormalities are rare. The treatment of Gila monster bites is largely local wound care and systemic support of the patient (fluids, pain relief, antibiotics, antiemetics). No antivenin is available. Tetanus immunization should be current. A period of observation after the bite to assess the potential for systemic toxicity is warranted.

Crocodile and alligator attacks on humans are not uncommon in certain parts of the world. Saltwater crocodiles (*Crocodylus porosis*) are formidable predators in northern Australia. They are the largest of 23 species of crocodilians and are indigenous to southeast Asia and northern Australia. They are significantly larger than North American alligators or Nile crocodiles, averaging 5 meters in length versus 3 to 3.5 meters. The largest recorded was 8.5 meters in length and weighed 2 tons.[39a] Injuries sustained are primarily from the forceful jaws, conical teeth, and heavy skull, resulting in mangled extremities infected with gram-negative water-borne organisms. While humans are usually not strong enough to force open a crocodile jaw, the strategy of applying forceful pressure to the reptile's eyes may be more than folklore. Of course, shooting the beast or beating it with a large stick may also provoke a release of the victim. Prevention is the best form of treatment.

Venomous Spiders and Spider Bites

4 More than six genera of spiders in the United States can inflict painful bites and necrotic ulceration, but most widely known and ones of medical significance are *Loxosceles reclusa* (brown recluse spider), *Tegenaria agrestis* (hobo spider), and *Latrodectus mactans* (black widow spider).[60] In the United States, the brown recluse spider is native to the central South, whereas other *Loxosceles* species exist in the southwestern border state regions[39] (Fig. 31.2). Sighting of the brown recluse outside its native region is rare, is usually attributed to shipping of the spider in boxes of possessions or commerce, and is a single specimen only, not the typical large populations of spiders that exist when the habitat is conducive to their survival. The hobo spider is indigenous to the Northwest, whereas the black widow spider resides throughout the United States, except for Alaska.[40]

The brown recluse and hobo spiders can cause a painful, slow-healing, necrotic ulceration, but not all painful ulcerations should be attributed to spider bites. The complaint of "spider bite" commonly accompanies a cutaneous abscess. When a spider has not been positively identified as the offending agent, consideration should be given to other possible causes of necrotic ulceration.[39,41,42] Lyme disease (*Borrelia burgdorferi*) in particular can present with the classic "bull's eye" patterning characteristic of the brown recluse bite.[43] Lyme disease is caused by an *Ixodes* tick-borne spirochete and is most common in the Northeast, Middle Atlantic area, and upper Midwest. Lyme disease is important to distinguish because early treatment with antibiotics (doxycycline) is usually curative, whereas unrecognized infections can cause late arthritic and neurologic symptoms that may not respond to antibiotics.

T. agrestis was introduced to the Pacific Northwest in the early 1900s from Europe. It was first reported from Seattle in the 1930s and had become common by the 1960s. *T. agrestis* is long legged (40 mm resting length), is hairy, and ranges in color from light tan to dark brown. The cephalothorax (10 to 12 mm) is distinguished by two stripes and "butterfly" markings on the dorsal surface and two stripes marking the ventral surface. *T. agrestis* is a poor climber and hence is usually found in low places. Sometimes referred to as an "aggressive house spider," the hobo builds a funnel-shaped web that can be found in woodpiles, crawl spaces, barns, haystacks, and objects that have not been moved in a long time. The hobo spiders are active from spring through fall, and although not overtly aggressive, the most dangerous time to encounter the hobo spider is during the fall mating season; the nests should be avoided and not probed with a finger. A bite of the hobo spider causes a necrotic wound similar to that of the brown recluse spider, along with a characteristic persistent headache.[39] The ulcer is slow to heal, often leaving a central crater.

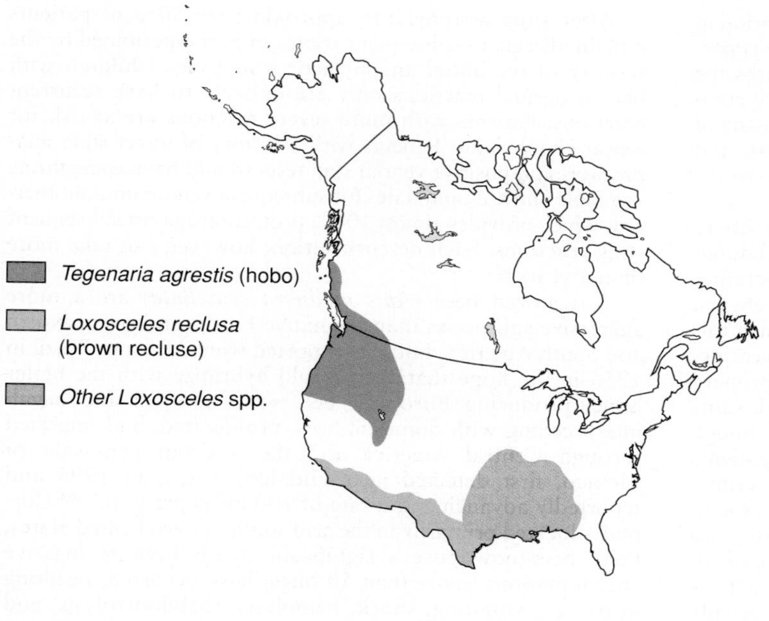

FIGURE 31.2. The geographic distribution of medically relevant spiders in North America.

The brown recluse spider is so named because it lives in dark, dry places, emerging only at night. This spider does not spin a web but catches prey by pursuit. It is small (body, 0.5 to 1 cm wide; leg span, 3 to 4 cm) and recognizable by the characteristic violin-shaped mark on the cephalothorax. When viewed under a microscope, it has three pairs of eyes rather than the two pairs most spiders have. Like most biting spiders, the brown recluse spider bites humans only when trapped or crushed against the skin. Brown recluse spider bites cause a complex and chronic soft tissue ulcer. Clinical signs begin first with an erythematous papule (2 to 8 hours), followed by white vasoconstriction (8 to 72 hours), ecchymosis (24 to 72 hours), and a hemorrhagic vesicle (48 to 96 hours).[39,41] Two to 7 days after the bite, an eschar develops over a characteristic crateriform ulcer, with surrounding soft tissue induration.[44] The eschar may conceal a progressive undermining necrosis that can persist for months. These wounds are most severe in the fatty parts of the body, such as the thighs and buttocks, perhaps because of the relatively poor blood supply to these tissues. There may also be a particular dermonecrotic factor in brown recluse venom. Sphingomyelinase D is present in the venom and appears to interact with the sphingomyelin of the red blood cell membrane and perhaps capillary endothelial cell membranes, causing cell destruction.[45] Histologically, the site of the bite is said to resemble a cutaneous Arthus reaction, with the mechanism involving interactions between complement neutrophils and the clotting system.[46] Investigations suggest the necrosis is completely dependent on the victim's neutrophils, yet these neutrophils are not activated by the venom. *Loxosceles* venom appears to be a novel yet potent endothelial cell agonist, stimulating the release of interleukin-8 and granulocyte-macrophage colony-stimulating factor and E-selectin expression.[47]

Significant systemic symptoms after a brown recluse bite occur infrequently, in fewer than 10% of cutaneous manifestations. The clinical spectrum includes fever, chills, malaise, arthralgia, nausea and vomiting, and a scarlatiniform rash but can progress to hemolytic anemia, renal failure, and DIC in rare cases, perhaps more commonly in children than adults.[48]

Treatment of brown recluse spider bites includes analgesics, wound care, antitetanus therapy, avoidance of early surgical débridement, and perhaps oral dapsone. Antibiotics are reserved for true associated cellulitis. Dapsone is thought to work as an inhibitor of polymorphonuclear leukocyte chemotaxis, but it can cause hemolysis in glucose-6-phosphate dehydrogenase–deficient patients and can produce methemoglobinemia. Some studies show dapsone effective in reducing the size of the skin lesion and limiting the need for surgical débridement,[49,50] whereas other studies demonstrate no benefit in animal models,[51] and no prospective study in humans supports its use.[52] The most common dose is 50 to 100 mg (0.7 mg/kg) twice daily for 3 days to 2 weeks, although it is not approved for this use by the U.S. Food and Drug Administration. One controlled trial of dapsone, electric shock therapy, or no therapy in guinea pigs injected with 30 mg of spider venom demonstrated efficacy of dapsone in reducing lesion induration and necrosis area 72 hours after envenomation.[53] Electric shock therapy had no benefit. Hyperbaric oxygen treatment of model envenomation in rabbits and pigs also failed to demonstrate any effect on lesion healing time or superficial appearance, although hyperbaric treatments seemed to have decreased the amount of undermining necrosis visualized histologically on day 24 after envenomation.[54,55] A trial of hyperbaric oxygen, dapsone, and cyproheptadine in rabbits also failed to demonstrate any significant difference in lesion size, ulcer size, or histopathologic ranking up to 10 days after injection of toxin.[55] Local injections of lidocaine, phentolamine, and systemic steroids and antihistamines have been widely used in the past but have no demonstrable benefit. Systemic corticosteroids probably have a role only in the rare case of systemic loxoscelism, which has minimal skin changes but produces massive hemolysis.[44] Surgical excision of the lesion itself has no clear benefit.[56]

Commercial antivenin for the brown recluse spider is not available in the United States, although a rabbit antivenin for *L. laeta* is available in South America.[39] Equine-derived antivenin has been shown effective in mice and rabbits, and pepsin treatment to isolate the $F(ab')_2$ monoclonal fragment has been attempted. However, studies to date fail to demonstrate any advantage to antivenin, with or without dapsone, particularly if there is a few-hour delay in administering the antivenin. In areas where Loxosceles spiders are endemic, vaccination might hold promise.[60]

Few living creatures invite such poetic fascination and fear as the black widow spider. Its name, coloring, carnivore diet, and the disconcerting habit of the female eating her sexual partner invite such fascination. And although both the male and female spider possess potent venom, only the female is dangerous to humans because the male is smaller and thus its bite cannot penetrate human skin. The mature female has a black body, approximately 6 mm in diameter, with a characteristic red hourglass mark on the ventral aspect of the thorax. This mark is not always present and may consist only of two red dots. The black widow prefers a dry, protected, dimly lit area with access to flies and other insects, such as an outdoor privy. During the period in which the female *L. mactans* is guarding an egg sac, she is particularly aggressive and will attack the male if he disturbs the web, hence earning the particularly dark and descriptive common name *black widow*.[49] The diet most commonly consists of insects of any size, but reportedly includes mice, toads, and tarantulas that wander into the dense web and succumb to the poisonous bite and organ liquefaction.

Black widow venom has a systemic neurotoxin, the primary effect of which is chest pain and abdominal pain. The abdominal pain may mimic an abdominal crisis, with marked cramping and a rigid abdomen. The neurologic signs of hyperreflexia, paresthesia, and cutaneous hyperesthesia help distinguish this from a true intra-abdominal catastrophe. Profuse sweating, hypertension, and tachycardia are also common.[57] The primary treatment is supportive care and narcotics and muscle relaxants (methocarbamol or benzodiazepine) for pain control, although antivenin therapy also provides effective pain relief in patients with severe envenomations.[58] Antivenin is a horse serum–derived immunoglobulin therapy, usually suggested for use in young patients (<6 years of age), very infirm patients, and patients with a severe reaction. The usual dose is 1 ampule in 50 mL of normal saline. Calcium gluconate, 10 mL of a 10% solution given intravenously over 15 to 20 minutes, has usually been considered the first-line treatment of severe envenomations, although one report disputes its efficacy at pain relief.[58] Most black widow spider bite symptoms resolve within 1 day, but recurrent symptoms may persist for 2 to 3 days. Antivenin has been reported to be effective up to 30 hours after a bite.[59] The reported mortality rate is 2% to 6%, usually as a result of severe acute or delayed hypersensitivity reactions with paralysis, hemolysis, renal failure, and coma.

Venomous Hymenoptera Species and Bites

The more than 100,000 species of Hymenoptera consist of the well-known families of bees, wasps, and hornets but also include the fire ants, a nonwinged Hymenoptera present in the southeastern United States.[61] More envenomations and deaths (approximately 40 annually) in the United States are caused by Hymenoptera stings than by snakebites, emphasizing the fact that the venom of most Hymenoptera is as toxic as the rattlesnake's venom, the difference being the volume administered. The venom is primarily a hemolysin and neurotoxin, known for triggering anaphylactic reactions. Bee venom also contains melittin, phospholipase A_2, and hyaluronidase, which when given in adequate volume can cause endothelial disruption, cell breakdown, and tissue necrosis. It is estimated that approximately 0.4% of the human population is at risk for anaphylaxis from Hymenoptera stings.[62] Fortunately, most sting reactions are mild, involving dermal manifestations (e.g., hives, edema) only. The clinical effects are related both to the local toxic effects and to the anaphylactic systemic effects. The local toxic effects include significant pain, swelling, and pruritus. If a significant amount of toxin is injected, the patient may experience nausea, emesis, and muscle spasms.

Most deaths from Hymenoptera stings are a result of severe anaphylactic reaction, which can occur at any age, but is relatively more common in adults. In this reaction, a preformed immunoglobulin E antibody activates mast cells, leading to degranulation with massive histamine release and prompting laryngeal and pulmonary edema, vasodilation, and vascular collapse. The treatment for Hymenoptera bites and stings is to remove the stinger, treat the local wound with ice and possibly an enzymatic meat tenderizer, and treat the anaphylactic reactions aggressively with antihistamines (diphenhydramine, 50 to 100 mg intramuscularly or intravenously) or epinephrine (1:1,000 dilution, 0.3 to 0.5 mL intramuscularly or subcutaneously). Patients also require supplemental oxygen and intravenous fluids.

After sting anaphylaxis, approximately 50% of patients remain allergic to subsequent stings, in part determined by the severity of the initial anaphylactic symptoms. Children with benign dermal reactions only are unlikely to have recurrent reactions. Patients with more severe reactions are at risk for repeat anaphylaxis. Patients with a history of insect sting anaphylaxis and positive venom skin tests should have epinephrine available and are candidates for subsequent venom immunotherapy, which provides almost 100% protection against subsequent sting reactions. Such desensitization, however, can take more than 3 years.[62]

Africanized bees (*Apis mellifera scutellata*) are a more aggressive subspecies than the native European bees of North and South America. Initially imported from Africa to Brazil in 1956 in the hope that they would hybridize with the better honey-producing European bee, some escaped and began interbreeding with domestic bees, proliferated, and migrated through Central America and the Yucatan peninsula of Mexico, first detected near Hidalgo, Texas, in 1993 and reportedly advancing at a rate of 100 miles per year.[63,64] Currently located primarily in the arid southwestern United States, these bees now pose a significant threat because massive envenomations (more than 50 bites) have occurred, resulting in nausea, vomiting, shock, hemolysis, rhabdomyolysis, and DIC; coma and renal failure may follow. Rarely, in patients initially complaining only of pain after multiple bee stings, a delayed (6 to 48 hours) toxic reaction has been reported. Some poison centers now recommend a 24-hour hospitalization for pediatric patients, older patients, and patients with underlying medical problems after an envenomation of 50 or more stings because such patients have an increased risk of delayed severe systemic reaction.[65] Laboratory studies on patients sustaining massive envenomations should be performed on presentation and 6 hours later to rule out hemolysis, thrombocytopenia, liver function abnormalities, and rhabdomyolysis.

Two species of imported fire ants now infest large areas of the Gulf Coast states.[66] The most aggressive species, *Solenopsis invicta,* has adapted well to environmental conditions in the southern United States, where it has become a considerable agricultural pest and a significant public health problem. Sting reactions typically include a dermal wheal-and-flare reaction followed by sterile pustules at sting sites. Occasionally, large local dermal reactions and pyoderma, or even life-threatening anaphylaxis, can occur. Caplan et al.[67] have shown that residents of Augusta, Georgia, an endemic area, had a 17% incidence of fire ant–specific immunoglobulin E compared with a 7.5% incidence of peanut-specific immunoglobulin E, posing a significant risk of potential fatal anaphylaxis.[67] Four venom allergens have been isolated and characterized. Clinical studies under way are designed to compare the safety and efficacy of fire ant venom with whole-body extract for diagnosis and treatment of fire ant allergy.[66] Additionally, biologic control of fire ants by the release of multiple species of decapitating flies has shown promise in keeping the fire ant population under control.[68]

Scorpions and Scorpion Stings

More than 650 types of scorpions can be found worldwide. In the United States, most scorpion stings are not lethal and the sting results primarily in local effects. In parts of Brazil, Mexico, North Africa, India, and Israel, however, the scorpion sting may be lethal. The venom toxicity depends greatly on the species, season, and age of the scorpion. In a fatal response, the venom induces a sympathetic storm, resulting in hypertension, tachycardia, and high-output cardiac failure.[69] Serum biochemistry reveals increased potassium and glucose, decreased sodium, and markedly elevated catecholamine levels. The treatment is specific antivenin therapy and systemic support directed at controlling hypertension and acute pulmonary edema. The outcome in the United States is usually excellent, with complete resolution of local effects; however, in some parts of Brazil, the mortality rates for a scorpion sting have been reported to be as high as 12% in adults and 60% in children.[70] In India, of 34 children admitted to a hospital after scorpion sting, 14 had hypertension, nine had acute pulmonary edema, five had myocardial failure, and four died.[69] In one report from Israel, respiratory distress was the main feature in 17 of 54 children with scorpion stings, but only three required mechanical ventilation; two patients died, but both failed to receive antivenin.[71] However, another report from Israel evaluated the treatment of 104 children with scorpion envenomation, noting that since 1989 they had discontinued using antivenin, with similar, if not better, results in the no-antivenin group.[72] The antivenin in this report, however, is prepared from donkeys treated with the venom of the yellow scorpion (*Leiurus quinquestriatus*), which is not the same as that of the North American bark scorpion (*Centuroides exilicauda*) antivenin.

Clinically significant scorpion envenomation by *Centruroides sculpturatus* produces a dramatic neuromotor syndrome and respiratory insufficiency that often necessitate intensive supportive care, particularly in children. In a randomized, double-blind study, the efficacy of scorpion-specific F(ab')2 antivenom was compared with placebo in 15 children ages 6 months to 18 years of age who were admitted to a pediatric intensive care unit in Tucson, Arizona, with clinically significant signs of scorpion envenomation.[71a] The clinical syndrome resolved more rapidly among recipients of the antivenom than among recipients of placebo, with a resolution of symptoms in all eight antivenom recipients versus one of seven placebo recipients within 4 hours after treatment (p = 0.001). Plasma venom concentrations were undetectable in all eight antivenom recipients but in only one placebo recipient 1 hour after treatment (p = 0.001). As of this writing, this antivenom is commercially available in Mexico, but only available in the United States through an investigational new drug application.

ENVIRONMENTAL INJURIES

Hypothermia

5 Because humans are homeotherms, we attempt to maintain a constant body temperature despite changes in environmental temperature. Normal body temperature depends on the site of measurement and is 37°C sublingually, 38°C in the rectum, 32°C at the skin, and 38.5°C deep in the liver. Even minor deviation from normal leads to important symptoms and disability.[73] Humans have a remarkable capacity to dissipate heat by evaporating body water; however, our tropical evolutionary heritage has provided us with far less ability to cope with cold conditions. As a result, hypothermia can occur in a variety of clinical settings and from a number of causes (Table 31.4).

To allow for the normal circadian temperature variation of 0.5°C to 1°C, hypothermia is considered to be present in humans if the core temperature drops below 35°C (95°F). Hypothermia is usually classified by temperature zones as mild (32°C to 35°C), moderate (28°C to 32°C), or severe (<28°C).[73] Primary accidental hypothermia is defined as a decrease in core temperature that occurs as a result of overwhelming environmental cold stress. It most often occurs as a result of recreational misadventures that lead to cold-water immersion or prolonged environmental exposure. Secondary accidental hypothermia occurs in patients with abnormal heat production or thermoregulation, who become cold despite only mild cold stress. The most significant risk factors are advanced age, mental impairment, and substance abuse, in particular, of alcohol, although hypothyroidism, hypoadrenalism, trauma, and hypoglycemia are other risk factors.[74,75] Chronic hypothermia develops in patients with impaired heat generation (i.e., the elderly and infirm) who live in unheated apartments, are under continual cold stress, and after a time are found always to have a low temperature as if they have autoregulated to a new set temperature. A multicenter review of 428 cases of accidental hypothermia reported an overall mortality rate of 17%,[76] although other reports document mortality rates as high as 80%, primarily a result of infection and underlying illness.

From 1979 to 2002, a total of 16,555 deaths in the United States, an average of 689 per year (range 417 to 1,021), were attributed to exposure to excessive natural cold (Fig. 31.3).[75] In 2002, a total of 646 hypothermia-related deaths were reported, with an annual death rate of 0.2 per 100,000 population. Most reported hypothermia-related deaths (66%)

TABLE 31.4

CLINICAL DEFINITIONS OF HYPOTHERMIA AND EXAMPLES OF SETTINGS IN WHICH THEY OCCUR

■ TYPE	■ SETTINGS
Accidental	Recreational environmental exposure, cold-water immersion
Therapeutic	Treatment of Reye syndrome, cardiopulmonary bypass, organ preservation
Drug induced	Alcohol, anesthetics, barbiturates, phenothiazines, morphine, other drugs
Central nervous system dysfunction	Transection of spinal cord, hypopituitarism, cerebrovascular accidents
Hypothalamic dysfunction	Wernicke encephalopathy, anorexia nervosa, head trauma, pinealoma, other tumors
Metabolic	Hypoglycemia, hypothyroidism, hypoadrenalism, malnutrition
Dermal dysfunction	Burns, erythrodermas
Traumatic	Occurs after any major injury

Adapted from Jurkovich GJ. Hypothermia in the trauma patient. *Adv Trauma* 1989;4:111–140.

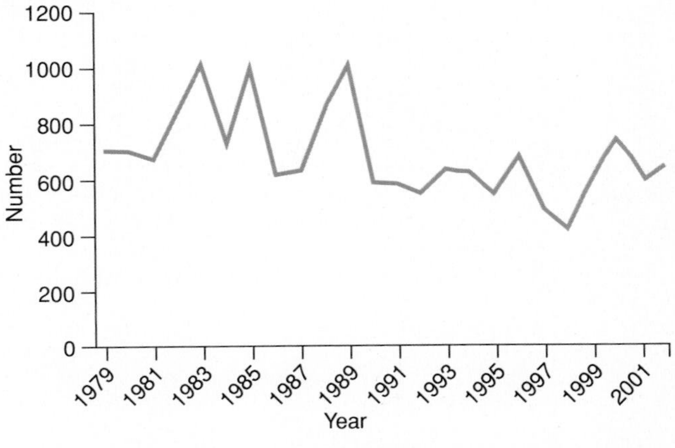

FIGURE 31.3. Number of hypothermia-related deaths by year in the United States, 1979–2002. (After Hypothermia-related deaths—United States, 2003–2004. *MMWR Morb Mortal Wkly Rep* 2005;54:173–175.)

TRAUMA

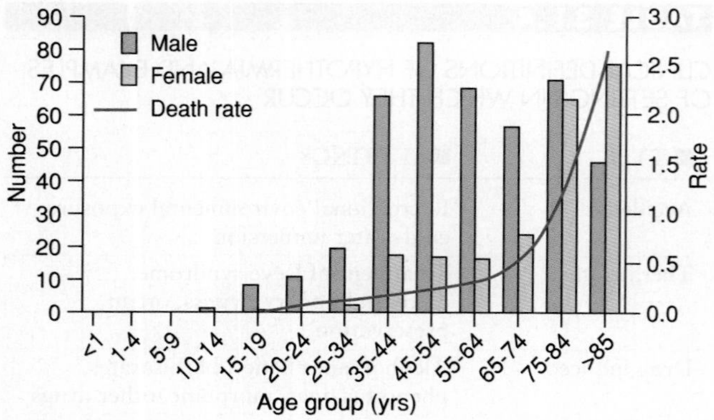

FIGURE 31.4. Number and rate (per 100,000 population) of hypothermia-related deaths, by age group and gender, in the United States, 1979–2002. (After Hypothermia-related deaths United States, 2003–2004. *MMWR Morb Mortal Wkly Rep* 2005;54:173–175.)

occurred in males (Fig. 31.4), but the overall death rate (0.5 per 100,000 population) was the same for both males and females. Hypothermia-related deaths are commonly reported by states with characteristically milder climates that experience rapid temperature changes (e.g., North Carolina [0.4] and South Carolina [0.4]) and by western states that have high elevations and experience considerable changes from daytime to nighttime temperatures (e.g., Arizona [0.3]). States with the greatest overall death rates caused by hypothermia are Alaska, New Mexico, North Dakota, and Montana.

The physiologic response to hypothermia is one of transitional changes, with few exact temperature-dependent responses (Fig. 31.5). Broadly speaking, the transition from a "safe zone" of hypothermia (in which physiologic adaptations to heat loss are working) to a "danger zone" of hypothermia (in which shivering is abolished, metabolism decreases, and heat loss is passively accepted) occurs between 33°C and 30°C. 6 The initial effects of hypothermia mimic intense sympathetic stimulation, with tremulousness, profound vasoconstriction, and tremendous increases in metabolic rate, oxygen consumption, and minute ventilation.[77]

The initial cardiovascular response includes tachycardia, followed by progressive bradycardia, which starts at approximately 34°C and results in a 50% heart rate decrease at 28°C.

FIGURE 31.5. Zones of hypothermia and corresponding physiologic responses. Wide biologic variability accounts for physiologic changes rarely occurring at the exact temperatures noted. (After Jurkovich GJ. Hypothermia in the trauma patient. *Adv Trauma* 1989; 4:111–140.)

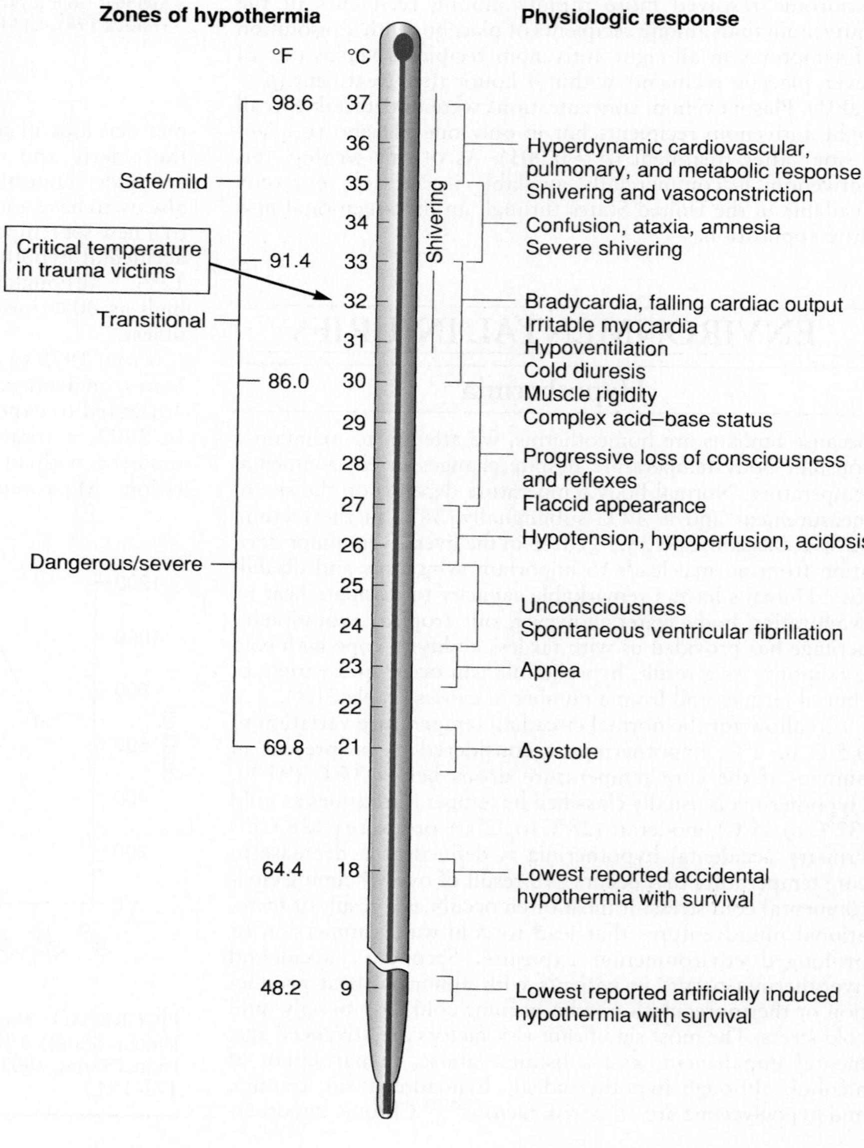

Cardiac output initially increases with the tachycardia, then progressively decreases, with a concomitant fall in blood pressure. The cardiac conduction system is particularly sensitive to hypothermia: the PR interval, then the QRS complex, and finally the QT interval become progressively prolonged.[78] As temperature falls below 30°C, atrial fibrillation, bradycardia, and ventricular dysrhythmia become common, with asystole occurring at temperatures below 25°C.[79] Because palpating pulses or measuring blood pressure in cold, stiff, hypothermic patients is difficult, the presence of an organized cardiac electrical rhythm should be taken as a sign of life that contraindicates cardiopulmonary resuscitation chest compressions, despite the absence of a palpable pulse. Such a rhythm may provide diminished but sufficient circulation in patients with severely reduced metabolism, and it is likely that vigorous chest compressions will convert this perfusing rhythm to fibrillation. Rewarming with close monitoring of rhythm, pulse, and blood pressure is indicated. If cardiac arrest occurs, extracorporeal cardiopulmonary bypass for perfusion and rewarming is indicated.[80–82] One report noted excellent long-term functional outcomes in 15 of 32 young patients successfully rewarmed in this manner.[81] All patients were intubated and ventilated and had received ongoing cardiac massage during transportation, and all 15 survivors had documented circulatory arrest (ventricular fibrillation or asystole) and fixed, dilated pupils. The mean interval from discovery of the patient to rewarming with cardiopulmonary bypass was 141 ± 50 minutes; the mean temperature was 21.8°C ± 2.5°C. A report from Finland documents a 61% (14 of 23) survival to hospital discharge for adults undergoing cardiopulmonary bypass after a mean of 70 minutes of cardiopulmonary resuscitation following hypothermic arrest primarily from cold-water immersion or exposure.[82]

Respiratory drive is increased during the early stages of hypothermia, but below 33°C progressive respiratory depression occurs, resulting in a decrease in minute ventilation. This decrease is not usually a significant problem until temperatures below 29°C are reached. Occasionally, hypothermia results in the production of a large amount of mucus (cold bronchorrhea).[83] This development predisposes to atelectasis and aspiration because ciliary action and the cough reflex are also depressed. Noncardiogenic pulmonary edema is also occasionally reported, especially in elderly patients and especially after prolonged periods of hypothermia.[84]

The effect of core hypothermia on arterial blood gas interpretation warrants a comment. Arterial blood gas samples are typically warmed to 37°C before measurement. A nomogram of Severinghaus mathematical corrections is then used to estimate the blood gas values at the patient's actual body temperature. With each 1°C temperature reduction, the partial pressure of carbon dioxide (PCO_2) decreases by 4.4% and the partial pressure of oxygen (PO_2) decreases by 7.2%. Thus, a blood gas measured at 37°C with a PCO_2 of 40 mm Hg and a PO_2 of 70 mm Hg in a 32°C patient is reported as having a PCO_2 of 32 mm Hg and a PO_2 of 48 mm Hg after temperature correction.

The decrease in partial pressure is related to the increased solubility of gases in cold fluids and is not a result of a change in carbon dioxide content, oxygen content, or serum bicarbonate level. Clinicians often assume that the normal PCP_2 and PO_2 at 37°C are the values that should be attained at all temperatures. However, if normothermic endpoints for PCO_2 are attained in a hypothermic patient, they would have increased total body CO_2 stores, which would manifest by a rising PCO_2 and a falling pH during rewarming. Likewise, attempts at increasing a PO_2 that reflects normal oxygen content at a lower
7 temperature are also inappropriate. A far simpler strategy is to assess the blood gases at 37°C without temperature correction. Values that are normal and acceptable when reported at 37°C correspond to normal values and contents when "corrected" for hypothermic temperatures.

Temperature correction of blood gases for pH management is also unnecessary. A pH of 7.40 at 37°C would be temperature corrected to 7.47 in a 32°C patient. At 37°C, the acid–base balance of water is neutral (pH is equal to pOH) when the pH is 6.8, and the body functions optimally when its pH is offset 0.6 pH units above the neutral point of water and has a relatively alkaline pH of 7.40. The pH of water rises with cooling, causing the pH of blood to rise by 0.015 pH units/°C, without a change in bicarbonate content.[85–87] Treating a patient with a temperature of 30°C with a pH of 7.40 instead of 7.47 fails to maintain the normal pH offset above the neutral point of water (relative alkalinity) and results in an acidotic cellular and chemical environment that has a multiplicity of effects on enzyme systems. Because blood with a pH of 7.40 assessed at 37°C is reported as having a pH of 7.47 when temperature is corrected to 32°C, the simplest strategy when confronted with a patient with a temperature of 32°C is to assess the blood gas at 37°C only and to use the 37°C uncorrected pH value for management.[87,88]

The neurologic response to hypothermia is heralded by progressive loss of lucidity and deep tendon reflexes and, eventually, by flaccid muscular tone. Patients are often amnestic below 32°C, and between 31°C and 27°C they usually lose consciousness. Pupillary dilatation and loss of cerebral autoregulation occur at temperatures below 26°C, and electroencephalography becomes silent at 19°C to 20°C.[89] These findings, combined with an unobtainable pulse and apparent rigor mortis, may cause the patient to appear dead. It is important to remember that patients have been revived from core temperatures as low as 14°C,[90] hence the saying "No one is dead until they are warm and dead." An exception to this admonition probably includes the patient who has sustained an anoxic event while still normothermic and has a serum potassium level greater than 10 mmol/L.[82,91] The reduction in blood pressure and cardiac output decreases glomerular filtration rate, but urinary output is maintained because of an impairment in renal tubular Na^+ reabsorption (cold diuresis).[92,93] Vasoconstriction also results in an initial increase in central blood volume that prompts a diuresis. Ileus, bowel wall edema, depressed hepatic drug detoxification, punctate gastric erosions (Wischnewsky ulcers), hyperamylasemia, and, rarely, hemorrhagic pancreatitis are hallmarks of the intestinal response to hypothermia. Hypothermia inhibits insulin release and insulin uptake at receptor sites, making hyperglycemia a relatively common finding, especially at temperatures below 30°C.[94] Exogenous insulin administration is unwarranted because it may result in rebound hypoglycemia during rewarming. Serum electrolyte changes are unpredictable, but serum potassium is often slightly increased in hypothermic patients because of renal tubular dysfunction, acidosis, sodium wasting, and the breakdown of liver glycogen.[95] Hypothermia also appears to affect endothelial cell adhesion molecule function and neutrophil recruitment and bactericidal activity, which may partially explain increased infectious complications in hypothermic patients.[96] Only a 1.9°C core hypothermia triples the incidence of surgical wound infection following colon resection and increases the duration of hospitalization by 20%.[97]

Body temperature has a significant effect on oxygen uptake. Oxygen consumption (VO_2) increases dramatically with any fall in body temperature. When involuntary muscle contractions in the form of shivering occur, oxygen consumption increases by as much as threefold to fivefold.[98,99] However, this process is inefficient because shivering produces heat near the surface of the body, causing most of the heat to be lost to the environment, with less than 45% being retained by the patient. In addition, shivering cannot be maintained due to the enormous energy requirements.

The thermoregulatory drive is such a powerful one that it takes precedence over many other homeostatic functions. The resultant increase in oxygen utilization may result in anaerobic metabolism, acidosis, and significant cardiopulmonary stress. One study noted a 35% increase in oxygen consumption and a 65% increase in CO_2 production in postoperative patients after resolution of anesthesia, when the thermostatic drive reappeared.[100] In another study, a core temperature decrease of as little as 0.3°C in postoperative patients was associated with a 7% increase in VO_2, and temperature reductions between 0.3°C and 1.2°C were associated with a 92% increase in VO_2, with proportional increases in minute ventilation.[101] Further details of the specific organ system responses to hypothermia are beyond the scope of this chapter, but the interested reader is referred to several excellent in-depth monographs.[73,101–103]

Hypothermia in Trauma Patients. Mild hypothermia is very common after traumatic injury. When ambient temperature falls below the thermoneutral temperature (i.e., the temperature at which no thermogenesis or heat dissipation is necessary), which is 28°C (82.5°F) for humans, an increase in heat production is required to maintain a normal body temperature. Combustion is the only source of endogenous heat production, and this process requires an increase in energy and oxygen utilization. After shock or injury, however, oxygen supplies are often limited and further heat loss occurs owing to cold emergency department and operating room environments, cold fluid resuscitation, and open thoracic and abdominal cavities. This is further aggravated by anesthetic and neuromuscular blocking agents that prevent the heat-producing shivering response. Thus, the occurrence of hypothermia in surgical or critically injured patients is most often a form of secondary unintentional hypothermia.

One study found that 57% of trauma patients admitted to a level 1 trauma center were hypothermic at some time and that temperature loss was most significant in the emergency department.[104] Another study reported that the average initial temperature for 94 intubated major trauma victims was 35°C, with no seasonal variation.[105] Of patients in this study, 66% were hypothermic on admission: 43% were mildly hypothermic (34°C to 36°C) and 23% had temperatures below 34°C. Likewise, Jurkovich et al.[106] reported that 42% of 71 adult trauma victims with an Injury Severity Score (ISS) of 25 or higher had core temperatures below 34°C and in 13% the core temperature fell below 32°C. Importantly, there were no survivors when core body temperature was below 32°C. Both mortality rate and the incidence of hypothermia increase with higher ISS, massive fluid resuscitation, and the presence of shock, but even controlling for these variables still demonstrates that the mortality rate of the hypothermic trauma patient is greater than that of the warm trauma patient.[106,107]
8 Although the mortality rate for moderate (28°C to 32°C) degrees of primary incidental hypothermia is approximately 20%,[76] moderate levels of hypothermia in trauma and critically ill patients are associated with a much higher mortality rate. Rutherford et al.[108] reported that 9.4% of surgical intensive care unit patients had a core body temperature less than 35°C; the mortality rate of the hypothermic trauma patients was 53%. In fact, compared with other patient populations, the mortality rate associated with hypothermia in the trauma victim is so high that the definition of mild, moderate, and severe hypothermia in the trauma patient warrants special reclassification (Table 31.5).[73]

TABLE 31.5 **CLASSIFICATION**

ZONES OF SEVERITY FOR HYPOTHERMIA

■ ZONE	■ TEMPERATURE
Mild hypothermia	36°C–34°C (<96.8°F–93.2°F)
Moderate hypothermia	34°C–32°C (<93.2°F–89.6°F)
Severe hypothermia	<32°C (<89.6°F)

Hypothermia appears to occur primarily in victims of relatively severe trauma. Little and Stoner,[109] reporting on a heterogeneous group of 82 trauma patients, observed that hypothermia occurred only in those patients with an ISS greater than 12. Skin temperature fell from 32.0°C to 31.7°C, whereas core temperature fell from 37.3°C to 36.5°C. Hypothermia did not occur in less severely injured patients, and shivering, which should be expected, was noted in only one of the hypothermic patients. Mild degrees of injury have, in fact, been associated with small elevations in core body temperature, particularly when the shivering response mechanism has not been abated.[73,110]

The detrimental effect of hypothermia in the human trauma victim is contrasted by a large body of experimental evidence in animals, suggesting that hypothermia has a protective role in shock. This extensive body of literature is reviewed elsewhere,[73] but in general, animals subjected to combined hypothermia and shock (hemorrhage, burn, blunt trauma) usually survive longer than similarly injured but actively warmed animals. Blalock and Mason[111] were among the first in modern times to recognize the ability of hypothermia to prolong survival times after shock, but they emphasized that the overall survival rate was unchanged, an observation reaffirmed in 2003.[112] However, other investigators have shown increases in both survival times and survival rates in a number of animal models of induced hypothermia after hemorrhagic shock.[113,114] The protective effects of hypothermia in preventing ischemia–reperfusion injury have been described in a number of models, including muscle, intestine, and rabbit ear.[115–118]

Hypothermia has also been suggested to protect the traumatically injured brain. The use of therapeutic hypothermia in a patient with traumatic brain injury was first reported in 1943[119] and sporadically over the ensuing two decades.[120] More recently, a randomized, multicenter, controlled trial of core body hypothermia in trauma patients with severe closed head injury (Glasgow Coma Scale scores of 3 to 7) was conducted.[121] Select trauma patients with severe head injury were intentionally cooled within 6 hours of injury to 32°C to 33°C for 48 hours after injury and then rewarmed. The outcome was poor (defined as severe disability, a vegetative state, or death) in 57% of the patients in both groups. Mortality was 28% in the hypothermia group and 27% in the normothermia group ($p = 0.79$). The patients in the hypothermia group had more hospital days with complications than the patients in the normothermia group. The authors concluded that treatment with hypothermia is not effective in improving outcomes in patients with severe brain injury. Other authors have also reported higher rates of pneumonia and diabetes insipidus in a small study of induced hypothermia in severely head-injured patients (Glasgow Coma Scale scores of 3 to 7) with no effect on neurologic outcome.[122] Evidence further supporting the harmful effect of hypothermia in the trauma patient is provided by a prospective randomized trial of rapid rewarming versus conventional rewarming of 57 multiple-trauma patients.[123] In this study, trauma patients who were rapidly rewarmed with continuous arteriovenous rewarming from less than 34.5°C to greater than 36°C required less resuscitation fluid volume and had a lower early mortality rate than those rewarmed more slowly. Failure to rewarm in either group was uniformly fatal. The survival rate at 3 days after injury was 82% in the rapid rewarm group versus 62% in conventionally managed patients. Approximately 50% of the patients in both groups had a severe head injury, defined as a head Abbreviated Injury Severity score of 3 or greater. In this well-controlled study, maintenance of hypothermia not only failed to confer an advantage but also was detrimental to early survival.

The role of hypothermia in the injured patient remains unresolved. It is apparent that the physiologic consequence of severe trauma is a drop in core body temperature. It remains unclear, however, whether this response is a protective response to shock or the result of diminished heat production caused by failing metabolism. The frequent presence of lactic acid accumulation in cold, seriously injured patients supports the latter hypothesis. Clinical studies indicate that even mild hypothermia in the trauma patient is predictive of a poor outcome. Hypothermia does diminish metabolic demands and oxygen consumption in anesthetized patients, but the price appears to be malfunction of enzymes and physiologic systems necessary to recover from injury.

The systems most affected by hypothermia in victims of injury are those involved in clotting. Reports of coagulation abnormalities in patients with apparently normal clotting factor levels surfaced shortly after the introduction of hypothermic cardioplegia for cardiac surgery.[124,125] Although hemodilution with volume expanders deficient in clotting factors and platelets is the usual cause of nonsurgical bleeding, cold platelets are known to undergo morphologic changes that affect adherence, including loss of shape, cytoplasmic swelling, and dissolution of cytoplasmic microtubules necessary for normal motility.[126] Platelet activation is also associated with activation of cell membrane phospholipases that hydrolyze phospholipids to arachidonic acid, a precursor to prostaglandin endoperoxides and thromboxane A_2, a potent vasoconstrictor necessary for normal platelet aggregation[127] Valeri et al.[128] induced systemic hypothermia to 32°C in baboons, but kept one forearm warm using heating lamps and a warming blanket. Simultaneous bleeding time measurements in the warm and cold arm were 2.4 and 5.8 minutes, respectively. This effect, which was reversible with rewarming, appeared to be mediated by cold-induced slowing of the enzymatic reaction rates. A recent report suggests that bleeding observed at mildly reduced temperatures (33°C to 37°C) results primarily from a platelet adhesion defect and not reduced enzyme activity or platelet activation; however, at temperatures below 33°C, both reduced platelet function and enzyme activity likely contribute to the coagulopathy,[129] perhaps helping to explain why 32°C is such a critical temperature for survival in the coagulopathic injured patient.

As with blood gases, clinical tests of coagulation are temperature standardized to 37°C. Fibrometers contain a thermal block that heats the plasma and reagents to 37°C before initiating the assay. Thus, tests of coagulation reflect clotting factor deficiencies but are corrected for any potential effect of hypothermia on clotting factor function. A detailed study of the kinetic effects of hypothermia on clotting factor function has been undertaken by Reed et al.,[130] who performed clotting tests (PT, PTT, and thrombin time) on reference human plasma-containing normal clotting factor levels at temperatures ranging from 25°C to 37°C. The results showed a significant slowing of all coagulation tests at temperatures below 35°C that was proportional to the degree of hypothermia. The prolongation of clot formation occurred at clinically relevant levels of hypothermia and was equivalent to that seen in normothermic patients with significant clotting factor depletion. For example, assays conducted at 35°C, 33°C, and 31°C prolonged the PTT to the same extent as would occur in a euthermic patient with reductions in factor IX levels to 66%, 32%, and 7% of normal, respectively.

Clotting factor supplementation is not the answer to a hypothermia-induced coagulopathy; rewarming is. However, in many seriously injured patients, clotting factor depletion exists in conjunction with hypothermia. A potentiating effect of hypothermia on coagulation dysfunction occurs in plasma of patients with deficient clotting factor levels, although there does not appear to be synergy between the two conditions.[131] Hypothermic, coagulopathic trauma patients still benefit from coagulation profile testing. If prolongation of PT and PTT is evident in plasma warmed to 37°C, clotting factor replacement is indicated. If PT and PTT are near normal, rewarming alone reverses the clinically relevant coagulopathy.

9 **Treatment.** Rewarming techniques are usually classified as passive external rewarming, active external rewarming, or active core rewarming.[132] Passive external rewarming simply implies allowing spontaneous rewarming to occur with the patient removed from a hypothermic environment and is usually used only for the mildly hypothermic patient. Active external rewarming techniques include surrounding the patient with warm blankets or heating pads, infrared heating lights, or immersion in warm water. Active core rewarming includes heated intravenous fluids, as well as heated peritoneal or thoracic lavage; heated gastric, bladder, or colonic lavage; heated and water-saturated inhaled air; and extracorporeal circulatory rewarming. Blood rewarming is currently limited to a maximum temperature of 42°C by the American Association of Blood Banks, but rewarming to 49°C with inline microwave blood rewarmers has been reported as safe, as has intravenous fluid rewarming to 65°C.[133,134]

The advantages and disadvantages of each technique are regularly debated, particularly regarding the role of external versus core rewarming. It is clear, however, that the rate of heat transfer to the hypothermic patient is greatest using active core rewarming, particularly extracorporeal circulation rewarming. This may be a critical factor in surgical patients for whom rapid restoration of clotting and cardiac function is necessary.

The technique of rewarming the hypothermic victim by extracorporeal circulation has been described by numerous authors, based primarily on small personal experiences.[81,82] This technique has appeal in cases of primary accidental hypothermia, in which maintenance of circulation, correction of hypoxia, and replenishment of intravascular volume may play a role as large as correcting the temperature change itself. The need for systemic anticoagulation has, however, generally limited the usefulness of full cardiopulmonary bypass rewarming in the trauma patient.

A simplified technique of extracorporeal active core rewarming is continuous arteriovenous rewarming (CAVR).[135] This technique makes use of the patient's own blood pressure to drive an extracorporeal circuit through an efficient but small countercurrent heat-exchange device (Sims Level 1, Rockland, Massachusetts). Systemic anticoagulation is not necessary if the tubing is heparin bonded and trauma patients are relatively anticoagulated. The relative ease of use made this device widely applicable in rewarming severely hypothermic patients with an intact circulation and, in a prospective randomized trial of rewarming trauma patients, demonstrated its efficacy by improved surival.[123] Unfortunately, as of 2007, the single manufacturing company for the tubing needed for CAVR halted production.

Direct intracirculation rewarming can be accomplished with commercially available devices that employ an intra–vena caval countercurrent heat exchange device (InnerCool Therapies, San Diego, California; Alsius Corporation, Irvine, California). While initially developed to cool patients for neurosurgical procedures and for induced resuscitative hypothermia following cardiac arrest, rewarming can be accomplished by simply changing the temperature of the closed-loop circulating fluid. Requirements are the commercial bedside console and specialized endovascular temperature control catheter, inserted via the femoral vein to the vena cava via an 11- to 12-French introducer. Preliminary data on rewarming cold patients suggest that rewarming can occur rapidly, up to 3°C per hour.[123a]

The use of body cavity lavage with warm solutions is a simple, less invasive method of accomplishing active core rewarming; however, rewarming rates with body cavity lavage vary greatly based on initial core temperature, dialysate temperature, infusion rate, and dwell time. Several studies support the notion that active core rewarming by peritoneal lavage is preferable to active external rewarming.[136] Moss[74] examined three techniques of rewarming hypothermic and cardiac-arrested dogs, concluding that both peritoneal lavage (55°C dialysate) and partial extracorporeal circulation were faster than active external rewarming with a heating blanket.[74] A frequently stated disadvantage of external rewarming is that the peripheral tissues are rewarmed in advance of the still cool "core," resulting in peripheral vasodilation. In the presence of inadequate volume resuscitation, this rewarming method may result in vascular collapse ("rewarming shock") and a subsequent fall in central temperature ("afterdrop") as the cold peripheral blood returns to the core. Volume contraction caused by vasoconstriction, cold diuresis, and cellular swelling coupled with inadequate fluid resuscitation may be a more appropriate explanation for circulatory collapse during rewarming.

The thermodynamic principles of heat transfer to the hypothermic patient are reviewed in greater detail elsewhere, but a sense of rewarming rates and quantity of heat transferred by various techniques is instructional.[132,137] Ventilating a patient with a core temperature of 32°C with water-saturated air at 41°C results in a maximum heat transfer rate of 9 kcal/h. For comparison, basal metabolic heat generation produces approximately 70 kcal/h, and shivering produces up to 250 kcal/h. Given the specific heat of the body (0.083 kcal/kg per °C), 58 kcal is required to raise the temperature of a 70-kg patient by 1°C. Thus, more than 6 hours would be required to warm a 32°C patient using 41°C humidified inspired air.

Heat transfer rates using body cavity lavage can be similarly calculated based on the specific heat of water (1 kcal/kg per °C). If 1 L of 44°C water infused into a body cavity dwells long enough to exit at 40°C, 4 kcal of heat will have been transferred to the patient. Thus, over 14 L of fluid is needed to increase core temperature by 1°C. However, warming becomes less efficient as the patient rewarms because a longer dwell time is required to reduce the temperature of the infusate to 40°C.

Warming by cardiopulmonary bypass or continuous arteriovenous rewarming is the most efficient method of core heating. With flow rates of 15 to 30 L/h, it is possible to deliver 120 to 240 kcal/h if the reinfused blood is heated to 40°C, a rate of heat transfer over 10 times that of the other methods. In each case, the urgency with which rewarming must be accomplished depends on how adversely the hypothermia is affecting the patient. With the exception of extracorporeal circulatory methods, most rewarming techniques serve primarily to prevent further loss of endogenously generated heat and are ineffective in circumstances during which rapid rewarming is indicated. Early and direct attention to the mechanisms of heat loss is necessary to optimize prevention of heat loss and the metabolic and hemorrhagic complications associated with hypothermia in surgical patients.

Cold Injury and Frostbite

Cold injuries limited to digits, extremities, or exposed surfaces are the result of either direct tissue freezing (frostbite) or more chronic exposure to an environment just above freezing (chilblain [pernio], trench foot). Cold injury has been a major cause of morbidity during war experiences. It resulted in more than 7 million lost soldier fighting days by Allied forces in World War II and was reportedly the most common major injury sustained by British soldiers in the Falklands expedition.[138]

The terms *chilblain* and *pernio* describe a form of local cold injury characterized by pruritic, red-purple papules, macules, plaques, or nodules on the skin. The lesions are often associated with edema or blistering and are caused by a chronic vasculitis of the dermis[139]; this entity does not appear to be related to hereditary protein C or S deficiency.[140] This pathologic process is provoked by repeated exposure to cold, but not freezing, temperatures. This injury typically occurs on the face, the anterior surface of the tibia, or the dorsum of the hands and feet, areas poorly protected or chronically exposed to the environment. With continued exposure, ulcerative or hemorrhagic lesions may appear and progress to scarring, fibrosis, and atrophy. Treatment consists of sheltering the patient, elevating the affected part on sheepskin, and allowing gradual rewarming at room temperature. Rubbing and massage are contraindicated because they can cause further damage and secondary infection.

Trench foot or cold immersion foot (or hand) describes a nonfreezing injury of the hands or feet, typically in sailors, fishermen, or soldiers, that is caused by chronic exposure to wet conditions and temperatures just above freezing.[141] It appears to involve an alternating arterial vasospasm and vasodilatation, with the affected tissue first cold and anesthetic and then hyperemic after 24 to 48 hours of exposure. With the hyperemia comes an intense, painful burning and dysesthesia, and tissue damage is characterized by edema, blistering, redness, ecchymosis, and ulceration. Complications of local infection or cellulitis, lymphangitis, and gangrene may occur. A posthyperemic phase occurs 2 to 6 weeks later and is characterized by tissue cyanosis with increased sensitivity to cold. Treatment is best started during or before the reactive hyperemia state and consists of immediate removal of the extremity from the cold, wet environment with exposure of the feet (or hands) to warm, dry air. Elevation to minimize edema, protection of pressure spots, and local and systemic measures to combat infection are indicated. Massage, soaking of the feet, or rapid rewarming is not indicated. Demyelination of nerves, muscle atrophy, fallen arches, and osteoporosis may all present long-term complications, and a tendency toward marked vasospasm during subsequent exposure to cold develops in some patients.[142]

Frostnip is the mildest form of cold injury. It is characterized by initial pain and pallor, with subsequent numbness of the affected body part. Skiers and other winter outdoor enthusiasts are most likely to experience this cold injury to the nose, ears, or tips of digits. The injury is reversible and warming of the cold tissue results in return of sensation and function with no tissue loss.

Frostbite is a more severe and common form of cold injury. Frostbite damage is caused by direct ice crystal formation at the cellular level with cellular dehydration and microvascular occlusion. Frostbite is traditionally classified into four grades of injury severity (Table 31.6).

The affected body part nearly always initially appears hard, cold, white, and anesthetic, regardless of the depth of injury. Because the appearance of the lesion changes frequently during the course of treatment and because the initial treatment regimen is applicable for all degrees of insult,[143] some authorities suggest discarding this classification as a prognostic impossibility and simply classifying frostbite as either superficial or deep.[144]

Weather conditions, altitude, degree of protective clothing, duration of exposure, and degree of tissue wetness are all contributing external factors to the development of frostbite injury. Because sensory nerve activity is abolished at 7°C to 9°C, the

TABLE 31.6 **CLASSIFICATION**

CLASSIFICATION OF FROSTBITE

DEGREE	DESCRIPTION OF FROSTBITE
First	Tissue freezing with hyperemia and edema but without blistering
Second	Tissue freezing with hyperemia, edema, and characteristic large, clear blisters
Third	Tissue freezing with death of subcutaneous tissues and skin, resulting in hemorrhagic vesicles that are in general smaller than second-degree blisters
Fourth	Tissue necrosis, gangrene, and eventual full-thickness tissue loss

disappearance of pain is an early warning sign of cold injury. Acclimation to cold may be protective, whereas a previous history of frostbite probably predisposes to another cold tissue injury. Smoking and a history of arterial disease also are contributing factors. In urban environments, more than 50% of frostbite injuries are alcohol related and a significant portion of these patients (16%) have an underlying psychiatric illness.[145]

10 Evidence suggests that frostbite injury has two components—the initial freeze injury and a reperfusion injury that occurs during rewarming. The initial response to tissue cooling is vasoconstriction and arteriovenous shunting, intermittently relieved (every 5 to 7 minutes) by vasodilation, the so-called hunting response.[146] With prolonged exposure, this response fails, and the temperature of the freezing tissue approximates ambient temperature until –2°C. At this point, extracellular ice crystals form, and as these crystals enlarge the osmotic pressure of the interstitium increases, resulting in movement of intracellular water into the interstitium. Cells begin to shrink and become hyperosmolar, disrupting cellular enzyme function. If freezing is rapid (>10°C/min), intracellular ice crystal formation occurs, resulting in immediate cell death.[138] Intravascularly, endothelial cell disruption and red cell sludging result in cessation of circulation.

During rewarming, red cell, platelet, and leukocyte aggregation is known to occur and results in patchy thrombosis of the microcirculation. These accumulated blood elements are thought to release, among other products, the toxic oxygen free radicals and the arachidonic acid metabolites PGF_{2a} and thromboxane A_2, which further aggravate vasoconstriction and platelet and leukocyte aggregation.[147,148] However, the exact mechanism of tissue destruction and death after freeze injury remains poorly defined. Animal studies suggest that vascular injury in the form of endothelial cell damage and subsequent interstitial edema, but not vessel thrombosis, predominate as initial events in rewarming injury.[149,150] A substantial component of severe cold injury may be neutrophil mediated, as suggested by the observation that a monoclonal antibody to neutrophil–endothelial and neutrophil–neutrophil adherence can markedly ameliorate the pathologic process of a severe cold injury.[151] In this rabbit model, animals treated with anti-CD11/CD18 adhesion molecule after cold injury (30 minutes at –15°C) but before rewarming (39°C water bath) had significantly less tissue loss and edema. The implication of these observations is that much of the injury of severe frostbite occurs during rewarming or reperfusion, although recent evidence of the efficacy of intra-arterial thrombolytic therapy suggests that endovascular clotting does occur and can be reversed.[151a]

Treatment

Prehospital or field care of the victim of cold injury should focus on removing the patient from the hostile environment and protecting the injured body part from further damage. Rubbing or exercising the affected tissue does not augment blood flow and risks further cold injury or mechanical trauma. Because repeated bouts of freezing and thawing worsen the injury, it is preferable for the patient with frostbite of the hands or feet immediately to seek definitive shelter and care rather than rewarm the tissue in the field and risk refreezing. Although the initial symptoms may be mild and overlooked by the patient, severe pain, burning, edema, and even necrosis and gangrene may appear with rewarming. With severe injury the range of motion progressively decreases and edema becomes prominent. The injury may progress to numbness and, eventually, to loss of all sensation in the affected tissue.

The emergency room treatment of a frostbite victim should first focus on the basic ABCs (airway, breathing, and circulation) of trauma resuscitation and then systemic hypothermia should be identified and corrected. Most patients are dehydrated, and resuscitation with warm fluids is an important part of early management. Fractures are often accompanied by frostbite in mountaineers, and although manipulation may be required to treat vascular compromise, open reduction is hazardous, and application of traction should be delayed until after postthawing edema has been assessed.

Rapid rewarming is the goal. Gradual, spontaneous rewarming is inadequate, particularly for deeper injuries, and rubbing the injured part in ice or snow often delays warming and results in marked tissue loss.[152] Rapid rewarming should be achieved by immersing the tissue in a large water bath of 40°C to 42°C (104°C to 108°F). The water should feel warm, but not hot, to the normal hand. The bath should be large enough to prevent rapid loss of heat, and the water temperature should be maintained. Dry heat is not advocated because it is difficult to regulate, and the result of using excessive heat is often disastrous. The rewarming process should take approximately 30 to 45 minutes for digits, with the affected area appearing flushed when rewarming is complete and good circulation has been reestablished. Narcotics are required because the rewarming process can be quite painful.

The skin should be gently but meticulously cleansed and air dried and the affected area elevated to minimize edema. A tetanus toxoid booster should be administered as indicated by immunization history. Sterile cotton is placed between toes or fingers to prevent skin maceration and extreme care taken to prevent infection and avoid even the slightest abrasion. The affected tissue should be protected by a tent or cradle, and pressure spots must be prevented. In one review, infection developed in 13% of urban frostbite victims, but one half of these infections were present at time of admission.[145] Most clinicians reserve antibiotics for identified infections.[153]

After rewarming, the treatment goals are to prevent further injury while awaiting the demarcation of irreversible tissue destruction. All patients should be hospitalized and affected tissue gently cleansed once or twice a day in warm (38°C) whirlpool baths, with some clinicians adding an antiseptic such as chlorhexidine or an iodophor to the bath. Based on the findings of arachidonic acid metabolites in the blisters of frostbite victims, some authors advocate the use of topical aloe vera (thromboxane inhibitor) and systemic ibuprofen or aspirin. Heggers et al.[154] report on a nonrandomized trial in which 56 patients treated with these agents, plus prophylactic penicillin, had less tissue loss, a lower amputation rate, and a shorter hospital stay than 98 patients treated with warm saline, silver sulfadiazine, or Sulfamylon dressings (Bertek Pharmaceuticals, Research Triangle Park, North Carolina).[154] Another report on frostbite treatment in rabbits demonstrated improved tissue viability when systemic pentoxifylline and topical aloe vera cream were used.[155] Uninfected blebs should be left intact because they provide a sterile biologic dressing for 7 to 10 days and protect underlying epithelialization. After resolution of edema, digits should be exercised during the whirlpool bath and physical therapy begun. Tobacco, nicotine, and other vasoconstrictive agents must be withheld. Weight bearing is prohibited until complete resolution of edema.

Numerous adjuvants have been suggested and tried in an effort to restore blood supply to frostbitten areas. The intense vasoconstrictive effect of cold injury has focused attention on increased sympathetic tone. Sympathetic blockade and even surgical sympathectomy continues to be advocated by some authors based on the theory that it releases the vasospasm that precipitates thrombosis in the affected tissue.[156,157] This method of treatment has produced inconsistent results and is difficult to evaluate clinically, with no prospective randomized trials available. Although sympathectomy appears to mollify the pain, hyperhidrosis, and vasospasm of cold injuries, it may increase vascular shunting and adversely affect healing. In one series, a more proximal demarcation of injury in sympathectomized

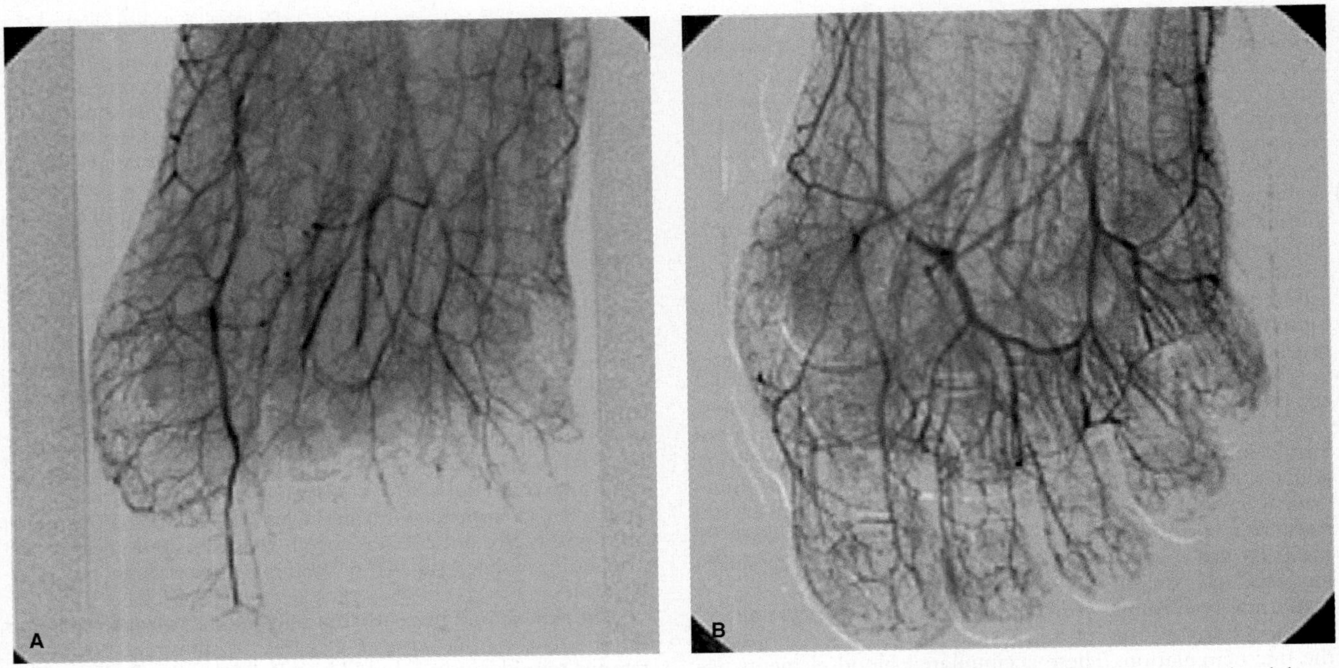

FIGURE 31.6. Digital angiography of a 19-year-old woman who sustained bilateral lower extremity frostbite following vehicle breakdown. **A:** The image demonstrates poor distal perfusion to the left toes. **B:** Following administration of tissue plasminogen activator via bilateral femoral catheters, angiography demonstrates return of perfusion. All 10 of her toes were saved. (Reproduced with permission from Bruen KJ, Ballard JR, Morris SE, et al. Reduction of the incidence of amputation in frostbite injury with thrombolytic therapy. *Arch Surg* 2007;142:546–553.)

limbs was noted than in nonsympathectomized ones, despite apparently equal bilateral injury.[152]

Experience with intra-arterial vasodilating drugs such as reserpine and tolazoline has also been unrewarding. Bouwman et al.[157] demonstrated in a controlled clinical study that immediate (mean 3 hours) ipsilateral intra-arterial reserpine infusion coupled with early (mean 3 days) ipsilateral operative sympathectomy failed to alter the natural history of acute frostbite injury compared with the contralateral limb. Heparin, thrombolytic agents, and hyperbaric oxygen have also failed to demonstrate any substantial treatment benefit, whereas low-molecular-weight dextran alleviated postthawing circulatory obstruction as late as 2 hours after thawing and markedly reduced tissue loss in rabbit feet.[158]

The most recent adjunct to the management of frostbite is the intra-arterial infusion of tissue plasminogen activator (tPA). In a nonrandomized study of a small number ($n = 7$) of patients who received intra-arterial tPA, the burn team at the University of Utah demonstrated that tPA infusion improved tissue perfusion and reduced amputations (10% vs. 41%) when administered within 24 hours of injury (six of the seven), as compared with 25 patients managed in a more traditional fashion.[151a] Candidates for this therapy should have minimal risk of bleeding from other injuries; have the tPA administered (intra-arterially or intravenously) within 24 hours of frostbite, with no episodes of rewarming or refreezing between injury and treatment; and have clear evidence of full-thickness tissue involvement, as well as abnormal perfusion on either angiogram or pyrophosphate scanning (Fig. 31.6; Table 31.7).

The difficulty in determining the depth of tissue destruction in cold injury has led to a conservative approach to the care of frostbite injuries.[153,159,160] As a general rule, amputation and surgical débridement are delayed for 2 to 3 months unless infection with sepsis intervenes, hence the adage: "frostbit in

TABLE 31.7

AMPUTATION OUTCOMES OF PATIENTS TREATED WITH TISSUE PLASMINOGEN ACTIVATOR (tPA) COMPARED WITH ALL OTHER PATIENTS BY FROSTBITE

AGENT	NO. OF PATIENTS	NO. OF INVOLVED EXTREMITIES	EXTREMITIES REQUIRING AMPUTATION, NO. (%)			NO. OF DIGITS AMPUTATED/TOTAL DIGITS INVOLVED (%)
			NONE	PROXIMAL	DIGITS ONLY	
No agent[a]	26	57	25 (45)	14 (25)	18 (29)	97/234 (41)
tPA administration, <24 h	6	13	10 (77)	0	3 (23)	6/59 (10)[b]
Total	32	70	35 (50)	14 (20)	21 (30)	103/293 (35)

[a]Includes one patient who received tPA starting 48 h after exposure.
[b]$p < 0.50$ using Mann-Whitney U test.
Reproduced with permission from Bruen KJ, Ballard JR, Morris SE, et al. Reduction of the incidence of amputation in frostbite injury with thrombolytic therapy. *Arch Surg* 2007;142:546–553.

January, amputate in June." The natural history of a full-thickness frostbite injury is the gradual demarcation of the injured area with dry gangrene or mummification clearly delineating nonviable tissue. Often the permanent tissue loss is much less than originally suspected. In an Alaskan series, only 10.5% of patients required amputation, usually involving only phalanges or portions of phalanges.[141] The need for emergency surgery is unusual, but vigilance should be maintained during the rewarming phase for the development of a compartment syndrome requiring fasciotomy. Open amputations are indicated in patients with persistent infection and sepsis that is refractory to débridement and antibiotics. Mills[161] convincingly demonstrated that of all the factors in the treatment of frostbite that may influence outcome, premature surgical intervention by any means, in any amount, was by far the greatest contributor to poor results.

The use of technetium-99m methylene diphosphonate bone scanning has shown some promise in the early detection of eventual bone and soft tissue viability,[162] as has the use of magnetic resonance imaging.[163] Technetium-99m "triple-phase" scanning (at 1 minute, 2 hours, and 7 hours) performed beginning 48 hours after admission has been used to assess early tissue perfusion and viability, in an attempt to define the extent of fatally damaged tissues and to allow for early débridement and wound closure.[164,165] The utility of this diagnostic modality continues to evolve, however, with one recent study suggesting that the moderate to severe frostbite lesion identified by technetium-99m scans can be "hibernating" (viable) tissue, which can show improvement up to 6 months following injury.[153,166]

Frostbitten tissues seldom recover completely. Some degree of cold insensitivity invariably remains. Hyperhidrosis (in up to 72% of patients), neuropathy, decreased nail and hair growth, and a persistent Raynaud phenomenon in the affected part are frequent sequelae to cold injury.[167] The affected tissue remains at risk for reinjury and should be carefully protected during any cold exposure. As mentioned previously, chilblain (or chronic pernio) is a specific form of a dermopathy secondary to cold-induced skin vasculitis. Treatment with antiadrenergic agents (prazosin hydrochloride, 1 to 2 mg/d) or calcium channel blockers (nifedipine, 30 to 60 mg/d) and careful protection from further exposure are often helpful.[139,167] However, few therapies afford significant relief to the chronic symptoms after tissue freeze injury, although β- and α-adrenergic blocking agents, calcium channel blockers, topical and systemic steroids, and a host of home remedies have been tried with occasional individual success.

References

1. Gold BS, Barish RA, Dart RC. North American snake envenomation: diagnosis, treatment, and management. *Emerg Med Clin North Am* 2004;22(2):423–443.
2. Russell FE. Medical problems of snakebite: epidemiology. In: Russell FE, ed. *Snake Venom Poisoning*. Great Neck, NY: Scholium International; 1983:250–258.
3. Litovitz TL, Klein-Schwartz W, White S, et al. Annual report of the American Association of Poison Control Centers Toxic Exposure Surveillance System. *Am J Emerg Med* 2001;19:337–395.
4. Centers for Disease Control and Prevention. National Institute for Occupational Safety and Health topic: Venomous Snakes. http://www.cdc.gov. Accessed May 28, 2005.

4a. Walter FG, Stolz U, Shirazi F, et al. Epidemiology of severe and fatal rattlesnake bites published in the American Association of Poison Control Center's Annual Reports. *Clin Toxicol* 2009;47(7):663–669.

4b. Seifert SA, Boyer LV, Benson BE, et al. AAPCC database characterization of native U.S. venomous snake exposures, 2001–2005. *Clin Toxicol* 2009;47(4):327–335.

5. Gold BS, Dart RC, Barish RA. Bites of venomous snakes. *N Engl J Med* 2002;347(5):347–356.
6. Curry SC, Horning D, Brady P, et al. The legitimacy of rattlesnake bites in central Arizona. *Ann Emerg Med* 1989;18:658–663.
7. Wingert WA, Chan L. Rattlesnake bites in southern California and rationale for recommended treatment. *West J Med* 1988;148:37–44.
8. Davidson TM. Intravenous rattlesnake envenomation. *West J Med* 1988; 148:45–47.
9. Russell FE. Snake venom poisoning in the United States. *Annu Rev Med* 1980;31:247–259.
10. Hutton RA, Warrell DA. Action of snake venom components on the haemostatic system. *Blood Rev* 1993;7:176–189.

10a. Norris RL, Pfalzgraf RR, Laing G. Death following coral snake bite in the United States – first documented case (with ELISA confirmation of envenomation) in over 40 years. *Toxicon* 2009;53(6):693–697.

11. Arnold R. Treatment of venomous snakebites in the Western Hemisphere. *Mil Med* 1984;149:361–365.
12. Guisto JA. Severe toxicity from crotalid envenomation after early resolution of symptoms. *Ann Emerg Med* 1995;26:387–388.
13. Gomez HF, Davis M, Phillips S, et al. Human envenomation from a wandering garter snake. *Ann Emerg Med* 1994;23:1119–1122.
14. White RR, Weber RA. Discussion of poisonous snakebite in central Texas: possible indicators for antivenin treatment. *Ann Surg* 1991;213: 466–472.
15. Garfin SR, Castilonia RR, Mubarak SJ, et al. The effect of antivenin on intramuscular pressure elevations induced by rattlesnake venom. *Toxicon* 1985;23:677–680.
16. Downey DJ, Omer GE, Moneim MS. New Mexico rattlesnake bites: demographic review and guidelines for treatment. *J Trauma* 1991;31: 1380–1386.
17. Glass TJ Jr. Early débridement in pit viper bites. *JAMA* 1976;235: 2513–2516.
18. Nelson BK. Snake envenomation: incidence, clinical presentation, and management. *Med Toxicol* 1989;4:17–31.
19. Bucher B, Canonge D, Thomas L, et al. Clinical indicators of envenoming and serum levels of venom antigens in patients bitten by Bothrops lanceolatus in Martinique. *Trans R Soc Trop Med Hyg* 1997;91:186–190.
20. Minton SA. Present tests for detection of snake venom: clinical applications. *Ann Emerg Med* 1987;16:932–937.

20a. McCullough N, Gennaro J. Evaluation of venomous snake bite in southern United States. *J Fla Med Assoc* 1963;40:959–967.

21. Kunkel DB. Bites of venomous reptiles. *Emerg Med Clin North Am* 1984;2:563–577.
22. Treatment of snakebite in the United States. *Med Lett* 1982:87–90.
23. Clark RW. Cryotherapy and corticosteroids in the treatment of rattlesnake bite. *Mil Med* 1971;136:42–44.
24. Jurkovich GJ, Luterman A, McCullar K, et al. Complications of Crotalidae antivenin therapy. *J Trauma* 1988;28:1032–1037.
25. Cribari C. *Management of Poisonous Snakebites*. Chicago, IL: American College of Surgeons Committee on Trauma Poster; 2004.
26. McCullough N, Gennaro J Jr. Treatment of venomous snake bites in the United States. *Clin Toxicol* 1970;3:483–500.
27. Wood JT, Hoback WW, Green TW. Treatment of snake venom poisoning with ACTH and cortisone. *Va Med Monthly* 1955;82:130–135.
28. Dart RC, Hurlbut KM, Garcia RA, et al. Validation of a severity score for the assessment of crotalid snakebite. *Ann Emerg Med* 1996;27:321–326.
29. Dart RC, Seifert SA, Boyer LV, et al. A randomized multicenter trial of Crotalinae polyvalent immune Fab (ovine) antivenom for the treatment of crotaline snakebite in the United States. *Arch Intern Med* 2001;161: 2030–2036.
30. Consroe P, Egen NB, Russell FE, et al. Comparison of a new ovine antigen binding fragment (Fab) antivenin for United States Crotalidae with the commercial antivenin for protection against venom-induced lethality in mice. *Am J Trop Med Hyg* 1995;53:507–510.
31. Garfin SR, Castilonia RR, Mubarak SJ, et al. Rattlesnake bites and surgical decompression: results using a laboratory model. *Toxicon* 1984;22: 177–182.
32. Curry SC, Kraner JC, Kunkel DB, et al. Noninvasive vascular studies in management of rattlesnake envenomations to extremities. *Ann Emerg Med* 1985;14:1081–1084.
33. Chippaux JP, Goyffon M. Venoms, antivenoms, and immunotherapy. *Toxicon* 1998;36:823–846.
34. Bornstein AC, Russell FE, Sullivan JB. Negative pressure suction in field treatment of rattlesnake bite. *Vet Hum Toxicol* 1985;25:297–299.
35. Hooker KR, Caravati EM, Hartsell SC. Gila monster envenomation. *Ann Emerg Med* 1994;24:731–735.
36. Cantrell FL. Envenomation by the Mexican beaded lizard: a case report. *J Toxicol Clin Toxicol* 2003;41:241–244.
37. Giannoukakis N. Exenatide. Amylin/Eli Lilly. *Curr Opin Investig Drugs* 2003;4:459–465.
38. Preston CA. Hypotension, myocardial infarction, and coagulopathy following Gila monster bite. *J Emerg Med* 1989;7:37–40.
39. Swanson DL, Vetter RS. Bites of brown recluse spiders and suspected necrotic arachnidism. *N Eng J Med* 2005;352:700–707.

39a. Gruen R. Crocodile attacks in Australia: challenges for injury prevention and trauma care. *World J Surg* 2009;33:1554–1561.

40. Centers for Disease Control and Prevention (CDC). Necrotic arachnidism—Pacific Northwest, 1988–1996. *MMWR Morb Mortal Wkly Rep* 1996;45:433–436.
41. Walker JS, Hogan DE. Bite to the left leg: clinical pearls. *Acad Emerg Med* 1995;2:223–237.
42. Russell F. A confusion of spiders. *Emerg Med* 1986;18:8–13.
43. Edlow JA. Lyme disease and related tick-borne illnesses. *Ann Emerg Med* 1999;33:680–693.

44. Wilson DC, King LE Jr. Spiders and spider bites. *Dermatol Clin* 1990;8:277–286.
45. Wasserman G. Wound care of spider and snake envenomations. *Ann Emerg Med* 1988;17:1331–1335.
46. Futrell JM. Loxoscelism. *Am J Med Sci* 1992;304:261–267.
47. Patel KD, Modur V, Zimmerman GA, et al. The necrotic venom of the brown recluse spider induces dysregulated endothelial cell-dependent neutrophil activation: differential induction of GM-CSF, IL-8, and E-selectin expression. *J Clin Invest* 1994;94:631–642.
48. Ginsberg C, Weinberg A. Hemolytic anemia and multiorgan failure associated with localized cutaneous lesion. *J Pediatr* 1988;112:496–499.
49. Pennell TC, Babu SS, Meredith JW. The management of snake and spider bites in the southeastern United States. *Am Surg* 1987;53:198–204.
50. DeLozier JB, Reaves L, King LE, et al. Brown recluse spider bites of the upper extremity. *South Med J* 1988;81:181–184.
51. Hobbs GD, Anderson AR, Greene TJ, et al. Comparison of hyperbaric oxygen and dapsone therapy for *Loxosceles* envenomation. *Acad Emerg Med* 1996;3:758–761.
52. Bryant SM, Pittman LM. Dapsone use in *Loxosceles reclusa* envenomations: is there an indication? *Am J Emerg Med* 2003;21:89–90.
53. Barrett SM, Romine-Jenkins M, Fisher DE. Dapsone or electric shock therapy of brown recluse spider envenomation? *Ann Emerg Med* 1994;24:21–25.
54. Strain GM, Snider TG, Tedford BL, et al. Hyperbaric oxygen effects on brown recluse spider *(Loxosceles reclusa)* envenomation in rabbits. *Toxicology* 1991;29:989–996.
55. Phillips S, Kohn M, Baker D, et al. Therapy of brown spider envenomation: a controlled trial of hyperbaric oxygen, dapsone, and cyproheptadine. *Ann Emerg Med* 1995;25:363–368.
56. Rees R, Altenbern D, Lynch J, et al. Brown recluse spider bites: a comparison of early surgical excision versus dapsone and delayed surgical excision. *Ann Surg* 1985;202:659–663.
57. Muller GJ. Black and brown widow spider bites in South Africa: a series of 45 cases. *S Afr Med J* 1993;83:399–405.
58. Clark RF, Wethern-Kestner S, Vance MV, et al. Clinical presentation and treatment of black widow spider envenomation: a review of 163 cases. *Ann Emerg Med* 1992;21:782–787.
59. Suntorntham S, Roberts J, Nilsen G. Dramatic clinical response to the delayed administration of black widow spider antivenin [Letter]. *Ann Emerg Med* 1994;24:1198–1199.
60. Saucier JR. Arachnid envenomation. *Emerg Med Clin North Am* 2004;22:405–422.
61. Freeman TM. Imported fire ants: the ants from hell! *Allergy Proc* 1994;15:11–15.
62. Reisman RE. Stinging insect allergy. *Med Clin North Am* 1992;76:883–894.
63. Schumacher M. Significance of Africanized bees for public health: a review. *Arch Intern Med* 1995;155:2038–2043.
64. Kim KT, Oguro J. Update on the status of Africanized honey bees in the western states. *West J Med* 1999;170:220–222.
65. Kolecki P. Delayed toxic reaction following massive bee envenomation. *Ann Emerg Med* 1999;33:114–116.
66. Stafford CT. Fire ant allergy. *Allergy Proc* 1992;13:11–16.
67. Caplan EL, Ford JL, Young PF, et al. Fire ants represent an important risk for anaphylaxis among residents of an endemic region. *J Allergy Clin Immunol* 2003;111:1274–1277.
68. Williams DF, deShazo RD. Biological control of fire ants: an update on new techniques. *Ann Allergy Asthma Immunol* 2004;93:15–22.
69. Bawaskar HS, Bawaskar PH. Cardiovascular manifestations of severe scorpion sting in India (review of 34 children). *Ann Trop Paediatr* 1991;11:381–387.
70. Yarom R. Scorpion venom: a tutorial review of its effects in man and experimental animals. *Clin Toxicol* 1970;3:561–569.
71. Dudin AA, Rambaud–Cousson A, Thalji A, et al. Scorpion sting in children in the Jerusalem area: a review of 54 cases. *Ann Trop Paediatr* 1991;11:217–223.
71a. Boyer LV, Theodorou AA, Berg RA, et al. Antivenom for critically ill children with neurotoxicity from scorpion stings. *N Eng J Med* 2009;360(20):2090–2098.
72. Sofer S, Shahak E, Gueron M. Scorpion envenomation and antivenom therapy. *J Pediatr* 1994;124:973–978.
73. Jurkovich GJ. Hypothermia in the trauma patient. *Adv Trauma* 1989;4:111–140.
74. Moss J. Accidental severe hypothermia. *Surg Gynecol Obstet* 1986;162:501–513.
75. Centers for Disease Control and Prevention (CDC). Hypothermia-related deaths—United States, 2003–2004. *MMWR Morb Mortal Wkly Rep* 2005;54(7):173–175.
76. Danzl D, Pozos R, Auerbach P, et al. Multicenter hypothermia survey. *Ann Emerg Med* 1987;16:1042–1055.
77. Brantigan C, Patton B. Clinical hypothermia, accidental hypothermia, and frostbite. In: Goldsmith H, ed. *Lewis' Practice of Surgery.* New York: Harper & Row; 1978.
78. Trevino A, Razi B, Beller BM. The characteristic electrocardiogram of accidental hypothermia. *Arch Intern Med* 1971;127:470–473.
79. Ferguson N. Urban hypothermia. *Anaesthesia* 1985;40:651–654.
80. Hauty MG, Esrig BC, Hill JG, et al. Prognostic factors in severe accidental hypothermia: experience from the Mt. Hood tragedy. *J Trauma* 1987;27:1107–1112.
81. Walpoth BH, Walpoth-Aslan BN, Mattle HP, et al. Outcome of survivors of accidental deep hypothermia and circulatory arrest treated with extracorporeal blood warming. *N Engl J Med* 1997;337:1500–1505.
82. Silfvast T, Pettila V. Outcome from severe accidental hypothermia in Southern Finland—a 10-year review. *Resuscitation* 2003;59(3):285–290.
83. Cohen DJ, Cline JR, Lepinski SM, et al. Resuscitation of the hypothermic patient. *Am J Emerg Med* 1988;6:475–478.
84. Ledingham IM, Mone JG. Treatment of accidental hypothermia: a prospective clinical study. *BMJ* 1980;1:1102–1105.
85. Rahn H, Reeves RB, Howell BJ. Hydrogen ion regulation, temperature, and evolution. *Am Rev Respir Dis* 1975;112:165–172.
86. Ream AK, Reitz BA, Silverberg G. Temperature correction of $PaCO_2$ and pH in estimating acid-base status: an example of emperor's new clothes? *Anesthesiology* 1982;56:41–44.
87. White FN. A comparative physiologic approach to hypothermia. *J Thorac Cardiovasc Surg* 1982;82:821–831.
88. Hansen JE, Sue DY. Should blood gas measurements be corrected for the patient's temperature? [Letter]. *N Engl J Med* 1980;303:341.
89. Orlowski JP, Erenberg G, Lüders H, et al. Hypothermia and barbiturate coma for refractory status epilepticus. *Crit Care Med* 1984;12:367–372.
90. Dobson JA, Burgess JJ. Resuscitation of severe hypothermia by extracorporeal rewarming in a child. *J Trauma* 1996;40:483–485.
91. Schaller MD, Fischer AP, Perret CH. Hyperkalemia: a prognostic factor during acute severe hypothermia. *JAMA* 1990;264:1842–1845.
92. Moyer J, Morris GJ, DeBakey M. Effect on renal hemodynamics and excretion of water and electrolytes in dog and man. *Ann Surg* 1957;145:26–40.
93. Anderson M, Nielsen KC. Renal function under experimental hypothermia in rabbits. *Acta Med Scand* 1955;151:191–199.
94. Curry DL, Curry KP. Hypothermia and insulin secretion. *Endocrinology* 1970;87:750–755.
95. Axelrod DR, Bass DE. Electrolytes and acid base balance in hypothermia. *Am J Physiol* 1956;186:31–34.
96. Haddix TL, Pohlman TH, Noel RF, et al. Hypothermia inhibits human E-selectin transcription. *J Surg Res* 1996;64:176–182.
97. Kurz A, Sessler DI, Lenhardt R, et al. Perioperative normothermia to reduce the incidence of surgical-wound infection and shorten hospitalization. *N Engl J Med* 1996;334:1209–1215.
98. Iampietro PF, Vaughan JA, Goldman RF, et al. Heat production from shivering. *J Appl Physiol* 1960;15:632–634.
99. Pozos R, Wittmers L. *The Nature and Treatment of Hypothermia.* Minneapolis, MN: University of Minnesota Press; 1983.
100. Zwischenberger JB, Kirsh MM, Dechert RE, et al. Suppression of shivering decreases oxygen consumption and improves hemodynamic stability during postoperative rewarming. *Ann Thorac Surg* 1987;43:428–431.
101. Roe C, Goldberg M, Blair C, et al. The influence of body temperature on early postoperative oxygen consumption. *Surgery* 1966;60:85–92.
102. Gentilello L. Practical approaches to hypothermia. *Adv Trauma Crit Care* 1994:39–79.
103. Paton B. Accidental hypothermia. *Pharmacol Ther* 1983;22:331–337.
103a. Reuler J. Hypothermia: pathophysiology, clinical settings, and management. *Ann Intern Med* 1978;89:519–527.
104. Gregory J, Townsend M, Cloutier C, et al. Timing and incidence of hypothermia (T < 36°C) in operated trauma patients. Paper presented at the American Association for the Surgery of Trauma 50th Annual Meeting, 1990, Tucson, AZ.
105. Luna GK, Maier RV, Pavlin EG, et al. Incidence and effect of hypothermia in seriously injured patients. *J Trauma* 1987;27:1014–1018.
106. Jurkovich GJ, Greiser WB, Luterman A, et al. Hypothermia in trauma victims: an ominous predictor of survival. *J Trauma* 1987;27:1019–1024.
107. Psarras P, Ivatury R, Rohman M, et al. Hypothermia in trauma: incidence and prognostic significance. Paper presented at the meeting of the Eastern Association for the Surgery of Trauma, 1988, Longboat Key, FL.
108. Rutherford EJ, Fusco MA, Nunn CR, et al. Hypothermia in critically ill trauma patients. *Injury* 1998;29:605–608.
109. Little RA, Stoner HB. Body temperature after accidental injury. *Br J Surg* 1981;68:221–224.
110. Hardy J, Randini I. Some physiologic aspects of surgical trauma. *Am Surg* 1952;136:345.
111. Blalock A, Mason M. A comparison of the effects of heat and those of cold in the prevention and treatment of shock. *Arch Surg* 1945;42:1054–1059.
112. Wu X, Stezoski J, Safar P, et al. After spontaneous hypothermia during hemorrhagic shock, continuing mild hypothermia (34 degrees C) improves early but not late survival in rats. *J Trauma* 2003;55(2):308–316.
113. Sori AJ, El-Assuooty A, Rush BF, et al. The effect of temperature on survival in hemorrhagic shock. *Am Surg* 1987;53:706–710.
114. Alam HB, Bowyer MW, Koustova E, et al. Learning and memory is preserved after induced a sanguineous hyperkalemic hypothermic arrest in a swine model of traumatic exsanguination. *Surgery* 2002;132(2):278–288.
115. Cornejo CJ, Kierney PC, Vedder NB, et al. Mild hypothermia during reperfusion reduces injury following ischemia of the rabbit ear. *Shock* 1998;9:116–120.
116. Jurkovich GL, Pitt RM, Curreri PW, et al. Hypothermia prevents increased capillary permeability following ischemia-reperfusion injury. *J Surg Res* 1988;44:514–521.

117. Wright J, Kerr J, Valeri C, et al. Regional hypothermia protects against ischemia-reperfusion injury in isolated canine gracilis muscle. *J Trauma* 1988;28:1027–1031.
118. Childs EW, Udobi KF, Hunter FA. Hypothermia reduces microvascular permeability and reactive oxygen species expression after hemorrhagic shock. *J Trauma* 2005;58:271–277.
119. Fay T. Observations on generalized refrigeration in cases of severe cerebral trauma. *Assoc Res Nerv Ment Dis Proc* 1943;24:611–619.
120. Milde LN. Clinical use of mild hypothermia for brain protection: a dream revisited. *J Neurosurg Anesthesiol* 1992;4:211–215.
121. Clifton GL, Miller ER, Choi SC, et al. Lack of effect of induction of hypothermia after acute brain injury. *N Engl J Med* 2001;344:556–563.
122. Shiozaki T, Kato A, Taneda M, et al. Little benefit from mild hypothermia therapy for severely head injured patients with low intracranial pressure. *J Neurosurg* 1999;91:185–191.
123. Gentilello LM, Jurkovich GJ, Stark MS, et al. Is hypothermia in the victim of major trauma protective or harmful? A randomized, prospective study. *Ann Surg* 1997;226:439–449.
123a. Laniewicz J, Lyn-Knew K, Silberglelt R. Rapid endovascular rewarming for profound hypothermia. *Ann Emerg Med* 2008;51(2):160–163.
124. Bachmann F, McKenna, Cole ER, et al. The hemostatic mechanism after open heart surgery: I. Studies on plasma coagulation factors and fibrinolysis in 512 patients after extracorporeal circulation. *J Thorac Cardiovasc Surg* 1975;79:76–85.
125. Harker LA, Malpass TW, Branson HE, et al. Mechanism of abnormal bleeding in patients undergoing cardiopulmonary bypass: acquired transient platelet dysfunction associated with selective alpha-granule release. *Blood* 1980;56:824–834.
126. Kattlove HE, Alexander B. The effect of cold on platelets: 1. Cold-induced platelet aggregation. *Blood* 1971;38:39–48.
127. Patt A, McCroskey BL, Moore EE. Hypothermia-induced coagulopathies in trauma. *Surg Clin North Am* 1988;68:775–785.
128. Valeri CR, Feingold H, Cassidy G, et al. Hypothermia induced reversible platelet dysfunction. *Ann Surg* 1987;205:175–181.
129. Wolberg AS, Meng ZH, Monroe DM III, et al. A systematic evaluation of the effect of temperature on coagulation enzyme activity and platelet function. *J Trauma* 2004;56:1221–1228.
130. Reed RL II, Bracey AW Jr, Hudson JD, et al. Hypothermia and blood coagulation: dissociation between enzyme activity and clotting factor levels. *Circ Shock* 1990;32:141–152.
131. Gubler KD, Gentilello LM, Hassantash SE, et al. The impact of hypothermia on dilutional coagulopathy. *J Trauma* 1994;36:847–851.
132. Gentilello L, Jurkovich G, Moujaes S. Hypothermia and injury: thermodynamic principles of prevention and treatment. In: Levine B, ed. *Perspectives in Surgery.* St. Louis, MO: Quality Medical; 1991:25–55.
133. Sheaff CM, Fildes JJ, Keogh P, et al. Safety of 65°C intravenous fluid for the treatment of hypothermia. *Am J Surg* 1996;172:52–55.
134. Herron DM, Grabowy R, Connolly R, et al. The limits of bloodwarming: maximally heating blood with an inline microwave bloodwarmer. *J Trauma* 1997;43:219–228.
135. Gentilello LM, Cortes V, Moujaes S, et al. Continuous arteriovenous rewarming: experimental results and thermodynamic model simulation of treatment for hypothermia. *J Trauma* 1990;30:1436–1449.
136. Patton JF, Doolittle WH. Core rewarming by peritoneal dialysis following induced hypothermia in the dog. *J Appl Physiol* 1972;33:800–804.
137. Gentilello LM, Moujaes S. Treatment of hypothermia in trauma victims: thermodynamic considerations. *J Intensive Care Med* 1995;10:5–14.
138. Britt LD, Dascombe WH, Rodriguez A. New horizons in management of hypothermia and frostbite injury. *Surg Clin North Am* 1991;71:345–370.
139. Jacob JR, Weisman MH, Rosenblatt SI, et al. Chronic pernio: a historical perspective of cold-induced vascular disease. *Arch Intern Med* 1986;146:1589–1592.
140. Benchikhi H, Roujeau JC, Levent M, et al. Chilblains and Raynaud phenomenon are usually not a sign of hereditary protein C and S deficiencies. *Acta Derm Venereol* 1998;78:351–352.
141. Auerbach P. Disorders due to physical and environmental agents. In: Mills J, Ho MT, Salber PR, et al., eds. *Current Emergency Diagnosis and Treatment.* Los Altos, CA: Lange Medical; 1985.
142. Francis T, Golden FSC. Non-freezing cold injury: the pathogenesis. *J R Nav Med Serv* 1985;71:3–8.
143. Lloyd E. *Hypothermia and Cold Stress.* Rockville, MD: Aspen Publications; 1986:84–85.
144. Mills WJ Jr. Frostbite: a discussion of the problem and a review of the Alaskan experience [1973 classical article]. *Alaska Med* 1993;35:28–49.
145. Urschel JD. Frostbite: predisposing factors and predictors of poor outcome. *J Trauma* 1990;30:340–342.
146. Dana H, Rex I, Samitz M. The hunting reaction. *Arch Dermatol* 1969;99:441–450.
147. Mjurphy JV, Banwell PE, Roberts AH, et al. Frostbite: pathogenesis and treatment. *J Trauma* 2000;48:171–178.
148. Ozyazgan I, Tercan M, Melli M, et al. Eicosanoids and inflammatory cells in frostbitten tissue: prostacyclin, thromboxane, polymorphonuclear leukocytes, and mast cells. *Plast Reconstr Surg* 1998;101:1881–1886.
149. Bourne M, Piepkorn M, Clayton F, et al. Analysis of microvascular changes in frostbite injury. *J Surg Res* 1986;40:26–35.
150. Zook H, Hussmann J, Brown R, et al. Microcirculatory studies of frostbite injury. *Ann Plast Surg* 1998;40:246–253.
151. Mileski WJ, Raymond JF, Winn RK, et al. Inhibition of leukocyte adherence and aggregation for treatment of severe cold injury in rabbits. *J Appl Physiol* 1993;74:1432–1436.
151a. Bruen KJ, Ballard JR, Morris SE, et al. Reduction of the incidence of amputation in frostbite injury with thrombolytic therapy. *Arch Surg* 2007;142:546–553.
152. Mills WJ Jr, Whaley R. Frostbite: experience with rapid rewarming and ultrasonic therapy: part I and II [1960 classical article]. *Alaska Med* 1993;35:6–18.
153. Petrone P, Kuncir EJ, Asensio JA. Surgical management and strategies in the treatment of hypothermia and cold injury. *Emerg Med Clin North Am* 2003;21:1165–1178.
154. Heggers J, Robson M, Weingarten M, et al. Experimental and clinical observations on frostbite. *Ann Emerg Med* 1987;16:1056–1062.
155. Miller MB, Koltai PJ. Treatment of experimental frostbite with pentoxifylline and aloe vera cream. *Arch Otolaryngol Head Neck Surg* 1995;121:678–680.
156. Rakower S, Shahgoli S, Wong SL. Doppler ultrasound and digital plethysmography to determine the need for sympathetic blockade after frostbite. *J Trauma* 1978;18:713–718.
157. Bouwman DL, Morrison S, Lucas CE, et al. Early sympathetic blockade for frostbite—is it of value? *J Trauma* 1980;20:744–749.
158. Purdue G, Hunt J. Cold injury: a collective review. *J Burn Care Rehabil* 1986;7:331–342.
159. Edlich R, Chang D, Birk K, et al. Cold injuries: comprehensive therapy. *Compr Ther* 1989;15:13–21.
160. Mills W Jr. Comment and recapitulation. *Alaska Med* 1993;35:69–87.
161. Mills W Jr. Summary of treatment of the cold injured patient: hypothermia [1980 classical article.] *Alaska Med* 1993;35:50–53.
162. Mehta RC, Wilson MA. Frostbite injury: prediction of tissue viability with triple-phase bone scanning. *Radiology* 1989;170:511–514.
163. Barker JR, Haws MJ, Brown RE, et al. Magnetic resonance imaging of severe frostbite injuries. *Ann Plast Surg* 1997;38:275–279.
164. Greenwald D, Cooper B, Gottlieb L. An algorithm for early aggressive treatment of frostbite with limb salvage directed by triple-phase scanning. *Plast Reconstr Surg* 1998;102:1069–1074.
165. Cauchy E, Marsigny B, Allamel G, et al. The value of technetium 99 scintigraphy in the prognosis of amputation in severe frostbite injuries of the extremities: a retrospective study of 92 severe frostbite injuries. *J Hand Surg* 2000;25:969–978.
166. Bhatnagar A, Sarker BB, Sawroop K, et al. Diagnosis, characterisation and evaluation of treatment response of frostbite using pertechnetate scintigraphy: a prospective study. *Eur J Nucl Med Mol Imaging* 2002;29:170–175.
167. Rustin M, Newton J, Smith N, et al. The treatment of chilblains with nifedipine: the results of a pilot study, a double-blind placebo-controlled randomized study and a long-term open trial. *Br J Dermatol* 1989;120:267–275.

CHAPTER 32 ■ TERRORISM

ERIC R. FRYKBERG

KEY POINTS

1. Terrorism is random and ruthless violence against people—usually innocent civilians—and property to intimidate societies and governments for political or ideologic purposes. Terrorism has increased greatly and is the most common cause of mass casualties today. In the United States, complacency and apathy of health care providers are the greatest impediments to effective response to terrorism.
2. The major goals of terrorism are maximal casualties and lethality using, most frequently "weapons of mass destruction" of biologic, nuclear or radiologic, incendiary, chemical, and explosive (BNICE) agents.
3. Biologic weapons use microorganisms or their toxins to inflict disease. Useful because of easy deployment over wide areas, delay in onset, variability in recognition for containment, and proven effectiveness in nature (e.g., influenza epidemics), biologic weapons have been used in war since at least the Roman Empire.
4. Major biologic agents include anthrax (*Bacillus anthracis*), botulinum toxin (*Clostridium botulinum*), bubonic plague, tularemia, small pox, and viral hemorrhagic fever, caused by four viral groups. However, their development is dangerous, expensive, and difficult, explaining their rare use.
5. Chemical agents are aerosolized or gaseous, ingested as contaminated food, or absorbed by direct contact and have been used frequently during wars in the 20th century. Response requires recognition, treatment (including decontamination and protection of caregivers), and specific antidotes.
6. Dispersal of radioactive agents has severe theoretical risk but is primarily a psychological and panic effect. Penetration by ionizing radiation causes severe damage but is limited in range (square of the distance), and containment is relatively easy and nontransmittable. Care is supportive, treating dermal burns and gastrointestinal and hematopoietic damage.
7. Terrorist attacks are, by far, implemented most commonly using conventional weapons and confirm the need of a system to treat the casualties of bombings. The magnitude of energy achieved, the ease of technology required, and cost effectiveness support an ongoing increase in risk of mass casualties.
8. Explosion injuries are caused by the primary blast wave–induced disruption of organs with air–liquid interfaces (lung, bowels, eyes, and ears); secondary blast injury from flying objects, particularly shrapnel placed in bombs and suicide bomber body parts; tertiary blast injury from displacement of the victim's body; and quaternary blast injury from indirect causes such as building collapse.
9. Response to mass casualty events requires triage of victims to effectively utilize resources, including the paradigm shift from greatest good for the individual to greatest good for the greatest number, with need for preemptive planning, coordination, and practice of an Incident Command System to respond optimally.

THE CHALLENGE

1 Terrorism is defined as the unlawful exercise of random and ruthless violence against people, usually innocent civilians including women and children, and property to intimidate governments or societies for political or ideologic purposes.[1] Over the past few decades, terrorist attacks on civilian populations worldwide have ranked among the most common and most prominent causes of mass casualty disasters. These attacks have increasingly confronted health care providers with the unique demands of mass casualty management and have demonstrated the importance of developing a basic knowledge and skill set for disaster planning and management within the medical community.

Among the greatest impediments to a successful response to terrorist-related disasters are the complacency and apathy that pervade the mindset of most health care providers in the United States because of the low probability of these events and the belief that this country is well protected from such attacks. Disaster and mass casualty management has never been included in medical school or residency training. Even though most terrorist attacks involve bodily injury, surgeons in particular have largely abrogated their natural leadership role in disaster planning and management to other nonsurgical specialists and even to nonmedical organizations, agencies, and personnel.[2] The inaccuracy of these perceptions has been repeatedly demonstrated by the suboptimal medical response to such prominent disasters as the 1993 World Trade Center bombing in New York City; the 1995 bombing of the Alfred P. Murrah Federal Building in Oklahoma City; the Centennial Olympics bombing in Atlanta, Georgia, in 1996; and the jetliner attacks on and collapse of the World Trade Center twin towers on September 11, 2001, among many others.[3–6]

2 The two major goals of most terrorist attacks are maximal casualty generation and maximal lethality.[7] These goals are best achieved by the "weapons of mass destruction" of biologic, nuclear or radiologic, incendiary, chemical, and explosive (BNICE) agents. Even the mere threat of these weapons is sufficient in many settings to achieve the public chaos and societal disruption that terrorists seek. It is essential that surgeons be fully prepared to meet these threats by learning the associated history, epidemiology, pathophysiology, and injury patterns, so as to allow appropriate preparation and practice for their medical management.

BIOLOGIC WEAPONS

3 The term *biologic weapons* as agents of terrorism refers to the deliberate use of microorganisms, or toxins derived from them, to intentionally inflict disease and death on large populations.[8] Biologic agents have a number of features that theoretically

make them useful weapons. The most prominent such feature is that they can easily be deployed silently and anonymously over wide areas. Their incubation period results in a delayed time interval after initial exposure before the effects, and any suspicion of a terrorist attack, become manifest. A large number of casualties may occur before the medical community is able to initiate containment measures. Also, most biologic pathogens are widely available, are readily disseminated over large geographic areas, and have a historically proved capability to cause widespread disease and death (i.e., bubonic plague and influenza epidemics). In contrast, only a relatively few pathogens are believed to be suitable for potential use in terrorist attacks, and their development into effective weapons is quite expensive and difficult, which is confirmed by the extreme rarity of their use for this purpose.[9]

There is a long history of the use of biologic pathogens as weapons of war and terrorism. The contamination of drinking water with animal carcasses or human feces dates back at least as far as the Roman Empire. In 1346, the corpses of victims of an outbreak of bubonic plague among Tartar invaders of the port city of Caffa (now Feodosiya, Ukraine) on the Black Sea were catapulted into the city, which spread the disease among the Genoese defenders. It is believed that these Genoese carried this disease back to Europe to begin the Black Death epidemic that killed one third of Europe's population. During the French and Indian War in North America, the British caused an outbreak of smallpox among Native Americans by giving them gifts of disease-ridden blankets. In recent decades, countries such as Japan, Iraq, the United States, and the Soviet Union developed large-scale weaponization of anthrax, smallpox, and botulinum toxin.[9–12]

The level of threat of any biologic agent for use as a bioterrorist weapon is dependent on four factors: (a) the public health impact, in terms of its virulence, communicability, and susceptibility in exposed populations and its lethality; (b) the ease of production, delivery, and dissemination to large populations; (c) the requirements for surveillance, diagnosis, and stockpiling of treatments and antidotes; and (d) the potential for fear, panic, and societal disruption based on public perceptions. 4 The U.S. Centers for Disease Control and Prevention (CDC) has developed three categories of threat of bioterrorist agents (A, B, and C), with the six pathogens in category A posing the greatest risks.[13] Frontline medical providers must be aware of the clinical manifestations and treatment of these six organisms and should have a high index of suspicion for their deliberate use to contain an attack as early as possible.

High-risk Biologic Agents

Anthrax is carried by the gram-positive rod *Bacillus anthracis* and is considered the most likely agent to be used in a bioterrorist attack. Its spores can be produced easily in large quantities with little training, they can be stored for many years without loss of potency, they are undetectable by human senses, and they are easily spread in air by such delivery mechanisms as sprayers, bombs, and missiles. Conversely, a relatively high dose of 10,000 to 50,000 spores is necessary to cause infection, and the infection cannot be transmitted from person to person.[14,15] An accidental release of anthrax spores from a Soviet military facility in 1979 led to 66 human deaths within a 4-km radius.[16] One report estimates that an aerosolized release of 100 kg of anthrax spores could result in 130,000 to 3 million deaths in the Washington, D.C. area.[15] Reports conflict as to how easily or cheaply weapons-grade anthrax can be produced, because the most virulent form requires that the anthrax particles be less than 5 microns in size with minimal clumping, which is difficult and expensive to achieve.

The incubation period of anthrax is between 2 and 6 days and manifests in three clinical forms: cutaneous, gastrointestinal, and pulmonary. The cutaneous form is the most common, representing 95% of all reported cases. It occurs naturally, from exposure to infected animals, and has a 20% case fatality rate. The gastrointestinal form results from ingestion of contaminated meat and has a higher mortality rate due to its delayed recognition. It manifests nonspecific symptoms of abdominal pain, fever, nausea, vomiting, and gastrointestinal bleeding and peritonitis. The pulmonary form is the most lethal and is believed to be the most likely form to be used in a terrorist attack from an aerosolized spread. This form is 100% fatal if untreated and 80% fatal if treated after the onset of symptoms. The antibiotics ciprofloxacin and doxycycline are the treatments of choice for both active infection and prophylaxis. Vaccination is considered to be 92% effective when given after exposure.[15]

Botulinum toxin is a highly lethal neurotoxin produced by the organism *Clostridium botulinum*, causing a neuromuscular blockade that leads to respiratory failure. Although most commonly contracted from ingestion of contaminated food, aerosolized forms have been developed that could be especially effective as lethal weapons through inhalation. Standard gas masks provide protection from this agent, and treatment involves supportive care with mechanical ventilation until the effects subside. Antitoxins may shorten the duration of clinical effects, and vaccines are available for high-risk individuals in research and the military.[15]

Bubonic plague and tularemia are bacterial diseases, and smallpox is a virulent viral pathogen; all have a high case fatality rate and an established history of causing millions of deaths. Although bubonic plague and tularemia are usually spread through the bite of infected organisms (i.e., mosquitoes, fleas) and smallpox is spread by contact with infected body fluids, all can be effectively transmitted by aerosolized airborne dissemination. Bubonic plague and tularemia are treated with streptomycin as the antibiotic of choice. Vaccination is the only effective measure against smallpox and must be administered as soon as possible after exposure to prevent or minimize its consequences.[15,17–19]

Viral hemorrhagic fever is a clinical syndrome that manifests symptoms of fever, myalgias, headaches, and malaise in association with evidence of neurovascular collapse (shock, mucous membrane hemorrhages). Viral hemorrhagic fever is caused by the four major viral groups of filoviruses (Ebola and Marburg), arenaviruses (Lassa fever), bunyaviruses (Rift Valley fever), and flaviviruses (yellow fever and dengue). Filoviruses are considered bioterrorist threats because of their ability to infect via aerosolized dissemination, their ease of replication in culture for large-scale production, and their virulence, with mortality rates ranging up to 90%. Treatment is supportive, and contact and droplet precautions are generally adequate for infection control. Antiviral drugs have shown some promise, and a vaccine is available only for yellow fever.[20]

CHEMICAL WEAPONS

Toxic chemicals have a proven capability to cause widespread morbidity, mortality, and societal disruption among large populations and thus pose a major threat as terrorist weapons. Their deadly effects could be imparted through inhalation of aerosolized and gaseous agents, ingestion of contaminated foods, and direct contact with the skin, mucous membranes, and eyes (Table 32.1).

5 Poison gases have been used extensively in warfare, especially in the 20th century. In World War I, about 4% of all casualties (about 1 million people) were caused by these agents, which included 26% of all American casualties.[21] The worst chemical disaster in history involved the accidental release of 40 tons of methyl isocyanate gas in Bhopal, India, in 1984, resulting in 2,500 deaths and an additional 200,000 casualties.[22] These devastating results demonstrate how effective these agents could be in the hands of terrorists. The bomb

TABLE 32.1 **DIAGNOSIS AND TREATMENT**

CHEMICAL AGENTS THAT POSE A THREAT AS TERRORIST WEAPONS

■ CATEGORY	■ AGENTS	■ TREATMENT/ANTIDOTE
Pulmonary irritants	Phosgene, chlorine, ammonia, mace	Decontamination, water cleansing, bronchodilators, mechanical ventilation
Incapacitating agents (anticholinergics)	Benzene	Intravenous hydration, physostigmine
Vesicants (blistering agents)	Mustard, lewisite, phosgene oxime	Decontamination, hypochlorite, dimercaprol
Nerve agents	Tabun, sarin, soman, *VX*	Atropine, 2-Pam, diazepam, airway control, decontamination
Blood agents	Cyanide	Decontamination, hyperbaric oxygen, amyl nitrite

that exploded in the World Trade Center in New York City in 1993 contained enough cyanide to contaminate the entire building, but it was destroyed by the blast.[23] In 1995, the gaseous release of the nerve agent sarin in the Tokyo subway system caused 12 deaths and 5,000 injuries, representing the first terrorist use of this agent on a civilian population.[24]

The initial phase of response to intentional chemical attacks, as well as biologic and radiologic attacks, is known as *consequence detection.* Early detection is essential if casualties and death are to be minimized and can occur from either the discovery of the source of environmental release or exposure, or the diagnosis of the afflicted casualties. Patterns of large numbers of patients with similar symptom clusters must be recognized, which requires a knowledge of the classic symptoms of chemical poisoning, including coughing and choking from pulmonary agents such as chlorine and phosgene, dry mouth and mucous membranes, seizures, eye irritation, and the cholinergic symptoms of nerve agent poisoning described by the mnemonic DUMBBELS (diarrhea, urination, miosis, bronchospasm, bronchorrhea, emesis, lacrimation, and salivation).

The response phase that involves organization and cleanup of the disaster scene and medical and psychological treatment of the casualties is termed *consequence management.* The identified source of contamination and exposure must be neutralized to prevent further damage. Health care workers must wear personal protective equipment to prevent their exposure to hazardous materials (HAZMAT), including the prevention of inhalation of toxic fumes from off-gassing that may emanate from the tissues or clothing and belongings of afflicted victims.

Triage and decontamination of casualties must be established outside the hospital, and away from the disaster scene, to prevent health care providers and hospital facilities from being contaminated and rendered useless for further treatment of casualties. Decontamination should furthermore take place at a site that is uphill and upwind from the scene for this purpose. A *hot zone* must be established for contaminated casualties, to be clearly demarcated from the *warm zone,* where decontamination takes place, and the *cold zone,* where casualties are considered fully decontaminated and ready to undergo re-triage and medical treatment. All casualties must undergo decontamination as early as possible to minimize adverse effects. Simply removing their clothing and showering with soap and water removes more than 90% of all contaminating agents, a process known as *gross decontamination.* The more intensive *technical decontamination* then follows for specific forms of exposure, such as hypochlorite solutions for mustard agents, and copious eye irrigation with saline solution. Poison control centers, public health officials, pharmacologists, and toxicologists are important resources and personnel who should be involved in the planning and management of chemical terrorist disasters.

NUCLEAR/RADIOLOGIC WEAPONS

Dispersal of radioactive substances poses a significant potential for a terrorist attack because of the theoretical damage that could be inflicted on large populations, although such a deliberate attack on civilian populations has never occurred outside of war. These agents also carry the potential of widespread psychosocial effects and panic caused by the mystique that is associated with radiation among the general population. The dangers of these agents are largely overestimated, however, and result from poor understanding of radiation biology. These misperceptions are as common among health care providers as among the lay public and represent a major barrier to effective management. In fact, major radiation exposure from a terrorist attack should be easier to manage than biologic or chemical events because of easy detection methods with Geiger counters and dose-rate meters; the large number of hospital, industrial, and government personnel who regularly deal with radiation; and the well-known clinical effects that can be monitored with simple laboratory tests.[25,26]

Radiation is categorized as nonionizing and ionizing, and may consist of particles or waves, each of which has specific implications for injury in mass casualty scenarios. Nonionizing radiation, such as infrared and visible light, has little if any
6 injurious effects on living organisms. Ionizing radiation represents the major radiologic threat from terrorist events, as it causes damage to living cells and tissues from its direct energy as well as from the indirect effects of the unstable and toxic hyperoxide molecules it creates. These effects are long term, as they continue far beyond the time of exposure. γ-Rays and x-rays, which are examples of wave radiation, have high tissue penetrance and cause the greatest tissue damage, especially to rapidly dividing cells (gastrointestinal tract and bone marrow). Neutrons are particles that behave much like γ- and x-rays as they also have high penetrance with severe tissue damage. α (Helium nuclei) and β (electrons) particle radiation have low tissue penetrance and damage potential and are easily shielded, but cause highly lethal damage if ingested or if they gain access through open wounds.[25]

The major factors that determine the severity of radiation exposure are time, distance, and shielding. The absorbed radiation dose rapidly decreases with shortened duration of exposure and with the square of the distance from the source, so that quadrupling the distance reduces the dose rate to one sixteenth of the original exposure. In doses of less than 1 Gy

(1 Gy = 100 rads), the biologic effects are not clinically significant, although long-term malignant transformation is always possible. The handling of highly radioactive sources or fallout of radioactive dust from α or β particles results in local skin exposure with thermal burns that are characterized by erythema, desquamation, and blistering. Treatment of these low levels of exposure includes prophylactic antibiotics and standard burn wound care.[25–27]

The effects of whole-body exposure from highly penetrating wave and particle sources (γ-rays, x-rays, and neutrons) are dose and duration dependent. Nausea, vomiting, diarrhea, and pancytopenia, especially lymphocyte count depression (termed *acute radiation syndrome*), begin at doses greater than 1.0 Gy. The LD_{50} of radiation exposure, which is the dose range that will kill 50% of the afflicted casualties, is 3.0 to 4.5 Gy. An absorbed dose of 10 Gy is considered to be the highest survivable dose if maximal medical therapy is provided. Symptoms develop in less than 5 minutes following doses greater than 10 Gy, and doses greater than 30 Gy inevitably lead to death from cardiovascular and nervous system collapse in 24 to 72 hours.[27] Thus, the timing of onset of gastrointestinal symptomatology and lymphocyte depression can serve as accurate and easily discerned determinants of mortality risk, which greatly aids in the triage of mass casualties from a radiologic event.

The two major forms that a nuclear or radiologic terrorist attack could take are the dispersal of radioactive materials that are commonly used in industry and medicine (i.e., cobalt-60, cesium-137, iridium-192, iodine-131), most likely using conventional explosives (*dirty bombs*), and the atmospheric release of large amounts of intense ionizing radiation through the sabotage of nuclear power plants or the detonation of nuclear bombs. Dirty bombs are easy to construct with little training. They could spread contamination over a few city blocks at most and cause bodily injuries from the blast as well as fear and panic in the population. Property damage and radiation exposure are unlikely to be extensive, and the relatively small area of contamination should be easily monitored and contained for long-term cleanup. In contrast, nuclear sabotage and explosions require significant technical expertise and money to develop and execute and are therefore considered relatively unlikely to be used by terrorists. However, they threaten substantial property destruction as well as injury and death to people over a range of hundreds of miles because of the physical effects of the blast, the thermal and blinding effects of the ensuing fireball, and the high levels of ionizing radiation thrown into the atmosphere.[28–30]

The appropriate medical care of casualties from a radiologic incident first requires an understanding of the distinction between radiation *exposure* and radiologic *contamination*. Exposure to ionizing radiation results in damage to body tissues, and the clinical manifestations of the victim and their timing provide a reliable guide to their absorbed dose. Exposure alone does not make a casualty "radioactive," does not require decontamination, and offers no danger whatever to medical providers. *Contamination* refers to radioactive material that is found on the clothing or body of a victim, which can be spread to medical providers and the environment and requires decontamination to reduce such spread. Treatment of these casualties is largely supportive, involving the management of the skin, gastrointestinal, and hematopoietic signs and symptoms, after removing them from the source. Internal contamination through inhalation, ingestion, or skin or open wound absorption is treated by minimizing absorption and through the use of dilution, blockage, displacement, stimulation of renal and gastrointestinal elimination, and chelation methods. Most of these approaches are largely unproved and ineffective, including bone marrow transplantation or stem cell augmentation, or they have some beneficial effect only against specific radioisotopes. There is no "antiradiation" drug or agent. Potassium iodide does effectively block thyroid uptake of radioactive iodine, but this isotope is found only after nuclear explosions or nuclear plant leaks. Also, potassium iodide is effective only if given within 4 hours of exposure and is of benefit only in children.[26,28]

External contamination of clothing and exposed skin is easily managed by simply removing clothing and showering with water and detergent, which should remove more than 90% of the contamination. Technical decontamination can then follow with removal or intensive cleansing of all hair and through scrubbing of the body, guided by the use of radiation dose meters to detect residual radiation. All clothing and fluid runoff is bagged and carefully disposed of to control the spread of radioactive materials. Open contaminated wounds must be washed and débrided according to standard aseptic principles, and wound excision should be considered for contamination with long-lived radionuclides (e.g., α emitters). After whole-body exposure of greater than 1.0 Gy, open wounds should be closed as soon as possible to prevent them from becoming portals of entry for lethal internal contamination. External radiologic contamination does not constitute a medical emergency for either victims or medical providers. It is best to consider radioactive contamination as nothing more than dirt, something that is preferably cleaned off before treatment or hospitalization but that should *not* cause any delay in treatment of life-threatening injuries or the withholding of appropriate medical care for fear of exposure. Life-threatening injuries that require urgent medical management should not await extensive decontamination, although removal of clothing and a quick shower can usually be accommodated. Medical personnel and hospital facilities will not be overexposed even with the highest levels of exposure and contamination of casualties, and medical personnel should simply wear protective gowns, caps, masks, and gloves in accordance with standard universal precautions.[25–27,29] There should be no reason for hospital-based providers to ever wear any more protective gear than this for any toxic contamination. Not only is it unwarranted for radiologic contamination, but also no chemically contaminated casualty should be allowed to enter the hospital until fully decontaminated.

The overall response to a radiologic or nuclear disaster should include proper planning and preparation, training of personnel, and on-scene triage and evacuation of casualties on the assumption of hazardous internal exposure. Triage officers must be familiar with the clinical effects and treatment of radiation injury.[29,30] National government resources should be contacted for guidance on the recognition and management of radiation exposure.[26] Severely injured casualties with radiation exposure should be triaged for definitive care to different facilities from those who are not seriously injured, and all possible measures to contain further contamination should be undertaken. Medical personnel should wear standard protective gear in accordance with universal precautions and treat all emergent medical and surgical problems without consideration of the radioactive contamination and exposure. Resources and procedures for dealing with the stress and psychosocial effects that are inevitably associated with radiologic incidents, in both casualties and medical providers, should be in place.[26,29]

EXPLOSIVE WEAPONS

7 Explosive attacks by terrorists have typically been characterized among conventional weapons, but the magnitude of energy that terrorist bombings have achieved over the past three decades and the thousands of resulting casualties make it clear that these agents belong as much in the category of unconventional weapons of mass destruction as those discussed previously. Furthermore, explosive devices have historically been and currently are the most common weapons of terrorism by far and therefore remain overwhelmingly the

TABLE 32.2 **RESULTS**

PROMINENT TERRORIST BOMBINGS WORLDWIDE

■ EVENT	■ YEAR(S)	■ EXPLOSIVE AGENT (*BUILDING COLLAPSE)
Irish Republican Army bombings, U.K.	1970s	TNT, dynamite
Bologna train terminal	1980	TNT
Beirut airport	1983	Ammonium nitrate(*)
Paris bombings	1986	TNT
World Trade Center, NY	1993	Ammonium nitrate
AMIA building, Buenos Aires	1994	Ammonium nitrate(*)
Oklahoma City	1995	Ammonium nitrate(*)
Atlanta Olympics	1996	TNT
U.S. Embassies, Africa	1998	TNT(*)
USS *Cole*, Yemen	2000	TNT
World Trade Center, NY; Pentagon, VA	2001	Jet air liner crashes(*)
Israel suicide bombings	2001–present	TNT, C-4
U.N. Baghdad headquarters	2003	Ammonium nitrate(*)
Madrid train terminals, Spain	2004	TNT
London subways and bus, U.K.	2005	TNT

most prominent and most likely threat for which civilian populations must be prepared in the future. This has important implications for the role of surgeons in disaster planning and management because the casualties of explosive disasters will be afflicted predominantly with traumatic injuries for which surgical expertise and support are necessary. The technology required for large-scale casualty generation and lethality with this mechanism is easily learned, and its cost effectiveness is unsurpassed by any other method.[31,32] These factors have resulted in a dramatic worldwide increase in frequency of these incidents with each passing year (Table 32.2).[7]

Historical Perspective

An analysis of two major accidental explosions of the 20th century serves to demonstrate the devastation of civilian populations that can result from large-magnitude explosive agents and provides important lessons in the planning for and prevention of their disastrous consequences. On December 6, 1917, in Halifax harbor, Nova Scotia, the Belgian ship *Imo* collided with the French munitions ship *Mont Blanc*, causing a fire on the top deck of *Mont Blanc* from the ignition of 35 tons of benzene. Hundreds of first-responder city firefighters and civilian onlookers then flocked to the scene. After 15 minutes, the fire ignited a cargo below decks consisting of 2,300 tons of picric acid, 10 tons of gun cotton, 300 rounds of ammunition, and 200 tons of trinitrotoluene (TNT). The ensuing explosion, the largest nonnuclear manmade explosion ever to occur, was followed by a 150-foot tidal wave, which leveled more than 2.5 km^2 of the city, blew the ship 1 mile high and vaporized it, threw its 1,100-pound anchor 2 miles away and a cannon 3.5 miles away, shattered windows 100 km away, and was heard in Boston. The resulting smoke plume rose 4 miles into the air. This delayed explosion wiped out the hundreds of curious citizens and firefighters who initially responded to the fire. There were 2,000 deaths, 9,000 injured, and more than 20,000 left homeless in a city with a population of only 50,000, and all medical facilities were destroyed.[33]

In the port of Texas City, Texas, on April 16, 1947, the freighter *Grand Camp* caught fire, again attracting the entire city's firefighters and hundreds of onlookers. Its cargo below decks of several tons of ammonium nitrate fertilizer was ignited 20 minutes later, creating an explosion with a 2,000-foot-high smoke plume and hurling the ship's anchor 2 miles away. A second more powerful blast occurred a short time later, causing widespread fires and a 150-foot tidal wave. This disaster resulted in 600 deaths in a city of only 16,000 population, including, again, the city's entire fire department and dozens of citizens initially attracted to the fire.[34]

These disasters demonstrate how devastating explosions can be and how effectively they can achieve the terrorist aims of casualty generation and lethality with relatively little cost or training. In Texas City, simple ammonium nitrate fertilizer caused one of the largest manmade explosions ever. It is quite likely that terrorists have studied these and similar events. With the ever-increasing use of bombings as instruments of terror in subsequent years, it is clear that lessons learned from these accidental disasters have been used. Ammonium nitrate–based fuel-air explosives have been used in several major terrorist attacks to generate explosions of great magnitude (see Table 32.2). Another effective and commonly used technique in terrorist bombings has been the "second hit," so well demonstrated in both Halifax and Texas City, in which an initial event draws in onlookers and first responders, who are then wiped out by a second deliberate event—another explosion, sniper fire, or a building collapse.[6,32,35,36] In this way, to further expand injury, death, and panic among their target population, terrorists exploit the natural and predictable urge of people to help others. This second-hit phenomenon is best combated by restricting access to any disaster scene, especially to medical personnel who have no training to manage that scene, whose help and skills are best used in the protected and resource-rich environment of hospitals, and whose deaths will further and needlessly magnify the risk to surviving casualties. The noble but emotional, ego-driven, and misguided urge to run to a scene to "help" must be restrained by a disciplined and rational analysis of how help can best be delivered.

Terrorist bombings increased dramatically in the 20th century, with 5,075 such events documented worldwide between 1973 and 1983, causing 3,689 deaths and 7,991 injuries. There was a 10-fold increase in these incidents between 1968 and 1980 as their success became evident.[37] In the United States alone, 12,216 terrorist bombings occurred between 1980 and 1990, with 1,582 bombings causing 222 injuries and 27 deaths occurring in 1990 alone.[38] From 1988 to 1997, the number of actual and attempted terrorist bombings increased by 127% within the United States, with 17,579 incidents causing 4,063 injuries and 427 deaths.[39] Between 1991 and 2000, 88% of all disasters involving more than 30 casualties were due to explosions.[40] Since then, major bombings of U.S. embassies in Tanzania and Kenya in 1998 and the USS *Cole* in Yemen in 2000, the jet airliner crashes into the World Trade Center and Pentagon in 2001, the Madrid train terminal bombings in 2004, the London subway and bus bombings in 2005, and the ongoing suicide bombings in Israel and Iraq have shown that explosive weapons remain the most likely mass casualty threat that must be confronted by surgeons in coming years. Analysis of these many events and an understanding of the pathophysiology of blast provide a valuable insight into the patterns of injury around which planning and management can be formulated.

Biodynamics of Blast

Terrorist bombings typically employ high-energy detonations that generate a pressure pulse wave, called a *blast wave*, which travels through air at supersonic speeds. The edge of this radially propagating wave is known as the *blast front*. Immediately following detonation, a *peak overpressure* phase, lasting only a fraction of a second, involves the sudden rise of air pressure far above ambient levels. This instantaneous rise in pressure imparts to the blast wave the characteristic of *brisance*, or shattering ability. The peak overpressure is followed by a more gradual ebbing of pressure lasting up to 10 times longer, which ends in a negative-pressure phase into which air and debris can be sucked (Fig. 32.1). This negative-pressure phase accounts for the implosion of some surrounding structures, as well as the creation of tidal waves in coastal areas, as happened after both the Halifax and Texas City explosions. The term *blast wind* refers to these rapid back-and-forth movements of air. Underwater blasts are generally three times more powerful in blast wave propagation than those in air because of the greater density of water.[41–43]

The four factors that determine the force of a blast and the severity of injuries it causes are the size of the explosive charge, the distance from the blast, indoor or outdoor location, and the surrounding medium of air or water. The magnitude of an

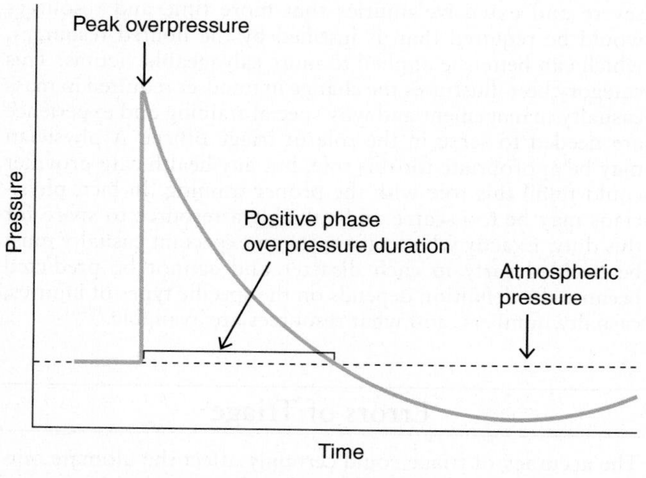

FIGURE 32.1. The Friedlander curve demonstrating the pressure characteristics of a blast wave over time.

air blast tends to dissipate rapidly according to the cube of the distance from the blast, so that moving three times the distance away reduces the energy by 27-fold. Indoor detonations cause the blast energy to be magnified rather than dissipated as the blast wave is reflected off walls, floors, and ceilings, causing greater damage than open-air blasts. This magnification of destructive force explains why terrorists seek to detonate bombs in confined spaces, such as in buses in Israel, rather than open air.[44,45]

8 The medical management of casualties of terrorist bombings requires an understanding of the three categories of injury that result from explosions. Primary blast injury is caused by the passage of the blast wave through the body, which causes a disruptive turbulence, called *spalling*, in the tissues of organs with air-to-liquid interfaces, such as the lung, bowels, eyes, and ears. For this reason, tympanic membrane rupture is quite common among casualties of explosive events and should be viewed as a sensitive marker for more severe internal effects of primary blast injury.[46] The lung is the most common visceral organ damaged in air blasts, whereas bowel disruption is found primarily in underwater blasts. Most victims of primary blast lung injury die immediately because such injuries require that they be so close to the blast that they suffer lethal bodily harm. Only 0.6% of survivors of major terrorist bombings have been found to have blast lung injury, but more than 10% of these victims ultimately die, indicating that this injury should also be considered a marker of severity that requires urgent treatment.[34] Blast lung is characterized by progressive pulmonary insufficiency, with radiologic and pathologic findings typical of blunt pulmonary contusion. Death is caused by cerebral and coronary air embolism.[41,47,48] A higher incidence of blast lung injury is found among survivors of urban bombings as compared with bombings in rural and isolated locales as a result of the rapid triage and transport of victims and abundant medical resources available in larger cities.[49]

Secondary blast injury is caused by the impact on the body of flying objects and debris set in motion by the blast. Tertiary blast injury involves the displacement of the victim's body to impact other objects. Both of these forms of blast injury cause the standard forms of blunt trauma that predominate among survivors of terrorist bombings and that surgeons typically manage in routine practice.[31,32,43,44,47,48,50] Secondary blast injury has also increasingly included penetrating trauma from destructive shrapnel placed in the bombs, as well as from body parts of suicide bombers that become embedded in the victim.[5,51,52] An especially bizarre implication of these latter injuries to both casualties and medical care providers is that the embedded terrorist body parts have been shown to carry chronic diseases, such as hepatitis and acquired immunodeficiency syndrome (AIDS), that are transmitted to surviving casualties and serve to further magnify the level of injury and terror.[53]

Quaternary, or miscellaneous, blast injuries are indirect consequences of explosive events, including burns, crush injuries from falling debris or structural collapse, inhalational injuries from dust and toxic chemicals, and ocular injuries. The dissemination of biologic, chemical, and radiologic agents in dirty bombs falls into this category and is also called *combined blast injury*.[2]

Patterns of Injury, Severity, and Mortality

Terrorist bombings result in consistent and predictable patterns of injury and mortality in all published reports.[3,31,32,47,48,50,54] The incidence of immediate deaths and critical injuries among survivors is related to the magnitude of the explosion, whether it occurs indoors or outdoors or in urban or isolated locales, and the association with building collapse. By exploding a bomb within a large building, the probability of complete structural collapse is increased, which greatly magnifies the casualty generation and lethality beyond the blast itself.[32] This

TABLE 32.3 **RESULTS**

IMPACT OF BUILDING COLLAPSE ON THE OUTCOME OF THE 1995 TERRORIST BOMBING IN OKLAHOMA CITY, OK[a]

CASUALTY LOCATION	NO. CASUALTIES	NO. DEAD	NO. SURVIVORS	NO. SURVIVORS HOSPITALIZED
Collapsed	175	153 (87%)	22	18 (82%)
Uncollapsed	186	10 (5%)	176	32 (18%)
Total	361	163 (45%)	198	50 (25%)

[a]Includes only 361 casualties inside the Alfred P. Murrah Federal Building stratified by portion of building in which they were located.
Adapted from data in Mallonee S, Shariat S, Stennies G, et al. Physical injuries and fatalities resulting from the Oklahoma City bombing. *JAMA* 1996;276:382–387.

is another reason why terrorists seek to place explosives in buildings. In the suicide bombing of the U.S. Marine barracks in Beirut, Lebanon, in 1983, with an ammonium nitrate fuel-air explosive imparting an estimated explosive force of 6 to 10 tons of TNT, the complete collapse of the four-story building resulted in the immediate death of 68% of all 346 casualties.[55] A terrorist bombing in Buenos Aires, Argentina, in 1994, caused the complete collapse of a seven-story building, resulting in the immediate death of 29% of all casualties but of 94% of casualties within the building.[54] In the 1995 bombing in Oklahoma City, the partial collapse of the nine-story Alfred P. Murrah Federal Building, also caused by an ammonium nitrate bomb constructed as a fuel-air explosive imparting a 2-ton TNT equivalent blast force,[3] resulted in significantly greater injury and death among victims in the collapsed portion of the building (Table 32.3). This is remarkably different from the 3.3% immediate death rate among the 574 casualties of the Khobar Towers bombing in Saudi Arabia in 1996, in which there was no building collapse.[56] These observations emphasize the preventive value of both barricading major buildings to prevent vehicular access and improving structural design of buildings to withstand major blasts without collapsing.

Most survivors of terrorist bombings are not critically injured. Generally only 10% to 20% of survivors require urgent treatment for severe injuries, a pattern that is typical of most mass casualty disasters from any mechanism. The most common injuries found in immediate fatalities involve the head, chest, abdomen, blast lung, and traumatic amputation. These same severe injuries are found in only a small minority of survivors (0.5% to 2%) but contribute to a disproportionately high mortality among those survivors (10% to 50%) and therefore must be considered important markers of severity that require urgent attention. The great majority of survivors have noncritical soft tissue and skeletal injuries, for which care may be delayed for hours or days if necessary to maximize casualty flow and the immediate care of critical injuries.[3,5,6,31,32,56,57]

TRIAGE AND HOSPITAL CASUALTY MANAGEMENT

The prioritizing of patients according to injury severity, their need for immediate care, and available resources is called *triage*. In societies and geographic areas with an abundance of medical resources, such as the United States, triage is seldom necessary or practical because all injured individuals are brought to hospitals and provided with maximal care. In true
9 mass casualty disasters, however, such as those resulting from terrorism, triage must assume major importance on the part of medical providers because of the limited resources available to the large casualty numbers. The difficulty of triage in this setting lies in the need to rapidly identify that small minority of critically injured casualties who require and are expected to respond to immediate care from among the large majority of casualties who have noncritical or untreatable injuries, but who tend to rapidly inundate medical facilities. Although this rationing of care, and the possibility of denying care to some victims because of limited resources, is antithetical to current medical training and moral values, it may nonetheless be essential to maximize casualty survival. Disaster triage thus requires a paradigm change in mindset and approach to medical care, which in turn mandates that medical providers be educated in these principles that are so different from the routine approach to medical care.[32] The goal of management must shift from the greatest good for each individual to the greatest good for the greatest number, with the population taking priority over the individual. Triage officers not only must be experienced in the care of those injuries expected in any form of disaster (i.e., trauma in explosive events), but also must understand how to assess and treat these injuries within the unique context of mass casualties.[58,59]

The five categories of triage that are generally accepted are immediate, delayed, minimal or walking wounded, expectant, and dead. In the first triage performed at a disaster scene, the only decision made is that of who is alive and who is dead. Living casualties are then removed from the dangers of the scene to one or more *casualty collection points*, where the only decision to be made is who needs immediate care and hospital transport and who does not.[36,58] It is best not to evacuate casualties directly to the hospital from the scene, so as to allow a systematic reevaluation and distribution of those needing hospital care among all available facilities, to avoid overloading any one hospital. As secondary and tertiary triage is performed later in the hospital, more discrimination can be applied.

The expectant category includes those casualties with such severe and extensive injuries that more time and resources would be required than is justified by the limited resources, which can better be applied to more salvageable victims. This category best illustrates the change in mindset required in mass casualty management and why special training and experience are needed to serve in the role of triage officer. A physician may be appropriate for this role, but any health care provider could fulfill this role with the proper training. In fact, physicians may be too scarce and valuable a resource to spare for this duty. Exactly what constitutes an expectant casualty must be decided early in each disaster and cannot be predicted because the definition depends on the specific types of injuries, casualty numbers, and what resources are available.[58–61]

Errors of Triage

The accuracy of triage could certainly affect the ultimate outcome of surviving casualties. Improper assignment to a delayed category of critically ill or injured casualties who require urgent care, termed *undertriage*, is the most important

TABLE 32.4 **RESULTS**

RELATION OF OVERTRIAGE TO CRITICAL MORTALITY IN TERRORIST BOMBING SURVIVORS

EVENT	YEAR	NO. SURVIVORS	NO. CRITICALLY INJURED (%)[a]	NO. OVERTRIAGE (%)[b]	NO. CRITICAL MORTALITY (%)[c]
Cu Chi, Vietnam[67]	1969	34	3 (9)	9 (75)	1 (33)
Craigavon, Northern Ireland[66]	1970s	339	113 (33)	29 (20)	5 (4)
Old Bailey, London, U.K.[63]	1973	160	4 (2.5)	15 (79)	1 (25)
Guildford pubs, U.K.[43]	1974	64	22 (34)	2 (8.3)	0
Birmingham, U.K.[65]	1974	119	9 (8)	12 (57)	2 (22)
Tower of London, U.K.[64]	1974	37	10 (27)	9 (47)	1 (10)
Bologna train station, Italy[50]	1980	218	48 (22)	133 (73.5)	11 (23)
Beirut, Lebanon[55]	1983	112	19 (17)	77 (80)	7 (37)
AMIA building, Buenos Aires, Argentina[54]	1994	200	14 (7)	47 (56)	4 (29)
Oklahoma City, OK[3]	1995	597	52 (9)	31 (37)	5 (10)
Total		1,880	294 (16)	364 (53)	37 (12.6)

[a]Percentage of total survivors.
[b]Number of noncritical survivors triaged to immediate care as a percentage of all casualties triaged to immediate care.
[c]Number and percentage of all critically injured survivors who died.
Adapted from Frykberg, ER. Medical management of disasters and mass casualties from terrorist bombings: how can we cope? *J Trauma* 2002;53: 201–212.

to avoid and imparts an obvious potential for preventable death in all settings. The term *overtriage* describes the assignment of noncritical casualties to immediate care. In the routine management of trauma patients, with small numbers arriving at any given time, overtriage is an economic, logistical, and administrative burden that does not affect casualty outcome and is considered necessary to minimize undertriage.[62]

However, the published results of 10 major mass casualty disasters from terrorist bombings that relate the overtriage rate to the mortality among critically injured survivors (Table 34.4) confirms a direct impact of overtriage on the *critical mortality rate* in this setting (Fig. 32.2).[3,43,50,54,55,63–67] This impact occurs because the inundation of a hospital with large numbers of casualties all at once, most of whom are not critically injured, impedes the ability of medical personnel to rapidly detect that small minority who require immediate care, thus increasing the risk of preventable deaths.[32] It is reasonable to postulate that this principle probably applies to all mass casualty events of any mechanism, as the essential element of this problem is the overwhelming casualty load. This emphasizes the critical importance of accurate triage discrimination in all disasters to minimize both overtriage and undertriage.[59]

Hospital Care Considerations

The system of casualty flow and treatment within the hospital following a mass casualty explosive event is a major factor in

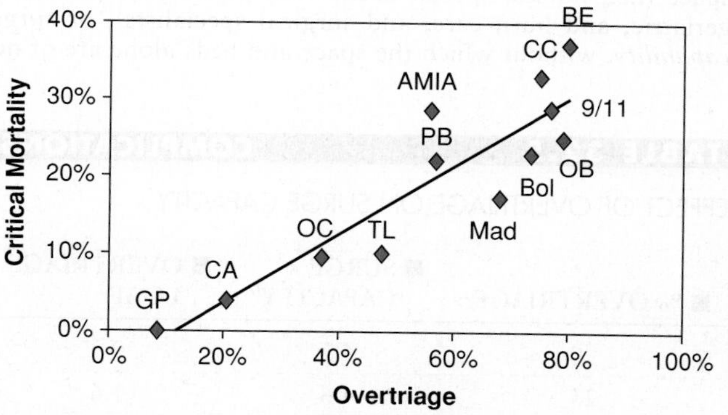

FIGURE 32.2. Relationship of overtriage to critical mortality rate in survivors of major terrorist bombings, from data in Table 34.4 ($r = 0.92$). GP, Guildford pubs U.K.; CA, Craigavon, Northern Ireland; OC, Alfred P. Murrah Federal Building, Oklahoma City, OK, U.S.; TL, Tower of London, U.K.; BP, Birmingham pubs, U.K.; AMIA, AMIA building, Buenos Aires, Argentina; Bol, Bologna train terminal, Italy; OB, Old Bailey, London, U.K.; CC, Cu Chi, Vietnam; BE, Beirut airport, Lebanon. (Adapted from Frykberg ER. Medical management of disasters and mass casualties from terrorist bombings: how can we cope? *J Trauma* 2002;53:201–212.)

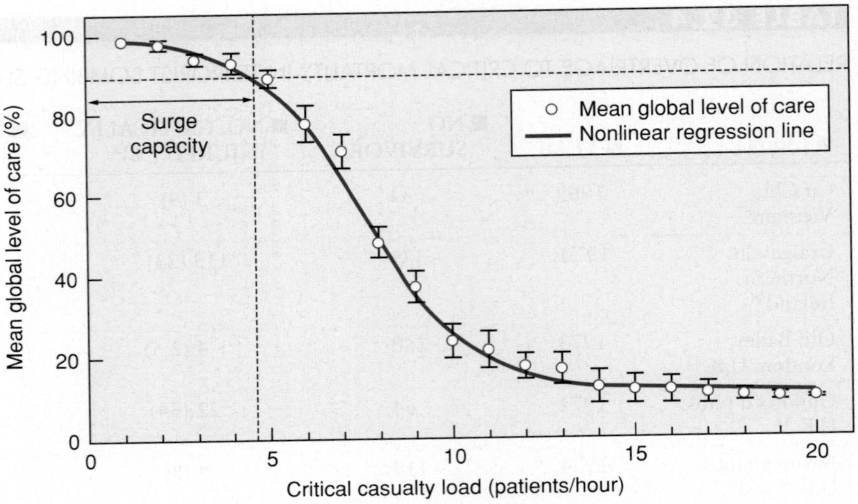

FIGURE 32.3. Relationship of hospital casualty arrival rate to quality of medical care following urban terrorist bombings. (Adapted from Hirshberg A, Scott BG, Granchi T, et al. How does casualty load affect trauma care in urban bombing incidents? A quantitative analysis. *J Trauma* 2005;58(4):686–695.)

the outcome of these casualties. The abundant published information on the hospital management of terrorist bombing casualties can be extrapolated to the expected demands from disasters of all kinds.[31,32,36,68]

Hospitals must restrict access of casualties to all but those most seriously injured in order to conserve their scarce resources and allow them to be applied to those most in need. No casualty should be allowed into a hospital before being both decontaminated and triaged. The three hospital resources most in demand in this setting are the emergency room (ER) where casualties are first received and evaluated, the operating room (OR), and the intensive care unit (ICU). Each of these units should have a designated *controller*, who is not involved directly in medical care but is responsible for the proper admission, movement, and disposition of all casualties to optimize rapid and efficient casualty handling. Casualties should always move forward through hospital spaces, never returning or going backward, thereby minimizing traffic gridlock and confusion.[36,40,60,61,69,70]

Developing the space to accommodate the added casualty load, or *surge capacity*, is the first thing that a hospital must accomplish following a mass casualty event, and this must be done within a matter of minutes. More important is the provision of the ability to care for the casualties brought into this space (i.e., nurses; special needs such as dialysis, pediatric, geriatric, and burn care; and surgical specialists), or *surge capability*, without which the space and beds alone are of no benefit. The most appropriate and realistic definition of surge capacity and capability is a functional one. An evidence-based computer modeling study by Hirshberg et al., using data from urban terrorist bombings, defines surge capacity as the *arrival rate* of critically injured casualties per hour that would allow at least 90% of the optimal quality of medical care to be delivered to each casualty.[71] They showed the relationship between casualty arrival rate and quality of hospital care to be best described by a sigmoid curve, and that there was a precipitous decline in the quality of medical care delivered to individual casualties at more than five critical casualties arriving per hour (Fig. 32.3). This could be improved (i.e., the curve moved to the right) by effective planning and preparation. However, the quality of medical care declines more precipitously (i.e., the curve moves to the left) with increasing levels of overtriage, defined as the arrival rate of noncritical casualties who do not require hospital care, presumably because overtriage delays the recognition and treatment of the critical casualties (Table 32.5). This further emphasizes the importance of minimizing overtriage in mass casualty events.

TABLE 32.5 **COMPLICATIONS**

EFFECT OF OVERTRIAGE ON SURGE CAPACITY

■ % OVERTRIAGE[a]	■ SURGE CAPACITY[b]	■ OVERTRIAGE LOAD[c]
0	4.7	0
25	4.6	1.6
50	3.8	3.8
75	2.7	8.1

[a]Percentage of casualties arriving at hospital not requiring hospital care.
[b]Number of critically injured casualties per hour.
[c]Number of noncritically injured casualties per hour.
Reprinted with permission from Hirshberg A, Scott BG, Granchi T, et al. How does casualty load affect trauma care in urban bombing incidents? A quantitative analysis. *J Trauma* 2005;58(4):686–695.

PLANNING AND REPORTING

Advance preparations are immensely important for the success of any disaster response because disasters are completely random, unexpected, and unpredictable. However, their magnitude requires a rapid, organized, and comprehensive response involving a number of disparate elements that do not usually work together, and a medical approach that is quite different from routine patient care.[70] Such a response cannot occur without plans in place that have been extensively rehearsed.

Disasters are rare events, requiring that planning be based on the abundant literature that documents experience from past disasters. Although every disaster is different in several specific factors, consistent patterns have clearly been established that are common to most disasters, allowing for realistic planning. Every plan must also have a built-in flexibility to allow adaptation to unique contingencies of a specific event. Terrorist bombings, in view of their frequency, should be considered as the universal model for disaster management, and planning can be based on the well-established patterns of injury and mortality previously described. It is possible to anticipate resource needs and distribution from knowledge of the prognostic factors of these events that can be gleaned from the literature (Table 32.6).[32] It is also possible to optimize the success of disaster plans by learning from the patterns and trends of major pitfalls described in past disasters (Table 32.7).[72]

TABLE 32.6 **RESULTS**

PROGNOSTIC FACTORS THAT AFFECT THE CASUALTY OUTCOME FOR TERRORIST BOMBINGS

Magnitude of explosion
Triage accuracy
Time interval to treatment
Anatomic injuries
Location
Confined space vs. open air
Rural vs. urban
Building collapse
Immediate presence of surgical capability

The Incident Command System has been widely adopted as the best organizational and functional scheme for a comprehensive and successful disaster response. The five major components of this system are command, planning, logistics, operations, and finance/administration. This integration of resources into a unified command has been shown to avoid the major barriers and to promote the most effective interaction of the several components of a disaster response.[72,73]

It is essential that surgeons be integrally involved in disaster planning and management by participating in their local hospital disaster committee, their hospital disaster drills, and community disaster exercises. The care of trauma patients and rapid decision making for large numbers of patients are what surgeons are trained to do and what they regularly practice. In fact, U.S. trauma centers and the nationwide trauma systems should logically serve as the template for a national disaster response system in view of their extensive resources, collective expertise, and already established liaisons with most of the elements necessary in a disaster response (i.e., prehospital assets, search and rescue, air medical transport, law enforcement, fire services, public health, media, local and state government health services).[74–76] It is also important that the results of a disaster be analyzed and reported in the surgical literature as the only means by which health care providers can be educated. This analysis also allows a postevent debriefing on the part of those involved in a disaster, which should result in a revision of the disaster plan to correct any deficiencies identified. These goals all require that an effective method of record keeping be in place to allow patient tracking and data accumulation during the disaster, from which a comprehensive analysis of results can be derived. A successful disaster response can be achieved only through intensive education, research, self-analysis, reassessment, and practice.

TABLE 32.7 **COMPLICATIONS**

MOST COMMON BARRIERS TO A SUCCESSFUL DISASTER RESPONSE

Failure of communications
Security failures at the scene and hospital
Failure to designate authority and responsibility
Ineffective and inefficient system of medical care of casualties
Failure of original disaster plan
Failure to manage and control volunteers
Lack of education and training among responders

References

1. US Department of State. *International Terrorism. Selected Documents, No. 24*. Washington, DC: US Government Printing Office; 1986.
2. Ciraulo DL, Frykberg ER, Feliciano DV, et al. A survey assessment of the level of preparedness for domestic terrorism and mass casualty incidents among Eastern Association for the Surgery of Trauma members. *J Trauma* 2004;56:1033–1041.
3. Mallonee S, Shariat S, Stennies G, et al. Physical injuries and fatalities resulting from the Oklahoma City bombing. *JAMA* 1996;276:382–387.
4. Quenemoen LE, Davis YM, Malilay J, et al. The World Trade Center bombing: injury prevention strategies for high-rise building fires. *Disasters* 1996;20:125–132.
5. Feliciano DV, Anderson GV, Rozycki GS, et al. Management of casualties from the bombing at the Centennial Olympics. *Am J Surg* 1998;176: 538–543.
6. Cushman JG, Pachter HL, Beaton HL. Two New York City hospitals' surgical response to the September 11, 2001 terrorist attack in New York City. *J Trauma* 2003;54:147–155.
7. Slater MS, Trunkey DD. Terrorism in America: an evolving threat. *Arch Surg* 1997;132:1059–1066.
8. Mobley JA. Biological warfare in the twentieth century: lessons from the past, challenges for the future. *Mil Med* 1995;160:547–553.
9. Kortepeter MG, Parker GW. Potential biological weapons threats. *Emerg-ing Inf Dis* 1999;5:523–527.
10. Derbes VJ. DeMussis and the Great Plague of 1348, a forgotten episode of bacteriological warfare. *JAMA* 1966;196:179–182.
11. Christopher GW, Cieslak TJ, Pavlin JJ, et al. Biological warfare, a historical perspective. *JAMA* 1997;278:412–417.
12. Zilinskas RA. Iraq's biological weapons, the past as future? *JAMA* 1997; 278:418–424.
13. Khan AS, Ashford DA, Craven RB, et al. Biological and chemical terrorism: strategic plan for preparedness and response. Recommendations of the CDC strategic planning workgroup. *MMWR Morb Mortal Wkly Rep* 2000;49:1–14.
14. Inglesby TV, Henderson DA, Bartlett JG, et al. Anthrax as a biological weapon: medical and public health management. *JAMA* 1999;281: 1735–1745.
15. Eachempati SR, Flomenbaum N, Barie PS. Biological warfare: current concerns for the health care provider. *J Trauma* 2002;52:179–186.
16. Meselson M, Gillemin J, Hugh-Jones M, et al. The Sverdlovsk anthrax outbreak of 1979. *Science* 1994;209:1202–1208.
17. Henderson DA, Inglesby TV, Bartlett JG, et al. Smallpox as a biological weapon: medical and public health management. *JAMA* 1999;281: 2127–2137.
18. Inglesby TV, Dennis DT, Henderson DA, et al. Plague as a biological weapon: medical and public health management. *JAMA* 2000;283: 2281–2290.
19. Dennis DT, Inglesby TV, Henderson DA, et al. Tularemia as a biological weapon. *JAMA* 2001;285:2763–2773.
20. Centers for Disease Control and Prevention. Management of patients with suspected viral hemorrhagic fever. *MMWR Morb Mortal Wkly Rep* 1988; 37:1–16.
21. Smart JK. History of chemical and biological warfare: an American perspective. In: *Medical Aspects of Chemical and Biological Warfare*. Bethesda, MD: Office of the Surgeon General; 1997:11–42.
22. Anderson N. Disaster epidemiology: lessons from Bhopal. In: Murray V, ed. *Major Chemical Disasters—Medical Aspects of Management*. London, UK: Royal Society of Medicine Services, Limited; 1990:183–195.
23. Jenkins BM. Understanding the link between motives and methods. In: Roberts B, ed. *Terrorism with Chemical and Biological Weapons: Calibrating Risks and Responses*. Alexandria, VA: Chemical and Biological Arms Control Institute; 1997:43–52.
24. Lillibridge SR, Sidell FR. *A Report on the Casualties from the Tokyo Subway Incident by the U.S. Medical Team*. Atlanta, GA: Centers for Disease Control and Prevention; 1995.
25. *Management of Terrorist Events Involving Radioactive Material*. NCRP report no. 138. Bethesda, MD: National Council on Radiation Protection and Measurement; 2001.
26. Mettler FA, Voelz GL. Major radiation exposure—what to expect and how to respond. *N Engl J Med* 2002;346:1554–1560.
27. Brill AB, ed. *Low Dose Radiation Effects: A Fact Book*. New York: Society of Nuclear Medicine; 1982.
28. Reeves GI. Radiation injuries. *Crit Care Clin North Am* 1999;2:457–472.
29. Fong F, Schrader DC. Radiation disasters and emergency department preparedness. *Emerg Med Clin North Am* 1996;14:349–369.
30. Reeves GI, Jarrett DG, Seed TM, et al, eds. *Triage of Irradiated Personnel*. Bethesda, MD: Armed Forces Radiology Research Institute; 1998.
31. Frykberg ER, Tepas JJ. Terrorist bombings: lessons learned from Belfast to Beirut. *Ann Surg* 1988;208:569–576.
32. Frykberg ER. Medical management of disasters and mass casualties from terrorist bombings: how can we cope? *J Trauma* 2002;53:201–212.
33. Bird M. *The Town That Died: The True Story of the Greatest Man-Made Explosion Before Hiroshima*. Halifax, NS: Nimbus Publishing; 1995.
34. Stephens HW. *Texas City Disaster, 1947*. Austin, TX: University of Texas Press; 1996.

35. Jacobs LM, Ramp JM, Breay JM. An emergency medical system approach to disaster planning. *J Trauma* 1979;19:157–162.
36. Stein M, Hirshberg A. Medical consequences of terrorism: the conventional weapon threat. *Surg Clin North Am* 1999;79:1537–1552.
37. Rignault DP, Deligny MC. The 1986 terrorist bombing experience in Paris. *Ann Surg* 1989;209:368–373.
38. Karmy-Jones R, Kissinger D, Golocovsky M, et al. Bomb-related injuries. *Mil Med* 1994;159:536–539.
39. Federal Bureau of Investigation. *1997 Bomb Summary*. Washington, DC: U.S. Department of Justice; 1997.
40. Arnold JL, Tsai M-C, Halpern P, et al. Mass-casualty, terrorist bombings: epidemiological outcomes, resource utilization, and time course of emergency needs (Part I). *Prehosp Disaster Med* 2003;18:220–234.
41. Clemedsson CJ. Blast injury. *Physiol Rev* 1956;36:336–354.
42. Hill JF. Blast injury with particular reference to recent terrorist bombing incidents. *Ann R Coll Surg Engl* 1979;61:4–11.
43. Cooper GJ, Maynard RL, Cross NL, et al. Casualties from terrorist bombings. *J Trauma* 1983;23:955–967.
44. DePalma RG, Burris DG, Champion H, et al. Current concepts: blast injuries. *N Engl J Med* 2005;352:1335–1342.
45. Lebovici D, Gofrit ON, Stein M, et al. Blast injuries: bus versus open-air-bombings—a comparative study of injuries in survivors of open-air versus confined-space explosions. *J Trauma* 1996;41:1030–1035.
46. Ciraulo DL, Frykberg ER. The surgeon and acts of civilian terrorism: blast injuries. *J Am Coll Surg* 2006;203:942–950.
47. Nelson TJ, Clark T, Stedje-Larsen ET, et al. Close proximity blast injury patterns from improvised explosive devices in Iraq: a report of 18 cases. *J Trauma* 2008;65:212–217.
48. Ramasamy A, Harrisson SE, Clasper JC, et al. Injuries from roadside improvised explosive devices. *J Trauma* 2008;65:910–914.
49. Gutierrez de Caballos JP, Turegano-Ruentes F, Perez-Diaz D, et al. Casualties treated at the closest hospital in the Madrid, March 11, terrorist bombings. *Crit Care* 2004;9:104–111.
50. Brismar B, Bergenwald L. The terrorist bomb explosion in Bologna, Italy, 1980: an analysis of the effects and injuries sustained. *J Trauma* 1982;22:216–220.
51. Boffard KD, MacFarlane C. Urban bomb blast injuries: patterns of injury and treatment. *Surg Ann* 1993;25:29–47.
52. Almogy G, Belzberg H, Mintz Y, et al. Suicide bombing attacks: update and modifications to the protocol. *Ann Surg* 2004;239:295–303.
53. Braverman I, Wexler D, Oren M. A novel mode of infection with hepatitis B: penetrating bone fragments due to the explosion of a suicide bomber. *Isr Med Assoc J* 2002;4:528–529.
54. Biancolini CA, Del Bosco CG, Jorge MA. Argentine Jewish community institution bomb explosion. *J Trauma* 1999;47:728–732.
55. Frykberg ER, Tepas JJ, Alexander RH. The 1983 Beirut airport terrorist bombing: injury patterns and implications for disaster management. *Am Surg* 1989;55:134–141.
56. Thompson D, Brown S, Mallonee S, et al. Fatal and non-fatal injuries among U.S. Air Force personnel resulting from the terrorist bombing of the Khobar Towers. *J Trauma* 2004;57:208–215.
57. Davis TP, Alexander BA, Lambert EW, et al. Distribution and care of shipboard blast injuries (USS Cole DDG-67). *J Trauma* 2003;55:1022–1028.
58. Kluger Y. Bomb explosions in acts of terrorism—detonation, wound ballistics, triage and medical concerns. *Isr Med Assoc J* 2003;5:235–240.
59. Frykberg ER. Triage: principles and practice. *Scand J Surg* 2005;94:272–278.
60. Almogy G, Luria Tal, Richter E, et al. Can external signs of trauma guide management? Lessons learned from suicide bombing attacks in Israel. *Arch Surg* 2005;140:390–393.
61. Hirshberg A, Stein M, Walden R. Surgical resource utilization in urban terrorist bombing: a computer simulation. *J Trauma* 1999;47:545–550.
62. American College of Surgeons Committee on Trauma. Field categorization of trauma patients (field triage). *Bull Am Coll Surg* 1986;71:17–21.
63. Caro D, Irving M. The Old Bailey bomb explosion. *Lancet* 1973;1:1433–1435.
64. Tucker K, Lettin A. The Tower of London bomb explosion. *BMJ* 1975;3:287–290.
65. Waterworth TA, Carr MJT. Report on injuries sustained by patients treated at the Birmingham General Hospital following the recent bomb explosions. *BMJ* 1975;2:25–27.
66. Pyper PC, Graham WJH. Analysis of terrorist injuries treated at Craigavon Area Hospital, Northern Ireland, 1972–1980. *Injury* 1982;14:332–338.
67. Henderson JV. Anatomy of a terrorist attack: the Cu Chi mess hall incident. *J World Assoc Emerg Dis Med* 1986;2:69–73.
68. Einav S, Feigenberg Z, Weissman C, et al. Evacuation priorities in mass casualty terror-related events: implications for contingency planning. *Ann Surg* 2004;239:304–310.
69. Einav S, Aharonson-Daniel L, Weissman C, et al. In-hospital resource utilization during multiple casualty incidents. *Ann Surg* 2006;243:533–540.
70. Lucci EB. Civilian preparedness and counter-terrorism: conventional weapons. *Surg Clin North Am* 2006;86:579–600.
71. Hirshberg A, Scott BG, Granchi T, et al. How does casualty load affect trauma care in urban bombing incidents? A quantitative analysis. *J Trauma* 2005;58:686–695.
72. Klein JS, Weigelt JA. Disaster management: lessons learned. *Surg Clin North Am* 1991;71:257–266.
73. Irwin RL. The incident command system (ICS). In: Auf der Heide E, ed. *Disaster Response: Principles of Preparation and Coordination*. St. Louis, MO: Mosby; 1989:133–163.
74. Jacobs LM, Goody M, Sinclair A. The role of a trauma center in disaster management. *J Trauma* 1983;23:697–701.
75. Ammons MA, Moore EE, Pons PT, et al. The role of a regional trauma system in the management of a mass disaster: an analysis of the Keystone Colorado chairlift accident. *J Trauma* 1988;28:1468–1471.
76. Jacobs LM, Burns KJ, Gross RI. Terrorism: a public health threat with a trauma system response. *J Trauma* 2003;55:1014–1021.

SECTION B

TRANSPLANTATION & IMMUNOLOGY

CHAPTER 33 TRANSPLANTATION IMMUNOLOGY

JEFFREY L. PLATT AND MARILIA CASCALHO

KEY POINTS

1. Development of the vascular anastomosis and immunosuppression were the key technologic advances that allowed clinical application of transplantation.
2. The condition of the donor and ischemia and reperfusion of the transplant impact directly on grafts and on the immune response to grafts.
3. The genetic relationship between the recipient and the donor determine the outcome of a transplant, especially susceptibility to rejection.
4. Transplantation provokes immune responses by T cells and B cells.
5. Modern immunosuppressive agents and regimens effectively prevent acute rejection.
6. The impact of T-cell and B-cell responses on a graft depends to the greatest extent on whether a transplant consists of cells, tissues, or an organ.
7. Transplanted organs but not transplanted cells and tissues are susceptible to various types of humoral rejection; all transplants are susceptible to cellular rejection.
8. Chronic rejection is the most common cause of loss of organ transplants.

Transplantation refers to the transfer of living cells, tissues, or organs from one individual to another. Envisioned from a theoretical perspective throughout history, transplantation has been attempted surgically since the early years of the twentieth century. Today, transplantation is the preferred method to replace the function of the heart, lungs, kidneys, liver, and bone marrow and, in some circumstances, the islets of Langerhans of the pancreas. Applications may soon be expanded if transplantation of stem cells or the derivatives of stem cells become part of clinical practice. Transplants have shed light on such fundamental principles of biology and immunology as the genetic differences between individuals in a population, the principle that organs are integral biologic structures, the major histocompatibility complex, and tolerance. Many terms have been applied to transplants based on the genetic relationship between the source and recipient of transplants. Some of these terms are listed and defined in Table 33.1.

THE VASCULAR ANASTOMOSIS AND FIRST LESSONS OF TRANSPLANTATION

The field of clinical transplantation was launched by the advent of the vascular anastomosis. The development of surgical techniques for repair and anastomosis of blood vessels met a widely recognized and urgent need for repair of traumatic and surgical wounds.[1,2] Development of the vascular anastomosis taught technical lessons such as the importance of asepsis and protection of vascular intimae. It taught that restoring blood flow could avert gangrene distal to a vascular lesion. It taught that some organs such as the kidney function as integral units (the kidney can be removed and reimplanted) and that function is not dependant on anatomic location (the kidney can be implanted in a heterotopic location). The greatest excitement was generated by the possibility that the vascular anastomosis might allow the replacement of a diseased or 1 injured organ with a healthy one. Ultimately, the vascular anastomosis was one of two advances critical to the clinical application of organ transplantation, the other advance being the discovery of immunosuppression.

Successful application of the vascular anastomosis for transplantation of the kidneys was reported by Alexis Carrel in 1908.[2] Carrel was awarded a Nobel Prize in 1912 for having developed the vascular anastomosis and using it to launch the field of transplantation. However, Carrel's collaborator, Charles Guthrie, actually perfected the technique of vascular suture, which Carrel applied.[3,4,5]

The outcome of the first transplants is illustrated in Figure 33.1.[5] Although Carrel claimed the transplants to be successful, all of the recipients died during the ensuing 5 weeks. This result contrasts with the outcome of transplants performed into the same animals from which the kidneys were harvested, termed *autografts*. These results illustrate several points. Organs transplanted into unrelated individuals (*allotransplants*) almost invariably fail, while organs transplanted into oneself or into a genetically identical recipient, an isograft, survive indefinitely. This chapter will consider the biologic reasons why transplanted tissues and organs fail.

INJURY FROM HARVESTING, ISCHEMIA-REPERFUSION, AND OTHER "TECHNICAL" PROBLEMS

2 The medical condition of the source of the transplant and the donor and the procedures associated with harvesting, preserving, transplanting, and reperfusing a graft influence the outcome of transplantation, sometimes profoundly.[6] The surgical removal or "harvesting" of organs and tissues for transplantation, like any surgical procedure, damages cells and extracellular structures (Fig. 33.2). The utmost haste and meticulous technique cannot avoid completely this injury. Because these problems vary with the organ and tissue transplanted, we focus

TABLE 33.1

TERMINOLOGY OF TRANSPLANTATION

■ TERM	■ DEFINITION
Autograft	Transplant to oneself
Allograft	Transplant from one individual to another in a species
Homograft	Allograft
Isograft	Transplant to a genetically identical individual
Xenograft	Transplant from an individual of one species to an individual of another species
Heterograft	Xenograft

here on the properties and impact of ischemia-reperfusion injury common to all organs and tissues.

Severe surgical trauma, such as prolonged ischemia or failed anastomosis, can condemn an organ or tissue. Such severe injury may underlie some early deaths after transplantation illustrated in Figure 33.1 and described in Carrel's seminal report.[2] Such technical failures are still observed, but fortunately far less often. The disruption of blood flow deprives tissues of oxygen and allows wastes to accumulate; physical injury triggers aggregation of platelets and activation of coagulation and complement cascades. Severe ischemia-reperfusion injury of organ and tissue transplants can cause immediate failure of grafts to function. Even mild ischemia-reperfusion injury activates endothelium and inflammatory cells, which in turn promote immunity to grafts. By means yet uncertain, ischemia-reperfusion injury may eventuate in changes over months and years, sometimes referred to as *chronic rejection.*

Ischemia-reperfusion injury refers to tissue damage seen after disruption and subsequent restoration of blood flow to a tissue or organ. The term reflects complexity of the pathogenesis; absence of flow causes some damage, restoration of flow causes other damage. Ischemia-reperfusion injury to the heart (myocardial infarction) and brain (stroke) are leading causes of death and disability. Organs differ in the extent to which they are damaged by ischemia-reperfusion. Lung, liver, and heart are more susceptible than kidney. The risk of severe ischemia-reperfusion injury limits the time that organs can be "preserved" prior to transplantation and hence the matching of organs to the recipients most in need.

The mechanisms by which ischemia-reperfusion injures tissues remain uncertain. Table 33.2 lists some factors implicated in the pathogenesis of ischemia-reperfusion injury. Inhibition or absence of these factors can prevent or decrease ischemia-perfusion injury. Since inhibition of many different factors decreases or eliminates ischemia-reperfusion injury, those factors must function in series or in a limiting way in parallel, with injury critically dependent on the sum of independent insults. How these factors orchestrate the pathology and pathophysiology of ischemia-reperfusion injury is a question of central importance in the field of transplantation.

The factors that initiate ischemia-reperfusion injury remain unclear and are the focus of much inquiry. Surgical harvesting deprives organs and tissues of the flow of blood. Severe injury and/or prolonged deprivation of blood cause changes in small blood vessels that prevent re-establishment of perfusion, a condition referred to as *no reflow,* and directly cause necrosis.[7] Mild injury and shorter periods of ischemia cause transient changes in structure and function. Deprivation of oxygen might initiate many of the reversible changes in ischemia-reperfusion injury.[8] Reperfusion of a graft also contributes to tissue injury, perhaps to a greater extent than ischemia.

Nearly every factor that contributes to tissue injury can also protect against it.[9,10] For example, activation of complement in subtoxic amounts causes cells to acquire resistance to toxic amounts of complement.[11] Similarly, while inhibiting interleukin-1 (IL-1) decreases ischemia-reperfusion injury, treatment with IL-1 in advance of reperfusion protects against damage.[12,13] This antithesis of injury and protection suggests that ischemia-reperfusion injury may cause damage in some circumstances but may be protective in others. As only one example, ischemia-reperfusion injury may help to sequester the

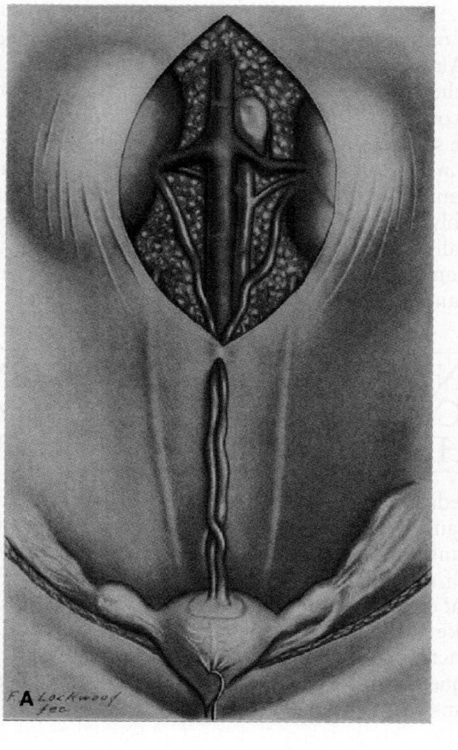

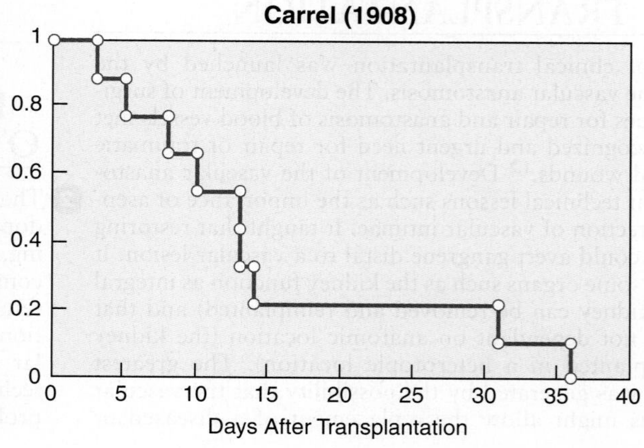

FIGURE 33.1. Method (A) and outcome (B) of the initial "successful" transplants reported by Carrel in 1908.[2] All recipients died over a period of weeks. In contrast, a few autografts performed by the same surgeon functioned for years. The difference between the outcome of autografts and allografts illustrates the preeminence of the immunologic barrier to transplantation. ([A] from Carrel A. © Originally published in *The Journal of Experimental Medicine.* 1908;10:98–140.)

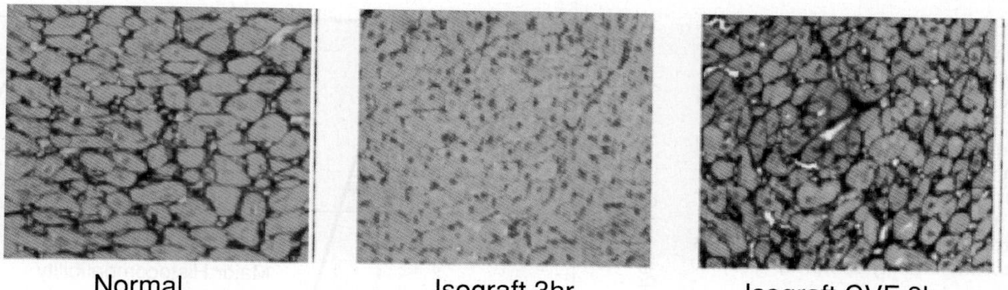

FIGURE 33.2. Impact of ischemia-reperfusion on the structure of a graft. The figure depicts heparan sulfate, a sugar that supports most of the normal functions of blood vessels, by silver staining in a normal heart (**left**) and in hearts transplanted heterotopically into genetically identical guinea pigs (**middle and right**). The micrograph on the right is from a recipient in which complement was inhibited by treatment with cobra venom factor (CVF). The figure shows that transplantation under optimal surgical conditions causes loss of all detectable heparan sulfate in a complement-dependant manner.

microorganisms through vasoconstriction and coagulation and at the same time may allow activation of antigen-presenting cells and delivery to lymphoid organs, thus promoting host defense.[14] Because the factors contributing to ischemia-reperfusion also contribute to tissue repair and host defense, the solution to the problem of reperfusion injury may not reside in complete inhibition of the processes activated by it.

GENETIC DETERMINANTS

3 The genetic relationship between the source (donor) and the recipient determines the fate of transplants that survive ischemia-reperfusion injury and technical complications of the procedure. The nature of this genetic relationship, termed *histocompatibility,* occupies a central place in the field of transplantation. Because transplants with novel genetic properties may soon enter practice, we consider in some detail the classic rules governing acceptance and failure of grafts.

Evidence for the importance of genetics in the fate of transplants emerged in the early years of the twentieth century. C.O. Jensen, a Danish biologist, discovered that tumors arising in an inbred strain of mouse could be maintained by transplanting pieces of tumor tissue between members of that strain; however, pieces of tumor transplanted into common mice would grow for a period of days and then regress and disappear. Transplanted into a mouse in which the tumor had previously regressed, the tumor would disappear almost immediately. Jensen speculated that regression of the tumor might be caused by immunity, and his observations sparked efforts in a number of laboratories to generate resistance to tumors by the transfer of serum from resistant mice. These efforts were futile and, Peter Medawar, reflecting on this period, later commented that "nearly everyone who supposed that he was using transplantation to study tumors was in fact using tumors to study transplantation—not always to very good effect."[15]

Jensen's contemporary, Leo Loeb, observed that spontaneous mammary adenocarcinomas in Japanese "waltzing" mice, so named because of a neurologic defect that made them twirl when stimulated, survived transplantation and grew in waltzing mice but never in mice of other stocks.[16] Tumors from waltzing mice grew in offspring of crosses between waltzing mice and other strains and thus appeared to be governed by the "rules" of Mendelian inheritance.[17] Tumors would not grow in mice of the F2 generation or in mice derived by crossing F1 with the resistant parent. If susceptibility to the tumor was conferred by a single genetic locus, then three fourths of the F2 generation and one half of the backcrosses should have been susceptible. This observation refuted Mendelian inheritance. From a large number of matings, a small fraction of the F2 generation and of backcrosses accepted the tumors, indicating that acceptance of tumors was governed by multiple independently segregating codominant traits.[18,19]

Investigators used congenic strains to explore in detail the role of histocompatibility or "H" genes in tumor transplantation (Fig. 33.3). Genes varied in their impact on the outcome of transplants, and the "strength" of different H genes was a specific feature of the gene. Incompatibility of strong histocompatibility genes, now known to be products of the major histocompatibility complex, inevitably caused resistance to tumors. Incompatibility of weak histocompatibility genes, now called *minor histocompatibility genes,* led sometimes but not always to resistance to tumors. Moreover, when incompatibility of weak histocompatibility genes led to tumor resistance, the tumors would often grow to larger size and over a longer period of time before resistance was manifest. Immunization with tissue incompatible for weak histocompatibility genes sometimes could make the immunized mouse resist tumors as fully as if the tumors carried strong histocompatibility disparities. Immunity to tumors was akin to immunity to normal tissues.[20] Histocompatibility, defined genetically, corresponds with immune responses and immunity aroused by transplantation of foreign tumors also recognizes nonmalignant cells of the same foreign source.[21]

The H-2 locus is a strong histocompatibility locus because tumors disparate at H-2 always regress and transplants disparate at H-2 are always rejected and the rejection reaction proceeds rapidly.[22,23] The strong histocompatibility locus was

TABLE 33.2

FACTORS CONTRIBUTING TO ISCHEMIA-REPERFUSION INJURY

■ FACTOR	■ MECHANISM
Hypoxia	Hypoxia-inducible factor
Complement	Senses injury; activates endothelium and leukocytes
Natural antibodies	Activate complement
Oxidants	Activate endothelium and damage cells
Apoptosis	Disrupts endothelium
Toll-like receptors	Activates endothelium and leukocytes
Cell adhesion molecules	Facilitate leukocyte migration
T cells	Unknown

TRANSPLANTATION

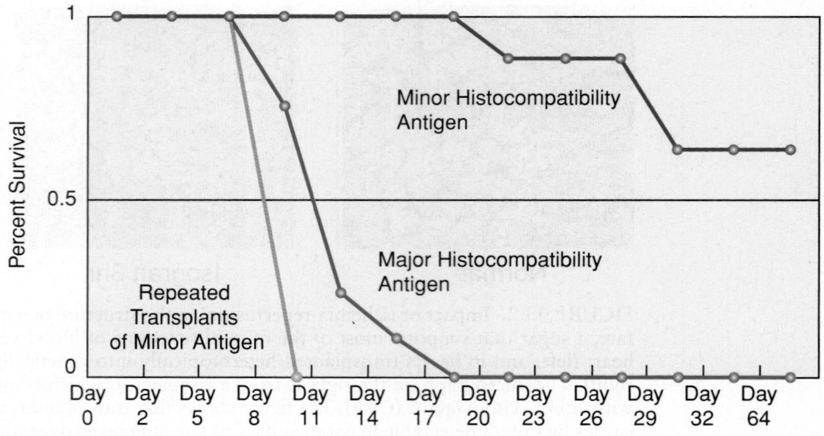

FIGURE 33.3. The outcome of transplants incompatible at strong and weak histocompatibility loci. The figure shows that incompatibility of strong histocompatibility genes causes rapid and universal rejection of allografts. Incompatibility of weak histocompatibility genes causes rejection to occur in some but not all transplants and at a relatively slow rate. Prior exposure to a transplant incompatible for a weak gene causes the response to be universal and more rapid. The locus of the strong histocompatibility genes is called the major histocompatibility complex.

later found to be a complex of genes called the *major histocompatibility complex* (MHC). Transplants matched for MHC might still undergo rejection, albeit at a slower tempo; this type of rejection was attributed to "weaker" histocompatibility antigens, later called "minor" antigens.

In 1958, Jean Dausset discovered that human patients who had received multiple transfusions of blood were subject to transfusion reactions, and contained in their serum antibodies specific for leukocyte alloantigens.[24] These antigens, ultimately called *human leukocyte antigens* (HLAs), were encoded by genes analogous to the murine H-2 genes.

The field of histocompatibility has struggled to address the nature of the genetic determinants of tissue individuality, the factors that condition recipient immune responses to foreign tissues, and the mechanisms mediating those responses. A central question has been whether antigens encoded by MHC ("MHC antigens") function only as passive targets of immune responses or whether MHC antigens participate in some way in the physiology of the immune system.[25] Another question has been what distinguishes the "strong" histocompatibility barrier posed by antigens encoded by MHC versus the weaker barrier posed by minor antigens. Yet another question concerned the nature of MHC genes and the proteins they encode that enable this system to confer uniqueness to each member of an outbred population. Only recently have answers to these questions emerged and the biologic role of histocompatibility determinants in the initiation and regulation of immune responses in normal animals been determined.

IMMUNITY AND THE REJECTION OF TRANSPLANTS

Initial efforts to connect immunity with the destruction of transplants failed. This failure stemmed from the belief that immunity was manifest only by production of antibodies and every effort to transfer immunity to transplants with immune serum failed. In the early 1940s, Landsteiner and Chase demonstrated that the cells but not the serum of sensitized animals could transfer delayed-type hypersensitivity reactions from one individual to another.[26] The existence of cellular immunity and pertinence for the rejection of transplants were appreciated by the demonstration that immunity to a transplant can be transferred by cells.[27] How the lymphoid cells, later called "T" lymphocytes because they originate in the thymus, might recognize foreign tissues became an issue of widespread interest. Those who studied transplants also failed to appreciate that antibodies have far more impact on organ grafts than on cell and tissue grafts.

The conceptual hurdles to connecting immunity with the failure of transplants were overcome by Thomas Gibson and Peter Medawar in 1943.[28] Skin allografts were thought to fail either because of local incompatibility leading to inflammation or because of immunity. Since immunity was thought only to be humoral, and since transfer of immune sera had no impact on grafts, immunity was not the favored explanation. Gibson, a surgeon, and Medawar, a biologist, asked whether immunity might cause the failure of skin grafts between different individuals (allografts). The question was urgent because surgeons were called upon to treat extensive burn wounds and skin grafting could prevent the loss of water, infection, and contractures caused by such wounds. Gibson and Medawar carried out a series of skin grafts on one human subject with extensive burns. A "first set" of skin grafts from the patient herself (autografts) and from the patient's brother (allografts) was performed. On the 10th day, the autografts and allografts appeared normal to the eye but biopsies revealed inflammation in the allografts. On the 15th day, a "second set" of autografts and allografts was performed. On the 23rd day, the first set of autografts appeared normal but the first set of allografts had deteriorated markedly. The second set of allografts (now in their eighth day) had not taken; some were detached and some appeared white and not perfused. The fate of the second set of allografts, accelerated destruction, pointed to immunity rather than a local reaction as the cause of graft loss. Medawar followed up on this initial clinical study with extensive work in rabbits.[29–31] This work confirmed irrefutably that the reaction to transplantation of foreign tissue causes the destruction of allografts and has the fundamental characteristics of an immune response. The reaction (a) is systemic, (b) is specific (e.g., the second set reaction does not afflict third-party grafts), (c) is generalized (e.g., the same reaction aroused by tumors is aroused by skin), and (d) exhibits memory. The recipient thus rejects the graft and the immune system is the vehicle of that process.

CHARACTERISTICS OF TRANSPLANT IMMUNITY

If the first 40 years of transplantation (~1906–1946) proved that Mendelian genetics and immunity govern the fate of transplants the exact mechanisms of governance are still incompletely understood. 4 Both T lymphocytes and B lymphocytes respond to transplantation, but the impact of these cells and their products varies profoundly depending on whether the transplant is an intact organ, which is attacked by both T cells and antibodies, or cells and tissues, which are attacked mainly by T cells (See Impact on Transplants below). In many cases clinicians define immune responses to transplantation based on graft injury or rejection. While the presence of graft injury may prove the existence of a destructive immune response, all immune responses to transplantation are not destructive and some may actually protect grafts.

PRODUCTS OF THE MAJOR HISTOCOMPATIBILITY COMPLEX

The immune response to products of the major histocompatibility complex (i.e., MHC) dominates the immune response to transplantation, except transplants between some siblings or inbred animals matched at the MHC.[21,22,24,32] Antigens encoded by the MHC dominate transplant immunity in part because the antigens are highly polymorphic, meaning all individuals in a species can be assumed to differ from all others at one or more loci of the MHC, and be highly antigenic.

Major Histocompatibility Complex Class I Molecules

MHC class I molecules consist of a 45-kD α chain and β_2-microglobulin, a 12-kD glycoprotein not encoded by the MHC complex (Fig. 33.4A). The MHC class I molecule has four extracellular domains, a transmembrane region, and a cytoplasmic "tail." Each MHC class I molecule has a groove that harbors an antigenic peptide. Correct folding of the class I MHC proteins depends on the presence of the peptide. The peptide and polymorphic regions of the α_1 and α_2 domains bind to the T-cell receptor. A nonpolymorphic region of the α_3 domain binds to CD8.

The peptides presented by MHC class I molecules are 8 to 10 amino acids in length and join the MHC class I molecule during assembly in the endoplasmic reticulum.[33] The peptides derive from degradation of cytoplasmic proteins by proteasomes made up of low-molecular-proteins encoded in the class II region of HLA in close linkage with genes encoding the peptide transporters for both class I and class II molecules and by other proteases. These transporters carry the peptides into the endoplasmic reticulum where the class I assembly takes place.[24] The major transporter of peptide destined to associate with MHC class I molecules is the *transporter associated with antigen processing* (TAP). The ability of the TAP to attach to a peptide determines in part the immunogenicity of the peptide. In the endoplasmic reticulum, the peptide is affixed to MHC class I molecules by a complex of proteins called the *peptide-loading complex*. This complex can promote exchange of bound peptides, further determining immunogenicity.

The peptides bound to MHC class I molecules in most cells originate either from endogenous proteins or proteins produced by viruses and other intracellular organisms. This limitation would seem to ensure that the cellular targets of cytotoxic T cells, which recognize MHC class I, include only those cells harboring intracellular microorganisms. However, this rule is violated by antigen-presenting cells, which can transform peptides derived from exogenous proteins into MHC class I molecules. This process is called *cross-presentation* (or *cross-priming*). Cross-presentation may occur in several ways; most involve the fusion of endosomes containing the products of phagocytosis, both proteins and cellular fragments, with the endoplasmic reticulum. Cross-presentation is essential for the development of cytotoxic responses against tumor cells, allogeneic cell transplants, and cells infected by viruses.

Major Histocompatibility Complex Class II Molecules

MHC class II molecules are heterodimers consisting of a 34-kD α chain and 29-kD β chain (Fig. 33.4B). MHC class II molecules are expressed mainly by specialized antigen-presenting cells such as macrophages and dendritic cells. In humans, endothelial cells also express MHC class II molecules. MHC class II molecules have four extracellular domains, a transmembrane region, and a cytoplasmic "tail." The tertiary structure of MHC class II antigens provides a pocket or antigen-binding cleft between the two polypeptide chains.[34] The assembly of MHC class II molecules in the endoplasmic reticulum requires

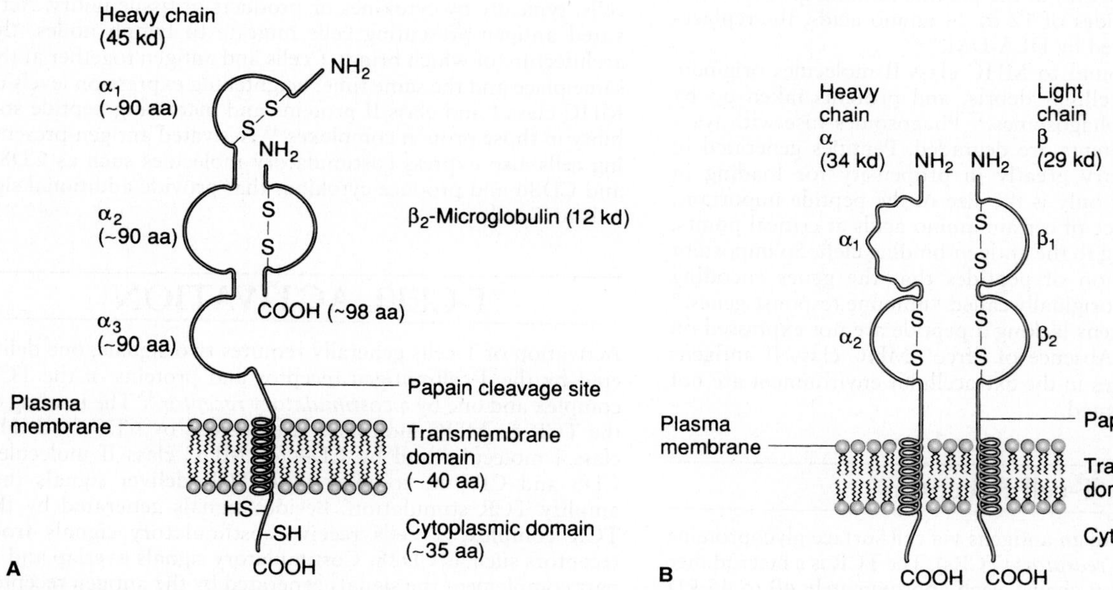

FIGURE 33.4. A: Human leukocyte antigen (HLA) class I molecule. The polymorphic heavy chain (45 kD) of the class I polypeptide is noncovalently bound to the invariant light chain, β_2-microglobulin (12 kD). The heavy chain consists of five domains—three extracellular domains (α_1, α_2, and α_3), a transmembrane domain, and a cytoplasmic domain. The α_1 and α_2 domains contain the most polymorphic residues responsible for antigen binding and form the side walls of the peptide-binding groove; the transmembrane portion anchors the molecule to the plasma membrane; and the β_2-microglobulin stabilizes the conformation of the extracellular domains. **B:** Human leukocyte antigen (HLA) class II molecule. The two chains, α (29 kD) and β (34 kD), are noncovalently associated and are made up of four domains—two extracellular domains, a transmembrane domain, and a cytoplasmic domain. Most of the allelic variance is contained in the β chain. The peptide-binding site is believed to be in the groove between the α_1 and β_1 domains.

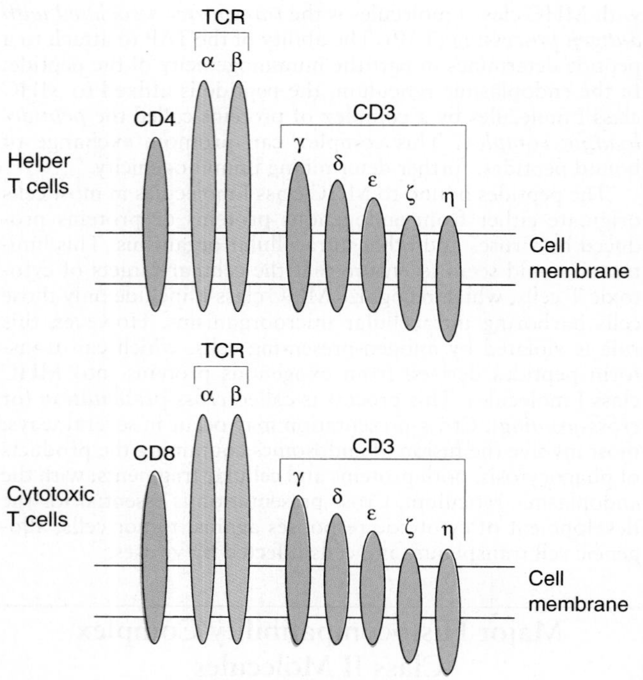

FIGURE 33.5. T-cell receptor (TCR) complex in the cell membrane composed of TCR $\alpha\beta$, CD3, CD4, and CD8 chains.

the presence of *invariant chain* or Ii, which stabilizes the tertiary structure until it is replaced by a peptide. The invariant chain also directs the traffic of MHC class II proteins from the endoplasmic reticulum to a specialized endosomal compartment known as the MHC class II compartment. There, the invariant chain is degraded, leaving *class II–associated invariant chain peptide* (CLIP) in the peptide-binding groove. CLIP is replaced by peptides of 12 to 24 amino acids, the replacement being facilitated by HLA-DM.[35,36]

The peptides bound to MHC class II molecules originate with intact cells, cellular debris, and proteins taken up by phagocytosis into phagosomes.[37] Phagosomes fuse with lysosomes and the contents are degraded. Peptides generated in phagolysosomes vary greatly in propensity for loading in MHC class II. Not only is the size of the peptide important, but also the presence of certain amino acids at critical points, which allow binding to the antigen-binding cleft. So important is this discrimination of peptides that the genes encoding MHC class II were originally called "immune response genes." MHC class II antigens lacking a peptide are not expressed on the cell surface.[38] Absence of "free" MHC class II antigens ensures that peptides in the extracellular environment are not inadvertently presented.

T-cell Receptors

T cells recognize foreign antigens via cell surface glycoproteins called *T-cell antigen receptors* (TCRs). The TCR is a heterodimer consisting of α and β chains, each approximately 40 to 45 kD and resembling immunoglobulins in three-dimensional structure (Fig. 33.5). TCRs reside in complexes with co-receptor proteins including CD3 and CD4 or CD8 that facilitate cellular signaling. While TCRs resemble immunoglobulins, they do not bind to "free" antigens as immunoglobulins do but only bind to antigens that are associated with MHC class I or class II molecules. TCR genes are assembled in T-cell precursors in the thymus by recombination of a constant region gene segment C with one each of a number of V, D, and J gene segments in the case of β chains and V and J segments in the case of α chains. Much of the diversity of the TCR repertoire is engendered by the inexact selection of the ends of the segments to be so spliced (i.e., from junctional diversity). The joining of various V, D, and J segments to form a T-cell antigen receptor gene could yield 10^{12} to 10^{16} specificities. However, from the repertoire of cells bearing TCRs actually assembled ($\sim10^{12}$ different cells), a much smaller repertoire ($\sim10^{9}$), which can bind to self-MHC proteins plus peptide, is "selected" to proceed toward maturity. This process ensures that all T cells can recognize self-MHC. Fashioning of the final T-cell repertoire in the thymus is also based on the general rule that the T cells that recognize peptides complexed with MHC class II molecules express CD4 glycoproteins; T cells that recognize MHC class I molecules express CD8 glycoproteins. The final T-cell repertoire is also fashioned by elimination of thymocytes with TCRs that bind too aggressively to self-MHC, a process called *negative selection.*

ANTIGEN PROCESSING AND PRESENTATION

Recognition of foreign antigen by T cells begins with the processing and presentation of antigen by *antigen-presenting cells.*[39] Phagocytic cells of all types, especially dendritic cells and B cells, process and present antigen. Antigen-presenting cells engulf and digest antigens (Fig. 33.6). Because cells generate many different peptides from endogenous proteins and proteins ingested into cells, relatively few peptides from any given source and of any given sequence will be presented on the cell surface at any point in time. Since activation of a T cell requires at least 200 peptides of a given type to be presented, effective presentation of peptide to a T cell capable of recognizing it is highly improbable.[40] Thus, under normal conditions, antigen-presenting cells do not effectively present peptides in association with MHC. Effective presentation of antigenic peptides requires activation of antigen-presenting cells, typically by cytokines or products of tissue injury. Activated antigen-presenting cells migrate to lymph nodes, the architecture of which brings T cells and antigen together at the same place and the same time, heightening expression levels of MHC class I and class II proteins and increasing peptide stability in those protein complexes.[41] Activated antigen-presenting cells also express costimulatory molecules such as CD80 and CD86 and produce cytokines that provide additional signals to T cells.

T-CELL ACTIVATION

Activation of T cells generally requires two signals, one delivered by the T-cell antigen receptor and proteins of the TCR complex and one by a *costimulatory receptor.*[42] The binding of the TCR to MHC molecules is enhanced by CD8 for MHC class I molecules and by CD4 for MHC class II molecules. CD8 and CD4 in complex with TCR deliver signals that amplify TCR stimulation. Besides signals generated by the TCR complex, T cells receive costimulatory signals from receptors such as CD28. Costimulatory signals overlap and in part complement the signals generated by the antigen receptor complex.[43,44] Signals delivered by the antigen receptor and by costimulatory receptors can be suppressed by stimulation of *controlling receptors* such as cytotoxic T-lymphocyte antigen-4 (CTLA-4). Both types of signals are modified further by other signals, such as those delivered by cytokines.

The biochemistry of T-cell activation and control is complex, but the biologic impact can be summarized as follows. Moderate signals delivered through the TCR complex in the

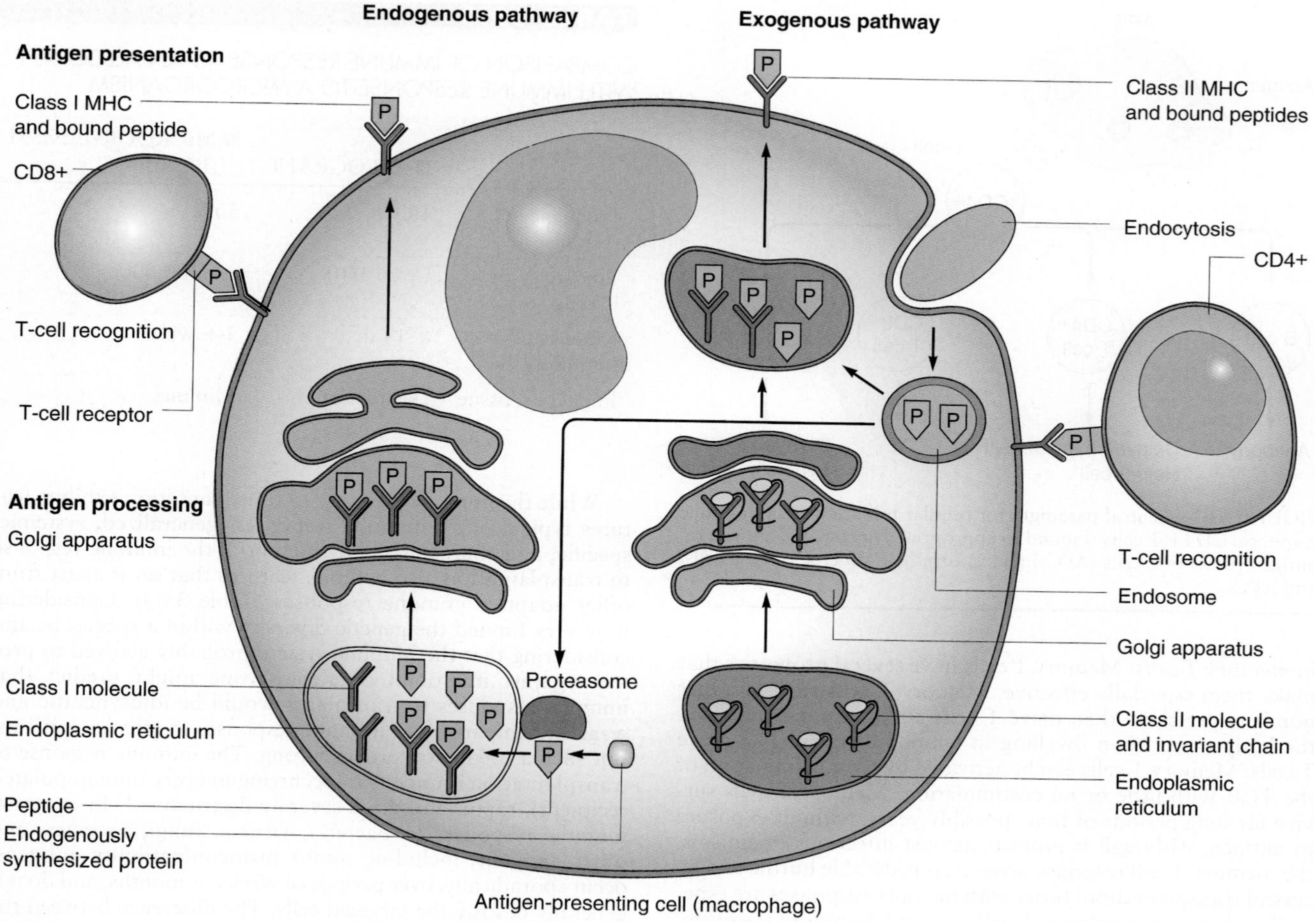

FIGURE 33.6. Antigen processing and presentation. Endogenously synthesized or intracellular proteins (e.g., viral gene products) are degraded into peptides that are transported to the endoplasmic reticulum. These peptides bind to class I major histocompatibility complex (MHC) molecules and are transported to the surface of the antigen-presenting cell. CD8+ T cells recognize the foreign peptide bound to class I MHC by way of the T-cell receptor complex. Exogenous antigen (e.g., bacterial) is endocytosed and broken down into peptide fragments in endosomes. Class II molecules are transported to the endosome in association with the invariant chain, bound to the peptide, and delivered to the surface of the antigen-presenting cell, where they are recognized by CD4+ cells.

presence of costimulatory receptors activate T cells, leading to proliferation and manifestation of effector functions such as secretion of cytokines and cytotoxicity. Moderate signals delivered through the TCR alone induce anergy, a condition in which T cells are transiently inured to delivery of full signaling. Strong signals delivered through the TCR can activate T cells without costimulation. Some allospecific T cells may be activated in this way. Finally, the survival of mature T cells depends on frequent weak signaling through the TCR; such signals reflect interaction of the TCR with MHC plus self-peptide.

Besides the specific signals delivered to T cells, the survival, activation, and apoptosis of T cells depend on the total level of signaling. Thus, the sum of many weak signals might evoke an activating response like a few strong signals. The impact of many weak signals may be especially pertinent in transplantation when T cells confront allogeneic antigen-presenting cells. The properties of the stimulated lymphocyte thus depend not only on the nature and strength of the antigenic stimulus, but also on the nature and strength of other sources of stimulation and the microenvironment in which the lymphocyte resides. For example, activation of T cells in the blood requires much more potent stimulation than activation of T cells in lymphoid tissues. Activation of T cells in lymphoid tissues may lead to a full immunologic response, whereas activation in the blood may lead to a limited response or to tolerance. To understand how T cells become activated and what governs the response of T cells, one must consider how T cells recognize antigen, the function of *accessory cells* that present antigen to T cells, and the surrounding microenvironment.

Some T cells activated by alloantigen can directly attack a graft. However, most T cells so activated provide "help" for other leukocytes that will exert the attack. These other leukocytes include B cells, CD4+ effector cells, CD8+ cytotoxic cells, and activated phagocytes like APC (Fig. 33.7).

IMMUNOLOGIC MEMORY

Protective immune responses by T cells and B cells generally reflect immunologic memory. The first encounter with foreign antigen may or may not activate naïve T cells, with activation occurring over an extended period of time (weeks). Consequently, defense against microorganisms and toxins on first encounter depends on innate immunity. Defense against subsequent encounters with microorganisms and toxins can be dominated by *immunologic memory*, which is more rapid, specific, and effective than innate immunity. The vigorous and reliable memory response to minor transplantation antigens was described earlier. For cellular immunity, memory resides

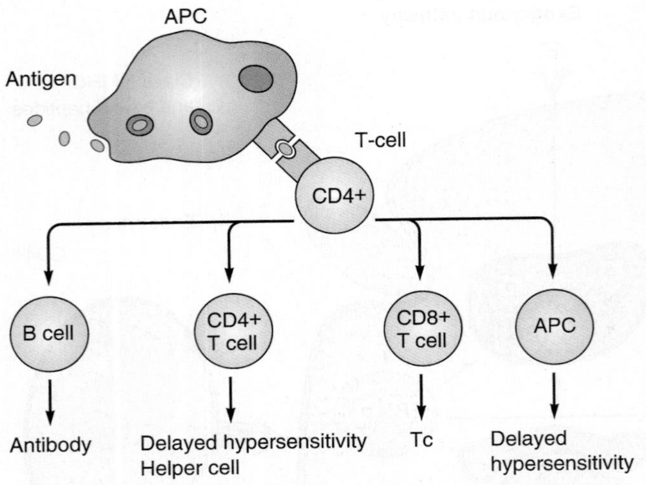

FIGURE 33.7. Central paradigm for cellular initiation of an immune response. CD4+ T cells respond to appropriately presented antigen on antigen-presenting cells (APCs) and in turn help other T cells, B cells, and APCs.

in *memory T cells.* Memory T cells have several properties that make them especially effective. Memory T cells exist in larger numbers per clone than naïve T cells and migrate throughout the body rather than dwelling in lymphoid organs like naïve T cells. Memory T cells can be activated by weak stimulation of the TCR with little or no costimulation. Memory T cells survive for long periods of time, possibly years, without exposure to antigen. Although it protects against infectious organisms, the memory T-cell response poses a considerable hurdle to successful transplantation: those with memory responses are especially prone to accelerated cellular and humoral rejection. Because primary immune responses to allogeneic stimulation are so powerful, detecting memory responses can be challenging. Allospecific antibodies against a transplant donor suggest that such a response might exist.

UNIQUE FEATURES OF THE IMMUNE RESPONSE TO TRANSPLANTATION

While recognition by T cells of foreign histocompatibility antigens might offer one explanation for the specificity of allogeneic responses, how transplants activate T cells is not so obvious. Under the best conditions, transplantation generates little costimulation. Some ischemia may be inevitable, but it is not clear that this amount would suffice to induce immunity rather than tolerance. Experimental models in which costimulation is entirely lacking reveal no diminution in rejection.[45] Thus, activation of T cells by transplants appears to violate rules governing immunity versus tolerance.

Activation of T cells by allogeneic cells poses another challenge. T cells recognize immunizing antigens if they are expressed by histocompatible cells.[25,46] Foreign antigens form a complex with self-MHC molecules, and this complex is recognized as *altered self*. Such a model allows allogeneic MHC molecules to serve as "altered self." This concept has been validated by the determination of the three-dimensional structure of the TCR in conjunction with allogeneic MHC. Thus, histocompatibility antigens are no longer thought of as mere markers of individuality but as cellular tools for the processing of antigenic peptides and the transmission of information between sets of functionally distinct immune cells. The function of MHC molecules in antigen presentation is one element of the central role of MHC antigens' alloimmune responses.

TABLE 33.3

COMPARISON OF IMMUNE RESPONSE TO AN ALLOGRAFT WITH IMMUNE RESPONSE TO A MICROORGANISM

	■ ALLOGRAFT	■ MICROORGANISM (BCG)
Frequency of response	100%	50%
Frequency of T cells	Up to 1/10	~1/100,000
Kinetics of immunity	8–14 d	3–6 wk
Impact on tissue	Destruction	Minimal

While the immune response to transplantation exhibits features typical of all immune responses (generalized, systemic, specific, and characterized by memory), the immune response to transplantation also exhibits features that set it apart from other adaptive immune responses (Table 33.3). Considering how very limited the genetic diversity within a species is, and considering that the immune system probably evolved to protect against microbial organisms, one might predict that immune responses to transplants would be idiosyncratic and weak in comparison to immune responses to microorganisms. But such a prediction proves wrong. The immune response to transplantation is universal (occurring in every unmanipulated recipient), rapid, and quite severely destructive.[47] In contrast, immune responses to bacteria, viruses, fungi, vaccines, and other antigens, including minor histocompatibility antigens, occur sporadically, over periods of weeks or months, and do not generally destroy the targeted cells. The difference between the immune response to allografts and to all other antigenic challenges could reflect the peculiar way in which antigens encoded by the major histocompatibility complex are presented, or it could reflect unanticipated immunologic memory.[48,49]

The mechanism by which T cells recognize allogeneic cells might explain the universal, rapid, and highly destructive allogeneic response. T cells can recognize allogeneic cells "directly"; T cells recognize intact allogeneic MHC expressed on allogeneic antigen-presenting cells. By direct recognition, a T cell can engage a large fraction of a given MHC on antigen-presenting cells.[50,51] Hence, direct recognition activates up to 30% of T cells.[52] In contrast, T cells recognize other antigens, such as toxins and bacterial and viral proteins, as degraded foreign peptides associated with MHC on autologous antigen-presenting cells. When T cells indirectly recognize antigen on autologous antigen-presenting cells, only a small fraction of MHC complexes on the autologous cells contain a given peptide. Hence, indirect recognition activates only a small fraction of 1% of T cells; in some cases no activation ensues.

Grafts consisting of allogeneic cells and tissues are fed by blood vessels of the recipient, and the immunologic reaction seems to be directed mainly against these blood vessels.[52–54] Recognition of these blood vessels must involve the indirect pathway. Yet these grafts are rejected universally, rapidly, and severely. Eliminating allogeneic MHC from the surface of all donor cells does not prevent or slow the course of allograft rejection.[55]

If peptides of allogeneic MHC presented indirectly can eventuate powerful rejection reactions, then the immune system might recognize peptides of allogeneic MHC differently than other proteins. The immune system is predisposed to respond aggressively to allogeneic MHC.[55] Heightened immunogenicity of MHC-derived peptides indicates that peptides from MHC efficiently load on MHC complexes.[56,57] MHC with MHC-derived peptides also interacts distinctly with T-cell receptors.

Besides efficient loading, peptides from MHC might be recognized in some special way. This idea may explain the distinct structure of TcRs bound to MHC-peptide complexes.

As still another explanation for the universal, rapid, and severe response to allotransplantation, one might postulate that the allogeneic response is actually a manifestation of immunologic memory. Generally, a protective response occurs weeks and sometimes months after the first exposure to antigen, if it occurs at all, and full protection is only exhibited upon re-exposure to antigen. On the other hand, responses on first exposure to cells bearing allogeneic MHC can be detected within a few days. The speed and intensity of the allogeneic response thus resembles the speed and intensity of the response on re-exposure to antigen. Consistent with this possibility, many of the T cells that respond to allogeneic cells in human adults are memory T cells.[58] This explanation would place alloimmune responses within the framework of conventional immune responses. Some T-cell clones for peptides of cytomegalovirus and intestinal flora also respond to allogeneic MHC. Allogeneic grafts in the newborn sometimes generate immunity and sometimes do not. Consistent with the concept, newborn mice do not reject tumor grafts acutely but can still be primed to generate second set responses, as if the antigens were minor rather than major.[60]

One practical implication of the difference in antigen recognition in alloimmune versus conventional responses is that alloimmune responses can be detected in cell cultures if allogeneic antigen-presenting cells are mixed with allogeneic T cells. For conventional antigens, primary responses are not detected in cell culture systems; only "memory" responses can be detected in this way.

The rapid kinetics of alloimmune responses probably reflects several factors. To the extent that peptides play a nominal role as antigenic targets, antigen-presenting cells of the donor are fully able to evoke alloimmune responses without antigen uptake processing and presentation. The large number of cells committed to alloimmune responses limits the amount of T-cell proliferation needed before a sizable response is achieved. Especially important, the effecter functions of the alloimmune response follow directly from activation of naïve T-cells.

REGULATION OF ALLOIMMUNE RESPONSES

The immune system must potentially recognize all microorganisms, every species of animal and plant, toxins of many types, and cells with histocompatibility antigens foreign at one or only a few amino acids. Given this diversity of recognition and destructiveness, how autoreactivity is avoided has been a question of importance for more than 100 years.[61,62] Freemartins are fraternal twins in cattle.[63] Freemartins have two kinds of erythrocytes, those that bear blood group antigens of autologous hematopoietic cells and those that bear the blood group antigens of the twin, thus making the freemartin hematopoietic chimeras. The existence of such chimerism shows that blood and hematopoietic precursor cells have been exchanged between twins sharing the same placenta. Such chimerism results from the failure to mount an immunologic response against the "foreign" blood cells; this failure is evidence of induced acceptance of a genetically distinct intrauterine graft, in other words, tolerance.[64] Thus, the discrimination between self and non-self is learned and not just inherited.

Today, one can think of tolerance at molecular, cellular, and systemic levels, yet the mechanism that avoids self-reactivity, or at least injury from self-reactivity, is incompletely known. A few aspects pertinent to transplantation immunology are mentioned and are summarized in Table 33.4. For T cells, the first and most important steps in avoiding self-reactivity take place in the thymus. Positive selection ensures that thymocytes bearing receptors that bind to anything other than MHC die. Negative selection destroys thymocytes that recognize self-MHC, and thymocytes that react to self-peptides too strongly also die. Tolerance of T cells during development in the thymus is referred to as *central tolerance.*

TABLE 33.4

MECHANISMS OF PERIPHERAL TOLERANCE

■ MECHANISM	■ EXAMPLE
Shape the repertoire to eliminate reactive lymphocytes	Peripheral deletion
Conditional responses	Anergy
Suppression	Regulatory T cells
Prevent immune-mediated injury	Accommodation

Some T cells capable of recognizing self-antigen inevitably emerge from the thymus. What prevents these cells from reacting with self has been the focus of much investigation. B cells stimulated only through the antigen receptor are not activated, and these cells are anergic.[65] B cells stimulated through the antigen receptor and by a second receptor are fully activated. Thus, activation of lymphocytes is conditional. A lymphocyte confronted with self-antigen without a second stimulus might become anergic and ultimately die; this process could shape the lymphocyte repertoire functionally and structurally to avoid self-responses. This concept of conditional responses has been supported by discovery of receptors such as CTLA-4 that deliver signals that suppress lymphocyte responses. Advances in understanding the function of antigen-presenting cells have further enriched the concept. Antigen-presenting cells confronting conditions of tissue injury heighten expression of MHC, express peptides enduringly, and express costimulatory agonists.[66] Thus, the concept of conditional responses of T cells can be used to explain how the immune system discriminates self from non-self.[67]

Anergy and conditional signaling cannot explain why transplant recipients do not become tolerant to their grafts. Vigorous immune responses are aroused by transplants under conditions in which danger signals are absent, and normal individuals suffer many small traumas every day without arousing autoimmunity to antigens in damaged tissue. Conditional immunity must depend on other controls.

Transplant immunologists in the 1970s and 1980s found that establishment of a graft for a period of time was associated with the development of suppressor cells. Perhaps lymphocytes could themselves suppress immune responses to self. This idea was not widely embraced until the 1990s, when T cells with a specific phenotype (CD25+) and functional properties (the cells proliferated slowly and did not exert effector properties) were found. The cells were called *regulatory T cells.* As further support for this mechanism, a transcription factor, foxP3, was found characteristically in these cells and was found to be essential for their function. Unfortunately, some of the immunosuppression regimens impair the function of regulatory T cells.[68]

If no theory of tolerance fully explains the lack of toxicity from self-recognition, a theory directed at the targets of immunity might do so. In the 1980s, a few transplants were performed across ABO blood group barriers in recipients temporarily depleted of anti–blood group antibodies.[69–71] Contrary to expectations, these transplants continued to function after antibodies specific for blood groups carried by the grafts returned to the circulation. The transplants were found to survive because they had acquired resistance to injury by antibody and complement.[72] This resistance was called *accommodation.*[73] The concept of accommodation has been extended to protection of tissues from T cells and inflammation.[73] If the immune system avoids self-reactivity imperfectly, cells and tissues have a way of avoiding immune-mediated injury.

Accommodation may yet prove integral to defend against invasive organisms.

PREVENTING AND TREATING TRANSPLANT REJECTION

Matching Histocompatibility Genes

Although the products of the major histocompatibility locus are extraordinarily polymorphic, MHC genes, located on the short arm of chromosome 6, can be matched. If the source and recipient are related, for example, a brother and sister, the MHC can potentially be identical. If the source and recipient are unrelated, typically if a deceased donor is the source, HLA type of both can be determined at various levels of approximation.[74] HLA typing was once performed by serology using sera of known specificity. Presently, MHC genes are identified using DNA amplified by polymerase chain reaction. Several methods are used to determine HLA-A, -B, and -DR at various levels of resolution, including sequencing of the most variable regions as necessary.

One might expect that matching a donor and recipient for MHC would minimize alloimmune responses and improve the outcome of transplantation, potentially allowing transplantation without use of immunosuppressive drugs. Consistent with this possibility, surveys in the 1980s showed that HLA compatibility improved the outcome of organ transplantation.[75–77] HLA matching takes time, thus lengthening the period before harvesting of organs or increasing ischemia-reperfusion injury. HLA matching also decreases the discretion of the clinician to find the best organ independent of HLA for each recipient. For example, matching might eclipse such considerations as matching for size or presence of viruses such as cytomegalovirus in the donor and recipient. Further, the benefit of matching is also decreased by improvements in immunosuppressive drugs.

Even where full matching of MHC can be accomplished, as in transplants between HLA-matched siblings, immunosuppressive therapy is still needed. What accounts for rejection of MHC-compatible grafts? Even with MHC typing performed by high-resolution methods, MHC sequences are not fully determined and may differ between the donor and recipient. If the donor of the transplant is infected with a virus, such as cytomegalovirus, that virus may be recognized as an alloantigen, generating an alloimmune-like response. Grafts matched with the recipient for MHC are still unmatched for other histocompatibility antigens because every protein exists as an allotype, and thus might potentially arouse an alloimmune response. In allotransplantation of the cornea, matching may actually increase the risk and/or severity of rejection, presumably because cornea antigens are presented through the indirect pathway in which alloantigen is presented as a peptide on self-MHC. With the indirect pathway, antigen presentation is best using self-MHC to present foreign peptide. To what extent this counterintuitive explanation—better matching worsens graft outcome owing to better antigen presentation—applies in cell and tissue transplantation is yet to be determined.

Besides determining HLA type, histocompatibility laboratories test would-be recipients of transplants for alloreactive antibodies. Three types of assays are performed.

The cross match tests the serum of a recipient for antibodies against a particular donor. The cross match can be performed by applying serum of the recipient to cells of the donor and testing for complement-mediated lysis or for binding by fluorescent-activated cell sorting (FACS). A strongly positive cross match indicates significant risk of hyperacute rejection, and is an absolute contraindication to transplantation.[78] The FACS cross match test can be quite sensitive, and the meaning of a weakly positive cross match is a current subject of debate.

The panel reactive antibody (PRA) test tests the serum of the recipient for antibodies against a panel of cells or antigen targets representing the broad population of potential donors. This test predicts how difficult the effort to find a cross match–negative donor for a given recipient will be. The test also predicts the risk of rejection in general, since the recipient with antibodies against many potential donors is more likely to mount a strong immune response to any transplant.

The blood type of the donor and recipient is determined. Where possible, donor and recipient are matched for ABO antigens.

IMMUNOSUPPRESSION FOR TRANSPLANTATION

Transplantation of organs and tissues in clinical subjects was attempted at various times during the first five decades of the twentieth century. With the exception of a few kidneys transplanted between identical twins, these clinical allografts always failed.[79] What allowed transplantation to succeed was the development of immunosuppressive drugs. Today, immunosuppressive drugs and regimens are so effective that many centers report success rates exceeding 90%. Some comments pertinent to the immunology of transplantation will be offered here; detailed consideration will be found in sections devoted to each type of organ transplant and in recent reviews.[68,80]

5 Immunosuppressive therapy sometimes begins with *induction therapy*. Induction therapy is delivered at the time of transplantation and usually consists of administration of antibodies, such as thymoglobulin, anti-CD3, or anti-CD25, which deplete or block the function of T cells. These treatments decrease the likelihood of early severe cellular rejection. Induction therapy might also limit ischemia-reperfusion injury, to which T cells may contribute. Because induction therapy acts directly and rapidly on many T cells, the treated individual is highly susceptible to infection and to dissemination of viruses and fungi.

The recipients of transplants are always treated with maintenance immunosuppressive therapy. Agents used for maintenance therapy are listed in Table 33.5. Combinations of agents listed in the table are usually employed to limit the complications of the drugs, because the drugs act synergistically, or both.

Given the strength and the quality of alloimmune responses, one might reasonably question why immunosuppression is effective and why the clinical course of those treated effectively is not dominated by infection. Table 33.3 compares features of the alloimmune response with features of the response against

TABLE 33.5

SOME AGENTS USED FOR MAINTENANCE IMMUNOSUPPRESSION

■ CLASS OF AGENT	■ MECHANISM[a]	■ EXAMPLES
Glucocorticoids	Regulate gene transcription	Prednisone
Calcineurin inhibitors	Inhibit protein kinases and phosphatases	Cyclosporine, tacrolimus, rapamycin
Antimetabolites	Inhibit de novo synthesis of nucleic acids	Azathioprine, mycophenolate mofetil, leflunomide

[a]The mechanisms listed predominate for class of immunosuppressive agent; however, immunosuppressive agents often act through several mechanisms, of which only one is listed.

Bacillus Calmette-Guérin (BCG). If the immune response to BCG is weaker and less predictable than the immune response to a transplant, one might predict that the response to BCG should be suppressed at lower doses of immunosuppression than immunity to transplantation. The surprising efficacy of immunosuppression for transplantation might be explained as an example of differential susceptibility of naïve and memory T cells to suppression. Thus, protective immunity conferred by memory T cells is not much abrogated by immunosuppression, and subjects presensitized to a given donor often require more immunosuppression and even then are much more susceptible to severe rejection than naïve recipients.

Immunosuppressive drugs are also used to treat established episodes of rejection. Therapeutic regimens often consist of the anti–T-cell antibodies used for induction and/or higher doses of corticosteroids. The drugs most effective for maintenance immunosuppression, particularly the calcineurin inhibitors, are not effective for treatment of established episodes of rejection. The ineffectiveness of calcineurin inhibitors for treatment of rejection is consistent with the concept that maintenance immunosuppression inhibits differentiation of naïve T cells into effector memory T cells and that cells so differentiated are less susceptible to immunosuppression.

INDUCTION OF TOLERANCE

The induction of tolerance for transplantation has been a central goal of transplantation immunology for five decades.[81,82] How to accomplish this goal without exerting undue toxicity has been difficult. Two general approaches have been proposed.

One approach to inducing allogeneic tolerance involves elimination of mature lymphocytes and other hematopoietic cells and provision of hematopoietic stem cells of the would-be transplant source, which would potentially rebuild an immune system lacking responsiveness to the hematopoietic cell source. If the source (transplant donor) is fully allogeneic, the approach should fail.[83] The thymus of the treated individual would select T cells, the function of which are restricted to the MHC of the treated individual, while the antigen-presenting cells would express incompatible MHC. In practice, however, the approach could work since fully allogeneic human thymus is capable of selecting T cells cross-reactive with allogeneic MHC.[84] Regardless, the problem of incompatible MHC can be overcome by administering hematopoietic stem cells of both the donor and the recipient.[85] The main deterrent to applying this approach to tolerance resides in the need to eliminate mature T cells and B cells. In the absence of mature lymphocytes, especially memory cells, the treated individual lacks the ability to protect against infection and the thymus of the mature individual may allow this defect to be repaired only slowly, if at all.

Another approach to inducing tolerance involves administration of inhibitors of costimulation, such as blockers of CD80, CD86, CD40, and CD40 ligand.[68,86] This approach prevents naïve T cells from being activated but avoids the eradication of memory lymphocytes and hence maintains acquired host defense. However, full tolerance is not induced and in some experimental model systems ongoing treatment is needed. The limitations may prove even more challenging because the approach does not inhibit memory T cells to any great extent and because T cells that protect against some infectious agents such as cytomegalovirus also recognize HLA.

B CELLS IN TRANSPLANTATION

B cells develop in the fetal liver and in the bone marrow of adult mammals from multipotent hematopoietic stem cells. In contrast to T cells, B cells are produced continuously throughout life. The most important feature of B-cell development is the assembly of a functional B-cell receptor, which is a membrane-bound immunoglobulin. Immunoglobulins are composed of two equal heavy and two equal light chains. Heavy and light chains have two functional domains: the variable region, which confers antigen-binding properties to the immunoglobulin, and the constant region, which confers the functional properties associated with antibodies. Immunoglobulins, like T-cell receptors, differ from most proteins in that their genes are not preformed in the germline. Immunoglobulin (Ig) heavy (H) and light (L) chain variable region exons are encoded by fragmented gene segments, variable (H+L), diversity (H), and joining (H+L) segments that must be joined by a process called *V(D)J recombination,* to generate a functional variable exon. The constant region exons are preformed in the germline. Following rearrangement of the variable gene exon, the IgH locus originates transcripts encoding Ig μ and Ig δ, containing the μ and δ HC constant region exons, which are produced by alternative splicing of a single transcript. The μ and δ heavy chains associate with light chains to produce IgM and IgD, which mark naïve B cells.

Upon activation, B cells secrete antibody as they lose membrane-bound Ig. Secretion of antibody is brought about by engaging an earlier transcription termination sequence, which excludes the membrane-encoding exons from the mature transcript. Activation of B cells also causes somatic hypermutation of the variable region exons and isotype class switch recombination. Somatic hypermutation consists of the introduction of frequent point mutations in the DNA encoding the heavy and light chain variable gene exons. Some mutations inserted in the variable region exons cause amino acid changes that modify the affinity of the antibody to its antigen. Because B cells that bind antigen better have a selective advantage, increased antibody affinity increases the likelihood of survival and favors the development of B-cell memory by creating long-lived quiescent memory B cells and long-lived antibody-secreting cells.

The various IgH isotypes are generated following B-cell activation by recombination between specialized genomic regions upstream of the constant heavy chain exons following class switch recombination. Briefly, isotype class switch consists of replacing the DNA encoding μ and δ constant regions with DNA encoding γ, α, or ε constant regions. The exchange is caused by recombination between specialized highly repetitive regions called the *switch regions* located in the intron upstream of the first exon of each constant region, with the exception of δ. Recombination involves loop-out and deletion of the intervening sequences, making class switch recombination an irreversible process. For example, once a cell produces IgG, it can no longer revert to producing IgM from the same allele.

While completely distinct processes, somatic hypermutation and class switch recombination share one necessary initiation factor, an enzyme called the *activation-induced cytidine deaminase* (AID). AID is required for somatic hypermutation and for class switch recombination.[87] AID deaminates cytidines to form uracyl (U), which is not a normal base in DNA. Introduction of U opposite a G in DNA creates a mismatch, which is resolved by DNA repair components to create point mutations or eventuating in recombination between switch regions.[88,89] It has been suggested that repair of the U-containing lesion necessarily originates DNA breaks that promote either error-prone repair, causing point mutations, or class switch recombination.[88–90]

TYPES OF B-CELL RESPONSES

Naïve B cells that come in contact with their cognate antigen differentiate into antibody-producing plasma cells or into memory cells. The path to the plasma cell differs according to the type of antigen. B cells responding to T-independent antigens differentiate into plasma cells without T-cell help but do not generate memory cells. B cells responding to T cell–dependent antigens require T-cell help to differentiate into plasma cells or into memory cells.

Transplants, blood transfusions, and pregnancy evoke humoral responses, the immunizing antigen being the donor blood group antigens, allogeneic MHC, and occasionally other foreign proteins. Blood group antigens are polysaccharides and evoke antibody responses that do not require T-cell help and are therefore called *T cell–independent responses.* Because blood group sugars are inserted onto a protein backbone, B cells that internalize part of the protein that serves as an anchor to the blood group can mount T cell–dependent antibody responses by engaging help of T cells specific to the protein backbone. Thus, T cell–dependent anti–blood group antibody responses require the activation of T cells that are specific to the allogeneic determinants of the protein bound to the blood group. Anti–blood group antibodies are often referred to as "natural" antibodies. The designation "natural" refers to the fact that these antibodies are found prior to exposure to the blood group to which they bind. Because the sugar residues that form the blood groups are abundantly present as part of bacteria walls, it is widely believed that anti–blood group antibodies are evoked in response to commensal bacteria, explaining their universal presence.

T cell–independent (TI) B-cell responses originate through one of two pathways. T cell–independent type 1 (TI-1) responses are initiated by *polyclonal activators,* such as lipopolysaccharide, which stimulate B cells through toll-like receptors.[91] T cell–independent type 2 (TI-2) responses are initiated by polysaccharide antigens and evoke antibodies that are important in the clearance of encapsulated bacteria and enteroviruses. TI-2 antigens have high molecular weight and repetitive epitopes and can thus stimulate B cells through extensive cross-linking of their surface Ig, which probably overcomes the need for T-cell help.

While it is generally accepted that antibody responses to soluble polysaccharides may be evoked in the absence of T-cell help and CD40/CD40L interaction, T cells and CD40/CD40L interaction enhance IgM and IgG antipolysaccharide responses.[92–96] In contrast, CD8+ T cells depress antipolysaccharide responses. How polysaccharides activate T cells is an unresolved question. Because polysaccharides resist degradation in vivo, they may persist in the animal, stimulating continuous B-cell activation and long-lived antibody responses.

All allotransplants may potentially evoke anti-MHC T cell–dependent antibodies, the impact of which varies profoundly with the type of transplant. T cell–dependent (TD) responses originate with the activation of T-helper cells and then proceed through the interaction of protein antigens with the B-cell receptor. Activation of B cells in this way depends absolutely on cognate T-cell help. B cells activated by protein antigens in the presence of T-cell help migrate to lymphoid follicles and form germinal centers. Here they are induced by T cells to proliferate, differentiate and hypermutate the variable region of Ig genes, switch Ig class, and give rise to plasma cells and long-lived memory B cells. Because the sequential activation of T cells and B cells in the T cell–dependent response takes time, TD antibody responses generally take much longer than T cell–independent antibody responses and are often too late to clear primary infections. However, because TD antibody responses generate high-affinity antibodies and long-lasting memory, antigens or organisms carrying TD antigens are rapidly and effectively neutralized by the memory responses. In transplantation, B-cell memory responses are one of the most vexing challenges. Memory B cells and long-lived plasma cells are resistant to B cell–depleting strategies, which effectively block antibody production de novo.

B-CELL MEMORY

The raison d'être of adaptive immunity is immunologic memory, and memory was the first feature of the immune system to be recognized. B-cell memory is characterized by a faster and more effective antibody response following a repeated antigen encounter, and is manifested by heightened clearance of the antigen. B-cell memory relies on persisting long-lived plasma cells that reside in the bone marrow or de novo generation of short-lived plasma-cells from long-lived memory B cells.[97–99] Long-lived plasma cells may be insufficient to maintain antibody levels because they may not last as long as the individual and because they must compete with newly formed plasma cells for the niches supporting their survival.[100] Thus, long-lasting humoral immunity may depend on the continuous differentiation of plasma cells from memory B cells in response to persisting antigen, to polyclonal stimuli such as nonmethylated CpG DNA acting on the TLR9 receptor, to noncognate T-cell help, or to cross-reactivity with self-antigens, or in response to stimulation by anti-idiotypic antibodies.[101,102] Whether B-cell memory requires persistence of antigen remains controversial.

B-CELL TOLERANCE

Humoral tolerance defines specific absence of a humoral immune response following an adequate stimulus in an individual fully able to respond to other immune stimuli. This definition has three critical parts. First, *tolerance* refers to the immune response and not its impact. Second, the stimulus must be adequate to induce a perceptible response; all foreign proteins are not immunogenic. Third, nonresponsiveness must be specific for the tolerizing antigen; absence of response in an immunosuppressed or immune-incompetent subject may not reflect tolerance.

Clonal deletion, receptor editing, and anergy establish tolerance in immature B cells or when the autoantigen is present during development. Elimination of self-reactive B cells is called *clonal deletion.* Membrane-bound antigens and complex autoantigens, such as DNA, that possess repetitive epitopes, with the potential to cross-link the B-cell receptor, induce central and/or peripheral deletion of antigen-specific B cells.[103]

Bone marrow B cells may also become self-tolerant by receptor editing. Receptor editing postulates that low-affinity/avidity self-antigen binding on immature B cells induces rearrangements of the immunoglobulin genes changing the cell specificity from self to non-self and presumably rescuing it from death. This salvage mechanism was first postulated to occur in immature B cells in the bone marrow.

Tolerance to soluble autoantigens is achieved by functional inactivation of self-reactive B cells. Anergic B cells express decreased amounts of surface IgM and have decreased responsiveness to B-cell receptor–mediated stimulation and shortened lifespan. Anergic B cells undergo apoptosis induced by Fas.

The mechanisms that establish tolerance of immature B cells are less efficient at precluding antibody production from mature B cells, as well illustrated by the fate of ABO-incompatible cardiac grafts in human subjects. While spontaneous tolerance occurs to A and B blood group antigens in infants with cardiac transplants, the same does not occur later in life. Infants lack the ability to produce antipolysaccharide antibodies including anti–blood group antibodies. Thus, without preexisting antibodies, the newborn becomes tolerant probably through deletion of B cells committed to producing anti–blood group antibodies upon exposure to a graft carrying these antigens. In contrast, adults who receive organ transplants carrying foreign blood group antigens continue to make anti–blood group antibodies because mature B cells are not susceptible to mechanisms that would eradicate or inactivate immature B cells.

IMPACT OF IMMUNITY ON TRANSPLANTS

Why the alloimmune response is more destructive than other immune responses is not fully understood. Alloimmune

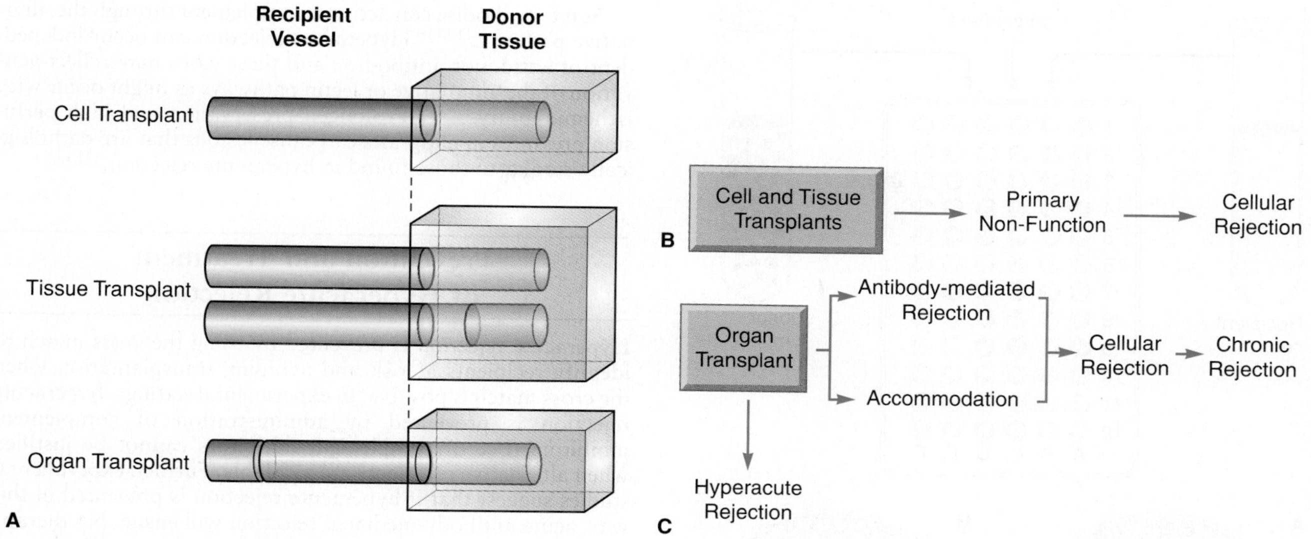

FIGURE 33.8. **A:** The origin of blood vessels in cell, tissue, and organ grafts. Both cell and tissue grafts are fed at least in part by blood vessels of the recipient. Organ grafts depend entirely on blood vessels of the donor. The consequences of this difference are shown in panels B and C. **B:** Cell and tissue transplants. Fed by blood vessels of the recipient, cell and tissue transplants are susceptible mainly to early nonfunction, perhaps owing to ischemia and cellular rejection. Antibodies and complement of the recipient penetrate poorly through blood vessel walls and hence do not injure these grafts. **C:** Organ transplants. An organ transplant is fed entirely by vessels of the transplant donor. Consequently, antibodies made by the recipient can bind to the blood vessel walls and cause injury manifest as hyperacute or acute vascular rejection and chronic rejection. Under some circumstances antibodies can cause an organ graft to resist immunological injury. This condition is called accommodation.

responses mainly attack blood vessels.[29,53,54] The targeted cells rapidly impair blood flow to transplanted organs and tissues. Since all donor blood vessels and many recipient blood vessels are affected, the impact is diffuse and profound and the viability of the transplant is rapidly compromised. As a related consideration, the direct attack of T cells, antibodies, and complement on transplanted cells may preclude the development of accommodation.

6 The impact of immunity on transplants depends to the greatest extent on whether transplants consist of cells, tissues, 7 or organs (Fig. 33.8).[104] All transplants are susceptible to cellular rejection. However, transplants differ profoundly in susceptibility to humoral immunity. The differential susceptibility to humoral immunity reflects in large part the way in which the transplant receives its vascular supply.

Isolated cells, such as hepatocytes, derive their vascular supply entirely from the host.[105] Antibodies of the recipient do not bind to blood vessels in these grafts, and very limited amounts of antibody penetrate the vessels to reach the allografted cells. The level of complement outside of vascular lumina is much lower than inside. Hence, blood vessels of the recipient of a cellular transplant shield the transplant from antibody- and complement-mediated injury.

Free tissues, such as skin and pancreatic islets, derive their vascular supply both by the in-growth of blood vessels of the recipient and by spontaneous anastomosis of graft and host capillaries. Antibodies of the recipient can bind to donor segments of these vessels and in doing so may cause focal ischemia in some types of grafts via vascular reactions.[106,107] Vascularization of tissue grafts by blood vessels of the recipient provides a parallel supply of blood and a partial shield against humoral injury.

Organ grafts such as heart, kidney, liver, and lung derive blood flow from the surgical anastomosis of donor and recipient vessels. The graft is thus fed entirely through a vascular system that is foreign to the immune system of the recipient. Antibodies of the recipient can bind to these foreign vessels. Antibody-mediated injury is observed in organ grafts to a much greater extent than in cell or tissue grafts. Furthermore, because immunoglobulins are largely confined to vascular spaces, alloreactive antibodies have minimal direct impact on parenchymal cells.[105,108]

HYPERACUTE REJECTION

Hyperacute rejection occurs within 24 hours of reperfusion and is characterized by immediate loss of graft function and by a pathologic picture of interstitial hemorrhage, thrombosis, and varying extents of inflammation. Hyperacute rejection is thought to be caused by antidonor antibodies binding to blood vessels and activating the complement system in a newly transplanted organ. The development of hyperacute rejection depends absolutely on the activation of complement, and inhibition of complement nearly always prevents hyperacute rejection.[73]

Anti-HLA antibodies most often cause hyperacute rejection of clinical allografts. Hyperacute rejection occurs in up to 80% of the kidneys transplanted into recipients with cytotoxic antibodies detected by cytotoxic cross match[78] (Fig. 33.9). Hyperacute rejection is now observed rarely because assays for anti-HLA antibodies identify subjects at risk and transplantation is avoided. FACS methods are especially sensitive but they may also exclude from transplantation recipients with very low levels of anti-HLA antibodies or non–complement-fixing antibodies who might safely receive a transplant.[109] The lymphocytotoxic cross match illustrated in Figure 33.9 is less sensitive, but a positive result may predict hyperacute rejection with more confidence.

Antibodies directed at blood group A and B antigens in a graft can also cause hyperacute rejection. Gleason reported that 46% of ABO-incompatible allografts never gained function and at 12 months only 1 of 24 ABO-incompatible renal transplants continued to function, whereas only 9% of a large group of ABO-compatible grafts did not show early function.[110] Whether anti–blood group antibodies cause hyperacute rejection depends on such factors as the antibody levels and the affinity and susceptibility of the graft to injury. For example, the A2 antigen interacts less well with anti-A antibodies; hence, organs expressing A2 transplanted into recipients of blood group O are less susceptible to destruction by humoral responses.[111]

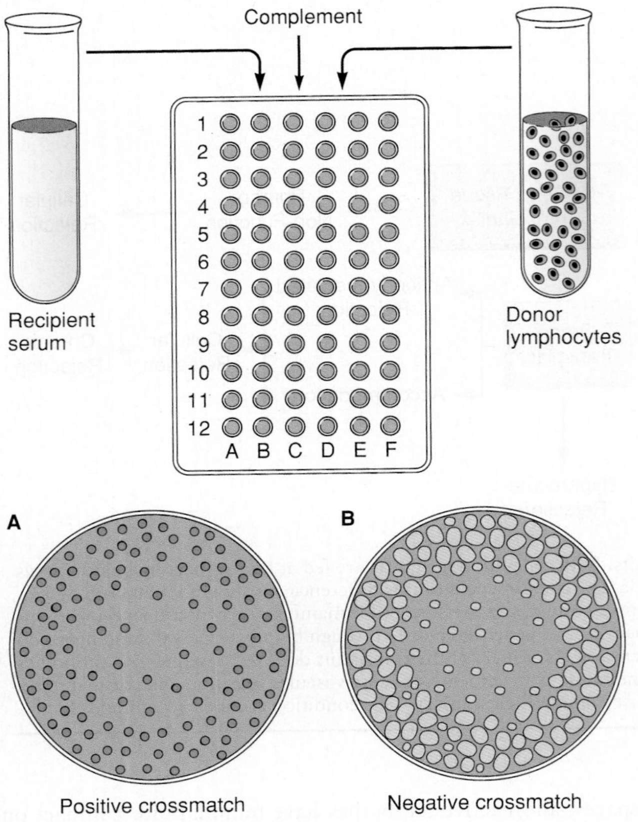

FIGURE 33.9. Lymphocytotoxicity cross match. Recipient serum is incubated with donor lymphocytes and complement in microtiter plates. If donor-specific lymphocytotoxic antibodies are present in the recipient serum, antibody binding results in complement fixation and lysis of the donor lymphocytes. This is detected by the addition of a dye that is taken up through the damaged cell membrane, and a positive cross match is noted (**A**). If no antibodies are present, cells remain viable and do not take up the dye (**B**). This is a negative cross match. A more sensitive approach to cross matching involves use of the fluorescence activated cell sorter (FACS) (not shown). This device detects antibody binding with great sensitivity but does not detect whether binding would be injurious.

ABO-incompatible organs vary in susceptibility to hyperacute rejection, liver transplants being less susceptible than kidney or heart transplants. The 3-year graft survival rate for ABO-compatible liver grafts and ABO-incompatible grafts is remarkably similar, 39% and 36%, respectively.[112] Differences in the size of the vascular beds may explain the varying susceptibility, as a given amount of antibody and complement would be deposited less densely in the liver than in a smaller organ such as the kidney. The liver also intrinsically resists injury by complement.[73,113]

Hyperacute rejection sometimes occurs in recipients lacking detectable antidonor antibodies. In some cases, antibody capable of causing rejection is present in the blood but is not detected by assays in which leukocytes are used as the target. For example, the major histocompatibility complex class I–related chain A is not expressed on leukocytes but is expressed on endothelial cells, and antibodies against that antigen have been postulated to cause some cases of hyperacute rejection in recipients with a negative cross match.[114,115] Similarly, antibodies against yet undefined endothelial antigens have also been linked to rejection of transplants between HLA-identical sibling transplants.[116] In other cases, the recipient may truly lack antidonor antibodies and the alternative or lectin pathways without the involvement of antibody may activate complement.

Some antibodies can activate complement through the alternative pathway.[117,118] Hyperacute rejection can occur independent of antidonor antibodies, and these cases may reflect activation of the alternative or lectin pathways as might occur with ischemic injury.[119,120] Prolonged preservation and high perfusion pressures in allografts can cause lesions that are pathologically similar to those found in hyperacute rejection.[121,122]

Prevention and Treatment of Hyperacute Rejection

Hyperacute rejection is prevented by using the cross match to identify recipients at risk and avoiding transplantation when the cross match is positive. In experimental settings, hyperacute rejection is prevented by administration of complement inhibitors. Use of complement inhibitors cannot be justified when alternative recipients are available. Further, experimental studies suggest that if hyperacute rejection is prevented in this way, acute antibody-mediated rejection will ensue. No therapy has proven effective for hyperacute rejection once it has begun.

ANTIBODY-MEDIATED REJECTION

Antibody-mediated rejection is a vexing condition.[123,124] Previously known as "humoral rejection" and before that as "acute vascular rejection," antibody-mediated rejection has been considered very difficult and expensive to reverse. Most cases appear to be caused by antibodies and therefore the term *antibody-mediated rejection* is used.

Antidonor antibodies such as those directed at MHC antigens likely trigger antibody-mediated rejection. The timing of antibody-mediated rejection after transplantation depends mainly on when antidonor antibodies are produced. In the absence of immunosuppression, antibody-mediated rejection can begin within 24 hours of transplantation and proceed over days if the recipient is sensitized to donor antigen. In immunosuppressed recipients, antibody-mediated rejection usually appears weeks or months after transplantation.

Evidence of antibody-mediated rejection can be found in 20% to 30% of episodes of acute rejection, but the diagnosis of antibody-mediated rejection is sometimes challenging.[125] Although antibodies specific for the donor are sometimes found in the circulation, such antibodies are not often found at high levels. The absence of antidonor antibodies does not exclude antibody-mediated rejection, because an organ graft can absorb tremendous amounts of antibody, leaving little or none in the blood.[126] Also, the antibodies found in the blood may be of lower affinity and thus may not represent the antibodies bound to the graft and those that cause tissue injury.

Because of the limited value of measuring antidonor antibodies, pathologists have turned to the detection of C4d as diagnostic evidence of antibody-mediated rejection.[127] C4d deposits in peritubular capillaries of transplant recipients with circulating donor-specific antibodies strongly suggest that C4d is a specific and reliable indication of antibody-mediated rejection following kidney transplantation.[128] Formed by cleavage of C4b covalently bound to target cells, C4d is functionally inert and hence a relatively enduring footprint of complement activation. Since C4 can be cleaved during activation of the classic pathway, the presence of C4d on the endothelium of a graft is taken as evidence that antidonor antibody has bound to that site. C4d is also generated during activation of the lectin pathway; hence, it might be found in some conditions in which antidonor antibodies do not exist. C4d can also be found in accommodation, a condition in which the graft resists injury caused by antibody and complement. Given these considerations, detection of C4d should not be taken by itself to mark antibody-mediated rejection; other evidence is needed to make that diagnosis.

Antibody-mediated rejection is characterized pathologically by focal ischemia, severe injury to the endothelial cells lining blood vessels in the graft, and intravascular coagulation. Antibody-mediated rejection is thought to be caused by endothelial cell activation in the graft.[129,130] Normally, resting endothelial cells inhibit coagulation through expression of such anticoagulant molecules as thrombomodulin and heparan sulfate proteoglycan.[131,132] The binding of antidonor antibodies to endothelium in the graft and the activation of complement disrupt the quiescent state and cause the endothelium to become activated. Activated endothelial cells promote coagulation by shedding thrombomodulin and heparan sulfate proteoglycan and subsequently expressing tissue factor and plasminogen activator inhibitor type 1.[133] Inflammation is promoted by activated endothelial cells, which induce expression of cell adhesion molecules and cytokines.[134] Complement-induced coagulation and inflammation both appear to be governed by transcription and production of IL-1α and by the availability of that cytokine to act in local blood vessels.[135,136] Coagulation and inflammation impair the flow of blood through regions of the vasculature, and this impairment probably accounts for the pathologic manifestations of antibody-mediated rejection, which are most consistent with ischemia.

Prevention and Treatment of Antibody-mediated Rejection

For many years, antibody-mediated rejection was thought to be inseparable from cellular rejection, but unlike cellular rejection, it resisted all therapeutic efforts. Recently, better approaches to treatment have emerged. Plasmapheresis, sometimes used in conjunction with administration of cytotoxic drugs, can effectively overcome established episodes of antibody-mediated rejection. This therapy engenders risk and is quite expensive. Administration of γ-globulin, sometimes in conjunction with plasmapheresis, has also proven effective. Gamma-globulin inhibits production of antibodies, blocks Fc receptors, and diverts activated fragments of complement away from endothelium. Anti–B cell antibodies, such as anti-CD20, have been used in some cases of antibody-mediated rejection with anecdotal claims of success. If confirmed, the success of these antibodies might point to functions of B cells other than antibody production, since plasma cells, which do not express CD20, probably produce most alloreactive antibodies.

CHRONIC REJECTION

8 Chronic rejection, more than any other condition, limits the long-term success of solid organ transplantation. Chronic rejection or chronic graft dysfunction may be caused by a number of processes, particularly repeated inflammation and injury from both immune- and non–immune-mediated causes. In the kidney, chronic rejection is sometimes called *chronic allograft nephropathy*; in the heart, *accelerated arteriosclerosis*; in the lung, *bronchiolitis obliterans*; and in the liver, *vanishing bile duct syndrome*. The term *chronic rejection* might best be applied to chronic graft dysfunction caused by an immunologic reaction and chronic allograft dysfunction caused by drug toxicity, ischemia, aging, and other nonimmunologic processes. While the clinical signs are organ specific, the result of chronic rejection is similar for all solid organ allografts - inexorable loss of function. Obliterative vasculopathy, infiltration of leukocytes, luminal occlusion, and a marked fibrotic response are common to many types of chronic rejection and are believed to account for loss of function.

Antidonor antibodies cause up to 60% of chronic dysfunction of organ transplants.[137] Circulating antidonor HLA antibodies correlate strongly with chronic rejection.[138] De novo anti-HLA antibodies are always present prior to graft failure. Whether antidonor antibodies actually cause chronic rejection or reflect a response to a damaged graft caused by other factors has not been determined.

The presence of C4d deposits seen in chronic graft dysfunction has been taken to implicate humoral immunity in the loss of graft function; 64% of subjects with chronic rejection have C4d deposits in graft biopsies.[139] In one report, all with donor-specific antibodies at the time of biopsy also had C4d deposits, and 90% of those positive for C4d also had antidonor antibodies.[137] C4d deposits precede and predict the development of chronic allograft glomerulopathy.[140] No treatment has proven effective for chronic rejection.

ACCOMMODATION

Accommodation refers to acquired resistance of an organ graft to humoral injury. Accommodation was first described and later named based on observations of the outcome of ABO-incompatible kidney transplants.[72,73,141] In the mid-1980s, several investigators observed that if anti–blood group antibodies were removed from the circulation at the time of transplantation, kidneys transplanted across blood group A or blood group B barriers could survive and function.[70,71] This suggested that incompatibility of blood groups was not an absolute barrier to transplantation and prompted the question of how these kidneys survived. Some recipients had antibodies specific for donor blood groups and the transplanted kidneys continued to express donor antigen, but graft injury and compromise of function did not occur. This observation suggested that the survival of the graft must reflect some change in the graft itself. Accommodation may be more frequent than currently assumed.[142] Healthy organs can absorb antidonor antibodies in large amounts, removing these antibodies from the circulation, and hence more recipients may make antidonor antibodies than surveys of the prevalence of antibodies would suggest.

Accommodation might reflect a change in the properties of the antibody or the antigen. Both of these mechanisms have been observed in experimental models. Under some conditions, the Ig subclass of antidonor antibodies does not efficiently fix complement and may even block the binding of complement-fixing antibodies.[142,143] In other conditions, carbohydrate antigen may be shed or undergo biochemical change and therefore might be less avidly bound.[144–146]

While these models may apply in some cases, most studies suggest that accommodation reflects resistance to injury. Exposure of an organ to heme induces heme oxygenase, which can protect the organ against lethal injury by various toxins.[147] Xenografts and allografts with accommodation express a number of "protective," antiapoptotic genes.[148,149] Products of these genes may prevent cells of the graft from undergoing apoptosis that otherwise would be triggered by humoral immunity. Consistent with this concept, exposure to xenoreactive antibodies induces expression of antiapoptotic genes in endothelial cells.[150] Anti-HLA antibodies likewise induce such genes.[151] Further understanding of how accommodation is induced and by what mechanisms it is manifest and maintained could have a profound impact on transplantation in general and perhaps on other fields.

CELLULAR REJECTION

All allografts are subject to cellular rejection, and the clinical application of transplantation depends absolutely on suppressing or eradicating cellular immune responses to the transplant source. Accordingly, no subject in transplantation has been studied more thoroughly than cellular rejection. Most research has focused on the mechanisms by which T cells are activated and the antigenic target of activated T cells. Much less has been elucidated about how cellular immunity, once induced, destroys transplants and why such destruction is more violent and complete than the tissue injury seen in autoimmune diseases.

Cellular rejection is directed against small blood vessels of the graft, at least initially. The blood vessels appear to be targeted by two fundamental mechanisms.[152,153] One mechanism involves the action of cytotoxic T cells. The importance of cytotoxic T cells is suggested by the observation that in grafts consisting of mixtures of allogeneic and isogeneic cells, the allogeneic cells are destroyed and the isogeneic cells are spared.[154] In grafts consisting of both allogeneic and syngeneic islets of Langerhans, the allogeneic islets were destroyed, while syngeneic islets, even those adjacent to allogeneic islets, survived.[155] However, early in the course, rejecting allografts do not contain many dead cells. This inconsistency raises the possibility that some function of cytotoxic cells other than killing may account for tissue injury. One potential effector is perforin, a pore-forming protein. Perforin and other pore-forming proteins activate endothelial cells and in so doing could evoke focal ischemia, inflammation, and thrombosis.[156] One concern about implicating cytotoxic T cells in the pathogenesis of cellular rejection is the observation repeated in many laboratories that rejection of allografts can be brought about by helper cells alone and proceeds fully when cytotoxic cells are eliminated.[157] These observations can be explained by the extraordinary extent to which immunity is aroused by allotransplantation; far more effector cells are activated than are needed for rejection.

The second mechanism of tissue injury in cellular rejection can be likened to delayed-type hypersensitivity. Helper T cells and some cytotoxic T cells secrete cytokines that modify the functions of blood vessels to promote leukocyte migration, thrombosis, and ischemia. Cellular rejection departs from delayed-type hypersensitivity in several respects. First, cellular rejection is often dominated by cytotoxic cells (CD8+) and delayed-type hypersensitivity by helper cells (CD4+).[158,159] Cellular rejection is associated with microvascular injury and thrombosis, whereas delayed-type hypersensitivity is characterized by edema and relatively uninjured blood vessels. Both allograft rejection and delayed-type hypersensitivity may be driven by products secreted by T cells, although the products may differ. Alloreactive T cells may preferentially secrete cytokines and other agonists when the TCR is stimulated by an adjacent allogeneic cell—the same mechanism that ensures specificity of cytoxic cells for their targets may ensure specificity of helper cells for theirs.

CONCLUDING REMARKS

This chapter reviews the immunology of transplantation as it is practiced in the first decade of the 21st century and elucidated over the past century. However, the practice of transplantation may soon change, as transplants consisting of stem cells, stem cell derivatives, and engineered tissues are used. Stem cells interact with the immune system in ways, very different from mature cells and organs. These differences will become important as surgeons turn increasingly to regenerative medicine and novel approaches to organ replacement for the treatment of disease.

References

1. Watts SH. VIII. The suture of blood vessels. Implantation and transplantation of vessels and organs. An historical and experimental study. *Ann Surg* 1907;46:373–404.
2. Carrel A. Transplantation in mass of the kidneys. *J Exp Med* 1908;10: 98–140.
3. Guthrie CC. On misleading statements. *Science* 1909;29:29–31.
4. Guthrie CC. *Blood-Vessel Surgery and Its Applications*. New York: Longmans, Green & Co; 1912.
5. Carrel A. The ultimate result of a double nephrectomy and the replantation of one kidney. *J Exp Med* 1911;14:124–125.
6. Jamieson RW, Friend PJ. Organ reperfusion and preservation. *Front Biosci* 2008;13:221–235.
7. Vanlangenakker N, Berghe TV, Krysko DV, et al. Molecular mechanisms and pathophysiology of necrotic cell death. *Curr Mol Med* 2008;8: 207–220.
8. Walshe TE, D'Amore PA. The role of hypoxia in vascular injury and repair. *Annu Rev Pathol* 2008;3:615–643.
9. Holzknecht ZE, Platt JL. The fine cytokine line between graft acceptance and rejection. *Nat Med* 2000;6:497–498.
10. Holzknecht ZE, Platt JL. Accommodation and the reversibility of biological systems. *Transplantation* 2001;71:594–595.
11. Shin ML, Carney DF. Cytotoxic action and other metabolic consequences of terminal complement proteins. *Prog Allergy* 1988;40:44–81.
12. Saadi S, Takahashi T, Holzknecht RA, et al. Pathways to acute humoral rejection. *Am J Pathol* 2004;164:1073–1080.
13. Brown JM, White CW, Terada LS, et al. Interleukin 1 pretreatment decreases ischemia/reperfusion injury. *Proc Natl Acad Sci U S A* 1990;87: 5026–5030.
14. Saadi S, Wrenshall LE, Platt JL. Regional manifestations and control of the immune system. *FASEB J* 2002;16:849–856.
15. Medawar PB. The immunology of transplantation. *Harvey Lect Ser* 1956–1957;52:144–176.
16. Loeb L. Über enstehung eines Sarkoms nach Transplantation eines Adenocarcinoms einer japanischen maus. *Z Krebsforsch* 1908;7:80–110.
17. Tyzzer EE. A study of inheritance in mice with reference to their susceptibility to transplantable tumors. *J Med Res* 1909;22:519–573.
18. Little CC, Tyzzer EE. Further experimental studies on the inheritance of susceptibility to a transplantable tumor, carcinoma (J.W.A.) of the Japanese Waltzing mouse. *J Med Res* 1916;33:393–453.
19. Little CC. The genetics of tissue transplantation in mammals. *Cancer Res* 1924;8:75–95.
20. Woglom WH. Immunity to transplantable tumors. *Cancer Rev* 1929;4: 129–214.
21. Gorer P. The genetic and antigenetic basis of tumor transplantation. *J Pathol Bacteriol* 1937;44:691–697.
22. Gorer PA, Lyman S, Snell GD. Studies on the genetic and antigenic basis of tumour transplantation. Linkage between a histocompatibility gene and "fused" in mice. *Proc R Soc Lond B Biol Sci* 1948;135:499–505.
23. Barth R, Counce S, Smith P, et al. Strong and weak histocompatibility gene differences in mice and their role in the rejection of homografts of tumors and skin. *Ann Surg* 1956;144:198–204.
24. Dausset J. Iso-leuco-anticorps. *Acta Haematol* 1958;20:156–166.
25. Doherty PC, Zinkernagel RM. A biological role for the major histocompatibility antigens. *Lancet* 1975;1:1406–1409.
26. Landsteiner K, Chase MW. Experiments on transfer of cutaneous sensitivity to simple compounds. *Proc Soc Exp Biol Med* 1942;49:688–690.
27. Mitchison NA. Passive transfer of transplantation immunity. *Nature* 1953;171:267–268.
28. Gibson T, Medawar PB. The fate of skin homografts in man. *J Anat* 1943; 77:299–310.
29. Medawar PB. A behaviour and fate of skin autografts and skin homografts in rabbits. *J Anat* 1944:78:176–199.
30. Medawar PB. A second study of the behaviour and fate of skin homografts in rabbits. *J Anat* 1945;79:157–176.
31. Medawar PB. Immunity to homologous grafted skin: the relationship between the antigens of blood and skin. *Br J Exp Pathol* 1946;27:15–24.
32. Dausset J, Nenna A. Presence d'une leuco-agglutinine dans le serum d'un can d'agranulocytose chronique. *C R Seances Soc Biol Fil* 1952;146: 1539–1541.
33. Jensen PE. Recent advances in antigen processing and presentation. *Nat Immunol* 2007;8:1041–1048.
34. Brown JH, Jardetzky TS, Gorga JC, et al. Three-dimensional structure of the human class II histocompatibility antigen HLA-DR1. *Nature* 1993; 364:33–39.
35. Sadegh-Nasseri S, Chen M, Narayan K, et al. The convergent roles of tapasin and HLA-DM in antigen presentation. *Trends Immunol* 2008;29: 141–147.
36. Ferrante A, Anderson MW, Klug CS, et al. HLA-DM mediates epitope selection by a "compare-exchange" mechanism when a potential peptide pool is available. *PLoS ONE* 2008;3:e3722.
37. Vyas JM, Van der Veen AG, Ploegh HL. The known unknowns of antigen processing and presentation. *Nat Rev Immunol* 2008;8:607–618.
38. Nelson CA, Petzoid SJ, Unanue ER. Peptides determine the lifespan of MHC class II molecules in the antigen-presenting cell. *Nature* 1994;371: 250–252.
39. Germain R. MHC-dependent antigen processing and peptide presentation: providing ligands for T lymphocyte activation. *Cell* 1994;76:287–299.
40. Harding CV, Unanue ER. Quantitation of antigen-presenting cell MHC class II/peptide complexes necessary for T-cell stimulation. *Nature* 1990; 346:574–577.
41. Stoll S, Delon J, Brotz TM, et al. Dynamic imaging of T cell-dendritic cell interactions in lymph nodes. *Science* 2002;296:1873–1876.

42. Song J, Lei FT, Xiong X, et al. Intracellular signals of T cell costimulation. *Cell Mol Immunol* 2008;5:239–247.
43. Torgersen KM, Aandahl EM, Tasken K. Molecular architecture of signal complexes regulating immune cell function. *Handb Exp Pharmacol* 2008: 327–363.
44. Liston A, Enders A, Siggs OM. Unravelling the association of partial T-cell immunodeficiency and immune dysregulation. *Nat Rev Immunol* 2008;8: 545–558.
45. Bingaman AW, Ha J, Waitze SY, et al. Vigorous allograft rejection in the absence of danger. *J Immunol* 2000;164:3065–3071.
46. Zinkernagel RM, Doherty PC. Restriction of in vitro T cell-mediated cytotoxicity in lymphocytic choriomeningitis within a syngeneic or semiallogeneic system. *Nature* 1974;248:701–702.
47. Platt JL, Rubinstein P. Mechanisms and characteristics of allograft rejection. In: Sabiston DC Jr, Lyerly HK, eds. *Textbook of Surgery. The Biological Basis of Modern Surgical Practice*. Philadelphia: W.B. Saunders; 1997: 400–408.
48. Cascalho M, Ma A, Lee S, et al. A quasi-monoclonal mouse. *Science* 1996;272:1649–1652.
49. AbuAttieh M, Rebrovich M, Wettstein PJ, et al. Fitness of cell-mediated immunity independent of repertoire diversity. *J Immunol* 2007;178: 2950–2960.
50. Matzinger P, Bevan MJ. Hypothesis: why do so many lymphocytes respond to major histocompatibility antigens? *Cell Immunol* 1977;29:1–5.
51. Felix NJ, Donermeyer DL, Horvath S, et al. Alloreactive T cells respond specifically to multiple distinct peptide-MHC complexes. *Nat Immunol* 2007;8:388–397.
52. Suchin EJ, Langmuir PB, Palmer E, et al. Quantifying the frequency of alloreactive T cells in vivo: new answers to an old question. *J Immunol* 2001; 166:973–981.
53. Dvorak HF, Mihm MC Jr, Dvorak AM, et al. Rejection of first-set skin allografts in man. The microvasculature is the critical target of the immune response. *J Exp Med* 1979;150:322–337.
54. Pober JS, Bothwell AL, Lorber MI, et al. Immunopathology of human T cell responses to skin, artery and endothelial cell grafts in the human peripheral blood lymphocyte/severe combined immunodeficient mouse. *Springer Semin Immunopathol* 2003;25:167–180.
55. Auchincloss H, Lee R, Shea S, et al. The role of "indirect" recognition in initiating rejection of skin grafts from major histocompatibility complex class II-deficient mice. *Proc Natl Acad Sci U S A* 1993;90:3373–3377.
56. Chicz RM, Urban RG, Lane WS, et al. Predominant naturally processed peptides bound to HLA-DR1 are derived from MHC-related molecules and are heterogeneous in size. *Nature* 1992;358:764–768.
57. João CM, Ogle BM, Gay-Rubenstein C, et al. B cell-dependent TCR diversification. *J Immunol* 2004;172:4709–4716.
58. Lombardi G, Sidhu S, Daly M, et al. Are primary alloresponses truly primary? *Int Immunol* 1990;2:9–13.
59. Billingham RE, Brent L, Medawar PB. Actively acquired tolerance of foreign cells. *Nature* 1953;172:603.
60. Ando K, Hasegawa T, Nakashima I, et al. Ontogeny of the transplantation immunity of mice for rejecting ascitic allogeneic tumors. *Dev Comp Immunol* 1985;9:701–708.
61. Ehrlich P, Morgenroth J. On hæmolysins. Fifth communication. In: Himmelweit F, ed. *The Collected Papers of Paul Ehrlich*. London, UK: Pergamon; 1957:246–255.
62. Landsteiner K. Cell antigens and individual specificity. *J Immunol* 1928; 15:589–600.
63. Gamadia LE, Remmerswaal EB, Surachno S, et al. Cross-reactivity of cytomegalovirus-specific CD8+ T cells to allo-major histocompatibility complex class I molecules. *Transplantation* 2004;77:1879–1885.
64. Billingham RE, Lampkin GH, Medawar PB, et al. Tolerance to homografts, twin diagnosis, and the freemartin condition in cattle. *Heredity* 1952;6: 201–212.
65. Bretscher P, Cohn M. A theory of self-nonself discrimination. *Science* 1970; 169:1042–1049.
66. Gallucci S, Matzinger P. Danger signals: SOS to the immune system. *Curr Opin Immunol* 2001;13:114–119.
67. Matzinger P. The danger model: a renewed sense of self. *Science* 2002;296: 301–305.
68. Krensky A, Vincenti F, Bennett W. Immunomodulators: immunosuppressive agents, tolerogens, and immunostimulants. In: Brunton L, Lazo J, & Parker K, eds. *Goodman & Gilman's The Pharmacological Basis of Therapeutics*. Philadelphia, PA: McGraw-Hill; 2005:1405–1431.
69. Alexandre GPJ, Squifflet JP, De Bruyere M, et al. Splenectomy as a prerequisite for successful human ABO-incompatible renal transplantation. *Transplant Proc* 1985;17:138–143.
70. Alexandre GPJ, Squifflet JP, De Bruyere M, et al. Present experiences in a series of 26 ABO-incompatible living donor renal allografts. *Transpl Proc* 1987;19:4538–4542.
71. Chopek MW, Simmons RL, Platt JL. ABO-incompatible renal transplantation: initial immunopathologic evaluation. *Transplant Proc* 1987;19: 4553–4557.
72. Bannett AD, McAlack RF, Morris M, et al. ABO incompatible renal transplantation: a qualitative analysis of native endothelial tissue ABO antigens after transplant. *Transplant Proc* 1989;21:783–785.
73. Snell GD. The major histocompatibility complex: its evolution and involvement in cellular immunity. *Harvey Lect* 1980;74:49–80.
74. Sheldon S, Poulton K. HLA typing and its influence on organ transplantation. *Methods Mol Biol* 2006;333:157–174.
75. Festenstein H, Doyle P, Holmes J. Long-term follow-up in London Transplant Group recipients of cadaver renal allografts. The influence of HLA matching on transplant outcome. *N Engl J Med* 1986;314:7–14.
76. Dyer PA, Johnson RW, Martin S, et al. Evidence that matching for HLA antigens significantly increases transplant survival in 1001 renal transplants performed in the northwest region of England. *Transplantation* 1989; 48:131–135.
77. Opelz G, Wujciak T, Dohler B, et al. HLA compatibility and organ transplant survival. Collaborative Transplant Study. *Rev Immunogenet* 1999;1: 334–342.
78. Patel R, Terasaki PI. Significance of the positive crossmatch test in kidney transplantation. *New Engl J Med* 1969;280:735–739.
79. Merrill JP, Murray JE, Harrison H, et al. Successful homotransplantation of the human kidney between identical twins. *J Am Med Assoc* 1958;160: 277–282.
80. Allison AC. Immunosuppressive drugs: the first 50 years and a glance forward. *Immunopharmacology* 2000;47:63–83.
81. Medawar PB. Immunological tolerance. *Science* 1961;133:303–306.
82. Burnet FM. Immunological recognition of self. *Science* 1961;133: 307–311.
83. Ildstad ST, Sachs DH. Reconstitution with syngeneic plus allogeneic or xenogeneic bone marrow leads to specific acceptance of allografts or xenografts. *Nature* 1984;307:168–170.
84. Markert ML, Boeck A, Hale LP, et al. Transplantation of thymus tissue in complete DiGeorge syndrome. *N Engl J Med* 1999;341:1180–1189.
85. Kawai T, Cosimi AB, Colvin RB, et al. Mixed allogeneic chimerism and renal allograft tolerance in cynomolgus monkeys. *Transplantation* 1995; 59:256–262.
86. Gudmundsdottir H, Turka LA. T cell costimulatory blockade: new therapies for transplant rejection. *J Am Soc Nephrol* 1999;10:1356–1365.
87. Muramatsu M, Kinoshita K, Fagarasan S, et al. Class switch recombination and hypermutation require activation-induced cytidine deaminase (AID), a potential RNA editing enzyme. *Cell* 2000;102:553–563.
88. Cascalho M. Advantages and disadvantages of cytidine deamination. *J Immunol* 2004;172:6513–6518.
89. Imai K, Zhu Y, Revy P, et al. Analysis of class switch recombination and somatic hypermutation in patients affected with autosomal dominant hyper-IgM syndrome type 2. *Clin Immunol* 2005;115:277–285.
90. Petersen-Mahrt SK, Harris RS, Neuberger MS. AID mutates E. coli suggesting a DNA deamination mechanism for antibody diversification. *Nature* 2002;418:99–103.
91. Medzhitov R. Toll-like receptors and innate immunity. *Nat Rev Immunol* 2001;1:135.
92. Kawabe T, Naka T, Yoshida K, et al. The immune responses in CD40-deficient mice: impaired immunoglobulin class switching and germinal center formation. *Immunity* 1994;1:167–178.
93. Renshaw BR, Fanslow WC III, Armitage RJ, et al. Humoral immune responses in CD40 ligand-deficient mice. *J Exp Med* 1994;180:1889–1900.
94. Foy TM, Aruffo A, Bajorath J, et al. Immune regulation by CD40 and its ligand GP39. *Annu Rev Immunol* 1996:14:591–617.
95. Wu ZQ, Shen Y, Khan AQ, et al. The mechanism underlying T cell help for induction of an antigen-specific in vivo humoral immune response to intact Streptococcus pneumoniae is dependent on the type of antigen. *J Immunol* 2002;168:5551–5557.
96. Jeurissen A, Wuyts M, Kasran A, et al. Essential role for CD40 ligand interactions in T lymphocyte-mediated modulation of the murine immune response to pneumococcal capsular polysaccharides. *J Immunol* 2002;168: 2773–2781.
97. Slifka MK, Ahmed R. Long-lived plasma cells: a mechanism for maintaining persistent antibody production. *Curr Opin Immunol* 1998;10:252–258.
98. Manz RA, Cassese G, Thiel A, et al. Long-lived plasma cells survive independent of antigen. *Curr Top Microbiol Immunol* 1999;246:71–74; discussion 74–75.
99. Bernasconi NL, Traggiai E, Lanzavecchia A. Maintenance of serological memory by polyclonal activation of human memory B cells. *Science* 2002;298:2199–2202.
100. Sze DM-Y, Toellner KM, Garcia de Vinuesa C, et al. Intrinsic constraint on plasmablast growth and extrinsic limits of plasma cell survival. *J Exp Med* 2000;192:813–821.
101. Shoenfeld Y, George J. Induction of autoimmunity. A role for the idiotypic network. *Ann N Y Acad Sci* 1997;815:342–349.
102. Grandien A, Andersson J, Portnoi D, et al. An example of idiotypic mimicry. *Eur J Immunol* 1997;27:1808–1815.
103. Nemazee DA, Burki K. Clonal deletion of B lymphocytes in a transgenic mouse bearing anti-MHC class I antibody genes. *Nature* 1989;337: 562–566.
104. Platt JL. New directions for organ transplantation. *Nature* 1998;392:11–17.
105. Nagata H, Ito M, Cai J, et al. Treatment of cirrhosis and liver failure in rats by hepatocyte xenotransplantation. *Gastroenterology* 2003;124:422–431.
106. Jooste SV, Colvin RB, Soper WD, et al. The vascular bed as the primary target in the destruction of skin grafts by antiserum. I. Resistance of freshly placed xenografts of skin to antiserum. *J Exp Med* 1981a;154:1319–1331.
107. Jooste SV, Colvin RB, Winn HJ. The vascular bed as the primary target in the destruction of skin grafts by antiserum. II. Loss of sensitivity to antiserum in long-term xenografts of skin. *J Exp Med* 1981b;154:1332–1341.
108. Platt JL, Fox IJ. Xenotransplantation and the liver. In: Busuttil RW, Klintmalm GB, eds. *Transplantation of the Liver*. Philadelphia, PA: Elsevier; 2005:1365–1377.

109. Sumitran-Holgersson S. HLA-specific alloantibodies and renal graft outcome. *Nephrol Dial Transplant* 2001;16:897–904.
110. Gleason RE, Murray JE. Report from kidney transplant registry: analysis of variables in the function of human kidney transplants. *Transplantation* 1967;5:343–359.
111. Brynger H, Rydberg L, Samuelsson BE, et al. Experience with 14 renal transplants with kidneys from blood group A (subgroup A_2) to O recipients. *Transplant Proc* 1984;16:1175.
112. Gordon RD, Iwatsuki S, Esquivel CO, et al. Liver transplantation across ABO blood groups. *Surgery* 1986;100:342–348.
113. Collins BH, Chari RS, Magee JC, et al. Mechanisms of injury in porcine livers perfused with blood of humans with fulminant hepatic failure. *Transplantation* 1994;58:1162–1171.
114. Zou Y, Mirbaha F, Lazaro A, et al. MICA is a target for complement-dependent cytotoxicity with mouse monoclonal antibodies and human alloantibodies. *Hum Immunol* 2002;63:30–39.
115. Zwirner NW, Marcos CY, Mirbaha F, et al. Identification of MICA as a new polymorphic alloantigen recognized by antibodies in sera of organ transplant recipients. *Hum Immunol* 2000;61:917–924.
116. Kalil J, Guilherme L, Neumann J, et al. Humoral rejection in two HLA identical living related donor kidney transplants. *Transplant Proc* 1989; 21:711–713.
117. Devine DV, Rosse WF. Regulation of the activity of platelet-bound C3 convertase of the alternative pathway of complement by platelet factor H. *Proc Natl Acad Sci U S A* 1987;84:5873–5877.
118. Lutz HU, Jelezarova E. Complement amplification revisited. *Mol Immunol* 2006;43:2–12.
119. Vakeva AP, Agah A, Rollins SA, et al. Myocardial infarction and apoptosis after myocardial ischemia and reperfusion: role of the terminal complement components and inhibition by anti-C5 therapy. *Circulation* 1998;97:2259–2267.
120. Zhou W, Farrar CA, Abe K, et al. Predominant role for C5b-9 in renal ischemia/reperfusion injury. *J Clin Invest* 2000;105:1363–1371.
121. Spector D, Limas C, Frost JL, et al. Perfusion nephropathy in human transplants. *N Engl J Med* 1976;295:1217–1221.
122. Cerra FB, Raza S, Andres GA, et al. The endothelial damage of pulsatile renal preservation and its relationship to perfusion pressure and colloid osmotic pressure. *Surgery* 1977;81:534–541.
123. Takemoto SK, Zeevi A, Feng S, et al. National conference to assess antibody-mediated rejection in solid organ transplantation. *Am J Trans* 2004;4:1033–1041.
124. Solez K, Colvin RB, Racusen LC, et al. Banff '05 meeting report: differential diagnosis of chronic allograft injury and elimination of chronic allograft nephropathy ('CAN'). *Am J Trans* 2007;7:518–526.
125. Mauiyyedi S, Colvin RB. Humoral rejection in kidney transplantation: new concepts in diagnosis and treatment. *Curr Opin Nephrol Hypertens* 2002;11:609–618.
126. Parker W, Lin SS, Platt JL. Antigen expression in xenotransplantation: how low must it go? *Transplantation* 2001;71:313–319.
127. Feucht HE, Felber E, Gokel MJ, et al. Vascular deposition of complement-split products in kidney allografts with cell-mediated rejection. *Clin Exp Immunol* 1991;86:464–470.
128. Collins AB, Schneeberger EE, Pascual MA, et al. Complement activation in acute humoral renal allograft rejection: diagnostic significance of C4d deposits in peritubular capillaries. *J Am Soc Nephrol* 1999;10:2208–2214.
129. Bustos M, Saadi S, Platt JL. Platelet-mediated activation of endothelial cells: implications for the pathogenesis of transplant rejection. *Transplantation* 2001;72:509–515.
130. Miyata Y, Platt JL. The role of complement in acute vascular rejection: lessons from the inhibition of C1rs activity. *Transplantation* 2002;73:675.
131. Marcum JA, Rosenberg RD. Anticoagulantly active heparan sulfate proteoglycan and the vascular endothelium. *Semin Thromb Hemost* 1987;13: 464–474.
132. Ihrcke NS, Wrenshall LE, Lindman BJ, et al. Role of heparan sulfate in immune system-blood vessel interactions. *Immunol Today* 1993;14: 500–505.
133. Saadi S, Platt JL. Transient perturbation of endothelial integrity induced by natural antibodies and complement. *J Exp Med* 1995;181:21–31.
134. Saadi S, Platt JL. Endothelial cell responses to complement activation. In: Volanakis JE, Frank MM, eds. *The Human Complement System in Health and Disease*. New York: Marcel Dekker, Inc.; 1998:335–353.
135. Brunn GJ, Saadi S, Platt JL. Differential regulation of endothelial cell activation by complement and interleukin 1alpha. *Circ Res* 2006;98:793–800.
136. Brunn GJ, Saadi S, Platt JL. Constitutive repression of IL-1alpha in endothelial cells. *Circ Res* 2008;102:823–830.
137. Mauiyyedi S, Pelle PD, Saidman S, et al. Chronic humoral rejection: identification of antibody-mediated chronic renal allograft rejection by C4d deposits in peritubular capillaries. *J Am Soc Nephrol* 2001;12:574–582.
138. Piazza A, Poggi E, Borrelli L, et al. Impact of donor-specific antibodies on chronic rejection occurrence and graft loss in renal transplantation: post-transplant analysis using flow cytometric techniques. *Transplantation* 2001;71:1106–1112.
139. Lederer SR, Kluth-Pepper B, Schneeberger H, et al. Impact of humoral alloreactivity early after transplantation on the long-term survival of renal allografts. *Kidney Int* 2001;59:334–341.
140. Platt JL, Vercellotti GM, Dalmasso AP, et al. Transplantation of discordant xenografts: a review of progress. *Immunol Today* 1990;11:450–456.
141. Bannett AD, McAlack RF, Raja R, et al. Experiences with known ABO-mismatched renal transplants. *Transplant Proc* 1987;19:4543–4546.
142. Saadi S, Holzknecht RA, Patte CP, et al. Complement-mediated regulation of tissue factor activity in endothelium. *J Exp Med* 1995;182:1807–1814.
143. McCurry KR, Kooyman DL, Alvarado CG, et al. Human complement regulatory proteins protect swine-to-primate cardiac xenografts from humoral injury. *Nat Med* 1995;1:423–427.
144. Cozzi E, Yannoutsos N, Langford GA, et al. Effect of transgenic expression of human decay-accelerating factor on the inhibition of hyperacute rejection of pig organs. In: Cooper DKC, Kemp E, Platt JL, et al., eds. *Xenotransplantation: The Transplantation of Organs and Tissues Between Species*. Berlin, Germany: Springer; 1997:665–682.
145. Pruitt SK, Kirk AD, Bollinger RR, et al. The effect of soluble complement receptor type 1 on hyperacute rejection of porcine xenografts. *Transplantation* 1994;57:363–370.
146. Lin SS, Weidner BC, Byrne GW, et al. The role of antibodies in acute vascular rejection of pig-to-baboon cardiac transplants. *J Clin Invest* 1998;101:1745–1756.
147. Nath KA, Balla G, Vercellotti GM, et al. Induction of heme oxygenase is a rapid, protective response in rhabdomyolysis in the rat. *J Clin Invest* 1992;90:267–270.
148. Bach FH, Ferran C, Hechenleitner P, et al. Accommodation of vascularized xenografts: expression of "protective genes" by donor endothelial cells in a host Th2 cytokine environment. *Nat Med* 1997;3: 196–204.
149. Hancock WW, Buelow R, Sayegh MH, et al. Antibody-induced transplant arteriosclerosis is prevented by graft expression of anti-oxidant and anti-apoptotic genes. *Nat Med* 1998p;4:1392–1396.
150. Delikouras A, Fairbanks LD, Simmonds AH, et al. Endothelial cell cytoprotection induced in vitro by allo- or xenoreactive antibodies is mediated by signaling through adenosine A2 receptors. *Eur J Immunol* 2003;33: 3127–3135.
151. Jindra PT, Zhang X, Mulder A, et al. Anti-HLA antibodies can induce endothelial cell survival or proliferation depending on their concentration. *Transplantation* 2006;82:S33–S35.
152. Rocha PN, Plumb TJ, Crowley SD, et al. Effector mechanisms in transplant rejection. *Immunol Rev* 2003;196:51–64.
153. Alegre ML, Florquin S, Goldman M. Cellular mechanisms underlying acute graft rejection: time for reassessment. *Curr Opin Immunol* 2007;19: 563–568.
154. Mintz B, Silvers W. "Intrinsic" immunological tolerance in allophenic mice. *Science* 1967;158:1484–1487.
155. Sutton R, Gray D, McShane P, et al. The specificity of rejection and the absence of susceptibility of pancreatic islet B cells to nonspecific immune destruction in mixed strain islets grafted beneath the renal capsule in the rat. *J Exp Med* 1989;170:751–762.
156. Saadi S, Holzknecht RA, Patte CP, et al. Endothelial cell activation by pore forming structures: pivotal role for IL-1α. *Circulation* 2000;101: 1867–1873.
157. Rosenberg AS, Singer A. Cellular basis of skin allograft rejection: an in vivo model of immune-mediated tissue destruction. *Ann Rev Immunol* 1992;10:333–358.
158. Platt JL, LeBien TW, Michael AF. Interstitial mononuclear cell populations in renal graft rejection: identification by monoclonal antibodies in tissue sections. *J Exp Med* 1982;155:17–30.
159. Platt JL, Grant BW, Eddy AA, et al. Immune cell populations in cutaneous delayed-type hypersensitivity. *J Exp Med* 1983;158:1227–1242.

CHAPTER 34 ■ ORGAN PRESERVATION

ROBERT M. MERION

KEY POINTS

1. Much of the injury to transplanted organs occurs not during the period of ischemia but during organ reperfusion.
2. The general attributes of an acceptable organ donor include pronouncement of donor death, previously good general health, and relative hemodynamic stability from the time of the precipitating event leading to death until organ procurement is complete.
3. The following requirements must be met to make a firm diagnosis of brain death: the presence of reversible causes of coma should be excluded; clinical criteria establishing the loss of all functions of the entire brain must be met (deep coma, absence of brainstem function, absence of spontaneous respiration); and a confirmatory diagnostic test must be carried out (electroencephalogram, nuclear brain blood flow study, four-vessel cerebral arteriography).
4. All transplant candidates within the United States are entered into a computer system, and an allocation system is used to determine the appropriate potential recipient for a given donor organ.

PATHOPHYSIOLOGY OF ORGAN PRESERVATION INJURY

The removal, storage, and transplantation of a solid organ from a donor results in profound alterations in homeostatic control of the *milieu interieur* of that organ. These effects manifest themselves in the degree to which the return of normal organ function is delayed or prevented once the recipient transplantation procedure is completed. The injury sustained by an organ during the processes of procurement, preservation, and transplantation occurs primarily as a result of ischemia and hypothermia, the former being customarily classified as warm or cold ischemia. Warm ischemia and its consequences are associated with normothermic events that occur before removal of the organ from the body. Cold ischemia refers to events occurring during the interval between initial organ cooling and revascularization in the recipient.

The principles of modern organ preservation are to provide for hypothermia, prevent cellular swelling, and avoid biochemical injury.[1,2] These principles are intended to interfere with the loss of cellular integrity, changes in ionic composition, and disruption of cellular energy systems that occur during organ storage. The following discussion describes these phenomena. Finally, the effects of oxygen-derived free radicals, cytokines, and nitric oxide at the time of reperfusion are discussed.

Structural Integrity

The cell membrane plays a crucial physical protective role and provides an active interface with the extracellular environment. Receptors, ion regulation, and enzyme systems linked to the cell membrane complex contain extracellular, transmembrane, and intracellular components essential to their function. The interrelation of such systems with the membrane itself is highly dependent on a stable configuration of the lipid bilayer and on tight control of temperature, pH, and osmolarity. Organ ischemia and preservation disrupt all these relations. Lowering the temperature through the phase transition of lipids results in profound changes in conformation and stability of the membrane in addition to drastically altering the function of membrane-bound enzymes. Physicochemical membrane changes induced by hypothermia result in increased permeability, which in turn adds to the burden of maintaining a stable intracellular environment and contributes to cell swelling. Organ preservation solutions have historically therefore been hypertonic to minimize these alterations.

Ionic Composition

The foregoing membrane changes are compounded by crippling of the Na^+-K^+-adenosine triphosphatase (ATPase) pump caused by the lack of ATP production and by generation of excess hydrogen ion resulting from anaerobic metabolism during ischemia. When the Na^+-K^+-ATPase pump is paralyzed, potassium diffuses down its concentration gradient to the extracellular environment while sodium, normally present at a low concentration in the cell, pours in. Modern preservation solutions have typically had electrolyte compositions similar to that inside the cell with high potassium and low sodium concentrations. Osmotic gradients are, therefore, minimized, and the cellular ionic charge remains relatively constant.

Hydrogen ion production continues in ischemic organs and may result in cellular damage. Intracellular pH gradually falls without replenishment of buffering capabilities, and under conditions requiring a switch from aerobic to anaerobic glycolysis, the production of lactic acid also increases. The liver appears to be especially susceptible to this type of injury. A plausible mechanism has been described whereby glucokinase in the liver phosphorylates glucose (endogenous or provided in preservation solution) to glucose-6-phosphate.[3] The normal metabolic pathway for glucose-6-phosphate results in production of pyruvate and ultimately lactate by lactic dehydrogenase (Fig. 34.1). Unlike the kidney, the hepatic isozyme of lactic dehydrogenase, M4, functions particularly well under acidotic conditions in the presence of high concentrations of lactic acid. These biochemical differences underlie the range of acceptable cold ischemia time for various organs.

Calcium ion permeability is increased with ischemia, and a rapid influx of calcium may overwhelm mitochondrial buffering capacity. There is increased activity of calmodulin, a cytoplasmic calcium-binding protein, and a cascade of enzyme activation events, including the upregulation of

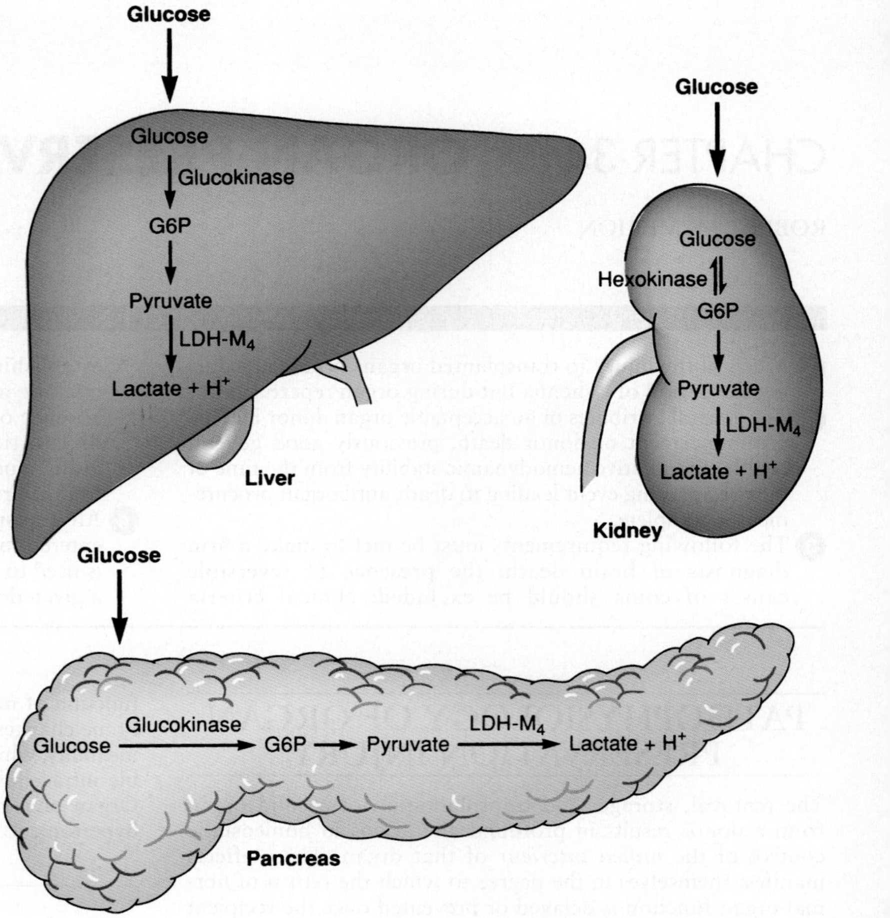

FIGURE 34.1. The effects of acidosis on glucose metabolism are organ specific. For example, the M4 isozyme of lactate dehydrogenase (LDH) functions well in an acidotic environment in the presence of high concentrations of lactic acid. G6P, glucose-6-phosphate. (Adapted with permission from Belzer FO, Southard JH. Principles of solid-organ preservation by cold storage. *Transplantation* 1988;45:673–676.)

phospholipases and subsequent production of prostaglandin derivatives, results in mitochondrial and cell membrane injury. Vascular smooth muscle myofibrillar contraction may be initiated by increased cellular calcium concentrations, with the resulting vasospasm contributing to ischemic damage. Endothelin, a 21-amino-acid peptide with potent vasoconstrictor properties, has been recognized as another factor that plays a role in preservation injury by inducing vasospasm after revascularization.[4,5]

Cellular Energy

The energy requirements of aerobic cells are provided by a combination of the enzymatic breakdown of glucose (glycolysis) and by the process of cellular respiration, encompassing the transfer of electrons from organic molecules to molecular oxygen (electron transport and oxidative phosphorylation) (Fig. 34.2). Hypothermia results in decreased metabolic rate and slows the rate at which enzymes degrade cellular components, but metabolism is not completely suppressed. It has been calculated that cooling from 37°C to 0°C results in a 12-fold reduction of cellular metabolism.[1] Although metabolism is slowed and utilization of cellular energy stores is slowed, ATP and adenosine diphosphate (ADP), the major sources of cellular metabolic energy, are gradually depleted during hypothermia. This depletion is presumably a result of residual energy requirements that exceed the capacity of the cell to produce ATP.

During ischemia and organ preservation, the glycolytic pathway is sidetracked to lactate production as the Krebs tricarboxylic acid cycle and mitochondrial respiration are impaired. Although some of the enzymes of the Krebs cycle may be found in the extramitochondrial cytoplasm, the inner compartment of the mitochondrion is where the enzymatic reactions of the cycle occur. Mitochondrial dysfunction, therefore, is responsible for most of the changes in cellular energy associated with ischemia and organ preservation.

Hypothermic preservation results in reduced activity of mitochondrial enzymes. Cellular respiration, which requires adenine nucleotide substrates, is reduced. For ADP to be transported into the mitochondrion as a substrate for conversion to high-energy ATP, a membrane adenine nucleotide translocase is required. Hypothermia unfavorably alters the relation between the enzyme and the inner mitochondrial membrane within which it resides, reducing substrate delivery.[6] Phospholipid hydrolysis by phospholipases increases levels of free fatty acids, acyl derivatives of which may also affect membrane structure and the function of the translocase. Cannibalization of ADP sequestered in the extramitochondrial cytoplasm by adenylate kinase for conversion to ATP results in accumulation of adenosine monophosphate as a byproduct, which reduces purine synthesis and results in the loss of ATP precursors from the cell.

Reperfusion Injury

1 It is apparent that much of the injury to transplanted organs occurs not during the period of ischemia per se but upon organ reperfusion. This realization has led to many advances in organ preservation. Furthermore, some of the events that occur during reperfusion may result in enhanced

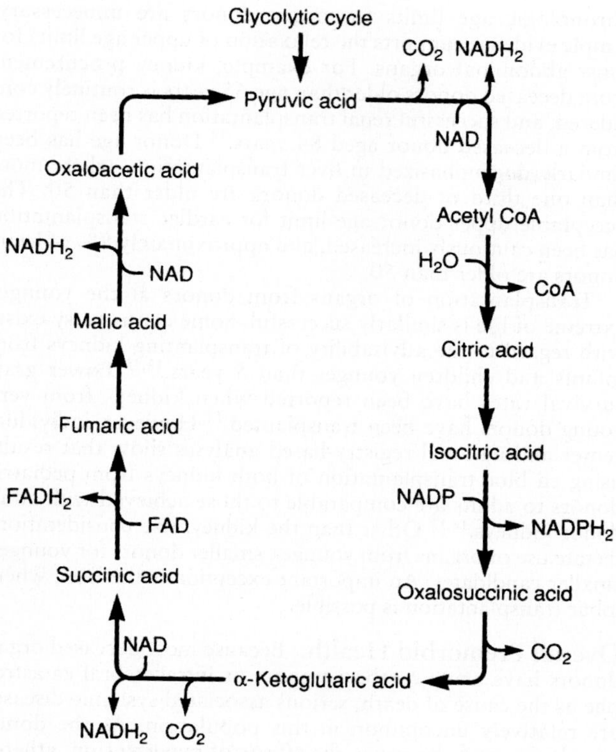

FIGURE 34.2. Cellular energy requirements are met largely through the processes of glycolysis, the Krebs tricarboxylic acid cycle, and oxidative phosphorylation. CoA, coenzyme A; $NADH_2$, reduced form of nicotinamide adenine dinucleotide; NAD, nicotinamide adenine dinucleotide; NADP, nicotinamide-adenine dinucleotide phosphate; $NADPH_2$, reduced form of NADPH; FAD, flavin adenine dinucleotide; $FADH_2$, reduced form of FAD.

immunogenicity of the graft. A better understanding of these events will hopefully lead to the development of preservation methods that decrease the propensity for allograft rejection at a later date.

Oxygen Free Radical–mediated Effects

The mechanisms by which reactive species of oxygen are produced in biologic systems and the effects of these molecules on various cells and tissues were elucidated in the 1970s and 1980s.[7] The best-studied model involves the production of superoxide anion (O_2^-) as a byproduct of the enzymatic catabolism of the purine metabolites hypoxanthine and xanthine to uric acid by xanthine oxidase (Fig. 34.3). During ischemic states, a cytosolic enzyme is activated by increased intracellular calcium, resulting in the conversion of xanthine dehydrogenase to xanthine oxidase. Both xanthine dehydrogenase and xanthine oxidase catabolize hypoxanthine and xanthine to uric acid. Xanthine oxidase utilizes molecular oxygen as an electron acceptor and forms (O_2^-) as a result. Superoxide anion rapidly reacts with itself to form hydrogen peroxide, a potent oxidant capable of injuring the cell by oxidizing lipid membranes and cellular proteins. Hydrogen peroxide then produces a cascade of oxygen free radicals, including hydroxyl radical (OH•) and singlet oxygen, that are even more potent oxidants. The damaging effects of oxygen free radicals begin upon reperfusion of the organ. During ischemic conditions, tissue oxygen levels fall below the threshold needed to allow xanthine oxidase to metabolize xanthine and hypoxanthine.

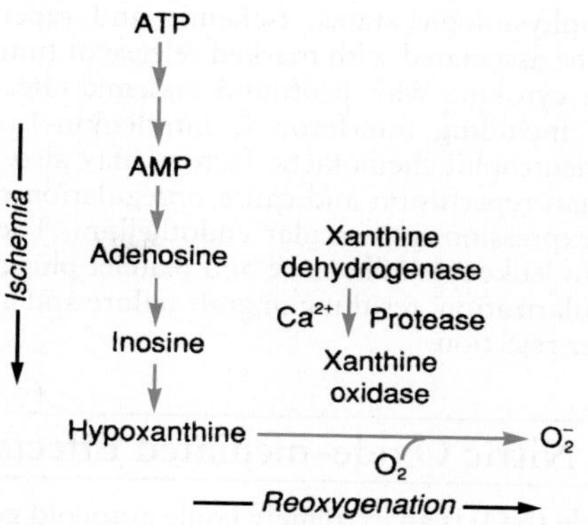

FIGURE 34.3. The classic pathway of superoxide anion generation by the metabolism of purines by xanthine oxidase. ATP, adenosine triphosphate; AMP, adenosine monophosphate; Ca^{2+}, calcium; O_2, oxygen; O_2^-, superoxide anion.

This allows the intracellular concentration of these metabolites to rise. Upon reperfusion, oxygen is suddenly available and metabolism proceeds rapidly, resulting in a dramatic and sudden production of reactive oxygen intermediates. The cellular defenses against peroxidation are overwhelmed and injury occurs.[8]

Agents that reduce oxygen free radical generation, or scavenge them once they are formed, have been used to determine the contribution of these molecular species to preservation-related reperfusion injury and have the ability to decrease peroxidation due to oxygen free radicals during reperfusion. Allopurinol, an inhibitor of xanthine oxidase, has been shown to have protective effects when used before the ischemic insult in a variety of experimental systems. Unfortunately, allopurinol has other effects, such as vasodilatation and preservation of the purine nucleotide pool, making it a less-than-ideal agent for defining oxygen free radical effects. Other studies using superoxide dismutase have clearly demonstrated a role for oxygen radicals in reperfusion injury in transplantation.[9] Similarly, desferrioxamine, an iron chelator, removes an essential metal cofactor for the generation of the extremely reactive hydroxyl radical, resulting in decreased oxidative injury.

Indirect evidence of oxygen free radical effects rests on the documentation of lipid peroxidation. In this process, interaction of highly reactive oxygen species with polyunsaturated fatty acids in the cell membrane starts a chain reaction that may ultimately destroy cellular integrity and result in cell death. The products of this reaction can be measured by several different assays. The magnitude of lipid peroxidation appears to be inversely related to levels of glutathione, which functions as an endogenous free radical scavenger. Glutathione and other agents that protect against peroxidation are, therefore, useful in organ preservation solutions to attenuate reperfusion injury.

Production of oxygen free radicals also initiates production of prostaglandins including leukotriene B_4 by direct activation of phospholipase A_2. This chemoattractant causes leukocyte adherence to vascular endothelium. These neutrophils may contribute to local injury by plugging the microcirculation and by degranulation, resulting in proteolytic damage to the organ.

Cytokine-mediated Effects

Cytokines are a recently described group of intercellular messenger molecules that may be produced in a variety of normal and pathophysiologic states. Ischemia and reperfusion are known to be associated with marked release of tumor necrosis factor-α, a cytokine with profound systemic effects.[10] Other cytokines, including interferon-γ, interleukin-1, and interleukin-8 (neutrophil chemotactic factor), may also be released during organ reperfusion and cause upregulation of adhesion molecule expression on vascular endothelium. These changes may lead to leukocyte adherence and platelet plugging following revascularization, resulting in graft failure and an increased risk of later rejection.

Nitric Oxide–mediated Effects

Nitric oxide (NO) is an extremely labile autocoid generated by nitric oxide synthase from L-arginine. It has potent vasodilatory effects on microvasculature and is responsible for a wide variety of physiologic effects. Evidence suggests that NO production is induced by inflammatory cytokines including tumor necrosis factor-α, interferon-γ, and interleukin-1. In the setting of ischemia-reperfusion, NO may, therefore, mediate injury to organs directly as a result of cytokine release. Inhaled nitric oxide has been demonstrated to attenuate reperfusion injury in transplanted lungs.[11] Increased NO synthesis also correlates with acute rejection.[12]

CONTEMPORARY CLINICAL PRACTICE

The science of transplantation has developed rapidly during the past 40 years. Improved understanding of the immune response to allografts and better appreciation of the complexity of organ ischemia and preservation-related injury have contributed to greatly improved graft and patient survival results. Most solid organ transplants are now performed as the therapeutic option of choice, and in many cases transplantation offers the only definitive treatment for a given disease entity. As a result, an ever-widening list of indications for solid organ transplantation has emerged, placing increasing pressure on an already limited supply of donor organs. As of December 2006, there were 93,820 patients awaiting deceased donor organ transplantation in the United States, almost double the number listed in 1997.[13] Each year, more patients are placed on the waiting lists than are transplanted, resulting in thousands of waiting list deaths and increasing waiting time.

Determination of Suitability for Deceased Donor Organ Donation

2 **General Considerations.** The characteristics of a suitable deceased organ donor can be divided into those that are general in nature and those that are organ specific. Broadly stated, the general attributes of an acceptable organ donor include pronouncement of donor death, previously good general health, and relative hemodynamic stability from the time of the precipitating event leading to death until organ procurement is complete. Informed consent from the donor's next of kin is required before organ procurement. The concepts of brain death and the renewed practice of donation after cardiac death (DCD) are discussed in detail later. A detailed understanding of these conditions and their associated pathophysiology is essential for the successful procurement and subsequent transplantation of solid organs from deceased donors. A detailed medical history should be sought by contacting family members or friends of the potential donor.

Age. As experience has been gained with donors considered less than ideal, it has become apparent that arbitrarily defined chronologic age limits for organ donors are unnecessary. Ample evidence supports the relaxation of upper age limits for most abdominal organs. For example, kidney procurement from deceased donors older than age 65 years is routinely considered, and successful renal transplantation has been reported from a deceased donor aged 84 years.[14] Donor age has been similarly de-emphasized in liver transplantation, where more than one third of deceased donors are older than 50. The acceptable upper donor age limit for cardiac transplantation has been cautiously increased, and approximately 8% of heart donors are older than 50.

Transplantation of organs from donors at the younger extreme of life is similarly successful. Some controversy exists with regard to the advisability of transplanting kidneys from infants and children younger than 5 years.[13,15] Lower graft survival rates have been reported when kidneys from very young donors have been transplanted.[13] However, individual center and national registry-based analyses show that results using en bloc transplantation of both kidneys from pediatric donors to adults are comparable to those achieved with adult donor kidneys.[16,17] Other than the kidney, size considerations dictate use of organs from younger, smaller donors for younger, smaller candidates. An important exception is the liver, where lobar transplantation is possible.

Overall Premorbid Health. Because most deceased organ donors have acute cerebral trauma or intracerebral catastrophe as the cause of death, serious associated systemic diseases are relatively uncommon in this population. As the donor population ages, however, the effects of hypertension, atherosclerosis, and other diseases associated with advancing age are more common. Thus, careful screening to ascertain that the donor was previously in good health is mandatory. Common disorders, such as hypertension and diabetes mellitus, do not automatically disqualify a person from organ donation, but the duration, severity, and treatment of such conditions should be evaluated for their potential effects on individual organs.

Hemodynamic Stability. Cardiovascular instability and eventual cardiopulmonary collapse eventually occur in all brain-dead patients. Thus, hemodynamic management is one of the most important aspects of donor management once brain death has been established and consent for organ donation has been obtained. Many potential organ donors sustain significant hypotension or even cardiac arrest during the initial stages of their illness or as the presenting signs of intracerebral catastrophe. Knowledge of the course and management of these episodes is helpful in predicting damage to the various organs and in guiding the workup of the donor for suitability of the organs for transplantation. In terms of specific organs, the kidneys appear to tolerate transient hypotension best, whereas the liver and pancreas may be more severely damaged by such episodes. The cardiac response to hypotension or actual cardiac arrest depends on the cause of the hemodynamic instability and the magnitude of direct cardiac injury sustained as a result of cardiac compressions during cardiopulmonary resuscitation.

Contraindications

Sepsis. Active systemic infection has traditionally been an absolute contraindication to organ donation. However, these tenets are being re-examined because of the current organ shortage. A history of diseases such as tuberculosis or human immunodeficiency virus (HIV) infection clearly renders a person unsuitable for donation. Pneumonia (except for lung donors) and urinary tract infection are no longer considered to be problematic in the absence of systemic sepsis. Even in the presence of bacteremia, the risk of transmission of infectious agents by organ transplantation appears to be small.[18] In all cases, appropriate antibiotic therapy should be initiated before the procurement procedure.

Viral Infection. All potential organ donors, regardless of whether they are considered high risk, are tested for evidence of infection with HIV. Although the incidence of false-positive results may be a problem, the high sensitivity of the test ensures that the potential for transmission of this virus is minimized. Nucleic acid testing for HIV is increasingly available by organ procurement organizations, which further reduces the so-called window period for false-negative test results. Screening for human T-lymphotropic virus (HTLV-1 and HTLV-2) has been done routinely for deceased donors, but concerns about false-positive rates, which result in otherwise suitable organs being discarded, and the recently announced removal from the market of the most commonly used U.S. Food and Drug Administration (FDA)-approved assay, have complicated decision making about testing for this virus. Testing is also routinely performed for evidence of hepatitis B and C virus infection. History of viral hepatitis or serologic evidence of past infection has previously been considered an absolute contraindication to organ donation. Many centers are now reconsidering this issue in selected situations. Some organs from donors who have evidence of past infection with the hepatitis B virus are able to transmit the virus. However, these organs may be considered for recipients who have longstanding infection with this virus or have received the recombinant hepatitis B vaccine and have serologic immunity. In addition, in medically appropriate circumstances, organs may be used from donors who test positive for hepatitis B core antibody and negative for hepatitis B surface antigen. In such cases, recipients are generally treated with lamivudine or other similar antiviral agents. Organs from donors with evidence of past infection with the hepatitis C virus are possible sources of infectious virus. The risk of infection is small, however, and these organs are now being considered for patients with known preexisting exposure to the hepatitis C virus.[19] Other viral titers that are frequently determined during workup of a donor include members of the herpesvirus family, such as cytomegalovirus (CMV), Epstein-Barr virus, and herpes simplex virus. Evidence of previous infection with these viruses does not preclude organ donation but may require additional therapy in the recipient, such as valganciclovir prophylaxis or hyperimmune globulin administration in the case of CMV.

Cancer. Cancer, whether treated or not, has long been considered to contravene organ donation based on the knowledge that tumor cells may circulate widely even in patients with malignant lesions thought to be localized. The transplantation of even a small number of malignant cells into a recipient who is heavily immunosuppressed carries the threat of dissemination and a disastrous outcome. The only exception to this rule has been the donor with a primary malignancy of the central nervous system. It has long been thought that as long as the blood–brain barrier is intact, these tumors are rarely capable of systemic spread. Although transmission of central nervous system tumors of donor origin to transplant recipients has been reported, the rate of transmission is dependent on the organ transplanted and the type of malignancy involved.[20] These cases must be considered on an individual basis.

Specific Organ Dysfunction.

The condition of particular organs of interest in great measure dictates their individual suitability for transplantation. With appropriate emphasis on the overall maintenance of donor homeostasis, most if not all transplantable organs should be procured from most donors. A history of longstanding hypertension may result in fixed damage to the kidneys as a result of hypertensive scarring and secondary to the effects of aortic and renal atherosclerosis. Similarly, insulin-dependent diabetes mellitus produces a well-known renal lesion. These changes may be reversible, however, after transplantation into a nondiabetic recipient.[21] The kidneys are relatively resilient organs, and simple measures usually suffice to identify serious renal dysfunction. Measurements of hourly urinary output, coupled with determinations of the central venous pressure, are useful monitors of the adequacy of volume repletion in potential donors. Significant volume depletion is the combined result of intentional volume contraction to treat cerebral edema and the effects of diabetes insipidus accompanying lethal brain injury. Serum creatinine is measured as a global, if imperfect, indicator of renal function. Significant elevation of the serum creatinine level during the course of the donor hospitalization may be a sign of renal injury, predisposing to delayed graft function after transplantation, although eventual outcomes may be very acceptable in the face of acute tubular necrosis in young and otherwise uncomplicated donors.[22,23]

Preexisting liver disease usually can be identified before organ procurement. A history of cirrhosis precludes donation. Prior cholecystectomy for uncomplicated cholelithiasis is not a contraindication to liver donation. Standard liver function tests, such as serum alanine aminotransferase, aspartate aminotransferase, alkaline phosphatase, and bilirubin, may be helpful in identifying gross injury to the donor liver resulting from traumatic, metabolic, or hemodynamic causes, but the absolute levels of these tests are poor indicators of the likelihood of immediate, life-sustaining graft function in the recipient. Hepatic synthetic function as assessed by prothrombin time may also be deceiving because of the effects of severe brain injury on the coagulation cascade.[24] An increasing incidence of obesity has led to higher rates of nonrecovery and discard of donor livers due to steatosis. Bedside donor liver biopsy is increasingly utilized to avoid the high cost of unnecessarily dispatching procurement teams to donor hospitals.

The pancreas may be difficult to assess until the time of organ procurement. Hyperglycemia and hyperamylasemia are common in patients who sustain brain death, particularly if the cause is traumatic. A careful history establishing the absence of preexisting diabetes mellitus and pancreatitis provides the most useful information. A history of alcohol abuse alone does not correlate well with the finding of chronic pancreatitis pathology at laparotomy. Computed tomographic examination of the abdomen may be indicated if the donor sustained any abdominal injury. It is more appropriate to examine the organ at the time of multiple organ procurement to determine if it is suitable for transplantation rather than making a decision on the basis of historical or laboratory information alone.

Intestinal donation still occurs quite uncommonly. Fewer than 200 candidates are on the waiting list in the United States at any given time, and many of these are children for whom appropriate size matching is required.

Cardiac dysfunction resulting in arrhythmia or the need for high-dose inotropic support suggests that the heart may be unsuitable for transplantation. Transient supraventricular tachycardias, ventricular arrhythmia associated with severe hemodynamic instability, or cardiac arrest requires investigation before acceptance as a cardiac donor. Significant valvular disease and wall motion abnormalities can be readily identified by bedside echocardiographic examination, a study that is routinely obtained by many transplant centers. In many cases the fluid management of the donor radically affects the apparent cardiac function since over- or underhydration will markedly reduce effective cardiac output. Urine output can be extremely misleading due to the loss of antidiuretic hormone secretion from the hypothalamus. Measurements of central venous pressure or pulmonary artery wedge pressure may allow for more accurate management of fluid replacement. Determination of cardiac output using a flow-directed balloon-tipped pulmonary artery catheter is also helpful and complements echocardiographic findings. In questionable cases, cardiac catheterization may be required to exclude significant coronary artery disease.

Pulmonary donation is dependent upon satisfactory gas exchange parameters and an absence of major lung disease history. In the setting of conditions that lead to deceased organ donation, oxygen saturation and arterial oxygen tension (PaO_2) may be suboptimal. However, lung resuscitation protocols have resulted in greater likelihood of successful placement of donor lungs for transplant.

Brain Death

3 **Definition.** The concept of brain death was crystallized in the 1968 Report of the Ad Hoc Committee of Harvard Medical School developed to examine the definition of brain death.[25] This document established the following clearly defined criteria that were reliably predictive of irreversibility: (a) unreceptivity and unresponsivity, (b) absence of spontaneous muscular movement, (c) absence of reflexes, and (d) silent electroencephalogram. Since the publication of the so-called Harvard Criteria, the prerequisites for the diagnosis of brain death have been refined. Most hospitals have constituted a Brain Death Committee that is responsible for making uniform determinations of brain death according to locally established specific criteria while conforming generally to the Harvard Criteria. The following requirements must be met to make a firm diagnosis of brain death: (a) the presence of reversible causes of coma should be excluded, (b) clinical criteria establishing the loss of all functions of the entire brain must be met (deep coma, absence of brainstem function, absence of spontaneous respiration), and (c) a confirmatory diagnostic test must be carried out (electroencephalogram, nuclear brain blood flow study, four-vessel cerebral arteriography).

Reversible causes of coma include sedation, hypothermia below 32.2°C, neuromuscular blockade, and shock. Coma should be deep and fixed, without perception or response to external stimuli, including deep pain. Decerebrate and decorticate responses should not be present. Occasionally, spinal reflexes may be present. Absence of brainstem function can be documented by confirming the absence of pupillary light response, corneal reflex, oculocephalic reflex, oculovestibular reflex, and spontaneous respiration.

An apnea test should be performed to assess spontaneous respiration. Ventilation of the patient with 100% oxygen for 10 minutes before the test reduces the risk of hypoxemia and subsequent cardiovascular collapse. After the period of pre-oxygenation, passive flow of oxygen into the endotracheal tube is continued, and the patient is monitored for evidence of respiratory effort. During this interval, hypercarbia with a arterial carbon dioxide tension ($PaCO_2$) greater than 60 mm Hg should be documented by arterial blood gas testing.

The confirmatory test of choice is an electroencephalogram documenting electrocerebral silence or absence of brain blood flow by nuclear scintigraphy. The electroencephalogram may be done 6 hours after the initial clinical determination of brain death and, when accompanied by a second clinical determination, is diagnostic of brain death. Nuclear scintigraphic determination of brain blood flow is a satisfactory method to provide definitive confirmation of brain death. This test has the advantage that it can be done as a portable examination at the patient's bedside in the intensive care unit (ICU) or emergency department, avoiding the risk of unnecessarily transporting a potentially unstable patient. Alternatively, four-vessel cerebral arteriography demonstrating cessation of blood flow to the brain may be used within an hour of the clinical brain death declaration.

Etiology. Any condition that results in an overwhelming cerebral insult may be sufficient to cause brain death. In general, these conditions fall into the broad categories of subarachnoid or intracerebral hemorrhage, direct cerebral trauma, primary malignancy of the central nervous system, and other rare and miscellaneous entities. Subarachnoid hemorrhage may result from rupture of an intracranial aneurysm. Other cerebrovascular accidents including hypertensive hemorrhagic stroke can be lethal. These entities are responsible for most cases of brain death that lead to organ donation. Brain injury after trauma, either vehicular or related to firearms, is also common.

Pathophysiology

Cardiovascular Instability. During the events that lead to brain death, there is usually progressive intracranial hypertension. Important pathophysiologic responses are evident before the actual occurrence of brain death, including the development of marked systemic hypertension associated with vastly increased sympathetic activity and the massive release of catecholamines. Arrhythmia may become manifest at any time during the process of tentorial herniation. Bradyarrhythmia may be associated with the systemic hypertensive response to intracranial hypertension (Cushing reflex), but ventricular and supraventricular tachyarrhythmia may also be seen in the presence of high levels of catecholamines.

Once herniation is complete and brain death has occurred, a high proportion of donors manifest a hypotensive response related to the loss of sympathetic tone and the failure to maintain circulating catecholamine levels. It has been reported that 62% of brain-dead patients sustain cardiac arrest within 24 hours and 87% by 72 hours in the absence of specific donor maintenance measures.[26] Even with aggressive donor support, about 10% of donors manifest cardiopulmonary arrest during the interval between the determination of brain death and the procurement of organs.[27]

Central Hormonal Failure. As the brain and brainstem cease to function, failure of the central hormonal axis occurs. Pituitary hormones cease to be produced, and diabetes insipidus ensues. Without antidiuretic hormone, urinary output may increase to astonishing rates, sometimes well in excess of 1 L/h. The urine becomes extremely dilute, resulting in increasing serum osmolarity and hypernatremia. The resultant hypovolemia may contribute to cardiovascular collapse if untreated.

The influence of other aspects of central hormonal function is less well understood. There is experimental evidence of reduced circulating levels of triiodothyronine, cortisol, and insulin after brain death in pigs and baboons.[28,29] These factors may contribute to the hemodynamic instability, cardiovascular collapse, and hyperglycemia so often seen in association with brain death and have led some to advocate using combinations of these compounds before organ procurement. Confirmatory studies in humans have not shown these hormonal systems to play major roles in the pathophysiology of the hypotensive state following brain death, although use of these agents is still common in clinical practice.

Request for Permission from Next of Kin. All states and the federal government have passed legislation requiring that relatives of deceased patients be asked whether they are willing to permit organ or tissue donation. Unfortunately, the contribution of such laws to an increase in the actual supply of donor organs is less than clear. What is far more important than required request is the careful training, uniform deployment, and empathetic demeanor of the individuals who actually approach the family. In many hospitals, trained donor coordinators are on call to discuss the option of organ donation with bereaved families. Such people may come from a variety of fields, including medicine, nursing, social work, or pastoral care. Refusal of consent by the family is one of the biggest stumbling blocks to increasing the supply of organs actually donated. It has also been suggested that the discussion of possible organ donation should occur at a time subsequent to and separate from informing the family of the patient's death.

The use of the term *brain death* may be confusing to laypeople and professionals alike; it implies that brain death

TABLE 34.1

CLASSIFICATION HIERARCHY FOR PERMISSION FOR ORGAN DONATION FROM NEXT OF KIN

1. Spouse
2. Adult son or daughter
3. Either parent
4. Adult brother or sister
5. Guardian
6. Any other person authorized to dispose of the body

is different from other kinds of death. Obviously, the distinction is intended to differentiate this modality of dying from cardiac death but not to indicate that the person is any less dead. Phrases such as "keeping the organs alive so they can be transplanted" are as misleading and confusing as they are incorrect.

According to the Uniform Anatomical Gift Act, a signed and witnessed organ donor card is a legally binding indication of the decedent's wishes, but throughout North America and most European countries, the family's consent is routinely obtained before organ procurement. Although it is desirable that the entire family be in agreement about donating, the legal next of kin is required to agree to the donation and grant signed permission (Table 34.1).

Donor Maintenance

Tissue Perfusion. Most donors are maintained with a minimum of fluids to prevent increased cerebral edema, and, therefore, one of the first priorities in donor maintenance should be the prompt restoration of intravascular volume. Depending on the duration of the donor's underlying illness, this process may require from 3 to 10 L of volume resuscitation. In general, the dosage of pressor agents required to support blood pressure can be progressively decreased as the central venous pressure is raised to 10 to 12 cm H_2O. Crystalloid may be used, and lactated Ringer solution is often given because its slightly lower sodium concentration counteracts the concentrating effects of diabetes insipidus. If the latter condition has resulted in severe hypernatremia, the addition of free water may be necessary. Colloid and blood should be used to restore and maintain osmotic pressure and normovolemia. The hematocrit should be kept around 35 volume percent to replace traumatic losses and to maintain oxygen-carrying capacity. Enough volume should be administered to achieve a urine output of at least 100 mL/h and a systolic arterial pressure of 90 to 120 mm Hg. Higher levels of arterial blood pressure are usually unnecessary because the loss of sympathetic tone accompanying brain death facilitates tissue perfusion at lower pressure.

If diabetes insipidus is severe, exogenous vasopressin must be given. Available in a variety of forms, desmopressin acetate, a synthetic analog of 8-arginine vasopressin, appears to have the least splanchnic vasoconstrictive effect compared with its antidiuretic action. This agent can be given by a variety of routes, including intranasally, subcutaneously, or intravenously. The usual dosage is 20 μg intranasally or 2 to 4 μg intravenously or subcutaneously.

Oxygenation and Ventilation. Arterial blood gases should be checked regularly and appropriate adjustments of the ventilator made to optimize gas exchange and acid–base balance. Oxygen supply should be adequate to maintain an arterial oxygen saturation of greater than 95% and mixed venous oxygen saturation above 70%. Low levels of positive end-expiratory pressure may facilitate achieving a balanced oxygen supply and demand.

Inotropic Support. Most donors are hypovolemic at the time of brain death and are receiving inotropic support in lieu of volume to support their blood pressure. Dopamine hydrochloride is the most commonly used agent. The need for dosages above 10 μg/kg/min usually indicates persistent hypovolemia, and the restoration of normovolemia is almost always accompanied by a reduction in dopamine requirements. High doses of dopamine maintained for long periods before organ procurement may be associated with increased rates of acute tubular necrosis and hepatic allograft failure. Cardiac procurement is often abandoned if high doses of inotropic support are required despite adequate volume status.

Other inotropic agents, such as isoproterenol, epinephrine, norepinephrine, and phenylephrine, are occasionally used, but the use of these agents should be discouraged because of their peripheral vasoconstrictive effects. Dobutamine is sometimes used in conjunction with low doses of dopamine.

Prevention of Hypothermia. Thermoregulatory homeostatic mechanisms are destroyed with the occurrence of brain death, and the development of severe hypothermia may lead to ventricular arrhythmia and cardiac arrest. Warming blankets should be used above and below the donor to keep body temperature above 35°C, and exposure for the purposes of examination or intervention should be kept to a minimum. If maintenance of normal body temperature is problematic, intravenous fluids may be prewarmed before administration, and a heated humidifier circuit can be added to the ventilator.

Multiple Organ Procurement

The Organ Procurement and Transplantation Network and the Coordination of Surgical Teams. When brain death has been declared, the person has been identified as a suitable organ donor, and permission has been given by the next of kin, the logistics of organ procurement must be arranged. Since passage of the National Organ Transplantation Act, a national Organ Procurement and Transplantation Network (OPTN) has been organized. The federal contract for this important function is held by the United Network for Organ Sharing (UNOS). The OPTN is responsible for the fair and equitable distribution of deceased donor organs throughout the United States. The 50 states and U.S. territories and possessions are divided into 11 regions (Fig. 34.4). Within each region, federally certified local organ procurement organizations (OPOs) are responsible for maintaining the list of
4 potential recipients for their catchment area. All transplant candidates within the United States are entered into a computer system, and an allocation system is used to determine the appropriate potential recipient for a given donor organ. In general, offers are made first to candidates listed with transplant centers in the local OPO service area, then to suitable candidates in the region, and finally to any candidate in the nation. In each case, priority is ordered by the existing allocation system designed for that organ.[30] An important exception to these general rules relates to renal transplant recipients who share six antigens with the donor. These kidneys are automatically shared nationwide even if suitable local recipients are available.

Recipients of the various organs may reside in geographically distant locations. Because the recipient transplant teams must be given considerable detailed information about the donor to decide whether to use a particular organ for a particular recipient, a finite period of time is required to assemble the necessary donor retrieval teams. A national computerized system (DonorNet) provides all relevant medical information simultaneously to multiple prospective accepting programs. The coordinating OPO contacts accepting teams, facilitates logistical arrangements and communications for travel to the donor hospital, and makes arrangements for the

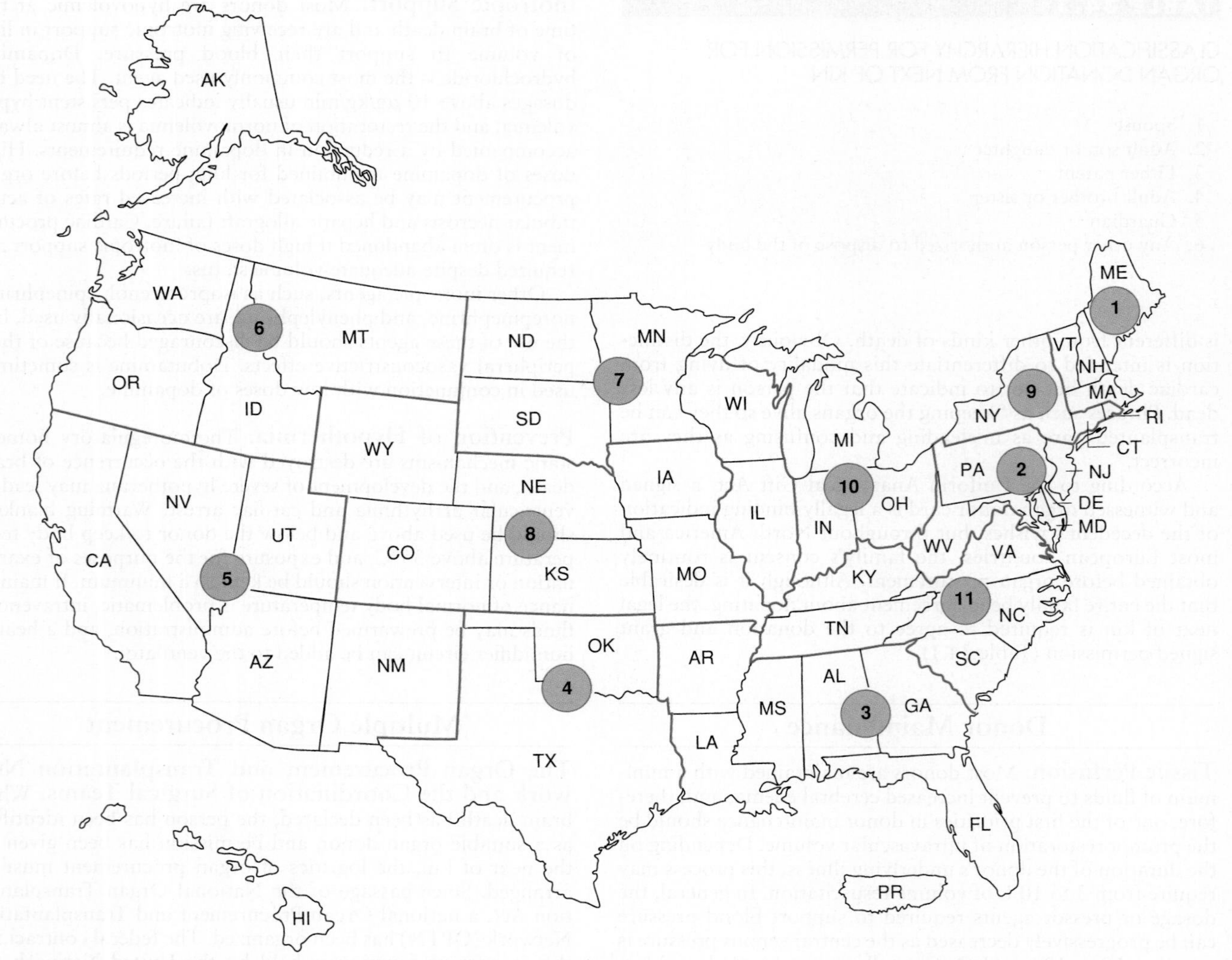

FIGURE 34.4. The 50 United States are divided into 11 regions of approximately equal populations for purposes of administration of organ procurement, distribution, and educational objectives.

donor operating room to be available at an appropriate time. When all teams are on site at the donor hospital, the donor is transferred to the operating room for the actual procurement procedure.

Surgical Technique for Multiple Organ Procurement.

Techniques of multiple organ procurement allow for the removal of the heart, lungs, kidneys, liver, intestine, and pancreas from a single donor for transplantation into multiple recipients. The following discussion details the methods used to remove all these organs from a donor.

The heart-beating donor is brought to the operating room from the ICU or emergency department with appropriate hemodynamic and electrocardiographic monitoring. Oxygen is delivered by hand bagging at 100% inspired concentration. Inotropic drug infusions are continued during transport and procurement. The anesthesiologist should maintain close communication with the procurement teams to avoid the development of cardiac arrhythmia, hypotension, and hypoxemia. The procuring surgical teams should each confirm documentation of the declaration of death, valid consent for organ donation, and ABO blood typing.

The steps in the procedure can be categorized as follows: (a) incision, (b) exploration and inspection, (c) individual organ mobilization, (d) in situ perfusion, (e) removal of organs, and (f) closure of the incision. Postprocurement processing, packaging, and transport to the recipient centers are the final steps.

The entire torso is prepared with an iodine-containing solution, and a field is draped from the neck to the pubis. A long, midline incision is made from the suprasternal notch to the pubis. The sternum is split with an electrical or air-powered saw if available, although manual methods using a Lebsche knife or Gigli saw work perfectly well. Exposure of the abdominal organs may be facilitated by the addition of cruciate incisions (Fig. 34.5). A general exploration is carried out to ascertain that no unexpected conditions are present that would preclude donation, such as tumor, infection, or specific organ damage. In general, a "no-touch" technique is used to minimize trauma to the organs during the procurement procedure.

For the so-called rapid technique of organ procurement, relatively little in the way of mobilization of individual organs is necessary. Preparation for in situ perfusion consists of a complete Kocher maneuver, with mobilization of the right colon, duodenum, and small bowel in a cephalad direction to the patient's left (Fig. 34.6). The aorta is exposed from the bifurcation distally to the level of the left renal vein

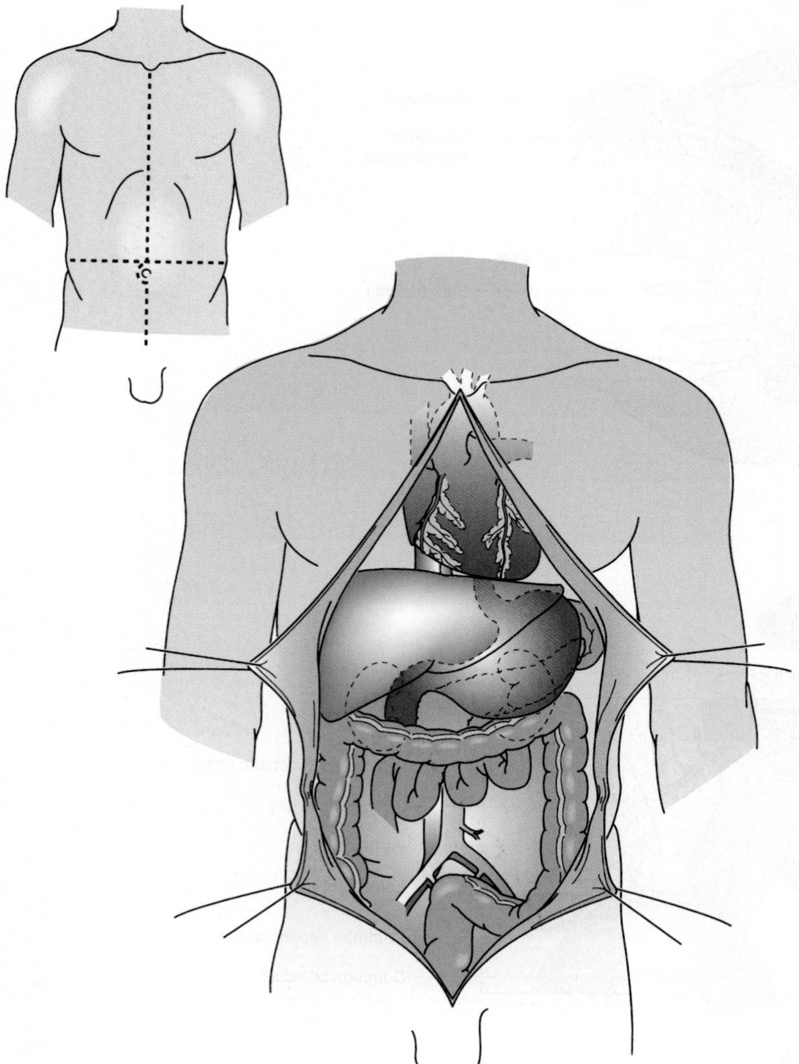

FIGURE 34.5. A complete midline incision from suprasternal notch to pubis is made for multiple organ procurement. The sternum is split. If necessary, cruciate abdominal incisions are added to facilitate exposure of the intra-abdominal organs.

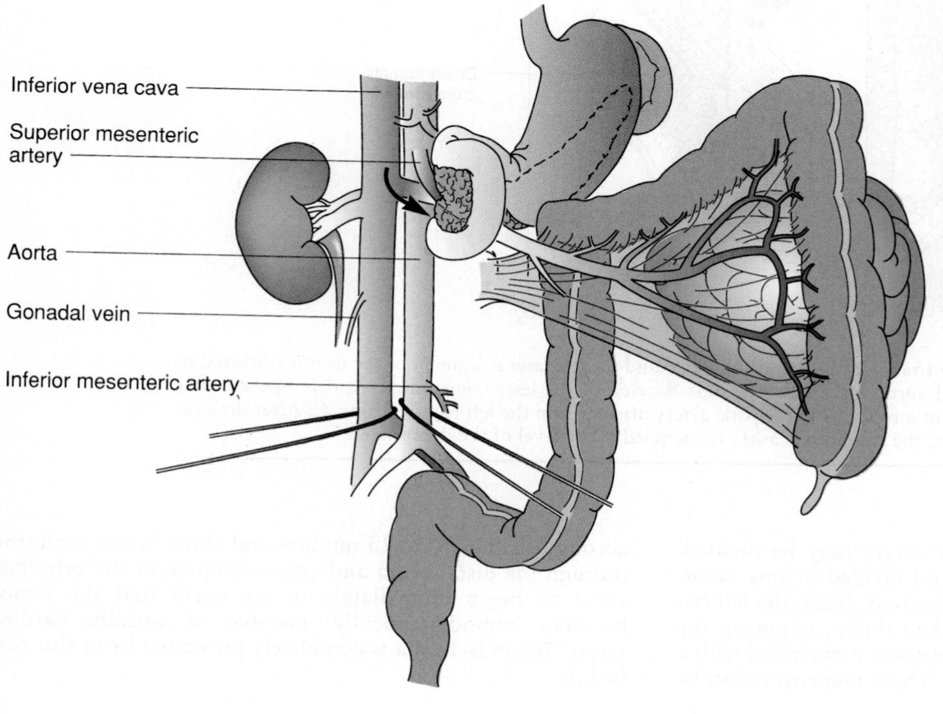

FIGURE 34.6. The Kocher maneuver is used to mobilize completely the right colon and duodenum, exposing the retroperitoneum, including the aorta, from the level of the superior mesenteric artery to the bifurcation and the inferior vena cava from the iliac veins to the edge of the liver.

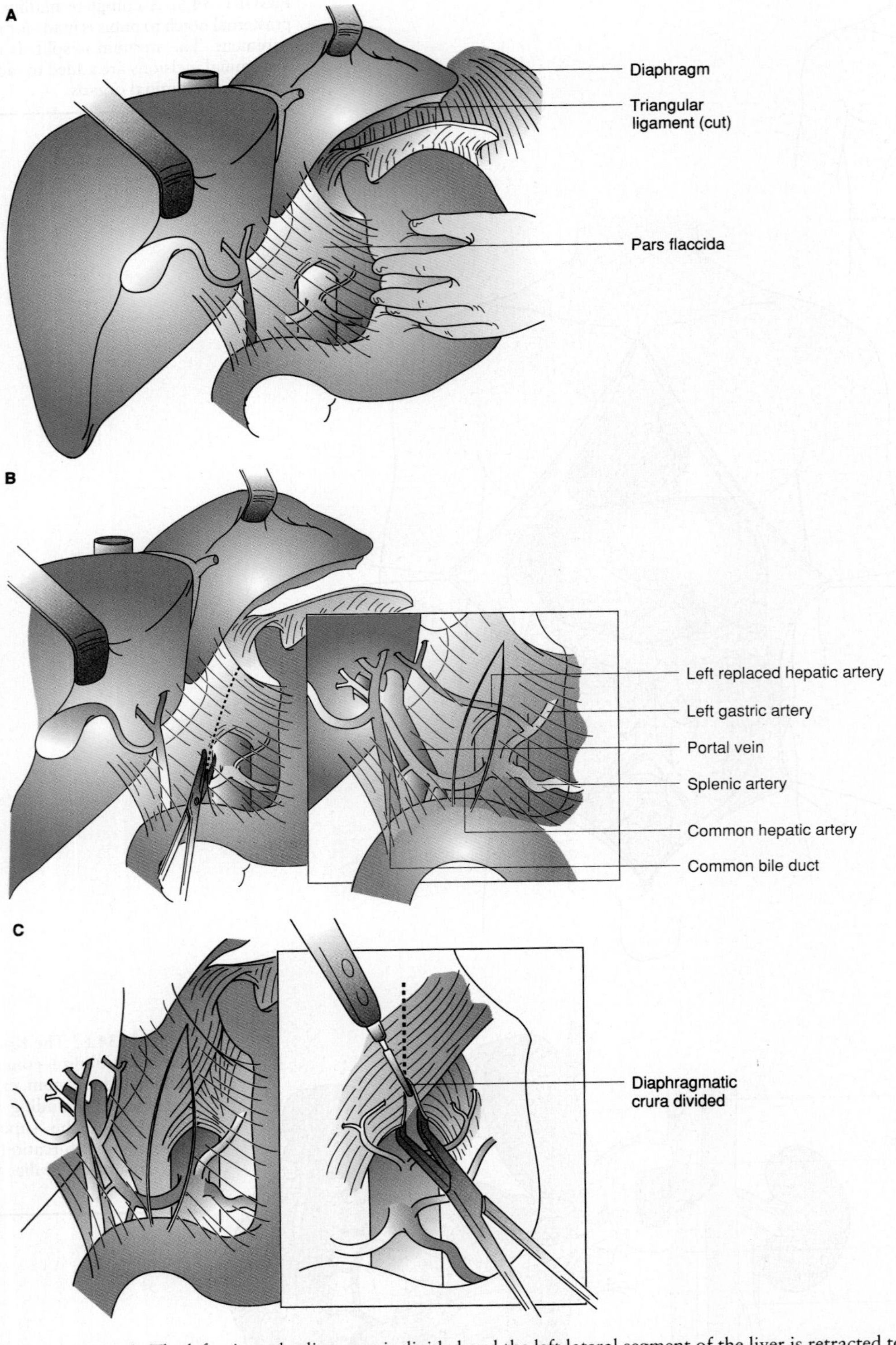

FIGURE 34.7. **A:** The left triangular ligament is divided and the left lateral segment of the liver is retracted to expose the esophagus and aortic hiatus. **B:** The pars flaccida of the lesser omentum is widely opened after checking for the presence of a replaced left hepatic artery arising from the left gastric artery. **C:** After division of the diaphragmatic crura, the supraceliac aorta is encircled at the level of the diaphragm.

proximally. The inferior mesenteric artery may be divided. Lumbar branches may be ligated and divided at this point. The inferior vena cava is similarly exposed. Next, the left triangular ligament of the liver is taken down, exposing the crural fibers at the aortic hiatus. The aorta is encircled with a tape at the diaphragm (Fig. 34.7A). These maneuvers can be accomplished in 10 to 15 minutes and allow in situ perfusion through the distal aorta and cross-clamping of the proximal aorta to begin immediately in the event that the donor becomes hemodynamically unstable or sustains cardiac arrest. Warm ischemia is completely prevented by in situ perfusion.

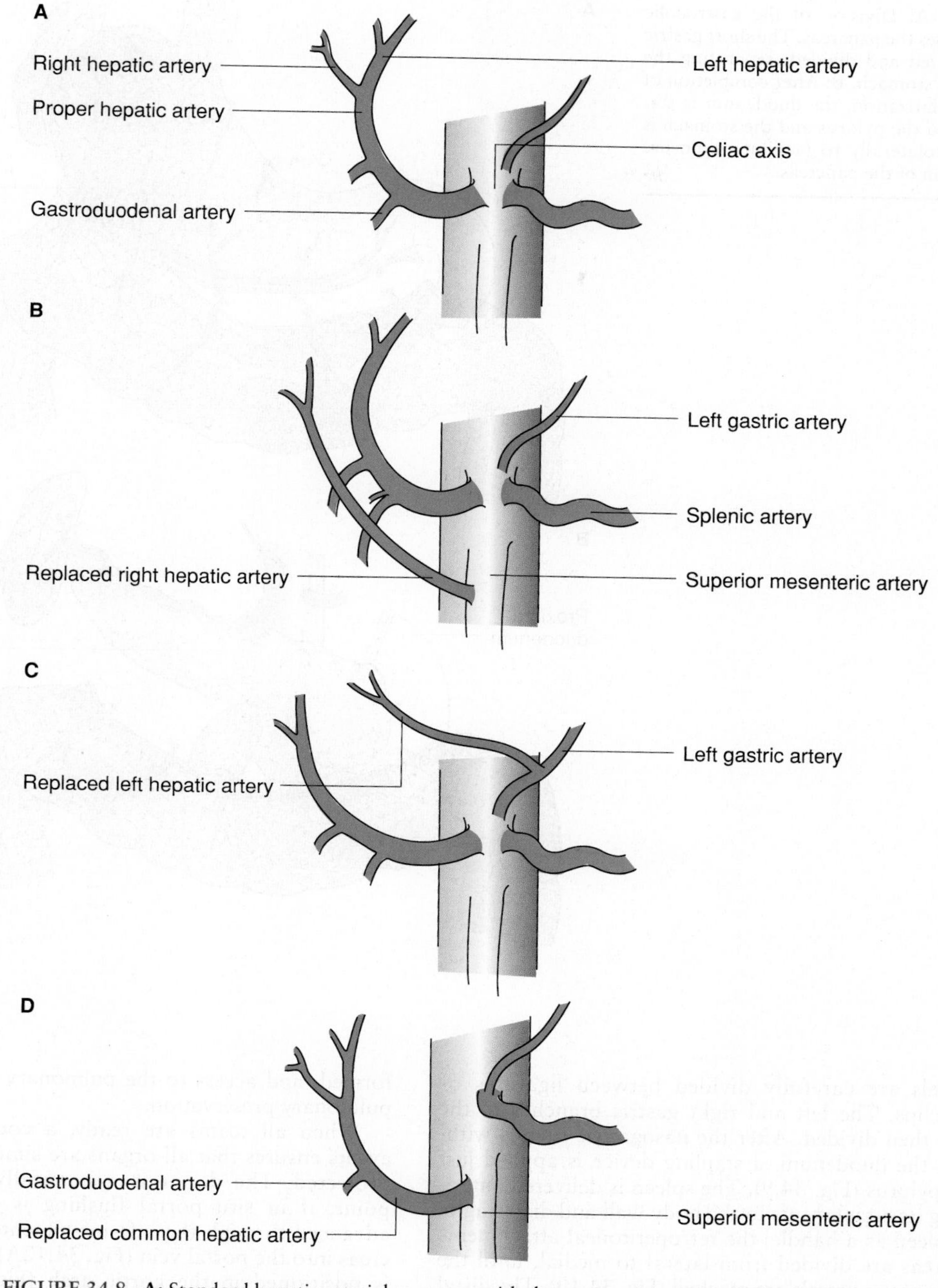

FIGURE 34.8. **A:** Standard hepatic arterial anatomy, with the artery arising as a single vessel as a branch of the celiac axis. **B:** Aberrant hepatic arterial anatomy, with a replaced right hepatic artery arising from the superior mesenteric artery and ascending posterior to the common bile duct and anterolateral to the portal vein. **C:** A replaced left hepatic artery arising from the left gastric artery is usually visible and palpable crossing the pars flaccida of the lesser omentum from the lesser curvature of the stomach. **D:** A completely replaced common hepatic artery arising from the superior mesenteric artery.

Stable donors afford the luxury of further preparation before in situ flushing. The inferior mesenteric vein is isolated as it enters the retroperitoneum behind the pancreas. This vein provides convenient access for in situ portal flushing by means of a small catheter. If pancreas and/or intestinal procurement is also planned, the portal flush can be done after removal. The pars flaccida of the lesser omentum should be inspected for evidence of a replaced left hepatic artery arising from the left gastric artery, and minimal dissection of the hepatic artery is necessary (Fig. 34.7B). The portal triad should be palpated carefully for evidence of a replaced right hepatic artery arising from the superior mesenteric artery. This vessel, when present, can be palpated as it courses toward the liver posterior to the common bile duct and along the right side of the portal vein as it emerges from its origin off the superior mesenteric artery posterior to the pancreas (Fig. 34.8).

If the pancreas is to be procured, 250 mL of an iodine-containing solution, followed by instillation of an antifungal agent, is administered via the nasogastric tube into the duodenum. After the gastrocolic omentum is divided, the short

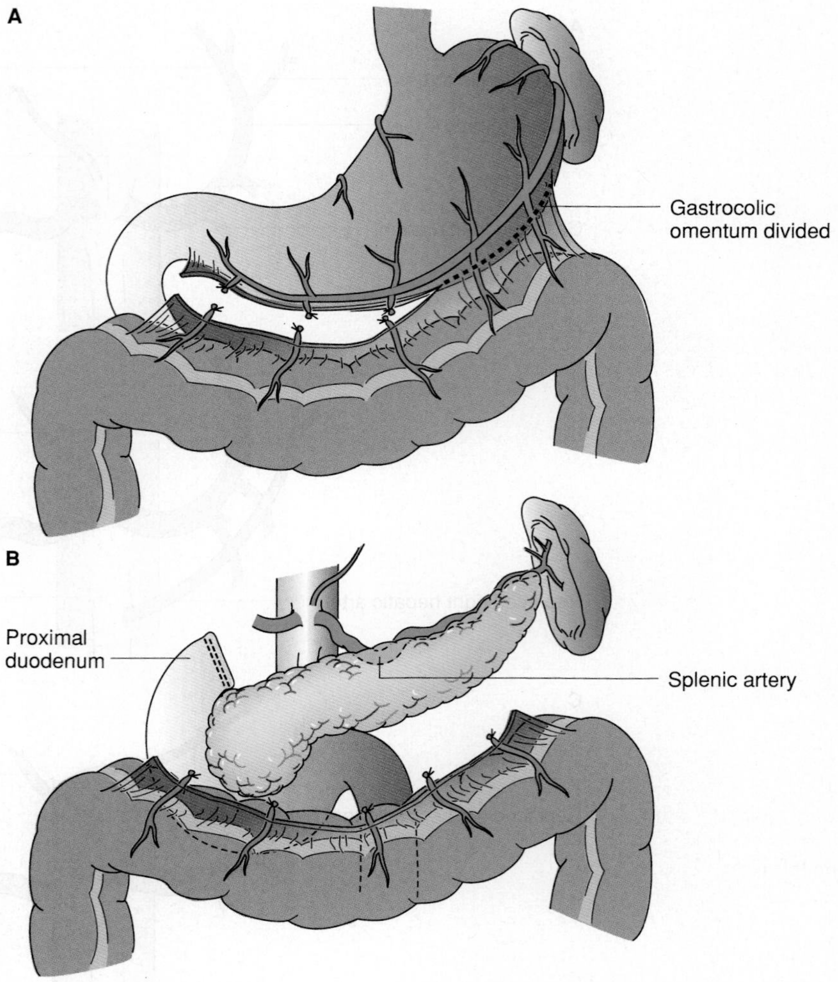

FIGURE 34.9. **A:** Division of the gastrocolic omentum exposes the pancreas. The short gastric vessels are ligated and divided, separating the spleen from the stomach. **B:** After completion of gastric devascularization, the duodenum is stapled just beyond the pylorus and the stomach is retracted superolaterally to facilitate exposure and mobilization of the pancreas.

gastric vessels are carefully divided between ligatures or hemostatic clips. The left and right gastric branches to the stomach are then divided. After the nasogastric tube is withdrawn from the duodenum, a stapling device is applied just beyond the pylorus (Fig. 34.9). The spleen is delivered anteriorly, dividing its attachments to the body wall and diaphragm. Using the spleen as a handle, the retroperitoneal attachments of the pancreas are divided from lateral to medial, until the superior mesenteric vessels are reached (Fig. 34.10). The distal duodenum is divided with a stapler near the Treitz ligament just before or after aortic cross-clamping.

If the intestine is to be procured for an isolated small bowel transplant, the only additional dissection required is to separate the distal ileum near the ileocecal valve from the colon. The small bowel is transected here using a stapling device.[31]

The course of the ureters should be identified. The Gerota fascia is widely incised to allow topical cooling with iced slush solution to supplement the in situ perfusion. Complete mobilization of the kidneys before in situ flushing is unnecessary and risks damage to the renal vessels or inadvertent division of accessory renal arteries.

The heart and lungs can be readied for removal by a team working simultaneously with the abdominal retrieval team. The superior and inferior vena cavae are mobilized, and the aortic arch is dissected sufficiently for the placement of a cross-clamp at the time of infusion of aortic root cardioplegia (Fig. 34.11). Preliminary mobilization of the lungs is usually performed, and access to the pulmonary artery is necessary for pulmonary preservation.

When all teams are ready, a coordinated sequence of events ensures that all organs are simultaneously cooled and protected. The donor is systemically heparinized. At this point, if in situ portal flushing is desired, a catheter is advanced through the inferior mesenteric vein near the pancreas into the portal vein (Fig. 34.12A). A cardioplegia needle is positioned in the aortic arch (Fig. 34.12B). The distal abdominal aorta is cannulated for retrograde in situ perfusion of the kidneys, liver, pancreas, and intestine, and an exsanguination cannula is placed in the distal inferior vena cava (Fig. 34.12C). Alternatively, the inferior vena caval–right atrial junction may be divided in the chest with suction catheters placed in the caval lumen and right thoracic cavity to decompress the venous circulation at the moment of aortic cross-clamping.

The aortic arch and the abdominal aorta at the diaphragm are simultaneously cross-clamped. Cardioplegia solution is infused under pressure into the aortic root, perfusing the coronary arteries and arresting the heart. Ventilation is ceased. Portal and distal aortic perfusion are initiated with ice-cold preservation solution. Topical iced slush is placed in the abdomen and chest to assist the cooling process. The heart and lungs are then removed. The clamp is removed from the distal vena caval cannula for exsanguination and to preclude venous congestion. The liver and pancreas are removed en bloc. The diaphragm surrounding the suprahepatic inferior

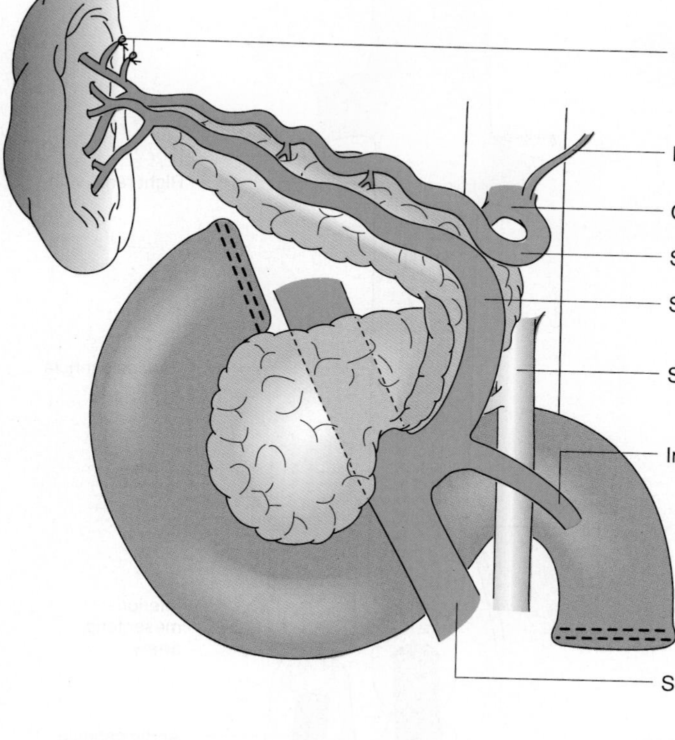

FIGURE 34.10. The pancreas is reflected anteriorly and to the right to the level of the superior mesenteric vein near the confluence with the splenic vein. The aortic origins of the celiac axis and superior mesenteric arteries are identified.

vena cava and adjacent to the bare area of the liver is divided. The infrahepatic inferior vena cava is divided just cephalad to the left renal vein. The liver and pancreas unit is now attached only by the distal superior mesenteric vessels coursing to the small bowel and by the aortic origins of the superior mesenteric artery and celiac axis. The superior mesenteric artery and vein emerging from the uncinate process are ligated and divided, and a cylinder of aorta is removed encompassing the superior mesenteric artery and celiac axis. The distal superior mesenteric artery and vein provide blood supply to the small intestinal graft, which is removed next. The liver and pancreas are separated as a bench procedure, retaining the celiac

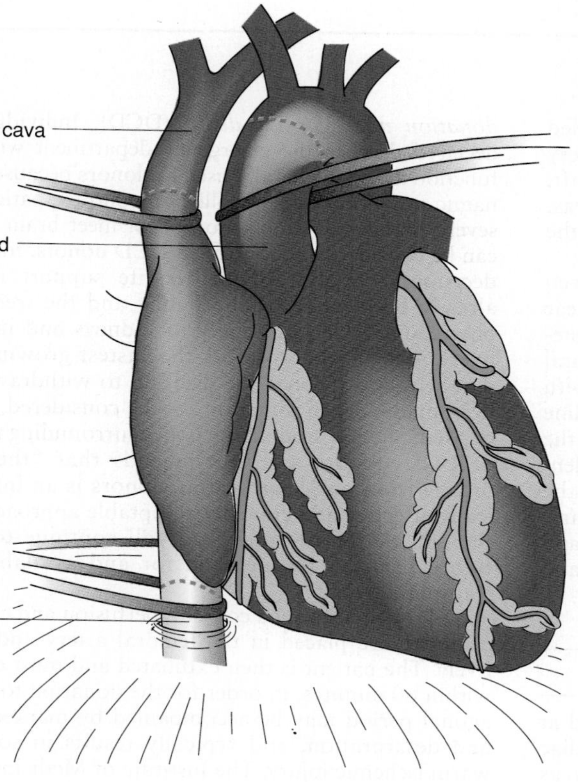

FIGURE 34.11. Preparation of the heart for cardioplegia. Minimal dissection is necessary. The venae cavae are encircled, and the aorta is separated from the pulmonary artery.

TRANSPLANTATION

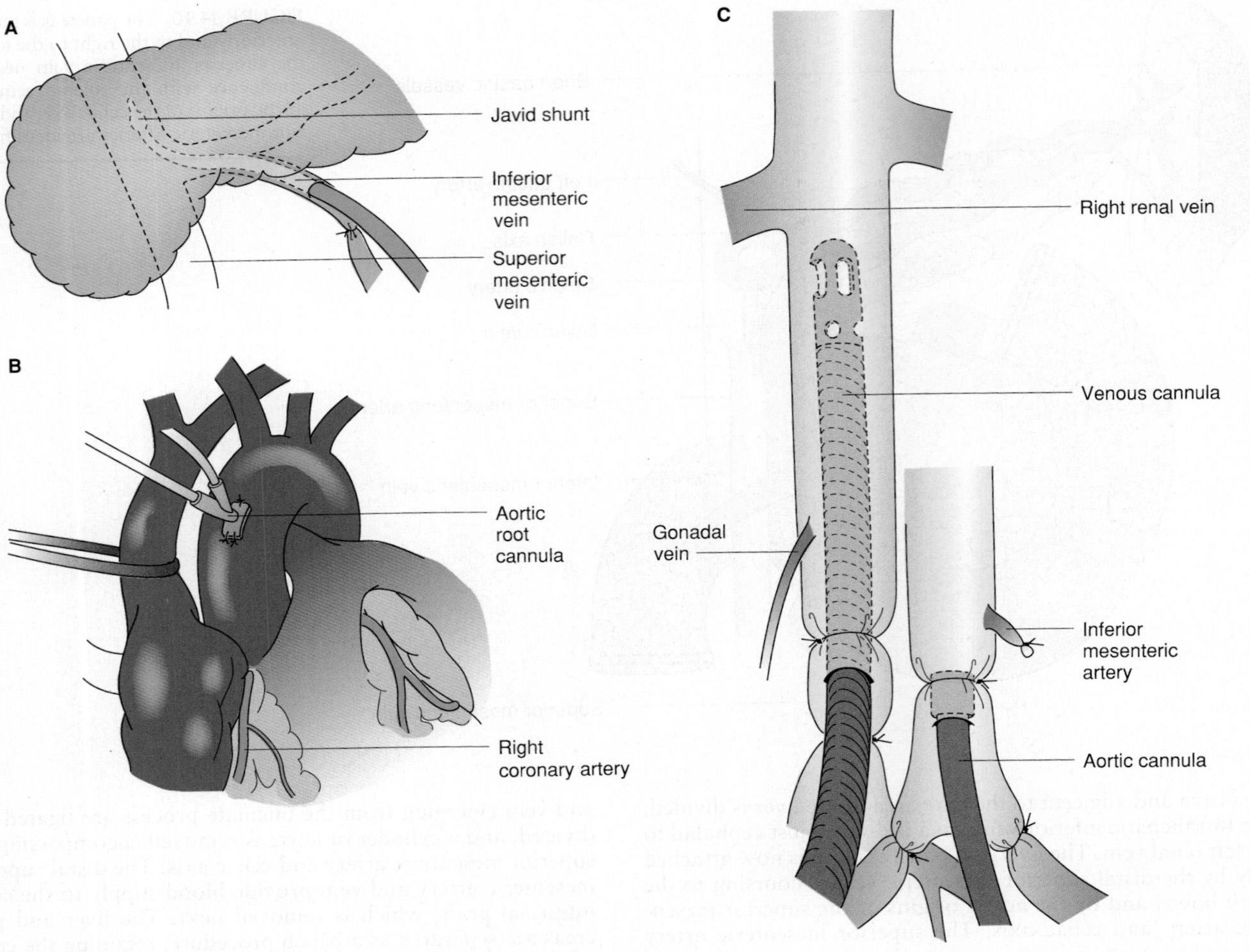

FIGURE 34.12. In situ perfusion set-up. **A:** A cannula is placed into the portal vein through the inferior mesenteric vein for portal venous perfusion. **B:** A needle is placed in the aortic root for perfusion of the coronary arteries with cardioplegia solution. **C:** A cannula is placed in the distal aorta for retrograde perfusion with cold preservation solution. Another cannula is placed in the distal vena cava for venous decompression and exsanguination.

axis with the liver (Fig. 34.13). The splenic artery is divided at its origin. This vessel and the superior mesenteric artery are reconstructed with a bifurcated donor iliac artery graft. The portal vein is divided about 1 cm from the pancreas. The common bile duct is divided at the superior edge of the pancreas.

The kidneys are also removed en bloc. The ureters are given wide berth to avoid devascularization and are divided near their entrance into the bladder. Dissection is carried out posterior to the aorta and vena cava in the plane of the prevertebral fascia. Once removed, the left renal vein is divided flush with the vena cava (Fig. 34.14). The aorta is opened in the midline to identify the orifices of the renal arteries from within the lumen. In this way, multiple renal arteries can be readily identified and kept on a single aortic Carrel patch. Once the abdominal and thoracic organs have been removed, a sampling of lymph nodes and spleen is taken for tissue typing and cross match testing. The chest and abdomen are closed, and standard postmortem care is given.

Donation after Cardiac Death

The profound shortage of organs has led to efforts aimed at utilizing organs from patients who die as a result of cardiac standstill rather than brain death. This process is referred to as *donation after cardiac death* (DCD). Individuals who are declared dead in the emergency department without cardiac function are not generally used as donors because the hemodynamic situation is uncontrolled. In contrast, patients who have severe brain injury but who do not meet brain death criteria can be considered as controlled DCD donors. In this setting, a decision to withdraw further life support measures has already been made by the family and the treating team of physicians. DCD, especially of kidneys and increasingly of livers, has become one of the fastest-growing sources of donor organs.[32] Once the decision to withdraw support has been made, organ donation can be considered. The Institute of Medicine has studied the issues surrounding the utilization of DCD donors and recommends that "the recovery of organs from non-heartbeating donors is an important medically effective and ethically acceptable approach to reducing the gap that exists now and will continue to exist in the future between the demand for and available supply for transplantation."[33]

Following informed consent, perfusion and exsanguination cannulae are placed in the femoral artery and vein, respectively. The patient is then extubated and must expire, usually within 60 minutes, in order for the donation to proceed. This agonal period may be accompanied by marked hypotension and desaturation, and typically results in some degree of warm ischemic injury. The Institute of Medicine recommends

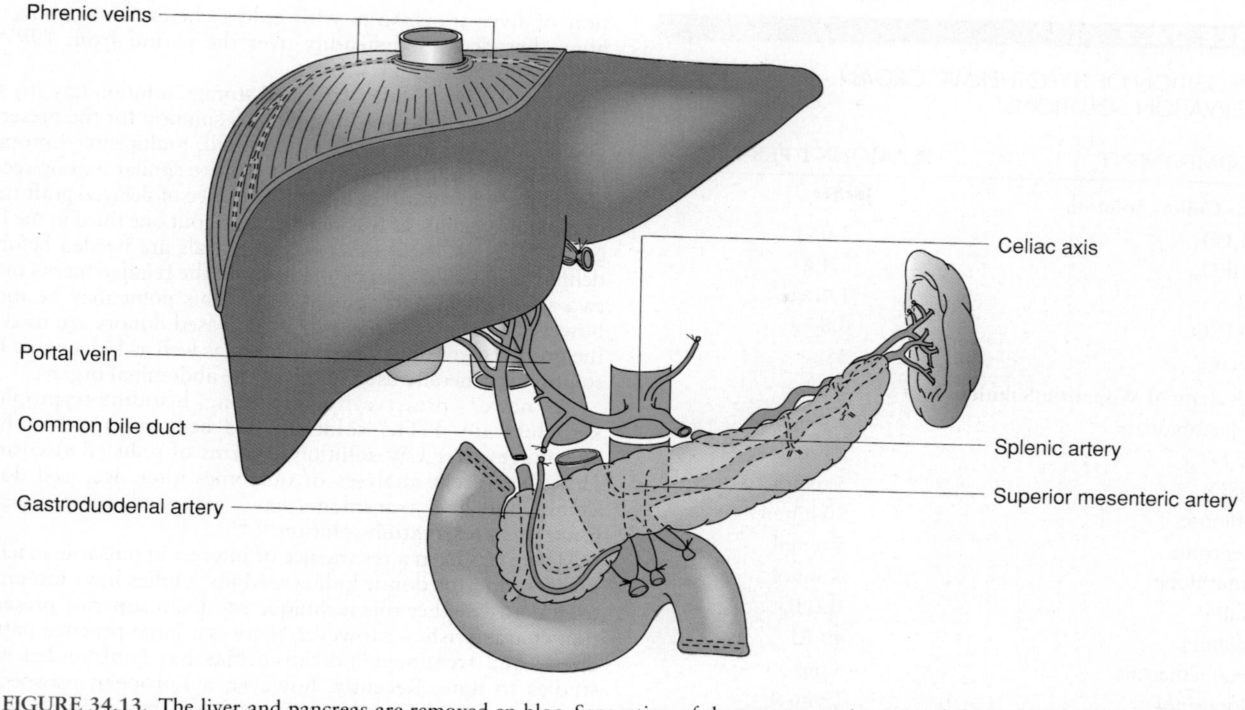

FIGURE 34.13. The liver and pancreas are removed en bloc. Separation of the two organs is accomplished as a bench procedure. The celiac axis is retained with the liver, dividing the splenic artery just beyond its origin. The gastroduodenal artery is ligated and divided. The portal vein is divided approximately 1 cm from the superior edge of the pancreas, and the common bile duct is divided just superior to its entrance into the pancreas.

waiting an additional 5 minutes after cessation of effective cardiac function and pronouncement of death before proceeding with organ procurement.

At this point, the organs are rapidly cooled by infusing cold preservation fluid via the previously placed cannula. Simultaneously, the abdomen and chest are opened and a standard organ procurement procedure is carried out. Growing experience demonstrates that outcomes of kidneys transplanted from DCD donors are comparable with those from brain-dead donors, with the exception of a higher incidence of delayed graft function.[34] However, DCD livers have been noted to develop ischemic-type biliary strictures, and significantly worse outcomes from livers from DCD versus brain-dead donors have been reported.[35]

Current Preservation Techniques and Results

Kidneys, Liver, and Pancreas. For many years, the primary solution used for cold storage preservation of the kidneys was Euro-Collins solution (Table 34.2). This formulation provides a hyperosmolar environment with intracellular electrolyte composition that is intended to reduce cellular swelling. In combination with hypothermia, kidneys can be safely stored in this solution for 36 to 48 hours before transplantation.

In the 1980s, the advent of new immunosuppressive agents, such as cyclosporine, meant that for the first time extrarenal organs could be transplanted with good success rates, and the

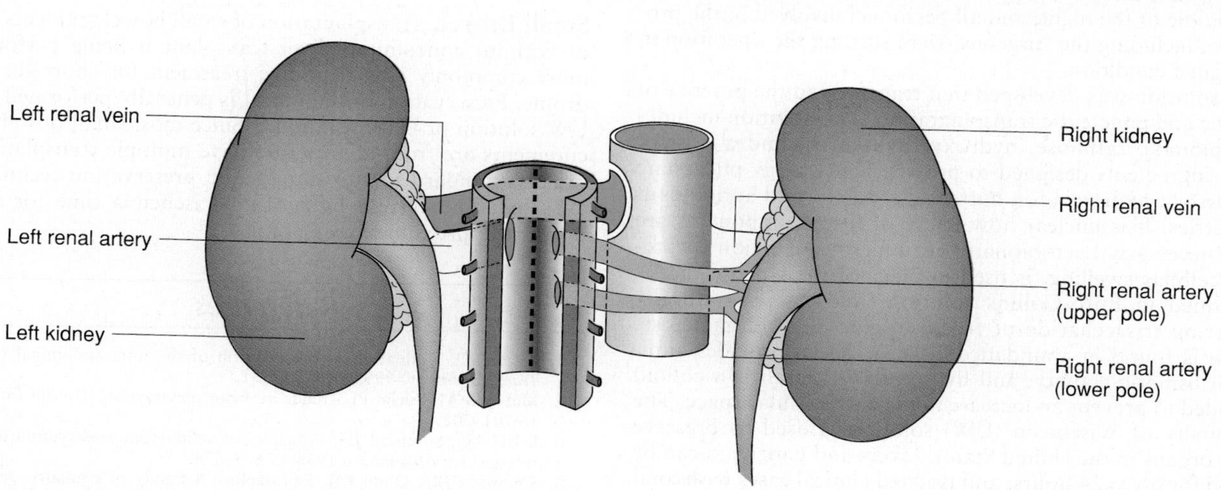

FIGURE 34.14. The kidneys are removed en bloc and separated on the back bench. Safe division is ensured by viewing the kidneys posteriorly. The aorta is divided between the paired lumbar arteries, and renal arterial orifices can be viewed directly from within the aortic lumen. This avoids any hilar dissection with the accompanying risk of injury to renal arteries. The left renal vein is divided at its entrance to the inferior vena cava, leaving the entire vena cava with the shorter right renal vein.

TABLE 34.2

COMPOSITION OF HYPOTHERMIC ORGAN PRESERVATION SOLUTIONS

■ COMPONENT	■ AMOUNT PER LITER
Euro-Collins Solution	
KH_2PO_4	2.05 g
K_2HPO_4	7.4 g
KCl	1.12 g
$NaHCO_3$	0.84 g
Glucose	35 g
University of Wisconsin Solution	
K^+-lactobionate	100 mmol
KH_2PO_4	25 mmol
$MgSO_4$	5 mmol
Raffinose	30 mmol
Adenosine	5 mmol
Glutathione	3 mmol
Insulin	100 IU
Penicillin	40 IU
Dexamethasone	8 mg
Allopurinol	1 mmol
HTK Solution	
NaCl	15 mmol
KCl	9 mmol
KH-2-ketoglutarate	1 mmol
$MgCl_2$	4 mmol
Histidine hydrochloride	18 mmol
Histidine	180 mmol
Tryptophan	2 mmol
Mannitol	30 mmol
$CaCl_2$	0.015 mmol

need for more effective preservation became apparent. Cold ischemia limitations of about 8 hours for the liver and pancreas meant that donor and recipient teams had to be exquisitely coordinated; complex recipient operations requiring a multitude of ancillary support services had to be organized in the middle of the night; and all personnel involved in the procedure, including the surgeons, were starting the operation in a fatigued condition.

A solution was developed that transformed the practice of hepatic and pancreatic transplantation. This solution includes lactobionate, raffinose, hydroxyethyl starch, and a host of other ingredients designed to provide high-energy phosphate precursors, hydrogen ion buffering capacity, and antioxidant properties. It is unclear how many of these components are truly necessary. Lactobionate, an impermeant anion to prevent cellular swelling, is used in place of the glucose that is contained in Euro-Collins solution; raffinose, a naturally occurring trisaccharide of fructose, glucose, and galactose, which is found in abundance in sugar beets, provides additional osmotic activity; and hydroxyethyl starch is a colloid intended to prevent an increase in the extracellular space. The University of Wisconsin (UW) solution is used to preserve most organs in the United States. Livers and pancreata can be stored for up to 24 hours, and isolated clinical cases with total cold ischemia times in excess of 30 hours have been reported.[36,37] However, although livers will function in terms of hepatocellular metabolism, evidence is accumulating that cold ischemia times of greater than 12 hours may be associated with a higher incidence of biliary strictures. The proportion of liver transplants with cold ischemia time above 10 hours has decreased steadily over the period from 1997 to 2006 from 23% to 11%.[13]

It is not clear whether UW cold storage solution has any significant advantages over Euro-Collins solution for the preservation of kidneys. In a large, randomized, multicenter European trial, patient and graft survival rates were similar among recipients of the two solutions, but the incidence of delayed graft function requiring dialysis was reduced by about one third in the UW group. The results of other ongoing trials are needed before a definitive statement can be made about the relative merits of the two solutions in renal preservation. This point may be moot, however, because the majority of deceased donors are used for the procurement of extrarenal organs as well as kidneys, so UW solution is generally used for all of the abdominal organs.

A newer preservative solution, histidine-tryptophan-ketoglutarate (HTK) solution, has been reported to have advantages over UW solution in terms of reduced viscosity.[38] However, recent analyses of outcomes after deceased donor kidney and liver transplants have suggested inferior results using this preservation solution.[39,40]

There has been a resurgence of interest in pulsatile machine preservation for donor kidneys. Many studies have attempted to discern whether this technique results in superior preservation characteristics. However, there is a large practice pattern effect, and treatment indication bias has confounded most studies to date. Recently, however, a European prospective randomized trial has shown significantly better results using machine preservation.[41] However, because of the added expense and logistical requirements for machine preservation, further studies are needed to identify which donor kidneys are best suited to this technique.

Heart and Lungs. Cardiac preservation has changed relatively little in recent years. Crystalloid cardioplegia solution is used at 4°C, and 4 hours is the generally accepted limit of cold ischemia. For this reason, donor and recipient operations must be finely coordinated. Recently, machine perfusion preservation has been explored as an alternative to simple cold storage, but this modality is still considered experimental.

A comprehensive review of pulmonary preservation has recently been published.[42] Hypothermia is used along with intracellular-type solutions such as Euro-Collins or UW solution. Pulmonary inflation is also important. The optimal vascular perfusate for the lungs remains unknown, however, and results with pulmonary transplantation are still limited by deficiencies in the quality and duration of preservation.

Small Bowel. Transplantation of small bowel segments with or without concomitant liver transplant is being performed more commonly as a definitive treatment for short-gut syndrome. Preservation of the bowel is generally performed with UW solution or HTK solution.[43] Since most small bowel procurements are from donors that have multiple transplantable organs, standard in situ intra-aortic preservation techniques are used. The current limit of cold ischemia time for small bowel is approximately 12 hours.[44]

References

1. Belzer FO. Evaluation of preservation of the intra-abdominal organs. *Transplant Proc* 1993;25:2527–2531.
2. McLaren AJ, Friend PJ. Trends in organ preservation. *Transpl Int* 2003; 16:701–708.
3. Belzer FO, Southard JH. Principles of solid-organ preservation by cold storage. *Transplantation* 1988;45:673–676.
4. Simonson MS, Dunn MJ. Endothelins: a family of regulator peptides. State-of-the-art lecture. *Hypertension* 1991;17:856–863.
5. Wilhelm SM, Simonson MS, Robinson AV, et al. Cold ischemia induces endothelin gene upregulation in the preserved kidney. *J Surg Res* 1999;85: 101–108.
6. Southard JH, Senzig KA, Belzer FO. Effects of hypothermia on canine kidney mitochondria. *Cryobiology* 1980;17:148–153.

7. McCord JM. Oxygen-derived free radicals in postischemic tissue injury. *N Engl J Med* 1985;312:159–163.
8. Clavien PA, Harvey RP, Strasberg SM. Preservation and reperfusion injuries in liver allografts. *Transplantation* 1992;53:957–978.
9. Koyama I, Bulkley GB, Williams GM, et al. The role of oxygen free radicals in mediating the reperfusion injury of cold preserved ischemic kidneys. *Transplantation* 1985;40:590–595.
10. Colletti LM, Burtch GD, Remick DG, et al. The production of tumor necrosis factor alpha and the development of a pulmonary capillary injury following hepatic ischemia/reperfusion. *Transplantation* 1990;49:268–272.
11. Sturber M, Harringer W, Ernst M, et al. Inhaled nitric oxide as a prophylactic treatment against reperfusion injury. *Thorac Cardiovasc Surg* 1999; 47:179–182.
12. Devlin J, Palmer RMJ, Gonde CE, et al. Nitric oxide generation. *Transplantation* 1994;58:592–595.
13. 2007 U.S. Organ Procurement and Transplantation Network and the Scientific Registry for Transplant Recipients Annual Report: Transplant Data 1997–2006: Department of Health and Human Services, Health Resources and Services Administration, Office of Special Programs, Division of Transplantation, Rockville, MD; United Network for Organ Sharing, Richmond, VA; University Renal Research and Education Association. Ann Arbor, MI; 2008.
14. The 11th report of the human renal transplant registry. *JAMA* 1973;226: 1197–1204.
15. Zhou YC, Cecka JM. Effect of age on kidney transplants. In: Terasaki PI, ed. *Clinical Transplants 1989*. Los Angeles, CA: UCLA Tissue Typing Laboratory; 1989:369–378.
16. Pelletier SJ, Guidinger MK, Merion RM, et al. Recovery and utilization of deceased donor kidneys from small pediatric donors. *Am J Transplant* 2006;6:1646–1652.
17. Sanchez-Fructuoso AI, Prats D, Perez-Contin MJ, et al. Increasing the donor pool using en bloc pediatric kidneys for transplant. *Transplantation* 2003;76:1180–1184.
18. Freeman RB, Giatras I, Falagas ME, et al. Outcome of transplantation of organs procured from bacteremic donors. *Transplantation* 1999;68: 1107–1111.
19. Roth D, Fernandez JA, Babischkin S, et al. Detection of hepatitis C virus among cadaver organ donors: evidence for low transmission of disease. *Ann Intern Med* 1992;117:470–475.
20. Kauffman HM, Cherikh WS, McBride MA, et al. Deceased donors with a past history of malignancy: an Organ Procurement and Transplantation Network/United Network for Organ Sharing update. *Transplantation* 2007;84:272–274.
21. Abouna GM, Al-Adnani MS, Kremer GD. Reversal of diabetic nephropathy in human cadaveric kidneys after transplantation into non-diabetic recipients. *Lancet* 1983;2:1274–1276.
22. Port FK, Bragg-Gresham JL, Metzger RA, et al. Donor characteristics associated with reduced graft survival: an approach to expanding the pool of kidney donors. *Transplantation* 2002;74:1281–1286.
23. Kayler LK, Garzon P, Magliocca J, et al. Outcomes and utilization of kidneys from deceased donors with acute kidney injury. *Am J Transplant* 2009;9:367–373.
24. Kaufman HH, Hui KS, Mattson JC, et al. Clinicopathologic correlations of disseminated intravascular coagulation in patients with head injury. *Neurosurgery* 1984;15:34–42.
25. A definition of irreversible coma. Report of the Ad Hoc Committee of Harvard Medical School to examine the definition of brain death. *JAMA* 1968;205:337–340.
26. Jorgensen EO. Spinal man after brain death. *Acta Neurochir (Wien)* 1973; 28:259–273.
27. Emery RW, Cork RC, Levinson MM, et al. The cardiac donor: a six-year experience. *Ann Thorac Surg* 1986;41:356–362.
28. Novitzky D, Wicomb WN, Cooper DKC, et al. Electrocardiographic, hemodynamic and endocrine changes occurring during experimental brain death in the Chacma baboon. *Heart Transplant* 1984;4:63–69.
29. Novitzky D, Wicomb WN, Cooper DKC, et al. Improved cardiac function following hormonal therapy in brain dead pigs: relevance to organ donation. *Cryobiology* 1987;24:1–10.
30. The Organ Procurement and Transplantation Network. Policies. Available at: http://optn.transplant.hrsa.gov/policiesAndBylaws/policies.asp. Accessed March 12, 2010.
31. Yersiz H, Renz JF, Hisatake GM, et al. Multivisceral and isolated intestinal procurement techniques. *Liver Transpl* 2003;9:881–886.
32. Tuttle-Newhall JE, Krishnan SM, Levy MF, et al. Organ donation and utilization in the United States: 1998–2007. *Am J Transplant* 2009;9(Part 2): 879–893.
33. The Institute of Medicine. *Non-heartbeating Organ Transplantation: Medical and Ethical Issues in Procurement*. Washington, DC: National Academy Press; 1997:1.
34. Cho YW, Terasaki PI, Cecka JM, et al. Transplantation of kidneys from donors whose hearts have stopped beating. *N Engl J Med* 1999;338: 221–225.
35. Merion RM, Pelletier SJ, Goodrich NP, et al. Donation after cardiac death as a strategy to increase deceased donor liver availability. *Ann Surg* 2006;244:555–562.
36. Todo S, Nery J, Yanaga K, et al. Extended preservation of human liver grafts with UW solution. *JAMA* 1989;261:711–714.
37. D'Alessandro AM, Sollinger HW, Hoffmann RM, et al. Experience with Belzer UW cold storage solution in simultaneous pancreas-kidney transplantation. *Transplant Proc* 1990;22:532–534.
38. Pokorny H, Rasoul-Rockenschaub S, Langer F, et al. Histidine-tryptophan-ketoglutarate solution for organ preservation in human liver transplantation—a prospective multi-centre observation study. *Transpl Int* 2004;17:256–260.
39. Stewart ZA, Lonze BE, Warren DS, et al. Histidine-tryptophan-ketoglutarate (HTK) is associated with reduced graft survival of deceased donor kidney transplants. *Am J Transplant* 2009;9:1048–1054.
40. Stewart ZA, Cameron AM, Singer AL, et al. Histidine-tryptophan-ketoglutarate (HTK) is associated with reduced graft survival in deceased donor livers, especially those donated after cardiac death. *Am J Transplant* 2009;9: 286–293.
41. Moers C, Smits JM, Maathuis MH, et al. Machine perfusion or cold storage in deceased-donor kidney transplantation. *N Engl J Med* 2009;360:7–19.
42. Conte JV, Baumgartner WA. Overview and future practice patterns in cardiac and pulmonary preservation. *J Card Surg* 2000;15:91–107.
43. Kokudo Y, Furuya T, Takeyochi I, et al. Comparison of University of Wisconsin, Euro-Collins, and lactated Ringer's solutions in rat small bowel preservation for orthotopic small bowel transplantation. *Transplant Proc* 1994;26:1492–1493.
44. Furukawa H, Casavilla A, Abu-Elmagd K, et al. Basic considerations for the procurement of intestinal grafts. *Transplant Proc* 1994;26:1470.

CHAPTER 35 ■ RENAL TRANSPLANTATION

CHRIS FREISE AND PETER STOCK

KEY POINTS

1. The major barriers to successful renal transplantation include ABO compatibility and the HLA system.
2. Before a renal transplant is undertaken, histocompatibility of the donor and recipient are determined.
3. Methods to expand the donor pool of kidneys include the use of donation after cardiac death and expanded criteria donors.
4. The etiology of kidney disease resulting in end-stage failure, and the necessity for transplantation is led by glomerulonephritis, diabetes, and hypertension.
5. Surgical complications of kidney transplantation include vascular, urologic, lymphocele, and wound problems.
6. The kidney transplant is heterotopically placed in the extraperitoneal iliac fossa.
7. Hyperacute rejection is humorally mediated by preformed anti-HLA antibodies. Hyperacute rejection occurs within minutes to hours following reperfusion of the kidney.
8. Acute cell-mediated rejection most typically occurs between 1 week and 3 months following transplantation.
9. Chronic rejection leads to loss of graft function over the course of months to several years.

Renal transplantation has evolved to become the preferred therapeutic modality for patients with end-stage renal failure. Improved patient survival and quality of life as compared with dialysis has been established, with cost effectiveness achieved after a minimum of 18 months of allograft function. The importance of minimizing time on dialysis, compounded by the exponential growth of patients on the wait list, has led to several strategies to increase the number of deceased and living donor organs in an effort to decrease waiting time and mortality on the wait list. These new strategies have been the focus of clinical research in kidney transplantation and will be discussed in this chapter. Other important topics that will be reviewed include immunologic considerations specific to kidney transplantation; preoperative assessment of kidney allograft recipients; the standard surgical approach in kidney transplantation and advances in laparoscopic technology for the donor; current strategies in immunosuppression; management of the technical and immunosuppressive complications; and future trends.

IMMUNOLOGY OF RENAL TRANSPLANTATION

The immunologic response to allografted tissue is well defined and under the influence of both T-cell– and B-cell–derived reactions. The cells and cytokines responsible for rejection vary with time posttransplant (hyperacute, acute, and chronic rejection) and have a differential response to currently available immunosuppressive agents.

1 The major barriers to successful renal transplantation include ABO compatibility and the human leukocyte antigen (HLA) system. In general, renal transplantation is done between ABO-compatible donor and recipients using the same guidelines as for blood transfusion. However, because of the shortage of donors, cadaver kidneys are nearly always used in recipients of identical blood type. Recently, ABO-incompatible living-donor transplants have been performed on an experimental basis secondary to excessive wait times for ABO-compatible deceased-donor transplants.[1,2]

The HLA system is made up of well-defined antigens present on most cell types that are genetically determined for each patient and are termed the *major histocompatibility complex*. These genes reside on chromosome 6 and are distributed in a Mendelian fashion to offspring. The HLA system includes several loci, but the most commonly characterized are the HLA-A, HLA-B, and HLA-D regions. Given that each human has two alleles for each locus, there are six potential HLA antigens of clinical significance. These are characterized using tissue typing techniques and can be used to determine the degree of matching between a donor and potential recipient, i.e., one-antigen match to six-antigen match. Improved results of graft survival are seen when the degree of matching reaches the six-antigen level, and long-term results may be better with matching to a lesser degree.

Class I antigens include the HLA antigens A, B, and C, whereas class II antigens include the D and DR loci. Class I antigens act as targets for cytotoxic T lymphocytes, and class II antigens are important for antigen presentation. Class II antigens are also responsible for triggering lymphocyte proliferation in the mixed lymphocyte culture system.

2 Before a renal transplant is undertaken, histocompatibility of the donor and recipient are determined. Standard testing consists of two procedures. Donors and recipients first undergo tissue typing, which involves characterization of their respective HLA type. Recipient serum is tested against a panel of antigens that contain the known HLA types, to identify anti-HLA antibodies. The sensitivity for detecting anti-HLA antibodies continues to improve, and newer technology uses single antigen beads to detect antibodies against a specific HLA antigen. The amount of reactivity that a potential recipient has against a panel of HLA antigens is indicative of the degree of sensitization. Based on the number of anti-HLA antibodies detected, a calculated percent reactive antibodies (cPRA) can be estimated. A cPRA of 70% would suggest that the potential recipient would have anti-HLA antibodies against 70% of the potential donor pool. Sensitization to HLA antigens occurs as a result of previous exposure to foreign HLA antigen either from pregnancy, previous blood transfusion, or a previous organ transplant. A patient who is highly sensitized is more difficult to transplant because of the greater likelihood of having antibodies to a potential donor.

The second test performed prior to transplantation is commonly known as the *final cross-match*. Several recipient serum samples collected at different times are mixed with donor lymphocytes in a culture system. This assay will detect preformed cytotoxic antibodies that would result in a hyperacute rejection if the transplantation were performed (see Rejection, later). A more sensitive method of detecting these antibodies uses a fluorescent activated cell scanner and is commonly used when evaluating potential recipients who are highly sensitized or receiving second transplants. In the near future, many transplant centers will be adopting a "virtual cross-match" based on the detection of anti-HLA antibodies present in a given recipient. The most sensitive technology will be used to detect the presence of anti-HLA antibodies in a given recipient. Based on these antibodies, each recipient will have a list of unacceptable donor antigens. Compatability with each donor will be determined in the absence of the final cross-match by eliminating a potential donor based on the presence of unacceptable antigens. This strategy facilitates an expedited transplant and minimization of cold ischemia times, as it avoids the additional time and expense associated with the final cross-match. Widespread acceptance of the virtual cross-match will require further confirmation that all donor antigens are sufficiently identified using the single antigen bead technology.

THE DONOR POOL: LIVING DONORS, DECEASED DONORS, DONATION AFTER CARDIAC DEATH

There is marked improvement in graft survival for both living and deceased donors when a transplant can be completed before the initiation of dialysis.[3] The significantly better outcomes achieved with preemptive transplantation and minimization of dialysis times have given rise to several strategies to increase the number of available kidneys.

Living Donors

The first long-term success in renal transplantation over 50 years ago involved a live donor transplant between twin brothers. The number of living donors has increased significantly in the last few years, in part as a result of the increased use of the laparoscopic technique for donor nephrectomies. For the first time, in 2001 the number of living donors exceeded the number of deceased donors, although deceased donor transplants still represent the majority of kidney transplants done today.[4] This trend toward increased live donation may also be the result of the excessive waiting times for deceased donor transplants, now more than 7 years for blood type O and B recipients in many parts of the United States. Despite initial concerns about the safety and efficacy of the laparoscopic technique for the donor procedure, morbidity and mortality rates (0.03%) remain low and comparable with those of the open technique.[5,6]

The evaluation of a potential living kidney donor begins with a brief overall assessment of physical condition because potential donors must be in good health with normal kidney function. Diabetes, hypertension, and cardiovascular disease generally rule out a potential donor. ABO is also determined before further workup, because ABO incompatibility has been a relative contraindication to donation. A cross-match test is usually performed at this time to ensure donor and recipient immunologic compatibility. After this initial screen, a careful medical and psychosocial screen takes place to confirm donor suitability. Following a normal physical examination, further studies should include chest radiography, electrocardiogram, urinalysis, and blood work. During this phase, any conditions that could predispose to later renal insufficiency need to be ruled out. For example, donors from families with a history of type II diabetes are at a significant risk for the development of diabetes, and glucose tolerance testing is justified as part of the screening process. A history of renal stones warrants stone analysis to assess likelihood for recurrent stones. Any inherited disorders of kidney disease must also be ruled out, particularly in potential living-related donors when the recipient has polycystic kidney disease.

The psychosocial history is directed at assessing the motivation of the donor, and to ensure that there are adequate resources for the donor to proceed with the surgery and recovery. Many centers require a relationship between the donor and intended recipient, although it is becoming increasingly common to have general members of the public show interest in being evaluated as a donor, with no particular recipient identified. These nondirected donors require the same careful scrutiny as any living donor, and the psychosocial evaluation is especially important. The motivation for donation should be clear and not be connected in any way to financial gain. It is also the duty of the physician evaluating the potential donor to review the current statistics on morbidity and mortality, and the potential donor should be provided with the opportunity to speak to the transplantation team privately to address issues of reluctance or coercion. To allow for an unbiased assessment of the donor, it is now required that an independent donor advocate be part of the evaluation team, and by definition this person should have no role in the care of an intended recipient.

The final testing of a potential donor involves anatomic definition of the two kidneys and is typically done with either a computed tomography angiogram or MR angiogram, both of which avoid the needle stick and catheters associated with a conventional angiogram. The results of these studies are used to detect any anatomic abnormalities that would exclude a donor and to decide which kidney will be removed. In general, the left kidney is favored for transplant because it has a longer renal vein.

Several strategies are currently being considered to increase the frequency of living donation. Potential donors with well-controlled hypertension on a single antihypertensive agent are being considered, although this remains controversial. Controversy also exists regarding the potential reimbursement for living donors, specifically providing financial compensation regarding lost wages during the donation. Consideration is also being given to providing health insurance to living donors for complications related to the donor procedure. The extent of the reimbursement provided to living donors continues to be debated by medical ethicists and
3 transplant professionals. Finally, a national exchange system is currently being designed that matches living donors who were incompatible with their intended recipient with other recipients with incompatible living donors. Such exchange systems have already been successful on a regional level, and extending this to a national system will permit many more successful exchanges and further expand the living donor pool.

Deceased Donors

Procurement of kidneys from brain-dead deceased donors has not increased at the same pace as the rapid growth of the national wait list (Fig. 35.1). Although most deceased donors are brain dead, there has been an increased use of kidneys from donors who do not meet the strict definitions of brain death but have cardiopulmonary support withdrawn because of a severe brain injury or high spinal cord injury, with little hope of living without the use of ongoing mechanical ventilation and/or the possibility of existing in a persistent vegetative state. Organs are recovered after withdrawal of support, once the heart stops beating, hence the terminology of *donors by cardiac death* or *DCD donors*. Usually support is withdrawn in a controlled setting so that the time of warm ischemia and poor organ perfusion can be minimized. Minimizing the time from cessation of the heart to perfusion of organs with preservation fluid requires an experienced procurement team, and the successful use of these organs is dependent on rapid procurement. Although the use of livers from DCD donors appears to be associated with a higher incidence of biliary tract complications following transplantation, kidneys procured from DCD donors are proving to be an important source of donor kidneys.[7] Several studies from the United States and Japan have demonstrated comparable graft success between kidneys procured from DCD donors and brain-dead donors. The percentage of DCD donors in the United States has progressively increased over the last decade and presently represents about 10% of deceased donors.

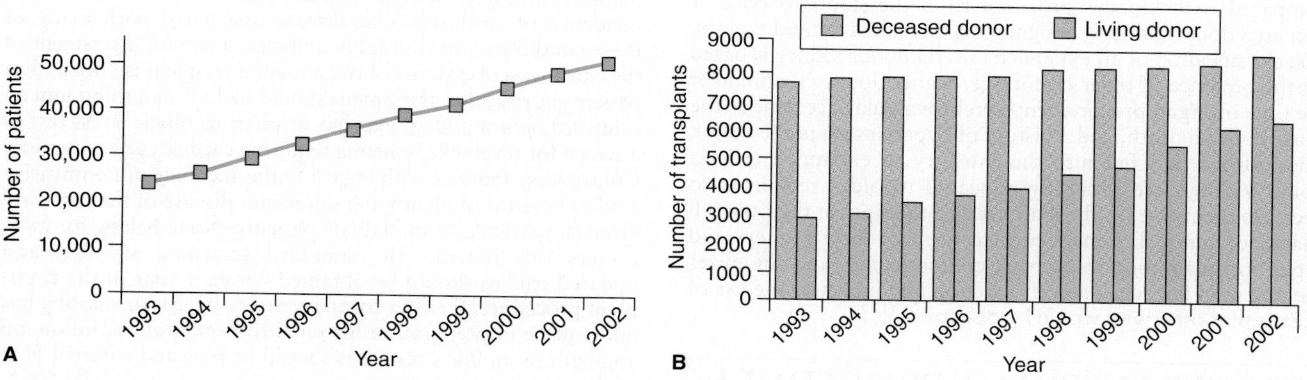

FIGURE 35.1. The growth in the number of patients awaiting transplant (A) has exceeded the relatively stagnant rate of deceased donor kidney transplants leading to progressively increasing waiting times over the last decade. Living donors have had a slight increase, which may be in part due to the introduction of the laparoscopic donation procedure. There has been an increase in the proportion of recipients aged 50 years and older on both the wait list and receiving transplants (B). (Adapted from Wolfe RA, Merion RM, Roys EC, et al. Trends in organ donation and transplantation in the United States, 1998–2007. *Am J Transplant* 2009;9:869–878, with permission.)

Placement of deceased donor kidneys is guided by a series of complex allocation rules established by the United Network for Organ Sharing (UNOS). Unfortunately, the number of people being added to waiting lists continues to be significantly greater than the number of people being removed following transplantation. As a result, waiting times in many parts of the country for blood type O kidneys are exceeding 7 years, and are getting longer each year. To accommodate the increasing size of the waiting lists, the UNOS kidney committee is in the process of establishing a new algorithm for the allocation of deceased donor kidneys. The current system is driven principally by waiting time, with a much smaller component driven by HLA-DR matching. A newer system is being developed that will address the changing demographics of both the patients on the waiting lists and deceased donors, most notably the increasing age of both donors and recipients. At the same time, a new allocation system must balance the conflicting goals of all the stakeholders involved in transplant process, while striking the best balance between justice and utility. As a result of the conflicting goals of all the stakeholders involved in kidney transplantation, the development of a new allocation system continues to be a hot topic of debate within UNOS and the transplant community.[8]

Further Strategies for Increasing the Number of Donor Kidneys

Many of the unique approaches for increasing the number of potential donors have come from Japan, where cultural beliefs have limited the number of available deceased donor transplants. Several groups have reported successful kidney transplantation across ABO blood group barriers, using aggressive pretransplant immunosuppression, plasmapheresis to decrease anti-ABO titers, and in some cases splenectomy.[1,2] This strategy has been implemented with increasing frequency in the United States as a result of the marked increases in the waiting times for blood group O and B recipients.[9]

An important strategy currently being implemented in the United States as well as internationally involves the use of intravenous gammaglobulin to facilitate transplantation across a known positive anti-HLA cross-match. This protocol could potentially impact the increasing number of sensitized patients on waiting lists with little hope of finding a compatible donor.[10]

Further strategies have recently been implemented to expand the availability of kidneys procured from deceased donors. In addition to the use of kidneys from DCD donors described earlier, another strategy recently implemented by UNOS involves expedited placement of kidneys from donors that are less than optimal. These kidneys are designated as *expanded criteria donors* (ECD) and are expected to have decreased graft survival compared with kidneys procured from the standard pool of deceased donor kidneys, designated as *standard criteria donors*. The classification of an expanded criteria donor kidney is based on the presence of older donor age, higher donor creatinine at the time of organ procurement, cerebrovascular accident as the cause of brain death, and a history of hypertension in the donor. The kidneys that fall into the category of expanded criteria donor kidneys are generally allocated to older recipients to decrease their time on the wait list and to improve their overall chance of survival. Expedited placement of these kidneys and rapid transplantation to decrease cold-ischemia time minimizes the potential for delayed graft function and increases the use of organs that otherwise would be discarded.[11,12]

THE TRANSPLANT PROCEDURE

Recipient Preoperative Assessment

4 The etiologies of kidney disease resulting in end-stage failure and the necessity for transplantation are led by glomerulonephritis, diabetes, and hypertension (Table 35.1).[13] Because of the high incidence of cardiovascular disease associated with many of these conditions, most notably diabetes, a careful assessment of the cardiovascular status of the potential recipient is critical. For patients at risk, this assessment should include at a minimum an echocardiogram and an exercise or pharmacologic stress test as a screen for reversible ischemia requiring cardiac catheterization. Controversy remains with regard to the accuracy of noninvasive studies in terms of identifying significant disease of the coronary arteries, particularly in diabetic patients. Nonetheless, for most centers this remains the standard screening strategy, and updated studies should be obtained within 1 year of the transplant procedure. If either coronary artery bypass or stenting has taken place in preparation for renal transplantation, follow-up angiograms and/or stress tests should be repeated within 1 year of the actual transplant.

Although the evaluation of potential recipients is focused on the assessment of cardiovascular status, further studies must exclude malignancies and infections that would contraindicate transplantation and immunosuppression. Potential kidney recipients who are infected with hepatitis C should be

TABLE 35.1 ETIOLOGY

ETIOLOGY OF RENAL DISEASE AS INDICATIONS FOR RENAL TRANSPLANTATION, RANKED IN ORDER OF PREVALENCE

Diabetes mellitus (types I and II)
Hypertension
Polycystic kidney disease
IgA nephropathy
Chronic glomerulonephritis
Focal sclerosis
Systemic lupus
Membranous glomerulonephritis
Pyelonephritis
Focal segmental glomerulosclerosis
Congenital obstructive uropathy
Nephritis
Alport syndrome
Hypoplasia, dysplasia
Wegener granulomatosis
Postinfectious glomerulonephritis
Obstructive uropathy
Hemolytic uremia
Membranoproliferative glomerulonephritis
Goodpasture syndrome
Membranous nephropathy
Analgesic nephropathy
Prune belly syndrome
Medullary cystic disease
Henoch-Schönlein purpura
Nephronophthisis
Scleroderma
Sickle cell anemia
Amyloidosis
Oxalosis

Adapted from Cecka JM. The OPTN/UNOS Renal Transplant Registry. In Cecka JM, Terasaki PI, eds. *Clinical Transplants 2003*. Los Angeles: UCLA Immunogenetics Center; 2004:1–12, with permission.

evaluated by a hepatologist to determine the risks of immunosuppression causing progression to end-stage liver disease. Potential kidney recipients with evidence of advanced liver disease should be evaluated for a combined liver and kidney transplant. For patients with less advanced liver disease, consideration could be given to interferon therapy before proceeding with kidney transplantation to provide the opportunity for viral clearance. Kidney transplantation was previously contraindicated in people with HIV infection secondary to concerns of exacerbating an already immunologically compromised state. Recent advances in antiretroviral therapy and the ability to provide effective prophylaxis against opportunistic infections has prompted several centers to perform transplantation in people with end-stage renal disease and HIV infection. Early results suggest that progression of HIV to AIDS has not been seen following transplantation and immunosuppression, with early allograft success rates comparable to those in non–HIV-positive recipients.[14] Potential patients with a previous history of tuberculosis or conversion to purified protein derivative positivity should be evaluated for active disease.

Colonoscopy, mammography, and Pap smear should be performed as dictated by age-specific standard guidelines. For most malignancies, with the exception of nonmelanoma skin cancers and early-stage renal cancers, a disease-free interval of 5 years is recommended before kidney transplantation.

For patients with congenital abnormalities as the cause of renal failure, a complete workup of the genitourinary systems is necessary, including urodynamics and voiding cystourethrograms. These studies are particularly important in children with end-stage disease resulting from posterior urethral valves, to ensure that the bladder will serve as an adequate conduit for the kidney transplant. For patients with severe reflux disease and chronic pyelonephritis, native nephroureterectomy may be required to prevent posttransplant infection secondary to chronic reflux into the native ureters. For patients with inadequate bladder capacity and function, pretransplant reconstructive procedures such as ileal augmentation or ileal conduits may be required.

For patients with suspected clotting disorders based on a previous history of thromboembolic events (frequent clotting problems with dialysis access) or diseases associated with an increased frequency of clotting disorders (i.e., lupus), a hematologic workup is necessary to determine the necessity for anticoagulation at the time of the transplant. This workup should include a determination of serum levels of protein C, protein S, anticardiolipin antibody, factor V Leiden, antithrombin III levels, and the G20210 A prothrombin gene mutation.

Living Donor Nephrectomy: Open and Laparoscopic

A living kidney donor operation is a unique surgical procedure for two reasons. First, the donor has no medical reason to be in the operating room, and the process is driven only by his or her willingness to help another person with the gift of donation. Second, the removed tissue must be in perfect condition because it will be reimplanted into the recipient. These two features, therefore, necessitate that the donor operation is done safely and done well. The original donor operation was done through a generous flank incision, allowing for good exposure and careful dissection of the renal vessels. Unfortunately, this flank approach generally left a large incision, with its accompanying morbidity, pain, and sometimes adverse cosmetic result. The development of the laparoscopic procedure to remove kidneys has revolutionized the field, although its initial introduction was met with trepidation because of concerns over donor safety. With the explosive growth and dissemination of this procedure, it has now become the standard for donor nephrectomy.

The procedure is most commonly done through a transperitoneal approach, although some surgeons prefer to remain retroperitoneal. Once the operative space is expanded with carbon dioxide gas and the scope is inserted, two to three additional ports are placed to allow for the passage of instruments to dissect the kidney (Fig. 35.2). Some centers also favor the use of a gastight "hand-port," which allows placement of the surgeon's hand in the operative space to assist in exposure and to have available if sudden bleeding is encountered. Once the kidney vessels are transected and the vessel stumps are controlled by laparoscopic staples, the kidney can be removed through a 2- to 3-inch incision, which can be placed in a position that leaves minimal scarring and avoids cutting muscle tissue. Most commonly this is via a Pfannenstiel incision, and recently the use of natural orifice approaches (NOTES) has been described. Donors who undergo the laparoscopic procedure typically have reduced pain medicine requirements, have a slightly shorter hospital stay, and are able to return to their usual activities sooner.[5,6]

The safety of this relatively new procedure has been established, in addition to the demonstration that kidneys recovered through a laparoscopic approach function as well as kidneys removed in an open operation. It is important that there seems to have been an increased interest in live donation, coincident with the introduction of the laparoscopic procedure, suggesting that this procedure has removed some of the disincentives of the donation process.

Recipient Operative Procedure

5 The kidney transplant is heterotopically placed in the extraperitoneal iliac fossa. Although this is a less technically demanding procedure than either liver or pancreas transplants, attention to detail is imperative to optimize immediate graft function and avoid technical complications resulting in loss of the kidney transplant.

The operation is initiated by exposure of the iliac fossa through a curvilinear incision and can be done on either the right or left side. The incision extends from 1 cm above the symphysis pubis to approximately 2 cm lateral to the anterior iliac spine (Fig. 35.3). The fascia is divided along the lateral border of the rectus sheath, and the contents of the peritoneal cavity are reflected cephalad and medially, exposing the iliac vessels in the retroperitoneum. Lymphatics overlying the iliac vessels are ligated and divided to prevent the development of lymphoceles. In males, the spermatic cord is secured with a vessel loop and can be retracted away from the operative field. In females, the round ligament is suture ligated and divided. The inferior epigastric artery and vein are typically divided to prevent potential compression of the transplanted ureter. Placement of a mechanical retractor should avoid compression of the iliac artery and vein as well as the femoral nerve to prevent neurapraxias.

The living or deceased donor kidney is inspected for the presence of multiple vessels, duplication of the urinary collecting system, and parenchymal abnormalities. The artery and vein are dissected from surrounding structures to provide the necessary length for transplantation. In the case of multiple arteries, a decision must be made as to whether to perform ex vivo reconstruction to achieve a single implantable conduit versus implanting the vessels separately. This decision is in part dependent on the quality of the recipient vessels and an assessment as to whether the anastomosis of multiple vessels directly into the recipient would require an unacceptable period of warm ischemia to the kidney. In general, in an adult the anastomosis of the renal artery and vein are performed in an end-to-side fashion to the external iliac vessels, although occasionally the presence of atherosclerotic disease requires transplantation to the common iliac vessels. In children who weigh less than 20 kg, or for third transplants in adults, an

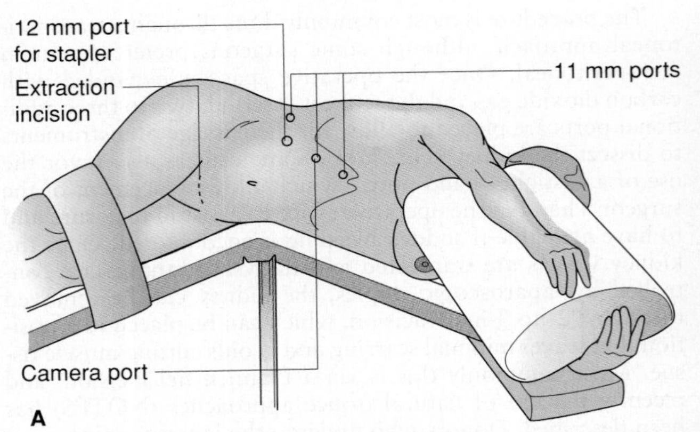

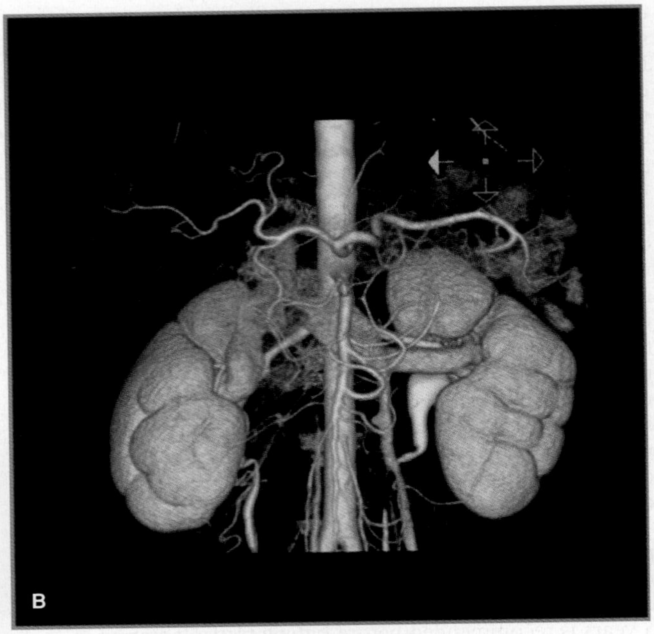

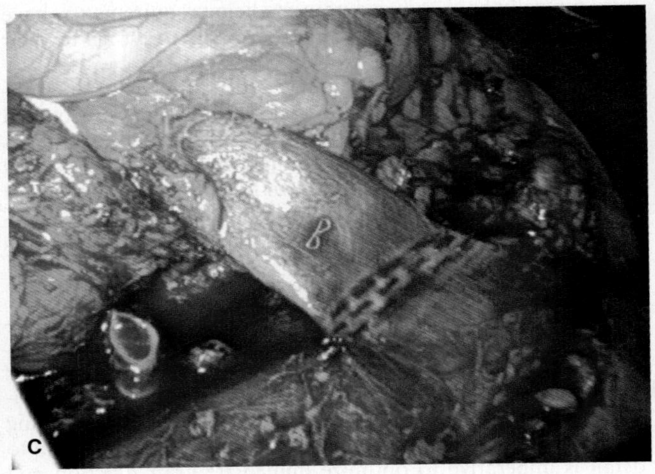

FIGURE 35.2. **A:** The laparoscopic donor procedure is performed with the donor in a lateral position, typically using three to four ports, with extraction of the kidney through a 6- to 8-cm incision. **B:** Preoperative computed tomography angiogram revealing the arterial and venous anatomy. **C:** Intraoperative photograph of laparoscopic view of right kidney just prior to transection of the renal vein. The artery has already been divided.

intraperitoneal approach is used and the vascular anastomoses are frequently performed to the aorta and inferior vena cava. For kidneys from deceased donors, a Carrel patch of aorta is used to prevent stenosis and to provide a common patch for multiple arteries. Warm ischemia time should be minimized to prevent delayed graft function. Ensuring adequate intravascular volume and stable hemodynamics at the time of reperfusion is extremely important to achieve optimal function of the transplant.

The reimplantation of the ureter is most frequently performed through an extravesicular technique. Following positioning of the revascularized kidney in the iliac fossa and assurance of hemostasis, the ureter is shortened to permit a tension-free anastomosis with adequate blood supply to the distal ureter. In men, the ureter is placed under the spermatic cord to prevent ureteral obstruction. The bladder is distended with an antibiotic solution to identify a suitable area for ureteral implantation on the dome of the bladder, and a

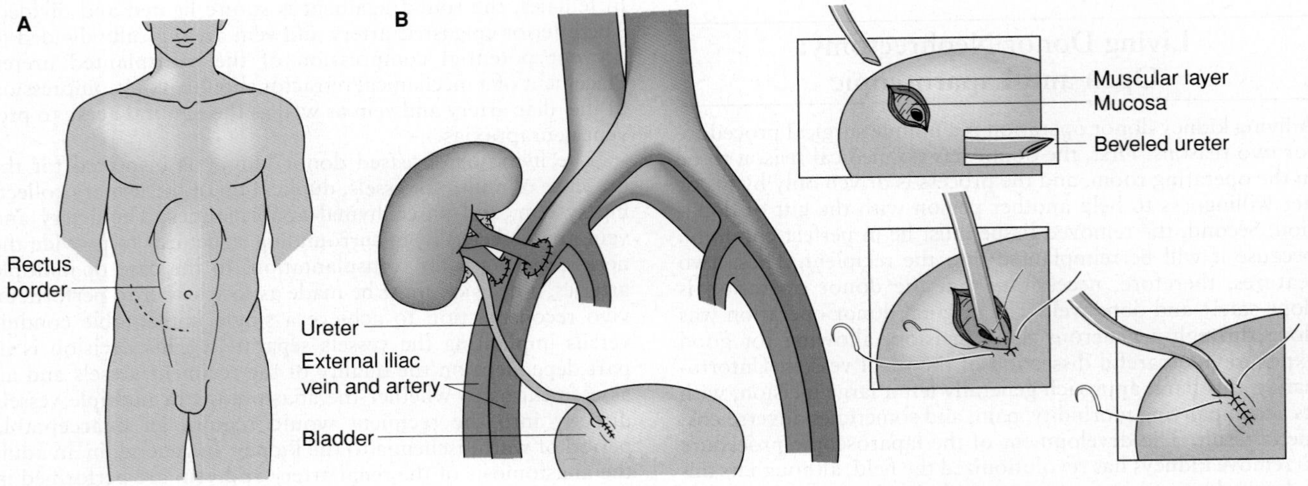

FIGURE 35.3. **A:** Curvilinear iliac fossa incision used for the kidney transplant recipient procedure. **B:** Vascular anastomoses completed between the recipient external iliac artery and vein and donor renal artery and vein. *Insets:* ureteral anastomosis performed using the external ureteroneocystostomy technique.

cystotomy is made at this site. An anastomosis between the mucosa of the bladder and transplanted ureter is constructed using an absorbable suture to prevent stone formation. A second layer of the bladder musculature is closed over the distal portion of the ureter to prevent reflux during micturition.

There are alternative techniques to reimplant the ureter, including the Politano-Leadbetter transvesical ureteroneocystostomy. This technique involves tunneling the ureter through the bladder wall from the inside of the bladder. This technique is still preferred by some surgeons who believe the long-term prevention of reflux is superior with the transvesicular approach. However, this technique requires a second cystotomy, and posttransplant hematuria is more common than with the extravesicular technique. A third technique for ureteral implantation in recipients with normal native ureters is uretero-ureterostomy over a double-J stent. In general, this technique is reserved as a salvage procedure for reimplantation of transplanted ureters with distal strictures secondary to ischemia. It can also be used as a primary technique if there are questions regarding the blood supply to the distal ureter at the time of transplant. This technique is preferred if the donor ureter was damaged or inadvertently stripped of its blood supply at the time of procurement but is dependent on the availability of normal native ureters to serve as an adequate conduit.

COMPLICATIONS

Early Graft Dysfunction

Most kidneys begin to function right after implantation, especially in the case of a living donor. When the initial function results in only a slow drop in serum creatinine, the diagnosis of slow graft function is made. When dialysis is needed in the first week because of poor function, the diagnosis of delayed graft function is made. Delayed graft function typically occurs in 15% to 30% of deceased donor transplants. The diagnosis of slow graft function or delayed graft function is important to establish because other problems, such as rejection, vascular occlusion, or ureteral obstruction, can also result in low urine output and need for dialysis. These other causes must be eliminated before the diagnosis of slow graft function or delayed graft function can be made.

In the immediate postoperative period, careful attention to fluid status is critical. In cases of immediate graft function, fluid orders should include replacement for urine output as well as a maintenance fluid rate. This approach ensures that the patient does not become volume depleted and compromise perfusion to the new kidney. In cases of delayed graft function, fluid should be restricted and dialysis instituted when electrolyte imbalance or fluid overload are evident.

A decrease in urine output in the early postoperative period requires immediate diagnostic and therapeutic intervention. A stepwise approach to diagnosing the etiology of oliguria is shown in Algorithm 35.1. Once mechanical obstruction of the indwelling Foley catheter has been excluded by irrigation, the volume status of the patient should be assessed, preferably with a central venous pressure line or pulmonary artery catheter. Fluid replacement to restore intravascular volume should be initiated in the volume-depleted patient.

Radiologic evaluation using various imaging techniques is required if urine output remains low in the face of adequate volume status. Ultrasonography is most helpful to diagnose ureteral obstruction caused by technical complications at the

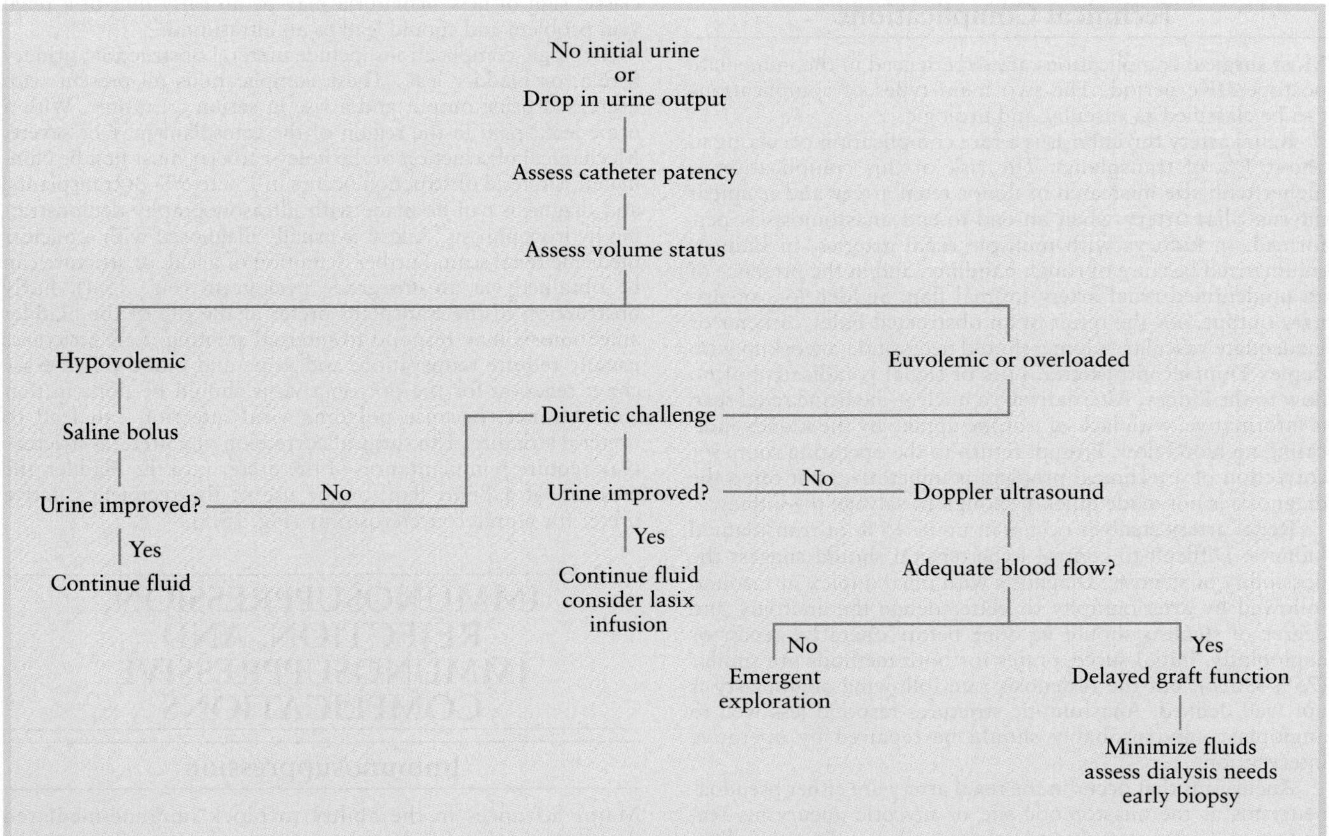

ALGORITHM 35.1

ALGORITHM 35.1. Stepwise approach to the management of decreased low urine output posttransplant.

anastomosis or fluid collections that may be obstructing the ureter by extrinsic compression. With the addition of duplex and color Doppler imaging, blood flow to the kidney can be evaluated and technical problems with the vessels can be assessed. Nuclear medicine techniques are also valuable for assessing renal function. Technetium 99m diethylenetriamine pentaacetic acid (DTPA) and iodine-131 iodohippurate (Hippuran) are the two major radionuclides used in the evaluation of renal allograft function. DTPA renal scans evaluate the vascular flow pattern of the kidney as well as the gross anatomy of the ureter and bladder. Scans are performed over 30 minutes, with uptake of contrast within 6 seconds indicating adequate flow to the graft. Peak activity in the parenchyma should be reached within 2 minutes, followed by a gradual decline in radioactivity in the renal parenchyma and an increase in radioactivity in the urinary collecting system and bladder. Iodine-131 iodohippurate scans are more sensitive in evaluating renal function. Peak activity is also reached in 2 to 4 minutes, with gradual decline over the next 30 minutes. In rejection, acute tubular necrosis and drug toxicity as well as poor uptake and poor excretion are the typical findings with a nuclear medicine scan.

If these imaging techniques do not indicate an explanation for the poor urine output, the diagnosis of delayed graft function is made. Immunosuppression can then be adjusted to minimize or avoid the calcineurin inhibitors, which can prolong the recovery from delayed graft function, and also to initiate antibody therapy to protect the kidney from rejection. The combination of delayed graft function and early rejection is clearly associated with worse outcome in the long term, and an early biopsy of the kidney that is functioning poorly is helpful to diagnose rejection and guide therapy.

Technical Complications

6 Most surgical complications are experienced in the immediate postoperative period. The two main types of complications can be classified as vascular and urologic.

Renal artery thrombosis is a rare complication occurring in about 1% of transplants. The risk of this complication is higher with size mismatch of donor renal artery and recipient internal iliac artery when an end-to-end anastomosis is performed, in kidneys with multiple renal arteries, in kidneys traumatized because of rough handling, and in the presence of an unidentified renal artery intimal flap. Sudden loss of urinary output, not the result of an obstructed Foley catheter or inadequate vascular volume, should necessitate a workup with duplex Doppler ultrasound. Loss of signal is indicative of no flow to the kidney. Alternatively, a nuclear medicine renal scan is informative, with lack of isotope uptake by the kidney indicating no blood flow. Prompt return to the operating room for correction of a technical problem is imperative, but often the diagnosis is not made quickly enough to salvage the kidney.

Renal artery stenosis occurs in up to 15% of transplanted kidneys. Difficult-to-control hypertension should suggest the possibility of stenosis. Diagnosis with renal duplex ultrasound followed by arteriography to better define the anatomy and degree of stenosis should be done before operative repair or angioplasty. Initial success rates for both methods are similar (75%–80%), but the restenosis rate following angioplasty is not well defined. Anastomotic strictures respond less well to angioplasty and probably should be repaired by operative intervention.

Aneurysms that occur in the renal artery are either pseudoaneurysms at the anastomotic site or mycotic aneurysms secondary to bacterial or fungal infection. A rapidly expanding, tender pulsatile mass in the region of the kidney suggests a mycotic aneurysm. Arteriography is confirmatory for diagnosis. Treatment consists of appropriate antibiotics and removal of the transplanted kidney.

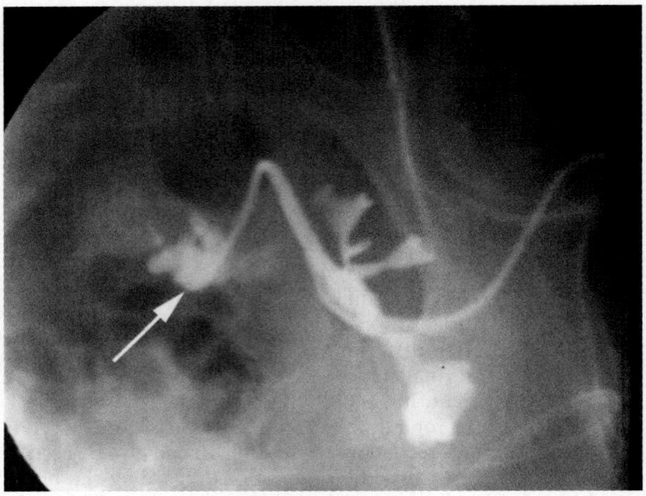

FIGURE 35.4. Percutaneous nephrostogram revealing a urine leak from the ureterovesical anastomosis.

Venous complications are less frequent, with thrombosis occurring in 1% to 4% of transplants. Causative factors include intimal damage during retrieval, kinking at the iliac vein anastomosis, or pressure secondary to a lymphocele, urinoma, or hematoma. Occasionally, severe rejection can result in venous occlusion. Heparin infusion for incomplete occlusion and transplant nephrectomy for complete occlusion are the indicated therapies. Occasionally, graft salvage is possible if the diagnosis is made before progression of clot into the kidney itself. The classic sign of new hematuria may be an early hint of a renal vein problem and should lead to an ultrasound.

Urologic complications include ureteral obstruction, urinary fistula, or bladder leak. These complications all present with decreased urine output and a rise in serum creatinine. With a urine leak, pain in the region of the transplant may be severe. Mechanical obstruction of the Foley catheter must first be eliminated. Ureteral obstruction occurs in 1% to 9% of transplants, and diagnosis can be made with ultrasonography demonstrating hydronephrosis. A leak is usually diagnosed with a nuclear medicine renal scan. Further definition of a leak or stricture can be obtained via an antegrade pyelogram (Fig. 35.4). Early obstruction of the transplant ureter at the site of the bladder anastomosis may respond to internal stenting. Late strictures usually require reoperation, and urine and blood polymerase chain reaction for the polyoma virus should be done in that circumstance, because polyoma viral infection can lead to ureteral stricture. The surgical correction of a ureteral stricture may require reimplantation of the ureter into the bladder, the creation of a Boari flap, or the use of the recipient's native ureter for a ureteroureterostomy (Fig. 35.5).

IMMUNOSUPPRESSION, REJECTION, AND IMMUNOSUPPRESSIVE COMPLICATIONS

Immunosuppression

Major advances in the ability to block immune-mediated destruction of the kidney have taken place in the past few years, resulting in a significant decrease in the incidence of acute rejection and improvement in long-term allograft survival rates.[13] This advance is the result of numerous agents that have been added during the past decade to the

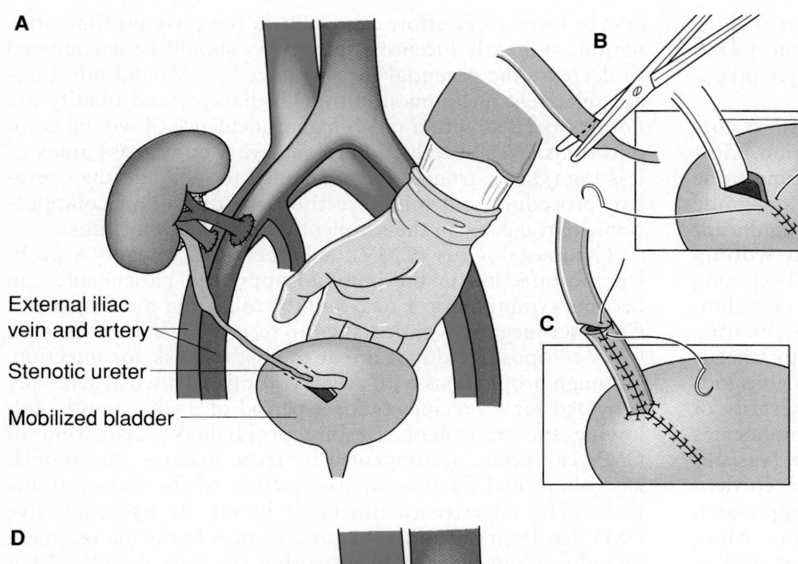

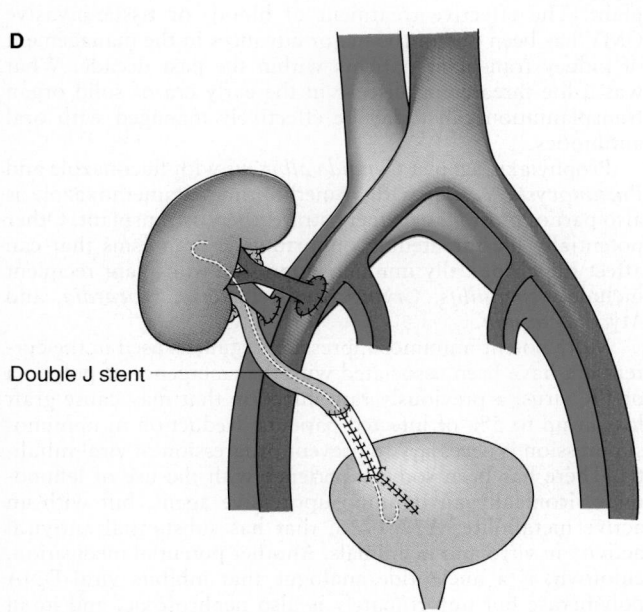

FIGURE 35.5. **A:** Reconstruction of a stenotic donor ureter, showing resection of the stenotic segment and mobilization of the bladder. **B to D:** A Boari flap is constructed from a tabularized segment of bladder wall and anastomosed end-to-end to the proximal donor ureter.

immunosuppressive armamentarium of prednisone, azathioprine, and cyclosporine A. These agents include tacrolimus, mycophenolate mofetil, sirolimus, anti-interleukin-2 receptor blockers, antithymocyte globulin (a polyclonal anti-T-cell agent), rituximab (an anti-CD20 monoclonal agent), and most recently costimulatory blockade with CTLA4-Ig. The addition of various newer drugs targeting different pathways in the alloimmune cascade has permitted the development of regimens that are less dependent on the calcineurin inhibitors or prednisone.[15]

Newer strategies in the immunosuppressive pipeline are targeted to block: costimulatory pathways; signaling pathways that activate T cells and T-cell proliferation; and trafficking and recruitment of immune cells. The most promising biologic agents targeted to block the costimulatory pathways include a second-generation CTLA4Ig (LEA29Y), a humanized anti-CD11-a (anti-LFA1), and a humanized anti-B7.1/B7.2. Promising agents designed to block T-cell activation and proliferation are the inhibitors of the Janus protein tyrosine kinase (JAK3) and the leflunomide analog FK778. Finally, drugs to block the trafficking and recruitment of immune cells are antagonists against the chemokine receptors CCR1, CXCR3, and CCR5. The chemokine antagonists have been effective in experimental transplantation and will likely be transitioned to clinical trials in the near future.[16]

Rejection

7 Hyperacute rejection is extremely rare and is humorally mediated by preformed anti-HLA antibodies. Hyperacute rejection occurs within minutes to hours following reperfusion of the kidney, whereas classic cell-mediated rejection typically does not occur until 1 to 2 weeks after the transplant. In hyperacute rejection, the anti-HLA antigens bind to the vascular endothelium of the kidney transplant, resulting in activation of the complement cascade and rapid graft thrombosis. The kidney appears blue-black with poor tissue turgor despite adequate blood flow. The characteristic histologic appearance includes the triad of polymorphonuclear leukocytes in the glomerular capillary loops, fibrin deposition, and platelet thrombi. The kidney cannot be salvaged, and a transplant nephrectomy is necessary. The presence of anti-HLA antibodies should be detected in the pretransplant cross-match, and with the sensitivity of current immunologic assays, hyperacute rejection is usually a result of technical or clerical errors in the cross-match procedure. A more common and less intense form of humoral rejection occurring within a few days of transplantation is a result of reactivation of memory B cells following reexposure to alloantigen. The histologic findings are defined by positive C4d staining on vascular endothelium, although lymphocytic infiltrates consistent with classic cell-mediated rejection can be

present. Treatment of this aggressive rejection can include plasmapheresis, the anti B-cell agent rituximab (anti-CD20 monoclonal antibody), and polyclonal antilymphocyte preparations (antithymocyte globulin).

8 Classic acute cell-mediated rejection typically occurs between 1 week and 3 months following transplantation. Most patients with rejection episodes present with decreasing urine volumes and increases in serum creatinine values. Low-grade fever and allograft tenderness may be present, but significant physical symptoms frequently are absent. Immediate workup of increasing serum creatinine should be initiated, beginning with an ultrasound to rule out ureteral obstruction or technical vascular complications as the cause of the deteriorating function. Similarly, toxicity from calcineurin inhibitors needs to be determined by checking drug levels. A percutaneous kidney biopsy is performed to confirm rejection. The severity of the rejection episode is based on the presence of lymphocytes in renal tubules (tubulitis) and vascular endothelium (vasculitis). Mild rejection is generally treated with pulse corticosteroids and maximizing the maintenance immunosuppression to ensure therapeutic levels of calcineurin inhibitors. More severe rejection with both tubulitis and vasculitis, as well as steroid-resistant rejection, is treated with antilymphocyte antibody preparations, most frequently muromonab-CD3 (a monoclonal agent directed against the CD3 receptor) or rabbit polyclonal antilymphocyte preparations. If the rejection episode occurred while the patients had therapeutic drug levels, maintenance therapy is frequently altered following the antibody therapy. For example, if maintenance therapy consisted of cyclosporine A, the calcineurin inhibitor could be switched to tacrolimus. Other potential strategies include the addition of sirolimus to the immunosuppressive regimen, particularly for cases where there is evidence of calcineurin inhibitor toxicity on biopsy.

Each rejection episode takes a toll on long-term function of the kidney transplant. Even well-controlled acute rejection episodes initiate a cascade of events leading to interstitial fibrosis and proliferative changes affecting the vascular endothelium. 9 These histologic and progressive degenerative changes are classified as chronic rejection or chronic allograft nephropathy. These changes lead to loss of graft function over the course of months to several years. Current strategies minimizing calcineurin inhibitor nephrotoxicity are being used to prolong function in kidneys with these chronic changes and involve the addition of sirolimus to replace the calcineurin inhibitors. It remains unclear whether the marked decrease in acute rejection episodes, from greater than 50% to less than 20% observed in the past 5 years, will translate to better long-term function of transplants. Nonetheless, it is evident that immunosuppression strategies minimizing prednisone and calcineurin inhibitors are providing safer and more effective immunosuppression for kidney transplant recipients while decreasing long-term toxicities associated with immunosuppression.

Immunosuppressive Complications

It would be naïve to assume that the intensification of immunosuppressive regimens resulting in decreased acute and chronic rejection rates can be accomplished without sequelae. Infections and malignancy remain significant complications associated with long-term immunosuppression and are the driving force for drug-minimization strategies. Early infections during the perioperative period are commonly iatrogenic and involve bladder infections or intravenous catheter use. Higher doses of immunosuppressive drugs used in the early postoperative period predispose patients to these infections and emphasize the importance of maintaining sterility during Foley catheter placement and insertion of intravenous catheters. Pneumonia related to mechanical ventilation and poor postoperative inspiratory effort can occur in the early postoperative period, and early incentive spirometry should be encouraged to decrease the potential for this infection. Wound infections are relatively uncommon, although diabetes and obesity are both associated with a much higher incidence of wound complications. Weight reduction to achieve a body mass index of less than 35 is strongly recommended to facilitate the operative procedure and minimize the risks of wound complications, particularly in the recipient with diabetes mellitus.

Cytomegalovirus (CMV), a herpesvirus, remains a problematic infection in the immunosuppressed patient and can become symptomatic 1 to 2 months following the transplant. CMV-seronegative patients who receive a kidney from a CMV-seropositive donor are at the highest risk for infection, although prophylaxis with acyclovir or ganciclovir is generally provided for all recipients for a period of 3 to 6 months following the transplant. Despite prophylaxis, activation of CMV can occur, accompanied by fever, malaise, pneumonia, gastrointestinal distress, or dysfunction of the kidney transplant. The effective treatment of blood- or tissue-invasive CMV has been one of the major advances in the management of kidney transplant patients within the past decade. What was a life-threatening disease in the early era of solid organ transplantation can today be effectively managed with oral antibiotics.

Prophylaxis against *Candida albicans* with fluconazole and *Pneumocystis carinii* with trimethoprim-sulfamethoxazole is also part of most management strategies posttransplant. Other potentially life-threatening opportunistic organisms that can affect the chronically immunosuppressed transplant recipient include *Aspergillus, Cryptococcus, Listeria, Nocardia,* and *Mycobacterium*.

More potent immunosuppression regimens used in the current era have been associated with the emergence of polyoma or BK virus, a previously rare infection that may cause graft loss in up to 5% of infected patients. Reduction in immunosuppression is necessary to prevent progression of viral tubulitis. There has been some experience with the use of leflunomide, ironically an immunosuppressive agent, but with an active metabolite, A77 1726, that has substantial antiviral activity in vitro and in animals. Another potential medication, cidofovir, is a nucleotide analogue that inhibits viral DNA polymerase but unfortunately is also nephrotoxic, and its in vivo efficacy has not been proved. Probably the best method to prevent graft loss due to polyoma is the use of monitoring of urine and serum levels of BK virus, with lowering of immunosuppression when early evidence of polyoma is detected.

Patients with a previous history of active tuberculosis or conversion to purified protein derivative (PPD) positivity should receive appropriate prophylaxis for 6 months to 1 year following the transplant procedure.

More potent immunosuppression regimens will also have an impact on the development of neoplasms following transplantation.[17] Skin cancers are the most common malignancy following transplantation, with more than 90% being squamous or basal cell cancers. The incidence of skin cancers is staggering, with 50% or more of white recipients ultimately developing lesions. The immunosuppressed patient also has a higher incidence of nodal spread, and educating the patient about the importance of avoiding direct sun exposure is essential. Other malignancies that have a particularly high incidence in transplant recipients include non-Hodgkin lymphomas and carcinomas of the anogenital areas. The etiology of anogenital carcinoma is related to the presence of human papilloma virus.

Posttransplant lymphoproliferative disease is the second most common form of malignancy in transplant recipients and is associated with Epstein-Barr virus. These lymphoproliferative syndromes present as a spectrum of pathology, extending from polyclonal lymphoproliferation to monoclonal B-cell lymphomas. Polyclonal disease has been managed by decreasing or withdrawing immunosuppression, whereas progression

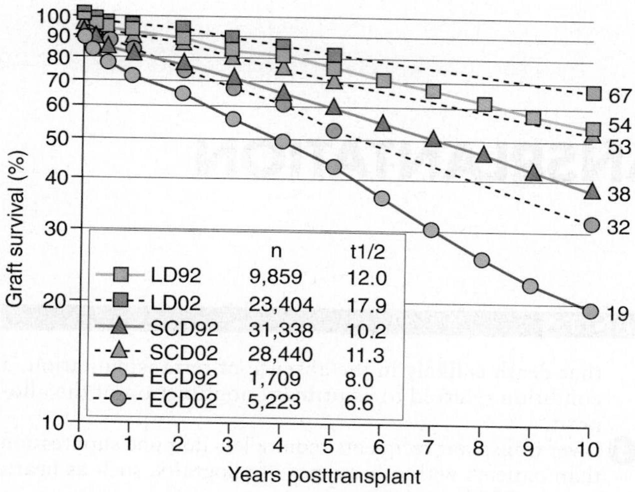

FIGURE 35.6. Comparison of graft survival and graft half-life ($t_{1/2}$) in 1992 and 2002 for different donor types (age >60 years in 1992 group, age >50 years with hypertension, elevated creatinine, or donor death from cerebrovascular accident in 2002 group). There has been an improvement in survival for all donor types, with the best long-term results with living donor kidneys. ECD, extended criteria donor; LD, living donor; SCD, standard deceased donor.

to monoclonal lymphomas has required chemotherapy. CD20-positive lymphomas have been successfully managed with rituximab, an anti-CD20 antibody, with no significant side effects.

CURRENT RESULTS AND FUTURE TRENDS

Over the past three decades, progressive improvement has been made in patient and graft survival, independent of donor source. This progression is best shown in Figure 35.6 for the period of time spanning 1992 to 2002. Overall graft survival, as well as the half-life of the graft, improved incrementally for live donor transplants, standard deceased donor transplants, and even deceased donor transplants using suboptimal or extended criteria donors.[13] This change is related to improved organ preservation, perfected operative technique, and most important, improved immunosuppressive agents. Current 1-year actuarial graft survival rates for living and deceased donor transplants are 94.8% and 88.9%, respectively.[18] These remarkable 1-year results continue to be overshadowed by the specter of late graft loss due to chronic rejection. This problem remains unsolved in renal transplantation, and future improvement in long-term survival will be achieved only when the mechanisms of this process are understood.

The exponential growth in waiting lists compounded by the ongoing critical shortage of organs will continue to stimulate creative means of increasing both the living and deceased donor pools. Expansion in the number and types of immunosuppressive agents has resulted in marked decreases in the incidence of acute rejection, which it is hoped will translate to prolongation in the long-term function of kidney transplants. Newer strategies in immunosuppressive regimens that minimize nephrotoxic cyclosporine and tacrolimus by adding non-nephrotoxic agents will also benefit the long-term function of transplanted kidneys. The effect of ischemia-reperfusion injury on both early and late graft function, as well as its impact on the development of chronic rejection and transplant glomerulopathy, is an area of active research, and potential therapeutic interventions to minimize this injury are being evaluated. The induction of tolerance to foreign antigen remains the "holy grail" of transplantation. A paucity of tolerizing regimens have been applied clinically, although the use of donor bone marrow or stem cells will likely have a future role in achieving the elusive goal of transplantation tolerance.

References

1. Tanabe K, Tokumoto T, Ishida H, et al. Excellent outcome of ABO-incompatible living kidney transplantation under pretransplantation immunosuppression with tacrolimus, mycophenolate mofetil, and steroid. *Transplant Proc* 2004;36:2175–2177.
2. Takahashi K, Saito K, Takahara S, et al. Excellent long-term outcome of ABO-incompatible living donor kidney transplantation in Japan. *Am J Transplant* 2004;4:1089–1096.
3. Meier-Kriesche HU, Kaplan B. Waiting time on dialysis as the strongest modifiable risk factor for renal transplant outcomes: a paired donor kidney analysis. *Transplantation* 2002;74:1377–1381.
4. Rosendale JD. Organ Donation in the United States: 1998–2002. In: Cecka JM, Terasaki PI, eds. *Clinical Transplants 2003*. Los Angeles: UCLA Immunogenetics Center; 2004:65–76.
5. Melcher M, Carter JT, Posselt A, et al. More than 500 consecutive laparoscopic donor nephrectomies without conversion or repeated surgery. *Arch Surg* 2005;140(9):835–839.
6. Nogueira JM, Jacobs SC, Haririan A, et al. A single center comparison of long-term outcomes of renal allografts procured laparoscopically versus historic controls procured by the open approach. *Transpl Int* 2008;21(9):908–914.
7. Cooper JT, Chin LT, Krieger NR, et al. Donation after cardiac death: the University of Wisconsin experience with renal transplantation. *Am J Transplant* 2004;4:1490–1494.
8. Bromberg J, Gill J. Heavy LYFTing: KASting Pearls Before Swine. *Am J Transplant* 2009;9:1489–1490.
9. Warren DS, Zachary AA, Sonnenday CJ, et al. Successful renal transplantation across simultaneous ABO incompatible and positive crossmatch barriers. *Am J Transplant* 2004;4:561–568.
10. Jordan SC, Tyan D, Stablein D, et al. Evaluation of intravenous immunoglobulin as an agent to lower allosensitization and improve transplantation in highly sensitized adult patients with end-stage renal disease: report of the NIH IG02 trial. *J Am Soc Nephrol* 2004;15:3256–3262.
11. Metzger RA, Delmonico FL, Feng S, et al. Expanded criteria donors for kidney transplantation. *Am J Transplant* 2003;3(suppl 4):114–125.
12. Port FK, Bragg-Gresham JL, Metzger RA, et al. Donor characteristics associated with reduced graft survival: an approach to expanding the pool of kidney donors. *Transplantation* 2002;74:1281–1286.
13. Cecka JM. The OPTN/UNOS Renal Transplant Registry. In: Cecka JM, Terasaki PI, eds. *Clinical Transplants 2003*. Los Angeles: UCLA Immunogenetics Center; 2004:1–12, 14.
14. Roland ME, Barin B, CarlsonL, et al. HIV-infected liver and kidney transplant recipients: 1- and 3-year outcomes. *Am J Transplant* 2008;8(2):355–365.
15. Vincenti F. Immunosuppression minimization: current and future trends in transplant immunosuppression. *J Am Soc Nephrol* 2003;14:1940–1948.
16. Vincenti F, Kirk AD. What's next in the pipeline. *Am J Transplant* 2008;8(10):1972–1981.
17. Morath C, Mueller M, Goldschmidt H, et al. Malignancy in renal transplantation. *J Am Soc Nephrol* 2004;15:1582–1588.
18. Wynn JJ, Distant DA, Pirsch JD, et al. Kidney and pancreas transplantation. *Am J Transplant* 2004;4(suppl 9):72–80.

CHAPTER 36 ■ HEPATIC TRANSPLANTATION

THEODORE H. WELLING AND SHAWN J. PELLETIER

KEY POINTS

1. The main indication for liver transplantation is end-stage liver disease, defined as the clinical scenario in which a pathologic process or multiple processes have resulted in a damaged liver that has minimal function and no potential for recovery.
2. The Organ Procurement and Transplantation Network uses the Model of End-stage Liver Disease (MELD) score as a method of prioritizing liver transplant recipients. The MELD score is an integer value based on three objective laboratory studies: creatinine, bilirubin, and the international normalized ratio.
3. The degree of preoperative debilitation and the complexity of the operative procedure make complications following hepatic transplantation very common.
4. Approximately 2% to 10% of transplanted livers function so poorly in the immediate postoperative period that death is likely in the absence of retransplantation, a condition referred to as primary nonfunction of the allograft.
5. Liver transplant recipients require less immune suppression than patients with other types of allografts, such as heart, lung, and kidney recipients.
6. Typical acute rejection in liver transplant recipients is usually cell mediated.
7. Chronic rejection is characterized by relentless immune attack on small bile ducts. Histologically, small bile ducts are obliterated or completely absent, termed *vanishing bile duct syndrome*.
8. The patient survival rate following liver transplantation in the United States at 1 year is more than 85% for adults and nearly 90% for children.

Liver transplantation has evolved over the past four decades to be the standard treatment for patients with a variety of acute and chronic liver diseases. The first successful liver transplant was performed on a moribund child with a hepatoma by Dr. Thomas Starzl at the University of Colorado in 1967.[1] This child lived more than a year before succumbing to recurrent tumor. Over the next 12 years, liver transplants continued to be performed at a modest rate. Despite 1-year survival rates of less than 50%, it was clear that some patients benefited from the procedure.

In 1979, cyclosporine was introduced into clinical organ transplantation by Sir Roy Calne.[2] Almost immediately, 1-year patient survival rates jumped to over 70%. As a result, liver transplantation programs began to appear worldwide. Today more than 10,000 liver transplants are performed annually in the United States, and survival rates exceed 85% at 1 year and 70% at 5 years, primarily varying on liver disease indication.[3,4]

The clinical expanse of liver transplantation is now primarily limited by the availability of suitable donor organs. Every year more patients are listed for liver transplantation than receive transplants. In the future it is likely that this problem will worsen because of the large number of individuals with chronic hepatitis C infection, a significant portion of whom will eventually develop cirrhosis and hepatocellular carcinoma (HCC), and the expanding numbers of patients with either HCC or nonalcoholic steatohepatitis (NASH).[5] Attention continues to be focused on methods to increase the available supply of livers for transplantation. Notable efforts to improve the supply of available organs include the work by the Department of Health and Human Services, which recently took up the cause of organ donation vigorously. This effort, termed the Organ Donation Breakthrough Collaborative,[6] focused on improving the success rate of organ donation efforts at the hospitals that have most potential organ donors nationwide. The Centers for Medicare and Medicaid Services also joined the effort by declaring specific Conditions of Participation for all hospitals that treat Medicare patients in the United States.[7] This effort focused on encouraging methods of approaching donor families that have been shown to be optimally effective.

Many other methods to increase the number of donor livers are currently being practiced. These methods include the utilization of older liver donors and steatotic donor livers, the development of techniques to allow a single liver graft to be split into two grafts, and the utilization of liver grafts from donors that die of cardiac death (DCD). Recently, many centers have continued the development of safe surgical techniques that allow healthy, living volunteers to donate a segment of their liver to a recipient in need of a liver transplant.[8,9]

GENERAL INDICATIONS FOR HEPATIC TRANSPLANTATION

1 The most common indication for liver transplantation is end-stage liver disease. The term *end stage* refers to the clinical scenario in which a pathologic process or multiple processes have resulted in a damaged liver that has minimal function and no potential for recovery. The diagnosis of end-stage liver disease is made primarily on the basis of clinical findings. Additional information about the etiology of the liver disease and thus its natural history can often be obtained by supplementary investigations including serologic studies and histologic examination of a liver biopsy specimen. It is important that potential liver transplant recipients are evaluated by a specialist with expertise in end-stage liver disease, because many other diseases may present similar clinical pictures.

The severity of liver disease in an individual is highly variable, from mild cirrhosis and no symptoms to severe decompensation resulting in deterioration of mental status and frank renal failure. The rate of progression of liver disease from a functional state to invalidism to death is variable and may be rapid or may take several years. The challenge facing liver transplant professionals is to identify patients who will benefit from transplantation. Hepatic transplantation may result in wonderful and dramatic results, but at the same time it is always a high-risk procedure. In situations in which patients enjoy full performance status, and are only

TABLE 36.1

FORMULAS TO CALCULATE MELD AND PELD SCORES

MELD score	$= 0.957 \times \text{Log}_e$ (Creatinine [mg/dL]) $+ 0.378 \times \text{Log}_e$ (Total bilirubin [mg/mL]) $+ 1.120 \times \text{Log}_e$ (INR) $+ 0.643$
PELD score	$= 0.436$ (Age younger than 1 year = 1, Older = 0) $- 0.687 \times \text{Log}_e$ (Albumin [g/dL]) $+ 0.480 \times \text{Log}_e$ (Total bilirubin [mg/mL]) $+ 1.857 \times \text{Log}_e$ (INR) $+ 0.667$ (Growth failure = 1)

INR, international normalized ratio; MELD, Model of End-stage Liver Disease; PELD, Pediatric End-stage Liver Disease.

TABLE 36.2

URGENT LISTING CRITERIA FOR LIVER TRANSPLANTATION

Status 1A	*Fulminant hepatic failure* (encephalopathy within 8 wk of liver disease and ICU status with ventilator dependence, renal replacement therapy, INR >2.0, or acute Wilson disease)
	Hepatic artery thrombosis of liver transplant (AST >3,000 U/mL and INR >2.5 or acidosis within 7 d)
	Primary nonfunction of liver transplant (AST >3,000 U/mL and INR >2.5 or acidosis within 7 d)
	Anhepatic state (graft removal for any reason)
Status 1B	Age <18, chronic liver disease in ICU with MELD/PELD >25 plus one of following: ventilator dependence, GI bleeding, renal replacement therapy, Glasgow Coma Score <10

AST, aspartate aminotransferase; GI, gastrointestinal; ICU, intensive care unit; INR, international normalized ratio; MELD, Model of End-stage Liver Disease; PELD, Pediatric End-stage Liver Disease.

minimally symptomatic, transplantation is an inappropriate therapeutic measure. A liver transplant is a major surgical procedure on a profoundly ill individual with unavoidable risk that also requires chronic, lifelong immunosuppression. Despite advances in immunosuppressive medications developed over the past four decades, immunosuppression remains a treatment that induces a state of vulnerability in the recipient by virtue of the fact that the recipient's natural resistance to infection and malignancy is compromised. It is thus critical that patients be carefully selected as to who will benefit from the procedure.

How is it possible to properly select patients and properly time transplantation so that the benefit of transplantation is
2 assured? In 2002, the Organ Procurement and Transplantation Network began using the Model of End-stage Liver Disease (MELD)[10] score as a method of prioritizing liver transplant recipients. The MELD score is an integer value based on three objective laboratory studies: creatinine, bilirubin, and the international normalized ratio (INR) (Table 36.1). This has been adapted to pediatric patients as well (Pediatric End-stage Liver Disease [PELD]) utilizing the variables in MELD along with albumin instead of creatinine and including age as well as the presence of growth failure (Table 36.1). Analysis done by the Scientific Registry of Transplant Recipients (SRTR) has shown that patients with MELD scores of less than 15 have a mortality rate on the waiting list that is less than the mortality of the transplant procedure in the same population.[11] This suggests that patients with a MELD score of less than 15 do not receive an absolute survival benefit from transplantation, whereas patients with higher MELD scores have the potential to receive a survival benefit with liver transplantation. In other words, there is no evidence that patients who are too ill from liver disease to benefit from liver transplantation are being transplanted, but patients who have stable, mild liver disease should not receive a transplant until their disease has progressed to a more severe state.

Surprisingly, MELD more accurately predicts mortality than clinical factors that were previously thought to be ominous signs of reduced (6 months or less) survival. Such factors, including the presence of ascites, hepatic encephalopathy, spontaneous bacterial peritonitis, and variceal hemorrhage, do not add to the predictive value of MELD.[10] This finding may be related to the difficult nature of accurately quantifying clinical variables in registry databases or to the fact that MELD is such an accurate way of measuring functional hepatic capacity that no additional clinical variables are more relevant.

As will be discussed later, the transplant community has agreed upon certain exceptions to the MELD score for patients with chronic liver disease. It is generally supported that patients with diseases such as HCC, hepatopulmonary syndrome (HPS), primary oxaluria, and familial amyloidosis benefit from additional MELD points by regional review boards. Other diseases or complications such as portal vein thrombosis or portal pulmonary hypertension (PPHTN) remain less clear and are handled on a case-by-case basis.[12]

The improved ability to predict mortality for patients with liver failure allowed the development of national allocation policies that direct livers to those patients who will benefit. Importantly, the implementation of the MELD system of allocation for livers from deceased donors has been associated with a decrease in the death rate on the waiting list.[13] Further refinements of our understanding will undoubtedly occur as improved long-term follow-up data on waiting list mortality become available and as quality-of-life considerations are added to the analysis.

These considerations apply to the chronic forms of liver failure, but not to the important emergency decisions about transplantation that must be made when a patient presents with fulminant hepatic failure (FHF), which is defined as the progression from good health to liver failure with hepatic encephalopathy within 8 weeks. Without transplantation, the mortality rate for fulminant hepatic failure is approximately 75%.[14] Death often occurs rapidly once patients progress to stage II (confusion), stage III (stuporous), or stage IV (unresponsive) hepatic encephalopathy. In these cases, the decision to perform transplantation is based on clinical grounds. Current liver transplant allocation policy allows for the rapid transplantation of patients with fulminant hepatic failure. These patients can be listed as status 1A (Table 36.2), which gives them higher priority for available livers than patients with chronic liver disease who are prioritized based on MELD score.

Contraindications to Liver Transplantation

The number of absolute contraindications to hepatic transplantation has steadily decreased during the past several years as experience with the procedure has increased. Many clinical situations once considered to be absolute contraindications for transplantation are now either no longer considered to be contraindications or to be only relative contraindications. A thrombosed portal vein is no longer a contraindication to transplantation because techniques have been devised to effectively deal with this condition (see later).[15] The presence of juvenile-onset diabetes mellitus formerly precluded transplantation. In current practice, this is not usually the case, depending on the patient's physiologic status at the time of evaluation. Similarly, advanced age causes concern, but in most centers the physiologic state of the patient is a more important consideration than the chronologic age.

The inability to withstand the operative procedure, usually for cardiovascular or pulmonary reasons, is considered to be a contraindication to liver transplantation. Specific examples include patients with depressed ejection fraction secondary to ischemic cardiomyopathy, significant pulmonary hypertension, and significant chronic obstructive pulmonary disease. Cardiac disease that is not amenable to percutaneous therapy poses a particular problem because these patients are frequently unable to withstand a corrective cardiac procedure because of their severe liver disease. In highly selected patients it may be possible to perform combined heart and liver transplantation or combined lung and liver transplantation.

Recent intracranial hemorrhage is almost always a contraindication because during the liver transplant procedure, coagulopathy is often present along with significant alterations in arterial blood pressure. The risk of a catastrophic exacerbation of intracranial bleeding during a transplant is therefore high in this setting. However, the meaning of "recent" is not defined in either the transplant or the neurosurgical literature. Profound, irreversible neurologic impairment is also considered to be a contraindication, but mild mental retardation is not necessarily problematic as long as a social support network exists to ensure compliance with posttransplant regimens. Active substance abuse remains a contraindication, as is the lack of the necessary social support network.

Human immunodeficiency virus (HIV) infection, long considered a contraindication, is no longer an absolute exclusion due to the development of highly effective antiretroviral therapies.[16,17] Active sepsis or untreated infection and active extrahepatic malignancy continue to be contraindications.

Although renal insufficiency increases the risk of liver transplantation, it is not a contraindication. Patients who have hepatorenal syndrome (HRS) frequently experience recovery of renal function following liver transplantation. However, patients who have longstanding hepatorenal failure and patients with known renal parenchymal disease requiring renal replacement therapy are often best served by combined liver/kidney transplantation.

TABLE 36.3

LIVER DISEASE COMPLICATIONS AND LIVER-SPECIFIC METABOLIC DISEASES

Complications:
Ascites
Encephalopathy
Refractory variceal hemorrhage or portal gastropathy
Hepatocellular carcinoma
Hepatopulmonary syndrome (HPS)
Portopulmonary hypertension (PPHTN)
Fulminant hepatic failure (FHF)
Metabolic diseases:
Wilson disease
α_1-Antitrypsin disease
Familial amyloidosis
Urea cycle enzyme deficiencies
Glycogen storage disease
Tyrosemia
Primary oxaluria

DISEASE-SPECIFIC INDICATIONS AND OUTCOMES

While the MELD score assessment plays a critical role in evaluating and listing patients who might benefit from liver transplantation, patients who develop liver disease–specific complications, regardless of MELD, are also appropriate to consider for liver transplantation. Some of these complications along with other liver-specific metabolic diseases are listed in Table 36.3. Hepatitis C is the most common disease for which liver transplantation is currently performed in the United States (33%) (Fig. 36.1). Alcoholic liver disease, NASH, and cholestatic liver diseases are the next most common ranging from 10% to 14% of cases. However, this trend is believed to be changing with a greater proportion of liver transplants being performed for NASH (Fig. 36.2).[5] Outcomes following liver transplantation are best for pediatric patients with biliary atresia, while patients with cholestatic liver diseases experience the best survival among adults (Fig. 36.3). Patients with hepatitis C or HCC experience worse survival secondary to disease recurrence. Disease-specific indications, outcomes, and considerations will be discussed in the following sections.

Alcoholic Liver Disease

Excessive alcohol consumption can lead to several hepatic abnormalities, ranging from alcoholic hepatitis to steatosis, hepatic fibrosis, and cirrhosis. Alcoholic liver disease was once thought to occur only in individuals who consumed large quantities of alcohol over long periods of time. It has recently become recognized that even moderate amounts of alcohol consumption can induce liver injury, suggesting that hereditary and/or environmental factors are probably important. Hepatitis C viral infection, found in 15% to 25% of patients with alcoholic liver disease, appears to exacerbate alcohol-induced liver injury and vice versa.

When liver transplantation emerged as a standard therapy for end-stage liver disease in the 1980s, intense debates occurred surrounding the issue of offering liver transplantation. There were two broad areas of concern. First, many were skeptical that patients with a history of longstanding alcoholism would be able to successfully comply with the rigorous long-term medical treatment required of patients who receive lifelong immunosuppression. On a broader level, concern was expressed that scarce societal resources should not be used to treat patients with "self-induced" diseases. With more experience in this area, it has been recognized that the incidence of recidivism after transplantation is low, and both short- and long-term results in this category are as good as for non–alcohol-related

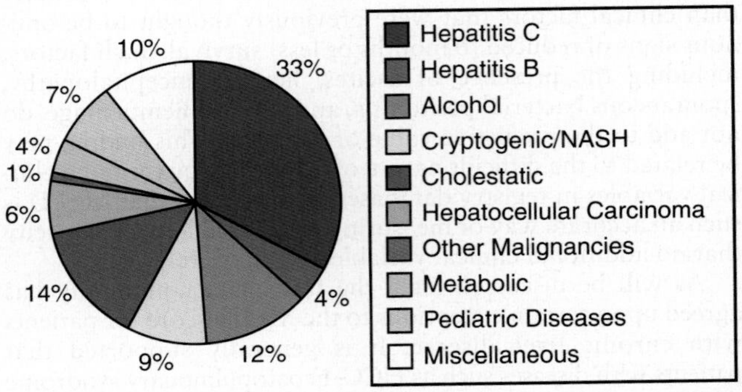

FIGURE 36.1. Percentage of liver transplants for each etiology. (Reproduced with permission from O'Leary JG, Lepe R, Davis GL. Indications for liver transplantation. *Gastroenterology* 2008;134: 1764–1776.)

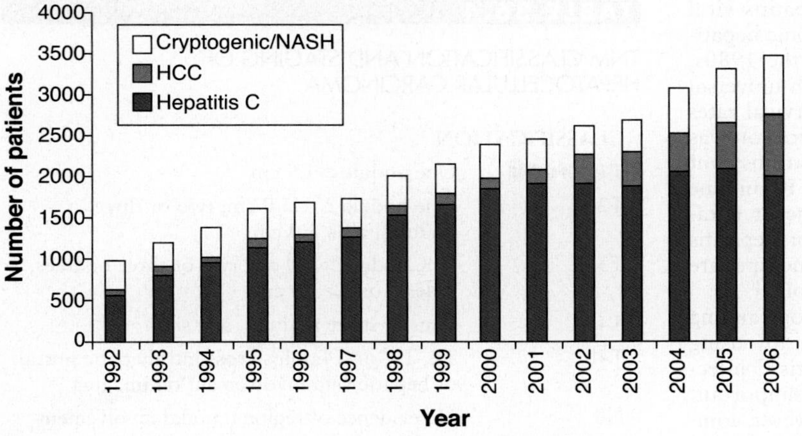

FIGURE 36.2. Changing incidence of liver transplantation for nonalcoholic steatohepatitis (NASH), hepatocellular carcinoma (HCC), and hepatitis C. (Reproduced with permission from O'Leary JG, Lepe R, Davis GL. Indications for liver transplantation. *Gastroenterology* 2008;134:1764–1776.)

categories. It has also become understood that determining worthiness for receiving a lifesaving organ by making a judgment about past behavior is neither ethical nor possible.

Today, the same methods of determining suitability for transplantation are used for patients with alcoholic liver disease as with other diagnoses with one proviso. Unlike other disorders that tend to be universally progressive, alcohol-induced liver injury frequently regresses following cessation of alcohol consumption as long as cirrhosis is not yet present. Patients with a history of recent alcohol abuse should therefore be observed for a minimum of 6 months to ensure that their hepatic dysfunction is not reversible. In addition, all patients with a history of substance abuse must be evaluated by individuals with expertise in addiction and found to have good insight into their past self-destructive behavior and a stable social support network for the posttransplant phase.

Viral Hepatitis

Most patients who become infected with hepatitis B develop an immunologic response to the virus that results in complete

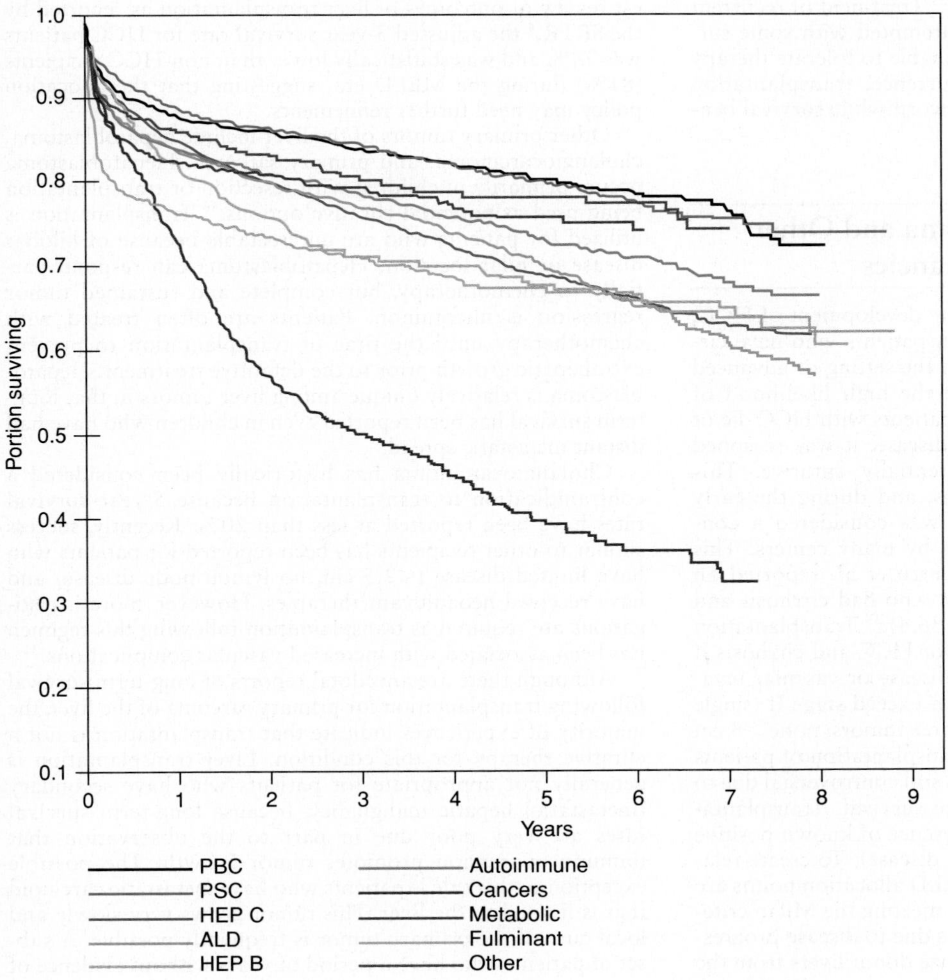

FIGURE 36.3. Disease-specific survival following liver transplantation. (Reproduced with permission from Roberts MS, Angus DC, Bryce CL, et al. Survival after liver transplantation in the United States: a disease-specific analysis of the UNOS database. *Liver Transpl* 2004;10:886–897.)

viral clearance. Patients who do not clear the hepatitis viral antigen may persist as carriers or may develop chronic hepatitis, which progresses to fibrosis and cirrhosis. In the 1980s, transplantation for hepatitis B was associated with universal recurrence of viral infection posttransplant and survival rates were poor. Fortunately, transplantation for this indication was revolutionized by the development of effective posttransplant prophylaxis using long-term, high-dose, hepatitis B immune globulin and the nucleoside inhibitors lamivudine or entacavir.[18,19] Today, outcomes for transplantation for hepatitis B–induced liver failure, while varying based on genotype, are equivalent to or better than those for other conditions.[20]

Hepatitis C has become the most common etiology among patients receiving liver transplants.[5] Antiviral therapy using pegylated interferon and ribavirin for early hepatitis C infection has been demonstrated to have clinically important responses seen in over half of patients treated. However, complete clearance of hepatitis C from serum can only be achieved in a minority of patients, which is largely related to viral genotype and whether significant toxicities to therapy develop.[21,22]

Following liver transplantation, recurrence of hepatitis C in the transplanted liver occurs universally unless the virus was eradicated pretransplant with therapy.[23] Although some patients experience an indolent course, most patients experience a more rapid progression to liver failure once cirrhosis has developed posttransplant. These patients can progress to end-stage liver failure within 6 months.[24] Short-term results of transplantation for this disease are comparable to those for the other noninfectious conditions. However, approximately 25% of patients develop recurrent cirrhosis within 5 years posttransplant, and long-term survival is less likely compared with patients who do not have hepatitis C infection. Use of livers from donors of increased age is thought to contribute to poorer results in hepatitis C patients.[25] Treatment of recurrent hepatitis C posttransplant is often attempted with some survival benefit, but many patients are unable to tolerate therapy or fail to respond.[24,26] Despite recurrence, transplantation appears to provide a substantial and worthwhile survival benefit to most patients with hepatitis C.

Hepatocellular Carcinoma and Other Hepatic Malignancies

Cirrhosis is a major risk factor for the development of HCC, and the majority of HCCs develop in patients who have cirrhosis. Curative resection is unsafe in the setting of advanced cirrhosis, and it does not eliminate the high likelihood of recurrent malignancy. Because most patients with HCC die of liver failure, rather than metastatic disease, it was reasoned that transplantation would be potentially curative. This approach yielded poor survival rates, and during the early 1990s primary hepatic malignancy was considered a contraindication to liver transplantation by many centers. This circumstance changed when Mazzaferro et al. reported an 85% 4-year survival rate for patients who had cirrhosis and either stage I or stage II HCC (Table 36.4).[27] Transplantation is now considered standard therapy for HCC and cirrhosis if there is no evidence of extrahepatic disease or vascular invasion and if the tumor burden does not exceed stage II (single tumor <5 cm in diameter, or two to three tumors, none >3 cm in diameter). While some advocate transplantation of patients with larger tumors,[28,29] this practice is still controversial due to concerns of overall lower disease-free survival. Transplantation is clearly not beneficial in the presence of known positive nodal or distant metastases (stage IV disease). To create relative equality for a scarce resource, MELD allocation points are standardly allocated to HCC patients meeting the Milan criteria so as to minimize waitlist dropouts due to disease progression and at the same time not overutilize donor livers from the remainder of the recipient candidate pool. However, in the latest review of outcomes of liver transplantation as reported by the SRTR,[4] the adjusted 3-year survival rate for HCC patients was 74% and was statistically lower than non-HCC recipients (81%) during the MELD era, suggesting that the allocation policy may need further refinements.

TABLE 36.4

TNM CLASSIFICATION AND STAGING OF HEPATOCELLULAR CARCINOMA

CLASSIFICATION	
T1	One nodule ≤1.9 cm
T2	One nodule 2.0–5.0 cm; two or three nodules, all <3.0 cm
T3	One nodule >5.0 cm; two or three nodules, at least one >3.0 cm
T4a	Four or more nodules, any size
T4b	T2, T3, or T4a plus gross intrahepatic portal or hepatic vein involvement on imaging
N0	No evidence of regional nodal involvement
N1	Regional (porta hepatitis) nodal involvement
M0	No evidence of metastatic disease
M1	Evidence of metastatic disease
STAGE GROUPING	
Stage I	T1
Stage II	T2
Stage III	T3
Stage IV A1	T4a
Stage IV A2	T4b
Stage IV B	Any N1, any M1

Other primary tumors of the liver include hepatoblastoma, cholangiocarcinoma, and primary sarcoma. Hepatoblastoma occurs primarily in children with resection or transplantation being used as potential curative options.[30] Transplantation is utilized for patients who are unresectable because of bilobar disease or hilar location. Hepatoblastoma can respond partially to chemotherapy, but complete and sustained tumor regression is uncommon. Patients are often treated with chemotherapy until the time of transplantation to prevent extrahepatic growth prior to the definitive treatment. Hepatoblastoma is relatively unique among liver tumors in that long-term survival has been reported even in children who have had distant metastatic spread.

Cholangiocarcinoma has historically been considered a contraindication to transplantation because 5-year survival rates have been reported at less than 20%. Recently, success similar to other recipients has been reported for patients who have limited disease (<2.5 cm, no lymph node disease) and have received neoadjuvant therapies. However, more investigations are required as transplantation following this regimen has been associated with increased vascular complications.[31]

Although there are anecdotal reports of long-term survival following transplantation for primary sarcoma of the liver, the majority of experiences indicate that transplantation is not a curative therapy for this condition. Liver transplantation is generally not appropriate for patients who have secondary (metastatic) hepatic malignancy, because long-term survival rates are very poor due in part to the observation that immunosuppression promotes tumor growth. The possible exception to this rule is patients who have metastatic carcinoid that is limited to the liver. This tumor grows very slowly and local cure of the primary tumor is frequently possible. A subset of patients who have a period of years without evidence of tumor growth anywhere else but in the liver will have long-term disease-free survival following liver transplantation.[32]

Nonalcoholic Fatty Liver Disease

NASH may be the most common liver disease in the United States. It has a high incidence in obese patients and those with adult-onset diabetes mellitus. The disease resembles alcoholic liver disease, but patients do not report a significant history of alcohol use. The degree of hepatic injury varies from benign elevations of serum hepatic transaminases in association with hepatic steatosis or steatohepatitis to fibrosis and cirrhosis. A majority of patients previously classified as having cryptogenic cirrhosis probably have longstanding steatohepatitis. It is estimated that at least two thirds of the obese population in the United States have hepatic steatosis and close to one fifth have steatohepatitis.[33] Patients who develop cirrhosis and progress to end-stage liver disease are appropriate candidates for liver transplantation. Recurrence of steatohepatitis leading to graft dysfunction is possible. Recipient diabetes and obesity appear to be independent negative prognostic indicators for survival after liver transplantation.[33]

Fulminant Hepatic Failure

Acute hepatic failure, defined as the development of altered mental status, coagulopathy, and hepatic dysfunction within 8 weeks of the onset of an acute hepatic disease, is a rare but lethal disease.[14,34] There are over 2,000 cases of acute hepatic failure per year in the United States. The mortality rate approaches 80% in patients who do not receive liver transplants. The causes of acute hepatic failure include viral hepatitis, toxins such as aflatoxins from the poisonous mushroom family *Amanita phalloides*, acute fatty liver of pregnancy, acute Budd-Chiari syndrome, and drug toxicities. Drug toxicities include both idiosyncratic reactions and drugs with predictable toxicity when taken in excess. Drugs that have been reported to induce idiosyncratic liver failure include isoniazid, halothane, valproate, disulfiram, and phenytoin, among many others. The over-the-counter analgesic acetaminophen causes dose-dependent hepatic failure and is now the single most common cause of acute hepatic failure in the United States.

The most generally accepted criteria for transplantation of patients with fulminant hepatic failure were described by the group at the King's College hospital in London, England (Table 36.5).[35] While the King's College criteria have been separately validated in other studies, more recent studies have begun to evaluate whether other scoring systems may have improved abilities to measure severity of illness. MELD has come under recent investigation in this regard and has been found to be additive to the King's College criteria in predicting outcome following fulminant hepatic failure.[36,37] The current United Network for Organ Sharing (UNOS) listing criteria for patients with fulminant hepatic failure is in Table 36.2. The outcomes following transplantation have shown overall higher perioperative mortality, compared to other diseases, with overall similar long-term survival (Fig. 36.3).[3]

TABLE 36.5

KING'S COLLEGE CRITERIA FOR LIVER TRANSPLANTATION

■ ACETAMINOPHEN	■ NONACETAMINOPHEN
pH <7.3	PT >100 s (INR >6.5)
Or all three of:	Or any three of:
Grade 3–4 encephalopathy	Age <10 or >40 y
PT >100 s (INR >6.5)	Etiology (non-A, non-B hepatitis, halothane, drug reaction, Wilson disease)
Cr >3.4 mg/dL	Period of transition from jaundice to encephalopathy >7 d
	PT >50 s (INR >3.5)
	Total bilirubin >17.5 mg/dL

Cr, creatinine; INR, international normalized ratio; PT, prothrombin time.

Biliary Atresia

Biliary atresia is a congenital disorder of infants that is characterized by biliary obstruction resulting from obliteration or discontinuity of the extrahepatic biliary system resulting in progressive hyperbilirubinemia, cirrhosis, and hepatic failure. The etiology is unknown yet is the most common indication for hepatic transplantation in pediatric patients. Standard treatment includes creation of a portoenterostomy (Kasai procedure), if this can be done before 3 months of age. After this point, success rates diminish markedly. Response to the portoenterostomy procedure is highly variable. Patients may develop cirrhosis within the first 6 months of life or live into their twenties before developing synthetic dysfunction and portal hypertension. Approximately 75% of children will require transplantation by 6 years of age.

It is critical that these patients are managed by an experienced pediatric gastroenterologist so that the correct window for effective transplantation can be identified and so they receive appropriate attention to their specialized nutritional needs. Specifically, deficiencies of fat-soluble vitamins that depend on bile for absorption are common and treatable. Transplantation is appropriate when children manifest growth and nutritional failure, when ascites develops, and when portal hypertension progresses to the point of variceal hemorrhage. Recurrent cholangitis is also thought to be an indication for liver transplantation. Transplantation for this population overall has had excellent results, with greater than 85% 10-year survival being achieved in the United States.[38] Factors that have been associated with improved survival include living donor transplants and older recipient age. Patients with significant growth failure generally have poorer outcomes.

Primary Biliary Cirrhosis

Primary biliary cirrhosis (PBC), thought to be autoimmune in nature, is characterized by gradually increasing serum bilirubin levels, progressive fatigue, and cirrhosis. Early stages of the disease are usually asymptomatic, and disease progression may evolve over 20 years. Treatment with ursodeoxycholic acid appears to slow the progression of the disease, but immunosuppression does not. It was once thought that primary biliary cirrhosis does not recur; however, histologic analysis has shown that the incidence of recurrence is approximately 15% within 5 years of transplantation.[39] Eventual progression to graft failure requiring retransplantation is possible, though rare.

Primary Sclerosing Cholangitis

Primary sclerosing cholangitis (PSC) is an autoimmune disease that is characterized by gradually progressive inflammation of the biliary tree, eventually resulting in cirrhosis. PSC is associated with ulcerative colitis, but removal of the colon does not affect progression of the disease. In most cases, colectomy for associated inflammatory bowel disease is done after successful transplantation because the failing liver makes the patient a poor candidate for a large abdominal procedure. PSC is also associated with the development of cholangiocarcinoma. Patients who experience a course that becomes rapidly progressive should be examined by endoscopic retrograde cholangiopancreatography (ERCP) with brushings to evaluate for cholangiocarcinoma. In addition to the usual considerations about the timing of transplantation, it is important to note that these patients are susceptible to bacterial cholangitis, which can cause systemic sepsis and rapid hepatic decompensation. Episodes of cholangitis that do not respond to suppressive antibiotic therapy should prompt early consideration for transplantation. Overall, patients with PBC or PSC experience the best outcomes with transplantation when compared to adults with other diseases; however, disease recurrence remains higher in PSC patients than in PBC patients.[3,40]

Inherited Metabolic Disorders

Numerous inherited metabolic disorders are treatable by liver transplantation (Table 36.3). Some enzymatic deficiencies in this group result in destruction of the liver, so transplantation may resolve the liver failure as well as supply the missing enzyme. Disorders in this category include Wilson disease, α_1-antitrypsin deficiency, tyrosinemia, and type I glycogen storage disease. In other cases, the liver is not affected by the disease, either structurally or functionally. In these circumstances transplantation is undertaken solely as enzyme replacement therapy. Diseases that have been cured by hepatic transplantation in this category include hemophilia A or B, homozygous familial hypercholesterolemia, Niemann-Pick disease, oxalosis, familial amyloid polyneuropathy, and numerous enzymatic deficiencies of urea cycle metabolism.[41] Transplantation depends on determining that transplantation will cure the disease, or at least halt its progression, and that the consequences of the disease without transplantation are devastating, making transplantation appropriate.

Budd-Chiari Syndrome

Budd-Chiari syndrome is characterized by obliteration of the hepatic veins. It may be due to congenital webs of the hepatic veins or suprahepatic cava or may be caused by spontaneous thrombosis of the hepatic veins. The latter condition is associated with polycythemia vera and other hypercoagulable states. Diagnosis is made by inferior vena cavagram or magnetic resonance venography. The classic presentation is a triad of right upper quadrant pain, hepatomegaly, and ascites. Patients may present with fulminant hepatic failure during acute Budd-Chiari and have symptoms of encephalopathy and coagulopathy, or they may present in a more indolent fashion with ascites as the predominant feature. The natural history of the indolent form of Budd-Chiari syndrome is the eventual development of cirrhosis.

Patients who present with intact hepatic function should undergo an assessment to determine whether the liver has evidence of cirrhosis. A transjugular intrahepatic portosystemic shunt (TIPS) is the preferred therapy for patients who do not have evidence of synthetic failure and have not yet developed cirrhosis. Transplantation is reserved for cases where portal decompressive shunting is not possible or for patients who have advanced cirrhosis. Long-term anticoagulation to prevent recurrent hepatic vein thrombosis in the liver graft is routinely recommended.

Other Considerations

HPS and PPHTN are two other manifestations of cirrhosis whereby transplantation is justified. Similar to HCC, these two diseases can occur in cirrhosis despite overall preserved hepatic function and appear to involve dysregulation of vasoactive mediators such as nitric oxide. Therefore, MELD exception scores are often sought when either HPS or PPHTN are present.[12] HPS is diagnosed on the basis of unexplained hypoxia in the presence of cirrhosis along with a positive "bubble" study for pulmonary shunt on echocardiography. PPHTN is diagnosed on the basis of pulmonary hypertension in the setting of cirrhosis without any other explainable etiology such as underlying pulmonary pathology. Recipient selection and management is critical to achieve reasonable success with liver transplantation. Patients with HPS experience the best outcomes if the preoperative partial pressure of arterial oxygen (PaO_2) is greater than 50 mm Hg.[42] Patients with PPHTN likewise must have mean pulmonary artery pressures less than 35 mm Hg with or without medical therapy to experience a reasonable chance of recovery following liver transplantation.[43,44]

In addition to isolated liver disease, liver transplantation is occasionally considered along with other solid organ transplantation. The two most notable examples are combined kidney and liver transplantation as well as combined liver and intestine transplantation.[4] Intestine transplantation is usually performed in cases where intestinal failure is present along with progressive cholestatic liver failure secondary to hyperalimentation.[45] Since hepatorenal syndrome frequently occurs with advanced cirrhosis and also frequently resolves with successful liver transplantation, the indications for combined liver and kidney transplantation are more controversial.[46] It is widely accepted that preexisting end-stage renal disease along with significant cirrhosis or the existence of hepatorenal syndrome requiring 8 or more weeks of renal replacement therapy warrants consideration of combined liver and kidney transplantation. Ongoing investigations are required to define patients with hepatorenal syndrome who are less likely to recover renal function following liver transplantation.

LIVER TRANSPLANTATION: SURGICAL PROCEDURE

Anesthetic Management

An anesthesiologist with experience in liver transplantation is invaluable to the transplant team, and liver transplant anesthesiology is rapidly becoming a subspecialty. Proper anesthetic management and effective communication between the surgery and anesthesiology teams is necessary to optimize patient care during the surgical procedure. While an extensive outpatient preoperative evaluation is usually performed, including cardiac risk stratification, many liver candidates report from home when a liver becomes available. If adequate time for fasting has not occurred, consideration of rapid sequence induction should be given to prevent aspiration. After induction and intubation, general anesthesia is maintained with a combination of inhalational agents and the administration of paralytic agents and analgesics. For adult patients, cardiac monitoring is often performed either by pulmonary artery catheterization or intraoperative transesophageal echocardiography. An arterial catheter is placed for blood pressure monitoring. Adequate vascular access, often including central venous catheters, is required for the administration of blood products and the potential for rapid resuscitation in the case of massive blood loss. A device for rapid infusion and the ability to warm blood products or intravenous fluids is advisable. Low central venous pressures maintained during the hepatectomy phase of the procedure may help avoid excess bleeding.

Intraoperative Management of Coagulopathy

Liver transplantation has the potential for massive blood loss for several reasons. Liver transplant candidates with cirrhosis often have synthetic deficiencies in circulating coagulation factors as well as severe portal hypertension associated with thrombocytopenia and extensive venous collaterals. Intraoperative coagulopathy may be worsened during the anhepatic phase of the procedure. Finally, liver transplantation involves extensive dissection of major vascular structures including the inferior vena cava, portal vein, and hepatic artery, all with an inherent risk for torrential bleeding.

Intraoperatively, coagulation is monitored by frequent determination of standard parameters including prothrombin time, partial thromboplastin time, platelet count, and fibrinogen. Abnormalities of these laboratory values associated with intraoperative bleeding are often corrected with fresh frozen plasma, platelets, or cryoprecipitate. Normal coagulation is also helped by maintaining normal pH, calcium levels, and normothermia. Intraoperative thromboelastography (TEG) can facilitate decision making by rapidly identifying which components of the coagulation cascade are deficient or by identifying the presence of a fibrinolytic state. However, the device for TEG can be fragile and overly sensitive, which may limit its practical use in the clinical setting. The decrease in excessive bleeding in the modern era of liver transplantation has led to many programs abandoning the routine use of TEG. While the administration of recombinant factor VII intraoperatively can rapidly and effectively stop nonsurgical bleeding, its use has a theoretical risk of postoperative thrombotic complications including hepatic arterial thrombosis. In addition, no definitive data have been demonstrated to decrease the need for intraoperative blood transfusions.[47,48] Therefore, its use is only recommended in emergent situations.

Following reperfusion of the donor liver, a fibrinolytic state may be encountered. This is related to the lack of production of fibrinolysis inhibitors during the anhepatic phase and the inability of the liver to metabolize profibrinolytic compounds. This state may be identified either by thromboelastography, recurrence of bleeding where hemostasis had been previously obtained (such as the wound edge), or extensive and refractory bleeding after revascularization. This state may be treated with the use of antithrombolytic agents including ε-aminocaproic acid, tranexamic acid, or aprotinin. Because therapy with antithrombolytic agents has been associated with intravascular thrombus formation, it should not be used routinely and should be discontinued when no longer needed.

Surgical Technique

Transplantation of the liver is among the most technically demanding surgical procedures. During induction and placement of the appropriate monitoring lines by the anesthesiology team, the donor liver is prepared on the back table for implantation (Fig. 36.4). Bench preparation includes resection of the donor diaphragm and adrenal gland off of the bare area of the liver and vena cava. Meticulous ligation of tributaries from the vena cava (adrenal vein, phrenic vein, and lumbar branches) is performed. The artery is dissected free from the Carrel patch of the aorta up to the gastroduodenal artery. Dissection near the right or left hepatic arteries is avoided to prevent unnecessary injury. The portal vein is circumferentially dissected free. The gallbladder may be removed at this stage or following reperfusion. Tissues surrounding the common bile duct are left intact to avoid injury of the blood supply.

Following this, the recipient's abdomen and bilateral groins are prepped and draped in a standard fashion. The most commonly used incision is a bilateral subcostal incision with a midline extension to the xiphoid process (Fig. 36.4B). After dividing the fascia, ascites, which can occasionally be present in a large volume, is evacuated. The ligamentum teres hepatis is carefully divided between clamps and ligated because a large recannulized umbilical vein is often present in patients with severe portal hypertension. After dividing the falciform ligament with cautery, a mechanical retractor is used to retract the bilateral costal margins anteriorly and superiorly for excellent exposure of the upper abdomen. The abdominal cavity and liver are then inspected for any abnormalities including unsuspected malignancy, particularly within the cirrhotic liver, which is a risk factor for hepatocellular carcinoma. Following this, liver transplantation occurs in three stages: (a) recipient hepatectomy, (b) anhepatic phase, and (c) postrevascularization.

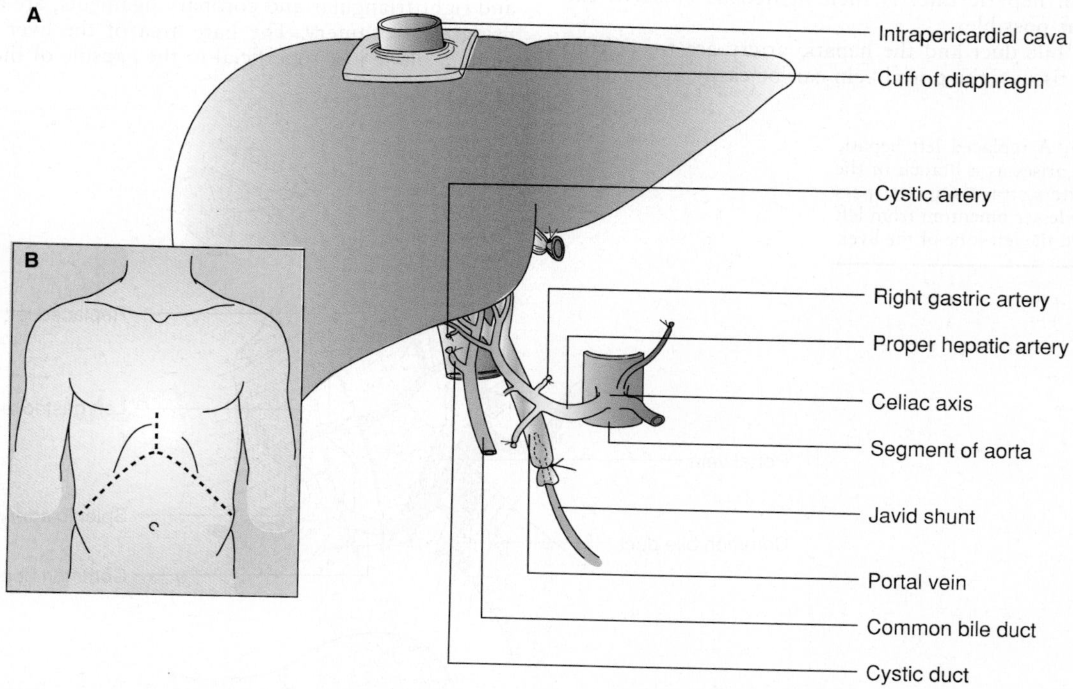

FIGURE 36.4. **A:** The donor liver after excision and before transplantation. **B:** Bilateral subcostal incision with a subxiphoid extension.

Recipient Hepatectomy

During the recipient hepatectomy phase, the liver is mobilized from its ligamentous attachments and the porta hepatis is skeletonized. Attention is first directed to dissecting and skeletonizing the structures of the portal triad. The peritoneum overlying the portal triad is divided with electrocautery near the liver edge. The right and left hepatic arteries are dissected free, ligated, and divided, leaving adequate length to form a branch patch for the arterial anastomosis. The proper hepatic artery is also dissected free to the level of the gastroduodenal artery allowing enough length for clamping during the anastomosis. Because portal venous flow of blood to the liver may be hepatofugal (away from the liver), division of the artery may leave the patient functionally anhepatic. If a prolonged period of time is expected for mobilization of the liver, such as when extensive adhesions are present, the artery may be dissected free but left in continuity to allow whatever synthetic capacity the native liver has to continue. A replaced or accessory right hepatic artery, which arises as a branch off the superior mesenteric artery and travels in a posterior position to the common bile duct and lateral to the portal vein, can usually be palpated if present and can be ligated and divided. When the replaced right hepatic artery is relatively large and the proper hepatic artery is diminutive in size, the replaced right hepatic artery can be left long and used for arterial inflow for the donor liver. A replaced or accessory left hepatic artery arises from the left gastric artery if present and can be identified by inspection of the pars flaccida of the lesser omentum along the lesser curvature of the stomach (Fig. 36.5).

Conceptually, the common bile duct and common hepatic duct should be dissected free with as much length as possible and without injuring the blood supply to the bile duct. Leaving the recipient bile duct as long as possible allows the length of the donor bile duct, which may have a tenuous blood supply, to be shorter and still avoid tension at the time of anastomosis. This is accomplished by first ligating and dividing the cystic duct. The common bile duct and common hepatic duct are then circumferentially dissected free leaving the surrounding tissue to preserve the bile duct blood supply. The common hepatic duct is then ligated as close to the native liver as possible.

Once the bile duct and the hepatic artery are freed from surrounding tissues, the portal vein can be easily approached from its anterior, medial, and lateral aspects. In general, the portal vein is freed circumferentially from the edge of the duodenum up to its bifurcation of the right and left portal veins. Small branches may arise near the pancreas and excessive bleeding may arise if these are inadvertently injured. Most patients with severe portal hypertension will not develop hypotension, small bowel edema, or ischemia if the portal vein is clamped and divided because of the presence of portal venous collaterals. However, patients without portal hypertension, such as those undergoing liver transplantation for fulminant hepatic failure or metabolic deficiency or those who have had a TIPS for a prolonged period of time, may develop extensive small bowel edema or hypotension when the portal vein is clamped. Small bowel edema can lead to limited exposure in the right upper quadrant, making implantation of the liver extremely difficult. In these situations, the portal vein should be left in continuity for as long as possible, particularly when the use of venovenous bypass is not intended. For those patients with portal vein thrombosis, portal venous flow can be restored in most cases. Often, the thrombus can be evacuated with the use of forceps or by placing a Yankauer suction tip within the lumen of the portal vein. If the thrombus is more mature, an eversion endovenectomy may be necessary.[49] If these maneuvers are unsuccessful, the junction of the splenic vein and superior mesenteric vein may be patent. Dissection of the portal vein behind the pancreas to this junction can then be performed to allow for future anastomosis. Dissection to the confluence of the splenic and superior mesenteric veins is sometimes necessary in pediatric recipients because of the small caliber of the portal vein within the porta hepatis. In rare cases, all of these maneuvers may be unsuccessful and a venous bypass graft from the superior mesenteric vein may be necessary. If the superior mesenteric vein is also occluded, the inferior vena cava can be used for portal inflow, a procedure termed cavoportal hemitransposition.[50] This procedure is associated with acceptable outcome despite the fact that portal hypertension may not be alleviated. A fourth option is arterialization of the portal vein, using a conduit created by anastomosing donor iliac vessels to the recipient aorta and connecting this to the donor portal vein.[51]

The ligamentous attachments of the liver, including the left and right triangular and coronary ligaments, are then divided using electrocautery. The bare area of the liver is dissected along a plane just superficial to the capsule of the liver. Care

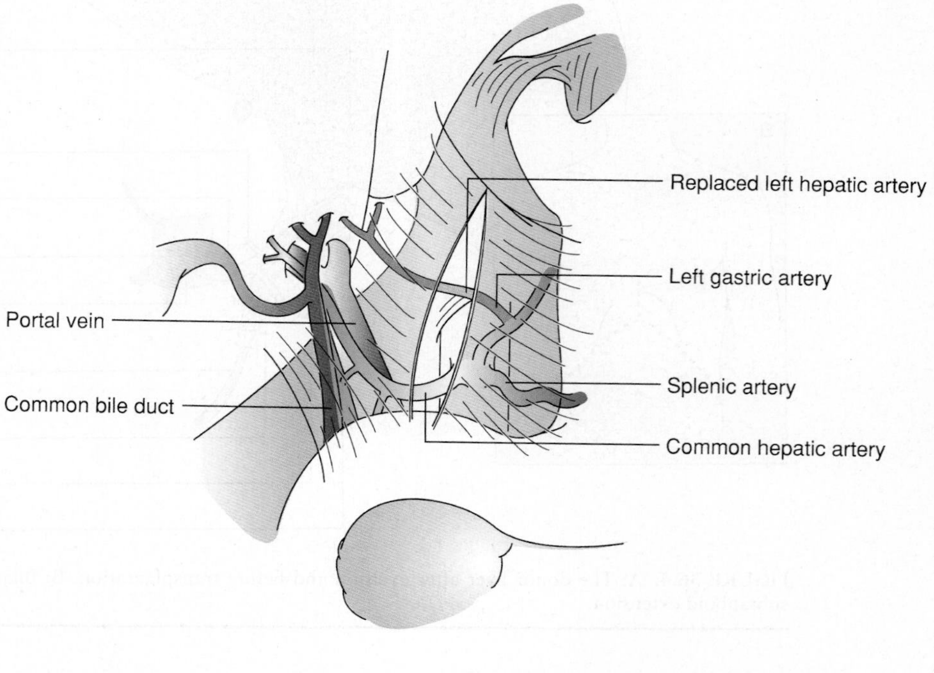

FIGURE 36.5. A replaced left hepatic artery usually arises as a branch of the left gastric artery, traversing the pars flaccida of the lesser omentum from left to right toward the left lobe of the liver.

must be taken to avoid injury to the phrenic or hepatic veins when freeing the suprahepatic inferior vena cava where it traverses the diaphragm. The hepatocaval ligament along the right lateral aspect of the vena cava can be divided using a combination of cautery and ligation as a phrenic venous branch is often present within this ligament. The liver is then dissected off of the anterior aspect of the inferior vena cava. Small venous branches from the inferior vena cava to the caudate lobe are ligated and divided. Larger branches, such as an accessory right hepatic vein, are clamped, divided, and oversewn. Division of the portal vein facilitates exposure for this dissection but is not required. The liver may be gradually retracted and dissected from either the right or left aspects until the right, middle, and left hepatic veins are reached. If a bicaval venous anastomosis technique will be used, the vena cava can be circumferentially mobilized near the diaphragm above the hepatic veins as well as in an infrahepatic position. However, if a piggyback or cavocavostomy (side-to-side caval anastomosis) technique is intended, the dissection of the posterior aspect of the vena cava should be avoided to prevent encountering unnecessary bleeding from collateral or lumbar venous branches in this area.

Anhepatic Phase and Implantation of the Donor Liver

At this point, the liver has been completely mobilized except for its attachments of the hepatic veins to the inferior vena cava and, in some cases, the portal vein. The decision should now be made whether to use venovenous bypass. Most patients will tolerate clamping of both the portal vein and the inferior vena cava without difficulty.[52] At this point, communication with the anesthesiologist is essential and the vena cava should be test clamped before division to make sure that adequate cardiac filling and blood pressure can be maintained. If the patient becomes hypotensive during test clamping, the clamp should be removed and additional volume or pressor support can be administered. Occasionally, patients will require venovenous bypass, but its use is no longer routine at most centers.

If necessary, venovenous bypass can be accomplished from both the portal vein and inferior vena cava simultaneously, or a single cannula in either the portal vein or the inferior vena cava may be used (Fig. 36.6). There are several accepted methods of placing cannulas for venovenal bypass. Cannulas may be placed percutaneously in the internal jugular vein and femoral vein prior to beginning the procedure. These cannulas are advanced into the superior and inferior vena cava, respectively. Alternatively, one or both of the bypass cannulas may be placed by cutdown on the axillary and/or greater saphenous vein. Inferior vena caval and mesenteric blood is delivered to the superior vena cava by a centrifugal pump. The cannulas, tubing, and centrifugal pump head are heparin bonded to reduce the chance of thrombus formation and subsequent embolism without the use of anticoagulation. Flow rates of 1 to 2 L/min are usual.

Once venovenous bypass has been established or the decision to forego bypass has been made, the recipient hepatectomy is completed. If still intact, the portal vein is divided as high in the hilum as possible. Three methods are commonly used for orthotopic liver transplantation: (a) the bicaval technique, (b) the piggyback technique, and (c) cavocavostomy (side-to-side caval technique).

1. For the bicaval technique, the recipient liver is excised en bloc with the retrohepatic inferior vena cava after caval clamps have been placed in a suprahepatic and infrahepatic position. The hepatic veins are divided within the substance

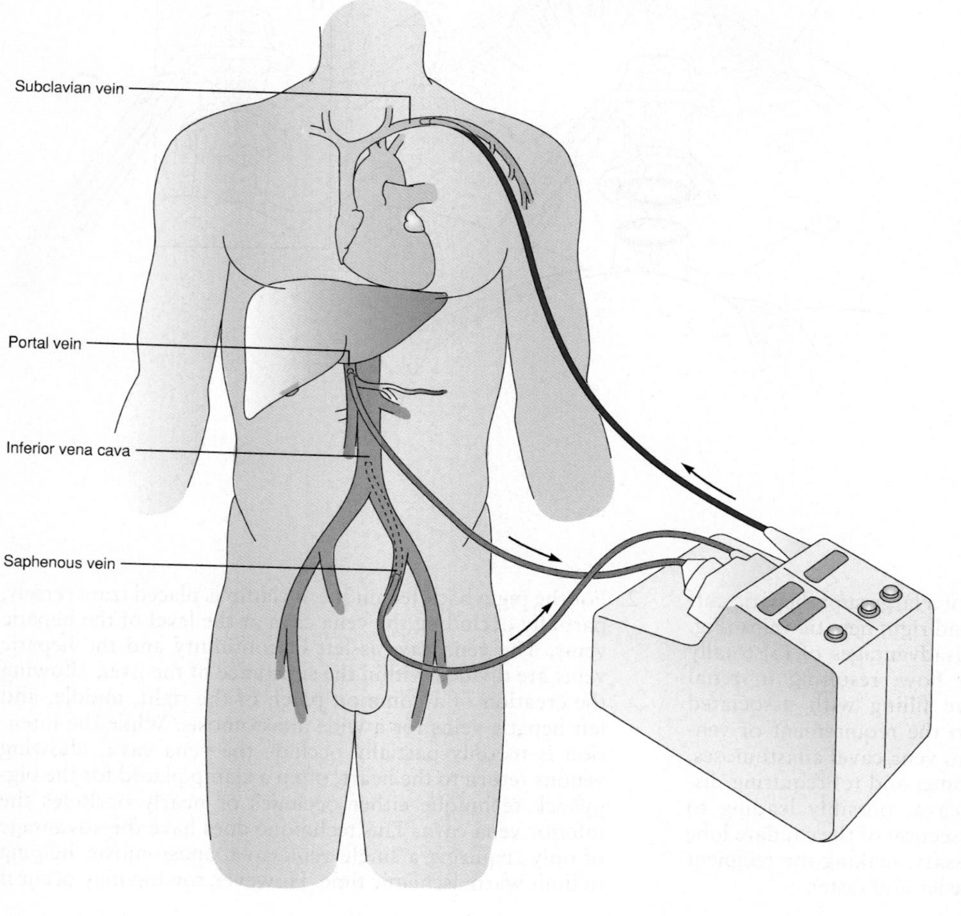

FIGURE 36.6. Setup for venovenous bypass during hepatic transplantation. Cannulas are placed into the portal vein to decompress the splanchnic bed and inferior vena cava (through the greater saphenous vein) to decompress the lower extremities and kidneys during the anhepatic phase of the transplantation. A centrifugal pump is used to deliver bypassed blood to the central circulation by means of a cannula passed into the axillary vein.

FIGURE 36.7. **A:** The diseased recipient liver is removed by incising the liver below the level of the hepatic veins. **B:** The hepatic veins are then opened to form a large suprahepatic cuff for anastomosis. The suprahepatic vena caval anastomosis: posterior suture line (C) and anterior suture line (D).

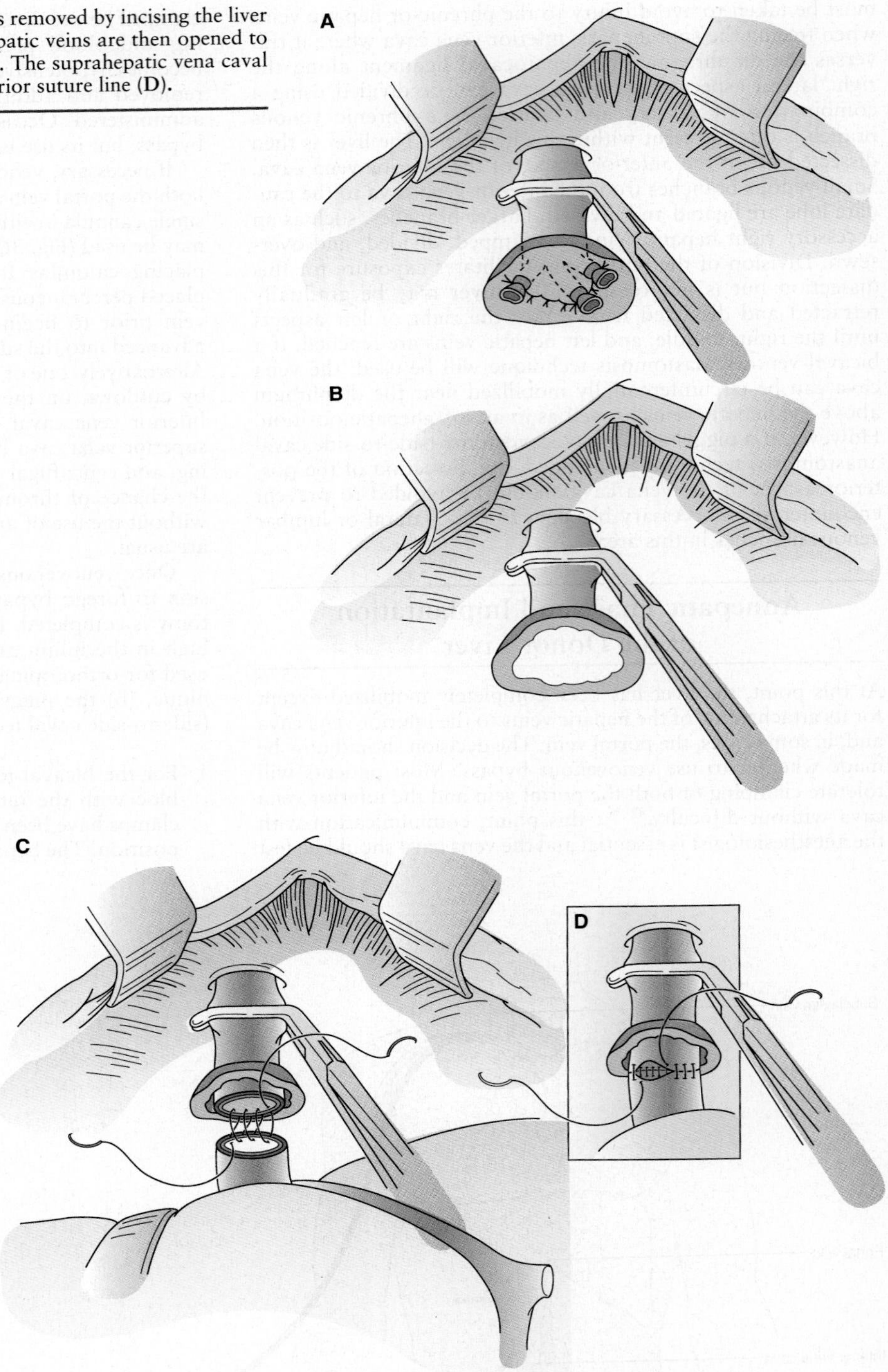

of the liver to allow the creation of a large suprahepatic cuff compromising the left, middle, and right hepatic veins (Fig. 36.7). This technique has the disadvantages of (a) totally obstructing inferior vena cava flow, resulting in renal ischemia and decreased cardiac filling with associated hypotension, possibly leading to the requirement of venovenous bypass; (b) requiring two vena caval anastomoses, prolonging the warm ischemic time; and (c) requiring dissection posterior to the vena cava, possibly leading to bleeding. However, complete dissection of the caudate lobe off of the vena cava is not necessary, making the recipient hepatectomy phase somewhat easier and faster.

2. For the piggyback technique, a clamp is placed transversely, partially occluding the vena cava at the level of the hepatic veins. The vena cava is left in continuity and the hepatic veins are divided within the substance of the liver, allowing the creation of a common patch of the right, middle, and left hepatic veins for a wide anastomosis. While the intention is to only partially occlude the vena cava, allowing venous return to the heart, often a clamp placed for the piggyback technique either occludes or nearly occludes the inferior vena cava. This technique does have the advantage of only requiring a single vena caval anastomosis, helping to limit warm ischemic time. However, torsion may occur if

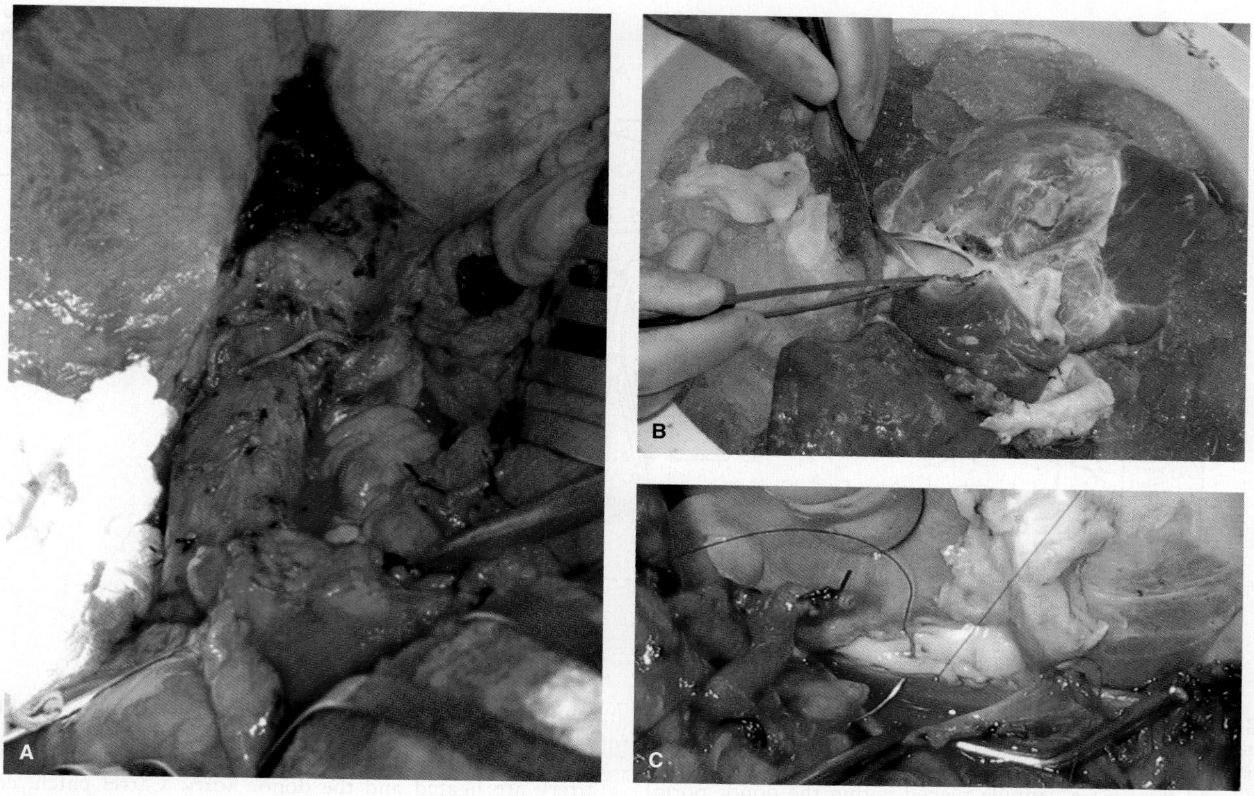

FIGURE 36.8. Cavocavostomy. A: The recipient right and junction of the middle and left hepatic veins are stapled and the inferior vena cava is left in continuity. B: The supra- and infrahepatic vena cavae are stapled and a venotomy is made longitudinally on the posterior aspect of the donor liver. C: A side-to-side caval anastomosis is performed with a running suture.

the right upper quadrant is relatively large, such as when a large volume of ascites is present, and the donor right hepatic lobe is relatively small. This may lead to right hepatic vein or inferior vena caval stenosis.

3. For the cavocavostomy technique, clamps can be placed on the right hepatic vein as well as the junction of the left and middle hepatic veins. The liver is excised and these venous branches are oversewn and the clamps are removed. Alternatively, the hepatic veins can be divided using an Endo GIA stapler (Fig. 36.8). Advantages of the cavocavostomy anastomosis include (a) minimalization of the time that the vena cava is clamped; (b) the vena caval clamp is placed longitudinally, only occluding the anterior third of the vena cava, leading to minimal or no changes in the recipient's hemodynamics; (c) a cavoplasty is performed, limiting the likelihood of caval stenosis; (d) a long anastomosis is performed, often over 6 cm in length, minimizing the risk for hepatic vein outflow complications; and (e) exposure during suturing of the anastomosis is considerably improved compared to the piggyback or bicaval technique.

After removal of the recipient liver, the right upper quadrant is carefully inspected and hemostasis is obtained. Complete hemostasis in the bare area is essential at this time because this region is easily visualized when the liver is absent but may be relatively inaccessible once the donor liver is implanted, especially if the donor liver is relatively large or the recipient is obese. Argon beam coagulation can also be used to aid in hemostasis at this point.

The donor liver is then brought onto the operative field. The vascular anastomoses are performed using a running monofilament polypropylene suture. If a bicaval technique is planned, two caval anastomoses are required. The suprahepatic vena caval anastomosis is first performed by suturing the posterior walls from within the lumen using an imbricating technique (Fig. 36.7). The anterior wall is then completed. The infrahepatic anastomosis is then completed in a similar fashion. Redundancy in the donor vena cava is avoided to prevent the potential for kinking. The completion of the anastomosis may be left until the time of hepatic revascularization to provide a vent for air and acidotic or hyperkalemic blood and for residual preservation solution. Venting of blood prior to reperfusion is most important if preservative solutions containing a high concentration of potassium, such as University of Wisconsin solution, are used. Venting of blood is less critical if preservative solutions that do not contain high concentrations of potassium are used, but care must still be taken to avoid the rapid bolus of air or cold blood to the heart. For the piggyback technique, the donor infrahepatic vena cava is either oversewn or stapled. The donor infrahepatic vena cava is then sewn in an end-to-side fashion to the recipient hepatic vein cuff (Fig. 36.9). As described earlier, an imbricating suture technique is often helpful to prevent gaps in the anastomosis and to compensate for size discrepancies. Venting at the time of reperfusion can either be performed through the suprahepatic anastomosis or at the donor infrahepatic vena cava. For the side-to-side caval technique, a clamp is placed longitudinally on the anterior third of the recipient vena cava. A longitudinal venotomy is made on the anterior surface of the recipient vena cava. The donor suprahepatic and infrahepatic vena cavae are either oversewn or stapled closed. A longitudinal posterior venotomy is then made matching the length of the recipient venotomy. The liver is then placed in the right upper quadrant and the left lateral segment is elevated. The two vena cavae are then sutured in a side-to-side fashion with the lateral wall sutured from within the lumen and the medial wall sutured from outside the lumen

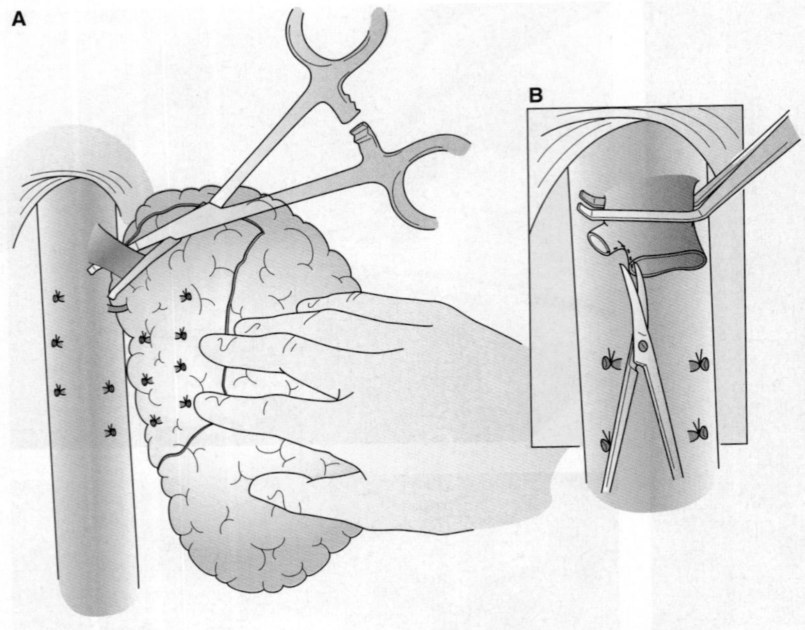

FIGURE 36.9. **A:** Recipient liver is dissected off the native inferior vena cava by dividing veins draining directly into the inferior vena cava up to the level of the hepatic veins. **B:** Clamp is placed on recipient hepatic veins in preparation of excision of the recipient's native liver and performance of a piggyback anastomosis.

(Fig. 36.8). Venting can be performed from either the suprahepatic donor vena cava or the medial wall of the anastomosis. During the caval anastomosis, the donor liver may be perfused with cold fluid via a cannula placed within the donor portal vein to wash out the preservation solution and to help maintain the cold temperature of the liver. This step is not required but may be considered if the liver was preserved with a solution containing a high concentration of potassium or if a prolonged warm ischemic time is anticipated.

Once the caval anastomosis or anastomoses are completed, either the portal anastomosis, arterial anastomosis, or both can be performed prior to reperfusion. In theory, reperfusion with arterial blood would limit the extent of warm ischemia to the biliary tree, which, unlike the remainder of the liver, receives its blood supply exclusively from the arterial blood and not along with portal venous blood. However, neither sequence has been clearly shown to be an advantage over the other, so the choice is made based on the surgeon's preference and the patient's anatomy. Most commonly, the portal venous anastomosis is completed and the liver is reperfused. If portal bypass has been used, the portal limb of the venovenous bypass circuit is removed. The portal anastomosis is usually performed in an end-to-end fashion using a running technique. To avoid narrowing, an air knot is used when the suture is tied.

At the time of revascularization, flow is restored to the liver through the portal vein and/or the hepatic artery. The first several hundred milliliters of blood may be vented through the infrahepatic vena cava and the knot can be tied completing the caval anastomosis. Alternatively, the caval clamp can be "flashed" and the anastomosis inspected for bleeding and repaired if present. If blood is not vented through the infrahepatic cava, portal blood should be restored gradually to minimize cardiac irritability, bradycardia, and hypotension, all of which routinely result from cold blood circulating through the donor liver and going directly into the right atrium. Close coordination between the surgeon and anesthesiologist is necessary during this phase as hypotension and bradycardia are routinely encountered and cardiac arrest may rarely occur. If venovenous bypass has been used during the anhepatic phase, it can now be discontinued.

Once hemostasis is obtained and the patient has stabilized, attention can now be turned toward the arterial anastomosis if it has not already been performed. Conceptually, the arterial anastomosis can be performed in one of two ways. The anastomosis can be performed with the artery being long, which allows the artery to lie with a smooth and gentle curve or loop (Fig. 36.10). For this technique, all branches on the donor artery are ligated and the donor aortic Carrel patch, celiac artery, or branch patch of the celiac and splenic artery is anastomosed in an end-to-end fashion to a branch patch of the recipient right and left hepatic arteries (Fig. 36.11). Alternatively, the artery can be cut to just the right length and sewn in an end-to-end fashion. This is often performed by forming branch patches between the donor and recipient proper hepatic and gastroduodenal arteries and performing the anastomosis in an end-to-end fashion. However, when the retractor is released, the liver may shift position and kinking of the artery may occur. Therefore, judging the proper length of the arteries may be difficult and this technique may be more technically demanding than the method that leaves the artery way too long. If the artery is somewhat long but not long enough to allow a gentle or smooth curve or loop, kinking and obstruction to blood flow may occur. For both techniques, the anastomosis can be performed using a fine, nonabsorbable, monofilament, running suture. If the recipient arterial inflow is inadequate, an aortic conduit may be constructed. This is often performed using a

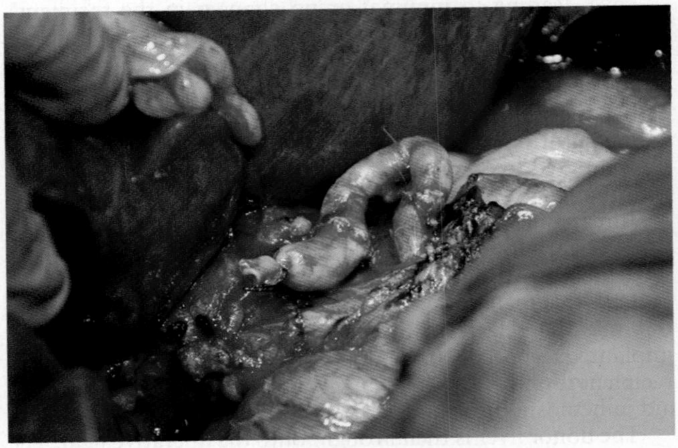

FIGURE 36.10. Hepatic artery anastomosis where the artery is left long to allow for a gentle loop or curve to form.

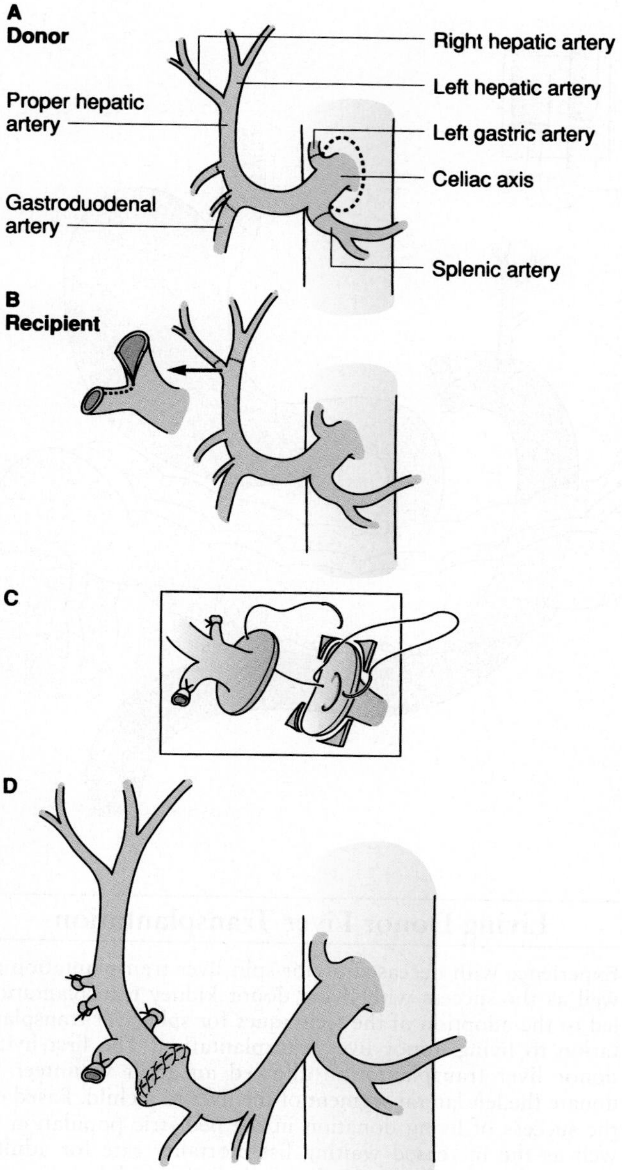

FIGURE 36.11. **A:** The donor hepatic artery is procured with a Carrel patch of aorta. **B:** The recipient hepatic artery bifurcation is used to fashion a branch patch for a larger anastomosis. **C:** The anastomosis is carried out using continuous monofilament suture material. **D:** The completed anastomosis.

graft consisting of the donor common and external (or internal) iliac artery. A partially occluding aortic clamp can either be placed in a supraceliac or infrarenal position and the common iliac artery is sutured in an end-to-side fashion to the recipient aorta. The donor Carrel patch can then be sutured in an end-to-end fashion to the external iliac artery of the conduit.

Postrevascularization Phase

Following revascularization, the liver should assume a normal color and consistency within several minutes. If the liver remains pale or is overly soft, problems with portal inflow should be considered. Alternatively, if the liver becomes edematous and overly firm, outflow obstruction should be excluded. Bile production should be seen while in the operating room and is among the first evidence for liver function. In contrast, watery or milky fluid from the bile duct raises concern for primary nonfunction. Inspection for surgical bleeding should be performed and entails examination of the vascular anastomoses as well as a search for branches of the major vessels that may not have been ligated. If bleeding continues after all surgical bleeding has been resolved, attention should be directed toward correction of coagulopathy as described earlier.

While biliary reconstruction does not carry the same risk for intraoperative disaster when compared to the recipient hepatectomy and reperfusion, it is associated with considerable postoperative morbidity and mortality and requires the same diligence and attention as other steps of the operation. Because of the relatively high complication rate associated with biliary reconstruction, it has been referred to as the "Achilles heel" of liver transplantation. There are several options for biliary reconstruction. In the past, the Calne conduit, or the use of the donor gallbladder, was used but has been abandoned due to the high rate of biliary complications associated with it. The simplest and most common technique is currently an end-to-end choledochocholedochostomy from the donor to the recipient bile duct (Fig. 36.12). If a size discrepancy exists, the narrower duct can be spatulated. Running or interrupted sutures can be used. Absorbable monofilament suture is most commonly used to avoid a nidus for future stone formation within the bile duct. While T-tubes were commonly used in the past to stent the anastomosis, evidence now suggests that more leaks or strictures develop as a result of the T-tube than are prevented. Internal biliary stents may be used and may help prevent leaks or strictures.[53] Alternative biliary reconstruction methods may be necessary for those with a bile duct of inadequate quality or size or in those whose primary disease is biliary pathology such as primary sclerosing cholangitis or biliary atresia. The most common option employed in these situations includes a standard Roux-en-Y choledochojejunostomy. If a choledochojejunostomy had been performed in the past, the limb of small bowel used may often be salvaged and used for biliary drainage of the new liver. Placement of drains is optional but may help identify and treat biliary leaks. Abdominal wall and skin closure is then performed in the standard fashion.

Technique for Reduced-size and Split Liver Transplantation

In the 1980s, the waiting list mortality for small, pediatric liver candidates was relatively high because the number of suitably sized small liver donors was inadequate. As a result, techniques to reduce the size of an adult liver, based on Couinaud's segmental anatomy (Fig. 36.13), were developed so that the left lobe, left lateral segment, or even a single segment could be used for a recipient more than 10 times smaller by weight than the donor.[54,55] During the early experience, the donor hepatectomy was performed in a standard fashion and the liver was brought back to the recipient hospital. The needed segments of the liver were cut down on the back table with the organ on ice, the vessels were left intact to the future transplant graft, and the remainder of the liver was discarded. Techniques have now developed so that both sides of the liver can be transplanted into two recipients, either a child and an adult or two adults.[56,57] In addition, the liver may be split in situ at the donor hospital, allowing coagulation of the cut edge of the liver so that bleeding is minimized following reperfusion. Perfusion to both sides of the liver can be inspected prior to flushing, ensuring that blood flow to all segments of each future graft has been preserved. Because of technical and practical issues, both the cut-down technique and in situ splitting of the liver are still employed. Split liver transplantation has been

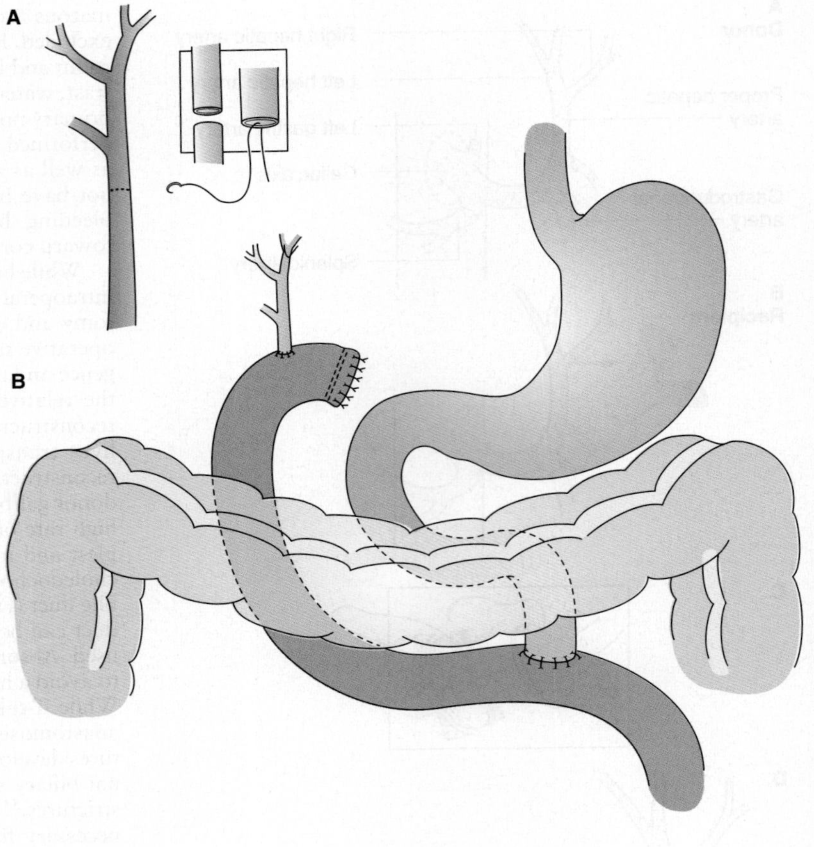

FIGURE 36.12. A: In most cases, a choledochocholedochostomy is performed, possibly over an internal stent. B: Patients with a diseased or unsuitable common bile duct require biliary reconstruction with a Roux-en-Y choledochoenterostomy.

associated with a decreased survival rate and the potential for increased risk of complications, including primary nonfunction, hepatic artery thrombosis, and biliary complications. Because of this, while widespread adoption of allocation policies to encourage greater utilization of split liver grafts in the adult population has been suggested, split liver transplantation only accounts for a small proportion of transplants performed. In addition, only grafts from "ideal donors" are thought to be suitable for this form of transplantation. Criteria supported by UNOS for splitting currently include that the donor be less than 40 years of age, be on a single pressor or no pressors, have transaminases no greater than three times normal, and have a body mass index of 28 or less.

Living Donor Liver Transplantation

Experience with deceased donor split liver transplantation as well as the success with living donor kidney transplantation led to the adoption of the techniques for split liver transplantation to living donor liver transplantation. The first living donor liver transplantation allowed an adult volunteer to donate the left lateral segment of the liver to a child. Based on the success of living donation in the pediatric population as well as the increased waiting list mortality rate for adults, these techniques have also been applied to adult recipients receiving either the right or left lobe from an adult volunteer.[58]

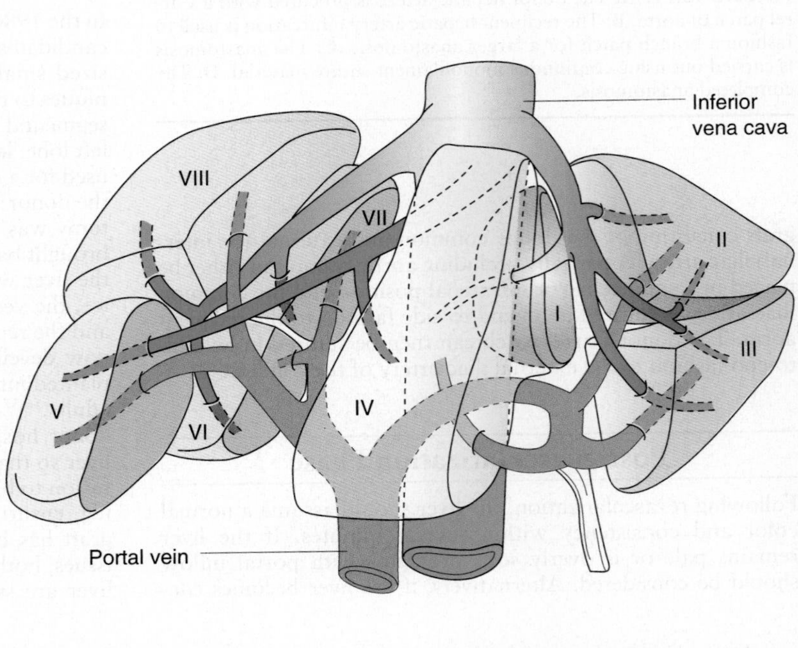

FIGURE 36.13. Segmental anatomy of the liver as based on Couinaud's nomenclature.

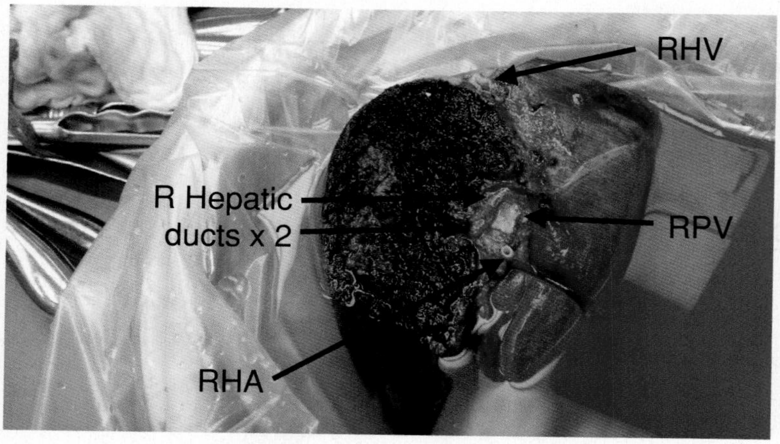

FIGURE 36.14. Living donor right hepatic lobe allograft demonstrating the right hepatic vein (RHV), right portal vein (RPV), right hepatic artery (RHA), and two right hepatic ducts.

Living donor liver transplantation was progressively developing in the United States until a well-publicized donor mortality occurred.[59] Living donor liver transplantation now accounts for approximately 5% of all liver transplants performed in the United States. In Japan and other areas of the Far East, where deceased donor transplantation has developed more slowly because of cultural difficulties with the concept of brain death, living donor transplant is the rule rather than the exception.

In many respects, transplantation of a graft from a living donor is similar to transplantation of a whole liver from a deceased donor. However, a bicaval technique is not possible given that the donor vena cava is not available for replacement of the recipient's retrohepatic inferior vena cava (Fig. 36.14). Therefore, the recipient vena cava must be left intact. A direct hepatic vein to vena caval anastomosis is used (Figs. 36.15 and 36.16). Establishing adequate outflow of hepatic venous blood

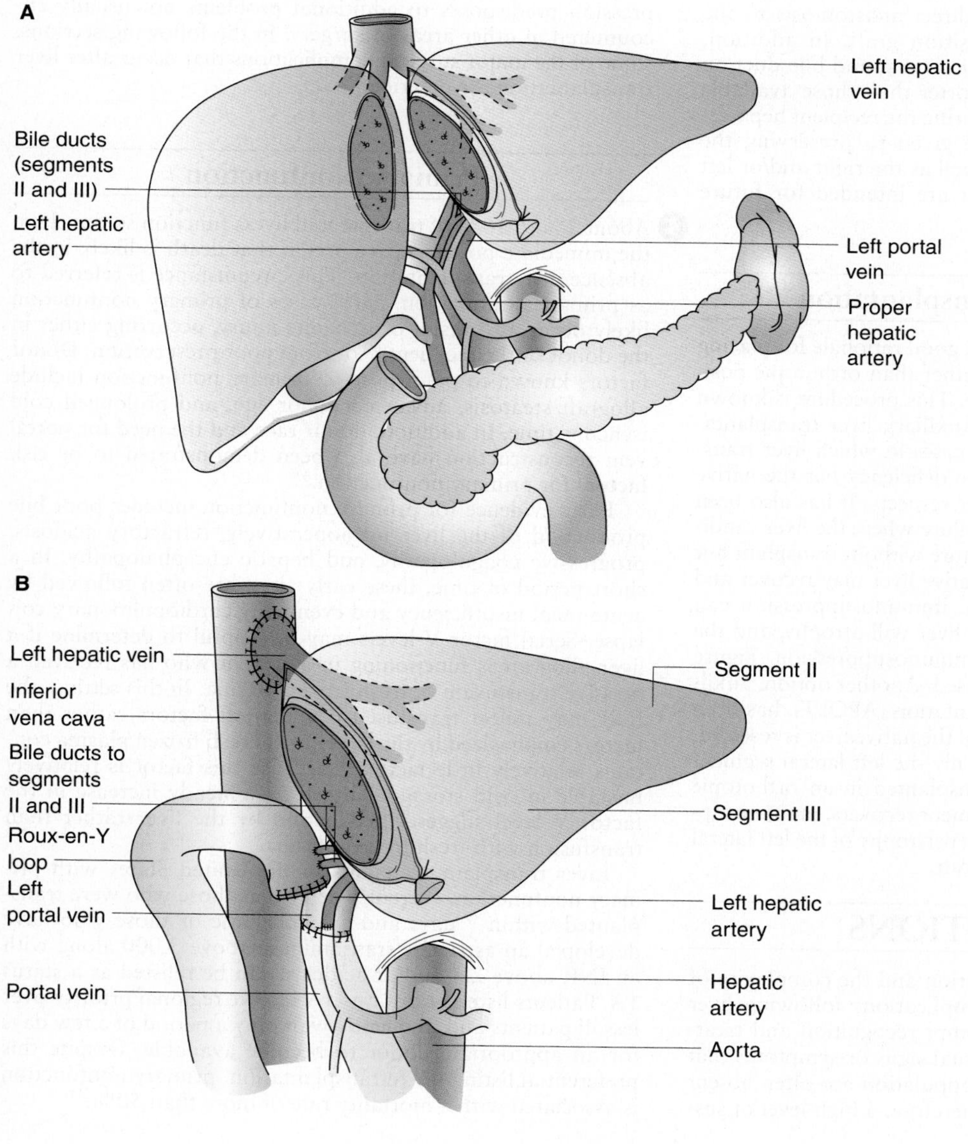

FIGURE 36.15. Left lateral segment (segments II and III) living donor transplantation. **A:** Donor operation. **B:** Recipient operation completed.

TRANSPLANTATION

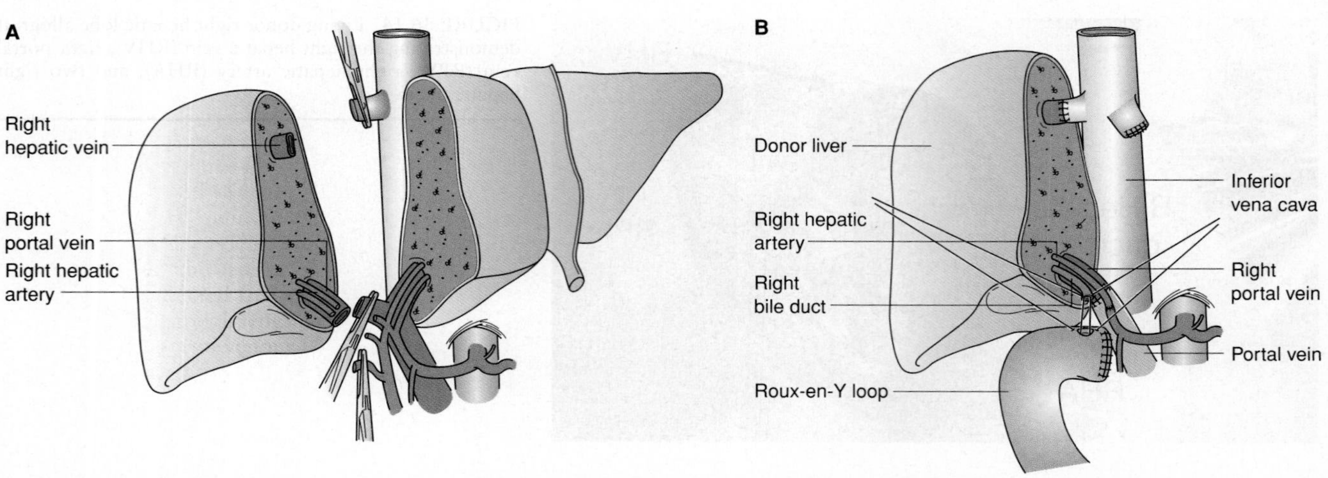

FIGURE 36.16. Right lobe (segments V to VIII) living donor transplantation. **A:** Donor operation. **B:** Recipient operation completed.

is necessary to prevent edema of inadequately drained segments of the liver possibly leading to small-for-size syndrome. Therefore, any accessory veins greater than 5 mm in diameter should be reconstructed either by direct anastomosis to the vena cava or by using an interposition graft. In addition, the lengths of the portal vein, hepatic artery, and bile duct on the donor graft are considerably shorter than those available from a deceased donor. Therefore, during the recipient hepatectomy, considerable care should be given to preserving the length of the recipient bile duct as well as the right and/or left hepatic artery and portal vein that are intended for future anastomosis.

Auxiliary Liver Transplantation

Under select circumstances, there is a good rationale for placing the donor allograft in heterotopic rather than orthotopic position, leaving the native liver in place. This procedure is known as auxiliary liver transplantation. Auxiliary liver transplantation has occasionally been used for cases in which liver transplantation is indicated for enzymatic deficiency but the native liver is otherwise normal in all other respects. It has also been used in cases of fulminant hepatic failure where the liver candidate is expected to die in the near future without transplant but if adequate time was allowed, the native liver may recover and return to normal. In this situation, immunosuppression can slowly be weaned, the transplanted liver will atrophy, and the recipient can be taken off of all immunosuppression. Figure 36.17 demonstrates one technique used. Another option, auxiliary partial orthotopic liver transplantation (APOLT), has been developed. For this technique, part of the native liver is resected, often the right trisegment, leaving only the left lateral segment intact. The donor liver is then transplanted in an orthotopic position. If the native left lateral segment recovers, immunosuppression can be weaned, leading to hypertrophy of the left lateral segment and involution of the allograft.

COMPLICATIONS

3 The degree of preoperative debilitation and the complexity of the operative procedure make complications following liver transplantation very common. Prompt recognition and treatment are essential. However, the usual signs or symptoms that would be expected in the general population are often absent or present to a lesser degree, and therefore, a high level of suspicion must be maintained. Early warnings, such as fever, leukocytosis, or pain, may be suppressed as a result of immunosuppression. In addition, the burden of immunosuppression predisposes to additional problems not usually encountered in other areas of surgery. In the following sections, some of the major surgical complications that occur after liver transplantation are described.

Primary Nonfunction

4 About 2% to 10% of transplanted livers function so poorly in the immediate postoperative period that death is likely in the absence of retransplantation. This circumstance is referred to as primary nonfunction. Most cases of primary nonfunction likely occur as a result of ischemic injury, occurring either in the donor or the recipient,[60] or from poor preservation. Donor factors known to predispose to primary nonfunction include allograft steatosis, advanced donor age, and prolonged cold ischemic time. In addition, donor race and the need for portal vein reconstruction have also been demonstrated to be risk factors for primary nonfunction.[61]

Early evidence for primary nonfunction includes poor bile production of the liver intraoperatively, refractory acidosis, progressive coagulopathy, and hepatic encephalopathy. In a short period of time, these early signs are often followed by acute renal insufficiency and eventually cardiopulmonary collapse. Serial factor V levels may be helpful to determine if a liver allograft is functioning in a patient who has received a massive transfusion of fresh frozen plasma. In this setting, the INR may reflect transfused coagulation factors rather than factors emphasized by the liver graft. Fresh frozen plasma contains relatively little factor V because this factor is relatively unstable in cold storage. Therefore, a steady increase in the factor V level suggests production by the liver rather than transfusion with fresh frozen plasma.

Liver transplant recipients in the United States with primary nonfunction, currently defined as those who were transplanted within 7 days and are anhepatic or those who have developed an aspartate transaminase above 3,000 along with an INR above 2.5 and/or acidosis, can be relisted as a status 1A. Patients listed as a status 1A receive regional priority over less ill patients and frequently wait only a period of a few days for an appropriate donor to become available. Despite this preferential listing for retransplantation, primary nonfunction is associated with a mortality rate of more than 50%.[61]

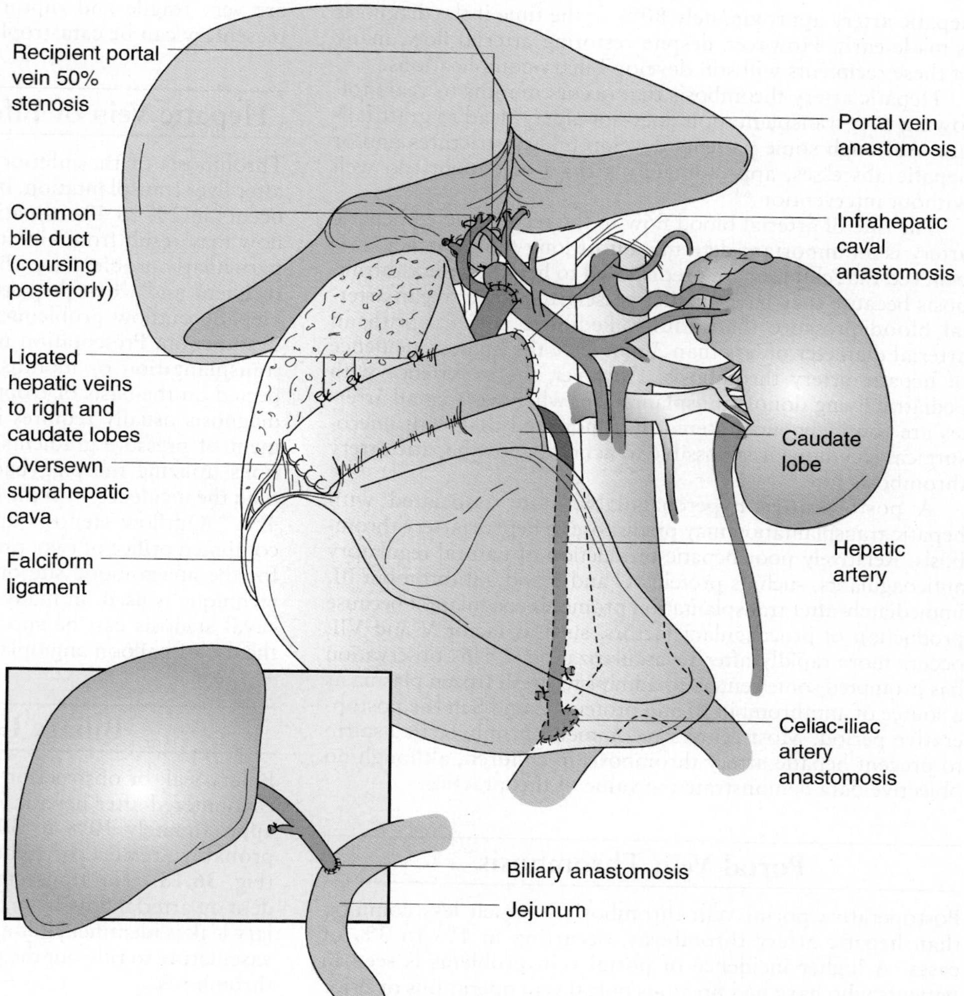

FIGURE 36.17. Heterotopic auxiliary liver transplantation using a reduced-size allograft.

Postoperative Hemorrhage

Postoperative hemorrhage requiring laparotomy occurs in approximately 5% to 15% of liver transplant recipients. Postoperative bleeding should be suspected in any liver recipient during the immediate posttransplant period who develops tachycardia, volume-dependent hypotension, oliguria, and abdominal distention. Because many liver transplant recipients may have had a large volume of ascites preoperatively (sometimes more than 10 to 20 L), a considerable amount of bleeding may occur before developing an abdominal compartment syndrome. In general, attempts to correct coagulopathy should be made and reexploration should occur in patients with refractory hypotension, abdominal compartment syndrome, or ongoing need for blood transfusion. At exploration, a specific bleeding point often cannot be identified, suggesting that bleeding may be related more to coagulopathy than failure of surgical hemostasis. Therefore, waiting until coagulopathy is corrected before reexploration may be wise, assuming that the recipient is otherwise reasonably stable.

Hepatic Artery Thrombosis

The incidence of hepatic artery thrombosis ranges from 1% to 2% up to 10% in some populations. The incidence of hepatic artery thrombosis is higher in pediatric recipients and recipients of living donors or split livers. Other risk factors include receiving a liver from a donor who is significantly smaller than the recipient, the need for reconstructive arterioplasty in the presence of nonstandard donor anatomy, acute rejection within the first week posttransplant, placement of cytomegalovirus (CMV)-positive organs into CMV-negative recipients, and a recipient history of smoking.[62] The association between rejection and hepatic artery thrombosis may be the result of a decrease in hepatic arterial flow that occurs when the liver is swollen and edematous or of release of procoagulations into the microcirculation in association with the inflammatory injury of graft rejection.

Hepatic artery thrombosis can occur in the early period, arbitrarily defined as within 30 days, or late posttransplant period. Early hepatic artery thrombosis is usually identified within the first 10 days posttransplant. The diagnosis is suspected in the setting of unexpectedly high liver enzymes, an elevation in liver enzymes rather than a gradual decline, or poor synthetic function during the first week to 10 days posttransplant. Other signs of biliary ischemia from hepatic arterial thrombosis include the development of biliary leaks, strictures, or intrahepatic abscesses. Doppler ultrasonography is usually used to confirm flow within the extrahepatic and intrahepatic arteries. If inappropriate waveforms or no flow is identified, the diagnosis can be confirmed by angiography or reexploration. At exploration, flow can be restored within the

TRANSPLANTATION

hepatic artery approximately 80% of the time if the diagnosis is made early. However, despite restoring arterial flow, many of these recipients will still develop biliary complications.

Hepatic artery thrombosis that occurs months to years following liver transplantation does not always lead to graft failure. Although some patients develop biliary strictures and/or hepatic abscesses, approximately a third of patients do well without intervention.[63]

The rate of arterial blood flow in the reconstructed hepatic artery is an important determinant of long-term patency. It is believed that children are predisposed to hepatic artery thrombosis because they have smaller vessels and lower mean arterial blood pressure than adults. Pediatric patients with an arterial diameter of less than 3 mm have the highest incidence of hepatic artery thrombosis. However, the experience with pediatric living donor transplantation, where very small arteries are routinely encountered, has indicated that with microsurgical technique it is possible to achieve a low hepatic artery thrombosis rate.[64]

A postoperative hypercoagulable state associated with hepatic transplantation may predispose to hepatic artery thrombosis. Relatively poor hepatic production of natural regulatory anticoagulants, such as proteins C and S and antithrombin III, immediately after transplantation promotes coagulation because production of procoagulant factors, such as factor V and VII, occurs more rapidly after revascularization.[65] This observation has prompted some centers to administer fresh frozen plasma as a source of antithrombin III and proteins C and S in the postoperative period. Most centers recommend prophylactic aspirin to prevent hepatic artery thrombosis in children, although no objective data demonstrate the value of this practice.

Portal Vein Thrombosis

Postoperative portal vein thrombosis is much less common than hepatic artery thrombosis, occurring in 1% to 3% of cases. A higher incidence of portal vein problems is seen in patients who have had previous portal vein operations or prior thrombosis of the portal system. Factors that decrease antegrade portal flow also predispose to portal vein thrombosis. Patients with chronic portal hypertension often spontaneously develop large retroperitoneal collaterals from the portal venous system to the renal vein and inferior vena cava. A previous surgically created splenorenal shunt should be disconnected at the time of transplantation because it usually is associated with reduced flow through the portal vein. This can be accomplished easily during a liver transplant by dissecting down the vena cava and ligating the left renal vein at its origin. This maneuver does not compromise the function of the left kidney. This maneuver can also be useful to improve portal flow if preoperative imaging discloses large spontaneous portal-systemic shunts to the left renal vein.

Portal vein thrombosis should be suspected when the recipient develops symptoms of portal hypertension or ascites that is unusually difficult to control. Doppler ultrasound examination is usually the first diagnostic tool, but magnetic resonance imaging is also an option, as are standard mesenteric arteriography with portal phase views and direct percutaneous transhepatic portography. Transhepatic portography is particularly useful if a stenosis, rather than thrombosis, is identified because it is possible to both measure the pressure gradient across a stenotic area and treat a stenotic area with angioplasty and/or stent placement.

When portal vein thrombosis is identified in the immediate postoperative period, reexploration and attempted thrombectomy are usually indicated. Thrombectomy is more likely to be successful if a technical flaw in the anastomosis is present and can be corrected. When performing thrombectomy, it is advisable to avoid using balloon embolectomy catheters to remove clot from the mesenteric venous system, because these veins are very fragile and rupture of mesenteric veins deep in the mesentery can be catastrophic.

Hepatic Vein or Inferior Vena Cava Stenosis

Thrombosis of the inferior vena cava is a rare complication after liver transplantation, but hepatic vein outflow obstruction occurs in 2% to 4% of patients. Restrictions of hepatic blood flow may result from kinking of the suprahepatic cava. This is particularly problematic when the donor is small relative to the recipient and when the suprahepatic anastomosis is left long. Hepatic outflow problems can present with ascites and renal dysfunction. Presentation may be early in the first week after transplantation or months later. The diagnosis may be suspected on the basis of Doppler ultrasonography, but definitive diagnosis usually requires inferior cavography with measurement of pressure gradients. The incidence of caval complications utilizing the piggyback technique appears to be higher than the incidence with the bicaval technique, at approximately 4%.[66] Outflow stenosis appears to be more common if the combined orifice of two, rather than three, hepatic veins is used for the anastomotic site on the recipient when the piggyback technique is used. In many cases, hepatic vein or suprahepatic caval stenosis can be successfully treated noninvasively with the use of balloon angioplasty and stenting.[67,68]

Biliary Leak or Stricture

Biliary leak or obstruction is a common surgical complication encountered after hepatic transplantation with an incidence of approximately 10% to 30%.[53,69] Most biliary complications probably relate to ischemia of the donor biliary tree (Fig. 36.18). The transected donor bile duct is totally dependent on arterial flow from the liver graft. Therefore, when a biliary leak is identified, it is appropriate to interrogate the hepatic vasculature to rule out the presence of hepatic artery stenosis or thrombosis.

Although anastomotic biliary complications can result in mortality from sepsis, they most commonly lead to short-term morbidity. The initial management of biliary complications can

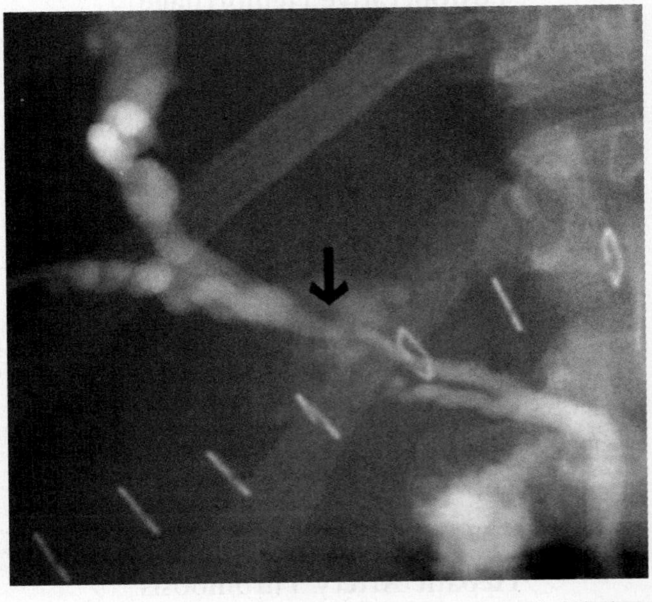

FIGURE 36.18. Bile leak (*arrow*) from the choledochocholedochostomy after hepatic transplantation.

generally be nonoperative. In most cases, the problem can be both diagnosed and treated by endoscopic retrograde cholangiopancreatography (ERCP). If the biliary reconstruction was made using a Roux-en-Y hepaticojejunostomy, or if ERCP is unsuccessful, biliary leaks must be diagnosed and treated by interventional radiology using percutaneous transhepatic cholangiography and percutaneous placement of a biliary stent. In addition to stenting the anastomosis, it may be necessary to place a percutaneous drain if there is a significant extrahepatic collection of bile. In cases where initial studies show a large defect and in cases where the leak is not controlled through percutaneous measures, operative repair using a Roux-en-Y hepaticojejunostomy may be indicated.

Biliary obstruction resulting from anastomotic strictures can also generally be managed nonoperatively by using percutaneous cholangioplasty or ERCP. When anastomotic strictures persist beyond two attempts at balloon dilatation and stent replacement, operative repair may be an option as long as the entire biliary stricture is extrahepatic and there are no intrahepatic strictures.

While anastomotic strictures are less likely to cause long-term morbidity, intrahepatic biliary strictures, also referred to as intrahepatic cholangiopathy, can be progressive and lead to allograft dysfunction, cholangitis, and, ultimately, either death or retransplantation. Intrahepatic cholangiopathy is largely related to ischemic injuries, occurs in the setting of hepatic artery thrombosis, and occurs in approximately 20% of donation following cardiac death (DCD) liver recipients.

Intra-abdominal Sepsis

Intra-abdominal sepsis presents as diffuse peritonitis or localized abscess and occurs in about 5% of patients who undergo liver transplantation. The most common cause of peritonitis is leakage of the biliary anastomosis. Abscesses may also develop spontaneously in the right upper quadrant or elsewhere in the abdomen. Most isolated infected fluid collections can be managed by percutaneous placement of drains guided by ultrasound or computed tomography (CT) scanning, along with broad-spectrum intravenous antibiotics. Generalized infected ascitic fluid is managed with paracentesis and antibiotics. Surgical drainage may be necessary if leakage of enteric contents is suspected based on the finding of extravasated oral contrast in the peritoneal cavity on CT scan, or if the patient does not respond to percutaneous drainage.

Neurologic Complications

A number of preoperative and postoperative factors predispose to impaired consciousness and seizure activity after transplantation. Patients who have significant preoperative encephalopathy are more likely to suffer from postoperative neurologic symptoms. In the extreme, patients who are in hepatic coma from fulminant liver failure can sometimes take weeks to regain complete consciousness. Patients undergoing liver transplants are also at risk for watershed infarcts if significant intraoperative hypotension occurs. The effects of transient cerebral ischemia are worsened by the large amount of intravenous fluids that are often necessary during and after transplantation, which can exacerbate cerebral edema. Air embolism is also a risk if venous bleeding occurs from the cava or hepatic veins at a time when the patient is relatively hypovolemic. If the patient has a patent foramen ovale, air embolism can result in cerebral ischemia if large bubbles lodge in the cerebral circulation. If the patient fails to awaken promptly after transplantation, and particularly if the transplant is functioning well, an urgent CT scan of the head should be obtained to rule out intracranial hemorrhage and to assess the degree of cerebral edema.

Seizures are reasonably common after transplantation. The calcineurin inhibitors cyclosporine and tacrolimus both lower seizure threshold and are associated with seizures following liver transplantation. Patients with a history of seizures are particularly predisposed to postoperative seizure activity. Seizures are treated with benzodiazepines acutely. The use of many long-term anticonvulsants alter the metabolism of calcineurin inhibitors. Therefore, levetiracetam is often used. To prevent recurrence of seizure activity, it is usually necessary to decrease the dosage of calcineurin inhibitor to a lower target blood level. Frequently it is also necessary to change to a different calcineurin inhibitor altogether, or even to change the patient's maintenance immunosuppression to a regimen that does not include a calcineurin inhibitor.

REJECTION AND IMMUNOSUPPRESSION

5 For reasons that are only partly understood, liver transplant recipients require less immune suppression than patients with other types of allografts, such as heart, lung, and kidney recipients. This is somewhat surprising given that the mass of the liver is so great compared with the mass of the other organs. With current immunosuppressive therapy, graft loss from rejection is rare.

Antibody-mediated Rejection

The liver is relatively resistant to injury from recipient antibodies, regardless of whether they are present at the time of transplant or develop later. This is very different compared with renal and cardiac recipients who experience rapid graft destruction, termed *hyperacute rejection*, if performed in a patient who has complement fixing antibodies directed against the donor organ in significant concentrations at the time of transplantation. Hepatic graft injury from preexisting antibodies directed at donor ABO determinants does occur, but in a much less pronounced fashion than in the context of renal transplantation. The overall results of ABO-incompatible liver transplants are somewhat inferior to those of ABO-compatible transplantations, but only by about a 10% to 20% decrease in 1-year graft survival rates compared to ABO-compatible grafts. Some of this decrease in graft survival rate may be due to the fact that ABO-incompatible transplants are usually performed only in dire circumstances where the patient is so ill that he or she may not survive the wait for a compatible organ. Because preformed antibodies do not seem to be clinically important, most transplantation programs do not perform prospective cross matches between recipient serum and donor cells before transplantation, and determination of recipient and donor HLA type is no longer considered mandatory.

Why the liver is less susceptible to antibody-mediated destruction than the kidney is not clearly understood. One factor may be the vastly different microcirculation that the liver has compared with the kidney, with a preponderance of sinusoidal channels and a smaller capillary network. It is probable that antibody-mediated injury affects blood flow through the delicate capillary network of the kidney more than it does liver sinusoids. In addition, each hepatocyte is exposed to two sinusoidal channels, presumably permitting survival if only one sinusoid is occluded. Finally, differences in HLA antigen expression are known to exist in the two organs, with the kidney the more antigenic of the two.

Cell-mediated Rejection

6 Typical acute rejection in liver transplant recipients is usually cell mediated and occurs frequently but is effectively blunted

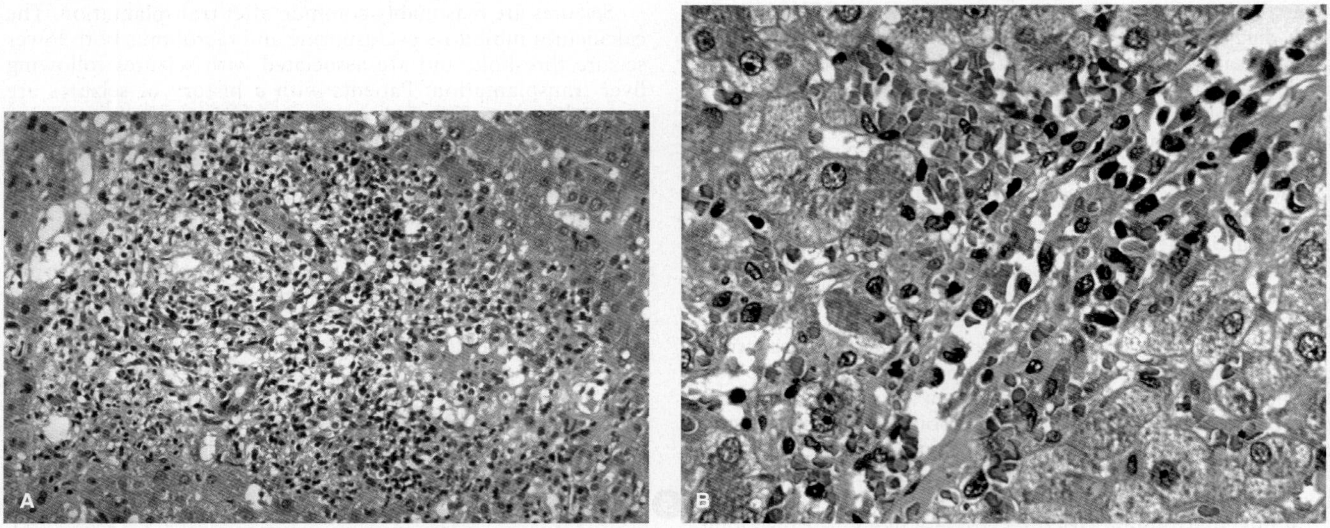

FIGURE 36.19. Acute rejection of a liver transplant. **A:** A portal tract is expanded by a polymorphous inflammatory infiltrate consisting of large and small lymphocytes, plasma cells, macrophages, and neutrophils. The bile ducts (*arrows*) are damaged and inflamed. **B:** A central vein from the same biopsy exhibits endothelialitis, characterized by swollen endothelial cells and infiltrating lymphocytes. (Reproduced with permission from Thung SN, Gerber MA. Histopathology of liver transplantation. In: Fabry TL, Klion FM, eds. *Guide to Liver Transplantation.* New York: Igaku-Shoin Medical Publishers; 1988.)

by antirejection therapy. Acute rejection occurs most commonly in the first 2 postoperative months. In modern practice, cell-mediated rejection is a less common cause of graft loss than is primary nonfunction or hepatic artery thrombosis. Still, the effectiveness of antirejection treatment assumes a relatively early diagnosis and treatment of acute rejection, which is in turn the result of careful monitoring by the transplantation physician and compliance by the patient with frequent laboratory testing. Treatment of acute rejection with enhanced immunosuppressive therapy is highly effective, and an episode of rejection does not affect long-term graft survival. This is very different from renal transplantation, where an episode of rejection decreases long-term graft survival markedly.

The diagnosis of cell-mediated rejection is made primarily on a histologic basis. Clinical features can include low-grade fever and malaise, but frequently the patient is completely asymptomatic. Laboratory evaluation of peripheral blood may demonstrate leukocytosis and occasionally eosinophilia. Biochemical changes associated with rejection include elevated and rising levels of serum transaminases and alkaline phosphatase. A prolonged serum prothrombin time and an abnormal serum bilirubin also suggest the possibility of rejection, but frequently these parameters are normal if rejection is detected early. Any of these findings should prompt a biopsy.

The diagnosis of cell-mediated rejection rests on the finding of a triad of portal lymphocytosis, endotheliitis (subendothelial deposits of mononuclear cells), and bile duct infiltration and damage (Figs. 36.19 and 36.20). Various classification schemes have been devised to grade the severity of the rejection process based on the degree of cellular involvement or injury in these areas. Cell characterization studies have documented that the cells in the portal triads are primarily T cells, with fewer macrophages and neutrophils. Bile duct epithelial cells appear to be a prime target of immune attack, and they are known to express large amounts of class II HLA antigen.

If the recipient has hepatitis C, it is critical that recurrent hepatitis C is differentiated from acute rejection. At times the difference can be subtle, and a pathologist with experience in the interpretation of allograft biopsies is extremely valuable. Enhanced immunosuppression is associated with accelerated rates of hepatitis C viral replication; it is, therefore, important that immunosuppression is kept to a minimum for these patients.

Chronic Rejection

7 Chronic rejection is characterized by relentless immune attack on small bile ducts. Clinically, the pattern is one of gradual elevation of alkaline phosphatase and bilirubin, in the absence of obstruction of the large bile ducts. Histologically, small bile ducts are obliterated or completely absent, with a less pronounced cellular infiltrate than is seen with acute rejection. This finding has been termed *vanishing bile duct syndrome* when bile ducts are absent in 15 of 20 portal triads examined.[70] The loss of small bile ducts is partly the result of lymphocyte-directed attack on biliary epithelium. Relative to other cells in the liver, biliary epithelium tends to express more class I antigen. Thus, biliary epithelial cells are vulnerable targets for host attack because of their antigenicity. Loss of bile ducts may also occur indirectly as the result of ischemia

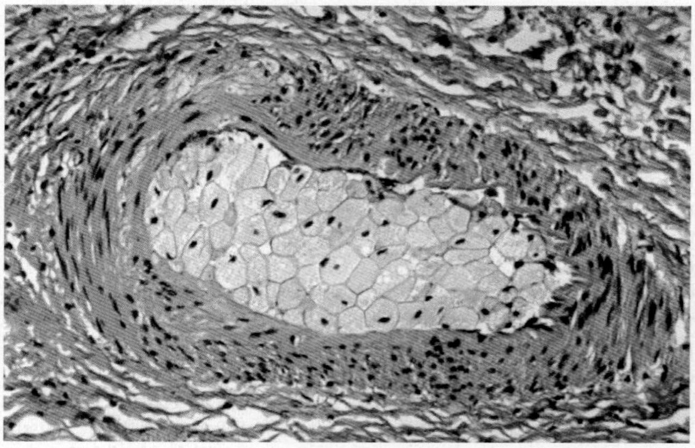

FIGURE 36.20. Arterial lesion of chronic hepatic rejection. Subintimal foam cells, intimal sclerosis, and myointimal hyperplasia obliterate the arterial lumen. (Reproduced with permission from Rubin E, Farber JL. *Pathology*, 3rd ed. Philadelphia, PA: Lippincott Williams & Wilkins; 1999.)

secondary to immune-mediated obliteration of small to medium arteries. As in the case of renal transplantations, there is no effective treatment for chronic rejection except retransplantation.

Immunosuppression Induction and Maintenance

Multiple immunosuppressive protocols achieve acceptable suppression of allograft rejection for liver transplant recipients. Induction with antithymocyte globulin is no longer considered to be mandatory but is used at some centers. Similarly, prednisone therapy, once considered a mainstay of a successful immunosuppressive protocol, is no longer considered absolutely necessary and when used is often tapered rapidly. Treatment with a calcineurin inhibitor, either cyclosporine or tacrolimus, is still considered to be imperative for most liver transplant recipients. These agents are associated with significant long-term morbidity, particularly the development of chronic renal failure. Dosages of these agents have gradually been reduced both to prevent renal insufficiency and to avoid the rapid and aggressive recurrence of hepatitis C infection. Induction antibody therapy with either polyclonal antilymphocyte preparations or with inhibitors of the receptor for interleukin 2 is still used commonly in the perioperative setting to avoid the nephrotoxicity associated with the immediate use of calcineurin inhibitors.

Because immunosuppression predisposes to infection, prophylactic anti-infective drugs are usually administered. Trimethoprim-sulfamethoxazole, dapsone, or pentamidine is recommended to prevent *Pneumocystis carinii* infection. Oral Mycostatin or fluconazole therapy is used to prevent fungal infections, particularly esophageal *Candida albicans*. Either ganciclovir or valganciclovir is prescribed for patients who are at risk for CMV infection, which includes any patient exposed to CMV in the past and any patient transplanted with organs from a donor who has been exposed to CMV. Patients who are CMV negative who receive CMV-negative organs are not at risk for CMV infection but should still receive prophylaxis against disseminated herpes simplex infections with acyclovir therapy. The duration of prophylactic anti-infective therapy has not been rigorously defined by evidence-based trials and is therefore dependent on each center's experience with the prevalence of these infections in its patient population.

Treatment of Acute Rejection

Despite the overall effectiveness of the regimen described, acute rejection does occur and must be treated promptly. Several options are available for treatment of acute rejection, depending on the clinical circumstances. Traditionally, high doses of methylprednisolone are administered (usually 500 mg to 1 g) intravenously on a daily basis for 3 days. This treatment is effective in reversing most acute rejection episodes. Alternatively, increased doses of a calcineurin inhibitor or the addition of an antimetabolite drug, such as mycophenolate mofetil, will also reverse most episodes of rejection, particularly if the rejection is mild. Rejection that is resistant to these maneuvers is treated with antilymphocyte therapy, either a monoclonal antibody directed at the T3 determinant common to all mature T cells (Orthoclone, OKT3) or polyclonal antilymphocyte treatments such as Atgam or thymoglobulin. These treatments are typically administered daily for 5 to 10 days. These agents are highly effective, and it is unusual to lose an allograft secondary to acute rejection. However, these treatments are associated with profound and long-lasting immunosuppression, and it is usually advisable to restart prophylactic anti-infective therapies when they are initiated.

RESULTS

8 The patient survival rate following liver transplantation in the United States at 1 year is more than 85% for adults and nearly 90% for children. Patients who survive the first year following a liver transplantation experience approximately a 3% annual mortality rate thereafter, so 3-year survival rates for adults and children are currently 78% and 83%, respectively.

The most important predictors of survival following liver transplantation are whether the patient has previously undergone transplantation and whether the patient was in the intensive care unit at the time of transplantation. Although not as important as the condition of the patient at transplantation, the cause of liver failure is also an important determinant of success. Five-year survival varies from approximately 60% for patients transplanted for malignancy to 70% for patients transplanted for viral and alcoholic cirrhosis. The best 5-year survival rates of around 80% are seen with patients transplanted for metabolic liver disease, biliary atresia, and cholestatic liver diseases (primary biliary cirrhosis and primary sclerosing cholangitis).[37] The volume of liver transplants performed at a given transplant center is also associated with patient survival, with higher-volume programs exhibiting higher adjusted overall patient survival rates.[71]

References

1. Starzl TE, Groth CG, Brettschneider L, et al. Orthotopic homotransplantation of the human liver. *Ann Surg* 1968;168(3):392–415.
2. Calne RY, Rolles K, White DJ, et al. Cyclosporin a initially as the only immunosuppressant in 34 recipients of cadaveric organs: 32 kidneys, 2 pancreases, and 2 livers. *Lancet* 1979;2(8151):1033–1036.
3. Roberts MS, Angus DC, Bryce CL, et al. Survival after liver transplantation in the United States: a disease-specific analysis of the UNOS database. *Liver Transpl* 2004;10(7):886–897.
4. Freeman RB Jr, Steffick DE, Guidinger MK, et al. Liver and intestine transplantation in the United States, 1997–2006. *Am J Transplant* 2008;8(4 Pt 2): 958–976.
5. O'Leary JG, Lepe R, Davis GL. Indications for liver transplantation. *Gastroenterology* 2008;134(6):1764–1776.
6. Punch JD, Hayes DH, LaPorte FB, et al. Organ donation and utilization in the United States, 1996–2005. *Am J Transplant* 2007;7(5 Pt 2): 1327–1338.
7. Medicare and Medicaid programs; conditions for coverage for organ procurement organizations (OPOs). Final rule. *Fed Regist* 2006;71(104): 30981–31054.
8. Olthoff KM, Merion RM, Ghobrial RM, et al. Outcomes of 385 adult-to-adult living donor liver transplant recipients: a report from the A2ALL Consortium. *Ann Surg* 2005;242(3):314–323, discussion 323–325.
9. Trotter JF, Wachs M, Everson GT, et al. Adult-to-adult transplantation of the right hepatic lobe from a living donor. *N Engl J Med* 2002;346(14): 1074–1082.
10. Kamath PS, Wiesner RH, Malinchoc M, et al. A model to predict survival in patients with end-stage liver disease. *Hepatology* 2001;33(2): 464–470.
11. Merion RM, Schaubel DE, Dykstra DM, et al. The survival benefit of liver transplantation. *Am J Transplant* 2005;5(2):307–313.
12. Freeman RB, Gish RG, Harper A, et al. Model for end-stage liver disease (MELD) exception guidelines: results and recommendations from the MELD exception study group and conference (MESSAGE) for the approval of patients who need liver transplantation with diseases not considered by the standard MELD formula. *Liver Transpl* 2006;12: S128–S136.
13. Freeman RB, Wiesner RH, Edwards E, et al. Results of the first year of the new liver allocation plan. *Liver Transpl* 2004;10(1):7–15.
14. Sass DA, Shakil AO. Fulminant hepatic failure. *Liver Transpl* 2005;11(6): 594–605.
15. Stieber AC, Zetti G, Todo S, et al. The spectrum of portal vein thrombosis in liver transplantation. *Ann Surg* 1991;213(3):199–206.
16. Roland ME, Barin B, Carlson L, et al. HIV-infected liver and kidney transplant recipients: 1- and 3-year outcomes. *Am J Transplant* 2008;8(2): 355–365.
17. Mindikoglu AL, Regev A, Magder LS. Impact of human immunodeficiency virus on survival after liver transplantation: analysis of United Network for Organ Sharing database. *Transplantation* 2008;85(3):359–368.
18. Wong SN, Chu CJ, Wai CT, et al. Low risk of hepatitis B virus recurrence after withdrawal of long-term hepatitis B immunoglobulin in patients receiving maintenance nucleos(t)ide analogue therapy. *Liver Transpl* 2007; 13(3):374–381.

19. Chu CJ, Fontana RJ, Moore C, et al. Outcome of liver transplantation for hepatitis B: report of a single center's experience. *Liver Transpl* 2001;7(8): 724–731.
20. Gaglio P, Singh S, Degertekin B, et al. Impact of the hepatitis B virus genotype on pre- and post-liver transplantation outcomes. *Liver Transpl* 2008; 14(10):1420–1427.
21. Bruno S, Stroffolini T, Colombo M, et al. Sustained virological response to interferon-alpha is associated with improved outcome in HCV-related cirrhosis: a retrospective study. *Hepatology* 2007;45(3):579–587.
22. Manns MP, McHutchison JG, Gordon SC, et al. Peginterferon alfa-2b plus ribavirin compared with interferon alfa-2b plus ribavirin for initial treatment of chronic hepatitis C: a randomised trial. *Lancet* 2001;358(9286): 958–965.
23. Everson GT, Trotter J, Forman L, et al. Treatment of advanced hepatitis C with a low accelerating dosage regimen of antiviral therapy. *Hepatology* 2005;42(2):255–262.
24. Terrault NA, Berenguer M. Treating hepatitis C infection in liver transplant recipients. *Liver Transpl* 2006;12(8):1192–1204.
25. Lake JR, Shorr JS, Steffen BJ, et al. Differential effects of donor age in liver transplant recipients infected with hepatitis B, hepatitis C and without viral hepatitis. *Am J Transplant* 2005;5(3):549–557.
26. Berenguer M, Palau A, Aguilera V, et al. Clinical benefits of antiviral therapy in patients with recurrent hepatitis C following liver transplantation. *Am J Transplant* 2008;8(3):679–687.
27. Mazzaferro V, Regalia E, Doci R, et al. Liver transplantation for the treatment of small hepatocellular carcinomas in patients with cirrhosis. *N Engl J Med* 1996;334(11):693–699.
28. Onaca N, Davis GL, Goldstein RM, et al. Expanded criteria for liver transplantation in patients with hepatocellular carcinoma: a report from the International Registry of Hepatic Tumors in Liver Transplantation. *Liver Transpl* 2007;13(3):391–399.
29. Schwartz M. Liver transplantation for hepatocellular carcinoma. *Gastroenterology* 2004;127(5)(suppl 1):S268–S276.
30. Finegold MJ, Egler RA, Goss JA, et al. Liver tumors: pediatric population. *Liver Transpl* 2008;14(11):1545–1556.
31. Mantel HT, Rosen CB, Heimbach JK, et al. Vascular complications after orthotopic liver transplantation after neoadjuvant therapy for hilar cholangiocarcinoma. *Liver Transpl* 2007;13(10):1372–1381.
32. Frilling A, Malago M, Weber F, et al. Liver transplantation for patients with metastatic endocrine tumors: single-center experience with 15 patients. *Liver Transpl* 2006;12(7):1089–1096.
33. Burke A, Lucey MR. Non-alcoholic fatty liver disease, non-alcoholic steatohepatitis and orthotopic liver transplantation. *Am J Transplant* 2004;4(5):686–693.
34. Mas A, Rodes J. Fulminant hepatic failure. *Lancet* 1997;349(9058): 1081–1085.
35. O'Grady JG, Alexander GJ, Hayllar KM, et al. Early indicators of prognosis in fulminant hepatic failure. *Gastroenterology* 1989;97(2): 439–445.
36. Dhiman RK, Jain S, Maheshwari U, et al. Early indicators of prognosis in fulminant hepatic failure: an assessment of the Model for End-Stage Liver Disease (MELD) and King's College Hospital criteria. *Liver Transpl* 2007; 13(6):814–821.
37. Yantorno SE, Kremers WK, Ruf AE, et al. MELD is superior to King's college and Clichy's criteria to assess prognosis in fulminant hepatic failure. *Liver Transpl* 2007;13(6):822–828.
38. Barshes NR, Lee TC, Balkrishnan R, et al. Orthotopic liver transplantation for biliary atresia: the U.S. experience. *Liver Transpl* 2005;11(10): 1193–1200.
39. Sylvestre PB, Batts KP, Burgart LJ, et al. Recurrence of primary biliary cirrhosis after liver transplantation: histologic estimate of incidence and natural history. *Liver Transpl* 2003;9(10):1086–1093.
40. Maheshwari A, Yoo HY, Thuluvath PJ. Long-term outcome of liver transplantation in patients with PSC: a comparative analysis with PBC. *Am J Gastroenterol* 2004;99(3):538–542.
41. Kayler LK, Rasmussen CS, Dykstra DM, et al. Liver transplantation in children with metabolic disorders in the United States. *Am J Transplant* 2003;3(3):334–339.
42. Arguedas MR, Abrams GA, Krowka MJ, et al. Prospective evaluation of outcomes and predictors of mortality in patients with hepatopulmonary syndrome undergoing liver transplantation. *Hepatology* 2003;37(1): 192–197.
43. Ashfaq M, Chinnakotla S, Rogers L, et al. The impact of treatment of portopulmonary hypertension on survival following liver transplantation. *Am J Transplant* 2007;7(5):1258–1264.
44. Swanson KL, Wiesner RH, Nyberg SL, et al. Survival in portopulmonary hypertension: Mayo Clinic experience categorized by treatment subgroups. *Am J Transplant* 2008;8(11):2445–2453.
45. Pomfret EA, Fryer JP, Sima CS, et al. Liver and intestine transplantation in the United States, 1996–2005. *Am J Transplant* 2007;7(5 Pt 2): 1376–1389.
46. Eason JD, Gonwa TA, Davis CL, et al. Proceedings of consensus conference on simultaneous liver kidney transplantation (SLK). *Am J Transplant* 2008;8(11):2243–2251.
47. Lodge JP, Jonas S, Jones RM, et al. Efficacy and safety of repeated perioperative doses of recombinant factor VIIa in liver transplantation. *Liver Transpl* 2005;11(8):973–979.
48. Planinsic RM, van der Meer J, Testa G, et al. Safety and efficacy of a single bolus administration of recombinant factor VIIa in liver transplantation due to chronic liver disease. *Liver Transpl* 2005;11(8):895–900.
49. Dumortier J, Czyglik O, Poncet G, et al. Eversion thrombectomy for portal vein thrombosis during liver transplantation. *Am J Transplant* 2002; 2(10):934–938.
50. Tzakis AG, Kirkegaard P, Pinna AD, et al. Liver transplantation with cavoportal hemitransposition in the presence of diffuse portal vein thrombosis. *Transplantation* 1998;65(5):619–624.
51. Charco R, Margarit C, Lopez-Talavera JC, et al. Outcome and hepatic hemodynamics in liver transplant patients with portal vein arterialization. *Am J Transplant* 2001;1(2):146–151.
52. Lerut J, Ciccarelli O, Roggen F, et al. Cavocaval adult liver transplantation and retransplantation without venovenous bypass and without portocaval shunting: a prospective feasibility study in adult liver transplantation. *Transplantation* 2003;75(10):1740–1745.
53. Welling TH, Heidt DG, Englesbe MJ, et al. Biliary complications following liver transplantation in the model for end-stage liver disease era: effect of donor, recipient, and technical factors. *Liver Transpl* 2008;14(1):73–80.
54. Otte JB, de Ville de Goyet J, Alberti D, et al. The concept and technique of the split liver in clinical transplantation. *Surgery* 1990;107(6):605–612.
55. Brolsch CE, Stevens LH, Whitington PF. The use of reduced-size liver transplants in children, including split livers and living related liver transplants. *Eur J Pediatr Surg* 1991;1(3):166–171.
56. Emond JC, Whitington PF, Thistlethwaite JR, et al. Transplantation of two patients with one liver. Analysis of a preliminary experience with 'split-liver' grafting. *Ann Surg* 1990;212(1):14–22.
57. Humar A, Khwaja K, Sielaff TD, et al. Technique of split-liver transplant for two adult recipients. *Liver Transpl* 2002;8(8):725–729.
58. Marcos A, Fisher RA, Ham JM, et al. Right lobe living donor liver transplantation. *Transplantation* 1999;68(6):798–803.
59. Miller C, Florman S, Kim-Schluger L, et al. Fulminant and fatal gas gangrene of the stomach in a healthy live liver donor. *Liver Transpl* 2004; 10(10):1315–1319.
60. Strasberg SM, Howard TK, Molmenti EP, et al. Selecting the donor liver: risk factors for poor function after orthotopic liver transplantation. *Hepatology* 1994;20(4 Pt 1):829–838.
61. Oh CK, Sawyer RG, Pelletier SJ, et al. Independent predictors for primary non-function after liver transplantation. *Yonsei Med J* 2004;45(6): 1155–1161.
62. Pungpapong S, Manzarbeitia C, Ortiz J, et al. Cigarette smoking is associated with an increased incidence of vascular complications after liver transplantation. *Liver Transpl* 2002;8(7):582–587.
63. Bhattacharjya S, Gunson BK, Mirza DF, et al. Delayed hepatic artery thrombosis in adult orthotopic liver transplantation—a 12-year experience. *Transplantation* 2001;71(11):1592–1596.
64. Furuta S, Ikegami T, Nakazawa Y, et al. Hepatic artery reconstruction in living donor liver transplantation from the microsurgeon's point of view. *Liver Transpl Surg* 1997;3(4):388–393.
65. Stahl RL, Duncan A, Hooks MA, et al. A hypercoagulable state follows orthotopic liver transplantation. *Hepatology* 1990;12(3 Pt 1):553–558.
66. Parrilla P, Sanchez-Bueno F, Figueras J, et al. Analysis of the complications of the piggy-back technique in 1,112 liver transplants. *Transplantation* 1999;67(9):1214–1217.
67. Borsa JJ, Daly CP, Fontaine AB, et al. Treatment of inferior vena cava anastomotic stenoses with the Wallstent endoprosthesis after orthotopic liver transplantation. *J Vasc Interv Radiol* 1999;10(1):17–22.
68. Frazer CK, Gupta A. Stenosis of the hepatic vein anastomosis after liver transplantation: treatment with a heparin-coated metal stent. *Australas Radiol* 2002;46(4):422–425.
69. Feller RB, Waugh RC, Selby WS, et al. Biliary strictures after liver transplantation: clinical picture, correlates and outcomes. *J Gastroenterol Hepatol* 1996;11(1):21–25.
70. Wiesner RH, Batts KP, Krom RA. Evolving concepts in the diagnosis, pathogenesis, and treatment of chronic hepatic allograft rejection. *Liver Transpl Surg* 1999;5(5):388–400.
71. Axelrod DA, Guidinger MK, McCullough KP, et al. Association of center volume with outcome after liver and kidney transplantation. *Am J Transplant* 2004;4(6):920–927.

CHAPTER 37 ■ CARDIAC TRANSPLANTATION

RICHARD N. PIERSON III

KEY POINTS

1. Over the past 50 years, heart transplantation has evolved from public spectacle to accepted therapeutic modality based on improved tools to diagnose rejection and infection and an expanded armamentarium of treatment options.
2. Heart transplantation is offered to patients for whom no other reasonable treatment options exist and who are at higher risk of death without transplant than with it, while excluding those whose comorbid conditions are likely to significantly limit length or quality of life.
3. The mortality rate for patients awaiting transplant has improved significantly over the past decade due to improvements in (a) patient selection, (b) medical therapy of patients awaiting transplantation, (c) mechanical support as a bridge to transplant, and (d) donor management and allocation algorithms.
4. Of the four techniques for performing heart transplantation, orthotopic transplant using bicaval right atrial connections has emerged as the most popular.
5. A "triple-drug" regimen including a calcineurin inhibitor, an antimitotic agent, and a steroid, with or without antilymphocyte "induction," is employed to prevent graft injury due to acute rejection.
6. Prophylaxis against opportunistic infections includes agents targeted at common bacterial, viral, and protozoal pathogens.
7. Although the number of heart transplants performed worldwide has declined due to a donor organ shortage, operative survival has improved over the past 20 years, and both patient and graft 1-year survival rates exceed 87% for adults.
8. Rejection and infection together account for most of the mortality during the first year, whereas long-term survival is limited by cardiac allograft vasculopathy (a manifestation of chronic rejection) and malignancy.
9. Current initiatives in the field include development of improved immunosuppression (perhaps leading to graft "tolerance") and alternatives to heart allotransplantation, such as "destination" mechanical support or heart xenografts from genetically modified pigs.

1 Since 1964, cardiac transplantation has evolved from a sensational, perilous experiment to become conventional therapy for end-stage heart disease, the paradigm of successful but expensive "high-tech" medicine. This remarkable transformation stemmed from fundamental surgical innovations supported by incremental improvements in the diagnosis and management of common problems. Current challenges revolve around donor supply and allocation, improving long-term outcomes, developing alternative therapies, and related ethical issues.

HISTORICAL PERSPECTIVE

Based on significant contributions by many surgical pioneers,[1–8] the first clinical heart transplant was performed in 1964 by Hardy, who attempted to salvage a man dying from cardiogenic shock by replacing his heart with one from a chimpanzee.[9] Then, before the concept of brain death achieved wide social or legal acceptance, in 1967 Christian Barnard et al. captured the imagination of the world with the first operative survival, using the heart of a resuscitated cadaveric donor.[10] This case, and many others that were performed shortly thereafter, demonstrated not only the physiologic capacity of the transplanted human heart allograft to support the recipient's circulation but also the difficulty of managing subsequent immunologic and infectious complications. After a worldwide flurry of activity, generally dismal outcomes at many prominent cardiac surgery centers made clear the need for more thoughtful approaches to what was clearly a difficult constellation of problems beyond effective circulatory support.

A few pioneering programs persisted in cautious clinical application supported by parallel laboratory investigation. Recognizing the need for a more sensitive and specific diagnostic technique to diagnose rejection, Phillip Caves, working with Shumway et al. at Stanford, developed the technique of transvenous endomyocardial biopsy.[11] Frequent, representative surveillance sampling of the graft allowed early detection of pathogenic host immune responses. Perivascular lymphocytic infiltrates were found to accurately diagnose acute cellular rejection in its presymptomatic phase; when detected early, rejection usually responded to enhanced immunosuppression. Equally important, when rejection was not seen, immunosuppression could be tapered to minimize drug toxicities and reduce the incidence of opportunistic infection. Coupled with important advances in the diagnosis, prevention, and treatment of infectious pathogens in immunosuppressed patients and in selection and management of patients with end-stage heart failure, patient survival at 1 year improved gradually, from about 20% in the 1960s to about 70% by 1980.[12]

However, even as recently as the early 1980s, when rejection persisted or recurred despite high-dose steroids, alternative treatments (total lymphoid irradiation, intramuscular antilymphocyte preparations, thoracic duct ligation, splenectomy) were often toxic or invasive and accompanied by a high incidence of major short- and long-term complications. In this context the discovery and clinical development of cyclosporin A[13,14] catalyzed the next major improvement in outcomes. Because the primary mechanism of action (inhibition of calcineurin-dependent cellular activation events) and toxicity profile were fundamentally different from those of azathioprine, an antimitotic agent, or anti-inflammatory steroids, combination "triple" therapy allowed each agent to be used more safely. Meanwhile, antithymocyte and antilymphocyte preparations were adapted for safe intravenous use, either as prophylactic induction therapy ("quadruple therapy") or as treatment for steroid-resistant rejection. Based primarily on these pharmacologic innovations in the regulation of the immune response, expected 1-year survival following heart transplant gradually rose from about 70% to almost 88% between 1980 and 2008 despite increasing reliance on older donors for older and sicker recipients.[15,16]

CANDIDATE EVALUATION

End-stage heart failure is the primary indication for heart transplantation in adults, with coronary artery occlusive disease and myopathy of various etiologies each accounting for about 45% of cases. Congenital heart disease is the primary indication for infants, whereas myopathy predominates in older children.

2 The heart transplant evaluation process seeks to identify patients for whom no other reasonable treatment options exist and who are at higher risk of death without transplant than with it, while excluding those whose comorbid conditions are likely to significantly limit length or quality of life. In 1993, a National Institutes of Health consensus conference developed recipient selection guidelines for cardiac transplantation, based on objective criteria known to predict poor outcome without transplantation[17]; these guidelines (Tables 37.1 through 37.3) continue to evolve in the context of improving heart failure therapy.[18–20] Among patients with heart failure symptoms, maximal oxygen consumption (MVO_2) is more sensitive and specific than ejection fraction in gauging prognosis, and blunted cardiac output response to exercise may further stratify patients into high- and low-risk groups.[18]

When no clear survival advantage is apparent for transplantation or an alternative management strategy, quality of life and other subjective factors are weighed. Contemporary studies defining relative risks, along with basic considerations in the medical management of end-stage heart failure, are well summarized in recent reviews.[19,20]

TABLE 37.2

SELECTION CRITERIA FOR STRATIFYING RISK AND SURVIVAL RESULTS

Survival benefit established
MVO_2 <10 mL/kg/min
Class IV CHF symptoms despite maximal medical therapy
Requiring mechanical circulatory support
Refractory angina without therapeutic alternative
Refractory ventricular arrhythmia without alternative
Survival benefit likely
MVO_2 10–14 with blunted CO response to exercise
Instability of fluid balance or renal function despite documented compliance
EF <20% with class III HF symptoms on maximal medical therapy
Survival benefit not established
MVO_2 10–14 with preserved CO response to exercise
MVO_2 >14, EF <20% without other indication
History of CHF or arrhythmia, controlled with medical therapy
Quality-of-life considerations may influence selection of recipients for whom survival benefit is not established.

CHF, congestive heart failure; CO, carbon monoxide; EF, ejection fraction; MVO_2, maximal oxygen consumption.

TABLE 37.1

INDICATIONS FOR HEART TRANSPLANT

General indications
End-stage heart disease without lower-risk alternative
Absence of any noncardiac condition likely to:
1) limit survival independent of cardiac function
2) preclude safe administration of adequate immunosuppression
3) predispose to life-threatening infection with immunosuppression
Specific indications
1) Heart failure of various etiologies
a) Myopathy: ischemic, idiopathic, viral, familial, restrictive
b) Valvular
c) Congenital
d) Failed transplant
Early: Primary nonfunction, acute rejection
Late: Cardiac allograft vasculopathy
2) Other indications
a) Angina not amenable to revascularization
b) Arrhythmia, failed conventional therapy
c) Hypertrophic cardiomyopathy
d) Restrictive cardiomyopathy
e) Primary cardiac tumor (completely resectable)

DONOR SELECTION AND MANAGEMENT

The ideal donor is a young, previously healthy individual without cardiac disease or hypertension, who is well matched in size to the intended recipient and whose hemodynamics have been carefully managed during the evolution of his or her lethal central nervous system (CNS) injury. Some programs have advocated use of older donors, donors who may transmit infection or malignancy to the recipient, and grafts with hypertensive myocardial hypertrophy for particular recipients.[21] Some aggressive programs have even proposed that hemodynamically significant coronary stenoses can be bypassed at the time of transplant.[22] These approaches to donor selection are associated with less favorable short- and long-term outcomes,[15,23,24] but the increased risk may be considered acceptable for patients in whom the short-term prognosis is poor without transplant.

Donor management requires skill and experience to successfully address the complex physiologic perturbations associated with brain death. Reflex hypertensive and hypotensive responses to intracranial pressure changes, fluid and electrolyte imbalances consequent to the diabetes insipidus from pituitary death, and additional stresses related to hemorrhage, trauma, and surgery often cause hemodynamic and metabolic instability, which may injure a previously healthy heart. The neurohumoral milieu of CNS catastrophe may also adversely affect other fundamental cell regulatory functions, such as those dependent on thyroid hormone. Despite controversy regarding the mechanisms involved, thyroid hormone is often administered to the donor as a continuous infusion, hoping to correct a "sick euthyroid" syndrome and optimize cardiac metabolism prior to explant. Although evidence to date is largely anecdotal, inotrope requirements can often be reduced after thyroid infusion is begun, and donor hemodynamic

TABLE 37.3

CONTRAINDICATIONS TO CARDIAC TRANSPLANTATION

Absolute contraindications
High pulmonary vascular resistance[a]
Transpulmonary gradient >15, fixed
Pulmonary vascular resistance index >5–6 Woods Units
Irreversible renal insufficiency (CrCl <40)[a]
Active infection (viral or bacterial)
Active peptic ulcer disease
Diabetes with end-organ damage, renal insufficiency, neuropathy, retinopathy
Symptomatic extracardiac vascular disease
CVOD with recent TIA, CVA
PVOD with claudication, rest pain, or tissue loss
Current malignancy or recent treatment (<2 y) for life-threatening malignancy
Disease of another organ system that would probably limit survival
Established cirrhosis, cardiac or other etiology
Symptomatic COPD; chronic bronchitis
High risk for inability to comply with complex medical regimen
Not firmly committed to transplantation
Inadequate cognitive capacity to comply with postop regimen, coupled with inadequate compensatory social support
Documented psychiatric instability
Recurrent drug or alcohol abuse
Demonstrated noncompliance with therapeutic recommendations
Relative contraindications
Age over 65
Established renal failure
Diabetes without end-organ disease
Asymptomatic or previously treated extracardiac vascular disease
COPD with FEV_1 or DLCO <60% predicted without referable symptoms
Remote malignancy, in remission (>4 y with no evidence of disease)
High pulmonary vascular resistance, reversible
Disease of another organ system that would limit quality of life
Difficulty complying with complex medical regimen

COPD, chronic obstructive pulmonary disease; CrCl, creatinine clearance; CVA, cardiovascular accident; CVOD, cerebrovascular obstructive disease; DLCO, carbon monoxide diffusing capacity; FEV_1, forced expiratory volume in 1 second; PVOD, pulmonary veno-occlusive disease; TIA, transient ischemic attack.
[a]On optimal medical therapy.

lability is less common, suggesting improved cardiac and vasoregulatory function.[25,26]

Cardiac echocardiography has become a standard component of donor assessment to measure ejection fraction and to exclude structural abnormalities or hypertrophy suggestive of hypertensive myopathy. Cardiac catheterization may be requested for donors over age 45, especially for those with a strong family history of coronary artery disease, for smokers, or when regional wall motion abnormalities are appreciated on echocardiography.

MATCHING DONOR TO RECIPIENT

Once a potential donor is identified, priority among blood type–compatible recipients is determined first by relative severity of illness ("status") and then by length of time on the waiting list among those at each status in the donor's geographic area. In the United States, this information is currently tracked and collated by a central, national registry operated by the United Network for Organ Sharing. The heart is first offered to the program whose candidate has priority on the list and whose registered height and weight range include the potential donor. Donor inotrope requirements and functional assessment, recipient pulmonary vascular resistance, possible infection transmission risks (known hepatitis or potential human immunodeficiency virus [HIV] exposure in the donor), and other logistical considerations (expected graft ischemic time) influence the recipient team's decision regarding acceptance of an organ for an individual patient. If the first program declines the offer for the first patient, the process is repeated for the patient next on the list until the heart is accepted.

Tissue typing, the time-consuming process by which donor and recipient are matched for shared transplant antigens, is not currently used for hearts. The probability is low of identifying a "close" match among the relatively small number of blood type–compatible potential recipients within the geographic radius (usually <1,500 miles) defined by a 4-hour projected ischemic time. In addition, the demonstrated benefit of partial human leukocyte antigen (HLA) matching is small relative to the added risk of prolonged graft ischemia, a risk augmented by increasing donor age.[16,27]

RECIPIENT MANAGEMENT BEFORE TRANSPLANT

3 The medical therapy of patients awaiting transplantation has improved significantly over the past decade, centered around aggressive afterload reduction and diuresis, anticoagulation, and beta blockade.[18–20] This trend, coupled with improved mechanical support and improved donor allocation algorithms (discussed later), has reduced the mortality rate for patients awaiting transplantation. As waiting lists have grown faster than the donor pool and average time waiting has similarly escalated, cardiac decompensation among patients on the waiting list is frequent. In most areas of the United States and Europe, the majority of hearts go to patients who are sick enough to require hospitalization for intensive diuresis and intravenous inotrope administration.[15,16]

When inotropic therapy proves inadequate, as gauged by progressive deterioration in renal and other end-organ function, temporary intra-aortic balloon pump counterpulsation and mechanical ventilation can stabilize some patients. These interventions are associated with important risks; the relative risk of death is increased threefold in patients who are ventilator dependent at the time of transplant.[15,16]

In contrast, mechanical circulatory support using ventricular assist devices has emerged as an effective bridging strategy. Although some bridged patients incur serious complications (stroke, renal or hepatic failure, systemic infection) that preclude transplantation, about three quarters are successfully transplanted, with excellent outcomes relative to patients not requiring this intervention.[16] Patients with biventricular failure can be supported with either implanted or paracorporeal pulsatile left ventricular support, with or without addition of temporary right heart support. Various total artificial heart devices can be implanted in place of the native heart and have been applied successfully in small numbers.[28] This approach is most likely to find a niche as an alternative to heart transplantation in patients not supportable with a left ventricular assist device, such as those with fixed pulmonary hypertension. Intravascular axial flow devices and other nonpulsatile assist systems have shown promise in clinical trials.[29,30]

HEART PROCUREMENT

Cardiac allograft protection depends primarily on hypothermia, which reduces myocardial energy requirements while the heart graft has no nutritive coronary blood flow. Other important principles include avoidance of distention and warm ischemia in both the donor and the recipient and induction of diastolic (flaccid) cardiac arrest. These goals are accomplished by interrupting systemic venous return for decompression, placing a clamp across the distal ascending aorta, and infusing a hyperkalemic preservation solution proximal to the clamp, and thus selectively into the coronary arteries. Both the inferior vena cava and left atrium are incised ("vented") to prevent distention of either ventricle. Some preservation solutions incorporating free radical scavenging molecules or other cytoprotective agents are associated with improved early graft function.[31,32]

Every effort is made to limit the ischemic interval, the time between initial interruption of coronary flow by aortic cross-clamping in the donor and removal of the cross-clamp in the recipient, to less than 4 hours. Although laboratory studies and isolated clinical reports suggest that good results may be expected with storage times of 8 hours or more using various preservation solutions, increased ischemic time remains a strong and important independent risk factor for poor recipient outcome.[15,16]

OPERATIVE RECIPIENT MANAGEMENT

Timing of the recipient operation requires careful coordination with the procurement team. Anesthesia is induced after the donor heart is visually inspected and found suitable. Venous access is obtained, which will permit rapid volume resuscitation and invasive cardiac monitoring after the new heart is implanted. Prior cardiac surgery may complicate coordination of operative timing and is associated with increased risk of bleeding.

If appropriate, Coumadin effects are reversed with fresh frozen plasma and vitamin K. Aprotinin or ε-aminocaproic acid are often used to inhibit fibrinolysis and prevent coagulopathic bleeding after prior cardiac surgery or associated with hepatic congestion. Increased inotropic infusion, antiarrhythmic agents, or mechanical circulatory support may be required

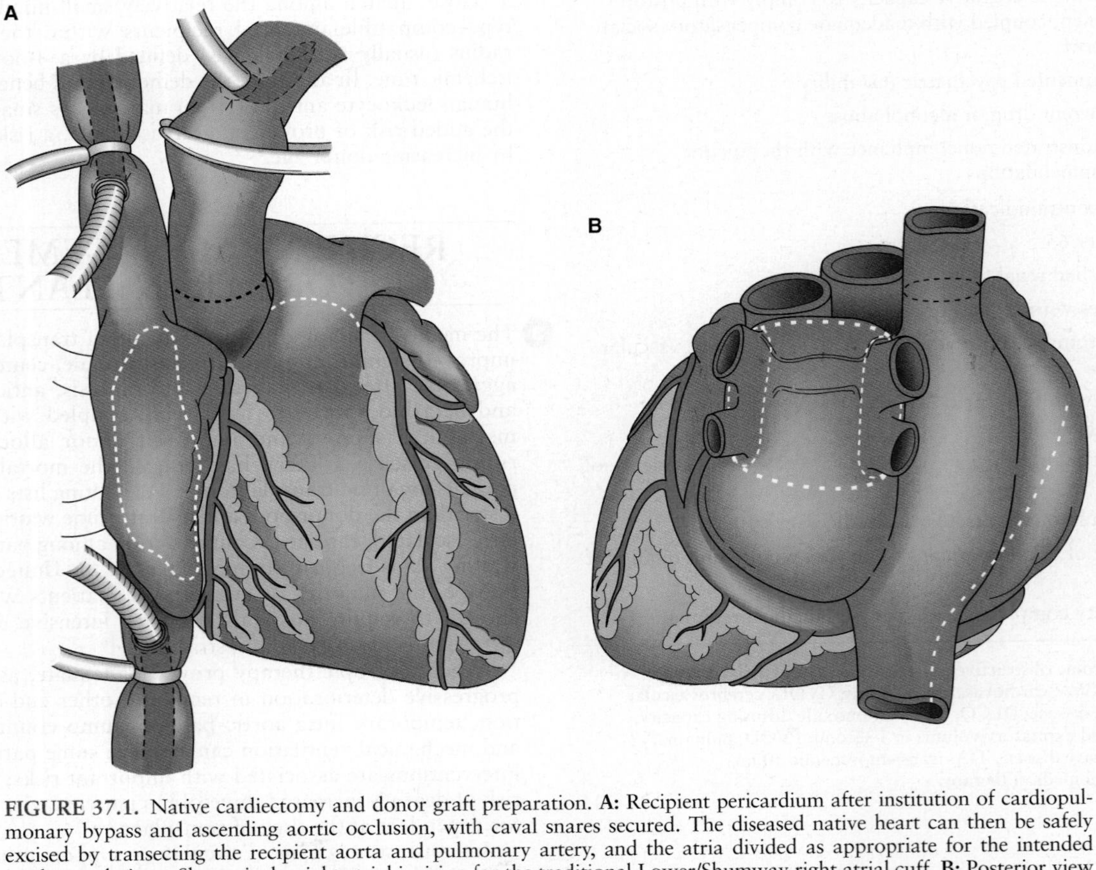

FIGURE 37.1. Native cardiectomy and donor graft preparation. **A:** Recipient pericardium after institution of cardiopulmonary bypass and ascending aortic occlusion, with caval snares secured. The diseased native heart can then be safely excised by transecting the recipient aorta and pulmonary artery, and the atria divided as appropriate for the intended implant technique. Shown is the right atrial incision for the traditional Lower/Shumway right atrial cuff. **B:** Posterior view of the explanted donor heart, indicating various incisions used for atrial cuff preparation. Donor atrial cuff incisions made in preparation for traditional Lower/Shumway biatrial implant are indicated by the heavy white dashed line. The superior vena cava (SVC) is ligated or oversewn. Right and left pulmonary vein (*light white dashed line*) and superior vena cava (*black dashed line*) incisions are indicated for the total atrioventricular implant technique. For the bicaval technique, the donor SVC (*black dashed line*) and inferior vena cava are retained as for the total atrioventricular technique (Fig. 37.4), and the donor left atrial cuff trimmed as for the traditional biatrial approach (*heavy white dashed line*).

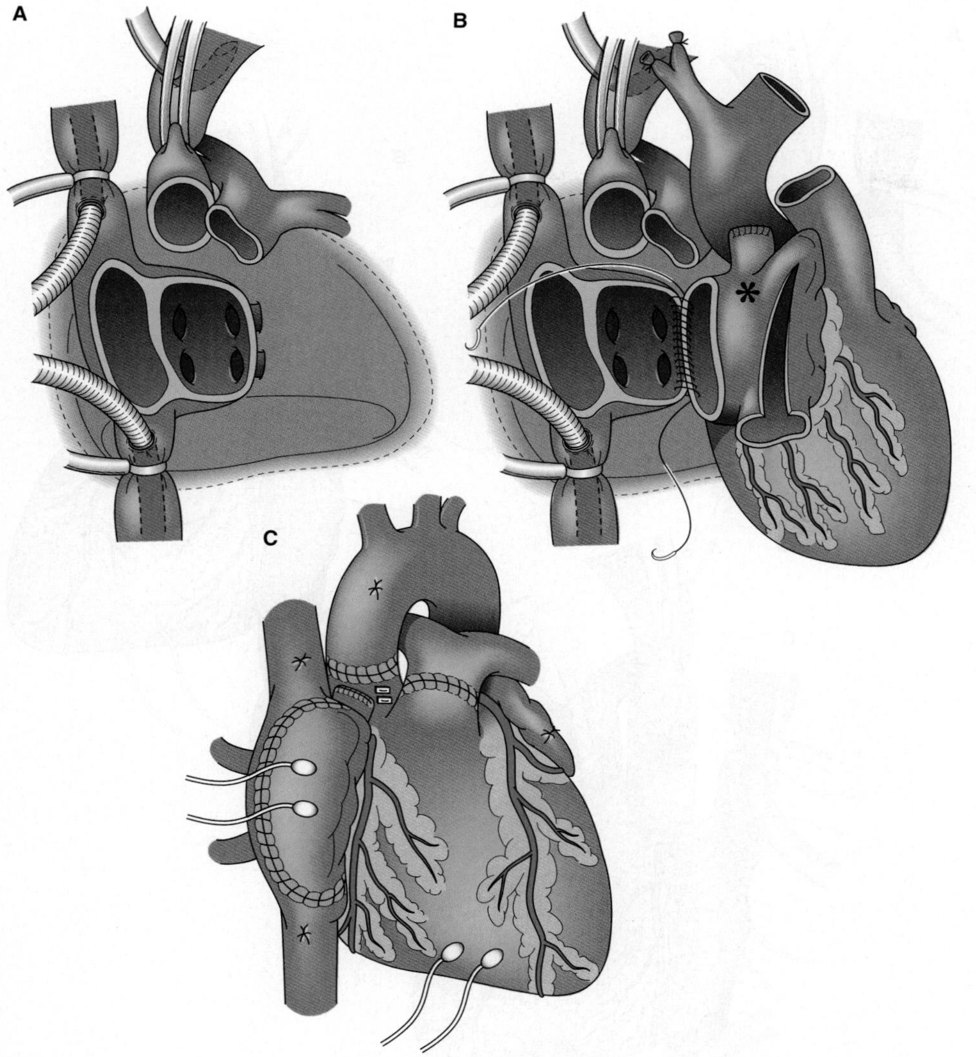

FIGURE 37.2. Traditional Lower/Shumway biatrial technique. **A:** Recipient cuffs, prepared for bicaval atrial implant technique. After completion of the left atrial anastomosis (**B**), the right atrial cuffs are joined. Care is taken to avoid carrying the right atrial incision or suture line close to the donor sinoatrial node, at the superior vena cava/right atrial junction (*asterisk*). **C:** Appearance of the operative field after completion of great vessel anastomoses, weaning from cardiopulmonary bypass, and decannulation.

to maintain adequate systemic perfusion prior to institution of cardiopulmonary bypass.

Vascular access for bypass is accomplished by cannulation of the superior and inferior vena cavae so as to completely divert systemic venous blood to the cardiopulmonary bypass circuit. The ascending aorta, common femoral, or subclavian artery is used for arterial return from the circuit to the patient. Technical misadventures, such as entry into the heart or great vessels before bypass is established or induction of ventricular arrhythmias, are more common with reoperative procedures and can greatly complicate the intraoperative course and postoperative management.

Once the proximate arrival of the donor heart is ensured, the recipient is placed on bypass and cooled. Snares are secured around the caval cannulae, the ascending aorta clamped, and the native heart excised (Fig. 37.1A). Vascular cuffs are preserved, which are appropriate for implantation of the donor heart (Figs. 37.2A, 37.3A, and 37.4A). The donor heart is then prepared according to the implant technique to be used (Fig. 37.1B).

Implant techniques and the sequence of vascular anastomosis vary widely between surgeons, as do strategies used to protect the ischemic organ during implantation. The biatrial orthotopic heart transplant technique is simple, easy to teach, and still used by many surgeons[8] (Fig. 37.2A–C). The donor atria are spatulated open, trimmed if necessary, and laid over the recipient's atrial remnants. The left atrial suture line is everted to achieve endothelial apposition and to avoid leaving epicardial fat or muscle exposed in the lumen as a potential nidus for thromboemboli. Sinoatrial node dysfunction can usually be prevented by keeping the donor right atriotomy well anterior on the right atrial appendage, away from the sinoatrial node and its blood supply (Fig. 37.2B), and by optimizing graft preservation.[32] Even if most of the dilated native atrium is excised, atrioventricular (AV) valve annular geometry may be distorted, causing regurgitation, or the area around the sinus node may be placed under tension, leading to atrial arrhythmias or sinus node dysfunction.

4

During the 1990s, these considerations led to evaluation of alternate atrial anastomotic techniques, including bicaval right atrial connections (Fig. 37.3A–C) and total atrioventricular replacement (two caval and two pulmonary vein anastomoses) (Fig. 37.4A, B). In a prospective, randomized trial (bicaval[33]) and several retrospective analyses,[34,35] the incidence of atrial arrhythmias and AV valve regurgitation was reduced, and hemodynamic results and survival were improved with either the bicaval or total atrioventricular technique.

Independent of whether the aorta or pulmonary artery connection is performed first, the anterior aspect of the pulmonary artery anastomosis is usually left open or vented, to allow decompression of the right heart after reperfusion (Fig. 37.3C). The size mismatch between donor and recipient aortas is often dramatic, but can usually be accommodated by beveling the smaller vessel (usually the more pliable donor) to increase its effective circumference and by distributing the discrepancy evenly over the length of each anastomosis. Occasionally it is

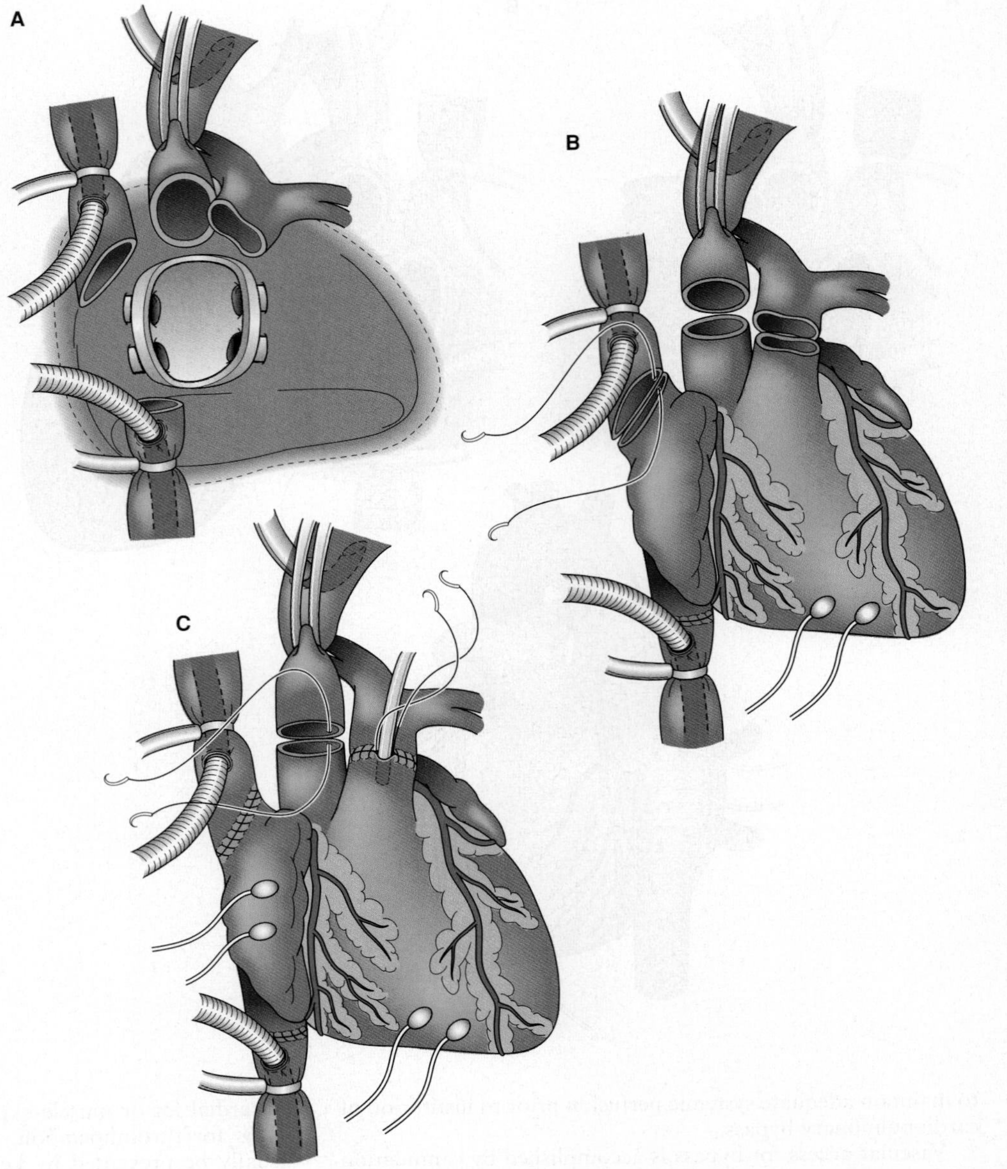

FIGURE 37.3. Bicaval right atrial implant technique. **A:** During explantation of the native heart, the interatrial septum may be excised, for end-to-end anastomosis of the cavae (**B**), or left in place (as in Fig. 37.2A), allowing the back walls of the donor cavae to be laid into those of the recipient. **C:** Technique for pulmonary artery venting through an opening in the anterior aspect of this anastomosis, which is useful for deairing and decompressing the right heart. Alternatively, the aorta may be anastomosed earlier in the operation to minimize graft ischemic time.

necessary to tailor down the larger vessel or to replace an aneurysmal ascending aorta with donor tissue or a prosthetic graft. Functional pulmonary stenosis is avoided by trimming back both donor and recipient sufficiently to prevent redundancy.

An alternate "heterotopic" implantation technique places a second heart in the circulation, in parallel with the retained native heart.[36] In principle, leaving the native heart affords protection in the event that the graft fails. The operation is technically demanding, usually produces compressive atelectasis in the right lung, and is associated with a high risk of stroke, perhaps due to stasis of blood in the native heart.[37] Not withstanding, this surgical approach may be considered for patients with high pulmonary vascular resistance unresponsive to vasodilators, and may in the future also find a role in the initial application of cardiac xenografts.

After completion of the anastomoses, the heart is reperfused and allowed to resume contracting without being required to function as a pump ("rested") as the recipient is rewarmed. Atrial and ventricular pacing wires are placed. Cardiac output of the denervated transplant is highly dependent on rate. In addition, the shorter cardiac filling time associated with higher heart rate prevents graft distention. Isoproterenol is initiated prior to weaning from bypass at a dose of 0.005 to 0.02 μg/kg per minute and titrated to achieve a heart rate of about 110 beats per minute.

Patients with high preoperative pulmonary vascular resistance may be particularly difficult to wean from cardiopulmonary bypass, even with excellent function of the donor heart, as the "normal" donor right ventricle may acutely dilate and fail when confronted by a high-resistance pulmonary vascular bed. Resting the recently ischemic heart on cardiopulmonary bypass, establishing a stable sinus or AV sequentially paced rhythm, instituting inotropic support, and intra-aortic balloon counterpulsation are useful in managing this problem. Traditional pharmacologic approaches to reducing pulmonary vascular resistance, such as prostaglandins E_1 or I_2 and sodium nitroprusside, may cause transpulmonary shunting of deoxygenated blood; these agents also reduce systemic vascular resistance and thus coronary perfusion pressure. Inhaled nitric oxide selectively dilates the pulmonary vascular bed before being rapidly inactivated by hemoglobin in the blood. We and others have found this very helpful to selectively reduce pulmonary vascular resistance without adverse effects on oxygenation or heart

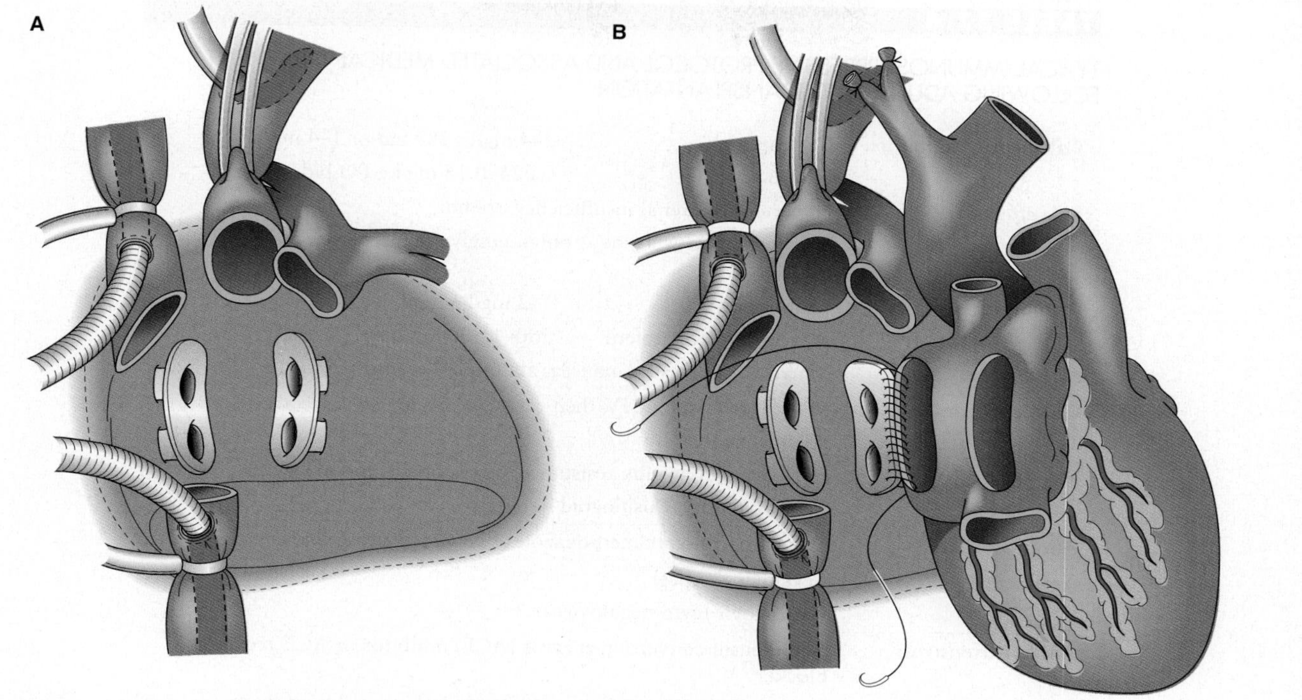

FIGURE 37.4. Total atrioventricular transplant technique. A: Recipient pericardial well after preparation of bilateral pulmonary vein pedicles and caval cuffs, for total atrioventricular heart transplant. B: Construction of left pulmonary vein anastomosis. As with other left atrial anastomotic approaches, atrial walls or vein cuffs are everted to minimize exposure of thrombogenic fat or muscle to the blood.

function, and this drug has recently been approved by the U.S. Food and Drug Administration for clinical use.[38] Poor function of either or both ventricles may necessitate institution of mechanical support as a bridge to graft recovery or to retransplantation.

Postoperatively, ventilator and inotropic support is weaned, immunosuppression is instituted, and diuretic and antihypertensive agents are initiated as necessary. Isoproterenol is continued for about 5 days and replaced with theophylline if needed to sustain a resting heart rate over 70. The first surveillance endomyocardial biopsy is performed 7 to 10 days after surgery and repeated as an outpatient procedure about every 2 weeks for the first 3 months. Patient and caregiver education with regard to medication schedules and physiologic monitoring facilitates early discharge for patients without complications. Biologic monitoring of peripheral blood gene or protein expression and electrical approaches to monitor the immune response to the graft have shown promise to supplant routine invasive monitoring.[39–41]

IMMUNOSUPPRESSION

The goal of immunosuppressive therapy is to prevent immune-mediated injury to the graft while minimizing associated com-
5 plications, including opportunistic infection. Most programs employ a "triple-drug" regimen, including a calcineurin inhibitor, an antimitotic agent, and steroids. This approach allows each individual drug to be used within its therapeutic window (Table 37.4). Some centers add antibody "induction" with anti-CD3, polyclonal antilymphocyte serum, or anti–interleukin-2 (anti-IL-2) receptor antibodies.[42–47] The mechanisms of action and side effect profiles of these agents are well described in an earlier section of this chapter.

Medical management after heart transplantation is focused on anticipation and prevention of common complications. Hypertension and hyperlipidemia are prevalent due to predisposition in the recipient patient population and as side effects
6 of various immunosuppressive agents. Prophylaxis against opportunistic infections includes agents targeted at common protozoal and viral pathogens (Table 37.4). Surveillance biopsies are performed according to a scheduled routine, and additional biopsies are performed to exclude rejection in the event of hemodynamic instability or unexplained fever. Typically, patients are able to leave the hospital within 10 days of uncomplicated operation, to be followed regularly in outpatient clinic. Monitored physical rehabilitation facilitates optimal cardiovascular and musculoskeletal recuperation,[48] and occupational rehabilitation may offer important psychological and social benefits.

COMPLICATIONS

Complications of antirejection therapy relate primarily to the side effects of the specific immunosuppressive agents currently used. Infections tend to occur in patients with the greatest degree of preoperative debility and malnutrition, or in conjunction with additional stressors such as perioperative bleeding or hepatorenal dysfunction. Bacterial pathogens are common in the first several weeks, particularly in the lung and related to surgical or vascular access sites. Opportunistic viral and fungal infections usually predominate later. Increasingly effective prophylaxis for cytomegalovirus and herpes infections has markedly reduced the morbidity associated with these common pathogens. When infection occurs, immunosuppression is tapered as aggressively as possible based on myocardial biopsy results.

Acute rejection occurs in the majority of patients and is graded histologically according to standardized criteria developed by the International Society for Heart and Lung Transplantation (ISHLT). When detected at an early histologic stage

TABLE 37.4

TYPICAL IMMUNOSUPPRESSIVE PROTOCOL AND ASSOCIATED MEDICAL TREATMENT FOLLOWING ADULT HEART TRANSPLANTATION

Calcineurin inhibitors:	Cyclosporine	2–4 mg/kg PO bid or 1–4 mg/h IV
	FK506	0.025–0.15 mg/kg PO bid
Side effects:	Hypertension, renal insufficiency, tremor,	
	Hirsutism (cyclosporine A only), gingival hyperplasia, diabetes (FK only)	
Antimitotic agents:	Azathioprine	1–2 mg/kg/d qd
	Mycophenolate mofetil	500–1,500 mg/d bid
Side effects:	Marrow suppression, nausea, abdominal cramps, diarrhea	
Glucocorticoids:	Methylprednisolone IV, then	
	Prednisone PO	
Side effects:	Hypertension, insulin resistance, osteoporosis, mood swings	
	Central obesity, Cushingoid habitus	
Antiprotozoal:	Trimethoprim-sulfamethoxazole (*Pneumocystis*; toxoplasmosis)	
Antiviral:	Acyclovir (herpes)	
	Ganciclovir (cytomegalovirus)	
Antihypertensives:	Angiotensin-converting enzyme (ACE) inhibitor or ACE-receptor blocker	
	Diltiazem (retards cyclosporine A metabolism, reducing drug requirement)	
	α-Receptor blockers	
Antilipid agents:	Statin class agent	

(ISHLT grade 1, Fig. 37.5) in an asymptomatic patient on surveillance biopsy, rejection will often respond to augmented oral steroids and/or an increased dose of calcineurin inhibitor. When a higher grade of rejection is found (Fig. 37.6), when the infiltrate fails to resolve in response to initial interventions, or in the setting of depressed cardiac function or shock, high-dose intravenous steroids are administered and antilymphocyte therapy often added. Inotropic or mechanical support is instituted as needed in hopes of rescuing graft and patient. Antibody-mediated "vascular" rejection is a controversial entity that, when documented by immunohistochemical techniques, may warrant introduction of cyclophosphamide or other agents with increased activity against B cells.

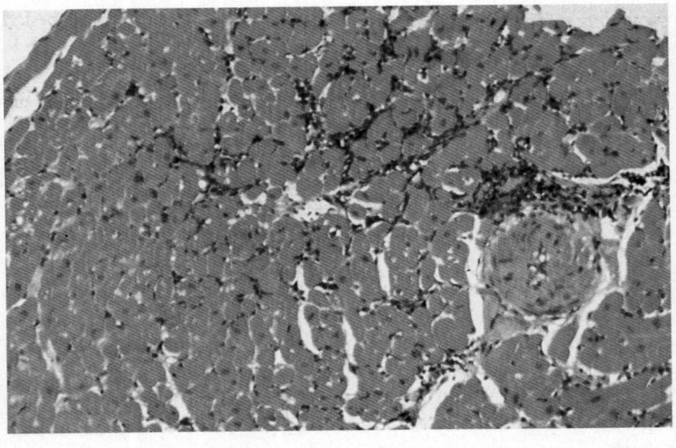

FIGURE 37.5. International Society for Heart and Lung Transplantation grade 1R—diffuse interstitial or focal perivascular infiltrate with rare or absent myocyte damage is characteristic of mild acute cellular rejection.

Bradycardia is prevalent in the denervated heart for the first weeks after transplant, but a resting heart rate over 70 can usually be achieved by initiating a β-agonist such as theophylline. Persistent bradycardia may be caused by ischemic, surgical, or immunologic injury to the sinus or AV nodes or by amiodarone leaching from stores accumulated preoperatively in body fat; pacemaker implantation may be necessary. Atrial flutter or fibrillation may occur spontaneously or herald acute rejection. This dysrhythmia can be difficult to manage because vagal denervation attenuates digoxin modulation of the

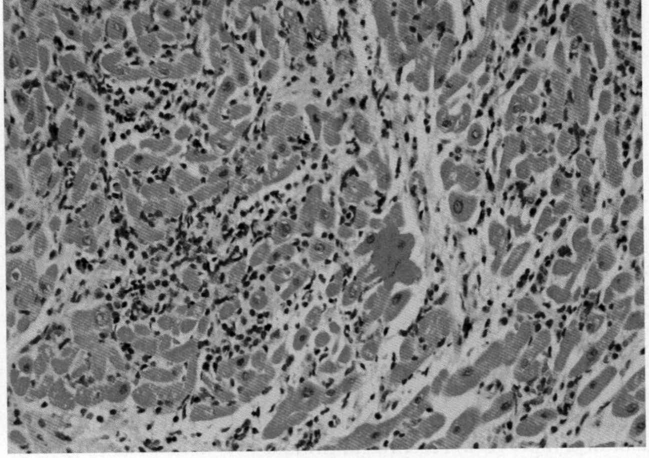

FIGURE 37.6. International Society for Heart and Lung Transplantation grade 3R—multifocal cellular infiltrate with focal myocyte necrosis, typical of severe acute cellular rejection.

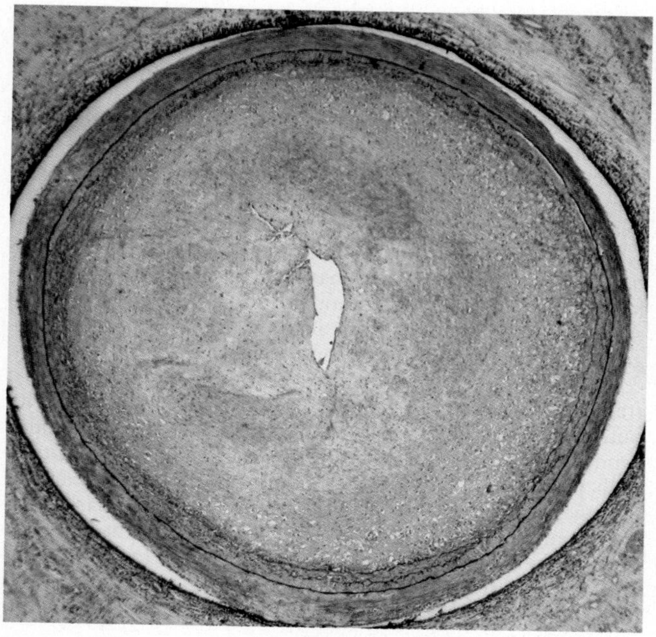

FIGURE 37.7. Autopsy specimen of an epicardial coronary artery demonstrating a moderately severe concentric fibroproliferative intimal lesion characteristic of cardiac allograft vasculopathy. (Courtesy of Dr. James Atkinson, Vanderbilt University School of Medicine, Nashville, TN.)

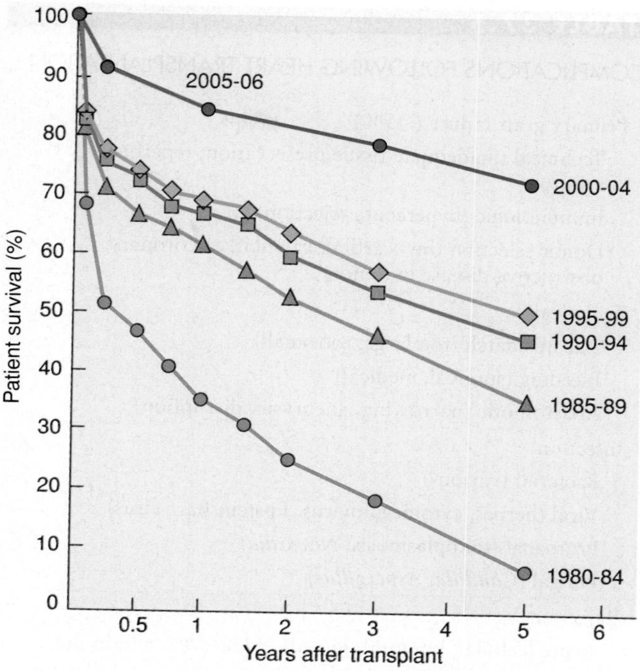

FIGURE 37.8. Heart Transplant Survival, 1980–2006. Survival following heart transplantation in recipients, grouped by era of operation, analyzed by the Kaplan-Meier method. Operative survival accounts for much of the steady improvement in outcomes over the past two decades. The subsequent rate of attrition appears to have changed little over the past 20 years, likely reflecting the effect of competing influences such as an older recipient population and improving patient management strategies. (Figure created from data provided by the United Network for Organ Sharing, including follow-up information available as of 12/10/09.) Current demographics and statistics may be found at International Society for Heart and Lung Transplantation website (www.ishlt.org).

typical rapid ventricular response. Most other agents traditionally used to treat atrial arrhythmias depress AV node conduction or myocardial contractility, particularly undesirable side effects in a recent heart recipient. Amiodarone is generally better tolerated, controls heart rate and promotes conversion to sinus rhythm, and has been used widely in this circumstance.

Among patients who survive beyond the first year, the primary limits to long-term survival are cardiac allograft vasculopathy (CAV) and malignancy[15,16,24] (Fig. 37.7). Current understanding of the pathogenesis of CAV is incomplete.[49–51] Widely presumed to be a consequence of "chronic rejection," this process has an incidence of approximately 5% per year. CAV may cause progressive insufficiency of coronary flow, myocardial infarction, and ultimately death. Recent research has drawn attention to the importance of donor stress associated with brain death and ischemia/reperfusion injury in the incidence and severity of CAV in animal models.[52] In contrast to the usual pattern of focal proximal lesions in conventional atherosclerosis, coronary arteries are diffusely involved, and conventional revascularization techniques are not generally feasible. In the future, new immunosuppressive or antiproliferative agents may prevent this process or delay its progression.[53] Both CAV and increased risk of malignancy would likely be prevented if efforts to accomplish durable tolerance are successful, but this obstacle is proving stubborn.[54]

RESULTS

7 Due to a decline in the number of donor hearts that are considered acceptable, the number of heart transplants performed worldwide has declined, from a peak of about 4,070 in 1995 to fewer than 3,200 reported in each year since 2000, a 20% decrease. While some decrease in reporting from European centers may have resulted from the absence of an incentive to contribute to international registries, reported U.S. activity—which is federally mandated by organ allocation regulations—decreased by about 15% between 1997 and 2004 despite a steady increase in average donor age.[15,24] A recent trend upward in U.S. heart transplant activity (from 2,000 to 2,200 cases annually) may reflect the influence of the Health Resources and Services Administration organ donor initiative,[15,55,56] implementation in 2006 of a donor allocation algorithm that emphasizes disease acuity over proximity to donor hospital or other factors.

Operative survival in adults has improved over the past 20 years to above 90%, and both patient and graft 1-year survival rates exceed 87%[15,16] (Fig. 37.8). The most important risk factors for death within the first year include previous transplant, increased donor age (with age older than 60 conferring greater risk than age older than 45), need for ventilator or left ventricular assist device support before transplant, and
8 recipient age older than 60. Among common complications, rejection and infection together account for most of the mortality during the first year and contribute approximately equally (Table 37.5). Beyond the first year, malignancy, including posttransplant lymphoproliferative disease, and chronic rejection emerge as prominent additional factors limiting long-term survival. Extrapolating from current early results, more than 50% of recent recipients can expect to be alive 10 years after transplant, with actuarial graft half-life over 12 years.[16,24,27]

Repeat heart transplantation accounts for less than 2% of all heart transplants done. When performed within the first 6 months, typically for early failure of the first graft, 1-year survival is less than 50%. When performed later, usually for cardiac allograft vasculopathy, 1-year survival is over 80%, and

TABLE 37.5

COMPLICATIONS FOLLOWING HEART TRANSPLANTATION

Primary graft failure (<5%)
Technical (inadequate tissue preservation; reperfusion injury)
Immunologic (hyperacute rejection)
Donor selection (myocardial, valvular, or coronary obstructive disease in donor)
Technical
Size mismatch (too large, too small)
Bleeding (surgical, medical)
Anastomotic (narrowing, aneurysm, disruption)
Infection
Bacterial (various)
Viral (herpes, cytomegalovirus, Epstein-Barr virus)
Protozoal (toxoplasmosis, *Nocardia*)
Fungal (*Candida, Aspergillus*)
Rejection
Acute (cellular, humoral, mixed) (24%–34% within first year)
Chronic (cardiac allograft vasculopathy) (53% by 10 years)
Treatment effects
Hypertension (99% by 10 years)
Hyperlipidemia (93% by 10 years)
Diabetes (37% by 10 years)
Renal failure (acute; chronic) (39% by 10 years; 6% dialysis or transplant recipient)
Malignancy (31% by 10 years)
Skin
Visceral (lung, colon, prostate/breast, other)
Lymphoproliferative disease

has improved significantly over the past decade. Overall, actuarial graft half-life following retransplant is about 4.6 years, and is over 9 years in those who survive the first year.[16] While these outcomes are significantly inferior to other transplant indications, retransplantation offers significant survival advantage for carefully selected patients.

Adolescent (11- to 17-year-olds) pediatric heart transplantation recipients fare better (>80% 1-year survival) than do younger children (1- to 10-year-olds: ~77%) or infants (younger than 1 year old: ~68%). Less favorable short-term outcomes may be ascribed to pulmonary hypertension and anatomic challenges posed by congenital heart disease, and to monitoring and compliance challenges characteristic of these age groups. Nonetheless, the graft half-life for pediatric patients (11.4 to 13 years) is similar to that for adults.[15,16,24,27]

ETHICS

Ethical considerations are important to every aspect of heart transplantation. The donor pool is limited and appears to be shrinking despite extended donor acceptance criteria, restricting the number of patients who can undergo transplantation. This shortage forces consideration of ways to limit recipient candidacy (age limits), to increase the donor pool (presumed consent, advertising initiatives, community outreach), and to develop alternatives (mechanical devices, xenografts).[57–59]

The heart transplant community has taken the lead in standardizing patient selection and management guidelines and has established policies for equitable organ allocation. Those given an opportunity to receive the "gift of life" are chosen from a much larger population who might benefit. Recipient candidacy decisions are made by a multidisciplinary group based on objective and subjective input from many individuals who come to know the patient and family in depth. Some recipient selection criteria are fundamentally arbitrary: age is retained as a criterion because of the limited supply of donor organs and based on the consensus view that younger patients deserve preferred access. Recipient selection criteria only become unfair if they are applied unequally or inconsistently at different programs or between various regions of the country.

Some of the most difficult decisions made by the heart transplant team involve medically marginal candidates with outstanding and effective social support or medically suitable candidates with marginal social support. While the majority of such patients will do well, outcomes in either case can, on average, be expected to fall below outcome benchmarks. For every marginal patient transplanted, a candidate who meets all the criteria may die. Thus, the "right" decision for an individual patient is difficult or impossible to know in advance and may conflict with the best interests of the population of potential recipients.

CURRENT ISSUES

Quantifiable, objective measures of efficacy beyond survival, such as improvement in exercise capacity, freedom from complications, and reduced costs, are becoming the standards by which individual heart transplantation programs are judged. Most important to the patient are subjective factors such as quality of life and productivity, for which standardized measurement tools are being developed. Meanwhile, the efficacy of any proposed alternative to transplantation must be measured against survival, cost, and quality-of-life benchmarks established by this once-experimental procedure.[60,61]

The most important factor currently restricting the application of heart transplantation is the limited supply of donor organs. Consent is obtained from the donor's legal representatives in only about 25% to 50% of cases where hearts are appropriate based on acceptable physiologic parameters. Various proactive approaches, such as institution of presumed consent, have been associated with high per capita donation rates in some countries. However, presumed consent is ethically dubious and may violate basic cultural or religious precepts of individuals or ethnic groups. An adverse societal response to imposition of this unpopular approach as national policy might paradoxically cripple efforts to maintain organ donation even at current levels. Well-conceived efforts to increase the rate of consent, by passing laws requiring hospitals to facilitate and document the request, by allowing trained individuals to manage the request process, and by educating the public about "the gift of life," have boosted per capita donation in several U.S. organ procurement regions.

9 Efforts to develop improved immunosuppressive drugs are important and are likely to yield incremental near-term improvements in the incidence of chronic rejection. Ideally, one could induce tolerance—permanent graft acceptance without requirement for indefinite immunosuppressive therapy. Modulation, rather than suppression, of host responses to donor antigens may allow achievement of this goal.[62,63]

Even if every physiologically suitable donor heart were available, only a minority of patients for whom transplantation would offer a survival advantage could be cared for using this modality. As technical issues related to transcutaneous power delivery, thromboembolism, infection risk, and reliability are addressed, mechanical assist devices are likely to emerge as definitive "destination" therapy for some patients.[57]

Progress has also been made toward use of porcine "xenografts" in man, and the initial immunologic barrier, hyperacute rejection, appears surmountable using organs from pigs genetically modified to express human complement regulatory proteins or "knocked out" for the gene encoding Gal α1,3Gal, the main carbohydrate target recognized by human antipig antibodies.[64–66] Control of subsequent cellular and antibody responses has proven difficult in animal models, but life-supporting function of renal xenografts for 3 months and heart xenografts for 1 month have been demonstrated in primates using an intensive regimen of "conventional" immunosuppressive agents.[67,68]

Heart transplantation is one of the most resource-intensive modalities in modern medicine when assessed as cost per year of life saved. The procedure itself, the in-hospital care before transplantation, and maintenance of program infrastructure are very expensive. Ongoing pharmacy charges and surveillance procedure costs are also substantial. Paradoxically, patients physically able to return to work often cannot do so because they rely on medical disability benefits to pay for medications and follow-up care. Whether heart transplantation will continue to receive wide support is a function of societal acceptance of these costs, as currently reflected by coverage policies established by public and private health care insurers.[60] In the future the application of heart transplantation and related technologies may be limited more by what society chooses to afford, rather than what is medically possible.

References

1. Carrel A, Guthrie CC. The transplantation of veins and organs. *Am Med (Philadelphia)* 1905;10:1101.
2. Carrel A. The surgery of blood vessels. *Bull Johns Hopkins Hosp* 1907;18:18.
3. Neptune WB, Cookson BA, Bailey CP, et al. Complete homologous heart transplantation. *Arch Surg* 1953;66:174–178.
4. Webb WR, Howard HS, Neely WA. Practical methods of homologous cardiac transplantation. *J Thorac Surg* 1959;37:361–366.
5. Goldberg M, Berman EF, Akman LC. Homologous transplantation of the canine heart. *J Int Coll Surg* 1958;30:575–586.
6. Cass MH, Brock R. Heart excision and replacement. *Guys Hosp Rep* 1959;108:285–290.
7. Demikhov VP. *Experimental Transplantation of Vital Organs* [in Russian]. Haigh B, trans-ed. New York: Consultant's Bureau; 1962.
8. Lower RR, Stofer RC, Shumway NE. Homovital transplantation of the heart. *J Thorac Cardiovasc Surg* 1961;41:196–204.
9. Hardy JD, Chavez CM, Kurrus FE, et al. Heart transplantation in man: developmental studies and report of a case. *JAMA* 1964;188:1132–1140.
10. Barnard CN. The operation. A human cardiac transplant: an interim report of a successful operation performed at Groote Schuur Hospital, Cape Town. *S Afr Med J* 1967;41:1271–1274.
11. Caves PK, Stinson EB, Braham AF, et al. Percutaneous transvenous endomyocardial biopsy. *JAMA* 1973;225:288.
12. Kaye MP, Elcombe SA, O'Fallon WM. The international heart transplantation registry. The 1984 report. *J Heart Transplant* 1985;4(3):290–292.
13. Calne RY, White DJ, Rolles K, et al. Prolonged survival of pig orthotopic heart grafts treated with cyclosporin A. *Lancet* 1978;1:1183.
14. Reitz BA, Bieber CP, Raney AA, et al. Orthotopic heart and combined heart and lung transplantation with cyclosporin-A immune suppression. *Transplant Proc* 1981;13:393.
15. Mulligan MS, Shearon TH, Weill D, et al. Heart and lung transplantation in the United States, 1997–2006. *Am J Transplant* 2008;8(4):977–987.
16. Taylor DO, Edwards LB, Aurora P, et al. Registry of the international society for heart and lung transplantation: twenty-fifth official adult heart transplant report—2008. *J Heart Lung Transplant* 2008;27(9):943–956.
17. O'Connell JB, Gunnar RM, Evans RW, et al. Task force 1: organization of heart transplantation in the US. *J Am Coll Cardiol* 1993;22:8.
18. Chomsky DB, Lang CC, Rayos GH, et al. Hemodynamic exercise testing. A valuable tool in the selection of cardiac transplantation candidates. *Circulation* 1996;94(12):3176–3183.
19. Butler J, Khadim G, Paul KM, et al. Selection criteria for cardiac transplantation in the current era of heart failure therapy. *J Am Coll Cardiol* 2004;43(5):787–793.
20. Mehra MR, Kobashigawa J, Starling R, et al. Listing criteria for heart transplantation: International Society for Heart and Lung Transplantation guidelines for the care of cardiac transplant candidates—2006. *J Heart Lung Transplant* 2006;25(9):1024–1042.
21. Jeevanandam V, Furukawa S, Prendergast TW, et al. Standard criteria for an acceptable donor heart are restricting heart transplantation. *Ann Thorac Surg* 1996;62(5):1268–1275.
22. Drinkwater DC, Laks H, Blitz A, et al. Outcomes of patients undergoing transplantation with older donor hearts. *J Heart Lung Transplant* 1996; 15(7):684–691.
23. Tenderich G, Koerner MM, Stuettgen B, et al. Extended donor criteria: hemodynamic follow-up of heart transplant recipients receiving a cardiac allograft from donors > or = 60 years of age. *Transplantation* 1998; 66(8):1109–1113.
24. Pierson RN III, Barr ML, McCullough KP, et al. SRTR report on the state of transplantation: thoracic organ transplantation. *Am J Transplant* 2004; 4(suppl 9):93–105.
25. Novitsky D, Cooper DKC, Reichart B. Hemodynamic and metabolic responses to hormonal therapy in brain-dead potential organ donors. *Transplantation* 1987;43:852–854.
26. Rosengard BR. Donor management initiative. *Chimera* 1999;10(3):12–13.
27. Opelz G. Results of cardiac transplantation and factors influencing survival based on the collaborative heart transplant study. In: Cooper DKC, Miller LW, Patterson GA, eds. *The Transplantation and Replacement of Thoracic Organs,* 2nd ed. Hingham, MA: Kluwer Academic Press; 1996: 417–427.
28. Copeland JG, Smith RG, Arabia FA, et al. CardioWest Total Artificial Heart Investigators. Cardiac Replacement with a total artificial heart as a bridge to transplantation. *N Engl J Med* 2004;351(9):859–867.
29. John R, Kamdar F, Liao K, et al. Improved survival and decreasing incidence of adverse events with the HeartMate II left ventricular assist device as bridge-to-transplant therapy. *Ann Thorac Surg* 2008;86(4):1227–1234.
30. Esmore D, Kaye D, Spratt P, et al. A prospective, multicenter trial of the VentrAssist left ventricular assist device for bridge to transplant: safety and efficacy. *J Heart Lung Transplant* 2008;27(6):579–588.
31. Vega JD, Ochsner JL, Jeevanandam V, et al. A multicenter, randomized controlled trial of Celsior for flush and hypothermic storage of cardiac allografts. *Ann Thorac Surg* 2001;71(5):1442–1447.
32. Jeevanandam V, Barr ML, Auteri JS, et al. University of Wisconsin solution versus crystalloid cardioplegia for human donor heart preservation. A randomized blinded prospective clinical trial. *J Thorac Cardiovasc Surg* 1992; 103(2):194–198.
33. el Gamel A, Yonan NA, Grant S, et al. Orthotopic cardiac transplantation: a comparison of standard and bicaval Wythenshawe techniques. *J Thorac Cardiovasc Surg* 1995;109(4):721–729.
34. Aziz T, Burgess M, Khafagy R, et al. Bicaval and standard techniques in orthotopic heart transplantation: medium-term experience in cardiac performance and survival. *J Thorac Cardiovasc Surg* 1999;118(1):115–122.
35. Trento A, Takkenberg JM, Czer LS, et al. Clinical experience with one hundred consecutive patients undergoing orthotopic heart transplantation with bicaval and pulmonary venous anastomoses. *J Thorac Cardiovasc Surg* 1996;112(6):1496–1550.
36. Cooper DKC, Taniguchi S. Heterotopic heart transplantation—indications, surgical techniques and special considerations. In: Cooper DKC, Miller LW, Patterson GA, eds. *Transplantation and Replacement of Thoracic Organs,* 2nd ed. Hingham, MA: Kluwer Academic Press; 1996:353–365.
37. Tagusari O, Kormos RL, Kawai A, et al. Native heart complications after heterotopic heart transplantation: insight into the potential risk of left ventricular assist device. *J Heart Lung Transplant* 1999;18(11):1111–1119.
38. Maxey TS, Smith CD, Kern JA, et al. Beneficial effects of inhaled nitric oxide in adult cardiac surgical patients. *Ann Thorac Surg* 2002;73(2): 529–532.
39. Marboe CC, Billingham M, Eisen HJ, et al. Refining pathological classification of acute rejection in cardiac allograft recipients: a multicenter study using peripheral blood gene expression profiling. *J Heart Lung Transplant* 2004;23(2S):S42.
40. Pham MX, Teuteberg JJ, Kfoury AG, et al.; Image study group. Gene-expression profiling for rejection surveillance after cardiac transplantation. *N Engl J Med* 2010;362(20):1890–1900.
41. Knosalla C, Grauhan O, Muller J, et al. Intramyocardial electrogram recordings (IMEG) for diagnosis of cellular and humoral mediated cardiac allograft rejection. *Ann Thorac Cardiovasc Surg* 2000;6(2):89–94.
42. Starnes VA, Oyer PE, Stinson EB, et al. Prophylactic OKT3 used as induction therapy for heart transplantation. *Circulation* 1989;80(5 Pt 2): III79–III83.
43. van Gelder T, Baan CC, Balk AH, et al. Blockade of the interleukin (IL)-2/IL-2 receptor pathway with a monoclonal anti-IL-2 receptor antibody (BT563) does not prevent the development of acute heart allograft rejection in humans. *Transplantation* 1998;65(3):405–410.
44. Carey JA, Frist WH. Use of polyclonal antilymphocytic preparations for prophylaxis in heart transplantation. *J Heart Transplant* 1990;9(3 Pt 2): 297–300.
45. Miller LW, Naftel DC, Bourge RC, et al. Infection after heart transplantation: a multiinstitutional study. Cardiac Transplant Research Database Group. *J Heart Lung Transplant* 1994;13:381–392.
46. Swinnen LJ, Costanzo-Nordin MR, Fisher SG, et al. Increased incidence of lymphoproliferative disorder after immunosuppression with the monoclonal antibody OKT3 in cardiac-transplant recipients. *N Engl J Med* 1990;323(25):1723–1728.
47. Hammond EH, Wittwer CT, Greenwood J, et al. Relationship of OKT3 sensitization and vascular rejection in cardiac transplant patients receiving OKT3 rejection prophylaxis. *Transplantation* 1990;50(5):776–782.
48. Kobashigawa JA, Leaf DA, Lee N, et al. A controlled trial of exercise rehabilitation after heart transplantation. *N Engl J Med* 1999;340(4):272–277.

49. Pierson RN III, Miller GM. Late graft failure: lessons from clinical and experimental thoracic organ transplantation. *Graft* 2000;3(2):88–93.
50. Caforio AL, Tona F, Fortina AB, et al. Immune and nonimmune predictors of cardiac allograft vasculopathy onset and severity: multivariate risk factor analysis and role of immunosuppression. *Am J Transplant* 2004;4(6): 962–970.
51. Valantine H. Cardiac allograft vasculopathy after heart transplantation: risk factors and management. *J Heart Lung Transplant* 2004:23(5S): S187–S193.
52. Schmid C, Heemann U, Tilney NL. Factors contributing to the development of chronic rejection in heterotopic rat heart transplantation. *Transplantation* 1997;64(2):222–228.
53. Kaufman DB, Shapiro R, Lucey MR, et al. Immunosuppression: practice and trends. *Am J Transplant* 2004;4(suppl 9):38–53.
54. Pierson RN 3rd. Tolerance after heart transplantation: the Holy Grail, or an attainable goal? *Heart Fail Clin* 2007;3(1):17–29.
55. Marks WH, Wagner D, Pearson TC, et al. Organ donation and utilization, 1995–2004: entering the collaborative era. *Am J Transplant* 2006;6(5): 1101–1110.
56. Shafer TJ, Wagner D, Chessare J, et al. US organ donation breakthrough collaborative increases organ donation. *Crit Care Nurse Q* 2008;31(3): 190–210.
57. Rose EA, Gelijns AC, Moskowitz AJ, et al. Long-term mechanical left ventricular assistance for end-stage heart failure. *N Engl J Med* 2001;345(20): 1435–1443.
58. Cooper DKC, Keogh AM, Brink J, et al. Report of the Xenotransplantation Advisory Committee of the International Society for Heart and Lung Transplantation: the present status of xenotransplantation and its potential role in the treatment of end-stage cardiac and pulmonary diseases. *J Heart Lung Transplant* 2000;19:1125–1165.
59. Cooper DKC, Dorling A, Rees M, et al. α1,3-galactosyltransferase gene-knockout pigs: where do we go from here? *Transplantation* 2007;84(1):1–7.
60. Evans RW. Socioeconomic aspects of heart transplantation. *Curr Opin Cardiol* 1995;10(2):169–179.
61. Evans RW. The economics of big game hunting: using a rifle to get a clear shot at transplantation. *Transplantation* 75(10):1626–1627.
62. Weaver TA, Charafeddine AH, Kirk AD. Costimulation blockade: towards clinical application. *Front Biosci* 2008;13:2120–2139.
63. Matthews JB, Ramos E, Bluestone JA. Clinical trials of transplant tolerance: slow but steady progress. *Am J Transplant* 2003;3(7):794–803.
64. Cozzi E, White DJ. The generation of transgenic pigs as potential organ donors for humans. *Nat Med* 1995;1(9):964–966.
65. McGregor CG, Davies WR, Oi K, et al. Cardiac xenotransplantation: recent preclinical progress with 3-month median survival. *J Thorac Cardiovasc Surg* 2005;130(3):844–851.
66. Kuwaki K, Tseng YL, Dor FJMF, et al. Transplantation of hearts from α1,3-galactosyl-transferase gene-knockout (GalT-KO) pigs into baboons. *Nat Med* 2005;11:29–31.
67. Zaidi A, Schmoeckel M, Bhatti F, et al. Life-supporting pig-to-primate renal xenotransplantation using genetically modified donors. *Transplantation* 1998;65(12):1584–1590.
68. Schmoeckel M, Bhatti FN, Zaidi A, et al. Orthotopic heart transplantation in a transgenic pig-to-primate model. *Transplantation* 1998;65(12): 1570–1577.

CHAPTER 38 ■ PULMONARY TRANSPLANTATION

RAJA S. MAHIDHARA, JULES LIN, AND ANDREW C. CHANG

KEY POINTS

1. Long-term survival after lung transplant is lower in comparison to outcomes in the transplantation of other solid organs. The lack of effective medical therapy for acute and chronic rejection remains a barrier.
2. Candidates for pulmonary transplantation have significant functional impairment that interferes with activities of daily living. In patients with restrictive or obstructive disease, abnormal gas exchange is the major problem and essentially all require supplemental oxygen. In patients with pulmonary vascular disease, the manifestations of right ventricular failure predominate.
3. A paradigm shift in the allocation of donor lungs has decreased lung waitlist times and waitlist mortality. The effect of the Lung Allocation Score on short-term and long-term mortality remains to be seen.
4. Advances in donor management and lung preservation have been shown (a) to minimize lung injury, (b) to increase the number and quality of recoverable donor lungs, and (c) likely to be responsible for the dramatic increase in the number of lung transplants performed over the last 10 years.
5. It is believed that posttransplant lung injury results not only from the ischemic insult and the host immunologic response but also from reperfusion of the ischemic organ and other mediators of non–alloimmune-related injury.
6. Airway anastomotic healing remains a concern following transplantation but has been ameliorated by improvements in operative technique and postoperative management.
7. By the end of the first year after transplantation, approximately 80% of recipients report no limitations in activity.

INTRODUCTION

1 With nearly 18,000 lungs implanted, pulmonary transplantation comprises only 4% of the organs transplanted in the United States between 1988 and 2008. Since the first lung transplant was performed in 1963,[1] outcomes for this operation have improved dramatically, but even with advances in immunosuppression, surgical technique, and perioperative and posttransplant care, long-term survival following pulmonary transplantation remains less than that of other solid organ transplant recipients. The major problems limiting durable pulmonary transplantation have been infection, acute rejection, impaired anastomotic healing,[2] and chronic rejection, manifested in lung transplant recipients as the onset of bronchiolitis obliterans.[3]

In the lung, unlike other solid organs, systemic arterial blood supply is limited to the bronchial arteries. Because the bronchial artery anatomy and caliber vary greatly, most transplant surgeons have not advocated reanastomosis of these vessels primarily to avoid prolonged total organ ischemia time, particularly when bilateral sequential transplantation is planned. Consequently, the bronchial anastomosis is more profoundly ischemic after transplantation and susceptible to airway dehiscence, typically within 3 weeks after transplantation. The combination of anastomotic ischemia and other factors such as infection and post-reperfusion edema hampered initial efforts to develop successful clinical programs in pulmonary transplantation.

The first combined heart and lung transplantation was performed successfully in 1981, but this procedure currently is rarely performed, with only 50 or fewer performed annually in the United States since 2000. Combined cardiac and pulmonary transplantation introduced a series of new problems related to transplanting two organs, including those associated with heart transplantation, especially accelerated coronary artery atherosclerosis. Tracheal anastomotic healing presents less of a problem, possibly because the bronchial artery collaterals in the subcarinal space are preserved. The discrepancy between available organ donors and the increasing number of patients on the waiting list for either heart or lung transplantation as well as the observation that both short- and intermediate-term survival appears to be worse among heart–lung transplant recipients than among individuals receiving one or the other thoracic organ likely are major factors mitigating against widespread use of heart–lung transplantation.

Recognizing the potential advantage of single-lung transplantation, investigators experimentally defined the factors contributing to failure in pulmonary transplantation.[4] They demonstrated the significant detrimental effect that corticosteroids exert on airway healing and showed that cyclosporine did not have this adverse effect. Delaying the administration of maintenance corticosteroids proved advantageous. It was later suggested that wrapping the bronchial anastomosis with a pedicle of gastrocolic omentum resulted in early capillary ingrowth and revascularization of the airway promoting healing, although this practice has not correlated with a reduction in anastomotic dehiscence.[5]

Another significant factor contributing to the improved success of single-lung transplantation was the recognition of the importance of careful recipient selection. Most early attempts at pulmonary transplantation involved severely ill, ventilator-dependent patients who had already suffered significant nutritional depletion and muscle wasting. It then became apparent that a more suitable candidate for single-lung transplantation was an individual with end-stage restrictive disease (pulmonary fibrosis), in which the allograft would receive preferential ventilation and perfusion due to increased compliance and relatively decreased pulmonary vascular resistance in the transplanted lung. Ultimately, the importance of assessing preoperative ambulatory status and of implementing intense pretransplantation pulmonary rehabilitation was recognized. Thorough patient evaluation and preparation in addition to advances in both operative techniques and immunosuppression have broadened considerably the indications for pulmonary transplantation.

As lung transplantation has become accepted more widely in the treatment of patients with end-stage lung diseases, the increasing disparity between donor organ availability and patients listed for transplantation has resulted in increasing waitlist mortality. Initial lung allocation policies were based on ABO blood type compatibility, geographic proximity to the organ donor hospital, and the amount of accumulated waiting time since listing. In 1998, the Final Rule was issued by the U.S. Department of Health and Human Services requiring increased organ sharing and development of an organ allocation system that would be more equitable and that would reduce the use of waitlist time as a criterion for allocation. In developing an allocation system, the chief priority of the Organ Procurement and Transplantation Network (OPTN) was "to reduce the number of deaths among potential and actual lung transplant candidates."[6] In 2005, based on analyses performed by the Lung Allocation Subcommittee of the OPTN Thoracic Organ Transplantation Committee, the Lung Allocation Score (LAS) was implemented to address the points of the Final Rule, incorporating waiting list mortality and posttransplant survival probabilities, in order to minimize waiting list mortality, increase the benefit of transplantation among recipients, and ensure equitable allocation of lungs to lung transplantation candidates.[6] Although the impact on long-term survival remains undetermined, since implementation of the LAS (spring 2005), as indicated in the 2007 OPTN/Scientific Registry of Transplant Recipients (SRTR) Annual Report 1997–2006 (Health and Human Services [HHS]/Health Resources and Services Administration [HRSA]/Healthcare Systems Bureau [HSB]/Division of Transplantation [DOT]), there has been a dramatic reduction in the duration of median waiting list time prior to transplantation, from 792 days in 2004 to 199 and 132 days in 2005 and 2006, respectively.[7] In addition, waiting list mortality has declined from 134.6 per 1,000 patient-years in 2004 to 114.9 per 1,000 patient-years and 97.2 per 1,000 patient-years in 2005 and 2006, respectively.

INDICATIONS

2 Transplantation is indicated for patients with isolated organ dysfunction who have limited life expectancy despite maximal medical therapy. A patient should be referred for lung transplantation when expected survival after transplant exceeds the expected survival without transplantation. While this may seem like an obvious statement, validated data are limited with respect to the natural history of even the more common subtypes of end-stage lung disease categories including emphysema/chronic obstructive pulmonary disease (COPD), fibrotic or interstitial lung disease such as interstitial pulmonary fibrosis (IPF), or infectious lung disease, particularly cystic fibrosis. In addition, substantive changes in patient selection, operative techniques, organ preservation, immunosuppression, and other aspects of posttransplant management have led to progressively better survival after transplantation over the last 18 years.

Since the overall median survival after transplantation is approximately 5 years, the timing of transplant is an important consideration for maximizing transplant benefit. Prior to May 2005, allocation of donor lungs was based on time on the waiting list. With the large discrepancy between the number of listed transplant candidates and the limited availability of donor lungs, referral for transplant often occurred well before patients had become severely debilitated from poor respiratory function.

Lung transplantation can provide considerable palliation for dyspnea. Due to the limited availability of donors, quality-of-life improvement has been considered secondary to survival benefit, although improved outcomes in terms of factors such as oxygen dependence, physical activity, and return to work remain important in assessing the success of pulmonary transplantation.

CONTRAINDICATIONS

Table 38.1 lists absolute and relative contraindications to lung transplant. The absolute contraindications are self-explanatory and consistent with the risks associated with immunosuppression and the physical and social rigors of maintaining a complex medical regimen after transplantation of any organ. With respect to body mass index (BMI), extremes in weight have been shown to confer lower short-term survival in heart transplant patients.[8] These findings have been reinforced by studies of lung transplantation where extremes in BMI have been shown to confer a three- to fivefold increase in 90-day mortality.[9,10]

Overall survival for patients over the age of 65 is significantly lower than younger cohorts.[11] Despite this, the number of transplants in older patients has increased from less than 1% prior to 1994 to approximately 5% since 2000. Single-institution studies have demonstrated equivalent short- and intermediate-term survival in highly selected older patients.[12,13]

Convalescence after lung transplant can be particularly grueling. Postoperative incisional pain, impaired ventilatory mechanics, malnutrition, and deconditioning impact directly on lung function as with any pulmonary operation. In the earlier eras of lung transplantation, ventilator-dependent, malnourished patients or those with immune suppression–related myopathy and osteoporosis experienced very poor survival. Recipients had marked improvement in survival in the late 1980s and early 1990s due to the recognized value of preoperative pulmonary rehabilitation and improved selection of

TABLE 38.1 INDICATIONS/CONTRAINDICATIONS

CONTRAINDICATIONS TO LUNG TRANSPLANTATION

ABSOLUTE CONTRAINDICATIONS
Recent malignancy other than nonmelanoma skin cancer
End-stage extrapulmonary organ dysfunction (i.e., cirrhosis, dialysis-dependent renal insufficiency)
Active sepsis
Active HIV infection
Active hepatitis B or C infection with histologic evidence of liver damage
Current or recent tobacco use
History of alcohol or drug abuse/addiction
Severe psychiatric illness
History of noncompliance with medical therapies
Malnutrition (BMI <18)
RELATIVE CONTRAINDICATIONS
Age >65
Debilitation (6-minute hall walk <150 meters)
Mechanical ventilation
Extrapulmonary organ dysfunction
Coronary artery disease
Gastroesophageal reflux disease
Osteoporosis
Poorly controlled chronic medical conditions (e.g., diabetes, hypertension)
Chronic high-dose steroid dependence
Chest or spinal deformity
Obesity (BMI >32)
Severe pleural disease including empyema, fungal infection, and pleurodesis
Chronic infection with HIV or hepatitis B or C

BMI, body mass index; HIV, human immunodeficiency virus.

TABLE 38.2 INDICATIONS/CONTRAINDICATIONS

DISEASE-SPECIFIC CONSIDERATIONS FOR LUNG TRANSPLANTATION

COPD
BODE index >7 or hospitalization for exacerbation with hypercapnia (PCO_2 >50 mm Hg)
Pulmonary hypertension
FEV_1 <20% and either DLCO <20% or non–upper-lobe-predominant emphysema
IPF
Histologic or radiographic evidence of UIP and
DLCO <39%
>10% decrease in FVC on 6-month follow-up
SaO_2 <88% during a 6-min walk test
"Honeycombing" on HRCT (fibrosis score ≥2)
CF
FEV_1 <30% or rapid decline in FEV_1 on follow-up
Exacerbation requiring ICU stay
Increasing frequency of exacerbations
Refractory or recurrent pneumothorax
Increasing oxygen requirements
Hypercapnia
Pulmonary hypertension
PAH
NYHA class III or IV on maximal therapy
Low or declining 6-min walk test
Cardiac index <2.0
Right atrial pressure >15

BODE, *b*ody mass, airflow *o*bstruction, degree of *d*yspnea, and *e*xercise tolerance; CF, cystic fibrosis; DLCO, carbon monoxide diffusing capacity; FEV_1, forced expiratory volume in 1 second; HRCT, high-resolution computed tomography; IPF, interstitial pulmonary fibrosis; NYHA, New York Heart Association; PAH, pulmonary artery hypertension; UIP, usual interstitial pneumonia.
Taken from Orens JB, Estenne M, Arcasoy S, et al. International guidelines for the selection of lung transplant candidates: 2006 update—a consensus report from the Pulmonary Scientific Council of the International Society for Heart and Lung Transplantation. *J Heart Lung Transplant* 2006;25(7):745–755.

ambulatory patients. Pulmonary transplantation still may be suitable in highly selected nonambulatory or ventilator-dependent patients as demonstrated in small single-center series[14] including patients who have had rapid deterioration in lung function and who have had only brief periods of debilitation. Although patients with end-stage extrapulmonary organ dysfunction are not candidates for lung transplant, limited experience has demonstrated acceptable survival in patients with surgically or percutaneously correctable coronary artery disease.[15]

Disease-Specific Indications

Disease-specific indications for lung transplantation are listed in Table 38.2.

Chronic Obstructive Pulmonary Disease. COPD is the most common indication for lung transplantation, accounting for 51% of single-lung and 37% of bilateral lung transplants since 1995.[11] Advances in the medical therapy of patients with emphysema that can prolong survival include smoking cessation, long-acting bronchodilators, oxygen supplementation, optimization of nutrition, pulmonary rehabilitation, and vaccination for pneumonia and influenza. In addition, lung volume reduction surgery has been shown to confer survival benefit in patients with upper lobe–predominant disease, impaired exercise capacity, and the absence of high-risk factors including forced expiratory volume in 1 second (FEV_1) less than 20% or carbon monoxide diffusing capacity (DLCO) less than 20%.[16] Referral for transplantation should occur for patients who deteriorate despite maximal therapy and who are not candidates for lung volume reduction.

Factors associated with poor survival in patients with COPD include respiratory exacerbation with hypercapnia, hypoxia, pulmonary hypertension, increasing age, decreasing FEV_1, decreasing DLCO, and increased BMI.[17] A prospectively validated index based on *b*ody mass, airflow *o*bstruction, degree of *d*yspnea, and *e*xercise tolerance (BODE) has been proposed as a robust predictor of mortality in patients with COPD. A BODE index of greater than 7 on a scale from 0 to 10 was associated with a median survival of 3 years.[18]

Idiopathic Pulmonary Fibrosis. Usual interstitial pneumonia (UIP) is the pathologic correlate of IPF and is the most common subtype of interstitial pneumonia. Pulmonary fibrosis has been the second most common indication for lung transplantation, accounting for 28% of single-lung transplants and 14% of bilateral lung transplants since 1995.[11] In 2006, IPF accounted for 32% of all lung transplants performed.

Although the options for effective medical therapy of patients with IPF are limited and patient mortality is high with median survival of 3 to 4 years following diagnosis, patients experience a varying clinical course, with some patients progressing rapidly and others following a more indolent deterioration. Risk factors for poor survival include a pathologic diagnosis of UIP (vs. other type of interstitial pneumonia), severe fibrosis by high-resolution computed tomography, the presence and severity of pulmonary hypertension, and acute pulmonary exacerbations.

Assessment of pulmonary function and exercise capacity also can be used to identify subgroups of patients with pulmonary fibrosis at higher risk for mortality. A baseline DLCO of less than 39% and greater than 10% decrement of DLCO or forced vital capacity (FVC) over a 6- to 12-month period are associated with an increased risk of death.[19,20] Oxygen desaturation and shorter walk distance during 6-minute walk testing independently predicted increased mortality in patients diagnosed with pulmonary fibrosis.[21]

Cystic Fibrosis/Bronchiectasis/Infection-related End-stage Lung Disease. Cystic fibrosis (CF) is the third most common indication for lung transplantation, accounting for 20% of lung transplants performed in 2006, with most recipients undergoing bilateral transplantation.[11] Colonization of the airway with resistant organisms is common in these patients and is not an absolute contraindication to transplantation, although overt sepsis is an absolute contraindication to transplantation. Single-institution studies have identified colonization with *Burkholderia cepacia* genomovar III (redesignated as *Burkholderia cenocepacia*) to be associated with a 30% to 40% increase in posttransplant mortality, although this finding has not been validated in a multi-institutional setting.

Among patients with pulmonary disease due to cystic fibrosis, the time course of respiratory deterioration is highly variable. As a consequence, the criteria for pulmonary transplantation in this population have been difficult to define by risk modeling, although deterioration of FEV_1 to below 30% of predicted remains an indication for referral to evaluation, although not for immediate listing.[22,23] Other factors to consider include increasing oxygen requirement, hypercapnia, and pulmonary hypertension.[24]

Pulmonary Artery Hypertension. Idiopathic pulmonary artery hypertension (PAH) has a median survival of less than 3 years if untreated. Although a more common indication for transplantation in the past, effective medical therapies including vasodilator therapy and continuous intravenous epoprostenol have prolonged survival in this population. Patients with a history of right heart failure or poor pretreatment functional status and those who, despite vasodilator therapy, have demonstrated either no response or functional deterioration should be referred for pulmonary transplantation. Modern guidelines emphasize progressive deterioration of right heart function despite maximal medical therapy as an appropriate indication for referral.[24] Patients with left ventricular heart failure requiring inotropic support may not be suitable candidates for pulmonary transplantation alone but instead should be considered for en bloc heart–lung transplantation.

LUNG ALLOCATION AND TRANSPLANT BENEFIT

3 Perhaps the most significant change in the practice of lung transplantation over the last 10 years has been a paradigm shift in the process of donor allocation. Prior to 2005, recipients were prioritized by length of time spent on the waiting list as well as other factors including size, ABO compatibility, and geographic location. In compliance with the Final Rule mandate of 1998 to allocate organs based on urgency (risk of dying without a transplant) and utility (minimizing transplantation of patients with low transplant survival), the Lung Allocation Score was developed by the Thoracic Committee of the OPTN.

Prior existing data to determine transplant benefit were conflicting. An analysis of all transplant patients with COPD, IPF, and CF from 1992 to 1994 demonstrated a survival benefit for patients with IPF and CF but not with COPD.[25] A similarly powered analysis of the European transplant experience demonstrated survival benefit for all lung transplant groups.[26] Recent studies also had called into question the transplant benefit for children with cystic fibrosis listed between 1992 and 2002 for pulmonary transplantation.[27] In this latter study, evaluating patients listed before implementation of the new LAS system, over half of the patients had a predicted median survival of greater than 5 years at the time of operation.

Egan et al. for the SRTR[6] analyzed over 4,000 patients on the UNOS lung transplant waiting list in order to identify markers of waitlist mortality. The listing diagnoses for these patients—COPD, IPF, CF, and PAH—accounted for 80% of the transplants performed at the time. Striking differences in waitlist mortality were noted, with patients listed for emphysematous diseases experiencing a 1-year waitlist mortality of less than 14% compared with 1-year waitlist mortality between 28% and 33% among patients listed with the other three primary diagnoses. Transplant candidate demographics, hemodynamic parameters, measures of pulmonary function, and other clinical variables were used to create a regression model. Similarly, a predictive model for posttransplant survival was developed. When these models were applied to evaluate survival in 2,484 patients with the aforementioned four primary diagnoses, factors including increasing recipient age, intensive care unit (ICU) admission, and need for mechanical ventilation were significant predictors for 1-year survival. Variables included in the LAS calculator are listed in Table 38.3. The normalized

TABLE 38.3 **STAGING**

SELECTED COMPONENTS OF THE LUNG ALLOCATION SCORE

Age
Diagnosis code
Functional status
Diabetes
Assisted ventilation
Supplemental oxygen
FVC% predicted
PA systolic
PA mean
PA wedge
PCO_2
Highest
Lowest
Change %
Six-min walk
Creatinine

FVC, forced vital capacity; PA, pulmonary artery.
http://www.unos.org/resources/frm_LAS_Calculator.asp

TRANSPLANTATION

lung allocation score ranges from 0 (lowest priority) to 100 (highest priority) with the intent of balancing urgency (waitlist mortality) and benefit (posttransplantation survival).

The LAS has been implemented for over 4 years and has had a clear impact on outcomes in lung transplantation. The number of active waitlist patients has declined by 54% as early listing confers no advantage. Waiting time to transplantation has decreased from 792 days in 2004 to 141 days in 2007. Death rates on the waiting list have been consistently declining over the past decade and have continued to decrease since implementation of the LAS. The death rate did not, however, decline as much as might be expected, possibly as a consequence of an overall increase in the acuity of the waiting list.

Overall early survival (30-day and 1-year) has enjoyed a slow but steady improvement since 1995, which has carried through the implementation of the LAS in 2005. The impact of the LAS on intermediate- and long-term outcomes is not yet evaluable. An increasing LAS score, however, is associated with lower 1-year survival. Transplanted patients with an LAS score less than 35 had a 1-year survival of 85.7%, whereas those with an LAS score greater than 60 had a 1-year survival of 71.3%.[28] The impact of the LAS on maximizing transplant benefit is not clear at this time. Reevaluation and revision of the criteria that determine the LAS remains one of the objectives of the Thoracic Organ Transplantation Committee of the OPTN.

DONOR CONSIDERATIONS

Donor Selection

The shortage of acceptable donors for lung transplantation is highlighted by the observation that although the number of lung transplants has steadily increased (1,465 in 2007) and waitlist times and waitlist death rates have decreased, the total number of registrants on the wait list has remained the same.[28] The reasons that fewer lungs are offered or accepted compared to other organs is manifold. Death from head injury or bleeding may lead to neurogenic pulmonary edema, while chest trauma can result in contusion or pneumothorax. All brain-dead donors are intubated and at risk for aspiration and nosocomial pneumonia, especially if there is a prolonged interval between hospitalization and declaration of brain death. Finally, hemodynamic instability, whether from herniation or trauma, often results in significant volume resuscitation that can contribute to acute lung injury.

Bronchoscopy allows for direct examination of the bronchial tree and for microbiologic examination of bronchial secretions, the results of which may influence later treatment of the recipient. Chest radiography and computed tomography are useful to evaluate for effusions or pulmonary infiltrates, consolidation, and contusion that might be contributing to donor hypoxemia. Unlike other solid organ transplants, lungs are unique in carrying a relatively high risk of intrinsic infection (i.e., pneumonia) following transplant. Infiltrates typically preclude donor candidacy. A small infiltrate in one lung without evidence of purulent secretions may still allow this lung to be used in conjunction with a contralateral normal lung in a bilateral lung transplant. Moreover, a pulmonary infiltrate does not necessarily preclude use of the contralateral lung for single-lung transplant.[29] Not infrequently, the lungs of a particular donor may not be suitable because of infiltrates when all other organs are acceptable. Because all brain-dead patients have endotracheal tubes and are on mechanical ventilation, there is a high likelihood that the airway is either colonized with bacteria or that there is ongoing invasive pulmonary infection. With pulmonary infection, an infiltrate often is present on the screening chest radiograph.

Aspiration at the time of the insult that resulted in brain death is a common cause of pulmonary infiltrates in potential donors. Signs of aspiration may not be evident on a chest radiograph for 24 to 48 hours, underscoring the importance of the bronchoscopic examination when evaluating donor candidacy. Characteristic early bronchoscopic evidence of aspiration includes erythematous tracheobronchial mucosa, purulent secretions, and occasionally the presence of food particles.

Major pulmonary contusion resulting from blunt chest trauma also may eliminate lungs from donor consideration, but minor to moderate contusions unilaterally are often acceptable. Evaluating the full extent of contusion at the time of donor retrieval can be difficult because the interval from injury to determination of brain death and donation may be short. Although the detrimental effect on gas exchange caused by a pulmonary contusion is usually transient, further bleeding into the lung parenchyma could occur if cardiopulmonary bypass is required to perform the transplantation. Pulmonary edema may occur as a result of massive head injury and may be exacerbated by donor management protocols directed at maintaining satisfactory nonpulmonary organ perfusion and function.

The well-recognized limitation of donor organ availability is compounded by the relatively fewer usable lungs per donor. Criteria for an acceptable donor lung are particularly stringent, as listed in Table 38.4.[30] This consensus statement highlights the dearth of data available to validate these criteria. Multiple single-institution retrospective reports looking at "extended criteria" donors (those who do not meet one or more ideal criterion) have been published with conflicting results on nearly every single criterion with respect to postoperative, short, and long-term outcomes. Clinically, these selection criteria provide an overall gestalt of the quality of the donor. If one aspect of the donor is marginal, the donor lungs can still be acceptable; however, when multiple criteria are not met, the risk of transplanting such lungs might be increased. There are several caveats that have come into "standard" practice. Although leukocytes or occasional bacteria on sputum Gram stain can be acceptable, the presence of gross pus or fungal elements confers a high risk of perioperative complications.[31] In the annual report of lung transplant outcomes, increasing donor age modestly increased the risk of 5-year mortality.[11] Analysis of a large cohort of more than 750 lung and heart–lung recipients demonstrated significantly worse long-term survival with ischemic times greater than 330 minutes. Hazard ratios for death were threefold higher in patients with ischemic times of 8 hours and nearly eightfold higher when ischemia reached 10 hours.[32] The detrimental effects of older donor age and longer ischemic times appear to be additive.[33]

TABLE 38.4 **MANAGEMENT**

CRITERIA FOR IDEAL LUNG DONORS

Age <55y
ABO compatibility
Height match within 20% of recipient
Clear chest radiograph
PaO_2 >300 on FiO_2 of 1.0, PEEP 5 cm H_2O
Tobacco history of <20 y
Absence of chest trauma
No evidence of aspiration or pulmonary sepsis
No previous cardiothoracic surgery
Negative sputum Gram stain
Absence of purulent secretions

PEEP, positive end-expiratory pressure.

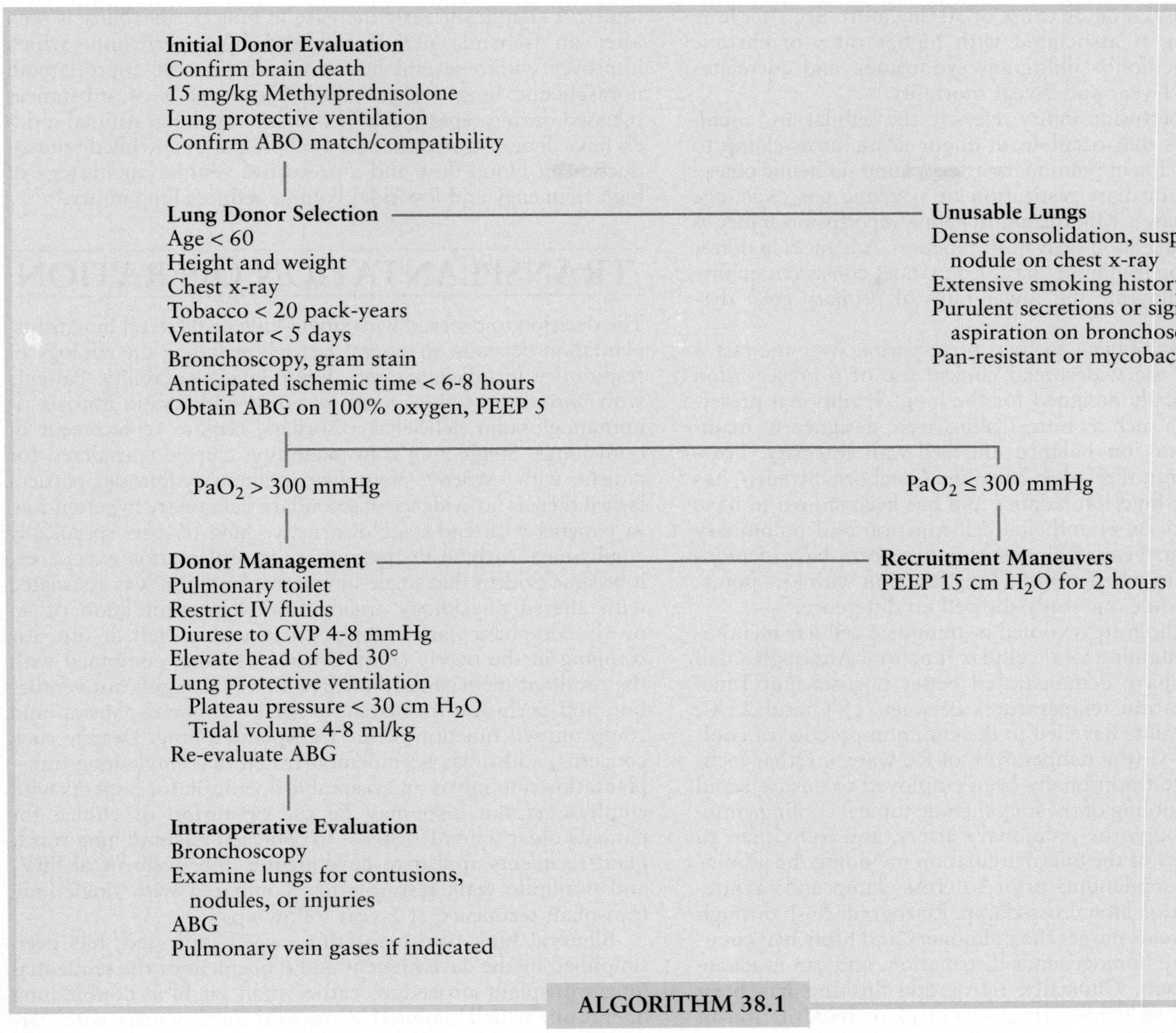

ALGORITHM 38.1. University of Michigan donor management algorithm.

Donor Management

4 Despite the inability to identify "extended" donor criteria that reliably provide acceptable grafts, donor management optimization has allowed an increase in donor recovery and is likely responsible for the increase in the overall number of transplants performed over the last decade. Algorithm 38.1 outlines the donor management algorithm used at the University of Michigan. Key principles include the early use of steroids and thyroxine to prevent neurogenic pulmonary edema and to maintain cardiovascular stability, alveolar recruitment with high positive end-expiratory pressure (PEEP) and aggressive endotracheal lavage for patients with partial pressure of arterial oxygen (PaO_2) less than 300 mm Hg, optimization of intravascular volume, maneuvers to prevent aspiration, and lung-protective ventilation utilizing high frequency, low tidal volumes, and high PEEP to prevent volutrauma and barotrauma to the lungs. These maneuvers have been shown to double the organ recovery rate without detrimental effects on 30-day or 1-year survival.[34] The presence of a dense infiltrate or purulent secretions in one lung does not preclude the use of the contralateral lung for single-lung transplant.

Investigators at the Texas Organ Sharing Alliance identified 330 potential lung donors over a 4-year period preceding initiation of an active donor management protocol and 381 potential donors managed on the protocol in the subsequent 4 years.[34] Overall, 1.7 organs per donor were procured in 19% (136/711) of potential donors. Prior to initiation of the management protocol, organ procurement occurred in only 12% (38/330), recovering 1.6 lungs per donor. In contrast, with lung-protective donor management, organ procurement occurred in 26% (98/381), recovering 1.7 organs per donor.

Following initial organ acceptance, the lungs are declined when the procurement team identifies significant purulent secretions during bronchoscopy or when arterial blood gases deteriorate significantly between the time of acceptance and when the procuring team reassesses the donor upon arrival at the donor hospital. On-site measurement of pulmonary vein blood gases at the time of donor sternotomy can aid the procuring team in determining whether donor hypoxemia is due to unilateral or bilateral organ compromise.[35] Size of the donor lungs is less important when the recipient suffers from emphysema, in which each hemithorax is very large, compared with pulmonary fibrosis, in which the hemithorax can be significantly contracted. The most important size consideration is a reasonable match between donor and recipient height.

Lung Preservation

Unlike the kidney, liver, or pancreas, immediate acceptable function of the transplanted lung is vital for survival of the recipient. Primary graft dysfunction occurs in 10% to 25% of cases, is the most common cause of 30-day mortality after lung transplantation, is associated with higher rates of chronic rejection (bronchiolitis obliterans syndrome), and correlates with increased 1-year and 5-year mortality.[36]

Ischemia-reperfusion injury refers to the cellular and architectural changes that occur from donor aortic cross-clamp to release of the recipient pulmonary artery clamp (ischemic phase) through the immediate restitution of systemic gas exchange (reperfusion phase). Minimizing ischemia-reperfusion injury is crucial in ensuring good early graft function. Advances in donor lung preservation techniques have led to more consistent quality of the donor allograft and lower rates of primary graft dysfunction.

A major development in lung preservation over the last 5 years has been the widespread clinical use of a preservation solution specifically designed for the lung. Traditional preservation solutions such as Euro-Collins were designed to maintain intracellular ion balance and cell-wall integrity. Low-potassium dextran (Perfadex, Vitrolife, Goteborg, Sweden) has an extracellular fluid ion balance and has been shown to have beneficial effects on endothelial cell function and pulmonary microcirculation. Five single-institution reports have demonstrated significantly better initial lung function with low-potassium dextran, while one study showed no difference.[37]

The donor allograft is cooled to minimize cellular metabolism while maintaining vital cellular function. Although small animal studies have demonstrated better postischemic function at preservation temperatures between 15°C and 23°C, practical constraints have led to the common practice of cooling to 4°C to 8°C (the temperature of ice water). Other techniques that have traditionally been employed to ensure rapid homogeneous cooling of the lung include topical cooling, antegrade flush through the pulmonary artery, and techniques to maintain patency of the microcirculation including the administration of prostaglandins prior to cross-clamp and maintenance of ventilation after cross-clamp. Retrograde flush through the pulmonary veins purges the pulmonary and bronchial circulations, has more homogeneous distribution, and can evacuate clot or fat emboli. Clinically, retrograde flushing has been shown to improve immediate posttransplant oxygenation in combination with antegrade flush.[38]

Optimizing storage technique has also evolved. After flushing of the pulmonary circulation, the lungs are recruited to expand atelectatic areas and the trachea is stapled and divided prior to separation from the donor and storage for transport. Methods of lung recruitment have been studied in animal models and have shown that ventilation with less than 50% oxygen and maintenance of airway pressure between 15 and 20 cm H_2O have beneficial effects on capillary leak, lipid peroxidation, and barotrauma.[39–41]

5 It is believed that lung injury results not only from the ischemic insult but also from reperfusion of the ischemic organ. Several experimental models of acute lung injury implicate oxygen free radicals as a factor in the genesis of reperfusion injury. A significant early increase in lung permeability is seen after an ischemic period followed by reperfusion, which improves within several hours. Changes in the contralateral, nonischemic lung are presumably the result of substances released during reperfusion of the ischemic lung. Animal models have demonstrated that gradual pressure-controlled reintroduction of blood flow and a protective ventilation strategy of high frequency and low tidal volume reduces lung injury.[42,43]

TRANSPLANTATION OPERATION

The decision to proceed with single-lung or bilateral lung transplantation depends on several factors, including the etiology of respiratory insufficiency and donor lung availability. Patients with chronic infection, such as those with cystic fibrosis or immunoglobulin deficiency disorders, require replacement of both lungs. Single-lung transplantation can be considered for patients with restrictive physiology (pulmonary fibrosis), particularly if there is no evidence of secondary pulmonary hypertension. In patients with end-stage obstructive lung disease, specifically emphysema, early in the pulmonary transplantation experience, it became evident that single-lung transplantation was associated with altered physiology arising from hyperventilation of an overly compliant native emphysematous lung left in situ. Air trapping in the overly compliant native lung, combined with the resultant mediastinal shift, resulted in a significant ventilation and perfusion mismatch, as well as poor expansion and compromised function of the transplanted lung. Despite such concerns, it also has been demonstrated that single-lung transplantation not only is an acceptable operation for patients with emphysema but also may be the operation of choice for patients older than 50 years.[44] In contrast, bilateral lung transplant recipients appear to have greater improvement of FEV_1 and 6-minute walk testing when compared with single-lung transplant recipients, at 1-year follow-up.[45]

Bilateral lung transplantation, when indicated, has been simplified by the development and refinement of the sequential lung transplant procedure rather than en bloc double-lung operation, which required a tracheal anastomosis with cardiopulmonary bypass and resulted in significant perioperative cardiac morbidity and mortality.[46] Bilateral sequential lung transplant can be approached either by median sternotomy or bilateral thoracotomies and with or without cardiopulmonary bypass depending on the indication for transplantation. A bilateral thoracosternotomy incision ("clamshell") permits easier completion of the recipient pneumonectomies than median sternotomy, but the clamshell incision tends to be more painful. A candidate's past history of chest operations does not alone preclude eligibility for bilateral lung transplantation.

In patients with pulmonary hypertension, single-lung transplantation historically had been felt to be adequate to unload the right ventricle, reduce pulmonary artery pressure, and thus lead to improved right ventricular function (Table 38.5). Currently,

TABLE 38.5 **COMPLICATIONS**

TYPICAL HEMODYNAMICS DATA FOR SINGLE-LUNG TRANSPLANTATION IN PATIENTS WITH PULMONARY HYPERTENSION

■ MEASUREMENT	■ PRETRANSPLANT	■ POSTTRANSPLANT
Pulmonary artery pressure		
Mean	58 mm Hg	16 mm Hg
Systolic	94 mm Hg	28 mm Hg
Right ventricular ejection fraction	25%	52%
Cardiac output	4 L/min	7 L/min
Pulmonary vascular resistance	1,302 dyne/cm^5/s	161 dyne/cm^5/s

although no significant survival benefit is demonstrable between patients treated with single-lung, bilateral lung, or heart–lung transplantation, most patients receive predominantly bilateral sequential transplantation, unless there is evidence for inotrope-dependent heart failure.[47] Patients with pulmonary arterial hypertension listed for lung transplantation tend to be younger, and thus may be more likely to obtain more durable improvement in lung function following bilateral lung transplantation. In addition, perioperative management and improved hemodynamic performance appear to be facilitated by bilateral rather than single-lung transplantation. Although seemingly contradictory, bilateral lung transplantation for this population also might improve organ utilization, since marginal lungs likely are more readily available than a single "ideal" donor lung.

OPERATIVE TECHNIQUE

Single-lung Transplantation

The performance of the donor operation does not vary because one always attempts to use both lungs, either for single-lung replacement on two recipients or for distribution in another transplant medical center. This practice provides the most efficient use of limited donor organs. In the recipient operation, a standard fourth intercostal space posterolateral thoracotomy is performed. In patients with emphysematous disease, muscle-sparing axillary thoracotomy can be performed, but this approach might not afford suitable exposure for patients who have significant volume loss due to severe pulmonary fibrosis, previous thoracotomy, or pleurodesis. The hilar dissection (Fig. 38.1) differs from that of a pneumonectomy in that the main pulmonary artery should be mobilized and divided distal to the origin of the first segmental trunk and the pulmonary veins should be divided at the main segmental tributaries as they return to the superior or inferior veins. Care should be taken to preserve lymphatic and areolar tissue at the point of division of the mainstem bronchus in order to maintain its vascular supply. When the donor lung arrives in the operating room, the recipient pneumonectomy is performed by dividing the hilar vessels as far *distally* as possible and the bronchus at the level of the upper lobe take-off.

The implantation procedure begins with construction of an anastomosis between the donor and recipient bronchus. End-to-end anastomosis, with running suture approximation of the membranous airway and figure-of-eight suture approximation of the cartilaginous airway using monofilament absorbable suture, appears to reduce bronchial anastomotic complications and permits adjustment for potential donor–recipient size mismatch, particularly when completing the cartilaginous portion.[48,49] The peribronchial areolar and lymphatic tissue can be reapproximated between the donor and recipient, particularly anteriorly, in order to separate the bronchial and pulmonary arterial anastomoses. Advocates of bronchial arterial bypass with a native internal mammary have demonstrated decreased bronchial anastomotic complications in small series, but this technique has not received widespread acceptance.[50–52]

The vascular anastomoses are then performed sequentially using running nonabsorbable monofilament sutures. Our preference has been to first perform the pulmonary arterial anastomosis and then the left atrial anastomosis. The recipient left atrial cuff is typically prepared by cross-clamp of the left atrium and unifocalization of the branch pulmonary veins. Once the vascular anastomoses are constructed, clamps are removed and blood flow is reestablished as the lung is inflated, with care taken to de-air the left atrial anastomosis prior to securing the anastomotic suture line. The chest is closed in standard fashion. Either the right or left lung can be transplanted, and the decision of which side to transplant is based on both donor lung availability and recipient quantitative perfusion lung scan data. If one lung receives most of the perfusion, the opposite lung typically is transplanted.

Bilateral Lung Transplantation

The technique of double-lung transplantation has evolved considerably since the late 1980s from en bloc replacement to bilateral, sequential lung replacement.[46,53] With the patient in the supine position, this operation can be performed through sternotomy, bilateral thoracosternotomy (clamshell) incision (Fig. 38.2), bilateral anterior thoracotomies without sternal division, or bilateral muscle-sparing axillary thoracotomies. The bilateral thoracosternotomy incision provides the broadest exposure to the hemithoraces, facilitating dissection and mobilization of hilar structures. This exposure is particularly important in recipients with diffuse dense adhesions between the visceral and parietal pleural surfaces, as is often seen in patients with chronic infection and bronchiectasis, such as those with cystic fibrosis.

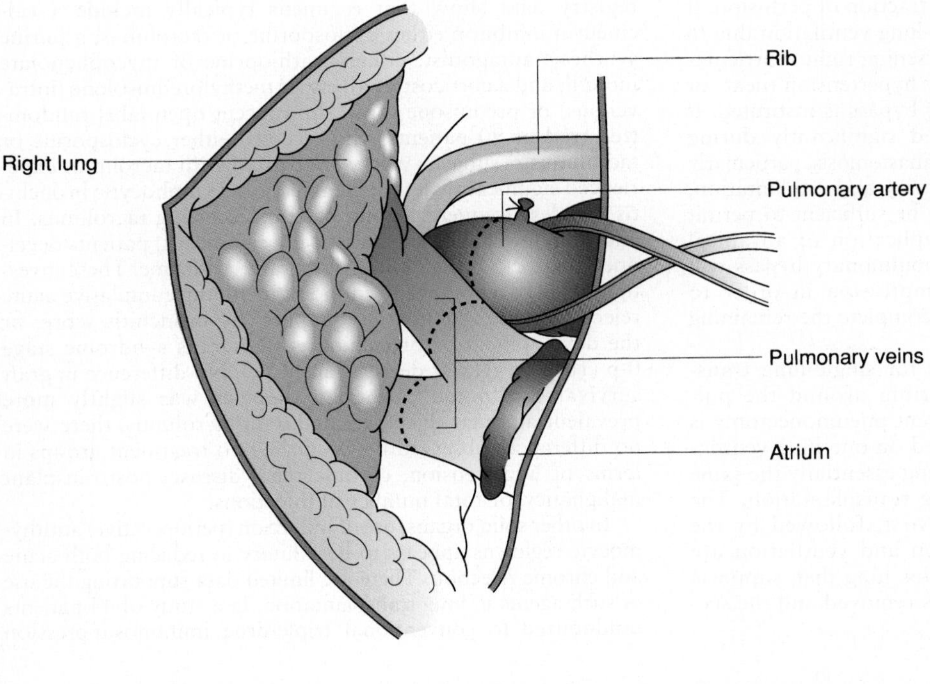

FIGURE 38.1. Mobilization of the hilum of the right lung demonstrating the encircled pulmonary artery with the first branch ligated and divided. The superior and inferior pulmonary veins have been exposed. Both the artery and veins are taken as close to the lung as possible. The bronchus is divided at the level of the take-off of the upper lobe.

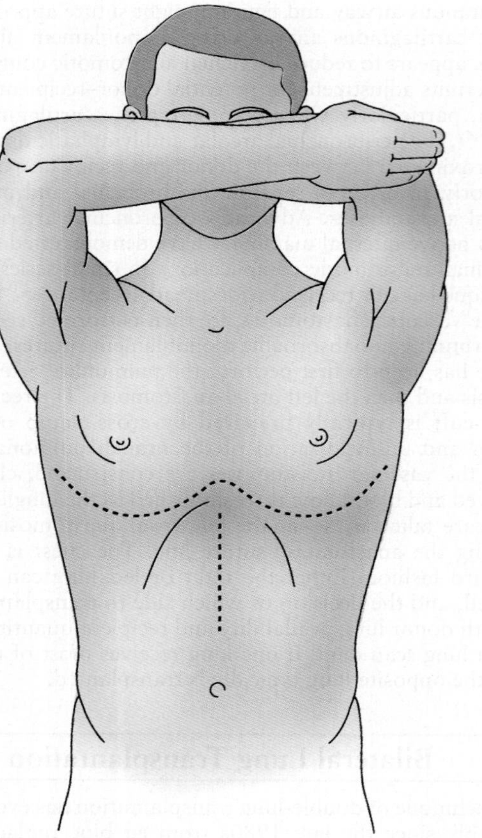

FIGURE 38.2. Patient positioning for bilateral, sequential pulmonary transplantation operation. The chest incision, a bilateral thoracosternotomy, is seen, as is the separate midline incision used to expose the omentum (if necessary). The sternum is divided transversely, and the fourth intercostal space on each side is entered.

Although both lungs are replaced, the operation often can be performed without cardiopulmonary bypass unless the recipient has significant pulmonary hypertension or severely limiting DLCO. By replacing the lung with the least function first, patient oxygenation and ventilation are maintained by the native lung that receives the major fraction of perfusion. If the patient is unable to tolerate single-lung ventilation due to either inadequate gas exchange or worsening right ventricular dysfunction and worsening pulmonary hypertension (near- or suprasystemic), then cardiopulmonary bypass is instituted. If recipient hemodynamics are impaired significantly during retraction and exposure of the left atrial anastomosis, particularly during left lung recipient pneumonectomy and implantation, opening the recipient pericardium can be sufficient to permit safe manual cardiac retraction or application of an apical cardiac stabilizer.[54] Initiation of cardiopulmonary bypass will also provide sufficient cardiac decompression in order to obtain adequate and safe exposure to complete the remaining anastomoses.

The donor lungs are separated as for single-lung transplantation, leaving a cuff of left atrium around the pulmonary veins on each side. The recipient pneumonectomy is carried out with the patient maintained on one-lung ventilation. Each donor lung is implanted using essentially the same technique as described for single-lung transplantation. The bronchial anastomosis is completed first, followed by the vascular anastomoses. Once perfusion and ventilation are restored to the first implanted lung, this lung then supports the patient while the remaining lung is removed and the second lung is implanted.

RESULTS

The Registry of the International Society of Heart and Lung Transplantation (ISHLT) has recorded 24,904 lung transplants between 1985 and 2006.[11] Currently, 147 centers actively perform lung transplants, but only 23 centers perform more than 30 per year. Of the 2,168 lung transplants performed captured by the ISHLT in 2006, over 67% of patients transplanted received bilateral lung transplants. The single most common indication for transplant was emphysema either as a result of α_1-antitrypsin deficiency (4% of cases) or idiopathy (32% of cases). Most of the so-called idiopathic cases of emphysema are related to cigarette smoking. Pulmonary fibrosis, the indication first treated successfully by lung transplantation, accounted for 26%, while cystic fibrosis accounted for 16%.

Overall, survival after transplant has steadily improved with time. In the era between 1988 and 1994, median survival was 3.9 years, while survival from 2000 to 2006 has increased to 5.5 years. In this most recent epoch of lung transplant, the overall 1-year survival rate following lung transplant is 81.4% and the 5-year survival is 53.5%. Patients receiving bilateral lung transplant survive significantly longer than patients after single-lung transplant (median survival of 6.2 vs. 4.5; $p < 0.0001$). In general, younger recipients enjoy longer survival than older patients. Patients with cystic fibrosis have the best median survival (6.4 years) as they comprise a younger population and in general will receive two lungs secondary to infectious lung disease. Median survival for patients with pulmonary fibrosis is significantly lower at 4.1 years, and that of patients with COPD is 5 years.

For all recipients, the factors associated with the highest risk of 1-year mortality were the era in which patients were transplanted, intravenous inotropes, and mechanical ventilation. The most significant risk factor, by far, for 5-year mortality was development of bronchiolitis obliterans syndrome within the first year of transplant.[11] Outcomes in lung transplant have clearly improved over time. The impact of changes in lung allocation in the United States on early and late outcomes remains to be seen.

IMMUNOSUPPRESSION

Immunosuppression is initiated in the immediate perioperative period and continued for the rest of the recipient's life. UNOS registry data show that regimens typically include a calcineurin inhibitor, either cyclosporine or tacrolimus; a purine synthesis antagonist, either azathioprine or mycophenolate mofetil; and a corticosteroid, either methylprednisolone (intravenous) or prednisone (oral). In a recent open-label randomized trial of 90 patients who received either cyclosporine or tacrolimus,[55] subjects who were treated with tacrolimus experienced significantly less acute rejection. Lymphocytic bronchitis was less frequent among patients receiving tacrolimus. In addition, fewer (but not statistically significant) patients developed stage 0-p bronchiolitis obliterans syndrome. These investigators used a composite endpoint including cumulative acute rejection score, cumulative lymphocytic bronchitis score, or the development of bronchiolitis obliterans syndrome stage 0-p (10% or greater decrease in FEV_1). No difference in graft survival was noted. Although diabetes was slightly more prevalent among subjects treated with tacrolimus, there were no differences observed between the two treatment groups in terms of hypertension, chronic renal disease, posttransplant malignancy, or total number of infections.

In other solid organs, use of induction (perioperative) antithymocyte regimens appears to be salutary in reducing both acute and chronic rejection. There are limited data supporting the use of such agents in lung transplantation. In a study of 44 patients randomized to conventional triple-drug immunosuppression with or without rabbit antithymocyte globulin, a significant reduction in early acute rejection from 41% to 5% was observed with the use of rabbit antithymocyte globulin, but there was no apparent effect on the total number of rejection episodes. Time to onset of bronchiolitis obliterans syndrome was earlier, and graft survival worse, with conventional treatment only, but these differences were not statistically significant. Several studies comparing antithymocyte globulin with T-cell–specific interleukin-2 (IL-2) receptor (CD25) monoclonal antibody suggest that outcomes, including early acute rejection and freedom from rejection, are equivalent[56] if not worse[57,58] for patients treated with IL-2–receptor antibody. Treatment-related complications, particularly cytomegalovirus infection, appear to be equivalent for these induction agents. These studies do not provide sufficient evidence, and likely lack sufficient power, to determine whether their use is beneficial for the prevention of acute or chronic rejection. Two important issues regarding standard immunosuppressive therapy are the myriad side effects associated with these agents and their numerous interactions with other commonly prescribed medications.[59]

Rapamycin (sirolimus) is a serine/threonine kinase inhibitor that can be used as a second-line agent for treatment of acute rejection, sometimes in combination with calcineurin inhibitors, but such use is considered off-label and not recommended. In addition, rapamycin is contraindicated absolutely in the early posttransplantation period because of its association with fatal bronchial anastomotic dehiscence.

COMPLICATIONS

Complications resulting from pulmonary transplantation occur frequently, may be severe, and occasionally result in death. Intraoperative complications include technical problems with the vascular or bronchial anastomoses, injury to the phrenic or recurrent laryngeal nerves, and myocardial infarction. Early postoperative complications include primary graft dysfunction, infection, and problems with airway healing and acute rejection. The most common late complications are infection and bronchiolitis obliterans (chronic rejection). Intra-abdominal complications are not uncommon. Wound infection is noted rarely. Noninfectious, nonpulmonary complications related to immunosuppression are common. The cumulative prevalence within 5 years after transplant of hypertension, renal insufficiency, hyperlipidemia, and diabetes is 85.3%, 37.0%, 53.6%, and 35.5%, respectively.[11] Finally, there is a three- to fourfold higher risk of malignancy in patients after transplant.[60]

Causes of recipient death can be categorized according to the time frame in which they occur. Early deaths (sooner than 30 days following transplant) most commonly result from primary graft failure (28.2%).[11] Infection is the second most common cause of early death (20.3%), followed by heart failure (11.1%). Rejection accounts for 4.3% of deaths in the early posttransplantation period. Hemorrhage and airway dehiscence each are responsible for 8.3% of early postoperative deaths. Infection accounts for about 39.5% of deaths within the first year of transplant (after 90 days). About one third of deaths result from manifestations of chronic rejection and obliterative bronchiolitis, the single biggest impediment to long-term survival following lung transplantation. Respiratory failure and malignancy are the next most common causes of late mortality. Despite the major strides made in the operation itself and early postoperative care, the complications resulting from chronic immunosuppression continue to plague transplant patients.

Primary Graft Dysfunction

Mild, transient pulmonary edema is a common feature of the freshly transplanted allograft. In approximately 15% of cases, the injury is sufficiently severe to cause a form of acute respiratory distress syndrome termed *primary graft failure*. Primary graft failure is presumed to reflect ischemia-reperfusion injury, but surgical trauma and lymphatic disruption may be contributing factors. The diagnosis rests on the presence of widespread infiltrates on chest radiographs, severe hypoxemia within 72 hours after transplantation, and the exclusion of other causes of graft dysfunction, such as volume overload, pneumonia, rejection, occlusion of the venous anastomosis, and aspiration. Treatment is supportive, relying principally on conventional mechanical ventilation. Independent lung ventilation, inhaled nitric oxide, and extracorporeal membrane oxygenation have been used as adjunctive measures. Mortality rates of up to 60% have been reported, and among those who survive, the recovery period is often protracted, but achievement of normal allograft function is possible. The results of emergency retransplantation in such cases have been poor.[59,61,62]

TABLE 38.6 **STAGING**

GRADING OF PRIMARY GRAFT DYSFUNCTION SEVERITY

■ GRADE	■ PaO_2/FiO_2	■ RADIOGRAPHIC INFILTRATE CONSISTENT WITH PULMONARY EDEMA
0	>300	Absent
1	>300	Present
2	200–300	Present
3	<200	Present

The impact of primary graft dysfunction on outcomes has been muddied by variability in the definition of this syndrome historically. A consensus statement by the ISHLT in 2005 sought to standardize the definition and severity of primary graft dysfunction (Table 38.6).[63] Studies examining outcome utilizing the current grading system have demonstrated a direct correlation with severity of primary graft dysfunction and ICU mortality, in-hospital mortality, 1-year survival, and freedom from bronchiolitis obliterans syndrome.[64,65]

Rejection

With few exceptions, acute rejection episodes occur soon after transplantation, usually between posttransplantation days 5 and 7. Often, two or three rejection episodes occur within the first month. Mild temperature elevation, perihilar fluffy infiltrates, or a minimal decrease in blood oxygenation as measured by arterial oxygen tension may herald rejection. Because rejection occurs so frequently during this period, the distinction between infection and rejection may be difficult. Often, the distinguishing factor between these two entities is that rejection responds positively to the administration of corticosteroids. Treatment of early rejection episodes involves the use of bolus corticosteroid administration given on 3 consecutive days. Within 12 to 18 hours after the first corticosteroid dose, symptoms relating to rejection usually resolve, including clearing of infiltrates on chest radiograph.

The diagnostic experience using transbronchial biopsy to diagnose and monitor rejection at some centers after cardiopulmonary transplantation is impressive, but the number of biopsies required to maximize specificity is large. One group recommends obtaining 18 separate transbronchial biopsy specimens to achieve 95% specificity. The risks and potential complications of transbronchial lung biopsy do not justify its routine performance because suspected rejection episodes respond so well to corticosteroids. Transbronchial lung biopsy can be used when the issue of rejection versus infection is not resolved after steroid administration. Flexible bronchoscopy can be performed at the bedside, and 6 to 10 separate biopsies can be obtained under fluoroscopic guidance. When symptoms or signs of rejection persist despite adequate treatment, open lung biopsy may be considered.

Infection

Infection in the posttransplantation period continues to be a significant cause of morbidity and mortality. Posttransplant prophylaxis strategies targeting gram-positive and gram-negative bacteria, *Pneumocystis pneumoniae*, cytomegalovirus, and *Aspergillus* have been shown to decrease the morbidity and mortality from this category of complication. Bacterial pneumonia usually responds to appropriate antibiotic therapy, and patients are maintained on broad-spectrum antibiotics until specificities are determined by culture of the donor and recipient bronchus. Antibiotic administration is particularly important if one predominant organism is grown from the donor lung cultures obtained at organ harvest. If a specific organism is grown from donor bronchial washings, the recipient is maintained on an appropriate antibiotic or combination of antibiotics for at least 1 week. The most common organism recovered from donor bronchial washings is *Staphylococcus aureus*. In a series of 32 transplants, this organism was recovered from donors 11 times and subsequently from 4 transplant recipients.[66] Other commonly recovered pathogens include *Enterobacter* species and *Candida albicans*. The presence of organisms cultured from donor bronchial washings, however, does not absolutely predict the development of invasive infection in recipients. Less than half of recipients from whom organisms were recovered went on to develop invasive infection.

The second most significant pathogen is cytomegalovirus (CMV). The diagnosis of CMV is usually made from culture of bronchoalveolar lavage fluid or tissue obtained from transbronchial lung biopsy. In the pulmonary transplantation population, CMV pneumonitis is the predominant form of CMV infection, although CMV enteritis and retinitis also occur. This experience corresponds to that seen in cardiac and cardiopulmonary transplant recipients. About half of lung recipients develop documented CMV infection. Ganciclovir has proved particularly effective and is the drug of choice for CMV infection in this circumstance. The drug is well tolerated in most patients, with neutropenia accounting for most of the toxicity. CMV prophylaxis with ganciclovir can be used for CMV-positive recipients or in those recipients who receive a lung from a CMV-positive donor. The mortality rate from life-threatening CMV infections treated with ganciclovir has been reported at 10%, far better than the 40% or greater mortality reported before this agent was available.[67] Life-threatening CMV infection can occur in CMV-negative recipients who receive a lung from a CMV-positive donor (primary infection) or in recipients who are already CMV positive (secondary infection). Cytolytic therapy especially with muromonab-CD3 is associated with an increased risk and severity of CMV infection. Attempts to match a CMV-negative recipient with a CMV-negative donor lung, given the shortage of donor organs, can prolong candidate waiting time.

A recent analysis of UNOS outcomes data demonstrated that donor–recipient CMV serologic mismatch, particularly donor-positive/recipient-negative (D+/R–) serologic status, was a significant adverse risk factor for posttransplantation mortality in earlier eras (1990–1994 and 1995–1999) but not in a more recent era (2000–2004) of pulmonary transplantation, when compared with donor-negative/recipient-negative transplants.[68] Mismatched donor–recipient CMV status also appears to be a significant univariate risk factor for mortality following retransplantation.[69] These findings suggest that donor–recipient CMV mismatch can be an adverse factor for posttransplant survival but also that this deleterious effect may be abrogated with the introduction of more effective CMV antiviral therapy.[70]

Infection with *Aspergillus* species is the most common fungal infection after lung transplant. It occurs in 15% to 35% of recipients. Overall mortality is high (52%), especially with invasive infections (80%).[71] Preemptive antifungal therapy has been shown to decrease the incidence of clinical fungal infection from 69% to 31%.[72]

Airway Complications

Airway complications can be categorized by the time course of occurrence (early vs. late) and the type of complication (stenosis, dehiscence, granulation, fistula, or infection). The incidence of airway complications has decreased substantially over time. This is likely due to improvements in lung preservation, surgical technique, and antibiotic prophylaxis.

6 During the early pulmonary transplantation experience, problems with airway healing resulted in a significant percentage of deaths. Patients often did well for the first 3 weeks after transplantation, and then the bronchial anastomosis split, often with erosion into the pulmonary artery. Bronchial anastomotic healing initially was facilitated by withholding maintenance corticosteroids until after the first posttransplantation week and using an omental pedicle wrapped around the anastomosis. Historically, most problems with airway healing occurred after the en bloc double-lung operation, which involves a tracheal anastomosis. Double-lung transplantation required extensive dissection in the subcarinal space, resulting in the disruption of a number of bronchial collateral vessels. Since this operation was modified to one involving bilateral, sequential lung replacement using two bronchial anastomoses, airway problems are infrequent and now are rarely if ever implicated in recipient deaths. Partial bronchial dehiscences often heal without sequelae.

The use of a telescoping bronchial anastomosis, in which the donor bronchus is intussuscepted into the recipient bronchus or vice versa, obviated the need for the omental pedicle wrap, allowed for immediate use of corticosteroids, and reduced anastomotic dehiscence rates. However, the telescoping anastomosis can increase the rate of anastomotic stenosis. Recently there has been a trend toward the use of primary end-to-end anastomosis using figure-of-eight sutures, and initial results demonstrate a lower incidence of stenosis with an equivalent rate of dehiscence (about 2%).[48,49]

Bronchiolitis Obliterans

Bronchiolitis obliterans remains the leading cause of late mortality following lung transplantation, with nearly 30% of deaths beyond the first year of transplantation attributed to the fibroproliferative changes and airway destruction of this disorder. Bronchiolitis obliterans syndrome, the clinical correlate of this complication, occurs in over 40% of patients who survive beyond 90 days of operation, and remains a significant cause of morbidity, occurring in one third of patients surviving at least 5 years. Following heart–lung transplantation, nearly 50% of deaths beyond the first year are attributable to bronchiolitis obliterans and pulmonary graft failure.[73]

Bronchiolitis obliterans syndrome is defined as decline in FEV_1 of greater than 20% from baseline, as determined by at least two separate measurements obtained at least 3 weeks apart.[74] The histologic appearance of bronchiolitis obliterans is characterized by progressive small airway destruction, airway deposition with an inflammatory exudate, and, finally, fibrosis. This complication is likely a form of chronic rejection, although its exact etiology remains unknown. If diagnosed early, enhancing immunosuppression may either halt the process or slow the progression. It has been hypothesized that the development of obliterative bronchiolitis in cardiopulmonary transplantation patients is related to a human major histocompatibility complex (human leukocyte antigen)–A2 antigen mismatch. Others postulate that CMV infection or early lung injury, such as that arising from primary graft dysfunction,[75] may be implicated. Once diagnosed, it is imperative to increase immunosuppression to prevent what is usually an insidiously progressive disorder. Unfortunately, in patients who have developed obliterative bronchiolitis and then undergo retransplantation, the pathology can recur in the newly transplanted lungs. Obliterative bronchiolitis remains the major problem in patients surviving for greater than 2 years following transplantation. Overall, long-term survival for lung transplantation is not likely to improve significantly until effective strategies for the prevention and treatment of obliterative bronchiolitis and bronchiolitis obliterans syndrome are identified.

POSTTRANSPLANTATION PHYSIOLOGY

Pulmonary transplantation has afforded an opportunity to observe changes in pulmonary physiology that are not seen under ordinary circumstances. It is important to examine these changes relative to the type of transplantation operation.

The development of bilateral, sequential lung replacement provides the opportunity to indirectly assess lung function by perfusion lung scan. Because the newly implanted lungs have different ischemic times, the immediate posttransplantation perfusion scan would be expected to demonstrate less perfusion to the side with the longer ischemic time. Indeed, this situation does occur, especially when ischemic times exceed 6 hours; however, the relative perfusion to each side usually equalizes within 24 to 48 hours.

Performing single-lung transplants in patients with pulmonary hypertension has been particularly illustrative in demonstrating the potential for reversing right ventricular dysfunction. As soon as the lung is implanted, the morphology of the right ventricle changes significantly, as assessed by transesophageal echocardiography. The interventricular septum, previously bulging into the left ventricle, immediately assumes a normal position. An increase in contractility of the right ventricle occurs with significant decrease in dilatation. The pulmonary artery pressure immediately decreases and is essentially normal by the time the patient leaves the operating room (Table 38.7). Late catheterization studies (2 years posttransplantation) in patients undergoing this operation show continued normal hemodynamics.

TABLE 38.7 INDICATIONS/CONTRAINDICATIONS

INDICATIONS FOR PULMONARY TRANSPLANTATION

	SINGLE LUNG (%)	DOUBLE LUNG (%)
Emphysema	53.0	23.0
α_1-Antitrypsin	8.5	9.5
Cystic fibrosis	2.3	31.0
Idiopathic pulmonary fibrosis	24.0	9.7
Primary pulmonary hypertension	1.1	7.6
Retransplant	2.0	1.7

Adapted with permission from Trulock EP, Edwards LB, Taylor DO, et al. The Registry of the International Society for Heart and Lung Transplantation: twenty-first official adult heart transplant report—2004. *J Heart Lung Transplant* 2004;23:804–815.

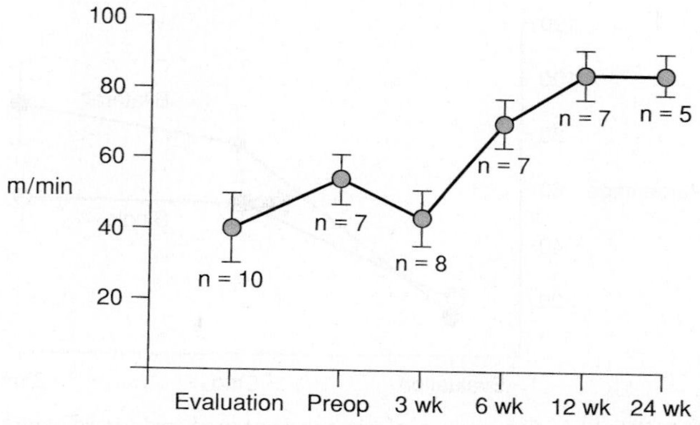

FIGURE 38.3. Mean 6-minute walk data for a group of patients undergoing single-lung transplantations for emphysema. Marked improvement is seen at the 6-week level, with continued improvement at 12 weeks.

The situation after single-lung transplantation in patients with emphysema is also illustrative. One would expect a significant ventilation/perfusion (V/Q) mismatch to occur, with ventilation to the native lung occurring preferentially because the native lung is significantly more compliant. Conversely, there is significantly greater differential perfusion to the newly transplanted lung, particularly at rest, with greater differences in perfusion observed in patients undergoing transplantation for emphysema compared with pulmonary fibrosis. With exercise, perfusion to the native lung tends to increase.[76] Despite significant perfusion to the nontransplanted lung, patients undergoing single-lung transplantation do well from a functional standpoint (Fig. 38.3) and do not typically have persistent carbon dioxide retention after transplantation. Physiologic dead space (V_D/V_T) decreases with work, with a shift in ventilation toward the transplanted side. By 3 months after transplantation, the V/Q mismatch narrows (Fig. 38.4). From a clinical standpoint, improvement in pulmonary function is seen almost immediately after transplantation. Spirometric improvement is noted within 2 weeks of operation, increasing significantly within 6 months and then remaining stable after 3 years following transplantation (Fig. 38.5). Improvement after bilateral lung replacement is slightly better.[77]

Exercise studies show modest, if any, improvement after lung transplantation, with no significant differences apparent in exercise tolerance between patients with bilateral or single-lung

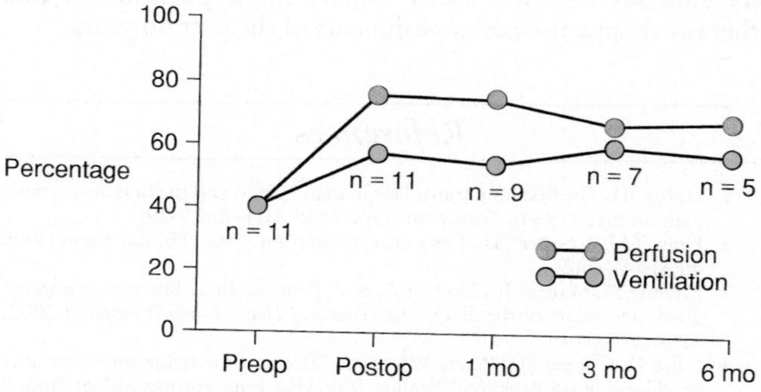

FIGURE 38.4. Mean values for ventilation and perfusion for patients undergoing single-lung transplantation for emphysema. Note the ventilation-perfusion mismatch that occurs, as expected, after transplantation.

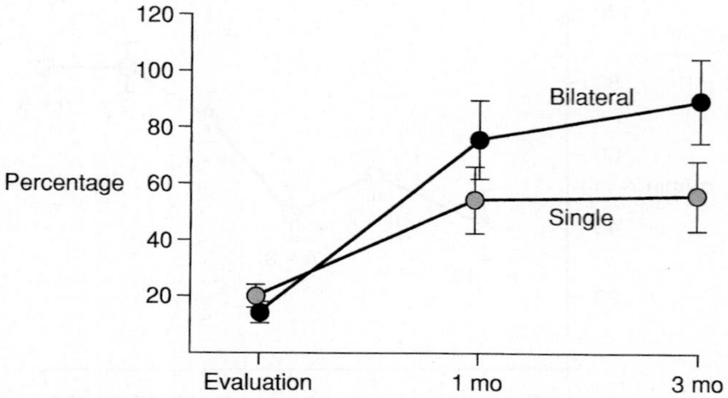

FIGURE 38.5. Comparison of percentage of predicted forced expiratory volume in 1 second in 14 patients undergoing single and 10 patients undergoing bilateral sequential pulmonary transplantation for chronic obstructive pulmonary disease.

transplants.[78,79] Maximum oxygen consumption, maximum work, peak ventilation, and anaerobic threshold are increased after lung transplantation but remain well below normal values.[80] This may be due in large part to an accompanying abnormal cardiovascular response to exercise and peripheral muscle weakness.[81] By the end of the first year after transplantation, approximately 80% of recipients report no limitations in activity.[59] On average, after transplantation, the distance a patient can cover during a standard 6-minute walk test is doubled that achieved preoperatively. Recipients of bilateral lung transplants can walk farther in 6 minutes than recipients of single-lung transplants, but this difference may reflect the younger age of the bilateral transplant recipients.[59,82]

7

FUTURE CONSIDERATIONS

Pulmonary transplantation has slowly evolved from an experimental therapy to standard of care for patients with respiratory failure, although many fewer patients undergo these operations compared with other solid organ transplants. Donor availability remains a limiting issue and will likely continue to be an obstacle despite efforts to improve both donor management and organ procurement efforts at a societal level. Lung volume reduction surgery has demonstrated some benefit in a select group of COPD patients but has not had as significant an impact on quality of life as lung transplant has for patients with emphysema. Questions about long-term impact and preservation of lung function remain to be answered. Other considerations including posttransplantation quality of life and cost–utility analyses also will likely impact the application of this therapy despite the accomplishments of the past 40 years.

References

1. Hardy JD. The first lung transplant in man (1963) and the first heart transplant in man (1964). *Transplant Proc* 1999;31(1–2):25–29.
2. Egan TM, Cooper JD. Lung transplantation. *Ann Thorac Surg* 1989; 48(5):741–742.
3. Estenne M, Maurer JR, Boehler A, et al. Bronchiolitis obliterans syndrome 2001: an update of the diagnostic criteria. *J Heart Lung Transplant* 2002; 21(3):297–310.
4. Lima O, Cooper JD, Peters WJ, et al. Effects of methylprednisolone and azathioprine on bronchial healing following lung autotransplantation. *J Thorac Cardiovasc Surg* 1981;82(2):211–215.
5. Khaghani A, Tadjkarimi S, al-Kattan K, et al. Wrapping the anastomosis with omentum or an internal mammary artery pedicle does not improve bronchial healing after single lung transplantation: results of a randomized clinical trial. *J Heart Lung Transplant* 1994;13(5):767–773.
6. Egan TM, Murray S, Bustami RT, et al. Development of the new lung allocation system in the United States. *Am J Transplant* 2006;6(5 Pt 2): 1212–1227.
7. Mulligan MS, Shearon TH, Weill D, et al. Heart and lung transplantation in the United States, 1997–2006. *Am J Transplant* 2008;8(4 Pt 2): 977–987.
8. Grady KL, White-Williams C, Naftel D, et al. Are preoperative obesity and cachexia risk factors for post heart transplant morbidity and mortality: a multi-institutional study of preoperative weight-height indices. *J Heart Lung Transplant* 1999;18(8):750–763.
9. Culver DA, Mazzone PJ, Khandwala F, et al. Discordant utility of ideal body weight and body mass index as predictors of mortality in lung transplant recipients. *J Heart Lung Transplant* 2005;24(2):137–144.
10. Madill J, Gutierrez C, Grossman J, et al. Nutritional assessment of the lung transplant patient: body mass index as a predictor of 90-day mortality following transplantation. *J Heart Lung Transplant* 2001;20(3):288–296.
11. Hertz MI, Aurora P, Christie JD, et al. Registry of the International Society for Heart and Lung Transplantation: a quarter century of thoracic transplantation. *J Heart Lung Transplant* 2008;27(9):937–942.
12. Mahidhara R, Bastani S, Ross DJ, et al. Lung transplantation in older patients? *J Thorac Cardiovasc Surg* 2008;135(2):412–420.
13. Smith PW, Wang H, Parini V, et al. Lung transplantation in patients 60 years and older: results, complications, and outcomes. *Ann Thorac Surg* 2006;82(5):1835–1841.
14. Baz MA, Palmer SM, Staples ED, et al. Lung transplantation after long-term mechanical ventilation. *Chest* 2001;119(1):224–227.
15. Patel VS, Palmer SM, Messier RH, et al. Clinical outcome after coronary artery revascularization and lung transplantation. *Ann Thorac Surg* 2003; 75(2):372–377.
16. National Emphysema Treatment Trial Research Group. A randomized trial comparing lung-volume-reduction surgery with medical therapy for severe emphysema. *N Engl J Med* 2003;348(21):2059–2073.
17. Oga T, Nishimura K, Tsukino M, et al. Analysis of the factors related to mortality in chronic obstructive pulmonary disease: role of exercise capacity and health status. *Am J Respir Crit Care Med* 2003;167(4): 544–549.
18. Celli BR, Cote CG, Marin JM, et al. The body-mass index, airflow obstruction, dyspnea, and exercise capacity index in chronic obstructive pulmonary disease. *N Engl J Med* 2004;350(10):1005–1012.
19. Latsi PI, du Bois RM, Nicholson AG, et al. Fibrotic idiopathic interstitial pneumonia: the prognostic value of longitudinal functional trends. *Am J Respir Crit Care Med* 2003;168(5):531–537.
20. Mogulkoc N, Brutsche MH, Bishop PW, et al. Pulmonary function in idiopathic pulmonary fibrosis and referral for lung transplantation. *Am J Respir Crit Care Med* 2001;164(1):103–108.
21. Lama VN, Flaherty KR, Toews GB, et al. Prognostic value of desaturation during a 6-minute walk test in idiopathic interstitial pneumonia. *Am J Respir Crit Care Med* 2003;168(9):1084–1090.
22. Kreider M, Kotloff RM. Selection of candidates for lung transplantation. *Proc Am Thorac Soc* 2009;6(1):20–27.
23. Kerem E, Reisman J, Corey M, et al. Prediction of mortality in patients with cystic fibrosis. *N Engl J Med* 1992;(18):1187–1191.
24. Orens JB, Estenne M, Arcasoy S, et al. International guidelines for the selection of lung transplant candidates: 2006 update—a consensus report from the Pulmonary Scientific Council of the International Society for Heart and Lung Transplantation. *J Heart Lung Transplant* 2006;25(7): 745–755.
25. Hosenpud JD, Bennett LE, Keck BM, et al. Effect of diagnosis on survival benefit of lung transplantation for end-stage lung disease. *Lancet* 1998; 351(9095):24–27.
26. De Meester J, Smits JMA, Persijn GG, et al. Lung transplant waiting list: differential outcome of type of end-stage lung disease, one year after registration. *J Heart Lung Transplant* 1999;18(6):563–571.
27. Liou TG, Adler FR, Cox DR, et al. Lung transplantation and survival in children with cystic fibrosis. *N Engl J Med* 2007;357(21):2143–2152.
28. McCurry KR, Shearon TH, Edwards LB, et al. Lung transplantation in the United States, 1998–2007. *Am J Transplant* 2009;9(4 Pt 2):942–958.
29. Puskas JD, Winton TL, Miller JD, et al. Unilateral donor lung dysfunction does not preclude successful contralateral single lung transplantation. *J Thorac Cardiovasc Surg* 1992;103(5):1015–1017.
30. Orens JB, Boehler A, de Perrot M, et al. A review of lung transplant donor acceptability criteria. *J Heart Lung Transplant* 2003;22(11):1183–1200.
31. Zenati M, Dowling RD, Dummer JS, et al. Influence of the donor lung on development of early infections in lung transplant recipients. *J Heart Transplant* 1990;9(5):502–508.
32. Thabut G, Mal H, Cerrina J, et al. Graft ischemic time and outcome of lung transplantation: a multicenter analysis. *Am J Respir Crit Care Med* 2005;171(7):786–791.
33. Weill D. Donor criteria in lung transplantation: an issue revisited. *Chest* 2002;121(6):2029–2031.
34. Angel LF, Levine DJ, Restrepo MI, et al. Impact of a lung transplantation donor-management protocol on lung donation and recipient outcomes. *Am J Respir Crit Care Med* 2006;174(6):710–716.
35. Botha P, Trivedi D, Searl CP, et al. Differential pulmonary vein gases predict primary graft dysfunction. *Ann Thorac Surg* 2006;82(6):1998–2002.
36. Arcasoy SM, Fisher A, Hachem RR, et al. Report of the ISHLT Working Group on primary lung graft dysfunction part V: predictors and outcomes. *J Heart Lung Transplant* 2005;24(10):1483–1488.

37. de Perrot M, Keshavjee S. Lung preservation. *Semin Thorac Cardiovasc Surg* 2004;16(4):300–308.
38. Venuta F, Rendina EA, Bufi M, et al. Preimplantation retrograde pneumoplegia in clinical lung transplantation. *J Thorac Cardiovasc Surg* 1999; 118(1):107–114.
39. Haniuda M, Hasegawa S, Shiraishi T, et al. Effects of inflation volume during lung preservation on pulmonary capillary permeability. *J Thorac Cardiovasc Surg* 1996;112(1):85–93.
40. DeCampos KN, Keshavjee S, Liu M, et al. Optimal inflation volume for hypothermic preservation of rat lungs. *J Heart Lung Transplant* 1998; 17(6):599–607.
41. Fukuse T, Hirata T, Ishikawa S, et al. Optimal alveolar oxygen concentration for cold storage of the lung. *Transplantation* 2001;72(2):300–304.
42. de Perrot M, Imai Y, Volgyesi GA, et al. Effect of ventilator-induced lung injury on the development of reperfusion injury in a rat lung transplant model. *J Thorac Cardiovasc Surg* 2002;124(6):1137–1144.
43. Pierre AF, DeCampos KN, Liu M, et al. Rapid reperfusion causes stress failure in ischemic rat lungs. *J Thorac Cardiovasc Surg* 1998;116(6): 932–942.
44. Kaiser LR, Cooper JD, Trulock EP, et al. The evolution of single lung transplantation for emphysema. The Washington University Lung Transplant Group. *J Thorac Cardiovasc Surg* 1991;102(3):333–339.
45. Pochettino A, Kotloff RM, Rosengard BR, et al. Bilateral versus single lung transplantation for chronic obstructive pulmonary disease: intermediate-term results. *Ann Thorac Surg* 2000;70(6):1813–1819.
46. Pasque MK, Cooper JD, Kaiser LR, et al. Improved technique for bilateral lung transplantation: rationale and initial clinical experience. *Ann Thorac Surg* 1990;49(5):785–791.
47. Toyoda Y, Thacker J, Santos R, et al. Long-term outcome of lung and heart-lung transplantation for idiopathic pulmonary arterial hypertension. *Ann Thorac Surg* 2008;86(4):1116–1122.
48. Garfein ES, Ginsberg ME, Gorenstein L, et al. Superiority of end-to-end versus telescoped bronchial anastomosis in single lung transplantation for pulmonary emphysema. *J Thorac Cardiovasc Surg* 2001;121(1):149–154.
49. Schroder C, Scholl F, Daon E, et al. A modified bronchial anastomosis technique for lung transplantation. *Ann Thorac Surg* 2003;75(6): 1697–1704.
50. Baudet EM, Dromer C, Dubrez J, et al. Intermediate-term results after en bloc double-lung transplantation with bronchial arterial revascularization. Bordeaux Lung and Heart-Lung Transplant Group. *J Thorac Cardiovasc Surg* 1996;112(5):1292–1299.
51. Sundset A, Tadjkarimi S, Khaghani A, et al. Human en bloc double-lung transplantation: bronchial artery revascularization improves airway perfusion. *Ann Thorac Surg* 1997;63(3):790–795.
52. Pettersson G, Norgaard MA, Arendrup H, et al. Direct bronchial artery revascularization and en bloc double lung transplantation—surgical techniques and early outcome. *J Heart Lung Transplant* 1997;16(3): 320–333.
53. Lau CL, Patterson GA. Technical considerations in lung transplantation. *Chest Surg Clin N Am* 2003;13(3):463–483.
54. Lau CL, Hoganson DM, Meyers BF, et al. Use of an apical heart suction device for exposure in lung transplantation. *Ann Thorac Surg* 2006;81(4): 1524–1525.
55. Hachem RR, Yusen RD, Chakinala MM, et al. A randomized controlled trial of tacrolimus versus cyclosporine after lung transplantation. *J Heart Lung Transplant* 2007;26(10):1012–1018.
56. Mullen JC, Oreopoulos A, Lien DC, et al. A randomized, controlled trial of daclizumab vs anti-thymocyte globulin induction for lung transplantation. *J Heart Lung Transplant* 2007;26(5):504–510.
57. Burton CM, Andersen CB, Jensen AS, et al. The incidence of acute cellular rejection after lung transplantation: a comparative study of anti-thymocyte globulin and daclizumab. *J Heart Lung Transplant* 2006;25(6):638–647.
58. Hachem RR, Chakinala MM, Yusen RD, et al. A comparison of basiliximab and anti-thymocyte globulin as induction agents after lung transplantation. *J Heart Lung Transplant* 2005;24(9):1320–1326.
59. Arcasoy SM, Kotloff RM. Lung transplantation. *N Engl J Med* 1999; 340(14):1081–1091.
60. Amital A, Shitrit D, Raviv Y, et al. Development of malignancy following lung transplantation. *Transplantation* 2006;81(4):547–551.
61. Christie JD, Kotloff RM, Ahya VN, et al. The effect of primary graft dysfunction on survival after lung transplantation. *Am J Respir Crit Care Med* 2005;171(11):1312–1316.
62. Novick RJ, Stitt LW, Al-Kattan K, et al. Pulmonary retransplantation: predictors of graft function and survival in 230 patients. Pulmonary Retransplant Registry. *Ann Thorac Surg* 1998;65(1):227–234.
63. Christie JD, Carby M, Bag R, et al. Report of the ISHLT Working Group on Primary Lung Graft Dysfunction part II: definition. A consensus statement of the International Society for Heart and Lung Transplantation. *J Heart Lung Transplant* 2005;24(10):1454–1459.
64. Prekker ME, Nath DS, Walker AR, et al. Validation of the proposed International Society for Heart and Lung Transplantation grading system for primary graft dysfunction after lung transplantation. *J Heart Lung Transplant* 2006;25(4):371–378.
65. Whitson BA, Prekker ME, Herrington CS, et al. Primary graft dysfunction and long-term pulmonary function after lung transplantation. *J Heart Lung Transplant* 2007;26(10):1004–1011.
66. Low DE, Kaiser LR, Haydock DA, et al. The donor lung: infectious and pathologic factors affecting outcome in lung transplantation. *J Thorac Cardiovasc Surg* 1993;106(4):614–621.
67. Ettinger NA, Bailey TC, Trulock EP, et al. Cytomegalovirus infection and pneumonitis. Impact after isolated lung transplantation. Washington University Lung Transplant Group. *Am Rev Respir Dis* 1993;147(4): 1017–1023.
68. Russo MJ, Sternberg DI, Hong KN, et al. Postlung transplant survival is equivalent regardless of cytomegalovirus match status. *Ann Thorac Surg* 2007;84(4):1129–1135.
69. Novick RJ, Schäfers H-J, Stitt L, et al. Recurrence of obliterative bronchiolitis and determinants of outcome in 139 pulmonary retransplant recipients. *J Thorac Cardiovasc Surg* 1995;110(5):1402–1414.
70. Monforte V, Lopez C, Santos F, et al. A multicenter study of valganciclovir prophylaxis up to day 120 in CMV-seropositive lung transplant recipients. *Am J Transplant* 2009;9(5):1134–1141.
71. Solé A, Salavert M. Fungal infections after lung transplantation. *Transplant Rev* 2008;22(2):89–104.
72. Husain S, Zaldonis D, Kusne S, et al. Variation in antifungal prophylaxis strategies in lung transplantation. *Transpl Infect Dis* 2006;8(4): 213–218.
73. Trulock EP, Edwards LB, Taylor DO, et al. Registry of the International Society for Heart and Lung Transplantation: Twenty-second Official Adult Lung and Heart-Lung Transplant Report–2005. *J Heart Lung Transplant* 2005;24(8):956–967.
74. Sato M, Keshavjee S. Bronchiolitis obliterans syndrome: alloimmune-dependent and -independent injury with aberrant tissue remodeling. *Semin Thorac Cardiovasc Surg* 2008;20(2):173–182.
75. Daud SA, Yusen RD, Meyers BF, et al. Impact of immediate primary lung allograft dysfunction on bronchiolitis obliterans syndrome. *Am J Respir Crit Care Med* 2007;175(5):507–513.
76. Starobin D, Shitrit D, Steinmetz A, et al. Quantitative lung perfusion following single lung transplantation. *Thorac Cardiovasc Surg* 2007;55(01): 48–52.
77. Mason DP, Rajeswaran J, Murthy SC, et al. Spirometry after transplantation: how much better are two lungs than one? *Ann Thorac Surg* 2008; 85(4):1193–1201.
78. Gerbase MW, Spiliopoulos A, Rochat T, et al. Health-related quality of life following single or bilateral lung transplantation: a 7-year comparison to functional outcome. *Chest* 2005;128(3):1371–1378.
79. Oelberg DA, Systrom DM, Markowitz DH, et al. Exercise performance in cystic fibrosis before and after bilateral lung transplantation. *J Heart Lung Transplant* 1998;17(11):1104–1112.
80. Schwaiblmair M, Reichenspurner H, Muller C, et al. Cardiopulmonary exercise testing before and after lung and heart-lung transplantation. *Am J Respir Crit Care Med* 1999;159(4):1277–1283.
81. Reinsma GD, ten Hacken NHT, Grevink RG, et al. Limiting factors of exercise performance 1 year after lung transplantation. *J Heart Lung Transplant* 2006;25(11):1310–1316.
82. Bavaria JE, Kotloff R, Palevsky H, et al. Bilateral versus single lung transplantation for chronic obstructive pulmonary disease. *J Thorac Cardiovasc Surg* 1997;113(3):520–527.

CHAPTER 39 ■ PANCREAS AND ISLET TRANSPLANTATION

RANDALL S. SUNG

KEY POINTS

1. The Diabetes Control and Complications Trial demonstrated that tight control of blood glucose and minimization of hemoglobin A1C delays the progression of secondary complications of diabetes.
2. Recipients with functioning pancreas transplants have normal glycemic control without the need for exogenous insulin, and pancreas transplantation has a beneficial impact on diabetic complications.
3. Most pancreas transplants are performed in patients with end-stage renal disease, either concomitant with or following a kidney transplant.
4. Pancreas transplant outcome is dependent on the careful selection of donors and on meticulous pancreas procurement technique.
5. Pancreas graft survival rates are greater than 80% at 1 year.
6. In contrast to kidney transplants, the effect of a pancreas transplant on patient survival is probably only modest.
7. Islet transplantation does not require an operative procedure.
8. Although early outcomes are excellent at major islet centers, long-term islet transplant outcomes are inferior to those of whole-pancreas transplants, with most recipients returning to insulin within 2 years.

Diabetes mellitus is a spectrum of impaired glucose tolerance that ranges from gestational glucose intolerance to severe hyperglycemia and ketoacidosis. Diabetes, which affects approximately 8% of the U.S. population, can be divided into two major classifications. Type 1, previously referred to as insulin-dependent diabetes, is an autoimmune disease characterized by the eventual loss of all pancreatic β-cell function. Type 2, previously referred to as non–insulin-dependent diabetes or adult-onset diabetes, characteristically presents in obese patients over age 40[1]; many of these individuals eventually require insulin therapy. The incidence of type 2 diabetes is increasing as the prevalence of obesity increases, especially in younger age groups. While the mean age of onset is in the early teenage years, the disease may present as early as the first year of life. Type 1 diabetes afflicts approximately 1 in every 400 to 500 children and adolescents.[2] Patients may present as late as the fourth decade of life, and these patients may be misclassified as type 2 diabetics, despite clearly possessing the physiology of type 1 diabetes. The disease classically presents in a lean patient with polyuria, polydipsia, and polyphagia. It may present at the time of a concurrent illness. While there may be a brief "honeymoon" period after presentation where insulin is not required, exogenous insulin is always required to replace that lost by the complete destruction of β-cell mass. While hyperglycemic episodes from poorly controlled diabetes or hypoglycemic events from insulin may be life-threatening, the major morbidity of type 1 diabetes stems from the myriad long-term manifestations of the disease, particularly those that are due to accelerated atherosclerosis.

PATHOPHYSIOLOGY

The classic pathophysiology of diabetes is that of insulin secretory failure in type 1 diabetes and peripheral insulin resistance in patients with type 2 diabetes. However, the etiology, epidemiology, and pathogenesis of diabetes is much more complex than is reflected in early characterizations of the disease. Type 1 diabetes is classically described as an autoimmune disorder manifest by destruction of β-cells, with proinsulin being the most likely primary target.[3] There is multigenic susceptibility, with known genes at the human leukocyte antigen (HLA) class II genotype, the 5′ flanking region of the insulin gene, and the CTLA4 gene; however, many genetic susceptibility loci have been demonstrated but not completely characterized. The possibility that these many genes may individually only have weak effects makes them more difficult to identify precisely, and may explain the heterogeneity of inheritance of type 1 diabetes. This genetic susceptibility background is thought to interact with environmental triggers, perhaps infectious, that lead to autoimmunity and insulitis, the characteristic pathologic lesion of type 1 diabetes, although definitive proof of these triggers is lacking. In type 2 diabetes, while β-cell hypersecretion initially may exist, ultimately loss of β-cell mass ensues. β-Cell apoptosis is mediated by glucotoxicity from insulin resistance, and is exacerbated by fatty acids, lipoproteins, leptins, and cytokines, all of which are elevated in type 2 diabetes and obesity.[4] Because of peripheral insulin resistance, many patients require insulin in amounts that exceed 1 unit/kg, far greater than typically required by type 1 diabetics.

The observation that type 1 and type 2 diabetes frequently co-occur in the same family has raised the possibility that they are opposite ends of the same disease spectrum, and ample evidence exists that suggests the two are more similar than initially believed.[5,6] Families with mixed diabetes histories tend to have an intermediate diabetes phenotype: insulin resistance in type 1 and lower body mass index (BMI) and C-peptide concentrations in type 2 patients. β-Cell destruction is common to both types, and obesity and insulin resistance have both been shown to be risk factors for childhood type 1 as well as type 2 diabetes. The "accelerator hypothesis" of diabetes proposes three determinants of disease in all types of diabetes: the intrinsic rate of β-cell apoptosis, insulin resistance, and autoimmunity (which would apply only to a subset). Genetic studies suggest there may be a common predisposition. However, the cytokines, signal transduction pathways, and other soluble mediators of apoptosis are quite different between the insulitis of type 1 diabetes and the lipotoxic or glucotoxic processes of type 2 diabetes, and thus at minimum represent distinct mechanisms of β-cell destruction.[7]

The relatively recent discovery of the replicative potential of a variety of adult tissue types, and their roles in the pathogenesis of disease, has raised questions about the relevance to the pathogenesis of diabetes. In such a model, diabetes occurs due to a failure of regeneration of β cells, and individual variation in the ability to regenerate β cells is an important determinant of diabetes development. This is partially supported by the finding of associations of type 2 diabetes with genes having identified roles in cellular development. While it is broadly agreed that failure of β-cell replication is an important contributor to diabetes development, this is largely attributed more to an increased susceptibility of replicating β cells to apoptosis, which in a proapoptotic environment leads to loss of β-cell mass, rather than individual variations in replication. There is also evidence that deficits of β-cell secretion are as important as those of replication. Furthermore, the range of β-cell mass in adult diabetic and nondiabetic humans is very wide, and exceeds the apparent capacity for expansion of β-cell mass in response to regenerative stimuli. Thus, it appears more likely that insufficient growth of β-cell mass during development may be more likely to have a role in the predisposition to diabetes than specific deficits in regeneration.[8]

SECONDARY COMPLICATIONS OF DIABETES

Diabetes mellitus is responsible for tens of thousands of deaths each year in the United States. The high incidence of cardiovascular complications in diabetics is primarily responsible for the twofold increase in the risk of death in diabetics compared with those without diabetes.[2] Clinical complications of diabetes include end-stage renal disease, retinopathy, peripheral vascular disease, coronary artery disease, and neuropathy. Diabetic nephropathy is responsible for nearly half of all cases of end-stage renal disease; diabetes is also the leading cause of blindness and amputations in the United States.[9] The estimated cost of providing care for diabetes and its complications is over $150 billion per year.[1]

While diabetic complications have a multifactorial etiology, they are ultimately secondary to structural alterations in nerves, blood vessels, and connective tissue. Excess glucose is converted to sorbitol by aldose reductase, leading to the reduction of cellular content of myoinositol, abnormal phosphoinositide metabolism, and reduction in Na^+-K^+-adenosine triphosphatase (ATPase) activity. In experimental animals aldose reductase inhibitors prevent diabetic neuropathy, cataracts, and retinopathy.[10] The accumulation of advanced glycosylation end products (AGEs), due to abnormal nonenzymatic glycosylation of proteins and extensive cross-linking of these proteins, is likely to be pathogenic.[11] Ligation of endothelial cell receptors by AGEs results in the release of proinflammatory cytokines and activation of the coagulation cascade. Microangiopathy is characterized by thickening of capillary basement membranes, which increases with the duration of disease, and altered capillary permeability.

1 The Diabetes Control and Complications Trial (DCCT) demonstrated that tight control of blood glucose prevents and delays the progression of secondary complications of diabetes.[12,13] This study, in which patients with type 1 diabetes were randomized to conventional treatment with one or two doses of daily insulin versus intensive treatment with three or more injections per day, demonstrated a dramatic reduction in the risk of progression of retinopathy, microalbuminuria, albuminuria, peripheral neuropathy, and cardiovascular disease in the subjects randomized to intensive treatment. However, the major side effect of intensive treatment was a threefold increase in the risk of severe hypoglycemic episodes; approximately 10% of patients in the intensive insulin therapy cohort experienced five or more episodes of seizure or coma during the study period. Even in the absence of overt brain injury, multiple episodes of severe hypoglycemia have been associated with cerebral perfusion abnormalities and poor neuropsychiatric performance. In addition, there is a significant risk of accident during hypoglycemic episodes. Frequently, as hypoglycemia becomes more frequent and autonomic neuropathy worsens, patients may develop a syndrome of unawareness to hypoglycemia where the typical symptoms of tremor and anxiety do not occur. Such patients with hypoglycemic unawareness may develop profound hypoglycemia, especially if left unsupervised, and risk severe neurologic and traumatic injury.

The overall management of diabetes is focused on maintaining blood glucose as close to normal range as possible while attempting to minimize significant hypoglycemic episodes. Although the frequency and extent of hyperglycemia is important in the assessment of glucose management, long-term glycemic control is best assessed by evaluation of blood levels of hemoglobin A1C, which measures the extent of glycosylation of hemoglobin. Although the incidence of diabetes is increasing, the overall treatment efficacy has improved. The use of subcutaneous insulin pumps is being increasingly employed; inhaled insulin has been used in selected patients; and infusion devices, which also assess serum glucose and automatically adjust insulin dose accordingly, are being developed.[14,15] However, in practice it is a rare diabetic who can maintain tight glucose control without hypoglycemic complications. In fact, in a study of type 2 diabetics designed to reduce cardiovascular complications through normalization of glycemic control, intensive therapy was associated with increased early mortality and no reduction of cardiovascular events.[16] Most type 1 diabetics, even if on optimal insulin therapy, are unable to maintain hemoglobin A1C levels in the normal range, and most will ultimately develop progressive diabetic complications.

PANCREAS TRANSPLANTATION

Overview

Pancreas transplantation, while not technically a cure, represents the only option for insulin elimination for many type 1
2 diabetics. Recipients with functioning pancreas transplants have normal glycemic control without the need for exogenous insulin. Initial experience with pancreas transplantation, from the first pancreas transplant performed by Kelly and Lillehei in 1966 until the 1980s, was marked by low success rates and high mortality.[17] In 1980, the 1-year graft survival rate for pancreas transplantation was only 21%, and there was tremendous skepticism about the utility of the procedure prior to the advent of cyclosporine. Advances in surgical technique and immunosuppression have dramatically improved current graft survival rates to greater than 85% at 1 year. In addition to the development of cyclosporine, the introduction of bladder drainage of the donor pancreas, first introduced by Sollinger in 1985 using a button of donor duodenum, and subsequently modified by Corry in 1986 using an entire segment of duodenum anastomosed to the urinary bladder, dramatically improved the results of pancreas transplantation (Fig. 39.1).[18,19] Graft survival continued to improve throughout the 1980s and 1990s, especially for isolated pancreas transplantation (pancreas transplant alone, or pancreas after kidney transplantation), the results of which have been historically inferior to simultaneous kidney–pancreas transplants. Both short- and long-term survival of pancreas transplants has remained relatively stable in the current decade. Because bladder drainage is associated with significant morbidity, in recent years there has been a shift toward enteric drainage into the recipient jejunum. Currently, most pancreas transplants are performed with enteric exocrine drainage and venous drainage into the systemic circulation. However, pancreas transplantation

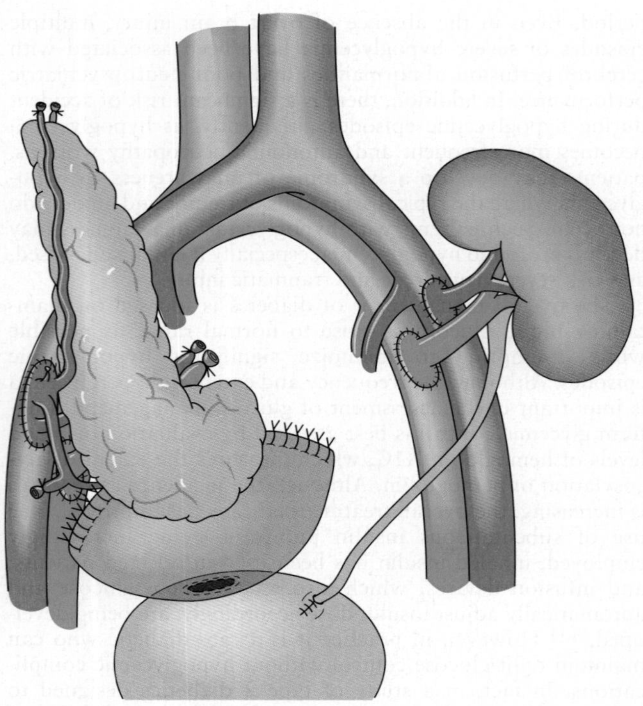

FIGURE 39.1. Simultaneous pancreas–kidney transplantation performed with drainage of the pancreatic exocrine secretions into the urinary bladder (bladder drainage). This technique has been predominant until recently. Note that a segment of the second portion of the duodenum is left attached to the pancreas. Despite its heterotopic location, the transplanted pancreas responds to gastrointestinal hormones with a marked increase in secretion of pancreatic juice that has very high bicarbonate content. Also note that the portal vein drains into the iliac vein (i.e., systemic venous drainage). In healthy individuals 50% of the secreted insulin is extracted from the circulation in the first pass through the liver. Transplant recipients with systemic venous drainage have peripheral insulin levels two to two and one half times higher than normal.

may also be performed by draining pancreatic venous blood into the recipient portal circulation, usually via the superior mesenteric vein.

Patient Selection

Pancreas transplantation is usually performed in patients with type 1 diabetes. The diagnosis of type 1 diabetes is relatively straightforward for most individuals. A history of juvenile or young adult onset, diabetic ketoacidosis, a lean body habitus, and a low insulin requirement (<0.7 units/kg) all support the diagnosis of type 1 diabetes. In contrast, older age of onset, obesity, an interval of treatment with diet or oral agents, or high insulin requirements are all suggestive of type 2 diabetes. A subset of adult-onset diabetics will display characteristics otherwise associated with type 1 diabetes, including absence of insulin production. Whether these individuals are properly classified as type 1 or type 2 diabetics may be subject to debate, but these individuals may certainly benefit from pancreas transplantation. Individuals with type 1 physiology but adult age of onset and low but detectable C-peptide secretion (so-called "type 1.5 diabetics") may also be considered for pancreas transplantation. Approximately 5% of pancreas transplant recipients are reported as having type 2 diabetes, and outcomes for these recipients are similar to those with type 1 diabetes.[20] These are likely to be highly selected individuals without significant insulin resistance; most type 2 diabetics would not be considered candidates. Some type 1 diabetics may develop insulin resistance as a result of years of insulin therapy; this is frequently accompanied by increased body weight and insulin requirements. While such patients, if transplanted, may be helped by oral agents typically used for type 2 diabetics, they are at higher risk for remaining on insulin after pancreas transplantation.[21] While provocative tests for insulin resistance exist, they are not commonly employed.

A small percentage of pancreas transplant recipients do not have type 1 diabetes, but have diabetes from other causes. Several have undergone pancreatectomy for chronic pancreatitis or other conditions.[22] Some pancreas transplants (<1%) are performed as part of a mutivisceral transplant that includes liver and small intestine in patients who do not have diabetes; in these transplants, the pancreas is included in the graft to facilitate the technical conduct of the operation and to reduce complications.[23]

3 Most individuals evaluated for pancreas transplantation have chronic renal disease. These patients may present prior to onset of dialysis, while currently receiving dialysis, or following kidney transplantation. For individuals without a functioning kidney transplant, potential options include simultaneous deceased donor kidney–pancreas transplantation (SPK), living donor kidney transplantation followed by deceased donor pancreas transplantation (PAK), simultaneous living donor kidney–deceased donor pancreas transplantation (SPLK), or simultaneous living donor kidney–pancreas transplantation. Of these options, the former two are by far the most common.

Simultaneous Kidney–Pancreas Transplantation

SPK from a deceased donor is the most commonly performed pancreas transplant option, with the number exceeding all other types combined. An SPK transplant has the advantage of requiring only one operation for both transplants. Since alloreactivity against the transplanted pancreas tends to be concordant with activity against the kidney, pancreas rejection may be heralded by signs of kidney rejection, which are more sensitive and present earlier. Consequently, SPK pancreas outcomes have been historically superior to those of solitary pancreas transplants.

Pancreas after Kidney Transplantation

If a living kidney donor is available, candidates have the option of receiving a living donor transplant, followed by a deceased donor pancreas transplant. This approach has the disadvantage of requiring two separate operations, but the recipient enjoys the benefit of a living donor kidney transplant that in many circumstances occurs sooner than would an SPK from a deceased donor. Since the primary survival benefit of the kidney–pancreas transplant comes from the restoration of renal function, this is a significant advantage. However, since a PAK is essentially a solitary pancreas transplant immunologically distinct from the kidney transplant, pancreas outcomes are worse than for SPK.

Simultaneous Living Donor Kidney–Deceased Donor Pancreas Transplantation

SPLK is another option performed at a few centers.[24] Candidates with identified living donors are listed for deceased donor pancreas transplantation. When a deceased donor pancreas becomes available, the living kidney donor transplant is performed at the same time as the pancreas transplant. This approach has the advantages of sequential living donor kidney followed by PAK transplants while requiring only one operation.

It does require that the potential living donor be available around the clock, a requirement that excludes some donors from this approach. It also has the disadvantage of potentially delaying a kidney transplant for the recipient if the waiting time for a deceased donor pancreas is long. However, since waiting times for solitary pancreas in some areas of the country can be quite short, the advantages may be substantial.

Living Donor Kidney–Pancreas Transplantation

A few centers perform living donor kidney–pancreas transplantation, with a single living donor donating the tail of the pancreas as well as the kidney (Fig. 39.2). This approach has all the advantages of a single operation, a single donor, and no waiting time. Results have been comparable to deceased donor SPK transplants.[25,26] Widespread adoption of this approach has been limited by concerns about donor morbidity from the pancreatectomy. Serious complications such as pancreatitis, fistula, abscess, or pseudocyst occur in nearly 10% of pancreas donors. Glucose intolerance and frank diabetes have occurred, although this problem has largely abated with more stringent donor selection criteria.[26]

Pancreas transplant candidates with renal failure may be counseled in a variety of ways depending on the availability of a living donor. How individuals are counseled depends in part on factors particular to the potential living donor and recipient, and also on the expected waiting time for SPK and PAK transplantation, which vary greatly by geographic region.

A

B

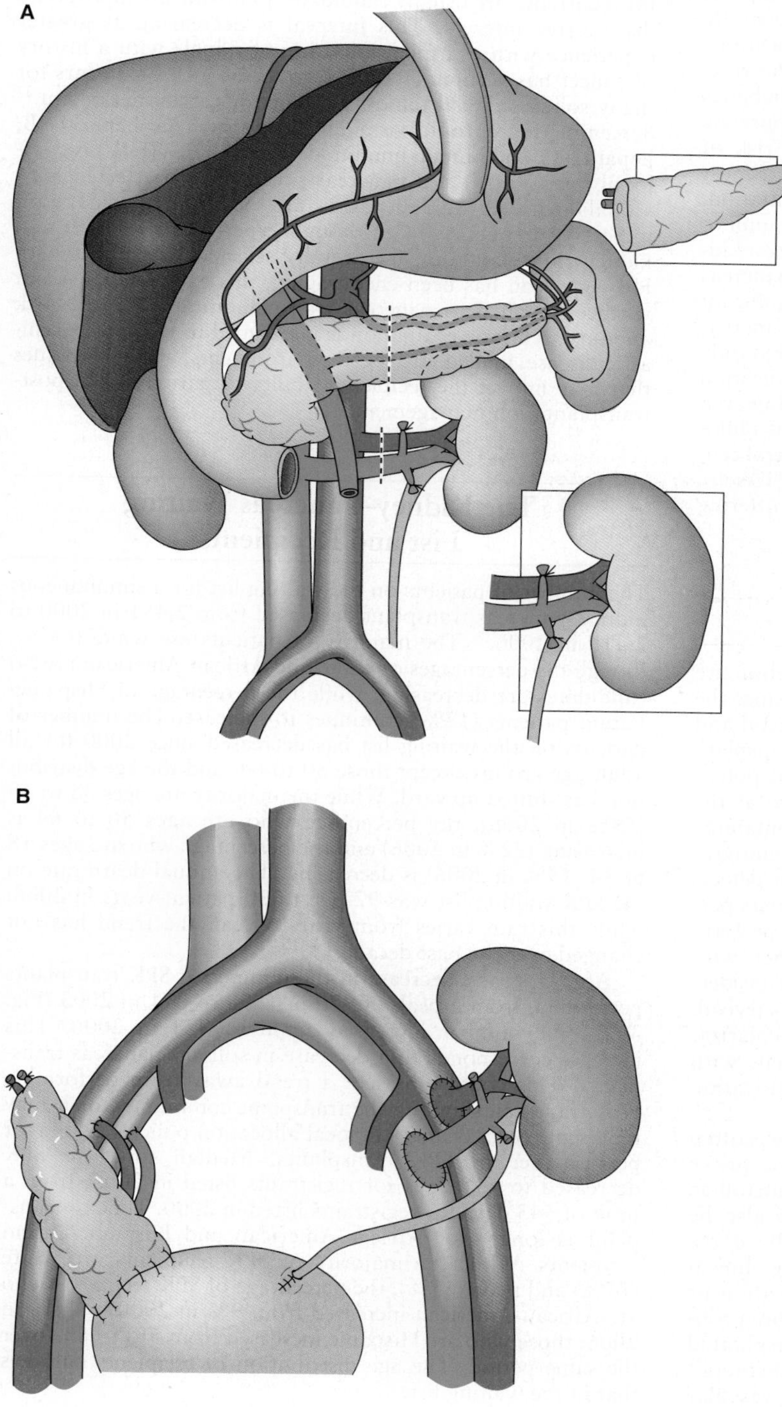

FIGURE 39.2. Live donor pancreas and kidney transplantation. **A:** Provided that the donor has a normal glucose tolerance test, a living donor may donate the segment of the pancreas that is to the left of the superior mesenteric vessels. **B:** Transplantation of the tail of the pancreas is based on the splenic artery and vein.

Since the mortality benefit of a kidney–pancreas transplant derives primarily from the kidney transplant, priority is generally given to achieving kidney transplantation expeditiously. In geographic regions where the waiting time for SPK is long (5 years is not unusual), living donor kidney transplantation is advised. Recipients of living donor kidney transplant can then be listed for PAK, which can be performed following recovery from the living donor kidney transplant. Individuals without living donors or those with borderline living donors in areas with short waiting times can be listed for SPK.

Pancreas Alone Transplantation

A small number of type 1 diabetics are evaluated for pancreas transplantation alone (PTA). These individuals are generally extremely labile diabetics who have progressive complications but do not have nephropathy. In these individuals the risk-benefit equation is quite different than that of uremic diabetics evaluated for kidney–pancreas transplantation. For nonuremic diabetics evaluated for pancreas transplantation the risk of immunosuppression in addition to the surgical procedure must be weighed against the potential benefits from transplantation. This contrasts to uremic diabetics, where the risk of immunosuppression is already assumed by virtue of the need for a kidney transplant. As will be discussed later, whether pancreas transplantation alone for type 1 diabetes results in a significant mortality benefit is controversial. For this reason, pancreas transplantation alone in most centers is generally offered only in the most exceptional cases, the most common indication being frequent life-threatening hypoglycemic events. However, several transplant programs exist that have a different philosophical outlook on the benefits of PTA, and these referral centers generally perform large numbers of PTAs. Most PTAs are from deceased donors, with a small number of centers offering living donor PTAs.

Evaluation and Screening

In general, eligibility criteria for pancreas transplantation are more stringent than for kidney transplantation alone, since the operation and potential complications are more stressful and the benefits less pronounced compared with kidney transplantation. All candidates, in addition to assessment of the potential benefit of pancreas transplantation, should have at the least noninvasive cardiac stress testing such as dobutamine stress echocardiography or adenosine thallium stress scintigraphy. Potential candidates with reversible myocardial defects should undergo coronary angiography, and many centers perform angiography on all candidates. The decision to perform pretransplantation coronary revascularization, either with angioplasty, stenting, or bypass, must be made with consideration of both peritransplant mortality and long-term survival. Although practices vary, a history of coronary revascularization is not necessarily a contraindication; individuals with extensive myocardium at risk and without revascularization options are frequently excluded.

Screening for peripheral vascular occlusive disease is often performed. Although distal peripheral vascular occlusive disease is characteristic of longstanding diabetes, aortoiliac disease and femoral popliteal vascular disease may also be pres-ent. Mild femoral popliteal disease is generally not a contraindication to transplantation, unless there are clinical signs of arterial insufficiency such as severe claudication or nonhealing ulcers. The presence of iliac disease is more problematic, as it can compromise inflow to the transplanted organs or increase the risk for postoperative arterial complications. In addition, diabetics may have significant vascular calcification, which could preclude transplantation even in the absence of flow abnormalities. Screening for peripheral vascular occlusive disease, in addition to a thorough physical exam, may include noninvasive flow studies, magnetic resonance angiography, conventional angiography, and pelvic radiography and/or computed tomography (CT) scanning to evaluate vascular calcification. Candidates with a history or exam findings suggestive of cerebrovascular disease should be screened for hemodynamically significant carotid occlusive disease.

Other evaluations, as with other types of transplant, are tailored to the individual medical history, and differ among centers. Screening for malignancy commonly includes mammography and Pap smears for women, prostate-specific antigen levels in men, and colonoscopy. Individuals with a prior history of treated cancer and who are judged to be at low risk for recurrence are usually candidates following an appropriate disease-free interval. This interval is decreasing as greater experience with transplantation in individuals with a history of cancer has accumulated, and can be as little as 2 years for many solid epithelial tumors to none for carcinoma in situ.[27] Screening for chronic viral infections such as hepatitis B, hepatitis C, and human immunodeficiency virus (HIV) is commonly performed, and pancreas transplants in selected individuals with chronic hepatitis are being performed with increasing frequency.[28,29] Although experience with liver and kidney transplantation in carefully selected individuals with HIV infection has been encouraging, this experience has not yet been applied to pancreas transplantation.[30] Social work and/or psychiatric evaluation is performed to rule out psychiatric disease, inadequate social environments, and other issues that may impact the recipient's ability to participate in post-transplantation management.

The Kidney–Pancreas Waiting List and Recipients

The number of patients on the waiting list for a simultaneous kidney–pancreas transplant decreased from 2,451 in 2000 to 2,416 in 2006.[31] The majority of patients are white (68%), though the percentages of white and African-American (16%) candidates are decreasing, while the percentage of Hispanic/Latino patients (12%) continues to increase. The number of patients on the waiting list has decreased since 2000 for all adult age groups except those 50 to 64, and the age distribution has shifted upward. While the majority are ages 35 to 49 (59% in 2006), the percentage who are ages 50 to 64 is increasing (22% in 2006) and the percentage who are ages 18 to 34 (19% in 2006) is decreasing. The annual death rate on the SPK waiting list was 97 per 1,000 patient-years in 2006; while this rate varies from year to year, the trend has not changed over the past decade.

After a steady decrease in the number of SPK transplants performed, from a peak of 970 in 1998 to 871 in 2003 (Fig. 39.3), the number increased again to 924 in 2006. This increase corresponds to a decrease in solitary pancreas transplants. This could represent a trend away from performing PAK transplants among the transplant community, or it may represent recent changes in local allocation policies that favor performance of SPK transplants. Median times to SPK decreased to 451 days for registrants listed in 2005, from a peak of 543 days for registrants listed in 2000. Time to transplant is longer for African-American and Hispanic/Latino recipients. While the majority of SPK recipients are white (75%) and male (65%), the percentage of SPK recipients who are African-American increased from 9% in 2000 to 15% in 2006; those who are Hispanic increased from 5% to 8% over the same period. The age distribution of recipients parallels that of the waiting list.

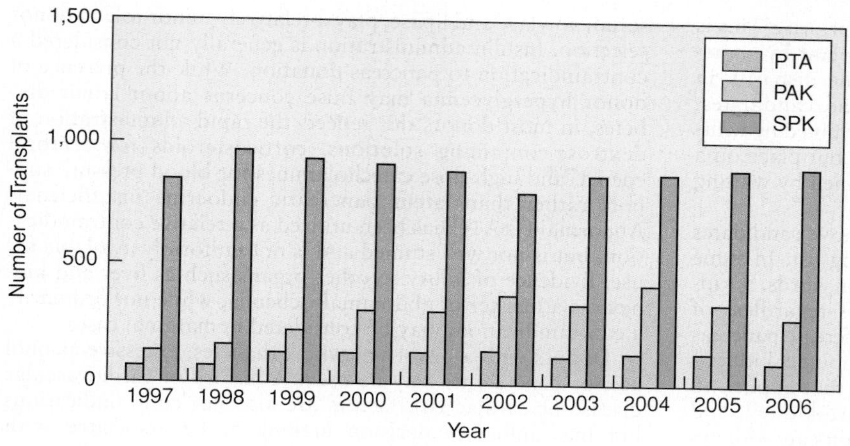

FIGURE 39.3. Number of U.S. simultaneous pancreas–kidney (SPK), pancreas after kidney transplantation (PAK), and pancreas transplantation alone (PTA) transplants performed by year. (Data from Scientific Registry of Transplant Recipients. *2007 Annual Report.* Rockville, MD: Health Resources and Services Administration, Department of Health and Human Services; 2008.)

The Pancreas Transplant Waiting List and Recipients

The number of patients awaiting isolated pancreas transplants in 2006 continued to increase, with 609 patients awaiting PTA versus 412 in 2002, and 1,007 awaiting PAK versus 786 in 2002.[31] The increase in the number of patients waiting for isolated pancreas transplants in the last 5 years is largely due to a decrease in the numbers of transplants performed rather than an impact of new registrations, which increased modestly for PTA but has decreased for PAK.

The great majority of patients awaiting isolated pancreas transplants are white (83% for PTA, 81% for PAK); there have been significant increases in the percentage of African-Americans on the PAK and PTA lists over the last several years. Although women continued to constitute 57% of the PTA waiting list in 2003, they were only 46% of the PAK waiting list. The majority of patients awaiting both PTA and PAK are between 35 and 49 years old, but as with SPK candidates, the percentage of older patients listed for PAK and PTA has increased, with 16% and 22%, respectively, of the waiting list in 2006 being between the ages of 50 and 64 years.

The median time to transplant for PAK has gradually increased over the last 5 years, with the mean waiting time for candidates registered in 2004 being 562 days. This is greater than the median time to transplant for SPK registrants. Wait times for PTAs have remained around 1 year since 2002, which suggests that solitary pancreata are more available than SPKs. PAK and PTA patients with blood group types O and B have historically had longer waiting times than those with types A and AB, a pattern observed in both kidney and SPK recipients.

The age and race of recipients of solitary pancreas transplants reflect the waiting list. In 2006, 88% of PAK and PTA recipients were white, reflecting an ongoing disparity in racial distribution of solitary pancreas transplants, which is even more marked than that for SPK transplants. The reasons for this disparity are uncertain, but likely reflect access to these procedures. More PAK recipients (54%) were male, but more PTA recipients (54%) were women, although the gender gap has closed in the past 5 years. The age at transplant has remained relatively consistent over the last several years, with a slight shift to younger patients receiving PTA.

Deceased Donor Pancreas Allocation

As with many organs, deceased donor pancreas allocation is determined primarily by geography, with most organs offered to centers in the donation service area (DSA) of donor origin. The base organ allocation unit is the organ procurement organization (OPO), which serves the population within the DSA. The 58 DSAs are organized into 11 regions, which serve as the second tier of organ allocation. In contrast to other organs, however, most pancreata are allocated according to locally determined policies set by the OPO; however, certain national rules exist.[32] There is mandatory sharing of pancreata to highly sensitized candidates that are completely matched to the donor. SPKs are allocated to these kidney–pancreas candidates first locally, then regionally, then nationally. If the pancreas is not allocated to an SPK candidate, then the solitary pancreata are similarly allocated to completely matched candidates.[32]

A number of utilization issues specific to pancreas transplantation influence allocation. Pancreata are significantly underutilized compared to other solid organs such as liver and kidney. Restrictions on cold ischemia time for whole-pancreas transplantation and particularly for islet transplantation make the placement of pancreata that are not used by the recovering center difficult. There is significant geographic variation in pancreas use, which correlates with activity by local transplant centers.[33] The allocation of pancreata is also complicated by the fact that pancreas donor selection criteria for islet transplant and whole-organ transplant overlap, leading to competition among certain types of pancreata. Allocation of kidneys to SPK candidates prevents allocation to kidney-alone candidates. This may lead to disagreement between transplant centers with and without pancreas transplant programs over allocation policies. Solitary pancreata are more difficult to place compared with SPK because their outcomes are slightly worse, but are more easily shared voluntarily since OPOs have no obligation to share kidneys along with pancreas for outside SPK candidates; since pancreas donors are carefully selected, the kidneys from these donors are usually able to be transplanted into a local kidney candidate.

In determining whether a given pancreas will be allocated to a solid organ or islet transplant candidate, donor age and BMI are considered. Donors under age 50 and with a BMI less than 30 are allocated for whole-organ pancreas transplant locally. If there is no local acceptance, the pancreas is offered regionally and then nationally. If there is no candidate for whole pancreas, the pancreas is then allocated for islets. For donors older than age 50 or with a BMI greater than 30, whose pancreata are rarely used for whole-organ transplant, the organ is first offered for pancreas transplant locally; if there are no local candidates, the pancreas is then offered for islets.[32]

Local policies vary widely. In some OPOs, SPK candidates have priority over candidates for isolated pancreas transplant, which increases the numbers of SPK and thus the overall benefit from transplantation to pancreas transplant candidates. In addition, because SPKs are easier to place, it is believed that this increases overall pancreas utilization. In other localities isolated pancreas transplant candidates receive priority. This is meant to encourage living donor kidney transplant by shortening wait times for PAK, and to decrease the disparity in waiting times between SPK and kidney-alone candidates. Within groups, status on the waiting list is determined by waiting time. In other systems no priority is given, but place on a combined SPK/PAK/PTA waiting list is determined by waiting time only.

Pancreas allocation is also influenced by how candidates are prioritized on the kidney transplant waiting list. In some cases, the kidney follows the pancreas; in other words, a kidney transplant is allocated to SPK candidates regardless of their place on the kidney list. This is thought to increase pancreas utilization by encouraging allocation of combined kidney–pancreas. This practice is also consistent with that applied to other multiorgan transplants such as heart–kidney and liver–kidney. Some OPOs will preferentially allocate kidneys to higher-priority kidney transplant candidates, such as highly sensitized or pediatric candidates, over SPK candidates. In other OPOs the pancreas follows the kidney; that is, pancreas allocation for an SPK candidate is dependent on the kidney match run. Since waiting times for kidney candidates exceed that for pancreas candidates, this tends to discourage SPK.

Donor Evaluation

4 The selection of appropriate pancreas donors is perhaps the most important determinant of successful pancreas transplantation. Many of the early complications of pancreas transplantation are thought to be secondary to processes related to organ quality and preservation, rather than the technical conduct of the recipient operation. While the ideal donor is young, nonalcoholic, and nonobese, very few donors meet this description, and the surgeon frequently needs to consider pancreata from imperfect donors. Donor selection criteria may vary among surgeons and transplant centers, and may depend on past experience, waiting time, and recent outcomes. Primary criteria are the age of the donor, donor BMI, donor cause of death, and gross appearance of the organ at the time of recovery. Additional information that may influence the decision includes aspects of the medical and social history, donor hemodynamics, laboratory values, HLA matching, and anticipated preservation time. As with donor selection with other organs, the decision-making process often involves consideration of multiple factors in aggregate.

The importance of donor age on graft outcomes has been confirmed by multiple studies, and the maximum age threshold is significantly lower than for liver and kidney transplantation.[34,35] Many centers use an age threshold, which may range from 40 to 50, above which donors are selected very carefully. Only 7% of pancreas transplants in 2006 were from donors over the age of 50.[31] The mechanism by which age affects outcomes is not firmly established: age appears to influence both early technical and late graft loss.[35,36]

Donor BMI has been found to be a determinant of graft failure by single-center and transplant registry analyses.[37,38] Very few pancreata from donors with BMIs greater than 30 are used for solid organ transplant, and are more likely to be recovered for islet transplant.[33] Interestingly, for overweight but not obese donors (BMI 25 to 30), a large single-center study found a higher rate of technical failure for donors that also had a cerebrovascular attack as cause of death.[37] It is not known whether associations with BMI relate to fatty infiltration of the pancreas or a separate mechanism.

The circumstances of death and the condition of the donor influence donor selection. Pancreata from donors with stroke as a cause of death have reduced graft survival. Although experience from donors after cardiac death (DCDs) is limited, a small number of centers have published good outcomes with careful donor selection.[39,40] Laboratory values, including serum amylase and lipase, play a relatively minor role in donor selection. Insulin administration is generally not considered a contraindication to pancreas donation. While the presence of donor hyperglycemia may raise concerns about latent diabetes, in most donors this reflects the rapid administration of dextrose-containing solutions, corticosteroids for cerebral edema, and high-dose catecholamines for blood pressure support rather than latent pancreatic endocrine insufficiency. Abnormal HbA1C has been utilized as a relative contraindication, but is not well studied and is not uniformly available for use. Evidence of injury to other organs such as liver and kidneys as a marker of abdominal ischemia, while not ordinarily a contraindication, may be considered in marginal cases.

Donors with a history of type 2 diabetes, excessive alcohol use, or pancreatitis may be used. A history of cardiovascular disease or cardiac risk factors are also not contraindications but may influence decision making or be associated with mesenteric atherosclerotic disease. A social history that suggests an increased risk of transmission of hepatitis or HIV should be evaluated, as with other organs, in the context of the degree of perceived risk relative to the benefit of the transplant.

Intraoperative evaluation of the donor organ is said to be the most important determinant of donor selection. Evidence of inflammation or fibrosis, which may manifest as focal or diffuse firmness to palpation, is considered to be a contraindication. Fatty infiltration of the pancreas, trauma, and pancreatic edema are also adverse findings, although the latter may be correctable with donor management. Traumatic injury to the pancreas or hematoma within the substance of the pancreas would preclude transplantation. However, a prior splenectomy is not a contraindication, provided that the tail can be dissected atraumatically.

Factors not intrinsic to the donor may bear on the decision to perform a transplant. The higher risk of graft failure–associated solitary pancreas transplants leads some centers to have more stringent selection criteria for PTA and PAK. While little data exist to suggest a definitive effect of cold ischemia, in practice shorter times are preferred, and those transplanted with clinical islet transplantation approaching 24 hours are more likely to be carefully selected. Attention to HLA matching varies widely by center; the many analyses performed suggest that any relationships between matching and graft outcome that may exist are not likely to be very significant.[36,38,41]

Procurement Technique

The importance of the pancreatic procurement cannot be overstated. It is thought by many pancreas transplant surgeons to be more critical to the success of the transplant than the recipient procedure. Because the pancreas is susceptible to traumatic injury, it must be carefully dissected and manipulated to avoid injury to the pancreatic parenchyma. Typically the pancreas is procured along with the liver and kidneys. This is performed in standard fashion through a midline incision that extends from the sternal notch to the pubic symphysis. After a generous Kocher maneuver, mobilization of the right colon, and isolation of the distal and supraceliac aorta to prepare these vessels for clamping, the pancreas is mobilized. This is most commonly achieved by entering the lesser sac, dividing the gastrocolic omentum. This dissection continues with division of the short gastric vessels and the avascular gastrosplenic ligament. The pancreas is dissected from the pancreatic bed using the spleen as a handle. The tail is lifted from the pancreatic bed using blunt dissection and the occasional use of electrocautery. The proximal jejunum is dissected at the ligament of Treitz. An antibiotic and/or Betadine-containing solution is frequently instilled into the duodenum through a nasogastric tube for decontamination. The duodenum is divided both at the ligament of Treitz and at the pylorus using a stapler. Division of the middle colic vessels permits exposure of the proximal small

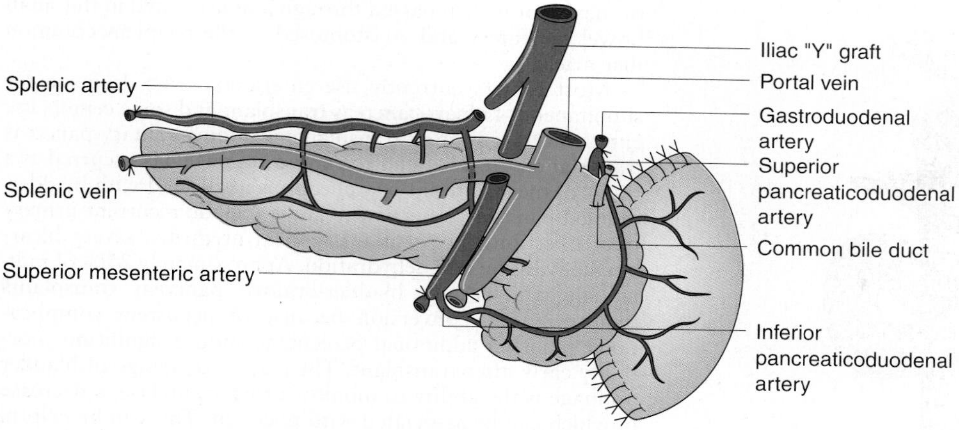

FIGURE 39.4. Back-table preparation of the pancreas. Before transplantation, the pancreas must be prepared in a slush-filled basin to maintain cold preservation. Preparation includes unifying the arterial blood supply of the pancreas by anastomosis of the donor external iliac artery to the superior mesenteric artery and the donor internal iliac artery to the splenic artery. The donor common iliac artery is used for anastomosis to the recipient iliac artery. During back-table preparation, donor splenectomy is performed.

bowel mesentery, which is divided distal to the pancreas with a vascular stapler. The mobilization of the pancreas may be performed either prior to or following the aortic perfusion procedure described later.

Perfusion of the pancreas is generally achieved through an intra-arterial cannula placed in the distal aorta following clamping of the supraceliac aorta and the aortic bifurcation. This is typically achieved with approximately 3 L of University of Wisconsin solution while the entire abdominal organs are packed in saline slush. Recent experience with HTK (histidine-tryptophan-ketoglutarate) in pancreas transplantation suggests no increase in risk of adverse outcomes with use of this preservation solution.[38,42] Some centers will also perfuse the abdominal viscera with a portal perfusion cannula, typically through the inferior mesenteric vein, although some surgeons maintain that overperfusion of either the arterial or particularly the venous circulation may result in pancreatic edema and an increased risk of complications.

The pancreas can be removed either en bloc with the liver and kidneys, en bloc with the liver, or separately, following removal of the liver. Whatever the technique, the portal triad is dissected out in cooperation with the liver procurement team. Typically the portal vein is shared by dividing it at the level of the coronary vein. Only in the rarest of circumstances should there be any difficulty using both the liver and the pancreas from the same donor even in the presence of hepatic arterial anomalies. In the presence of a replaced right hepatic artery, the superior mesenteric artery can be divided just distal to the replaced right hepatic artery, leaving a very short cuff of superior mesenteric artery on the pancreas. Alternatively, the replaced right hepatic artery, if large enough to be safely reconstructed by the liver transplant team without a cuff of superior mesenteric artery, can be transected as it exists superiorly from behind the head of the pancreas. The bile duct and gastroduodenal artery are ligated on the pancreas side and divided on the liver side. Dissection then proceeds along the superior aspect of the pancreas along the proper hepatic artery. The splenic artery, which constitutes the other arterial blood supply to the pancreas, is divided a few millimeters from its origin to allow for adequate length on the pancreas while allowing the stump to be oversewn without compromising flow to the liver. Once the pancreas is removed or split from the liver, the pancreas is packed in preservation solution; the entire common iliac artery and its two main branches, the internal and external iliac arteries, are packaged along with the pancreas for back-table reconstruction. A graft of donor iliac vein is also included in case the portal vein needs to be extended, which is done by some surgeons. Although most centers transplant the pancreas as soon as possible, up to 24 hours of cold ischemia time (time between perfusate infusion and organ reperfusion) has not been associated with reduced graft survival.[36]

Back-table Preparation of the Pancreas

The pancreas is placed on ice and remains cold at all times on the back table. The spleen is removed by dividing all vessels near the spleen, taking care to avoid injury to the tail of the pancreas, which should be clearly identified. Some surgeons elect to wait until reperfusion of the pancreas in the recipient to remove the spleen. Significant peripancreatic fat, if left on at the time of procurement, should be trimmed. Both ends of the distal duodenum are shortened to the point where they are immediately adjacent to the head of the pancreas. Both stapled ends of the duodenum may be oversewn with silk or polypropylene sutures. Some surgeons elect to reinforce the mesenteric staple line by oversewing with polypropylene suture. The iliac artery Y-graft is typically attached by anastomosis of the internal iliac artery to the splenic artery and anastomosis of the external iliac artery to the superior mesenteric artery (SMA, Fig. 39.4). In the absence of a Y-graft, the splenic artery may be implanted in end-to-side fashion to the SMA. The portal vein is mobilized by freeing from surrounding adventitial tissue to the confluence of the splenic vein and superior mesenteric vein. This should allow an adequate length of portal vein for anastomosis, as only 1 to 2 cm of portal vein length is generally needed.

Recipient Operation

The pancreas transplant is typically performed through a midline incision, although a lower quadrant incision similar to a kidney transplant incision may be used. The recipient should receive broad-spectrum antibiotics preoperatively. The pancreas transplant, for systemic venous drainage, is placed in the iliac fossa, preferably on the right side. After dissection of the iliac artery and vein, the portal vein is anastomosed in an end-to-side fashion to the external iliac vein. The common iliac vein or distal inferior vena cava may also be used; the recipient vein segment should be mobile enough for the portal vein to reach without tension. The common iliac artery component of the donor Y-graft is then anastomosed in an end-to-side fashion to either the recipient external iliac artery or common iliac artery; the distal aorta can also serve as the site of anastomosis. A pancreas placed on the left side in the recipient may be placed either medial or lateral to the sigmoid colon. Multiple variations have been described.

Because of concerns about the systemic hyperinsulinemia that invariably develops with systemically drained pancreas transplants, portal venous drainage is also utilized (Fig. 39.5). As 50% of insulin is removed with the first pass through the liver, systemic drainage leads to elevated peripheral insulin levels, which is not observed following portal venous drainage. Since hyperinsulinemia has been associated with dyslipidemia

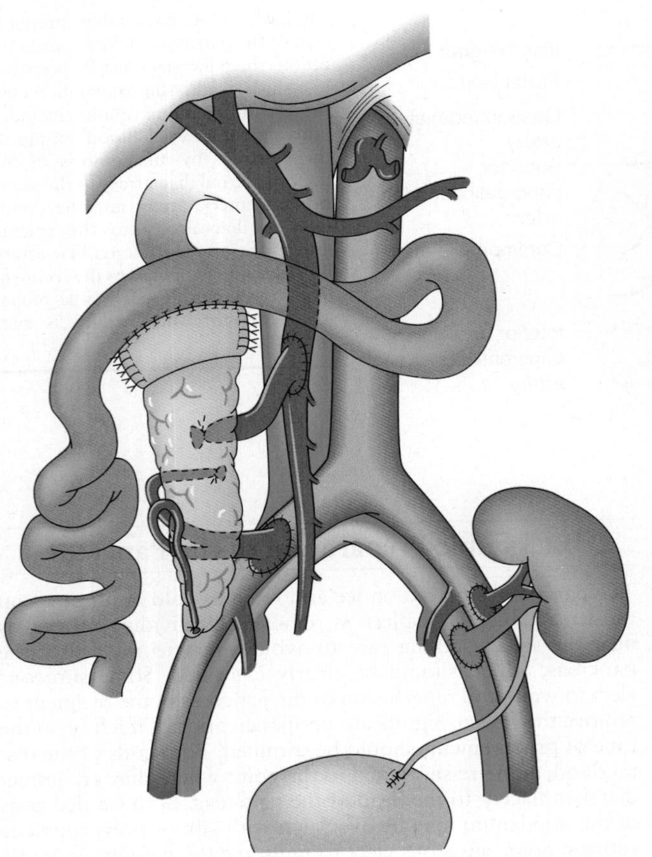

FIGURE 39.5. Simultaneous pancreas–kidney transplantation performed with drainage of the pancreatic exocrine secretions into the proximal jejunum (enteric drainage). This technique has been adopted by most transplant centers in the United States for simultaneous pancreas–kidney transplants. For solitary pancreas transplantation, some centers still utilize bladder drainage to allow monitoring of the urinary amylase. Note that the donor portal vein drains into the recipient superior mesenteric vein (portal venous drainage), preventing peripheral hyperinsulinemia. Many centers continue to place the pancreas in the pelvis, combining enteric drainage and systemic venous drainage. This placement requires enteric anastomosis to a more distal segment of jejunum or ileum.

and accelerated atherosclerosis, portal venous drainage theoretically ought to decrease cardiovascular risk compared with systemic drainage.[43] Portal drainage is associated with stimulation of the insulinlike growth factor I (IGF-I)/growth hormone (GH) axis, contributing to glucose control despite lower insulin levels.[44] However, despite a nearly 10-year experience with the procedure, no effect on cardiac morbidity or mortality has been shown, although equivalent graft and patient survival has been demonstrated.[45,46]

Although the type of venous drainage typically depends on the preferences of individual surgeons or transplant centers, the decision to perform portal or systemic drainage may also depend on the anatomy of an individual patient. Patients with multiple previous abdominal operations or who have a thickened mesentery may be more suited for systemic venous drainage. Alternatively, patients who have had multiple transplants or other operations on the iliac vessels may be candidates for portal venous drainage.

For portal venous drainage the superior mesenteric vein is dissected out just below the transverse mesocolon.[47] The right common iliac artery is almost completely dissected. An end-to-side anastomosis of the donor portal vein to the recipient superior mesenteric vein is performed with the duodenum oriented superiorly and the tail pointed inferiorly. The iliac artery graft of the donor is then passed through a hole created in the small bowel mesentery and anastomosed to the recipient common iliac artery.

Most centers currently use enteric exocrine drainage for simultaneous kidney–pancreas transplant and some centers use enteric drainage for all transplants including solitary pancreas transplantation. This shift to enteric drainage has occurred as a result of the significant complications associated with bladder-drained pancreas transplants. These include recurrent urinary tract infections, hematuria, chemical urethritis, severe bicarbonate wasting, and dehydration. Approximately 25% of individuals who receive bladder-drained pancreas transplants require enteric conversion because of persistent complications,[48] but an additional percentage endure significant morbidity early after transplant. The major advantage of bladder drainage is the ability to monitor urinary amylase, a decrease in which can be associated with rejection. This can be helpful in solitary pancreas transplants, but is perhaps not as important for simultaneous pancreas–kidney transplants where graft function may be monitored by serum creatinine. Improved immunosuppression and an increased utilization of biopsy to diagnose rejection have led to a decreased reliance on urinary amylase.[49]

Enteric drainage is achieved by creating a side-to-side or end-to-side anastomosis of donor duodenum to recipient jejunum. This may be a loop of jejunum, or a Roux-en-Y configuration may be created. For bladder drainage, a side-to-side anastomosis between the donor duodenum and the bladder is performed. Enteric drainage is always used for pancreas transplants with portal venous drainage because the orientation of the pancreas precludes anastomosis of the duodenum to the bladder.

If a simultaneous kidney–pancreas transplant is performed, the kidney transplant is usually placed in the left iliac fossa. The anastomoses, as with a kidney transplant via a retroperitoneal incision, are typically to the external iliac artery and external iliac vein. The kidney is typically placed in an intraperitoneal location, which increases the potential for torsion of the kidney on its vascular pedicle compared with kidney-alone transplants, which are usually placed in a retroperitoneal location. Some surgeons prefer to raise a retroperitoneal flap to place the kidney retroperitoneally after implantation. Advantages to this approach include improved percutaneous access should biopsy be required and a decreased risk of postbiopsy hemorrhage.

Following revascularization of the pancreas, attention is paid to bleeding from the pancreas, which can be quite brisk. These are controlled with ties or suture ligatures. Since thrombosis is a common complication of pancreas transplantation, anticoagulation in the perioperative period is frequently employed, particularly for solitary pancreas transplantation. Thrombosis is less frequent in simultaneous pancreas–kidney transplantation, where uremic platelet dysfunction is protective. The extent of anticoagulation may range from the intraoperative administration of heparin prior to clamping of vessels, followed up by low-dose heparin infusion and warfarin anticoagulation, to more conservative approaches such as the use of low-dose heparin for a limited interval postoperatively, or the use of aspirin or other antiplatelet agents. Hypercoagulability states may predispose to graft thrombosis in a significant number of individuals, although definitive data are lacking, and anticoagulation is not commonly individualized based on risk.[50] Whatever the approach, patients should be monitored for bleeding, since as many as 5% of patients experience postoperative hemorrhage requiring reoperation.[51]

Following revascularization, serum glucose levels are obtained hourly. It is common for the blood glucose to decline significantly following revascularization, and it is not uncommon for it to fall to normal levels soon after the patient's arrival in the recovery room. At some point intravenous fluids should be converted to dextrose-containing solution in order to prevent hypoglycemia. Pancreas transplant recipients with enteric drainage require only maintenance fluid with consideration of third-space losses. Simultaneous kidney–pancreas transplant recipients require the additional fluid replacement that would be administered following kidney transplantation alone. Individuals who receive bladder-drained pancreas transplants require replacement of pancreatic exocrine losses, which can be quite profound in the early postoperative period.

Immunosuppression

The immunogenicity of a pancreas transplant is considered to be greater than the majority of solid organ transplants because of the extensive lymphoid component of the gland. In addition, the difficulty in diagnosing rejection compared to other solid organ transplants makes the choice of immunosuppression perhaps more significant for pancreas transplants. Most centers use some form of triple maintenance therapy utilizing a calcineurin inhibitor, an antiproliferative agent, and steroids, although steroid-free regimens are becoming more common. According to data from the Scientific Registry of Transplant Recipients, 92% of kidney–pancreas recipients in 2006 received tacrolimus as maintenance therapy, compared to only 6% who received cyclosporine.[31] Mycophenolate mofetil is the antiproliferative agent of choice in pancreas transplantation, although the use of sirolimus has increased from virtually nil in 1999 to nearly 16% in 2006. The use of steroids for combined kidney transplantation is also decreasing; whereas in 1999, 97% of kidney–pancreas recipients received steroids as part of initial maintenance immunosuppression, this has decreased to 67% in 2006. This pattern of usage is similar to that employed for solitary pancreas transplantation, either PTA or PAK.

The use of induction therapy to inhibit lymphocyte function is common. Two large randomized multicenter trials utilizing diverse agents such as T-cell–depleting antibody induction (OKT3, ATGAM, and thymoglobulin) and interleukin-2 (IL-2) receptor antibody inhibition (daclizumab and basiliximab) showed a reduction in the incidence of acute rejection but failed to demonstrate a significant effect on patient or graft survival.[52,53] Despite this modest impact on overall graft outcome, 83% of kidney–pancreas transplant recipients received induction therapy in 2006.[31] Of these, approximately three quarters received thymoglobulin; the remaining were split between anti–IL-2 receptor and Campath induction therapy. For pancreas after kidney transplants, fewer recipients received induction (78%), with a similar proportion receiving thymoglobulin over anti–IL-2 receptor agents or Campath. The International Pancreas Transplant Registry (IPTR) has demonstrated a lower risk of pancreas graft loss in all categories of pancreas transplantation with the use of tacrolimus, and also demonstrated similar associations with the use of mycophenolate mofetil.[36] Consistent with the multicenter trials, IPTR analyses also fail to demonstrate a beneficial effect of induction therapy on patient and graft survival.

Several groups have reported excellent intermediate-term patient and graft outcomes utilizing steroid minimization protocols.[54–56] These protocols generally employ an induction agent (usually a depleting T-cell antibody or Campath), tacrolimus, and either mycophenolate mofetil or sirolimus. Steroids are given for a maximum of 3 days. These steroid minimization protocols, as in kidney transplantation, aim to avoid the significant short- and long-term side effects associated with corticosteroids. Regimens employing maintenance monotherapy have also been successfully employed, although long-term outcomes are not yet established.[57]

Complications

Thrombosis of the pancreas transplant is the most common cause of graft loss in the early postoperative period. Why pancreas transplants are more prone to thrombosis than other solid organ transplants is uncertain. The most likely mechanism is that ischemia-reperfusion injury in the pancreas, characterized by the release of cytokines and activation of pancreatic enzymes, leads to accelerated injury and a procoagulant state. Diabetic patients have impaired fibrinolysis and are therefore relatively hypercoagulable. The relatively low venous flow through the portal vein, which leads to diminished flow velocity, may be contributory. Thrombosis is more common in solitary pancreas transplantation than in SPK, probably due to the absence of uremic platelet dysfunction present in SPK recipients. The risk of thrombosis has been associated with donor factors such as older patient age, BMI, and cerebrovascular cause of death.[35,58]

Pancreas transplant thrombosis is usually heralded by a sudden rise in blood glucose in a pancreas that was previously functioning. Confirmation of the diagnosis is usually obtained with duplex ultrasound. Although anecdotal reports have described successful surgical and angiographic thrombectomy or thrombolysis in restoring flow to the pancreas,[59,60] the usual treatment is removal of the infarcted pancreas. While this usually occurs immediately after diagnosis, some centers opt to relist the patient urgently and wait until another pancreas transplant becomes available. Depending on the waiting time for another pancreas, the added morbidity of delaying the graft pancreatectomy is usually not significant. Because of the high risk of thrombosis, anticoagulation is frequently employed. It is likely due to these efforts and improvements in immunosuppression that the thrombosis rate has decreased to less than 5% for simultaneous pancreas–kidney transplants and to less than 10% for isolated pancreas transplants.

Bleeding is another frequent cause for reoperation in the early postoperative period. Because of the large number of vessels that enter and exit the pancreas, bleeding following reperfusion is not unusual. While readily controllable, it is not uncommon for bleeding points to emerge later in the procedure, and postoperatively. This can be minimized by meticulous attention to ligating vascular structures during pancreas procurement. The use of anticoagulation in the perioperative period, as described earlier, adds to the bleeding risk. Pancreas transplant recipients are monitored carefully in the early postoperative period for signs and symptoms of intra-abdominal hemorrhage.

The other major early complication is leak from the donor duodenum. Duodenal leaks occur in approximately 10% of cases, usually 1 to 2 weeks after the transplant.[61] A leak may present as fever, abdominal pain, leukocytosis, lower abdominal tenderness, and persistent ileus. The diagnosis may be supported by the finding of a focal fluid collection near the head of the pancreas on CT scanning or ultrasound. Alternatively, diffuse peritonitis may reflect disseminated contamination. For bladder-drained pancreas transplants, the diagnosis may be made by cystography.

The management of a suspected duodenal leak is operative. Peripancreatic sepsis or abscess can occur in the absence of a frank duodenal leak. This is caused by the growth of organisms transmitted into the peritoneal cavity during performance of the duodenal anastomosis. The peritoneum should be lavaged and all necrotic debris removed and débrided. If a leak is present, it is usually at the stapled end of the duodenum rather than at the anastomosis. The likelihood of success for repair of a duodenal leak depends on the viability of the duodenum at the point of the leak, the patient's overall hemodynamic stability, and the degree of surrounding inflammation. Usually one attempt at repair is made, but failure may necessitate removal of the pancreas in order to control life-threatening sepsis. Some surgeons have adopted a practice of managing leaks from duodenal enteric anastomoses by conversion to bladder drainage. This minimizes the risk of recurrent contamination of the peritoneal cavity with enteric contents and allows for Foley catheter decompression of the duodenum, but has the morbidity associated with bladder drainage. Occasionally a fluid collection or leak that presents late can be treated with percutaneous CT-guided drainage.[62] In addition, drainage of infection without primary repair of the duodenal leak has been successfully employed in situations where inflammation is so profound that the leak could not be primarily repaired. However, the morbidity associated with these duodenal fistulas dictates that these options be employed only when definitive repair is not possible.

In contrast to renal transplantation, the complications of pancreas transplantation can be severe and life threatening if not properly managed. Even in the most experienced centers, occasional patients who suffer extended intensive care unit stays and even death are not unusual. This is a consequence of both the tenuous medical status of longstanding diabetics and the substantial morbidity of pancreas transplant complications. Therefore, given the limited survival benefit of pancreas transplantation, particularly compared with kidney transplantation, patients should be counseled frankly about the potential magnitude of these complications so that they have a realistic expectation of outcomes. Even with honest discussion and informed consent, most individuals will elect pancreas transplantation, and many will pursue multiple pancreas transplants even with a history of significant complications from previous pancreas transplants.

Diagnosis and Treatment of Rejection

The timely and accurate diagnosis of pancreas transplant rejection is one of the most important and challenging aspects of posttransplant management. As noninvasive means of diagnosing rejection are neither sensitive nor specific, the diagnosis of rejection is best made with the histologic examination of a pancreatic biopsy specimen.[63] The pancreas graft in SPK transplants may be monitored by following the serum creatinine, as the concordance rate for rejection between kidney and pancreas grafts is believed to be high.[64,65] Improvements in the outcome of solitary pancreas transplants are largely attributable to not only improvements in the overall quality of immunosuppression, but also the ability to more accurately diagnose and treat pancreas rejection.

The technique of pancreas transplant biopsy has evolved over the years. In the era of bladder-drained pancreas transplants, cystoscopic biopsy of both the pancreas and transplant duodenum was common.[66] As more enteric-drained pancreas transplants have been performed, a greater reliance on percutaneous biopsy has developed, using either ultrasound or CT-guided techniques.[67] Laparoscopic-assisted or open pancreas biopsy may be utilized for patients whose pancreas transplant may not be accessible to percutaneous approaches, although the need for operative biopsy is decreasing as the percutaneous procedure has become more routine.[68] The indications for pancreatic biopsy include hyperamylasemia, hyperlipasemia, hyperglycemia, or unexplained pain in the vicinity of the pancreas transplant. The differential diagnosis includes pancreatitis, cytomegalovirus infection, toxicity from calcineurin inhibitors, and, in the early postoperative period, peripancreatic infection. The histologic grading system developed at the University of Maryland for determining rejection grade in pancreas biopsies is generally used (Table 39.1).[69] Indeterminate rejection may be treated with increases in calcineurin inhibitor dose or pulse corticosteroids. More substantial rejection is generally treated with depleting antilymphocyte antibody therapy, either OKT3 or Thymoglobulin.

As long-term survival of pancreas transplants becomes more commonplace, chronic rejection is emerging as an important problem.[70] Chronic rejection is histologically characterized as expansion of fibrous septa within the pancreatic parenchyma. This may progress to lobular atrophy or loss of both acini and β cells. Although there are parallels to chronic allograft nephropathy, whether chronic calcineurin inhibitor toxicity contributes to chronic pancreas rejection is unknown.

Recurrent Autoimmunity

Selective β-cell destruction in pancreas transplants may occur in a pattern similar to the insulitis seen in type 1 diabetes. This pattern is histologically distinct from cellular rejection. Although recurrent autoimmunity has been documented in both immunosuppressed pancreas transplant recipients and nonimmunosuppressed living donor recipients from identical twin siblings, well-documented case series have been infrequent. A variety of

TABLE 39.1 **CLASSIFICATION**

PROPOSED BANFF CLASSIFICATION FOR GRADING PANCREAS ALLOGRAFT ACUTE CELLULAR REJECTION

■ GRADE	■ SEVERITY	■ FINDINGS
	Normal	Absent inflammation or inactive septal, mononuclear inflammation not involving ducts, veins, arteries, or acini. There is no graft sclerosis. The fibrous component is limited to normal septa and its amount is proportional to the size of the enclosed structures (ducts and vessels). The acinar parenchyma shows no signs of atrophy or injury.
	Indeterminate	Septal inflammation that appears active but the overall features do not fulfill the criteria for mild cell-mediated acute rejection
I	Mild	(a) Active septal inflammation (activated, blastic lymphocytes ± eosinophils) involving septal structures: venulitis (subendothelial accumulation of inflammatory cells and endothelial damage in septal veins), ductitis (epithelial inflammation and damage of ducts); neural/perineural inflammation and/or (b) focal acinar inflammation: no more than two inflammatory foci per lobule with absent or minimal acinar cell injury
II	Moderate	(a) Multifocal (but not confluent or diffuse) acinar inflammation (three or more foci per lobule) with spotty (individual) acinar cell injury and drop-out and/or (b) minimal intimal arteritis
III	Severe	(a) Diffuse (widespread, extensive) acinar inflammation with focal or diffuse multicellular/confluent acinar cell necrosis and/or (b) moderate or severe intimal arteritis and/or (c) transmural inflammation: necrotizing arteritis

From Drachenberg CB, Odorico J, Demetris AJ, et al. Banff schema for grading pancreas allograft rejection: working proposal by a multi-disciplinary international consensus panel. *Am J Transplant* 2008;8(6):1237–1249.

associations have been suggested with autoantibodies to glutamic acid decarboxylase (GAD-65) and islet cells (IA-2), but patterns of autoantibody expression have not proven reliable enough to establish their etiologic relevance or prognostic value.

Posttransplant Viral Infections. The higher level of immunosuppression given to pancreas transplant recipients compared with kidney transplant recipients, particularly with respect to lymphocyte-depleting induction therapy, places pancreas transplant recipients at risk for conditions known to be influenced by overall immunosuppressive exposure. While rates of cytomegalovirus (CMV) infection are generally higher than for kidney recipients, especially when the donor is known to carry the virus, the use of intravenous and oral ganciclovir over the past decade has reduced the incidence of significant CMV-associated disease.[71,72] The incidence of CMV disease may also be lower in those recipients receiving steroid-free immunosuppression.[72] Data are mixed with respect to the incidence of polyoma-associated, or BK, nephropathy, with some analyses suggesting a higher rate and others an equivalent incidence in SPK recipients compared with kidney-alone recipients.[73,74] As with kidney-alone recipients, those SPK recipients with BK nephropathy have inferior kidney graft survival. Posttransplant lymphoproliferative disorder (PTLD), often associated with Epstein-Barr virus (EBV) infection, has a 5-year incidence of approximately 2%, which is similar to kidney recipients.[75] However, pancreas recipients with PTLD may have a worse prognosis than other abdominal organ transplant recipients with PTLD.

Results of Kidney–Pancreas Transplantation

There were 6,832 recipients of SPK transplants alive with functioning grafts at the end of 2005.[31] Current kidney graft survival at 1 and 5 years following SPK transplantation is 93% and 78%, respectively. African-Americans have somewhat poorer five-year graft survival (71%) than whites (79%). Kidneys from older donors have the poorest graft survival; 5-year graft survival from donors older than 50 is 68% compared with approximately 80% from donors aged 11 to 34. As opposed to previous decades, 5-year kidney graft survival is not associated with HLA matching.

5 Pancreas graft survival at 1 and 5 years following SPK transplantation is 86% and 73%, respectively (Fig. 39.6).

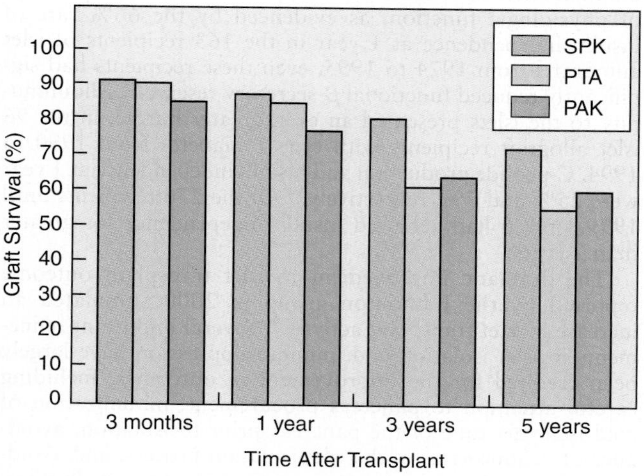

FIGURE 39.6. Pancreas graft survival for U.S. transplants. Cohorts are transplants performed during 2005 for 3-month and 1-year survival; 2003 for 3-year survival; and 2001 for 5-year survival. (Data from Scientific Registry of Transplant Recipients. *2007 Annual Report*. Rockville, MD: Health Resources and Services Administration, Department of Health and Human Services; 2008.)

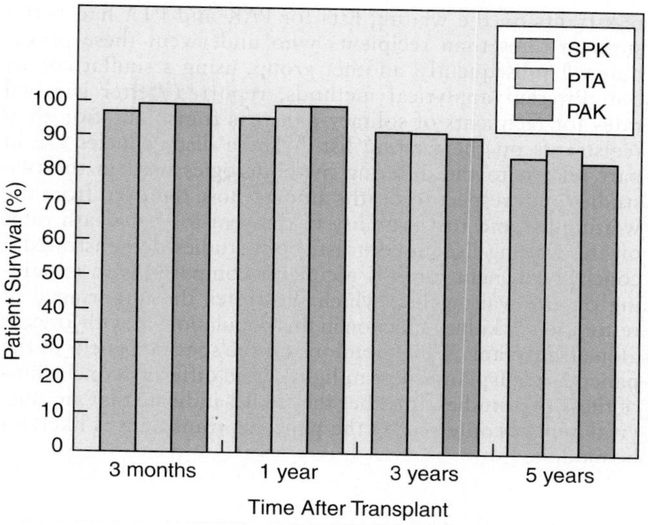

FIGURE 39.7. Patient survival for U.S. pancreas transplant recipients. Cohorts are transplants performed during 2005 for 3-month and 1-year survival; 2003 for 3-year survival; and 2001 for 5-year survival. (Data from Scientific Registry of Transplant Recipients. *2007 Annual Report*. Rockville, MD: Health Resources and Services Administration, Department of Health and Human Services; 2008.)

Worse 5-year graft survival is seen in African-American (68%) recipients compared with whites (73%). Five-year graft survival from donors over age 50 years (66%) is significantly lower than those from donors under 35 years (74%), including those under 10 years of age. Recipients with a previous transplant (kidney, pancreas, or both) have worse pancreas graft survival. As with kidney survival, there is no difference in 5-year pancreas graft survival with increasing levels of HLA mismatch.

Registry analyses demonstrate a mortality benefit of SPK transplantation compared with dialysis[76] or kidney transplantation alone.[77] Patient survival at 1 year and 5 years following SPK transplantation is 95% and 85%, respectively (Fig. 39.7). Race, ethnicity, sex, and transplant center volume are not associated with decreased patient survival at 5 years, and patient survival has improved since 1995 but not appreciably in the past 5 years. Death rates for recipients continue to be lower than the corresponding death rates for candidates on the SPK waiting list. Older (ages 50 to 64) and African-American recipients tend to have higher death rates in the first year following transplantation.

Results of Solitary Pancreas Transplantation

The 1-year pancreas graft survival for recipients of a PAK transplant has improved in the last 5 years, although the 1-year unadjusted graft success decreased from 82% for PAK transplants performed in 2001 to 78% for PAK transplants performed in 2005.[32] The graft survival for PAK at 3 years and 5 years is currently 64% and 60%, respectively. Patient survival for PAK recipients is excellent, 98% and 83% at 1 and 5 years, respectively.

One-year pancreas graft survival for PTA has improved in the last 5 years to 85% for transplants performed in 2005. The unadjusted graft survival for PTA at 3 and 5 years is 60% and 54%, respectively. Graft survival rates for PTA are better than PAK early but the rate of graft failure in the long term is greater for PTA than for PAK. Patient survival rates for PTA recipients are 98% at 1 year and 87% at 5 years.

Whether pancreas transplantation positively impacts patient mortality is controversial. One study reported that

registrants on the waiting lists for PAK and PTA had better survival rates than recipients who underwent these procedures.[76] Subsequently, another group, using a similar cohort but different analytical methods, reported better survival rates for recipients of solitary pancreas transplantation than registrants on the waiting list.[78] These discrepancies are in part related to the differing methodologies used in the two studies with respect to deaths among those removed from the waiting list and to variability in the year-to-year death rates on the waiting list. In contrast, both studies demonstrated a conclusive benefit for SPK recipients compared with remaining on the waiting list, which illustrates the importance of restoration of kidney function in this population, as with kidney-
6 alone transplant. While opinions on the specific benefit of the pancreas transplant differ in light of the differing conclusions of these two studies, together the studies indicate that any survival benefit conferred by the pancreas transplant is likely to be modest.

Effect of Pancreas Transplantation on Secondary Complications of Diabetes Mellitus

There are data that clearly demonstrate the impact of pancreas transplantation on the course of secondary complications of diabetes. This could to some extent be predicted from the results of the DCCT, in that pancreas transplantation leads to a complete normalization of blood glucose and glycosylated hemoglobin levels that are vastly superior to those achievable by intensive insulin therapy. Therefore, it should not be surprising that pancreas transplantation has an impact on diabetic complications.

For example, while type 1 diabetic recipients of kidney transplants alone show typical findings of diabetic nephropathy following transplantation, SPK transplantation prevents the development of recurrent diabetic nephropathy.[79] In addition, native diabetic nephropathy has been demonstrated to reverse 10 years following successful isolated pancreas transplantation.[80] These reports demonstrate convincingly that pancreas transplantation has a significant impact on diabetic nephropathy. Effects on diabetic neuropathy have also been documented using nerve conduction studies, which are significantly improved following pancreas transplantation.[81] Small corneal nerve fiber regeneration can be detected.[82] Furthermore, clinical progression of diabetic neuropathy is significantly diminished compared to nontransplanted controls. However, no study has been able to demonstrate clinical improvement in existing diabetic neuropathy following transplantation. There is also an impact on autonomic neuropathy, with clinical improvement in epinephrine responses to hypoglycemia.[83] While the DCCT demonstrated a relationship between glycemic exposure and retinopathy, the effect of pancreas transplantation on retinopathy is only modest. While stabilization of moderate retinopathy has been demonstrated, long-term graft function (>3 years) is required.[84,85] Many pancreas transplant candidates have advanced retinopathy, and an effect has not been demonstrated in these individuals. Early acceleration of retinopathy, a phenomenon that has been noted with other methods of improving glycemic control, can occur in the first 6 to 12 months following transplant. Despite the findings of the DCCT trial, an assessment of the impact of pancreas transplantation on the progression of atherosclerosis is lacking a definitive large-scale study. Smaller single-center studies are mixed, with some centers demonstrating a positive impact on peripheral vascular occlusive disease, and others demonstrating a worsening of disease.[86,87]

Regardless of the magnitude of objectively demonstrable benefits of pancreas transplantation, most recipients enjoy a dramatic improvement in quality of life.[65,88,89] While many diabetics can adapt quite well to the dramatic glucose fluctuations and the associated morbidity of diabetes, the freedom from insulin and the avoidance of hyper- and hypoglycemia offered by a functioning pancreas transplant is a primary motivator for many recipients. The fervor with which many candidates pursue pancreas transplantation, especially retransplantation, is an indication of the enormous benefit on quality of life for these individuals.

ISLET TRANSPLANTATION

Overview

The notion that insulin-producing β cells could be physically separated from the pancreas and transplanted for the treatment of diabetes has long been recognized. Islet transplantation, as a cellular transplant, has significant potential advantages over
7 whole-organ pancreas transplantation. Islet transplantation does not require an operative procedure.[90] In addition, the potential ability to preserve islets without impairment of graft function opens up possibilities with regard to distribution, allocation, transportation, and preparation of the islet recipient. Pretreatment of the graft to reduce immunogenicity or enhance survival and function is also possible.[91] Recipients of successful islet transplants can have glucose metabolism and insulin secretion profiles that are close to normal and maintain metabolic control in a manner equivalent to whole-pancreas transplantation.[92] Although effects on mortality and progression of diabetic complications are unproven, these benefits are also anticipated. From a long-range perspective, the development of islet transplantation sets some of the procedural, technical, and regulatory groundwork for the eventual establishment of stem cell–derived β-cell transplantation.

History

The development of islet transplantation was historically limited by poor graft survival. The first human islet allograft in a type 1 diabetic was performed in 1974 by the University of Minnesota.[93] The first islet autograft for the treatment of chronic pancreatitis was performed at Minnesota in 1977. Despite intense research in islet transplantation over three decades, until 2000, clinical islet transplantation met with minimal success.[94] While the transplanted islets were capable of physiologic function, as evidenced by the 66% rate of insulin independence at 1 year in the 163 recipients of islet autografts from 1974 to 1995, even these recipients had significantly reduced functional β-secretory reserve.[95] Alloimmunity to the islets presented an even greater hurdle; in the 96 islet allograft recipients with type 1 diabetes from 1990 to 1994, C-peptide production and insulin independence at 1 year were 25% and 7%, respectively.[94] Of the 270 recipients until 1999, only 6 had achieved insulin independence for greater than 2 years.

The dramatic improvement in islet transplant outcome reported by the Edmonton group in 2000 stimulated an increase in islet transplant activity.[96] Several important refinements in islet isolation and immunosuppression have largely been credited for the improvement in outcomes, including careful attention to pancreas procurement, minimization of cold ischemia time of the pancreas prior to isolation, avoidance of xenoproteins in the islet isolation process, and avoidance of steroids in the immunosuppressive regimen. Furthermore, the use of sequential infusions to achieve insulin independence has been critical to success for many centers. The enthusiasm that accompanied this recent success has been tempered recently by the inability for many new centers to replicate the success of more established centers,[97] the disappointing long-term survival of the transplants,[98] and the costs

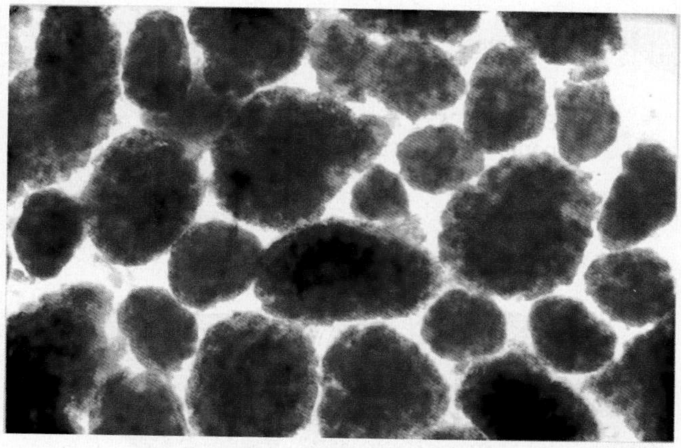

FIGURE 39.8. Isolated, purified human islets. Islets are stained red with diphenylthiocarbazone. (Adapted from Robertson PR. Islet transplantation as a treatment for diabetes: a work in progress. *N Engl J Med* 2004;350:694–705.)

associated with islet transplants, which are not routinely reimbursed by insurers.[99] As a result, the volume of islet transplants has contracted in the past few years.[100]

Islet Isolation

The precise separation of the islets from the other tissues of the pancreas (exocrine cells, lymphatics, vascular structures) is perhaps the most important determinant of successful islet transplantation (Fig. 39.8). One of the limitations of islet isolation is the difficulty in getting a large number of high-quality islets, and consistent success in islet isolation is a combination of science, art, and experience. Although a variety of methods have been utilized, most currently employ some modification of the semiautomated method described by Ricordi in 1988.[101] This method combines mechanical distention with enzymatic digestion of the pancreas. After cleaning the pancreas of surrounding fat, the pancreatic duct is cannulated with an angiocatheter and the pancreas is distended and loaded with warm collagenase solution, which digests the pancreas.[102] The pancreas is then placed into a sterile chamber, which also contains a number of stainless steel or glass spheres. Additional collagenase solution is added, and the chamber is attached to a shaking apparatus or agitated by hand. The collagenase solution is recirculated and kept at 37°C as the chamber is agitated. Agitation of the chamber allows the spheres to continue to disrupt the structural integrity of the pancreas as it digests. Following digestion, the separation of islets from nonislet tissue is performed via density gradient centrifugation. After suspension in culture media, islets are counted and assessed for sterility, purity, viability, and functional capacity. As islet isolation in the United States is regulated by the U.S. Food and Drug Administration, stringent product release criteria are in place to ensure the quality of the transplanted islets. The percentage of islet isolations that result in a transplantable preparation varies widely among centers, between 25% and 70%, and depends on both donor selection practices and the experience and expertise of the particular center.

Patient Selection

Candidates for islet transplantation are selected in a similar manner as for whole-organ pancreas transplantation. Islet transplantation is currently limited to adult type 1 diabetics with progressive diabetic complications who have failed intensive insulin therapy. Because islet transplantation remains experimental therapy with limited availability, the procedure is offered only to ideal candidates with minimal medical conditions other than diabetes. Most centers require evaluation and/or a period of treatment by an experienced endocrinologist specializing in diabetes. Candidates with coronary artery disease; chronic infections, including hepatitis B and C; or a prior solid organ transplant are excluded. Nonuremic candidates must be free of renal insufficiency, due to concerns about aggravation of nephropathy by calcineurin inhibitors. Since efficacy of the islet transplant appears to be related to the number of islets transplanted per kilogram of recipient body weight, only lean (<70 kg or BMI <28) recipients are selected. Although most islet transplants are currently performed in nonuremic diabetics, islet transplants either concurrent with or following kidney transplantation are also performed.[103,104]

Donor Selection, Procurement, and Preservation

Donor selection for islet isolation differs from that for whole-pancreas transplantation in several respects. While the ideal donor for islet isolation is still young and healthy, the age and weight criteria are less stringent than for whole-pancreas transplantation. Donors older than age 50, donors on vasopressors, and especially obese donors are all perfectly suitable for islet isolation. Since the ideal pancreas is easily distensible and digestible, fatty pancreata are felt to be especially suitable, whereas fibrotic pancreata are not. As previously mentioned, pancreata from older and obese donors (which are infrequently used for whole pancreas) are preferentially allocated for islet transplantation rather than for regional and national sharing for whole-pancreas transplantation.[33]

The pancreas is procured in a manner similar to whole-pancreas transplantation. However, less attention to preservation of vascular structures is required. Attention is paid to surface cooling following flushing of preservation solution, and avoidance of pancreatic injury. A number of reports have highlighted the importance of a dedicated team trained in pancreas procurement in the success of islet isolation.[105,106] Expanded use of the two-layer technique of pancreas preservation, using both standard preservation solution (University of Wisconsin solution or HTK) and oxygenated perfluorocarbon solution, has resulted in increased islet yields.[107–109] The two-layer technique also permits the successful use for islet transplantation of pancreata subjected to prolonged cold ischemia as long as 18 hours. Success with pancreata from DCDs has been reported.[110]

Transplant Techniques

The portal circulation of the liver is currently the preferred site for islet transplantation (Fig. 39.9).[111] This can be performed by a minilaparotomy, with infusion of the islets into a peripheral mesenteric vein. However, most centers utilize interventional radiology techniques, avoiding both a surgical incision and general anesthesia. Percutaneous transhepatic portal vein catheterization is done under ultrasound and fluoroscopic guidance, with usually a small-gauge (4-French) catheter. The islets are infused into the portal vein through the catheter by either gravity from an infusion bag or by hand injection, and the islets lodge in the hepatic parenchyma. Portal vein pressure is monitored intermittently throughout the procedure. Following infusion of the islets, hemostasis is usually achieved using a combination of coils and Gelfoam. Recipients receive heparin in the islet preparation, systemically during the procedure, and in the perioperative period as prophylaxis against portal vein thrombosis, a now rare but serious complication.

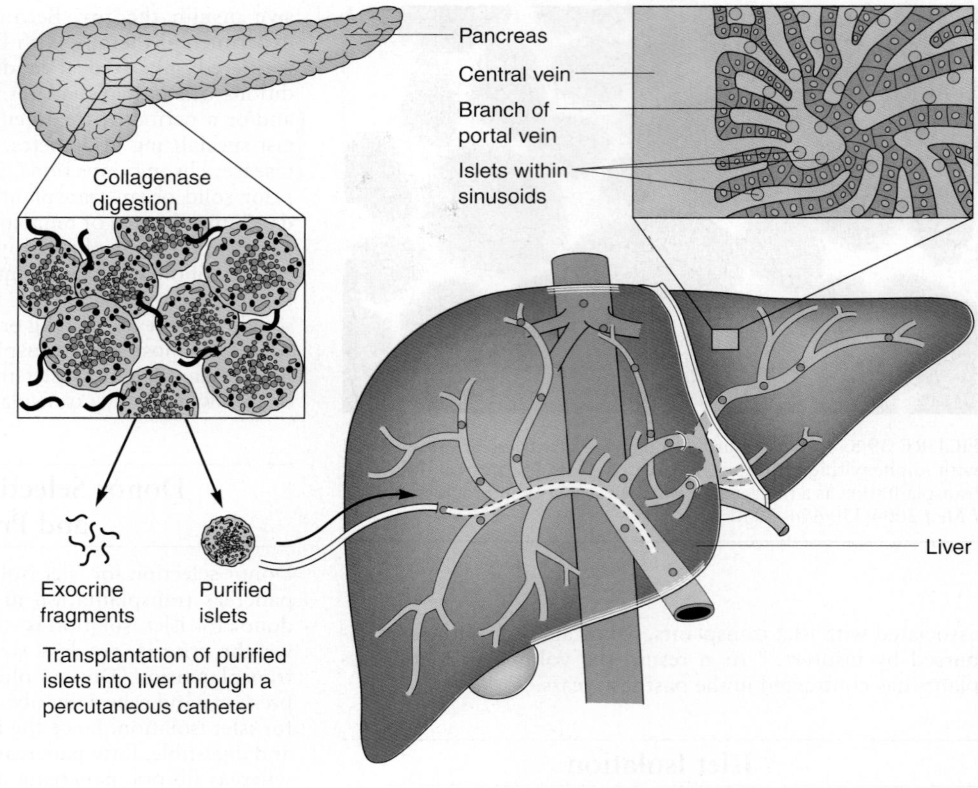

FIGURE 39.9. Islet transplantation. The pancreas is procured as a whole organ from the donor. The islets are isolated from the pancreas and are purified and infused into a cannula placed in a branch of the recipient's portal vein.

Perioperative Care

Although islet transplantation is in theory an outpatient procedure, it is not uncommon for recipients to receive a few days of inpatient care for monitoring purposes. Immediately following the islet transplant, patients are maintained on bed rest for a short interval and monitored for bleeding. Liver function tests are monitored, and a liver ultrasound is frequently done to assess portal venous flow and to check for hematoma. It has been demonstrated that intensive glycemic control with insulin in the immediate posttransplant period is beneficial for islet function.[112] Hence, many centers will give insulin postoperatively to keep the serum glucose tightly controlled, in order to "rest" the islets. Additional adjuncts to prevent nonspecific inflammation may include antioxidants such as vitamin E, antibodies against tumor necrosis factor-α, pentoxifylline, and others.

Immunosuppression

Current thinking focuses on the importance of the elimination of steroids from the immunosuppressive regimen, which typically uses basiliximab induction, and maintenance therapy with low-dose tacrolimus and sirolimus. Regimens employing mycophenolate mofetil and cyclosporine are also used, and thymoglobulin is an alternative induction agent. The best results for islet–kidney transplantation are cases where steroids are avoided or eliminated at the time of islet transplantation. Long-term effects of either the islet transplant or steroid elimination on kidney function are not known, and steroid avoidance in kidney transplant recipients is becoming increasingly common.[31]

Metabolic Control

Islet recipients show significant improvement in metabolic function and glycemic reserve. Although hormonal counterregulation to hypoglycemia is diminished, actual hypoglycemic events are rare.[113] However, islet recipients have significantly more diminished β-cell reserve than do recipients of whole-pancreas transplants, which may account for their reduced long-term survival.[114] Analyses of the impact on diabetic complications and mortality await further experience.

Complications

Morbidity from islet transplantation is substantial but much less than for whole-pancreas transplantation. The most common serious complication is bleeding (1% to 5%). Most cases of bleeding can be managed nonoperatively with adjustments in anticoagulation, though occasionally laparotomy is required. The side effects of immunosuppression, such as hyperlipidemia and mouth ulcers in sirolimus-containing regimens, are much more common and can significantly affect quality of life.[115] Renal insufficiency is an uncommon but serious consequence.[98] Transient elevations of portal venous pressure during islet infusion and elevations of liver function tests following infusion are common and usually well tolerated.[116,117] Recently, the demonstration of late steatosis has raised concerns about chronic liver disease; to date, this has not occurred.[118] Cytomegalovirus infection is rare. Sensitization to alloantigen does occur, although perhaps to a lesser extent than for whole-organ transplants.[98] Mortality is virtually nil.

Results

8 The short-term results of islet transplantation at high-volume centers are approaching that of whole-pancreas transplantation. The most successful centers achieve insulin independence rates of 80% to 90% at 1 year.[96,119,120] In the Immune Tolerance Network multicenter trial of the Edmonton Protocol, success rates at the most successful centers (Edmonton, Minnesota, and Miami) were significantly higher than at the other

centers.[97] However, long-term rates of insulin independence are significantly worse than whole-pancreas transplants: in most centers less than 50% of recipients are insulin-free at 3 years, and at the University of Alberta the median insulin-free interval was 15 months.[98]

One of the shortcomings of islet transplantation compared with whole-pancreas transplantation is the inability to reverse diabetes with the islets from one pancreas. Most of the recipients in the modern era have required two or more islet infusions to achieve insulin independence. However, some centers have successfully employed single-donor islet transplantation by utilizing careful donor and recipient selection, usually by transplanting islets from pancreata from large donors into small recipients.[119,121,122] However, as long-term outcome appears to be related to β-cell mass, which is likely to be lower for single-donor infusions, these recipients may return to insulin or require retransplants earlier.[123]

The ability to maximize the use of islets and minimize islet requirements and pancreas utilization for an individual recipient is critical if islet transplantation is to compare favorably with whole-pancreas transplantation.

Graft Failure

Graft failure appears to occur earlier than for whole-pancreas transplants. This may be related to a lower initial islet mass or the inability to histologically diagnose and treat islet rejection, since the islets are scattered about the liver parenchyma. Attempts to identify immunologic markers of rejection or recurrent autoimmunity, or metabolic indicators of impending graft failure are not of sufficient predictive value for clinical application.[124,125] Recipients with prior graft function who have returned to insulin are candidates for retransplantation. In fact, some centers have used transplanted islets from isolations where yields are insufficient for a primary transplant as retransplants, where the islet requirement may be less.

THE FUTURE OF PANCREAS AND ISLET TRANSPLANTATION

Many challenges remain in determining the ideal insulin replacement therapy for type 1 diabetics. While the current allocation system designed to maximize whole-pancreas transplantation ensures the most efficient use of donor pancreata, improvements in the efficiency of islet isolation may require that further refinements be made to allocation policy. Current outcomes support the prioritization of whole-pancreas transplantation over islet transplantation, and sufficient long-term survival reproducible among a larger number of centers may be required before islet transplantation can move further into the mainstream. If this occurs, the reduced morbidity of islet transplantation may mean that a large number of candidates who are not surgical candidates for pancreas transplantation may be islet candidates in the future. Many centers have taken the philosophical step to offer islet transplantation primarily to diabetics who would not otherwise receive immunosuppression (i.e., nonuremic diabetics). This is somewhat in contrast to PTA transplantation, which is offered to only the most exceptional candidates. Taken further, islet transplantation could theoretically be open to a large number of type 1 diabetics who would surely exhaust the limited supply of human donor pancreata. However, the experience gained by the development of islet transplantation would surely apply to technologies not affected by donor supply, such as islet xenografts or engineered β cells, which could have a profound impact on the devastating effects of diabetes on the public health worldwide.

References

1. American Diabetes Association. *National Diabetes Statistics*. Available at: http://www.diabetes.org/diabetes-statistics.jsp. Accessed December 1, 2008.
2. Engelgau MM, Geiss LS, Saaddine JB, et al. The evolving diabetes burden in the United States. *Ann Intern Med* 2004;140:945–950.
3. Faideau B, Larger E, Lepault F, et al. Role of beta-cells in type 1 diabetes pathogenesis. *Diabetes* 2005;54(suppl 2):S87–S96.
4. Donath MY, Ehses JA, Maedler K, et al. Mechanisms of β-cell death in type 2 diabetes. *Diabetes* 2005;54(suppl 2):S108–S113.
5. Tuomi T. Type 1 and type 2 diabetes. What do they have in common? *Diabetes* 2005;54(suppl 2):S40–S45.
6. Boitard C, Efendic S, Ferrannini E, et al. A tale of two cousins: type 1 and type 2 diabetes. *Diabetes* 2005;54(suppl 2):S1–S3.
7. Cnop M, Welsh N, Jonas J-C, et al. Mechanisms of pancreatic β-cell death in type 1 and type 2 diabetes. *Diabetes* 2005;54(suppl 2): S97–S107.
8. Butler PC, Meier JJ, Butler AE, et al. The replication of β-cells in normal physiology, in disease and for therapy. *Nat Clin Pract Endocrinol Metab* 2007;3(11):758–768.
9. Rubin RJ, Altman WM, Mendelson DN. Health care expenditures for people with diabetes mellitus, 1992. *J Clin Endocrinol Metab* 1994;78: 809A–809F.
10. Greene DA, Lattimer S, Ulbrecht J, et al. Glucose-induced alterations in nerve metabolism: current perspective on the pathogenesis of diabetic neuropathy and future directions for research and therapy. *Diabetes Care* 1985;8:290–299.
11. Sheetz MJ, King GL. Molecular understanding of hyperglycemia's adverse effects for diabetic complications. *JAMA* 2002;288:2579–2588.
12. DCCT Research Group. The effect of intensive treatment of diabetes on the development and progression of long-term complications in insulin-dependent diabetes mellitus. *N Engl J Med* 1993;329:977–986.
13. Nathan DM, Cleary PA, Backlund JY, et al. Diabetes Control and Complications Trial/Epidemiology of Diabetes Interventions and Complications (DCCT/EDIC) Study Research Group. Intensive diabetes treatment and cardiovascular disease in patients with type 1 diabetes. *N Engl J Med* 2005;353(25):2643–2653.
14. Garg S, Zisser H, Schwartz S, et al. Improvement in glycemic excursions with a transcutaneous, real-time continuous glucose sensor: a randomized controlled trial. *Diabetes Care* 2006;29(1):44–50.
15. Ceglia L, Lau J, Pittas AG. Meta-analysis: efficacy and safety of inhaled insulin therapy in adults with diabetes mellitus. *Ann Intern Med* 2006; 145(9):665–675.
16. Gerstein HC, Miller ME, Byington RP, et al.; Action to Control Cardiovascular Risk in Diabetes Study Group. Effects of intensive glucose lowering in type 2 diabetes. *N Engl J Med* 2008;358(24):2545–2559.
17. Kelly WD, Lillehei R, Merkel F, et al. Allotransplantation of the pancreas and duodenum along with the kidney in diabetic nephropathy. *Surgery* 1967;61:827–837.
18. Sollinger HW, Cook K, Kamps D, et al. Clinical and experimental experience with pancreaticocystostomy for exocrine pancreatic drainage in pancreas transplantation. *Transplant Proc* 1984;16:749–751.
19. Nghiem DD, Corry RJ. Technique of simultaneous renal pancreatoduodenal transplantation with urinary drainage of pancreatic secretion. *Am J Surg* 1987;153:405–406.
20. Nath DS, Gruessner AC, Kandaswamy R, et al. Outcomes of pancreas transplants for patients with type 2 diabetes mellitus. *Clin Transplant* 2005;19:792–797.
21. Dean PG, Kudva YC, Larson TS, et al. Posttransplant diabetes mellitus after pancreas transplantation. *Am J Transplant* 2008;8(1): 175–182.
22. Gruessner RWG, Sutherland DER, Drangstveit MB, et al. Pancreas allotransplants in patients with a previous total pancreatectomy for chronic pancreatitis. *J Am Coll Surg* 2008;206:458–465.
23. Scientific Registry of Transplant Recipients. *Special Analysis for the Organ Procurement and Transplantation Network Pancreas Committee*. 2008.
24. Farney AC, Cho E, Schweitzer EJ, et al. Simultaneous cadaver pancreas living-donor kidney transplantation: a new approach for the type 1 diabetic uremic patient. *Ann Surg* 2000;232:696–703.
25. Gruessner RW, Kendall DM, Drangstveit MB, et al. Simultaneous pancreas-kidney transplantation from live donors. *Ann Surg* 1997;226: 471–482.
26. Gruessner RWG. Living donor pancreas transplantation. In: Gruessner RWG, Sutherland DER, eds. *Transplantation of the Pancreas*. New York: Springer; 2004:429.
27. Morath C, Mueller M, Goldschmidt H, et al. Malignancy in renal transplantation. *J Am Soc Nephrol* 2004;15:1582–1588.
28. Stehman-Breen CO, Psaty BM, Emerson S, et al. Association of hepatitis C virus infection with mortality and graft survival in kidney-pancreas transplant recipients. *Transplantation* 1997;64:281–286.
29. Honaker MR, Stratta RJ, Lo A, et al. Impact of hepatitis C virus status in pancreas transplantation: a case controlled study. *Clin Transplant* 2002; 16:243–251.
30. Stock P, Roland M, Carlson L, et al. Solid organ transplantation in HIV-positive patients. *Transplant Proc* 2001;33:3646–3648.

31. Scientific Registry of Transplant Recipients. *2007 Annual Report*. Rockville, MD: Health Resources and Services Administration, Department of Health and Human Services; 2004.
32. Organ Procurement and Transplantation Network. *Organ Distribution: Pancreas Allocation*. Policy 3.8.
33. Stegall MD, Dean PG, Sung RS, et al. The rationale for the new deceased donor pancreas allocation schema. *Transplantation* 2007;83:1156–1162.
34. Douzdjian V, Gugliuzza KG, Fish JC. Multivariate analysis of donor risk factors for pancreas allograft failure after simultaneous pancreas-kidney transplantation. *Surgery* 1995;118:73–81.
35. Humar A, Ramcharan T, Kandaswamy R, et al. Technical failures after pancreas transplants: why grafts fail and the risk factors–a multivariate analysis. *Transplantation* 2004;78:1188–1192.
36. Gruessner AC, Gruessner RW. Pancreas transplant outcomes for United States (US) and non-US cases as reported to the United Network for Organ Sharing (UNOS) and the International Pancreas Transplant Registry (IPTR) as of June 2004. *Clin Transplant* 2005;19:433–455.
37. Humar A, Ramcharan T, Kandaswamy R, et al. The impact of donor obesity on outcomes after cadaver pancreas transplants. *Am J Transplant* 2004;4:605–610.
38. Scientific Registry of Transplant Recipients. *Final Analysis for Data Request for the Outcomes Model Review Sub-Committee of the OPTN Pancreas Transplantation Committee Meeting of March 5, 2008*.
39. Salvalaggio PR, Davies DB, Fernandez LA, et al. Outcomes of pancreas transplantation in the United States using cardiac-death donors. *Am J Transplant* 2006;6:1059–1065.
40. Fernandez LA, Di Carlo A, Odorico JS, et al. Simultaneous pancreas-kidney transplantation from donation after cardiac death: successful long-term outcomes. *Ann Surg* 2005;242(5):716–723.
41. Berney T, Malaise J, Morel P, et al.; the Euro SPK Study Group. Impact of HLA matching on the outcome of simultaneous pancreas–kidney transplantation. *Nephrol Dial Transplant* 2005;20:ii48–ii53.
42. Fridell JA, Agarwal A, Milgrom ML, et al. Comparison of histidine-tryptophan-ketoglutarate solution and University of Wisconsin solution for organ preservation in clinical pancreas transplantation. *Transplantation* 2004;77:1304–1306.
43. Rosenlof LK, Earnhardt RC, Pruett TL, et al. Pancreas transplantation. An initial experience with systemic and portal drainage of pancreatic allografts. *Ann Surg* 1992;215:586–597.
44. Frystyk J, Ritzel RA, Maubach J, et al. Comparison of pancreas-transplanted type 1 diabetic patients with portal-venous versus systemic-venous graft drainage: impact on glucose regulatory hormones and the growth hormone/insulin-like growth factor-I axis. *J Clin Endocrinol Metab* 2008; 93:1758–1766.
45. Petruzzo P, Lefrancois N, Berthillot C, et al. Impact of pancreatic venous drainage site on long-term patient and graft outcome in simultaneous pancreas-kidney transplantation. *Clin Transplant* 2008;22:107–112.
46. Stratta RJ, Shokouh-Amiri MH, Egidi MF, et al. A prospective comparison of simultaneous kidney-pancreas transplantation with systemic-enteric versus portal-enteric drainage. *Ann Surg* 2001;233:740–751.
47. Gaber AO, Shokouh-Amiri H, Grewal HP, et al. A technique for portal pancreatic transplantation with enteric drainage. *Surg Gynecol Obstet* 1993;177:417–419.
48. Sollinger HW, Sasaki TM, D'Alessandro AM, et al. Indications for enteric conversion after pancreas transplantation with bladder drainage. *Surgery* 1992;112:842–846.
49. Benedetti E, Najarian JS, Gruessner AC, et al. Correlation between cystoscopic biopsy results and hypoamylasuria in bladder-drained pancreas transplants. *Surgery* 1995;118:864–872.
50. Adrogue HE, Matas AJ, McGlennon RC, et al. Do inherited hypercoagulable states play a role in thrombotic events affecting kidney/pancreas transplant recipients? *Clin Transplant* 2007:21:32–37.
51. Troppmann C, Gruessner AC, Dunn DL, et al. Surgical complications requiring early relaparotomy after pancreas transplantation: a multivariate risk factor and economic impact analysis of the cyclosporine era. *Ann Surg* 1998;227:255–268.
52. Stratta RJ, Alloway RR, Lo A, et al. Two-dose daclizumab regimen in simultaneous kidney-pancreas transplant recipients: primary endpoint analysis of a multicenter, randomized study. *Transplantation* 2003;75: 1260–1266.
53. Kaufman DB, Iii GW, Bruce DS, et al. Prospective, randomized, multicenter trial of antibody induction therapy in simultaneous pancreas-kidney transplantation. *Am J Transplant* 2003;3:855–864.
54. Freise CE, Kang SM, Feng S, et al. Excellent short-term results with steroid-free maintenance immunosuppression in low-risk simultaneous pancreas-kidney transplantation. *Arch Surg* 2003;138:1121–1126.
55. Kaufman DB, Leventhal JR, Koffron AJ, et al. A prospective study of rapid corticosteroid elimination in simultaneous pancreas-kidney transplantation: comparison of two maintenance immunosuppression protocols: tacrolimus/mycophenolate mofetil versus tacrolimus/sirolimus. *Transplantation* 2002;73:169–177.
56. Kaufman DB, Leventhal JR, Gallon LG, et al. Alemtuzumab induction and prednisone-free maintenance immunotherapy in simultaneous pancreas-kidney transplantation comparison with rabbit antithymocyte globulin induction—long-term results. *Am J Transplant* 2006;6:331–339.
57. Thai NL, Khan A, Tom K, et al. Alemtuzumab induction and tacrolimus monotherapy in pancreas transplantation: one- and two-year outcomes. *Transplantation* 2006;82:1621–1624.
58. Troppmann C, Gruessner AC, Benedetti E, et al. Vascular graft thrombosis after pancreatic transplantation: univariate and multivariate operative and nonoperative risk factor analysis. *J Am Coll Surg* 1996;182: 285–316.
59. Gilabert R, Fernandez-Cruz L, Real MI, et al. Treatment and outcome of pancreatic venous graft thrombosis after kidney-pancreas transplantation. *Br J Surg* 2002;89:355–360.
60. Ciancio G, Julian JF, Fernandez L, et al. Successful surgical salvage of pancreas allografts after complete venous thrombosis. *Transplantation* 2000; 70:126–131.
61. Sollinger HW, Odorico JS, Knechtle SJ, et al. Experience with 500 simultaneous pancreas-kidney transplants. *Ann Surg* 1998;228:284–296.
62. Nath DS, Gruessner A, Kandaswamy R, et al. Late anastomotic leaks in pancreas transplant recipients—clinical characteristics and predisposing factors. *Clin Transplant* 2005:19:220–224.
63. Kuo PC, Johnson LB, Schweitzer EJ, et al. Solitary pancreas allografts. The role of percutaneous biopsy and standardized histologic grading of rejection. *Arch Surg* 1997;132:52–57.
64. Bartlett ST, Schweitzer EJ, Johnson LB, et al. Equivalent success of simultaneous pancreas kidney and solitary pancreas transplantation. A prospective trial of tacrolimus immunosuppression with percutaneous biopsy. *Ann Surg* 1996;224:440–452.
65. Sutherland DER, Gruessner RWG, Dunn DL, et al. Lessons learned from more than 1,000 pancreas transplants at a single institution. *Ann Surg* 2001; 233(4):463–501.
66. Carpenter HA, Engen DE, Munn SR, et al. Histologic diagnosis of rejection by using cystoscopically directed needle biopsy specimens from dysfunctional pancreatoduodenal allografts with exocrine drainage into the bladder. *Am J Surg Pathol* 1990;14:837–846.
67. Atwell TD, Gorman B, Larson TS, et al. Pancreas transplants: experience with 232 percutaneous US-guided biopsy procedures in 88 patients. *Radiology* 2004;231:845–849.
68. Kayler LK, Merion RM, Rudich SM, et al. Evaluation of pancreatic allograft dysfunction by laparoscopic biopsy. *Transplantation* 2002;74: 1287–1289.
69. Drachenberg CB, Odorico J, Demetris AJ, et al. Banff schema for grading pancreas allograft rejection: working proposal by a multi-disciplinary international consensus panel. *Am J Transplant* 2008;8(6):1237–1249.
70. Humar A, Khwaja K, Ramcharan T, et al. Chronic rejection: the next major challenge for pancreas transplant recipients. *Transplantation* 2003; 76:918–923.
71. Ricart MJ, Malaise J, Moreno AN, et al.; the Euro-SPK Study Group. Cytomegalovirus: occurrence, severity, and effect on graft survival in simultaneous pancreas–kidney transplantation. *Nephrol Dial Transplant* 2005;20(suppl 2):ii25–ii32.
72. Axelrod D, Leventhal JR, Gallon LG, et al. Reduction of CMV disease with steroid-free immunosuppression in simultaneous pancreas–kidney transplant recipients. *Am J Transplant* 2005;5:1423–1429.
73. Gupta G, Shapiro R, Thai N, et al. Low incidence of BK virus nephropathy after simultaneous kidney pancreas transplantation. *Transplantation* 2006;82:382–388.
74. Lipshutz GS, Mahanty H, Feng S, et al. BKV in simultaneous pancreas-kidney transplant recipients: a leading cause of renal graft loss in first 2 years post-transplant. *Am J Transplant* 2005;5:366–373.
75. Paraskevas S, Coad JE, Gruessner A, et al. Posttransplant lymphoproliferative disorder in pancreas transplantation: a single-center experience. *Transplantation* 2005;80:613–622.
76. Venstrom JM, McBride MA, Rother KI, et al. Survival after pancreas transplantation in patients with diabetes and preserved kidney function. *JAMA* 2003;290:2817–2823.
77. Reddy KS, Stablein D, Taranto S, et al. Long-term survival following simultaneous kidney-pancreas transplantation versus kidney transplantation alone in patients with type 1 diabetes mellitus and renal failure. *Am J Kidney Dis* 2003;41:464–470.
78. Gruessner RWG, Sutherland DER, Gruessner AG. Mortality assessment for pancreas transplants. *Am J Transplant* 2006;4(12):2018–2026.
79. Bilous RW, Mauer SM, Sutherland DE, et al. The effects of pancreas transplantation on the glomerular structure of renal allografts in patients with insulin-dependent diabetes. *N Engl J Med* 1989;321:80–85.
80. Fioretto P, Steffes MW, Sutherland DE, et al. Reversal of lesions of diabetic nephropathy after pancreas transplantation. *N Engl J Med* 1998;339: 69–75.
81. Kennedy WR, Navarro X, Goetz FC, et al. Effects of pancreatic transplantation on diabetic neuropathy. *N Engl J Med* 1990;322:1031–1037.
82. Mehra S, Tavakoli M, Kallinikos PA, et al. Corneal confocal microscopy detects early nerve regeneration after pancreas transplantation in patients with type 1 diabetes. *Diabetes Care* 2007;30:2608–2612.
83. Kendall DM, Rooney DP, Smets YF, et al. Pancreas transplantation restores epinephrine response and symptom recognition during hypoglycemia in patients with long-standing type I diabetes and autonomic neuropathy. *Diabetes* 1997;46:249–257.
84. Walsh AW. Effects of pancreas transplantation on secondary complications of diabetes: retinopathy. In: Gruessner RWG, Sutherland DER, eds. *Transplantation of the Pancreas*. New York: Springer; 2004:462–470.
85. Giannarelli R, Coppelli A, Sartini MS, et al. Pancreas transplant alone has beneficial effects on retinopathy in type 1 diabetic patients. *Diabetologia* 2006;49:2977–2982.

86. Morrissey PE, Shaffer D, Monaco AP, et al. Peripheral vascular disease after kidney-pancreas transplantation in diabetic patients with end-stage renal disease. *Arch Surg* 1997;132:358–362.
87. Knight RJ, Schanzer H, Guy S, et al. Impact of kidney-pancreas transplantation on the progression of peripheral vascular disease in diabetic patients with end-stage renal disease. *Transplant Proc* 1998;30:1947–1949.
88. Nakache R, Tyden G, Groth CG. Quality of life in diabetic patients after combined pancreas-kidney or kidney transplantation. *Diabetes* 1989; 38(suppl 1):40–42.
89. Gross CR, Limwattananon C, Matthees BJ. Quality of life after pancreas transplantation: a review. *Clin Transplant* 1998;12:351–361.
90. Owen RJ, Ryan EA, O'Kelly K, et al. Percutaneous transhepatic pancreatic islet cell transplantation in type 1 diabetes mellitus: radiologic aspects. *Radiology* 2003;229:165–170.
91. Lau H, Reemtsma K, Hardy MA. Prolongation of rat islet allograft survival by direct ultraviolet irradiation of the graft. *Science* 1984;223: 607–609.
92. Ryan EA, Lakey JR, Paty BW, et al. Successful islet transplantation: continued insulin reserve provides long-term glycemic control. *Diabetes* 2002; 51:2148–2157.
93. Sutherland DE, Matas AJ, Goetz FC, et al. Transplantation of dispersed pancreatic islet tissue in humans: autografts and allografts. *Diabetes* 1980; 29(suppl 1):31–44.
94. Brendel MD, Hering BJ, Schultz AO, et al., eds. *International Islet Transplant Registry 2001*. 2001;8:5.
95. Teuscher AU, Kendall DM, Smets YF, et al. Successful islet autotransplantation in humans: functional insulin secretory reserve as an estimate of surviving islet cell mass. *Diabetes* 1998;47:324–340.
96. Shapiro AM, Lakey JR, Ryan EA, et al. Islet transplantation in seven patients with type 1 diabetes mellitus using a glucocorticoid-free immunosuppressive regimen. *N Engl J Med* 2000;343:230–238.
97. Shapiro AM, Ricordi C, Hering BJ, et al. International trial of the Edmonton protocol for islet transplantation. *N Engl J Med* 2006;355(13): 1318–1330.
98. Ryan EA, Paty BW, Senior PA, et al. Five year follow-up after clinical islet transplantation. *Diabetes* 2005;54:2060–2069.
99. Markmann JF, Kaufman DB, Ricordi C, et al. Financial issues constraining the use of pancreata recovered for islet transplantation: a white paper. *Am J Transplant* 2008;8(8):1588–1592.
100. Close N, Alejandro R, Hering B, et al. Second annual analysis of the Collaborative Islet Transplant Registry. *Transplant Proc* 2007;39:179–182.
101. Ricordi C, Lacy PE, Firike EH, et al. Automated method for isolation of human pancreatic islets. *Diabetes* 1988;37:413–420.
102. Linetsky E, Bottino R, Lehmann R, et al. Improved human islet isolation using a new enzyme blend, Liberase™. *Diabetes* 1997;46:1120–1123.
103. Gerber PA, Pavlicek V, Demartines N, et al. Simultaneous islet-kidney vs pancreas-kidney transplantation in type 1 diabetes mellitus: a 5 year single centre follow-up. *Diabetologia* 2008;51(1):110–119.
104. Kaufman DB, Baker MS, Chen X, et al. Sequential kidney/islet transplantation using prednisone-free immunosuppression. *Am J Transplant* 2002; 2:674–677.
105. Lakey JR, Warnock GL, Rajotte RV, et al. Variables in organ donors that affect the recovery of human islets of Langerhans. *Transplantation* 1996; 61:1047–1053.
106. Kneteman NM, Lakey JR, Kizilisik TA, et al. Cadaver pancreas recovery technique. Impact on islet recovery and in vitro function. *Transplantation* 1994;58:114–119.
107. Lakey JR, Tsujimura T, Shapiro AM, et al. Preservation of the human pancreas before islet isolation using a two-layer (UW solution-perfluorochemical) cold storage method. *Transplantation* 2002;74:1809–1811.
108. Ricordi C, Fraker C, Szust J, et al. Improved human islet isolation outcome from marginal donors following addition of oxygenated perfluorocarbon to the cold-storage solution. *Transplantation* 2003;75:1524–1527.
109. Hering BJ, Matsumoto I, Sawada T, et al. Impact of two-layer pancreas preservation on islet isolation and transplantation. *Transplantation* 2002; 74:1813–1816.
110. Markmann JF, Deng S, Desai NM, et al. The use of non-heart-beating donors for isolated pancreatic islet transplantation. *Transplantation* 2003; 75:1423–1429.
111. Weimar B, Rauber K, Brendel MD, et al. Percutaneous transhepatic catheterization of the portal vein: a combined CT- and fluoroscopy-guided technique. *Cardiovasc Intervent Radiol* 1999;22:342–344.
112. Bretzel RG, Brandhorst D, Brandhorst H, et al. Improved survival of intraportal pancreatic islet cell allografts in patients with type-1 diabetes mellitus by refined peritransplant management. *J Mol Med* 1999;77: 140–143.
113. Paty BW, Ryan EA, Shapiro AM, et al. Intrahepatic islet transplantation in type 1 diabetic patients does not restore hypoglycemic hormonal counterregulation or symptom recognition after insulin independence. *Diabetes* 2002;51:3428–3434.
114. Frank A, Deng S, Huang X, et al. Transplantation for type I diabetes: comparison of vascularized whole-organ pancreas with isolated pancreatic islets. *Ann Surg* 2004;240(4):631–640.
115. Hirshberg B, Rother KI, Digon BJ III, et al. Benefits and risks of solitary islet transplantation for type 1 diabetes using steroid-sparing immunosuppression: The National Institutes of Health experience. *Diabetes Care* 2003;26:3288–3295.
116. Casey JJ, Lakey JR, Ryan EA, et al. Portal venous pressure changes after sequential clinical islet transplantation. *Transplantation* 2002;74: 913–915.
117. Rafael E, Ryan EA, Paty BW, et al. Changes in liver enzymes after clinical islet transplantation. *Transplantation* 2003;76:1280–1284.
118. Markmann JF, Rosen M, Siegelman ES, et al. Magnetic resonance-defined periportal steatosis following intraportal islet transplantation: a functional footprint of islet graft survival? *Diabetes* 2003;52:1591–1594.
119. Hering BJ, Kandaswamy R, Harmon JV, et al. Transplantation of cultured islets from two-layer preserved pancreases in type 1 diabetes with anti-CD3 antibody. *Am J Transplant* 2004;4:390–401.
120. Froud T, Ricordi C, Baidal DA, et al. Islet transplantation in type 1 diabetes mellitus using cultured islets and steroid-free immunosuppression: Miami experience. *Am J Transplant* 2005;5(8):2037–2046.
121. Gangemi A, Salehi P, Hatipoglu B, et al. Islet transplantation for brittle type 1 diabetes: the UIC Protocol. *Am J Transplant* 2008;8:1250–1261.
122. Markmann JF, Deng S, Huang X, et al. Insulin independence following isolated islet transplantation and single islet infusions. *Ann Surg* 2003;237: 741–750.
123 Keymeulen B, Gillard P, Mathieu C, et al. Correlation between β-cell mass and glycemic control in type 1 diabetic recipients of islet cell graft. *Proc Natl Acad Sci U S A* 2006;103(46):17444–17449.
124. Han D, Xu X, Pastori RL, et al. Elevation of cytotoxic lymphocyte gene expression is predictive of islet allograft rejection in nonhuman primates. *Diabetes* 2002;51:562–566.
125. Shapiro AM, Hao EG, Lakey JR, et al. Novel approaches toward early diagnosis of islet allograft rejection. *Transplantation* 2001;71:1709–1718.

CHAPTER 40 ■ HEAD AND NECK

MATTHEW C. MILLER, JEFFREY S. MOYER, AND THEODOROS N. TEKNOS

KEY POINTS

1. Tobacco and alcohol are the best-recognized risk factors for head and neck cancers. Their effects are synergistic.
2. No head and neck examination is complete until all mucosal surfaces of the upper aerodigestive tract have been visualized.
3. Early recognition of and preparation for a potentially difficult airway may prevent it from becoming an emergency airway.
4. The most common neoplasm in the head and neck is squamous cell carcinoma.
5. Cystic neck masses in adults are metastatic oropharyngeal carcinoma until proven otherwise.
6. In any smoker aged 35 or older with hoarseness, a neck mass, or mucosal abnormality, carcinoma must be ruled out.

The head and neck is a complex and intricate region of the body, and surgical management of head and neck diseases is both challenging and rewarding. A wide variety of benign and malignant processes are encountered by the head and neck surgeon, and a comprehensive review of this material is well beyond the scope of this chapter. However, head and neck complaints are relatively common and it behooves the surgeon to familiarize himself or herself with the processes. With that in mind, the following chapter is designed to introduce the reader to head and neck diseases, provide a framework for diagnostic evaluation, and discuss the treatment strategies commonly employed.

EVALUATING THE PATIENT WITH A HEAD AND NECK COMPLAINT

Patient Presentation and History

Though a few patients will be referred to the head and neck surgeon for incidentally discovered abnormalities, the vast majority of patients will present with a specific head and neck complaint. As with any medical discipline, concise history taking begins with questions aimed at determining the onset, severity, location, and quality of the presenting symptom along with any exacerbating or alleviating factors. Once this is completed, a head and neck review of systems should be obtained. Pertinent positives and negatives in this category will help to narrow the differential diagnosis and might point to the presence of an underlying malignancy. Table 40.1 lists common signs and symptoms that are associated with head and neck cancers. When any of these are present—particularly in the context of tobacco use or other risk factors (Table 40.2)—malignancy must be strongly considered.

The social history is of vital importance in evaluating patients with head and neck complaints. Tobacco and alcohol
1 use history must be specific and detailed. Tobacco users have up to 25 times the risk of head and neck squamous cell carcinoma when compared to nonusers. These carcinogenic effects are increased synergistically among heavy consumers of alcohol.[1,2] Type, amount, and duration of use should be documented as well as any previous efforts to quit (including methods used). Any significant secondhand smoke exposure should also be documented. Passive smoking either at home or at work is often overlooked during the history, but its role in the pathogenesis of many head and neck cancers is becoming increasingly evident.[3]

Human papillomavirus (HPV) infection is now widely recognized as a risk factor for oropharyngeal cancer. HPV is transmitted sexually, and the risk of oropharyngeal cancers has been strongly correlated to the lifetime number of sexual partners.[4] Consequently, the sexual history has become an important component of the overall assessment if carcinoma is suspected—particularly in the absence of other risk factors.

Additional medical, surgical, family, and occupational history should also be documented at this point. While these items may or may not have direct implications to the presenting problem, they may be critical to the overall patient evaluation and therapeutic decision-making process.

Physical Examination

Once an appropriate patient history has been obtained, a comprehensive head and neck examination should be undertaken. Many of the techniques and equipment used in the head and neck exam are specialized and may be unfamiliar to some practitioners. However, the examiner must become facile with them to perform a complete and appropriate patient evaluation. At a minimum, physicians treating head and neck disorders should have at their disposal and be comfortable using a stethoscope, a pneumatic otoscope, an assortment of angled mirrors, and nasal specula. A headlight or head mirror should be worn. This allows for the use of both hands during examination and provides superior visualization as compared to the omnipresent "single hand and flashlight" technique. Though most of the upper aerodigestive tract is visible by direct or indirect (mirror) examination, portions of the nasal cavity, nasopharynx, hypopharynx, and larynx are often difficult to assess. The flexible fiberoptic nasopharyngolaryngoscope (NPL scope, or NPL) has become an indispensable tool for this purpose.

Physical examination need not follow a strict sequence per
2 se. However, the entire surface of the head, neck, and upper aerodigestive tract must be evaluated. It behooves the examiner to develop his or her own systematic approach to prevent inadvertent omissions. It is the authors' practice to progress sequentially from the least to the most invasive portions of the exam. This allows for a gradual building of rapport and trust during what can for many patients be a sensitive exam and an invasion of personal space. It generally begins by visually inspecting the patient's face, neck, and scalp—paying attention to any asymmetry or irregularity of natural contours, cutaneous lesions, neuromuscular deficits, scars, or other stigmata of previous surgery and/or radiation therapy. Palpation of the neck ensues,

TABLE 40.1

DIAGNOSIS PROGRESSIVE SIGNS AND SYMPTOMS THAT MAY INDICATE A HEAD AND NECK CANCER

Odynophagia
Dysphagia
Weight loss
Loose dentition
Oral fetor
Trismus
Otalgia
Neck mass
Serous otitis media
Nasal obstruction
Epistaxis
Facial pain
Cranial neuropathies
Secondary infections
Aspiration
Fistulization
Hemorrhage
Voice changes
Stridor
Airway obstruction

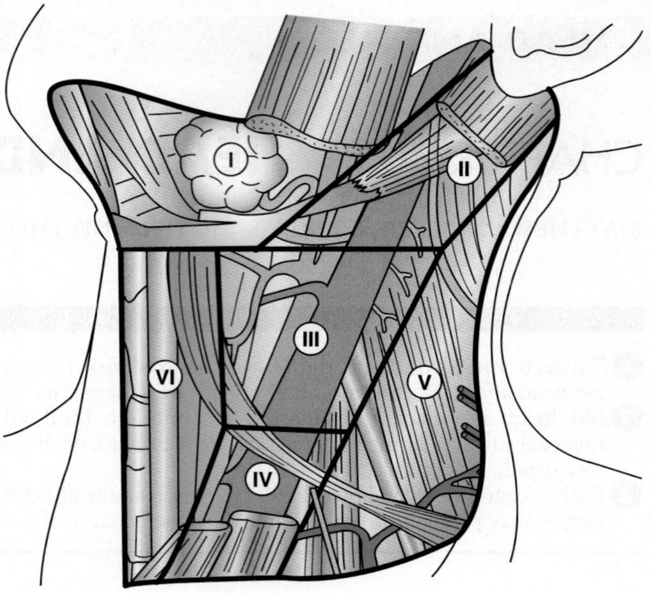

FIGURE 40.1. The cervical lymph nodes are divided into six groups, or levels. (Reproduced with permission from Robbins KT, Samant S. Chapter 116: Neck Dissection. In: *Cummings Otolaryngology-Head & Neck Surgery*, 4th ed. Philadelphia: Elsevier; 2003:2616.)

TABLE 40.2 **ETIOLOGY**

SELECTED RISK FACTORS FOR HEAD AND NECK MALIGNANCY

SKIN CANCER	**ORAL CARCINOMA**
Ultraviolet and ionizing radiation	Betel nut chewing
Neoprene inorganic arsenics	Snuff
Burns	Tobacco chewing
Riboflavin deficiencies	Reverse smoking
NOSE AND PARANASAL SINUS CARCINOMA	Syphilis
Wood dust	Vitamin B and riboflavin deficiencies
Leather manufacturing	Chronic irritation
Nickel refining	**LARYNGEAL AND HYPOPHARYNGEAL CARCINOMA**
Radium dial painting	Asbestos
Thorotrast and mustard gas	Coke oven exposure
NASOPHARYNGEAL CARCINOMA	Wood dust
Nitrosamine	Riboflavin deficiency
Salted fish	Gastroesophageal reflux disease
Epstein-Barr virus	Fanconi anemia
Vitamin deficiency	**SALIVARY GLAND CARCINOMAS**
Chinese heritage	Radiation exposure
Eskimo heritage	Eskimo heritage
	THYROID CARCINOMA
	Radiation exposure
	Iodine deficiency
	Genetic inheritance

TABLE 40.3 DIAGNOSIS

MOST COMMON PRIMARY SITES IN PATIENTS PRESENTING WITH NECK MASSES

NODAL LEVEL	PRIMARY SITE
I	Oral cavity
II	Oropharynx Nasopharynx Supraglottic larynx
III	Hypopharynx Larynx
IV	Thyroid Hypopharynx Larynx Subclavicular sites
V	Scalp Nasopharynx

TABLE 40.4 DIAGNOSIS

CLINICAL AND HISTORICAL ELEMENTS THAT MAY BE ASSOCIATED WITH DIFFICULT INTUBATION

Head and Neck Tumors (Both current and previously treated)
Trismus
Stridor
"Hot-potato" voice
Obesity
Sleep apnea
Micrognathia
Retrognathia
Macroglossia
Angioedema
Prior thyroid surgery
Prior orthognathic surgery
Facial fractures

with attention to the salivary glands, cervical lymph nodes, thyroid, trachea, and laryngeal cartilages. Auscultation of the neck and chest should also be accomplished. This is followed by formal cranial nerve assessment and pneumatic otoscopy. The remainder focuses on the mucosa-covered surfaces and should include a speculum exam of the nasal cavity, inspection of the oral cavity using a tongue blade in each hand to manipulate the soft tissues, bimanual palpation of the oral cavity and oropharynx, and indirect visualization of the nasopharynx, hypopharynx, and larynx with either the mirror or the NPL.

Documentation of the exam should include detailed descriptions and diagrammatic representations of any abnormality. Size, location, extent, and character should be included for any suspected neoplasm. When cervical adenopathy is present, the number, size, and anatomic level (Fig. 40.1) of the involved lymph nodes should be reported. The pattern of nodal spread from head and neck cancers is relatively predictable. In the presence of a neck mass, the nodal level involved may help to identify an occult primary tumor. Conversely, finding an unusual drainage pattern from a known primary tumor can alert the examiner to the presence of a second primary lesion (Table 40.3).[5]

The following sections review many of the conditions seen in a surgical head and neck practice. Coupled with the information garnered through the history and physical exam, it will provide a framework for generating and ultimately narrowing the differential diagnosis.

AIRWAY MANAGEMENT

Many conditions affecting the head and neck can result in upper airway obstruction. Obstruction may be chronic, as in the case of some neoplasms, or it may be acute, as in the case of hemorrhage or trauma. In either case, it is crucial that the surgeon be familiar with the techniques involved in securing an impaired airway.

3 *Management of the difficult airway begins with early recognition.* The historical and clinical elements listed in Table 40.4 may be associated with difficult intubation and/or airway obstruction. If attention is paid to these signs and symptoms, potentially hazardous situations may be anticipated and addressed in a controlled fashion before a difficult airway becomes an emergency airway. Orotracheal intubation remains the preferred means of accomplishing this goal. However, various conditions render the airway "difficult" and may preclude successful intubation. As a consequence, surgical intervention may become necessary.

Tracheostomy is the gold standard surgical airway. Elective tracheostomy is typically performed in a controlled setting (i.e., in the operating room). In an intubated patient, this procedure is undertaken under general anesthesia. If intubation cannot safely be performed, local anesthesia is used and tracheostomy is carried out on the awake, spontaneously breathing patient. Despite the anxiety and discomfort that may accompany this procedure, anxiolytics and sedatives must be used with caution. Continuous and detailed communication with the anesthesiologist is vital in the perioperative period and throughout the case. Figure 40.2 outlines the primary steps involved in elective tracheostomy.

In emergency situations, the procedure is identical with one significant distinction: Whereas elective tracheostomy uses a horizontal incision, emergent or urgent airway situations call for one that is vertically oriented along the midline of the neck (Fig. 40.2A). This reduces the risk of inadvertent injury to the anterior jugular veins and the associated increase in difficulty and time needed to secure the airway.

An alternative to the emergent tracheostomy is the cricothyrotomy. Cricothyrotomy has the advantage of being technically easier and faster to perform than tracheostomy. It is a means of rapidly securing the airway when the patient is in danger of imminent death because of mechanical respiratory obstruction. However, cricothyrotomy has the disadvantage of being a temporary solution. Instrumentation of the cricothyroid membrane may result in injury to the vocal folds as well as subglottic stenosis.[6] Consequently, the smallest endotracheal or tracheostomy tube that permits adequate ventilation should be used. Once the patient is stably ventilated, this should immediately be converted to a formal tracheostomy to prevent long-term damage to the larynx and proximal trachea.

NONNEOPLASTIC DISORDERS

Sialadenitis and Sialolithiasis

The three pairs of major salivary glands include the parotid, submandibular, and sublingual glands. In addition, there are hundreds of minor salivary glands situated diffusely throughout the oral cavity, pharynx, and larynx. A wide variety of nonneoplastic conditions can eventuate in swelling of either

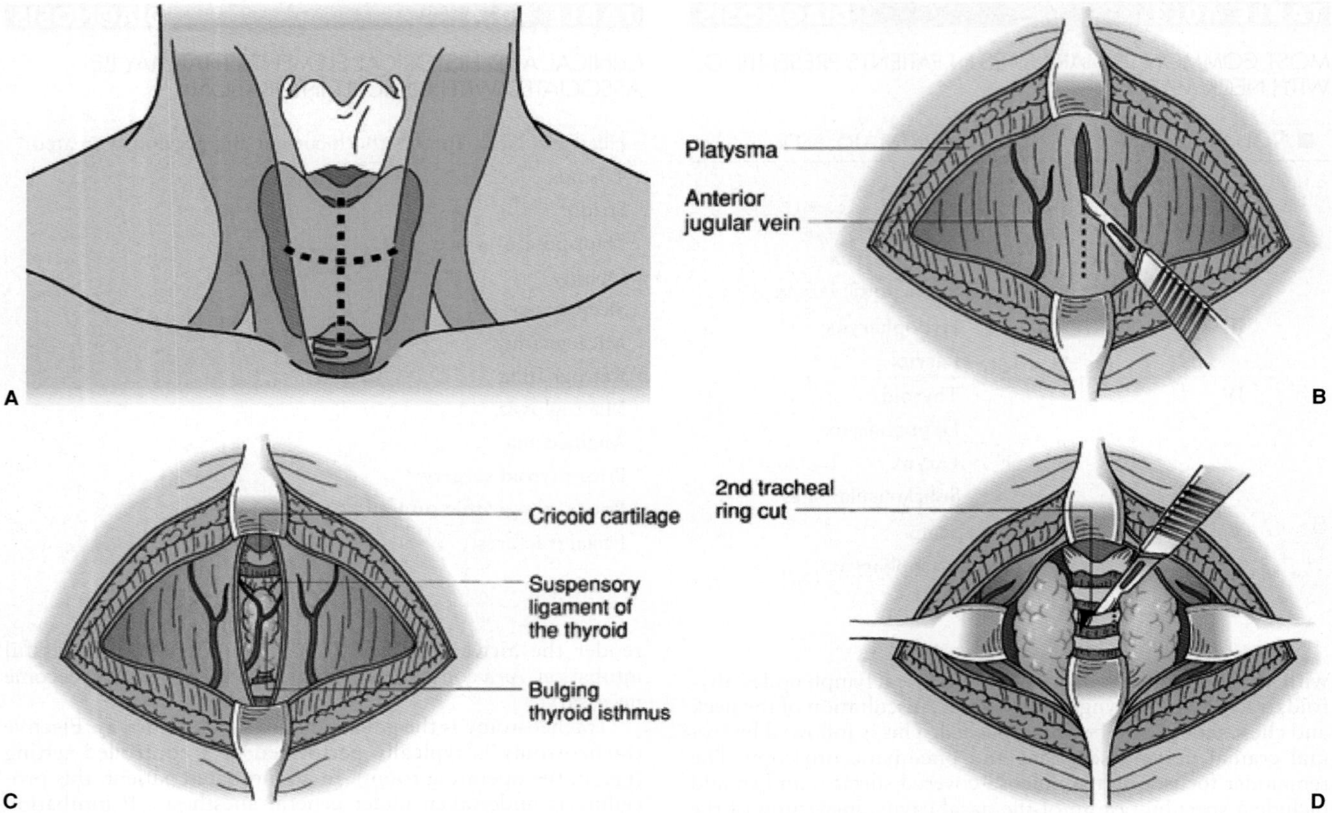

FIGURE 40.2. Tracheostomy. **A:** The incision for an elective tracheostomy is typically placed on a horizontal axis, approximately 2 finger breadths above the sternal notch. A vertical incision allows for less bleeding when the procedure must be performed emergently. **B:** The strap muscles are separated in the midline. The thyroid isthmus may bulge into the wound (**C**), necessitating inferior retraction or division (**D**). **E:** After the second tracheal ring is cleaned, an inferiorly based flap (i.e., Björk flap) is developed in the tracheal wall and sutured to the skin. This allows for easy access to the trachea while the tract is maturing.

the major or minor salivary glands—though they are most often observed in the paired major glands.[7] Table 40.5 lists several commonly encountered etiologic agents. Among these, infectious causes are most frequent. Mumps and other viruses may lead to diffuse bilateral swelling of the parotid and, to a lesser extent, the sublingual and submandibular glands.[7] Treatment is generally supportive.

Acute suppurative sialadenitis presents in a more fulminant fashion, with sudden onset of salivary gland pain and swelling. Acute sialadenitis is most often seen in the context of dehydration and xerostomia. The condition is commonly seen in the postoperative setting, particularly among patients undergoing gastrointestinal operations.[7] When compared to viral etiologies, bacterial sialadenitis is more often unilateral and is associated with a tense and tender gland. Purulent material may be expressed from the Wharton or Stensen duct during bimanual palpation. This material, when cultured, typically yields *Staphylococcus aureus*. However, other aerobic and anaerobic organisms have also been implicated.[8] Management is aimed at improving salivary flow through aggressive hydration, massage, warm compresses, and sialogogues such as sour candy and lemons. Antibiotic therapy should be initiated and should be broad enough to cover *S. aureus* and gram-positive aerobes. Rarely, parotitis may progress to an intraparotid abscess. This should be suspected in patients who are not responding to conservative therapy after 48 to 72 hours or in whom symptoms rapidly progress. Incision and drainage becomes a consideration in these patients, but should be undertaken with caution as the facial nerve and Stenson duct may be inadvertently injured during the procedure. Confirmatory imaging is a prerequisite to operative intervention in these cases.

TABLE 40.5 CLASSIFICATION

NONNEOPLASTIC SALIVARY DISORDERS

Congenital	
	First Branchial Cleft Cyst
	Lymphatic Malformation
	Vascular Malformation
Granulomatous	
	Sarcoidosis
Infectious	
	Mumps
	Hepatitis C
	CMV
	Tuberculosis
	Cat-scratch Disease
	Suppurative Sialadenitis
Other	
	Sialolithiasis
	Sialadenosis
	Juvenile Recurrent Parotitis

Adapted from: Kaplan M, Abemayor E. Major salivary glands. In: Fu Y, Wenig BM, Abemayor E, et al., eds. *Head and Neck Pathology with Clinical Correlations*. Philadelphia: Churchill Livingstone; 2001: 234, with permission.

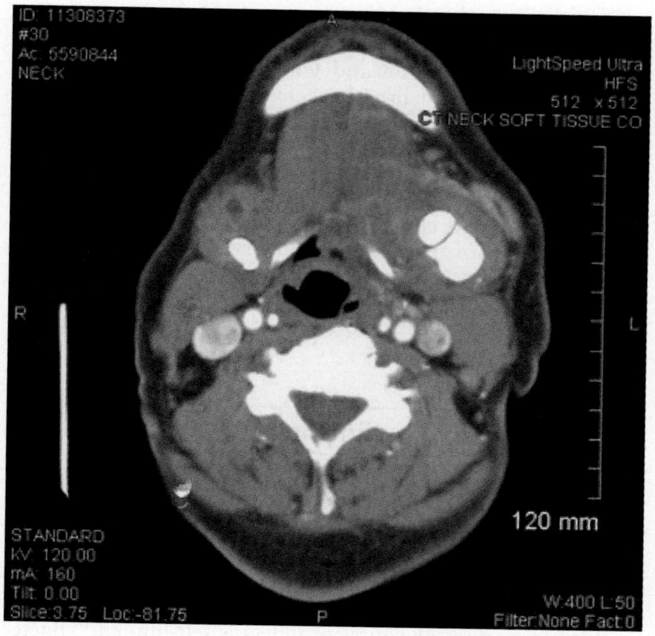

FIGURE 40.3. Axial CT scan demonstrating large bilateral hilar calculi of the submandibular glands. Stones of this size and location are generally not amenable to transoral or minimally invasive excision techniques. This patient underwent bilateral submandibular gland excision and recovered uneventfully.

Sialolithiasis is a disorder that merits special attention. Salivary stones are most commonly composed of calcium salts in the form of hydroxyapatite.[7,9] They are typically seen in the context of chronic sialadenitis, though their exact pathogenesis remains unclear. Calculi may form in any of the major salivary glands, though 80% to 90% are submandibular.[9] Patients typically present with recurrent, painful swelling of the submandibular region, often exacerbated at mealtimes. Noncontrast CT is the initial study of choice as nearly 90% of submandibular stones will be radio-opaque.[7,10]

Treatment depends on the size and location of the calculus. Occasionally, small calculi will pass through the Wharton duct spontaneously. Initial therapy for small, distally situated stones consists of observation and sialogogues. Dilatation of the papilla and proximal end of the Wharton duct and may also be performed. Stones located proximal to the mylohyoid muscle are less likely to be amenable to transoral removal. However, recent advances in fiberoptics have made transoral/transductal endoscopy (i.e., "sialendoscopy") possible. Several endoscopic techniques are now used for this purpose and have been successful in treating proximal stones.[9] Despite these advances, large, hilar, or intraglandular calculi are typically not amenable to transoral approaches (Fig. 40.3).[10] In these cases, formal submandibular gland excision is usually necessary.

Pharyngitis

Pharyngitis is one of the most common reasons for ambulatory care visits in the United States today. Strictly defined, pharyngitis is an inflammatory process affecting the mucosa and submucosal structures of the throat. Bacterial infection with group A beta-hemolytic streptococci (GABHS) has classically been associated with pharyngitis (i.e., strep throat). However, only 5% to 15% of all adult cases of pharyngitis can be attributed to GABHS. The vast majority of cases are viral in origin.[11,12] Other bacterial etiologies include non–group A

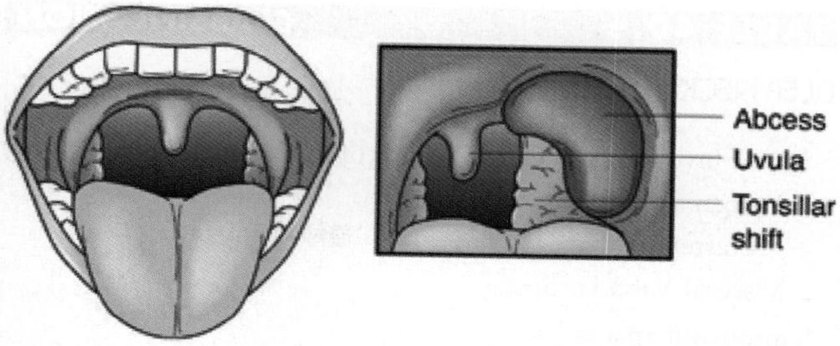

FIGURE 40.4. Schematic representation of a peritonsillar abscess. Purulence develops between the tonsillar capsule and the superior pharyngeal constrictor muscle. As a result, the palate bulges and the tonsil is deviated medially. Inflammation in the region of the pterygoid muscles results in pain and trismus, which may be significant.

streptococci, *Corynebacterium,* and *Neisseria* species, among others. Pharyngitis typically presents with sore throat and odynophagia. Bacterial tonsillitis is associated with purulent exudate, though this may also be seen in viral infections such as mononucleosis. Signs highly indicative of GABHS infection include fever, tonsillar exudates, tender cervical adenopathy, and the absence of a cough.[12] Patients with these signs and symptoms or in whom streptococcal testing is positive should be considered for antibiotic therapy with amoxicillin, erythromycin, or clindamycin.

Most pharyngitis is acute and self-limited, responding to supportive measures such as antipyretics, hydration, and, when indicated, antibiotics. However, bacterial pharyngitis may occasionally be complicated by a collection of purulent material in a potential space that lies between the tonsillar capsule and the superior constrictor muscle—the peritonsillar space. This space is contiguous with the retropharyngeal and parapharyngeal space.

Peritonsillar abscesses (PTAs) can potentially involve critical structures in these regions. Patients typically have a history of an antecedent pharyngitis. As pus collects in the peritonsillar space, symptoms may progress to severe sore throat, odynophagia, otalgia, and a "hot potato" voice.[13] On exam, the oropharynx has an asymmetric appearance, with uvular deviation, medial displacement of the tonsil, and bulging of the soft palate on the affected side (Fig. 40.4). Trismus is a common feature. The diagnosis is clinical, though contrast-enhanced CT scan may be used in equivocal cases or if repeated aspirations fail to alleviate the symptoms. Needle aspiration, incision and drainage (I&D), and tonsillectomy have each been successfully used in the initial management of PTA.[14] For cooperative adult patients without airway compromise, the authors favor a combination of bedside needle aspiration and I&D. After applying topical anesthesia, a 14-gauge needle is passed into the peritonsillar space and its contents aspirated. A number 11 scalpel is then used to create a cruciate incision centered on the needle entry point. This is enlarged and marsupialized using a hemostat. The remainder of the infected material is then evacuated. Antibiotic therapy with clindamycin or an extended-spectrum aminopenicillin is initiated.

Deep Neck Space Infections

The muscles and fascia of the neck divide it into a series of distinct but interconnected potential spaces commonly referred to as the deep neck spaces (Table 40.6). The intimate relationship that these spaces share with the airway, the great vessels, and the mediastinum underscores the importance of prompt recognition and management of deep neck infections (Fig. 40.5). Delays in diagnosis and treatment can be catastrophic as complications include airway obstruction, aspiration of ruptured

TABLE 40.6 CLASSIFICATION

DEEP NECK SPACES

Spaces Involving the Entire Length of the Neck
Danger Space
Prevertebral Space
Visceral Vascular Space
Suprahyoid Spaces
Pharyngomaxillary Space
Submandibular Space
Parotid Space
Masticator Space
Peritonsillar Space
Temporal Space
Infrahyoid Spaces
Anterior Visceral Space

Adapted from: Gadre AK, Gadre KC. Infections of the deep spaces of the neck. In: Bailey BJ, Johnson JT, eds. *Head & Neck Surgery—Otolaryngology,* 4th ed. Philadelphia: Lippincott Williams & Wilkins; 2006:670, with permission.

abscess material, mediastinitis, necrotizing cervical fasciitis, jugular vein thrombosis, and carotid artery aneurysm or rupture.[13] Fortunately, with the widespread use of antibiotics, the incidence of deep neck infections and their sequelae has declined.

Though classically associated with pharyngotonsillar disease, a growing number of deep neck infections are odontogenic in nature.[13] Other risk factors include diabetes mellitus, immunocompromise, intravenous drug abuse, and branchial anomalies.[13,15] A deep neck space infection should be suspected in any patient with the just-named risk factors who presents with neck pain and swelling.

The initial step in managing a patient with suspected deep neck infection is to ascertain the adequacy of the airway. Any signs of compromise should be addressed immediately by oral/nasal intubation or, alternatively, tracheostomy under

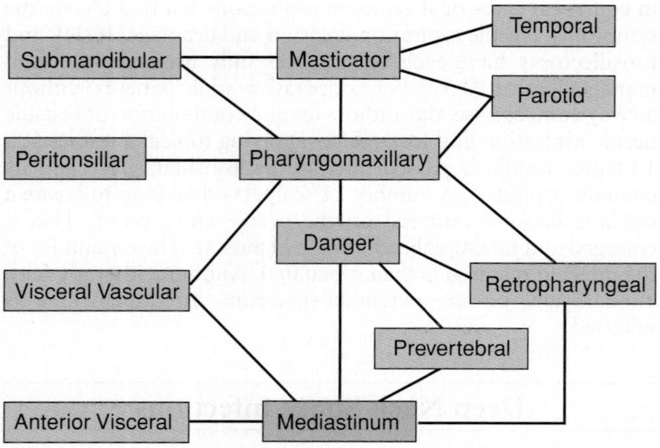

FIGURE 40.5. The deep spaces of the neck are distinct but interconnected compartments. Infections in any one of these may spread to involve other potential spaces and critical structures contained therein. (Adapted with permission from Gadre AK, Gadre KC. Infections of the deep spaces of the neck. In: Bailey BJ, Johnson JT, eds. *Head & Neck Surgery—Otolaryngology,* 4th ed. Philadelphia: Lippincott Williams & Wilkins; 2006:670.)

local anesthesia. Once a secure airway has been established, a contrast CT scan should be obtained. This will help to better characterize the infection and will aid in surgical planning. Empiric therapy with broad-spectrum antibiotics should be initiated. Coverage should include beta-lactamase–producing and anaerobic species. Though a few patients will respond completely to intravenous antibiotics, surgical drainage is the definitive therapy. This may be accomplished transorally or transcervically. The choice of approach depends on the exact anatomic locale of the infection, but should provide the most direct access to the affected space while minimizing risk to surrounding structures. It must also allow for the complete exposure and drainage of the involved space(s) and débridement of any necrotic tissue.

Sinusitis

Sinonasal complaints are among the most common reasons for ambulatory care visits. Patients present with headache, facial/retro-orbital pressure, nasal congestion, anosmia, and purulent rhinorrhea. Though these features are suggestive of acute bacterial rhinosinusitis, they are by no means pathognomonic. In most patients, the etiologic agent is a community-acquired viral infection and the course of illness is self-limited.[16] Bacterial growth is present in as few as one third of patients treated for sinusitis. The most common pathogens include *Streptococcus pneumoniae, Haemophilus influenzae, Moraxella catarrhalis,* and *S. aureus*.[16,17] Diagnosis is based on the constellation of symptoms and the presence of purulent material during nasal endoscopy.

Although there are significant effects on quality of life during bouts of acute and chronic sinusitis, most cases will resolve without antibiotics and the vast majority of patients will convalesce without long-term consequences.[16,18] However, the surgeon must be aware of the potential complications of acute suppurative sinusitis and their management. Complications of sinusitis may be grouped into three categories: local, orbital, and intracranial (Table 40.7).[19] A high index of suspicion is

TABLE 40.7 COMPLICATIONS

COMPLICATIONS OF SINUSITIS

Local
Mucocele
Pott's Puffy Tumor
Osteomyelitis
Orbital
Preseptal Cellulitis
Orbital (Postseptal) Cellulitis
Subperiosteal Abscess
Orbital Abscess
Cavernous Sinus Thrombosis
Intracranial
Meningitis
Epidural Abscess
Subdural Abscess
Intracerebral Abscess
Cavernous Sinus Thrombosis
Superior Sagittal Sinus Thrombosis

From: Epstein VA, Kern RC. Invasive fungal sinusitis and complications of sinusitis. *Otolaryngol Clin North Am* 2008;41:497, with permission.

vital since many of these conditions can lead to significant morbidity and even mortality if left untreated. The presence of high fever, facial swelling, mental status changes, cranial neuropathies, proptosis, chemosis, or vision changes should alert the clinician to the presence of a complicated sinusitis. High-resolution CT scan of the brain and sinuses should be obtained along with ophthalmologic and/or neurosurgical consultation. Treatment consists of parenteral antibiotics and prompt surgical intervention aimed at relieving sinus obstruction and draining the infected material.[19]

Sinusitis in the context of an immunocompromised patient presents a particular challenge. Individuals with diabetes mellitus, HIV, or myelosuppression owing to chemotherapy or transplantation are at risk of developing fulminant invasive fungal sinusitis. Failure to recognize and treat these individuals in a timely fashion results in rapid deterioration and death. Even among appropriately managed patients, the mortality rates may be as high as 80%. Patients with intracranial involvement fare worse, with the condition being almost universally fatal.[19] Diagnosis relies on clinical suspicion and the classic findings of black, necrotic tissue in the lateral nasal cavity on endoscopy. Biopsy and culture are required. The agents responsible for invasive fungal sinusitis include the Zygomycetes (*Mucor, Rhizopus,* and *Absidia* genera) and *Aspergillus* species. Histology reveals extensive necrosis and the presence of submucosal, perivascular, and intravascular hyphae on silver staining. The treatment involves aggressive surgical débridement that is extended until healthy, bleeding tissues are encountered. Craniotomy and orbital exenteration may be required. Long-term parenteral antifungal therapy and control of the underlying disease process are a must.

HEAD AND NECK NEOPLASIA

Neoplasms of the head and neck comprise a varied group of benign and malignant processes. While a handful of these diseases have no clear risk factors associated with them, a great number may be attributed to alcohol and tobacco use. Despite continued public health measures aimed at reducing the abuse of these substances, head and neck cancers remain prevalent throughout our society. Though there has been an overall reduction in the incidence rates over the past 30 years, mortality rates have shown more modest decreases during this period. In 2001, there were an estimated 75,000 new cases diagnosed and nearly 30,000 deaths attributable to head and neck cancers.[20]

Continued advances in diagnosis, treatment, and reconstruction have improved our ability to manage these diseases. However, the oncologic, functional, communicative, cosmetic, and psychosocial implications of head and neck neoplasms continue to be a challenge. A systematic approach is vital to achieving success in any of these areas.

The following sections will review the salient features of the most common head and neck neoplasms and their management strategies.

Salivary Neoplasms

Tumors of the salivary glands constitute 3% to 6% of all head and neck neoplasms. The parotid gland is most commonly affected, with 65% of all tumors arising in it. An additional 8% of tumors will be seen in the submandibular gland while 27% occur in minor salivary glands.[21] Most parotid and submandibular neoplasia is benign (75%–80% and 50%–60%, respectively). Conversely, more than 80% of all minor salivary gland tumors are malignant (Table 40.8). Patients with salivary tumors typically present with an asymptomatic mass. The presence of pain, trismus, or cranial neuropathy is suggestive of malignancy. Evaluation begins with a comprehensive history and physical examination. Given that most of these masses represent benign tumors of the superficial parotid gland, superficial parotidectomy with dissection and preservation of the facial nerve is often undertaken without additional workup. However, malignancy may be present in the absence of the previously mentioned signs and symptoms. As a consequence, fine-needle aspiration (FNA) cytology is often used prior to surgical intervention. This test has predictive values in excess of 90%, and the results may be useful in surgical planning and patient counseling.[22] MRI with contrast is the preferred imaging modality. This test can provide additional useful information about tumor size and position relative to the deep and superficial lobes of the parotid gland and may uncover multifocal disease (a feature present in nearly 10% of Warthin tumors).[7,22]

TABLE 40.8 **CLASSIFICATION**

COMMON SALIVARY NEOPLASMS

Benign
Pleomorphic adenoma (benign mixed tumor)
Warthin tumor (papillary cystadenoma lymphomatosum)
Basal cell adenoma
Oncocytoma
Malignant
Mucoepidermoid carcinoma
Adenoid cystic carcinoma
Acinic cell carcinoma
Salivary ductal adenocarcinoma
Carcinoma ex pleomorphic adenoma
Adenocarcinoma NOS

Among the benign salivary neoplasms, pleomorphic adenoma (benign mixed tumor) is the most common, accounting for nearly 70%.[7] Grossly, these appear as nodular, gray-tan masses. Though they appear to be well-circumscribed, histologic examination commonly reveals islands of tumor and pseudopodia extending into and beyond the capsule.[23] Simple enucleation of these tumors may result in their incomplete removal and eventuate in multifocal tumor recurrence. Appropriate surgical management therefore requires that they be widely excised to include a cuff of normal parotid tissue. The position of the facial nerve within the substance of the parotid gland necessitates its proximal identification and distal dissection during parotidectomy (Fig. 40.6). Superficial parotidectomy is the procedure of choice for nearly all benign parotid neoplasms.

Malignant salivary neoplasms are less frequent but require more aggressive therapy. They are staged according to their size and the degree of local extension (Table 40.9). Mucoepidermoid carcinoma is the most common malignancy of the parotid gland. These tumors are grouped by histologic grade, with low-grade tumors behaving in a more indolent fashion than intermediate and high-grade tumors. High-grade tumors demonstrate a prominent epidermoid component and smaller numbers of mucoid cells. Overall, high-grade mucoepidermoid carcinomas carry a poor prognosis. Rates of nodal and distant metastases may exceed 40% and 30%, respectively.[24]

Surgery for malignant parotid tumors involves total parotidectomy. The facial nerve should be preserved except in cases of direct tumor extension or preexisting facial paresis.[21,24]

Adenoid cystic carcinoma is the most common malignancy of the submandibular and minor salivary glands (Fig. 40.7).[21] These tumors are characterized by their propensity for

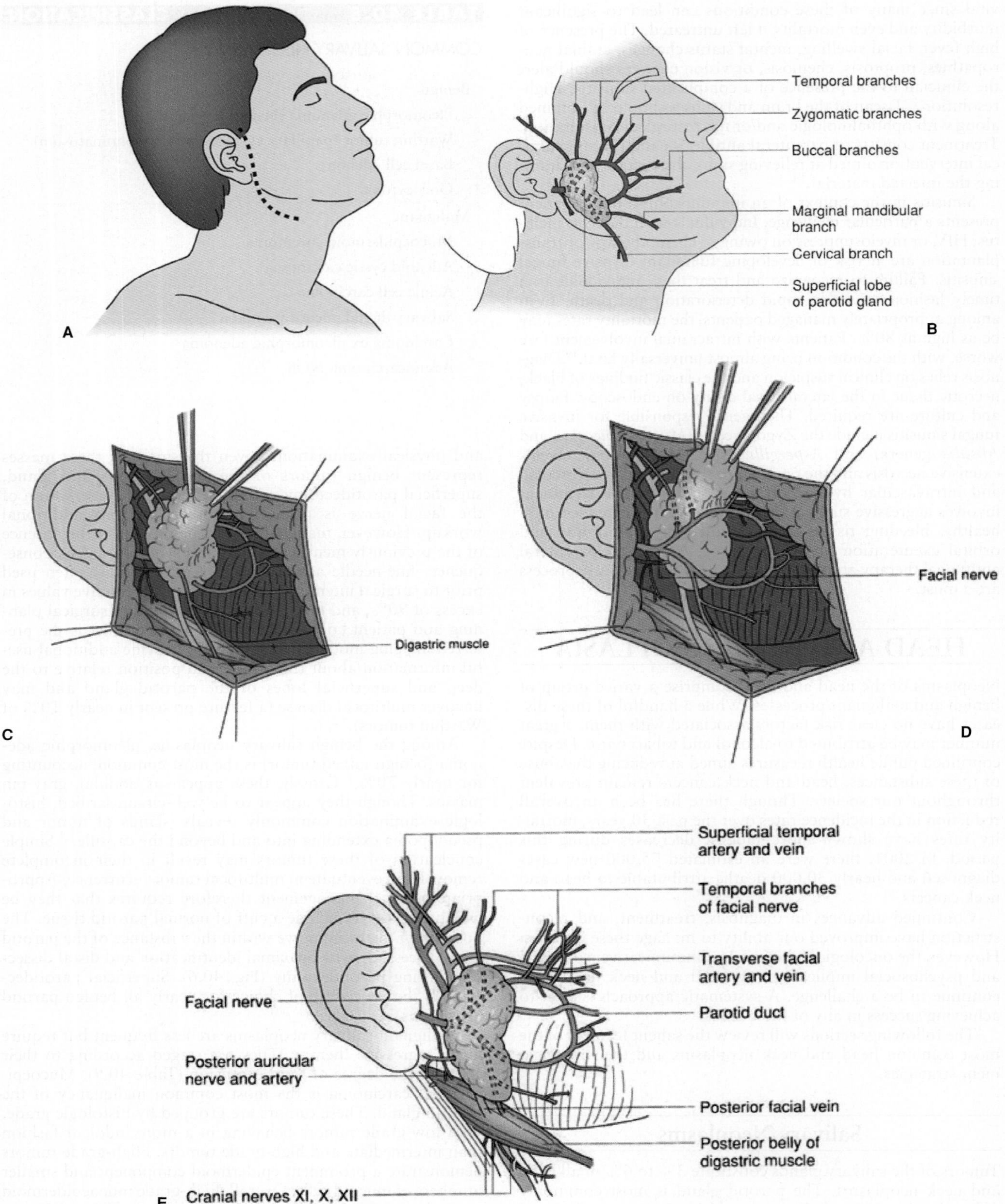

FIGURE 40.6. Superficial parotidectomy. A: The standard Blair incision or the cosmetically superior rhytidectomy incision may be used. B: Branches of the facial nerve course between the superficial and deep lobes of the parotid. C: The main trunk of the facial nerve is identified 8 mm deep to the tympanomastoid suture line and at the same level as the digastric muscle. D: The nerve is then dissected distally, separating it from the substance of the parotid. E: Schematic representation of the relationship between the parotid and surrounding structures.

TABLE 40.9 STAGING

AJCC STAGING FOR PRIMARY TUMORS OF THE MAJOR SALIVARY GLANDS

Tx	Tumor cannot be assessed
T0	No evidence of primary tumor
T1	Tumor < or = 2 cm in greatest dimension without extraparenchymal extension
T2	Tumor > 2 cm, but ≤ 4 cm in greatest dimension without extraparenchymal extension
T3	Tumor > 4 cm and/or having extraparenchymal extension
T4a	Tumor invades skin, mandible, ear canal, and/or facial nerve
T4b	Tumor invades skull base and/or pterygoid plates and/or encases the carotid artery

From: American Joint Committee on Cancer. *Cancer Staging Manual,* 6th ed. New York: Springer-Verlag; 2002, with permission.

TABLE 40.10 MANAGEMENT

GENERAL CONSIDERATIONS FOR TREATMENT OF SALIVARY GLAND MALIGNANCIES

Malignant tumors of the parotid gland warrant total parotidectomy.

The facial nerve should be sacrificed only in cases of direct tumor invasion or preexisting facial paralysis.

Patients with high-grade tumors should undergo elective neck dissection.

Postoperative radiotherapy is indicated for all high-grade tumors; close margins; recurrent disease; skin, bone, nerve, or extraparotid extension; positive nodes; and unresectable tumors.

perineural spread. Up to 70% will exhibit this feature and skip lesions are common, resulting in a high local recurrence rate.[24] Adenoid cystic carcinomas are also marked by their unique natural history. Patients may experience 10- to 20-year disease-free intervals followed by a sudden and aggressive recurrence. Lung metastases are common, occurring in nearly half of all patients. Treatment consists of aggressive local therapy and adjuvant radiation with electron or neutron beam radiation.[24,25] General principles regarding the management of salivary carcinomas are listed in Table 40.10.

Sinonasal Neoplasms

Various epithelial and mesenchymal tumors may arise within the sinonasal tract. Patients with sinonasal neoplasms will often present with recurrent epistaxis and unilateral nasal obstruction. Many will report having been treated for chronic sinusitis for several months prior to referral. Diagnosis is established by nasal endoscopy with biopsy. Imaging should include both high-resolution CT scan and a contrast-enhanced MRI. CT is used to evaluate for bony destruction whereas MRI is useful for differentiating tumor mass from inspissated secretions within the nose and sinuses. Approximately half of all sinonasal neoplasms are malignant, with squamous cell carcinoma accounting for nearly 80% of the cancers (these will be discussed in detail later in this chapter).[26] However, several benign lesions involving the nose and paranasal sinuses can exhibit aggressive behavior as well.

The most common benign sinonasal tumor is the papilloma. There are three categories of sinonasal papilloma (also known as schneiderian papillomas after the schneiderian mucosa lining the nasal wall): fungiform, cylindrical, and inverting.[27] Fungiform papillomas arise from the nasal septum, whereas cylindrical and inverting papillomas originate from the lateral nasal wall. Inverting papillomas are the most common variant. They are noteworthy for their significant propensity for recurrence

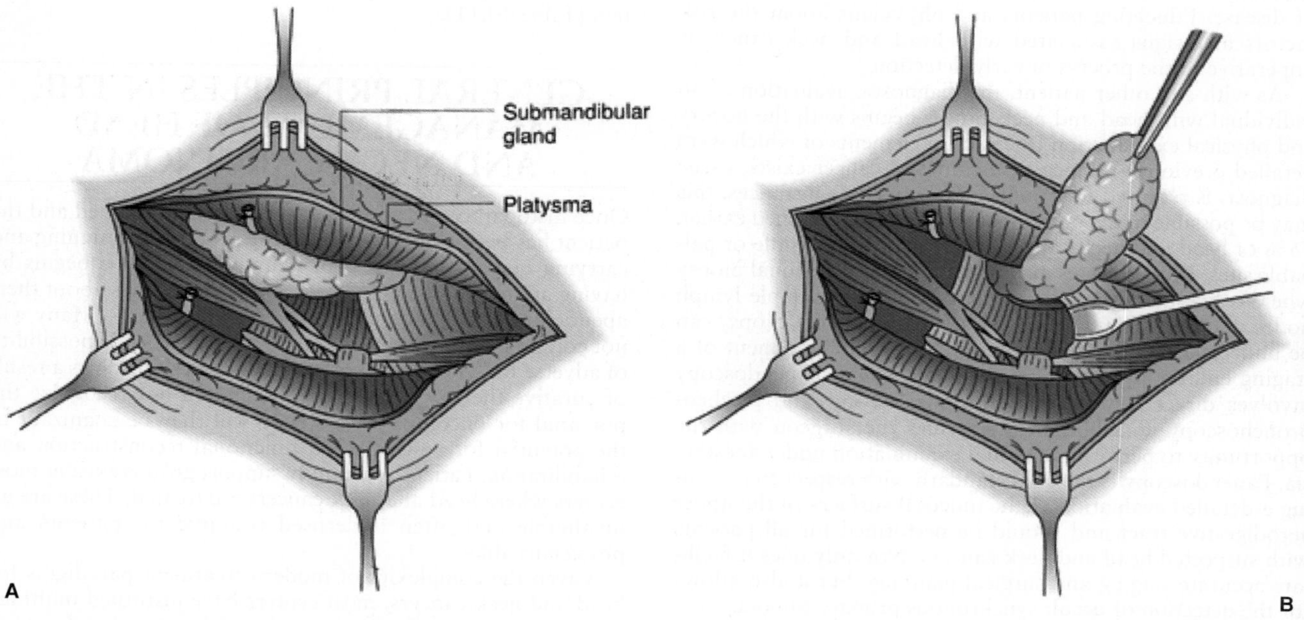

FIGURE 40.7. Excision of the submandibular gland. The skin incision usually is placed in a skin crease. **A:** After division of platysma, the ramus mandibularis is identified and retracted superiorly. **B:** Elevation of the gland allows identification of the lingual and hypoglossal nerves. After removal of the gland, the lingual nerve is in the base of the wound.

and for the fact that up to 20% will harbor in situ or invasive squamous cell carcinoma.[26] Consequently, removal of these lesions should be aggressive. Wide excision using a lateral rhinotomy approach and medial maxillectomy provides the greatest chance of cure, with recurrence rates ranging from 0 to 30%.[27] Advances in endoscopic instrumentation and techniques over the past decade have allowed for complete excision of these lesions through minimally invasive transnasal approaches. At centers experienced in endoscopic resection, the rates of disease control meet and in some cases exceed those achieved through open maxillectomy.[28]

Juvenile nasal angiofibromas (JNAs) are benign vascular tumors found in the adolescent male population. These patients present with unilateral nasal obstruction with recurrent bouts of epistaxis. Many will require repeat transfusions. Recurrent epistaxis in a young or adolescent male necessitates a formal endonasal and nasopharyngeal exam. On endoscopy, these appear as friable masses along the lateral nasopharyngeal wall. They are thought to originate near the sphenopalatine foramen. Though histologically benign, these lesions may expand into the pterygopalatine fossa, nasal cavity, orbit, and skull base—leading to pain, swelling, trismus, cranial neuropathies, and vision changes.[26,29] Management involves complete excision via a transpalatal or transmaxillary approach. Surgery is often complicated by profuse bleeding, and preoperative embolization is recommended. Endoscopic-transnasal approaches have demonstrated safety and efficacy in the management of JNA. These techniques continue to be investigated, but in expert hands it appears that they may impart better cosmetic outcomes, reduced blood loss, and shorter hospital stay.[30]

Squamous Cell Carcinoma

In many ways, squamous cell carcinoma has become synonymous with head and neck cancer. Indeed, 80% to 90% of nonthyroidal/nonsalivary head and neck cancers are squamous cell carcinomas.[2,20] Most of these tumors occur at readily visible or palpable sites.[20] Despite this, many patients delay seeking treatment and present with advanced disease—thereby dramatically reducing the chance of cure. With earlier diagnosis, many of these individuals might otherwise be rendered free of disease. Educating patients and physicians about the risk factors and signs associated with head and neck cancer is imperative to the process of early detection.

As with any other patient, the diagnostic evaluation of an individual with head and neck cancer begins with the history and physical examination (the critical elements of which were detailed previously). Once suspicion of a cancer exists, tissue diagnosis is required for confirmation. In some instances, this may be possible in the outpatient setting. As mentioned earlier, 75% of head and neck cancers occur at readily visible or palpable sites. Mucosal sites may be sampled by excisional biopsy whereas fine-needle aspiration may be used to sample lymph nodes or other subcutaneous masses. Alternatively, biopsy can be undertaken under general anesthesia as a component of a staging endoscopy procedure (*panendoscopy*). Panendoscopy involves direct laryngoscopy, esophagoscopy, and tracheobronchoscopy. In addition, it provides the surgeon with the opportunity to perform bimanual examination under anesthesia. Panendoscopy is the gold standard with respect to providing a detailed evaluation of the mucosal surfaces of the upper aerodigestive tract and should be performed for all patients with suspected head and neck cancers. Not only does it facilitate accurate staging and surgical planning, but it also allows for the detection of occult synchronous primary tumors.

Second primary tumors are common in the context of head and neck cancer and occur in approximately 20% of patients (published reports range from ~5%–~35%).[31] Second primary tumors are more likely in heavy tobacco users (>20 pack years), patients diagnosed before age 60 years, patients with oropharyngeal cancers, and among those with early-stage disease at initial presentation.[31,32] Among patients with nonlaryngeal primary head and neck tumors, synchronous lesions are most often found on the mucosal surface of other upper aerodigestive tract subsites. The lung and mainstem bronchi are the most frequently affected locations in the context of laryngeal carcinoma.[33] The development of a synchronous or metachronous primary tumor imparts a dismal prognosis. Mortality rates in excess of 80% can be expected in the presence of a second primary head and neck cancer. If the second primary tumor develops in the lung or esophagus, the probability of survival drops to less than 5%.[32]

The findings on panendoscopy are coupled with the outpatient examination and the results of imaging studies, and the patient is then staged according to the TNM classification and the American Joint Committee for Cancer (AJCC) staging system (Table 40.11).

TABLE 40.11 STAGING

AJCC STAGE GROUPING FOR CANCERS OF THE HEAD AND NECK (EXCLUDING THYROID AND NASOPHARYNX)

■ STAGE	■ STAGE GROUPING
0	Tis, N0, M0
I	T1, N0, M0
II	T2, N0, M0
III	T3, N0, M0
	T1–T3, N1, M0
IVA	T4a, N0–1, M0
	T1–T4a, N2, M0
IVB	T4b, Any N, M0
	Any T, N3, M0
IVC	Any T, Any N, M1

From: American Joint Committee on Cancer. *Cancer Staging Manual*, 6th ed. New York: Springer-Verlag; 2002, with permission.

GENERAL PRINCIPLES IN THE MANAGEMENT OF HEAD AND NECK CARCINOMA

Once histopathologic confirmation has been obtained and the patient has been clinically staged, the process of designing and carrying out a treatment plan is undertaken. This begins by having an open and frank discussion with patients about therapeutic options, risks, outcomes, and expectations. Many will not comprehend the gravity of their situation or the possibility of adverse functional and cosmetic outcomes arising as a result of curative therapy. Conversely, some will not recognize the potential for oncologic success nor will they be cognizant of the potential for aesthetic and functional reconstruction and rehabilitation. Patient and family support groups exist at most centers where head and neck cancers are treated. These are an invaluable and often underused resource for patients and physicians alike.

Given the complexity of modern treatment paradigms for head and neck cancers, most centers have instituted multidisciplinary tumor boards from which therapeutic plans are derived for each individual patient. Specific plans outlined will differ based on a given patient's tumor characteristics, functional status, potential for rehabilitation, and comorbidities.

Individual and institutional resources, customs, and biases also come into play. However, the principal goal in treating any head and neck cancer is to completely and permanently eradicate the disease. Treatment should be carried out in a manner that limits potential functional consequences to the greatest degree possible (without compromising the chance for cure).

The mainstays of treatment in head and neck cancer are surgery, external beam radiation therapy, and systemic chemotherapy. As a general rule, single-modality therapy is highly effective for early cancers (stages I and II). By definition, stages I and II carcinomas represent small, localized tumors without evidence of cervical metastases. This is true for all mucosal subsites within the head and neck. These are readily treated by surgery or radiation therapy and have a favorable prognosis. Among stages I and II head and neck tumors, survival rates exceed 80% after either definitive radiotherapy or surgery.[34] The decision to use surgery or radiation therapy depends on the tumor subsite, the expertise of the surgeon and radiation oncologist, and the preference of the patient. Surgical treatment provides immediate cure and allows radiation therapy to be reserved for future needs (i.e., recurrent disease, second primary tumors, etc.). Radiation carries with it a significant time requirement (standard head and neck protocols call for approximately 6 weeks of daily treatments). However, it avoids the removal or recontouring of anatomic structures that is associated with surgical resection. This has made radiation therapy a popular alternative for tumors in functionally sensitive areas such as the glottic larynx.

In contrast to stages I and II carcinomas, later-stage disease requires sequential or concomitant therapy using two and sometimes three different treatment modalities. In most cases, these tumors exhibit locally aggressive features or have metastasized to regional lymph nodes. Though radical resection is typically used with curative intent, there is a potential for microscopic residual disease even after all gross disease has been removed. In this context, adjuvant therapy is aimed at sterilizing any remaining viable tumor. Classically, external beam radiation therapy was used for this purpose. Indications for postoperative radiation therapy include locally advanced (T3 or T4) primary tumors, high-grade histology, perineural or vascular invasion, positive or close resection margins, N2 or N3 disease, and extracapsular nodal extension.[34] In 2004, the results of two separate prospective trials comparing the effects of adjuvant radiation therapy to adjuvant chemoradiotherapy were published simultaneously. Among high-risk head and neck cancers (i.e., with extracapsular nodal extension, multiple positive lymph nodes, or positive resection margins), both found that adjuvant chemoradiation significantly improved locoregional control. Survival was also improved in both, though to a statistically significant degree in only one of the two.[35,36]

In rare instances, tumor volume, invasiveness, or proximity to critical structures may render it unresectable. In such circumstances, the potential for morbidity and/or mortality exceeds the reasonable probability of cure. Examples include circumferential encasement of the common or internal carotid artery, extensive skull base masses with multilevel cranial nerve or brain parenchyma involvement, and invasion of the prevertebral fascia or cervical spine. Likewise, distant metastases (including isolated dermal metastases) point to the presence of an advanced disease state for which cure is unlikely. In selected cases, resection may be undertaken for palliative purposes. However, for the vast majority of these stages IVb and c cancers, palliative chemotherapy and/or radiation therapy is the most appropriate option.

Several factors contribute to the overall prognosis among head and neck cancer patients. Many of these are inherent to the TNM staging system. Tumor size and invasiveness correlate to the risk of nodal metastases and assist with determining the need for elective neck dissection. The number, size, and location of cervical metastases are predictive of regional recurrence and distant metastases. Distant metastases, in turn, are almost universally incurable. However, a recent report does demonstrate improved survival among patients undergoing resection of lung metastases versus those receiving conservative measures.[37] Though previous attempts at metastasectomy have not yielded positive results, these findings have sparked optimism and warrant further investigation.

Other patient and tumor characteristics associated with poor outcome include positive resection margins; perineural, vascular, or extracapsular nodal extension; African American race; malnutrition; anemia; and multiple medical comorbidities. Continued tobacco and alcohol use have significant effects on patient outcomes. Patients who abstain from tobacco have better locoregional control rates and are 2.5 times more likely to survive than those who continue to smoke. Smoking and alcohol cessation also significantly reduces the risk of second primary tumors.[38]

Management of the Neck in Head and Neck Cancers

Neck masses are among the most common presenting signs and symptoms in patients with head and neck cancer. After determining the site of the primary tumor, attention should be paid to the size, number, and location of cervical metastases. These are essential components of the TNM staging system (Table 40.12). The nodal stage of a tumor provides important prognostic information. In the presence of even a single cervical metastasis, the stage can be no lower than III—regardless of the primary tumor size. As the number of involved nodes increases, there is a significant and stepwise decrease in recurrence-free and overall survival that is highly statistically significant.[39]

Head and neck cancers have well-established lymphatic drainage patterns. In the absence of a known primary tumor, the location of cervical adenopathy may suggest the site of origin (Table 40.3). Alternatively, if the pattern of lymph node enlargement does not correspond to the mucosal site in question, the possibility of an occult second primary tumor should be considered.[5]

Much like primary tumors, early-stage cervical adenopathy (i.e., N0 or N1 disease) may be sterilized with single-modality therapy. In the N0 or N1 neck, surgery and radiation therapy are equally efficacious for this purpose. The neck must be addressed with one of these modalities when it is clinically positive (N1) or when the risk of occult metastases in an N0

TABLE 40.12 **STAGING**

AJCC STAGING SYSTEM FOR CERVICAL LYMPH NODE METASTASES

Nx	Nodal status cannot be assessed
N0	No evidence of nodal metastases
N1	Single ipsilateral lymph node metastasis < or = 3 cm
N2a	Single ipsilateral lymph node metastasis >3 cm but <=6 cm
N2b	Multiple ipsilateral lymph node metastases, none greater than 6 cm
N2c	Any bilateral or contralateral lymph node metastases, none greater than 6 cm
N3	Any nodal metastasis greater than 6 cm

From: American Joint Committee on Cancer. *Cancer Staging Manual*, 6th ed. New York: Springer-Verlag; 2002, with permission.

TABLE 40.13 MANAGEMENT

INDICATIONS FOR ELECTIVE TREATMENT OF THE NECK BASED ON ANATOMIC LOCALE AND T STAGE

■ SUBSITE	■ T STAGES WITH >20% RISK OF OCCULT NODAL METASTASES
Oral Cavity	T2, T3, T4
Oropharynx	T1, T2, T3, T4
Hypopharynx	T1, T2, T3, T4
Supraglottic Larynx	T1, T2, T3, T4
Glottic Larynx	T2, T3, T4

From: Frank DK, Sessions RB. Management of the Neck-Surgery. In: Harrison LB, Sessions RB, Hong WK, eds. *Head and Neck Cancer: A Multidisciplinary Approach*, 3rd ed. Philadelphia: Lippincott Williams & Wilkins; 2009:189, with permission.

patient exceeds 20%. This risk varies by T stage and subsite and will be discussed under the individual tumor site headings that follow. Table 40.13 provides general subsite and stage-specific indications for elective neck dissection in the context of a clinically negative neck. The decision to use radiation therapy or surgery depends to some extent on which modality has been chosen to treat the primary site. Radiation therapy avoids the potential risks of neck dissection and obviates the need for general anesthesia. However, selective neck dissection is acceptable in these cases. In experienced hands, selective neck dissections are of low morbidity and have the distinct advantage of providing tissue for accurate pathologic staging (Fig. 40.8).

In advanced nodal disease (N2 or N3) and in cases where extracapsular extension is present, combination therapy is used. More extensive neck dissection is required in these cases and is typically followed by adjuvant radiation or chemoradiation. The modified radical neck dissection is the procedure of choice for clinically positive disease. This procedure can take one of three forms, depending on the extent of the patient's disease.[40] Table 40.14 describes various neck dissections and the structures that are removed during each modification.

One unique entity that should be discussed is the cystic neck mass. When seen in adults, these are commonly assumed to be benign lesions such as branchial cleft cysts and are managed with simple excisional biopsy. However, a large series of patients with isolated cystic neck masses revealed that approximately 10% harbored squamous cell carcinoma. This number is significantly higher among patients older than 40 years of
5 age—approaching 25%.[41] Cystic cervical metastases are most often observed with primary tumors of the Waldeyer ring and strongly associated with HPV.[42] Fine-needle aspiration biopsy is the preferred initial diagnostic modality in these cases. If the cytology is benign, an open biopsy may be performed, but frozen section should be used. In the presence of carcinoma, the patient should undergo formal neck dissection and panendoscopy with directed biopsies and tonsillectomy *at that setting*.

HEAD AND NECK CANCER MANAGEMENT BY SUBSITE

Sinonasal Carcinomas

Squamous cell carcinomas (SCC) involving the sinonasal tract may occur in association with inverting papillomas or may be secondary to environmental exposures. In addition to tobacco smoke, occupational exposure to heavy metals such as nickel and hydrocarbons such as those used in the leather tanning and textile industries have been implicated. Chronic wood-dust exposure is associated with the development of sinonasal adenocarcinomas. However, these occur far less frequently than squamous cell cancers.[26,27] Most sinonasal SCCs (approximately 60%) arise in the maxillary sinuses. Approximately one third are found on the lateral nasal wall, whereas 10% are ethmoidal. Primary carcinomas of the frontal and sphenoid sinuses are rare and constitute less than 2% of all sinonasal cancers.[26] Staging of these tumors follows the AJCC criteria (Table 40.15). Surgical resection is the preferred treatment for cure of sinonasal cancers. Cervical lymph node metastases are rare except in advanced-stage disease. Elective treatment of the neck is not indicated for T1 and T2 tumors. The approach to and extent of surgical resection depends on the location and stage of the primary tumor. For maxillary sinus tumors, options include partial or total maxillectomy

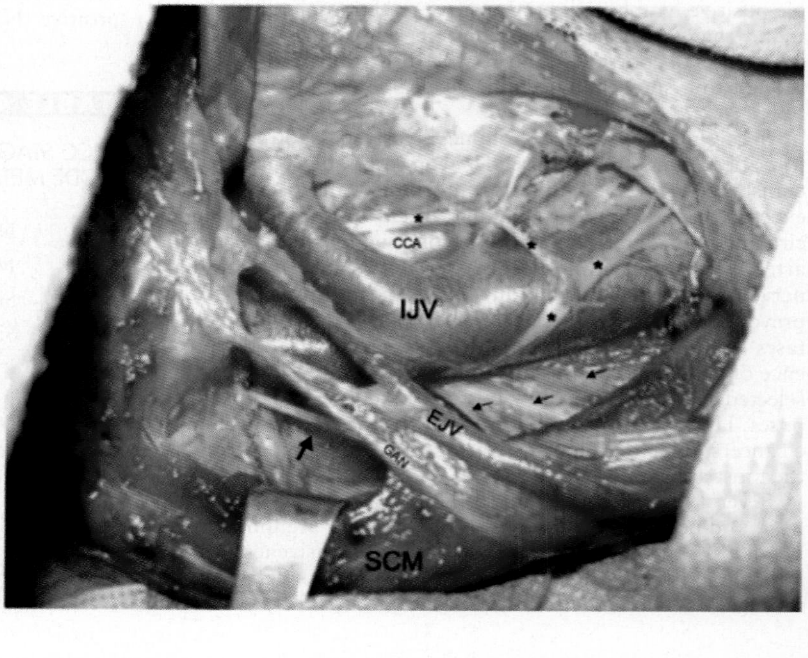

FIGURE 40.8. Intraoperative photograph demonstrating the left neck after performance of a selective (supraomohyoid) neck dissection. Selective neck dissection is generally a low-morbidity procedure. Vital structures such as the internal jugular vein (IJV), common carotid artery (CCA), and spinal accessory nerve (*large arrow*) are carefully preserved. In the context of an N0 neck, other nonvital structures such as the sternocleidomastoid muscle (SCM), external jugular vein (EJV), greater auricular nerve (GAN), cervical sensory rootlets (*small arrows*) and ansa cervicalis (*asterisks*) may also be spared.

TABLE 40.14 **CLASSIFICATION**

CLASSIFICATION OF NECK DISSECTIONS

Radical neck dissection	Lymph node levels I–V, SCM, IJV, and XI are removed
Modified radical neck dissection (MRND)	Node-bearing tissues from levels I–V are removed, but at least one of the above mentioned nonlymphatic structures is spared
MRND type I	Removal of levels I–V, SCM, IJV
MRND type II	Removal of levels I–V, IJV
MRND type III	Removal of levels I–V only
Selective neck dissections	Fewer than levels I–V are removed
Supraomohyoid neck dissection	
For N0 tumors of the oral cavity	Levels I–III
Anterolateral neck dissection	
For N0 tumors of the oropharynx	Levels I–IV
Lateral neck dissection	
For N0 tumors of the hypopharynx and larynx	Levels II–IV
Posterolateral neck dissection	
For N0 cutaneous malignancies of the temporal/scalp region	Levels II–V

SCM, sternocleidomastoid; IJV, internal jugular vein; XI, spinal accessory nerve.

with or without orbital exenteration. Ethmoidal tumors require external ethmoidectomy via anterior subcranial or midface degloving approaches. Significant cranial base involvement necessitates a combined approach with neurosurgery (i.e., craniofacial resection). The orbit may be preserved in cases without radiographic or clinical evidence of direct invasion. However, if the apex, orbital fat, extraocular muscles, or eyelids are involved, exenteration is indicated.[43] As with the benign sinonasal tumors, an increasing body of literature suggests that endoscopic surgery is a safe and effective alternative

TABLE 40.15 **STAGING**

AJCC STAGING CLASSIFICATION FOR TUMORS OF THE NASAL CAVITY AND PARANASAL SINUSES

Maxillary Sinus	
Tx	Primary tumor cannot be assessed
T0	No evidence of primary tumor
T1	Tumor limited to the maxillary sinus mucosa with no bony erosion
T2	Tumor erodes into the hard palate or middle meatus of the nose. Tumor does not involve the posterior maxillary wall or pterygoid plates
T3	Tumor invades any of the following: posterior wall of the maxillary sinus, subcutaneous tissues, floor or medial wall of the orbit, pterygoid fossa, or ethmoid sinuses
T4a	Tumor invades anterior orbital contents, skin of cheek, pterygoid plates, infratemporal fossa, cribriform plate, sphenoid sinus, or frontal sinus
T4b	Tumor invades any of the following: orbital apex, dura, brain, middle cranial fossa, cranial nerve other than V2, nasopharynx, or clivus
Nasal Cavity and Ethmoid Sinuses	
Tx	Primary tumor cannot be assessed
T0	No evidence of primary tumor
T1	Tumor restricted to any one subsite with or without bony invasion
T2	Tumor invading two subsites within a single region or extending to involve an adjacent region within the nasoethmoidal complex, with or without bony invasion
T3	Tumor invades the medial wall or floor of the orbit, maxillary sinus, palate, or cribriform plate
T4a	Tumor invades any of the following: anterior orbital contents, skin of nose or cheek, minimal invasion of anterior cranial fossa, pterygoid plates, sphenoid sinus, or frontal sinus
T4b	Tumor invades any of the following: orbital apex, dura, brain, middle cranial fossa, cranial nerves other than V2, nasopharynx, or clivus

From: American Joint Committee on Cancer. *Cancer Staging Manual*, 6th ed. New York: Springer-Verlag; 2002, with permission.

to open approaches.[44] Adjuvant radiation therapy is reserved for patients with advanced-stage disease (i.e., those with skull base, orbital, pterygopalatine fossa or infratemporal fossa invasion). Five-year disease-specific survival among these tumors is approximately 50%.[44]

Oral Cavity Carcinomas

Oncologically, the oral cavity extends from the vermillion border to the anterior tonsillar pillar. It is divided into eight distinct subsites including the lips, buccal mucosa, maxillary and mandibular alveoli, mobile tongue (i.e., tip of the tongue to the linea terminalis and circumvallate papillae), floor of mouth, hard palate, and retromolar trigone. The AJCC staging classification scheme for oral cavity tumors is presented in Table 40.16. Oral cavity carcinomas can be debilitating with regard to speech and deglutition. Functional and aesthetic reconstruction and rehabilitation present unique challenges among this patient population.

The oral tongue is the most common site of origin, accounting for 38% of all oral cavity carcinomas. This is followed by the floor of mouth and the lips (26% and 18%, respectively). Each of the remaining subsites constitutes a small overall percentage.[45] The following section reviews the management of the most frequently encountered oral cavity carcinomas.

Oral Tongue. Early-stage oral tongue lesions may be treated with transoral partial glossectomy. Given the lack of fascial barriers to spread within the tongue musculature, wide excision with 2-cm margins is advised. Advanced-stage tumors may require mandibulotomy for exposure or in some cases mandibulectomy and composite resection. Primary closure, healing by secondary intention, or split-thickness skin grafting may be used for small defects. Tethering of the tongue to the floor of the mouth should be avoided. To provide adequate bulk and mobility for speech and food bolus propulsion, hemitongue or larger defects should be reconstructed with regional or microvascular free flaps.

Because of its rich vascularity, lesions of the oral tongue tend to grow rapidly and develop early occult metastases. Nearly 40% of patients with T1 and T2 oral tongue carcinomas will have developed occult nodal disease at the time of presentation.[46] This may be related to the depth of tumor invasion as lesions with greater than 2 mm thickness have nearly four times the rate of nodal metastases of thinner tumors (47% vs. 12%).[47] At present, elective neck dissection is indicated for all but the most superficially invasive T1 tumors.[48] Bilateral lymphadenectomy should be performed for lesions approaching the midline. The prognostic significance of nodal metastases cannot be overstated. Five-year survival is approximately 75% among patients with localized disease. In the presence of advanced T-stage or regional nodal metastases, this drops to 25% to 48%.[45,49]

Floor of Mouth. As with the oral tongue, floor of mouth cancers have a high propensity for early nodal metastases. Though nearly 60% of patients will be clinically N0 at presentation,[50] nearly 21% with T1 disease and 62% with T2 tumors will harbor occult metastases.[51] Likewise, the risk of regional lymphatic spread is correlated to the depth of invasion at the primary site.[52] Elective neck dissection is thus advocated even in the case of T1 disease. Bilateral neck dissection should be performed for tumors approaching midline. In addition, bilateral neck dissection is recommended for patients with bulky (T3/T4) tumors and in patients with clinically positive ipsilateral nodes as the incidence of occult contralateral disease is approximately 21% and 36%, respectively.[53] Involvement of the submandibular gland may also occur in these tumors. This may result from direct invasion by bulky, aggressive tumors, but also indirectly along the submandibular duct. Many of these cancers are in close proximity to the Wharton duct papilla. This provides a preformed pathway for even the smallest floor of mouth lesions. Consequently, it is recommended that the ipsilateral submandibular gland be excised along with the primary tumor and neck contents.

Surgery is the treatment of choice for floor of mouth cancers. Local resection with or without adjuvant radiation therapy provides superior disease control to radiation therapy alone for early-stage tumors.[50] If the resection is limited to the mucosa and submucosa, split-thickness skin grafts may be used to resurface the floor of mouth and ventral tongue with excellent functional outcomes. In advanced disease, treatment typically involves composite resection—in many cases including glossectomy and mandibulectomy. Adjuvant radiation or chemoradiation is used in such cases. These patients typically require microvascular free flap reconstruction. Composite flaps such as the osteocutaneous fibular free flap are often used for this purpose, allowing for re-establishment of the bony mandibular contour and excellent functional outcomes. The 5-year disease-specific survival for floor of mouth carcinomas is 72% for stage I disease, 63% for stage II, 44% for stage III, and 47% for stage IV.[50]

Lip. The lip is the third most common site for cancer in the oral cavity.[45] Squamous cell carcinoma accounts for 90% of these lesions.[54] The lower lip is affected much more frequently than the upper lip, with nearly 95% of cases involving the former.[55,56] Most of these patients present with local disease, and the long-term prognosis is excellent. The actuarial 5-year overall survival for lip cancers is in excess of 90%.[45] Treatment is typically surgical and involves full-thickness resection with wide margins. If resection involves less than one third of the lip, primary closure or w-plasty may be used. However, larger defects that involve up to two thirds of the lip require local flaps such as the Karapandzic, Abbe, or Estlander. If more than two thirds of the lip is removed, more complex reconstruction such as the Bernard-Burrows, or, in some cases, microvascular free flaps are needed. The goal of lip reconstruction is to maintain oral competence while minimizing microstomia. Meticulous technique in reapproximating the vermillion border is a must.

Lymph node metastases in lip cancers are exceedingly rare. Most patients will present with T1 and T2 lesions, and among

TABLE 40.16 STAGING

AJCC STAGING CLASSIFICATION FOR TUMORS OF THE LIP AND ORAL CAVITY

Tx	Primary tumor cannot be assessed
T0	No evidence of primary tumor
T1	Tumor is 2 cm or less in greatest dimension
T2	Tumor is greater than 2 cm, but <=4 cm in greatest dimension
T3	Tumor is greater than 4 cm in greatest dimension
T4	(**Lip**) Tumor invades through cortical bone, inferior alveolar nerve, floor of mouth, or facial skin (cheek or nose)
T4a	(**Oral Cavity**) Tumor invades adjacent structures: e.g., through cortical bone, into deep (extrinsic) muscle of tongue (genioglossus, hyoglossus, palatoglossus, styloglossus), maxillary sinus, skin of face
T4b	(**Oral Cavity**) Tumor invades masticator space, pterygoid plates, or skull base and/or encases internal carotid artery

From: American Joint Committee on Cancer. *Cancer Staging Manual*, 6th ed. New York: Springer-Verlag; 2002, with permission.

these lesions, the incidence of occult nodal metastasis is less than 5%. However, in patients with T3 and T4 tumors, the rate nears 25%. Tumors involving the oral commissure also have elevated rates of occult cervical lymph node involvement that is independent of T stage.[55] Elective neck dissection should be performed for patients with clinical evidence of disease and also for those with bulky primary tumors and those involving the oral commissure.

Oropharyngeal Carcinomas

The oropharynx extends from the anterior tonsillar pillars and the junction of the soft and hard palate to the level of the hyoid bone. Oropharyngeal subsites include the palatine tonsils, base of tongue, soft palate, and posterior oropharyngeal wall. The current primary tumor staging is listed in Table 40.17. Nearly 90% of oropharyngeal cancers are squamous cell carcinomas.[54] The symptoms of oropharyngeal carcinomas are typically vague, and primary tumors may be difficult to assess. Consequently, delay in diagnosis is common and nearly 70% of patients will present with advanced disease.[45,54] Because of the rich vascularity of this region and bilateral lymphatic drainage patterns, these patients often develop bilateral or even contralateral nodal metastases. The tonsillar fossa is the most common site for primary tumors of the oropharynx, followed closely by the base of tongue. Primary tumors of the soft palate and posterior oropharyngeal wall occur much less frequently.

For early-stage, localized disease, surgery and radiation have approximately equal cure rates, with nearly 90% local control rates for the pooled group of oropharyngeal cancers.[57,58] Ablative surgery of the oropharynx—particularly the tongue base—can have significant effects on speech and swallowing. Radiation therapy results in less functional impairment and is in most cases the preferred initial treatment for T1 and T2 tumors. Advanced-stage disease is typically treated with multimodal therapy including surgery with adjuvant radiation or chemoradiation. Among all head and neck sites, surgical resections of the oropharynx are the most likely to result in functional morbidity with respect to speech, deglutition, and management of airway secretions. Historically, tongue base resections very often necessitated the performance of a total laryngectomy as a means to prevent chronic aspiration. For several years, pedicled pectoralis major myocutaneous flaps were used to offset some of these difficulties. However, these have fallen out of favor because of pedicle retraction, unpredictability of residual bulk, and their insensate nature. As reconstructive surgery has grown more sophisticated, microvascular free flaps have supplanted their use and have become the gold standard for oropharyngeal reconstruction. Microvascular free flaps have resulted in approximately 80% to 90% of patients returning to a normal diet. Conversely, this figure is approximately 40% to 50% after pedicled myocutaneous flaps.[59]

For patients with localized disease, the 5-year overall survival is approximately 73%. However, this drops to less than 40% among patients with regional lymph node involvement.[45] Five-year survival for tongue base carcinomas is approximately 67% for stages I and II, 66% for stage III, and 50% for stage IV.[58] These numbers are slightly better for tonsil carcinomas, where survival is approximately 80% among patients with stages I and II disease and 40% to 50% for stages III and IV.[60]

Recent data suggest that definitive chemoradiation may provide similar rates of disease control and survival to those historically observed for standard sequential therapy (surgery plus radiation).[61] This approach is thought to provide superior functional outcomes.[62] However, long-term quality of life scores are remarkably similar between chemoradiated patients and those treated with surgery followed by free flap reconstruction.[63]

An increasing body of evidence implicates human papilloma virus (HPV), particularly HPV-16, in the pathogenesis of oropharyngeal squamous cell carcinoma.[4,64] Approximately 50% of oropharyngeal cancers have been shown to contain HPV DNA. Though histologically similar, HPV-positive and HPV-negative squamous cell cancers differ with respect to their pathogenesis, patient characteristics, and clinical behavior. Patients with HPV-positive tumors tend to have a better overall prognosis. Cancer-related mortality may be reduced by up to 80% when compared to patients with HPV-negative tumors.[64] These data seem to suggest that HPV-positive and HPV-negative oropharyngeal cancers are distinct disease processes. However, the therapeutic implications of this are yet to be determined.

TABLE 40.17 STAGING

AJCC STAGING CLASSIFICATION FOR PRIMARY TUMORS OF THE OROPHARYNX

Tx	Primary tumor cannot be assessed
T0	No evidence of primary tumor
T1	Tumor is 2 cm or less in greatest dimension
T2	Tumor is greater than 2 cm but less than or equal to 4 cm in greatest dimension
T3	Tumor is greater than 4 cm in greatest dimension
T4a	Tumor invades the larynx, deep/extrinsic muscle of tongue, medial pterygoid, hard palate, or mandible
T4b	Tumor invades the lateral pterygoid muscle, pterygoid plates, lateral nasopharynx, or skull base or encases carotid artery

From: American Joint Committee on Cancer. *Cancer Staging Manual*, 6th ed. New York: Springer-Verlag; 2002, with permission.

Nasopharyngeal Carcinoma

Nasopharyngeal carcinoma (NPC) is a relatively uncommon diagnosis in the United States, though it is prevalent in other parts of the world—particularly in Southern China, where the disease is endemic. The risk of NPC remains elevated in patients who have emigrated from these areas, suggesting that both environmental and genetic factors contribute to its pathogenesis.[65] Environmental agents include nitrosamines such as those present in cured meats and fish, cigarette smoking, formaldehyde, wood dust, and polycyclic hydrocarbons.[66] However, Epstein-Barr virus (EBV) is the most widely implicated etiologic agent. More than 90% of endemic NPC and over 60% of cases worldwide are associated with EBV.[67–69] Though NPC is a squamous cell carcinoma, there are three distinct histologic classifications based on the degree of differentiation: keratinizing, nonkeratinizing, and undifferentiated. The World Health Organization (WHO) has designated these as types I, II, and III, respectively. WHO type III is the most common, accounting for 63% of North American cases and 95% of endemic cases in China. In China, types I and II account for less than 5% of all cases. However, WHO type I NPC occurs much more frequently in North America, where up to 40% of the cases may be of the keratinizing variety.[70,71] Endemic/EBV-associated NPC is typically WHO types II and III whereas sporadic NPC is most frequently keratinizing (type I). However, molecular detection methods have identified EBV DNA among a significant proportion of type I NPCs as well.[72]

The most common presenting symptom of a patient with NPC is a neck mass. This is followed closely by nasal obstruction and otologic complaints.[65,68,73] Advanced disease may be heralded by cranial neuropathies, headache, or mental status changes. These tumors most typically arise within the Fossa of Rosenmüller, an anatomic region situated in the superolateral nasopharynx—just above the torus tubarius. The close proximity of these masses to the eustachian tube orifice is responsible for the high prevalence of aural pressure, hearing loss, and serous otitis media among patients with NPC. Indeed, the presence of an unexplained unilateral middle ear effusion necessitates visualization of the nasopharynx (either via endoscopy or high-resolution imaging) to rule out NPC.

Diagnosis is confirmed by biopsy and should be followed by imaging of the temporal bones and skull base with MRI. This will allow for more accurate staging and treatment planning. The staging classification of NPC differs somewhat from that of other head and neck subsites, particularly with reference to cervical lymph node metastases (Table 40.18). Radiation therapy is the mainstay of treatment, though a recent phase III clinical trial suggests that concomitant chemoradiation provides improved locoregional control and disease-specific survival among patients with the endemic form of the disease.[74] Survival is strongly correlated to the histologic type, with WHO type III disease having a better prognosis than types II and I, respectively. Five-year overall survival is approximately 68% for type III, 56% for type II, and 46% for WHO type I NPC.[70]

TABLE 40.18 STAGING

AJCC STAGING CLASSIFICATION FOR PRIMARY TUMORS OF THE NASOPHARYNX

Tx	Primary tumor cannot be assessed
T0	No evidence of primary tumor
T1	Tumor confined to the nasopharynx
T2	Tumor extends to soft tissues
T2a:	Tumor extends to the oropharynx and/or nasal cavity without parapharyngeal extension
T2b:	Any tumor with parapharyngeal extension
T3	Tumor invades bony structures and/or paranasal sinuses
T4	Tumor with intracranial extension and/or involvement of cranial nerves, infratemporal fossa, hypopharynx, orbit, or masticator space
Nx	Regional lymph nodes cannot be assessed
N0	No evidence of regional lymph node metastasis
N1	Unilateral metastasis in lymph node(s), not more than 6 cm in greatest dimension, above the supraclavicular fossa
N2	Bilateral metastasis in lymph node(s), not more than 6 cm in greatest dimension, above the supraclavicular fossa
N3	Metastasis in a lymph node(s) larger than 6 cm and/or to supraclavicular fossa
N3a:	Larger than 6 cm
N3b:	Extension to the supraclavicular fossa

Stage Grouping	
Stage I	T1, N0, M0
Stage IIa	T2a, N0, M0
Stage IIb	T1, N1, M0
	T2, N0–1, M0
Stage III	T3, N0–1, M0
	T1–3, N2, M0
Stage IVa	T4, N0–2, M0
Stage IVb	Any T, N3, M0
Stage IVc	Any M1

From: American Joint Committee on Cancer. *Cancer Staging Manual*, 6th ed. New York: Springer-Verlag; 2002, with permission.

Hypopharyngeal Carcinomas

The hypopharynx is a region that extends from the hyoid bone to the esophageal inlet and includes the pyriform sinuses, postcricoid region, and posterior hypopharyngeal walls. Squamous cell carcinoma of the hypopharynx is extremely aggressive, and the prognosis is poor irrespective of the therapeutic regimen used. The use of tobacco and alcohol account for a great number of hypopharyngeal carcinomas. However, several other risk factors including Plummer-Vinson syndrome, Fanconi anemia, and gastroesophageal reflux disease have also been reported.[75–77] Patients will typically present with dysphagia, odynophagia, and otalgia. In addition, the hypopharynx has a rich lymphovascular supply and nodal metastases are common. Nearly 65% will present with N+ disease and more than three fourths of patients with clinically negative necks will harbor occult metastases.[78,79] Contralateral disease is frequent, especially among tumors approaching the midline and those with clinically positive disease on the ipsilateral side.[79]

Hypopharyngeal tumors are not readily visible on routine examination. Coupled with the vagueness of the symptoms, this often results in a delay in diagnosis. Nearly 80% will present with stage III or IV disease.[54] The primary tumor staging system may be seen in Table 40.19.

Early-stage disease may be treated using either definitive radiation therapy or open partial pharyngectomy/partial laryngopharyngectomy.[80] Advanced disease requires a combined approach using surgery and adjuvant radiation or chemoradiation. Surgery typically involves total laryngopharyngectomy and flap reconstruction. The submucosal lymphatic plexus of the hypopharynx is extensive and allows for proximal and distal spread of disease. This often necessitates a wide margin that may extend beyond the thoracic inlet. In these cases, resection includes not only total laryngopharyngectomy but also esophagectomy. Gastric pullup or jejunal free flap reconstruction is necessary in this circumstance.[81] Given the morbidity of these procedures and the dismal prognosis, organ-preservation

TABLE 40.19 STAGING

AJCC STAGING CLASSIFICATION FOR PRIMARY TUMORS OF THE HYPOPHARYNX

Tx	Primary tumor cannot be assessed
T0	No evidence of primary tumor
T1	Tumor involves one subsite of the hypopharynx and is less than or equal to 2 cm in greatest dimension
T2	Tumor involves more than one subsite of hypopharynx or adjacent site or measures >2 cm but not more than 4 cm in greatest diameter without fixation of hemilarynx
T3	Tumor measures >4 cm in greatest dimension or with fixation of hemilarynx
T4	Tumor invades thyroid/cricoid cartilage, hyoid bone, thyroid gland, esophagus, or central compartment soft tissues

From: American Joint Committee on Cancer. *Cancer Staging Manual*, 6th ed. New York: Springer-Verlag; 2002, with permission.

protocols are now frequently used in the management of advanced hypopharyngeal carcinomas. The overall survival is similar to that obtained after surgery and adjuvant radiation therapy.[82] Published 5-year overall survival rates are approximately 58%, 43%, 31%, and 13% for stages I, II, III, and IV, respectively.[83]

Laryngeal Carcinomas

Cancers of the larynx receive a great deal of attention among both the medical and the lay community. This is not surprising given the vital role that this organ plays in speech, swallowing, and respiration. The psychosocial implications of laryngeal disease and its varied therapies are significant. Indeed, quality of life issues are more evident here than perhaps for any other head and neck subsite. For this reason, functional preservation of the larynx has become central to treatment paradigms for laryngeal carcinomas. However, as with any head and neck tumor, eradication of disease remains the primary goal. Fortunately, modern protocols have allowed for organ preservation in a significant proportion of early and advanced laryngeal carcinomas. Among those patients who do undergo total laryngectomy, there are a host of options that provide for alaryngeal speech as well.

The larynx itself is divided into three subsites: the supraglottis, the glottis, and the subglottis. The supraglottic larynx extends from the root of the epiglottis in the vallecula down to the ventricle. It includes the epiglottis, aryepiglottic folds, arytenoid cartilages, and false vocal folds. The glottis is the space encompassed by the true vocal folds. Oncologically, this subsite includes the true vocal folds and the mucosal surfaces approximately 5 mm above and below them. The subglottis begins at the inferior extent of the glottis and extends 1 cm distally into the trachea.

Given that even small perturbations of normal laryngeal airflow will result in dysphonia, many laryngeal cancers will present at early stages. This is particularly true of glottic carcinomas. Given the relative ease of diagnosis and the curability of these early-stage lesions, any hoarseness present for more than 3 weeks should be evaluated by direct or indirect laryngoscopy. Other symptoms of laryngeal cancers include referred otalgia, hemoptysis, stridor, dysphagia, odynophagia, and a neck mass. Larger tumors may result in dyspnea and airway obstruction. Supraglottic and subglottic tumors are particularly prone to this, as they may not manifest (i.e., with hoarseness) until the primary tumor is at an advanced stage.

6

As a general rule, equal cure rates may be achieved for stages I and II disease using either radiation therapy or surgery as a single modality. Radiation therapy typically results in better functional outcomes and is typically the primary treatment of choice. Stages III and IV disease most often requires extended partial laryngectomy or total laryngectomy with adjuvant radiation or chemoradiation therapy. The functional and social consequences of total laryngectomy can be significant. As a consequence, organ-preservation protocols have been developed as an alternative to laryngectomy in these cases as well. The concept of organ preservation for laryngeal carcinoma was championed after the publishing of a landmark study conducted through the Department of Veterans Affairs.[84] This seminal study used induction chemotherapy (cisplatin plus 5-fluorouracil) and external-beam radiation therapy as an alternative to total laryngectomy with adjuvant radiation therapy for patients with advanced laryngeal carcinoma. The 5-year survival rates among the two groups were 42% and 46% (p = NS). However, it was found that nearly two thirds of the patients in the organ preservation arm had laryngeal preservation at 5 years. Subsequent studies have confirmed chemo/radiation as an oncologically equivalent but functionally superior treatment for advanced laryngeal carcinoma. Today, induction chemotherapy has largely been replaced by concurrent chemoradiation therapy as it was found to provide even greater rates of laryngeal preservation.[85] However, patients must be carefully selected for organ preservation protocols as there is speculation that their indiscriminate use may be responsible for an overall decrease in survival observed in recent years.[86]

Supraglottic Carcinoma. The supraglottic larynx accounts for approximately 32% of all laryngeal carcinomas.[86] Staging of these tumors is outlined in Table 40.20. Unlike other head and neck cancers, laryngeal tumor stage is not based on size. Rather, it includes information regarding the number of subsites involved, degree of functional impairment of the vocal folds, and involvement of surrounding structures. Even small tumors of the supraglottis may be advanced-stage lesions if they invade the pre-epiglottic space or cause vocal fold fixation. The supraglottis has a rich lymphovascular supply, which facilitates early bilateral nodal metastases even among small primary tumors. Although more than two thirds of patients will be clinically N0 at presentation,[87] the rate of occult metastases is 20%, 25%, and 40% among T2, T3, and T4 tumors, respectively.[88]

Management of early supraglottic carcinomas may be through single-modality therapy with either radiation or surgery. Disease-specific survival for stage I and II supraglottic cancers are approximately 79% and 76%, respectively. Surgery for T1 and T2 supraglottic carcinoma involves open supraglottic laryngectomy. In recent years transoral laser resection has emerged as an alternative to the open procedure. Local control rates and disease-specific survival for T1 and T2 disease are equivalent to historical controls undergoing open supraglottic laryngectomy.[89,90] Advanced-stage supraglottic carcinomas should be treated with a multimodal approach. Surgery with adjuvant radiation/chemoradiation or definitive chemoradiation may be used. Surgical resection classically involved total laryngectomy. Alternatively, selected T1 to T3 glottic, supraglottic, and transglottic tumors may be surgically addressed via the supracricoid laryngectomy. This procedure is a form of partial laryngectomy that involves removal of the entire thyroid cartilage, true vocal folds, and supraglottic larynx. The cricoid cartilage and at least one arytenoid cartilage are preserved. This allows for preservation of a limited but functional voice. However, these patients must be carefully selected as nearly all will experience some degree of chronic aspiration. Contraindications to supracricoid laryngectomy are fixation of the arytenoid, subglottic extent, cricoid invasion, extralaryngeal spread, and poor pulmonary reserve. In carefully selected patients at experienced centers, oncologic and functional results are similar to those obtained after total laryngectomy.[91] Disease-specific survival rates for stages III and IV supraglottic carcinoma are 64% and 50%, respectively.[87]

Glottic Carcinoma. Glottic carcinomas account for 51% of all laryngeal cancers.[86] Given that even small glottic tumors can have a significant impact on the voice, patients will frequently present with early-stage disease. The glottic larynx is devoid of lymphatics, and the incidence of nodal metastases is low in T1 and T2 disease. Elective neck dissection is reserved for patients with advanced primary tumors. Therapeutic neck dissection should be used for any clinically positive nodes. For early glottic cancers, radiation therapy or surgery may be used with equal cure rates. Disease-specific survival among T1 tumors ranges from 89% to 100%. Patients with T2 tumors fare slightly worse, with published survival rates ranging between 75% and 90%.[86,92] From a surgical standpoint, open partial laryngectomy is the gold standard, with local control rates approaching 95% for T1 disease and 80% to 90% for T2.[92] However, transoral laser resection results in similar rates of disease control with less overall morbidity. Voice outcomes tend to be similar after radiation or laser excision of T1 tumors, though radiation is superior in this regard when the

TABLE 40.20 **STAGING**

AJCC STAGING CLASSIFICATION FOR PRIMARY TUMORS OF THE LARYNX

Supraglottis	
Tx	Primary tumor cannot be assessed
T0	No evidence of primary tumor
T1	Tumor limited to one subsite of supraglottis with normal vocal fold mobility
T2	Tumor invades mucosa of more than one adjacent subsite of supraglottis or glottis or region outside supraglottis (e.g., mucosa of base of tongue, vallecula, medial wall of pyriform sinus) without fixation of the hemilarynx
T3	Tumor limited to larynx with vocal cord fixation and/or invades any of the following: postcricoid area, preepiglottic space, and/or minor cartilage erosion (e.g., inner cortex)
T4a	Tumor invades through the thyroid cartilage and/or invades tissues beyond the larynx (e.g., trachea, soft tissues of neck including deep extrinsic muscle of tongue, strap muscles, thyroid, or esophagus)
T4b	Tumor invades prevertebral space, encases carotid artery, or invades mediastinal structures
Glottis	
Tx	Primary tumor cannot be assessed
T0	No evidence of primary tumor
T1a	Tumor limited to one vocal fold with normal vocal fold motion
T1b	Tumor involves both vocal folds with normal vocal fold motion
T2	Tumor extends to supraglottic or subglottic larynx or with impaired vocal fold motion
T3	Tumor limited to the larynx with vocal cord fixation and/or invades paraglottic space, and/or minor thyroid cartilage erosion (e.g., inner cortex)
T4a	Tumor invades through the thyroid cartilage and/or invades tissues beyond the larynx (e.g., trachea, soft tissues of neck including deep extrinsic muscle of tongue, strap muscles, thyroid, or esophagus)
T4b	Tumor invades prevertebral space, encases carotid artery, or invades mediastinal structures
Subglottis	
Tx	Primary tumor cannot be assessed
T0	No evidence of primary tumor
T1	Tumor limited to subglottis
T2	Tumor extends to vocal folds with normal or impaired mobility
T3	Tumor limited to larynx with vocal cord fixation
T4a	Tumor invades through the thyroid cartilage and/or invades tissues beyond the larynx (e.g., trachea, soft tissues of neck including deep extrinsic muscle of tongue, strap muscles, thyroid, or esophagus)
T4b	Tumor invades prevertebral space, encases carotid artery, or invades mediastinal structures

From: American Joint Committee on Cancer. *Cancer Staging Manual*, 6th ed. New York: Springer-Verlag; 2002, with permission.

primary tumor is larger.[92] Stages 3 and 4 lesions are managed similar to supraglottic tumors. Total laryngectomy and, in selected cases, supracricoid laryngectomy with bilateral neck dissection and adjuvant radiation/chemoradiation or definitive chemoradiation (in selected cases) may be used. Five-year survival for locally advanced stages III and IV glottic carcinoma is 60% and 53%, respectively. In the presence of regional nodal disease, these numbers decrease significantly.[86]

Subglottic Carcinoma. Subglottic cancers represent 2% of all malignant laryngeal tumors. Consequently, there are limited data with regard to treatment and outcomes. The literature suggests that most patients present with advanced-stage disease and that the prognosis is dismal. Current recommendations for stages I and II disease is definitive radiation therapy, with local control and survival rates of approximately 65% to 70%.[93,94] Advanced disease often involves the thyroid gland, paratracheal lymph nodes, trachea, and other structures of the superior mediastinum. Total laryngectomy with tracheal resection and adjuvant radiation/chemoradiation are advocated. Despite aggressive local and systemic therapy, the prognosis is poor, with overall survival nearing 25%.[94]

References

1. Maier H, Dietz A, Gewelke U, et al. Tobacco and alcohol and the risk of head and neck cancer. *Clin Investig* 1992;70(3–4):320.

2. Marur S, Forastiere A. Head and neck cancer: changing epidemiology, diagnosis, and treatment. *Mayo Clin Proc* 2008;83(4):489.
3. Lee YA, Boffetta P, Sturgis E, et al. Involuntary smoking and head and neck cancer risk: pooled analysis in the international head and neck cancer Epidemiology Consortium. *Cancer Epidemiol Biomarkers Prev* 2008;17(8): 1974.
4. D'Souza G, Kreimer AR, Viscidi R, et al. Case-control study of human papillomavirus and oropharyngeal cancer. *N Engl J Med* 2007;356:1944.
5. Shah JP. Patterns of cervical lymph node metastasis from squamous carcinomas of the upper aerodigestive tract. *Am J Surg* 1990;160(4):405.
6. Cole RR, Aguilar EA III. Cricothyroidotomy versus tracheotomy: an otolaryngologist's perspective. *Laryngoscope* 1988;98(2):131.
7. Rice DH. Nonneoplastic diseases of the salivary glands. In: Bailey BJ, Johnson JT, eds. *Head & Neck Surgery—Otolaryngology,* 4th ed. Philadelphia: Lippincott Williams & Wilkins; 2006:545.
8. Brook I. Acute bacterial suppurative parotitis: microbiology and management. *J Craniofac Surg* 2003;14(1):37.
9. Marchal F, Dulguerov P. Sialolithiasis management: the state of the art. *Arch Otolaryngol Head Neck Surg* 2003;129:951.
10. Yousem DM, Kraut MA, Chalian AA. Major salivary gland imaging. *Radiology* 2000;216(1):19.
11. Bisno AL. Acute pharyngitis. *N Engl J Med* 2001;344(3):205.
12. Snow V, Mottur-Pilson C, Cooper RJ, et al. Principles of appropriate antibiotic use for acute pharyngitis in adults. *Ann Intern Med* 2001;134: 506.
13. Vieira F, Allen SM, Stocks RM, et al. Deep neck infection. *Otlaryngol Clin North Am* 2008;41:459.
14. Johnson RF, Stewart MG, Wright CC. An evidence-based review of the treatment of peritonsillar abscess. *Otolaryngol Head Neck Surg* 2003;128: 332.
15. Gadre AK, Gadre KC. Infections of the deep spaces of the neck. In: Bailey BJ, Johnson JT, eds. *Head & Neck Surgery—Otolaryngology,* 4th ed. Philadelphia: Lippincott Williams & Wilkins; 2006:665.
16. Meltzer EO, Hamilos DL, Hadley JA, et al. Rhinosinusitis: establishing definitions for clinical research and patient care. *Otolaryngol Head Neck Surg* 2004;131:s1.
17. Sokol W. Epidemiology of sinusitis in the primary care setting: results from the 1999–2000 respiratory surveillance program. *Am J Med* 2001;111: 19s.
18. Linder JA, Singer DE. Health-related quality of life of adults with upper respiratory tract infections. *J Gen Intern Med* 2003;18:802.
19. Epstein VA, Kern RC. Invasive fungal sinusitis and complications of sinusitis. *Otolaryngol Clin North Am* 2008;41:497.
20. Davies L, Welch HG. Epidemiology of head and neck cancer in the United States. *Otolaryngol Head Neck Surg* 2006;135:451.
21. Shah JP, Patel SG. Salivary glands. In: Shah JP, ed. *Head & Neck Surgery & Oncology,* 3rd ed. Philadelphia: Mosby; 2003:439.
22. Kaplan M, Abemayor E. Major salivary glands: I. Clinical considerations for the diseases of the salivary glands. In: Fu YS, Wenig BM, Abemayor E, et al., eds. *Head and Neck Pathology: With Clinical Correlations.* New York: Churchill-Livingstone; 2001:231.
23. Eversole L. Manor salivary glands: II. Salivary gland pathology. In: Fu YS, Wenig BM, Abemayor E, et al., eds. *Head and Neck Pathology: With Clinical Correlations.* New York: Churchill-Livingstone; 2001:242.
24. Futran N, Parvathaneni U, Martins RG, et al. Malignant salivary gland tumors. In: Harrison LB, Sessions RB, Hong WK, eds. *Head and Neck Cancer: A Multidisciplinary Approach*, 3rd ed. Philadelphia: Lippincott Williams & Wilkins; 2009:589.
25. Oh YS, Eisele DW. Salivary gland neoplasms. In: Bailey BJ, Johnson JT, eds. *Head & Neck Surgery—Otolaryngology,* 4th ed. Philadelphia: Lippincott Williams & Wilkins; 2006:1515.
26. Wang M, Osguthorpe D, Abemayor E. Nasal cavity and paranasal sinuses: I. Clinical considerations for the diseases of the nasal cavity and paranasal sinuses. In: Fu YS, Wenig BM, Abemayor E, et al., eds. *Head and Neck Pathology: With Clinical Correlations.* New York: Churchill-Livingstone; 2001:113.
27. Zimmer LA, Carrau RL. Neoplasms of the nose and paranasal sinuses. In: Bailey BJ, Johnson JT, eds. *Head & Neck Surgery—Otolaryngology,* 4th ed. Philadelphia: Lippincott Williams & Wilkins; 2006:1481.
28. Mirza S, Bradley PJ, Acharya A, et al. Sinonasal inverted papillomas: recurrence and synchronous and metachronous malignancies. *J Laryngol Otol* 2007;121:857.
29. Zimmer LA, Carrau RL, Snyderman CH, et al. Endoscopic management of neoplasms of the nose and paranasal sinuses. In: Bailey BJ, Johnson JT, eds. *Head & Neck Surgery—Otolaryngology,* 4th ed. Philadelphia: Lippincott Williams & Wilkins; 2006:447.
30. Pryor SG, Moore EJ, Kasperbaure JL. Endoscopic versus traditional approaches for excision of juvenile nasopharyngeal angiofibroma. *Laryngoscope* 2005;115:1201.
31. Wenig BM, Cohen JM. General principles of head and neck pathology. In: Harrison LB, Sessions RB, Hong WK, eds. *Head and Neck Cancer: A Multidisciplinary Approach*, 3rd ed. Philadelphia: Lippincott Williams & Wilkins; 2009:1.
32. Schwartz LH, Ozsahin M, Zhang GN. Synchronous and metachronous head and neck carcinomas. *Cancer* 1994;74:1933.
33. Sturgis EM, Miller RH. Second primary malignancies in the head and neck cancer patient. *Ann Otol Rhinol Laryngol* 1995;104:946.
34. Chong LM. Principles of radiation oncology. In: Shah JP, ed. *Head & Neck Surgery & Oncology,* 3rd ed. Philadelphia: Mosby; 2003:643.
35. Cooper JS, Pajak TF, Forastiere AA, et al. Postoperative concurrent radiotherapy and chemotherapy in high-risk squamous-cell carcinoma of the head and neck. *N Engl J Med* 2004;350:1937.
36. Bernier J, Domenge C, Ozsahin M, et al. Postoperative irradiation with or without concomitant chemotherapy for locally advanced head and neck cancer. *N Engl J Med* 2004;350:1945.
37. Winter H, Meimarakas G, Hoffman G, et al. Does surgical resection of pulmonary metastases of head and neck cancer improve survival? *Ann Surg Oncol* 2008;15:2915.
38. Smith BD, Haffty BG. Prognostic factors in patients with head and neck cancer. In: Harrison LB, Sessions RB, Hong WK, eds. *Head and Neck Cancer: A Multidisciplinary Approach*, 3rd ed. Philadelphia: Lippincott Williams & Wilkins; 2009:51.
39. Kowalski LP, Bagietto R, Lara JRL, et al. Prognostic significance of the distribution of neck node metastasis from oral carcinoma. *Head Neck* 2000; 22:207.
40. Robbins KT, Clayman G, Levine PA, et al. Neck dissection classification update. *Arch Otolaryngol Head Neck Surg* 2002;128:751.
41. Gourin CG, Johnson JT. Incidence of unsuspected metastasis in lateral cervical cysts. *Laryngoscope* 2000;110:1637.
42. Goldenberg D, Begum S, Westra WH, et al. Cystic lymph node metastasis in patients with head and neck cancer: an HPV-associated phenomenon. *Head Neck* 2008;30:898.
43. Persky MS, Tabaee A. Cancer of the nasal vestibule, nasal cavity, and paranasal sinuses: surgical management. In: Harrison LB, Sessions RB, Hong WK, eds. *Head and Neck Cancer: A Multidisciplinary Approach*, 3rd ed. Philadelphia: Lippincott Williams & Wilkins; 2009:454.
44. Piero N, Battaglia P, Bignami M, et al. Endoscopic surgery for malignant tumors of the sinonasal tract and adjacent skull base: a 10-year experience. *Am J Rhinol* 2008;22:308.
45. SEER Cancer Database. http://seer.cancer.gov; Accessed 1 November, 2008.
46. Spiro RH, Alfonso AE, Farr HW, et al. Cervical node metastases from epidermoid carcinoma of the oral cavity and oral pharynx: a critical assessment of current staging. *Am J Surg* 1974;128:562.
47. Spiro RH, Huvos AG, Wong GY, et al. Predictive value of tumor thickness in squamous carcinoma confined to the tongue and floor of the mouth. *Am J Surg* 1986;152:345.
48. Sparano A, Weinstein G, Chalian A, et al. Multivariate predictors of occult neck metastasis in early oral tongue cancer. *Otolaryngol Head Neck Surg* 2004;131:472.
49. Sessions DG, Spector GJ, Lenox J, et al. Analysis of treatment results for oral tongue cancer. *Laryngoscope* 2002;112:616.
50. Sessions DG, Spector GJ, Lenox J, et al. Analysis of treatment results for floor of mouth cancer. *Laryngoscope* 2000;110:1764.
51. Hicks WJ, Loree TR, Garcia RI, et al. Squamous cell carcinoma of the floor of the mouth: a 20-year review. *Head Neck* 1997;19:400.
52. Wallwork BD, Anderson SR, Coman WB. Squamous cell carcinoma of the floor of the mouth: tumor thickness and the rate of cervical metastasis. *ANZ J Surg* 2007;77:761.
53. Koo BS, Lim YC, Lee JS, et al. Management of the contralateral N0 neck in oral cavity squamous cell carcinoma. *Head Neck* 2006;28:896.
54. Hoffman HT, Karnell LH, Funk GF, et al. The national cancer database report on cancer of the head and neck. *Arch Otolaryngol Head Neck Surg* 1998;124:951.
55. Vartanian JC, Carvalho AL, Filho MJ, et al. Predictive factors and distribution of lymph node metastasis in lip cancer patients and their implications on the treatment of the neck. *Oral Oncol* 2004;40:223.
56. Campbell JP. Surgical management of lip carcinoma. *J Oral Maxillofac Surg* 1998;56:955.
57. Fein DA, Lee WR, Amos WR, et al. Oropharyngeal carcinoma treated with radiotherapy: a 30-year experience. *Int J Radiat Oncol Biol Phys* 1996;34:289.
58. Mendenhall WM, Morris CG, Amdur RJ, et al. Definitive radiotherapy for squamous cell carcinoma of the base of tongue. *Am J Clin Oncol* 2006; 29:32.
59. Rieger JM, Zalmanowitz JG, Li SY, et al. Functional outcomes after surgical reconstruction of the base of tongue using radial forearm free flap in patients with oropharyngeal carcinoma. *Head Neck* 2007;29:1024.
60. Shirazi HA, Sivanandan R, Goode R, et al. Advanced-stage tonsillar squamous carcinoma: organ preservation versus surgical management of the primary site. *Head Neck* 2006;28:587.
61. Denis F, Garaud P, Bardet E, et al. Final results of the 94–01 French head and neck oncology and radiotherapy group randomized trial comparing radiotherapy alone with concomitant radiochemotherapy in advanced-stage oropharynx carcinoma. *J Clin Oncol* 2004;22:69.
62. Gillespie MB, Brodsky MB, Day TA, et al. Laryngeal penetration and aspiration during swallowing after the treatment of advanced oropharyngeal cancer. *Arch Otolaryngol Head Neck Surg* 2005;131:615.
63. Mowry SE, Ho A, LoTempio MM, et al. Quality of life in advanced oropharyngeal carcinoma after chemoradiation versus surgery and radiation. *Laryngoscope* 2006;116:1589.
64. Fakhry C, Gillison ML. Clinical implications of human papillomavirus in head and neck cancers. *Clin Oncol* 2006;24:2606.
65. Wei WI, Sham J. Nasopharyngeal carcinoma. *Lancet* 2005;365:2041.
66. Yu MC, Yuan JM. Epidemiology of nasopharyngeal carcinoma. *Sem Cancer Biol* 2002;12:421.
67. Liu FF, Frappier L, Kim J, et al. East-West symposium on nasopharyngeal cancer. *Int J Radiat Oncol* 2007;67:703.

68. Dickson RI. Nasopharyngeal carcinoma: an evaluation of 209 patients. *Laryngoscope* 1981;91:333.
69. Neal HB, Pearson GR, Taylor WF. Antibodies to Epstein-Barr virus in patients with nasopharyngeal carcinoma in comparison groups. *Ann Otol Rhinol Laryngol* 1984;93:477.
70. Ou SH, Zell JA, Ziogas A, et al. Epidemiology of nasopharyngeal carcinoma in the United States: improved survival of Chinese patients within the keratinizing squamous cell carcinoma histology. *Ann Oncol* 2007; 18:29.
71. Nicholls JM. Nasopharyngeal carcinoma: classification and histological appearances. *Adv Anat Pathol* 1997;4:71.
72. Raab-Traub N, Flynn K, Pearson G, et al. The differentiated form of nasopharyngeal carcinoma contains Epstein-Barr virus DNA. *Int J Cancer* 1987;39:25.
73. Neal HB. Nasopharyngeal carcinoma: clinical presentation, diagnosis, treatment, and prognosis. *Otolaryngol Clin North Am* 1985;18:47.
74. Lin JC, Jan JS, Hsu CY, et al. Phase III study of concurrent chemoradiotherapy versus radiotherapy alone for advanced nasopharyngeal carcinoma: positive effect on overall and progression-free survival. *J Clin Oncol* 2003;21:631.
75. Kutler DI, Auerbach AD, Satagopan J, et al. High incidence of head and neck squamous cell carcinoma in patients with Fanconi anemia. *Arch Otolaryngol Head Neck Surg* 2003;129:106.
76. Rezaii J, Tavakoli H, Esfandiari K, et al. Association between *Helicobacter pylori* infection and laryngopharyngeal carcinoma: a case-control study and review of the literature. *Head Neck* 2008;30:1624.
77. Galli J, Cammarota G, Calo L, et al. The role of acid and alkaline reflux in laryngeal squamous cell carcinoma. *Laryngoscope* 2002;112:1861.
78. Cole I, Hughes L. The relationship of cervical lymph node metastases to primary sites of carcinoma of the upper aerodigestive tract: a pathological study. *Aust N Z J Surg* 1997;67:860.
79. Koo BS, Lim YC, Lee JS, et al. Management of contralateral N0 neck in pyriform sinus carcinoma. *Laryngoscope* 2006;116:1268.
80. Amdur RJ, Mendenhall WM, Stringer SP, et al. Organ preservation with radiotherapy for T1-T2 carcinoma of the pyriform sinus. *Head Neck* 2001;23:353.
81. Triboulet J, Mariette C, Chevalier D, et al. Surgical management of carcinoma of the hypopharynx and cervical esophagus. *Arch Surg* 2001;136: 1164.
82. Lee M, Ho H, Hsiao S, et al. Treatment results and prognostic factors in locally advanced hypopharyngeal cancer. *Acta Otolaryngol* 2008;128:103.
83. Rabbani A, Amdur RJ, Mancuso AA. Definitive radiotherapy for T1-T2 squamous cell carcinoma of the pyriform sinus. *Int J Radiat Oncol* 2008; 72:351.
84. Wolf GT, Hawn WK, Fisher SG, et al. Induction chemotherapy plus radiation compared with surgery plus radiation in patients with advanced laryngeal cancer. *N Engl J Med* 1991;324:1685.
85. Forastiere AA, Goepfert H, Maor M, et al. Concurrent chemotherapy and radiotherapy for organ preservation in advanced laryngeal cancer. *N Engl J Med* 2003;349:209.
86. Hoffman HT, Porter K, Karnell LH, et al. Laryngeal cancer in the United States: changes in demographics, patterns of care, and survival. *Laryngoscope* 2006;116(suppl 11):1.
87. Sessions DG, Lenox J, Spector GJ. Supraglottic laryngeal cancer: analysis of treatment results. *Laryngoscope* 2005;115:1402.
88. Redaelli de Zinis LO, Nicolai P, Tomenzoli D, et al. The distribution of lymph node metastases in supraglottic squamous cell carcinoma: therapeutic implications. *Head Neck* 2002;24:913.
89. Cabanillas R, Rodrigo JP, Llorente JL, et al. Oncologic outcomes of transoral laser surgery of supraglottic carcinoma compared with a transcervical approach. *Head Neck* 2008;30:750.
90. Rodrigo JP, Suarez C, Silver CE, et al. Transoral laser surgery for supraglottic cancer. *Head Neck* 2008;30:658.
91. Laudadio P, Presutti L, Dall'Olio D, et al. Supracricoid laryngectomies: long-term oncological and functional results. *Acta Otolaryngol* 2006;126: 640.
92. Mendenhall WM, Wernig JW, Hinerman RW, et al. Management of T1-T2 glottic carcinomas. *Cancer* 2004;100:1786.
93. Paisley S, Warde PR, O'Sullivan B, et al. Results of radiotherapy for primary subglottic squamous cell carcinoma. *Int J Radiat Oncol* 2002;52:1245.
94. Garas J, McGuirt WF. Squamous cell carcinoma of the subglottis. *Am J Otolaryngol* 2006;27:1.

SECTION D

ESOPHAGUS

CHAPTER 41 ESOPHAGEAL ANATOMY AND PHYSIOLOGY AND GASTROESOPHAGEAL REFLUX DISEASE

JEFFREY H. PETERS, VIRGINIA R. LITTLE, AND THOMAS J. WATSON

KEY POINTS

1. The lymphatics of the esophagus form a rich submucosal network draining into regional lymph nodes in the periesophageal connective tissue; thus, little barrier exists to the longitudinal spread of esophageal cancer.
2. The diagnosis of gastroesophageal reflux based on symptoms alone is correct in only approximately two thirds of patients because the symptoms are often nonspecific and can be caused by other conditions.
3. The three characteristics of the lower esophageal sphincter that maintains its resistance or "barrier" function to intragastric and intra-abdominal pressure challenges are pressure, overall length, and length exposed to the positive-pressure environment of the abdomen.
4. An important complication of gastroesophageal reflux is the development of reflux-induced respiratory symptoms either with or without heartburn.
5. Antireflux surgery improves respiratory symptoms in nearly 90% of children and 70% of adults with asthma and reflux disease.
6. Factors predisposing to the development of Barrett esophagus include early-onset gastroesophageal reflux disease, abnormal lower esophageal and esophageal body physiology, and mixed reflux of gastric and duodenal contents into the esophagus.
7. Proton pump inhibitor therapy, both to relieve symptoms and to control esophagitis, is an acceptable treatment, although most patients will require life-long treatment.
8. Progression of nondysplastic Barrett epithelium occurs with 5% to 10% of patients per year progressing to dysplasia and 0.5% to 1% per year progressing to adenocarcinoma.
9. Until recently, esophagectomy was considered the standard of care for patients with high-grade dysplasia. With the Western acceptance of an Eastern modality, endoscopic mucosal resection is becoming an increasingly attractive option for patients with high-grade dysplasia and intramucosal cancers.
10. The standard of care for the treatment of confirmed Barrett esophagus with high-grade dysplasia has been esophagectomy because approximately 35% of patients will harbor invasive adenocarcinoma. Where expertise exists, endoscopic therapies such as endoscopic resection or mucosal ablation are being increasingly utilized in highly selected patients with high-grade dysplasia or early esophageal carcinoma.
11. The mainstay of maintenance medical therapy is acid suppression. Patients with persistent symptoms should be given proton pump inhibitors, such as omeprazole. In doses as high as 40 mg/d, they can effect an 80% to 90% reduction in gastric acidity. Such a regimen usually heals mild esophagitis, but healing may occur in only three fourths of patients with severe esophagitis.
12. Three factors predictive of a successful outcome following antireflux surgery are (a) an abnormal score on 24-hour esophageal pH monitoring; (b) the presence of typical symptoms of gastroesophageal reflux disease, namely, heartburn or regurgitation; and (c) symptomatic improvement in response to acid suppression therapy prior to surgery.

ANATOMY

A detailed knowledge of the anatomic relationships of the esophagus is essential for the surgeon to plan and perform safe surgery, as well as to understand the significance of abnormalities detected on studies such as upper endoscopy, barium roentgenography, or computed tomography.[1] In this section, the embryology of the esophagus is first described, then the topographic relations of the esophagus are covered, and finally the conduct of investigations that yield anatomic information is addressed.

The embryology of the esophagus is important in understanding the pathogenesis of congenital malformations of the esophagus and trachea. The embryonic esophagus forms when paired longitudinal grooves appear on each side of the laryngotracheal diverticulum. These grooves subsequently grow medially and fuse to form the tracheoesophageal septum. This septum divides the foregut into the ventral laryngotracheal tube and the dorsal esophagus. Incomplete fusion of the two lateral grooves was thought to be the major factor in the pathogenesis of congenital tracheoesophageal fistula, but the anomaly is now attributed to abnormal growth and differentiation of the lung buds. Initially the esophagus is short, but elongation occurs rapidly, and the final relative length is attained by the seventh gestational week. This is followed by endodermal proliferation, resulting in near obliteration of the esophageal lumen and subsequent recanalization by the development of large vacuoles that coalesce. The striated muscle of the upper esophagus is derived from the caudal branchial arches and is innervated by the vagus nerve and its recurrent laryngeal branches. The smooth muscle of the lower esophagus arises from splanchnic mesenchyme and is supplied by a visceral nerve plexus derived from neural crest cells. The adult position of the vagus nerves on the esophagus is the result of unequal growth of the greater curve of the stomach relative to the lesser curve, resulting in rotation of the left vagus anteriorly and the right vagus posteriorly.

The *cervical esophagus* begins below the cricopharyngeus muscle, which itself is a continuation of the inferior constrictor of the pharynx. The potential space between these muscles posteriorly is the site where Zenker diverticulum develops. The cervical esophagus is about 5 cm long. It begins at the level of C6 and extends to the lower border of T1, curving slightly to the left in its descent. Anteriorly, it abuts against the trachea and posterior larynx and can be dissected off both organs if necessary. Posteriorly, the retroesophageal space is continuous with the retropharyngeal space above and the superior mediastinum below. Laterally, the omohyoid muscle crosses it obliquely and is usually divided to gain access to the esophagus. The carotid sheaths lie laterally and the lobes of the thyroid and the strap muscles anteriorly. The recurrent laryngeal nerves lie in the grooves between the esophagus and the trachea. The right recurrent nerve runs a more oblique course and is more prone to anatomic variants. Consequently, although the surgical approach to this portion of the esophagus may be from either side of the neck through an incision along the anterior border of sternocleidomastoid muscle, the left side is chosen if possible.

The *thoracic esophagus* in its upper part is closely related to the posterior wall of the trachea. This close relation is responsible for the early spread of cancer of the upper esophagus into the trachea, and it limits the ability of the surgeon to perform an en bloc resection of such a tumor. Above the level of the tracheal bifurcation, the esophagus moves to the right of the descending aorta. It then moves to the left, passes behind the tracheal bifurcation and the left main bronchus, and descends to the diaphragm. In its lower third, the esophagus courses anteriorly and to the left to pass through the diaphragmatic hiatus. The lower esophagus is covered only by flimsy mediastinal pleura on the left, and it is this portion that is most commonly the site of perforation in Boerhaave syndrome. The azygos vein is closely related to the esophagus as it arches from its paraspinal position over the right main bronchus to enter the superior vena cava. The thoracic duct ascends behind and to the right of the distal esophagus, but at the level of T5 it passes posterior to the aorta and ascends on the left side of the esophagus and posterior to the left subclavian artery.

Throughout its length, the attachments of the esophagus to its adjacent structures other than the posterior trachea are flimsy. This accounts for the ease with which the esophagus may be bluntly mobilized out of the mediastinum during transhiatal esophagectomy. In general, the lower esophagus is most easily approached through the left chest, but access to the supra-aortic esophagus is restricted. Thus, a left thoracotomy is most useful for performing Heller myotomy, transthoracic fundoplication, or resection of an epiphrenic diverticulum. Access to the entire thoracic esophagus can be obtained only from the right chest, but access to the intra-abdominal organs is restricted by the liver and normally requires a separate upper abdominal incision.

The abdominal esophagus begins as the esophagus enters the abdomen through the diaphragmatic hiatus (Fig. 41.1). It is surrounded by a fibroelastic membrane, the phrenoesophageal ligament, which arises from the subdiaphragmatic fascia (Fig. 41.2). The lower limit of the phrenoesophageal membrane anteriorly is marked by a prominent fat pad, which corresponds to the gastroesophageal (GE) junction. The lower esophageal sphincter (LES) is a zone of high pressure 3 to 5 cm long at the lower end of the esophagus.[2] Although it does not correspond to any macroscopic anatomic structure, its function appears to be related to the microscopic architecture of the muscle fibers. The esophageal hiatus is formed by the right and left crura, which form a sling of muscular fibers arising by tendinous bands from the anterolateral surface of the first four lumbar vertebrae. The relative contributions of the right and left crura to the sling are variable. Surgeons name the crura from their relation to the esophagus, whereas anatomists name them from their relation to the aorta. Thus, both right and left "surgical" crura originate from the right "anatomic" crus. Caudally, the crura are united by a tendinous arch, the median arcuate ligament, just anterior to the aorta at the level of the celiac axis.

The blood supply and venous drainage are largely segmental. The inferior thyroid artery provides the main blood supply to the cervical portion of the esophagus. This becomes important in a patient with a previous thyroidectomy, although ligation is usually performed distal to the esophageal branch. The thoracic portion of the esophagus receives its blood supply from two sources. Usually, branches from two to three

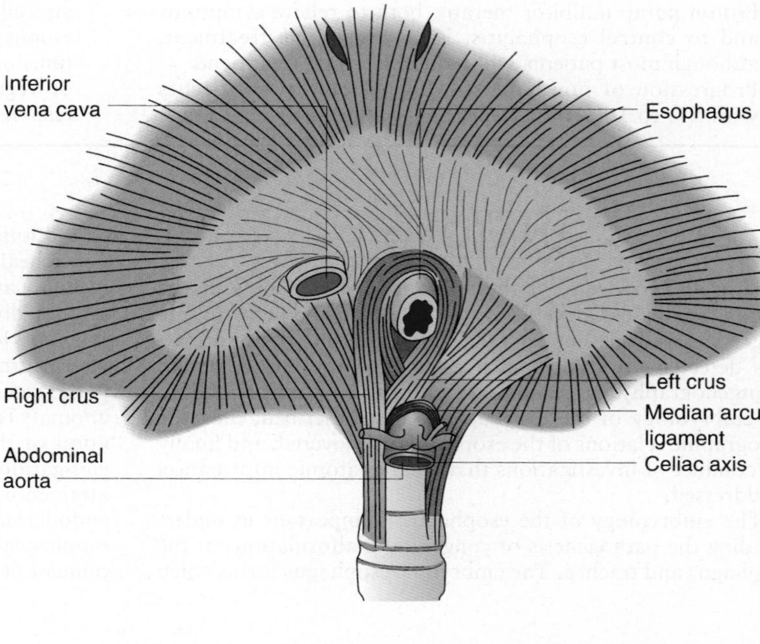

FIGURE 41.1. The diaphragm and esophageal hiatus viewed from below.

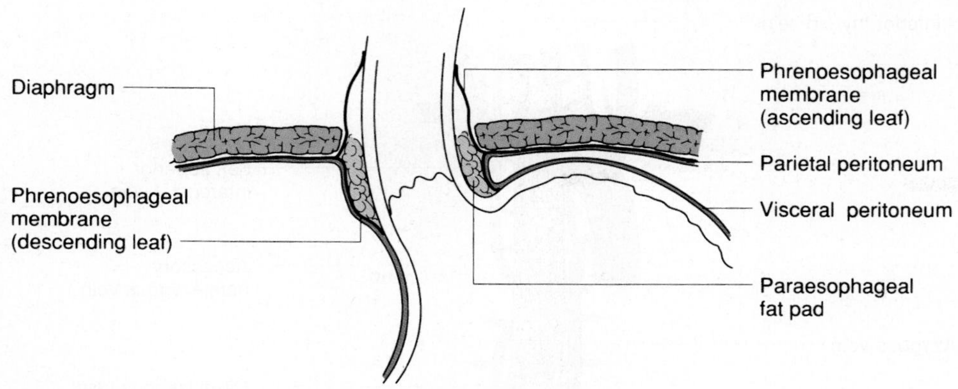

FIGURE 41.2. Attachments of the phrenoesophageal membrane.

bronchial arteries provide the proximal arterial supply, and branches directly from the aorta supply the more distal thoracic esophagus. The upper of these aortic branches arises between the sixth and seventh thoracic vertebrae; the lower one arises between the eighth and ninth thoracic vertebrae. Intrathoracic mobilization of the esophagus during the performance of antireflux procedures often requires ligation of these branches. The abdominal esophagus receives its blood supply from branches of the left gastric artery and inferior phrenic arteries (Fig. 41.3). A particularly constant artery at the base of the left surgical crus connects the inferior phrenic artery to branches of the left gastric artery and is sometimes called the Belsey artery. It is often seen during the crural dissection in performing laparoscopic fundoplication. Once the vessels have

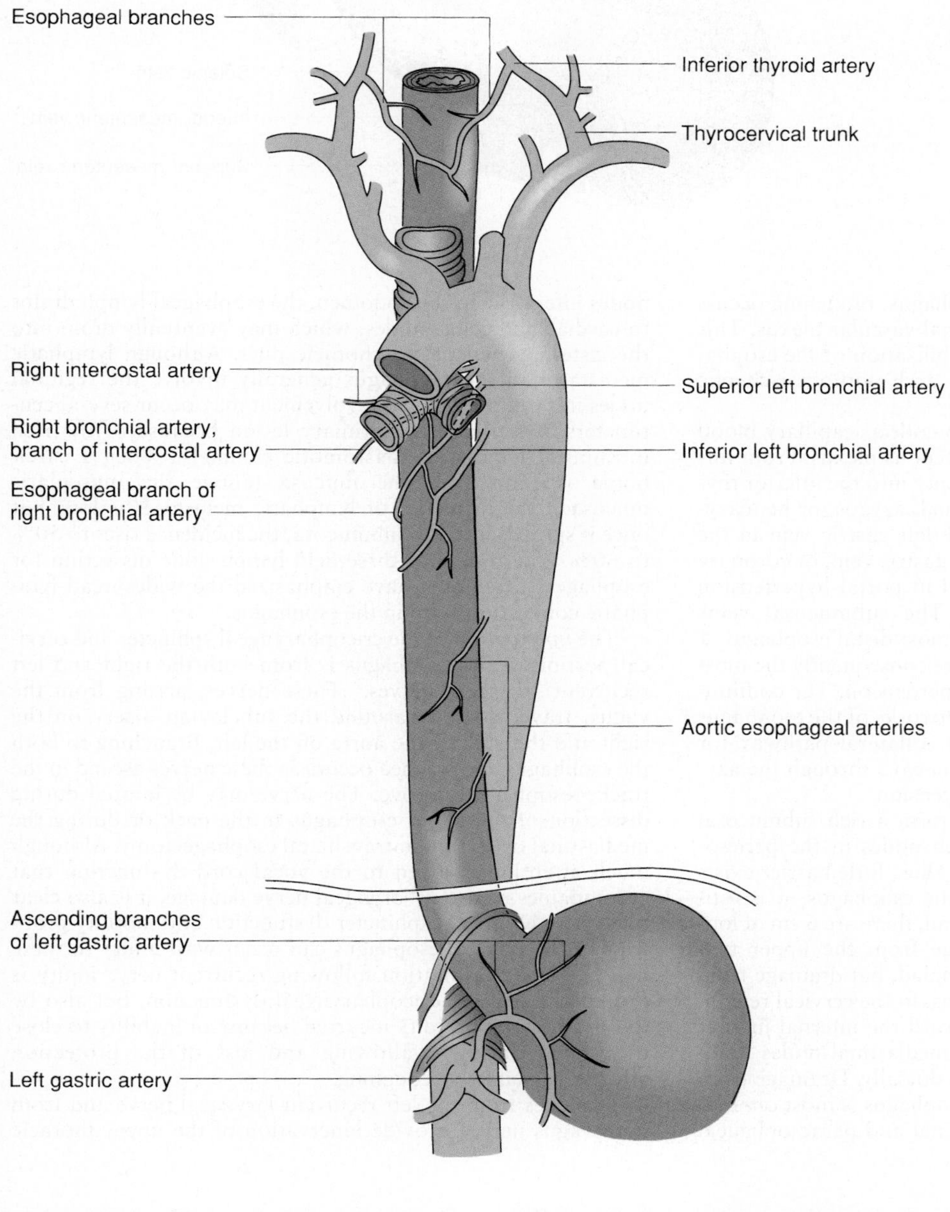

FIGURE 41.3. Arterial blood supply of the esophagus.

HEAD AND NECK

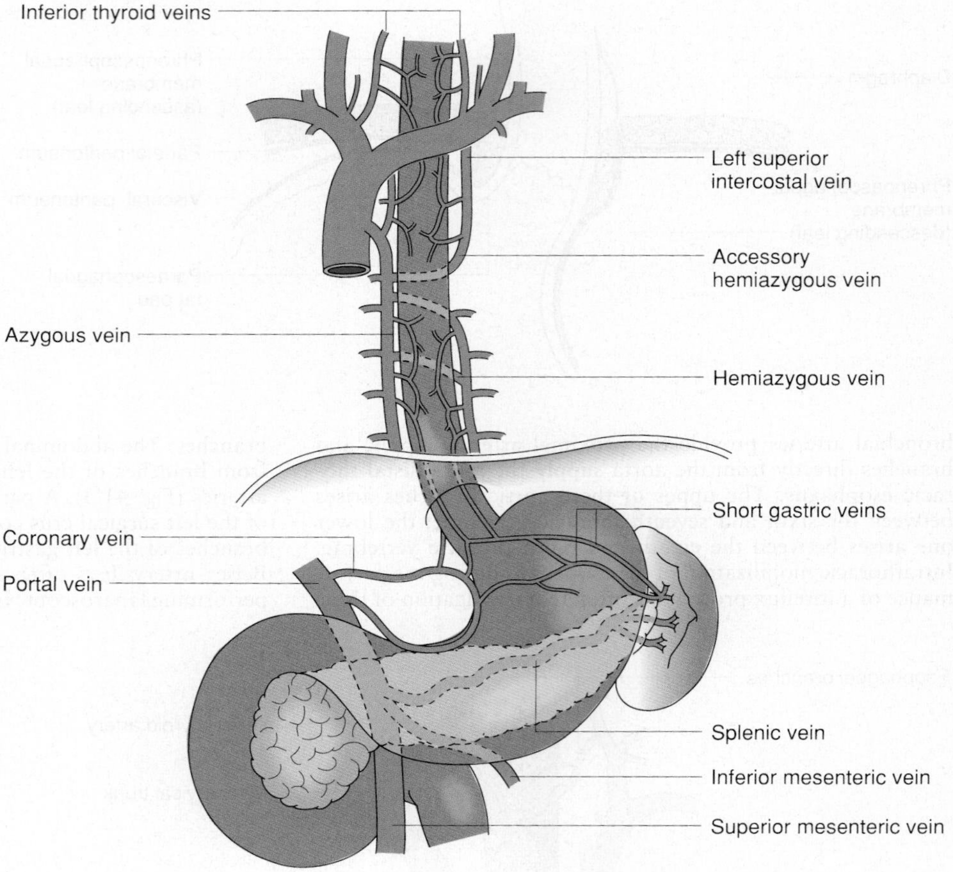

FIGURE 41.4. Venous drainage of the esophagus.

entered the muscular wall of the esophagus, branching occurs at right angles to provide a longitudinal vascular plexus. This anatomic arrangement allows for mobilization of the esophagus from the stomach to the aortic arch without ischemic injury.

A venous plexus in the submucosa collects capillary blood and delivers it into a periesophageal venous plexus. From this plexus, esophageal veins arise that empty into the inferior thyroid vein proximally; into the bronchial, azygos, or hemiazygos veins in the thorax; and into the left gastric vein in the abdominal region (Fig. 41.4). The left gastric vein, or coronary vein, provides the principal collateral in portal hypertension when esophageal varices develop. The submucosal veins become much more superficial in the most distal esophagus, 1 to 2 cm above the GE junction, and are consequently the most common site of bleeding in portal hypertension. The continuity between the submucosal venous networks of the esophagus and stomach provides an additional collateral pathway for portal blood to enter the superior vena cava through the azygos vein in patients with portal hypertension.

1 The *lymphatics* of the esophagus form a rich submucosal network draining into regional lymph nodes in the periesophageal connective tissue (Fig. 41.5). Thus, little barrier exists to longitudinal spread of cancer in the esophagus; it is estimated that for every 1 cm of axial spread, there are 6 cm of longitudinal spread. Lymphatic drainage from the upper two thirds of the esophagus is usually cephalad, but drainage from the lower one third is in both directions. In the cervical region, esophageal lymphatic drainage is toward the internal jugular and upper tracheal nodes. Posterior mediastinal nodes drain the thoracic portion of the esophagus dorsally. Drainage from the anterior portion of the thoracic esophagus is most often to tracheal nodes superiorly and subcarinal and paraesophageal nodes inferiorly. In the abdomen, the esophageal lymph drains to cardiac and celiac nodes, which may eventually drain into the cisterna chyli or the thoracic duct. Although lymphatic metastases in the esophagus generally involve the regional nodes in proximity, nodal involvement may occur several centimeters away from the primary lesion because of the rich intramural lymphatic anastomotic channels. When a carcinoma is limited to the mucosa (above the muscularis mucosae), the incidence of lymphatic metastases is low, but once it spreads into the submucosa, the incidence rises to 50% to 60%. The results of three-field lymph node dissection for esophageal carcinoma have emphasized the widespread lymphatic connections within the esophagus.

The *innervation* of the cricopharyngeal sphincter and cervical portion of the esophagus is from both the right and left recurrent laryngeal nerves.[2] These nerves, arising from the vagus, travel dorsally around the subclavian artery on the right and the arch of the aorta on the left. Branching to both the esophagus and trachea occurs as these nerves ascend in the tracheoesophageal groove. The nerve may be injured during dissection of the upper esophagus in the neck or during the mediastinal dissection in transhiatal esophagectomy. Although much attention is given to the vocal cord dysfunction that accompanies recurrent laryngeal nerve damage, it is also clear that cricopharyngeal sphincter dysfunction and motility problems of the cervical esophagus can occur with injury to these nerves. Serious aspiration following recurrent nerve injury is caused not only by cricopharyngeal dysfunction, but also by the additional morbidity incurred because of inability to close the glottis during swallowing and loss of the protection afforded by effective coughing.

Branches from the left recurrent laryngeal nerve and from both vagus nerves provide innervation of the upper thoracic

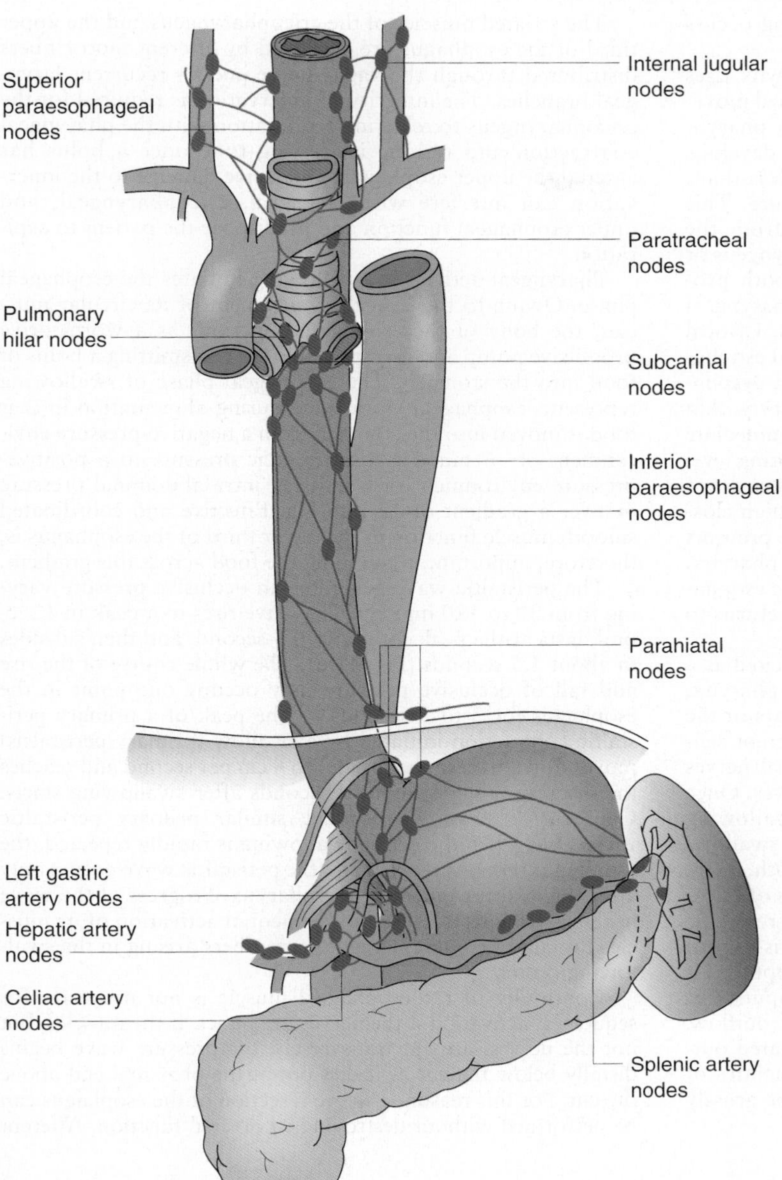

FIGURE 41.5. Lymphatic drainage of the esophagus.

esophagus. The esophageal plexus on the anterior and posterior wall of the esophagus provides innervation for the lower esophagus. The esophageal plexus also receives fibers from the thoracic sympathetic chain. The single trunks located distally contain fibers from both right and left original vagus nerves.

Efferent preganglionic sympathetic fibers supplying the esophagus arise from the fourth to sixth thoracic spinal cord segments and terminate in the cervical and thoracic sympathetic ganglions. Fibers from the superior cervical ganglion arrive at the pharyngeal plexus by way of vagal nerves. The postganglionic fibers reach the esophagus by branches from the cervical and thoracic sympathetic chain. The distal esophageal segments also receive direct sympathetic fibers from the celiac ganglion.

Afferent visceral sensory pain fibers from the esophagus terminate without synapsing in the first four segments of the thoracic spinal cord, following both sympathetic and vagal pathways. Pain fibers from the heart also travel in this same pathway, which explains the similarity of the symptoms in many esophageal and cardiac diseases.

PHYSIOLOGY

The act of alimentation requires the passage of food and drink from the mouth into the stomach. Food is taken into the mouth in a variety of bite sizes, where it is broken up, mixed with saliva, and lubricated. Swallowing, once initiated, is entirely a reflex. When food is ready for swallowing, the tongue, acting like a piston, moves the bolus into the posterior oropharynx and forces it into the hypopharynx.[3] Concomitantly with the posterior movement of the tongue, the soft palate is elevated, thereby closing the passage between the oropharynx and nasopharynx. This partitioning prevents pressure generated in the oropharynx from being dissipated through the nose. When the soft palate is paralyzed, as following a cerebral vascular accident, food is commonly regurgitated into the nasopharynx. During swallowing, the hyoid bone moves upward and anteriorly, elevating the larynx and opening the retrolaryngeal space, bringing the epiglottis under the tongue. The backward tilt of the epiglottis covers the opening of the larynx to prevent aspiration. The whole pharyngeal part of swallowing occurs within 1.5 seconds.

During swallowing, the pressure in the hypopharynx rises abruptly to at least 60 mm Hg because of the backward movement of the tongue and contraction of the posterior pharyngeal constrictors. A sizable pressure difference develops between the hypopharyngeal pressure and the less-than-atmospheric mid-esophageal or intrathoracic pressure. This pressure gradient speeds the movement of food from the hypopharynx into the esophagus when the cricopharyngeus or upper esophageal sphincter relaxes. The bolus is both propelled by peristaltic contraction of the posterior pharyngeal constrictors and sucked into the thoracic esophagus. Critical to receiving the bolus is the compliance of the cervical esophagus; when compliance is lost due to muscle pathology, dysphagia can result. The upper esophageal sphincter closes within 0.5 second of the initiation of the swallow, with the immediate closing pressure reaching approximately twice the resting level of 30 mm Hg. The postrelaxation contraction continues down the esophagus as a peristaltic wave (Fig. 41.6). The high closing pressure and the initiation of the peristaltic wave prevents reflux of the bolus from the esophagus back into the pharynx. After the peristaltic wave has passed further down the esophagus, the pressure in the upper esophageal sphincter returns to its resting level.

Swallowing can be started at will, or it can be elicited as a reflex by the stimulation of areas in the mouth and pharynx, among them the anterior and posterior tonsillar pillars or the posterior lateral walls of the hypopharynx. The afferent sensory nerves of the pharynx are the glossopharyngeal nerves and the superior laryngeal branches of the vagus nerves. Once aroused by stimuli entering via these nerves, the swallowing center in the medulla coordinates the complete act of swallowing by discharging impulses through the 5th, 7th, 10th, 11th, and 12th cranial nerves, as well as the motor neurons of C1 to C3. Discharges through these nerves occur in a rather specific pattern and last for approximately 0.5 second. Little is known about the organization of the swallowing center except that it can trigger swallowing after a variety of different inputs, but the response is always a rigidly ordered pattern of outflow. Following a cerebral vascular accident, this coordinated outflow may be altered, causing mild to severe abnormalities of swallowing. In more severe injury, swallowing can be grossly disrupted, leading to repetitive aspiration.

The striated muscles of the cricopharyngeus and the upper third of the esophagus are activated by efferent motor fibers distributed through the vagus nerve and its recurrent laryngeal branches. The integrity of innervation is required for the cricopharyngeus to relax in coordination with the pharyngeal contraction and resume its resting tone once a bolus has entered the upper esophagus. Operative damage to the innervation can interfere with laryngeal, cricopharyngeal, and upper esophageal function and predispose the patient to aspiration.

Pharyngeal activity in swallowing initiates the esophageal phase. Owing to the helical arrangement of its circular muscles, the body of the esophagus functions as a worm drive propulsive pump and is responsible for transmitting a bolus of food into the stomach. The esophageal phase of swallowing represents esophageal work done during alimentation in that food is moved into the stomach from a negative-pressure environment of −6 mm Hg intrathoracic pressure to a positive-pressure environment of 6 mm Hg intra-abdominal pressure or over a gradient of 12 mm Hg. Effective and coordinated smooth muscle function in the lower third of the esophagus is, therefore, important in pumping the food across this gradient.

The peristaltic wave generates an occlusive pressure varying from 30 to 120 mm Hg. The wave rises to a peak in 1 second, lasts at the peak for about 0.5 second, and then subsides in about 1.5 seconds (Fig. 41.6). The whole course of the rise and fall of occlusive pressure may occupy one point in the esophagus for 3 to 5 seconds.[4,5] The peak of a primary peristaltic contraction initiated by a swallow (primary peristalsis) moves down the esophagus at 2 to 4 cm per second and reaches the distal esophagus about 9 seconds after swallowing starts. Consecutive swallows produce similar primary peristaltic waves, but when the act of swallowing is rapidly repeated, the esophagus remains relaxed and the peristaltic wave occurs only after the last movement of the pharynx. Progress of the wave in the esophagus is caused by sequential activation of its muscles initiated by efferent vagal nerve fibers arising in the swallowing center.

Continuity of the esophageal muscle is not necessary for sequential activation if the nerves are intact. If the muscles, but not the nerves, are cut transversely, the pressure wave begins distally below the cut as it dies out at the proximal end above the cut. For this reason, a sleeve resection of the esophagus can be performed without destroying its normal function. Afferent

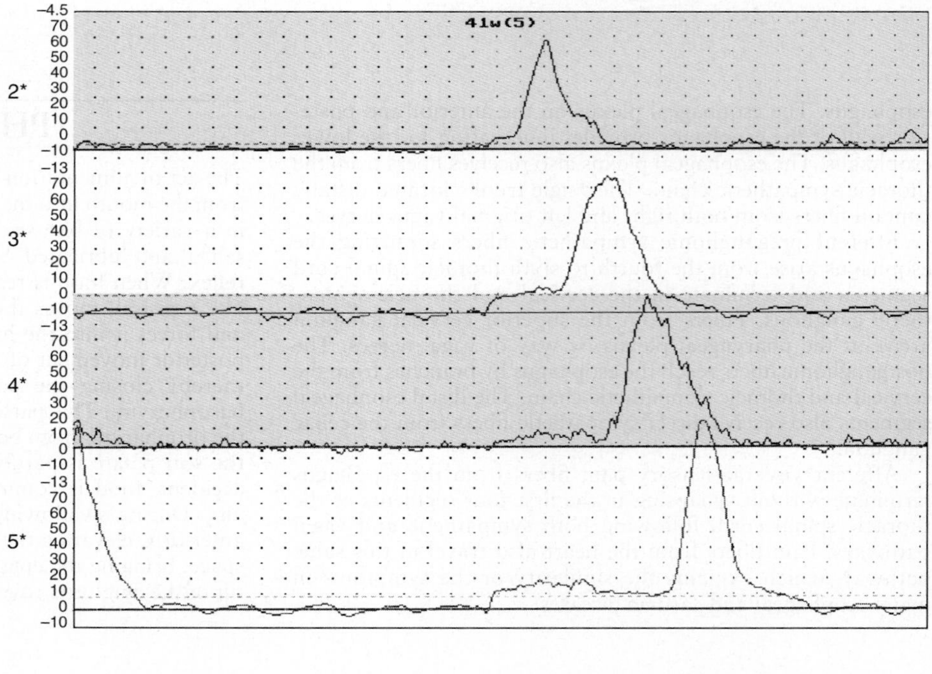

FIGURE 41.6. Representative example of manometric tracing of an esophageal peristaltic wave. Channel 2 is in the proximal esophagus and channel 5 is in the distal esophagus. The channels are 5 cm apart. The wave can be seen to progress in time down the esophagus.

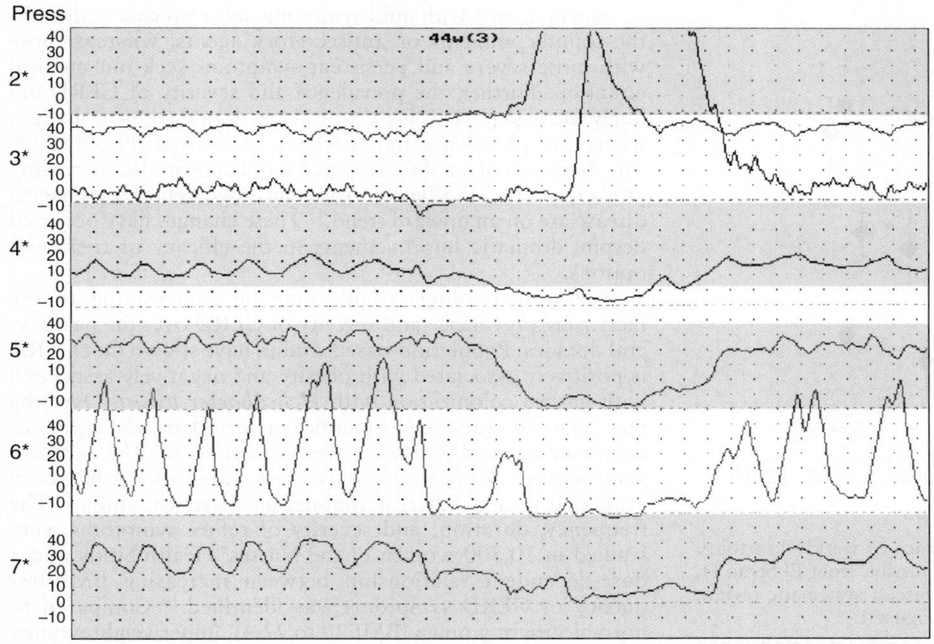

FIGURE 41.7. Representative example of a manometric tracing of lower esophageal sphincter relaxation. Channels 2 and 3 are in the distal esophagus and show a peristaltic wave progressing downward. The lower four channels are all at the same level within the lower esophageal sphincter and oriented radially at 12, 3, 6, and 9 o'clock. The dotted lines below each tracing represent gastric baseline pressures. The lower four tracings each relax to gastric baseline at the initiation of the swallow.

impulses from receptors within the esophageal wall are not essential for progress of the coordinated wave. Afferent nerves, however, do go to the swallowing center from the esophagus, because if the esophagus is distended at any point, a contractual wave begins with a forceful closure of the upper esophageal sphincter and sweeps down the esophagus. This secondary contraction occurs without any movements of the mouth or pharynx. Secondary peristalsis can occur as an independent local reflex to clear the esophagus of ingested material left behind after the passage of the primary wave. Current studies suggest that secondary peristalsis is not as common as once thought.

Despite the rather powerful occlusive pressure, the propulsive force of the esophagus is relatively feeble. If a subject attempts to swallow a bolus attached by a string to a counterweight, the maximum weight that can be overcome is 5 to 10 g. Orderly contractions of the muscular wall and anchoring of the esophagus at its inferior end are necessary for efficient aboral propulsion to occur. Loss of the inferior anchor, as occurs with a large hiatal hernia, can lead to inefficient propulsion.

The LES provides a pressure barrier between the esophagus and stomach. Although an anatomically distinct LES has been difficult to identify, microdissection studies show that, in humans, the sphincterlike function is related to the architecture of the muscle fibers at the junction of the esophageal tube with the gastric pouch. The sphincter actively remains closed to prevent reflux of gastric contents into the esophagus and opens by a relaxation that coincides with a pharyngeal swallow (Fig. 41.7). The LES pressure returns to its resting level after the peristaltic wave has passed through the esophagus. Consequently, reflux of gastric juice that may occur through the open valve during a swallow is cleared back into the stomach.

If the pharyngeal swallow does not initiate a peristaltic contraction, then the coincident relaxation of the LES is unguarded and reflux of gastric juice can occur. This may be an explanation for the observation of spontaneous LES relaxation, thought by some to be a causative factor in gastroesophageal reflux disease (GERD). The power of the esophageal body is insufficient to force open a valve that does not relax. In dogs, a bilateral cervical parasympathetic blockade abolishes the relaxation of the LES that occurs with pharyngeal swallowing or distention of the esophagus. Consequently, vagal function appears to be important in coordinating the relaxation of the LES with esophageal contraction.

The LES has intrinsic myogenic tone, which is modulated by neural and hormonal mechanisms.[6,7] α-Adrenergic neurotransmitters or beta-blockers stimulate the LES, and alpha-blockers and β stimulants decrease its pressure. It is not clear to what extent cholinergic nerve activity controls LES pressure. The vagus nerve carries both excitatory and inhibitory fibers to the esophagus and sphincter. The hormones gastrin and motilin have been shown to increase LES pressure; cholecystokinin, estrogen, glucagon, progesterone, somatostatin, and secretin decrease LES pressure. The peptides bombesin, B-enkephalin, and substance P increase LES pressure; calcitonin gene–related peptide, gastric inhibitory peptide, neuropeptide Y, and vasoactive intestinal polypeptide decrease LES pressure. Some pharmacologic agents such as antacids, cholinergics, domperidone, metoclopramide, and prostaglandin F_2 are known to increase LES pressure; anticholinergics, barbiturates, calcium channel blockers, caffeine, diazepam, dopamine, meperidine, prostaglandin E_1 and E_2, and theophylline decrease LES pressure. Peppermint, chocolate, coffee, ethanol, and fat are all associated with decreased LES pressure and may be responsible for esophageal symptoms after a sumptuous meal.

During 24-hour esophageal pH monitoring, healthy individuals have occasional episodes of GE reflux. This physiologic reflux is more common when a person is awake and in the upright position than during sleep in the supine position. When reflux of gastric juice occurs, normal subjects rapidly clear the acid gastric juice from the esophagus regardless of their position.

GASTROESOPHAGEAL REFLUX DISEASE

Definition and Epidemiology

Developing an accurate definition of gastroesophageal reflux disease is surprisingly difficult. The disease can be associated with myriad common gastrointestinal (GI) and respiratory symptoms and there is no fully accurate diagnostic test that can be relied upon. In an effort to provide a consensus definition, a group of experts came together in Montreal in 2004 and concluded that GERD can be best defined as "a condition

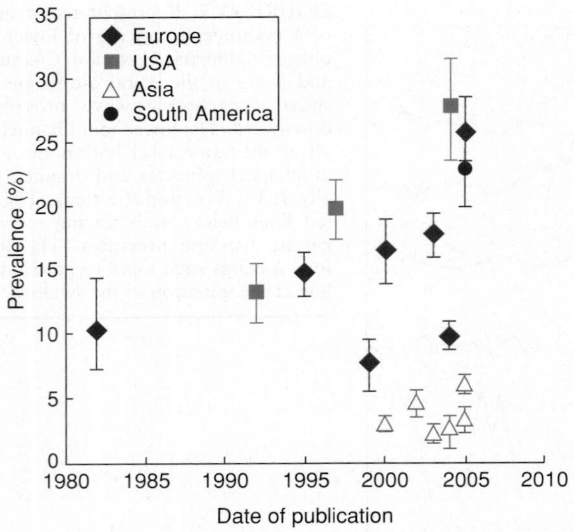

FIGURE 41.8. Time trends for the prevalence of weekly heartburn from 1980 to 2005. (Reproduced with permission from El-Serag H. Time trends of gastroesophageal reflux disease: a systematic review. *Clin Gastroenterol Hepatol* 2007;5:17–26, Figure 1.)

which develops when the reflux of stomach contents causes troublesome symptoms and/or complications."[8]

GERD is a very common disease. Population-based studies have reported that one third of Western populations experience the symptoms of GERD at least once a month, with 4% to 7% of the population experiencing daily symptoms.[9,10] Its prevalence varies considerably around the globe and is highest in North America, Australia, and Western Europe and lowest in Africa and Asia.[11] It is also likely that both the prevalence and severity of GERD are increasing in many parts of the world. Time trend analyses have shown that the prevalence of GERD symptoms has increased progressively in most longitudinal studies, including those from the United States, Singapore, and China (Fig. 41.8).[12] Further, recent data reported by the Agency for Healthcare Research and Quality (AHRQ) indicate a marked increase (103%) in hospitalizations for treating disorders caused by GERD; a 216% increase in hospitalization of patients who, in addition to the ailment for which they were admitted, have milder forms of GERD; and a 39% increase in admission for GERD with severe symptoms including anemia, weight loss, and vomiting.[13] These data suggest that the current therapeutic approach to GERD may be inadequate.

Most patients with mild symptoms self-medicate with over-the-counter antacids or antisecretory agents, whereas those with more severe and persistent symptoms seek out medical attention. Further, the prevalence and severity of GERD are likely increasing. This is in contrast to duodenal ulcer disease, where the prevalence has markedly decreased (Fig. 41.9).[14] The diagnosis of a columnar-lined esophagus is also increasing at a rapid rate, and deaths from end-stage benign esophageal disease are on an upward trend.[15] These changes have occurred despite dramatic improvements in the efficacy of treatment options.

Two epidemiologic trends may be contributing to the increasing prevalence and severity of GERD over the past several decades. Population-based studies have shown that GERD is positively associated with obesity and negatively associated with gastric colonization with *Helicobacter pylori.* Over the past 20 to 30 years, the former has increased and the latter has decreased markedly in most Western countries. The relationship between GERD and body mass index (BMI) has been evaluated in a number of well-designed clinical studies. The frequency, duration, and severity of reflux symptoms were studied in 10,500 women of the Nurses' Health Study and a dose-dependent relationship between increasing BMI frequency of GERD symptoms was identified.[16] Compared to normal-weight women (BMI 20 to 22.4), underweight women (BMI <20) were one-third less likely and overweight women (BMI 25 to 27.4) two times more likely to have frequent GERD symptoms. Obese women (BMI >30) had a nearly three times higher risk of frequent GERD symptoms (Fig. 41.10). Recent meta-analyses confirm these findings, with studies from the United States demonstrating an association between increasing BMI and the presence of GERD.[17] High-resolution motility studies have shown a significant correlation with BMI and both intragastric pressure and gastroesophageal pressure gradients, providing a physiologic explanation for the BMI–GERD association.[18] These studies suggest that obese subjects are more likely to have esophagogastric junction disruption and abnormal pressure gradients favoring the development of reflux. Finally, the risk of Barrett esophagus has been correlated with the presence of central obesity. Measures of central obesity, including waist circumference and waist-to-hip ratios, were associated with both short- and long-segment Barrett esophagus, with a 4.1 higher odds ratio of long-segment Barrett in patients with a high waist-to-hip ratio.[19]

The possible pathogenic role of helical-shaped bacteria found in gastric fluids was first suggested in the late 19th century by the Polish scientist Walery Jaworski of the University of Krakow.[20] It was the publication of two Australian scientists in 1983 that convincingly demonstrated the pathogenic role of *H. pylori.*[21] These pioneering studies of Barry Marshall and

FIGURE 41.9. Trends in hospitalization for duodenal ulcer and gastroesophageal reflux disease from the 1970s to 1990s in U.S. veterans. (Reproduced with permission from El-Serag HB, Sonnenberg A. Opposing time trends of peptic ulcer and reflux disease. *Gut* 1998;43:327.)

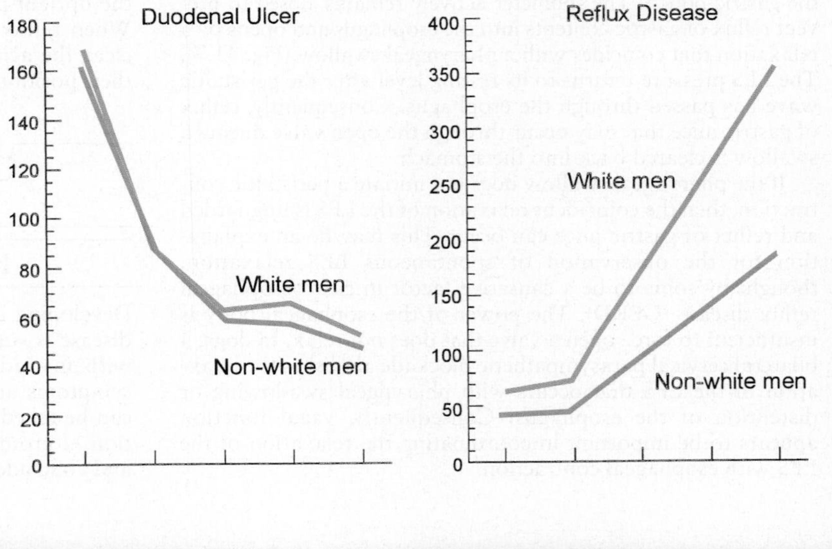

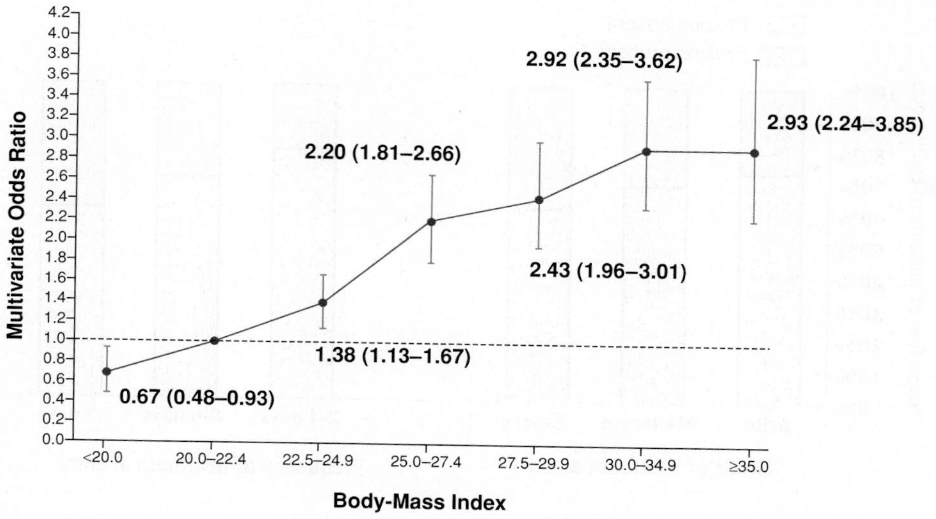

FIGURE 41.10. Association between body mass index and the risk of frequent symptoms of GERD. (Reproduced with permission from Jacobson B, Somers SC, Fuchs CS, et al. Body-mass index and symptoms of gastroesophageal reflux in women. *N Eng J Med* 2006;354:2340–2348, Figure 1.)

Robin Warren from Perth, Australia, included self-experiments and were later awarded the Nobel Prize. *H. pylori* induces a significant inflammatory and immune response in the affected host, resulting in persistent inflammation in virtually all infected subjects.

The relationship between *H. pylori* and GERD has been of interest for decades. The observation that gastric mucosal atrophy was less frequent in patients with reflux esophagitis was made well before the *H. pylori* era. Evolutionary hypotheses assume, and the majority of available epidemiologic data show, that the decline of *H. pylori* infection is one of the reasons behind the increasing incidence of GERD-related diseases including esophageal and cardia adenocarcinoma in the Western world. This inverse relationship is strongest between *H. pylori* and esophageal adenocarcinoma, although significant evidence relates *H. pylori* and the development of Barrett esophagus and GERD. Over the period from 1970 to 1995, the incidence of both duodenal ulcer, compared to erosive esophagitis, and distal gastric cancer, compared to gastric cardia cancer, displays strikingly opposing time trends. It has been postulated that *H. pylori*–induced chronic corpus gastritis may protect against the development of gastroesophageal reflux disease and its malignant transformation. A detailed report by Labenz et al. in 1997 provided some of the first evidence in support of this theory.[22] In a case-control study of 460 duodenal ulcer patients, new-onset GERD symptoms were significantly higher in patients who had successful *H. pylori* eradication than in those with persisting infection. Although a number of subsequent studies have raised doubts as to whether a true relationship exists, the available evidence suggests that the prevalence of *H. pylori* infection in patients with GERD is lower than non-GERD control populations and that there is likely an inverse epidemiologic relationship between GERD and *H. pylori*.

The relationship of Barrett esophagus to gastric *H. pylori* colonization is also debated, although most studies show an even stronger inverse relationship than that of GERD alone. Bowrey et al. reported an *H. pylori* prevalence of 27% in patients with Barrett esophagus compared to 41% in healthy control subjects.[23] Werdmuller and Loffeld also found significantly lower *H. pylori* infection rates in Barrett than non-Barrett patients (23% vs. 51%), whereas Loffeld et al. reported very high rates (62%) in a retrospective analysis of 107 consecutive patients with columnar-lined esophagus.[24,25] Investigations focused on the role of subpopulations of *H. pylori* have implicated cagA$^+$ strains as particularly relevant to the development of GE reflux and its complications.[26] Vicari et al. demonstrated that in patients with *H. pylori* infection, the prevalence of cagA$^+$ strains progressively decreased with the severity of GERD, including Barrett esophagus and esophageal adenocarcinoma.[27] Other studies have confirmed an inverse relationship between the presence of cagA positivity and adenocarcinoma of the esophagus and the GE junction.[28] Most authors postulate that cagA$^+$ strains may protect from the development of adenocarcinoma by inducing more severe mucosal inflammation and atrophic gastritis and thereby decreasing acid reflux. Present data regarding gastric acid secretion are conflicting, however, and further studies are required to test whether this hypothesis is true.

Studies on the natural history of GERD are rare. The few that do exist usually involve patients who were receiving some form of therapy. One of the most detailed studies on the natural history of the disease comes from investigators in Europe.[29] The progression or regression of GERD complications was assessed in a cohort of nearly 4,000 patients with predominant heartburn over a 2-year period. After 2 years, 25% of patients with nonerosive GERD progressed to erosive disease, 1.6% with mild erosive esophagitis worsened to more severe esophagitis, and nearly 8% progressed to Barrett esophagus, the latter predominantly in patients with Los Angeles grade C/D erosive disease at baseline. On the other hand, 50% to 60% of patients with baseline esophagitis improved to a milder grade or no erosive disease and 22% were off medications at 2 years. Given that virtually all patients were receiving significant antisecretory therapy, the study shows that a substantial minority of patients will continue to worsen despite pharmacologic treatment. Investigators in Lausanne, Switzerland, reported an intensive endoscopic follow-up of a defined population of 959 patients over a 30-year period.[30] The study involved only patients who had endoscopic esophagitis and did not include those who had symptoms without mucosal injury. Esophagitis was an isolated episode and did not return while on acid suppression therapy in roughly half of the patients. In the remaining patients, esophagitis intermittently recurred on acid suppression therapy, and in 42% it progressed on therapy to more severe mucosal injury. This latter group makes up roughly one quarter of the initial population of patients with esophagitis, similar to that reported in the Labenz study outlined previously. The study also showed that as many as 18% of the initial population may have acquired, while on therapy, a columnar-lined lower esophagus with intestinal metaplasia.

Clinical Presentation

The most common complaints in patients with GERD are heartburn, regurgitation, and dysphagia or difficulty swallowing. These represent the so-called typical symptoms of GERD. Although none of these are specific to GERD, dysphagia is

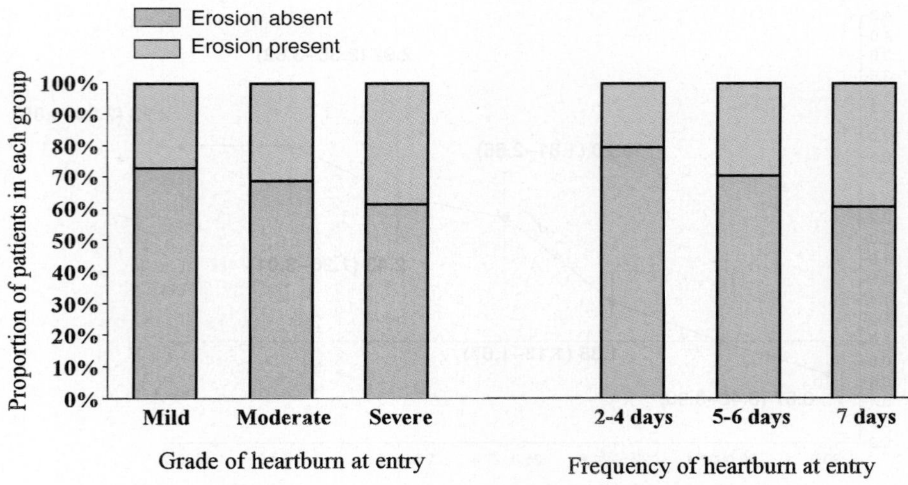

FIGURE 41.11. Prevalence of erosive esophagitis in 994 patients with varying severity and frequency of reflux symptoms. (Reproduced with permission from Venables TL, Newland RD, Patel AC, et al. Omeprazole 10 milligrams once daily, omeprazole 20 milligrams once daily, or ranitidine 150 milligrams twice daily, evaluated as initial therapy for the relief of symptoms of gastro-oesophageal reflux disease in general practice. *Scand J Gastroenterol* 1997;32:965.)

more commonly a sign of serious underlying pathology, including esophageal carcinoma, and should always be investigated promptly and thoroughly.

Heartburn is characterized as a substernal "burning" discomfort often radiating from the epigastrium to sternal notch. Occasionally patients will refer to it as "chest pain" rather than heartburn, and the two can be difficult to distinguish. Even the location can be variable with patients occasionally experiencing discomfort in the epigastrium, base of the neck, back, or other areas. Heartburn is typically made worse by "spicy" foods such as tomato sauce, citrus juices, chocolate, coffee, and alcohol. It occurs 1 to 2 hours after eating, often at night, and is relieved by antacids and antisecretory agents such as the over-the-counter histamine-2 blockers. It is well recognized that the severity of symptoms is not necessarily related to the severity of the underlying disease (Fig. 41.11).

Regurgitation is the spontaneous return of gastric contents proximal to the GE junction. Its spontaneous nature distinguishes it from vomiting. The patient often gets a sensation that fluid or food is returning into the esophagus, even if it does not reach as high as the pharynx or mouth. It is typically worse at night in the recumbent position or when lying down after a meal. Patients commonly compensate by not eating late at night or by sleeping partially upright with several pillows or in a chair. This symptom is often less well relieved with antacids and antisecretory agents, although it may change in character from acid to a more "bland" nature.

Dysphagia is present in up to 40% of patients with GERD. It is generally manifested by a sensation of food hanging up in the lower esophagus (esophageal dysphagia) rather than difficulty transferring the bolus from the mouth to the esophageal inlet (oropharyngeal dysphagia). Classically, dysphagia limited to only solid food, with normal passage of liquids, suggests a mechanical disorder such as a large hernia, stricture, or tumor, whereas difficulty with both solids and liquids suggests a functional or motor disorder. It often develops slowly enough that the patient may adjust his or her eating habits and not necessarily notice that it is happening. Thus, a thorough esophageal history includes an assessment of the patient's dietary history. Questions should be asked regarding the consistency of food that is typically eaten and whether the patient requires liquids with the meal, is the last to finish, has interrupted a social meal, chokes or vomits with eating, or has been admitted on an emergency basis for food impaction. These assessments, in addition to the ability to maintain nutrition, help to quantify the dysphagia and are important in determining the indications for surgical therapy.

Many patients with GE reflux often manifest "atypical" symptoms, such as cough, asthma, hoarseness, and noncardiac chest pain. Atypical symptoms are the primary complaint in 20% to 25% of patients with GERD and are secondarily present in association with heartburn and regurgitation in many more. It is considerably more difficult to prove a cause-and-effect relationship between atypical symptoms and GE reflux than it is to do so for the typical symptoms. Consequently, the results of surgical therapy have been correspondingly less good. That is not to say that patients with atypical symptoms are not good candidates for antireflux surgery, because many will benefit greatly, but that in these patients it should be applied cautiously. Often a trial of high-dose proton pump inhibitors (PPIs) is helpful. Given atypical symptoms, the outcome of antireflux surgery is optimal in patients with a good response to medical treatment rather than in those who fail to respond.

2 The diagnosis of GERD based on symptoms alone is correct in only approximately two thirds of patients.[31] This is because these symptoms are not specific for GE reflux and can be caused by other diseases such as achalasia, diffuse spasm, esophageal carcinoma, pyloric stenosis, cholelithiasis, gastritis, gastric or duodenal ulcer, and coronary artery disease. This fact underscores the need for objective diagnosis before the decision is made for surgical treatment.

Physiology of the Antireflux Barrier

The common denominator for virtually all episodes of gastroesophageal reflux, whether physiologic or pathologic, is the loss of the normal gastroesophageal high-pressure zone and the resistance it imposes to the flow of gastric juice from an environment of higher pressure, the stomach, to an environment of lower pressure, the esophagus. This barrier, composed of both anatomic (flap valve and diaphragm) and physiologic (LES) components, acts to prevent reflux during stressed and unstressed conditions. The key determinates of the barrier include:

1. The frequency of swallow- and non–swallow-induced transient relaxations of the LES
2. The structural integrity of the LES
3. Anatomic alterations of the diaphragmatic crura and gastroesophageal flap valve represented by the angle of His

The presence or absence of pathologic esophageal acid exposure (i.e., abnormal 24-hour pH studies) is not only influenced by the degree of barrier loss but also by esophageal and gastric functional characteristics including esophageal clearance, intra-abdominal pressure, and gastric emptying abnormalities.

TABLE 41.1

NORMAL MANOMETRIC VALUES OF THE DISTAL ESOPHAGEAL SPHINCTER IN 50 SUBJECTS

■ PARAMETER	■ MEDIAN VALUE	■ 2.5TH PERCENTILE	■ 97.5TH PERCENTILE
Pressure (mm Hg)	13	5.8	27.7
Overall length (cm)	3.6	2.1	5.6
Abdominal length (cm)	2	0.9	4.7

Transient Relaxation of the Lower Esophageal Sphincter

The lower esophageal high-pressure zone is normally present except in two situations: (a) after a swallow, when it momentarily relaxes to allow passage of food into the stomach, and (b) when the fundus is distended with gas, and it is reflexly relaxed to allow venting of the gas (a belch). In 1982, Dodds et al. reported that non–swallow-induced transient relaxations of the lower esophageal sphincter (TLESRs) were a significant mechanism of gastroesophageal reflux in normal individuals and patients with gastroesophageal reflux disease.[32] These spontaneous relaxations occurred without pharyngeal contraction, were prolonged (>10 seconds), and, when reflux occurred, were associated with relaxation of the crural diaphragm. Underscoring the importance of the crural diaphragm to barrier integrity, Mital et al. later showed that pharmacologic elimination of lower esophageal sphincter pressure to zero did not result in reflux unless crural diaphragmatic contraction was also absent.[33] Gastric distention, upright posture, and meals high in fat have all been shown to increase the frequency of TLESRs.[33,34] The latter observations suggest that unfolding of the sphincter may be responsible for the loss of sphincter pressure.

As a result of these findings, TLESRs became commonly accepted as the major mechanism of gastroesophageal reflux regardless of the underlying severity of disease, despite evidence to the contrary. The facts that in over 80% of patients with symptomatic gastroesophageal reflux a hiatal hernia could be identified and that most patients with erosive esophagitis and Barrett esophagus had incompetent lower esophageal sphincter characteristics at rest were largely ignored by many. When these facts are taken into account, particularly in association with the known characteristics of TLESRs, it seems likely that transient relaxations are (a) a physiologic response to gastric distention by food or gas, (b) the mechanism of belching, and (c) responsible for physiologic reflux episodes in individuals with normal lower esophageal sphincter and hiatal anatomy, but not the primary mechanism of gastroesophageal reflux disease. Evidence supporting this has been provided via studies of Van Herwaarden et al., in which ambulatory esophageal manometry and esophageal pH monitoring were performed on patients with and without hiatal hernia.[35] Patients with hiatal hernia had greater esophageal acid exposure and more reflux episodes, but the frequency of TLESRs, and the proportion associated with reflux, was similar in both groups. They concluded that excess reflux in patients with GERD and hiatal hernia is caused by a combination of low LES pressure, swallow-induced relaxation, and straining.

Structural Integrity of the Lower Esophageal Sphincter

In humans, a zone of high pressure can be identified at the junction of the esophagus and stomach. This lower esophageal "sphincter" provides an important component of the barrier between the esophagus and stomach that normally prevents gastric contents from entering the esophagus. It has no anatomic landmarks, but its presence can be identified by a rise in pressure over gastric baseline as a pressure transducer is pulled from the stomach into the esophagus.

3 There are three characteristics of the lower esophageal sphincter that maintain its resistance or barrier function to intragastric and intra-abdominal pressure challenges. They are its pressure, its overall length, and the length exposed to the positive-pressure environment of the abdomen (Table 41.1). The tonic resistance of the lower esophageal sphincter is a function of both its pressure and the length over which this pressure is exerted.[36] The shorter the overall length of the high-pressure zone, the higher the pressure must be to maintain sufficient resistance to remain competent (Fig. 41.12). Consequently, a short overall sphincter length can nullify a normal sphincter pressure.[37] Further, as the stomach fills, the length of the sphincter decreases, rather like the neck of a balloon shortening as the balloon is inflated. If the overall length of the sphincter is abnormally short when the stomach is empty, then with minimal gastric distention there will be insufficient sphincter length for the existing pressure to maintain sphincter competency, and reflux will occur.

The third characteristic of the lower esophageal sphincter is its position, in that a portion of the overall length of the high-pressure zone should be exposed to positive intra-abdominal pressure. During periods of increased intra-abdominal pressure, the resistance of the lower esophageal sphincter would be

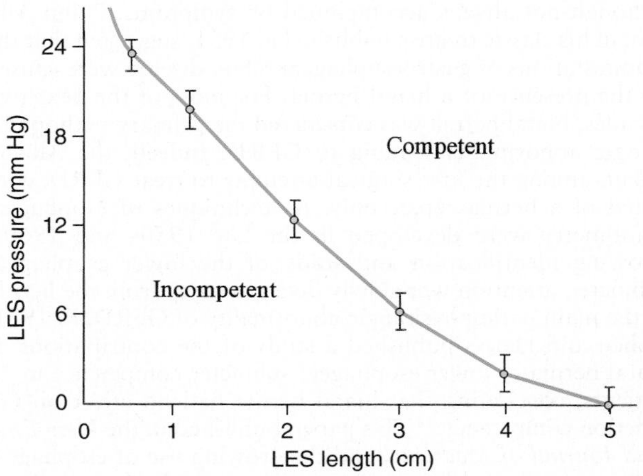

FIGURE 41.12. The relationship between the magnitude of pressure in the high-pressure zone measured at the respiratory inversion point and the overall length of the zone to the resistance to the flow of fluid through the zone. Competent, no flow. Incomplete, flow of varied volumes. Note that the shorter the overall length of the high-pressure zone, the higher the pressures must be to maintain sufficient resistance to remain competent.

overcome if the abdominal pressure were not applied equally to the high-pressure zone and stomach. This is akin to sucking on a soft soda straw immersed in a bottle of Coke; the hydrostatic pressure of the fluid and the negative pressure inside the straw due to sucking cause the straw to collapse instead of allowing the liquid to flow up the straw in the direction of the negative pressure. If the abdominal length is inadequate, the sphincter cannot respond to an increase in applied intra-abdominal pressure by collapsing, and reflux is more liable to result. If the high-pressure zone has an abnormal low pressure, a short overall length, or minimal exposure to the abdominal pressure environment in the fasting state, then there is a permanent loss of lower esophageal sphincter resistance and the unhampered reflux of gastric contents into the esophagus throughout the circadian cycle. This is referred to as a *permanently defective sphincter* and is identified by having one or more of the following characteristics: a high-pressure zone with an average pressure of less than 6 mm Hg, an average overall length of 2 cm or less, and an average length exposed to the positive-pressure environment of the abdomen of 1 cm or less.[38] Compared with normal subjects, these values are below the 2.5th percentile for each parameter. The most common cause of a permanently defective sphincter is an inadequate abdominal length, most likely a consequence of the development of a hiatal hernia. It is important to note that an inadequate abdominal length or an abnormally short overall length can nullify the efficiency of a sphincter with a normal pressure.

The presence of a permanently defective sphincter has several implications. First, it is commonly associated with esophageal mucosal injury and predicts that the patient's symptoms may be difficult to control with medical therapy.[39,40] It is now accepted that when the sphincter is permanently defective, it is irreversible, even when the associated esophagitis is healed. The presence of a permanently defective sphincter is commonly associated with reduced esophageal body function,[41] and if the disease is not brought under control, the progressive loss of effective esophageal clearance can lead to severe mucosal injury, repetitive regurgitation, aspiration, and pulmonary failure.

Anatomic Alterations

With the advent of clinical roentgenology, it became evident that a hiatal hernia was a relatively common abnormality although not always accompanied by symptoms. Philip Allison, in his classic treatise published in 1951, suggested that the manifestations of gastroesophageal reflux disease were caused by the presence of a hiatal hernia. For most of the next two decades, hiatal hernia was considered the primary pathophysiologic abnormality leading to GERD. Indeed, the Allison repair, among the first surgical attempts to treat GERD, consisted of a hernia repair only. As techniques of esophageal manometry were developed in the late 1950s and 1960s, allowing identification and study of the lower esophageal sphincter, attention was slowly diverted away from the hernia as the main pathophysiologic abnormality of GERD. In 1971, Cohen and Harris published a study of the contributions of hiatal hernia to lower esophageal sphincter competence in 75 patients, concluding that hiatal hernia had no effect on GE junction competence.[42] This paper, published in the *New England Journal of Medicine*, and the growing use of esophageal manometry shifted the emphasis away from the hernia almost exclusively toward features of the lower esophageal sphincter as the primary abnormality in symptomatic GERD.

Perhaps serendipitously, studies of the phenomenon of TLESRs identified the diaphragmatic crura as an important factor in preventing reflux during periods of loss of LES pressure.[43] In normal subjects, even with absent LES pressure, reflux does not occur without relaxation of the crural diaphragm. Coincidentally, Hill et al. stressed the importance of the physiologic flap valve created by the angle of His as a barrier to gastroesophageal reflux.[44] The endoscopic appearance of the flap valve can be correlated with abnormal esophageal acid exposure, emphasizing that the geometry of the gastroesophageal region is also important to barrier competence.[45] If mechanical forces set in play by gastric distention are important in pulling on the terminal esophagus and shortening the length of the high-pressure zone or "sphincter," then the geometry of the cardia, that is, the presence of a normal acute angle of His or the abnormal dome architecture of a sliding hiatus hernia, should influence the ease with which the sphincter is pulled open. Evidence that this occurs was provided by Ismail et al., who showed a close relationship between the degree of gastric distention necessary to overcome the high-pressure zone (yield pressure) and the morphology of the cardia (Fig. 41.13).[46] No relationship between the yield pressure and lower esophageal sphincter resting pressure and length was found. A higher intragastric pressure was needed to open the sphincter in patients with an intact angle of His when compared to patients with a hiatal hernia. The presence of a hiatal hernia also disturbs esophageal clearance mechanisms likely due to loss of anchorage of the esophagus in the abdomen. Kahrilas et al. have shown that complete esophageal emptying was achieved in 86% of swallows in control subjects without a hiatal hernia, 66% in patients with a reducing hiatal hernia, and only 32% of patients with a nonreducing hiatal hernia.[47] Impaired clearance in patients with nonreducing hiatal hernias further supports the contribution of hiatal hernia to the pathogenesis of gastroesophageal reflux disease. Thus, present evidence is overwhelming that hiatal hernia does indeed play a significant, if not primary, role in the pathophysiology of gastroesophageal reflux disease.

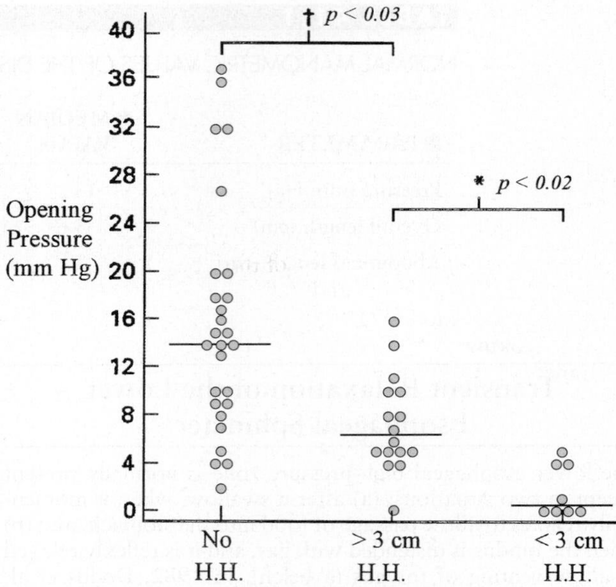

FIGURE 41.13. The intragastric pressure at which the lower esophagus endoscopically opened in response to gastric distention by air during endoscopy. Note that the dome architecture of a hiatus hernia (HH) influences the ease with which the sphincter can be pulled open by gastric distention. (Reproduced with permission from Ismail T, Bancewicz J, Barlow J. Yield pressure, anatomy of the cardia and gastro-oesophageal reflux. *Br J Surg* 1995;82:943.)

A transient loss of the high-pressure zone can also occur and usually results from a functional problem of the gastric reservoir.[48] Excessive air swallowing or food can result in gastric dilatation and, if the active relaxation reflex has been lost, an increased intragastric pressure. When the stomach is distended, the vectors produced by gastric wall tension pull on the GE junction with a force that varies according to the geometry of the cardia; that is, the forces are applied more directly when a hiatal hernia exists than when a proper angle of His is present. The forces pull on the terminal esophagus, causing it to be "taken up" into the stretched fundus and thereby reducing the length of the high-pressure zone or "sphincter." This process continues until a critical length is reached, usually about 1 to 2 cm, when the pressure drops precipitously and reflux occurs. The mechanism by which gastric distention contributes to shortening of the length of the high-pressure zone, so that its pressure drops and reflux occurs, provides a mechanical explanation for "transient relaxations" of the LES without invoking a neuromuscular reflex. Rather than a "spontaneous" muscular relaxation, there is a mechanical shortening of the high-pressure zone, secondary to progressive gastric distention, to the point where it becomes incompetent. These "transient sphincter" shortenings occur in the initial stages of GERD and are the mechanism for the early complaint of excessive postprandial reflux. After gastric venting, the length of the high-pressure zone is restored and competence returns until distention again shortens it and encourages further venting and reflux. This sequence results in the common complaints of repetitive belching and bloating in patients with GERD. The increased swallowing frequency seen in patients with GERD contributes to gastric distention and is due to their repetitive ingestion of saliva in an effort to neutralize the acid refluxed into their esophagus.[49] Thus, GERD may begin in the stomach, secondary to gastric distention resulting from overeating and the increased ingestion of fried foods, which delay gastric emptying. Both characteristics are common in Western society and may explain the high prevalence of the disease in the Western world.

A recent series of studies from Glasgow assesses the nature of the acid environment at the GE junction,[50] including possible inciting factors in the development of cardia and distal esophageal adenocarcinoma. The studies were initiated to investigate a long-recognized observation that esophageal pH monitoring reveals postprandial esophageal acidification at the same time as the gastric contents are alkalinized. This paradox is hard to explain given that reflux of gastric content into the esophagus is the primary mechanism underlying GERD. Hypothesizing that acidic material must be present somewhere in the upper stomach, the investigators studied luminal pH at 1-cm increments across the upper stomach and lower esophagus in healthy volunteers before and after meals. Surprisingly, they identified a "pocket" of acid at the GE junction unaffected by the buffering action of the meal, which extended across the squamocolumnar junction an average of 1.8 cm into the lumen of the esophagus (Fig. 41.14). The authors concluded that this was the source of postprandial esophageal acid exposure. They expanded these initial studies, confirming that the same process occurs in patients with endoscopy-negative dyspepsia and normal conventional esophageal pH monitoring 5 cm above the upper border of the LES.[51] Perhaps more important, they also identified that dietary nitrate consumed in the form of green vegetables results in the generation of concentrations of nitric oxide at the GE junction high enough to be potentially mutagenic (Fig. 41.15).[52] These observations provide the fundamental basis for the observations of inflammation and other alterations in the epithelium long known to occur at the squamocolumnar junction in both overt and unrecognized GERD.

The data support the likelihood that GERD begins in the stomach. Fundic distention occurs because of overeating and delayed gastric emptying secondary to the high-fat Western diet. The distention causes the sphincter to be "taken up" by the expanding fundus, exposing the squamous epithelium with the high-pressure zone, which is the distal 3 cm of the esophagus, to gastric juice. Repeated exposure causes inflammation of the squamous epithelium, columnarization, and carditis.

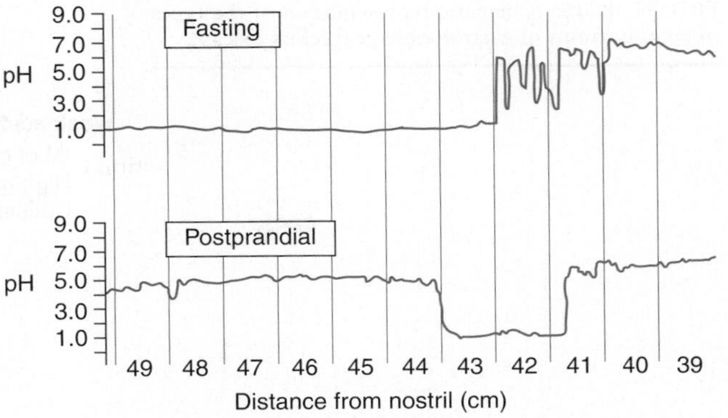

FIGURE 41.14. Fasting and postprandial gastric and esophageal pH measurements in 1-cm increments during a pull through the gastroesophageal junction. The postprandial tracing reveals an "acid pocket" from 44 to 41 cm from the nares. The fasting tracing reveals this to be the same area as the pH "step-up" corresponding to the transition from the stomach to the esophagus. (Reproduced with permission from Fletcher J, Wirz A, Young J, et al. Unbuffered highly acidic gastric juice exists at the gastroesophageal junction after a meal. *Gastroenterology* 2001;121:775.)

This is the initial step and explains why in early disease the esophagitis is mild and commonly limited to the very distal esophagus. The patient compensates by increased swallowing, allowing saliva to bathe the injured mucosa and alleviate the discomfort induced by exposure to gastric acid. Increased swallowing results in aerophagia, bloating, and repetitive belching. The distention induced by aerophagia leads to further exposure and repetitive injury to the terminal squamous epithelium and the development of cardiac-type mucosa. This is an inflammatory process, commonly referred to as "carditis," and explains the complaint of epigastric pain so often registered by patients with early disease. The process can lead to a fibrotic mucosal ring at the squamocolumnar junction and explains the origin of a Schatzki ring. Extension of the inflammatory process into the muscularis propria causes a progressive loss in the length and pressure of the distal esophageal high-pressure zone associated with an increased esophageal exposure to gastric juice and the

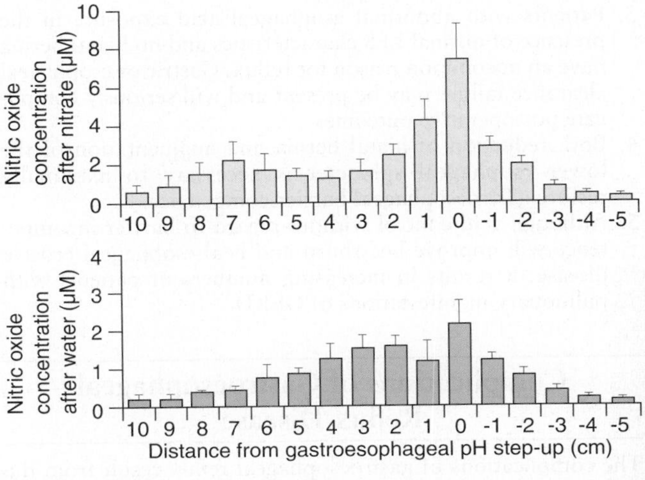

FIGURE 41.15. Mean (±SEM) nitric oxide concentrations in the upper stomach and lower esophagus after administration of water with 2 mmol nitrate (upper tracing) and water alone (lower tracing) (**$p < 0.01$, *$p < 0.05$ compared with value at gastroesophageal junction pH step-up). (Reproduced with permission from Iljima K, Henry E, Moriya A, et al. Dietary nitrate generates potentially mutagenic concentrations of nitric oxide at the gastroesophageal junction. *Gastroenterology* 2002;122:1248.)

FIGURE 41.16. Schematic representation of the types of complications of gastroesophageal reflux disease.

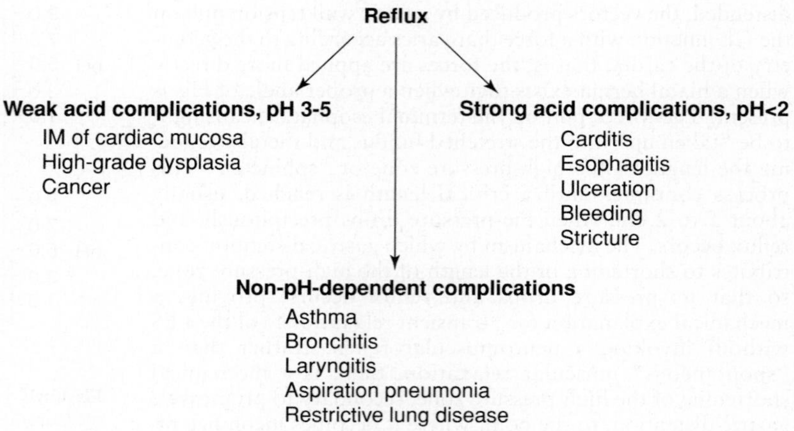

symptoms of heartburn and regurgitation. The loss of the barrier occurs in a distal-to-proximal direction and eventually results in the permanent loss of LES resistance and the explosion of the disease into the esophagus with all the clinical manifestations of severe esophagitis. This accounts for the observation that severe esophageal mucosal injury is almost always associated with a permanently defective sphincter. At any time during this process and under specific luminal conditions or stimuli, such as exposure time to a specific pH range, intestinalization of the cardiac-type mucosa can occur and set the stage for malignant degeneration.

Implications

Implications of recognizing anatomic alterations as component of GE barrier:

1. Transient lower esophageal sphincter relaxation is the likely underlying mechanism of belching and physiologic reflux. It does not play a major role in patients with symptomatic gastroesophageal reflux, particularly those with erosive disease, those with Barrett esophagus, or those referred for surgery.
2. Efforts to augment the gastroesophageal barrier either pharmacologically or endoscopically will commonly fail when a hiatal hernia is present.
3. Patients with abnormal esophageal acid exposure in the presence of normal LES characteristics and no hiatal hernia have an uncommon reason for reflux. Gastric or esophageal clearance failure may be present and will seriously complicate postoperative outcome.
4. Both reduction of hiatal hernia and augmentation of the lower esophageal sphincter is necessary to maximally restore gastroesophageal barrier competence.
5. Although acid control without regard to barrier incompetence will improve heartburn and heal esophageal erosive disease, it results in increasing numbers of patients with pulmonary manifestations of GERD.

Complications of Gastroesophageal Reflux Disease

The complications of gastroesophageal reflux result from the damage inflicted by gastric juice on the esophageal mucosa or laryngeal or respiratory epithelium (Fig. 41.16). These can be conceptually divided into (a) mucosal complications such as esophagitis and stricture; (b) extraesophageal or respiratory complications such as chronic cough, asthma, and pulmonary fibrosis; and (c) metaplastic (Barrett esophagus) and neoplastic (adenocarcinoma). The prevalence and severity of complications is related to the degree of loss of the gastroesophageal barrier, defects in esophageal clearance, and the content of refluxed gastric juice (Fig. 41.17).

Mucosal Complications. The potential injurious components that reflux into the esophagus include gastric secretions, such as acid and pepsin; biliary and pancreatic secretions that regurgitate from the duodenum into the stomach; and toxic compounds generated in the mouth, esophagus, and stomach by the action of bacteria on dietary substances.

Our current understanding of the role of the various ingredients of gastric juice in the development of esophagitis is based on classic animal studies performed by Lillimoe et al.[53,54] These studies have shown that acid alone does minimal damage to the esophageal mucosa, but the combination of acid and pepsin is highly deleterious. Hydrogen ion injury to the esophageal squamous mucosa occurs only at a pH below 2. In acid refluxate, the enzyme pepsin appears to be the major injurious agent. Similarly, the reflux of duodenal juice alone does little damage to the mucosa, while the combination of duodenal juice and gastric acid is particularly noxious. Reflux of bile and pancreatic enzymes into the stomach can either protect or augment esophageal mucosal injury. For instance, the reflux of duodenal contents into the stomach may prevent the development of peptic esophagitis in a patient whose gastric acid secretion maintains an acid environment, because the bile salts would attenuate the injurious effect of pepsin and the acid would inactivate the trypsin. Such a patient would have

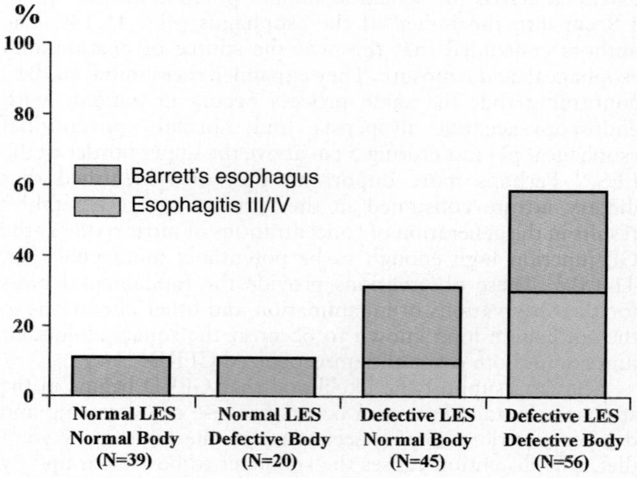

FIGURE 41.17. Prevalence of esophageal mucosal injury related to the presence of a defective lower esophageal sphincter, esophageal body motility, or both.

bile-containing acid gastric juice that, when refluxed, would irritate the esophageal mucosa but cause less esophagitis than if it were acid gastric juice containing pepsin. In contrast, the reflux of duodenal contents into the stomach of a patient with limited gastric acid secretion can result in esophagitis, because the alkaline intragastric environment would support optimal trypsin activity and the soluble bile salts with a high pK_a would potentiate the enzyme's effect. Hence, duodenal-gastric reflux and the acid-secretory capacity of the stomach interrelate by altering the pH and enzymatic activity of the refluxed gastric juice to modulate the injurious effects of enzymes on the esophageal mucosa.

This disparity in injury caused by acid and bile alone as opposed to the gross esophagitis caused by pepsin and trypsin provides an explanation for the poor correlation between the symptom of heartburn and endoscopic esophagitis. The reflux of acid gastric juice contaminated with duodenal contents could break the esophageal mucosal barrier, irritate nerve endings in the papillae close to the luminal surface, and cause severe heartburn. Despite the presence of intense heartburn, the bile salts present would inhibit pepsin, the acid pH would inactivate trypsin, and the patient would have little or no gross evidence of esophagitis. In contrast, the patient who refluxed alkaline gastric juice may have minimal heartburn because of the absence of hydrogen ions in the refluxate but have endoscopic esophagitis because of the bile salt potentiation of trypsin activity on the esophageal mucosa. This is supported by recent clinical studies that indicate that the presence of alkaline reflux is associated with the development of mucosal injury.[55]

Although numerous studies have suggested the reflux of duodenal contents into the esophagus in patients with gastroesophageal reflux disease, few have measured this directly. The components of duodenal juice thought to be most damaging are the bile acids, and as such, they have been the most commonly studied. Most studies have implied the presence of bile acids using pH measurements. Studies using either prolonged ambulatory aspiration techniques (Fig. 41.18) or spectrophotometric bilirubin measurement have shown that, as a group, patients with gastroesophageal reflux disease have greater and more concentrated bile acid exposure to the esophageal mucosa than normal subjects.[39,40] This increased exposure occurs most commonly during the supine period while asleep and during the upright period following meals. Most studies have identified the glycine conjugates of cholic, deoxycholic, and chenodeoxycholic acids as the predominant bile acids aspirated from the esophagus of patients with GERD, although appreciable amounts of taurine conjugates of these bile acids were also found. Other bile salts were identified but in small concentrations. This is as one would expect because glycine conjugates are three times more prevalent than taurine conjugates in normal human bile.

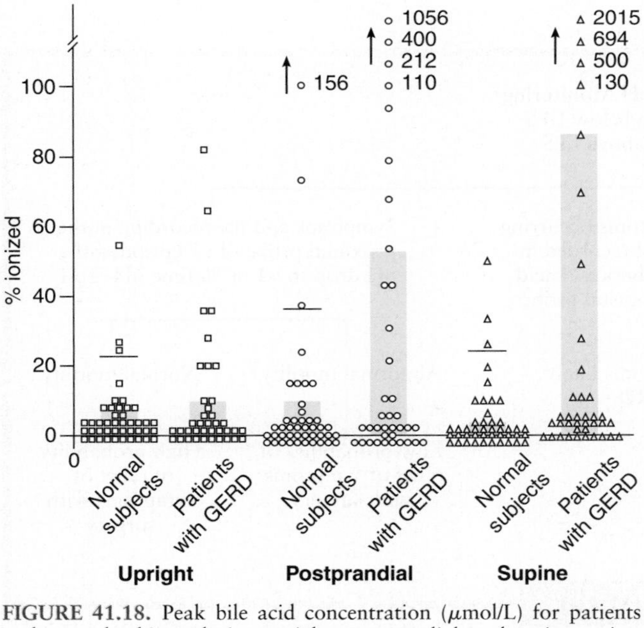

FIGURE 41.18. Peak bile acid concentration (μmol/L) for patients and normal subjects during upright, postprandial, and supine aspiration periods. The shaded area represents the mean and the bar the 95th percentile values.

The potentially injurious action of toxic compounds either ingested or newly formed on the mucosa of the gastroesophageal junction and distal esophagus has long been postulated. Until recently, however, few studies have substantiated this possibility. Expanding upon studies of acid exposure at the gastroesophageal junction, investigators from Glasgow, Scotland, have recently shown that dietary nitrate consumed in the form of green vegetables and food contaminated by nitrate-containing fertilizers results in the generation of nitric oxide at the gastroesophageal junction in concentrations high enough to be potentially mutagenic.[52] Previous studies have shown that nitrate ingested in food is reabsorbed in the small bowel, with approximately 25% resecreted into the mouth via the salivary glands. Oral bacteria chemically transforms the relatively innocuous nitrate to the more toxic nitrite, which is swallowed and subsequently converted to nitric oxide and other toxic nitroso-compounds by acid and ascorbic acid in the stomach. Whether this mechanism in fact contributes to injury and/or neoplastic transformation in the upper stomach, gastroesophageal junction, and distal esophagus is currently unknown.

4 **Respiratory Complications.** It is increasingly recognized that a significant proportion of patients with gastroesophageal reflux will have either primary respiratory symptoms or respiratory symptoms in association with more prominent heartburn and regurgitation.[56] Reflux has been implicated as causative of asthma and idiopathic pulmonary fibrosis (IPF) and can complicate advanced lung diseases including chronic obstructive pulmonary disease (COPD) and cystic fibrosis (CF). Thirty-five to fifty percent of asthmatics have been shown to have abnormal esophageal pH, esophagitis, and a hiatal hernia.[57] Others have shown that the prevalence of reflux symptoms exceeded 50% in patients with asthma and CF.[58,59] In addition, patients with COPD and gastroesophageal reflux are twice as likely to have significant COPD exacerbations than their nonreflux counterparts,[60] and reflux symptoms correlate with airway obstruction in COPD patients. These reports suggest that the frequency of dual pathology is higher than would be expected by chance alone.

Pathophysiology of Reflux-induced Respiratory Symptoms. Two mechanisms have been proposed as the pathogenesis of reflux-induced respiratory symptoms. The first, the so-called "reflux" theory, maintains that respiratory symptoms are the result of the aspiration of gastric contents. The second or "reflex" theory maintains that vagally mediated bronchoconstriction follows acidification of the lower esophagus.

The evidence supporting a *reflux* mechanism was shown in animals in the 1950s to 1970s, with studies of acid instillation in the lungs resulting in pneumonitis,[61,62] epithelial damage,[63] and increased airway resistance.[64] The evidence in humans can be categorized as follows. First, there is radiographic evidence. Patients with pulmonary fibrosis have an increased prevalence of hiatal hernia on upper GI series,[65,66] while elderly patients with large hiatal hernias have a significantly increased frequency of pleural scarring on chest computed tomography (CT) scans.[67] Second, erosive esophagitis was found at a high frequency in a large series of Veterans Affairs patients with asthma, pneumonia, chronic bronchitis, and pulmonary fibrosis.[56] Third, patients with chronic lung diseases, including asthma and pulmonary fibrosis in particular, have a significantly higher frequency of positive 24-hour pH studies.[67,68] With dual pH monitoring of the proximal and distal esophagus, prolonged exposure of the proximal esophagus to gastric juice occurs at a higher frequency in patients with gastroesophageal reflux and respiratory symptoms than in patients without respiratory complaints.[69,70] Fourth, simultaneous tracheal and esophageal pH monitoring in patients with reflux disease have documented tracheal acidification in concert with esophageal acidification.[64] Finally, medications used to treat chronic lung diseases, in particular, bronchodilators, relax esophageal sphincter tone.[71]

A *reflex* mechanism is primarily supported by the fact that bronchoconstriction occurs following the infusion of acid into the lower esophagus.[72–74] This can be explained by the common embryologic origin of the tracheoesophageal tract and its shared vagal innervation.

The primary challenge in implementing treatment for reflux-associated respiratory symptoms lies in establishing the diagnosis. In those patients with predominantly typical reflux symptoms and secondary respiratory complaints, the diagnosis may be straightforward. However, in a substantial number of patients with reflux-induced respiratory symptoms, the respiratory symptoms dominate the clinical scenario. Gastroesophageal reflux in these patients is often silent and is only uncovered when investigation is initiated.[68,75] A high index of suspicion is required, notably in patients with poorly controlled asthma in spite of appropriate bronchodilator therapy. Supportive evidence for the diagnosis can be gleaned from endoscopy and stationary esophageal manometry. Endoscopy may show erosive esophagitis or Barrett esophagus. Manometry may indicate a hypotensive lower esophageal sphincter or ineffective body motility, defined by 30% or more contractions in the distal esophagus of less than 30 mm Hg in amplitude.[76] D'Ovidio et al. studied 78 patients awaiting lung transplant for IPF, scleroderma, COPD, or CF and found that 72% had a hypotensive lower esophageal sphincter, 33% abnormal esophageal body motility, and 38% abnormal 24-hour pH testing,[77] although, interestingly, patients with IPF in other series have been shown to have normal manometry.[70]

The current "gold standard" for the diagnosis of reflux-induced respiratory complaints is ambulatory dual-probe pH monitoring, often combined with multichannel intraluminal impedance (MII-pH). One probe is positioned in the distal esophagus and the other at a more proximal location. Sites for proximal probe placement have included the trachea, pharynx, and proximal esophagus. Most authorities would agree that the proximal esophagus is the preferred site for proximal probe placement. While ambulatory esophageal pH monitoring allows a direct correlation between esophageal acidification and respiratory symptoms, the chronologic relationship between reflux events and bronchoconstriction is complex.

Nonrespiratory Extraesophageal Complications. Other extraesophageal manifestations of gastroesophageal reflux range from laryngitis, pharyngitis, hoarseness, and sinusitis to sleep disturbance and dental erosions.[78,79] Nearly half of patients referred for antireflux surgery may have nongastrointestinal symptoms. The term *laryngopharyngeal reflux* (LPR) is used for a broad category of atypical symptoms of gastroesophageal reflux, respiratory and nonrespiratory. Mechanisms for these symptoms are difficult to prove and substantial evidence remains lacking.[80]

Treatment of Extraesophageal Complications. Once gastroesophageal reflux is suspected or thought to be responsible for extraesophageal symptoms, treatment may be with either prolonged PPI therapy or antireflux surgery. Initially, a 3- to 6-month trial of high-dose PPI therapy (b.i.d. or t.i.d. dosing) may help confirm (by virtue of symptom resolution) the fact that reflux is partly or completely responsible for the symptoms. If symptoms are improved, patients can be treated with maintenance medical therapy or may be offered surgical treatment to control the reflux. The persistence of symptoms despite PPI treatment, however, does not necessarily rule out reflux as being a potential contributor. Algorithm 41.1 bases clinical decisions on the results of dual-probe 24-hour pH monitoring and is a useful starting point.

Based on reported observations, relief of respiratory symptoms can be anticipated for 25% to 50% of patients with reflux-induced asthma treated with antisecretory medications,[81–83] although patients with pulmonary fibrosis in particular may have an inherent resistance to standard-dose PPIs.[84] Fewer than 15% of asthmatics with symptom relief, however, can be expected to have objective improvements in their pulmonary

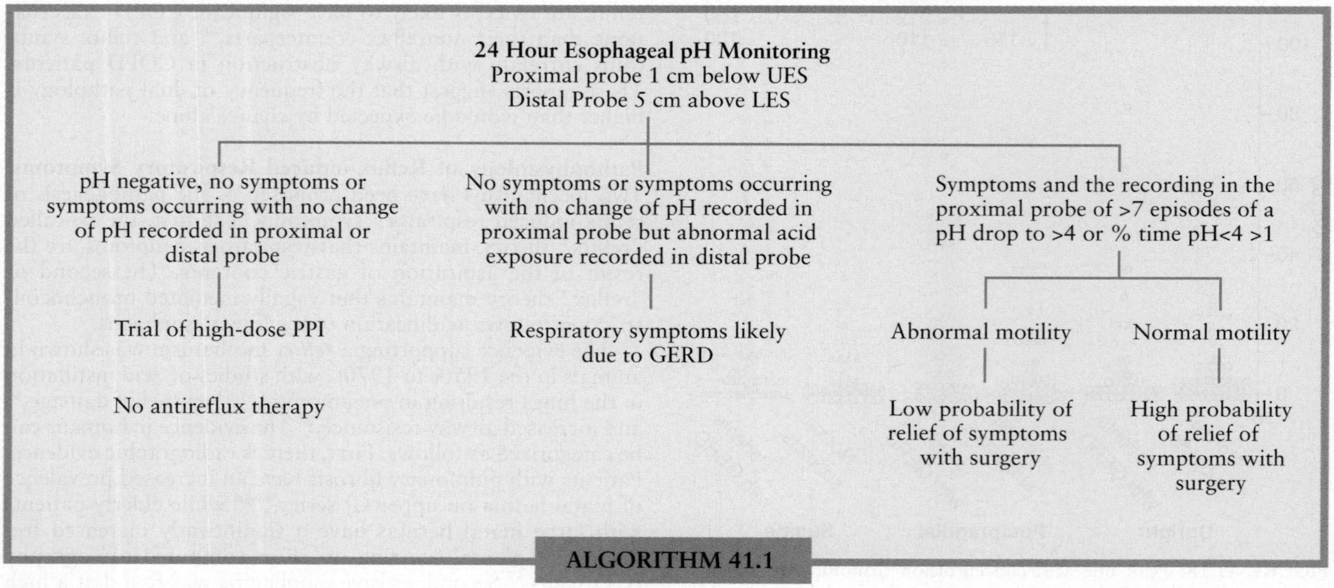

ALGORITHM 41.1. Algorithm of clinical decision making based on outcome of dual-probe 24-hour pH testing and esophageal manometry in patients with respiratory symptoms thought secondary to gastroesophageal reflux disease.

function. The reason for this apparent paradox may be that most studies employed relatively short courses of antisecretory therapy (<3 months). This time period may have been sufficient for symptomatic improvement but insufficient for recovery of pulmonary function. The chances of success with medical treatment are likely directly related to the extent of reflux elimination. The conflicting findings of reports of antisecretory therapy may well be due to inadequate control of gastroesophageal
5 reflux in some studies. The literature indicates that antireflux surgery improves respiratory symptoms in nearly 90% of children and 70% of adults with asthma and reflux disease.[83,85] Improvements in pulmonary function were demonstrated in around one third of patients. Comparison of the results of uncontrolled studies of each form of therapy and the evidence from the two randomized controlled trials of medical versus surgical therapy indicate that fundoplication is the most effective therapy for reflux-induced asthma.[85] The superiority of the surgical antireflux barrier over medical therapy is probably most noticeable in the supine posture, which corresponds with the period of acid breakthrough with PPI therapy and is the time in the circadian cycle when asthma symptoms and peak expiratory flow rates are at their worst.

More convincing data establishing the benefit of antireflux surgery in improving respiratory symptoms and pulmonary function tests derives from the lung transplantation literature. Bronchiolitis obliterans syndrome (BOS), synonymous with chronic rejection of the transplanted lung, is diagnosed by a greater than 20% decline in pulmonary function tests from posttransplant baseline. Lau et al. showed in the early 2000s that 67% of 18 patients with BOS had an improvement in their pulmonary function tests after antireflux surgery.[86] More recently, several groups have reported improvements in oxygen requirements and stabilization of declining pulmonary function tests when pre–lung transplant patients underwent antireflux surgery.[87,88] In addition, pulmonary and other extraesophageal symptoms can improve after laparoscopic Nissen fundoplication with minimal perioperative morbidity.[89]

It is also important to realize that, in asthmatic patients with a non–reflux-induced motility abnormality of the esophageal body, performing an antireflux operation may not prevent the aspiration of orally regurgitated, swallowed liquid or food. This can result in respiratory symptoms and airway irritation that may elicit an asthmatic reaction. This factor may be the explanation why surgical results appear to be better in children than adults, since disturbance of esophageal body motility is more likely in adult patients.

Metaplastic (Barrett) and Neoplastic (Adenocarcinoma) Complications. The condition whereby the tubular esophagus is lined with columnar epithelium rather than squamous epithelium was first described by Norman Barrett in 1950 (Fig. 41.19).[90] He incorrectly believed it to be congenital in origin. It is now realized that it is an acquired abnormality, occurring in 7% to 10% of patients with gastroesophageal reflux disease, and represents the end stage of the natural history of this disease.[91] It is also understood to be distinctly different from the congenital condition in which islands of mature gastric columnar epithelium are found in the upper half of the esophagus.

The definition of Barrett esophagus has evolved considerably over the past decade.[90–93] Traditionally, Barrett esophagus was identified by the presence of any columnar mucosa extending at least 3 cm into the esophagus. Recent data indicating that specialized intestinal-type epithelium is the only tissue predisposed to malignant degeneration, coupled with the finding of a similar risk of malignancy in segments of intestinal metaplasia less than 3 cm long, have resulted in the diagnosis of Barrett esophagus, given any length of endoscopically visible tissue that is intestinal metaplasia on histology (Fig. 41.20). Whether to call long segments of columnar mucosa without intestinal metaplasia Barrett esophagus is unclear. The hallmark of intestinal metaplasia is the presence of goblet cells. Recent studies have identified a high prevalence of biopsy-proven intestinal metaplasia at the cardia, in the absence of endoscopic evidence of a columnar-lined esophagus. The significance and natural history of this finding remain unknown. The term *Barrett esophagus* should currently be used in the setting of an endoscopically visible segment of intestinal metaplasia of any length or columnar replacement of the esophagus of 3 cm or more.

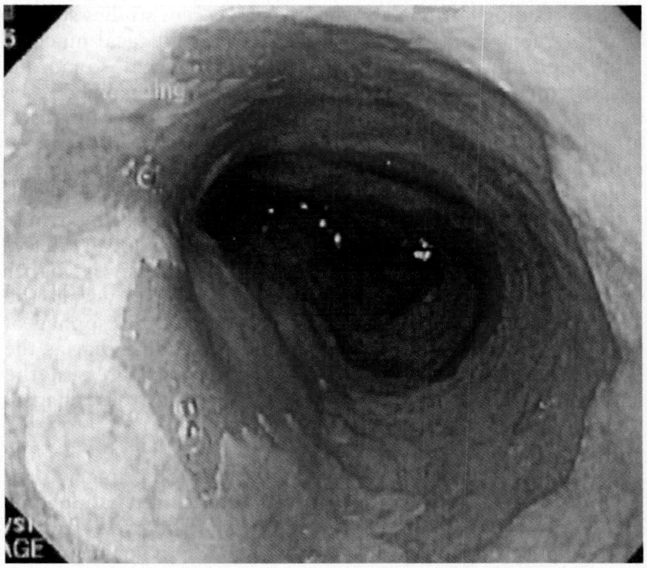

FIGURE 41.19. Endoscopic appearance of Barrett esophagus. Note the pink metaplastic mucosa as opposed to the normal whitish squamous lining of the esophagus.

6 Factors predisposing to the development of Barrett esophagus include early-onset GERD, abnormal lower esophageal sphincter and esophageal body physiology, and mixed reflux of gastric and duodenal contents into the esophagus.[93] Direct measurement of esophageal bilirubin exposure as a marker for duodenal juice has shown that 58% of the patients with gastroesophageal reflux disease have increased esophageal exposure to duodenal juice and that this exposure is most dramatically related to Barrett esophagus.[94]

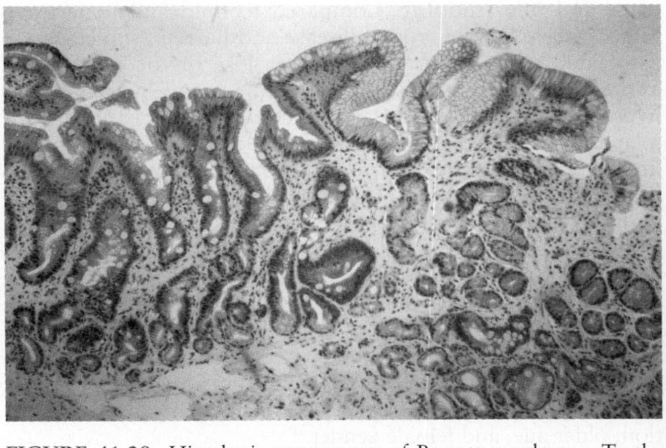

FIGURE 41.20. Histologic appearance of Barrett esophagus. To the left of the photograph, columnar mucosa with abundant goblet cells is seen. This is intestinal metaplasia, which is the histologic hallmark of Barrett esophagus. To the right of the photomicrograph, cardiac epithelium is present.

Pathophysiology of Barrett Metaplasia. Recent studies suggest that the metaplastic process at the gastroesophageal junction may begin by conversion of distal esophageal squamous mucosa to cardiac-type epithelium, heretofore presumed to be a normal finding.[92] This is likely due to exposure of the distal esophagus to excess acid and gastric contents via prolapse of esophageal squamous mucosa into the gastric environment. This results in inflammatory changes at the gastroesophageal junction and/or a metaplastic process, both of which may result in the loss of muscle function and a mechanically defective sphincter allowing free reflux with progressively higher degrees of mucosal injury. Intestinal metaplasia within the sphincter may result, as in Barrett metaplasia of the esophageal body. This mechanism is supported by the finding that as the severity of gastroesophageal reflux disease progresses, the length of columnar lining above the anatomic gastroesophageal junction is increased.

Treatment. The relief of symptoms remains the primary force driving antireflux surgery in patients with Barrett esophagus. Healing of esophageal mucosal injury and the prevention of disease progression are important secondary goals. In this regard, patients with Barrett esophagus are no different than the broader population of patients with gastroesophageal reflux. Antireflux surgery should be considered when patient factors suggest severe disease or predict the need for long-term medical management, both of which are almost always true in patients with Barrett esophagus.

7 PPI therapy, both to relieve symptoms and to control any coexistent esophagitis or stricture, is an acceptable treatment option in patients with Barrett esophagus. Once initiated, however, most patients with Barrett esophagus will require life-long treatment. Complete control of reflux with PPI therapy can be difficult, however, as has been highlighted by studies of acid breakthrough while on therapy. Katzka and Castell, and Ouatu-Lascar and Triadafilopoulos have shown that 40% to 80% of patients with Barrett esophagus continue to experience abnormal esophageal acid exposure despite up to 20 mg twice daily of PPI.[95,96] Ablation trials have shown that mean doses of 56 mg of omeprazole are necessary to normalize 24-hour esophageal pH studies.[97] Antireflux surgery likely results in more reproducible and reliable elimination of reflux of both acid and duodenal content, although long-term outcome studies suggest that as many as 25% of patients postfundoplication will have persistent pathologic esophageal acid exposure confirmed by 24-hour pH studies.[98]

An important consideration is that patients with Barrett esophagus generally have severe GERD, with its attendant sequelae such as large hiatal hernia, stricture, shortened esophagus, and poor motility. Compared to mild and nonerosive reflux disease, severe erosive disease and Barrett esophagus are associated with significantly greater loss of the mechanical antireflux barrier because of associated hiatal hernias and a hypotensive lower esophageal sphincter. Surgical treatment with a laparoscopic Nissen fundoplication reduces the hiatal hernia, improves the antireflux barrier, and consequently provides similarly excellent symptom control.[99] Large studies in patients with typical acid reflux symptoms have been published from the United States and Europe.[100–103] In patients having laparoscopic Nissen fundoplication at Emory University, relief of heartburn and regurgitation occurred in 90%, and 70% were off all reflux medications at a mean follow-up of 11 years.[104] These results emphasize the durability of the procedure as well as the persistent relief of typical symptoms. Risk factors for persistent use of antacids after antireflux surgery include a partial fundoplication, older age, and female gender.[105]

Studies focusing on the symptomatic outcome following antireflux surgery in patients with Barrett esophagus document excellent to good results in 72% to 95% of patients at 5 years following surgery.[98–100] The outcome of laparoscopic Nissen fundoplication in patients with Barrett esophagus has been assessed at 1 to 3 years after surgery. Hofstetter et al. reported the experience at the University of Southern California (USC) in 85 patients with Barrett esophagus at a median of 5 years after surgery. Fifty-nine had long- and 26 short-segment Barrett esophagus and 50 underwent a laparoscopic antireflux procedure.[98] Reflux symptoms were absent postoperatively in 79% of the patients. Postoperative 24-hour pH was normal in 17 of 21 patients (81%). Ninety-nine percent of the patients considered themselves cured or improved and 97% were satisfied with the surgery. In addition to symptomatic improvement in reflux after surgery, there is evidence that mediators of esophageal inflammation implicated in carcinogenesis are decreased as well. Cyclooxygenase-2 (COX-2) gene expression is elevated in the distal esophagus of reflux patients, but the expression of COX-2 and another inflammatory mediator, interleukin 8, can be decreased in the distal esophageal mucosa after a fundoplication.[106–108]

The Development of Dysplasia in Barrett Esophagus. The prevalence of dysplasia at diagnosis in patients presenting with Barrett esophagus ranges from 15% to 25%, and approximately 5% of patients will develop dysplasia each year. The identification of dysplasia in Barrett epithelium rests on histologic examination of biopsy specimens. The cytologic and tissue architectural changes are similar to those described in ulcerative colitis (Fig. 41.21). By convention, Barrett metaplasia is currently classified into four broad categories:

1. No dysplasia
2. Indefinite for dysplasia
3. Low-grade dysplasia
4. High-grade dysplasia

8 There are few prospective studies documenting the progression of nondysplastic Barrett epithelium to low- or high-grade dysplasia. Those that are available suggest that 5% to 6% per year will progress to dysplasia and 0.5% to 1% per year to adenocarcinoma (Table 41.2). Once identified, Barrett esophagus complicated by dysplasia should undergo aggressive therapy. Patients whose biopsies are interpreted as indefinite for dysplasia should be treated with a medical regimen consisting of 60 to 80 mg of PPI therapy for 3 months and rebiopsied. Importantly, esophagitis should be healed prior to interpretation of the presence or absence of dysplasia. The presence of severe inflammation makes the microscopic interpretation of dysplasia difficult. The purpose of acid suppression therapy is to resolve inflammation that may complicate the interpretation of the biopsy specimen. If the

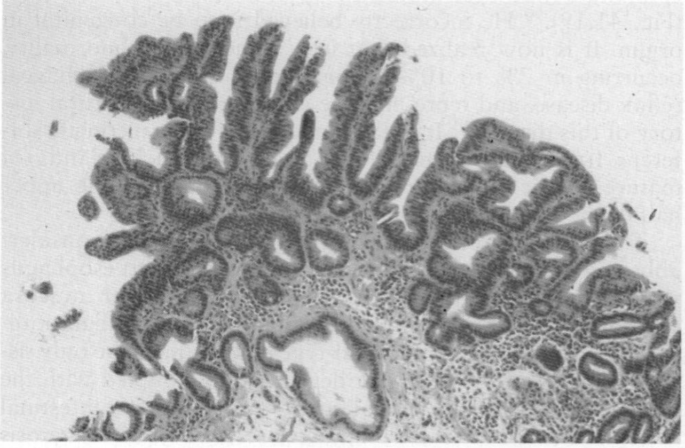

FIGURE 41.21. Histologic appearance of high-grade dysplasia. The cellular architecture and structure of the glands are becoming disorganized.

TABLE 41.2 **DIAGNOSIS**

DEVELOPMENT OF DYSPLASIA: PROSPECTIVE EVALUATION OF 62 PATIENTS

■ INITIAL DIAGNOSIS	■ FINAL DIAGNOSIS				
	■ NO.	■ METAPLASIA	■ I/LGD	■ HGD	■ CA
Metaplasia	39	27	10	1	1
I/LGD	20	4	8	3	2
HGD	3			1	2

CA, carcinoma; HGD, high-grade dysplasia; I, indeterminate; LGD, low-grade dysplasia.
From Reid BJ, Blount PL, Rubin CE, et al. Flow-cytometric and histological progression to malignancy in Barrett's esophagus: prospective endoscopic surveillance of a cohort. *Gastroenterology* 1992;102:1212–1219.

diagnosis remains indefinite, the patient should be treated as if low-grade dysplasia were present with continued medical therapy or antireflux surgery and repeat biopsy every 6 months.

High-grade dysplasia should be confirmed by two pathologists knowledgeable in GI pathology. Once high-grade dysplasia is confirmed, observation is less than optimal as more than 50% of patients will progress to multifocal high-grade
9 dysplasia or cancer.[109] Until recently, esophagectomy was considered the standard of care for patients with high grade dysplasia. With the Western acceptance of an Eastern modality, endoscopic mucosal resection (EMR) is becoming an increasingly attractive option for patients with high-grade dysplasia and intramucosal cancers. The aim of EMR is to excise the area of interest including the mucosal and submucosal layers down to the lamina muscularis propria allowing optimal histologic interpretation. Reports from specialized centers combining EMR with mucosal ablation using either photodynamic or radiofrequency energy are encouraging, with a high prevalence of eradication of dysplasia/neoplasia.[110–115] Ell et al. initially showed that EMR is feasible and safe; however, in one of their earlier reports, recurrent or metachronous carcinomas were found in 14% of 64 patients during 1-year follow-up.[116]

Longer success rates with EMR for early Barrett cancer have been reported from the experienced centers. The largest study comes from Wiesbaden, Germany, involving over 300 patients with high-grade dysplasia or intramucosal cancers and a mean follow-up of over 5 years.[117] A complete response was achieved in 97% of patients, and surgery was necessary in 3.7% after endoscopic therapy failed. Metachronous lesions developed during the follow-up in 21% of the patients. The risk factors most frequently associated with recurrence were piecemeal resection, long-segment Barrett esophagus, and multifocal lesions.[118]

Traditionally, high-grade dysplasia has been considered a marker for the presence of invasive carcinoma in nearly half of patients, as confirmed in esophagectomy reports from the University of Southern California, Mayo Clinic, Johns Hopkins, and other centers.[119–122] It is not possible with present technology, including endoscopic ultrasound, to differentiate the patients who harbor a cancer from those who do not. Furthermore, esophageal adenocarcinoma associated with high-grade dysplasia, identified by surveillance endoscopy, is generally highly curable. We and others have documented 5-year survival rates of 90% after potentially curative esophagectomy.
10 Although on average 30% to 40% of patients with the preoperative diagnosis of high-grade dysplasia will harbor invasive cancer when the esophagus is examined in its entirety, removal of the lesion via EMR, histologic assessment including the submucosa, and the addition of mucosal ablation of residual Barrett epithelium are shifting the treatment paradigm. However, the standard of care for treatment of high-grade dysplasia and intramucosal carcinoma outside a specialized esophageal center, particularly in younger patients or those unable to undergo consistent endoscopic surveillance, remains esophagectomy.

Treatment of Gastroesophageal Reflux Disease

Medical Treatment. GERD is one of the most prevalent conditions encountered in general medical practice. As a result, medications for control of GERD comprise one of the largest pharmaceutical markets in the United States and abroad. Since PPIs were introduced in the United States in 1989, a number of different agents have emerged, each with substantial penetration in the marketplace. Data from the year 2004 reveal that, of the top 10 expenditures for medications in the United States, the third highest dollar amount was spent on Prevacid (lansoprazole, TAP Pharmaceutical Products, Inc., Lake Forest, Illinois; $4.0 billion), while the fourth highest was on Nexium (esomeprazole magnesium, AstraZeneca Pharmaceuticals, Wilmington, Delaware; $3.6 billion).[123,124]

GERD is such a common condition that most patients with mild symptoms carry out self-medication, particularly now that generic and over-the-counter H_2-receptor antagonists (H_2RAs) and PPIs have become widely available. When first seen with symptoms of heartburn or regurgitation without obvious complications, patients can reasonably be placed on 8 to 12 weeks of acid suppression therapy before extensive investigations are carried out. In many situations, symptoms successfully resolve. Patients should be advised to elevate the head of the bed; avoid tight clothing; eat small, frequent meals; avoid eating their nighttime meal shortly before retiring; lose weight; and avoid alcohol, coffee, chocolate, and peppermints, which may aggravate the symptoms. Medications to promote gastric emptying, such as metoclopramide, are beneficial in early disease but of little value in more severe disease.

11 The mainstay of maintenance medical therapy is acid suppression. Patients with persistent symptoms should be given PPIs, such as omeprazole. In doses as high as 40 mg/d, they can effect an 80% to 90% reduction in gastric acidity. Such a regimen usually heals mild esophagitis, but healing may occur in only three fourths of patients with severe esophagitis. It is important to realize that in patients who reflux a combination of gastric and duodenal juice, inadequate acid suppression therapy may give symptomatic improvement while still allowing mixed reflux to occur. This can result in an environment that allows persistent mucosal damage in an asymptomatic patient. Unfortunately, within 6 months of discontinuation of any form of medical therapy for GERD, 80% of patients have a recurrence of symptoms.[125]

In patients with reflux disease, esophageal acid exposure is reduced by up to 80% with H_2RAs and up to 95% with PPIs. Despite the superiority of the latter class of drug over the former, periods of acid breakthrough still occur.[126,127] Breakthrough occurs most commonly at nighttime and is some justification for a split rather than a single dosing regimen. Katzka et al.[126] studied 45 patients with breakthrough reflux symptoms while on omeprazole 20 mg b.i.d. and found that 36 patients were still refluxing, defined by a total distal esophageal acid exposure greater than 1.6%. Peghini et al.[127] employed intragastric pH monitoring in 28 healthy volunteers and 17 patients with reflux disease and found that nocturnal recovery of acid secretion (more than 1 hour) occurred in 75% of the individuals. Recovery of acid secretion occurred within 12 hours of the oral evening dose of PPI, the median recovery time being 7.5 hours. This is particularly pertinent because it is during the nighttime and early morning that asthma symptoms are most pronounced and that peak expiratory flow rate is at its lowest. Ranitidine 300 mg at bedtime appears superior to omeprazole 20 mg at bedtime in preventing acid breakthrough, likely due to the abolition of histamine-mediated acid secretion in the fasting state.

An accumulating body of literature suggests potential adverse consequences to long-term acid suppressive therapy. A population-based cohort study from the Netherlands covering the years 1995–2002 revealed higher incidence rates of community-acquired pneumonia in patients using H_2RAs or PPIs compared to those who never used them or those who had used them previously but stopped.[128] The risk was most pronounced for PPIs and showed a clear dose-response relationship. Other studies have focused on the association between acid suppression and the development of osteoporosis-related fractures.[129–131] Of note, a population-based study from the United Kingdom assessed the risk of hip fractures from long-term PPI therapy.[129] The study covered the years 1987–2003 and compared users of PPI therapy to nonusers of any acid suppressive medication. The risk of hip fracture was significantly increased in patients prescribed long-term high-dose PPI, and the strength of the association increased with increasing duration of PPI therapy. The authors conjectured that calcium malabsorption secondary to chronic acid suppression may potentially explain the positive association.

Failure of acid suppression to control symptoms or immediate return of symptoms after stopping treatment suggests that either the diagnosis is incorrect or the patient has relatively severe disease. Endoscopic examination at this stage of the patient's evaluation provides the opportunity for assessing the severity of mucosal damage and the presence of Barrett esophagus. Both of these findings on initial endoscopy predict a high risk for medical failure. A measurement of the degree and pattern of esophageal exposure to gastric juice, with 24-hour pH monitoring, should be obtained at this point. The status of the LES and the function of the esophageal body should also be assessed. These studies identify features that predict a poor response to medical therapy, frequent relapses, and the development of complications and include supine reflux, poor esophageal contractility, erosive esophagitis, a columnar-lined esophagus, and a structurally defective sphincter. Patients who have these risk factors should be given the option of surgery as a primary therapy with the expectation of long-term control of symptoms and complications.

Antireflux Surgery

Indications. Antireflux surgery is indicated for the treatment of objectively documented, relatively severe GERD. Candidates for surgery include not only patients with erosive esophagitis, stricture, and Barrett esophagus but also those without severe mucosal injury who are dependent on PPIs for symptom relief. Patients with atypical or respiratory symptoms who have a good response to intensive medical treatment are also candidates. The option of antireflux surgery should be given to all patients who have demonstrated the need for long-term medical therapy, particularly if escalating doses of PPIs are needed to control symptoms. Antireflux surgery may be the preferred option in patients younger than 50 years, those who are noncompliant with their drug regimen, those for whom medications are a financial burden, and those who favor a single intervention over long-term drug treatment. It may be the treatment of choice in patients who are at high risk of progression despite medical therapy. Although this population is not well defined, risk factors that predict progressive disease and a poor response to medical therapy include (a) nocturnal reflux on 24-hour esophageal pH study, (b) a structurally deficient LES, (c) mixed reflux of gastric and duodenal juice, and (d) mucosal injury at presentation.[132]

Preoperative Evaluation. Successful antireflux surgery is largely defined by two objectives: the achievement of long-term relief of reflux symptoms and the absence of complications or complaints after the operation. In practice, achieving these two deceptively simple goals is difficult. Both are critically dependent on establishing that the symptoms for which the operation is performed are the result of excess esophageal exposure to gastric juice, as well as the proper performance of the appropriate antireflux procedure. Success can be expected in the vast majority of patients if these two criteria are met. The status of the LES is not as important a factor as in the days of open surgery. Patients with normal resting sphincters are often selected for antireflux surgery in the era of laparoscopic fundoplication. The outcome is not dependent on sphincter function. There are four important goals of the diagnostic approach to patients suspected of having GERD and being considered for antireflux surgery (Table 41.3).

The introduction of laparoscopic access, coupled with the growing recognition that surgery is a safe and durable treatment for GERD, has dramatically increased the number of patients being referred for laparoscopic fundoplication compared to the prelaparoscopic era. Recent data suggest that the peak use of antireflux surgery in the United States occurred in 1999, with an estimated 15.7 cases per 100,000 adults at that time.[133] Since then, the frequency of antireflux surgery has declined, such that an estimated 11 antireflux procedures were performed per 100,000 adults in 2003. This recent decline may reflect the availability of generic and over-the-counter PPIs, a constantly evolving menu of endoscopic antireflux therapies, increased utilization of Roux-en-Y gastric bypass for control of GERD in morbidly obese individuals, and the long-term efficacy of fundoplication being called into question. Given the various therapies for GERD, each with its potential advantages and shortcomings, accurate and contemporary data regarding outcomes after antireflux surgery are necessary as a basis against which other established and novel therapies must be judged.

TABLE 41.3 DIAGNOSIS

GOALS OF THE DIAGNOSTIC APPROACH TO PATIENTS SUSPECTED OF HAVING GERD AND BEING CONSIDERED FOR ANTIREFLUX SURGERY

Establish that GERD is the underlying cause of the patient's symptoms.
Estimate the risk of progressive disease.
Determine the presence or absence of esophageal shortening.
Evaluate esophageal body function and, occasionally, gastric emptying function.

GERD, gastroesophageal reflux disease.

TABLE 41.4

PREDICTORS OF OUTCOME AFTER LAPAROSCOPIC FUNDOPLICATION: STEPWISE LOGISTIC REGRESSION RESULTS OF 199 PATIENTS

PREDICTOR	STATUS	ADJUSTED ODDS RATIO (95% CONFIDENCE INTERVALS)	WALD'S p VALUE
Composite acid score	Increased	5.4 (1.9–15.3)	<0.001
	Normal	—	—
Symptom	Typical	5.1 (1.9–13.7)	<0.001
	Atypical	—	—
Response to medical therapy	Complete/partial	3.3 (1.3–8.7)	0.02
	Minor/none	—	—

Odds ratios and corresponding p values are adjusted for age and for all other factors in the model.
From Campos GMR, Peters JH, DeMeester TR, et al. Multivariate analysis of the factors predicting outcome after laparoscopic Nissen fundoplication. *J Gastrointest Surg* 1999;3:292–300.

Given the large number of surgical referrals, the importance of selecting patients for surgery who are likely to have a successful outcome cannot be overemphasized. Although a Nissen fundoplication will reliably and reproducibly halt the return of gastroduodenal juice into the esophagus, little benefit is likely if the patient's symptoms are not caused by this specific pathophysiologic derangement. Thus, in large part, the anticipated success rate of laparoscopic fundoplication is directly proportional to the degree of certainty that GERD is the underlying cause of the patient's complaints.

12 Three factors predictive of a successful outcome following antireflux surgery have emerged (Table 41.4).[134] These are (a) an abnormal score on 24-hour esophageal pH monitoring; (b) the presence of typical symptoms of GERD, namely, heartburn or regurgitation; and (c) symptomatic improvement in response to acid suppression therapy prior to surgery. It is immediately evident that each of these factors helps to establish that GERD is indeed the cause of the patient's symptoms and that they have little to do with the severity of the disease.

Endoscopic Assessment. Endoscopic visualization of the esophagus equates to the physical examination of the foregut and is a critical part of the preoperative evaluation of patients with GERD. Its main aim is to detect complications of GE reflux, the presence of which may influence therapeutic decisions.

In every patient, the locations of the diaphragmatic crura, the GE junction, and the squamocolumnar junction are determined. These anatomic landmarks are commonly at three different sites in patients with GERD. The crura are usually evident and can be confirmed by having the patient sniff during the examination. The anatomic GE junction is identified as the point where the gastric rugal folds meet the tubular esophagus and is often below the squamocolumnar junction, even in patients without otherwise obvious Barrett esophagus.

Endoscopic esophagitis is defined by the presence of mucosal erosions (Table 41.5). When present, the grade and length of esophageal mucosal injury are recorded. The presence and length of columnar epithelium extending above the anatomic GE junction is also noted. Columnar-lined esophagus (CLE) is suspected at endoscopy when there is difficulty in visualizing the squamocolumnar junction at its normal location and by the appearance of a velvety red luxuriant mucosa. The presence of Barrett esophagus is confirmed by biopsy evidence of specialized intestinal metaplasia involving the tubular esophagus and is considered histologic evidence of GERD. Endoscopic visualization of columnar lining without histologic confirmation of specialized intestinal metaplasia is not considered Barrett esophagus and likely has no premalignant potential. Multiple biopsies should be taken in a cephalad direction to determine the level at which the junction of Barrett epithelium and normal squamous mucosa occurs. Barrett esophagus is susceptible to ulceration, bleeding, stricture formation, and malignant degeneration. Dysplasia is the earliest sign of malignant change. Because dysplastic changes typically occur in a random distribution within the distal esophagus, a minimum of four biopsies (each quadrant) every 2 cm should be obtained from the metaplastic epithelium. Particular attention must be paid to the squamocolumnar junction in these patients, where a mass, ulcer, nodularity, or inflammatory tissue is always considered suspicious for malignancy and requires thorough biopsy or endoscopic resection. The GE junction is defined endoscopically where the tubular esophagus meets gastric rugal folds, and the squamocolumnar junction is where there is an obvious change from the velvety and darker columnar epithelium to the lighter squamous epithelium.

After completion of the esophageal examination, the first and second portions of the duodenum and the stomach are systematically inspected. This is commonly done on withdrawal of the endoscope. When the antrum is visualized, the incisura angularis appears as a constant ridge on the lesser curve. Turning the lens of the scope 180 degrees allows inspection of the fundus and cardia. Attention is paid to the frenulum (angle of His) of the esophagogastric junction and to the closeness with which the cardia grips the scope. Hill et al.[135] have graded the appearance of this valve on a scale from I to IV according to the

TABLE 41.5 **CLASSIFICATION**

MODIFIED LOS ANGELES CLASSIFICATION OF ESOPHAGITIS

GRADE	LESION
A	One (or more) mucosal break of longer than 5 mm that does not extend between the tops of two mucosal folds
B	One (or more) mucosal break more than 5 mm long that does not extend between the tops of two mucosal folds
C	One (or more) mucosal break that is continuous between the tops of two or more mucosal folds but that involves <75% of the circumference
D	One (or more) mucosal break that involves at least 75% of the esophageal circumference

degree of unfolding or deterioration of the normal valve architecture. This grading system has been correlated with the presence of increased esophageal acid exposure, occurring predominantly in patients with a grade III or IV valve.

A hiatal hernia is endoscopically confirmed by finding a pouch lined with gastric rugal folds lying 2 cm or more above the margins of the diaphragmatic crura. A prominent sliding hernia is frequently associated with increased esophageal exposure to gastric juice. When a paraesophageal hernia exists, particular attention is given to exclude a gastric ulcer or gastritis within the pouch. The term *Cameron erosions* refers to such mucosal erosions occurring in large sliding or paraesophageal hernias, typically at the level of the diaphragmatic hiatus. The intragastric retroflex or "J" maneuver is important in evaluating the full circumference of the mucosal lining of the herniated stomach. As the endoscope is removed, the esophagus is again examined and biopsies taken. The location of the cricopharyngeus is identified and the larynx and vocal cords are visualized. Acid reflux may result in inflammation of the larynx. Vocal cord movement is recorded both as a reference for subsequent surgery and an assessment of the patient's ability to protect the airway.

Twenty-four Hour Ambulatory pH Monitoring. The most direct method of assessing the relationship between symptoms and GERD is to measure the esophageal exposure to gastric juice with an indwelling pH electrode. Miller[136] first reported prolonged esophageal pH monitoring in 1964, although it was not until 1973 that its clinical applicability and advantages were demonstrated by Johnson and DeMeester.[137] Ambulatory pH testing is considered by many to be the "gold standard" for the diagnosis of GERD, because it has the highest sensitivity and specificity of all tests currently available. Some experts have suggested that 24-hour pH monitoring be used selectively, limited to patients with atypical symptoms or no endoscopic evidence of GE reflux. Given present-day referral patterns, more than half of the patients referred for antireflux surgery will have no endoscopic evidence of mucosal injury. For these patients, 24-hour pH monitoring provides the only objective measure of the presence of pathologic esophageal acid exposure. Although it is true that most patients with typical symptoms and erosive esophagitis have a positive 24-hour pH result, the pH study provides other useful information. It quantifies the actual time that the esophageal mucosa is exposed to gastric juice, measures the ability of the esophagus to clear refluxed acid, and correlates esophageal acid exposure with the patient's symptoms. It is the only way to quantitatively express the overall degree and pattern of esophageal acid exposure, both of which may impact the decision toward surgery.[138] Patients with nocturnal or bipositional reflux have a higher prevalence of complications and failure of long-term medical control. For these reasons, we continue to advocate the routine use of pH monitoring in clinical practice.

Present technology includes both transnasal catheter-based pH probes and an implantable capsule (Bravo pH system, Medtronic Corporation, Minneapolis, Minnesota) placed under endoscopic guidance.[138–140] The units used to express esophageal exposure to gastric juice are (a) cumulative time the esophageal pH is below a chosen threshold, expressed as the percent of the total, upright, and supine monitored time; (b) frequency of reflux episodes above a chosen threshold, expressed as number of episodes per 24 hours; and (c) duration of the episodes, expressed as the number of episodes greater than 5 minutes per 24 hours and the time in minutes of the longest episode recorded. Table 41.6 shows the normal values for these components of the 24-hour record at the whole number pH threshold derived from 50 normal, asymptomatic subjects. The upper limits of normal were established at the 95th percentile. Most centers use pH 4 as the threshold. Combining the result of the six components into one expression that reflects the overall esophageal acid exposure below a pH threshold, a pH score was calculated by using the standard deviation of the mean of each of the six components measured.

Several limitations exist, however, to standard pH monitoring: nonacid reflux events are not detected, the height and quantity of refluxate above the gastroesophageal junction are not defined, and the physical nature of the refluxed material (i.e., liquid, gas, or a mixture) cannot be differentiated. As reflux symptoms such as regurgitation and cough may be present in the absence of demonstrable reflux of acid, improved modalities for detection of nonacid refluxate may be clinically important.

Ambulatory Combined Impedance–pH Monitoring. New technology has been introduced into clinical practice that allows for detection of both acid and nonacid refluxate. The Sleuth system (Sandhill Scientific, Denver, Colorado) combines pH monitoring and intraluminal impedance measurements using a single catheter (Fig. 41.22). The technology identifies refluxate via changes in impedance caused by the presence of a bolus in the esophagus, and the reflux event can be categorized as acid or nonacid by the contemporaneous change in intraluminal pH. Multichannel intraluminal impedance (MII) has been validated as an appropriate method for the evaluation of gastrointestinal function and reflux.[141] All episodes of gastroesophageal reflux can be detected using this technology without regard to their chemical composition. Surprisingly, recent studies using this technology have shown that, in normal subjects, PPI therapy does not alter the number of reflux episodes; it simply converts them to neutral pH.[142] This observation may have important implications in the treatment of gastroesophageal reflux disease.

TABLE 41.6

NORMAL VALUES FOR ESOPHAGEAL EXPOSURE TO pH <4 IN 50 SUBJECTS

COMPONENT	MEAN	STANDARD DEVIATION	95TH PERCENTILE
Total time pH <4	1.51	1.36	4.45
Upright time pH <4	2.34	2.34	8.42
Supine time pH <4	0.63	1.0	3.45
No. episodes	19.00	12.76	46.9
No. >5 min	0.84	1.18	3.45
Longest episode	6.74	7.85	19.8

From Johnson LF, DeMeester TR. Development of the 24-hour intraesophageal pH monitoring composite scoring system. *J Clin Gastroenterol* 1986;8(suppl 1):52–58.

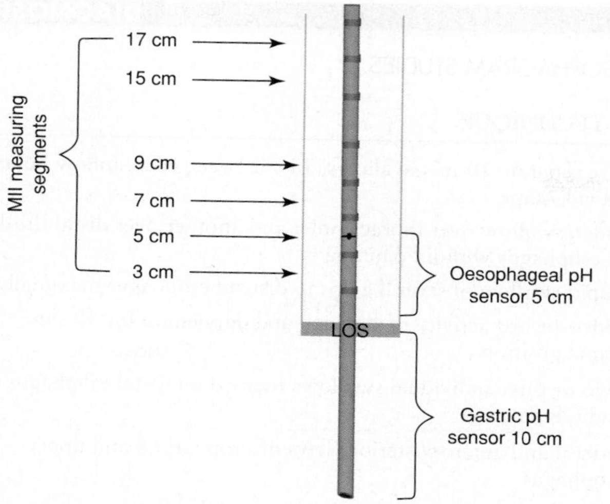

FIGURE 41.22. Combined multichannel intraluminal impedance–pH catheter. (Reproduced with permission from Mainie I, Tutuian R, Agrawal A, et al. Combined multichannel intraluminal impedance-pH monitoring to select patients with persistent gastro-oesophageal reflux for laparoscopic Nissen fundoplication. *Br J Surg* 2006;93:1483–1487.)

Combined MII-pH monitoring has recently been used to select patients, both with typical and atypical manifestations of GERD and who are resistant to medical treatment, for fundoplication.[143] Patients with a positive symptom index, as assessed by combined MII-pH testing while on PPI therapy, were noted to respond well to surgery. Another recent trial demonstrated that combined MII-pH testing is more accurate for the preoperative assessment of GERD in patients off of PPI therapy compared to pH monitoring alone.[144]

Assessment of Esophageal Length. Esophageal shortening is a consequence of scarring and fibrosis associated with repetitive esophageal injury. Anatomic shortening of the esophagus can compromise the ability to perform an adequate tension-free fundoplication and may result in an increased incidence of breakdown or thoracic displacement of the repair. Esophageal length is best assessed preoperatively using video roentgenographic contrast studies and endoscopic findings. Endoscopically, hernia size is measured as the difference between the diaphragmatic crura, identified by having the patient sniff, and the GE junction, identified as the loss of gastric rugal folds. We consider the possibility of a short esophagus in patients with strictures or those with large hiatal hernias (>5 cm), particularly when the latter fail to reduce in the upright position on a video barium esophagram.[145]

The definitive determination of esophageal shortening is made intraoperatively when, after thorough mobilization of the esophagus, the GE junction cannot be reduced below the diaphragmatic hiatus without undue tension on the esophageal body. Surgeons performing fundoplication have reported varying incidences of esophageal shortening, attesting to the judgment inherent in defining and recognizing "undue tension." An advantage of transthoracic fundoplication is the ability to mobilize the esophagus extensively from the diaphragmatic hiatus to the aortic arch. With the GE junction marked with a suture, esophageal shortening is defined by an inability to position the repair beneath the diaphragm without tension. In this situation, a Collis gastroplasty coupled with either a partial or complete fundoplication may be performed.[146]

Potential pitfalls of laparoscopic fundoplication include the elevation of the diaphragm due to pneumoperitoneum, potentially contributing to a false impression that esophageal length is adequate, and the limited ability to mobilize the esophagus relative to the transthoracic approach.[147] In our experience, the failure to appreciate esophageal shortening is a major cause of fundoplication failure and is often the explanation for the "slipped" Nissen fundoplication. In many such instances, the initial repair is incorrectly constructed around the proximal tubularized stomach rather than the terminal esophagus. Surgeons opting to perform fundoplication laparoscopically in the setting of potential esophageal shortening must be vigilant of esophageal tension, technically facile at extensive mediastinal mobilization of the esophagus while preserving vagal integrity, and able to perform a laparoscopic or open transabdominal Collis gastroplasty should esophageal lengthening be necessary.

Radiographic Evaluation. Radiographic assessment of the anatomy and function of the esophagus and stomach is one of the most important parts of the preoperative evaluation. Critical issues are assessed, including the presence of esophageal shortening (Fig. 41.23), the size and reducibility of a hiatal hernia, and the propulsive function of the esophagus for both liquids and solids.

The definition of radiographic GE reflux varies depending on whether reflux is spontaneous or induced by various maneuvers. In only about 40% of patients with classic symptoms of GERD is spontaneous reflux observed by the radiologist (i.e., reflux of barium from the stomach into the esophagus with the patient in the upright position). In most patients who show spontaneous reflux on radiography, the diagnosis of increased esophageal acid exposure is confirmed by 24-hour esophageal pH monitoring. Therefore, the radiographic demonstration of spontaneous regurgitation of barium into the esophagus in the upright position is a reliable indicator that reflux is present. On the contrary, failure to see radiographic reflux does not prove the absence of reflux disease.

A carefully performed video esophagram can provide an enormous amount of information on the structure and function of the esophagus and stomach. The modern barium

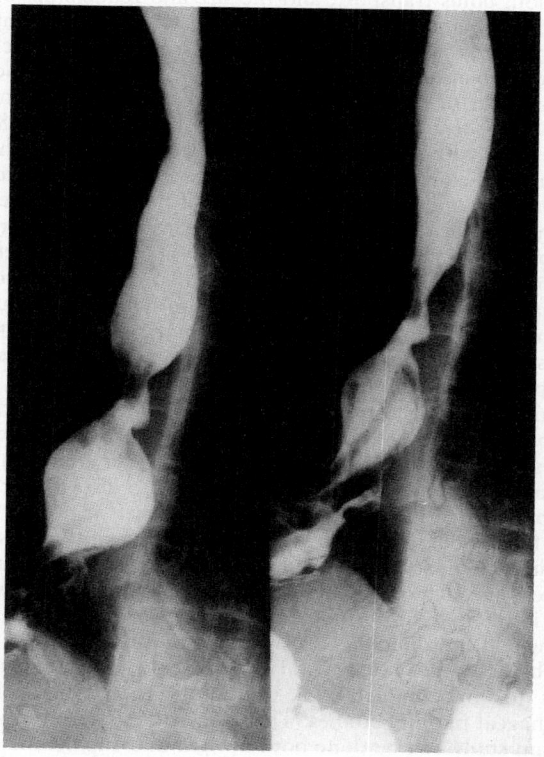

FIGURE 41.23. Barium-filled esophagogastric segment in a patient with a short esophagus. Note that the gastroesophageal junction is well above the hiatus.

TABLE 41.7 **DIAGNOSIS**

UNIVERSITY OF SOUTHERN CALIFORNIA PROTOCOL FOR VIDEO ESOPHAGRAM STUDIES

■ PATIENT POSITION	■ PURPOSE	■ TECHNIQUE
Prone RAO	Esophageal body function	Five separate 10-mL swallows, 15 s between each, follow bolus on videotape
		Video swallow over thoracic inlet and another over distal third of esophagus without panning
	Esophageal diameter	Rapid swallow of several gulps to distend esophagus maximally
	Gastric function	Video-record activity of stomach and duodenum for 30 s in prone position
Supine	Relationship of GE junction to hiatus	Two or three individual swallows focused on distal esophagus and GE junction
Erect	Cricopharyngeal function	Lateral and anteroposterior views of oropharynx and upper esophagus
	Mucosal injury	Spot of collapsed esophagus for mucosal detail
	Reducibility of hernia	Video images of one or two swallows focused on distal esophagus and GE junction
	Gas distention of distal esophagus	
Erect	Solid bolus transport	Record video images of passage of two contrast-coated hamburger boluses from oropharynx to stomach

GE, gastroesophageal; RAO, right anterior oblique.

swallow emphasizes motion recording (video), utilizes a tightly controlled examination protocol (Table 41.7), and requires an understanding of esophageal physiology.

Videotaping the study greatly aids the evaluation, providing the surgeon with a real-time assessment of swallowing function, bolus transport, and the size and reducibility of an associated hiatal hernia. Given routine review before antireflux surgery, the value of the study becomes increasingly clear. The examination provides structural information including the presence of obstructing lesions and anatomic abnormalities of the foregut. A hiatal hernia is present in more than 80% of patients with GE reflux and is best demonstrated with the patient in the prone position, which causes increased abdominal pressure and promotes distention of the hernia above the diaphragm. The presence of a hiatal hernia is an important component of the underlying pathophysiology of GE reflux. Other relevant findings include a large (>5 cm) or irreducible hernia, suggesting the presence of a shortened esophagus; a tight crural "collar" that inhibits barium transit into the stomach, suggesting a possible cause of dysphagia; and the presence of a paraesophageal hernia.

Lower esophageal narrowing resulting from a ring, stricture, or obstructing lesion is optimally viewed with full distention of the esophagogastric region. A full-column technique with distention of the esophageal wall can be used to discern extrinsic compression of the esophagus. Mucosal relief or double-contrast films should be obtained to enhance the detection of small esophageal neoplasms, mild esophagitis, and esophageal varices. The pharynx and upper esophageal sphincter are evaluated in the upright position, and an assessment of the relative timing and coordination of pharyngeal transit is possible.

The assessment of peristalsis on video esophagram often adds to, or complements, the information obtained by esophageal motility studies. This is in part because the video barium study can be done both upright and supine and with liquid and solid bolus material, which is not true of a stationary motility examination. This is particularly true with subtle motility abnormalities. During normal swallowing, a stripping wave (primary peristalsis) is generated that completely clears the bolus. Residual material can stimulate a secondary peristaltic wave, but usually a second pharyngeal swallow is required. Motility disorders with disorganized or simultaneous esophageal contractions have "tertiary waves" and provide a segmented appearance to the barium column, often referred to as beading or corkscrewing. In dysphagic patients, a barium-impregnated marshmallow, bread, or hamburger is a useful adjunct, which can discern a functional esophageal transport disturbance not evident on the liquid barium study. Reflux is not easily seen on video esophagram, and motility disorders that cause retrograde barium transport may be mistaken for reflux.

Assessment of the stomach and duodenum during the barium study is a necessity for proper preoperative evaluation of the patient with GERD. Evidence of gastric or duodenal ulcer, neoplasm, or poor gastroduodenal transit has obvious importance in the proper preoperative evaluation.

Assessment of Esophageal Function. The presence of poor esophageal body function can impact the likelihood of relief of regurgitation, dysphagia, and respiratory symptoms following surgery and may influence the decision to undertake a partial rather than a complete fundoplication. When peristalsis is absent or severely disordered, many surgeons would opt for a partial fundoplication, although recent studies would suggest a complete fundoplication may be appropriate even in this setting. The less favorable response of atypical, compared with typical, reflux symptoms after fundoplication may be related to persistent poor esophageal propulsive function and the continued regurgitation of esophageal contents.[148,149]

The function of the esophageal body is assessed with esophageal manometry. Conventional water-perfused or solid-state manometry is performed with five pressure transducers located in the esophagus (Fig. 41.24). To standardize the procedure, the most proximal pressure transducer is located 1 cm below the well-defined cricopharyngeal sphincter. With this method, a pressure response along the entire esophagus can be obtained during one swallow. The study consists of recording 10 wet swallows with 5 mL of water. Amplitude, duration,

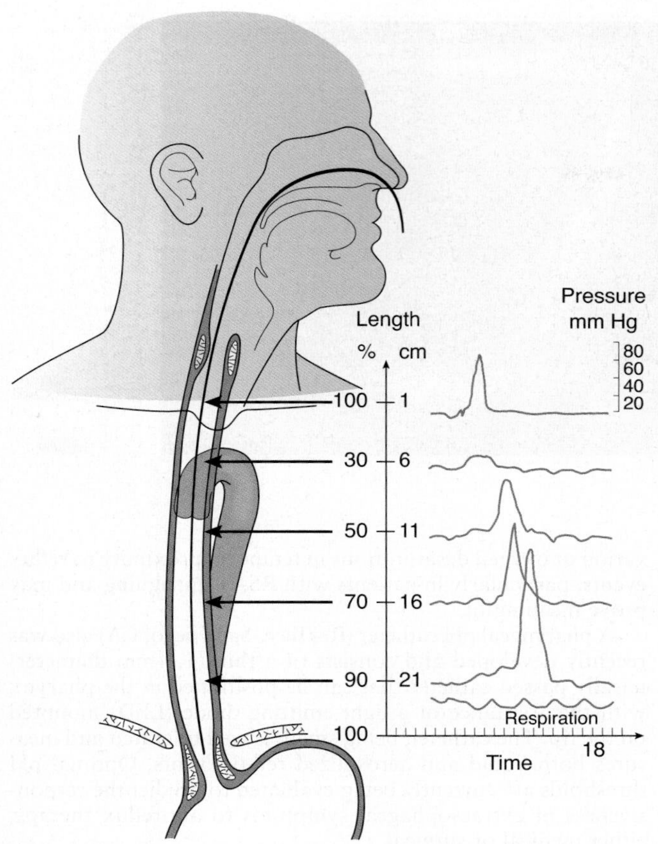

FIGURE 41.24. Illustration of the position of a five-channel esophageal motility catheter during the esophageal body portion of the study.

and morphology of contractions following each swallow are all calculated at the five discrete levels within the esophageal body (Fig. 41.25). The delay between onset or peak of esophageal contractions at the various levels of the esophagus is used to calculate the speed of wave propagation and represents the degree of peristaltic activity.

Recently, high-resolution manometry (ManoScan[360], Sierra Scientific Instruments, Los Angeles, CA) has been introduced into clinical practice and may possess several advantages over the other manometric systems currently available.[150] The high-resolution catheter is 4.2 mm in diameter and has 36 solid-state transducers spaced at 1-cm intervals, compared to the standard 3- to 5-cm spacing of traditional water-perfused or solid-state catheters. Pressure transduction technology allows each of the sensors to detect pressure over a length of 2.5 mm in 12 radially dispersed sectors. The pressure of each sector is averaged, making each of the 36 sensors a circumferential pressure detector. This construct allows a more thorough and precise evaluation of esophageal function than standard manometry. In addition, given the number and span of transducers across the length of the catheter, the upper esophageal sphincter, esophageal body, and lower esophageal sphincter can be assessed simultaneously without moving the catheter. Thus, the study can be performed more quickly and with improved patient comfort compared to conventional manometry in that multiple repositionings of the catheter are not required to complete the evaluation. The experience in our laboratory has been that high-resolution manometry takes, on average, only 8.1 minutes to complete, whereas standard manometry with a solid-state catheter takes 24.4 minutes ($p < 0.0001$).[150] Finally, the color-coded readouts allow for a better, more intuitive, graphic description of the motor activity of the esophagus, the characteristics of the lower esophageal sphincter, and the presence of a hiatal hernia compared to the other technologies (Fig. 41.26). The catheter, however, is expensive with a high replacement cost should it break. With increasing experience and further study, the pros and cons of this new technology will continue to be elucidated.

Assessment of Gastric Function. Esophageal disorders are frequently associated with abnormalities of duodenogastric function. Symptoms suggestive of gastroduodenal pathology include nausea, epigastric pain, anorexia, and early satiety. Abnormalities of gastric motility or increased gastric acid secretion can be responsible for increased esophageal exposure to gastric juice. If not identified before surgery, unrecognized gastric motility abnormalities are occasionally "unmasked" by an antireflux procedure, resulting in disabling postoperative symptoms.[151] Considerable experience and judgment are necessary to identify the patient with occult gastroduodenal

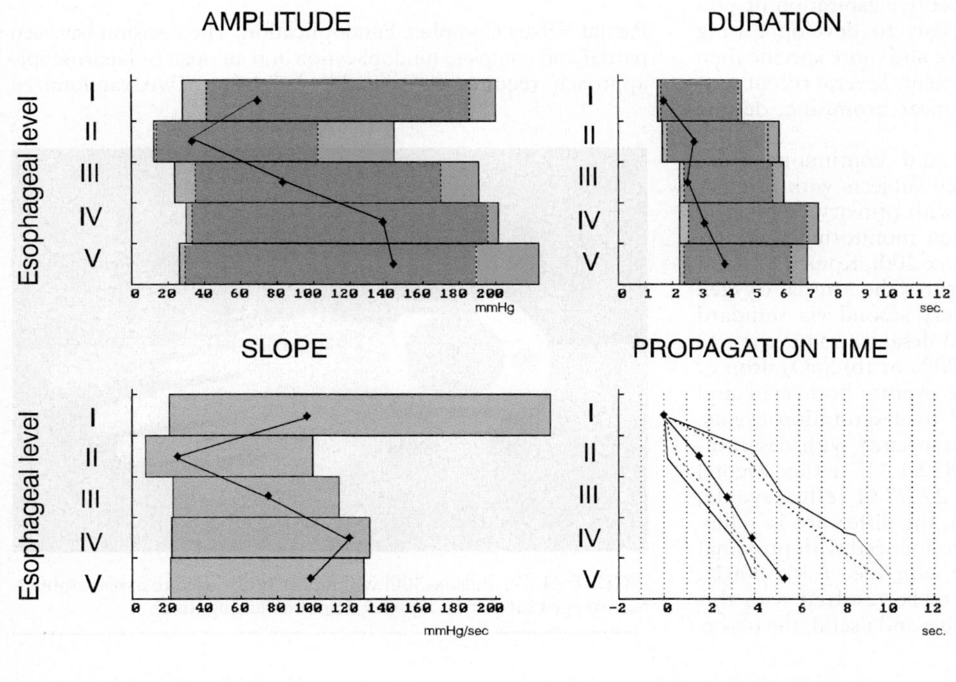

FIGURE 41.25. Computer-generated graphic representation of esophageal body contraction amplitudes, duration of contraction, and wave progression.

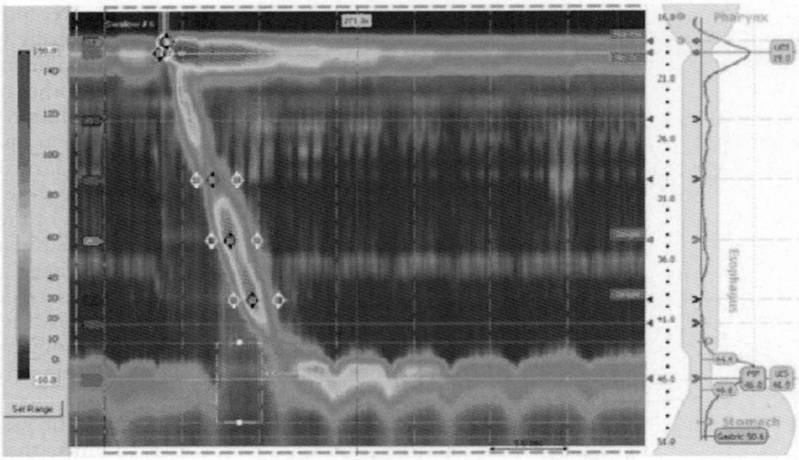

FIGURE 41.26. High-resolution manometry (HRM) display. Note the color-coded graphic description of esophageal body wave amplitudes and lower esophageal sphincter function.

dysfunction. The surgeon should maintain a keen awareness of this possibility and investigate the stomach given any suggestion of problems. Tests of duodenogastric function that are helpful when investigating the patient with GE reflux include gastric emptying studies, gastric acid analysis, 24-hour gastric pH monitoring, and ambulatory bilirubin monitoring of the esophagus and stomach.

Poor gastric emptying or transit can provide for reflux of gastric contents into the distal esophagus. Standard gastric emptying studies are performed with radionuclide-labeled meals. They are often poorly standardized and difficult to interpret. Emptying of solids and liquids can be assessed simultaneously when both phases are marked with different tracers. After ingestion of a labeled standard meal, gamma camera images of the stomach are obtained at 5- to 15-minute intervals for 1.5 to 2 hours. After correction for decay, the counts in the gastric area are plotted as percentage of total counts at the start of the imaging. The resulting emptying curve can be compared with data obtained in normal volunteers. In general, normal subjects will empty 59% of a meal within 90 minutes.

Evolving Technologies for Assessment of Extraesophageal Manifestations of GERD. Given the difficulty inherent in proving that GERD is etiologic to extraesophageal symptoms, such as cough, sore throat, or hoarseness, or to more chronic and insidious conditions, such as repetitive aspiration or pulmonary fibrosis, a great interest exists to develop testing modalities that are both more sensitive and more specific than the technologies widely utilized at present. Several recent testing paradigms have emerged that appear promising, despite lacking extensive data.

Simultaneous 24-hour MII-pH and continuous pulse oximetry recently was evaluated in 20 subjects with primary respiratory symptoms (RSs) and 10 with primary esophageal symptoms (ESs).[152] Oxygen saturation monitoring was performed using a finger clip probe (Pulsox-300i, Konica Minolta Sensing, Inc., Ramsey, NJ) that measures the arterial oxygen saturation (SpO_2) and pulse rate every second via standard photometrics (Fig. 41.27). An oxygen desaturation event was defined by either (a) SpO_2 less than 90% or (b) SpO_2 drop of 6% or greater (Fig. 41.28). Reflux events, both acid and nonacid, were temporally correlated to desaturation events. Markedly more reflux events were associated with desaturation in patients with RSs (74.5%, 832/1,117 reflux events) than in patients with ESs (30.4%, 223/734 reflux events, $p < 0.0001$) (Fig. 41.29). In addition, the difference in reflux desaturation association was more pronounced with proximal reflux (80.3% with RSs vs. 20.4% with ESs, $p < 0.0001$). While a number of issues still need to be resolved with this technique for it to be considered reliable and useful, the observation of oxygen desaturations in temporal proximity to reflux events, particularly in patients with RSs, is intriguing and may prove meaningful.

A pharyngeal pH catheter (ResTech, San Diego, CA) also was recently developed and consists of a thin (1.5-mm diameter) nasally passed catheter that can be positioned in the pharynx with the assistance of a light-emitting diode (LED) mounted on the tip. The catheter, being small, is well tolerated and measures both liquid and aerosolized reflux events. Optimal pH thresholds are currently being evaluated to predict the responsiveness of extraesophageal symptoms to antireflux therapy, either medical or surgical.

Finally, several centers have investigated the utility of salivary/sputum or laryngoscopic biopsy specimen assays for pepsin as a marker for underlying GERD.[153–155] As pepsin is produced only in the gastric mucosa, its presence in the sputum or larynx reflects gastric reflux. Pepsin assays, when compared to ambulatory pH monitoring, showed a high correlation to proximal reflux events. Positive assays were also highly correlated with the presence of laryngopharyngeal reflux symptoms. Still lacking are data showing that a positive sputum or laryngeal pepsin assay predicts a successful symptomatic response to antireflux therapy. With additional study, the utility and reliability of each of these modalities will be determined in the clinical marketplace.

Partial Versus Complete Fundoplication. The decision between partial and complete fundoplication and an open or laparoscopic approach requires considerable judgment. Two randomized

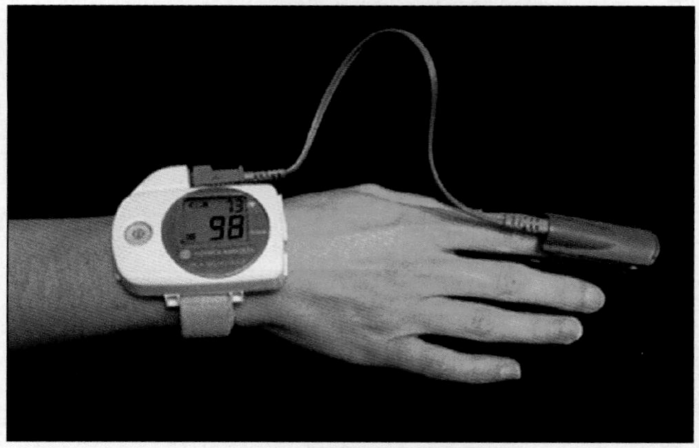

FIGURE 41.27. Pulsox-300i with finger probe used to assess ambulatory oxygen saturation (Konica Minolta Sensing, Inc.).

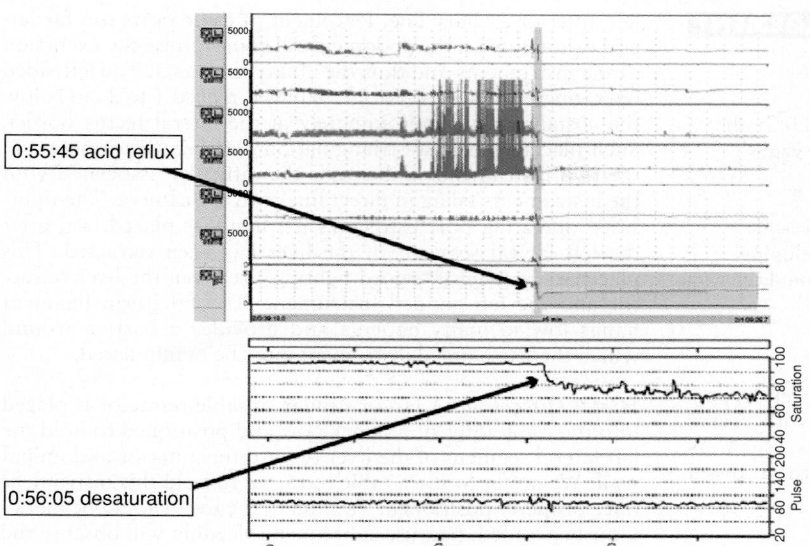

FIGURE 41.28. Example of the association between a reflux episode detected by multichannel intraluminal impedance–pH study and oxygen desaturation detected by pulse oximetry. (Reproduced with permission from Salvador R, Watson TJ, Herbella F, et al. Association of gastroesophageal reflux and O_2 desaturation: a novel study of simultaneous 24-h MII-pH and continuous pulse oximetry. *J Gastrointest Surg* 2009; 13:854–861.)

studies of unselected patients undergoing laparoscopic fundoplication have shown equivalence of complete and partial fundoplications, anterior in one study[156] and posterior in the other,[83] in terms of operative time, perioperative morbidity, and hospital stay. Watson et al.[156] noted that resting and residual LES pressures were greater after complete fundoplication and that esophageal clearance of liquid radioisotope was prolonged in these patients compared with after partial fundoplication. Six months after operation, partial fundoplication was linked to a greater overall level of patient satisfaction manifested by a lower incidence of the symptoms of dysphagia, inability to belch, and excessive flatus. Laws et al.[157] did not identify any difference in symptomatic outcome between patients treated by complete and those treated by posterior partial fundoplication at a mean follow-up time of 27 months.

Hagedorn et al. reported on the results of a randomized, controlled trial comparing total (Nissen-Rosetti) and posterior

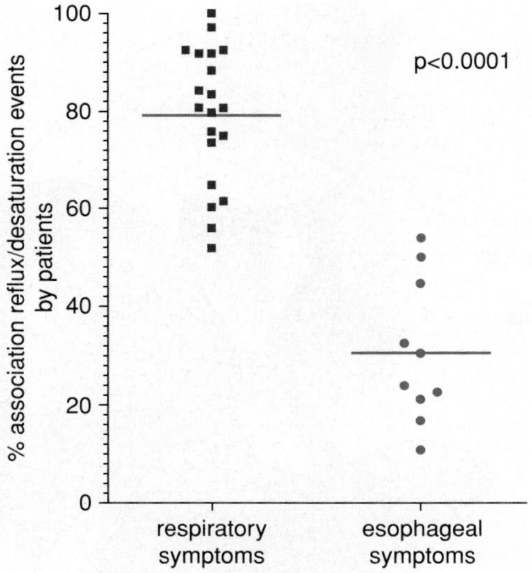

FIGURE 41.29. Scatterplot of association between reflux episodes and desaturation events by patient group. The prevalence of reflux-associated desaturations was remarkably different between the two groups ($p < 0.0001$). (Reproduced with permission from Salvador R, Watson TJ, Herbella F, et al. Association of gastroesophageal reflux and O_2 desaturation: a novel study of simultaneous 24-h MII-pH and continuous pulse oximetry. *J Gastrointest Surg* 2009;13:854–861.)

partial (Toupet) fundoplication in which long-term efficacy was assessed.[158] A total of 110 patients (54 undergoing a total wrap, 56 a partial wrap) completed a median follow-up of 11.5 years. No significant differences were observed between the groups in terms of heartburn, regurgitation, or dysphagia scores. A significant difference, however, was noted in the prevalence of rectal flatus and postprandial fullness, which were reported more often by those having undergone a total fundoplication.

A recent prospective, randomized trial from Australia comparing laparoscopic Nissen fundoplication to an anterior 180-degree partial fundoplication similarly revealed no significant differences between the two groups with regard to reflux symptoms, dysphagia, abdominal bloating, ability to belch, and overall satisfaction at 10 years' follow-up.[159]

These observations, however, must be tempered by reports questioning the durability of partial fundoplications. Jobe et al. found that 51% of patients studied by 24-hour esophageal pH monitoring after Toupet fundoplication still had pathologic acid exposure.[160] Disturbingly, only 40% of the refluxers were symptomatic. Two studies have identified the presence of a defective LES function, an aperistaltic distal esophagus, and higher grades of esophagitis (Savary-Miller grades 2 to 4) as risk factors for partial fundoplication failure.[158,160] Bell et al. reported recurrent reflux in 14% after Toupet fundoplication.[161] The presence of mild esophagitis and a normal LES were associated with a 3-year success rate of 96%, whereas the presence of complicated esophagitis or a defective LES lowered this value to 50% (Fig. 41.23).

These findings highlight an apparent paradox, in that partial fundoplications afford suboptimal reflux protection in those most at risk from the effects of unabated GERD. The question arises, therefore, whether total fundoplication should be applied more liberally to patients with severe reflux disease and associated esophageal dysmotility. Patti et al. recently reported on 357 patients undergoing antireflux surgery, 235 undergoing a "tailored approach" with either a partial or total fundoplication depending on the results of preoperative manometry, and 122 more recent patients undergoing a total fundoplication regardless of the quality of esophageal peristalsis.[161] In the first group, heartburn from pathologic reflux, confirmed by postoperative ambulatory esophageal pH monitoring, recurred in 19% after partial fundoplication and in 4% after total fundoplication. In the latter group, heartburn recurred in 4% after total fundoplication. Importantly, the incidence of postoperative dysphagia was similar in the two groups. This recent evidence, as well as our own experience, has led us to utilize the complete fundoplication more readily,

TABLE 41.8 MANAGEMENT

ELEMENTS OF LAPAROSCOPIC FUNDOPLICATION

1. Crural dissection, identification and preservation of both vagi including the hepatic branch of the anterior vagus
2. Circumferential dissection of the esophagus
3. Crural closure
4. Fundic mobilization by division of short gastric vessels
5. Creation of a short, loose fundoplication by enveloping the anterior and posterior wall of the fundus around the lower esophagus

particularly in patients with Barrett esophagus. Currently, partial fundoplication is best reserved for patients with severe esophageal dysmotility approaching aperistalsis, such as occurs in scleroderma, or in combination with a distal esophageal myotomy for achalasia.[162]

Laparoscopic Nissen Fundoplication. The performance of laparoscopic fundoplication should include the steps identified in Table 41.8.

Port Placement. Five ports are used (Fig. 41.30). The camera is placed above and to the left of the umbilicus, roughly one third of the distance to the xiphoid process. In most patients, placement of the camera in the umbilicus is too low to allow adequate visualization of the hiatal strictures once dissected. A transrectus location is preferable to midline to minimize the prevalence of port site hernia formation. Two lateral retracting ports are placed, one for the liver retractor in the right midabdomen (anterior axillary line), at or slightly below the camera port. This allows the proper angle toward the left lateral segment of the liver and thus the ability to push the retractor toward the operating table, lifting the liver. A second retraction port is placed slightly above the level of the umbilicus, in the left anterior axillary line. Placement of these ports too far lateral or too low on the abdomen will compromise the excursion of the instruments and thus the ability to retract. The left-sided operating port (surgeon's right hand) is placed 1 to 2 cm below the costal margin approximately at the lateral rectus border. Such placement allows triangulation between the camera and the two instruments and avoids the difficulty associated with the instruments being in direct line with the camera. The right-sided operating port (surgeon's left hand) is placed last, after the left lateral segment of the liver has been retracted. This placement prevents "sword fighting" between the liver retractor and the left-handed instrument. The falciform ligament hangs low in many patients and provides a barrier around which the left-handed instrument must be manipulated.

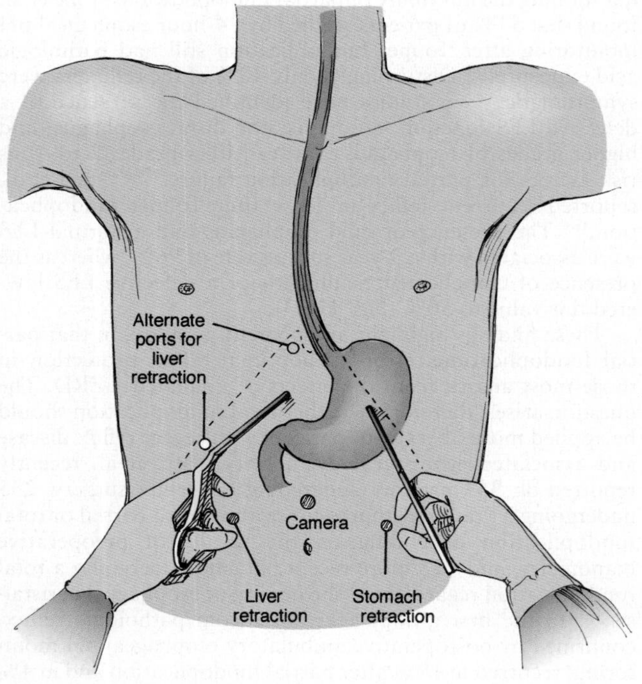

FIGURE 41.30. Trocar placement for laparoscopic antireflux surgery. The patient is placed with the head elevated 45 degrees in the modified lithotomy position. The surgeon stands between the patient's legs and the procedure is completed via five abdominal access ports.

Hiatal Dissection. A fan or similar suitable retractor is placed into the right anterior axillary port and positioned to hold the left lateral segment of the liver toward the anterior abdominal wall. We prefer to use a table retractor to hold this instrument once properly positioned. Trauma to the liver should be meticulously avoided, because subsequent bleeding will obscure the field. Mobilization of the left lateral segment by division of the triangular ligament is not necessary. A Babcock or fundus clamp placed through the left anterior axillary port is used to grasp the GE fat pad and retract the stomach toward the patient's left foot. This maneuver exposes the esophageal hiatus. Commonly a hiatal hernia will need to be reduced. Atraumatic clamps should be used and care taken not to grasp the stomach too vigorously, as gastric perforations can occur.

Crural Dissection. Crural dissection begins with identification of the right crus. Metzenbaum-type scissors and fine grasping forceps are preferred for dissection. In all except the most obese patients, there is a very thin portion of the gastrohepatic omentum overlying the caudate lobe of the liver. The dissection is begun by incising the portion of the gastrohepatic omentum above and below the hepatic branch of the anterior vagal nerve (which some authors routinely spare). A large left hepatic artery arising from the left gastric artery is present in up to 25% of patients (Fig. 41.31); it should be identified and avoided. A right crural branch is occasionally seen, which can

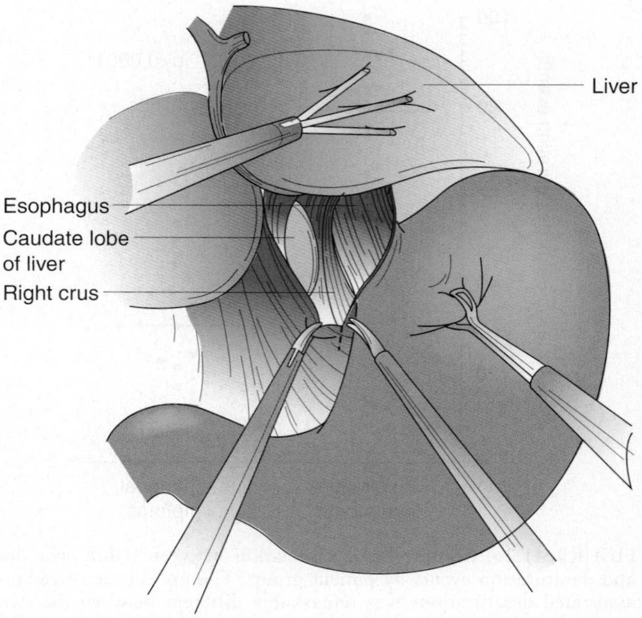

FIGURE 41.31. Illustration of the initial dissection of the esophageal hiatus. The right crus is identified and dissected toward its posterior confluence with the left crus.

be divided. After incising the gastrohepatic omentum, the outside of the right crus will become evident. The peritoneum overlying the anterior aspect of the right crus is incised with scissors and electrocautery, and the right crus dissected from anterior to posterior as far as possible. The medial portion of the right crus leads into the mediastinum and is entered by blunt dissection with both instruments.

At this juncture the esophagus usually becomes evident. The right crus is retracted laterally with the surgeon's left-handed grasper and a modest dissection of the tissues posterior to the esophagus is performed. In most patients it is best not to dissect behind the GE junction at this time. Meticulous hemostasis is critical. Blood and fluid tend to pool in the hiatus and are difficult to remove. Irrigation should be avoided. Modest bleeding can be controlled by placing a 4 × 4 sponge into the abdomen. A large hiatal hernia often makes this portion of the procedure easier because it accentuates the diaphragmatic crura. On the other hand, dissection of a large mediastinal hernia sac can be difficult.

Following dissection of the right crus, attention is turned toward the anterior crural confluence. The tissues anterior to the esophagus are held upward by the left-handed grasper and the esophagus is swept downward and to the right, separating it from the left crus (Fig. 41.32). The anterior crural tissues are then divided and the left crus identified. The anterior vagus nerve often "hugs" the left crus and can be injured in this portion of the dissection if not carefully searched for and protected. The left crus is dissected as completely as possible, including taking down the angle of His and the attachments of the fundus to the left diaphragm (Fig. 41.33). A complete dissection of the lateral and inferior aspect of the left crus and fundus of the stomach is the key maneuver allowing circumferential mobilization of the esophagus. Failure to do so will result in difficulty encircling the esophagus, particularly if approached from the right. Repositioning of the Babcock retractor toward the fundic side of the stomach facilitates retraction for this portion of the procedure. The posterior vagus nerve may be encountered in the low left crural dissection and should be protected.

A window behind the GE junction can generally now be easily created. Attention is returned to the right side of the esophagus where the left-handed instrument is used to retract the esophagus anteriorly. This allows the right hand to perform the dissection behind the esophagus. The posterior vagus nerve should be identified and left on the esophagus. The left crus is identified and the dissection kept caudal to it. There is a tendency to dissect into the mediastinum and left pleura. In the presence of severe esophagitis, transmural inflammation,

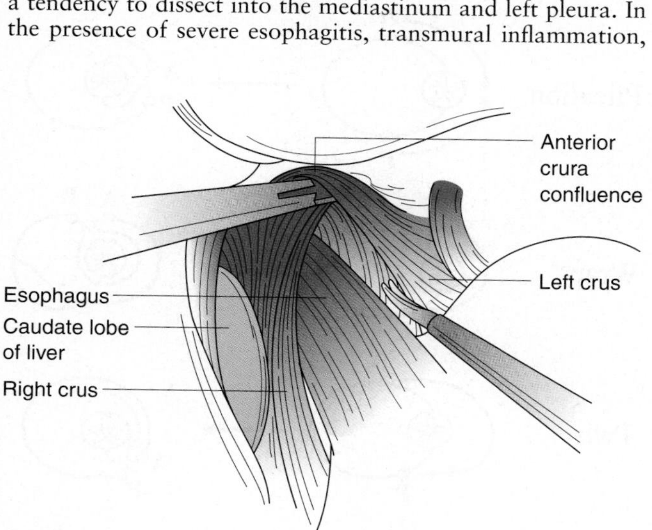

FIGURE 41.32. Artistic depiction of division of the anterior crural fibers and mobilization of the esophagus off the left crus.

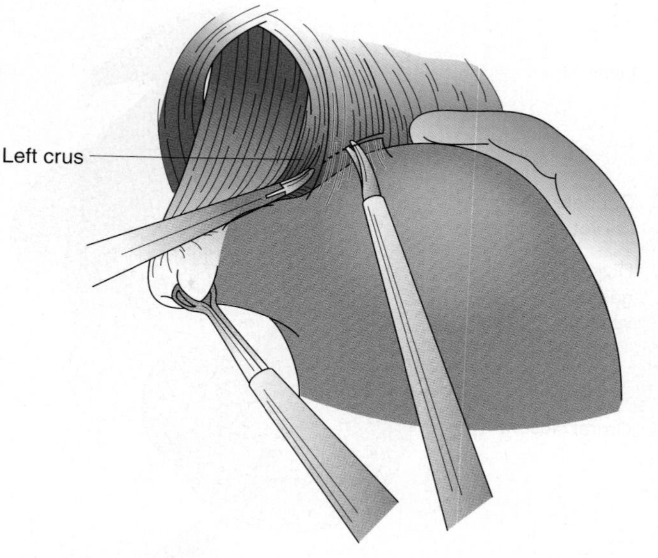

FIGURE 41.33. Left-sided crural dissection. The left crus is dissected as completely as possible and the attachments of the fundus of the stomach to the diaphragm are taken down.

esophageal shortening, or a large posterior fat pad, this dissection may be particularly difficult. If unduly difficult, abandon this route of dissection and approach the hiatus from the left side by dividing the short gastric vessels at this point in the procedure rather than later. After completing the posterior dissection, pass a grasper (through the surgeon's left-handed port) behind the esophagus and over the left crus and pull a Penrose drain around the esophagus to be used as an esophageal retractor for the remainder of the procedure.

Fundic Mobilization. Complete fundic mobilization allows construction of a tension-free fundoplication. This is best done by suspending the gastrosplenic omentum anteroposteriorly, in a clothesline fashion via two Babcock forceps, and opening into the lesser sac approximately one-third the distance down the greater curvature of the stomach (Fig. 41.34). The short

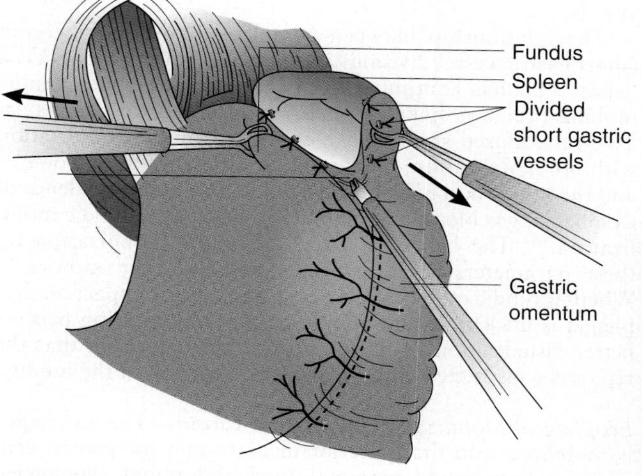

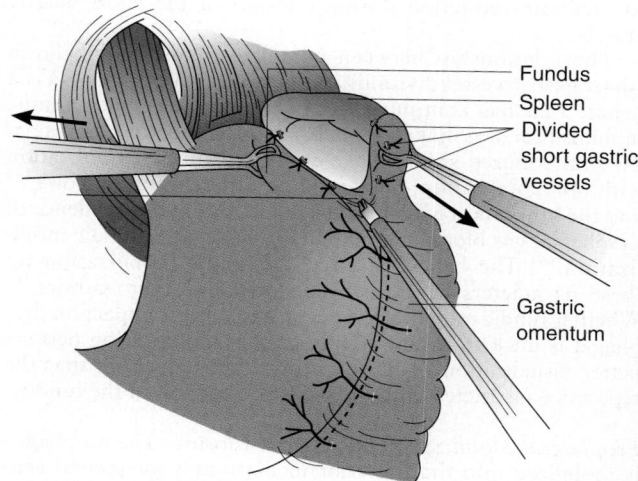

FIGURE 41.34. Illustration of the proper retraction of the gastrosplenic omentum facilitating the initial steps in short gastric division. Complete fundic mobilization is continued by retraction of the stomach rightward and the spleen and omentum left and downward. These maneuvers allow opening of the lesser sac and facilitate division of the high short gastric vessels.

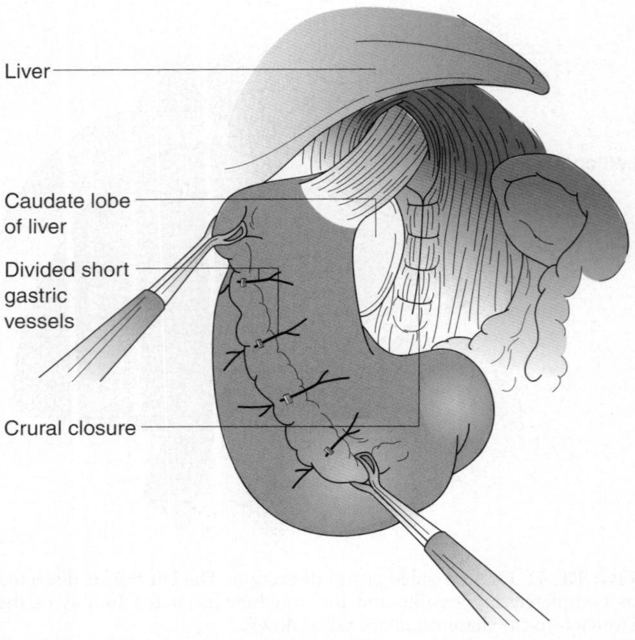

FIGURE 41.35. The fundic mobilization is continued to include pancreaticogastric branches as well as the short gastric branches. Dissection continues until the crura and the caudate lobe can be seen from left posterior.

gastric vessels can then be sequentially dissected and divided with the aid of ultrasonic shears (Ethicon Endosurgery, Cincinnati, Ohio). An anterior-posterior rather than medial-to-lateral orientation of the vessels is preferred, with the exception of those close to the spleen. The dissection includes pancreaticogastric branches posterior to the upper stomach and continues until the right crus and caudate lobe can be seen from the left side (Fig. 41.35). With caution and meticulous dissection, the fundus can be completely mobilized in virtually all patients. Although generally possible via the right- and left-handed surgeon's access ports, occasionally this dissection requires removal of the liver retractor and placement of a second Babcock forceps through the right anterior axillary port to facilitate retraction during division of the short gastric vessels.

The relationship between complete fundic mobilization (short gastric vessel division) and postoperative dysphagia is a debate that has continued from the open era, when fundic mobilization was linked to a lower incidence of dysphagia. Two randomized studies have compared fundic mobilization with nonmobilization; one found no difference in outcome[163] and the other showed significant reductions in the incidence of dysphagia, gas bloat, and inability to belch after fundic mobilization.[164] The beneficial effect of fundic mobilization on these parameters has also been noted by other authors.[165] Whether fundic mobilization per se has a direct impact on dysphagia is unclear. It may simply be that mobilization permits better visualization of the procedure, thus ensuring that the repair is constructed with the posterior portion of the fundus.

Esophageal Mobilization and Crural Closure. The esophagus is mobilized into the posterior mediastinum for several centimeters to provide maximal intra-abdominal esophageal length. Posterior and right lateral mobilization is readily accomplished. In performing the anterior and left lateral mobilization, the surgeon must take care not to injure the anterior vagus nerve. Gentle traction on the Penrose drain around the GE junction facilitates exposure. The right and left pleural reflection often come into view and should be avoided. Continue the crural dissection to enlarge the space behind the GE junction as much as possible. Following mobilization and an assessment of intra-abdominal esophageal length, the hiatus is closed in all patients. The esophagus is held anterior and to the left and the crura approximated with two to four interrupted figure-of-eight 0-Ethibond sutures, starting just above the aortic decussation and working anterior. The authors prefer a large needle (CT1) passed down the left upper 10-mm port to facilitate a durable crural closure. Because space is limited, it is often necessary to use the surgeon's left-handed (nondominant) instrument as a retractor, facilitating placement of single bites through each crus with the surgeon's right hand. The aorta may be punctured while suturing the left crus. Identification of the anterior aortic surface and retracting the left crus via the left-handed grasper will help avoid inadvertent aortic puncture. The authors prefer extracorporeal knot tying using a standard knot pusher or a "tie knot" device (LSI Solutions, Victor, New York), although tying within the abdomen is perfectly appropriate. More recently, we have inspected the crural closure at the completion of the procedure following creation of the fundoplication and removal of the bougie. Doing so will often reveal that the bougie has dilated the hiatal opening such that a final stitch should be placed to further approximate it. Although there have been no randomized studies evaluating the role of routine crural closure, there is compelling evidence to indicate that closure should be standard. Watson et al.[166] identified paraesophageal herniation in 17 of 253 patients (7%), the frequency being 3% in those who had undergone crural repair and 11% in those who had not.

Creation of the Fundoplication. A short, loose fundoplication is fashioned with particular attention to the geometry of the wrap (Fig. 41.36). The midposterior fundus is grasped and passed left to right behind the esophagus rather than pulling right to left. This ensures that the posterior fundus is used for the posterior aspect of the fundoplication. This is accomplished by placing a Babcock clamp through the left lower port and grasping the midportion of the posterior fundus (Fig. 41.37). One should gently bring the posterior fundus behind the esophagus to the right side with an upward, rightward, and clockwise twisting motion. This maneuver can be difficult, particularly for the novice. If so, placement of a 0-silk suture in the midposterior fundus and grasping it from the right side facilitates bringing the posterior fundus around to create the

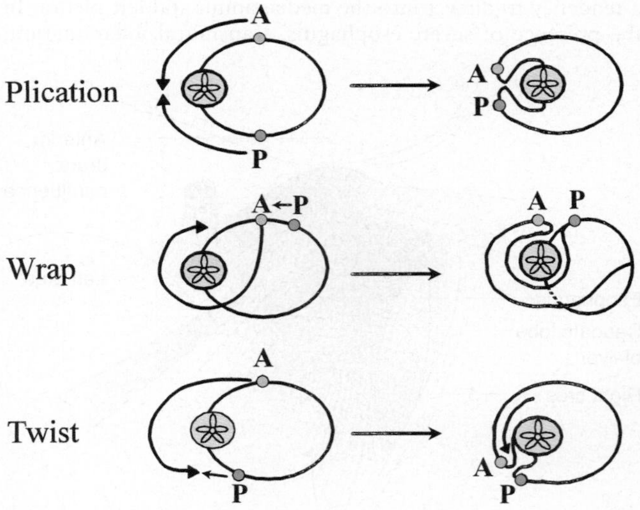

FIGURE 41.36. Schematic representations of the various possibilities of orientation of a Nissen fundoplication. The top set of figures represents the preferred approach, whereas the bottom two sets can be seen to result in twisting of the fundoplication.

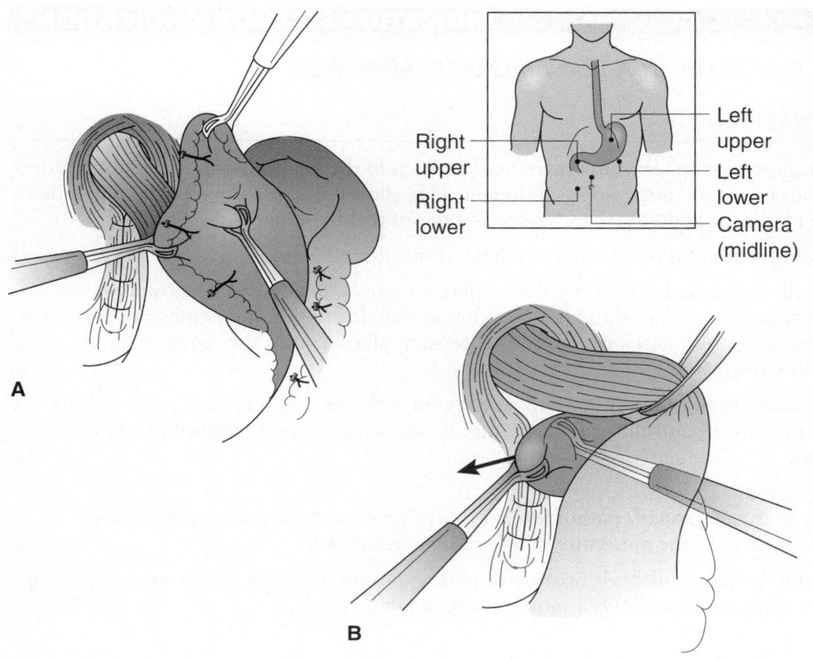

FIGURE 41.37. Placement of Babcock on the posterior fundus in preparation for passing it behind the esophagus to create the posterior or right lip of the fundoplication. *Inset:* To achieve the proper angle for passage, the Babcock is placed through the left lower trocar. The posterior fundus is passed left to right and grasped from the right via a Babcock through the right upper trocar. **A:** Location of posterior fundus for passage to the right side. **B:** The posterior fundus passed underneath the esophagus and grasped on the right.

fundoplication. The anterior wall of the fundus is then folded over the esophagus to meet the posterior at about the 10 to 11 o'clock position above the supporting Penrose drain.

The posterior and anterior fundic lips should be maneuvered (as in a "shoe shine") to allow the fundus to envelope the esophagus without twisting. Laparoscopic visualization has a tendency to exaggerate the size of the posterior opening that has been dissected. Consequently, the space for the passage of the fundus behind the esophagus may be tighter than thought and the fundus relatively ischemic when brought around. If the right lip of the fundoplication has a bluish discoloration, the stomach should be returned to its original position and the posterior dissection enlarged. A 60-French bougie is passed to properly size the fundoplication, and the "lips" of the fundoplication sutured utilizing a single U-stitch of 2–0 Prolene buttressed with felt pledgets. The most common error is an attempt to grasp the anterior portion of the stomach to construct the right lip of the fundoplication rather than the posterior fundus. The esophagus should comfortably lie in the untwisted fundus prior to suturing. Finally, two anchoring sutures of 2–0 silk or Ethibond are placed above and below the U-stitch to complete the fundoplication. When finished, the suture line of the fundoplication should be facing in a right anterior direction (Fig. 41.38). The abdomen is then irrigated, hemostasis checked, and the bougie, Penrose drain, and any sponges placed into the abdomen removed.

Transthoracic Nissen Fundoplication. The indications for performing an antireflux procedure by a transthoracic approach are given in Table 41.9.

In the thoracic approach the hiatus is exposed through a left posterior lateral thoracotomy incision in the sixth intercostal space (i.e., over the upper border of the seventh rib). When necessary, the diaphragm is incised circumferentially 2 to 3 cm from the lateral chest wall for a distance of approximately 10 to 15 cm. The esophagus is mobilized from the level of the diaphragm to underneath the aortic arch. Mobilization up to the aortic arch is usually necessary to place the repair in a patient with a shortened esophagus into the abdomen without undue tension. Failure to do this is one of the major causes for subsequent breakdown of a repair and return of symptoms. The cardia is then freed from the diaphragm. When all the attachments between the cardia and diaphragmatic hiatus are divided, the fundus and part of the body of the stomach are drawn up through the hiatus into the chest. The vascular fat pad that lies at the GE junction is excised. Crural sutures are then placed to close the hiatus though are not tightened until later. The fundoplication is constructed by enveloping the fundus around the distal esophagus in a manner similar to that described for the abdominal approach. When complete, the fundoplication is placed into the abdomen by compressing the fundic ball with the hand and manually maneuvering it through the hiatus. The previously placed crural stitches are then tightened and knotted.

Collis Gastroplasty. In patients with a short esophagus secondary to a stricture, Barrett esophagus, or a large hiatal hernia,

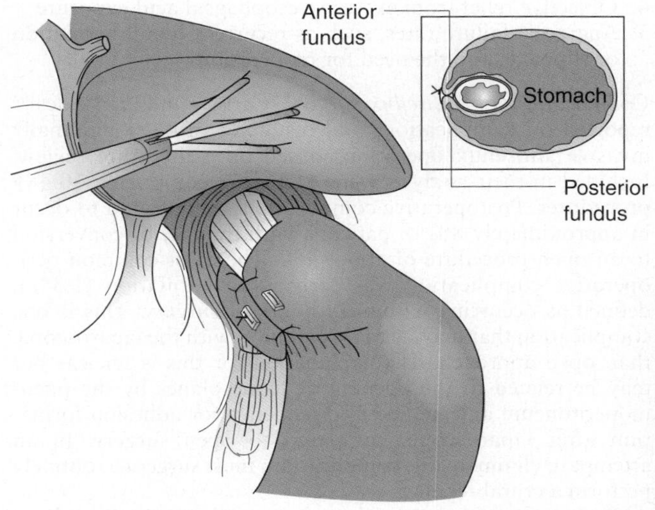

FIGURE 41.38. Fixation of the fundoplication. The fundoplication is sutured in place with a single U-stitch of 2–0 Prolene pledgeted on the outside. A 60-French mercury-weighted bougie is passed through the gastroesophageal junction prior to fixation of the wrap to ensure a floppy fundoplication. Inset illustrates the proper orientation of the fundic wrap.

TABLE 41.9 **INDICATIONS/CONTRAINDICATIONS**

INDICATIONS FOR PERFORMING AN ANTIREFLUX PROCEDURE BY A TRANSTHORACIC APPROACH

■ INDICATION	■ EXPLANATION
Previous hiatal hernia repair	In this situation, a peripheral circumferential incision in the diaphragm is made to provide simultaneous exposure of the upper abdomen. This allows safe dissection of the previous repair from both the abdominal and thoracic sides of the diaphragm.
Concomitant procedure	Concomitant esophageal myotomy for achalasia or diffuse spasm.
Short esophagus	This is usually associated with a stricture or Barrett esophagus. In this situation, the thoracic approach is preferred to allow maximum mobilization of the esophagus, the performance of a Collis gastroplasty, or, if necessary, placement of the repair without tension below the diaphragm.
Sliding hiatal hernia that does not reduce below the diaphragm during a roentgenographic barium study in the upright position	This can indicate esophageal shortening and, again, a thoracic approach is preferred for maximum mobilization of the esophagus and, if necessary, the performance of a Collis gastroplasty.
Associated pulmonary pathology	The nature of the pulmonary pathology can be evaluated and the proper pulmonary surgery, in addition to the antireflux repair, can be performed.
Obesity	The abdominal repair is difficult because of poor exposure, whereas the thoracic approach gives better exposure and allows a more precise repair.

the esophagus is lengthened with a Collis gastroplasty. The gastroplasty lengthens the esophagus by forming a gastric tube or "neoesophagus" along the lesser curvature. The procedure allows a tension-free construction of a total or partial fundoplication around the newly formed gastric tube, with placement of the repair in the abdomen. A gastroplasty can be readily performed via either an abdominal or thoracic approach. A number of techniques have been reported for the laparoscopic performance of Collis gastroplasty, and the surgeon opting to manage the shortened esophagus laparoscopically must be able to perform such a procedure should the need arise.[167]

Outcomes Following Antireflux Surgery. Any discussion regarding results following fundoplication must consider:

1. Perioperative morbidity and mortality
2. Control of typical and atypical symptoms
3. Side effects
4. Objective relief from excessive esophageal acid exposure
5. Anatomic failure rates, such as recurrent hiatal herniation or slippage, and the need for reoperation

Complications of Antireflux Surgery. Carlson and Frantzides[168] reported on complications and results of primary minimally invasive antireflux operations based on a literature review. Included in their analysis were 41 papers comprising 10,489 procedures. Postoperative complications were found to occur in approximately 8% of patients, with the rate of conversion to an open procedure of about 4%. The most common perioperative complication was early wrap herniation (1.3%), defined as occurring within 48 hours of surgery. This is one complication that may be more common with the laparoscopic than open approach. The explanation for this is unclear but may be related to the opening of tissue planes by the pneumoperitoneum and the reduced tendency for adhesion formation after laparoscopic compared to open surgery. In an attempt to eliminate this complication, most surgeons routinely perform a crural repair.

Both pneumothorax and pneumomediastinum have been reported. The occurrence of pneumothorax is related to breach of either pleural membrane, usually the left, during the hiatal dissection. Chest drain insertion is usually not required because accumulated carbon dioxide rapidly dissipates following release of pneumoperitoneum by a combination of positive-pressure ventilation and absorption.

As with any laparoscopic procedure, instrumental perforation of the hollow viscera may occur. Early esophageal perforation may arise during passage of the bougie, during the retroesophageal dissection, or during suture pull-through. Late esophageal perforation is related to diathermy injury at the time of mobilization. Gastric perforations usually result from excessive traction on the fundus for retraction purposes. Recognition of the problem at the time of surgery requires repair, which may be performed either laparoscopically or by an open technique.

Hemorrhage during the course of laparoscopic fundoplication usually arises from the short gastric vessels or spleen. Rarer causes include retractor trauma to the liver, injury to the left inferior phrenic vein, an aberrant left hepatic vein, or the inferior vena cava. Cardiac tamponade as a result of right ventricular trauma has also been reported. Major vascular injury mandates immediate conversion to an open procedure to achieve hemostasis. One complication that has been virtually eliminated since the advent of laparoscopic fundoplication is incidental splenic injury necessitating splenectomy (0.06%), which occurred with a frequency of around 2% to 5% during the open era. The mortality rate for primary minimally invasive antireflux surgery has fortunately been quite low, reported at 0.08%.

Symptomatic Outcomes Following Antireflux Surgery. Studies of long-term outcome following both open and laparoscopic fundoplication document the ability of laparoscopic fundoplication to relieve typical reflux symptoms (heartburn, regurgitation, and dysphagia) in more than 90% of patients at follow-up intervals averaging 2 to 3 years and 80% to 90% of patients 5 years or more following surgery.[169–177] The data include evidence-based reviews of antireflux surgery,[174] prospective randomized trials comparing antireflux surgery to PPI therapy[175] and open to laparoscopic fundoplication,[176] and analysis of U.S. national trends in utilization and outcomes.[177] The results of laparoscopic fundoplication compare favorably with those of the "modern" era of open fundoplication. They also indicate the less predictable outcome of atypical reflux symptoms (cough, asthma, laryngitis) after surgery being relieved in only two thirds of patients.[178]

A few recent trials deserve emphasis. Results were updated on a prospective, randomized trial comparing PPI therapy to antireflux surgery.[179] The outcome of the study previously had been reported at a follow-up of 5 years,[175] while the latest update provided follow-up of at least 7 years. The proportion of patients in whom treatment did not fail during the 7 years was significantly higher in the surgical arm than in the medical arm. A smaller difference in outcomes was noted after dose adjustments in the medical group. More patients in the surgical cohort, however, complained of side effects such as dysphagia, inability to belch or vomit, and hyperflatulence. Disease control was essentially stable between 5 and 7 years of follow-up. The authors concluded that surgery was more effective in controlling overall GERD symptoms, though postfundoplication side effects were a concern.

Another prospective trial from the United Kingdom compared laparoscopic Nissen fundoplication to PPI and reported follow-up at a median of 6.9 years.[180] Some patients initially randomized to PPI therapy were offered the opportunity to undergo surgery. While both the medical and surgical cohorts reported an improvement in GERD-related symptoms after 12 months, further symptomatic improvement was noted in those patients subsequently undergoing surgery despite optimal PPI therapy.

A multicenter, European, prospective randomized trial comparing laparoscopic antireflux surgery (LARS) to medical therapy with esomeprazole is ongoing (the LOTUS trial). Three-year outcomes in 288 patients assigned to LARS and 266 assigned to medical therapy were reported in 2008.[181] The proportion of patients remaining in symptomatic remission was similar between the two groups (90% for LARS, 93% for medical therapy in an intention-to-treat analysis, $p = 0.25$). No major perioperative complications were noted and esomeprazole appeared to be well tolerated.

Recent reports have called attention to the observation that many patients are prescribed acid suppression medications after antireflux surgery. Spechler et al. reported on the long-term follow-up of patients with complicated GERD enrolled in the Department of Veterans Affairs randomized trial of medical versus surgical therapies.[182,183] In the first report, almost half (46.9%) of the patients treated by fundoplication had taken acid suppression medications at some point during the 11- to 13-year follow-up period.[182] In the second report, 62% of the surgically treated patients had used medications.[183]

Lord et al.[184] reported on 86 patients who had symptoms after Nissen fundoplication severe enough to warrant evaluation with 24-hour ambulatory esophageal pH monitoring. Thirty-seven (43%) of these patients were taking acid suppression medications, and only 9 of them (24%) were found to have abnormal pH scores. Heartburn and regurgitation were the only symptoms that were significantly associated with an abnormal pH study. Multivariable logistic regression analysis showed that patients with a disrupted, abnormally positioned fundoplication had a 52.6 times increased risk of abnormal esophageal acid exposure. Based on these data, most patients using acid suppression medications after antireflux surgery do not have abnormal esophageal acid exposure. Objective evidence of reflux should be obtained in patients who complain of postoperative symptoms.

The goal of surgical treatment for GERD is to relieve the symptoms of reflux by re-establishing the GE barrier. The challenge is to accomplish this without inducing dysphagia or other untoward side effects. Dysphagia that existed prior to surgery usually improves following laparoscopic fundoplication. Temporary dysphagia is common after surgery and generally resolves within 3 months. Dysphagia persisting beyond 3 months has been reported in up to 10% of patients. In our experience, dysphagia, manifested by occasional difficulty in swallowing solids, was present in 7% of patients at 3 months, 5% at 6 months, 2% at 12 months, and a single patient at 24 months following surgery.[170] Others have observed a similar improvement in postoperative dysphagia with time. Induced dysphagia is usually mild, does not require dilatation, and is temporary. It can be induced by technical misjudgments, but this explanation does not hold in all instances. In experienced hands, its prevalence should be less than 3% at 1 year. Other side effects common to antireflux surgery include the inability to vomit and increased flatulence. Most patients cannot vomit through an intact wrap, though this is rarely clinically relevant. Hyperflatulence is a common and noticeable problem, likely related to increased air swallowing that is present in most patients with reflux disease.

Objective Outcomes Following Antireflux Surgery. Laparoscopic fundoplication results in a significant increase in LES pressure and length, generally restoring these values to normal. The ability of an antireflux operation to restore esophageal acid exposure to normal depends on the type of fundoplication performed. Complete (Nissen) fundoplications generally are more reliable and durable than partial (e.g., Toupet) fundoplications at preventing pathologic acid reflux. Objective studies have shown that more than 90% of patients will have normal pH studies at 1 to 3 years following complete fundoplication, whereas only 50% of patients will have normal esophageal acid exposure following a partial fundic wrap.[160]

Quality-of-life analyses have become an important part of surgical outcome assessment, with both generic and disease-specific questionnaires in use, in an attempt to quantitate quality of life before and after surgical intervention. In general, these measures relate the effect of disease management to the overall well-being of the patient.[185] Most studies have utilized the Short Form 36 (SF-36) instrument, because it is rapidly administered and well validated. This questionnaire measures 12 different health-related quality-of-life parameters encompassing mental and physical well-being. Data from Los Angeles indicate significant improvements in scores for the area of bodily pain and in a portion of the general health index.[170] Most other measures were improved but failed to achieve statistical significance. Trus et al.[186] have also analyzed SF-36 scores before and after laparoscopic antireflux surgery. In contrast to our data, scores in all fields were significantly better after surgery. In this study, preoperative scores were dramatically lower than were found in our study. Thus, the difference is likely to be secondary to the relatively high scores of our patients prior to surgery (perhaps reflecting good disease control on medical therapy) and to our small sample size.

Other investigators have also reported improvement in quality of life following antireflux surgery. Glise et al.[187] utilized two standardized and validated questionnaires, the Psychological General Well-Being Index and the Gastrointestinal Symptom Rating Scale, to evaluate quality of life in a cohort of 40 patients following laparoscopic antireflux surgery. Scores with both instruments were improved following antireflux surgery and better than in untreated patients. Of particular note was that scores were as good as or better than those of patients receiving optimal medical therapy. Velonovich et al.,[188] using a 10-item health-related quality-of-life questionnaire specific for GERD, have also shown an improvement in quality of life following antireflux surgery.

Fernando et al.[189] reported on quality of life after antireflux surgery compared with nonoperative management for severe GERD. Follow-up quality of life was measured using the SF-36, and heartburn severity was measured using the Health-Related Quality of Life (QOL) scale. Detailed outcomes were available for 101 surgical patients and 37 medical patients. Mean QOL scores were better in the surgical group. More of the medical patients were dissatisfied with therapy. SF-36 scores were better in six of eight domains for surgical patients. These data support the notion that antireflux surgery, performed on properly selected patients, can significantly improve quality of life and may outperform medical therapy in this regard.

Anatomic Failure Following Antireflux Surgery. An important and often underemphasized point is that the rate of failure of fundoplication is largely dependent upon the size of the underlying hiatal hernia. Repair of large sliding and paraesophageal hernias (PEHs) is associated with a higher risk of recurrent hiatal herniation compared to fundoplication for GERD in the setting of no or small hiatal hernias. Multiple potential explanations exist to explain this differential, including the presence of a widened hiatus with weakened or attenuated crural fibers that must be brought together under tension, the coexistence of esophageal body shortening, the generally older and frailer nature of patients with a PEH, and underlying anatomic, muscular, or connective tissue deficits that contributed to the pathogenesis of the hernia. In particular, the association between kyphosis and intrathoracic stomach is becoming increasingly recognized, as skeletal abnormalities likely are contributory to the pathogenesis of paraesophageal hiatal herniation.[190]

The need for reoperation after fundoplication for GERD is only approximately 5% over the patient's lifetime, whereas the risk can run as high as 42% after repair of a giant PEH.[191] In a trial from Finland, objective outcomes were assessed by endoscopy and demonstrated a 40% disruption rate following open Nissen fundoplication and a 13% disruption rate following a laparoscopic procedure.[192] Despite these relatively high rates of objective breakdown, only 8% of patients in the open group and 2% in the laparoscopic group had undergone repeat operation for fundoplication failure.

A recent trial compared two techniques of laparoscopic PEH repair, with or without the use of a biologic prosthesis placed at the esophageal hiatus.[193] At 6 months, 9% of patients with the prosthesis and 24% of patients without mesh reinforcement had developed a recurrent hiatal hernia as assessed by a barium upper gastrointestinal examination, underscoring the potential for failure when operation is undertaken for PEHs.

Some surgeons routinely add a Collis gastroplasty as an esophageal lengthening procedure in the setting of fundoplication for giant PEHs given the high incidence of acquired esophageal body shortening associated with this condition.[194] Methods to reduce the risk of recurrent hiatal herniation following repair of giant PEHs, such as gastroplasty, mesh reinforcement, extensive esophageal mobilization, or use of open surgical approaches rather than laparoscopy, are areas of active ongoing investigation.

FUTURE DIRECTIONS

Medical therapy for GERD and antireflux surgery both have inherent drawbacks. Major limitations of acid suppressive medications include the inability to prevent regurgitation of weakly acidic or nonacidic refluxate and the need for chronic, continual therapy, not to mention the cost, inconvenience, potential side effects, and need for ongoing dietary and lifestyle modifications. In addition, current therapy does not address the main pathophysiologic contributor to the presence of GERD, the mechanically defective LES. Fundoplications, while intended to permanently restore the LES, suffer from the potential for perioperative complications, a high initial cost, the risks inherent in general anesthesia, possible short- and long-term side effects, and inconsistent reflux control across centers. In addition, proper patient selection is critical and the operative technique is not well standardized, perhaps adversely affecting outcomes, particularly in inexperienced hands.

For all of these reasons, an interest remains to create means of restoring LES competence by medical or less invasive surgical or endoscopic techniques that are easily applied and highly reproducible. Medications such as baclofen, a γ-aminobutyric $acid_B$ receptor agonist, have been utilized to decrease TLESRs, thereby decreasing GERD.[195] Similar investigational drugs are in the pipeline and likely will reach clinical practice soon. A number of endoluminal therapies have been devised and tested to date, including endoscopically injected agents for bulking of the LES, endoluminal suturing or valvuloplasty, and radiofrequency energy application to the LES, though most have been withdrawn from the marketplace.[196]

Despite these notable recent failures, new devices continue to emerge and offer potential improvements over prior technologies. A transoral endoscopic fundoplication device (EsophyX, EndoGastric Solutions, Inc., Redmond, Washington) has been trialed in animal models and a limited number of human GERD patients.[197] Another device that creates an endoscopic, anterior partial fundoplication (Medigus SRS, Medigus, Ltd., Omer, Israel) has been tested in Europe, Australia, and India and is in early U.S. trials as of this time. Finally, magnetic augmentation of the LES via a laparoscopically placed ring of small magnets (TORAX Medical, Inc., Shoreview, Minnesota) is in clinical trials and offers the potential for a quick, highly reproducible, and effective means of chronic GERD control with low risk.[198] The long-term safety profile, as well as the symptomatic and objective success rates, of each of these devices awaits further study.

References

1. Patti MG, Gantert W, Way LW. Surgery of the esophagus; anatomy and physiology. *Surg Clin North Am* 1997;77:959.
2. Gray SW, Rowe JS Jr, Skandalakis JE. Surgical anatomy of the gastroesophageal junction. *Am Surg* 1979;45:575.
3. Dua KS, Ren J, Bardan E, et al. Coordination of deglutitive glottal function and pharyngeal bolus transport during normal eating. *Gastroenterology* 1997;112:73.
4. Pouderoux P, Shi G, Tatum RP, et al. Esophageal solid bolus transport; studies using concurrent videofluoroscopy and manometry. *Am J Gastroenterol* 1999;94:1457.
5. Pouderoux P, Lin S, Kahrilis PJ. Timing, propagation, coordination and effect of esophageal shortening during peristalsis. *Gastroenterology* 1997; 112:1147.
6. Mittal RK, Balaban DH. The esophagogastric junction. *N Engl J Med* 1997;336:924.
7. Clave P, Gonzalez A, Moreno A, et al. Endogenous cholecystokinin enhances postprandial gastroesophageal reflux in humans through extrasphincteric receptors. *Gastroenterology* 1998;115:597.
8. Vakil N, van Zanten SV, Kahrilas P, et al. The Montreal definition and classification of gastroesophageal reflux disease; a global evidence-based consensus. *Am J Gastroenterol* 2006;101:1900–1920.
9. Locke GR, Talley NJ, Fett SL, et al. Prevalence and clinical spectrum of gastroesophageal reflux; a population-based study in Olmsted County Minnesota. *Gastroenterology* 1997;112:1448.
10. Isolauri J, Laippala P. Prevalence of symptoms suggestive of gastroesophageal reflux disease in an adult population. *Ann Med* 1995;27: 67.
11. Sharma P, Wani S, Romero Y, et al. Racial and geographic issues in gastroesophageal reflux disease. *Am J Gastroenterol* 2008;103:2669–2680.
12. El-Serag H. Time trends of gastroesophageal reflux disease: a systematic review. *Clin Gastroenterol Hepatol* 2007;5:17–26.
13. Agency for Healthcare Research and Quality. Hospitalizations for problems caused by severe acid reflux increase by 103 percent. *AHRQ News and Numbers*. Rockville, MD: Agency for Healthcare Research and Quality; 2008. Available at: http://www.ahrq.gov/news/nn/nn010208.htm. Accessed January 2009.
14. El-Serag HB, Sonnenberg A. Opposing time trends of peptic ulcer and reflux disease. *Gut* 1998;43:327.
15. Panos MZ, Walt RP, Stevenson C, et al. Rising death rate from non-malignant disease of the oesophagus (NMOD) in England and Wales. *Gut* 1995;36:488.
16. Jacobson BC, Somers SC, Fuchs CS, et al. Body-mass index and symptoms of gastroesophageal reflux in women. *N Eng J Med* 2006;354:2340–2348.
17. Corely DA, Kubo A. Body mass index and gastroesophageal reflux disease: a systematic review and meta-analysis. *Am J Gastroenterol* 2006;108: 2619–2628.
18. Pandolfino JE, El-Serag HB, Zhang Q, et al. Obesity: a challenge to esophagogastric junction integrity. *Gastroenterology* 2006;130:639–649.
19. Edlestein ZR, Farrow DC, Bronner MP, et al. Central obesity and risk of Barrett's esophagus. *Gastroenterology* 2007;133:403–411.
20. Konturek JW. Discovery by Jaworski of Helicobacter pylori and its pathogenetic role in peptic ulcer, gastritis and gastric cancer. *J Physiol Pharmacol* 2003;54(suppl 3):23–41.
21. Marshall BJ, Warren JR. Unidentified curved bacilli in the stomach of patients with gastritis and peptic ulceration. *Lancet* 1984;1:1311–1315.
22. Labenz J, Blum AL, Bayerdorffer E, et al. Curing Helicobacter pylori infection in patients with duodenal ulcer may provoke reflux esophagitis. *Gastroenterology* 1997;112:1442–1447.
23. Bowrey DJ, Williams GT, Clark GW. Interactions between Helicobacter pylori and gastroesophageal reflux disease. *Dis Esophagus* 1998;11: 203–209.
24. Werdmuller BF, Loffeld RJ. Helicobacter pylori infection has no role in the pathogenesis of reflux esophagitis. *Dig Dis Sci* 1997;42:103–105.

25. Loffeld RJ, Ten Tije BJ, Arends JW. Prevalence and significance of Helicobacter pylori in patients with Barrett's esophagus. *Am J Gastroenterol* 1992;87:1598–1600.
26. Weel JF, van der Hulst RW, Gerrits Y, et al. The interrelationship between cytotoxin-associated gene A, vacuolating cytotoxin, and Helicobacter pylori-related diseases. *J Infect Dis* 1996;173:1171–1175.
27. Vicari JJ, Peek RM, Falk GW, et al. The seroprevalence of cagA-positive Helicobacter pylori strains in the spectrum of gastroesophageal reflux disease. *Gastroenterology* 1998;115:50–57.
28. Chow WH, Blaser MJ, Blot WJ, et al. An inverse relation between cagA+ strains of Helicobacter pylori infection and risk of esophageal and gastric cardia adenocarcinoma. *Cancer Res* 1998;58:588–590.
29. Labenz J, Nocon M, Lind T, et al. Prospective follow-up data for the ProGERD study suggest that GERD is not a categorical disease. *Am J Gastroenterol* 2006;101:2457–2462.
30. Monnier Ph, Ollyo JB, Fontolliet C, et al. Epidemiology and natural history of reflux esophagitis. *Semin Laparosc Surg* 1995;2:2.
31. Costantini M, Crookes PF, Bremner RM, et al. The value of physiologic assessment of foregut symptoms in a surgical practice. *Surgery* 1993;114:780.
32. Dodds WJ, Dent J, Hogan WJ, et al. Mechanisms of gastroesophageal reflux in patients with reflux esophagitis. *N Engl J Med* 1982;307:1547–1552.
33. Mittal RK, Holloway R, Dent J. Effect of atropine on the frequency of reflux and transient lower esophageal sphincter relaxation in normal subjects. *Gastroenterology* 1995;109:1547–1554.
34. Mittal RK, Hollaway RH, Penagini R, et al. Transient lower esophageal sphincter relaxation. *Gastroenterology* 1995;109:601–610.
35. Van Herwaarden MA, Samson M, Smout AJP. Excess gastroesophageal reflux in patients with hiatal hernia is caused by mechanisms other than transient LES relaxations. *Gastroenterology* 2000;119:1439–1446.
36. O'Sullivan GC, DeMeester TR, Joelsson BE, et al. The interaction of the lower esophageal sphincter pressure and length of sphincter in the abdomen as determinants of gastroesophageal competence. *Am J Surg* 1982;143:40.
37. Bonavina L, Evander A, DeMeester TR, et al. Length of the distal esophageal sphincter and competency of the cardia. *Am J Surg* 1986;151:25.
38. Zaninotto G, DeMeester TR, Schwizer W, et al. The lower esophageal sphincter in health and disease. *Am J Surg* 1988;155:104.
39. Stein HJ, Barlow AP, DeMeester TR, et al. Complications of gastroesophageal reflux disease: role of the lower esophageal sphincter, esophageal acid and acid/alkaline exposure, and duodenogastric reflux. *Ann Surg* 1992;216:35.
40. Kuster E, Ros E, Toledo-Pimentel V, et al. Predictive factors of the long term outcome in gastro-oesophageal reflux disease: six year follow up of 107 patients. *Gut* 1994;35:8.
41. Stein HJ, Eypasch EP, DeMeester TR, et al. Circadian esophageal motor function in patients with gastroesophageal reflux disease. *Surgery* 1990;108:769.
42. Cohen S, Harris LD. Does hiatus hernia affect competence of the gastroesophageal sphincter. *N Engl J Med* 1971;284:1053–1056.
43. Mittal RK, Fisher MJ. Electrical and mechanical inhibition of the crural diaphragm during transient relaxation of the lower esophageal sphincter. *Gastroenterology* 1990;99:1265–1268.
44. Hill LD, Kozarek RA, Kraemer SJM, et al. The gastroesophageal flap valve: in vitro and in vivo observations. *Gastrointest Endosc* 1996;44:541–547.
45 Oberg S, Peters JH, DeMeester TR, et al. Endoscopic grading of the gastroesophageal valve in patients with symptoms of gastroesophageal reflux disease (GERD). *Surg Endosc* 1999;13:1184–1188.
46. Ismail T, Bancewicz J, Barlow J. Yield pressure, anatomy of the cardia and gastroesophageal reflux. *Br J Surg* 1995;82:943.
47. Kahrilas PJ, Wu S, Shezhang L, et al. Attenuation of esophageal shortening during peristalsis with hiatus hernia. *Gastroenterology* 1995;109:1818–1825.
48. DeMeester TR, Ireland AP. Gastric pathology as an initiator and potentiator of gastroesophageal reflux disease. *Dis Esoph* 1997;10:1.
49. Bremner RM, Hoeft SF, Costantini M, et al. Pharyngeal swallowing: the major factor in clearance of esophageal reflux episodes. *Ann Surg* 1993;218:364.
50. Fletcher J, Wirz A, Young J, et al. Unbuffered highly acidic gastric juice exists at the gastroesophageal junction after a meal. *Gastroenterology* 2001;121:775.
51. Fletcher J, Wirz A, Henry E, et al. Studies of acid exposure immediately above the gastroesophageal squamocolumnar junction: evidence of short segment reflux. *Gut* 2004;53:168.
52. Iljima K, Henry E, Moriya A, et al. Dietary nitrate generates potentially mutagenic concentrations of nitric oxide at the gastroesophageal junction. *Gastroenterology* 2002;122:1248.
53. Lillimoe KD, Johnson LF, Harmon JW. Role of the components of the gastroduodenal contents in experimental acid esophagitis. *Surgery* 1982;92:276–284.
54. Lillimoe KD, Johnson LF, Harmon JW. Alkaline esophagitis: a comparison of the ability of components of gastroduodenal contents to injure the rabbit esophagus. *Gastroenterology* 1983;85:621–628.
55. Kauer WKH, Peters JH, DeMeester TR, et al. Mixed reflux of gastric juice is more harmful to the esophagus than gastric juice alone. The need for surgical therapy reemphasized. *Ann Surg* 1995;222:525–533.
56. El-Serag HB, Sonnenberg A. Comorbid occurrence of laryngeal or pulmonary disease with esophagitis in United States Military Veterans. *Gastroenterology* 1997;113:755–760.
57. Havemann BD, Henderson CA, El-Serag HB. The association between gastro-oesophageal reflux disease and asthma: a systematic review. *Gut* 2007;56:1654–1664.
58. Sontag SJ. The spectrum of pulmonary symptoms due to gastroesophageal reflux. *Thorac Surg Clin* 2005;15:353–368.
59. Blondeau K, Dupont L, Mertens V, et al. Gastroesophageal reflux and aspiration of gastric contents in adult patients with cystic fibrosis. *Gut* 2008;57:1049–1055.
60. Rascon-Aguilar IE, Pamer M, Wludyka P, et al. Role of gastroesophageal reflux symptoms in exacerbations of COPD. *Chest* 2006;130:1096–1101.
61. Hamelberg W, Bosomworth PP. Aspiration pneumonitis: experimental studies and clinical observations. *Anesth Analg Curr Res* 1964;170:74–86.
62. Greenfield LJ, Singleton RP, McCaffree DR, et al. Pulmonary effects of experimental graded aspiration of hydrochloric acid. *Ann Surg* 1969;170:74–86.
63. Glauser FL, Millen JE, Falls R. Effects of acid aspiration on pulmonary alveolar epithelial membrane permeability. *Chest* 1979;76:201–205.
64. Tuchman DN, Boyle JT, Pack AI, et al. Comparison of airway responses following tracheal or esophageal acidification in the cat. *Gastroenterology* 1984;87:872–881.
65. Pearson JE, Wilson RS. Diffuse pulmonary fibrosis and hiatus hernia. *Thorax* 1971;26:300–305.
66. Mays EE, Dubois JJ, Hamilton GB. Pulmonary fibrosis associated with tracheobronchial aspiration: a study of the frequency of hiatal hernia and gastroesophageal reflux in interstitial fibrosis of obscure etiology. *Chest* 1976;69:512–515.
67. Raiha I, Manner R, Hietanen E. Radiographic pulmonary changes of gastro-oesophageal reflux disease in elderly patients. *Age Ageing* 1992;21:250–255.
68. Tobin RW, Pope CE, Pellegrini CA. Increased prevalence of gastroesophageal reflux in patients with idiopathic pulmonary fibrosis. *Am J Respir Crit Care Med* 1988;158:1804–1808.
69. Kauer WK, Stein HJ, Möbius C, et al. Assessment of respiratory symptoms with dual pH monitoring in patients with gastro-oesophageal reflux disease. *Br J Surg* 2004;91:867–871.
70. Raghu G, Freudenberger TD, Yang S, et al. High prevalence of abnormal acid gastro-oesophageal reflux in idiopathic pulmonary fibrosis. *Eur Respir J* 2006;27:136–142.
71. Crowell MD, Zayat EN, Lacy BE, et al. The effects of an inhaled beta(2)-adrenergic agonist on lower esophageal function: a dose-response study. *Chest* 2001;120:1184–1189.
72. Mansfield LE, Hameister HH, Spaulding HS, et al. The role of the vagus nerve in airway narrowing caused by intraesophageal hydrochloric acid provocation and esophageal distention. *Ann Allergy* 1981;47:431–434.
73. Wright RA, Miller SA, Corsello BF. Acid-induced esophagobronchial-cardiac reflexes in humans. *Gastroenterology* 1990;99:71–73.
74. Schan CA, Harding SM, Haile JM, et al. Gastroesophageal reflux-induced bronchoconstriction. An intraesophageal acid infusion study using state-of-the-art technology. *Chest* 1994;106:731–737.
75. Sweet MP, Patti MG, Leard LE, et al. Gastroesophageal reflux in patients with idiopathic pulmonary fibrosis referred for lung transplantation. *J Thorac Cardiovasc Surg* 2007;133:1078–1084.
76. Sweet MP, Herbella FAM, Leard L, et al. The prevalence of distal and proximal gastroesophageal reflux in patients awaiting lung transplantation. *Ann Surg* 2006;244:491–497.
77. D'Ovidio F, Singer LG, Hadjiliadis D, et al. Prevalence of gastroesophageal reflux in end-stage lung disease candidates for lung transplant. *Ann Thoracic Surg* 2005;80:1254–1261.
78. Frank L, Kleinman L, Ganoczy D, et al. Upper gastrointestinal symptoms in North America: prevalence and relationship to healthcare utilization and quality of life. *Dig Dis Sci* 2000;45:809–818.
79. Jailawala JA, Shaker R. Oral and pharyngeal complications of gastroesophageal reflux disease: globus, dental erosions, and chronic sinusitis. *J Clin Gastroenterol* 2000;30(3 suppl):S35–S38.
80. Hungin AP, Raghunath AS, Wiklund I. Beyond heartburn: a systematic review of the extra-oesophageal spectrum of reflux-induced disease. *Fam Pract* 2005;22:591–603.
81. Levin TR, Sperling RM, McQuaid KR. Omeprazole improves peak expiratory flow rate and quality of life in asthmatics with gastroesophageal reflux. *Am J Gastroenterol* 1998;93:1060–1063.
82. Boeree MJ, Peters FTM, Postma DS, et al. No effects of high-dose omeprazole in patients with severe airway hyperresponsiveness and symptomatic gastro-oesophageal reflux. *Eur Respir J* 1998;11:1070–1074.
83. Harding SM, Richter JE, Guzzo MR, et al. Asthma and gastroesophageal reflux: acid suppressive therapy improves asthma outcome. *Am J Med* 1996;100:395–405.
84. Raghu G, Yang ST, Spada C, et al. Sole treatment of acid gastroesophageal reflux in idiopathic pulmonary fibrosis: a case series. *Chest* 2006;129:794–800.
85. Sontag SJ, O'Connell S, Khandelwal S, et al. Asthmatics with gastroesophageal reflux: long term results of a randomized trial of medical and surgical antireflux therapies. *Am J Gastroenterol* 2003;98:987–999.
86. Lau CL, Palmer SM, Howell DN, et al. Laparoscopic antireflux surgery in the lung transplant population. *Surg Endosc* 2002;16:1674–1678.

87. Linden PA, Gilbert RJ, Yeap BY, et al. Laparoscopic fundoplication in patients with end-stage lung disease awaiting transplantation. *J Thorac Cardiovasc Surg* 2006;131:438–446.
88. Patti MG, Tedesco P, Golden J, et al. Idiopathic pulmonary fibrosis: how often is it really idiopathic? *J Gastrointest Surg* 2005;9:1053–1056.
89. Fernando HC, El-Sherif A, Landreneau RJ, et al. Efficacy of laparoscopic fundoplication in controlling pulmonary symptoms associated with gastroesophageal reflux disease. *Surgery* 2005;138:612–616.
90. Spechler SJ. The columnar lined esophagus: history, terminology and clinical issues. *Gastroenterol Clin North Am* 1997;26:455–466.
91. Peters JH, Hagen JA, DeMeester SR. Barrett's esophagus. *J Gastrointest Surg* 2004;8:1–17.
92. Chandrasoma P. Norman Barrett: so close, yet 50 years away from the truth. *J Gastrointest Surg* 1999;3:7–14.
93. Campos GMR, DeMeester SR, Peters JH, et al. Predictive factors of Barrett's esophagus: multivariate analyses of 502 patients with GERD. *Arch Surg* 2001;136:1267–1273.
94. Kauer WK, Stein HJ. Bile reflux in the constellation of gastroesophageal reflux disease. *Thorac Surg Clin* 2005;15:335–340.
95. Katzka DA, Castell DO. Successful elimination of reflux symptoms does not insure adequate control of acid reflux in patients with Barrett's esophagus. *Am J Gastroenterol* 1994;89:989–991.
96. Ouatu-Lascar R, Triadafilopolous G. Complete elimination of reflux symptoms does not guarantee normalization of intraesophageal acid reflux in patients with Barrett's esophagus. *Am J Gastroenterol* 1998;93:711–716.
97. Sampliner RE, Fennerty B, Garewal HS. Reversal of Barrett's esophagus with acid suppression and multipolar electrocoagulation: preliminary results. *Gastrointest Endos* 1996;44:532–535.
98. Hofstetter WA, Peters JH, DeMeester TR, et al. Long term outcome of antireflux surgery in patients with Barrett's esophagus. *Ann Surg* 2001;234:532–539.
99. Lord RV, DeMeester SR, Peters JH, et al. Hiatal hernia, lower esophageal sphincter incompetence, and effectiveness of Nissen fundoplication in the spectrum of gastroesophageal reflux disease. *J Gastrointest Surg* 2009;13:602–610.
100. Farrell TM, Smith CD, Metreveli RE, et al. Fundoplication provides effective and durable symptom relief in patients with Barrett's esophagus. *Am J Surg* 1999;178:18–21.
101. Oelschlager BK, Barreca M, Chang L, et al. Clinical and pathologic response of Barrett's esophagus to laparoscopic antireflux surgery. *Ann Surg* 2003;238:458–466.
102. Mehta S, Bennett J, Mahon D, et al. Prospective trial of laparoscopic Nissen fundoplication versus proton pump inhibitor therapy for gastroesophageal reflux disease: seven-year follow-up. *J Gastrointest Surg* 2006;10:1312–1316.
103. Dallemagne B, Weerts J, Markiewicz S, et al. Clinical results of laparoscopic fundoplication at ten years after surgery. *Surg Endosc* 2006;20:159–165.
104. Morgenthal CB, Shane MD, Stival A, et al. The durability of laparoscopic Nissen fundoplication: 11-year outcomes. *J Gastrointest Surg* 2007;11:693–700.
105. Wijnhoven BP, Lally CJ, Kelly JJ, et al. Use of antireflux medication after antireflux surgery. *J Gastrointest Surg* 2008;12:510–517.
106. Lurje G, Vallbohmer D, Collet PH, et al. COX-2 mRNA expression is significantly increased in acid-exposed compared to nonexposed squamous epithelium in gastroesophageal reflux disease. *J Gastrointest Surg* 2007;11:1105–1111.
107. Vallböhmer D, DeMeester SR, Oh DS, et al. Antireflux surgery normalizes cyclooxygenase-2 expression in squamous epithelium of the distal esophagus. *Am J Gastroenterol* 2006;101:1458–1466.
108. Oh DS, DeMeester SR, Vallböhmer D, et al. Reduction of interleukin 8 gene expression in reflux esophagitis and Barrett's esophagus with antireflux surgery. *Arch Surg* 2007;142:554–559.
109. Weston AP, Sharma P, Topalovski M, et al. Long term follow-up Barrett's high grade dysplasia. *Am J Gastroenterol* 2000;95:1888–1893.
110. Overholt BF, Panjehpour M, Halberg DL. Photodynamic therapy for Barrett's esophagus with dysplasia and/or early stage carcinoma; long term results. *Gastrointest Endosc* 2003;58:183–188.
111. Pacifico RJ, Wang KK, Wongkeesong LM, et al. Combined endoscopic mucosal resection and photodynamic therapy versus esophagectomy for management of early adenocarcinoma in Barrett's esophagus. *Clin Gastroenterol Hepatol* 2003;1:252–257.
113. Seewald S, Akaraviputh T, Seitz U, et al. Circumferential EMR and complete removal of Barrett's epithelium: a new approach to management of Barrett's esophagus containing high-grade intraepithelial neoplasia and intramucosal carcinoma. *Gastrointest Endosc* 2003;57:854–859.
114. Pech O, Behrens A, May A, et al. Long-term results and risk factor analysis for recurrence after curative endoscopic therapy in 349 patients with high-grade intraepithelial neoplasia and mucosal adenocarcinoma in Barrett's oesophagus. *Gut* 2008;57:1200–1206.
115. Pouw RE, Gondrie JJ, Sondermeijer CM, et al. Eradication of Barrett esophagus with early neoplasia by radiofrequency ablation, with or without endoscopic resection. *J Gastrointest Surg* 2008;12:1627–1636.
116. Ell C, May A, Gossner L, et al. Endoscopic mucosal resection of early cancer and high-grade dysplasia in Barrett's esophagus. *Gastroenterology* 2000;118:670–677.
117. Pech O, May A, Rabenstein T, et al. Endoscopic resection of early oesophageal cancer. *Gut* 2007;56:1625–1634.
118. Ell C, May A, Pech O, et al. Curative endoscopic resection of early esophageal adenocarcinomas (Barrett's cancer). *Gastrointest Endosc* 2007;65:3–10.
119. Peters JH, Clark GWB, Ireland AP, et al. Outcome of adenocarcinoma arising in Barrett's esophagus in endoscopically surveyed and non-surveyed patients. *J Thorac Cardiovasc Surg* 1994;108:813–822.
120. Altorki NK, Sunagawa M, Little AG, et al. High-grade dysplasia in the columnar-lined esophagus. *Am J Surg* 1991;161:99–100.
121. Pera M, Trastek VF, Carpenter HA, et al. Barrett's esophagus with high grade dysplasia: an indication for esophagectomy. *Ann Thorac Surg* 1992;54:199–204.
122. Ferguson MK, Naunheim KS. Resection for Barrett's mucosa with high-grade dysplasia: implications for prophylactic photodynamic therapy. *J Thorac Cardiovasc Surg* 1997;114:824–829.
123. www.drugs.com. Accessed September 12, 2006.
124. www.rxlist.com. Accessed September 12, 2006.
125. Sandmark S, Carlsson R, Fausa O, et al. Omeprazole or ranitidine in the treatment of reflux esophagitis. *Scand J Gastroenterol* 1988;23:625.
126. Katzka DA, Paoletti V, Leite L, et al. Prolonged ambulatory pH monitoring in patients with persistent gastroesophageal reflux disease symptoms: testing while on therapy identifies the need for more aggressive anti-reflux therapy. *Am J Gastroenterol* 1996;91:2110.
127. Peghini PL, Katz PO, Bracy NA, et al. Nocturnal recovery of gastric acid secretion with twice-daily dosing of proton pump inhibitors. *Am J Gastroenterol* 1998;93:763.
128. Laheij RJF, Sturkenboom MCJM, Hassing R-J, et al. Risk of community-acquired pneumonia and use of gastric acid-suppressive drugs. *JAMA* 2004;292:1955–1960.
129. Yang Y-X, Lewis JD, Epstein S, et al. Long-term proton pump inhibitor therapy and the risk of hip fracture. *JAMA* 2006;296:2947–2953.
130. Roux C, Briot K, Gossec L, et al. Increase in vertebral fracture risk in postmenopausal women using omeprazole. *Calcif Tissue Int* 2009;84:13–19.
131. Targownik LE, Lix LM, Metge CJ, et al. Use of proton pump inhibitors and risk of osteoporosis-related fractures. *CMAJ* 2008;179:319–326.
132. Campos GM, Peters JH, DeMeester TR, et al. The pattern of esophageal acid exposure in GERD influences the severity of the disease. *Arch Surg* 1999;134:882.
133. Finks JF, Wei Y, Birkmeyer JD. The rise and fall of antireflux surgery in the United States. *Surg Endosc* 2006;20:1698–1701.
134. Campos GMR, Peters JH, DeMeester TR, et al. Multivariate analysis of the factors predicting outcome after laparoscopic Nissen fundoplication. *J Gastrointest Surg* 1999;3:292–300.
135. Hill LD, Kozarek RA, Kraemer SJM, et al. The gastroesophageal flap valve. In vitro and in vivo observations. *Gastrointest Endosc* 1996;44:541.
136. Miller FA. Utilization of inlying pH-probe for evaluation of acid-peptic diathesis. *Arch Surg* 1964;89:199.
137. Johnson LF, DeMeester TR. Development of the 24-hour intraesophageal pH monitoring composite scoring system. *J Clin Gastroenterol.* 1986;8(suppl 1):52.
138. Jamieson JR, Stein HJ, DeMeester TR, et al. Ambulatory 24-h esophageal pH monitoring: normal values, optimal thresholds, specificity, sensitivity, and reproducibility. *Am J Gastroenterol* 1992;87:1102.
139. Pandolfino JE, Richter JE, Ours T, et al. Ambulatory esophageal pH monitoring using a wireless system. *Am J Gastroenterol* 2003;98:740–749.
140. Wenner J, Johansson J, Johnsson F, et al. Optimal thresholds and discriminatory power of 48-h wireless esophageal pH monitoring in the diagnosis of GERD. *Am J Gastroenterol* 2007;102:1862–1869.
141. Tutuian R, Vela MF, Shay SS, et al. Multichannel intraluminal impedance in esophageal function testing and gastroesophageal reflux monitoring. *J Clin Gastroenterol* 2003;37:206–215.
142. Vela MF, Camacho-Lobato L, Srinivasan R, et al. Simultaneous intraesophageal impedance and pH measurement of acid and nonacid gastroesophageal reflux: effect of omeprazole. *Gastroenterology* 2001;120:1599–1606.
143. Mainie I, Tutuian R, Agrawal A, et al. Combined multichannel intraluminal impedance-pH monitoring to select patients with persistent gastro-oesophageal reflux for laparoscopic Nissen fundoplication. *Br J Surg* 2006;93:1483–1487.
144. Gruebel C, Linke G, Tutuian R, et al. Prospective study examining the impact of multichannel intraluminal impedance on antireflux surgery. *Surg Endosc* 2008;22:1241–1247.
145. Gastal OL, Hagen JA, Peters JH, et al. Short esophagus: analysis of predictors and clinical implications. *Arch Surg* 1999;134:633.
146. Ritter MP, Peters JH, DeMeester TR, et al. Treatment of advanced gastroesophageal reflux disease with Collis gastroplasty and Belsey partial fundoplication. *Arch Surg* 1998;133:523.
147. DeMeester SR, Sillin LF, Lin HW, et al. Increasing esophageal length: a comparison of laparoscopic versus transthoracic esophageal mobilization with and without vagal trunk division in pigs. *J Am Coll Surg* 2003;197:558.
148. Stein HJ, Feussner H, Siewart JR. Failure of antireflux surgery: causes and management. *Am J Surg* 1996;171:36.
149. Johnson WE, Hagen JA, DeMeester TR, et al. Outcome of respiratory symptoms after antireflux surgery on patients with gastroesophageal reflux disease. *Arch Surg* 1996;131:489.
150. Salvador R, Dubecz A, Polomsky M, et al. A new era in esophageal diagnostics: the image-based paradigm of high-resolution manometry. *J Am Coll Surg* 2009;208:1034–1044.

151. Schwizer W, Hinder RA, DeMeester TR. Does delayed gastric emptying contribute to gastroesophageal reflux disease? *Am J Surg* 1989;157:74.
152. Salvador R, Watson TJ, Herbella F, et al. Association of gastroesophageal reflux and O2 desaturation: a novel study of simultaneous 24-h MII-pH and continuous pulse oximetry. *J Gastrointest Surg* 2009;13:854–861.
153. Potluri S, Friedenberg F, Parkman HP, et al. Comparison of a salivary/sputum pepsin assay with 24-hour esophageal pH monitoring for detection of gastric reflux into the proximal esophagus, oropharynx, and lung. *Dig Dis Sci* 2003;48:1813–1817.
154. Johnston N, Knight J, Dettmar PW, et al. Pepsin and carbonic anhydrase isoenzyme III as diagnostic markers for laryngopharyngeal reflux disease. *Laryngoscope* 2004;114:2129–2134.
155. Kim TH, Lee KJ, Yeo M, et al. Pepsin detection in the sputum/saliva for the diagnosis of gastroesophageal reflux disease in patients with clinically suspected atypical gastroesophageal reflux disease symptoms. *Digestion* 2008;77:201–206.
156. Watson DI, Jamieson GG, Pike GK, et al. Prospective randomized double-blind trial between laparoscopic Nissen and anterior partial fundoplication. *Br J Surg* 1999;86:123.
157. Laws HL, Clements RH, Swillie CM. A randomized, prospective comparison of the Nissen fundoplication versus the Toupet fundoplication for gastroesophageal reflux disease. *Ann Surg* 1997;225:647.
158. Hagedorn C, Lonroth H, Rydberg L, et al. Long-term efficacy of total (Nissen-Rossetti) and posterior partial (Toupet) fundoplication: results of a randomized clinical trial. *J Gastrointest Surg* 2002;6:540.
159. Cai W, Watson DI, Lally CJ, et al. Ten-year clinical outcome of a prospective randomized clinical trial of laparoscopic Nissen versus anterior 180° partial fundoplication. *Br J Surg* 2008;95:1501–1505.
160. Jobe BA, Wallace J, Hansen PD, et al. Evaluation of laparoscopic Toupet fundoplication as a primary repair for all patients with medically resistant gastroesophageal reflux. *Surg Endosc* 1997;11:1080.
161. Bell RC, Hanna P, Mills MR, et al. Patterns of success and failure with laparoscopic partial fundoplication. *Surg Endosc* 1999;13:1189.
161. Patti MG, Robinson T, Galvani C, et al. Total fundoplication is superior to partial fundoplication even when esophageal peristalsis is weak. *J Am Coll Surg* 2004;198:863.
162. Horvath KD, Jobe BA, Herron DM, et al. Laparoscopic Toupet is an inadequate procedure for patients with severe reflux disease. *J Gastrointest Surg* 1999;3:583.
163. Watson DI, Pike GK, Baigrie RJ, et al. Prospective double-blind randomized trial of laparoscopic Nissen fundoplication with division and without division of short gastric vessels. *Ann Surg* 1997;226:642.
164. Dalenbäck J, Lönroth H, Blomqvist A, et al. Improved functional outcome after laparoscopic fundoplication by complete gastric fundus mobilization. *Gastroenterology* 1998;114:A1384.
165. Hunter JG, Swanstrom L, Waring JP. Dysphagia after laparoscopic antireflux surgery. The impact of operative technique. *Ann Surg* 1996;224:51.
166. Watson DI, Jamieson GG, Devitt PG, et al. Paraoesophageal hiatus hernia: an important complication of laparoscopic Nissen fundoplication. *Br J Surg* 1995;82:521.
167. Terry ML, Vernon A, Hunter JG. Stapled-wedge Collis gastroplasty for the shortened esophagus. *Am J Surg* 2004;188:195.
168. Carlson MA, Frantzides CT. Complications and results of primary minimally invasive antireflux procedures: a review of 10,735 reported cases. *J Am Coll Surg* 2001;193:429.
169. Hinder RA, Filipi CJ, Wetscher G, et al. Laparoscopic Nissen fundoplication is an effective treatment for gastroesophageal reflux disease. *Ann Surg* 1994;220:472.
170. Peters JH, DeMeester TR, Crookes P, et al. The treatment of gastroesophageal reflux disease with laparoscopic Nissen fundoplication. Prospective evaluation of 100 patients with "typical" symptoms. *Ann Surg* 1998;228:40.
171. DeMeester TR, Bonavina L, Albertucci M. Nissen fundoplication for gastroesophageal reflux disease—evaluation of primary repair in 100 consecutive patients. *Ann Surg* 1986;204:9.
172. Bammer T, Hinder RA, Klaus A, et al. Five- to eight-year outcome of the first laparoscopic Nissen fundoplications. *J Gastrointest Surg* 2001; 5:42.
173. Granderath FA, Kamolz T, Schweiger UM, et al. Long-term results of laparoscopic antireflux surgery: surgical outcomes and analysis of failure after 500 laparoscopic antireflux procedures. *Surg Endosc* 2002;16: 753.
174. Catarci M, Gentileschi P, Papi C, et al. Evidence-based appraisal of antireflux fundoplication. *Ann Surg* 2004;239:325.
175. Lundell L, Miettinen P, Myrvold HE, et al. Continued (5-year) follow-up of a randomized clinical study comparing antireflux surgery and omeprazole in gastroesophageal reflux disease. *J Am Coll Surg* 2001; 192:172.
176. Nilsson G, Wenner J, Larsson S, et al. Randomized clinical trial of laparoscopic versus open fundoplication for gastroesophageal reflux. *Br J Surg* 2004;91:552.
177. Finlayson SRG, Laycock WS, Birkmeyer JD. National trends in utilization and outcomes of antireflux surgery. *Surg Endosc* 2003;17:864.
178. So JB, Zeitels SM, Rattner DW. Outcomes of atypical symptoms attributed to gastroesophageal reflux treated by laparoscopic fundoplication. *Surgery* 1998;124:28.
179. Lundell L, Miettinen P, Myrvold HE, et al. Seven-year follow-up of a randomized clinical trial comparing proton-pump inhibition with surgical therapy for reflux oesophagitis. *Br J Surg* 2007;94:198–203.
180. Mehta S, Bennett J, Mahon D, et al. Prospective trial of laparoscopic Nissen fundoplication versus proton pump inhibitor therapy for gastroesophageal reflux disease: seven-year follow-up. *J Gastrointest Surg* 2006;10:1312–1317.
181. Lundell L, Attwood SE, Ell C, et al. Comparing laparoscopic antireflux surgery with esomeprazole in the management of patients with chronic gastro-oesophageal reflux disease: a 3-year interim analysis of the LOTUS trial. *Gut* 2008;57:1207–1213.
182. Spechler SJ. Comparison of medical and surgical therapy for complicated gastroesophageal reflux disease in veterans. The Department of Veterans Affairs Gastroesophageal Reflux Disease Study Group. *N Engl J Med* 1992;326:786.
183. Spechler SJ, Lee E, Ahnen D, et al. Long-term outcome of medical and surgical therapies for gastroesophageal reflux disease: follow-up of a randomized controlled trial. *JAMA* 2001;285:2331.
184. Lord RVN, Kaminski A, Oberg S, et al. Absence of gastroesophageal reflux disease in a majority of patients taking acid suppression medications after Nissen fundoplication. *J Gastrointest Surg* 2002;6:3.
185. Testa MA, Simonson DC. Assessment of quality-of-life outcomes. *N Engl J Med* 1996;334:835.
186. Trus TL, Laycock WS, Waring JP, et al. Improvement in quality of life measures following laparoscopic antireflux surgery. *Ann Surg* 1999;229: 331.
187. Glise H, Hallerbäck B, Johansson B. Quality-of-life assessments in evaluation of laparoscopic Rosetti fundoplication. *Surg Endosc* 1995;9:183.
188. Velonovich V, Vallance SR, Gusz JR, et al. Quality of life scale for gastroesophageal reflux disease. *J Am Coll Surg* 1996;183:217.
189. Fernando HC, Schauer PR, Rosenblatt M, et al. Quality of life after antireflux surgery compared with nonoperative management for severe gastroesophageal reflux disease. *J Am Coll Surg* 2002;194:23.
190. Polomsky M, Siddall KA, Salvador R, et al. Association of kyphosis and spinal skeletal abnormalities with intrathoracic stomach: a link toward understanding its pathogenesis. *J Am Coll Surg* 2009;208:562–569.
191. Hashemi M, Peters JH, DeMeester TR, et al. Laparoscopic repair of large type III hiatal hernia: objective follow-up reveals high recurrence rate. *J Am Coll Surg* 2000;190:553–560.
192. Salminen PTP, Hiekkanen HI, Rantala APT, et al. Comparison of long-term outcome of laparoscopic and conventional Nissen fundoplication: a prospective randomized study with an 11-year follow-up. *Ann Surg* 2007;246:201–206.
193. Oelschlager BK, Pellegrini CA, Hunter J, et al. Biologic prosthesis reduces recurrence after laparoscopic paraesophageal hernia repair: a multicenter, prospective, randomized trial. *Ann Surg* 2006;244:481–490.
194. Pierre AF, Luketich JD, Fernando HC, et al. Results of laparoscopic repair of giant paraesophageal hernias: 200 consecutive patients. *Ann Thorac Surg* 2002;74:1909–1916.
195. Rosen R, Nurko S, Furuta GT. Impeding gastroesophageal refluxate: a new application of an old medication. *Gastroenterology* 2003;125: 984–985.
196. Watson TJ, Peters JH. Lower esophageal sphincter injections for the treatment of gastroesophageal reflux disease. *Thorac Surg Clin* 2005;15:405–415.
197. Jobe BA, O'Rourke RW, McMahon BP, et al. Transoral endoscopic fundoplication in the treatment of gastroesophageal reflux disease: the anatomic and physiologic basis for reconstruction of the esophagogastric junction using a novel device. *Ann Surg* 2008;248:69–76.
198. Bonavina L, Saino GI, Bona D, et al. Magnetic augmentation of the lower esophageal sphincter: results of a feasibility clinical trial. *J Gastrointest Surg* 2008;12:2133–2140.

CHAPTER 42 ■ ESOPHAGUS: TUMORS AND INJURY

PHILIP A. RASCOE, JOHN C. KUCHARCZUK, AND LARRY R. KAISER

KEY POINTS

1. The high fat content of the esophageal submucosa leads to mobility of the overlying mucosa; therefore, care must be taken that every anastomotic suture transfixes the submucosa to prevent anastomotic leak.
2. The incidence of esophageal perforation has increased over recent decades due to the increasing use of invasive endoscopic procedures, such that iatrogenic injury by instrumentation accounts for more than 50% of all cases.
3. The management of esophageal perforation is dictated by the location and extent of the perforation, the clinical condition of the patient, and the presence or absence of underlying esophageal pathology.
4. Perforations of the upper third of the esophagus down to the level of the carina are treated by cervical drainage, most commonly via a left neck incision.
5. The management of an esophageal perforation associated with endoscopic dilatation for achalasia includes primary repair of the injury, a vertical esophageal myotomy performed 180 degrees opposite the injury, and a noncircumferential wrap such as a Belsey fundoplication.
6. The incidence of esophageal adenocarcinoma in the United States has increased in the last 25 years greater than the incidence of any other major malignancy.
7. The goal of surgical resection for esophageal cancer is cure, as effective palliation can be obtained with chemotherapy, radiation therapy, and endoscopic interventions such as stenting and laser fulguration.
8. Data concerning improved survival following neoadjuvant chemotherapy and radiation for esophageal cancer are inconclusive and must be considered in light of the associated toxicity of multimodality therapy.
9. Advantages of transhiatal esophagectomy are less surgical trauma by avoidance of a thoracotomy and placement of the anastomosis in the neck, which minimizes the morbidity of an anastomotic leak.
10. The intent of palliation of unresectable esophageal cancer is to maintain comfort, restore swallowing function if possible, and support nutrition.

The role of the esophagus is to propel food and secretions from the pharynx to the stomach. As such, it is primarily an organ of motility with no absorptive capacity. It also provides an important barrier function, isolating the mediastinum from the bacteria present in the mouth and external environment.

The esophageal anatomy is discussed in the previous chapter. Nevertheless, several specific anatomic points need to be highlighted when discussing surgery for injuries and tumors of the esophagus. First, indentations made on the esophagus by external mediastinal structures are clinically important. These indentations can be seen readily on esophagram (Fig. 42.1). The cricopharyngeus causes the first constriction of the esophagus and is a common location for iatrogenic perforations caused by instrumentation. The second indentation seen to the left of the esophagus is the aortic arch, which is a common location for food or foreign body impaction. The third indentation is the left mainstem bronchus.

In the adult, esophageal length is variable depending on upper body length. Nevertheless, the overall average length from the upper esophageal sphincter to the lower one approximates 24 cm or 10 inches. Because endoscopy plays an important role in the localization of esophageal injuries and tumors, esophageal locations are usually referenced relative to the distance from the incisors. Thus, on average, the esophagus begins at 16 cm from the incisors and ends at 38 to 40 cm from the incisors.

Externally, the esophagus is composed of an outer layer of longitudinal muscle and an inner layer of circular muscle. There is no serosal layer as ensheathes all other parts of the gastrointestinal tract. Transmural invasion by esophageal carcinoma is common because the tumor is not limited by overlying serosa or pleura. This is in contrast to other gastrointestinal cancers, which usually extend to, but not through, the peritoneum. (1) Another important anatomic feature of the esophagus is the unique submucosal layer. This layer has a high fat content, which accounts for the mobility of the overlying mucosa. Because of this arrangement, care must be taken to ensure that every anastomotic suture transfixes the submucosa; if it does not "an anastomotic leak will occur when the mucosa retracts proximally and an accurate apposition of the mucosa is not achieved."[1]

The esophageal blood supply is segmental. The esophagus is vascularized by numerous arteries coursing through the lateral attachments, and it has an extensive submucosal collateral circulation. The cervical esophagus receives blood from the superior and inferior thyroid arteries. Multiple aortic esophageal arteries supply the intrathoracic esophagus and through collaterals connect with the inferior thyroid, intercostal, bronchial, inferior phrenic, and left gastric arteries. Improper control of these vessels during a transhiatal esophagectomy can result in significant blood loss.

The intramural lymphatic network of the esophagus is predominantly located within the submucosa. However, there are lymphatic channels within the lamina propria of the mucosa. This explains the occasional presence of nodal metastasis arising from superficial cancers.

The esophagus is innervated by the autonomic nervous system. The cervical esophagus receives parasympathetic innervation through the recurrent laryngeal branches of the vagus nerve. Thus, injury to the recurrent laryngeal nerve not only produces hoarseness and a poor cough but may also result in upper esophageal sphincter dysfunction predisposing to life-threatening aspiration following esophagectomy.

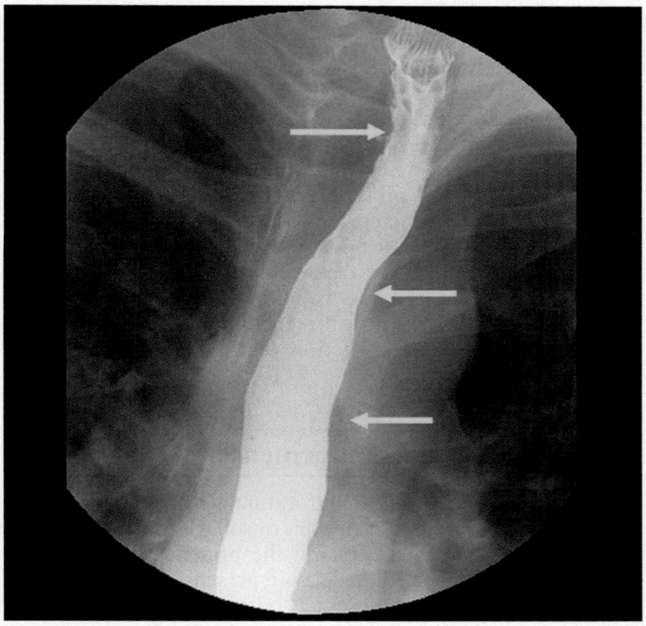

FIGURE 42.1. Barium contrast esophagography showing the constriction caused by the cricopharyngeal muscle, aortic arch, and the left mainstem bronchus. Indentations of the esophagus made by external structures are important anatomic landmarks and are often the sites of perforation due to instrumentation.

SURGICAL APPROACHES TO THE ESOPHAGUS

Multiple factors influence the surgical approach to the esophagus. These include the nature of the injury or neoplasm (benign vs. malignant), the overall health of the patient, and the expertise of the surgeon.

A complete working knowledge of the anatomic relationships between the esophagus and adjacent structures is vital to planning surgical therapy. The upper thoracic esophagus is in contact with the posterior membranous trachea, the left mainstem bronchus, and the aortic arch. Patients with cancers involving the upper thoracic esophagus must undergo preoperative bronchoscopy to rule out invasion of the posterior membranous trachea, because this precludes resection. Although flexible bronchoscopy may demonstrate gross airway invasion, rigid bronchoscopy is much more sensitive in determining adherence to the membranous trachea. Loss of the normal ripple effect as the rigid scope slides over the membranous trachea suggests the tumor is fixed to the airway and is not resectable. This is equally important where the esophagus passes under the left mainstem bronchus.

From a surgical perspective, the esophagus is divided into thirds. The upper third can be reached through a cervical incision. The middle third is best approached through the right chest, as access to the middle third of the esophagus from the left chest is obscured by the aorta. The distal third of the esophagus is best approached through the left chest. The short segment of intra-abdominal esophagus may be approached through the upper abdomen.

When esophagectomy is required, several surgical approaches have been described. These include the transhiatal approach,[2] the transabdominal transthoracic approach (Ivor Lewis),[3] the three-stage or "three-hole" approach (McKeown),[4] the thoracoabdominal approach, and the minimally invasive approach. Each approach has its own set of risks and benefits as well as outspoken opponents and proponents. Selection of the appropriate approach requires experienced surgical judgment. Despite the rhetoric, several studies have shown equivalent outcomes among the multiple approaches. It appears that the experience of the surgeon[5] and the number of cases performed at a particular institution are the leading factors determining outcome.[6] Clearly, failures in technique that occur during the performance of an esophagectomy are associated with increased length of hospital stay and increased in-hospital mortality and are predictive of a poorer overall long-term survival.[7]

ESOPHAGEAL INJURY

Perforation

Despite decades of clinical experience and surgical innovation, perforation of the esophagus continues to present diagnostic and therapeutic challenges. Accurate diagnosis and early treatment are essential to the successful management of patients with esophageal perforation. Outcome is determined by the cause and location of the injury, the presence of concomitant esophageal disease, and the interval between perforation and initiation of therapy.

The causes of esophageal perforation are listed in Table 42.1. Over the past decade, the incidence of esophageal perforation 2 has increased, and the most common etiology has become iatrogenic, due to the increasing use of invasive diagnostic and therapeutic endoscopic procedures. In our review of the literature, we found that iatrogenic injury to the esophagus by instrumentation accounted for 59% of all cases and spontaneous perforations accounted for only 15%.[8]

Other, less common injuries include foreign body ingestion (12%) and trauma (9%). Ingestion of foreign bodies or caustic materials can produce perforation most commonly in areas of anatomic narrowing including the cricopharyngeus, the segment where the aortic arch and left mainstem bronchus impinge on the esophagus, and at the distal esophageal sphincter. External penetrating trauma causes perforations mainly in the cervical esophagus, the portion not protected by the

TABLE 42.1 **ETIOLOGY**

CAUSES OF ESOPHAGEAL PERFORATION

INSTRUMENTAL
Endoscopy
Dilation
Intubation
Sclerotherapy
Laser therapy
NONINSTRUMENTAL
Barogenic trauma
Postemetic (Boerhaave syndrome)
Blunt chest or abdominal trauma
Other (e.g., labor, convulsions, defecation)
Penetrating neck, chest, or abdominal trauma
Operative trauma
Esophageal reconstruction (anastomotic disruption)
Vagotomy, pulmonary resection, hiatal hernia repair, esophagomyotomy
Corrosive injuries (acid or alkali ingestion)
Erosion by adjacent infection
Swallowed foreign body

HEAD AND NECK

thoracic cage. The morbidity and mortality of penetrating esophageal trauma is usually the result of the associated injuries including major vascular and airway injuries.[9] Blunt traumatic perforation is exceedingly rare but may be evident following motor vehicle accident or performance of the Heimlich maneuver.

Spontaneous, or barogenic, esophageal perforation results from a sudden increase in intraesophageal pressure. This has been associated with hyperemesis, childbirth, seizure, prolonged coughing, or weightlifting. Of special historical note are patients with Boerhaave syndrome. These patients develop perforation of the distal esophagus after the excessive ingestion of food and alcohol followed by violent emesis resulting in disruption of the distal esophagus with soilage into the left pleural cavity. This syndrome is named after Herman Boerhaave who, in 1723, provided a detailed account with postmortem correlation of the esophageal perforation of the High Admiral of the Dutch Navy, Baron Van Wassenaer.[10] The admiral had attempted to relieve his postprandial discomfort by self-induced vomiting after having feasted richly on roast duck and beer.

Clinical Features

The presenting clinical features of esophageal perforation depend on the location of the perforation and the time interval between injury and presentation. Patients with cervical perforations generally present with cervical dysphagia, neck pain, dysphonia, and subcutaneous cervical emphysema. This is in distinction to patients with intrathoracic perforations, who often present with signs and symptoms of mediastinitis. These include tachycardia, tachypnea, fever, and leukocytosis. Perforations of the intra-abdominal esophagus result in soilage of the peritoneal cavity and present as an acute abdomen. As with thoracic perforations, patients present with tachycardia, tachypnea, fever, and leukocytosis. Systemic sepsis, rapid deterioration, and shock are common.

Diagnosis

The diagnosis of esophageal perforation begins with a high level of suspicion. Esophageal perforation must be ruled out in any patient presenting with cervical, thoracic, or abdominal pain following endoscopy. Contrast esophagography remains the gold standard for diagnosis, as it both confirms the diagnosis and localizes the site of perforation. Water-soluble contrast (e.g., Gastrografin) is the initial agent used for contrast esophagography. These agents demonstrate extravasation in 50% of cervical perforations and 80% of perforations located within the chest.[11] If no extravasation is seen with Gastrografin, thin barium should be used because it will demonstrate 60% of cervical perforations and 90% of intrathoracic perforations.[12] In patients with known or suspected aspiration risk, or in cases of suspected airway-esophageal fistula, barium contrast should be used alone because the hyperosmolar water-soluble contrast agents may cause rapid pulmonary edema and ventilatory collapse.

Flexible esophagoscopy may be used to directly visualize and localize the area of perforation. It has a sensitivity of 100% and a specificity of 80%.[13] Proponents of flexible esophagoscopy use this technique for confirmation of the injury and in planning the surgical approach. Opponents of this practice argue that air insufflation enlarges the injury and results in further bacterial contamination. One particular case that warrants special discussion is a mucosal or submucosal tear without perforation. Clearly, endoscopy is contraindicated in these patients as air insufflation may convert this to a full-thickness injury, thus converting a problem that could be managed conservatively to one that requires surgical intervention. We routinely perform flexible endoscopy in the operating room for localization in patients requiring operative management of their perforation. In the small subset of patients who will be treated conservatively, we avoid the practice.

Computed tomography (CT) scan is useful in localizing collections in the pleural space or mediastinum; it is not used to localize the primary site of perforation. We do not generally obtain this study on presentation, although many patients have this study performed prior to surgical consultation. Commonly, the recognition of pneumomediastinum on a CT scan obtained in the emergency department prompts surgical consultation. However, the real value of CT scanning is in the patient who remains septic following drainage and repair. The CT scan may reveal a collection requiring percutaneous or operative drainage.

Management

3 The treatment of esophageal perforation is dictated by the location of the perforation, the amount of soilage present, the clinical condition of the patient, and the presence of underlying esophageal pathology. While delay in presentation is associated with increased mortality, it is not a contraindication to definitive surgical repair. The goal of treatment is to stabilize the patient, stop ongoing soilage, control infection, and reestablish esophageal continuity. Our current protocol for management of esophageal perforations is outlined in Algorithm 42.1.

Nonoperative Treatment. In practice, only a very small subset of patients with esophageal perforation are appropriate for nonoperative treatment. The successful use of nonoperative therapy requires careful patient selection, sound surgical judgment, and repeated clinical evaluation. Because the stakes are so high, it must be recognized that operative treatment really is the more conservative approach. Selecting the wrong patient or making a poor judgment will lead to local complications, continued sepsis, and a potentially devastating outcome.

The first reported series of nonoperative treatment of esophageal perforation appeared in 1965 and included 18 patients with instrument perforations of the thoracic esophagus; there was only one death.[14] In 1979, Cameron et al.[15] established a set of criteria to aid in the selection of patients for nonoperative management. Currently, nonoperative management is appropriate for the treatment of all intramural dissections without evidence of frank full-thickness perforation. For transmural perforations, however, the approach can be considered only if (a) the perforation is well contained, (b) there is no associated esophageal malignancy, (c) the perforation is not in the abdominal cavity, (d) there is no simultaneous obstructive esophageal disease, and (e) there are no signs or symptoms of systemic sepsis.[16]

Nonoperative management begins with the administration of broad-spectrum antibiotics, the suspension of oral intake, and the institution of alternative nutrition either parenterally or enterally via a gastric or jejunal feeding tube. Vigilant monitoring for fever, tachycardia, and leukocytosis is necessary, as these findings are indicative of impending sepsis. Any clinical deterioration suggests failure of this approach and should prompt expedient operative intervention. From a practical standpoint, it is best to think in terms of operative management whenever esophageal perforation is suspected.

Stent Placement. Endoscopic placement of an endoluminal stent to palliate inoperable esophageal malignancy was first described in the 1970s.[17] The past three decades have seen expanded indications and improved technology for esophageal stenting. There are an increasing number of small case series in the literature detailing stent placement for esophageal perforations. Attempts to stent the cervical esophagus cause dysphagia and aspiration, whereas stenting the distal esophagus and

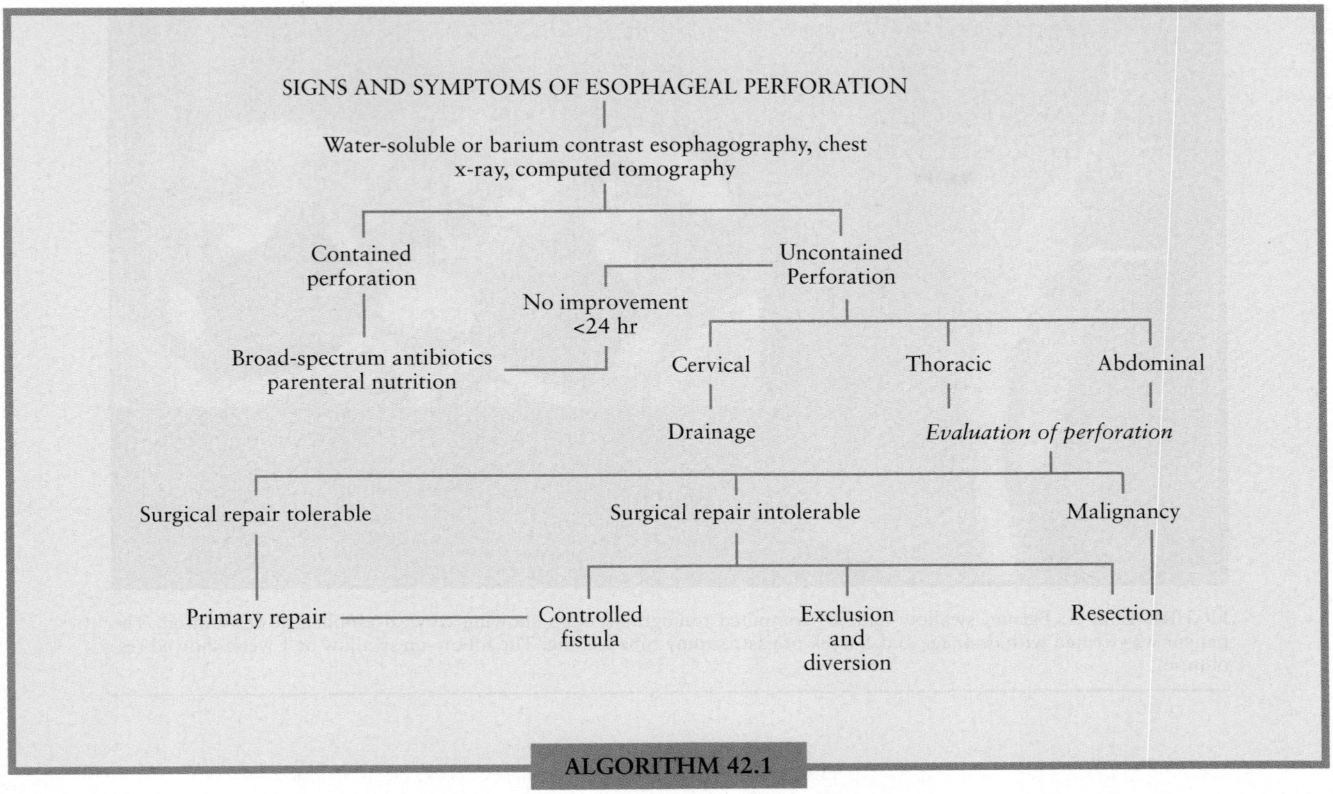

ALGORITHM 42.1. Evaluation and treatment of esophageal perforation. (Adapted with permission from Brinster CJ, Singhal S, Lawrence L, et al. Evolving options in the management of esophageal perforation. *Ann Thorac Surg* 2004;77:1475.)

esophagogastric junction is plagued by gastroesophageal reflux and stent migration. It appears that iatrogenic midthoracic perforations in patients without underlying esophageal pathology are most amenable to stenting. In a report of 17 such patients, leak occlusion occurred in 94% as confirmed by contrast esophagram.[18] Of note, all patients underwent simultaneous endoscopic or surgical procedures, and 18% of patients required repeat endoscopy for replacement or repositioning due to stent migration. In our opinion, highly selected patients may be candidates for stenting but should be cared for by a thoracic surgeon and managed expectantly in case urgent surgical exploration is clinically mandated.

Operative Treatment. The operative management of esophageal perforation is dictated by the location of the perforation, the extent of injury, and the presence or absence of underlying esophageal pathology. Approaches include drainage alone, primary reinforced repair, esophagectomy with immediate reconstruction, and exclusion or resection with diversion.

Although the anatomic relationships of the neck and mediastinum had been previously described, Herman Pearse's 1938 publication[19] regarding cervicomediastinal fascial continuity and the surgical prevention and management of mediastinitis following cervical suppuration was indeed landmark. Pearse noted that approximately 20 percent of cases of suppurative mediastinitis resulted from descending cervical infections, most as a result of cervical esophageal perforation. He identified the retrovisceral space as the most common path of dependent spread and advocated early operative drainage via cervical mediastinotomy in such cases, noting 35% mortality in patients operated on as compared to 85% mortality in the nonoperative group.[19] Air within the retrovisceral space may be detected by lateral roentogram of the neck. The typical radiographic studies of a patient with cervical esophageal perforation are shown in
4 Figure 42.2. Perforations of the upper third of the esophagus down to the level of the carina are treated by cervical drainage. This is easily performed through a left neck incision as depicted in Figure 42.3. Usually it is not necessary to find or close the perforation. However, ensuring complete drainage by opening the prevertebral fascia is of paramount importance. If the perforation is easily seen, it can be sutured with minimal difficulty. In all patients, we place a Penrose drain alongside the esophagus into the posterior mediastinum and bring it out through the inferior aspect of the neck incision. A gastrostomy or jejunostomy tube is placed for enteral feeding during the recovery period. Oral intake is prohibited for 1 week, and then the patient is restudied with contrast esophagography. If no extravasation is noted, the diet is advanced, the drain is removed, and the patient is discharged. If a leak persists, oral intake is again prohibited, enteral feeding is continued, and the patient is studied at 1-week intervals until resolution occurs. As long as there is no underlying distal esophageal pathology, essentially all adequately drained esophageal perforations will heal spontaneously.

Perforations of the middle third are best approached through a right fifth intercostal space thoracotomy. We favor a buttressed primary repair whenever possible, even in delayed presentations.[20] Material for buttressing the repair includes flaps of pleura, pericardium, diaphragm, omentum, or muscle. For small- to moderate-size repairs, we prefer an intercostal muscle flap. This is a reliable pedicled muscle flap based on the intercostal vessels. It should be harvested at the start of the procedure prior to the placement of retractors to avoid damage to the vascular pedicle. Once harvested, the chest is opened, all pleural collections are drained, and the perforation is localized. Necrotic tissue around the perforation is débrided. A vertical myotomy is performed to fully expose the rent in the

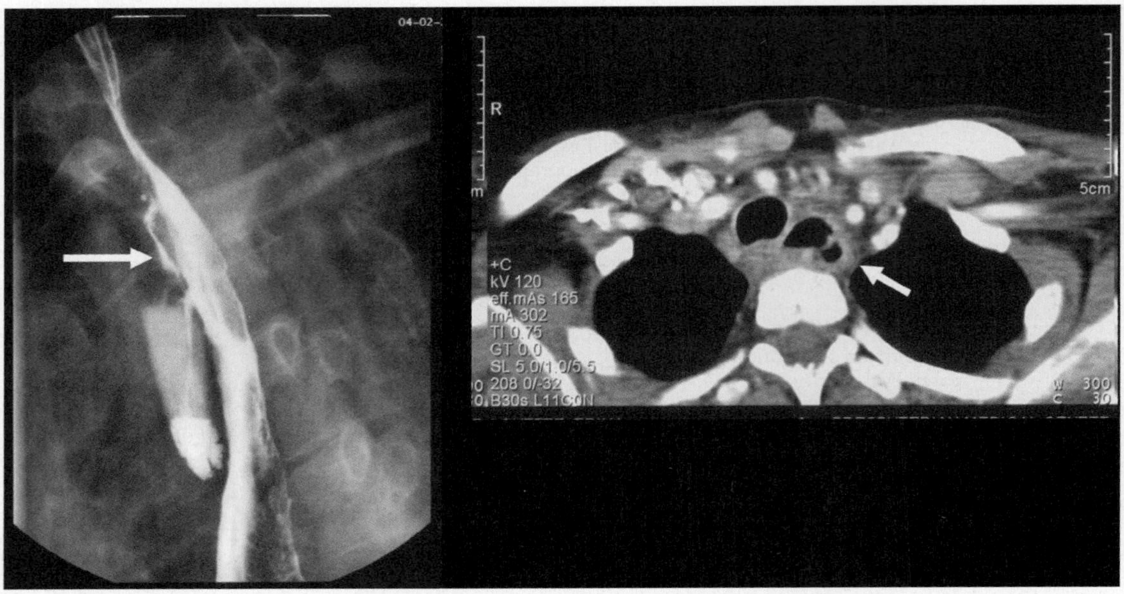

FIGURE 42.2. A: Barium swallow and (B) computed tomography scan showing cervical esophageal perforation. The patient was treated with drainage and 1 week of gastrostomy tube feeding. The follow-up swallow at 1 week showed resolution.

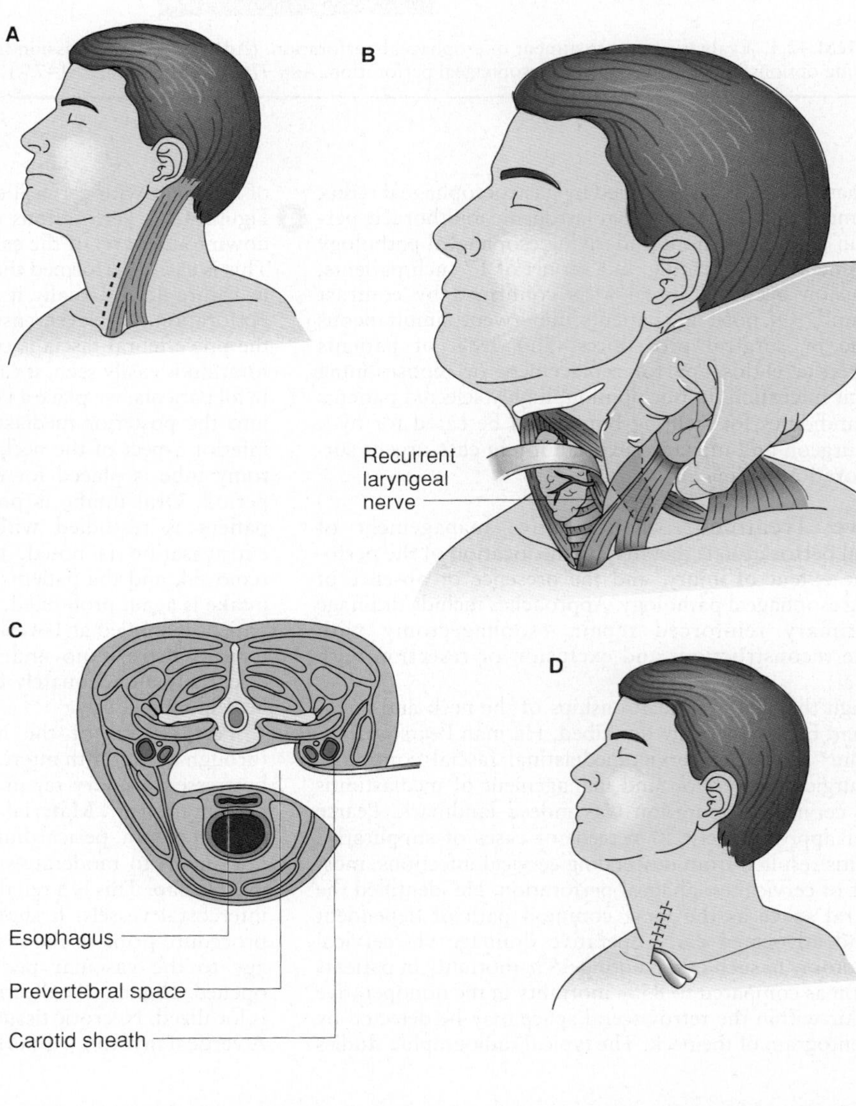

FIGURE 42.3. Approach for drainage of a cervical esophageal perforation. **A:** Skin incision parallel to the anterior border of the left sternocleidomastoid muscle, extending from the level of the cricoid cartilage to the sternal notch. **B:** With the sternocleidomastoid muscle and carotid sheath retracted laterally and the trachea and thyroid gland medially, blunt dissection along the prevertebral fascia in the superior mediastinum is carried out. Injury to the recurrent laryngeal nerve in the tracheoesophageal groove must be avoided. **C:** Schematic drawing of the prevertebral space drained by this cervical approach. **D:** Two 1-in. rubber drains placed into the superior mediastinum are brought out through the neck wound to allow establishment of an esophagocutaneous fistula, which usually heals spontaneously. (Adapted with permission from Orringer MB. The mediastinum. In: Nora PH, ed. *Operative Surgery,* 3rd ed. Philadelphia: WB Saunders; 1990:370.)

MALIGNANT NEOPLASMS

Malignant neoplasms of the esophagus include adenocarcinoma, squamous cell carcinoma, small cell carcinoma, leiomyosarcoma, rhabdomyosarcoma, fibrosarcoma, liposarcoma, lymphomas, and metastatic lesions from distant primary sites. Adenocarcinoma and squamous cell carcinoma are the most frequent malignant lesions, and adenocarcinoma has emerged in recent years as the more common lesion (Fig. 42.8). 6 In fact, the incidence of esophageal adenocarcinoma has increased in the last 25 years greater than the incidence of any other major malignancy in the United States (Fig. 42.9).[30] Most thoracic surgeons will complete an entire career without seeing the less common types of esophageal malignancies.

7 The goal of esophageal resection, whether as primary treatment or as part of a multimodality plan, is cure, though this goal remains elusive. Palliative esophagectomy is associated with mortality rates in excess of 20% and morbidity rates as high as 50% and should therefore be avoided.[31] Very effective palliation can be obtained with chemotherapy, radiation therapy, and endoscopic interventions such as stenting. Surveillance, epidemiology and end results (SEER) data from the National Cancer Institute estimate that 16,470 Americans will be diagnosed with and 14,280 will die of esophageal cancer annually. The lifetime risk of developing esophageal cancer is about 0.5%, being slightly higher for men than women.

Tobacco, alcohol, and obesity are all risk factors associated with the development of esophageal cancer. Table 42.4 shows the additional risk factors associated with esophageal cancer and their contributions to the development of either squamous cell carcinoma or adenocarcinoma.

Although many have postulated a genetic predisposition to esophageal cancer, tylosis is the only recognized familial syndrome that predisposes to the development of esophageal cancer. This is an autosomal dominant disorder that has been mapped to chromosome 17q25.[32] Patients have hyperkeratosis of the palms of their hands and the soles of their feet. The risk of developing squamous cell carcinoma of the esophagus by age 70 is 95% in this cohort of patients.[33]

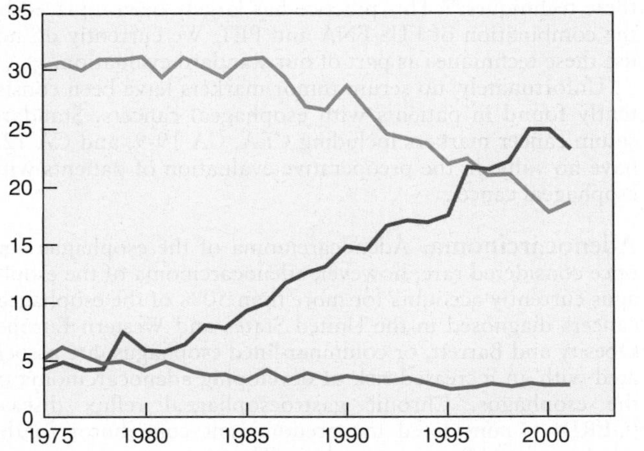

FIGURE 42.8. Histology and esophageal cancer incidence (1975–2001). Data from the National Cancer Institute's Surveillance, Epidemiology, and End Results program with age-adjustment using the 2000 U.S. standard population. *Blue line*, adenocarcinoma; *orange line*, squamous cell carcinoma; *green line*, not otherwise specified. (Adapted with permission from Pohl H, Welch G. The role of overdiagnosis and reclassification in the marked increase of esophageal adenocarcinoma incidence. *J Natl Cancer Inst* 2005;97:142–146.)

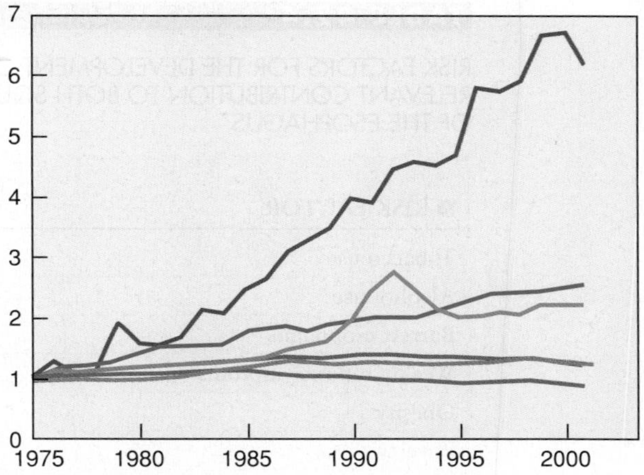

FIGURE 42.9. Relative change in incidence of esophageal adenocarcinoma and other malignancies (1975–2001). Data from the National Cancer Institute's Surveillance, Epidemiology, and End Results program with age-adjustment using the 2000 U.S. standard population. Baseline was the average incidence between 1973 and 1975. *Blue line*, esophageal adenocarcinoma; *green line*, melanoma; *orange line*, prostate cancer; *yellow line*, breast cancer; *purple line*, lung cancer; *red line*, colorectal cancer. (Adapted with permission from Pohl H, Welch G. The role of overdiagnosis and reclassification in the marked increase of esophageal adenocarcinoma incidence. *J Natl Cancer Inst* 2005;97:142–146.)

Diagnosis

Unfortunately, early esophageal carcinomas are largely asymptomatic. As a distensible muscular tube, a significant portion of the esophageal lumen must be obstructed to impede passage of a food bolus and produce symptoms. Dysphagia is the primary manifestation of esophageal cancer in 80% of patients, and up to 20% have odynophagia. Vague symptoms of retrosternal discomfort and transient dysphagia are often overlooked by the patient and the physician. On retrospective evaluation, many patients have significantly altered their eating habits by avoiding foods such as meats and breads while increasing their intake of semisolid foods and liquids. About one half of patients have significant weight loss. Weight loss of more than 10% of body mass is an independent predictor of poor prognosis.[34]

Pulmonary symptoms may be caused by aspiration of regurgitated food or by direct invasion of the airway by esophageal tumor. Direct airway invasion can occur with locally advanced lesions at the location where the left mainstem bronchus passes anterior to the esophagus. New hoarseness due to vocal cord paralysis is indicative of left recurrent nerve involvement and suggests unresectability. The Virchow node, a palpable left supraclavicular lymph node, may be apparent in some patients. Fine-needle aspiration with positive cytology confirms the pathologic involvement of the Virchow node, which is considered distant metastatic disease and precludes resection.

The evaluation of a patient with suspected esophageal cancer involves securing the diagnosis, clinically staging the patient, and determining the medical operability of patients with stage-appropriate lesions for resection. Barium swallow and esophagoscopy remain the most important diagnostic tools for assessing the patient with esophageal symptoms. Barium swallow is usually the first study obtained. It provides both anatomic and functional information. Flexible esophagoscopy is used to precisely locate the lesion and provide tissue confirmation of malignancy. In patients considered for surgical resection, endoscopic ultrasonography (EUS) is the single most

TABLE 42.4 **ETIOLOGY**

RISK FACTORS FOR THE DEVELOPMENT OF ESOPHAGEAL CANCER WITH THEIR RELEVANT CONTRIBUTION TO BOTH SQUAMOUS CELL AND ADENOCARCINOMA OF THE ESOPHAGUS

RISK FACTOR	SQUAMOUS CELL CARCINOMA	ADENOCARCINOMA
Tobacco use	+++	++
Alcohol use	+++	—
Barrett esophagus	—	++++
Weekly reflux symptoms	—	+++
Obesity	—	++
Poverty	++	—
Achalasia	+++	—
Caustic injury to the esophagus	++++	—
Nonepidermolytic palmoplantar keratoderma (tylosis)	++++	—
Plummer-Vinson syndrome	++++	—
History of head and neck cancer	++++	—
History of breast cancer treated with radiotherapy	+++	+++
Frequent consumption of extremely hot beverages	+	—
Prior use of beta-blockers, anticholinergic agents, or aminophyllines	—	±

+, Increase in the risk by a factor of less than two; ++, increase by a factor of two to four; +++, increase by a factor of more than four to eight; ++++, increase by a factor of more than eight; ±, conflicting results have been reported; —, no proven risk.

Reproduced with permission from Enzinger C, Mayer J. Esophageal cancer. *N Engl J Med* 2003; 349:2241

valuable test in determining tumor size and depth of penetration (T stage). EUS successfully predicts the T stage in greater than 80% of cases confirmed at surgery and generally performs better for advanced (T4) than local (T1) disease. Regional lymph nodes are also visualized during EUS and can be sampled by FNA to determine the cytologic presence or absence of metastatic nodal disease (N stage). The sensitivity of EUS alone to predict N stage is 85% and improves to greater than 95% with FNA.[35] Figure 42.10 shows an example of EUS for esophageal cancer.

A computed tomographic (CT) scan of the chest, abdomen, and pelvis with intravenous contrast is valuable for assessing lung and liver metastasis. However, it is not accurate for determining T stage or assessing regional lymph node involvement.

Positron emission tomography (PET) with 18 F-fluorodeoxyglucose (FDG) is a physiologic test unique in its ability to detect increased metabolic activity within tissues. It is increasingly used to detect distant metastasis (M stage) in patients with esophageal cancer. It has been reported that PET will detect otherwise radiographically occult metastatic disease in up to 15% of patients who were thought to have only localized disease by conventional studies, thus making them more appropriately managed by non-surgical interventions.[36] We now routinely obtain a PET scan as part of the preoperative staging evaluation in patients under consideration for esophagectomy. Increasingly, PET is being used to restage patients and evaluate response after neoadjuvant chemoradiation. Several studies have shown promising results in demonstrating that decreased FDG-avidity after neoadjuvant therapy predicts pathologic response and increased survival.[37,38]

The use of combined thoracoscopy and laparoscopy for preoperative staging has been advocated by some centers. Periesophageal mediastinal lymph nodes and celiac lymph nodes can be sampled with a high degree of accuracy using these techniques.[39] This practice has largely been replaced by the combination of EUS-FNA and PET. We currently do not use these techniques as part of our standard evaluation.

Unfortunately, no serum tumor markers have been consistently found in patients with esophageal cancers. Standard serum cancer markers including CEA, CA 19-9, and CA 125 have no value in the preoperative evaluation of patients with esophageal cancer.

Adenocarcinoma. Adenocarcinoma of the esophagus was once considered rare; however, adenocarcinoma of the esophagus currently accounts for more than 50% of the esophageal cancers diagnosed in the United States and Western Europe. Obesity and Barrett, or columnar-lined esophagus, are associated with an increased risk of developing adenocarcinoma of the esophagus. Chronic gastroesophageal reflux disease (GERD) is considered the predominant contributor to the development of Barrett metaplasia. The frequency, severity, and duration of reflux symptoms are correlated with an increased risk of developing esophageal adenocarcinoma.[40] Patients with recurring symptoms of reflux have an eightfold increase in the risk of esophageal adenocarcinoma.

A Barrett esophagus develops in about 5% of patients with GERD. Endoscopically, it is recognized by inflamed salmon-colored mucosa extending proximally from the GE junction. Often there are intervening areas of normal-appearing mucosa,

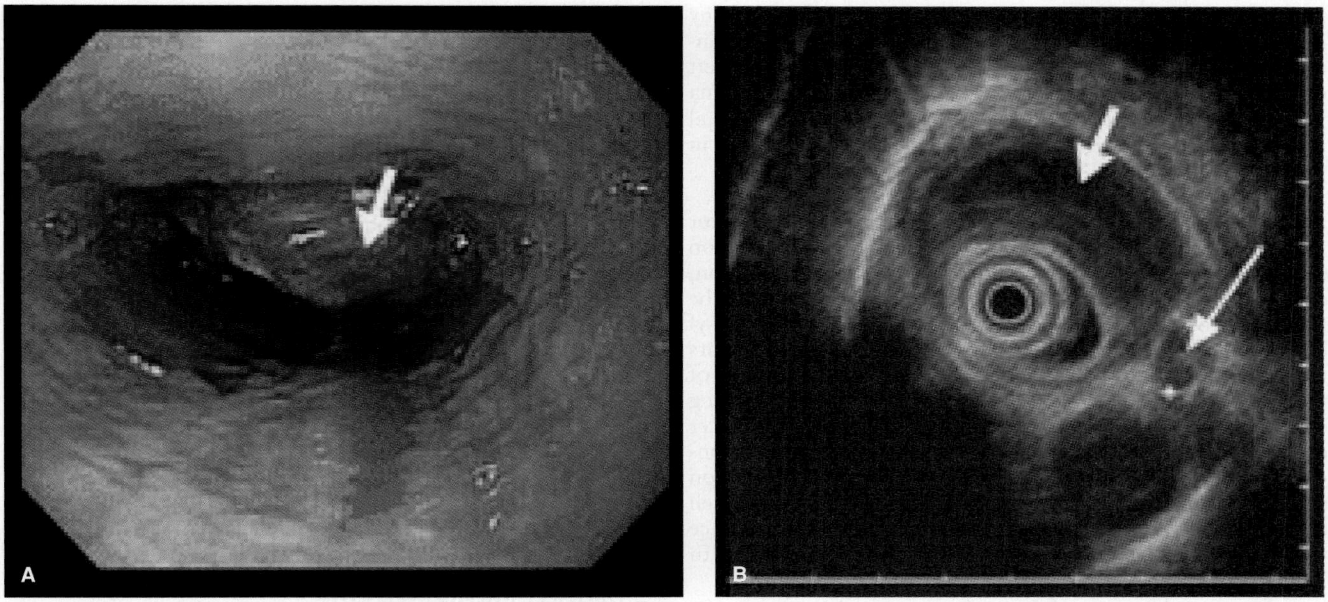

FIGURE 42.10. Endoscopic image (**A**) and endoscopic ultrasound (**B**) showing a transmural adenocarcinoma of the esophagus associated with a Barrett esophagus (*short arrows*), with lymph node metastasis (*long arrow*). (Reproduced with permission from Enzinger C, Mayer J. Esophageal cancer. *N Engl J Med* 2003;349:2245. Copyright © 2003 Massachusetts Medical Society. All rights reserved.)

or so-called skip areas. Figure 42.11A shows the typical endoscopic appearance; Figure 42.11B shows the same patient with methylene blue vital stain, which can be used to highlight the mucosal changes. Microscopic evaluation reveals replacement of the normal stratified squamous epithelium of the esophagus with columnar epithelium more typical of other parts of the gastrointestinal tract. Thus, these changes are often referred to as "intestinalization" of the mucosa. With progression to dysplasia, the nuclei become crowded and the normal glandular architecture is lost. Histologically, patients with high-grade dysplasia carry a significant risk for esophageal carcinoma and should be considered candidates for resection. Ten percent to thirty percent of patients with high-grade dysplasia will develop invasive adenocarcinoma within 5 years of the initial

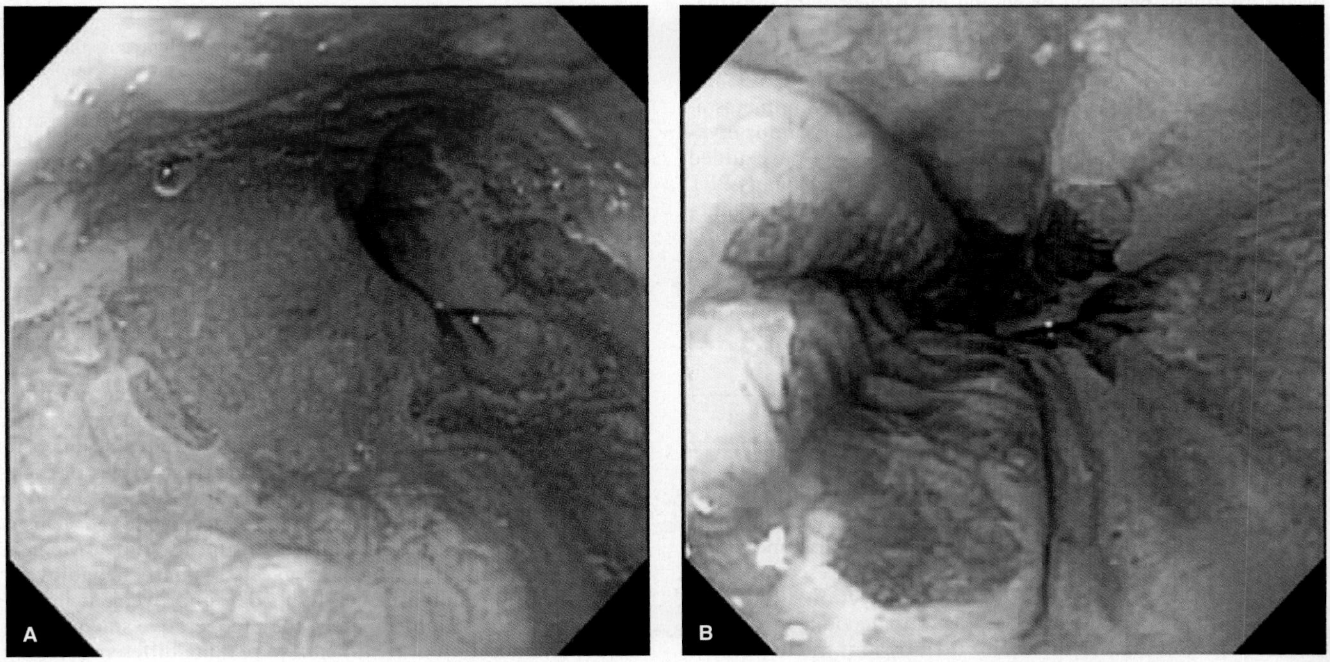

FIGURE 42.11. **A:** The typical endoscopic appearance of Barrett changes at the gastroesophageal (GE) junction. Note the salmon-colored areas of erosion extending from the GE junction. Also note the intervening areas of normal appearing mucosa. **B:** Vital staining with methylene blue. Vital stains are used to highlight the mucosal changes at the time of endoscopy. (Courtesy of Michael L. Kochman, M.D., University of Pennsylvania, Philadelphia.)

diagnosis; moreover, in patients undergoing esophagectomy for presumed high-grade dysplasia, invasive carcinoma is identified in 30% to 40% of the pathologic specimens.[41] A Barrett esophagus increases the risk of esophageal adenocarcinoma when compared with the general population.[42] The annual rate of neoplastic transformation to adenocarcinoma in patients with Barrett is 0.5%.[43]

Squamous Cell Carcinoma. The primary risk factor for squamous cell carcinoma of the esophagus is chronic irritation of the esophageal mucosa. Prolonged alcohol consumption, especially in combination with tobacco exposure, appears to be the major contributing factor. Nitrosamines and other nitrosyl compounds found in smoked meats are also important factors in native populations who rely on them for their main source of nutrition. In some Asian countries, there appears to be strong correlation between the development of squamous cell cancer of the esophagus and ingestion of hot beverages. Medical conditions including achalasia, caustic strictures, Plummer-Vinson syndrome, and tylosis also increase the risk of squamous cell carcinoma. Patients with tylosis have a 40% lifetime incidence of squamous cell carcinoma of the esophagus.[32] The risk with long-standing achalasia approximates 7%.[44]

Staging of Esophageal Cancers

Esophageal cancers are staged according to the American Joint Committee on Cancer (AJCC) TNM staging system.[45] The current (sixth edition) AJCC definitions are shown in Table 42.5. The stage groupings and current recommended treatment strategy for each stage are displayed in Table 42.6. The staging system for esophageal cancer has recently undergone revision and should be published soon. Pathologic stage according to the updated system will be dependent on the number of nodes containing metastasis, tumor grade, tumor location, and histologic cell type.

It is clear that the outcome in esophageal cancer is strongly associated with the stage of the disease. Thus, accurate clinical staging is of paramount importance in formulating an appropriate treatment plan and providing the patient with information regarding prognosis. The preoperative evaluation is intended to define the extent of disease and thus the clinical stage. All patients should have a CT scan of the chest and abdomen. In the absence of lung, liver, or other distant metastatic disease, EUS is performed to define the depth of tumor invasion and assess regional lymph nodes. Recently, we have added PET scanning to the standard preoperative evaluation as PET is a complementary modality to the CT scan and in conjunction with CT is very sensitive at detecting distant metastatic disease. In stage-appropriate candidates, plans are made to optimize the patient from a medical standpoint and proceed to resection. The role of preoperative therapy followed by operation remains ill defined and hotly debated.

TABLE 42.5 STAGING

AMERICAN JOINT COMMITTEE ON CANCER (AJCC) STAGING OF ESOPHAGEAL CANCER

STAGE	DESCRIPTION
PRIMARY TUMOR (T)	
TX	Primary tumor cannot be assessed
T0	No evidence of primary tumor
Tis	Carcinoma in situ
T1	Tumor invades lamina propria or submucosa
T2	Tumor invades muscularis propria
T3	Tumor invades adventitia
T4	Tumor invades adjacent structures
REGIONAL LYMPH NODES (N)	
NX	Regional lymph nodes cannot be assessed
N0	No regional lymph node metastasis
N1	Regional lymph node metastasis
DISTANT METASTASIS (M)	
MX	Distant metastasis cannot be assessed
M0	No distant metastasis
M1	Distant metastasis
TUMORS OF THE LOWER THORACIC ESOPHAGUS	
M1a	Metastasis in celiac lymph nodes
M1b	Other distant metastasis
TUMORS OF THE MIDTHORACIC ESOPHAGUS[a]	
M1a	Not applicable
M1b	Nonregional lymph nodes and/or other distant metastasis
TUMORS OF THE UPPER THORACIC ESOPHAGUS	
M1a	Metastasis in cervical nodes
M1b	Other distant metastasis

[a]For tumors of midthoracic esophagus, use only M1b because these tumors with metastasis in nonregional lymph nodes have an equally poor prognosis as those with metastasis in other distant sites. Reproduced with permission from American Joint Committee on Cancer. *AJCC Cancer Staging Manual,* 6th ed. New York: Springer; 2002:91–98.

Neoadjuvant Therapy

8 The current information on neoadjuvant treatment can be divided into studies evaluating preoperative radiation, preoperative chemotherapy, and combined preoperative chemoradiation therapy. In operable patients with resectable tumors, the results of any preoperative therapy followed by resection must be compared with the results of primary resection alone. It is important that this analysis must take into account the toxicities associated with multimodality therapy and the impact on the intended resection and quality of life.

Several randomized trials have failed to show any benefit from preoperative radiation therapy alone. Proponents of preoperative radiotherapy argue that the trials are too small to demonstrate the advantages of this approach. A meta-analysis of available randomized trials comprising 1,147 patients, however, found no improvement in survival with preoperative radiotherapy alone in patients with resectable esophageal cancer.[46] At this time, there is no indication for preoperative radiation therapy alone followed by resection.

The utility of preoperative chemotherapy alone is much more poorly defined. A large multicenter randomized trial in the United States (Intergroup Trial) of 440 patients failed to show any improvement in survival after three cycles of combined cisplatin and fluorouracil followed by surgery and two postoperative cycles when compared to surgery alone.[47] This is in contrast to a large randomized European study (Medical Research Council), which suggested that neoadjuvant chemotherapy resulted in nearly a 10% improvement in survival at 2 years.[48] Unfortunately, the preoperative staging techniques and duration of treatments were quite different, making the two studies difficult to compare. More recently, another European neoadjuvant chemotherapy trial (MAGIC trial) demonstrated improved survival with perioperative chemotherapy versus surgery alone (36% vs. 23% at 5 years).[49] Of note, 75% of the MAGIC trial participants had gastric cancer, while

TABLE 42.6 **STAGING**

AMERICAN JOINT COMMITTEE ON CANCER (AJCC) STAGE GROUPING WITH RECOMMENDED TREATMENT STRATEGY AND PREDICTED 5-YEAR SURVIVAL

STAGE	TNM DESIGNATION	TREATMENT	5-YR SURVIVAL (%)
0	Tis, N0, M0	Surgery alone	95
I	T1, N0, M0	Surgery alone	75
IIA	T2, N0, M0 T3, N0, M0	Surgery alone	30
IIB	T1, N1, M0	Surgery alone or surgery +/− preop chemo/XRT under investigation	20
	T2, N1, M0		
III	T3, N1, M0	Surgery for T3 lesions with or without preoperative chemo/XRT under investigation	10–15
	T4, any N, M0	Palliation (chemo, XRT, stenting, or combination)	
IVA	Any T, any N, M1a	Palliation (chemo, XRT, stenting, or combination)	5
IVB	Any T, any N, M1b	Palliation (chemo, XRT, stenting, or combination)	1

chemo, chemotherapy; XRT, radiation therapy.

only 25% had either distal esophageal or GE junction adenocarcinoma. Also, only 41.6% of patients randomized to perioperative chemotherapy were able to complete all six prescribed cycles of therapy. In the most recent Cochrane review of the topic, 11 randomized controlled trials with 2,051 patients suggested that preoperative chemotherapy plus surgery may offer a survival advantage compared to surgery alone for resectable esophageal cancer.[50] There was no demonstrable difference in the rate of resection, tumor recurrence, or postoperative morbidity. There was some chemotherapy-related morbidity. Presumably based on the relative success of the MRC and MAGIC trials, chemotherapy alone is used quite commonly as neoadjuvant therapy in Europe, whereas combined chemotherapy and radiation is used more commonly in the United States.

Several small randomized trials have evaluated combined preoperative chemoradiation followed by surgical resection. The most widely cited trial to justify the use of combined treatment followed by surgery was published by Walsh et al.[51] in 1996. This study projected a 3-year survival of 32% in the neoadjuvant treatment group as compared to 6% in the surgery alone group for patients with adenocarcinoma. Critics were quick to point out the lack of appropriate staging, the poor survival in the surgical group as compared with other surgical series, and the small study size. A more recent study found equivalent median and 3-year survival in patients with squamous cell carcinoma of the esophagus randomized to either preoperative chemoradiation followed by surgery or surgery alone.[52] An increased complication rate was noted in the patients undergoing preoperative chemoradiation therapy. A recent meta-analysis of 10 randomized controlled trials of neoadjuvant chemoradiotherapy versus surgery alone demonstrated an absolute survival advantage of 13% at 2 years favoring neoadjuvant therapy.[53] Despite a paucity of conclusive data, there seems to be an evolving consensus at most centers that patients with T3 and/or N1 disease should receive neoadjuvant chemoradiation. This issue remains unresolved, and operation remains the standard treatment for localized esophageal cancer outside of a clinical trial. At this time we consider neoadjuvant chemoradiotherapy to be investigational. Unfortunately, a large intergroup trial designed to answer this question was closed because of poor accrual.

Operative Management

Approaches to Esophagectomy. There are several surgical approaches to esophagectomy. Selecting the appropriate procedure for an individual patient depends on the overall medical condition of the patient, the location of the tumor, and the expertise and experience of the surgeon. Possible approaches include the transhiatal approach, the transabdominal transthoracic approach (Ivor Lewis), the three-stage or "three-hole" approach (McKeown), the thoracoabdominal approach, and the minimally invasive approach. Options for reconstruction include a gastric tube, a colonic interposition, and in selected cases small intestinal free graft. Because of its ample blood supply, ease of mobilization, and sufficient length to reach the neck, the gastric tube is the usual conduit of choice for reconstruction. The use of colon is more complex and has increased morbidity when compared to gastric pull-up.[54] We reserve the use of colon or jejunum for patients with an unusable stomach due to previous surgery, tumor extension, or other technical considerations.

The esophageal anastomosis requires meticulous attention. Many esophageal operations are plagued by high anastomotic leak rates and a significant number of postoperative strictures. At present, the modified stapled anastomosis as described by Orringer et al.[55] appears to have the lowest leak rate, about 3% as compared with sutured techniques, which are as high as 15%. The technique is shown in Figure 42.12; many thoracic surgeons have adopted this anastomotic technique.

The Transhiatal Approach. The transhiatal esophagectomy was reintroduced by Orringer and Sloan[2] in 1978 and continues to be refined.[56,57] The procedure is performed through an

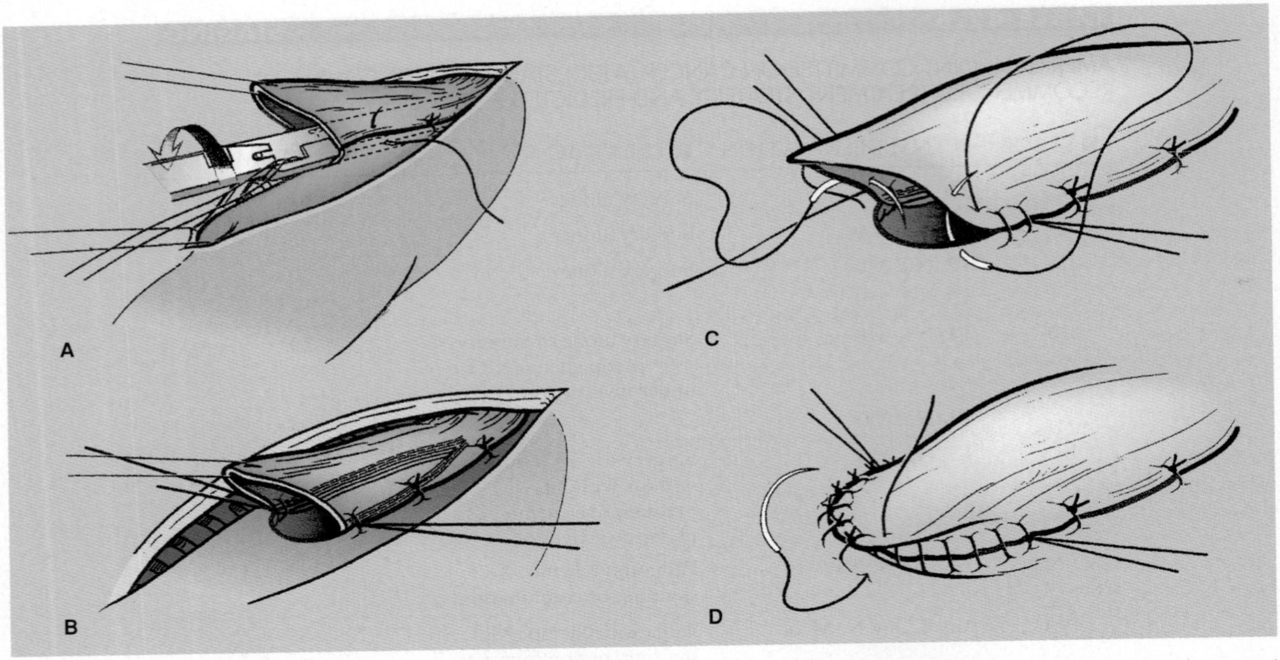

FIGURE 42.12. The stapled technique for cervical esophageal anastomosis. This technique results in lower anastomotic leak rates and fewer postoperative strictures. (Adapted with permission from Orringer MB, Marshall B, Iannettoni MD. Eliminating the cervical esophagogastric anastomotic leak with a side-to-side stapled anastomosis. *J Thorac Cardiovasc Surg* 2000;119:277.)

upper midline laparotomy and left cervical incision as shown in Figure 42.13. A gastric conduit based on the right gastroepiploic artery is used to establish gastrointestinal continuity. The completed operation is depicted in Figure 42.14. If the stomach is unusable, a colonic interposition can be performed.

Today, the transhiatal esophagectomy is the preferred approach by many surgeons. Nevertheless, debate continues over whether this approach has lower morbidity and mortality than other approaches involving thoracotomy and whether it
9 provides an optimal cancer operation. Proponents argue that this approach results in less surgical trauma by avoiding thoracotomy and thus less postoperative morbidity, especially pulmonary complications. Furthermore, with placement of the anastomosis in the neck, a leak, should it occur, can be treated by simple bedside cervical drainage. In contrast, a leak in the chest is far more likely to result in severe mediastinitis and more devastating complications.

The Ivor Lewis Approach. The transabdominal transthoracic approach to esophagectomy as initially described is often referred to as the Ivor Lewis esophagectomy.[3] This approach includes an upper midline laparotomy for mobilization of the stomach with creation of a gastric tube in the same manner used for the transhiatal esophagectomy. Once the stomach has been mobilized, the hiatus is opened and the GE junction and distal esophagus are mobilized. At this point the abdomen is closed, the patient is repositioned, and a right fifth intercostal space thoracotomy is performed. The intrathoracic esophagus is mobilized under direct vision up to the level of the azygous vein. The esophagogastric anastomosis is performed at the level of the divided azygous vein. The advantage of this approach is that the intrathoracic esophagus is mobilized directly with full exposure of the mediastinum and surrounding structures. This may be of value in avoiding injury to the airway or other mediastinal structures, especially with bulky tumors in the middle third of the esophagus at the level of the carina. Unfortunately, these patients are subject to increased early postoperative pulmonary complications due to the thoracotomy incision. In addition, placing the anastomosis in the chest can lead to life-threatening mediastinitis should an anastomotic leak occur. Additionally, a large amount of thoracic esophagus is retained with this approach and may be at risk of recurrent disease, specifically in the setting of severe Barrett esophagus.

Three-Field Esophagectomy. This approach is carried out through separate laparotomy, right thoracotomy, and cervical incisions.[4] Proponents of this approach fall into two categories. The first group uses this approach to resect large intrathoracic lesions of the midesophagus. Exposure especially at the level of the carina and left mainstem bronchus is superior as compared with the transhiatal approach. Because visualization is improved, the injury rate to nearby structures, especially the airway and azygous vein, is lower. The second group uses this approach to perform a complete two- or three-field lymph node dissection, suggesting that this approach provides a more complete resection and thus improves long-term survival. This approach has been shown to have acceptable morbidity and mortality as compared with other approaches; however, the often-cited report was from a single U.S. center.[58] On the other hand, a large randomized Dutch trial comparing transhiatal resection with extended transthoracic resection showed that the transhiatal approach was associated with a lower morbidity and no statistically different overall, disease-free, and quality-adjusted survival.[59] Patients who underwent thoracotomy had an increased incidence of chyle leak and pulmonary complications, as well as longer ventilator dependence, ICU stay, and hospital stay (Table 42.7). In a recent retrospective review of 2,303 esophageal cancer patients treated with R0 resection without adjuvant or neoadjuvant therapy, the number of nodes removed was an independent predictor of survival. The authors concluded that to maximize this survival benefit, a minimum of 23 nodes should be removed at esophagectomy.[60] The true value of extensive lymphadenectomy in esophageal cancer remains undefined.

The Thoracoabdominal Approach. The left thoracoabdominal approach is probably the least used of all approaches to

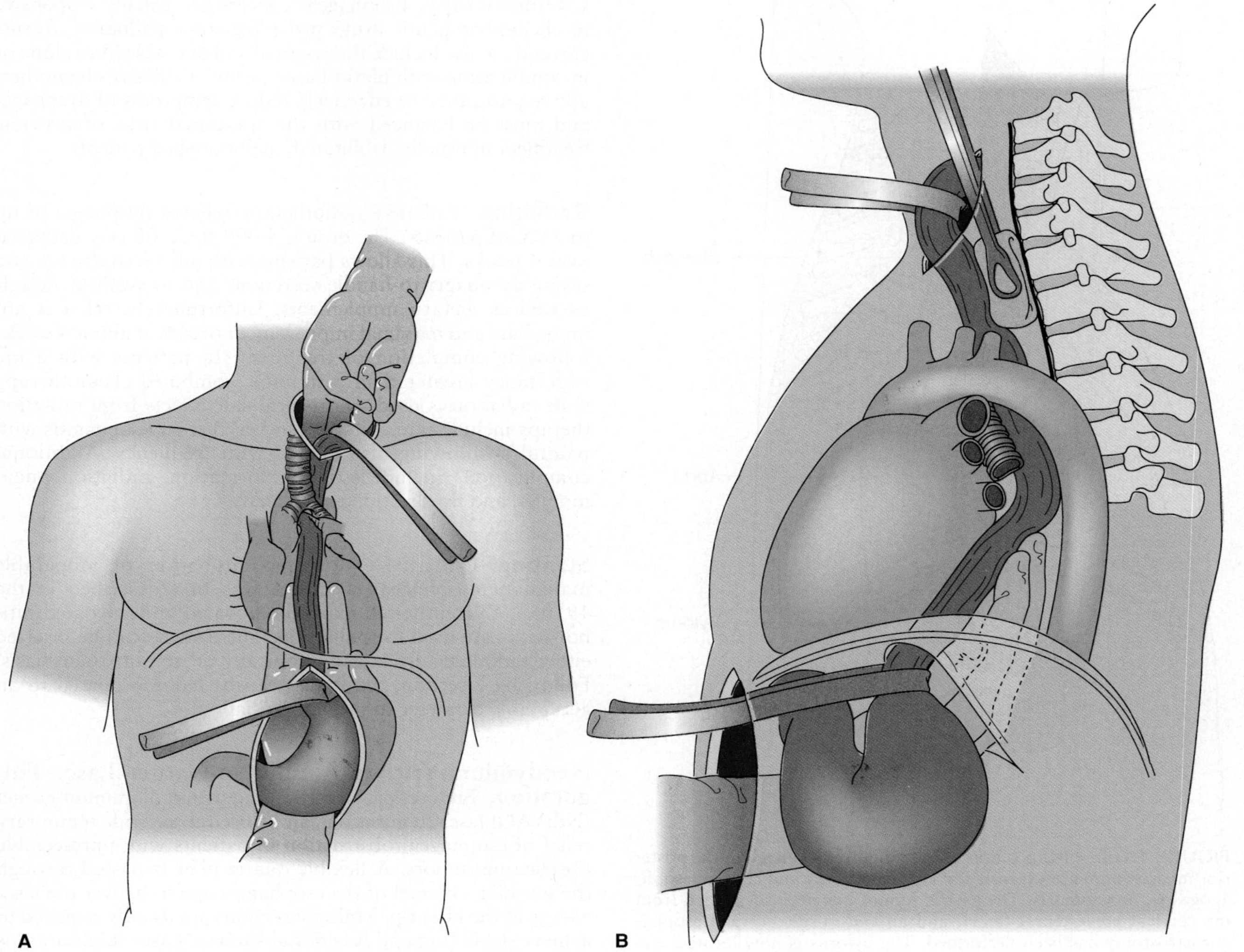

FIGURE 42.13. **A:** Transhiatal mobilization of the thoracic esophagus from the posterior mediastinum with the use of blunt dissection and traction on rubber drains placed around the esophagogastric junction and cervical esophagus. The volar aspects of the fingers are kept against the esophagus to reduce the risk for injury to adjacent structures. **B:** Lateral view showing transhiatal mobilization of the esophagus away from the prevertebral fascia. Half of a sponge on a stick is inserted through the cervical incision and advanced until it makes contact with the hand inserted from below through the diaphragmatic hiatus. Arterial pressure is monitored as the heart is displaced forward by the hand in the posterior mediastinum. (Adapted with permission from Orringer MB. Surgical options for esophageal resection and reconstruction with stomach. In: Baue AE, Geha AS, Hammond GL, eds. *Glenn's Thoracic and Cardiovascular Surgery*, 5th ed. Norwalk, CT: Appleton & Lange; 1991:799.)

the esophagus. It is performed by making an oblique incision from the midpoint between the xiphoid and umbilicus across the costal arch to the tip of the scapula. The abdomen is opened, the costal arch is divided, and the chest is entered through the seventh intercostal space. The diaphragm is opened in a circumferential manner along the chest wall to avoid any damage to the phrenic nerve branches. At least a 2-cm rim of diaphragm is preserved on the chest wall to aid in reconstruction of the diaphragm at the completion of the procedure. This approach offers superior exposure to the left upper quadrant, including the hiatus, and is our approach of choice in patients with previous extensive hiatal or proximal gastric surgery. For patients with distal tumors and inadequate conduit for total esophageal replacement, the anastomosis can be placed in the left chest below the inferior pulmonary vein or up to the level of the aortic arch. For those with adequate conduit, a separate left cervical incision can be made and the cervical esophagogastric anastomosis can be placed in the neck. A consecutive case series of 64 thoracoabdominal esophagectomies reported no anastomotic leaks and a 2% mortality rate.[61]

The Minimally Invasive Approach. Various minimally invasive techniques to esophagectomy have been described. These include laparoscopic, hand-assisted, thoracoscopic, and robotic-assisted esophagectomy. The hope of these procedures is that minimizing the incision size will decrease the morbidity of the operation while at the same time providing adequate resection. The largest study included 217 patients from the University of Pittsburgh who underwent esophagectomy via thoracoscopy, laparoscopy, and a left neck incision.[62] The investigators observed equivalent results as compared to open techniques and suggest development of a multicenter trial to define the role of minimally invasive esophagectomy. At present, the advantage of this approach remains to be determined.

Cervical Esophageal Cancer.

Cervical esophageal cancer represents a very small subset of primary esophageal cancers.

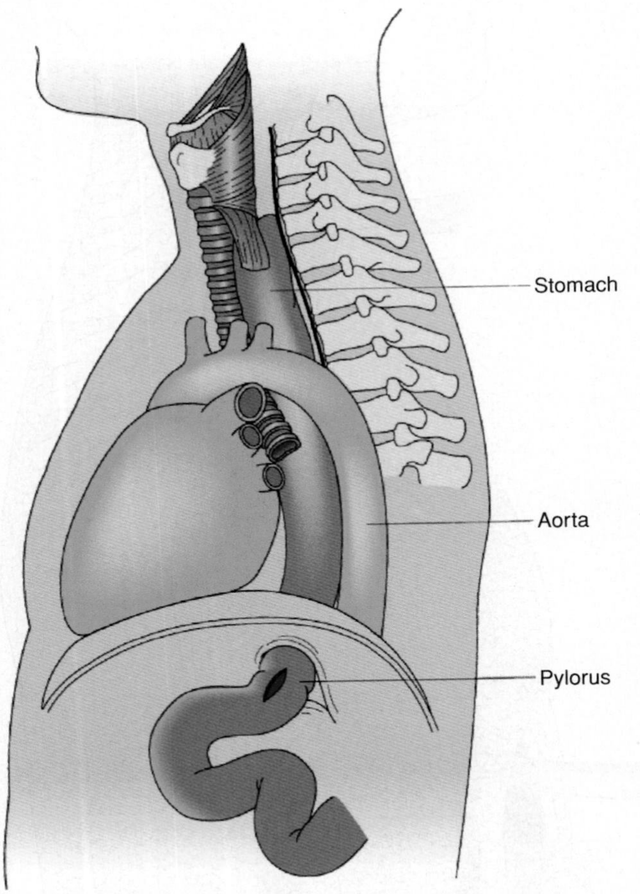

FIGURE 42.14. Final position of the mobilized stomach in the posterior mediastinum after transhiatal esophagectomy and cervical esophagogastric anastomosis. The gastric fundus has been suspended from the cervical prevertebral fascia, and an end-to-side cervical esophagogastrostomy has been performed. The pylorus is now located several centimeters below the level of the diaphragmatic hiatus. (Adapted with permission from Orringer MB, Sloan H. Esophagectomy without thoracotomy. *J Thorac Cardiovasc Surg* 1978;76:643.)

Direct extension into the cervical esophagus from a primary laryngeal or thyroid malignancy is much more common. Unfortunately, all are difficult to treat. Traditional methods of treatment have relied on definitive chemoradiation therapy. A small subset of patients may be candidates for salvage resection, which usually includes laryngectomy with permanent tracheostomy, esophagectomy, and gastric transposition to reconstitute the gastrointestinal tract.

Palliation

Several palliative therapies are available for patients who have unresectable disease, have metastatic disease, or are medically
10 unfit for surgery. The intent of palliation is to maintain comfort, restore swallowing function if possible, and support nutrition.

Establishment of alternative enteral access is helpful in maintaining nutritional status and hydration. When possible, this is provided by a percutaneous gastrostomy (PEG) tube placed under endoscopic guidance. For patients with bulky obstructing lesions who cannot undergo PEG, an open gastrostomy or jejunostomy tube is required.

Chemotherapy. Esophageal cancers are usually responsive to chemotherapeutic drugs providing some palliation. Agents currently in use include fluorouracil and taxanes either alone or in combination with platin-based agents. Palliative chemotherapy requires time to effectively reduce symptoms of dysphagia and must be balanced with the associated risks of systemic treatment in usually debilitated, malnourished patients.

Radiation. Palliative radiotherapy relieves dysphagia in up to 75% of patients. The dose is 4,000 to 5,000 cGy delivered over 4 weeks. This allows patients with advanced disease and severe dysphagia to handle secretions and to swallow liquids as well as dietary supplements. Unfortunately, relief is not immediate and maximal improvement occurs at about 4 weeks following completion of treatment. In patients with a life expectancy greater than 3 months, combined chemotherapy with radiation is used. Short-term side effects from radiation therapy include skin irritation and erythema. Esophagitis with painful swallowing also occurs with frequency. Additional complications include stricture formation, radiation pneumonitis, and fistulization to the airway.

Stenting. Palliative endoscopic intubation of inoperable malignant esophageal strictures was first described in the 1970s.[17] Currently, self-expanding coated and uncoated nitinol stents are used for palliation. These stents can be inserted either radiologically or endoscopically on an outpatient basis. Following insertion, the lumen can be balloon dilated to an acceptable diameter to provide palliation.

Neodymium:Yttrium-Aluminum-Garnet Laser Fulguration. Endoscopic neodymium:yttrium-aluminum-garnet (Nd:YAG) laser fulguration can be used to provide temporary relief of esophageal obstruction in patients with unresectable obstructing tumors. A flexible quartz fiber is passed through the working channel of the esophagoscope to deliver the laser energy at the fiber tip. Multiple sessions are usually required to achieve debulking and functional success. Laser fulguration is often combined with endoluminal stenting and radiation therapy. It can also be useful in patients who have undergone uncovered stenting procedures with ingrow of tumor through the stent.

Photodynamic Therapy. Intraluminal photodynamic therapy (PDT) is a nonthermal ablative technique that can be used to palliate patients. This technique requires the systemic administration of a hematoporphyrin, which is concentrated within the malignant cells. Approximately 48 hours after administration of the photosensitizer, patients undergo endoscopy and an argon-pump dye-laser is used to deliver endoluminal light at a wavelength of 630 nm. This results in the generation of oxygen radicals, which quickly lead to tumor necrosis. The depth of penetration is relatively limited, and this decreases the risk of full-thickness necrosis with perforation. Unfortunately, the photosensitizing agents are retained by the reticuloendothelial system in skin; thus, patients are sensitive to infrared wavelength light, including sunlight, radiant heat, fluorescent light, and strong incandescent light. Depending on the photosensitizing agent used, this sensitivity can persist up to 3 months, a challenging problem in patients with short life expectancies.

A recent series of 215 patients treated with palliative endoluminal PDT revealed a procedure-related mortality rate of 1.8%, effective palliation for patients with obstructing cancers in 85% of the treatment courses, and median survival of 4.8 months.[63] Some patients in this series also required stenting, suggesting that PDT has a role in multimodality palliation of obstructing esophageal cancers.

TABLE 42.7

COMPLICATIONS

	TRANSTHORACIC ($n = 114$)	TRANSHIATAL ($n = 106$)	P VALUE
Pulmonary complications	57%	27%	<0.001
Chylothorax	10%	2%	0.02
Ventilator time (days)			<0.001
Median	2	1	
Range	0–76	0–19	
Intensive care unit stay (days)			<0.001
Median	6	2	
Range	0–79	0–38	
Hospital stay (days)			<0.001
Median	19	15	
Range	7–154	4–63	
Anastomotic leak	16%	14%	0.85
Vocal cord paralysis	21%	13%	0.15

Reproduced with permission from Hulscher JB, van Sandick JW, de Boer AG, et al. Extended transthoracic resection compared with limited transhiatal resection for adenocarcinoma of the esophagus. *N Engl J Med* 2002;374:1662.

References

1. Orringer MB. Complications of esophageal surgery and trauma. In: Greenfield LJ, ed. *Complications in Surgery and Trauma*, 3rd ed. Philadelphia: JB Lippincott Co; 1990:302.
2. Orringer MB, Sloan H. Esophagectomy without thoracotomy. *J Thorac Cardiovasc Surg* 1978;76:643.
3. Lewis I. The surgical treatment of carcinoma of the esophagus with special reference to a new operation for growths of the middle third. *Br J Surg* 1946;34:18.
4. McKeown KC. Total three-stage esophagectomy for cancer of the esophagus. *Br J Surg* 1976;51:259.
5. Bolton JS, Teng S. Transthoracic or transhiatal esophagectomy for cancer of the esophagus—does it matter? *Surg Oncol Clin N Am* 2002;11:365.
6. Dimick JB, Pronovost PJ, Cowan JA, et al. Surgical volume and quality of care for esophageal resection: do high-volume hospitals have fewer complications? *Ann Thorac Surg* 2003;75:337.
7. Rizk NP, Bach PB, Schrag D, et al. The impact of complications on outcomes after resection for esophageal and gastroesophageal junction carcinoma. *J Am Coll Surg* 2004;198:42.
8. Brinster CJ, Singhal S, Lawrence L, et al. Evolving options in the management of esophageal perforation. *Ann Thorac Surg* 2004;77:1475.
9. Weiman DS, Walker WA, Brosnan KM, et al. Noniatrogenic esophageal trauma. *Ann Thorac Surg* 1995;59:845; discussion 849.
10. Barrett N. Spontaneous perforation of the esophagus: review of the literature and a report of three new cases. *Thorax* 1946;1:48.
11. Foley MJ, Ghahremani GG, Rogers LF. Reappraisal of contrast media used to detect upper gastrointestinal perforations: comparison of ionic water-soluble media with barium sulfate. *Radiology* 1982;144:231.
12. Gollub MJ, Bains MS. Barium sulfate: a new (old) contrast agent for diagnosis of postoperative esophageal leaks. *Radiology* 1997;202:360.
13. Horwitz B, Krevsky B, Buckman RF Jr, et al. Endoscopic evaluation of penetrating esophageal injuries. *Am J Gastroenterol* 1993;88:1249.
14. Mengold L, Klassen KP. Conservative management of esophageal perforation. *Arch Surg* 1965;91:232.
15. Cameron JL, Kieffer RF, Hendrix TR, et al. Selective nonoperative management of contained intrathoracic esophageal disruptions. *Ann Thorac Surg* 1979;27:404.
16. Altorjay A, Kiss J, Voros A, et al. Nonoperative management of esophageal perforations. Is it justified? *Ann Surg* 1997;225:415.
17. Atkinson M, Ferguson R. Fibreoptic endoscopic palliative intubation of inoperable oesophagogastric neoplasms. *Br Med J* 1997;1:266–267.
18. Freeman RK, Van Woerkom JM, Ascioti AJ. Esophageal stent placement for the treatment of iatrogenic intrathoracic esophageal perforation. *Ann Thorac Surg* 2007;83:2003–2008.
19. Pearse HE. Mediastinitis following cervical suppuration. *Ann Surg* 1938; 108(4):588–611.
20. Port JL, Kent MS, Korst RJ, et al. Thoracic esophageal perforations: a decade of experience. *Ann Thorac Surg* 2003;75:1071.
21. Hugh TB, Kelly MD. Corrosive ingestion and the surgeon. *J Am Coll Surg* 1999;189:508.
22. Seremetis MG, Lyons WS, deGuzman VC, et al. Leiomyomata of the esophagus. An analysis of 838 cases. *Cancer* 1976;38:2166.
23. Postlethwait RW, Musser AW. Changes in the esophagus in 1,000 autopsy specimens. *J Thorac Cardiovasc Surg* 1974;68:953.
24. Taylor FH, Christenson W, Zollinger RW II, et al. Multiple leiomyomas of the esophagus. *Ann Thorac Surg* 1995;60:182.
25. Stelow EB, Jones DR, Shami VM. Esophageal leiomyosarcoma diagnosed by endoscopic ultrasound-guided fine-needle aspiration. *Diagn Cytopathol* 2007;35(3):167–170.
26. Bonavina L, Segalin A, Rosati R, et al. Surgical therapy of esophageal leiomyoma. *J Am Coll Surg* 1995;181:257–262.
27. Lee LS, Singhal S, Brinster CJ, et al. Current management of esophageal leiomyoma. *J Am Coll Surg* 2004;198:136.
28. Kent M, d'Amato T, Nordman C, et al. Minimally invasive resection of benign esophageal tumors. *J Thorac Cardiovasc Surg* 2007;134(1): 176–181.
29. Schuhmacher C, Becker K, Dittler HJ, et al. Fibrovascular esophageal polyp as a diagnostic challenge. *Dis Esophagus* 2000;13:324.
30. Pohl H, Welch G. The role of overdiagnosis and reclassification in the marked increase of esophageal adenocarcinoma incidence. *J Natl Cancer Inst* 2005;97:142–146.
31. Orringer MB. Substernal gastric bypass of the excluded esophagus—results of an ill-advised operation. *Surgery* 1984;96:467.
32. Risk JM, Mills HS, Garde J, et al. The tylosis esophageal cancer (TOC) locus: more than just a familial cancer gene. *Dis Esophagus* 1999;12:173.
33. Ellis A, Field JK, Field EA, et al. Tylosis associated with carcinoma of the oesophagus and oral leukoplakia in a large Liverpool family—a review of six generations. *Eur J Cancer B Oral Oncol* 1994;30:102.
34. Fein R, Kelsen DP, Geller N, et al. Adenocarcinoma of the esophagus and gastroesophageal junction: prognostic factors and results of therapy. *Cancer* 1985;56:2512.
35. Puli SR, Reddy JB, Bechtold ML, et al. Staging accuracy of esophageal cancer by endoscopic ultrasound: a meta-analysis and systematic review. *World J Gastroenterol* 2008;14(10):1479–1490.
36. Flamen P, Lerut A, Van Cutsem E, et al. Utility of positron emission tomography for the staging of patients with potentially operable esophageal carcinoma. *J Clin Oncol* 2000;18:3202.
37. Swisher SG, Maish M, Erasmus JJ, et al. Utility of PET, CT, and EUS to identify pathologic responders in esophageal cancer. *Ann Thorac Surg* 2004;78:1152–1160.
38. Cerfolio RJ, Bryant AS, Buddhiwardhan O, et al. The accuracy of endoscopic ultrasonography with fine-needle aspiration, integrated positron emission tomography with computed tomography, and computed tomography in restaging patients with esophageal cancer after neoadjuvant chemoradiotherapy. *J Thorac Cardiovasc Surg* 2005;129:1232–1241.
39. Krasna MJ, Flowers JL, Attar S, et al. Combined thoracoscopic/laparoscopic staging of esophageal cancer. *J Thorac Cardiovasc Surg* 1996;111: 800; discussion 806.

40. Lagergren J, Bergström R, Lindgren A, et al. Symptomatic gastroesophageal reflux as a risk factor for esophageal adenocarcinoma. *N Engl J Med* 1999;340:825.
41. Spechler SJ. Dysplasia in Barrett's esophagus: limitations of current management strategies. *Am J Gastroenterol* 2005;100(4):927–935.
42. Solaymani-Dodaran M, Logan RF, West J, et al. Risk of oesophageal cancer in Barrett's oesophagus and gastro-oesophageal reflux. *Gut* 2004;53:1070.
43. Shaheen N, Ransohoff DF. Gastroesophageal reflux, Barrett esophagus, and esophageal cancer: scientific review. *JAMA* 2002;287:1972.
44. Aggestrup S, Holm JC, Sørensen HR. Does achalasia predispose to cancer of the esophagus? *Chest* 1992;102:1013.
45. Esophagus. In: American Joint Committee on Cancer. *AJCC Cancer Staging Manual*, 6th ed. New York: Springer; 2002:91–98.
46. Arnott SJ, Duncan W, Gignoux M, et al; (Oeosphageal Cancer Collaborative Group). Preoperative radiotherapy for esophageal carcinoma. *Cochrane Database Syst Rev* 2005 Oct 19;(4): CD001799.
47. Kelsen DP, Ginsberg R, Pajak TF, et al. Chemotherapy followed by surgery compared with surgery alone for localized esophageal cancer. *N Engl J Med* 1998;339:1979.
48. Medical Research Council Oesophageal Cancer Working Group. Surgical resection with or without postoperative chemotherapy in oesophageal cancer: a randomised controlled trial. *Lancet* 2002;359:1727.
49. Cunningham D, Allum WH, Stenning SP, et al. Perioperative chemotherapy versus surgery alone for resectable gastroesophageal cancer. *N Engl J Med* 2006;355(1):11–20.
50. Malthaner RA, Collin S, Fenlon D. Preoperative chemotherapy for resectable thoracic esophageal cancer. *Cochrane Database Syst Rev* 2006 Jul 19;(3):CD001556.
51. Walsh T, Noonan N, Hollywood D, et al. A comparison of multimodal therapy and surgery for esophageal adenocarcinoma. *N Engl J Med* 1996;335:462.
52. Bosset J-F, Gignoux M, Triboulet J-P, et al. Chemoradiotherapy followed by surgery compared with surgery alone in squamous-cell cancer of the esophagus. *N Engl J Med* 1997;337:161.
53. Gebski V, Burmeister B, Smithers BM, et al. Survival benefits from neoadjuvant chemoradiotherapy or chemotherapy in oesophageal carcinoma: a meta-analysis. *Lancet Oncol* 2007;8:33–34.
54. Davis PA, Law S, Wong J. Colonic interposition after esophagectomy for cancer. *Arch Surg* 2003;138:303.
55. Orringer MB, Marshall B, Iannettoni MD. Eliminating the cervical esophagogastric anastomotic leak with a side-to-side stapled anastomosis. *J Thorac Cardiovasc Surg* 2000;119:277.
56. Orringer MB, Marshall B, Iannettoni MD. Transhiatal esophagectomy: clinical experience and refinements. *Ann Surg* 1999;230:392; discussion 400.
57. Orringer MB, Marshall B, Chang AC, et al. Two thousand transhiatal esophagectomies: changing trends, lessons learned. *Ann Surg* 2007;246:363–374.
58. Altorki N, Kent M, Ferrara C, et al. Three-field lymph node dissection for squamous cell and adenocarcinoma of the esophagus. *Ann Surg* 2002;236:177.
59. Hulscher JB, van Sandick JW, de Boer AG, et al. Extended transthoracic resection compared with limited transhiatal resection for adenocarcinoma of the esophagus. *N Engl J Med* 2002;374:1662.
60. Peyre CG, Hagen JA, DeMeester SR, et al. The number of lymph nodes removed predicts survival in esophageal cancer: an international study on the impact of extent of surgical resection. *Ann Surg* 2008;248:549–556.
61. Heitmiller RF. Results of standard left thoracoabdominal esophagogastrectomy. *Semin Thorac Cardiovasc Surg* 1992;4:314.
62. Luketich JD, Alvelo-Rivera M, Buenaventura PO, et al. Minimally invasive esophagectomy: outcomes in 222 patients. *Ann Surg* 2003;238:486.
63. Litle VR, Luketich JD, Christie NA, et al. Photodynamic therapy as palliation for esophageal cancer: experience in 215 patients. *Ann Thorac Surg* 2003;76:1687.

CHAPTER 43 ■ GASTRIC ANATOMY AND PHYSIOLOGY

MICHAEL W. MULHOLLAND

KEY POINTS

1. The stomach is an extremely well-vascularized organ, supplied by a number of major arteries and protected by a large number of extramural and intramural collaterals.
2. Oxyntic glands occupy the fundus and body of the stomach and contain the oxyntic or parietal cells, which are the sites of acid production. Oxyntic glands also contain chief cells, the site of gastric pepsinogen synthesis.
3. The most important stimulant of gastrin release is a meal. Postprandial luminal pH also strongly affects gastrin secretion.
4. Ghrelin is the only known circulating hormone that causes the sensation of hunger and stimulates oral intake.
5. The basolateral membrane of the parietal cell contains specific receptors for histamine, gastrin, and acetylcholine, the three major stimulants of acid production.
6. Pepsins are a heterogeneous group of proteolytic enzymes that are secreted by the gastric chief cells.
7. The gastric mucosa is the site of production of intrinsic factor, which is necessary for the absorption of cobalamin from the ileal mucosa. Total gastrectomy is regularly followed by cobalamin malabsorption, as is resection of the proximal stomach or atrophic gastritis that involves the oxyntic mucosa.

GROSS ANATOMY

The stomach and duodenum, along with the esophagus, liver, bile ducts, and pancreas, are derived from the embryonic foregut. During the fifth week of gestation, the future stomach is marked as a dilation in the caudal portion of the foregut. Cranial to this dilation, the trachea forms as a bud from the future esophagus. At this time, the primitive stomach is invested with both ventral and dorsal mesenteries. The embryonic ventral mesentery is represented in postnatal life by the falciform ligament and by the gastrohepatic and hepatoduodenal mesenteries that form the lesser omentum. The celiac artery, the major blood supply to the foregut, passes within the dorsal mesentery. The primitive dorsal mesentery ultimately forms three structures: the gastrocolic ligament, the gastrosplenic ligament, and the gastrophrenic ligament.

During the sixth and seventh weeks of gestation, the typical morphology of the stomach is established. Accelerated growth of the left gastric wall, relative to the right, establishes the greater and lesser curvatures. This unequal growth also rotates the stomach and causes the left vagal nerve trunk to assume its anterior position, whereas the right vagal trunk is located posteriorly. The growth of structures cephalad to the stomach causes the organ to descend. During the sixth week, the primitive stomach lies between the T10 and T12 vertebral segments. By the eighth week, the stomach is located between the T11 and the L4 segments. In adult life, the stomach is most commonly located between the T10 and the L3 vertebral segments.

The stomach can be divided into anatomic regions based on external landmarks (Fig. 43.1). Although this division is commonly referred to in surgical texts and is useful in discussing gastric resective procedures, it does not necessarily reflect the secretory or motor functions of the mucosal and muscular layers of the stomach. The gastric cardia is the region of the stomach just distal to the gastroesophageal junction. The fundus is the portion of the stomach above and to the left of the gastroesophageal junction. The corpus constitutes the region between the fundus and the antrum. The margin between the corpus and antrum is not distinct externally but can be defined arbitrarily by a line from the incisura angularis on the lesser curvature to a point one-fourth the distance from the pylorus to the esophagus along the greater curvature. The gastric antrum is bounded distally by the pylorus, which can be appreciated by palpation as a thickened ring of smooth muscle.

The stomach is mobile in most people and is fixed at only two points, proximally by the gastroesophageal junction and distally by the retroperitoneal duodenum. Therefore, the position of the stomach varies and depends on the habitus of the person, the degree of gastric distention, and the position of the other abdominal organs. Anteriorly, the stomach is in contact with the left hemidiaphragm, the left lobe and the anterior segment of the right lobe of the liver, and the anterior parietal surface of the abdominal wall. The posterior surface of the stomach is related to the left diaphragm; the left kidney and left adrenal gland; the neck, tail, and body of the pancreas; the aorta and celiac trunk; and the periaortic nerve plexuses. The greater curvature of the stomach is near the transverse colon and the transverse colonic mesentery. The concavity of the spleen contacts the left lateral portion of the stomach.

1 The stomach is an extremely well-vascularized organ, supplied by a number of major arteries and protected by a large number of extramural and intramural collaterals. Gastric viability can be preserved after ligation of all but one primary artery, an advantage that can be exploited during gastric reconstructive procedures. Also, the rich network of anastomosing vessels means that gastric hemorrhage cannot be controlled by the extramural ligation of gastric arteries. Most gastric blood flow is ordinarily derived from the celiac trunk (Fig. 43.2). The lesser curvature is supplied by the left gastric artery, which is the first major branch of the celiac trunk, and by the right gastric artery, which is derived from the hepatic artery. Branches of the left gastric artery also supply the lowermost portion of the esophagus. The greater curvature is supplied by the short gastric and left gastroepiploic arteries, which are branches of the splenic artery, and by the right gastroepiploic

FIGURE 43.1. Topographic relations of the stomach.

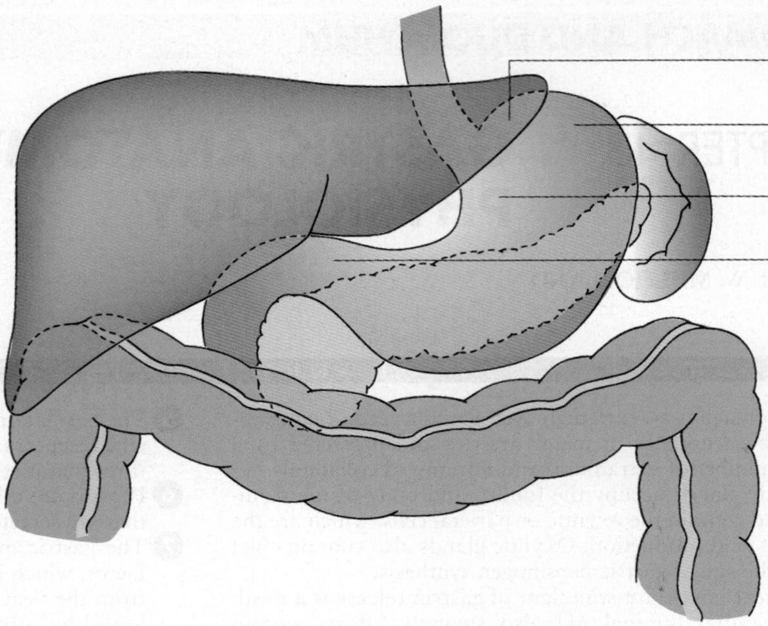

artery, a branch of the gastroduodenal artery. In instances of celiac trunk occlusion, gastric blood flow is usually maintained from the superior mesenteric artery collaterally by way of the pancreaticoduodenal arcade. In general, venous effluent from the stomach parallels the arterial supply. The venous equivalent of the left gastric artery is the coronary vein.

As a first approximation, the lymphatic drainage of the stomach parallels gastric venous return (Fig. 43.3). Lymph from the proximal portion of the stomach along the lesser curvature first drains into superior gastric lymph nodes surrounding the left gastric artery. The distal portion of the lesser curvature drains through suprapyloric nodes. The proximal portion of the greater curvature is supplied by lymphatic vessels that traverse pancreaticosplenic nodes, whereas the antral portion of the greater curvature drains into the subpyloric and omental nodal groups. Secondary drainage from each of these systems eventually traverses nodes at the base of the celiac axis. These discrete anatomic groupings are misleading. The lymphatic drainage of the human stomach, like its blood supply, exhibits extensive intramural ramifications and a number of extramural communications. As a consequence, disease processes that involve the gastric lymphatics often spread

FIGURE 43.2. Arterial blood supply of the stomach.

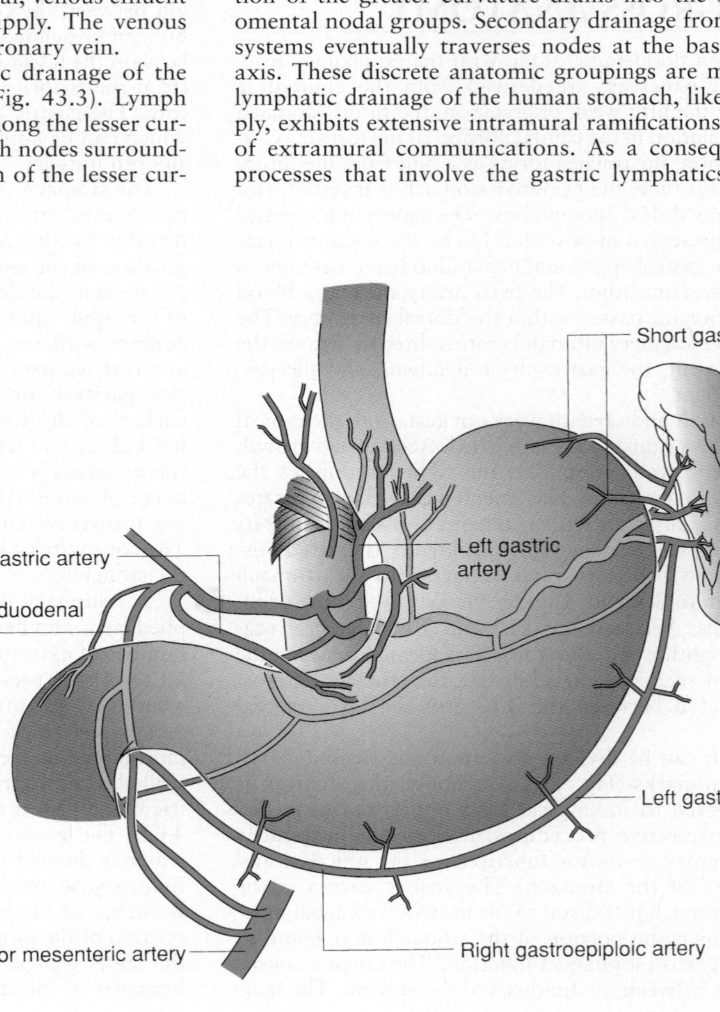

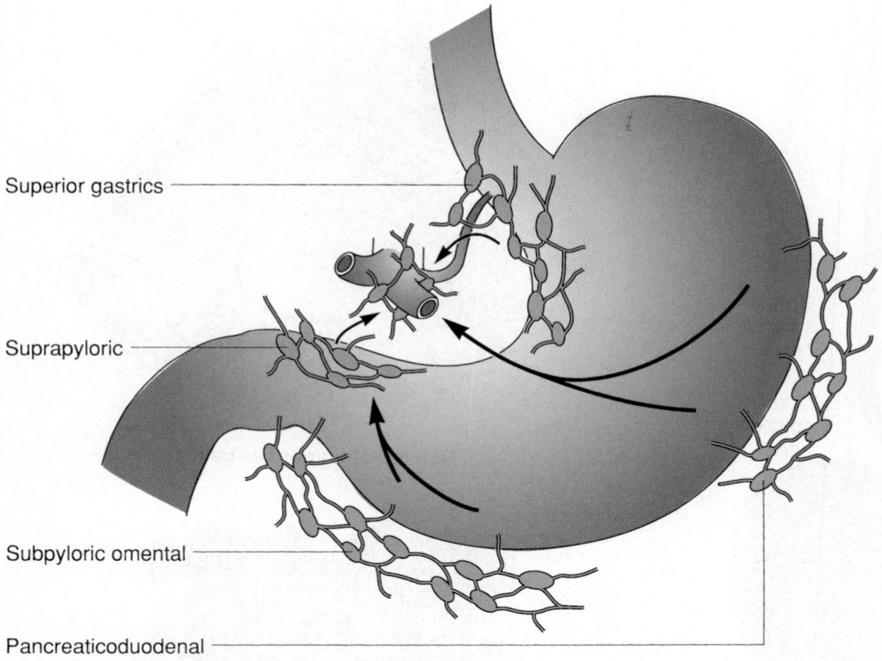

FIGURE 43.3. Lymphatic drainage of the stomach.

intramurally beyond the region of origin and to nodal groups at a distance from the primary lymphatic zone.

The left and right vagal nerves descend parallel to the esophagus within the thorax before forming a periesophageal plexus between the tracheal bifurcation and the diaphragm. From this plexus, two vagal trunks coalesce before passing through the esophageal hiatus of the diaphragm (Fig. 43.4). The left vagal trunk is usually closely applied to the anterior surface of the esophagus, whereas the posterior vagal trunk is often midway between the esophagus and the aorta. The anterior vagus supplies a hepatic division, which passes to the right in the lesser omentum before innervating the liver and biliary tract. The remainder of the anterior vagal fibers parallel the lesser curvature of the stomach, branching to the anterior gastric wall. The posterior vagus nerve branches into the celiac division, which passes to the celiac plexus, and a posterior gastric division, which innervates the posterior gastric wall.

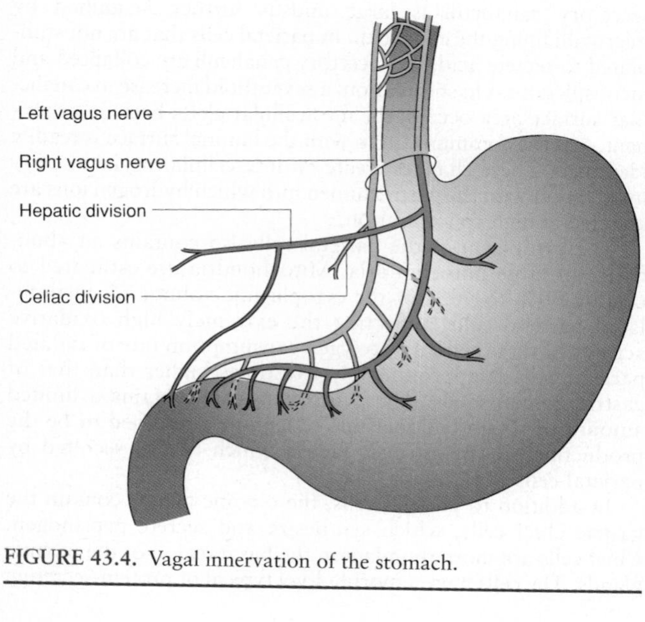

FIGURE 43.4. Vagal innervation of the stomach.

Approximately 90% of the fibers in the vagal trunks are afferent, transmitting information from the gastrointestinal tract to the central nervous system (CNS). Parasympathetic afferent fibers are not responsible for the sensation of gastric pain. Only 10% of vagal nerve fibers are motor or secretory efferents. Parasympathetic efferent fibers contained in the vagus originate in the dorsal nucleus of the medulla. Vagal efferent fibers pass without synapse to contact postsynaptic neurons in the gastric wall in the myenteric and submucous plexuses. Secondary neurons directly innervate gastric smooth muscle or epithelial cells. Acetylcholine is the neurotransmitter of primary vagal efferent neurons.

The gastric sympathetic innervation is derived from spinal segments T5 through T10. Sympathetic fibers leave the corresponding spinal nerve roots by way of gray rami communicantes and enter a series of bilateral prevertebral ganglia (Fig. 43.5). From these ganglia, presynaptic fibers pass through the greater splanchnic nerves to the celiac plexus, where they synapse with secondary sympathetic neurons. Postsynaptic sympathetic nerve fibers enter the stomach in association with blood vessels. Afferent sympathetic fibers pass without synapse from the stomach to dorsal spinal roots. Pain of gastroduodenal origin is sensed through afferent fibers of sympathetic origin.

MICROSCOPIC ANATOMY

The glandular portions of the stomach are lined by a simple columnar epithelium composed of surface mucous cells. The luminal surface, visualized by scanning electron microscopy, appears cobblestoned, interrupted at intervals by gastric pits. Opening into the gastric pits are one or more gastric glands that impart functional significance to the gastric mucosa. The mucosa of the human stomach is composed of three distinct types of gastric glands—cardiac, oxyntic, and antral.

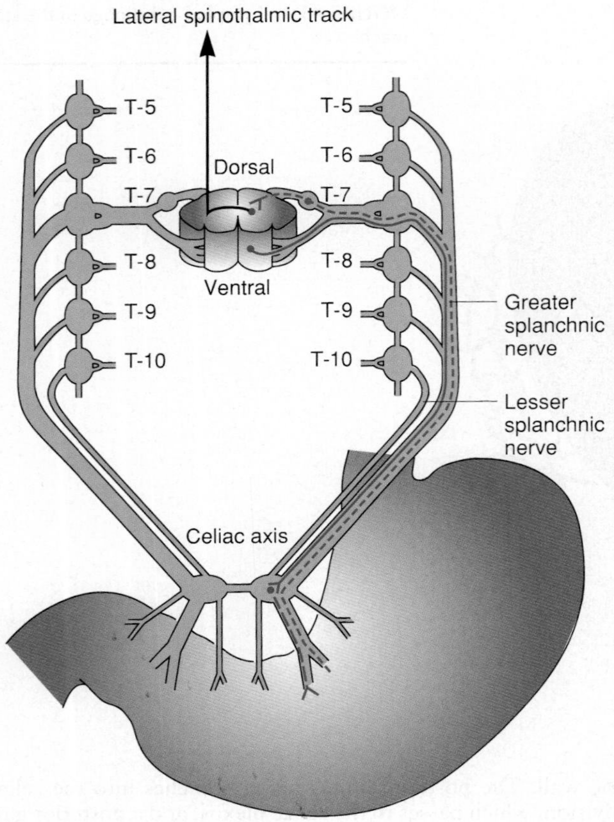

FIGURE 43.5. Derivation of gastric sympathetic innervation.

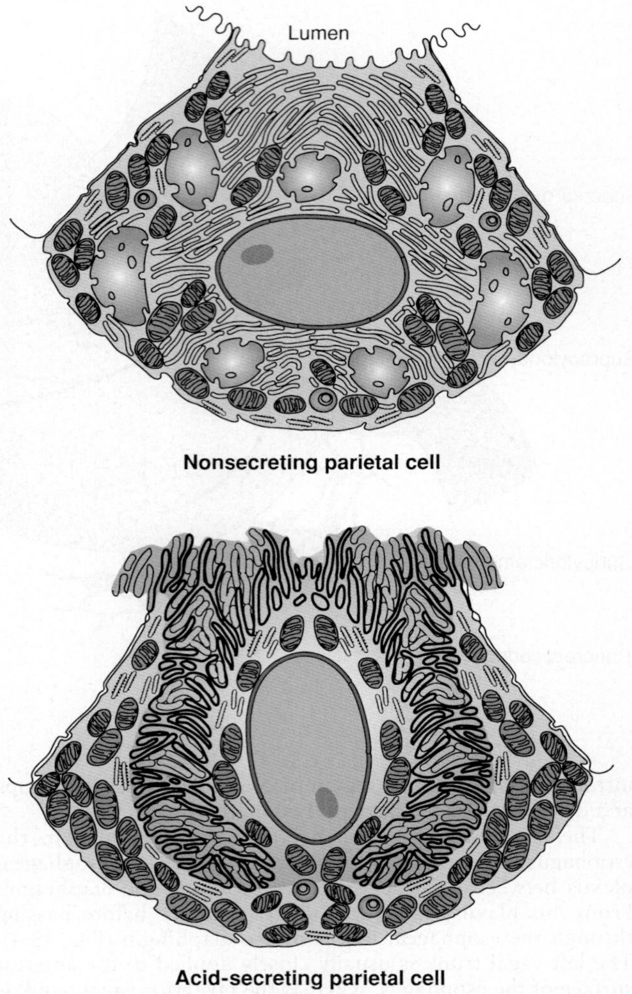

FIGURE 43.6. Resting and stimulated parietal cell, emphasizing morphologic transformation with increase in secretory canalicular membrane surface area that occurs with acid secretion.

In humans, cardiac glands occupy a narrow zone adjacent to the esophagus and mark a transition from the stratified squamous epithelium of the esophagus to the simple columnar epithelium of the stomach. The surface and gastric pit mucous cells of the cardia are not distinguishable from those in other areas of the stomach. Cardiac glands contain mucous and undifferentiated and endocrine cells but not the parietal or chief cells that are prominent in the adjacent oxyntic mucosa. Cardiac glands are usually branched and connect with relatively short gastric pits. The functional properties of cardiac glands include the secretion of mucus.

2 Oxyntic glands are the most distinctive feature of the human stomach. They occupy the fundus and body of the stomach and contain the oxyntic or parietal cells, which are the sites of acid production. Oxyntic glands also contain chief cells, the site of gastric pepsinogen synthesis. The tubular oxyntic glands are usually relatively straight but sometimes branch; several glands may empty into a single gastric pit. The glands are divided into three regions: (a) the isthmus, containing surface mucous cells and a few scattered parietal cells; (b) the neck, with a heavy concentration of parietal cells and a few neck mucous cells; and (c) the base of the gland, containing chief cells, undifferentiated cells, a few parietal cells, and some mucous neck cells. Endocrine cells are scattered throughout all three regions of oxyntic glands.

The most distinctive cell of the gastric mucosa is the acid-secreting parietal cell. Parietal cells have an unusual ultrastructural specialization in the form of intracellular canaliculi, a network of clefts extending to the basal cytoplasm and often encircling the nucleus, which is continuous with the gland lumen (Fig. 43.6). The surface area provided by the intracellular secretory canaliculi is large and is further magnified by microvilli lining the canaliculi. In parietal cells that are not stimulated to secrete acid, the secretory canaliculi are collapsed and inconspicuous. On stimulation, a severalfold increase in canalicular surface area occurs, the intracellular clefts become prominent, and the communication with the luminal surface is readily identified. These changes create an intracellular space in communication with the gastric lumen into which hydrogen ions are secreted at high concentration.

The cytoplasm of the parietal cell also contains an abundance of large mitochondria. Mitochondria are estimated to occupy 30% to 40% of the cytoplasmic volume of unstimulated parietal cells, reflecting the extremely high oxidative activity of these cells. The oxygen consumption rate of isolated parietal cells is approximately five times higher than that of gastric mucous cells. The cytoplasm also contains a limited amount of rough endoplasmic reticulum, presumed to be the production site of intrinsic factor, which is also secreted by parietal cells.

In addition to parietal cells, the oxyntic glands contain the gastric chief cells, which synthesize and secrete pepsinogen. Chief cells are most abundant in the basal region of the oxyntic glands. The cells have a morphology typical of protein-secreting

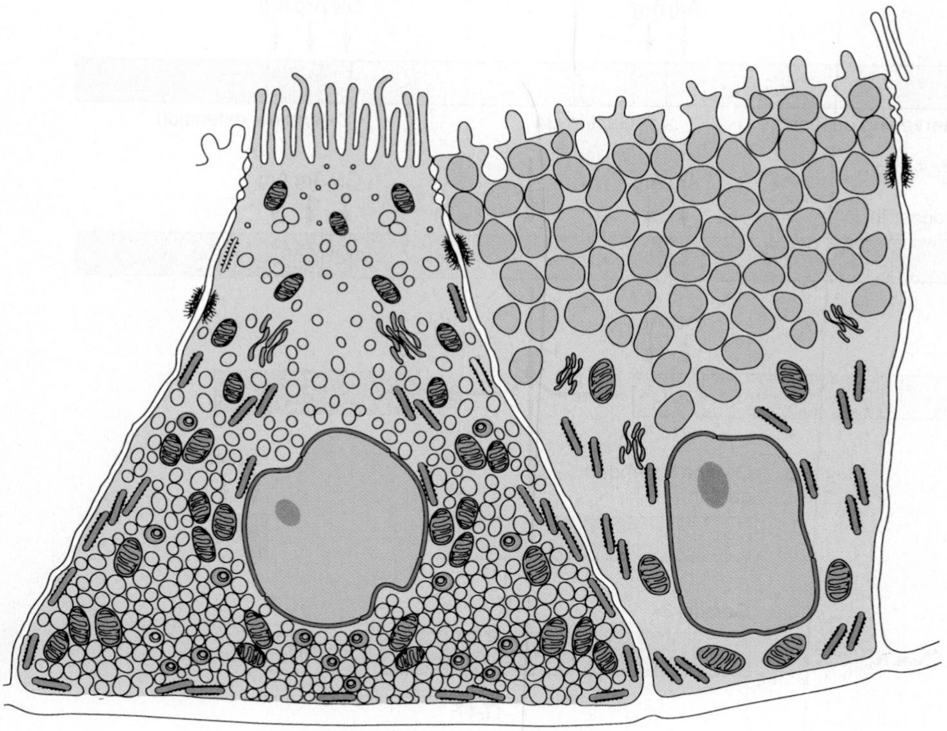

FIGURE 43.7. Contrasting morphology of antral gastrin cell (*left*) with basally oriented secretory granules, and gastric mucous cell (*right*) with apical mucous granules.

exocrine cells and are similar in ultrastructural appearance to pancreatic acinar cells. Rough endoplasmic reticulum is abundant in the cytoplasm and extends between secretory granules. Zymogen granules containing pepsinogen are most concentrated in the apical cytoplasm. Pepsinogen is released by exocytosis from secretory granules at the apical surface of chief cells.

Antral glands occupy the mucosa of the distal stomach and pyloric channel. Antral glands are relatively straight and often empty through deep gastric pits. Although most cells in the antral glands are mucus secreting, gastrin cells are the distinctive feature of this mucosa. Gastrin cells are pyramid shaped, with a narrow area of luminal contact apically and a broad surface overlying the lamina propria basally (Fig. 43.7). Gastrin cells are identified immunocytochemically by the presence of the peptide. Granules ranging from 150 to 400 nm in diameter are the sites of gastrin storage and are most numerous in the basal cytoplasm. Gastrin is released by exocytotic fusion of the secretory granule with the plasma membrane. In contrast to secretion from chief cells, emptying of gastrin-containing granules occurs at the basal membrane rather than at the apical region of the cell. Gastrin thus released diffuses to and enters submucosal capillaries in close apposition to the lamina propria.

GASTRIC PEPTIDES

The stomach contains a number of biologically active peptides in nerves and mucosal endocrine cells, including gastrin, somatostatin, ghrelin, gastrin-releasing peptide, vasoactive intestinal polypeptide (VIP), substance P, glucagon, and calcitonin gene–related peptide. The peptides with the greatest importance to human disease and clinical surgery are gastrin, somatostatin, and ghrelin.

Gastrin

The synthesis, secretion, and action of gastrin have been extensively studied, and many aspects of the biology of gastrin appear to be shared by other gastrointestinal peptide hormones.[1] The gene that encodes for gastrin has been isolated using a human DNA library. The human gastrin gene contains three exons; two exons consist of coding sequences. The major active product is encoded by a single exon. In adults, the gastrin gene is expressed primarily in mucosa cells of the gastric antrum, with lower levels of expression in the duodenum, pituitary, and testis. During embryonic development, the gastrin gene is transiently active in pancreatic islets and colonic mucosa.

The human gene encompasses approximately 4,100 base pairs and directs the synthesis of a peptide of 101 amino acids (Fig. 43.8). The resulting peptide, preprogastrin, contains the sequence of gastrin within its amino acid sequence. Preprogastrin consists of a signal peptide of 21 amino acids, an intervening peptide of 37 amino acids, the 34-residue region of the gastrin molecule, and a carboxyl-terminal extension of nine amino acids. Gastrin is derived from its preprohormone by the sequential enzymatic cleavage of the signal peptide, the intervening peptide, and the carboxyl-terminal extension.

The signal peptide region of preprogastrin consists of a series of hydrophobic amino acids that direct the nascent peptide into the endoplasmic reticulum as it is translated from messenger RNA. After directing the preprogastrin molecule into the rough endoplasmic reticulum, the signal peptide is removed. The remaining peptide is termed *progastrin.* Progastrin is further processed as it traverses the endoplasmic reticulum to mature secretory vesicles. Enzymatic cleavage at a pair of basic amino acid residues proximal to the gastrin 34 (G_{34}) sequence removes the intervening peptide. A similar cleavage removes a six-amino-acid fragment at the carboxyl-terminal end. The peptide that remains has a Gly-Arg-Arg sequence at

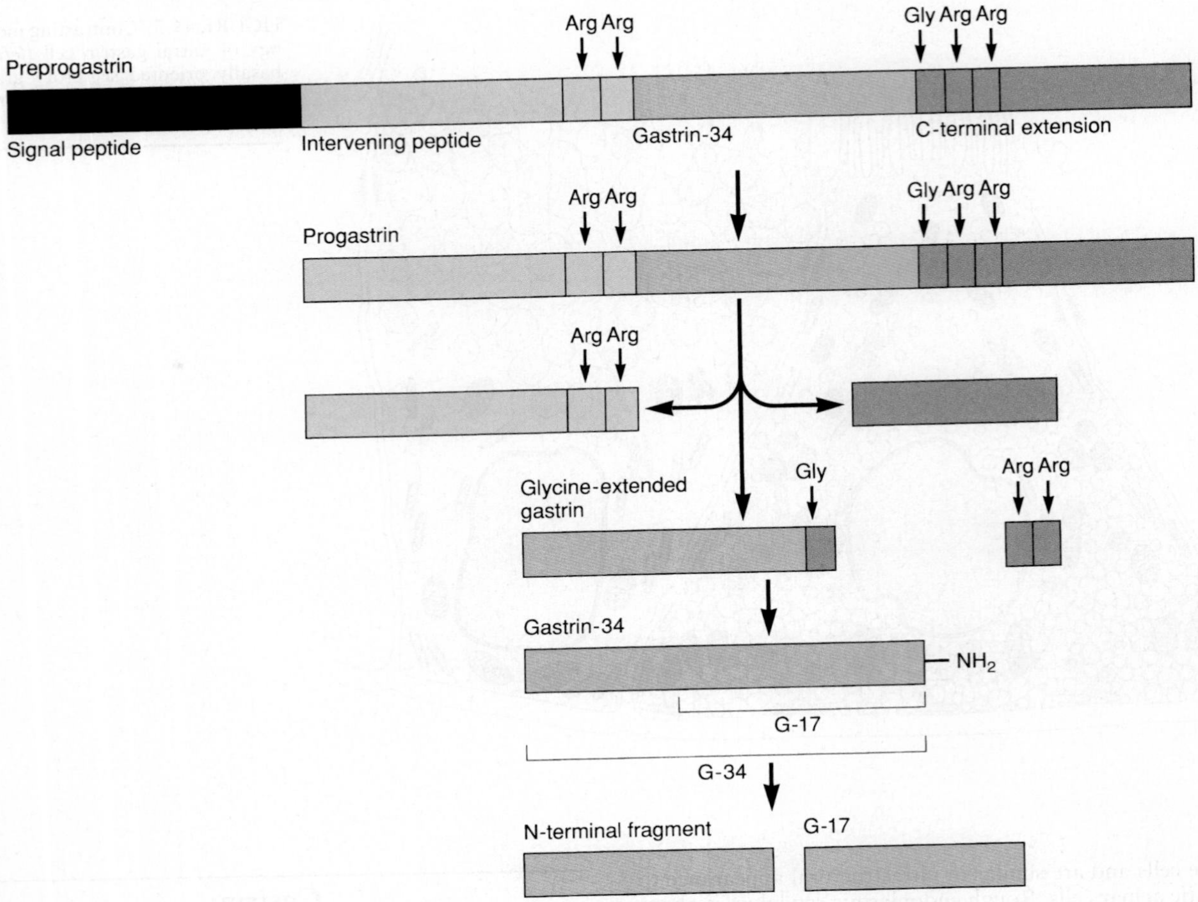

FIGURE 43.8. Sequential processing of preprogastrin molecule.

the carboxyl terminus. Carboxypeptidase cleaves the Arg residues, and the peptide that results is termed *glycine-extended gastrin.* G_{34} is formed by cleavage of the Gly-Arg-Arg sequence and amidation of the carboxyl-terminal phenylalanine. Gastrin, like most gastrointestinal peptide hormones, requires terminal amidation for biologic activity. Gastrin 17 (G_{17}), the most abundant form of gastrin in the human antrum, is formed by further processing that removes the first 17 amino acids at the amino terminus of G_{34}. G_{34} is the predominate molecular form of gastrin in the duodenum.

3 The most important stimulant of gastrin release is a meal. Small peptide fragments and amino acids that result from intragastric proteolysis are the most important food components that stimulate gastrin release. The most potent gastrin-releasing activities are demonstrated by the amino acids tryptophan and phenylalanine. Ingested fat and glucose do not cause gastrin release. Gastric distention by a meal activates cholinergic neurons and stimulates gastrin release. As the meal empties and distention diminishes, VIP-containing neurons are activated, which stimulate somatostatin secretion and thus attenuate gastrin secretion.

Postprandial luminal pH also strongly affects gastrin secretion. Gastrin release is inhibited when acidification of an ingested meal causes the intraluminal pH to fall below 3.0. Conversely, maintaining intragastric pH above 3.0 potentiates gastrin secretion after ingestion of protein or amino acids.[2] Pernicious anemia and atrophic gastritis, which produce chronic achlorhydria, are associated with fasting hypergastrinemia and an exaggerated gastrin meal response. Release of mucosal somatostatin occurs with gastric acidification, and this peptide has been implicated in the inhibition of gastrin release that occurs when luminal pH falls.

The vagus nerve appears to both stimulate and inhibit gastrin release.[3] In humans, vagally mediated stimulation of gastrin release can be demonstrated by sham feeding, insulin-induced hypoglycemia, and administration of the vagal stimulant ψ-aminobutyric acid. In contrast to these stimulatory vagal effects, hypergastrinemia, observed after vagotomy, suggests that inhibitory vagal effects on gastrin release may also exist. Cholinergic neurons stimulate gastrin secretion directly by actions on gastrin cells. By decreasing somatostatin secretion, cholinergic neurons also indirectly stimulate gastrin release. Evidence suggests that vagal stimulation of gastrin release is mediated by bombesin or its mammalian equivalent, gastrin-releasing peptide, acting as a neurotransmitter in the gastric wall. Adrenergic stimulation has also been noted to increase gastrin release.

Chronic gastric infection with *Helicobacter pylori* causes increased acid secretion by altering gastrin release.[4,5] *H. pylori* has been observed to upregulate proinflammatory cytokines, including interleukin (IL)-6, IL-8, and tumor necrosis factor-α (TNF-α). Several inflammatory mediators have been demonstrated to stimulate gastrin release from isolated gastrin cells. The putative gastrin secretagogues include IL-1, IL-8, TNF-α, interferon-ψ, and leukotrienes C4 and D4. The same factors that affect gastrin release also influence gastrin mRNA expression. Food ingestion increases gastrin mRNA abundance, whereas fasting and somatostatin decrease gastrin mRNA production. Chronic achlorhydria, as seen in pernicious anemia, increases gastrin mRNA production.

In addition to stimulating acid secretion from gastric parietal cells (detailed later in this chapter), gastrin has important physiologic actions in the control of gastrointestinal mucosal growth. The acid-secreting oxyntic mucosa is particularly sensitive to the trophic actions of gastrin, but the mucous membranes of the duodenum, colon, and pancreatic parenchyma are also affected. Stimulation of mucosal growth by gastrin is enhanced by the presence of solid food in the diet. The 17- and 34-amino-acid forms of gastrin are equipotent in stimulating mucosal growth. In humans, the relative importance of gastrin and other influences, such as the composition and form of the diet and the actions of other trophic hormones, have not been completely established. Prolonged stimulation by high levels of gastrin, as seen in the Zollinger-Ellison syndrome, is associated with hypertrophy of the gastric mucosa. Smaller increases in circulating gastrin, such as those that follow vagotomy, do not cause mucosal hypertrophy.

Somatostatin

Somatostatin, like gastrin, is very significant in gastric physiology. Somatostatin was first isolated from hypothalamic tissues and was named for its ability to inhibit the release of growth hormone. The peptide was subsequently localized in neurons in central and peripheral nervous systems, and in endocrine cells in the pancreas, stomach, and intestine. The wide tissue distribution of somatostatin suggested important regulatory functions, a concept validated by many investigations.

The human somatostatin gene is located on chromosome 3 and encodes for a precursor of 116 amino acids (Fig. 43.9). The somatostatin molecule is contained in the carboxyl-terminal sequence of this preprohormone. The first 24 amino acids of the amino terminus of preprosomatostatin constitute a signal peptide; cleavage of this signal peptide leaves prosomatostatin. Enzymatic cleavage of an additional 64-amino-acid segment from prosomatostatin forms somatostatin 28. Further processing of somatostatin 28 to somatostatin 14 is tissue-specifically regulated. In the stomach, most somatostatin exists as the shorter peptide.

Gastric somatostatin release responds to luminal, hormonal, and neural signals. Luminal acidification is associated with increased somatostatin release, whereas somatostatin release decreases when luminal pH is increased. A number of peptides have been demonstrated experimentally to release somatostatin from the stomach, including gastrin, cholecystokinin, and secretin. β-Adrenergic agonists have also been shown to release somatostatin. In contrast, electrical stimulation of vagal nerves inhibits somatostatin release, as does the cholinergic agonist methacholine.

The most important gastric function of somatostatin appears to be regulation of acid secretion and gastrin release. Circulating somatostatin appears to be important in modulating gastric acid secretion; locally released somatostatin functions to regulate gastrin release. In each instance, somatostatin serves an inhibitory function, decreasing acid secretion and diminishing the release of gastrin. In animals, antral or duodenal acidification has been associated with an increase in circulating somatostatin. Increases in circulating somatostatin are followed, in turn, by decreased gastric acid secretion. Infusion of exogenous somatostatin in doses that produce somatostatin levels similar to those observed postprandially has also been shown to inhibit acid secretion. In humans, concentrations of somatostatin capable of inhibiting acid secretion can do so without altering serum gastrin levels, indicating a direct action on the acid-secreting fundic mucosa.

Somatostatin is believed to influence gastrin secretion through a locally active intramucosal mechanism. Local actions of somatostatin are supported by ultrastructural studies of antral somatostatin cells, which demonstrate long cytoplasmic processes that make intimate cell-to-cell contact with antral gastrin cells. The presence of somatostatin at these sites of cellular contact implies that somatostatin cells influence the function of gastrin cells through local release of the peptide. Somatostatin can also reach neighboring gastrin cells through diffusion or local blood flow. A number of experiments have suggested that release of somatostatin and gastrin is functionally, although reciprocally, linked. For example, in anesthetized animals, an increase in gastric pH or ingestion of a meal is associated with increases in gastrin and decreases in somatostatin in antral venous blood. Cholinergic agents stimulate gastrin release while inhibiting somatostatin release. Prostaglandin E_2, in contrast, inhibits gastrin release and stimulates somatostatin secretion. These and similar observations suggest that increases in somatostatin release are often associated with decreased gastrin secretion. A family of five somatostatin receptors has been cloned. Inhibition of gastrin-stimulated gastric acid secretion is mediated by somatostatin receptor subtype 2.

Ghrelin

The control of feeding behavior and nutrient intake is an extremely important, and highly regulated, biologic process.

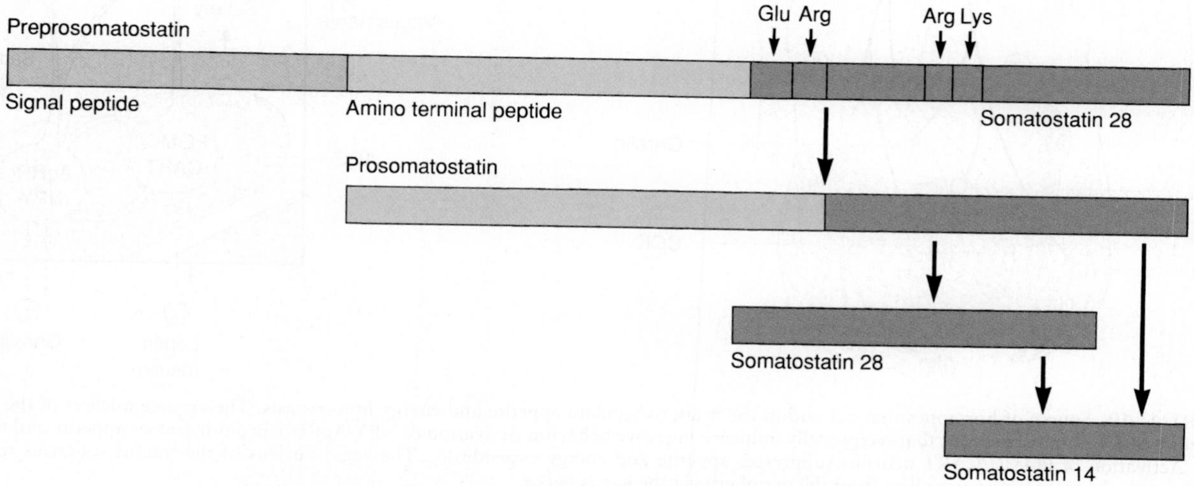

FIGURE 43.9. Derivation of somatostatin 14 from preprosomatostatin precursor.

The control of caloric intake is centered in the hypothalamus, which integrates information on nutritional status, environment, and energy expenditure. This process is regulated by both central and peripheral orexigenic and anorexigenic signals. Peripheral messengers include adiposity signals such as leptin, and a variety of gut peptides. The stomach has recently been recognized as the site of production of an important stimulant of feeding, ghrelin.

Ghrelin is a gastric peptide that is localized to oxyntic glands. Gastric ghrelin cells represent about one fourth of endocrine cells within the gastric mucosa. Ghrelin-expressing cells have no microscopic contact with the gastric lumen, and are presumed to sense signals relevant to feeding from the basolateral side. Ghrelin-positive cells are accordingly closely associated with capillaries in the lamina propria. The hormone is also produced in the hypothalamus.

The ghrelin receptor is a member of the family of G protein–coupled receptors and contains seven transmembrane domains. Ghrelin receptors are widely distributed among both central and peripheral tissues, including the pituitary gland, hypothalamus, pancreas, stomach, and intestine. Ghrelin causes growth hormone secretion following either peripheral or central administration, and release of growth hormone from cultured pituitary cells.

Ghrelin plays an important role in the control of food
4 intake and energy metabolism.[6,7] Ghrelin is the only orexigenic hormone identified to date. In humans, the intravenous administration of ghrelin at physiologic concentrations induces the sensation of hunger and stimulates oral intake. Circulating ghrelin levels peak just prior to meal initiation and decline rapidly postprandially. Ghrelin secretion is increased by weight loss and by restriction of caloric intake. Serum ghrelin levels are increased in anorexic individuals and depressed in obese subjects.[8,9] In animals, ghrelin administration has been found to stimulate food intake, to induce growth of adipose tissues, and to increase body weight. Administration of ghrelin antibody or ghrelin receptor antagonists blunts ghrelin-induced weight gain and positive energy balance.

Ghrelin is a circulating hormone with CNS effects. The arcuate nucleus of the hypothalamus is a crucial site for the integration of fasting and feeding signals.[10] Two types of neurons, with opposing actions on feeding behavior, have been identified in the arcuate nucleus. Neurons that express proopiomelanocortin (POMC) and cocaine and amphetamine-related transcript (CART) suppress food intake, reduce body weight, and increase energy expenditure. In contrast, neurons producing neuropeptide Y and agouti gene–related transcript (AgRP) are orexigenic. These cells act to stimulate food intake and reduce energy expenditure. Ghrelin directly mediates the activities of these two types of neurons, as depicted in Figure 43.10. Direct peripheral effects of ghrelin on peripheral tissues that contribute to the regulation of body weight and energy homeostasis may also exist.

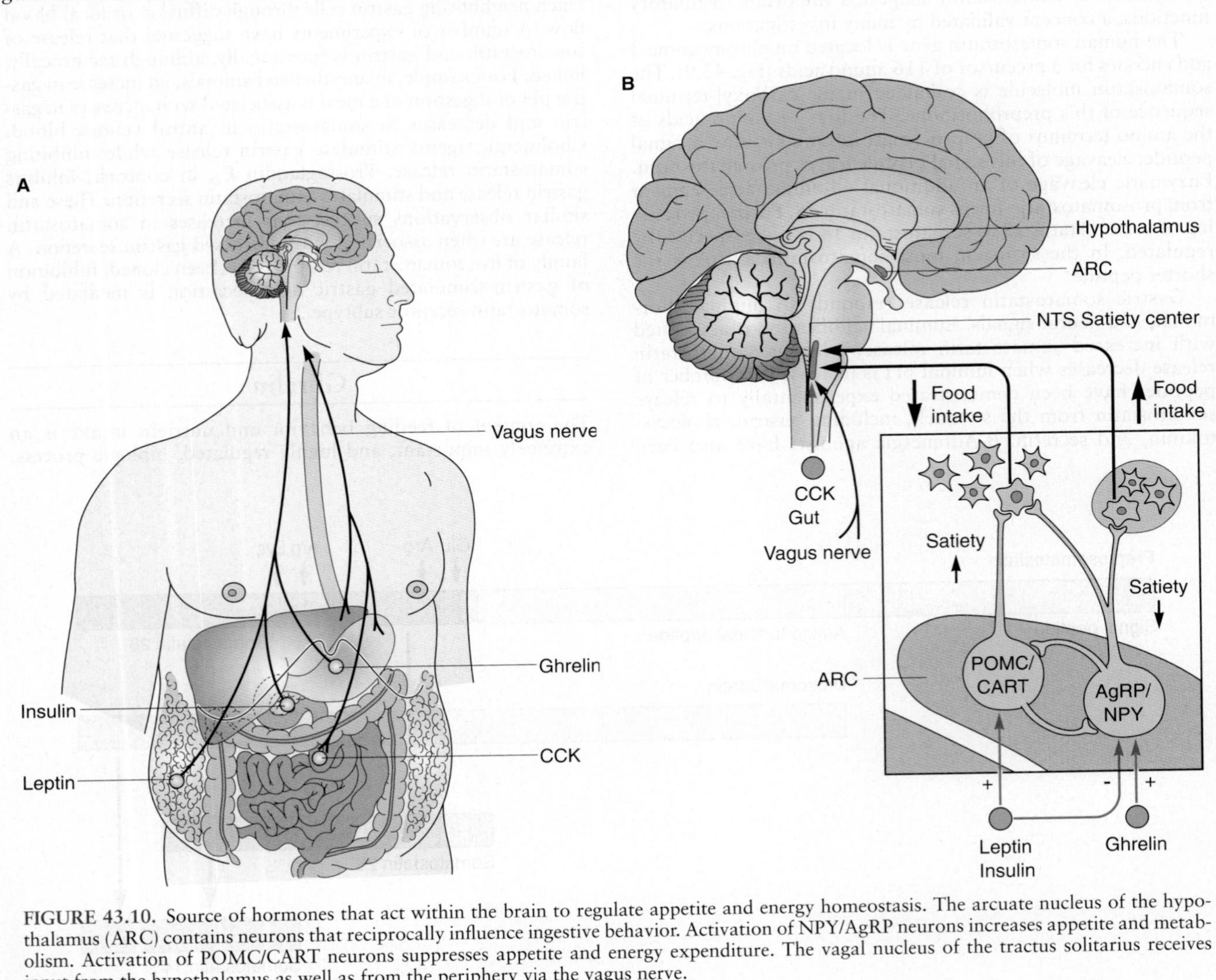

FIGURE 43.10. Source of hormones that act within the brain to regulate appetite and energy homeostasis. The arcuate nucleus of the hypothalamus (ARC) contains neurons that reciprocally influence ingestive behavior. Activation of NPY/AgRP neurons increases appetite and metabolism. Activation of POMC/CART neurons suppresses appetite and energy expenditure. The vagal nucleus of the tractus solitarius receives input from the hypothalamus as well as from the periphery via the vagus nerve.

GASTRIC ACID SECRETION

Cellular Events

An appreciation of the mechanisms that control gastric acid formation is essential to a discussion of gastric disease. An understanding of the cellular basis of acid secretion by the gastric parietal cell also provides a foundation for discussing the pharmacologic treatment of acid–peptic diseases. The basolateral membrane of the parietal cell contains specific receptors for histamine, gastrin, and acetylcholine, the three major stimulants of acid production.[11] Each stimulant reaches the parietal cell by a different route. Histamine is released from mast-like cells within the lamina propria and diffuses to the mucosa, acetylcholine is released in close proximity to the parietal cells from cholinergic nerve terminals, and gastrin is delivered by the systemic circulation to the fundic mucosa from its source in the antrum and proximal duodenum (Fig. 43.11), activating protein kinase A, which in turn catalyzes protein phosphorylation. The target protein molecules for this phosphorylation, in turn, stimulate acid production.

5 Acetylcholine and related cholinergic agonists activate parietal cells after binding to muscarinic receptors. The stimulatory effects of acetylcholine and its congeners can be abolished by atropine. The action of acetylcholine is mediated by muscarinic receptor subtype 3 (M_3). Studies suggest that cholinergic stimulation of parietal cell function is coupled to enhanced mobilization of intracellular calcium. The resultant transient increases in intracellular calcium activate mechanisms that stimulate acid secretion (Fig. 43.12). Evidence also indicates that occupation of acetylcholine receptors increases turnover of specific membrane phospholipids termed *phosphatidylinositides*. Acetylcholine–receptor binding is followed by activation of membrane-associated phospholipase C. Phospholipase C acts on phosphatidylinositol-4,5-bisphosphate (PIP_2) within the plasma membrane to liberate water-soluble inositol triphosphate (IP_3) and diacylglycerol. A major action of IP_3 is to increase intracellular calcium, mainly from intracellular stores in the endoplasmic reticulum. The resulting increased cytosolic calcium interacts with calmodulin or other calcium-binding proteins. Calmodulin kinase type II is involved in parietal cell activation by acetylcholine. Intracellular calcium in this form is postulated to modulate parietal cell function through protein phosphorylation or enzyme activation. Diacylglycerol, the second product released by hydrolysis of PIP_2, activates a class of protein kinases that are phospholipid dependent and Ca^{2+} activated, protein kinase C. Protein kinase C in turn acts to phosphorylate a set of proteins that are distinct from those affected by the calmodulin-dependent system. The ultimate result of this protein phosphorylation is parietal cell activation and hydrogen ion secretion.

Parietal cells can also be activated by occupation of specific gastrin receptors. As with cholinergic stimulation, gastrin exposure increases membrane PIP_2 turnover (see Fig. 43.12). Like acetylcholine, the actions of gastrin depend highly on increases in intracellular calcium and activation of protein kinase C.

Although histamine, acetylcholine, and gastrin occupy separate receptors on the parietal cell and activate differing second-messenger systems, each secretagogue ultimately acts by means of a specialized ion transport system called the *parietal cell proton pump*. This membrane-bound protein is located in the secretory canaliculus of the parietal cell; the peptide has not been identified in other gastric cells or in significant amounts in other organs. The proton pump is an H^+-K^+-adenosine triphosphatase (ATPase) that electroneutrally exchanges cytosolic H^+ for luminal K^+. Hydrogen ions are concentrated 2.5-million-fold within the secretory canaliculus, and the hydrolysis of ATP is the energy source for transport against the steep electrochemical gradient generated. For each H^+ ion transported to the luminal

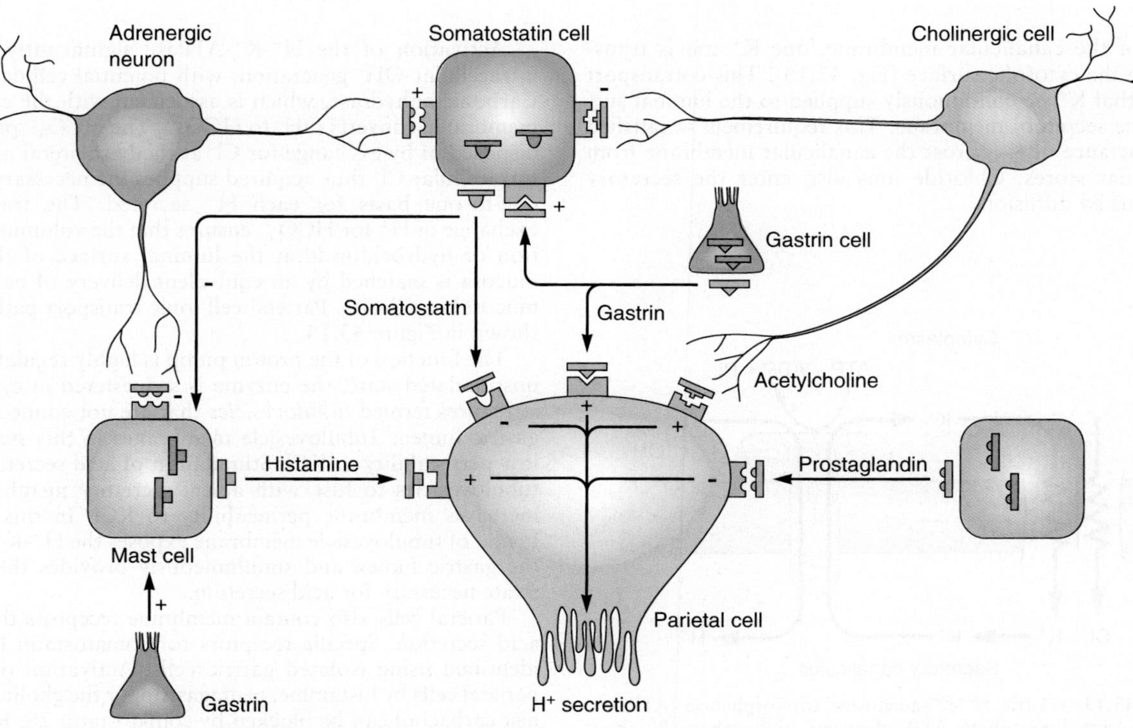

FIGURE 43.11. Interactions of cell types that affect parietal cell acid secretion.

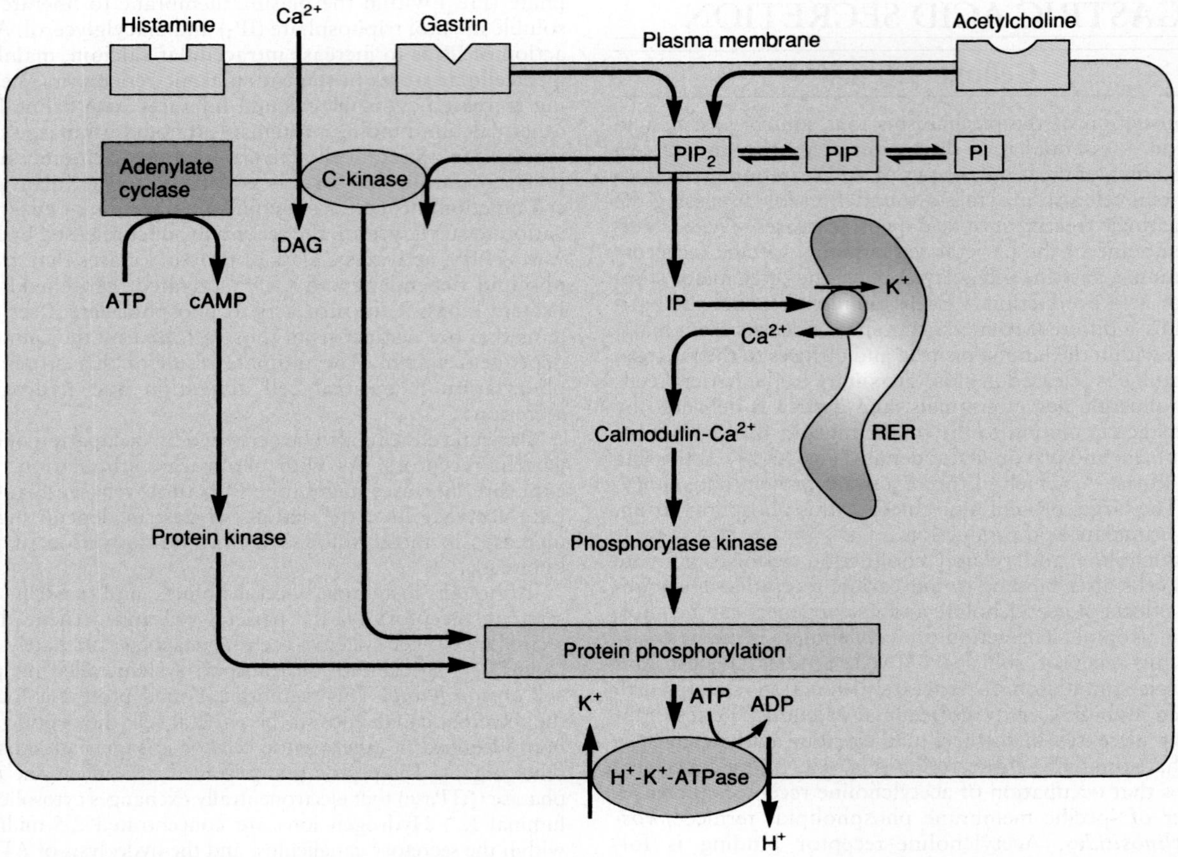

FIGURE 43.12. Cellular mechanisms controlling parietal cell acid secretion. ADP, adenosine diphosphate; ATP, adenosine triphosphate; cAMP, cyclic adenosine monophosphate; PI, phosphatidylinositol; PIP, phosphatidylinositol-4,5-phosphate; PIP_2, phosphatidylinositol-4,5-bisphosphate; RER, rough endoplasmic reticulum.

surface of the canalicular membrane, one K^+ ion is transported to the cytosolic surface (Fig. 43.13). This cotransport requires that K^+ be continuously supplied to the luminal surface of the secretory membrane. This requirement is satisfied by conductance of K^+ across the canalicular membrane from intracellular stores. Chloride ions also enter the secretory canaliculus by diffusion.

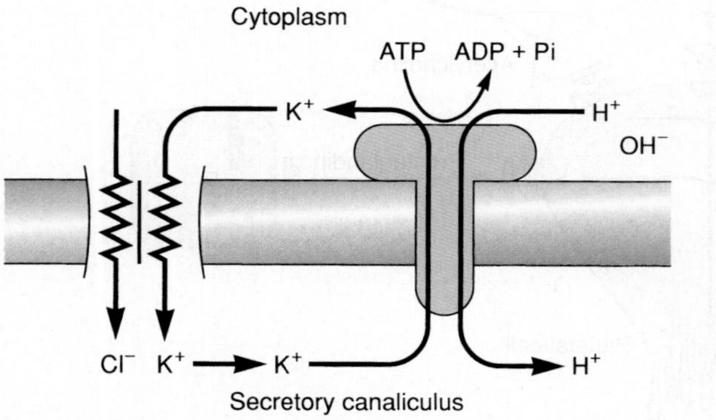

FIGURE 43.13. Gastric H^+-K^+-adenosine triphosphatase (ATPase). ADP, adenosine diphosphate; ATP, adenosine triphosphate; Pi, phosphate ion.

Activation of the H^+-K^+-ATPase significantly increases intracellular OH^- generation, with potential cellular toxicity. Carbonic anhydrase, which is associated with the canalicular membrane, converts OH^- to HCO_3^-. The HCO_3^- produced is disposed of by exchange for Cl^- at the basolateral membrane. Intracellular Cl^- thus acquired supplies the necessary Cl^- on a one-to-one basis for each H^+ secreted. The transcellular exchange of H^+ for HCO_3^- ensures that the voluminous secretion of hydrochloride at the luminal surface of the gastric mucosa is matched by an equivalent delivery of base to submucosal capillaries. Parietal cell ionic transport pathways are shown in Figure 43.14.

The function of the proton pump is highly regulated. In the unstimulated state, the enzyme is sequestered in cytoplasmic structures termed *tubulovesicles* that are not connected to the gastric lumen. Tubulovesicle membranes in this state have a low permeability to KCl. Stimulation of acid secretion causes tubulovesicles to fuse with apical secretory membranes and increases membrane permeability to KCl. In this way, the fusion of tubulovesicle membrane exposes the H^+-K^+ pump to the gastric lumen and simultaneously provides the K^+ substrate necessary for acid secretion.

Parietal cells also contain membrane receptors that inhibit acid secretion. Specific receptors for somatostatin have been identified using isolated gastric cells. Activation of isolated parietal cells by histamine, pentagastrin, or the cholinergic agonist carbachol can be blocked by somatostatin 28. In the case of histamine activation, the inhibitory effects appear to be mediated by the ability of somatostatin to block the production

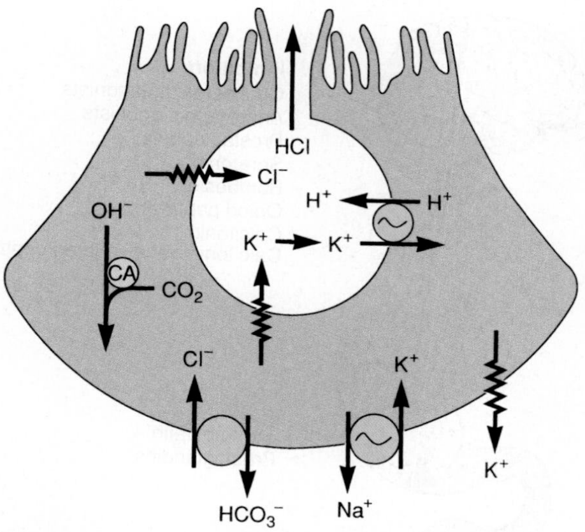

FIGURE 43.14. Ionic fluxes associated with acid secretion by the parietal cell.

of cyclic adenosine monophosphate (cAMP). Somatostatin appears to inhibit the actions of these agonists at a point distal to second-messenger generation. Gastric parietal cells also contain receptors for prostaglandins, notably prostaglandin E_2 and its derivatives. Prostaglandin E_2 is a potent inhibitor of histamine-stimulated parietal cell activation, probably by a mechanism that inhibits formation of cAMP. Prostaglandin inhibition is specific for histamine; the actions of gastrin or carbachol are not affected. Epidermal growth factor and transforming growth factor-α also inhibit histamine-stimulated acid secretion through effects on cAMP production.

These considerations of the cellular basis of acid production demonstrate how parietal cell function can be altered pharmacologically. Gastric acid production can be blocked by receptor antagonists for each of the three primary stimulants—gastrin, acetylcholine, and histamine. Direct inhibition of acid production can be effected by derivatives of somatostatin or prostaglandin E_2. All forms of stimulated acid production can be blocked by agents that act as inhibitors of the parietal cell proton pump. Agents that act at each of these points have been developed, and their appropriate clinical applications are discussed in subsequent chapters.

Regulation of Acid Secretion

Given the multiple receptors on parietal cells, it is not surprising that a great deal of secretagogue interdependence, both stimulatory and inhibitory, exists in humans. Parietal cell activation, and the resultant acid secretion, is greater in response to a combination of agonists than it is in response to the total effect of agents used singly. This increase in responsiveness is defined as *potentiation.* Potentiating interactions are most apparent when agents are used that act by way of different second-messenger systems. Thus, histamine strongly potentiates the acid-secretory response to pentagastrin or to carbachol in humans. Conversely, blockade of receptors to one stimulant also decreases responsiveness to the other agonists. For example, blocking histamine receptors with agents such as cimetidine decreases responsiveness to pentagastrin, even though gastrin receptors are not directly affected. These inhibitory interactions are exploited therapeutically in the treatment of acid–peptic diseases.

Humans normally secrete 2 to 5 mEq/h of hydrochloride in the fasting state, constituting basal acid secretion. Both vagal tone and ambient histamine secretion are presumed to be important in determining the rate of basal acid secretion. In humans, truncal vagotomy decreases basal secretion by approximately 85%. Similarly, H_2-receptor antagonists also inhibit basal acid secretion by approximately 80%. Gastrin does not have an important role in determining basal acid secretion in normal people.

Stimulated acid secretion begins with the thought, sight, or smell of food (Fig. 43.15). This cephalic phase of gastric acid secretion is mediated by the vagus nerve. Vagal discharge directs a cholinergic mechanism, and the cephalic phase of acid secretion can be inhibited by administering atropine. Vagal discharge secondary to cephalic stimulation also inhibits the release of somatostatin. Diminished secretion of somatostatin further augments stimulatory vagal effects, presumably by eliminating tonic inhibition of acid secretion exerted by somatostatin. The cephalic component of acid secretion can be measured in normal people by sham feeding and is approximately 10 mEq/h. The cephalic phase approximates 40% of the maximal acid-secretory response to gastrin infusion.

The gastric phase of acid secretion begins when food enters the stomach. The presence of partially hydrolyzed food constituents, gastric distention, and the buffering capacity of food all stimulate acid secretion. Gastrin is the most important mediator of the gastric phase of acid secretion. In normal humans, acid-secretory rates after a mixed meal average 15 to 25 mEq/h, approximately 75% of the maximal response achieved with infusion of exogenous gastrin or histamine. The meal response is less than the maximal response to exogenous stimulants because food also causes the release of somatostatin and initiates other inhibitory responses. In humans, 90% of meal-stimulated acid secretion is mediated by gastrin release.[12]

The inhibitory regulation of gastric acid secretion is accomplished by CNS, gastric, and intestinal mechanisms. Stimulated acid secretion can be inhibited experimentally by administering various neuropeptides into the lateral cerebral ventricles, including gastrin-releasing peptide (bombesin), corticotropin-releasing factor, and calcitonin gene–related peptide. Although the relevance of these observations to human physiology remains to be determined, it is likely that CNS inhibition of acid secretion exists in humans. In this regard, the vagus nerve has both a stimulatory and an inhibitory role in acid secretion and gastrin release. Vagotomy causes fasting and postprandial hypergastrinemia, indicating that an inhibitory regulation of gastrin release normally exists. Hypergastrinemia is sustained long term after vagotomy by hyperplasia of antral gastrin cells. The vagal fibers to the oxyntic region of the stomach appear to mediate this inhibitory effect.

In humans, the most important and clearly established gastric inhibitory influence is the suppression of gastrin release when the antral mucosa is exposed to acid. When luminal pH falls to 2.0, gastrin release stops. Antral acidification also suppresses the gastrin response to an ingested meal. Somatostatin acting locally in the gastric mucosa as a paracrine agent may mediate this important inhibitory response. Release of gastric somatostatin is reciprocally linked to that of gastrin; acidification of the antrum causes increases in somatostatin release and decreases in gastrin secretion. Antral distention also inhibits stimulated acid secretion.

The entry of digestive products into the intestine begins intestinal-phase inhibition of gastric acid secretion. Acidification of the duodenal bulb inhibits acid secretion, and although exogenous secretin also can inhibit acid secretion, this effect appears to be independent of the release of secretin from the duodenal mucosa. Hyperosmolar solutions and those containing fat also potently inhibit acid secretion. Several peptides,

FIGURE 43.15. Regulation of acid secretion in vivo. TRH, thyroid-releasing hormone.

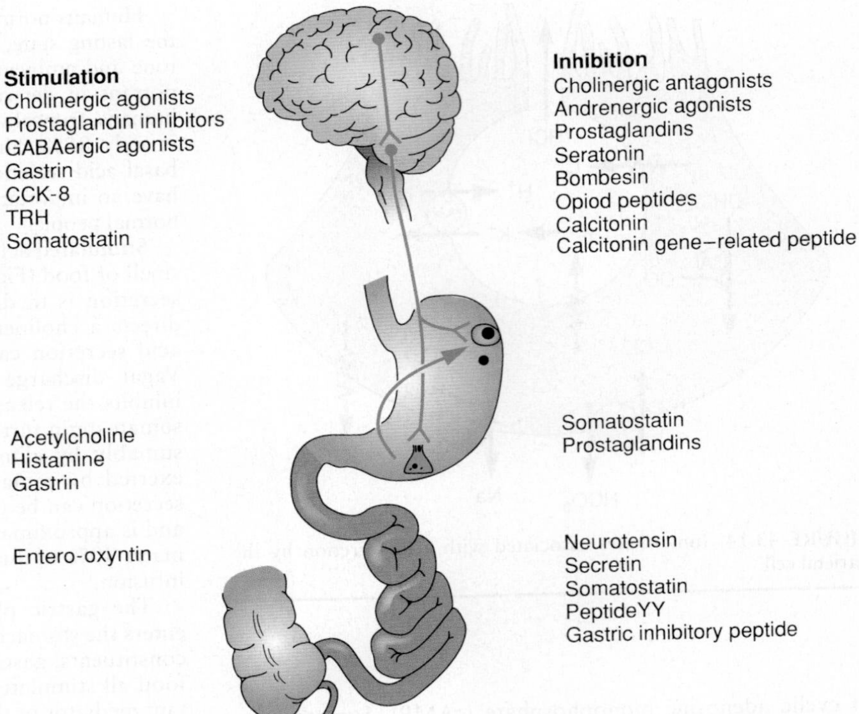

including secretin, somatostatin, peptide YY, gastric inhibitory peptide, and neurotensin, have been proposed as mediators of the intestinal phase effects.

PEPSIN

6 Pepsins are a heterogeneous group of proteolytic enzymes that are secreted by the gastric chief cells. Pepsin is derived under acidic conditions from pepsinogen by the autocatalytic loss of a variable amino-terminal sequence of the parent compound. This conversion occurs slowly at pH values of 5.0 to 6.0 and occurs rapidly when luminal pH approximates 2.0. Pepsin catalyzes the hydrolysis of a wide variety of peptide bonds that contain acidic residues, with a pH optimum for hydrolysis between 1.5 and 2.5. Once activated, pepsin is sensitive to ambient pH values; it is irreversibly denatured at pH 7.0 or greater.

The most important stimulus for pepsinogen secretion is cholinergic stimulation. Acetylcholine and its derivatives stimulate pepsinogen secretion by a mechanism that can be antagonized by atropine, indicating a muscarinic receptor. The receptor is an M_1 type. Endogenous cholinergic stimulation through the vagal nerve results in the formation of a gastric secretion that is rich in pepsin. Although both exogenous histamine and gastrin can stimulate pepsin secretion, their actions appear to be indirectly due to the concomitant secretion of gastric acid rather than to direct stimulation of chief cells. Chief cells have also been shown to possess cholecystokinin receptors, and cholecystokininlike peptides appear to have a direct stimulatory action on chief cells. The oxyntic mucosa contains somatostatin cells near chief cells. Pepsinogen secretion in response to a variety of stimuli has been demonstrated to be inhibited by somatostatin.

The major physiologic function of pepsin is to initiate protein digestion. Pepsin is highly active against collagen and may be important in the digestion of animal protein. Intragastric protein hydrolysis by pepsin is incomplete, and relatively large peptides enter the intestine, although amino acids and small peptide fragments are released. These products of partial hydrolysis are important signals for gastrin and cholecystokinin release, which in turn regulate digestive processes. In this way, pepsin also contributes to the overall coordination of the digestive process.

INTRINSIC FACTOR

7 The gastric mucosa is the site of production of intrinsic factor, which is necessary for the absorption of cobalamin from the ileal mucosa. Total gastrectomy is regularly followed by cobalamin malabsorption, as is resection of the proximal stomach or atrophic gastritis that involves the oxyntic mucosa.

Autoradiographic and immunocytochemical techniques have confirmed the parietal cell as the site of intrinsic factor synthesis and storage in humans. Intrinsic factor secretion, like acid secretion, is stimulated by histamine, acetylcholine, and gastrin. Unlike acid production, intrinsic factor secretion peaks rapidly after stimulation and then returns to baseline. The amount of intrinsic factor secreted usually greatly exceeds the amount needed to bind and absorb available dietary cobalamin.

GASTRIC BICARBONATE PRODUCTION

It is generally agreed that the gastric mucosa secretes HCO_3^- in addition to acid. The cells responsible for HCO_3^- production are presumed to be the surface mucous cells facing the gastric lumen, and HCO_3^- transport has been postulated to protect against damage from luminal acid. In theory, H^+ ions diffusing from luminal bulk fluids toward the gastric mucosa could be neutralized by secreted HCO_3^- near the surface (Fig. 43.16).

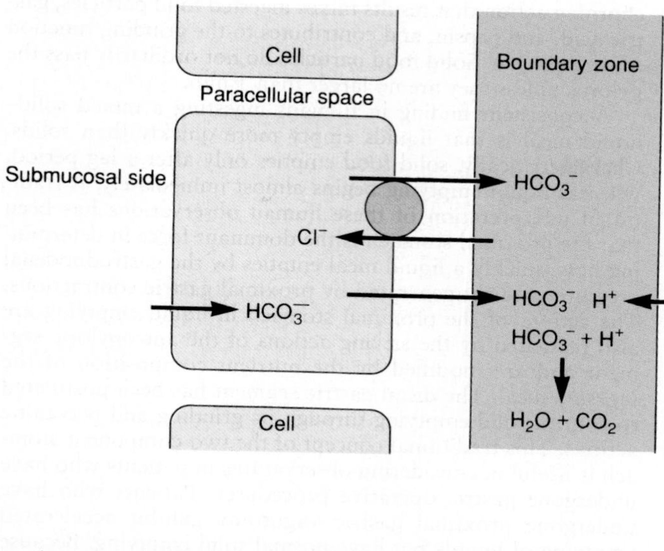

FIGURE 43.16. Schematic representation of mucosal bicarbonate secretion showing neutralization of luminal hydrogen ions immediately above the mucosal surface.

In this way, nearly neutral pH can be maintained at the mucosal surface, even if the total amount of hydrochloride secreted greatly exceeds gastric HCO_3^- production. The occurrence of pH gradients at the surface of the gastric mucosa have been demonstrated in humans using microelectrodes. Drugs or chemicals that inhibit bicarbonate secretion result in acidification of the mucosal surface.

The degree of luminal acidity, reflected by pH, required to stimulate bicarbonate secretion is greater in the stomach than in the duodenum. Direct exposure of the gastric mucosa to pH levels of 2.0 or more increases bicarbonate secretion. In the duodenum, exposure of the mucosa to pH 5.0 doubles bicarbonate secretion, whereas exposure to pH 2.0 increases alkaline secretion 10-fold.

Cholinergic agonists, vagal nerve stimulation, and sham feeding have all been shown to increase gastric HCO_3^- production. The effects of cholinergic stimulation can be blocked by atropine. In the human stomach, exposure to luminal perfusates at pH 2.0 has been associated with increased release of prostaglandin E_2. Prostaglandin E_2 and its synthetic derivatives are also potent stimulants of gastric bicarbonate secretion. Because mucosal bicarbonate production can be decreased in experimental models by indomethacin, endogenous prostaglandins are thought to be important in the mucosal alkaline response.

GASTRIC BLOOD FLOW

Because the gastric mucosa is metabolically highly active, control of mucosal blood flow is of great physiologic importance. In addition, studies have implicated perfusion abnormalities in the development of mucosal lesions during periods of stress. Mucosal blood flow is regulated by neural, hormonal, and locally active influences.

Postganglionic sympathetic nerve fibers reach the stomach in association with its blood supply and richly innervate small mucosal arteries. Mucosal capillaries do not receive adrenergic innervation. Electrical stimulation of sympathetic nerves supplying the stomach is followed by decreased total gastric blood flow, decreased flow in celiac and gastroepiploic vessels, and diminished blood flow to the mucosa. Studies in animals demonstrate that vasoconstriction of the gastric vascular bed is mediated by α-adrenergic receptors and that vasodilation is mediated by β-adrenergic receptors.

Stimulation of the vagus nerve is followed by a prompt increase in blood flow, suggesting a dilatory effect of parasympathetic nerves. The effects of vagal stimulation on mucosal blood flow are complicated by accompanying increases in acid secretion. Almost all stimuli that increase acid production also increase blood flow secondarily.

A number of gastrointestinal peptide hormones affect gastric blood flow, most because of their ability to increase or decrease acid secretion. Thus, gastrin, because it is a potent stimulant of acid secretion, also increases mucosal blood flow. Cholecystokinin appears to have direct vasodilatory effects on the gastric vasculature. Vasopressin has been well demonstrated to have direct vasoconstrictor activity.

Nitric oxide modulates basal gastric vascular tone and controls gastric vasodilation and hyperemia. Nitric oxide mediates the hyperemic response that accompanies increases in acid secretion, although the molecule has no direct stimulatory role in acid production.

Prostaglandins are important mucosally produced compounds that have clear effects on the gastric vasculature. Prostaglandins of the E class have been shown in animals and humans to increase gastric blood flow at doses that decrease acid secretion. Indomethacin, in doses sufficient to inhibit prostaglandin formation, decreases the diameter of submucosal blood vessels and reduces basal blood flow. Complete inhibition of cyclooxygenase activity causes an approximate 50% reduction in resting blood flow. These studies suggest that endogenous, locally produced prostaglandins are crucial to maintaining basal gastric blood flow in humans and probably act in concert with endogenous nitric oxide.

GASTRIC MOTILITY

Gastric Smooth Muscle

Consideration of gastric motility requires that the stomach be viewed in functional terms as two different regions, the proximal one third and the distal two thirds. These areas are distinct in terms of smooth muscle anatomy, electrical activity, and contractile function. The regions do not correspond to the traditional anatomic divisions of fundus, corpus, and antrum.

In the proximal stomach, three layers of gastric smooth muscle can be distinguished: an outer longitudinal layer, a middle circular layer, and an inner oblique layer. In the distal two thirds of the stomach, the longitudinal layer is most clearly defined, and the inner oblique layer is usually not distinct. The gastric smooth muscle ends at the pylorus.

The smooth muscle of the proximal stomach is electrically stable, whereas the smooth muscle of the distal stomach demonstrates spontaneous, repeated electrical discharges. Gastric smooth muscle exhibits myoelectric activity that is based on a highly regular pattern called the *slow wave*.[13] In the stomach, slow waves occur with a frequency of three cycles per minute. Slow waves do not, by themselves, lead to gastric contractions, but they do set the maximum rate of contractions at three per minute. Gastric contractions occur when action potentials are phase locked with the crest of the slow wave.

Extracellular electrical recording from the serosal surface of the stomach also demonstrates the intrinsic electrical activity of the distal stomach in the form of pacesetter potentials. Pacesetter potentials reflect partial depolarization of the gastric smooth muscle cell and are recorded during relatively long periods (2 or 3 seconds). Pacesetters originate along the greater curvature at a point in the proximal third of the stomach. Pacesetter potentials, discharging at a rate of three times per minute in humans, drive cells located distally. Spread of the pacesetter potentials is faster along the greater curvature, so that a ring of electrical activity reaches the pylorus simultaneously along both curvatures. The pacesetter potentials do not result in smooth muscle contraction unless an additional depolarization is superimposed in the form of an action potential. When action potentials occur, a ring of smooth muscle contraction moves peristaltically along the distal stomach toward the pylorus.

Duodenal slow-wave frequency and maximum rate of phasic contractions are higher than those observed in the stomach. The duodenal rate is approximately 12 cycles per minute; the contraction rate declines progressively to nine cycles per minute in the distal ileum.

The smooth muscle activity of the proximal stomach is fundamentally different from that of the distal stomach. There are no pacesetter or action potentials in the proximal stomach. As a result, peristalsis does not occur. Proximal gastric contraction is tonic and prolonged, and increases in luminal pressure are often sustained for several minutes.

Coordination of Contraction

Important vagally mediated reflexes influence intragastric pressure, presumably by affecting contractile activity of smooth muscle in the proximal stomach. The most important reflex is termed *receptive relaxation* and occurs with ingestion of a meal. Increasing gastric volumes are accommodated with little increase in intragastric pressure by relaxation of the proximal stomach. This receptive relaxation allows the proximal stomach to act as a storage site for ingested food in the immediate postprandial period. Afferent impulses, presumed to originate from stretch receptors in the gastric wall, are carried along vagal fibers; efferent vagal discharges are inhibitory. Receptive gastric accommodation is lost after either truncal or proximal gastric vagotomy. After the meal has been ingested, proximal contractile activity increases; alterations in proximal gastric tone cause the compressive movement of gastric content from the fundus to the antrum.

Food that enters the antrum from the proximal stomach is propelled peristaltically toward the pylorus. A number of observations indicate that the pylorus closes 2 or 3 seconds before the arrival of the antral contraction ring. This coordinate closing of the pylorus allows a small bolus of liquid and suspended food particles to pass while retropulsing the main mass of gastric contents back into the proximal antrum. The churning action that results mixes ingested food particles, gastric acid, and pepsin, and contributes to the grinding function of the stomach. Solid food particles do not ordinarily pass the pylorus unless they are no larger than 1 mm.

A consistent finding in humans ingesting a mixed solid–liquid meal is that liquids empty more quickly than solids. Characteristically, solid food empties only after a lag period, whereas liquid emptying begins almost immediately. A traditional interpretation of these human observations has been that the proximal stomach is the dominant force in determining how quickly a liquid meal empties by the gastroduodenal pressure gradient generated by proximal gastric contractions. The actions of the proximal stomach in liquid emptying are also regulated by the sieving actions of the antropyloric segment and are modified by the nutrient composition of the ingested meal. The distal gastric segment has been postulated to control solid emptying through its grinding and peristaltic actions. This traditional concept of the two-component stomach is useful in considering observations in patients who have undergone gastric operative procedures. Patients who have undergone proximal gastric vagotomy exhibit accelerated emptying of liquids but have normal solid emptying. Because of loss of receptive relaxation, the denervation of the proximal stomach is presumed to increase intragastric pressure and accelerate liquid emptying while leaving the distal gastric segment unaffected. Conversely, vagal denervation of the antrum interrupts gastric emptying of solids to a greater degree than liquids. Although this model of gastric emptying oversimplifies the many mechanisms (gastric, pyloric, and intestinal) that work in concert to control gastric emptying, it provides a useful framework for considering the effects of gastric surgical procedures.

References

1. Dockray GJ, Varro A, Dimaline R. Gastric endocrine cells: gene expression, processing, and targeting of active products. *Phys Rev* 1996;76:767–798.
2. Magee DF. Pyloric antral inhibition of gastrin release. *J Gastroenterol* 1996; 31:758–763.
3. Debas HT, Carvajal SH. Vagal regulation of acid secretion and gastrin release. *Yale J Biol Med* 1994;67:145–151.
4. DeValle J. The stomach as an endocrine organ. *Digestion* 1997;58(suppl 1):4–7.
5. Sachs G, Meyer-Rosberg K, Scott DR, et al. Acid secretion and Helicobacter pylori. *Digestion* 1997;58(suppl 1):8–13.
6. Date Y, Kojima M, Hosoda H, et al. Ghrelin, a novel growth hormone-releasing acylated peptide, is synthesized in a distinct endocrine cell type in the gastrointestinal tracts of rats and humans. *Endocrinology* 2000;141: 4255–4261.
7. van der Lely AJ, Tschop M, Heiman ML, et al. Biological, physiological, and pathophysiological aspects of ghrelin. *Endocr Rev* 2004;25:426–457.
8. Otto B, Cuntz U, Fruehauf E, et al. Weight gain decreases elevated plasma ghrelin concentrations of patients with anorexia nervosa. *Eur J Endocrinol* 2001;145:669–673.
9. Cummings DE, Weigle DS, Frayo RS, et al. Plasma ghrelin levels after diet-induced weight loss or gastric bypass surgery. *N Engl J Med* 2002;346: 1623–1630.
10. Gao Q, Horvath TL. Neuronal control of energy homeostasis. *FEBS Lett* 2008;582:132–141.
11. Urushidani T, Forte JG. Signal transduction and activation of acid secretion in the parietal cell. *J Membr Biol* 1997;59:99–111.
12. Waldum HL, Brenna E, Kleveland PM, et al. Gastrin—physiological and pathophysiological role: clinical consequences. *Dig Dis* 1995;13:25–38.
13. Quigley EM. Gastric and small intestinal motility in health and disease. *Gastroenterol Clin North Am* 1996;25:113–145.

CHAPTER 44 ■ GASTRODUODENAL ULCERATION

MICHAEL W. MULHOLLAND

GASTROINTESTINAL

KEY POINTS

1. Mucosal infection with *Helicobacter pylori* is the factor that contributes to ulcer pathogenesis in most patients.
2. *H. pylori* virulence factors include vacuolating cytotoxin A (VacA) and cytotoxin-associated gene A (CagA).
3. As a group, patients with duodenal ulcers have an increased capacity for gastric acid secretion relative to normal people.
4. Current treatment of peptic ulceration involves a combination of an antisecretory drug, usually a proton pump inhibitor, with antibiotics.
5. Hemorrhage is the leading cause of death associated with peptic ulcer. Patients with recurrent hemorrhage and elderly patients are at greatest risk of death.
6. For perforation, current therapy includes omental patch closure with postoperative anti–*H. pylori* therapy. Minimally invasive approaches are becoming standard practice.
7. Major trauma accompanied by shock, sepsis, respiratory failure, hemorrhage, or multiorgan injury is often accompanied by acute stress gastritis.

EPIDEMIOLOGY

Peptic ulceration remains a major public health problem worldwide. Some 300,000 new cases of peptic ulcer are diagnosed in the United States each year, and 4 million people receive some form of ulcer treatment. In the United States, ulcer mortality and hospitalization rates have fallen since the early 1980s, but physicians are now treating a cohort of older patients with frequent comorbidity and ulcer disease of greater chronicity. Mortality attributed to peptic ulceration remains substantial; ulcer disease is listed as a contributing cause of death in more than 10,000 cases annually.

The surgical treatment of peptic ulcer has changed fundamentally. New insights into disease pathogenesis, especially the realization that gastric infection has a role in most cases of peptic ulceration, have been especially exciting. Antibiotics are now front-line antiulcer therapy. A number of powerful antisecretory drugs have been introduced into clinical practice. Medical, endoscopic, and surgical therapies are frequently integrated in the care of individual patients.

No clear racial predilection for the development of duodenal ulceration exists, but genetic factors can be important. Hyperpepsinogenemia I, with autosomal dominant inheritance, is common in duodenal ulcer, although the relation of this trait to the development of ulceration remains obscure. A number of rare familial syndromes associated with peptic ulceration have been described.

PATHOPHYSIOLOGY

The pathogenesis of peptic ulceration is complex and multifactorial but increasingly understood. Approximately 85% of peptic ulcer cases are caused by *Helicobacter pylori*, with almost all other cases due to use of nonsteroidal anti-inflammatory drugs (NSAIDs).[1] The development of peptic ulceration is often depicted as a balance between chronic inflammatory injury, acid–peptic secretion, and mucosal defense, with the equilibrium shifted toward disease. Although acid–peptic secretion is crucial in the development of ulcers, (1) usually a defect in mucosal defense induced by bacterial infection also exists to tip the balance away from health. Mucosal infection with *H. pylori* is the factor that contributes to ulcer pathogenesis in most patients.

Helicobacter pylori

The relation between *H. pylori* infection and ulceration is inferential but overwhelmingly strong; a causal relation between *H. pylori* infection and peptic ulceration has not been tested directly. Because *H. pylori* infection is difficult to eradicate with certainty, and because of the potentially serious consequences of infection, the intentional exposure of humans to the organism to establish such a relation is not justified.

Many lines of evidence establish *H. pylori* as a factor in the pathogenesis of duodenal ulceration:

- *H. pylori* is the primary cause of chronic active gastritis, characterized by nonerosive inflammation of the gastric mucosa. Antral gastritis is nearly always present histologically in patients with duodenal ulcer, and *H. pylori* can be isolated from gastric mucosa in almost all cases.
- Gastric metaplasia is extremely common in duodenal epithelium surrounding areas of ulceration. *H. pylori* binds only to gastric-type epithelium, regardless of location; metaplastic gastric epithelium can become colonized by *H. pylori* from gastric sources. Gastric metaplasia of the duodenal bulb is a nonspecific response to damage and is the means by which antral gastritis with *H. pylori* is converted to active chronic duodenitis.
- Eradication of *H. pylori* with antimicrobials that have no effect on acid secretion leads to ulcer healing rates superior to those seen with acid-suppressing agents.
- Relapse of duodenal ulcer after antimicrobial therapy is preceded by reinfection of the gastric mucosa by *H. pylori*.

In addition, half of patients evaluated for dyspepsia, but without ulceration, have histologic evidence of mucosal bacterial infection. Furthermore, 20% of healthy volunteers harbor the bacteria; the incidence of bacterial carriage in the healthy, asymptomatic population increases with age. The occurrence of peptic ulcers in only a small proportion of people who carry the organism suggests that other factors must also act to induce ulceration. The ability of *H. pylori* infection to induce alterations in gastric acid secretion is a prerequisite for ulcer development in most patients.

H. pylori is the most common bacterial infection worldwide. *H. pylori* infection is usually *acquired in childhood and lasts lifelong absent specific therapy.* Epidemiologic studies suggest that *H. pylori* infection occurs via person-to-person contact, usually among family members. Transmission is believed to occur during a bout of gastroenteritis; the highest risk is associated with vomiting.

H. pylori is the only human bacterium to persistently infect the stomach.[2] The organism is actually somewhat fragile, being killed by exposure to high levels of oxygen and to the low pH found in the acidic lumen of the stomach. To avoid the bactericidal activity of the stomach, the organism has evolved mechanisms to move within the gastric environment, to adhere to gastric mucosa, and to protect itself from the harmful effects of acid. Over 300 genes of *H. pylori* are regulated by acid.

H. pylori bacteria are spiral shaped with polar flagella. Most bacilli are free-swimming within the mucous layer covering the gastric epithelium. The organisms orient according to a pH gradient, moving away from the lower pH of the lumen toward the epithelium. The majority of organisms remain motile within the mucous layer, but contact promotes adherence to epithelial cells, particularly in the region of intercellular junctions. The products of more than 30 genes are expressed on the outer membrane of the bacterium and function as adhesins to promote attachment to the gastric cells' surface. The best-characterized adhesin binds to the Lewis blood group antigen b. Adhesion triggers the expression of other bacterial genes, including bacterial virulence factors.

2 All strains of *H. pylori* cause persistent infection and all strains induce gastric inflammation. Yet, only 15% of infected individuals develop peptic ulceration and only 1% develop gastric adenocarcinoma. Differential expression of bacterial virulence factors is presumed to account for these observations. Two virulence factors are best characterized: vacuolating cytotoxin A (VacA) and cytotoxin-associated gene A (CagA)[3] (Table 44.1).

VacA is a pore-forming cytotoxin. VacA is expressed in all strains of *H. pylori* but is polymorphic with marked variation in two regions. The VacA protein is 88 kD. Upon secretion from the bacterium, the protein moves to the host cell membrane, where it forms a ring structure in the shape of a flower.[4] This ring complex inserts into the membrane of the host cell, creating a pore. VacA pores are permeable to anions and small neutral molecules, including urea. Pore formation may be a mechanism by which the organism obtains nutrients from gastric epithelial cells.

VacA also inserts into endosomal membranes, leading to osmotic swelling. VacA induces gastric cell death through apoptosis. This action is thought to occur via pore formation in mitochondrial membranes. VacA has been reported to interfere with immune T-cell activation and proliferation. This activity may inhibit clearance of the organism by immune mechanisms.

The second major virulence factor in *H. pylori* is termed *CagA*. The CagA gene is part of a region of DNA that is inserted into the genome of more virulent strains of *H. pylori*, termed a *pathogenicity island*.[5] The genes in this island that are adjacent to the CagA gene encode proteins, which function as microscopic needles for the transfer of bacterial products into host gastric cells. CagA is transferred to host cells through this injection mechanism.

After CagA protein is transferred to host cells, it becomes phosphorylated on tyrosine residues by host cell kinases. Phosphorylated CagA activates a number of cellular signaling pathways involved in cellular polarity, cytoskeletal protein function, and cellular proliferation and differentiation. As a consequence, infected gastric cells change shape and become more elongated. Apical junctions between cells become disrupted, gaps develop between epithelial cells, and epithelial barrier function is lost. CagA protein also stimulates transcription factors involved in regulation of cellular proliferation. Disturbance of cellular function in favor of apoptosis affects epithelia restitution and may inhibit ulcer healing.

Acid-secretory Status

3 The formation of duodenal ulcers depends on gastric secretion of acid and pepsin. As a group, patients with duodenal ulcers have an increased capacity for gastric acid secretion relative to normal people (Table 44.2). The maximal acid output of normal men is approximately 20 mEq/h in response to intravenous histamine stimulation, whereas patients with duodenal ulcer secrete an average of approximately 40 mEq/h. Considerable overlap exists between these two groups, and the values for most people with duodenal ulcer fall within the normal range. The increase in acid secretion in some patients with duodenal ulcer has been postulated to be due to an increase in the mass of parietal cells in the acid-secreting

TABLE 44.1

HELICOBACTER PYLORI VIRULENCE FACTORS

Vacuolating cytotoxin A (VacA)
Forms ring structure in the shape of a flower
Inserts into gastric cell membrane, forming pore
Inserts into endosomal membranes, causing cellular swelling
Damages mitochondrial membranes
Causes leakage of ions and small molecules
Cytotoxin-associated gene A (CagA)
Contained within pathogenicity island DNA sequence
Injected into host cells
Phosphorylated by cellular oncogenes
Activates growth factor receptor–like signaling
Disturbs normal proliferation, adhesion, cytoskeletal function
Disturbs intercellular junctions, causing disruption of epithelial permeability
Elicits inflammatory response

TABLE 44.2 ETIOLOGY

PATHOGENESIS OF PEPTIC ULCER

Helicobacter pylori infection
ENDOCRINE CONSEQUENCES
■ Increased basal serum gastrin
■ Increased gastrin response to a meal
■ Increased responsiveness to gastrin-releasing peptide
■ Production of N^{α}-methylhistamine
■ Decreased density of somatostatin cells
■ Decreased mucosal somatostatin content
GASTRIC ACID SECRETION
■ Increased acid = secretory capacity
■ Increased basal secretion
■ Increased pentagastrin-stimulated output
■ Increased meal response
■ Abnormal gastric emptying
MUCOSAL DEFENSE
■ Decreased duodenal bicarbonate production
■ Decreased gastric mucosal prostaglandin production
■ Increased apoptosis of epithelial cells
■ Disruption of epithelial barrier function
■ Inhibited epithelial restitution

gastric mucosa or to an increased sensitivity to circulating gastrin.

Groups of patients with duodenal ulcer demonstrate a prolonged and larger acid-secretory response to a mixed meal than do groups of normal subjects. As with histamine-stimulated acid output, overlap exists between patients with duodenal ulcer and normal subjects. Disturbances in gastric motility can exacerbate meal-stimulated acid-secretory abnormalities.

Patients with duodenal ulcer have accelerated emptying of gastric contents, particularly liquids, after a meal, and duodenal acidification fails to slow emptying appropriately. In such patients, the duodenal mucosa can be exposed to low pH for prolonged periods relative to normal subjects.

Groups of patients with duodenal ulcer also demonstrate increased basal secretion of acid. Increased basal secretion can be demonstrated by nocturnal collection of gastric secretions.

Studies indicate that most of these secretory abnormalities are a direct consequence of *H. pylori* infection. Ironically, the earliest stages of *H. pylori* infection are accompanied by a marked decrease in gastric acid secretion. Acute antral gastritis is followed by fundal inflammation. Fundal inflammation is associated with mucosal production of a number of cytokines, including interleukin (IL)-1β, IL-6, IL-8, and tumor necrosis factor-α (TNF-α). IL-1β is a potent inhibitor of gastric acid secretion. Investigators have postulated that acute reduction in gastric acid secretion facilitates further gastric colonization with *H. pylori*. Acute hypochlorhydria resolves despite persistence of *H. pylori* and is followed by a state of chronically increased acid secretion.

Basal and peak acid outputs are increased in patients with duodenal ulcer infected with *H. pylori* relative to uninfected healthy volunteers. With eradication of *H. pylori* infection, basal acid output returns to normal within 4 weeks, and peak acid output declines to the normal range by 6 months. Peak acid output reflects parietal cell mass; the slow return to normal levels suggests that *H. pylori* infection may stimulate increases in the parietal cell mass.

Abnormalities in acid secretion and parietal cell mass appear to be due to *H. pylori*–induced hypergastrinemia.[6] *H. pylori*–infected patients have increased basal serum gastrin levels, increased gastrin responses to meal stimulation, and an augmented gastrin response to intravenous gastrin-releasing peptide. Eradication of *H. pylori* infection causes serum gastrin levels to return to baseline. Gastric mucosal inflammatory cells and epithelial cells are activated by *H. pylori* infection to release cytokines such as IL-8, interferon-γ, and TNF-α. These cytokines are stimulants of gastrin release from cultured canine gastrin cells.

H. pylori expresses N^{α}-histamine methyltransferase activity. This enzyme produces N^{α}-methylhistamine, an abnormal analogue of histamine that can act as a gastric acid–secretory stimulant.

The concentration of somatostatin in the antral mucosa and the number of somatostatin-producing cells in the antrum are diminished in *H. pylori*–infected patients. Treatment of *H. pylori* infection is followed by increases in numbers of somatostatin cells and in mucosal somatostatin messenger RNA levels. These observations suggest that alterations in mucosal somatostatin metabolism may also contribute to the hypergastrinemia seen in *H. pylori*–infected patients by removing the inhibitory effects that somatostatin exerts on gastrin release. Somatostatin release is also suppressed by N^{α}-methylhistamine.

Mucosal Defense against Peptic Injury

Investigative attention has also focused on the ability of the duodenal mucosa to resist the injurious effects of luminal acid and pepsin. Because many patients with duodenal ulcer secrete normal amounts of acid and pepsin, it is attractive to postulate that abnormalities of mucosal defense might result in ulceration. In addition, several agents that are useful in the treatment of peptic ulceration are cytoprotective, which is defined as the ability to protect the mucosa from injury at doses lower than the threshold dose needed to inhibit acid secretion. The ability of cytoprotective agents to heal ulcers has suggested that abnormalities in mucosal defense are responsible for some instances of ulceration. Most investigative efforts have focused on the role of mucosally secreted bicarbonate and on mucosal prostaglandin production.

Gastric surface epithelial cells secrete mucus and bicarbonate, creating a pH gradient within the mucous layer that is nearly neutral at the mucous cell surface, even when the lumen is highly acidic. Failure of normal bicarbonate secretion locally would, in theory, result in exposure of surface epithelial cells to the peptic activity of gastric secretions at low pH. Patients with duodenal ulcers have been demonstrated to have significantly lower basal bicarbonate secretion in the proximal duodenum than normal subjects. In addition, in response to a physiologically relevant amount of hydrochloric acid instilled into the duodenal bulb, stimulated bicarbonate output was approximately 40% of the normal response. Abnormalities in duodenal bicarbonate secretion normalize after elimination of *H. pylori* in infected patients. These results suggest one mechanism by which ulceration could occur, even in patients secreting normal amounts of acid.

Diminished mucosal prostaglandin production has also been proposed to exist in subsets of patients with duodenal ulcer. Prostaglandins and prostaglandin analogues have been shown to exert cytoprotective effects, to accelerate healing of established duodenal ulcers, and to decrease acid secretion. In the duodenum, locally produced prostaglandins stimulate mucosal bicarbonate secretion. In patients with active duodenal ulceration, gastric mucosal production of prostaglandin E_2 and other prostanoids has been shown to be diminished. An increase in prostanoid synthesis within the gastric mucosa characterizes ulcer healing. Duodenal bicarbonate responses to prostaglandin E_2 are impaired in patients with duodenal ulcer.

Inflammatory responses to *H. pylori* infection are central to the pathogenesis of peptic ulceration. While *H. pylori* infection always induces inflammation, the patterns of response are not uniform. Three major patterns have been recognized.[7] The most common pattern is a mild to moderate inflammation of all regions of the stomach. This form is not associated with major alterations in gastric acidity and most individuals are asymptomatic and do not develop peptic ulceration. Approximately 15% of infected individuals develop an antral-predominant form of gastritis. These individuals exhibit an intense inflammation limited to the antrum without involvement of the mucosa of the gastric corpus. Gastrin levels are elevated and acid secretion is high. Inhibitory control of gastric acid production is impaired in this form of gastritis. As a result, duodenal and prepyloric ulcers are common. The third form of inflammatory response, occurring in 1% of infected individuals, is least common but most serious. This form is characterized by corpus-predominant gastritis, hypochlorhydria, and gastric atrophy. This form of inflammatory response is considered a precursor state for gastric cancer. Individuals with the third pattern of inflammation demonstrate hypergastrinemia, low acid secretion, and diminished secretion of pepsinogen.

Environmental Factors

Substantial evidence implicates cigarette smoking as an additive risk factor in the development of duodenal ulcers. Cigarette smoking impairs ulcer healing and increases the recurrence of ulcers. Continued smoking attenuates the effectiveness of active ulcer therapy. Cigarette smoking increases both the probability that surgery will be required and the risks of operative therapy. Cessation of smoking is a key element of antiulcer therapy.

NSAIDs have emerged as a significant risk factor for the development of acute ulceration.[8] Although acute mucosal injury caused by NSAIDs is more common in the stomach than in the duodenum, NSAID-induced ulcer complications occur with equal frequency in these two sites. NSAIDs produce a variety of lesions, ranging from hemorrhage, to superficial mucosal erosions, to deeper ulcerations. In the duodenum, it appears likely that invasive NSAID-associated ulcers result from underlying peptic ulcer diathesis compounded by the direct injurious effects of these drugs.

The ulcerogenic actions of NSAIDs have been attributed to their systemic suppression of prostaglandin production. Numerous experimental models have demonstrated the ability of NSAIDs to injure the gastroduodenal mucosa. Ulcers resembling those caused by NSAIDs can be produced experimentally by antibodies to prostaglandins. Conversely, NSAID-associated gastric ulcers can be prevented by the coadministration of prostaglandin analogues. Ulcers associated with NSAIDs usually heal rapidly when the drug is withdrawn, corresponding to the reversal of antiprostaglandin effects. All available NSAIDs appear to pose the hazard of gastroduodenal ulceration. Clinically important ulceration (of both the stomach and duodenum) is estimated by the U.S. Food and Drug Administration to occur at a rate of 2% to 4% per patient-year. The risks inherent with NSAID use appear to be increased by a history of *H. pylori* infection, by cigarette smoking, and by alcohol use. The incidence of NSAID-caused ulcer complications is highest in older patients, as is the attendant mortality rate. Peptic ulcer disease is rare in individuals who are *H. pylori* negative and who are not receiving NSAID medications.

A role of NSAIDs in upper gastrointestinal (GI) hemorrhage is widely recognized. The risk of bleeding is particularly acute for peptic ulceration. In three reports, spanning two decades, NSAIDs were linked to 50% to 75% of bleeding peptic ulcers, one third of deaths due to hemorrhage, and 30% of hospitalizations.[8–10] Use of NSAIDs increases the risk of bleeding from peptic ulcer threefold for those under 65 years of age, but by eightfold for individuals over 75 years of age. The odds ratio for bleeding is 13 for patients with a prior history of bleeding ulcer.

Because of the risk of gastrointestinal side effects, a selective class of cyclooxygenase-2 (COX-2) inhibitors was developed for long-term pain relief and anti-inflammatory therapy. Selective COX-2 inhibitors have reduced potential to injure the gastrointestinal mucosa relative to standard NSAIDs.[11] The incidence of upper GI bleeding for celecoxib or rofecoxib therapy was reported to be fourfold less than standard NSAID therapy. Nonetheless, a definite risk for upper GI hemorrhage is still present, and is higher in aged patients. Concurrent use of aspirin with COX-2 inhibitors significantly undermines the safety advantages of the COX-2 agents, as does smoking. An increased incidence of adverse cardiovascular events caused the withdrawal of rofecoxib and valdecoxib from the market.

DIAGNOSIS

The cardinal feature of duodenal ulceration is epigastric pain. The pain is usually confined to the upper abdomen and is described as burning, stabbing, or gnawing. Unless perforation or penetration into the head of the pancreas has occurred, referral of pain is not common. Many patients report pain on arising in the morning. Ingestion of food or antacids usually provides prompt relief. In uncomplicated cases, abnormal physical findings are minimal. The differential diagnosis is broad and includes a variety of diseases originating in the upper gastrointestinal tract. The most common disorders to be distinguished include nonulcerative dyspepsia, gastric neoplasia, cholelithiasis and related diseases of the biliary system, and both inflammatory and neoplastic disorders of the pancreas. In dyspeptic patients, the principal diagnoses that must be differentiated definitively are peptic ulceration and gastric cancer.

The evaluation of patients with suspected peptic ulceration usually involves endoscopy, the standard against which other diagnostic modalities are measured. Endoscopy is employed because it permits biopsy of the esophagus, stomach, and duodenum. Endoscopy must be recommended with discretion because of associated morbidity (approximately 1 per 5,000 cases) and higher costs.

Duodenal ulcer is characterized by lesions that are erosive to the bowel wall. When viewed endoscopically, the ulcers have a typical appearance. The edges are usually sharply demarcated and the underlying submucosa is exposed. The ulcer base is often clean and smooth, although acute ulcers and those with recent hemorrhage can demonstrate eschar or adherent exudate. Surrounding mucosal inflammation is common. The most frequent site for peptic ulceration is the first portion of the duodenum, with the second portion less commonly involved. Ulceration of the third or fourth portions of the duodenum is unusual, and occurrence in these sites should arouse suspicion of an underlying gastrinoma. Ulceration in the pyloric channel or the prepyloric area is similar in endoscopic appearance to duodenal ulceration, and ulcers in these areas demonstrate other clinical features similar to duodenal ulcers. Endoscopic demonstration of a duodenal ulcer should prompt mucosal biopsy of the gastric antrum to demonstrate the presence of *H. pylori* and guide subsequent therapy.

The hallmarks of the histologic appearance of duodenal ulcers are chronicity and invasiveness. Chronic injury is suggested by surrounding fibrosis; collagen is deposited in the submucosa during each round of ulcer relapse and healing. The adjacent mucosa often demonstrates evidence of chronic injury with infiltration of acute and chronic inflammatory cells. Gastric metaplasia, in which the duodenum exhibits histologic features of gastric mucosa, is common in the surrounding nonulcerated mucosa. The ulcer can extend for a variable distance through the wall of the duodenum, including the full thickness of the bowel in cases of perforation.

DRUG TREATMENT OF ULCER DISEASE

In the absence of active treatment, *H. pylori* infection is lifelong. Spontaneous healing of infected mucosa is very rare,
4 occurring in less than 0.5% per patient-year. Current treatment of peptic ulceration involves a combination of an antisecretory drug, usually a proton pump inhibitor, with antibiotics.[12] This therapy is rational for most patients who are *H. pylori* positive and results in a high rate of sustained ulcer healing.

A large number of drug regimens have been described, but the most widely used treatment protocols combine a proton pump inhibitor, usually omeprazole, with two antibiotics, usually clarithromycin and metronidazole or amoxicillin. A combination of antibiotics is more effective than one antibiotic alone in almost all series. This triple therapy is administered for 7 or 14 days. Triple-drug therapy is cost effective and associated with a low rate of side effects, low rates of antibiotic resistance, and acceptable levels of patient compliance. *H. pylori* eradication rates of greater than 90% have been reported.

After elimination of *H. pylori*, ulcer recurrence rates reflect the rate of reinfection. In developed countries, reinfection rates of less than 10% at 5 years have been reported. Eradication of

H. pylori improves quality of life, as measured by symptoms, drug prescriptions, physician visits, and days of missed employment. To date, antibiotic resistance has been low, approximately 5% worldwide, but it is likely to increase with ongoing use of macrolide antibiotics.

HISTAMINE-RECEPTOR ANTAGONISTS

Histamine, released into the interstitial fluid by cells in the fundic mucosa, diffuses to the mucosal parietal cell. Histamine stimulates acid production by occupying a membrane-bound receptor and activating parietal cell adenylate cyclase. Histamine is released in response to a number of physiologic stimuli; blockade of histamine receptors inhibits most forms of stimulated acid secretion in humans. Parietal cell histamine receptors are classified as H_2 receptors because they are activated by agonists such as 4-methylhistamine and are selectively blocked by agents such as cimetidine. Some H_2 receptor antagonists also possess nongastric actions by binding to androgen receptors, by interacting with the hepatic microsomal oxidase system, and by crossing the blood–brain barrier. All clinically useful gastric histamine receptor antagonists are of the H_2 type.

H_2-receptor antagonists bind competitively to parietal cell H_2 receptors to produce a reversible inhibition of acid secretion. An enormous worldwide experience has accumulated with the use of H_2-receptor antagonists. The agents are effective and safe when used in the treatment of peptic ulcer. The various compounds have similar efficacy in terms of ulcer healing when used in doses that produce similar reductions in acid output. It is clear that H_2-receptor blockers do not affect the underlying ulcer diathesis; if H_2-receptor antagonists are stopped, recurrent ulceration occurs in more than half of patients within 1 year. The current understanding of the role of *H. pylori* in ulcer pathogenesis has changed the role of H_2-receptor antagonists from primary therapy to that of a substitute for proton pump inhibitors in conjunction with antibiotic treatment.

PROTON PUMP BLOCKERS

Acid secretion by the gastric parietal cells is due to the active transport of hydrogen ions from the parietal cell cytoplasm into the secretory canaliculus in exchange for potassium. Because this so-called *proton pump* is tissue specific, being present only in gastric mucosa, its blockade would be expected to have minimal effects on nongastric functions. Omeprazole is representative of a family of compounds that selectively block the parietal cell proton pump.

Omeprazole is a weak base, with a pKa of approximately 4. The drug is nonionized and lipid soluble at neutral pH, but it becomes ionized and activated at a pH of less than 3. In its activated state, omeprazole binds to the membrane-bound H^+-K^+-adenosine triphosphatase (ATPase) of the parietal cell. Because the compound is a weak base, omeprazole accumulates selectively within the acidic environment of the parietal cell secretory canaliculus; 4 hours after administration, the drug is detectable in appreciable quantities only in the gastric mucosa. If enough drug is administered to occupy all parietal cell–binding sites, anacidity can be produced. Omeprazole, in doses from 20 to 30 mg, causes nearly complete inhibition of stimulated gastric acid secretion within 6 hours. At 24 hours after drug administration, a 60% to 70% reduction in acid secretion persists.

Repeated daily dosing with omeprazole results in increasing inhibitory action on gastric secretion and thus in decreased intragastric degradation of the drug. Acid suppression stabilizes after approximately 3 days. Because of tissue accumulation, the secretory actions of omeprazole do not correlate with plasma levels. Several studies have demonstrated a significant inhibition of peak acid output, marked relief of epigastric pain, and decreased use of supplemental antacids during omeprazole therapy. Direct comparisons with H_2-receptor antagonists have generally favored omeprazole in terms of pain relief and rate of ulcer healing.

SUCRALFATE

Sucralfate is the aluminum salt of sulfated sucrose. In the acidic environment of the stomach, sucralfate polymerizes, becoming viscous and adhering to the gastroduodenal mucosa. Coating of the ulcer base by the polymer has been claimed to provide a protective barrier, binding bile salts and inhibiting the actions of pepsin. Sucralfate also stimulates the production of mucus. Sucralfate stimulates increased mucosal prostaglandin E_2 production and increases bicarbonate secretion. Sucralfate binds epidermal growth factor and may protect the mitogen from acid degradation. Sucralfate stimulates epithelial proliferation at the ulcer margin. The drug has almost no buffering capacity. Virtually no systemic absorption occurs, and because of this property, sucralfate is safe for the treatment of peptic ulcer in pregnancy.

OPERATIVE TREATMENT OF ULCER DISEASE

Surgical Goals

Operative intervention is reserved for the treatment of complicated ulcer disease. Three complications are most common and constitute the indications for peptic ulcer surgery—hemorrhage, perforation, and obstruction.[13] The first goal in the surgical treatment of the complications of ulcer disease is treatment of coexisting anatomic complications, such as pyloric stenosis or perforation. The second major goal should be patient safety and freedom from undesirable chronic side effects. To achieve these goals, the gastric surgeon can direct therapy through endoscopic or operative means, the appropriate choice depending on the clinical circumstances.

Operative Procedures

A number of operative procedures have been used to treat peptic ulcer, but with decreasing frequency in the past decade. There is currently no indication for surgical treatment of uncomplicated ulcer disease. Operative treatment of gastric outlet obstruction has decreased by approximately 50%. Most surgical patients are now treated emergently for the complications of bleeding or perforation.

Three procedures—truncal vagotomy and drainage, truncal vagotomy and antrectomy, and proximal gastric vagotomy—have been widely used in the past in the operative treatment of peptic ulcer disease. With increasing frequency, surgical therapy of peptic ulcer is directed exclusively at correction of the immediate problem (e.g., closure of duodenal perforation) without gastric denervation. The underlying ulcer diathesis is then addressed after surgery by antibiotic therapy directed at *H. pylori*. This approach is applicable to most patients with peptic ulcer undergoing emergent operation and predicts a rapidly diminishing role for vagotomy in the future.

Division of both vagal trunks at the esophageal hiatus—truncal vagotomy—denervates the acid-producing fundic mucosa as well as the remainder of the vagally supplied viscera (Fig. 44.1). Because denervation impedes normal pyloric coordination and can result in impairment of gastric emptying,

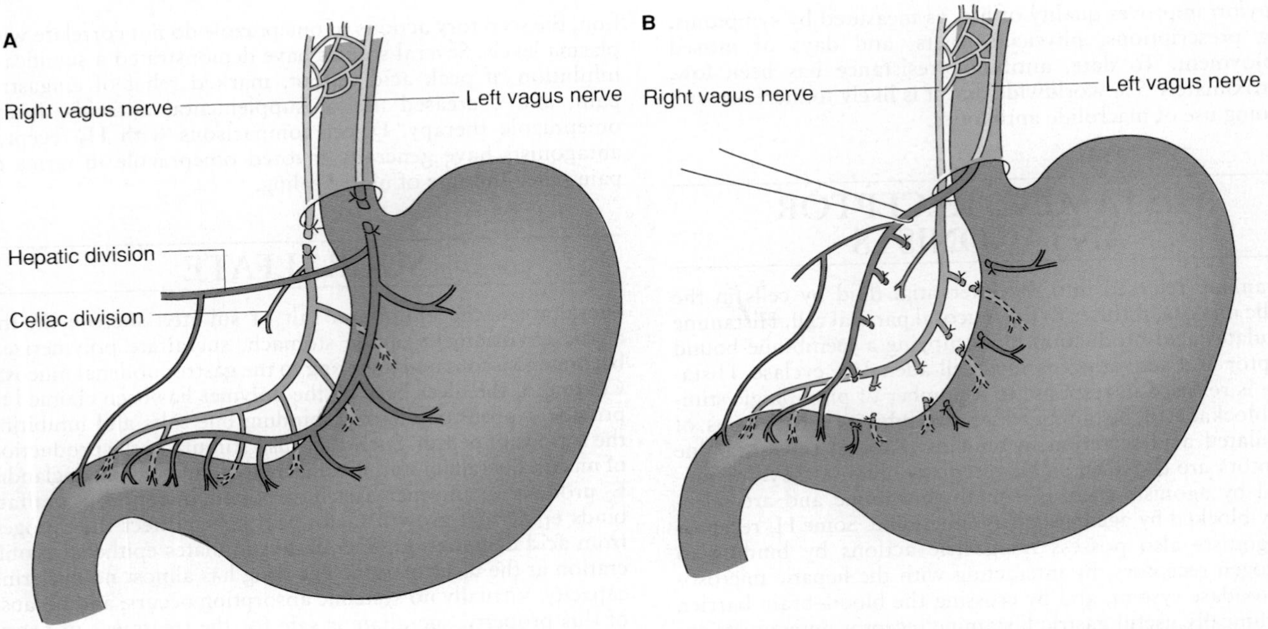

FIGURE 44.1. Truncal vagotomy and proximal gastric vagotomy. **A:** With truncal vagotomy, both nerve trunks are divided at the level of the diaphragmatic hiatus. **B:** Proximal gastric vagotomy involves division of the vagal fibers that supply the gastric fundus. Branches to the antropyloric region of the stomach are not transected, and the hepatic and celiac divisions of the vagus nerves remain intact.

truncal vagotomy must be combined with a procedure to eliminate pyloric sphincteric function. Usually, gastric drainage is ensured by performance of a pyloroplasty (Fig. 44.2).

Truncal vagotomy can also be combined with resection of the gastric antrum to effect a further reduction in acid secretion, presumably by removing antral sources of gastrin. The limits of antral resection are usually defined by external landmarks, rather than the histologic transition from fundic to antral mucosae. The stomach is divided proximally along a line from a point above the incisura angularis to a point along the greater curvature midway from the pylorus to the gastroesophageal junction. Restoration of gastrointestinal continuity by a gastroduodenostomy is termed a Billroth I reconstruction. A Billroth II procedure uses a gastrojejunostomy (Fig. 44.3).

Proximal gastric vagotomy differs from truncal vagotomy in that only the nerve fibers to the acid-secreting fundic mucosa are divided (see Fig. 44.1). Vagal nerve fibers to the antrum and pylorus are left intact, and the hepatic and celiac divisions are not transected. The operation has also been called parietal cell vagotomy to emphasize its most important functional consequence.

The role of vagotomy in clinical surgery diminished significantly in the 1990s. In 1998, only 7,000 vagotomies were performed in the United States, of more than 41 million operative procedures.[14]

Physiologic Consequences of Operation

Division of efferent vagal fibers directly affects acid secretion by reducing cholinergic stimulation of parietal cells. In addition, vagotomy also diminishes parietal cell responsiveness to gastrin and histamine. Basal acid secretion is reduced by approximately 80% in the immediate postoperative period. Acid secretion increases slightly within months of surgery but remains unchanged thereafter. The maximal acid output in response to exogenously administered stimulants such as pentagastrin is reduced by approximately 70% in the early period after surgery. After 1 year, pentagastrin-stimulated maximal acid output rebounds to 50% of prevagotomy values but

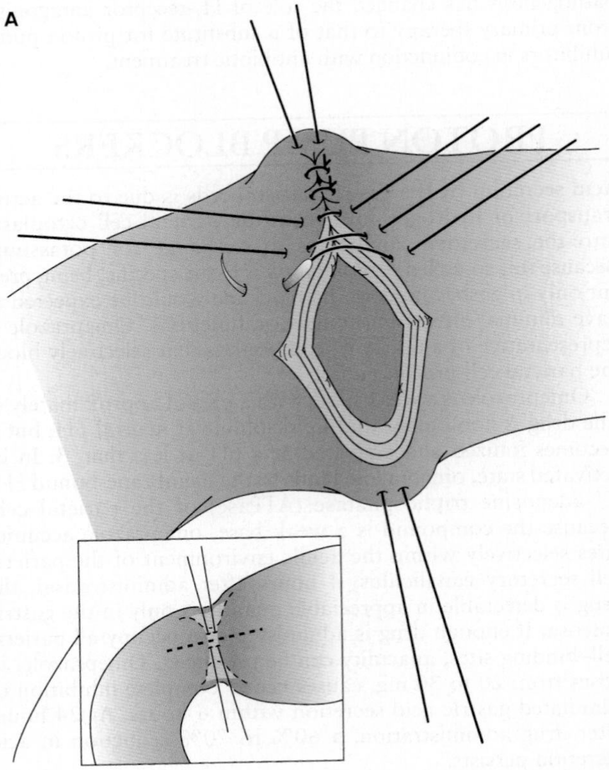

FIGURE 44.2. Pyloroplasty formation. **A:** A Heineke-Mikulicz pyloroplasty involves a longitudinal incision of the pyloric sphincter followed by a transverse closure. (*continued*)

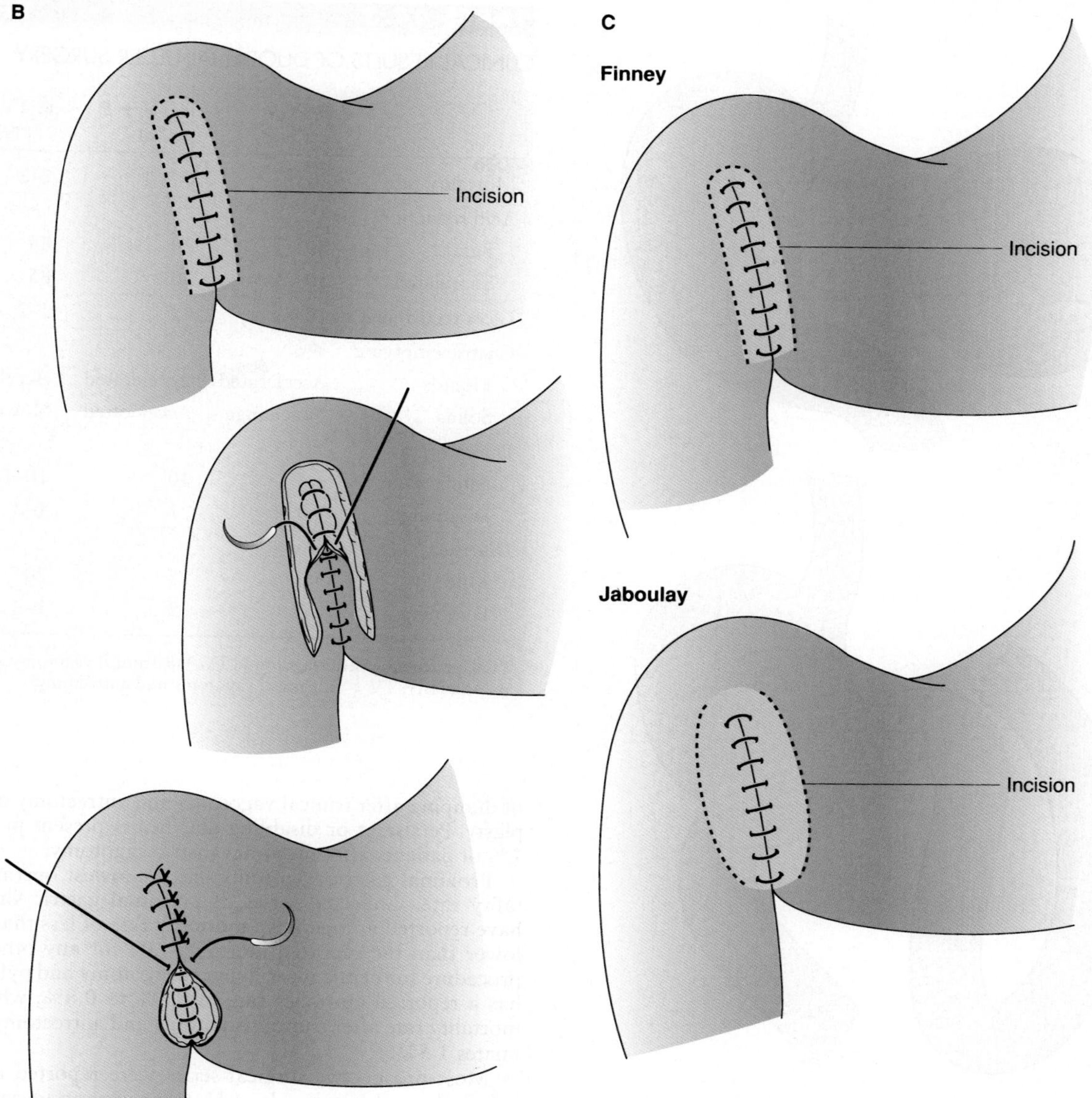

FIGURE 44.2. (*Continued*) **B:** The Finney pyloroplasty is performed as a gastroduodenostomy with division of the pylorus. **C:** The Jaboulay pyloroplasty differs from the Finney procedure in that the pylorus is not transected.

remains at this level on subsequent testing. Acid secretion due to endogenous stimulation by a liquid meal is reduced by 60% to 70% relative to normal subjects.

The inclusion of antrectomy with truncal vagotomy causes further reductions in acid secretion. Pentagastrin-stimulated maximal acid output is reduced by 85% relative to values recorded before surgery. Little rebound in acid secretion occurs with the passage of time.

Truncal vagotomy and proximal gastric vagotomy both cause postoperative hypergastrinemia. Fasting gastrin values are elevated to approximately twice preoperative levels, and the postprandial response is exaggerated. Immediately after vagotomy, hypergastrinemia appears to be due to decreased luminal acid, with loss of feedback inhibition of gastrin release. Loss of vagal inhibitory pathways can also be important. Chronic hypergastrinemia, sustained long term in most cases, is caused by gastrin cell hyperplasia in addition to loss of inhibitory feedback. When antrectomy is added to vagotomy, circulating gastrin levels are decreased. Basal gastrin values are reduced by approximately half and postprandial gastrin levels by two thirds. The major form of circulating hormone after antrectomy is gastrin 34, released from the duodenum.

Operations that involve vagotomy alter gastric emptying. Proximal gastric denervation abolishes vagally mediated receptive relaxation. Thus, for any given volume ingested, the intragastric pressure rise is greater and the gastroduodenal pressure gradient higher than in normal subjects. As a result, emptying of liquids, which depends critically on the gastroduodenal pressure gradient, is accelerated after proximal gastric vagotomy. Because nerve fibers to the antrum and pylorus are preserved, the function of the distal stomach to mix and triturate solid food is preserved, and emptying of solids is nearly normal in patients who have undergone proximal gastric vagotomy. Truncal vagotomy affects the motor activities of both the proximal and distal

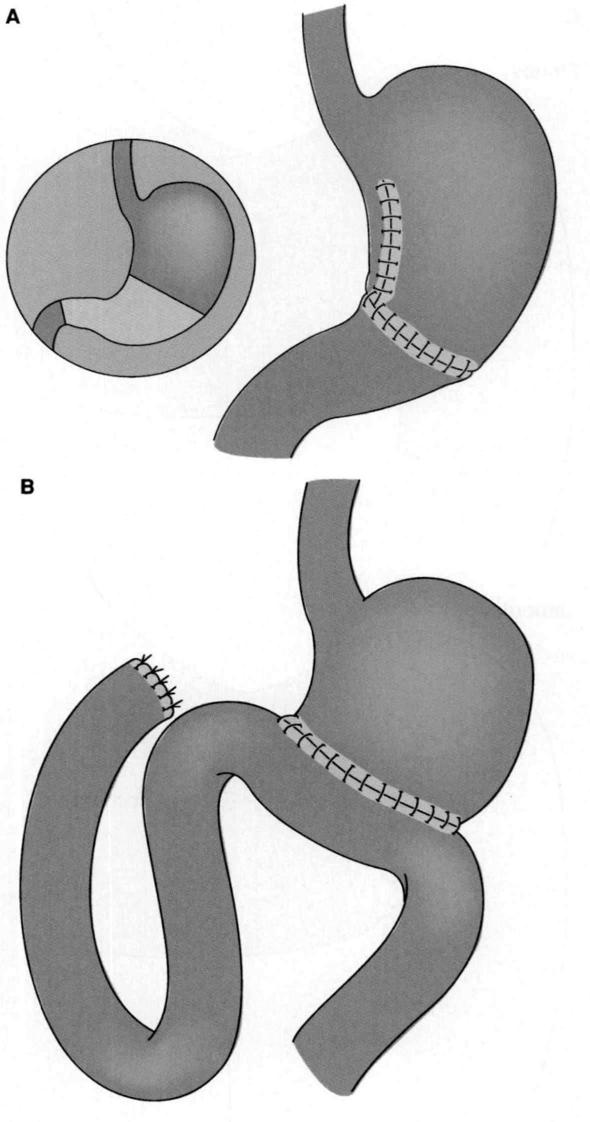

FIGURE 44.3. Antrectomy involves resection of the distal stomach (pink area in inset). Restoration of gastrointestinal continuity may be accomplished as a Billroth I gastroduodenostomy (**A**) or Billroth II gastrojejunostomy (**B**) reconstruction.

TABLE 44.3 **RESULTS**

CLINICAL RESULTS OF DUODENAL ULCER SURGERY

	■ PGV (%)	■ TV + P (%)	■ TV + A (%)
Mortality rate	0	0.5–1	1–2
Acid reduction			
Basal	80	70	85
Stimulated	50	50	85
Ulcer recurrence	10	12	1–2
Gastric emptying			
Liquids	Accelerated	Accelerated	Accelerated
Solids	No change	Accelerated	Slowed
Dumping			
Mild	<5	10	10–15
Disabling	0	1	1–2
Diarrhea			
Mild	<5	25	20
Disabling	0	2	1–2

PGV, proximal gastric vagotomy; TV + P, truncal vagotomy and pyloroplasty; TV + A, truncal vagotomy and antrectomy.

stomach. Solid and liquid emptying rates are usually increased when truncal vagotomy is accompanied by pyloroplasty.

A number of prospective, randomized trials have compared the various surgical options in terms of postoperative symptoms, including dumping, diarrhea, weight loss, and disturbance of lifestyle (Table 44.3). In most comparisons, proximal gastric vagotomy has proved superior to other operations in these measures. Dumping, a postprandial symptom complex of abdominal discomfort, weakness, and vasomotor symptoms of sweating and dizziness, occurs in 10% to 15% of patients with truncal vagotomy and antrectomy in the early postoperative period and is chronically disabling in 1% to 2%. After truncal vagotomy and pyloroplasty, dumping is present initially in 10%, and remains severe in approximately 1%. Permanent symptoms of dumping are rare after proximal gastric vagotomy. The incidence of diarrhea, which is presumably caused by denervation of the pylorus and small bowel and by elimination of pyloric function, parallels the incidence of dumping after truncal vagotomy and antrectomy or pyloroplasty. Persistent or disabling diarrhea is present in less than 1% of patients after proximal gastric vagotomy.

Proximal gastric vagotomy has the lowest operative mortality rate. Collected series of proximal gastric vagotomies have reported an operative mortality rate of less than 0.05%, lower than the reported mortality rate for any other gastric procedure for peptic ulcer. Truncal vagotomy and pyloroplasty has a reported mortality rate of 0.5% to 0.8%, whereas the mortality rate after truncal vagotomy and antrectomy approximates 1.5%.

Most prospective surgical series were reported in the era before the pathogenic role of *H. pylori* was appreciated. With appropriate use of postoperative antimicrobials directed against *H. pylori*, ulcer recurrence rates are currently much lower than historical standards. Although recurrence rates (without *H. pylori* treatment) as low as 5% have been reported, a more generally accepted figure is 10%.[15] This rate is similar to that of reinfection with *H. pylori* after its successful eradication. The reported ulcer recurrence rates after proximal gastric vagotomy can be adversely affected by the inclusion of prepyloric and pyloric channel ulcers. For reasons that are not clear, proximal gastric vagotomy is significantly less effective when used to treat ulcers in this position than when used for duodenal ulceration.

Hemorrhage

5 Hemorrhage is the leading cause of death associated with peptic ulcer, and the incidence of this complication has not changed since the introduction of H_2-receptor antagonists. The lifetime risk of hemorrhage for patients with duodenal ulcer who have not had surgery and who do not receive continuing maintenance drug therapy approximates 15% at 5 years.[16] Most hemorrhages occur during the initial episode of ulceration or during a relapse, and patients who have hemorrhaged previously have a higher risk of bleeding again. Contin-

ued or recurrent bleeding occurs in 20% to 30% of patients, and when this happens, mortality varies between 10% and 40%. Patients with recurrent hemorrhage and elderly patients are at greatest risk of death, and these two groups should be resuscitated vigorously, investigated promptly, and treated aggressively.[17]

The contemporary risk of mortality from bleeding ulcer approximates 10% to 20%. Operative risk is increased in patients who have shock at admission, recurrent bleeding, delay in operative intervention, or coexisting medical illnesses. Surgical delay may lead to recurrent hypovolemia and, subsequently, multisystem organ failure.

Upper gastrointestinal endoscopy is the appropriate initial diagnostic test when hemorrhage from duodenal ulceration is suspected. Endoscopy can correctly determine the site and cause of bleeding in more than 90% of patients. An ulcer should be accepted as the bleeding source only if it has one of the stigmata of active or recent hemorrhage. Active hemorrhage is defined by an arterial jet, active oozing, or oozing beneath an adherent clot. The signs of recent hemorrhage include an adherent clot without oozing, an adherent slough in the ulcer base, or a visible vessel in the ulcer. The ability of these endoscopic findings to accurately predict recurrent hemorrhage has been extensively validated. Approximately 30% of patients who have stigmata of recent hemorrhage experience rebleeding, and most of the patients who experience recurrent hemorrhage require emergency treatment. These stigmata are not sufficiently accurate to be used alone as indications for surgery. Rather, they serve as a warning that aggressive therapy is needed and close follow-up mandatory. The occurrence of hypovolemic shock, rebleeding during hospitalization, and a posteroinferior location of the ulcer are additional clinical features that have been associated with increased risks of recurrent bleeding. The role of gastric acidity as a cause for in-hospital rebleeding appears to be inconsequential, and reduction of acid secretion by H_2-receptor antagonists or omeprazole is not sufficient to prevent recurrent hemorrhage.

The ability to visualize bleeding duodenal ulcers endoscopically has led to development of methods to treat hemorrhage endoscopically. There are many different methods of endoscopic therapy, but the most established consist of thermal coagulation, injection of alcohol, or sclerosants. Thermal coagulation can be achieved by bipolar electrocoagulation or direct application of heat through a heater probe.[18] Injection of epinephrine into the base of the bleeding ulcer is also effective in control of ulcer hemorrhage.

Proof of efficacy, in the form of lowered rebleeding rates and avoidance of operation, has been convincingly demonstrated for all of these methods of endoscopic hemostasis. The analysis of reports of endoscopic treatment of hemorrhage is complicated by the 70% rate of spontaneous, although sometimes temporary, cessation of bleeding without intervention. In addition to endoscopic stigmata, hemodynamic instability, need for continuing transfusion, red stool or hematemesis, age older than 60 years, and serious medical comorbidity are clinical features that mandate endoscopic therapy. Rebleeding during hospitalization and the endoscopic findings of visible vessel, oozing, or bleeding associated with an adherent clot are other indications for endoscopic hemostasis. Ulcers with clean bases require no treatment. Failure of endoscopic hemostasis is usually due to inaccessibility because of scarring, to rapid active bleeding obscuring the endoscopic view, or to an adherent clot. Patients treated endoscopically should be observed closely for further hemorrhage. Patients who rebleed within 72 hours of initial endoscopic control may be successfully retreated without increasing the risk of mortality.[19]

The efficacy of endoscopy is dependent on timing. Early endoscopy correctly identifies patients at low risk for recurrent hemorrhage and permits safe avoidance of hospitalization. Early endoscopy also benefits high-risk patients by directing active hemostatic therapy. Patients treated in this way have been demonstrated to have fewer episodes of rebleeding, lower rates of operation, and shorter hospitalizations.

TABLE 44.4 INDICATIONS/CONTRAINDICATIONS

SITUATIONS IN WHICH OPERATIVE INTERVENTION IS APPROPRIATE

Massive hemorrhage leading to shock or cardiovascular instability
Prolonged blood loss requiring continuing transfusion
Recurrent bleeding during medical therapy or after endoscopic therapy
Recurrent hemorrhage requiring hospitalization

Table 44.4 lists situations in which operative intervention is appropriate. The need for emergency surgery significantly increases surgical risks; mortality rates are increased approximately 10-fold. Operative therapy should consist of duodenotomy with direct ligation of the bleeding vessel in the ulcer base.

Postoperatively, patients should receive antibiotics directed against *H. pylori*. This treatment paradigm is based on the observation that peptic ulcer hemorrhage recurs in 20% of patients in whom *H. pylori* is not eradicated, whereas rebleeding is reduced to 3% in patients who receive *H. pylori* eradication therapy[20] (Algorithm 44.1). The studies that support this practice were not specifically designed to evaluate postoperative hemorrhage, but the results are so definitive that they support this application (Fig. 44.4).

Perforation

The lifetime risk for perforation in patients with duodenal ulceration who do not receive therapy approximates 10%. In contrast, ulcer perforation is unusual if initial ulcer healing has been achieved.

Perforation of a duodenal ulcer is usually accompanied by sudden and severe epigastric pain. The pain, caused by the

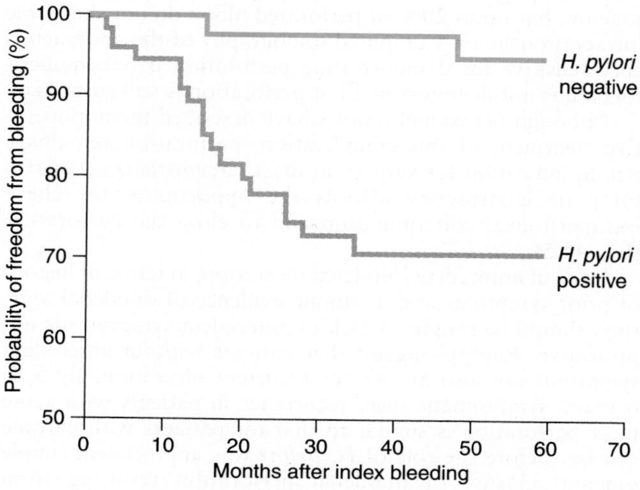

FIGURE 44.4. Probability of freedom from recurrent hemorrhage according to posttreatment *Helicobacter pylori* status.

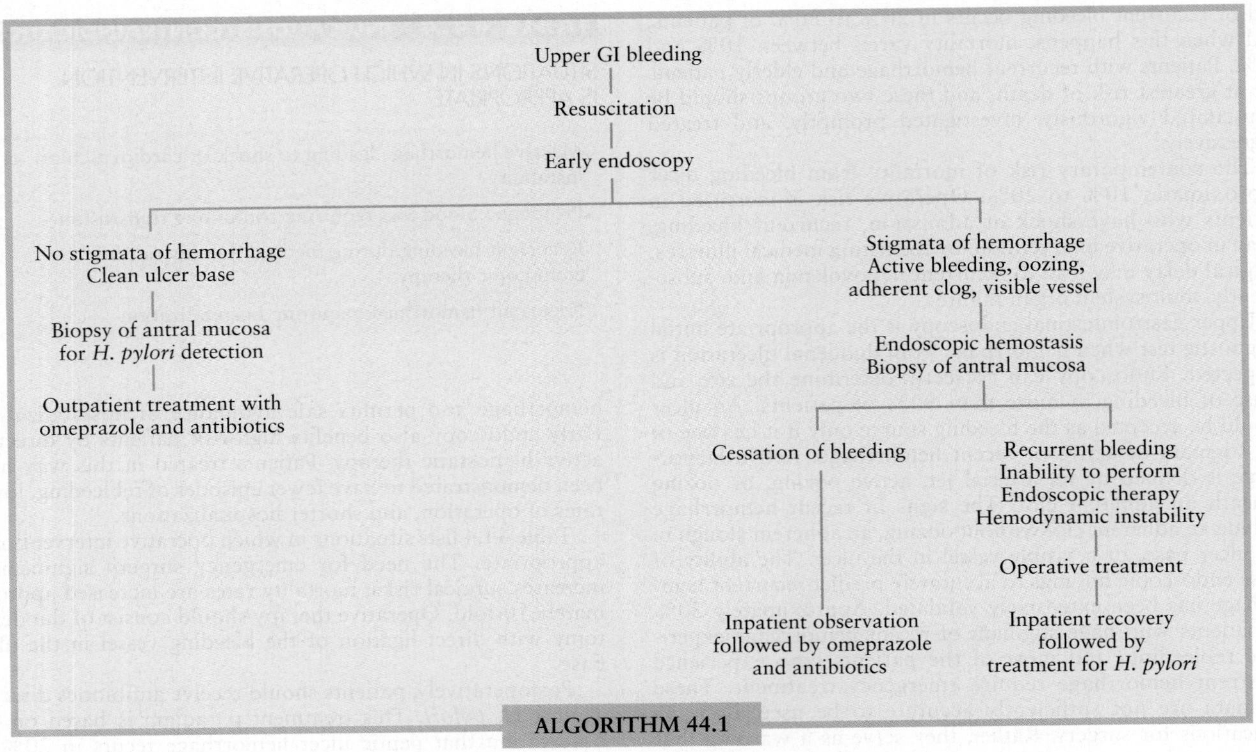

ALGORITHM 44.1 Treatment of bleeding duodenal ulceration.

spillage of highly caustic gastric secretions into the peritoneum, rapidly reaches peak intensity and remains constant. Radiation to the right scapular region is common because of right subphrenic collection of gastric contents. Occasionally, pain is sensed in the lower abdomen if gastric contents travel caudally through the paracolic gutter. Peritoneal irritation is usually intense, and most patients avoid movement to minimize discomfort.

Physical examination reveals low-grade fever, diminished bowel sounds, and rigidity of the abdominal musculature. Usually, upright abdominal radiographs reveal pneumoperitoneum, but up to 20% of perforated ulcers do not show free intraperitoneal air. Computed tomography of the abdomen is very sensitive for demonstrating perforation if pneumoperitoneum is not demonstrated but perforation is still suspected.

Although occasional reports have described the nonoperative treatment of this complication, perforation remains a strong indication for surgery in most circumstances. Laparotomy or laparoscopy affords the opportunity to relieve intraperitoneal contamination and to close the perforation (Fig. 44.5).

Signs of antecedent duodenal ulceration, in terms of history of prior symptoms and anatomic evidence of duodenal scarring, should be sought. A lack of antecedent symptoms is not protective. Reports suggest that patients without antecedent symptoms are also at risk for recurrent ulceration. By 5 to 6 years, symptomatic ulcer recurrence in patients with acute ulcer perforation is similar to that for patients with chronic disease. Before the role of *H. pylori* was appreciated, simple omental closure of duodenal perforation resulting from chronic ulceration did not provide satisfactory long-term results; up to 80% of patients so treated had recurrent ulceration, and 10% experienced reperforation if untreated. Approximately four fifths of all patients with perforation have

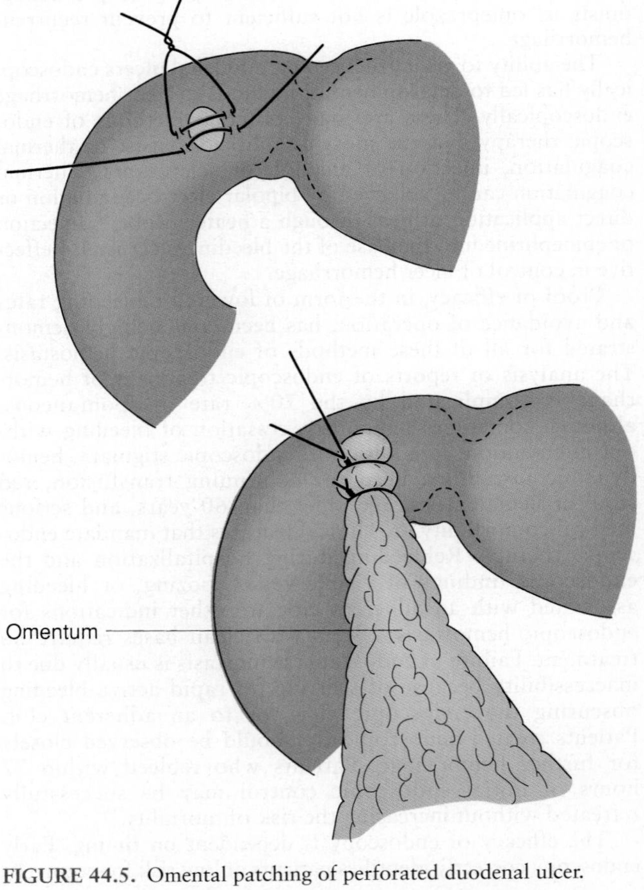

FIGURE 44.5. Omental patching of perforated duodenal ulcer.

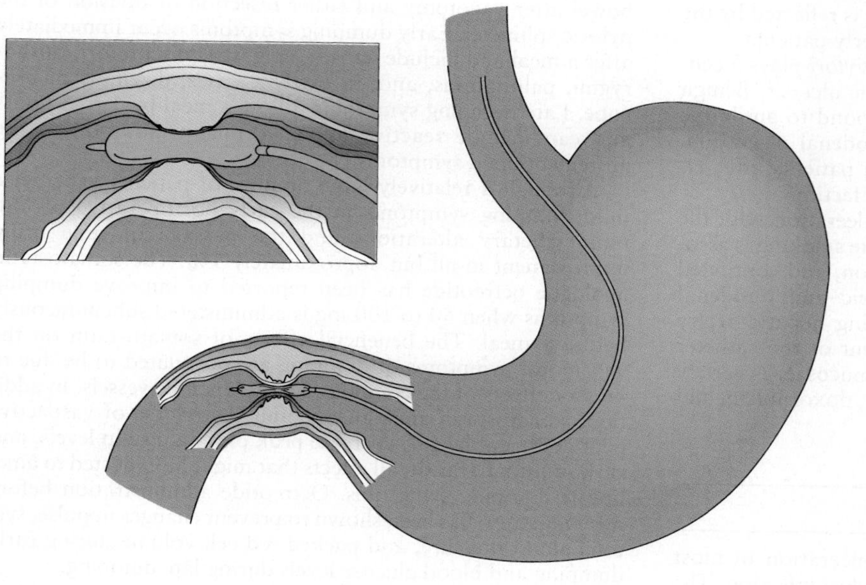

FIGURE 44.6. Schematic representation of balloon dilatation of pyloric stenosis.

H. pylori infestation and therefore are at risk of recurrent disease.

The mortality of emergent ulcer operations is most clearly correlated with the following circumstances: preoperative shock, coexisting medical illness, and presence of perforation for more than 48 hours.[21]

6 Current reports advocate omental patch closure only, often laparoscopically, with postoperative anti–*H. pylori* therapy. This approach presumes that most duodenal ulcers are caused by *H. pylori*, that secure closure of the perforation can be obtained, and that further surgical therapy will be obviated by the effects of medical therapy. Minimally invasive approaches are becoming standard practice.

Two meta-analyses of surgical treatment of perforated peptic ulcer have compared open surgical therapy with laparoscopic approaches.[22,23] In terms of operative time, there is no clear superiority of one approach over the other, but all trials reported after 2001 have favored laparoscopic repair. While in-hospital analgesic use is less in laparoscopically treated patients, the more important variable of hospital length of stay was not significantly shorter for these patients. Overall rates of postoperative complications were not statistically different between the two approaches. A lower rate of wound infection in the laparoscopic group approached significance. Return to normal daily activities and work favored the laparoscopic group. The pooled estimate of mortality favored laparoscopic repair.

Obstruction

Gastric outlet obstruction can occur acutely or chronically in patients with duodenal ulcer disease. Acute obstruction is caused by edema and inflammation associated with ulcers in the pyloric channel and the first portion of the duodenum. Pyloric obstruction is suggested by recurrent vomiting, dehydration, and hypochloremic alkalosis due to loss of gastric secretions. Acute gastric outlet obstruction is treated with nasogastric suction, rehydration, and intravenous administration of antisecretory agents. In most instances, acute obstruction resolves with such supportive measures within 72 hours.

Repeated episodes of ulceration and healing can lead to pyloric scarring and a fixed stenosis with chronic gastric outlet obstruction.[23] In cases of untreated duodenal ulceration, the lifetime risk of chronic pyloric stenosis approximates 10%.

Upper endoscopy is indicated to confirm the nature of the obstruction and to exclude neoplasm. Endoscopic hydrostatic balloon dilatation of pyloric stenoses can also be attempted at this time (Fig. 44.6). Approximately 85% of pyloric stenoses are amenable to balloon dilatation. Only 40% of patients with gastric stenoses have sustained improvement by 3 months after balloon dilatation. Recurrent stenoses are presumably due to residual scarring in the pyloric channel. Thus, although pyloric dilatation is occasionally palliative, in most cases operative correction is required.

Operative management of gastric outlet obstruction should be focused on relief of the anatomic abnormality. Antrectomy has been used with success in this circumstance, with low ulcer recurrence rates and with satisfactory restoration of gastric emptying.

GASTRIC ULCER

Benign gastric ulcers are a form of peptic ulcer disease, occurring with one-third the frequency of benign duodenal ulceration. In the United States, gastric ulcer is somewhat more common in men than in women and occurs in a patient cohort approximately 10 years older than for duodenal ulceration.

Endoscopic Diagnosis

Upper gastrointestinal endoscopy is the preferred method for diagnosing gastric ulceration. The ulcer base in benign disease is commonly smooth and flat and often covered by a gray, fibrous exudate. The margin is usually slightly raised, erythematous, and friable. Differentiation of benign and malignant gastric ulcers is reliably made only by histologic examination. Visual endoscopic differentiation of benign from malignant ulcers is not reliable. All gastric ulcers should have multiple biopsies taken from the perimeter of the lesion. The addition of lesional brushings to biopsy increases diagnostic accuracy to approximately 95%.

Benign gastric ulcers may occur in any location in the stomach, but approximately 60% are located along the lesser curvature proximal to the incisura angularis. Less than 10% of benign gastric ulcers are located on the greater curvature. Virtually all gastric ulcers lie within 2 cm of the histologic transition between fundic and antral mucosa. With increasing age, this mucosal transition zone moves proximally along the lesser curvature. Movement of this transition zone is reflected by the greater prevalence of proximal ulcers in elderly patients.

As with benign duodenal ulceration, *H. pylori* plays a central role in the pathogenesis of benign gastric ulcers.[25] Benign gastric ulcers associated with *H. pylori* respond to antibiotic therapy at a rate equivalent to that of duodenal ulceration. The recurrence rate of ulcerations in these patients after *H. pylori* eradication is equal to the rate of reinfection.

A strong association of benign gastric ulceration with the use of NSAIDs has been recognized. Cigarette smoking is associated with development of gastric ulceration, and continued smoking impedes medical therapy. Gastric and duodenal ulcers have been noted in patients receiving hepatic artery chemotherapy in whom improper placement of the catheter permits perfusion of gastric and duodenal mucosae. A variety of agents, including 5-fluorouracil, cisplatin, doxorubicin, and mitomycin C, have been implicated.

Therapy

The primary therapy for benign gastric ulceration in most patients is antimicrobial treatment of *H. pylori* infection. The treatment protocols are similar to those used for benign duodenal ulceration. For many patients, cessation of NSAID therapy is also required.

Indications for surgical treatment of gastric ulcer include hemorrhage, perforation, failure of a recurrent ulcer to respond to medical therapy, and inability to exclude malignant disease.

For benign gastric ulcers, the elective operation of choice is usually a distal gastrectomy with gastroduodenal (Billroth I) anastomosis. The ulcer should be included in the gastrectomy specimen. With this approach, operative mortality rates of 2% to 3%, with ulcer recurrence rates of less than 5%, have been reported. Because benign gastric ulcers are not associated with gastric acid hypersecretion, inclusion of vagotomy is not necessary.

The occurrence of a gastric ulcer near the gastroesophageal junction represents a difficult surgical problem. When possible, the ulcer should be excised. This usually requires a distal gastrectomy with an extension along the lesser curvature near the esophageal wall and reconstruction with gastrojejunostomy.

Emergency operations performed for hemorrhage or perforation require ulcer excision. Distal gastrectomy, performed with gastroduodenal reconstruction, is usually the procedure of choice. Operative mortality rates average 10% to 20% in the presence of hemorrhage or perforation.

POSTGASTRECTOMY SYNDROMES

A number of syndromes have been described that are associated with distressing symptoms after gastric operations performed for peptic ulcer or gastric neoplasm. The occurrence of severe postoperative symptoms is fortunately low, perhaps 1% to 3% of cases, but the disturbances can be disabling. The two most common postgastrectomy syndromes, categorized according to predominant manifestation, are dumping and alkaline reflux gastritis.

Dumping

The term *dumping* denotes a clinical syndrome with both gastrointestinal and vasomotor symptoms. The precise cause of dumping is not known but is believed to relate to the unmetered entry of ingested food into the proximal small bowel after vagotomy and either resection or division of the pyloric sphincter. Early dumping symptoms occur immediately after a meal and include nausea, epigastric discomfort, borborygmi, palpitations, and, in extreme cases, dizziness or syncope. Late dumping symptoms follow a meal by 1 to 3 hours and can include reactive hypoglycemia in addition to the aforementioned symptoms.

Although a relatively large number of patients experience mild dumping symptoms in the early postoperative period, minor dietary alterations and the passage of time bring improvement in all but approximately 1%. The somatostatin analogue octreotide has been reported to improve dumping symptoms when 50 to 100 mg is administered subcutaneously before a meal. The beneficial effects of somatostatin on the vasomotor symptoms of dumping are postulated to be due to pressor effects of the compound on splanchnic vessels. In addition, somatostatin analogues inhibit the release of vasoactive peptides from the gut, decrease peak plasma insulin levels, and slow intestinal transit, all effects that might be expected to ameliorate dumping symptoms. Octreotide administration before meal ingestion has been shown to prevent changes in pulse, systolic blood pressure, and packed red cell volume during early dumping and blood glucose levels during late dumping.

Alkaline Reflux Gastritis

The term *alkaline reflux gastritis* should be reserved for patients who demonstrate the clinical triad of postprandial epigastric pain often associated with nausea and vomiting, evidence of reflux of bile into the stomach, and histologic evidence of gastritis. One or more of these findings occur transiently in 10% to 20% of patients after gastric resection, but they persist in only 1% to 2%.

The differential diagnosis for a patient with postoperative epigastric pain includes recurrent ulceration, biliary and pancreatic disease, afferent loop obstruction, and esophagitis in addition to alkaline reflux gastritis. Gastric acid analysis shows basal hypochlorhydria with little increase with pentagastrin stimulation. Serum gastrin measurements should be determined to exclude Zollinger-Ellison syndrome and retained gastric antrum. Endoscopic examination is essential to exclude recurrent ulcer.

Endoscopically, the gastric mucosa appears red, friable, and edematous. Gastric inflammation is patchy and nonulcerative. Histologic examination shows mucosal and submucosal edema and infiltration of acute and chronic inflammatory cells into the lamina propria. Glandular atrophy and intestinal metaplasia are frequent accompaniments.

No perfect solution to alkaline reflux gastritis exists. Antacids, H_2-receptor antagonists, bile acid chelators, and dietary manipulations have not been demonstrated definitely to be beneficial. The only proved treatment for alkaline reflux gastritis is operative diversion of intestinal contents from contact with the gastric mucosa. The most common surgical procedure used for this purpose is a Roux-en-Y gastrojejunostomy with an intestinal limb of 50 to 60 cm constructed to prevent reflux of intestinal contents (Fig. 44.7). This procedure is effective in eliminating bilious vomiting (nearly 100%), but recurrent or persistent pain is reported in up to 30% of patients, and up to 20% of patients are troubled with postoperative delayed gastric emptying.

STRESS GASTRITIS

7 Major trauma accompanied by shock, sepsis, respiratory failure, hemorrhage, or multiorgan injury is often accompanied by acute stress gastritis.[26] Acute stress gastritis is particularly prevalent after thermal injury with greater than 35% total surface area burned. A similar entity is also observed as a

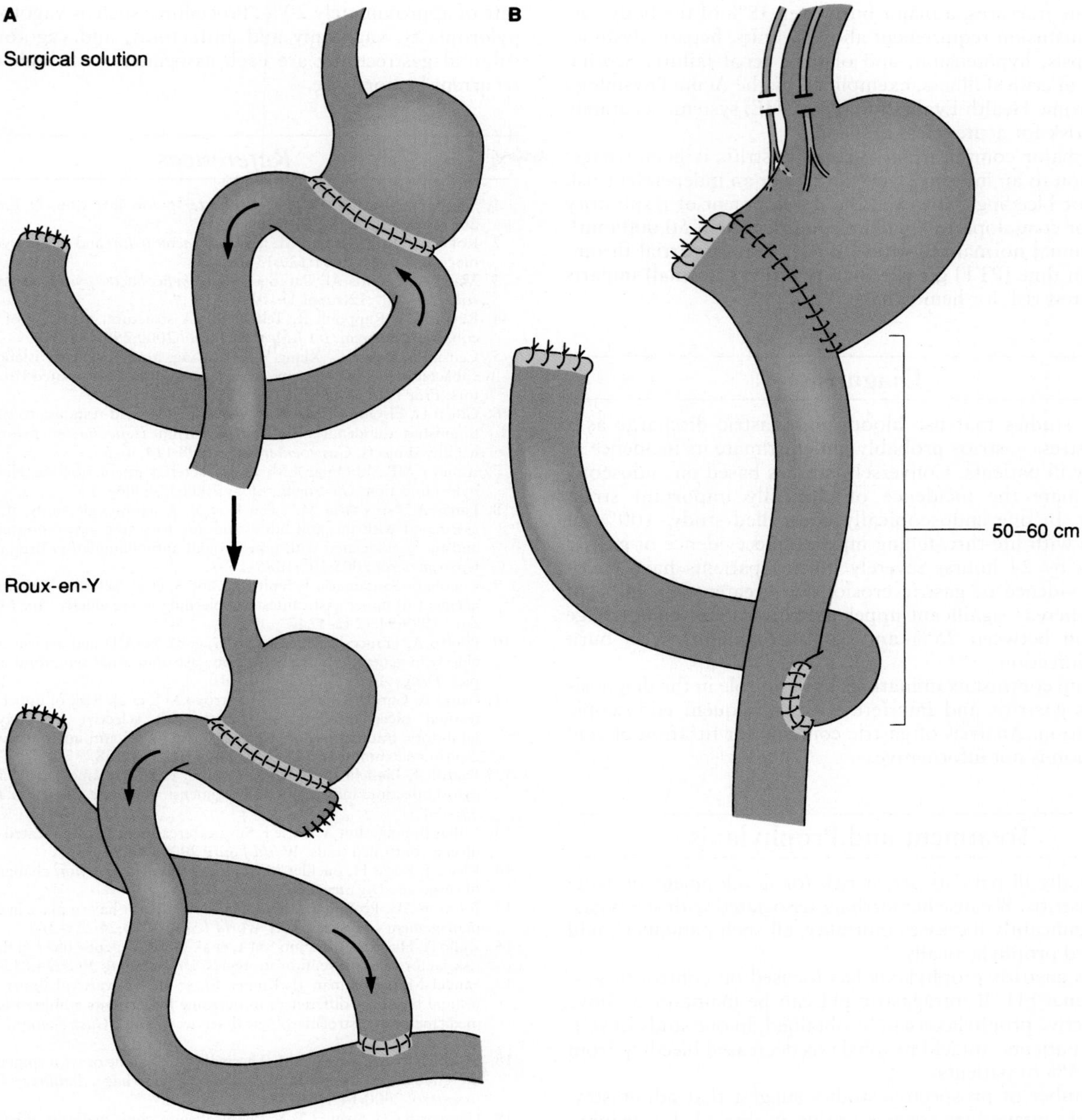

FIGURE 44.7. Conversion of Billroth II gastrojejunostomy to Roux-en-Y gastrojejunostomy. The afferent limb is divided (**A**), and intestinal continuity is re-established by anastomosis 50 to 60 cm downstream from the original gastrojejunostomy (**B**).

result of central nervous system injury or intracranial hypertension. Multiple superficial ulcerations and erosions are noted in the proximal, acid-secreting portion of the stomach, with fewer lesions in the antrum and only rare ulcerations in the duodenum.

The most sensitive diagnostic test for stress ulceration is endoscopic examination. If patients are examined within 12 hours of the onset of injury, acute mucosal ulcerations may be observed that appear as multiple, shallow areas of erythema and friability, often accompanied by focal hemorrhage. The lesions are progressive during the first 72 hours after injury. When lesions are examined histologically, they are seen to consist of coagulation necrosis of the superficial endothelium with infiltration of leukocytes into the lamina propria. Chronic disease, characterized by fibrosis and scarring, is not observed. With resolution of the underlying injury or sepsis, healing is accompanied by mucosal restitution and regeneration.

Clinical observations and a large number of experimental studies suggest that mucosal ischemia is the central event underlying the development of stress gastritis. In clinical practice, most patients who contract stress gastritis do so after an episode of sepsis, hemorrhage, or cardiac dysfunction accompanied by shock.[27] Experimental studies that cause depletion of high-energy phosphate compounds such as ATP predispose to the development of stress gastritis. Luminal gastric acid secretion, although not the sole cause of stress gastritis, appears to be a necessary concomitant process. A number of experimental observations suggest that a critical concentration of luminal acid is required to initiate injury in the setting of mucosal ischemia. The fall in mucosal energy supply permits proton back-diffusion into the mucosa; the resultant decrease in mucosal pH exacerbates ischemic damage.

Clinical risk factors that predict development of stress gastritis include adult respiratory distress syndrome, multiple long-bone fractures, a major burn over 35% of the body surface, transfusion requirement above 6 units, hepatic dysfunction, sepsis, hypotension, and oliguric renal failure. Scoring systems of critical illness, exemplified by the Acute Physiology and Chronic Health Evaluation (APACHE) system, accurately predict risk for acute stress gastritis.

The major complication of stress gastritis is hemorrhage. Admission to an intensive care unit is not an independent risk factor for bleeding. However, the development of respiratory failure or coagulopathy (platelet count less than 50,000/mm^3, international normalized ratio [INR] >1.5, or partial thromboplastin time [PTT] greater than two times normal) imparts the greatest risk for hemorrhage.

Diagnosis

Clinical studies that use bloody nasogastric discharge as a sign of stress gastritis probably underestimate its incidence in critically ill patients. Conversely, studies based on endoscopy overestimate the incidence of clinically important stress gastritis. In one endoscopically controlled study, 100% of patients with life-threatening injuries had evidence of gastric erosions by 24 hours. Severely burned patients have endoscopic evidence of gastric erosions in greater than 90% of cases, whereas significant upper gastrointestinal hemorrhage occurs in between 25% and 50% of patients with burn wound infection.

Barium contrast examinations have no role in the diagnosis of stress gastritis and interfere with subsequent endoscopic examination. Analysis of gastric contents for titration of acid production is not informative.

Treatment and Prophylaxis

All critically ill patients are at risk for development of acute stress gastritis. Because hemorrhage associated with stress gastritis significantly increases mortality, all such patients should be treated prophylactically.[28]

Stress gastritis prophylaxis has focused on control of gastric luminal pH. If intragastric pH can be maintained above 3.5, effective prophylaxis can be obtained. In one study of seriously ill patients, antacid prophylaxis decreased bleeding from 25% to 4% of patients.

A number of prospective studies suggest that administration of H_2 antagonists are as effective as antacids for prophylaxis of stress gastritis.[29] Infusion of an H_2 antagonist at a rate that maintains intraluminal gastric pH at greater than 3.5 is equally effective, relative to antacids, in terms of prevention of bleeding. Continuous-infusion H_2-receptor antagonist therapy appears to be equally effective relative to intermittent dosing with H_2 blockers or antacids. Proton pump inhibitors have also been shown to be effective as stress ulcer prophylaxis.

When stress gastritis causes gastrointestinal bleeding, endoscopic therapy is used as first-line treatment. Endoscopic examination is diagnostic and permits application of electrocautery or heater probe hemostasis.

Only a small minority of patients with acute stress gastritis and hemorrhage require operative therapy. The surgical approach should control acute bleeding, have a low risk of recurrent hemorrhage, and be associated with a low operative mortality rate. No procedure meets all of these criteria, and no large clinical experience is available to confirm the superiority of one procedure over another. Total gastrectomy is associated with the lowest risk of recurrent bleeding but has a mortality rate of approximately 20%. Procedures such as vagotomy and pyloroplasty, vagotomy and antrectomy, and vagotomy and subtotal gastrectomy are each associated with high risks of recurrent hemorrhage.

References

1. Suerbaum S, Michetti P. *Helicobacter pylori* infection. *N Engl J Med* 2002;347(15):1175–1186.
2. Kokoska ER, Kauffman GL Jr. *Helicobacter pylori* and the gastroduodenal mucosa. *Surgery* 2001;130:13–16.
3. Maeda S, Mentis AF. Pathogenesis of *helicobacter pylori* infection. *Helicobacter* 2007;12(suppl 1):10–14.
4. Reyrat JM, Rappouli R, Telford JL. A structural overview of the Helicobacter cytotoxin. *Int J Med Microbiol* 2000;290:375–379.
5. Censini S, Lange C, Xiang Z, et al. Cag, a pathogenicity island of Helicobacter pylori encodes type I-specific and disease-associated virulence factors. *Proc Natl Acad Sci U S A* 1996;93:1259–1264.
6. Gillen D, El-Omar EM, Wirz AA, et al. The acid response to gastrin distinguishes duodenal ulcer patients from *Helicobacter pylori*-infected healthy subjects. *Gastroenterology* 1998;114:50–57.
7. Amieva MR, El-Omar EM. Host-bacterial interactions in *Helicobacter pylori* infection. *Gastroenterology* 2008;134;306–323.
8. Lanas A, Perex-Aisa MA, Feu F, et al. A nationwide study of mortality associated with hospital admission due to severe gastrointestinal events and those associated with nonsteroidal antiinflammatory drug use. *Am J Gastroenterol* 2005;100:1685–1693.
9. Cebollaro-Santamaria F, Smith J, Gioe S, et al. Selective outpatient management of upper gastrointestinal bleeding in the elderly. *Am J Gastroenterol* 1999;94:1242–1247.
10. Pilotto A, Franceshi M, Leandro G, et al. NSAID and aspirin use by the elderly in general practice: effect on gastrointestinal symptoms and therapies. *Drugs Aging* 2003;20:701–710.
11. Lanas A, Garcia-Rodriguez LA, Arroyo MT, et al. Risk of upper gastrointestinal ulcer bleeding associated with selective cyclooxygenase-2 inhibitors, traditional non-aspirin non-steroidal anti-inflammatory drugs, aspirin and combinations. *Gut* 2006;55;1731–1738.
12. Bazzoli F, Bianchi Porro G, Maconi G, et al. Treatment of Helicobacter pylori infection: indications and regimens: an update. *Dig Liver Dis* 2002; 34:70–83.
13. Millat B, Fingerhut A, Borie F. Surgical treatment of complicated duodenal ulcers: controlled trials. *World J Surg* 2000;24:299–306.
14. Kleeff J, Friess H, Büchler MW. How *Helicobacter pylori* changed the life of surgeons. *Dig Surg* 2003;20:93–102.
15. Johnson AG. Proximal gastric vagotomy: does it have a place in the future management of peptic ulcer? *World J Surg* 2000;24:259–263.
16. Zullo A, Hassan C, Campo SMA, et al. Bleeding peptic ulcer in the elderly: risk factors and prevention strategies. *Drugs Aging* 2007;24:815–828.
17. Sandel MH, Kolkman JJ, Kuiper EJ, et al. Nonvariceal upper gastrointestinal bleeding: differences in outcome for patients admitted to internal medicine and gastroenterological services. *Am J Gastroenterol* 2000;95: 2357–2362.
18. Machicado GA, Jensen DM. Thermal probes alone or with epinephrine for the endoscopic haemostasis of ulcer haemorrhage. *Baillieres Clin Gastroenterol* 2000;14:443–458.
19. Hepworth CC, Swain CP. Mechanical endoscopic methods of haemostasis for bleeding peptic ulcers: a review. *Baillieres Clin Gastroenterol* 2000;14: 467–476.
20. Sharma VK, Sahai AV, Corder FA, et al. Helicobacter pylori eradication is superior to ulcer healing with or without maintenance therapy to prevent further ulcer haemorrhage. *Ailment Pharmacol Ther* 2001;15:1939–1947.
21. Boey J, Choi SKY, Alagaratnam TT, et al. Risk stratification for perforated duodenal ulcers: a prospective validation of predictive factors. *Ann Surg* 1987;205:22–28.
22. Lunevicius R, Morkevicius M. Systematic review comparing laparoscopic and open repair for perforated peptic ulcer. *Br J Surg* 2005;92:1195–1207.
23. Sanabria AE, Morales CH, Villegas MI. Laparoscopic repair for perforated peptic ulcer disease. *Cochrane Database Syst Rev* 2005:CD004778.
24. Ellis H. Pyloric stenosis complicating duodenal ulceration. *World J Surg* 1987;11:198–202.
25. Atherton JC. The pathogenesis of Helicobacter pylori-induced gastroduodenal disease. *Annu Rev Pathol* 2006;1:63–96.
26. Hiramoto JS, Terdiman JP, Norton JA. Evidence-based analysis: postoperative gastric bleeding: etiology and prevention. *Surg Oncol* 2003;12:9–19.
27. Mutlu GM, Mutlu EA, Factor P. GI complications in patients receiving mechanical ventilation. *Chest* 2001;119:1222–1238.
28. Tryba M. Role of acid suppressants in intensive care medicine. *Best Pract Res Clin Gastroenterol* 2001;15:447–461.
29. Yang Y, Lewis JD. Prevention and treatment of stress ulcers in critically ill patients. *Semin Gastrointest Dis* 2003;14:11–19.

CHAPTER 45 ■ MORBID OBESITY

REBECCA P. PETERSEN, CHRISTOPHER J. MYERS, AND ERIC J. DeMARIA

KEY POINTS

1. Overweight and obesity can be quantified by body mass index (BMI), which is calculated as weight in kilograms divided by the square of the height in meters.
2. Two thirds of the U.S. adult population is considered overweight (BMI $\geq$25 kg/m^2) and half of these are obese (BMI $\geq$30 kg/m^2).
3. Obesity is associated with numerous comorbidities including diabetes and atherosclerosis, respiratory and cardiac failure, venous thromboembolic disease, cholelithiasis, degenerative joint disease, pseudotumor cerebri, and nonalcoholic steatohepatitis.
4. Patients are considered eligible for surgical treatment of obesity if they have a BMI greater than or equal to 40 kg/m^2 without an obesity-related comorbidity or a BMI greater than or equal to 35 kg/m^2 with an obesity-related comorbidity (e.g., diabetes, respiratory insufficiency, pseudotumor cerebri).
5. A National Institutes of Health Technology Assessment Conference in 1992 concluded that dietary management of severe obesity, with or without behavioral modification, failed to provide acceptable evidence of long-term efficacy.
6. Adjustable gastric banding and gastroplasties are restrictive procedures that have been performed with either horizontal or vertical placement of the staples.
7. Gastric bypass combines restriction and malabsorption to assist weight loss.

1 Obesity and overweight have now reached epidemic proportions, and their associated conditions have serious implications for global health. Traditionally, categories of obesity and overweight have been defined using body mass index (BMI), which is calculated as weight in kilograms divided by the square of the height in meters. Thresholds to classify overweight, obesity, and morbid obesity have been created based on long-term outcome.

2 According to this classification, more than two thirds of the U.S. adult population is overweight and half of these are obese, which has important public health implications because obesity is clearly associated with increased morbidity and mortality.[1,2] In addition, this crisis now involves the developing world, and the World Health Organization (WHO) currently estimates that 1.7 billion people worldwide are overweight or obese.[3] Alarmingly, obesity has become increasingly prevalent in the pediatric population, and 30% of U.S. children have a BMI greater than the 85th percentile for their age.[4]

3 Severe obesity is associated with a large number of associated comorbidities, many of which are associated with an increased risk of mortality (Table 45.1) and include coronary artery disease, hypertension, heart failure, type 2 diabetes mellitus, obesity hypoventilation and sleep apnea syndromes, hypercoagulability and venous thromboembolic disease, necrotizing panniculitis, diverticulitis, and necrotizing pancreatitis. In addition, morbidly obese patients have an increased risk of colon, prostate, breast, and uterine carcinoma.

4 The 1991 National Institutes of Health (NIH) Consensus Panel (Table 45.2) established eligibility criteria for surgical management. In general, a BMI greater than or equal to 40 kg/m^2 without an associated comorbidity and a BMI greater than or equal to 35 kg/m^2 with an established comorbidity are considered general criteria for consideration of surgical management of obesity.

ETIOLOGY

The causes of morbid obesity are not entirely known but likely include a combination of genetic, endocrinologic, behavioral, and environmental factors. Multiple studies have identified a genetic predisposition to obesity, and several genetic markers have been described. In adoption studies, severity of obesity was found to be more concordant with the natural than the adoptive parents.[5,6] Furthermore, monozygotic twins have more similar weights than dizygotic twins, even if they grow up in different environments.[7,8]

Gastrointestinal and neuroendocrine peptides are involved in weight homeostasis, in conjunction with neural or humoral transmitters to the hypothalamic hunger or satiety centers, and the psychologically induced oral dependency drive. Ghrelin, a potent orexigenic peptide secreted by the stomach, increases in response to fasting and decreases postprandially. Ghrelin levels are decreased in obese individuals.[9] The adipocyte hormone leptin stimulates anorexigenic neuropeptides in the hypothalamus to inhibit food intake; obese individuals often have increased serum levels of leptin and may be resistant to leptin effects on food intake and energy expenditure.[10] This is supported by studies demonstrating that morbidly obese adults have been found to have a lower basal energy expenditure.[11]

The distribution of body fat is an important characteristic, as android or central obesity has been associated with significantly worse long-term health compared with gynoid or peripheral obesity. Anthropomorphic measurements such as the waist-to-hip ratio have been used to quantify central obesity; however, computed tomography scans have shown that abdominal circumference is a more accurate measurement of central fat distribution.[8] The increased metabolic activity of mesenteric fat is associated with increased metabolism of amino acids to carbohydrates, leading to hyperglycemia and hyperinsulinemia. Hyperinsulinemia gives rise to increased sodium absorption and hypertension and insulin resistance. Central abdominal obesity has also been associated with dyslipidemia, including low high-density lipoprotein (HDL) cholesterol and elevated triglycerides, increased systemic inflammation, and hypercoagulability. As these conditions tend to track together, collectively these conditions are referred to as the metabolic syndrome. Other conditions associated with obesity include increased fatty acid and cholesterol turnover with an increased risk of atherosclerosis

TABLE 45.1

MORBIDITY OF OBESITY

Cardiovascular dysfunction
Hypertension
Coronary artery disease
Heart failure
Type 2 diabetes mellitus (adult onset or non–insulin dependent)
Nonalcoholic steatohepatitis
Respiratory insufficiency of obesity (pickwickian syndrome)
Obesity hypoventilation syndrome
Obstructive sleep apnea syndrome
Increased intra-abdominal pressure
Stress overflow urinary incontinence
Gastroesophageal reflux
Venous disease
Thrombophlebitis
Stasis ulcers
Pulmonary embolism
Nephrotic syndrome
Pseudotumor cerebri
Degenerative osteoarthritis
Cholelithiasis
Infectious complications
Difficulty recognizing peritonitis
Necrotizing subcutaneous infections
Wound infections or dehiscence
Sexual hormone dysfunction
Polycystic ovary (Stein-Leventhal) syndrome

and cholelithiasis, polycystic ovary (Stein-Leventhal) syndrome, and nonalcoholic steatohepatitis.[7]

CONDITIONS ASSOCIATED WITH MORBID OBESITY

An important consequence of central obesity is increased intra-abdominal pressure, which contributes to many of the conditions associated with morbid obesity. In addition to the conditions in this section, gastroesophageal reflux, stress or urge urinary incontinence, nephrotic syndrome, and incisional and inguinal hernias are common problems in obese patients.[12,13]

TABLE 45.2 INDICATIONS/CONTRAINDICATION

CRITERIA FOR PATIENT SELECTION FOR BARIATRIC SURGERY

Body mass index >40 kg/m^2
Body mass index >35 kg/m^2 with coexisting comorbidities
Failure of nonsurgical methods of weight reduction
Psychological stability
Absence of drug and alcohol abuse

Respiratory Disorders Associated with Obesity

There are two components of respiratory dysfunction in obesity—obstructive sleep apnea syndrome (OSA) and obesity hypoventilation syndrome (OHS)—and collectively these conditions comprise the pickwickian syndrome. Both of these conditions may be present before operation but may be exacerbated by a surgical procedure. Following gastric surgery for obesity, OSA and OHS can completely resolve.[14]

OSA is a potentially fatal complication of morbid obesity and is characterized by frequent daytime somnolence and heavy snoring. The frequent episodes of apnea result in inadequate stage IV and rapid eye movement (REM) sleep, leading to somnolence during the day. Patients with suspected sleep apnea syndrome should undergo preoperative polysomnography at a sleep center to confirm the diagnosis and to guide therapy. During surgical procedures, patients with OSA are at great risk for acute upper airway obstruction and respiratory arrest at the time of anesthetic induction. In severe cases, it may be worthwhile to consider elective tracheostomy prior to bariatric surgery.

Obesity Hypoventilation Syndrome

OHS is a condition in which an obese patient suffers from hypoxemia and hypercapnia when breathing room air while awake but resting.[15] As many alveolar units are collapsed at end expiration, considerable ventilation/perfusion (V/Q) mismatch occurs, leading to shunting, hypoxemia, and hypercapnia. The condition is not directly associated with the degree of obesity, and among patients undergoing gastric bypass surgery, no statistically significant difference in weight was found between those who had OHS and those who did not.[14] The diagnosis can be confirmed with spirometry and arterial blood gas analysis.

Chronic pulmonary arterial hypoxemia leads to severe pulmonary hypertension and subsequent right-sided heart failure, manifested by jugular venous distention, tricuspid valve regurgitation, right upper quadrant tenderness due to acute hepatic engorgement, and massive peripheral edema.[16,17]

Cardiac Dysfunction

Cardiac dysfunction in the morbidly obese patient is often associated with respiratory disorders of obesity.[10] Elevated pulmonary pressures are secondary to hypoxemia-induced pulmonary arterial vasoconstriction and increased pleural pressures transmitted by elevated intra-abdominal pressure (IAP).[16,18,19] In obese patients, circulating blood volume, plasma volume, and cardiac output increase in proportion to body weight, but massively obese patients may occasionally present with high-output heart failure, which is likely due to the enormous circulatory and metabolic requirements of such patients.[20] Significant weight loss has been demonstrated to correct pulmonary hypertension as well as left ventricular dysfunction associated with respiratory insufficiency.[16,21]

Venous Thromboembolic Disease

Morbidly obese individuals are markedly predisposed to venous thromboembolic disease, as they tend to be sedentary and have a large amount of abdominal weight resting on the inferior vena cava and have increased intrapleural pressure, which impedes venous return.[17,18] Low levels of antithrombin may also increase the tendency toward venous thrombosis.[22]

Venous stasis ulcers in patients with morbid obesity are almost impossible to cure due to elevated venous pressure. In addition to standard treatments for stasis ulcers, a critical goal in obese patients is weight loss. Significant improvements in weight almost invariably lead to healing of the ulcer and are probably the result of decreased IAP and venous pressure.[23]

Gallstones

Approximately one third of morbidly obese patients have cholelithiasis. Many have either had a cholecystectomy or had gallstones noted during another intra-abdominal operative procedure. In addition, rapid weight loss has been associated with development of gallstones in 25% to 40% of patients who undergo gastric bypass procedures. The risk of cholelithiasis in this setting can be reduced to 2% by administering ursodeoxycholic acid, 300 mg orally twice daily.[24]

Preoperative evaluation of the gallbladder may be technically quite difficult in morbidly obese patients because gallstones may be missed with transcutaneous ultrasonography. Among patients with symptoms of cholelithiasis, intraoperative sonography is a useful procedure to characterize cholelithiasis. Consideration should be given to cholecystectomy in a patient undergoing gastric operation for obesity.

Pseudotumor Cerebri

Pseudotumor cerebri is an unusual complication of morbid obesity that is associated with benign intracranial hypertension, papilledema, blurred vision, headache, and elevated cerebrospinal fluid pressures.[25] Currently, there is no evidence that patients with pseudotumor cerebri are at any additional perioperative risk, and cerebrospinal fluid does not have to be removed or shunted before anesthesia and major abdominal operations. Importantly, successful weight reduction will lead to resolution of pseudotumor cerebri.[26,27]

Degenerative Osteoarthritis

Degenerative osteoarthritis of the knees, hips, and back is a common complication of morbid obesity. In addition, podiatric pain is quite common. Weight reduction alone may greatly reduce the pain and immobility that afflict these patients, although many patients may require total joint replacement. Of note, joint replacement in patients who weigh more than 250 lb is associated with an unacceptable incidence of loosening, highlighting the importance of weight reduction prior to aggressive orthopedic interventions in morbidly obese patients.[28] Given the significant limitations of conservative weight loss programs in patients with severe degenerative joint disease, weight reduction by means of a gastric bariatric operation may be the most sensible initial approach, followed by repeat orthopedic evaluation if pain and dysfunction persist.

MEDICAL MANAGEMENT OF MORBID OBESITY

There are many dietary programs for weight reduction, including hospital-supervised programs, psychiatric behavioral modification programs, commercial organizations, commercial diets, protein-sparing fast programs, and medications. Unfortunately, while many people can lose weight successfully through dietary manipulation, only 5% to 10% of patients with extreme obesity are able to sustain significant
5 weight reduction.[29] An NIH Technology Assessment Conference in 1992 concluded that dietary management of severe obesity, with or without behavioral modification, failed to provide acceptable evidence of long-term efficacy.[23] Pharmacotherapy includes orlistat, a pancreatic lipase inhibitor that blocks fat absorption, and sibutramine, which works as an appetite suppressant. These agents provide only modest weight loss and are inadequate therapy for the morbidly obese patient.[24]

SURGICAL MANAGEMENT OF MORBID OBESITY

Eligibility for Obesity Surgery

The mortality risk for patients undergoing gastric bypass can now be assessed by the Obesity Surgery Mortality Risk Score (OS-MRS), which is composed of five independent, preoperative clinical variables and predicts 90-day mortality after gastric bypass surgery (Table 45.3). The OS-MRS was derived from 2,075 patients undergoing gastric bypass surgery at a single institution, and validation of the OS-MRS has been completed in a multicenter study involving 4,431 patients from four institutions. The OS-MRS is a valuable tool that can be used to stratify risk and aid in surgical decision making and patient discussion in bariatric surgery.[6]

While morbid obesity does impose greater perioperative risk, the risk can be markedly reduced by appropriate preoperative and postoperative care. Specifically, these risks include wound infection, dehiscence, thrombophlebitis, pulmonary embolism, anesthetic calamities, acute postoperative asphyxia in patients with OSA, acute respiratory failure, right ventricular or biventricular cardiac failure, and missed acute catastrophes of the abdomen, such as an anastomotic leak (Table 45.4).

Periprocedure Considerations

Morbidly obese patients are at significant risk of coronary artery disease as a result of the increased prevalence of coronary risk factors including systemic hypertension, dyslipidemia, insulin resistance, and diabetes. Thus, preoperative

TABLE 45.3

THE OBESITY SURGERY MORTALITY RISK SCORE

Body mass index >50 kg/m^2	
Male gender	
Hypertension	
Increased risk of pulmonary embolus:	
Previous thrombosis	
Previous pulmonary embolus	
Inferior vena caval filter	
Right heart failure	
Obesity hypoventilation syndrome	
Age ≥45 years	
Mortality Assessment	
Score[a]	**Mortality Risk**
0–1	0.2%
2–3	1.1%
4–5	2.4%

[a]The presence of each variable is equal to 1 point, resulting in a score of 0–5.

TABLE 45.4

COMPLICATIONS OF BARIATRIC OPERATIONS

Wound infection
Incisional hernia
Thrombophlebitis
Pulmonary embolism
Acute postoperative asphyxia
Acute respiratory failure
Cardiac failure
Marginal ulcer
Anastomotic leak
Death

electrocardiography should be performed on all obese patients 30 years of age or older, and abnormal findings worrisome for underlying coronary artery disease should be pursued.

Morbidly obese patients with a history of pulmonary disease or a BMI greater than 50 kg/m^2 should have preoperative determinations of blood gas values. If arterial blood gas (ABG) measurement reveals severe hypoxemia (partial pressure of arterial oxygen [PaO_2] ≤55 mm Hg), severe hypercapnia (partial pressure of arterial carbon dioxide [$PaCO_2$] ≥47 mm Hg), or both, consideration should be given to right heart catheterization prior to surgery. Morbidly obese patients may also have significantly elevated pulmonary artery wedge pressure (PAWP), which may indicate left ventricular dysfunction.[16] It is highly probable that some of the elevated pulmonary artery pressure (PAP) and PAWP measurements are caused by the increased IAP in the morbidly obese.[18,30] Typically, this is manifested by an elevated diaphragm, which in turn increases intrapleural pressure and subsequently PAP and PAWP. Pleural pressure can be measured with an esophageal transducer in conjunction with a right heart catheter and the transmyocardial pressure can be estimated. For this reason, these patients may require a markedly elevated PAWP to maintain an adequate cardiac output, and excessive diuresis may lead to hypotension.

If PAWP is greater than or equal to 18 mm Hg, diuresis with intravenous furosemide should be administered before elective operation. In some cases, low cardiac output and hypotension may follow diuresis. These patients may require higher than normal ventricular filling pressures, requiring some volume reexpansion. It is important to identify the optimal filling pressures for patients based on relative changes in cardiac output in response to either volume challenge or diuresis in morbidly obese patients.

Morbidly obese patients should be placed in the reverse Trendelenburg position to maximize diaphragmatic excursion and to increase residual lung volume.[31] In a supine position, these patients will often complain of air hunger and respiratory distress, and breaking of the bed at the waist may exacerbate the problem by pushing the abdominal contents into the chest by raising the diaphragm and further reducing lung volumes.

During surgical procedures, patients with OSA are at great risk for acute upper airway obstruction and respiratory arrest at the time of anesthetic induction. Obese patients with respiratory disorders pose the greatest challenge because they often have a short neck with considerable adipose tissue and a heavy chest wall, both of which create challenges for successful intubation and adequate ventilation. If endotracheal intubation proves too difficult, these patients can be well ventilated with a mask. Awake intubation can be performed, with or without fiberoptic aids, but is quite unpleasant and rarely necessary.

An oral airway is strongly recommended after muscle paralysis due to the redundant tissue of the soft palate. In general, it is useful if one anesthetist is responsible for airway positioning, including two-handed seal of the mask, and the second anesthetist is responsible for adequate ventilation, including two-hand compression of the ventilation reservoir bag. Intubation should only be attempted after ventilation with 100% oxygen for several minutes and attempts at intubation should be limited to no longer than 30 seconds. If the patient has severe OSA and continuous positive airway pressure (CPAP) is ineffective or cannot be tolerated, a tracheostomy should be considered. Often, an extra-long tracheostomy tube is necessary due to excess adipose tissue.

Three high-risk complications of chronic and severe hypoxemia for OHS patients are polycythemia, pulmonary arterial vasoconstriction, and pulmonary hypertension. Polycythemia further increases the already significant risk for venous thrombosis and pulmonary embolism, and in general if the hemoglobin (Hb) concentration is greater than or equal to 16 g/dL, phlebotomy to a concentration of 15 g/dL should be performed to reduce the postoperative risk of venous thrombosis. In patients with OHS, oxygen administration is occasionally associated with worsening CO_2 retention and hypoventilation, potentially prolonging intubation and mechanical ventilation. Because pulmonary disease is typically restrictive rather than obstructive, obese patients are often easy to ventilate without high peak airway pressures. In considering extubation, achieving normal arterial blood gas values is not necessary; only a return to the baseline preoperative values is needed. In patients undergoing a major open upper abdominal operation, this can be achieved on average 4 days postoperatively when patients experience a decrease in incisional pain, particularly with the laparoscopic technique.[32]

In the periprocedure setting, obese patients are most at risk for thromboembolic events when immobilized in the supine position for long periods. Although respiratory function in the morbidly obese patient is greatly enhanced with the reverse Trendelenburg position, this position decreases venous pressure and predisposes to deep venous thrombus formation. All patients should make every attempt to walk during the evening after operation and deep venous thrombosis prophylaxis using standard or low-molecular-weight heparin should be administered subcutaneously 30 minutes before the start of the operation and for at least 2 days or until the patient is ambulatory. Intermittent sequential venous compression boots are also useful to counteract the increased venous stasis and the propensity for clotting. It is important to initiate this treatment before induction of anesthesia and throughout the operative procedure. Compression boots are usually part of a standard preoperative protocol in gastric procedures for weight control and should also be used for both elective and emergency procedures on morbidly obese patients.

Patients with severe venous stasis disease, manifested by pretibial stasis ulcers or bronze edema, are at particularly high risk for fatal pulmonary embolism (PE).[23] If mean pulmonary arterial pressure is greater than or equal to 40 mm Hg, consideration should be given to prophylactic insertion of an inferior vena caval filter because of the high risk of a fatal pulmonary embolism in these patients.[33]

Jejunoileal Bypass

The first popular surgical procedure for morbid obesity was the jejunoileal bypass. This operation produced an obligatory malabsorption state through bypass of a major portion of the absorptive surface of the small intestine. The procedure connected a short length of proximal jejunum (8 to 14 inches) to the distal ileum (4 to 12 inches) as an end-to-end or end-to-side anastomosis. The end-to-end procedures, which were associated with a better weight loss, required decompression of the bypassed small intestine into the colon. The jejunoileal bypass was associated with a number of early and late complications. The most serious postoperative complication was cirrhosis due to either protein–calorie malnutrition or absorption of degradation products from bacterial overgrowth in the bypassed intestine. Other complications include cholelithiasis, urolithiasis, metabolic acidosis, chronic diarrhea with electrolyte depletion, iron deficiency anemia, and vitamin K deficiency resulting from bacterial overgrowth.[24] Randomized prospective studies have shown that the gastric bypass operation is associated with a comparable weight loss and a significantly lower complication rate than jejunoileal bypass.[25] Because of the significant complication rate, standard jejunoileal bypass should no longer be performed.

Gastric Procedures for Morbid Obesity

In 1969, investigators reported the results of weight loss after division of the stomach into a small upper pouch connected to a loop gastroenterostomy. The concept for this procedure was based on the observation of weight loss that sometimes followed subtotal gastrectomy for duodenal ulcer disease. There was initial concern that peptic ulcers would develop in the bypassed stomach or duodenum, and although these have occurred, the incidence is low. The technique for gastric bypass was simplified with the use of stapling instruments. The concept of gastroplasty was then proposed as a safer, easier method for restricting food intake. In gastroplasty, the stomach is only stapled and not divided, leaving a small opening to permit the normal passage of food into the distal stomach and duodenum. Thus, weight loss can be assisted through pure restrictive gastric procedures (gastroplasty or gastric banding) or a combination of restriction and malabsorption (gastric bypass, biliopancreatic diversion).

Gastroplasty

6 Gastroplasties are purely restrictive procedures that have been performed with either horizontal or vertical placement of the staples. Horizontal gastroplasty usually requires ligation and division of the short gastric vessels between the stomach and spleen, and it carries the risk of devascularization of the gastric pouch or splenic injury. The failure rate (loss of <40% of excess weight) of horizontal gastroplasty ranges from 42% to 71%.[26] The vertical banded gastroplasty is a procedure in which a stapled opening is made in the stomach with a circular stapler 5 cm from the cardioesophageal junction. Two applications of a 90-mm stapling device are made between this opening and the angle of His, and a 1.5×5-cm strip of polypropylene mesh is wrapped around the stoma on the lesser curvature and sutured to itself but not to the stomach. Erosion of the mesh into the stomach has been an unusual complication of this procedure. Pouch enlargement and stomal dilation are less common with the vertical technique, although staple line disruption occurs in up to 35% of cases. Some surgeons now recommend transecting the stomach to decrease the incidence of this complication.

Gastric Bypass

7 Gastric bypass combines restriction and malabsorption to assist weight loss. A small (15- to 30-mL) gastric pouch is created along the lesser curve with staplers, followed by construction of a gastrojejunostomy (most commonly Roux-en-Y configuration) with a 1-cm stoma to drain the pouch. With the Roux technique, a 40- to 50-cm jejunal limb provides moderate malabsorption and limits bile reflux (Fig. 45.1). Significantly improved weight loss has been achieved in the superobese population (BMI ≥50 kg/m^2) with a 150-cm Roux limb (long-limb gastric bypass).[27]

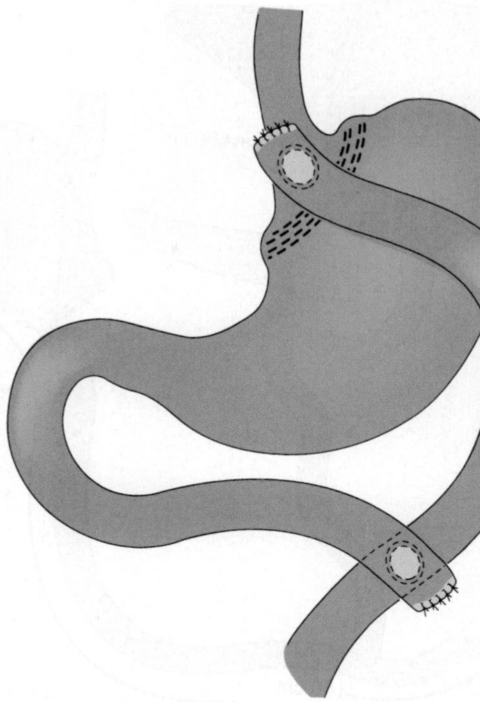

FIGURE 45.1. Open proximal Roux-en-Y gastric bypass.

Gastroplasty Versus Gastric Bypass

Roux-en-Y gastric bypass provides significantly improved weight loss over vertical banded gastroplasty. Reduction in excess body weight at 2 years ranges from 60% to 70% with gastric bypass compared with 40% to 50% with vertical banded gastroplasty. Gastric bypass carries a higher incidence of stomal ulcer, stomal stenosis, vitamin B_{12} deficiency, and, in menstruating women, iron deficiency anemia than does gastroplasty. Gastric bypass is, however, more effective than vertical banded gastroplasty in correcting glucose intolerance in patients without overt type 2 diabetes mellitus. "Sweet eaters" tend to achieve greater weight reduction with gastric bypass, likely from the development of dumping syndrome symptoms.[28]

Weight reduction failures nonetheless occur with gastric bypass. Although regained weight could be the result of staple disruption, pouch expansion, or stomal dilation, these findings are not observed in the majority of patients. Approximately 10% to 15% regain lost weight or fail to achieve an acceptable weight loss. The cause for this failure appears to be excessive, constant nibbling on foods with high caloric density.

Partial Biliopancreatic Diversion

The partial biliopancreatic diversion was developed as both a gastric restrictive procedure and a malabsorptive procedure that does not have a blind intestinal limb for bacterial overgrowth.[34] In this operation (Fig. 45.2), the quantity of food ingested is partially restricted and then passes down the intestine mostly undigested and unabsorbed until it reaches the bile and pancreatic juices, 0.5 meter from the ileocecal valve, where digestion and absorption take place. Treated patients usually pass four to six stools per day, which are foul smelling

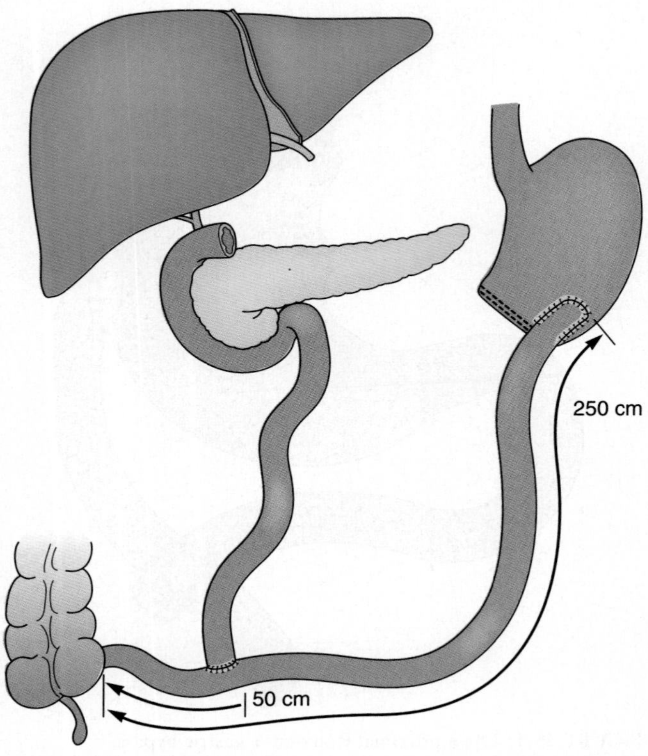

FIGURE 45.2. Biliopancreatic diversion. A distal gastrectomy is performed, followed by division of the distal small bowel 250 cm proximal to the ileocecal valve. The proximal bypassed bowel is anastomosed to the ileum 50 cm from the ileocecal valve.

and float, reflecting malabsorption of fat. Reduction in excess weight approximates 70% to 80%.

As with the proximal or standard gastric bypass, patients with the biliopancreatic diversion are at risk for iron deficiency anemia and vitamin B_{12} deficiency. In addition, they are at risk for protein deficiency, osteoporosis secondary to calcium and vitamin D malabsorption, night blindness and skin eruptions secondary to vitamin A deficiency, and problems with the other fat-soluble vitamins, E and K.[34] Italian patients—the operation was developed in Italy—appear to have less malabsorption and nutritional deficiencies than U.S. patients, probably because of a much lower fat content in the Italian diet. The duodenal switch operation is a modification of the partial biliopancreatic bypass but still may be associated with malnutrition and fat-soluble vitamin and calcium deficiencies.[35]

Laparoscopic Obesity Surgery

The adjustable silicone gastric band has been developed to be placed laparoscopically. The procedure involves placing the band around the proximal stomach to create a 15-mL pouch (Fig. 45.3). The amount of restriction is adjusted by injecting saline into a subcutaneously implanted port. This procedure has become very popular in Europe, where loss of up to 50% of excess weight at 2 years has been reported. This device was approved by the U.S. Food and Drug Administration in 2001, but American trials have yielded varied results.[36,37] Long-term studies validating its safety and efficacy are needed. Complications include band slippage, gastric obstruction, port malfunction or infection, and band erosion.

Laparoscopic Roux-en-Y gastric bypass is being performed with increasing frequency in the United States. This is a technically demanding procedure with a steep learning curve. Five or six ports are utilized (Fig. 45.4). A linear cutting stapler is used to create a stapled side-to-side jejunojejunostomy after measuring a 50-cm Roux limb. This alimentary limb can be tunneled through the mesocolon (retrocolic) or allowed to pass anterior to the colon and stomach (antecolic). The proximal lesser curvature 15- to 20-mL gastric pouch is created with the linear cutting stapler with care to avoid injury to the spleen or esophagus. The gastrojejunostomy is formed with a stapled posterior row and a hand-sewn anterior row (Fig. 45.5). The anastomosis is tested with insufflation via a gastroscope. Drainage and postoperative radiographs to assess for

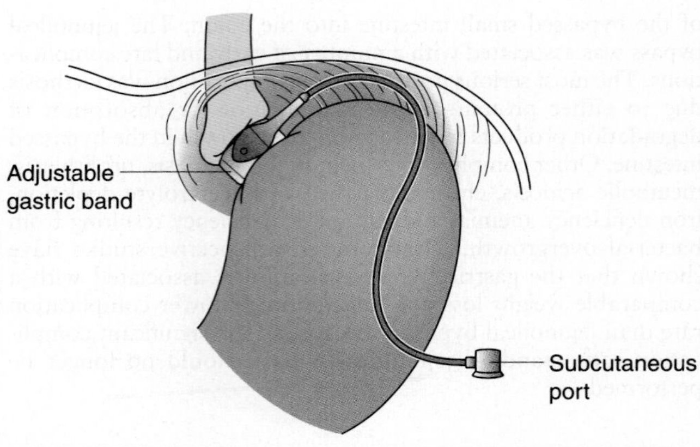

FIGURE 45.3. Schematic representing laparoscopic adjustable gastric banding. The buckle would be oriented medially, and anterior gastrogastric sutures would be placed proximal and distal to the band to prevent gastric herniation.

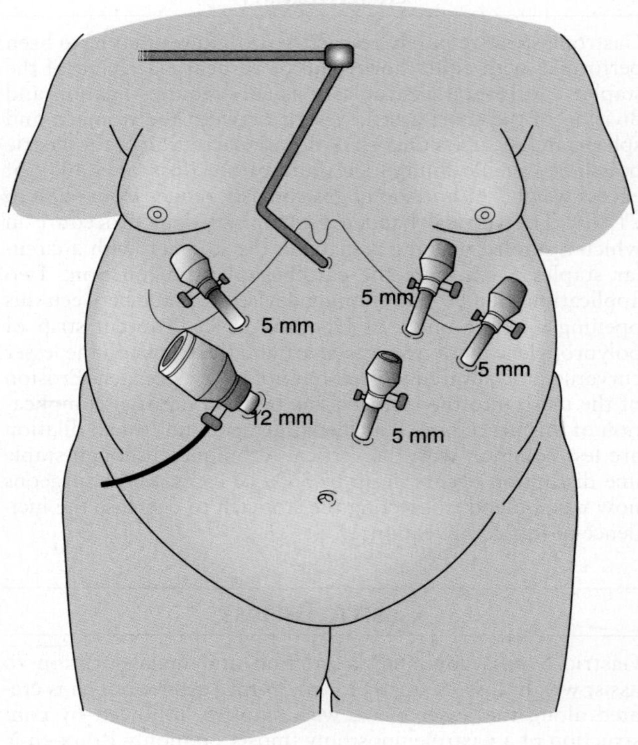

FIGURE 45.4. Trocar placement for laparoscopic Roux-en-Y gastric bypass.

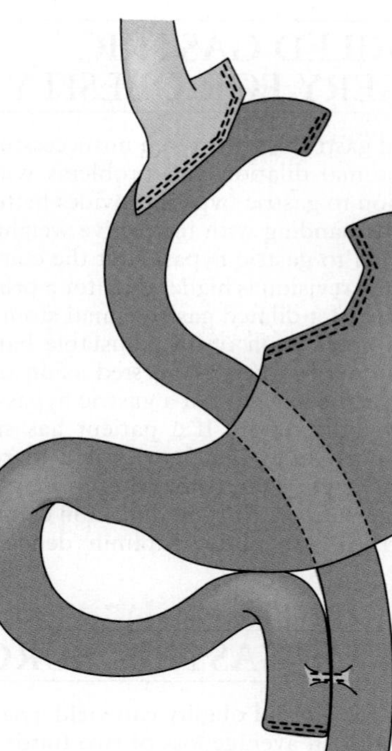

FIGURE 45.5. Laparoscopic proximal Roux-en-Y gastric bypass (retrocolic, retrogastric).

leaks can be performed routinely or selectively according to surgeon preference.

Although the laparoscopic technique is associated with increases in operative time, operative cost, and incidence of gastrojejunal stricture, advantages include decreased hospital length of stay, decreased incidence of wound infection and incisional hernia, and reductions in perioperative blood transfusions. Internal hernias may increase in frequency with the laparoscopic technique as a result of decreased severity of adhesions (Fig. 45.6). In terms of weight loss, laparoscopic

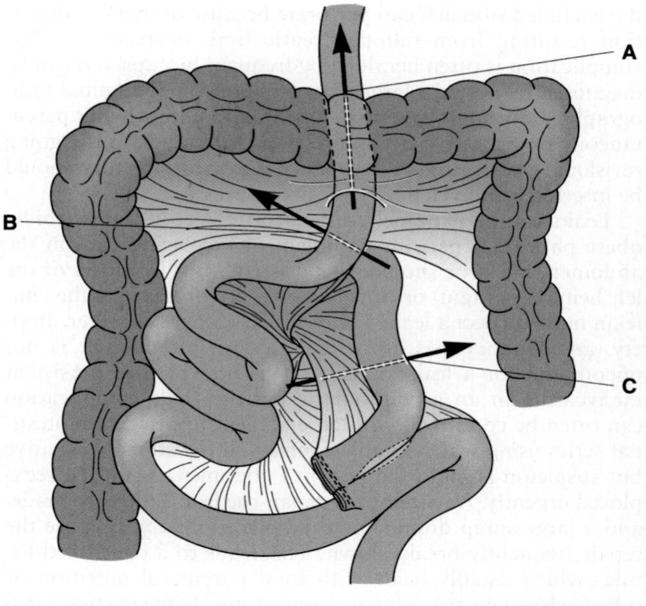

FIGURE 45.6. Potential sites of internal hernia following Roux-en-Y gastric bypass: mesocolic defect (*A*), Petersen defect (*B*), and jejunojejunal (*C*).

gastric bypass offers similar short-term reductions in excess body weight when compared with the open technique in randomized prospective trials.[38]

COMPLICATIONS OF GASTRIC SURGERY FOR MORBID OBESITY

The most feared complication of gastric surgery for morbid obesity is gastrointestinal leak (Algorithm 45.1). This occurs most commonly at the gastrojejunostomy, although other potential sites include the jejunojejunostomy, excluded stomach, and inadvertent enterotomies. Following gastric bypass,

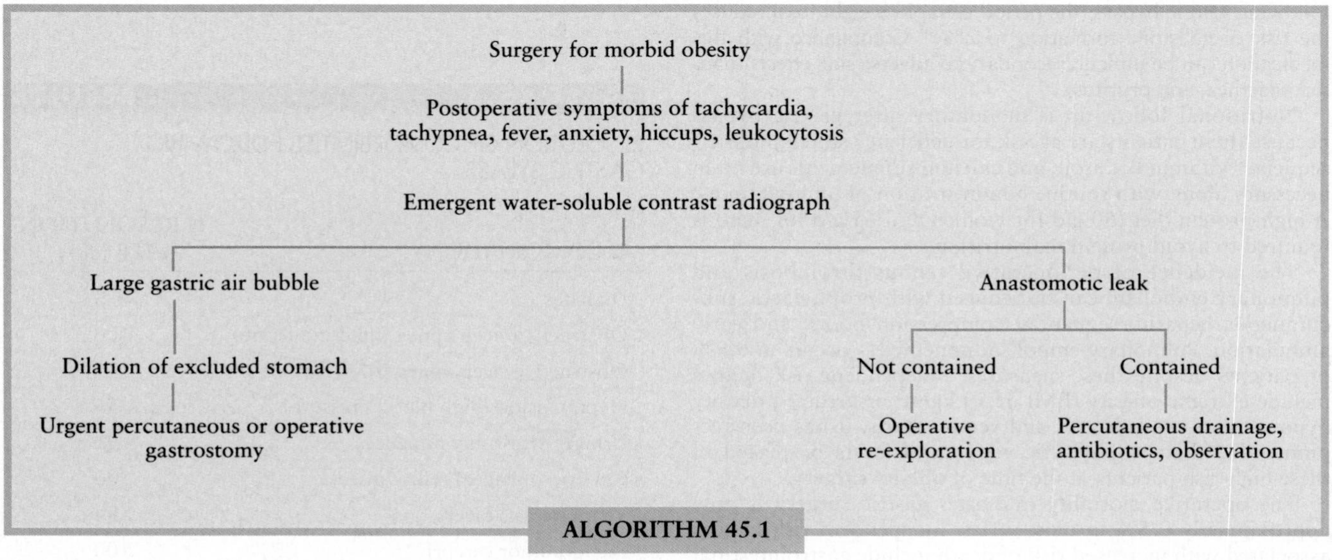

ALGORITHM 45.1. Management of anastomotic leak after gastric surgery for obesity.

the excluded stomach can perforate because of marked dilatation resulting from biliopancreatic limb obstruction. This complication is often heralded by frequent hiccups and can be diagnosed by noting a large gastric bubble on abdominal radiographs. Impending gastric perforation requires urgent percutaneous or operative decompression. In patients undergoing revisional gastric surgery for obesity, a gastrostomy tube should be inserted prophylactically for decompression.

Leaks can be extremely difficult to detect in the morbidly obese patient. If patients complain of increasing pain in the abdomen, back, or shoulder (consistent with irritation of the left hemidiaphragm) or of pelvic pressure or hiccups, the clinician must suspect a leak. Tachycardia, tachypnea, fever, anxiety, and leukocytosis are often present, although it is not uncommon for a leak to manifest as unexplained persistent tachycardia in an asymptomatic patient. This complication can often be confirmed with an emergent upper gastrointestinal series using water-soluble contrast. If the study is negative but suspicion is high, the patient's abdomen should be reexplored urgently. An attempt to repair the leak should be made, and a large sump drain should be placed nearby because the repair frequently breaks down. This leads to a controlled fistula, which usually heals with total parenteral nutrition or tube feeds via gastrostomy or jejunostomy. Some gastrojejunal leaks can be managed nonoperatively in situations where the leak is drained (via a drain placed at the time of operation or radiographically guided) or contained; in either circumstance, Algorithm 45.1 is appropriate only in stable patients without signs of systemic toxicity. Factors associated with leak include increasing age, revisional surgery, male gender, and sleep apnea.[39]

Marginal ulcers develop in approximately 10% of patients with gastric bypass even when treated with postoperative acid suppression. This complication usually responds to additional medical therapy with proton pump inhibitors. Stomal stenosis can occur following gastric bypass or vertical banded gastroplasty. Outpatient endoscopic dilatation is usually successful in patients with gastric bypass, although more than one treatment may be necessary.

Rapid weight loss following bariatric surgery is associated with a high incidence (up to 35%) of gallstone formation and need for subsequent cholecystectomy for biliary colic or acute cholecystitis. Some surgeons recommend prophylactic cholecystectomy at the time of bariatric surgery, whereas others perform cholecystectomy only if sonographic evidence of gallstones is identified. Ursodeoxycholic acid (300 mg orally twice daily) administered for 6 months following gastric bypass (the period of rapid weight loss) reduces the risk of gallstone formation to 2%.[40] Compliance with this medication can be difficult secondary to adverse side effects (nausea, diarrhea, and pruritus).

Nutritional follow-up is mandatory after gastric bypass because these patients are at risk for deficiency states and their sequelae. Vitamin B_{12}, iron, and calcium supplements are often necessary along with routine administration of multivitamins. A high-protein diet (50 g/d for women and 65 g/d for men) is required to avoid protein malnutrition.

The incidence of perioperative venous thrombosis and pulmonary embolism can be reduced with prophylactic subcutaneous heparin, sequential compression boots, and early ambulation. Pulmonary embolism nonetheless occurs in 0.9% of patients despite these measures; independent risk factors include extreme obesity (BMI of 50 kg/m^2 or greater), obesity hypoventilation syndrome, and venous stasis. It has been recommended that prophylactic vena caval filters be placed in these high-risk patients at the time of obesity surgery.

The operative mortality rate after gastric surgery is now approximately 0.5% in most series. Independent risk factors associated with increased risk of death include gastrointestinal leak, pulmonary embolus, hypertension, and preoperative weight.[41]

FAILED GASTRIC SURGERY FOR OBESITY

Revision of a failed gastroplasty is often unsuccessful because of recurrence of stomal dilation and problems with gastric emptying; conversion to gastric bypass provides better results. Laparoscopic gastric banding with ineffective weight loss can likewise be converted to gastric bypass, but the complication rate with this and any revision is higher than for a primary gastric bypass. Revision of a dilated gastrojejunal stoma has not been effective, but application of an adjustable band to the pouch above the stoma has been suggested as an option for this problem. Most patients who fail a gastric bypass do so as a result of dietary indiscretion. If a patient has significant obesity-related comorbidities that have failed to resolve or have returned with weight gain, conversion to long-limb gastric bypass can be performed. This modification can be associated with steatorrhea, fat-soluble vitamin deficiency, and osteoporosis.

OVERVIEW OF GASTRIC SURGERY

Gastric procedures for morbid obesity can yield a satisfactory weight reduction, with an average loss of two thirds of excess weight within 1 to 1.5 years. Weight becomes stable at this level in most patients as the reduced caloric intake meets caloric expenditure. The patients must be followed carefully to ensure adequate protein, vitamin, and other micronutrient levels.

Numerous comorbidities associated with morbid obesity resolve following gastric bypass (Table 45.5). Weight loss completely corrects type 2 diabetes mellitus in three fourths of cases, hypertension in two thirds of patients, and headaches associated with cerebrospinal fluid pressure elevation in almost all patients with pseudotumor cerebri. OSA resolves with weight loss in approximately 80% of cases. Hypoxemia and hypercarbia seen in OHS return toward normal with weight reduction.[42] Elevated pulmonary artery and pulmonary capillary wedge pressures also improve significantly after weight loss with correction of abnormal arterial blood gases. The loss of weight usually corrects female sexual hormone abnormalities, permits healing of chronic venous stasis ulcers associated with venous insufficiency, prevents reflux esophagitis, relieves stress overflow urinary incontinence, and improves low back pain as well as joint-related pain. Weight loss can

TABLE 45.5 **RESULTS**

RESOLUTION OF COMORBIDITIES FOLLOWING GASTRIC BYPASS

■ COMORBIDITY	■ RESOLUTION RATE (%)
Diabetes	73
Obstructive sleep apnea (mild/moderate)	100
Obstructive sleep apnea (severe)	75
Hypertension (high blood pressure)	56
Urinary stress incontinence	91
Gastroesophageal reflux disease	90
Venous stasis ulcers	94
Pseudotumor cerebri	100
Joint pain	71

permit successful total artificial joint replacement. Patient self-image is often markedly improved after gastric surgery for obesity.

Treatment of morbidly obese patients requires a multidisciplinary approach including psychologists, nutritionists, and experienced physicians and ward personnel. Patients must be willing to make a lifelong commitment to behavioral modification, regular exercise, and long-term medical follow-up.

References

1. National Center for Health Statistics NHANES IV report. Available at: http://www.cdc.gov/nchs/product/pubs/pubd/hestats/obes/obese99.htm2002. Accessed November 29, 2004.
2. Fontaine KR, Redden DT, Wang C, et al. Years of life lost due to obesity. *JAMA* 2003;289:187–193.
3. Deitel M. Overweight and obesity worldwide now estimated to involve 1.7 billion people. *Obes Surg* 2003;13:329–330.
4. Ogden CL, Flegal KM, Carroll MD, et al. Prevalence and trends in overweight among US children and adolescents, 1999–2000. *JAMA* 2002;288: 1728–1732.
5. Stunkard AJ, Sorensen TA, Hanis C, et al. An adoptive study of human obesity. *N Engl J Med* 1986;314:193–198.
6. Vogler GP, Sorensen TI, Stunkard AJ, et al. Influences of genes and shared family environment on adult body mass index assessed in an adoption study by a comprehensive path model. *Int J Obes Relat Metab Disord* 1995;19:40–45.
7. Stunkard AJ, Harris JR, Pedersen NL, et al. The body-mass index of twins who have been reared apart. *N Engl J Med* 1990;322:1483–1487.
8. Austin MA, Friedlander Y, Newman B, et al. Genetic influences on changes in body mass index: a longitudinal analysis of women twins. *Obes Res* 1997;5:326–331.
9. Neary NM, Small CJ, Bloom SR. Gut and mind. *Gut* 2003;52:918–921.
10. Jequier E. Leptin signaling, adiposity, and energy balance. *Ann N Y Acad Sci* 2002;967:379–388.
11. van Gemert WG, Westerterp KR, van Acker BA, et al. Energy, substrate and protein metabolism in morbid obesity before, during and after massive weight loss. *Int J Obes Relat Metab Disord* 2000;24:711–718.
12. Sugerman H, Windsor A, Bessos M, et al. Intra-abdominal pressure, sagittal abdominal diameter, and obesity co-morbidity. *J Intern Med* 1997;241: 71–79.
13. Sugerman H, Windsor A, Bessos M, et al. Effects of surgically induced weight loss on urinary bladder pressure, sagittal abdominal diameter, and obesity co-morbidity. *Int J Obes Relat Metab Disord* 1998;22: 230–235.
14. Bjorntorp P, Rosmond R. The metabolic syndrome—a neuroendocrine disorder? *Br J Nutr* 2000;83:S49–S57.
15. Sugerman HJ, Felton WL III, Salvant JB, et al. Effects of surgically induced weight loss on idiopathic intracranial hypertension in morbid obesity. *Neurology* 1995;45:1655–1659.
16. Wong CY, O'Moore-Sullivan T, Leano R, et al. Alterations of left ventricular myocardial characteristics associated with obesity. *Circulation* 2004; 110:3081–3087.
17. Alpert MA. Obesity cardiomyopathy: pathophysiology and evolution of the clinical syndrome. *Am J Med Sci* 2001;321:225–236.
18. Wang TJ, Parise H, Levy D, et al. Obesity and the risk of new-onset atrial fibrillation. *JAMA* 2004;292:2471–2477.
19. Frey WC, Pilcher J. Obstructive sleep-related breathing disorders in patients evaluated for bariatric surgery. *Obes Surg* 2003;13:676–683.
20. Rubino F, Gagner M, Gentileschi P, et al. The early effect of the Roux-en-Y gastric bypass on hormones involved in body weight regulation and glucose metabolism. *Ann Surg* 2004;240:236–242.
21. Sugerman HJ, Sugerman EL, Wolfe L, et al. Risks and benefits of gastric bypass in morbidly obese patients with severe venous stasis disease. *Ann Surg* 2001;234:41–46.
22. Bump RC, Sugerman HJ, Fantl JA, et al. Obesity and lower urinary tract function in women: effect of surgically induced weight loss. *Am J Obstet Gynecol* 1992;167:392–397.
23. NIH Technology Assessment Conference Panel. NIH conference: methods for voluntary weight loss and control. *Ann Intern Med* 1992;116: 942–949.
24. Hocking MP, Duerson MC, O'Leary JP, et al. Jejunoileal bypass for morbid obesity. Late follow-up in 100 cases. *N Engl J Med* 1983;308:995–999.
25. Griffen WO Jr, Young VL, Stevenson CC. A prospective comparison of gastric and jejunoileal bypass procedures for morbid obesity. *Ann Surg* 1977;186:500–509.
26. Sugerman HJ, Wolper JL. Failed gastroplasty for morbid obesity. Revised gastroplasty versus Roux-Y gastric bypass. *Am J Surg* 1984;148:331–336.
27. Brolin RE, Kenler HA, Gorman JH, et al. Long-limb gastric bypass in the superobese. A prospective randomized study. *Ann Surg* 1992;215: 387–395.
28. Sugerman HJ, Starkey J, Birkenhauer R. A randomized prospective trial of gastric bypass versus vertical banded gastroplasty for morbid obesity and their effects on sweets versus non-sweets eaters. *Ann Surg* 1987;205: 613–624.
29. Fisher BL, Schauer P. Medical and surgical options in the treatment of severe obesity. *Am J Surg* 2002;184:9S–16S.
30. Alpert MA, Terry BE, Mulekar M, et al. Cardiac morphology and left ventricular function in normotensive morbidly obese patients with and without congestive heart failure, and effect of weight loss. *Am J Cardiol* 1997; 80:736–740.
31. Sugerman HJ, Baron PL, Fairman RP, et al. Hemodynamic dysfunction in obesity hypoventilation syndrome and the effects of treatment with surgically induced weight loss. *Ann Surg* 1988;207:604–613.
32. Huang B, Rodreiguez BL, Burchfiel CM, et al. Associations of adiposity with prevalent coronary heart disease among elderly men: the Honolulu Heart Program. *Int J Obes Relat Metab Disord* 1997;21:340–348.
33. Sugerman HJ, DeMaria EJ, Felton WL III, et al. Increased intra-abdominal pressure and cardiac filling pressures in obesity associated pseudotumor cerebri. *Neurology* 1997;49:507–511.
34. Scopinaro N, Gianetta E, Civalleri D, et al. Two years of clinical experience with biliopancreatic bypass for obesity. *Am J Clin Nutr* 1980;33: 506–514.
35. Hess DS, Hess DW. Biliopancreatic diversion with a duodenal switch. *Obes Surg* 1998;8:267–282.
36. Ren CJ, Weiner M, Allen JW. Favorable early results of gastric banding for morbid obesity: the American experience. *Surg Endosc* 2004;18:543–546.
37. DeMaria EJ, Sugerman HJ, Meador JG, et al. High failure rate after laparoscopic adjustable silicone gastric banding for treatment of morbid obesity. *Ann Surg* 2001;233:809–818.
38. Nguyen NT, Goldman C, Rosenquist CJ, et al. Laparoscopic versus open gastric bypass: a randomized study of outcomes, quality of life, and costs. *Ann Surg* 2001;234:279–289.
39. Fernandez AZ Jr, DeMaria EJ, Tichansky DS, et al. Experience with over 3,000 open and laparoscopic bariatric procedures: multivariate analysis of factors related to leak and resultant mortality. *Surg Endosc* 2004;18: 193–197.
40. Sugerman HJ, Brewer WH, Shiffman ML, et al. A multicenter, placebo-controlled, randomized, double-blind, prospective trial of prophylactic ursodiol for the prevention of gallstone formation following gastric-bypass-induced rapid weight loss. *Am J Surg* 1995;169:91–96.
41. Fernandez AZ Jr, Demaria EJ, Tichansky DS, et al. Multivariate analysis of risk factors for death following gastric bypass for treatment of morbid obesity. *Ann Surg* 2004;239:698–702.
42. Buchwald H, Avidor Y, Braunwald E, et al. Bariatric surgery: a systematic review and meta-analysis. *JAMA* 2004;292:1724–1737.
43. Jones DB, Provost DA, DeMaria EJ, et al. Optimal management of the morbidly obese patient SAGES appropriateness conference statement. *Surg Endosc* 2004;18:1029–1037.

CHAPTER 46 ■ GASTRIC NEOPLASMS

REBECCA M. MINTER

KEY POINTS

1. The presence of a gastric adenomatous polyp is a marker of increased risk for the development of cancer in the remaining gastric mucosa, and therefore these patients should be enrolled in an appropriate endoscopic surveillance program.
2. *Helicobacter pylori* infection is the predominant risk factor for gastric carcinogenesis; however, additional cofactors also play an important role and likely drive the progression from a premalignant condition to adenocarcinoma in most individuals.
3. The symptoms produced by gastric cancer are not specific and can mimic those associated with several nonneoplastic gastroduodenal diseases, especially benign gastric ulcer.
4. The extent of gastric resection is determined by the need to obtain a resection margin free of microscopic disease, and a minimum of 15 nodes are required for adequate nodal sampling and staging.
5. Multimodality treatment should be the standard of care for treating locally advanced resectable gastric cancer.
6. Low-grade gastric MALT lymphomas are usually effectively treated with eradication of *H. pylori* infection alone.
7. Almost all (95%–99%) gastrointestinal stromal tumors express the KIT antigen.

Gastric cancer is a relatively common, frequently lethal affliction and remains a serious and unsolved problem in general surgery. The disease often is not recognized until it is at an advanced stage. Gastric cancer usually cannot be controlled by surgery alone, and surgical cure rates have remained disappointingly low. Increasingly, a multidisciplinary approach is being applied to these difficult neoplasms, with some modest improvements in outcome finally being observed. Technical innovations and basic scientific investigations continue to be applied to this disease, and cautious optimism for the future is appropriate.

ADENOCARCINOMA

Epidemiology

Starting in 1930, the incidence of gastric cancer declined dramatically in the United States (Fig. 46.1). By 1980, the incidence of gastric cancer (10 cases per 100,000 population) was approximately one fourth the incidence recorded in 1930. The incidence of the disease remained relatively constant in the decades from 1980 to 2000.[1] By 1997, reported new cases of gastric cancer had declined to 22,000. While this is a small number relative to the 150,000 estimated deaths from cancer of the lung,[2] gastric cancer remains among the top 10 causes of cancer-related deaths for both men and women in the United States. In 2008, it is estimated that 21,500 new cases of gastric cancer will be diagnosed in the United States—thus the incidence remains fairly stable over the last decade.[3] An increase in the proportion of proximal gastric cancers has been observed, with young white men being much more likely to present with proximal gastric cancers whereas distal cancers are more likely to occur in Asian, African American, and Hispanic patients.[4] While the reasons for the decline in the incidence of gastric cancer in the 1930s are not entirely known (though some attribute the decreased incidence to the introduction of refrigeration and widespread access to fresh fruits and vegetables), we now have a better understanding of the factors contributing to its persistence.

The worldwide incidence and death rates for gastric cancer vary markedly. The highest age-adjusted death rate for gastric cancer occurs in Japan, where the disease accounts for approximately 50% of cancer-related deaths in men and 40% of cancer deaths in women. High incidence rates are also reported in South Korea, Chile, Costa Rica, Hungary, Portugal, Singapore, and Romania, a geographically and ethnically diverse group. It had been widely assumed that exposure to environmental carcinogens accounted for the increased disease frequency observed in these populations. A high intake of salt and nitrite-containing preserved foods and a relative lack of fresh fruits and vegetables have been implicated. The supposition that environmental carcinogens play a role in gastric carcinogenesis is supported by studies of immigrant populations; migration from an area at high risk to one at low risk is associated with a decreased probability of developing gastric cancer. The predominant risk factor for gastric carcinogenesis is now generally regarded as infection with the organism *Helicobacter pylori*.

Premalignant Lesions. The risk for development of gastric cancer is greater in stomachs that harbor polyps. Risk is related most closely to polyp histologic type, size, and number. Variations in these three factors account for the wide range in reported risk associated with gastric polyps. In terms of malignant potential, gastric polyps can be divided into two broad categories—hyperplastic polyps and adenomatous polyps.

Hyperplastic polyps are common, occurring in 0.5% to 1% of the general population and accounting for 70% to 80% of all gastric polyps. The hyperplastic polyp contains an overgrowth of histologically normal-appearing gastric epithelium. Atypia is rare. Hyperplastic gastric polyps are considered to have no neoplastic potential. Most people with hyperplastic polyps are asymptomatic. Dyspepsia and vague epigastric discomfort are the most common complaints, although coexistent gastroduodenal disease is also frequently identified. Complications are unusual, and gastrointestinal hemorrhage occurs in less than 20% of patients. When hyperplastic polyps are discovered, endoscopic removal for histologic examination is indicated and is sufficient treatment. Subsequent surveillance is also not necessary given the lack of neoplastic potential in these polyps.

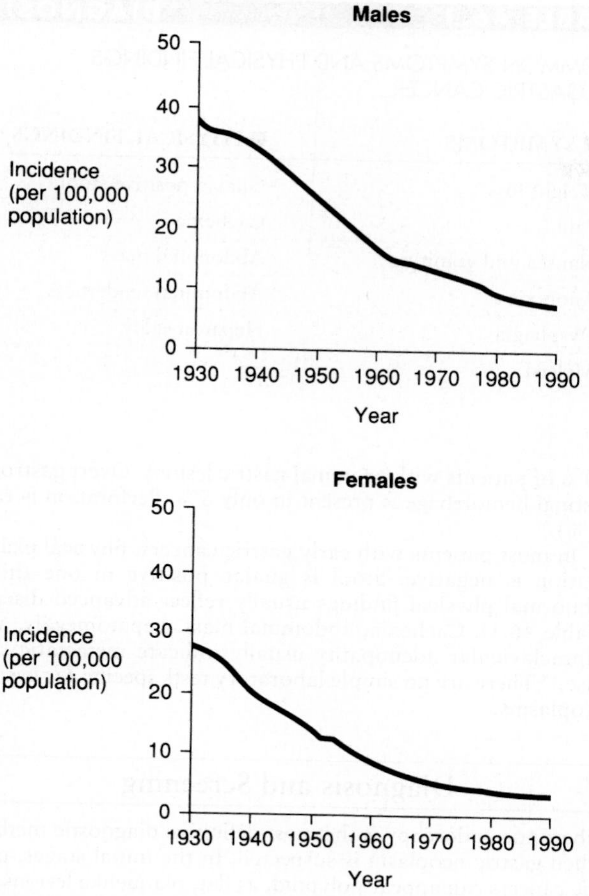

FIGURE 46.1. Incidence of gastric cancer deaths in the United States.

1 Adenomatous polyps, in contrast, have a distinct risk for the development of malignancy.[5] Mucosal atypia is frequent, and mitotic figures are more common than in hyperplastic polyps. Dysplasia and carcinoma in situ have developed in adenomatous polyps observed over time. The risk for the development of carcinoma has been estimated at 10% to 20% and is greatest for polyps more than 2 cm in diameter. Multiple adenomatous polyps increase the risk of cancer. The presence of an adenomatous polyp is also a marker indicating an increased risk for the development of cancer in the remainder of the gastric mucosa.

Symptoms are similar to those for hyperplastic polyps. Endoscopic removal is indicated for pedunculated lesions and is sufficient if the polyp is completely removed and shows no evidence of invasive cancer on histologic examination. Operative excision is recommended for sessile lesions larger than 2 cm, for polyps with biopsy-proved invasive carcinoma, and for polyps complicated by pain or bleeding. After removal, endoscopic surveillance of the remaining gastric mucosa is indicated.

Gastritis. The incidence of both gastric cancer and atrophic gastritis increases with age. Chronic gastritis is frequently associated with intestinal metaplasia and mucosal dysplasia, and these histologic features are often observed in mucosa adjacent to gastric cancer. Gastritis is frequently progressive and severe in the gastric mucosa of patients with cancer.

Gastric malignancy seems to be increased in patients with chronic gastritis associated with pernicious anemia, although the risk appears to have been overstated in the past. This disease, characterized by fundic mucosal atrophy, loss of parietal and chief cells, hypochlorhydria, and hypergastrinemia, is present in 3% of people older than 60 years. For people in whom pernicious anemia has been active for more than 5 years, the risk of gastric cancer is twice that of age-matched control subjects. Evidence also indicates an increased risk of gastric carcinoid development in patients with pernicious anemia. This increased risk warrants aggressive investigation of new symptoms in patients with long-standing pernicious anemia, but it is not high enough to justify repeated endoscopic surveillance.

Intestinal metaplasia, the presence of intestinal glands within the gastric mucosa, is also commonly associated with both gastritis and gastric cancer. The evolution from metaplasia to dysplasia to carcinoma to invasive cancer has been demonstrated in other organs and in adenocarcinoma arising in the gastroesophageal junction. However, no direct evidence can be provided for this progression in gastric cancer.

2 ***Helicobacter Pylori.*** As outlined earlier, *Helicobacter pylori* has been unequivocally associated with chronic inflammatory conditions in the stomach, and this association has stimulated interest in the role of chronic infection by this organism in gastric carcinogenesis. Childhood acquisition of *H. pylori* infection is frequent in areas of high gastric cancer incidence, and high rates of infection have been identified in patients with premalignant lesions and invasive cancer.

In the United States, seropositivity for *H. pylori* increases the risk for cancer development approximately threefold.[6] Infection with *H. pylori* is associated with an increased risk of adenocarcinoma of both major histologic types and for tumors arising in the body or antrum of the stomach. In contrast, *H. pylori* infection is not a risk factor for cancers of the gastroesophageal junction, which are frequently associated with mucosal abnormalities of Barrett esophagus and which seem to follow the metaplasia to dysplasia to carcinoma pattern of development.

The presumed mechanism of carcinogenesis related to *H. pylori* infection stems from the known association between chronic atrophic gastritis and inflammation, and the subsequent development of gastric adenocarcinoma. Despite this known association, *H. pylori* cannot solely account for gastric carcinogenesis. For patients chronically infected with *H. pylori*, only about 1% will develop the gastric cancer phenotype, which consists of corpus-predominant gastritis, multifocal atrophic gastritis, high gastrin levels, hypochlorhydria/achlorhydria, and low pepsinogen I/II ratio. Most subjects infected with *H. pylori* will develop the simple gastritis phenotype that is not associated with any significant clinical outcome, or the duodenal ulcer phenotype (10%–15% of infected subjects), which consists of antral predominant gastritis, high gastrin and acid secretion, and actually provides protection from developing gastric cancer.[7] There is variable distribution of these three phenotypes geographically, with particular prevalence of the gastric cancer phenotype in certain parts of Asia where gastric cancer is common.[8] Currently worldwide it is estimated that approximately 50% to 75% of the mortality from gastric cancer is attributable to *H. pylori* infection.[9] Other cofactors such as bacterial virulence factors, environmental exposures, and host genetic factors also clearly play an important role in the pathogenesis of gastric carcinogenesis following infection-related gastritis.[7,10]

Previous Gastric Surgery. Several uncontrolled reports have suggested that gastric cancer is more likely to develop in people who have undergone previous partial gastrectomy, with patients who have undergone a gastrojejunal (Billroth II) anastomosis seeming to be at higher risk for carcinogenesis than those reconstructed with a gastroduodenal anastomosis (Billroth I).[11,12] The so-called *gastric remnant cancer* is a true clinical entity, although the risk for development of this gastric neoplasm appears to have been overestimated. Several large, prospective studies with long-term follow-up indicate that the relative risk is not increased for up to 15 years after gastric resection, likely due to surgical removal of mucosa at risk for development of gastric cancer, followed by modest increases in cancer risk (three times the control value) observed only after 25 years.[13–16]

The cellular mechanisms that contribute to the development of neoplasia in the remnant stomach are unknown. Decreased luminal pH, bacterial overgrowth with increased production of *N*-nitroso carcinogens, and reflux of bile acids into the stomach have been postulated to promote cancer development, but remain unproved. Vagotomy, often performed in conjunction with gastric surgery for benign disease, does not appear to promote cancer development. A population-based study from Sweden of 7,198 vagotomized patients followed for up to 18 years did not report increased risk.[14]

A recent study explored genetic alterations in gastric remnant cancer and found that the microsatellite instability high (MSI-H) phenotype frequency was much higher (43%) in gastric remnant cancers than in sporadic gastric cancers (6%), and that this incidence was much higher in patients who had undergone a Billroth II anastomosis (67%) as compared to those who had undergone a Billroth I anastomosis (11%). Additionally, these MSI-H phenotype tumors were significantly associated with a lack of expression of hMLH1 and hMSH2—two important DNA mismatch repair genes. The significance of this relationship is not yet clear; however, it is postulated that this unfavorable phenotype may account in part for the poor prognosis associated with these tumors.[17] Reported 5-year survival ranges from 7% to 33% for gastric remnant cancers, though this poor prognosis is most likely due to the fact that these cancers are usually diagnosed at an advanced stage when treatment options are limited.

Clinical Features

3 The symptoms produced by gastric cancer are not specific and unfortunately can closely mimic those associated with a number of nonneoplastic gastroduodenal diseases, especially benign gastric ulcer (Fig. 46.2). In early gastric cancers, epigastric pain is present in over 70% of patients.[18] The pain is often constant, nonradiating, and unrelieved by food ingestion. In a surprising number of patients, pain can be relieved, at least temporarily, by antacids or gastric antisecretory drugs. Anorexia, nausea, and weight loss are present in less than 50% of patients with early gastric cancers but become increasingly common with disease progression. Dysphagia is present in

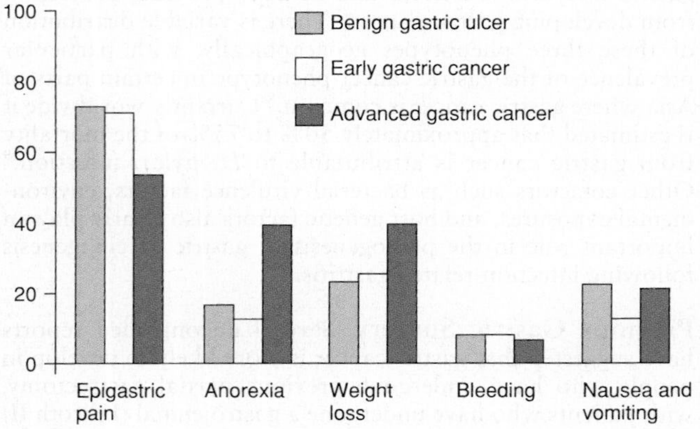

FIGURE 46.2. Clinical symptom frequency in benign gastric ulcer, early gastric cancer, and advanced gastric cancer. (Adapted with permission from Meyer WC, Damiano RJ, Postlethwait RW, et al. Adenocarcinoma of the stomach: changing patterns over the past four decades. *Ann Surg* 1987;205:18.)

TABLE 46.1 DIAGNOSIS

COMMON SYMPTOMS AND PHYSICAL FINDINGS IN GASTRIC CANCER

■ SYMPTOMS	■ PHYSICAL FINDINGS
Weight loss	Guaiac-positive stool
Pain	Cachexia
Nausea and vomiting	Abdominal mass
Anorexia	Abdominal tenderness
Dysphagia	Hepatomegaly
Melena	—

20% of patients with proximal gastric lesions. Overt gastrointestinal hemorrhage is present in only 5%. Perforation is rare (1%).

In most patients with early gastric cancers, physical examination is negative. Stool is guaiac positive in one third. Abnormal physical findings usually reflect advanced disease (Table 46.1). Cachexia, abdominal mass, hepatomegaly, and supraclavicular adenopathy usually indicate metastatic disease.[19] There are no simple laboratory tests specific for gastric neoplasms.

Diagnosis and Screening

Fiberoptic endoscopy is the most definitive diagnostic method when gastric neoplasm is suspected. In the initial stages, gastric cancers can appear polypoid, as flat, plaquelike lesions, or as shallow ulcers. Advanced lesions are typically ulcerated. The ulcer border can have an irregular, beaded appearance because of infiltrating cancer cells, and the base is frequently necrotic and shaggy. The ulcer can appear to arise from an underlying mass. Although each of these features suggests a malignant ulcer, differentiation of benign from malignant gastric ulcers can be made definitively only with gastric biopsy. Accuracy of diagnosis can exceed 95% if multiple biopsy specimens are obtained. False-negative results occur in approximately 10% of patients, usually as the result of sampling error or due to the absence of a mucosal abnormality as can occur with linitis plastica; false-positive results are rare. Diagnostic accuracy can be further enhanced by the addition of direct brush cytology and with the use of endoscopic ultrasound with fine-needle aspiration biopsy for infiltrative tumors involving the wall of the stomach without obvious mucosal abnormalities.

The ability to diagnose gastric adenocarcinoma endoscopically has prompted screening programs for populations at high risk. Mass screening has been performed in Japan since the 1960s with the use of fiberoptic endoscopy. The overall yield for the Japanese screening program has been 0.12%,[20] and has decreased the gastric cancer mortality by two thirds in compliant patients.[9] The proportion of early cancers identified (defined as tumors whose growth is confined to the mucosa and submucosa regardless of the presence or absence of metastatic disease in the perigastric lymph nodes) steadily increased during the study period. Currently, greater than 60% of gastric malignancies detected by this program are early cancers, and early detection has translated directly into improved survival (Fig. 46.3). The Japanese findings that early detection and identification of early gastric cancer can improve survival has been confirmed by European investigations, in which patients with early gastric cancers have been shown to have survival rates equivalent to those of patients with benign gastric ulcer[18] (Fig. 46.4). Despite the success of the Japanese

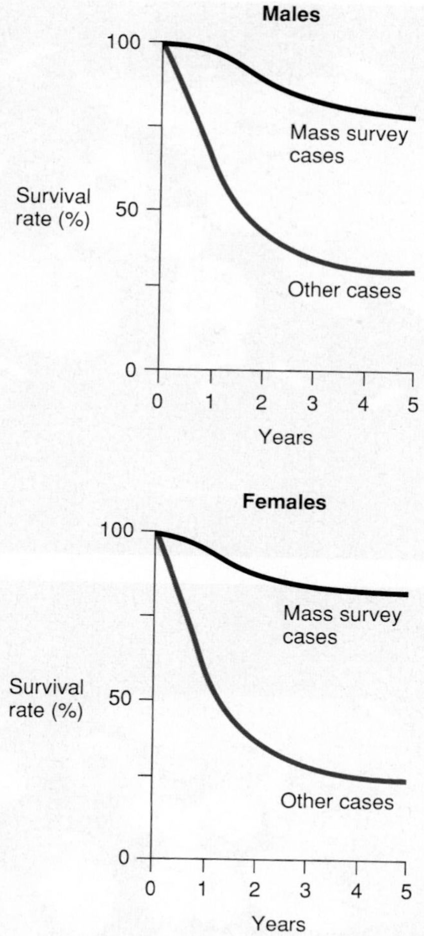

FIGURE 46.3. Early cancer survival rate in Japan.

screening program, mass screening for gastric adenocarcinoma has not been advocated in the United States or Canada. With incidence rates approximately one fifth of those observed in Japan, detection rates are too low to justify such a program economically. It will be interesting to observe over time whether the Japanese screening program continues to be cost

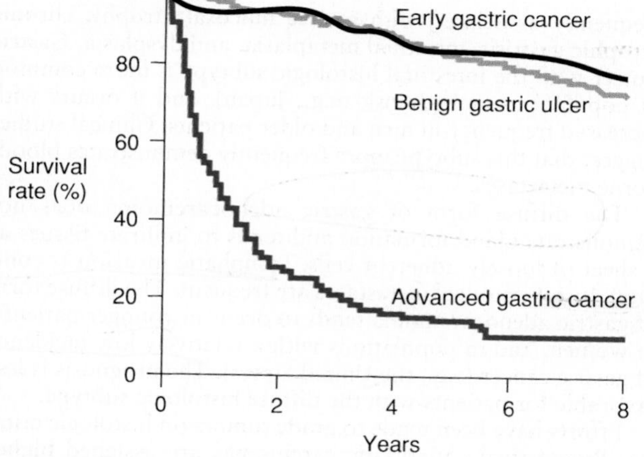

FIGURE 46.4. Early cancer survival rate in Europe.

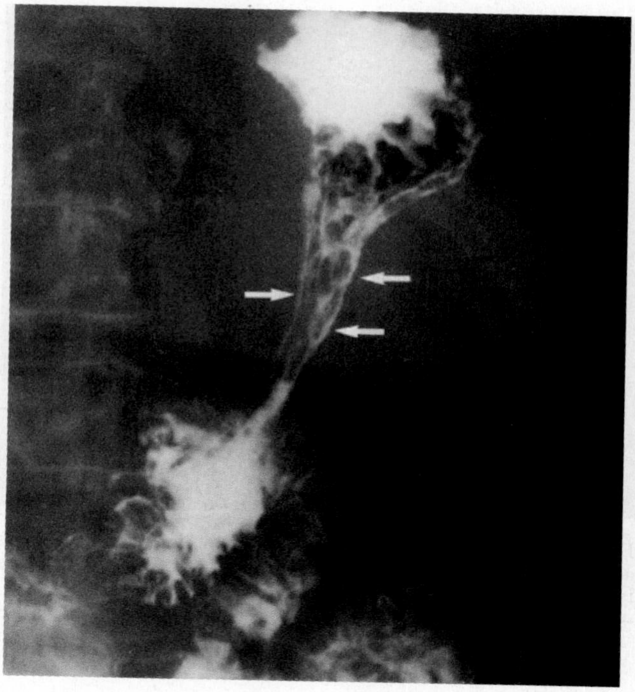

FIGURE 46.5. Barium contrast radiograph demonstrating extensive involvement of the gastric body by infiltrating adenocarcinoma (linitis plastica). The gastric silhouette is narrowed (*arrows*), and the stomach is nondistensible.

effective given the significant decrease in the rate of chronic *H. pylori* infection in persons now under the age of 30 in Japan (25% vs. 60% as compared to their parents).[9]

Barium contrast radiographs have, in the past, been the standard method for diagnosing gastric neoplasm. Single-contrast examinations have a diagnostic accuracy of 80%. This diagnostic yield increases to approximately 90% when double-contrast (air and barium) techniques are used. Typical findings include ulceration, the presence of a gastric mass, loss of mucosal detail, and distortion of the gastric silhouette (Fig. 46.5). Contrast radiography has been largely supplanted by endoscopy because of the ability to obtain biopsy material by the latter technique.

Computed tomography (CT) has been used both as a primary diagnostic method and to assess for extragastric spread of disease. When performed with intraluminal and intravenous contrast, CT can reliably demonstrate infiltration of the gastric wall by tumor, gastric ulceration, and the presence of hepatic metastases (Figs. 46.6 and 46.7). The technique is less reliable with regard to invasion of adjacent organs or the presence of lymphatic metastases. In most series, involvement of adjacent organs has been overestimated by CT scanning (false-positive). Conversely, metastases to regional or distant lymph nodes have been underestimated (false-negative). One review estimated a 40% to 50% accuracy rate in preoperative local staging of gastric carcinoma for CT scanning.[21]

Endoscopically directed ultrasound is another useful method of preoperative evaluation for local staging and diagnosis. Endoscopic ultrasound (EUS) is excellent at delineating subepithelial lesions that may be confused with gastric cancer, and to guide biopsy of submucosal tumors within the wall of the stomach. Investigation of submucosal masses, infiltrative gastric disorders, enlarged gastric epithelial folds, and differentiation of gastric lymphoma from gastric adenocarcinoma are each aided by endoscopic ultrasound. This technique has the ability to assess the depth and pattern of gastric wall penetration by the tumor as well as relationship to adjacent structures,

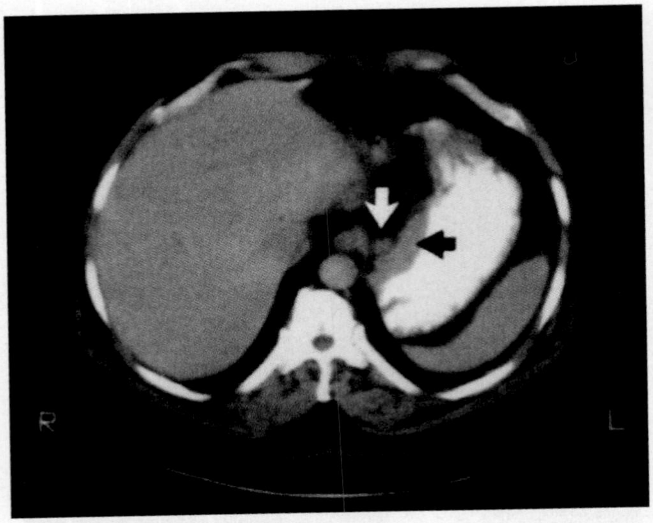

FIGURE 46.6. Computed tomography scan demonstrating mass along lesser curvature of the stomach (*black arrow*) and associated lymph node enlargement (*white arrow*).

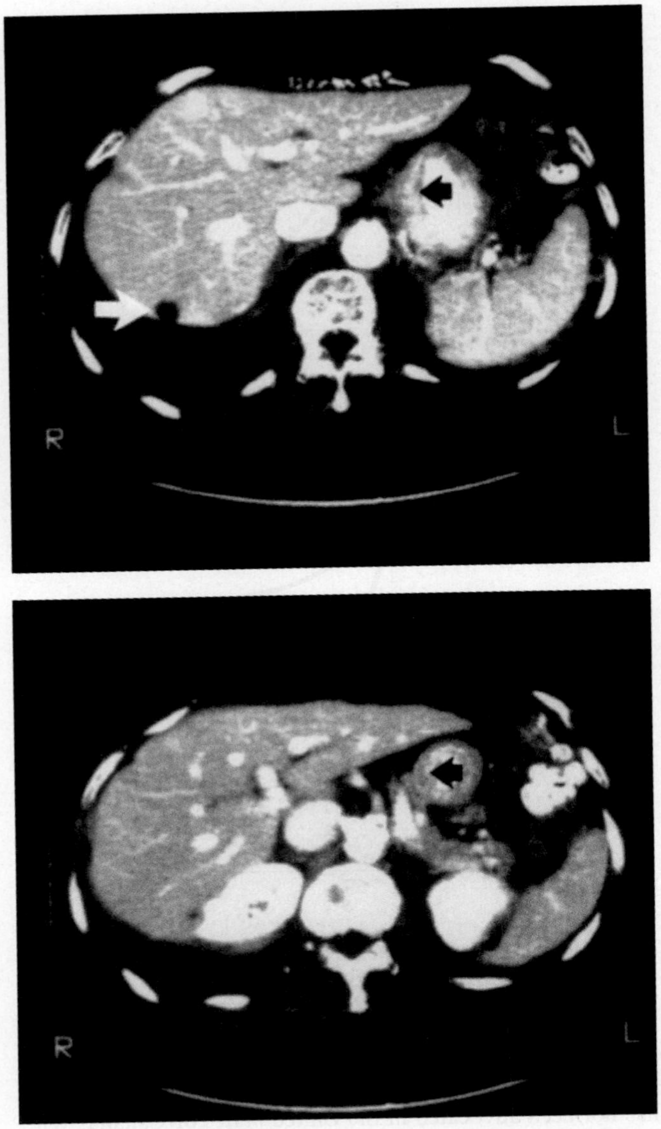

FIGURE 46.7. Computed tomography scans of the upper abdomen showing extensive thickening of the gastric wall (*black arrows*) caused by infiltrating adenocarcinoma and associated hepatic metastasis (*white arrow*).

and has good correlation with intraoperative assessment and histologic findings. Perigastric lymph nodes involved with tumor are also reliably identified by endoscopic ultrasound, and therefore EUS provides the most accurate assessment of local stage of disease (TN status), with an accuracy of 57–83% for staging depth of tumor invasion and 50–78% for nodal involvement.[3] Because of a limited depth of tissue penetration, however, endoscopic ultrasound is unable to detect hepatic metastases; this inability is its major limitation in preoperative staging of patients with gastric cancer. Therefore, EUS serves as an adjunct to cross-sectional methods of radiologic imaging and is only indicated as a staging method for patients with gastric adenocarcinoma who are potentially resectable (e.g. have no evidence of distant metastases on cross-sectional imaging).

Metabolic Imaging

Metabolic imaging with positive emission tomography (PET) using 18 F-fluorodeoxyglucose has been found to be less accurate than cross-sectional imaging and EUS for staging locoregional involvement, but more sensitive for detecting distant metastases in patients with gastric cancer.[3] A metanalysis comparing PET, ultrasound, CT, and magnetic resonance imaging (MRI) found that PET scan was the most sensitive imaging modality for detecting hepatic metastases.[22] A separate study found that tumors which responded metabolically on PET to neoadjuvant chemotherapy correlated highly with histopathologic response and improved patient survival.[23] Therefore, current recommendations regarding the use of PET for staging gastric cancer are for selective use for patients with locally advanced tumors where the metastatic potential is high, and in cases where neoadjuvant therapy is being considered.[3]

Pathology

Gastric adenocarcinoma occurs in two distinct histologic subtypes—intestinal and diffuse. These subtypes are characterized by differing pathologic and clinical features and by differing patterns of metastatic spread.

In the intestinal form of gastric cancer, the malignant cells tend to form glands. The intestinal form of malignancy is more frequently associated with gastric mucosal atrophy, chronic atrophic gastritis, intestinal metaplasia, and dysplasia. Gastric cancer with the intestinal histologic subtype is more common in populations at high risk (e.g., Japan), and it occurs with increased frequency in men and older patients. Clinical studies suggest that this subtype more frequently demonstrates bloodborne metastases.

The diffuse form of gastric adenocarcinoma does not demonstrate gland formation and tends to infiltrate tissues as a sheet of loosely adherent cells. Lymphatic invasion is common. Intraperitoneal metastases are frequent. The diffuse form of gastric adenocarcinoma tends to occur in younger patients, in women, and in populations with a relatively low incidence of gastric cancer (e.g., the United States). The prognosis is less favorable for patients with the diffuse histologic subtype.

Efforts have been made to grade tumors on histologic criteria. Progressively anaplastic carcinomas are assigned higher grades. Not surprisingly, histologic grade correlates closely with 5-year survival; only 11% of grade IV patients survive

5 years, whereas 66% of grade I patients are alive 5 years after operation.

Sporadic gastric adenocarcinomas demonstrate a number of chromosomal and genetic abnormalities. Cytometric analysis reveals that gastric tumors with a large fraction of aneuploid cells (with a greater-than-normal amount of nuclear DNA) tend to be more highly infiltrative and have a poorer prognosis. Amplifications of both the HER-2/*neu* and *K-ras* protooncogenes have been consistently detected in gastric adenocarcinomas, and in a small percentage of tumors a lack of expression of the tumor suppressor gene *MKK4* is robustly associated with poor survival.[24] The exact mechanisms by which these genetic abnormalities contribute to gastric oncogenesis is currently unclear. Additionally, a number of growth factors, including epidermal growth factor, platelet-derived growth factor, and transforming growth factor-β, are overexpressed in gastric carcinoma cells.[25]

In the United States the incidence of proximal gastric cancer has been increasing; such that in 2001 the rate of proximal cancers, defined as cancers arising in the cardia and fundus, exceeded that of distal cancers, defined as cancers arising in the antrum and pylorus. Based on this data, collected by the National Cancer Database, proximal cancers are more likely to occur in young white men and distal cancers are more likely to occur in Asian, African American, and Hispanic patients within the United States. The proportion of tumors involving the proximal stomach has dramatically increased over the past decades; in the 1960s, only 16% involved this region, and a clear explanation for this rise in proximal disease remains elusive. In 10% of the cases, the stomach is diffusely involved at the time of diagnosis.[19] Prognosis is distinctly less favorable for tumors arising from the proximal stomach or for those with diffuse involvement of the organ relative to distal tumors, and these patients are much more likely to undergo neoadjuvant and adjuvant therapy.[4,26] The need to resect other organs in the upper abdomen, in addition to gastric resection, is also an unfavorable prognostic factor,[27] and postoperative morbidity increases as more organs are resected in order to achieve negative surgical margins.

The gastric cancer staging format used by the American Joint Committee on Cancer is presented in Table 46.2. The staging system is oriented toward surgical and pathologic examinations but also accurately reflects prognosis (Fig. 46.8). A consideration of staging data illustrates the high frequency with which lymph node metastases are present at the time of diagnosis in the United States, and the severe impact lymphatic involvement has on survival. Even early gastric cancers (tumors restricted to the mucosa and submucosa) have a 15% prevalence of nodal metastasis.

TABLE 46.2 CLASSIFICATION AND STAGING

TNM CLASSIFICATION FOR STAGING OF GASTRIC ULCER

PRIMARY TUMOR	
TX	Tumor cannot be assessed
T0	No evidence of primary tumor
Tis	Carcinoma in situ; intraepithelial tumor without invasion of the lamina propria
T1	Tumor invades lamina propria or submucosa
T2a	Tumor invades muscularis propria
T2b	Tumor invades subserosa
T3	Tumor penetrates serosa without invasion of adjacent structures
T4	Tumor invades adjacent structures
REGIONAL LYMPH NODE INVOLVEMENT	
NX	Regional lymph node(s) cannot be assessed
N0	No regional nodal metastasis
N1	Metastasis to 1–6 regional lymph nodes
N2	Metastasis to 7–15 regional lymph nodes
N3	Metastasis in more than 15 regional lymph nodes
DISTANT METASTASIS	
MX	Distant metastasis cannot be assessed
M0	No distant metastasis
M1	Distant metastasis
Stage Grouping	
Stage 0	Tis N0 M0
Stage IA	T1 N0 M0
Stage IB	T1 N1 M0
	T2 N0 M0
Stage II	T1 N2 M0
	T2 N1 M0
	T3 N0 M0
Stage IIIA	T2 N2 M0
Stage IIIB	T3 N1 M0
	T4 N0 M0
	T3 N2 M0
Stage IV	T4 N1 M0
	T1 N3 M0
	T2 N3 M0
	T3 N3 M0
	T4 N2 M0
	T4 N3 M0
	Any T Any N M1

Reproduced with permission from Greene FL, Page DL, Fleming ID, et al. *AJCC Cancer Staging Manual*, 6th ed. New York: Springer; 2002.

Curative Treatment

Surgical resection is the only hope for cure in gastric cancer, but an advanced stage of disease at the time of diagnosis precludes curative resection for most patients. The surgical objectives in gastric cancer must, therefore, be two: (a) to maximize chances for cure in patients with localized tumor

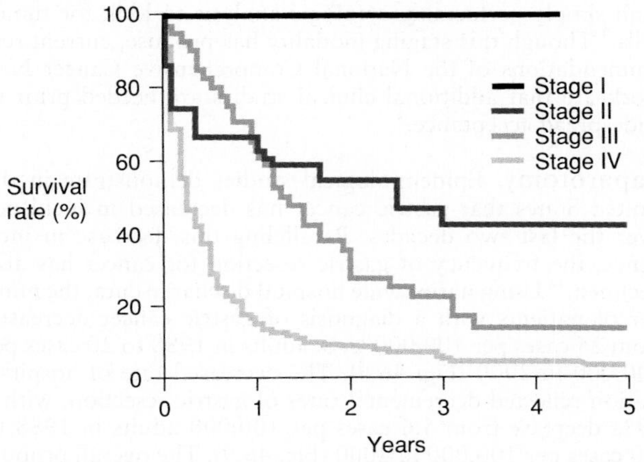

FIGURE 46.8. Survival rates of gastric cancer by stage.

and (b) to provide effective and safe palliation to patients with advanced malignancy. Evolution of the surgical approach to gastric adenocarcinoma has focused on the following six issues: the ability of preoperative tests to detect metastatic disease, the extent of gastric resection needed for potentially curable lesions, the extent of perigastric lymphadenectomy, the adequacy of proximal and distal resection margins, the role of splenectomy, and the implications of involvement of adjacent organs.

Staging Laparoscopy. The ability of CT scanning to detect metastatic disease is limited, especially when tumor deposits are small. The surface of the liver, the omentum, and the peritoneal surfaces are common sites for gastric cancer metastasis that are difficult to evaluate preoperatively by CT scanning. In prospective studies, diagnostic laparoscopy has been superior to preoperative CT or percutaneous ultrasound in detection of peritoneal, hepatic, or lymphatic metastasis. Diagnostic laparoscopy can also be combined with laparoscopic ultrasound to further increase diagnostic yield. Preoperative endoscopic ultrasound and operatively performed laparoscopic ultrasound are complementary techniques. When combined, 100% sensitivity in detecting inoperable cancers has been reported.[28]

Accurate staging and detection of incurable lesions is crucial because the mean life expectancy of affected patients is only 3 to 9 months. In 10–25% of patients, laparoscopy will detect distant disease that precludes curative resection.[29–31] Relative to laparotomy, the shorter hospitalization and reduced operative trauma following laparoscopy are obvious benefits to individuals with a short life expectancy. Most patients with systemic metastasis can be treated without the need for palliative surgical resection. In one study, no patients deemed incurable by laparoscopy required subsequent operation.[32]

In addition to visual inspection of the abdominal organs and peritoneal surfaces, some have also advocated for the routine use of peritoneal cytological analysis at the time of laparoscopy to further increase the accuracy of staging prior to proceeding with radical surgical resection. A number of retrospective studies have identified positive peritoneal cytology as an indicator of both early recurrence and poor survival. In a recent large series, outcomes for patients with positive peritoneal cytology without gross metastatic disease were not significantly different than for patients found to have gross metastatic disease at the time of laparoscopy,[33] and similar findings have been observed in other smaller series. A current limitation of this approach is that the overall incidence of positive peritoneal cytology in the absence of gross disease is low (6–15%). To try to improve the sensitivity and specificity of this approach, some investigators are exploring the use of advanced diagnostic technologies to identify specific tumor markers on the cells from the peritoneal lavage fluid rather than simply performing cytologic analysis to look for tumor cells.[3] Though this staging modality has promise, current recommendations of the National Comprehensive Cancer Network are that additional clinical studies are needed prior to widespread acceptance.[3]

Laparotomy. Epidemiological studies demonstrate in the United States that gastric cancer has decreased in incidence over the last two decades. Paralleling this decrease in incidence, the frequency of gastric resection for cancer has also declined.[34] Using nationwide hospital discharge data, the number of patients with a diagnosis of gastric cancer decreased from 25 cases per 100,000 U. S. adults in 1988 to 20 cases per 100,000 in 2000 (Fig. 46.9). The decreased rate of hospitalization reflected decremental rates of gastric resection, with a 29% decrease from 5.6 cases per 100,000 adults in 1988 to 4.0 cases per 100,000 in 2000 (Fig. 46.9). The overall proportion of hospitalized gastric cancer patients undergoing gastric resection remained constant at 22%.

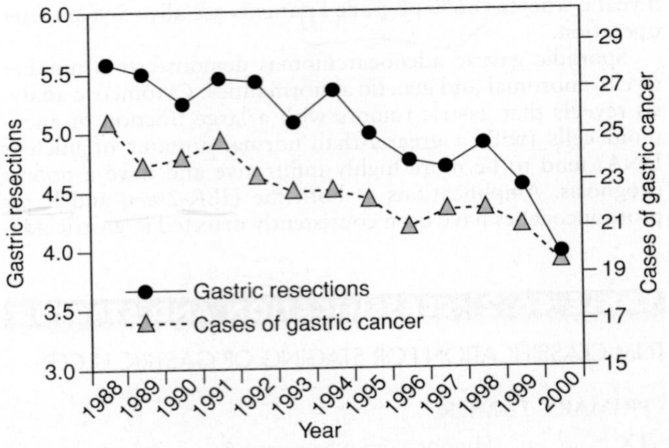

FIGURE 46.9. Incidence of gastric cancer and gastric cancer resection in the United States, per 100,000 adults, over the time period 1988 through 2000.

Gastric resection for cancer has a relatively high rate of postoperative complications and significant operative mortality. From 1988 to 2000, in-hospital mortality did not significantly change, with an overall mortality rate of 7.4% for the nationwide group. Complication rates were not uniform, however, and varied in relation to hospital experience with gastric surgery. Low-volume centers had an 8.3% mortality rate, medium-volume hospitals had a 7.1% death rate, and high-volume centers had a 6.5% mortality rate (Fig. 46.10). The safety of gastric resection improved progressively from 1988 to 2000 at high-volume medical centers. A decline in mortality was not observed at low- or medium-volume hospitals. Despite no significant change in overall complication rates, patients are spending less time in the hospital after gastric resection (Fig. 46.11). Shorter hospital stays likely reflect improved efficiency with better use of hospital resources, but may also derive from societal efforts to curtail health-care costs.

Since the mid-1990s, the surgical treatment of gastric cancer has continued to evolve, with minimally invasive approaches increasingly pursued for early cancers and increasingly radical operations for advanced tumors. Japanese surgeons have reported the largest experience with early gastric cancer. The Japanese Gastric Cancer Association defines early

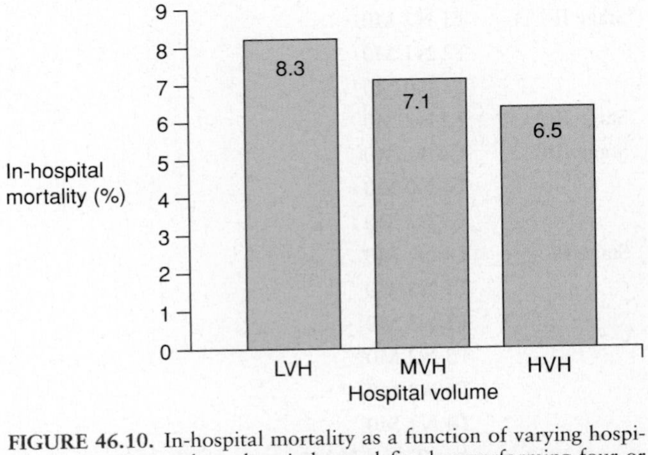

FIGURE 46.10. In-hospital mortality as a function of varying hospital volume. Low-volume hospitals are defined as performing four or fewer resections per year. Medium-volume hospitals are defined as performing five to eight resections per year. High-volume hospitals are defined as performing nine or more resections per year.

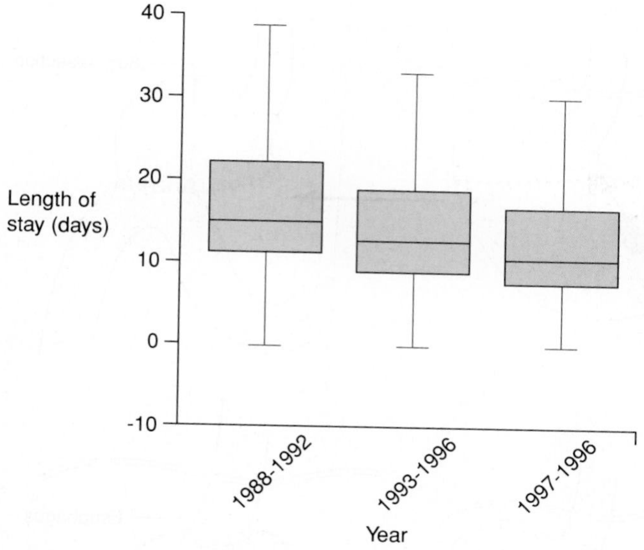

FIGURE 46.11. Length of stay after gastric resection by time period from 1988 through 2000.

gastric cancer as tumor in which invasion is restricted to the mucosa or submucosa.[35] The presence or absence of lymph node metastasis is not considered in this classification. While the presence of lymphatic metastasis cannot be correctly judged by endoscopic findings, it is critically important in prognosis. For tumors confined to the mucosa, lymphatic metastasis is present in 1% to 3% of cases; with submucosal involvement, the rate of nodal positivity increases to 14% to 20%.[36,37]

For well-differentiated mucosal tumors of less than 3 cm without ulceration, endoscopic mucosal resection has been performed. With this approach, postoperative bleeding or perforation has been reported in 5%, and in 17% histologic examination revealed submucosal invasion that required further operative treatment.[38] Reports that suggest underestimation of tumor invasion in 45% and missed lymphatic metastasis in 9% urge caution before widespread acceptance of this technique.[39]

Laparoscopic gastrectomy has also been reported for treatment of gastric malignancy, with advantages of reduced pain, shorter hospitalization, and improved quality of life.[40] Studies from Japan, Korea, and Italy have demonstrated that distal, subtotal, and total gastrectomy with lyphadenectomy are feasible with acceptable morbidity and mortality. However, the majority of patients in these studies had early gastric cancer.[3] A multi-center non-randomized study demonstrated acceptable oncologic outcomes following laparoscopic gastrectomy for early gastric cancers in Japan (99% 5-year disease-free survival for Stage I disease and 86% for Stage II disease);[41] however, the non-randomized nature of this study precludes declaration of equivalency of a laparoscopic approach to open surgery due to uncontrolled patient selection bias. A single institution randomized prospective trial for laparoscopic versus open subtotal gastrectomy for distal gastric cancer (in patients with both early and locally advanced gastric cancer) did report equivalent lymph node retrieval (33.4±7.4 in the open group versus 30±14.9 in the laparoscopic group), as well as similar rates of peri-operative morbidity and mortality as outlined in Table 46.3. Five-year overall and disease-free survival were also similar for both groups, 55.7% and 54.8% for the laparoscopic group versus 58.9% and 57.3% for the open group.[42] However, the lack of a multi-center study design precludes generalizability of this data to all centers, and a true multi-center randomized prospective trial is still needed to truly define the equivalency or superiority of this approach to open surgery.

4 Since the early 1980s, radical operations have been performed for the treatment of gastric cancer, including total gastrectomy, extended subtotal gastrectomy with *en bloc* resection of celiac and splenic lymph nodes, splenectomy, and distal pancreatectomy. With time, it has become apparent that radical operations, in general, increase operative morbidity without improving survival. For early lesions (N0–1, M0) of the antrum or middle stomach, distal subtotal gastrectomy including 80% of the stomach provides satisfactory 5-year survival rates without increasing operative morbidity. Proximal gastric lesions or larger middle stomach lesions may require total gastrectomy or esophagogastrectomy to encompass the tumor (Figs. 46.12 and 46.13). For tumors involving the cardia without involvement of the gastroesophageal junction, some have advocated proximal gastrectomy. While this operation appears to afford equivalent oncologic outcomes compared to total gastrectomy, there is a significantly higher incidence of anastomotic stricture and severe reflux esophagitis with proximal gastrectomy.[3] Regardless of the extent of gastric resection, patients with more advanced tumors fare poorly because of the increased likelihood of lymphatic and hematogenous spread.

TABLE 46.3 **COMPLICATIONS**

PERIOPERATIVE MORTALITY AND MORBIDITY FOR OPEN VERSUS LAPAROSCOPIC SUBTOTAL GASTRECTOMY FOR DISTAL GASTRIC CANCER

	■ OPEN GROUP [no. (%)]	■ LAPAROSCOPIC GROUP [no. (%)]
Perioperative mortality	2 (6.7%)	1 (3.3%)
Overall morbidity	8 (27.6%)	7 (23.3%)
Duodenal stump leak	1 (12.5%)	0
Edematous pancreatitis	0	1 (14.3%)
Pleural effusion	3 (37.5%)	3 (42.8%)
Bronchopneumonia	2 (25%)	1 (14.3%)
Wound infection	2 (25%)	2 (28.6%)

Reproduced with permission from Huscher CG, Mingoli A, Sgarzini G, et al. Laparoscopic versus open subtotal gastrectomy for distal gastric cancer: five-year results of a randomized prospective trial. *Ann Surg* 2005;241(2):232–237.

FIGURE 46.12. Surgical options for resection of gastric neoplasms. A: Subtotal gastrectomy with gastrojejunal reconstruction. B: Total gastrectomy with esophagojejunostomy. C: Esophagogastrectomy with anastomosis in cervical or thoracic position.

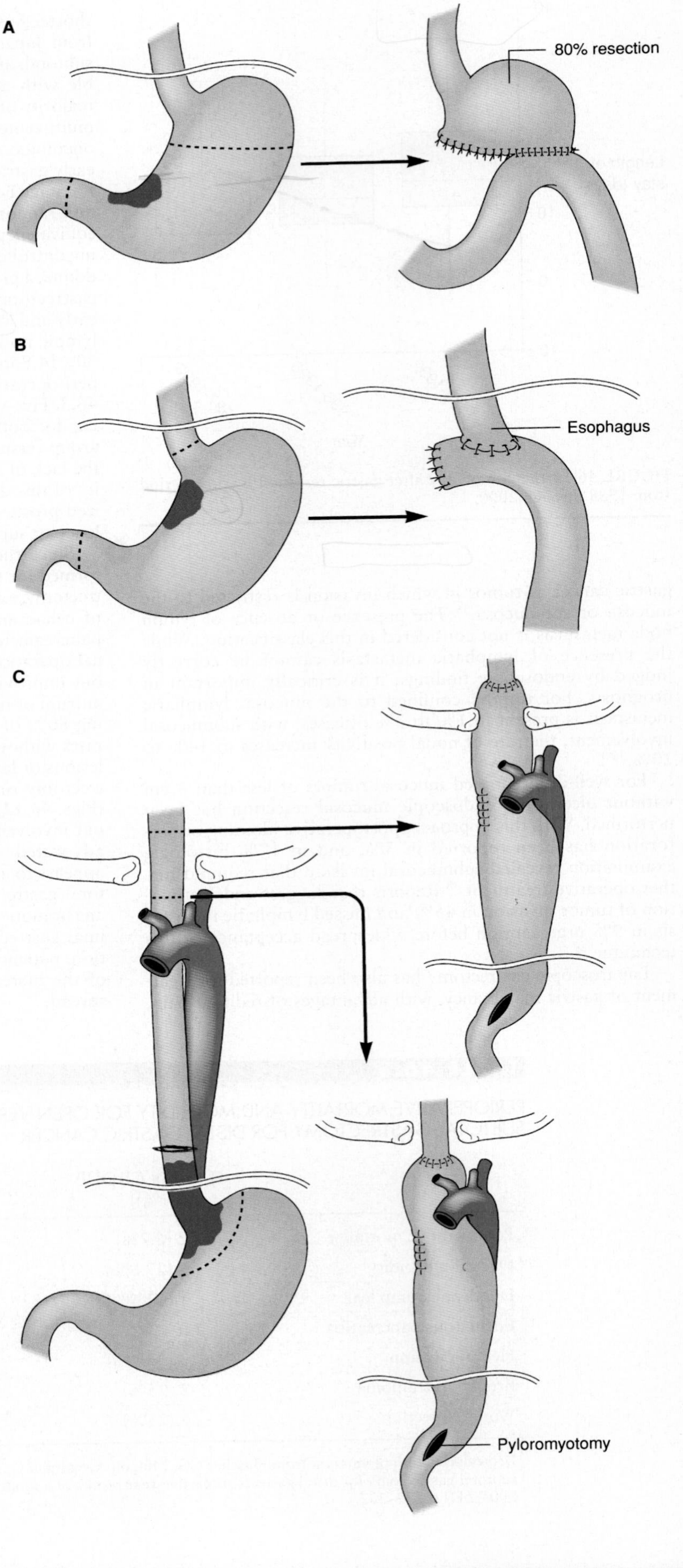

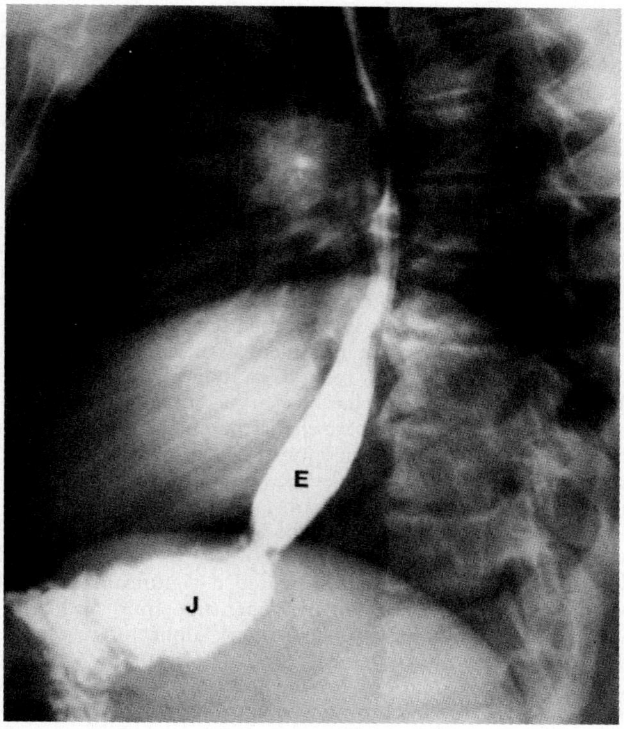

FIGURE 46.13. Postoperative radiograph after total gastrectomy with esophagojejunal anastomosis, showing esophagus (E) and jejunum (J).

The extent of gastric resection is determined, in part, by the need to obtain a resection margin free of microscopic disease. Microscopic involvement of the resection margin by tumor cells is associated with poor prognosis.[19] Patients with positive surgical margins are at high risk for development of recurrent disease, and histologically positive margins are strongly correlated with the development of anastomotic recurrence. In the setting of ≥5 positive nodes, however, margin positivity does not impact survival.[43] In contrast to colon cancer, gastric cancer frequently demonstrates extensive intramural spread. The propensity for intramural metastasis is related, in part, to the extensive anastomosing capillary and lymphatic network in the wall of the stomach. Retrospective studies suggest that when performing a subtotal gastrectomy, a margin of 6 cm from the tumor mass proximally and 3–5.9 cm distally is necessary to ensure a low rate of anastomotic recurrence.[44] Efforts to achieve even larger margins, however, have not translated into improved survival. Regardless of the type of resection or length of margins, most surgeons obtain a frozen section evaluation of margin prior to proceeding with reconstruction to try to improve the probability that an R0 resection can be achieved.

Radical gastric operations can be performed with acceptable morbidity and low mortality rates in the older age groups at greatest risk for gastric cancer. Mortality rates for total gastrectomy range from 3% to 7%.[45] Nutritional support in the immediate postoperative period is an important adjunctive measure as patients resume oral intake,[46] and many surgeons place a jejunal feeding tube at the time of total gastrectomy to ensure that optimal enteral nutrition can be delivered in the post-operative period. Surgical reconstructions that interpose a small intestinal reservoir between the esophagus and the jejunum have been advocated after total gastrectomy, but provide no clear-cut nutritional benefit.[47–50]

Because gastric cancer metastasizes so frequently to lymph nodes, radical extirpation of draining lymph nodes has both therapeutic and staging implications.[51] The value of routine extended lymphadenectomy beyond the peri-gastric lymph nodes in the treatment of gastric adenocarcinoma, however, is controversial. The first favorable experience was reported by Japanese surgeons and the Japanese Research Society for Gastric Cancer.[52,53] Resections in the original Japanese system are shown in Table 46.4, and the current nomenclature used to define extent of lymphadectomy is shown in Table 46.5. Only retrospective studies of extended perigastric lymphadenectomy have been reported from Japan. Initial reports suggested an improvement of approximately 10%, stage for stage, for patients with advanced disease treated with R2 or R3 operations.[52–55] The benefits of extended lymphadenectomy have not been confirmed in non-Japanese centers, and several randomized trials have failed to show a survival benefit for extended lymphadenectomy when the entire patient population was analyzed.[56–60]

The safety of extended lymphadenectomy is disputed. Data from a national Japanese registry indicate a contemporary mortality of less than 1%.[61] Low mortality risks have been reported from multiinstitutional trials conducted in Italy and Germany.[60,62] Investigations from the United States, Britain, and the Netherlands have been less optimistic, indicating increased short-term morbidity and in-hospital mortality.[56,57]

TABLE 46.4 MANAGEMENT

LYMPHADENECTOMY RESECTIONS IN THE ORIGINAL SYSTEM OF THE JAPANESE RESEARCH SOCIETY FOR GASTRIC CANCER

■ LEVEL	■ DESCRIPTION
R1	Resection of stomach, omentum, and perigastric lymph nodes
R2	Resection of stomach, omentum, and en bloc removal of the superior leaf of the transverse mesocolon, the pancreatic capsule, and lymph nodes along the branches of the celiac artery and in the infraduodenal and supraduodenal areas
R3	Resection of the above structures plus lymph nodes along the aorta and esophagus, along with the spleen and the tail of the pancreas, and skeletonization of vessels in the porta hepatis

TABLE 46.5 MANAGEMENT

CURRENT NOMENCLATURE USED TO DESCRIBE THE EXTENT OF LYMPHADENECTOMY PERFORMED IN CONJUNCTION WITH GASTRECTOMY

■ LEVEL	■ DESCRIPTION
D0	Any lymph node removal that is less than D1
D1	Resection of greater and lesser omenta—which includes the perigastric nodes along the right and left cardiac regions, lesser and greater curves, suprapyloric along the right gastric artery, and infrapyloric
D2	D1 dissection plus the anterior leaf of the transverse mesocolon and all of the nodes along the left gastric artery, common hepatic artery, celiac artery, splenic hilum, and splenic artery
D3	D2 dissection plus the para-aortic lymph nodes

One effect of extended lymphadenectomy appears to be "up-staging" of tumors; as more lymph nodes are removed, additional micrometastatic disease is discovered, and patients are correctly placed in higher-stage categories with worse prognoses.[63,64] Reciprocally, some patients who do not undergo extended lymphadenectomy will have undetected micrometastases and, because of progressive disease, will decrease the survivorship of the staging group to which they are assigned.

In the United States, greater emphasis has been placed on the total number of nodes removed and histologically examined rather than the location of the nodes (e.g., D1 vs. D2 lymphadenectomy). Current recommendations of the American Joint Committee on Cancer (AJCC) staging for gastric cancer require that a minimum of 15 nodes be evaluated for accurate staging.[65]

Histologically positive lymph nodes are frequently present in the splenic hilum and along the splenic artery, and routine splenectomy has been practiced in some centers. Splenectomy has not been demonstrated to improve outcome for similarly staged patients.[66,67] Likewise, resection of the tail or body of the pancreas has not been demonstrated to improve survival. Thus, associated splenectomy or pancreatosplenectomy is only beneficial when there is direct extension or bulky adenopathy at the splenic hilum.[68] Resection of adjacent organs may be required for local control if direct invasion has occurred. In this circumstance, operative morbidity is increased and the long-term survival rate is approximately 25%.[69]

Palliative Treatment

When preoperative evaluation demonstrates disseminated disease, palliation of symptoms becomes a primary consideration. Palliation does not usually require surgery. Obstruction and bleeding can be managed nonoperatively by the use of endoscopic laser fulguration in selected patients. Dysphagia and bleeding caused by proximal lesions can also be controlled in 80% of patients using this modality. Successful application of laser treatment requires adequate visualization, and is hampered by circumferential tumor growth that impedes passage of the endoscope, by sharp angulation of the esophagogastric junction, and by lesions more than 6 cm long.

In the setting of metastatic gastric cancer, palliative resection does not improve survival. Nonetheless, resection appears to provide superior relief of symptoms, particularly dysphagia, as compared with surgical bypass. Bypass of obstructing distal gastric cancers without resection provides relief to less than half of patients, and mean survival is less than 6 months. For proximal obstructing lesions, total gastrectomy with Roux-en-Y esophagojejunal reconstruction may be necessary. An operative mortality rate of less than 5% has been reported, and introduction of stapling devices has reduced the rate of anastomotic leaks to less than 5% in several series. Mean survival after palliative gastric resection approximates 9 months. For symptomatic unresectable gastric adenocarcinoma, radiation therapy with or without concomitant chemotherapy can also provide significant palliation.

5 **Neoadjuvant and Adjuvant Therapy.** Given the largely disappointing outcomes in Western countries with radical surgery and peri-operative treatment with multiple chemotherapeutic agents for the management of localized gastric cancer, significant interest has been generated for exploring the use of chemoradiation as either a neoadjuvant or adjuvant therapy. Two trials have recently re-defined standard clinical practice for fit patients with resectable locally advanced gastric cancer who can tolerate multi-modality therapy.

The first of these trials was the US Intergroup Trial (SWOG-9008/INT0116), initiated in 1991 to evaluate whether the addition of 5-fluorouracil (5FU), leukovorin, and external beam radiation following gastrectomy would improve survival over surgery alone for locally advanced gastric cancer. After a median follow-up period of 5 years, disease-free survival and overall survival were significantly improved with multi-modality therapy. Median time to relapse was 30 months in the multimodality treatment group versus 19 months in the surgery alone group, $p < 0.001$, and overall survival was 36 months in the chemoradiation group versus 27 months in the surgery alone group, $p = 0.005$.[70] The primary criticism of this trial was that the extent of lymphadectomy was not standardized, and a less than D1 lymph node dissection was performed in 54% of the patients. Additionally, due to the morbid nature of gastrectomy, approximately one third of the patients were unable to complete their adjuvant chemoradiation due to perioperative complications or treatment associated toxicities; in fact three patients died related to complications of the chemoradiation therapy. It has been argued that improved radiation techniques and less toxic chemotherapeutic regimens can lessen the toxicity of the therapy; the issue of post-operative disability and diminished tolerance of adjuvant chemoradiation following gastrectomy remains.

More recently, the results of the Medical Research Council Adjuvant Gastric Infusional Chemotherapy (MAGIC) trial were published, which demonstrated a significant survival benefit in patients receiving peri-operative (pre- and postoperative) chemotherapy versus surgery alone for resectable gastric cancer, with a five-year survival rate of 36% versus 23%.[71] Though extent of lymphadenectomy was improved as compared to the US Intergroup trial, only 42% of patients completed all courses of chemotherapy and optimal additional study arms were not evaluated—namely the inclusion of a neoadjuvant chemoradiation treatment arm. Additionally, given the results of the Intergroup trial, it would not be considered standard practice to treat a patient with surgery alone for locally advanced gastric cancer and this was the primary comparison group.

Despite the limitations of these studies, the improved survival observed in both trials makes it clear that a multi-modality approach is superior to surgery alone; patients with locally advanced resectable gastric cancer are optimally treated in a center where a collaborative multi-disciplinary treatment approach can be devised and executed (Algorithm 46.1).

GASTRIC LYMPHOMA

Clinical Features

The stomach is the site of more than half of gastrointestinal lymphomas and is the most common organ involved in extranodal lymphomas. Non-Hodgkin's lymphomas account for approximately 5% of malignant gastric tumors; lymphoma represents an increasing proportion of gastric neoplasms diagnosed currently. Patients are considered to have primary gastric lymphoma if initial symptoms are gastric and the stomach is exclusively or predominantly involved with the tumor. Patients who do not fulfill these criteria are considered to have secondary gastric involvement from systemic lymphoma.

Gastric lymphoma is distinctly uncommon in children and young adults. The peak incidence is in the sixth and seventh decades. Symptoms are indistinguishable from those of gastric adenocarcinoma. Epigastric pain, weight loss, anorexia, nausea, and vomiting are common.[72] Although gross bleeding is uncommon, occult hemorrhage and anemia are observed in more than half of patients. Patients rarely have spontaneous perforation.

Diagnosis

Radiologic findings are similar to those for adenocarcinoma. Endoscopic examination has become the diagnostic method of

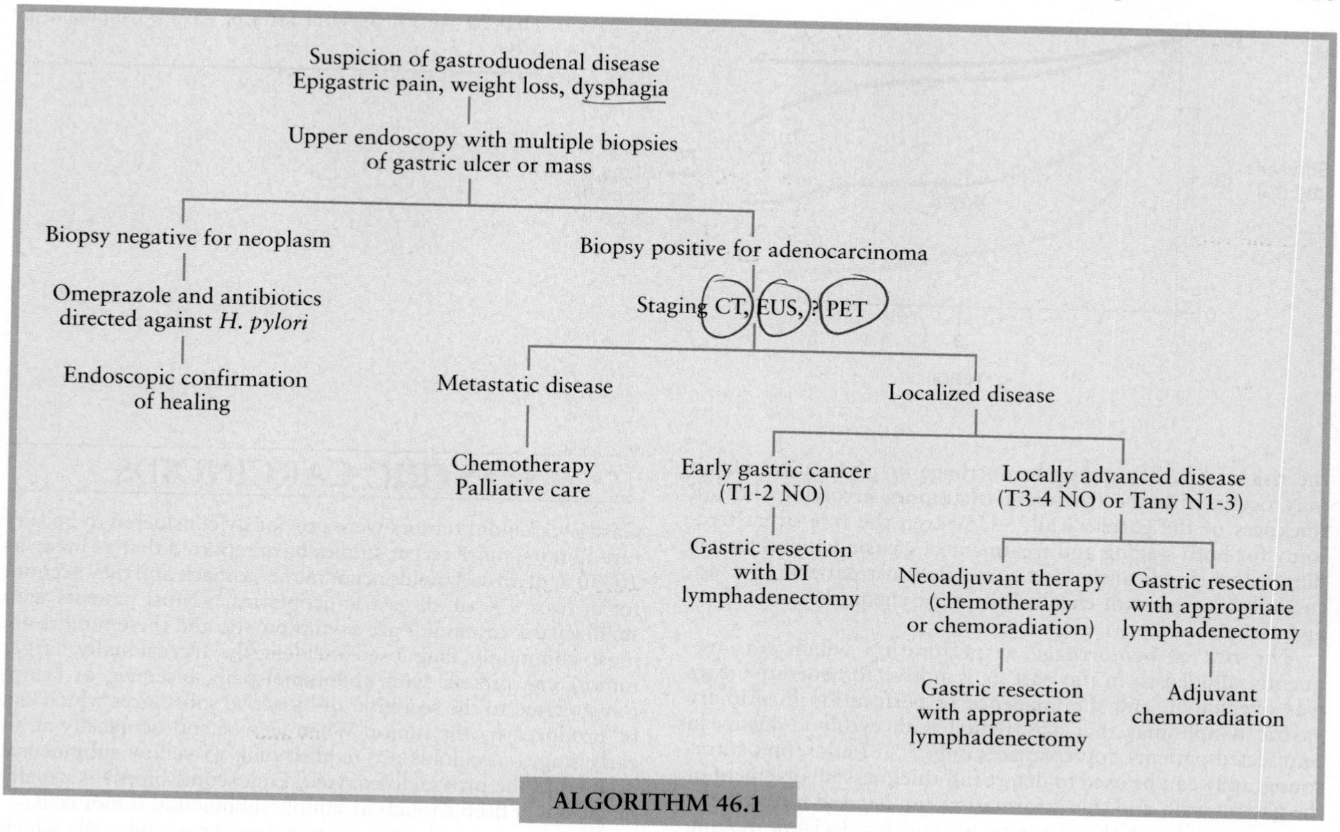

ALGORITHM 46.1. Treatment of gastric adenocarcinoma.

choice. The endoscopic appearance of lesions may be ulcerated, polypoid, or infiltrative. Gastric lymphoma is most commonly localized to the middle or distal stomach and unusually involves the proximal stomach, in contrast to gastric adenocarcinoma. Endoscopic biopsy, combined with endoscopic brush cytology and ultrasonography, provides positive diagnosis in 90% of cases. Submucosal growth without ulceration of the overlying mucosa can occasionally render endoscopic biopsy nondiagnostic. Endoscopic ultrasound-guided biopsy is useful in this circumstance.

When gastric lymphoma is first diagnosed by endoscopic means, evidence of systemic disease should be sought. CT of the chest and abdomen (to detect lymphadenopathy), bone marrow biopsy, and biopsy of enlarged peripheral lymph nodes are all appropriate.

6 Mucosa-associated Lymphoma Tissue. The concept that low-grade gastric lymphomas have features resembling mucosa-associated lymphoid tissue (MALT) is a major advance in the understanding of gastric lymphomas. The gastric submucosa does not ordinarily contain lymphoid tissue, and the development of lymphoid tissue resembling small intestinal Peyer's patches is believed to occur in response to infection with *H. pylori*.[73] A number of observations support a causal relationship between chronic *H. pylori* infection and lymphoma development. *H. pylori* is present in the stomachs of more than half of patients with gastric lymphoma.[74] As with gastric adenocarcinoma, geographic regions with a high prevalence of *H. pylori* also have a high incidence of gastric lymphoma. Infection with *H. pylori* has been noted to precede development of gastric lymphoma.[75]

After development of gastric lymphoid tissue, low-grade lymphoma is postulated to occur as a result of monoclonal B-cell proliferation. Initially, B-cell proliferation depends on interleukin-2 production by antigenically stimulated nonneoplastic T cells. Progressive genetic rearrangements lead to B-cell proliferation that is independent of *H. pylori*—stimulated interleukin-2. With cumulative genetic defects, low-grade MALT lymphoma progresses to high-grade MALT lymphoma.

Low-grade MALT lymphomas resemble Peyer's patches. Lymphoma cells invade between follicles and into gastric epithelium; invasion of gastric glands forms characteristic lymphoepithelial lesions. Low-grade lesions are often multifocal. Low-grade MALT lesions are less likely than high-grade tumors to invade transmurally, involve perigastric lymph nodes, or invade adjacent organs.[75] Approximately 40% of gastric lymphomas are low-grade MALT lymphomas.[76] High-grade MALT lymphomas cannot be distinguished histologically from non-MALT, high-grade B-cell lymphomas.

The concept that low-grade lymphoma depends on continued *H. pylori* antigenic stimulation supports eradication of *H. pylori* with antibiotics as first-line antineoplastic therapy. Complete regression of low-grade MALT lymphomas with antibiotic treatment has been reported in 70% to 100% of cases.[77,78] The median time to complete response averaged 5 months.[79] Most patients with partial responses were subsequently determined also to have foci of high-grade lymphoma. Radiation and chemotherapy have been proposed as salvage for antibiotic treatment failures.

Non-MALT Lymphomas. In the past, a multimodality treatment program was used in most centers for primary gastric lymphomas, with gastrectomy as the first step in the therapeutic strategy.[80] This approach evolved empirically, and prospective data to support it were lacking. Several advantages of this approach had been cited: (a) more accurate histologic evaluation was possible; (b) in cases with localized tumor, the procedure could be curative; and (c) gastrectomy eliminated

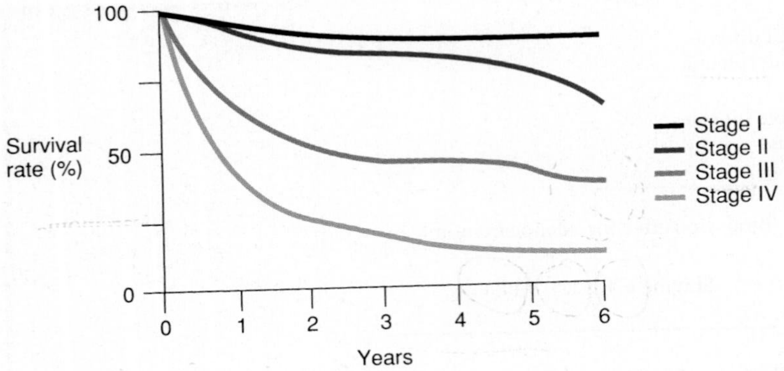

FIGURE 46.14. Survival rates of gastric lymphoma by stage.

the risk of life-threatening hemorrhage or perforation which may occur with the treatment of tumors involving the full thickness of the gastric wall.[81] However, the role of gastrectomy for both staging and treatment of gastric lymphoma has diminished significantly; and currently most patients are successfully treated with chemotherapy or chemoradiation therapy alone.

The risk of hemorrhage or perforation which was frequently alluded to in the past as a motive for operative care was overstated, and the incidence of perforation in primary gastric lymphomas that are treated with cytolytic agents in unresected patients approximates only 5%. Endoscopic ultrasonography can be used to detect full-thickness involvement of the gastric wall, and this information can be used to counsel a patient regarding risks of treatment and for decision making regarding risk of perforation.

More than 30% of patients who present with stage II primary gastric lymphoma who undergo apparently adequate surgery and radiation therapy, will develop disease recurrence outside of the treatment field. Patients with stage II primary gastric lymphoma should, therefore, be considered to have systemic disease and to require systemic therapy in addition to surgery or radiation therapy for local management of the primary gastric lymphoma. Survival for gastric lymphoma is closely linked to stage at diagnosis (Fig. 46.14). A recent prospective, randomized study has demonstrated that complication-free survival is highest in patients treated with chemotherapy alone consisting of cyclophosphamide, vincristine, doxorubicin, and prednisone (Fig. 46.15).[82]

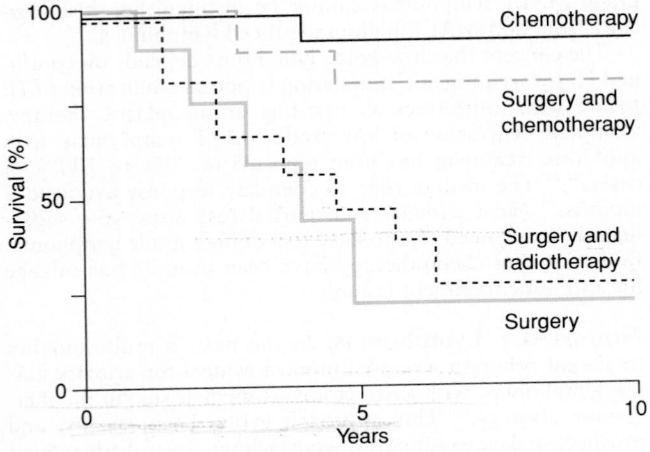

FIGURE 46.15. Actuarial curves of complication-free survival, according to stage.

GASTRIC CARCINOIDS

Gastric carcinoid tumors were previously considered to be very rare tumors; more recent studies have reported that as many as 10–30% of all carcinoids occur in the stomach and they account for at least 1% of all gastric neoplasms.[83] Most patients with small gastric carcinoids are asymptomatic and these tumors are most commonly diagnosed incidentally. Occasionally, larger tumors can present with abdominal pain, bleeding, or symptoms related to the secretion of bioactive substances which can be produced by the tumor. When viewed endoscopically at an early stage, carcinoids are reddish-pink to yellow submucosal nodules in the proximal stomach. Endoscopic biopsy is usually diagnostic if deep enough to sample submucosal tumor cells.

Gastric carcinoids arise from enterochromaffin cells which mediate the secretion of histamine, which in turn stimulates parietal cells to secrete acid. Hypergastrinemia is thought to cause enterochromaffin cell hyperplasia, and may lead to the development of gastric carcinoids over time.[84] Four types of gastric carcinoids have been described. Type I is the most common, and is associated with chronic atrophic gastritis and pernicious anemia. These tumors tend to be slow growing with less malignant potential. Type II tumors are described as having an intermediate malignant potential and occur in patients with Zollinger Ellison syndrome and multiple endocrine neoplasia I. Both Type I and Type II gastric carcinoid tumors are associated with hypergastrinemia. These tumors tend to be small (<1 cm) and are often multi-focal. Type III gastric carcinoids tend to be larger, solitary lesions, are associated with normal gastrin levels, and behave much more aggressively.[84] Type IV are also larger, solitary, aggressive lesions which are associated with parietal cell hyperplasia. Histologically, the tumors appear as nests of monotonous hyperchromatic cells originating in the submucosa or in the basal area of gastric glands.

A recent review of 1,543 patients with gastric carcinoid identified from the Surveillance Epidemiology and End Results (SEER) database found that the mean tumor size was 1.73 cm, with 12% and 7.9% of patients presenting with lymph node metastasis and distant metastasis, respectively.[84] Greater depth of tumor invasion and the presence of lymph node or distant metastasis adversely affected survival. Overall, 5-year survival for Types I and II gastric carcinoids is 81% (>95% for Type I lesions), while Type III and IV tumors have only a 33% overall 5-year survival.[83] Given the potential for invasion by all gastric carcinoids, attempts at curative resection with appropriate gastric resection and lymphadenectomy is indicated in all patients deemed fit for surgery.

GASTROINTESTINAL STROMAL TUMORS OF THE STOMACH

Gastrointestinal stromal tumors (GIST) were historically misclassified as leiomyomas, leiomyosarcomas, and leiomyoblastomas due to a mistaken belief that they arose from the smooth muscle in the bowel wall. It is now recognized that GISTs represent a distinct mesenchymal tumor type, and arise from the interstitial cells of Cajal, an intestinal pacemaker cell located in and around the myenteric plexus in the bowel wall. Additionally, 95–99% of GISTs also express the CD117 antigen (*KIT*), and express the *c-kit* receptor. *c-kit* is the receptor for the *KIT* ligand, also known as cytokine stem cell factor. *c-kit* is a tyrosine kinase that acts as a growth factor or developmental antigen receptor; occupation of the receptor acts to stimulate cellular proliferation; positive staining for *c-kit* is diagnostic of a GIST.

While GISTs can arise anywhere within the gastrointestinal tract, approximately 50% of these tumors are found in the stomach. With a slight male predominance, GIST most commonly are identified in individuals in the fourth to eighth decades of life, with a median presentation of approximately 60 years of age. The majority of these tumors are asymptomatic, and are most commonly identified incidentally during endoscopy performed for other reasons. Endoscopically, they typically appear as a submucosal mass. If these tumors become large, they may present with symptoms of abdominal pain and bleeding. GISTs frequently have prominent extraluminal growth patterns, and central necrosis is common as these tumors become large and outgrow their blood supply (Fig. 46.16). If the majority of the growth is extraluminal, endoscopic examination may be unrevealing or only demonstrate umbilication of the mucosa possibly indicate an underlying mass. Endoscopic ultrasound or CT imaging may be helpful for diagnosis in these cases. With large tumors, symptoms related to mass effects with compression of adjacent structures are most common. Additionally, ulceration of the overlying gastric mucosa may occur with tumor necrosis, and these patients may present with significant and intermittent gastrointestinal hemorrhage.

Determination of whether an isolated primary GIST is benign or malignant is difficult, and only the evidence of metastatic disease is diagnostic of a malignant tumor. Certain morphologic features have been identified as being associated with increased risk of local recurrence or distant metastasis. Tumor size (>2 cm) and mitotic index (>5–10 mitoses/high power field) are the most important prognostic variables, as well as site of origin within the gastrointestinal tract; however, all GISTs should be viewed as having malignant potential with the possible exception of very small tumors measuring <1 cm.[85] As compared to other sites of origin, gastric GISTs tend to have a more favorable prognosis.

If GISTs do metastasize, it is by a hematogenous route (most commonly to peritoneal surfaces and the liver), therefore, associated lymphadenectomy is typically not performed

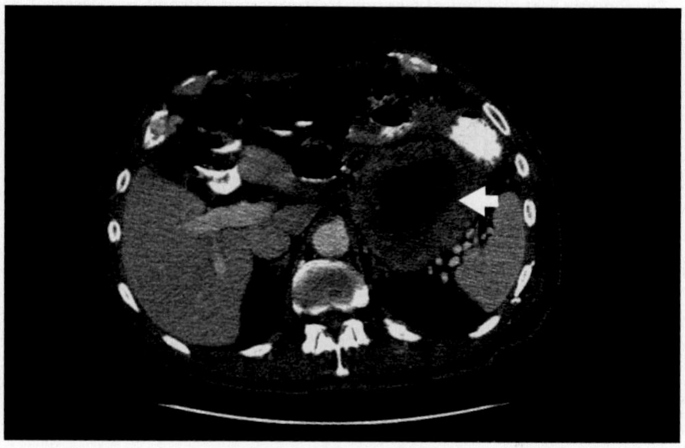

FIGURE 46.16. CT scan of GIST of stomach arising from lesser curvature. The *arrow* indicates central tumor necrosis. The lesion caused mucosal erosion with gastrointestinal hemorrhage.

at the time of gastric resection for GIST. Additionally, unlike adenocarcinoma, GISTs do not present with an intramural growth pattern and thus gross margins of 1–2 cm are deemed adequate for resection of a GIST. Ultimately the goal of resection is a negative microscopic margin. If the tumor involves adjacent structures, then en bloc resection of nonvital structures should be performed whenever possible. Due to the less radical nature of surgery required for appropriate oncologic resection of these tumors as compared to adenocarcinoma of the stomach, minimally invasive surgical techniques have become widely accepted as an appropriate and acceptable operative approach for these tumors.

For patients presenting with metastatic GIST or locally advanced disease, the use of neoadjuvant or palliative targeted molecular therapy should be considered. Imatinib mesylate (Gleevec, Novartis Pharmaceuticals) is a small molecule tyrosine kinase inhibitor which targets *KIT*, and approximately 80% of patients with metastatic GIST will demonstrate at least a partial response to imatinib mesylate therapy. Unfortunately, complete or lasting responses are rare as approximately half of the patients who demonstrate initial responses eventually develop resistance to the drug.[86] Due to these failures, several second generation tyrosine kinase inhibitors are currently under study for treatment of imatinib-resistant GISTs. The role of imatinib mesylate as a neoadjuvant agent prior to surgical resection for locally advanced tumors is being explored in clinical trials.

References

1. Silverberg E, Boring CC, Squires TS. Cancer statistics, 1990. *CA Cancer J Clin* 1990;40(1):9–26.
2. Boring CC, Squires TS, Tong T. Cancer statistics, 1993. *CA Cancer J Clin* 1993;43(1):7–26.
3. Ly QP, Sasson AR. Modern surgical considerations for gastric cancer. *J Natl Compr Canc Netw* 2008;6(9):885–894.
4. Wilkinson NW, et al. Differences in the pattern of presentation and treatment of proximal and distal gastric cancer: results of the 2001 gastric patient care evaluation. *Ann Surg Oncol* 2008;15(6):1644–1650.
5. Harju E. Gastric polyposis and malignancy. *Br J Surg* 1986;73(7):532–533.
6. Parsonnet J, et al. *Helicobacter pylori* infection and the risk of gastric carcinoma. *N Engl J Med* 1991;325(16):1127–1131.
7. Amieva MR, El-Omar EM. Host-bacterial interactions in *Helicobacter pylori* infection. *Gastroenterology* 2008;134(1):306–323.
8. Naylor GM, et al. Why does Japan have a high incidence of gastric cancer? Comparison of gastritis between UK and Japanese patients. *Gut* 2006; 55(11):1545–1552.
9. Marshall BJ, Windsor HM. The relation of *Helicobacter pylori* to gastric adenocarcinoma and lymphoma: pathophysiology, epidemiology, screening, clinical presentation, treatment, and prevention. *Med Clin North Am* 2005;89(2):313–344, viii.
10. Forman D, Pisani P. Gastric cancer in Japan—honing treatment, seeking causes. *N Engl J Med* 2008;359(5):448–451.
11. Caygill CP, et al. Mortality from gastric cancer following gastric surgery for peptic ulcer. *Lancet* 1986;1(8487):929–931.
12. Lundegardh G, et al. Stomach cancer after partial gastrectomy for benign ulcer disease. *N Engl J Med* 1988;319(4):195–200.
13. Hansson LE. Risk of stomach cancer in patients with peptic ulcer disease. *World J Surg* 2000;24(3):315–320.
14. Lundegardh G, et al. Gastric cancer risk after vagotomy. *Gut* 1994;35(7): 946–949.
15. Tersmette AC, et al. Long-term prognosis after partial gastrectomy for benign conditions. Survival and smoking-related death of 2633 Amsterdam postgastrectomy patients followed up since surgery between 1931 and 1960. *Gastroenterology* 1991;101(1):148–153.
16. von Holstein CS. Long-term prognosis after partial gastrectomy for gastroduodenal ulcer. *World J Surg* 2000;24(3):307–314.
17. Aya M, et al. Carcinogenesis in the remnant stomach following distal gastrectomy with Billroth II reconstruction is associated with high-level microsatellite instability. *Anticancer Res* 2006;26(2B):1403–1411.
18. Moreaux J, Bougaran J. Early gastric cancer. A 25-year surgical experience. *Ann Surg* 1993;217(4):347–355.
19. Wanebo HJ, et al. Cancer of the stomach. A patient care study by the American College of Surgeons. *Ann Surg* 1993;218(5):583–592.
20. Endo M, Habu H. Clinical studies of early gastric cancer. *Hepatogastroenterology* 1990;37(4):408–410.
21. Rösch T, Classen M. Staging gastric cancer: the Munich experience. In: Van Dam J, Sivak MV, eds. *Gastrointestinal Endosonography*. New York: WB Saunders; 1999:195–199.

22. Kinkel K, et al. Detection of hepatic metastases from cancers of the gastrointestinal tract by using noninvasive imaging methods (US, CT, MR imaging, PET): a meta-analysis. *Radiology* 2002;224(3):748–756.
23. Ott K, et al. Early metabolic response evaluation by fluorine-18 fluorodeoxyglucose positron emission tomography allows in vivo testing of chemosensitivity in gastric cancer: long-term results of a prospective study. *Clin Cancer Res* 2008;14(7):2012–2018.
24. Cunningham SC, et al. MKK4 status predicts survival after resection of gastric adenocarcinoma. *Arch Surg* 2006;141(11):1095–1099; discussion 1100.
25. Katano M, et al. Prognostic value of platelet-derived growth factor-A (PDGF-A) in gastric carcinoma. *Ann Surg*1998;227(3):365–371.
26. Harrison LE, Karpeh MS, Brennan MF. Proximal gastric cancers resected via a transabdominal-only approach. Results and comparisons to distal adenocarcinoma of the stomach. *Ann Surg*1997;225(6):678–683; discussion 683–685.
27. Kodama I, et al. Gastrectomy with combined resection of other organs for carcinoma of the stomach with invasion to adjacent organs: clinical efficacy in a retrospective study. *J Am Coll Surg*1997;184(1):16–22.
28. Mortensen MB, et al. Combined endoscopic ultrasonography and laparoscopic ultrasonography in the pretherapeutic assessment of resectability in patients with upper gastrointestinal malignancies. *Scand J Gastroenterol* 1996;31(11):1115–1119.
29. Blackshaw GR, et al. Laparoscopy significantly improves the perceived preoperative stage of gastric cancer. *Gastric Cancer* 2003;6(4):225–229.
30. Lowy AM, et al. Laparoscopic staging for gastric cancer. *Surgery* 1996; 119(6):611–614.
31. Sarela AI, et al. Clinical outcomes with laparoscopic stage M1, unresected gastric adenocarcinoma. *Ann Surg* 2006;243(2):189–195.
32. D'Ugo DM, et al. Immediately preoperative laparoscopic staging for gastric cancer. *Surg Endosc* 1996;10(10):996–999.
33. Badgwell B, et al. Does neoadjuvant treatment for gastric cancer patients with positive peritoneal cytology at staging laparoscopy improve survival? *Ann Surg Oncol* 2008;15(10):2684–2691.
34. Wainess RM, et al. Epidemiology of surgically treated gastric cancer in the United States, 1988–2000. *J Gastrointest Surg* 2003;7(7):879–883.
35. Adachi Y, Shiraishi N, Kitano S. Modern treatment of early gastric cancer: review of the Japanese experience. *Dig Surg* 2002;19(5):333–339.
36. Kunisaki C, et al. Prognostic factors in early gastric cancer. *Hepatogastroenterology* 2001;48(37):294–298.
37. Nakamura K, et al. An early gastric carcinoma treatment strategy based on analysis of lymph node metastasis. *Cancer* 1999;85(7):1500–1505.
38. Ono H, et al. Endoscopic mucosal resection for treatment of early gastric cancer. *Gut* 2001;48(2):225–229.
39. Korenaga D, et al. Pathological appearance of the stomach after endoscopic mucosal resection for early gastric cancer. *Br J Surg* 1997;84(11): 1563–1566.
40. Cuschieri A. Laparoscopic gastric resection. *Surg Clin North Am* 2000; 80(4):1269–1284, viii.
41. Kitano S, et al. A multicenter study on oncologic outcome of laparoscopic gastrectomy for early cancer in Japan. *Ann Surg* 2007;245(1):68–72.
42. Huscher CG, et al. Laparoscopic versus open subtotal gastrectomy for distal gastric cancer: five-year results of a randomized prospective trial. *Ann Surg* 2005;241(2):232–237.
43. Kim SH, et al. Effect of microscopic resection line disease on gastric cancer survival. *J Gastrointest Surg* 1999;3(1):24–33.
44. Bozzetti F, et al. Adequacy of margins of resection in gastrectomy for cancer. *Ann Surg* 1982;196(6):685–690.
45. Schwarz RE, Karpeh MS, Brennan MF. Factors predicting hospitalization after operative treatment for gastric carcinoma in patients older than 70 years. *J Am Coll Surg* 1997;184(1):9–15.
46. Daly JM, et al. Enteral nutrition during multimodality therapy in upper gastrointestinal cancer patients. *Ann Surg* 1995;221(4):327–338.
47. Bozzetti F, et al. Comparing reconstruction with Roux-en-Y to a pouch following total gastrectomy. *J Am Coll Surg* 1996;183(3):243–248.
48. Chareton B, et al. Prospective randomized trial comparing Billroth I and Billroth II procedures for carcinoma of the gastric antrum. *J Am Coll Surg* 1996;183(3):190–194.
49. de Almeida AC, dos Santos NM, Aldeia FJ. Long-term clinical and endoscopic assessment after total gastrectomy for cancer. *Surg Endosc* 1993; 7(6):518–523.
50. Nakane Y, et al. Jejunal pouch reconstruction after total gastrectomy for cancer. A randomized controlled trial. *Ann Surg* 1995;222(1):27–35.
51. Shiu MH, et al. Influence of the extent of resection on survival after curative treatment of gastric carcinoma. A retrospective multivariate analysis. *Arch Surg* 1987;122(11):1347–1351.
52. Maruyama K, Okabayashi K, Kinoshita T. Progress in gastric cancer surgery in Japan and its limits of radicality. *World J Surg* 1987;11(4): 418–425.
53. Noguchi Y, et al. Radical surgery for gastric cancer. A review of the Japanese experience. *Cancer* 1989;64(10):2053–2062.
54. Adachi Y, et al. Role of lymph node dissection and splenectomy in node-positive gastric carcinoma. *Surgery* 1994;116(5):837–841.
55. Baba H, et al. Effect of lymph node dissection on the prognosis in patients with node-negative early gastric cancer. *Surgery* 1995;117(2):165–169.
56. Bonenkamp JJ, et al. Extended lymph-node dissection for gastric cancer. *N Engl J Med* 1999;340(12):908–914.
57. Cuschieri A, et al. Postoperative morbidity and mortality after D1 and D2 resections for gastric cancer: preliminary results of the MRC randomised controlled surgical trial. The Surgical Cooperative Group. *Lancet* 1996; 347(9007):995–999.
58. Maeta M, et al. A prospective pilot study of extended (D3) and superextended para-aortic lymphadenectomy (D4) in patients with T3 or T4 gastric cancer managed by total gastrectomy. *Surgery* 1999;125(3):325–331.
59. Robertson CS, et al. A prospective randomized trial comparing R1 subtotal gastrectomy with R3 total gastrectomy for antral cancer. *Ann Surg* 1994;220(2):176–182.
60. Siewert JR, et al. Relevant prognostic factors in gastric cancer: ten-year results of the German Gastric Cancer Study. *Ann Surg* 1998;228(4): 449–461.
61. Lee JS, Douglass HO Jr. D2 dissection for gastric cancer. *Surg Oncol* 1997;6(4):215–225.
62. Pacelli F, et al. Extensive versus limited lymph node dissection for gastric cancer: a comparative study of 320 patients. *Br J Surg* 1993;80(9): 1153–1156.
63. Kodera Y, et al. The number of metastatic lymph nodes: a promising prognostic determinant for gastric carcinoma in the latest edition of the TNM classification. *J Am Coll Surg* 1998;187(6):597–603.
64. Maehara Y, et al. Clinical significance of occult micrometastasis lymph nodes from patients with early gastric cancer who died of recurrence. *Surgery* 1996;119(4):397–402.
65. Greene FL, Page DL, Fleming ID, et al. *AJCC Cancer Staging Manual*, 6th ed. New York: Springer; 2002.
66. Otsuji E, et al. End results of simultaneous splenectomy in patients undergoing total gastrectomy for gastric carcinoma. *Surgery* 1996;120(1): 40–44.
67. Stipa S, et al. Results of curative gastrectomy for carcinoma. *J Am Coll Surg* 1994;179(5):567–572.
68. Kunisaki C, et al. Impact of splenectomy in patients with gastric adenocarcinoma of the cardia. *J Gastrointest Surg* 2007;11(8):1039–1044.
69. Shchepotin IB, et al. Extended surgical resection in T4 gastric cancer. *Am J Surg* 1998;175(2):123–126.
70. Macdonald JS, et al. Chemoradiotherapy after surgery compared with surgery alone for adenocarcinoma of the stomach or gastroesophageal junction. *N Engl J Med* 2001;345(10):725–730.
71. Cunningham D, et al. Perioperative chemotherapy versus surgery alone for resectable gastroesophageal cancer. *N Engl J Med* 2006;355(1):11–20.
72. Isaacson PG. Gastrointestinal lymphoma. *Hum Pathol* 1994;25(10): 1020–1029.
73. Isaacson PG. Gastric lymphoma and *Helicobacter pylori*. *N Engl J Med* 1994;330(18):1310–1311.
74. Parsonnet J, et al. *Helicobacter pylori* infection and gastric lymphoma. *N Engl J Med* 1994;330(18):1267–1271.
75. Montalban C, et al. Gastric B-cell mucosa-associated lymphoid tissue (MALT) lymphoma. Clinicopathological study and evaluation of the prognostic factors in 143 patients. *Ann Oncol* 1995;6(4):355–362.
76. Yoon SS, et al. The diminishing role of surgery in the treatment of gastric lymphoma. *Ann Surg* 2004;240(1):28–37.
77. Bayerdorffer E, et al. Regression of primary gastric lymphoma of mucosa-associated lymphoid tissue type after cure of *Helicobacter pylori* infection. MALT Lymphoma Study Group. *Lancet* 1995;345(8965):1591–1594.
78. Neubauer A, et al. Cure of *Helicobacter pylori* infection and duration of remission of low-grade gastric mucosa-associated lymphoid tissue lymphoma. *J Natl Cancer Inst* 1997;89(18):1350–1355.
79. Pinotti G, et al. Clinical features, treatment and outcome in a series of 93 patients with low-grade gastric MALT lymphoma. *Leuk Lymphoma* 1997; 26(5–6):527–537.
80. Stephens J, Smith J. Treatment of primary gastric lymphoma and gastric mucosa-associated lymphoid tissue lymphoma. *J Am Coll Surg* 1998; 187(3):312–320.
81. Bartlett DL, et al. Long-term follow-up after curative surgery for early gastric lymphoma. *Ann Surg* 1996;223(1):53–62.
82. Aviles A, et al. The role of surgery in primary gastric lymphoma: results of a controlled clinical trial. *Ann Surg* 2004;240(1):44–50.
83. Modlin IM, et al. Current status of gastrointestinal carcinoids. *Gastroenterology* 2005;128(6):1717–1751.
84. Landry CS, et al. A proposed staging system for gastric carcinoid tumors based on an analysis of 1,543 patients. *Ann Surg Oncol* 2009;16(1):51–60.
85. Gold JS, Dematteo RP. Combined surgical and molecular therapy: the gastrointestinal stromal tumor model. *Ann Surg* 2006;244(2):176–184.
86. Antonescu CR. Targeted therapies in gastrointestinal stromal tumors. *Semin Diagn Pathol* 2008;25(4):295–303.

GASTROINTESTINAL

CHAPTER 47 ■ ANATOMY AND PHYSIOLOGY OF THE SMALL INTESTINE

ERIC T. KIMCHI, NIRAJ J. GUSANI, AND JUSSUF T. KAIFI

KEY POINTS

1. The normal adult anatomy of the small intestine is the result of a complex cascade of embryological events, which results in 270 degrees of total rotation of the bowel around its axis. A failure of these precise steps produces a spectrum of anatomical variants that are grouped together as malrotation of the intestinal tract.
2. There is no clear anatomic boundary between the jejunum and ileum. The proximal two fifths of the small intestine distal to the ligament of Treitz has been arbitrarily defined as *jejunum* and the distal three fifths as ileum.
3. The enteric nervous system contains two major plexuses. The first is the myenteric (Auerbach's) plexus, located between the longitudinal and circular muscle layers.
4. The second major plexus of the enteric nervous system is the submucosal (Meissner's) plexus.
5. The small intestine is the largest endocrine organ in the human body. The secretion of these numerous hormones and neurotransmitters is specific to distinct anatomic zones within the small intestine.
6. The coordination of movements of the gastrointestinal tract is necessary for the proper digestion of food. Well-timed contraction and relaxation patterns are initiated in the gastrointestinal nervous system causing coordinated electrical activity and muscular movements.
7. The lumen of the gastrointestinal tract is connected to the outside environment and comes in direct contact with many potentially pathogenic microorganisms. Consequently, the small intestine has a complex defense mechanism to battle against these exposures in different ways.
8. The small intestine reabsorbs nearly 80% of the fluid that passes through it. This dynamic process is accomplished by a rapid bidirectional movement of fluid in the intestinal lumen. This ebb and flow of fluid in the intestinal lumen is critical in maintaining normal homeostasis. Minor changes in intestinal permeability or rate of flow of the intestinal contents can result in net secretion and diarrheal states.

The small intestine's intrinsic design serves to provide a maximum amount of surface area for absorption of nutrients, water, and electrolytes. Specialized areas provide neurohormonal stimulation to the digestive tract. Its structure and vast surface area also provide an important physical barrier to potential pathogens, and certain areas are critical in immune surveillance.

GROSS ANATOMY AND EMBRYOLOGY

The small intestine spans from the pylorus to the ileocecal valve and includes three distinct regions: the duodenum, the jejunum, and the ileum. These areas combined measure, on average, approximately 5 meters and comprise nearly 62% of the entire length of the alimentary tract. The gastrointestinal tract is formed from the endodermal layer of the developing embryo. The small intestine is derived from the distal foregut (proximal duodenum), the midgut, and the adjacent splanchnic mesenchyme. Epithelium and glands develop from the embryonic endoderm, while connective tissue, muscle, and serosa develop from the mesoderm. During the fifth and sixth weeks of development, the duodenal lumen is temporarily obliterated due to proliferation of its mucosal lining. During the subsequent weeks, luminal vacuolization and degeneration of some of the proliferating cells result in recanalization of the
1 duodenal lumen. From the 4th to the 10th week of development, a large portion of the midgut is herniated through the umbilicus. This may be due to the rapid growth of the intestinal tract at this time in relation to the abdominal cavity. At approximately 8 weeks of gestation, the midgut begins to rotate in a counterclockwise manner 90 degrees around the axis of the mesenteric vasculature. The extra-abdominal portion of the gut returns to the abdominal cavity approximately 2 weeks later. Around this time point an additional 180-degree rotation occurs. These two rotations provide 270 degrees of total rotation and result in the typical anatomy that is found in humans. A failure of these precise steps produces a spectrum of anatomic variants that are grouped together as malrotation of the intestinal tract.[1]

Duodenum

The duodenum makes up the first portion of the small intestine and plays an important role in connecting the foregut organs to the midgut. It anatomically begins at the duodenal bulb, which is immediately adjacent to the pylorus and terminates at the ligament of Treitz, where it joins the jejunum. The duodenum is approximately 20 to 30 cm in length and is divided into four distinct areas.

The first portion of the duodenum is approximately 5 cm in length and is referred to as the bulb or cap. This area is directly attached to the pylorus and extends laterally and cephalad. It serves as an attachment for the hepatoduodenal ligament and traverses over the common bile duct, portal vein, pancreatic head, and gastroduodenal artery. The mucosal surface of the duodenal bulb is smooth until its junction with the second portion of the duodenum, where the concentric Kerckring folds begin. This portion of the duodenum is prone to ulceration, with approximately 90% of duodenal ulcers occurring here. Unfortunately, due to its anatomic positioning, these ulcers may erode into the gastroduodenal artery, which lies

FIGURE 47.1. Arterial blood supply to the duodenum.

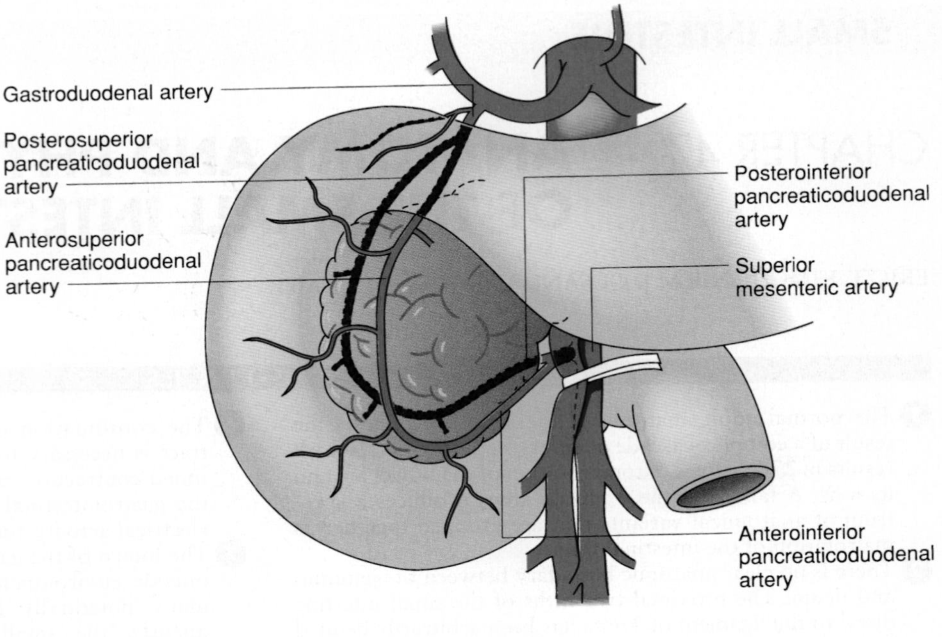

directly posterior to the duodenum, causing potentially life-threatening bleeding.

The second portion of the duodenum (descending duodenum) extends from the origin of the Kerckring folds to the beginning of the transverse duodenum and travels over the right renal vasculature, over the medial aspect of Gerota fascia, over the inferior vena cava, and to the right of the L1 and L2 vertebra. It is approximately 10 cm in length and 3 to 5 cm in diameter. The Kerckring folds (plicae circulares) are concentric mucosal folds that are 1 to 2 mm thick and 2 to 4 mm high and are separated by 2 to 4 mm of smooth, flat mucosa. This portion of the duodenum serves as an entry point for pancreatic and biliary secretions into the gastrointestinal tract. This is typically through the major papilla (ampulla of Vater), which is a valvular structure that arises in the midportion of the descending duodenum, approximately 7 to 10 cm from the pylorus. Through this point the confluence of the common bile duct and the main pancreatic duct (duct of Wirsung) join the duodenum. The valvular function of the papilla is regulated through the muscular sphincter of Oddi. The minor pancreatic duct (duct of Santorini) enters through a minor papilla proximal to the ampulla of Vater in 50% to 60% of patients and endoscopically appears as a 1- to 3-mm polypoid structure.

The second portion of the duodenum is important surgically as it represents the entry of the duodenum into the retroperitoneum. Surgical evaluation of this part of the duodenum requires mobilization from its posterior and lateral attachments, described as a Kocher maneuver. This allows for further evaluation of the duodenum, pancreatic head, and bile duct.

The third (transverse) and fourth (ascending) portion of the duodenum complete the duodenal sweep. The third portion of the duodenum is about 10 cm in length and courses transversely from right to left, crossing the midline anterior to the spine, aorta, and inferior vena cava. This portion is closely attached to the uncinate process of the pancreas. The superior mesenteric artery (SMA) and vein (SMV) course anterior to the third portion of the duodenum to provide blood supply to the gut. The transition between the third and fourth portion of the duodenum is marked by the passage of the SMA in front of the duodenum. The SMA forms an acute angle as it originates from the aorta. An abnormally narrow angle can result in obstruction of the duodenum at this location (SMA syndrome). The fourth portion of the duodenum is approximately 5 cm long and courses upward and obliquely to reach the ligament of Treitz, marking the end of the duodenum and the return of the small bowel to the peritoneal cavity.

Following its embryologic origins, the vascular supply to the duodenum arises from branches of the celiac trunk for the foregut portion, whereas the distal (midgut origin) duodenum is supplied by branches of the SMA (Fig. 47.1). Venous drainage includes a series of pancreaticoduodenal veins that drain into the SMV–portal vein system. Lymphatic drainage follows the vascular supply with drainage to the pancreaticoduodenal nodes. From here, lymph drains superiorly to the hepatic nodes or inferiorly to the superior mesenteric nodes.

Jejunum and Ileum

2 Distal to the ligament of Treitz, the jejunum and ileum form the remainder of the small intestine. The boundary between the two is arbitrarily determined such that 40% of the intraperitoneal small intestine is composed of jejunum and 60% is composed of ileum. This portion of the bowel is suspended within the peritoneal cavity by a thin, broad-based mesentery that is attached to the posterior abdominal wall. The jejunum and ileum are freely mobile within the peritoneal cavity. The jejunum is the widest portion of the small intestine, whose caliber progressively decreases as it approaches the ileocecal valve. The mucosa of the jejunum has a thick lining and is characterized by prominent plicae circulares that become shorter and less frequent in the ileum. The total length of jejunum and ileum varies, but is usually 3 to 7 meters, with an average length of 5 meters. The small intestine terminates in the right lower quadrant at the ileocecal valve. The ileocecal valve exhibits motor characteristics separate from the terminal ileum and colon, postulated to prevent reflux of fecal material from the colon into the small intestine.[2]

The arterial blood supply of the jejunum and the ileum arises from the superior mesenteric artery. The main vascular branches form arcades within the mesentery. The vasa recta, intestinal arterial branches, enter into the intestinal wall without anastomosing. The vasa recta of the jejunum are straight and long, in contrast to the vasa recta of the ileum, which are shorter with greater arborization (Fig. 47.2). The venous and lymphatic drainage follow the arterial supply. The main venous outflow is through the superior mesenteric vein, which, along with the splenic vein, becomes the portal vein.

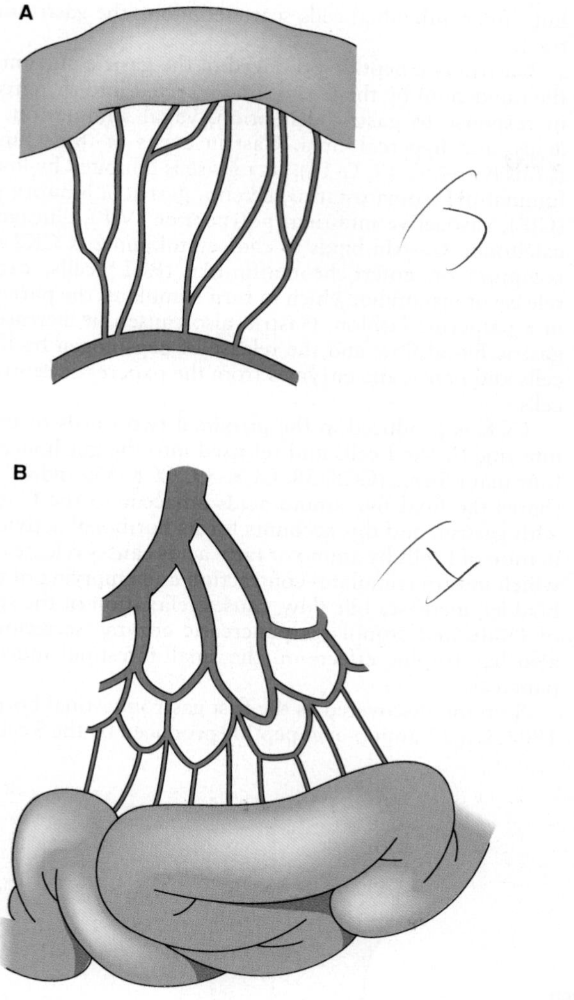

FIGURE 47.2. The superior mesenteric artery supplies blood flow into the small intestinal arteries (vasa recta), which branch within the mesentery. In the jejunum (A), the vasa recta are straight and long, in contrast to the vasa recta within the ileum (B), which are shorter with greater arborization.

MICROSCOPIC ANATOMY

General Considerations

The wall of the small intestine is composed of four distinct layers: mucosa, submucosa, muscle, and serosa. The role of the mucosa is absorption and secretion. The luminal mucosal surface forms circular folds known as plica circularis or valvulae conniventes in all segments of the small intestine distal to the first portion of the duodenum. The submucosa contains an elaborate network of blood vessels, lymphatics,
3 and nerves. The muscular portion of the wall includes outer longitudinal and inner circular muscle layers. Between the muscle layers lies the myenteric (Auerbach) plexus. The muscular layers are responsible for coordinating peristaltic movements. The outermost layer, the serosa, is composed of a thin layer of mesothelial cells overlying loose connective tissue. The serosa covers only the anterior surface of the retroperitoneal segments of small bowel, but it completely covers the portions of small bowel that are invested with mesentery.

Mucosa

The mucosa lines the luminal surface of the small intestine. It consists of three layers: epithelial cells, lamina propria, and a narrow layer of smooth muscle, the muscularis mucosae. The basic structural units of the mucosa are crypts and villi. Villi are fingerlike projections of mucosa 0.5 to 1 mm high extending into the intestinal lumen that have a columnar epithelial surface and a cellular connective tissue core of lamina propria. Each villus contains a central lacteal (lymphatic) and a vascular network consisting of a small artery, vein, and capillaries. Ninety percent of the cells of the villi are columnar epithelial cells responsible for absorption and secretion. These cells are 22 to 25 μm high with basally located nuclei. The apices of these cells have microvilli, produced by numerous folds in the apical membrane, which account for the brush border appearance. Microvilli are approximately 1 μm long and 0.08 μm wide. Their surface is coated by glycoproteins rooted in the cell membrane. These glycoprotein filaments are referred to as the glycocalyx and are essential for digestion and absorption.[3] The lateral membranes of neighboring enterocytes are connected by tight junctions, an apparent fusion of adjoining plasma membranes just below the level of the brush border. Movement of ions and water can occur by either a transmembrane or a paracellular route through tight junctions, which behave as selective pores.

Between the villi lie the crypts of Lieberkühn. Stem cells within the crypts of Lieberkühn are the source of the four major types of differentiated cells: the absorptive enterocyte, goblet cells, enteroendocrine cells, and Paneth cells. Absorptive enterocytes differentiate as they migrate from the crypt compartment up toward the tip of the intestinal villus. Cells then undergo apoptosis and are shed into the intestinal lumen. Most of the intestinal lining is renewed over a period of approximately 5 days. Despite the rapid rate of cellular turnover, intestinal epithelial cells exhibit complex patterns of gene expression that vary according to their location on the two main spatial axes of the gut, the vertical (crypt–villus) and horizontal (proximal to distal) axes. For example, cells destined to become enterocytes do not begin to express a variety of genes important in digestion and absorption until the cells have migrated out of the crypt and up the villus. In addition, many epithelial cell genes are selectively expressed in the proximal small intestine, whereas other genes are specifically expressed only in the ileum.[4]

Several other cell types are present in the mucosa. Mucus-secreting goblet cells are present in both the crypts and villi. Goblet cells have a narrow base containing the nucleus and a wide apical membrane with a large number of granules containing mucin. Mucin is secreted in a combination of merocine and apocrine fashion by the goblet cell, functions as a lubricant, and has a cytoprotective function.[5]

Paneth cells are pyramidal cells that reside in the crypt base. They contain large eosinophilic secretory granules located at their apical surface. It is thought that Paneth cells play a role in host defense based on their abundant expression of lysozymes and defensins, a family of small peptides that are also found in human neutrophils and exhibit microbicidal activity toward many different bacterial organisms in vitro. However, examination of the role of Paneth cells in the small intestine by lineage ablation in transgenic mice revealed no alteration in host defense mechanisms; thus, the actual function of Paneth cells has yet to be delineated.[6]

Enteroendocrine (also referred to as *amine precursor uptake and decarboxylation*, or *APUD*) cells may reside in either the crypts or the villi, depending on the particular neuroendocrine substance they produce. Specific areas of the small intestine have higher concentrations of specific neuroendocrine substances than other areas. These cells do not contact the intestinal lumen, unlike exocrine cells, and their secretory granules are located below the nucleus near the basement membrane. This suggests that these cells secrete their contents into the circulation rather than into the intestinal lumen.

Submucosa

4 The submucosa is a dense connective tissue layer with a rich network of blood vessels, nerves, and lymphatics. The submucosa contains the Meissner plexus and is the strongest layer of the intestinal wall. Brunner glands are found in the submucosa of the duodenum and secrete mucus and bicarbonate into the intestinal lumen. These secretions aid in the neutralization of the gastric acid load that enters the duodenum. Peyer patches are localized collections of lymphoid follicles that are most prominent in the submucosa of the ileum. These are typically 8 to 10 mm in diameter and are most abundant early in life, gradually disappearing with age.

PHYSIOLOGY

5 The small intestine plays important physiologic roles in motility, blood flow, growth, digestion, absorption, immune function, and endocrine secretion. In fact, the small intestine is the largest endocrine organ in the human body.[7] The secretion of these numerous hormones and neurotransmitters is specific to distinct anatomic zones within the small intestine (Fig. 47.3). There is no specific cell mass that produces these hormones, but rather individual cells scattered along the gastrointestinal tract.

Gastrin is a peptide produced in the gastric antrum and in the duodenum by the G cells and secreted into the circulation in response to gastric distention, vagal stimulation, amino acids, and hypercalcemia. Gastrin exists in three functional forms (G-34, G-17, G-14). Its release is inhibited by low intraluminal pH, somatostatin, secretin, gastric inhibitory peptide (GIP), vasoactive intestinal polypeptide (VIP), glucagon, and calcitonin. Gastrin binds to cholecystokinin 2 (CCK2)/gastrin receptors on enterochromaffin-like (ECL) cells, causing a release of histamine, which in turn stimulates the parietal cells in a paracrine fashion. Gastrin also causes an increase in the gastric blood flow and the release of pepsinogen by the chief cells and pancreatic enzymes from the pancreatic centroacinar cells.

CCK is produced in the proximal two thirds of the small intestine by the I cells and released into the gut lumen. It has four main forms (CCK-58, CCK-39, CCK-33, and CCK-8). It shares the final five amino acids adjacent to the C-terminus with gastrin, and this accounts for its hormonal activity. Stimulation of I cells by amino or fatty acids causes release of CCK, which in turn stimulates contraction and emptying of the gallbladder, increases bile flow, causes relaxation of the sphincter of Oddi, and stimulates pancreatic enzyme secretion. CCK also has trophic effects on the small-intestinal mucosa and pancreas.

Secretin, discovered as the first gastrointestinal hormone in 1902, is a 27-amino-acid peptide produced by the S cells of the

FIGURE 47.3. Distribution of peptide hormones in the gastrointestinal tract.

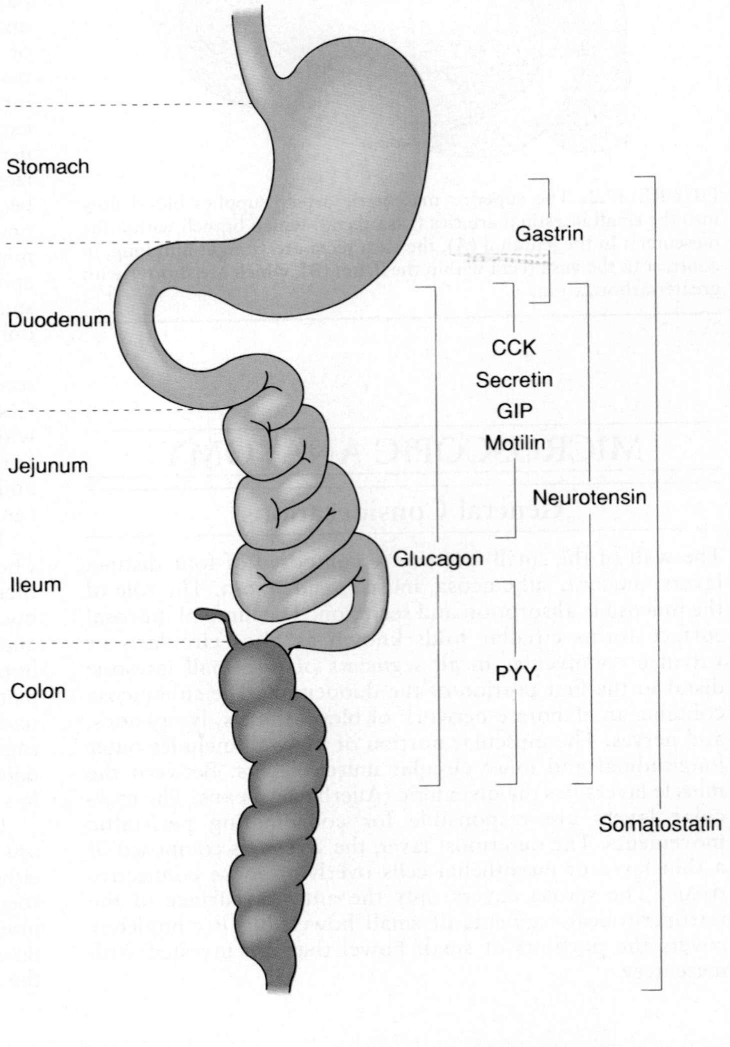

duodenum and jejunum. Secretin is released into the circulation and intestinal lumen in response to low intraluminal pH, fatty acids, and bile salts. Water and bicarbonate are secreted by the pancreas in response to secretin. Bicarbonate is also released from the biliary ductal epithelium and Brunner's glands in response to secretin. In turn, pancreatic enzymes are released from the pancreas. The increased pH and the presence of pancreatic enzymes aids in the digestion of lipids. The increased pH also provides a negative feedback loop to inhibit further production of secretin. Secretin produces a paradoxical release of gastrin in patients with gastrinomas, but does not produce this effect on normal individuals.

Somatostatin is a peptide hormone consisting of 14 or 28 amino acids and is produced by D cells in the pancreatic islets, gastric antrum, and duodenum. Its primary role is inhibition of other gastrointestinal hormones and inhibition of pancreatic, biliary, and gastric secretion. In addition, somatostatin decreases splanchnic and portal blood flow. Somatostatin is stimulated by the presence of fat, proteins, acid, glucose, amino acids, and cholecystokinin. Octreotide, a long-acting synthetic somatostatin analogue, is used in the treatment of variceal bleeding, hormone-secreting neuroendocrine tumors, carcinoid syndrome, and enterocutaneous and pancreatic fistulas.[8]

Gastrin-releasing peptide, the mammalian homologue of bombesin, is a 27-amino-acid peptide that is produced by the small intestine and is released in response to vagal stimulation. It is a prostimulatory molecule that causes the release of most gastrointestinal hormones, with the exception of secretin. It also has a promotility effect and stimulates endothelial proliferation. GIP or glucose-dependent insulinotropic peptide is a 42-amino-acid peptide produced by the K cells of the duodenum and jejunum. It is released in response to glucose, fat, protein, and adrenergic stimulation. It stimulates secretion of insulin and inhibits gastric acid and pepsin production. Type 2 diabetics are resistant to the effects of GIP.

Motilin is a 22-amino-acid peptide produced by the enteroendocrine cells in the duodenum and jejunum. Release of motilin occurs during the interdigestive and fasting periods. Release may also be related to alkalinization of the duodenum. Motilin's main function is to stimulate the migrating myoelectric complex. Motilin agonists such as erythromycin are used clinically as stimulants of gastrointestinal motility.

VIP is a 28-amino-acid peptide that is produced by gastrointestinal tract neurons. It serves as a neurotransmitter stimulating pancreatic exocrine and intestinal secretion. Conversely, it has an inhibitory effect on gastric acid secretion. VIP is a potent vasodilator and relaxant of smooth muscle.

Neurotensin is a 13-amino-acid peptide that is produced by the N cells primarily in the ileum, but also in the proximal small intestine and colon in response to the presence of intraluminal fat. It stimulates pancreatic bicarbonate secretion and intestinal motility. Neurotensin also serves as a trophic factor on the small-intestinal mucosa and inhibits gastric secretion.

Pancreatic glucagon and enteroglucagon are 29- and 37-amino-acid peptides produced by the α-islet cells of the pancreas and the L cells of the small intestine, respectively. Pancreatic glucagon is released in response to low serum glucose and subsequently induces glycogenolysis, lipolysis, gluconeogenesis, and ketogenesis. Enteroglucagon is released in response to the presence of a mixed meal and inhibits gastric emptying and small-bowel motility.

Motility

6 The coordination of movements of the gastrointestinal tract is necessary for the proper digestion of food. Well-timed contraction and relaxation patterns are initiated in the gastrointestinal nervous system causing coordinated electrical activity and muscular movements. This may be influenced by both internal and external factors. The small intestine has motor functions that are distinct from the other parts of the gastrointestinal tract. The intrinsic nerves (myenteric or Auerbach plexus) provide the basis for coordinating the circular and longitudinal smooth muscles of the small intestine. Extrinsic sympathetic (epinephrine) stimulation slows motility, while parasympathetic (acetylcholine) stimulation increases motility (Fig. 47.4).

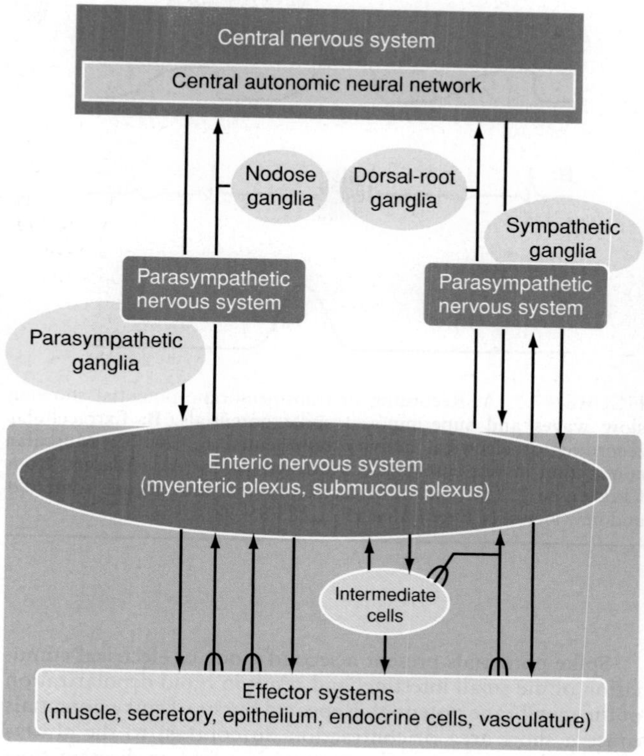

FIGURE 47.4. Innervation of the gastrointestinal tract. The neural plexuses in the gut represent an independently functioning network, the enteric nervous system, which is connected to the central autonomic neural network in the central nervous system by parasympathetic and sympathetic nerves. The enteric nervous system may influence the effector system in the gut directly, or indirectly through its actions on intermediate cells, which include endocrine cells and cells of the immune system. The cell bodies of the primary vagal and primary splanchnic afferent neurons are located in the nodose ganglia and dorsal root ganglia, respectively; each carries distinct information from the gut to the central nervous system. The *pitchfork* symbols represent afferent nerve endings, and the *arrows* show the direction of neural transmission. (Adapted from Goyal RK, Hirano I. Mechanisms of disease: the enteric nervous system. *N Engl J Med* 1996;334:1106–1115.)

The intrinsic electrical activity of the small intestine is based on the intestinal smooth muscle normal resting potential. This normally is −50 to −70 mV and is maintained by Na^+-K^+-ATPase activity.[9] The resting potential varies by 5 to 15 mV and results in a phasic depolarization, which is referred to as slow waves, basic electrical rhythm, or pacemaker potential. These depolarizations occur at regular intervals of approximately 11 to 13 times per minute in the duodenum and decrease to 8 to 10 times in the ileum, but do not directly lead to muscular contractions. The electrical activity is coupled to muscular contraction at the level of gap junctions, which are low-resistance cell-to-cell connections. These gap junctions become less regular in the midjejunum and in the distal small intestine. This causes slowing of the frequency of contractions distally, allowing for absorption of more slowly digested intestinal contents, including fats and bile salts.

GASTROINTESTINAL

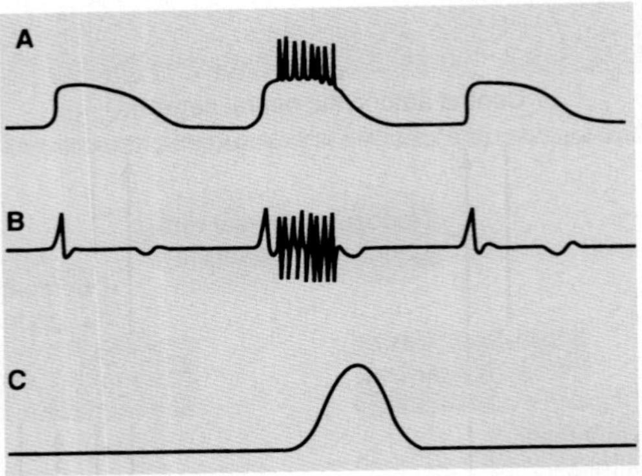

FIGURE 47.5. **A:** Recording of transmembrane potential showing slow waves and superimposed spike potentials. **B:** Extracellular recording of electrical activity represented in (A). **C:** Muscular contraction in response to electrical activity in (A). (Adapted from Christensen J. The control of gastrointestinal movements: some old and new views. *N Engl J Med* 1971;285:85–98.)

Spike potentials present a second mode of electrical stimulation of the small intestine, and result in rapid depolarization of the membrane potential. Repeated bursts of spike potentials cause a short area of contraction. In contrast to the always present slow waves, spike potentials occur at discrete time intervals. The coordination of a slow wave and a spike potential leads to the initiation, duration, and frequency of rhythmic migratory small-intestinal contractions (Fig. 47.5).

During the interdigestive period between feeding, the small intestine follows a well-defined rhythmic pattern. This pattern consists of muscular contractions that migrate from the stomach or duodenum, continue on to the terminal ileum, and are regulated by the migrating motor complex (MMC). This pattern can be broken down into four distinct phases. Phase I is a period of relative quiescence, phase II is a period of accelerated irregular electrical spiking and muscular activity, phase III is a series of high-amplitude rapid electrical spikes corresponding to rhythmic gut contractions, and phase IV is a period of subsiding activity. This process occurs over a period of 90 to 120 minutes and progresses from the proximal small bowel and terminates in the ileum. Once the MMC reaches the terminal ileum, the process starts over again in the proximal small bowel. The circular muscles provide segmental contraction over a 1-cm length of small intestine. These contractions occur approximately 11 to 13 times per minute in the duodenum and decrease to 8 to 10 times in the ileum. This creates functional compartments where prolonged exposure to the mucosa and mixing of the intestinal chyme occur, aiding the process of digestion and absorption. The circular muscles are also responsible for the peristaltic waves, which propagate regularly at a rate of 1 to 2 cm per second. These regular waves may be interspersed with rushes of contractions followed by periods of no motor activity. This rate becomes progressively slower in the distal small intestine. These peristaltic movements serve as a method of propelling chyme through the length of the small intestine. The total transit time from the duodenum to the terminal ileum is approximately 220 minutes (± 53 minutes).[10] Serum motilin levels have been found to mirror the activity of the MMC. Exogenous motilin administration has been found to increase MMC activity.

During and immediately following times of feeding, the intestinal movements are not rhythmic, with complexes of peristaltic and antiperistaltic contractions. This is thought to be a disruption of the MMC from bolus feeding. This seemingly random pattern of movements allows for effective mixing of chyme. Hormonal changes are thought to play a role in this process. Physiologic doses of neurotensin, insulin, gastrin, and CCK cause an alteration in the MMC similar to bolus feeding. Visual and olfactory feeding cues can also cause a disruption of the MMC. The MMC is more significantly inhibited by fatty meals as opposed to protein or carbohydrate meals of similar caloric value. The intrinsic nervous plexus or Meissner plexus innervating the submucosa helps to regulate mucosal absorption and secretion, but has no control on motility.

Immunology

7 **Principles of Gut Immunology.** The lumen of the gastrointestinal tract is connected to the outside environment and comes in direct contact with many potentially pathogenic microorganisms. Lymphocytes, macrophages, polymorphic granulocytes, and other cells that take part in the immune response are distributed throughout the whole gut. The commensal microflora have many benefits to the host by supporting digestion and keeping the appropriate balance among different microbial species.[11] The immune system is highly effective at responding selectively to invading pathogens yet on the other hand tolerating a much larger number of harmless food antigens and commensal organisms. Many bacteria, viruses, and parasites are digested and enter the small intestine every day.[12] Consequently, the small intestine needs a complex defense mechanism to battle against these exposures in different ways.[13]

While the immune system in the small intestine is important for host defense, other mechanisms within the small intestine also participate in host defense. Proteolytic and lipolytic enzymes are produced in high concentrations by extraintestinal cells in the pancreas and degrade different pathogenic agents at an early phase of digestion. In addition, mucin is produced by the enterocytes, which protects them and inhibits bacterial growth. Actively increased peristalsis functions to mechanically get rid of pathogenic agents and potentially dangerous gut content. In addition, tight junctions between epithelial cells prevent penetration of bacteria in between cells. Potential pathogens vary greatly in size, from very small viruses that are nanometers in size to parasites such as helminths that are macroscopically visible and quite large. To put this into the broader picture of evolution, a large range of defense mechanisms is essential for survival of each individual.

The primary cellular barrier in the gut that prevents antigens from encountering the immune system is the single layer of gut epithelium. The total surface area of the small intestine is 400 m^2, due not only to intestinal length but also to the formation of millions of villi in the small bowel, which contribute significantly to the overall surface area.[14] In the upper small intestine, the bulk of antigen exposure comes from the diet, whereas in the ileum and colon, the additional antigenic load of an abundant and highly complex commensal microflora is prevalent. The epithelial cells of the gut mucosa have developed features that make the intestinal epithelium an active immunologic as well as anatomic barrier. For example, these nonclassical immune cells express major histocompatibility complex (MHC) class I and II molecules, consistent with their ability to participate in adaptive immune recognition of pathogenic bacteria. Small-intestinal epithelial cells also express Toll-like receptors on their apical surface that enables them to detect bacterial products and to initiate an innate immune response. Antigen-presenting dendritic cells (DCs) also send processes between gut epithelial cells without disturbing tight junction integrity and sample commensal and pathogenic gut bacteria.[15,16] The gut epithelial barrier therefore represents a highly flexible structure that limits antigens from entering the systemic circulation.

The gut-associated immune system represents one of the largest immunologic compartments in the body. Lymphoid tissue in the gastrointestinal tract is a major part of the whole body immune system and consists of both aggregated (lymphoid follicles, Peyer patches) and nonaggregated (luminal, intraepithelial, and in lamina propria) immune cells. Under physiologic circumstances, oral administration of protein antigens induces systemic unresponsiveness when the same antigen is given parenterally (a phenomenon known as oral tolerance). In animal models, oral tolerance appears to be a specific consequence of the immune environment in the gut, which favors the generation of regulatory T cells.

Nonaggregated and Aggregated Lymphoid Tissue.

The gut epithelium and its mucous layer form a major barrier to trap pathogens, which are then eliminated when the gut epithelium is shed and replaced by new cells deriving from stem cells in the crypts. Several different cell types face antigenic exposure present in the intestinal lumen and include the epithelium, neutrophils, lymphocytes, and macrophages. These luminal cells represent an initial effector mechanism in the first front directed toward an antigenic exposure. In addition, there are also intraepithelial lymphocytes, which migrate and are found between epithelial cells beneath the tight junctions. Local defense depends in part on these T lymphocytes that are nestled among gut epithelial cells. These T cells modulate homeostasis of the gut epithelium through local production of cytokines and have cytolytic effects. In fact, the number of intraepithelial lymphocytes can increase dramatically in response to inflammation or infection. After exposure to antigens, these cells reenter the circulation to initiate a systemic immune response. The lamina propria contains nonaggregated, diffusely distributed lymphoid tissue, including different types of immune cells (Fig. 47.6). B cells in the lamina propria undergo cytokine-induced differentiation in the lamina propria to become active producers of immunoglobulin A (IgA), which is secreted into the gut lumen. T cells in the lamina propria may have a different role in a helper–inducer function for immunoglobulin production rather than a cytolytic function. Mast cells and eosinophils are also present in the lamina propria in small numbers. They exhibit an important role in allergic and hypersensitivity reactions as well as defense against parasites. Parasites including worms are recognized and tagged using monovalent IgE, which is mostly bound to host cell surfaces. Actual parasite killing depends on toxic proteins secreted by eosinophils.

There are also large aggregates of lymphoid tissue found in the small intestine. These so-called Peyer patches are localized collections of lymphoid follicles that are most prominent and macroscopically visible in the submucosa of the ileum. Peyer patches are most prominent in children and gradually disappear with age. Along with the nonaggregated immune system, the enormous quantity and diversity of antigens present within the gut are also processed via Peyer patches in the lamina propria and the mucosa-associated lymphoid tissue (MALT), which in total contains about 70% of the body's lymphoid cells. Another often used term to describe the immune system within the small intestine is gut-associated lymphoid tissue (GALT). Peyer patches do not have any villi, and so-called microfold (M) cells concentrated within the epithelium allow the selective uptake of food antigens and microorganisms (Fig. 47.7). M cells are specific cells in the intestinal epithelium over lymphoid follicles that endocytose antigens. M cells transport them into the underlying tissue, where they are taken up by local dendritic cells and macrophages.[17] Dendritic cells and macrophages that receive antigens from M cells present them to T cells in the gut-associated lymphoid tissue, leading ultimately to the appearance of IgA-secreting plasma cells in the mucosa. B-lymphocyte precursors proliferate in germinal centers within the Peyer patches. Dendritic cells below the epithelium can also take up luminal antigens by pushing pseudopods up between epithelial cells.

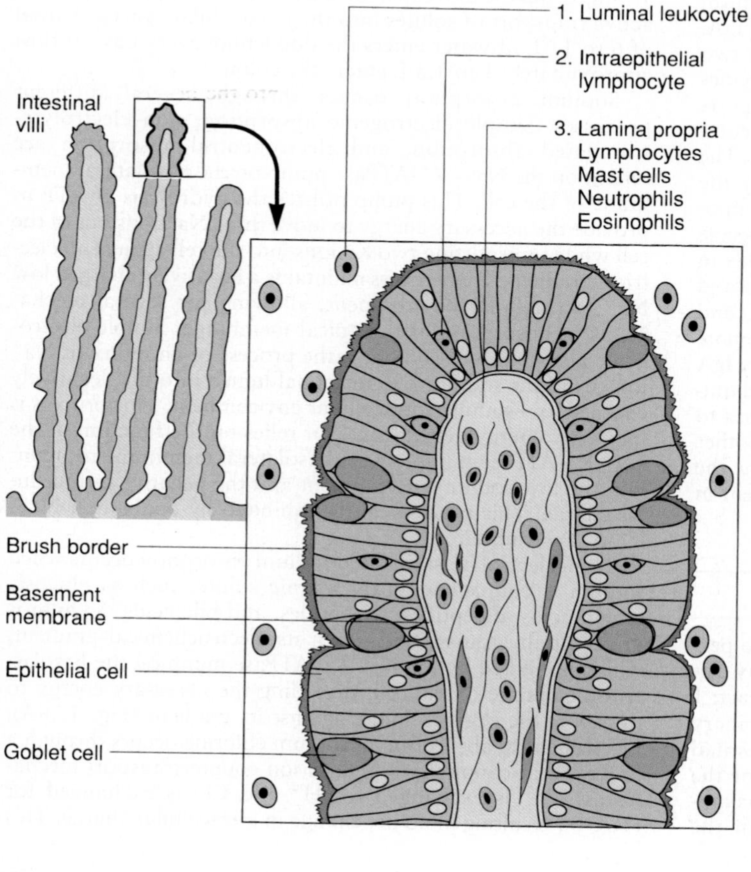

FIGURE 47.6. Small-intestinal villus with associated immunologic cells.

FIGURE 47.7. Epithelial anatomy in the area of Peyer patches.

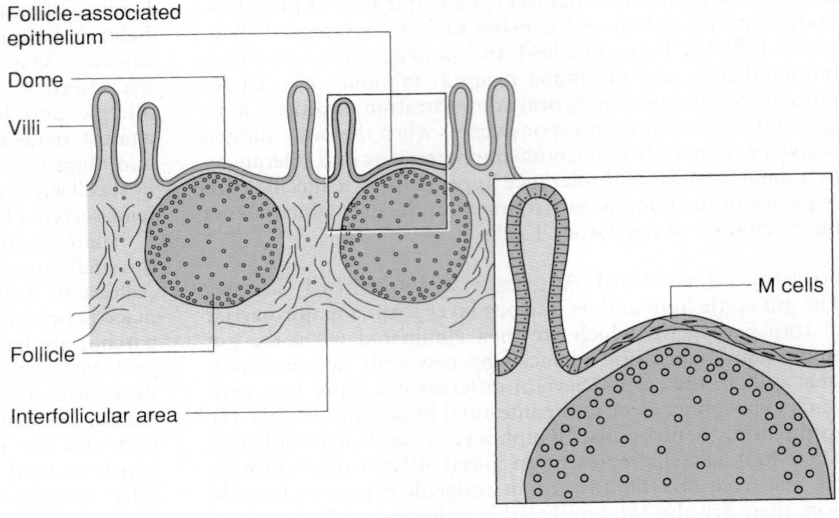

Immunoglobulin Secretion. At an early level of exposure at the gut epithelium, M cells take up antigen and transport it transcellularly using an endocytic mechanism into the underlying lymphoid tissues of Peyer patches. Lymphocyte activation ensues, and these activated lymphocytes migrate into afferent lymphatics, pass through mesenteric lymph nodes, and enter the systemic circulation through the thoracic duct. During this process, the lymphocytes mature into B and T lymphoblasts with an enriched population of IgA-producing B cells.[18] Passage of viable bacteria from the intact gastrointestinal tract to the mesenteric lymph node and beyond has been termed *bacterial translocation*, possibly explaining septic complications and multiple organ failure in peritonitis, burn, and trauma patients. The immunogenic integrity of the mucosa is significantly damaged by systemic injury of different kinds. A major protective mechanism of the intestinal immune system is synthesis and secretion of IgA. In the intestine, IgA exists as a dimer that is linked with two additional molecules—the J chain—linking two IgA molecules and the polymeric immunoglobulin receptor, which transports the IgA complex across the cell and allows release of the complex, termed *secretory component,* into the intestinal lumen. The transmembrane immunoglobulin receptor is produced by the intestinal epithelial cell. It is thought that the secretory component may prevent proteolytic degradation of the IgA molecule and may stabilize the structure of the polymeric IgA complex in an environment containing numerous proteolytic enzymes and bacteria that would otherwise rapidly degrade it. Unlike IgG and IgM, IgA does not activate complement and does not promote cell-mediated opsonization. The major function of secretory IgA in host defense is protection against bacteria, viruses, and luminal antigens. Secretory IgA inhibits the adherence of bacteria to epithelial cells. It is well known that a breast-feeding mother transfers secretory IgA to her nursing infant, protecting the infant from bacteria and viruses that were originally present in the mother's gastrointestinal tract.

Digestion and Absorption

Absorption of Water and Electrolytes. An average person consumes approximately 1 to 1.5 L of water per day. An additional 5 to 10 L is secreted by the gastrointestinal tract: 1 to 2 L of saliva, 2 to 3 L of gastric secretions, 0.5 L of biliary secretions, 1 to 2 L of pancreatic juice, and 1 L of intestinal secretions. The small intestine reabsorbs nearly 80% of the fluid that passes through it. This dynamic process is accomplished by a rapid bidirectional movement of fluid in the intestinal lumen. This ebb and flow of fluid in the intestinal lumen is critical in maintaining normal homeostasis. Minor changes in intestinal permeability or rate of flow of the intestinal contents can result in net secretion and diarrheal states.

8

The tonicity of the intraluminal contents determines the overall net movement of water. In general, after a meal is consumed, the addition of large amounts of saliva, gastric juice, and hypotonic chyme enters the proximal small intestine. Acid gastric contents are neutralized by the secretion of bicarbonate, creating NaCl and water and decreasing the osmotic pressure. The jejunum is effective at passively reabsorbing water in a paracellular fashion due to its relatively large intercellular pores. As the chyme travels through the length of the small intestine, the intercellular channels become more tightly arranged and the movement of water becomes dependent on the active transport of solutes into the paracellular spaces. A total of 6 to 11 L of water enters the duodenum every day; of this, approximately 1 to 1.5 L enters the colon.

Sodium absorption occurs through several different processes. Simple electrogenic absorption, non–electrolyte-stimulated absorption, and electroneutral absorption are reliant on the Na^+- K^+-ATPase pump on the basolateral membrane of the cell. This pump utilizes the hydrolysis of ATP to provide the necessary energy to move three Na^+ ions out of the cell while transporting two K^+ ions into the cell against an electrical gradient. This process maintains a negatively charged low Na^+ intracellular environment, allowing for several mechanisms of absorption at the apical membrane. Simple electrogenic absorption of sodium is the process of an influx of Na^+ ions from the sodium-rich intestinal lumen into the negatively charged low-sodium intracellular environment. This process is indirectly energy dependent, as it relies on the function of the Na^+-K^+-ATPase pump on the basolateral membrane to maintain the low-sodium environment and the negative intracellular charge. This process can be inhibited by ouabain, a Na^+-K^+-ATPase inhibitor.[19]

Non–electrolyte-stimulated sodium absorption occurs when sodium is coupled with an organic solute, such as glucose, amino acids, dipeptides, tripeptides, and bile acids. Sodium is preferentially transported down its electrochemical gradient, which is created by the Na^+-K^+-ATPase pump on the basolateral membrane of the cell, providing the necessary energy to transport the organic solute against its gradient (Fig. 47.8A). Electroneutral absorption of sodium chloride occurs through a process that couples two neutral ion countertransport mechanisms. Na^+ is exchanged for H^+ and Cl^- is exchanged for HCO_3^-, resulting in no net change in intracellular charge. This

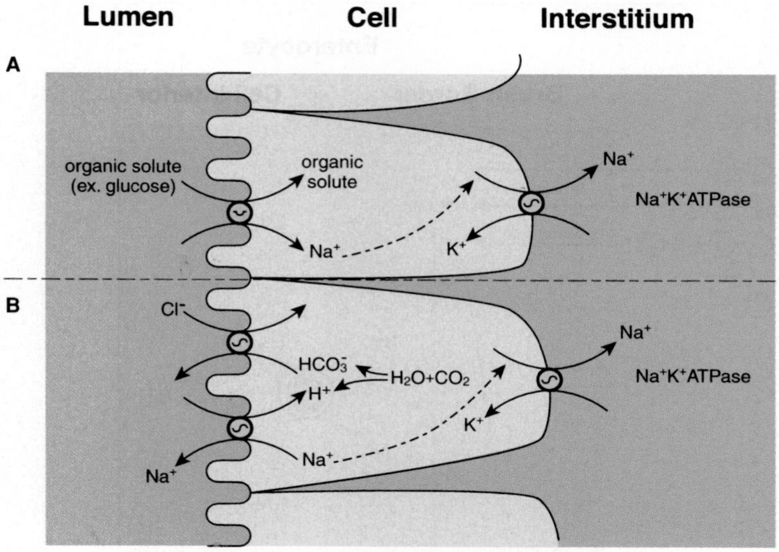

FIGURE 47.8. Mechanisms of sodium absorption in the small intestine: solute-coupled Na^+ absorption (**A**) and electroneutral NaCl absorption (**B**).

process provides an influx of NaCl in exchange for H^+/HCO_3^- efflux. This electroneutral transfer of ions allows for intracellular pH regulation and for sodium and chloride transport (Fig. 47.8B).

While the majority of chloride is absorbed by electroneutral transfer, chloride is also absorbed by passive diffusion in a paracellular fashion. This is due to the slightly positive interstitium when compared to the gut lumen, allowing the negatively charged chloride ions to be absorbed. An additional important source of chloride transport involves the reabsorption of chloride ions contained within gastric hydrochloric acid secretions. Chloride is a major determinant of the regulation of fluid secretion into the small intestine and in intestinal hydration.[20]

Bicarbonate absorption occurs primarily in the jejunum and requires the formation of carbon dioxide in the intestinal lumen from HCO_3^- and H^+. This creates an increase in the partial pressure of carbon dioxide in the intestinal lumen. Carbon dioxide subsequently diffuses back into the enterocyte and is enzymatically cleaved into H^+ and HCO_3^- by the action of carbonic anhydrase. HCO_3^- diffuses into the interstitium and H^+ is resecreted in exchange for other cations, predominantly Na^+. In the duodenum and ileum, HCO_3^- is secreted in exchange for Cl^-. This efflux of HCO_3^- provides a mechanism to neutralize gastric acid entering into the duodenum. HCO_3^- secretion in the ileum most likely helps maintain acid–base equilibrium, although this process is not well understood.[21]

Approximately 90 mEq/d of potassium is ingested in a normal diet, of which 90% is absorbed. An equal amount of potassium is excreted in the urine as is absorbed in the intestine, allowing maintenance of potassium homeostasis. The majority of absorption occurs in the small intestine, mainly through passive mechanisms.[22] This process is thought to occur through intercellular pores or through a H^+-K^+ exchange pathway facilitated by the intracellular electrochemical gradient that is created predominantly by the basolateral ATPase pump. Intracellular K^+ then diffuses across the basolateral membrane by a K^+ channel or carrier.

Mineral Absorption. Mineral absorption is necessary for the proper form and function of the human body. These inorganic elements are responsible for approximately 4% to 6% of a person's mass. Calcium accounts for approximately 50% of this mass, phosphate provides an additional 25%, and a variety of other minerals constitute the remaining 25%. Many of these minerals are best absorbed in their ionized forms, which is aided by the presence of hydrochloric acid in the gastric lumen. Calcium, phosphate, magnesium, sulfur, sodium, chloride, and potassium are considered macrominerals, with daily requirements exceeding 100 mg/d. Microminerals (trace minerals) include iron, zinc, copper, manganese, iodine, selenium, fluoride, molybdenum, chromium, and cobalt with daily requirements of less than 15 mg/d.

Approximately 1 g of calcium is consumed per day, mainly from dairy products. Once in its ionized form, calcium is primarily absorbed in the duodenum, although this process occurs throughout the length of the small intestine. When calcium is present intraluminally at low levels, it is transported across the apical membrane of the enterocyte by carrier-mediated facilitated diffusion. Once calcium is in the cytoplasm, it is bound to calcium-binding proteins and delivered to the basal membrane. Calcium is then transferred into the interstitium by a Ca^{2+}-ATPase pump. This process is indirectly regulated by parathyroid hormone (PTH). PTH in low-calcium states promotes conversion of vitamin D to its active form, $1{,}25(OH)_2$ vitamin D. This activated form of vitamin D causes an increase in the expression of both calcium-binding proteins and Ca^{2+}-ATPase, causing an increase in the absorption of calcium by the small intestine.[23,24] When intraluminal calcium is in excess of its capacity to be actively transferred by the apical membrane's carrier-mediated mechanism, passive paracellular calcium absorption occurs in the distal small intestine.

Absorbable dietary sources of iron are typically either contained within a protein, such as heme, or as a ferrous Fe^{2+} ion. Iron-containing proteins are usually from ingested meats, whereas ferrous forms are typically present in vegetables, grains, and fruits. Vitamin C (ascorbic acid) increases iron absorption by reducing the ferric (Fe^{3+}) ion into the more soluble ferrous state. Absorption of iron is facilitated by carrier-mediated translocation across the apical membrane of the enterocyte in the duodenum and proximal jejunum. Once in the cytoplasm, the ferrous ion is released by enzymatic cleavage. Ferrous ions may be stored intracellularly by ferritin or transported into the circulation by transferrin. The process of iron absorption is regulated in the enterocyte by hypoxia-inducible factor signaling and iron-regulatory proteins. Systemically, the central iron-regulatory hormone is hepatic hepcidin. Hepatic hepcidin regulates iron absorption and mobilization from systemic stores by inhibiting ferroportin, a cellular iron exporter.[25]

Carbohydrate Digestion and Absorption. Carbohydrates are a staple in many diets and provide a major source of

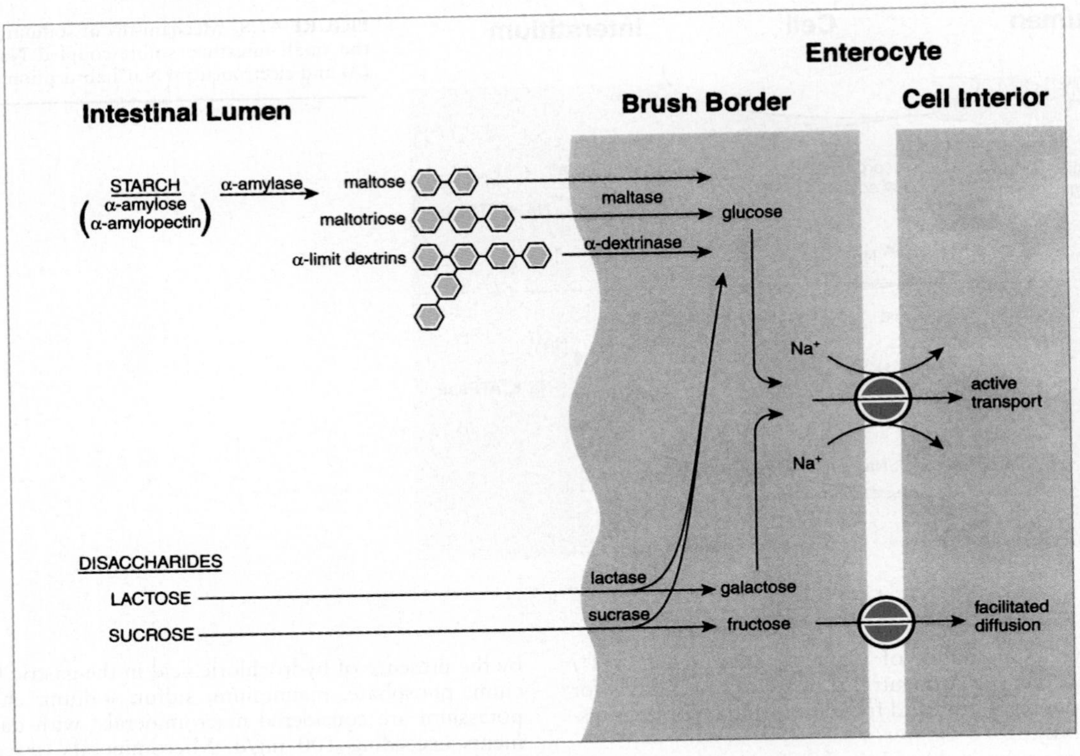

FIGURE 47.9. Digestion and absorption of carbohydrates.

daily caloric intake. In Western diets 400 g of carbohydrates are consumed by the average adult daily, providing 1,600 kcal (4 kcal/g of carbohydrate). Carbohydrates are present in three main digestible forms: complex starches, disaccharides, and simple sugars. Complex starches account for approximately 60% of daily carbohydrate intake. The most common form is amylopectin, which consists of glucose linked in a linear fashion with $\alpha(1,4)$-glycosidic bonds with branch points consisting of $\alpha(1,6)$-glycosidic linkages occurring after approximately every 20 to 26 glucose moieties. Amylose is a long linear grouping of glucose molecules connected with $\alpha(1,4)$-glycosidic bonds without branch points. Disaccharides, mainly sucrose and lactose, are the next most common source of dietary carbohydrates, representing nearly a third of daily intake. Sucrose disaccharides are composed of glucose-fructose dimers, whereas lactose disaccharides consist of glucose-galactose dimers.

The complex starches amylopectin and amylose are digested with the aid of salivary and pancreatic amylase. Salivary amylase contributes a small amount to this process as it is inactivated by gastric acid, leaving the remainder of this process to be completed by pancreatic amylase. This process yields maltose, which is a glucose dimer with $\alpha(1,4)$-glycosidic bonds, and maltotriose, which is a glucose trimer with $\alpha(1,4)$-glycosidic bonds. In addition, α-dextrins are produced with an average of six glucose moieties with $\alpha(1,4)$-glycosidic bonds and side branches linked by $\alpha(1,6)$-glycosidic bonds. This digestive process is usually completed before the carbohydrate bolus leaves the duodenum. These small oligosaccharides along with ingested disaccharides, typically sucrose and lactose, are then further digested by the brush border saccharidases in the jejunum.

The brush border of the small bowel contains specific enzymes that through catalytic reactions hydrolyze these oligo- and disaccharides into their component monosaccharide moieties, such as glucose, galactose, and fructose. Once broken down into their basic subunits, these monosaccharides can be transported across the apical cell membrane. A sodium-dependent hexose transporter (SGLUT-1) is required for the transport of glucose and galactose as they utilize the same carrier mechanism. The cotransportation of these monosaccharides with sodium is dependent on the Na^+-K^+-ATPase pump on the basolateral membrane to maintain a sodium gradient allowing for this influx. Fructose is transported in a carrier-mediated diffusion-dependent manner by GLUT5 and does not require sodium as a cotransporter (Fig. 47.9). The movement of monosaccharides into the cellular cytoplasm provides an additional gradient by which water is absorbed by the enterocytes from the intestinal lumen. The monosaccharides are then transported across the basolateral membrane by GLUT2. This hexose transporter allows for the diffusion of all three monosaccharides into the extracellular space and ultimately into the portal blood flow. A small portion of these monosaccharides may be used by the enterocyte, but the majority are transported through the cell.

Nondigestible carbohydrates (dietary fiber) such as cellulose are thought to be an important part of a normal diet even though they do not provide dietary calories. Dietary fiber is present in grains, vegetables, and pulpy fruits. Dietary fiber helps decrease bowel transit time by absorbing water in the intestinal lumen. In addition, fiber can absorb organic materials such as lipids and bile salts and inorganic minerals such as zinc, calcium, and magnesium. These actions of fiber are thought to play a role preventing carcinogenesis and in helping to maintain normal serum lipid profiles. Unfortunately, fiber is underrepresented in most Western diets.

Protein Digestion and Absorption. Protein consumption is essential to the daily diet. An average adult requires 0.75 g/kg of protein per day, although this requirement may be significantly increased during childhood, pregnancy, and times of significant illness. Protein provides an important caloric energy source as well as the essential building blocks for production of new proteins. A nearly equal amount of protein is ingested daily from dietary sources (70 to 100 g) as is provided by endogenous proteins (50 to 60 g of protein per day) in the small intestine from secreted enzymes, desquamated cells, and plasma protein leakage. Nearly 90% of this protein load is metabolized in a similar fashion to dietary proteins.

The initial digestion of protein begins with the activation of pepsinogen to pepsin in the acid environment of the stomach. Pepsin hydrolyzes protein into its component amino acids; however, this action only represents a small part of overall protein digestion. The majority of protein digestion occurs in the small intestine by pancreatic peptidases and proteases. Pancreatic enzymes flow into the duodenum, initiating this phase of protein digestion. These pancreatic proteases are initially released as proenzymes (zymogens). These zymogens are inactive and require a further catalytic process to occur for their activation. This is initiated by the brush border enzyme enteropeptidase (enterokinase) in the duodenum. Endopeptidase cleaves trypsinogen into the active enzyme trypsin. Trypsin in turn activates the other zymogens into their active endopeptidases (trypsin, chymotrypsin, and elastase), which hydrolyze internal peptide bonds. Additional protein digestion is performed by exopeptidases (carboxypeptidase A and B), which are able to cleave amino acids from the C-terminal ends of proteins. Seventy percent of the process results in short oligopeptides of two to six amino acids and the remaining 30% produces single amino acids.

Short oligopeptides are further digested by enzymes in the brush border of the small intestine or within the cell cytoplasm. Single amino acids, dipeptides, and tripeptides are able to diffuse through the apical membrane into the cytoplasm. Single amino acids are cotransported into the cytoplasm with sodium along an electrochemical gradient. This electrochemical gradient is maintained by the Na^+-K^+-ATPase pump on the basolateral cell membrane. At least four separate transport mechanisms exist for the various electrochemical properties of amino acids that are transported (neutral, dibasic, acidic, and imino). Peptides greater than three amino acids in length are broken down into smaller peptides by enzymes in the brush border. The resultant dipeptides and tripeptides are then moved into the cytoplasm along with H^+ by a cotransporter PepT1, where they are hydrolyzed by specific peptidases into their component amino acids. Transport of amino acids into the cytosol provides an osmotic gradient by which water is further absorbed from the intestinal lumen. A small portion of the processed amino acids is utilized by the enterocyte, and the vast majority are shuttled into the portal blood flow via amino acid transporters on the basolateral membrane.

Fat Digestion and Absorption. Forty percent of the average daily caloric intake (60 to 90 g) in a Western diet is in the form of fat. Ninety percent of these ingested fats are triglycerides, while the remainder is composed of cholesterol, phospholipids, and fat-soluble vitamins. The initiation of lipid digestion occurs when CCK is stimulated by the presence of fatty acids on the duodenal mucosa. CCK in turn stimulates pancreatic secretion of lipase and its cofactor colipase. Lipase hydrolyzes triglycerides at the 1 and 3 position of the glycerol backbone, yielding two fatty acids and a monoglyceride (a fatty acid esterified to glycerol). Cholesterol and fat-soluble vitamins are hydrolyzed by pancreatic cholesterol esterase and phospholipids by phospholipase A_2. The products of lipolysis interact with bile salts to form water-soluble micelles. Mixed micelles are 50 to 400 Å in diameter and are a combination of fatty acids, bile salts, and monoglycerides. The structure of a micelle is composed of an inward-facing hydrophobic region and a hydrophilic region facing outward toward the aqueous environment of the intestinal lumen. Due to the hydrophobic core, cholesterol, phospholipids, and fat-soluble vitamins can reside within the micelle structure. Micelles are able to interact with the mucosal cells and empty their contents into the cytoplasm. This occurs by the process of dissolution of the micelles into the lipid bilayer of the mucosal cell. Once this is completed, the components of the micelle are ready to re-form with new lipid components to repeat this process. There is no energy consumed directly in the transfer of lipids into the cell cytoplasm.

Once in the cytoplasm, long-chain fatty acids and β-monoglycerides are carried by cytosolic fatty acid–binding proteins to the smooth endoplasmic reticulum (SER). In the SER, resynthesis of triglycerides occurs. These triglycerides are further processed in the Golgi apparatus where a phospholipid and an apoprotein coat are added to form a chylomicron. Chylomicrons are 90% triglyceride; the remaining 10% is composed of phospholipid, cholesterol, and protein. These large particles are 750 to 6,000 Å in diameter. Before exiting the Golgi apparatus, the chylomicrons are packaged into secretory vesicles. They exit the cell membrane by exocytosis and enter the central lacteal of the villus and the intestinal lymphatic system. In addition, enterocytes also produce smaller lipoprotein particles, very-low-density lipoproteins, which contain a higher cholesterol/triglyceride ratio and provide the major route of entry for dietary cholesterol into the lymphatic system.

Short-chain fatty acids contain less than eight carbon atoms and are water soluble. This allows these molecules to enter and exit the enterocyte by simple diffusion independent of bile micelles or chylomicrons. Medium-chain triglycerides consist of 6 to 12 carbon atoms and can be absorbed by simple diffusion or through the previously mentioned process of transport of long-chain fatty acids via the formation of bile micelles and chylomicrons. Both short- and medium-chain fatty acids may enter the portal circulation without entering into the lymphatics. The majority of dietary fat is processed and absorbed in the duodenum and upper jejunum.

Absorption of Bile Salts. Approximately 95% of the bile salts secreted into the intestine are reabsorbed and returned to the liver through the portal circulation. Once in the liver, these bile salts are reprocessed and secreted and stored in the gallbladder in preparation for the next meal. This process of recycling bile salts is referred to as the enterohepatic circulation. This reabsorption occurs by both passive and active means. A small amount of bile salts are passively reabsorbed along the entire length of the small intestine. The majority of bile salts, however, are reabsorbed though an active Na^+-dependent transport mechanism in the terminal ileum. Bile, which is not reabsorbed, passes into the colon where it is deconjugated by bacteria. This process increases the solubility of the bile and promotes further passive absorption. High concentrations of bile salts within the colon inhibit sodium and water reabsorption, resulting in diarrhea. Patients who have undergone resection of their ileum may suffer from diarrhea due to this process. These patients may be treated with the bile-binding resin cholestyramine to help alleviate their symptoms.

Vitamin Absorption. Fat-soluble vitamins (A, D, E, and K) are incorporated into micelles along with fats in order to pass into the enterocyte. These vitamins are then processed and packaged into chylomicrons so that they can exit into the lymphatic system. Water-soluble vitamins are absorbed in the jejunum and ileum through a variety of mechanisms. Vitamin C (ascorbic acid), biotin, and niacin are transported by Na^+-dependent mechanisms. Folate, vitamin B_1 (thiamine), and vitamin B_2 (riboflavin) are absorbed by Na^+-independent mechanisms, and vitamin B_6 is absorbed by passive diffusion.[26]

Vitamin B_{12} (cobalamin) absorption is dependent on the presence of intrinsic factor, a glycoprotein produced by the gastric parietal cells. One molecule of intrinsic factor binds two molecules of cobalamin to form a complex that attaches to a specific membrane receptor in the terminal ileum. Unbound cobalamin cannot be absorbed. Cobalamin becomes unbound from its complex in the enterocyte and exits from the cell into the portal circulation with the aid of B_{12}-binding proteins called transcobalamins. Cobalamin is essential for DNA synthesis, and a deficiency usually presents with megaloblastic anemia. Inability to absorb sufficient amounts of cobalamin may be due to lack of intrinsic factor after proximal or total gastrectomy, autoimmunity to gastric parietal cells or intrinsic factor, or atrophic gastritis. In addition, cobalamin–intrinsic factor complexes may fail to be absorbed due to distal ileal disease or resection, and cobalamin deficiency may occur from bacterial overgrowth due to bacterial overconsumption of cobalamin.

References

1. Kluth D, Jaeschke-Melli S, Fiegel H. The embryology of gut rotation. *Semin Pediatr Surg* 2003;12:275–279.
2. Cohen S, Harris LD, Levitan R. Manometric characteristics of the human ileocecal junctional zone. *Gastroenterology* 1968;54:72–75.
3. Holmes R, Lobley RW. Intestinal brush border revisited. *Gut* 1989;30:1667–1678.
4. Rubin DC. Spatial analysis of transcriptional activation in fetal rat jejunal and ileal gut epithelium. *Am J Physiol* 1992;263:G853–G863.
5. Trier JS. Studies on small intestinal crypt epithelium. I. The fine structure of the crypt epithelium of the proximal small intestine of fasting humans. *J Cell Biol* 1963;18:599–620.
6. Garabedian EM, Roberts LJ, McNevin MS, et al. Examining the role of Paneth cells in the small intestine by lineage ablation in transgenic mice. *J Biol Chem* 1997;272:23729–23740.
7. Englander E, Greeley J. *Postpyloric Gastrointestinal Peptides*. San Diego: Elsevier; 2005.
8. Weckbecker G, Lewis I, Albert R, et al. Opportunities in somatostatin research: biological, chemical and therapeutic aspects. *Nat Rev Drug Discov* 2003;2:999–1017.
9. Casteels R. *Membrane Potential in Smooth Muscle Cells*. Austin, TX: University of Texas Press; 1981.
10. Ofori-Kwakye K, Fell JT, Sharma HL, et al. Gamma scintigraphic evaluation of film-coated tablets intended for colonic or biphasic release. *Int J Pharm* 2004;270:307–313.
11. Xavier RJ, Podolsky DK. Microbiology. How to get along—friendly microbes in a hostile world. *Science* 2000;289:1483–1484.
12. Kraehenbuhl JP, Corbett M. Immunology. Keeping the gut microflora at bay. *Science* 2004;303:1624–1625.
13. Macdonald TT, Monteleone G. Immunity, inflammation, and allergy in the gut. *Science* 2005;307:1920–1925.
14. Hayday A, Viney JL. The ins and outs of body surface immunology. *Science* 2000;290:97–100.
15. Niess JH, Reinecker HC. Lamina propria dendritic cells in the physiology and pathology of the gastrointestinal tract. *Curr Opin Gastroenterol* 2005;21:687–691.
16. Pasare C, Medzhitov R. Toll-like receptors: balancing host resistance with immune tolerance. *Curr Opin Immunol* 2003;15:677–682.
17. Niess JH, Brand S, Gu X, et al. CX3CR1-mediated dendritic cell access to the intestinal lumen and bacterial clearance. *Science* 2005;307:254–258.
18. Macpherson AJ, Uhr T. Induction of protective IgA by intestinal dendritic cells carrying commensal bacteria. *Science* 2004;303:1662–1665.
19. Charney AN, Donowitz M. Functional significance of intestinal Na+-K+-ATPase: in vivo ouabain inhibition. *Am J Physiol* 1978;234:E629–636.
20. Barrett KE, Keely SJ. Chloride secretion by the intestinal epithelium: molecular basis and regulatory aspects. *Annu Rev Physiol* 2000;62:535–572.
21. Minhas BS, Sullivan SK, Field M. Bicarbonate secretion in rabbit ileum: electrogenicity, ion dependence, and effects of cyclic nucleotides. *Gastroenterology* 1993;105:1617–1629.
22. Agarwal R, Afzalpurkar R, Fordtran JS. 1994. Pathophysiology of potassium absorption and secretion by the human intestine. *Gastroenterology* 1993;107:548–571.
23. Cai Q, Chandler JS, Wasserman RH, et al. Vitamin D and adaptation to dietary calcium and phosphate deficiencies increase intestinal plasma membrane calcium pump gene expression. *Proc Natl Acad Sci U S A* 1993; 90:1345–1349.
24. Walters JR. Calbindin-D9k stimulates the calcium pump in rat enterocyte basolateral membranes. *Am J Physiol* 1989;256:G124–G128.
25. Zhang AS, Enns CA. Molecular mechanisms of normal iron homeostasis. *Hematology Am Soc Hematol Educ Program* 2009;207–214.
26. Said HM. Recent advances in carrier-mediated intestinal absorption of water-soluble vitamins. *Annu Rev Physiol* 2004;66:419–446.

CHAPTER 48 ■ ILEUS AND BOWEL OBSTRUCTION

DAVID I. SOYBEL AND WENDY B. LANDMAN

KEY POINTS

1. In simple obstruction the intestinal lumen is partially or completely occluded without compromise of intestinal blood flow. Simple obstructions may be complete, meaning that the lumen is totally occluded, or incomplete, meaning that the lumen is narrowed but permitting distal passage of some fluid and air. In strangulation obstruction, blood flow to the obstructed segment is compromised and tissue necrosis and gangrene are imminent.
2. The four key symptoms that are associated with acute mechanical bowel obstruction include abdominal pain, vomiting, distention, and obstipation.
3. Peritoneal adhesions account for more than half of small-bowel obstruction cases.
4. Ileus denotes underlying alterations in motility of the gastrointestinal tract, leading to functional obstruction.
5. Postoperative ileus can be differentiated from small-bowel obstruction with the use of contrast computed tomography and enteroclysis imaging techniques.
6. Postoperative ileus (POI) is often self-limiting; less frequent interventions are required for prolonged POI if proper precautions have been taken during surgery.

INTRODUCTION AND HISTORICAL PERSPECTIVE

The purpose of this chapter is to provide an overview of the pathophysiology, natural history, diagnosis, and management of acute obstruction and ileus of the small and large intestines. The development of the modern approach to intestinal obstruction and ileus paralleled the development of techniques for safe abdominal surgery. Chief among these accomplishments were the discovery of safe general anesthetics, the popularization of aseptic methods in the operating room and in the management of wounds, and the development of techniques for intestinal resection, intestinal anastomosis, and colostomy. The foundations of the recognition and management of intestinal obstruction and ileus are attributed to Frederick Treves.[1–3] In 1884, he published a detailed discussion of the etiologies (including adhesions) and surgical management of mechanical intestinal obstruction.[1] Treves also distinguished mechanical from nonmechanical (i.e., paralytic) causes of intestinal distention, classifying the latter causes under the term *ileus*. From 1880 to 1925, proximal intestinal decompression was recognized to provide relief from the symptoms of mechanical obstruction or ileus.[3] In 1933, Wangensteen and Paine reported the efficacy of gastrointestinal intubation in relieving symptoms of intestinal distention caused by intestinal obstruction or from the ileus that resulted from laparotomy.[4,5] Subsequently, Wangensteen and Rea provided experimental evidence that the source of gaseous distention in cases of obstruction or ileus was swallowed air.[6] The value of intravenous fluid resuscitation in experimental models of intestinal obstruction was recognized as early as 1912[7] and became a principle of care of the patients with intestinal obstruction in the late 1920s. By 1920, plain abdominal radiographs were used in diagnosis of intestinal obstruction.[3] Thus, the principles of early diagnosis, rapid intravenous fluid resuscitation, gastrointestinal decompression, and early operation to avoid intestinal gangrene and peritonitis were established well before the advent of antibiotic therapy, invasive hemodynamic monitoring, and parenteral nutrition.[8] These early developments were most important in reducing morbidity and mortality of mechanical intestinal obstruction and ileus.[9]

MECHANICAL OBSTRUCTION OF THE INTESTINES

Terminology and Classification

The term *mechanical obstruction* means that luminal contents cannot pass through the gut tube because the lumen is blocked. This obstruction is in contrast with *neurogenic* or *functional* obstruction in which luminal contents are prevented from passing because of disturbances in gut motility that prevent coordinated peristalsis from one region of the gut to the next. This latter form of obstruction is commonly referred to as *ileus* in the small intestine and *pseudo-obstruction* **1** in the large intestine. In *simple* obstruction the intestinal lumen is partially or completely occluded without compromise of intestinal blood flow. Simple obstructions may be *complete*, meaning that the lumen is totally occluded (Fig. 48.1), or *incomplete*, meaning that the lumen is narrowed but permitting distal passage of some fluid and air. In *strangulation*

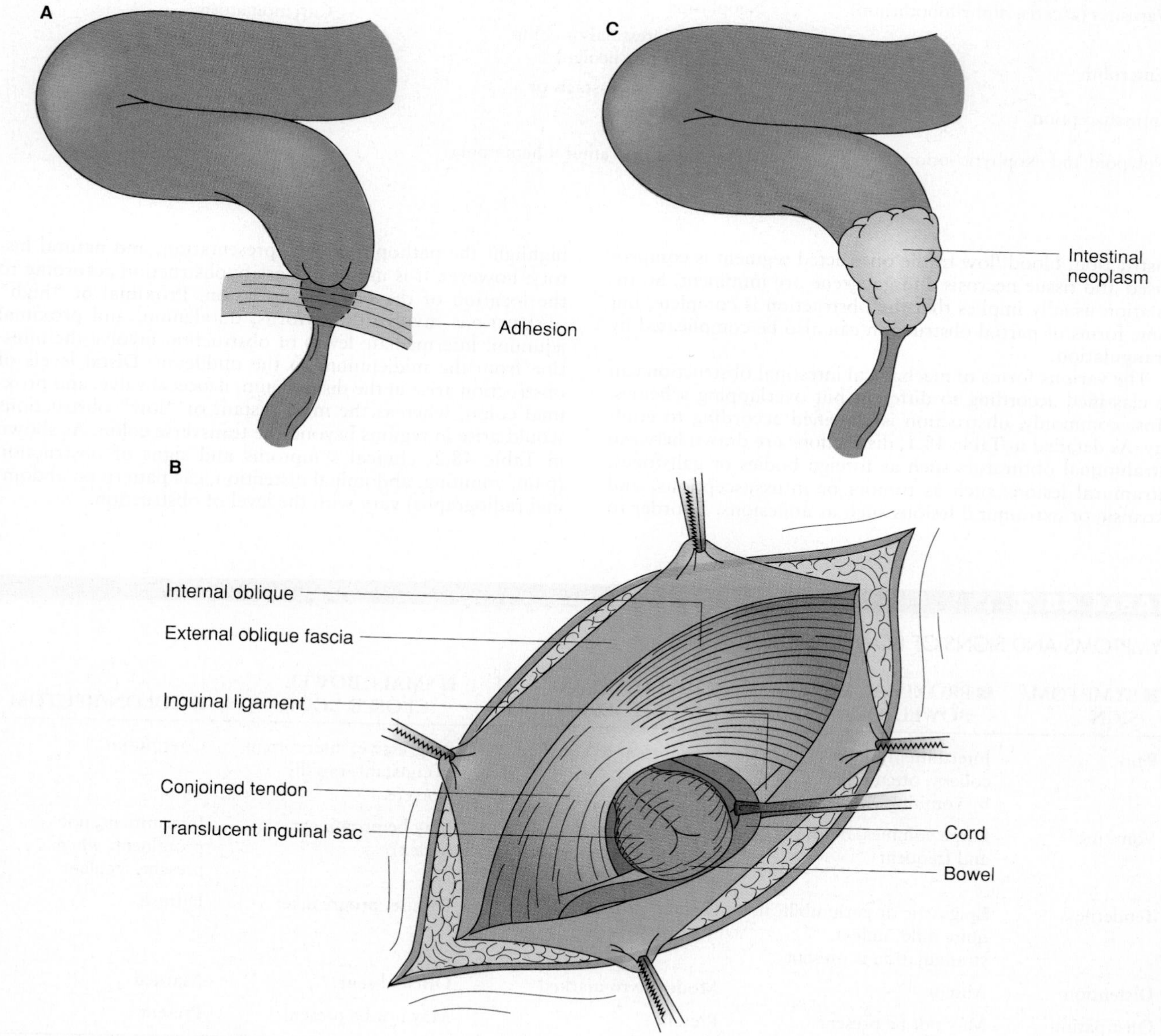

FIGURE 48.1. Schematic illustration of different forms of simple mechanical obstruction. Simple obstruction is most often due to adhesion (**A**), groin hernia (**B**), or neoplasm (**C**). The hernia can act as a tourniquet, causing a closed-loop obstruction and strangulation.

TABLE 48.1

CLASSIFICATION OF ADULT MECHANICAL INTESTINAL OBSTRUCTIONS

■ INTRALUMINAL	■ INTRAMURAL	■ EXTRINSIC
Foreign bodies	Congenital (rare in adult)	Adhesions
	Atresia, stricture, or stenosis	Congenital: Ladd or Meckel bands
Barium inspissation (colon)	Web	Postoperative
	Intestinal duplication	Postinflammatory (after pelvic inflammatory disease)
Bezoar	Meckel diverticulum	
Inspissated feces	Inflammatory process	Hernias
	Crohn disease	Abdominal wall
	Diverticulitis	Internal
Gallstone ileus	Stricture from ischemia	Volvulus
	Radiation enteritis or stricture	External mass effect
Meconium (cystic fibrosis)	Medication induced (nonsteroidal anti-inflammatory drugs, KCl tablets)	Abscess
		Annular pancreas
		Pancreatic pseudocyst
Parasites (ascaris, diphyllobothrium)	Neoplasms	Carcinomatosis
	Primary intestinal or colon (malignant or benign)	Endometriosis
Enterolith		Pregnancy
	Secondary (metastasis or carcinomatosis)	
Intussusception		
Polypoid and exophytic lesions	Trauma (e.g., intramural hematoma)	

obstruction, blood flow to the obstructed segment is compromised and tissue necrosis and gangrene are imminent. Strangulation usually implies that the obstruction is complete, but some forms of partial obstruction can also be complicated by strangulation.

The various forms of mechanical intestinal obstruction can be classified according to different but overlapping schemes. Most commonly, obstruction is classified according to etiology. As detailed in Table 48.1, distinctions are drawn between intraluminal obturators such as foreign bodies or gallstones, intramural lesions such as tumors or intussusceptions, and extrinsic or extramural lesions such as adhesions. In order to highlight the pathophysiology, presentation, and natural history, however, it is useful to classify obstruction according to the location of the obstructing lesion. Proximal or "high" obstructions involve the pylorus, duodenum, and proximal jejunum. Intermediate levels of obstruction involve the intestine from the midjejunum to the midileum. Distal levels of obstruction arise in the distal ileum, ileocecal valve, and proximal colon, whereas the most distant or "low" obstructions would arise in regions beyond the transverse colon. As shown in Table 48.2, clinical symptoms and signs of obstruction (pain, vomiting, abdominal distention, gas pattern on abdominal radiographs) vary with the level of obstruction.

TABLE 48.2

SYMPTOMS AND SIGNS OF BOWEL OBSTRUCTION

■ SYMPTOM/SIGN	■ PROXIMAL SMALL BOWEL (OPEN LOOP)	■ DISTAL SMALL BOWEL (OPEN LOOP)	■ SMALL BOWEL (CLOSED LOOP)	■ COLON/RECTUM
Pain	Intermittent, intense, colicky, often relieved by vomiting	Intermittent to constant	Progressive, intermittent to constant, rapidly worsens	Continuous
Vomiting	Large volumes, bilious and frequent	Low volume and frequency, progressively feculent with time	May be prominent (reflex)	Intermittent, not prominent; when present, feculent
Tenderness	Epigastric or periumbilical; quite mild, unless strangulation is present	Diffuse, progressive	Diffuse, progressive	Diffuse
Distention	Absent	Moderate to marked	Often absent	Marked
Obstipation	May not be present	Present	May not be present	Present

Adapted from Schuffler MD, Sinanan MN. Intestinal obstruction and pseudo-obstruction. In: Sleisenger MH, Fordtran JS, eds. *Gastrointestinal Disease*, 5th ed. Philadelphia, PA: WB Saunders; 1993:898–916.

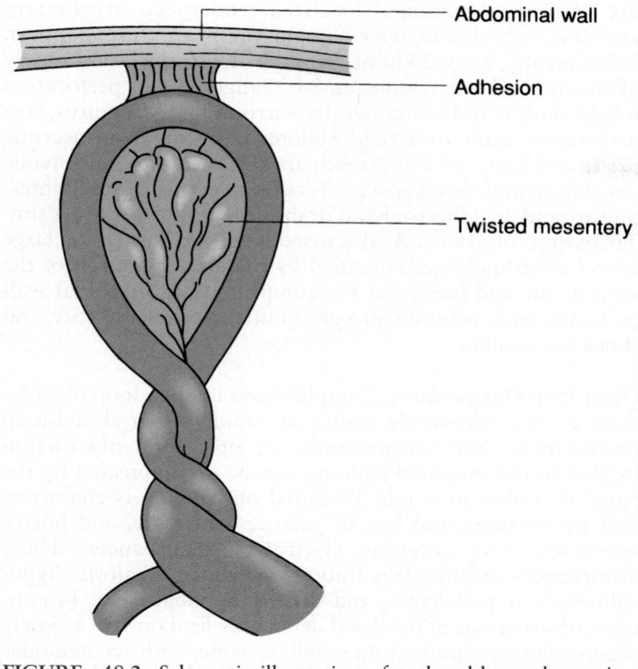

FIGURE 48.2. Schematic illustration of a closed-loop obstruction. The small intestine twists around its mesentery, compromising inflow and outflow of luminal contents from the loop. Also, the vascular supply to the loop may be compromised due to the twisting of the mesentery. The risk of strangulation is high.

It is also important to distinguish between *open-loop* and *closed-loop* obstructions. An open-loop obstruction occurs when intestinal flow is blocked but proximal decompression is possible through vomiting. A closed-loop obstruction occurs when inflow to the loop of bowel and outflow from the loop are both blocked. This obstruction permits gas and secretions to accumulate in the loop without a means of decompression, proximally or distally. Examples of closed-loop obstructions are torsion of a loop of small intestine around an adhesive band (Fig. 48.2), incarceration of the bowel in a hernia, volvulus of the cecum or colon, and development of an obstructing carcinoma of the colon with a competent ileocecal valve. The primary symptoms of a closed-loop obstruction of the small intestine are sudden, severe abdominal pain and vomiting, whereas symptoms of the large intestine are pain and sudden abdominal distention. This pain often occurs before associated findings of localized abdominal tenderness or involuntary guarding. When physical findings develop, there is a high level of suspicion that the viability of the bowel is compromised. When bowel obstruction is the most likely diagnosis, "abdominal pain out of proportion to physical findings" represents a surgical emergency.

Pathophysiology of Intestinal Obstruction

Local Effects of Bowel Obstruction. When a loop of bowel becomes obstructed, intestinal gas and fluid accumulate. Stasis of luminal content favors bacterial overgrowth, alters intestinal fluid transport properties and motility, and causes variations in intestinal perfusion and lymph flow. Luminal contents and volume, bacterial proliferation, and alterations in motility and perfusion work in concert to determine the rate at which symptoms and complications develop. Each of these factors merits discussion in some detail.

Intestinal Gas. Approximately 80% of the gas seen on plain abdominal radiographs is attributable to swallowed air.[6] Approximately 70% of the gas in the obstructed gut is inert nitrogen.[10] Oxygen accounts for 10% to 12%, CO_2 for 6% to 9%, hydrogen for 1%, methane for 1%, and hydrogen disulfide for 1% to 10%. In the setting of acute pain and anxiety, patients with intestinal obstruction may swallow excessive amounts of air. Passage of such swallowed air distally is prevented by nasogastric suction.

Intestinal Flora. An important contribution to normal digestive function comes from its bacterial population. In patients with normal gastric acid secretion, the chyme entering the duodenum is sterile. The small numbers of bacteria that are found in the stomach and proximal intestine are aerobic, gram-positive species found in the oropharynx. Distally, in the ileum and colon, gram-negative aerobes are present and anaerobic organisms predominate. Total bacterial counts in normal feces reach 10^{11} organisms per gram of fecal matter. Control of the bacterial populations depends on intact motor activity of the intestines and the interactions of all species present. This ecology can be disturbed by antibiotic therapy or by surgical reconstructions that result in stasis within intestinal segments. Intestinal bacteria serve several functions, including metabolism of fecal sterols, releasing the small-chain fatty acids that are an important food source for colonocytes; metabolism of fecal bile acids, fat-soluble vitamins (e.g., vitamin K), and vitamin B_{12}; and breakdown of complex carbohydrates and organic matter, leading to formation of CO_2, H_2, and CH_4 gases.[9] Considerable evidence suggests that the normal flora may contribute to baseline levels of intestinal secretion and, perhaps, normal intestinal motility. Under baseline conditions, the small intestines in germ-free animals are frequently dilated, fluid filled, and without peristalsis.[11,12]

In recent years, the role of bacterial toxins in mediating the mucosal response to obstruction has received increasing attention. In germ-free dogs, luminal accumulation of fluid is not observed and absorption continues.[12] In addition, it is well recognized that bacterial endotoxins can stimulate secretion, possibly via release or potentiation of activity of neuroendocrine substances and prostaglandins.[11] Finally, since a substantial part of systemic microvascular and hemodynamic responses to endotoxemia appears to be attributable to heightened synthesis of nitric oxide,[13,14] it seems likely that mucosal response to local inflammation and endotoxin release will also be altered by conditions modifying the synthesis or activity of nitric oxide. The role of nitric oxide in mucosal fluid and electrolyte movements is currently under active investigation.[15,16]

Intestinal Fluid. Classical experimental studies established that fluid accumulates intraluminally with open- or closed-loop small-intestinal obstruction.[9,17] Factors contributing to the accumulation of fluid include intraluminal distention and pressure, release of prosecretory and antiabsorptive hormones and paracrine substances, changes in mesenteric circulation, and elaboration and luminal release of bacterial toxins. Experimental studies and clinical investigation[18,19] demonstrated that elevation of luminal pressures above 20 cm H_2O inhibits absorption and stimulates secretion of salt and water into the lumen proximal to an obstruction. In closed-loop obstructions, luminal pressures may exceed 50 cm H_2O and may account for a substantial proportion of luminal fluid accumulation.[20] In simple, open-loop obstructions, distention of the lumen by gas rarely leads to luminal pressures higher than 8 to 12 cm H_2O.[21] Thus, in open-loop obstructions, the contributions of high luminal pressures to hypersecretion may not be important.

The release of endocrine/paracrine substances remains relatively uncharacterized in states of mechanical bowel obstruction.[22,23] Suggestions have been made that vasoactive intestinal polypeptide (VIP) may be released from the submucosal and myenteric plexuses within the gut wall, promoting epithelial secretion and inhibiting absorption.[23] Use of prostaglandin synthesis inhibitors has also implicated excess release of prostaglandins.[22] Further work may be expected to focus on the role of luminal factors such as irritative bile acids, proinflammatory agents such as endotoxin and platelet-activating factor, and messengers such as nitric oxide in coordinating responses of mucosal secretory and absorptive functions during intestinal obstruction.

Intestinal Blood Flow. Microvascular responses to intestinal obstruction may also play an important role in determining the hydrostatic gradients for fluid transfer across the mucosa into the lumen. In response to heightened luminal pressure, total blood flow to the bowel wall may initially increase.[24] The breakdown of epithelial barrier structures and enzymatic breakdown of stagnant intestinal contents leads to increased osmolarity of luminal contents. In addition to secretory stimulation and absorptive inhibition of the mucosa, the simultaneous changes in hydrostatic and osmotic pressures on the blood and lumen sides of the mucosa favor flow of extracellular fluid into the lumen. Perfusion is then compromised as luminal pressures increase, bacteria invade, and inflammation leads to edema within the bowel wall.

Intestinal Motility. Obstruction of the intestinal lumen does not simply block distal passage of luminal contents. The accumulation of fluid and gas in the obstructed lumen also elicits changes in myoelectrical function of the gut, proximal and distal to the obstructed segment. In response to this distention, the obstructed segment itself may dilate, a process known as *receptive relaxation*.[25] Such changes ensure that, despite accumulation of air and fluid, intraluminal pressures do not amplify easily to the point of compromising blood flow to the intestinal mucosa. At sites proximal and distal to the obstruction, changes in myoelectrical activity are time dependent. Initially, there may be intense periods of activity and peristalsis. Subsequently, myoelectrical activity is diminished and the interdigestive migrating myoelectrical complex pattern is replaced by ineffectual and seemingly disorganized clusters of contractions.[26–28] Similar alterations have been observed in experimental models of large-bowel obstruction. Subsequent patterns of myoelectrical quiescence may correspond to increasing accumulation of fluid and air proximally and the attempt to prevent luminal pressures from rising. It is likely that many factors contribute to the rate at which these changes in myoelectrical activity occur. These factors would include neurohumoral milieu, bacterial products, and luminal constituents.

Complications and Systemic Effects of Bowel Obstruction

Closed-loop Obstructions. The complications of closed-loop obstructions evolve rapidly. The reasons for this rapid evolution are best understood by considering the simplest and most common form of closed-loop obstruction, appendicitis. When a fecalith obstructs the blind-ended appendix, secretion of mucus and enhanced peristalsis represent the initial attempt to clear the blockage. Intense crampy abdominal pain focused at the umbilicus results. Nausea and vomiting are not uncommon as a result of luminal obstruction but as a reflexive response to hyperperistalsis and stretching of the mesentery. Over the next 8 to 18 hours, continued secretion of mucus to high intraluminal pressures, stasis, bacterial overgrowth, mucosal disruption, and elevation of luminal pressures convert intermittent cramps to constant and worsening pain. When luminal pressure exceeds mural venous pressure and then capillary perfusion pressures, inflammatory cells are recruited from surrounding peritoneal structures. This sequence of events leads to intense inflammation, release of exudate in the area of the appendix, and the first localization of pain from the umbilicus to the area of peritoneum lying nearest the inflamed appendix. Peritoneal findings (localized tenderness, involuntary guarding, rebound or referred tenderness) and fevers appear. Subsequently, 20 to 24 hours into the illness, the blood supply of the appendix is compromised. Gangrene and perforation follow and, if not contained by surrounding structures, free perforation leads to a rigid abdomen. Toxins from necrotic tissue and bacterial overgrowth are released into the systemic circulation and shock ensues. Torsion of a loop of small intestine around an adhesive band or inside a hernia leads to a similar pattern of events. As discussed later, torsions of the large bowel are usually accompanied by massive distention of the loop by air and feces, but the compromise of intestinal wall perfusion and evolution into peritonitis, systemic toxicity, and shock are similar.

Open-loop Obstructions. Complications in open-loop obstructions do not necessarily evolve as rapidly as in closed-loop obstructions. Not uncommonly, an open-loop obstruction located in the proximal jejunum can be decompressed by the patient's ability to vomit. Proximal obstruction is characterized by vomiting and loss of gastric, pancreatic, and biliary secretions, with resulting electrolyte disturbances. These disturbances include dehydration, metabolic alkalosis, hypochloremia, hypokalemia, and usually hyponatremia. In contrast, obstructions of the distal ileum may lead only to a slowly progressing distention of the small intestine, with accommodation by intestinal myoelectrical function and minor alterations in fluid and electrolyte balances. Open-loop obstructions located in the midgut are often complicated by events similar to those seen in closed-loop obstructions or combinations of events seen in high and low obstructions (Table 48.2). Patients with distal jejunal obstruction tend to present with a combination of complications resulting from loss of intestinal contents from vomiting, as well as distention and compromise of intestinal wall perfusion.

Clinical Presentation and Differential Diagnosis

2 The four key symptoms associated with acute mechanical bowel obstruction are abdominal pain, vomiting, distention, and obstipation. Colon obstruction is usually accompanied by varying levels of pain with massive abdominal distention and obstipation. As noted earlier, the signs and symptoms of acute but simple small-intestinal obstructions are related to the level of the obstruction and the closed- or open-loop nature of the obstruction. Other abdominal conditions, such as appendicitis, diverticulitis, perforated peptic ulcer, cholecystitis, or choledocholithiasis, can usually be distinguished from small-bowel obstruction by clinical examination and basic laboratory data. It should be emphasized that bowel obstruction can complicate any of these abdominal conditions. The presence of another abdominal process does not exclude the complication of small-bowel obstruction.

Over the years, numerous attempts have been made to use groupings of clinical criteria to establish the diagnosis of complete and irreversible intestinal obstruction, as distinguished from partial intestinal obstruction that might improve without operative intervention or other abdominal pathology. In recent studies, computer-assisted analysis has been used to identify such criteria.[29] Key factors in the history and clinical examination include previous abdominal surgery, quality of pain (colic/intermittent vs. steady), abdominal distention, and hyperactivity of bowel sounds. Not surprisingly, the use of such computer-assisted algorithms confirms that the most important clues to the diagnosis of simple obstruction of the small intestine are obtained in a complete and careful history and physical examination. As discussed later, the role of plain abdominal radiographs and other imaging studies is to confirm the clinical diagnosis of simple obstruction. It should be emphasized that, in simple obstruction, laboratory studies do not play a direct role in diagnosis, but aid in understanding the extent of complications such as dehydration, strangulation, and sepsis.

Strangulation obstruction is accompanied by symptoms and signs suggesting peritonitis, large fluid shifts, or systemic toxicity. These symptoms and signs include abdominal tenderness or involuntary guarding localizing to the area of the strangulated loop of bowel, decreasing urine output, fever, and tachycardia. There have been attempts to use common clinical and laboratory test criteria to identify the likelihood that the obstruction is associated with strangulation. Stewardson et al.[30] observed that the risk of strangulation was low in patients with partial (i.e., incomplete) or complete small-bowel obstruction if fever, tachycardia, localized abdominal tenderness, or leukocytosis were not present. These authors suggested that, in a setting consistent with bowel obstruction, any one of these four cardinal signs indicated a small risk for strangulation. The presence of any two of these signs increased the risk of strangulation so high as to warrant immediate surgery. These authorities and others have stressed, however, that when complete obstruction is present, no satisfactory clinical criteria are available to reliably exclude the possibility of strangulation.[30–33]

Different laboratory tests have been advocated for early detection of strangulated intestine. Metabolic (i.e., lactic) acidosis and increases in serum amylase, inorganic phosphate, hexosaminidase, intestinal fatty acid–binding protein, and serum D-lactate levels have all been associated with intestinal ischemia.[34,35] Such laboratory abnormalities may be helpful in diagnosing established strangulation in a small group of patients where the diagnosis of necrotic bowel is not clear. However, a noninvasive and rapid test has not yet been developed that can provide information to suggest that tissue necrosis is imminent but not yet established.

Radiographs and Imaging

Plain Films. The role of plain abdominal radiographs and imaging studies is to confirm the diagnosis of bowel obstruction, locate the site of obstruction, and gain insight into the lesion responsible for the obstruction. On plain radiographs of the abdomen, the key findings of small-bowel obstruction reflect the accumulation of air and fluid proximal and clearance of fluid and air distal to the point of obstruction. Dilated loops of small intestine are defined as those greater than 3 cm in diameter. Free air represents perforation of a viscus and mandates immediate operation. Such findings include dilated loops of small bowel on the flat plate (Fig. 48.3) and multiple air–fluid levels located at different levels on the upright film or lateral decubitus film (Fig. 48.4). Based on these criteria, plain abdominal radiography is diagnostic in 67% to 80% of patients.[36,37] In complete obstruction of the small intestine, the colon loops and rectum do not contain air. If there is air in the colon, the obstruction may be complete but early, or it may be incomplete.

In the colon, tight closed-loop obstructions (i.e., volvulus of the cecum, transverse colon, or sigmoid colon) are accompanied by distention of the obstructed segment (Fig. 48.5). The proximal colon is considered dilated when it reaches 8 to 10 cm; the sigmoid colon is considered dilated at 4 to 5 cm. In contrast, obstruction by carcinoma or diverticulitis presents with massive distention of the entire colon from the point of obstruction to the ileocecal valve. From this standpoint, any large-bowel obstruction may represent a "closed loop" as long as the ileocecal valve is competent. Although plain film findings can be used to differentiate obstruction of the small bowel from that of the large bowel, they are not accurate for localizing the specific site of obstruction.

A number of findings on plain films are highly suggestive of the nature of the offending lesion. These findings will be discussed later in relation to specific causes of intestinal obstruction. One point needs to be stressed, however, and that is the appearance of plain films in the patient with a closed-loop obstruction of the small intestine. Such a loop of bowel may contain fluid and very little gas. Thus, in a plain film, it may not be visible or only barely visible as a minimally dilated "sentinel loop" that remains unchanged in position on films

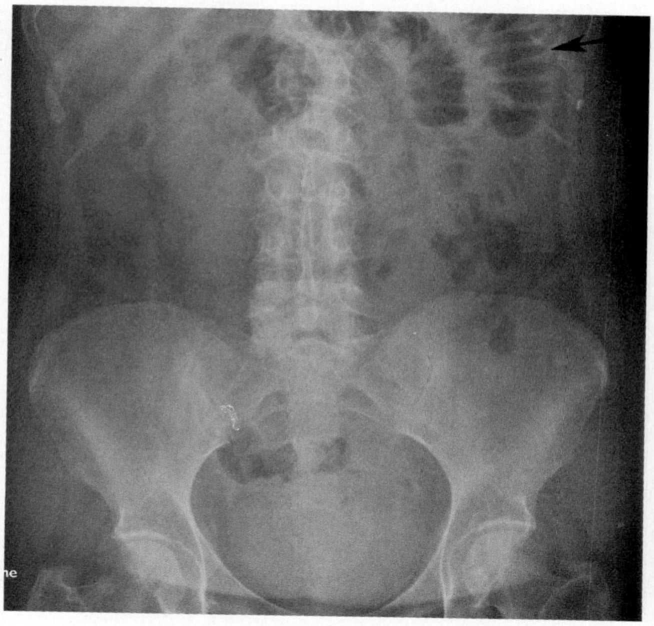

FIGURE 48.3. Plain supine abdominal film of a patient with small-intestinal obstruction. Note the multiple dilated loops of small intestine (*black arrow*) in the left upper quadrant, characterized by complete markings of the plicae. Also note absence of air in colon and rectum.

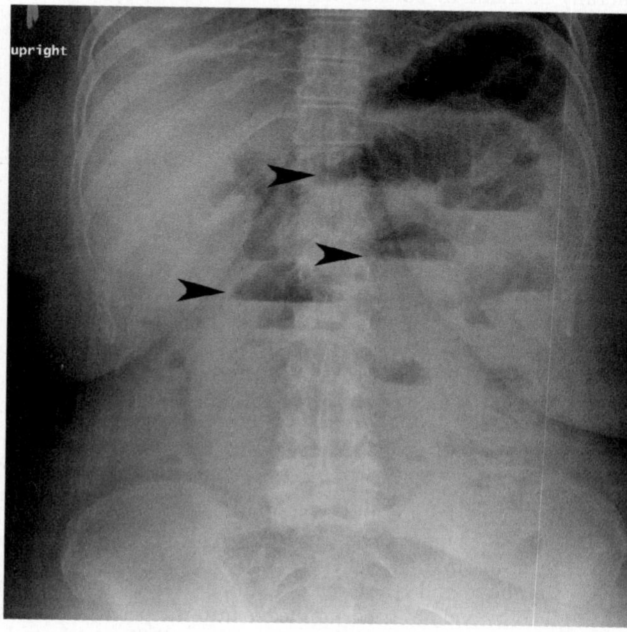

FIGURE 48.4. Plain upright abdominal film of a patient with small-intestinal obstruction. Note the air–fluid levels in the stomach and multiple dilated loops of small intestine (*black arrows*), and absence of air in the colon or rectum.

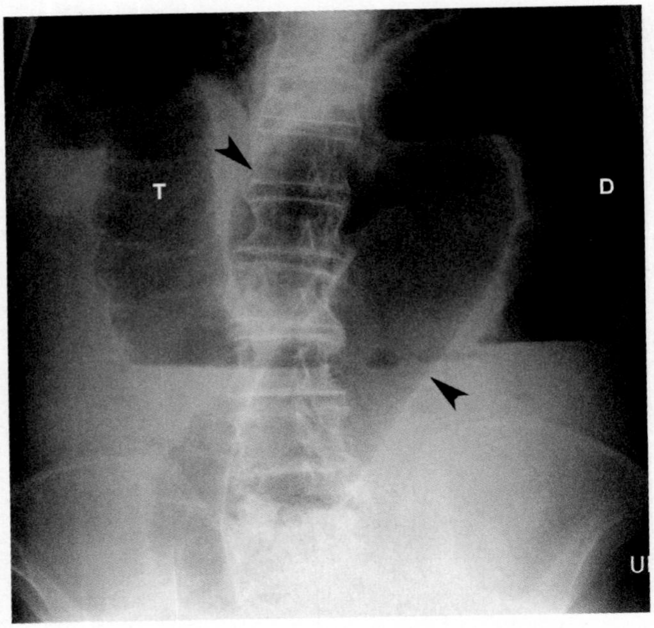

FIGURE 48.5. Plain upright abdominal film of a patient with sigmoid volvulus. The dilated centrally located sigmoid loop is seen (*arrowheads*). The proximal colon is dilated and gas filled. (T, transverse colon; D, descending colon.)

that are performed in different projections. Because such patients generally present early after the onset of symptoms, the loops proximal to the closed loop will not have had time to fill with air and the remainder of the abdomen may appear gasless. In the setting of "abdominal pain out of proportion to physical findings," a "normal" plain film does not exclude a closed-loop obstruction.

Contrast Studies. The diagnosis of bowel obstruction can generally be made by considering the clinical history, physical examination, laboratory, and plain radiograph findings. Contrast studies (i.e., small-bowel follow-through, enteroclysis, contrast enema) may provide specific localization of the point of obstruction and the nature of the underlying lesion. When obstruction of the small intestine is not progressing or resolving, a small-bowel follow-through may be performed to confirm the presence and location of the obstruction. Also, even under acute circumstances, diagnosis and management of colonic obstructions are generally enhanced by the use of a contrast enema. Under some circumstances, however, contrast studies are unnecessary and may be contraindicated. For example, in the classic setting of abdominal pain, nausea, vomiting, and a plain film indicating multiple air–fluid levels in the small intestine and colonic collapse, the diagnosis of acute obstruction can be made clinically. Failure to improve in a short period of time will mandate operation and contrast studies are unnecessary. When strangulation or perforations are strongly suspected, contrast studies are contraindicated.

The choice of contrast materials includes water-insoluble suspensions of barium and water-soluble agents such as Gastrografin or Hypaque. Barium studies provide the clearest images, in both small-bowel studies in which the contrast is given from above and colon/rectum studies in which the contrast is given by enema. If barium leaks into the peritoneum, it elicits intense peritonitis. If there is any possibility of bowel perforation or gangrene, barium should not be used. Water-soluble agents such as sodium amidotrizoate/meglumine amidotrizoate diatrizoate oral solution (Gastrografin) or diatrizoate sodium/diatrizoate meglumine (Hypaque) are hyperosmotic and can elicit fluid translocation into the gut. When the obstruction of the small intestine is incomplete (as discussed later), the use of these agents may facilitate resolution. In two randomized trials, diagnostic and therapeutic use of water-soluble contrast agents such as Gastrografin reduced the need for operation by 74%.[38,39] Gastrografin is hyperosmolar and causes mobilization of fluid into the bowel lumen and occasionally is therapeutic in cases of incomplete obstruction. Assalia et al.[38] divided 99 patients including 107 episodes of adhesive partial small-bowel obstruction into two groups: conservative management versus administration of 100 mL of Gastrografin via nasogastric tube. The group of patients who received Gastrografin had their first bowel movement, on average, in 6 hours versus 23 hours in the control group. Operative intervention was required in only 10% of the Gastrografin group (six episodes) compared with 21% (10 episodes) in the control group. The mean intervals of hospital stay were 2.2 days and 4.4 days, respectively. The authors suggested that orally administered Gastrografin is safe and therapeutic in adhesive partial small-bowel obstruction, though further studies were required to confirm the significance of the reduction in need for an operation.

Computed Tomography and Other Imaging Modalities. The potential benefits of **computed tomography** (CT) scanning in diagnosis of bowel obstruction include the following[40–42]: first, using dilute barium for luminal contrast, the obstructing segment may be localized and characterized as complete or incomplete. Second, the nature of the obstructing lesion, especially if it is malignant, can be established. Third, additional abdominal pathology (e.g., metastases, ascites, parenchymal liver abnormalities) may be identified. There is also evidence that, in special circumstances, CT may improve preoperative detection of strangulation.[33,42] CT findings indicating the site of obstruction and impending ischemia include beaklike narrowing, mesenteric edema, vascular engorgement, and moderate to severe intestinal wall thickening (>2 mm) (Fig. 48.6). In addition, high attenuation of bowel wall on unenhanced CT scans, low or reduced attenuation of bowel wall on intravenous contrast CT scans, and presence of intramural air (pneumatosis) or portal venous gas are CT findings suggestive of strangulation. Attenuation reflects increased energy absorption, scattering, beam divergence, and other causes of energy loss. Thus, areas of high attenuation appear darker than areas of low attenuation.

It has also been suggested that real-time abdominal sonography could aid in the diagnosis of strangulation obstruction. In studies conducted in two different institutions, Ogata et al.[43,44] demonstrated that the presence of significant amounts of peritoneal fluid and of an akinetic and dilated loop of bowel were strongly associated with the presence of strangulation. In patients who had strangulation but were thought to have simple obstruction only, these finding helped to make the preoperative diagnosis of infarction.

It should be emphasized that when the clinical picture suggests strangulation, unnecessary imaging studies should not delay resuscitation or expeditious movement to the operating room. Such studies will not necessarily be helpful when clinical criteria and basic abdominal radiographs have indicated the presence of a simple and complete obstruction. By itself, this diagnosis mandates urgent exploration and the information sought should be weighed against the risk of delay in going to the operating room. The message of the literature on imaging is not that the clinical picture can be misleading; in fact, in most studies evaluating the impact of imaging on diagnosis and timing of intervention, clinical diagnosis is seldom incorrect—it is highly specific when multiple clinical signs (tenderness, peritoneal signs, leukocytosis, profound dehydration) of strangulation are present. However, such a picture represents advanced disease and use of CT scan may detect strangulation before such signs are manifest. These findings

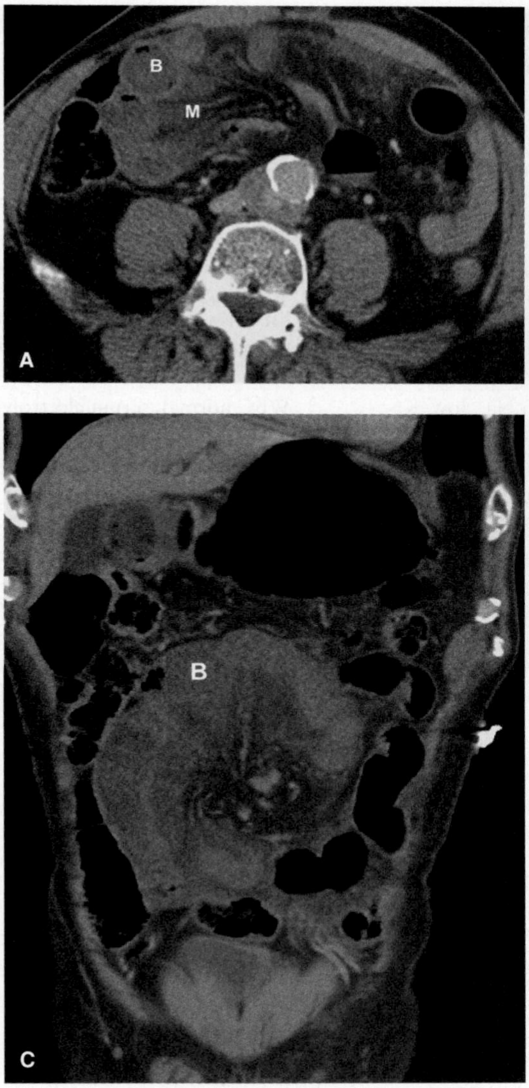

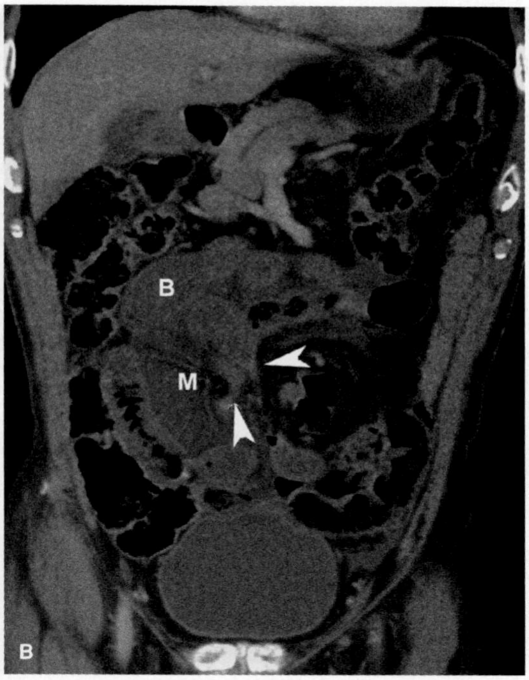

FIGURE 48.6. Axial (**A**) and coronal (**B**) images of a closed-loop obstruction with strangulated small bowel secondary to a volvulus from an adhesive band. Distended fluid-filled loops of small bowel (B) in a radial distribution converge toward the point of torsion (*white arrows*). There is edema within the mesentery (M). Shown in **C** is a coronal view of vascular engorgement and mesenteric edema in a closed-loop obstruction.

reinforce the dictum that when there are clinical signs of strangulation, surgery should be performed without additional imaging studies. In patients with equivocal findings or uncertain clinical diagnosis, CT can be highly useful in confirming the diagnosis, localizing the site, and detecting the cause of intestinal obstruction and strangulation.[42]

General Considerations in Management of the Patient with Bowel Obstruction

Patients with obstruction of the large bowel present with abdominal pain, distention, and obstipation. Vomiting and electrolyte imbalances are sometimes prominent, though usually delayed. Elderly patients, in particular, are prone to dehydration. The presentation of small-bowel obstruction depends on level of obstruction, open- or closed-loop nature, and interval since onset of symptoms. Symptoms and signs of pain, vomiting, obstipation, and distention are present in variable degrees. The overall picture, however, is usually one of a patient with abdominal symptoms that are evolving and getting worse. In the settings described previously, the following questions must be addressed as expeditiously as possible.

1. *Is the abdominal pain disproportionate to the physical findings and laboratory studies?*
2. *How rapidly are the symptoms and signs evolving: minutes, hours, or less acutely?*
3. *Does the patient suffer from dehydration, electrolyte imbalance, and acid–base disturbance?*
4. *Is the obstruction complete or incomplete?*
5. *Is there a possibility of strangulation?*

Clinical data and basic laboratory studies will provide reliable information to answer the first three questions. Answering questions 4 and 5 will often depend on close clinical observation and reexamination in the first hours or days after presentation. Abdominal radiographs and imaging studies are frequently used to provide additional information to help answer these latter questions and to identify the obstructing lesion.

Summarized in Table 48.3 are thumbnail sketches of different, but typical, kinds of patients presenting with symptoms and signs consistent with obstruction of the small intestine. The principles of diagnosis and management of each of these patients begin with clinical information that indicates the likelihood of a bowel obstruction. Laboratory studies and plain abdominal films are used to confirm the diagnosis of obstruction and determine the extent of physiologic impairment. The patient's history and clinical course in the first few hours of observation are used to determine the likelihood of strangulation. Indications for surgery include rapid evolution of symptoms and signs and the diagnosis that the obstruction is complete. Contrast or imaging studies are used only when symptoms

TABLE 48.3

MANAGEMENT OF BOWEL OBSTRUCTION IN THREE HYPOTHETICAL PATIENTS

	■ PATIENT I *CLOSED-LOOP OBSTRUCTION*	■ PATIENT II *INTESTINAL OBSTRUCTION WITH STRANGULATION*	■ PATIENT III *OPEN-LOOP OBSTRUCTION OF THE DISTAL SMALL INTESTINE OR CECUM*
Clinical:	Crampy periumbilical pain worsening over last 12 h. Two to three episodes of emesis. No distention, minimal flatus	Diffuse, crampy abdominal pain over 2 d with many episodes of vomiting. No bowel movements or flatus. T 100°F, P 100, dehydrated. Mild distention; local tenderness lower abdomen	Progressive abdominal distention over previous 2 wk. Mild discomfort. No vomiting. Few bowel movements and little flatus. Distention prominent, mild tenderness, no peritoneal findings
Lab:	No leukocytosis, pH, or electrolyte disturbances	WBC 16K. Serum Na^+ low, K^+ low, Cl^- low, pH alkalotic	WBC normal, serum electrolytes mildly decreased
Radiography:	Nonspecific gas pattern on plain film	Multiple dilated loops and air–fluid levels. No gas in colon	Multiple dilated small bowel loops and air–fluid levels. Some gas and stool in proximal colon
Differential Dx:	Broad: includes appendicitis, closed-loop SBO, pancreatitis, nonsurgical conditions	Narrow: complete SBO likely, strangulation cannot be excluded	Narrow: distal small bowel or proximal colon obstruction likely, possibly incomplete
Initial Rx:	Admit with q3–4h reevaluation by clinical exam, WBC. Repeat films q8–12h. NG tube if vomiting persists. IVFs	Admit for rapid resuscitation with IVFs, IV antibiotics. Urinary catheter and NG intubation indicated	Admit for IVFs, NG intubation. Hypaque enema followed by barium to evaluate colon. CT if malignancy suspected
Indications for surgery:	If pain worsens, local tenderness or peritoneal signs evolve, WBC rises, urine output falls	Already present. Patient should be scheduled and brought to OR after adequate resuscitation (dramatic improvement with resuscitation may permit observation for 4 h)	Surgery performed when evaluation is complete or if clinical course deteriorates during evaluation

CT, computed tomography; Dx, diagnosis; IVF, intravenous fluids; NG, nasogastric; OR, operating room; P, pulse; T, temperature; SBO, small-bowel obstruction; WBC, white blood cell.

are not evolving rapidly and when identification of the underlying lesion might alter the operative strategy (see specific lesions later).

The initial management of all patients with suspected bowel obstruction includes designating the patient "NPO" and starting intravenous fluids composed of isotonic Ringer or normal saline solutions. Restoration of fluid and electrolyte balance is a priority, often requiring frequent evaluation of serum electrolytes and pH. In rapidly evolving cases or patients with significant dehydration, an indwelling urinary catheter should be placed to monitor urine output. Invasive hemodynamic monitoring (e.g., a Swan-Ganz catheter) may be necessary to monitor the response to fluid resuscitation in patients with underlying cardiac, pulmonary, or renal insufficiency. Nasogastric decompression is indicated in most cases. The nasogastric tube, typically a 16- or 18-French sump tube, serves to prevent distal passage of swallowed air and minimizes the discomfort of refluxing intestinal content. The use of longer tubes has been advocated in certain settings, especially for patients with chronic but intermittent obstruction arising from Crohn disease, peritoneal carcinomatosis, radiation enteritis, or many previous laparotomies for obstruction. The underlying rationale is that advancement of the tip of the long tube to the obstructed loop would permit more effective decompression, perhaps resulting in relaxation of the loop and relief of the obstruction. Although this concept is appealing, there is no evidence to suggest a benefit for the use of a long tube in such settings.[45,46]

The use of intravenous antibiotics in the initial management of bowel obstruction should be discussed as well. Clinically, it has been recognized that antibiotics can ameliorate the evolution of symptoms and signs of strangulation in closed-loop obstruction and appendicitis. Studies in humans have demonstrated that, even in simple obstruction, bacterial counts in succus rise from under 10^6 organisms/L to over 10^9 organisms/L[47] and are not necessarily reduced with short-term administration of antibiotics.[48] Moreover, experimental studies indicate that bacteria can translocate across the intestinal mucosa, passing into lymph channels.[49] Further studies have demonstrated that germ-free animals can survive strangulation obstruction longer than normal animals and that luminal fluid taken from obstructed segments in germ-free animals is much less toxic than fluid taken from normal animals.[50,51]

For all these reasons, it is a well-established practice to administer antibiotics perioperatively, in order to reduce wound infection and abdominal sepsis rates in patients undergoing operation to relieve intestinal obstruction, simple or strangulated. Once the decision has been made to proceed with surgery, broad-spectrum antibiotics, covering gram-negative aerobes and anaerobes, should be given. A second-generation cephalosporin or a combination of a first-generation cephalosporin and metronidazole is rational practice for perioperative coverage in both simple and strangulation obstruction. Nevertheless, the use of antibiotics in patients who have not yet been committed to operation has not been evaluated systematically. Giving antibiotics to patients who are being observed can obscure the underlying process and, in the end, delay optimal therapy.

The decision to perform abdominal exploration to relieve intestinal obstruction should be made expeditiously, but not in the absence of critical information or before adequate resuscitation. Indications for surgery are outlined in Table 48.3, for each of the thumbnail vignettes. It should be emphasized that once a diagnosis of complete obstruction is made, simple or strangulated, the operation should proceed without undue delay. It is reasonable to commit the patient to a period of observation when the diagnosis is uncertain (i.e., there is a possibility of a nonsurgical diagnosis or that the obstruction is not complete). A practical point is that obstruction occurring in a patient without a previous history of laparotomy is not likely to be caused by peritoneal adhesions. This is known as de novo obstruction and, whatever the underlying cause, will not usually resolve without operation.

Specific Types of Bowel Obstruction

3 **Chronic Adhesions.** Peritoneal adhesions account for more than half of small-bowel obstruction cases. Lower abdominal procedures such as appendectomy, hysterectomy, colectomy, and abdominoperineal resection are common precursor operations to adhesive obstruction. Adhesions form after any abdominal procedure, however, including cholecystectomy, gastrectomy, and abdominal vascular procedures. In long-term follow-up, about 5% of patients undergoing laparotomy will develop adhesive obstruction; of these, 10% to 30% will suffer from additional episodes.[52,53] Up to 80% episodes of small-bowel obstruction due to adhesions may resolve nonoperatively.[30,31,38,45] However, an index episode and three recurrences indicate a likelihood of over 80% that there will be more recurrences.[52] Surgical management of an acute episode appears to reduce subsequent recurrence rates from ~15% to ~6%,[53] but no studies have been able to establish whether the immediate benefit of laparotomy for any given episode of simple adhesive obstruction outweighs the overall benefit of expectant management and operation only for serial recurrences. Thus, a previous history of a laparotomy simply provides a reasonable basis for expectant management of patients in whom it is not yet possible to diagnose a complete obstruction. Ultimately, patients who present with signs and symptoms from bowel obstruction are managed according to the CT findings and clinical course.

The pathobiology of adhesion formation has been the subject of considerable investigation. Histologic examination of chronic adhesions reveals foreign body reaction, usually to talc, starch, lint, intestinal content, or suture. Talc and starch are found less commonly now than previously, because of improvements in techniques of manufacture and sterilization of surgical gloves. Mesothelial cells are the presumed origin of tissue plasminogen activator (TPA). TPA binds fibrin and plasminogen, thereby preventing adhesion formation. In early studies, inflammatory cells, including mast cells,[54] were implicated in the process that produces adhesions. Recent studies[55,56] have emphasized the role of various cytokines in exacerbating or inhibiting adhesion formation in different animal models. Biologically active substances that might prove useful in preventing postoperative adhesions include transforming growth factor-β (TGF-β) and vascular endothelial growth factor (VEGF), both of which may be targeted for inhibition with less fear of compromising the response to bacterial infection.[55,56]

Current strategies to prevent adhesions after a first laparotomy include targeting the fibrinolytic system, which enhances rapid healing and appears to minimize formation of peritoneal adhesions.[55] Attempts to minimize or prevent adhesion formation have resulted in development of a hyaluronic acid–carboxymethylcellulose membrane (Seprafilm, Genzyme, Cambridge, MA). This compound mechanically prevents adhesion formation by physically separating adjoining tissues. It is absorbed by the body in 7 days and thus is present only during the phase of fibrosis, and not as a persistent foreign body. Randomized trials have suggested that this compound prevents, minimizes severity, and decreases density and vascularity of adhesions.[55,57] Other trials corroborate decreased severity, density, and vascularity of adhesions but not total prevention of adhesions or reduction of the incidence of subsequent bowel obstruction.[58] Seprafilm and similar barriers have been advocated for use in patients in whom a second abdominal procedure is planned or significant adhesions anticipated (e.g., Hartmann procedure, ileal pouch anal anastomosis with protecting ileostomy, pelvic surgery, gynecologic procedures, and colon surgery), though it has been proposed for all surgeries by the manufacturers. Meta-analyses in gynecologic procedures support claims that numbers and density of adhesions are reduced, without necessarily improving the incidence of subsequent intestinal obstruction.

More important than pharmacologic approaches, however, are the efforts of the surgeon to pay meticulous attention to hemostasis and surgical technique, and to carefully inspect for and remove foreign material from the peritoneal cavity. It is also possible that the use of monofilament sutures for fascial closure and avoidance of closure of the peritoneum as a separate layer may lower the formation of adhesions between viscera and the abdominal wall.[59]

Early Postoperative Adhesions. Obstruction in the immediate period following abdominal surgery is uncommon but may occur in up to 1% of patients in the 4 weeks following laparotomy. Adhesions are responsible for approximately 90% of such cases and hernias for approximately 7%.[60] Intussusception, abscess, or technical errors may be responsible for the remainder of cases.[61,62] Most cases occur after surgery of the colon, especially abdominoperineal resections, or operations in the lower abdomen. It is rare for upper abdominal surgery to cause such obstructions. A common scenario is that a patient will undergo colectomy uneventfully, pass flatus, and have bowel sounds by postoperative day 3. On the fourth postoperative day the patient suddenly becomes distended and uncomfortable, and stops passing flatus and stool. Patients with acutely evolving symptoms and signs represent complete obstruction and should be managed as such. In this latter setting, the mortality may be as high as 15% due to delays in recognition and operative intervention. The loss of bowel sounds after a short period of normal or hyperactive activity is worrisome for ischemia of the obstructed segment. The vast majority of such cases may be treated as partial intestinal obstruction; nasogastric suction and intravenous fluids will help resolve symptoms within a few days (Algorithm 48.1). When the clinical course does not demand earlier intervention, a nonoperative approach may be tried for 10 to 14 days and will resolve the obstruction in over 75% of such cases.[60,62,63]

Hernia. Hernias of all types are second only to adhesions as the most frequent causes of obstruction in western countries. External hernias such as inguinal (Fig. 48.7) or femoral hernias may present with the symptoms of obstruction and will not be diagnosed unless sought.[64] Femoral hernias are particularly prone to incarceration and bowel necrosis due to the small size of the hernia inlet.[64] Other hernias such as umbilical, incisional, paracolostomy, or lumbar hernias are obvious. Still others such as internal hernias are usually diagnosed at laparotomy for obstruction. These include obturator hernias, paraduodenal hernias (Fig. 48.8), and hernias through the foramen of Winslow or mesenteries. When hernia has been identified as the cause of the obstruction, the patient is quickly resuscitated, given antibiotics, and taken to the operating room. The hernia is then reduced and the viability of the bowel assessed. If viable, the bowel is left alone; if not, it is resected. The hernia defect is then repaired. One important consideration is the Richter hernia (Fig. 48.9).[65] In this variant, only a portion of the wall of the bowel is incarcerated and thus incarceration and strangulation may not be associated with complete obstruction. These most frequently occur in association with femoral or inguinal hernias. Complete obstruction can occur if more than half of the bowel circumference is incarcerated.

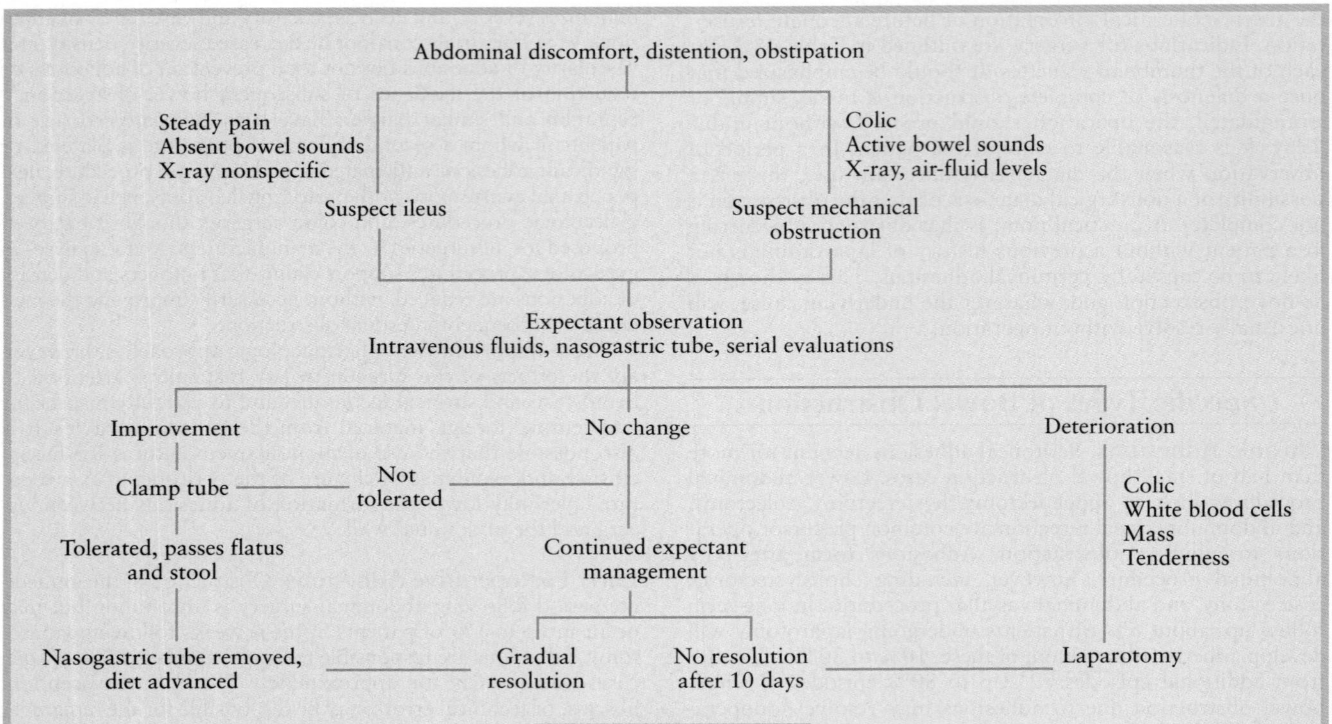

ALGORITHM 48.1

ALGORITHM 48.1. Approach to recognition and management of early postlaparotomy obstruction of the small intestine. (Adapted from Welch JP. *Bowel Obstruction: Differential Diagnosis and Clinical Management*. Philadelphia, PA: WB Saunders; 1989.)

For external (abdominal wall) hernias, it may be possible to perform *taxis,* that is, the manual reduction of an incarcerated/irreducible hernia. Taxis is usually successful in reduction of an irreducible hernia. Occasionally, taxis results in reduction of the contents of the hernia sac en mass (still obstructed), reduction of strangulated bowel resulting in generalized peritonitis, or reduction of an obstructed Richter hernia. This is one reason for using circumspection in relying on taxis as a mode of treatment for incarcerated inguinal, femoral, and incisional hernias. In general, taxis should be followed expeditiously by operative repair.

Gallstone Ileus. As a result of intense inflammation surrounding a gallstone, a fistula may develop between the biliary tree and the small or large intestine. Most fistulas develop between the gallbladder fundus and duodenum. If the stone is greater than 2.5 cm in diameter, it can lodge in the narrowest

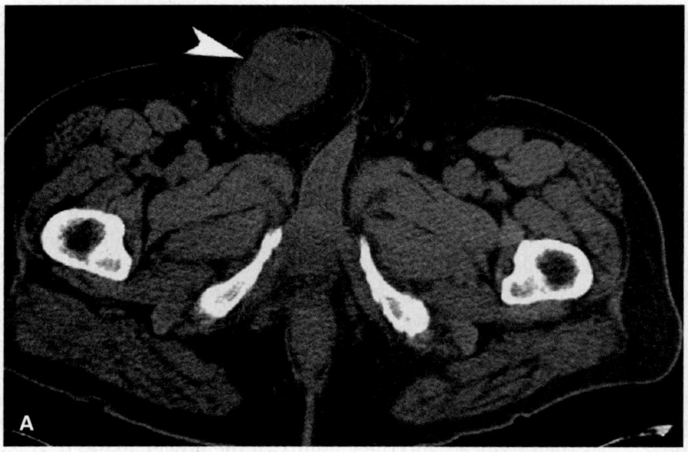

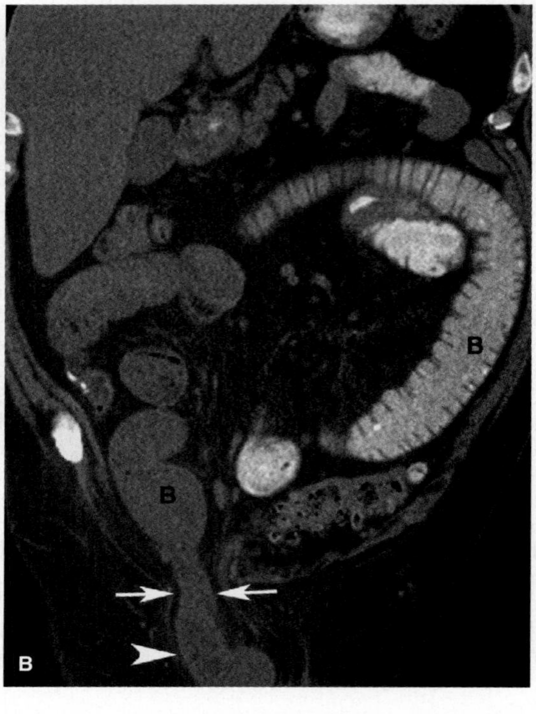

FIGURE 48.7. Computed tomography images of an inguinal hernia. Axial (**A**) and coronal CT scan (**B**) images showing incarcerated right inguinal hernia with air and fluid filled loop of small bowel (*arrowhead*) in the right inguinal canal (*arrow*) causing small bowel obstruction with dilated loops of proximal small bowel (**B**).

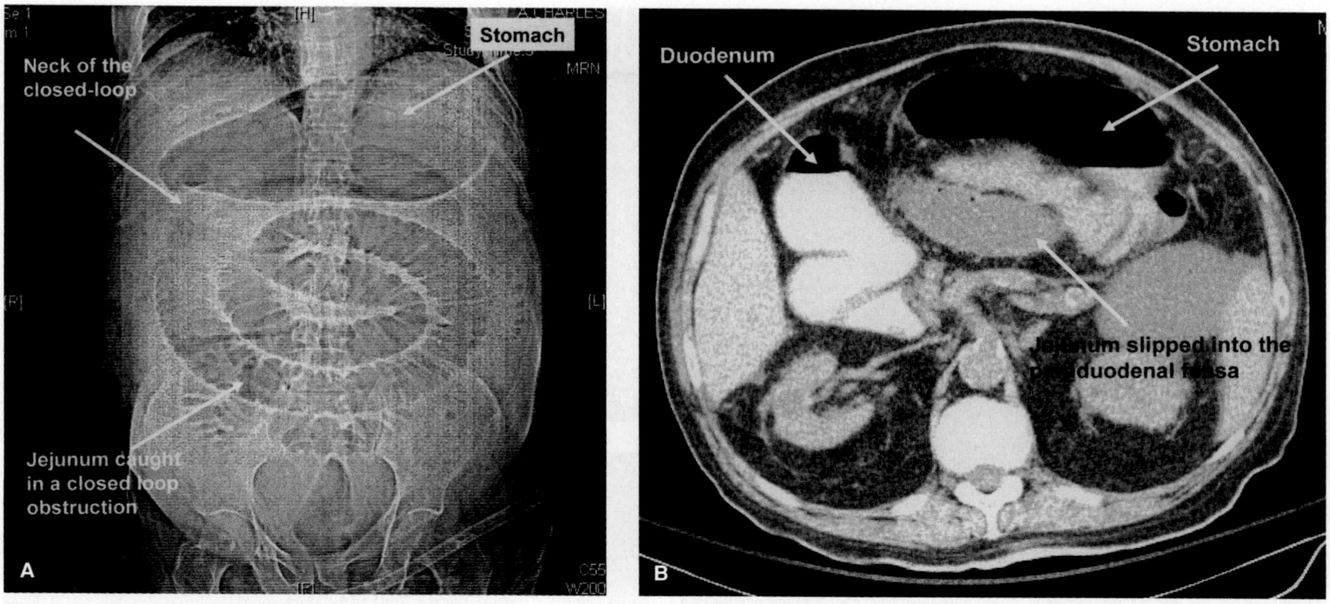

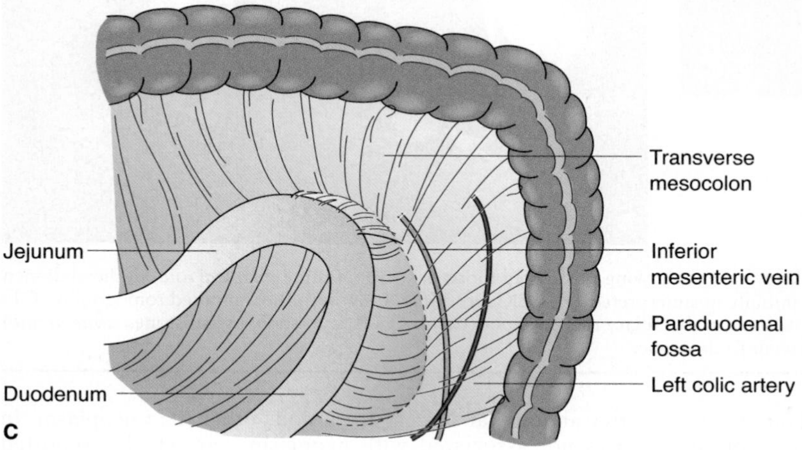

FIGURE 48.8. Paraduodenal hernia. **A:** Plain film of closed-loop obstruction with neck of the closed loop in the right upper abdomen. **B:** Computed tomography scan showing slippage of the jejunum behind the stomach, with dilatation and obstruction of the duodenum. **C:** Schematic diagram showing relationships of the paraduodenal fossa and transverse mesocolon. (Adapted from Skandalakis G. *Embryology for Surgeons*, 2nd ed. Baltimore: Williams and Wilkins; 1994:131–149.)

portion of the terminal ileum, which is just proximal to the ileocecal valve. This complication is rare, accounting for less than 6 in 1,000 cases of cholelithiasis and no more than 3% of cases of intestinal obstruction. Typically, the patient is elderly and presents with intermittent symptoms over several days, as the stone tumbles distally toward the ileum. The classic findings on plain radiographs include those of intestinal obstruction, a stone lying outside the right upper quadrant, and air in the biliary tree (Fig. 48.10). Treatment includes removal of the stone and resection of the obstructed segment only if there is evidence of tissue

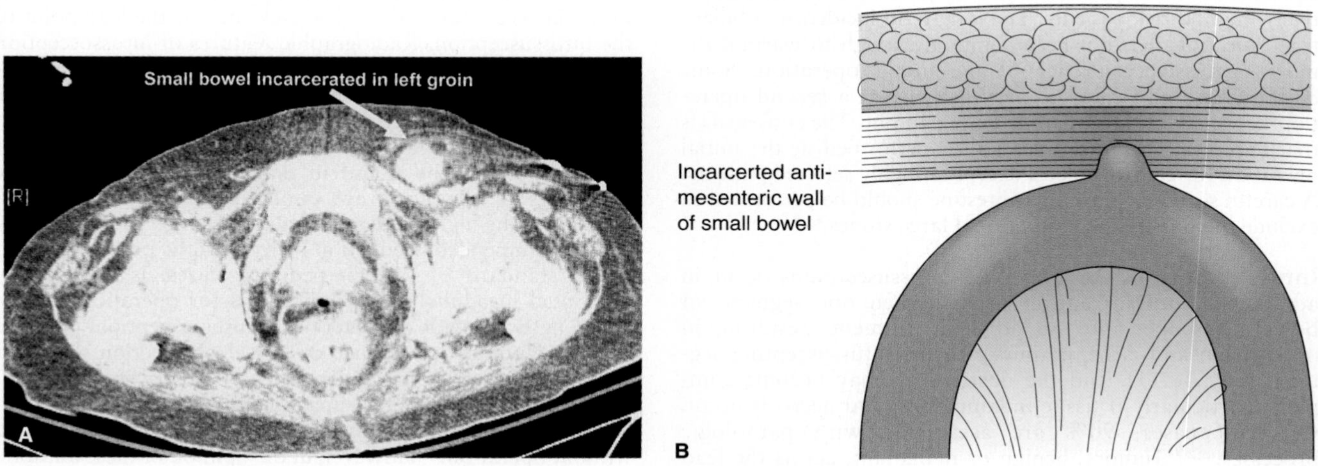

FIGURE 48.9. Richter hernia. **A:** Computed tomography scan showing contrast and air in the incarcerated segment within the left groin. **B:** Schematic diagram showing Richter hernia, in which the antimesenteric border (but not the whole wall) of the intestine is incarcerated.

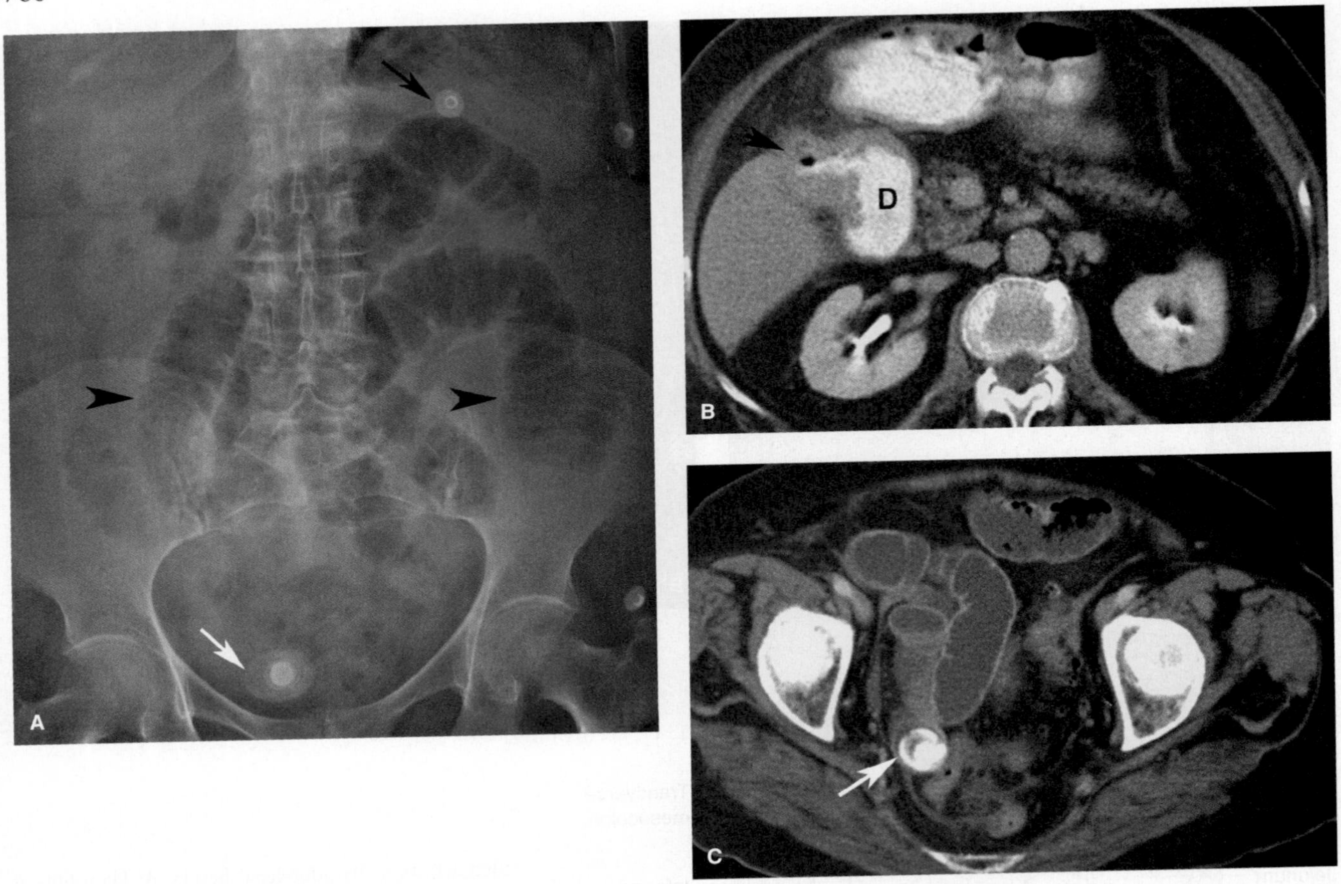

FIGURE 48.10. **A:** Plain radiograph of a patient with gallstone ileus, showing obstructed loops of small intestine (*black arrow*) in the abdomen and a gallstone (*white arrow*) in the pelvis (gallstone was initially misinterpreted as an EKG lead [*black arrow*]). **B:** Computed tomography (CT) scan showing a cholecystoduodenal fistula (*black arrow*) with air in the biliary tree (D, duodenum). **C:** CT scan showing gallstone (*white arrow*) in the distal ileum and fecalization of luminal content adjacent to the stone.

necrosis. The risk of a recurrent gallstone ileus is about 5% to 10%.[66,67] Such recurrences usually occur within 30 days of the initial episode and are usually due to stones in the small intestine that were missed at the original operation.

The difficult decisions in management of gallstone ileus focus on the fistula. The arguments in favor of disconnecting the fistula and removing the gallbladder have been the possibility of recurrence of gallstone ileus and the risk of cholangitis due to reflux of intestinal content into the biliary tree. When the latter operation is included, the mortality may be doubled as compared to simple removal of the gallstone. It is used selectively in good-risk patients. The long-term incidence of biliary tract infections has not been common enough to warrant the more aggressive approach at the initial operation. Some authors have advocated cholecystectomy at a second operation, especially if the patient is young and fit. The consensus is that cholecystectomy should not be performed at the initial operation for gallstone ileus, except in highly selected patients. A careful search of the entire intestine should be performed to exclude the possibility of additional large stones.[66,67]

Intussusception. About 5% of intussusceptions occur in adults. An intussusception occurs when one segment of bowel telescopes into an adjacent segment, resulting in obstruction and ischemic injury to the intussuscepting segment (Fig. 48.11), and the obstruction may become complete, particularly if tissue inflammation and necrosis occur. Of adult cases, 90% are associated with pathologic processes.[68,69] Tumors, benign or malignant, act as the lead point of intussusception in more than 65% of adult cases. A significant proportion of cases have been reported to occur after abdominal surgery for lesions other than neoplasm. In cases not associated with neoplasm, Sarr et al.[69] reported that approximately 20% were related to the suture line, approximately 30% to adhesions, and approximately 60% to intestinal tubes. Intussusception related to long tubes can occur when the tube is withdrawn, but most frequently occurs with the tube in place. Perioperative intussusception frequently subsides without intervention.

Four types of intussusception are recognized: enteric (Fig. 48.12), ileocolic, ileocecal, and colonic. In the ileocolic form, the ileum telescopes into the colon past a fixed ileocecal valve. In the ileocecal form, the valve itself may be the lead point of the intussusception. Radiographic features of intussusception are not specific. Plain films reveal evidence of partial or complete obstruction. Occasionally, a sausage-shaped soft tissue density will be seen, outlined by two strips of air. Recently, in both pediatric and adult cases, it has been suggested that sonography may be useful in diagnosis. Nevertheless, the mainstays of diagnosis are contrast studies or CT scan. Because of the high incidence of tumors, surgery has generally been recommended. Reduction by hydrostatic pressure, which is the standard of care in pediatric cases, is not usually attempted in adults. Clear indications for operation include long length and wide diameter of the intussusception, presence of a lead point, or evidence of bowel obstruction.[68] Recent studies have called into question the need to operate in all cases detected on sensitive imaging studies such as CT scan, arguing that a number of these patients can be safely managed without operation.[68] However, in the opinion of these authors, it is difficult to advise expectant management except in unusual circumstances.

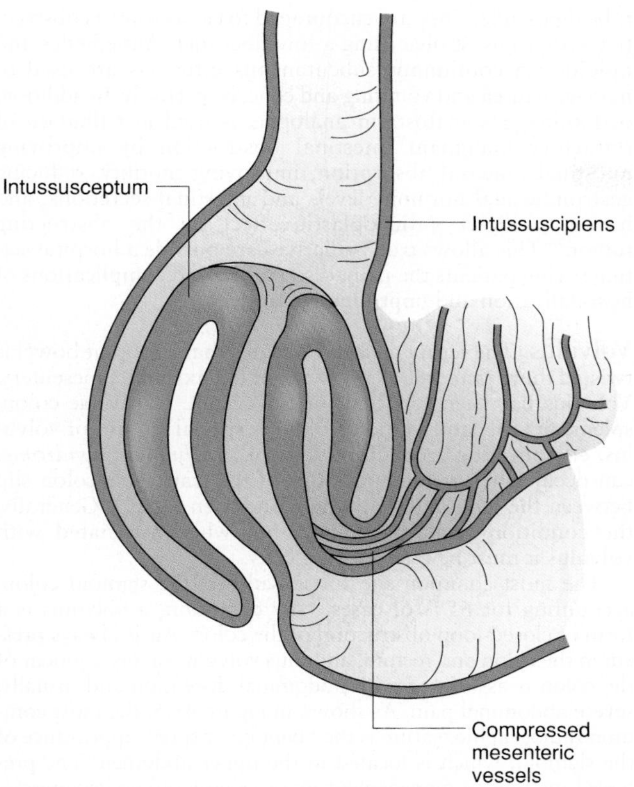

FIGURE 48.11. Anatomy of intussusception. The intussusceptum is the segment of bowel that invaginates into the intussuscipiens.

Crohn Disease. Indications for surgery in Crohn disease are discussed elsewhere in this book. In this disease, obstruction occurs under two different sets of circumstances.[70] When the disease has flared acutely, the lumen may be narrowed by a reversible inflammatory process. The result is an open-loop obstruction that may respond first to intravenous hydration and nasogastric decompression, and ultimately to therapy with corticosteroids or other anti-inflammatory regimens. Alternatively, obstruction may occur in the setting of a chronic stricture. Such strictures will not respond to conservative measures and, once diagnosed, operative therapy should not be delayed. One important clinical point is that about 7% of strictures in the colon, and an uncertain proportion of those in the small intestine, are malignant.[70] Extent of resection is thus based on intraoperative findings, that is, to margins beyond visibly diseased bowel and not necessarily including enlarged lymph nodes in the mesentery. If there is suspicion for malignancy, a lymphadenectomy is performed.

A second clinical point is that Crohn-affected bowel may not be dilated proximal to the obstruction but can be complicated by a small perforation. Such a microperforation may not be large enough to be associated with free air on plain films. The patient may thus present with significant abdominal pain and tenderness. A CT scan is likely to be the most sensitive imaging modality for obtaining evidence that differentiates conditions that require immediate surgery (closed-loop obstruction, microperforation) from simple obstruction that would otherwise be observed. In the absence of clinical progression of symptoms and signs, however, extended conservative management is warranted before the patient is committed to surgery.

Malignant Obstruction. Obstruction can complicate malignancies of the small and large bowel in a number of settings. Studies have documented that 10% to 28% of patients with colorectal cancer and 20% to 50% of patients with ovarian cancer will present with a malignant bowel obstruction at some point during the course of their disease.[71] Most commonly, a primary lesion such as an adenocarcinoma or lymphoma will enlarge until the lumen of the intestine is blocked. The lesion then presents with symptoms and signs associated with the level of obstruction and is managed accordingly.

A second setting involves a patient who previously has undergone surgery for malignancy and now returns with evidence of bowel obstruction. The likelihood that the obstruction is due to recurrent disease is based on several factors,

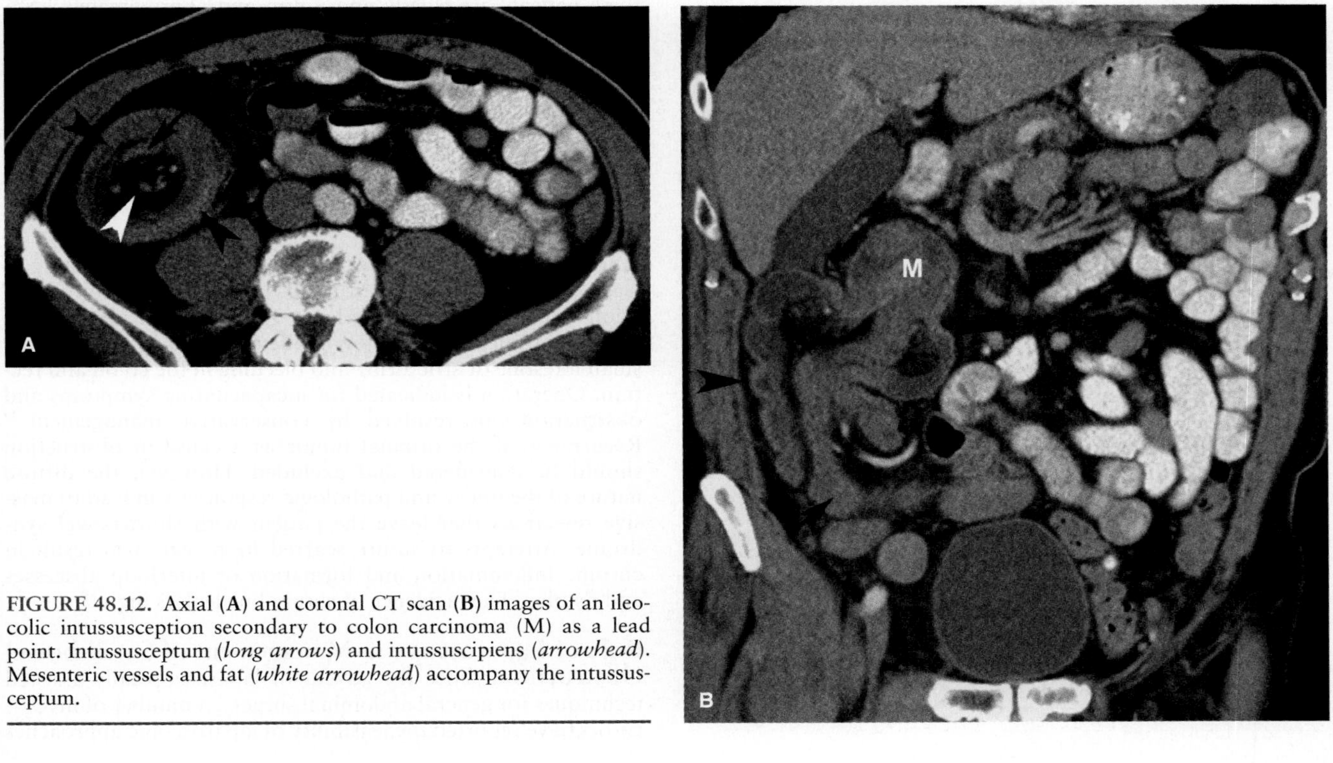

FIGURE 48.12. Axial (**A**) and coronal CT scan (**B**) images of an ileocolic intussusception secondary to colon carcinoma (M) as a lead point. Intussusceptum (*long arrows*) and intussuscipiens (*arrowhead*). Mesenteric vessels and fat (*white arrowhead*) accompany the intussusceptum.

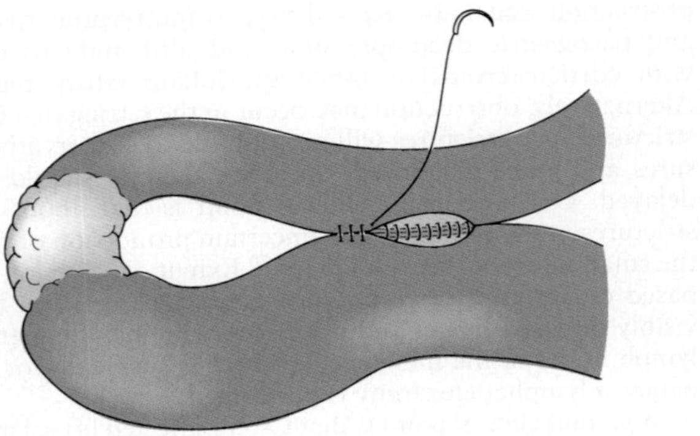

FIGURE 48.13. Significant palliation can be achieved in a patient with obstructing but unresectable malignancy. Enteroenterostomy is performed to bypass the obstructing segment.

including the origin of the primary malignancy, the stage of the primary malignancy, and the designation of the original surgery as curative or palliative. Gastric and pancreatic carcinomas often present with or are subsequently complicated by peritoneal carcinomatosis and thus the subsequent obstruction is most likely due to malignancy. With respect to colon and rectal carcinomas, as many as 50% of cases presenting with obstruction after resection of the primary malignancy may be due to adhesions and not recurrent malignancy.[71,72] In addition, even if the obstruction is due to now unresectable disease, significant palliation can be obtained through bypass or enterostomy in up to 75% of patients (Fig. 48.13). However, the underlying diagnosis of cancer in this patient population mandates careful attention be paid to patient selection prior to any surgical intervention and risk factors for poor outcome (Table 48.4, Algorithm 48.2). In patients presenting with gastroduodenal and colorectal obstructing lesions who are not candidates for surgical bypass or enterostomy, endoscopic management options including percutaneous endoscopic gastrostomy tube (PEG) placement and self-expanding metallic stent (SEMS) placement are available (Algorithm 48.2). These options have been associated with symptomatic relief in more than 75% of patients.[71]

Management of incurable malignant obstruction may require an approach that moves away from classical surgical teaching of nothing by mouth, nasogastric tube, intravenous fluids, and serial radiographs.[73] Patients with advanced malignant obstruction in the absence of a solitary or correctable obstructing lesion are generally managed without surgery (Algorithm 48.2). Patients are managed without a nasogastric tube if possible. They are encouraged to eat as soon as obstructive symptoms resolve using a low-fiber diet. Antiemetics and opioids via continuous subcutaneous infusions are used to manage nausea and vomiting and colic, respectively. In addition, octreotide, a somatostatin analogue, is used in palliation of refractory malignant intestinal obstruction by improving intestinal mucosal absorption, improving motility, reducing gastrointestinal hormone levels and intestinal secretions, and having a direct antineoplastic effect on the obstructing tumor.[74] This allows true palliative care outside a hospital setting saving patients the pain, discomfort, and complications of hospitalization and unproductive surgery.[73]

TABLE 48.4

RISK FACTORS FOR UNFAVORABLE OUTCOME IN MALIGNANT OBSTRUCTIONS

Advanced age (biologic/physiologic)
Poor performance status
Advanced stage of primary malignancy (previous treatments, availability of anticancer options, life expectancy)
Malnutrition/cachexia
Comorbidities
Absence of psychosocial support
Ascites (>100 mL associated with poor outcome)
Single vs. multiple sites of obstruction
Carcinomatosis (believed to respond poorly to surgical intervention)

Volvulus. The term *volvulus* indicates that a loop of bowel is twisted more than 180 degrees about the axis of its mesentery. Volvulus has been reported for the cecum, transverse colon, splenic flexure, and sigmoid colon. A special variant of volvulus, complicating a condition known as *Chilaiditi syndrome*, can occur when redundant loops of the transverse colon slip between the liver and diaphragm and then torse.[75] Generally, the condition is asymptomatic, but when associated with volvulus it must be relieved surgically.

The most common site for volvulus is the sigmoid colon, accounting for 65% of cases.[76] By definition, a volvulus is a form of closed-loop obstruction of the colon. Air is always present in the colon and rectum, and thus volvulus of any segment of the colon is associated with abdominal distention and, usually, severe abdominal pain. As shown in Figure 48.5, the most common radiographic feature is the "bent inner tube" appearance of the sigmoid, which is located in the upper abdomen. The preferred method of management involves endoscopic decompression. A rigid or flexible proctosigmoidoscope is advanced gently into the rectum until a rush of air and feces indicate that the loop has been untorsed. A rectal tube is then advanced well into the loop as a stent to prevent retorsion. Gangrene of the colon does not usually complicate the picture if the patient is seen and treated promptly. This conservative approach resolves the volvulus in 85% to 90% of cases and elective resection or fixation of the redundant segment can then be planned. Following endoscopic decompression, recurrence of the volvulus is higher than 60%.[77] Thus, an operation to remove the sigmoid should be performed if the patient is fit for surgery.[78] However, a majority of these patients are elderly and infirm and approximately 15% have a history of psychiatric disorder. As a result, the patient may present with peritoneal findings, sepsis, and shock. In this setting, rapid resuscitation followed by urgent resection and colostomy is warranted. Other forms of volvulus generally cannot be detorsed without operation. Fixation of the torsed segment (e.g., via cecostomy or cecopexy) is generally a less satisfactory solution than resection of the involved segment and is not generally recommended.[76]

Radiation Enteritis. After asymptomatic periods lasting at least 10 years, chronic intestinal obstruction can result. Radiation injury elicits an underlying vasculitis and fibrosis that lead to chronic, recurring low-grade partial obstruction of the small intestine or stricturing and bleeding in the colon and rectum. Operation is indicated for incapacitating symptoms and obstruction not resolved by conservative management.[79] Recurrence of the original tumor as a cause of obstruction should be considered and excluded. However, the diffuse nature of the injury and pathologic responses can lead to massive resections that leave the patient with short-bowel syndrome. Attempts to suture scarred loops can also result in chronic inflammation and formation of interloop abscesses and fistulas. The incidence of suture line leak is high.[80]

Role of Laparoscopy in Management of Small-bowel Obstruction. Since the advent of laparoscopically assisted techniques for general abdominal surgery, a number of investigators have reported the feasibility of laparoscopic approaches

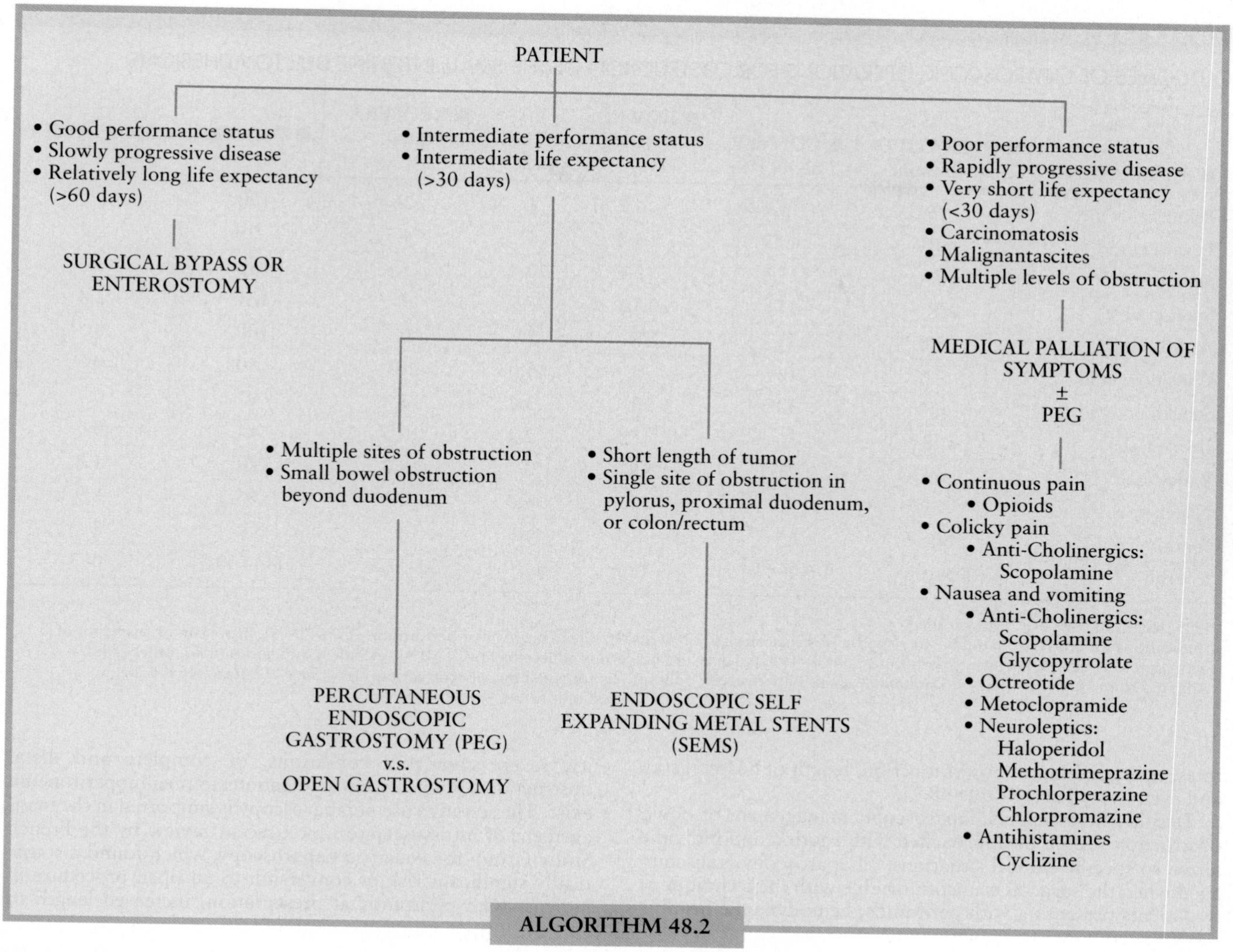

ALGORITHM 48.2. Algorithm for management of malignant obstruction. (Contributed by William Peranteau, M.D.)

to small- and large-bowel obstruction. Such approaches have been used, with varying degrees of success, to manage obstruction from a number of different etiologies (Table 48.5).[81–83] Laparoscopic management of bowel obstruction provides many potential benefits including quicker recovery of bowel function, shorter hospital stay, and fewer postoperative complications including a decreased incidence of wound infection and pneumonia. Additionally, as suggested by both clinical and experimental studies in animal models, laparoscopy is associated with less postoperative adhesion formation than open surgery.[84] Thus, laparoscopic management of bowel obstruction may result in a decreased lifetime risk for recurrent bowel obstruction. An appealing hypothesis, this long-term benefit of laparoscopic surgery has not yet been proven clinically.

In adults, the most common etiology for which laparoscopic versus open surgical management of bowel obstruction has been evaluated is adhesive bowel obstruction.[83,85–94] Studies of laparoscopic lysis of adhesions for small-bowel obstruction indicate that it is feasible, with acceptable operative times, length of hospital stay, and conversion and complication rates (Table 48.6). Studies directly comparing laparoscopic to open surgical management of adhesive small-bowel obstruction highlight the benefits of the laparoscopic approach as indicated by statistically significant decreases in complication

TABLE 48.5

FORMS OF INTESTINAL OBSTRUCTION SELECTIVELY AMENABLE TO LAPAROSCOPIC MANAGEMENT

Diaphragmatic (hiatal) hernia	Gallstone ileus
Inguinal hernia	Intussusception
Incisional hernia	Adenocarcinoma of colon
Femoral hernia	Diverticulitis
Spigelian hernia	Colitis (ischemic, radiation)
Internal hernia	Volvulus
Adhesions	Benign colon tumors
Crohn disease	Periappendicular abscess
Small-bowel tumor	Carcinomatosis
Meckel diverticula	Ogilvie syndrome
Ingested foreign body	Bezoar

Table prepared by William Peranteau, M.D.

TABLE 48.6

OUTCOMES OF LAPAROSCOPIC OPERATIONS FOR OBSTRUCTION OF THE SMALL INTESTINE DUE TO ADHESIONS

REFERENCES	OPERATIVE TIME (min)	CONVERSION (%)[a]	BOWEL INJURY (%)	LOS (d)	REOPERATION (%)	SUCCESS (%)	MORTALITY (%)
Pekmezci et al.[85]	99	6.7	6.7	4	0	100	0
Levard et al.[83]	NR	40.9	8.4	4	4.5	95	2.2
Sato et al.[86]	105	17.6	17.6	10.4	5.8	88	0
Suter et al.[87]	NR	43	15.6	5.9	9	NR	2.4
Al-Mulhim[88]	58	32	NR	5	0	100	0
Chosidow et al.[89]	71.7	16	3	5.03	NR	80	0
Strickland et al.[90]	68	32.5	10	3.6	5	97	0
Leon et al.[91]	108	35	7.5	2.9	17.5	81	0
Bailey et al.[92]	64	21.5	NR	3	10.8	NR	1.8
Navez et al.[93]	77	40	9	6.6	2.9	85.3	2.9
Ibrahim et al.[94]	NR	15	9.1	NR	3	NR	3
Overall	58–108	6.7–43	3–17.6	2.9–10.4	0–17.5	80–100	0–3

LOS, length of stay; NR, not recorded.
[a]Indications for conversion: unable to visualize obstruction site (22%–49%), bowel necrosis or perforation (19%–23%), neoplasm or suspicion of neoplasm (3%–25%), iatrogenic perforation (14%–19%), dense and numerous adhesions (14%–50%), technical difficulties (6%), other (5%).
Adapted from Nagle A, Ujiki M, Denham W, et al. Laparoscopic adhesiolysis for small bowel obstruction. *Am J Surg* 2004;187:464–470.

rates, time to return of bowel function, length of hospital stay, and even overall cost (Table 48.7).

Despite these benefits, laparoscopic management of bowel obstruction should be approached with caution and individualized to specific clinical situations.[95] Laparoscopy is discouraged when the surgeon is uncomfortable with the technique or in patients presenting with peritonitis, hemodynamic instability, severe comorbid conditions, or complete and distal obstruction, or when contraindications to pneumoperitoneum exist. The selective use of laparoscopy is supported in the management of intussusception by a recent review by the French Study Group for Pediatric Laparoscopy, which found a statistically significant risk of conversion to an open procedure in patients with peritonitis at presentation, increased length of

TABLE 48.7

OUTCOMES, COMPLICATIONS, AND COSTS IN LAPAROSCOPIC MANAGEMENT OF INTESTINAL OBSTRUCTION DUE TO ADHESIONS

REFERENCE	CONVERSION (%)		COMPLICATION (%)	TIME TO RBF (d)	LOS (DAYS)	OPERATIVE TIME (min)	COST ($)
Wullstein et al.[f]	52[a]	Laparoscopic	Intraop: 29[b] $P = 0.156$ Postop: 19.2[c] $P = 0.032$	3.5 $p = 0.001$	11.3 $p < 0.001$	103 $p > 0.05$	NR
		Open	Intraop: 15[d] Postop: 40.4[e]	4.4	18.1	84	NR
Mancini et al.[g]	17.2	Laparoscopic	19.2 $p = 0.008$	NR	6 $p = 0.0001$	NR	9,412 $p = 0.0003$
		Open	30.1	NR	9	NR	11,858

LOS, length of stay; RBF, return to bowel function.
[a]Indications for conversion: need for resection (14.8%), extent of adhesions or problems in view (37%), uncertain viability of small bowel (22.2%), small bowel perforation (25.9%).
[b]Laparoscopic intraoperative complications: perforation (26.9%), hemorrhage (1.9%).
[c]Laparoscopic postoperative complications: pulmonary (1.9%), wound infection (5.8%), anastomotic leak (3.8%).
[d]Open intraoperative complications: perforation (13.5%), mesenteric injury (1.9%).
[e]Open postoperative complications: pulmonary (3.8%), cardiac (3.8%), deep venous thrombosis (1.9%), death (3.8%), wound infection (11.5%).
Table prepared by William Peranteau, M.D.
[f]Wullstein C, Gross E. Laparoscopic compared with conventional treatment of acute adhesive small bowel obstruction. *Br J Surg* 2003;90: 1147–1151.
[g]Mancini GJ, Petroski GF, et al. Nationwide impact of laparoscopic lysis of adhesions in the management of intestinal obstruction in the US. *J Am Coll Surg* 2008;207:520–526.

time between the onset of symptoms and diagnosis (1.6 vs. 3.1 days), and the presence of a pathologic lead point.[96] Although these early retrospective studies are encouraging, prospective studies evaluating laparoscopic management of small-bowel obstruction are required to definitively document its benefits over the traditional open approach.

ILEUS AND PSEUDO-OBSTRUCTION

Ileus

4 **Etiologic Factors.** An ileus or *eileos* (Greek for "twisting") reflects a loss of forward peristalsis and coordination of the motility of the different regions of the gastrointestinal tract. A functional obstruction results.[97] Clinically, bowel sounds, passage of flatus, and bowel movements have been used to signal the return of bowel function and coordination of peristalsis. Liquid contrast and radiolabeled marker studies suggest that effective duration of ileus varies in different regions of the alimentary tract.[98,99] A postoperative ileus (POI) may last for 0 to 24 hours in the small intestine, 24 to 48 hours in the stomach, and 48 to 72 hours in the large bowel.[100,101] The type of surgery and the wide variety of endpoints used to measure gut recovery often decide the duration of ileus. There is no consensus as to which one is most clinically meaningful. Duration of ileus is therefore primarily dependent on the return of colonic motility and its coordination with other regions of the gastrointestinal tract. A typical period of ileus is thus self-limited and easily tolerated. Factors implicated in ileus (Table 48.6) are outlined in the following sections.

Neurohumoral Peptides. Increases in endogenous opioid release and other peptides such as calcitonin gene–related peptide, motilin, substance P, VIP, and substance P have all been established as inhibitory neurotransmitters in the intrinsic gut nervous system. Antagonists to VIP, substance P, and inhibitors of nitric oxide (NO) synthesis improve postoperative bowel motility.[102,103] Calcitonin gene–related peptide inhibits postoperative gastric emptying and gastrointestinal transit.[104,105] The use of anticholinergic medications delays recovery of an ileus.[106]

One group of neurohumoral substances that are particularly important in this regard are the opioids, both synthetic and endogenous. Opioids are established neurotransmitters in the central and peripheral nervous systems, and it is well established that their use delays gastric emptying and promotes nonpropulsive smooth muscle contraction with an increase in intraluminal pressure throughout the entire gastrointestinal tract.[107,108] Over the years, a series of experimental studies have indicated that recovery of ileus is accelerated during administration of specific antagonists to κ or μ opioid receptors,[109,110] suggesting that endogenous opioid release modulates recovery from ileus.

Inflammation. A relatively recent series of experimental and clinical investigations have focused attention on the role of inflammatory cells and mediators of inflammation in the development of prolonged ileus. Surgical intervention results in elevated levels of interleukin-6 (IL-6), cyclooxygenase-2 (COX-2), and inducible nitric oxide synthetase (iNOS), all mediators of inflammation from macrophages.[111,112] In experimental animals, focal manipulation of the bowel may result in a panenteric inflammation and ileus.[112] In experimental animals and human subjects, activated macrophages have been found in the muscularis of the small bowel as early as 3 hours after laparotomy.[113] Increased COX-2 expression leads to prostaglandin release. Jejunal contractility appears to be impaired, an effect blocked in COX-2 knockout mice and by the administration of selective COX-2 inhibitors. In related studies both in experimental animals and human subjects, Kalff et al.[113] found that NO synthesis is stimulated in activated macrophages in the muscular layer of the small intestine following surgical intervention. More recently, degranulation of mast cells has also been implicated in the pathogenesis of ileus after laparotomy,[114,115] with mast cell destabilizers having been shown to prevent mechanically induced intestinal inflammation and dysmotility.

Inhibitory Neural Reflexes. Noxious spinal afferent signals are thought to increase inhibitory sympathetic activity in the gastrointestinal tract.[116] Blockade of spinal afferents with epidural local anesthetics or with topical capsaicin has been shown to accelerate resolution of ileus in experimental studies.[104,105] In clinical studies of patients undergoing complex abdominal operations through conventional laparotomy incisions, it appears that conventional intramuscular injections are less likely to be associated with prolonged ileus than strategies utilizing patient-controlled intravenous injection.[117,118] Moreover, utilization of epidural analgesia tends to decrease recovery times from ileus in this group of patients,[119–121] suggesting that autonomic pathways coursing through the spinal cord may serve as control points for ileus.

Central responses have also been observed as a result of laparotomy[116] and have been linked to activation of afferent pathways in the vagus nerve and a general response of the organism to stress and release of corticotrophin-releasing factor.[122] Very recently, the efferent pathways in the vagus have also been implicated as possible modulators or control points for the inflammatory response. A series of experimental studies[123,124] has suggested that the vagus participates in suppression of certain macrophage activities, leading to earlier resolution of intestinal ileus.[124] These observations offer the possibility of a multidimensional understanding of ileus, both in individuals who are recuperating normally and in those who are not and have no specific risk factors for protracted ileus (e.g., undrained sepsis, overuse of narcotics, spinal cord injury, severe pelvic fractures, and retroperitoneal inflammation).

5 **Diagnosis.** It is important to distinguish between a normal *postoperative ileus* and a *paralytic ileus*. The distinction is predominantly one of time since operation and based on circumstance. Postoperative ileus is less severe, self-limiting (lasts 2 to 3 days vs. 3 to 5 days), and usually an indicator of colonic dysmotility, whereas a paralytic ileus represents inhibition of small-bowel activity. A prolonged POI (PPOI) occurs with protracted signs or symptoms of abdominal distention, bloating, diffuse and persistent abdominal pain, nausea, vomiting, and an inability to pass flatus or tolerate an oral diet.

It is also important to distinguish between a PPOI from a mechanical small-bowel obstruction (SBO). Clinically, the presence of intense colicky pain, feculent emesis, or rapidly progressing pain or distention is more suggestive of SBO than PPOI. Localized tenderness, fever, tachycardia, and peritoneal signs suggest bowel ischemia or perforation, necessitating emergent surgical intervention.[10]

A variety of clinical circumstances and laboratory tests may also increase suspicion for prolonged ileus and lessen concern for mechanical obstruction and associated complications. In addition to opiates, a number of medications have been associated with slow recovery of intestinal motor function (Table 48.8). Isolated metabolic disturbances such as ketoacidosis, hypomagnesemia, hypercalcemia, and hypokalemia can prolong ileus. Ileus can be caused and perpetuated by systemic inflammatory responses to sepsis, abscess, and pancreatitis.

When the patient's postoperative ileus has extended beyond the expected period, plain films of the abdomen reveal gas in segments of both small and large bowel (Fig. 48.14). At this point, the patient may begin to experience some discomfort and distention, as swallowed air fills loops that do not have effective peristalsis. Bowel sounds may be present, if hypoactive. The differential diagnosis now includes the possibility of mechanical obstruction from early postoperative adhesions

TABLE 48.8

FACTORS CONTRIBUTING TO PROLONGED ILEUS

■ NEUROGENIC	■ METABOLIC	■ PHARMACOLOGIC	■ INFECTIOUS
Spinal cord lesions or injury	Hypokalemia Uremia	Anticholinergics Opiates	Systemic sepsis Pneumonia
Retroperitoneal process hematoma, tumor	Ca^{2+}, Mg^{2+} imbalance	Autonomic blockers	Peritonitis
Ureteral colic	Hypothyroidism Diabetic coma or ketoacidosis	Antihistamines Psychotropics Phenothiazines Haloperidol Tricyclic antidepressants Clonidine Vincristine	Herpes zoster Tetanus Bacterial overgrowth (blind loop)

(see earlier). To differentiate early postoperative obstruction from ileus, contrast studies or a CT scan is helpful. The latter may be useful if other abdominal pathology such as an abscess could be contributing to the clinical picture. CT with oral contrast has a sensitivity and specificity of 90% to 100% in distinguishing ileus from a complete postoperative SBO.[125] However, it is less reliable in distinguishing ileus from a partial SBO.[125] If the diagnosis is uncertain after CT, upper gastrointestinal contrast studies (enteroclysis) with water-soluble radiopaque contrast material (e.g., Gastrografin) are especially helpful in distinguishing ileus from partial SBO (which more closely mimics ileus than complete SBO) and in identifying the severity of partial obstruction.[125]

6 **Management.** A normal POI is usually self-limiting. Nevertheless, there are a number of interventions that are effective

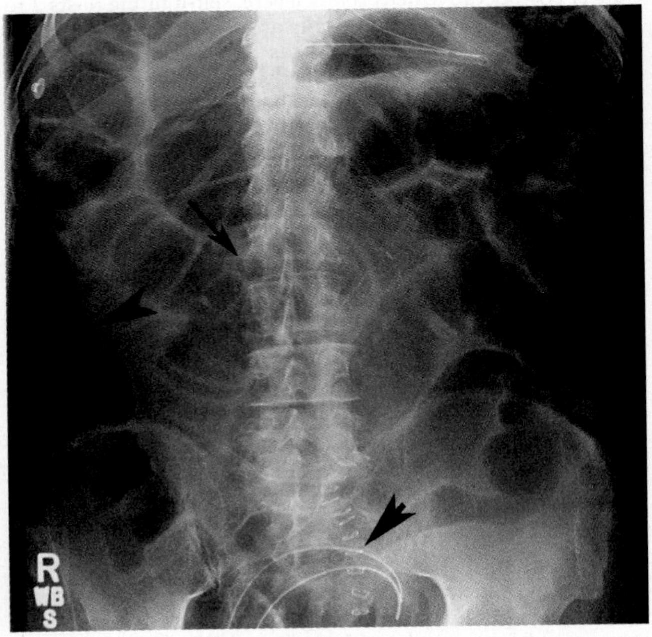

FIGURE 48.14. Plain supine abdominal radiograph of a patient with ileus. Air–fluid levels are present in the small intestine (*thin arrow*). Gas is seen in the colon (*thick arrowhead*). These findings are characteristic of, but not specific for, ileus. Surgical drains in the pelvis and skin staples (*short arrow*).

in reducing the duration of a normal postlaparotomy ileus (Table 48.9). Midthoracic epidurals with neuraxial local anesthetics have been shown to hasten the return of bowel function compared to systemic or epidural opioids.[119–121] Midthoracic local anesthetic epidurals block nociceptive afferent signals from the surgical site as well as sympathetic efferent outflow; this is useful for 48 to 72 hours postoperatively.

The goals in management in the normal period of postoperative ileus are to prevent uncomfortable distention, vomiting, and aspiration. Classic studies[6,10] indicate that flatus and the air accumulating during intestinal distention is derived largely from swallowing. Under normal circumstances, flatus is passed as early as 30 minutes after a "test bolus" of air is administered by tube into the stomach. Thus, passage of flatus is used, in reliable patients, as the index indicating coordination of all segments of the gastrointestinal tract and resolution of ileus.

For many years, the mainstay of therapy was the use of nasogastric suction to prevent accumulation of swallowed air and secreted fluids in an alimentary tract not yet coordinating flow distally. Subsequent studies have demonstrated that the putative benefit does not compensate for risks of aspiration and discomfort of the tube. Thus, in routine abdominal cases such as colectomy, nasogastric tubes are used selectively[126,127] in patients who are felt to be at risk for complications of ileus, based on the surgeon's judgments about intraoperative findings or manipulations—prolonged handling and packing of the bowel, anticipation of intensive use of narcotics or other antikinetic agents, presence of sepsis or peritonitis, or extensive blood loss. Otherwise, a nasogastric tube is used for a short postoperative period or never placed, with the expectation that a small percentage of patients will require placement for symptoms.[127] In these cases, the patient is allowed nothing by mouth or to have sips until there is evidence (by listening for bowel sounds or the patient's report of "rumbles") that ileus is likely resolving. Intravenous fluids are necessary until the patient can be advanced to full intake of his or her requirements, usually after flatus is passed.

In addition, correctable conditions such as electrolyte disturbances or uremia are investigated and rectified. Mobilization has other benefits in reducing morbidity.[128,129] Early feeding is thought to stimulate gastrointestinal hormones, secretions and motility, and coordinated propulsive activity. In addition, early feeding may improve immune function and reduce infectious and catabolic complications.[97,130] Despite the use of laxatives with prokinetic agents, no controlled trial exists to assess the possible beneficial effects of laxatives on postoperative ileus.[97]

One treatment, gum chewing, has attracted attention as a simple and inexpensive method of accelerating return of bowel

TABLE 48.9 **MANAGEMENT**

TREATMENT FOR POSTOPERATIVE ILEUS

■ TREATMENT	■ BENEFIT	■ DRAWBACK
Nasogastric tube	■ Possible relief of vomiting and bloating	■ Does not shorten duration of ileus ■ May contribute to fever, atelectasis, and aspiration ■ Discomfort
Early postoperative feeding	■ Stimulates reflex for propulsive bowel motility and enzyme secretion ■ Stimulates immune system ■ Reduces postoperative and posttraumatic infectious complications ■ Reduces risk of anastomotic dehiscence, wound infection, and pneumonia	■ Patients may not tolerate feeding
Opioid antagonists (alvimopan)	■ Peripheral acting ■ FDA approved to hasten postoperative ileus following partial large- or small-bowel resection with primary anastomosis	■ Possible cardiovascular or neoplastic risk ■ Currently restricted to in-patient use only
Laparoscopic procedures	■ Earlier return of bowel function and discharge from hospital ■ Minimal skin incision, minimal mechanical bowel manipulation	■ Not all patients and procedures are amenable to laparoscopic approach
Epidural anesthetics/analgesics	■ Reduced duration of ileus vs. systemic opioid ■ Increases splanchnic blood flow ■ Anti-inflammatory	■ Risks associated with epidural catheter placement
Gum chewing	■ May shorten duration of ileus ■ Simple and inexpensive	■ Limited data
Laxatives	■ May shorten duration of ileus ■ Inexpensive	■ Limited data on efficacy
Nonsteroidal anti-inflammatory drugs (COX-2 inhibitors)	■ Decreases opioid needed for pain control ■ May increase motility by acting as an anti-inflammatory	■ Possible increased risk of postoperative bleeding ■ Other adverse effects

COX-2, cyclooxygenase-2; FDA, U.S. Food and Drug Administration.
Adapted from Table 2 in Luckey A, Livingston E, Tache Y. Mechanisms and treatment of postoperative ileus. *Arch Surg* 2003;138(2):206–214.
Prepared by Zain Khalpey, M.D.

function. Mastication stimulates the vagal cholinergic pathways that increase gastrointestinal hormone secretion such as gastrin, pancreatic polypeptide, and neurotensin, which affect gastrointestinal motility.[131,132] Since the initial publication of one small and underpowered study,[133] a number of prospective randomized trials have been conducted to test the hypothesis that gum chewing results in earlier passage of flatus and bowel movement in patients undergoing laparoscopic colectomy.[134,135] No conclusive evidence has been obtained to demonstrate a clear benefit of gum chewing, although subgroup analysis suggests some patients may benefit.[135] According to one hypothesis, sorbitol and other hexitols, the key gradients of "sugar-free" chewing gums, may also play a role in the earlier recovery of postoperative ileus.[136] This hypothesis and its putative benefits are intriguing.

Salt and water disturbances in the body also may influence return of bowel function following laparotomy. In one initial study, patients undergoing colectomy received a restricted perioperative fluid resuscitation regimen or a standard, more liberal fluid resuscitation. The "restricted" group had a quicker passage of flatus and moved their bowels earlier, leading in part to shorter hospital stays.[137] Subsequent studies[138,139] have not uniformly suggested that recovery from ileus is faster with temperance in fluid resuscitation, or have indicated that there is a benefit from fluid restriction protocols but have not reported return of gastrointestinal function as an endpoint.[140] However, this benefit, as well as others, may be more clearly observed when fluid therapy is directed by physiologic assessments of volume status, such as esophageal Doppler monitoring of the great vessels and heart chambers.[141,142]

Experimental evidence of pharmacologic interventions specifically directed at abnormal surges of neurotransmitters or hormones that might prolong ileus has provided a useful insight into the pathophysiology of postoperative ileus. Opioid antagonists, somatostatin analogues, sympatholytics, injection of local anesthetics into mesenteric nerve roots, and nonsteroidal anti-inflammatory agents, such as ketorolac, appear to promote faster recovery to normal myoelectric activity and intestinal transit times.[106,143,144] In contrast, nonspecific adrenergic receptor blockers such as propranolol have been found to be ineffective.[145] Opioid antagonists such as alvimopan and methylnaltrexone are peripherally acting opioid antagonists and do not cross the blood–brain barrier.[146] In many, but not all, studies, alvimopan has been shown to hasten postoperative gastrointestinal recovery following bowel surgery and abdominal hysterectomy.[146] In one study where an overall benefit was not observed,[147] subgroup analysis showed that there was a benefit in patients who received patient-controlled, intravenously administered opiate analgesia, suggesting that prolonged ileus may be shortened if opiates are being used regularly to control pain. However, cardiovascular and neoplastic risks with the use of alvimopan have precluded its widespread use, limiting U.S. Food and Drug Administration approval following partial large- or small-bowel resections with primary anastomosis.[146] Additional studies[148] have suggested a benefit in fast-track pathways of care and routine use for accelerating recovery of ileus following laparotomy may be recommended under circumstances in which opiates are used liberally for pain control.

Prokinetic agents such as metoclopramide, cisapride (presently not approved by the U.S. Food and Drug Administration), and erythromycin have been evaluated for their efficacy in shortening the duration of POI. For ileus following upper gastrointestinal procedures (e.g., pancreaticoduodenectomy), such medications may be effective in promoting gastric emptying.[112] For general abdominal procedures involving the small intestine, colon, and retroperitoneal structures such as the aorta, there has been limited success in using such agents to shorten recovery times.[113,114] In multiple controlled studies, metoclopramide did not have significant impact on the duration of ileus.[114,118] In other studies, no benefit was observed when patients were given erythromycin.[113,119] Promising results have been observed with cisapride, which significantly reduced the duration of ileus. The results would depend on the route of its administration.[120–128] However, this medication is no longer approved for use in the United States due to the occurrence of potentially fatal arrhythmias.[129]

Along with pharmacologic measures, it should be emphasized that, in otherwise routine laparotomy or laparoscopy, gentle handling of tissues, meticulous attention to hemostasis, and applications of sound principles of wound management are likely to have the greatest impact on optimizing recovery from ileus and minimizing the incidence of prolonged ileus. Efforts to reduce incision size and time spent handling the intestines through the use of laparoscopic approaches clearly improve recovery from ileus in some, if not all, patients undergoing standardized intra-abdominal procedures such as appendectomy[149] and colectomy.[150] Even in open procedures,[151] standardization of management and effective communication help expedite clinical fast-track pathways and facilitate earlier recovery of bowel function and discharge from hospital.[97,142,148] Currently effective measures to minimize the prolongation of ileus are summarized in Table 48.10.

TABLE 48.10 MANAGEMENT

MEASURES TO PREVENT PROLONGATION OF ILEUS

- Minimization of trauma to tissues; using proper technique in the operating room with gentle handling of bowel during surgery
- Minimal use of narcotics for analgesia, for any route of administration (intravenous, intramuscular, epidural)
- Use of opioid antagonists (alvimopan)
- Generous use of midthoracic epidural anesthesia with local anesthetic use
- Use of nonsteroidal anti-inflammatory (cyclooxygenase-2 inhibitors) agents for analgesia
- Early feeding
- Correction of any electrolyte or metabolic imbalances
- Early recognition of septic complications (e.g., abdominal abscess, pneumonia, central line sepsis) that may contribute to prolongation beyond the expected period for ileus

Colonic Pseudo-obstruction (Ogilvie Syndrome)

Etiologic Factors. Acute pseudo-obstruction of the colon, also known as *Ogilvie syndrome*,[152] is a paralytic ileus of the large bowel, characterized by rapidly progressive abdominal distention, often painless.[153] Although the distention of the colon is not due to mechanical obstruction, the wall of the bowel, particularly that of the cecum, can become sufficiently distended so that its blood supply is compromised. Gangrene, perforation, peritonitis, and shock can follow. In 95% of the cases, there is an underlying disease.[153,154]

Major risk factors for development of Ogilvie syndrome include traumatic injury (11%); infections such as pneumonia and sepsis (10%); obstetric/gynecologic conditions (10%); myocardial infarction and congestive heart failure (10%); abdominal and pelvic surgery (9%); neurologic conditions such as Parkinson disease, spinal cord injury, multiple sclerosis, and Alzheimer disease (9%); orthopedic procedures (7%); other medical conditions including metabolic imbalances (e.g., hypokalemia, hypocalcemia, hypomagnesemia) (32%); and other surgical conditions (12%).[152,154] Evidence suggests that Ogilvie syndrome is thought to be related, at least in part, to sympathetic nervous overactivity or interference with sacral parasympathetic efferents, although there is little direct experimental evidence for this.[153] It is postulated that the distal colon becomes atonic on interruption of the S2 to S4 parasympathetic nerve fibers.

Diagnosis. This syndrome is commonly encountered in patients hospitalized over 3 to 7 days, often in men older than 60 years of age. Primary manifestations include gastrointestinal symptoms such as nausea, vomiting, abdominal pain, constipation, or even diarrhea with great variability.[153,154] Labored breathing, caused by abdominal distention, is often part of the clinical picture. Other than distention, there are no characteristic physical or laboratory findings for this syndrome. The abdomen resonates with percussion. Sounds from the small intestine are present and may not be high pitched, as they are in intestinal obstruction.

Laboratory findings associated with this syndrome may include hypokalemia, hypocalcemia, and hypomagnesemia, which are implicated as etiologic factors. Leukocytosis, elevation of the sedimentation rate, or C-reactive protein is also present if inflammation is initiated or perforation is impending.

The diagnosis is usually apparent from plain films. Radiographs of the abdomen may reveal air in the small bowel and distention of discrete segments of the colon (i.e., cecum or transverse colon often up to the splenic flexure) or the entire abdominal colon. Haustral markings disappear with increasing distention. In doubtful cases in which bowel necrosis is not a significant worry, a Hypaque contrast enema can establish the nonmechanical nature of the dilatation. Alternatively, colonoscopy can be diagnostic as well as therapeutic. Features suggesting the complication of bowel ischemia may include localized tenderness, worsening leukocytosis, metabolic acidosis, evidence of sepsis, or a rapidly deteriorating clinical course.

It is important to differentiate this syndrome from toxic megacolon and mechanical obstruction before establishing a final diagnosis. Mechanical obstruction of the colon, occurring in volvulus or obturator obstructions from cancer or diverticular disease, presents with acute pain along with distention. In contrast, pseudo-obstruction is less often associated with acute pain and more likely to present with discomfort due to distention. However, lack of pain in postoperative patients on opiates or elderly patients cannot exclude mechanical obstruction. In plain radiographs, the pathognomonic signs of mechanical obstruction such as lack of gas in the distal colon or rectum and air–fluid levels in the small intestine can also be

TABLE 48.11 MANAGEMENT

TREATMENT FOR PSEUDO-OBSTRUCTION

■ TREATMENT	■ BENEFIT
Nasogastric tube	■ Prevention of swallowed air from passing distally
Neostigmine	■ Increase motility through its parasympathomimetic action ■ Premedication with colonoscopic decompression adding benefits
Erythromycin	■ Increases intestinal motility through motilin receptors in intestinal wall
Colonoscopic decompression	■ Prevention of complications such as perforation
Surgical interventions: total colectomy, Hartmann procedure, percutaneous endoscopic cecostomy	■ Required in case of refractory medical therapy

seen in Ogilvie syndrome. CT scan is currently the standard method for identifying colon pseudo-obstruction and excluding other forms of obstruction.[153] Patients with toxic megacolon may manifest typically with symptoms such as fever, tachycardia, abdominal tenderness, bloody diarrhea, or other manifestations of chronic inflammatory bowel disease along with evidence of "thumb printing" on an abdomen x-ray film in upright posture. Flexible sigmoidoscopy is contraindicated if toxic megacolon is thought to be likely, but it or contrast enemas[153] can be useful diagnostically and therapeutically if toxic megacolon is thought unlikely.

Management. Initial management includes resuscitation and correction of any underlying metabolic or electrolyte imbalances (Table 48.11). A physical examination and serial plain abdominal radiographs should be performed to evaluate colonic diameter in order to determine which patients may need colonoscopic decompression or surgery. If the patient is not very uncomfortable and the colonic distention is no greater than 12 cm, conservative treatment can be continued for 1 to 2 days. It may be helpful to place the patient in a prone position or at the knee-chest position with hips held high, alternating right and left lateral decubitus position each hour. A nasogastric tube is helpful if the patient is vomiting and will prevent swallowed air from passing distally. When bowel ischemia is suspected, surgery is indicated. If bowel necrosis is found, the affected segment is resected and an ileostomy or colostomy should be performed. If the bowel is viable, a cecostomy is placed to vent the colon and prevent distention.

If, initially, the distention is painless and the patient shows no signs of toxicity or bowel ischemia, expectant management is successful in about 50% of cases.[153,155] The risk of spontaneous perforation is approximately 3%, with attendant mortality of 50%. In most patients acute colonic pseudo-obstruction usually resolves within 3 days.[153,156] If worsening and cecal diameter increases beyond 10 to 12 cm or if it persists for more than 48 hours, intervention is recommended. The duration of distention may be more important than the absolute size of the cecum with respect to spontaneous perforation. Colonoscopy should only be performed by experienced endoscopists. Endoscopic decompression is successful in 60% to 90% of cases, but the condition can recur in up to 40%. This rate of recurrence may be decreased by placement of a decompressive tube. Recurrence would require repeated colonoscopic decompression in approximately 40% of cases after initial successful decompression. The placement of a decompression with the aid of a guidewire at the time of colonoscopy may reduce the need for repeated colonoscopic decompression. Rectal tubes are ineffective as primary modalities in managing distention of the proximal colon. Such tubes may be useful in promoting passage of air and feces after colonoscopy but should not be used as a substitute for colonoscopic decompression. Percutaneous endoscopic left-sided colostomy (PEC), a minimally invasive technique, can be used to treat pseudo-obstruction provided these cases are carefully selected in the hands of a skilled endoscopist because of a high failure rate caused by infection.[157]

In anecdotal reports, prokinetic agents such as cisapride and erythromycin have been used to treat Ogilvie syndrome with some success. Erythromycin acts by binding to motilin receptors in the small intestine, causing intestinal smooth muscle contraction and perhaps better coordination with colonic motor function. Anecdotal reports have suggested the success of erythromycin treatment on either intravenous route for 3 days or oral route for 10 days.[158,159] However, the relative paucity of motilin receptors in colon smooth muscle may explain why erythromycin is only anecdotally effective in relieving colonic pseudo-obstruction. Successful resolution of pseudo-obstruction has been reported with sympatholytic agents or spinal sympathetic block. The efficacies of these modalities have not been systematically evaluated.[153,160]

Neostigmine, a parasympathomimetic, is used in the treatment of acute colonic pseudo-obstruction. The decompression with this drug has been achieved in 80% to 100% with a recurrence rate of 5%.[153] Neostigmine may be a viable alternative to colonoscopy in pregnant women, provided mechanical obstruction is properly excluded. The administration of a polyethylene glycol electrolyte balanced solution after initial resolution of colonic dilation may reduce the recurrence rate with use of neostigmine.[161]

Neostigmine has expected cardiovascular side effects such as bradycardia, hypotension, and dizziness and is excreted via the kidneys. The few relative contraindications to its use in treatment of acute colonic pseudo-obstruction are a baseline heart rate of less than 60 beats per minute or systolic blood pressure of less than 90 mm Hg, active bronchospasm requiring medication, a history of colon cancer or partial colonic resection, active gastrointestinal bleeding, pregnancy, or a serum creatinine concentration of greater than 3 mg/dL (265 μmol/L). Other side effects would include mild to moderate crampy abdominal pain, excessive salivation, and vomiting. Side effects such as increasing airway secretions and bronchospasm can be reduced by concomitant use of glycopyrrolate without reduction of colonic response.[162,163] Ponec et al.[164] recommend use of neostigmine prior to colonoscopy, based on its easy administration, lower expense, and superior results in comparison to colonoscopy. Reported rates of response to treatment with neostigmine are 91% (single administration) and 100% (second administration) in a group of 21 randomized patients.[153,164] Colonoscopy is associated with morbidity of 3% and mortality of 1%. Further studies of this combination therapy are warranted. It should be emphasized, however, that patients should undergo immediate exploration if they exhibit signs of clinical deterioration or bowel perforation (peritoneal signs on physical examination or free air on radiographs).

Surgery is reserved for patients not responding to medical and endoscopic management and for patients who develop signs of peritonitis or perforation. Percutaneous endoscopic cecostomy can also be performed if conservative measures fail.[165] Cecostomy tubes are often poorly tolerated because of issues related to skin breakdown; in the authors' opinion, this approach is advisable only when more extensive surgical procedures are considered too risky. Procedures such as total colectomy, ileostomy, and Hartmann procedure are taken into consideration in case of perforation.[153]

References

1. Treves F. *Intestinal Obstruction: Its Varieties, with Their Pathology, Diagnosis, and Treatment*. Philadelphia, PA: H.C. Lea's Son and Co; 1884.
2. Ballantyne GH. The meaning of ileus. Its changing definition over three millennia. *Am J Surg* 1984;148:252–256.
3. Welch JP. History. In: *Bowel Obstruction: Differential Diagnosis and Clinical Management*. Philadelphia, PA: W.B. Saunders Co; 1990:3–27.
4. Wangensteen OH, Paine JR. Treatment of acute intestinal obstruction by suction with a duodenal tube. *JAMA* 1933;101:1532–1539.
5. Paine JR, Carlson HA, Wangensteen OH. Postoperative control of distension, nausea and vomiting; clinical study with reference to employment of narcotics, cathartics, and nasal catheter suction-siphonage. *JAMA* 1933;100: 1910–1917.
6. Wangensteen OH, Rea CE. The distension factor in simple intestinal obstruction: an experimental study with exclusion of swallowed air by cervical esophagostomy. *Surgery* 1939;5:327–329.
7. Hartwell HJ, Woods JA. Experimental intestinal obstruction in dogs with special reference to the cause of death and the treatment by large amounts of normal saline solution. *JAMA* 1912;59:82–87.
8. Milamed DR, Hedley-Whyte J. Contributions of the surgical sciences to a reduction of the mortality rate in the United States for the period 1968 to 1988. *Ann Surg* 1994;219:94–102.
9. Wangensteen OH. *Intestinal Obstructions*. Springfield, VA: Charles C. Thomas; 1955.
10. Ellis H. *Intestinal Obstruction*. New York: Appleton Crofts; 1982.
11. Roscher R, Oettinger W, Beger HG. Bacterial microflora, endogenous endotoxin, and prostaglandins in small bowel obstruction. *Am J Surg* 1988;155:348–355.
12. Heneghan JB, Robinson JW, Menge H, et al. Intestinal obstruction in germ-free dogs. *Eur J Clin Invest* 1981;11:285–290.
13. Stark ME, Szurszewski JH. Role of nitric oxide in gastrointestinal and hepatic function and disease. *Gastroenterology* 1992;103:1928–1949.
14. Caplan MS, Hedlund E, Hill N, et al. The role of endogenous nitric oxide and platelet-activating factor in hypoxia-induced intestinal injury in rats. *Gastroenterology* 1994;106:346–352.
15. Barry MK, Aloisi JD, Pickering SP, et al. Nitric oxide modulates water and electrolyte transport in the ileum. *Ann Surg* 1994;219:382–388.
16. Kubes P. Nitric oxide modulates epithelial permeability in the feline small intestine. *Am J Physiol* 1992;262:G1138–G1142.
17. Shields R. The absorption and secretion of fluid and electrolytes by the obstructed bowel. *Br J Surg* 1965;52:774–779.
18. Wright HK, O'Brien JJ, Tilson MD. Water absorption in experimental closed segment obstruction of the ileum in man. *Am J Surg* 1971;121:96–99.
19. Sung DT, Williams LF Jr. Intestinal secretion after intravenous fluid infusion in small bowel obstruction. *Am J Surg* 1971;121:91–95.
20. Ruf W, Suehiro GT, Suehiro A, et al. Intestinal blood flow at various intraluminal pressures in the piglet with closed abdomen. *Ann Surg* 1980;191: 157–163.
21. Ohman U. Studies on small intestinal obstruction. I. Intraluminal pressure in experimental low small bowel obstruction in the cat. *Acta Chir Scand* 1975;141:413–416.
22. Ohman U. The effects of luminal distension and obstruction on the intestinal circulation. In: *Physiology of the Intestinal Circulation*. New York: Raven Press; 1984.
23. Basson MD, Fielding LP, Bilchik AJ, et al. Does vasoactive intestinal polypeptide mediate the pathophysiology of bowel obstruction? *Am J Surg* 1989;157:109–115.
24. Enochsson L, Nylander G, Ohman U. Effects of intraluminal pressure on regional blood flow in obstructed and unobstructed small intestines in the rat. *Am J Surg* 1982;144:558–561.
25. Fondacaro J. *Intestinal Blood Flow and Motility*. New York: Raven Press; 1984.
26. Frank JW, Sarr MG, Camilleri M. Use of gastroduodenal manometry to differentiate mechanical and functional intestinal obstruction: an analysis of clinical outcome. *Am J Gastroenterol* 1994;89:339–344.
27. Camilleri M. Jejunal manometry in distal subacute mechanical obstruction: significance of prolonged simultaneous contractions. *Gut* 1989;30: 468–475.
28. Summers RW, Yanda R, Prihoda M, et al. Acute intestinal obstruction: an electromyographic study in dogs. *Gastroenterology* 1983;85:1301–1306.
29. Eskelinen M, Ikonen J, Lipponen P. Contributions of history-taking, physical examination, and computer assistance to diagnosis of acute small-bowel obstruction. A prospective study of 1333 patients with acute abdominal pain. *Scand J Gastroenterol* 1994;29:715–721.
30. Stewardson RH, Bombeck CT, Nyhus LM. Critical operative management of small bowel obstruction. *Ann Surg* 1978;187:189–193.
31. Sarr MG, Bulkley GB, Zuidema GD. Preoperative recognition of intestinal strangulation obstruction. Prospective evaluation of diagnostic capability. *Am J Surg* 1983;145;176–182.
32. Pain JA, Collier DS, Hanka R. Small bowel obstruction: computer-assisted prediction of strangulation at presentation. *Br J Surg* 1987;74:981–983.
33. Jancelewicz T, Vu LT, Shawo AE, et al. Predicting strangulated small bowel obstruction: an old problem revisited. *J Gastrointest Surg* 2009;13:93–99.
34. Gollin G, Marks WH. Early detection of small intestinal ischemia by elevated circulating intestinal fatty acid binding protein (I-FABP). *Surg Forum* 1991;42:118–119.
35. Murray MJ, Barbose JJ, Cobb CF. Serum D(-)-lactate levels as a predictor of acute intestinal ischemia in a rat model. *J Surg Res* 1993;54:507–509.
36. Silen W, Hein MF, Goldman L. Strangulation obstruction of the small intestine. *Arch Surg* 1962;85:121–129.
37. Maglinte DD, Balthazar EJ, Kelvin FM, et al. The role of radiology in the diagnosis of small-bowel obstruction. *AJR Am J Roentgenol* 1997;168: 1171–1180.
38. Assalia A, Schein M, Kopelman D, et al. Therapeutic effect of oral Gastrografin in adhesive, partial small-bowel obstruction: a prospective randomized trial. *Surgery* 1994;115:433–437.
39. Choi HK, Chu KW, Law WL. Therapeutic value of Gastrografin in adhesive small bowel obstruction after unsuccessful conservative treatment: a prospective randomized trial. *Ann Surg* 2002;236:1–6.
40. Balthazar EJ, George W. Holmes lecture. CT of small-bowel obstruction. *AJR Am J Roentgenol* 1994;162:255–261.
41. Frager D, Medwid SW, Baer JW, et al. CT of small-bowel obstruction: value in establishing the diagnosis and determining the degree and cause. *AJR Am J Roentgenol* 1994;162:37–41.
42. Mallo RD, Salem L, Lalani T, et al. Computed tomography diagnosis of ischemia and complete obstruction in small bowel obstruction: a systematic review. *J Gastrointest Surg* 2005;9:690–694.
43. Ogata M, Imai S, Hosotani R, et al. Abdominal ultrasonography for the diagnosis of strangulation in small bowel obstruction. *Br J Surg* 1994;81: 421–424.
44. Ogata M, Mateer JR, Condon RE. Prospective evaluation of abdominal sonography for the diagnosis of bowel obstruction. *Ann Surg* 1996;223: 237–241.
45. Brolin RE, Krasna MJ, Mast BA. Use of tubes and radiographs in the management of small bowel obstruction. *Ann Surg* 1987;206:126–133.
46. Fleshner PR, Siegman MG, Slater GI, et al. A prospective, randomized trial of short versus long tubes in adhesive small-bowel obstruction. *Am J Surg* 1995;170:366–370.
47. Sykes PA, Boulter KH, Schofield PF. The microflora of the obstructed bowel. *Br J Surg* 1976;63:721–725.
48. Elmes ME, Howells CH, Lowe GH. Mucosal flora of the small intestine and the effect of pre-operative antibiotics. *J Clin Pathol* 1984;37: 1272–1275.
49. Deitch EA. Simple intestinal obstruction causes bacterial translocation in man. *Arch Surg* 1989;124:699–701.
50. Cohn I Jr, Floyd CE, Dresden CF, et al. Strangulation obstruction in germfree animals. *Ann Surg* 1962;156:692–702.
51. Amundsen E, Gustafsson BE. Results of experimental intestinal strangulation obstruction in germfree rats. *J Exp Med* 1963;117:823–832.
52. Fevang BT, Fevang J, Lie SA, et al. Long-term prognosis after operation for adhesive small bowel obstruction. *Ann Surg* 2004;240:193–201.
53. Duron JJ, Silva NJ, du Montcel ST, et al. Adhesive postoperative small bowel obstruction: incidence and risk factors of recurrence after surgical treatment: a multicenter prospective study. *Ann Surg* 2006;244:750–757.
54. Liebman SM, Langer JC, Marshall JS, et al. Role of mast cells in peritoneal adhesion formation. *Am J Surg* 1993;165:127–130.
55. Attard JA, MacLean AR. Adhesive small bowel obstruction: epidemiology, biology and prevention. *Can J Surg* 2007;50:291–300.
56. Cahill RA, Redmond HP. Cytokine orchestration in post-operative peritoneal adhesion formation. *World J Gastroenterol* 2008;14:4861–4866.
57. Beck DE. The role of Seprafilm bioresorbable membrane in adhesion prevention. *Eur J Surg Suppl* 1997;577:49–55.
58. Vrijland WW, Tseng LN, Eijkman HJ, et al. Fewer intraperitoneal adhesions with use of hyaluronic acid-carboxymethylcellulose membrane: a randomized clinical trial. *Ann Surg* 2002;235:193–199.
59. O'Leary DP, Coakley JB. The influence of suturing and sepsis on the development of postoperative peritoneal adhesions. *Ann R Coll Surg Engl* 1992;74:134–137.
60. Ellozy SH, Harris MT, Bauer JJ, et al. Early postoperative small-bowel obstruction: a prospective evaluation in 242 consecutive abdominal operations. *Dis Colon Rectum* 2002;45:1214–1217.
61. Stewart RM, Page CP, Brender J, et al. The incidence and risk of early postoperative small bowel obstruction. A cohort study. *Am J Surg* 1987;154: 643–647.
62. Sajja SB, Schein M. Early postoperative small bowel obstruction. *Br J Surg* 2004;91:683–691.
63. Pickleman J, Lee RM. The management of patients with suspected early postoperative small bowel obstruction. *Ann Surg* 1989;210:216–219.
64. Ihedioha U, Alani A, Modak P, et al. Hernias are the most common cause of strangulation in patients presenting with small bowel obstruction. *Hernia* 2006;10:338–340.
65. Skandalakis PN, Zoras O, Skandalakis JE, et al. Richter hernia: surgical anatomy and technique of repair. *Am Surg* 2006;72:180–184.
66. Reisner RM, Cohen JR. Gallstone ileus: a review of 1001 reported cases. *Am Surg* 1994;60:441–446.
67. Vagefi PA, Ferguson CM, Hall JF. Recurrent gallstone ileus: third time is the charm. *Arch Surg* 2008;143:1118–1120.
68. Rea JD, Lockhart ME, Yarbrough DE, et al. Approach to management of intussusception in adults: a new paradigm in the computed tomography era. *Am Surg* 2007;73:1098–1105.
69. Sarr MG, Nagorney DM, McIlrath DC. Postoperative intussusception in the adult: a previously unrecognized entity? *Arch Surg* 1981;116:144–148.
70. Strong SA, Koltun WA, Hyman NH, et al. Practice parameters for the surgical management of Crohn's disease. *Dis Colon Rectum* 2007;50: 1735–1746.

71. Ripamonti CI, Easson AM, Gerdes H. Management of malignant bowel obstruction. *Eur J Cancer* 2008;44:1105–1115.
72. Soybel DI, Bliss DP Jr, Wells SA Jr. Colon and rectal carcinoma. *Curr Probl Cancer* 1987;11:257–356.
73. Glare PA, Dunwoodie D, Clark K, et al. Treatment of nausea and vomiting in terminally ill cancer patients. *Drugs* 2008;68:2575–2590.
74. Mystakidou K, Tsilika E, Kalaidopoulou O, et al. Comparison of octreotide administration vs conservative treatment in the management of inoperable bowel obstruction in patients with far advanced cancer: a randomized, double-blind, controlled clinical trial. *Anticancer Res* 2002;22: 1187–1192.
75. Saber AA, Boros MJ. Chilaiditi's syndrome: what should every surgeon know? *Am Surg* 2005;71:261–263.
76. Oren D, Atamanalp SS, Aydinli B, et al. An algorithm for the management of sigmoid colon volvulus and the safety of primary resection: experience with 827 cases. *Dis Colon Rectum* 2007;50:489–497.
77. Wertkin MG, Aufses AH Jr. Management of volvulus of the colon. *Dis Colon Rectum* 1978;21:40–45.
78. Peoples JB, McCafferty JC, Scher KS. Operative therapy for sigmoid volvulus. Identification of risk factors affecting outcome. *Dis Colon Rectum* 1990;33:643–646.
79. Regimbeau JM, Panis Y, Gouzi JL, et al. Operative and long term results after surgery for chronic radiation enteritis. *Am J Surg* 2001;182: 237–242.
80. Meissner K. Late radiogenic small bowel damage: guidelines for the general surgeon. *Dig Surg* 1999;16:169–174.
81. Franklin ME, Gonzalez JJ, Miter DB, et al. Laparoscopic diagnosis and treatment of intestinal obstruction. *Surg Endosc* 2004;18:26–30.
82. Kirshtein B, Roy-Shapira A, Lantsberg L, et al. Laparoscopic management of acute small bowel obstruction. *Surg Endosc* 2005;19:464–467.
83. Levard H, Boudet MJ, Msika S, et al. Laparoscopic treatment of acute small bowel obstruction: a multicentre retrospective study. *ANZ J Surg* 2001;71:641–646.
84. Gutt CN, Oniu T, Schemmer P, et al. Fewer adhesions induced by laparoscopic surgery? *Surg Endosc* 2004;18:898–906.
85. Pekmezci S, Altinli E, Saribeyoglu K, et al. Enteroclysis-guided laparoscopic adhesiolysis in recurrent adhesive small bowel obstructions. *Surg Laparosc Endosc Percutan Tech* 2001;12:165–170.
86. Sato Y, Ido K, Kumagai M, et al. Laparoscopic adhesiolysis for recurrent small bowel obstruction: long-term follow-up. *Gastrointest Endosc* 2001; 54:476–479.
87. Suter M, Zermatten P, Halkic N, et al. Laparoscopic management of mechanical small bowel obstruction: are there predictors of success or failure? *Surg Endosc* 2000;14:478–484.
88. Al-Mulhim AA. Laparoscopic management of acute small bowel obstruction. Experience from a Saudi teaching hospital. *Surg Endosc* 2000;14: 157–160.
89. Chosidow D, Johanet H, Montariol T, et al. Laparoscopy for acute small-bowel obstruction secondary to adhesions. *J Laparoendosc Adv Surg Tech A* 2000;10:155–159.
90. Strickland P, Lourie DJ, Suddleson EA, et al. Is laparoscopy safe and effective for treatment of acute small-bowel obstruction? *Surg Endosc* 1999;13: 695–698.
91. Leon E, Metzger A, Tsiotos GG, et al. Laparoscopic management of small bowel obstruction: indications and outcomes. *J Gastrointest Surg* 1998;2: 132–140.
92. Bailey IS, Rhodes M, O'Rourke N, et al. Laparoscopic management of acute small bowel obstruction. *Br J Surg* 1998;85:84–87.
93. Navez B, Arimont JM, Guit P. Laparoscopic approach in acute small bowel obstruction. A review of 68 patients. *Hepatogastroenterology* 1998; 45:2146–2150.
94. Ibrahim IM, Wolodiger F, Sussman B, et al. Laparoscopic management of acute small bowel obstruction. *Surg Endosc* 1996;10:1012–1015.
95. Ghosheh B, Salameh JR. Laparoscopic approach to acute small bowel obstruction: review of 1061 cases. *Surg Endosc* 2007;21:1945–1949.
96. Bonnard A, Demarche M, Dimitriu C, et al. Indications for laparoscopy in the management of intussusception: a multicenter retrospective study conducted by the French Study Group for Pediatric Laparoscopy (GECI). *J Pediatr Surg* 2008;43:1249–1253.
97. Kehlet H. Postoperative ileus: an update on preventive techniques. *Nat Clin Pract Gastroenterol Hepatol* 2008;5:552–558.
98. Waldhausen JH, Shaffrey ME, Skenderis BS, et al. Gastrointestinal myoelectric and clinical patterns of recovery after laparotomy. *Ann Surg* 1990; 211:777–784; discussion 785.
99. Condon RE, Cowles VE, Ferraz AA, et al. Human colonic smooth muscle electrical activity during and after recovery from postoperative ileus. *Am J Physiol* 1995;269:G408–G417.
100. Nadrowski L. Paralytic ileus: recent advances in pathophysiology and treatment. *Curr Surg* 1983;40:260–273.
101. Condon RE, Frantzides CT, Cowles VE, et al. Resolution of postoperative ileus in humans. *Ann Surg* 1986;203:574–581.
102. Espat NJ, Cheng G, Kelley MC, et al. Vasoactive intestinal peptide and substance P receptor antagonists improve postoperative ileus. *J Surg Res* 1995;58:719–723.
103. De Winter BY, Robberecht P, Boeckxstaens GE, et al. Role of VIP1/PACAP receptors in postoperative ileus in rats. *Br J Pharmacol* 1998;124: 1181–1186.
104. Zittel TT, Lloyd KC, Rothenhofer I, et al. Calcitonin gene-related peptide and spinal afferents partly mediate postoperative colonic ileus in the rat. *Surgery* 1998;123:518–527.
105. Zittel TT, Reddy SN, Plourde V, et al. Role of spinal afferents and calcitonin gene-related peptide in the postoperative gastric ileus in anesthetized rats. *Ann Surg* 1994;219:79–87.
106. Frantzides CT, Cowles V, Salaymeh B, et al. Morphine effects on human colonic myoelectric activity in the postoperative period. *Am J Surg* 1992; 163:144–148; discussion 148–149.
107. Thorn SE, Wattwil M, Lindberg G, et al. Systemic and central effects of morphine on gastroduodenal motility. *Acta Anaesthesiol Scand* 1996;40: 177–186.
108. Ferraz AA, Cowles VE, Condon RE, et al. Opioid and nonopioid analgesic drug effects on colon contractions in monkeys. *Dig Dis Sci* 1995;40: 1417–1419.
109. Kurz A, Sessler DI. Opioid-induced bowel dysfunction: pathophysiology and potential new therapies. *Drugs* 2003;63:649–671.
110. Riviere PJ, Pascaud X, Chevalier E, et al. Fedotozine reverses ileus induced by surgery or peritonitis: action at peripheral kappa-opioid receptors. *Gastroenterology* 1993;104:724–731.
111. Schwarz NT, Kalff JC, Türler A, et al. Prostanoid production via COX-2 as a causative mechanism of rodent postoperative ileus. *Gastroenterology* 2001;121:1354–1371.
112. Schwarz NT, Kalff JC, Türler A, et al. Selective jejunal manipulation causes postoperative pan-enteric inflammation and dysmotility. *Gastroenterology* 2004;126:159–169.
113. Kalff JC, Turler A, Schwarz NT, et al. Intra-abdominal activation of a local inflammatory response within the human muscularis externa during laparotomy. *Ann Surg* 2003;237:301–315.
114. de Jonge WJ, The FO, van der Coelen D, et al. Mast cell degranulation during abdominal surgery initiates postoperative ileus in mice. *Gastroenterology* 2004;127:535–545.
115. The FO, Bennink RJ, Ankum WM, et al. Intestinal handling-induced mast cell activation and inflammation in human postoperative ileus. *Gut* 2008;57:33–40.
116. Barquist E, Bonaz B, Martinez V, et al. Neuronal pathways involved in abdominal surgery-induced gastric ileus in rats. *Am J Physiol* 1996;270: R888–R894.
117. Petros JG, Realica R, Ahmad S, et al. Patient-controlled analgesia and prolonged ileus after uncomplicated colectomy. *Am J Surg* 1995;170: 371–374.
118. Stanley BK, Noble MJ, Gilliland C, et al. Comparison of patient-controlled analgesia versus intramuscular narcotics in resolution of postoperative ileus after radical retropubic prostatectomy. *J Urol* 1993;150:1434–1436.
119. Block BM, Liu SS, Rowlingson AJ, et al. Efficacy of postoperative epidural analgesia: a meta-analysis. *JAMA* 2003;290:2455–2463.
120. Moraca RJ, Sheldon DG, Thirlby R. The role of epidural anesthesia and analgesia in surgical practice. *Ann Surg* 2003;238:663–673.
121. Marret E, Remy C, Bonnet F, et al. Meta-analysis of epidural analgesia versus parenteral opioid analgesia after colorectal surgery. *Br J Surg* 2007;94:665–673.
122. Taché Y, Bonaz Y. Corticotropin-releasing factor receptors and stress-related alterations of gut motor function. *J Clin Invest* 2007;11733– 11740.
123. The FO, Boeckxstaens GE, Snoek SA, et al. Activation of the cholinergic anti-inflammatory pathway ameliorates postoperative ileus in mice. *Gastroenterology* 2007;133:1219–1228.
124. de Jonge WJ, van der Zanden EP, The FO, et al. Stimulation of the vagus nerve attenuates macrophage activation by activating the Jak2-STAT3 signaling pathway. *Nat Immunol* 2005;6:844–851.
125. Frager DH, Baer JW, Rothpearl A, et al. Distinction between postoperative ileus and mechanical small-bowel obstruction: value of CT compared with clinical and other radiographic findings. *AJR Am J Roentgenol* 1995;164: 891–894.
126. Sagar PM, Kruegener G, MacFie J. Nasogastric intubation and elective abdominal surgery. *Br J Surg* 1992;79:1127–1131.
127. Cheatham ML, Chapman WC, Key SP, et al. A meta-analysis of selective versus routine nasogastric decompression after elective laparotomy. *Ann Surg* 1995;221:469–476; discussion 476–468.
128. Waldhausen JH, Schirmer BD. The effect of ambulation on recovery from postoperative ileus. *Ann Surg* 1990;212:671–677.
129. Rao SS, Beaty J, Chamberlain M, et al. Effects of acute graded exercise on human colonic motility. *Am J Physiol* 1999;276:G1221–G1226.
130. Moore FA, Feliciano DV, Andrassy RJ, et al. Early enteral feeding, compared with parenteral, reduces postoperative septic complications. The results of a meta-analysis. *Ann Surg* 1992;216:172–183.
131. Soffer EE, Adrian TE. Effect of meal composition and sham feeding on duodenojejunal motility in humans. *Dig Dis Sci* 1992;37:1009–1014.
132. Katschinski M, Dahmen G, Reinshagen M, et al. Cephalic stimulation of gastrointestinal secretory and motor responses in humans. *Gastroenterology* 1992;103:383–391.
133. Asao T, Kuwano H, Nakamura J, et al. Gum chewing enhances early recovery from postoperative ileus after laparoscopic colectomy. *J Am Coll Surg* 2002;195:30–32.
134. Matros E, Rocha F, Zinner MJ, et al. Does gum chewing ameliorate postoperative ileus? Results of a prospective, randomized, placebo-controlled trial. *J Am Coll Surg* 2006;202:773–778.
135. Purkayastha S, Tilney HS, Darzi AW, et al. Meta-analysis of randomized studies evaluating chewing gum to enhance postoperative recovery following colectomy. *Arch Surg* 2008;143:788–793.

136. Tandeter H. Hypothesis: hexitols in chewing gum may play a role in reducing postoperative ileus. *Med Hypotheses* 2009;72:39–40.
137. Lobo DN, Bostock KA, Neal KR, et al. Effect of salt and water balance on recovery of gastrointestinal function after elective colonic resection: a randomised controlled trial. *Lancet* 2002;359:1812–1818.
138. MacKay G, Fearon K, McConnachie A, et al. Randomized clinical trial of the effect of postoperative intravenous fluid restriction on recovery after elective colorectal surgery. *Br J Surg* 2006;93:1469–1474.
139. Holte K, Foss NB, Andersen J, et al. Liberal or restrictive fluid administration in fast-track colonic surgery: a randomized, double-blind study. *Br J Anaesth* 2007;99:500–508.
140. Brandstrup B, Tønnesen H, Beier-Holgersen R, et al. Effects of intravenous fluid restriction on postoperative complications: comparison of two perioperative fluid regimens: a randomized assessor-blinded multicenter trial. *Ann Surg* 2003;238:641–648.
141. Wakeling HG, McFall MR, Jenkins CS, et al. Intraoperative oesophageal Doppler guided fluid management shortens postoperative hospital stay after major bowel surgery. *Br J Anaesth* 2005;95:634–642.
142. Abbas SM, Hill AG. Systematic review of the literature for the use of oesophageal Doppler monitor for fluid replacement in major abdominal surgery. *Anaesthesia* 2008;63:44–51.
143. Cullen JJ, Eagon JC, Dozois EJ, et al. Treatment of acute postoperative ileus with octreotide. *Am J Surg* 1993;165:113–119; discussion 119–120.
144. Garcia-Caballero M, Vara-Thorbeck C. The evolution of postoperative ileus after laparoscopic cholecystectomy. A comparative study with conventional cholecystectomy and sympathetic blockade treatment. *Surg Endosc* 1993;7:416–419.
145. Ferraz AA, Wanderley GJ, Santos MA Jr, et al. Effects of propranolol on human postoperative ileus. *Dig Surg* 2001;18:305–310.
146. Becker G, Blum HE. Novel opioid antagonists for opioid-induced bowel dysfunction and postoperative ileus. *Lancet* 2009;373:1198–1206.
147. Büchler MW, Seiler CM, Monson JR, et al. Clinical trial: alvimopan for the management of post-operative ileus after abdominal surgery: results of an international randomized, double-blind, multicentre, placebo-controlled clinical study. *Aliment Pharmacol Ther* 2008;28:312–325.
148. Ludwig K, Enker WE, Delaney CP, et al. Gastrointestinal tract recovery in patients undergoing bowel resection: results of a randomized trial of alvimopan and placebo with a standardized accelerated postoperative care pathway. *Arch Surg* 2008;143:1098–1105.
149. Bennett J, Boddy A, Rhodes M. Choice of approach for appendicectomy: a meta-analysis of open versus laparoscopic appendicectomy. *Surg Laparosc Endosc Percutan Tech* 2007;17:245–255.
150. Abraham NS, Byrne CM, Young JM, et al. Meta-analysis of non-randomized comparative studies of the short-term outcomes of laparoscopic resection for colorectal cancer. *Aust N Z J Surg* 2007;77:508–516.
151. Basse L, Hjort Jakobsen D, Billesbolle P, et al. A clinical pathway to accelerate recovery after colonic resection. *Ann Surg* 2000;232:51–57.
152. Ogilvie WH. Large-intestine colic due to sympathetic deprivation. A new clinical syndrome. *Dis Colon Rectum* 1987;30:984–987.
153. De Giorgio R, Knowles CH. Acute colonic pseudo-obstruction. *Br J Surg* 2009;96:229–239.
154. Vanek VW, Al-Salti M. Acute pseudo-obstruction of the colon (Ogilvie's syndrome). An analysis of 400 cases. *Dis Colon Rectum* 1986;29:203–210.
155. Strodel WE, Nostrant TT, Eckhauser FE, et al. Therapeutic and diagnostic colonoscopy in nonobstructive colonic dilatation. *Ann Surg* 1983;197:416–421.
156. Sloyer AF, Panella VS, Demas BE, et al. Ogilvie's syndrome. Successful management without colonoscopy. *Dig Dis Sci* 1988;33:1391–1396.
157. Cowlam S, Watson C, Elltringham M, et al. Percutaneous endoscopic colostomy of the left side of the colon. *Gastrointest Endosc* 2007;65:1007–1014.
158. Armstrong DN, Ballantyne GH, Modlin IM. Erythromycin for reflex ileus in Ogilvie's syndrome. *Lancet* 1991;337:378.
159. Jiang DP, Li ZZ, Guan SY, et al. Treatment of pediatric Ogilvie's syndrome with low-dose erythromycin: a case report. *World J Gastroenterol* 2007;13:2002–2003.
160. Lee JT, Taylor BM, Singleton BC. Epidural anesthesia for acute pseudo-obstruction of the colon (Ogilvie's syndrome). *Dis Colon Rectum* 1988;31:686–691.
161. Sgouros SN, Vlachogiannakos J, Vassiliadis K, et al. Effect of polyethylene glycol electrolyte balanced solution on patients with acute colonic pseudo obstruction after resolution of colonic dilation: a prospective, randomised, placebo controlled trial. *Gut* 2006;55:638–642.
162. Korsten MA, Rosman AS, Ng A, et al. Infusion of neostigmine-glycopyrrolate for bowel evacuation in persons with spinal cord injury. *Am J Gastroenterol* 2005;100:1560–1565.
163. Child CS. Prevention of neostigmine-induced colonic activity. A comparison of atropine and glycopyrronium. *Anaesthesia* 1984;39:1083–1085.
164. Ponec RJ, Saunders MD, Kimmey MB. Neostigmine for the treatment of acute colonic pseudo-obstruction. *N Engl J Med* 1999;341:137–141.
165. Lynch CR, Jones RG, Hilden K, et al. Percutaneous endoscopic cecostomy in adults: a case series. *Gastrointest Endosc* 2006;64:279–282.

CHAPTER 49 ■ CROHN DISEASE*

FABRIZIO MICHELASSI AND SHARON L. STEIN

KEY POINTS

1. Crohn disease is a chronic inflammatory disorder of the gastrointestinal tract with varied presentations.
2. Although no cure exists for Crohn disease, symptoms can be ameliorated with medical therapy, and surgical intervention is reserved for when medical treatment fails or to treat complications of disease.
3. Understanding medical therapies for Crohn disease is imperative for the appropriate perioperative care of patients.
4. Indications for surgical intervention in Crohn disease include failure of medical management, obstruction, and septic complications.
5. The recurrent nature of Crohn disease requires preservation of bowel length with each surgical intervention to prevent complications of malabsorption and decreased intestinal length.

(1) Crohn disease is a chronic inflammatory disorder of the gastrointestinal tract that can affect patients from the mouth to the anus. Crohn disease was first described by Dalziel in 1913[1] but derives its name from Burill Crohn, the first author of the (2) now classic paper published in 1932.[2] Although much has been discovered regarding the etiology and treatment of Crohn disease in recent years, there remains no medical or surgical cure for this disease. Treatment of Crohn disease consists primarily of medical management and modulation of symptoms, with surgical involvement when complications or escalations of symptoms occur. The course and severity of Crohn disease is affected by its location and disease characteristics, and are difficult to generalize. Patterns of disease and involved segments vary from ileocolic disease, the most common surgical manifestation, to colon disease, to pan-intestinal tract disease. Over 70% of patients will require a surgical intervention at some point in their lives and over half of patients will require (3) multiple surgical interventions. A comprehensive understanding of the disease process and surgical options is imperative for appropriate treatment of the disease.

*This chapter has been adapted from the fourth edition of *Greenfield's Surgery* and the authors are grateful for the contributions of previous authors Roger D. Hurst and Alessandro Fichera.

EPIDEMIOLOGY

Current estimates are that 400,000 to 600,000 Americans are affected by Crohn disease and four new patients are diagnosed with Crohn disease annually per 100,000 people in the United States.[3] Traditionally, the United States and Europe have a higher prevalence than Asia, South America, or Africa. Patients of Ashkenazi Jewish descent have higher rates than people from other ethnic groups. Within the United States and Europe, there is variation in concentration of cases; Crohn disease is almost twice as prevalent in northern populations.[4]

A familial predilection for Crohn disease exists; one of five patients has a relative with ulcerative colitis or Crohn disease. Additionally, the presence of a first-degree relative with inflammatory bowel disease increases the risk of developing Crohn disease 6- to 10-fold.[5] No direct mendelian pattern of inheritance has been discovered.

ETIOLOGY OF CROHN DISEASE

The exact etiology of Crohn disease remains unknown. Strong associations between Crohn disease and immunologic, genetic, bacterial, and epidemiologic factors exist and have been the focus of significant research.

Current theory centers on the altered immune response of patients with Crohn disease. Affected patients appear to lack the ability to respond appropriately to periodic bacterial penetration from the gastrointestinal lumen to the circulatory system. The normal immunologic response is to upregulate inflammatory mediators in response to bacterial incursions and downregulate these systems when they are no longer needed. Patients with Crohn disease lack variable regulation and differentiation, resulting in an uncontrolled inflammatory state and chronic changes in the intestinal wall.[6]

Research into the source of this altered inflammatory response has focused on the discovery of genomic changes.[7] The NOD2 gene, located in the pericentromeric region of chromosome 16, is a gene of particular interest. NOD2 appears to have a role in bacterial sensing and links to the muramyl dipeptide protein present on virtually all bacterial cell walls. Mutations at this locus result in loss of function affecting innate cell response to bacteria and may be partly responsible for the immunologic changes seen in Crohn disease.[8]

Other theories have focused on infectious sources as the etiology of Crohn disease. Associations with specific infectious agents including *Mycobacterium paratuberculosis, Helicobacter pylori, Escherichia coli,* and various viral agents exist. Bacterial and viral markers have been found in surgical specimens. However, no single bacterial or viral source has been a consistent finding as the etiology of the disease.

Epidemiologic factors of disease variance have led to hypotheses regarding social and dietary sources of Crohn disease. It has been hypothesized that colonization of bacteria secondary to water sources, food preservation, or dietary choices places individuals at increased risk for Crohn disease. These theories are supported by epidemiologic factors; antibiotics successfully treat symptoms, immigrants match the incidence rates of their adopted geographic locale, and dietary modifications improve symptoms. Smokers are at increased risk for contracting Crohn disease, and smoking exacerbates Crohn disease. No specific component within cigarettes has been shown to act as a clear aggravating or inciting factor.[9]

DIAGNOSIS

Diagnosis is based on a combination of clinical history, physical examination, and laboratory, endoscopic, and radiographic findings, but no definitive test for Crohn disease exists. The

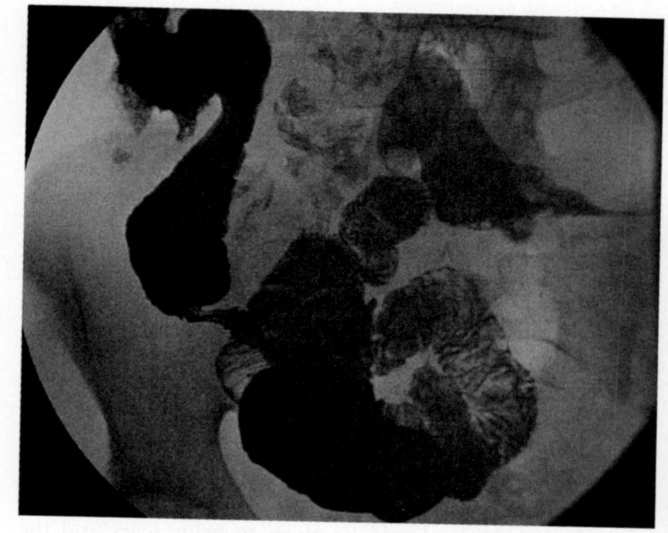

FIGURE 49.1. Small-bowel follow-through demonstrating stenosis in the jejunum of a patient with Crohn disease. Dilation is noted upstream of the narrowed segment.

varied location and pathologic features may complicate diagnosis. Approximately 60% of patients have involvement of the ileum, with or without cecal disease. Colonic disease presents in 15% to 20% of patients. Ten percent of patients have proximal small bowel involvement and 15% of patients have multiple sites of disease throughout the gastrointestinal tract.[10] The peak age of diagnosis is between 15 and 25 years of age with a second peak between 55 and 65 years. Crohn disease is uncommon prior to the age of 6 years.

DISEASE PATTERNS

Crohn disease is categorized by three general disease categories: inflammatory disease, stricturing disease, and perforating disease. It is believed that these patterns do not represent distinct disease entities but rather a continuum of the disease. An inflammatory disease pattern is typically characterized by mucosal ulceration and thickening of the bowel wall, resulting in narrowing of the intestinal lumen (Fig. 49.1). Symptoms of the inflammatory pattern of disease are characteristic of chronic obstruction and include weight loss, nausea, abdominal pain, bloating, and change in bowel habits. A stricturing disease pattern is characterized by intestinal luminal narrowing, forming cicatricial strictures surrounded by fibrotic scar tissue. Unlike the inflammatory pattern, stricturing disease is rarely amenable to medical management.

Perforating disease is characterized by the macroscopic or microscopic presence of fistulas and abscesses. Perforating disease typically begins on the mesenteric portion of the intestinal lumen and bores through the bowel wall. Tracks may penetrate for only a short distance and form blind tracks or sinuses, or continue into an adjacent segment of intestine, into an abdominal organ, or through the abdominal wall. Abscesses may cause obstructive symptoms, fevers, abdominal pain, or sepsis. Fistulas are often asymptomatic but, depending on the location, can result in diarrhea, fecaluria, pneumaturia, or enteric drainage through the abdominal wall or the vagina.

CLINICAL PRESENTATION

Patients with Crohn disease most frequently present with abdominal pain. The location of pain varies by disease location, but abdominal pain and anorexia are common regardless of location. Postprandial crampy abdominal pain and bloating are characteristic of obstructive disease, while septic complications are usually associated with steady pain and localized tenderness. Weight loss and fatigue secondary to anemia are frequent complaints. Right lower quadrant pain mimicking appendicitis is a frequent presentation of ileocolic disease. Patients with Crohn colitis may also present with diarrhea, which may be bloody. Increased fecal urgency and incontinence often coexist with colorectal disease. Delayed gastric emptying may signify gastroduodenal disease. A history of prior appendectomy, irritable bowel syndrome, and food allergies is common. A complete history of patients with Crohn disease includes questioning for secondary symptoms of Crohn disease, such as rashes, mouth ulcers, uveitis, liver abnormalities, and musculoskeletal problems.

Examination of a patient with Crohn disease should assess signs of diffuse or localized peritonitis secondary to perforation, abscess, and toxic megacolon, necessitating prompt surgical intervention. Physical examination should note signs of obstruction, such as abdominal distention and abnormal bowel sounds. Masses and tenderness are frequent findings. Particular attention should be given to prior scars and the presence of abdominal or vaginal drainage, which may signify enterocutaneous or enterovaginal fistulas. Rectal examination should evaluate perianal disease, skin tags, abscesses, fissures, scarring or fistulas, and sphincter tone. An atypical location of perianal disease, such as lateral fissures, or recurrence of perianal disease should raise a suspicion for Crohn disease and warrant further evaluation, even without other intestinal symptoms.

Laboratory testing of patients with Crohn disease may reveal metabolic derangement, acute infection, and malnutrition. Electrolyte disturbances and renal insufficiency are common in patients with severe diarrhea. An elevated white blood cell count, elevated sedimentation rates, and elevated C-reactive protein levels are indicators of acute inflammatory disease or infection. Patients are often anemic, with decreased folate and vitamin B_{12} levels secondary to ileal disease and malabsorption. Albumin, prealbumin, and transferrin testing can demonstrate evidence of malnutrition secondary to acute or chronic weight loss. Although no definitive laboratory testing exists for Crohn disease, the presence of perinuclear antineutrophil cytoplasmic antibodies (pANCAs) and absence of antisaccharomyces cerevisiae antibodies (ASCAs) may help differentiate Crohn disease from indeterminate colitis or ulcerative colitis.

EXTRAINTESTINAL DISEASE

Extraintestinal manifestations of Crohn disease occur in up to 25% of patients with Crohn disease and are most likely to occur in patients with ileal disease.[11] Patients may present with dermatologic disorders, ocular disease, arthralgias, hepatic dysfunction, and deep venous thrombosis. Some other manifestations, including peripheral arthritis, episcleritis, aphthous ulcers, and erythema nodosum, which generally parallel the activity of the intestinal disease, and symptoms often regress with successful medical or surgical treatment. Surgical intervention is occasionally advocated when these extraintestinal manifestations fail to resolve. Ankylosing spondylitis, uveitis, pyoderma gangrenosum, and primary sclerosing cholangitis do not correlate with bowel disease activity, and their clinical course is not attenuated by surgical resection of intestinal Crohn disease.

ENDOSCOPY

The evaluation of Crohn disease should survey the entire gastrointestinal tract. Endoscopic evaluation includes upper endoscopy for evaluation of gastroduodenal ulcers and colonoscopy with ileal intubation to investigate colonic and ileal disease. Findings typical of Crohn disease include ulcerations, cobblestoning, and skip lesions. The presence of ileal disease may differentiate Crohn disease from ulcerative colitis, though backwash ileitis (present in ulcerative colitis) may make differentiating the two entities challenging. Rectal sparing or fistulous perianal disease may help differentiate Crohn disease from ulcerative colitis. The presence of aphthous ulcers, cobblestoning, and strictures are highly suggestive of Crohn disease.

SMALL-BOWEL RADIOGRAPHY

Small-bowel follow-through and enteroclysis were traditionally used to evaluate the small bowel between the duodenum and the terminal ileum. In both these studies, oral contrast is ingested and serial radiographic imaging is performed with fluoroscopy or still images. Radiographic findings may be distinctive.[12] Mucosal granularity, ulceration, and blunting of normal intestinal architecture may be seen. Abnormal spacing of bowel loops on enterography is characteristic of mesenteric and bowel wall thickening found in Crohn disease. Fistulas may be demonstrated between loops of bowel; strictures and skip lesions may also be visualized.

COMPUTED TOMOGRAPHY

Computed tomography (CT) allows for identification of extraluminal pathology, unavailable on traditional small-bowel studies. CT can evaluate ureteric obstruction, air within the urinary bladder, inflammatory masses, and abscesses. Information provided by the CT scan is integral for planning percutaneous drainage of abscesses. Recent advancements in the use of CT enterography have increased the sensitivity of CT scan for intraluminal pathology. Using a multidetector CT scanner with oral and intravenous (IV) contrast, CT enterography can evaluate the bowel wall for enhancement and the presence or absence of strictures and fistulas. The sensitivity and specificity of CT enterography still falls behind that of traditional small-bowel follow-through and enteroclysis, but are improving with increasing experience.[13]

CAPSULE ENDOSCOPY

Capsule endoscopy is a recent advancement in gastrointestinal endoscopy. Patients swallow a small capsule, which transmits continuous images to a monitor, which is placed on the patient for the duration of the study. This provides direct imaging of the small bowel between the ligament of Treitz and ileocecal valve, not previously accessible by endoscopy. Patients who undergo capsule endoscopy should first be evaluated for the presence of strictures and chronic obstruction, as cases of retained capsule requiring surgical retrieval have been reported.

PATHOLOGY

Pathologic findings of Crohn disease tend to progress from small aphthous ulcers to full-thickness inflammation and fistulas. Aphthous ulcers are small red spots or depressions in the intestine that represent mucosal ulceration over microscopic lymphoid aggregates and are the earliest manifestation of Crohn disease.[14] As the disease progresses, the ulcers enlarge, forming longitudinal ulcerations on the mesenteric aspect of the bowel wall. Further disease progression leads to a serpiginous network of thin, linear ulcerations surrounding islands of edematous mucosa, producing a classic "cobblestone" appearance. Pseudopolyps, which are actually formed by the paucity of normal surrounding mucosa secondary to severe disease, may be seen in Crohn disease (Fig. 49.2A).

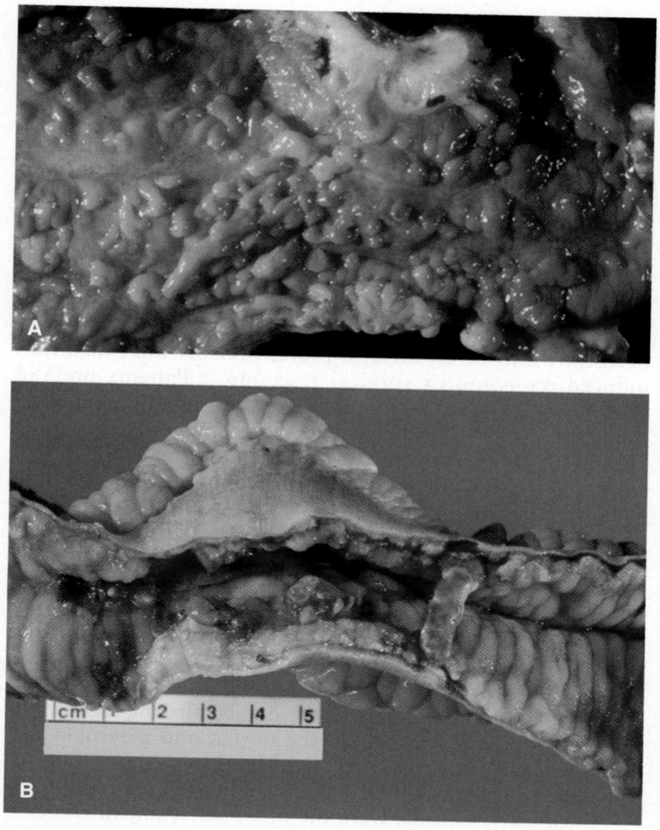

FIGURE 49.2. **A:** Pseudopolyps and full-thickness ulceration in a patient with Crohn disease of the ileum. **B:** Fat wrapping or "creeping fat" is seen extending over the serosal surface of the bowel of a stenotic, diseased segment of ileum. Fibrotic changes are noted on the cut surface of ileum, extending to all layers of the bowel wall.

Gross pathologic findings including an inflamed thickened mesentery and enlarged regional lymph nodes are found in the majority of patients with Crohn disease. Fatty tissue develops from the mesentery and extends over the serosal surface of the small bowel, resulting in a phenomenon known as "fat wrapping" or "creeping fat" (Fig. 49.2B). Early in the disease progression the bowel wall is hyperemic and boggy, but as inflammation progresses, fibrotic scarring develops and the bowel becomes thickened and leathery.

The inflammation of Crohn disease eventually extends through all layers of the bowel wall. Mucosal ulcerations progress and penetrate through the bowel wall, resulting in abscesses, fistulas, or sinuses (Fig. 49.3A). Lymphoid aggregates in the submucosa thicken and extend through the muscularis propria (Fig. 49.3B). Well-developed lymphoid aggregates in edematous or fibrotic submucosa or subserosa are virtually diagnostic of Crohn disease. Noncaseating granulomas are found in up to 50% of surgically resected specimens but are rarely seen in specimens obtained endoscopically (Fig. 49.3C). Although granulomas are a valuable diagnostic feature of Crohn disease, their presence is not pathognomonic and they do not imply activity.

DIFFERENTIAL DIAGNOSIS

The differential diagnosis of Crohn disease includes a wide variety of abdominal pathologies. Infectious, ischemic, inflammatory, and functional disorders can all mimic Crohn disease.

Differentiating Crohn disease from appendicitis is a common diagnostic dilemma. Young, otherwise healthy patients with right lower quadrant pain, mild leukocytosis, and inflammation on CT are common to both diseases. Careful CT evaluation can be suggestive of disease primarily arising from the appendix, with appendiceal occlusion, versus inflammation arising from the cecum or terminal ileum. Occasionally, the diagnosis of Crohn disease is made intraoperatively, when a

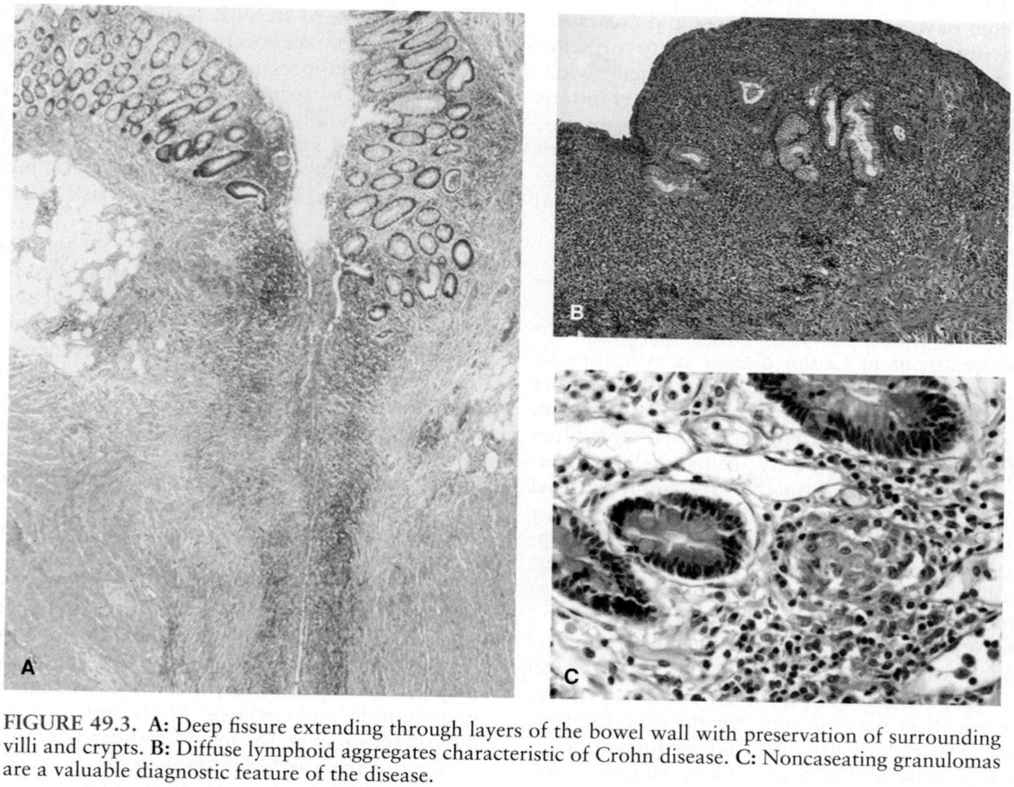

FIGURE 49.3. **A:** Deep fissure extending through layers of the bowel wall with preservation of surrounding villi and crypts. **B:** Diffuse lymphoid aggregates characteristic of Crohn disease. **C:** Noncaseating granulomas are a valuable diagnostic feature of the disease.

normal appendix and inflamed ileum are noted. If the cecum is normal, performing an appendectomy may be appropriate to prevent future diagnostic dilemmas, but the ileum is not typically resected in this acute setting unless obstruction is complete or medical therapy has failed. Should the ileum require immediate resection, ileocecal resection is suggested. Infectious ileal diseases such as *Yersinia*, tuberculosis, and *Salmonella* are uncommon but can present with similar clinical scenarios.

Noninfectious colitis, most commonly ulcerative colitis, can be confused with Crohn colitis. It is believed that ulcerative colitis and Crohn disease may exist on a spectrum of inflammatory bowel disease rather than as distinct disease entities. Crohn disease is typically distinguished from ulcerative colitis by endoscopic, anatomic, and pathologic findings. Endoscopically, ulcerative colitis tends to start at the rectum and progress proximally. Rectal sparing and skip lesions, common in Crohn disease, are unusual in ulcerative colitis. The presence of perianal and small-intestinal disease is common in Crohn disease and rare in ulcerative colitis. Backwash ileitis, a phenomenon associated with an incompetent ileocecal valve, may confuse the diagnosis, but the presence of ulcers, cobblestoning, fistulas, and disease in the proximal ileum are highly suggestive of Crohn disease. Pathologic findings of transmural inflammation or granulomas are characteristic of Crohn disease and rarely found in ulcerative colitis.

Crohn colitis can be mimicked by other colitides, such as infections (*Clostridium difficile, Salmonella*, cytomegalovirus) or ischemic colitis, but endoscopic, bacteriologic, or pathologic findings usually differentiate between diseases. Radiation or nonsteroidal anti-inflammatory drug (NSAID)-induced colitis or enteritis may affect the large or small bowel and can be similar in presentation. History and location may help to differentiate between etiologies.

TREATMENT

Neither medical nor surgical therapy is curative for Crohn disease. Management of Crohn disease is focused on the relief of
5 symptoms and prevention of recurrence. As patients with Crohn disease often have multiple recurrences and escalation of symptoms, avoidance of surgical resection to preserve bowel length is an important component in treatment. Medical therapy represents first-line treatment for most symptoms of Crohn disease and is based on the severity of symptoms. The understanding of medical treatments for patients with Crohn disease is imperative for the surgeon, as many medications affect postoperative physiology and risks for surgical complications.

MEDICAL MANAGEMENT

The first line of treatment in Crohn disease is symptomatic supportive care. Many patients find that a bland, low-fiber diet may alleviate the symptoms of bloating and abdominal pain. Bowel rest can decrease disease activity, but remission is often transient. Antidiarrheal and antimotility agents, such as diphenoxylate, loperamide, and diluted tincture of opium, are used for chronic diarrhea related to colitis, ileal disease, or prior bowel resection. These medications decrease intestinal cramping and diarrhea by decreasing intestinal motility. In the presence of severe colitis, these medications are contraindicated as they may precipitate toxic megacolon.

Patients with severe malnutrition may benefit from parenteral nutrition. Data extrapolated from the literature on cancer patients suggest that 1 week to 10 days of preoperative total parenteral nutrition may prevent weight loss, improve nitrogen balance, and reduce perioperative complications.[15] The risks of total parenteral nutrition must be weighed carefully against the benefits of nutritional optimization.

Aminosalicylates or 5-aminosalicylic acid (5-ASA) derivatives are commonly used as first-line treatment for patients with mild to moderate Crohn disease of the large and small intestine. These medications inhibit proinflammatory mediators and are designed to deliver medications to a specific bowel segment. Diffusion-dependent medications (Pentasa) target the distal small intestine and are effective in patients with diarrhea. pH-dependent medications (Asacol) are effective in the terminal ileum and ascending colon where the bowel pH reaches 6 to 7. Flora-dependent derivatives (Colazal, sulfasalazine) rely on colonic flora to break the diazobond and work most effectively in the colon.

Aminosalicylates may be taken orally or rectally and have been shown to be effective to prevent relapse after medically induced remission or surgical resection.[16] Patients on ASA derivatives are not at increased risk of postoperative complications and may be started early in the postoperative period to help decrease recurrence rates and maintain remission.[17] It is critical that 5-ASA derivatives not be confused with acetylsalicylic acid (aspirin) or other NSAIDs frequently used in postoperative patients. NSAIDs have the potential to exacerbate disease activity and should be avoided in patients with Crohn disease.[18]

Antibiotics have been demonstrated to improve symptoms of Crohn disease. They are used to treat intra-abdominal and perianal infection and abscesses and to obtain and retain remission in inflammatory and fistulizing disease.[19] The mechanism of action is theorized to be due to altering indigenous luminal bacteria and modifying the aerobic and anaerobic bacteria concentrations in the gastrointestinal tract. Fluoroquinolones, metronidazole, and rifaximin are used commonly.

Historically, steroids were the first-line treatment of acute flares of Crohn disease and were used for medically refractory disease. Recent medical literature has de-emphasized the use of steroids in favor of antibiotics and biologic and immunologic pharmacotherapies. Multiple studies have demonstrated that steroids may be helpful in achieving remission, but only about 30% of patients will maintain remission without continued steroids.[20] Steroids may be administered orally, intravenously, or rectally.

A limitation of steroids is the extensive side effect profile, which includes osteonecrosis, diabetes, myopathy, infection, and adrenal suppression. Intravenous and oral medications with systemic absorption have a high risk of steroid-induced side effects. Orally available budesonide and topical enemas have decreased systemic absorption and side effects. In general, chronic use of doses of 20 mg/d or higher portends a worse prognosis, with an increased risk of surgical intervention.[21]

The thiopurines azathioprine (AZA) and 6-mercaptopurine (6-MP) are used for treatment of moderate to severe disease and have been particularly useful for patients with fistulizing disease. Studies have shown 6-mercaptopurine and azathioprine to be effective in decreasing recurrence, ameliorating fistulizing disease, and maintaining remission.[22] The mechanism of action is induction of apoptosis and inhibition of ribonucleotide synthesis. Side effects of these agents include bone marrow suppression, hepatitis, pancreatitis, and lymphoma, which can be severe and limit usage. Approximately 20% of patients are intolerant to the medications. These medications are not thought to be a major risk factor for patients undergoing surgical intervention.

Methotrexate has been used in patients to facilitate weaning from steroids, particularly in patients intolerant to 6-MP/AZA. Studies in Crohn disease demonstrate an increased rate of remission and ability to wean steroids when compared to placebo.[23] Side effects include bone marrow suppression, pneumonitis, and cirrhosis. Methotrexate is not thought to be a particular risk factor for postoperative complications.

One of the most important recent advances in the medical treatment of Crohn disease is the use of biologic agents. Infliximab

(Remicade) was the first such agent to be introduced. It is a monoclonal antibody directed against tumor necrosis factor-α (TNF-α). While infliximab was initially used only in patients with severe fistulizing disease, its use has been broadened to patients with moderate to severe inflammatory disease, fistulizing disease, and medically refractory disease. Practitioners advocate its use in patients with severe disease as a first-line "top-down" approach. This theory advocates starting patients on traditionally second- or third-line drugs to induce a quicker remission. Studies have demonstrated increased rates of clinical remission and improvement of fistulizing disease.[24] Similar agents, including adalimumab (TNF antibody), Visilizumab (CD3 antibody), and certolizumab (TNF), are increasingly available and approved for use in Crohn disease. Significant side effects include rare opportunistic infections and reports of lymphoma. Patients may develop severe anaphylaxis during administration and may form antibodies to these medications. Immunosuppressive therapy is also believed to increase the risk of postoperative infectious complications.

INDICATIONS FOR OPERATION

The indications for surgical intervention in patients with Crohn disease are listed in Table 49.1.

Failure of Medical Management

4 Failure of medical management is the most common indication for surgical intervention.[25] Failure can occur in a number of ways: patients may continue to worsen, despite maximal medical therapy; medical management can fail to induce remission or quell signs of acute flare; or side effects of medical treatment such as pancreatitis, hepatitis, diabetes, lymphoma, anaphylaxis, and psychosis may limit its use. Alternatively, patients may be unwilling to start or continue medications secondary to the risk of side effects. Each of these reasons may be an indication for surgical intervention.

Intestinal Obstruction

Intestinal obstruction generally occurs secondary to inflammatory or stricturing disease. Partial or complete obstruction is a common indication for surgery in patients with Crohn disease,[10] but acute obstruction is rare. Initial treatment usually involves bowel rest, antibiotics, and supportive therapy. Partial small-bowel obstruction related to acute inflammation can often be managed with medical therapy. Traditionally steroids were used, but recently, new therapies such as infliximab and adalimumab have proven useful in inflammatory disease. Stricturing disease is less likely to respond to medical treatment. Patients with Crohn disease may also have obstruction secondary to adhesions, or volvulus or herniation secondary to prior surgical intervention and should be treated accordingly.

Short-segment strictures may be considered for endoscopic dilation if they are endoscopically accessible in the duodenum, ileum, or colon. Endoscopic dilation has been shown to be safe and efficacious in several studies[26] and may be performed with or without simultaneous local treatment with steroid injection.[27] If this approach is used, repeated procedures are often necessary.

Failure to resolve, escalation of symptoms, or signs of sepsis are indications for surgical treatment. Most cases of obstruction will eventually require surgical treatment. Obstruction can be treated with resection, strictureplasty, or a combination of the techniques.

TABLE 49.1 INDICATIONS

SURGICAL INDICATIONS IN CROHN DISEASE

Failure of medical management
Intestinal obstruction
Abscess/inflammatory masses
Fistulas
Perforation
Hemorrhage
Cancer
Toxic colitis
Growth retardation

Abscess and Inflammatory Masses

Intra-abdominal abscesses and inflammatory masses are frequent indications for surgical intervention. Abscesses result from a localized, contained perforation or fistulization of diseased bowel; small abscesses are often contained in inflammatory masses. Often the reactive serositis will facilitate adhesions to normal bowel wall and form an inflammatory mass to prevent generalized peritonitis and perforation. Abscesses and inflammatory masses may present with an indolent course of low-grade fevers, abdominal pain, and leukocytosis. Abdominal examination may demonstrate a tender mass.

Most abscesses are amenable to antibiotics and drainage. An unstable patient who fails to respond to initial resuscitation and has free perforation or peritonitis should undergo immediate surgical intervention. In a stable patient, a CT scan can evaluate the abscess size, location, and accessibility to percutaneous drainage (Fig. 49.4). Intramesenteric and intraloop abscesses are often inaccessible to drainage. Percutaneous drainage improves clinical symptoms[28] and reduces the risk of enterocutaneous fistula.[29] However, the source of the abscess is typically severely diseased intestine and most patients will progress to require surgical intervention. Drainage, antibiotics, and parenteral nutrition may reduce inflammation and facilitate a more limited intestinal resection.

Enteric Fistulas

Fistulization is a common manifestation of Crohn disease and results from full-thickness rupture into an adjacent hollow organ or through the abdominal wall. Fistulas may occur at the site of prior anastomoses; ileocolic resection often fistulizes to the duodenum, and colon resections can fistulize to the stomach. Crohn disease may form symptomatic fistulas between proximal and distal loops of bowel or between the small bowel and colon. Enteric fistulas may be found in as many as one third of patients with Crohn disease, but constitute an indication for surgery in only a small minority of patients. Immunologics such as anti-TNF chimeric monoclonal antibody (infliximab) may be used for the medical treatment of fistulous disease.[30]

Most fistulas between loops of bowel are asymptomatic and are noted incidentally at the time of surgery or on radiographic studies. Up to two thirds of ileosigmoid fistulas are not diagnosed prior to surgery, and the surgeon and patient should be prepared for this possibility.[31] Occasionally, fistulas may be symptomatic and warrant surgical intervention or escalation of medical therapy. Most commonly this occurs when a large-diameter fistula forms between the ileum and sigmoid secondary to the proximity of these loops of bowel. The large-diameter fistulas may cause shunting of the fecal stream and significant diarrhea. Often, the sigmoid is only secondarily

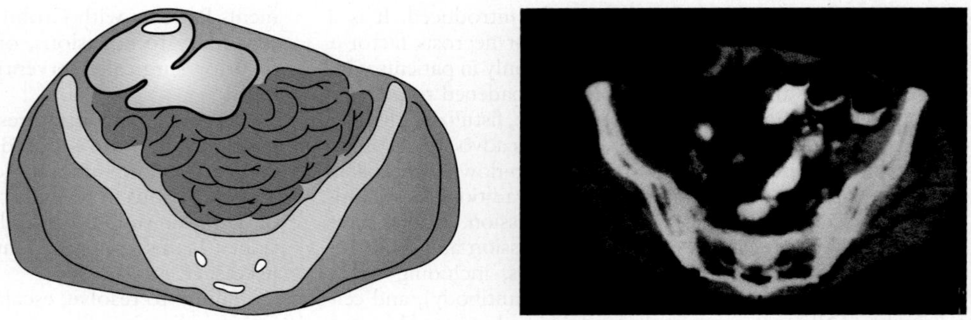

FIGURE 49.4. Computed tomogram showing an abscess in the right lower quadrant of the abdomen resulting from Crohn disease of the terminal ileum.

involved and may be separated from the primary loop and repaired primarily; in cases with severe inflammation or primary sigmoid disease, wedge or segmental resection of the sigmoid colon along with ileal resection should be considered.

Urinary and Gynecologic Fistulas

Enterovesical fistulas are encountered in 5% of patients with Crohn disease[32] and often in patients with a concomitant ileosigmoid fistula.[33] Patients with this complication present with pneumaturia, fecaluria, and frequent urinary tract infections. An abdominopelvic CT scan may demonstrate air within the bladder, but direct visualization of the fistula is rare. Most surgeons and gastroenterologists agree that patients with urinary fistulas warrant surgery to prevent renal damage from chronic urinary tract infections. Fistulas most frequently track to the dome of the bladder and can be primarily repaired.

Fistulas may occur to the vagina, the fallopian tube, or the uterus. Patients may complain of malodorous, feculent discharge per vagina, causing significant embarrassment and discomfort. Enterovaginal fistulas occur most commonly in patients with prior hysterectomy. Surgical treatment of the fistula is resection of involved intestine and extirpation of the fistulous tract. Associated abscesses should be drained adequately. Enterosalpingeal fistulas are rare and treatment often requires resection of the affected area. Fistulas to the uterus may be treated with bowel resection and débridement of the uterine opening to preserve fertility; in severe cases a hysterectomy may be necessary.

Enterocutaneous Fistulas

Enterocutaneous fistulas occur in approximately 4% of patients with Crohn disease,[32] typically from direct penetration of a sinus through the abdominal wall or rupture of a superficial abscess. Prior scars are common sites of drainage. Evaluation of the fistulas with radiographic imaging may demonstrate the existence of an abscess requiring drainage or an obstruction preventing spontaneous healing. The presence of an enterocutaneous fistula does not necessarily dictate the need for surgical intervention; sepsis must be cleared, abscesses drained, and nutritional support supplied if necessary. Enterocutaneous fistulas are often slow to heal, and surgery is ultimately required in many cases. The general principles of management include resection of diseased segment and débridement of the fistulous tract and abdominal wall.

Perforation

Free perforation with peritonitis is a rare complication of Crohn disease, occurring in 1% of patients, and is a clear indication for urgent operation.[34] Perforation can occur in the large or small bowel. Resection of the diseased segment is favored over simple suture repair. Depending on patient stability, the duration of perforation, and the overall medical condition of the patient, a primary anastomosis, diverted anastomosis, or creation of an end stoma may be indicated.

Hemorrhage

Hemorrhage is an uncommon complication of Crohn disease. Massive gastrointestinal hemorrhage occurs more frequently in Crohn colitis than in small-bowel disease. Often, hemorrhage can be managed with endoscopic or interventional therapies and does not require surgical intervention. Hemorrhage in small-bowel disease tends to be more indolent, with episodes of chronic bleeding that require intermittent transfusion.[32] Uncontrolled hemorrhage requires localization and resection.

Cancer and Suspected Cancer

Patients with Crohn disease are at increased risk for the development of adenocarcinoma of the colon and small intestine. Current estimates indicate an observed prevalence of 0.3% for small-bowel adenocarcinoma and 1.8% for large-intestinal adenocarcinoma. Small-intestinal carcinoma should be suspected in patients with a sudden change in disease symptoms or acute high-grade obstruction. Nonfunctional bowel excluded from the fecal stream seems to be at particular risk for malignancy. Therefore, bypass surgery should not be performed for Crohn disease of the small bowel. Any stricture treated surgically should be biopsied, if suspicious, prior to performing a strictureplasty.[35] Adenocarcinomas in the setting of Crohn disease tend to be multifocal and poorly differentiated. Segmental resection is appropriate treatment.

Screening colonoscopy with random biopsies should be performed for patients with long-standing colonic Crohn disease. It may be difficult to distinguish neoplastic from inflammatory strictures, and approximately 7% of colonic strictures are malignant. When adenocarcinoma is suspected or histologically proven, surgical treatment is indicated.[36] Unlike ulcerative colitis, the recommended treatment for colon cancer in the setting of Crohn disease does not clearly favor total colectomy over segmental resection.

Toxic Colitis

Patients with Crohn disease occasionally develop severe colitis. Severe colitis is defined by Truelove and Witts[37] as dilation on radiography (typically defined as transverse colon >5.5 cm in diameter), abdominal tenderness, more than 10 bloody bowel movements per day, fever, tachycardia, anemia, and elevated sedimentation rate. Failure to respond to medical therapy or progression on medical therapy is accepted as an indication for therapy. Subtotal colectomy with ileostomy should be performed.

Growth Retardation

Normal growth is retarded in up to 25% of children affected by Crohn disease. If growth retardation persists despite adequate medical and nutritional therapy, prompt surgical treatment should be carried out before puberty as meaningful growth will not occur after epiphyseal closure. Resection of the affected segment should be performed to enable a decrease of medications and improved physiologic development.

General Principles of Crohn Surgery

Abdominal Exploration. Whether approached laparoscopically or with an open technique, initial evaluation of the entire abdomen should be performed in all patients with Crohn disease. The surgeon should closely examine the small bowel from the ligament of Treitz to the ileocecal valve. Areas of disease, recognizable by dilation and narrowing (chain of lakes), encroachment of mesenteric fat along the serosal surface of the bowel (creeping fat), serosal hyperemia (corkscrew vessels), fistulas, and their exact location from the ligament of Treitz, should be noted. The total length of small bowel should be measured. Bowel downstream to an obstruction must be carefully evaluated for stricture; failure to treat downstream strictures is one cause of early postoperative recurrence.

Resection. Small-bowel resection, specifically ileocolic resection, is the most common surgical procedure performed for Crohn disease. In general, resection should encompass grossly abnormal bowel. Resection of additional bowel to obtain negative microscopic margins has not been shown to decrease the risk of recurrence and microscopically positive margins have not been shown to adversely affect long-term results.[38]

Division of the mesentery in Crohn disease can be challenging. The mesentery may be massively thickened and traditional transection and ligation techniques may prove inadequate. Often it is difficult to fashion vascular pedicles for simple ligation and attempts to separate mesentery into segments appropriate for clamping may cause inadvertent bleeding. Hematomas in the mesentery further complicate ligation and may cause undermining of the vascular supply to normal intestine. Vessel-sealing devices may be problematic secondary to thickened tissue and provide inadequate hemostasis. Overlapping clamps on either side of the intended line of transection with suture ligation or mattress sutures are a safe method to ensure hemostasis (Fig. 49.5).

A wide variety of anastomotic techniques following bowel resection may be applied. Standard stapling techniques are safe on healthy, pliable bowel, but in the case of severely edematous or hypertrophied intestine, a hand-sewn technique may provide greater versatility. A recent meta-analysis of techniques demonstrated that end-to-end anastomosis is associated with an increased anastomotic leak rate when compared to other anastomotic techniques, and side-to-side anastomosis may provide a decreased anastomotic leak rate, decreased postoperative complication rates, and shorter hospital stay.[39] Regardless of the technique employed, the basic premises of a safe anastomosis include ensuring an adequate blood supply, tension-free anastomosis, and waterproof anastomotic seal. Patients with severe malnutrition, anemia, or fecal contamination may not be appropriate for primary anastomosis and a colostomy, diverting stoma, or end ileostomy may be necessary.

Strictureplasty. Intestinal strictureplasty is an alternative approach to resection that preserves bowel length by surgically reconfiguring narrowed segments of bowel to allow passage of enteric contents. The presence of active fistulizing disease, acute inflammation, and phlegmon are contraindications to

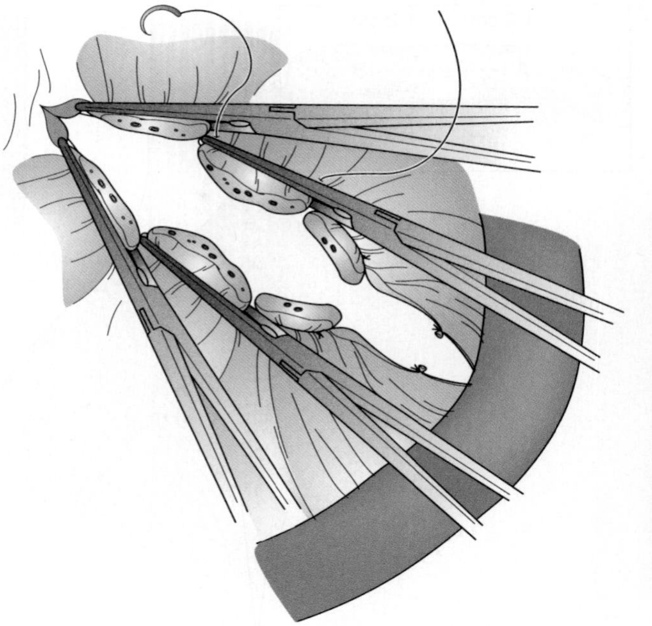

FIGURE 49.5. Technique for safe suture ligation and division of thickened and friable mesentery in a patient with Crohn disease. (Adapted from Walsh CJ, Lavery IC. Ileocecectomy. In: Michelassi F, Milsom JW, eds. *Operative Strategies in Inflammatory Bowel Disease.* New York: Springer-Verlag; 1999:294–302.)

strictureplasty. Additionally, very long segments of severe, high-grade strictures may not be amenable to current strictureplasty techniques. Most importantly, malignancy in the diseased segment is an absolute contraindication to strictureplasty. Any candidate intestinal segment should be opened and examined for signs of malignancy prior to repair.

The *Heineke-Mikulicz* (Fig. 49.6) and the *Finney* (Fig. 49.7) strictureplasty are both techniques derived from pyloroplasty. The Heineke-Mikulicz is appropriate for diseased segments 7 cm or less in length. A longitudinal incision is made on the antimesenteric border of the bowel and closed in a transverse fashion, increasing the luminal width of the bowel. The Finney strictureplasty can be used for diseased segments up to 15 cm in length. In this technique, the bowel is folded into a U shape, and a longitudinal incision is made between mesenteric and antimesenteric borders. Sutures are placed on the posterior wall of the enterostomy, beginning at the apex, and continued the entire length of the enterostomy. Functionally, the Finney strictureplasty creates a diverticulum on the lateral edge of the bowel, which may cause stagnation of the fecal stream and lead to bacterial overgrowth. The Finney strictureplasty is used less frequently than the Heineke-Mikulicz strictureplasty.

More recently, the side-to-side isoperistaltic strictureplasty (Fig. 49.8) has been used for diseased segments longer than 15 to 20 cm in length. In this technique, the mesentery of the diseased segment is divided at its midpoint and the small bowel is transected. The proximal loop is staggered in respect to the distal loop to allow narrowed segments in one loop to be approximated to dilated segments of the second loop of bowel. A two-layered hand-sewn closure is created in a side-to-side fashion. A multicenter, international study recently demonstrated the efficacy and safety of this technique.[40]

Strictureplasty has been demonstrated to have similar perioperative morbidity and reduction in recurrence rates when compared to conventional resections.[41] The most common postoperative complication after strictureplasty is hemorrhage from diseased newly sewn segments of bowel occurring in up to 9% of cases. In most cases, bleeding stops spontaneously

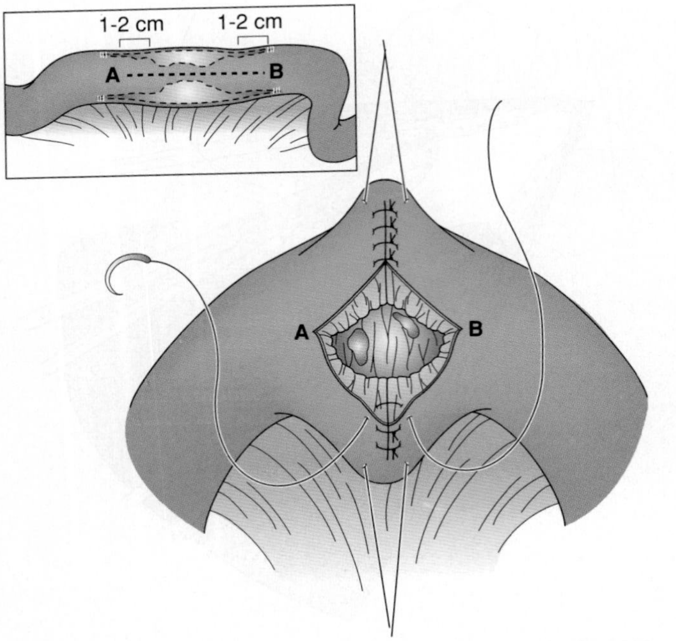

FIGURE 49.6. Heineke-Mikulicz strictureplasty. This technique is limited to patients with short-segment disease in close proximity. (Adapted from Milsom JW. Strictureplasty and mechanical dilation in strictured Crohn's disease. In: Michelassi F, Milsom JW, eds. *Operative Strategies in Inflammatory Bowel Disease*. New York: Springer-Verlag; 1999:259–267.)

with observation alone. Occasionally, arteriography has been used to infuse localized vasopressin into branches of the superior mesenteric artery. Rarely is surgical intervention required to control postoperative hemorrhage. Sepsis and anastomotic dehiscence occur postoperatively in only 2% of strictureplasties. Several small studies seem to demonstrate reduced recurrence rates, but no randomized controlled trial has compared resection versus strictureplasty. Recent studies suggest normalization of endoscopic and radiographic features in previously diseased segments of bowel following strictureplasty; these findings suggest a possible restitution of function in diseased segments that would have significant implications for preservation of bowel length in patients with Crohn disease.[42]

Minimally Invasive Surgery. Resections of Crohn disease throughout the large and small intestine can successfully be accomplished laparoscopically. Benefits of laparoscopic surgery include reduced length of ileus and decreased postoperative stay in several studies.[43,44] Long-term follow-up has not demonstrated an increased rate of surgical recurrence or intervention in patients who underwent laparoscopic resection. A long-term follow-up series demonstrated that as many as 50% of patients with Crohn disease who had their operation performed laparoscopically were able to undergo a second surgery laparoscopically.[45] Many patients with Crohn disease are young healthy patients and the cosmetic advantages of a laparoscopic approach can be considerable.

Laparoscopic surgery for Crohn disease may be challenging. Thickened mesentery, abscesses, and fistulas may make dissection difficult. Conversion rates are typically higher in Crohn surgery than other types of laparoscopic bowel surgery, with rates of conversion cited between 4.8% and 29.2%.[42] It is estimated that surgeons require 10 to 50 cases per year to obtain minimum proficiency, and laparoscopic cases for Crohn disease are recommended only for experienced laparoscopic surgeons.[46]

SPECIFIC SCENARIOS OF CROHN DISEASE

Crohn Disease of the Upper Gastrointestinal Tract

Crohn disease of the duodenum is a relatively rare entity and may be stratified into primary and secondary disease. Primary duodenal involvement occurs in 4% of patients and is generally inflammatory in nature, whereas secondary disease is typically the result of perforating disease from an intestinal segment following prior surgical resection.[47] Half of all patients with duodenal disease have concomitant disease elsewhere requiring simultaneous surgical intervention.[48]

Primary disease of the duodenum manifests with symptoms due to ulceration and edema, such as heartburn, obstruction, and weight loss. Symptoms can initially be managed with anti-inflammatory and antacid medications, but 90% of patients will eventually require surgical intervention.[49] The optimal surgical strategy depends on the individual pattern of disease. The Heineke-Mikulicz strictureplasty is best employed for disease involving the proximal duodenum, while a Finney strictureplasty is better suited for disease involving the fourth portion of the duodenum.[50] If the duodenal stricture is lengthy or rigid and unyielding, an intestinal bypass procedure should be performed. Simple side-to-side retrocolic gastrojejunostomy can be performed for obstructing disease of the duodenum. Improved antiulcer medications such as proton pump inhibitors have minimized the need for simultaneous vagotomy to prevent marginal ulcers. Vagotomy

FIGURE 49.7. Finney strictureplasty. (Adapted from Hurst RD, Michelassi F. Management of small bowel Crohn's disease. *World J Surg* 1998;22:359–363.)

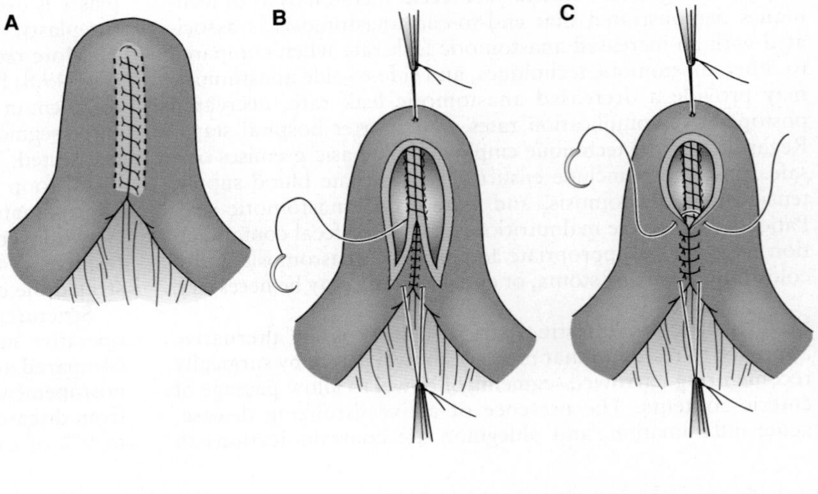

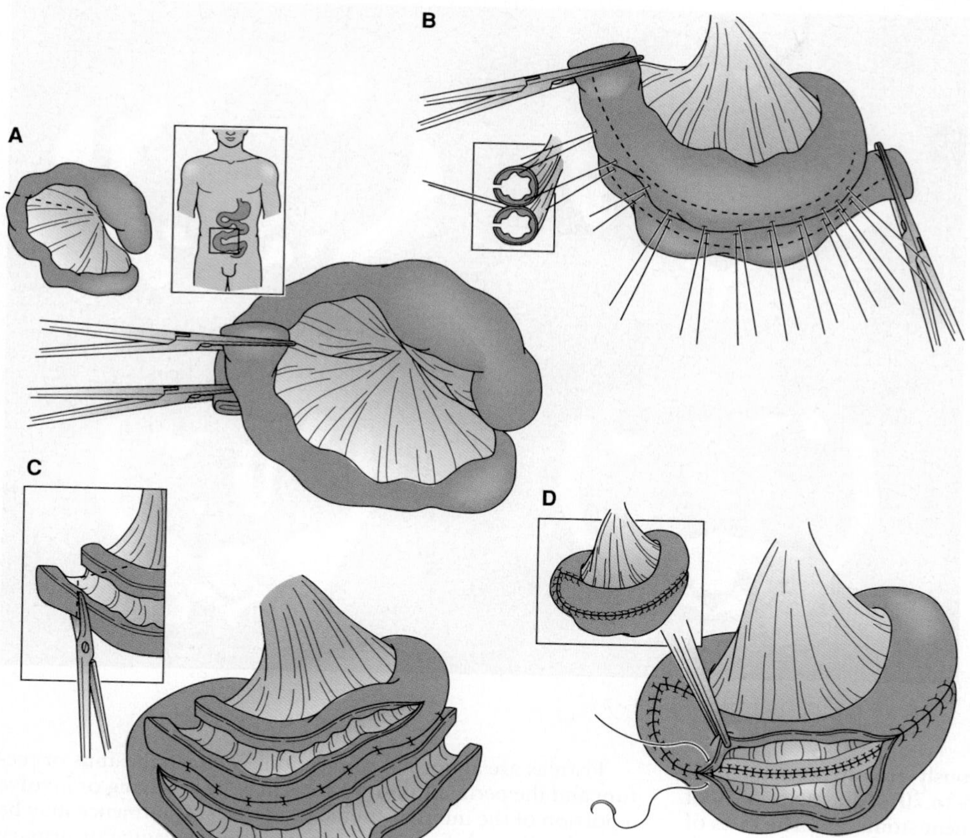

FIGURE 49.8. Side-to-side isoperistaltic strictureplasty. (Adapted from Michelassi F. Side-to-side isoperistaltic stricturoplasty for multiple Crohn's strictures. *Dis Colon Rectum.* 1996;39:345–349.)

has been associated with the occurrence or worsening of diarrhea in patients with Crohn disease.[48] Distal duodenal disease may be amenable to Roux-en-Y duodenojejunostomy. Both of these procedures can be performed using either an open or laparoscopic technique with a high rate of success. Surgical resection is generally avoided secondary to a high rate of complications.

Secondary involvement of the second or third portion of the duodenum typically occurs from recurrent disease in the neoterminal ileum after a prior ileocolic anastomosis. Secondary disease of the fourth portion of the duodenum or the stomach usually occurs from primary disease of the transverse colon. Although most fistulas are asymptomatic, shunting of enteric contents may cause malabsorption and diarrhea. Surgical management involves resection of the primary diseased intestine. The duodenum or stomach edges may be débrided to healthy bowel and repaired primarily. In cases of large defect or tension on the repair site, closure with jejunal serosal patch or duodenojejunostomy may be necessary.

Ileal and Small-Intestinal Disease

Ileal and small-bowel disease is common in Crohn disease. As mentioned previously, the bowel should be evaluated for abscesses, fistulas, and strictures. Surgical resection is generally recommended in short-segment disease; strictureplasty may be preferred in focal circumferential strictures, longer diseased segments, and patients with prior resections to preserve bowel length (Fig. 49.9). Small-bowel disease may be resected using either laparoscopic or open techniques. Adhesions and fistulas may make the laparoscopic approach quite challenging.

The small bowel and ileum are common sites for disease recurrence. Crohn disease is most likely to recur close to the previously resected intestinal segment. The length of small bowel involved in recurrent disease generally corresponds to the length of bowel originally resected.[51] Diffuse disease, multiple resections, or symptomatic fistulas can lead to malabsorptive syndromes. Most common is the loss of bile salts normally absorbed by the terminal ileum. Bile salts hinder absorption in the colon, leading to increased frequency of stools and frank diarrhea. Bile salt diarrhea is treated with oral cholestyramine, which binds unabsorbed bile acids. More significantly, patients with severe disease may be unable to meet nutritional needs secondary to rapid transit and decreased functional intestinal length, either from disease or resection. These patients may require parental nutritional supplementation on a long- or short-term basis. Fortunately, this occurs only when less than 100 cm of bowel remains. A surgeon should be aware of this issue and attempt to preserve bowel length by minimizing resection and considering strictureplasty, where appropriate.

Crohn Disease of the Colon and Rectum

Approximately 25% of patients with Crohn disease have isolated colonic involvement, with 5% of these patients with disease isolated to the anorectum.[52] Careful examination of the anus and rectum is vital, because the procedure of choice for treatment of colonic Crohn disease is determined by extent of involvement and fecal incontinence.

Segmental colitis with rectal and anal sparing occurs in up to 50% of patients with Crohn colitis. Segmental resection has been advocated to spare patients from having a permanent colostomy and maintain absorptive length of the colon. Although patients may have several years of success with segmental resection or ileal rectal anastomosis, colon disease has

FIGURE 49.9. Computed tomography (CT) scan demonstrates a long segment of disease in the terminal ileum. Near-obliteration of the intestinal lumen is demonstrated by minimal passage of contrast. The loop of ileum in the right pelvis is also severely diseased, with mucosal changes apparent on CT scan.

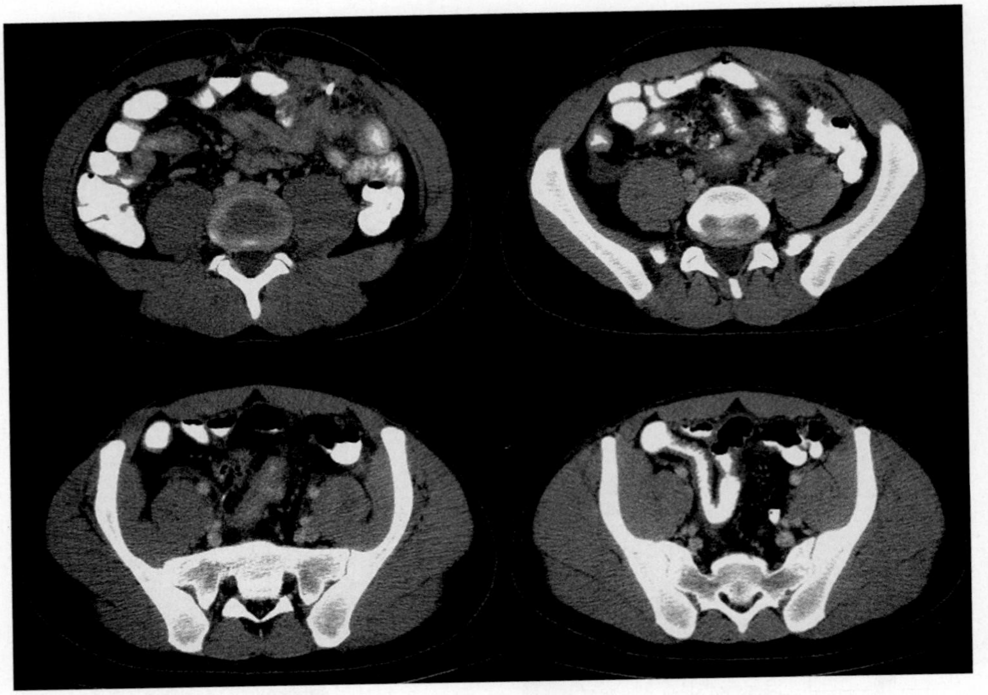

high recurrence rates even in previously grossly normal colon. Long-term recurrence rates are 30% to 70%, and up to 25% of patients eventually require a permanent stoma.[53,54] The rates of recurrence are similar for total abdominal colectomy with ileoanal anastomosis. Although ileal pouch anal anastomosis is commonly performed in ulcerative colitis, the recurrent nature of Crohn disease renders restorative procedures more risky and therefore this procedure is generally not recommended.

Patients who require emergency colon surgery for toxic megacolon or sepsis should undergo subtotal colectomy with end ileostomy. Subtotal colectomy defers difficult rectal dissection in an acutely ill patient and allows for conversion to an ileorectal anastomosis at a later date. In addition, patients who are acutely ill, malnourished, and immunosuppressed are more likely to develop difficult wound infections and pelvic sepsis from rectal dissection.[55] Placement of the rectal stump above the fascia prevents intrapelvic or intra-abdominal perforation and should be performed any time the rectal stump appears to carry a high likelihood of dehiscence.[56]

The surgical treatment of Crohn disease of the rectum requires proctectomy with creation of a permanent stoma. Crohn proctitis often occurs with extensive Crohn colitis requiring total proctocolectomy. Care should be taken to preserve pelvic sympathetic and parasympathetic nerves; in benign disease the dissection may be undertaken close to the rectal wall to limit risk of nerve injury. In the absence of significant perianal disease, intersphincteric resection with preservation of the external sphincter decreases the risk of a large perineal wound and adequately removes diseased mucosa of the rectum and anus. If perianal abscesses, complex fistulas, and dense scarring are present, a wide perineal excision is required. In severe cases, the perineal wound may require closure with gracilis or rectus muscle flaps.

Crohn Disease of the Anus

Perianal disease, in the form of abscesses, fistulas, ulcers, strictures, and hypertrophic skin tags, occurs in approximately 30% of patients with Crohn disease, although rarely in isolation. Crohn disease of the anus tends to be recurrent, complex, and progressive in nature.

Fistulas are abnormal connections between the anus or rectum and the perianal skin. Fistulas may be low lying or involve a portion of the internal sphincter muscles. Continence may be severely affected. Fistulas may extend to the vagina or urinary tract. Patients with abscesses should have surgical drainage and treatment with antibiotics including metronidazole and ciprofloxacin. Placement of setons, in the form of suture material or plastic loops, through the fistulous tract can stent the track and prevent formation of abscesses (Fig. 49.10).

Recent advances in medical therapies such as anti-TNF antibody (infliximab) have been shown to be effective in promoting the healing of complex Crohn perianal fistulas. Although short-term data show improvement, longer follow-up shows a low rate of sustained healing, even when combined with surgical drainage of abscess.[57] Local injection of immunologics may also be used, especially in the setting of painful skin tags and fissures.

When medical therapy fails to improve symptoms, or in the case of fistulizing disease to the vagina, surgical therapy is advocated. Fistulotomies, or laying open of the fistulous tract, may be used for low-lying fistulas, but the risk of incontinence limits its use in Crohn patients at risk for recurrent fistulas.

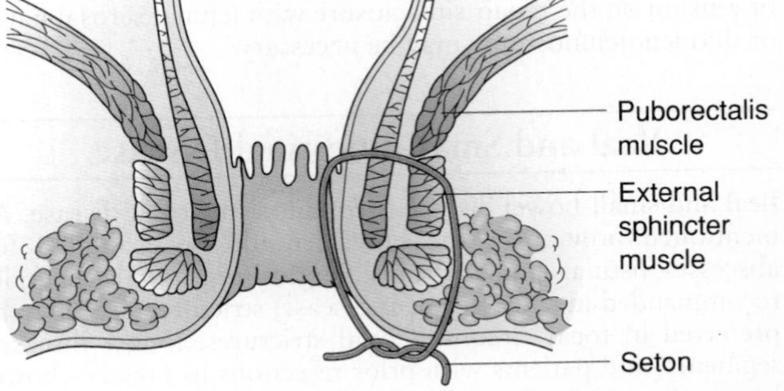

FIGURE 49.10. Placement of a seton suture through a transsphincteric fistula-in-ano. (Adapted from Gordon PH, Nivatvongs S, eds. *Principles and Practice of Surgery for the Colon, Rectum, and Anus.* St. Louis, MO: Quality Medical; 1992:221–265.)

Creation of rectal mucosal advancement flaps is appropriate when the rectal mucosa is not grossly affected with Crohn disease. Recent alternative approaches include fibrin-based glue and submucosal xenograft plug, with successful closure in up to 80% of initial studies.[58] One of the benefits of this technique is the low risk of incontinence or worsening of symptoms after these procedures.

Ultimately, a temporary stoma to divert the fecal stream may be appropriate to facilitate the healing of complex perianal disease such as severe fistulizing disease or rectovaginal fistulas or following creation of a rectal advancement flap. Up to 30% of patients with perianal disease may require permanent or temporary fecal diversion for treatment of their disease. Temporary fecal diversion is sometimes employed in conjunction with rectal advancement flaps to assist in the healing of particularly difficult cases. In severe cases of perianal disease that do not respond to aggressive medical and surgical treatment, fecal diversion typically results in significant relief of local sepsis and inflammation. Unfortunately, disease activity typically recurs rapidly in these cases after reestablishment of the fecal stream.

RECURRENCE

The most common long-term complication following surgery for Crohn disease is recurrent disease. Reported recurrence rates vary greatly. Endoscopic recurrence, which is often asymptomatic, has been reported to vary from 28% to 73% at 1 year and from 77% to 85% at 3 years after ileal resection.[59] Symptomatic recurrence occurs in 60% of patients at 5 years and 75% to 95% of patients at 20 years. Reports vary, but the rate of reoperation to treat recurrent disease is approximately 20% at 5 years, 33% at 10 years, and 50% at 20 years.[60]

Research has focused on the prevention of recurrence. Some evidence indicates that the use of NSAIDs or nicotine both promote recurrence of disease. All patients with Crohn disease should be strongly advised to refrain from smoking cigarettes or taking NSAIDs.

Patients are often placed on maintenance therapy within days or weeks of surgery. The most common maintenance therapies recommended are controlled-release 5-ASA (Pentasa) and 6-MP, but newer regimens include the use of metronidazole and infliximab. The degree to which postsurgical maintenance therapy lessens the risk for recurrent disease is in some cases only marginal. The effects on long-term quality of life and the cost-effectiveness of postoperative maintenance therapy have not been fully determined. Thus, the decision to recommend maintenance therapy must be individualized for each patient.

References

1. Dalziel TK. Chronic interstitial enteritis. *Br Med J* 1913;2:1068–1070.
2. Crohn's BB, Ginzburg L, Oppenheimer GD. Regional ileitis: a pathological and clinical entity. *JAMA* 1932;99:1323–1329.
3. Sandler RS, Glenn ME. Epidemiology of inflammatory bowel disease. In: Kirsner JB, ed. *Inflammatory Bowel Disease*, 5th ed. Philadelphia: WB Saunders; 2000:89–112.
4. Economou M, Pappas G. New global map of Crohn's disease: genetic, environmental and socioeconomic correlations. *Inflamm Bowel Dis* 2008; 14:709–720.
5. Yang H, McElree C, Roth MP, et al. Familial empiric risks for inflammatory bowel disease: differences between Jews and non-Jews. *Gut* 1993;34: 517–524.
6. Sands BR. Inflammatory bowel disease: past present and future. *J Gastroenterol* 2007;42:16–25.
7. Schreiber S, Hampe J. Genomics and inflammatory bowel disease. *Curr Opin Gastroenterol* 2000;16:297–305.
8. Inohara N, Ogura Y, Fontalba A, et al. Host recognition of bacterial muramyl dipeptide mediated through NOD2. Implications for Crohn's disease. *J Biol Chem* 2003;278:5509–5512.
9. Thomas GA, Rhodes J, Green JT. Inflammatory bowel disease and smoking—a review. *Am J Gastroenterol* 1998;93:144–149.
10. Michelassi F, Balestracci T, Chappell R, et al. Primary and recurrent Crohn's disease. Experience with 1379 patients. *Ann Surg* 1991;214: 230–238; discussion 238–240.
11. Vesolo FT, Carvalho J, Magro F. Immune-related systemic manifestations of inflammatory bowel disease. A prospective study of 792 patients. *J Clin Gastroenterol* 1996;23:29–34.
12. Carlson HC. Perspective: the small bowel examination in the diagnosis of Crohn's disease. *AJR Am J Roentgenol* 1986;147:63–65.
13. Vogel J, Moreira AL, Baker M, et al. CT enterography for Crohn's disease: accurate preoperative diagnostic imaging. *Dis Colon Rectum* 2007;50: 1761–1769.
14. Block GE, Michelassi F, Tanaka M, et al. Crohn's disease. *Curr Probl Surg* 1993;30:173–265.
15. Campos AC, Meguid MM. A critical appraisal of the usefulness of perioperative nutritional support. *Am J Clin Nutr* 1992;55:117–130.
16. McLeod RS, Wolff BG, Steinhart AH, et al. Prophylactic mesalamine treatment decreases postoperative recurrence of Crohn's disease. *Gastroenterology* 1995;109:404–413.
17. Ardizzone S, Maconi G, Sampietro GM, et al. Azathioprine and mesalamine for prevention of relapse after conservative surgery for Crohn's disease. *Gastroenterology* 2004;127:730–740.
18. Takeuchi K, Smale S, Premchand P, et al. Prevalence and mechanism of nonsteroidal anti-inflammatory drug-induced clinical relapse in patients with inflammatory bowel disease. *Clin Gastroenterol Hepatol* 2006;4: 196–202.
19. Rutgeerts P, Hiele M, Geboes K, et al. Controlled trial of metronidazole treatment for prevention of Crohn's recurrence after ileal resection. *Gastroenterology* 1995;108:1617–1621.
20. Faubion WA, Loftus EV, Harmsen WS, et al. The natural history of corticosteroid therapy for inflammatory bowel disease: a population-based study. *Gastroenterology* 2001;121:255–260.
21. Munkohlm P, Langholz E, Davidsen M, et al. Frequency of glucocorticoid resistance and dependency in Crohn's disease. *Gut* 1994;35:360–362.
22. Chelbi JM, Gaburri PD, De Souza AF, et al. Long-term results with azathioprine therapy in patients with corticosteroid-dependent Crohn's disease: open-label prospective study. *J Gastroenterol Hepatol* 2007;22: 268–274.
23. Panaccione R, Rutgeerts P, Sandborn WJ, et al. Review article: treatment algorithms to maximize remission and minimize corticosteroid dependence in patients with inflammatory bowel disease. *Aliment Pharmacol Ther* 2008;28:674–688.
24. Sands BE, Anderson FH, Berstein CN, et al. Infliximab maintenance therapy for fistulizing Crohn's disease. *N Engl J Med* 2004;350:876–885.
25. Hurst RD, Molinari M, Chung TP, et al. Prospective study of the features, indications, and surgical treatment in 513 consecutive patients affected by Crohn's disease. *Surgery* 1997;122:661–667; discussion 667–668.
26. Singh VV, Draganov P, Valentine J. Efficacy and safety of endoscopic balloon dilation of symptomatic upper and lower gastrointestinal Crohn's disease strictures. *J Clin Gastroenterol* 2005;39:284–290.
27. Brooker JC, Beckett CG, Saunders BP, et al. Long-acting steroid injection after endoscopic dilation of anastomotic Crohn's strictures may improve outcome: a retrospective case series. *Endoscopy* 2003;35:333–337.
28. Doemeny JM, Burke DR, Meranze SG. Percutaneous drainage of abscesses in patients with Crohn's disease. *Gastrointest Radiol* 1988;13:237–241.
29. Sahai A, Belair M, Gianfelice D, et al. Percutaneous drainage of intra-abdominal abscess in Crohn's disease: short and long term outcome. *Am J Gastroenterol* 1997;92:275–278.
30. Present DH, Rutgeerts P, Targan S, et al. Infliximab for the treatment of fistulas in patients with Crohn's disease. *N Engl J Med* 1999;340:1398–1405.
31. Block GE, Schraut WH. The operative treatment of Crohn's enteritis complicated by ileosigmoid fistula. *Ann Surg* 1982;196:356–360.
32. Michelassi F, Stella M, Balestracci T, et al. Incidence, diagnosis, and treatment of enteric and colorectal fistulae in patients with Crohn's disease. *Ann Surg* 1993;218:660–666.
33. Schraut WH, Chapman C, Abraham VS. Operative treatment of Crohn's ileocolitis complicated by ileosigmoid and ileovesical fistulae. *Ann Surg* 1988;207:48–51.
34. Caravan C, Abrams KR, Mayberry J. Meta-analysis: colorectal and small bowel cancer risk in patients with Crohn's disease. *Aliment Pharmacol Ther* 2006;23:1097–1104.
35. Jaskowiak NT, Michelassi F. Adenocarcinoma at a strictureplasty site in Crohn's disease: report of a case. *Dis Colon Rectum* 2001;44:284–287.
36. Yamazaki Y, Ribiero MB, Sachar DB, et al. Malignant colorectal strictures in Crohn's disease. *Am J Gastroenterol* 1991;86:882–885.
37. Truelove SC, Witts LF. Cortisone in ulcerative colitis: final report on a therapeutic trial. *BMJ* 1955;2:1041–1048.
38. Fazio VW, Marchetti F, Church M, et al. Effect of resection margins on the recurrence of Crohn's disease in the small bowel. A randomized controlled trial. *Ann Surg* 1996;224:563–571; discussion 571–573.
39. Similiis C, Purkayastha S, Yamamoto T, et al. A meta-analysis comparing conventional end-to-end anastomosis vs. other anastomotic configurations after resection in Crohn's disease. *Dis Colon Rectum* 2007;50:1674–1687.
40. Michelassi F, Taschieri A, Tonelli F, et al. An international multicenter prospective observational study of the side-to-side isoperistaltic strictureplasty in Crohn's disease. *Dis Colon Rectum* 2006;50:277–284.
41. Fichera A, Locadina S, Rubin M, et al. Patterns and operative treatment of recurrent Crohn's disease: a prospective longitudinal study. *Surgery* 2006; 140(4):649–654.

42. Poggioli G, Stocchi L, Laureti S, et al. Conservative surgical management of terminal ileitis. *Dis Colon Rectum* 1997;40:234–239.
43. Tan JJY, Tjandra JJ. Laparoscopic surgery for Crohn's disease: a meta-analysis. *Dis Colon Rectum* 2007;50:576–585.
44. Milsom JW, Hammerhofer KA, Bohm B, et al. Prospective randomized trial comparing laparoscopy vs conventional surgery for refractory ileocolic Crohn's disease. *Dis Colon Rectum* 2001;44:1–9.
45. Stocchi L, Milsom JW, Vazio VW. Crohn's disease: follow up of a prospective randomized trial. *Surgery* 2008;144:622–628.
46. Evans J, Poritz L, MacRae H. Influence of experience on laparoscopic ileocolic resection for Crohn's disease. *Dis Colon Rectum* 2002;45:1595–1600.
47. Harold KL, Kelly KA. Duodenal Crohn disease. *Probl Gen Surg* 1999;16:50–57.
48. Shapiro M, Greenstein AJ, Byrn J, et al. Surgical management and outcomes of patients with duodenal Crohn's disease. *J Am Coll Surg* 2008;207:36–42.
49. Nugent FW, Roy MA. Duodenal Crohn's disease: an analysis of 89 cases. *Am J Gastronetol* 1989;84:249–254.
50. Poggioli G, Stocchi L, Laureti S, et al. Duodenal involvement of Crohn's disease: three different clinicopathologic patterns. *Dis Colon Rectum* 1997;40:179–183.
51. D'Haens G, Baert F, Gasparaitis A, et al. Length and type of recurrent ileitis after ileal resection correlate with presurgical features in Crohn's disease. *Inflamm Bowel Dis* 1997;3:249–253.
52. Farmer RG, Hawk WA, Turbull RG. Clinical patterns of Crohn's disease: a statistical study of 615 cases. *Gastroenterology* 1975;68:627–635.
53. Longo WE, Ballantyne GH, Cahow E. Treatment of Crohn's colitis. Segmental of total colectomy? *Arch Surg* 123;588–590.
54. Prabhakar LP, Laramee C, Nelson H, et al. Avoiding a stoma: role for segmental or abdominal colectomy in Crohn's colitis. *Dis Colon Rectum* 1997;40:71–78.
55. Moscovitz I, Belin BM, Wexner SD. Colonic Crohn's disease. *Tech Coloproctol* 2000;4:39–44.
56. Trickett JP, Tilney HS, Gudgeon AM, et al. Management of the rectal stump after emergency subtotal colectomy: which surgical option is associated with the lowest morbidity? *Colorectal Dis* 2005;7:519–522.
57. Hyder SA, Travis SPL, Jewell DP, et al. Fistulizing anal Crohn's disease: results of combined surgical and infliximab treatment. *Dis Colon Rectum* 2006;49:1837–1841.
58. O'Connor L, Champagne BJ, Ferguson MA, et al. Efficacy of anal fistula plug in closure of Crohn's anorectal fistulas. *Dis Colon Rectum* 2006;49:1569–1573.
59. Mekhjian HS, Switz DM, Watts HD, et al. National Cooperative Crohn's Disease Study: factors determining recurrence of Crohn's disease after surgery. *Gastroenterology* 1979;77(4 Pt 2):907–913.
60. Post S, Herfarth C, Bohm E, et al. The impact of disease pattern, surgical management, and individual surgeons on the risk for relaparotomy for recurrent Crohn's disease. *Ann Surg* 1996;223:253–260.

CHAPTER 50 ■ SMALL-INTESTINAL NEOPLASMS

DOUGLAS J. TURNER, AJAY JAIN, AND BARBARA L. BASS

KEY POINTS

1. Although the small bowel accounts for 75% of the length and 90% of the mucosal surface of the gastrointestinal tract, it is the site of only 1% to 3% of gastrointestinal malignancies.
2. As in the colon, small-bowel adenomas may be histologically classified as tubular, tubulovillous, or villous. Adenomas occur predominantly in the duodenum with the majority found in the periampullary region.
3. Like adenomas, adenocarcinomas have a predilection for the duodenum, with a marked decrease in frequency moving axially along the small bowel. Approximately 80% of tumors are located in the duodenum or proximal jejunum.
4. The gastrointestinal tract is the site of 4% to 20% of all non-Hodgkin lymphomas, being the most common extranodal site. The stomach harbors the most lymphomas, followed by the small bowel and then the colon.
5. Carcinoids are indolent malignant neuroendocrine tumors that arise from the enterochromaffin cells at the base of the crypts of Lieberkühn.
6. Gastrointestinal stromal tumors are characterized by expression of c-kit and PDGFRα gene mutations. While surgical resection is the only curative treatment, adjuvant therapy with imatinib and other tyrosine kinase antagonists can decrease the risk of relapse in patients after resection of high-risk tumors.

Small-bowel tumors, both benign and malignant, are uncom-
1 mon. Although the small bowel accounts for 75% of the length and 90% of the mucosal surface of the gastrointestinal tract, less than 5% of primary gastrointestinal malignancies arise from the small intestine.[1] Although they are unusual, benign small-bowel lesions have been incidentally discovered in 0.2% to 0.3% of autopsy specimens, 15 times more than the number discovered in surgical specimens, attesting to the frequently asymptomatic nature of these neoplasms.[2] Recent data have reported an increase in the incidence of small-intestinal tumors, a factor at least partly due to improved imaging modalities and to an increasing number of immunocompromised patients.[1,3] Small-intestinal tumors may originate from cells of epithelial origin (adenomas, adenocarcinomas, or carcinoids), lymphatic tissues (lymphomas), or mesenchymal or neural elements (gastrointestinal stromal tumors, leiomyomas, lipomas, hemangiomas, neuromas, and a wide variety of sarcomas). From 1975 to 2000, the rates increased by almost 50%. This trend reflected increases for adenocarcinomas, malignant carcinoid tumors, and lymphomas in men, and for carcinoid tumors and lymphomas in women.[4] The small intestine is also a rare site for metastasis from other primary tumors.

EPIDEMIOLOGY

While the relative incidence rates of small-bowel tumors in the United States appear to be increasing,[3] there are clearly geographic variations in incidence worldwide. Carcinoid tumors are virtually nonexistent in Asian populations, yet represent about 30% of malignant small-bowel neoplasms in Western series.[3,5,6] The proportion of benign small-bowel tumors varies from 14% to 52% in various international series, a disparity likely explained by failure to detect the typically asymptomatic benign lesions. Reported rates of non-Hodgkin lymphoma of the small bowel vary from 27% to 72%, a discrepancy due in part to inconsistent categorization of lymphomas as primary or metastatic tumors, but also due partly to geographic variation. Given the rarity of small-bowel tumors and the wide variety of histologies, there are no large case series for any specific histologic subtype in the world literature, making comparisons difficult and definitive incidence rates difficult to confirm.[7]

Although generalizations regarding these rare tumors can be difficult to formulate, certain patterns can be discerned. Small-bowel neoplasms are less common in women than in men: a male preponderance (3:2 ratio) is reported for both benign and malignant neoplasms. Most patients with small-bowel neoplasms present in their sixth to seventh decade of life. Except for adenocarcinoma, which has a predilection for the duodenum, malignant small-bowel tumors are more common in the distal small bowel. Approximately 20% of tumors arise in the duodenum, 30% in the jejunum, and 50% in the ileum.[8]

PATHOGENESIS

Several hypotheses have been proposed to explain the low incidence of small-bowel tumors, particularly those derived from cells of the intestinal epithelium. These hypotheses postulate that small-bowel neoplasms may arise from disruption of normal small-bowel flora, pH, transit times, or mucosal integrity. Although none of these hypotheses have been verified, they are plausible given what is known about the pathogenesis of other gastrointestinal tumors. The dilute alkaline liquid contents of healthy small bowel are potentially less capable of inducing direct mechanical mucosal injury and disruption than the more solid contents of the colon. The luminal content of the healthy small-bowel lumen does not harbor pathogenic bacteria and their potentially toxic metabolites are not present to induce the genetic alterations implicated in colon carcinogenesis. Rapid transit time through the small-bowel lumen, normally 30 minutes to 2 hours, may limit mucosal exposure to potential carcinogens, whereas the presence of the enzyme benzopyrene hydroxylase in the brush border of the small intestine may provide protection against mucosal damage by detoxifying the carcinogen benzopyrene. The greater concentration and distribution of lymphoid tissue in the intestinal epithelium and submucosa and high levels of luminal immunoglobulin A may provide an immunologic protective mechanism against neoplasia. Some investigators suggest that the high rate of metachronous primary malignancies, observed in up to 20% of patients, and the frequency of multicentric small-bowel malignancies support an alteration in host defenses or a breakdown in this immunologic protective mechanism as an important etiologic factor.

CONDITIONS ASSOCIATED WITH INCREASED RISK FOR SMALL-BOWEL TUMORS

Although the small bowel develops few tumors, risk factors for the development of malignant lesions have been identified. As shown in Table 50.1, several conditions carry an increased risk of neoplasia.

Crohn Disease

Crohn disease is associated with up to a 10- to 12-fold increased risk of developing small-bowel adenocarcinoma,[9] with carcinoma developing in diseased segments of the bowel with preexisting dysplasia. Three quarters of these small-intestinal cancers arise in the ileum, the area most commonly involved with Crohn disease but the segment of small bowel least commonly affected by adenocarcinoma in healthy individuals. The remaining small-intestinal tumors in patients with Crohn disease are found in the duodenum and the jejunum, following the usual distribution of sporadic carcinoma, which tends to develop in the duodenum. Crohn-associated carcinomas carry a particularly poor prognosis because the tumors are frequently diagnosed at an advanced stage, likely because the abdominal symptoms of the tumor are initially attributed to the underlying inflammatory bowel disease.[10]

TABLE 50.1 **ETIOLOGY**

CONDITIONS ASSOCIATED WITH AN INCREASED RISK OF NEOPLASIA

■ PREEXISTING CONDITION	■ POTENTIAL MALIGNANCY
Adenomatous polyps	Adenocarcinoma
Familial adenomatous polyposis	Adenocarcinoma
Peutz-Jeghers syndrome/ hamartomatous polyps	Adenocarcinoma
Leiomyomas	Possible leiomyosarcoma
Neurofibromatosis	Leiomyosarcoma, carcinoid, adenocarcinoma
Crohn disease	Adenocarcinoma
Celiac sprue	Lymphoma, adenocarcinoma
Immunosuppression	Lymphoma
Human immunodeficiency virus infection	Lymphoma, Kaposi sarcoma
Helicobacter pylori infection	Low-grade lymphoma (mucosal-associated lymphoid tissue)
Epstein-Barr virus infection	Lymphoma

Familial Adenomatous Polyposis

Also at risk for the development of adenocarcinoma, primarily of the duodenum, are patients with familial adenomatous polyposis (FAP).[11] Close to 100% of FAP patients will eventually develop adenomatous polyps in the duodenum, and the risk of duodenal carcinoma in these patients has been estimated to be 300-fold over that of the healthy population.[11] Duodenal and periampullary adenocarcinomas are the leading cause of cancer death in FAP patients who have previously had a colectomy. Careful screening with periodic esophagogastroduodenoscopy and prompt local resection of adenomas is of paramount importance in this patient population. Endoscopic polypectomy is appropriate for small or pedunculated lesions, whereas larger villous tumors, which have a greater risk for adenocarcinoma, particularly in the periampullary region, may require pancreaticoduodenectomy for adequate treatment.

Other Conditions with Increased Risk for Small-bowel Malignancy

Celiac sprue is associated with lymphoma, and to a lesser degree adenocarcinoma, occurring in up to 14% of patients.[12] It is impossible to determine whether patients with celiac disease will develop cancer, but about 8% to 10% of patients with severe small-bowel mucosa biopsy changes develop lymphoma, and this figure has remained remarkably constant.[13–15] Patients who are diagnosed with celiac disease late in life tend to have a higher incidence of lymphoma than patients who are diagnosed early on. Some have suggested that this discrepancy may be attributed to initiation of a protective gluten-free diet at a much younger age.[15] It remains unclear, however, whether a gluten-free diet decreases the risk of gastrointestinal lymphoma. Dietary compliance did not show a decreased risk of malignancy in a recent study.[16]

The neurofibromas of von Recklinghausen disease may undergo malignant transformation, as may leiomyomas of the small bowel. In Peutz-Jeghers syndrome, hamartomas develop throughout the gastrointestinal tract and may carry a risk of malignant transformation to adenocarcinoma.[17] Whether these malignancies, especially in the duodenum, actually arise from preexisting hamartomas has been poorly documented. Sporadic benign adenomatous polyps are at risk for malignant transformation and should be removed when identified.

Bile acids and their metabolites may have a possible role in the pathogenesis of small-bowel adenocarcinoma. In one study of all patients with small-intestinal malignancy, 12% had a history of cholecystectomy, and of those with duodenal adenocarcinoma, 25% had prior cholecystectomy, although a causative relationship between cholecystectomy and small-intestinal adenocarcinoma remains unproven. Within the duodenum, the periampullary region is the most frequent site of primary carcinoma, although a link between this finding and pancreaticobiliary secretions is unexplored.

Immunosuppression, both iatrogenic following organ transplantation or secondary to disease, places a patient at increased risk for small-bowel malignancy, primarily lymphoma and sarcoma. After solid organ transplantation, patients maintained on immunosuppressive regimens have an incidence rate 45 to 100 times higher than that of nontransplanted persons for non-Hodgkin lymphoma (NHL), a condition termed *posttransplant lymphoproliferative disorder* (PTLD).[18] PTLD accounts for 30% of all malignancies in cyclosporine-treated patients but accounts for only 12% of malignancies in patients without cyclosporine in their regimen. PTLD tends to develop rapidly, often within 12 months of transplantation in cyclosporine-treated patients. The level of immunosuppression appears to influence the incidence of PTLD; patients who require high degrees of immunosuppression to sustain their graft, such as patients with small-bowel, heart, liver, or lung transplants, show rates of lymphoma as high as 30%. In contrast, only 5% of kidney transplant recipients (who generally require less immunosuppression) develop lymphoproliferative tumors. Reduction of immunosuppression remains the mainstay of treatment of PTLD. This can be challenging since reduction of immunosuppression increases the risk of allograft rejection. Additional treatment options include systemic chemotherapy or rituximab.[19] For localized disease, there may also be a role for surgical resection and/or radiation.[20] Human immunodeficiency virus (HIV) infection (another form of immunosuppression) is also associated with lymphoma. Lymphoma is the second most common malignancy, after Kaposi sarcoma, in these patients. As life expectancy for patients with HIV infection has lengthened with improved antiviral medications, the rates of lymphoma have increased such that the risk at 3 years now approaches 30%. Two thirds of these lymphomas are extranodal and the gastrointestinal tract is involved in 10% to 25% of cases.

CLINICAL PRESENTATION

There are no pathognomonic signs or symptoms of small-bowel tumors. Complaints, if reported, are nonspecific. As shown in Table 50.2, the most common symptoms—abdominal pain, weight loss, anemia, nausea, and vomiting—do not suggest specific localization and are usually present in about 45% of patients. These vague complaints often lead to diagnostic delay before the correct diagnosis of small-bowel neoplasm is established. Tumor location may influence the time required for detection. Smaller lesions often present earlier in the ileum, where the lumen is narrower and obstruction more likely to develop. As tumors enlarge, symptoms are more likely to develop. Of all lesions measuring at least 4 cm, 75% will cause symptoms, whereas 92% of malignant lesions of that size will be symptomatic. Overall, malignant lesions tend to be more symptomatic than benign lesions, eliciting complaints of abdominal pain and weight loss. In contrast, benign tumors more often present with acute hemorrhage as the primary symptom or are identified as an incidental finding on a radiologic examination or at laparotomy.

TABLE 50.2 **DIAGNOSIS**

CLINICAL PRESENTATION OF PRIMARY SMALL-BOWEL TUMORS

■ SIGNS AND SYMPTOMS	■ FREQUENCY (%)
Benign Neoplasms	
Asymptomatic	47–60
Abdominal pain	24–50
Acute gastrointestinal hemorrhage	29–44
Anemia	28–58
Intermittent obstruction	12–28
Malignant Neoplasms	
Asymptomatic	6–12
Abdominal pain	62–83
Weight loss	38–55
Nausea/vomiting	23–64
Acute gastrointestinal hemorrhage	6–31
Anemia	12–38
Abdominal mass	5–32

Because of their ill-defined symptoms, both benign and malignant small-bowel tumors frequently present late in their course. Tumors are often diagnosed at the time of emergency surgical exploration for intestinal obstruction, perforation, or massive gastrointestinal hemorrhage. Only in hindsight may a history of abdominal complaints be elicited.

DIAGNOSIS

Diagnosis of a small-bowel neoplasm can be challenging. In most series, the average duration of symptoms prior to diagnosis ranges from weeks to many months. Diagnosis is hindered by the infrequency of these tumors and failure to consider small-bowel neoplasm in the differential diagnosis for patients with nonspecific abdominal complaints. More importantly, diagnosis is delayed because imaging modalities available to study the small bowel are limited. Accurate preoperative diagnosis is rarely established prior to surgery.[1]

Plain abdominal radiography is rarely helpful unless the patient presents with obstructive symptoms. For patients being evaluated for gastrointestinal complaints or gastrointestinal bleeding, the diagnosis of small-bowel tumor is usually considered after negative endoscopic evaluation of the foregut and colon. The diagnostic workup should then proceed to computed tomography (CT) scan of the abdomen. In addition to readily identifying bulky mass lesions, imaging allows detection of subtle findings that are highly suggestive of small-bowel tumors. Neoplastic disease must be strongly suspected if the small bowel wall is thicker than 1.5 cm or if there are discrete mesenteric lymph nodes or masses greater than 1.5 cm in diameter. The CT scan may reveal a transition zone, demarcating dilated proximal bowel from decompressed distal bowel. If associated with bowel wall thickening, a tumor is likely, except in patients with clinical characteristics more typical of Crohn disease or those who carry a known diagnosis of Crohn disease.

Tumors of the distal small bowel may show CT findings of ileocolic or jejunoileal intussusception. Diagnosis of intussusception in adult patients warrants operative intervention without further delay. During intussusception, the small-bowel tumor serves as the lead point to pull the small bowel into the distal small bowel or colonic lumen; the mass lesion precludes spontaneous reduction. In adults, radiographic attempts to reduce an intussusception should not be attempted. Rather, prompt surgical exploration and resection of the nonreduced intussuscepted bowel segment with mesenteric resection should be completed.

If abdominal CT imaging fails to reveal evidence of a small-bowel tumor, one should proceed to the next steps in the diagnostic algorithm for small-bowel lesions, which have changed in recent years due to the greater availability of two new technologies to visualize and assess the small-bowel lumen: interventional methods in endoscopy, endoscopic ultrasound, and now video capsule endoscopy (VCE) and double-balloon enteroscopy (DBE). Prior to the development of these technologies, luminal contrast studies were the next diagnostic step, and there is a place for these studies where expertise in newer technologies remains unavailable. Luminal radiographic contrast studies and upper gastrointestinal and small-bowel follow-through (UGI and SBFT) remain useful to identify areas of partial obstruction and to identify patients in whom VCE may be contraindicated due to the presence of strictures that would prevent passage of the capsule. However, interpretation of subtle findings on UGI and SBFT for the evaluation of possible small-bowel tumors remains challenging, and diagnostic accuracy is only 60% to 70% in most series.

Endoscopic examination of the duodenum is readily accomplished and the diagnostic procedure of choice. Endoscopy also offers optimal means for tissue diagnosis with forceps biopsy, snare polypectomy, or fine-needle aspiration. Endoscopic ultrasound has expanded the diagnostic and therapeutic assessment of mucosal and mural lesions of the small bowel, and is widely utilized to provide structural characteristics of lesions of the duodenum. Accurate staging of depth of mucosal-based lesions is enhanced and identification of submucosal extension can confirm malignancy and dictate a resectional therapeutic approach as opposed to a luminal submucosal excision. Lesions confined to the mucosa but too large for snare polypectomy may be removed with endoscopic techniques and devices that allow endoscopic mucosal resection (EMR), offering both diagnostic and therapeutic efficacy.

Given these poor detection rates, some radiologists support enteroclysis as the primary study of choice for imaging the small bowel distal to the ligament of Treitz. Enteroclysis is a dynamic contrast technique that uses a combination of barium and methylcellulose infused into the small bowel via a nasoduodenal tube to uniformly distend the small bowel without abolishing peristalsis. Expertise in this procedure is important for success and is rapidly losing favor as a diagnostic test given the newer technologies of VCE and DBE. It can be a useful study, however, as in one series, enteroclysis identified 90% of cases compared to 33% by SBFT in the same cohort of patients.

In addition to these techniques that attempt to visualize intraluminal pathology, other modalities are useful in specific situations. Selective visceral angiography may be helpful in the diagnosis of patients with acute or chronic gastrointestinal hemorrhage. Massive hemorrhage is most common with benign smooth muscle tumors and arteriography may provide both diagnostic and temporizing therapeutic advantages if selective embolization of a bleeding vessel can be achieved. Benign vascular lesions, including hemangioma, are more likely to present with occult gastrointestinal blood loss.

Small-bowel Enteroscopy

Endoscopic modalities include push enteroscopy, intraoperative enteroscopy, VCE, and DBE. The older modality of Sonde pull-through enteroscopy is no longer in clinical use. "Push" enteroscopy utilizes a pediatric colonoscope for direct examination of the mucosa of the proximal small bowel.[21] Biopsy of identified lesions can be performed with this instrument, although the examination is limited to visualization of only the proximal 2 to 3 feet of small bowel. Performed in the endoscopy suite with intravenous sedation, the procedure is not well tolerated by all patients.

Intraoperative enteroscopy—a combined procedure including an endoscopist who navigates the enteroscope though the lumen on the bowel, which is facilitated by manipulation of the bowel by a surgeon, using laparoscopic, hand-assist, or open approaches—allows full visualization of the small-bowel mucosal surface and the opportunity to surgically treat identified lesions.

VCE with a wireless video capsule endoscope is being employed increasingly in the diagnosis of small-bowel tumors with negative CT scan and upper endoscopy. The device is an ingestible 11 × 26-mm capsule that the patient swallows; it contains a miniature video camera, light source, battery, and transmitter that sends images (up to 60,000 overall) to a recording device worn by the patient.[22,23] The patient simply swallows the capsule and subsequently passes the device; no sedation is required. VCE is a good test to identify potential small-bowel lesions; however, it does not have the capacity for biopsies, nor can precise localizations along the bowel be determined. Relative contraindications to VCE include obstructive symptoms, motility disorders, and pacemakers. The major complication is capsule retention, which can occur at a stricture; the incidence of this in healthy patients is close to 0%; however, it can be as high as 10% to 25% in patients with small-bowel tumors.[22] A dissolvable test capsule is in development to identify those patients in whom the capsule is most likely to be retained. While retention of the capsule may not be considered a complication in those patients requiring surgery for an identified obstructing tumor, it is a much more serious complication in patients who would otherwise be managed conservatively, such as those with Crohn disease (where retention rates have been reported at 5% to 13%).[22] VCE has been useful in the identification of all mucosal-based lesions, including neoplasms, of the small bowel. The diagnostic rates are lower with submucosal lesions such as gastrointestinal stromal tumors. The major limitation of VCE is that it can only roughly identify the location of the lesion within the length of the small bowel and it does not offer any therapeutic impact or ability to sample tissue.

DBE is an endoscopic procedure that utilizes a therapeutic endoscope coupled to a pair of inflatable balloons. Sequential inflation and deflation of the balloons allows the endoscope to be pulled through the lumen of the small bowel. The entire mucosal surface can be visualized in antegrade (per oral) or retrograde (per anus) fashion. The procedure requires deep sedation or general anesthesia and considerable technical expertise and experience for successful execution. The major advantage of the procedure over the less complex and safer procedure of VCE is that tissue diagnosis and therapeutic capacity exists with DBE. In a large registry study from Japan, of 1,045 patients undergoing DBE, 144 (14%) were found to have small-bowel tumors. Biopsy confirmed the diagnosis of tumor type in 85 patients including gastrointestinal stromal tumors, lymphoma, and carcinoid tumors. In 45 patients interventional procedures were completed including endoscopic mucosal resection, clipping or coagulation for bleeding, and stent placement. Complications occurred in 3% of patients, including perforation requiring subsequent surgical management.

Despite these multiple diagnostic modalities, more than half of patients with small-bowel neoplasms present with a surgical emergency, and more than half of patients with malignant disease have metastatic spread at the time of operation.

SURGICAL MANAGEMENT

Surgical approaches have changed as laparoscopic procedures for abdominal conditions have been disseminated throughout the surgical community. Laparoscopic approaches are suitable for isolated benign and nonbulky tumors. Hand-assist ports facilitate these procedures using tactile palpation to identify smaller lesions, particularly in obese patients where the tumors may not be readily identified. Abdominal wall seeding has not been described, although most advocate removal of the tumor in a specimen retrieval bag to avoid tissue contact.

Mesenteric resection is important in tumors characterized by lymphatic spread including adenocarcinoma, carcinoid, and lymphoma. Open procedures, to ensure adequate wide mesenteric resection, may be more appropriate for these tumors. During the surgical procedure, it is essential to carefully examine the entire small bowel, because multiple lesions occur in up to 20% of patients depending on tumor type. Assessment for metastatic disease elsewhere in the abdomen including the liver is also essential.

BENIGN TUMORS OF THE SMALL INTESTINE

Accounting for 30% to 50% of primary neoplasms of the small bowel, benign tumors are poorly characterized. Half the patients with benign tumors are symptom free, even in retrospect, until the need for emergency surgery. Up to 60% of benign small-bowel tumors will be diagnosed at the time of presentation with a surgical emergency including obstruction, massive gastrointestinal hemorrhage, or perforation. For patients who do present with symptoms necessitating evaluation, vague abdominal pain and recurrent gastrointestinal bleeding are the most common. In one series,[2] 29% of patients with benign lesions presented with an acute hemorrhage and 40% in another series,[8] a feature that may help differentiate benign from malignant lesions, the latter of which bleed less often. Many more lesions are never identified because they elicit no symptoms.

As noted previously, the diagnostic workup is challenging. In patients with symptoms, investigations should proceed as outlined previously. The sequelae of the neoplasms (obstruction, hemorrhage, perforation) will dictate the pathway of evaluation.

Regardless of the location, the treatment of benign small-bowel tumors is local excision or limited resection. As gross appearance in the operating room may not definitively establish a small-bowel tumor as benign, segmental resection is often the most appropriate surgical approach. Endoscopic resection or submucosal excision via operative enterotomy may be appropriate for small lesions with obvious benign-appearing features such as a lipoma or for multiple symptomatic lesions as occurs with Peutz-Jeghers syndrome[24]; however, segmental limited resection is usually the most appropriate intervention. Intraoperative examination of the small bowel with careful palpation, including the possible use of intraoperative enteroscopy for evaluation of suspected abnormalities, is essential to rule out synchronous lesions.

ADENOMAS

Unique to the duodenum, Brunner gland adenomas are rare tumors of the proximal duodenum.[25] Brunner glands are normally found in the duodenal submucosa and secrete an alkaline bicarbonate-rich fluid and mucus that aids in the neutralization of gastric acid. The pathogenesis of the glandular hyperplasia that is linked to adenoma formation remains unknown. Brunner gland adenomas appear to have minimal, if any, malignant potential. Once identified, local resection via endoscopic means or duodenotomy with submucosal excision should be performed to prevent intussusception or biliary obstruction as the adenoma grows.

2 As in the colon, small-bowel adenomas may be histologically classified as tubular, tubulovillous, or villous. Adenomas occur predominantly in the duodenum with the majority found in the periampullary region, but they may also be found in the proximal jejunum. Because roughly 25% of these villous and tubulovillous adenomas harbor malignancy, it is important to identify and resect these tumors when they are identified.[26] Submucosal resection (SMR) via DBE has been described for these smaller lesions. It is the preferred approach when technical expertise with these modalities is available. All adenomas are associated with potential risk for malignant transformation, a risk that presumably increases with size, although relative risks of transformation are difficult to determine given the low number of reported cases. Nonetheless, adenomas larger than 2 cm should be considered worrisome for malignancy.

Approximately one third of adenomas in the duodenum present with obstructive jaundice or small-bowel obstruction, leading to ultrasound and abdominal radiography as the initial diagnostic studies. Without these physical signs to direct the workup, appropriate initial diagnostic studies of the duodenum include double-contrast upper gastrointestinal series or esophagogastroduodenoscopy, both of which are equally sensitive in most series. Adenomas appear usually as small intraluminal filling defects and are frequently pedunculated on a stalk (Fig. 50.1). For those few patients subjected to contrast series prior to esophagogastroduodenoscopy, the pathognomonic finding for villous adenoma is a "soap bubble" or "paint brush" sign, in which rounded radiolucent areas are intermixed with a meshwork of contrast material. Esophagogastroduodenoscopy should follow a positive upper gastrointestinal study incorporating endoscopic ultrasound to detect depth of the lesion, potential for invasive disease, and lymphadenopathy. Treatment requires either endoscopic excision or surgical resection for larger invasive lesions. The surgical choices include transduodenal local excision for small lesions, pancreas-sparing duodenectomy for lesions confined to the mucosa, or pylorus-preserving pancreaticoduodenectomy

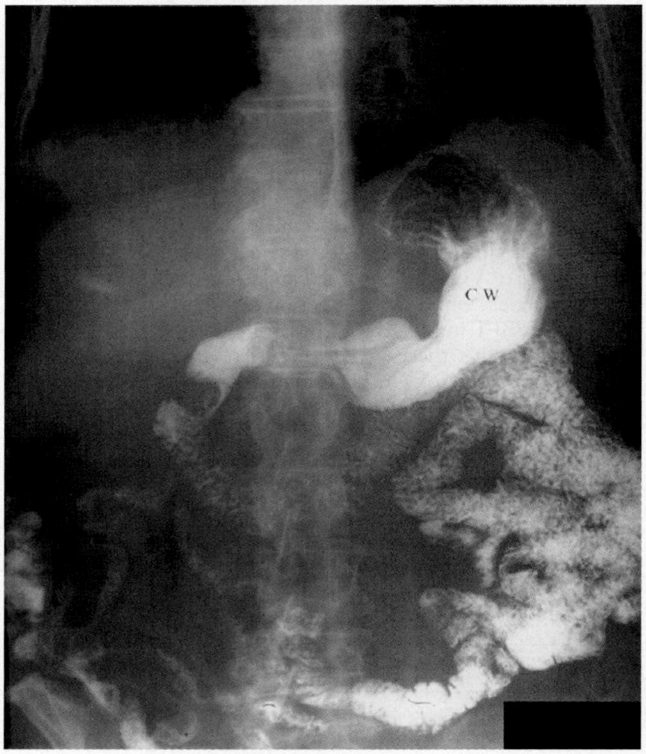

FIGURE 50.1. A 64-year-old woman with a polypoid lesion in the second portion of her duodenum on upper gastrointestinal series, found to be a benign adenoma at operation.

for larger lesions or periampullary tumors. Duodenal villous tumors demonstrate local recurrence rates of 40% at 10 years, 25% of which are malignant. Based on these retrospective data, pancreaticoduodenectomy is recommended as an appropriate surgical option for benign lesions in selected patients. As mentioned previously, patients with FAP are at particularly high risk for developing duodenal polyps with potential for malignant transformation. After the colon, the duodenum is the second most common site of polyp formation in FAP, and duodenal cancer is the second most common cancer after colon cancer in FAP patients. FAP patients have a 100- to 300-fold greater risk of developing duodenal cancer than the general population.[27] Because of this high risk of local recurrence, those patients in whom local excision is performed require annual surveillance with endoscopy.[28] In FAP patients with multiple polyps that cannot be completely excised or in patients with dysplastic changes, pancreaticoduodenectomy should be offered.[27]

LIPOMAS

Lipomas are true fatty neoplasms of the small bowel that are typically asymptomatic. These tumors are most often found incidentally on abdominal CT scans completed for evaluation of other clinical conditions. Lipomas are identified as well-circumscribed lesions of fat density on CT imaging. Unless associated with bleeding or obstruction, small tumors under 2 cm can be safely observed, while larger lesions or growing lesions should be resected to rule out malignant liposarcoma. Because these tumors are polypoid, compressible intraluminal lesions, they are predisposed to induce intussusception. If surgery is performed either for a complication of the lipoma or an unrelated condition, local excision is adequate treatment.

HAMARTOMAS

Peutz-Jeghers syndrome (PJS) is an autosomal dominant condition characterized by multiple gastrointestinal hamartomas and mucocutaneous pigmentation. The polyps arise predominantly in the jejunum and ileum and often present as an intussusception. Although hamartomas rarely if ever undergo malignant transformation, the condition is associated with the development of adenocarcinoma.[17] Double-balloon enteroscopy and video capsule endoscopy have provided effective screening technologies for patients with PJS. Endoscopic mucosal resection of hamartomas or polyps in patients with PJS via double-balloon enteroscopy has been described. Surveillance is recommended with endoscopic removal of lesions when they are identified. Patients who are diagnosed with PJS are at increased risk for developing a number of cancer types, including colorectal, gastric, small-bowel, ovarian/testicular, and pancreatic cancer. Patients who are diagnosed with this disease should undergo genetic counseling and have first-degree relatives screened. Screening for duodenal and small-bowel tumors in patients who are positive for the genetic mutation that causes PJS can include interval esophagogastroduodenoscopy and small-bowel contrast studies beginning in childhood (as early as age 8).[24] Although no consensus exists regarding the exact screening guidelines for these patients, close follow-up by a gastroenterologist is warranted given the high risk for a number of malignancies.

HEMANGIOMAS

Hemangiomas are rare lesions of the small bowel, developing predominantly in the jejunum and ileum. They are congenital lesions that grow slowly, typically coming to medical attention in the third decade of life because of acute or chronic blood loss. Arising from the submucosal vascular plexuses, hemangiomas are classified as capillary, cavernous, or mixed depending on what size vessel primarily is affected. They are usually solitary lesions and malignant degeneration is exceedingly rare. Depending on size, hemangiomas may be locally excised or resected with a laparoscopic approach with limited small-bowel resection. Efforts to manage hemangiomas with endoscopic or operative sclerotherapy or coagulation and operative or angiographic interruption of arterial supply have been minimally successful.

MALIGNANT NEOPLASMS

Malignant neoplasms in the small bowel are either primary or metastatic. Primary malignancies include adenocarcinoma, gastrointestinal stromal tumors (GISTs), leiomyosarcoma, non-Hodgkin lymphoma (NHL), and carcinoid tumors, with rare reports of other lesions including liposarcoma, myxoliposarcoma, and lymphangiosarcoma. Metastatic tumors of the small bowel have been reported from many primary solid tumors, but melanoma and lymphoma are the most common. Compared with benign tumors, malignant lesions are more likely to present with pain, weight loss, and anorexia. Although nonspecific, these findings are more ominous than other symptoms shared with benign tumors, such as nausea and vomiting and acute or chronic blood loss. As a group, patients with malignant small-bowel tumors present at advanced stages and have a poor prognosis. High rates of metastatic spread are noted on initial surgical operation.

The diagnosis of small-bowel malignancy should prompt a thorough diagnostic evaluation. Second primary malignancies are found in 20% to 30% of patients. This association is especially relevant for carcinoid tumors, where the incidence rate of second primaries is as high as 30% to 50%. The second primary cancer may arise in any organ, but the most frequent second primary sites are the colorectum and breast.[29]

ADENOCARCINOMA

Epidemiology

3 Adenocarcinoma accounts for about 30% of small-bowel tumors.[1] Like adenomas, sporadic adenocarcinomas have a predilection for the duodenum, with a marked decrease in frequency moving axially along the small bowel.[3] Approximately 80% of tumors are located in the duodenum or proximal jejunum. Most studies report a slight male preference.

There are several risk factors for the development of adenocarcinoma. Malignant transformation of villous and tubulovillous adenomas is likely the most important and occurs predominantly in the periampullary region of the duodenum. Crohn disease increases the risk up to 100-fold and predisposes to cancer in the more distal small bowel in regions of dysplasia.

Clinical Presentation

The presenting symptoms of small-bowel adenocarcinoma depend on the location and size of the tumor. Because tumors tend to arise in the proximal small bowel and to encompass the bowel wall, adenocarcinomas cause obstruction with associated anorexia. The majority of tumors cause crampy abdominal pain. Periampullary duodenal adenocarcinomas may cause obstructive jaundice or pancreatitis as they grow. In this case, the physical complaints and findings help guide the direction of the diagnostic evaluation. Often, the only complaint is vague, persistent abdominal pain.

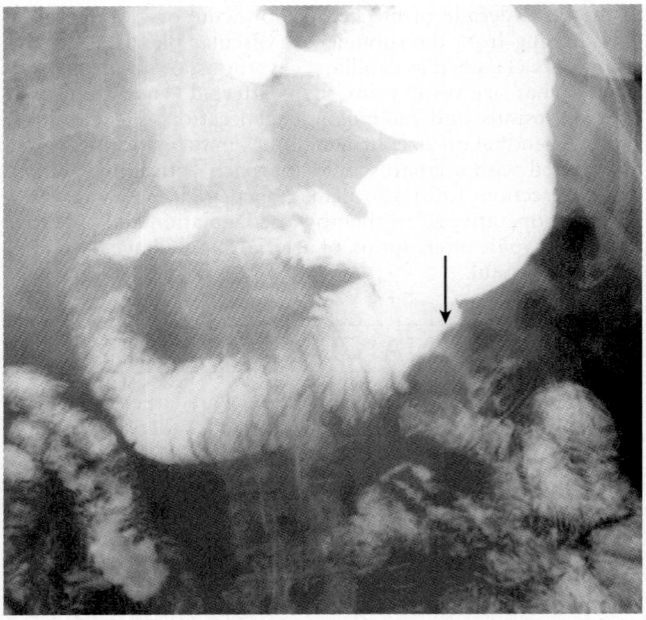

FIGURE 50.2. A 73-year-old woman who presented with gastric outlet obstruction was found on this small-bowel follow-through study to have apple-core lesion of the proximal jejunum. At exploration, she was found to have jejunal adenocarcinoma.

Diagnosis

If obstruction is present, plain abdominal films may reveal gastric distention or near-complete proximal small-bowel obstruction. More commonly, however, these films are unrevealing. For the jaundiced patient, ultrasound or abdominal CT or magnetic resonance cholangiopancreatography may demonstrate the duodenal mass and site of biliary obstruction. Esophagogastroduodenoscopy is the diagnostic modality of choice, with diagnostic rates of 85% to 90%.

Of small-bowel adenocarcinomas, 70% are polypoid, 20% are ulcerated, and 10% are infiltrative. Comparable to other segments of the gastrointestinal tract, adenocarcinomas of the jejunum and ileum are usually annular constricting tumors seen as apple-core lesions, as demonstrated on luminal contrast studies or esophagogastroduodenoscopy (Fig. 50.2). Long lesions, especially when ulcerated, may be mistaken for lymphomas. On CT scan, adenocarcinomas may attenuate heterogenously and have moderate contrast enhancement. Again, usually only a short segment of small bowel is involved, and occasionally they are associated with an ulcer. Despite the array of diagnostic modalities, preoperative diagnosis remains infrequent, achieved in only 20% to 50% of cancers.

Management

The only potential cure for adenocarcinoma is complete surgical resection. At operation, the resectability rate for cure approaches 60%. For proximal and midduodenal lesions, pancreaticoduodenectomy is necessary to completely resect the tumor and lymphatic basin. In the third and fourth portions of the duodenum and in the mesenteric small bowel, a segmental resection with lymphadenectomy should be performed to attempt surgical cure. In patients with metastatic or unresectable disease, palliative procedures to relieve obstruction or control hemorrhage should be considered. Segmental resection or intestinal bypass is appropriate in some patients. Duodenal obstruction may be palliated with endoscopic placement of expandable stents, although recurrent obstruction and hemorrhage may complicate this procedure. Consideration should be given to placement of gastrojejunal or gastrostomy tubes in patients with carcinomatosis or unresectable disease found at the time of surgery for palliative decompression or nutritional support and hydration.

Staging and Prognosis

The American Joint Committee on Cancer (AJCC) staging system for small-bowel adenocarcinoma is similar to those for gastric and colon carcinoma. The staging system applies only to adenocarcinoma of the small bowel and not to other malignant neoplasms of the small intestine. Carcinoma of the ampulla of Vater is also staged separately. As in other gastrointestinal malignancies, the tumor classification (T) describes depth of invasion, with T1 and T2 both contained within the bowel wall and T3 and T4 describing gradations of penetration through the wall. Unlike colon cancer, the node classification (N) in small-bowel carcinoma is classified only by presence or absence of lymph node metastases, and not by numbers of positive nodes. Distant metastases are classified (M). The TNM classification for small-bowel adenocarcinoma is summarized in Table 50.3. As shown, prognosis is grim for patients presenting with stage III or IV disease, the most frequent stages at diagnosis.

Factors that affect long-term survival in small-bowel adenocarcinoma vary slightly by study and tumor location. For duodenal tumors, negative resection margins and tumors in the first and second portions seem to favorably affect prognosis, whereas nodal status and size and differentiation of the tumor do not.[30] In contrast, ampullary tumors are associated with better prognosis if lymph nodes are not involved and the tumor does not infiltrate the pancreas.[26] One study evaluating prognostic factors for all small-bowel malignancies, exclusive of periampullary lesions, demonstrated poor survival in node-positive patients regardless of curative resection. Studies examining cancers of the jejunum and ileum are limited by their small sizes; however, a recent study concluded that among the factors for survival were positive margins, extramural venous spread, positive lymph nodes, and history of Crohn disease.[31]

Chemotherapy (typically 5-fluorouracil [5-FU] alone or in combination with other agents such as doxorubicin, cisplatin, mitomycin C, cyclophosphamide, and oxaliplatin) is often administered to patients with adenocarcinoma of the small intestine based on regimens administered for other gastrointestinal cancer. Unfortunately, chemotherapy and/or radiation therapy has not been shown to confer a survival advantage or prolonged disease-free interval.[31] It should be noted, however, that no adequate clinical trials have been conducted to delineate the efficacy of adjuvant chemotherapy for adenocarcinoma of the small intestine, so at the present time it is not possible to definitively comment on its role in the treatment of small-intestinal adenocarcinoma.[32]

NON-HODGKIN LYMPHOMA

4 NHL of the gastrointestinal tract represents 4% to 20% of all NHLs, with the gastrointestinal tract being the most common extranodal site for NHL to occur. In the gastrointestinal tract, NHL is most commonly located in the stomach, followed by the small bowel and then the colon. Of all gastrointestinal NHLs, 25% to 35% of cases occur within the small bowel. The distribution pattern is marked by relative sparing of the duodenum and equal frequency in the jejunum and ileum.

Many retrospective reviews of small-bowel cancer exclude primary NHL from analysis because of the difficulties in differentiating primary small-bowel lymphomas from those that originated outside of the gastrointestinal tract. Specific criteria must be met to establish the diagnosis of primary gastrointestinal NHL. In order to definitively make this diagnosis, there must be no evidence of lymphoma outside of the gastrointestinal tract.

TABLE 50.3 **STAGING**

TNM CLASSIFICATION AND STAGING OF SMALL-BOWEL ADENOCARCINOMA

TNM	CARCINOMA PENETRATION	STAGE	5-YEAR SURVIVAL RATE
Tx	Unknown primary		
T0	No evidence of primary		
Tis	Carcinoma in situ	0	
T1	Tumor invades lamina propria or submucosa	I	70%
T2	Tumor invades muscularis propria		
T3	Tumor extends <2 cm into subserosa or into nonperitonealized perimuscular tissue (mesentery in jejunum or ileum, retroperitoneum in duodenum)	II	50%
T4	Tumor penetrates visceral peritoneum or directly invades >2 cm into adjacent structures		
Nx	Regional lymph nodes not assessed		
N0	No regional lymph node involvement		
N1	Regional lymph nodes involved		
Mx	Distant metastases not assessed	III	20%
Mo	No distant metastases		
M1	Distant metastases present	IV	10%

On physical examination, there should be no superficial adenopathy, and chest radiograph (CT or x-ray) should reveal no mediastinal adenopathy. Peripheral blood cell counts must be normal, and there may be no evidence of splenic or hepatic involvement. Finally, at laparotomy, disease must be restricted to the primary tumor with mesenteric lymph node involvement.

Multiple histologic variations of lymphoma exist, showing significant geographic variability. The majority of primary intestinal NHLs are of the B-cell type, with T-cell lymphoma comprising only 10% to 25% of cases. Further classifications of B-cell and T-cell tumors have been proposed, but none has been uniformly adopted. A significant number of gastrointestinal lymphomas appear to be low-grade lymphomas derived from mucosal-associated lymphoid tissue. These lymphomas arise predominantly in the stomach but also occur in the small bowel. In the stomach they are associated with *Helicobacter pylori* infection and may regress with treatment of this infection. In the small bowel these low-grade lymphomas should be resected. T-cell lymphomas tend to have a worse prognosis than B-cell tumors.

Clinical Presentation

Similar to other small-bowel malignancies, the majority of patients with NHL present with abdominal pain that is nonspecific and unlocalized. Malabsorption, obstruction, and evidence of a palpable mass may be present. Although rare, perforation is a more common presentation for gastrointestinal NHL than for adenocarcinoma, possibly related to a lack of a vigorous desmoplastic response in lymphoma. Signs that are common in nodal lymphoma, such as adenopathy and splenomegaly, are unusual in primary gastrointestinal NHL.

Diagnosis

Most small-bowel lymphomas will be demonstrable on CT scan, as these lymphomas may grow to be quite large. CT scan will demonstrate the mass as well as marked luminal dilatation, bowel wall thickening, and displacement of neighboring loops (Figs. 50.3 and 50.4). Short strictures are more suggestive of adenocarcinoma but may occasionally be seen with lymphoma. Small-bowel follow-through will reveal multifocal lesions in 10% to 25% of patients. To make a tissue diagnosis, biopsies must be obtained from the submucosa, as the overlying mucosa often demonstrates no evidence of tumor infiltration. CT-guided biopsy may be diagnostic, although proximal lesions are best diagnosed with endoscopic submucosal biopsy.

Staging and Prognosis

Unlike other solid tumors of the gastrointestinal tract, the TNM system does not apply to staging of gastrointestinal NHL. Rather, staging is based on site involvement, outlined in Table 50.4. Like tumors elsewhere in the small bowel, lymphomas are typically diagnosed late, with almost half of patients presenting as stage III or IV disease. Fewer than 30% of patients have surgically resectable tumors. Patients with stage I tumors have a 40% to 60% 5-year survival, whereas those with stage II disease have a 20% 5-year survival. The long-term survival for patients with stages III and IV disease remains negligible, despite the aggressive use of chemoradiation therapy.

Treatment

With no randomized series and small numbers of cases at single institutions, the optimal treatment of gastrointestinal NHL remains controversial. Previously, surgical resection of localized gastrointestinal lymphomas followed by systemic chemotherapy was considered to be standard first-line therapy.[33–35] The data regarding the efficacy of primary surgical therapy with or without adjuvant chemotherapy versus systemic therapy alone are limited since gastrointestinal lymphomas are relatively rare. In many case series reporting outcomes after surgical resection of gastrointestinal lymphoma, the diagnosis of lymphoma was not known preoperatively and discovered only after intervention for a symptomatic small-bowel lesion. It is not clear, however,

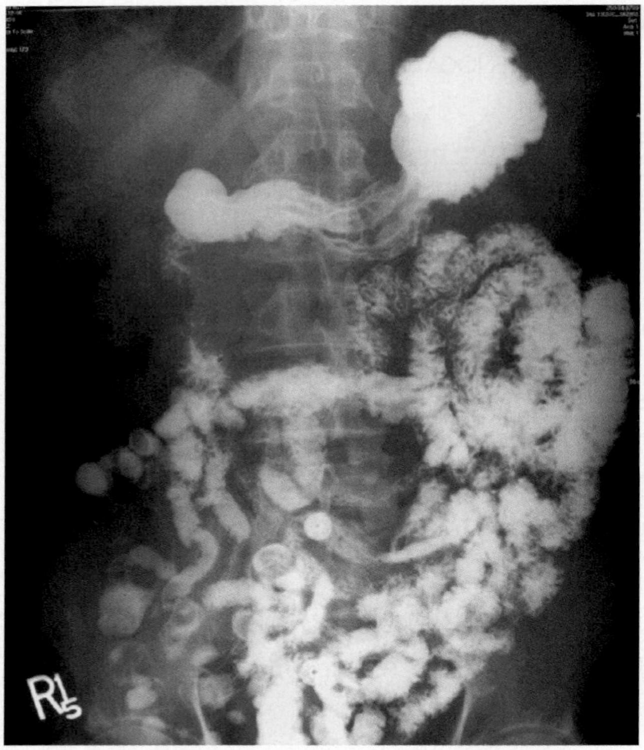

FIGURE 50.3. This small-bowel follow-through was performed on a 71-year-old man with chronic symptoms of partial small-bowel obstruction. It demonstrated a persistently dilated small-bowel loop in the terminal ileum with a thickened wall. The computed tomography scan in Figure 50.4 was obtained.

whether surgery should be the first line of treatment if a diagnosis of lymphoma can be made prior to any operative interventions. Indeed, for most lymphomas, systemic therapy and/or radiation has been considered to be standard first-line therapy, rather than surgical resection, because lymphoma is recognized to have the potential for systemic dissemination. For other gastrointestinal lymphomas, such as gastric lymphoma, chemotherapy and/or radiation is now considered to be the first-line therapy of choice, with surgical interventions being reserved for complications such as bleeding, perforation, obstruction, or failure to respond. Indeed, non-Hodgkin, diffuse B-cell lymphoma is the most common type of gastric lymphoma, and it is now

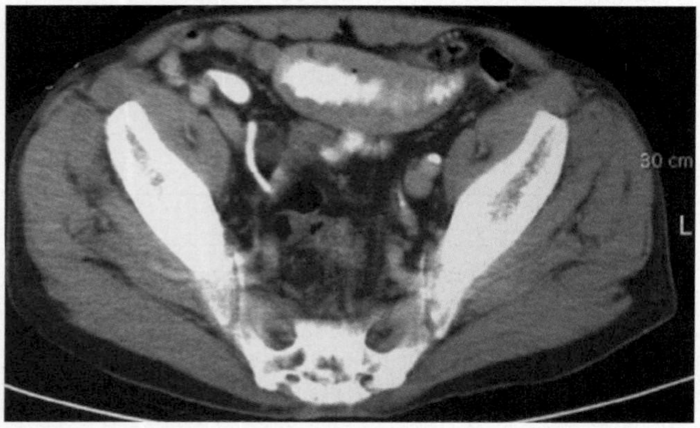

FIGURE 50.4. The computed tomography scan similarly demonstrated a thickened ileal loop with dilatation. No adenopathy was noted. At surgery, the patient was found to have a primary lymphoma of the small bowel.

TABLE 50.4 STAGING

STAGING OF NON-HODGKIN LYMPHOMA OF THE GASTROINTESTINAL TRACT

■ STAGE	■ EXTENT OF DISEASE
I	Tumor confined to the gastrointestinal tract, either as single primary site or multiple noncontiguous lesions
II	Tumor extends from primary gastrointestinal site, either to lymph nodes or direct invasion. Confined to below the diaphragm
IIE	Tumor penetrates serosa to involve adjacent structures
II_1	Local nodal involvement
II_2	Distant nodal involvement
III	Evidence of supradiaphragmatic disease
IV	Disseminated disease above and below the diaphragm

routinely treated primarily with anthracycline-based chemotherapy regimens, in combination with monoclonal-based antibody therapies such as rituximab and/or irradiation.[36] The majority of small-bowel lymphomas are also large-cell, non-Hodgkin, B-cell–type lymphomas. Although they may appear to be localized, biologically these tumors tend to be more aggressive and often require systemic therapy for definitive management. Increasingly, systemic therapy is considered to be the mainstay for management of these lesions. Surgical intervention can still be considered for patients who are refractory to chemotherapy or as primary therapy for localized small-bowel lymphoma with favorable histology.[37] Decisions regarding the management of small-bowel lymphomas that do not require emergent surgical management should be made in a multidisciplinary setting with input from surgeons, medical oncologists, and pathologists, as there is currently no definitive consensus regarding standard first-line therapy for small-bowel lymphomas.[3,37–39]

CARCINOID TUMORS

5 Carcinoids are indolent malignant neuroendocrine tumors that arise from the enterochromaffin cells at the base of the crypts of Lieberkühn. These cells are part of the amine precursor uptake and decarboxylation (APUD) system and can secrete peptides responsible for the carcinoid syndrome. Although 80% of carcinoids arise in the gastrointestinal tract, 10% of primary carcinoids occur in the bronchus or lung. Other sites, such as the ovaries, testicles, pancreas, and kidney, are far less common. Within the gastrointestinal tract, carcinoids are most often identified in the appendix, followed by the small bowel, which harbors approximately 30% of all gastrointestinal carcinoids. Almost half of these arise in the distal 2 feet of ileum.

A recently published series (the largest to date) evaluated all small-bowel malignancies reported to the National Cancer Database from 1985 to 2005. Analysis of 67,000 patients with small-intestinal tumors revealed that the incidence of small-bowel cancer of all histologies has increased, but most of the change is a result of a more than fourfold increase in the incidence of carcinoid tumors. In this particular series, carcinoid tumors accounted for the majority of small-intestinal cancers, surpassing adenocarcinoma of the small intestine.[3] Of all the patients evaluated, 25,339 patients (37.4%) had carcinoid tumors and 25,053 patients (36.9%) had adenocarcinomas. In various series, carcinoid tumors comprise 30% to 35% of small-bowel neoplasms, and carcinoids are found slightly more often in men than in women.[3,40] The mean age of presentation is 60 years. The tumors are frequently asymptomatic; in fact, the autopsy rate in one study was over 2,000 times that of the annual incidence rate, indicating the potential for long-standing slow growth. When symptomatic, carcinoids typically present with pain or obstructive symptoms. Because these tumors are typically slow growing, symptoms may be present for 2 to 20 years prior to diagnosis. Ulceration is rare in carcinoids, so gastrointestinal bleeding is uncommon. Patients present with carcinoid syndrome in up to 40% of cases and only in the presence of symptoms of carcinoid syndrome is the diagnosis consistently made preoperatively.

There are five histologic patterns that correlate embryologically with the location of the tumor.[41] The foregut, or duodenal, lesions usually demonstrate a trabecular or ribbon pattern. An insular pattern predominates in the midgut or small-bowel lesions, and a mixed pattern is typical of the hindgut or colorectal lesions. The least common patterns are glandular or tubular and undifferentiated, both of which have a much poorer prognosis than the three more common variations. The histologic pattern does not affect treatment, but with other factors, appears to impact on long-term survival.

Clinical Presentation and Diagnosis

The most common presenting symptom for patients with a small-bowel carcinoid tumor is abdominal pain. As carcinoids grow, the polypoid lesions may serve as a lead point for intussusception. Intussusception is characterized by intermittent abdominal symptoms and signs of obstruction. Abdominal films often demonstrate a distal small-bowel obstruction. The CT findings of intussusception are distinctive, demonstrating a multilayer ringed structure in the ileocolic region (Figs. 50.5 and 50.6).

Unlike in the appendix where multicentricity is rare, carcinoids of the small bowel are multiple 30% to 40% of the time.[42] In addition, 30% to 50% of small-bowel carcinoids are associated with second primary malignancies, most frequently of the breast and colon. Gastrointestinal carcinoids have the capacity to elicit a marked desmoplastic reaction. The mesentery of the small bowel becomes fibrotic and foreshortened, leading to kinking of the bowel or even intestinal ischemia as a result of sclerosis of the mesenteric blood vessels. The exact mechanism of this fibrosis, which is not only peritumoral but also distant in the heart and lungs, is still unknown.[43] This finding is readily identified on CT scan[44] and is sometimes

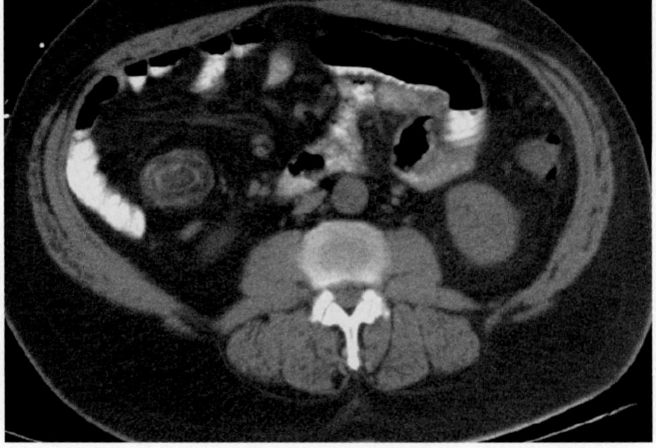

FIGURE 50.5. A 63-year-old man presented with a short history of abdominal pain that he described as similar to his pancreatitis pain. A computed tomography scan demonstrated an ileal carcinoid tumor as the lead point for an intussusception into the cecum.

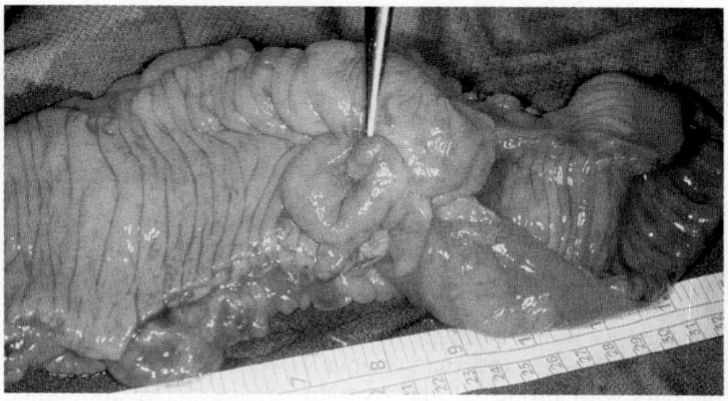

FIGURE 50.6. Resection of ileocolic segment of bowel in the patient shown in Figure 50.5 to have an intussusception. Here carcinoid tumor can be seen as the lead point for intussusception through the ileocecal valve.

associated with calcifications while the small bowel appears fixed and angulated.

Stage and Prognosis

Tumor size is proportional to the risk for metastatic spread at initial diagnosis and must be considered in directing surgical strategies. In comparison to appendiceal carcinoids, which may cause appendicitis at a small size prior to lymph node metastasis, small-bowel lesions often remain asymptomatic long enough to allow not only lymph node spread but also hepatic metastasis. For lesions smaller than 1 cm, there is a 20% to 30% incidence of nodal and hepatic spread. Tumors 1 to 2 cm in size have nodal spread in 60% to 80% and hepatic disease in 20%. The rate of nodal and hepatic metastasis for tumors larger than 2 cm is greater than 80% and 40% to 50%, respectively.[40] These figures must guide the choice of operation. Whereas a small lesion less than 1 cm may be adequately treated with local excision, anything larger must be presumed to be metastatic and a wide resection with lymphadenectomy and careful examination of the liver is necessary.

Carcinoid Syndrome

Carcinoid syndrome refers to vasomotor, gastrointestinal, and cardiac manifestations induced by systemic circulation of a variety of peptides elaborated by carcinoid tumors. The amine precursor uptake and decarboxylation cells of carcinoid tumors can produce vasoactive products including serotonin, histamine, kallikrein, bradykinin, and prostaglandins, although the specific mediator or mediators of the syndrome remain unknown. Carcinoid syndrome is most reliably confirmed by finding elevated 24-hour 5-hydroxyindoleacetic acid (5-HIAA) urinary excretion, the primary stable metabolite of serotonin.

Attacks are initiated by stimuli including stress, alcohol, a large meal, or sexual intercourse, all of which manipulate the liver in some capacity. Flushing is the most common finding and affects approximately 80% of syndrome patients. The flush varies slightly by the location of the tumor, but in midgut carcinoids the flush is usually short-lived, lasting 5 to 10 minutes. Classically, the erythematous flush begins on the face and spreads to the trunk and limbs. Diarrhea, found in 75% of patients, seems to be caused by serotonin release. The diarrhea is intermittent, watery, and at times explosive. It may be associated with abdominal cramps and the patient may experience a certain degree of malabsorption. Cardiac manifestations are present in 60% to 70% of patients due to tricuspid and pulmonary valve fibrosis, possibly secondary to high levels of 5-hydroxyindoleacetic acid. As the disease progresses, the fibrotic plaque stiffens, leading eventually to right heart failure.

Patients with gastrointestinal carcinoid tumors who present with carcinoid syndrome have metastatic disease in either the liver or retroperitoneum. The liver contains large amounts of monoamine oxidase, which deactivates serotonin, the major effector hormone. Hence, to develop carcinoid syndrome, a patient must either have tumor in a location that does not primarily drain into the portal circulation, such as a bronchial carcinoid or retroperitoneal tumor, or have hepatic metastases of a magnitude that overwhelms the capacity of monoamine oxidase to break down serotonin. The bioactive products from a small volume of hepatic metastases may be cleared by the hepatocytes, but a larger tumor burden allows release of these products into the hepatic veins and the systemic circulation. It follows that patients with bronchial and ovarian carcinoids, or abdominal disease that has penetrated the retroperitoneum, which drains directly into the systemic circulation, can manifest carcinoid syndrome from primary disease. Patients with gastrointestinal carcinoids, which drain into the portal circulation, must have metastatic disease prior to the development of the syndrome.

Management of patients with carcinoid syndrome may be approached surgically, radiologically, and medically, and often requires a combination of all three modalities. Surgical debulking of extensive hepatic disease with segmental resection or ablation or formal hepatic resection for resectable metastases may improve symptoms and prolong life. For patients with residual abdominal tumor and hepatic metastases, 5- and 10-year survival rates approached 60%, so although in general the initial surgery should involve attempts to debulk as much tumor as possible, it must also avoid catastrophic injuries such as those to the superior mesenteric vessels that may lead to short-gut syndrome.[45] Hepatic artery embolization or radiofrequency ablation may be more appropriate for widespread hepatic metastases and in small series have been shown to give marked symptomatic relief and durable tumor control.[46–48] Medical therapy relies primarily on the use of a variety of somatostatin analogues (octreotide) including short- and long-acting peptides for relief of carcinoid syndrome symptoms. Carcinoid tumors express somatostatin receptors and the somatostatin analogues inhibit vasoactive peptide release from these tumors. Efficacy of treatment can be documented by following excretion of the tumor marker 5-hydroxyindoleacetic acid. Palliation of symptoms is effective in 90% of patients with octreotide and some studies have even demonstrated a tumorostatic or tumor reduction effect after the administration of somatostatin, although these latter findings have not been consistently observed. Serotonin antagonists are useful in the management of gastrointestinal symptoms including rapid transit and diarrhea.

Chemotherapeutic agents for the treatment of metastatic carcinoid tumor have been used singly and in combination in an effort to halt progression of disease as well as to promote tumor regression; however, objective responses to chemotherapy are limited. Studies testing single-agent chemotherapy (5-FU, doxorubicin, actinomycin D, dacarbazine, and streptozocin) demonstrated no beneficial effect.[48a,49] Combination regimens have also been studied in phase II trials including 5-FU and streptozocin with or without cyclophosphamide. Responses to streptozocin-based combined chemotherapy regimens were evident in approximately 8% to 25% of patients.[49] Cytotoxic treatment in patients with malignant carcinoid tumors. Preliminary reports on the use of novel targeted radiotherapeutic agents have been presented. These are synthetic somatostatin analogues that can bind to somatostatin receptors on carcinoid tumors with high affinity. After binding receptors on the tumor, the ligand–receptor complex is internalized. These analogues can be conjugated to radioactive surface isotopes, effectively generating a "smart bomb" that can theoretically deliver radiation specifically to carcinoid cells. In an early-phase study, ^{111}indium-labeled pentetreotide induced a greater tumor regression response compared to unlabeled somatostatin analogue.[50] Further investigations are ongoing.

GASTROINTESTINAL STROMAL TUMORS

Although GISTs are the most common nonepithelial cell tumors of the small bowel, they are rare tumors of the gastrointestinal tract, representing only about 5,000 cases nationwide per year.[51] Approximately 25% of GISTs arise in the small bowel, with 50% gastric, 15% rectal, and 10% colonic in origin.[52] GISTs are diagnosed equally in men and women, with a median age at onset of 64 years. Arising from the interstitial cell of Cajal, the pacemaker cells of the gastrointestinal tract situated between the intramural neurons and the smooth muscle cells, GISTs are characterized by the presence of activating c-kit mutations, a transmembrane receptor tyrosine kinase involved in the regulation of cellular proliferation, apoptosis, and differentiation. More than 95% of GISTs express kit (CD117) mutations.[51] This molecular marker allows for distinction of GISTs from histologically similar mesenchymal tumors of the small bowel including leiomyomas, leiomyosarcomas, and schwannomas. This molecular feature has led to reclassification of up to 70% of small-bowel tumors as GISTs that had previously been classified as a variety of mesenchymal tumors. Those GISTs that do not express c-kit mutations may express a mutation in another tyrosine kinase receptor, platelet-derived growth factor receptor-α (PDGFR-α).[53] Present in approximately 5% to 7% of GISTs, these activating mutations also result in abnormal cellular proliferation.

Like other primary small-bowel tumors, GISTs are characterized by indolent clinical symptoms including vague abdominal pain, weight loss, and occult gastrointestinal bleeding. Although acute hemorrhage, perforation, or obstruction may lead to an emergency presentation, GISTs may grow to a massive size prior to surgical presentation. Usually they grow insidiously as extraluminal masses from their submucosal origin in a noninvasive manner, characteristically pushing adjacent organs away from the expanding mass.

Diagnostic strategies are the same as for other tumors of the small bowel. Given the propensity of GIST to grow to a large size prior to diagnosis, CT scan is most likely to be the initial positive test. A characteristic finding is the presence of a large space-occupying mass, occasionally with calcification and hypervascularity and often with evidence of central necrosis and compression of adjacent organs (Fig. 50.7A). Smaller tumors are detected with esophagogastroduodenoscopy in the stomach and duodenum and with video capsule endoscopy or double-balloon enteroscopy in the small bowel. ^{18}F-fluorodeoxyglucose (^{18}F-FDG) positron emission tomography (PET) testing has also been utilized for assessing response to adjuvant therapies but is not employed generally for initial staging of the disease.[51]

All GISTs should be considered to be malignant.[54] Malignant potential is based on two major criteria, as reported from the National Institutes of Health consensus workshop: tumor size and mitotic rate (Table 50.5). Biologically aggressive tumors are large lesions with a high mitotic index, whereas tumors with benign features are small and exhibit a low mitotic index. Tumors are thus classified into very-low- to high-risk lesions for malignant potential, a classification that has prognostic significance. Additional reports have suggested negative factors for prognosis including high Ki-67 index and male gender, but these parameters have not consistently been predictive.[51]

Treatment

Surgery is the primary therapeutic option with the goal being complete resection. Preoperative biopsy is controversial, and a presumed diagnosis of GIST is enough to warrant surgery if the disease appears resectable. At operation, wide local excision of the primary tumor with in continuity resection of adherent organs is appropriate to attain curative resection

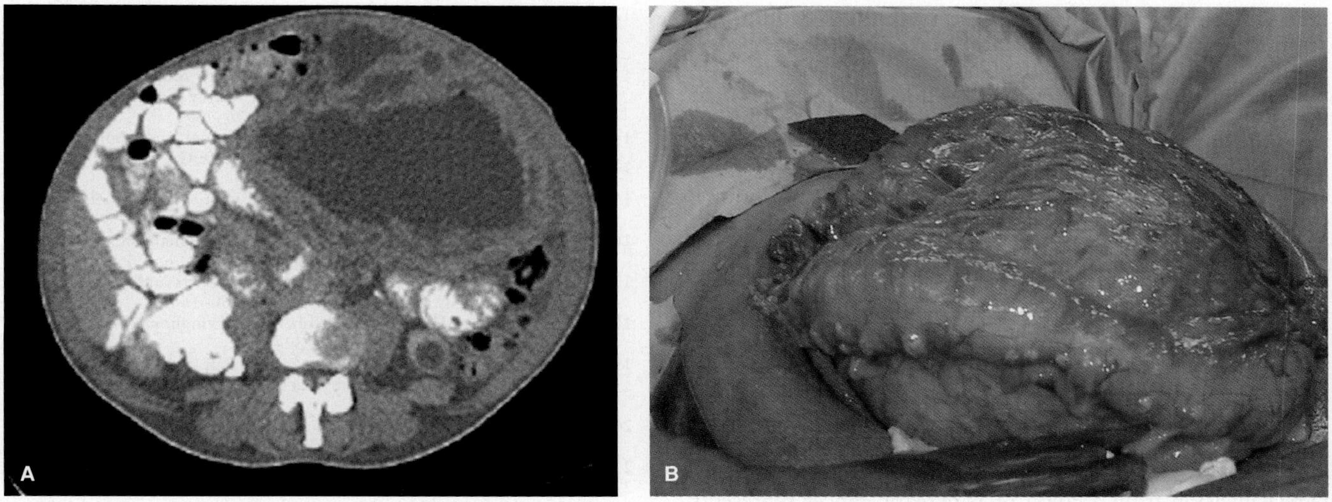

FIGURE 50.7. **A:** Computed tomography image of a 76-year-old man with abdominal distention demonstrating a complex abdominal mass with varying degrees of thickness, central necrosis, and compression of adjacent organs. This was found to be a gastrointestinal stromal tumor with markedly increased mitotic activity. **B:** Intraoperative photograph of the same patient, showing displacement of adjacent organs.

(Fig. 50.7B). For small and localized lesions, laparoscopic resection appears to be safe and effective. Lymph node metastases are rare, but if bulky mesenteric adenopathy is noted, wide mesenteric resection is indicated.

Molecular Therapeutics and Gastrointestinal Stromal Tumor

6 The discovery of the pathognomonic constitutively activated mutations in the tyrosine kinases c-kit and PDGFR-α in GIST has stimulated development of therapeutic agents targeting these moieties. Activation of c-kit leads to phosphorylation of a receptor substrate protein initiating an intracellular phosphorylation cascade. This cytoplasmic cascade ultimately leads to nuclear activation of transcription events culminating in cell proliferation and survival. Imatinib mesylate is a small molecule that occupies the adenosine triphosphate–binding pocket of the c-kit kinase domain, blocking phosphorylation of the receptor and intracellular signaling. This binding arrests cellular proliferation and survival signaling.

Imatinib is now commonly used to manage unresectable or metastatic GISTs, or as adjuvant therapy in those at high risk for recurrence. The American College of Surgeons Oncology Group (ACOSOG) conducted a phase II intergroup trial (Z9000) examining adjuvant imatinib (400 mg/d for 12 months) after complete macroscopic resection in patients with high-risk primary GISTs (five or more tumors, tumor size ≥10 cm, or intraperitoneal tumor rupture or hemorrhage). One hundred and six patients were treated using imatinib (400 mg/d) for 1 year. Eighty three percent of the accrued patients were able to compete the full year of imatinib therapy. Three-year survival in these imatinib-treated patients was 97%, which was concluded to be better than historic controls. A separate double-blind, phase III ACOSOG trial (Z9001) testing the efficacy of adjuvant imatinib preventing GIST recurrence in patients with completely resected GISTs at least 3 cm in size had to be terminated at a median follow-up of 13 to 14 months due to significantly better recurrence-free survival in the treatment versus placebo group (97% vs. 83%).[55] Imatinib is well tolerated and highly effective for patients with metastatic GISTs. Although complete regression of tumor is rare, partial regression of disease and arrest of progression of disease can be achieved for durable intervals with continuous treatment in up to 80% of patients.[51] Efficacy of treatment can be predicted and followed using ^{18}F-FDG PET scanning; these highly biologically active tumors will become metabolically silent with imatinib therapy in those patients with responsive tumors. With greater clinical experience with imatinib, resistant clones have been identified with eventual progression of disease. For these patients, a newer

TABLE 50.5

MALIGNANT POTENTIAL AND PROGRESS OF GASTROINTESTINAL STROMAL TUMORS

■ RISK CLASSIFICATION	■ SIZE	■ MITOTIC RATE	■ 10-YEAR SURVIVAL
High	Any size	>10/50 HPF	30%
	>10 cm	Any rate	
	>5 mm	>5/50 HPF	
Intermediate	5–10 cm	<5/50 HPF	60%
	<5 cm	6–10/50 HPF	
Low	2–5 cm	<5/50 HPF	75%
Very low	<2 cm	<5/50 HPF	80%
Normal population	—	—	80%

HPF, high power field.

multitarget receptor tyrosine kinase inhibitor, sunitinib, has recently been introduced for clinical trials. This inhibitor has a broader spectrum of activity than imatinib and has shown early promise in patients with progression of disease on imatinib or in those relatively few patients who cannot tolerate imatinib.[54]

Use of imatinib in the neoadjuvant setting for unresectable or locally aggressive tumors has been reported recently[56] with response rates near 75%,[51] and about 25% of unresectable lesions are converted to resectable lesions.[56] The efficacy of imatinib in the adjuvant setting for high-risk or partially resected tumors is also being evaluated in ongoing trials.

METASTATIC LESIONS TO THE SMALL BOWEL

The small bowel is the site of metastatic disease from multiple other primary sites. Metastatic spread can occur by direct invasion, hematogenous spread, or intraperitoneal seeding. Direct invasion from a colon or pancreatic cancer represents the most common mode of involvement. Hematogenous spread arises most frequently from bronchogenic or breast carcinoma or malignant melanoma. Peritoneal seeding has been documented from primary tumors of the stomach, liver, ovary, appendix, and colon.

A CT scan often demonstrates not only the degree of involvement of the small bowel but also the primary tumor. In metastatic small-bowel tumors, one may see bowel wall thickening as well as lesions in the mesentery or retroperitoneal fat. For small lesions, CT scan may be negative, while video capsule endoscopy or double-balloon enteroscopy may reveal a luminal mass. Carcinomatosis may be difficult to identify even on body CT imaging.

Optimal management is based on clinical criteria. Palliative intestinal resection or bypass to relieve hemorrhage, obstruction, or pain is indicated except in the most terminal stages of disease. Case reports of prolonged survival after intestinal resection of solitary metastases have been reported, although progression of metastatic disease is more common.[57]

Management of patients with carcinomatosis, regardless of tumor origin, remains difficult. Palliative measures to maintain intestinal continuity and liberal use of decompressive gastrostomy tubes are indicated.

References

1. Hatzaras I, Palesty JA, Abir F, et al. Small-bowel tumors: epidemiologic and clinical characteristics of 1260 cases from the Connecticut tumor registry. *Arch Surg* 2007;142:229–235.
2. Ciresi DL, Scholten DJ. The continuing clinical dilemma of primary tumors of the small intestine. *Am Surg* 1995;61:698–702; discussion 702–703.
3. Bilimoria KY, Bentrem DJ, Wayne JD, et al. Small bowel cancer in the United States: changes in epidemiology, treatment, and survival over the last 20 years. *Ann Surg* 2009;249:63–71.
4. Schottenfeld D, Beebe-Dimmer JL, Vigneau FD. The epidemiology and pathogenesis of neoplasia in the small intestine. *Ann Epidemiol* 2009;19: 58–69.
5. Matsuo S, Eto T, Tsunoda T, et al. Small bowel tumors: an analysis of tumor-like lesions, benign and malignant neoplasms. *Eur J Surg Oncol* 1994;20:47–51.
6. Minardi AJ Jr, Zibari GB, Aultman DF, et al. Small-bowel tumors. *J Am Coll Surg* 1998;186:664–668.
7. Johnson AM, Harman PK, Hanks JB. Primary small bowel malignancies. *Am Surg* 1985;51:31–36.
8. Serour F, Dona G, Birkenfeld S, et al. Primary neoplasms of the small bowel. *J Surg Oncol* 1992;49:29–34.
9. Xie J, Itzkowitz SH. Cancer in inflammatory bowel disease. *World J Gastroenterol* 2008;14:378–389.
10. Freeman HJ. Colorectal cancer risk in Crohn's disease. *World J Gastroenterol* 2008;14:1810–1811.
11. Howe JR, Karnell LH, Menck HR, et al. The American College of Surgeons Commission on Cancer and the American Cancer Society. Adenocarcinoma of the small bowel: review of the national cancer data base, 1985–1995. *Cancer* 1999;86:2693–2706.
12. O'Boyle CJ, Kerin MJ, Feeley K, et al. Primary small intestinal tumours: increased incidence of lymphoma and improved survival. *Ann R Coll Surg Engl* 1998;80:332–334.
13. Freeman HJ. Failure of added dietary gluten to induce small intestinal histopathological changes in patients with watery diarrhea and lymphocytic colitis. *Can J Gastroenterol* 1996;10:436–439.
14. Freeman HJ. Lymphoproliferative and intestinal malignancies in 214 patients with biopsy-defined celiac disease. *J Clin Gastroenterol* 2004;38: 429–434.
15. Freeman HJ. Malignancy in adult celiac disease. *World J Gastroenterol* 2009;15:1581–1583.
16. Green PH, Fleischauer AT, Bhagat G, et al. Risk of malignancy in patients with celiac disease. *Am J Med* 2003;115:191–195.
17. Dong K, Li B. Peutz-Jeghers syndrome: case reports and update on diagnosis and treatment. *Chin J Dig Dis* 2004;5:160–164.
18. Crump M, Gospodarowicz M, Shepherd FA. Lymphoma of the gastrointestinal tract. *Semin Oncol* 1999;26:324–337.
19. Svoboda J, Kotloff R, Tsai DE. Management of patients with post-transplant lymphoproliferative disorder: the role of rituximab. *Transpl Int* 2006;19:259–269.
20. Everly MJ, Bloom RD, Tsai DE, et al. Posttransplant lymphoproliferative disorder. *Ann Pharmacother* 2007;41:1850–1858.
21. Waye JD. Small-bowel endoscopy. *Endoscopy* 2003;35:15–21.
22. Rondonotti E, Villa F, Mulder CJ, et al. Small bowel capsule endoscopy in 2007: indications, risks and limitations. *World J Gastroenterol* 2007;13: 6140–6149.
23. Ersoy O, Sivri B, Bayraktar Y. How helpful is capsule endoscopy to surgeons? *World J Gastroenterol* 2007;13:3671–3676.
24. Calva D, Howe JR. Hamartomatous polyposis syndromes. *Surg Clin North Am* 2008;88:779–817, vii.
25. Zangara J, Kushner H, Drachenberg C, et al. Iron deficiency anemia due to a Brunner's gland hamartoma. *J Clin Gastroenterol* 1998;27:353–356.
26. Beger HG, Treitschke F, Gansauge F, et al. Tumor of the ampulla of Vater: experience with local or radical resection in 171 consecutively treated patients. *Arch Surg* 1999;134:526–532.
27. Brosens LA, Keller JJ, Offerhaus GJ, et al. Prevention and management of duodenal polyps in familial adenomatous polyposis. *Gut* 2005;54:1034–1043.
28. Farnell MB, Sakorafas GH, Sarr MG, et al. Villous tumors of the duodenum: reappraisal of local vs. extended resection. *J Gastrointest Surg* 2000;4:13–21, discussion 22–23.
29. Cunningham JD, Aleali R, Aleali M, et al. Malignant small bowel neoplasms: histopathologic determinants of recurrence and survival. *Ann Surg* 1997;225:300–306.
30. Sohn TA, Lillemoe KD, Cameron JL, et al. Adenocarcinoma of the duodenum: factors influencing long-term survival. *J Gastrointest Surg* 1998;2:79–87.
31. Abrahams NA, Halverson A, Fazio VW, et al. Adenocarcinoma of the small bowel: a study of 37 cases with emphasis on histologic prognostic factors. *Dis Colon Rectum* 2002;45:1496–1502.
32. Singhal N, Singhal D. Adjuvant chemotherapy for small intestine adenocarcinoma. *Cochrane Database Syst Rev* 2007:CD005202.
33. Koniaris LG, Drugas G, Katzman PJ, et al. Management of gastrointestinal lymphoma. *J Am Coll Surg* 2003;197:127–141.
34. Huang WT, Hsu YH, Yang SF, et al. Primary gastrointestinal follicular lymphoma: a clinicopathologic study of 13 cases from Taiwan. *J Clin Gastroenterol* 2008;42:997–1002.
35. Yamaguchi T, Takahashi H, Kagawa R, et al. Surgical resection combined with chop chemotherapy plus rituximab for a patient with advanced mesenteric diffuse large B cell lymphoma. *Hepatogastroenterology* 2008; 55:891–894.
36. Psyrri A, Papageorgiou S, Economopoulos T. Primary extranodal lymphomas of stomach: clinical presentation, diagnostic pitfalls and management. *Ann Oncol* 2008;19:1992–1999.
37. Cheung MC, Housri N, Ogilvie MP, et al. Surgery does not adversely affect survival in primary gastrointestinal lymphoma. *J Surg Oncol* 2009;100:59–64.
38. Pandey M, Wadhwa MK, Patel HP, et al. Malignant lymphoma of the gastrointestinal tract. *Eur J Surg Oncol* 1999;25:164–167.
39. Gollub MJ. Imaging of gastrointestinal lymphoma. *Radiol Clin North Am* 2008;46:287–312, ix.
40. Horton KM, Kamel I, Hofmann L, et al. Carcinoid tumors of the small bowel: a multitechnique imaging approach. *AJR Am J Roentgenol* 2004; 182:559–567.
41. Memon MA, Nelson H. Gastrointestinal carcinoid tumors: current management strategies. *Dis Colon Rectum* 1997;40:1101–1118.
42. Yantiss RK, Odze RD, Farraye FA, et al. Solitary versus multiple carcinoid tumors of the ileum: a clinical and pathologic review of 68 cases. *Am J Surg Pathol* 2003;27:811–817.
43. Modlin IM, Shapiro MD, Kidd M. Carcinoid tumors and fibrosis: an association with no explanation. *Am J Gastroenterol* 2004;99:2466–2478.
44. Sheth S, Horton KM, Garland MR, et al. Mesenteric neoplasms: CT appearances of primary and secondary tumors and differential diagnosis. *Radiographics* 2003;23:457–473; quiz 535–536.
45. Soreide JA, van Heerden JA, Thompson GB, et al. Gastrointestinal carcinoid tumors: long-term prognosis for surgically treated patients. *World J Surg* 2000;24:1431–1436.
46. Schell SR, Camp ER, Caridi JG, et al. Hepatic artery embolization for control of symptoms, octreotide requirements, and tumor progression in metastatic carcinoid tumors. *J Gastrointest Surg* 2002;6:664–670.

47. Roche A, Girish BV, de Baere T, et al. Trans-catheter arterial chemoembolization as first-line treatment for hepatic metastases from endocrine tumors. *Eur Radiol* 2003;13:136–140.
48. Roche A, Girish BV, de Baere T, et al. Prognostic factors for chemoembolization in liver metastasis from endocrine tumors. *Hepatogastroenterology* 2004;51:1751–1756.
48a. Moertel et al. *Proc Am Soc Clin Oncol* 1982.
49. Modlin IM, Kidd M, Latich I, et al. Current status of gastrointestinal carcinoids. *Gastroenterology* 2005;128:1717–1751.
50. Anthony LB, Woltering EA, Espenan GD, et al. Indium-111-pentetreotide prolongs survival in gastroenteropancreatic malignancies. *Semin Nucl Med* 2002;32:123–132.
51. Hueman MT, Schulick RD. Management of gastrointestinal stromal tumors. *Surg Clin North Am* 2008;88:599–614, vii.
52. Miettinen M, Lasota J. Gastrointestinal stromal tumors–definition, clinical, histological, immunohistochemical, and molecular genetic features and differential diagnosis. *Virchows Arch* 2001;438:1–12.
53. Heinrich MC, Corless CL, Duensing A, et al. PDGFRa activating mutations in gastrointestinal stromal tumors. *Science* 2003;299:708–710.
54. von Mehren M. New therapeutic strategies for soft tissue sarcomas. *Curr Treat Options Oncol* 2003;4:441–451.
55. Kingham TP, DeMatteo RP. Multidisciplinary treatment of gastrointestinal stromal tumors. *Surg Clin North Am* 2009;89:217–233, x.
56. Andtbacka RH, Ng CS, Scaife CL, et al. Surgical resection of gastrointestinal stromal tumors after treatment with imatinib. *Ann Surg Oncol* 2007;14:14–24.
57. Cipollone G, Santarelli G, Quitadamo S, et al. Small bowel metastases from lung cancer. *Chir Ital* 2004;56:639–648.

CHAPTER 51 PANCREAS ANATOMY AND PHYSIOLOGY

TAYLOR S. RIALL

KEY POINTS

1. The pancreas is both an endocrine and exocrine organ.
2. Congenital anomalies of the pancreas largely result from failure of rotation or fusion of the ventral and dorsal pancreatic buds.
3. The two major components of the exocrine pancreas, the acinar cells and the ductular network, constitute 80% to 90% of the pancreatic mass, whereas the endocrine pancreas constitutes only 2% of the pancreatic mass.
4. The pancreatic islets of Langerhans are composed of four major cell types—alpha (A), beta (B), delta (D), and pancreatic polypeptide (PP or F) cells, which secrete glucagon, insulin, somatostatin, and PP, respectively.
5. B cells constitute 70% of the islet mass.
6. The different types of islet cells are not evenly distributed throughout the pancreas, so resection of different parts of the pancreas has differing endocrine effects.
7. Knowledge of the relationship of the pancreas to surrounding structures including the stomach, duodenum, distal bile duct, hepatic arterial blood supply, splenic artery and vein, celiac axis, superior mesenteric artery and vein, portal vein, spleen, adrenal glands, colon, and kidneys is critical in preventing injury to these structures during pancreatic surgery.
8. Progressive destruction of the afferent sensory fibers occurs during recurrent episodes of pancreatitis, which contributes to chronic pain.
9. The location within the pancreas, the pancreatic blood supply, and lymphatic drainage of the pancreas dictate the operation performed in patients with pancreatic malignancies.
10. Secretin is the major stimulant for pancreatic bicarbonate secretion, whereas pancreatic enzyme secretion is regulated through hormonal (cholecystokinin) and neural factors.
11. Somatostatin inhibits nearly all peptide hormones as well as gastric, pancreatic, and biliary secretions.
12. Tests of pancreatic exocrine function include the secretin test, 24-hour fecal fat determination, dimethadione (DMO) test, Lundh test meal, triolein breath test, and para-aminobenzoic acid (PABA) test. These tests help differentiate steatorrhea due to pancreatic insufficiency from other digestive disorders.

The pancreas is an elongated digestive organ that lies transversely in the retroperitoneum at the level of the second
1 lumbar vertebra. It is a glandular organ that has both exocrine and endocrine function. The exocrine pancreas is composed of acinar cells and ductal networks that function to deliver alkaline solution (pH >8.0) containing over 20 enzymes and zymogens to the small intestine daily. The pancreatic secretions provide the optimal pH for the enzymes and zymogens to carry out the major digestive activity of the small intestine.

The endocrine pancreas is composed of islets of Langerhans. The islets secrete hormones including insulin, glucagon, and somatostatin directly into the bloodstream in endocrine fashion. These hormones regulate glucose homeostasis and also play a role in the complex regulation of pancreatic secretion and digestion.

The pancreas is divided anatomically into four parts: the pancreatic head, neck, body, and tail (Fig. 51.1). The pancreatic head includes the uncinate process, which is an extension of the pancreatic head wrapping posterior to the superior mesenteric vessels. An understanding of the close relationship of the pancreas to adjacent organs (duodenum, stomach, spleen, transverse colon, bile duct, and left adrenal gland) and major vessels (celiac axis, superior mesenteric artery, superior mesenteric vein, splenic artery and vein, portal vein, inferior mesenteric vein, and vena cava) is critical when performing surgical procedures on the pancreas. In addition, understanding of the embryology is critical for recognizing congenital anomalies, understanding their significance, and treating them appropriately. Knowledge of the normal pancreatic physiology provides insight into the pathologic processes and subsequent treatments that can affect the normal function of the pancreas.

EMBRYOLOGY

Normal Pancreatic Embryology

During the fifth week of gestation, the pancreas begins forming at the junction of the foregut and midgut. The formation begins as two endodermal pancreatic buds, the dorsal bud and the ventral bud, which eventually fuse to form the pancreas (Fig. 51.2). Both the acinar cells and islet cells differentiate from the endodermal cells found in the embryonic buds. The endocrine function of the pancreas begins between 10 and 15 weeks' gestation, whereas the exocrine function does not begin until after birth.

The dorsal and ventral buds are composed of endoderm covered in splanchnic mesoderm. The splanchnic mesoderm eventually develops into the dorsal and ventral mesentery. The dorsal bud forms first and is larger. It ultimately forms much of the head, body, and tail of the pancreas. As the duodenum grows and rotates, the ventral bud rotates clockwise (Fig. 51.2) and fuses with the dorsal bud, forming the uncinate process and inferior head of the pancreas. In the majority of cases, the duct in the ventral bud fuses with the duct in the dorsal bud to become the main pancreatic duct (duct of Wirsung), which drains the majority of the pancreas into the duodenum through the major papilla, or ampulla of Vater. The proximal duct of the dorsal bud forms the lesser or minor pancreatic duct

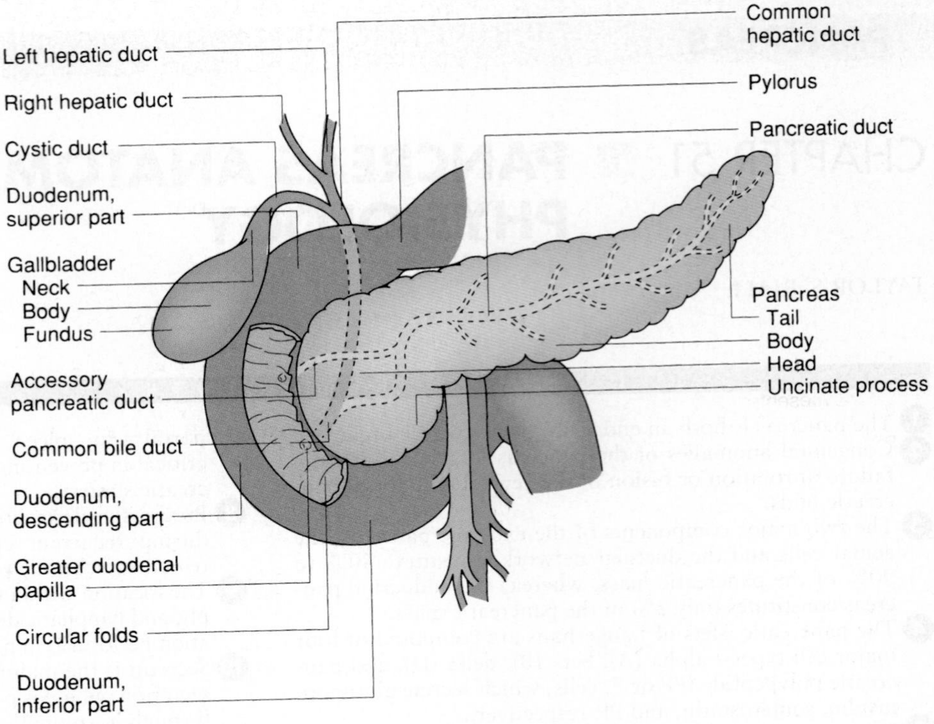

FIGURE 51.1. Relationship of the pancreas to the duodenum and extrahepatic biliary system. The head of the pancreas lies within the C loop of the duodenum. The common bile duct courses through the head of the pancreas, emptying into the duodenum at the greater duodenal papilla (ampulla of Vater). (After Woodburne RT. *Essentials of Human Anatomy.* New York: Oxford University Press; 1973.)

(duct of Santorini), which drains into the duodenum through the minor papilla superior to the major papilla.

Surgical Significance of Abnormalities during Pancreatic Development

2 Abnormalities in the rotation and fusion of the pancreas during embryonic development can result in specific congenital anomalies that have surgical significance (Table 51.1). Approximately 60% of the time, rotation and fusion occur normally, resulting in the classic anatomy seen in Figure 51.3A. The dorsal and ventral ducts fuse to form the main pancreatic duct, which drains the majority of the pancreas into the ampulla of Vater. The lesser duct, formed from the proximal duct of the dorsal bud, drains into the duodenum at the minor papilla.

In 30% of cases, the ventral and dorsal ducts fuse and drain normally into the duodenum at the ampulla of Vater. However, there is atrophy of the accessory or minor duct with a blind end and no minor papilla, or drainage into the duodenum (Fig. 51.3B). As this blind duct still communicates with

TABLE 51.1

CONGENITAL DISORDERS RESULTING FROM ABNORMALITIES IN THE ROTATION OR FUSION OF THE DEVELOPING PANCREAS

■ DISORDER	■ DESCRIPTION	■ PRESENTATION	■ TREATMENT
Pancreas divisum	The lesser duct drains the entire pancreas through minor papilla; caused by incomplete fusion of the ventral and dorsal pancreatic ducts during development	Often asymptomatic Adults: recurrent acute pancreatitis, chronic pancreatitis, or chronic abdominal pain	Operative or endoscopic sphincteroplasty of the minor papilla and accessory duct in symptomatic patients
Annular pancreas	Thin band of pancreatic parenchyma surrounding duodenum and causing varying degrees of duodenal stenosis; caused by abnormal fusion of ventral bud to duodenum, leading to improper rotation of ventral bud[a]	In utero: polyhydramnios Infancy: duodenal obstruction, low birth weight, feeding intolerance Adults: often asymptomatic and found incidentally	Duodenal bypass (duodenoduodenostomy or gastrojejunostomy)
Heterotopic pancreas	Functional pancreatic tissue found in locations outside the pancreas including, but not limited to, the stomach, duodenum, ileum, umbilicus, colon, appendix, and gallbladder; usually submucosal	Often an incidental finding Can present with ulceration, obstruction, intussusception	Treatment directed at presenting symptoms

[a]Ikeda Y, Irving IM. Annular pancreas in a fetus and its three-dimensional reconstruction. *J Pediatr Surg* 1984;19(2):160–164.

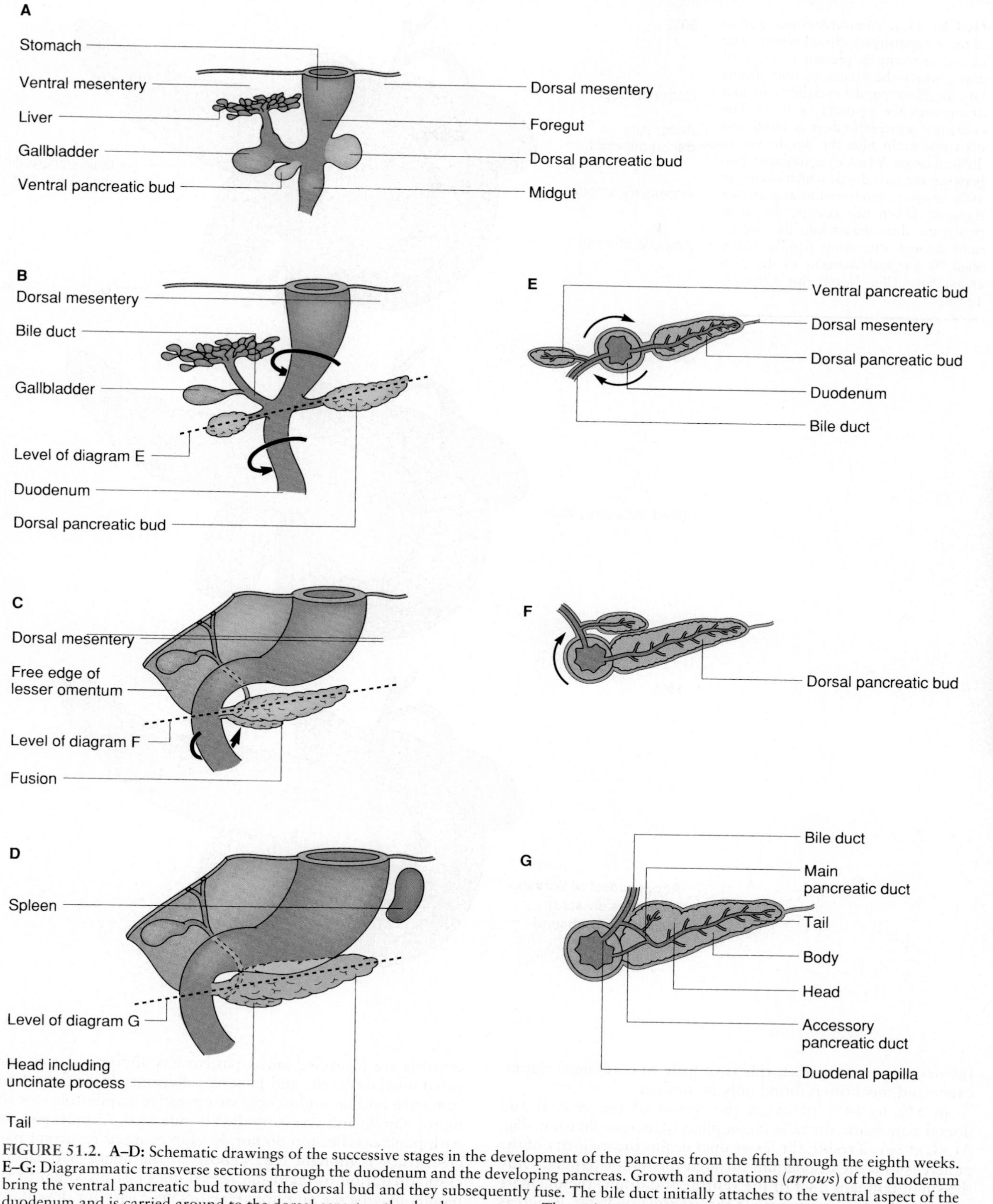

FIGURE 51.2. **A–D:** Schematic drawings of the successive stages in the development of the pancreas from the fifth through the eighth weeks. **E–G:** Diagrammatic transverse sections through the duodenum and the developing pancreas. Growth and rotations (*arrows*) of the duodenum bring the ventral pancreatic bud toward the dorsal bud and they subsequently fuse. The bile duct initially attaches to the ventral aspect of the duodenum and is carried around to the dorsal aspect as the duodenum rotates. The main pancreatic duct is formed by the union of the distal part of the dorsal pancreatic duct and the entire ventral pancreatic duct. (After Moore KL. *The Developing Human,* 3rd ed. Philadelphia, PA: WB Saunders; 1982.)

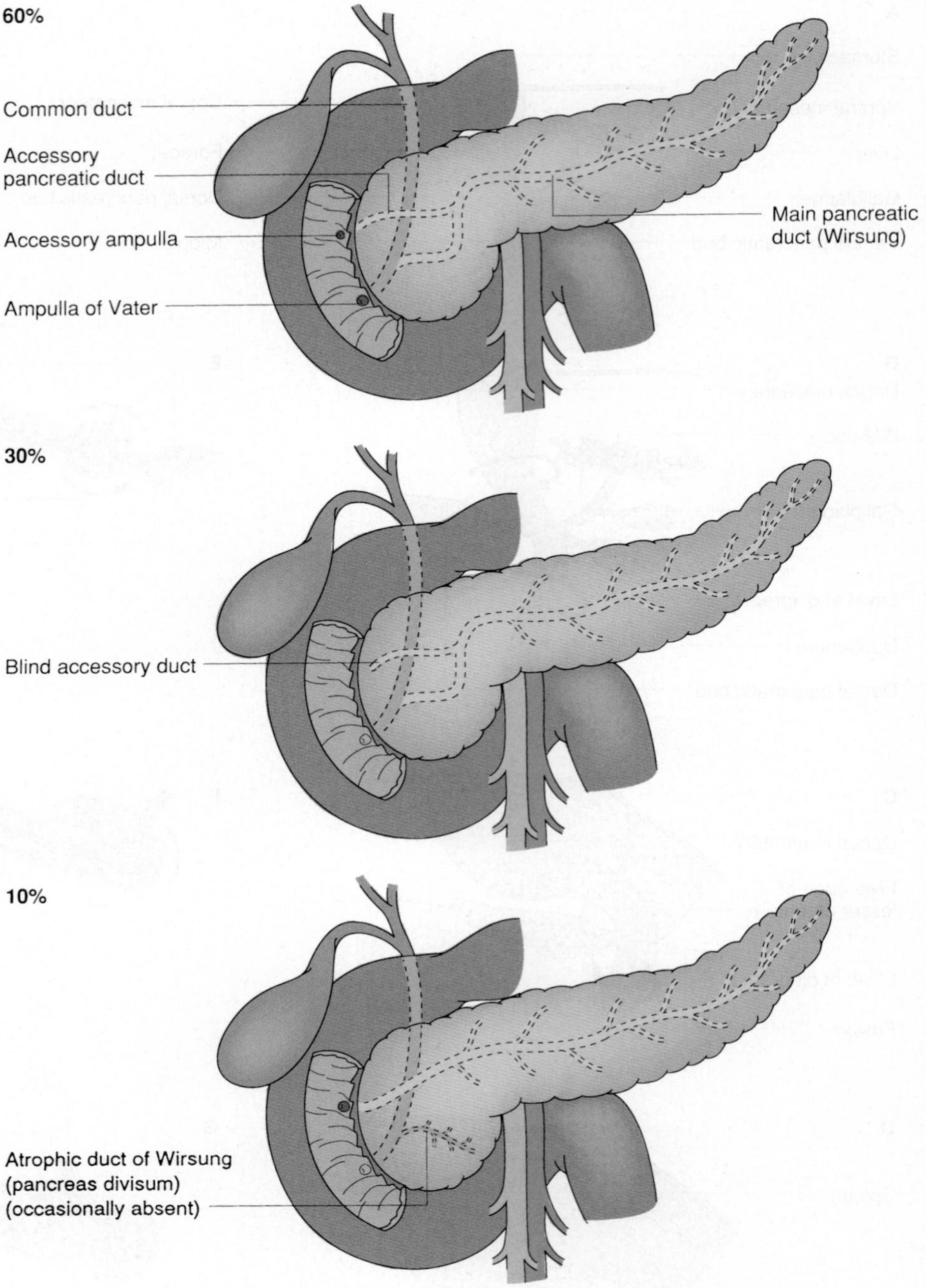

FIGURE 51.3. Anatomic configuration of the intrapancreatic ductal system. The classic anatomy is present in 60% of cases, where the accessory duct drains into the minor papilla and the main duct drains into the ampulla of Vater. The accessory pancreatic duct is blind and does not drain into the duodenum in 30% of cases. A lack of communication between the two ducts, which occurs in 10% of cases, is referred to as *pancreas divisum*. When this occurs, the main pancreatic duct drains into the duodenum through the minor papilla. (After Silen W. Surgical anatomy of the pancreas. *Surg Clin North Am* 1964;44:1253.)

the main pancreatic duct, this is of little to no clinical significance and most often found only at autopsy.

In 5% to 14% of cases, the fusion of the ventral and dorsal pancreatic ducts is incomplete (pancreas divisum, Fig. 51.3C).[1–3] As a result, the lesser duct drains the majority of the pancreas into the duodenum through the minor papilla. Only the small remnant duct of the ventral bud drains the uncinate process into the duodenum via the ampulla of Vater. Pancreas divisum is often asymptomatic. Whether this anomaly is causative in producing pancreatitis and abdominal pain is unclear.[1,4,5] However, there is evidence that inadequate drainage of the pancreas associated with mucosal stenosis of the minor papilla is associated with amylase elevations and abdominal pain.[1,6,7] Patients can have recurrent episodes of acute pancreatitis or chronic pancreatitis with chronic pain, most often seen in young females. If no other causes of pancreatitis are identified and a patient has abdominal pain, elevated amylase levels, and pancreas divisum, this is considered causative and an endoscopic or operative papillotomy of the minor papilla and accessory duct is indicated. As most patients with pancreas divisum do not develop acute or recurrent pancreatitis, it is thought that stenosis at the minor papilla or a cystic dilatation of the distal dorsal duct just proximal to the papilla may be the additional factors necessary for developing pancreatitis in the setting of pancreas divisum.[8]

Annular pancreas is a rare congenital anomaly of the pancreas first recognized in 1818. Early autopsy and surgical series estimate the incidence to be approximately 3 in 20,000.[9,10] However, with better imaging modalities such as computed tomography (CT), magnetic resonance cholangiopancreatography (MRCP), and endoscopy, the incidence is thought to be closer to 1 in 1,000.[11–13] People with annular pancreas have a

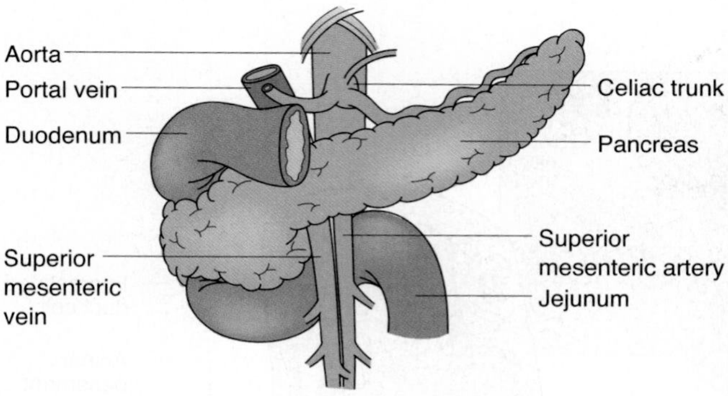

FIGURE 51.4. Annular pancreas. The ring of pancreatic tissue surrounds the duodenum. This ring contains a large duct and may be heavily fixed to the duodenal musculature. The duodenum beneath the annulus is often stenosed. As a result, dividing the ring of pancreatic tissue may not provide relief of duodenal obstruction. There is also the danger of creating a pancreatic fistula or duodenal perforation. Duodenojejunostomy bypassing the annulus is the procedure of choice for duodenal obstruction caused by annular pancreas. (After Gray SW, Skandalakis JE. *Atlas of Surgical Anatomy for General Surgeons.* Baltimore, MD: Williams and Wilkins; 1985.)

thin band of normal pancreatic parenchyma completely surrounding the second portion of the duodenum. This band is in continuity with the head of the pancreas and causes variable degrees of duodenal compression and stenosis (Fig. 51.4). In 1910, Lecco postulated that annular pancreas resulted from abnormal fusion of the ventral pancreatic bud to the duodenum, leading to improper rotation of the ventral bud around the duodenum.[14]

Annular pancreas represents a spectrum of disease, presenting at varying time points from in utero to adulthood. The disease differs significantly in adults and children.[13] When annular pancreas presents in childhood, it tends to be severe, presenting at a median age of 1 day. In children it is more commonly associated with other congenital anomalies including Down syndrome, cardiac anomalies, and other intestinal anomalies. When diagnosed in utero, the most common presentation is polyhydramnios due to duodenal obstruction. Newborns present most commonly with duodenal obstruction as evidenced by low birth weight and feeding intolerance. Duodenal bypass (duodenoduodenostomy or gastrojejunostomy) is the treatment of choice in children.

Fifty percent of cases of annular pancreas occur in adults. Adults are less likely to have significant obstruction and less likely to require surgical intervention. In adults, annular pancreas is more commonly associated with pancreas divisum and pancreatic neoplasia than in children.[13] This abnormal ring of pancreatic tissue may contain a pancreatic duct. Therefore, the surgeon must be aware of this anomaly since division of the abnormal ring can result in pancreatic fistula or obstruction of pancreatic ductal drainage.

Heterotopic pancreas is pancreatic tissue outside the bounds of the normal pancreas without anatomic or vascular connections to the pancreas itself. Heterotopic pancreas occurs in 0.5% to 14% of autopsy series. The heterotopic pancreatic tissue is functional and can occur in a variety of sites including the stomach, duodenum, ileum, umbilicus, colon, appendix, and gallbladder, and even within a Meckel diverticulum. This tissue is usually submucosal and uniformly contains acini and ducts. Up to one third contain islet cells. Heterotopic pancreas is usually an incidental finding, but can present with ulceration, obstruction, or intussusception, in which case treatment is directed at the presenting symptoms and may require resection. In incidental and asymptomatic cases, no treatment is required. The pancreas is susceptible to the same diseases as normal pancreas and can even undergo malignant transformation.[15,16]

STRUCTURE AND HISTOLOGY

3 The pancreas has two major components: the exocrine structure and the endocrine structure. The exocrine structure of the pancreas accounts for 80% to 90% of the pancreatic mass, while the endocrine structure accounts for approximately 2% of the pancreatic mass. The remainder of the pancreas is composed of extracellular matrix, blood vessels, and major ductal structures. The exocrine component secretes the enzymes responsible for digestion, and the endocrine component is critical in glucose homeostasis.

Exocrine Structure

The exocrine structure of the pancreas is composed of two main components: the acinar cells and the ductal network. The acinar cells produce and secrete the enzymes responsible for digestion. The acinar cells are pyramidal cells with an apex that faces the pancreatic ductal network. Within the apex of the cells there are numerous zymogen granules, which contain the digestive enzymes for secretion into the ductal system. There are approximately 20 to 40 acinar cells that cluster together to form the functional unit called an acinus (Fig. 51.5A, B). A second cell type in the acinus, the centroacinar cell, functions to secrete fluid and electrolytes of the correct pH into the pancreatic ductal system. The role of the ductal system is to carry the digestive secretions to the duodenum. The acinus drains into small intercalated ducts, which join to form interlobular ducts that also secrete fluid and electrolytes (Fig. 51.5A). These interlobular ducts form secondary ducts that drain into the main pancreatic ductal system and eventually the duodenum at the ampulla of Vater.

Endocrine Structure

The pancreatic islet cells are of neural crest origin and part of the family of amine precursor uptake and decarboxylation (APUD) cells. The most critical role of the pancreatic islet cells is the secretion of insulin and glucagon to maintain glucose homeostasis, although the islets secrete other hormones with varying roles in digestion. Each pancreatic islet is approximately 40 to 900 mm and contains an average of 3,000 cells.
4 The islets are composed of four cell types. Alpha (A) cells secrete glucagon, beta (B) cells secrete insulin and amylin,[17] delta (D) cells secrete somatostatin, and F cells secrete pancreatic polypeptide.

5 B cells are located centrally within the islets and constitute approximately 70% of the islet cell mass. F cells and A cells are located peripherally within the islets and constitute 15% and 10% of the islet cell mass, respectively. D cells are located both centrally and peripherally and constitute 5% of the islet
6 cell mass.[18] The distribution of endocrine cell types is not uniform throughout the pancreas. B and D cells are uniformly distributed throughout the gland. However, A cells are concentrated in the body and tail of the pancreas, and F cells are concentrated in the uncinate process. This distribution is important clinically, since resection of different parts of the pancreas will have varying endocrine effects.

The islet cells have a rich blood supply with the afferent arteriole entering the islet in an area of discontinuity in the non-B cells surrounding the periphery. The afferent arteriole then breaks into a capillary bed within the islet and then exits the islet through an efferent arteriole (Fig. 51.6). The hormones from the islet cells are secreted directly into this rich capillary network within the islet.

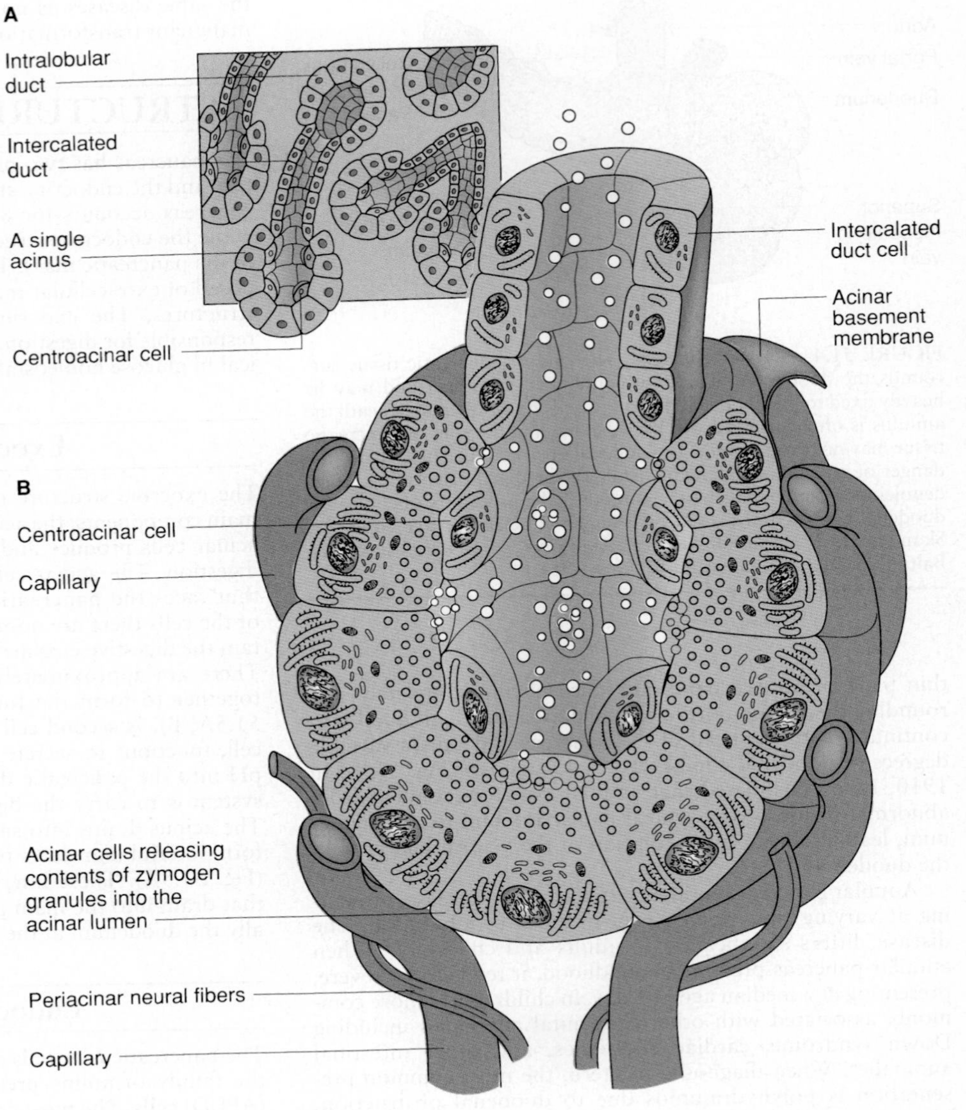

FIGURE 51.5. Histologic anatomy of the acinus. A: Low-magnification view of a portion of the pancreas. B: High-magnification view of a single acinus. The acinar cells, containing zymogen granules, are pyramidal cells with an apex that faces the pancreatic ductal network. Twenty to 40 acinar cells cluster together to form the functional unit called an acinus. The centroacinar cell, also present within the acinus, functions to secrete fluid and electrolytes of the correct pH into the pancreatic ductal system. The acinus drains into small intercalated ducts, which join to form interlobular ducts that also secrete fluid and electrolytes. These interlobular ducts form secondary ducts that drain into the main pancreatic ductal. (After Krstic RV. *Die Gewebes des Menschen und der Saugetiere*. Berlin, Germany: Springer-Verlag;1978.)

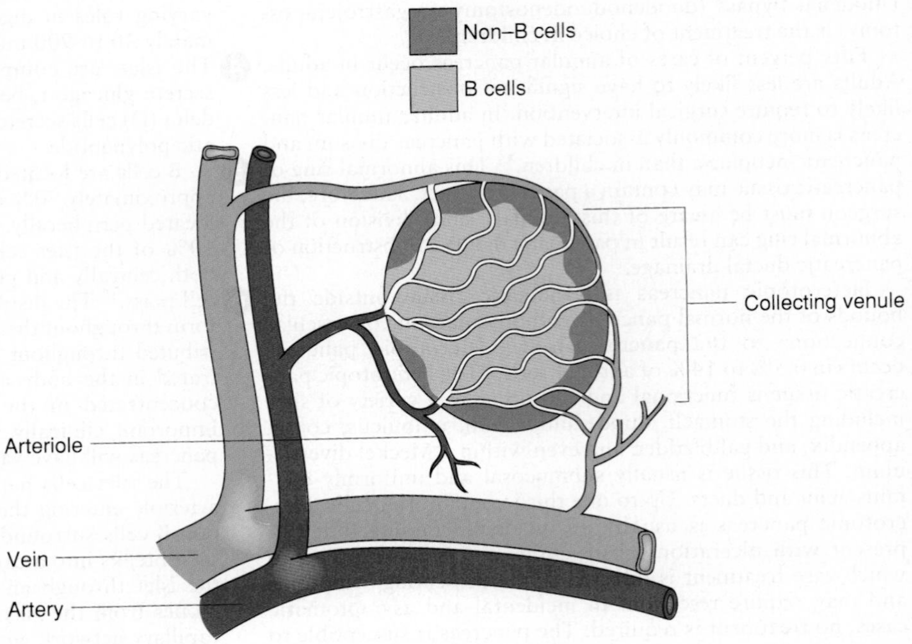

FIGURE 51.6. Diagram of a typical islet. Afferent arterioles enter the islet through discontinuities of the mantle of non-B cells and break into capillaries, most of which traverse the B-cell mass and pass through the mantle as efferent vessels. Occasionally, a capillary passes at the interface of the B cell and non-B cells and never enters the B-cell core. In larger islets, the efferent capillaries coalesce at the edge of the islet and pass along the mantle as collecting venules before draining into a vein. (After Bonner-Weir S, Orci L. New perspectives on the microvasculature of the islets of Langerhans in the rat. *Diabetes* 1982;31:883.)

PANCREATIC ANATOMY

The pancreas lies in the retroperitoneum at the level of the second lumbar vertebra. It lies obliquely and transversely from its most caudal point at the duodenal C loop on the right to its most cranial point in the splenic hilum on the left. The pancreas is composed of four anatomic parts: the head (including the uncinate process), neck, body, and tail (Fig. 51.1).

Relationship to Adjacent Structures

7 The understanding of the pancreatic anatomy in relation to adjacent structures is critical when performing operative procedures on the pancreas or surrounding structures including the duodenum, bile duct, and spleen. The pancreatic head, further subdivided into the head and uncinate process, is embraced by the C loop of the duodenum (Fig. 51.1). The pancreatic head is the portion of the pancreas extending to the right of the superior mesenteric vessels. The uncinate process is a projection from the inferior portion of the pancreas head that extends medially to the left, posterior to the superior mesenteric vessels. The head of the pancreas is attached to the medial aspect of the descending duodenum and its horizontal third portion, and the two organs share a blood supply. Posterior to the pancreatic head lie the inferior vena cava, right renal artery and vein, and left renal vein. In order for these structures to be exposed, the pancreas must be mobilized out the retroperitoneum (Kocher maneuver). The bile duct runs through the posterior and superior aspect of the pancreatic head, joining the pancreatic duct and draining into the duodenum medially at the ampulla of Vater.

The pancreatic neck is the 1.5 to 2.0 cm of pancreatic tissue that overlies the superior mesenteric artery and vein anteriorly. These vessels form a vascular groove in the posterior aspect of the gland. The anterior surface of the pancreatic neck is covered by peritoneum and lies directly posterior to the pylorus of the stomach. The splenic vein joins the superior mesenteric vein posterior to the pancreatic neck forming the portal vein, which drains the intestinal blood supply to the liver.

The body of the pancreas continues left from the pancreatic neck. The anterior surface of the pancreatic body is covered with peritoneum and forms the floor of the omental bursa within the lesser sac. The stomach overlies the pancreatic body/lesser sac anteriorly. The posterior surface of the pancreatic body is not peritonealized and directly contacts the aorta, left adrenal gland, left kidney, and left renal artery and vein. The body of the pancreas is the portion overlying the second lumbar vertebrae.

The tail of the pancreas begins anterior the left kidney and extends superolaterally to the hilum of the spleen. The splenic artery and vein run along the posterior surface of the pancreas. The tail of the pancreas is in close proximity to the spleen and splenic flexure of the colon.

Pancreatic Ductal Anatomy

The main pancreatic duct, or duct of Wirsung, begins in the pancreatic tail. It most commonly runs within the posterior aspect of the pancreatic parenchyma, midway between the superior and inferior border of the gland. In the head of the pancreas, the pancreatic duct turns inferiorly at the genu of the pancreatic duct and joins the common bile duct, draining into the duodenum at the ampulla of Vater 7 to 10 cm distal to the pylorus. The common channel between the common bile duct and main pancreatic duct varies in length. At the level of the ampulla of Vater, the pancreatic duct is anterior and inferior to the common bile duct. There are over 20 secondary branches of the main pancreatic duct throughout the pancreas providing drainage of acinar units.

The main pancreatic duct is 2 to 4 mm in diameter and has a ductal pressure of approximately 15 to 30 mm Hg. This is higher than the pressure in the common bile duct, 7 to 17 mm Hg, thereby preventing reflux of bile into the pancreatic ductal system. At the ampulla of Vater, the sphincter of Oddi prevents reflux of duodenal contents into the bile duct and pancreatic duct. This sphincter is controlled by a variety of neural and hormonal factors that regulate relaxation and constriction.

The accessory pancreatic duct, or duct of Santorini, is more variable than the main pancreatic duct (Fig. 51.3). It typically drains the uncinate process and inferior portion of the pancreatic head into the duodenum at the minor papilla, proximal to the ampulla of Vater.

Arterial Blood Supply

The pancreas has a rich blood supply derived from both the celiac axis and superior mesenteric artery. The celiac axis arises from the abdominal aorta and most commonly gives rise to the splenic artery, the left gastric artery, and the common hepatic artery (Fig. 51.7A). The splenic artery courses along the posterior surface of the pancreatic body and tail and gives rise to more than 10 branches that supply the pancreatic body and tail. Three of these branches are named branches. The first is the dorsal pancreatic artery, which arises close to the origin of the splenic artery and supplies blood to the proximal body. The great pancreatic artery arises more distally and supplies the midportion of the body. Finally, the caudal pancreatic artery arises more distally and supplies the pancreatic tail. Near the head of the pancreas, branches arising from the splenic artery form collaterals with the inferior pancreaticoduodenal arcades.

The gastroduodenal artery is the first branch off the common hepatic artery. Distal to the first portion of the duodenum, the gastroduodenal artery becomes the superior pancreaticoduodenal artery and divides into anterior and posterior branches.

The superior mesenteric artery gives rise to the inferior pancreaticoduodenal artery, which also gives rise to anterior and posterior branches. The inferior and superior pancreaticoduodenal arcades form an extensive collateral network with the superior pancreaticoduodenal arcades, supplying both the duodenum and head of the pancreas. Anteriorly, these arcades lie in the groove between the pancreas and duodenum. Posteriorly, they cross the common bile duct.

Variations or anomalies in the pancreatic and biliary blood supply are found in 20% to 30% of people and mainly consist of portions of the hepatic arterial blood supply being replaced. In these cases, all or part of the hepatic arterial blood supply does not arise from the celiac axis. As much of the pancreatic blood supply is derived from the hepatic arterial blood supply, these variations lead to variations in the pancreatic blood supply. The most common anomaly is a replaced right hepatic artery arising from the superior mesenteric artery (SMA; Fig. 51.7D). This variation is seen in approximately 20% of patients. The replaced right hepatic artery arises from the proximal SMA in the retropancreatic position and traverses the upper edge of the uncinate process, then runs posterolateral to the portal vein. The right hepatic artery can also originate from the right gastric artery in 2% of cases or from the gastroduodenal artery in 6% of cases.

Anomalies in the common hepatic artery also exist, with the most common being a common hepatic artery originating from the SMA instead of the celiac axis (Fig. 51.7C). In this case, there is no hepatic arterial pulse medially in the hepatoduodenal ligament. The replaced common hepatic artery runs anterior to the portal vein but posterior to the bile duct and gives rise to a gastroduodenal branch, which is also posterior to the bile duct. In approximately 10% of cases, the left hepatic artery can be aberrant, most commonly arising from the left gastric artery instead of the proper hepatic artery.

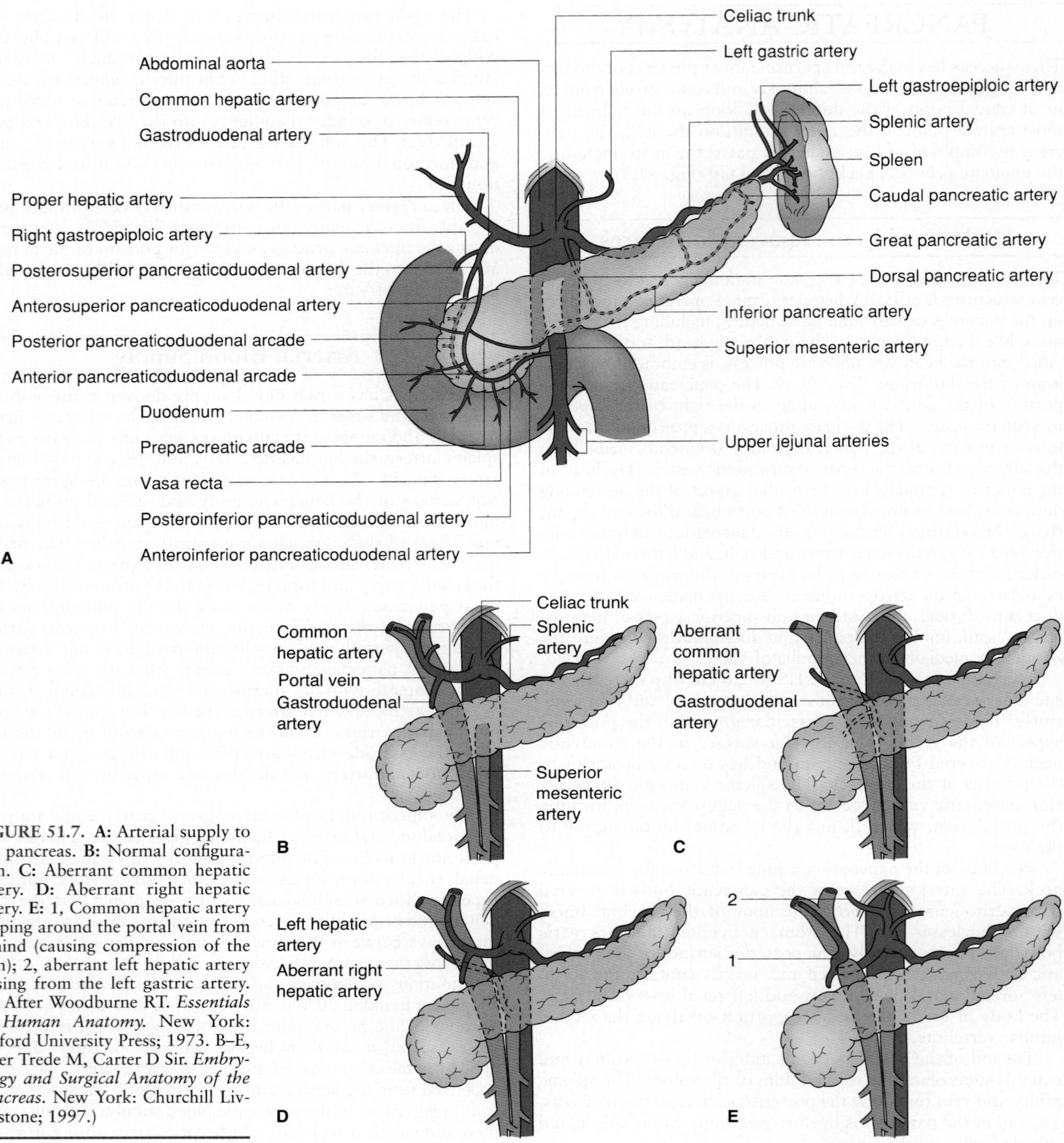

FIGURE 51.7. A: Arterial supply to the pancreas. B: Normal configuration. C: Aberrant common hepatic artery. D: Aberrant right hepatic artery. E: 1, Common hepatic artery looping around the portal vein from behind (causing compression of the vein); 2, aberrant left hepatic artery arising from the left gastric artery. (A, After Woodburne RT. *Essentials of Human Anatomy.* New York: Oxford University Press; 1973. B–E, After Trede M, Carter D Sir. *Embryology and Surgical Anatomy of the Pancreas.* New York: Churchill Livingstone; 1997.)

The arterial blood supply of the ampulla of Vater is from three pedicles off the superior and inferior pancreaticoduodenal arteries. The posterior pedicle, located at 11 o'clock, arises from the superior pancreaticoduodenal artery. The ventral commissural pedicle, located at 1 o'clock, arises from both arcades. Finally, the inferior pedicle, located at 6 o'clock, arises from the anterior branch of the inferior pancreaticoduodenal artery.

Venous Drainage

The venous drainage of the pancreas follows the arterial blood supply and is eventually returned to the portal circulation and delivered back to the liver. There are four main routes of venous drainage in the pancreas. In the pancreatic head, superior venous arcades drain either directly into the suprapancreatic portal vein or laterally into the retropancreatic portal vein. The anterior and inferior branches of the pancreaticoduodenal arcades of the pancreatic head drain directly into the infrapancreatic superior mesenteric vein. There are rarely any anterior branches from the pancreatic head and neck into the superior mesenteric and portal veins. When they do occur, it is most commonly at the superior border of the pancreatic neck. The body and tail of the pancreas have many venous tributaries that drain into the splenic vein, which joins the superior mesenteric vein posterior to the pancreatic neck, forming the portal vein. The three named tributaries of the splenic vein are the inferior pancreatic vein, the caudal pancreatic vein, and the great pancreatic vein. The inferior mesenteric vein does not drain the pancreas, but joins the splenic vein posterior the pancreatic body.

Lymphatic Drainage

Throughout the pancreas there is a rich periacinar network of lymphatic vessels that drain to five major nodal groups.[19] The first is the superior nodal group along the superior border of the pancreas and celiac trunk. These lymph nodes drain the superior portion of the pancreatic head. The inferior nodal group along the inferior border of the head and body of the pancreas drains the inferior pancreatic head and uncinate process, eventually draining to the superior mesenteric and para-aortic lymph nodes. The anterior lymphatics drain to the prepyloric and infrapyloric nodes. The posterior lymph nodes include the distal common bile duct and ampullary lymphatics and drain directly into the para-aortic lymph nodes. Lastly, the splenic lymph nodes drain the lymphatics of the pancreatic body and tail into the interceliomesenteric lymph nodes.

The Japanese Pancreas Society has classified the pancreatic lymphatic drainage into 18 lymph node stations.[20] The greater and lesser curves of the stomach drain into lymph node stations 1 through 4. The anterior lymphatics described earlier drain into lymph node stations 5 and 6. The superior nodal group includes lymph node stations 7 through 9 along the left gastric artery, common hepatic artery, and celiac axis. The splenic lymph node group corresponds to lymph node stations 10 and 11. The posterior lymph nodes include lymph node stations 12 (and all subdivisions) and 13, while the inferior nodal group includes lymph node stations 14 through 18. This classification system is commonly used to describe the extent of nodal dissection in pancreatic surgery.

Innervation

The innervation to the pancreas is derived from the vagus and thoracic splanchnic nerves as well as peptidergic neurons that secrete amines and peptides.[21] Parasympathetic and sympathetic fibers reach the pancreas by passing along the arteries from the celiac axis and superior mesenteric arteries (Fig. 51.8). These fibers give rise to periacinar plexuses within the pancreatic parenchyma, which send fibers directly to the acinar cell group. The pancreatic islets and islet vasculature are similarly innervated. The parasympathetic nerves stimulate both exocrine and endocrine secretion, while the sympathetic fibers have a predominantly inhibitory effect (Fig. 51.9).[22] The peptidergic neurons secrete hormones including somatostatin, vasoactive intestinal peptide (VIP), calcitonin gene–related peptide (CGRP), and galanin. While the peptidergic neurons influence exocrine and endocrine secretion, their precise physiologic role is unclear. The pancreas also has a rich network of afferent sensory fibers.

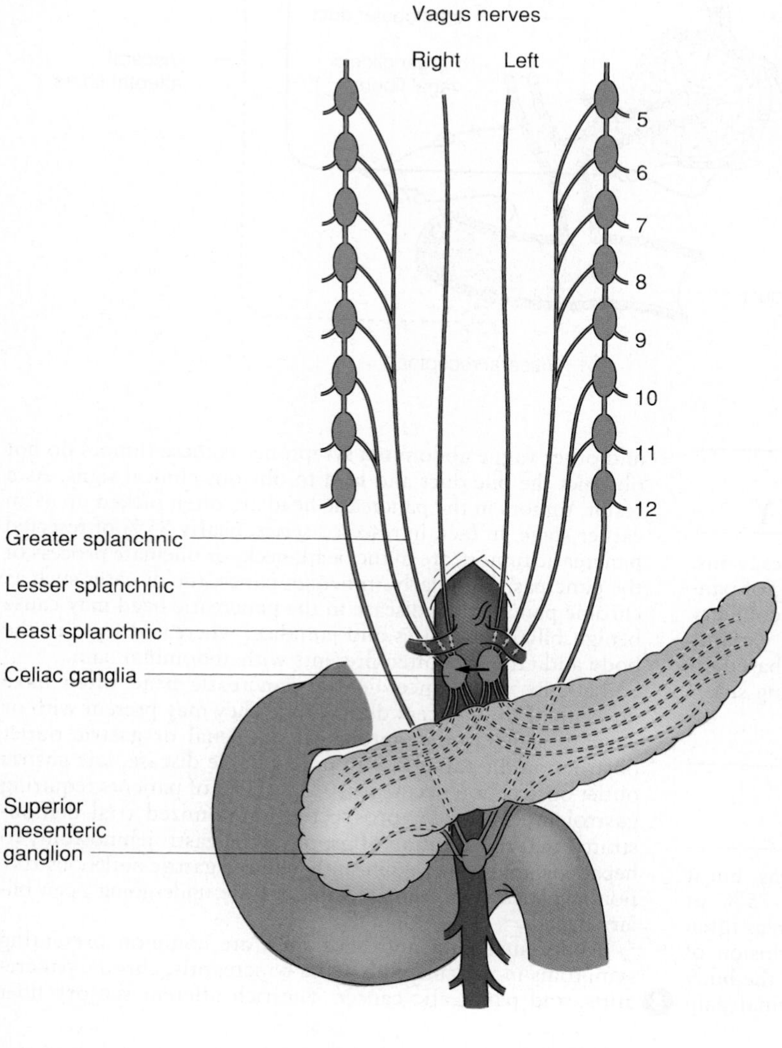

FIGURE 51.8. Diagram of the autonomic nerve supply to the pancreas. The innervation to the pancreas is derived from the vagus and thoracic splanchnic nerves. Parasympathetic and sympathetic fibers reach the pancreas by passing along the arteries from the celiac axis and superior mesenteric arteries. (After Skandalakis JE, Gray SW, Rowe JS Jr, et al. Anatomical complications of pancreatic surgery. *Contemp Surg* 1979;15:17.)

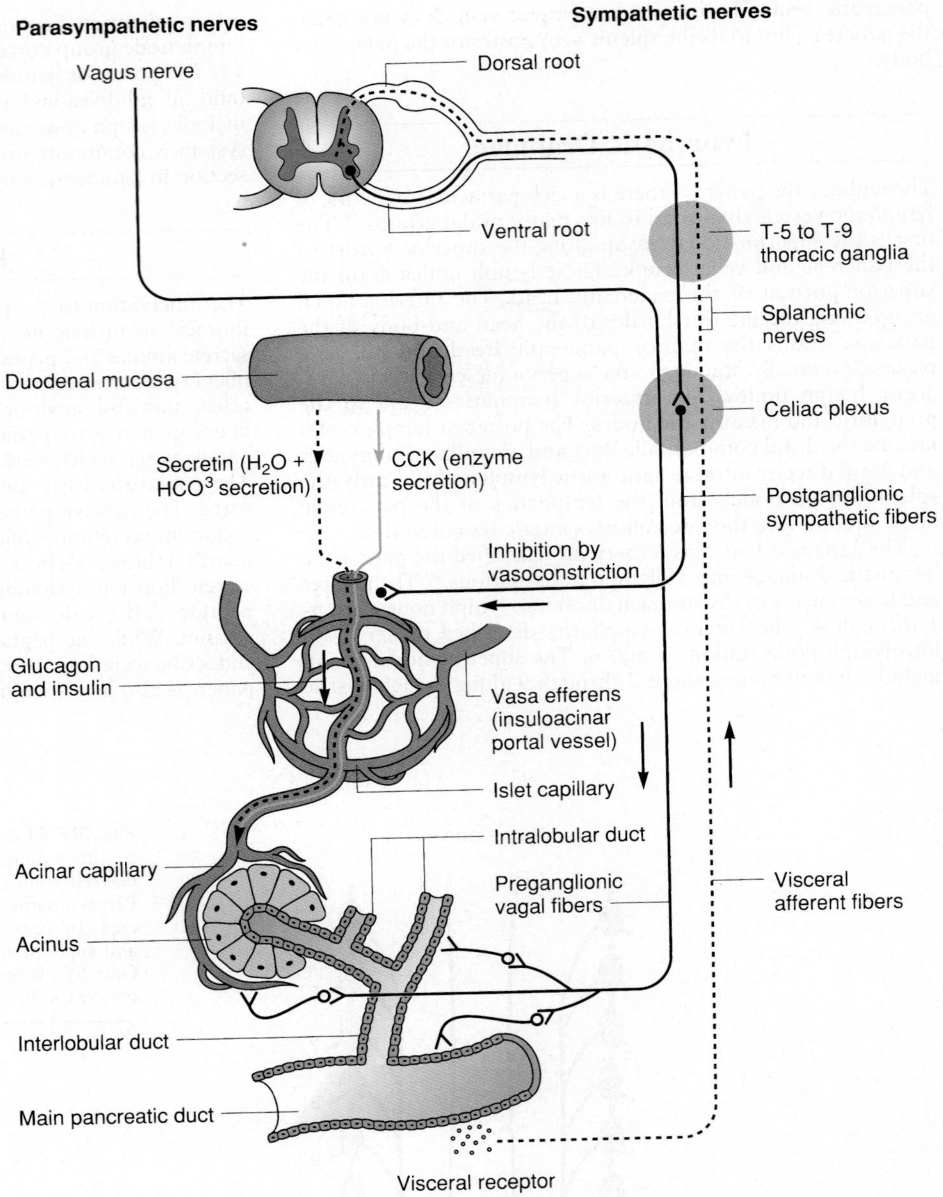

FIGURE 51.9. Schematic diagram of the neurohormonal control of the exocrine cells. Visceral receptors line the ductule system and carry the sensation of pain to the spinal cord. Sympathetic fibers first synapse in the celiac plexus after traveling through the thoracic ganglia and splanchnic nerves. Postganglionic fibers then synapse on intrapancreatic arterioles. Parasympathetic preganglionic fibers travel through the celiac plexus after leaving the vagus nerves and course with vessels and ducts to synapse on postganglionic fibers near acinar cells, islet cells, and smooth muscle cells of major ducts. Stimulation of these parasympathetic fibers results in an immediate release of pancreatic enzymes. Secretin and cholecystokinin (CCK) first enter the pancreas through the capillary network of the islet cells, then enter the separate capillary network of the acinar tissue through the insuloacinar portal vessels. Glucagon, somatostatin, pancreatic polypeptide, and insulin from the islet cells reach the acinar tissue immediately after release. In this way, the islet cells can influence the acinar tissue responses to CCK and secretin. (After Tompkins RK, Traverso LW. The exocrine cells. In: Keynes WM, Keith RG, eds. *The Pancreas*. New York: Appleton-Century-Crofts; 1981.)

SURGICAL SIGNIFICANCE OF PANCREATIC ANATOMY

The proximity of the pancreas to major visceral arteries, veins, and other abdominal organs makes the understanding of pancreatic anatomy critical for the general and pancreaticobiliary surgeon. Knowledge of the anatomy and anatomic variants can give clues to the diagnosis of pancreatic disease based on signs and symptoms and prevent injury to surrounding structures in the operating room.

Presenting Signs and Symptoms of Pancreatic Disease

Pancreatic cancer can occur anywhere in the pancreas, but it occurs in the pancreatic head in approximately 75% of cases.[23] Patients with cancer in the head of the pancreas often present with obstructive jaundice secondary to occlusion of the intrapancreatic bile duct. Patients with cancer in the body and tail of the pancreas often present with abdominal pain and other vague abdominal symptoms as these tumors do not obstruct the bile duct and lead to obvious clinical signs. As a result, tumors in the pancreatic head are often picked up at an earlier stage. In fact, in resected series, nearly 85% of resected pancreatic tumors are in the head, neck, or uncinate process of the pancreas.[24] Similarly, in benign pancreatic diseases such as chronic pancreatitis, disease in the pancreatic head may cause benign biliary strictures and jaundice, whereas disease in the body and tail more often presents with abdominal pain.

Patients with cancer in the pancreatic head often have invasion of the adjacent duodenum. They may present with or develop signs and symptoms of duodenal or gastric outlet obstruction. In patients with unresectable disease, late gastric outlet obstruction occurs in 10% to 20% of patients requiring gastrojejunostomy. A prospective randomized trial demonstrated that the addition of prophylactic gastrojejunostomy to hepaticojejunostomy significantly reduced gastric outlet obstruction in patients with unresectable disease undergoing open biliary bypass.[25]

8 Abdominal pain and back pain are common presenting symptoms in patients with acute pancreatitis, chronic pancreatitis, and pancreatic cancer. The rich afferent sensory fiber

network within the pancreas likely contributes to the pain associated with pancreatic disease processes including pancreatic cancer and chronic pancreatitis. In addition, as pancreatic cancer progresses, the nervous plexuses along the celiac axis in the retroperitoneum can be invaded by tumor, causing the characteristic intractable back pain. Celiac ganglion blockade (sympathectomy) or neurolysis using alcohol can provide significant pain relief by interrupting these somatic fibers. A celiac block can be performed endoscopically, percutaneously, or intraoperatively. Endoscopic ultrasound (EUS)- or CT-guided celiac plexus neurolysis should be considered first-line therapy in patients with pain secondary to unresectable, locally advanced pancreatic cancer.[26] In addition, intraoperative celiac blockade has been shown to reduce pain in patients with unresectable pancreatic cancer undergoing operative bypass procedures for obstructive jaundice and duodenal obstruction.[27] The use of celiac plexus blockade as routine therapy for pain in chronic pancreatitis is currently not recommended since only 50% of patients experience reduction in pain and the beneficial effect lasts only several months.[26]

Resectability and Involvement of Adjacent Structures

9 Resectability of pancreatic cancers depends on two things: the presence or absence of distant metastases and the extent of local invasion. Liver or lung metastases from hematogenous spread, peritoneal carcinomatosis, or lymphatic involvement outside of the resection field such as around the celiac axis or root of the mesentery is considered unresectable.

Pancreatic cancers in the head, neck, or uncinate process often involve the intrapancreatic bile duct and/or duodenum given their close proximity. Assuming no distant metastases, pancreatic head cancers are resectable if they do not involve the major vascular structures. Involvement of the celiac axis or superior mesenteric artery precludes surgical resection. In addition, occlusion or circumferential involvement of the superior mesenteric–portal vein confluence is considered a contraindication to surgical resection by most surgeons. However, resection of the portal vein–superior mesenteric vein confluence and reconstruction has been advocated by some groups for select patients with locally advanced disease who are good surgical candidates.[28–32] The results have been mixed, but most studies show that limited venous resection and reconstruction is safe and has similar 5-year survival when compared to patients not undergoing venous resection. However, a recent systematic review of 52 nonduplicated studies suggests that cure is unlikely in patients with major vascular involvement. Such patients had high rates of concurrent lymph node metastases and low 5-year survival rates following pancreatectomy with major venous resection.[33]

Pancreatic head cancer may also involve adjacent organs including the hepatic flexure of the colon, the gallbladder, or the stomach. If there are no distant metastases, resection of these organs en bloc is indicated.

For cancers in the body and tail without distant metastasis, involvement of the splenic artery and/or vein does not preclude resection, as these vessels are normally taken during the operation. However, involvement of the celiac axis or superior mesenteric artery precludes resection. Involvement of adjacent organs including the left kidney, left adrenal, spleen, and left colon can be resected if involved with tumor and there is no distant disease.

Blood Supply

Knowledge of the normal pancreatic blood supply is critical in order to perform an adequate cancer operation. As the duodenum and head of the pancreas share a blood supply, it is necessary to remove these organs en bloc when performing an operation for carcinoma. While the duodenum can be preserved in resections performed for benign disease (duodenum-preserving pancreatic head resection), this is not the case in patients with cancer. Likewise, for cancers in the body and tail of the pancreas, it is necessary to resect the spleen and its blood supply since it shares a blood supply with the tail of the pancreas. For benign diseases of the pancreatic tail, the spleen can be preserved.

Extent of Lymphatic Resection

There has been significant debate regarding the extent of lymph node dissection necessary in patients undergoing curative resection for pancreatic cancer. Knowledge of the lymph node station numbers used by the Japanese Pancreas Society is useful in understanding the difference between standard pancreaticoduodenal resection and "extended" or "radical" dissection involving a more extensive lymphadenectomy. The results of a randomized trial reported in 2005 showed no difference in survival with standard compared to radical resection.[34,35] Table 51.2 shows the difference in the extent of lymphadenectomy between the standard and radical procedures. The standard procedure includes the bile duct (station 12b2) and cystic duct lymph nodes (station 12c), the posterior (station 13) and anterior (station 17) pancreaticoduodenal lymph nodes, the superior mesenteric vein nodes (station 14v), and the nodes on the right side of the superior mesenteric artery (station 14b). Radical resection adds a distal gastrectomy (stations 3, 4, 5, and 6) and a retroperitoneal dissection extending from the right renal hilum to the left lateral border of the aorta horizontally with samples of celiac nodes, and from the portal vein to below the third portion of the duodenum vertically (lymph node stations 16a1, 16b2, and 9).

Aberrant Vascular Anatomy

Awareness of the common anatomic variants in biliary and pancreatic arterial supply is necessary to prevent major vascular injury and damage to the hepatic blood supply during pancreatic resection. The gastroduodenal artery (GDA) is the largest named artery taken during pancreaticoduodenectomy. In the normal case, the GDA arises from the common hepatic artery (Fig. 51.7A), entering the head of the pancreas anterior and medial to the bile duct. In the case of a replaced right hepatic artery arising from the superior mesenteric artery, the GDA arises from this replaced vessel and enters the pancreas posterior to the bile duct. In addition, this replaced right hepatic artery courses to the liver lateral to the bile duct and can easily be injured during dissection of the pancreatic uncinate process off of the superior mesenteric vessels. This replaced vessel can often supply the entire right lobe of the liver, causing significant hepatic ischemia if injured. In the case of a replaced right hepatic artery, there will still be a pulse medially in the hepatoduodenal ligament from the left hepatic artery, but this will supply only the left lobe of the liver.

In the case of a replaced common hepatic artery, there will be no pulse medially in the hepatoduodenal ligament and the entire hepatic blood supply will be from the superior mesenteric artery. The replaced vessel will again be posterior and lateral to the bile duct and at risk of injury if not correctly identified. Given the closer proximity of the replaced vessels to the pancreatic head and uncinate process, these vessels may also be more prone to direct involvement by tumor. If injured or involved with tumor and resected, these often require reconstruction to restore adequate hepatic blood supply.

Blunt Pancreatic Injury

The pancreas lies deep in the retroperitoneum. The pancreatic body lies anterior to the second lumbar vertebra. In cases of

TABLE 51.2

JAPANESE LYMPH NODE STATIONS

STATION NUMBER	NAME	STANDARD	RADICAL
3	Gastric lesser curve	No[a]	Yes[b]
4	Gastric greater curve	No[a]	Yes[b]
5	Superior pyloric	No[a]	Yes
6	Inferior pyloric	No[a]	Yes
8	Common hepatic artery	No	No
9	Celiac origin	No	Yes[c]
12	Hepatoduodenal ligament		
12a2	Proper hepatic artery near GDA	No[d]	No[d]
12b2	Bile duct below cystic duct	Yes[e]	Yes[e]
12c	Around cystic duct	Yes	Yes
12p2	Retro portal vein below cystic duct	No[d]	No[d]
13	Posterior pancreaticoduodenal	Yes	Yes
14	SMA and SMV nodes		
14a	Origin of SMA	No	No
14b	Right side of SMA	Yes[e]	Yes[e]
14c	Anterior SMA at middle colic	No	No
14d	Left side of SMA at first jejunal branch	No	No
14v	SMV nodes	Yes[e]	Yes[e]
16	Aortocaval nodes		
16a2	Celiac to left renal vein	No	Yes[f]
16b1	Left renal vein to IMA	No	Yes
17	Anterior pancreaticoduodenal	Yes	Yes

GDA, gastroduodenal artery; IMA, inferior mesenteric artery; SMA, superior mesentery artery; SMV, superior mesenteric vein.
[a]Unless a distal gastrectomy is performed as part of standard resection.
[b]Some of these nodes may accompany the distal gastrectomy specimen.
[c]Sampled only.
[d]Not formally resected.
[e]Some of these nodes may accompany the pancreaticoduodenectomy specimen.
[f]Some of these nodes, cephalad to the left renal vein, but not required to dissect the celiac axis origin.
Reproduced with permission from Yeo CJ, Cameron JL, Lillemoe KD, et al. Pancreaticoduodenectomy with or without distal gastrectomy and extended retroperitoneal lymphadenectomy for periampullary adenocarcinoma, part 2: randomized controlled trial evaluating survival, morbidity, and mortality. *Ann Surg* 2002;236:355–368.

blunt abdominal trauma, specifically deceleration injury, the pancreatic body is crushed against the second vertebral body and can be transected at this point. In trauma patients with elevated amylase and lipase levels, the trauma surgeon should be aware of this possibility and obtain cross-sectional pancreatic imaging to rule out ductal disruption. In the case of complete ductal disruption, distal pancreatectomy or drainage of the pancreas into the intestine may be necessary.

PANCREATIC PHYSIOLOGY

Exocrine Function

The pancreas secretes 1.5 to 3 liters of a colorless, odorless, isosmotic, and alkaline solution daily containing over 20 enzymes and zymogens. The enzymes and zymogens play a major role in the digestive activity of the gastrointestinal tract. The alkaline solution secreted by the pancreas ranges in pH from 7.6 to 9.0. It carries the proteolytic enzymes to the duodenum in their inactive state, where it then serves to neutralize gastric acid and provides an optimal milieu for the function of these enzymes. Pancreatic secretion is regulated via an intimate interaction of both hormonal and neural pathways.

Gastric acid is the primary stimulus for release of secretin, which then stimulates the secretion of pancreatic fluid rich in water, electrolytes, and bicarbonate. In response to the presence of long-chain fatty acids, some essential amino acids (methionine, valine, phenylalanine, and tryptophan), and gastric acid, the duodenum and jejunum release cholecystokinin (CCK). CCK then stimulates enzyme-rich secretion from the pancreas. The presence of bile salts in the intestine also stimulates pancreatic secretion, integrating the function of the pancreas, biliary tract, and small intestine. Vagal (parasympathetic) afferent and efferent pathways strongly affect pancreatic secretion. In fact, the secretion of enzyme-rich fluid is largely dependent on the vagal stimulation, whereas fluid and electrolyte secretion are more dependent on the direct hormonal effects of secretin and CCK. Parasympathetic stimulation also causes the release of VIP, which also serves to stimulate secretin secretion.[36]

Many neuropeptides also influence pancreatic secretion in an inhibitory fashion. These include somatostatin, pancreatic polypeptide, peptide YY, calcitonin gene–related peptides, neuropeptide Y, pancreastatin, enkephalin, glucagon, and galanin. While these neuropeptides are known to play a role in the regulation of pancreatic secretion, the mechanisms of action and the intricate interplay between the neuropeptides are not fully understood.[36]

Bicarbonate Secretion

Bicarbonate is the most physiologically important ion secreted by the pancreas. Bicarbonate is formed from carbonic acid by the enzyme carbonic anhydrase. The secretion of water and electrolytes originates in the centroacinar and intercalated duct cells (Fig. 51.5). These cells secrete 20 mmol of bicarbonate per liter in the basal state and up to 150 mmol/L in the maximally stimulated state.[36] The bicarbonate secreted from the ductal cells is primarily derived from the plasma and not from intracellular metabolism. Chloride efflux through the cystic fibrosis transmembrane conductance regulator (CFTR) leads to depolarization and bicarbonate entry through the sodium bicarbonate cotranporter.[36] As a result, chloride secretion varies inversely with bicarbonate secretion, with the sum of these two anions balancing the sodium and potassium cations and remaining constant and equal to that of the plasma.

10 Both secretin and VIP stimulate bicarbonate secretion by increasing intracellular cyclic adenosine monophosphate, which acts on the CFTR.[36] Secretin is released from the duodenal mucosa in response to a duodenal lumen pH of less than 3.0 due to gastric acid. CCK is a weak direct stimulator of bicarbonate secretion, but it acts as a neuromodulator and potentiates the stimulatory effects of secretin. Gastrin and acetylcholine are also weak stimulators of bicarbonate secretion.[37] Bicarbonate secretion is inhibited by atropine (vagal stimulation) and can be reduced by 50% after truncal vagotomy.[38] Islet peptides including somatostatin, pancreatic polypeptide, glucagon, galanin, and pancreastatin are thought to inhibit exocrine secretion.

Enzyme Secretion

Pancreatic enzymes originate in the acinar cells, which are highly compartmentalized. Proteins are synthesized in the rough endoplasmic reticulum, processed in the Golgi apparatus, then targeted to the appropriate cell compartment (zymogen granules, lysosomes, etc.). The acinar cells secrete enzymes that fall into three major enzyme groups: amylolytic enzymes, lipolytic enzymes, and proteolytic enzymes. Amylolytic enzymes such as amylase hydrolyze starch to oligosaccharides and the disaccharide maltose. Lipolytic enzymes such as lipase, phospholipase A, and cholesterol esterase function work in conjunction with bile salts to digest fats and cholesterol. Proteolytic enzymes include endopeptidases (trypsin and chymotrypsin), which act on the internal peptide bonds of proteins and polypeptides, and exopeptidases (carboxypeptidases), which act on the free carboxy- and amino-terminal ends of proteins. The proteolytic enzymes are secreted as inactive precursors. Enterokinase cleaves the lysine–isoleucine bond in trypsinogen to create the active enzyme trypsin. Trypsin then activates the other proteolytic enzyme precursors.[36]

The enzyme groups are not secreted in a fixed ratio. Dietary alterations and stimulation by specific nutrients can result in changes in the relative amounts of each enzyme type. When enzyme secretion is absent or impaired, malabsorption or incomplete digestion occurs, leading to fat and protein loss through the gastrointestinal tract. This is seen in patients with acute and chronic pancreatitis (who have destruction of the exocrine pancreas) and in patients who have undergone surgical resection of all or part of the pancreas. These patients often present with weight loss and steatorrhea. These signs and symptoms can be corrected by oral replacement of pancreatic enzymes with meals.

The nervous system initiates pancreatic enzyme secretion. This involves extrinsic innervation by the vagus nerve and subsequent innervation by the intrapancreatic cholinergic fibers. The neurotransmitters, acetylcholine, and gastrin-releasing peptides activate calcium-dependent release of zymogen granules.[36] CCK is also a predominant regulator of enzyme secretion, doing so through activation of specific membrane-bound receptors and calcium-dependent second messenger pathways. Secretin and VIP weakly stimulate acinar cell secretion independently, but they potentiate the effect of CCK on acinar cells. Insulin is required locally and serves in a permissive role for secretin and CCK to promote exocrine secretion (Fig. 51.10).[36]

Through the secretion of the three classes of enzymes, the pancreas regulates complete digestion of carbohydrates, fats,

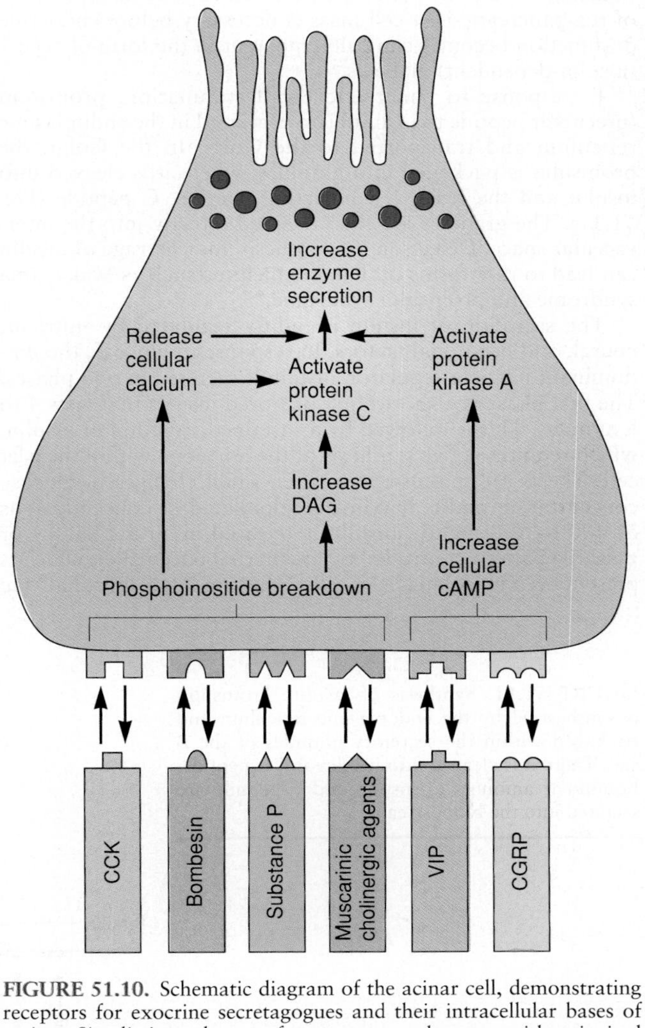

FIGURE 51.10. Schematic diagram of the acinar cell, demonstrating receptors for exocrine secretagogues and their intracellular bases of action. Six distinct classes of receptors are known, with principal ligands shown. CCK, cholecystokinin; CRGP, calcitonin gene–related peptide; DAG, diacylglycerol; VIP, vasoactive intestinal peptide.

and proteins. Autodigestion of the pancreas by these proteolytic enzymes is prevented by packaging of proteases in an inactive precursor form and by the synthesis of protease inhibitors including pancreatic secretory trypsin inhibitor (PSTI), serine protease inhibitor kazal type 1 (SPINK1), and protease serine 1 (PRSS1). These enzymes are found in the acinar cell and loss of these protective mechanisms can lead to activation, autodigestion, and acute pancreatitis. Mutations in the SPINK1 and PRSS1 genes are known to cause one of the aggressive familial forms of chronic pancreatitis, leading to recurrent episodes of pancreatitis with associated exocrine and endocrine insufficiency.[39,40]

Endocrine Function

Insulin Synthesis, Secretion, and Action. Insulin is a 56-amino-acid polypeptide with a molecular weight of 6 kD. It consists of two polypeptide chains (A and B) joined by two disulfide bridges. The amino acid sequence varies among species, but the location of the disulfide bridges are highly conserved and are critical for its biologic activity. Insulin is synthesized by the B cells within the islets of Langerhans. Insulin functions to promote glucose transport in all cells except B cells, hepatocytes, and central nervous system cells. Insulin inhibits glycogenolysis and fatty acid breakdown but stimulates protein synthesis. There is a significant secretory reserve of insulin within the pancreas. Destruction or removal of 80% of the pancreatic islet cell mass is necessary before endocrine dysfunction becomes clinically apparent in the form of type 1 (insulin-dependent) diabetes.[41]

In response to pancreatic B-cell stimulation, proinsulin (precursor peptide to insulin) is synthesized in the endoplasmic reticulum and transported to the Golgi. In the Golgi, the proinsulin is packaged into granules, where it is cleaved into insulin and the residual connecting peptide, C peptide (Fig. 51.11). The granules are then released directly into the intervascular space. Defects in the synthesis and cleavage of insulin can lead to rare forms of diabetes mellitus such as Wakayama syndrome and proinsulin syndrome.[42]

The secretion of insulin is tightly regulated by nutrient, neural, and hormonal factors. In response to glucose, the predominant nutrient regulator, insulin is secreted in two phases. The first phase is a short burst of stored insulin that lasts 4 to 6 minutes. This is followed by a sustained secretion of insulin, which requires active synthesis of the hormone within the islet cell. The B cell is sensitive to even small changes in glucose concentration and is maximally stimulated at concentrations of 400 to 500 mg/dL. Insulin is released in an oscillatory or pulsatile pattern controlled by an internal pacemaker, which is present even in isolated islet cells.[43] Insulin has a short half-life of 7 to 10 minutes after secretion, when it is primarily metabolized by the liver. Forty percent to 70% of insulin secreted into the portal venous system is cleared by hepatocytes on the first pass through the liver. Excess insulin is then slowly metabolized by the liver, kidneys, and skeletal muscles. Both brain cells and red blood cells do not take up insulin.

Like all hormones, insulin binds to specific cell surface receptors that have been isolated and well characterized. The insulin receptor is a 300-kD glycoprotein. Stimulation of the insulin receptor is dependent on insulin concentration. Insulin resistance, present in type 2 diabetes, can be the result of decreased numbers of receptors or a decreased affinity for insulin.

Glucose is actively transported across cell membranes throughout the body by 55-kD membrane-bound facilitator peptides called glucose transporters (Fig. 51.12). There are several classes of glucose transporters with varying affinities for glucose. The GLUT-2 transporter located on B cells has a low affinity for glucose. This results in a low rate of transport at physiologic concentrations of glucose but an increased rate of transport at higher concentrations, with subsequent higher insulin secretion rates.[44] The loss of B-cell GLUT-2 transporter can contribute to the development of diabetes mellitus.[45]

Orally administered glucose has a greater effect on insulin secretion than an equivalent amount of glucose administered intravenously. This effect is called the enteroinsular axis and is related to the release of enteric hormones in response to glucose that also potentiate insulin secretion. Gastric inhibitory polypeptide (GIP) is an important regulator of this effect.[46] Additional gut peptides and hormones that stimulate insulin secretion include glucagon, glucagonlike peptide-1, and CCK, while somatostatin, amylin, and pancreastatin inhibit insulin secretion. Nutrients including certain amino acids (arginine, lysine, and leucine) and free fatty acids also regulate insulin secretion. Sulfonylurea compounds, which act independently of glucose concentration, also stimulate insulin secretion and are used in the treatment of type 2 diabetes, where the primary defect is peripheral insulin resistance, not insulin production or decreased islet cell mass.

B cells are also neuronally regulated. Both cholinergic and b-sympathetic fibers stimulate insulin secretion, whereas a-sympathetic fibers are inhibitory. A loss of pancreatic innervation in the setting of pancreatic transplantation can therefore result in changes in the pattern and quality of insulin secretion.

Glucagon Synthesis, Secretion, and Action. Glucagon, secreted by the islet A, is a single-chain, 29-amino-acid polypeptide with a molecular weight of 3.5 kD. Glucagon elevates blood glucose levels through stimulation of glycogenolysis and gluconeogenesis in the hepatocytes. Like epinephrine, cortisol, and growth hormone, glucagon is considered a stress

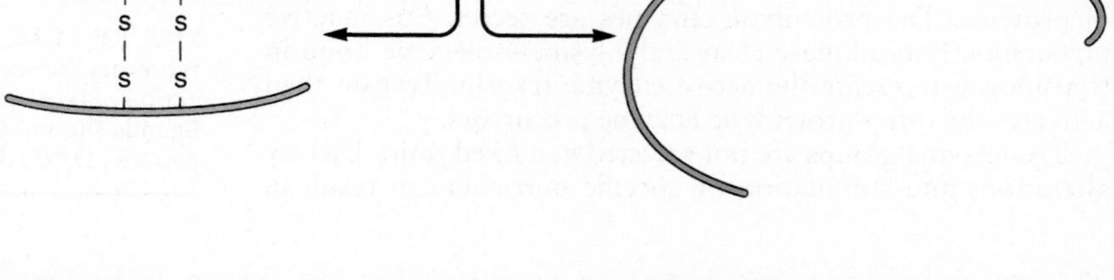

FIGURE 51.11. Synthesis of insulin. Proinsulin is synthesized by the endoplasmic reticulum and packaged within the secretory granules of the B cell. There it is cleaved into insulin and C-peptide. Equimolar amounts of insulin and C-peptide are secreted into the bloodstream.

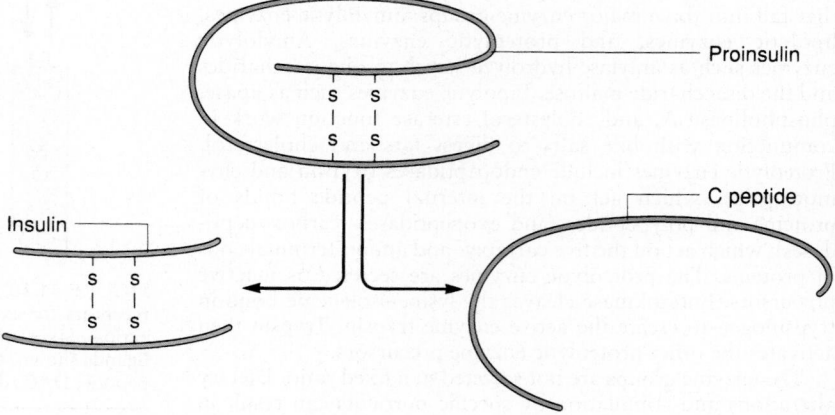

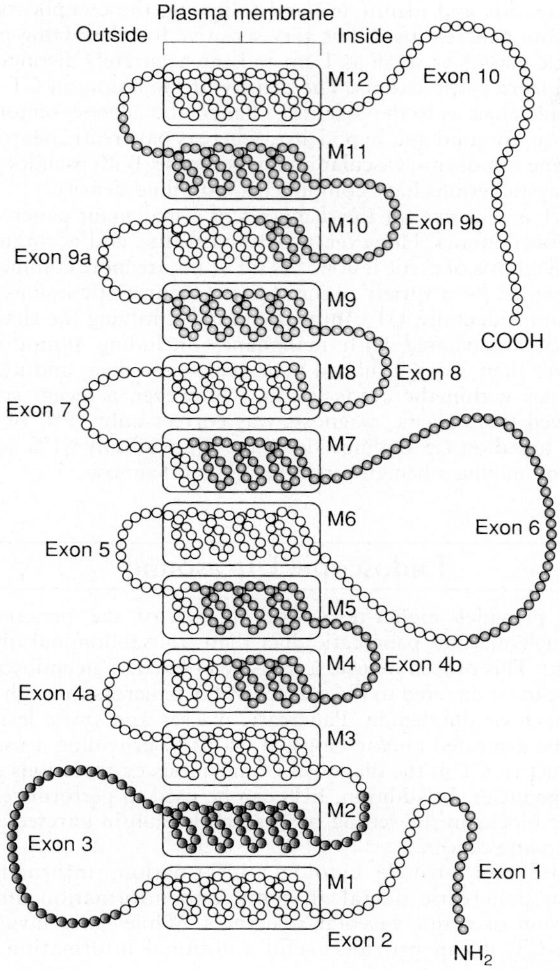

FIGURE 51.12. Model of the basic structure of a membrane-bound glucose transporter peptide, encoded by the gene divided into 10 exon regions. Membrane-spanning β-helical peptide chains are numbered M1 through M12. Mutations of the promoter region of the gene or the synthesis of an abnormal form of the protein could result in altered transport of glucose. For the B-cell GLUT-2 transporter, this could cause reduced sensitivity to glucose. For the muscle and fat cell GLUT-4 transporter, this could result in decreased peripheral uptake of glucose. (After Bell GI, Kayano T, Buse JB, et al. Molecular biology of mammalian glucose transporters. *Diabetes Care* 1990;86:1615.)

hormone because it increases metabolic fuel in the form of glucose during stress. Secretion of pancreatic glucagon is tightly controlled by neural, hormonal, and nutrient factors. Like insulin, glucose is the primary regulator, but the two hormones respond to glucose in reciprocal fashion. It has a strong suppressive effect on glucagon secretion. The two hormones are counterregulatory and function together to tightly control blood glucose levels. Excess glucagon can lead to hyperglycemia, whereas insufficient glucagon can lead to profound hypoglycemia. For this reason, the diabetes resulting from total pancreatectomy is very brittle and difficult to control due to the lack of endogenous glucagon to balance exogenously administered insulin.

Glucagon secretion is also stimulated by the amino acids arginine and alanine. Through paracrine effects within the islets, both insulin and somatostatin have a suppressive effect on glucagon secretion. The neural regulation of glucagon parallels that of insulin, with cholinergic fibers being strongly stimulatory, B-sympathetic fibers being weakly stimulatory, and A-sympathetic fibers being inhibitory.

Dysfunctional A-cell secretion of glucagon may play a role in the elevation of blood sugar in diabetes. Suppression of glucagon with somatostatin has been shown to improve glucose control in type 1 (insulin-dependent) diabetes.[47]

Somatostatin Synthesis, Secretion, and Action.

11 Somatostatin is a 14-amino-acid polypeptide that inhibits the release of growth hormone. While endogenous somatostatin has not proven to directly influence the secretion of other peptide hormones from islet cells, exogenous administration of somatostatin has been shown to inhibit the release of insulin, glucagon, and pancreatic polypeptide (PP). It has also been shown to inhibit gastric, pancreatic, and biliary secretion.

A synthetic octapeptide that mimics somatostatin pharmacologically (Octreotide, Novartis, East Hanover, NJ) has been developed. It is a more potent inhibitor of growth hormone, glucagon, and insulin secretion than the natural hormone. The potent inhibitory effect of octreotide has been used to treat both exocrine and endocrine disorders of the pancreas. For example, in hormone-producing islet cell tumors that express somatostatin receptors, octreotide can effectively suppress the hormonal symptoms associated with the disease process.[48] Although still controversial due to mixed results, a recent meta-analysis has shown that prophylactic octreotide reduces pancreatic fistula formation following elective pancreatic surgery.[49] It has also been shown to decrease iatrogenic pancreatic fistula output once a fistula has developed.

Pancreatic Polypeptide Synthesis, Secretion, and Action. PP is a 36-amino-acid polypeptide secreted by the F cells of the pancreatic islet. The physiologic role of PP remains unclear. It has been shown to inhibit pancreatic exocrine secretion and gallbladder emptying. Cholinergic innervation predominantly regulates PP secretion. As a result, surgical vagotomy ablates the increased PP response normally observed after meals. In diabetes and normal aging, PP secretion is increased, resulting in increased circulating PP levels.

Other Peptide Products

Other peptides are secreted within the pancreatic islet. These include neuropeptides such as VIP, galanin, and serotonin, which are believed to play a role in the regulation of islet cell secretion. Amylin, a 36-amino-acid polypeptide, is secreted by the B cells, but not in equimolar amounts to proinsulin. Amylin inhibits secretion of insulin and its uptake in the periphery. Amylin has been found to be deposited in the pancreas of patients with type 2 diabetes and has been implicated in the pathogenesis of the disease. Pancreastatin is another peptide found in large amounts in the pancreas. It is a derivative of chromogranin A, but its physiologic significance is unknown.

DIAGNOSTIC APPROACH TO PATIENTS WITH PANCREATIC DISEASE

Pancreatic Imaging (Studies of Pancreatic Structure)

If pancreatic disease is suspected, the pancreas can be imaged by several radiographic modalities including plain abdominal radiographs, upper gastrointestinal series, abdominal ultrasonography, CT, MRCP, endoscopic retrograde cholangiopancreatography (ERCP), and EUS.

Abdominal Plain Films

Plain films of the abdomen may be useful in patients with acute and chronic pancreatitis. In patients with acute pancreatitis, the most common findings on plain film include a generalized ileus with air–fluid levels, a localized ileus or "sentinel loop" of jejunum or duodenum in the area of the inflamed pancreas, or a cutoff of the colon due to distention of the transverse colon. In the setting of acute pancreatic fluid collections or pseudocysts, you can see an actual mass on plain film with displacement of the stomach or duodenum.[50] These findings are not sensitive or specific for acute pancreatitis, but in the setting of elevated amylase and lipase and associated abdominal symptoms, they can provide support for the diagnosis and an indication for more sensitive pancreatic imaging studies.

In the setting of chronic pancreatitis, the most common finding on plain film is the presence of calcifications within the pancreas. These are most commonly seen at the level of the second lumbar vertebra, where the pancreas lies in the retroperitoneum.

Upper Gastrointestinal Series

In the setting of a mass or mass effect on plain film, an upper gastrointestinal series can demonstrate displacement of the stomach or duodenum by a retroperitoneal mass. Displacement or narrowing of the duodenal C loop suggests the presence of a pancreatic mass. However, the character of the mass (inflammatory, neoplastic, cystic, etc.) cannot be further defined on upper gastrointestinal series.[50] For this reason, the upper gastrointestinal series has been largely replaced by ultrasound and other three-dimensional imaging modalities such as CT or MRCP.

Ultrasonography

Abdominal ultrasound can be useful in the setting of acute pancreatitis, chronic pancreatitis, pancreatic cystic lesions, pancreatic pseudocysts, and pancreatic cancer. In acute pancreatitis, the abdominal ultrasound may demonstrate gallstones, suggesting a potential etiology. In addition, the ultrasound can identify an enlarged pancreas, pancreatic edema, and peripancreatic fluid collections consistent with the diagnosis of acute pancreatitis. Ultrasound can also identify pancreatic pseudocysts, cystic lesions, and other pancreatic masses.[50] Pancreatic pseudocysts usually appear as a smooth, round fluid collection without acoustic shadowing. A pancreatic cancer is more likely to distort the underlying pancreatic anatomy and appear as a localized, solid lesion on ultrasound, also without acoustic shadowing. Cystic neoplasms of the pancreas can have both solid and cystic components. They can be uniloculated or multiloculated and contain cysts of varying size.

Ultrasound examination can be limited by obesity, overlying bowel gas, and recently performed barium contrast studies. Small masses or fluid collections can be easily missed. The presence of a mass on ultrasound is an indication for more extensive workup via CT or MRCP imaging.

Computed Tomography

Contrast-enhanced, helical three-dimensional CT is the most commonly performed study for the detection and characterization of pancreatic solid and cystic tumors. It is also useful in defining the pancreatic anatomy in the presence of chronic pancreatitis and identifying and following the complications of acute pancreatitis. CT is very sensitive for identifying pancreatic masses as small as 1 cm and can accurately distinguish solid from cystic lesions. The density of the lesion on CT can provide clues as to the diagnosis. Pancreatic adenocarcinomas are usually solid and hypodense, whereas pancreatic neuroendocrine tumors are vascular and hyperdense. Both pseudocysts and cystic lesions have components with fluid density.

CT is sensitive for the diagnosis of a malignant pancreatic adenocarcinoma. However, it is less sensitive and accurate in the diagnosis of cystic lesions. As CT scans are more commonly performed for a variety of indications, many cystic lesions are found incidentally. CT can be useful in identifying the characteristics associated with malignancy including tumor size greater than 3 cm, a dilated main pancreatic duct, and mural nodules within the cystic lesion.[51] However, a recent study showed that specific diagnosis was correct only 39% of the time based on CT findings alone and CT was only 61% accurate in making a benign versus malignant diagnosis.[52]

Endoscopic Ultrasound

EUS provides higher-resolution images of the pancreatic parenchyma and pancreatic duct than transabdominal ultrasound. This procedure uses a transducer fixed to an endoscope that can be directed to the surface of the pancreas through the stomach or duodenum. Pancreatic masses and cystic lesions can be aspirated and/or biopsied via EUS, providing a useful adjunct to CT in the diagnosis of mucinous cystic lesions and malignancies. In addition, EUS can be used to perform celiac nerve blocks in the setting of intractable pain in unresectable pancreatic cancer.

EUS can provide cytologic information, information about pancreatic ductal anatomy, and information about invasion of major vascular structures. While more invasive than CT, it can provide useful additional information. In addition, it can provide information about pancreatic ductal anatomy without invasive pancreatography (ERCP), which can cause severe pancreatitis. As with any endoscopic procedure, the risks include perforation of the stomach and/or duodenum.

A list of 11 EUS criteria have been defined for the diagnosis of chronic pancreatitis. The ductal criteria include pancreatic duct stones, echogenic ductal walls, irregular ductal walls, pancreatic duct strictures, visible side branches, and ductal dilatation. The parenchyma criteria include echogenic strands, echogenic foci, calcifications, lobular contour, and pancreatic cysts. Recent studies have determined that three or more EUS criteria provide the best balance of sensitivity and specificity for histologic pancreatic fibrosis.[53]

Magnetic Resonance Cholangiopancreatography

MRCP using three-dimensional turbo spin-echo techniques is now being used more commonly as a noninvasive way to image both the bile duct and pancreatic duct. This imaging modality can provide excellent images and detect abnormalities of the common bile duct and main pancreatic duct, but it is more limited in its ability to detect abnormalities in the secondary ducts. This noninvasive imaging technique is very useful in high-risk patients and pregnant patients. It is also useful in diagnosis, especially in settings where interventions such as biopsy or biliary drainage are unnecessary. MRCP can be a good modality for defining pancreatic ductal anatomy in patients with chronic pancreatitis and pancreatic pseudocysts to help plan operative management.

Endoscopic Retrograde Cholangiopancreatography

Like MRCP and EUS, ERCP can provide useful information about pancreatic ductal anatomy. Pancreatic cancer is characterized by obstruction or stenosis of the pancreatic duct and/or common bile duct (double duct sign). In chronic pancreatitis, the pancreatic duct may have irregularities including stenosis, dilation, sacculation, and ectasia. Pancreatic duct stones may be present within the pancreatic duct. Similar ductal changes can be observed immediately following acute attacks of pancreatitis.

As with any endoscopic procedure, perforation of the gastrointestinal tract is a potential complication of ERCP. Five to 20% of patients develop clinical pancreatitis after ERCP and 25% to 75% have elevated amylase and lipase levels.[50] There is no way to prevent post-ERCP pancreatitis; however, high-pressure injection of the pancreatic duct is thought to contribute. ERCP is performed less commonly since much of the information can now be obtained with CT and/or EUS. However, ERCP is still useful in the palliation of obstructive jaundice with endostent placement, neither of which can be achieved using the other modalities.

Tests of Pancreatic Exocrine Function

Several tests are useful in the assessment of pancreatic exocrine function. When pancreatic disease is suspected, the measurement of serum amylase and lipase levels serves as a useful screening test. As amylase is found in organs other than the pancreas (salivary glands, liver, small intestine, kidneys, fallopian tubes), serum amylase levels may be elevated in both pancreatic and nonpancreatic diseases (Table 51.3). Assays for the isoenzymes of amylase can be performed but are unreliable in determining whether the source of amylase is pancreatic or nonpancreatic and are not widely used. It has been shown that serum lipase is a more accurate biomarker of acute pancreatitis than serum amylase, with 19% of patients with acute pancreatitis having normal serum amylase levels, but only 3% having normal serum lipase levels.[54] Unlike amylase and lipase, serum trypsinogen is made only by the pancreas and may serve as a better marker for acute pancreatitis. Trypsinogen can also be measured in the urine and serves as a specific screening test for acute pancreatitis.[55,56] All three markers are cleared by the kidneys, so in the setting of acute renal failure, all may be falsely elevated.

TABLE 51.3

PANCREATIC AND NONPANCREATIC CAUSES OF HYPERAMYLASEMIA

Pancreatic Diseases Causing Elevated Amylase Levels
Acute, uncomplicated pancreatitis
Pancreatic pseudocyst
Acute peripancreatic fluid collections
Pancreatic ascites
Pancreatic necrosis and/or abscess (infected pancreatic necrosis)
Pancreatic injury/trauma
Ductal obstruction in pancreatic cancer, pancreatic cystic neoplasms, or chronic pancreatitis
Nonpancreatic Diseases Causing Elevated Amylase Levels
Perforated duodenal ulcer
Duodenal ulcer penetrating pancreas
Small-bowel obstruction
Ruptured ectopic pregnancy
Peritonitis
Salivary gland lesions (mumps, salivary duct stones, sialadenitis, iatrogenic ductal obstruction)
Other cancers (lung, esophagus, breast, ovarian)
Burns
Diabetic ketoacidosis
Renal insufficiency
Pregnancy

In the case of acute pancreatitis, serum amylase and lipase levels are usually elevated and peak within 24 hours of the onset of symptoms and return to normal within 2 to 4 days if the inflammation resolves. In cases of severe necrotizing pancreatitis, pancreatic ductal obstruction, and pseudocyst formation, amylase and lipase levels can remain elevated for much longer periods of time. While amylase and lipase levels are elevated in over 85% of patients with acute pancreatitis, their elevation is far less common in chronic pancreatitis, where the exocrine function of the pancreas may be impaired. Amylase levels may be normal in patients with acute pancreatitis if there is a delay in their diagnosis or if their pancreatitis is related to hypertriglyceridemia, which can falsely decrease the serum amylase levels.[50]

12 Several tests of pancreatic exocrine function require duodenal intubation: the secretin test, the dimethadione test (DMO), and the Lundh test. The classic test of pancreatic endocrine function is the secretin test.[57] A patient fasts overnight. A double-lumen tube is then placed in the duodenum. Basal collections are performed for 20 minutes and analyzed for total volume, bicarbonate output, and enzyme secretion. An intravenous bolus of 2 units of secretin per kilogram is given and four 20-minute collections are performed and analyzed as discussed earlier.

Normal values for the standard secretin stimulation test are 2.0 mL of pancreatic fluid per kilogram per hour, bicarbonate concentration of 80 mmol/L, bicarbonate output of greater than 10 mmol/L in 1 hour, and amylase secretion of 6 to 18 IU/kg. The maximal bicarbonate concentration provides the greatest discrimination between normal subjects and patients with chronic pancreatitis.[58] The results of the secretin stimulation test for different pancreatic disease processes is shown in Table 51.4.

The pancreas is known to metabolize the anticonvulsant drug trimethadione to its metabolite, DMO. To test pancreatic exocrine function, patients are given 0.45 g of trimethadione three times daily for 3 days. A double-lumen tube is placed in the duodenum and secretin is given to maximally stimulate pancreatic secretion. The duodenal output of DMO correlates well with exocrine function.[59]

Likewise, a Lundh test requires duodenal intubation, but this test measures pancreatic enzyme secretion directly in response to a meal of carbohydrate, fat, and protein. A patient fasts overnight, then has a double-lumen duodenal tube placed. Basal duodenal fluid collection is performed and patients are then given a meal consisting of 18 g of corn oil, 15 g of casein, and 40 g of glucose in 300 mL of water. Duodenal fluid is collected every 30 minutes for 2 hours and analyzed for trypsin, amylase, and lipase. This test relies on endogenous secretin and CCK secretion and may be abnormal in diseases involving the intestinal mucosa.

The triolein breath test is a noninvasive test of exocrine insufficiency.[60] Twenty-five grams of 14C-labeled corn oil (triglycerides) is given to the patient orally. The metabolite, 14C carbon dioxide, can be measured in the breath 4 hours after administration. Patients with disorders of fat digestion or absorption exhale less than 3% of the dose per hour. The test can be repeated after pancreatic enzyme replacement. Patients

TABLE 51.4

CHARACTERISTIC RESULTS OF SECRETIN TESTING: VOLUME, BICARBONATE CONCENTRATION, AND ENZYME SECRETION CHANGES IN PANCREATIC DISEASE PROCESSES

■ DISORDER	■ PATTERN	■ TOTAL VOLUME	■ MAXIMUM BICARBONATE SECRETION	■ ENZYME SECRETION
End-stage pancreatitis	Total insufficiency	Decreased	Decreased	Decreased
Advanced pancreatic cancer	Total insufficiency	Decreased	Decreased	Decreased
Chronic pancreatitis	Qualitative insufficiency	Normal	Decreased	Normal
Pancreatic cancer	Quantitative insufficiency	Decreased	Normal	Normal
Malnutrition[a]	Isolated enzyme deficiency	Normal	Normal	Decreased
Hemochromatosis, Zollinger-Ellison syndrome, cirrhosis	Hypersecretion	Increased	Normal	Normal

[a]Sprue, ulcerative colitis, and Crohn disease.
Adapted from Table 53.3 in "Pancreatic Anatomy and Physiology" chapter in last edition.
Originally from Dreiling DA, Wolfson P. New insights into pancreatic disease revealed by the secretion test. In: Berk JE, ed. *Developments in Digestive Diseases,* vol 2. Philadelphia, PA: Lea and Febiger; 1979:155.

with pancreatic insufficiency will achieve a normal rate of excretion of 14C carbon dioxide, whereas patients with enteric disorders show no improvement.

N-benzoyl-1-tyrosyl-para-aminobenzoic acid (BT-PABA) is cleaved by chymotrypsin to form para-aminobenzoic acid (PABA), which is then excreted in the urine. The PABA test is performed by administering 1 g of BT-PABA in 300 mL of water orally. Urine is then collected for 6 hours. Patients with chronic pancreatitis excrete less than 60% of the ingested dose of PT-PABA.

Suspected pancreatic disease can also be confirmed giving patients a test meal and measuring serum levels of the islet cell hormone pancreatic polypeptide. Basal and meal-stimulated levels of serum PP are reduced in severe chronic pancreatitis and after extensive pancreatic resection. After an overnight fast, a test meal of 20% protein, 40% fat, and 40% carbohydrate is ingested. The normal basal range of PP is 100 to 250 pg/mL. In severe chronic pancreatitis, the basal levels are often less than 50 pg/mL. The normal response to a meal is a rise in PP levels to 700 to 1,000 pg/mL for 2 to 3 hours after the meal. In severe disease, this response is decreased to less than 250 pg/mL. PP release depends on intact pancreatic innervation and can also be decreased after truncal vagotomy or antrectomy or in the setting of diabetic autonomic neuropathy.

The fecal fat test measures intraluminal digestion products and is used to distinguish between pancreatic dysfunction and malabsorption due to enteric disease. Many tests can help differentiate the two types of steatorrhea (Table 51.5). Steatorrhea from pancreatic dysfunction is the result of lipase deficiency and is usually not present until lipase secretion is reduced by 90%. Fecal fat content is measured over a 24-hour time period. If the fecal fat is elevated to more than 20 g, this indicates pancreatic insufficiency, whereas steatorrhea in the presence of low levels of fecal fat (<20 g) indicates intestinal

TABLE 51.5

DIFFERENTIAL DIAGNOSIS OF INTESTINAL AND PANCREATIC STEATORRHEA

■ PARAMETER	■ INTESTINAL STEATORRHEA	■ PANCREATIC INSUFFICIENCY
24-hour fecal fat	<20 g; soapy consistency	>20 g; only seepage
D-xylose	Abnormal (low)	Normal
Secretin test	Normal	Abnormal
Small-bowel series	Abnormal	Normal
Small-bowel biopsy	Abnormal	Normal
PABA test	Normal	Abnormal
PP response to meal	Normal	Abnormal
Vitamin B_{12} and folate	Abnormal (low)	Normal
Treatment with pancreatic enzymes	No change	Improvement

PABA, para-aminobenzoic acid; PP, pancreatic polypeptide.

dysfunction. A reduction of fecal fat can be used to demonstrate adequate replacement of pancreatic enzymes in patients with endocrine insufficiency. However, this test is time consuming and disliked by patients, and pancreatic enzyme replacement is often titrated based on symptom relief once the diagnosis of pancreatic insufficiency is made.

Tests of Pancreatic Endocrine Function

The most widely used test of pancreatic endocrine function is the oral glucose tolerance test. This test, used to test for diabetes, measures the body's ability to utilize glucose. The oral glucose tolerance test provides an indirect assessment of the insulin response to an oral glucose load as it measures the glucose profile and not the actual insulin response. After an overnight fast, two basal blood samples are drawn and glucose levels are analyzed. Patients are then given an oral glucose load of 40 g/m^2 over 10 minutes. Blood samples are then drawn every 30 minutes for 2 hours. The fasting glucose level should be less than 110 mg/dL. Fasting levels between 110 and 126 mg/dL are considered borderline diabetes, and fasting levels above 126 mg/dL are diagnostic of diabetes. The 2-hour glucose level should be below 140 mg/dL. Two-hour levels between 140 and 200 mg/dL are borderline, and 2-hour levels over 200 mg/dL are again diagnostic of diabetes mellitus. The insulin response to oral glucose can be affected by enteric factors including hormones involved in the enteroinsular axis (GIP, glucagonlike peptide-1, CCK). The test can also be affected by antecedent diet, drug use, exercise, and patient age.

The intravenous glucose tolerance test can be used to eliminate the gastrointestinal influences of glucose metabolism experienced in the oral test. This test measures the disappearance of plasma glucose after administration of an intravenous glucose bolus, which indirectly reflects both the secretion and action of insulin. This test is performed in similar fashion to the oral glucose tolerance test, except the glucose load is delivered as an intravenous bolus of 0.5 g/kg over 2 to 5 minutes. Blood is then drawn every 10 minutes for an hour. The disappearance of glucose per minute (K value) is calculated. A K value of 1.5 or higher is normal. The response to this test decreases with age, so the results should be age adjusted.

The intravenous arginine test and tolbutamide response test are used to help in diagnosis of hormone-secreting tumors. Arginine is known to stimulate the secretion of islet cell hormones. After an overnight fast, a patient is given a 30-minute intravenous infusion of 0.5 g/kg of arginine. Blood samples are taken every 10 minutes and radioimmunoassay are performed for the hormone in question. This test is most useful for glucagon-secreting tumors. Elevations of plasma glucagon levels to over 400 pg/mL are diagnostic for glucagonoma.

Tolbutamide is a sulfonylurea that stimulates insulin secretion. After the patient fasts overnight, blood samples are drawn and the patient is given 1 g of tolbutamide intravenously. Blood glucose is monitored for 1 hour and blood samples are drawn to determine levels of the hormone of interest. Sustained hypoglycemia with hypersecretion of insulin is diagnostic of insulinoma. Somatostatin levels more than twice as high as the normal values of the particular assay used are considered diagnostic of somatostatinoma.

In making the diagnosis of insulinoma, surreptitious exogenous administration of insulin must be ruled out. Both insulin and C-peptide levels can be measured in the bloodstream and should be present in a 1:1 ratio. Surreptitious administration of exogenous insulin can be differentiated from insulinoma by the absence of C-peptide in the case of the exogenously administered insulin. The "gold standard" for diagnosis of insulinoma is the 72-hour monitored fast. This test attempts to document the Whipple triad of hypoglycemia, neuroglycopenic symptoms concurrent with hypoglycemia, and resolution of symptoms with administration of glucose. Patients are fasted in a monitored setting. All nonessential medications are stopped and patients can only drink water; black, decaffeinated coffee; and diet sodas. Glucose and insulin levels are closely monitored. The criteria for discontinuing the fast include serum glucose levels less than 45 mg/dL, and the patient must be symptomatic. The 72-hour fast is highly sensitive for insulinoma and a patient rarely finishes this test without an unequivocal diagnosis.

References

1. Klein SD, Affronti JP. Pancreas divisum, an evidence-based review: part II, patient selection and treatment. *Gastrointest Endosc* 2004;60(4):585–589.
2. Levy MJ, Geenen JE. Idiopathic acute recurrent pancreatitis. *Am J Gastroenterol* 2001;96(9):2540–2555.
3. Testoni PA. Aetiologies of recurrent acute pancreatitis: acute or chronic relapsing disease? *JOP* 2001;2(6):357–367.
4. Delhaye M, Engelholm L, Cremer M. Pancreas divisum: controversial clinical significance. *Dig Dis* 1988;6(1):30–39.
5. Delhaye M, Engelholm L, Cremer M. Pancreas divisum: congenital anatomic variant or anomaly? Contribution of endoscopic retrograde dorsal pancreatography. *Gastroenterology* 1985;89(5):951–958.
6. Cotton PB. Congenital anomaly of pancreas divisum as cause of obstructive pain and pancreatitis. *Gut* 1980;21(2):105–114.
7. Khalid A, Slivka A. Approach to idiopathic recurrent pancreatitis. *Gastrointest Endosc Clin N Am* 2003;13(4):695–716, x.
8. Manfredi R, Costamagna G, Brizi MG, et al. Pancreas divisum and "santorinicele": diagnosis with dynamic MR cholangiopancreatography with secretin stimulation. *Radiology* 2000;217(2):403–408.
9. Ravitch MM, Woods AC Jr. Annular pancreas. *Ann Surg* 1950;132(6):1116–1127.
10. Theodorides T. Annular Pancreas. *J Chir (Paris)* 1964;87:445–462.
11. Chevillotte G, Sahel J, Raillat A, et al. Annular pancreas. Report of one case associated with acute pancreatitis and diagnosed by endoscopic retrograde pancreatography. *Dig Dis Sci* 1984;29(1):75–77.
12. Glazer GM, Margulis AR. Annular pancreas: etiology and diagnosis using endoscopic retrograde cholangiopancreatography. *Radiology* 1979; 133 (2):303–306.
13. Zyromski NJ, Sandoval JA, Pitt HA, et al. Annular pancreas: dramatic differences between children and adults. *J Am Coll Surg* 2008;206(5):1019–1025; discussion 1025–1017.
14. Ikeda Y, Irving IM. Annular pancreas in a fetus and its three-dimensional reconstruction. *J Pediatr Surg* 1984;19(2):160–164.
15. Guillou L, Nordback P, Gerber C, et al. Ductal adenocarcinoma arising in a heterotopic pancreas situated in a hiatal hernia. *Arch Pathol Lab Med* 1994;118(5):568–571.
16. Makhlouf HR, Almeida JL, Sobin LH. Carcinoma in jejunal pancreatic heterotopia. *Arch Pathol Lab Med* 1999;123(8):707–711.
17. Cooper GJ, Day AJ, Willis AC, et al. Amylin and the amylin gene: structure, function and relationship to islet amyloid and to diabetes mellitus. *Biochim Biophys Acta* 1989;1014(3):247–258.
18. Kleinman R, Gingerich R, Wong H, et al. Use of the Fab fragment for immunoneutralization of somatostatin in the isolated perfused human pancreas. *Am J Surg* 1994;167(1):114–119.
19. Cubilla AL, Fortner J, Fitzgerald PJ. Lymph node involvement in carcinoma of the head of the pancreas area. *Cancer* 1978;41(3):880–887.
20. Japanese Pancreas Society. *Classification of Pancreatic Carcinoma*, 1st English ed. Tokyo: Kanehara and Complany, Ltd.; 1996.
21. Ahren B, Taborsky GJ Jr, Porte D Jr. Neuropeptidergic versus cholinergic and adrenergic regulation of islet hormone secretion. *Diabetologia* 1986; 29(12):827–836.
22. Havel PJ, Taborsky GJ Jr. The contribution of the autonomic nervous system to changes of glucagon and insulin secretion during hypoglycemic stress. *Endocr Rev* 1989;10(3):332–350.
23. Yeo TP, Hruban RH, Leach SD, et al. Pancreatic cancer. *Curr Probl Cancer* 2002;26(4):176–275.
24. Sohn TA, Yeo CJ, Cameron JL, et al. Resected adenocarcinoma of the pancreas-616 patients: results, outcomes, and prognostic indicators. *J Gastrointest Surg* 2000;4(6):567–579.
25. Lillemoe KD, Cameron JL, Hardacre JM, et al. Is prophylactic gastrojejunostomy indicated for unresectable periampullary cancer? A prospective randomized trial. *Ann Surg* 1999;230(3):322–328; discussion 328–330.
26. Michaels AJ, Draganov PV. Endoscopic ultrasonography guided celiac plexus neurolysis and celiac plexus block in the management of pain due to pancreatic cancer and chronic pancreatitis. *World J Gastroenterol* 2007; 13(26):3575–3580.
27. Lillemoe KD, Cameron JL, Kaufman HS, et al. Chemical splanchnicectomy in patients with unresectable pancreatic cancer. A prospective randomized trial. *Ann Surg* 1993;217(5):447–455; discussion 456–447.
28. Tseng JF, Tamm EP, Lee JE, et al. Venous resection in pancreatic cancer surgery. *Best Pract Res Clin Gastroenterol* 2006;20(2):349–364.

29. Al-Haddad M, Martin JK, Nguyen J, et al. Vascular resection and reconstruction for pancreatic malignancy: a single center survival study. *J Gastrointest Surg* 2007;11(9):1168–1174.
30. Yekebas EF, Bogoevski D, Cataldegirmen G, et al. En bloc vascular resection for locally advanced pancreatic malignancies infiltrating major blood vessels: perioperative outcome and long-term survival in 136 patients. *Ann Surg* 2008;247(2):300–309.
31. Illuminati G, Carboni F, Lorusso R, et al. Results of a pancreatectomy with a limited venous resection for pancreatic cancer. *Surg Today* 2008;38(6): 517–523.
32. Adham M, Mirza DF, Chapuis F, et al. Results of vascular resections during pancreatectomy from two European centres: an analysis of survival and disease-free survival explicative factors. *HPB (Oxford)* 2006;8(6): 465–473.
33. Siriwardana HP, Siriwardena AK. Systematic review of outcome of synchronous portal-superior mesenteric vein resection during pancreatectomy for cancer. *Br J Surg* 2006;93(6):662–673.
34. Yeo CJ, Cameron JL, Lillemoe KD, et al. Pancreaticoduodenectomy with or without distal gastrectomy and extended retroperitoneal lymphadenectomy for periampullary adenocarcinoma, part 2: randomized controlled trial evaluating survival, morbidity, and mortality. *Ann Surg* 2002;236(3): 355–366; discussion 366–368.
35. Riall TS, Cameron JL, Lillemoe KD, et al. Pancreaticoduodenectomy with or without distal gastrectomy and extended retroperitoneal lymphadenectomy for periampullary adenocarcinoma–part 3: update on 5-year survival. *J Gastrointest Surg* 2005;9(9):1191–1204; discussion 1204–1206.
36. Greenberger N, Toskes P. Acute and chronic pancreatitis. In: Fauci AS, Braunwald E, Kasper DL, et al., eds. *Harrison's Principles of Internal Medicine*, 17th ed. New York: McGraw-Hill; 2008.
37. Valenzuela JE, Weiner K, Saad C. Cholinergic stimulation of human pancreatic secretion. *Dig Dis Sci* 1986;31(6):615–619.
38. Konturek SJ, Becker HD, Thompson JC. Effect of vagotomy on hormones stimulating pancreatic secretion. *Arch Surg* 1974;108(5):704–708.
39. Oh HC, Kim MH, Choi KS, et al. Analysis of PRSS1 and SPINK1 mutations in Korean patients with idiopathic and familial pancreatitis. *Pancreas* 2008;38:180–183.
40. Masamune A, Kume K, Shimosegawa T. Differential roles of the SPINK1 gene mutations in alcoholic and nonalcoholic chronic pancreatitis. *J Gastroenterol* 2007;42(suppl 17):135–140.
41. Leahy JL, Bonner-Weir S, Weir GC. Abnormal glucose regulation of insulin secretion in models of reduced B-cell mass. *Diabetes* 1984;33(7): 667–673.
42. Nanjo K, Sanke T, Miyano M, et al. Diabetes due to secretion of a structurally abnormal insulin (insulin Wakayama). Clinical and functional characteristics of [LeuA3] insulin. *J Clin Invest* 1986;77(2): 514–519.
43. Opara EC, Atwater I, Go VL. Characterization and control of pulsatile secretion of insulin and glucagon. *Pancreas* 1988;3(4):484–487.
44. Bell GI, Kayano T, Buse JB, et al. Molecular biology of mammalian glucose transporters. *Diabetes Care* 1990;13(3):198–208.
45. Orci L, Unger RH, Ravazzola M, et al. Reduced beta-cell glucose transporter in new onset diabetic BB rats. *J Clin Invest* 1990;86(5): 1615–1622.
46. Ebert R, Creutzfeldt W. Gastrointestinal peptides and insulin secretion. *Diabetes Metab Rev* 1987;3(1):1–26.
47. Gerich JE. Somatostatin and diabetes. *Am J Med* 1981;70(3):619–626.
48. Mulvihill S, Pappas TN, Passaro E Jr, et al. The use of somatostatin and its analogs in the treatment of surgical disorders. *Surgery* 1986;100(3): 467–476.
49. Alghamdi AA, Jawas AM, Hart RS. Use of octreotide for the prevention of pancreatic fistula after elective pancreatic surgery: a systematic review and meta-analysis. *Can J Surg* 2007;50(6):459–466.
50. Toskes PP GN. Approach to the patient with pancreatic disease. In: Fauci AS, Braunwald E, Kasper DL, et al., eds. *Harrison's Principles of Internal Medicine*, 17th ed. New York: McGraw-Hill; 2008.
51. Tanaka M, Chari S, Adsay V, et al. International consensus guidelines for management of intraductal papillary mucinous neoplasms and mucinous cystic neoplasms of the pancreas. *Pancreatology* 2006;6(1–2):17–32.
52. Fisher WE, Hodges SE, Yagnik V, et al. Accuracy of CT in predicting malignant potential of cystic pancreatic neoplasms. *HPB (Oxford)* 2008; 10(6):483–490.
53. Chong AK, Hawes RH, Hoffman BJ, et al. Diagnostic performance of EUS for chronic pancreatitis: a comparison with histopathology. *Gastrointest Endosc* 2007;65(6):808–814.
54. Smith RC, Southwell-Keely J, Chesher D. Should serum pancreatic lipase replace serum amylase as a biomarker of acute pancreatitis? *ANZ J Surg* 2005;75(6):399–404.
55. Kemppainen E, Hedstrom J, Puolakkainen P, et al. Increased serum trypsinogen 2 and trypsin 2-alpha 1 antitrypsin complex values identify endoscopic retrograde cholangiopancreatography induced pancreatitis with high accuracy. *Gut* 1997;41(5):690–695.
56. Kemppainen EA, Hedstrom JI, Puolakkainen PA, et al. Rapid measurement of urinary trypsinogen-2 as a screening test for acute pancreatitis. *N Engl J Med* 1997;336(25):1788–1793.
57. Dreiling D, Wolfson P. New insights into pancreatic disease revealed by the secretin test. In: Berk JE, ed. *Developments in Digestive Diseases*, vol 2. Philadelphia, PA: Lea and Febiger; 1979:155.
58. Toskes P, Greenberger N. Approach to the patient with pancreatic disease. In: Fauci AS, Braunwald E, Kasper DL, et al., eds. *Harrison's Principles of Internal Medicine*, 17th ed. New York: McGraw-Hill; 2008.
59. Noda A, Hayakawa T, Kondo T, et al. Clinical evaluation of pancreatic excretion test with dimethadione and oral BT-PABA test in chronic pancreatitis. *Dig Dis Sci* 1983;28(3):230–235.
60. Goff JS. Two-stage triolein breath test differentiates pancreatic insufficiency from other causes of malabsorption. *Gastroenterology* 1982;83(1 Pt 1): 44–46.

CHAPTER 52 ■ ACUTE PANCREATITIS

JASON S. GOLD AND EDWARD E. WHANG

KEY POINTS

1. In the United States, more than 75% of cases of acute pancreatitis are attributable to either gallstones or alcohol.
2. Approximately 80% of cases of acute pancreatitis are mild, are associated with minimal systemic derangements, and generally resolve within 5 to 7 days, even with minimal therapy.
3. Severe acute pancreatitis accounts for about 20% of cases and is defined as acute pancreatitis associated with one or more of the following: pancreatic necrosis, distant organ failure, and the development of local complications such as hemorrhage, abscess, or pseudocyst.
4. The mortality rate associated with severe acute pancreatitis ranges from 10% to 20%, with half of the deaths in the first 2 weeks as the result of systemic inflammatory response syndrome–induced multisystem organ failure and the remaining occurring later as the result of pancreatic necrosis/infection.
5. Computed tomography scanning is the most important imaging test for acute pancreatitis and is useful in confirming the diagnosis, assessing disease severity, and detecting complications.
6. The most important component of initial management of acute pancreatitis is fluid resuscitation.
7. Early endoscopic retrograde cholangiopancreatography with sphincterotomy and stone extraction has been shown in randomized controlled trials to benefit the subset of patients with gallstone pancreatitis who have associated obstructive jaundice and/or cholangitis.
8. Infection of pancreatic and peripancreatic necrosis complicates 30% to 70% of cases of acute necrotizing pancreatitis and most commonly becomes established during the second to third weeks after onset of disease.
9. Infected pancreatic necrosis can be diagnosed by fine-needle aspiration and is most effectively treated with mechanical débridement.
10. Treatment options for pancreatic pseudocysts include percutaneous aspiration, percutaneous drainage, internal drainage (performed surgically or endoscopically), or resection; surgical therapy is the best validated procedure and is associated with high efficacy and a low recurrence rate.

TABLE 52.1 CLASSIFICATION

TERMS USED IN THE CLASSIFICATION OF ACUTE PANCREATITIS

■ TERM	■ DEFINITION
Mild acute pancreatitis	Acute inflammation of the pancreas with minimal distant organ dysfunction and an uneventful recovery
Severe acute pancreatitis	Acute pancreatitis associated with pancreatic necrosis, distant organ failure, and/or the development of local complications, such as hemorrhage, abscess, or pseudocyst
Acute fluid collections	Fluid collections that occur early in the course of acute pancreatitis, are located in or near the pancreas, and lack a wall of granulation or fibrous tissue
Pancreatic necrosis	Diffuse or focal areas of nonviable pancreatic parenchyma, typically associated with peripancreatic fat necrosis
Pseudocyst	Collection of pancreatic secretions enclosed by a wall of fibrous or granulation tissue arising as a consequence of acute pancreatitis, chronic pancreatitis, or trauma to the pancreas
Pancreatic abscess	Collection of pus, usually near the pancreas, containing little or no pancreatic necrosis; arises as a consequence of acute pancreatitis or trauma to the pancreas

Acute pancreatitis is an acute inflammatory process of the pancreas with variable involvement of other regional tissues or remote organ systems.[1] In the United States, more than 200,000 patients are hospitalized annually with acute pancreatitis as the primary diagnosis.[2] It is the principal cause of approximately 3,200 deaths per year and a contributing factor in an additional 4,000 deaths. The direct cost attributable to acute pancreatitis exceeds $2 billion per year in the United States.

CLASSIFICATION AND DEFINITIONS

A useful and widely accepted system for defining and classifying the severity and complications of acute pancreatitis was developed during a multidisciplinary symposium held in 1992.[1] The clinically based definitions reached by consensus are shown in Table 52.1. Efforts to refine this classification system are currently under way.[3]

PATHOLOGY AND PATHOPHYSIOLOGY

The typical pathologic correlate of mild acute pancreatitis is *interstitial (edematous) pancreatitis*, in which the pancreatic parenchyma is edematous and infiltrated with inflammatory cells. Gross architectural features are preserved. In contrast, severe acute pancreatitis (SAP) can be associated with *necrotizing pancreatitis*, in which variable amounts of pancreatic parenchyma and peripancreatic fat have undergone tissue necrosis, with vascular inflammation and thrombosis being prominent features.

Studies using experimental models suggest that prototypical molecular and cellular derangements lead to pancreatic injury, regardless of the specific etiology or inciting event that triggers an episode of acute pancreatitis. Among the earliest of these derangements appears to be abnormal activation of proteolytic enzymes within pancreatic acinar cells.[4] Under normal conditions, trypsinogen and other digestive zymogens are stored in granules that are segregated from lysosomal enzymes (e.g., cathepsin B) and acid. Early in the course of acute pancreatitis, cytoplasmic vacuoles containing activated proteolytic enzymes appear. How the digestive enzymes are activated, and what role these vacuoles play, has been the subject of much investigation. In the prevailing model, trypsinogen is believed to be activated to yield trypsin either by colocalization with the lysosomal hydrolase cathepsin B[5] or through autoactivation due to a moderately acidic pH.[6] Recently, it has been noted that the cytoplasmic vacuoles appearing in the acinar cell in experimental acute pancreatitis share expression of proteins with autophagosomes. Autophagosomes are vacuoles that degrade cellular components such as organelles in the process of autophagy. Highlighting the possible importance of autophagy in the development of pancreatitis, mice lacking expression of the autophagy-related gene *Atg5* in the pancreas fail to exhibit prototypical features of acute pancreatitis.[7]

Acinar cell injury induced by active trypsin allows it to be released into the pancreatic parenchyma (Fig. 52.1), where it activates more trypsin and other digestive enzymes (e.g., chymotrypsin, phospholipase, and elastase). Trypsin can also activate the complement, kallikrein-kinin, coagulation, and fibrinolysis cascades within the pancreatic parenchyma. Activation of these enzymes is believed to initiate a vicious cycle in which

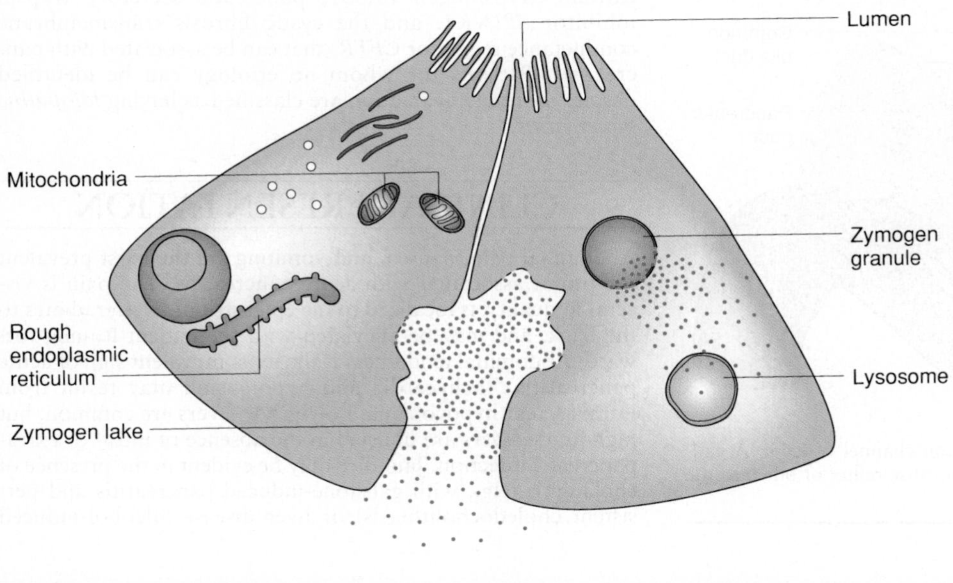

FIGURE 52.1. Schematic diagram depicting activation of proteolytic enzymes, possibly through colocalization of zymogen granules and lysosomes, and subsequent rupture of zymogen granules releasing the activated enzymes into the cytoplasm of the pancreatic acinar cell. The activated enzymes then undergo disordered basolateral discharge from the acinar cell into the pancreatic parenchyma.

activated enzymes cause cellular injury, an event that leads to the release of even more destructive enzymes. This cycle can overwhelm defense mechanisms that normally serve to limit the injurious consequences of premature trypsin activation within the pancreas (e.g., pancreatic secretory trypsin inhibitor–mediated inhibition of trypsin activity).

As injury progresses, the pancreatic parenchyma becomes infiltrated with macrophages and polymorphonuclear leukocytes, resulting in the release of a broad range of proinflammatory mediators (e.g., tumor necrosis factor; interleukins 1, 6, and 8; prostaglandins; platelet-activating factor; leukotrienes; and reactive oxygen species). The result of these events is pancreatic autodigestion, with injury to the vascular endothelium, interstitium, and acinar cells. Increases in vascular permeability lead to interstitial edema. Vasoconstriction, thrombosis, and capillary stasis can lead to ischemic (and perhaps ischemia-reperfusion injury) and the development of pancreatic necrosis. With severe pancreatic injury, the systemic inflammatory response syndrome (SIRS) and distant organ failure can occur. The systemic complications are believed to be mediated by digestive enzymes and inflammatory mediators released from the injured pancreas. For example, activated phospholipase A–induced digestion of lecithin (an important component of pulmonary surfactant) may play a role in the pathogenesis of acute respiratory distress syndrome (ARDS) that occurs in the setting of acute pancreatitis. In addition, the circulatory and inflammatory effects induced by acute pancreatitis are postulated to impair intestinal epithelial barrier function, allowing for the translocation of bacteria from the intestinal lumen into the systemic circulation. This phenomenon has been demonstrated to occur in animal models and may account for the pathogenesis of pancreatic and peripancreatic infection that can complicate necrotizing pancreatitis.

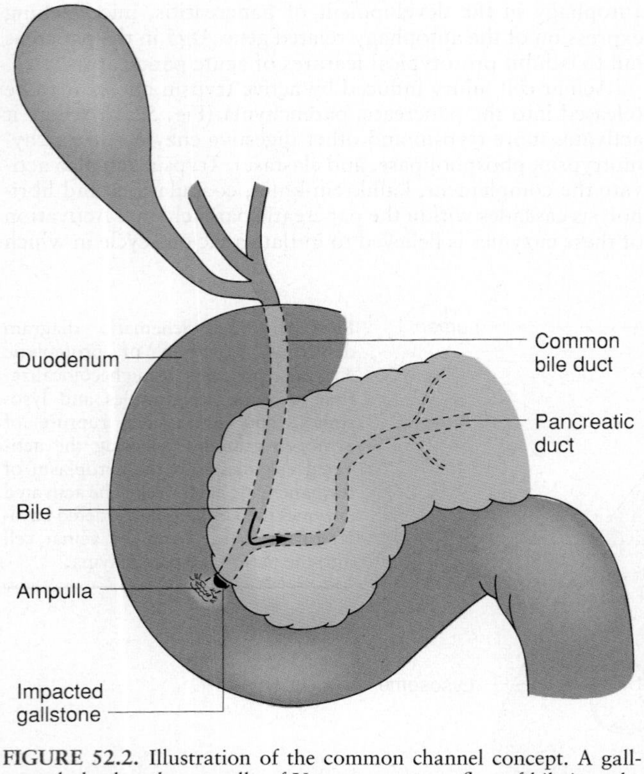

FIGURE 52.2. Illustration of the common channel concept. A gallstone lodged at the ampulla of Vater can cause reflux of bile into the pancreatic duct.

ETIOLOGY

1 Although many etiologies of acute pancreatitis have been described, in the United States, more than 75% of cases are attributable to either gallstones or alcohol.

Gallstones

Gallstones cause approximately 35% of episodes of acute pancreatitis in the United States. In a mechanistic model proposed over a century ago, a gallstone lodged at the papilla of Vater occludes the ampullary orifice, leading to retrograde reflux of bile into the pancreatic duct through a common channel shared by the common bile duct and the pancreatic duct (Fig. 52.2). Although elements of this model have been challenged, the prevailing view is that transient or persistent obstruction of the ampullary orifice by a gallstone or edema induced by stone passage is the inciting factor in the pathogenesis of gallstone-induced pancreatitis. *Microlithiasis* refers to aggregates (<5 mm in diameter) of cholesterol monohydrate crystals or calcium bilirubinate granules detected as "sludge" within the gallbladder on ultrasonography or on examination of bile obtained during endoscopic retrograde cholangiopancreatography (ERCP). An etiologic role for microlithiasis in acute pancreatitis remains unproved; however, data derived from case-control studies suggest that cholecystectomy or endoscopic sphincterotomy can reduce the risk of recurrent acute pancreatitis in patients with microlithiasis.

Alcohol

Ethanol causes approximately 40% of cases of acute pancreatitis in the United States. Most patients with alcohol-induced acute pancreatitis also have underlying chronic pancreatitis. Potential mechanisms by which alcohol induces pancreatitis include sphincter of Oddi spasm, obstruction of small pancreatic ductules by proteinaceous plugs, alcohol-induced metabolic abnormalities (e.g., hyperlipidemia), and direct toxic effects induced by alcohol and its metabolites (e.g., acetaldehyde, acetate, and nonesterified fatty acids).

Other Etiologies

A wide range of other etiologies of acute pancreatitis have been identified (Table 52.2). Ongoing investigations are beginning to reveal specific gene abnormalities (e.g., mutations in cationic trypsinogen *PRSS1*, pancreatic secretory trypsin inhibitor *SPINK1*, and the cystic fibrosis transmembrane conductance regulator *CFTR*) that can be associated with pancreatitis. Patients for whom no etiology can be identified despite thorough evaluation are classified as having *idiopathic pancreatitis*.

CLINICAL PRESENTATION

Abdominal pain, nausea, and vomiting are the most prevalent symptoms associated with acute pancreatitis. The pain is visceral in quality, is localized to the epigastrium, often radiates to the back, and may be alleviated with the patient leaning forward. Abdominal tenderness is the most prevalent sign of acute pancreatitis. Tachycardia and hypotension may result from intravascular hypovolemia. Low-grade fevers are common, but high-grade fevers are unusual in the absence of intra- or extra-pancreatic infection. Jaundice may be evident in the presence of cholangitis (e.g., with gallstone-induced pancreatitis and persistent choledocholithiasis) or liver disease (alcohol-induced

TABLE 52.2 **ETIOLOGY**

ETIOLOGY OF ACUTE PANCREATITIS

Gallstones
Ethanol
Iatrogenic causes ERCP Abdominal and nonabdominal operations Cardiopulmonary bypass
Trauma
Neoplasms (e.g., pancreatic cancer)
Pancreas divisum
Sphincter of Oddi spasm
Medications
Toxins Parathion Scorpion venom
Hyperlipidemia
Hypercalcemia
Infectious agents Viruses (e.g., mumps and Coxsackie B viruses, HIV) Bacteria (e.g., *Salmonella* and *Shigella* species; hemorrhagic *Escherichia coli*) Biliary parasites (e.g., *Ascaris lumbricoides*)
Genetic causes Cationic trypsinogen *PRSS1* mutations Pancreatic secretory trypsin inhibitor *SPINK1* mutations Cystic fibrosis transmembrane conductance regulator *CFTR* mutations
Autoimmune pancreatitis (lymphoplasmacytic sclerosing pancreatitis)
Vasculitis (e.g., systemic lupus erythematosus and polyarteritis nodosa)
Ischemia
Pregnancy

ERCP, endoscopic retrograde cholangiopancreatography; HIV, human immunodeficiency virus.

pancreatitis in a patient with cirrhosis). Evidence of retroperitoneal hemorrhage may become apparent if blood dissects into the subcutaneous tissues of the flanks (Grey-Turner sign), umbilicus (Cullen sign), or inguinal region (Fox sign); however, these findings are unusual.

2 Approximately 80% of cases of acute pancreatitis are mild, are associated with minimal systemic derangements, and generally resolve within 5 to 7 days, even with minimal therapy. The mortality rate associated with mild acute pancreatitis is less than 1%.

3 Approximately 20% of cases are classified as *severe acute pancreatitis* (SAP), defined as acute pancreatitis associated with one or more of the following: (a) necrosis of greater than one third of the pancreas; (b) distant organ failure (indicated by systolic blood pressure $\leq$90 mm Hg, serum creatinine $>$2.9 mg/dL, gastrointestinal blood loss exceeding 500 mL in volume within a 24-hour period, and/or partial pressure of arterial oxygen [PaO_2] $\leq$60 mm Hg); and/or (c) the development of local complications, such as hemorrhage, abscess, or pseudocyst.[1] 4 The mortality rate associated with SAP ranges from 10% to 20% in contemporary series.[8,9] One half of deaths occur within the first 2 weeks after the onset of symptoms; these deaths are primarily the result of SIRS-induced multisystem organ failure. Most of the remaining deaths occur 2 to 3 weeks after presentation and result from complications of pancreatic necrosis, especially infection.

DIAGNOSIS

The differential diagnosis of acute pancreatitis includes other conditions causing acute upper abdominal pain, such as biliary colic and cholecystitis, acute mesenteric ischemia, small-bowel obstruction, visceral perforation, and ruptured aortic aneurysm. Acute exacerbations of chronic pancreatitis can also be associated with clinical features resembling those of acute pancreatitis. The diagnosis of acute pancreatitis usually can be made by confirming biochemical evidence of pancreatic injury. Imaging tests should be used selectively to rule out other diagnoses and for the indications discussed later.

Laboratory Tests

With pancreatic injury, a variety of digestive enzymes escape from acinar cells and enter the systemic circulation. Of these enzymes, amylase is the most widely assayed to confirm the diagnosis of acute pancreatitis. Amylase levels rise within several hours after onset of symptoms and typically remain elevated for 3 to 5 days during uncomplicated episodes of mild acute pancreatitis. Because of the short serum half-life of amylase (10 hours), levels can normalize as soon as 24 hours after disease onset. The sensitivity of this test depends on what threshold value is used to define a positive result (90% sensitivity with a threshold value just above the normal range vs. 60% sensitivity with a threshold value at three times the upper limit of normal). Specificity (which also varies with the threshold values selected) is limited because a wide range of disorders can cause elevations in serum amylase concentration. Assays that detect increases in the serum concentration of amylase of pancreatic origin (P-isoamylase) alone are associated with greater specificity. Increased urinary amylase concentrations and amylase-to-creatinine clearance ratios occur with acute pancreatitis; however, these parameters offer no advantage over serum amylase concentrations, except in the evaluation of macroamylasemia (in which urinary amylase excretion is not increased despite elevations in serum amylase concentration).

Serum lipase concentrations increase with kinetics similar to those of amylase. It has a longer serum half-life than amylase, however, and may be useful for diagnosing acute pancreatitis late in the course of an episode (at which time serum amylase concentrations may have already normalized). Although lipase is more specific than amylase in the diagnosis of acute pancreatitis, note that lipase is produced at a range of nonpancreatic sites, including the intestine, liver, biliary tract, stomach, and tongue.

The magnitude of the increases in amylase or lipase concentrations has no correlation with severity of pancreatitis. In general, the magnitude of increases in amylase concentrations tends to be greater in patients with gallstone pancreatitis than in those with alcohol-induced pancreatitis; however, this finding is unreliable in distinguishing between these two etiologies.

Imaging Tests

Findings on plain radiographs associated with acute pancreatitis are nonspecific and include ileus that may be generalized or localized to a segment of small intestine ("sentinel loop") or transverse colon ("colon cut-off sign"), psoas muscle margins that are obscured by retroperitoneal edema, an

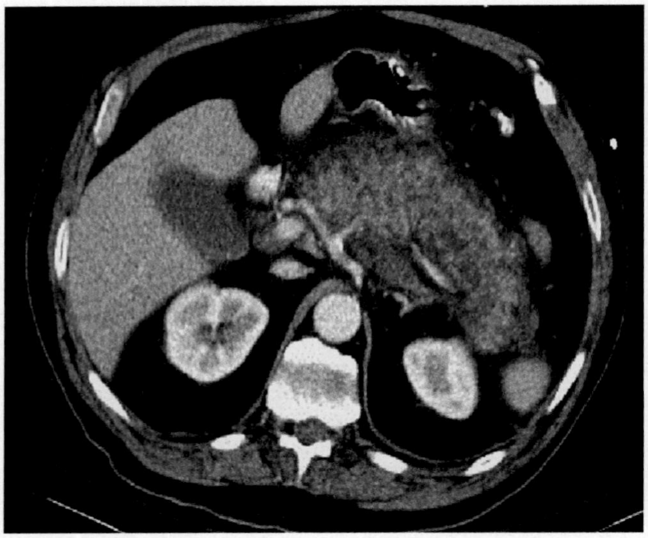

FIGURE 52.3. Computed tomography scan of acute interstitial pancreatitis.

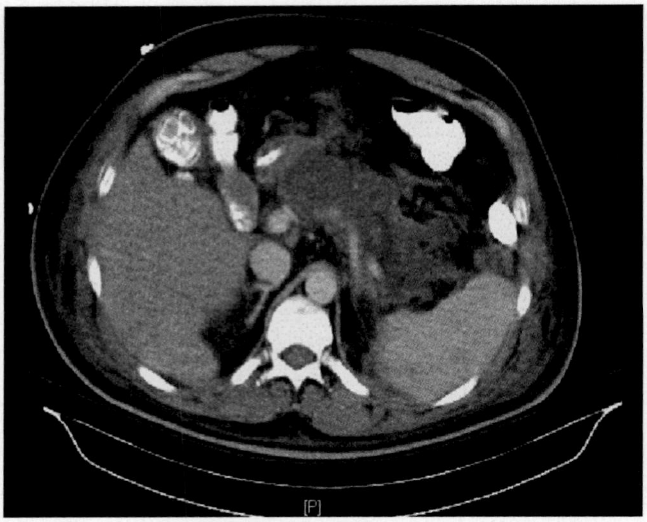

FIGURE 52.4. Computed tomography scan of acute necrotizing pancreatitis.

elevated hemidiaphragm, pleural effusions, and basilar atelectasis.

Ultrasonography may reveal a diffusely enlarged, hypoechoic pancreas. However, overlying bowel gas (particularly prominent with ileus) limits visualization of the pancreas in a large percentage of cases. Although ultrasonography has poor sensitivity in the diagnosis of acute pancreatitis, it plays an important role in the identification of the etiology of pancreatitis (e.g., the detection of gallstones).

5 Computed tomography (CT) scanning is the most important imaging test in the evaluation of acute pancreatitis. CT findings of mild acute pancreatitis include pancreatic enlargement and edema, effacement of the normal lobulated contour of the pancreas, and stranding of peripancreatic fat (Fig. 52.3). In addition, dynamic CT scanning performed after the bolus administration of intravenous contrast can demonstrate regions of pancreas that have poor or no perfusion, as seen with pancreatic necrosis (Fig. 52.4). Detection of necrosis plays an important role in assessment of disease severity, as discussed further later.

Magnetic resonance imaging (MRI) and magnetic resonance cholangiopancreatography (MRCP) are being used with increasing frequency in patients with acute pancreatitis. These examinations have the potential to offer better definition of pancreatic and biliary ductal abnormalities than CT scanning, and they are applicable in patients for whom ionizing radiation or iodinated intravenous contrast agents used in CT scanning are contraindicated. Disadvantages of MRI include high cost, limited availability, and the long duration of examinations.

ASSESSMENT OF DISEASE SEVERITY

Accurate prediction of severity early in the course of disease offers potential benefits in that complications can be anticipated and detected early through the use of intensive monitoring and frequent clinical assessment, and early and aggressive therapies can be instituted to attempt to prevent these complications. Routine clinical assessment at the time of admission is associated with low sensitivities (<50%) in identifying patients with SAP.[10] Therefore, alternative methods for assessing disease severity based on scoring systems, CT scanning, and serum markers have been widely studied. In addition to these methods, hemoconcentration and obesity have been reported to be predictive of severe disease.[11]

Scoring Systems

The Ranson criteria (Table 52.3) are easily tabulated, and the resulting scores are well correlated with morbidity and mortality rates.[12] The presence of three or more of these criteria is indicative of SAP. Important limitations of the Ranson criteria are that the predictive score cannot be determined prior to 48 hours following admission and that it can only be used once. Furthermore, because these criteria were developed using a cohort of patients for whom alcohol was the predominant etiology of pancreatitis, their generalizability may be limited. A similar predictive scoring system developed in Glasgow using a cohort of patients for whom gallstones were the predominant etiology of pancreatitis is available.[13]

TABLE 52.3 **STAGING**

RANSON CRITERIA FOR ASSESSING SEVERITY OF PANCREATITIS

AT ADMISSION	
Age	>55 y
WBC count	>16,000/mm^3
Glucose	>200 mg/dL
LDH	>350 IU/L
AST	>250 IU/L
WITHIN 48 H	
Hematocrit decrease	>10 pt
BUN increase	>5 mg/dL
Calcium	<8 mg/dL
PaO_2	<60 mm Hg
Base deficit	>4 mEq/L
Fluid requirement	>6 L

AST, aspartate aminotransferase; BUN, blood urea nitrogen; LDH, lactate dehydrogenase; PaO_2, partial pressure of arterial oxygen; WBC, white blood cell.

Acute Physiology and Chronic Health Evaluation (APACHE) II scores, which are based on patient age, indices of chronic health, and physiologic parameters, can be determined at any time after admission, can be updated continuously during the course of disease, and may have greater predictive power than Ranson scores.[14] However, the complexity of calculating APACHE II (or related APACHE III) scores limits its application in routine clinical practice.

Computed Tomography Scanning

The diagnostic application of CT scanning was discussed previously. For assessment of disease severity, dynamic intravenous contrast-enhanced CT scanning should be obtained. This technique is associated with greater than 90% sensitivity in the detection of pancreatic necrosis, a finding that is predictive of severe disease, and is indicated if clinical deterioration occurs or if one of the scoring systems discussed earlier suggests severe disease (e.g., presence of three or more Ranson criteria or APACHE II score ≥8). Because necrosis takes time to develop, a contrast-enhanced CT scan obtained too early in the disease course (e.g., at the time of admission) is unlikely to have predictive value. In addition, concerns that early administration of iodinated intravenous contrast agents used in CT scanning may exacerbate pancreatic injury have been raised, although these agents have not been shown to cause or exacerbate pancreatitis in humans.[15]

Serum and Urinary Markers

C-reactive protein (CRP) is an easily assayed marker for which serum concentrations are well correlated with disease severity. However, CRP levels do not become significantly elevated until 48 hours after onset of disease; therefore, this marker is not useful for early prediction of disease severity. Serum concentrations of neutrophil elastase and interleukin 6 and urinary concentrations of TAP (a product of trypsinogen activation) are also correlated with disease severity. Because these markers become elevated within 24 hours of disease onset, they may be relevant to early prediction strategies in the future. Currently, however, assays for these markers are not widely available.

MANAGEMENT

The goals of management for patients with acute pancreatitis are summarized next.

Correcting Pathophysiologic Derangements and Ameliorating Symptoms

6 The most important component of initial management is fluid resuscitation. Third-space fluid losses can be large, with up to one third of plasma volume being sequestered. An indwelling urinary catheter should be placed, intravascular volume should be frequently assessed, and aggressive fluid and electrolyte replacement should be ensured.

Patients with SAP, as well as those for whom initial resuscitation fails, are best managed in a dedicated intensive care unit (ICU). Central venous monitoring may facilitate fluid management. Patients should be closely monitored for development of distant organ failure, particularly respiratory, cardiovascular, and renal failure, so that supportive management of these conditions (positive-pressure ventilation, administration of vasopressor agents, and hemodialysis, respectively) can be instituted without delay.

Abdominal pain is usually ameliorated with intravenous narcotics. In the past, morphine was avoided because of concerns that morphine-induced increases in sphincter of Oddi pressure might exacerbate an episode of pancreatitis. However, there is no clinical evidence that morphine can induce or exacerbate acute pancreatitis. Other analgesic agents commonly used in patients with acute pancreatitis include meperidine and fentanyl. Evacuation of gastric contents using a nasogastric tube should be instituted if vomiting is a prominent symptom; otherwise, it is unnecessary.

Minimizing Progression of Pancreatic Inflammation and Injury

Identification of strategies for interrupting the inflammatory cascades that induce pancreatic injury and distant organ failure is an area of active investigation. Currently, the only method used in routine clinical practice is bowel rest (nothing by mouth). The rationale underlying this approach is that avoidance of bolus oral nutrient intake may limit stimulation of pancreatic exocrine secretion induced by the presence of nutrients in the intestine, particularly the duodenum.

Patients with mild acute pancreatitis generally need no nutritional support, as their disease typically resolves within 1 week. In contrast, patients with SAP usually have a more prolonged disease course and should begin to receive nutritional support as early as feasible. Although these patients traditionally have been administered total parenteral nutrition (TPN), accumulating evidence suggests that enteral nutrition is safe, is less costly, and may be associated with a lower complication rate than TPN.[16] Administration of enteral nutrition is also associated with the theoretical advantage of helping to maintain the integrity of the intestinal mucosal barrier, thus potentially limiting or preventing bacterial translocation. Enteral nutrients have typically been delivered to the jejunum through nasojejunal tubes to avoid stimulating pancreatic exocrine secretion; however, randomized controlled trials indicate that continuous feedings delivered through nasogastric tubes are equally safe and effective.[17] TPN is still required in many patients who do not tolerate enteral nutrition due to ileus.

Clinical trials of agents that inhibit activated pancreatic enzymes, inhibit pancreatic secretion, or interrupt the inflammatory cascade have yielded disappointing results. Meta-analyses of clinical trials of gabexate mesylate (a proteinase inhibitor), somatostatin, and octreotide suggest these agents have limited, if any, efficacy in improving outcomes in acute pancreatitis. A platelet-activating factor antagonist, lexipafant, showed promise in an initial study but not in a subsequent larger trial and is not currently recommended. Other adjuncts for which clinical trials have failed to demonstrate efficacy in limiting pancreatic injury in patients with acute pancreatitis include glucagon, anticholinergics, fresh frozen plasma, and peritoneal lavage.

Treating the Underlying Cause

This discussion is particularly relevant to patients with gallstone pancreatitis. There is both theoretical and experimental rationale to believe that removal of gallstones impacted at the ampulla of Vater early in the course of an episode of acute gall-
7 stone pancreatitis might limit disease severity. The efficacy of early ERCP to accomplish this goal has been subjected to prospective, randomized clinical trials.[18,19] These studies show that early ERCP with stone extraction and sphincterotomy benefits the subset of patients with gallstone pancreatitis who have obstructive jaundice and/or cholangitis. In the absence of these features, early ERCP is associated with high complication rates but no apparent benefits and is therefore not recommended.

There is a 25% incidence of recurrent pancreatitis or other gallstone-related complications during the 6-week period following an episode of gallstone pancreatitis in patients who do not undergo cholecystectomy. Indeed, there is a substantial incidence of recurrent pancreatitis and gallstone-related complications in patients with biliary pancreatitis whose cholecystectomy is delayed even 2 weeks after hospital discharge.[20] Therefore, cholecystectomy should be performed during the same hospitalization for most patients with mild gallstone pancreatitis. In severe biliary pancreatitis, the risk of deferring surgery needs to be balanced against the risk of performing early surgery in patients who are debilitated and nutritionally compromised. Endoscopic sphincterotomy is another option; however, the high risk of recurrent gallstone-related complications and the higher mortality compared to cholecystectomy suggest that this strategy should be reserved for patients with severe comorbidities precluding safe surgery.[21]

Examples of other measures directed at correcting the underlying cause of pancreatitis include cessation of drugs known to cause pancreatitis and treatment of hypercalcemia or hyperlipidemia.

Preventing and Treating Complications

Complications of acute pancreatitis include pancreatic abscesses and infected necrosis, acute fluid collections and pseudocysts, pancreatic ascites and fistulas, splenic vein thrombosis, and arterial pseudoaneurysms (Table 52.4). Infected necrosis and pseudocysts are discussed in detail next.

8 **Infected Necrosis.** Infection of pancreatic and peripancreatic necrosis complicates 30% to 70% of cases of acute necrotizing pancreatitis and most commonly becomes established during the second to third weeks after onset of disease. Historical data suggest that mortality rates associated with untreated
9 infected necrosis approach 100%. The diagnosis of infected necrosis is made based on cultures of aspirates of fluid or necrotic tissue obtained during CT-guided fine-needle aspiration (FNA) or specimens collected during surgery. The concordance rate between bacteriologic results of FNA and those of surgical specimens is greater than 95%.[22] In addition, the visualization of air bubbles within necrotic tissue on CT scans is highly suggestive of infection. Because the presence or absence of infection has a strong impact on surgical decision making, FNA should be obtained in patients with acute necrotizing pancreatitis who exhibit clinical features of sepsis or whose clinical course deteriorates beyond 1 to 2 weeks after onset of disease.

If FNA indicates the presence of infected necrosis, surgical intervention is indicated. Infected necrosis consists of thick and tenacious material that is most effectively treated with mechanical débridement. Traditionally, the abdomen is entered through a vertical midline or bilateral subcostal incision. The anterior surface of the pancreas can be exposed by dividing the gastrocolic ligament (greater omentum) and entering the lesser sac. If inflammatory changes have obliterated the lesser sac, this approach may be hazardous. In such cases, an alternative route to the pancreas is achieved by dividing avascular portions of the transverse mesocolon, with care taken to preserve the middle colic vessels. Clearly nonviable tissue should be débrided bluntly. Anatomic resections should be avoided to minimize potential for removing viable pancreatic parenchyma. The débridement field is irrigated with several liters of sterile saline, after which large-bore drains are placed. Postoperatively, the drains are left in place at least 7 days and until the effluent becomes clear. If more prolonged drainage is necessary because a pancreatic fistula develops, the surgically placed drains should be replaced with soft, smaller-bore drains to minimize potential for bowel erosion.

TABLE 52.4 **COMPLICATIONS**

LOCAL COMPLICATIONS OF ACUTE PANCREATITIS

Infected necrosis
Acute fluid collections
Pancreatic abscesses
Pancreatic pseudocyst
Pancreatic ascites
Enteric or colonic fistula
Splenic vein thrombosis
Arterial pseudoaneurysm
Hemorrhage

The procedure described previously is known as *necrosectomy with closed drainage.* In a variant of this procedure, both gauze packing and drains are placed at the time of surgery and gradually withdrawn postoperatively. Other procedures include *necrosectomy with open packing* and *necrosectomy with planned, staged relaparotomy* in which the initial operation is followed by repeat laparotomies, during which gauze packing is changed or additional débridement is performed, every 2 days until all necrotic tissues have been removed. Another option is *necrosectomy with continuous lavage* in which high-volume lavage of the lesser sac is performed, using drains placed at the time of surgery, until the effluent becomes clear and the patient's clinical course improves. These latter procedures are resource intensive but may be necessary if necrosectomy is performed early in the course of disease, before clear demarcation between necrotic and viable tissues has occurred. Modern mortality rates associated with necrosectomy performed for infected necrosis range from 10% to 20%.[8,9] On long-term follow-up, approximately 25% of survivors develop exocrine insufficiency, and 30% develop endocrine insufficiency.

Recently, less invasive approaches to necrosectomy have been reported. Percutaneous catheter drainage has been attempted. While this technique has become standard for pancreatic abscess, complete removal of all necrotic tissues often is difficult to achieve with drainage alone. A few centers have reported promising results using a video-assisted technique for mechanical débridement. This technique, called minimally invasive pancreatic necrosectomy, is usually accomplished through a retroperitoneal approach via flank incisions. Irrigation is usually continued postoperatively through surgically placed drains.[23] In a recently reported randomized controlled trial, patients with infected pancreatic necrosis were randomized to undergo primary open necrosectomy or a step-up approach consisting of percutaneous or endoscopic drainage followed, in most cases (65%), by *minimally invasive pancreatic necrosectomy*. Although mortality between the two groups did not differ, primary open necrosectomy was associated with a higher incidence of major complications.[24] Additional ongoing studies are evaluating the efficacy and safety of this and related approaches.

Although surgical débridement is clearly indicated for infected necrosis, its role in sterile necrosis has undergone evolution. In the past, early necrosectomy was recommended for patients with necrotizing pancreatitis, even in the absence of documented infection. The rationale for this approach was to prevent infection from developing and to remove the source of toxins and inflammatory mediators. Today, most authors recommend avoiding surgery in patients without documentation of infected necrosis, based on favorable outcomes reported using this conservative approach.[8,9] However, there remains a subset of patients with sterile necrosis who, despite prolonged supportive care, have persistent problems, including pain, malaise, and gastric outlet obstruction. If necrosectomy is performed to provide symptomatic palliation, it should be delayed until at least 4 weeks after onset of disease, to maximize the probability of clear-cut demarcation between viable and nonviable tissues.

Because of the high morbidity and mortality rates associated with infected necrosis, there has been much investigation into the use of antibiotics as prophylaxis against infection.

Initial clinical trials failed to demonstrate a benefit of prophylactic antibiotics; however, these studies were flawed by the inclusion of patients with mild disease who were at low risk for developing infected necrosis and the use of antibiotics with poor penetration into the pancreas. Trials were published in the 1990s showing a significant reduction in the incidence of pancreatic infection among patients receiving antibiotic prophylaxis, and based on this evidence, the use of antibiotic prophylaxis in patients documented to have necrotizing pancreatitis has become a widespread practice. Several recent trials that failed to show a benefit for prophylactic antibiotics have now been published.[25,26] Similarly, recent meta-analyses of the available trials have failed to demonstrate a benefit for patients receiving prophylactic antibiotics.[27,28] Disadvantages of using prophylactic antibiotics include the risks of fungal superinfection and the selection of resistant organisms. Another strategy for prophylaxis against infection in patients with acute pancreatitis has been the administration of probiotic bacteria to reduce the load of pathogenic bacteria in the bowel; however, prospective evaluation has yielded disappointing results.[29]

An algorithm for the general management of acute pancreatitis and pancreatic necrosis is shown in Algorithm 52.1.

Pseudocysts. *Acute fluid collections* develop in up to 30% to 50% of patients with acute pancreatitis. As most resolve spontaneously, no specific treatment directed at acute fluid collections is necessary in the absence of evidence that the fluid is infected. However, in up to 10% of patients with acute pancreatitis, these fluid collections progress to develop a wall of fibrous granulation tissue, at which point they are classified as *pseudocysts*. The walls of pseudocysts generally require at least 4 weeks from the onset of pancreatitis to develop. Pseudocysts are distinguished from true cysts, which have epithelium-lined walls.

Most pseudocysts are asymptomatic; however, they can cause upper abdominal pain, gastric outlet obstruction, and obstructive jaundice. They also have the potential to rupture, to bleed, and to become infected.

Pseudocysts are usually diagnosed on ultrasonography or CT scanning (Fig. 52.5). It is important to distinguish pseudocysts from cystic neoplasms of the pancreas, as these lesions can be malignant or have malignant potential. These lesions are being

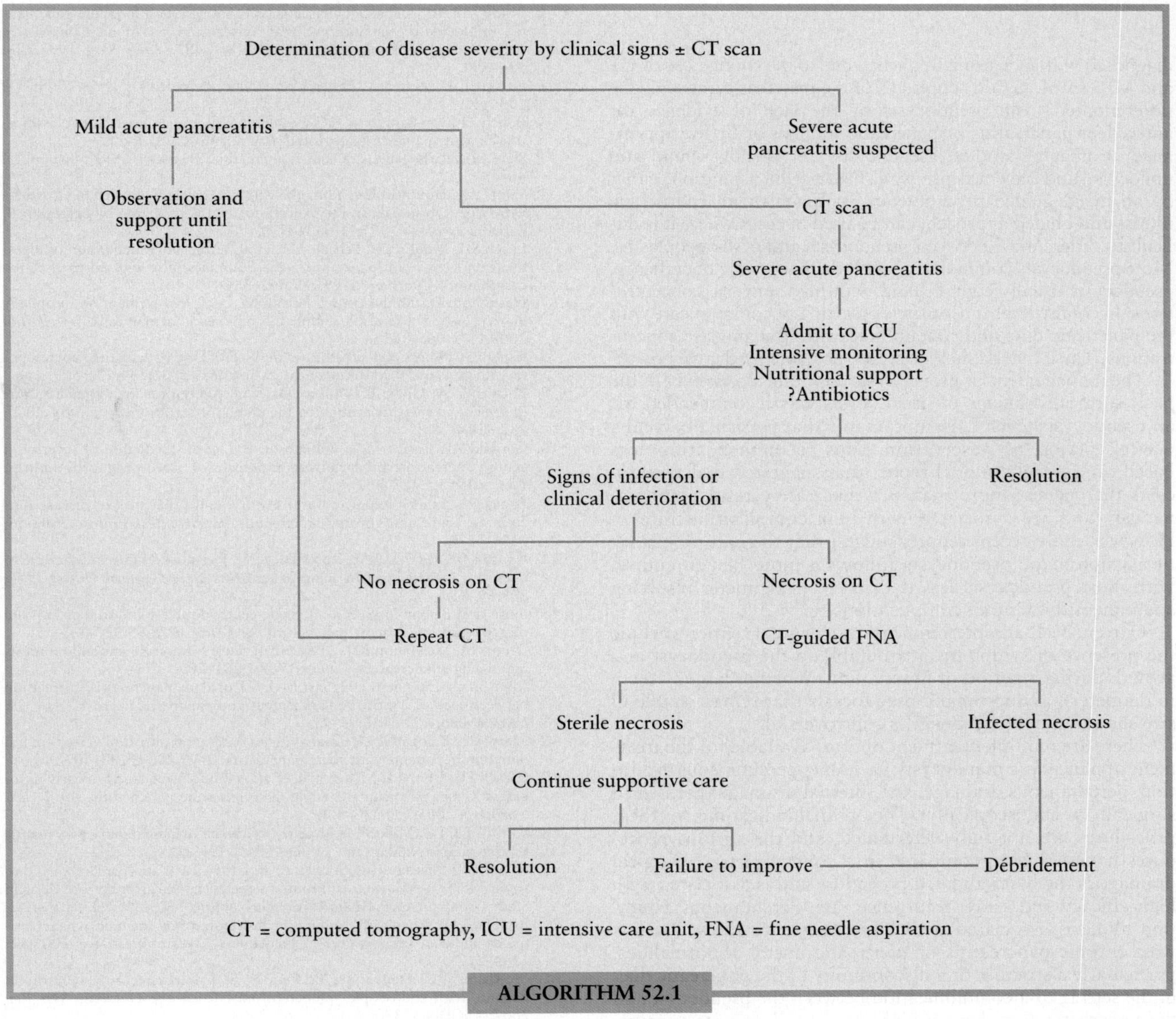

ALGORITHM 52.1. Algorithm for the management of acute pancreatitis.

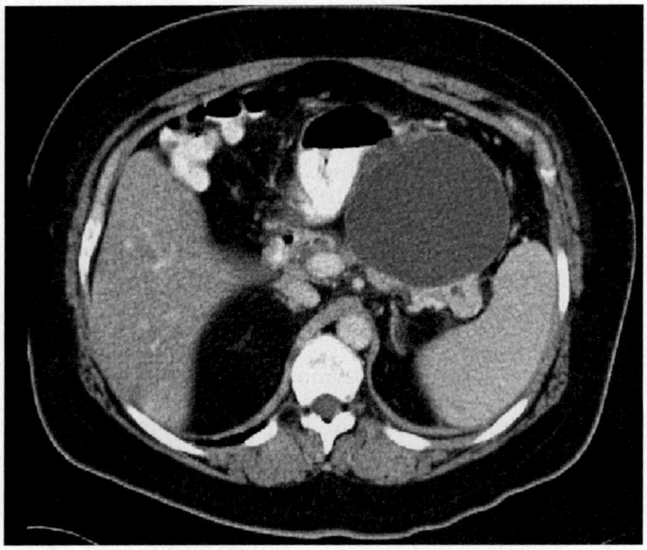

FIGURE 52.5. Computed tomography scan of pancreatic pseudocyst.

diagnosed with increasing frequency due to the routine use of CT and MRI scans. Cystic neoplasms of the pancreas can usually be differentiated from pseudocysts by the lack of evidence for antecedent pancreatitis or pancreatic trauma, or by the appearance on imaging studies. Pseudocysts are typically round and unilocular and have a dense wall. Fine-needle aspiration, either by an image-guided percutaneous approach or an endoscopic ultrasound-guided approach, can be used in cases where it is difficult to differentiate between pseudocysts and cystic neoplasms. Most pseudocysts communicate with the pancreatic duct; hence, pseudocysts usually contain fluid with high amylase concentrations. In contrast, most neoplastic cysts do not communicate with the pancreatic duct and contain fluid with low amylase concentrations. These criteria, however, lack absolute predictive power.

The management of pseudocysts continues to evolve. In the past, surgical drainage of pseudocysts was recommended for all pseudocysts (even if asymptomatic) that persisted beyond a 6-week period of observation. This recommendation was based on a widely quoted report that suggested that pseudocysts that persist more than 6 weeks rarely resolve spontaneously and are associated with high complication rates.[30] However, more recent reports suggest that the natural history of asymptomatic pseudocysts follows a more benign course, with most pseudocysts less than 6 cm in diameter resolving spontaneously without complications.[31,32]

Current well-accepted indications for intervention include the presence of symptoms attributable to the pseudocyst and growth during a period of observation. Whether large (>6 cm in diameter), asymptomatic pseudocysts that remain stable in size should undergo drainage is controversial.

10 There are multiple treatment options available for the treatment of pancreatic pseudocysts, including percutaneous aspiration, percutaneous drainage, and internal drainage (performed surgically or endoscopically). The optimal indications for these procedures are not fully determined, and the various procedures have not been compared in a controlled trial. Surgical drainage is the best validated procedure and is associated with high efficacy and a low recurrence rate. Percutaneous aspiration alone is associated with high recurrence rates. Patients with chronic pancreatitis or pancreatic ductal abnormalities, particularly a stricture or a discontinuity of the pancreatic duct in the setting of a communication between the pseudocyst and the pancreatic duct, have a high rate of failure with percutaneous drainage. Percutaneous drainage alone should be avoided in these circumstances.[33] Endoscopic cystgastrostomy is an option for patients in whom the pseudocyst is intimately adherent to the posterior wall of the stomach; however, high rates of bleeding-related complications have been reported in some series. Avoidance of surgical drainage was achieved in just under half of patients through the use of endoscopic and percutaneous procedures in one series. Operations performed on patients who were initially treated nonoperatively were associated with a greater morbidity rate than cases in which surgery was the initial pseudocyst intervention.[34]

The most commonly performed surgical procedures used to treat pseudocysts include cystgastrostomy, cystoduodenostomy, and Roux-en-Y cystjejunostomy. Cystgastrostomy or cystoduodenostomy applicable if a portion of the pseudocyst wall is adherent to the stomach or duodenum respectively allowing for the creation of anastomosis. Otherwise, the cyst wall can be anastomosed to a Roux limb of jejunum. These procedures, which can be performed as open or laparoscopic operations, should be delayed until pseudocyst wall maturation occurs. Mortality rates associated with surgical drainage procedures average less than 5%, with pseudocyst recurrence rates averaging 10%.

References

1. Bradley EL III. A clinically based classification system for acute pancreatitis. Summary of the International Symposium on Acute Pancreatitis, Atlanta, Ga, September 11 through 13, 1992. *Arch Surg* 1993;128: 586–590.
2. Frossard JL, Steer ML, Pastor CM. Acute pancreatitis. *Lancet* 2008;371: 143–152.
3. Bollen TL, van Santvoort HC, Besselink MG, et al. The Atlanta classification of acute pancreatitis revisited. *Br J Surg* 2008;95:6–21.
4. Steer ML. Pathogenesis of acute pancreatitis. *Digestion* 1997;58(suppl 1): 46–49.
5. Saluja AK, Donovan EA, Yamanka K, et al. Cerulein-induced in vitro activation of trypsinogen in rat pancreatic acini is mediated by cathepsin B. *Gastroenterology* 1997;113:304–310.
6. Leach SD, Modlin IM, Scheele GA, et al. Intracellular activation of digestive zymogens in rat pancreatic acini. Stimulation by high doses of cholecystokinin. *J Clin Invest* 1991;87:362–366.
7. Hashimoto D, Ohmuraya M, Hirota M, et al. Involvement of autophagy in trypsinogen activation within the pancreatic acinar cells. *J Cell Biol* 2008;181:1065–1072.
8. Ashley SW, Perez A, Pierce EA, et al. Necrotizing pancreatitis: contemporary analysis of 99 consecutive cases. *Ann Surg* 2001;234:572–579.
9. Büchler MW, Gloor B, Muller CA, et al. Acute necrotizing pancreatitis: treatment strategy according to the status of infection. *Ann Surg* 2000; 232:619–626.
10. Corfield AP, Cooper MJ, Williamson RC, et al. Prediction of severity in acute pancreatitis: prospective comparison of three prognostic indices. *Lancet* 1985;2:403–407.
11. Banks PA. Epidemiology, natural history, and predictors of disease outcome in acute and chronic pancreatitis. *Gastrointest Endosc* 2002;56: S226–S230.
12. Ranson JH, Rifkind KM, Roses DF, et al. Prognostic signs and the role of operative management in acute pancreatitis. *Surg Gynecol Obstet* 1974; 139:69–81.
13. Imrie CW, Benjamin IS, et al. A single-centre double-blind trial of Trasylol therapy in primary acute pancreatitis. *Br J Surg* 1978;65:337–341.
14. Larvin M, McMahon MJ. APACHE-II score for assessment and monitoring of acute pancreatitis. *Lancet* 1989;2:201–205.
15. Johnson CD, Stephens DH, Sarr MG. CT of acute pancreatitis: correlation between lack of contrast enhancement and pancreatic necrosis. *AJR Am J Roentgenol* 1991;156:93–95.
16. Marik PE, Zaloga GP. Meta-analysis of parenteral nutrition versus enteral nutrition in patients with acute pancreatitis. *BMJ* 2004;328:1407.
17. Eatock FC, Chong P, Menezes N, et al. A randomized study of early nasogastric versus nasojejunal feeding in severe acute pancreatitis. *Am J Gastroenterol* 2005;100:432–439.
18. Fan ST, Lai EC, Mok FP, et al. Early treatment of acute biliary pancreatitis by endoscopic papillotomy. *N Engl J Med* 1993;328:228–232.
19. Fölsch UR, Nitsche R, Lüdtke K, et al. Early ERCP and papillotomy compared with conservative treatment for acute biliary pancreatitis. The German Study Group on Acute Biliary Pancreatitis. *N Engl J Med* 1997;336:237–242.
20. Ito K, Ito H, Whang EE. Timing of cholecystectomy for biliary pancreatitis: do the data support current guidelines? *J Gastrointest Surg* 2008;12: 2164–2170.
21. McAlister VC, Davenport E, Renouf E. Cholecystectomy deferral in patients with endoscopic sphincterotomy. *Cochrane Database Syst Rev* 2007;(4):CD006233.
22. Gerzof SG, Banks PA, Robbins AH, et al. Early diagnosis of pancreatic infection by computed tomography-guided aspiration. *Gastroenterology* 1987;93:1315–1320.

23. Carter CR, McKay CJ, Imrie CW. Percutaneous necrosectomy and sinus tract endoscopy in the management of infected pancreatic necrosis: an initial experience. *Ann Surg* 2000;232:175–180.
24. van Santvoort HC, Besselink MG, Bakker OJ, et al. A step-up approach or open necrosectomy for necrotizing pancreatitis. *N Engl J Med* 2010;362:1491–1502.
25. Isenmann R, Runzi M, Kron M, et al. Prophylactic antibiotic treatment in patients with predicted severe acute pancreatitis: a placebo-controlled, double-blind trial. *Gastroenterology* 2004;126:997–1004.
26. Dellinger EP, Tellado JM, Soto NE, et al. Early antibiotic treatment for severe acute necrotizing pancreatitis: a randomized, double-blind, placebo-controlled study. *Ann Surg* 2007;245:674–683.
27. de Vries AC, Besselink MG, Buskens E, et al. Randomized controlled trials of antibiotic prophylaxis in severe acute pancreatitis: relationship between methodological quality and outcome. *Pancreatology* 2007;7:531–538.
28. Bai Y, Gao J, Zou DW, et al. Prophylactic antibiotics cannot reduce infected pancreatic necrosis and mortality in acute necrotizing pancreatitis: evidence from a meta-analysis of randomized controlled trials. *Am J Gastroenterol* 2008;103:104–110.
29. Besselink MG, van Santvoort HC, Buskens E, et al. Probiotic prophylaxis in predicted severe acute pancreatitis: a randomised, double-blind, placebo-controlled trial. *Lancet* 2008;371:651–659.
30. Bradley EL, Clements JL Jr, Gonzalez AC. The natural history of pancreatic pseudocysts: a unified concept of management. *Am J Surg* 1979;137: 135–141.
31. Vitas GJ, Sarr MG. Selected management of pancreatic pseudocysts: operative versus expectant management. *Surgery* 1992;111:123–130.
32. Yeo CJ, Bastidas JA, et al. The natural history of pancreatic pseudocysts documented by computed tomography. *Surg Gynecol Obstet* 1990;170:411–417.
33. Nealon WH, Walser E. Main pancreatic ductal anatomy can direct choice of modality for treating pancreatic pseudocysts (surgery versus percutaneous drainage). *Ann Surg* 2002;235:751–758.
34. Ito K, Perez A, Ito H, et al. Pancreatic pseudocysts: is delayed surgical intervention associated with adverse outcomes? *J Gastrointest Surg* 2007;11:1317–1321.

CHAPTER 53 ■ CHRONIC PANCREATITIS

NICHOLAS J. ZYROMSKI AND THOMAS J. HOWARD

PANCREAS/LIVER

KEY POINTS

1. Habitual alcohol use is responsible for 70% of chronic pancreatitis cases in the Western world; however, the precise pathophysiology of this disease is complex, incompletely understood, and almost certainly multifactorial.
2. Up to 90% of patients with chronic pancreatitis will experience pain at some point in their disease process. In contrast, 10% of patients will have painless pancreatitis.
3. Abdominal computed tomography is an excellent first test in the diagnosis of chronic pancreatitis; other diagnostic modalities include magnetic resonance imaging (MRI), endoscopic retrograde pancreatography (ERP), and endoscopic ultrasonography (EUS).
4. Medical treatment of chronic pancreatitis involves abstinence from ethanol and tobacco, as well as pancreatic enzyme replacement.
5. Surgical therapy may be required to treat mechanical complications of chronic pancreatitis such as biliary and duodenal stricture; however, the most common surgical indication is for treatment of pain.
6. Pancreatic anatomic changes in chronic pancreatitis are widely heterogeneous; selecting the proper operation for individual patients is crucial to obtain excellent outcomes.
7. Pancreas-directed operations may involve resection (pancreaticoduodenectomy, distal pancreatectomy, Beger operation), drainage (lateral pancreaticojejunostomy), or a combination of both resection and drainage (Frey operation).

Chronic pancreatitis (CP) has been defined by the Cambridge International Workshop on Pancreatitis as a "continuing inflammatory disease of the pancreas typically characterized by irreversible morphologic change and typically causing pain and/or permanent loss of function" [of the pancreas].[1] In 2010, the pathogenesis of CP is poorly understood, and no one ideal treatment currently exists. This vexing disease challenges clinicians and researchers alike; nevertheless, a significant number of patients afflicted with CP require medical attention. Surgical intervention targets the complications of CP; the heterogeneous nature of the disease mandates good clinical judgment to match the appropriate operation with the pathologic anatomy. In well-selected patients, the appropriate operation can provide durable relief of symptoms.

EPIDEMIOLOGY

The lack of a simple, consistent definition of CP hinders epidemiologic research. Estimates of CP incidence are widely variable—ranging from 1.6/100,000 new cases per year in Switzerland to as many as 14/100,000 new cases per year in the Cantabria region of Spain.[2,3] In the United States, it has been estimated that the incidence and prevalence of CP are 4/100,000 and 13/100,000, respectively.[4] With more widespread use of contemporary imaging modalities and a better understanding of underlying genetic predisposition to CP, future estimates will likely reveal an increased incidence and prevalence of chronic pancreatitis.

ETIOLOGY AND PATHOGENESIS

1 The principal cause of CP in the Western world is habitual alcohol use (up to 70% of patients).[4] Contemporary investigation supports the concept that the etiopathology of CP is complex and almost certainly multifactorial. Recognition of the fact that alcohol alone seldom causes CP and that only a small percentage (5%) of alcohol abusers will ever develop CP, in conjunction with the discovery of pancreatitis-associated gene mutations,[5] led to the proposal of the TIGAR-O classification system (*t*oxic/metabolic factors; *i*diopathic, *g*enetic predispositions; *a*utoimmune, *r*ecurrent, and severe acute pancreatitis; and *o*bstructive pancreatitis). This system allows organization and assessment of individual interacting risk factors and provides a framework for instituting risk-reduction strategies and specific therapy. Individual components of the TIGAR-O system are shown in Table 53.1.

Over the past 50 years, several theories have been proposed to explain the development of CP. In 1946, Comfort et al.[6] from the Mayo Clinic reported 29 patients with CP, concluding that

TABLE 53.1

CLASSIFICATION OF CHRONIC PANCREATITIS BY THE TIGAR-O SYSTEM

T	*Toxic and metabolic factors*
	Alcohol—increasing incidence of CP with duration of alcohol use
	Tobacco—etiology unknown
I	*Idiopathic*
	Early onset—mean age 20; pain predominant; calcification rare
	Late onset—mean age 56; relatively painless; calcification, endocrine, and exocrine insufficiency present
	Minimal change—abdominal pain syndrome; minimal pancreatic changes on imaging studies
	Tropical pancreatitis—tropical calcific and fibrocalculous pancreatic diabetes
G	*Genetic predispositions*
	PRSS1—cationic trypsinogen cannot be inactivated
	CFTR—cystic fibrosis transmembrane conductance regulator mutation; cannot hydrolyze mucus
	SPINK1—inactivates trypsin inhibitor
A	*Autoimmune*
	Lymphoplasmacytic sclerosing pancreatitis; increased IgG-4; increased association with other autoimmune diseases
R	*Recurrent and severe acute pancreatitis*
	Recurrent bouts of acute pancreatitis lead to chronic pancreatitis
O	*Obstructive*
	Stricture in main pancreatic duct leads to upstream (to the tail) ductal dilation, acinar atrophy, and chronic pancreatitis
	Caused by trauma, sphincter of Oddi dysfunction, pancreas divisum, sequelae of acute pancreatitis

Reproduced with permission from Etemad B, Whitcomb DC. Chronic pancreatitis: diagnosis, classification, and new genetic developments. *Gastroenterology* 2001;120(3):682–707.

the disease was caused by repeated bouts of acute pancreatitis. Nearly 20 years later, the consensus conference on CP in Marseille proposed that chronic pancreatic ductal obstruction (with proteinaceous and calcium plugs) was the underlying factor precipitating CP.[7] More recently, a hypothesis was advanced suggesting that toxic metabolites in the form of free oxygen radicals lead to increased lipid peroxidation and oxidative stress.[8] Clinical and basic investigations have supported this hypothesis. Nearly 50 years after the work of Comfort, their idea was revisited in the form of the necrosis-fibrosis hypothesis.[9] This hypothesis suggests that repeated bouts of acute pancreatitis lead to focal areas of necrosis, which are eventually replaced by fibrotic tissue. The central role of pancreatic stellate cells has received significant attention in this regard.[10]

Significant insight into CP pathophysiology has been gained from seminal work defining hereditary pancreatitis. In 1996, Whitcomb et al.[5] discovered a point mutation in the cationic trypsinogen gene (PRSS1). This mutation eliminates a fail-safe hydrolysis site in the trypsin molecule, subsequently rendering the molecule immune to inactivation by autolysis. Two other genetic mutations have subsequently been identified in patients with idiopathic CP. These genes encode the cystic fibrosis transmembrane conductance regulator (CFTR) and the pancreatic secretory trypsin inhibitor (SPINK1).[11–13] These discoveries provide insight into the molecular mechanisms of CP and advance diagnostic possibilities.

CLINICAL PRESENTATION

The clinical presentation of patients with CP involves pain, malabsorption (exocrine insufficiency), and diabetes mellitus (endocrine insufficiency). It is surprising that the interval between symptom onset and time of CP diagnosis ranges from 30 to 60 months.[14] Several factors likely play a role in this delay in diagnosis, including (i) unreliability of alcoholic patients (the most common etiology of CP); (ii) nonspecificity of abdominal pain; (iii) difficulty in diagnosing idiopathic CP; and (iv) difficulty in diagnosing the small percentage (7%) of patients with painless CP. It is not unusual for morphologic changes of CP to exist for some time before symptoms occur.

2 The vast majority of patients with CP experience abdominal pain. Typical CP pain is described as located in the epigastrium and boring through the abdomen to the midback. In some cases, the pain is felt to wrap around the right or left flank in a bandlike nature. The pain may or may not be exacerbated by eating and is often worse at night.

More than 90% of acinar function must be lost before symptoms of malabsorption appear.[15] Steatorrhea (fat malabsorption) usually precedes azotorrhea (protein malabsorption). Patients with steatorrhea complain of loose foul-smelling stools that appear greasy and float on the surface of the toilet bowl. Fat malabsorption may be accompanied by crampy abdominal pain and bloating. Weight loss and protein-calorie malnutrition commonly accompany malabsorption.

Most patients with CP will experience glucose intolerance at some point of their disease, and up to 60% will require insulin replacement. Endocrine insufficiency is due to a combination of decreased insulin production (as disease progresses and islet cell volume decreases) as well as a blunted insulin response. Diabetic ketoacidosis is rare; it seems that only a small amount of endogenous insulin/glucagon is necessary to prevent brittle diabetes.

DIAGNOSIS

The diagnosis of chronic pancreatitis is notoriously difficult in the early stages of the disease. The ideal gold standard for diagnosis of CP is histologic tissue analysis. Biopsy of the pancreas, however, is hazardous and not commonly available. Four principal modalities are currently used to image the pancreatic duct and pancreatic parenchyma: abdominal computed tomography (CT), magnetic resonance imaging (MRI), endoscopic retrograde pancreatography (ERP), and endoscopic ultrasound (EUS).

Radiologic Imaging

Identification of pancreatic calcification either on plain abdominal x-ray or on abdominal CT is pathognomonic for the disease; in this situation, the diagnosis of CP may be made with
3 90% confidence.[4] Abdominal CT is the first noninvasive imaging test of choice in diagnosis and should be performed with a specific pancreas protocol—i.e., with water as gastrointestinal contrast and scanning both without intravenous contrast (to detect calcification) as well as with intravenous contrast in the arterial and portal venous phase. This test is widely available, easy to interpret, and allows visualization of the entire pancreas and surrounding structures (Fig. 53.1).

Recent advances in MRI technique, including the application of secretin-stimulated imaging, have led to increased utility of this noninvasive test, particularly at dedicated pancreatic centers. Like CT, MRI allows visualization of the entire pancreas and peripancreatic tissues in cross section. In addition,

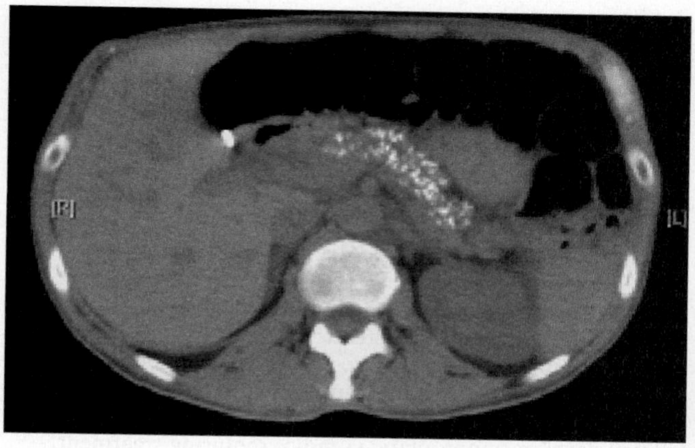

FIGURE 53.1. Abdominal computed tomography scan without contrast in a patient with chronic pancreatitis demonstrating marked parenchymal calcification.

image reformatting allows performance of magnetic resonance cholangiopancreatography (MRCP), which offers a specific view of the pancreatic ductal system (Fig. 53.2). Magnetic resonance imaging is noninvasive and avoids the use of ionizing radiation. However, this test is simply diagnostic and does not afford the potential for intervention offered by endoscopic imaging tests.

Endoscopic Imaging

Historically, ERP has played an important role not only in diagnosis but also in treatment of patients with chronic pancreatitis. Changes in the pancreatic ducts observed on ERP include dilation and irregularity of side branches in early disease, with significant main duct changes (stricturing, irregularity, tortuosity, calcification, and cysts) occurring as CP progresses (Fig. 53.3). The small but significant potential for complications (bleeding, perforation, acute pancreatitis) accompanying ERP must be weighed against the potential benefits of diagnosis (in more difficult cases) and the ability to provide therapeutic intervention.

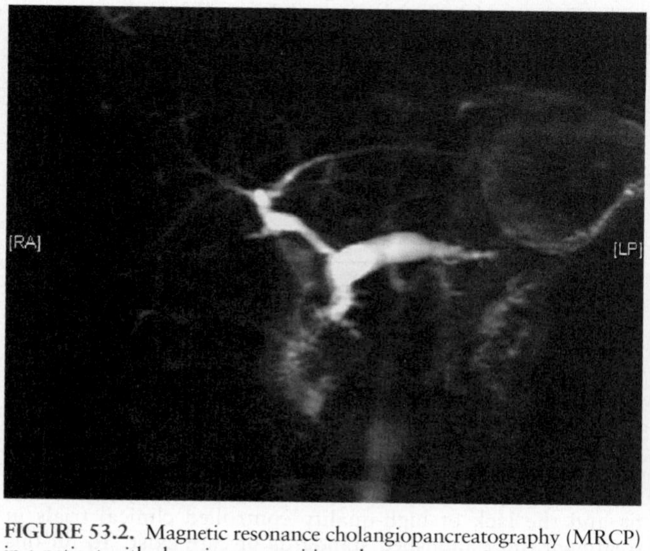

FIGURE 53.2. Magnetic resonance cholangiopancreatography (MRCP) in a patient with chronic pancreatitis and a narrow main pancreatic duct stricture downstream in the head. Note moderate biliary dilatation, marked main pancreatic duct dilatation, and dilation of side-branch pancreatic ducts in the uncinate process and tail of the gland.

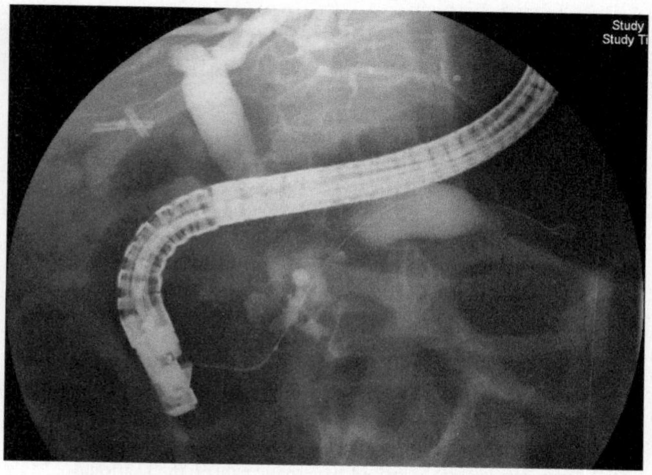

FIGURE 53.3. Endoscopic retrograde pancreatogram (ERP) in the same patient presented in Figure 53.2. This patient was treated successfully by pancreatic duct stenting.

Tremendous recent advances in the technique and application of endoscopic ultrasound have led to its increased use for diagnosing CP. Sonographic features of CP include irregularity of the pancreatic duct, hyperechoic duct margins, and hyperechoic stranding in the pancreatic parenchyma (Fig. 53.4). Data are accumulating that attempt to correlate these changes with parenchymal histology.[16] Advantages of EUS include its relative noninvasive nature, the ability to biopsy discrete lesions with great precision, and the ability to collect tissue (by fine-needle or core-needle biopsy) and pancreatic juice. The major disadvantage of EUS is the potential for significant intraobserver variability. Nevertheless, as further work to standardize definitions of sonographic CP evolves, it is likely that EUS will play an increasingly important role in the future.

Functional Tests

Pancreatic exocrine insufficiency invariably accompanies chronic pancreatitis; however, it is not necessarily diagnostic of CP. Tests of pancreatic exocrine function are mostly invasive

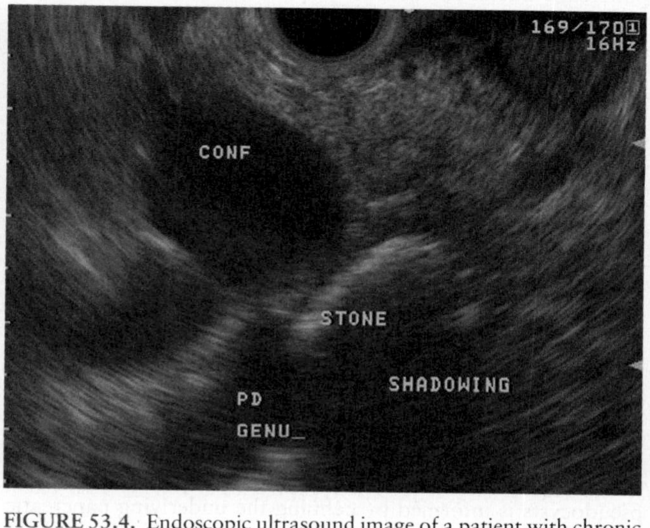

FIGURE 53.4. Endoscopic ultrasound image of a patient with chronic pancreatitis. Note hyperechoic pancreatic duct edges and large stone (stone) with posterior shadowing in the pancreatic head. Conf, confluence of superior mesenteric and splenic vein; PD, pancreatic duct; genu, genu of pancreatic duct.

TABLE 53.2

COMPLICATIONS OF CHRONIC PANCREATITIS

Pain	90%
Pseudocyst	25%–30%
Biliary stricture	10%–15%
Mesenteric venous thrombosis	5%–10%
Duodenal stricture	4%–5%
Pseudoaneurysm	2%–3%
Pancreatic adenocarcinoma	2%–4%[a]
Extrapancreatic malignancy	10%–15%

[a]Risk of pancreatic cancer is 2% after 10 years and 4% after 20 years with chronic pancreatitis; Lowenfels AB, Maisonneuve P, Cavallini G, et al. Pancreatitis and the risk of pancreatic cancer. International Pancreatitis Study Group. *N Engl J Med* 1993;328(20):1433–1437.

(i.e., collecting pancreatic juice by ERP before and after secretin stimulation), and are performed only at a few major pancreatic centers. In addition, results of these tests have been difficult to compare between centers. In general, pancreatic function tests have a limited role in diagnosing CP.

COMPLICATIONS

A wide variety of symptomatic and anatomic complications accompany the progression of CP. Of these complications, pain, pseudocyst, and biliary stricture are the most common (Table 53.2).

Pain

More than 90% of patients with CP have symptoms of abdominal pain at some point during the course of their disease. The mechanisms responsible for CP pain are incompletely understood but likely involve multiple factors including acute and chronic inflammation of pancreatic nerves as well as increased pancreatic ductal and interstitial pressure.[17]

Exocrine/Endocrine Insufficiency

Virtually all patients with CP demonstrate impaired exocrine function. This exocrine insufficiency is generally mild in the early course of the disease process. Patients with moderate to severe exocrine insufficiency should be treated by pancreatic enzyme replacement. Glucose intolerance appears later in the course of the disease (usually after 8–10 years). Patients with CP should undergo regular screening for endocrine insufficiency.

Pseudocyst

The true incidence of pseudocyst complicating CP is difficult to accurately identify, but likely ranges from 25% to 30%.[18,19] Pseudocysts by definition arise after disruption of main or side-branch ducts and may be solitary or multiple. Treatment of pseudocysts is informed by defining the underlying pancreatic ductal anatomy. It is worth mention that the classic teaching that all pseudocysts greater than 5 to 6 mm in size should be treated is no longer accepted by most pancreatic surgeons. Currently, indications for treating pseudocysts are related strictly to symptoms.[20]

Pseudoaneurysm

Pseudoaneurysms of the visceral arterial tree are generally seen in patients with concomitant pseudocysts. Interventional radiologic treatment (i.e., transarterial coiling) is successful in arresting hemorrhage in almost 100% of cases.

Biliary Stricture

Chronic inflammation and scarring in the pancreatic head leads to stricture of the intrapancreatic bile duct in up to 50% of patients. Many of these strictures are mild (in fact, clinical jaundice is generally preceded by asymptomatic elevation of alkaline phosphatase); however, between 10% and 15% of patients with CP will develop symptomatic jaundice requiring treatment.

Duodenal Obstruction

Pancreatic head inflammatory changes and/or compression by pseudocysts lead to duodenal obstruction in 4% to 5% of patients with CP.

Mesenteric Venous Thrombosis

The true incidence of splenic vein thrombosis in the setting of CP is unknown but may occur in as many as 5% to 10% of patients. Splenic vein thrombosis leads to left-sided (sinistral) portal hypertension, and clinically significant upper gastrointestinal hemorrhage from gastric varices may ensue. Most contemporary pancreatic surgeons reserve treatment of splenic vein thrombosis (i.e., splenectomy) for patients who have suffered a significant bleeding episode; prophylactic splenectomy has fallen out of favor.[21] Similarly, it is difficult to estimate the incidence of superior mesenteric vein and extrahepatic portal vein thrombosis in CP. Collateral veinous formation (cavernous transformation) in this setting significantly complicates operations targeting the pancreatic head.

Cancer

The specter of pancreatic cancer looms large in all patients with CP. Lowenfels et al.[22] showed the incidence of pancreatic cancer to be 1.8% after 10 years with CP and 4% after 20 years. Chronic inflammatory changes and fibrosis of the pancreatic parenchyma make the diagnosis of pancreatic cancer quite difficult in the setting of CP. It is notable that CP patients have a significantly elevated risk of developing extrapancreatic malignancy (10%–15%), primarily in the upper and lower airway and gastrointestinal tract.

THERAPY

Pain is the main symptom in CP, and although concomitant treatment of the physiologic derangements that occur in these patients such as diabetes mellitus (endocrine insufficiency) and steatorrhea (exocrine insufficiency) are important factors in improving an individual's overall quality of life, pain control remains the central focus for most patients. Due to the poorly understood nature of pain in patients with chronic pancreatitis and the lack of high-quality controlled clinical trials in treatment, no established standards of care exist. To fill this void, the American Gastroenterological Association developed an algorithm for treatment guidelines progressing from less-
4 invasive to more-invasive therapies.[23] The first step in management of patients with CP should be targeted at lifestyle

changes, specifically the avoidance of alcohol and tobacco. Total abstinence of alcohol can result in pain relief in up to 50% of patients, albeit mainly those with mild to moderate disease.[24] Miyake et al.[25] demonstrated pain relief in 60% of those patients who discontinued or reduced alcohol intake, whereas in the group of patients who continued drinking, spontaneous pain relief was only 26%. Similarly, cigarette smoking is associated with a higher risk of developing chronic pancreatitis and increases the likelihood of developing pancreatic calcifications, a structural change that may influence the yearly number of painful relapses.[26,27] Tobacco cessation in patients with established chronic pancreatitis reduces the risk of developing pancreatic calcifications.[28]

5 Treating patients with supplemental pancreatic enzymes has been hypothesized to work by stimulating receptors in the proximal small intestine to trigger a negative-feedback loop that suppresses baseline pancreatic enzyme secretion, decreasing ductal pressures and thereby decreasing pain. Several studies have been published with widely varying enzyme preparations, dosages, and outcome measurements. To date, the exact efficacy of this frequently used treatment modality remains unclear.[29,30]

If lifestyle modifications and medical treatment including pancreatic enzyme supplementation and the judicious use of narcotic and nonnarcotic analgesics fail to control symptoms, more invasive endoscopic and percutaneous techniques should be considered. The role of endoscopic therapy for pain in patients with CP involves sphincterotomy, lithotripsy, and pancreatic duct stenting.[31] While some of these interventions have shown significant promise, these results are largely confined to small cohorts of patients in specialized centers and have focused specifically on short-term outcome measurements. Celiac plexus blockade with a steroid (triamcinolone) plus an anesthetic agent (bupivacaine) or complete neurolysis (absolute alcohol) has been used both percutaneously and via endoscopic ultrasound (EUS) as a method of blocking the transmission of pain impulses from the celiac plexus to the central nervous system in patients with pancreatic cancer and CP.[32] While it appears that EUS is more efficacious than percutaneous methods due presumably to better visualization of the celiac plexus leading to a more targeted injection of neurolytic agent, these techniques require further evaluation in well-designed clinical trials.[33]

SURGERY FOR COMPLICATIONS OF CP

Biliary Obstruction

This local complication of CP results from either fibrotic stricturing of the distal common bile duct as it traverses the head of the pancreas or through compression of the intrapancreatic biliary segment by the inflammatory enlargement and microcystic disease in the pancreatic head. It is reported to occur in approximately 6% (3%–32%) of hospitalized patients with CP and is found in 35% (15%–60%) of patients undergoing surgical intervention for CP.[34] Significant biliary obstruction is commonly defined as an elevated alkaline phosphatase greater than two times the upper limit of normal values in the laboratory used associated with radiographic evidence of biliary dilatation. Although it is tempting to manage these fibrotic biliary strictures initially with endoscopic therapy, the long-term success rates with this modality are disappointing.[35] Self-expanding metal stents have been used in a highly selected population of 13 patients unable to undergo operative bypass, with good results reported after a mean of 50 months.[36] Choledochoduodenostomy or hepaticojejunostomy Roux-en-Y are the operations of choice to simply relieve the biliary tract obstruction,[34] although most surgeons would employ a pancreatic head resection as described below to treat both the inflammatory pancreatic head mass as well as the concomitant biliary tract obstruction.

Duodenal Obstruction

Obstruction of the duodenum due to CP is either acute or chronic. Acute obstruction is usually transient and related to the severe inflammatory process occurring in the pancreas and retroperitoneum during an acute attack and as such, has the potential to resolve once the pancreatic inflammation subsides. Chronic duodenal obstruction occurs from repeated inflammatory insults resulting in cicatricial stenosis and fibrosis of the duodenum. These structural alterations will not resolve when the pancreatic inflammation subsides. Although chronic duodenal obstruction is a rare complication, occurring in 1.2% (0.5%–13%) of hospitalized patients with CP, it can be found in up to 13% (2%–36%) of patients requiring surgical intervention.[34] Similar to biliary obstruction, its specific treatment is a gastrojejunostomy, although most surgeons would relieve this obstruction using a pancreatic head resection.

Pancreatic Pseudocysts\Pseudoaneurysms

Complicated pseudocysts that frequently occur in patients with CP are commonly associated with an underlying pancreatic duct abnormality, and their surgical treatment should take these facts into account.[18] Patients with pseudocysts and CP should not be treated by cyst drainage solely, as is often the case in patients with a pseudocyst following a bout of acute pancreatitis, because the underlying anatomic and morphologic abnormalities are left untreated, leading to a high incidence of recurrence.[19] Patients with CP frequently require some form of pancreatic duct drainage, and at times, a parenchymal resection to treat the underlying anatomic abnormality that contributed to the formation of the pancreatic pseudocyst.

Less common complications occur as a consequence of fibrotic stricturing of adjacent organs including the biliary tract (elevated alkaline phosphatase, transaminases, and a dilated common bile duct) or duodenum (early satiety, weight loss, inability to eat); most of these complications can be addressed by the judicious application of one of the aforementioned operative procedures.

Pseudoaneurysms that occur as a consequence of severe inflammation and in patients with chronic pancreatitis are commonly related to a pseudocyst. Their presentation is that of bleeding, either into an established pseudocyst causing an increase in abdominal pain, or rarely through the ampulla of Vater (hemosuccus pancreaticus) or freely into the abdominal cavity (hemoperitoneum). Mesenteric angiography can detect the source of bleeding from the splenic, gastroduodenal, superior and inferior pancreaticoduodenal arteries in 94% of cases.[37] Angiographic embolization for control is generally the treatment of choice. Following control of hemorrhage and stabilization of the patient's clinical course, formal pancreatic resection of the involved pancreas may be carried out.

Incapacitating Abdominal Pain

Failure of both medical management and minimally invasive measures of pain control require careful counseling with the patient regarding the options for continued management. Some evidence exists that spontaneous pain relief occurs during the clinical course of the disease with progressive glandular destruction resulting in endocrine and exocrine insufficiency, although this may take up to 15 years from diagnosis.[38] The duration of pain, however, remains woefully unpredictable, limiting the enthusiasm for "watchful waiting."[39] Recently, two randomized controlled trials (RCT) in patients with chronic pancreatitis were published, which demonstrated a relative equivalence between surgical and endoscopic therapy in short-term pain relief, with surgery having a significant advantage in durability of pain reduction.[40,41] Given these findings, perhaps surgical therapy should not be viewed as the last resort in patients with painful chronic pancreatitis.

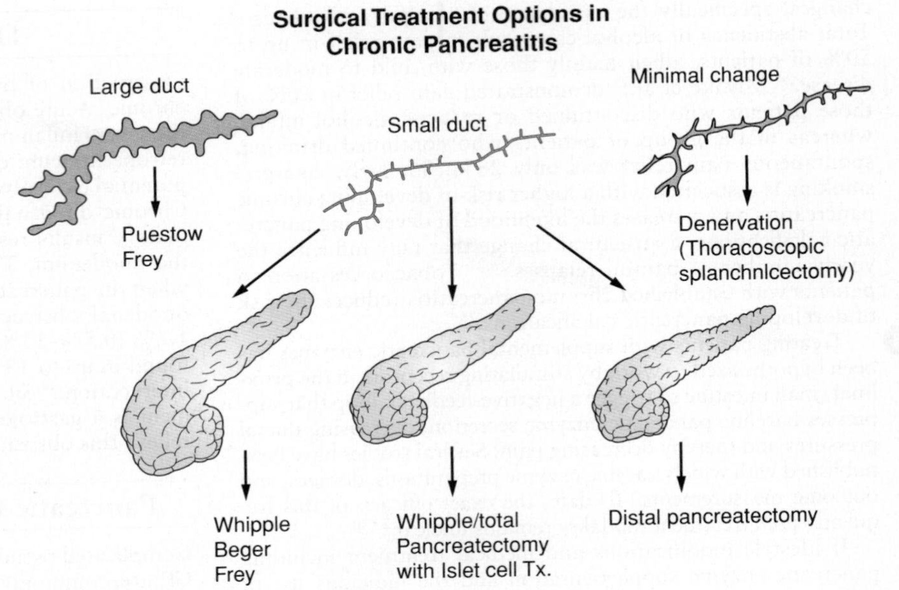

FIGURE 53.5. Surgical treatment options in patients with chronic pancreatitis based on pancreatic ductal morphology.

6 Operations for patients with chronic pancreatitis can be divided into four basic types: resection, drainage, combined resection and drainage, and denervation. Due to the morphologic heterogeneity of the disease in different patients, choosing the correct operation for any individual patients with chronic pancreatitis comes from interpreting the results of published clinical experience when applied to different anatomic and morphologic subsets. Dominant anatomic abnormalities found in patients with chronic pancreatitis can be broken down into three groups, either large duct, small duct, or minimal change variants based on the anatomic configuration of their main pancreatic duct (Fig. 53.5). Large duct variants have a cross-sectional diameter of their main pancreatic duct of 7 mm whereas small duct variants have a main pancreatic duct diameter of less than this.[42] Minimal change pancreatitis describes a group of patients who have symptoms of the disease but few or no anatomic changes in their gland or duct to confirm this.[43] In the small duct variant of chronic pancreatitis, there are three specific subgroups: large pancreatic head, small pancreatic head, and obstructive pancreatitis. The precise measurements of a large, hypertrophic pancreatic head have not been specifically defined, but enlargement is generally considered to be greater than 3 cm when measured in AP diameter on cross-sectional imaging.[44] Obstructive pancreatitis occurs in the setting of a physiologically significant stricture of the main pancreatic duct with upstream (toward the spleen) changes of pancreatic duct dilatation, blunted side branches, and parenchymal inflammation.[45]

For some anatomic subsets, several different operations may be successfully applied. An example is in patients with small duct, enlarged head chronic pancreatitis where either pancreaticoduodenectomy or the Beger or Frey-type duodenal preserving pancreatic head resection can be successfully used depending on the specific patient characteristics and surgeon preferences. The following paragraphs provide a brief description of the operations currently available to treat patients with chronic pancreatitis.

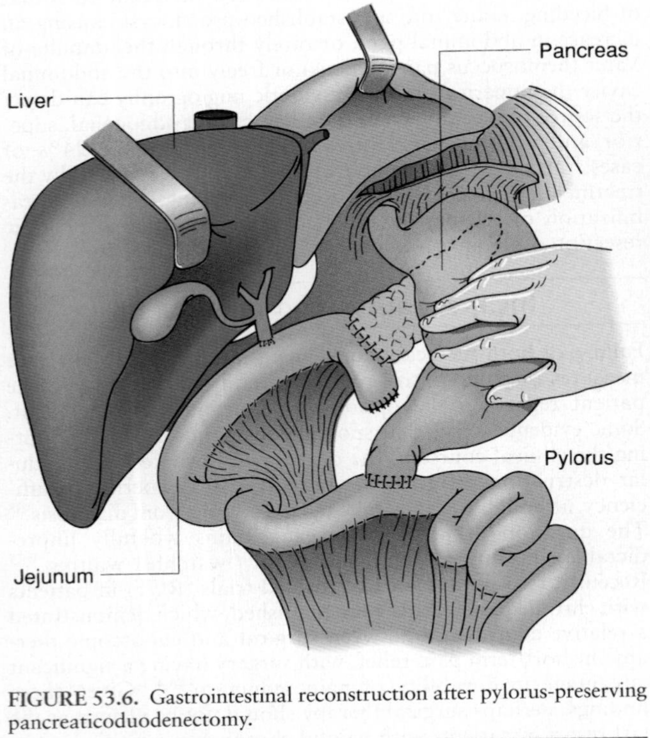

FIGURE 53.6. Gastrointestinal reconstruction after pylorus-preserving pancreaticoduodenectomy.

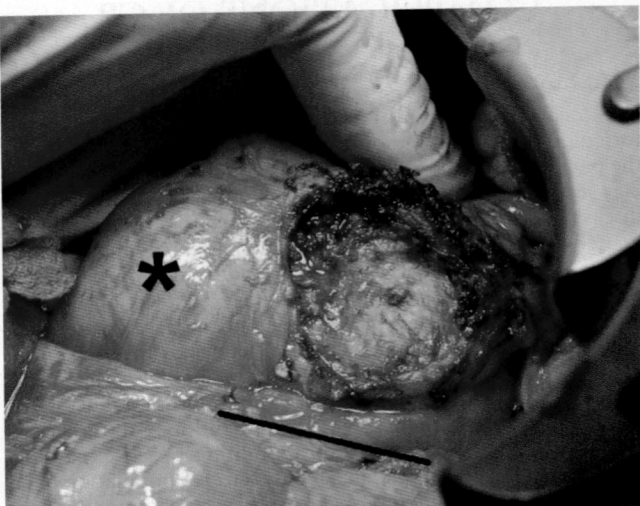

FIGURE 53.7. Operative photograph demonstrating the "cored-out" pancreatic head and uncinate process in a patient undergoing the Beger operation. The patient's head is to the right, the *asterisk* is at the junction of the second and third portion of the duodenum; the *line* parallels the superior mesenteric vein/portal vein path.

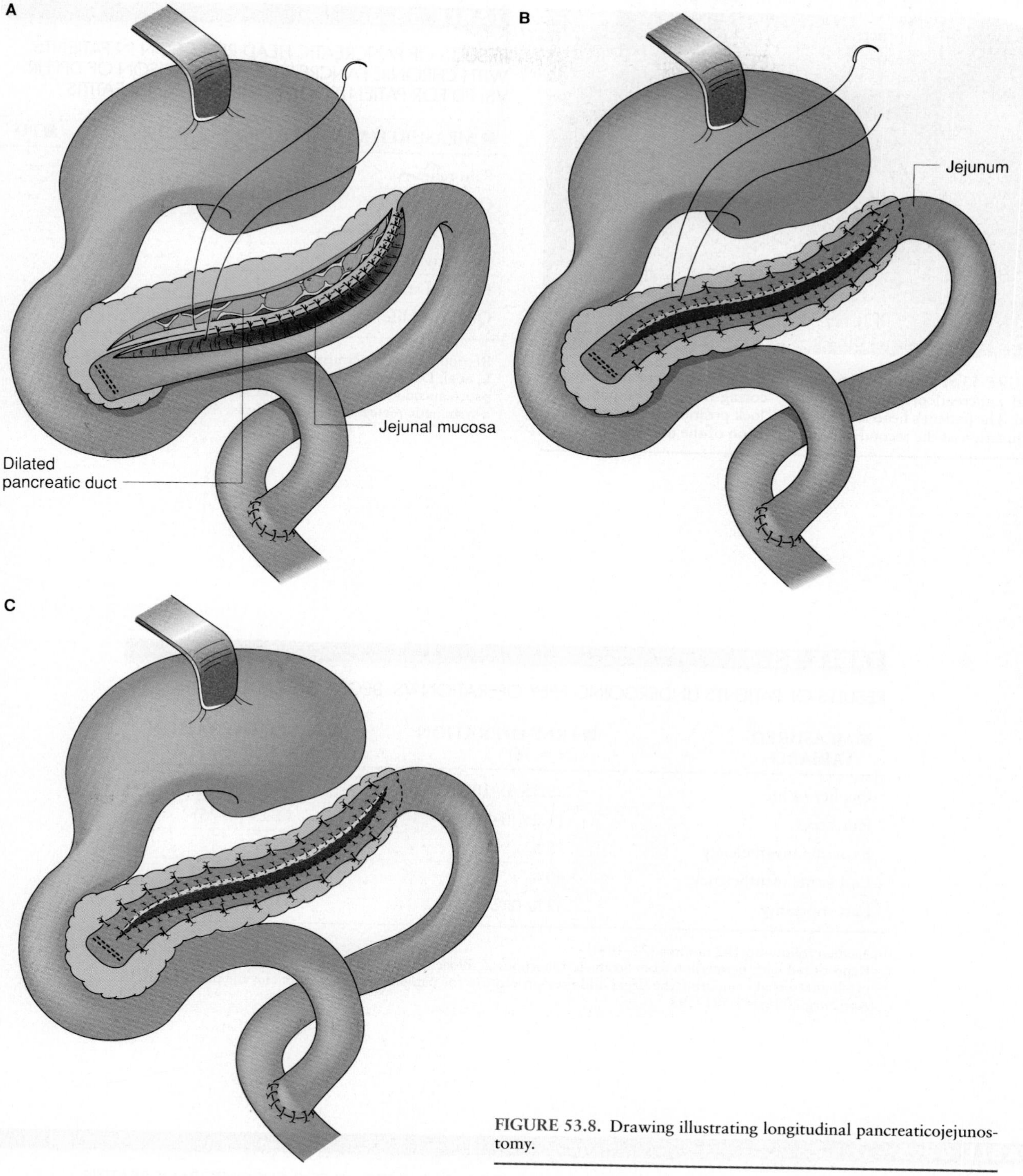

FIGURE 53.8. Drawing illustrating longitudinal pancreaticojejunostomy.

Resection Operations. Pancreaticoduodenectomy (PD), either the classic or pylorus-preserving variant, is the traditional resection operation used in patients with chronic pancreatitis.[46] It removes the head of the pancreas, duodenum, and distal common bile duct, a region of the pancreas that has been regarded as the "pacemaker" of the disease (Fig. 53.6). This operation is generally applied to small duct variants and has the flexibility to be used in both large and small head subtypes.

The Beger operation, termed one of the duodenal-preserving pancreatic head resection (DPPHR) procedures, involves transecting the pancreatic neck followed by a subtotal resection of the pancreatic head, removing diseased tissue in the head and uncinate process (Fig. 53.7) while preserving the normal relationship and function of the duodenum and distal common bile duct.[47] This operation is applied to patients with small duct chronic pancreatitis and a large, hypertrophic pancreatic head. It has also been selectively used with good overall results in patients with small duct chronic pancreatitis and normal pancreatic heads (pancreas divisum).[48]

Distal pancreatectomy removes pancreatic parenchyma to the left of the confluence of the splenic vein with the portal vein (body and tail of the pancreas). This operation is used very selectively in patients with obstructive chronic pancreatitis.[45,49]

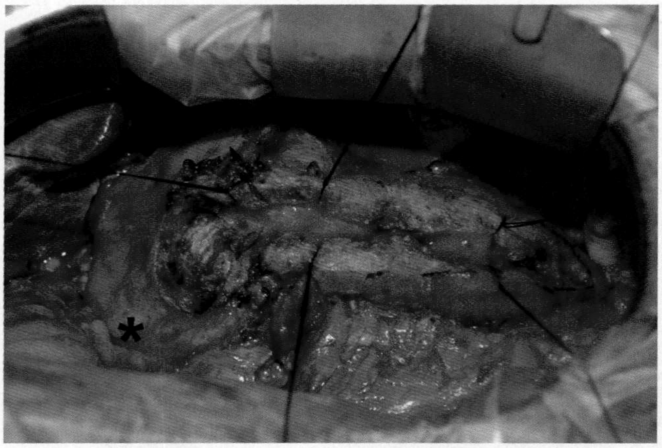

FIGURE 53.9. Operative photograph of the Frey operation: longitudinal pancreaticojejunostomy with "coring-out" of the pancreatic head. The patient's head is at the 12 o'clock position; the *asterisk* is on the junction of the second and third portion of the duodenum.

TABLE 53.3

RESULTS OF PANCREATIC HEAD RESECTION IN PATIENTS WITH CHRONIC PANCREATITIS; COMPARISON OF DPPHR VS. PD FOR PATIENTS WITH CHRONIC PANCREATITIS

MEASURED VARIABLE	DPPHR	PD
Pain relief	=	=
Overall morbidity	=	=
Endocrine insufficiency	=	=
Operative time	+++	–
Hospital stay	+	–
Quality of life	++	–

Reproduced with permission from Diener MK, Rahbari NN, Fischer L, et al. Duodenum-preserving pancreatic head resection versus pancreaticoduodenectomy for surgical treatment of chronic pancreatitis: a systematic review and meta-analysis. *Ann Surg* 2008;247:950–960.

TABLE 53.4

RESULTS OF PATIENTS UNDERGOING FREY OPERATION VS. BEGER OPERATION

MEASURED VARIABLE	FREY OPERATION (*N* = 36)	BEGER OPERATION (*N* = 38)
Quality of life	58.35 (0–100)	66.7 (0–100)
Pain score	11.25 (0–99.75)	11.25 (0–75)
Exocrine insufficiency	78%	88%
Endocrine insufficiency	60%	56%
Late mortality	32% (8/25)	31% (8/26)

Median follow-up 102 months (72–144).
Reproduced with permission from Strate T, Taherpour Z, Bloechle C, et al. Long-term follow-up of a randomized trial comparing the Beger and Frey procedures for patients suffering from chronic pancreatitis. *Ann Surg* 2005;241:591–598.

TABLE 53.5

RESULTS OF PATIENTS SUBJECTED TO LONGITUDINAL PANCREATICOJEJUNOSTOMY FOR CHRONIC PANCREATITIS

REFERENCE	NO. PATIENTS	COMPLETE OR PARTIAL PAIN RELIEF (%)	MORTALITY (%)	MEAN F/U (mos)
Greenlee et al.[53]	86	80	3	95
Adloff et al.[59]	105	93	2	65
Adams et al.[60]	85	55	0	76
Sielezneff et al.[61]	57	84	0	65
Sakorafas et al.[62]	120	81	0	96
Mean results	453	72	1	79

TABLE 53.6

RESULTS OF PATIENTS UNDERGOING THORASCOPIC SPLANCHNICECTOMY FOR CHRONIC PANCREATITIS

REFERENCE	NO. PATIENTS	MEAN F/U (mos)	COMPLETE OR PARTIAL PAIN RELIEF (%)
Moodley et al.[63]	17	12	94
Ihse et al.[64]	21	43	50
Buscher et al.[65]	44	36	46
Howard et al.[55]	55	32	35
Hammond et al.[66]	20	15	60
Mean results	157	30	50

A high-grade pancreatic duct stricture in the body or tail of the pancreas with upstream (toward the spleen) side-branch changes and evidence of pancreatic inflammation is the key to diagnosis. Care should be taken to evaluate these strictures for the possibility of pancreatic cancer.

Extended distal pancreatectomy (95% pancreatectomy) was advanced in the 1970s and 1980s as a better option for patients with CP.[50] Careful follow-up of these patients showed poor long-term outcomes, particularly with regard to brittle diabetes, and this operation has been abandoned.[51] It is worthwhile to note that experience gained performing 95% pancreatectomy led to the development of the Frey duodenal preserving pancreatic head resection described later.

Total pancreatectomy with or without islet cell transplantation removes the entire pancreas and is currently limited in its applicability to patients with chronic pancreatitis outside of clinical trials using salvage procedures for the pancreatic islets with isolation and reinfusion as an islet cell transplant, or for patients with no other therapeutic options.[52] It is used optimally in patients with small duct or minimal change chronic pancreatitis who have not undergone prior resection or drainage procedures.

Drainage Operation. The Partington-Rochelle modification of the Puestow procedure, a longitudinal pancreaticojejunostomy is the classic operation used to treat patients with large duct pancreatitis by decompressing the entire length of the pancreatic duct (head to tail) into a defunctionalized (Roux-en-Y) limb of jejunum (Fig. 53.8).[53]

Combined Resection and Drainage. The Frey operation is the other procedure termed as a duodenal-preserving pancreatic head resection (DPPHR), but in contrast to the Beger operation, the pancreatic neck is not transected. The surgeon identifies the pancreatic duct in the neck of the pancreas and then opens the duct longitudinally by following it down into the pancreatic head and out to the tail. In the pancreatic head, the surgeon then cores out pancreatic tissue from the pancreatic duct outward until just a thin rim of tissue remains around the head of the pancreas contiguous with the duodenum. A defunctionalized limb of jejunum (Roux-en-Y) is then anastomosed side to side to the pancreatic duct in the body and tail and to the remaining rim of pancreatic tissue in the head to effect complete drainage of the entire gland (Fig. 53.9). This operation is perhaps the most versatile as it can be applied to patients with either small or large duct chronic pancreatitis as well as patients with either large or normal pancreatic head size.[54]

Denervation Operations. Bilateral thoracoscopic splanchnicectomy is a minimally invasive approach to splanchnic denervation used to treat pain in patients with chronic pancreatitis.[55] Candidates are generally patients with no other surgical targets (i.e., minimal change pancreatitis) who have been shown to have a splanchnic mediated pain pathway based on their response to a differential epidural anesthetic.

Clinical Results following Operation in Patients with CP

In measuring the results of surgery in patients with chronic pancreatitis, long-term success is typically defined by a thorough clinical follow-up of at least 5 years' duration.[56] When restricting data to long-term outcome measures, the results for pancreatic head resections (DPPHR and PD) are as shown in Table 53.3. In a recent meta-analysis, DPPHRs have been shown to be equivalent in outcome to pancreaticoduodenectomy (PD) in the measured variables of pain relief, overall morbidity, and incidence of postoperative endocrine insufficiency.[57] In this same analysis, DPPHRs were judged to be superior to PD in terms of operative time, postoperative hospital stay, and overall quality of life measures.

In a comparison of the two most common DPPHRs, the Beger operation and the Frey operation, no significant differences were found in a controlled randomized clinical trial when patients were followed for more than 8 years (Table 53.4).[58]

Outcomes of patients with chronic pancreatitis treated by longitudinal/lateral pancreaticojejunostomy (drainage operation) are shown in Table 53.5. After a mean follow-up of 79 months, 72% of patients experienced either complete or partial pain relief following operation with a mean perioperative mortality rate in this group of patients of only 1%.

A surgical denervation procedure as exemplified by bilateral thoracoscopic splanchnicectomy is a minimally invasive treatment of chronic pancreatitis with low perioperative morbidity and mortality rates. Based on currently available data, complete or partial pain relief is achieved in only 50% of patients during long-term clinical follow-up (Table 53.6).

CONCLUSION

Various operations are available to treat the heterogeneous complications of chronic pancreatitis. Surgeons who accept care of these challenging patients must be well versed in several therapeutic strategies, and committed to following these patients closely for the long term to ensure optimal clinical outcomes. Future advances in the therapy of chronic pancreatitis will be predicated on obtaining a better understanding of the underlying pathophysiology.

References

1. Sarner M, Cotton PB. Classification of pancreatitis. *Gut* 1984;25(7): 756–759.
2. Andersen BN, Pedersen NT, Scheel J, et al. Incidence of alcoholic chronic pancreatitis in Copenhagen. *Scand J Gastroenterol* 1982;17(2):247–252.
3. De las Heras G, Pons F. Epidemiologia y aspectos etiopatogenicos de la pancreatitis alcoholica cronica. *Rev Esp Enferm Dig* 1993;84:253–258.
4. Etemad B, Whitcomb DC. Chronic pancreatitis: diagnosis, classification, and new genetic developments. *Gastroenterology* 2001;120(3):682– 707.
5. Whitcomb DC, Gorry MC, Preston RA, et al. Hereditary pancreatitis is caused by a mutation in the cationic trypsinogen gene. *Nat Genet* 1996; 14(2):141–145.
6. Comfort M, Gambill E, Baggenstoss A. Chronic relapsing pancreatitis: a study of twenty-nine cases without associated disease of the biliary or gastro-intestinal tract. *Gastroenterology* 1946;6(4):239–408.
7. Sarles H, Sahel J. Pathology of chronic calcifying pancreatitis. *Am J Gastroenterol* 1976;66(2):117–139.
8. Bordalo O, Goncalves D, Noronha M, et al. Newer concept for the pathogenesis of chronic alcoholic pancreatitis. *Am J Gastroenterol* 1977;68(3): 278–285.
9. Kloppel G, Maillet B. The morphological basis for the evolution of acute pancreatitis into chronic pancreatitis. *Virchows Arch A Pathol Anat Histopathol* 1992;420(1):1–4.
10. Shimizu K. Pancreatic stellate cells: molecular mechanism of pancreatic fibrosis. *J Gastroenterol Hepatol* 2008;23(suppl 1):S119–S121.
11. Witt H, Luck W, Hennies HC, et al. Mutations in the gene encoding the serine protease inhibitor, Kazal type 1 are associated with chronic pancreatitis. *Nat Genet* 2000;25(2):213–216.
12. Sharer N, Schwarz M, Malone G, et al. Mutations of the cystic fibrosis gene in patients with chronic pancreatitis. *N Engl J Med* 1998;339(10): 645–652.
13. Cohn JA, Friedman KJ, Noone PG, et al. Relation between mutations of the cystic fibrosis gene and idiopathic pancreatitis. *N Engl J Med* 1998; 339(10):653–658.
14. Lankisch PG. The problem of diagnosing chronic pancreatitis. *Dig Liver Dis* 2003;35(3):131–134.
15. DiMagno EP, Go VL, Summerskill WH. Relations between pancreatic enzyme outputs and malabsorption in severe pancreatic insufficiency. *N Engl J Med* 1973;288(16):813–815.
16. Wiersema MJ, Hawes RH, Lehman GA, et al. Prospective evaluation of endoscopic ultrasonography and endoscopic retrograde cholangiopancreatography in patients with chronic abdominal pain of suspected pancreatic origin. *Endoscopy* 1993;25(9):555–564.
17. Sarr MG, Sakorafas GH. Incapacitating pain of chronic pancreatitis: a surgical perspective of what is known and what needs to be known. *Gastrointest Endosc* 1999;49(3 Pt 2):S85–S89.
18. Nealon WH, Walser E. Duct drainage alone is sufficient in the operative management of pancreatic pseudocysts in patients with chronic pancreatitis. *Ann Surg* 2003;237:614–620.
19. Nealon WH, Walser E. Surgical management of complications associated with percutaneous and\or endoscopic management of pseudocysts of the pancreas. *Ann surg* 2005;241:948–957.
20. Vitas GJ, Sarr MG. Selected management of pancreatic pseudocysts: operative versus expectant management. *Surgery* 1992;111(2):123–130.
21. Heider TR, Azeem S, Galanko JA, et al. The natural history of pancreatitis-induced splenic vein thrombosis. *Ann Surg* 2004;239(6):876–880; discussion 880–882.
22. Lowenfels AB, Maisonneuve P, Cavallini G, et al. Pancreatitis and the risk of pancreatic cancer. International Pancreatitis Study Group. *N Engl J Med* 1993;328(20):1433–1437.
23. AGA treatment Guidelines. American Gastroenterological Association Medical Position Statement: treatment of pain in chronic pancreatitis. *Gastroenterology* 1998;115:763–764.
24. Ihse I, Lankisch PG. Treatment of chronic pancreatitis. Current status. *Acta Chir Scand* 1988;154:553–558.
25. Miyake H, Harada H, Kunichika K, et al. Clinical course and prognosis of chronic pancreatitis. *Pancreas* 1987;2:378–385.
26. Maisonneuve P, Lowenfels AB, Mullhaupt B, et al. Cigarette smoking accelerates progression of alcoholic chronic pancreatitis. *Gut* 2005;54: 510–514.
27. Talamini G, Bassi C, Falconi M, et al. Pain relapses in the first 10 years of chronic pancreatitis. *Am J Surg* 1996;171:565–569.
28. Talamini G, Bassi C, Galconi M, et al. Smoking cessation at the clinical onset of chronic pancreatitis and risk of pancreatic calcifications. *Pancreas* 2007;35:320–326.
29. Dominguez-Munoz JE, Hieronymus C, Sauerbruch T, et al. Fecal elastase test: evaluation of a new noninvasive pancreatic function test. *Am J Gastroenterol* 1995;90(10):1834–1837.
30. Winstead NS, Wilcox CM. Clinical trials of pancreatic enzyme replacement for painful chronic pancreatitis—a Review. *Pancreatology* 2009;9: 344–350.
31. Attasaranya S, Abdel Aziz AM, Lehman GA. Endoscopic management of acute and chronic pancreatitis. *Surg Clin North Am* 2007;87:1379–1402.
32. Michaels AJ, Draganov PV. Endoscopic ultrasonography guided celiac plexus neurolysis and celiac plexus block in the management of pain due to pancreatic cancer and chronic pancreatitis. *World J Gastroenterol* 2007; 13:3575–3580.
33. Santosh D, Lakhtakia S, Gupta R, et al. Clinical trial: a randomized trial comparing fluoroscopically guided percutaneous tchnique vs. endoscopic ultrasound guided technique of celiac plexus bock for treatment of pain in chronic pancreatitis. *Aliment Pharmacol Ther* 2009;29:979–984.
34. Vijungco JD, Prinz RA. Management of biliary and duodenal complications of chronic pancreatitis. *World J Surg* 2003;27:1258–1270.
35. Smits ME, Rauws EA, Van Gulik TM, et al. Long-term results of endoscopic stenting and surgical drainage for biliary stricture due to chronic pancreatitis. *Br J Surg* 1996;83:764–768.
36. Van Berkel AM, Cahen DL, van Westerloo DF, et al. Self-expanding metal stents in benign biliary strictures due to chronic pancreatitis. *Endoscopy* 2004;36:381–384.
37. Balachandra S, Siriwardena AK. Systematic appraisal of the management of major vascular complications of pancreatitis. *Am J Surg* 2005;190: 489–495.
38. Amman RW, Akovbiantz A, Largiader F, et al. Course and outcome of chronic pancreatitis. Longitudinal study of a mixed medical-surgical series of 245 patients. *Gastroenterology* 1984;86:820–828.
39. Lankisch PG, Happe-Loehr A, Otto J, et al. Natural course in chronic pancreatitis. Pain, exocrine and endocrine pancreatic insufficiency and prognosis of the disease. *Digest* 1993;54:148–155.
40. Dite P, Ruzicka M, Zboril V, et al. A prospective, randomized trial comparing endoscopic and surgical therapy for chronic pancreatitis. *Endoscopy* 2003;35:553–558.
41. Cahen DL, Gouma DJ, Nio Y, et al. Endoscopic versus surgical drainage of the pancreatic duct in chronic pancreatitis. *New Engl J Med* 2007;356: 676–684.
42. Warshaw AL. Conservation of pancreatic tissue by combined gastric, biliary, and pancreatic duct drainage for pain from chronic pancreatitis. *Am J Surg* 1985;149:563–569.
43. Walsh TN, Rode J, Theis BA, et al. Minimal change chronic pancreatitis. *Gut* 1992;33:1566–1571.
44. Keck T, Marjanovic G, Fernández-del Castillo C, et al. The inflammatory pancreatic head mass: significant differences in the anatomic pathology of German and American patients with chronic pancreatitis determine very different surgical strategies. *Ann Surg* 2009;249:105–110.
45. Howard TJ, Maiden CL, Smith HG, et al. Surgical treatment of chronic obstructive pancreatitis. *Surgery* 1995;118:727–735.
46. Traverso LW, Kozarek RA. Pancreaticoduodenectomy for chronic pancreatitis: anatomic selection criteria and subsequent long-term outcome analysis. *Ann Surg* 1997;226:429–435.
47. Beger HR, Büchler M, Bittner R, et al. Duodenum-preserving resection of the head of the pancreas in severe chronic pancreatitis. Early and late results. *Ann Surg* 1989;209:273–248.
48. Schlosser W, Rau BM, Poch B, et al. Surgical treatment of pancreas divisum causing chronic pancreatitis: the outcome benefits of duodenum-preserving pancreatic head resection. *J Gastrointest Surg* 2005;9:710–715.
49. Sakorafas GH, Sarr MG, Rowland CM, et al. Postobstructive chronic pancreatitis: results with distal resection. *Arch Surg* 2001;136:643–648.
50. Fry WJ, Child CG III. Ninety-five per cent distal pancreatectomy for chronic pancreatitis. *Ann Surg* 1965;162(4):543–549.
51. Frey CF, Child CG, Fry W. Pancreatectomy for chronic pancreatitis. *Ann Surg* 1976;184(4):403–413.
52. Blondet JJ, Carlson AM, Kobayashi T, et al. The role of total pancreatectomy and islet autotransplantation for chronic pancreatitis. *Surg Clin North Am* 2007;87:1477–1501.
53. Greenlee HB, Prinz RA, Aranha GV. Long-term results of side-to-side pancreaticojejunostomy. *World J Surg* 1990;14:70–76.
54. Frey CF, Amikura K. Local resection of the head of the pancreas combined with longitudinal pancreaticojejunostomy in the management of patients with chronic pancreatitis. *Ann Surg* 1994;220:492–507.
55. Howard TJ, Swofford JB, Wagner DL, et al. Quality of life after bilateral thoracoscopic splanchnicectomy: long-term evaluation in patients with chronic pancreatitis. *J Gastrointest Surg* 2002;6:845–854.
56. Frey CF, Pitt HA, Yeo CJ, et al. A plea for uniform reporting of patient outcome in chronic pancreatitis. *Arch Surg* 1996;131:233–234.
57. Diener MK, Rahbari NN, Fischer L, et al. Duodenum-preserving pancreatic head resection versus pancreaticoduodenectomy for surgical treatment of chronic pancreatitis: a systematic review and meta-analysis. *Ann Surg* 2008;247:950–960.
58. Strate T, Taherpour Z, Bloechle C, et al. Long-term follow-up of a randomized trial comparing the Beger and Frey procedures for patients suffering from chronic pancreatitis. *Ann Surg* 2005;241:591–598.
59. Adloff M, Schloegel M, Arnaud JP, et al. Role of pancreaticojejunostomy in the treatment of chronic pancreatitis. A study of 105 operated patients. *Chirurgie* 1991;117:251–256.
60. Adams DB, Ford MC, Anderson MC. Outcome after lateral pancreaticojejunostomy for chronic pancreatitis. *Ann Surg* 1994;219:481–487.
61. Sielezneff I, Malouf A, Salle E, et al. Long term results of lateral pancreaticojejunostomy for chronic alcoholic pancreatitis. *Eur J Surg* 2000;166: 58–64.
62. Sakorafas GH, Farnell MB, Farley DR, et al. Long-term results after surgery for chronic pancreatitis. *Int J Pancreatol* 2000;27:131–142.
63. Moodley J, Singh B, Shaik AS, et al. Thoracoscopic splanchnicectomy: Ppilot evaluation of a simple alternative for chronic pancreatic pain control. *World J. Surg* 1999;23:688–692.
64. Ihse I, Zoucas E, Gylistedt E, et al. Bilateral thoracoscopic splanchnicectomy: effects on pancreatic pain and function. *Ann Surg* 1999;230: 785–791.
65. Buscher HCJL, Jansen JJMB, van Goor H. Bilateral thoracoscopic splanchnicectomy in patients with chronic pancreatitis. *Scand J Gastroenterol* 1999;34(suppl 230):29–34.
66. Hammond B, Vitale GC, Rangnekar N, et al. Bilateral thoracoscopic splanchnicectomy for pain control in chronic pancreatitis. *Am Surg* 2004; 70:546–549.

CHAPTER 54 ■ NEOPLASMS OF THE EXOCRINE PANCREAS

ATTILA NAKEEB AND KEITH D. LILLEMOE

KEY POINTS

1. There is increasing evidence that ductal pancreatic cancer arises from precursor lesions referred to as pancreatic intraepithelial neoplasia (PanIN) with progression from proliferative lesions without nuclear abnormality to carcinoma in situ, known as PanIN-3.
2. Intraductal papillary mucinous neoplasms (IPMNs) are intraductal mucin-producing tumors that range from benign adenomas to invasive carcinoma and should be considered for resection.
3. Spiral computed tomography scan is the preferred noninvasive imaging test for the diagnosis and staging of pancreatic cancer demonstrating the primary lesion and its relationship to adjacent visceral vessels as well as metastatic disease to the liver and peritoneum.
4. Perioperative mortality rates following pancreaticoduodenectomy have fallen to the range of 2% to 5%, although perioperative complications occur in approximately 40% of patients.
5. The survival rate after pancreaticoduodenectomy for pancreatic cancer is approximately 20%, with factors influencing survival including tumor size, margin status, and node status.
6. Although some controversy exists, most data support the role for adjuvant therapy, either chemotherapy or chemoradiation, for patients following resection of pancreatic cancer.
7. Surgical palliation of patients with pancreatic cancer located in the head found to be unresectable at laparotomy includes biliary bypass, gastrojejunostomy, and chemical splanchnicectomy to palliate the symptoms of jaundice, duodenal obstruction, and pain, respectively.

In the United States, it is estimated that nearly 42,470 new cases of pancreas cancer will be diagnosed, with almost 35,240 people dying of the disease in 2009. Pancreatic cancer is the fourth leading cause of cancer death in this country.[1] Currently, only 15% to 20% of patients diagnosed with pancreatic adenocarcinoma are candidates for pancreatic resection. Five-year survival averages 15% to 20% for patients with resected disease and only 3% for all stages combined.[2] The nonspecific symptoms associated with early pancreatic cancer, the inaccessibility of the pancreas to examination, the aggressiveness of the tumors, and the technical difficulties associated with pancreatic surgery make pancreatic cancer one of the most challenging diseases treated by general surgeons. In recent years, significant advances have been made in our understanding of the pathogenesis and clinical management of pancreatic cancer. This chapter will review the epidemiology and risk factors associated with pancreatic cancer, discuss recent developments in the field of molecular genetics, and provide an update on the current clinical management of pancreatic cancer.

EPIDEMIOLOGY AND RISK FACTORS

In the United States, approximately 11 new cases of pancreatic cancer are diagnosed per 100,000 population annually.[1] Although the incidence rate of pancreatic cancer has been relatively stable during the last two decades, it has increased nearly threefold since the beginning of the last century (Fig. 54.1). It has been argued that the apparent increase in the incidence of pancreatic cancer may represent a misclassification of pancreatic cancer as other types of upper gastrointestinal cancer, particularly gastric cancer, in the past. However, several analyses indicate that a portion of the threefold increase in the incidence of pancreatic cancer has been real. The risk for the development of pancreatic cancer is related to age, race, sex, tobacco use, diet, and specific genetic syndromes (Table 54.1). The incidence increases with advancing age. More than 80% of cases occur in persons between the ages of 60 and 80 years, and pancreatic cancer is rare in people younger than 40 years. The incidence and mortality rates for pancreatic cancer in African Americans of both sexes are higher than those in whites. The gender differences in pancreatic cancer have been equalizing during recent years. Pancreatic cancer is still more common in men than in women, but the incidence and mortality rates have increased in women, while they have stabilized or slightly decreased in men.[1]

Environmental and dietary factors have also been implicated as risk factors for the development of pancreatic cancer. The most consistently observed environmental risk for the development of pancreatic cancer is cigarette smoking. It has been estimated that cigarette smoking can increase the risk for pancreatic cancer between one and a half and five times. The mechanism is unknown, but carcinogens in cigarette smoke have been shown to produce pancreatic cancers in laboratory animals. In addition, autopsy studies have documented hyperplastic changes in pancreatic ductal cells with atypical nuclear patterns in smokers. Alcohol consumption does not seem to be a risk factor for pancreatic cancer despite conflicting past reports. Recent studies suggest that past studies linking pancreatic cancer to alcohol use may have been confounded by tobacco use. Similarly, coffee consumption and exposure to ionizing radiation have been shown not to be associated with an increased pancreatic cancer risk.

Several epidemiologic investigations have suggested that diet may play an important role in the development of pancreatic cancer. An apparent association has been noted between pancreatic cancer and an increased consumption of total calories, carbohydrate, cholesterol, meat, salt, dehydrated food,

FIGURE 54.1. U. S. age-adjusted death rates for pancreatic carcinoma.

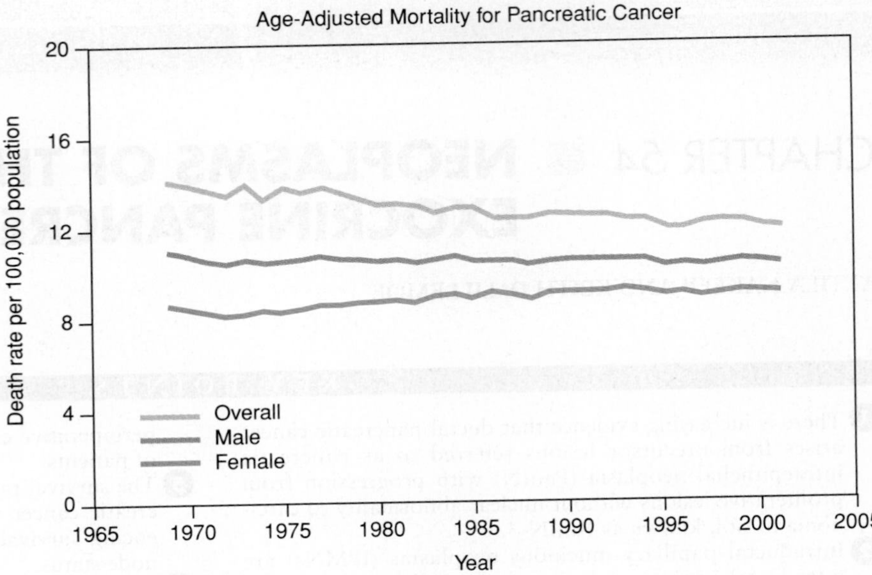

fried food, refined sugar, soy beans, and nitrosamines. The risks are unproven for the ingestion of fat, β-carotene, and coffee. A protective effect has been reported for dietary fiber, vitamin C, fruits, and vegetables.[3]

In addition to well-defined genetic syndromes, a number of common conditions have been thought to be etiologic factors in the development of pancreatic cancer. An apparent association between diabetes and pancreatic cancer has been suggested. Approximately 80% of patients diagnosed with pancreatic cancer have impaired glucose metabolism, impaired glucose tolerance, or diabetes mellitus. It is unclear if alterations in glucose tolerance/metabolism are a causative factor for pancreatic cancer or represent reaction to an enlarging malignancy in the pancreas. Among patients with newly diagnosed diabetes, 0.85% went on to be diagnosed with pancreatic cancer within 3 years.[4] Type 2 diabetes of at least 5 years' duration has been shown to increase the risk of pancreas cancer twofold.

The risk of pancreatic cancer has been shown to increase as body mass index increases. Examination of data from the Nurses' Health Study and the Health Professionals' follow-up study show a 1.72 relative risk (95% confidence interval [CI], 1.19–2.48) of pancreatic cancer in patients with a body mass index (BMI) greater than 30 kg/m^2 as compared to individuals with a BMI less than 23 kg/m^2.[5]

Chronic pancreatitis of any cause has been associated with a 25-year cumulative risk for the development of pancreatic cancer of approximately 4%. Other conditions for which a possible association with pancreatic cancer has been demonstrated include thyroid and other benign endocrine tumors, cystic fibrosis, and pernicious anemia.

TABLE 54.1

RISK FACTORS FOR PANCREATIC CANCER

	■ INCREASED RISK	■ POSSIBLE RISK	■ UNPROVED RISK
Demographic factors	Advancing age Male sex Black race	Geography	Socioeconomic status Migrant status
Host factors	Hereditary nonpolyposis colorectal cancer Familial breast cancer Peutz-Jeghers syndrome Ataxia-telangiectasia Familial atypical multiple mole melanoma Hereditary pancreatitis		Peptic ulcer surgery
Environmental factors	Tobacco	Diet Occupation	Alcohol Coffee Radiation

Modified from Gold EB, Goldin SB. Epidemiology of and risk factors for pancreatic cancer. *Surg Oncol Clin North Am* 1998;7:67.

TABLE 54.2

GENETIC SYNDROMES ASSOCIATED WITH HEREDITARY PANCREATIC CANCER

■ SYNDROME	■ MODE OF INHERITANCE	■ GENE	■ FOLD INCREASE IN RISK	■ MANIFESTATION OF PANCREATIC CANCER
Peutz-Jeghers	AD	*STKll*	140×	Hamartomatous polyps of the gastrointestinal tract; mucocutaneous melanin macules
Hereditary pancreatitis	AD	*PRSSl*	60×	Recurrent episodes of severe pancreatitis starting at a young age
Familial pancreatic cancer	Unknown	Unknown	18×	At least one pair of first-degree relatives with pancreatic cancer
FAMMM	AD	p16	20×	Multiple nevi, atypical nevi, melanomas
Familial breast cancer 2	AD	*BRCA2*	10×	Breast, ovarian, and pancreatic cancer
HNPCC	AD	*MSH2* *HLHl*	Unknown	Colonic, endometrial, and gastric cancers; mutator phenotype

AD, autosomal dominant; FAMMM, familial atypical multiple mole melanoma; HNPCC, hereditary nonpolyposis colorectal cancer.

Most cases of pancreatic cancer have no obvious predisposing factors. However, it is believed that between 5% and 10% of pancreatic cancers arise because of a familial predisposition. Six genetic syndromes have been associated with an increased risk for the development of pancreatic cancer (Table 54.2). These include hereditary nonpolyposis colon cancer, familial breast cancer associated with the *BRCA2* mutation, Peutz-Jeghers syndrome, ataxia-telangiectasia syndrome, familial atypical multiple mole melanoma syndrome, and hereditary pancreatitis.

MOLECULAR GENETICS

Tremendous advances have been made in understanding the molecular genetics of pancreatic cancer in recent years. In general, the genes involved in the pathogenesis of pancreatic cancer can be divided into three categories: tumor-suppressor genes, oncogenes, and DNA mismatch-repair genes (Table 54.3).

Tumor-suppressor genes normally function to control cellular proliferation. When these genes are inactivated by genetic events such as mutation, deletion, chromosome rearrangements, or mitotic recombination, their function as growth suppressors can be lost, and abnormal growth regulation is the result. The tumor-suppressor genes *p53, p16, DPC4*, and *BRCA2* are frequently inactivated in sporadic adenocarcinoma of the pancreas. The function of *p53* appears to be inactivated in up to 75% of all pancreatic cancers. The *p53* gene product is a DNA-binding protein that acts as both a cell cycle checkpoint and an inducer of apoptosis. Inactivation of the *p53* gene in pancreatic cancer leads to the loss of two important controls of cell growth: regulation of cellular proliferation and induction of cell death. The *p16* gene encodes a protein that binds cyclin to cyclin D–Cdk4 complexes. When the *p16* gene product binds to these complexes, it inhibits the phosphorylation of a number of growth and regulatory proteins. Inactivation of *p16* leads to the loss of an important cell cycle checkpoint and therefore relatively unchecked proliferation. *DPC4* is a tumor-suppressor gene that has been identified on chromosome 18q. This chromosome has been shown to be missing in nearly 90% of pancreatic cancers. The *DPC4* gene is inactive in almost 50% of pancreatic carcinomas. The mutation appears to be a homozygous deletion in 30% of pancreatic cancers and a point mutation in another 20% of tumors. *DPC4* mutations are more specific than *p53* or *p16* mutations for pancreatic cancer. The function of *BRCA2* has not been established, but the gene product appears to be a tumor suppressor participating in DNA damage repair. Mutations in *BRCA2* have been linked to hereditary breast and ovarian cancers. Recent studies also suggest a significantly increased risk of pancreatic cancer development in patients with germline *BRCA2* mutations.

Oncogenes are derived from normal cellular genes called *proto-oncogenes*. When overexpressed or activated by mutation, oncogenes encode proteins with transforming properties. Activating point mutations in the K-*ras* oncogene is the most common genetic alteration in pancreatic cancer. Point mutations in

TABLE 54.3

GENETIC ALTERATIONS IN PANCREATIC ADENOCARCINOMAS

■ GENE	■ CHROMOSOME LOCUS	■ FREQUENCY (%)
ONCOGENES		
K-*ras*	12	90
TUMOR-SUPPRESSOR GENES		
p16	9p	95
p53	17p	50–75
DPC4	18q	55
BRCA2	13q	7
LKB1	17p	4
MKK4	19p	5
ALK4	12q	2
Genome maintenance 4 genes *bMSH2*, *bMLH1*	2P, 3P	

Reproduced with permission from Hruban RH. Pancreatic cancer: from genes to patient care. *J Gastrointest Surg* 2001;5:583.

PANCREAS/LIVER

codons 12, 13, or 61 of the K-*ras* oncogene impair the intrinsic guanosine triphosphatase activity of its gene product; the result is a protein that is constitutively active in signal transduction. Mutations of K-*ras* have been found in 80% to 100% of pancreatic cancers and therefore may prove useful in the development of a molecular screening test for pancreatic cancer.

Mismatch-repair genes function to ensure the accuracy of DNA replication, and when these genes are mutated, errors in DNA replication are not repaired. The human mismatch-repair genes are *hMSH2, hMLH1, hPMS1, hPMS2, hMSH6/GTBP*, and *hMSH3*. The enzymes encoded by these genes repair single base-pair changes and small insertions and deletions that occur during DNA replication. Approximately 4% of pancreatic cancers can be characterized by disorders of DNA mismatch-repair genes.[6]

PATHOLOGY

Tumors of the exocrine pancreas can be classified based on their cell of origin (Table 54.4). The most common neoplasms of the exocrine pancreas are ductal adenocarcinomas. Approximately 65% of pancreatic ductal cancers arise in the head, neck, or uncinate process of the pancreas; 15% originate in the body or the tail of the gland; and 20% diffusely involve the whole gland.

Solid Epithelial Tumors

Ductal Adenocarcinomas. Ductal adenocarcinomas account for more than 75% of all nonendocrine pancreatic cancers. Grossly, they are white–yellow, poorly defined, hard masses that often obstruct the distal common bile duct or main pancreatic duct. They are often associated with a desmoplastic reaction that causes fibrosis and chronic pancreatitis. Microscopically, they contain infiltrating glands of varying size and shape surrounded by dense, reactive fibrous tissue (Fig. 54.2). The epithelial cells sometimes form papillae and cribriform structures, and they frequently contain mucin. The nuclei of the cells can show marked pleomorphism, hyperchromasia, loss of polarity, and prominent nucleoli.

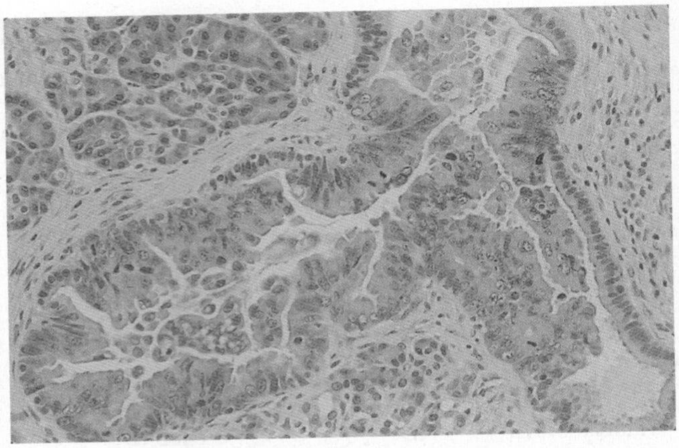
FIGURE 54.2. Microscopic appearance of ductal adenocarcinoma of the head of the pancreas demonstrating glands from an adenocarcinoma embedded in a fibrous matrix.

TABLE 54.4 CLASSIFICATION

HISTOLOGIC CLASSIFICATION OF 645 CASES OF PRIMARY NONENDOCRINE CANCER OF THE PANCREAS

■ CLASSIFICATION	■ NUMBER
Duct cell origin	572 (89%)
Duct cell adenocarcinoma	494
Giant cell carcinoma	28
Adenosquamous carcinoma	20
Microadenocarcinoma	16
Mucinous carcinoma	9
Mucinous cystadenocarcinoma	5
Acinar cell origin	8 (1%)
Acinar cell carcinoma	7
Cystadenoma	1
Uncertain histogenesis	61 (9%)
Pancreaticoblastoma	1
Papillary and cystic neoplasm	1
Mixed type—duct and islet cells	1
Unclassified	58
Connective tissue origin	4 (1%)

Reproduced with permission from Bell RH. Neoplasms of the exocrine pancreas. In: Greenfield LJ, Mulholland MW, Oldham KT, eds. *Surgery: Scientific Principles and Practice*, 2nd ed. Philadelphia: Lippincott–Raven; 1997:901.

Ductal adenocarcinomas tend to infiltrate into vascular, lymphatic, and perineural spaces. At the time of resection, most ductal carcinomas have already metastasized to regional lymph nodes. In addition to the lymph nodes, pancreatic ductal adenocarcinomas frequently metastasize to the liver (80%), peritoneum (60%), lungs and pleurae (50% to 70%), and adrenal glands (25%). They also can directly invade the duodenum, stomach, transverse mesocolon, colon, spleen, and adrenal glands.

The histologic examination of a pancreas resected for cancer frequently reveals the presence of precursor lesions in the
1 pancreatic ducts and ductules adjacent to the cancers.[7] This suggests that much like colon cancer, which arises from benign adenomas, pancreatic cancer may also demonstrate progression to malignant from benign precursor lesions. These precursor lesions are referred to as pancreatic intraepithelial neoplasia (PanIN). Briefly, PanIN-1A and PanIN-1B are proliferative lesions without remarkable nuclear abnormality that have a flat and papillary architecture, respectively. PanIN-3 is associated with severe architectural and cytonuclear abnormalities, but invasion through the basement membrane is absent. The older term for PanIN-3 includes carcinoma in situ (CIS). PanIN-2 is an intermediate category between PanIN-1 and PanIN-3 and is associated with a moderate degree of architectural and cytonuclear abnormality.[8] Several lines of evidence suggest that PanINs are precursors of infiltrating pancreatic cancer: PanINs are often found in association with ductal adenocarcinomas, three-dimensional mapping techniques have demonstrated a stepwise transformation from mild dysplasia to severe dysplasia in pancreatic duct lesions, and PanINs demonstrate some of the same genetic changes seen in infiltrating adenocarcinomas, most notably activating point mutations in codon 12 of K-*ras* and mutations in the *p16* and *p53* tumor-suppressor genes.

Adenosquamous Carcinomas. Adenosquamous carcinoma is a rare variant of ductal adenocarcinoma that shows both glandular and squamous differentiation. This variant appears to be more common in patients who have undergone previous chemoradiation therapy. The biologic behavior of adenosquamous carcinoma appears to be similar to that of ductal adenocarcinoma, with similar rates of perineural invasion, lymph node metastases, and dissemination.

Acinar Cell Carcinomas. Acinar cell carcinomas account for only 1% of pancreatic exocrine tumors. Acinar tumors are typically smooth, fleshy, lobulated, hemorrhagic, or necrotic. Histologically, they form acini, and the cells display an eosinophilic, granular cytoplasm. Immunohistochemical staining demonstrates expression of trypsin, lipase, chymotrypsin, or amylase. These tumors are more common in males, with a male-to-female predominance of approximately 3:1. The age of diagnosis is usually in the fifth to seventh decades. These tumors tend to be larger than ductal adenocarcinomas, often being larger than 10 cm. Although data are limited, it appears that patients with acinar cell carcinoma have a slightly better prognosis than patients with ductal carcinoma.[9] Therefore, surgical resection is the treatment of choice.

Giant Cell Carcinomas. Giant cell carcinomas account for fewer than 1% of nonendocrine pancreatic cancers. They tend to be large, with average diameters greater than 15 cm. Microscopically, they contain large, uninucleated or multinucleated tumor cells, many of which are pleomorphic. The nuclei contain prominent nucleoli and numerous mitotic figures. Giant cell carcinomas are associated with a poorer prognosis than ductal adenocarcinomas. There is a variant of giant cell carcinoma termed *giant cell carcinoma with osteoclastlike giant cells*. These lesions tend to be well circumscribed with nonpleomorphic giant cells and are less aggressive than standard giant cell carcinomas.

Pancreatoblastoma. Pancreatoblastomas occur primarily in children ages 1 to 15 years. Pancreatoblastomas contain both epithelial and mesenchymal elements. The epithelial component appears to arise from acinar cells. The tumors are typically larger than 10 cm and often contain areas of degeneration and hemorrhage. The prognosis appears to be more favorable than that for typical ductal adenocarcinoma if the tumor can be resected.

Cystic Epithelial Tumors

Cystic neoplasms also arise from the exocrine pancreas. Cystic neoplasms are less common than ductal adenocarcinomas, tend to occur in women, and are evenly distributed throughout the gland. Many pancreatic and peripancreatic cysts are actually benign inflammatory pseudocysts. It is important to identify cystic neoplasms because their management is very different from that of nonneoplastic cysts. With advancements in imaging technology, cystic lesions of the pancreas are being detected with increased frequency. As many as 1% of individuals undergoing cross-sectional abdominal imaging are found to have pancreatic cysts. Although many of these lesions are small and asymptomatic, they can have malignant potential. Therefore, the management of these patients is complex, and knowledge of pancreatic cyst natural history and predictors of neoplasia are important.

Serous Cystic Neoplasms. Serous cysts are epithelial neoplasms composed of uniform cuboidal glycogen-rich cells that usually form numerous small cysts containing serous fluid. Serous cystadenomas or microcystic adenomas are more common in women than in men (2:1 preponderance). These tumors can vary from a few centimeters to more than 10 cm in size. Twenty-five percent to 30% of patients are asymptomatic; however, most patients present with symptoms such as abdominal or epigastric pain, dyspepsia, nausea, or vomiting. Serous cystadenomas can be located anywhere in the pancreas—head, body, or tail—and usually do not communicate with the pancreatic ducts. Plain computed tomography (CT) shows a honeycomb pattern of microlacunae, with thin septa separating different segments. Serous cystic neoplasms can have a sunburst pattern of central calcification, which is seen in 10% to 30% of cases. Grossly, they appear as spongy, well-circumscribed, multiloculated cysts. Microscopically, they consist of a layer of simple cuboidal cells separated by dense fibrous bands. Most serous cystic neoplasms are benign, although malignant behavior has been reported rarely (i.e., metastases to the liver or peripancreatic lymph nodes). Symptomatic cysts or cysts that cannot be differentiated from other potentially malignant cysts should undergo surgical excision. Recently, it has been suggested that cysts greater than 4 cm in size should also be resected since they demonstrate a significant increased growth rate compared to smaller cysts.[10]

Mucinous Cystic Neoplasms. Mucinous cystic neoplasms (MCNs) are neoplasms composed of mucin-producing epithelial cells associated with an ovarian type of stroma. These cysts usually do not communicate with the larger pancreatic ducts. MCNs are relatively uncommon but account for almost 30% of all cystic neoplasms. The mean age at diagnosis is between 40 and 50 years. MCNs are more common in women, with a female-to-male ratio of 9:1. Most patients with MCNs present with vague abdominal symptoms that include epigastric pain or a sense of abdominal fullness. The majority (70% to 90%) of MCNs arise in the body or tail of the pancreas, and only a minority (10% to 30%) involve the head of the gland. Microscopically, the cysts are lined by tall, columnar, mucin-producing epithelium. These columnar cells have basal nuclei and abundant intracytoplasmic apical mucin and can form flat sheets or papillae. The walls of the cysts contain a very distinctive "ovarian-type" stroma. This stroma is composed of densely packed spindle cells with sparse cytoplasm and uniform elongated nuclei. All MCNs are considered to be premalignant lesions and should be completely resected to prevent progression to malignancy.

Invasive mucinous cystadenocarcinomas are MCNs associated with an invasive carcinoma, whereas noninvasive mucinous neoplasms can be categorized into mucinous cystic neoplasms with low-grade dysplasia (adenoma), mucinous cystic neoplasms with moderate dysplasia (borderline), and mucinous cystic neoplasms with high-grade dysplasia (carcinoma in situ) based on the degree of architectural and cytologic atypia of the epithelial cells. Approximately one third of all MCNs are associated with invasive carcinoma. Patients with mucinous cystadenocarcinomas tend to be 5 to 10 years older than patients with benign MCNs. The extent of invasive and in situ carcinomas in MCNs can be very focal. Therefore, a benign diagnosis cannot be established on biopsy alone and the lesions should be completely resected. The prognosis for patients with resected benign or borderline tumors is excellent. Patients with mucinous cystadenocarcinoma tend to do better than patients with ductal adenocarcinoma, with a 5-year survival of approximately 50%.

2 **Intraductal Papillary-Mucinous Neoplasms.** Intraductal papillary-mucinous neoplasms (IPMNs) are intraductal mucin-producing neoplasms with tall, columnar, mucin-containing epithelium with or without papillary projections. These neoplasms extensively involve the main pancreatic ducts and/or major side branches. In addition, IPMNs lack the ovarian stroma characteristic of MCNs. Similar to the well-defined adenoma–carcinoma sequence in pancreatic ductal adenocarcinoma (PanIN to invasive ductal carcinoma), IPMNs seem to follow a similar pattern progressing from IPMN adenoma, to borderline IPMN with dysplasia, to IPMN with CIS, and eventually to invasive carcinoma. Microscopically, they consist of papillary projections lined by columnar

TABLE 54.5 DIAGNOSIS

COMPARISON BETWEEN MUCINOUS CYSTIC NEOPLASM (MCN) AND INTRADUCTAL PAPILLARY MUCINOUS NEOPLASM (IPMN)

	■ MCN	■ IPMN
Age (y)	40–50	60–80
Gender	More common in females	More common in males
Location	Body/tail	Head
Communicates with pancreatic duct	No	Yes
Mucin at ampulla	No	Yes
Ovarianlike stroma	Yes	No

mucin-secreting cells. They show varying degrees of cellular atypia. The mean age of patients with invasive carcinoma is approximately 5 years older than patients with noninvasive IPMNs, suggesting an approximate 5-year lag period for progression to malignancy.

IPMNs are subclassified as main- and branch-duct types and as a mixed type that contains elements of both. Main-duct IPMN is characterized by involvement of the duct of Wirsung, which is dilated to more than 1 cm in diameter. Branch-duct IPMN originates in the side branches of the pancreatic ductal system and appears as a multilobular cystic lesion communicating with a nondilated main pancreatic duct. Typically, branch-duct IPMN occurs in the uncinate process or head of the gland, but it can also be seen in the neck and distal pancreas. If the main duct is dilated with synchronous involvement of the branch ducts, it is described as a mixed IPMN.

IPMNs are usually found in individuals in their 60s to 80s. Some patients may experience symptoms that include abdominal pain, steatorrhea, weight loss, jaundice, diabetes, and chronic pancreatitis. A substantial number of these lesions are also detected as incidental findings on cross-sectional imaging studies performed for other indications. IPMNs appear to be more common in the head, neck, and uncinate process of the pancreas but can be found diffusely throughout the whole gland. CT scans will typically reveal a cystic mass in the head of the pancreas that appears to communicate with the pancreatic ductal system. On endoscopy, mucin can be seen oozing from the ampulla of Vater. Endoscopic retrograde cholangiopancreatography (ERCP) can be used to confirm that the cysts communicate with the pancreatic ducts.

MCNs are the main entity to consider in the differential diagnosis of IPMNs (Table 54.5). Two morphologic features distinguish IPMNs from MCNs: IPMNs communicate with ducts, while mucinous cysts do not; IPMNs also lack an ovarian stroma that is present in mucinous cysts. In addition, mucinous cysts are usually seen in the tail of the pancreas and occur in middle-aged women, whereas IPMNs are found in the head of the pancreas and occur in older individuals of either sex.

As noted, IPMNs represent a continuum of disease from benign to malignant. In a large series of resected IPMNs from the Johns Hopkins Hospital,[11] the prognosis for the benign forms of the disease appears to be significantly better than for invasive IPMNs with 1-, 2-, and 5-year actuarial survivals of 97%, 94%, and 77%, respectively. Although invasive IPMNs are associated with disease progression and death, the prognosis remains markedly better than for invasive ductal carcinoma of the pancreas with survivals of 72%, 58%, and 43% at 1, 2, and 5 years, respectively. It is unclear whether this fact is due to earlier presentation or differences in tumor biology.

International consensus guidelines for the management of IPMNs have been developed.[12] The guidelines suggest that patients with a main-duct component to their IPMN (i.e., main and mixed types) should be optimally managed with surgical resection since at least 60% of these lesions have evidence of malignancy (either carcinoma in situ or invasive cancer) in the resected specimen. The management of branch-type IPMNs, however, remains controversial. The guidelines suggest that branch-type IPMNs less than 3 cm can be safely observed if they are asymptomatic and have no concerning radiographic or cytopathologic evidence of malignancy (mural nodules or abnormal cytology of cyst fluid). The guidelines further suggest a management strategy for branch-type IPMNs based on size. For lesions less than 1 cm in size, management entails serial cross-sectional imaging. For lesions 1 to 3 cm, management entails cross-sectional imaging, endoscopic ultrasound, and cytology. In patients with lesions 1 to 3 cm in size, surgical management is considered for symptoms or concerning radiographic (e.g., mural nodules, main-duct dilation) or cytopathologic evidence of malignancy. For lesions greater than 3 cm, surgical management is recommended even in the absence of other concerning features of malignancy. Again, the decision to resect must be individualized based on a variety of considerations. These include patient age, patient compliance for a surveillance program, and the quality of a surveillance program, which can vary according to available resources.

The goal of surgical therapy for IPMNs should be a complete surgical resection yielding negative margins for all invasive and noninvasive disease. Unlike those patients with completely resected noninvasive MCNs (who are routinely cured), patients with completely resected noninvasive IPMNs should undergo careful follow-up and surveillance for the development of recurrent disease. Furthermore, patients with resected invasive IPMNs should also undergo careful follow-up and surveillance as they, too, remain at risk for the development of recurrent disease.

Solid Pseudopapillary Tumor. Solid pseudopapillary tumors (SPTs), also termed solid and cystic tumors, papillary cystic tumors, *Hamoudi tumors,* and *Frantz tumor,* occur primarily in women in their third to fourth decade of life. Grossly, the masses range from 5 to 15 cm in diameter. The tumors show solid, cystic, and papillary components. Although most patients are cured after resection, metastases have been reported in a small number of cases.

CLINICOPATHOLOGIC STAGING

Accurate pathologic staging of pancreatic cancer is important for providing prognostic information to patients and for

TABLE 54.6 **STAGING**

AMERICAN JOINT COMMITTEE ON CANCER STAGING OF PANCREATIC CANCER

STAGE	T	N	M	5-Y SURVIVAL (%)
IA	T1	N0	M0	20–30
IB	T2	N0	M0	20–30
IIA	T3	N0	M0	10–25
IIB	T1, T2, T3	N1	M0	10–15
III	T4	Any N	M0	0–5
IV	Any T	Any N	M1	—

TUMOR (T)

TX: Primary tumor cannot be assessed

T0: No evidence of primary tumor

Tis: Carcinoma in situ

T1: Tumor limited to the pancreas, 2 cm or less in greatest dimension

T2: Tumor limited to the pancreas, more than 2 cm in greatest dimension

T3: Tumor extends beyond the pancreas but without involvement of the celiac axis or the superior mesenteric artery

T4: Tumor involves the celiac axis or the superior mesenteric artery (unresectable primary tumor)

REGIONAL LYMPH NODES (N)

NX: Regional lymph nodes cannot be assessed

N0: No regional lymph node metastasis

N1: Regional lymph node metastasis

DISTANT METASTASIS (M)

MX: Distant metastasis cannot be assessed

M0: No distant metastasis

M1: Distant metastasis

Adapted from American Joint Committee on Cancer. Exocrine pancreas. In: *AJCC Cancer Staging Manual*, 6th ed. New York: Springer; 2002:157.

comparing the results of various therapeutic trials. The American Joint Committee on Cancer (AJCC) staging for pancreatic cancer is shown in Table 54.6. This system, based on the TNM classification, takes into account the extent of the primary tumor (T), the presence or absence of regional lymph node involvement (N), and the presence or absence of distant metastatic disease (M).

DIAGNOSIS

Clinical Presentation

Many of the difficulties associated with the management of pancreatic cancer result from our inability to make the diagnosis at an early stage. The early symptoms of pancreatic cancer include anorexia, weight loss, abdominal discomfort, and nausea. Unfortunately, the nonspecific nature of these symptoms often leads to a delay in the diagnosis. Specific symptoms usually develop only after invasion or obstruction of nearby structures has occurred. Most pancreatic cancers arise in the head of the pancreas, and obstruction of the intrapancreatic portion of the common bile duct leads to progressive jaundice, acholic stools, darkening of the urine, and pruritus. Pain is a common symptom of pancreatic cancer. The pain usually starts as vague upper abdominal or back pain that is often ignored by the patient or attributed to some other cause. It is usually worse in the supine position and is often relieved by leaning forward. Pain may be caused by invasion of the tumor into the splanchnic plexus and retroperitoneum and by obstruction of the pancreatic duct. Other digestive symptoms are also common in pancreatic cancer (Table 54.7).

Occasionally, pancreatic cancer may be discovered in an unusual manner. The onset of diabetes may be the first clinical feature in 10% to 15% of patients. An episode of acute pancreatitis may also be the initial presentation of pancreatic cancer if the tumor partially obstructs the pancreatic duct. It is important to consider a pancreatic cancer in patients presenting with acute pancreatitis, especially those without an obvious cause for their pancreatitis (alcohol or gallstones).

The most common physical finding at the initial presentation is jaundice (Table 54.8). Hepatomegaly and a palpable gallbladder may be present in some patients. In cases of advanced disease, cachexia, muscle wasting, or a nodular liver, consistent with metastatic disease, may be evident. Other physical findings in patients with disseminated cancer include left supraclavicular adenopathy (Virchow node), periumbilical adenopathy (Sister Mary Joseph node), and pelvic drop metastases (Blumer shelf). Ascites can be present in 15% of patients.

Laboratory Studies

In patients with cancer of the head of the pancreas, laboratory studies usually reveal a significant increase in serum total bilirubin, alkaline phosphatase, and γ-glutamyl transferase,

TABLE 54.7 **DIAGNOSIS**

SYMPTOMS OF PANCREATIC CANCER

■ SYMPTOM	■ PATIENTS (%)
HEAD	
Weight loss	92
Jaundice	82
Pain	72
Anorexia	64
Dark urine	63
Light stools	62
Nausea	45
Vomiting	37
Weakness	35
Pruritus	24
Diarrhea	18
Melena	12
Constipation	11
Fever	11
Hematemesis	8
BODY AND TAIL	
Weight loss	100
Pain	87
Weakness	43
Nausea	43
Vomiting	37
Anorexia	33
Constipation	27
Hematemesis	17
Melena	17
Jaundice	7
Fever	7
Diarrhea	3

TABLE 54.8 **DIAGNOSIS**

SIGNS OF PANCREATIC CANCER

■ SIGN	■ PATIENTS (%)
HEAD	
Jaundice	87
Palpable liver	83
Palpable gallbladder	29
Tenderness	26
Ascites	14
Abdominal mass	13
BODY AND TAIL	
Palpable liver	33
Tenderness	27
Abdominal mass	23
Ascites	20
Jaundice	13
Diarrhea	3

indicating bile duct obstruction. The transaminases can also be elevated but usually not to the same extent as the alkaline phosphatase. In patients with localized cancer of the body and tail of the pancreas, laboratory values are frequently normal early in the course. Patients with pancreatic cancer may also demonstrate a normochromic anemia and hypoalbuminemia secondary to the nutritional consequences of the disease. In patients with jaundice, the prothrombin time can be abnormally prolonged. This usually is an indication of biliary obstruction, which prevents bile from entering the gastrointestinal tract and leads to malabsorption of fat-soluble vitamins and decreased hepatic production of vitamin K–dependent clotting factors. The prothrombin time can usually be normalized by the administration of parenteral vitamin K. Serum amylase and lipase levels are usually normal in patients with pancreatic cancer.

A wide variety of serum tumor markers have been proposed for use in the diagnosis and follow-up of patients with pancreatic cancer. The most extensively studied of these is CA 19–9, a Lewis blood group–related mucin glycoprotein. Approximately 5% of the population lacks the Lewis gene and therefore cannot produce CA 19–9. When a normal upper limit of 37 U/mL is used, the accuracy of the CA 19–9 level in identifying patients with pancreatic adenocarcinoma is only about 80%. When a higher cutoff value of more than 90 U/mL is used, the accuracy improves to 85%, and increasing the cutoff value to 200 U/mL increases the accuracy to 95%.[13] The combined use of CA 19–9 and ultrasonography, CT, or ERCP can improve the accuracy of the individual tests, so that the combined accuracy approaches 100% for the diagnosis of pancreatic cancer. Levels of CA 19–9 have also been correlated with prognosis and tumor recurrence. In general, higher CA 19–9 values before surgery indicate an increased size of the primary tumor and increased rate of unresectability. In addition, the CA 19–9 level has been used to monitor the results of neoadjuvant and adjuvant chemoradiation therapy in patients. Increasing CA 19–9 levels usually indicate recurrence or progression of disease, whereas stable or declining levels indicate a stable tumor burden, absence of recurrence on imaging studies, and an improved prognosis.

Radiologic Investigations

Radiologic imaging plays a crucial role in the diagnosis, staging, and follow-up of patients with pancreatic cancer. In addition to identifying the primary tumor, the goals of imaging include the assessment of local and regional invasion, evaluation of lymph nodes and vascular structures, identification of distant metastatic disease, and determination of tumor resectability. Ultrasonography, CT, and magnetic resonance imaging (MRI) are all useful noninvasive tests in the patient suspected of having a pancreatic cancer.

Transabdominal ultrasonography is operator dependent but can demonstrate dilated intrahepatic and extrahepatic bile ducts, liver metastases, pancreatic masses, ascites, and enlarged peripancreatic lymph nodes. Pancreatic cancer typically appears as a hypoechoic mass on ultrasonography. Ultrasonography will reveal a pancreatic mass in 60% to 70% of patients with cancer. Because helical CT is just as sensitive as ultrasonography and provides more complete information about surrounding structures and the local and distant extent of the disease, transabdominal ultrasonography has been largely replaced by CT.

3 Helical or spiral CT is currently the preferred noninvasive imaging test for the diagnosis of pancreatic cancer. Pancreatic cancer usually appears as an area of pancreatic enlargement with a localized hypodense lesion (Fig. 54.3). For pancreatic lesions, a dual-phase intravenous contrast study is ideal. Thin cuts are obtained through the pancreas and liver during both an arterial phase and portal venous phase after the administration

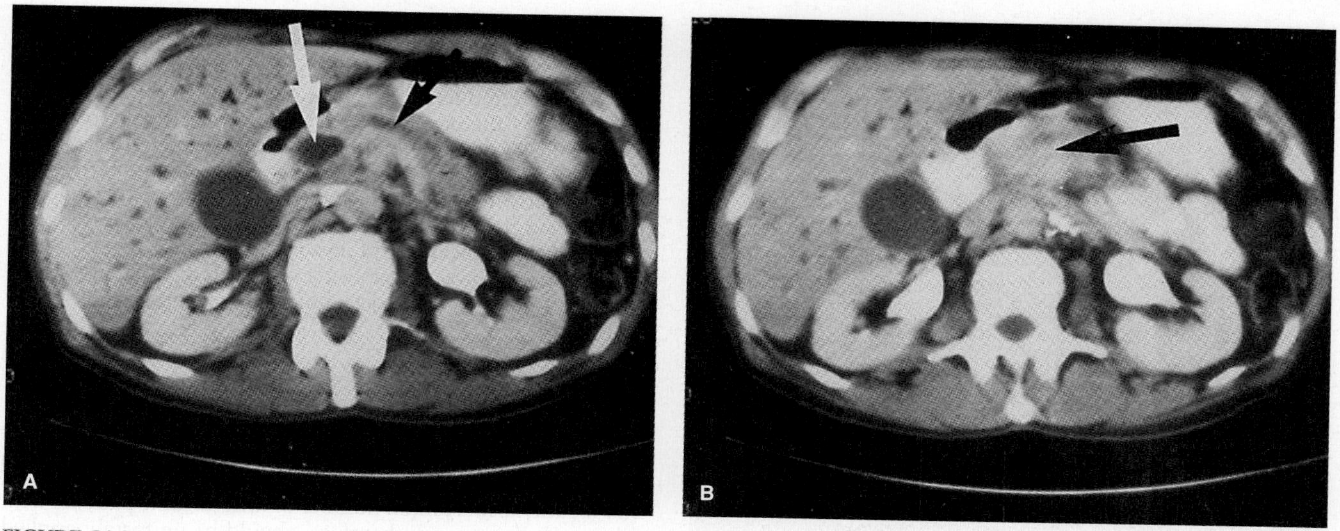

FIGURE 54.3. Computed tomogram of the abdomen of a patient with adenocarcinoma of the pancreas. **A:** The obstructed and dilated common bile duct (*light arrow*) and pancreatic duct (*dark arrow*) can be seen. In the adjacent cross section (**B**), a large mass is present in the head of the pancreas (*arrow*).

of intravenous contrast. In addition to determining the primary tumor size, CT is used to evaluate invasion into local structures or metastatic disease.

In general, MRI offers no significant advantages over CT because of a low signal-to-noise ratio, motion artifacts, lack of bowel opacification, and low spatial resolution. MRI can be considered an alternative preoperative staging exam in patients with allergies to iodinated contrast agents and in patients with renal insufficiency. On MRI, a typical pancreatic adenocarcinoma appears hypointense on T1-weighted, unenhanced images, and has a variable appearance on T2-weighted sequences. The T2 signal of the tumor is often dependent on the amount of desmoplastic response associated

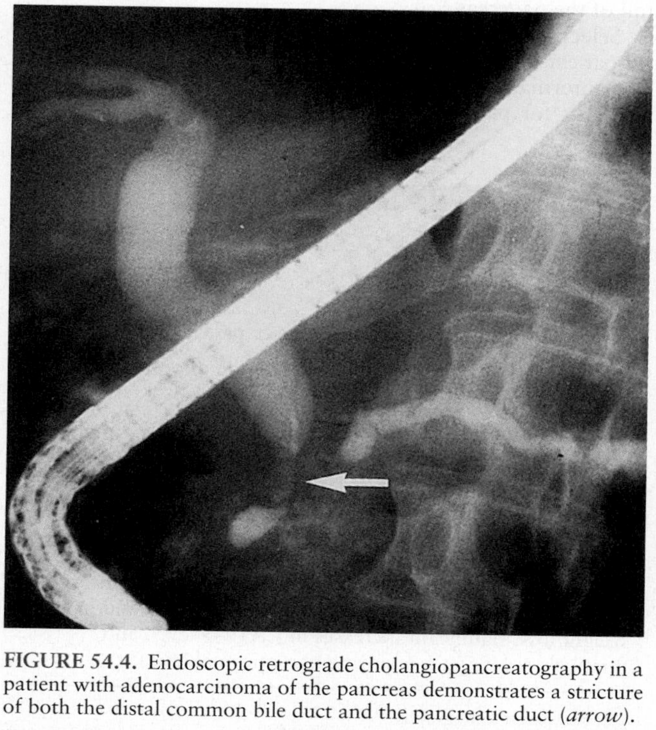

FIGURE 54.4. Endoscopic retrograde cholangiopancreatography in a patient with adenocarcinoma of the pancreas demonstrates a stricture of both the distal common bile duct and the pancreatic duct (*arrow*).

with the tumor. On dynamic imaging following a gadolinium contrast injection, an adenocarcinoma enhances relatively less than the background pancreatic parenchyma in the early phase and then reveals progressive enhancement in the subsequent phases. Magnetic resonance imaging with magnetic resonance cholangiopancreatography (MRCP) is currently indicated for noninvasive diagnostic imaging to evaluate the biliary and pancreatic ducts and may be the optimal method to survey patients with IPMN and the pancreatic remnant after surgery.

Traditionally, the next step in the evaluation of the jaundiced patient has been cholangiography, either by the endoscopic or by the percutaneous route. If the endoscopic approach is used, the duodenum and ampulla can be visualized and biopsy specimens obtained if necessary. In addition, ERCP allows for direct imaging of the pancreatic duct. The sensitivity of ERCP for the diagnosis of pancreatic cancer approaches 90%. The finding of a long, irregular stricture in an otherwise normal pancreatic duct is highly suggestive of a pancreatic cancer (Fig. 54.4). Often, the pancreatic duct will be obstructed with no distal filling. Although ERCP is reliable in confirming the presence of a clinically suspected pancreatic cancer, it should not be used routinely. Diagnostic ERCP should be reserved for patients with presumed pancreatic cancer and obstructive jaundice in whom no mass is demonstrated on CT, symptomatic but nonjaundiced patients without an obvious pancreatic mass, and patients with chronic pancreatitis who develop jaundice.

PREOPERATIVE STAGING

The goal of preoperative staging of pancreatic cancer is to determine the feasibility of surgery and the optimal treatment for each individual patient. In many cases, dynamic CT with oral and intravenous contrast may provide all the information necessary. With objective, specific anatomy-based CT criteria, patients with pancreatic cancer can be stratified into three distinct groups: (a) metastatic, defined by CT evidence of distant metastatic spread to the liver, peritoneum, or lung; (b) locally advanced, which is defined by CT evidence of arterial encroachment of the celiac axis or superior mesenteric artery or venous involvement or occlusion of the superior mesenteric or portal veins; and (c) potentially resectable, which is defined

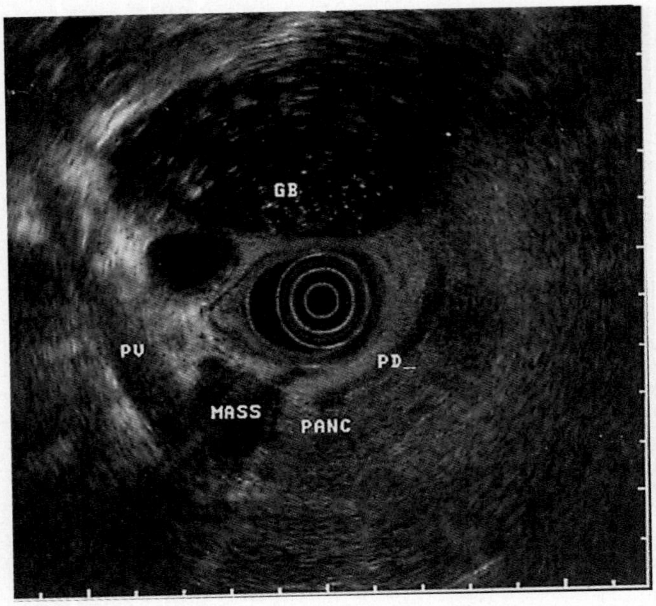

FIGURE 54.5. Endoscopic ultrasonogram of a 2.2-cm mass in the head of the pancreas. The transducer tip is located in the duodenum. The dilated common bile duct and gallbladder (GB) can be seen at the top of the image. The pancreatic duct (PD) is also dilated. The mass involves the portal vein (PV).

as no CT evidence of extrapancreatic disease, a patent superior mesenteric vein (SMV)–portal vein confluence, and no evidence of direct tumor extension to the celiac axis or superior mesenteric artery. Up to 85% of potentially resectable patients can be resected, whereas only 20% of patients with locally advanced pancreatic cancer can be successfully resected.[14] For tumors of the head, neck, or uncinate process of the pancreas, occlusion of the SMV or portal vein along with the presence of periportal collateral vessels is a sign of unresectability and typically precludes resection for cure. In contrast, for tumors of the body and tail of the pancreas, occlusion of the splenic vein with perigastric collaterals does not always preclude resection and should not be considered a sign of unresectability.

Endoscopic ultrasonography (EUS) is a minimally invasive technique in which a high-frequency ultrasonographic probe is placed into the stomach and duodenum endoscopically and the pancreas is imaged. Tumors appear as hypoechoic areas in the pancreatic substance (Fig. 54.5). The strengths of EUS techniques for pancreatic cancer are the clarification of small lesions (<2 cm) when CT findings are questionable or negative, detection of malignant lymphadenopathy, detection of vascular involvement, and the ability to perform EUS-guided fine-needle aspiration (FNA) for definitive diagnosis and staging. EUS is not effective in assessing metastatic disease to the liver. In patients for whom a tissue diagnosis is required (poor operative candidates or undergoing neoadjuvant therapy), EUS-guided FNA has been used to acquire tissue samples for cytologic analysis. This approach may avoid the risks of tumor seeding from percutaneous biopsy. The accuracy of EUS without FNA averages 85% for determining T-stage and 70% for determining N-stage disease. The combination of EUS and FNA has a sensitivity of 93% and a specificity of 100% for T-stage and an accuracy of 88% for N-stage disease.[15] At the time of diagnosis, only 10% of patients have tumors confined to the pancreas, 40% have locally advanced disease, and more than 50% have distant spread.

Percutaneous FNA of pancreatic masses is helpful in selected patients. The technique is safe and generally reliable but is of limited use in patients in whom surgical exploration for attempted resection or palliation is planned. The reasons for not using FNA or percutaneous biopsy in potentially resectable lesions are twofold. First, even after repeated sampling, a negative result does not exclude malignancy; in fact, it is the smaller and likely more curable tumors that are likely to be missed by the needle. The second concern is the potential for seeding of the tumor, either along the needle tract or with intraperitoneal spread. Percutaneous biopsy is primarily indicated in patients with unresectable cancers based on preoperative staging to direct palliative chemoradiation therapy or in patients with cancer in the head of the pancreas for whom neoadjuvant protocols are being considered. Currently, however, EUS is the preferred technique when possible in either situation.

STAGING LAPAROSCOPY

The use of diagnostic laparoscopy in pancreatic cancer remains controversial. Proponents believe that laparoscopy can identify a substantial number of unresectable patients with advanced disease and, therefore, should be uniformly applied to all patients with potentially resectable tumors.[16] On the other hand, opponents believe that the inherent cost of such a practice far outweighs the benefit to the small number of patients in whom diagnostic laparoscopy is useful. The liver and peritoneum are the most common sites of distant spread of pancreatic carcinoma. Once distant metastases have developed, survival is so limited that a conservative approach is usually indicated. Liver metastases larger than 1 cm in diameter can usually be detected by CT, but approximately 30% of these metastases are smaller and therefore may not be routinely detected. Moreover, peritoneal and omental metastases are usually only 1 to 2 mm in size and frequently can be detected only by direct visualization. With the recent improvements in CT imaging, the rate of unsuspected positive peritoneal findings approaches 10% to 15% for all patients. The percentage, however, varies with tumor location. Patients presenting with obstructive jaundice secondary to tumors in the head of the pancreas typically have only a 15% to 20% incidence of unexpected intraperitoneal metastasis after routine staging studies. In contrast, unexpected peritoneal metastasis is found in up to 50% of patients with cancer of the body and tail of the pancreas.[17]

Selective use of staging laparoscopy should be considered for patients at high risk of occult metastatic disease (Table 54.9). The information gained from preoperative staging provides the basis for planning therapy for each individual patient. If

TABLE 54.9 **DIAGNOSIS**

SIGNS OF HIGH RISK OF OCCULT METASTATIC DISEASE

Large primary tumors
Lesions in the neck, body, or tail of the pancreas
Equivocal radiographic findings suggestive of occult distant metastatic disease
Low-volume ascites
CT findings indicating possible carcinomatosis
Small hypodense regions in the hepatic parenchyma that suggest hepatic metastases that are not amenable to percutaneous biopsy
Subtle clinical and laboratory findings suggesting more advanced disease (e.g., marked hypoalbuminemia and/or weight loss, significant increases in CA19–9 level, and relatively severe pain requiring narcotic analgesia)

CT, computed tomography.

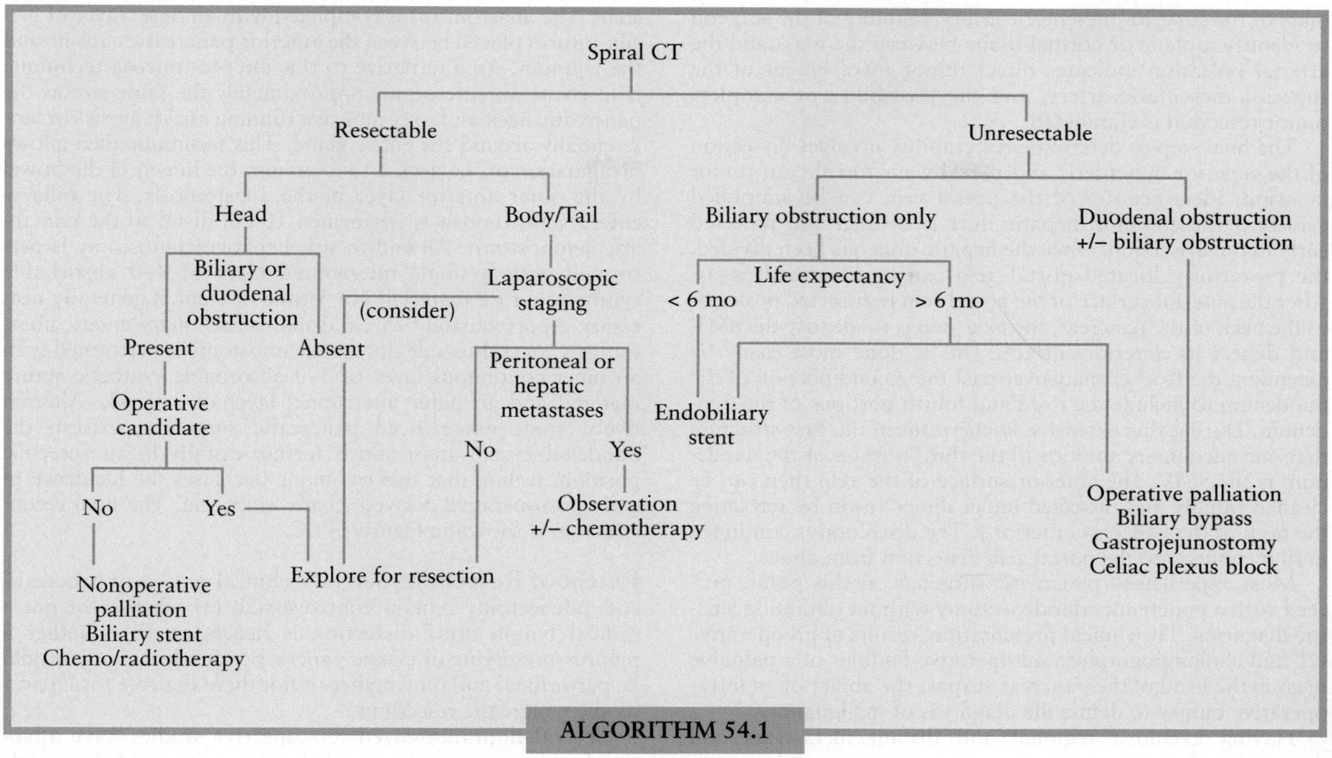

ALGORITHM 54.1. Diagnosis and management of pancreatic cancer. (After Tsiotis GG, Sarr MG. Diagnosis and clinical staging of pancreatic cancer. In: Howard JM, Idezuki Y, Ihse I, et al., eds. *Surgical Disease of the Pancreas,* 3rd ed. Baltimore: Williams & Wilkins; 1998:510.)

the results of preoperative staging with CT/MRI and laparoscopy show localized disease, resectability rates may approach 90% for tumors in the head of the pancreas. A decision tree for the clinical staging of suspected pancreatic cancer is shown in Algorithm 54.1.

RESECTION OF PANCREATIC CARCINOMA

Carcinoma of the Head, Neck, or Uncinate Process

In 1912, Kaush[18] reported the first successful resection of the duodenum and a portion of the pancreas for an ampullary cancer. In 1935, Whipple et al.[19] described a technique for radical excision of a periampullary carcinoma. The operation was originally performed in two stages. A cholecystogastrostomy to decompress the obstructed biliary tree and a gastrojejunostomy to relieve gastric outlet obstruction comprised the first stage. The second stage was performed several weeks later when the jaundice had resolved and the nutritional status had improved. During the second stage, an en bloc resection of the second portion of the duodenum and head of the pancreas was performed without reestablishing pancreatic–enteric continuity. Although earlier contributions had been made, the report by Whipple et al. began the modern-day approach to the treatment of pancreatic carcinoma.

Since Whipple's original description, pancreaticoduodenal resection has undergone numerous modifications and technical refinements. Unfortunately, during most of the first 50 years when the procedure was performed, the reported morbidity and mortality rates were unacceptably high, and long-term survival rates were disappointing. During the late 1960s and 1970s, the high operative morbidity and mortality and poor long-term survival rates led some surgeons to suggest that the Whipple procedure be abandoned. However, during the last two decades, a number of reports have documented improved operative results and long-term survival rates for patients with periampullary tumors following the Whipple procedure, so that a resurgence in its popularity has occurred.

The operative management of pancreatic cancer consists of two phases: first, assessing tumor resectability and then, if the tumor is resectable, completing a pancreaticoduodenectomy and restoring gastrointestinal continuity. After the abdomen has been opened through an upper midline or bilateral subcostal incision, a careful search for tumor outside the limits of a pancreaticoduodenal resection should be carried out. The liver, omentum, and peritoneal surfaces are inspected and palpated, and suspect lesions are sampled and specimens submitted for frozen section analysis. Next, regional lymph nodes are evaluated for tumor involvement. The presence of tumor in the periaortic lymph nodes of the celiac axis indicates that the tumor is beyond the limits of normal resection. However, the presence of tumor-bearing lymph nodes that normally would be incorporated within the resection specimen do not constitute a contraindication to resection.

Once distant metastases have been excluded, the primary tumor is assessed in regard to resectability. Local factors that preclude pancreaticoduodenal resection include retroperitoneal extension of the tumor to involve the inferior vena cava or aorta or direct involvement or encasement of the superior mesenteric artery, hepatic artery, and celiac axis. Involvement of the SMV or portal vein can be managed with venous resection and reconstruction in select cases. The technical aspects of determining local resectability begin with a Kocher maneuver and mobilization of the duodenum and head of the pancreas from the underlying inferior vena cava and aorta. Once the duodenum and head of the pancreas are mobilized sufficiently, the surgeon's hand can be placed under the duodenum and head of the pancreas to palpate the relationship of the tumor mass to the superior mesenteric artery. Inability of the surgeon to identify a plane of normal tissue between the mass and the arterial pulsation indicates direct tumor involvement of the superior mesenteric artery, and the possibility of complete tumor resection is eliminated.

The final step to determine resectability involves dissection of the superior mesenteric and portal veins to rule out tumor invasion. Identification of the portal vein can be simplified greatly if the common hepatic duct is divided and reflected early in the dissection. Once the hepatic duct has been divided, the posteriorly located portal vein can be identified easily. After the anterior surface of the portal vein is dissected posterior to the neck of the pancreas, the next step is to identify the SMV and dissect its anterior surface. This is done most easily by extending the Kocher maneuver past the second portion of the duodenum to include the third and fourth portions of the duodenum. During this extensive kocherization, the first structure that one encounters anterior to the third portion of the duodenum is the SMV. The anterior surface of the vein then can be cleaned rapidly and dissected under direct vision by retracting the neck of the pancreas anteriorly. The dissection is continued until it connects to the portal vein dissection from above.

Most experienced pancreatic surgeons, at this point, proceed with a pancreaticoduodenectomy without obtaining a tissue diagnosis. The clinical presentation, results of preoperative CT and cholangiography, and operative findings of a palpable mass in the head of the pancreas surpass the ability of an intraoperative biopsy to define the diagnosis of malignancy.

Having excluded regional and distant metastases and demonstrated no tumor involvement in major vascular structures, the surgeon can proceed with pancreaticoduodenectomy with a high degree of certainty that the tumor is resectable. In the pylorus-preserving modification of pancreaticoduodenectomy, the duodenum is first mobilized and divided approximately 2 cm distal to the pylorus. If a classic Whipple procedure is to be performed, the stomach is divided to include approximately 40% to 50% of the stomach with the resected specimen. The gastroduodenal artery is exposed, ligated, and divided near its origin at the common hepatic artery. It is always important to confirm, before ligation, that the structure to be ligated is indeed the gastroduodenal artery and not a replaced right hepatic artery. Next, the neck of the pancreas is divided, with care taken to avoid injury to the underlying superior mesenteric and portal veins. The portal and superior mesenteric veins are then dissected from the uncinate process and head of the pancreas. At this point, the fourth portion of the duodenum and the proximal jejunum are mobilized, with the proximal jejunum divided approximately 10 cm distal to the ligament of Treitz. The proximal jejunum and fourth portion of the duodenum are passed under the superior mesenteric vessels to the right, and the uncinate process is dissected from the superior mesenteric artery. The course of the superior mesenteric artery should be clearly identified to avoid injury to this structure. At this point, the specimen consisting of the gallbladder and common bile duct; the head, neck, and uncinate process of the pancreas; the entire duodenum; and the proximal jejunum (and the distal stomach for a traditional Whipple procedure) is freed completely and removed from the operative field (Fig. 54.6).

There are a number of techniques for restoring gastrointestinal continuity after a pancreaticoduodenal resection. Our preferred technique is to bring the end of the divided jejunum through the transverse mesocolon in a retrocolic fashion and perform an end-to-side pancreaticojejunostomy. The anastomosis is begun by placing a series of interrupted 3–0 silk sutures between the side of the jejunum and the posterior capsule of the end of the pancreas. A small enterotomy is then made in the jejunum to match the size of the pancreatic duct and an inner layer of interrupted 5–0 absorbable monofilament sutures is used to create a duct-to-mucosa anastomosis. A short segment of a pediatric feeding tube may be placed across the anastomosis to be used as a temporary indwelling stent. The anastomosis is completed with an outer layer of 3–0 silk sutures placed between the anterior pancreatic capsule and the jejunum. An alternative to this duct-to-mucosa technique is to create an enterotomy approximately the same size as the pancreatic neck and to complete a running anastomosis circumferentially around the entire gland. This technique then allows invagination of the neck 1 to 2 cm into the lumen of the bowel by the outer anterior layer of the anastomosis. The biliary-enteric anastomosis is performed 10 cm distal to the pancreaticojejunostomy. An end-to-side hepaticojejunostomy is performed with a single interrupted layer of 4–0 absorbable synthetic suture material. No T-tube or stent is generally necessary. Approximately 15 cm distal to the biliary-enteric anastomosis, an end-to-side duodenojejunostomy is performed with an inner continuous layer of 3–0 absorbable synthetic suture material and an outer interrupted layer of 3–0 silk. Alternatively, some experienced pancreatic surgeons perform the duodenal-jejunal anastomosis further distally in an antecolic position, feeling that this technique decreases the incidence of early postoperative delayed gastric emptying. The final reconstruction is shown in Figure 54.6C.

Extent of Resection. Several technical aspects of pancreaticoduodenectomy remain controversial: (a) whether or not a radical lymph node dissection is necessary, (b) whether a pylorus-preserving or classic pancreaticoduodenectomy should be performed, and (c) whether or not there is a role for laparoscopic pancreatic resections.

Several nonrandomized retrospective studies have advocated adding a radical (extended) retroperitoneal lymph node dissection to pancreaticoduodenectomy in an attempt to improve survival. However, results from four randomized prospective trials[20–23] (Table 54.10) have shown extended lymph node dissections not to be beneficial. The prospective trial performed by Pedrazzoli et al.[20] suggested a survival advantage to extended retroperitoneal lymph node dissection in patients with positive lymph nodes. Eighty-one patients with pancreatic adenocarcinoma were randomized to either standard or radical lymphadenectomy over 3 years at six different institutions. While the two groups were similar with respect to preoperative parameters, operative morbidity, and overall survival, a subgroup analysis of the 48 patients with positive lymph nodes showed a statistically significant survival advantage for patients undergoing the extended lymph node dissection. However, the largest prospective randomized trial from the Johns Hopkins Hospital failed to demonstrate a survival advantage for a radical resection as compared with a classic pancreaticoduodenectomy.[21] Two hundred and ninety-four patients undergoing resection for periampullary adenocarcinoma were randomized between a standard resection (pylorus-preserving pancreaticoduodenectomy with en bloc resection of the anterior and posterior pancreaticoduodenal lymph nodes, lower hepatoduodenal lymph nodes, and nodes along the right lateral aspect of the superior artery and vein) and a radical resection (standard resection plus distal gastrectomy and retroperitoneal lymph node dissection extending from the right renal hilum to the left lateral border of the aorta and from the portal vein to the inferior mesenteric artery). The groups did not differ with respect to age, gender, site of primary tumor, lymph node status, or margin status. There were no significant differences in 1-, 3-, or 5-year and median survival when comparing the standard and radical groups (Fig. 54.7). However, the radical group had a higher overall morbidity (43% vs. 29%) with significantly higher rates of delayed gastric emptying and pancreatic fistula in addition to a longer postoperative hospital stay.

In 1978, Traverso and Longmire[24] popularized the pylorus-preserving modification of the Whipple procedure. Preserving antral and pyloric function, the pylorus-preserving Whipple procedure reduces the incidence of troublesome postgastrectomy symptoms. A number of studies have documented that

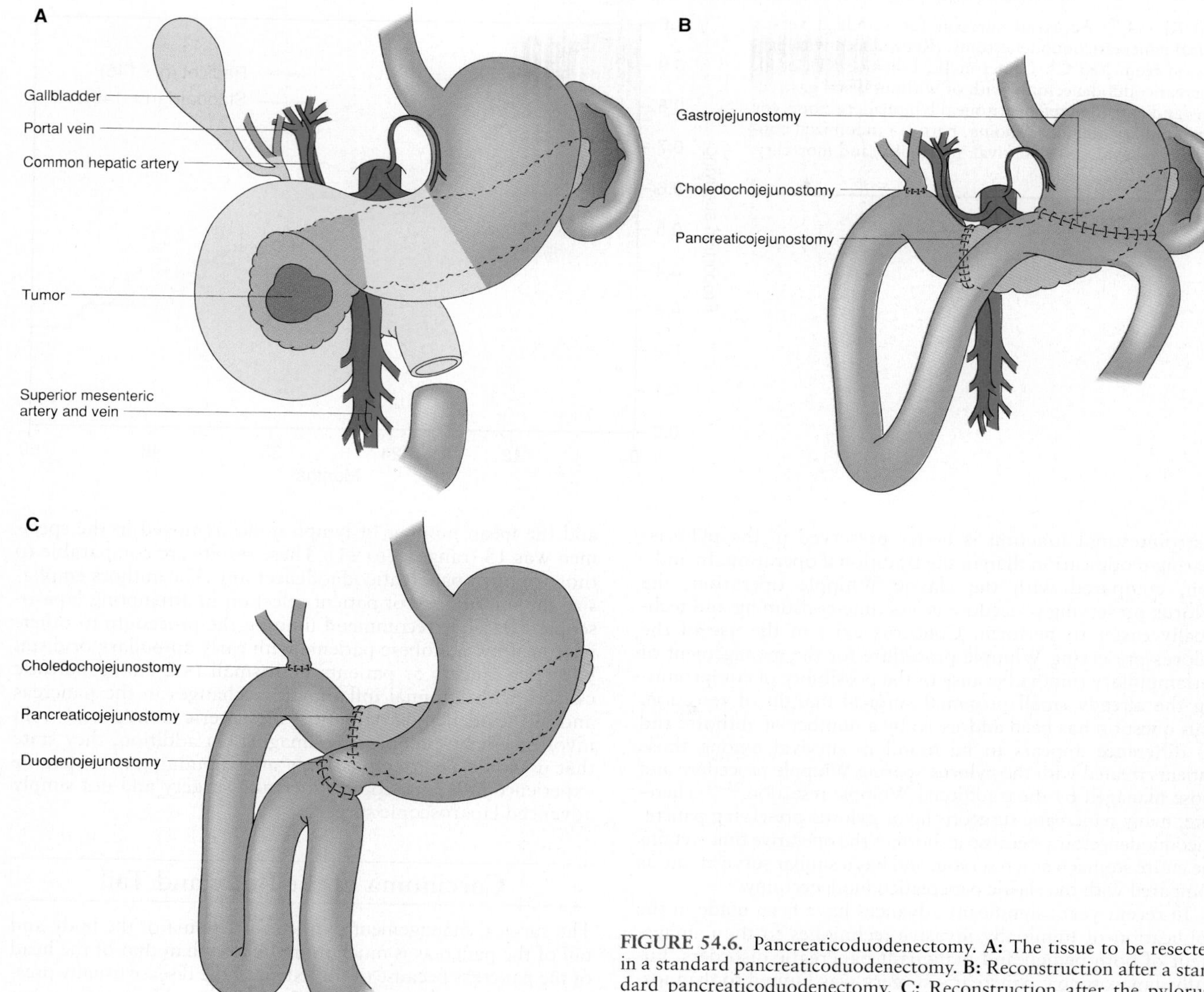

FIGURE 54.6. Pancreaticoduodenectomy. **A:** The tissue to be resected in a standard pancreaticoduodenectomy. **B:** Reconstruction after a standard pancreaticoduodenectomy. **C:** Reconstruction after the pylorus-sparing variation.

TABLE 54.10 **TREATMENT**

RANDOMIZED PROSPECTIVE TRIALS OF STANDARD VERSUS EXTENDED LYMPHADENECTOMY FOR PANCREATIC CANCER

■ AUTHOR	■ YEAR	■ PROCEDURE	■ *n*	■ OP TIME (h)	■ MORBIDITY (%)	■ MORTALITY (%)	■ 3-Y SURVIVAL (%)
Pedrazzoli et al.[20]	1998	Standard	40	6.2	35	5	12
		Extended	41	6.6	45	5	6
Yeo et al.[21]	2002	Standard	146	5.9	29	4	36
		Extended	148	6.4	43	2	38
Nimura et al.[22]	2004	Standard	51	7.0	12	0	29
		Extended	50	9.0	20	2	17
Farnell et al.[23]	2005	Standard	34	6.2	35	0	41
		Extended	31	7.6	45	2.6	25

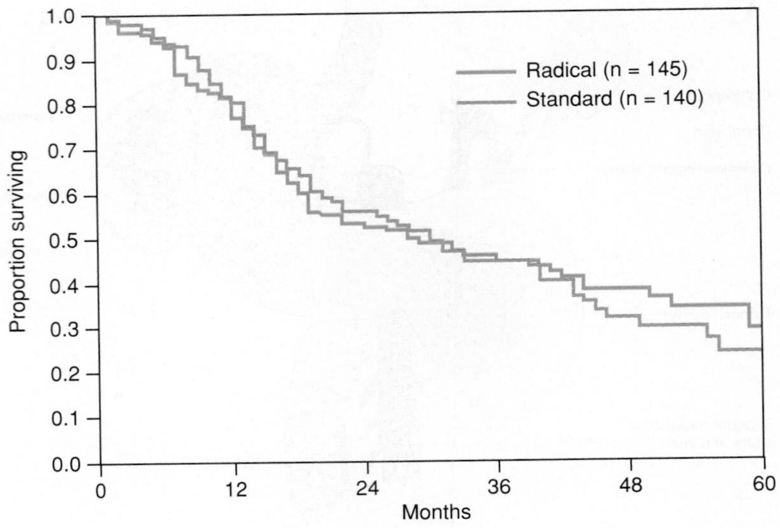

FIGURE 54.7. Actuarial survival for standard versus radical pancreaticoduodenectomy. (Reproduced with permission from Yeo CJ, Cameron JL, Lillemoe KD, et al. Pancreaticoduodenectomy with or without distal gastrectomy and extended retroperitoneal lymphadenectomy for periampullary adenocarcinoma, part 2: randomized controlled trial evaluating survival, morbidity, and mortality. *Ann Surg* 2002;236:355.)

gastrointestinal function is better preserved in the pylorus-sparing modification than in the traditional operation. In addition, compared with the classic Whipple operation, the pylorus-preserving procedure is less time-consuming and technically easier to perform. Concerns exist in the use of the pylorus-preserving Whipple procedure for the management of periampullary tumors because of the possibility of compromising the already small proximal surgical margin of resection. This question has been addressed by a number of authors, and no difference appears to be found in survival among those patients treated with the pylorus-sparing Whipple procedure and those managed by the traditional Whipple resection.[25–27] Therefore, many pancreatic surgeons favor pylorus-preserving pancreaticoduodenectomy because it shortens the operative time, retains the entire stomach as a reservoir, and has a similar survival rate as compared with the classic pancreaticoduodenectomy.

In recent years significant advances have been made in the application of minimally invasive techniques to the management of both benign and malignant pancreatic disorders. Initially, laparoscopic pancreatic surgery was limited to diagnostic staging in patients with pancreatic cancer prior to resection. More recently minimally invasive techniques have been used to manage benign and malignant lesions of the pancreas. While laparoscopic distal pancreatic resections are being performed with increasing frequency,[28] the role of laparoscopic pancreaticoduodenectomy (PD) remains controversial. Laparoscopic PD is a technically demanding procedure due to the retroperitoneal location of the pancreas, its intimate association with surrounding gastrointestinal and major vascular structures, and the need for three separate anastomoses to complete the reconstruction. In addition, it is unclear whether an adequate cancer operation can be performed with respect to lymph node harvest and margin status in patients with malignancy. Currently, laparoscopic PD is only performed in a handful of specialized centers. The procedures are performed as either pure laparoscopic, hand assisted or as laparoscopic-assisted procedures with the resection being performed laparoscopically and the reconstruction being completed via a "mini" laparotomy or through a hand port.

Palanivelu et al.[29] describe 42 patients who successfully underwent laparoscopic PD for ampullary carcinoma (n = 24), pancreatic cystadenocarcinoma (n = 4), pancreatic adenocarcinoma (n = 9), distal cholangiocarcinoma (n = 3), and chronic pancreatitis (n = 2). All of the procedures were able to be completed with a totally laparoscopic technique and there were no conversions to open. There was one perioperative mortality (2.4%) and the complication rate was 31%. The operative time averaged 370 minutes and the postoperative length of stay was 10.1 days. All patients underwent an R0 resection and the mean number of lymph nodes removed in the specimen was 13 (range, 8 to 21). These results are comparable to those of open pancreaticoduodenectomy. The authors emphasize the importance of patient selection in attempting laparoscopic PD. They recommend limiting the procedure to otherwise healthy, nonobese patients with early ampullary or distal bile duct cancers or patients with small (<2 cm) pancreatic cancers with minimal inflammatory changes in the pancreas and no evidence of superior mesenteric vein/portal vein involvement by preoperative imaging. In addition, they state that it should be attempted only after obtaining considerable experience in laparoscopic pancreatic surgery and not simply advanced laparoscopic surgery.

Carcinoma of the Body and Tail

The surgical management of adenocarcinoma of the body and tail of the pancreas is much more limited than that of the head of the pancreas because of the extent of the disease usually present at the time of symptomatic presentation. Most patients are unable to undergo resection, based on findings of major vascular involvement on CT or peritoneal or liver metastases on laparoscopy. If an attempt at open exploration for possible cure is undertaken, the exploration should be started with a search for evidence of either metastatic disease to the liver or peritoneal implants. If this is not the case, the lesser sac is opened, and the SMV is identified as it passes under the neck of the pancreas. If this vessel is normal, and if the splenic vein does not appear to be obstructed preoperatively, a distal pancreatectomy with splenectomy is performed. The spleen is mobilized, as is the distal pancreas, and an en bloc resection of the structure, including the mass, is obtained. The resection should be extended as proximally as possible, with the transected pancreas simply oversewn. The tumor bed should be marked with the placement of clips for postoperative radiation therapy. If, as in most cases, the tumor cannot be resected, a tissue biopsy should be performed, in addition to a chemical splanchnicectomy with alcohol for pain management. In some cases, a prophylactic gastrojejunostomy may be indicated because of the potential for obstruction by tumor at the ligament of Treitz.

Postoperative Results

4 During the 1960s and 1970s, many centers reported operative mortality following pancreaticoduodenectomy in the range of 20% to 40%, with postoperative morbidity rates as high as 40% to 60%. During the last two decades, a dramatic decline

TABLE 54.11 **COMPLICATIONS**

COMPLICATIONS AFTER PANCREATICODUODENECTOMY

COMMON	
Delayed gastric emptying	
Pancreatic fistula	
Intra-abdominal abscess	
Hemorrhage	
Wound infection	
Metabolic	
	Diabetes
	Pancreatic exocrine insufficiency
UNCOMMON	
Fistula	
	Biliary
	Duodenal
	Gastric
Organ failure	
	Cardiac
	Hepatic
	Pulmonary
	Renal
Pancreatitis	
Marginal ulceration	

From Yeo CJ, Cameron JL. Pancreatic cancer. *Curr Probl Surg* 1999; 36:61, with permission.

in operative morbidity and mortality following pancreaticoduodenectomy has been reported at a number of centers, with operative mortality rates in the range of 2% to 5%.[30–32] The reasons behind this decline appear to be the following: (a) fewer, more experienced surgeons are performing the operation on a more frequent basis; (b) preoperative and postoperative care has improved; (c) anesthetic management has improved; and (d) large numbers of patients are being treated at high-volume centers.[33]

Although the operative mortality rates for pancreatic cancer have been reduced significantly, the complication rates approach 40% (Table 54.11). Pancreatic fistula remains the most frequent serious complication following pancreaticoduodenectomy, with an incidence ranging from 5% to 15%. In the past, the development of pancreatic fistula after pancreaticoduodenectomy was associated with mortality rates of 10% to 40%. Although the incidence of pancreatic fistula following pancreaticoduodenectomy remains stable, the overall associated mortality rate has diminished owing to improved management. Important supportive measures include careful maintenance of fluid and electrolyte balance, parenteral nutrition, and controlling the pancreatic leak with percutaneous or intraoperative drainage.

Long-term Survival

Historically, 5-year survival rates for patients undergoing resection for adenocarcinoma of the head of the pancreas were reported to be in the range of 5%. However, recent studies have suggested an improved survival for patients following pancre-
5 aticoduodenectomy. In 2006, Winter et al.[34] reported on 1,175 patients with cancer of the pancreas managed by resection. The actuarial 5-year survival for these patients was 18%, with a median survival of 18 months (Fig. 54.8). In this study, factors found to be important predictors of survival included tumor diameter (<3 cm), negative resection margin status, well/moderate tumor differentiation, and postoperative chemoradiation treatment. Patients who underwent resection with negative margins had a median survival of 20 months and a 5-year survival of 21%, whereas those with positive margins fared significantly worse, with a median survival of 14 months and a 5-year survival of 12%. The outcome was particularly favorable in the subgroup of patients with small tumors (<3 cm) who underwent margin-negative, node-negative resections; the median survival was 44 months and the 5-year survival was 43%.

ADJUVANT AND NEOADJUVANT THERAPY

At present, the general consensus of most surgeons treating patients with pancreatic carcinoma is that any future improvement in survival for this disease will involve improvements in adjuvant therapy. Despite advances in surgery and perioperative care that have resulted in markedly reduced postoperative mortality after pancreaticoduodenectomy, the median survival for pancreatic cancer patients has changed minimally over the past two decades. Even with optimal surgical management, 5-year survival averages 15% to 20% for resectable disease and 3% for all stages combined. Approximately 85% of patients with resected pancreatic cancer will ultimately have a recurrence and die of their disease. This suggests that in most cases pancreatic cancer is a systemic disease at the time of diagnosis, making surgical resection alone inadequate therapy. The results of the most important randomized prospective trials of adjuvant therapy for pancreatic cancer are summarized in Table 54.12.

6 In 1985, the Gastrointestinal Tumor Study Group (GITSG) reported encouraging results from a prospective randomized trial to evaluate the efficacy of adjuvant radiation and chemotherapy following curative resection for adenocarcinoma of the head of the pancreas.[35] Forty-three patients were randomized to either adjuvant therapy with radiation and 5-fluorouracil (5-FU) or no adjuvant therapy. The median survival for the 21 patients who received adjuvant therapy was 20 months, and three (14%) survived 5 years or longer. For the 22 patients who received no adjuvant therapy, the median survival was 11 months, and only one patient (4.5%) survived 5 years.

The randomized trial conducted by the European Organization for Research and Treatment of Cancer (EORTC)[36] sought to recapitulate the results of the GITSG study in 114 patients with pancreatic head lesions (observation, $n = 54$; adjuvant treatment, $n = 60$). However, chemotherapy (5-FU) given during radiation was given as a continuous infusion (rather than via bolus) during each radiation sequence, depending on toxicity, for up to 5 days. No chemotherapy was given postchemoradiation. Fifty-six percent of patients received the intended chemotherapy dose during radiation. Patients in the chemoradiation arm had a median survival of 17.1 months versus 12.6 months in the observation arm ($p = 0.099$); 2- and 5-year overall survivals were 37% and 20%, respectively, for the experimental arm and 23% and 10%, respectively, for the control arm.

The European Study Group for Pancreatic Cancer (ESPAC-1) trial published in 2004 analyzed 289 patients recruited from 53 hospitals in a 2 × 2 factorial design.[37] The four study groups included (a) surgery only ($n = 69$); (2) chemotherapy only ($n = 73$) consisting of 5-FU, 425 mg/m^2, and leucovorin, 20 mg/m^2, given daily for 5 days every 4 weeks for six cycles of treatment; (c) radiation therapy and 5-FU given ($n = 75$) according to the

PANCREAS/LIVER

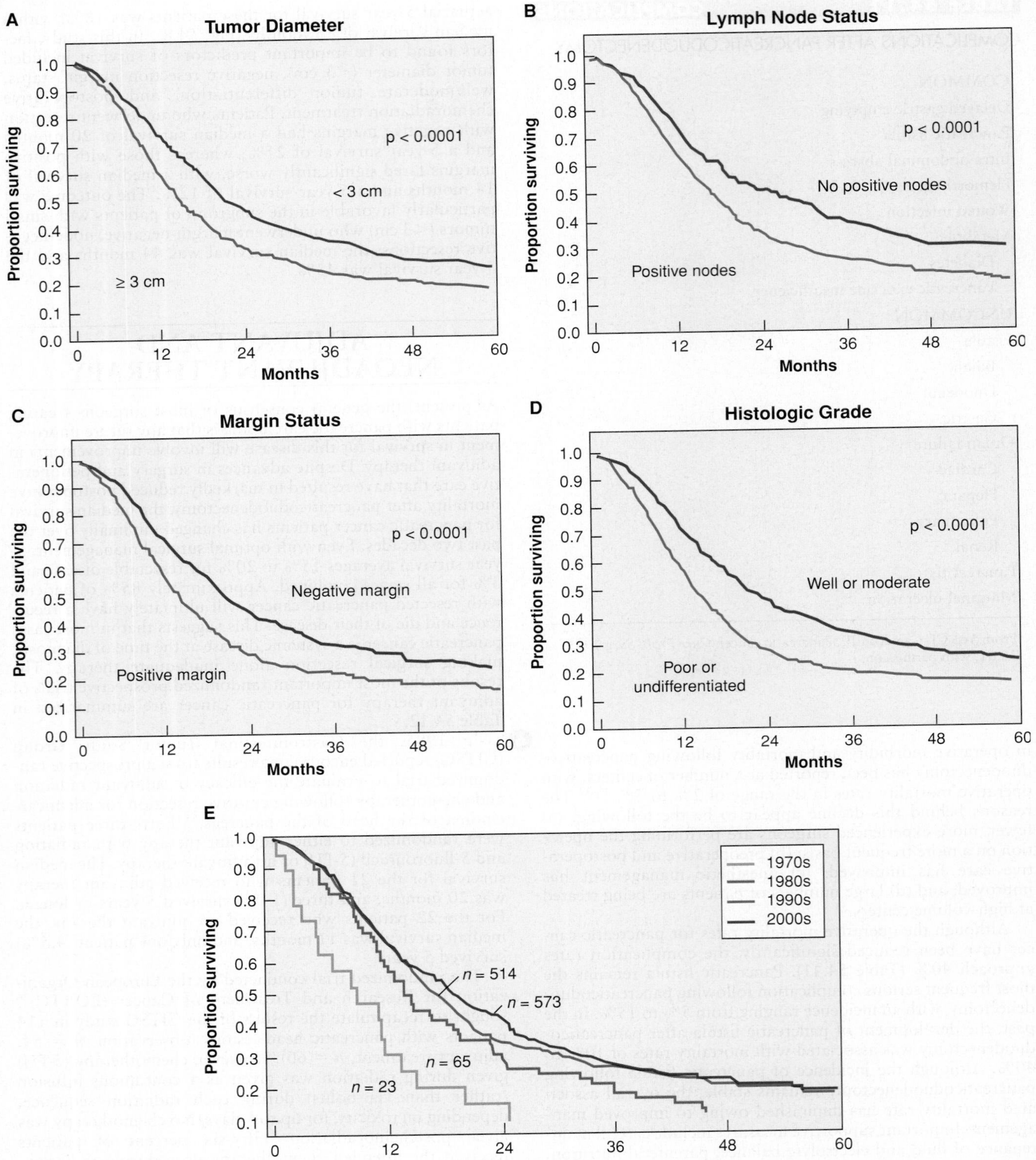

FIGURE 54.8. Survival of patients with pancreaticoduodenectomy based on tumor size (A), lymph node status (B), margin status (C), histologic grade (D), and historical context (E). (Reproduced with permission from Winter JM, Cameron JL, Campbell KA, et al. 1,423 pancreaticoduodenectomies for pancreatic cancer: a single-institution experience. *J Gastrointest Surgery* 2006;10:1199–1210.)

TABLE 54.12 **TREATMENT**

RANDOMIZED PROSPECTIVE TRIALS OF ADJUVANT THERAPY FOR PANCREATIC CANCER

STUDY	TREATMENT ARM	MEDIAN SURVIVAL (mo)	2-Y OVERALL SURVIVAL (%)	5-Y OVERALL SURVIVAL (%)
GITSG[35]	Surg	11	18	0
	Surg, XRT, 5-FU	18	43	19
EORTC[36]	Surg	13	23	10
	Surg, XRT, 5-FU	17	37	20
ESPAC-1[37]	Surg	17	—	11
	Surg, 5-FU	20	40	21
	Surg, XRT, 5-FU	16	29	10
RTOG[38]	Surg, XRT, 5-FU	17	21 (3 y)	—
	Surg, XRT, Gemcitabine	19	31 (3 y)	—
CONKO[39]	Surg	20	42	12
	Surg, Gemcitabine	22	48	23

5-FU, 5-fluorouracil; EORTC, European Organization for Research and Treatment of Cancer; ESPAC, European Study Group for Pancreatic Cancer; GITSG, Gastrointestinal Tumor Study Group; Surg, surgical; ROTC, Radiation Therapy Oncology Group; XRT, radiation therapy.

original GITSG method; and (d) both treatments (n = 73, chemoradiation followed by chemotherapy). The major study conclusions were the 5-year overall survival comparisons between patients who received chemotherapy versus those who did not (21% vs. 8%, $p = 0.009$) and those who received radiation therapy versus those who did not (10% vs. 20%, $p = 0.05$). The authors concluded that adjuvant chemotherapy had a beneficial effect in resected pancreas cancer, whereas chemoradiation had a deleterious effect. A quality-of-life questionnaire showed no difference between those who received chemotherapy and those who did not and those who received chemoradiation and those who did not. Thus, the survival benefit of adjuvant chemoradiation for pancreatic cancer patients remains unclear, and the optimal regimen has yet to be determined.

The Radiation Therapy Oncology Group (RTOG) 9704 trial, presented in abstract form in 2006,[38] contained 442 eligible patients who received adjuvant chemoradiation (5,040 cGy) given as continuous fractions with radiosensitizing doses of 5-FU. The comparisons were with the addition of either three cycles of 5-FU (one prechemoradiation, two postchemoradiation for 12 weeks) or four cycles of gemcitabine (one prechemoradiation, three postpostchemoradiation). Although the study showed no overall difference in aggregate survival, when pancreatic head lesions only were considered (eliminating study results from resected lesions in the pancreatic body or tail), both median survival (16.7 vs. 18.8 months) and overall survival at 3 years (21% vs. 31%) favored the gemcitabine arm ($p = 0.047$). The study concluded that the addition of adjuvant gemcitabine to postoperative 5-FU chemoradiation was superior to the addition of 5-FU.

The CONKO-1 trial,[39] conducted in Germany and Austria, represented a randomization of 368 patients following R0 or R1 resection to either observation or an experimental arm of gemcitabine. After a median follow-up time of 53 months, the median disease-free survival was 13.9 months in the gemcitabine arm versus 6.9 months in the observation arm ($p < 0.001$). There was no difference in overall survival for the gemcitabine arm versus the control group—median survival was 22 versus 20 months. Although survival was not different, the authors concluded that postoperative gemcitabine significantly delayed the development of recurrent disease after complete resection of pancreatic cancer compared with observation alone and, thus, was supported as adjuvant therapy in resectable pancreatic cancer.

At present, many centers are utilizing preoperative neoadjuvant chemoradiation for the treatment of pancreatic cancer (Table 54.13). Neoadjuvant therapy offers several

TABLE 54.13 **TREATMENT**

SELECTED NEOADJUVANT TRIALS FOR POTENTIALLY RESECTABLE PANCREATIC CANCER

AUTHOR	YEAR	n	REGIMEN	RESECTED (%)	MEDIAN SURVIVAL (mo)
Spitz et al.[40]	1997	91	XRT, 5-FU	45	19
Hoffman et al.[41]	1998	53	XRT, 5-FU, Mitomycin C	45	16
Pisters et al.[42]	2002	37	XRT, Paclitaxel	54	19
Wolff et al.[43]	2002	86	XRT, Gemcitabine	73	36
Talamonti et al.[44]	2006	20	XRT, Gemcitabine	85	26

5-FU, 5-fluorouracil; XRT, radiation therapy.

potential benefits, including (a) delivery of treatment to well-oxygenated tissue, which enhances efficacy of chemoradiation; (b) downstaging, which can enhance ability to achieve a negative margin resection and thereby reduce local recurrence; and (c) avoidance of surgery in patients with rapidly progressive disease. Neoadjuvant therapy can be completed without increasing the subsequent morbidity and mortality of surgical resection. The group from the M.D. Anderson Cancer Center has reported on the multimodality treatment of 142 consecutive patients with localized adenocarcinoma of the pancreatic head.[40] A subset of 41 patients treated by preoperative chemoradiation and pancreaticoduodenectomy were compared with 19 patients receiving pancreaticoduodenectomy and postoperative adjuvant chemoradiation. Surgery was not delayed for any patient who received preoperative chemoradiation because of chemoradiation toxicity, but 24% of the eligible patients did not receive their intended postoperative chemoradiation because of delayed recovery following pancreaticoduodenectomy. The patients treated with rapid fractionation were reported to have a significantly shorter duration of treatment (median, 62.5 days) than patients who received postoperative chemoradiation (median, 98.5 days). In early follow-up, no patient who received preoperative chemoradiation experienced a local recurrence, and peritoneal recurrence developed in only 10% of these patients. Local or regional recurrence developed in 21% of patients who received postoperative chemoradiation. The overall survival curves were similar for both cohorts.

Wolff et al.[43] examined 86 patients treated with weekly gemcitabine at a dose of 400 mg/m^2 and 30 Gy of radiation. Sixty-one patients ultimately underwent resection (71%). The median survival in the resected patients was 36 months, which is significantly longer than those seen in regimens using 5-FU or paclitaxel as the radiation sensitizer. Analysis of the specimens revealed two pathologic complete responses and more than 50% nonviable tumor cells in 36 (59%). A gemcitabine-based regimen was also used in a multi-institutional study of 20 patients reported by Talamonti et al.[44] This group used full-dose gemcitabine and limited-field radiation to 36 Gy (2.4 Gy/fraction). The authors described 14 patients as resectable and six as borderline resectable. Ultimately, all patients were explored and 17 resected (85%), again representing a very high rate of resectability. A single pathologic complete response was observed and, in 24% of tumors, greater than 90% of the tumor cells were felt to be nonviable. Also notable was the low incidence, 6%, of margin positivity in this trial. The median survival in the resected patients was 26 months. Based on the results of these initial trials, gemcitabine-based neoadjuvant regimens remain of considerable interest.

PALLIATION

7 Unfortunately, it has been the experience nationwide that only a minority of patients with carcinoma of the pancreas can undergo resection for possible cure at the time diagnosis is made. Therefore, the optimal palliation of symptoms to maximize quality of life is of primary importance in most patients with pancreatic cancer. Both operative and nonoperative options are available for the palliation of pancreatic cancer.

Jaundice

Obstructive jaundice is present in most patients who have pancreatic cancer. If left untreated, it can result in progressive liver dysfunction, hepatic failure, and early death. In addition, the pruritus associated with obstructive jaundice can be debilitating and usually does not respond to medication. When patients undergo exploration for possible cure and are found to have unresectable disease, a biliary bypass should be performed.

Traditionally, surgeons have performed either choledochojejunostomy or cholecystojejunostomy for the relief of malignant biliary obstruction. Both procedures are effective in relieving jaundice, but it appears that the rate of recurrent jaundice after cholecystojejunostomy is approximately 10%. Therefore, our preference for the palliation of obstructive jaundice is a hepaticojejunostomy or choledochojejunostomy reconstructed with a Roux-en-Y limb of jejunum. The surgical palliation of jaundice can be accomplished safely, with a mortality rate of less than 3% and an overall morbidity rate of 30% to 40%.[45] In recent years, nonoperative palliation has become available as an option for managing patients who are deemed unresectable by preoperative staging. Plastic or metal stents can be placed across the biliary obstruction by either an endoscopic or a percutaneous technique. For pancreatic cancer, the endoscopic approach is usually preferred. The overall morbidity rate for endoscopic stenting ranges up to 35%, but the rate of major procedure-related morbidity is less than 10%. Early complications include cholangitis, pancreatitis, and bile duct or duodenal perforation. The major late complications of stent placement are cholecystitis, duodenal perforation, and stent migration. Stent occlusion can result in episodes of cholangitis and recurrent jaundice. For most patients, an exchange of stents is required every 3 to 6 months. The newer metal stents appear to remain patent for longer periods.

Nonoperative palliation appears to be associated with lower complication rates, lower procedure-related mortality rates, and shorter initial periods of hospitalization in comparison with surgical palliation. However, the rate of recurrent jaundice is higher. No advantage with respect to long-term survival has been noted for either approach. Therefore, nonoperative palliation should be offered to patients with advanced disease or poor performance status. Surgical palliation should be considered for patients with an anticipated life expectancy of at least 6 months.

Duodenal Obstruction

At the time that pancreatic cancer is diagnosed, approximately one third of patients have symptoms of nausea or vomiting. Although true mechanical obstruction of the duodenum seen by radiologic or endoscopic examination is much less frequent, duodenal obstruction develops in almost 20% of patients before they die as the disease progresses.[46] Duodenal obstruction can be caused in the C-loop by cancers of the head or at the ligament of Treitz by cancers of the body and tail. In patients with evidence of duodenal obstruction or impending obstruction, a gastrojejunostomy is indicated for palliation. This is typically performed as a retrocolic, isoperistaltic loop gastrojejunostomy with a loop of jejunum 20 to 30 cm distal to the ligament of Treitz.

In patients with unresectable pancreatic cancer who do not have symptoms of gastric outlet obstruction, whether or not to perform a prophylactic gastric bypass at the time of biliary bypass is a matter of debate. Surgeons who do not perform a prophylactic bypass feel that it needlessly increases the postoperative length of stay and can be associated with delayed gastric emptying and increased morbidity and mortality. However, data from a prospective randomized trial of prophylactic gastrojejunostomy in patients with unresectable cancer do not support this view.[47] In this study, 44 patients were randomized to a gastrojejunostomy, and 43 did not undergo gastric bypass. No mortality occurred in either group. No difference was observed in either the

TABLE 54.14

MANAGEMENT

PROSPECTIVE RANDOMIZED TRIAL OF PROPHYLACTIC GASTROJEJUNOSTOMY IN PATIENTS WITH UNRESECTABLE PERIAMPULLARY CANCER

	PATIENTS (no.)	MORBIDITY (%)	MORTALITY (%)	POSTOPERATIVE LENGTH OF STAY (d)	LATE GASTRIC OUTLET OBSTRUCTION (%)
Gastrojejunostomy	44	32	0	8.5	0
No gastrojejunostomy	43	33	0	8.0	19

Adapted from Lillemoe KD, Cameron JL, Hardacre JM, et al. Is prophylactic gastrojejunostomy indicated for unresectable periampullary cancer? *Ann Surg* 1999;230:322–330.

complication rate or the postoperative length of stay (Table 54.14). However, late duodenal obstruction developed in 19% of the patients who did not undergo bypass. A recent multicenter prospective randomized controlled trial has confirmed these results.[48] Therefore, we believe that a prophylactic gastrojejunostomy should be performed in patients undergoing surgical palliation for unresectable pancreatic carcinoma.

Pain

Tumor-associated pain can be incapacitating in patients with unresectable pancreatic cancer. The postulated causes of tumor-associated pain are many and include tumor infiltration into the celiac plexus, increased parenchymal pressure caused by pancreatic duct obstruction, pancreatic inflammation, gallbladder distention resulting from biliary obstruction, and gastroduodenal obstruction. The management of pain in patients dying of carcinoma of the pancreas is one of the most important aspects of their care. The appropriate use of oral agents can be successful in most patients. Patients with significant pain should receive their medication on a regular schedule and not an "as needed" basis. The use of long-acting morphine derivative compounds appears to be best suited for such treatment. Percutaneous neurolytic block of the celiac axis, performed under either fluoroscopic or CT guidance, is also successful in the majority of patients at eliminating pain. Patients with unresectable cancer at the time of surgical exploration should receive a chemical splanchnicectomy, with 20 mL of 50% alcohol injected on either side of the aorta at the level of the celiac axis.[49]

Summary

The decision to perform nonoperative versus surgical palliation for pancreatic cancer is influenced by a number of factors, including the patient's symptoms, overall health status, predicted procedure-related morbidity and mortality, and projected survival. Surgical palliation can be completed with acceptable perioperative morbidity and mortality and postoperative length of stay. The avoidance of late complications of recurrent jaundice, duodenal obstruction, and disabling pain would strengthen the argument in favor of surgical palliation in those patients expected to survive 6 months or more. Nonoperative methods of palliation should be considered for patients in whom preoperative staging suggests distant metastatic disease or a locally unresectable tumor, patients who are not candidates for operative intervention, and those not expected to survive more than 3 months.

Radiation and Chemotherapy for Unresectable Pancreatic Carcinoma

Specific antitumor therapies in patients with advanced pancreatic carcinoma have been studied for years, with limited success. Trials evaluating the use of chemotherapy and radiation therapy both alone and in combination have shown a marginal improvement in survival, often with relatively high toxicity rates and some negative impact on quality of life. Recently gemcitabine, a deoxycytidine analogue capable of inhibiting DNA replication and repair, has become increasingly popular. When gemcitabine was compared with bolus 5-FU in a randomized phase III trial, it was shown to confer a significant survival benefit in advanced pancreatic cancer, increasing median survival from 4.4 months to 5.7 months and increasing 1-year survival from 2% to 18%, respectively.[50] A key endpoint in this study was "clinical benefit response," based on reducing pain, improving performance status, and inducing weight gain, which was attained in 24% of patients receiving gemcitabine compared with 5% for those receiving 5-FU. In patients with metastatic pancreatic cancer that had progressed with 5-FU and then been treated with gemcitabine, the median survival (in 63 of 74 patients enrolled) was 3.9 months.[51] Seventeen patients (27%) attained a clinical benefit response with a median duration of 14 weeks. Gemcitabine is generally well tolerated with a low incidence of significant toxicity and therefore seems to be a reasonable choice for palliative therapy.

In addition to gemcitabine, other agents are currently being studied for a role in the palliation of patients with pancreatic adenocarcinoma. Examples of such agents are paclitaxel (Taxol), matrix metalloproteinase inhibitors (e.g., marimastat, perillyl alcohol), and inhibitors of angiogenesis, such as TNP-470. The results of such studies are eagerly awaited.

References

1. American Cancer Society. Cancer Statistics, 2009. *CA Cancer J Clin* 2009; 59:225–249.
2. Sohn TA, Yeo CJ, Cameron JL, et al. Resected adenocarcinoma of the pancreas 616 patients: results, outcomes, and prognostic indicators. *J Gastrointest Surg* 2000;4:567.
3. Yeo CJ, Cameron JL. Pancreatic cancer. *Curr Probl Surg* 1999;36:61.
4. Chari ST, Leibson CL, Rabe KG, et al. Probability of pancreatic cancer following diabetes: a population based study. *Gastroenterology* 2005;129: 504–511.
5. Brune KA, Klein AP. Familial pancreatic cancer. In: Lowy Am, Leach SD, Philip PA, eds. *Pancreatic Cancer*. New York: Springer Science + Buisness; 2008:65–79.
6. Hruban RH. Pancreatic cancer: from genes to patient care. *J Gastrointest Surg* 2001;5:583.
7. Wilentz RE, Hruban RH. Pathology of cancer of the pancreas. *Surg Oncol Clin North Am* 1998;7:43.
8. Takaori K, Hruban RH, Maitra A, et al. Pancreatic intraepithelial neoplasia. *Pancreas* 2004;28:257.

9. Schmidt CM, Matos JM, Bentrem DJ, et al. Acinar cell carcinoma of the pancreas in the United States: prognostic factors and comparison to ductal adenocarcinoma. *J Gastrointest Surg* 2008;12:2078–2086.
10. Tseng JF, Warshaw AL, Sahani DV, et al. Serous cystadenoma of the pancreas: tumor growth rates and recommendations for treatment. *Ann Surg* 2005:242:413–419.
11. Sohn TA, Yeo CJ, Cameron JL, et al. Intraductal papillary mucinous neoplasms of the pancreas an updated experience. *Ann Surg* 2004; 239:788.
12. Tanaka M, Chari S, Adsay V, et al. International consensus guidelines for management of intraductal papillary mucinous neoplasms and mucinous cystic neoplasms of the pancreas. *Pancreatology* 2005;6:17–32.
13. Ritts RE, Pitt HA. CA 19–9 in pancreatic cancer. *Surg Oncol Clin North Am* 1998;7:93.
14. Pisters PWT, Lee JE, Vauthey, et al. Laparoscopy in the staging of pancreatic cancer. *Br J Surg* 2001;88:325.
15. Dye CE, Waxman I. Endoscopic ultrasound. *Gastroenterol Clin North Am* 2002;31:863.
16. Conlon KC, Dougherty E, Klimstra DS, et al. The value of minimal access surgery in the staging of patients with potentially resectable peripancreatic malignancy. *Ann Surg* 1996;223:134.
17. Barreiro CJ, Lillemoe KD, Koniaris LG, et al. Diagnostic laparoscopy for periampullary and pancreatic cancer: what is the true benefit? *J Gastrointest Surg* 2002;6:75.
18. Kausch W. Das Carcinom der Papilla Duodeni and seine radikale Entfeinung. *Beitragezur Klinische Chirurgie* 1912;78:439.
19. Whipple AO, Parsons WB, Mullins CR. Treatment of carcinoma of the ampulla of Vater. *Ann Surg* 1935;102:763.
20. Pedrazzoli S, DiCarlo V, Dionigi R, et al. Standard versus extended lymphadenectomy associated with pancreatoduodenectomy in the surgical treatment of adenocarcinoma of the head of the pancreas: a multicenter, prospective, randomized study. Lymphadenectomy Study Group. *Ann Surg* 1998;228:508–517.
21. Yeo CJ, Cameron JL, Lillemoe KD, et al. Pancreaticoduodenectomy with or without distal gastrectomy and extended retroperitoneal lymphadenectomy for periampullary adenocarcinoma, part 2: randomized controlled trial evaluating survival, morbidity, and mortality. *Ann Surg* 2002;236: 355.
22. Nimura Y, Nagino M, Kato H, et al. Regional vs extended lymph node dissection in radical pancreaticoduodenectomy for pancreatic cancer. A multicenter randomized controlled trial. *HPB (Oxford)* 2004;6 (suppl 1):2.
23. Farnell MB, Pearson RK, Sarr MG, et al. A prospective randomized trial comparing standard pancreatoduodenectomy with pancreatoduodenectomy with extended lymphadenectomy in resectable pancreatic head adenocarcinoma. *Surgery* 2005;138:618–630.
24. Traverso LW, Longmire WP Jr. Preservation of the pylorus in pancreaticoduodenectomy. *Surg Gynecol Obstet* 1978;146:959.
25. Kozuschek W, Reith HB, Waleczek H, et al. A comparison of long term results of the standard Whipple procedure and the pylorus preserving pancreatoduodenectomy. *J Am Coll Surg* 1994;178:443.
26. Takada T, Yasuda H, Amano H, et al. Results of a pylorus-preserving pancreatoduodenectomy for pancreatic cancer: a comparison with results of the Whipple procedure. *Hepatogastroenterology* 1997;44:1536.
27. Tran KT, Smeenk HG, van Eijck CH, et al. Pylorus-preserving pancreaticoduodenectomy versus standard Whipple procedure a prospective randomized multicenter analysis of 170 patients with pancreatic and periampullary tumors. *Ann Surg* 2004;240:738.
28. Kooby D, Gillespie T, Bentrem D, et al. Left-sided pancreatectomy: a multicenter comparison of laparoscopic and open approaches. *Ann Surg* 2008; 248:438–446.
29. Palanivelu C, Jani K, Senthilnathan P, et al. Laparoscopic pancreaticoduodenectomy: technique and outcomes. *J Am Coll Surg* 2007;205: 222–230.
30. Yeo CJ, Cameron JL, Lillemoe KD, et al. Pancreaticoduodenectomy for cancer of the head of the pancreas: 201 patients. *Ann Surg* 1995;221: 721–733.
31. Richter A, Neidergethmann M, Sturm JW, et al. Long-term results of partial pancreaticoduodenectomy for ductal adenocarcinoma of the pancreatic head: 25-year experience. *World J Surg* 2003;27:324.
32. Schmidt CM, Powell ES, Yiannoutsos CT, et al. Pancreaticoduodenectomy: a 20-year experience in 516 patients. *Arch Surg* 2004;139:718.
33. Sosa JA, Bowman HM, Gordon TA, et al. Importance of hospital volume in the overall management of pancreatic cancer. *Ann Surg* 1998; 228:320.
34. Winter JM, Cameron JL, Campbell KA, et al. 1423 pancreaticoduodenectomies for pancreatic cancer: a single-institution experience. *J Gastrointest Surg* 2006;10:1199–1210.
35. Gastrointestinal Tumor Study Group. Further evidence of effective adjuvant combined radiation and chemotherapy following curative resection of pancreatic cancer. *Cancer* 1987;59:2006–2010.
36. Kinkenbijl JH, Jeekel J, Sahmoud T, et al. Adjuvant radiotherapy and 5-fluorouracil after curative resection of cancer of the pancreas and periampullar region. *Ann Surg* 1999;230:776.
37. Neoptolemos JP, Stocken DD, Freiss H, et al. A randomized trial of chemoradiotherapy and chemotherapy after resection of pancreatic cancer. *N Engl J Med* 2004;350:1200.
38. Regine WF, Winter KW, Abrams R, et al. RTOG 9704 a phase III study of adjuvant pre and post chemoradiation (CRT) 5-FU vs. gemcitabine (G) for resected pancreatic adenocarcinoma. *J Clin Oncol* 2006;24(18 S pt 1): abstract 4007.
39. Oettle H, Post S, Neuhaus P, et al. Adjuvant chemotherapy with gemcitabine vs. observation in patients undergoing curative-intent resection of pancreatic cancer: a randomized controlled trial. *JAMA* 2007;297: 267–277.
40. Spitz FR, Abbruzzese JL, Lee JE, et al. Preoperative and postoperative chemoradiation strategies in patients treated with pancreaticoduodenectomy for adenocarcinoma of the pancreas. *J Clin Oncol* 1997;15:928.
41. Hoffman JP, Lipsitz S, Pisansky T, et al. Phase II trial of preoperative radiation therapy and chemotherapy for patients with localized, resectable adenocarcinoma of the pancreas: an Eastern Cooperative Oncology Group Study. *J Clin Oncol* 1998;16:317–323.
42. Pisters PW, Wolff RA, Janjan NA, et al. Preoperative paclitaxel and concurrent rapid-fractionation radiation for resectable pancreatic adenocarcinoma: toxicities, histologic response rates, and event-free outcome. *J Clin Oncol* 2002;20:2537.
43. Wolff RA, Evans DB, Crane CH. Initial results of preoperative gemcitabine-based chemoradiation for resectable pancreatic adenocarcinoma [abstract]. *Proc Am Soc Clin Oncol* 2002;21:130.
44. Talamonti MS, Small W Jr, Mulcahy MF, et al. A multi-institutional phase II trial of preoperative full-dose gemcitabine and concurrent radiation for patients with potentially resectable pancreatic carcinoma. *Ann Surg Oncol* 2006;13:150–158.
45. Sohn TA, Lillemoe KD, Cameron JL, et al. Surgical palliation of unresectable periampullary carcinoma in the 1990s. *J Am Coll Surg* 1999;188: 658.
46. Sarr MG, Cameron JL. Surgical management of unresectable carcinoma of the pancreas. *Surgery* 1982;91:123.
47. Lillemoe KD, Cameron JL, Hardacre JM, et al. Is prophylactic gastrojejunostomy indicated for unresectable periampullary cancer? *Ann Surg* 1999;230:322.
48. Van Heek NT, De Castro SM, van Eijck CH, et al. The need for a prophylactic gastrojejunostomy for unresectable periampullary cancer: a prospective randomized multicenter trial with special focus on assessment of quality of life. *Ann Surg* 2003;238:894.
49. Lillemoe KD, Cameron JL, Kaufman HS, et al. Chemical splanchnicectomy in patients with unresectable pancreatic cancer: a prospective randomized trial. *Ann Surg* 1993;217:447.
50. Burris HA, Moore MJ, Anderson J, et al. Improvements in survival and clinical benefit with gemcitabine as first-line therapy for patients with advanced pancreas cancer: a randomized trial. *J Clin Oncol* 1997;15:2403.
51. Rothenberg ML, Moore MJ, Cripps MC, et al. A phase II trial of gemcitabine in patients with 5-FU refractory pancreas cancer. *Ann Oncol* 1996; 7:347.

CHAPTER 55 ■ NEOPLASMS OF THE ENDOCRINE PANCREAS

EUGENE P. KENNEDY, JONATHAN R. BRODY, AND CHARLES J. YEO

KEY POINTS

1. Pancreatic endocrine neoplasms (PENs) originate from multipotential stem cells in pancreatic ductules. Therefore, use of the older terms *islet cell tumor* and *islet cell carcinoma* is now discouraged, in favor of the terms *pancreatic endocrine neoplasms* or *pancreatic endocrine tumors*.
2. PENs are best classified according to the size and the mitotic rate of the tumor into one of three categories: pancreatic endocrine microadenomas, well-differentiated pancreatic endocrine neoplasms, and poorly differentiated or high-grade endocrine carcinomas.
3. The World Health Organization classification divides well-differentiated PENs into well-differentiated endocrine tumors and well-differentiated endocrine carcinomas based on local invasion beyond the pancreas or metastatic spread to lymph nodes and/or distant locations, which results in classification as carcinoma.
4. The best initial imaging technique for a pancreatic endocrine neoplasm is a high-quality multidetector computed tomography scan.
5. Endoscopic ultrasonography is particularly useful in localizing tumors in patients with gastrinoma and insulinoma.
6. Insulinomas may present with either neuroglycopenic symptoms (confusion, seizure, obtundation, coma) or hypoglycemic-induced symptoms (palpitations, diaphoresis, tachycardia).
7. Ninety percent of insulinomas are solitary, 90% are sporadic, and 90% are benign with location evenly distributed throughout the pancreas.
8. Seventy-five percent of gastrinomas are sporadic (25% are associated with multiple endocrine neoplasia type 1 syndrome), and all should be considered to be of malignant potential.
9. Most gastrinomas are located in the *gastrinoma triangle* and may be intrapancreatic, within the wall of the duodenum, or in a peripancreatic lymph node, and in most cases local resection (enucleation) may be adequate therapy.
10. Glucagonomas usually present with a characteristic severe dermatitis (termed *necrolytic migratory erythema*) and are typically large and bulky and often with metastatic disease.

Pancreatic endocrine neoplasms (PENs) are rare tumors that account for 1% to 2% of pancreatic neoplasms.[1] First described by Nicholls in 1902 as a tumor arising from pancreatic islet cells, these "islet cell adenomas" were long thought to
1 arise from the islets of Langerhans.[2] Recent investigations have revealed that PENs more likely originate from multipotential stem cells in pancreatic ductules.[3,4] This non–islet cell origin has been further demonstrated in tumors arising in patients with multiple endocrine neoplasia type 1.[5] Therefore, use of the older terms *islet cell tumor* and *islet cell carcinoma* is now discouraged, in favor of the terms *pancreatic endocrine neoplasms* or *pancreatic endocrine tumors*.[6,7]

2 Overall, PENs are best classified according to the size and the mitotic rate of the tumor (Table 55.1). This system places PENs into one of three categories: pancreatic endocrine microadenomas, well-differentiated pancreatic endocrine neoplasms, and poorly differentiated or high-grade endocrine carcinomas. Additionally, they can be classified by the presence (i.e., functional tumors) or absence (i.e., nonfunctional tumors) of a syndrome due to hormone production. The production of certain hormones and the resulting syndromes lead to well-described clinical syndromes, which are detailed later in this chapter.

PENs less than 0.5 cm in diameter are classified as pancreatic endocrine microadenomas. Oncologically, they are considered to be benign lesions. Their prevalence is estimated to be as high as 10% of the population in autopsy series.[8,9] Most pancreatic endocrine microadenomas are noted as incidental findings in pancreata resected for other indications and, by definition, produce no neoplastic syndromes (i.e., are nonfunctional). Functional PENs less than 0.5 cm are classified with well-differentiated pancreatic endocrine neoplasms.

PENs measuring greater than 0.5 cm in diameter and having a low mitotic rate of less than 10 mitoses per 10 high-power fields are referred to as well-differentiated pancreatic endocrine neoplasms. This group comprises the large majority of clinically relevant PENs. They are uncommon, with an estimated incidence of approximately 1 out of 100,000 people.[10,11] Although rare in children, cases have been described at all ages, and the peak incidence occurs between the ages of 40 and 60 years.[6] Overall distribution is equal between men and women with some differences in ratio among different functional types.

No well-established staging system exists for PENs.[12] Multiple studies have been performed attempting to establish prognostic characteristics such as size, mitotic count, vascular and perineural invasion, nuclear polymorphisms, and Ki-67 label-
3 ing index.[13–16] The most recent World Health Organization (WHO) classification divides well-differentiated PENs into well-differentiated endocrine tumors and well-differentiated endocrine carcinomas based on their clinical behavior.[1] Any local invasion beyond the pancreas or metastatic spread to lymph nodes or distant locations results in classification as carcinoma. The WHO well-differentiated endocrine tumors are further subclassified as having predicted benign behavior or uncertain behavior. This subdivision (benign vs. uncertain) is based on size (<2 cm or ≥2 cm), mitotic count (less than two or two or more mitotic figures per 10 high-power fields), Ki-67 labeling index (<2% or ≥2%), and absence or presence of perineural and vascular invasion (Table 55.2).

Well-differentiated PENs can also be classified as functional or nonfunctional based on the presence or absence of an associated clinically recognizable syndrome (Table 55.3). These syndromes are the result of the secretion of biologically active

TABLE 55.1 CLASSIFICATION

CLASSIFICATION OF PANCREATIC ENDOCRINE NEOPLASMS

NEOPLASM	SIZE	MITOTIC RATE	CLINICAL BEHAVIOR
Pancreatic endocrine microadenomas	<0.5 cm	<2 per 10 HPF	Benign
Well-differentiated pancreatic endocrine neoplasms	>0.5 cm	<10 per 10 HPF	Indeterminate
High-grade endocrine carcinomas	Any	>10 per 10 HPF	Malignant

HPF, high-power fields.

hormones by the tumors and are confirmed by measurable elevations of the hormones in the blood. The most common functional PENs include insulinomas, gastrinomas, vasoactive intestinal polypeptide-omas (VIPomas), glucagonomas, and somatostatinomas. The incidence of these lesions ranges from 1 per 1 million for insulinomas to 1 per 40 million for somatostatinomas.[17] Even less common PENs secreting calcitonin,[18,19] parathyroid hormone–related protein,[20] growth hormone–releasing factor, and adrenocorticotropic hormone[21] have been reported. Nonfunctional PENs are classified as such due to their lack of an associated clinical syndrome. Some of the tumors in this group do secrete elevated amounts of hormones, including chromogranin A, which can be detected in either the serum or surgical specimens using immunohistochemistry.[22] These secreted hormones either produce no clinical syndromes, as is seen with tumors that secrete pancreatic polypeptide,[23] or secrete hormones in subclinical amounts or inactive forms. Traditionally, functional PENs were reported to comprise the majority of PENs. As methods of detecting these lesions and patterns of presentation have evolved, due primarily to the widespread use of high-quality cross-sectional imaging, nonfunctional PENs now comprise more than half of surgically resected cases.[13,24]

The least common group of PENs is the poorly differentiated or high-grade endocrine carcinomas. These are aggressive tumors characterized by their high mitotic count (>10 mitotic figures per 10 high-powered fields).[25] These tumors primarily occur in adults and have a male predominance. Some have been reported to be functional, producing varied clinical syndromes (commonly gastrinoma, VIPoma, glucagonoma, and, less frequently, insulinoma). Prognosis is often poor, with the clinical course varying from a rapid decline to a more indolent, prolonged survival.

MOLECULAR GENETICS

The majority of PENs are sporadic. Some of them, however, occur as part of inherited familial syndromes such as multiple endocrine neoplasia type 1 (MEN-1), von Hippel-Lindau (VHL) syndrome, neurofibromatosis (NF-1), and tuberous sclerosis (TSC) (Table 55.4). Recent technical advances in molecular biology have provided new insights into the genesis of PENs and possible reasons why certain tumors behave more aggressively than others. Further, recent studies analyzing the gross chromosomal changes found in PENs provide hope for markers for early diagnosis of this disease.

Familial Syndromes

Significant progress has been made in the genetic understanding of the MEN-1 syndrome in relation to PENs.[26] Chromosomal linkage studies have localized the genetic defect to the 11q13 locus, and studies of DNA markers have localized the MEN-1 gene between PYGM and D11S97. The gene contains 10 exons that code for a 610-amino-acid protein called menin, whose function is unknown, although it is classically labeled as a tumor suppressor gene. Some studies provide a possible explanation for loss of this gene in neuroendocrine tumors.[27] The menin protein is expressed in diverse tissues and is highly conserved evolutionarily. Menin is predominately a nuclear protein, which binds to JunD and may repress JunD-mediated transcription. Studies in patients with MEN-1 have shown allelic deletions at chromosome 11q13 in nearly 100% of parathyroid tumors, 85% of nongastrinoma islet cell tumors, and up to 40% of gastrinomas. In patients with sporadic tumors (without MEN-1), 11q13 deletions are seen in about 25%, 20%, and almost 50% of parathyroid tumors, nongastrinoma PENs, and gastrinomas, respectively. Recently it has been shown that a comprehensive genetic testing program for patients at risk for MEN-1 can identify patients harboring a MEN-1 mutation almost 10 years before the development of clinical signs or symptoms of disease.[28] Since MEN-1 loss has been detected in both the sporadic and the familial forms of PENs, the menin pathway is most likely involved in the pathogenesis of this disease.[27]

Less frequently than MEN-1, PENs may be associated with VHL syndrome. VHL syndrome is another autosomal dominant inheritance disease that includes many clinical disorders,[29] including retinal hemangioblastomas, cerebellar and medullary hemangioblastomas, and PENs. PENs are found in a small percentage of patients with VHL syndrome. A mutation in the VHL gene, a tumor suppressor located on chromosome 3p25–26,

TABLE 55.2 CLASSIFICATION

WHO CLASSIFICATION OF WELL-DIFFERENTIATED PANCREATIC ENDOCRINE TUMORS

CLINICAL BEHAVIOR	SIZE	MITOTIC COUNT	Ki-67 INDEX	PERINEURAL AND VASCULAR INVASION
Benign	<2 cm	<2 per 10 HPF	<2%	Absent
Uncertain	>2 cm	≥2 per 10 HPF	≥2%	Present

HPF, high-power fields; WHO, World Health Organization.

TABLE 55.3 CLASSIFICATION

CLASSIFICATION OF FUNCTIONAL PANCREATIC ENDOCRINE TUMORS

TUMOR (SYNDROME)	CLINICAL FEATURES	EXTRAPANCREATIC LOCATION	MALIGNANCY RATE
Insulinoma	Hypoglycemia Anabolic state	Rare	10%
Gastrinoma (Zollinger-Ellison)	Peptic ulcer Diarrhea	Frequent	50%
VIPoma (Verner-Morrison; WDHA; pancreatic cholera)	Watery diarrhea Hypokalemia Achlorhydria/acidosis	10%	Most
Glucagonoma	Hyperglycemia Catabolic state Dermatitis	Rare	Most
Somatostatinoma	Hyperglycemia Steatorrhea Gallstones	Rare	Most

WDHA, watery diarrhea, hypokalemia, and either achlorhydria or acidosis.

which regulates hypoxia-induced cell proliferation, is responsible. Although germline mutations with loss of heterozygosity (LOH) are associated with this disease, it has been proposed that other tumor suppressors most likely cooperate with VHL in order to form PENs.

NF-1 (von Recklinghausen disease) is an autosomal dominant disorder that produces a well-described clinical syndrome characterized by café-au-lait spots and neurofibromas. These patients may develop pancreatic somatostatinomas. The NF-1 gene is a tumor suppressor gene located on 17q11.2 that encodes for neurofibromin, a regulator of the mammalian target of rapamycin (mTOR) pathway. Loss of NF-1 results in mTOR activation and tumor development.[30]

Sporadic Pancreatic Endocrine Neoplasms

The genetic landscape of sporadic PENs has been explored. Up to half of malignant pancreatic endocrine tumors have been found to have clonal chromosomal abnormalities,[31] whereas, unlike with pancreatic ductal adenocarcinoma, k-ras oncogene mutations are absent in most of these tumors.[32] Gastrinoma has been shown to be associated with amplification of the HER2/neu proto-oncogene,[33] and a high level of expression of mRNA for the α subunit of G_s protein has been demonstrated in insulinoma.[34] MAGE1, a protein identified in a number of neoplastic cell types including testicular germ cell cancer, breast cancer, and melanoma, was found to be present in 86% of primary PENs as well as in lymph node metastases.

Additional recent discoveries have furthered our understanding of this diverse group of tumors. For instance, hypermethylation of hMLH1 in PENs leads to microsatellite instability and is associated with an improved prognosis.[35] However, the most promising and breakthrough work comes from two studies looking at genome-wide alterations in PENs.[36,37] Nagano et al.[37] found allelic imbalances by utilizing high-density single-nucleotide polymorphism (SNP) arrays. In short, they found that tumors with high allelic imbalances (more than four chromosomal aberrations) had a larger tumor size compared to PENs with minimal chromosomal abreactions ($p = 0.03$). The authors do point to the limitations in the number of tumors (15 patients) analyzed in the study and note the gross heterogeneity found in their samples.

Another intriguing study was performed by Jonker et al.,[36] which correlated the following molecular markers with clinical outcomes of PENs (stratifying insulinomas and noninsulinomas): Ki67, CK19, specific chromosomal alterations, gross chromosomal instability (CIN), and tumor size.[36] The authors

TABLE 55.4 ETIOLOGY

FAMILIAL GENETIC SYNDROMES ASSOCIATED WITH PANCREATIC ENDOCRINE NEOPLASMS (PENs)

SYNDROME	CHROMOSOMAL LOCATION	GENE PRODUCT	PEN TYPE
MEN-1	11q13	Menin	Gastrinoma Nonfunctional
VHL syndrome	3p25–26	VHL gene	Various
NF-1	17q11.2	Neurofibromin	Somatostatinomas

MEN-1, multiple endocrine neoplasia 1; NF, neurofibromatosis; VHL, von Hippel-Lindau.

found a strong correlation between CIN, specific chromosomal alterations, and metastatic disease and poor tumor-free survival in insulinomas and noninsulinomas. The authors also note that CK19 is a strong indicator of tumor-specific death in all PENs.[36] Other epigenetic studies have correlated altered methylation patterns in well-characterized tumor suppressor genes (e.g., APC, E-cadherin, p16) with tumor staging.[38] Further, Chan et al. assessed differences between methylation patterns in a similar set of genes between carcinoid and pancreatic endocrine tumors. This study found distinct differences between these uncommon tumor types.[39]

In summary, PENs are most likely difficult to characterize molecularly (and clinically) due to molecular and thus cellular heterogeneity within the tumor. Ongoing efforts to search for candidate genes that lay the foundation for CIN in these tumors will aid in unraveling the molecular etiology of this disease. It was suggested in one study that FANCD2 is a good candidate gene since it resides in a chromosomal region of loss for PENs (chromosome 3p25).[36,40] However, it should be noted that loss of FANCD2 has been shown previously to be lethal (i.e., counterproductive) to cancer cells.[41] Further studies are needed to explore the connection between the FANCD2 gene and PENs. Currently, using modern techniques such as comparative genomic hybridization (CGH) along with tumor sizing and markers such as CK19 may provide clinically relevant information.

PRESENTATION AND EVALUATION

There are three primary ways by which patients with PENs come to clinical attention: the incidental discovery of a mass in the pancreas during cross-sectional imaging, symptoms secondary to the mass effect of a lesion in the pancreas (i.e., obstructive jaundice or pain), and, as a consequence of the symptoms of, a syndrome associated with a functional PEN. As mentioned previously, incidentally detected nonfunctional PENs currently comprise the majority of clinically relevant tumors. They are typically hypervascular on imaging studies such as computed tomography (CT) or magnetic resonance imaging (MRI). In the absence of any clinical syndrome, these lesions can be managed as any other incidental pancreatic lesion. Typically, the size of a PEN at discovery guides decision making between three standard options: serial observation, endoscopic ultrasound-guided biopsy, or definitive surgical resection. Size greater than 2 cm is a standard stratification measure, with lesions larger than this usually managed in a more aggressive fashion. If a nonfunctional PEN is suspected, baseline serum levels of chromogranin A and pancreatic polypeptide can be useful diagnostic markers prior to surgical resection.

PENs presenting due to mass effect on surrounding structures resulting in jaundice, pain, or gastric outlet obstruction are uncommon. These lesions should be addressed as any other symptomatic pancreatic lesion with definitive surgical resection if clinically appropriate.

Patients presenting with symptoms from a functional PEN can be a diagnostic challenge. Three general principles apply to the diagnosis and treatment of patients with suspected functional neoplasms of the endocrine pancreas. One must first recognize the abnormal physiology or characteristic syndrome. Patients are often misdiagnosed or have their symptoms disregarded for years before an accurate diagnosis is reached. Characteristic clinical syndromes are well described for insulinoma, gastrinoma, VIPoma, and glucagonoma. The somatostatinoma syndrome is nonspecific, much more difficult to recognize, and exceedingly rare. Second is the detection of hormone elevations in the serum by radioimmunoassay. Such assays are readily available for measuring insulin, gastrin, vasoactive intestinal peptide (VIP), and glucagon. Assays for somatostatin, pancreatic polypeptide (PP), prostaglandins, and other hormonal markers are less commonly available but can be obtained from certain laboratories. The third step involves localizing and staging the tumor in preparation for possible operative intervention (Algorithm 55.1).

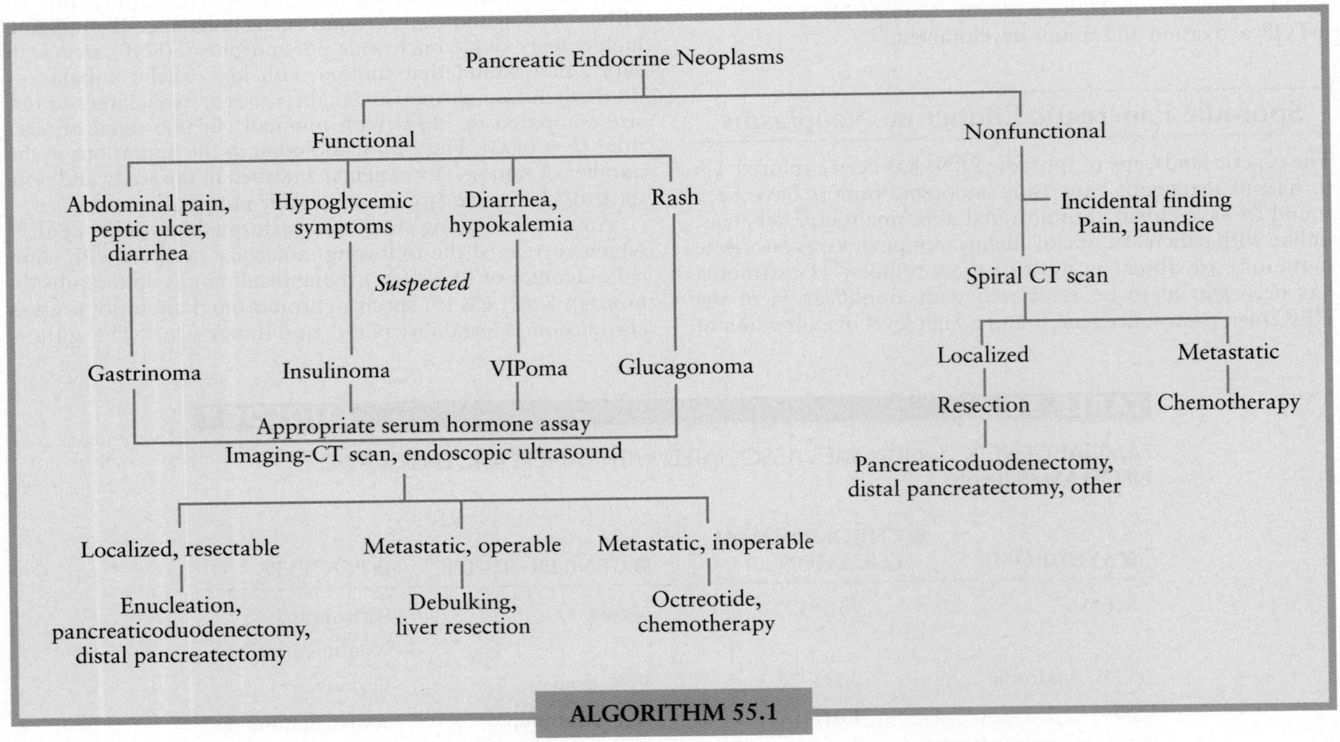

ALGORITHM 55.1. Diagnosis and management of pancreatic endocrine neoplasms.

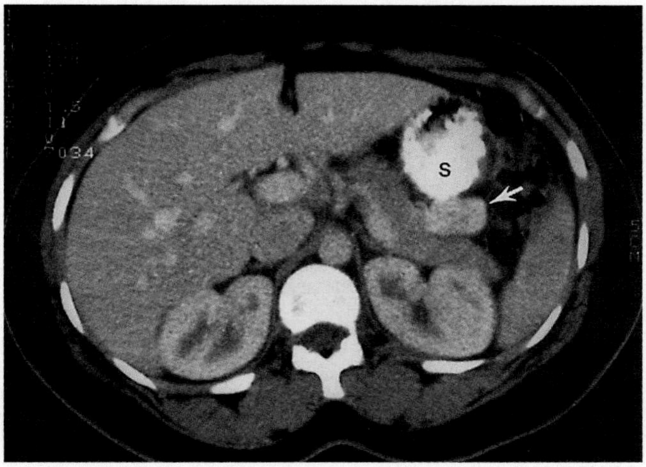

FIGURE 55.1. Computed tomography with oral and intravenous contrast in a patient with biochemical evidence of insulinoma. The neoplasm (*arrow*) is seen as a contrast-enhancing structure, 3 cm in diameter, in the tail of the pancreas posterior to the stomach (S). (From Yeo CJ. Islet cell tumors of the pancreas. In: Niederhuber JE, ed. *Current Therapy in Oncology*. St. Louis, MO: Mosby; 1993:272, with permission.)

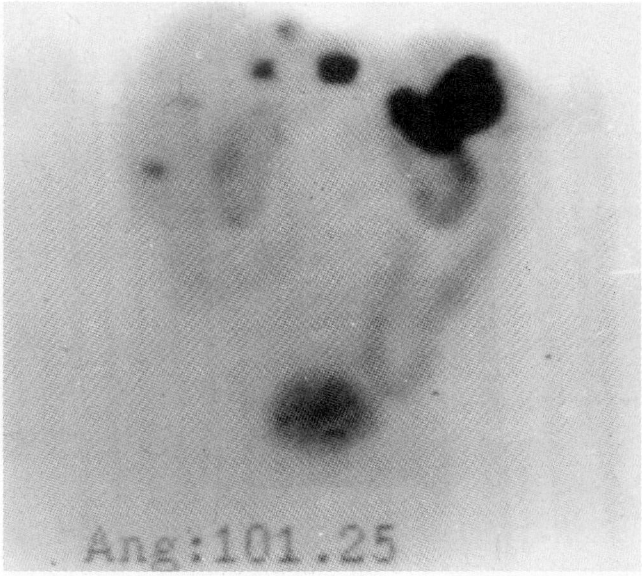

FIGURE 55.2. Octreotide scan (anterior view) in a patient with a large endocrine tumor in the tail of the pancreas (large dark mass, upper right) and several hepatic metastases (upper left quadrant). A small amount of the tracer is seen in the bladder (lower midline).

LOCALIZATION AND STAGING

Computed Tomography

4 The initial imaging technique used to localize a PEN and stage the disease is high-quality multidetector three-dimensional CT.[42] The accuracy of CT in detecting primary pancreatic endocrine neoplasms ranges from 64% to 82% and depends largely on the size of the tumor.[43,44] PENs are typically hyperdense on arterial phases of imaging. Lesions that are obvious during the early arterial phase can become isodense on later phases of imaging. Therefore, a multiphase approach is typically recommended.[45,46] CT is useful in assessing size and location of the primary tumor, proximity to visceral vessels, peripancreatic lymph node involvement, and the presence or absence of liver metastases (Fig. 55.1).

Magnetic Resonance Imaging

MRI is increasingly used in the detection of PENs, particularly small lesions. They are especially well visualized on T1- and T2-weighted images with fat suppression. MRI has the advantage of increased soft tissue contrast without the administration of intravenous contrast when compared to CT.[42] PENs characteristically have high signal intensity on T2-weighted images.[47] On dynamic contrast-enhanced T1-weighted images, the tumors show the same typical enhancement pattern as on CT scan. The sensitivity of MRI has been reported to be between 74% and 100%.[43,44]

Somatostatin Receptor Scintigraphy (Octreoscan)

Somatostatin receptor scintigraphy (SRS) also plays an important role in imaging patients with pancreatic endocrine tumors.[48–54] In this technique, the octapeptide analogue of somatostatin (Octreotide) labeled with indium-111 is administered intravenously to patients in whom a PEN is suspected. Because neuroendocrine tumors often express large numbers of somatostatin receptors on their cell surfaces (Fig. 55.2), the tracer preferentially identifies tumors. The overall sensitivity of SRS has been reported to range from 74% to near 100% depending on the functional type of PEN.[55] There is a significant false-negative rate, indicating that negative SRS findings in patients with pancreatic endocrine neoplasms should be viewed with caution. Nonfunctional tumors and insulinomas seem to be localized less frequently by SRS, while SRS performs well for gastrinoma, VIPoma, and glucagonoma. In addition, SRS appears to play a role in the evaluation of patients with metastatic pancreatic endocrine tumors, especially in identifying extrahepatic tumor spread. In a study by Frilling et al.,[54] 54% of patients with liver metastases had extrahepatic tumor spread detected by SRS that was not detected by alternate imaging techniques.

Endoscopic Ultrasound

5 Endoscopic ultrasonography (EUS) has also shown utility in localizing pancreatic endocrine neoplasms.[56–60] Rosch et al.[59] were able to localize 32 of 39 tumors (82%) correctly with EUS after CT had failed to locate the tumor (Fig. 55.3). In their experience, EUS was more sensitive than the combination of CT and visceral angiography. A more recent study by Proye et al.[61] evaluated preoperative EUS and SRS in 41 patients with insulinoma and gastrinoma. The sensitivity and positive predictive value of EUS were 77% and 94%, respectively, for pancreatic tumors; 40% and 100%, respectively, for duodenal gastrinomas; and 58% and 78%, respectively, for metastatic lymph nodes. These results indicate that EUS is best at detecting lesions in the head of the pancreas. It is less successful at evaluating the distal pancreas and the duodenal wall. Additionally, the procedure is operator dependent.[62] These results have been duplicated by others and have led some to suggest that EUS should serve as the initial localization procedure in patients with insulinoma and gastrinoma. Of note, the drawback to EUS is that it does not evaluate accurately for hepatic metastatic disease; rather, it is more sensitive than CT for

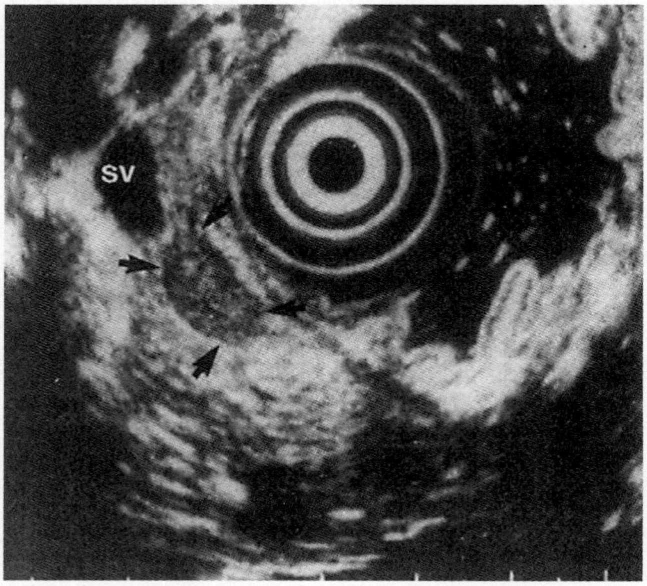

FIGURE 55.3. Endoscopic ultrasonographic image from a patient with an insulinoma (*arrows*) in the body of the pancreas. SV, splenic vein. (From Rosch T, Lightdale CJ, Botet JF, et al. Localization of pancreatic endocrine tumors by endoscopic ultrasonography. *N Engl J Med* 1992;326:1721, with permission.)

imaging the duodenal wall, pancreatic parenchyma, and peripancreatic lymph nodes.

Intraoperative Ultrasound

Historically, the primary methods of localizing PENs intraoperatively have been visualization and palpation. With the advent of laparoscopic exploration for PENs, intraoperative ultrasound has been substituted for palpation. Results have been promising, with sensitivities reported between 75% and 90%.[63,64]

Venous Sampling

Percutaneous transhepatic portal venous sampling (PTPVS) and arterial stimulation with venous sampling (ASVS) are two techniques that are used exclusively for the diagnosis and localization of PENs. In a small number of cases, CT, MRI, SRS, and EUS are unsuccessful at localizing a pancreatic endocrine neoplasm. When insulinoma or gastrinoma are suspected, PTPVS may help in localizing the occult neoplasm.[65–69] The technique involves placing a catheter percutaneously through the liver into the portal vein and then sequentially sampling for hormone levels in the splenic vein, superior mesenteric vein, and portal vein, thereby regionalizing the location of hormone production (Fig. 55.4). The overall accuracy of this test ranges from 70% to greater than 95% depending on the number of samples obtained, the persistence of autonomous hormone production by the tumor, and the careful handling and assaying of all samples. ASVS involves the selective visceral arterial injection of secretin or calcium with concurrent hepatic venous sampling for either gastrin or insulin.[70,71] Gastrinoma cells are known to respond to secretin by releasing gastrin,[72,73] and insulinoma cells are known to respond to calcium by releasing insulin. The provocative secretogogue is serially injected through an arterial catheter into at least three sites—the splenic, gastroduodenal, and inferior pancreaticoduodenal arteries. Samples are drawn from a hepatic vein catheter before

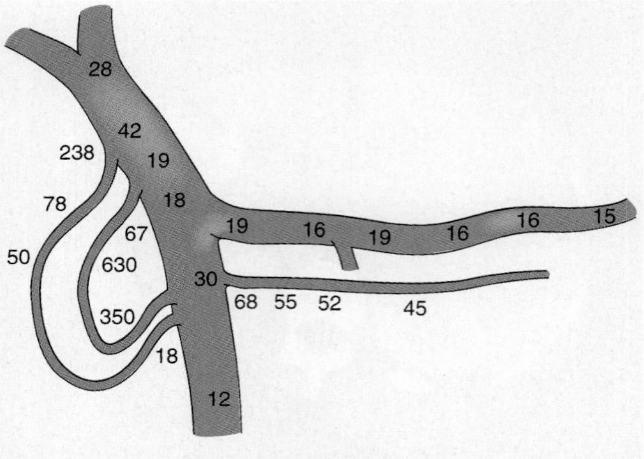

FIGURE 55.4. Schematic depiction of data from percutaneous transhepatic portal venous sampling (PTPVS) in a patient with an insulinoma. Insulin levels are given in microunits per milliliter. These data localize the neoplasm to the head of the pancreas. (Adapted from Norton JA, Sigel B, Baker AR, et al. Localization of an occult insulinoma by intraoperative ultrasonography. *Surgery* 1985;97:381.)

and immediately after each injection. The arterial supply to the occult tumor can then be deduced based on which selective secretogogue injection is followed by a large increase in hepatic vein hormone concentration (Fig. 55.5). This technique, particularly when combined with intraoperative ultrasonography, results in a sensitivity of greater than 90%, essentially obviating the need for blind resection in unlocalized insulinomas.[63,74]

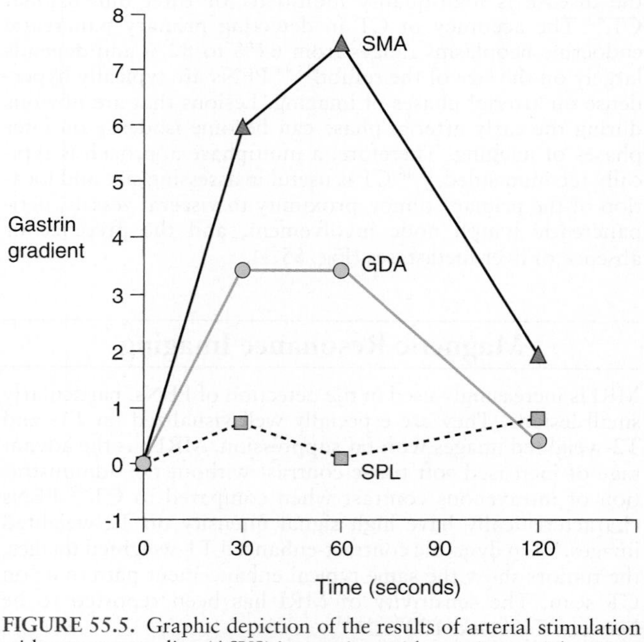

FIGURE 55.5. Graphic depiction of the results of arterial stimulation with venous sampling (ASVS) in a patient with gastrinoma. The rise in hepatic vein gastrin concentration (gastrin gradient) is plotted on the y-axis, and basal values are plotted on the x-axis: 1, 100% rise; 2, 200% rise; and so forth. A rise in the hepatic vein gastrin concentration observed after the injection of secretin into the superior mesenteric artery (SMA) and gastroduodenal artery (GDA) localizes the neoplasm to the head of the pancreas or duodenum. SPL, splenic artery. (Adapted from Thom AK, Norton JA, Doppman JL, et al. Prospective study of the use of intra-arterial secretin injection and portal venous sampling to localize duodenal gastrinomas. *Surgery* 1992;112:1002.)

Additionally, ASVS can differentiate the 5% of patients with nesidioblastosis from those with insulinoma.[75]

SURGICAL EXPLORATION

At the time of surgical exploration for PEN, a complete evaluation of the pancreas and peripancreatic regions is performed. The body and tail of the pancreas are exposed by dividing the gastrocolic ligament. This portion of the pancreas can be partially elevated out of the retroperitoneum by dividing the inferior retroperitoneal attachments to the gland. After the second portion of the duodenum has been elevated out of the retroperitoneum by means of the Kocher maneuver, the pancreatic head and uncinate process are palpated bimanually. The liver is carefully assessed for evidence of metastatic disease. Potential extrapancreatic sites of tumor are evaluated in all cases, with particular attention paid to the duodenum, splenic hilum, small intestine and its mesentery, peripancreatic lymph nodes, and reproductive tract in women. The goals of surgical therapy for pancreatic endocrine neoplasms include controlling the symptoms of hormone excess, safely resecting maximal tumor mass, and preserving maximal pancreatic parenchyma. Management strategies, including preoperative, intraoperative, and postoperative considerations, vary for the different types of endocrine neoplasms of the pancreas.

INSULINOMA

Insulinoma is the most common functional neoplasm of the endocrine pancreas (Table 55.5). The insulinoma syndrome is associated with the following features, known as Whipple's triad[76]:

1. Symptoms of hypoglycemia during fasting
2. Documentation of hypoglycemia, with a serum glucose level below 50 mg/dL
3. Relief of hypoglycemic symptoms following administration of exogenous glucose

6 Autonomous insulin secretion in insulinomas leads to spontaneous hypoglycemia, with symptoms that can be classified into two groups (see Table 55.5). Neuroglycopenic symptoms include confusion, seizure, obtundation, personality change, and coma. Hypoglycemia-induced symptoms, related to a surge in catecholamine levels, include palpitations, trembling, diaphoresis, and tachycardia. In most cases, patients consume carbohydrate-rich meals and snacks to relieve or prevent these symptoms.

Whipple's triad is not specific for insulinoma. The differential diagnosis of adult hypoglycemia is extensive and includes the following: reactive hypoglycemia, functional hypoglycemia associated with gastrectomy or gastroenterostomy, nonpancreatic tumors, pleural mesothelioma, sarcoma, adrenal carcinoma, hepatocellular carcinoma, carcinoid, hypopituitarism, chronic adrenal insufficiency, extensive hepatic insufficiency, and surreptitious self-administration of insulin or ingestion of oral hypoglycemic agents.

A common error made in evaluating a patient with suspected insulinoma is to begin with an oral glucose tolerance test. Instead, insulinoma is most reliably diagnosed by means of a monitored fast. During a monitored fast, blood is sampled for glucose and insulin determinations every 4 to 6 hours and when symptoms appear. Hypoglycemic symptoms typically occur when glucose levels are below 50 mg/dL, with concurrent serum insulin levels often exceeding 25 microunits/mL. Additional support for the diagnosis of insulinoma comes from the calculation of the insulin-to-glucose ratio at different times during the monitored fast. Normal persons have insulin-to-glucose ratios below 0.3, whereas patients with insulinoma typically demonstrate insulin-to-glucose ratios above 0.4 after a prolonged fast. Other measurable β-cell products synthesized in excess in patients with insulinoma include C peptide and proinsulin. Elevated levels of both are typically found in the peripheral blood of patients with insulinoma.

The possibility of the surreptitious administration of insulin or oral hypoglycemic agents should be considered in all patients with suspected insulinoma. Levels of C peptide and proinsulin are not elevated in patients who self-administer insulin. Additionally, patients self-administering either bovine or porcine insulin may demonstrate anti-insulin antibodies in circulating blood. The ingestion of oral hypoglycemic agents, such as sulfonylureas, can be assessed by means of standard toxicologic screening.

Insulinomas are evenly distributed throughout the pancreas, with one third found in the head and uncinate process, one third in the body, and one third in the tail of the gland.[77] Less than 3% are located outside the pancreas, with these lesions
7 located in the peripancreatic area.[78] Ninety percent are found to be benign solitary adenomas amenable to surgical cure. Ninety percent of insulinomas are sporadic, with approximately 10% being associated with the MEN-1 syndrome. In patients with MEN-1, the possibility of multiple insulinomas must be considered, and recurrence rates are higher. In approximately 10% of patients, insulinoma is metastatic to the peripancreatic lymph nodes or liver, making the diagnosis of malignant insulinoma.

After the diagnosis of insulinoma has been confirmed biochemically, the appropriate localization and staging studies described earlier are performed (typically CT and EUS). Once the lesion has been localized,[79] patients undergo surgical exploration, where the pancreas is assessed not only by operative palpation but also by intraoperative ultrasonography. This allows for confirmation of preoperative localization and evaluates for the presence or absence of multiple primary tumors. Small, benign tumors that are not close to the main pancreatic duct can be removed by enucleation[80] (Fig. 55.6), regardless of their location in the gland. Larger tumors in the neck or proximal body may be resected via central pancreatectomy.[81–83] In the body and tail of the pancreas, insulinomas more than 2 cm in diameter and those close to the pancreatic duct are most commonly removed via distal pancreatectomy. Large lesions in the head or uncinate process of the gland may not be amenable to local resection and may occasionally require pancreaticoduodenectomy for complete excision.[84,85] Increasingly, experienced surgeons are utilizing a laparoscopic approach to these tumors. Both laparoscopic pancreatectomy and enucleation are now performed on a routine basis with excellent results.[86–90]

In rare instances, preoperative localization studies and intraoperative ultrasound fail to identify the tumor. Intraoperative biopsy of the pancreatic tail may help make the diagnosis of nesidioblastosis as the cause of hyperinsulism. Some authors have recommended a "blind" distal pancreatic resection to the

TABLE 55.5 **DIAGNOSIS**

INSULINOMA

■ PARAMETER	■ DESCRIPTION
Symptoms	Neuroglycopenia causes confusion, personality change, coma
	Catecholamine surge causes trembling, diaphoresis, tachycardia
	Anabolic state: weight gain
Diagnostic tests	Monitored fast
	Insulin-to-glucose ratio
Anatomic localization	Evenly distributed throughout pancreas

PANCREAS/LIVER

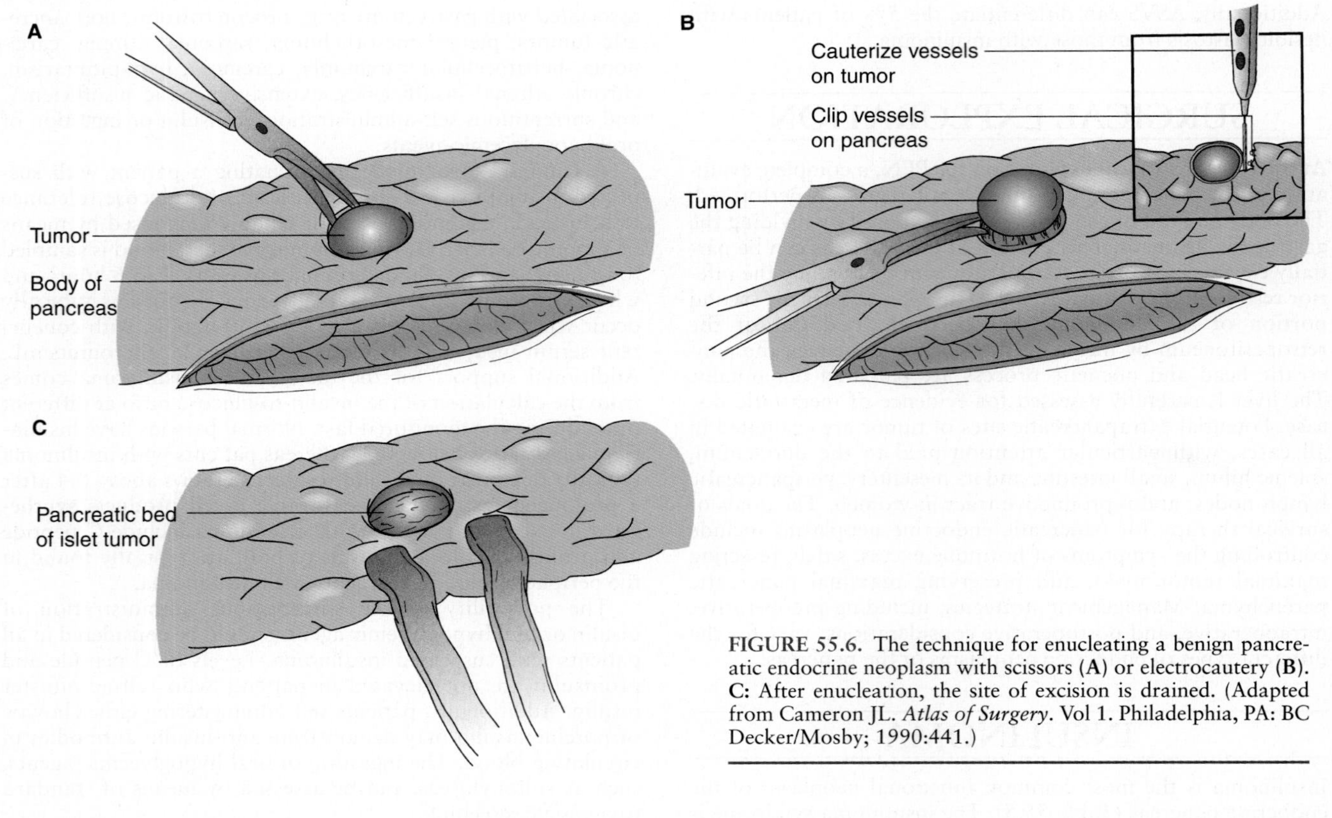

FIGURE 55.6. The technique for enucleating a benign pancreatic endocrine neoplasm with scissors (**A**) or electrocautery (**B**). **C**: After enucleation, the site of excision is drained. (Adapted from Cameron JL. *Atlas of Surgery*. Vol 1. Philadelphia, PA: BC Decker/Mosby; 1990:441.)

level of the superior mesenteric vein (60% to 70% pancreatectomy), in the hope of excising an unidentified insulinoma in the body and tail. Others have suggested blind pancreaticoduodenectomy, because the thickness of the gland in this region makes it more likely to harbor an occult neoplasm. The favored approach at the current time is to defer any blind resection, close the patient without pancreatectomy, and perform postoperative selective arterial calcium stimulation with hepatic venous insulin sampling to allow for specific tumor localization and directed surgical excision at a second operation.[91]

Approximately 10% of insulinomas are malignant, presenting with lymph node or liver metastases. In the presence of hepatic metastases, resection of the primary tumor and accessible metastases should be considered if it can be performed safely.[92–94] Such tumor debulking can be helpful in reducing hypoglycemic symptoms and improving long-term survival. In patients with unresectable disease, medications such as diazoxide and octreotide can be used to reduce insulin secretion from the tumor, minimizing hypoglycemia. One promising new treatment is everolimus, an oral rapamycin analogue that inhibits mammalian target of rapamycin (mTOR). In a pilot study of patients with refractory hypoglycemia due to metastatic insulinoma, everolimus resulted in improved glycemic control.[95] Dietary manipulations, including judicious spacing of carbohydrate-rich meals and the consumption of nighttime snacks, can also reduce the number of hypoglycemic episodes. Multiple chemotherapeutic regimens have been used including streptozocin, dacarbazine, doxorubicin, and 5-fluorouracil.[96–98] Combination chemotherapy has yielded the highest response rates but has not been shown to be curative.

GASTRINOMA (ZOLLINGER-ELLISON SYNDROME)

In 1955, Zollinger and Ellison described two patients with severe peptic ulcer disease and pancreatic endocrine tumors and postulated that an ulcerogenic agent originated from the pancreatic tumor.[99–101] It has been estimated that approximately 1 in 1,000 patients with primary duodenal ulcer disease and 2 in 100 patients with recurrent ulcer after ulcer surgery harbor gastrinomas.[102] Seventy-five percent of gastrinomas occur sporadically, and 25% are associated with the MEN-1 syndrome. Historically, the majority of gastrinomas were found to be malignant, with metastatic disease present at the time of initial workup. With increased awareness and screening for hypergastrinemia, the diagnosis of gastrinoma is made earlier and a higher percentage of patients present with benign and potentially curable neoplasms.[103]

8

The clinical symptoms of patients with gastrinoma are a direct result of increased levels of circulating gastrin (Table 55.6). Abdominal pain and peptic ulceration of the upper gastrointestinal (UGI) tract are seen in up to 90% of patients. Diarrhea is seen in 50% of patients, with 10% having diarrhea as their only symptom. Esophageal symptoms or endoscopic abnormalities resulting from gastroesophageal reflux are seen in up to half of patients. The diagnosis of gastrinoma should

TABLE 55.6 DIAGNOSIS

GASTRINOMA

■ PARAMETER	■ DESCRIPTION
Symptoms	Peptic ulcer disease Diarrhea Esophagitis
Diagnostic tests	Serum gastrin measurement Gastric acid analysis (or pH testing) Secretin stimulation test
Anatomic localization	Duodenum and head of pancreas (gastrinoma triangle)

TABLE 55.7 DIAGNOSIS

DISEASE STATES ASSOCIATED WITH HYPERGASTRINEMIA

Nonulcerogenic causes (normal to low gastric acid secretion)
Atrophic gastritis
Pernicious anemia
Previous vagotomy
Renal failure
Short-gut syndrome
Ulcerogenic causes (excess gastric acid secretion)
Antral G-cell hyperplasia or hyperfunction
Gastric outlet obstruction
Retained excluded gastric antrum
Zollinger-Ellison syndrome

be suspected in several clinical settings, including the initial diagnosis of peptic ulcer disease, recurrent ulcer after medical or surgical therapy, postbulbar ulcer, family history of ulcer disease, ulcer with diarrhea, prolonged undiagnosed diarrhea, MEN-1 kindred, nongastrinoma pancreatic endocrine tumors (high association of secondary hormone elevations), and prominent gastric rugal folds on UGI examination. Serum gastrin levels should be obtained in all of these settings.

In most patients with gastrinoma, the fasting serum gastrin level is greater than 200 pg/mL. Gastrin levels greater than 1,000 pg/mL in the setting of hyperacidity and ulcer disease are virtually pathognomonic for gastrinoma. Because hypergastrinemia can occur in other pathophysiologic states (Table 55.7), fasting hypergastrinemia alone is not sufficient for the diagnosis of gastrinoma. Gastric acid analysis (or at least gastric pH testing) is critical in differentiating between ulcerogenic (high levels of acid) and nonulcerogenic (low levels of acid) causes of hypergastrinemia. To obtain an accurate gastric acid analysis, patients must not be taking antisecretory medications including histamine (H_2)-receptor antagonists or proton pump inhibitors (PPIs). The diagnosis of gastrinoma is supported by a basal acid output above 15 mEq/h in nonoperated patients, a basal acid output exceeding 5 mEq/h in patients with previous vagotomy or ulcer operations, or a ratio of basal acid output to maximal acid output exceeding 0.6.

After documenting that hypergastrinemia and excessive acid secretion exist, provocative testing with secretin should be performed to differentiate between gastrinoma, antral G-cell hyperplasia or hyperfunction, and the other causes of ulcerogenic hypergastrinemia. This is achieved with a secretin stimulation test (Fig. 55.7). A baseline gastrin level is drawn. The patient is then stimulated with 2 units per kilogram of secretin as an intravenous bolus and subsequent gastrin samples are collected at 5-minute intervals for 30 minutes. An increase in the gastrin level by more than 200 pg/mL above the basal level supports the diagnosis of gastrinoma.

After the biochemical diagnosis of gastrinoma has been made, the gastric acid hypersecretion should be pharmacologically controlled. The PPIs are now considered the drugs of choice for doing so.[104,105] The dose is adjusted to achieve a nonacidic pH during the hour immediately before the next dose of the drug. Typically, PPI doses needed for acid control exceed usual dosing levels. After the initiation of antisecretory therapy, all patients should undergo imaging studies to localize the primary tumor and to assess for metastatic disease.

If localization studies reveal unresectable hepatic metastases, the patient should undergo percutaneous or laparoscopic-directed liver biopsy to obtain a definitive histologic diagnosis. These patients should be maintained on long-term PPI therapy. Virtually all patients can be rendered achlorhydric with an

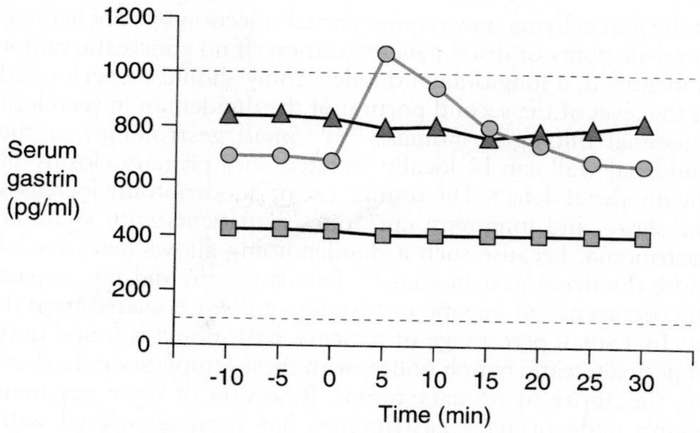

FIGURE 55.7. Results of intravenous secretin stimulation tests in patients with atrophic gastritis (*triangles*), gastric outlet obstruction (*squares*), and gastrinoma (*circles*). A positive test result, consistent with the presence of gastrinoma, is indicated by an increase over basal serum gastrin levels of at least 200 pg/mL. (Adapted from Wolfe MM, Jensen RT. Zollinger-Ellison syndrome: current concepts in diagnosis and management. *N Engl J Med* 1987;317:1200.)

appropriate dose of PPIs. Patients noncompliant with antisecretory therapy who experience complications related to their ulcer diathesis may require removal of the end organ (total gastrectomy) if tumor resection is not possible. However, total gastrectomy, once the operation of choice for gastrinoma, is now only rarely used.

If unresectable disease is not identified by staging studies, patients should be offered surgical exploration with curative intent. On exploration, the entire abdomen should be assessed for areas of extrapancreatic and extraduodenal gastrinoma. 9 Most gastrinomas are found in the *gastrinoma triangle*[77,106] (Fig. 55.8), the area to the right of the superior mesenteric vessels, in the head of the pancreas or in the duodenal wall. Both intraoperative ultrasound and intraoperative upper endoscopy may be helpful in tumor localization. Transillumination of the duodenum may help identify small duodenal gastrinomas.[107,108] Well-encapsulated tumors less than 2 cm in size and distant from the pancreatic duct can be enucleated. Those situated deep

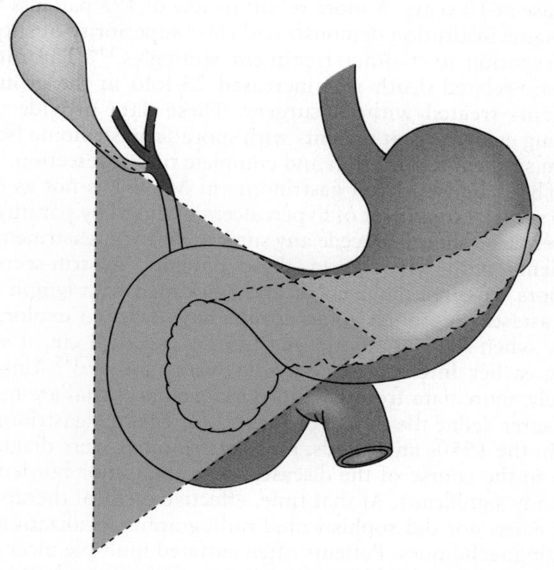

FIGURE 55.8. Most gastrinomas are found within the gastrinoma triangle. (Adapted from Stabile BE, Morrow DJ, Passaro E. The gastrinoma triangle: operative implications. *Am J Surg* 1984;147:26.)

in the parenchyma may require partial resection by pancreaticoduodenectomy or distal pancreatectomy. If no pancreatic tumor is identified, a longitudinal duodenotomy should be performed at the level of the second portion of the duodenum in search of duodenal microgastrinomas.[109,110] Small gastrinomas in the duodenal wall can be locally resected with primary closure of the duodenal defect. The routine use of duodenotomy increases the short- and long-term cure rates in patients with sporadic gastrinoma, because such a duodenotomy allows detection of more duodenal gastrinomas.[111] Duodenotomy did not impact the occurrence of hepatic metastases or disease-related mortality. In a small percentage of patients, gastrinoma is found only in peripancreatic lymph nodes, with these lymph nodes harboring the apparent primary tumor. Resection of these apparent lymph node primary gastrinomas has been associated with long-term eugastrinemia and biochemical cure in up to half of cases.[112] A review from the National Institutes of Health identified likely primary lymph node gastrinomas in 26 of 176 gastrinoma patients (14.7%), with 69% being eugastrinemic at a mean of 10 years after resection.[113]

Occasionally, preoperative localization studies may identify the tumor in the gastrinoma triangle, but at the time of exploration, the tumor is not demonstrable. Several surgical options are available at this point. First, a parietal cell vagotomy has been proposed as a way to reduce antisecretory drug dose requirements in patients on high-dose antisecretory drug therapy but without prior life-threatening complications.[114] However, this approach leaves behind potentially resectable gastrinoma and has lost favor as an option. A second option is total gastrectomy; however, the availability of PPIs has drastically reduced the need to perform this operation for gastrinoma. It may have a limited role in patients whose tumors cannot be localized, if they cannot or will not take their PPIs. Like parietal cell vagotomy, this leaves tumor behind. A third, controversial option in patients with localization to the gastrinoma triangle is blind pancreaticoduodenectomy. Some argue this should include distal gastrectomy, as duodenal gastrinomas may arise close to the pylorus and be left behind during a pylorus-preserving resection.

Patients with sporadic gastrinomas tend to fare better following resection than those with MEN-1. In a series of 151 patients reported by Norton et al.,[115] 123 had sporadic gastrinoma and 28 had MEN-1–associated gastrinoma. Of those with sporadic gastrinoma, 34% were free of disease 10 years following resection. None of the MEN-1 patients were free of disease at 10 years. A more recent review of 195 patients from the same institution demonstrated clear superiority of surgical intervention over other treatment strategies.[116] The rate of disease-related death was increased 23-fold in the group of patients treated without surgery. These data provide compelling evidence that patients with sporadic gastrinoma benefit from surgical exploration and complete tumor resection.

The management of gastrinoma in MEN-1 is not as clear. The surgical treatment of hypercalcemia caused by parathyroid hyperplasia should precede any surgery for hypergastrinemia in patients with MEN-1. In these patients, gastrin-secreting tumors are often multicentric and associated with lymph node metastases. Although some groups have favored exploration only when MEN-1 gastrinoma tumors exceed 3 cm, it seems that earlier intervention may be warranted.[117,118] Unfortunately, more data from an appropriate clinical trial are needed to better define the timing of surgery for MEN-1 gastrinoma.

In the 1950s and 1960s, most gastrinomas were diagnosed late in the course of the disease, when the tumor burden was already significant. At that time, effective medical therapy did not exist, nor did sophisticated radiographic localization and staging techniques. Patients often suffered multiple ulcer complications, required total gastrectomy to control the ulcer diathesis, and typically succumbed to continued tumor growth following gastrectomy. Recent reviews of patients with surgically treated gastrinoma provide room for optimism.[119–122] Currently, up to 35% of patients who undergo resection with curative intent have been rendered eugastrinemic at follow-up. Cure rates approach 60% to 70% when the extent of disease allows a complete resection.

Most patients with incurable metastatic disease eventually die of tumor growth and dissemination. Multiple modalities have been used to treat such patients. Chemotherapy including streptozocin, 5-fluorouracil, and doxorubicin provides response rates of less than 50%.[123] Hormonal therapy with octreotide may relieve symptoms, reduce hypergastrinemia, and diminish hyperchlorhydria.[124,125] In patients with hepatic metastases, aggressive resection for debulking,[126–129] hepatic transplantation,[130] hepatic artery embolization, and interferon therapy have all been used, with variable results.

VIPOMA (VERNER-MORRISON SYNDROME)

Synonyms for VIPoma include WDHA syndrome (watery diarrhea, hypokalemia, and either achlorhydria or acidosis) and pancreatic cholera syndrome (Table 55.8). Verner and Morrison[131] characterized this secretory diarrheal syndrome in a 1958 report. Patients characteristically present with intermittent, severe, watery diarrhea averaging up to 5 L/d. Hypokalemia results from fecal loss of large amounts of potassium. Low serum potassium levels lead to lethargy, muscle weakness, and nausea. A metabolic acidosis may be present, due to loss of bicarbonate in the diarrhea. Half of the patients may have hyperglycemia or hypercalcemia, and cutaneous flushing can be observed in a minority. The diagnosis of VIPoma is made after other common causes of diarrhea have been excluded (Table 55.9)[132] and an elevated serum VIP level is documented.

VIP secretion can be episodic, so repeated fasting levels should be measured if there is a strong clinical suspicion. Preoperative tumor localization is critical, because 10% of patients may have extrapancreatic tumors located in the retroperitoneum or chest. Most tumors are located in the distal pancreas where they are amenable to resection via distal pancreatectomy (Fig. 55.9). In most cases, hepatic metastases accompany the primary tumor. Therapies directed at debulking these metastases such as resection or ablative strategies are appropriate.

Surgical excision is appropriate in nearly all patients with Verner-Morrison syndrome. Prior to surgery, fluid and electrolyte imbalances must be corrected. Octreotide can serve as a treatment adjunct, reducing the levels of circulating VIP,

TABLE 55.8 DIAGNOSIS

VIPOMA

■ PARAMETER	■ DESCRIPTION
Symptoms	Watery diarrhea Weakness Lethargy Nausea
Diagnostic tests	Hypokalemia Achlorhydria Metabolic acidosis Serum VIP levels elevated
Anatomic localization	Most in body and tail of pancreas, with liver metastases

VIP, vasoactive intestinal peptide.

TABLE 55.9 DIAGNOSIS

DIFFERENTIAL DIAGNOSIS OF VERNER-MORRISON SYNDROME

■ ENTITY	■ WORKUP
Villous adenoma	Lower GI endoscopy
Laxative abuse	Stool examination for phenolphthalein
Celiac disease	Fecal fat measurement D-xylose tolerance test Small bowel biopsy
Parasitic and infectious diseases	Stool culture Ovum and parasite analysis *Clostridium difficile* toxin assay
Inflammatory bowel disease	Lower GI endoscopy Upper GI and small bowel series
Carcinoid syndrome	Urinary 5′-HIAA Upper GI and small bowel series Abdominal CT Serum serotonin measurement
Gastrinoma	Serum gastrin measurement Gastric acid analysis Secretin stimulation test

CT, computed tomography; GI, gastrointestinal; 5′-HIAA, 5′-hydroxyindoleacetic acid.

TABLE 55.10 DIAGNOSIS

GLUCAGONOMA

■ PARAMETER	■ DESCRIPTION
Symptoms	Dermatitis manifested as necrolytic migratory erythema Stomatitis Catabolic state: weight loss
Diagnostic tests	Hyperglycemia Hypoproteinemia Serum glucagon measurement Serum amino acid profile
Anatomic localization	Most in body and tail of pancreas, with liver metastases

with a resultant decrease in the volume of diarrhea. Octreotide is also useful for symptom control in the setting of unresectable disease. Chemotherapy specific for this disease has not been well studied.

GLUCAGONOMA

10 The most common findings in the glucagonoma syndrome are severe dermatitis, mild diabetes, stomatitis, anemia, and weight loss (Table 55.10). The dermatitis manifests as a characteristic skin rash termed *necrolytic migratory erythema*. This rash

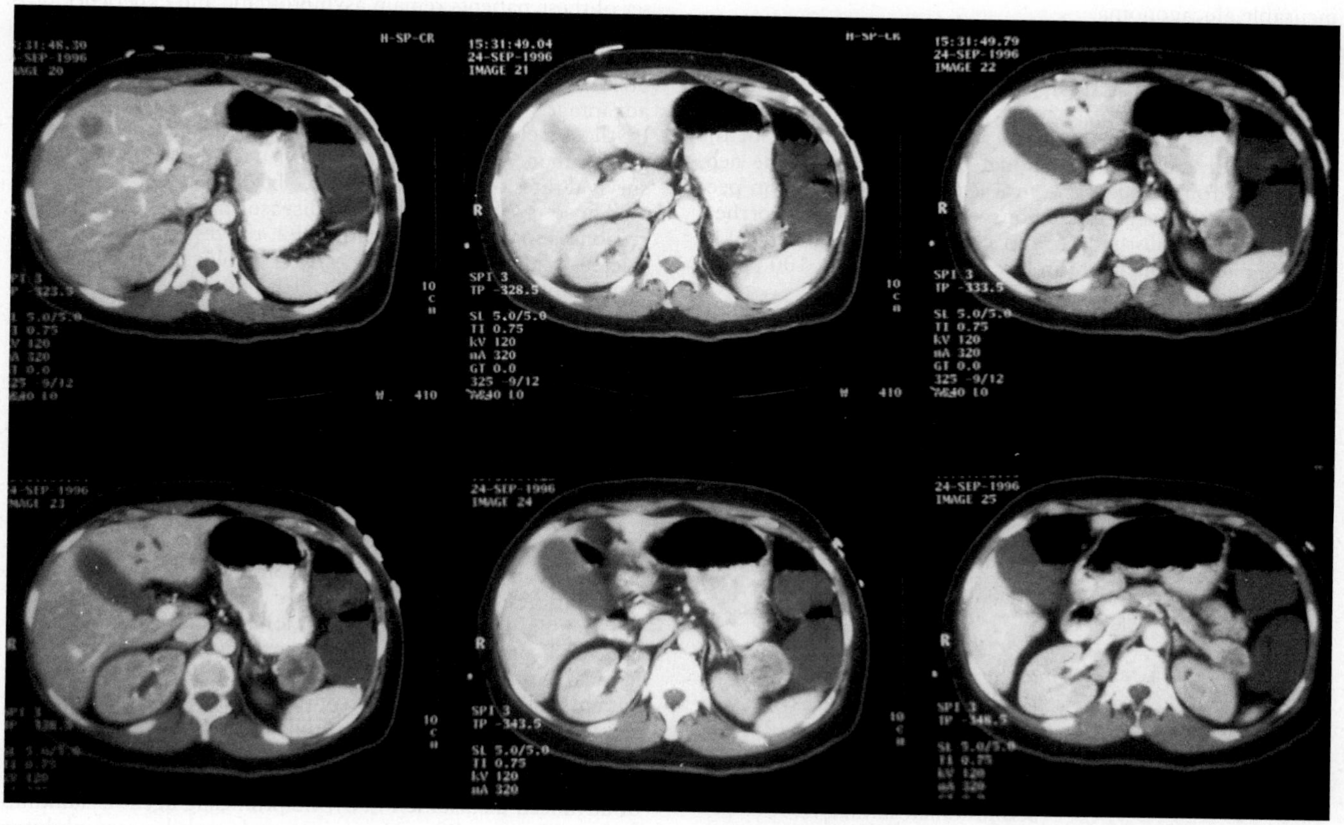

FIGURE 55.9. Several computed tomographic images from a patient with a primary vasoactive intestinal polypeptide-oma (VIPoma) in the tail of the pancreas. The tumor is nearly spherical. Its location is posterior to the stomach and adjacent to the spleen.

PANCREAS/LIVER

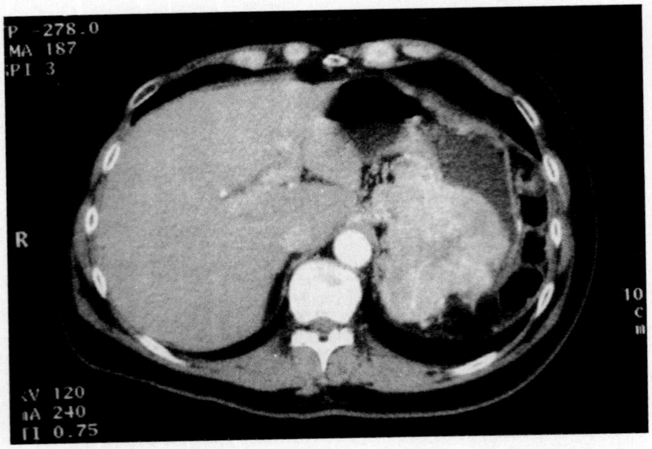

FIGURE 55.10. Computed tomography with oral and intravenous contrast in a patient with a glucagonoma. The large tumor appears to be posterior to the stomach and to the right of the aorta from the viewer's perspective.

exhibits cyclic migrations, and it has been theorized that the hypoaminoacidemia accompanying glucagonoma is the cause.

The diagnosis of glucagonoma is suggested by the clinical presentation and biopsy of the skin lesions but is secured by the documentation of high fasting levels of serum glucagon. Most glucagonomas are located in the body and tail of the gland. These tumors are typically large and bulky, and surgical resection requires distal pancreatectomy (Fig. 55.10). Metastases are found in most patients and safe debulking of these should be considered.[133] As in patients with VIPoma and insulinoma, octreotide can be useful in controlling the signs and symptoms (hyperglycemia and dermatitis) associated with incurable glucagonoma.

SOMATOSTATINOMA

The somatostatinoma syndrome is the least common of the five generally accepted functional pancreatic endocrine neoplasia syndromes, occurring in less than 1 in 40 million people. The clinical features are nonspecific including steatorrhea, diabetes, hypochlorhydria, and cholelithiasis (Table 55.11). Fasting plasma somatostatin levels of greater than 100 pg/mL can be used to confirm the diagnosis.

Most somatostatinomas are located in the pancreatic head or periampullary region.[134] Tumors are of variable size and are often easily localized. Metastatic disease may be present at the time of diagnosis. Safe resection of the primary tumor (often via pancreaticoduodenectomy) and careful debulking of hepatic metastases are indicated.

TABLE 55.11 DIAGNOSIS

SOMATOSTATINOMA

PARAMETER	DESCRIPTION
Symptoms	Steatorrhea Right upper quadrant pain
Diagnostic tests	Hyperglycemia Hypochlorhydria Gallstones Serum somatostatin level
Anatomic localization	Most in head or uncinate process of pancreas; often periampullary

NONFUNCTIONAL ISLET CELL TUMORS

Currently, the majority of patients with neoplasms of the endocrine pancreas have no defined clinical syndrome and no elevated hormone levels. One hormone that may be elevated in these patients is pancreatic polypeptide, but this is not associated with a clinical syndrome. Another elevated serum marker may be chromogranin A. A study by Mutch et al.[135] determined a relationship between fasting plasma PP levels in patients with MEN-1 and the presence of radiographically detectable pancreatic endocrine tumor. A PP level that is more than three times the age-specific normal value is 95% sensitive and 88% specific for an islet cell tumor that can be imaged. Patients with nonfunctional endocrine tumors typically present with abdominal pain, weight loss, and jaundice, caused by the space-occupying nature of the mass in the pancreas. Overall, nonfunctional tumors tend to grow more slowly and have a much more indolent course and a better survival rate than pancreatic ductal adenocarcinoma. Even patients with locally advanced disease have a median survival in excess of 5 years.[136,137] Patients with resectable disease should undergo resection for potential cure via pancreaticoduodenectomy or distal pancreatectomy, depending on tumor location.

METASTATIC PANCREATIC ENDOCRINE TUMORS

At least one third of patients with malignant PENs present with synchronous liver metastases at the time of diagnosis.[138] A subset of these patients remain asymptomatic and experience prolonged survival even without aggressive therapy.[96] However, overall 5-year survival with liver metastases is less than 50%.[139] PENs are one of the few tumors for which a survival advantage for surgical debulking has been shown.[127,138,140–142] In those selected patients where safe surgical resection of greater than 90% of the tumor burden can be achieved, 5-year survival rates of 60% to 75% have been reported.

Those with unresectable disease have shown partial responses to chemotherapy. In 1992, the results of a trial conducted by the Eastern Cooperative Oncology Group (ECOG) were published.[96] In this study, 105 patients with advanced nonfunctional endocrine tumors were randomly assigned to one of three groups. The lowest response rate (30%) was seen in patients receiving chlorozotocin alone, an intermediate response rate (45%) was seen in patients receiving the combination of streptozotocin plus 5-fluorouracil, and the highest response rate (69%) was noted in patients receiving streptozotocin plus doxorubicin. The last regimen also showed significant survival advantage in comparison with the other two treatments. More recent attempts to replicate these results have been disappointing.[143]

Somatostatin analogues are another approach to treating metastatic PENs. Results are more favorable in tumors that have high-affinity receptors (gastrinomas, VIPomas, glucagonomas, and some nonfunctional tumors) as compared to insulinomas. Symptomatic improvement occurs in 60% to 90% of patients. However, an objective tumor response is seen in only 5% to 15% of patients, with stabilization of disease in 50% or more of patients.[144–146]

Multiple investigational agents have been tried in the setting of advanced metastatic PEN. One promising agent is sunitinib malate (Sutent, Pfizer Inc.), an oral multikinase inhibitor approved for the treatment of advanced renal cell carcinoma and refractory gastrointestinal stromal tumors. Interim analysis of a phase III trial showed significant benefit in the group taking sunitinib and the trial was halted early.[147]

References

1. Heitz PU, Komminoth P, Perren A, et al. Tumors of the endocrine pancreas. In: DeLellis RA, Lloyd RV, Heitz PU, et al., eds. *Pathology and Genetics of Tumors of Endocrine Organs*. Lyon, France: IARC Press; 2004:175–208.
2. Nicholls AG. Simple adenoma of the pancreas arising from an island of Langerhans. *J Med Res* 1902;8:385–401.
3. Pour PM, Schmied B. The link between exocrine pancreatic cancer and the endocrine pancreas. *Int J Pancreatol* 1999;25(2):77–87.
4. Apel RL, Asa SL. Endocrine tumors of the pancreas. *Pathol Annu* 1995; 30:305–349.
5. Vortmeyer AO, Huang S, Lubensky I, et al. Non-islet origin of pancreatic islet cell tumors. *J Clin Endocrinol Metab* 2004;89(4):1934–1938.
6. Klimstra DS. Nonductal neoplasms of the pancreas. *Mod Pathol* 2007; 20(1):S94–S112.
7. Wick MR, Graeme-Cook F. Pancreatic neuroendocrine neoplasms. *Am J Clin Pathol* 2001;115:S28–S45.
8. Kimura W, Kuroda A, Morioka Y. Clinical pathology of endocrine tumors of the pancreas. *Dig Dis Sci* 1991;36(7):933–942.
9. Klimstra DS, Perren A, Oberg K, et al. Pancreatic endocrine tumors: nonfunctioning tumors and microadenomas. In: DeLellis RA, Lloyd RV, Heitz PU, et al., eds. *Pathology and Genetics of Tumours of Endocrine Origin*. Lyon, France: IARC Press; 2004:201–204.
10. Molder RE, Connelly RR. Epidemiology of pancreatic cancer in Connecticut. *Gastroenterology* 1968;55:677.
11. Eriksson B, Oberg K. Neuroendocrine tumors of the pancreas. *Br J Surg* 2000;87:129.
12. Frankel WL. Update on pancreatic endocrine tumors. *Arch Pathol Lab Med* 2006;130(7):963–966.
13. Hochwald SN, Zee S, Conlon KC, et al. Prognostic factors in pancreatic endocrine neoplasms: an analysis of 136 cases with a proposal for low-grade and intermediate-grade groups. *J Clin Oncol* 2002;20(11):2633–2642.
14. Capella C, Heitz PU, Hafler H, et al. Revised classification of neuroendocrine tumours of the lung, pancreas and gut. *Virchows Arch* 1995; 425(6):547–560.
15. La Rosa S, Sessa F, Capella C, et al. Prognostic criteria in nonfunctioning pancreatic endocrine tumours. *Virchows Arch* 1996;429(6):323–333.
16. Pelosi G, Bresaola E, Bogina G, et al. Endocrine tumors of the pancreas: Ki-67 immunoreactivity on paraffin sections is an independent predictor for malignancy: a comparative study with proliferating-cell nuclear antigen and progesterone receptor protein immunostaining, mitotic index, and other clinicopathologic variables. *Hum Pathol* 1996;27(11):1124–1134.
17. Goldin SB, Aston J, Wahi MM. Sporadically occurring functional pancreatic endocrine tumors: review of recent literature. *Curr Opin Oncol* 2008; 20(1):25–33.
18. McLeod MK, Vinik AI. Calcitonin immunoreactivity and hypercalcitoninemia in two patients with sporadic, nonfamilial, gastroenteropancreatic neuroendocrine tumors. *Surgery* 1992;111(5):484–488.
19. Howard JM, Gohara AF, Cardwell RJ. Malignant islet cell tumor of the pancreas associated with high plasma calcitonin and somatostatin levels. *Surgery* 1989;105(2 Pt 1):227–229.
20. Mao C, Carter P, Schaefer P, et al. Malignant islet cell tumor associated with hypercalcemia. *Surgery* 1995;117(1):37–40.
21. Aniszewski JP, Young WF Jr, Thompson GB, et al. Cushing syndrome due to ectopic adrenocorticotropic hormone secretion. *World J Surg* 2001;25(7): 934–940.
22. Mukai K, Grotting JC, Greider MH, et al. Retrospective study of 77 pancreatic endocrine tumors using the immunoperoxidase method. *Am J Surg Pathol* 1982;6(5):387–399.
23. Tomita T, Kimmel JR, Friesen SR, et al. Pancreatic polypeptide in islet cell tumors. Morphologic and functional correlations. *Cancer* 1985;56(7): 1649–1657.
24. Vagefi PA, Razo O, Deshpande V, et al. Evolving patterns in the detection and outcomes of pancreatic neuroendocrine neoplasms: the Massachusetts general hospital experience from 1977 to 2005. *Arch Surg* 2007;142(4):347–354.
25. Brodi C, Oberg K, Papotti M, et al. Pancreatic endocrine tumors: poorly differentiated endocrine carcinoma. In: DeLellis RA, Lloyd RV, Heitz PU, et al., eds. *Pathology and Genesis of Tumors of Endocrine Organs*. Lyon, France: IARC Press; 2004:207–208.
26. Marx S, Spiegel AM, Skarulis MC, et al. Multiple endocrine neoplasia type 1: clinical and genetic topics. *Ann Intern Med* 1998;129(6):484–494.
27. Toumpanakis CG, Caplin ME. Molecular genetics of gastroenteropancreatic neuroendocrine tumors. *Am J Gastroenterol* 2008;103(3):729–732.
28. Lairmore TC, Piersall LD, DeBenedetti MK, et al. Clinical genetic testing and early surgical intervention in patients with multiple endocrine neoplasia type 1 (MEN 1). *Ann Surg* 2004;239(5):637–645; discussion 645–647.
29. Halfdanarson TR, Rubin J, Farnell MB, et al. Pancreatic endocrine neoplasms: epidemiology and prognosis of pancreatic endocrine tumors. *Endocr Relat Cancer* 2008;15(2):409–427.
30. Johannessen CM, Reczek EE, James MF, et al. The NF1 tumor suppressor critically regulates TSC2 and mTOR. *Proc Natl Acad Sci U S A* 2005;102 (24):8573–8578.
31. Long PP, Hruban RH, Lo R, et al. Chromosome analysis of nine endocrine neoplasms of the pancreas. *Cancer Genet Cytogenet* 1994;77(1):55–59.
32. Yashiro T, Fulton N, Hara H, et al. Comparison of mutations of ras oncogene in human pancreatic exocrine and endocrine tumors. *Surgery* 1993; 114(4):758–763; discussion 763–764.
33. Evers BM, Rady PL, Sandoval K, et al. Gastrinomas demonstrate amplification of the HER-2/neu proto-oncogene. *Ann Surg* 1994;219(6):596–601; discussion 602–604.
34. Zeiger MA, Norton JA. Gs alpha–identification of a gene highly expressed by insulinoma and other endocrine tumors. *Surgery* 1993;114(2):458–462; discussion 462–463.
35. House MG, Herman JG, Guo MZ, et al. Prognostic value of hMLH1 methylation and microsatellite instability in pancreatic endocrine neoplasms. *Surgery* 2003;134(6):902–908; discussion 909.
36. Jonkers YM, Claessen SM, Perren A, et al. DNA copy number status is a powerful predictor of poor survival in endocrine pancreatic tumor patients. *Endocr Relat Cancer* 2007;14(3):769–779.
37. Nagano Y, Kim do H, Zhang L, et al. Allelic alterations in pancreatic endocrine tumors identified by genome-wide single nucleotide polymorphism analysis. *Endocr Relat Cancer* 2007;14(2):483–492.
38. House MG, Herman JG, Guo MZ, et al. Aberrant hypermethylation of tumor suppressor genes in pancreatic endocrine neoplasms. *Ann Surg* 2003; 238(3):423–431; discussion 431–432.
39. Chan AO, Kim SG, Bedeir A, et al. CpG island methylation in carcinoid and pancreatic endocrine tumors. *Oncogene* 2003;22(6):924–934.
40. Chung DC, Smith AP, Louis DN, et al. A novel pancreatic endocrine tumor suppressor gene locus on chromosome 3p with clinical prognostic implications. *J Clin Invest* 1997;100(2):404–410.
41. Gallmeier E, Hucl T, Calhoun ES, et al. Gene-specific selection against experimental Fanconi anemia gene inactivation in human cancer. *Cancer Biol Ther* 2007;6(5):654–660.
42. Tamm EP, Kim EE, Ng CS. Imaging of neuroendocrine tumors. *Hematol Oncol Clin North Am* 2007;21(3):409–432; vii.
43. Ichikawa T, Peterson MS, Federle MP, et al. Islet cell tumor of the pancreas: biphasic CT versus MR imaging in tumor detection. *Radiology* 2000;216(1): 163–171.
44. Vick C, Zech CJ, Hopfner S, et al. Imaging of neuroendocrine tumors of the pancreas. *Radiologe* 2003;43(4):293–300.
45. King AD, Ko GT, Yeung VT, et al. Dual phase spiral CT in the detection of small insulinomas of the pancreas. *Br J Radiol* 1998;71(841):20–23.
46. Van Hoe L, Gryspeerdt S, Marchal G, et al. Helical CT for the preoperative localization of islet cell tumors of the pancreas: value of arterial and parenchymal phase images. *AJR Am J Roentgenol* 1995;165(6):1437–1439.
47. Semelka RC, Cumming MJ, Shoenut JP, et al. Islet cell tumors: comparison of dynamic contrast-enhanced CT and MR imaging with dynamic gadolinium enhancement and fat suppression. *Radiology* 1993;186(3):799–802.
48. Termanini B, Gibril F, Reynolds JC, et al. Value of somatostatin receptor scintigraphy: a prospective study in gastrinoma of its effect on clinical management. *Gastroenterology* 1997;112(2):335–347.
49. Meko JB, Doherty GM, Siegel BA, et al. Evaluation of somatostatin-receptor scintigraphy for detecting neuroendocrine tumors. *Surgery* 1996; 120(6):975–983; discussion 983–984.
50. Kisker O, Bartsch D, Weinel RJ, et al. The value of somatostatin-receptor scintigraphy in newly diagnosed endocrine gastroenteropancreatic tumors. *J Am Coll Surg* 1997;184(5):487–492.
51. Schirmer WJ, O'Dorisio TM, Schirmer TP, et al. Intraoperative localization of neuroendocrine tumors with 125I-TYR(3)-octreotide and a handheld gamma-detecting probe. *Surgery* 1993;114(4):745–751; discussion 751–752.
52. Modlin IM, Tang LH. Approaches to the diagnosis of gut neuroendocrine tumors: the last word (today). *Gastroenterology* 1997;112(2):583–590.
53. Krausz Y, Bar-Ziv J, de Jong RB, et al. Somatostatin-receptor scintigraphy in the management of gastroenteropancreatic tumors. *Am J Gastroenterol* 1998;93(1):66–70.
54. Frilling A, Malago M, Martin H, et al. Use of somatostatin receptor scintigraphy to image extrahepatic metastases of neuroendocrine tumors. *Surgery* 1998;124(6):1000–1004.
55. Kwekkeboom DJ, Krenning EP. Somatostatin receptor imaging. *Semin Nucl Med* 2002;32(2):84–91.
56. Anderson MA, Carpenter S, Thompson NW, et al. Endoscopic ultrasound is highly accurate and directs management in patients with neuroendocrine tumors of the pancreas. *Am J Gastroenterol* 2000;95(9):2271–2277.
57. McLean AM, Fairclough PD. Endoscopic ultrasound in the localisation of pancreatic islet cell tumours. *Best Pract Res Clin Endocrinol Metab* 2005;19(2):177–193.
58. Glover JR, Shorvon PJ, Lees WR. Endoscopic ultrasound for localisation of islet cell tumours. *Gut* 1992;33(1):108–110.
59. Rosch T, Lightdale CJ, Botet JF, et al. Localization of pancreatic endocrine tumors by endoscopic ultrasonography. *N Engl J Med* 1992;326(26): 1721–1726.
60. Thompson NW, Czako PF, Fritts LL, et al. Role of endoscopic ultrasonography in the localization of insulinomas and gastrinomas. *Surgery* 1994; 116(6):1131–1138.
61. Proye C, Malvaux P, Pattou F, et al. Noninvasive imaging of insulinomas and gastrinomas with endoscopic ultrasonography and somatostatin receptor scintigraphy. *Surgery* 1998;124(6):1134–1143; discussion 1143–1144.
62. Mertz H, Gautam S. The learning curve for EUS-guided FNA of pancreatic cancer. *Gastrointest Endosc* 2004;59(1):33–37.

63. Grover AC, Skarulis M, Alexander HR, et al. A prospective evaluation of laparoscopic exploration with intraoperative ultrasound as a technique for localizing sporadic insulinomas. *Surgery* 2005;138(6):1003–1008; discussion 1008.
64. Zeiger MA, Shawker TH, Norton JA. Use of intraoperative ultrasonography to localize islet cell tumors. *World J Surg* 1993;17(4):448–454.
65. Norton JA, Shawker TH, Doppman JL, et al. Localization and surgical treatment of occult insulinomas. *Ann Surg* 1990;212(5):615–620.
66. Vinik AI, Moattari AR, Cho K, et al. Transhepatic portal vein catheterization for localization of sporadic and MEN gastrinomas: a ten-year experience. *Surgery* 1990;107(3):246–255.
67. Pedrazzoli S, Pasquali C, Miotto D, et al. Transhepatic portal sampling for preoperative localization of insulinomas. *Surg Gynecol Obstet* 1987;165(2):101–106.
68. Vinik AI, Delbridge L, Moattari R, et al. Transhepatic portal vein catheterization for localization of insulinomas: a ten-year experience. *Surgery* 1991;109(1):1–11; discussion 111.
69. Fraker DL, Norton JA. Localization and resection of insulinomas and gastrinomas. *JAMA* 1988;259(24):3601–3605.
70. Imamura M, Takahashi K, Adachi H, et al. Usefulness of selective arterial secretin injection test for localization of gastrinoma in the Zollinger-Ellison syndrome. *Ann Surg* 1987;205(3):230–239.
71. Rosato FE, Bonn J, Shapiro M, et al. Selective arterial stimulation of secretin in localization of gastrinomas. *Surg Gynecol Obstet* 1990;171(3):196–200.
72. Gower WR Jr, Buzogany JA Jr, Ellison EC, et al. Control of gastrin release in cultured gastrinoma-derived G cells. *Surgery* 1988;104(2):424–430.
73. Chiba T, Yamatani T, Yamaguchi A, et al. Mechanism for increase of gastrin release by secretin in Zollinger-Ellison syndrome. *Gastroenterology* 1989;96(6):1439–1444.
74. Brown CK, Bartlett DL, Doppman JL, et al. Intraarterial calcium stimulation and intraoperative ultrasonography in the localization and resection of insulinomas. *Surgery* 1997;122(6):1189–1193; discussion 1193–1194.
75. Pereira PL, Roche AJ, Maier GW, et al. Insulinoma and islet cell hyperplasia: value of the calcium intraarterial stimulation test when findings of other preoperative studies are negative. *Radiology* 1998;206(3):703–709.
76. Whipple AO, Frantz VK. Adenoma of islet cells with hyperinsulinism: a review. *Ann Surg* 1935;101(6):1299–1335.
77. Howard TJ, Stabile BE, Zinner MJ, et al. Anatomic distribution of pancreatic endocrine tumors. *Am J Surg* 1990;159(2):258–264.
78. Ectors N. Pancreatic endocrine tumors: diagnostic pitfalls. *Hepatogastroenterology* 1999;46(26):679–690.
79. Richards ML, Gauger PG, Thompson NW, et al. Pitfalls in the surgical treatment of insulinoma. *Surgery* 2002;132(6):1040–1049; discussion 1049.
80. Menegaux F, Schmitt G, Mercadier M, et al. Pancreatic insulinomas. *Am J Surg* 1993;165(2):243–248.
81. Sauvanet A, Partensky C, Sastre B, et al. Medial pancreatectomy: a multi-institutional retrospective study of 53 patients by the French pancreas club. *Surgery* 2002;132(5):836–843.
82. Efron DT, Lillemoe KD, Cameron JL, et al. Central pancreatectomy with pancreaticogastrostomy for benign pancreatic pathology. *J Gastrointest Surg* 2004;8(5):532–538.
83. Goldstein MJ, Toman J, Chabot JA. Pancreaticogastrostomy: a novel application after central pancreatectomy. *J Am Coll Surg* 2004;198(6):871–876.
84. Udelsman R, Yeo CJ, Hruban RH, et al. Pancreaticoduodenectomy for selected pancreatic endocrine tumors. *Surg Gynecol Obstet* 1993;177(3):269–278.
85. Phan GQ, Yeo CJ, Cameron JL, et al. Pancreaticoduodenectomy for selected periampullary neuroendocrine tumors: fifty patients. *Surgery* 1997;122(6):989–996; discussion, 996–997.
86. Fernandez-Cruz L, Blanco L, Cosa R, et al. Is laparoscopic resection adequate in patients with neuroendocrine pancreatic tumors? *World J Surg* 2008;32(5):904–917.
87. Jaroszewski DE, Schlinkert RT, Thompson GB, et al. Laparoscopic localization and resection of insulinomas. *Arch Surg* 2004;139(3):270–274.
88. Iihara M, Kanbe M, Okamoto T, et al. Laparoscopic ultrasonography for resection of insulinomas. *Surgery* 2001;130(6):1086–1091.
89. Ayav A, Bresler L, Brunaud L, et al.; SFCL (Societe Francaise de Chirurgie Laparoscopique), AFCE (Association Francophone de Chirurgie Endocrinienne). Laparoscopic approach for solitary insulinoma: a multicentre study. *Langenbecks Arch Surg* 2005;390(2):134–140.
90. Sweet MP, Izumisato Y, Way LW, et al. Laparoscopic enucleation of insulinomas. *Arch Surg* 2007;142(12):1202–1204; discussion 1205.
91. Thompson GB, Service FJ, van Heerden JA, et al. Reoperative insulinomas, 1927 to 1992: an institutional experience. *Surgery* 1993;114(6):1196–1204; discussion 1205–1206.
92. Carty SE, Jensen RT, Norton JA. Prospective study of aggressive resection of metastatic pancreatic endocrine tumors. *Surgery* 1992;112(6):1024–1031; discussion 1031–1032.
93. Modlin IM, Lewis JJ, Ahlman H, et al. Management of unresectable malignant endocrine tumors of the pancreas. *Surg Gynecol Obstet* 1993;176(5):507–518.
94. McEntee GP, Nagorney DM, Kvols LK, et al. Cytoreductive hepatic surgery for neuroendocrine tumors. *Surgery* 1990;108(6):1091–1096.
95. Kulke MH, Bergsland EK, Yao JC. Glycemic control in patients with insulinoma treated with everolimus. *N Engl J Med* 2009;360(2):195–197.
96. Moertel CG, Lefkopoulo M, Lipsitz S, et al. Streptozocin-doxorubicin, streptozocin-fluorouracil or chlorozotocin in the treatment of advanced islet-cell carcinoma. *N Engl J Med* 1992;326(8):519–523.
97. Moertel CG, Hanley JA, Johnson LA. Streptozocin alone compared with streptozocin plus fluorouracil in the treatment of advanced islet-cell carcinoma. *N Engl J Med* 1980;303(21):1189–1194.
98. Altimari AF, Badrinath K, Reisel HJ, et al. DTIC therapy in patients with malignant intra-abdominal neuroendocrine tumors. *Surgery* 1987;102(6):1009–1017.
99. Zollinger RM, Ellison EH. Primary peptic ulcerations of the jejunum associated with islet cell tumors of the pancreas. *Ann Surg* 1955;142(4):709–723; discussion, 724–728.
100. Zollinger RM, Ellison EC, Fabri PJ, et al. Primary peptic ulcerations of the jejunum associated with islet cell tumors. Twenty-five-year appraisal. *Ann Surg* 1980;192(3):422–430.
101. Ellison EC, Johnson JA. The Zollinger-Ellison syndrome: a comprehensive review of historical, scientific, and clinical considerations. *Curr Probl Surg* 2009;46(1):13–106.
102. Wolfe MM, Jensen RT. Zollinger-Ellison syndrome. Current concepts in diagnosis and management. *N Engl J Med* 1987;317(19):1200–1209.
103. Andersen DK. Current diagnosis and management of Zollinger-Ellison syndrome. *Ann Surg* 1989;210(6):685–703.
104. Maton PN, Vinayek R, Frucht H, et al. Long-term efficacy and safety of omeprazole in patients with Zollinger-Ellison syndrome: a prospective study. *Gastroenterology* 1989;97(4):827–836.
105. Metz DC, Pisegna JR, Fishbeyn VA, et al. Currently used doses of omeprazole in Zollinger-Ellison syndrome are too high. *Gastroenterology* 1992;103(5):1498–1508.
106. Stabile BE, Morrow DJ, Passaro E Jr. The gastrinoma triangle: operative implications. *Am J Surg* 1984;147(1):25–31.
107. Sugg SL, Norton JA, Fraker DL, et al. A prospective study of intraoperative methods to diagnose and resect duodenal gastrinomas. *Ann Surg* 1993;218(2):138–144.
108. Frucht H, Norton JA, London JF, et al. Detection of duodenal gastrinomas by operative endoscopic transillumination. A prospective study. *Gastroenterology* 1990;99(6):1622–1627.
109. Farley DR, van Heerden JA, Grant CS, et al. Extrapancreatic gastrinomas. Surgical experience. *Arch Surg* 1994;129(5):506–511; discussion 511–512.
110. Chiarugi M, Pucciarelli M, Goletti O, et al. Outcome of surgical treatment for extrapancreatic gastrinomas. *Surg Gynecol Obstet* 1993;177(2):153–157.
111. Norton JA, Alexander HR, Fraker DL, et al. Does the use of routine duodenotomy (DUODX) affect rate of cure, development of liver metastases, or survival in patients with Zollinger-Ellison syndrome? *Ann Surg* 2004;239(5):617–625; discussion 626.
112. Arnold WS, Fraker DL, Alexander HR, et al. Apparent lymph node primary gastrinoma. *Surgery* 1994;116(6):1123–1129; discussion 1129–1130.
113. Norton JA, Alexander HR, Fraker DL, et al. Possible primary lymph node gastrinoma: occurrence, natural history, and predictive factors: a prospective study. *Ann Surg* 2003;237(5):650–657; discussion 657–659.
114. Richardson CT, Peters MN, Feldman M, et al. Treatment of Zollinger-Ellison syndrome with exploratory laparotomy, proximal gastric vagotomy, and H2-receptor antagonists. A prospective study. *Gastroenterology* 1985;89(2):357–367.
115. Norton JA, Fraker DL, Alexander HR, et al. Surgery to cure the Zollinger-Ellison syndrome. *N Engl J Med* 1999;341(9):635–644.
116. Norton JA, Jensen RT. Role of surgery in Zollinger-Ellison syndrome. *J Am Coll Surg* 2007;205(4)(suppl 1):S34–S37.
117. Cadiot G, Vuagnat A, Doukhan I, et al. Prognostic factors in patients with Zollinger-Ellison syndrome and multiple endocrine neoplasia type 1. Groupe d'etude des neoplasies endocriniennes multiples (GENEM and groupe de recherche et d'etude du syndrome de zollinger-ellison (GRESZE). *Gastroenterology* 1999;116(2):286–293.
118. Lowney JK, Frisella MM, Lairmore TC, et al. Pancreatic islet cell tumor metastasis in multiple endocrine neoplasia type 1: correlation with primary tumor size. *Surgery* 1998;124(6):1043–1048; discussion 1048–1049.
119. Norton JA, Doppman JL, Jensen RT. Curative resection in Zollinger-Ellison syndrome. Results of a 10-year prospective study. *Ann Surg* 1992;215(1):8–18.
120. Fraker DL, Norton JA, Alexander HR, et al. Surgery in Zollinger-Ellison syndrome alters the natural history of gastrinoma. *Ann Surg* 1994;220(3):320–328; discussion 328–330.
121. Delcore R, Friesen SR. The place for curative surgical procedures in the treatment of sporadic and familial Zollinger-Ellison syndrome. *Curr Opin Gen Surg* 1994:69–76.
122. Zogakis TG, Gibril F, Libutti SK, et al. Management and outcome of patients with sporadic gastrinoma arising in the duodenum. *Ann Surg* 2003;238(1):42–48.
123. von Schrenck T, Howard JM, Doppman JL, et al. Prospective study of chemotherapy in patients with metastatic gastrinoma. *Gastroenterology* 1988;94(6):1326–1334.
124. Mozell E, Woltering EA, O'Dorisio TM, et al. Effect of somatostatin analog on peptide release and tumor growth in the Zollinger-Ellison syndrome. *Surg Gynecol Obstet* 1990;170(6):476–484.
125. Mozell EJ, Cramer AJ, O'Dorisio TM, et al. Long-term efficacy of octreotide in the treatment of Zollinger-Ellison syndrome. *Arch Surg* 1992;127(9):1019–1024; discussion 1024–1026.
126. Elias D, Lasser P, Ducreux M, et al. Liver resection (and associated extrahepatic resections) for metastatic well-differentiated endocrine tumors: a 15-year single center prospective study. *Surgery* 2003;133(4):375–382.
127. Sarmiento JM, Heywood G, Rubin J, et al. Surgical treatment of neuroendocrine metastases to the liver: a plea for resection to increase survival. *J Am Coll Surg* 2003;197(1):29–37.

128. Sarmiento JM, Que FG, Grant CS, et al. Concurrent resections of pancreatic islet cell cancers with synchronous hepatic metastases: outcomes of an aggressive approach. *Surgery* 2002;132(6):976–982; discussion 982–983.
129. Norton JA, Kivlen M, Li M, et al. Morbidity and mortality of aggressive resection in patients with advanced neuroendocrine tumors. *Arch Surg* 2003;138(8):859–866.
130. Florman S, Toure B, Kim L, et al. Liver transplantation for neuroendocrine tumors. *J Gastrointest Surg* 2004;8(2):208–212.
131. Verner JV, Morrison AB. Islet cell tumor and a syndrome of refractory watery diarrhea and hypokalemia. *Am J Med* 1958;25(3):374–380.
132. Schiller LR. Chronic diarrhea. *Gastroenterology* 2004;127(1):287–293.
133. Chu QD, Al-kasspooles MF, Smith JL, et al. Is glucagonoma of the pancreas a curable disease? *Int J Pancreatol* 2001;29(3):155–162.
134. House MG, Yeo CJ, Schulick RD. Periampullary pancreatic somatostatinoma. *Ann Surg Oncol* 2002;9(9):869–874.
135. Mutch MG, Frisella MM, DeBenedetti MK, et al. Pancreatic polypeptide is a useful plasma marker for radiographically evident pancreatic islet cell tumors in patients with multiple endocrine neoplasia type 1. *Surgery* 1997; 122(6):1012–1019; discussion 1019–1020.
136. Phan GQ, Yeo CJ, Hruban RH, et al. Surgical experience with pancreatic and peripancreatic neuroendocrine tumors: review of 125 patients. *J Gastrointest Surg* 1998;2(5):473–482.
137. Solorzano CC, Lee JE, Pisters PW, et al. Nonfunctioning islet cell carcinoma of the pancreas: survival results in a contemporary series of 163 patients. *Surgery* 2001;130(6):1078–1085.
138. House MG, Cameron JL, Lillemoe KD, et al. Differences in survival for patients with resectable versus unresectable metastases from pancreatic islet cell cancer. *J Gastrointest Surg* 2006;10(1):138–145.
139. Thompson GB, van Heerden JA, Grant CS, et al. Islet cell carcinomas of the pancreas: a twenty-year experience. *Surgery* 1988;104(6):1011–1017.
140. Chen H, Hardacre JM, Uzar A, et al. Isolated liver metastases from neuroendocrine tumors: does resection prolong survival? *J Am Coll Surg* 1998; 187(1):88–92; discussion 92–93.
141. Chamberlain RS, Canes D, Brown KT, et al. Hepatic neuroendocrine metastases: does intervention alter outcomes? *J Am Coll Surg* 2000;190(4): 432–445.
142. Touzios JG, Kiely JM, Pitt SC, et al. Neuroendocrine hepatic metastases: does aggressive management improve survival? *Ann Surg* 2005;241(5): 776–783; discussion 783–785.
143. Cheng PN, Saltz LB. Failure to confirm major objective antitumor activity for streptozocin and doxorubicin in the treatment of patients with advanced islet cell carcinoma. *Cancer* 1999;86(6):944–948.
144. Gorden P, Comi RJ, Maton PN, et al. NIH conference. Somatostatin and somatostatin analogue (SMS 201–995) in treatment of hormone-secreting tumors of the pituitary and gastrointestinal tract and non-neoplastic diseases of the gut. *Ann Intern Med* 1989;110(1):35–50.
145. Arnold R, Trautmann ME, Creutzfeldt W, et al. Somatostatin analogue octreotide and inhibition of tumour growth in metastatic endocrine gastroenteropancreatic tumours. *Gut* 1996;38(3):430–438.
146. Oberg K. Chemotherapy and biotherapy in the treatment of neuroendocrine tumours. *Ann Oncol* 2001;12(Suppl 2):S111–S114.
147. Sutent significantly increases progression free survival for patients with advanced pancreatic islet cell tumors, study stopped early [homepage on the Internet]. Pfizer. March 12, 2009. Available at: http://mediaroom.pfizer.com/news/pfizer/20090312005308/en. Accessed April 1, 2009.

CHAPTER 56 HEPATOBILIARY ANATOMY

RICHARD D. SCHULICK

KEY POINTS

1. The most widely accepted nomenclature for liver anatomy is based on Couinaud's description of eight anatomic segments of the liver.
2. There are three major hepatic veins, with most patients having a right hepatic vein that joins the right anterior wall of the inferior vena cava (IVC) and a middle and left hepatic vein that converge into a common trunk before joining the IVC.
3. Classic hepatic arterial anatomy exists in only approximately 50% of patients, with a replaced or accessory right hepatic artery arising from the superior mesenteric artery and a replaced or accessory left hepatic artery arising from the left gastric artery being the most common variants.
4. Callot's triangle is bounded by the common hepatic duct on the left, the cystic duct inferiorly, and the cystic artery superiorly.
5. The blood supply of the common bile duct is segmental in nature and consists of branches from the cystic, hepatic, and gastroduodenal arteries, which meet to form collateral vessels that run in the 3 o'clock and 9 o'clock positions.
6. Multiphase computerized tomography magnetic resonance imaging with intravenous contrast are commonly used to characterize hepatic lesions.
7. Magnetic resonance cholangiopancreatography is often used to view biliary anatomy as it involves no contrast agent and optimally can provide images that rival formal cholangiography.
8. Intraoperative ultrasonography is used routinely to assess the anatomy of the hepatic pedicles (portal vein, hepatic artery, bile duct) and hepatic veins and to identify and characterize hepatic lesions within the parenchyma and their relationships within the eight anatomic segments.
9. The portal pedicles are invested with the Glisson capsule and have a very echogenic covering to them on ultrasound in contrast to hepatic vein branches.
10. The steps involved in major hepatectomy include optimal exposure, vascular inflow control, vascular outflow control, and parenchymal transection.

A precise knowledge of the anatomy of the liver and biliary tract and their relationship to associated blood vessels is essential for the performance of hepatobiliary surgery. Every surgeon caring for a patient with a hepatobiliary problem should have a thorough understanding of the general anatomy and an absolute understanding of each individual patient's anatomy, because variations are common.

TOPOGRAPHIC ANATOMY

The normal adult liver is a large, wedge-shaped organ that occupies much of the right upper quadrant of the abdomen. Most of the liver bulk lays to the right of the midline where it molds to the undersurface of the right diaphragm, and where the lower border coincides with the right costal margin. The liver extends as a wedge to the left of the midline between the anterior surface of the stomach and the left dome of the diaphragm. The anterior surface of the liver is invested by visceral peritoneum that extends to the anterior abdominal wall in the midline from the ligamentum teres, or round ligament (the obliterated umbilical vessels), and by an obliquely oriented fusion of peritoneum known as the falciform ligament. Posteriorly, the investing peritoneum is contiguous with the peritoneum of the diaphragm and covers the liver, except for a *bare area* bounded by the *right and left triangular ligaments* (Fig. 56.1). The Glisson capsule is a thin, fibrous covering that envelops the liver deep to the peritoneum, sending fibrous septa into the hepatic parenchyma investing the portal structures.

Ordinarily, the liver can be separated from adjacent organs and structures by simply moving it or dividing loose areolar tissue (Fig. 56.2). Neoplastic or inflammatory conditions may obliterate these planes. Superiorly and anteriorly, the diaphragm or abdominal wall and liver may jointly be involved in a pathologic process. Posteriorly, the right adrenal gland or upper pole of the right kidney may involve or be involved by the liver. Inferiorly, the gallbladder, colon, duodenum, or periportal lymphatics may be involved. Cancers of the stomach or gastroesophageal junction may involve the left liver or vice versa.

MORPHOLOGIC AND FUNCTIONAL ANATOMY

The description and definition of the anatomic divisions of the liver have been revised and written about numerous times in the past 100 years.[1–8] At present, there is still confusion between the various hepatic anatomic nomenclatures in the English and French literature. Based only on morphologic criteria and surface anatomy, the liver can be divided into right and left halves by forming a plane through the gallbladder fossa (Cantlie line) and inferior vena cava (IVC) (Fig. 56.3). As will be shown later, this plane approximates the true division between the right and left halves using the more strict definition of a plane through the middle hepatic vein and IVC, but the middle hepatic vein is not obvious based solely on morphology and without ultrasound. Further subdivisions of the right half of the liver into a right anterior sector and a right posterior sector are not possible based only on surface anatomy. The left half of the liver can be further subdivided into a left medial section and left lateral section based on the umbilical fissure and falciform ligament. The caudate (tail-shaped) process of the liver is identified as lying posterior to the gastrohepatic ligament and emanating from a process of liver situated posterior to the main portal pedicle and anterior to the IVC.

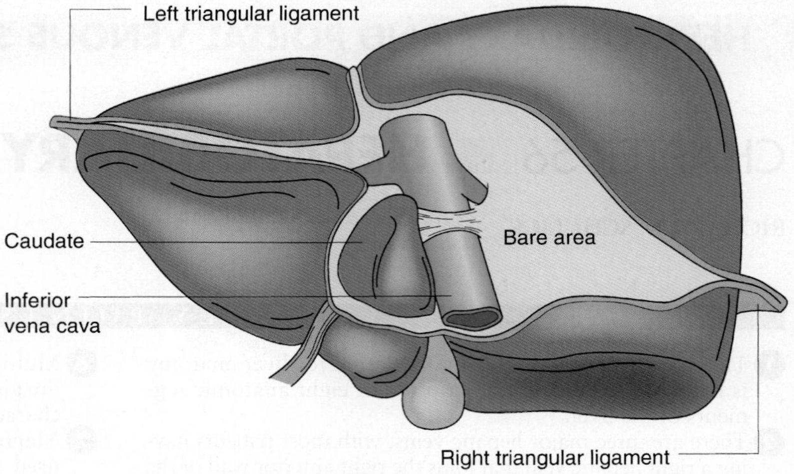

FIGURE 56.1. Posterior view of the liver, showing the level of peritoneal reflections.

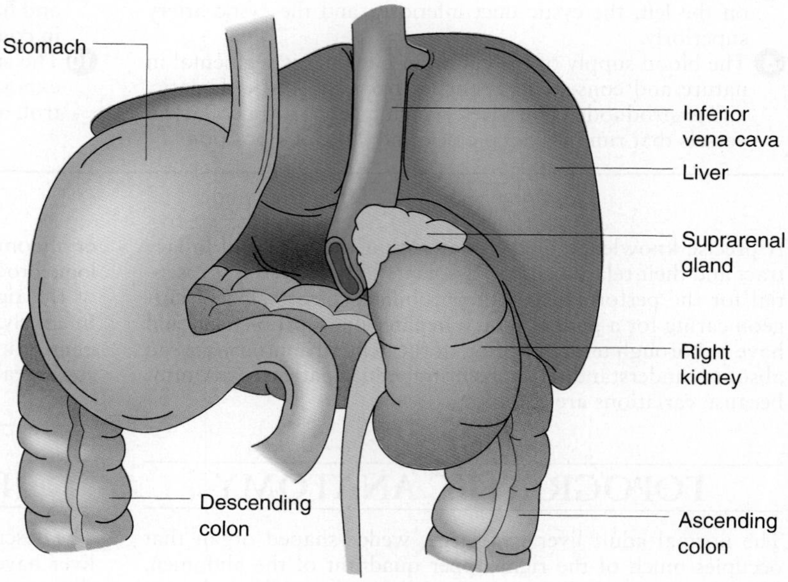

FIGURE 56.2. Posterior view of the liver, showing organs that produce impressions on its inferior surface.

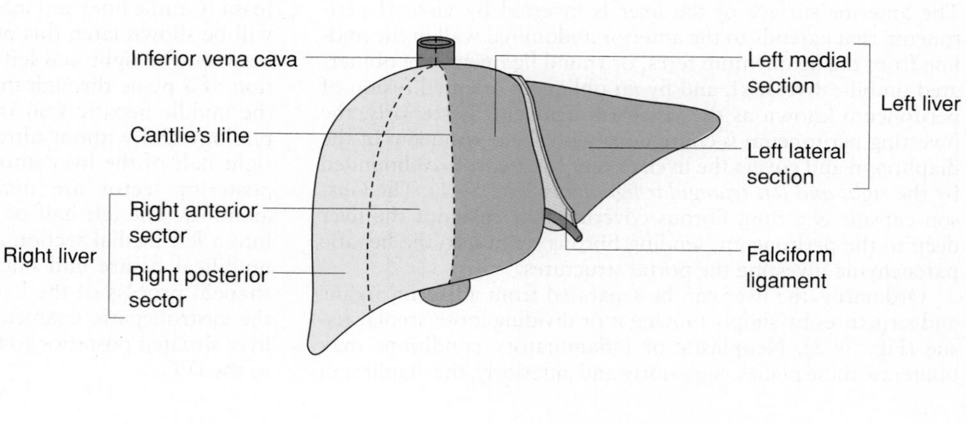

FIGURE 56.3. Anatomic division of the liver into right and left halves by a plane extending from the gallbladder fossa posteriorly to the inferior vena cava.

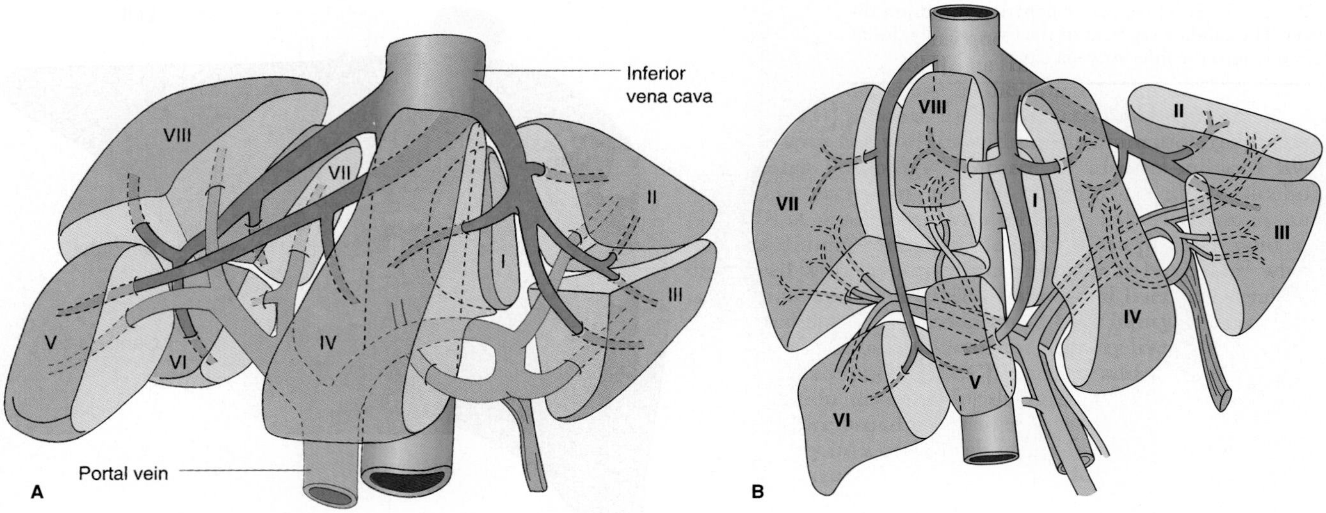

FIGURE 56.4. Functional divisions of the liver and liver segments according to Couinaud's nomenclature.

1 The most widely accepted nomenclature is based on Couinaud's description of the discrete anatomic segments of the liver (Fig. 56.4).[6] The eight segments of a liver can be determined using surface anatomy and location of the three main hepatic veins, the portal pedicle bifurcation into right and left, and the umbilical fissure and falciform ligament. As described, the right and left halves of the liver are delineated by a plane through the middle hepatic vein and IVC. Segments II, III, and IV lie to the left of this plane and form the left half of the liver. Segments V, VI, VII, and VIII lie to the right of this plane and form the right half of the liver. Segment I, or the caudate process, is morphologically distinct from the two halves of the liver and emanates from a process of liver lying posterior to the portal pedicle and anterior to the IVC. Whereas the right and left halves of the liver derive blood supply from the corresponding right and left portal veins and hepatic arteries, segment I derives blood supply from both. Additionally, the right half of the liver has venous drainage primarily through the right and middle hepatic veins, and the left half of the liver primarily through the left and middle hepatic veins. Segment I, however, drains directly via small branches into the IVC. The left liver and especially the right liver usually have small accessory hepatic venous branches draining directly into the inferior vena cava. Occasionally on the right, the accessory branch is significant in size.

The right half of the liver can be further subdivided using a plane through the right hepatic vein and the IVC. Liver anterior to this plane forms the right anterior sector, and liver posterior to this plane forms the right posterior sector. The right anterior sector of the liver is composed of segment V (inferior to the portal bifurcation) and segment VIII (superior to the portal bifurcation). The right posterior sector of the liver is composed of segment VI (inferior to the portal bifurcation) and segment VII (superior to the portal bifurcation).

The left half of the liver can be further subdivided using a plane through the umbilical fissure and falciform ligament. Liver medial to this plane forms the left medial section of the liver or segment IV, and liver lateral to this plane forms the left lateral section of the liver. The left medial section of the liver is sometimes divided into two halves, with IVa closer to the inferior vena cava and IVb farther. The left lateral section of the liver is further subdivided into segment II (which is superior) and segment III (which is inferior).

Hepatic Veins

2 Three major hepatic veins carry blood from the liver to the IVC. Most patients have a right hepatic vein that joins the right anterior wall of the IVC and a middle and left hepatic vein that converge into a common trunk about 1 cm from the IVC that enters the left anterior wall of the IVC (Fig. 56.5). In some patients, the three main hepatic veins join the IVC via three distinct trunks. These hepatic veins usually lie within the hepatic parenchyma. Usually, a definable extraparenchymal segment of the hepatic veins, especially the right, can be dissected out before it empties into the IVC, which makes outflow control safer and easier. Usually, multiple accessory right hepatic veins empty from the right half of the liver directly into the IVC as it courses posterior to the liver (Fig. 56.6). On occasion, these accessory right hepatic veins are sizable and may even support venous outflow should the native right hepatic vein need to be taken. Additionally, sometimes an umbilical vein can be appreciated running to the falciform ligament between the middle and left hepatic veins and emptying into the terminal portion of the left hepatic vein.

Portal Veins

The superior mesenteric and splenic veins join posterior to the neck of the pancreas to form the main portal vein. It receives pyloric and coronary vein branches as it courses cephalad and obliquely to the right to form the most posterior structure within the hepatoduodenal ligament (portal triad). In the hilus of the liver, the main portal vein bifurcates into a short oblique right portal vein and a longer, more transverse, and more superficial left portal vein (Fig. 56.7). These branches then enter the parenchyma and become invested along with the other components of the portal triad by extensions of the Glisson capsule. Both the right and left portal veins give off small branches to dually supply segment I. The right portal vein usually enters the hepatic parenchyma immediately and is quick to divide into a right anterior portal vein supplying segments V and VIII and a right posterior portal vein supplying segments VI and VII. The left portal vein may remain near the surface of the left half of the liver in the hilar plate for a significant distance as it courses to the umbilical fissure to give off medial branches to segment IV and lateral branches to segments II and III.

Hepatic Arteries

There is much variability in the hepatic arterial supply to the liver. The most common anatomy is a common hepatic artery that arises from the celiac trunk and courses near the superior border of the neck of the pancreas. After the origins of the

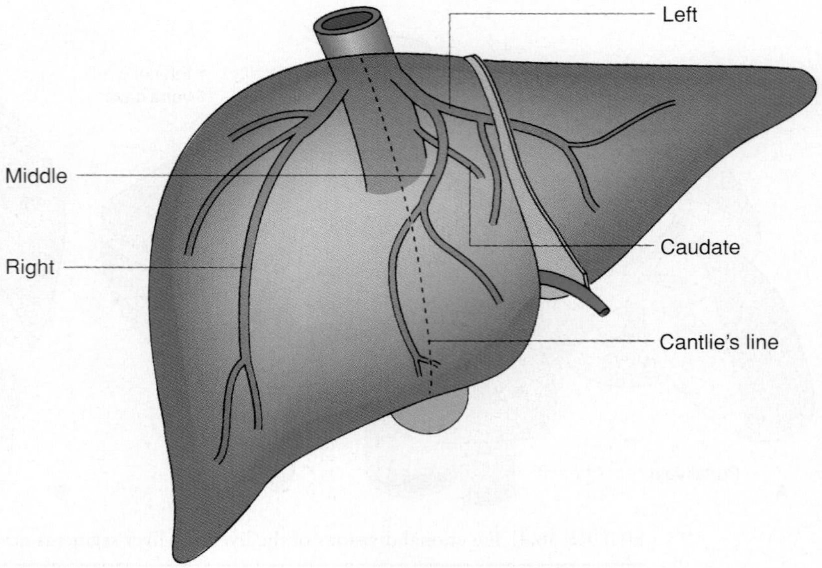

FIGURE 56.5. Three major hepatic veins drain the liver. The caudate segment of the liver usually drains directly into the inferior vena cava.

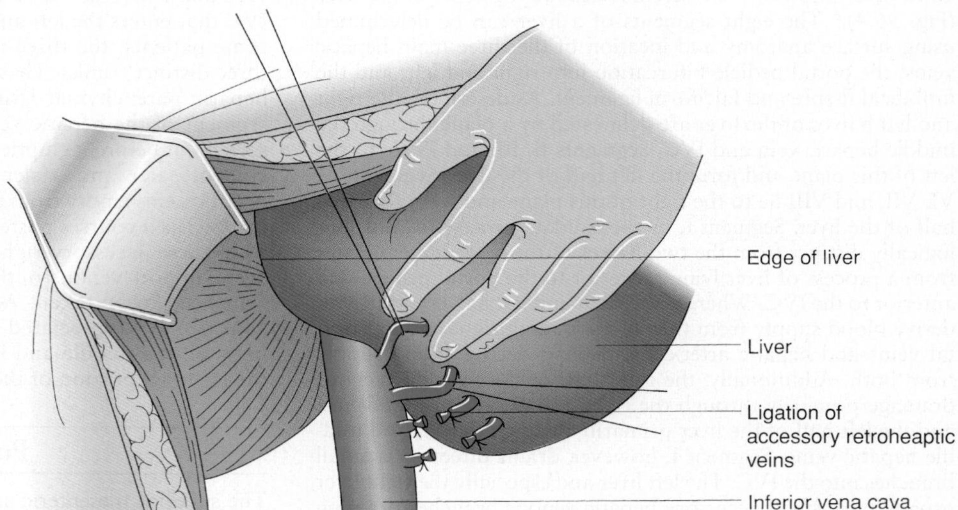

FIGURE 56.6. Retraction of right liver medially exposes small venous tributaries that drain the right liver directly into the retrohepatic vena cava. Several branches are ligated.

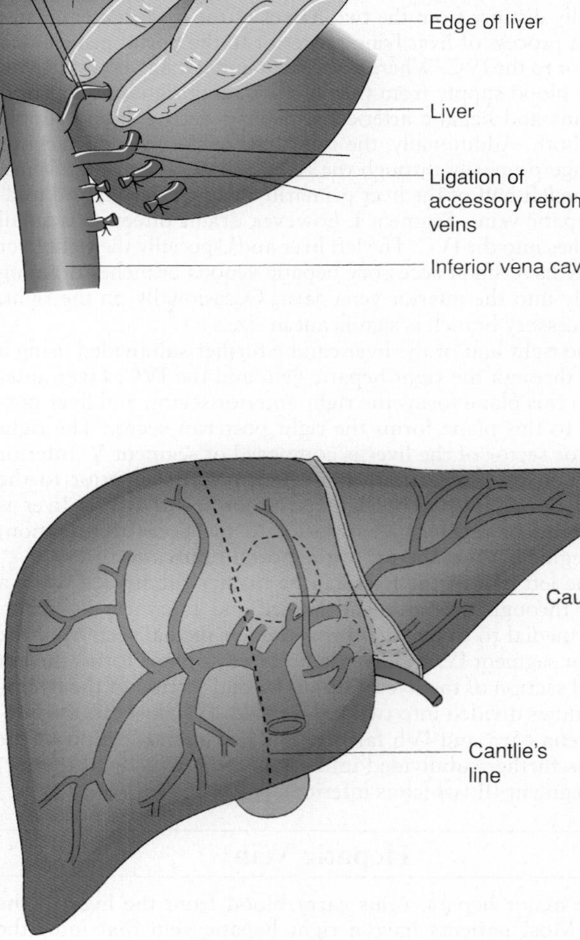

FIGURE 56.7. Intrahepatic divisions of the portal vein.

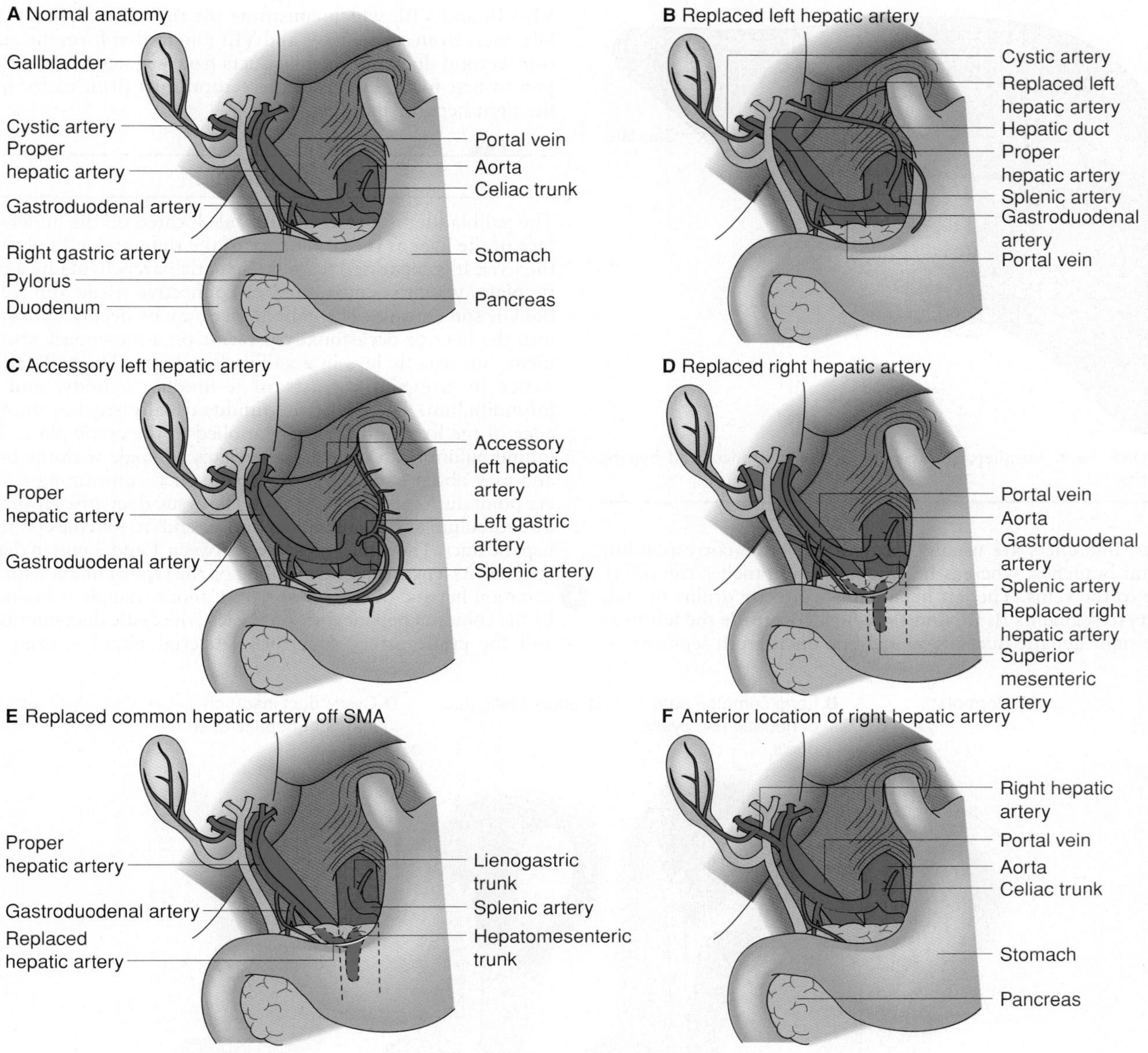

FIGURE 56.8. Variations in hepatic arterial anatomy.

gastroduodenal, supraduodenal, and right gastric arteries, the proper hepatic artery courses in the left anterior aspect of the hepatoduodenal ligament in front of the portal vein and to the left of the common hepatic duct. The proper hepatic artery usually bifurcates into right and left hepatic arteries outside the liver. The anatomy of the hepatic artery is variable and should be familiar to surgeons operating in this area (Fig. 56.8). Approximately 45% of people have variant hepatic arterial anatomy.[9] The right hepatic artery usually courses posterior to the common hepatic duct but anterior to the right portal vein to supply the right liver. The left hepatic artery usually remains extrahepatic until near the base of the umbilical fissure, where it enters the liver to give off branches to segments II, III, and IV. Small branches from near the bifurcation of the proper hepatic artery also supply segment I. A middle hepatic artery branch may arise from either the right or left hepatic arteries 3 after bifurcation. Although this anatomy is described as normal, it is found only in approximately 50% to 60% of patients. A replaced or accessory right hepatic artery may arise off of the superior mesenteric artery near its origin and course posteriorly or through the head of the pancreas to lie along the right posterior border of the hepatoduodenal ligament. A replaced or accessory left hepatic artery may arise off of the left gastric artery and course transversely toward the base of the umbilical fissure in the lesser omentum. In general, within the hepatic parenchyma, the hepatic arterial branches course closely with bile duct branches and fairly closely with portal venous branches, but not always, and anatomic variations should be suspected. The descriptions and frequency of hepatic arterial variants have been well characterized by Michels.[9]

Intrahepatic Biliary Tree

The right and left livers are respectively drained by the right and left hepatic ducts, whereas the caudate (segment I) is drained by several small ducts joining the bifurcation and the first several centimeters of both hepatic ducts. The intrahepatic ducts are tributaries of the corresponding hepatic ducts, which penetrate the liver invaginating the Glisson capsule at the

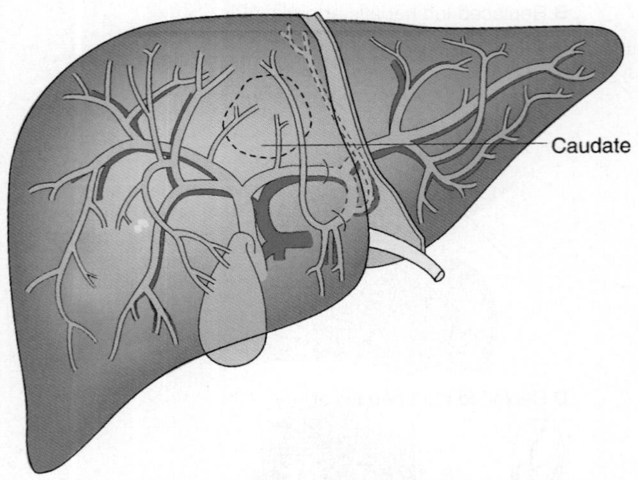

FIGURE 56.9. Intrahepatic divisions of the bile ducts and hepatic arteries.

hilus. Bile ducts are usually located above the corresponding portal branches, whereas hepatic arterial branches run inferiorly to the veins. The left hepatic duct directly drains the bile ducts to segments II, III, and IV, which constitute the left liver. The right hepatic duct drains the bile ducts from segments V, VI, VII, and VIII, which constitute the right liver. Usually, the bile ducts from segments V and VIII join to first form the anterior sectoral duct and the bile ducts from segments VI and VII join to first form the posterior sectoral duct prior to forming the right hepatic duct (Fig. 56.9).

Gallbladder

The gallbladder is a reservoir for bile located on the undersurface of the liver at the confluence of the right and left halves of the liver. It is separated from the hepatic parenchyma by a cystic plate, which is constituted of connective tissue applied to the Glisson capsule. The gallbladder may be deeply imbedded into the liver or occasionally presents on a mesenteric attachment, but usually lays in a gallbladder fossa. The gallbladder varies in size and consists of a fundus, a body, and an infundibulum. The tip of the fundus usually reaches the free edge of the liver and is closely applied to the cystic plate. The infundibulum of the gallbladder makes an angle with the body and may obscure the common hepatic duct, constituting a danger point during cholecystectomy. The cystic duct arises from the infundibulum of the gallbladder and extends to join the common hepatic duct. The lumen measures between 1 and 3 mm in diameter, and its length varies depending on the type of union with the
4 common hepatic duct (Fig. 56.10). Callot's triangle is bounded by the common hepatic duct on the left, the cystic duct inferiorly, and the cystic artery superiorly. Arterial blood reaches the

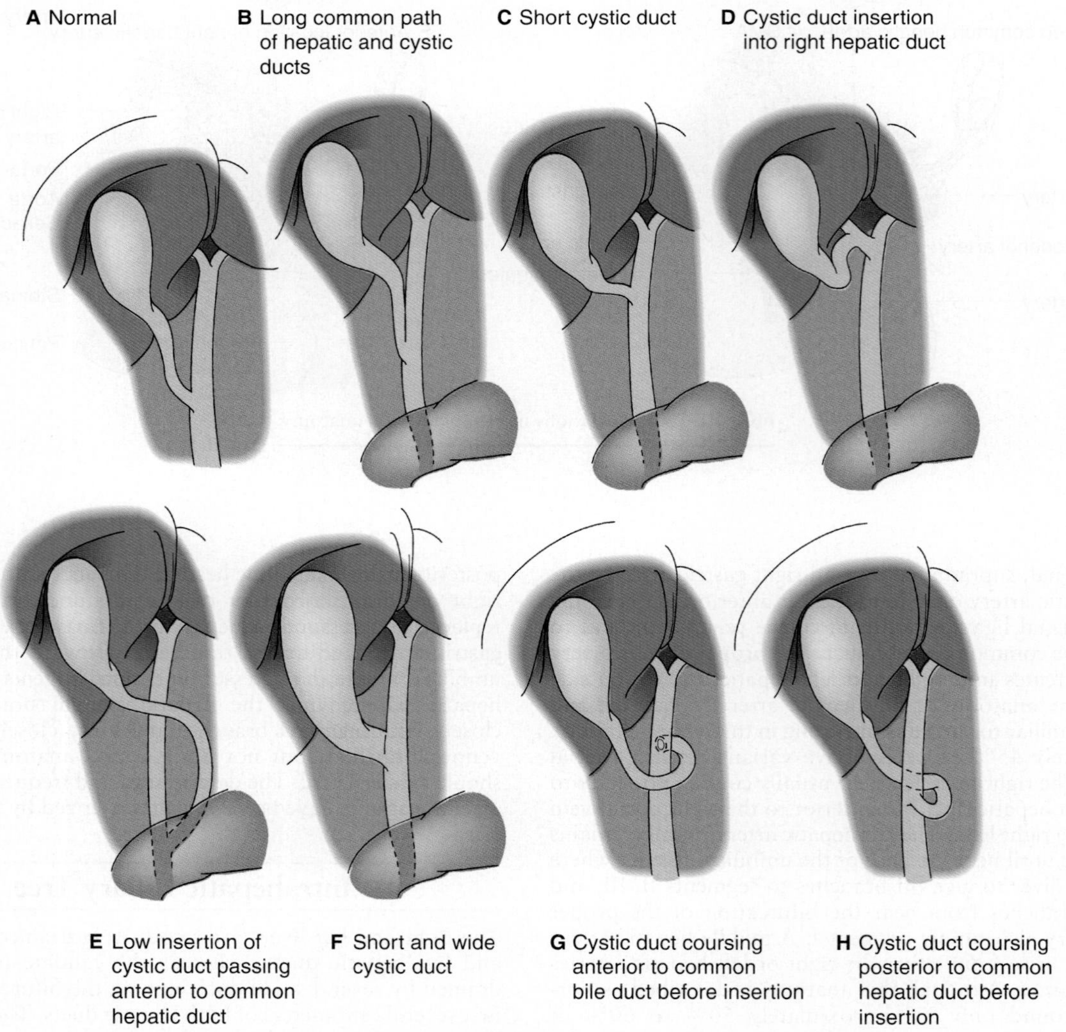

FIGURE 56.10. Variations in the junction of the cystic duct and common hepatic duct.

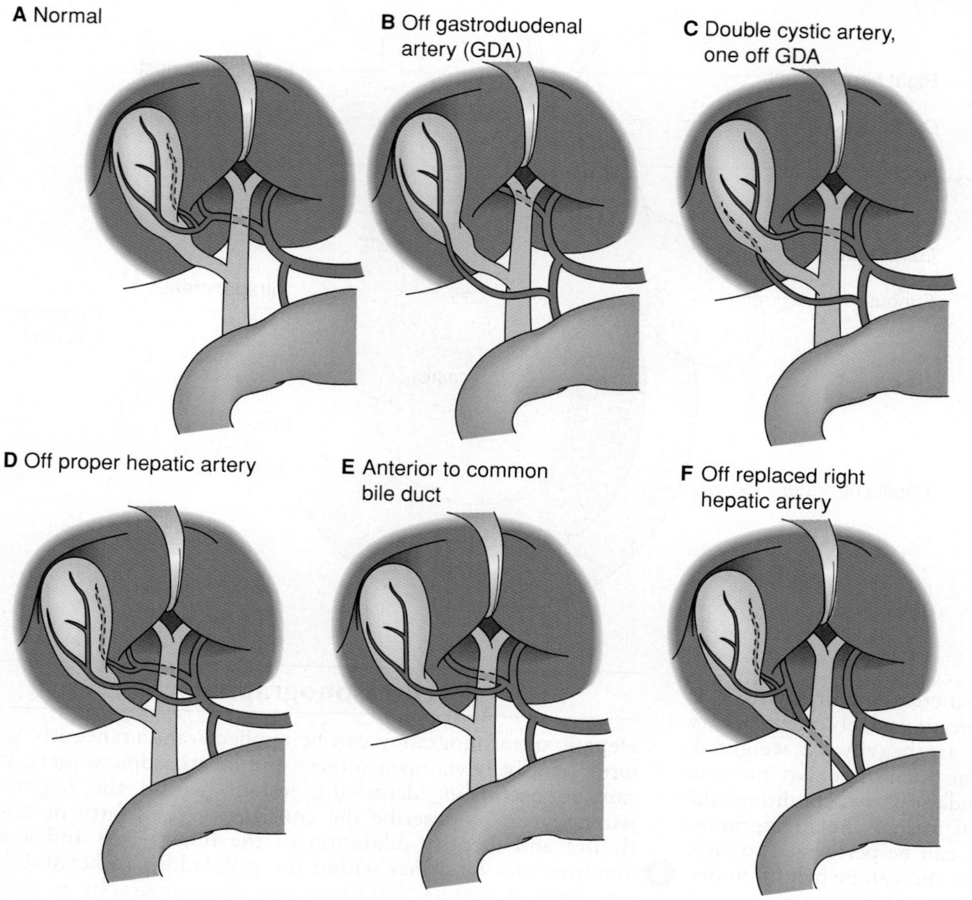

FIGURE 56.11. Variations of the cystic artery.

PANCREAS/LIVER

gallbladder via the cystic artery, which usually originates from the right hepatic artery. Several known variations in the origin and course of the cystic artery are illustrated in Figure 56.11. The venous drainage of the gallbladder is directly into the liver parenchyma or into the common bile duct plexus.

Common Bile Duct

The cystic and common hepatic ducts join to form the common bile duct. The common bile duct is approximately 8 to 10 cm in length and 0.4 to 0.8 cm in diameter. The common bile duct can be divided into three anatomic segments: supraduodenal, retroduodenal, and intrapancreatic (Fig. 56.12). The supraduodenal segment resides in the hepatoduodenal ligament lateral to the hepatic artery and anterior to the portal vein (Fig. 56.13). The course of the retroduodenal segment is posterior to the first portion of the duodenum, anterior to the inferior vena cava, and lateral to the portal vein. The pancreatic portion of the duct lies within a tunnel or groove on the posterior aspect of the pancreas. The common bile duct then enters the medial wall of the duodenum, courses tangentially through the submucosal layer for 1 to 2 cm, and terminates in the major papilla in the second portion of the duodenum (Fig. 56.12). The distal portion of the duct is encircled by smooth muscle that forms the sphincter of Oddi. The common bile duct usually joins the pancreatic duct to form a common channel before entering the duodenum at the ampulla of Vater. Some patients will have an accessory pancreatic duct emptying into the duodenum.

5 The blood supply of the common bile duct is segmental in nature and consists of branches from the cystic, hepatic, and gastroduodenal arteries. These meet to form collateral vessels that run in the 3 and 9 o'clock positions. The venous drainage forms a plexus on the anterior surface of the common bile duct that enters the portal system. The lymphatic drainage follows the course of the hepatic artery to the celiac nodes.

LIVER IMAGING

Computed Tomography

Computed tomography (CT) is widely available and quick and has become the main modality to initiate the assessment of hepatic processes. It also has the advantage of being able to quickly assess other organs within the abdominal cavity and chest. With the introduction of multidetector spiral CT, the resolution of hepatic lesions is quite good. This scanning technique allows total hepatic imaging in arterial, portal venous, and delayed phases after a rapid intravenous contrast bolus during a single breath hold by the patient (Fig. 56.14). In addition, three-dimensional reconstructions can be obtained to construct hepatic arteriograms that approach the quality of invasive angiography.

Magnetic Resonance Imaging

6 Magnetic resonance imaging (MRI) of the liver with gadolinium as a contrast agent is commonly used to help further characterize hepatic lesions. Resolution of some lesions may be slightly better with MRI. Additionally, certain lesions, such as hemangiomas and cysts, can easily be identified based on MRI characteristics when the CT characteristics are indeterminate (Fig. 56.15). The disadvantages of MRI are its increased cost, increased amount of time to perform, inability to quickly screen other organs and body cavities within the same session, and wide variability in quality from one imaging center to another.

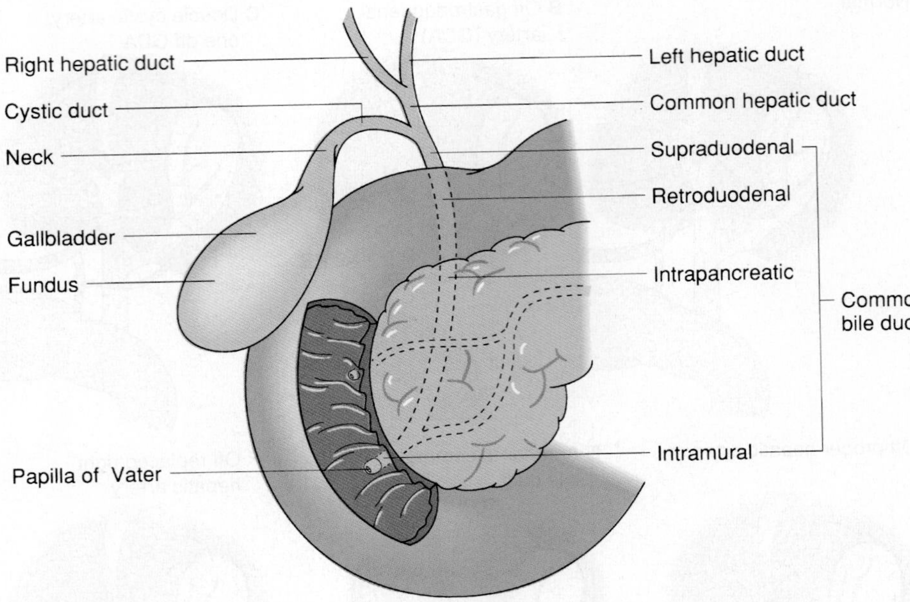

FIGURE 56.12. Anatomy of the extrahepatic biliary tree and pancreatic duct.

7 Magnetic resonance cholangiopancreatography (MRCP) is becoming more widely used to noninvasively view biliary anatomy (Fig. 56.16). The scans are heavily T2 weighted, which maximizes the signal from the biliary tree. No injection of contrast agent is needed, and under optimal conditions the resulting imaging can rival that of formal cholangiography. Three-dimensional reconstructions can be performed to view the biliary tree from multiple angles and can be helpful in distinguishing between stones, strictures, and neoplasms.

Ultrasonography

Hepatic ultrasonography can be applied transcutaneously or intraoperatively via open surgery and laparoscopic surgery. It can be useful in identifying lesions within the hepatic parenchyma, to describe the consistency (i.e., fatty or cirrhotic) and identify dilatation of the biliary tree and any
8 abnormalities or stones within the gallbladder. In hepatobiliary surgical centers, intraoperative ultrasonography is used

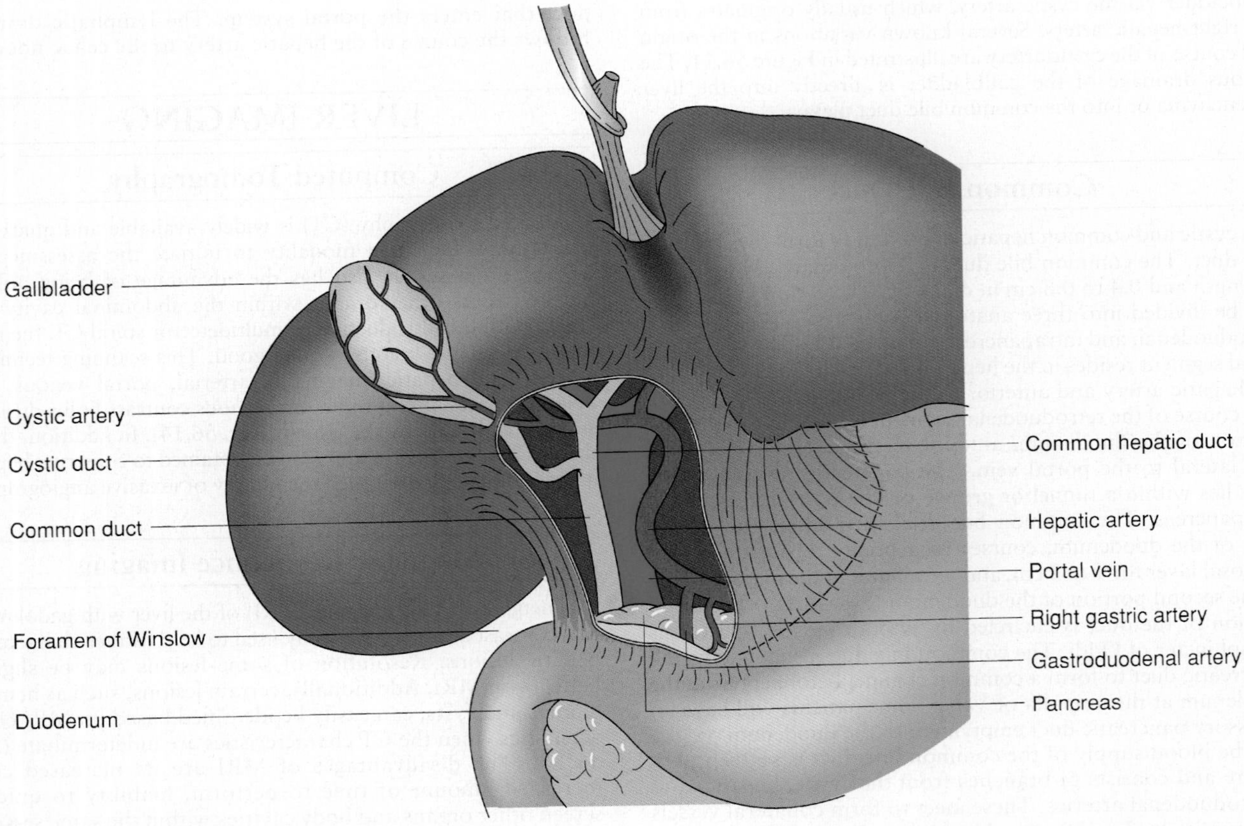

FIGURE 56.13. Relationship of structures within the hepatoduodenal ligament.

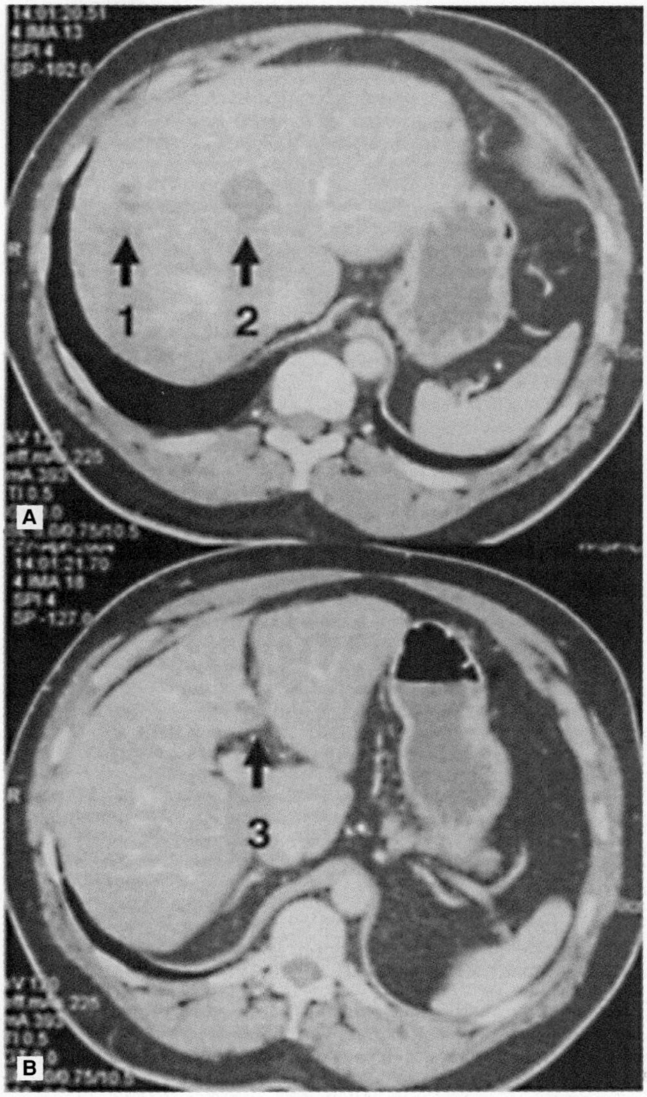

FIGURE 56.14. Portal venous phase of computed tomography (CT) scan from a patient with a history of colorectal cancer and three lesions in the liver. Lesion 1 in segment VIII is irregular and rim enhancing and was a colorectal cancer metastasis. Lesion 2 straddling segments IV and VIII has smooth borders, is not rim enhancing, and was found to be a cyst. Lesion 3 straddling segments IV and III across the umbilical fissure is irregular and rim enhancing and was a colorectal cancer metastasis.

routinely to assess the anatomy of the pedicles (portal vein, hepatic artery, bile duct), the hepatic veins, and the hepatic parenchyma. It is useful both to further identify and characterize lesions within the hepatic parenchyma and to delineate their relationships within the eight anatomic segments of the liver. Additionally, it is often helpful to delineate proximity of lesions to major vascular structures and to survey for abnormal anatomy in planning a resection.

With ablational therapies more commonly employed, ultrasound has become indispensable in directing the use of radiofrequency ablation. This ablational therapy can be performed percutaneously, laparoscopically, and during open surgery.

Typically, intraoperative assessment of the liver involves examining the portal pedicles. The main portal pedicle is identified within the hepatoduodenal ligament. It is followed superiorly to the portal bifurcation into the main right and
9 left pedicle. The portal pedicles are invested with the Glisson capsule and have a very echogenic covering to them in contrast to hepatic vein branches. The main right portal pedicle is followed toward the right where it gives off an anterior and posterior branch (Fig. 56.17A). The right anterior branch gives off separate pedicles to segment V (caudad) and to segment VIII (cephalad). The right posterior branch gives off separate pedicles to segment VI (caudad) and to segment VII (cephalad). The main left pedicle is usually much longer and courses intact to the base of the umbilical fissure before branching into various segmental pedicles (Fig. 56.17B). At the base of the umbilical fissure, the main left pedicle courses anteriorly toward the round ligament and gives off a pedicle to segment IV medially and pedicles to segments II and III laterally. Next, if the falciform ligament has been divided, the hepatic veins can easily be visualized using intraoperative ultrasonography (Fig. 56.17C). As described previously, usually a larger right hepatic vein can be delineated and smaller left and middle hepatic veins joining into a common trunk before emptying into the IVC are seen. Commonly, an umbilical hepatic vein branch can be identified coursing between the middle and left hepatic veins and running under the falciform ligament. Not uncommonly, significant accessory right hepatic veins can be seen emptying from the posterior surface of the right liver directly into the IVC as it courses posterior to the liver. The identification of these accessory right hepatic veins is potentially important for both vascular control and preservation of outflow from the liver (in occasional cases where outflow of the remnant right liver can be supported by a very large accessory vein). Lastly, the hepatic parenchyma is systematically scanned to identify lesions within the liver (Fig. 56.17D). It is sometimes useful to adjust the ultrasound settings on a known lesion defined preoperatively to maximize the echogenicity in the hopes of identifying other occult lesions not identified preoperatively.

Positron Emission Tomography

Positron emission tomography (PET), especially when combined with CT (PET-CT), has become a valuable tool in helping to select patients who will most benefit from aggressive liver resection. This technique is based on the increased metabolism of glucose in neoplastic tissues. A glucose analogue, fluorodeoxyglucose, that is tagged with fluorine 18 is injected intravenously before scanning and is retained preferentially in metabolically active tumors over normal tissue. Sometimes PET scans will identify areas of occult disease within the liver, but more importantly, they can identify areas of extrahepatic occult disease previously unsuspected. When combined with a CT scanner within the same machine and the ability to fuse images, the areas of increased activity can be more precisely anatomically identified (Fig. 56.18).

Correlation of Computed Tomographic Images with Segmental Anatomy

Preoperative CT remains the primary imaging modality used by most surgeons before hepatic resection. Figure 56.14 is provided to help correlate CT images to the segmental anatomy defined previously. The segments of the liver are defined using identifiable structures on the CT (Fig. 56.19).

PREOPERATIVE EVALUATION OF HEPATIC RESERVE

Whenever a surgical resection is planned, an important consideration is whether the remnant liver will be sufficient to regenerate and sustain the patient long term. In patients with

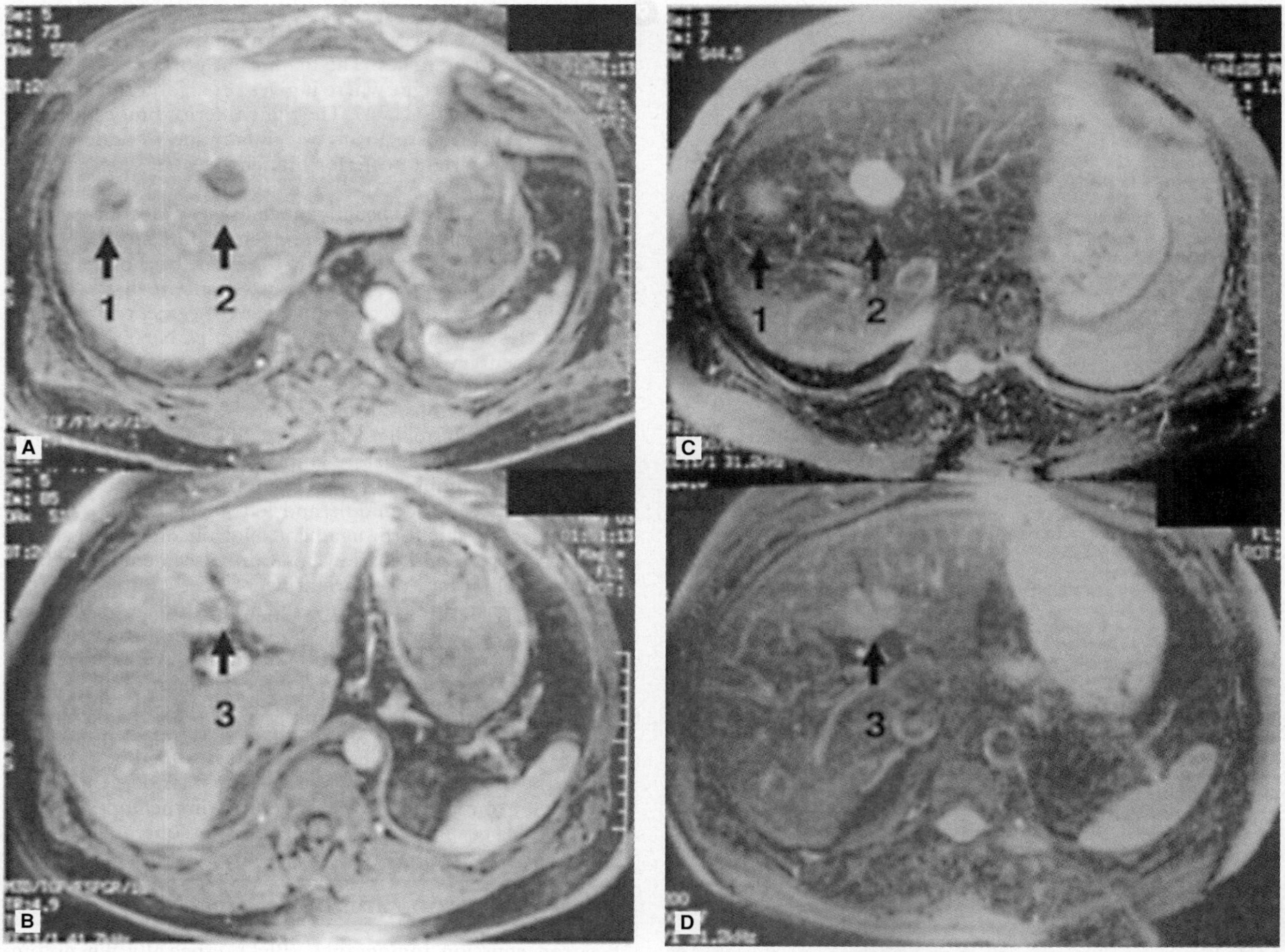

FIGURE 56.15. A, B: T1-weighted magnetic resonance imaging (MRI) with gadolinium from the same patient as in Figure 58.14 with history of colorectal cancer and three lesions in the liver. Lesion 1 in segment VIII is irregular and rim enhancing and was a colorectal cancer metastasis. Lesion 2 straddling segments IV and VIII has smooth borders, is not rim enhancing, and was found to be a cyst. Lesion 3 straddling segments IV and III across the umbilical fissure is irregular, rim enhancing, and was a colorectal cancer metastasis. C, D: T2-weighted MRI from same patient with history of colorectal cancer and three lesions in liver. Lesion 1 in segment VIII is irregular and mildly bright and was a colorectal cancer metastasis. Lesion 2 straddling segments IV and VIII has smooth borders, is very bright, and was found to be a cyst. Lesion 3 straddling segments IV and III across the umbilical fissure is mildly bright and was a colorectal cancer metastasis. Colorectal metastases and many tumors are mildly bright on T2-weighted MRI, whereas cysts and hemangiomas are typically very bright.

relatively normal hepatic parenchyma (without active hepatitis, cirrhosis, or metabolic defects), up to 75% of the hepatic volume can be resected with good recovery as long as the remnant liver has adequate portal venous and hepatic arterial inflow, adequate hepatic venous outflow, and adequate biliary drainage. Many groups around the world have used various strategies to predict hepatic reserve (Tables 56.1 and 56.2). None of these tests or strategies has been demonstrated to clearly better predict outcome than another. Many centers in the United States rely simply on the Child-Pugh score and the prediction of adequate liver remnant volume after resection. In select circumstances, it may be of benefit to perform portal vein embolization to the right or left half (rare) of the liver in the hopes of obtaining compensatory hypertrophy of the other side before resection. This is especially useful when the predicted liver remnant after resection is small or if the patient has an underlying hepatic dysfunction that may not allow the remnant to fully regenerate and sustain the patient long term. To gain maximal growth of the left lateral section of the liver, some centers will also embolize the portal vein branches to segment IV in addition the main right portal vein. The disadvantages of portal vein embolization include the need to wait 3 to 4 weeks before resection to allow the compensatory hypertrophy to occur and, for more central lesions, the need to commit to taking out one or the other side with an extended hepatectomy without the benefit of intraoperative evaluation.

TABLE 56.1

STRATEGIES TO PREDICT HEPATIC RESERVE

- Child-Pugh score (Table 56.2) to assess synthetic ability (albumin, prothrombin time, and ascites), bile cojugation and excretory function (total bilirubin), and metabolic function (changes in mental status from ammonia retention)
- Clearance of galactose or organic anionic dyes, such as indocyanine green
- Tests of microsomal function such as caffeine clearance, lidocaine clearance, or aminopyrine breath tests
- Volumetric measurements of the liver and prediction of liver remnant after resection based on three-dimensional reconstructions from computed tomography and magnetic resonance imaging

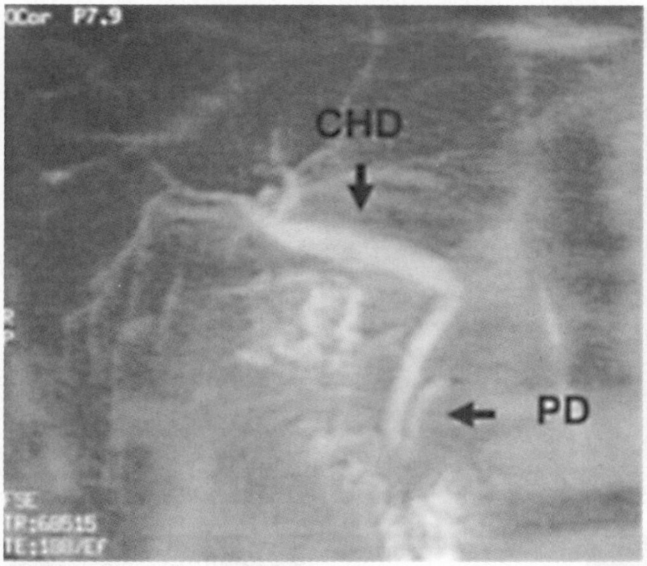

FIGURE 56.16. Magnetic resonance cholangiopancreatography (MRCP) of a patient after cholecystectomy with mild dilation of common hepatic duct (CHD). The pancreatic duct (PD) is also visible.

TABLE 56.2

CHILD-PUGH CLASSIFICATION

	■ 1 POINT	■ 2 POINTS	■ 3 POINTS
Bilirubin (mg/dL)	<2	2–3	>3
Albumin (g/dL)	>3.5	2.8–3.5	<2.8
Ascites	Absent	Moderate	Severe
Encephalopathy	Absent	Moderate	Severe
Prothrombin time			
Seconds prolonged	<4	4–6	>6
INR	<1.7	1.7–2.3	>2.3

INR, international normalized ratio.
A: 5–6 points; B: 7–9 points; C: 10–15 points.

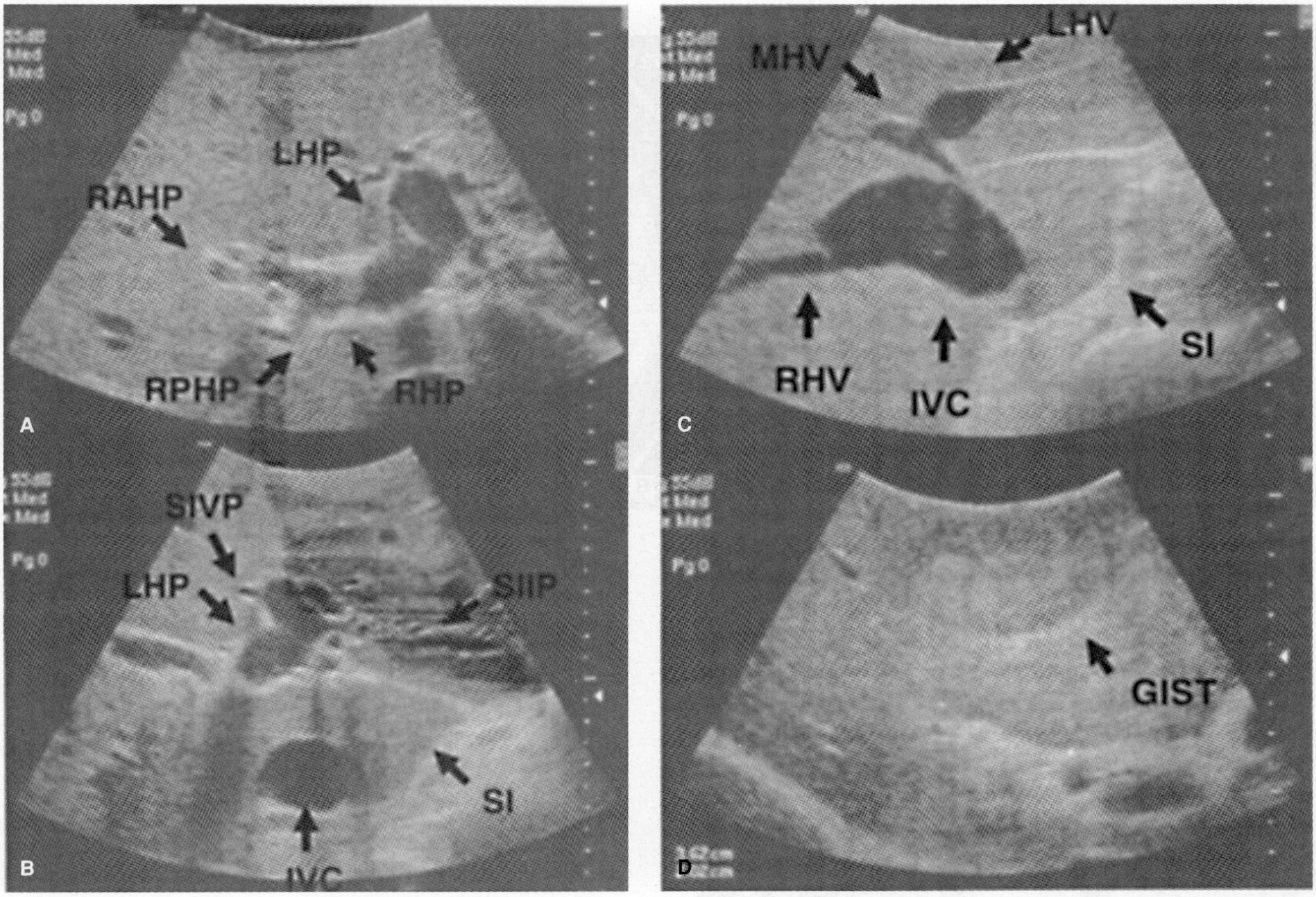

FIGURE 56.17. **A, B:** Intraoperative ultrasound images of liver demonstrating right hepatic pedicle (RHP), right anterior sector pedicle (RASP), right posterior sector pedicle (RPSP), left hepatic pedicle (LHP), segment II pedicle (SIIP), segment IV pedicle (SIVP), segment I (SI), and inferior vena cava (IVC). **C, D:** Intraoperative ultrasound images of liver demonstrating inferior vena cava (IVC), right hepatic vein (RHV), middle hepatic vein (MHV), left hepatic vein (LHV), segment I (SI), and a metastatic gastrointestinal stromal tumor lesion straddling segments IV and V of the liver.

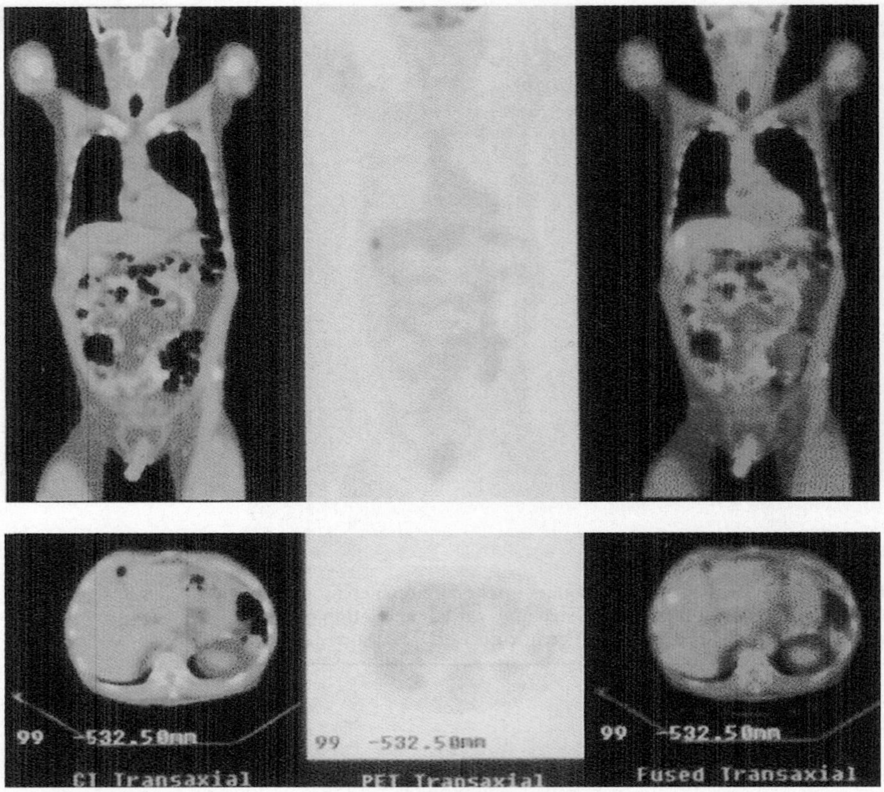

A
B

FIGURE 56.18. Positron emission tomography and computed tomography (PET-CT) scan images of patient in Figure 56.17B and C with solitary gastrointestinal stromal tumor metastasis straddling segments IV and V. Noncontrast CT images (*left*). PET images (*center*). Fusion images (*right*).

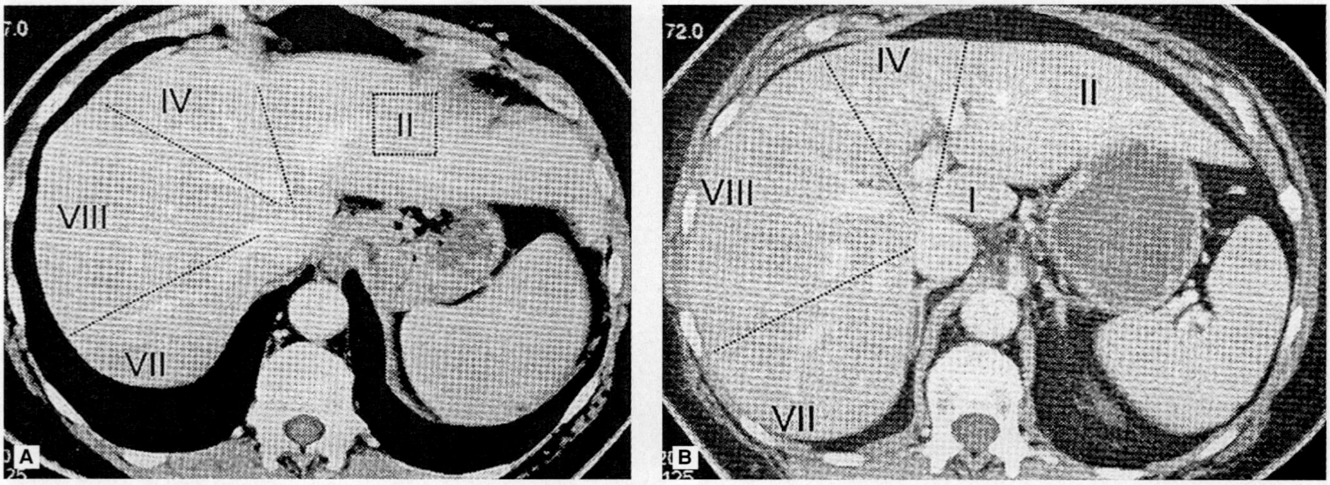

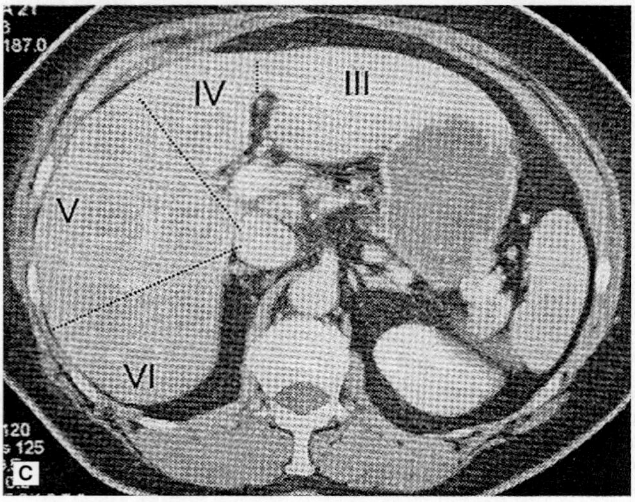

FIGURE 56.19. Computed tomography scan demonstrating segmental anatomy of the liver with cuts through the dome (**A**), just above the portal bifurcation (**B**), and below the portal bifurcation (**C**).

ONCOLOGIC CONSIDERATIONS IN HEPATIC RESECTION

The decision of when and whether to operate is often just as important as the technical details of successfully removing a liver lesion(s) identified in a patient. It is very important to consider the likely diagnosis in making the decision of whether to operate. For example, a solitary liver lesion presenting in an elderly patient with a rising carcinoembryonic antigen (CEA) and a recent history of a resected colon cancer should be treated differently from a young woman with a solitary lesion with radiologic characteristics of a focal nodular hyperplasia lesion. It is important to consider the biology of the tumor within the patient. For example, a patient who re-presents with a solitary hepatic colorectal cancer metastasis 4 years after resection of the primary tumor will more likely benefit from hepatic resection than another patient who presents with eight synchronous lesions in the liver at the time of diagnosis of the primary tumor. It is important to consider whether the goal of resection is curative or palliative. For example, patients with neuroendocrine tumor metastases of the liver may be debulked of hepatic metastases, but they are rarely totally eradicated of disease. If the tumor is functional and difficult to control medically, then there may be a benefit to debulking. Even if the tumor is not functional, some evidence indicates that surgical debulking of liver metastases in carefully selected patients may benefit long-term survival. It is important to exclude other distant extrahepatic disease with a reasonable number of preoperative tests. For example, before performing hepatic resection for colorectal cancer metastases, it is often helpful to obtain a PET scan to exclude extrahepatic metastases. This will allow better selection of patients most likely to benefit from hepatic resection and will allow patients with previously unsuspected systemic disease to get systemic therapy sooner.

The comorbid status of the patient is also important. Extended hepatic resections with or without biliary reconstruction can exert a toll on even very fit patients. It is important to identify patients who may have difficulties with hepatic regeneration (e.g., those with a history of hepatitis, cirrhosis, or metabolic disorders). Patients with suspected cardiopulmonary disease should undergo appropriate preoperative evaluation and treatment before hepatic resection. Lastly, other effective treatments and the optimal sequence of treatments should be considered. For example, in the treatment of hepatocellular carcinoma the possibilities include liver transplantation, liver resection, liver ablation (radiofrequency, cryotherapy, or ethanol), embolization, and systemic chemotherapies. A patient with very poor hepatic reserve because of chronic liver disease and a single small hepatocellular carcinoma may be best treated with liver transplantation, whereas a patient with normal liver parenchyma and a resectable lesion may be best treated with liver resection. Additionally, some patients may best be treated with ablative techniques, especially if they have very small lesions that are easily approached percutaneously. Some patients are treated with a combination of these modalities. For example, some centers will first treat patients with chemoembolization before liver transplantation or resection for hepatocellular carcinoma depending on the waiting time for a liver graft or to test the biology of the disease.

INTRAOPERATIVE ASSESSMENT

Incisions for hepatic resections usually involve a right subcostal incision. Significant exposure can be obtained with a trifurcated incision as shown in Figure 56.20. In the majority of cases, however, all that is needed is an extended right subcostal incision with a vertical extension to the base of the xiphoid. The xiphoid can be resected for better exposure. For bulky lesions on the left or if the left half of the liver extends significantly to the left upper quadrant, a left subcostal component can be added. In rare circumstances, especially for lesions high on the dome, an intercostal extension or even median sternotomy may improve exposure. This is especially true for lesions involving the hepatic vein and IVC confluences.

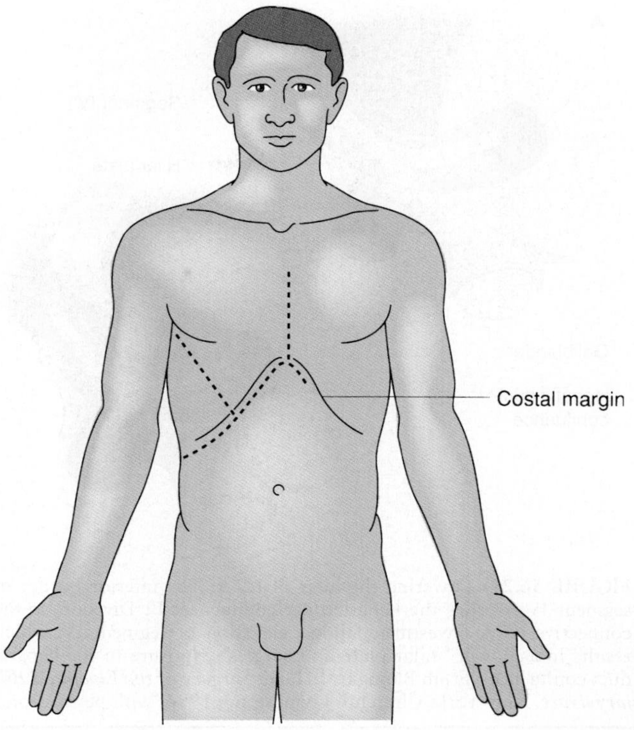

FIGURE 56.20. Incisions used for hepatic resection.

Several versions of self-retaining costal margin retractors or ringed retractors are available that provide good access to the subdiaphragmatic surface. For complete intraoperative ultrasonography and for major resections, complete mobilization of the involved side of the liver is required. The round ligament is divided and the falciform ligament divided. The right and/or left triangular ligaments are then divided to expose the bare areas of the liver. During exposure of the bare areas of the liver, care should be taken to avoid entering the right or left chest through the ligamentous portions of the diaphragm because this will cause excessive bellowing of the diaphragm and poor exposure until a chest tube is placed on that side or the hemithorax is "bubbled out" to remove the air and the diaphragm repaired. Additionally, the right and left phrenic veins are very superficial on the hemidiaphragms and can be injured. The right colon can be mobilized out of the field by dividing Gerota fascia over the right kidney and pulling the hepatic flexure inferiorly. To completely assess the caudate lobe, the overlying lesser omentum should be divided. Care should be taken to avoid inadvertently dividing a replaced or accessory left hepatic artery running in this space. After mobilization, a thorough bimanual examination should be performed and intraoperative ultrasonography used as previously described.

The porta hepatis is often dissected to identify the main bifurcations of the hepatic artery, bile duct, and portal vein. This allows individual ligation of the branches of these structures supplying one side of the liver while preserving the branches to the other side. Ligation of the hepatic artery and portal vein to one side also allows the liver parenchyma to demarcate a line of resection between the right and left liver. Greater exposure of the superior aspect of the hepatic hilum and exposure of a high or intraparenchymal bifurcation of a

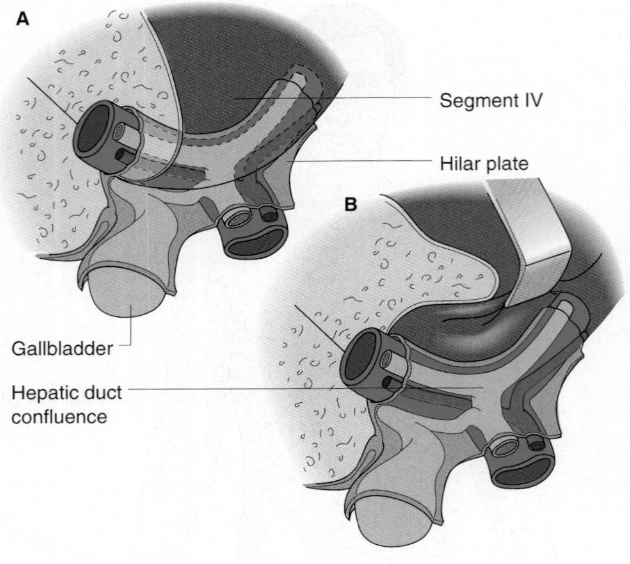

FIGURE 56.21. Lowering the hilar plate. **A:** The inferior border of segment IV overlies the hepatic duct confluence. **B:** Division of the connective tissue investment allows elevation of segment IV, which results in a "lower" hilar plate and surgical exposure to the hepatic duct confluence. (From Blumgart LH, ed. *Surgery of the Liver and Biliary Tract*. New York: Churchill Livingstone; 1994, with permission.)

portal triad structure may be aided by exposing the hilar plate (Fig. 56.21) and dividing the Glisson capsule at the most inferior border of segment IV. Inflow control to the liver can also be obtained by pedicle ligations in which small hepatotomies are made around the main right pedicle, main left pedicle, right anterior pedicle, or right posterior pedicle after identification with ultrasound (Fig. 56.22).[10] The pedicle of interest can be dissected out bluntly with a right angle or by palpation. The pedicle can then be clamped to confirm that it does indeed supply the area of liver of interest (i.e., right half, left half, right anterior section, or right posterior section). Once confirmed, the pedicle can be divided. Alternatively, the inflow pedicles can be divided as they are encountered while transecting hepatic parenchyma. With this technique, hemorrhage can be minimized by intermittent portal inflow occlusion, which is accomplished by gently clamping the main portal triad within the hepatoduodenal ligament ("Pringle maneuver").

Outflow control of the hepatic veins can be obtained before or after hepatic transection and should be decided on a case-by-case basis. When there is a significant extraparenchymal component to the hepatic vein(s), often it is easier to divide the hepatic vein(s) early and before parenchymal transection (but after inflow control) (Fig. 56.23). When the extraparenchymal component to the hepatic vein(s) is very short or absent and when the tumor margin is not near the junction of the hepatic vein(s) and IVC, it may be easier and safer to divide the hepatic vein(s) within the hepatic parenchyma after most of the parenchymal transection has been performed. The use of endoscopic vascular stapling devices has made the ligation of hepatic veins, whether extra- or intraparenchymally, much quicker and safer[10] (Fig. 56.24). It is often useful to keep the central venous pressure (CVP) of the patient low (<5 mm Hg) until after parenchymal transection as this will decrease bleeding from the IVC and hepatic vein branches.[11]

MAJOR HEPATECTOMIES

To develop a uniform nomenclature understood by all, the American and International Hepato-Pancreato-Biliary Associations (AHPBA and IHPBA) have adopted the Brisbane 2000 terminology of hepatic anatomy and resections. Right hepatectomy or right hemihepatectomy involves the resection of segments V through VIII. Left hepatectomy or hemihepatectomy involves the resection of segments II through IV. Either of these resections may or may not include resection of segment I, which should be stated. Extended right hepatectomy involves the resection of segments IV through VIII. Extended left hepatectomy involves the resection of segments II through V plus VIII. Again, either of these extended resections may or may not include resection of segment I, which should be stipulated.

Right anterior sectorectomy includes segments V and VIII. Right posterior sectorectomy includes segments VI and VII. Left medial sectionectomy removes segment IV. Left lateral sectionectomy includes segments II and III. A segmentectomy involves the resection of a single segment and a bisegmentectomy involves the resection of two contiguous segments.

10 The steps involved in each of these major hepatectomies include optimal exposure of the liver, vascular inflow control, vascular outflow control, and parenchymal transection. Vascular inflow control can be obtained by directly ligating the main right or left branches of the hepatic artery and portal vein in the hilum or by intermittent 10- to 20-minute intervals of a Pringle maneuver with 3 minutes in between to reestablish blood flow (or both). It is the author's preference to encircle the hepatoduodenal ligament twice with a quarter-inch Penrose drain that is tightened and clamped for a Pringle maneuver. Pedicle ligation can also be performed, as described previously, or the pedicles can be controlled as they are encountered during parenchymal transection. It is the author's preference to obtain vascular inflow by ligating the appropriate vessels in the hilum or by pedicle ligations and to supplement this with intermittent Pringle maneuvers, as necessary, during parenchymal transection. Often the Pringle maneuver is not required, but if bleeding from inflow vessels becomes significant, then it should be performed. Vascular outflow to the right or left liver can be obtained by exposing and ligating the hepatic veins, as previously described, or by ligating the vessels intraparenchymally during transection of the liver tissue. Parenchymal transection can be performed using a multitude of techniques including finger fracture, using a Kelly clamp to fracture, Cavitron Ultrasonic Surgical Aspirator (CUSA), harmonic

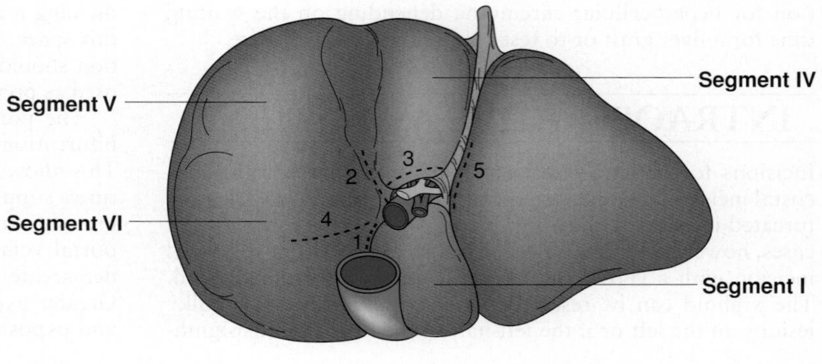

FIGURE 56.22. Hepatotomies to access pedicles for ligation: right hepatectomy, 1 and 2; left hepatectomy, 3 and 5; right anterior sectorectomy, 2 and 4; and right posterior sectorectomy, 1 and 4. (From Fong Y, Blumgart LH. Useful stapling techniques in liver surgery. *J Am Coll Surg* 1997;185:93–100, with permission.)

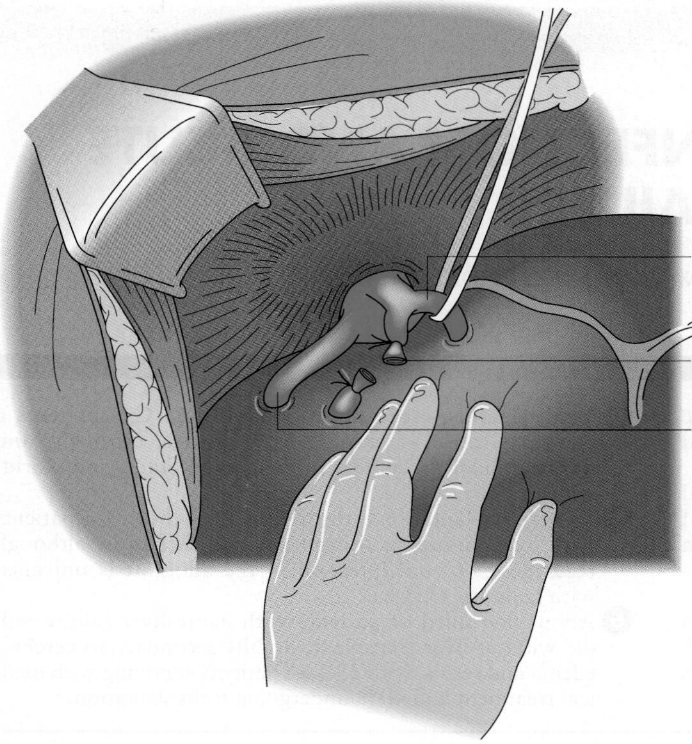

FIGURE 56.23. Caudal retraction of the left hepatic lobe with division of middle and left hepatic veins during left hepatic lobectomy. Often, the division of the middle and left hepatic veins is intraparenchymal.

scalpel, stapling devices, electrocautery devices with or without saline perfusion, high-pressure water jets, and radiofrequency planar arrays. The superiority of any one of these techniques has not been established, and all are used. With these techniques, individual blood vessels and bile ducts are cauterized, clipped, or sutured in rapid succession as they are encountered. Constant reevaluation of the direction of transection is important both to not injure vital structures to the remnant liver and to maintain a negative margin. After parenchymal transection and removal of the specimen, the raw surface of the liver is carefully inspected for bleeding and bile leakage, which can then be controlled by suture ligation and the use of argon beam coagulation. The author's preference is to selectively use closed suction drains near resected liver surfaces to monitor and drain unrecognized postoperative bile leaks. Some centers have decreased the use of closed suction drains in favor of radiologic intervention when necessary, because they often clog or do not actually drain the fluid collections that form.

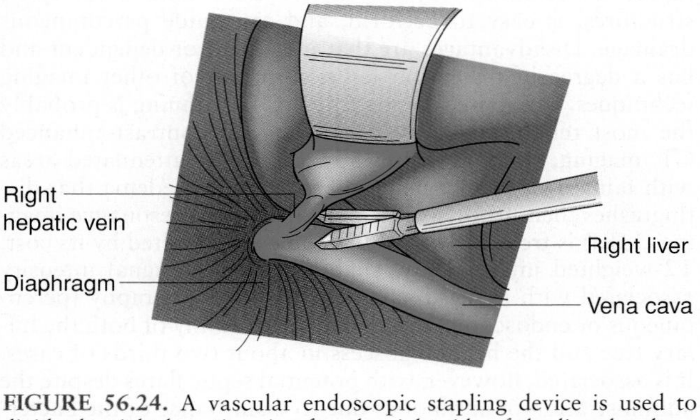

FIGURE 56.24. A vascular endoscopic stapling device is used to divide the right hepatic vein after the right side of the liver has been mobilized. (From Fong Y, Blumgart LH. Useful stapling techniques in liver surgery. *J Am Coll Surg* 1997;185:93–100, with permission.)

SEGMENTAL RESECTIONS

To maximize functional reserve, (multi)segmental or subsegmental (or nonanatomic) hepatectomies can be performed. For example, left lateral sectionectomy (segments II and III), central hepatectomy to remove the right anterior section (segments V and VIII) and left medial section (segment IV), right posterior sectionectomy (segments VI and VII), or caudate resection (segment I) are examples in which one, two, or three contiguous segments are removed to eradicate tumors within those regions of the liver. These resections are often done with intermittent Pringle maneuvers until the specific pedicles supplying these areas are controlled.

References

1. McIndoe AH, Counseller VX. A report on the bilaterality of the liver. *Arch Surg* 1927;15:589.
2. Hjörtsjö CH. The topography of the intrahepatic duct systems. *Acta Anat (Basel)* 1931;11:599–615.
3. Tung TT. La vascularixation veineuse du foie et ses applications aux resections hepatiques. *Thèse Hanoi*, 1939.
4. Healy JE, Schroy PC. Anatomy of the biliary ducts within the human liver. Analysis of the prevailing pattern of branchings and the major variations of the biliary ducts. *AMA Arch Surg* 1953;66:599–616.
5. Goldsmith NA, Woodvurne RT. Surgical anatomy pertaining to liver resection. *Surg Gynecol Obstet* 1957;195:310–318.
6. Couinaud C Le Foi. *Etudes anatomogiques et chirurgicales*. Paris: Masson; 1957.
7. Bismuth J, Houssin D, Castaing D. Major and minor segmentectomies–réglées–in liver surgery. *World J Surg* 1982;6:10–24.
8. Blumgart LH, Hann LE. Surgical and radiologic anatomy of the liver and biliary tract. In: Blumgart LH, Fong Y, eds. *Surgery of the Liver and Biliary Tract*, 3rd ed. New York: WB Saunders; 2000.
9. Michels NA. Newer anatomy of the liver and its variant blood supply and collateral circulation. *Am J Surg* 1966;112:337.
10. Fong Y, Blumgart LH. Useful stapling techniques in liver surgery. *J Am Coll Surg* 1997;185:93–100.
11. Melendez JA, Arslan V, Fischer ME, et al. Perioperative outcomes of major hepatic resections under low central venous pressure anesthesia: blood loss, blood transfusion, and the risk of postoperative renal dysfunction. *J Am Coll Surg* 1998;187:620–625.

CHAPTER 57 ■ HEPATIC INFECTION AND ACUTE HEPATIC FAILURE

ARUNA SUBRAMANIAN, AHMET GURAKAR, ANDREW KLEIN, AND ANDREW CAMERON

KEY POINTS

1. Gram-negative anaerobes account for two thirds of the cases of pyogenic liver abscesses, with anaerobes isolated in 30% of cases.
2. First-line treatment of hepatic amebic abscesses is oral metronidazole, with percutaneous drainage considered if there is a poor response to therapy or when superinfection is suspected.
3. The treatment of choice for hydatid cysts is surgical resection of the intact cyst, often preceded by injection of ethyl chloride, 95% ethanol, or 20% sterile saline solution. Surgery should occur after antiparasitic medication has begun.
4. Viral hepatitis, especially hepatitis B and C, represents a principal cause of chronic liver disease, cirrhosis, and hepatocellular carcinoma in the United States and worldwide.
5. Liver transplantation is the treatment of choice for patients with liver failure resulting from viral hepatitis, although recurrence of viral infection in the allograft is universal with hepatitis C virus.
6. About one third of patients with acute liver failure will die without liver transplant, usually secondary to cerebral edema and sepsis, with 25% of patients surviving with medical treatment and 40% undergoing transplantation.

PYOGENIC LIVER ABSCESS

Liver abscesses are broadly categorized as either pyogenic (of bacterial origin) or amebic (caused by *Entamoeba histolytica*). Pyogenic liver abscesses are infrequent, with an estimated incidence of 2.3 per 100,000 population, and a peak incidence in the fifth and sixth decades of life.[1] However, they are potentially lethal and outcomes correlate directly with prompt diagnosis and rapid intervention.

Over the past century, the pathogenesis of liver abscesses has changed. A classic study by Ochsner in the 1930s, prior to the introduction of antibiotics, reported that appendicitis and other intra-abdominal infections were the most frequent cause of pyogenic liver abscess. The route of infection was attributable to the portal vein in 43% of instances, whereas the biliary tree was the source of infection in only 14% of cases. Over the past 20 years, invasive procedures involving the liver, biliary tree, and pancreas have resulted in an increased incidence of pyogenic liver abscesses. Currently, cholangitis is the major cause of pyogenic liver abscess, due to obstruction from biliary malignancies and stone disease. The use of stents to treat both malignant and nonmalignant strictures is also a contributing factor. The portal vein serves as the conduit for infection from intraperitoneal sources in a minority of cases, and appendicitis has been replaced as the most frequent intraperitoneal source by infections associated with diverticulitis, perforated cancers, perforated ulcers, and inflammatory bowel disease. Hepatic abscesses that occur following liver transplantation should raise concern for the presence of hepatic artery thrombosis (Fig. 57.1). Direct extension from a contiguous source of infection can occur with cholecystitis, subphrenic abscess, or perinephric abscess. Fewer than 5% of pyogenic liver abscesses are due to trauma, and 20% to 40% are considered cryptogenic. Most pyogenic abscesses are solitary and polymicrobial and involve the right lobe of the liver. Abscesses in liver metastases usually result from superinfection of a central area of necrosis. Hepatic abscesses may be further complicated by rupture into the peritoneum or retroperitoneum, pleuropulmonary fistulas, rupture into the pericardial cavity, rupture into the gastrointestinal tract, and involvement of surrounding blood vessels.[2–4]

Individuals over 50 years of age, males, liver transplant patients, diabetics, and those with malignancies are at highest risk for pyogenic liver abscesses. Fever is the most frequent presenting symptom, often without other localizing signs and symptoms. Right upper quadrant pain, chills, anorexia, weight loss, malaise, jaundice, and weakness are usually present. Hepatomegaly is less frequent than in amebic abscesses.[1,2,4]

Laboratory studies show leukocytosis in approximately 70% of patients. Elevated serum bilirubin, elevated alkaline phosphatase, elevated transaminases, or low albumin levels are observed in approximately 50% of all cases.[2,3]

Chest radiographs are abnormal in half of patients with pyogenic liver abscesses, reflecting an underlying inflammatory process. The most frequent findings include a right pleural effusion, elevation of the right hemidiaphragm, and atelectasis of the base of the right lung. Gas within the abscess may be seen in 10% to 20% of patients. Ultrasound evaluation is diagnostic in over 90% of cases. Advantages are that it is rapid, is radiation-free, can differentiate solid from cystic structures, is easy to perform, and can guide percutaneous drainage. Disadvantages are that it is operator dependent and has a degree of resolution inferior to that of other imaging techniques. Computed tomography (CT) scanning is probably the most reliable diagnostic modality. In contrast-enhanced CT imaging, small abscesses appear as hypoattenuated areas with faint rim enhancement and surrounding edema that distinguishes them from hepatic cysts. Magnetic resonance imaging (MRI) is frequently used but somewhat limited by its cost. T2-weighted images show slightly increased signal intensity associated with perilesional edema. Cholangiography (percutaneous or endoscopic) can define the anatomy of both the biliary tree and the hepatic abscess in about two thirds of cases. It is associated, however, with potential septic flares despite the administration of antibiotics due to disturbance of the bacterial flora.[2,5,6]

1 Gram-negative aerobes are encountered in two thirds of patients. Among these pathogens, *Escherichia coli*, *Klebsiella*

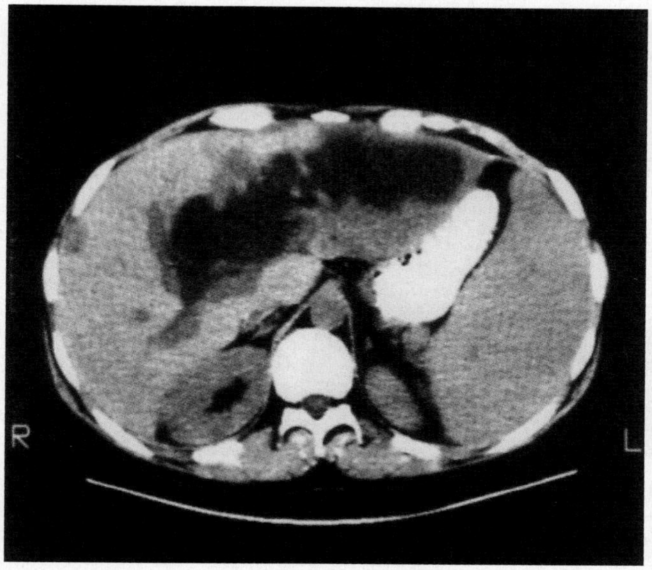

FIGURE 57.1. Computed tomogram of a pyogenic hepatic abscess in a liver transplant recipient with occlusion of the hepatic artery.

pneumoniae, and *Proteus* species are the ones most frequently isolated. These bacteria are frequently accompanied by enterococci in abscesses arising from a biliary source; anaerobes accompany the gram-negative aerobes when there is a colonic or pelvic source. Anaerobes (such as *Bacteroides fragilis*) are found in 30% of cases. Streptococci, including aerobic and anaerobic forms, are present in approximately one third of patients. Approximately 60% of patients have concordant results of blood and abscess cultures, and blood cultures should be obtained prior to antibiotic administration. Broad-spectrum antibiotics aimed at gram-negative aerobes, streptococci, and anaerobes are indicated until bacterial sensitivities have been clearly identified. A frequently used antibiotic combination is ampicillin, an aminoglycoside, and metronidazole. The ampicillin and aminoglycoside can be replaced with a third-generation cephalosporin (e.g., ceftriaxone) in patients at risk for renal toxicity, and those with β-lactam intolerance can be treated with a fluoroquinolone plus metronidazole. In instances of mixed pyogenic and fungal abscesses, antifungal agents should be considered early. Overall, the duration of the treatment should be based on clinical response, toxicity of the regimen, and characteristics of the abscesses. Intravenous antibiotics are usually administered for 14 days, followed by oral agents for a total of 6 weeks.[2,3,7–9]

In the past, surgical drainage was the treatment of choice. Currently, percutaneous drainage is considered the standard therapy. Its use, however, may be limited or contraindicated by the presence of ascites, multiple abscesses, a transpleural drainage route, large size of the abscess, and the presence of an intra-abdominal source requiring an open approach. Unless appropriate therapy is started as soon as the diagnosis is made, death is the usual outcome. Reported mortality ranges from 2.5% to over 30% and is highest in patients with multiple abscesses, with non–*K. pneumoniae* pathogens, with mixed bacterial and fungal abscesses, with respiratory symptoms, and with abscesses 5 cm or greater in diameter.[2,3,7,10,11]

AMEBIC LIVER ABSCESS

Amebic liver abscesses are caused by *E. histolytica*, a nonflagellated pseudopod-forming protozoan. Amebiasis is most prevalent in tropical and subtropical regions with poor sanitation, and it is estimated that 40 million to 50 million people are infected annually worldwide. In the United States, the highest incidence of infection is encountered in immigrants from and travelers to endemic areas. Most infection is asymptomatic, but amebic dysentery, amebic liver abscesses, and, rarely, pulmonary, cardiac, or brain involvement can occur. Hepatic abscesses occur in only 3% to 7% of individuals with amebiasis. The peak incidence of amebic abscesses is observed in patients in their third or fourth decade of life. Men are affected 7 to 10 times more frequently than women, and corticosteroid use is a risk factor for invasive amebiasis.[2,12]

Fecal-oral transmission is the most frequent route of infection. Ingested cysts, containing four nuclei, pass unaltered through the stomach and reach the intestine. Once in the intestine, the cyst wall is degraded by trypsin and eight trophozoites are released. These infective forms multiply in the colonic lumen, especially in the cecum. While living within the colonic lumen, *E. histolytica* may become tissue invasive. Invasion may range from superficial mucosal ulceration to perforation. Amebic trophozoites that enter the mesenteric veins or lymphatics reach other organs. The portal vein is the route via which they reach the liver, the most frequent site of extraintestinal involvement. Amebic trophozoites cause obstruction of venules, thrombosis and infarction of the corresponding areas of hepatic parenchyma, and eventually abscesses (Fig. 57.2). In the distal colon they become cystic, undergo two consecutive divisions, are excreted in the feces as tetranucleate cysts, and remain viable for 8 to 30 days after being shed. Cysts are susceptible to acetic acid, iodine, chlorine, and temperatures greater than 68°C.[2,6,12]

Liver abscesses range in size from several millimeters to gigantic masses (Fig. 57.3). Differential diagnosis is with pyogenic abscess and malignancies. Abscesses are encountered more frequently in the right lobe and tend to be single lesions. Amebic abscesses show slight inflammation on the periphery, and many times contain a dark hemorrhagic fluid known as "anchovy paste" (Fig. 57.4). Patients most frequently present with fever and right upper quadrant abdominal pain. Other findings include hepatomegaly, weight loss, diarrhea, chills, and afternoon and night sweats. Jaundice is less frequent than in pyogenic abscesses. Abscesses have been classified into acute

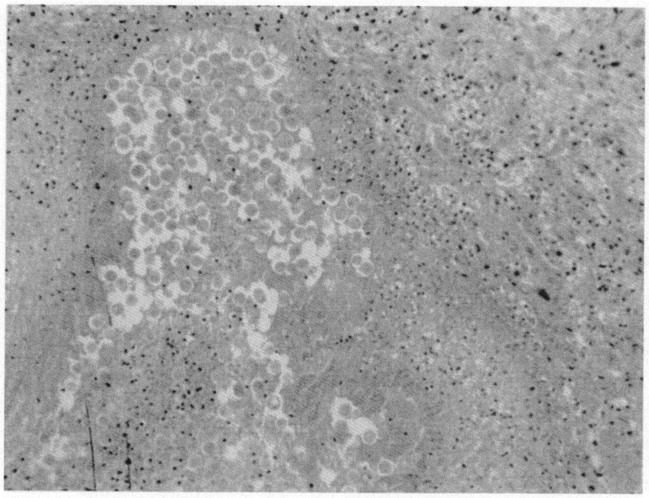

FIGURE 57.2. Amebic abscess of the liver. A photomicrograph of the margin of an amebic abscess shows fibroblastic proliferation surrounding the cavity and amebic trophozoites in the lumen. (Reproduced with permission from Rubin E, Farber JL. *Pathology,* 3rd ed. Philadelphia, PA: Lippincott Williams & Wilkins; 1999.)

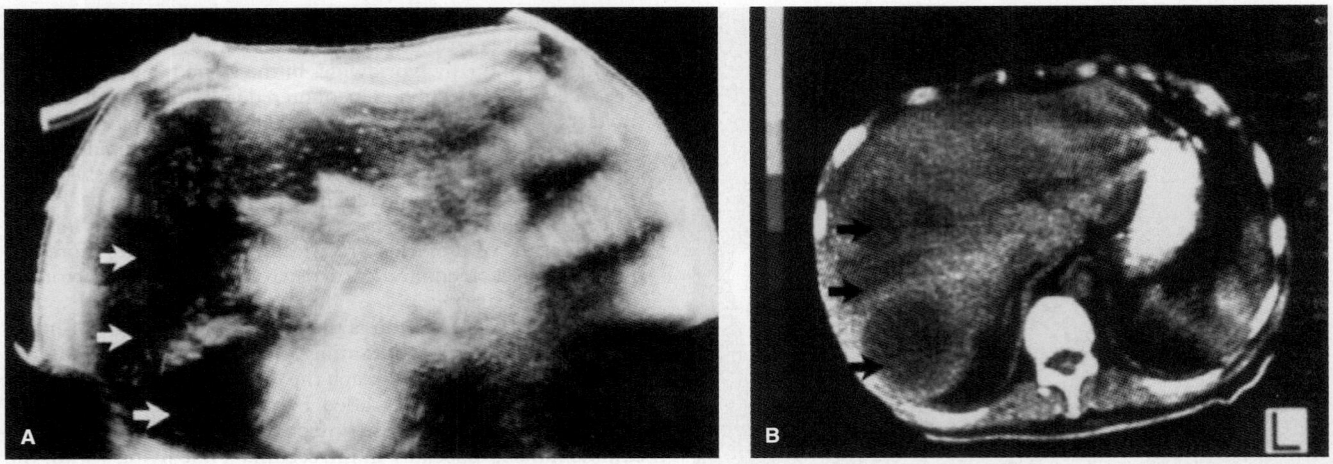

FIGURE 57.3. Sonogram (**A**) and computed tomogram (**B**) in a patient with multiple amebic abscesses (*arrows*).

or chronic and benign or aggressive. The most feared complication is rupture into surrounding tissues or spaces. Bacterial superinfection of initially amebic abscesses may occur.[1,2,4,6,12–14]

Most patients with amebic abscesses have elevated white blood cell counts with no eosinophilia. Serum alkaline phosphatase is elevated in approximately 75% of cases. Hypoalbuminemia may be seen, and serum bilirubin and transaminase levels are slightly elevated. *E. histolytica* is not found in fecal specimens of most patients with hepatic abscesses. Antibodies in serum are encountered in 92% to 99% of patients with amebic liver abscesses and are detectable 7 to 10 days after the appearance of symptoms. Indirect hemagglutination and enzyme-linked immunosorbent assay (ELISA) have reported sensitivities of 99% and 97.9% and specificities of 99.8% and 94.8%, respectively. Other available diagnostic tests include indirect immunofluorescence, latex agglutination, complement fixation, gel diffusion, and counterimmunoelectrophoresis. Gel diffusion and counterimmunoelectrophoresis remain positive for only 6 to 12 months after infection and are used to distinguish current from previous infection.[2,12,15]

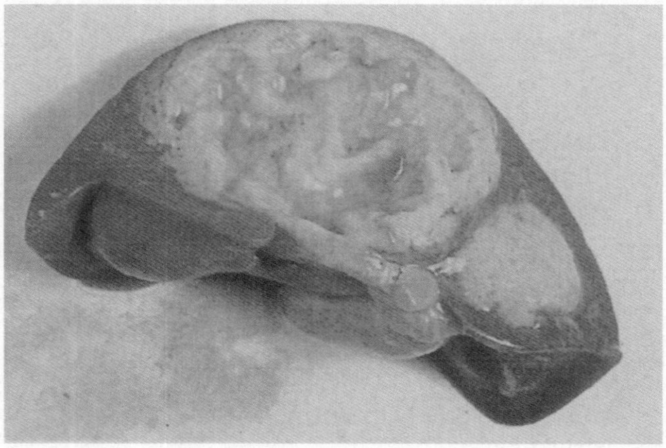

FIGURE 57.4. Amebic abscesses of the liver. The cut surface of the liver shows multiple abscesses containing "anchovy paste" material. (Reproduced with permission from Rubin E, Farber JL. *Pathology*, 3rd ed. Philadelphia, PA: Lippincott Williams & Wilkins; 1999.)

Chest radiographs are abnormal in the majority of patients with amebic hepatic abscesses. Findings include elevation of the right hemidiaphragm, right pleural effusion, atelectasis in the region of the base of the right lung, and a right pleural effusion. CT scanning is probably the imaging technique of choice, given the detailed information it provides. An enhancing wall and surrounding edema are usually observed in contrast-enhanced CT scans. Ultrasonography is very useful as well, but its accuracy is associated with the skills of the operator, is influenced by physiologic changes such as hepatic steatosis, and has a resolution inferior to that of CT scans. Amebic abscesses usually lack wall echoes by ultrasound. MRI shows homogeneous low signal intensity on T1- and high signal intensity on T2-weighted images. Technetium Tc99m nuclear scanning displays a photopenic area. Gallium scanning shows amebic abscesses as cold spots, because they do not contain leukocytes, which may aid in differentiating them from pyogenic abscesses.[2,6,12]

2 Treatment of hepatic amebic abscesses is based on amebicidal drugs. Metronidazole is the drug of choice. Standard dosing is 750 mg orally three times daily or 500 mg intravenously every 6 hours for 7 to 10 days, with oral administration being the preferred route. Metronidazole has been shown to effectively treat both intestinal and extraintestinal sites. In patients who are slow to respond to therapy or with relapsed disease, a prolonged course of metronidazole may be considered, or a nitroimidazole with a longer half-life (e.g., tinidazole) can be given at a dose of 2 g for 3 days. Following therapy for invasive amebiasis, a luminal agent must be given, such as paromomycin for 10 days or iodoquinol for 20 days. Amebic liver abscesses can almost always be treated with medical therapy alone. Percutaneous drainage is considered in cases of poor response to antiamebic agents, when superinfection is suspected, or when there is a risk of rupture. Open surgical drainage is almost never required and is recommended only in severe, complicated cases.[2,12,13]

ECHINOCOCCUS (HYDATID DISEASE)

Hydatid disease, caused by *Echinococcus granulosus*, *E. multilocularis*, and *E. vogeli*, is endemic in the Mediterranean basin and other regions with sheep-rearing economies but rare in the United States. *E. granulosus* is the species that most frequently results in liver involvement. Dogs are the definitive host, although the disease is endemic

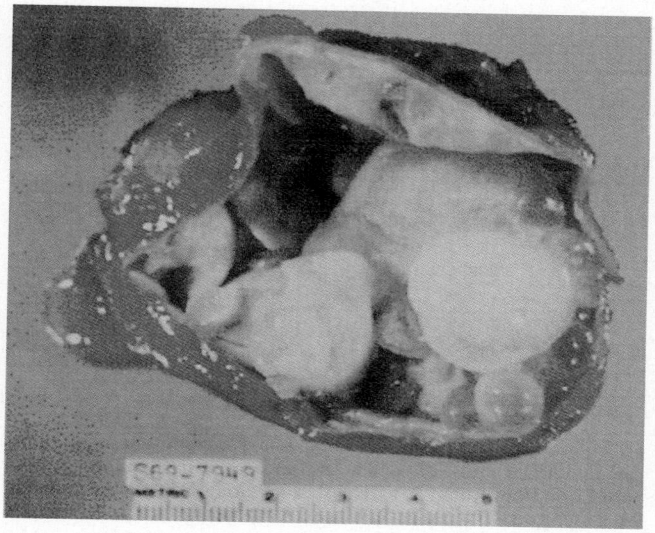

FIGURE 57.5. A partly opened hepatic hydatid cyst. Brood capsule and daughter cysts are visible in the cavity. (Reproduced with permission from Kean BH, Sun T, Ellsworth RM. *Color Atlas/Text of Ophthalmic Parasitology.* New York: Igaku-Shoin; 1991:188.)

in sheep and cattle farming regions. The life cycle of the organism is complete when the definitive host ingests infected viscera, and scoleces released in the intestine develop into adult worms. Humans are intermediate hosts and acquire echinococcal eggs by either ingestion of contaminated foods or contact with infected animals. The egg is digested in the duodenum and yields an embryo (oncospheres). Embryos invade the intestinal wall and reach the liver via the portal vessels. Although many embryos are destroyed in the liver, those that survive lodged in capillaries develop into hydatid cysts. The most frequent site of hydatid cysts is the liver (50% to 77% of cases), followed by the lungs (10% to 40% of cases).[6,16–18]

E. granulosus and *E. vogeli* cause liver cysts, while *E. multilocularis* is associated with tumorlike lesions or alveolar disease. Liver involvement may lead to venous obstruction, portal hypertension, sepsis, and cholangitis. Hydatid cysts are fluid filled and round and contain three layers of host tissue: an outer 2- to 4-mm-thick fibrous *pericyst* composed of compressed and fibrotic liver tissue, a 2-mm-thick middle anuclear hyaline layer or *ectocyst*, and an *internal germinal layer* or *endocyst* derived from the parasite. As the cyst matures, invagination of the germinal layer leads to development of daughter cysts in the periphery (Fig. 57.5). Calcifications may be observed in both viable and nonviable cysts.[6,17,18]

Cysts have an annual growth rate of 1 to 3 cm in diameter. Symptoms are caused by enlarging cysts that lead to abdominal pain (the most common presenting symptom), biliary obstruction, jaundice, and, rarely, portal hypertension. The only typical clinical finding of hepatic hydatid cyst is a palpable hepatic mass. Involvement of the biliary tree is seen in 12% to 80% of cases. Biliary findings may occur either as a result of communication between the pericyst and the biliary ducts or due to rupture of the cyst into the biliary tract. Fistulous communication of the cyst and bile ducts may be associated with secondary bacterial infection of the cyst, cholangitis, or biliary obstruction. Bacterial contamination occurs in 10% to 35% of cases. Occasionally, cysts spontaneously rupture into the peritoneal cavity and cause abdominal pain and anaphylaxis. Multiple intra-abdominal cysts may develop as a result of intraperitoneal leakage. Hepatic hydatid cysts may perforate the diaphragm and lead to empyema, pulmonary cysts, biliary-bronchial fistulas, or pericardial collections.[19]

Routine laboratory tests in patients with hydatid cysts may be normal or nonspecifically abnormal (e.g., showing features of obstructive jaundice). Eosinophilia is frequently present. Serologic screening tests (e.g., indirect hemagglutination, latex agglutination, ELISA) based on crude antigens are associated with high rates of false-positive and false-negative results. However, ELISA detection of specific antigens and immune complexes of the cyst has a much higher sensitivity, while ELISA and radioallergosorbent test (RAST) can also detect specific IgE antibodies. Antigen 5 (arc-5) and antigen B8 are the parasitic antigens of major diagnostic value. Confirmatory arc-5 immunoelectrophoresis has a reported positive rate of over 90%. Purified fractions enriched in antigens 5 and B8 and glycoproteins from hydatid fluid are reported to have sensitivity and specificity rates of 95% and 100%, respectively. Serology is less likely to be positive when the cyst is calcified or nonviable.[6,16]

Hydatid cysts have a typical appearance on imaging studies. Furthermore, imaging studies are useful in detecting associated complications. Ultrasound images may show daughter cysts, peripheral calcifications, or the so-called water lily sign of curved bands of delaminated endocyst. On CT scans, hydatid cysts are usually seen as hypoattenuating lesions. Daughter cysts are visualized in approximately 75% of cases and calcifications within the surrounding cyst wall in 50% of cases. MRI is the technique that best demonstrates pericyst, matrix or "hydatid sand" (free scoleces), and daughter cysts. The fibrous and calcified pericyst appears as a hypointense ring on both T1- and T2-weighted images. The hydatid matrix is hyperintense on T2-weighted images and hypointense on T1-weighted images. Daughter cysts are hypointense on both T1- and T2-weighted images. Endoscopic retrograde cholangiopancreatography (ERCP) is especially useful in cases involving the bile ducts.[6,16]

3 Open surgical resection is classically the treatment of choice in cases of symptomatic or complicated hepatic cysts (Fig. 57.6). The goals of surgery are to remove the cyst intact (without spillage of the internal contents) and to obliterate the cyst cavity; surgical resection lowers the rate of recurrence. Alternative methods have been developed, however. One of them is to aspirate the cyst contents after the operative field has been protected to prevent any potential contamination should spillage of the cyst contents occur. In cases in which the aspirate is clear, ethyl alcohol or 20% sterile

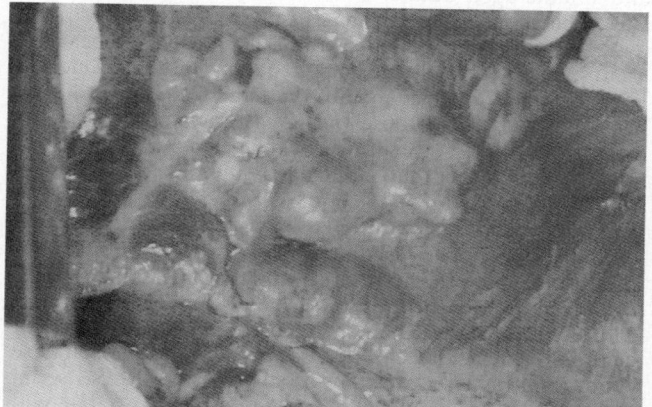

FIGURE 57.6. The external surface of the liver of a patient with echinococcosis before operation. (Reproduced with permission from Sun T. *Parasitic Disorders: Pathology, Diagnosis, and Management,* 2nd ed. Baltimore, MD: Lippincott Williams & Wilkins; 1999.)

saline solution is injected to kill remaining scoleces. The cyst contents and pericystic wall are subsequently removed. In cases in which the aspirate is bilious and a communication with the biliary tree is suspected, the cyst is resected without injecting alcohol to prevent sclerosing cholangitis. Laparoscopic resections have also been reported. A percutaneous technique referred to as PAIR (puncture, aspiration, injection, reaspiration) simultaneously with albendazole therapy has been employed successfully and found to have several advantages over surgical resection. In this modality, after ultrasound-guided percutaneous puncture and aspiration of the hydatid cyst, 20% sodium chloride solution or 95% ethanol is injected into the cavity and subsequently reaspirated. Therapy with albendazole and/or mebendazole is not usually a curative approach by itself but should precede and follow the resection whenever possible. Recent studies report postoperative morbidity and mortality rates of 3% to 24% and 0% to 4%, respectively. Recurrence rates after surgery or invasive procedures range from 0% to 15% and are usually associated with residual vesicles or spillage of hydatid cyst contents.[16–23]

SCHISTOSOMA

Schistosomiasis constitutes a health risk for inhabitants of endemic regions as well as for visitors to these sites. *Schistosoma mansoni, S. japonicum,* and *S. hematobium* are the species of this trematode fluke that most frequently infect humans. Liver disease, although encountered with all species, is especially severe with *S. mansoni, S. japonicum,* and *S. mekongi*. Endemic areas where these trematodes are encountered are also frequently associated with a high prevalence of hepatitis B and C. The life cycle of *Schistosoma* species alternates between sexual reproduction in humans and asexual multiplication in water snails. Cercariae enter the human host by penetrating the skin. An irritating maculopapular rash that lasts for several days is one of the early manifestations. Schistosomes live in the intestinal lumen. Eggs reach the liver via the portal circulation and cause an inflammatory reaction.[17,18,24]

Infection is characterized by the presence of inflammatory granulomata surrounding schistosomal eggs. Acute schistosomiasis is seen most frequently in nonimmune visitors to endemic areas. Inflammatory hepatic schistosomiasis causes hepatomegaly and severe splenomegaly, usually in children and adolescents. With very intense egg infestation, it can lead to widespread granulomatous necrosis of the liver and even death. In contrast, chronic schistosomiasis is seen in young and middle-aged adults. It is usually asymptomatic until variceal hemorrhage occurs as a result of presinusoidal portal hypertension. These patients exhibit hepatosplenomegaly, no ascites, and relatively normal hepatic synthetic function. Hepatomegaly involves mainly the left lobe. Severe decompensation tends to be observed in cases where schistosomal infections and viral hepatitis coexist. Hepatocellular carcinoma, colon cancer, and follicular lymphoma of the spleen have been reported in association with hepatic schistosomiasis.[6,17,18,25,26]

Active infection is usually diagnosed by the presence of schistosomal eggs in the stool (Kato-Katz smears), epidemiologic data, and biochemical or serologic findings. Laboratory features include eosinophilia, hypoalbuminemia, hypergammaglobulinemia, and elevated serum alkaline phosphatase. Serum transaminase levels are usually normal. ELISA serum antibody tests are highly sensitive but may not correlate with activity of the infection. Histologically, heavy infection can lead to prominent granulomata formation, normal liver architecture, and severe portal fibrosis (Symmers pipestem fibrosis). In mild infections small white granulomata, each with a schistosomal egg at its center, are observed throughout the liver (Fig. 57.7). The hepatic parenchyma is darker than usual as a result of regurgitated heme-derived pigments from the schistosome gut.[6,17,18,26]

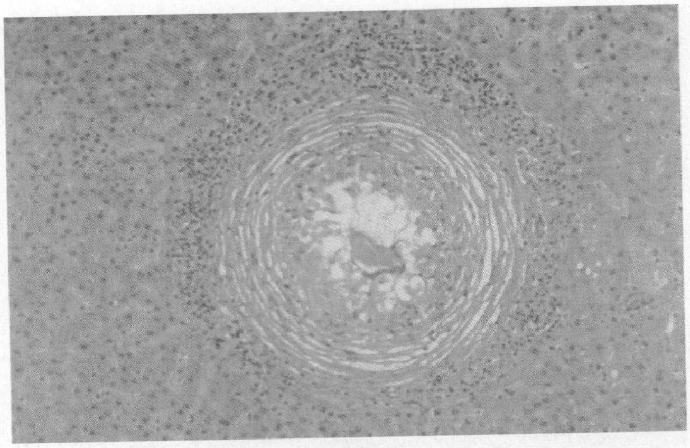

FIGURE 57.7. Hepatic schistosomiasis. A hepatic granuloma surrounds a degenerating egg of *Schistosoma mansoni*. (Reproduced with permission from Rubin E, Farber JL. *Pathology*, 3rd ed. Philadelphia, PA: Lippincott Williams & Wilkins; 1999.)

Imaging studies are not useful in the diagnosis of acute infection. Ultrasound examination in chronic *S. mansoni* infection shows echogenic thickening of the wall of the portal vein and its branches, in a bull's-eye pattern. Hypertrophy of the left hepatic lobe, splenomegaly, and engorged venous collaterals are also observed. On noncontrast CT scan the fibrosis around the portal vein branches presents as low-attenuation rings throughout the liver. Administration of intravenous contrast material leads to marked enhancement of the lesions. The periportal bands appear isointense on magnetic resonance T1-weighted images and hyperintense on T2-weighted images.[6]

The preferred treatment of schistosomiasis is administration of praziquantel, though this is ineffective in early infection. The reported cure efficacy is approximately 90%. It is essential that patients with chronic schistosomiasis undergo evaluation and treatment of esophageal varices.[17,18]

VIRAL HEPATITIDES

4 Viral hepatitis represents a principal cause of chronic liver disease, cirrhosis, and hepatocellular carcinoma. Infection is pandemic in the United States and worldwide, representing one of the significant global public health problems of our time.
5 Hepatitis C virus (HCV) has become the most common indication for liver transplant in the United States and recurrent HCV disease after transplant is a major unmet challenge in the field. Liver transplant for hepatitis B, in distinction, has shown greatly improved results in recent years due to improved pharmacologic treatment options.

The pathophysiology of liver injury is largely host response to noncytopathic virus. Table 57.1 summarizes the characteristics of the five viruses most commonly associated with clinical hepatitis, their modes of transmission, and the consequences of infection.

Hepatitis G virus (HGV) does not appear to be injurious to the liver and will not be considered further. Other viral infections can produce acute hepatitis in a fraction of patients (e.g., Epstein-Barr virus, cytomegalovirus, herpes simplex virus, and varicella virus). In some cases the hepatitis caused by these viruses generally associated with more systemic illness may be severe, and in fact liver involvement may be the dominant component of the infected patient's illness.

TABLE 57.1

CLASSIFICATION OF VIRAL HEPATITIS

	THE VIRAL HEPATITIDES				
VIRUS	HEP A PICORNAVIRUS (RNA)	HEP B HEPADNAVIRUS (DNA)	HEP C FLAVIVIRUS (RNA)	HEP D VIROID (RNA)	HEP E CALICIVIRUS (RNA)
Transmission	Fecal-oral	Parenteral	Parenteral	Parenteral	Fecal-oral
Acute disease	Common	Common	Uncommon	Common	Yes
Evolution to chronic disease	Never	Infrequent in adults	Frequent (70%)	Yes	Described in organ transplant recipients
New cases/year	180,000	180,000	40,000	Unknown, found in approximately 5% of cases of HBV infection	300
# Infected (U.S.)	—	1,250,000	4,000,000		Unknown, uncommon
Worldwide	—	350,000,000	170,000,000		
Treatment	None	Lamivudine Adefovir Entecavir	Interferon + Ribavirin	Treatment of HBV	Mainly sanitary preventative
Prophylaxis	Vaccine and Ig	Vaccine and Ig	None	Vaccinate against HBV	In development
Fulminant failure	Rare	Yes	Never	With HBV, as coinfection or superinfection	Especially in pregnant women

HBV, hepatitis B virus; Hep, hepatitis; Ig, immunoglobulin.

HEPATITIS A VIRUS

Molecular Structure

Hepatitis A virus (HAV) was identified in 1973.[27] HAV belongs to the Picornaviridae family, genus Hepatovirus. Four distinct genotypes have been identified, though no clinical difference between them has been appreciated and all four genotypes belong to a single serotype.[28] HAV is a single-stranded RNA virus. It is 27 nm in diameter and nonenveloped. The viral genome is 7,474 nucleotides in length and is divided into 5′ and 3′ untranslated regions and a single long open reading frame that encodes a 2,227-amino-acid polypeptide. Upon processing this peptide yields four structural and seven nonstructural proteins.

Epidemiology/Risk Factors for Transmission

Hepatitis A disease has been long known (*epidemic jaundice, catarrhal jaundice, campaign jaundice*) and continues to occur worldwide. The incidence in the United States has declined with effective vaccination but remains around 1.2 per 100,000.[29]

The major mode of transmission is fecal-oral spread and is more common in lower socioeconomic areas where sanitation is poor. Common risk factors in the United States are international travel, especially to Mexico or Central/South America; household contact with another infected with HAV; homosexual activity in men; foodborne or waterborne outbreaks; children in daycare centers; and injection drug use. Humans are the only host for HAV infection, and the only organ injured is the liver.

Community outbreaks due to contaminated food have been described.[30,31] Contaminated shellfish and green onions have been implicated in several outbreaks, as have frozen strawberries.

Clinical Features

Hepatitis A infection almost universally results in an acute self-limited illness and can produce either icteric or anicteric syndromes (Fig. 57.8). The incubation period is 28 days. The anicteric prodrome lasts from 2 days to 3 weeks and typically consists of fatigue, malaise, nausea, vomiting, anorexia, fever, and right upper quadrant pain; the diagnosis of hepatitis may be missed when it does not progress to jaundice. In cases where jaundice becomes manifest, it persists for 1 to 6 weeks. Transaminase levels are usually above 1,000 IU/mL and serum bilirubin (>10 mg/dL) and alkaline phosphatase values are elevated as well. Serum IgM antibodies are detected in 95% of patients and are the "gold standard" of diagnosis. IgG antibodies become elevated as jaundice subsides and may persist for years.

HAV infection leads to fulminant liver failure in 0.01% to 0.35% of cases of acute hepatitis A. This rare event mostly occurs in patients with underlying liver disease, especially hepatitis C and less commonly hepatitis B or alcoholic liver disease. The risk of fulminant failure is also higher in people over 40 years of age, intravenous drug users, homosexual men, and inhabitants of endemic areas.[32]

Treatment

Most patients with HAV infection recover with supportive care (approximately 20% require hospitalization in large outbreaks). Hygiene should be a top priority to prevent spread of

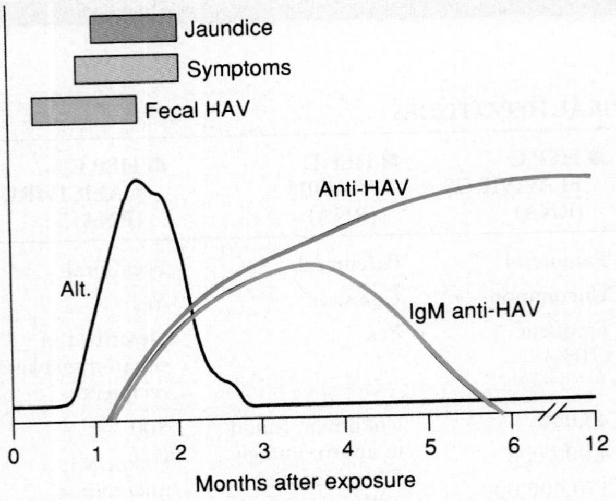

FIGURE 57.8. Clinical course of hepatitis A infection.

the virus, because fecal shedding of the virus occurs prior to the onset of symptoms and jaundice. Spontaneous survival in cases of acute liver failure may be as high as 50%. Liver transplantation is indicated in cases in which recovery is unlikely. Recurrence of HAV infection in the allograft may occasionally be encountered. This has led some to recommend administration of immunoglobulin in such instances.[32,33]

A formalin-inactivated HAV vaccine was found to be safe and to induce an immune response in almost all recipients after two doses. Vaccination as recommended by the Advisory Committee on Immunization Practices of the Centers for Disease Control and Prevention (CDC) includes children 2 years of age or older in states or counties with high rates of infection (20 or more cases per 100,000 population from 1987 to 1997) as well as high-risk persons 2 years of age or older. Immune globulin, administered intramuscularly at a dose of 0.02 mL/kg of body weight within the first 14 days after exposure, prevents disease in more than 85% of cases. Close contacts of patients with recent onset of the illness, people exposed to contaminated foods, and selected travelers to endemic areas benefit the most.[34]

HEPATITIS B VIRUS

Molecular Structure

Hepatitis B virus (HBV) is a DNA virus that belongs to the hepadnavirus family. It is the smallest DNA virus with the ability to infect humans. HBV virions are 40 to 42 nm in diameter, with a double shell and an outer lipoprotein envelope. The viral nucleocapsid, or core, contains a 3.2-kb partially duplex DNA and a polymerase. Replication resembles that of retroviruses, in which the viral DNA polymerase acts as a reverse transcriptase. The HBV polymerase lacks proofreading activity. This finding is associated with an estimated frequency of 10^5 to 10^6 mutations per nucleotide per year and the resultant development of mutant forms of the virus.[35–37]

Epidemiology/Risk Factors for Transmission

It is estimated that 350 million people are infected with HBV worldwide. Transmission is usually via nonsterile needles, intimate contacts, and blood transfusions. Infection by vertical transmission from mother to child is a serious problem in the developing world. There are no known animal reservoirs or evidence that insects are involved in transmission of the disease.

The hepatitis B virus replicates mainly in hepatocytes but is not itself cytotoxic. Hepatocyte injury is due to the resultant host immune response.

Clinical Features

The incubation period in cases of acute infection is approximately 8 weeks. The presence of serum hepatitis B surface antigen (HBsAg) may precede the clinical onset of jaundice. Acute infection is associated with serum HBV DNA, HBV DNA polymerase, hepatitis B early antigen (HBeAg), and liver HBV DNA and hepatitis B core antigen (HBcAg). HBeAg is a useful marker of viral replication, except in individuals infected with mutant viruses where it may be undetectable despite active viral replication (Fig. 57.9). In such circumstances, serum HBV DNA is detected by hybridization techniques. Serum anti-HBc IgM becomes detectable with the onset of jaundice. In most individuals, when HBV does not develop into chronic hepatitis, anti-HBc IgM becomes undetectable beyond 6 months. On occasion, however, it may persist for years after the acute infection or may recur as an amnestic phenomenon in reactivating chronic hepatitis B, thus limiting its usefulness as a marker of acute hepatitis B infection.

Although HBV accounts for 40% of cases of acute liver failure in developing countries, it is estimated that the incidence in the United States is approximately 10%. Hepatitis B becomes fulminant in approximately 1% of acute cases. Women, elderly individuals, and those who sustain superinfection with another virus (such as HCV) seem to be at greater risk. Furthermore, the risk of acute liver failure is directly proportional to the antibody titers to HBcAg and HBsAg. Some cases of acute liver failure may be due to reactivation of HBV in patients with chronic infection. In cases of reactivation, reappearance of HBc IgM antibodies (Abs) aids in the diagnosis. Spontaneous survival after HBV acute liver failure ranges from 15% to 36%.[38,39]

Most patients with acute HBV infection in the Western world (low carrier rates) recover completely. Approximately 25% of adult cases in the Western world develop clinical jaundice but do

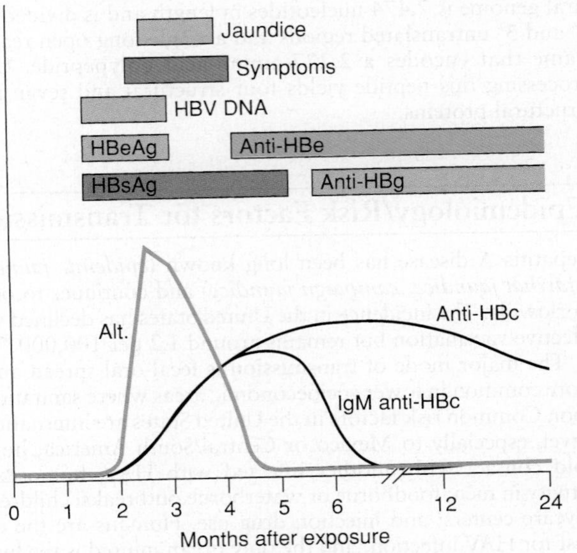

FIGURE 57.9. Clinical course of acute hepatitis B infection.

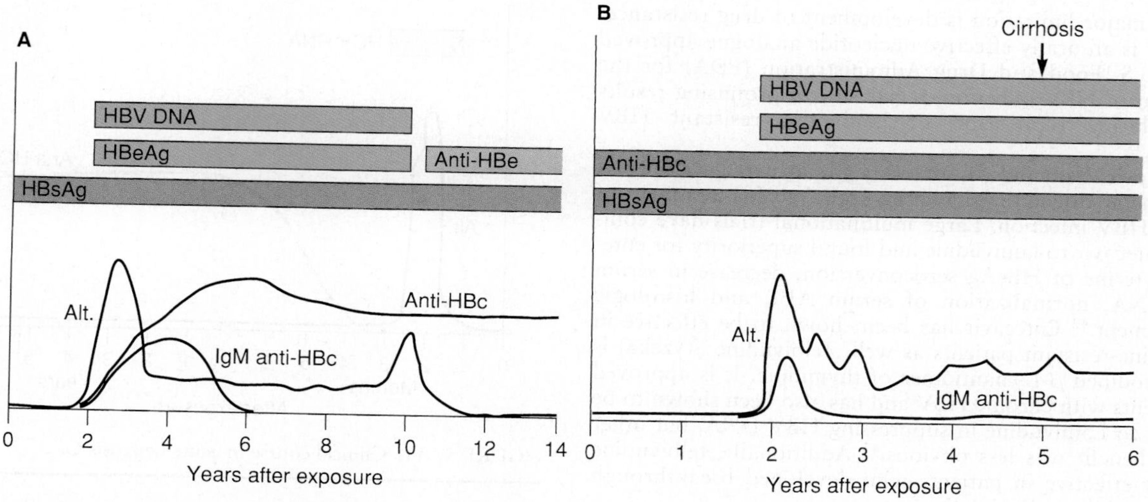

FIGURE 57.10. Clinical course of chronic hepatitis B. **A:** A benign chronic carrier has continued production of hepatitis B surface antigen but there is an absence of serum markers of viral replication. **B:** A pattern of continuing liver injury and serum markers of active viral replication.

not become HBV carriers. They usually retain HBcAb and HBsAb markers with no detectable HBsAg or HBV DNA. Approximately 10% of Western adults with acute HBV infection become chronic carriers, as determined by the presence of HBsAg in serum for more than 6 months (Fig. 57.10). Most HBV carriers have a benign state, with HBV DNA sequences integrating into their native genome. Histologically, these individuals show hepatocytes with ground-glass appearance resulting from cytoplasmic accumulation of HBsAg proteins. Portal triad inflammation may or may not be present. The remainder of HBV carriers develop ongoing liver injury and usually have detectable HBeAg or HBV DNA and have free episomal HBV sequences in addition to the ones integrated into their native genomes. Histologically, there is evidence of active inflammation.

In Western Europe and North America, the overall incidence of chronic infection is less than 1%. It is estimated that there are 1 million deaths each year as a result of cirrhosis and hepatocellular carcinoma associated with chronic hepatitis B worldwide. Cirrhosis develops in 10% to 30% of individuals with evidence of active viral replication within 5 years and is especially high in patients infected early in life, with persistent seropositivity for HBeAg or with increased serum alanine aminotransferase (ALT) levels after HBeAg seroconversion. Although imperfect, twice-a-year screening with hepatic ultrasound and/or α-fetoprotein levels to detect early hepatocellular cancers is recommended for chronically infected patients.[36,37,40]

Treatment

Primary prevention by means of vaccination constitutes the best treatment approach for HBV infection. Individuals at high risk include health care workers, visitors to highly endemic areas, sexual contacts of chronic carriers or acutely infected people, and household contacts of those at high risk of infection (intravenous drug users, hemophiliacs, patients with thalassemia). The hepatitis B vaccine is given as a series of three intramuscular doses and has an almost 100% efficacy among immunocompetent persons with antibody levels of at least 10 mIU/mL. Since the World Health Organization in 1991 called for all children to receive the vaccine, 116 countries have adopted it as a routine immunization. Hepatitis B immune globulin has a reported efficacy of 85% to 95% in the prevention of newborn infections and approximately 75% in cases of needle sticks or sexual infections in people exposed to the virus with no previous HBV immunity. It should be administered as soon as possible after exposure (for perinatal cases within 24 hours after birth, for needle sticks within 7 days, and for sexual exposures within 14 days) together with the first dose of the hepatitis B vaccine series. Additional doses of the vaccine should follow according to the regular schedule. Testing for HBsAg is warranted in pregnant women to reduce the risk of vertical transmission.[35]

Therapy is usually directed at HBeAg-positive cases that have an increased risk of cirrhosis and hepatocellular carcinoma. It seems that HBeAg-negative patients with viremias of greater than 10^5 molecules per milliliter and liver dysfunction may also benefit from antiviral therapy. At present, antiviral therapy is not offered to asymptomatic HBeAg-negative chronic carriers with viral loads under 10^5 molecules per milliliter and normal alanine aminotransferase values. Therapeutic success in HBeAg-positive cases is determined by seroconversion to HBeAb and reduction of viral loads. Cure of infection as determined by loss of HBsAg and absent viremia by polymerase chain reaction (PCR) analysis is achieved in only 1% to 5% of cases. Patients with chronic hepatitis B and cirrhosis or advanced fibrosis showed a reduction in the incidence of hepatic decompensation and the risk of hepatocellular carcinoma after continuous treatment with lamivudine.[36,40]

Interferon alfa (5 million to 10 million units subcutaneously three times per week, for at least 3 months) used to constitute the main therapy in cases of HBV, achieving a successful response in approximately 30% of cases. However, its multiple side effects (fever, myalgias, bone marrow suppression, and depression, among others) made it difficult to tolerate. Furthermore, the potential for overt liver failure made it a risky treatment in people with advanced liver disease. Lamivudine is an orally effective antiviral agent that competitively inhibits the viral DNA polymerase. Its administration is associated with a more rapid seroconversion to HBeAg-positive status, a more rapid loss of HBeAg, improved aminotransferase levels, and a 3- to 4-log reduction in circulating levels of HBV DNA in the first 3 months of therapy. It is also associated with improved liver histologic findings in cases of chronic hepatitis. Lamivudine tends to be tolerated well. Its major limitation is development of drug resistance. Adefovir is an orally effective nucleotide analogue approved by the U.S. Food and Drug Administration (FDA) for the treatment of HBV infection. It has shown promising results by inhibiting replication of lamivudine-resistant HBV mutants.[41]

Entecavir (Baraclude) is an orally administered cyclopentyl guanosine analogue that has been approved for treatment of chronic HBV infection. Large multinational trials have compared entecavir to lamivudine and found superiority for entecavir in terms of HBeAg seroconversion, decrease in serum HBV DNA, normalization of serum ALT, and histologic improvement.[42] Entecavir has been shown to be effective in lamivudine-resistant patients as well. Telbivudine (Tyzeka) is the unmodified β-L-enantiomer of thymidine. It is approved for patients with chronic HBV and has also been shown to be superior to Lamivudine in suppressing HBV DNA, but other clinical benefit was less obvious.[43] Additionally, telbivudine was not effective in patients who developed breakthrough infection while on lamivudine.

Liver transplantation is the treatment of choice in patients with hepatic failure. Recurrence of viral infection in the allograft can be as high as 80% in HBeAg-positive cases where no postoperative prophylaxis is administered. The combination of lamivudine and hepatitis B immune globulin posttransplantation reduced the reinfection rate to approximately 10%, and increased the 5-year HBV-free survival rate to approximately 80%.[36] Other posttransplant pharmacologic regimens are now being examined.

HEPATITIS C VIRUS

Molecular Structure

Hepatitis C virus (HCV) is a lipid-enveloped, 9.4-kb, single-stranded RNA virus of the family Flaviviridae, genus Hepacivirus. Six genotypes have been identified, which differ from one another by as much as 30% at the sequence level.[44] Quasispecies within genotypes demonstrate further genetic heterogeneity and reflect the high rate of mutation seen in viral replication. Over 70% of U.S. cases are due to genotype 1 virus.

Epidemiology/Risk Factors for Transmission

There are 4 million people infected with HCV in the United States, or approximately 1% of the population. Additionally, there are 170 million infected worldwide. The most commonly identified factors responsible for infection are exposure to blood or blood products prior to 1992 and intravenous drug use. Other less common risk factors include occupational exposure, nosocomial spread, sexual contacts, tattooing, and vertical transmission, each of which is a relatively inefficient and uncommon means of viral transmission.

Clinical Features

The usual incubation period is 5 to 10 weeks. Most acutely infected patients are asymptomatic and therefore the infection goes unappreciated. Initial laboratory findings after infection include hepatitis characterized by elevated ALT levels (500 to 1,000 IU/mL) and high HCV RNA titers (Fig. 57.11). HCV is thought to be cleared spontaneously in 20% of individuals following primary infection. Hepatitis C infection by itself is almost never associated with acute liver failure. Liver damage in the setting of chronic infection is due to host immune response rather than to viral hepatotoxicity. Ongoing chronic hepatic injury leads to progressive fibrosis and cirrhosis, in most cases undetected until the appearance of overt liver failure decades after the initial infection (Fig. 57.12). The incidence of hepatic decompensation (variceal hemorrhage, ascites, jaundice, encephalopathy) in the setting of cirrhosis is approximately 5% per year. Hepatitis C cirrhosis is strongly associated with the development of hepatocellular carcinoma. Extrahepatic manifestations of hepatitis C include membranoproliferative glomerulonephritis, cryoglobulinemia, diabetes, porphyria cutanea tarda, lichen planus, vitiligo, and non-Hodgkin lymphoma.[45]

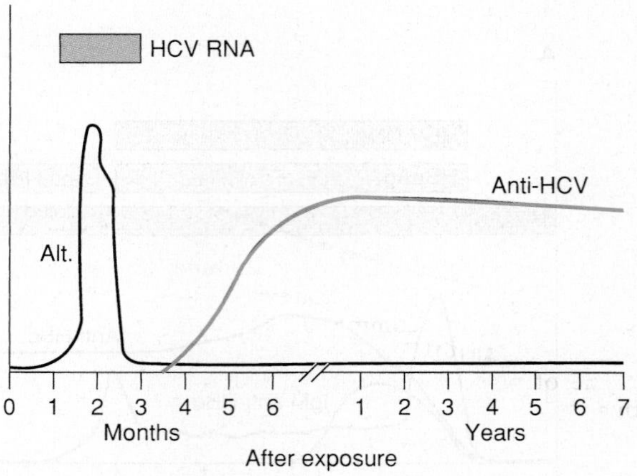

FIGURE 57.11. Clinical course in acute hepatitis C.

The diagnosis of hepatitis C is based on serologic demonstration of HCV RNA and/or antibodies. HCV RNA can be detected weeks earlier than antibodies, which are not observed until approximately 18 weeks after the initial illness.

Treatment

Therapy is indicated in cases of chronic hepatitis C with elevated serum aminotransferase concentrations and chronic hepatitis on liver biopsy. The current treatment of chronic hepatitis C is via a combination of pegylated interferon alfa and ribavirin. Pegylation of interferon alfa optimizes its pharmacodynamics and pharmacokinetics by providing sustained concentrations after single weekly injections. Its principal mechanism of action seems to be the immune clearance of infected cells, perhaps via mobilization of endogenous

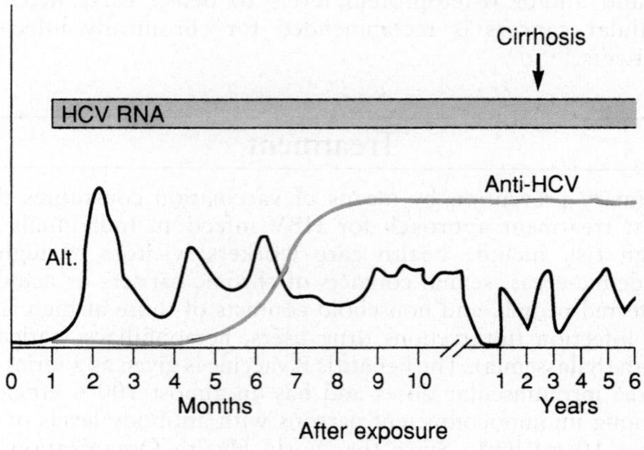

FIGURE 57.12. Clinical course in chronic hepatitis C.

microRNAs that participate in interference with HCV replication.[46] Ribavirin is a synthetic guanosine analogue that prevents relapses during and after therapy in patients who exhibit an initial response. Approximately 80% of patients with genotype 2 or 3 infection and 50% of patients with genotype 1 infection show sustained virologic response with therapy. Male sex, race, advanced age, chronic infection, fibrosis, and high body mass index are associated with diminished rates of sustained virologic response. Transplantation is the treatment of choice in terminal cases of hepatitis C where hepatic recovery is not expected and HCV cirrhosis has become the most common indication for orthotopic liver transplantation (OLT). Transplantation ameliorates the sequelae of portal hypertension and cancer risk associated with a cirrhotic liver, but viral reinfection after OLT is immediate and universal. Furthermore, HCV disease progression to graft cirrhosis is accelerated after transplant as opposed to the rate seen in native livers.[47]

HEPATITIS D VIRUS

Molecular Structure

The hepatitis D virus (HDV), or delta agent, is an incomplete RNA virus that requires the concomitant presence of HBV for viral assembly and propagation. The only enzymatic activity of HDV is a ribozyme that autocleaves the circular RNA and makes it linear. The HDV genome is a 1,680-nucleotide, single-stranded circular RNA.[48] Eight genotypes have been proposed.[49] A single HDV antigen is encoded, it is a structural component of the virion, and a lipoprotein envelope is provided by HBV.

Epidemiology/Risk Factors for Transmission

It is estimated that HDV is found in approximately 5% of HBV carriers. Due to its dependence on HBV, HDV always occurs in association with HBV infection. Transmission is similar to that of HBV, via parenteral or sexual exposure to blood or body fluids. HDV hepatitis occurs only in HBsAg-positive patients.

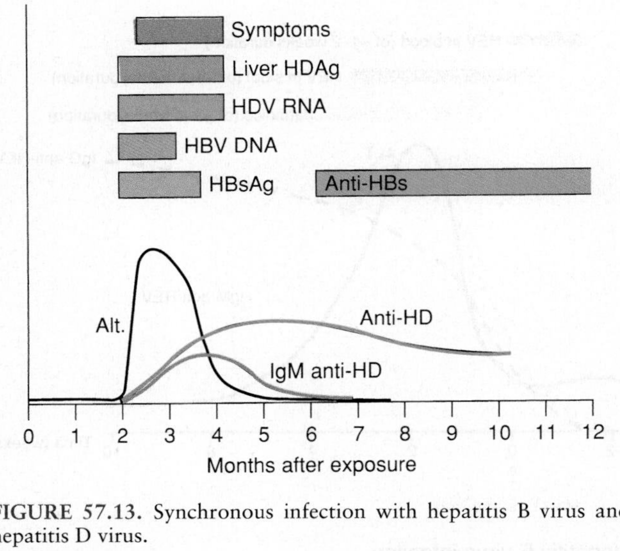

FIGURE 57.13. Synchronous infection with hepatitis B virus and hepatitis D virus.

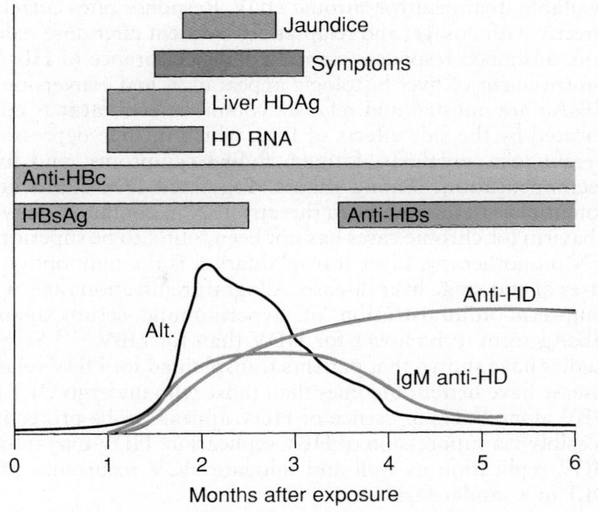

FIGURE 57.14. Superinfection of chronic hepatitis B carrier with hepatitis D.

Clinical Features

Acute infection is diagnosed by the presence of anti-HDV IgM. Anti-HBc IgM distinguishes coinfection from superinfection (Figs. 57.13 and 57.14). The diagnosis in patients with chronic liver disease is made by the presence of HBsAg and antibodies against HDV in the serum and confirmed by the presence of HDV antigen in the liver or HDV RNA in the serum (Fig. 57.15). Acute liver failure is seen with both coinfection (HDV and HBV simultaneously infect the host) and superinfection (HDV infects a host already infected with HBV). Superinfection seems to be associated with a higher mortality rate. Chronic HDV and HBV infection may coexist. Cirrhosis is observed in at least two thirds of patients and occurs at a younger age than in patients infected with HBV alone.[50,51]

Treatment

Treatment and prevention of HDV are associated with that of hepatitis B, with which it always coexists. Vaccination with the hepatitis B vaccine is contributing to the decline in the incidence of HDV. α-Interferon (IFN) is the only currently

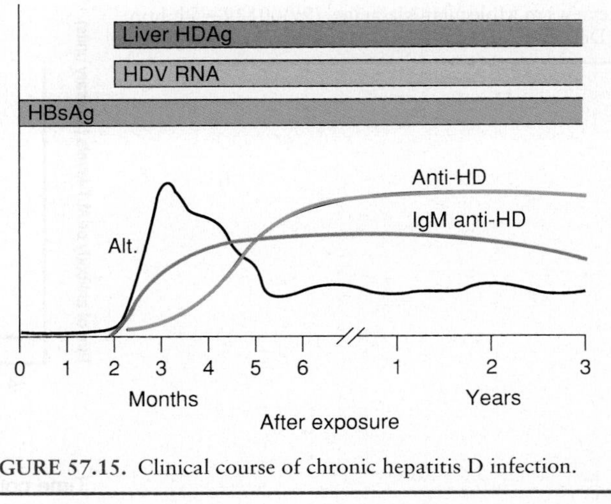

FIGURE 57.15. Clinical course of chronic hepatitis D infection.

available treatment for chronic HDV. Response rates correlate directly with dosage, and relapses are frequent after dose reduction. Sustained responses associated with clearance of HBsAg, improvement of liver histologic appearance, and conversion to HBsAb are unusual and relapses common. Treatment is complicated by the side effects of IFN, which include depression, weight loss, myalgias, fatigue, flulike symptoms, and liver decompensation, among others. Pegylated IFN could be a potentially useful long-term therapy. IFN in combination with ribavirin for chronic cases has not been found to be superior to IFN monotherapy. Liver transplantation is the only option in cases of end-stage liver disease. Allograft reinfection rates with long-term administration of hyperimmune serum against HBsAg seem to be lower for HDV than for HBV.[50,51] Several studies have shown that patients transplanted for HDV-related disease have better outcomes than those who undergo OLT for HBV alone.[52] The presence of HDV appears to be protective, possibly via suppression of HBV replication. HDV may inhibit HCV replication as well and mitigate HCV recurrence after OLT in a similar fashion.

HEPATITIS E VIRUS

Molecular Structure

Hepatitis E virus (HEV) is a nonenveloped single-stranded RNA virus. It is 30 nm in diameter and is most similar to other viruses of the Caliciviridae family. There are three large open reading frames, the first of which is 1,693 codons and codes for nonstructural proteins. The second is 660 codons and encodes structural proteins. The third is smaller and of undetermined function. There are thought to be four genotypes.[53]

Epidemiology/Risk Factors for Transmission

Hepatitis E is enterically transmitted (*waterborne hepatitis* or *enterically transmitted non-A, non-B hepatitis*) and is epidemiologically similar to HAV. Infection has been prominently observed in Asia, Africa, the Middle East, and Central America. In addition, vertical transmission from mother to child has been documented and can be a source of perinatal morbidity and mortality.

Clinical Features

HEV generally causes a self-limited acute infection, although chronic infection has been described in organ transplant recipients. The incubation period usually lasts 3 to 8 weeks, and most individuals recover without chronic findings after a transient cholestatic jaundice (Fig. 57.16). However, young adults and women in late stages of pregnancy may develop fulminant cases of hepatitis E. Mortality from HEV is 0.5% to 4% in the general population but up to 20% in pregnant women.[54–56] Diagnosis is aided by amplification of serum and fecal viral genomes during the acute phase. The presence of anti-HEV IgM or follow-up demonstration of IgG may be required.

Treatment

There is currently no specific treatment for HEV infection, although vaccines against HEV are in development and appear to be highly effective. Improving sanitation and purifying or boiling water can reduce the incidence of this disease.

CYTOMEGALOVIRUS

Cytomegalovirus (CMV) is a member of the β-Herpesviridae family. It is usually associated with mild hepatitis but may occasionally cause acute liver failure. Transmission can be intrauterine; perinatal or postnatal; through intimate contact of infected fluids such as blood, saliva, or urine; or through transplanted organs. Infection is lifelong due to latency of the virus and can be detected in up to 70% of individuals in U.S. urban cities. Organ injury can occur as a result of primary infection or reactivation of a latent infection. In the neonatal period, severe cases of congenital infection are usually generalized and can be fatal. In immunocompetent adults, liver dysfunction tends to be found in association with CMV mononucleosis. In immunosuppressed adults, infection leads to liver dysfunction with jaundice and at times liver failure. Acalculous gangrenous cholecystitis may also be encountered.[32,57,58]

Shell vial assay is a more sensitive and rapid method than conventional human fibroblast culture of saliva, urine, bronchoalveolar lavage fluid, or blood to detect infection. Currently, the use of CMV antigenemia assays and detection of CMV by PCR amplification from serum has greatly increased the rapidity and ease of diagnosis. Detection of IgM is helpful

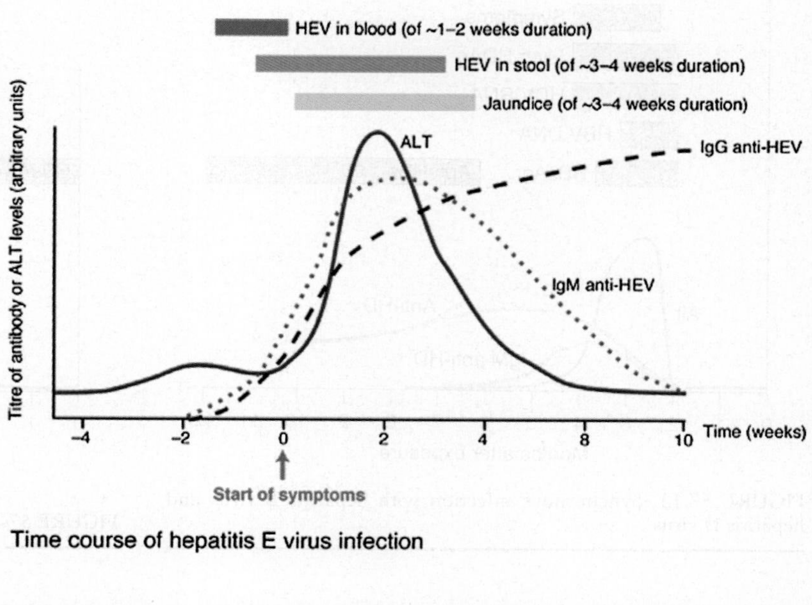

FIGURE 57.16. Clinical course of chronic hepatitis E infection. (Reproduced with permission from Expert Reviews in Molecular Medicine: (99)00129—5 h.htm; 6 December 1999.)

only in neonatal infection; serology is not useful as a diagnostic tool in adults. Liver biopsy is of importance to establish the diagnosis of hepatitis. Microscopic examination shows inflammation and injury ranging from fatty changes to necrosis to fibrosis. Giant multinucleated cells and large nuclear inclusions can be encountered in hepatocytes and bile duct epithelial cells.[32,57,58]

Several drugs are available for the systemic treatment of CMV, including ganciclovir, valganciclovir, foscarnet, and cidofovir; anti-CMV hyper–immune globulin is sometimes used as an adjunctive therapeutic modality.[41]

EPSTEIN-BARR VIRUS

Epstein-Barr virus (EBV) is a DNA virus and member of the Herpesviridae family. Infection persists for life due to latency of the virus, and is usually transmitted in the course of close personal or intimate contact via oral secretions. Some degree of liver involvement is encountered in almost all cases of EBV mononucleosis. It is usually mild, with no major clinical manifestations, and resolves spontaneously. The presence of jaundice may reflect either more severe hepatitis or an associated hemolytic anemia. Occasional cases of fatal acute liver failure have been reported in both immunocompromised and immunocompetent patients. Leukocytosis is usually present, with lymphocytosis and monocytosis. The monospot test is sensitive but not specific. Diagnosis is by detection of nucleic acids with in situ hybridization, Southern blot analysis, and PCR of involved organ biopsies. Detection of IgG and IgM antibodies improves sensitivity and specificity. No antiviral agent has so far proved effective in EBV hepatitis. Liver transplantation has been reported in life-threatening situations.[41,57,59,60]

HERPES SIMPLEX VIRUS

The prevalence of antibodies to herpes simplex virus 1 (HSV-1) in the populations of industrialized nations is 80% in lower socioeconomic strata (SES) and 50% in higher SES; prevalence of antibodies to herpes simplex virus 2 (HSV-2) is approximately 20%. Fulminant hepatitis is a rare complication of HSV infection, but those at risk include neonates and immunocompromised, malnourished, and pregnant adults. Fulminant hepatitis is usually associated with multiorgan involvement and carries a high (>80%) mortality rate. Clinical features include fever, anorexia with nausea, abdominal pain, leucopenia, and coagulopathy. Liver biopsy is of prime importance to establish the diagnosis, especially in pregnant women. Microscopic examination shows diffuse eosinophilic intranuclear inclusion bodies, multinucleated cells, widespread necrosis, and slight inflammation. Cowdry A-type intranuclear inclusions are typical. Confirmation is by means of HSV DNA detection by PCR. Approved antivirals include acyclovir, famciclovir, and valacyclovir. Treatment with intravenous acyclovir should be started prior to confirmation of the etiology, given that progression of the disease is extremely rapid and lethal. Liver transplantation can be considered even in selected cases of disseminated disease.[41,57,58]

VARICELLA ZOSTER VIRUS

Herpesvirus varicellae (also called varicella zoster virus [VZV]) is usually associated with mild hepatitis but may occasionally cause acute liver failure. Up to one fourth of children with varicella (chickenpox) may exhibit temporary mild biochemical liver abnormalities. Reye syndrome may be encountered during the convalescence period, especially in those who receive aspirin. In such cases, mortality can be as high as 30%. Fulminant fatal hepatic failure is uncommon, but generally affects immunocompromised patients. Confirmation of the diagnosis can be achieved by isolation of the virus from involved tissues. Varicella zoster immune globulin therapy should be considered after exposure to the virus by immunocompromised or pregnant patients who lack immunity to VZV. Current therapies for VZV infection in immunocompetent and immunocompromised hosts include acyclovir, valacyclovir, and famciclovir. CDC guidelines should be followed for infection control.[32,41,57]

ACUTE LIVER FAILURE

Definition

6 Acute liver failure (ALF) is an uncommon but serious condition, with approximately 2,000 to 2,300 cases per year in the United States,[61] which carries a high mortality rate of 60% to 80%.[62] It is characterized by rapid deterioration of liver function as well as coexistence of hepatic encephalopathy in a previously healthy individual without a known hepatopathy. Currently, emergency liver transplantation is the only therapeutic option available, and the King's College Criteria are widely accepted as the standard of guidance. ALF is responsible for about 6% of all liver-related deaths, and approximately 6% of adult liver transplant recipients undergo transplantation with this indication.[63]

The most widely accepted definition includes an international normalized ratio (INR) greater than or equal to 1.5 and any degree of mental alteration (encephalopathy) in a patient without preexisting cirrhosis and with an illness of less than 26 weeks' duration.[64] Patients with Wilson disease, vertically acquired hepatitis B, or autoimmune hepatitis can be considered to have ALF if the disease process has started within 26 weeks. Although the literature suggests hyperacute (<7 days) and subacute (>21 days but <26 weeks) forms, they do not have prognostic significance except with hyperacute failure, which may carry a better prognosis since it is mostly due to acetaminophen toxicity.[66]

Diagnosis

A high index of suspicion is vital in early recognition of the disease process. Patients with evidence of moderate to severe degrees of hepatitis and any degree of encephalopathy with or without coexistence of coagulopathy as evidenced by an INR greater than or equal to 1.5 require hospitalization, since that process may progress to death rapidly.[65] Likewise, early transfer to an intensive care unit (ICU) setting in a liver transplant center is important (especially before approaching grade III or IV encephalopathy), since worsening encephalopathy can potentially hamper transportation efforts because of concern over increased intracranial pressure.

Detailed history taking from accompanying persons, including medications/herbal supplements taken and recent social history, is essential. Stigmata of chronic liver disease need to be assayed during the physical examination, although jaundice might be a late manifestation of the disease process. The initial laboratory testing shown in Table 57.2 is recommended.[65]

Transjugular liver biopsy can be considered as part of the initial workup to rule out neoplastic infiltration or HSV/herpes zoster virus (HZV) hepatitis,[66] although its routine application is still considered controversial.

Etiology

It is important to elicit the etiology of ALF in an effort to administer the appropriate antidotes and to better anticipate

TABLE 57.2

MANAGEMENT IN ACUTE LIVER FAILURE: INITIAL LABORATORY EVALUATIONS

Serum chemistries	Sodium, potassium, chloride, bicarbonate, calcium, magnesium, phosphate, glucose, BUN, creatinine, amylase, lipase
Hepatic panel	AST, ALT, alkaline phosphatase, total bilirubin, albumin
Prothrombin time/INR	
Complete blood count	
Arterial blood gas, lactate, ammonia	
Toxicology screen	
Viral hepatitis serologies	Anti-HAV IgM, Hep B surface Ag, Anti-HBV core IgM, anti-HCV, anti-HEV IgM (if indicated)
Anti-VZV IgM, Anti-HSV IgM	
Autoimmune markers	ANA, ASMA, IgG levels, SPEP
Pregnancy test	
Serum ceruloplasmin level and 24-h urine copper collection	(if Wilson disease is suspected)

Ag, antigen; ALT, alanine aminotransferase; ANA, antinuclear antibody; ASMA, anti–smooth muscle antibody; AST, aspartate aminotransferase; BUN, blood urea nitrogen; HAV, hepatitis A virus; HBV, hepatitis B virus; HCV, hepatitis C virus; HEV, hepatitis E virus; HSV, herpes simplex virus; IgM, immunoglobulin M; INR, international normalized ratio; SPEP, serum protein electrophoresis; VZV, varicella zoster virus.

prognosis and hence the need for liver transplantation.[67] Etiology seems to have some geographic variances. In the United States, the etiology is reported to be acetaminophen overdose in 46% of cases, followed by indeterminate causes (14%), drug related (11%), HBV (7%), autoimmune hepatitis (5%), and Wilson disease (2%).[68] In the United Kingdom, acetaminophen toxicity is reported to be as high as 60.9%,[69] whereas in France, the reported etiologies are viral infection with hepatitis A and B (31%), acetaminophen toxicity (20%), other drug overdose (18%), and unknown (17%).[66]

Viral Hepatitis. In those with HAV, ALF occurs in up to 0.4% of cases; age over 40 years and preexisting liver disease represent a higher risk. In those with HBV, ALF occurs in up to 1.2% of cases. ALF may occur due to acute hepatitis or reactivation of a chronic carrier state. HDV coinfection and HEV should be suspected in endemic areas. VZV, HSV, and CMV are other rare viral causes.[67]

Drug-induced Liver Injury. Intrinsic hepatotoxins are usually dose dependent, while idiosyncratic responses are unpredictable and are not dose dependent. Acetaminophen is a good example of the dose-dependent form, generally greater than 10 g/d but sometimes reported to be as low as in the 3 to 4 g/d range. Glutathione becomes depleted with excess free NAPQI (a toxic byproduct of acetaminophen) reacting with hepatocytes, causing the liver injury.[67] In the presence of poor nutritional state or alcoholism, glutathione levels are chronically depleted, further contributing to acetaminophen toxicity. Stevens-Johnson syndrome, caused by phenytoin, amoxicillin-clavulanate, carbamazepine, and halothane, is a form of hypersensitivity idiosyncratic reaction, while isoniazid, valproate, and amiodarone mainly cause metabolic idiosyncratic reactions.

Other. Acute Budd-Chiari syndrome, veno-occlusive disease due to medications and herbs, and malignancies involving the liver (i.e., lymphoma, angiosarcoma) are less common causes of ALF.[65] Acute fatty liver of pregnancy (AFLP) and HELLP (hemolysis, elevated liver enzymes, low platelets) are important diagnoses to be considered among pregnant women presenting with manifestations of ALF. AFLP occurs during the third trimester due to deficiencies in long-chain 3-hydroxyacyl-CoA dehydrogenase in both the mother and the fetus with rapid deposition of triglycerides and free fatty acids into hepatocytes. HELLP also occurs during the third trimester or immediately postpartum. Autoimmune hepatitis (AIH) can present acutely with absence of autoimmune markers, where the diagnosis is made by exclusion and transjugular liver biopsy. In the fulminant form of Wilson disease, chelator treatment is ineffective and diagnosis is usually based on familial history of liver disease in a young adult with Coombs-negative hemolysis and low serum alkaline phosphatase or uric acid levels. Kayser-Fleischer rings are present in 50% of patients.[64] Diagnosis is usually confirmed by hepatic copper content greater than 250 μg/g in patients homozygous for Wilson disease, and the rate of urinary excretion may exceed 100 μg/24 h.[70] Heat stroke, mushroom ingestion, EBV, and parvovirus B19 may be considered as rare causes of ALF.[66]

Clinical Features, Management, and Treatment

Acute liver injury in the absence of hepatic encephalopathy is a reversible entity, unless an underlying chronic liver disease is present. Altered mental status accompanied by jaundice and elevated serum aminotransferases and prothrombin time (PT)/INR is the hallmark of the presentation. Rapid loss of liver mass can lead to multiorgan system failure and eventual death.[65] Liver transplantation needs to be considered and accomplished prior to reaching this moribund state. Therefore, early transfer to a liver transplant center ICU setting has paramount importance due to this time-limited window of opportunity for high-acuity ALF patients.[71] Encephalopathy may be accompanied by myopathy and neuropathy, loss of vascular tone with hypotension, cardiac dysfunction, acute lung injury, gastrointestinal bleeding, pancreatitis, acute renal failure, and/or disseminated intravascular coagulation and cholestasis.[71] Intracranial hypertension is recognized in 50% to 70% of patients in stage 4 coma. Therefore, neurocritical care, with ability to rapidly respond to hemodynamic changes, becomes an important issue in management. Other precepts are maintenance of normoxia, euglycemia, control of seizures, therapeutic hypothermia, osmotic therapy, and judicious hyperventilation.[71]

Initial management includes identification and treatment of infection, titration of intravascular volume expansion, and selection of fluids to minimize cerebral edema. Hypertonic saline may be considered to maintain serum sodium in the mildly hypernatremic range. Norepinephrine is the vasopressor of choice and early initiation of renal replacement therapy is important for tight control of intravascular volume. Mild reduction in blood CO_2 tension can also restore cerebral vasoreactivity and autoregulation.[71]

Advanced cerebral edema is associated with hyperventilation, hypertension, papillary abnormalities, decerebrate posturing, and ultimately uncal herniation and death. Arterial ammonia levels greater than 200 μg/dL may be correlated with herniation.[65] Although well-powered controlled trials are still needed to determine the role of intracranial pressure monitoring,[72] management should aim to keep the cerebral perfusion pressure (mean arterial pressure − intracranial pressure) over 50 mm Hg and the intracranial pressure below 25 mm Hg. Sustained pressures greater than these values for longer than 2 hours usually signifies irreversible brain damage.[65] Mannitol intravenous bolus doses of 0.5 to 1 g/kg are effective in decreasing cerebral edema by maintaining osmotic diuresis and can be repeated provided serum osmolarity does not exceed 320 mosm/L.[64] Profound coagulopathy (INR >7) and/or planned invasive procedures warrant correction of coagulopathy with fresh frozen plasma (FFP) in combination with recombinant activated factor VII (rFVIIa).[64]

Liver Transplantation

Establishing the cause of ALF is an important determinant of outcomes following liver transplantation, with the best results achieved for Wilson disease and the worst seen with idiosyncratic drug reactions. Overall, survival rates following transplantation at 1 year are 7% to 15% below those obtained for elective transplants in patients with chronic liver disease but are similar to survival of chronic liver disease patients going to liver transplantation from an ICU setting.[73]

Patients who are at high risk of death should be identified early in the course of ALF and listed and transplanted in a timely fashion. Therefore, it is also crucial to identify patients who are too sick to benefit from liver transplantation. Relative contraindications for liver transplantation can be summarized as (a) sustained cerebral hypoperfusion detected as cerebral perfusion pressure less than 40 mm Hg for longer than 2 hours, (b) arterial vasodilatation requiring more than 1 μg/kg per minute norepinephrine infusion, and (c) acute respiratory distress syndrome requiring fraction of inspired oxygen (FiO_2) at 60% and positive end-expiratory pressure (PEEP) at greater than 12 cm H_2O.[71]

TABLE 57.3 STAGING

KING'S COLLEGE CRITERIA OF POOR PROGNOSTIC INDICATORS

Acetaminophen-induced ALF:

Arterial pH <7.3 irrespective of coma grade

OR all of the following:

INR >6.5, creatinine >3.4 mg/dL (300 μmol/L), grade III/IV encephalopathy

Non–acetaminophen-induced ALF:

INR >6.5

OR any three of the following:

Age <10 or >40, drug toxicity or undetermined etiology, jaundice >7 days before encephalopathy, INR >3.5, bilirubin >17 mg/dL (300 μmol/L)

ALF, acute liver failure; INR, international normalized ratio.

Liver Support Systems

Various biologic and charcoal-based sorbent systems have been tested to date with no demonstrable clinical impact. Total plasma exchange has been studied retrospectively, in an attempt to stabilize the ALF patient until a liver graft is identified or self-regeneration occurs.[63] Sorbent systems have shown transient detoxification with no long-term benefit at the expense of worsening coagulopathy. Porcine cell–based and hepatoblastoma-derived extracorporeal systems, the Molecular Adsorbents Recirculating System (MARS),[74] and the Prometheus System[75] are available only for clinical trials and their future in the management of acute liver failure currently remains unclear.[64]

Meets Definition
- rapid deterioration of liver function tests with encephalopathy
- no previous liver disease (liver bx may help)

Etiology
- acetominophen tox most common, then acute viral Hep (B and A, not C)
- Less Common: drug reaction, Autoimmune Hepatitis, Wilson's

Managment
- Early transfer to Liver Transplant Center
- Treat infection, restrict IVF, ICP monitoring controversial
- Ultimately must decide: continude observation vs OLT

Outcomes
- 25-50% survival without OLT (depends on etiology/severity)
- 60-75% survival with OLT: lower outcomes than with other indications

ALGORITHM 57.1

ALGORITHM 57.1.

Differential Diagnosis ——
- pyogenic (bacterial origin) vs amebic
- most are solitary and in the right lobe

Workup ——
- Symptoms: fever +/– RUQ pain, jaundice
- Labs: elevated WBC, Bili, and LFTs
- US: 90% diagnostic, facilitates aspiration
- CT: most commonly used and reliable

Etiology ——
- 66% are gram negative: E Coil, Klebs, Proteus, 30% have anaerobes: B, frag
- Most are now due to cholangitis from obstruction/stenting: malignancy or stones
- also: diverticulitis, IBD, appendicitis

Treatment ——
- Percutaneous drainage
- Broad specrum abx with gram-/anearobic coverage
- 2 weeks IV + 4 more weeks PO for total of 6 wks abx

ALGORITHM 57.2

ALGORITHM 57.2.

Prognosis

Accurate prognosis in ALF is important to avoid unnecessary liver transplantation, and the traditionally accepted King's College Criteria are most commonly used for this purpose (Table 57.3). Of note is that the Model for End-Stage Liver Disease (MELD) system cannot be applied in ALF.[64]

ALF due to acetaminophen overdose, hepatitis A, shock liver, or pregnancy-related disease showed a 50% or more transplant-free survival, while most other etiologies have shown less than 25% transplant-free survival.[64] Other proposed but not widely accepted poor prognostic criteria have been α-fetoprotein levels, ratio of factor VIII and V, liver histology, and serum phosphate levels.

Recipients who underwent liver transplantation for drug-induced ALF in the United States from 1987 to 2006 were retrospectively studied, and the most common drug groups were identified as acetaminophen, antituberculosis medications, antiepileptics, and other nontuberculosis antibiotics. Patients age 7 years or younger with antiepileptic toxicity had the highest risk of death following liver transplantation compared to all other groups. Being on life support and elevated serum creatinine were identified as other predictors of poor survival after liver transplantation.[76]

References

1. Kaplan GG, Gregson DB, Laupland KB. Population-based study of the epidemiology of and the risk factors for pyogenic liver abscess. *Clin Gastroenterol Hepatol* 2004;2:1032–1038.
2. Webb TH, Lillemoe KD, Pitt HA. Liver abscess. *Hosp Phys* 1989;25:46–59.
3. Rahimian J, Wilson T, Oram V, et al. Pyogenic liver abscess: recent trends in etiology and mortality. *Clin Infect Dis* 2004;39:1654–1659.
4. Yang DM, Kim HN, Kang JH, et al. Complications of pyogenic hepatic abscess: computed tomography and clinical features. *J Comput Assist Tomogr* 2004;28:311–317.
5. Hanbidge AE, Buckler PM, O'Malley ME, et al. From the RSNA refresher courses: imaging evaluation for acute pain in the right upper quadrant. *Radiographics* 2004;24:1117–1135.
6. Mortele KJ, Segatto E, Ros PR. The infected liver: radiologic-pathologic correlation. *Radiographics* 2004;24:937–955.
7. Zibari GB, Maguire S, Aultman DF, et al. Pyogenic liver abscess. *Surg Infect (Larchmt)* 2000;1:15–21.
8. Lipsett PA, Huang CJ, Lillemoe KD, et al. Fungal hepatic abscesses: characterization and management. *J Gastrointest Surg* 1997;1:78–84.
9. Sharara AI, Rockey DC. Pyogenic liver abscess. *Curr Treat Options Gastroenterol* 2002;5:437–442.
10. Tan YM, Chung AY, Chow PK, et al. An appraisal of surgical and percutaneous drainage for pyogenic liver abscesses larger than 5 cm. *Ann Surg* 2005;241:485–490.
11. Yang CC, Yen CH, Ho MW, et al. Comparison of pyogenic liver abscess caused by non-Klebsiella pneumoniae and Klebsiella pneumoniae. *J Microbiol Immunol Infect* 2004;37:176–184.
12. Wells CD, Arguedas M. Amebic liver abscess. *South Med J* 2004;97:673–682.
13. Lucey MR. Hepatic infection and acute hepatic failure. In: Greenfield LJ, Mulholland ML, Oldham KT, et al., eds. *Surgery: Scientific Principles and Practice,* 3rd ed. Philadelphia, PA: Lippincott Williams & Wilkins; 2001;943–957.
14. Lodhi S, Sarwari AR, Muzammil M, et al. Features distinguishing amoebic from pyogenic liver abscess: a review of 577 adult cases. *Trop Med Int Health* 2004;9:718–723.
15. Ahsan T, Jehangir MU, Mahmood T, et al. Amoebic versus pyogenic liver abscess. *J Pak Med Assoc* 2002;52:497–501.
16. Sayek I, Tirnaksiz MB, Dogan R. Cystic hydatid disease: current trends in diagnosis and management. *Surg Today* 2004;34:987–996.
17. DiazGranados CA, Duffus WA, Albrecht H. Parasitic diseases of the liver. In: Zakim D, Boyer TD, eds. *Hepatology. A Textbook of Liver Disease,* 4th ed. Philadelphia, PA: WB Saunders; 2003:1073–1107.
18. Dunn MA. Parasitic diseases. In: Shiff ER, Sorrell MF, Maddrey WC, eds. *Schiff's Diseases of the Liver,* 8th ed. Philadelphia, PA: Lippincott Williams & Wilkins; 1999:1533–1548.
19. Kjossev KT, Losanoff JE. Classification of hydatid liver cysts. *J Gastroenterol Hepatol* 2005;20:352–359.
20. Bastid C, Ayela P, Sahel J. Percutaneous treatment of a complex hydatid cyst of the liver under sonographic control. Report of the first case. *Gastroenterol Clin Biol* 2005;29:191–192.
21. Chautems R, Buhler LH, Gold B, et al. Surgical management and long-term outcome of complicated liver hydatid cysts caused by Echinococcus granulosus. *Surgery* 2005;137:312–316.
22. Gollackner B, Längle F, Auer H, et al. Radical surgical therapy of abdominal cystic hydatid disease: factors of recurrence. *World J Surg* 2000;24:717–721.
23. Smego RA Jr, Sebanego P. Treatment options for hepatic cystic echinococcosis. *Int J Infect Dis* 2005;9:69–76.
24. Godyn JJ, Siderits R, Hazra A. Schistosoma mansoni in colon and liver. *Arch Pathol Lab Med* 2005;129:544–545.
25. Qiu DC, Hubbard AE, Zhong B, et al. A matched, case-control study of the association between *Schistosoma japonicum* and liver and colon cancers, in rural China. *Ann Trop Med Parasitol* 2005;99:47–52.
26. El-Zayadi AR. Curse of schistosomiasis on Egyptian liver. *World J Gastroenterol* 2004;10:1079–1081.

27. Feinstone SM, Kapikian AZ, Purceli RH. Hepatitis A: detection by immune electron microscopy of a virus like antigen associated with acute illness. *Science* 1973;182:1026.
28. Lemon SM, Jansen RW, Brown EA. Genetic, antigenic and biological differences between strains of hepatitis A virus. *Vaccine* 1992;10(suppl 1): S40.
29. Wasley A, Samandari T, Bell BP. Incidence of hepatitis A in the United States in the era of vaccination. *JAMA* 2005;294:194.
30. Dentinger CM, Bower WA, Nainan OV, et al. An outbreak of hepatitis A associated with green onions. *J Infect Dis* 2001;183:1273.
31. Wheeler C, Vogt TM, Armstrong GL, et al. An outbreak of hepatitis A associated with green onions. *N Engl J Med* 2005;353:890.
32. Sanyal AJ, Stravitz RT. Acute liver failure. In: Zakim D, Boyer TD, eds. *Hepatology. A Textbook of Liver Disease,* 4th ed. Philadelphia, PA: WB Saunders; 2003:445–496.
33. Gane E, Sallie R, Saleh M, et al. Clinical recurrence of hepatitis A following liver transplantation for acute liver failure. *J Med Virol* 1995;45: 35–39.
34. Craig AS, Schaffner W. Prevention of hepatitis A with the hepatitis A vaccine. *N Engl J Med* 2004;350:476–481.
35. Poland GA, Jacobson RM. Clinical practice: prevention of hepatitis B with the hepatitis B vaccine. *N Engl J Med* 2004;351:2832–2838.
36. Ganem D, Prince AM. Hepatitis B virus infection–natural history and clinical consequences. *N Engl J Med* 2004;350:1118–1129.
37. Wands JR. Prevention of hepatocellular carcinoma. *N Engl J Med* 2004; 351:1567–1570.
38. Schiodt FV, Atillasoy E, Shakil AO, et al. Etiology and outcome for 295 patients with acute liver failure in the United States. *Liver Transpl Surg* 1999;5:29–34.
39. Lee WM. Hepatitis B virus infection. *N Engl J Med* 1997;337: 1733–1745.
40. Liaw YF, Sung JJ, Chow WC, et al., for the Cirrhosis Asian Lamivudine Multicentre Study Group. Lamivudine for patients with chronic hepatitis B and advanced liver disease. *N Engl J Med* 2004;351: 1521–1531.
41. Hewlett G, Hallenberger S, Rubsamen-Waigmann H. Antivirals against DNA viruses (hepatitis B and the herpes viruses). *Curr Opin Pharmacol* 2004;4:453–464.
42. Chang TT, Gish RG, de Man R, et al. A comparison of entecavir and lamivudine for HBeAg-positive chronic hepatitis B. *N Engl J Med* 2006; 354:1001.
43. Lai CL, Gane E, Liaw YF, et al. Telbivudine versus lamivudine in patients with chronic hepatitis B. *N Engl J Med* 2007;357:2576.
44. Lauer GM, Walker BD. Hepatitis C virus infection. *N Engl J Med* 2001; 345(1):41–52.
45. El-Serag HB, Hampel H, Yeh C, et al. Extrahepatic manifestations of hepatitis C among United States male veterans. *Hepatology* 2002;36: 1439–1445.
46. Pedersen IM, Cheng G, Wieland S, et al. Interferon modulation of cellular microRNAs as an antiviral mechanism. *Nature* 2007;449(7164):919–922.
47. Cameron AM, Ghobrial RM, Hiatt JR, et al. Effect of nonviral factors on hepatitis C recurrence after liver transplantation. *Ann Surg* 2006;244(4): 563–571.
48. Bichko V, Netter HJ, Wu TT, et al. Pathogenesis associated with replication of hepatitis delta virus. *Infect Agents Dis* 1994;3:94.
49. Le Gal F, Gault E, Ripault MP, et al. Eighth major clade for hepatitis delta virus. *Emerg Infect Dis* 2006;12:1447.
50. Niro GA, Rosina F, Rizzetto M. Treatment of hepatitis D. *J Viral Hepat* 2005;12:2–9.
51. Kaymakoglu S, Karaca C, Demir K, et al. Alpha interferon and ribavirin combination therapy of chronic hepatitis D. *Antimicrob Agents Chemother* 2005;49:1135–1138.
52. Samuel D, Muller R, Alexander G, et al. Liver transplantation in European patients with the hepatitis B surface antigen. *N Engl J Med* 1993;329: 1842.
53. Lu L, Li C, Hagedorn CH. Phylogenetic analysis of global hepatitis E virus sequences: genetic diversity, subtypes and zoonosis. *Rev Med Virol* 2006; 16:5.
54. Enterically transmitted non-A, non-B hepatitis–East Africa. *MMWR Morb Mortal Wkly Rep* 1987;36:241.
55. Khuroo MS, Teli MR, Skidmore S, et al. Incidence and severity of viral hepatitis in pregnancy. *Am J Med* 1981;70:252.
56. Asher LV, Innis BL, Shrestha MP, et al. Virus-like particles in the liver of a patient with fulminant hepatitis and antibody to hepatitis E virus. *J Med Virol* 1990;31:229.
57. Yousfi MM, Douglas DD, Rakela J. Other hepatitis viruses. In: Zakim D, Boyer TD, eds. *Hepatology. A Textbook of Liver Disease,* 4th ed. Philadelphia, PA: WB Saunders; 2003:1063–1072.
58. Schiff GM. Hepatitis caused by other viruses. In: Shiff ER, Sorrell MF, Maddrey WC, eds. *Schiff's Diseases of the Liver,* 8th ed. Philadelphia, PA: Lippincott Williams & Wilkins; 1999:869–877.
59. Hinedi TB, Koff RS. Cholestatic hepatitis induced by Epstein-Barr virus infection in an adult. *Dig Dis Sci* 2003;48:539–541.
60. Feranchak AP, Tyson RW, Narkewicz MR, et al. Fulminant Epstein-Barr viral hepatitis: orthotopic liver transplantation and review of the literature. *Liver Transpl Surg* 1998;4:469–476.
61. Hoofnagle JH, Carithers RL Jr, Shapiro C, et al, Fulminant hepatic failure: summary of a workshop. *Hepatology* 1995;21:240–252.
62. Mas A, Rodes J. Fulminant hepatic failure. *Lancet* 1997;349:1081–1085.
63. Akdogan M, Camci C, Gurakar A, et al. The effect of total plasma exchange on fulminant hepatic failure. *J Clin Apheresis* 2006;21: 96–99.
64. Polson J, Lee WM. AASLD position paper: the management of acute liver failure. *Hepatology* 2005;41(5):1179–1197.
65. Larson AM. Acute liver failure. *Dis Mon* 2008;54:457–485.
66. Ichai P, Samuel D. Etiology and prognosis of fulminant hepatitis in adults. *Liver Transpl* 2008;14:S67–S79.
67. Sanyal AJ, Stravitz RT. Acute liver failure. In: Boyer TD, Wright TL, Manns MP, eds. *Zakim and Boyer's Hepatology: A Textbook of Liver Disease,* 5th ed. Philadelphia, PA: Saunders Elsevier; 2006:383–415.
68. Lee WM, Squires RH Jr, Nyberg SL, et al. Acute liver failure: summary of a workshop. *Hepatology* 2008;47:1401–1415.
69. Williams R, Wendon J. Indications for orthotopic liver transplantation in fulminant liver failure. *Hepatology* 1994;20:S5–S10.
70. Schilsky ML, Tavill AS. Wilson disease. In: Schiff ER, Sorrell MF, Maddrey WC, eds. *Schiff's Diseases of the Liver,* 9th ed. Philadelphia: Lippincott Williams & Wilkins; 2003:1169–1186.
71. Kramer DJ, Canabal JM, Arasi LC. Application of intensive care medicine principles in the management of the acute liver failure patient. *Liver Transpl* 2008;14:S85–S89.
72. Raschke RA, Curry S, Rempe S, et al. Results of a protocol for the management of patients with fulminant liver failure. *Crit Care Med* 2008; 36(8):2244–2213.
73. O'Grady JG. Postoperative issues and outcome for acute liver failure. *Liver Transpl* 2008;14:S97–S101.
74. Heeman U, Treichel U, Loock J, et al. Stange albumin dialysis in cirrhosis with superimposed acute liver injury. *J Hepatology* 2002;36(4 Pt 1): 949–958.
75. Rifai K, Ernst T, Kretschmer U, et al. Prometheus (R)-a new extracorporeal system for the treatment of liver failure. *J Hepatol* 2003;39(6): 984–990.
76. Mindikoglu AL, Magder LS, Regev A. Outcome of liver transplantation for drug induced acute liver failure in the United States: analysis of the United Network for Organ Sharing database. *Hepatology* 2008;48(4)(suppl): A351.

CHAPTER 58 ■ CIRRHOSIS AND PORTAL HYPERTENSION

MICHAEL R. MARVIN AND JEAN C. EMOND

KEY POINTS

1. Although the causes of cirrhosis and the morphologic and histologic changes seen in the liver overlap significantly, oxidative stress leading to chronic injury and inflammation appears to be a common theme.
2. The key mediator in alcohol-induced liver disease is acetaldehyde, which produces numerous deleterious effects on the liver.
3. Nonalcoholic fatty liver disease or nonalcoholic steatohepatitis (NASH) is characterized by infiltration of the liver with fat and is associated with obesity, hyperlipidemia, and non–insulin-dependent diabetes.
4. Viral hepatitis is the most common cause of cirrhosis worldwide, accounting for at least 50% of cases.
5. Budd-Chiari syndrome is a rare disease caused by mechanical obstruction of the hepatic veins owing to obstructing webs or membranes (most commonly in Asia and Africa) or thrombosis secondary to hypercoagulable states and neoplasms (most commonly in the West).
6. Hepatorenal syndrome is a complication of cirrhosis, usually associated with ascites, characterized by progressive renal failure in the absence of intrinsic renal disease.
7. Hepatic encephalopathy is a neuropsychiatric syndrome that occurs in the setting of hepatic disease and is characterized by variable alterations in mental status ranging from deficits detectable only by detailed psychometric tests to confusion, lethargy, and ultimately coma.
8. Portal hypertension is defined as a portal pressure above the normal range of 5 to 8 mm Hg and can be secondary to cirrhosis (hepatic), portal vein thrombosis (presinusoidal), or hepatic venous obstruction (postsinusoidal).
9. The Child-Turcotte-Pugh score is a scoring scale that incorporates clinical and laboratory data as a means to assess the functional status of the liver, estimate hepatic reserve, and predict morbidity and mortality of liver disease. The Model for End-stage Liver Disease (MELD) score is a highly reliable prognostic marker for cirrhosis, is calculated from standard laboratory tests, and has replaced the Child-Turcotte-Pugh score in liver transplant candidate stratification.
10. The use of the transjugular intrahepatic portosystemic shunt (TIPS) has become first-line therapy for refractory or recurrent bleeding esophageal varices, with 6-month and 1-year patency rates and prevention of rebleeding in 92% and 82% of patients, respectively.
11. Although the surgical interventions for treatment of bleeding varices are divided into three main types—liver transplantation, shunt procedures, and devascularization procedures—the only definitive procedure in patients with cirrhosis is orthotopic liver transplant.
12. Spontaneous bacterial peritonitis is a potentially lethal complication of unknown etiology associated with portal hypertension with ascites that occurs in up to 10% of patients.

CIRRHOSIS

Background and Definition

Cirrhosis is the end result of multiple, varied, repeated or chronic pathologic insults to the liver with subsequent repair that cause a derangement in the hepatic architecture; the primary histologic features are marked fibrosis, destruction of vascular and biliary elements, regeneration, and nodule formation (Fig. 58.1). In addition to progressive failure of hepatic function, portal hypertension is the most prominent clinical manifestation associated with cirrhosis, but it is possible to have portal hypertension in the absence of cirrhosis. The continuum of cirrhosis to liver cancer and its devastating clinical consequences requires us to consider hepatocellular carcinoma as a central complication of cirrhosis.

Pathophysiology

Cirrhosis is caused by a wide range of pathologic entities, including the viral hepatitides, alcohol, metabolic disorders, drug toxicity, and biliary obstruction, among others (Table 58.1). Triggered by the underlying cause, the liver is exposed to a broad range of pathologic injuries leading to hepatocyte death and the gradual loss of architectural integrity made permanent by the development of fibrosis. The capacity of the liver to regenerate is a distinct feature of the liver metaphorically represented in the Promethean myth, and the liver is able to absorb injury without structural alteration. However, the capacity of the liver to regenerate is finite, and understanding the deviation from successful regeneration with restoration of hepatocyte mass and normal architecture to the path leading to fibrogenesis and cirrhosis remains a central question in liver biology.[1] Significant progress in our understanding of the evolution of liver fibrosis, which ends with cirrhosis, has been gained in recent years.

❶ The pathway from the injuring agent to fibrosis is of growing interest, and the central role of oxidative stress in many forms of liver injury has received growing attention. Alcoholic liver disease has long been known to be associated with consequences of oxidative stress in the liver with failure of homeostatic mechanisms.[2] Obesity and metabolic syndrome, a major health problem in the United States, may produce hepatic injury and may potentiate the effects of viral injury.[3,4] In addition to direct oxidative stress, hepatocyte injury is mediated by a variety of mechanisms including proinflammatory cytokines[1] and failure of reparative or modulatory pathways.[5]

The failure of protective or reparatory mechanisms is also widely studied.[6] Over time, fibrosis is the inexorable consequence

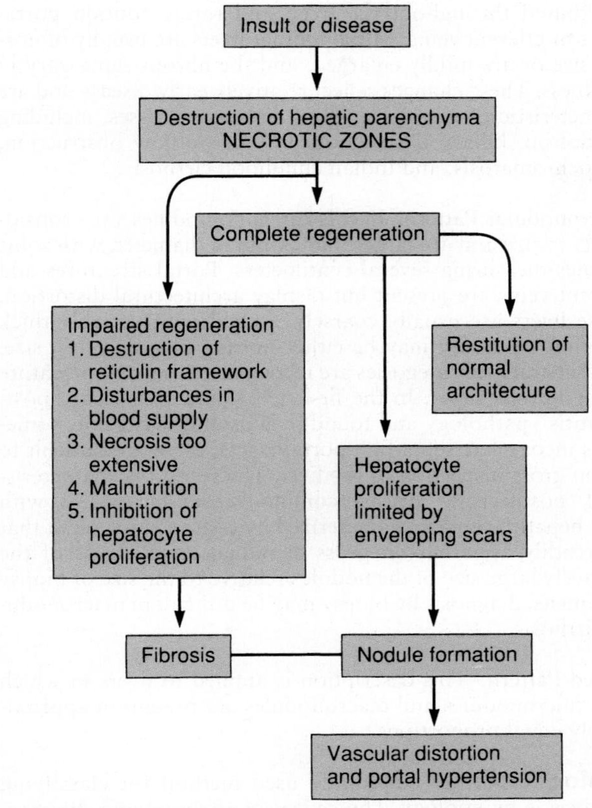

FIGURE 58.1. Evolution of cirrhosis. Fibrosis develops in nonregenerative necrotic areas, producing scars. The pattern of nodularity and scars reflects the type of response to injury (e.g., uniform vs. nonuniform necrosis) and the extent of injury.

TABLE 58.1 **CLASSIFICATION**

CLASSIFICATION OF CIRRHOSIS

Alcohol
Viral hepatitis
Biliary obstruction
Primary
Secondary
Veno-occlusive disease
Hemochromatosis
Wilson disease
Autoimmune
Syphilis
Drugs and toxins
α_1-Antitrypsin deficiency
Cystic fibrosis
Glycogen storage disease
Other metabolic diseases
Sarcoidosis
Copper
Small-bowel bypass
Idiopathic

of injury and the primary cell implicated in the formation of fibrosis is the hepatocyte stellate cell (HSC), located in the perisinusoidal space of Disse (Fig. 58.2).[7] In the normal liver, these cells are quiescent and are primarily responsible for the storage of vitamin A.[8] Injured hepatocytes release soluble factors that activate HSCs, as evidenced by cellular enlargement and proliferation, an increase in rough endoplasmic reticulum,

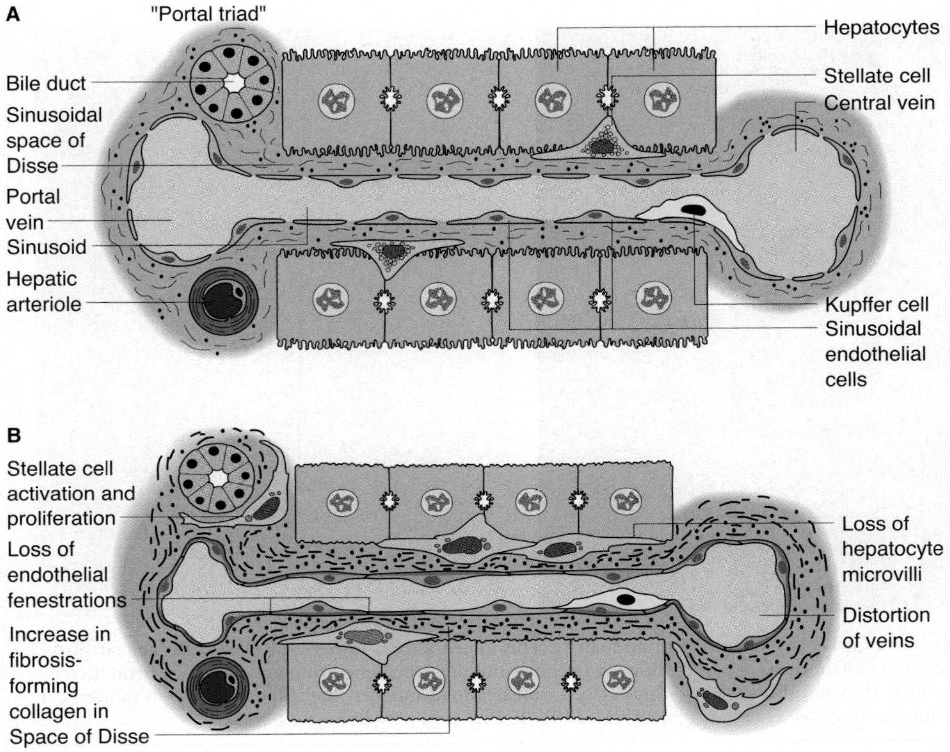

FIGURE 58.2. Matrix and cellular alterations in hepatic fibrosis. **A:** In normal liver, a modest amount of low-density matrix is present in the subendothelial space of Disse. **B:** In the fibrotic liver, the accumulation of fibril-forming matrix in this region leads to "capillarization" of the sinusoid and functional changes in all neighboring cell types. (From Friedman SL, Arthur MJP, Millward-Sadler GH. Cirrhosis and hepatic fibrosis. In: Wright R, et al., eds. *Liver and Biliary Disease*, 3rd ed. London: Bailliere Tindall, 1992: 822–881, with permission.)

loss of vitamin A droplets, expression of actin filaments, and increased expression of "fibril-forming" collagen types I, III, and V.[9] They also express components of the extracellular matrix, including heparan sulfate, dermatan, chondroitin sulfate,[10] laminin,[11] and fibronectin.[12] Macrophages within the liver (Kupffer cells) secrete transforming growth factor-β1 (TGF-β1), which appears to be critical for the activation of HSCs.[13,14] Both TGF-β and platelet-derived growth factor (PDGF) have been shown to enhance proliferation and fibrogenesis in animal models,[14–16] with TGF-β being the primary stimulator of collagen synthesis and fibrosis. Further evidence implicating TGF-β in the production of hepatic fibrosis is the observation that levels of TGF-β are reduced by therapy with interferon-α in patients who are positive for hepatitis C. This reduction has been correlated with a regression of hepatic fibrosis.[17] As a result of the activation of stellate cells and a subsequent enhancement in collagen and extracellular matrix synthesis, the space of Disse becomes thickened, so that "capillarization" develops and the normal fenestrated architecture of the sinusoidal endothelium is lost.[18] Obliteration of sinusoidal fenestrations may be the essential component of fibrosis-induced hepatocellular dysfunction in cirrhosis, preventing the normal flow of nutrients to hepatocytes and increasing vascular resistance.[19] In addition, production of endothelin-1, a potent vasoconstrictor, by endothelial or stellate cells can cause contraction of the myofilaments within the stellate cell, influencing blood flow to injured areas and contributing to portal hypertension.[20] Initially, fibrosis may be reversible if the inciting agents are removed. With sustained injury, the process of fibrosis becomes irreversible and leads to cirrhosis. Growing attention has been given to approaches that might disconnect hepatic injury from the inexorable path of fibrosis.[21]

Classification Systems

Morphology. In 1977, the World Health Organization divided cirrhosis into three categories based on the morphologic characteristics of hepatic nodules (Fig. 58.3).[22]

Micronodular Pattern. Nodules are almost always less than 3 mm in diameter, are relatively uniform in size, are regularly distributed throughout the liver, and rarely contain portal tracts or efferent veins. Micronodular livers are usually of normal size or are mildly enlarged, and the fibrous septa vary in thickness. These changes reflect relatively early disease and are characteristic of a wide range of disease processes, including alcoholism, biliary obstruction, venous outflow obstruction, hemochromatosis, and Indian childhood cirrhosis.

Macronodular Pattern. In this category, nodules vary considerably in size and are larger than 3 mm in diameter, with some nodules measuring several centimeters. Portal structures and efferent veins are present but display architectural distortion. These livers are usually coarsely scarred with variably thick and thin septa and may be either normal or reduced in size. Two separate subcategories are recognized based on the nature of the fibrous septa. In the first one, characteristic of "posthepatitis" pathology and found in Wilson disease, fine, sometimes incomplete septa link portal tracts; these are difficult to see on gross inspection of the liver. The second is characteristic of "postnecrotic" disease, commonly found in patients with viral hepatitis, and is characterized by coarse, thick septa that are readily apparent on gross examination. Because of the relatively large size of the nodules relative to the size of biopsy specimens, diagnosis by biopsy may be difficult in macronodular cirrhosis.

Mixed Pattern. This description is applied to livers in which both micronodules and macronodules are present in approximately equal proportions.

Etiology. Another commonly used method for classifying cirrhosis is by etiology. The causes of cirrhosis and the morphologic and histologic characteristics of the liver, however, overlap significantly. Oxidative stress leading to chronic injury and inflammation appears to be a common theme of these disorders, which leads to both scar formation and an increased risk of liver cancer.

Alcohol. The relationship between alcohol and liver disease has been well established. In 1849, Rokitansky, referring to the association of alcohol intake and liver disease, coined the term *Laennec cirrhosis*.[23] More than 50% of alcoholics with

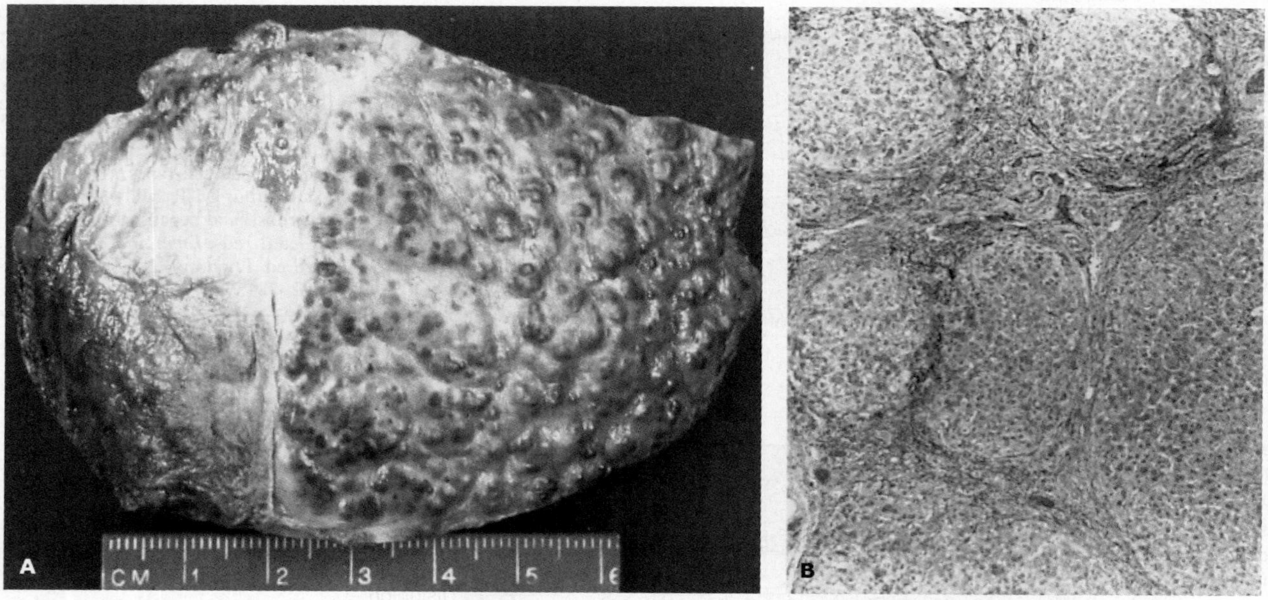

FIGURE 58.3. **A:** Small, shrunken liver and a fairly regular pattern of nodularity. This appearance is rather typical of end-stage cirrhosis, regardless of the cause. **B:** Photomicrograph of cirrhotic liver tissue, showing irregular nodules of regenerating hepatocytes surrounded by scar. Trichrome stain. (From Stal P, Broome U, Scheynius A, et al. Kupffer cell iron overload induces intercellular adhesion molecule-1 expression on hepatocytes in genetic hemochromatosis. *Hepatology* 1995;21:1308–1316.)

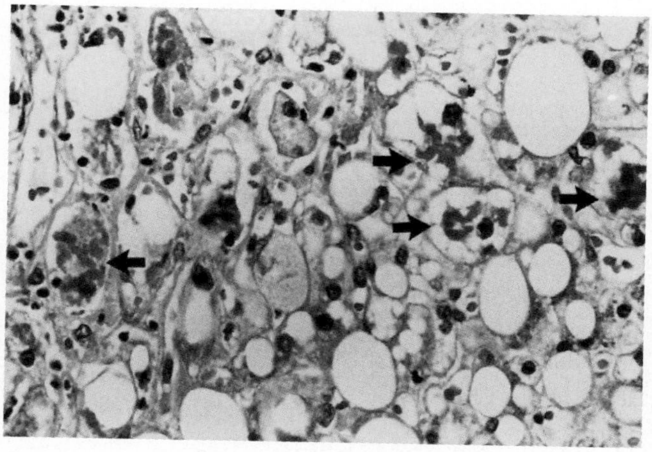

FIGURE 58.4. Alcoholic hepatitis. Mallory bodies (*arrows*) are evident within the swollen, clear cytoplasm of several hepatocytes. This hyaline material is chemotactic for leukocytes, many of which are seen within the field. Hematoxylin and eosin (H&E) stain × 470.

cirrhosis and two thirds of patients with alcoholic hepatitis and cirrhosis die within 4 years of diagnosis.[24] Cirrhosis, however, develops in only 10% to 30% of heavy drinkers.[25] The reasons why cirrhosis develops in some alcoholics but not in others are not clear and may depend on a variety of factors, such as genetic predisposition, nutritional effects, concomitant drug use, and viral infection.

Alcoholic liver disease usually begins with a transition of normal architecture to fatty liver and alcoholic hepatitis, indicated histologically by the presence of megamitochondria, Mallory bodies (eosinophilic accumulations of intermediate filaments with cytokeratin proteins), inflammation and necrosis, and ultimately fibrosis (Fig. 58.4). Classically, the morphology of alcoholic cirrhosis is a micronodular pattern.

2 Although alcohol may directly activate stellate cells to produce collagen independently of inflammation and necrosis,[26] the key mediator in alcohol-induced liver disease is acetaldehyde, the product of alcohol metabolism by the enzyme alcohol dehydrogenase. Acetaldehyde (ADH) produces numerous deleterious effects on the liver, including the following: direct activation of stellate cells[27]; inhibition of DNA repair[28]; depletion of glutathione, which impairs mitochondrial function and the ability to handle free radical production; damage to microtubules, which causes protein and water sequestration[25]; and formation of reduced nicotinamide adenine dinucleotide (NADH), which opposes gluconeogenesis and inhibits fatty acid oxidation, so that steatosis and hyperlipidemia develop.[25] ADH is most active in the perivenular/centrilobular zone 3 of the hepatic lobule; as a result, relatively high concentrations of acetaldehyde are found in this area of the liver. In addition, zone 3 is hypoxic because of its distance from portal venous and hepatic arterial inflow. These two factors are presumably responsible for the characteristic initial perivenular location of alcohol-induced liver disease.

Other effects of ADH include induction of lipid peroxidation with subsequent loss of integrity of cell membranes, which causes the characteristic "ballooning degeneration" of alcohol-induced liver disease. Necrosis and inflammation in the perivenular region activate the stellate cells in the space of Disse, so that fibrosis develops. With continued ingestion of alcohol and hepatic injury, expansion of the areas of fibrosis toward the periportal regions leads to bridging fibrosis and ultimately cirrhosis.

Nonalcoholic Fatty Liver Disease/Nonalcoholic Steatohepatitis. As noted earlier, this entity has become a major health problem in the United States and adds even further to

3 the litany of health consequences of obesity. Nonalcoholic steatohepatitis (NASH), as this disease was previously called, is only one stage in the nonalcoholic fatty liver disease (NAFLD) process.[29] It is characterized by infiltration of the liver with fat, with or without inflammation (hepatitis), that shares pathologic features of alcohol-induced liver injury but occurs in patients who do not abuse alcohol. NAFLD is associated with obesity, hyperlipidemia, and non–insulin-dependent diabetes.[30] Most patients who are diagnosed with cryptogenic cirrhosis have NAFLD,[31] which is the most common cause of abnormal liver test results in the United States.[32] In addition to liver injury and cirrhosis, NAFLD is a major risk factor for primary liver cancer (hepatocellular carcinoma [HCC]) and, in addition to hepatitis virus infection, accounts for the rapid rise in the incidence of HCC.[33] More broadly considered, recent reports have identified obesity as a major risk factor for cancer deaths with a 4.5-fold increase of the relative risk for liver cancer in obese subjects.[34]

4 **Hepatitis.** Viral hepatitis is the most common cause of cirrhosis worldwide, accounting for at least 50% of cases. Hepatitis A, B, C, D, and E have all been proved to cause acute hepatitis, characterized histologically by lymphocytic parenchymal and portal inflammation, focal necrosis, ballooning degeneration, cholestasis, Kupffer cell and macrophage hypertrophy and hyperplasia, and lobular disarray. Only hepatitis B, C, and D have been shown to progress to chronic hepatitis, defined by persistent liver cell necrosis and inflammation lasting longer than 6 months. Chronic infection with hepatitis B virus (HBV) develops in fewer than 5% of patients who experience acute HBV infection. The development of cirrhosis in approximately 10% to 20% of chronically infected persons produces an overall rate of cirrhosis of approximately 1%. Hepatitis B remains a major public health problem in Asian countries and Africa, with up to 10% of the population showing evidence of chronic infection. The widespread use of antiviral medications effective against hepatitis B effectively controls progression of the disease in most patients.[35] In addition, public health strategies with systematic vaccination of newborns should substantially decrease the incidence of new infections. In contrast, hepatitis C poses a much higher risk of chronic infection, and therapeutic strategies eradicate viral replication in a minority of patients. Of patients with hepatitis C virus (HCV), 90% become chronically infected, and chronic hepatitis develops in 60% of these. Of these patients with chronic hepatitis, 30% progress to cirrhosis,[23] so that the incidence of cirrhosis in patients initially infected with hepatitis C is approximately 10%.

Treatment of HCV hepatitis with interferon-α can completely eradicate infection in a small portion of patients (15% to 30%).[36] In patients who respond to interferon therapy, progression to cirrhosis is eliminated and it is generally thought that hepatocellular carcinoma does not develop. In patients who do not respond to interferon therapy, cirrhosis develops in approximately 40%, and hepatocellular carcinoma develops in 16% of these.[37] Combination therapy with interferon and ribavirin has improved response rates, producing sustained remissions in 30% to 40% of patients.[38] Recently, pegylation of interferon has resulted in new drug formulations that have allowed for once-weekly drug administration and improved sustained response rates to greater than 50%.[39] It should be noted that hepatitis C occurs naturally in multiple genotypes, of which types 2 and 3 respond well to treatment with sustained viral suppression in 70% to 80% of patients.[39] Most recently, trials of antiviral agents aimed at blocking replication have demonstrated marked reduction of HCV RNA, though the effect is not sustained.[40]

Hepatitis D virus (HDV) is an RNA virus that requires the presence of HBV to be pathogenic. Superinfection of HBV-positive patients with HDV leads to a more rapid clinical

PANCREAS/LIVER

TABLE 58.2

CAUSES OF CHOLESTASIS

Extrahepatic	Vanishing bile duct syndrome
Common bile duct stones	Allograft rejection
Cancers	Graft versus host disease
Pancreas	Alagille syndrome
Ampulla of Vater	Idiopathic adult ductopenia
Bile duct	Primary sclerosing cholangitis
Cysts	Hodgkin disease
Pancreatic	Cystic fibrosis
Choledochal	**Hepatocellular Cholestasis**
Infections	Genetic
Parasites	α-Antitrypsin deficiency
Acquired immunodeficiency syndrome	Benign recurrent intrahepatic cholestasis
Chronic pancreatitis	Byler syndrome
Bile duct strictures	Cholestasis of pregnancy
Benign	Abnormal bile acid synthesis
Ischemic	Porphyrias
Hodgkin disease	Acquired
Biliary atresia	Viral hepatitis
Intrahepatic	Drugs
Primary biliary cirrhosis	Alcoholic hepatitis
Space-occupying lesions	Bacterial infections
Primary or metastatic hepatic tumors	Total parenteral nutrition
Lymphoma	Renal carcinoma
Amyloidosis	Hodgkin disease
	Postoperative cholestasis

course, with progression to cirrhosis in 70% to 80% of patients.[41]

Among patients with compensated cirrhosis of viral origin, hepatocellular carcinoma developed in approximately 20% with HCV, 9% with HBV, and 41% with both HBV and HCV.[23] The progressive increase in hepatitis-infected individuals in the United States precedes an epidemic in HCC, which has been well documented and is expected to peak over the coming decade.[42]

Cholestasis. Cholestasis, defined as a decrease or absence of bile flow into the duodenum, may be caused by intrahepatic or extrahepatic biliary obstruction or defects in the ability of hepatocytes to excrete bile. Causes of cholestasis are presented in Table 58.2. Prolonged biliary obstruction leads to proliferation of bile ducts, formation of bile lakes caused by disruption of bile ducts, fibrosis, and ultimately secondary biliary cirrhosis as a result of the direct toxic effects of bile salts on hepatobiliary elements.

Immune or Inflammatory Cirrhosis. Although cholestasis is a generically toxic insult to the liver that can cause cirrhosis, several diseases that are characterized by cholestasis seem to be caused by underlying immune or inflammatory disorders affecting either small (primary biliary cirrhosis [PBC]) or large (primary sclerosing cholangitis [PSC]) bile ducts. Primary biliary cirrhosis is a chronic, slowly progressive disease that most commonly affects middle-aged women; it is characterized by portal inflammation, destruction of intrahepatic bile ducts, and progression to cirrhosis. Approximately 95% of patients are women, and 95% of these women express antimitochondrial antibodies in serum.[43] The autoimmune inflammatory process damages both the bile ducts and, eventually, the hepatocytes as a result of leakage of bile acids into surrounding parenchyma.[44] Patients present with fatigue, jaundice, and pruritus, but as many as 50% to 60% of patients may be asymptomatic.[45] PBC progresses in the majority of patients; median survival times are approximately 10 to 15 years in asymptomatic patients and 7 years in symptomatic patients.[46,47] Poor prognostic factors include hyperbilirubinemia, advanced age, hepatosplenomegaly, and symptomatic disease. Treatment options include cholestyramine, colchicine, and methotrexate for pruritus and fatigue, and ursodiol for slowing progression of the disease and delaying the need for transplant.[47,48] Liver transplantation is ultimately required as the definitive treatment in most patients, and the parameters for liver transplantation and its timing are relatively predictable and have been well studied.[49]

Primary sclerosing cholangitis is a chronic, progressive cholestatic liver disease of unknown cause characterized by diffuse segmental intrahepatic or extrahepatic biliary ductular strictures with associated fibrosis and inflammation. The disease has no cure and often leads to secondary biliary cirrhosis, portal hypertension, hepatic failure, and cholangiocarcinoma if hepatic transplantation is not performed. PSC is strongly associated with inflammatory bowel diseases, most commonly ulcerative colitis, and probably shares an underlying disturbance related to disturbed mucosal immunity of the gastrointestinal tract.[50] Approximately 70% of patients with PSC also have ulcerative colitis.[50] Conversely, approximately 5% of patients with ulcerative colitis have PSC, though subtler forms of the disease may be present but clinically asymptomatic. PSC is thought to be autoimmune in nature; elevated levels of autoantibodies and an increased expression of human leukocyte antigen (HLA) class II molecules on biliary epithelial cells have been observed.[51,52] Approximately two thirds of patients are male and younger than 45 years of age at the time of diagnosis.[53,54] Patients with PSC may be completely asymptomatic (up to 50%) or have signs of advanced disease at the time of diagnosis.[55] Commonly, the diagnosis is made in symptomatic patients after endoscopic retrograde cholangiopancreatography (ERCP) has been performed to evaluate elevated liver enzymes, including alkaline phosphatase and γ-glutamyltransferase. Symptomatic patients have a waxing and waning course and may present with complaints of fatigue (75%), pruritus (25% to 70%), jaundice (30% to 69%), abdominal pain (16% to 37%), and weight loss (10% to 34%).[50] Complications secondary to progression to cirrhosis are less common and include ascites, variceal bleeding, and acute cholangitis.

The diagnosis of PSC is suggested by a history of inflammatory bowel disease in the setting of elevated liver enzymes and is established by cholangiography. The disease process may range from a single dominant stricture to, more commonly, diffuse multifocal sclerosis of the intrahepatic and extrahepatic bile ducts. Pathologically, bile ductular proliferation, periductal fibrosis and inflammation, ductopenia, and, less commonly, obliterative fibrous cholangitis may be present. PSC may be considered a premalignant condition. Like ulcerative colitis, PSC confers a significant risk of malignant transformation of the biliary mucosa, which is one of the considerations in considering patients for transplantation.[56] Natural history studies suggest that cholangiocarcinoma occurs in up to one third of patients, although the risk increases with the duration of disease and the degree of cholestasis.[57] Screening for premalignant changes with ERCP and cytologic examination and serum testing of CA19-9 have been helpful, though both have limited specificity and sensitivity. Recently, it has been proposed that newer analysis methods of biliary material obtained at screening ERCP, including fluorescence in situ hybridization (FISH), may be used for chromosomal abnormalities associated with cancer with an increase in the sensitivity.[58] Transplantation should be performed before cancer develops and, generally, the discovery of cancer has been considered an absolute contraindication to transplantation because of poor outcomes. Highly selected patients with localized tumors may be transplanted with an acceptable survival rate with intensive preoperative therapy including radiation and chemotherapy, as proposed by Shaw and implemented on a larger scale by the Mayo group.[59]

Metabolic and Genetic Disorders. Some of these diseases are listed in Table 58.1. A description of all the metabolic disorders causing liver disease is beyond the scope of this chapter.

In hemochromatosis of the liver, an inborn error of metabolism causes an increased absorption of iron from the gastrointestinal tract. The pathophysiology of iron-induced hepatotoxicity is related to lipid peroxidation induced by iron in periportal regions of the liver. Activation of stellate cells by cytokines released from Kupffer cells that have phagocytosed necrotic hepatocytes injured by iron toxicity is also contributory.[60] Over time, the reaction progresses to bridging fibrosis and eventually to a mixed micronodular–macronodular cirrhosis. Treatment includes reduction of iron intake, repeated phlebotomy, and orthotopic liver transplantation.[61]

Wilson disease is an autosomal, recessively inherited disease caused by a deficiency in hepatocyte transport of copper into the bile. The disease is characterized biochemically by low serum ceruloplasmin levels and clinically by corneal pigmentation (Kayser-Fleischer rings), neuropsychiatric disease, and hepatic cirrhosis.[62] As copper accumulates in the liver, periportal inflammation develops that leads to piecemeal and lobular necrosis, bridging fibrosis, and a mixed micronodular–macronodular cirrhosis. Treatment options include chelating agents, such as penicillamine, trientine, zinc salts, and orthotopic liver transplantation.

Venous Outflow Obstruction. Cirrhosis may also result from obstruction of the hepatic veins. Causes include chronic right-sided heart failure as a result of severe tricuspid regurgitation, constrictive pericarditis, and the Budd-Chiari syndrome.

Hepatic dysfunction secondary to passive vascular congestion in the setting of right-sided heart failure and increased right-sided heart pressures is caused by the transmission of increased pressure to the hepatic venous system. This increased pressure leads to sinusoidal congestion, perivenular atrophy, hemorrhagic necrosis, and distortion and enlargement of sinusoidal fenestrations.[63] Increased pressure also causes perisinusoidal edema that eventually exceeds the clearance capabilities of hepatic lymphatics, so that ascites develops.[64] Grossly, the liver is described as having a "nutmeg" appearance in which areas of hemorrhage are interspersed with relatively normal yellowish parenchyma.[64] Histologically, perivenular fibrosis progresses to bridging fibrosis that spares the portal regions. Portal sparing is characteristic of "cardiac cirrhosis." In addition to causing ascites, chronic vascular congestion can lead to fibrosis in the space of Disse, which compromises nutrient delivery and contributes to portal hypertension and zone 3 hepatocellular injury.[65]

5 Budd-Chiari syndrome is a rare disease caused by mechanical obstruction of the hepatic veins (Table 58.3). Obstruction may occur at the level of the terminal hepatic veins, the major hepatic veins, or the vena cava and may be caused by obstructing webs or membranes (most commonly in Africa and Asia) or thrombosis secondary to hypercoagulable states and neoplasms (most commonly in the West).

The range of presentations is wide; some patients are completely asymptomatic, whereas acute hepatic failure or cirrhosis develops in others.[66] These variations in symptoms are related to the degree and rate of progression of hepatic outflow obstruction. Patients classically present with abdominal pain, hepatomegaly, and ascites. The diagnosis can be made by

TABLE 58.3 **ETIOLOGY**

ETIOLOGIC FACTORS IN BUDD-CHIARI SYNDROME

Idiopathic
Hematologic disorders
Polycythemia vera
Paroxysmal nocturnal hemoglobinuria
Myeloproliferative disorders
Antithrombin III deficiency
Circulating lupus anticoagulants
Oral contraceptives
Pregnancy and postpartum
Tumors
Hepatocellular carcinoma
Renal cell carcinoma
Adrenal carcinoma
Leiomyosarcoma of the inferior vena cava
Vena caval webs
Infections
Amebic abscess
Aspergillosis
Hydatid cyst
Phlebitis
Trauma
Veno-occlusive disease

TABLE 58.4 DIAGNOSIS

PHYSICAL FINDINGS IN CIRRHOSIS

PHYSICAL FINDINGS	INCIDENCE (%)
Palpable liver	96
Jaundice	68
Ascites	66
Spider angiomas	49
Dilated abdominal wall veins	47
Palpable spleen	46
Testicular atrophy	45
Palmar erythema	24
Noninfectious fever	22
Hepatic coma	18
Gynecomastia	15
Dupuytren contractures	5

duplex Doppler ultrasonography, which has a sensitivity of 85% to 95%.[67] Computed tomography (CT) and magnetic resonance imaging (MRI) offer optimal characterization of intrahepatic vascular anatomy and are currently used for the planning of complex interventions.[68]

Diagnosis

Although cirrhosis can be asymptomatic for decades, significant information can be obtained by performing a thorough history and physical examination. A history of alcohol abuse, hepatitis, toxin or drug exposure, upper gastrointestinal bleeding, enlarging hemorrhoids, infections, and alteration in mental status suggest the possibility of liver disease. Physical findings associated with cirrhosis are listed in Table 58.4. In addition to these findings, fetor hepaticus, purpura and bruising, decreased body hair, and white nails are common.

Laboratory tests of liver function are indicated if liver disease is suggested by the history and physical examination. Although levels of bilirubin, aspartate aminotransferase, alanine aminotransferase, and alkaline phosphatase are elevated in hepatic disease, the increases are not specific for liver pathology, and levels may be normal even in the setting of significant disease. A very common finding in patients with cirrhosis is thrombocytopenia, caused by hypersplenism and portal hypertension. The platelet growth factor thrombopoietin, which is produced by the liver, has been shown to be decreased in patients with cirrhosis, and this deficit may contribute to the thrombocytopenia associated with hepatic disease.[69]

The definitive diagnosis of cirrhosis usually requires biopsy, either percutaneous or operative, or gross inspection during laparoscopy or laparotomy. Noninvasive methods to diagnose cirrhosis include ultrasonography, CT, and MRI, which generally reveal an atrophic, nodular liver and an enlarged spleen. More recent work suggests that subtle changes in the hepatic veins may be early markers of cirrhosis.[68] Ultrasonographic criteria for cirrhosis include the demonstration of multiple nodular irregularities on the ventral liver surface that are clearly separate from the anterior abdominal wall. Parenchymal texture is altered in the setting of fibrosis, though this feature can be subtle. When these criteria are used, ultrasonography has been shown to have a sensitivity, specificity, and accuracy of approximately 90% in the diagnosis of cirrhosis.[70] Indirect evidence of cirrhosis includes endoscopically discovered varices of the esophagus, and the presence of splenomegaly detected by CT or MRI.

Manifestations

Renal. Renal complications in cirrhosis are intrinsic to functional dysregulation of vascular tone throughout the body.[71] Several elements come into play and renal dysfunction is characterized by avid sodium retention despite normovolemia or hypervolemia, dilutional hyponatremia secondary to free water overload, ascites, and ultimately renal failure and the hepatorenal syndrome (HRS). The paradoxical arterial vasoconstriction of the renal arterial bed in the face of global fluid overload is critical to the pathophysiology of HRS.[72] Among the complications of cirrhosis, HRS confers the highest risk of mortality.[73] Although HRS is the most dramatic renal complication of liver failure, renal dysfunction in patients with advanced liver disease is generally multifactorial.[72] Renal insufficiency may develop in a patient with cirrhosis as a direct consequence of the underlying condition (i.e., primary biliary cirrhosis, amyloidosis), as a consequence of excessive diuretic use in the treatment of ascites and fluid overload, or as a secondary reaction to the release of cytokines or hormones by the liver that alter renal function.

Much progress has been made in the understanding of the pathophysiology of HRS focusing on the dysregulation of arterial tone in the end stages of liver disease. Empiric observations that support a functional or "secondary effect" theory include the lack of anatomic renal abnormalities in patients with cirrhosis-related renal dysfunction, the normal function of previously dysfunctional kidneys transplanted into otherwise healthy recipients, and resolution of renal abnormalities after successful hepatic transplantation. Recent clinical studies have defined the critical role of optimizing colloid balance in the patient with cirrhosis[74] and the exploration of regulators of renal blood flow such as terlipressin in counteracting the deranged vascular tone.[75]

Sodium Retention. Patients with cirrhosis who do not have ascites have relatively normal sodium handling capabilities. Patients in whom ascites develops have a marked inability to excrete sodium. Because of this deficit, sodium intake in excess of renal excretion contributes to fluid overload. Three potential mechanisms have been invoked to explain the cause of sodium retention and the development of ascites in cirrhotic patients. The first is the "underfill" theory, whereby portal hypertension causes an increase in pressure in the splanchnic circulation. Ascites occurs when hepatic lymph production exceeds lymphatic return, with subsequent contraction of the blood volume and renal sodium retention. The second is the "overflow" theory, which suggests that the primary defect is inherent to the kidney. Abnormal renal retention of sodium leads to concomitant water retention, expansion of plasma volume, and subsequently edema and ascites.[76] The third explanation is the "arterial vasodilation hypothesis," which suggests that the responsible defect lies within the vascular system, with arterial hypotension as the primary event. Arterial vasodilation in the splanchnic circulation leads to relative peripheral hypovolemia and activation of the renin–angiotensin–aldosterone and sympathetic nervous systems. The effects, in turn, are a release of antidiuretic hormone (arginine vasopressin), enhancement of sodium and water conservation, an increase in effective circulating volume, and edema and ascites.[77,78] Most evidence supports the latter hypothesis.

The cause of the splanchnic vasodilation is unclear. Some evidence suggests that nitric oxide may be the key mediator. Elevations in portal venous nitric oxide have been reported in both animal and human studies,[79,80] and inhibitors of nitric oxide production have been shown to reduce the activity of vasoconstrictor systems and enhance renal hemodynamics.[79]

TABLE 58.5 **DIAGNOSIS**

DIFFERENTIAL DIAGNOSIS OF ACUTE AZOTEMIA IN PATIENTS WITH LIVER DISEASE

	PRERENAL AZOTEMIA	HEPATORENAL SYNDROME	ACUTE RENAL FAILURE
Urinary sodium	<10 mEq/L	<10 mEq/L	>30 mEq/L
Urine/plasma creatinine ratio	>30:1	>30:1	<20:1
Urine osmolality	100 mOsm, or more than plasma osmolality	100 mOsm, or more than plasma osmolality	Equal to plasma osmolality
Urine sediment	Normal	Normal	Casts: cellular debris

The exact role of nitric oxide activity in the pathophysiology of renal disease in cirrhosis remains to be determined.

Water Retention. Patients with cirrhosis and ascites may have a marked inability to handle free water. An increased production of antidiuretic hormone, decreased delivery of fluid to the diluting segments of the nephron, and reduced renal production of prostaglandins all may contribute.[76] Retention of water leads to dilutional hyponatremia (serum sodium 130 mEq/L), which can cause nausea, vomiting, lethargy, and seizures.[81]

6 **Hepatorenal Syndrome.** Hepatorenal syndrome is a complication of cirrhosis, most often with ascites, characterized by progressive renal failure in the absence of intrinsic renal disease. This syndrome occurs in 10% of hospitalized patients with cirrhosis and ascites.[82] Manifestations of the disease include progressive oliguria, with urine outputs of 400 to 800 mL/d, a rising serum creatinine level, increased cardiac output, and decreased arterial pressure. The disease process is highly variable and is associated with marked renal cortical vasoconstriction induced by activity of the renin–angiotensin–aldosterone and sympathetic nervous systems. In addition, the powerful endothelium-derived vasoconstrictor endothelin-1, combined with decreased renal production of vasodilator prostaglandins, may play a role.

Hepatorenal syndrome may develop as a result of infection, use of nonsteroidal anti-inflammatory drugs, variceal hemorrhage, or excessive diuretic use in patients who were previously well compensated. The differentiation of hepatorenal syndrome from acute renal failure is possible by the laboratory evaluation of urine and serum samples. Hepatorenal syndrome, however, is virtually indistinguishable by laboratory testing from prerenal azotemia. Both prerenal azotemia and hepatorenal syndrome are characterized by extremely low sodium concentrations in the urine, high urine osmolality, high urine-to-plasma ratios of creatinine, and normal urinary sediment (Table 58.5). Criteria for the diagnosis of hepatorenal syndrome are listed in Table 58.6.

The treatment of ascites in patients with cirrhosis requires sodium and water restriction in addition to the use of diuretics. Excessive use of these treatment modalities may lead to increases in serum creatinine that can be difficult to distinguish from those of hepatorenal syndrome. A failure to respond to cessation of diuretics and fluid challenge suggests hepatorenal syndrome. If liver transplantation cannot be performed, patients with hepatorenal syndrome usually die within months of the development of severe disease, defined as a serum creatinine level above 2 mg/dL.[73] Recent studies, however, have shown improvement in renal function in patients with hepatorenal syndrome after treatment with vasopressors and albumin.

Pulmonary. Many pathologic processes in patients with cirrhosis affect pulmonary function. Some reflect an underlying condition that causes both hepatic and pulmonary disease (i.e., cystic fibrosis, α_1-antitrypsin deficiency); others are primary pulmonary processes, such as interstitial lung disease, primary pulmonary hypertension (portopulmonary hypertension), and obstructive airway disease. Three main pulmonary manifestations of cirrhosis are discussed here; one is related to increased intra-abdominal pressure secondary to ascites, one is caused by intrapulmonary shunting and is known as the hepatopulmonary syndrome, and the last is portopulmonary hypertension.

The presence of copious ascitic fluid can lead to pulmonary dysfunction by compromising diaphragmatic excursion secondary to increases in intra-abdominal and intrapleural pressures. Ascites may also induce large pleural effusions because of the presence of lymphatic transdiaphragmatic communications between the abdomen and thorax.[83] Effusions can compress the

TABLE 58.6 **DIAGNOSIS**

DIAGNOSTIC CRITERIA FOR HEPATORENAL SYNDROME[a]

Major Criteria

1. Low glomerular filtration rate, as indicated by serum creatinine >1.5 mg/dL or 24-hour creatinine clearance 40 mL/min
2. Absence of shock, ongoing bacterial infection, fluid losses, and current treatment with nephrotoxic drugs
3. No sustained improvement in renal function (decrease in serum creatinine to ≤1.5 mg/dL or increase in creatinine clearance to 340 mL/min) following diuretic withdrawal and expansion of plasma volume with 1.5 L of a plasma expander
4. Proteinuria <500 mg/d and no ultrasonographic evidence of obstructive uropathy or parenchymal renal disease

Additional Criteria

1. Urine volume <500 mL/d
2. Urine sodium <10 mEq/L
3. Urine osmolality greater than plasma osmolality
4. Urine red blood cells <50 per high-power field
5. Serum sodium concentration <130 mEq/L

[a]All major criteria must be present for the diagnosis of hepatorenal syndrome. Additional criteria are not necessary for the diagnosis but provide supportive evidence.
From Arroyo V, Ginés P, Gerbes A, et al. Definition and diagnostic criteria of refractory ascites and hepatorenal syndrome in cirrhosis. *Hepatology* 1996;23:164.

pulmonary parenchyma and impair gas exchange, so that ventilation–perfusion mismatch and hypoxemia develop. Patients present with worsening pulmonary symptoms in the setting of increasing abdominal girth. Pulmonary function testing reveals decreases in functional residual capacity and total lung capacity.[84] Marked improvement in pulmonary function results from large-volume paracentesis.[85] This intervention decreases the work of breathing and relieves symptoms. With control of ascites, even in the presence of pleural effusions, no other interventions may be necessary.

Hepatopulmonary syndrome occurs in patients with mild to severe hepatic disease and in approximately 10% to 50% of patients with hepatic dysfunction.[86,87] The criteria for diagnosis include hepatic dysfunction; an oxygen tension below 70 mm Hg or a diffusion gradient above 20 mm Hg, or both; and the presence of pulmonary vascular dilation in patients with structurally normal lungs.[88] Other manifestations include platypnea (increased shortness of breath with movement from a supine to an erect position) and orthodeoxia (decreased oxygen tension on moving from a supine to an erect position). These two positional deficits in pulmonary function are related to the increased number of dilated capillaries in the basal areas of the lung; flow is increased in these vessels while the subject is standing, so that shunting is increased. Physical findings include clubbing and cyanosis of the nail beds and spider nevi.

Although the underlying cause of hypoxemia in these patients is right-to-left intrapulmonary shunting, ventilation–perfusion mismatch and impaired hypoxic vasoconstriction also play a role. Patients usually present with dyspnea and worsening hypoxemia without evidence of a primary pulmonary process. Initial diagnostic tools include pulse oximetry and arterial blood gas analysis. When significant hypoxemia is found, pulmonary function testing is useful to rule out obstructive or restrictive airway disease. A definitive diagnosis can be obtained by the use of contrast-enhanced echocardiography (bubble study), spiral CT, or angiography, which will confirm the presence of a shunt.[89] The only effective therapy for this disease is orthotopic liver transplantation.

Portopulmonary hypertension is defined as a mean pulmonary arterial pressure of greater than 25 mm Hg in the setting of liver disease. It is a relatively rare (<10%) complication of cirrhosis that, when severe, carries a substantial risk of mortality and is a relative contraindication to liver transplantation.[90,91] Screening of patients with cirrhosis by Doppler echocardiography will reveal evidence of elevated right heart pressures, which need to be confirmed by right heart catheterization. Although the high flow state of cirrhosis can elevate right-sided pressures, fixed obstruction of the pulmonary microcirculation is highly lethal and is not likely to improve with liver transplantation. The exact pathophysiology behind portopulmonary hypertension is not known, but portal hypertension is a necessary component of the disease process. The hyperdynamic state in portal hypertension may be the main contributory factor. Treatment with prolonged intravenous infusion of prostaglandins has been shown to be effective in improving pulmonary hemodynamics but does not prolong survival.[91]

Hepatic Encephalopathy

7 **Etiology.** Hepatic encephalopathy is a neuropsychiatric syndrome that occurs in the setting of hepatic disease. It is characterized by variable alterations in mental status, ranging from deficits detectable only by detailed psychometric tests to confusion, lethargy, and ultimately frank coma. The disease may present in association with acute hepatic failure, as a consequence of progression of chronic liver disease, or after the creation of a surgical portosystemic shunt. Usually, a precipitating cause, such as an acute variceal hemorrhage or infection, can be found.

The causative agent in hepatic encephalopathy has been the subject of much debate. Most evidence implicates ammonia in the development of this condition. Ammonia is produced during the bacterial digestion of proteins in the gut, is absorbed into the portal circulation, and usually undergoes extensive degradation in the liver.[92] Most researchers believe that encephalopathy is caused by products, such as ammonia, derived from the gastrointestinal tract that are usually metabolized by the liver. These agents reach the peripheral circulation as a result of poor hepatic metabolism or through portosystemic shunts that may be physiologic or the result of surgical procedures. In patients with cirrhosis, in addition to the accumulation of ammonia in the blood, the permeability of the brain to ammonia appears to be increased.[93] Other suggested etiologic agents for hepatic encephalopathy include γ-aminobutyric acid, endogenous benzodiazepines,[94] branched-chain amino acids (e.g., tryptophan),[95] neurotoxic short-chain fatty acids, mercaptans, phenols,[96] and endogenous opiates.[97]

The following observations suggest that ammonia is the key mediator in hepatic encephalopathy: (a) ammonia levels are increased in 80% to 90% of patients with the condition,[98] (b) factors that precipitate hepatic encephalopathy cause increases in ammonia levels, and (c) treatments that relieve hepatic encephalopathy lower ammonia levels.[99] Arguments against this hypothesis include the following: (a) levels of ammonia correlate poorly with the severity of hepatic encephalopathy, (b) high ammonia levels alone do not cause encephalopathy, (c) administration of ammonia to patients with cirrhosis but not hepatic encephalopathy does not cause encephalopathy, and (d) treatments that reduce ammonia levels also reduce the levels of other putative toxins.[99]

Clinical Features. A wide range of neurologic symptoms may occur in patients with hepatic dysfunction. Subtle deficits may include changes in personality, memory loss, alterations in sleep patterns, and minor decreases in intellectual function. Defects may be detectable only by detailed psychometric testing. If no known underlying liver disease is suspected, establishing the cause of an alteration in mental status may be difficult.

With progression of disease, asterixis, a rapid repetitive flexion–extension of the wrist that occurs in response to sustained extension of the forearm and fingers, may occur. In addition, stigmata of liver disease are usually evident, including fetor hepaticus and spider angiomas. The combination of asterixis, elevated ammonia levels, and altered mental status in a patient with known liver disease strongly suggests the diagnosis. Electroencephalographic changes are nonspecific and may occur in patients with a variety of other conditions.

Factors that commonly precipitate hepatic encephalopathy include impaired renal function, variceal hemorrhage, constipation, infection, excessive dietary protein, and drugs, especially benzodiazepines and barbiturates.

Treatment. Treatment options for hepatic encephalopathy include correction of the precipitating factors, alterations in diet, bowel cleansing, medications that reduce ammonia production and neutralize its effects, and medications to treat possible neurotransmitter and nutrient deficiencies.

A search for precipitating factors is imperative and includes cultures of urine, sputum, and ascitic fluid; determination of electrolyte abnormalities; screening for viral infection; assessment of overall volume status; drug history; and endoscopy (Table 58.7).

Therapy begins with a trial of volume expansion via intravenous hydration to relieve azotemia and reduce concentrations of toxic substances by dilution. The mainstays of treatment are directed at the removal of nitrogenous compounds from the gut. Most ammonia is produced within the small and large bowel by bacterial metabolism of dietary and endogenous protein. Orally administered cathartics and enemas are the best methods to achieve bowel cleansing, and these are combined with marked dietary restriction of protein.[100]

TABLE 58.7 **TREATMENT**

TREATMENT OF HEPATIC ENCEPHALOPATHY

Identify precipitating factors
Disordered carbohydrate metabolism
Narcotics
Infection
Hypotension
Hypoxia
Excess exogenous protein
Gastrointestinal bleeding
Electrolyte abnormalities
Alkalosis
Supportive therapy
Eliminate dietary nitrogen
Purge gastrointestinal tract to remove blood and other nitrogenous compounds
Nonabsorbable antibiotics (neomycin or metronidazole)
Lactulose or lactitol
Dopamine receptor agonists
L-Dopa and bromocriptine[a]
Branched-chain amino acid[b]
Temporary liver support
Orthotopic liver transplantation

[a]Arousal effect in selected patients may be secondary to enhanced renal function.
[b]High cost and equivocal benefits of intravenous amino acid mixtures make it difficult to justify routine use.

The cathartic of choice is lactulose, a nonabsorbable disaccharide that reaches the distal ileum and colon essentially unmetabolized. Many theories regarding the mechanism of action of lactulose have been proposed. Initially, the presumed mechanism of action was that on reaching the colon, lactulose is metabolized by colonic bacteria to acidic products that lower the pH of the colon. Lowering the pH inhibits the growth of ammonia- and urea-producing bacteria and promotes the growth of *Lactobacillus,* a bacterium with little proteolytic activity.[101] The validity of this theory has been questioned. It appears now that lactulose alters the metabolism of intestinal bacteria by providing carbohydrate, which enhances the bacterial uptake of ammonia.[102] Combined with the osmotic diarrhea caused by the cathartic activities of lactulose, this effect leads to an increased excretion of ammonia.

The dosage of lactulose, 45 to 90 g/d, is administered orally, divided into three or four doses. The dosage can be adjusted to produce two or three soft stools daily. Hourly doses of 30 to 45 mL can be used to induce more rapid improvement during the initial phase of therapy. Symptoms usually abate within 24 hours, but more than 48 hours may be required. Doses can be adjusted if side effects such as flatulence, diarrhea, and electrolyte abnormalities occur.

Nonabsorbable antibiotics have also been used to decrease the number and concentration of ammonia-forming bacteria in the gut. Most experience has accrued for neomycin and metronidazole. These antibiotics are active against gram-negative anaerobes such as *Bacteroides,* which are considered to be a major source of ammonia production.[103,104] The dosage of neomycin, 2 to 8 g/d, is divided into four doses and is continued for 4 to 10 days. Multiple double-blinded, randomized trials have determined the efficacy of antibiotics alone or in combination with lactulose. For acute hepatic encephalopathy, studies have shown that neomycin for 4 days is equally as effective as lactulose,[105] and metronidazole for 7 days is as effective as neomycin.[106] In addition, for chronic hepatic encephalopathy, neomycin for 10 days was equal to lactulose.[101] Although only small amounts (1% to 3%) of neomycin are absorbed, a risk for nephrotoxicity and ototoxicity still exists.[107] Rifaximin, a macrolide antibiotic not approved for use in the United States, has similar efficacy when compared with lactulose and neomycin.[108]

PORTAL HYPERTENSION

8 Portal hypertension is defined as a portal vein pressure above the normal range of 5 to 8 mm Hg. Portal hypertension may also be defined by the hepatic vein–portal vein pressure gradient, which is greater than 5 mm Hg in portal hypertensive states.[109] Pressures in the portal venous system are usually measured indirectly via the wedged hepatic venous pressure. The technique is similar to that used to determine pulmonary capillary wedge pressure by pulmonary arterial (Swan-Ganz) catheterization.

Anatomy

The venous anatomy of the portal system is relatively constant, with the "usual" anatomy present in 98% of the population (Fig. 58.5). The portal vein is formed by the confluence of the superior mesenteric and splenic veins behind the neck of the pancreas. The inferior mesenteric vein most often joins the splenic vein before the portal vein is formed, but approximately one third of the time the inferior mesenteric vein joins the superior mesenteric vein. The superior mesenteric vein may not be present, and the portal vein may be formed by multiple small branches from the mesenteric system that join the splenic vein.

Many branches of the portal venous system are affected when portal pressure rises. As pressure increases, blood flow decreases and the pressure in the portal system is transmitted to its branches. This transmission of pressure through branches of the portal system is beneficial in that it decreases overall portal pressure. It also is responsible for many of the complications of portal hypertension, however, because of the resulting dilation of venous tributaries.

The coronary or left gastric vein becomes highly significant in portal hypertension, by diverting portal blood to the veins of the lesser curve of the stomach and the esophagus, leading to the formation of varices. Other important collaterals include the inferior mesenteric vein, which connects with its rectal branches, which, when distended, form hemorrhoids; the umbilical vein in the ligamentum teres of the falciform ligament, which joins the left portal vein and causes abdominal wall veins around the paraumbilical plexus to dilate (caput medusae); the short gastric veins, branches of the splenic vein, which communicate with gastric veins and contribute to gastric varices; and the retroperitoneal veins of Retzius, which communicate with the gastrointestinal veins through the bare areas of the liver where no peritoneal layer separates the abdominal viscera from the retroperitoneum. The retroperitoneal collaterals can also form large splenorenal shunts that may decompress the portal system but are associated with severe encephalopathy.

Physiology

As in any vascular bed, portal hypertension is the product of blood flow and resistance. In nearly all cases, portal hypertension is caused by increased resistance to portal blood flow

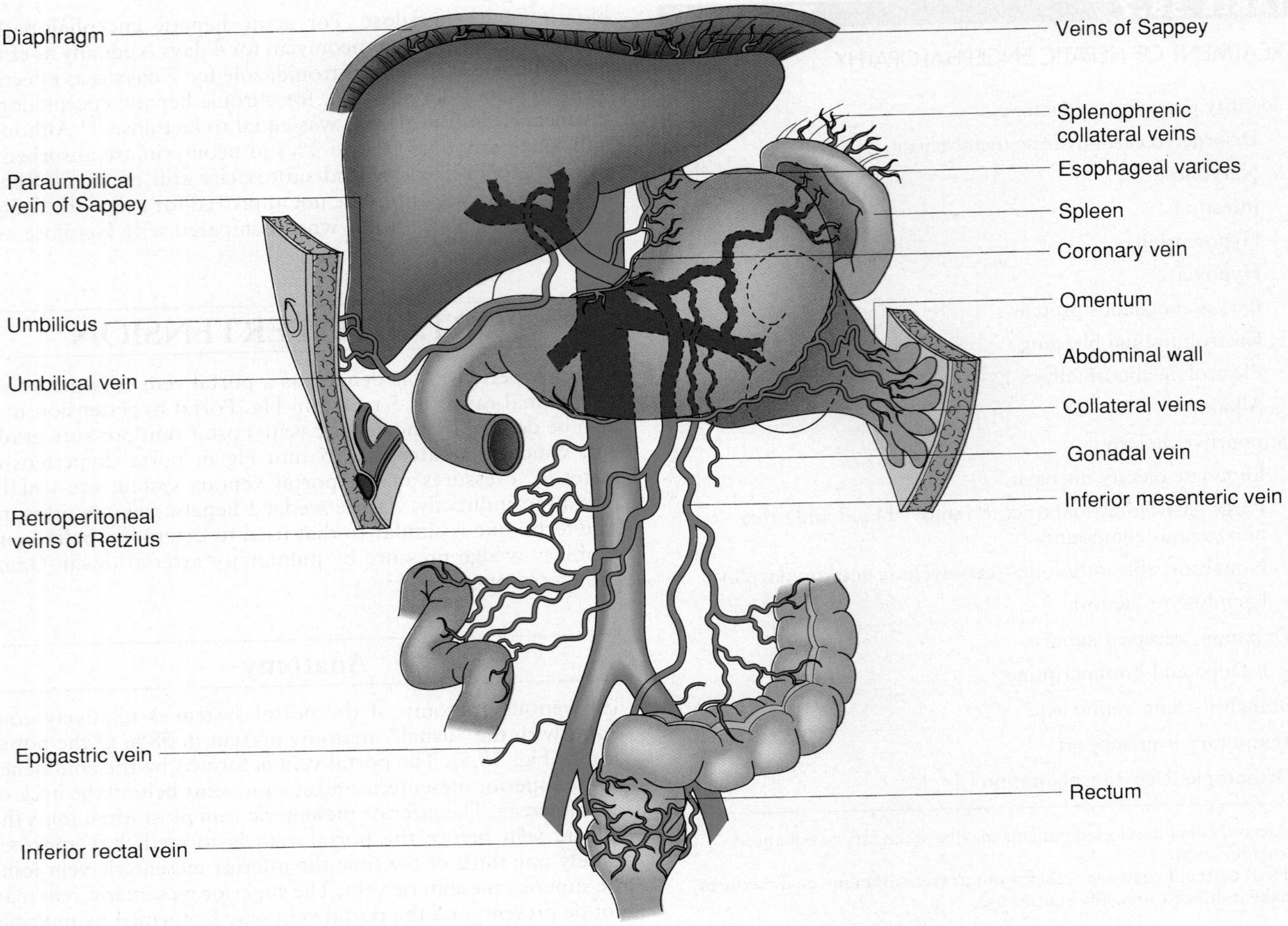

FIGURE 58.5. Potential venous collaterals that develop with portal hypertension. The veins of Sappey drain portal blood through the bare areas of the diaphragm and through paraumbilical vein collaterals to the umbilicus. The veins of Retzius form in the retroperitoneum and shunt portal blood from the bowel and other organs to the vena cava.

secondary to cirrhosis, portal vein thrombosis, or hepatic venous obstruction, though in rare instances, an arterioportal fistula may cause flow-related hypertension. Normally, the liver offers little resistance to portal flow because of the porous nature of the hepatic sinusoids and the capacity of the organ to expand. Moreover, the liver has no intrinsic control over portal blood flow; it is merely a passive recipient of splanchnic flow, the primary regulation of which occurs at the level of the splanchnic arterioles.[110] As discussed earlier, the deposition of collagen in the space of Disse (capillarization), in addition to the contractile properties of stellate cells, causes an increased resistance to portal blood flow in cirrhosis. In addition, various cytokines and hormones contribute to elevated portal pressures by inducing splanchnic vasodilation and an increase in splanchnic flow.

The increased blood flow through collateral vessels and subsequently increased venous return cause the characteristic hemodynamic features of portal hypertension, which include an increase in cardiac output and total blood volume and a decrease in systemic vascular resistance.[111] Arteriovenous shunts within the liver, stomach, and small intestine contribute to the augmented venous return and decreased peripheral vascular resistance. Early in the course of portal hypertension, blood pressure may be normal, but with progression of disease, blood pressure usually falls.[112]

The portal venous concentration of nitric oxide, a potent vasodilator, has been shown to be elevated in patients with cirrhosis and portal hypertension.[113] In addition to nitric oxide, many other vasodilators are elevated in portal hypertension, including prostacyclin, endotoxin, and glucagon.[114]

Etiology

Many pathologic processes can cause portal hypertension (Table 58.8). These are usually classified as prehepatic, hepatic, or posthepatic (presinusoidal, sinusoidal, or postsinusoidal) conditions. As noted above, in prehepatic and posthepatic conditions, portal hypertension in the result of mechanical venous obstruction at the level of the portal or hepatic veins, respectively, whereas cirrhosis is the main cause of hepatic portal hypertension.

Budd-Chiari Syndrome and Veno-occlusive Disease. The Budd-Chiari syndrome is caused by hepatic venous obstruction. The name of the syndrome is derived from two investigators, the first of whom (Budd)[115] described the classic presentation of abdominal pain, ascites, and hepatomegaly, and the second of whom (Chiari)[116] described the pathologic characteristics of the liver. The obstruction may occur at the level of the inferior vena cava, the hepatic veins, or the central veins within the liver itself and may be the result of congenital webs (most common in Africa and Asia), acute or chronic thrombosis (most common in the West), and malignancy. With occlusion of the hepatic veins, pressure increases in the central veins. As a result, centrilobular congestion, necrosis, and, with

TABLE 58.8 **ETIOLOGY**

COMMON CAUSES OF PORTAL HYPERTENSION

Disorders That Primarily Increase Resistance to Flow
Prehepatic
Congenital atresia
Extrinsic compression
Schistosomiasis
Portal, superior mesenteric, or splenic vein thrombosis
Hepatic
CHRONIC–CIRRHOTIC
Hepatitis B, C
α_1-Antitrypsin deficiency
Cryptogenic
Cystic fibrosis
Hemochromatosis
Nutritional (alcoholic)
Wilson disease
CHRONIC–NONCIRRHOTIC
Congenital hepatic fibrosis
Focal regenerative hyperplasia
Hepatic veno-occlusive disease
Idiopathic
Metastatic carcinoma
Sarcoidosis
Toxin and drug injuries
ACUTE DISEASE
Acute fatty liver
Alcoholic hepatitis
Fulminant hepatic failure
Posthepatic
Budd-Chiari syndrome
Chronic heart failure
Constrictive pericarditis
Vena cava webs
Disorders That Primarily Increase Flow
Hepatocellular carcinoma
Mesenteric arteriosclerotic or aneurysmal vascular disease
Osler-Weber-Rendu syndrome
Splenomegaly

chronic disease, fibrosis and cirrhosis with portal hypertension develop.

In the West, the most common causes of this syndrome are hypercoagulable states associated with polycythemia vera, myeloproliferative disorders, paroxysmal nocturnal hemoglobinuria, and defects in the coagulation cascade, as in conditions associated with high estrogen levels (e.g., pregnancy, use of birth control pills).[117,118] Neoplasms may cause hepatic venous obstruction by direct invasion and occlusion of the vessels, or by establishment of a prothrombotic milieu secondary to the malignancy itself. In the East, the major causes of obstruction of the vena cava and hepatic veins are membranous webs that directly occlude the vessels. The etiology of vena cava webs is unknown.

Veno-occlusive disease is characterized by obliterative endophlebitis of the intrahepatic veins (see Table 58.3). Causes of veno-occlusive disease include medications, toxins, and pyrrolizidine alkaloids.

Budd-Chiari syndrome may present with acute, subacute, or chronic symptoms and is often misdiagnosed. This is unfortunate, because early treatment will prevent the development of hepatic fibrosis, which can lead to end-stage liver disease. Nearly 50% of patients have had symptoms for more than 3 months.[119,120] Acute symptoms include hepatomegaly, right upper quadrant abdominal pain, nausea, vomiting, and ascites. In the chronic form of the disease, patients may present with the sequelae of cirrhosis and portal hypertension, including variceal bleeding, ascites, spontaneous bacterial peritonitis, fatigue, and encephalopathy. In the chronic form, the entire liver atrophies except for the caudate lobe, which may hypertrophy because its hepatic vein(s) enters the vena cava separately, so that venous outflow is not impeded.[67] The hypertrophy of the caudate lobe creates a longitudinal narrowing of the retrohepatic vena cava, which is surrounded by parenchyma, leading to secondary obstruction of the caval flow in the abdomen.

The diagnosis is most often made by ultrasonographic evaluation of the liver and its vasculature, which has a sensitivity of 85% to 95%.[117] Duplex scanning may reveal the location of the obstruction and characterize the flow within the vena cava and hepatic, portal, mesenteric, and splenic veins. Cross-sectional imaging using contrast-enhanced CT or MRI is helpful in defining the entire abdominal venous circulation and assessing the status of the liver and its individual lobes, which is essential in planning therapy. Traditionally, the "gold standard" for the diagnosis has been angiography, which provides detailed information on the location and degree of obstruction.

The management of patients with this syndrome has traditionally been surgical intervention. Liver biopsies are usually performed preoperatively. The response rates to medical therapy, which does not relieve the obstruction to portal outflow, are poor, and survival rates without surgical intervention are approximately 10%. Antithrombotic agents may be used in the rare patient who presents early with acute venous occlusion. Although major surgery has been favored in the past, including meso-atrial shunting[121,122] and even liver transplantation,[123] minimally invasive approaches are now preferred.[124] The mainstay of therapy is mechanical decompression with a side-to-side portosystemic shunt, optimally achieved with a percutaneous portocaval shunt. After shunt placement, the pressure on the vena cava by the caudate lobe is gradually relieved, leading to restoration of liver function.

A more direct solution, which is necessary in the face of complete caval obstruction, is the creation of a mesoatrial shunt, which was described by Cameron and Maddrey.[121] This radical procedure has been largely supplanted by percutaneous portocaval shunting (transjugular intrahepatic portosystemic shunt [TIPS]). The rates of postprocedural encephalopathy are usually not increased in patients with Budd-Chiari syndrome, because they have anatomically healthy livers that recover fully if decompression is achieved early prior to the establishment of cirrhosis. In patients with end-stage liver disease, liver transplantation may be performed.[123] The 5-year survival rate for patients with good hepatic function before the shunt procedure is approximately 60%, with a 34% to 88% survival for patients after liver transplantation.[125] Postoperatively, patients are treated with long-term anticoagulation to prevent recurrent thrombosis.

As noted, minimally invasive treatment using TIPS may be first-line therapy, and it has supplanted surgical shunting in our practice.[126,127] Case reports and small series have suggested efficacy for this technique,[128] and a recent larger study has indicated 1- and 5-year survival rates of 93% and 74%, respectively.[129] Many patients develop shunt occlusion, however, and further angiographic manipulation and long-term anticoagulation are required to maintain patency.

Portal Vein Thrombosis. Portal vein thrombosis is commonly associated with advanced cirrhosis, and may be the ominous portent of a hepatocellular carcinoma. Spontaneous portal vein thrombosis in the absence of cirrhosis is the cause of portal hypertension in fewer than 10% of adult patients but is the most common cause in children.[130] In contrast to patients with cirrhosis-induced portal hypertension, these patients have normal liver function and are not as susceptible to the development of complications, such as encephalopathy. Causes of portal vein thrombosis include umbilical vein infection (the most common cause in children), coagulopathies (protein C and antithrombin III deficiency), hepatic malignancy, myeloproliferative disorders, inflammatory bowel disease, pancreatitis, trauma, and previous splenorenal shunt.[131] Most cases in adults are idiopathic.

The diagnosis can be made by sonography, which reveals an echogenic lesion in the lumen of the portal vein and an absence of portal venous flow on duplex examination.[132] With time, cavernous transformation of the portal vein may occur, in which channels develop within the clotted portal vein.[130] CT and MRI are also useful in establishing the diagnosis. Often, the initial manifestation of portal vein thrombosis is variceal bleeding in a noncirrhotic patient with normal liver function. Splenomegaly is another common finding.

The initial therapeutic option for the control of hemorrhage caused by portal vein thrombosis is esophageal variceal ligation. If unsuccessful, the distal splenorenal shunt has been the traditional surgical treatment for patients with isolated portal vein thrombosis. In patients whose intrahepatic portal vein is patent (most commonly children), however, a shunt created by placing an internal jugular vein graft between the superior mesenteric vein and the patent left portal vein within the parenchyma of the liver (Rex shunt) may be the optimal therapeutic procedure for reestablishing physiologic portal flow.[133] This is the most elegant solution for portal obstruction because the portal pressure is reduced by restoring blood flow to the liver, preventing chronic hepatic atrophy and dysfunction, which can occur in a patient with long-standing portal decompression. In fact, in our practice, the Rex shunt is the first-line treatment and we reserve splenorenal shunting for patients who have no remnant intrahepatic portal system to receive the shunted blood.

Splenic Vein Thrombosis. Splenic vein thrombosis is most often caused by disorders of the pancreas, including acute and chronic pancreatitis, trauma, pancreatic malignancy, and pseudocysts. This association is related to the location of the splenic vein behind and close to the pancreas. Other causes include retroperitoneal masses, abscesses, and inflammatory bowel disease; the remaining cases are idiopathic. Gastric varices are present in approximately 80% of patients, and esophageal varices in 30% to 40%.[134] Isolated "sinistral" or left-sided portal hypertension occurs in the setting of normal liver function, and patients are readily cured with splenectomy, although observation for asymptomatic patients is acceptable. The main indication for splenectomy is variceal hemorrhage.

Complications of Portal Hypertension

The most important complications of portal hypertension are gastrointestinal bleeding secondary to esophageal and gastric varices, ascites, and hepatic encephalopathy. The mortality risk associated with portal hypertension is primarily related to the functional status of the cirrhotic liver. Child introduced a scoring system of liver function for the purposes of assessing prognosis after portosystemic shunt surgery in patients with cirrhosis, which has been subsequently modified several times
9 to the *Child-Turcotte-Pugh (CTP) score* (Table 58.9). These indices incorporate clinical and laboratory data as a means to assess the functional status of the liver, estimate hepatic reserve, and predict morbidity and mortality. They had been adopted by the United Network for Organ Sharing (UNOS) as a tool for stratifying pretransplant mortality risk for patients on the waiting list for liver transplantation.[135] Over the last decade, the use of these criteria in transplant have been replaced by the Model for End-stage Liver Disease (MELD)

TABLE 58.9 **CLASSIFICATION**

CHILD-TURCOTTE CRITERIA FOR HEPATIC FUNCTIONAL RESERVE

CRITERION	CLASS A	CLASS B	CLASS C
Encephalopathy	None	Minimal	Advanced
Ascites	None	Easily controlled	Poorly controlled
Bilirubin (mg/dL)	<2	2–3	>3
Albumin (g/gL)	>3.5	3–3.5	<3
Nutrition	Excellent	Good	Poor, "wasting"
Child-Turcotte-Pugh Grading of Severity of Liver Disease			
Score	1	2	3
Encephalopathy	None	1 or 2	3 or 4
Ascites	None	Mild	Moderate
Bilirubin (mg/dL)	1–2	2.1–3	≥3.1
Albumin (g/dL)	≥3.5	2.8–3.5	≤2.7
Prothrombin time (s)	1–4	4.1–6	≥6.1
or INR	<1.7	1.7–2.3	>2.3
Grade A, 5–6; grade B, 7–9; grade C, 10–15			

INR, international normalized ratio.
From Wantz GE, Payne MA. Experience with portacaval shunt for portal hypertension. *N Engl J Med* 1961;265:721, with permission.

score, which uses serum bilirubin, creatinine, and the international normalized ratio (INR) to produce a surprisingly robust prediction of 90-day mortality for patients with cirrhosis on the transplant list.[136] Though the CTP score produces a more complete assessment of the patient, its use of subjective clinical elements in the score made it unreliable as a verifiable element in assessment compliance with center behavior in national organ transplant policy.[137,138]

While the MELD score was initially developed for the prognosis of patients after TIPS, the CTP score has had long-standing use as a reliable predictor of mortality risk for shunt surgery and, by extension, mortality risk of patients with cirrhosis undergoing other types of abdominal surgery.[139,140] Patients with normal function, termed "Child A," have adequate hepatic reserve and survival rates similar to those of noncirrhotic patients, whereas Child C patients have mortality rates in excess of 50% and may not tolerate any intervention short of hepatic transplantation.

Varices. One of the most life-threatening complications of portal hypertension is bleeding from esophageal varices. Esophageal varices are dilated veins found most commonly in the distal 5 cm of the esophagus. In the normal esophagus, a venous plexus is located in the submucosa; it becomes more superficially located to the lamina propria in the distal esophagus.[141–143] This more superficial location in the distal esophagus is consistent with the known increased occurrence of bleeding varices in that location. In addition, 10% to 15% of patients with esophageal varices have gastric varices.

The pressure in the portal system is an important determinant of the likelihood for varices to develop. As noted earlier, portal pressure may be estimated from the hepatic vein wedge pressure, and the gradient between the wedge pressure and the free hepatic vein pressure is an indirect measure of the resistance across the liver. In general, varices do not develop in persons with hepatic vein–portal vein gradients below 12 mm Hg. Pressure gradients above 12 mm Hg are invariably present in patients with varices, but this pressure does not necessarily produce varices in all patients. Other, undetermined factors must play a role. The prevalence of varices in patients with cirrhosis varies from 25% to 70%, depending on the severity of their liver disease.

In approximately 10% of all patients presenting with acute upper gastrointestinal bleeding, esophageal varices are the cause of bleeding. Rates of bleeding from varices vary among studies. In a study of the natural history of varices in which patients were prospectively followed for 6 years, esophageal varices developed in approximately 8% of patients with cirrhosis each year during the first 2 years of observation; the percentage increased to 30% by 6 years. Of the patients who had small varices detected at initial endoscopy, large varices developed in 25%.[144] Other studies show an incidence of varices of up to 90% for patients with cirrhosis.[145,146] Once varices are present, bleeding occurs in 25% to 35% of cases, with the highest risk occurring within the first year after diagnosis.[146,147] Of patients who survive an episode of bleeding, 30% experience rebleeding within 6 weeks, and 70% at 1 year.[147,148] The correlation between severity of varices and derangement of hepatic function is inconstant, so mortality rates from bleeding varices range from 5% to 50%, with rates of 5%, less than 25%, and more than 50% for Child A, B, and C patients, respectively.[148]

The propensity for varices to bleed has been extensively studied. When combined with clinical data such as the presence of active alcohol consumption, certain endoscopic characteristics of varices have been correlated with initial episodes of bleeding (Table 58.10). These factors include variceal size, Child-Pugh class, and the presence of red wale markings (longitudinal dilated venules that resemble whip marks).[146] Direct and indirect measurements of portal pressure have been used

TABLE 58.10

ENDOSCOPIC SIGNS THAT CORRELATE WITH RISK FOR VARICEAL RUPTURE

Basic Color
White varices
Blue varices
Signs
Red color sign
Red wale marking
Cherry-red spot
Hematocystic spot
Diffuse redness
Form
Linear
Tortuous
Large

Adapted from Japanese Research Society for Portal Hypertension.

to predict the likelihood of bleeding, with hemorrhage occurring only in patients with portal–hepatic venous gradients above 12 mm Hg.[149,150]

Prevention of Initial Variceal Bleeding. Because of the severe consequences of variceal bleeding, methods to prevent first (primary prophylaxis) and recurrent (secondary prophylaxis) episodes of bleeding have been developed. These include control of the underlying cause of cirrhosis (i.e., alcohol consumption) and pharmacologic and surgical interventions to lower portal pressure. The next section discusses methods of primary prophylaxis to prevent initial episodes of bleeding (Table 58.11).

Beta Blockade. Use of nonspecific β-adrenergic blockade has been studied extensively in randomized controlled trials of the primary prophylaxis of variceal bleeding. The mechanism of action of these drugs (propranolol, nadolol) involves effects of both β_1-adrenergic and β_2-adrenergic blockade, including decreased cardiac output and increased splanchnic arteriolar vasoconstriction as a result of the loss of opposing β_2-adrenergic dilation.[150,151] The combined effects decrease portal blood flow and subsequently portal pressure.

These drugs are effective in portal hypertension associated with prehepatic, intrahepatic, and posthepatic conditions,[152] regardless of whether ascites is present.[153] Not all patients respond to therapy, however. Two meta-analyses have evaluated seven randomized controlled trials comparing propranolol or nadolol with placebo in the prevention of initial variceal bleeding. Both analyses concluded that beta blockade is significantly correlated with a reduced incidence of bleeding.[154,155] A reduction of 40% was noted overall after all trial results were combined, with bleeding developing in approximately 16% of treated and 27% of untreated patients. The goal of therapy is to reduce the hepatic vein–portal vein gradient to below 12 mm Hg or to more than 20% below baseline.[156]

In addition to reducing the number of first episodes of bleeding, beta blockade therapy has been shown to reduce mortality in most clinical trials.[157] However, the differences were significant in only one study. A meta-analysis of these studies concluded that mortality from bleeding is reduced in patients with large varices.

TABLE 58.11 TREATMENT

PREVENTION/TREATMENT OPTIONS FOR VARICEAL BLEEDING

DRUG	DOSE
Propranolol	10–20 mg bid titrated weekly to maximum of 160 mg bid
Nadolol	20 mg orally qd, titrated to reduction of HR by 20%–25%, absolute HR of 55–60, symptoms
Isosorbide-5-mononitrate	20 mg orally tid
Vasopressin with nitroglycerin	0.4 U/min to maximum of 1.0 U/min, titrated to maintain SBP at approximately 100 mm Hg
Octreotide	50-mg bolus, followed by 50 mg/h for 5 d or until definitive treatment

HR, heart rate; SBP, systolic blood pressure.
Adapted from Rikkers LF. Variceal hemorrhage: surgical therapy. *Gastroenterol Clin North Am* 1993; 22(4):821–842.

Nitrates. Organic nitrates such as isosorbide-5-mononitrate, a vasodilator, have been used to reduce portal pressures. The possible mechanisms of action may include the following: (a) reflex splanchnic vasoconstriction secondary to peripheral venodilation and venous pooling; (b) decreased collateral resistance by arterial vasodilation; and (c) decreased intrahepatic resistance, possibly as a result of inhibition of stellate cell contractility.[158] These agents may be used alone in patients with contraindications to beta-blocker therapy, such as chronic obstructive pulmonary disease and congestive heart failure, or in combination with beta blockade in patients who do not have contraindications but respond inadequately to beta-blocker therapy alone. Studies have indicated an enhanced reduction of portal pressure and a decreased incidence of bleeding in patients who receive combination therapy.[159] In the only study that compared combination therapy with beta-blocker therapy alone, approximately 8% of patients treated with the combined regimen experienced bleeding, compared with 18% of patients treated with beta-blocker therapy alone.[160] Thus, combination therapy may become the mainstay for prevention of bleeding in cirrhotic patients with varices.

Surgical Intervention. In the 1950s and 1960s, surgeons created prophylactic portosystemic shunts in an attempt to prevent variceal bleeding. These procedures were studied in a randomized controlled fashion and, although effective in preventing variceal bleeding, they caused an increased incidence of hepatic failure and encephalopathy and had no effect on overall survival.[160,161] These results provided clinical support for the notion that portal diversion accelerated the decline of liver function in patients with cirrhosis and they are no longer performed for this indication.

Endoscopic Sclerotherapy and Variceal Ligation. In the past, prophylactic sclerotherapy to prevent variceal bleeding was an accepted practice. An increased mortality in alcoholic patients treated with sclerotherapy, however, has been seen. Technical challenges of endoscopic sclerotherapy (ES) and esophageal and pulmonary complications have led to abandonment of ES for the primary prevention of variceal bleeding. Initial investigations of the effectiveness of endoscopic variceal ligation (EVL) as a method of primary prophylaxis to prevent initial bleeding in high-risk patients with esophageal varices reported mixed results.[162,163] In one study, no statistically significant differences in the incidence of initial bleeding and mortality were found in a comparison of patients after variceal ligation with controls,[164] though subgroup analysis revealed a significant decrease in the incidence of initial bleeding for Child-Pugh class B patients.[163] Furthermore, there seems to be a significant prognostic divergence related to variceal size. As data have accumulated, consensus recommendations regarding prophylaxis have emerged as presented in recent practice guidelines from the American Association for the Study of Liver Diseases (AASLD). Briefly summarized, patients with cirrhosis with small, low-risk varices should be managed with beta-blocker prophylaxis. Variceal ligation may be most appropriately indicated in primary prophylaxis in patients who do not tolerate beta-blocker therapy. Patients with high-risk varices need to be managed with pharmacologic protection supplemented by EVL, and the specific protocol of variceal obliteration is proposed in the guidelines.[164]

Treatment of Esophageal Variceal Bleeding

Initial Management. Initial management of the patient with acute variceal bleeding includes the following: (a) establishment and maintenance of an airway; (b) hemodynamic monitoring; (c) placement of large-bore intravenous lines; (d) full laboratory investigation, including measurement of hemoglobin and hematocrit, coagulation profile, liver function tests, measurement of electrolytes, and assessment of renal function; (e) administration of blood products as needed, including packed red cells, platelets, and fresh frozen plasma; and (f) intensive care unit monitoring.

Pharmacologic Therapy. Administration of vasoactive medications can be commenced almost immediately after patient presentation if the history and physical findings suggest variceal bleeding. This practice decreases the rate of bleeding and enhances the endoscopic ability to visualize the site(s) of bleeding.

Vasopressin (antidiuretic hormone) has potent splanchnic vasoconstrictive properties that decrease portal venous and collateral flow and reduce portal pressure. In randomized prospective trials, as well as in a meta-analysis, continuous intravenous administration of vasopressin has proved to reduce variceal bleeding, an observation initially made in 1962.[165–167] When vasopressin was compared with placebo, bleeding stopped in an average of 52% of patients who received vasopressin and 18% of patients who received placebo. Rates of rebleeding as high as 45% were noted, however. Because of coronary vasoconstrictive effects, vasopressin is often used in combination with a vasodilator, such as nitroglycerin. The combination provides protection from adverse cardiac events and increases the effectiveness of vasopressin by decreasing intrahepatic and collateral resistance.[168] A meta-analysis of three randomized controlled trials confirmed the

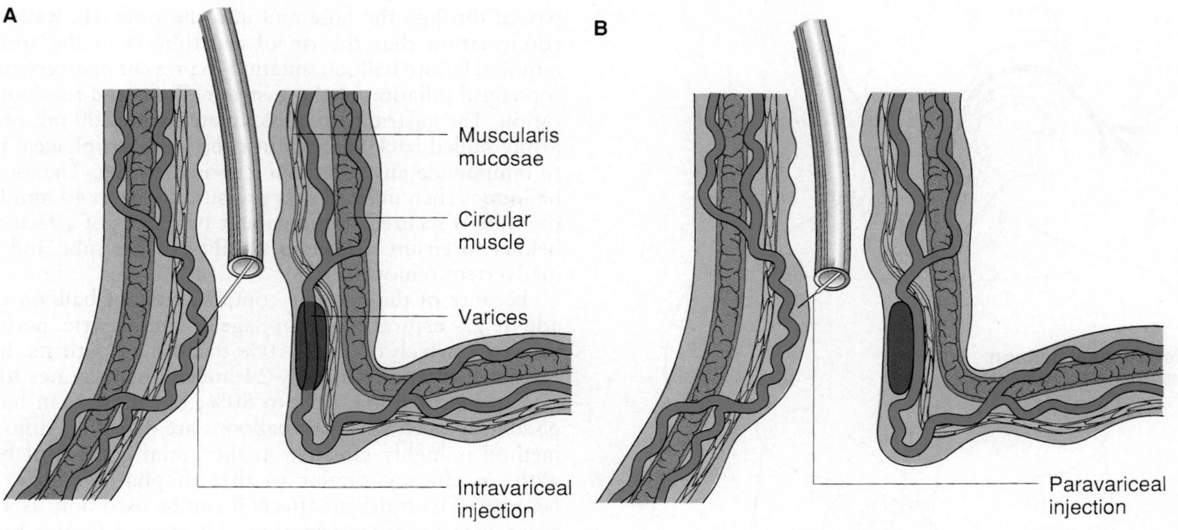

FIGURE 58.6. Techniques of intravariceal (**A**) and paravariceal (**B**) injection of esophageal varices.

increased effectiveness of vasopressin and nitroglycerin in comparison with vasopressin alone.[169] Somatostatin and octreotide, its longer-acting eight-amino-acid derivative, have been used extensively for the treatment of variceal bleeding. These agents decrease splanchnic blood flow indirectly by reducing the levels of other factors, such as glucagon, vasoactive intestinal peptide, and substance P, rather than by direct vasoconstriction.[170] The effects of somatostatin are limited to the splanchnic circulation, so that side effects are minimized.[171] A somatostatin and octreotide combination has proved to be as effective as vasopressin, sclerotherapy, and balloon tamponade in multiple studies.[172–174] Because of the lack of complications related to somatostatin therapy, octreotide is the initial drug of choice for the treatment of acute variceal hemorrhage.

Endoscopic Interventions. Esophageal variceal ligation has become the principal approach to the initial control and ongoing treatment of variceal bleeding; it is performed at the bedside in acute bleeding and has replaced variceal sclerosis in recent years. The technique of sclerotherapy (Fig. 58.6) entails performing upper gastrointestinal endoscopy with a flexible endoscope, visualizing the varices, and injecting 1 to 5 mL of sclerosing agent into or in close proximity to each varix. Sclerosing agents include sodium morrhuate, ethanolamine, polidocanol, and sodium tetradecyl sulfate. Total injection volume is 20 to 30 mL. The injections are begun at the distal esophagus and are continued circumferentially and proximally until all clinically relevant varices have been injected. Complications of sclerotherapy occur in 10% to 30% of patients and include fever, retrosternal chest pain (most common), dysphagia, and, more significantly, perforation with mediastinitis, bleeding from sclerosant-induced ulcers, esophageal stenosis, and sepsis. Overall, the treatment-related mortality rate is less than 2%. In the approximately 1% of patients in whom perforation occurs, the mortality rate may be as high as 50%. Success rates for initial control of variceal bleeding by endoscopy range from 60% to 90%, but more than one session is required to stop bleeding completely in up to 95% of cases.[175,176]

The technique of ligation (Fig. 58.7) includes placing an endoscope over a sheath (which allows multiple insertions and removal of the endoscope), suctioning of a varix into the lumen of a plastic channel, and then placing a rubber band around the tissue. The procedure is similar to the ligation of hemorrhoids. The tissue then sloughs in 1 to 3 days, leaving a shallow ulcer. Up to six bands can be placed at each session. Newer endoscopes allow for the placement of multiple bands without removal of the endoscope. The placement of bands follows the same pattern as in sclerotherapy.

Success rates for variceal ligation range from 80% to 100%, in comparison with 77% to 94% for sclerotherapy, in controlled trials.[177] A meta-analysis that examined these data and compared the results of seven randomized controlled trials indicated an equal or better success rate for variceal ligation than for sclerotherapy in eliminating esophageal variceal bleeding, with fewer complications. When patients who underwent ligation therapy were compared with patients who underwent sclerotherapy, a reduction of approximately 50% in the incidence of rebleeding (50% vs. 25%) and death from bleeding (17% vs. 10%) and a reduction of 30% in overall

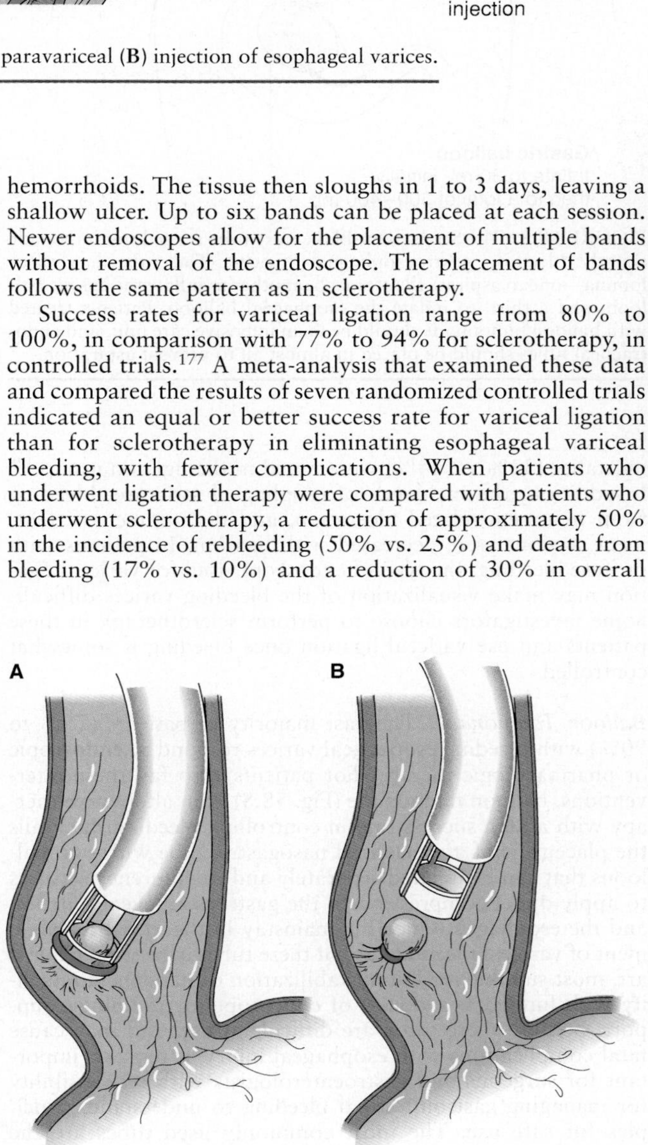

FIGURE 58.7. Endoscopic ligation of esophageal varices. The device used for ligation is based on the standard Barron-type ligator for the treatment of anal hemorrhoids. The esophageal varix is drawn up into the ligating device with suction (**A**), and the base of the varix is ligated with an O-ring (**B**). Up to six varices can be treated at a single session.

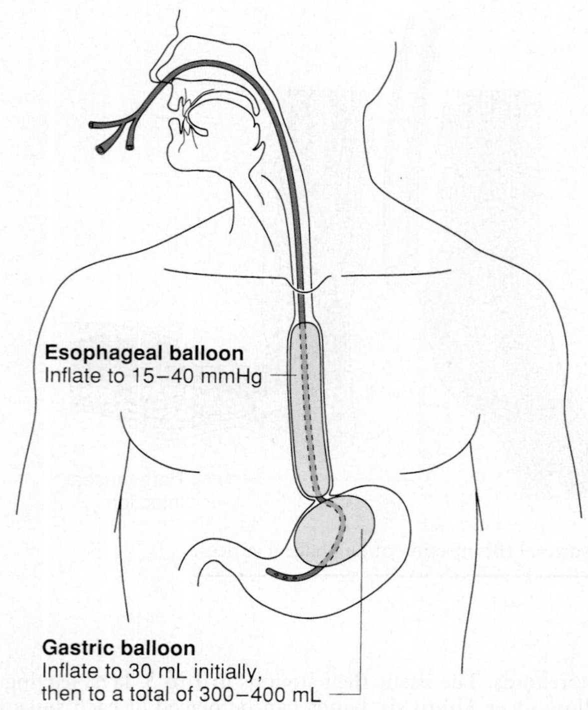

FIGURE 58.8. The Sengstaken-Blakemore tube is used to tamponade acutely bleeding gastroesophageal varices. The tube has three lumina—one to aspirate the stomach, another to inflate the gastric balloon, and a third to inflate the esophageal balloon. Patients treated with balloon tamponade should be in an intensive care unit, and endotracheal tubes should be placed in almost all to prevent aspiration.

mortality (32% vs. 24%) were noted in the ligation group.[178] In addition, the incidence of esophageal stricture, bleeding from treatment-related ulceration, and the number of treatment sessions were decreased with ligation. In patients with profuse bleeding, the type of endoscope used for variceal ligation may make visualization of the bleeding varices difficult. Some investigators choose to perform sclerotherapy in these patients and use variceal ligation once bleeding is somewhat controlled.

Balloon Tamponade. The vast majority of patients (75% to 90%) with bleeding esophageal varices respond to endoscopic or pharmacologic therapy. For patients who fail these interventions, balloon tamponade (Fig. 58.8) is an alternative therapy with a high success rate in controlling bleeding. It entails the placement of a specialized nasogastric tube with two balloons that can be inflated separately and to different pressures to apply direct compression to the gastroesophageal junction and the esophagus. Once the mainstay in the initial management of variceal bleeding, use of these tubes is becoming a lost art, most suitable for initial stabilization of patients in a facility with limited availability of endoscopic or radiologic support. Because these tubes are difficult to use, and may cause fatal complications with esophageal injury, it remains important for surgeons and gastroenterologists with responsibility for managing gastrointestinal bleeding to understand principles for safe use. The most commonly used tubes are the Sengstaken-Blakemore tube and the Minnesota tube. The former consists of a gastric balloon and an esophageal balloon with a sump port for gastric suctioning. The latter tube has an additional port above the esophageal balloon for the aspiration of saliva and other material from the esophagus and pharynx.

Placement of these tubes begins with the establishment of a safe airway by endotracheal intubation. The tube is then passed through the nose and into the stomach. Radiographic confirmation that the tip of the tube is in the stomach is required before balloon inflation to prevent inadvertent intraesophageal inflation of the gastric balloon and resultant perforation. The gastric balloon is inflated with 200 mL of air and firmly pulled backward against the gastroesophageal junction to tamponade any proximal gastric bleeding. The esophageal balloon is then inflated to a pressure of 30 to 40 mm Hg, and the tube is secured to the patient by means of a face mask or helmet to ensure adequate stability of the tube and prevent inadvertent removal.

Because of the possible complications of balloon tamponade (e.g., aspiration, esophageal and gastric perforation, necrosis), which occur in 10% to 20% of patients, its use is restricted to approximately 24 hours. Success rates for cessation of bleeding are 70% to 80%, but more than half of all patients rebleed when the balloons are deflated. Although this method is highly effective in the initial control of bleeding, with an efficacy similar to that of pharmacologic agents, because of its transient effects it can be used only as a temporizing measure in anticipation of a more definitive procedure (e.g., TIPS, placement of a surgical shunt, or transplantation) and is used only after endoscopic and pharmacologic therapies have failed.

Transjugular Intrahepatic Portosystemic Shunt. In the 10% to 20% of patients who continue to bleed or who have early rebleeding, a shunt procedure (to bypass the high-pressure hepatic vascular bed) may be indicated. The mortality rate associated with failure to control bleeding can be as high as 90%, and surgically created shunts in this setting are associated with a high morbidity and mortality rate.

The transjugular intrahepatic portosystemic shunt (Fig. 58.9) has become first-line treatment for bleeding esophageal varices when the aforementioned attempts fail.[179] After ultrasonographic confirmation of patency of the portal vein, the procedure is performed in the interventional radiology suite, where a wire-guided stent (8 to 12 mm in diameter) is placed percutaneously into the jugular vein. The wire is then guided through the superior vena cava, right atrium, and inferior vena cava into a hepatic vein, after which the catheter traverses the hepatic parenchyma and joins the hepatic vein to a portal vein. This connection effectively creates a side-to-side portacaval shunt. Success rates in the cessation of variceal bleeding are as high as 90% to 100%, with an incidence of recurrent bleeding of approximately 10%.[180,181]

As discussed earlier, the ideal portosystemic shunt lowers the pressure in the portal system without critically reducing liver perfusion, which may cause hepatic dysfunction and may accelerate the progression of cirrhosis. It is possible to readily measure the portal pressure during TIPS, and many authors have proposed these measurements as a guide to optimal management of the TIPS to balance control of bleeding with hepatic perfusion. To control bleeding, the therapeutic goal is to reduce the hepatic–portal venous pressure gradient to below 12 mm Hg. TIPS reduces the portosystemic pressure gradient to a mean of approximately 9 to 15 mm Hg (average, 10 mm Hg) or to 40% to 62% below baseline.[182–184] A recent study has indicated that a residual portal gradient less than 5 mm Hg is associated with a deleterious impact on hepatic flow.[185] Earlier studies documented high mortality (40% to 60% at 6 to 7 weeks) despite the relative noninvasiveness of the procedure, reflecting the gravity of the clinical condition of most patients requiring this intervention. One potential cause of the high mortality is a delay in instituting TIPS until multiple unsuccessful attempts at sclerotherapy or banding have been made. Since well-validated instruments predict the survival of patients after TIPS, the procedure should be used with caution in patients with high MELD scores, though TIPS has been used successfully to bridge patients to transplantation.[186,187] The use of TIPS in massive variceal bleeding in a patient with a high

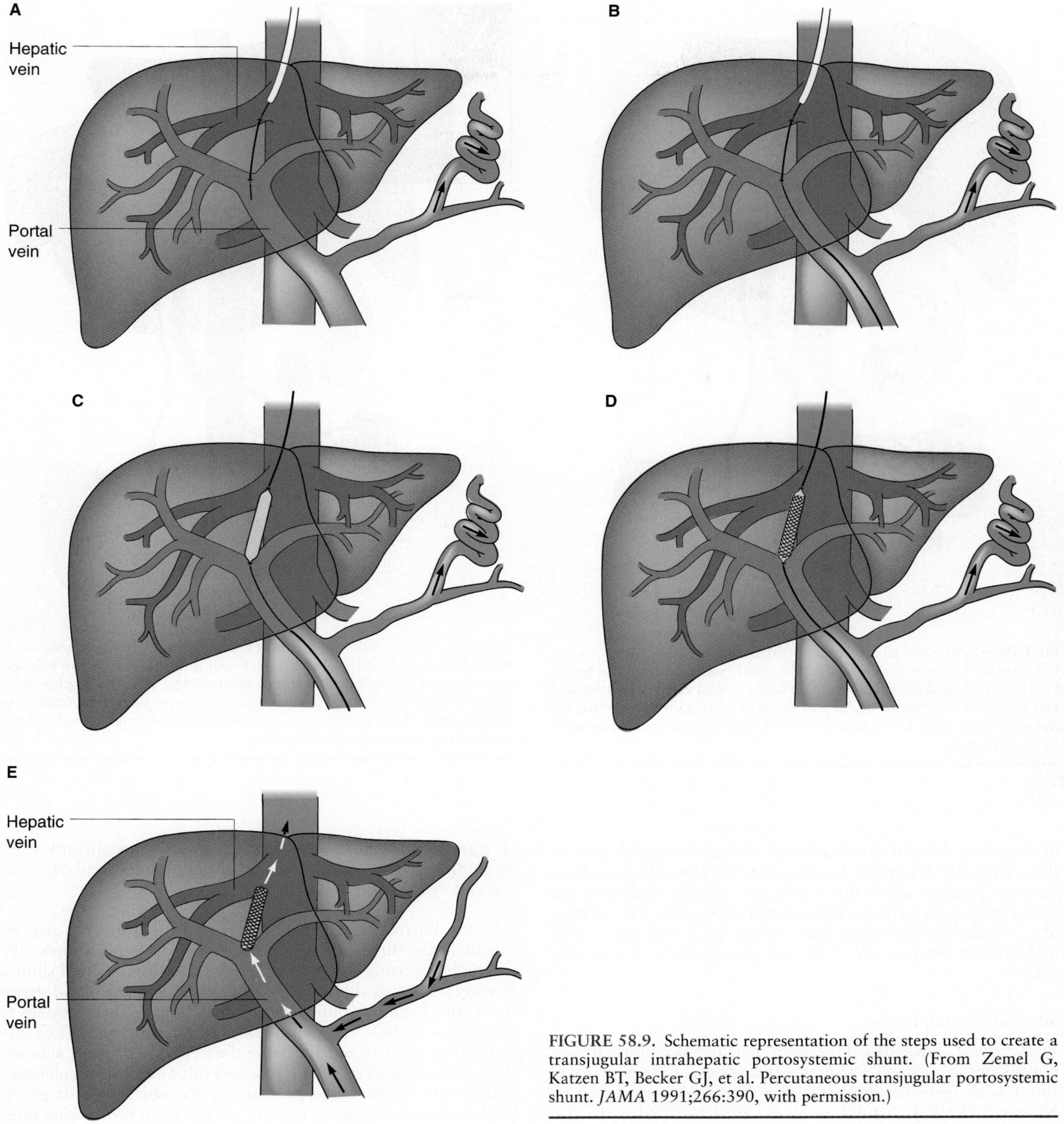

FIGURE 58.9. Schematic representation of the steps used to create a transjugular intrahepatic portosystemic shunt. (From Zemel G, Katzen BT, Becker GJ, et al. Percutaneous transjugular portosystemic shunt. *JAMA* 1991;266:390, with permission.)

MELD score who has contraindications to liver transplant should be regarded as a palliative intervention.

As with all portosystemic shunts, a significant complication of TIPS is the development of hepatic encephalopathy. After placement of a TIPS, the incidence of hepatic encephalopathy rises from 10% before treatment to 25%,[188] and the incidence of progression to accelerated liver failure is approximately 3% to 5%.

Although in early series stenoses or occlusion of the stent developed in up to 50% to 60% of patients in the first year, long-term patency can be maintained by ongoing surveillance of the shunt with redilatation, as needed. Shunt stenosis is managed angiographically with thrombolytic therapy, dilation, or replacement of the stent. The newest shunts are lined with polytetrafluoroethylene (PTFE) and have a much higher patency than the original permeable Wallstents.[189] Patients are usually followed at 3-month intervals by ultrasonography to
10 assess the patency of the shunt. At 6 months of follow-up, 92% of patients had had no episodes of rebleeding, and 82% were free of hemorrhage at 1 year. It is safe to assert that the TIPS is now the standard procedure used to halt bleeding in patients who fail medical therapy. The ability to effectively

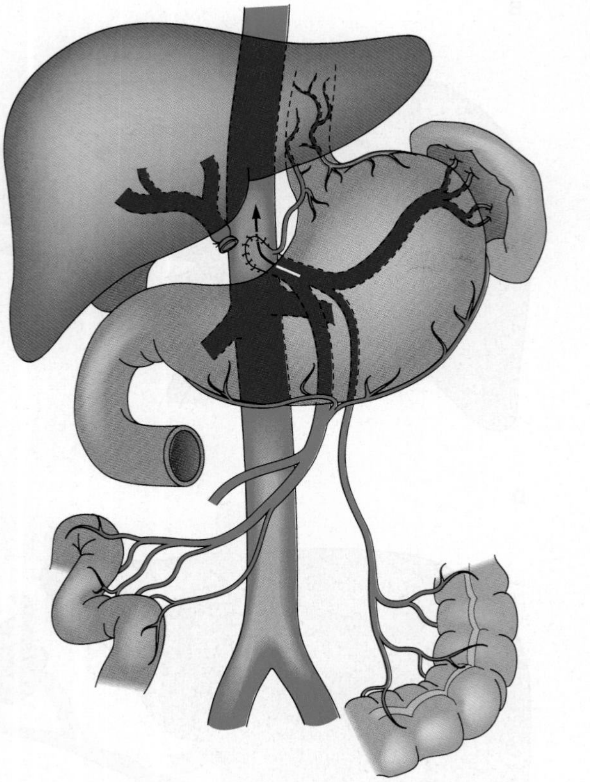

FIGURE 58.10. End-to-side portacaval shunt, also referred to as an Eck fistula. The portal vein is divided, the hepatic limb of the portal vein is ligated, and the splanchnic end of the portal vein is anastomosed end to side to the vena cava. All portal blood is necessarily diverted into the vena cava, and the hepatic limb of the portal vein cannot serve as an outflow tract.

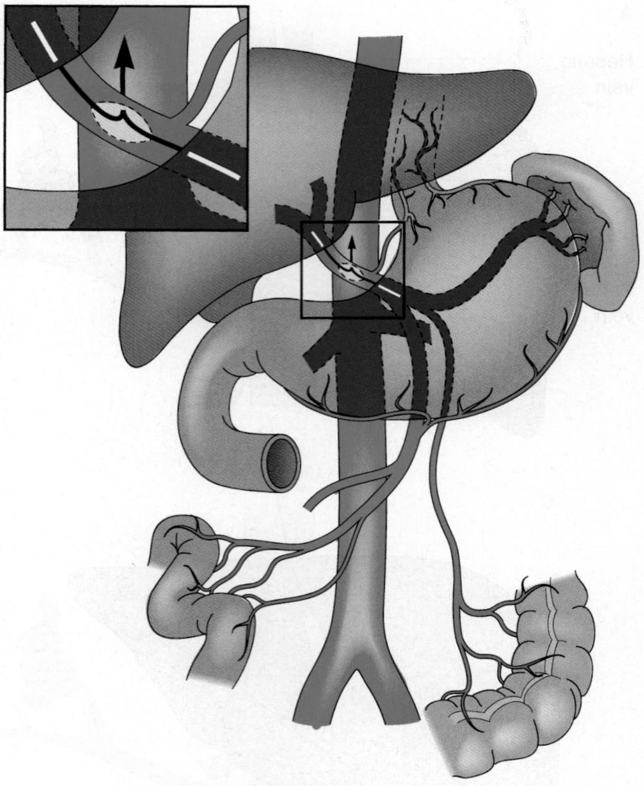

FIGURE 58.11. Side-to-side portacaval shunt. An anastomosis is made between the side of the portal vein and the side of the inferior vena cava. With a shunt of standard diameter, almost all splanchnic blood is diverted around the liver into the low-pressure vena cava. The hepatic limb of the portal vein serves as an outflow tract from the liver toward the low-pressure vena cava.

decompress the portal circulation without open surgery in these critically ill patients has transformed clinical hepatology. Patients become medically stable and can be evaluated for transplantation electively. Patients with reversible liver disease (e.g., abstinent alcoholics) may recover fully without further intervention because the TIPS will slowly close as the liver heals.

Surgical Decompression

Background. Surgeons have been performing shunt procedures since the 1800s. The first was an end-to-side portacaval shunt with ligation of the distal portal vein, performed by Nicolai Eck (Eck fistula) in dogs. In 1945, Whipple and Blakemore at the Columbia-Presbyterian Medical Center in New York performed this shunt for the first time for the indication of variceal bleeding.[190] This group was also responsible for the development of the tube for the tamponade of bleeding esophageal varices, which adopted the name of Blakemore, as discussed previously.

11 Surgical interventions for the treatment of bleeding varices are divided into three main types: (a) liver transplantation, (b) shunt procedures, and (c) devascularization procedures. The only definitive procedure for the treatment of portal hypertension caused by cirrhosis is orthotopic liver transplantation, and the success of this option during the past two decades has revolutionized the treatment of portal hypertension and its complications in patients with end-stage liver disease. However, for the treatment of portal hypertension in patients without cirrhosis or in those whose liver function does not warrant a transplant (e.g., patients with portal vein thrombosis), decompressive surgically created shunts or devascularization procedures may be performed.

Shunts. Portosystemic shunts created operatively can be divided into three categories: (a) totally diverting shunts, (b) partially diverting shunts, and (c) selective shunts. Total shunts are created by completely bypassing the flow of blood away from the liver by joining the portal vein to the vena cava. Examples include the end-to-side portacaval shunt (Eck fistula) (Fig. 58.10) and the large-diameter (>10 mm) side-to-side portacaval (Fig. 58.11), mesocaval, and central splenorenal shunts. Because the pressure in the portal vein is much higher than that in the vena cava (or the renal vein), large side-to-side shunts divert all blood flow through the path of least resistance, so that flow in the portal vein is reversed, creating "hepatofugal" flow, out of the liver and decreasing total hepatic perfusion. One of the causes of ascites in patients with portal hypertension is high pressure at the level of the hepatic sinusoids with protein-rich fluid leaking directly out of the swollen liver. The main difference between end-to-side and side-to-side shunts is that maintenance of high pressure with end-to-side shunts may worsen ascites, whereas side-to-side procedures effectively relieve this problem by reducing sinusoidal pressure. Complete portal blood flow diversion lowers portal pressure and is highly effective in the treatment of bleeding esophageal varices but, as noted earlier, may accelerate hepatic decompensation.

The main complications of totally diverting shunts are a worsening of liver function and hepatic encephalopathy as a

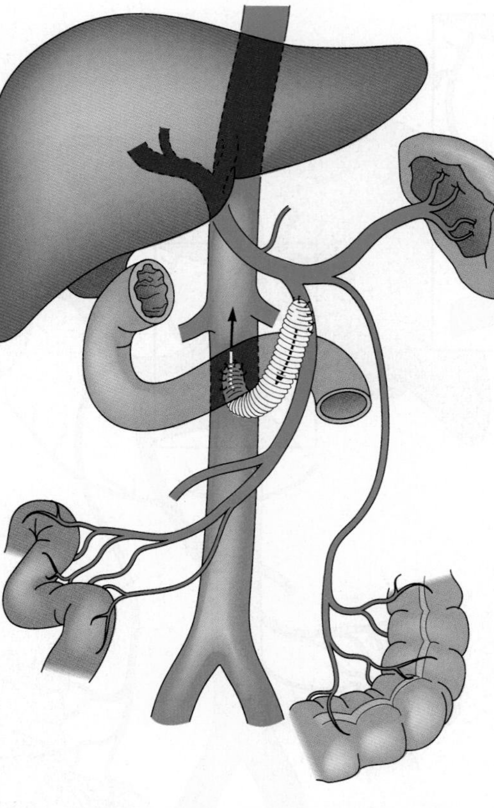

FIGURE 58.12. Interposition mesocaval shunt. A plastic prosthesis or an autogenous internal jugular vein is used for the shunt. One end is anastomosed to the inferior vena cava, and the other end is anastomosed to the trunk of the superior mesenteric vein. The shunt curves around the lower edge of the third portion of the duodenum and is sometimes called a C-shunt.

result of decreased flow through the liver and loss of hepatotropic factors from the mesenteric venous system. Another disadvantage of portocaval shunts is that the porta hepatis must be dissected, so that future surgical procedures in the area (e.g., liver transplantation) are more difficult.

Partially diverting shunts allow for the maintenance of hepatopetal flow while decompressing the high pressures in the portal system. The original shunts were larger than 10 mm in diameter and were able to create a gradient between the portal vein and vena cava that maintained some prograde hepatic flow. All these shunts, however, dilated over time and became complete shunts in that the portal vein–to–inferior vena cava pressure gradient disappeared. The small-diameter (8-mm) side-to-side mesocaval (Fig. 58.12) and portacaval (Sarfeh) (Fig. 58.13) shunts are performed with an interposition graft made of either expanded PTFE or Dacron. A significant component of the Sarfeh procedure is ligation of the coronary (left gastric), gastroepiploic, and other collateral veins. Bleeding from varices resolves in more than 90% of patients.[191,192] This smaller-diameter shunt has a higher resistance than the larger shunt, is synthetic and therefore does not dilate, can maintain hepatic perfusion, and is associated with a lower incidence of hepatic encephalopathy. With these shunts, portal pressure gradients can be reduced to the critical 12 mm Hg while hepatopetal flow is maintained in up to 80% to 90% of patients. In addition, the maintenance of mesenteric pressure at or relatively close to normal levels may prevent the hyperammonemia associated with total shunts. One relatively common complication is graft thrombosis, which occurs in up to 16% of patients.[192] Shunt thrombosis can usually be treated angiographically. Dissection at the porta hepatis leads to the formation of adhesions, which may compromise later liver transplantation.

Selective shunts are designed to create two separate drainage systems within the portal venous network. A high pressure is maintained within the mesenteric system and a low pressure is created in the esophagogastric system by shunting blood from the latter into the systemic circulation without decompressing the mesenteric network. The most traditional and most favored selective shunt is the distal splenorenal shunt (Fig. 58.14).[193] The distal splenorenal shunt selectively decompresses the gastroesophageal venous system through an anastomosis between the distal end of the splenic vein and the side of the renal vein. Decompression occurs through the short gastric veins, which are in continuity with the splenic vein. In addition, as in the small side-to-side shunts described earlier, collateral veins must be ligated.

Advantages to this procedure are the following: (a) control of bleeding is excellent in more than 90% of patients, (b) no dissection of the porta hepatis is required, (c) hepatopetal flow is maintained, and (d) the incidence of encephalopathy (5% to 24%) and the risk of progressive liver failure is lower.[194] Experience with this shunt has revealed that most patients have hepatopetal flow, with 84% of alcoholic and 90% of nonalcoholic patients having prograde flow at 4 years after surgery.[195] Some loss of prograde portal flow does occur as a result of either portal vein thrombosis (approximately 10% of patients) or increased flow through collaterals located along the pancreas. This latter mechanism can be prevented by complete dissection of the splenic vein from the posterior aspect of the pancreas (splenopancreatic disconnection),[196] but this additional technique adds to the complexity of the operative procedure and to the incidence of complications.

The distal splenorenal shunt is relatively contraindicated in patients with significant ascites. Because no portal venous decompression occurs, ascites may increase after a distal splenorenal shunt is created. In addition, ligation of collateral vessels and lymphatics during the procedure contributes to increased portal pressures and subsequent increase in ascites. Patients with small splenic veins (<8 mm) have a relatively high incidence of shunt thrombosis.

Several trials comparing side-to-side total shunts with the distal splenorenal shunt found that they are equally effective (>90%) in stopping variceal hemorrhage.[197] The incidence of hepatic encephalopathy is lower after the distal splenorenal shunt, with rates of 36% and 15% for the total and selective shunts, respectively. Rates of rebleeding were similar and ranged from zero to 30%, with no survival advantage for either procedure.

Investigators have also used the side-to-side nonselective total shunt for the emergency treatment of bleeding varices. Bleeding stopped in more than 90% of patients with medical therapy alone, although bleeding often restarted shortly thereafter. Bleeding stopped in all patients after surgery, and 99% of patients were completely free of episodes of rebleeding. The 5-year survival was approximately 80%, with the majority of deaths occurring during the first year after surgery as a result of progressive hepatic failure. Hepatic encephalopathy requiring recurrent intervention, including dietary restriction and lactulose or neomycin therapy, occurred in 8% of patients. These data support an aggressive, systematic approach to caring for these patients before, during, and after surgery, though most of these patients had alcoholic liver disease, which recovers rapidly with withdrawal of the alcohol.

Devascularization Procedures. Devascularization procedures are nonshunting techniques in which the venous drainage of the stomach and esophagus is disconnected from the liver and intestinal vessels. These procedures are relatively less technically demanding than shunting procedures and can be performed in

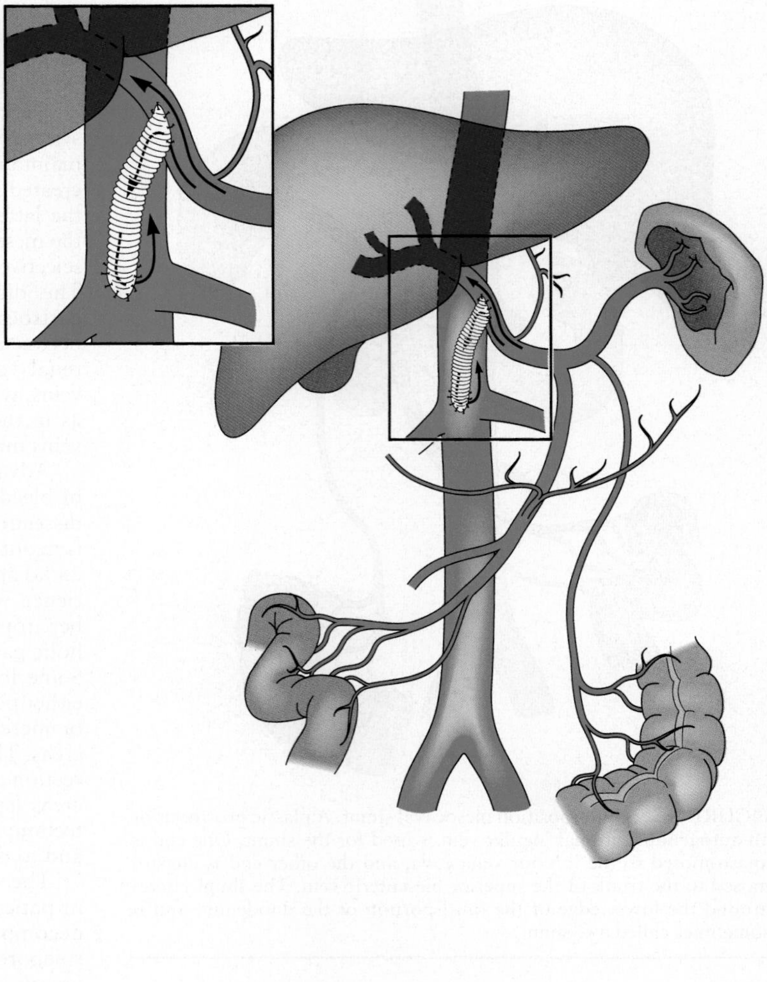

FIGURE 58.13. Small-diameter interposition portacaval Sarfeh shunt. A vascular prosthesis measuring 8 to 10 mm in diameter is interposed between the side of the vena cava and the side of the portal vein. The goal is to reduce portal pressure partially and thereby prevent variceal hemorrhage but still maintain sufficient pressure to permit the prograde flow of portal blood to the liver. This procedure is simpler to perform than that for the Warren shunt and theoretically avoids the problem of diversion of an increasing proportion of portal blood away from the liver over time, as occurs with the Warren shunt.

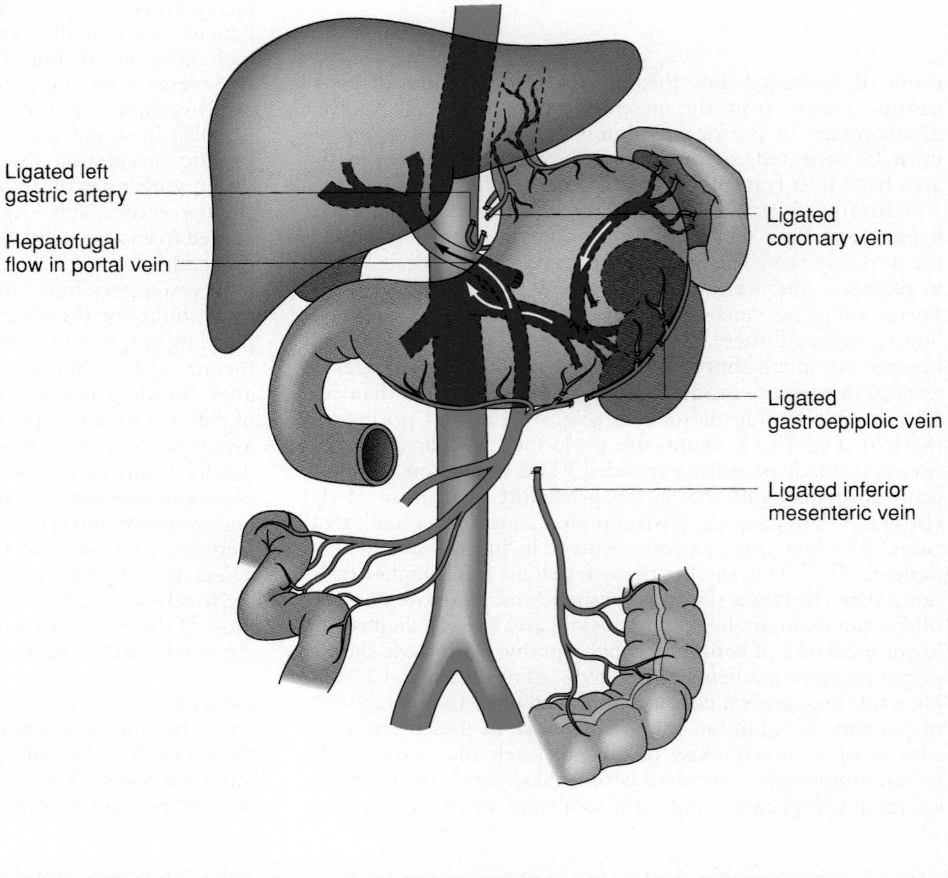

FIGURE 58.14. Distal splenorenal Warren shunt. The splenic vein is divided near its junction with the superior mesenteric vein. The distal end of the splenic vein is anastomosed to the renal vein. Varices are selectively decompressed through the stomach and short gastric veins into the splenic vein and then into the vena cava through the renal vein. Portal hypertension is maintained in the portal and superior mesenteric veins to provide enough pressure to drive portal blood through the diseased liver.

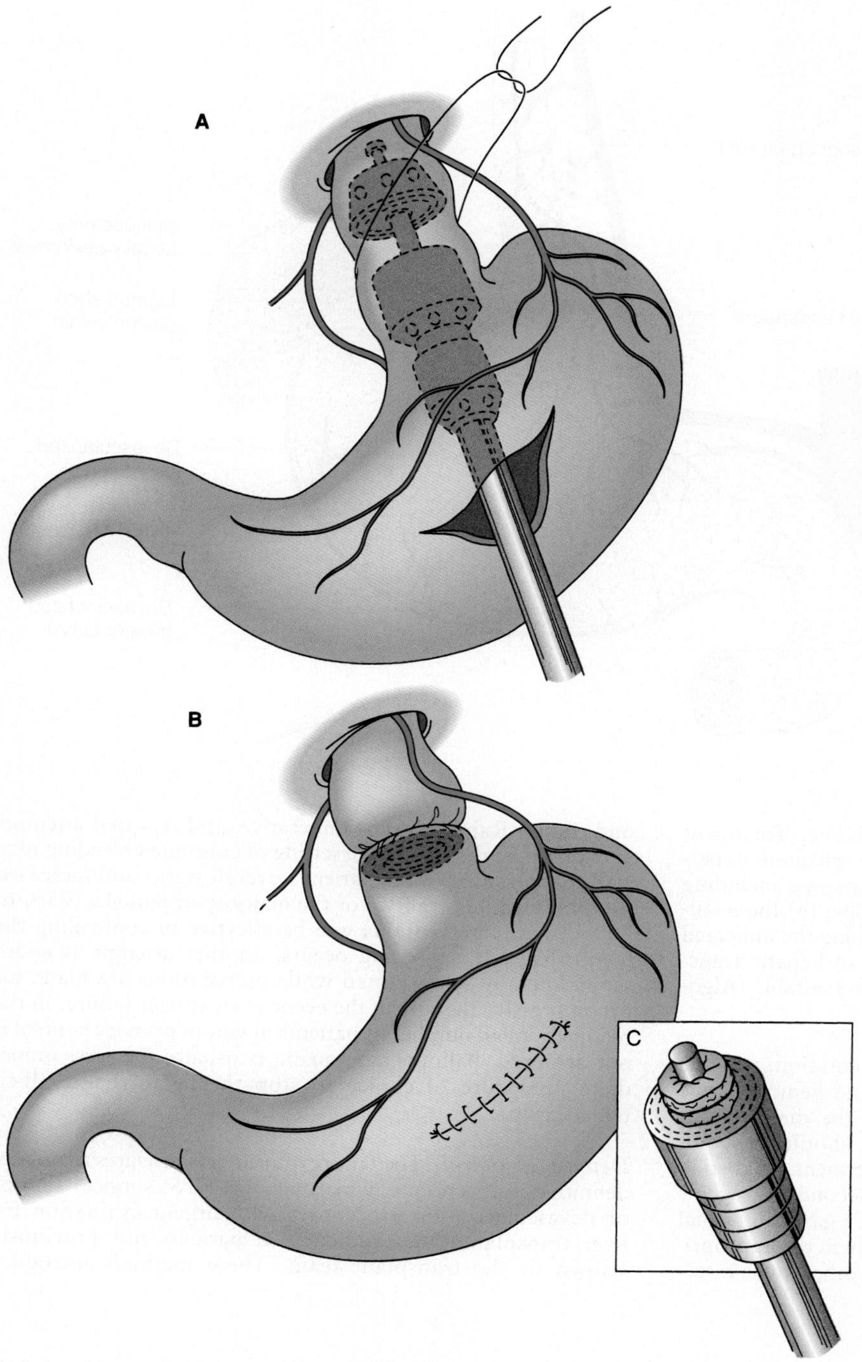

FIGURE 58.15. Transection and reanastomosis of the distal esophagus with the stapling device to control variceal hemorrhage. **A:** A stapling device is inserted through a small gastrotomy incision. **B:** When the device is fired, the esophagus is simultaneously transected and reanastomosed with staples. **C:** If the device fires correctly, a complete ring of esophageal tissue is excised.

patients with extensive portal thromboses that preclude other options. They do not interfere with hepatopetal blood flow and therefore do not increase the incidence of hepatic encephalopathy.

The procedures range in complexity from simple esophageal transection and reanastomosis with an end-to-end anastomosis (EEA) stapler combined with ligation of the coronary vein (Fig. 58.15) to the Sugiura procedure (Fig. 58.16). The Sugiura procedure requires both abdominal and thoracic incisions, through which a splenectomy, devascularization of the proximal stomach and esophagus, transection of the esophagus with reanastomosis, and ligation of all gastroesophageal collaterals are performed.[198] The latter procedure can also be performed via a single abdominal incision.[199] Bleeding recurs in fewer than 5% of patients in Japan, but rates of rebleeding range from 10% to 54% in other countries.[200] Operative mortality rates range from 10% to 35% and outcomes are certainly related to the severity of liver disease. In our practice, these procedures are not used in patients with liver disease, but exclusively in patients with diffuse portomesenteric thrombosis, in whom decompressive shunts cannot be made.

Hepatic Transplantation. Liver transplantation is the definitive therapy for portal hypertension and cirrhosis and the complications thereof, but is indicated for the overall management of end-stage liver disease and has no role in the control of acute variceal bleeding. When successful, transplantation treats both the underlying disease and any acute complication.

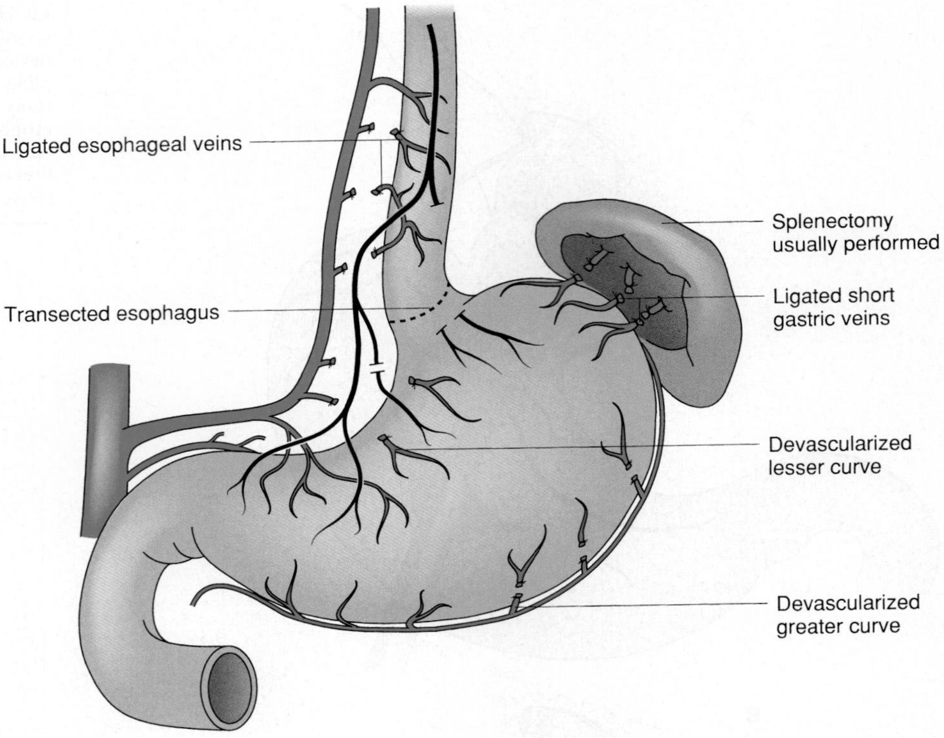

FIGURE 58.16. Sugiura esophageal transection and devascularization operation.

Algorithm for the Treatment of Variceal Bleeding. Treatment recommendations assume the following: (a) adequate expertise in all aspects of caring for cirrhotic patients, including expert endoscopy and interventional radiology; (b) the availability of trained surgeons capable of performing the indicated surgical procedures; and (c) the availability of hepatic transplantation or transfer to a center where it is available (Algorithm 58.1).

Resuscitation and Primary Control. At presentation, patients should immediately undergo resuscitation and hemodynamic monitoring, followed by establishment of the diagnosis of variceal bleeding. A pharmacologic agent should be commenced immediately in the emergency department, consisting of octreotide or beta blockade, or both. Second-tier agents include vasopressin and nitroglycerin. Upper gastrointestinal endoscopy should be performed expeditiously in the appropriate setting to attempt variceal ligation. Sclerotherapy is a second choice. Rapid triage is imperative, and repeated attempts at endoscopic therapy in the setting of continued bleeding may lead to worsening of the patient's overall status and increased morbidity and mortality. For the majority of patients (75% to 90%), these interventions will be effective in controlling the hemorrhage. If rebleeding occurs, another attempt at endoscopic therapy is warranted while preparations are made for decompressive therapy in the event of treatment failure. In the relatively small number of patients in whom primary control is not achieved, balloon tamponade is usually the next immediate procedure of choice to stop the hemorrhage, albeit temporarily.

Definitive Control. The failure of primary measures mandates definitive interventions, which include TIPS, surgical shunts, or devascularization procedures with urgent evaluation for liver transplantation candidacy in patients not previously known to the transplant team. These methods introduce

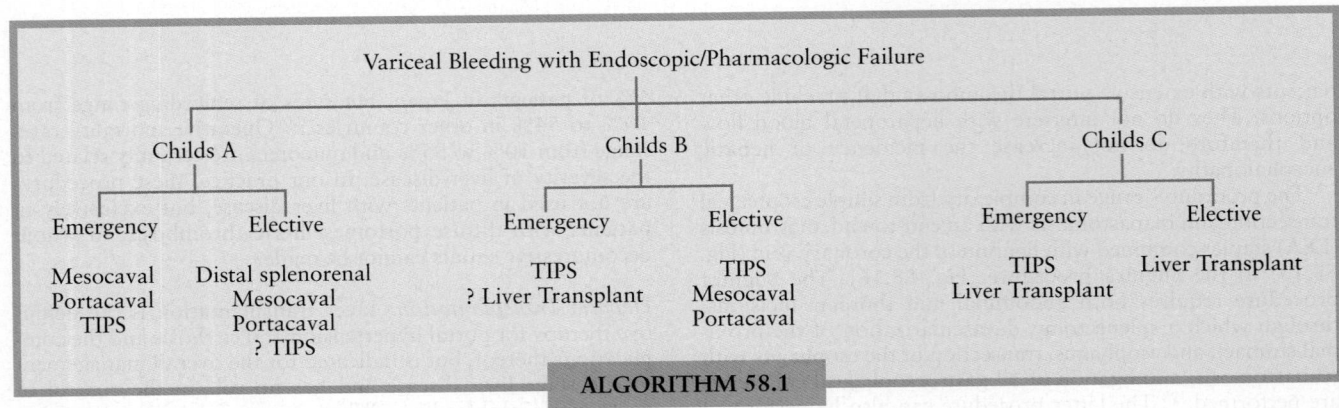

Variceal Bleeding with Endoscopic/Pharmacologic Failure

- Childs A
  - Emergency: Mesocaval, Portacaval, TIPS
  - Elective: Distal splenorenal, Mesocaval, Portacaval, ? TIPS
- Childs B
  - Emergency: TIPS, ? Liver Transplant
  - Elective: TIPS, Mesocaval, Portacaval
- Childs C
  - Emergency: TIPS, Liver Transplant
  - Elective: Liver Transplant

ALGORITHM 58.1

ALGORITHM 58.1. Suggested treatment options, in order of preference, for patients who fail medical management for variceal bleeding.

permanent mechanical alterations that may adversely affect liver function and are of varying practical utility in the emergency setting. Proper decision making requires primary stratification based on hepatic function and secondary stratification according to treatment setting (emergent vs. elective). It is critical that the issue of eligibility for hepatic transplantation be addressed before these interventions are undertaken because portal decompression can provoke hepatic failure. In patients who are not transplant candidates, the development of postoperative hepatic failure is a lethal event, and this must be discussed in detail with patients before intervention.

The question of which of the various types of surgical procedures should be used for emergency variceal bleeding has been studied in multiple trials. The number of publications on a given topic is not necessarily correlated with the general applicability of a specific surgical intervention and may reflect the referral pattern or hospital system in which the studies were performed. As in all complex operative procedures, the technical ability of an individual surgeon to perform a given procedure is crucial to its success and is correlated with complications. The following recommendations are based on the assumption that well-trained surgeons are performing these procedures.

Patients with well-compensated liver function (Child A) rarely fail to respond to pharmacologic and endoscopic therapy. Patients who continue to bleed should undergo TIPS, particularly if they are potential transplant candidates. TIPS does not disturb surgical anatomy and avoids the technical difficulty associated with transplantation in patients with previous shunts of any type. The rare patients with anticipated long-term survival without a transplant may be candidates for a distal splenorenal shunt. Excellent results have also been reported in this setting with small-diameter portacaval H-graft shunts. The arguments for the H-graft are that it is technically easier to perform and provides excellent control of bleeding. In addition, it is associated with high rates of long-term maintenance of prograde portal flow and patency and low rates of hepatic encephalopathy and mortality. Similar arguments can be made for the small-diameter mesocaval H-graft shunts. Mesocaval shunts have the added advantage of eliminating the need for portal dissection and subsequent adhesion formation.

In the hemodynamically unstable Child A cirrhotic patient, TIPS is the procedure of choice. If this is not an option, a nonselective side-to-side portacaval or mesocaval shunt can be performed for immediate control of bleeding, though this approach has been used only once in the last decade in hundreds of bleeding patients in our center. For patients who are noncompliant or live far from tertiary care medical centers capable of performing and maintaining the TIPS, a simple operation such as the side-to-side shunt, which requires comparatively little follow-up, may be more appropriate.

Child B patients with cirrhosis with high-risk varices who have failed endoscopic treatment are best treated with TIPS. If TIPS is technically impossible, a shunt may be considered for patients with contraindications to liver transplantation.

For Child C patients with cirrhosis with refractory bleeding, the options are much more limited. These patients should undergo TIPS, with the expectation that liver function will deteriorate and hepatic encephalopathy may worsen unless urgent transplant can be performed. In nontransplant candidates who fail nonoperative therapy and continue to bleed, TIPS may be lifesaving in the short term, but many patients will die of progressive liver failure.

Currently, the only indication for devascularization procedures is the presence of extensive thrombosis in the portal vessels, which precludes the use of a shunt.

In conclusion, open surgical intervention short of liver transplantation for patients with cirrhosis and portal hypertension is becoming a rarity. With the advent of TIPS, the indications for surgically created shunts are dwindling. Although some studies have shown an increased need for reintervention in patients who have undergone TIPS for variceal bleeding, the overwhelming efficacy and safety of TIPS has essentially settled the issue and today, even in large liver centers, open portal decompressive procedures are rarely performed.

Prevention of Recurrent Variceal Bleeding. The risk for rebleeding in untreated patients with a history of prior variceal bleeding ranges from 47% to 70%, with an associated mortality rate of 20% to 70%. The risk factors for subsequent bleeding from esophageal varices are the same as those for initial bleeding and include continued alcohol abuse, size of varices, Child class, and the presence of red markings on endoscopic evaluation.

Multiple randomized trials,[189] including a meta-analysis, have shown a reduction in rebleeding rates with the use of beta-blocker therapy in comparison with placebo. Mortality rates were reduced in most of those trials. All patients without a contraindication to beta-blocker therapy should be treated with one of these agents. In addition, combination therapy with beta blockade and nitrates reduces rates of rebleeding in comparison with either agent alone.[201]

As indicated in the section on treatment of bleeding varices, endoscopic variceal ligation has surpassed sclerotherapy in stopping bleeding. Moreover, in preventing rebleeding, variceal ligation has proved to be at least as effective as sclerotherapy, with fewer complications, and has become the endoscopic intervention of choice.

Almost 10 randomized trials have been performed to compare endoscopic intervention with TIPS.[202,203] The vast majority of data support the use of TIPS, which is associated with significantly decreased rates of rebleeding (approximately 25% less) and no increase in mortality. Because the incidence of significant encephalopathy is doubled, however, TIPS should be reserved for patients who fail other means of therapy.

In the older literature, many randomized trials have compared endoscopic sclerotherapy with elective shunt surgery to prevent recurrent bleeding from esophageal varices, but the importance of this comparison is now nearly irrelevant. The majority used the distal splenorenal shunt. Rates of rebleeding varied from 3% to 17% for shunts and from 35% to 60% for sclerotherapy, with no difference in overall survival. For good-risk patients without medically intractable ascites, the distal splenorenal shunt appears to be a better option to prevent recurrent variceal bleeding than repetitive sclerotherapy. TIPS is readily chosen in the face of recurrent bleeding in the setting of failed endoscopic therapy.

Gastropathy and Gastric Varices. Approximately 10% of patients with esophageal varices also have gastric varices. Conversely, about 90% of patients with gastric varices have esophageal varices.[204] Bleeding from gastric varices occurs in approximately 25% of affected patients, is usually more severe than bleeding from esophageal varices, and is poorly controlled by sclerotherapy. Rebleeding occurs in up to 30% of patients after an initial bleed.[205] The same pharmacologic interventions used for esophageal varices are used to treat gastric varices. Balloon tamponade may also be used. TIPS is the primary therapy for controlling gastric varices with the distal splenorenal shunt for the rare patient who cannot receive TIPS.

Portal hypertensive gastropathy is a condition characterized by dilation of the venules and capillaries of the gastric mucosa without associated inflammation. The major complication of gastropathy is bleeding; gastropathy accounts for 4% to 38% of all episodes of acute bleeding in patients with cirrhosis.[206] TIPS may provide therapeutic decompression in this setting as well.

Ascites. One of the most important consequences of hepatic dysfunction in cirrhosis and portal hypertension is ascites.

TABLE 58.12 **DIAGNOSIS**

DIFFERENTIAL DIAGNOSIS OF ASCITES

Portal Hypertension
Cirrhosis and other intrahepatic diseases
Hepatic congestion
Congestive heart failure
Constrictive pericarditis
Inferior vena cava obstruction
Budd-Chiari syndrome
Portal vein occlusion
Hypoalbuminemia
Nephrotic syndrome
Protein-losing enteropathy
Malnutrition
Miscellaneous Disorders
Myxedema
Ovarian disease (Meigs syndrome, struma ovarii)
Peritoneal carcinomatosis
End-stage renal disease
Chylous ascites
Bile ascites
Urine ascites

From Sleisenger MH, Fordran JS. *Gastrointestinal Disease: Pathophysiology, Diagnosis and Management*, 4th ed. Philadelphia, PA: WB Saunders; 1989:433.

This development portends a significant worsening of the patient's condition, with markedly decreased survival rates. Ascites is defined as the accumulation of free fluid within the abdominal cavity (normally <150 mL). Causes of ascites are listed in Table 58.12. In cirrhosis, the fluid is derived from a combination of hepatic (high in protein) and splanchnic (low in protein) lymph that cannot be absorbed as a result of the increased hydrostatic pressures within the liver and splanchnic systems secondary to cirrhosis and capillarization of the space of Disse.[207] Because of the loss of sinusoidal fenestrations and a subsequent decrease in their permeability, splanchnic lymph is more abundant than hepatic lymph in patients with advancing cirrhosis, so that the protein content of ascitic fluid is relatively low.[208] The main underlying pathophysiology in the development of ascites is renal sodium retention and associated water retention, which lead to fluid overload. Peripheral vasodilation and lower pressures are thought to be secondary to the dilator effects of nitric oxide, glucagon, and prostaglandins on nascent arteriovenous shunts present throughout the splanchnic vascular system, as well as in muscle, skin, and brain. The severity of liver disease is not uniformly correlated with the presence or absence of ascites.

Clinical and Laboratory Features. Ascites may be present in patients with cirrhosis who have no other overt signs or symptoms. Patients may present with subtle signs of weight gain and an inability to fit into clothes. Physical examination reveals shifting dullness to percussion (1.5 L of ascitic fluid), fluid waves (10 L), and bulging flanks.[209] With progression of disease and massive ascites, respiratory status may be compromised secondary to increased intra-abdominal pressure and pleural effusions, which are often present and usually located on the right side. The progression may be slow or more rapid after an inciting event, such as a variceal bleed or infection.

Stigmata of poor liver function include peripheral muscle wasting, palmar erythema, spider angiomas, peripheral edema, a palpable liver, and caput medusae (dilated periumbilical veins). With progressive ascites and increased abdominal pressure, umbilical and inguinal hernias often develop and may be difficult to manage. Abdominal distention may be caused by gastrointestinal gas rather than ascites. Gas can be differentiated from fluid by eliciting hyperresonance to percussion, secondary to gas, as opposed to dullness with fluid. The most widely used test for the diagnosis of ascites is ultrasonography, which can also be helpful in determining the best location for therapeutic and diagnostic paracentesis.

Diagnostic Paracentesis. The differential diagnosis of ascites is presented in Table 58.12. Determination of the character of the ascitic fluid is helpful in establishing the diagnosis. Paracentesis may be performed in the midline, midway between the umbilicus and the pubic symphysis. The fluid from patients with cirrhosis is usually straw-colored and clear; measurements of protein (usually <2 g/dL), quantitative cell counts, and microbiologic culture and determination of pH, amylase, glucose, and albumin levels should be obtained. The serum-to-ascitic fluid albumin gradient (SAG) is calculated by subtracting the albumin concentration in ascites from the level found in serum. This gradient is helpful in determining the cause of ascites; high values (>1.1 g/dL) are generally associated with portal hypertension, whereas lower levels may be associated with other disorders, including malignancy.[210]

Treatment. Initial therapy is usually directed at control of renal sodium and water retention, with bed rest and dietary manipulation. The upright position exacerbates sodium retention as a result of venous pooling and relative hypovolemia. Up to 15% of patients respond to this therapy alone with a natriuresis. A low-sodium diet is a critical part of the management of patients with cirrhosis (1 to 2 g of sodium per day or 45 to 90 mEq/d). A major problem with a strict low-sodium diet is lack of palatability and poor compliance. Fluid restriction is also an essential component of therapy in patients in whom hyponatremia develops (sodium concentration <125 mEq/L), with only 1,000 to 1,500 mL of fluid allowed each day.

For the 85% to 95% of patients who do not respond to bed rest and fluid and salt restriction, the mainstay of treatment is diuresis (Table 58.13). The loop diuretic furosemide and the potassium-sparing diuretic spironolactone are the two most widely used agents, and they can be combined to minimize side effects and maximize effectiveness. A diuresis of approximately 500 mL/d is the goal for patients with mild ascites and of up to 1 to 2 L/d for patients with both ascites and peripheral edema. More than 90% of patients respond to the combination of dietary manipulation and diuretics.[209,211]

Complications of the use of spironolactone include painful breast enlargement in males, hyperkalemia, and metabolic acidosis. Complications of the more potent furosemide include prerenal azotemia, which occurs in approximately 20% of patients as a result of excessive diuresis and hypovolemia.[209] Additional complications include hyponatremia and encephalopathy.

Large-volume paracentesis (removal of 4 to 6 L of ascitic fluid per day) and total paracentesis are techniques that can be used for patients with large amounts of fluid who are experiencing symptoms and are not responding to the aforementioned therapeutic endeavors. Patients requiring paracentesis usually have severe underlying liver disease and a 1-year survival rate of 25%.[212] The technique of paracentesis involves placing a catheter into the abdominal cavity, either in the lower midline or in one of the lower quadrants. Care is taken

TABLE 58.13 TREATMENT

TREATMENT OF ASCITES

Bed rest	
Sodium restriction	
	1–2 g/d (45–90 mEq/d)
Fluid restriction	
	1–1.5 L/d
Diuretics	
	Spironolactone
	50 mg PO q8h
	Maximum of 100 mg q6h
	Furosemide
	40–370 mg/d
Antibiotics	
	Cefotaxime
	2 g IV q12h
	Ofloxacin
	400 mg PO q12h
	Prophylaxis
	Norfloxacin
	400 mg/d while hospitalized
	Ciprofloxacin
	750 mg PO weekly
	Norfloxacin
	400 mg/d for 6 mo
	Trimethoprim/sulfamethoxazole
	One double-strength tablet five times a week

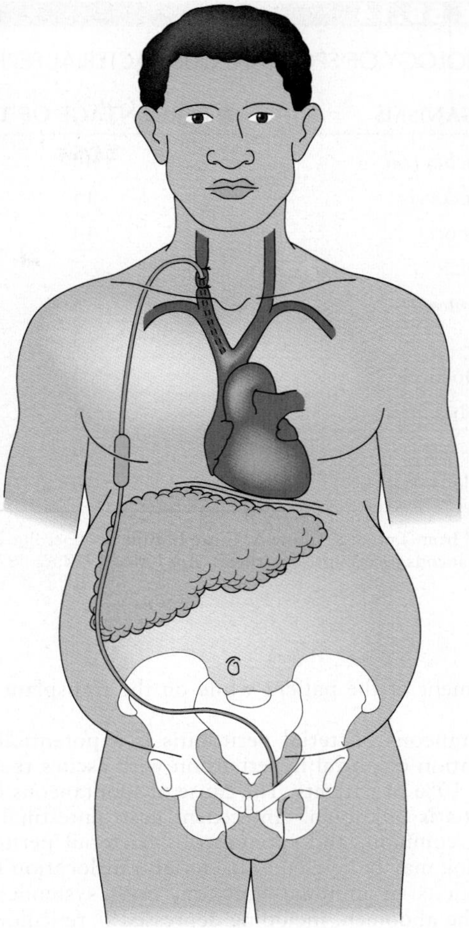

FIGURE 58.17. LeVeen peritoneovenous shunt used for routing ascitic fluid into the systemic circulation. The shunt consists of fenestrated tubing for insertion into the peritoneal cavity, a one-way valve, and a length of venous tubing for insertion into the superior vena cava.

to enter lateral to the rectus muscle and avoid the inferior epigastric artery. More than 30 L of fluid can be removed by means of total paracentesis, with 6 to 10 g of albumin infused for each liter of ascitic fluid removed.[209,211,212] The albumin commonly is administered in the form of 25% albumin (12.5 g/50 mL). Controversy exists regarding the need for albumin replacement therapy in patients undergoing total paracentesis and repetitive large-volume paracentesis. Patients who have less than 5 L of ascitic fluid removed do not require albumin replacement.[213]

The efficacy of paracentesis in the treatment of tense ascites has been studied extensively. Repetitive large-volume paracentesis has been shown to be as effective as diuretics in the treatment of moderate to severe ascites, with fewer systemic complications. A decreased length of hospital stay with no increase in the incidence of spontaneous bacterial peritonitis has been noted.[214] Paracentesis has become the therapy of choice for severe ascites.

Peritoneovenous shunts are surgically placed tubes that connect the peritoneal cavity with the superior vena cava via the internal jugular vein (Fig. 58.17). The two main types are the LeVeen shunt and the Denver shunt, both of which have a one-way valve that allows unidirectional movement of ascitic fluid from the peritoneal cavity into the systemic circulation. Although these shunts are effective in decreasing the volume of ascitic fluid, a significant number of major complications have been noted, including disseminated intravascular coagulation, heart failure, and sepsis,[212,215] and associated mortality rates are high (approximately 20%).[216] The shunt is occluded in approximately 50% of patients at 1 year, and no improvement in survival is noted.[212] The use of these shunts has drastically decreased with the development of the TIPS procedure. In addition to the use of TIPS, the placement of peritoneovenous shunts is now done percutaneously, further increasing the safety of these procedures.

Surgically created portosystemic shunts have been used in the past for the treatment of ascites. Because of high morbidity and mortality rates, an increase in encephalopathy and progression to liver failure, and the addition of the TIPS procedure to treatment options, surgically created shunts are now used infrequently for this indication alone. As discussed earlier, the TIPS is a total nonselective shunt that decompresses the portal system and reduces pressure at the hepatic sinusoids, thereby eliminating the drive for the production of ascitic fluid. In a study evaluating the use of TIPS for the treatment of medically refractory ascites, the ascites resolved completely in almost 75% of patients, and a partial response was noted in an additional 20%.[217] In addition, renal function improved during the 6 months of follow-up. TIPS in this group of patients, however, was associated with an increase in the number of cases of encephalopathy. Although survival appears to be unaffected by a TIPS procedure when compared with large-volume paracentesis, TIPS may simplify the

TABLE 58.14

BACTERIOLOGY OF SPONTANEOUS BACTERIAL PERITONITIS

ORGANISMS	PERCENTAGE OF TOTAL
Escherichia coli	40
Pneumococci	15
Streptococci	14
Klebsiella	7
Pseudomonas	3
Proteus	3
Staphylococci	3
Anaerobes	5
Other	20
Multiple isolates	10

Adapted from Targan S, Chow A, Gluze L. Role of anaerobic bacteria in spontaneous peritonitis of cirrhosis. *Am J Med* 1977;62:397.

management of the patient while on the transplant waiting list.

12 Spontaneous bacterial peritonitis is a potentially lethal complication of portal hypertension with ascites that occurs in up to 10% of patients. The cause of spontaneous bacterial peritonitis is unknown. Antecedent gastrointestinal hemorrhage is common, and spontaneous bacterial peritonitis in this setting may be related to bacterial translocation from the gut. Deficits in immune function, both systemically and within the abdomen, including depressed[218] reticuloendothelial function,[219–221] low ascitic protein concentration, and deficient ascitic opsonic activity, may play a role. Patients often present with abdominal pain and fever, but 10% to 20% of cases are discovered on routine paracentesis.[222–224] In addition, patients may present with other signs not clearly related to spontaneous bacterial peritonitis, including worsening encephalopathy and deteriorating renal function. The diagnosis is easily made by examination of the ascitic fluid obtained by paracentesis. An elevated number of white blood cells (>250/mm^3) is diagnostic. The vast majority of cases of spontaneous bacterial peritonitis are caused by a single organism, most commonly gram-negative enteric bacteria. Hematogenous spread may lead to infection with *Streptococcus pneumoniae* (Table 58.14). If more than one organism is present, the diagnosis of spontaneous bacterial peritonitis must be questioned, and a search for intra-abdominal disease (secondary peritonitis), such as a perforated viscus or diverticulitis, should be performed.

The treatment of spontaneous bacterial peritonitis consists of supportive care and broad-spectrum antibiotics, most commonly cefotaxime, a third-generation cephalosporin. Protein replacement has been shown to significantly reduce mortality in patients with spontaneous bacterial peritonitis and is complementary to other interventions as established in the landmark publication from Barcelona.[225] Other antibiotics with proved efficacy include ofloxacin, a quinolone. This antibiotic has potent activity against gram-negative organisms and reaches high levels in ascitic fluid. For patients who are clinically stable and able to take oral medications, this is the drug of choice. Cure can be achieved in 75% to 90% of cases, but mortality rates are high, ranging from 20% to 40%.[226,227] The poor prognosis associated with spontaneous bacterial peritonitis warrants consideration of liver transplantation.

Prophylactic oral or intravenous antibiotics are indicated for two distinct groups of patients with cirrhosis with ascites: (a) those with gastrointestinal hemorrhage and (b) those with low protein counts in the ascitic fluid (<10 to 15 g/L).[228] The antibiotics used in patients with hemorrhage are neomycin, colistin, and nystatin in combination, and ofloxacin alone. These antibiotics reduce the incidence of spontaneous bacterial peritonitis from approximately 15% to 20% to 3% to 9% and cause few side effects.[229–231] A meta-analysis evaluating the use of prophylactic antibiotics in patients with gastrointestinal hemorrhage confirmed the utility of prophylaxis, with an approximately 30% decrease in the incidence of infection, a 20% decrease in the incidence of spontaneous bacterial peritonitis and bacteremia, and a 10% improvement in overall survival.[232] In patients with low protein levels in the ascitic fluid, multiple regimens have proved effective in reducing the incidence of spontaneous bacterial peritonitis, from approximately 20% to less than 5%.[232–234]

Hernias and Ascites. Hernias of the anterior abdominal wall occur in up to 20% of patients with cirrhosis. The causes include increased intra-abdominal pressure and nutritional deficits, with muscular wasting and thinning of the fascia. If the hernias are left untreated, complications include incarceration, rupture, strangulation, and leakage. Patients with hernias and decompensated cirrhosis need to be evaluated for liver transplantation. In patients with stable liver function, hernias should be treated electively, with preoperative paracentesis to decrease intra-abdominal pressure. No increase in complication rates was noted in a study comparing the outcome of umbilical hernia repair in patients with and without ascites. A longer hospital stay and a significantly higher recurrence rate (73% vs. 14%) was noted, however, in the group of patients with ascites.[235–237] We favor the use of abdominal drains to remove the ascites until the incision is healed, thereby preventing ascites from leaking through the wound. Meticulous fluid management is essential during the postoperative period to prevent early reaccumulation of ascites.

In patients with severe ascites, TIPS should be performed before hernia repair to ensure a good result. Emergency repair of hernias complicated by skin breakdown with ascites leak or incarceration or strangulation are managed in a similar fashion with preoperative large-volume paracentesis, and aggressive control of ascites postoperatively.

References

1. Cataldegirmen G, Zeng S, Feirt N, et al. RAGE limits regeneration after massive liver injury by coordinated suppression of TNF-alpha and NF-kappaB. *J Exp Med* 2005;201:473–484.
2. Albano E. New concepts in the pathogenesis of alcoholic liver disease. *Expert Rev Gastroenterol Hepatol* 2008;2:749–759.
3. Vuppalanchi R, Chalasani N. Nonalcoholic fatty liver disease and nonalcoholic steatohepatitis: selected practical issues in their evaluation and management. *Hepatology* 2009;49:306–317.
4. Rafiq N, Younossi ZM. Interaction of metabolic syndrome, nonalcoholic fatty liver disease and chronic hepatitis C. *Expert Rev Gastroenterol Hepatol* 2008;2:207–215.
5. Enomoto N, Ikejima K, Bradford BU, et al. Role of Kupffer cells and gut-derived endotoxins in alcoholic liver injury. *J Gastroenterol Hepatol* 2000;15(suppl):D20–D25.
6. Baskol G, Baskol M, Kocer D. Oxidative stress and antioxidant defenses in serum of patients with non-alcoholic steatohepatitis. *Clin Biochem* 2007;40:776–780.
7. Friedman SL, Roll FJ, Boyles J, et al. Hepatic lipocytes: the principal collagen-producing cells of normal rat liver. *Proc Natl Acad Sci U S A* 1985;82:8681–8685.
8. Wake K. "Sternzellen" in the liver: perisinusoidal cells with special reference to storage of vitamin A. *Am J Anat* 1971;132:429–462.
9. Takahara T, Kojima T, Miyabayashi C, et al. Collagen production in fat-storing cells after carbon tetrachloride intoxication in the rat. Immunoelectron microscopic observation of type I, type III collagens, and prolyl hydroxylase. *Lab Invest* 1988;59:509–521.

10. Gressner AM, Bachem MG. Cellular sources of noncollagenous matrix proteins: role of fat-storing cells in fibrogenesis. *Semin Liver Dis* 1990;10:30–46.
11. Loreal O, Levavasseur F, Rescan PY, et al. Differential expression of laminin chains in hepatic lipocytes. *FEBS Lett* 1991;290:9–12.
12. Ramadori G, Knittel T, Odenthal M, et al. Synthesis of cellular fibronectin by rat liver fat-storing (Ito) cells: regulation by cytokines. *Gastroenterology* 1992;103:1313–1321.
13. Li Y, Schwabe RF, DeVries-Seimon T, et al. Free cholesterol-loaded macrophages are an abundant source of tumor necrosis factor-alpha and interleukin-6: model of NF-kappaB- and map kinase-dependent inflammation in advanced atherosclerosis. *J Biol Chem* 2005;280:21763–21772.
14. Friedman SL, Arthur MJ. Activation of cultured rat hepatic lipocytes by Kupffer cell conditioned medium. Direct enhancement of matrix synthesis and stimulation of cell proliferation via induction of platelet-derived growth factor receptors. *J Clin Invest* 1989;84:1780–1785.
15. Pinzani M, Gesualdo L, Sabbah GM, et al. Effects of platelet-derived growth factor and other polypeptide mitogens on DNA synthesis and growth of cultured rat liver fat-storing cells. *J Clin Invest* 1989;84:1786–1793.
16. Matsuoka M, Pham NT, Tsukamoto H. Differential effects of interleukin-1 alpha, tumor necrosis factor alpha, and transforming growth factor beta 1 on cell proliferation and collagen formation by cultured fat-storing cells. *Liver* 1989;9:71–78.
17. Tsushima H, Kawata S, Tamura S, et al. Reduced plasma transforming growth factor-beta1 levels in patients with chronic hepatitis C after interferon-alpha therapy: association with regression of hepatic fibrosis. *J Hepatol* 1999;30:1–7.
18. Schaffner F, Poper H. Capillarization of hepatic sinusoids in man. *Gastroenterology* 1963;44:239–242.
19. Reeves HL, Friedman SL. Activation of hepatic stellate cells–a key issue in liver fibrosis. *Front Biosci* 2002;7:d808–d826.
20. Oda M, Han JY, Yokomori H. Local regulators of hepatic sinusoidal microcirculation: recent advances. *Clin Hemorheol Microcirc* 2000;23:85–94.
21. DeLeve LD, Wang X, Kanel GC, et al. Prevention of hepatic fibrosis in a murine model of metabolic syndrome with nonalcoholic steatohepatitis. *Am J Pathol* 2008;173:993–1001.
22. Anthony PP, Ishak KG, Nayak NC, et al. The morphology of cirrhosis: definition, nomenclature, and classification. *Bull World Health Organ* 1977;55:521–540.
23. Chiaramonte M, Stroffolini T, Vian A, et al. Rate of incidence of hepatocellular carcinoma in patients with compensated viral cirrhosis. *Cancer* 1999;85:2132–2137.
24. Chedid A, Mendenhall CL, Gartside P, et al. Prognostic factors in alcoholic liver disease. VA Cooperative Study Group. *Am J Gastroenterol* 1991;86:210–216.
25. Lieber CS. Medical disorders of alcoholism. *N Engl J Med* 1995;333:1058–1065.
26. Friedman SL. Seminars in medicine of the Beth Israel Hospital, Boston. The cellular basis of hepatic fibrosis. Mechanisms and treatment strategies. *N Engl J Med* 1993;328:1828–1835.
27. Moshage H, Casini A, Lieber CS. Acetaldehyde selectively stimulates collagen production in cultured rat liver fat-storing cells but not in hepatocytes. *Hepatology* 1990;12:511–518.
28. Lieber CS. *Medical and Nutritional Complications of Alcoholism: Mechanisms and Management*. New York: Plenum; 1992.
29. Angulo P, Lindor KD. Non-alcoholic fatty liver disease. *J Gastroenterol Hepatol* 2002;17(suppl):S186–S190.
30. Serfaty L, Lemoine M. Definition and natural history of metabolic steatosis: clinical aspects of NAFLD, NASH and cirrhosis. *Diabetes Metab* 2008;34:634–637.
31. Browning JD, Kumar KS, Saboorian MH, et al. Ethnic differences in the prevalence of cryptogenic cirrhosis. *Am J Gastroenterol* 2004;99:292–298.
32. Mendes FD, Levy C, Enders FB, et al. Abnormal hepatic biochemistries in patients with inflammatory bowel disease. *Am J Gastroenterol* 2007;102:344–350.
33. Takamatsu S, Noguchi N, Kudoh A, et al. Influence of risk factors for metabolic syndrome and non-alcoholic fatty liver disease on the progression and prognosis of hepatocellular carcinoma. *Hepatogastroenterology* 2008;55:609–614.
34. Calle EE, Rodriguez C, Walker-Thurmond K, et al. Overweight, obesity, and mortality from cancer in a prospectively studied cohort of U.S. adults. *N Engl J Med* 2003;348:1625–1638.
35. Younger HM, Bathgate AJ, Hayes PC. Review article: nucleoside analogues for the treatment of chronic hepatitis B. *Aliment Pharmacol Ther* 2004;20:1211–1230.
36. Di Bisceglie AM, Martin P, Kassianides C, et al. Recombinant interferon alfa therapy for chronic hepatitis C. A randomized, double-blind, placebo-controlled trial. *N Engl J Med* 1989;321:1506–1510.
37. Shindo M, Ken A, Okuno T. Varying incidence of cirrhosis and hepatocellular carcinoma in patients with chronic hepatitis C responding differently to interferon therapy. *Cancer* 1999;85:1943–1950.
38. Fried MW, Shiffman ML, Reddy KR, et al. Peginterferon alfa-2a plus ribavirin for chronic hepatitis C virus infection. *N Engl J Med* 2002;347:975–982.
39. Davis GL. Treatment of chronic hepatitis C: impact of combination therapy. *Curr Gastroenterol Rep* 1999;1:9–14.
40. Brown NA. Progress towards improving antiviral therapy for hepatitis C with hepatitis C virus polymerase inhibitors. Part I: nucleoside analogues. *Expert Opin Investig Drugs* 2009;18:709–725.
41. Szakacs JG, Szakacs JE. Progress in diagnosis of hepatitis and the cirrhotic liver. *Ann Clin Lab Sci* 1999;29:87–103.
42. El-Serag HB. Epidemiology of hepatocellular carcinoma in USA. *Hepatol Res* 2007;37(suppl 2):S88–S94.
43. Kaplan MM. Primary biliary cirrhosis. *N Engl J Med* 1996;335:1570–1580.
44. Portmann B, Popper H, Neuberger J, et al. Sequential and diagnostic features in primary biliary cirrhosis based on serial histologic study in 209 patients. *Gastroenterology* 1985;88:1777–1790.
45. Tornay AS Jr. Primary biliary cirrhosis: natural history. *Am J Gastroenterol* 1980;73:223–236.
46. Balasubramaniam K, Grambsch PM, Wiesner RH, et al. Diminished survival in asymptomatic primary biliary cirrhosis. A prospective study. *Gastroenterology* 1990;98:1567–1571.
47. Mahl TC, Shockcor W, Boyer JL. Primary biliary cirrhosis: survival of a large cohort of symptomatic and asymptomatic patients followed for 24 years. *J Hepatol* 1994;20:707–713.
48. Heathcote EJ, Cauch-Dudek K, Walker V, et al. The Canadian multicenter double-blind randomized controlled trial of ursodeoxycholic acid in primary biliary cirrhosis. *Hepatology* 1994;19:1149–1156.
49. Wiesner RH, Porayko MK, Dickson ER, et al. Selection and timing of liver transplantation in primary biliary cirrhosis and primary sclerosing cholangitis. *Hepatology* 1992;16:1290–1299.
50. Angulo P, Lindor KD. Primary sclerosing cholangitis. *Hepatology* 1999;30:325–332.
51. Broome U, Glaumann H, Hultcrantz R, et al. Distribution of HLA-DR, HLA-DP, HLA-DQ antigens in liver tissue from patients with primary sclerosing cholangitis. *Scand J Gastroenterol* 1990;25:54–58.
52. Zauli D, Schrumpf E, Crespi C, et al. An autoantibody profile in primary sclerosing cholangitis. *J Hepatol* 1987;5:14–18.
53. Wiesner RH. Current concepts in primary sclerosing cholangitis. *Mayo Clin Proc* 1994;69:969–982.
54. Martin FM, Braasch JW. Primary sclerosing cholangitis. *Curr Probl Surg* 1992;29:133–193.
55. Okolicsanyi L, Fabris L, Viaggi S, et al. Primary sclerosing cholangitis: clinical presentation, natural history and prognostic variables: an Italian multicentre study. The Italian PSC Study Group. *Eur J Gastroenterol Hepatol* 1996;8:685–691.
56. Bergquist A, Glaumann H, Persson B, et al. Risk factors and clinical presentation of hepatobiliary carcinoma in patients with primary sclerosing cholangitis: a case-control study. *Hepatology* 1998;27:311–316.
57. Broome U, Lofberg R, Veress B, et al. Primary sclerosing cholangitis and ulcerative colitis: evidence for increased neoplastic potential. *Hepatology* 1995;22:1404–1408.
58. Levy MJ, Baron TH, Clayton AC, et al. Prospective evaluation of advanced molecular markers and imaging techniques in patients with indeterminate bile duct strictures. *Am J Gastroenterol* 2008;103:1263–1273.
59. De Vreede I, Steers JL, Burch PA, et al. Prolonged disease-free survival after orthotopic liver transplantation plus adjuvant chemoirradiation for cholangiocarcinoma. *Liver Transpl* 2000;6:309–316.
60. Stal P, Broome U, Scheynius A, et al. Kupffer cell iron overload induces intercellular adhesion molecule-1 expression on hepatocytes in genetic hemochromatosis. *Hepatology* 1995;21:1308–1316.
61. Wheeler CJ, Kowdley KV. Hereditary hemochromatosis: a review of the genetics, mechanism, diagnosis, and treatment of iron overload. *Compr Ther* 2006;32:10–16.
62. Schilsky ML, TA. Wilson's disease. In: Schiff ER, Sorrell M, Maddrey WC, eds. *Diseases of the Liver*, 8th ed. Philadelphia, PA: JB Lippincott; 1999:1091–1106.
63. Safran AP, Schaffner F. Chronic passive congestion of the liver in man. Electron microscopic study of cell atrophy and intralobular fibrosis. *Am J Pathol* 1967;50:447–463.
64. Dunn GD, Hayes P, Breen KJ, et al. The liver in congestive heart failure: a review. *Am J Med Sci* 1973;265:174–189.
65. Rosenberg PM, FL. The liver in circulatory failure. In: Schiff ER, Sorrell M, Maddrey WC, eds. *Diseases of the Liver*, 8th ed. Philadelphia, PA: JB Lippincott; 1999:1215–1227.
66. Tilanus HW. Budd-Chiari syndrome. *Br J Surg* 1995;82:1023–1030.
67. Gupta S, Barter S, Phillips GW, et al. Comparison of ultrasonography, computed tomography and 99mTc liver scan in diagnosis of Budd-Chiari syndrome. *Gut* 1987;28:242–247.
68. Zhang Y, Zhang XM, Prowda JC, et al. Changes in hepatic venous morphology with cirrhosis on MRI. *J Magn Reson Imaging* 2009;29:1085–1092.
69. Ishikawa T, Ichida T, Matsuda Y, et al. Reduced expression of thrombopoietin is involved in thrombocytopenia in human and rat liver cirrhosis. *J Gastroenterol Hepatol* 1998;13:907–913.
70. Simonovsky V. The diagnosis of cirrhosis by high resolution ultrasound of the liver surface. *Br J Radiol* 1999;72:29–34.
71. Ohsuga M, Moreau R, Hartleb M, et al. Blunted systemic, splanchnic, and renal hemodynamic responses to atrial natriuretic peptide in rats with cirrhosis. *J Hepatol* 1994;20:91–96.

72. Angeli P, Merkel C. Pathogenesis and management of hepatorenal syndrome in patients with cirrhosis. *J Hepatol* 2008;48(suppl 1):S93–S103.
73. Gines A, Escorsell A, Gines P, et al. Incidence, predictive factors, and prognosis of the hepatorenal syndrome in cirrhosis with ascites. *Gastroenterology* 1993;105:229–236.
74. Martin-Llahi M, Pepin MN, Guevara M, et al. Terlipressin and albumin vs albumin in patients with cirrhosis and hepatorenal syndrome: a randomized study. *Gastroenterology* 2008;134:1352–1359.
75. Sharma P, Kumar A, Shrama BC, et al. An open label, pilot, randomized controlled trial of noradrenaline versus terlipressin in the treatment of type 1 hepatorenal syndrome and predictors of response. *Am J Gastroenterol* 2008;103:1689–1697.
76. Lieberman FL, Reynolds TB. Plasma volume in cirrhosis of the liver: its relation of portal hypertension, ascites, and renal failure. *J Clin Invest* 1967;46:1297–1308.
77. Schrier RW, Arroyo V, Bernardi M, et al. Peripheral arterial vasodilation hypothesis: a proposal for the initiation of renal sodium and water retention in cirrhosis. *Hepatology* 1988;8:1151–1157.
78. P G. Renal complications. In: Schiff ER, Sorrell M, Maddrey WC, eds. *Diseases of the Liver*, 8th ed. Philadelphia, PA: JB Lippincott; 1999:453–464.
79. Martin PY, Gines P, Schrier RW. Nitric oxide as a mediator of hemodynamic abnormalities and sodium and water retention in cirrhosis. *N Engl J Med* 1998;339:533–541.
80. Sarela AI, Mihaimeed FM, Batten JJ, et al. Hepatic and splanchnic nitric oxide activity in patients with cirrhosis. *Gut* 1999;44:749–753.
81. Sterns RH, Cappuccio JD, Silver SM, et al. Neurologic sequelae after treatment of severe hyponatremia: a multicenter perspective. *J Am Soc Nephrol* 1994;4:1522–1530.
82. Rodes J, Bosch J, Arroyo V. Clinical types and drug therapy of renal impairment in cirrhosis. *Postgrad Med J* 1975;51:492–497.
83. Singer JA, Kaplan MM, Katz RL. Cirrhotic pleural effusion in the absence of ascites. *Gastroenterology* 1977;73:575–577.
84. Fitz G. Systemic complications of liver disease. In: Feldman M, ed. *Sleisenger and Fordtran's Gastrointestinal and Liver Disease*. Philadelphia, PA: WB Saunders; 1998:1340–1342.
85. Berkowitz KA, Butensky MS, Smith RL. Pulmonary function changes after large volume paracentesis. *Am J Gastroenterol* 1993;88:905–907.
86. Hopkins WE, Waggoner AD, Barzilai B. Frequency and significance of intrapulmonary right-to-left shunting in end-stage hepatic disease. *Am J Cardiol* 1992;70:516–519.
87. Hourani JM, Bellamy PE, Tashkin DP, et al. Pulmonary dysfunction in advanced liver disease: frequent occurrence of an abnormal diffusing capacity. *Am J Med* 1991;90:693–700.
88. Scott VL, Dodson SF, Kang Y. The hepatopulmonary syndrome. *Surg Clin North Am* 1999;79:23–41, vii.
89. McAdams HP, Erasmus J, Crockett R, et al. The hepatopulmonary syndrome: radiologic findings in 10 patients. *AJR Am J Roentgenol* 1996;166:1379–1385.
90. De Wolf AM, Begliomini B, Gasior TA, et al. Right ventricular function during orthotopic liver transplantation. *Anesth Analg* 1993;76:562–568.
91. Swanson KL, Wiesner RH, Nyberg SL, et al. Survival in portopulmonary hypertension: Mayo clinic experience categorized by treatment subgroups. *Am J Transplant* 2008;8:2445–2453.
92. Nomura F, Ohnishi K, Terabayashi H, et al. Effect of intrahepatic portal-systemic shunting on hepatic ammonia extraction in patients with cirrhosis. *Hepatology* 1994;20:1478–1481.
93. Lockwood AH, Yap EW, Wong WH. Cerebral ammonia metabolism in patients with severe liver disease and minimal hepatic encephalopathy. *J Cereb Blood Flow Metab* 1991;11:337–341.
94. Schafer DF, Jones EA. Hepatic encephalopathy and the gamma-aminobutyric-acid neurotransmitter system. *Lancet* 1982;1:18–20.
95. Mullen KD, Martin JV, Mendelson WB, et al. Could an endogenous benzodiazepine ligand contribute to hepatic encephalopathy? *Lancet* 1988;1:457–459.
96. Bengtsson F, Gage FH, Jeppsson B, et al. Brain monoamine metabolism and behavior in portacaval-shunted rats. *Exp Neurol* 1985;90:21–35.
97. Zieve L, Doizaki WM, Zieve J. Synergism between mercaptans and ammonia or fatty acids in the production of coma: a possible role for mercaptans in the pathogenesis of hepatic coma. *J Lab Clin Med* 1974;83:16–28.
98. Yurdaydin C, Karavelioglu D, Onaran O, et al. Opioid receptor ligands in human hepatic encephalopathy. *J Hepatol* 1998;29:796–801.
99. Schenker S, Hoyumpa AM Jr. Pathophysiology of hepatic encephalopathy. *Hosp Pract (Off Ed)* 1984;19:99–103, 7–8, 10–14 passim.
100. Schenker S, Breen KJ, Hoyumpa AM Jr. Hepatic encephalopathy: current status. *Gastroenterology* 1974;66:121–151.
101. Conn HO, Leevy CM, Vlahcevic ZR, et al. Comparison of lactulose and neomycin in the treatment of chronic portal-systemic encephalopathy. A double blind controlled trial. *Gastroenterology* 1977;72:573–583.
102. Mortensen PB. The effect of oral-administered lactulose on colonic nitrogen metabolism and excretion. *Hepatology* 1992;16:1350–1356.
103. Vince AJ, Burridge SM. Ammonia production by intestinal bacteria: the effects of lactose, lactulose and glucose. *J Med Microbiol* 1980;13:177–191.
104. Vince A, Zeegen R, Drinkwater JE, et al. The effect of lactulose on the faecal flora of patients with hepatic encephalopathy. *J Med Microbiol* 1974;7:163–168.
105. Atterbury CE, Maddrey WC, Conn HO. Neomycin-sorbitol and lactulose in the treatment of acute portal-systemic encephalopathy. A controlled, double-blind clinical trial. *Am J Dig Dis* 1978;23:398–406.
106. Morgan MH, Read AE, Speller DC. Treatment of hepatic encephalopathy with metronidazole. *Gut* 1982;23:1–7.
107. Kunin CM, Chalmers TC, Leevy CM, et al. Absorption of orally administered neomycin and kanamycin with special reference to patients with severe hepatic and renal disease. *N Engl J Med* 1960;262:380–385.
108. Pedretti G, Calzetti C, Missale G, et al. Rifaximin versus neomycin on hyperammonemia in chronic portal systemic encephalopathy of cirrhotics. A double-blind, randomized trial. *Ital J Gastroenterol* 1991;23:175–178.
109. Reynolds TB, Balfour DC Jr, Levinson DC, et al. Comparison of wedged hepatic vein pressure with portal vein pressure in human subjects with cirrhosis. *J Clin Invest* 1955;34:213–218.
110. Vorobioff J, Bredfeldt JE, Groszmann RJ. Increased blood flow through the portal system in cirrhotic rats. *Gastroenterology* 1984;87:1120–1126.
111. Moller S, Christensen E, Henriksen JH. Continuous blood pressure monitoring in cirrhosis. Relations to splanchnic and systemic haemodynamics. *J Hepatol* 1997;27:284–294.
112. Battista S, Bar F, Mengozzi G, et al. Hyperdynamic circulation in patients with cirrhosis: direct measurement of nitric oxide levels in hepatic and portal veins. *J Hepatol* 1997;26:75–80.
113. Jaffe DL, Chung RT, Friedman LS. Management of portal hypertension and its complications. *Med Clin North Am* 1996;80:1021–1034.
114. Gupta TK, Chen L, Groszmann RJ. Pathophysiology of portal hypertension. *Baillieres Clin Gastroenterol* 1997;11:203–219.
115. Budd BG. *On Diseases of the Liver*. London: John Churchill; 1845.
116. Chiari H. Über die selbstandige phlebitis obliterans der hauptstamme der venae hepaticae als todesursache. *Beitr Z Pathol Anat* 1899;26:1–18.
117. Gordon SC, Polson DJ, Shirkhoda A. Budd-Chiari syndrome complicating pre-eclampsia: diagnosis by magnetic resonance imaging. *J Clin Gastroenterol* 1991;13:460–462.
118. Valla D, Le MG, Poynard T, et al. Risk of hepatic vein thrombosis in relation to recent use of oral contraceptives. A case-control study. *Gastroenterology* 1986;90:807–811.
119. Mitchell MC, Boitnott JK, Kaufman S, et al. Budd-Chiari syndrome: etiology, diagnosis and management. *Medicine (Baltimore)* 1982;61:199–218.
120. Mitchell AW, Jackson JE. Budd-Chiari syndrome. *Clin Radiol* 1996;51:747–748.
121. Cameron JL, Maddrey WC. Mesoatrial shunt: a new treatment for the Budd-Chiari syndrome. *Ann Surg* 1978;187:402–406.
122. Cameron JL, Herlong HF, Sanfey H, et al. The Budd-Chiari syndrome. Treatment by mesenteric-systemic venous shunts. *Ann Surg* 1983;198:335–346.
123. Halff G, Todo S, Tzakis AG, et al. Liver transplantation for the Budd-Chiari syndrome. *Ann Surg* 1990;211:43–49.
124. Cura M, Haskal Z, Lopera J. Diagnostic and interventional radiology for Budd-Chiari syndrome. *Radiographics* 2009;29:669–681.
125. Shaked A, Goldstein RM, Klintmalm GB, et al. Portosystemic shunt versus orthotopic liver transplantation for the Budd-Chiari syndrome. *Surg Gynecol Obstet* 1992;174:453–459.
126. Rautou PE, Moucari R, Escolano S, et al. Prognostic indices for Budd-Chiari syndrome: valid for clinical studies but insufficient for individual management. *Am J Gastroenterol* 2009;104:1140–1146.
127. Carnevale FC, Szejnfeld D, Moreira AM, et al. Long-term follow-up after successful transjugular intrahepatic portosystemic shunt placement in a pediatric patient with Budd-Chiari syndrome. *Cardiovasc Intervent Radiol* 2008;31:1244–1248.
128. Blum U, Rossle M, Haag K, et al. Budd-Chiari syndrome: technical, hemodynamic, and clinical results of treatment with transjugular intrahepatic portosystemic shunt. *Radiology* 1995;197:805–811.
129. Rossle M, Olschewski M, Siegerstetter V, et al. The Budd-Chiari syndrome: outcome after treatment with the transjugular intrahepatic portosystemic shunt. *Surgery* 2004;135:394–403.
130. Orozco H, Takahashi T, Mercado MA, et al. Surgical management of extrahepatic portal hypertension and variceal bleeding. *World J Surg* 1994;18:246–250.
131. Cohen J, Edelman RR, Chopra S. Portal vein thrombosis: a review. *Am J Med* 1992;92:173–182.
132. Parvey HR, Raval B, Sandler CM. Portal vein thrombosis: imaging findings. *AJR Am J Roentgenol* 1994;162:77–81.
133. de Ville de Goyet J, Alberti D, Falchetti D, et al. Treatment of extrahepatic portal hypertension in children by mesenteric-to-left portal vein bypass: a new physiological procedure. *Eur J Surg* 1999;165:777–781.
134. Loftus JP, Nagorney DM, Ilstrup D, et al. Sinistral portal hypertension. Splenectomy or expectant management. *Ann Surg* 1993;217:35–40.
135. Brown RS Jr, Kumar KS, Russo MW, et al. Model for End-stage Liver Disease and Child-Turcotte-Pugh score as predictors of pretransplantation disease severity, posttransplantation outcome, and resource utilization in United Network for Organ Sharing status 2A patients. *Liver Transpl* 2002;8:278–284.
136. Forman LM, Lucey MR. Predicting the prognosis of chronic liver disease: an evolution from Child to MELD. Mayo End-stage Liver Disease. *Hepatology* 2001;33:473–475.
137. Botta F, Giannini E, Romagnoli P, et al. MELD scoring system is useful for predicting prognosis in patients with liver cirrhosis and is correlated with residual liver function: a European study. *Gut* 2003;52:134–139.

138. Sheth M, Riggs M, Patel T. Utility of the Mayo End-Stage Liver Disease (MELD) score in assessing prognosis of patients with alcoholic hepatitis. *BMC Gastroenterol* 2002;2:2.
139. Carbo J, Garcia-Samaniego J, Castellano G, et al. Liver cirrhosis and mortality by abdominal surgery. A study of risk factors. *Rev Esp Enferm Dig* 1998;90:105–112.
140. Mansour A, Watson W, Shayani V, et al. Abdominal operations in patients with cirrhosis: still a major surgical challenge. *Surgery* 1997;122:730–735; discussion 735–736.
141. Noda T. Angioarchitectural study of esophageal varices. With special reference to variceal rupture. *Virchows Arch A Pathol Anat Histopathol* 1984;404:381–392.
142. Kamath PS. Esophageal variceal bleeding: primary prophylaxis. *Clin Gastroenterol Hepatol* 2005;3:90–93.
143. Roberts LR, Kamath PS. Pathophysiology of variceal bleeding. *Gastrointest Endosc Clin N Am* 1999;9:167–174.
144. Cales P, Desmorat H, Vinel JP, et al. Incidence of large oesophageal varices in patients with cirrhosis: application to prophylaxis of first bleeding. *Gut* 1990;31:1298–1302.
145. North Italian Endoscopic Club for the Study and Treatment of Esophageal Varices. Prediction of the first variceal hemorrhage in patients with cirrhosis of the liver and esophageal varices. A prospective multicenter study. *N Engl J Med* 1988;319:983–989.
146. Graham DY, Smith JL. The course of patients after variceal hemorrhage. *Gastroenterology* 1981;80:800–809.
147. Polio J, Groszmann RJ. Hemodynamic factors involved in the development and rupture of esophageal varices: a pathophysiologic approach to treatment. *Semin Liver Dis* 1986;6:318–331.
148. Garcia-Tsao G, Groszmann RJ, Fisher RL, et al. Portal pressure, presence of gastroesophageal varices and variceal bleeding. *Hepatology* 1985;5:419–424.
149. Price HL, Cooperman LH, Warden JC. Control of the splanchnic circulation in man. Role of beta-adrenergic receptors. *Circ Res* 1967;21:333–340.
150. Braillon A, Moreau R, Hadengue A, et al. Hyperkinetic circulatory syndrome in patients with presinusoidal portal hypertension. Effect of propranolol. *J Hepatol* 1989;9:312–318.
151. Kiire CF. Controlled trial of propranolol to prevent recurrent variceal bleeding in patients with non-cirrhotic portal fibrosis. *BMJ* 1989;298:1363–1365.
152. Poynard T, Cales P, Pasta L, et al. Beta-adrenergic-antagonist drugs in the prevention of gastrointestinal bleeding in patients with cirrhosis and esophageal varices. An analysis of data and prognostic factors in 589 patients from four randomized clinical trials. Franco-Italian Multicenter Study Group. *N Engl J Med* 1991;324:1532–1538.
153. Feu F, Garcia-Pagan JC, Bosch J, et al. Relation between portal pressure response to pharmacotherapy and risk of recurrent variceal haemorrhage in patients with cirrhosis. *Lancet* 1995;346:1056–1059.
154. Andreani T, Poupon RE, Balkau BJ, et al. Preventive therapy of first gastrointestinal bleeding in patients with cirrhosis: results of a controlled trial comparing propranolol, endoscopic sclerotherapy and placebo. *Hepatology* 1990;12:1413–1419.
155. Ideo G, Bellati G, Fesce E, et al. Nadolol can prevent the first gastrointestinal bleeding in cirrhotics: a prospective, randomized study. *Hepatology* 1988;8:6–9.
156. Pascal JP, Cales P. Propranolol in the prevention of first upper gastrointestinal tract hemorrhage in patients with cirrhosis of the liver and esophageal varices. *N Engl J Med* 1987;317:856–861.
157. Prophylaxis of first hemorrhage from esophageal varices by sclerotherapy, propranolol or both in cirrhotic patients: a randomized multicenter trial. The PROVA Study Group. *Hepatology* 1991;14:1016–1024.
158. Angelico M, Carli L, Piat C, et al. Isosorbide-5-mononitrate versus propranolol in the prevention of first bleeding in cirrhosis. *Gastroenterology* 1993;104:1460–1465.
159. Vorobioff J, Picabea E, Gamen M, et al. Propranolol compared with propranolol plus isosorbide dinitrate in portal-hypertensive patients: long-term hemodynamic and renal effects. *Hepatology* 1993;18:477–484.
160. Grace ND, Muench H, Chalmers TC. The present status of shunts for portal hypertension in cirrhosis. *Gastroenterology* 1966;50:684–691.
161. D'Amico G, Pagliaro L, Bosch J. The treatment of portal hypertension: a meta-analytic review. *Hepatology* 1995;22:332–354.
162. Lo GH, Lai KH, Cheng JS, et al. Prophylactic banding ligation of high-risk esophageal varices in patients with cirrhosis: a prospective, randomized trial. *J Hepatol* 1999;31:451–456.
163. Svoboda P, Kantorova I, Ochmann J, et al. A prospective randomized controlled trial of sclerotherapy vs ligation in the prophylactic treatment of high-risk esophageal varices. *Surg Endosc* 1999;13:580–584.
164. Grace ND, Groszmann RJ, Garcia-Tsao G, et al. Portal hypertension and variceal bleeding: an AASLD single topic symposium. *Hepatology* 1998;28:868–880.
165. Fogel MR, Knauer CM, Andres LL, et al. Continuous intravenous vasopressin in active upper gastrointestinal bleeding. *Ann Intern Med* 1982;96:565–569.
166. Chojkier M, Groszmann RJ, Atterbury CE, et al. A controlled comparison of continuous intraarterial and intravenous infusions of vasopressin in hemorrhage from esophageal varices. *Gastroenterology* 1979;77:540–546.
167. Merigan TC Jr, Plotkin GR, Davidson CS. Effect of intravenously administered posterior pituitary extract on hemorrhage from bleeding esophageal varices. A controlled evaluation. *N Engl J Med* 1962;266:134–135.
168. Groszmann RJ, Kravetz D, Bosch J, et al. Nitroglycerin improves the hemodynamic response to vasopressin in portal hypertension. *Hepatology* 1982;2:757–762.
169. Tsai YT, Lay CS, Lai KH, et al. Controlled trial of vasopressin plus nitroglycerin vs. vasopressin alone in the treatment of bleeding esophageal varices. *Hepatology* 1986;6:406–409.
170. Bosch J, Kravetz D, Rodes J. Effects of somatostatin on hepatic and systemic hemodynamics in patients with cirrhosis of the liver: comparison with vasopressin. *Gastroenterology* 1981;80:518–525.
171. Lee HY, Lee HJ, Lee SM, et al. A prospective randomized controlled clinical trial comparing the effects of somatostatin and vasopressin for control of acute variceal bleeding in the patients with liver cirrhosis. *Korean J Intern Med* 2003;18:161–166.
172. Burroughs AK, McCormick PA, Hughes MD, et al. Randomized, double-blind, placebo-controlled trial of somatostatin for variceal bleeding. Emergency control and prevention of early variceal rebleeding. *Gastroenterology* 1990;99:1388–1395.
173. Jaramillo JL, de la Mata M, Mino G, et al. Somatostatin versus Sengstaken balloon tamponade for primary haemostasia of bleeding esophageal varices. A randomized pilot study. *J Hepatol* 1991;12:100–105.
174. Burroughs AK, Hamilton G, Phillips A, et al. A comparison of sclerotherapy with staple transection of the esophagus for the emergency control of bleeding from esophageal varices. *N Engl J Med* 1989;321:857–862.
175. Stiegmann GV, Goff JS, Michaletz-Onody PA, et al. Endoscopic sclerotherapy as compared with endoscopic ligation for bleeding esophageal varices. *N Engl J Med* 1992;326:1527–1532.
176. Goff JS, Reveille RM, Stiegmann GV. Three years experience with endoscopic variceal ligation for treatment of bleeding varices. *Endoscopy* 1992;24:401–404.
177. Young MF, Sanowski RA, Rasche R. Comparison and characterization of ulcerations induced by endoscopic ligation of esophageal varices versus endoscopic sclerotherapy. *Gastrointest Endosc* 1993;39:119–122.
178. Laine L, Cook D. Endoscopic ligation compared with sclerotherapy for treatment of esophageal variceal bleeding. A meta-analysis. *Ann Intern Med* 1995;123:280–287.
179. LaBerge JM, Ring EJ, Gordon RL, et al. Creation of transjugular intrahepatic portosystemic shunts with the Wallstent endoprosthesis: results in 100 patients. *Radiology* 1993;187:413–420.
180. Sanyal AJ, Freedman AM, Luketic VA, et al. Transjugular intrahepatic portosystemic shunts for patients with active variceal hemorrhage unresponsive to sclerotherapy. *Gastroenterology* 1996;111:138–146.
181. Miller-Catchpole R. Diagnostic and therapeutic technology assessment. Transjugular intrahepatic portosystemic shunt (TIPS). *JAMA* 1995;273:1824–1830.
182. Patel NH, Chalasani N, Jindal RM. Current status of transjugular intrahepatic portosystemic shunts. *Postgrad Med J* 1998;74:716–720.
183. Kerlan RK Jr, LaBerge JM, Gordon RL, et al. Transjugular intrahepatic portosystemic shunts: current status. *AJR Am J Roentgenol* 1995;164:1059–1066.
184. Radosevich PM, LaBerge JM, Gordon RL. Current status and future possibilities of transjugular intrahepatic portosystemic shunts in the management of portal hypertension. *World J Surg* 1994;18:785–789.
185. Chung HH, Razavi MK, Sze DY, et al. Portosystemic pressure gradient during transjugular intrahepatic portosystemic shunt with Viatorr stent graft: what is the critical low threshold to avoid medically uncontrolled low pressure gradient related complications? *J Gastroenterol Hepatol* 2008;23:95–101.
186. Ryu RK, Durham JD, Krysl J, et al. Role of TIPS as a bridge to hepatic transplantation in Budd-Chiari syndrome. *J Vasc Interv Radiol* 1999;10:799–805.
187. de Oliveira e Silva A, Cardoso ES, de Melo CR, et al. Transjugular intrahepatic portosystemic shunts (TIPS) as a bridge for liver transplantation. *Arq Gastroenterol* 1996;33:201–206.
188. Hernandez-Guerra M, Turnes J, Rubinstein P, et al. PTFE-covered stents improve TIPS patency in Budd-Chiari syndrome. *Hepatology* 2004;40:1197–1202.
189. Lebrec D, Poynard T, Bernuau J, et al. A randomized controlled study of propranolol for prevention of recurrent gastrointestinal bleeding in patients with cirrhosis: a final report. *Hepatology* 1984;4:355–358.
190. Whipple AO. The problem of portal hypertension in relation to the hepatosplenopathies. *Ann Surg* 1945;122:449–475.
191. Sarfeh IJ, Rypins EB. Partial versus total portacaval shunt in alcoholic cirrhosis. Results of a prospective, randomized clinical trial. *Ann Surg* 1994;219:353–361.
192. Rosemurgy AS, Goode SE, Zwiebel BR, et al. A prospective trial of transjugular intrahepatic portasystemic stent shunts versus small-diameter prosthetic H-graft portacaval shunts in the treatment of bleeding varices. *Ann Surg* 1996;224:378–384; discussion 384–386.
193. Hermann RE, Henderson JM, Vogt DP, et al. Fifty years of surgery for portal hypertension at the Cleveland Clinic Foundation. Lessons and prospects. *Ann Surg* 1995;221:459–466; discussion 466–468.
194. Orozco H, Mercado MA, Granados Garcia J, et al. Selective shunts for portal hypertension: current role of a 21-year experience. *Liver Transpl Surg* 1997;3:475–480.

195. Henderson JM, Warren WD, Millikan WJ, et al. Distal splenorenal shunt with splenopancreatic disconnection. A 4-year assessment. *Ann Surg* 1989; 210:332–339; discussion 339–341.
196. Jin G, Rikkers LF. Cause and management of upper gastrointestinal bleeding after distal splenorenal shunt. *Surgery* 1992;112:719–725; discussion 725–727.
197. Orloff MJ, Orloff MS, Orloff SL, et al. Three decades of experience with emergency portacaval shunt for acutely bleeding esophageal varices in 400 unselected patients with cirrhosis of the liver. *J Am Coll Surg* 1995;180: 257–272.
198. Sugiura M, Futagawa S. Esophageal transection with paraesophagogastric devascularizations (the Sugiura procedure) in the treatment of esophageal varices. *World J Surg* 1984;8:673–679.
199. Wexler MJ, Stein BL. Nonshunting operations for variceal hemorrhage. *Surg Clin North Am* 1990;70:425–448.
200. Cello JP, Crass R, Trunkey DD. Endoscopic sclerotherapy versus esophageal transection of Child's class C patients with variceal hemorrhage. Comparison with results of portacaval shunt: preliminary report. *Surgery* 1982;91:333–338.
201. Villanueva C, Balanzo J, Novella MT, et al. Nadolol plus isosorbide mononitrate compared with sclerotherapy for the prevention of variceal rebleeding. *N Engl J Med* 1996;334:1624–1629.
202. Sauer P, Theilmann L. Prevention of transjugular intrahepatic portosystemic stent shunt thrombosis. *Digestion* 1998;59(suppl 2):45–47.
203. Sauer P, Theilmann L, Stremmel W, et al. Transjugular intrahepatic portosystemic stent shunt versus sclerotherapy plus propranolol for variceal rebleeding. *Gastroenterology* 1997;113:1623–1631.
204. Sarin SK, Lahoti D, Saxena SP, et al. Prevalence, classification and natural history of gastric varices: a long-term follow-up study in 568 portal hypertension patients. *Hepatology* 1992;16:1343–1349.
205. Kim T, Shijo H, Kokawa H, et al. Risk factors for hemorrhage from gastric fundal varices. *Hepatology* 1997;25:307–312.
206. D'Amico G, Montalbano L, Traina M, et al. Natural history of congestive gastropathy in cirrhosis. The Liver Study Group of V. Cervello Hospital. *Gastroenterology* 1990;99:1558–1564.
207. Huet PM, Goresky CA, Villeneuve JP, et al. Assessment of liver microcirculation in human cirrhosis. *J Clin Invest* 1982;70:1234–1244.
208. Roberts LR, Kamath PS. Ascites and hepatorenal syndrome: pathophysiology and management. *Mayo Clin Proc* 1996;71:874–881.
209. Stanley MM, Ochi S, Lee KK, et al. Peritoneovenous shunting as compared with medical treatment in patients with alcoholic cirrhosis and massive ascites. Veterans Administration Cooperative Study on Treatment of Alcoholic Cirrhosis with Ascites. *N Engl J Med* 1989;321: 1632–1638.
210. Marshall JB. Finding the cause of ascites. The importance of accurate fluid analysis. *Postgrad Med* 1988;83:189–190, 195–198.
211. Bories P, Garcia Compean D, Michel H, et al. The treatment of refractory ascites by the LeVeen shunt. A multi-centre controlled trial (57 patients). *J Hepatol* 1986;3:212–218.
212. Aiza I, Perez GO, Schiff ER. Management of ascites in patients with chronic liver disease. *Am J Gastroenterol* 1994;89:1949–1956.
213. Gines P, Arroyo V, Quintero E, et al. Comparison of paracentesis and diuretics in the treatment of cirrhotics with tense ascites. Results of a randomized study. *Gastroenterology* 1987;93:234–241.
214. Sola R, Andreu M, Coll S, et al. Spontaneous bacterial peritonitis in cirrhotic patients treated using paracentesis or diuretics: results of a randomized study. *Hepatology* 1995;21:340–344.
215. Greig PD, Langer B, Blendis LM, et al. Complications after peritoneovenous shunting for ascites. *Am J Surg* 1980;139:125–131.
216. Ochs A, Rossle M, Haag K, et al. The transjugular intrahepatic portosystemic stent-shunt procedure for refractory ascites. *N Engl J Med* 1995; 332:1192–1197.
217. Sanyal AJ, Genning C, Reddy KR, et al. The North American study for the treatment of refractory ascites. *Gastroenterology* 2003;124:634–641.
218. Runyon BA. Low-protein-concentration ascitic fluid is predisposed to spontaneous bacterial peritonitis. *Gastroenterology* 1986;91:1343–1346.
219. Rimola A, Soto R, Bory F, et al. Reticuloendothelial system phagocytic activity in cirrhosis and its relation to bacterial infections and prognosis. *Hepatology* 1984;4:53–58.
220. Runyon BA, Squier S, Borzio M. Translocation of gut bacteria in rats with cirrhosis to mesenteric lymph nodes partially explains the pathogenesis of spontaneous bacterial peritonitis. *J Hepatol* 1994;21:792–796.
221. Runyon BA, Morrissey RL, Hoefs JC, et al. Opsonic activity of human ascitic fluid: a potentially important protective mechanism against spontaneous bacterial peritonitis. *Hepatology* 1985;5:634–637.
222. Runyon BA. Early events in spontaneous bacterial peritonitis. *Gut* 2004; 53:782–784.
223. Guarner C, Runyon BA. Spontaneous bacterial peritonitis: pathogenesis, diagnosis, and management. *Gastroenterologist* 1995;3:311–328.
224. Hoefs JC, Runyon BA. Spontaneous bacterial peritonitis. *Dis Mon* 1985; 31:1–48.
225. Sort P, Navasa M, Arroyo V, et al. Effect of intravenous albumin on renal impairment and mortality in patients with cirrhosis and spontaneous bacterial peritonitis. *N Engl J Med* 1999;341:403–409.
226. Guarner C, Runyon BA, Heck M, et al. Effect of long-term trimethoprim-sulfamethoxazole prophylaxis on ascites formation, bacterial translocation, spontaneous bacterial peritonitis, and survival in cirrhotic rats. *Dig Dis Sci* 1999;44:1957–1962.
227. Runyon BA, Borzio M, Young S, et al. Effect of selective bowel decontamination with norfloxacin on spontaneous bacterial peritonitis, translocation, and survival in an animal model of cirrhosis. *Hepatology* 1995;21: 1719–1724.
228. Runyon BA, McHutchison JG, Antillon MR, et al. Short-course versus long-course antibiotic treatment of spontaneous bacterial peritonitis. A randomized controlled study of 100 patients. *Gastroenterology* 1991;100: 1737–1742.
229. Soriano G, Guarner C, Tomas A, et al. Norfloxacin prevents bacterial infection in cirrhotics with gastrointestinal hemorrhage. *Gastroenterology* 1992;103:1267–1272.
230. Lin HC. Antibiotic prophylaxis for the prevention of bacterial infections in cirrhotic patients with gastrointestinal hemorrhage. *Zhonghua Yi Xue Za Zhi (Taipei)* 2002;65:361–362.
231. Bernard B, Grange JD, Khac EN, et al. Antibiotic prophylaxis for the prevention of bacterial infections in cirrhotic patients with ascites: a meta-analysis. *Digestion* 1998;59(suppl 2):54–57.
232. Grange JD, Roulot D, Pelletier G, et al. Norfloxacin primary prophylaxis of bacterial infections in cirrhotic patients with ascites: a double-blind randomized trial. *J Hepatol* 1998;29:430–436.
233. Singh N, Gayowski T, Yu VL, et al. Trimethoprim-sulfamethoxazole for the prevention of spontaneous bacterial peritonitis in cirrhosis: a randomized trial. *Ann Intern Med* 1995;122:595–598.
234. Rolachon A, Cordier L, Bacq Y, et al. Ciprofloxacin and long-term prevention of spontaneous bacterial peritonitis: results of a prospective controlled trial. *Hepatology* 1995;22:1171–1174.
235. McKay A, Dixon E, Bathe O, et al. Umbilical hernia repair in the presence of cirrhosis and ascites: results of a survey and review of the literature. *Hernia* 2009;13:461–468.
236. Douard R, Lentschener C, Ozier Y, et al. Operative risks of digestive surgery in cirrhotic patients. *Gastroenterol Clin Biol* 2009;33:555–564.
237. Youssef YF, El Ghannam M. Mesh repair of non-complicated umbilical hernia in ascitic patients with liver cirrhosis. *J Egypt Soc Parasitol* 2007; 37:1189–1197.

CHAPTER 59 ■ HEPATIC NEOPLASMS

CHRISTOPHER J. SONNENDAY, THEODORE H. WELLING, AND SHAWN J. PELLETIER

KEY POINTS

1. Evaluation of hepatic reserve, facilitated by assessment of the Child-Turcotte-Pugh classification and computed tomography volumetry, is essential to minimize the risk of postoperative liver failure following hepatectomy, particularly in patients with chronic liver disease and hepatic steatosis.
2. Surgical therapy of benign hepatic neoplasms should be confined to symptomatic patients and those patients with risk of malignant transformation (e.g., biliary cystadenoma, hepatic adenoma).
3. Treatment for hepatocellular cancer may include diverse modalities (resection, ablation, transplantation, systemic therapy), selected based on stage of disease and severity of underlying liver disease.
4. Liver transplantation for early-stage hepatocellular cancer can provide excellent patient survival, with long-term outcomes similar to patients undergoing liver transplantation for other indications.
5. Hepatic resection of colorectal metastases may be associated with 25% to 58% 5-year survival in appropriately selected patients. Patients most likely to benefit from metastasectomy include patients with small, solitary metastases and a prolonged disease-free interval since treatment of the primary tumor.
6. The number of hepatic neoplasms amenable to surgical therapy appears to be increasing in incidence, associated with increased diagnosis due to improved cross-sectional imaging, rising incidence of diseases (viral hepatitis, nonalcoholic fatty liver disease) associated with primary hepatic malignancies, and extension of surgical therapy to more patients with metastatic disease to the liver.
7. Portal vein embolization (PVE) prior to hepatic resection is an effective adjunct to increase the size of the future liver remnant, allowing expansion of major hepatectomy to patients with underlying liver disease. Failure to respond to PVE is a poor prognostic sign and contraindication to resection.
8. Laparoscopic liver resection has been demonstrated to be feasible and safe in properly selected patients, allowing extension of minimally invasive approaches to major hepatectomy and even living donor hepatectomy in highly experienced hands.
9. Advanced hepatobiliary techniques such as total vascular exclusion and hypothermic perfusion can be performed in select patients and experienced centers, allowing resection of tumors involving the inferior vena cava and/or hepatic veins with outcomes similar to other major hepatectomies.

The management of hepatic neoplasms is an increasingly complex and multidisciplinary area of medicine and surgery. Major hepatic resection, though an accepted therapy for appropriate indications, may carry significant risk of morbidity and mortality, especially in the setting of chronic liver disease. Increasingly, hepatic surgery is being performed by surgeons with subspecialty hepatobiliary and oncology training. Nevertheless, liver masses are commonly encountered by the general surgeon and proper management requires adherence to several key principles reviewed in the following text.

The surgical treatment of hepatic neoplasms was made possible by the evolution of understanding of hepatic physiology and anatomy over the past century. No person deserves more credit for the expansion of liver surgery than the French surgeon Claude Couinaud (Fig. 59.1).[1] He performed exhaustive anatomic studies of the segmental anatomy of the liver, facilitated by the examination of thousands of cadaver livers treated by injection of the common bile duct, hepatic artery, and portal and hepatic veins with polyvinyl acetate. Subsequent dissolution of the liver parenchyma with dilute acid left remarkable casts of the vascular and biliary anatomy of the liver. He subsequently translated his findings in the context of surgical procedures, identifying surface landmarks to segmental structures, describing the critical planes of the Glissonian sheaths, and identifying important anatomic variants that influenced the feasibility of resection procedures (Fig. 59.2).[2,3] His published studies and observations, originally appearing in 1954 and continuing until his death in 2008, are required reading for surgeons who desire to understand surgical anatomy of the liver.

DIAGNOSIS

Hepatic neoplasms may present in a protean manner, ranging from incidental lesions found at the time of imaging for other indications, to profound hepatic dysfunction in patients with advanced liver disease and malignancy, to symptoms such as pain or jaundice influenced by tumor size and location. Regardless of the presentation, the initial diagnostic steps in the evaluation of a patient with a liver mass include assessment of hepatic synthetic function, precise anatomic review, and understanding of the oncologic context of the lesion(s) in question. These principles will be repeated throughout the following text, and guide decision making regarding the most appropriate therapy for a given neoplasm.

History, Physical Examination, and Laboratory Evaluation

Assessment of the patient with a new diagnosis of a hepatic mass or neoplasm should begin with consideration of any underlying chronic liver disease. By far, the most important risk factor for primary hepatic malignancies is chronic liver disease of any cause. Viral hepatitis remains the most common cause of chronic liver disease and cirrhosis worldwide, and we are in the midst of the peak of the hepatitis C epidemic in the United States. Importantly, many carriers of chronic hepatitis B and C infection remain unaware of their disease. The World Health Organization estimates that more than 500 million people

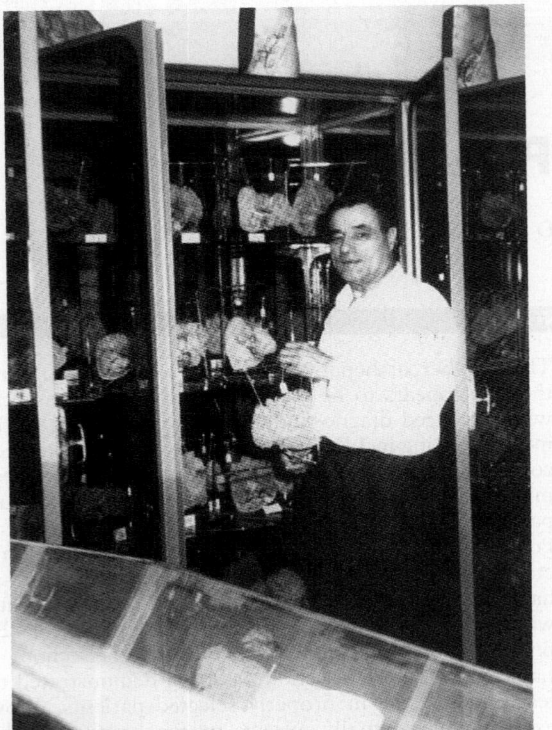

FIGURE 59.1. Claude Couinaud working with his collection of "liver casts" at the school of medicine in Paris, 1988. (Reprinted with permission from Francis Sutherland, MD, FSCRC.)

worldwide are infected with either hepatitis C (180 million) or hepatitis B (350 million).[4] Assessment of a patient with a new liver mass should include viral serologic testing, even when risk factors for infection may not be obvious. Nonalcoholic fatty liver disease (NAFLD) is likely to be the next epidemic cause of chronic liver disease in the developed world,[5] and it appears that primary liver cancer will remain an important potential consequence of this disease as it is with other chronic hepatitides. Cholestatic liver disease, particularly primary sclerosing cholangitis (PSC), is a primary risk factor for cholangiocarcinoma, and the distinction between benign and malignant strictures can be especially troubling in the advanced stages of PSC.

A careful history about past liver disease and current symptoms is critical. Symptoms of chronic liver disease may be subtle in initial stages of the disease (fatigue, weight loss, muscle wasting), but may even be difficult to discern in more advanced cases (splenomegaly, bleeding diatheses, mild jaundice). Clearly, any symptoms of decompensated cirrhosis or portal hypertension should be cause for pause in the evaluation of a patient with a liver tumor. Encephalopathy, ascites, variceal hemorrhage, and progressive cholestasis are ominous signs that may pose prohibitive risk for hepatic resection or other procedures. Physical examination should also focus on eliciting signs of chronic liver disease such as skin changes, ecchymoses, splenomegaly, anasarca, or ascites. In patients with malignant disease, careful assessment for evidence of extrahepatic disease should be performed, with attention paid to lymphadenopathy, pleural effusions, or other mass lesions.

In addition to appropriate tumor markers when indicated, laboratory evaluation should include appraisal of hepatic synthetic function. A comprehensive metabolic panel to include measurement of bilirubin, albumin, and transaminases is important. Attention should be paid to renal function, which can be compromised with advanced liver disease and carries an especially poor prognostic value. A complete blood count is necessary, with special attention paid to the platelet count. Thrombocytopenia can be indicative of advanced hypersplenism and portal hypertension, which may translate to increased risk for hepatic resection and other procedures. Measurements of coagulation parameters, especially prothrombin time (PT) and the associated international normalized ratio (INR), are also sensitive indicators of hepatic synthetic function.

Evaluation of Hepatic Reserve

1 In patients with documented chronic liver disease, a more refined evaluation of hepatic synthetic function and reserve is necessary. In addition, a careful consideration of underlying

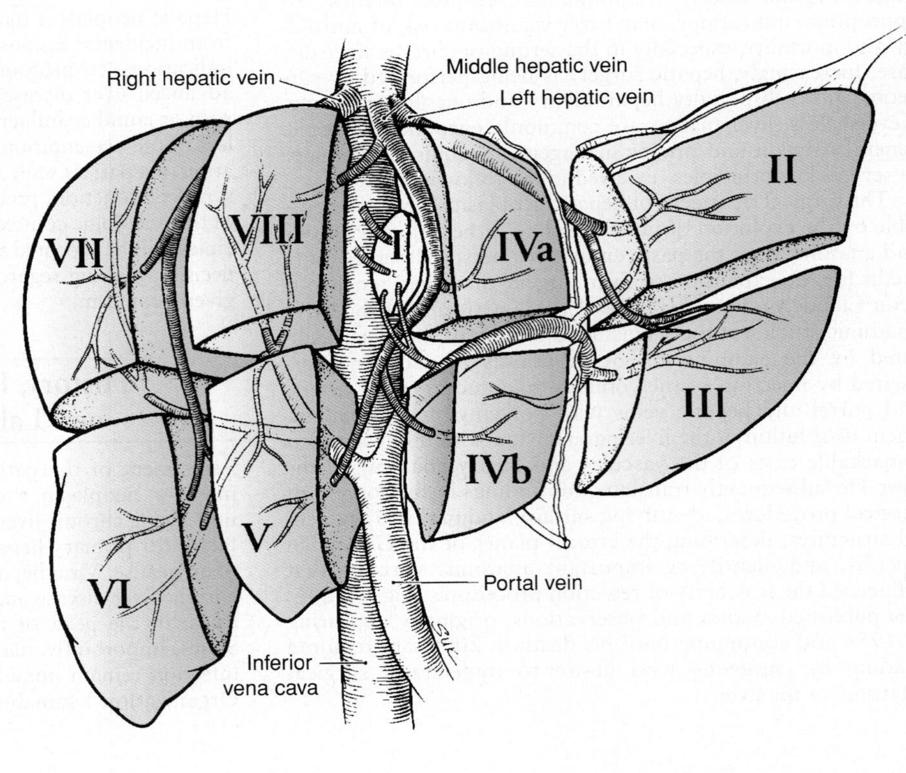

FIGURE 59.2. Couinaud's segmental anatomy of the liver. Segments II, III, and IV make up the left lobe and segments V, VI, VII, and VIII constitute the right lobe. Segment I is the caudate lobe.

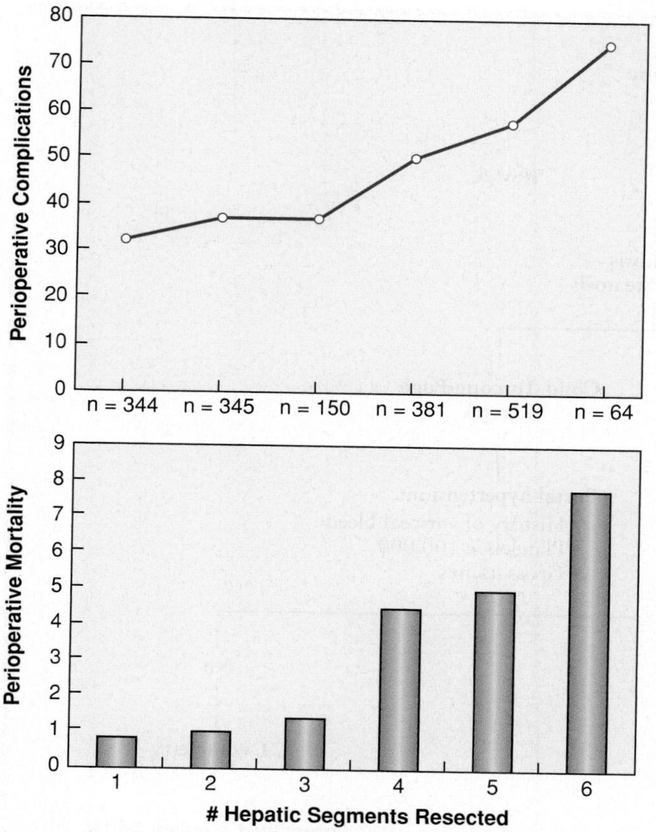

FIGURE 59.3. Perioperative complications and mortality among 1,803 patients undergoing hepatic resection at the Memorial Sloan Kettering Cancer Center (1991–2001), stratified by the number of hepatic segments resected. (Redrawn from Jarnagin WR, Gonen M, Fong Y, et al. Improvement in perioperative outcome after hepatic resection. *Ann Surg* 2002;236[4]:402.)

liver function should be performed in patients undergoing major hepatectomy (resection of three or more Couinaud segments), even in the absence of overt chronic liver disease, as the risk of perioperative morbidity and mortality rises substantially for such procedures (Fig. 59.3).[6] While multiple modalities and strategies may be employed to evaluate hepatic reserve prior to liver resection, a reasonable algorithm is included in Algorithm 59.1 and reviewed here.

A number of clinical classification methods to assess underlying chronic liver disease have been developed, with the Child-Turcotte-Pugh (CTP) classification recognized universally (Table 59.1).[7] Consensus exists that CTP class C patients should not undergo hepatic resection due to excessive perioperative morbidity and mortality, and CTP class B patients should only be considered for minor hepatic resections (resection of two or fewer Couinaud segments).[8,9] The evaluation of CTP class A patients for hepatic resection is more difficult, as these patients can vary substantially in their risk of perioperative mortality and postoperative liver failure.

In recent years, the Model for End-Stage Liver Disease (MELD) score has been shown to accurately predict mortality among patients undergoing transjugular intrahepatic portosystemic shunt (TIPS) procedures,[10] and is currently used in liver transplant allocation due to its accuracy in predicting transplant waitlist mortality.[11] Recently, investigators have advocated that MELD can be used to predict nontransplant surgical outcomes, particularly among cirrhotics undergoing hepatic resection.[12,13] Among a population of CTP class A patients with hepatocellular carcinoma (HCC), perioperative mortality for patients with a MELD score greater than 9 was 29%, whereas there were no perioperative deaths among patients with a MELD score under 9.[12] However, a large multi-institutional study of Veteran's Affairs patients utilizing National Surgical Quality Improvement Project (NSQIP) data refuted the value of the MELD in risk stratification prior to hepatic resection, with CTP score and American Society of Anesthesiologists (ASA) class proving to be better predictors of perioperative complications and 30-day mortality.[14]

Assessment of cirrhotic patients for evidence of significant portal hypertension is believed by most hepatobiliary surgeons to be a critical step in risk stratification for hepatic resection. Patients with clinical signs of portal hypertension, such as a history of variceal hemorrhage, esophageal or gastric varices

TABLE 59.1 **CLASSIFICATION**

CHILD-TURCOTTE-PUGH (CTP) CLASSIFICATION OF CHRONIC LIVER DISEASE

	■ POINTS		
■ CLINICAL CRITERIA	1	2	3
Albumin (g/dL)	>3.5	2.8–3.5	<2.8
Bilirubin (mg/dL)	<2.0	2.0–3.0	>3.0
Prothrombin time			
Seconds	<4	4–6	>6
International normalized ratio (INR)	<1.7	1.7–2.3	>2.3
Ascites	None	Moderate (or suppressed by medication, not requiring regular paracentesis)	Severe (tense ascites, refractory to medication, or requiring regular paracentesis)
Encephalopathy	None	Grade I–II (or suppressed by medication)	Grade III–IV (or refractory to medication)
CTP class A	5–6 points		
CTP class B	7–9 points		
CTP class C	10–15 points		

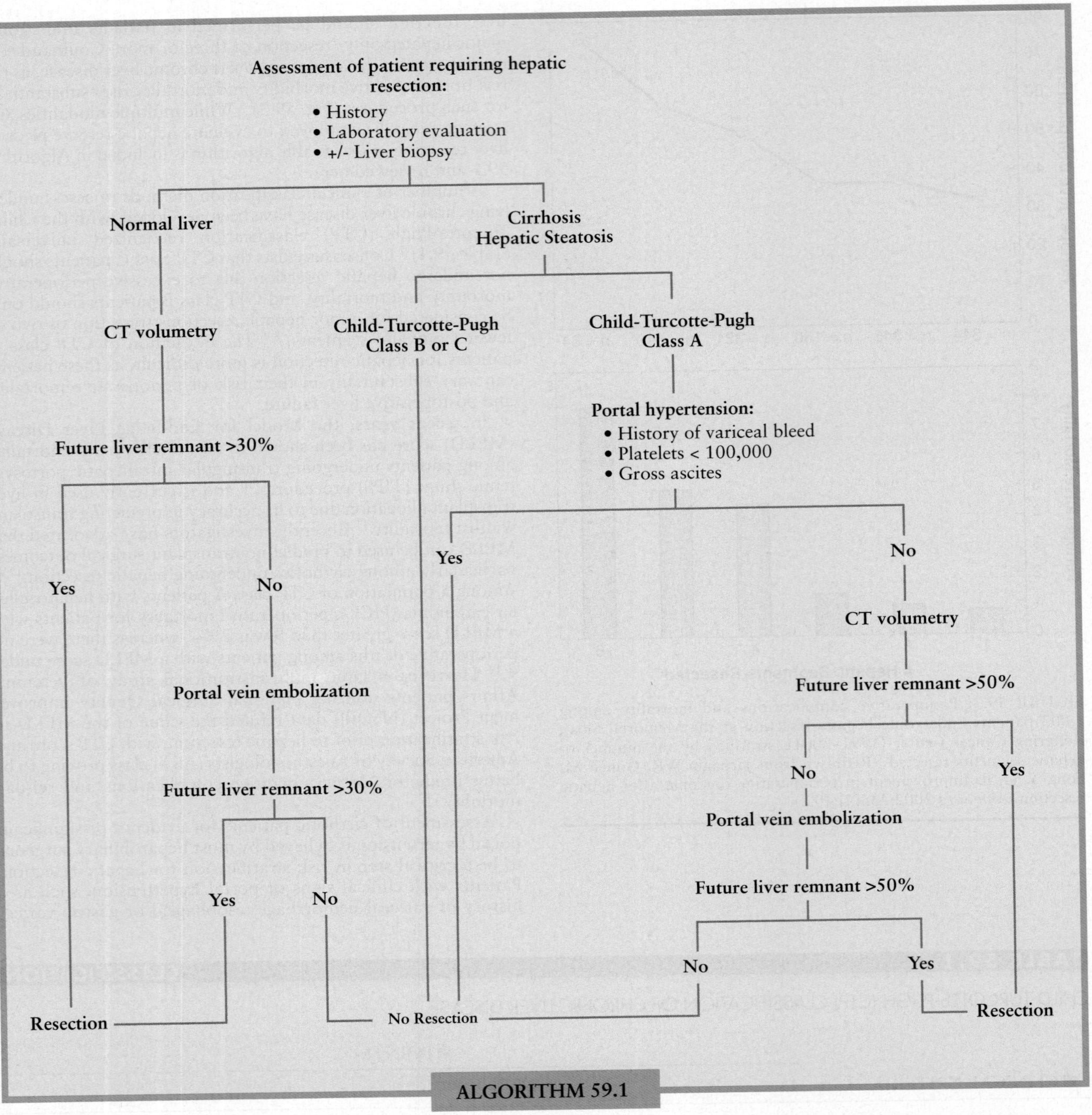

ALGORITHM 59.1. Proposed algorithm for evaluation of hepatic reserve in the patient being considered for hepatic resection. (Adapted from Clavien PA, Petrowsky H, DeOliveria ML, et al. Strategies for safer liver surgery and partial liver transplantation. *New Engl J Med* 2007;356:1553.)

on upper endoscopy, visible upper abdominal varices on cross-sectional imaging, or grossly apparent ascites, are not considered viable candidates for hepatic resection. Some centers have advocated direct measurement of the hepatic venous pressure gradient by percutaneous venous access with hepatic manometry,[15,16] although other surgeons have disputed the necessity of this study given the accuracy of clinical signs of portal hypertension and the relative invasiveness of the manometry procedure.[9] Thrombocytopenia is another critical clinical indicator of surgical risk with hepatic resection, reflecting the hypersplenism of advanced cirrhosis and portal hypertension.[17] A platelet count under 100,000 is considered a contraindication to major hepatectomy.

A number of quantitative liver function tests have been investigated to assess hepatic reserve prior to hepatic resection, including indocyanine green (ICG) clearance,[18] galactose elimination capacity,[19] and technetium-99m galactosyl human serum albumin scan,[20] among others. The ICG clearance study is the most commonly used internationally, though it is not commonly used or available in the United States. ICG retention at 15 minutes (ICGR-15) is believed to be the most accurate predictor of postoperative outcome among CTP class A patients, though this value may be affected by such factors as hepatic blood flow. Advocates of this method of risk stratification believe that an ICGR-15 under 14% is associated with acceptable outcomes following major hepatectomy, while an

ICGR-15 greater than 20% is a contraindication to such a resection.[21,22] Patients with an intermediate ICGR-15 of 14% to 20% must be considered selectively, with careful attention to remnant liver volume.[8,9]

Considerable attention has been paid in recent years to evaluation of remnant liver volume as a method to stratify risk of postoperative liver failure, and this method is the most common method of evaluating hepatic reserve among hepatobiliary centers in the United States.[23] This assessment relies on the use of computed tomography (CT) volumetry, produced by manual or automated serial measurement of cross-sectional liver volumes produced from a rapid-sequence, thin-section helical CT scan. The volume of the liver segments to be preserved following resection is then divided by the total estimated liver volume, producing a percentage of future liver remnant volume. In patients with normal liver parenchyma and function, a future liver remnant volume of 25% to 30% is considered adequate, especially if two contiguous Couinaud segments are preserved. In patients with chronic liver disease, cirrhosis, or documented hepatic steatosis, a future liver remnant volume of 40% to 50% is desired. In such patients, preoperative portal vein embolization, as discussed later in this chapter, should be considered if the liver remnant volume will not be adequate. Particular consideration should be given to patients undergoing major hepatectomy with no overt liver disease but prior exposure to prolonged chemotherapy, as this may be associated with the development of hepatic steatosis and adverse postoperative outcomes.[24] Compromise of hepatic venous return should be considered as equivalent to leaving a smaller liver remnant. For example, in the case of an extended right hepatectomy that leaves most of segment 4 intact but sacrifices the drainage of the middle hepatic vein, estimated future liver remnant volumes might be more accurate if they ignored the contribution of most of segment 4. Sacrifice of segmental vascular inflow, though collateralized in the liver parenchyma to some degree, should also be considered when determining the volume of future liver remnant.

Radiographic Evaluation and Imaging Techniques

Liver imaging is a rapidly evolving field, and the proliferation of new technologies affords the surgeon multiple modalities and techniques for defining the anatomy of a hepatic neoplasm. Familiarity with the technology available within one's community or hospital, as well as a close alliance with experienced radiologists, will aid in the selection of the imaging technique that best informs treatment decisions. While a comprehensive discussion of liver imaging techniques is beyond the scope of this text, some important principles about each of the primary modalities should be considered.

Ultrasound. Transcutaneous ultrasound is often the most accessible and least invasive diagnostic study available for evaluation of hepatic anatomy, and these characteristics make it particularly applicable to screening of high-risk populations for HCC.[25–27] Ultrasound is often the initial diagnostic modality in the evaluation of symptomatic liver masses, and is typically followed by dedicated cross-sectional imaging. In addition, ultrasound has important applications as a guide to percutaneous biopsy of liver lesions and to assist in the performance of percutaneous ablation or injection techniques.

As ultrasound may be limited in its ability to precisely evaluate the relationship of hepatic lesions to key vascular structures, most surgeons are more comfortable planning resection based on cross-sectional imaging. Nevertheless, ultrasound can be particularly useful in assessing specific lesions and may aid in narrowing a radiographic differential diagnosis. Cystic lesions in particular are well imaged by ultrasound, and characteristic lack of internal echoes and posterior acoustic enhancement (through-transmission) may be adequate to distinguish a simple cyst from other lesions that require more careful evaluation. Use of Doppler color imaging may also add to the exam, but is often not definitive in defining specific pathology. For example, clinicians may propose to use ultrasound with Doppler to identify the vascularity of a hemangioma. However, the Doppler signal in these lesions is often subtle as the flow in the tortuous vessels that make up these lesions is of low velocity. Metastatic lesions can often have a similar flow signal, thus making ultrasound with Doppler inadequate to diagnose hemangiomas definitively. Nevertheless, liver ultrasound in experienced hands can offer useful information about liver lesions and associated anatomy and can guide subsequent diagnostic testing.

Computed Tomography. CT is the dominant cross-sectional imaging technique in the developed world, and is often the source for initial recognition of incidental hepatic neoplasms, as well as an important diagnostic tool for hepatic lesions when ordered for cause (such as investigation of a finding on screening exam, or a follow-up exam in a patient with a known malignancy). While a dedicated liver CT can be the definitive study for much liver pathology, the quality of hepatic imaging varies significantly by technique and timing of contrast administration. A standard single-phase intravenous contrast CT may provide excellent images of hepatic lesions, but can underestimate the burden of disease based on slice thickness and the lack of a true arterial and delayed phase images. Numerous examples of standard CT techniques missing subtle lesions that could affect treatment decisions may be cited, especially in the case of metastatic disease or HCC in patients with chronic liver disease where multifocality is common. For that reason, careful attention must be paid to the ordering of dedicated liver imaging, and communication to radiology of the indication for imaging is essential.

As is true of magnetic resonance imaging (MRI), attention is often particularly paid to the behavior of identified lesions throughout the distinct contrast phases of a liver CT: arterial, portal venous, and systemic (hepatic) venous. Definitive diagnostic criteria for HCC may be achieved, as discussed later, avoiding the need for biopsy in the majority of patients.

Magnetic Resonance Imaging. MRI has become the definitive imaging study for liver tumors in many centers, demonstrating increased sensitivity and specificity to CT in comparison studies. Furthermore, the addition of magnetic resonance cholangiopancreatography (MRCP) to liver tumor studies in appropriate patients (e.g., cholangiocarcinoma) offers distinct advantage over the cross-sectional images of CT. Like CT, liver MRI is highly dependent on technique, with the difference between a critical and useless study often defined by timing of contrast administration, synchronization of imaging series with patient breath holding and movement, and proper reconstruction of distinct imaging series. Again, institutional experience and expertise often determine which cross-sectional imaging study is appropriate for treatment planning.

Positron Emission Tomography. Positron emission tomography (PET) may be a powerful adjunct to other liver imaging techniques in appropriately selected patients. PET is often best reserved for defining the nature of small indeterminate lesions, identifying multifocal disease, and characterizing liver metastases in the context of the presence or absence of extrahepatic disease. Given the strong background of glucose metabolism in the liver, more subtle lesions such as HCC, which may closely resemble normal liver parenchyma on a cellular level, are poorly identified on PET. In the case of metastatic colorectal cancer, PET has become established as an important addition to cross-sectional imaging in defining the extent of metastatic disease and aiding in treatment planning. PET, particularly when performed in combination with synchronized CT imaging, has been shown to alter treatment decisions by aiding in the detection of subtle hepatic metastases not well visualized on standard cross-sectional imaging studies and by adding sensitivity in the detection of extrahepatic metastases.[28,29]

BENIGN HEPATIC NEOPLASMS

Cystic Lesions

The increased use of cross-sectional imaging has led to a marked increase in the diagnosis of incidental hepatic masses and lesions. The distinction between solid and cystic lesions is important, as the vast majority of cystic lesions of the liver are benign in behavior. The majority of incidentally discovered cystic lesions of the liver are simple or congenital cysts, lesions that have no malignant potential and rarely become symptomatic. In some cases, a large or dominant simple cyst may become symptomatic as it stretches the adjacent liver capsule or compresses adjacent organs. These lesions are ideal for laparoscopic resection or marsupialization, a procedure that can be performed safely with excellent results and negligible recurrence in experienced hands (Fig. 59.4).[30] In the case of patients with polycystic liver disease (PCLD), an autosomal dominant disease with variable penetrance and presentation, a minority of patients will develop disabling cystic hepatomegaly. In these patients, a variety of percutaneous[31,32] and surgical methods[33,34] have been attempted to alleviate symptoms, with liver transplantation[35,36] reserved for select few patients with refractory symptoms and/or associated superinfection or hepatic dysfunction. Surgical resection and marsupialization of dominant cysts in PCLD can have reasonable results in well-selected patients, though the risk of complications and recurrence is higher than in similar patients with simple hepatic cysts.[37]

2 The majority of cystic lesions are asymptomatic, and treatment is only indicated for lesions where there is concern for malignancy, or malignant potential. While a variety of primary and secondary hepatic neoplasms can have cystic components or degeneration, biliary cystadenomas are the most important primary cystic neoplasms of the liver, accounting for approximately 5% of all cystic lesions of the liver.[38] These neoplasms arise from the biliary epithelium, typically present in middle-aged women, and can vary markedly in size. Cystadenomas have a propensity toward local recurrence and malignant degeneration to cystadenocarcinoma.[39,40] The diagnosis of cystadenoma can be made radiographically in select circumstances, as classic lesions will demonstrate internal septae with papillary projections.[41] Intratumoral hemorrhage or fine calcifications may be present. Contrast enhancement on CT or MRI can suggest the presence of cystadenocarcinoma, though the definitive distinction between cystadenoma and cystadenocarcinoma without a surgical specimen is typically not possible. Cyst fluid analysis by percutaneous aspiration may aid in the diagnosis of cystadenoma versus simple cyst, as elevated fluid CA 19–9 and carcinoembryonic antigen (CEA) levels may be present in cystadenoma, but again cannot reliably distinguish benign from malignant disease.[42] For this reason, surgical resection is recommended in all cases where biliary cystadenoma is suspected or cannot be definitively excluded.

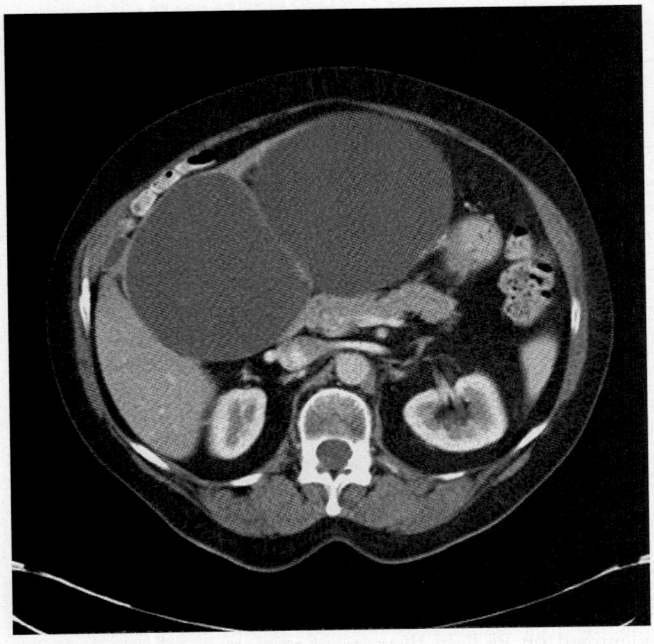

FIGURE 59.4. Contrast-enhanced computed tomography of a large bilobed simple hepatic cyst in a 73-year-old female who presented with an abdominal mass and early satiety. The patient underwent laparoscopic resection of the anterior cyst wall with complete resolution of symptoms. Pathology of the cyst wall was consistent with a simple cyst.

Solid Lesions

Solid mass lesions of the liver deserve more careful consideration in regards to surgical therapy and follow-up imaging. Dedicated liver MRI or CT can make the definitive diagnosis of a benign solid lesion, obviating the need for serial imaging in asymptomatic patients. While there are many benign solid lesions of the liver, the vast majority of clinical decision making for benign hepatic lesions relates to the proper distinction between hemangioma, hepatic adenoma, and focal nodular hyperplasia (FNH). Each of these lesions will be discussed here.

Hemangioma. Hemangiomata of the liver, like their relatives in other anatomic locations, are congenital tumors of disorganized vasculature with intervening fibrous tissue of variable quantities. The tumors are composed of multiple intertwined vessels, the size of capillaries, but may contain larger vascular channels with cavernous transformation. The vast majority are small in size (approximately 80% will be <4 cm),[43] though enormous lesions (>10 to 20 cm) may be encountered. Approximately 10% to 20% of persons with hepatic hemangioma will have multiple lesions.[43,44]

Hemangiomata represent the most common benign neoplasm of the liver, at least in clinical practice (subcentimeter biliary hamartomas are likely more prevalent). Autopsy studies suggest that hemangiomata are present in 4% to 20% of individuals.[45,46] Most hemangiomata are identified in individuals ages 40 to 60, though this age at presentation will likely fall with the increased use of abdominal ultrasound and cross-sectional imaging for other indications in younger patients. Hemangiomata, like other benign hepatic neoplasms, appear to be more common in women, with a female-to-male ratio of at least 2:1.[43] The use of female sex hormones for oral contraception or hormone replacement therapy is associated with a slight increase in hemangioma size at presentation, and appears to be more likely associated with a solitary hemangioma rather than multiple lesions.[44] In addition, ongoing sex hormone exposure appears to be associated with an increased incidence of enlargement in some women with hepatic hemangioma.

The majority of hepatic hemangiomata present as asymptomatic, incidental findings found on imaging studies performed for other indications. These lesions are also commonly identified incidentally at the time of operative exploration for another diagnosis. While there are reports of spontaneous or traumatic hemangioma rupture in exceptional cases (~30 cases in the surgical literature), there are no clear risk factors to predict this extremely rare occurrence.[47] Thus, the vast majority of hepatic hemangiomata can be left undisturbed, with surgical therapy reserved for the symptomatic hemangioma. Surgical dogma has

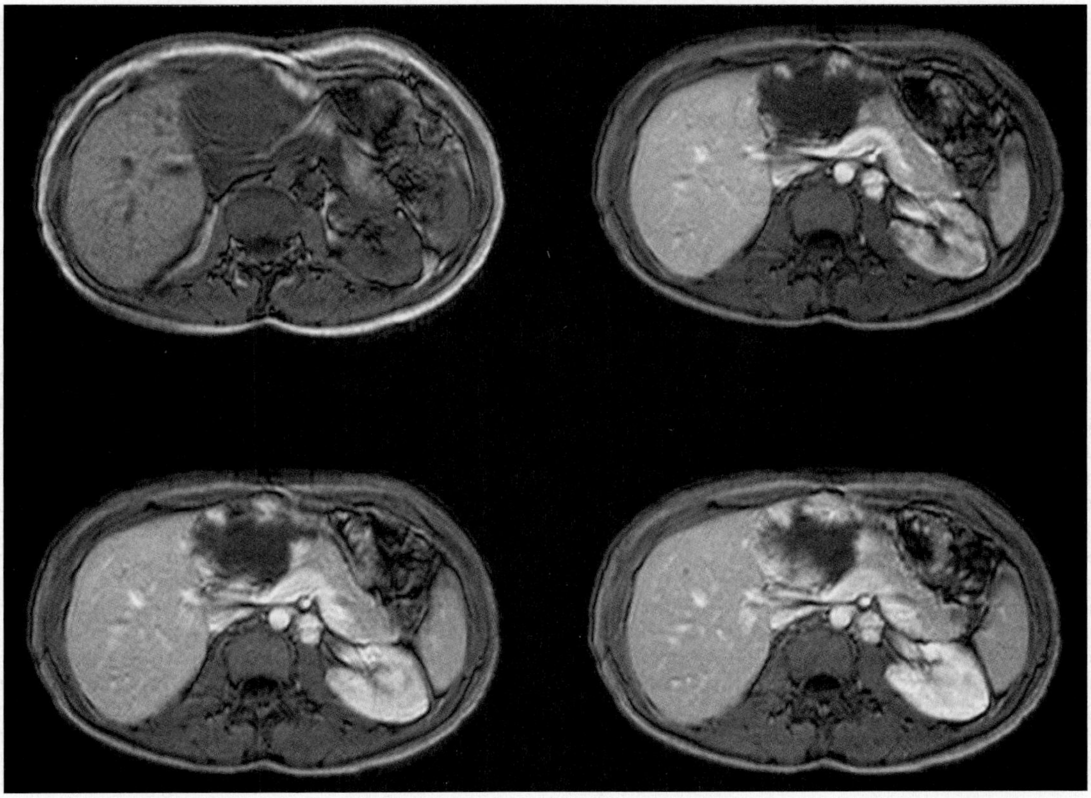

FIGURE 59.5. Magnetic resonance imaging of a hepatic hemangioma, demonstrating hypointensity on unenhanced images (*upper left*) and peripheral nodular enhancement with centripetal progression of enhancement on contrast-enhanced images (*upper right, lower left, lower right*). No treatment was recommended for this asymptomatic incidentally discovered lesion.

suggested that hemangiomata over 10 cm in size should be considered for excision, though again there are no clear data to support this practice in asymptomatic lesions. Radiographic follow-up of larger asymptomatic hemangiomata is also probably unnecessary, as size at presentation does not appear to predict any risk for growth.[44] The only potentially effective intervention for asymptomatic hemangiomata in appropriate female patients would be to recommend cessation of hormonal therapy.

Accurate radiographic diagnosis of a hepatic hemangioma is essential, as establishment of this diagnosis requires no additional intervention or test in almost all patients. MRI is now considered the most sensitive and specific imaging modality for hemangioma. Hemangiomata have a homogeneous high signal on T2-weighted images and demonstrate a pathognomonic pattern of initial peripheral, nodular enhancement following intravenous gadolinium administration with progressive infilling of the lesion on delayed sequences (Fig. 59.5).[48,49] Contrast-enhanced CT demonstrates a similar pattern of peripheral to central filling on delayed images. Ultrasound of hepatic hemangioma typically reveals a well-defined lobular lesion with increased echogenicity, though these characteristics may be less reliable in larger lesions. Historically, tagged red blood cell studies have been used to confirm the diagnosis of hemangioma, but this study is not necessary when the preferred high-quality MRI or CT is available. Biopsy, though not absolutely contraindicated when hemangioma is in the differential diagnosis,[50] should not be necessary with appropriate imaging.

Symptomatic hemangiomata of the liver may present with abdominal pain, evidence of intratumoral or intraperitoneal rupture, or Kasabach-Merritt syndrome (thrombocytopenia and consumptive coagulopathy associated with a massive cavernous hemangioma).[51] Symptomatic lesions tend to be large (>10 cm) and located on the periphery of the liver with stretching of the liver capsule that some surgeons believe accounts for the pain associated with these lesions. Care should be taken not to blame a small hemangioma for nonspecific abdominal pain; longitudinal studies seem to suggest that hemangioma under 5 cm are rarely, if ever, symptomatic.[43] Intratumoral hemorrhage noted on CT or MRI may also be associated with pain in some patients, and is a generally accepted indication for surgical excision. Significant ongoing hemorrhage is extremely rare, but case reports seem to indicate that an initial approach of hemodynamic stabilization, transcatheter intra-arterial embolization, and subsequent surgical excision is the preferred approach when resources are available.[52]

Elective surgical treatment of a symptomatic hemangioma may be accomplished by either enucleation or formal hepatic resection. Enucleation is often surprisingly simple to accomplish, as most large symptomatic lesions are exophytic to some degree and a pseudocapsular plane can be developed efficiently. Incision into the Glisson capsule adjacent to the hemangioma allows identification of the proper plane, which is truly distinct from the hepatic parenchyma. Progression along the pseudocapsule of the lesion may be accomplished with hydrodissection, an ultrasonic dissector, or blunt dissection. Multiple small feeding vessels appear to be far more common than a single large inflow vessel, and these vessels may be methodically controlled with ligatures, bipolar cautery, or other surgical energy devices. Inflow occlusion with a Pringle maneuver may be helpful to decompress an exceptionally large hemangioma, but is often not necessary with an enucleation procedure. A formal anatomic or nonanatomic hepatectomy may be accomplished in cases where enucleation is more difficult, such as the rare symptomatic intraparenchymal lesion.

Techniques of hepatectomy described later in this chapter, including liberal use of intraoperative ultrasound, would apply. Excellent outcomes should be the standard in the surgical therapy of patients with hemangiomata.[53] Symptomatic lesions in poor surgical candidates can be treated effectively with focal external beam radiation or embolization.

Hepatic Adenoma. Hepatocellular adenomas are rare benign tumors of the liver, with an estimated prevalence of approximately 1% on postmortem exams.[45] The incidence of adenoma has appeared to increase notably with the more common use of oral contraceptives, an association made by the famed hepatobiliary pathologist Gerald Klatskin and others in the late 1970s.[54] There appears to be a directly proportional relationship between oral contraceptive exposure and adenoma risk, with a fivefold increase in incidence among women on oral contraceptives for more than 5 years.[55] Adenomas have also been associated with anabolic steroid use and glycogen storage disease, but may occur sporadically. Hepatic adenomatosis, originally defined as greater than 10 hepatic adenomas, appears to be a distinct entity from hepatic adenoma with different implications for treatment.[56] Germline mutations in hepatocyte nuclear factor 1α may be associated with a subset of cases, with other genetic defects suspected in other forms of the disease.[57]

Adenomas are well-circumscribed lesions that contain sheets of hepatocytes without intervening biliary ductules or portal tracts. The hepatocytes are laden with glycogen and lipid, which contributes to their imaging characteristics. Adenomas are well vascularized, fed by the hepatic arterial tree. Adenomas may vary widely in size, but most historical series seem to indicate a median size of 4 to 8 cm.[58-61] Unlike the other more common benign hepatic lesions of hemangioma and FNH, adenoma appears to have a low but consistent risk of either rupture or malignant degeneration (Fig. 59.6). Thus, surgical resection is typically recommended in otherwise appropriate candidates. In small lesions (<4 to 5 cm) in women on oral contraception, some experts have recommended withdrawal of oral contraception with subsequent imaging at 6 to 12 months to document regression.[62,63] Tumors with regression in size may be observed if hormonal therapy can be avoided definitely. More recently, other surgeons have argued that the safety of hepatic resection, and the increasing use of minimally invasive hepatectomy, has lessened the risks and burdens of liver surgery such that all adenomas, and other lesions with any diagnostic uncertainty, should be resected.[64] While the risk of any hepatic surgical procedure should not be overly minimized, a strategy of surgical excision should be the default pathway in most patients with a diagnosis of hepatic adenoma.

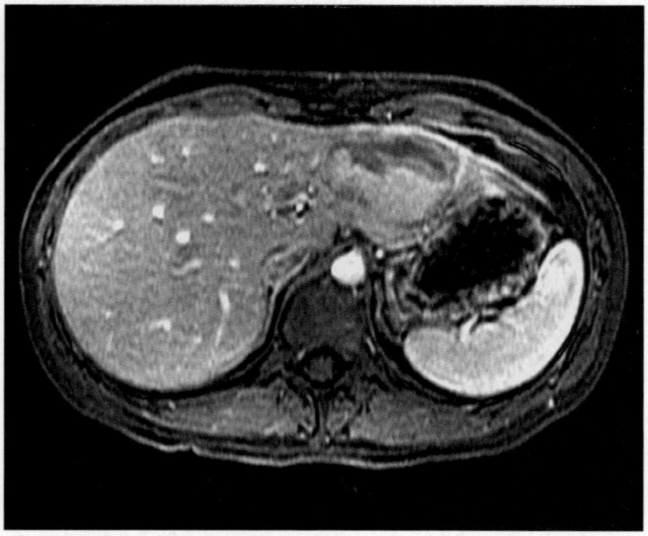

FIGURE 59.6. Magnetic resonance imaging of a hepatic adenoma consuming much of segments II and III, with intratumoral hemorrhage. This image, taken in the arterial phase following gadolinium administration, shows marked tumor enhancement, with the hemorrhagic component of the mass appearing hypointense to the tumor and surrounding liver. The patient was a healthy 25-year-old female on oral contraceptive pills who presented with acute epigastric pain. The lesion was resected with a laparoscopic left lateral segmentectomy.

With surgical excision the preferred approach for hepatocellular adenoma, the establishment of an accurate diagnosis for these lesions remains paramount. MRI provides the most definitive imaging study in the majority of patients. Adenomas are well-defined lesions with isointense or hyperintense (depending on the fat content of the lesion) features on T1- and T2-weighted images. With gadolinium administration, adenomas typically enhance markedly in a uniform manner on the arterial phase and disappear (become isointense) on the portal phase of imaging. CT imaging characteristics are similar, with a bright enhancement on the arterial phase of contrast administration. On ultrasound exam, adenomas are well circumscribed but have few other specific features to allow distinction from other hepatic neoplasms.

The distinction between adenoma and FNH can be difficult even with optimal cross-sectional imaging if the characteristic central scar and feeding artery of FNH are not visualized. Unfortunately, biopsy can sometimes be unreliable in this same diagnostic dilemma.[65] A 99m-technitium sulfur colloid scan can be considered in such cases, as an adenoma will not take up the radionuclide tracer due to the absence of Kupffer cells, while an FNH will typically demonstrate uptake. The failure to establish a definitive diagnosis of FNH is considered an indication for resection due to the risks associated with an undiagnosed adenoma. Patients with significant contraindications to surgical therapy should have oral contraception withdrawn and be enrolled in an annual surveillance program.

Focal Nodular Hyperplasia. FNH is often cited as the second most common benign neoplasm of the liver, after hemangioma. Clinical and autopsy series estimate that FNH occurs in 4% to 8% of individuals, with a strong predilection for women ages 20 to 50.[45,66–68] However, recent evidence suggests that calling FNH a neoplasm is perhaps a misnomer. Wanless et al. first suggested that FNH is a hyperplastic response of normal hepatic parenchyma to localized areas of increased arterial perfusion, facilitated by the existence of small arteriovenous malformations.[69] To that end, FNH is known to be associated with vascular diseases associated with arterial hyperperfusion of the liver, including hereditary hemorrhagic telangiectasia or congenital absence of the portal vein.[69–73]

FNH appears as a firm mass that is often slightly lighter in color than the surrounding hepatic parenchyma. Importantly, it lacks a true capsule, a characteristic that distinguishes FNH from adenoma or hemangioma. FNHs are usually located in the periphery of the liver, in a subcapsular position, and may be quite pedunculated. Histologically, the lesions consist of normal hepatic elements but the hepatocytes are not organized in normal cords around the sinusoids. Proliferating bile ductules may be present, but do not connect to the biliary tree proper.[68] Fibrous septae of various degrees of organization and maturity may be present, as well as areas of necrosis. These features account for the central stellate scar that may be seen radiographically in a large proportion of these lesions.[74]

The majority of FNHs are asymptomatic, found incidentally with abdominal imaging for other indications, or at laparotomy. Peripheral or pedunculated lesions that grow to significant size (5 to 10 cm) may be associated with abdominal pain or fullness in rare cases. Unlike adenoma, the risk of rupture and hemorrhage is extremely rare, though a handful of cases have been reported in the medical literature.[75] FNH is also not a premalignant lesion; thus, treatment should be reserved for patients with persistent symptoms not explained by another problem.

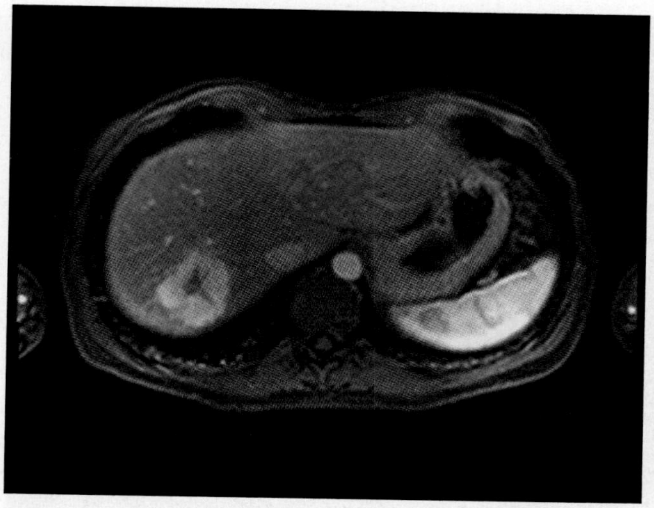

FIGURE 59.7. Gadolinium-enhanced magnetic resonance imaging of the liver, revealing a mass consistent with focal nodular hyperplasia. Note the bright contrast enhancement on the arterial phase, with prominent central scar that appears hypointense on this early phase of imaging.

Diagnosis of FNH can be established radiographically with current modalities. On unenhanced CT, FNH may be well defined with mass effect on adjacent vascular structures. The lesions are typically isoattenuated with normal liver and may have the characteristic hypoattenuated central scar. With contrast in the arterial phase, FNHs enhance brightly and become again isoattenuated to adjacent parenchyma in the portal phase. Small feeding vessels may be seen on the periphery of these lesions in the arterial phase. The central scar may enhance on delayed phases.

Similar enhancement patterns may be seen on a liver mass protocol MRI with gadolinium administration. FNHs appear typically isointense on T1-weighted sequences, and T2-weighted images will often reveal hyperintensity of the central scar. The entire lesion will enhance brightly and uniformly following gadolinium administration in the arterial phase, while the central scar will become hyperintense on delayed phases (Fig. 59.7). The intense and homogenous arterial enhancement of FNH helps distinguish the lesion from other hepatic masses that enhance in the arterial phase and become isointense in more delayed phases (e.g., HCC).[74]

Because of the typical indolent nature of FNH, its lack of malignant potential, and the characteristic radiographic features, the role of the surgeon in the management of this lesion is most often reduced to offering important reassurance to patients with incidental diagnoses. Indications for surgical resection should be limited to the rare patient with overt symptoms and the occasional case where the lack of classic imaging characteristics makes establishing a clear benign diagnosis difficult.[76] In the latter case, biopsy may also be confounding, as the normal cellular elements in FNH can make definitive diagnosis difficult, particularly if the fibrous scar elements are not sampled in the biopsy specimen.

PRIMARY HEPATIC MALIGNANCIES

Hepatocellular Carcinoma

HCC is the most common primary hepatic malignancy and is one of the most prevalent solid malignancies worldwide.[77] In the United States, its incidence is increasing the second fastest of any other tumors, believed to be related primarily to the hepatitis C (HCV) epidemic.[78] Risk factors for HCC include all problems causing chronic hepatitis or cirrhosis. HCV ranks the highest in risk, with a 3.7% to 7.1% annual incidence of HCC, and hepatitis B infection comes in at a close second, with a 2.2% to 4.3% annual incidence of the malignancy.[79] Other risk factors include alcohol, cirrhosis of any cause, aflatoxin, androgenic hormones, hemochromatosis, α_1-antitrypsin deficiency, glycogen storage diseases, hypercitrullinemia, porphyrias, hereditary tyrosinemia, Wilson disease, and any hepatic toxin exposure. Its incidence is certainly higher in areas of Asia and Africa where viral hepatitis or aflatoxin exposure is more endemic.

Screening for HCC has been examined in numerous trials, primarily focusing on the role of serum α-fetoprotein (AFP) determination and hepatic ultrasound.[25–27] While some controversy still exists about the frequency of screening and relative cutoff values for AFP, the American Association for the Study of Liver Disease (AASLD) has made guidelines regarding the use of these screening techniques based on the best existing evidence.[80] The AASLD currently recommends serial hepatic ultrasound and serum AFP every 6 to 12 months in at-risk populations (e.g., any patient with cirrhosis). However, a recent Chinese study evaluating primarily hepatitis B patients showed that the use of ultrasound and AFP could lower HCC-related mortality by 37%.[81] When a diagnosis of HCC is suspected, a contrast-enhanced three-phase MRI is more preferred than a CT in that there is an improved sensitivity and specificity of approximately 75% and 76%, respectively, compared to 61% and 66%, respectively, for CT.[82–84] The characteristic features of HCC on MRI or CT include arterial enhancement with early washout of contrast on the delayed phases of the scan (Fig. 59.8). These enhancement characteristics increase the specificity of the scan to greater than 95%.[85] Biopsy is reserved for cases in which the diagnosis is still in doubt following adequate imaging or in cases where it is thought to change management based on clinical suspicion.

3 Once the diagnosis of HCC is established, the choice of therapy must be individualized to each patient and based on tumor burden, degree of underlying liver disease, patient performance status, and the overall possibility of side effects or complications balanced with acceptable results. The therapeutic goals must also be individualized to either palliative or curative. Overall survival represents the best standard by which to judge most therapies as this measure incorporates much of the aforementioned patient-related factors. Therefore, the Barcelona Clinic Liver Cancer (BCLC) staging system (Algorithm 59.2) is considered the most current method to adequately stratify patients for specific therapies and has now been independently validated as superior to other staging systems used in the past.[86,87]

Resection is the treatment of choice for patients without liver disease; however, consideration of resection for cirrhotic patients requires greater scrutiny. Selection of patients for resection is critical and dependent on the following factors: degree of fibrosis, future liver remnant, patient performance status, tumor characteristics, and whether patients are similarly benefited by other therapies such as transplantation or radiofrequency ablation (RFA). In the best selected patients, survival rates at 5 years can vary from 38% to 70%, primarily depending on tumor stage.[88–90] Indeed, Child class B patients can have 5-year survival rates following resection of 20% to 50%, which approaches the survival rates of ablative therapies for tumors of similar size.[91–93] The perioperative mortality rate following resection for HCC is on the order of 4.0% to 4.7%, higher than mortality rates for benign disease or colorectal metastases,[94,95] reflecting the burden of chronic liver disease among patients with HCC.[96] Aside from liver disease burden, the presence of tumor vascular invasion is the single most important predictor of outcome following resection, decreasing

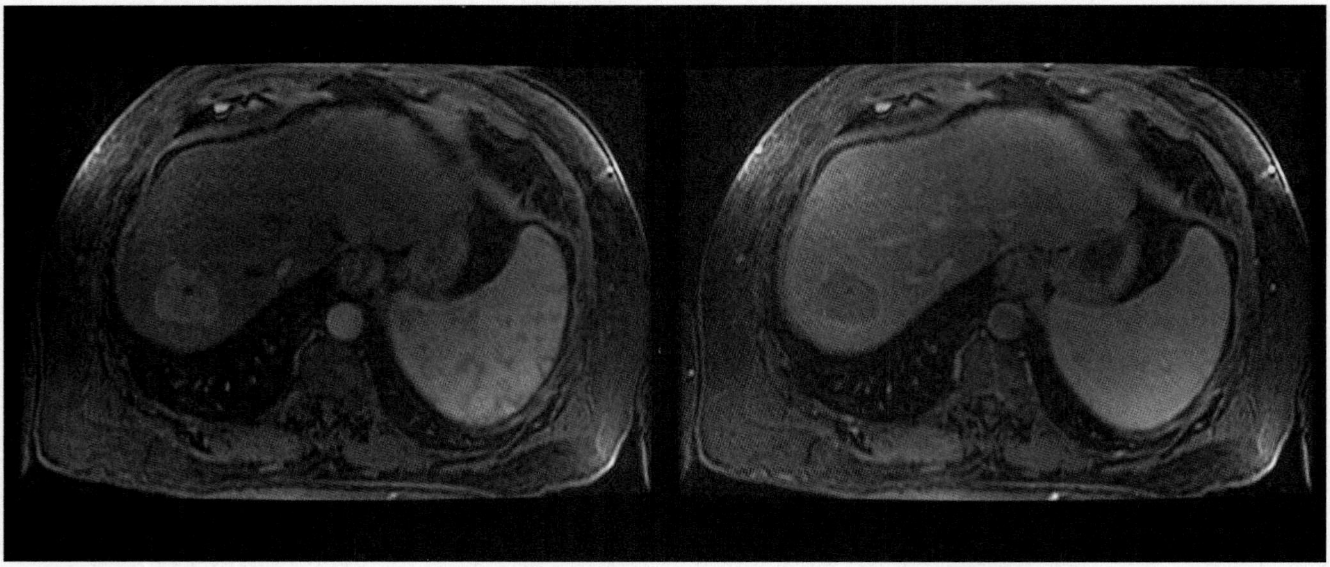

FIGURE 59.8. Magnetic resonance imaging of hepatocellular carcinoma, demonstrating characteristic enhancement on arterial phase imaging (*left panel*) with washout of contrast on delayed-phase imaging (*right panel*).

5-year survival from 41% to 57% to 15% to 34%.[90,97] Whether tumor size or tumor number is independently associated with worse outcomes is more controversial, as both of these factors are thought to have higher associations with vascular invasion as well.[97] In concordance, patients with very large HCCs, without vascular invasion or associated liver disease, can experience 5-year survival rates of 54% to 57.7% following resection.[98,99] Currently, there is no known benefit for adjuvant therapy following resection for HCC other than therapies aimed at treating the presence of viral hepatitis for

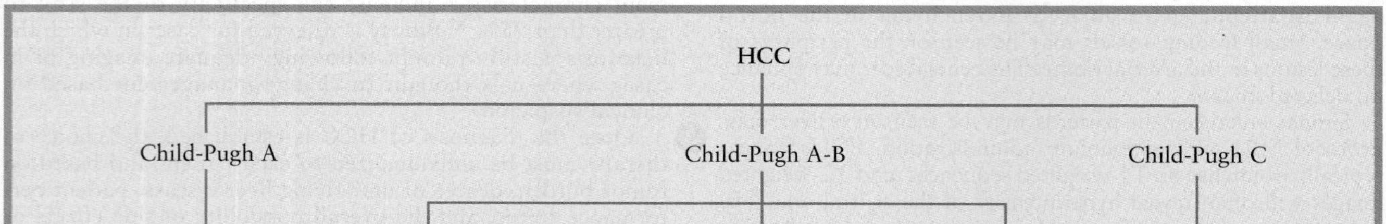

ALGORITHM 59.2. Algorithm for staging and treatment of hepatocellular carcinoma (HCC) according to the Barcelona Clinic Liver Cancer staging system and published as the American Association for the Study of Liver Diseases Practice Guidelines for HCC. (Adapted from Bruix J, Sherman M. *Hepatology* 2005;42[5]:1208–1236.)

acceptable candidates.[100] Therefore, this represents an area of ongoing research, especially as newer medications arrive.[101]

4 Liver transplantation is a useful consideration for patients not otherwise candidates for liver resection due to cirrhosis and with early-stage HCC as defined by Mazzaferro et al.[102] The staging definition set by these authors, now referred to as the Milan criteria, is defined as the absence of macrovascular invasion and a single tumor less than or equal to 5.0 cm or two to three tumors with none being greater than 3.0 cm. In the original study, patients experienced a 74% 4-year survival following liver transplantation. This survival rose to 85% when pathology on explant matched the preoperative imaging findings. Efforts to expand liver transplantation to patients with greater tumor burdens have met with mixed results and therefore more study is required before expanding this therapy to patients with greater stages of disease.[103,104] However, downstaging patients just above Milan stage before transplantation with the use of RFA or transarterial chemoembolization (TACE) is gaining popularity, with a 2-year survival rate of 81% following transplantation for patients successfully downstaged.[105] Patients meeting the Milan criteria who are otherwise acceptable candidates for liver transplantation are generally awarded MELD exception points so as to minimize waitlist dropouts due to progression of tumor disease.

Several locoregional therapies have been developed for the treatment of HCC and include RFA, TACE, microwave ablation, percutaneous ethanol ablation,[106] cryotherapy, radiotherapy, and yttrium-90 microspheres. Of the ablative therapies, RFA has proven to be superior, with less recurrence and fewer treatment sessions required.[107] RFA appears to be most beneficial for tumors less than 4.0 cm in size having a survival rate of 74% at 4 years and efficacy increasing for even smaller tumors.[108,109] Interestingly, a randomized controlled trial evaluating RFA versus resection for tumors less than 2.0 cm in size showed equivalent 4-year survival of 64% and 67.9%, respectively, and overall a decreased complication rate with RFA.[110] However, more trials are clearly needed to evaluate outcomes for small HCCs.

TACE is a very useful therapy for patients not eligible for other regional therapies as it has been proven in several randomized trials to provide a significant survival advantage, increasing median survival from 16 to 20 months in a meta-analysis of these trials, and with one large study showing a median survival of 34 months.[111] TACE is performed using angiographic techniques followed by selective embolization of the hepatic arterial supply to the tumor often with the addition of doxorubicin and cisplatin.[112,113] Relative contraindications to TACE include the presence of portal vein thrombosis or cirrhosis with many Child class B and all of Child class C patients being poor candidates due to risk of hepatic decompensation. Therefore, the best results are for patients with BCLC intermediate stage.[80,111]

Experience is accumulating with yttrium-90 microspheres, introduced transarterially, with a large single center demonstrating a median survival of 12 months in treated patients with BCLC intermediate and advanced stage.[114] External beam radiotherapy has also been used with one study showing a 75% tumor control rate at 2 years for large tumors not amenable to other treatments.[115] Both of these therapies hold promise but will require further study.

The only known systemic medical therapy for HCC with proven efficacy is sorafenib, a multikinase inhibitor with activity against the vascular endothelial growth factor (VEGF) receptor 2, platelet-derived growth factor (PDGF) receptor, c-kit receptor, and kinases in the b-Raf/Ras/mitogen-activated protein kinase kinase (MAPKK) pathway. Sorafenib was studied in the phase III, placebo-controlled Sorafenib HCC Assessment Randomized Protocol (SHARP) trial.[101] HCC patients not eligible for other therapies showed an increase in median survival with sorafenib therapy to 10.7 months when compared to placebo (7.9 months). Many other agents and compounds have been studied that have unfortunately shown no effect in randomized clinical trials. Other directed molecular therapies that are currently under clinical trial include bevacizumab (VEGF inhibitor), erlotinib (endothelial growth factor [EGF] receptor inhibitor), sunitinib (multikinase inhibitor), and gefitinib (EGF receptor inhibitor).[116]

Intrahepatic Cholangiocarcinoma

Intrahepatic cholangiocarcinoma (CCA) is the second most common primary hepatic malignancy. Unlike extrahepatic cholangiocarcinoma, its development is thought to derive from a common hepatic progenitor cell that may also give rise to HCC.[117] Indeed, some CCAs are characterized as a "mixed" histology with components of HCC and more classic CCA. Chronic liver disease or cirrhosis of varying etiologies is the only known risk factor for CCA, though many patients have no risk factors.[118] The prognosis of CCA compared to HCC is clearly worse following therapy. Patients are more likely to present with an advanced stage of disease such as intrahepatic metastases or lymph node metastasis, both of which portend a very poor prognosis following surgical resection.[119,120] Three-phase MRI and CT are the diagnostic modalities of choice, with biopsy being much more necessary as these lesions often appear hypointense on contrast-enhanced studies with no other clear primary gastrointestinal malignancies being noted. PET scanning is often helpful in contrast to extrahepatic CCA in evaluating for extrahepatic or intrahepatic metastases.[121,122] Surgical resection is the only known effective therapy. Results are generally poorer than resection for most other hepatic malignancies as 5-year survival ranges from 25% to 43% for patients with an R0 resection and no lymph node involvement, depending on the presence of vascular invasion (25% to 31%) or intrahepatic metastases/satellite nodules (9.9% to 40%).[119,120] The survival rate drops off dramatically for patients with positive lymph nodes, down to a 0% to 4% 5-year survival. Adjuvant therapy using radiation therapy or chemotherapy has shown no demonstrable benefit at the present time for this disease.

METASTATIC HEPATIC MALIGNANCIES

The management of metastatic disease confined to the liver is a rapidly evolving clinical challenge, particularly for metastatic colorectal cancer. As local and systemic therapies improve for various malignancies with a tendency to metastasize to the liver, the role of liver-directed therapy can in turn change considerably. In general terms, hepatic metastasectomy is best performed in two clinical scenarios:

5
1. Isolated hepatic metastasis in select patients with established locoregional control of their primary disease and good overall oncologic prognostic indicators (such as long disease-free interval, solitary or few hepatic lesions, and response to systemic therapy). Metastatic colorectal cancer is the most common example of this type of disease.
2. Hepatic metastasis in cancers where additional treatment options for metastatic disease are limited, disease may follow a protracted and indolent course, and patient performance status is favorable. Metastatic neuroendocrine cancer is an example of this category of disease, though many cancer types may meet this definition in select cases.

Given this framework, hepatic resection for poor-prognosis cancers with synchronous or metachronous metastatic lesions may subject patients to notable surgical risk without offering the benefit of improved survival. Examples of cancers for which hepatic metastasectomy has had such a limited role include gastric, pancreatic, lung, and breast. As hepatic metastases are typically asymptomatic, palliative hepatic resection is rarely, if ever, indicated.

Given the extensive collective surgical experience that has been gathered in the treatment of metastatic colorectal cancer, much of the rest of this section will be dedicated to the discussion of that disease, though the oncologic principles could be applied to select patients with other malignancies.

Metastatic Colorectal Cancer

More than 145,000 Americans will be diagnosed with colorectal cancer annually, and up to 50% of patients will develop hepatic metastases at some time during their disease course.[123] Several important trends appear to have increased the number of patients with metastatic colorectal cancer to the liver who are eligible for surgical therapy: improved colonoscopy screening programs have increased the number of patients presenting with early-stage disease, posttreatment surveillance programs have identified developing metastatic disease earlier and more efficiently, and systemic chemotherapy has improved notably for colorectal cancer, extending the survival of patients with advanced disease such that more aggressive surgical treatment of metastatic disease has become more appropriate.

Diagnosis. There are multiple imaging modalities that can play a role in the diagnosis and treatment planning for hepatic metastases from colorectal cancer.[124] Diagnosis of metastatic colorectal cancer is typically made by abdominal CT scan, performed either at the time of diagnosis or on surveillance imaging following treatment of a primary lesion. Hepatic metastases are slightly more common among patients with primary lesions in the rectum, and are clearly associated with regional lymph node disease. On standard single-phase intravenous contrast CT, hepatic metastases are typically more peripherally located low-attenuation lesions. Larger lesions may have central areas of necrosis or cystic degeneration. CT performed in three contrast phases (arterial, portal venous, systemic venous) may more sensitively identify subcentimeter lesions that are more difficult to identify in contrast to normal adjacent liver parenchyma. Hepatic metastases are often fed by the hepatic artery, and thus may enhance slightly on arterial phase, but remain less vascular than normal hepatic parenchyma. The lesions are of low attenuation in the portal phase. Mucin-containing lesions may have subtle calcifications. Contrast-enhanced liver MRI may offer additional sensitivity for small lesions and can be helpful in defining the extent of metastatic disease in patients with multiple small-volume lesions. Metastases typically have low signal intensity on T1-weighted images and high signal intensity on T2-weighted sequences. Contrast enhancement on MRI will give a similar appearance to metastases as with CT, with low signal intensity on unenhanced, arterial, and portal phases. PET has been advocated as an important study in the diagnosis of colorectal hepatic metastases and can play an important role in the evaluation for extrahepatic disease that may affect treatment decisions (Fig. 59.9). PET has

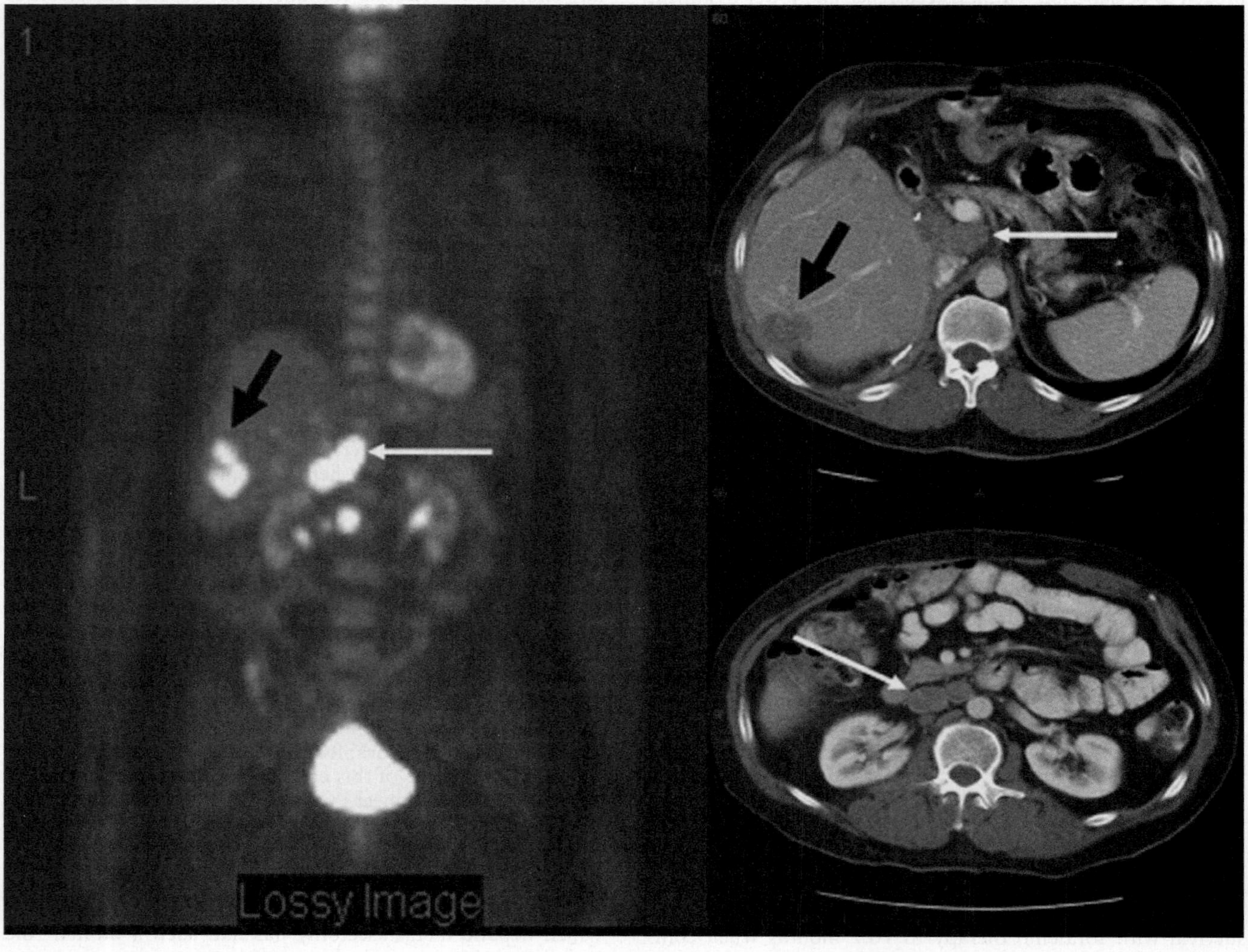

FIGURE 59.9. Positron emission tomography scan confirming hypermetabolic activity of lesions identified on corresponding computed tomography scans. *Black arrows* indicate hepatic metastases, and *white arrows* demonstrate portal and para-aortic lymph node metastases.

been demonstrated to change treatment decisions in up to 24% of cases when interpreted by experienced users.[28]

In patients with known colorectal cancer, the development of new hepatic lesions with characteristic imaging findings is sufficient for diagnosis without biopsy. Biopsy may be helpful in patients without previous comparison imaging or equivocal lesions, or in patients with synchronous metastases without a tissue diagnosis. The tumor marker CEA may aid in the diagnosis of metastatic disease, but should be interpreted cautiously as 20% to 40% of patients with metastatic disease may have normal or minimally elevated serum CEA levels.[125,126]

Treatment. Significant clinical experience in the surgical treatment of hepatic metastases from colorectal cancer has demonstrated the efficacy of hepatic resection (Algorithm 59.3). Multiple published series from high-volume centers have demonstrated 25% to 58% 5-year survival in select patients with surgically treated colorectal cancer metastatic to the liver (Table 59.2).[95,127–137] Review of national Medicare data reveals 25% 5-year survival for patients treated with hepatic resection for colorectal metastases, an impressive durable survival for elderly patients treated at centers of variable experience.[138] Recent analysis of Surveillance, Epidemiology,

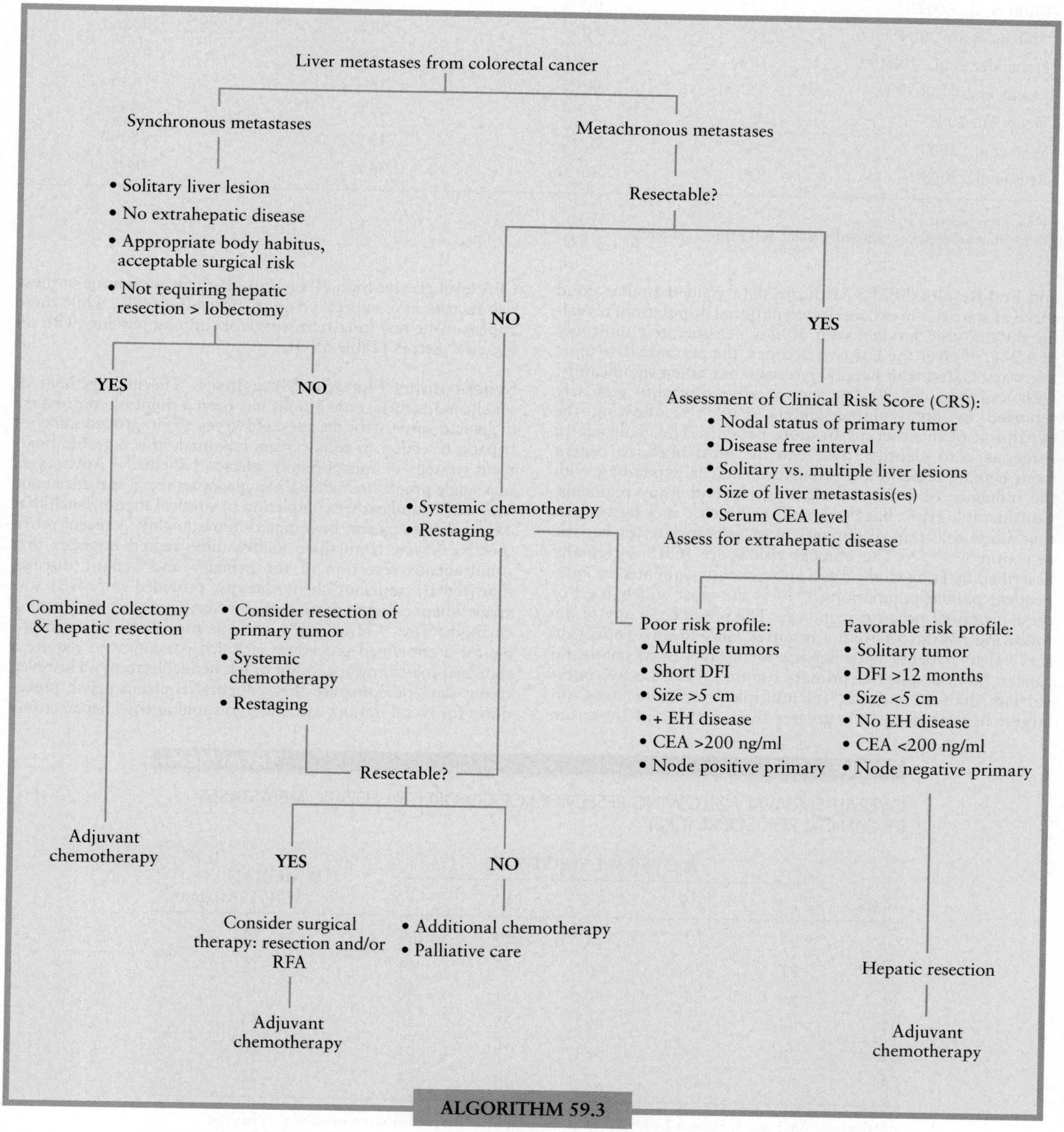

ALGORITHM 59.3. Algorithm for the management of colorectal cancer with hepatic metastases.

TABLE 59.2 **TREATMENT**

SURGICAL AND ONCOLOGIC OUTCOMES OF HEPATIC RESECTION FOR METASTATIC COLORECTAL CANCER

■ STUDY	■ *n*	■ 30-D MORTALITY	■ 5-Y OVERALL SURVIVAL	■ MEDIAN OVERALL SURVIVAL
Rosen et al., 1992[127]	280	2%	25%	34 mo
Scheele et al., 1995[128]	434	4.4%	34%	39 mo
Fong et al., 1999[130]	1,001	2.8%	37%	42 mo
Minagawa et al., 2000[131]	254	0%	38%	37 mo
Choti et al., 2002[132]	226	0.9%	40%	46 mo
Abdalla et al., 2004[133]	190	NR	58%	60 mo
Fernandez et al., 2004[134]	100	1%	58%	#
Pawlik et al., 2005[95]	557	0.9%	58%	74 mo
Wei et al., 2006[135]	395	1.7%	47%	68 mo
Shah et al., 2007[136]	841	3.5%	43%	48 mo
Rees et al., 2008[137]	929	1.3%	36%	42 mo

NR, not reported.
#, Median survival not reached; median follow-up 31 months.

and End-Results (SEER)-Medicare data yielded similar good survival statistics in an unselected national population, revealing 33% 5-year survival with 30-day perioperative mortality of 4.3%.[139] Over the last two decades, the perioperative mortality associated with hepatic resection has fallen significantly, with less than 2% 30-day perioperative mortality regularly reported by high-volume centers,[95,132,134,135] allowing the expansion of this therapy to more patients. The challenge to surgeons is to identify those patients most likely to benefit from hepatic resection, a population that is expanding with the influence of modern multidrug chemotherapy regimens. Considerable effort has been made to develop scoring systems that allow selection of patients most appropriate for hepatic resection.[130,140-142] The clinical risk score (CRS) originally described by Fong et al.[130] and subsequently validated in independent patient populations,[143,144] is the most widely used of these proposed prognostic indices. The presence of any of the following risk factors had a negative, and additive, effect on survival in patients with hepatic metastases from colorectal cancer: (a) node-positive primary tumor, (b) disease-free interval less than 12 months, (c) multiple liver metastases, (d) largest hepatic metastasis greater than 5 cm, and (e) serum CEA level greater than 200 ng/mL. Patients with none of these risk factors may expect a 5-year survival of 60%, while there appear to be few long-term survivors among patients with all five risk factors (Table 59.3).

Synchronous Hepatic Metastases. The management of synchronous metastatic lesions has been a point of controversy in general surgery for decades. However, the improved safety of hepatic resection in recent years has made this a viable treatment strategy in appropriately selected patients.[153] Advantages of a single procedure include a single laparotomy and anesthetic experience, and earlier completion of surgical therapy such that adjuvant therapy can be initiated more quickly. A recent retrospective review from three high-volume centers suggests that simultaneous resection of the primary and hepatic disease, followed by adjuvant chemotherapy, provided improved survival when compared to staged resections with intervening chemotherapy.[154] Historically, patients thought to be appropriate for a combined procedure included patients who require a standard colectomy (e.g., right or left hemicolectomy). However, recent data demonstrate that patients requiring pelvic procedures for rectal tumors can undergo simultaneous hepatectomy

TABLE 59.3 **TREATMENT**

OVERALL SURVIVAL FOLLOWING RESECTION OF COLORECTAL HEPATIC METASTASES BY CLINICAL RISK SCORE (CRS)

	■ OVERALL SURVIVAL					
CRS	1 Y	2 Y	3 Y	4 Y	5 Y	■ MEDIAN SURVIVAL (mo)
0	93	79	72	60	60	74
1	91	76	66	54	44	51
2	89	73	60	51	40	47
3	86	67	42	25	20	33
4	70	45	38	29	25	20
5	71	45	27	14	14	22

[a]Adopted from Fong Y, Fortner J, Sun RL, et al. Clinical score for predicting recurrence after hepatic resection for metastatic colorectal cancer: analysis of 1,001 consecutive cases. *Ann Surg* 1999;230:309–318; discussion 318–321.

with acceptable outcomes.[153,155] In contrast, the extent of the hepatectomy required can affect postoperative outcomes. Major hepatectomy (e.g., resection of at least three Couinaud segments) may best be handled in a staged fashion due to increased perioperative morbidity in patients undergoing simultaneous colorectal procedures.[153] Additional patient factors such as body habitus and comorbid disease should also influence surgical decision making in these cases.

Metachronous Hepatic Metastases. In metachronous metastatic disease, the appropriateness of hepatic resection may be dictated by patient comorbidity and prognostic indices such as the CRS.[130] The presence or absence of extrahepatic disease or local recurrence should be established with the use of cross-sectional imaging, PET, and colonoscopy. Presence of extrahepatic disease should influence treatment of hepatic metastases, as described later. In patients with good prognostic indicators (single small lesions, long disease-free interval), hepatic resection is most appropriate, followed by adjuvant chemotherapy. Patients with unresectable disease, or other poor prognostic indicators, should be considered for systemic chemotherapy, followed by restaging and consideration for surgical therapy.

Oligometastases. One particularly challenging group of patients with metastatic colorectal cancer include those with multiple hepatic metastases. If the patient otherwise has good risk factors and all the disease can be resected to a negative microscopic margin (R0), primary surgical therapy may be appropriate. Combination of radiofrequency ablation and resection in select patients may also be considered, though retrospective studies do appear to suggest that resection is superior to RFA when possible.[133,156,157] Patients with oligometastases appear to be most appropriate for treatment with systemic chemotherapy prior to an attempt at surgical resection, similar to the principles that may be applied to patients with unresectable hepatic metastases as discussed later.[158–161] This strategy provides several advantages, including the ability to observe the biology of the patient's cancer. Patients with progression of intrahepatic disease, or appearance of extrahepatic metastases, will exclude themselves from what is likely to be futile surgical therapy.[159] Response to chemotherapy appears to be an important prognostic factor for survival following hepatectomy.[162] Additional advantages of preoperative chemotherapy include the ability to downsize metastatic lesions, making R0 resections more likely.

Strategies to Expand Application of Hepatic Metastasectomy. As outcomes following metastasectomy for colorectal cancer have improved, strategies to expand the application of hepatic metastasectomy for colorectal cancer have continued to evolve. This evolution has been assisted by the improved efficacy of modern multidrug chemotherapy regimens, providing disease regression and stabilization that has facilitated progressive surgical approaches.

Unresectable Hepatic Metastases. In the case of patients with initially unresectable disease, either due to vascular involvement or the volume of liver parenchyma involved, neoadjuvant chemotherapy followed by reassessment of resectability has become common in experienced centers. Adam et al. reported a 12.5% resection rate among unresectable patients completing a multidrug regimen consisting typically of 5-fluorouracil/leucovorin and oxaliplatin (FOLFOX).[160] Despite the aggressive use of adjuvant surgical strategies including portal vein embolization (PVE), concomitant ablative procedures, and staged resections in 30% of patients, perioperative mortality was less than 1% with 33% 5-year survival, statistics that compare favorably to reported outcomes in more standard hepatic resection as described in Table 59.1. In a recent report by an Italian oncology cooperative, patients with unresectable hepatic colorectal metastases were treated with an aggressive regimen combining 5-fluorouracil/leucovorin, irinotecan, and oxaliplatin (FOLFOXIRI), which facilitated a 19% R0 resection rate without perioperative mortality.[163] Median survival among patients undergoing R0 resection was 30 months versus 14 months in patients who were unable to undergo an attempt at surgical therapy due to lack of tumor regression. While further prospective study is required to optimize chemotherapy regimens and patient selection, it is clear that select patients with unresectable hepatic metastases from colorectal cancer can be treated with curative surgical intent.

Staged Hepatic Resection. In cases where the degree of hepatic parenchyma involved by metastatic colorectal cancer precludes a single definitive resection, staged hepatectomy can be performed with acceptable outcomes. This strategy takes advantage of the regenerative response of the liver following surgical resection, increasing the size of the liver remnant such that a second definitive procedure can be performed. A recent French report describes a strategy of initial systemic chemotherapy (typically FOLFOX), followed by the first hepatectomy, intervening chemotherapy delayed 3 to 4 weeks to allow initiation of liver regeneration, restaging, and second hepatectomy in patients where imaging suggests the possibility of an R0 resection.[164] Of the 59 patients initially treated, 41 (69%) completed the second hepatectomy, while the remainder developed progressive disease. Three deaths occurred due to liver failure following the second hepatectomy, though survivors of the two-stage approach achieved 42% 5-year survival. Smaller series have reported similar results, demonstrating the feasibility of this approach by experienced hepatobiliary surgeons.[165,166]

Repeat Hepatic Resection. Patients with isolated hepatic recurrence following hepatectomy for metastatic colorectal cancer may be eligible for repeat resection in select cases. These procedures are typically more technically demanding, but published series suggest perioperative outcomes equivalent to primary hepatic resection.[167–169] Oncologic outcomes, while inferior to primary hepatic resection, are acceptable, with 5-year survival rates of 26% to 35%.[168,169] For these reasons, decisions about resection of recurrent hepatic disease should be made according to similar criteria as primary hepatic resection.

Treatment of Extrahepatic Metastatic Disease. Extrahepatic disease has traditionally been a contraindication to hepatic resection for metastatic colorectal cancer, and likely should remain so in the majority of patients. However, select patients with stable extrahepatic disease in addition to hepatic metastases may be appropriate for surgical therapy. Elias et al. reported a 29% 5-year survival among patients who underwent simultaneous resection of hepatic metastases and extrahepatic disease.[170] While published series have not been large enough to determine the prognostic significance of individual extrahepatic sites of disease, it appears that peritoneal metastases and multiple lesions portend worse survival. By far the greatest experience with extrahepatic metastasectomy for colorectal cancer exists for pulmonary resection, which can produce survival rates similar to hepatic metastasectomy in select patients.[171–173] Similarly, perihepatic regional lymph node disease that stabilizes or regresses during chemotherapy can be resected at the time of hepatic resection with acceptable overall survival.[174] Lymphadenectomy for metastatic disease should be confined to the hepatic pedicle, as celiac and periaortic retroperitoneal metastatic lymph node disease appears to be associated with poor long-term survival.

SURGICAL TREATMENT OF HEPATIC NEOPLASMS

Hepatic Resection

6 Recent years have seen the expansion in the number of hepatic resections performed for multiple indications, a trend that is

PANCREAS/LIVER

associated with increased diagnosis of hepatic lesions due to better imaging, improved outcomes of patients with primary or secondary hepatic malignancies and an associated increase in the willingness to be aggressive surgically, and enhanced safety of these operations due to the evolution of advanced hepatobiliary techniques and perioperative management. Nevertheless, hepatic resection remains an operation associated with significant perioperative risk, and thus an increasing majority of these procedures are being performed by surgeons with advanced hepatobiliary and/or surgical oncology training. Recent reports from national administrative data suggest that overall mortality following hepatic resection is higher than that reported from high-volume experienced centers, emphasizing the impact of specialized care following this major operation.[96,175,176]

Success in the operating room is created by careful preoperative planning. In addition to a standard medical evaluation, attention should be paid to factors that could make hepatectomy more complicated. Patients with significant hypervolemia (either due to renal or cardiac disease) or right heart failure with elevated central venous pressure (CVP) can pose particular challenges in liver surgery, as minimizing CVP has become a standard technique in liver surgery and is associated with decreased blood loss and improved outcomes.[177,178] Previous abdominal surgery can make hepatic procedures more complicated, and should be planned for accordingly. Most importantly, assessment for underlying liver dysfunction is essential as previously discussed.

Portal Vein Embolization. Assessment of each liver resection patient for adequate hepatic reserve is critical to achieving good patient outcomes, as reviewed earlier and outlined in
7 Algorithm 59.1. For the patient without an adequate predicted future liver remnant, PVE can be a necessary adjunct to expanding hepatic resection while avoiding postoperative liver failure. PVE takes advantage of the contralateral hypertrophy and ipsilateral atrophy that takes place in response to selective portal vein occlusion. Originally described in 1990, this technique has become a common procedure in high-volume hepatobiliary centers.[179] Portal vein ligation can be performed in an open or laparoscopic technique and can be used in staged hepatectomy procedures to induce hypertrophy prior to the second hepatectomy, but is most commonly performed via a percutaneous transhepatic approach. This allows access to lobar and segmental branches without manipulation of the portal supply to the future liver remnant. Repeat imaging is typically performed 3 to 4 weeks following embolization, with repeat liver volume estimates. Failure to respond to PVE portends a poor outcome following resection and should be considered a contraindication to proceeding with surgical therapy. Most centers will aim to operate on patients with an appropriate response at 21 to 30 days following PVE, capitalizing on the peak hypertrophic response at this time period. Published series report low rates of complications following PVE, with successful hypertrophy in the majority of patients.[180–182]

Operative Technique. Perioperative management of the hepatic resection patient can have a profound influence on outcomes. A dedicated anesthesia team, with experience in advanced hepatobiliary procedures, can be associated with improved patient outcomes. Establishment of large-bore venous access is essential, and arterial line placement for systemic blood pressure monitoring is also advised. Central venous access, which has been advocated both for large-volume resuscitation and for CVP monitoring, can be helpful in the most complex cases, but is probably not necessary in limited resection cases. Use of large-bore peripheral intravenous catheters (14 or 16 gauge) and conservative volume resuscitation can achieve similar goals.

In the case of open hepatectomy, incision choice is critical to exposure and efficiency. Left-sided hepatic lesions can be approached from an upper midline incision, but typically a right subcostal incision is preferred. A right subcostal incision with midline extension is a very versatile incision, allowing exposure to the suprahepatic vena cava, making a bilateral subcostal or Chevron incision necessary only for cases with difficult exposure due to body habitus or large tumors. In unusual cases with involvement of the suprahepatic vena cava or diaphragm, a median sternotomy or right thoracotomy extension may be necessary.[183] An appropriate retractor system, with bariatric blades for larger patients, can make a difficult case much easier.

As with all oncologic operations, the hepatectomy should begin with a thorough exploration of the abdomen, looking for extrahepatic disease that could change management of known intrahepatic disease. The liver should then be carefully inspected and palpated, with attention paid to any evidence of occult chronic liver disease or additional liver masses. Limited mobilization of the liver is then advisable prior to proceeding with the intraoperative ultrasound examination, as the exam is facilitated by mobilizing the liver such that the ultrasound probe has complete access to the hepatic parenchyma. However, if not necessary, leaving the ligamentous attachments of the future liver remnant intact can prevent torsion or compression of a small remnant. For example, in the case of a right trisegmentectomy, efforts should be made to preserve the left triangular ligament to keep the left lateral segment suspended in its typical anatomic relationship. In cases where it is necessary to take down such ligaments to facilitate exposure and mobility of the liver, the ligament can be reconstructed prior to abdominal closure.

Intraoperative ultrasound (IOUS) remains an irreplaceable tool in the surgical management of hepatic neoplasms, and has been shown to have increased sensitivity when compared to preoperative imaging.[184] Experienced hepatobiliary surgeons include the IOUS exam as a standard element of their operative exploration, typically following gross inspection and palpation of the abdomen and initial mobilization of the liver and placement of retractors. A careful IOUS should follow a reproducible and consistent three-step sequence, beginning with definition of the Couinaud segments based on the portal and hepatic venous anatomy. Attention is paid to important anatomic variants and anomalies, such as early or late division of the right portal pedicle or large accessory hepatic veins. The second phase of the IOUS exam should be a methodical scan through the entire liver parenchyma, with identification and measurement of all lesions. This is a critical step especially in operations where preoperative imaging identifies one dominant lesion; routine and thorough examination of the entire liver parenchyma is a crucial insurance against missing smaller synchronous lesions, which may be easily missed when distracted by a large known lesion. The whole liver scan should proceed in the same direction every time, typically in a cephalad to caudad position, moving slowly from the right to the left. Filling the upper abdomen with saline and removing any sponges from the field will prevent distracting echoes that can cause one to miss small peripherally based lesions. The final step in a comprehensive IOUS exam is planning of intended resection (or ablation), with note taken of the important critical vasculature to be included or avoided in a segmental resection. Mapping of the hepatic veins, for example, can be critical to avoid compromising venous drainage to the remnant liver in an extended resection.

The careful hepatobiliary surgeon will return to IOUS throughout the resection, ensuring that the resection margin is adequate and important vasculature is preserved. Caution often calls for temporary clamping of major portal branches, with subsequent Doppler IOUS confirmation of the intact flow to the liver remnant. A completion IOUS with Doppler to again demonstrate preserved inflow and outflow to the remnant liver should also be documented.

Once the plan of resection is confirmed by IOUS, the dissection phase is entered. The portion of the liver to be resected

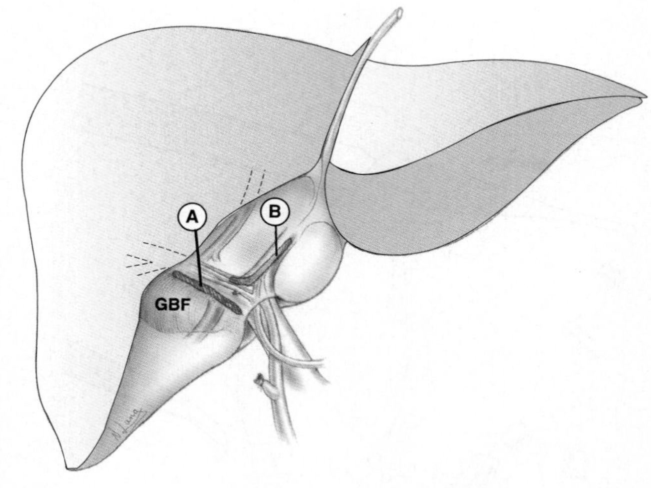

FIGURE 59.10. Identification of the extrahepatic structures during portal dissection. **A** indicates the right main portal triad; **B** indicates the left main portal triad, with its longer extrahepatic segment. (Copyright © 2003, the University of Texas M.D. Anderson Cancer Center.)

should be mobilized completely, freed from diaphragmatic attachments with division of the hepatic suspensory ligaments. The portal structures should be isolated by opening the pars flaccida (gastrohepatic ligament) and passing a finger through the foramen of Winslow such that the porta can be encircled with a tape. This maneuver facilitates quick access to the porta when necessary, and can facilitate episodic inflow occlusion. The amount of portal dissection necessary is then determined by the extent of hepatectomy planned (Fig. 59.10). A peripheral nonanatomic or segmental resection will not require much additional portal dissection. A formal or extended lobectomy may be approached with a formal portal dissection and pedicle control prior to parenchymal transection. Techniques of intrahepatic and extrahepatic pedicle control have been advocated by surgeons, depending on the tumor location and behavior.[185–187] Extrahepatic ligation of the portal vein and hepatic artery on the side of the lobectomy is typically best for lesions close to the portal plate, and can be accomplished safely. Alternatively, dissection of the portal structures to allow segmental inflow occlusion with subsequent division of the inflow vessels in the parenchyma is a method to provide definitive vascular control without depriving the liver remnant of inflow during parenchymal transection (i.e., a selective Pringle maneuver). The only hazard of extrahepatic pedicle control or division is the risk of injuring portal structures to the remnant liver, especially the biliary drainage. For example, when performing a right hepatic lobectomy, care should be taken to divide the right hepatic duct at or above the level of the portal plate, as the left hepatic duct may have a high insertion that can be compromised when the right duct is ligated near the bifurcation.

Control of the hepatic veins is most commonly performed within the liver as the final step of parenchymal transection, but vascular staplers have provided an efficient way to control hepatic veins at their origin with even a small window of extrahepatic vein at the level of the caval insertion (Fig. 59.11). This is easiest for the right hepatic vein, but with caution and experience, the middle and left hepatic veins can be divided separately as well. Care should be taken not to narrow the vena

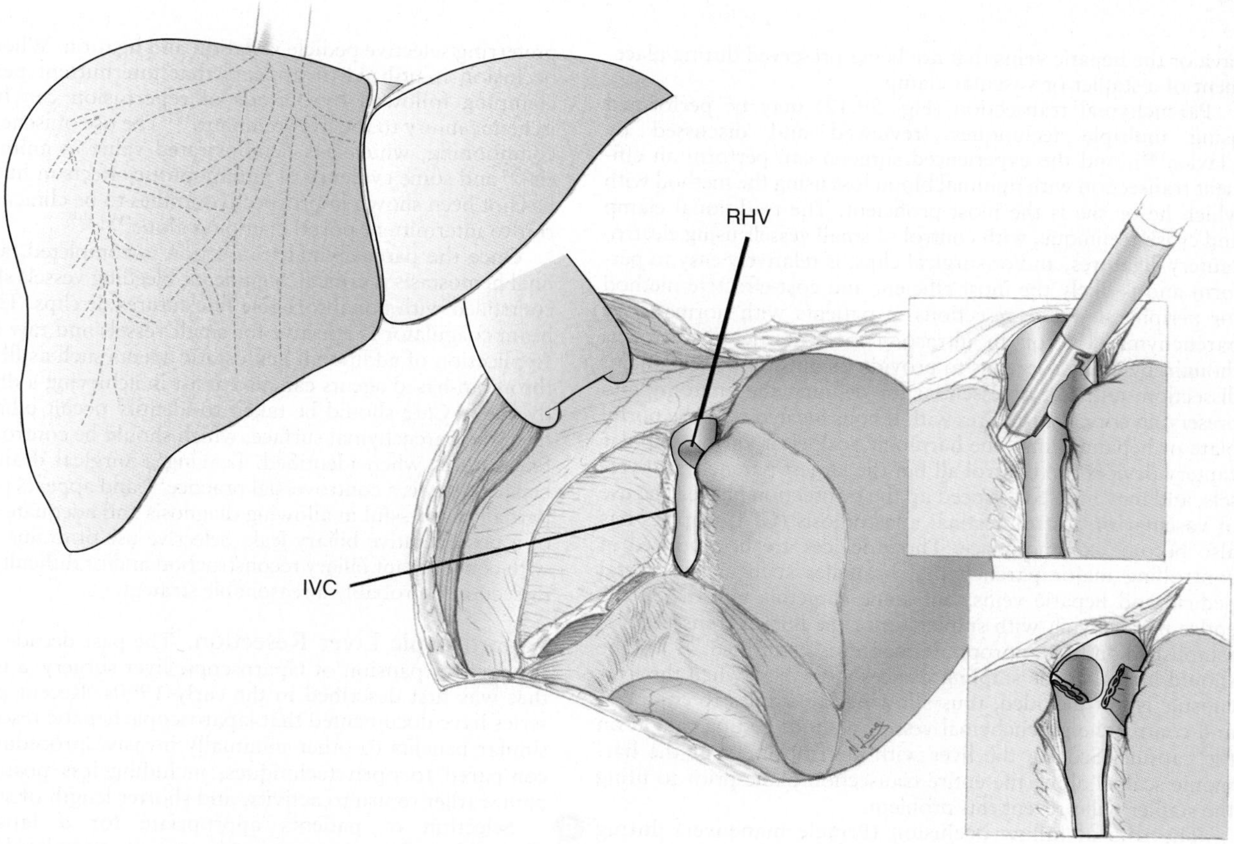

FIGURE 59.11. Exposure of the right hepatic vein for use of an endovascular stapler to ligate and divide the right hepatic vein. The liver is retracted medially and anteriorly after mobilization. (Copyright © 2003, the University of Texas M.D. Anderson Cancer Center.)

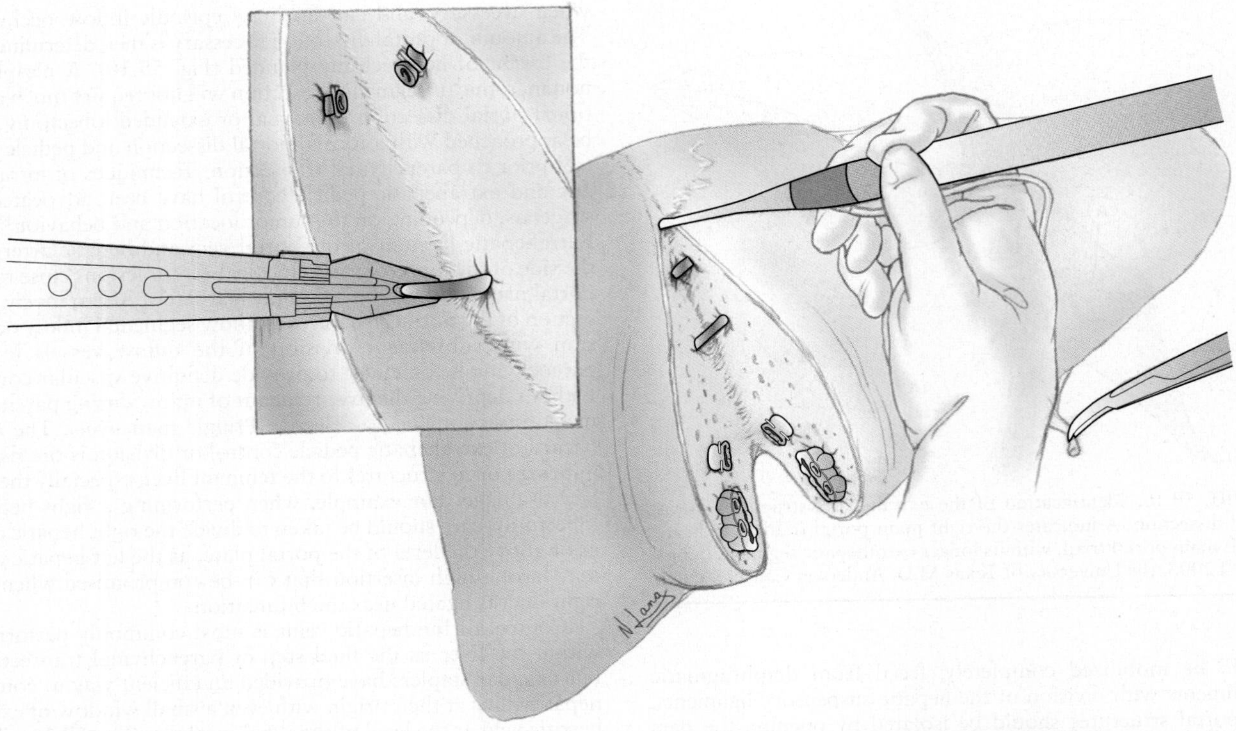

FIGURE 59.12. Parenchymal transection is carried out along the plane identified after vascular isolation. Parenchymal division can be performed by a number of different techniques, including coagulation dissecting devices or ultrasonic dissection. Large crossing ducts and vessels can be ligated with suture or clips, whereas smaller vessels are often readily coagulated with a variety of electrosurgical techniques. (Copyright © 2003, the University of Texas M.D. Anderson Cancer Center.)

cava or the hepatic veins that are being preserved during placement of a stapler or vascular clamp.

Parenchymal transection (Fig. 59.12) may be performed using multiple techniques (reviewed and discussed by Clavien[188]), and the experienced surgeon can perform an efficient transection with minimal blood loss using the method with which he or she is the most proficient. The traditional clamp and crush technique, with control of small vessels using electrocautery, ligatures, and/or surgical clips, is relatively easy to perform and is likely the most efficient and cost-effective method for peripheral wedge resections in patients with normal liver parenchyma. Use of an ultrasonic or water-jet dissector is thought by many surgeons to provide the most precise plane of dissection, and can be essential for defining the anatomy and preserving critical structures with lesions located near the portal plate or hepatic veins. The harmonic scalpel or various bipolar cautery devices can control all but the largest parenchymal vessels, and may be used to speed up the transection phase. The use of vascular or gastrointestinal anastomosis (GIA) staplers has also become commonplace. These devices are best utilized in controlling major parenchymal branches such as the portal pedicle and hepatic veins, but some surgeons will divide the entire parenchyma with staplers once the line of transection is established and an appropriate margin is confirmed.[189,190] One should note that the stapling devices work best when the liver capsule is not included, thus allowing the staples to compress and control the parenchymal vessels without getting caught on the capsule. Scoring the liver with electrocautery or the harmonic scalpel along the entire transection plane prior to firing the stapler will prevent this problem.

The role of inflow occlusion (Pringle maneuver) during parenchymal transection has been studied extensively and should be utilized to limit excessive blood loss when appropriate. While some surgeons use this technique routinely, others try to limit any potential ischemic injury to the liver remnant, preferring selective pedicle isolation and ligation. When inflow occlusion is utilized, it appears that intermittent periods of clamping followed by periods of reperfusion can limit the ischemic injury to the liver remnant.[191] The use of ischemic preconditioning, which has demonstrated value in animal models[192] and some evidence of antiapoptotic effects in humans,[193] has not been shown in prospective studies to be clinically superior to intermittent portal clamping alone.[194,195]

Once the parenchymal transection is completed, achieving final hemostasis is critical. Significant bleeding vessels should be controlled with nonabsorbable fine sutures or clips. The argon beam coagulator is effective for small vessels and raw surfaces. Application of additional hemostatic agents such as fibrin- and thrombin-based agents can also assist in achieving a dry operative field. Care should be taken to identify occult biliary leaks from the parenchymal surface, which should be controlled with fine sutures when identified. Leaving a surgical drain after a hepatectomy is a controversial practice[196] and appears to be only partially successful in allowing diagnosis and adequate drainage of a postoperative biliary leak. Selective use of drains for cases with concomitant biliary reconstruction and/or difficult perihilar dissection is probably a reasonable strategy.

Laparoscopic Liver Resection. The past decade has seen the rapid expansion of laparoscopic liver surgery, a technique that was first described in the early 1990s. Recent published series have documented that laparoscopic hepatic resection has similar benefits to other minimally invasive procedures when compared to open techniques, including less postoperative pain, earlier return to activity, and shorter length of stay.[198–201]

8 Selection of patients appropriate for a laparoscopic approach to hepatic resection is critical, and should be performed with honest consideration of surgeon experience. Limited wedge resections and left lateral segmentectomies (segments II and III) are becoming standard laparoscopic procedures, with

a limited role for open hepatic resection in patients with these lesions. Major liver resections (lobectomy, trisegmentectomy, central hepatectomy, and resection of the posterior segments VI and VII) are complex laparoscopic procedures that should not be approached laparoscopically by surgeons without significant laparoscopic liver surgery experience. While tumors located near the hilum of the liver or with involvement of the vena cava and hepatic vein orifices have been addressed laparoscopically in highly experienced centers, these procedures should generally not be considered candidates for a minimally invasive approach. As technology and surgical experience evolves, it is likely that the majority of hepatic resection procedures will gradually become minimally invasive procedures, though this evolution should occur only with assurance of patient safety and oncologic outcomes equivalent to open techniques.

Evolution of Laparoscopic Hepatic Resection. Historically, laparoscopy was only used in liver surgery for the staging of tumors, biopsy of the liver, and treatment of simple cysts. In 1994, Croce et al. performed hepatic wedge resections in four patients utilizing argon beam coagulation.[202] One of these four patients developed cardiac arrest due to a gas embolism, hindering the enthusiasm for this technique. Six succesful laparoscopic liver resections were reported in 1995 by Rau et al.[203] The first anatomic liver resection was a left lateral segmentectomy performed by Azagra et al. in 1996.[204] Kaneko et al. also reported laparoscopic left lateral segment resection during the same time period.[205] Other attempts by groups with extensive open liver resection were less successful, with conversion rates to open resection in 6 of 11 patients (55%), suggesting a steep learning curve with this technique.[206] Other early reports suggested a lower incidence of postoperative liver failure with laparoscopic approach (8% vs. 36%) along with improved 3-year survival (89% vs. 55%). While these findings were likely biased by patient selection, they did provide groundwork for the development of minimally invasive liver surgery.[207,208]

Since that time, large studies have demonstrated the feasibility of laparoscopic hepatic resection and successful outcomes.[209–211] In a comprehensive review of the literature, 75% of laparoscopic liver resections reported were performed totally laparoscopically and 17% were hand assisted. Conversion from laparoscopic to open occurred in 4% of patients. While wedge resections or segmentectomies were most common, formal right or left hepatectomies accounted for 16% of all cases reported.[211] However, prospective studies comparing a minimally invasive to an open approach have not been performed and will be difficult to plan because of the technically demanding nature of this technique, which is selectively performed at specialized centers.

Limitations of Laparoscopic Liver Surgery. The performance of laparoscopic liver surgery requires experience and expertise in both open complex liver surgery and advanced laparoscopy. Minimally invasive surgery on the liver faces unique challenges including retraction and mobilization of a relatively large and heavy organ, limiting hemorrhage while performing parenchymal transection, and identifying intrahepatic anatomy or pathology without anatomic markers on the surface of the liver. Methods must be immediately available to control hemorrhage, including the ability for laparoscopic suturing, stapling techniques, inflow occlusion, the use of hand-assisted laparoscopy, or the conversion to open surgery. In addition, techniques to limit the risk of air embolism under pneumoperitoneum should be utilized. Central lesions and bulky tumors that compromise laparoscopic working space may be difficult to resect laparoscopically.

The laparoscopic resection of liver malignancies remains controversial, and arguments for and against are similar to those of other gastrointestinal malignancies.[212,213] These arguments include concern for potential tumor cell exfoliation as well as port site metastases. In addition, concern for obtaining an inadequate margin has also been expressed. In a retrospective study that included 11 European centers, it was noted that almost one out of three patients did not meet a goal of a 1-cm margin on the specimen.[214] A more recent study has suggested that similar margins, recurrence rates, and long-term survival can be achieved in patients with malignant tumors using a laparoscopic approach when compared to open surgery.

These limitations and the constraints inherent in the utilization of evolving surgical devices should lead to the cautious adoption of laparoscopic liver resection, with laparoscopic major hepatectomy only performed by experienced surgeons. However, consensus appears to exist in the surgical community that laparoscopic approaches to liver surgery can produce equivalent outcomes to open hepatic surgery with appropriate patient selection and meticulous surgical technique.[215,216]

Hepatic Resection with Vascular Isolation, Resection, and/or Reconstruction. Improved outcomes with hepatic resection, advances with anesthetic and critical care management of the hepatectomy patient, and the increasing influence of hepatobiliary surgeons with liver transplant experience have all contributed to the extension of hepatic resection to include treatment of malignancies that were previously considered either impossible or unsafe to resect. This includes hepatic tumors involving the vena cava and/or hepatic vein orifices, neoplasms associated with the portal vein or its major branches, and retrohepatic neoplasms involving or displacing the hepatic vasculature such as retroperitoneal sarcomas. Select expert hepatobiliary centers have demonstrated that patients with tumors in these unfortunate locations can be offered resection as long as such procedures adhere to the principles of patient selection, evaluation of hepatic reserve, and comprehensive oncologic care that are applied to patients with more typical hepatic neoplasms.

9 Initial forays into isolation of the hepatic inflow and outflow to facilitate the resection of centrally based and/or large hepatic tumors were first described in the 1960s,[217] and the technique of TVE should be familiar to all surgeons performing major hepatectomy (Fig. 59.13).[218] Bismuth et al. described the largest

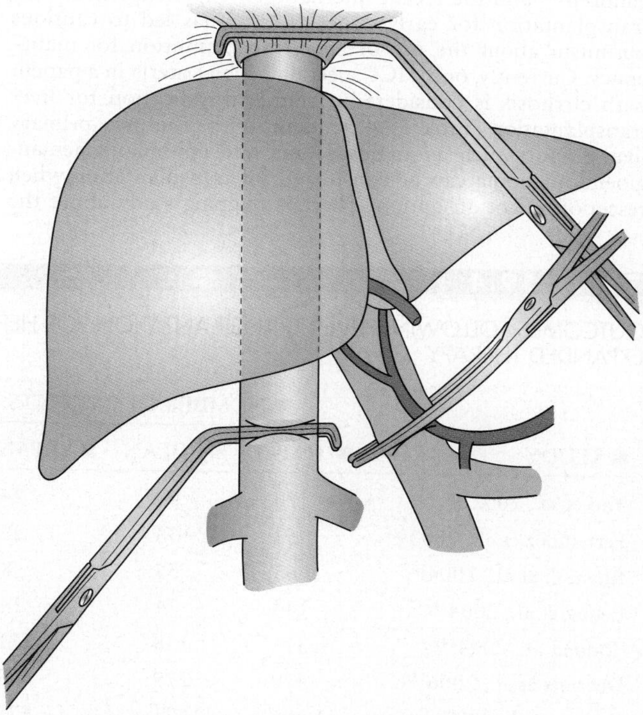

FIGURE 59.13. The technique of total vascular exclusion (TVE) can facilitate the safe resection of a large and centrally based tumor, particularly when the vena cava or hepatic veins are involved.

initial series utilizing this technique, demonstrating no increased rate of complications beyond major hepatectomy without TVE.[218] Increasing comfort with this technique has led some surgeons to suggest its use for all major hepatic resection procedures, though recent systematic reviews of the available published studies showed no benefit of routine TVE over intermittent hepatic inflow occlusion.[219,220] Nevertheless, TVE can be a lifesaving procedure in cases of massive hepatic hemorrhage, and may be necessary to allow the resection of tumors that involve or efface the vena cava or hepatic veins.

Recognition of the potential deleterious effects of the period of warm ischemia associated with TVE, which may be particularly injurious to steatotic or fibrotic livers,[197] led to interest in providing hypothermic perfusion of the liver during extended periods of TVE required for vascular resection and reconstruction. Azoulay et al. described the use of in situ hypothermic perfusion, demonstrating favorable results with no mortality in 20 patients.[221] The authors recommended consideration of hypothermic perfusion, either using in situ or ex vivo techniques, when TVE of more than 60 minutes would be required. Subsequent reports using this technique have described reconstruction of portal venous inflow to remnant liver segments,[222,223] resection and reconstruction of the vena cava and hepatic venous drainage for hepatic neoplasms,[224] and temporary total hepatectomy to facilitate resection and reconstruction of the vena cava for retroperitoneal tumors.[225] While these procedures should be reserved for only experienced hepatobiliary surgeons, it is clear that they can be considered safe in select patients.

Liver Transplantation

Total hepatectomy and replacement with a liver allograft has been considered as a treatment for hepatic tumors since the earliest days of liver transplantation.[226] Recognition of the profound impact that immunosuppression can have on tumor recurrence led to the conclusion that hepatic malignancy is a contraindication to liver transplantation. Experience with select tumors in rare circumstances, such as hepatoblastoma in children[227] and the recent international experience with liver transplantation for early-stage HCC,[102] has led to cautious optimism about the use of liver transplantation for malignancy. Currently, only HCC meeting Milan criteria in a patient with cirrhosis is considered a standard indication for liver transplantation (Table 59.4). Patients with other rare primary liver tumors such as angiosarcoma and epithelioid hemangioendothelioma can be considered for transplantation when resection is not an option. There is ongoing study about the role of liver transplantation in the treatment of hilar cholangiocarcinoma[228] and metastatic neuroendocrine tumors isolated to the liver.[229] To date, there is little evidence to support extension of liver transplantation to other more common hepatic malignancies, such as metastatic colorectal cancer.

Ablation of Liver Tumors

Ablative techniques have evolved extensively over the past few decades, extending surgical therapies to small tumors in patients not appropriate for surgical resection. Many of these techniques can increasingly be performed percutaneously, but surgical approaches remain important in patients where transcutaneous approaches are not possible or when ablation is combined with resection in the case of multiple hepatic tumors. Available ablation techniques include cryotherapy, microwave coagulation therapy, and laser-induced hyperthermic ablation. By far the greatest international experience exists with RFA.

RFA involves the application of a high-frequency alternating current from the tip of an electrode to the tissue surrounding that electrode. As the ions within the tissue move in response to this current, frictional heat is generated. As the temperature in the tissue increases above 60°C, cells begin to die, ultimately leading to coagulative necrosis.[230] Generally, ultrasound is used to guide the placement of the needle and ensure a complete therapeutic field. Once placed, RF energy is then applied across the needle electrode using an established protocol specific for the instrument (Figs. 59.14 and 59.15).[231] Smaller tumors can often be treated with one application, whereas larger tumors (>2.5 cm) will require more than one deployment of the electrode to ensure complete destruction of the lesion. Overlapping zones of coagulative necrosis are a key element in the use of RF ablative techniques requiring more than one deployment. To mimic a surgical margin of resectability, the electrode array is positioned so as to obtain a field of thermal necrosis including, when possible, a 1-cm perimeter of normal hepatic parenchyma surrounding each ablated lesion. After RF ablation, CT scans demonstrate cystic areas ideally larger than the original tumors. These ablation zones decrease in size over time.

Candidates for RF ablation of hepatic tumors are generally patients who do not meet criteria for resection of their disease but do not have evidence of extrahepatic disease.[231,232] In selected cases, patients with tumors that are usually associated with disseminated, systemic metastatic disease (e.g., breast or renal cell carcinoma) may be considered for RF ablation if they have received a prolonged period of effective chemotherapy

TABLE 59.4 **TREATMENT**

OUTCOMES FOLLOWING LIVER TRANSPLANTATION FOR HEPATOCELLULAR CARCINOMA USING MILAN AND EXPANDED THERAPY

STUDY	NUMBER OF PATIENTS: TOTAL	MILAN	EXPANDED	1-Y SURVIVAL: MILAN	EXPANDED	5-Y SURVIVAL: MILAN	EXPANDED
Yao et al., 2002[145]	70	46	24	91	71	72	57
Fernandez et al., 2003[146]	53	33	20	82	75	68	54
Ravaioli et al., 2004[147]	63	55	8	90	76	78	38
Leung et al., 2004[148]	144	74	14	86	—	51	—
Todo et al., 2004[149]	316	138	171	81	75	78	60
Decaens et al., 2006[150]	479	279	188	80	78	60	46
Onaca et al., 2007[103]	1,206	631	575	85	67	62	43
Duffy et al., 2007[151]	467	173	294	91	88	79	64

Adopted in part from Hoti E, Adam R. Liver transplantation for primary and metastatic liver cancers. *Transpl Int* 2008;21:1109.

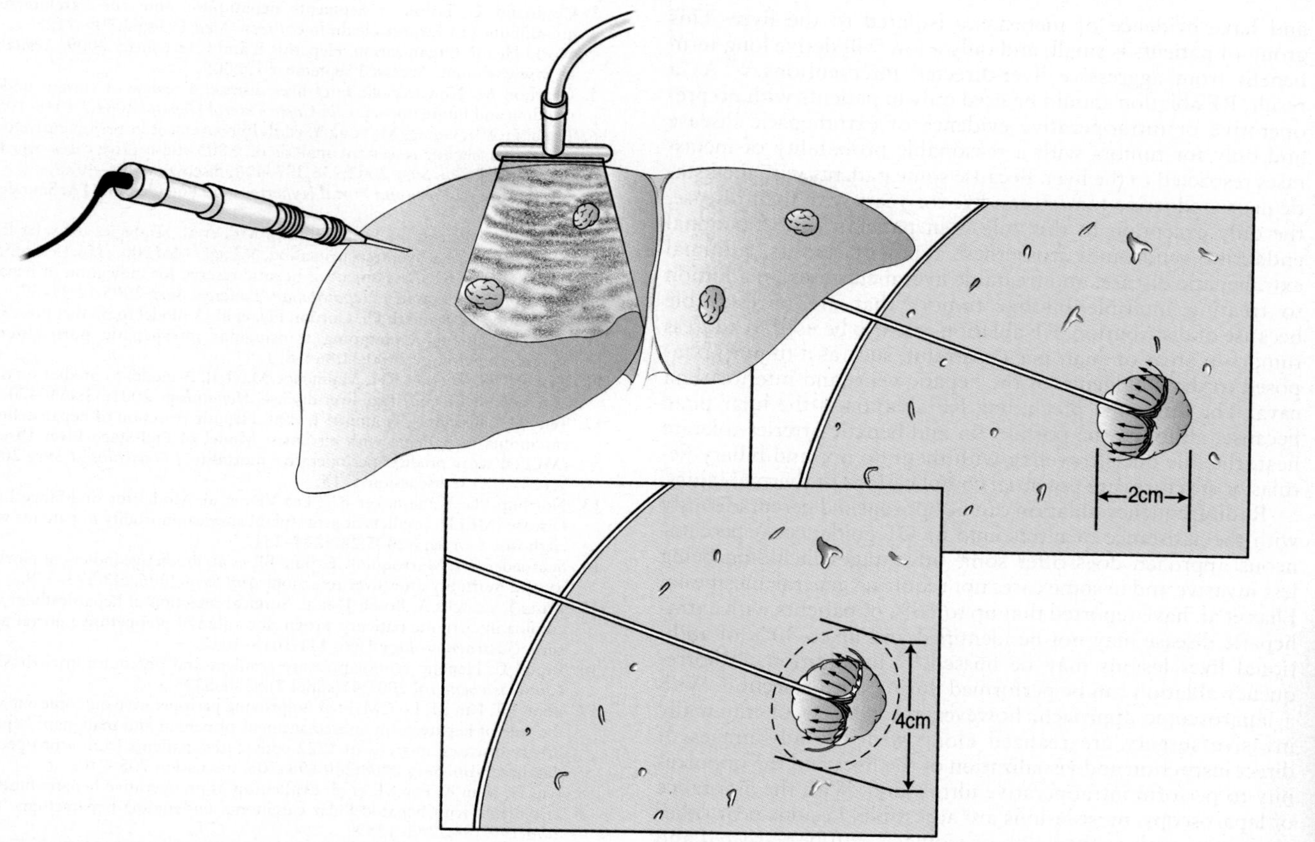

FIGURE 59.14. Technique for radiofrequency ablation. Using ultrasound guidance, the probe is inserted into a lesion and the array is opened so that it encompasses the entire lesion.

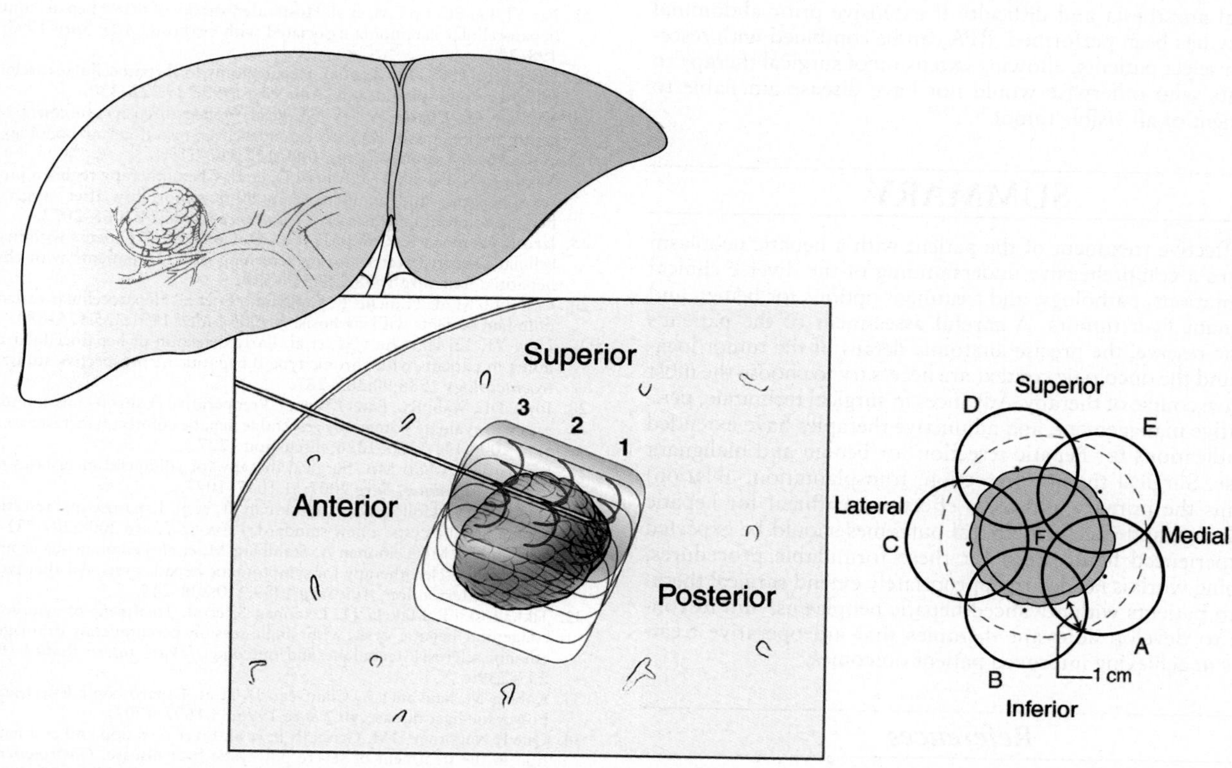

FIGURE 59.15. Technique for larger lesions. Overlapping ablations are performed so that the entire lesion, along with a margin of normal tissue, is submitted to the ablative current.

and have evidence of metastases isolated to the liver. This group of patients is small, and only a few will derive long-term benefit from aggressive liver-directed interventions.[233] As a result, RF ablation should be used only in patients with no preoperative or intraoperative evidence of extrahepatic disease and only for tumors with a reasonable probability of metastases restricted to the liver. Because some patients with metastatic neuroendocrine tumors can live for years with their disease, the only exception to this rule is in patients with functional endocrine syndromes from these types of tumors, minimal extrahepatic disease, and treatable liver metastases. In addition to treating multiple bilobar tumors that are unresectable because of distribution, RF ablation can also be used to address tumors in areas of anatomic constraint, such as a tumor juxtaposed to the confluence of the hepatic veins and inferior vena cava. The only area precluding RF ablation is the hilar plate because, although the portal vein and hepatic arteries tolerate heat, the bile ducts traveling with them do not and biliary fistulas or strictures are potential complications of thermal injury.

Radiofrequency ablation can be approached percutaneously with the assistance of ultrasound or CT guidance. A percutaneous approach does offer some advantages including being less invasive and in some cases not requiring general anesthesia. Elias et al. have reported that up to 16% of patients with extrahepatic disease may not be identified and up to 30% of additional liver lesions may be missed.[234] In addition, radiofrequency ablation can be performed during open resection. With a laparoscopic approach, however, the benefits of minimally invasive surgery are realized along with the advantages of direct inspection and visualization of the liver and the opportunity to perform intraoperative ultrasound. With the assistance of laparoscopy, most lesions are accessible. Lesions near other structures, such as the colon or stomach, can be retracted and radiofrequency ablation can be performed safely without injury to surrounding organs. In addition, when near major vascular structures, vascular inflow occlusion can also be used to prevent a heat-sink effect. Disadvantages of the laparoscopic radiofrequency ablation approach include the requirement for general anesthesia and difficulty if extensive prior abdominal surgery has been performed. RFA can be combined with resection in select patients, allowing extension of surgical therapy to patients who otherwise would not have disease amenable to treatment of all visible tumor.[133,156]

SUMMARY

The effective treatment of the patient with a hepatic neoplasm requires a comprehensive understanding of the diverse clinical presentations, pathology, and treatment options for benign and malignant liver tumors. A careful assessment of the patient's hepatic reserve, the precise anatomic details of the tumor location, and the oncologic context are necessary to choose the most effective course of therapy. Advances in surgical technique, perioperative management, and adjunctive therapies have extended the indications for hepatic resection for benign and malignant disease. Surgical therapy (resection, transplantation, ablation) remains the primary and most effective treatment for hepatic neoplasms, and excellent clinical outcomes should be expected in experienced hands even for these formidable procedures. Ongoing work is needed to appropriately extend surgical therapies to patients with advanced hepatic neoplasms, and to continue to develop adjuvant therapies that aid operative treatments in achieving improved patient outcomes.

References

1. Sutherland F, Harris J. Claude Couinaud: a passion for the liver. *Arch Surg* 2002;137:1305–1310.
2. Couinaud C. Anatomic principles of left and right regulated hepatectomy: technics. *J Chir (Paris)* 1954;70:933–966.
3. Couinaud C. Lobes et Segments hepatiques: note sur l'architecture anatomique et Chirurgicale du foie. *Presse Med* 1954;62:709–712.
4. World Health Organization. Hepatitis B and C fact sheet. 2009. Available at: www.who.int. Accessed September 1, 2009.
5. Charlton M. Nonalcoholic fatty liver disease: a review of current understanding and future impact. *Clin Gastroenterol Hepatol* 2004;2:1048–1058.
6. Jarnagin WR, Gonen M, Fong Y, et al. Improvement in perioperative outcome after hepatic resection: analysis of 1,803 consecutive cases over the past decade. *Ann Surg* 2002;236:397–406; discussion 406–407.
7. Child CG. *The Liver and Portal Hypertension*. Philadelphia, PA: Saunders; 1964.
8. Clavien PA, Petrowsky H, DeOliveira ML, et al. Strategies for safer liver surgery and partial liver transplantation. *N Engl J Med* 2007;356:1545–1559.
9. Poon RT, Fan ST. Assessment of hepatic reserve for indication of hepatic resection: how I do it. *J Hepatobiliary Pancreat Surg* 2005;12:31–37.
10. Malinchoc M, Kamath PS, Gordon FD, et al. A model to predict poor survival in patients undergoing transjugular intrahepatic portosystemic shunts. *Hepatology* 2000;31:864–871.
11. Kamath PS, Wiesner RH, Malinchoc M, et al. A model to predict survival in patients with end-stage liver disease. *Hepatology* 2001;33:464–470.
12. Teh SH, Christein J, Donohue J, et al. Hepatic resection of hepatocellular carcinoma in patients with cirrhosis: Model of End-Stage Liver Disease (MELD) score predicts perioperative mortality. *J Gastrointest Surg* 2005; 9:1207–1215; discussion 1215.
13. Northup PG, Wanamaker RC, Lee VD, et al. Model for End-Stage Liver Disease (MELD) predicts nontransplant surgical mortality in patients with cirrhosis. *Ann Surg* 2005;242:244–251.
14. Schroeder RA, Marroquin CE, Bute BP, et al. Predictive indices of morbidity and mortality after liver resection. *Ann Surg* 2006;243:373–379.
15. Bruix J, Castells A, Bosch J, et al. Surgical resection of hepatocellular carcinoma in cirrhotic patients: prognostic value of preoperative portal pressure. *Gastroenterology* 1996;111:1018–1022.
16. Ripoll C. Hepatic venous pressure gradient and outcomes in cirrhosis. *J Clin Gastroenterol* 2007;41(suppl 3):S330–S335.
17. Poon RT, Fan ST, Lo CM, et al. Improving perioperative outcome expands the role of hepatectomy in management of benign and malignant hepatobiliary diseases: analysis of 1222 consecutive patients from a prospective database. *Ann Surg* 2004;240:698–708; discussion 708–710.
18. Lau H, Man K, Fan ST, et al. Evaluation of preoperative hepatic function in patients with hepatocellular carcinoma undergoing hepatectomy. *Br J Surg* 1997;84:1255–1259.
19. Redaelli CA, Dufour JF, Wagner M, et al. Preoperative galactose elimination capacity predicts complications and survival after hepatic resection. *Ann Surg* 2002;235:77–85.
20. Mitsumori A, Nagaya I, Kimoto S, et al. Preoperative evaluation of hepatic functional reserve following hepatectomy by technetium-99 m galactosyl human serum albumin liver scintigraphy and computed tomography. *Eur J Nucl Med* 1998;25:1377–1382.
21. Fan ST, Lai EC, Lo CM, et al. Hospital mortality of major hepatectomy for hepatocellular carcinoma associated with cirrhosis. *Arch Surg* 1995;130: 198–203.
22. Fan ST, Lo CM, Liu CL, et al. Hepatectomy for hepatocellular carcinoma: toward zero hospital deaths. *Ann Surg* 1999;229:322–330.
23. Vauthey JN, Chaoui A, Do KA, et al. Standardized measurement of the future liver remnant prior to extended liver resection: methodology and clinical associations. *Surgery* 2000;127:512–519.
24. Vauthey JN, Pawlik TM, Ribero D, et al. Chemotherapy regimen predicts steatohepatitis and an increase in 90-day mortality after surgery for hepatic colorectal metastases. *J Clin Oncol* 2006;24:2065–2072.
25. Izzo F, Cremona F, Ruffolo F, et al. Outcome of 67 patients with hepatocellular cancer detected during screening of 1125 patients with chronic hepatitis. *Ann Surg* 1998;227:513–518.
26. Colombo M, de Franchis R, Del Ninno E, et al. Hepatocellular carcinoma in Italian patients with cirrhosis. *N Engl J Med* 1991;325:675–680.
27. Liaw YF, Tai DI, Chu CM, et al. Early detection of hepatocellular carcinoma in patients with chronic type B hepatitis. A prospective study. *Gastroenterology* 1986;90:263–267.
28. Joyce DL, Wahl RL, Patel PV, et al. Preoperative positron emission tomography to evaluate potentially resectable hepatic colorectal metastases. *Arch Surg* 2006;141:1220–1226; discussion 1227.
29. Pawlik TM, Choti MA. Surgical therapy for colorectal metastases to the liver. *J Gastrointest Surg* 2007;11:1057–1077.
30. Gamblin TC, Holloway SE, Heckman JT, et al. Laparoscopic resection of benign hepatic cysts: a new standard. *J Am Coll Surg* 2008;207:731–736.
31. Kairaluoma MI, Leinonen A, Stahlberg M, et al. Percutaneous aspiration and alcohol sclerotherapy for symptomatic hepatic cysts. An alternative to surgical intervention. *Ann Surg* 1989;210:208–215.
32. Tikkakoski T, Makela JT, Leinonen S, et al. Treatment of symptomatic congenital hepatic cysts with single-session percutaneous drainage and ethanol sclerosis: technique and outcome. *J Vasc Interv Radiol* 1996;7: 235–239.
33. Kabbej M, Sauvanet A, Chauveau D, et al. Laparoscopic fenestration in polycystic liver disease. *Br J Surg* 1996;83:1697–1701.
34. Que F, Nagorney DM, Gross JB Jr, et al. Liver resection and cyst fenestration in the treatment of severe polycystic liver disease. *Gastroenterology* 1995;108:487–494.
35. Kirchner GI, Rifai K, Cantz T, et al. Outcome and quality of life in patients with polycystic liver disease after liver or combined liver-kidney transplantation. *Liver Transpl* 2006;12:1268–1277.

36. Starzl TE, Reyes J, Tzakis A, et al. Liver transplantation for polycystic liver disease. *Arch Surg* 1990;125:575–577.
37. Li TJ, Zhang HB, Lu JH, et al. Treatment of polycystic liver disease with resection-fenestration and a new classification. *World J Gastroenterol* 2008;14:5066–5072.
38. Del Poggio P, Buonocore M. Cystic tumors of the liver: a practical approach. *World J Gastroenterol* 2008;14:3616–3620.
39. Wheeler DA, Edmondson HA. Cystadenoma with mesenchymal stroma (CMS) in the liver and bile ducts. A clinicopathologic study of 17 cases, 4 with malignant change. *Cancer* 1985;56:1434–1445.
40. Devaney K, Goodman ZD, Ishak KG. Hepatobiliary cystadenoma and cystadenocarcinoma. A light microscopic and immunohistochemical study of 70 patients. *Am J Surg Pathol* 1994;18:1078–1091.
41. Choi BI, Lim JH, Han MC, et al. Biliary cystadenoma and cystadenocarcinoma: CT and sonographic findings. *Radiology* 1989;171:57–61.
42. Koffron A, Rao S, Ferrario M, et al. Intrahepatic biliary cystadenoma: role of cyst fluid analysis and surgical management in the laparoscopic era. *Surgery* 2004;136:926–936.
43. Gandolfi L, Leo P, Solmi L, et al. Natural history of hepatic haemangiomas: clinical and ultrasound study. *Gut* 1991;32:677–680.
44. Glinkova V, Shevah O, Boaz M, et al. Hepatic haemangiomas: possible association with female sex hormones. *Gut* 2004;53:1352–1355.
45. Karhunen PJ. Benign hepatic tumours and tumour like conditions in men. *J Clin Pathol* 1986;39:183–188.
46. Lam KY. Autopsy findings in diabetic patients: a 27-yr clinicopathologic study with emphasis on opportunistic infections and cancers. *Endocr Pathol* 2002;13:39–45.
47. Corigliano N, Mercantini P, Amodio PM, et al. Hemoperitoneum from a spontaneous rupture of a giant hemangioma of the liver: report of a case. *Surg Today* 2003;33:459–463.
48. Adam A, Dixon AK, Grainger RG, et al. *Grainger & Allison's Diagnostic Radiology: A Textbook of Medical Imaging,* 5th ed. Philadelphia, PA: Churchill Livingstone/Elsevier; 2008.
49. Fulcher AS, Sterling RK. Hepatic neoplasms: computed tomography and magnetic resonance features. *J Clin Gastroenterol* 2002;34:463–471.
50. Tung GA, Cronan JJ. Percutaneous needle biopsy of hepatic cavernous hemangioma. *J Clin Gastroenterol* 1993;16:117–122.
51. Hall GW. Kasabach-Merritt syndrome: pathogenesis and management. *Br J Haematol* 2001;112:851–862.
52. Vassiou K, Rountas H, Liakou P, et al. Embolization of a giant hepatic hemangioma prior to urgent liver resection. Case report and review of the literature. *Cardiovasc Intervent Radiol* 2007;30:800–802.
53. Yoon SS, Charny CK, Fong Y, et al. Diagnosis, management, and outcomes of 115 patients with hepatic hemangioma. *J Am Coll Surg* 2003;197:392–402.
54. Klatskin G. Hepatic tumors: possible relationship to use of oral contraceptives. *Gastroenterology* 1977;73:386–394.
55. Prentice RL, Thomas DB. On the epidemiology of oral contraceptives and disease. *Adv Cancer Res* 1987;49:285–401.
56. Flejou JF, Barge J, Menu Y, et al. Liver adenomatosis. An entity distinct from liver adenoma? *Gastroenterology* 1985;89:1132–1138.
57. Greaves WO, Bhattacharya B. Hepatic adenomatosis. *Arch Pathol Lab Med* 2008;132:1951–1955.
58. Liu CL, Fan ST, Lo CM, et al. Hepatic resection for incidentaloma. *J Gastrointest Surg* 2004;8:785–793.
59. Reddy KR, Kligerman S, Levi J, et al. Benign and solid tumors of the liver: relationship to sex, age, size of tumors, and outcome. *Am Surg* 2001;67:173–178.
60. Terkivatan T, Hussain SM, De Man RA, et al. Diagnosis and treatment of benign focal liver lesions. *Scand J Gastroenterol Suppl* 2006;(243):102–115.
61. Weimann A, Ringe B, Klempnauer J, et al. Benign liver tumors: differential diagnosis and indications for surgery. *World J Surg* 1997;21:983–990; discussion 990–991.
62. van der Windt DJ, Kok NFM, Hussain SM, et al. Case-orientated approach to the management of hepatocellular adenoma. *Br J Surg* 2006;93:1495–1502.
63. Charny CK, Jarnagin WR, Schwartz LH, et al. Management of 155 patients with benign liver tumours. *Br J Surg* 2001;88:808–813.
64. Koffron A, Geller D, Gamblin TC, et al. Laparoscopic liver surgery: shifting the management of liver tumors. *Hepatology* 2006;44:1694–1700.
65. Nagorney DM. Benign hepatic tumors: focal nodular hyperplasia and hepatocellular adenoma. *World J Surg* 1995;19:13–18.
66. Nguyen BN, Flejou JF, Terris B, et al. Focal nodular hyperplasia of the liver: a comprehensive pathologic study of 305 lesions and recognition of new histologic forms. *Am J Surg Pathol* 1999;23:1441–1454.
67. Federle MP, Brancatelli G. Imaging of benign hepatic masses. *Semin Liver Dis* 2001;21:237–249.
68. Choi BY, Nguyen MH. The diagnosis and management of benign hepatic tumors. *J Clin Gastroenterol* 2005;39:401–412.
69. Wanless IR, Mawdsley C, Adams R. On the pathogenesis of focal nodular hyperplasia of the liver. *Hepatology* 1985;5:1194–1200.
70. Rebouissou S, Bioulac-Sage P, Zucman-Rossi J. Molecular pathogenesis of focal nodular hyperplasia and hepatocellular adenoma. *J Hepatol* 2008;48:163–170.
71. Altavilla G, Guariso G. Focal nodular hyperplasia of the liver associated with portal vein agenesis: a morphological and immunohistochemical study of one case and review of the literature. *Adv Clin Path* 1999;3:139–145.
72. Buscarini E, Danesino C, Plauchu H, et al. High prevalence of hepatic focal nodular hyperplasia in subjects with hereditary hemorrhagic telangiectasia. *Ultrasound Med Biol* 2004;30:1089–1097.
73. De Gaetano AM, Gui B, Macis G, et al. Congenital absence of the portal vein associated with focal nodular hyperplasia in the liver in an adult woman: imaging and review of the literature. *Abdom Imaging* 2004;29:455–459.
74. Heiken JP. Distinguishing benign from malignant liver tumours. *Cancer Imaging* 2007;7(Spec No A):S1–S14.
75. Demarco MP, Shen P, Bradley RF, et al. Intraperitoneal hemorrhage in a patient with hepatic focal nodular hyperplasia. *Am Surg* 2006;72:555–559.
76. Bonney GK, Gomez D, Al-Mukhtar A, et al. Indication for treatment and long-term outcome of focal nodular hyperplasia. *HPB (Oxford)* 2007;9:368–372.
77. Parkin DM, Bray F, Ferlay J, et al. Estimating the world cancer burden: Globocan 2000. *Int J Cancer* 2001;94:153–156.
78. El-Serag HB, Davila JA, Petersen NJ, et al. The continuing increase in the incidence of hepatocellular carcinoma in the United States: an update. *Ann Int Med* 2003;139:817–823.
79. Fattovich G, Stroffolini T, Zagni I, et al. Hepatocellular carcinoma in cirrhosis: incidence and risk factors. *Gastroenterology* 2004;127:S35–S50.
80. Bruix J, Sherman M. Management of hepatocellular carcinoma. *Hepatology* 2005;42:1208–1236.
81. Zhang BH, Yang BH, Tang ZY. Randomized controlled trial of screening for hepatocellular carcinoma. *J Cancer Res Clin Oncol* 2004;130:417–422.
82. Burrel M, Llovet JM, Ayuso C, et al. MRI angiography is superior to helical CT for detection of HCC prior to liver transplantation: an explant correlation. *Hepatology* 2003;38:1034–1042.
83. Krinsky GA, Lee VS, Theise ND, et al. Hepatocellular carcinoma and dysplastic nodules in patients with cirrhosis: prospective diagnosis with MR imaging and explantation correlation. *Radiology* 2001;219:445–454.
84. Rode A, Bancel B, Douek P, et al. Small nodule detection in cirrhotic livers: evaluation with US, spiral CT, and MRI and correlation with pathologic examination of explanted liver. *J Comput Assist Tomogr* 2001;25:327–336.
85. Marrero JA, Hussain HK, Nghiem HV, et al. Improving the prediction of hepatocellular carcinoma in cirrhotic patients with an arterially-enhancing liver mass. *Liver Transpl* 2005;11:281–289.
86. Llovet JM, Bru C, Bruix J. Prognosis of hepatocellular carcinoma: the BCLC staging classification. *Semin Liver Dis* 1999;19:329–338.
87. Marrero JA, Fontana RJ, Barrat A, et al. Prognosis of hepatocellular carcinoma: comparison of 7 staging systems in an American cohort. *Hepatology* 2005;41:707–716.
88. Chang CH, Chau GY, Lui WY, et al. Long-term results of hepatic resection for hepatocellular carcinoma originating from the noncirrhotic liver. *Arch Surg* 2004;139:320–325; discussion 326.
89. Cho CS, Gonen M, Shia J, et al. A novel prognostic nomogram is more accurate than conventional staging systems for predicting survival after resection of hepatocellular carcinoma. *J Am Coll Surg* 2008;206:281–291.
90. Vauthey JN, Lauwers GY, Esnaola NF, et al. Simplified staging for hepatocellular carcinoma. *J Clin Oncol* 2002;20:1527–1536.
91. Wayne JD, Lauwers GY, Ikai I, et al. Preoperative predictors of survival after resection of small hepatocellular carcinomas. *Ann Surg* 2002;235:722–730; discussion 730–731.
92. Tateishi R, Shiina S, Teratani T, et al. Percutaneous radiofrequency ablation for hepatocellular carcinoma. An analysis of 1000 cases. *Cancer* 2005;103:1201–1209.
93. Arii S, Yamaoka Y, Futagawa S, et al. Results of surgical and nonsurgical treatment for small-sized hepatocellular carcinomas: a retrospective and nationwide survey in Japan. The Liver Cancer Study Group of Japan. *Hepatology* 2000;32:1224–1229.
94. Parikh AA, Gentner B, Wu TT, et al. Perioperative complications in patients undergoing major liver resection with or without neoadjuvant chemotherapy. *J Gastrointest Surg* 2003;7:1082–1088.
95. Pawlik TM, Scoggins CR, Zorzi D, et al. Effect of surgical margin status on survival and site of recurrence after hepatic resection for colorectal metastases. *Ann Surg* 2005;241:715–722, discussion 722–724.
96. Asiyanbola B, Chang D, Gleisner AL, et al. Operative mortality after hepatic resection: are literature-based rates broadly applicable? *J Gastrointest Surg* 2008;12:842–851.
97. Pawlik TM, Delman KA, Vauthey JN, et al. Tumor size predicts vascular invasion and histologic grade: implications for selection of surgical treatment for hepatocellular carcinoma. *Liver Transpl* 2005;11:1086–1092.
98. Pandey D, Lee KH, Wai CT, et al. Long term outcome and prognostic factors for large hepatocellular carcinoma (10 cm or more) after surgical resection. *Ann Surg Oncol* 2007;14:2817–2823.
99. Shah SA, Wei AC, Cleary SP, et al. Prognosis and results after resection of very large (> or = 10 cm) hepatocellular carcinoma. *J Gastrointest Surg* 2007;11:589–595.
100. Kumada T, Nakano S, Takeda I, et al. Patterns of recurrence after initial treatment in patients with small hepatocellular carcinoma. *Hepatology* 1997;25:87–92.
101. Llovet JM, Ricci S, Mazzaferro V, et al. Sorafenib in advanced hepatocellular carcinoma. *N Engl J Med* 2008;359:378–390.
102. Mazzaferro V, Regalia E, Doci R, et al. Liver transplantation for the treatment of small hepatocellular carcinomas in patients with cirrhosis. *N Engl J Med* 1996;334:693–699.
103. Onaca N, Davis GL, Goldstein RM, et al. Expanded criteria for liver transplantation in patients with hepatocellular carcinoma: a report from the International Registry of Hepatic Tumors in Liver Transplantation. *Liver Transpl* 2007;13:391–399.
104. Schwartz M. Liver transplantation for hepatocellular carcinoma. *Gastroenterology* 2004;127:S268–S276.

105. Yao FY, Hirose R, LaBerge JM, et al. A prospective study on downstaging of hepatocellular carcinoma prior to liver transplantation. *Liver Transpl* 2005;11:1505–1514.
106. Zervos EE, Pearson H, Durkin AJ, et al. In-continuity hepatic resection for advanced hilar cholangiocarcinoma. *Am J Surg* 2004;188:584–588.
107. Galandi D, Antes G. Radiofrequency thermal ablation versus other interventions for hepatocellular carcinoma. *Cochrane Database Syst Rev* 2004;(2):CD003046.
108. Shiina S, Teratani T, Obi S, et al. A randomized controlled trial of radiofrequency ablation with ethanol injection for small hepatocellular carcinoma. *Gastroenterology* 2005;129:122–130.
109. Lin SM, Lin CJ, Lin CC, et al. Radiofrequency ablation improves prognosis compared with ethanol injection for hepatocellular carcinoma < or = 4 cm. *Gastroenterology* 2004;127:1714–1723.
110. Chen MS, Li JQ, Zheng Y, et al. A prospective randomized trial comparing percutaneous local ablative therapy and partial hepatectomy for small hepatocellular carcinoma. *Ann Surg* 2006;243:321–328.
111. Llovet JM, Bruix J. Systematic review of randomized trials for unresectable hepatocellular carcinoma: chemoembolization improves survival. *Hepatology* 2003;37:429–442.
112. Lo CM, Ngan H, Tso WK, et al. Randomized controlled trial of transarterial lipiodol chemoembolization for unresectable hepatocellular carcinoma. *Hepatology* 2002;35:1164–1171.
113. Llovet JM, Real MI, Montana X, et al. Arterial embolisation or chemoembolisation versus symptomatic treatment in patients with unresectable hepatocellular carcinoma: a randomised controlled trial. *Lancet* 2002;359:1734–1739.
114. Kulik LM, Carr BI, Mulcahy MF, et al. Safety and efficacy of 90Y radiotherapy for hepatocellular carcinoma with and without portal vein thrombosis. *Hepatology* 2008;47:71–81.
115. Bush DA, Hillebrand DJ, Slater JM, et al. High-dose proton beam radiotherapy of hepatocellular carcinoma: preliminary results of a phase II trial. *Gastroenterology* 2004;127:S189–S193.
116. Llovet JM, Bruix J. Novel advancements in the management of hepatocellular carcinoma in 2008. *J Hepatol* 2008;48(suppl 1):S20–S37.
117. Roskams T. Liver stem cells and their implication in hepatocellular and cholangiocarcinoma. *Oncogene* 2006;25:3818–3822.
118. Lee TY, Lee SS, Jung SW, et al. Hepatitis B virus infection and intrahepatic cholangiocarcinoma in Korea: a case-control study. *Am J Gastroenterol* 2008;103:1716–1720.
119. Okabayashi T, Yamamoto J, Kosuge T, et al. A new staging system for mass-forming intrahepatic cholangiocarcinoma: analysis of preoperative and postoperative variables. *Cancer* 2001;92:2374–2383.
120. Nathan H, Aloia TA, Vauthey JN, et al. A proposed staging system for intrahepatic cholangiocarcinoma. *Ann Surg Oncol* 2009;16:14–22.
121. Kim YJ, Yun M, Lee WJ, et al. Usefulness of 18F-FDG PET in intrahepatic cholangiocarcinoma. *Eur J Nucl Med Mol Imaging* 2003;30:1467–1472.
122. Kluge R, Schmidt F, Caca K, et al. Positron emission tomography with [(18)F]fluoro-2-deoxy-D-glucose for diagnosis and staging of bile duct cancer. *Hepatology* 2001;33:1029–1035.
123. Horner MJ, Ries LAG, Krapcho M, et al., eds. *SEER Cancer Statistics Review, 1975–2006*. Bethesda, MD: National Cancer Institute; 2009.
124. Kinkel K, Lu Y, Both M, et al. Detection of hepatic metastases from cancers of the gastrointestinal tract by using noninvasive imaging methods (US, CT, MR imaging, PET): a meta-analysis. *Radiology* 2002;224:748–756.
125. Glover C, Douse P, Kane P, et al. Accuracy of investigations for asymptomatic colorectal liver metastases. *Dis Colon Rectum* 2002;45:476–484.
126. Rocklin MS, Senagore AJ, Talbott TM. Role of carcinoembryonic antigen and liver function tests in the detection of recurrent colorectal carcinoma. *Dis Colon Rectum* 1991;34:794–797.
127. Rosen CB, Nagorney DM, Taswell HF, et al. Perioperative blood transfusion and determinants of survival after liver resection for metastatic colorectal carcinoma. *Ann Surg* 1992;216:493–504; discussion 504–505.
128. Scheele J, Stang R, Altendorf-Hofmann A, et al. Resection of colorectal liver metastases. *World J Surg* 1995;19:59–71.
129. Jamison RL, Donohue JH, Nagorney DM, et al. Hepatic resection for metastatic colorectal cancer results in cure for some patients. *Arch Surg* 1997;132:505–510; discussion 511.
130. Fong Y, Fortner J, Sun RL, et al. Clinical score for predicting recurrence after hepatic resection for metastatic colorectal cancer: analysis of 1001 consecutive cases. *Ann Surg* 1999;230:309–318; discussion 318–321.
131. Minagawa M, Makuuchi M, Torzilli G, et al. Extension of the frontiers of surgical indications in the treatment of liver metastases from colorectal cancer: long-term results. *Ann Surg* 2000;231:487–499.
132. Choti MA, Sitzmann JV, Tiburi MF, et al. Trends in long-term survival following liver resection for hepatic colorectal metastases. *Ann Surg* 2002;235:759–766.
133. Abdalla EK, Vauthey JN, Ellis LM, et al. Recurrence and outcomes following hepatic resection, radiofrequency ablation, and combined resection/ablation for colorectal liver metastases. *Ann Surg* 2004;239:818–825; discussion 825–827.
134. Fernandez FG, Drebin JA, Linehan DC, et al. Five-year survival after resection of hepatic metastases from colorectal cancer in patients screened by positron emission tomography with F-18 fluorodeoxyglucose (FDG-PET). *Ann Surg* 2004;240:438–447; discussion 447–450.
135. Wei AC, Greig PD, Grant D, et al. Survival after hepatic resection for colorectal metastases: a 10-year experience. *Ann Surg Oncol* 2006;13:668–676.
136. Shah SA, Bromberg R, Coates A, et al. Survival after liver resection for metastatic colorectal carcinoma in a large population. *J Am Coll Surg* 2007;205:676–683.
137. Rees M, Tekkis PP, Welsh FK, et al. Evaluation of long-term survival after hepatic resection for metastatic colorectal cancer: a multifactorial model of 929 patients. *Ann Surg* 2008;247:125–135.
138. Robertson DJ, Stukel TA, Gottlieb DJ, et al. Survival after hepatic resection of colorectal cancer metastases: a national experience. *Cancer* 2009;115:752–759.
139. Cummings LC, Payes JD, Cooper GS. Survival after hepatic resection in metastatic colorectal cancer: a population-based study. *Cancer* 2007;109:718–726.
140. Cady B, Stone MD, McDermott WV Jr, et al. Technical and biological factors in disease-free survival after hepatic resection for colorectal cancer metastases. *Arch Surg* 1992;127:561–568; discussion 568–569.
141. Iwatsuki S, Dvorchik I, Madariaga JR, et al. Hepatic resection for metastatic colorectal adenocarcinoma: a proposal of a prognostic scoring system. *J Am Coll Surg* 1999;189:291–299.
142. Poston GJ, Adam R, Alberts S, et al. OncoSurge: a strategy for improving resectability with curative intent in metastatic colorectal cancer. *J Clin Oncol* 2005;23:7125–7134.
143. Mala T, Bohler G, Mathisen O, et al. Hepatic resection for colorectal metastases: can preoperative scoring predict patient outcome? *World J Surg* 2002;26:1348–1353.
144. Kattan MW, Gonen M, Jarnagin WR, et al. A nomogram for predicting disease-specific survival after hepatic resection for metastatic colorectal cancer. *Ann Surg* 2008;247:282–287.
145. Yao FY, Ferrell L, Bass NM, et al. Liver transplantation for hepatocellular carcinoma: comparison of the proposed UCSF criteria with the Milan criteria and the Pittsburgh modified TNM criteria. *Liver Transpl* 2002;8:765–774.
146. Fernandez JA, Robles R, Marin C, et al. Can we expand the indications for liver transplantation among hepatocellular carcinoma patients with increased tumor size? *Transplant Proc* 2003;35:1818–1820.
147. Ravaioli M, Ercolani G, Cescon M, et al. Liver transplantation for hepatocellular carcinoma: further considerations on selection criteria. *Liver Transpl* 2004;10:1195–1202.
148. Leung JY, Zhu AX, Gordon FD, et al. Liver transplantation outcomes for early-stage hepatocellular carcinoma: results of a multicenter study. *Liver Transpl* 2004;10:1343–1354.
149. Todo S, Furukawa H. Living donor liver transplantation for adult patients with hepatocellular carcinoma: experience in Japan. *Ann Surg* 2004;240:451–459; discussion 459–461.
150. Decaens T, Roudot-Thoraval F, Hadni-Bresson S, et al. Impact of UCSF criteria according to pre- and post-OLT tumor features: analysis of 479 patients listed for HCC with a short waiting time. *Liver Transpl* 2006;12:1761–1769.
151. Duffy JP, Vardanian A, Benjamin E, et al. Liver transplantation criteria for hepatocellular carcinoma should be expanded: a 22-year experience with 467 patients at UCLA. *Ann Surg* 2007;246:502–509; discussion 509–511.
152. Hoti E, Adam R. Liver transplantation for primary and metastatic liver cancers. *Transpl Int* 2008;21:1107–1117.
153. Reddy SK, Pawlik TM, Zorzi D, et al. Simultaneous resections of colorectal cancer and synchronous liver metastases: a multi-institutional analysis. *Ann Surg Oncol* 2007;14:3481–3491.
154. Reddy SK, Zorzi D, Lum YW, et al. Timing of multimodality therapy for resectable synchronous colorectal liver metastases: a retrospective multi-institutional analysis. *Ann Surg Oncol* 2009;16:1809–1819.
155. Weber JC, Bachellier P, Oussoultzoglou E, et al. Simultaneous resection of colorectal primary tumour and synchronous liver metastases. *Br J Surg* 2003;90:956–962.
156. Pawlik TM, Izzo F, Cohen DS, et al. Combined resection and radiofrequency ablation for advanced hepatic malignancies: results in 172 patients. *Ann Surg Oncol* 2003;10:1059–1069.
157. Gleisner AL, Choti MA, Assumpcao L, et al. Colorectal liver metastases: recurrence and survival following hepatic resection, radiofrequency ablation, and combined resection-radiofrequency ablation. *Arch Surg* 2008;143:1204–1212.
158. Bismuth H, Adam R, Levi F, et al. Resection of nonresectable liver metastases from colorectal cancer after neoadjuvant chemotherapy. *Ann Surg* 1996;224:509–520; discussion 520–522.
159. Adam R, Pascal G, Castaing D, et al. Tumor progression while on chemotherapy: a contraindication to liver resection for multiple colorectal metastases? *Ann Surg* 2004;240:1052–1061; discussion 1061–1064.
160. Adam R, Delvart V, Pascal G, et al. Rescue surgery for unresectable colorectal liver metastases downstaged by chemotherapy: a model to predict long-term survival. *Ann Surg* 2004;240:644–657; discussion 657–658.
161. Adam R, Avisar E, Ariche A, et al. Five-year survival following hepatic resection after neoadjuvant therapy for nonresectable colorectal. *Ann Surg Oncol* 2001;8:347–353.
162. Pawlik TM, Abdalla EK, Ellis LM, et al. Debunking dogma: surgery for four or more colorectal liver metastases is justified. *J Gastrointest Surg* 2006;10:240–248.
163. Masi G, Loupakis F, Pollina L, et al. Long-term outcome of initially unresectable metastatic colorectal cancer patients treated with 5-fluorouracil/leucovorin, oxaliplatin, and irinotecan (FOLFOXIRI) followed by radical surgery of metastases. *Ann Surg* 2009;249:420–425.
164. Wicherts DA, Miller R, de Haas RJ, et al. Long-term results of two-stage hepatectomy for irresectable colorectal cancer liver metastases. *Ann Surg* 2008;248:994–1005.
165. Chun YS, Vauthey JN, Ribero D, et al. Systemic chemotherapy and two-stage hepatectomy for extensive bilateral colorectal liver metastases: perioperative safety and survival. *J Gastrointest Surg* 2007;11:1498–1504; discussion 1504–1505.

166. Togo S, Nagano Y, Masui H, et al. Two-stage hepatectomy for multiple bilobular liver metastases from colorectal cancer. *Hepatogastroenterology* 2005;52:913–919.
167. Tuttle TM, Curley SA, Roh MS. Repeat hepatic resection as effective treatment of recurrent colorectal liver metastases. *Ann Surg Oncol* 1997;4:125–130.
168. Adam R, Bismuth H, Castaing D, et al. Repeat hepatectomy for colorectal liver metastases. *Ann Surg* 1997;225:51–60; discussion 60–62.
169. Petrowsky H, Gonen M, Jarnagin W, et al. Second liver resections are safe and effective treatment for recurrent hepatic metastases from colorectal cancer: a bi-institutional analysis. *Ann Surg* 2002;235:863–871.
170. Elias D, Ouellet JF, Bellon N, et al. Extrahepatic disease does not contraindicate hepatectomy for colorectal liver metastases. *Br J Surg* 2003;90:567–574.
171. Inoue M, Kotake Y, Nakagawa K, et al. Surgery for pulmonary metastases from colorectal carcinoma. *Ann Thorac Surg* 2000;70:380–383.
172. Watanabe K, Nagai K, Kobayashi A, et al. Factors influencing survival after complete resection of pulmonary metastases from colorectal cancer. *Br J Surg* 2009;96:1058–1065.
173. Miller G, Biernacki P, Kemeny NE, et al. Outcomes after resection of synchronous or metachronous hepatic and pulmonary colorectal metastases. *J Am Coll Surg* 2007;205:231–238.
174. Adam R, de Haas RJ, Wicherts DA, et al. Is hepatic resection justified after chemotherapy in patients with colorectal liver metastases and lymph node involvement? *J Clin Oncol* 2008;26:3672–3680.
175. Dimick JB, Cowan JA Jr, Knol JA, et al. Hepatic resection in the United States: indications, outcomes, and hospital procedural volumes from a nationally representative database. *Arch Surg* 2003;138:185–191.
176. Dimick JB, Wainess RM, Cowan JA, et al. National trends in the use and outcomes of hepatic resection. *J Am Coll Surg* 2004;199:31–38.
177. Melendez JA, Arslan V, Fischer ME, et al. Perioperative outcomes of major hepatic resections under low central venous pressure anesthesia: blood loss, blood transfusion, and the risk of postoperative renal dysfunction. *J Am Coll Surg* 1998;187:620–625.
178. Jones RM, Moulton CE, Hardy KJ. Central venous pressure and its effect on blood loss during liver resection. *Br J Surg* 1998;85:1058–1060.
179. Makuuchi M, Thai BL, Takayasu K, et al. Preoperative portal embolization to increase safety of major hepatectomy for hilar bile duct carcinoma: a preliminary report. *Surgery* 1990;107:521–527.
180. Azoulay D, Castaing D, Smail A, et al. Resection of nonresectable liver metastases from colorectal cancer after percutaneous portal vein embolization. *Ann Surg* 2000;231:480–486.
181. Sugawara Y, Yamamoto J, Higashi H, et al. Preoperative portal embolization in patients with hepatocellular carcinoma. *World J Surg* 2002;26:105–110.
182. Farges O, Belghiti J, Kianmanesh R, et al. Portal vein embolization before right hepatectomy: prospective clinical trial. *Ann Surg* 2003;237:208–217.
183. Xia F, Poon RT, Fan ST, et al. Thoracoabdominal approach for right-sided hepatic resection for hepatocellular carcinoma. *J Am Coll Surg* 2003;196: 418–427.
184. Zacherl J, Scheuba C, Imhof M, et al. Current value of intraoperative sonography during surgery for hepatic neoplasms. *World J Surg* 2002;26:550–554.
185. Batignani G. Hilar plate detachment and extraglissonian extrahepatic anterior approach to the right portal pedicle for right liver resections. *J Am Coll Surg* 2000;190:631–634.
186. Machado MA, Herman P, Figueira ER, et al. Intrahepatic glissonian access for segmental liver resection in cirrhotic patients. *Am J Surg* 2006;192:388–392.
187. Strasberg SM, Linehan DC, Hawkins WG. Isolation of right main and right sectional portal pedicles for liver resection without hepatotomy or inflow occlusion. *J Am Coll Surg* 2008;206:390–396.
188. Clavien PA. Surgical techniques for liver resection. *J Gastrointest Surg* 2006;10:166–167.
189. Reddy SK, Barbas AS, Gan TJ, et al. Hepatic parenchymal transection with vascular staplers: a comparative analysis with the crush-clamp technique. *Am J Surg* 2008;196:760–767.
190. Smith DL, Arens JF, Barnett CC Jr, et al. A prospective evaluation of ultrasound-directed transparenchymal vascular control with linear cutting staplers in major hepatic resections. *Am J Surg* 2005;190:23–29.
191. Belghiti J, Noun R, Malafosse R, et al. Continuous versus intermittent portal triad clamping for liver resection: a controlled study. *Ann Surg* 1999; 229:369–375.
192. Peralta C, Prats N, Xaus C, et al. Protective effect of liver ischemic preconditioning on liver and lung injury induced by hepatic ischemia-reperfusion in the rat. *Hepatology* 1999;30:1481–1489.
193. Arkadopoulos N, Kostopanagiotou G, Theodoraki K, et al. Ischemic preconditioning confers antiapoptotic protection during major hepatectomies performed under combined inflow and outflow exclusion of the liver. A randomized clinical trial. *World J Surg* 2009;33:1909–1915.
194. Petrowsky H, McCormack L, Trujillo M, et al. A prospective, randomized, controlled trial comparing intermittent portal triad clamping versus ischemic preconditioning with continuous clamping for major liver resection. *Ann Surg* 2006;244:921–928; discussion 928–930.
195. Gurusamy KS, Kumar Y, Pamecha V, et al. Ischaemic pre-conditioning for elective liver resections performed under vascular occlusion. *Cochrane Database Syst Rev* 2009;(1):CD007629.
196. Fan ST, Lo CM, Liu CL. Technical refinement in adult-to-adult living donor liver transplantation using right lobe graft. *Ann Surg* 2000;231:126–131.
197. Emond J, Wachs ME, Renz JF, et al. Total vascular exclusion for major hepatectomy in patients with abnormal liver parenchyma. *Arch Surg* 1995;130:824–830; discussion 830–831.
198. Suh KS, Yi NJ, Kim T, et al. Laparoscopy-assisted donor right hepatectomy using a hand port system preserving the middle hepatic vein branches. *World J Surg* 2009;33:526–533.
199. Suh KS, Yi NJ, Kim J, et al. Laparoscopic hepatectomy for a modified right graft in adult-to-adult living donor liver transplantation. *Transplant Proc* 2008;40:3529–3531.
200. Koffron AJ, Kung R, Baker T, et al. Laparoscopic-assisted right lobe donor hepatectomy. *Am J Transplant* 2006;6:2522–2525.
201. Cherqui D, Soubrane O, Husson E, et al. Laparoscopic living donor hepatectomy for liver transplantation in children. *Lancet* 2002;359:392–396.
202. Croce E, Azzola M, Russo R, et al. Laparoscopic liver tumour resection with the argon beam. *Endosc Surg Allied Technol* 1994;2:186–188.
203. Rau HG, Meyer G, Cohnert TU, et al. Laparoscopic liver resection with the water-jet dissector. *Surg Endosc* 1995;9:1009–1012.
204. Azagra JS, Goergen M, Gilbart E, et al. Laparoscopic anatomical (hepatic) left lateral segmentectomy-technical aspects. *Surg Endosc* 1996;10:758–761.
205. Kaneko H, Takagi S, Shiba T. Laparoscopic partial hepatectomy and left lateral segmentectomy: technique and results of a clinical series. *Surgery* 1996;120:468–475.
206. Fong Y, Jarnagin W, Conlon KC, et al. Hand-assisted laparoscopic liver resection: lessons from an initial experience. *Arch Surg* 2000;135:854–859.
207. Laurent A, Cherqui D, Lesurtel M, et al. Laparoscopic liver resection for subcapsular hepatocellular carcinoma complicating chronic liver disease. *Arch Surg* 2003;138:763–769; discussion 769.
208. Cherqui D. Laparoscopic liver resection. *Br J Surg* 2003;90:644–646.
209. Koffron AJ, Auffenberg G, Kung R, et al. Evaluation of 300 minimally invasive liver resections at a single institution: less is more. *Ann Surg* 2007; 246:385–392; discussion 392–394.
210. Buell JF, Thomas MT, Rudich S, et al. Experience with more than 500 minimally invasive hepatic procedures. *Ann Surg* 2008;248:475–486.
211. Nguyen KT, Gamblin TC, Geller DA. World review of laparoscopic liver resection-2,804 patients. *Ann Surg* 2009;250:831–841.
212. Jayne DG, Guillou PJ, Thorpe H, et al. Randomized trial of laparoscopic-assisted resection of colorectal carcinoma: 3-year results of the UK MRC CLASICC Trial Group. *J Clin Oncol* 2007;25:3061–3068.
213. Fleshman J, Sargent DJ, Green E, et al. Laparoscopic colectomy for cancer is not inferior to open surgery based on 5-year data from the COST Study Group trial. *Ann Surg* 2007;246:655–662; discussion 662–664.
214. Gigot JF, Glineur D, Santiago Azagra J, et al. Laparoscopic liver resection for malignant liver tumors: preliminary results of a multicenter European study. *Ann Surg* 2002;236:90–97.
215. Buell JF, Cherqui D, Geller DA, et al. The international position on laparoscopic liver surgery: the Louisville statement, 2008. *Ann Surg* 2009;250:825–830.
216. Dagher I, O'Rourke N, Geller DA, et al. Laparoscopic major hepatectomy: an evolution in standard of care. *Ann Surg* 2009;250:856–860.
217. Heaney JP, Stanton WK, Halbert DS, et al. An improved technic for vascular isolation of the liver: experimental study and case reports. *Ann Surg* 1966;163:237–241.
218. Bismuth H, Castaing D, Garden OJ. Major hepatic resection under total vascular exclusion. *Ann Surg* 1989;210:13–19.
219. Gurusamy KS, Sheth H, Kumar Y, et al. Methods of vascular occlusion for elective liver resections. Cochrane Database Syst Rev 2009;(1):CD007632.
220. Rahbari NN, Koch M, Mehrabi A, et al. Portal triad clamping versus vascular exclusion for vascular control during hepatic resection: a systematic review and meta-analysis. *J Gastrointest Surg* 2009;13:558–568.
221. Azoulay D, Eshkenazy R, Andreani P, et al. In situ hypothermic perfusion of the liver versus standard total vascular exclusion for complex liver resection. *Ann Surg* 2005;241:277–285.
222. Hemming AW, Kim RD, Mekeel KL, et al. Portal vein resection for hilar cholangiocarcinoma. *Am Surg* 2006;72:599–604; discussion 604–605.
223. Hemming AW, Reed AI, Fujita S, et al. Role for extending hepatic resection using an aggressive approach to liver surgery. *J Am Coll Surg* 2008;206: 870–875; discussion 875–878.
224. Hemming AW, Reed AI, Langham MR Jr, et al. Combined resection of the liver and inferior vena cava for hepatic malignancy. *Ann Surg* 2004;239: 712–719; discussion 719–721.
225. Azoulay D, Andreani P, Maggi U, et al. Combined liver resection and reconstruction of the supra-renal vena cava: the Paul Brousse experience. *Ann Surg* 2006;244:80–88.
226. Starzl TE, Marchioro TL, Vonkaulla KN, et al. Homotransplantation of the liver in humans. *Surg Gynecol Obstet* 1963;117:659–676.
227. Faraj W, Dar F, Marangoni G, et al. Liver transplantation for hepatoblastoma. *Liver Transpl* 2008;14:1614–1619.
228. Rea DJ, Heimbach JK, Rosen CB, et al. Liver transplantation with neoadjuvant chemoradiation is more effective than resection for hilar cholangiocarcinoma. *Ann Surg* 2005;242:451–458; discussion 458–461.
229. Frilling A, Malago M, Weber F, et al. Liver transplantation for patients with metastatic endocrine tumors: single-center experience with 15 patients. *Liver Transpl* 2006;12:1089–1096.
230. McGahan JP, Brock JM, Tesluk H, et al. Hepatic ablation with use of radio-frequency electrocautery in the animal model. *J Vasc Interv Radiol* 1992;3:291–297.
231. Curley SA, Izzo F, Delrio P, et al. Radiofrequency ablation of unresectable primary and metastatic hepatic malignancies: results in 123 patients. *Ann Surg* 1999;230:1–8.
232. Curley SA, Izzo F, Ellis LM, et al. Radiofrequency ablation of hepatocellular cancer in 110 patients with cirrhosis. *Ann Surg* 2000;232:381–391.
233. Curley SA. Radiofrequency ablation of malignant liver tumors. *Oncologist* 2001;6:14–23.
234. Elias D, Sideris L, Pocard M, et al. Incidence of unsuspected and treatable metastatic disease associated with operable colorectal liver metastases discovered only at laparotomy (and not treated when performing percutaneous radiofrequency ablation). *Ann Surg Oncol* 2005;12:298–302.

CHAPTER 60 ■ CALCULOUS BILIARY DISEASE

HENRY A. PITT, STEVEN A. AHRENDT, AND ATTILA NAKEEB

KEY POINTS

1. Gallstones are classified by their cholesterol content as either cholesterol (70% to 80%) or pigment (20% to 30%), with pigment stones further classified as black or brown.
2. Biliary sludge refers to a mixture of cholesterol crystals, calcium bilirubinate granules, and a mucin gel matrix and is thought to serve as the nidus for gallstone growth.
3. The pathogenesis of cholesterol gallstones is clearly multifactorial but essentially involves four factors: (a) cholesterol supersaturation in bile, (b) crystal nucleation, (c) gallbladder dysmotility, and (d) gallbladder absorption/secretion.
4. Prophylactic cholecystectomy is generally not indicated in patients with asymptomatic gallstones, because studies show that only 20% to 30% will become symptomatic within 20 years and only 1% to 2% will develop serious complications per year.
5. Elective laparoscopic cholecystectomy is associated with a mortality rate of less than 0.3% and an overall complication rate of 10%, with less than 5% of patients requiring conversion to an open procedure.
6. Randomized trials have shown that early laparoscopic cholecystectomy performed for acute cholecystitis can result in a lower morbidity rate, shorter hospital stay, and quicker return to work than delayed cholecystectomy.
7. Chronic acalculous cholecystitis is associated with typical symptoms of biliary colic without evidence of gallstones and is diagnosed by cholescintigraphy with an ejection fraction of less than 35% in response to cholecystokinin.
8. Acute cholangitis results from the combination of significant bacterial concentration in bile and increased biliary pressure associated with biliary obstruction.
9. The strongest clinical indications for the presence of a common bile duct stone include a history of cholangitis, common bile duct stones identified on ultrasound, and jaundice; a patient with any one of these indicators has at least a 10 times increased risk of common bile duct stones.
10. Endoscopic cholangiography is the "gold standard" for the diagnosis of common bile duct stones, being successful in 90% to 95% of patients although associated with complications of cholangitis or pancreatitis in up to 5% of patients.

Calculous biliary disease is a major health care problem in developed countries as well as in many underdeveloped countries. In the United States, approximately 12% of the population or more than 30,000 Americans have gallstones. Currently more than 750,000 cholecystectomies are performed annually in the United States, and the cost of caring for these patients is estimated to be between $7 million and $10 million per year.[1] To properly manage these patients, surgeons should understand biliary physiology and gallstone pathogenesis, incidence, risk factors, and natural history as reviewed in the following discussion. In addition, this chapter reviews the diagnostic options, clinical manifestations, management options, and expected outcomes for calculous biliary disease.

BILIARY PHYSIOLOGY

Bile Flow

The bile ducts, gallbladder, and sphincter of Oddi act in concert to modify, store, and regulate the flow of bile. Approximately 600 to 750 mL of bile is produced daily. During its passage through the bile ductules, canalicular bile is modified by the absorption and secretion of electrolytes and water. The gastrointestinal hormone secretin increases bile flow primarily by increasing the active secretion of chloride-rich fluid by the bile ducts. Bile ductular secretion is also stimulated by other hormones such as cholecystokinin and gastrin. The bile duct epithelium is also capable of water and electrolyte absorption, which may be of primary importance in the storage of bile during fasting in patients who have previously undergone cholecystectomy. The main functions of the gallbladder are to concentrate and store hepatic bile during the fasting state and deliver bile into the duodenum in response to a meal. The usual capacity of the human gallbladder is approximately 40 to 50 mL. Only a small fraction of the 600 to 750 mL of bile produced each day would be stored were it not for its remarkable absorptive capacity. The gallbladder mucosa has the greatest absorptive capacity per unit of any structure in the body.

Bile Composition

Bile is usually concentrated 5- to 10-fold by the absorption of water and electrolytes, leading to a marked change in bile composition (Table 60.1). Active sodium chloride transport by the gallbladder epithelium is the driving force for the concentration of bile.[2] Water is passively absorbed in response to the osmotic force generated by solute absorption. The concentration of bile may affect the solubilities of two important components of gallstones, cholesterol and calcium. Although the gallbladder mucosa does absorb calcium, this process is not nearly as efficient as the absorption of sodium or water, leading to a greater relative increase in calcium concentration. As the gallbladder bile becomes concentrated, several changes occur in the capacity of bile to solubilize cholesterol. The solubility in the micellar fraction is increased, but the stability of phospholipid–cholesterol vesicles is greatly decreased. Because cholesterol crystal precipitation occurs preferentially by vesicular rather than micellar mechanisms, the net effect of concentrating bile is an increased tendency to form cholesterol crystals.

Bile facilitates the intestinal absorption of lipids and fat-soluble vitamins and represents the route of excretion for certain organic solids such as bilirubin and cholesterol. The major organic solutes in bile are bilirubin, bile salts, phospholipids,

TABLE 60.1

COMPOSITION OF HEPATIC AND GALLBLADDER BILE

CHARACTERISTIC	HEPATIC	GALLBLADDER
Sodium (mEq/L)	160	270
Potassium (mEq/L)	5	10
Chloride (mEq/L)	90	15
Bicarbonate (mEq/L)	45	10
Calcium (mEq/L)	4	25
Magnesium (mEq/L)	2	—
Bilirubin (mEq/L)	1.5	15
Protein (mEq/L)	150	—
Bile acids (mEq/L)	50	150
Phospholipids (mEq/L)	8	40
Cholesterol (mEq/L)	4	18
Total solids (mEq/L)	—	125
pH	7.8	7.2

and cholesterol. Bilirubin is the breakdown product of spent red blood cells and is conjugated with glucuronic acid prior to being excreted. Bile salts solubilize lipids and facilitate their absorption. Phospholipids are synthesized in the liver in conjunction with bile salt synthesis. The final major solute of bile is cholesterol, which is also produced primarily by the liver with little contribution from dietary sources. Cholesterol is highly nonpolar and insoluble in water and thus in bile as well.

Gallbladder Function

As a result of active absorption, the gallbladder stores concentrated bile that reenters the distal bile duct and is secreted into the duodenum in response to a meal. In addition to absorption and concentration, the gallbladder's mucosa actively secretes glycoproteins and hydrogen ions. Secretion of mucous glycoproteins occurs primarily from the glands of the gallbladder neck and cystic duct. The resultant mucin gel is believed to constitute an important part of the unstirred layer (diffusion-resistant barrier) that separates the gallbladder cell membrane from the luminal bile. This mucous barrier may be very important in protecting the gallbladder epithelium from the strong detergent effect of the highly concentrated bile salts found in the gallbladder. However, considerable evidence also suggests that mucin glycoproteins play a role as a pronucleating agent for cholesterol crystallization. The transport of hydrogen ions by the gallbladder epithelium leads to a decrease in bile pH through a sodium-exchange mechanism. Acidification of bile in the gallbladder promotes calcium solubility, thereby preventing its precipitation as calcium salts. The gallbladder's normal acidification process lowers the pH of entering hepatic bile from 7.5 to 7.8 down to 7.1 to 7.3.[2]

Biliary Motility

Gallbladder. Gallbladder filling is facilitated by tonic contraction of the ampullary sphincter, which maintains a constant pressure in the common bile duct (CBD) (10 to 15 mm Hg). However, the gallbladder does not simply fill passively and continuously during fasting. Rather, periods of filling are punctuated by brief periods of partial emptying (10% to 15% of its volume) of concentrated gallbladder bile. Emptying periods are coordinated with each passage through the duodenum of phase III of the migrating myoelectric complex (MMC). This process is mediated, at least in part, by the hormone motilin. Following a meal, the release of stored bile from the gallbladder requires a coordinated motor response of gallbladder contraction and sphincter of Oddi relaxation. One of the main stimuli to gallbladder emptying is the hormone cholecystokinin, which is released from the duodenal mucosa in response to a meal. When stimulated by eating, the gallbladder empties 50% to 70% of its contents within 30 to 40 minutes. Gallbladder refilling then occurs gradually over the next 60 to 90 minutes. Many other hormonal and neural pathways are also necessary for the coordinated action of the gallbladder and sphincter of Oddi. Defects in gallbladder motility, which increase the residence time of bile in the gallbladder, play a central role in the pathogenesis of gallstones.[3]

Sphincter of Oddi

The human sphincter of Oddi is a complex structure that is functionally independent from the duodenal musculature. Endoscopic manometric studies have demonstrated that the human sphincter of Oddi creates a high-pressure zone between the bile duct and the duodenum. The sphincter regulates the flow of bile and pancreatic juice into the duodenum and also prevents the regurgitation of duodenal contents into the biliary tract. These functions are achieved by keeping pressure within the bile and pancreatic ducts higher than duodenal pressure. The sphincter of Oddi also has very high-pressure phasic contractions, which may play a role in preventing the regurgitation of duodenal contents into the biliary tract.

Both neural and hormonal factors influence the sphincter of Oddi. In humans, sphincter of Oddi pressure and phasic wave activity diminish in response to cholecystokinin. Thus, sphincter pressure relaxes after a meal, allowing the passive flow of bile into the duodenum. During fasting, high-pressure phasic contractions of the sphincter of Oddi persist through all phases of the MMC. However, recent animal studies suggest that sphincter of Oddi phasic waves do vary to some degree in concert with the MMC. Thus, sphincter of Oddi activity is undoubtedly coordinated with the partial gallbladder emptying and increases in bile flow that occur during phase III of the MMC. This activity may be a preventative mechanism against the accumulation of biliary crystals during fasting.[4]

Neurally mediated reflexes link the sphincter of Oddi with the gallbladder and stomach to coordinate the flow of bile and pancreatic juice into the duodenum. The cholecystosphincter of Oddi reflex allows the human sphincter to relax as the gallbladder contracts. Similarly, antral distention causes both gallbladder contraction and sphincter relaxation.

GALLSTONE PATHOGENESIS

Gallstone Types

Gallstones represent a failure to maintain certain biliary solutes, primarily cholesterol, and calcium salts in a solubilized state. Gallstones are classified by their cholesterol content as either cholesterol or pigment stones. Pigment stones are further classified as either black or brown (Fig. 60.1). Pure cholesterol gallstones are uncommon (10%), with most cholesterol stones containing calcium salts in their center, or nidus. In most American populations, 70% to 80% of gallstones are cholesterol, and black pigment stones account for most of the remaining 20% to 30%.

An important biliary precipitate in gallstone pathogenesis is biliary "sludge," which refers to a mixture of cholesterol crystals, calcium bilirubinate granules, and a mucin gel matrix. Biliary sludge has been observed clinically in prolonged fasting states or with the use of long-term total parenteral nutrition

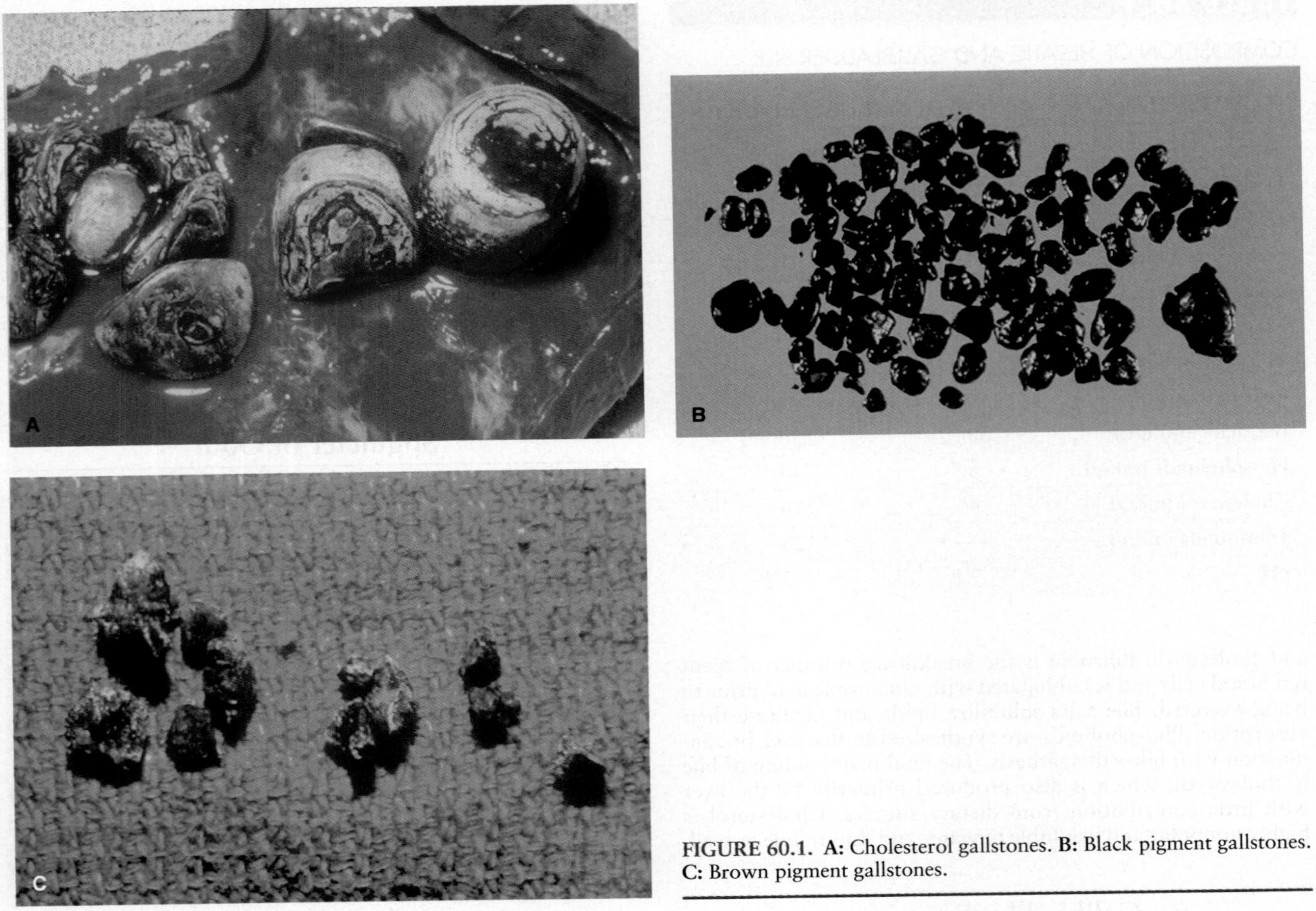

FIGURE 60.1. **A:** Cholesterol gallstones. **B:** Black pigment gallstones. **C:** Brown pigment gallstones.

(TPN). Both of these conditions are also associated with gallstone formation. The finding of macromolecular complexes of mucin and bilirubin, similar to biliary sludge in the central core of most cholesterol gallstones, suggests that sludge may serve as the nidus for gallstone growth.

3 **Cholesterol Gallstones.** The pathogenesis of cholesterol gallstones is clearly multifactorial but essentially involves four factors: (a) cholesterol supersaturation in bile, (b) crystal nucleation, (c) gallbladder dysmotility, and (d) gallbladder absorption/secretion. For many years, gallstones were thought to result primarily from a defect in the hepatic secretion of biliary lipids. More recently, it has become increasingly clear that gallbladder mucosal and motor function also play key roles in gallstone formation.

Biliary Lipids. The key to maintaining cholesterol in solution is the formation of both micelles, a bile salt–phospholipid–cholesterol complex, and cholesterol–phospholipid vesicles (Fig. 60.2). Present theory suggests that in states of excess cholesterol production, these large vesicles may also exceed their capability to transport cholesterol, and crystal precipitation may occur. Cholesterol solubility depends on the relative concentration of cholesterol, bile salts, and phospholipid. By plotting the percentages of each component on triangular coordinates, the micellar zone in which cholesterol is completely soluble can be demonstrated (Fig. 60.3). In the area above the curve, bile is supersaturated with cholesterol, and precipitation of cholesterol crystals can occur.

Cholesterol Crystallization. Cholesterol supersaturation is present in many normal humans without gallstones. As bile is concentrated in the gallbladder, a net transfer of phospholipids and cholesterol from vesicles to micelles occurs. The phospholipids are transferred more efficiently than cholesterol, leading to cholesterol enrichment of the remaining vesicles. These cholesterol-rich vesicles aggregate to form large multilamellar liquid vesicles that then precipitate cholesterol monohydrate crystals. Several pronucleating factors including mucin glycoproteins, immunoglobulins, and transferrin accelerate the precipitation of cholesterol in bile.

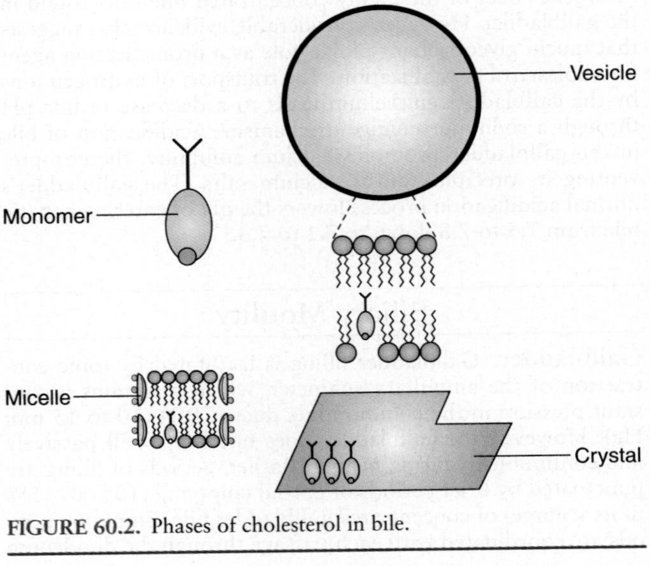

FIGURE 60.2. Phases of cholesterol in bile.

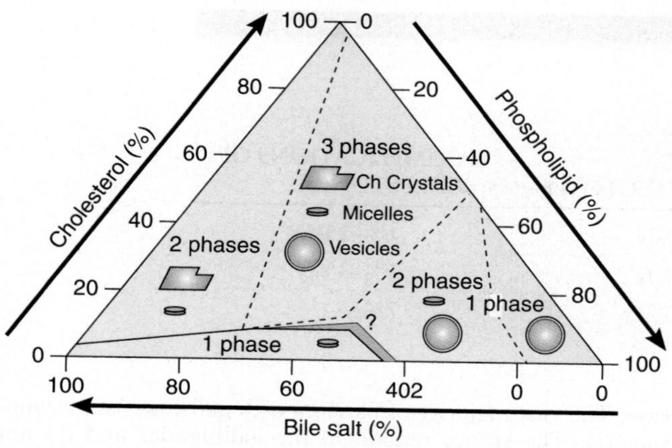

FIGURE 60.3. Equilibrium phase diagram for bile salt–lecithin–cholesterol–water at a concentration of 10% solids, 90% water. The monomeric phase is not depicted as a phase because it exists at the same concentration throughout. The one-phase zone contains only micelles. Several other zones exist, but only the two on the left above the one-phase zone apply to human gallbladder bile, and both contain cholesterol monohydrate crystals at equilibrium.

Gallbladder Motility. For gallstones to cause clinical symptoms, they must obtain a size sufficient to produce mechanical injury to the gallbladder or obstruction of the biliary tree. Growth of stones may occur in two ways: (a) progressive enlargement of individual crystals or stones by deposition of additional insoluble precipitate at the bile–stone interface, or (b) fusion of individual crystals or stones to form a larger conglomerate. In addition, defects in gallbladder motility increase the residence time of bile in the gallbladder, thereby playing a role in stone formation. Gallstone formation occurs in clinical states with gallbladder stasis, as seen with prolonged fasting, with the use of long-term parenteral nutrition, after vagotomy, in diabetic patients, and in patients with somatostatin-producing tumors or in those receiving long-term somatostatin therapy.

Gallbladder Absorption/Secretion. As noted previously, the gallbladder is a very effective absorptive organ, and a normal function of the gallbladder is to concentrate and acidify bile. For many years, three factors have been thought to be key in cholesterol gallstone pathogenesis: cholesterol supersaturation, cholesterol crystallization, and biliary motility. However, a fourth factor, gallbladder absorption/secretion, also may be key to gallstone formation. Alterations in sodium, chloride, bicarbonate, and water absorption may alter the milieu for cholesterol saturation and crystal formation as well as for calcium precipitation.[2]

Pigment Gallstones

Black Pigment Stones. With the recognition that calcium salts are present in most, if not all, cholesterol gallstones, renewed interest has developed in the events leading to the precipitation of calcium with the anions, bilirubin, carbonate, phosphate, or palmitate. Precipitation of these anions as insoluble calcium salts serves as a nidus for cholesterol stone formation. Furthermore, calcium bilirubinate and calcium palmitate also form major components of pigment gallstones. Pigment gallstones are classified as either black or brown pigment stones. Black pigment stones are typically tarry and frequently are associated with hemolytic conditions or cirrhosis. In hemolytic states, the bilirubin load and concentration of unconjugated bilirubin increase. These stones are usually not associated with infected bile and are located almost exclusively in the gallbladder.

Brown Pigment Stones. In contrast to black pigment stones, brown pigment stones are earthy in texture and are typically found in the bile ducts, especially in Asian populations. Brown stones often contain more cholesterol and calcium palmitate than black stones and occur as primary common duct stones in Western patients with disorders of biliary motility and associated bacterial infection. In these settings, bacteria-producing slime and bacteria containing the enzyme glucuronidase cause enzymatic hydrolysis of soluble conjugated bilirubin glucuronide to form free bilirubin, which then precipitates with calcium.

GALLSTONE INCIDENCE AND RISK FACTORS

Incidence

Cholesterol gallstones account for 70% to 80% of all stones in Western industrialized countries. Their prevalence increases with patient age. Stones are uncommon in patients younger than age 20 years, but a sharp increase is noted, especially in women, with each decade to approximately age 70 years (Fig. 60.4). Approximately 20% of women and 10% of men have stones by age 60 years. Collectively, approximately 12% of Americans or 36 million men and women harbor gallstones. In certain populations, such as Native Americans, the incidence is extremely high, especially in women. In Chileans and Bolivians of Indian ancestry, gallstones are also very common, and they are associated with a high incidence of gallbladder cancer. In fact, gallbladder cancer is the most common gastrointestinal cancer in these countries. In the United States, the prevalence of stones is highest in Mexican American women (26%), and the prevalence in white women (17%) is higher than in black women (14%).[5]

Risk Factors

Gallstones are more common in women, especially those who have had multiple pregnancies, are taking birth control pills, are obese, are undergoing rapid weight loss, or have elevated serum triglyceride levels. Diet plays an important role in cholesterol supersaturation. Cholesterol gallstones do not form in vegetarians. Cholesterol gallstones are common in populations consuming a Western diet, which is relatively high in overall calories as well as animal fats and carbohydrates. The incidence of cholesterol gallstones rises in a population as it shifts

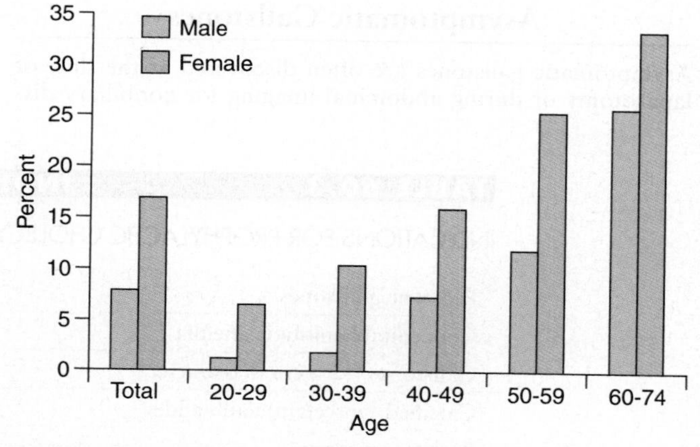

FIGURE 60.4. Influence of age and gender on gallstone incidence. (After the National Health and Nutrition Examination and Survey III [1988–1994]. The National Center for Health Statistics, Division of Health Examination Studies, Centers for Disease Control and Prevention, October 1996.)

TABLE 60.2

NATURAL HISTORY OF GALLSTONES

DEGREE OF SYMPTOMS	SYMPTOMS REQUIRING CHOLECYSTECTOMY	COMPLICATIONS OF GALLSTONES
Asymptomatic	1%–2%/y	1%–2%/y
Mild symptoms	6%–8%/y	1%–3%/y
Symptomatic	5%–30%/y	7%/y

to a higher consumption of dietary fat. Diabetic patients also have an increased incidence of gallstones, which may be caused, in part, by alterations in gallbladder motor function and/or absorption/secretion. Gallstones also are known to occur more frequently in certain families. However, the genetic factors underlying this phenomenon have not been elucidated. Nevertheless, current data suggest that approximately 30% of the risk for gallstone formation is hereditary whereas 70% is environmental, with diet being the primary environmental factor.[6]

As mentioned previously, prolonged fasting, TPN, ileal resection, vagotomy, hemolytic states, and cirrhosis are additional risk factors, and many of these factors lead to black pigment stone formation. Finally, bile duct stasis, as occurs with biliary strictures, congenital cysts, chronic pancreatitis, sclerosing cholangitis, and perivaterian duodenal diverticula, is the primary risk factor for brown pigment stone formation.

NATURAL HISTORY OF GALLSTONES

An understanding of the natural history of gallstone disease is necessary for the appropriate management of patients with cholelithiasis. The presence or absence of symptoms remains the most important factor in the determination of the natural history of gallstones. Gallstone disease can be considered as a spectrum of clinical entities that includes asymptomatic gallstones, symptomatic gallstones, and complicated gallstone disease. The complications of gallstone disease include (a) acute cholecystitis, (b) choledocholithiasis with or without cholangitis, (c) gallstone pancreatitis, (d) gallstone ileus, and (e) gallbladder carcinoma.

Asymptomatic Gallstones

Asymptomatic gallstones are often discovered at the time of laparotomy or during abdominal imaging for nonbiliary disease. The vast majority of patients with gallstones are asymptomatic. The stones remain in the gallbladder and do not obstruct the cystic duct. As a result, the gallbladder fills and empties normally, and the gallstones remain silent. Over time, asymptomatic gallstones can progress to symptomatic disease. Symptomatic gallstones usually present with what is termed *biliary colic*, right upper quadrant or epigastric abdominal pain that typically develops postprandially and may be associated with nausea and vomiting. The pain results from the impaction of a gallstone at the neck of the gallbladder or cystic duct. 4 Studies that have followed asymptomatic patients have shown that 20% to 30% of patients become symptomatic within 20 years.[7,8] Approximately 1% to 2% of asymptomatic individuals with gallstones per year develop serious symptoms or complications related to their gallstones (Table 60.2). The longer stones remain silent, the less likely symptoms are to develop. In addition, almost all patients will develop symptomatic disease before developing one of the complications of gallstones. Therefore, prophylactic cholecystectomy is not generally indicated in patients with asymptomatic gallstones.

In select groups of patients, however, prophylactic cholecystectomy should be considered (Table 60.3). Children with gallstones almost always develop symptoms and should be considered for early cholecystectomy. In patients with sickle cell disease, cholecystitis can precipitate a crisis with substantial operative risks. Therefore, these patients are best treated with elective cholecystectomy. A nonfunctioning gallbladder usually indicates advanced disease with more than 25% of these patients developing symptoms that require cholecystectomy. Large gallstones (>2.5 cm) are more frequently associated with acute cholecystitis and gallbladder carcinoma, and prophylactic cholecystectomy may also be indicated in these patients. In the past, the presence of a porcelain gallbladder (calcified gallbladder wall) was thought to be associated with a 25% risk of malignant transformation, and prophylactic cholecystectomy has been recommended. More recent data suggest that the true risk may be less than 5%,[9,10] but is still high enough to justify cholecystectomy. Patients with a long

TABLE 60.3 **INDICATIONS/CONTRAINDICATIONS**

INDICATIONS FOR PROPHYLACTIC CHOLECYSTECTOMY

Pediatric gallstones
Congenital hemolytic anemia
Gallstones >2.5 cm in diameter
Calcified (porcelain) gallbladder
Bariatric surgery
Incidental gallstones found during intra-abdominal surgery
Long common channel of bile and pancreatic ducts
No access to medical care

common channel between the bile and pancreatic ducts also are at significant risk for gallbladder cancer and should undergo prophylactic cholecystectomy.

In obese patients in whom gallstones have already developed and who undergo bariatric surgery, cholecystectomy may be indicated because in a large number of these patients symptoms develop that are difficult to distinguish from symptoms caused by complications of their primary operation. Moreover, in 36% of patients who require gastric bypass operations for morbid obesity who did not have gallstones previously, gallstones developed within 6 months of their operation during the period of rapid weight loss.[11] Even more remarkable is that symptoms develop in 40% of these patients and 28% require cholecystectomy during the first year after operation. Prophylactic cholecystectomy adds minimal morbidity and mortality risks to most bariatric operations and is clearly indicated in patients with gallstones. Finally, acute cholecystitis is a potentially life-threatening condition in immunosuppressed patients. For this reason, prophylactic cholecystectomy has been recommended prior to major organ transplantation.

Prophylactic cholecystectomy is not indicated in patients with diabetes and asymptomatic gallstones. Although diabetic patients have an increased risk of surgery with emergent cholecystectomy, recent studies have shown that they also have an increased risk with elective cholecystectomy. This increased risk is related to comorbid conditions, not to the diabetes itself. Furthermore, no evidence suggests that asymptomatic diabetics are at increased risk to develop complications of gallstone disease.

Symptomatic Gallstones

Patients with mild symptoms (intermittent biliary colic) are at higher risk for developing gallstone-related complications or requiring cholecystectomy than asymptomatic patients who have gallstones. Approximately 1% to 3% of mildly symptomatic patients per year will develop gallstone-related complications, and at least 6% to 8% per year will require a cholecystectomy to manage their gallbladder symptoms. The diagnosis of symptomatic gallstones requires the presence of characteristic symptoms and the documentation of gallstones on diagnostic imaging.

The primary symptom associated with chronic cholecystitis or symptomatic cholelithiasis is pain. This pain is often referred to as *biliary colic*, a term that is inaccurate and suggests that the pain related to gallstones is intermittent and spasmodic like other colicky pain. In fact, obstruction of the cystic duct results in a progressive increase in tension in the gallbladder wall, leading to constant pain in the majority of patients. The pain is usually located in the right upper quadrant and/or epigastrium and frequently radiates to the back and right scapula. The intensity of the pain is often severe enough that patients often seek immediate medical attention with the first episode. Classically, the pain of biliary colic occurs following fatty meals, although this situation does not occur in most cases. An association with meals is present in only 50% of patients, and in these patients, the pain often develops more than 1 hour after eating. In the remaining patients, the pain is not temporally related to meals and often begins at nighttime, waking the patient from sleep.

The duration of pain is typically 1 to 5 hours. The attacks rarely persist for more than 24 hours and are rarely shorter than 1 hour. Pain lasting beyond 24 hours suggests that acute inflammation or cholecystitis is present. The attacks are often discrete and severe enough that the patient can accurately recall and number them. The episodes of biliary colic are usually less frequent than one episode per week. Other symptoms such as nausea and vomiting often accompany each episode (60% to 70% of cases). Bloating and belching are also present in 50% of patients. Fever and jaundice occur much less frequently with simple biliary colic.

Atypical pain is common. Sometimes the pain is continuous rather than episodic. The pain may be located predominantly in the back or the left upper or right lower quadrant. Not all attacks are necessarily severe, and some patients do not relate their pain to meals or time of day. The less typical the pain, the more carefully the clinician should search for another cause, even in the presence of stones—causes such as renal colic, peptic ulcer disease, hiatal hernia, abdominal wall hernia, liver tumors, and disease of the small and large intestine. Treatment of atypical biliary colic is appropriate when other causes of pain have been eliminated.

Complicated Gallstones

Acute cholecystitis occurs in approximately 10% to 20% of patients with symptomatic gallstones and results from occlusion of the cystic duct by one or more gallstones. Obstruction of the cystic duct incites an inflammatory response in the gallbladder and can lead to significant complications, including gangrene, empyema, emphysematous cholecystitis, perforation, or cholecystenteric fistula. Historically, choledocholithiasis (CBD stones) was present in 8% to 15% of patients with symptomatic gallstones. However, with the advent of laparoscopic cholecystectomy, the median age for cholecystectomy and the incidence of choledocholithiasis have reduced. The incidence of CBD stones varies with age and is less than 5% in younger patients and more than 20% in older patients with gallstones. CBD stones typically develop in the gallbladder and subsequently enter the CBD via the cystic duct. CBD stones may cause secondary biliary cirrhosis, cholangitis, and pancreatitis.

DIAGNOSTIC IMAGING

Abdominal Plain Films

In general, abdominal plain films have a low yield in diagnosing biliary tract problems. Plain films are most useful in diagnosing other causes of acute abdominal pain such as a perforated viscus or a bowel obstruction. Only approximately 15% of gallstones contain sufficient calcium to appear radiopaque on a plain radiography. Rarely, abdominal films may show a calcified gallbladder wall or pneumobilia that may aid in the diagnosis of biliary disease.

Ultrasound

Transabdominal ultrasound is the radiologic procedure of choice for identifying gallstones and bile duct dilation. Ultrasound is noninvasive, inexpensive, and widely available. Patients should receive nothing by mouth for several hours prior to performing an ultrasound examination so that the gallbladder is fully distended. Gallstones create echoes that are reflected back to the ultrasound probe. The ultrasound waves cannot penetrate the stones; therefore, acoustic shadowing is seen posterior to the stones (Fig. 60.5). In addition, gallstones that are free-floating in the gallbladder will move to a dependent position when the patient is repositioned during scanning. When these two features are present, the accuracy of ultrasound at diagnosing gallstones approaches 100%. Echoes without shadows may be caused by gallbladder polyps.

Several features lower the diagnostic accuracy of ultrasound in detecting gallstones. Small gallstones may not demonstrate an acoustic shadow. Furthermore, a lack of fluid (bile) around the gallstones (stone impacted in cystic duct, gallbladder filled with gallstones) also impairs their detection. In addition, an ileus with increased abdominal gas as occurs with acute cholecystitis may hamper gallbladder visualization. Overall, the false-negative rate for ultrasound in detecting

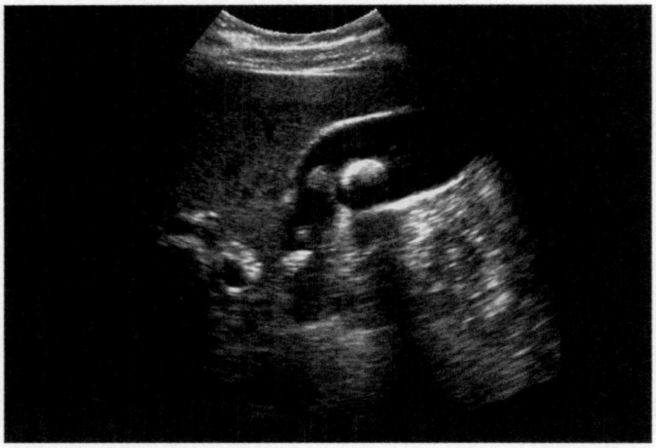

FIGURE 60.5. Abdominal ultrasound of gallbladder with multiple echogenic gallstones.

gallstones is approximately 5% but may increase to 15% with acute cholecystitis.

Ultrasound also can demonstrate dilatation of the intrahepatic or proximal extrahepatic bile ducts with at least an 80% accuracy rate.[12] The normal extrahepatic bile duct diameter is less than 10 mm, and normal intrahepatic duct diameter is less than 4 mm. Dilated ducts may signify the presence of stones in the CBD.

Cholescintigraphy

Cholescintigraphy provides a noninvasive evaluation of the liver, gallbladder, bile duct, and duodenum with both anatomic and functional information. ^{99m}Technetium-labeled iminodiacetic acid derivatives (hepatic 2,6-dimethyl-iminodiacetic acid [HIDA], diisopropyl-acetanilidoiminodiacetic acid, P-isopropylacetanilido-imidodiacetic acid) are injected intravenously, rapidly extracted from the blood, and excreted into the bile. These radionuclide scans provide functional information about the liver's ability to excrete radiolabeled substances into a nonobstructed biliary tree. Uptake by the liver, gallbladder, CBD, and duodenum should all be present after 1 hour. Slow uptake of the tracer by the liver suggests hepatic parenchymal disease. Filling of the gallbladder and CBD with delayed or absent filling of the intestine suggests an obstruction at the ampulla.

The primary use of cholescintigraphy is in the diagnosis of acute cholecystitis. Although used less frequently for this indication because of the availability and accuracy of ultrasound, cholescintigraphy demonstrates the presence of cystic duct obstruction, which is invariably present in acute cholecystitis. Nonvisualization of the gallbladder 1 hour after the injection of the radioisotope with filling of the CBD and duodenum is consistent with total or partial cystic duct obstruction and acute cholecystitis. The sensitivity and specificity of cholescintigraphy for diagnosing acute cholecystitis are each about 95%. False-positive results are increased in the setting of gallbladder stasis as in critically ill patients or in patients on parenteral nutrition.

Computed Tomography/Magnetic Resonance Imaging

Abdominal computed tomography (CT) is less sensitive in diagnosing gallstones than ultrasound. Calcified gallstones are visualized in approximately 50% of patients. The role of CT scanning is primarily limited to the diagnosis of complications of gallstone disease such as acute cholecystitis (gallbladder wall thickening, pericholecystic fluid), choledocholithiasis (intrahepatic and extrahepatic bile duct dilation), pancreatitis (pancreatic edema and inflammation), and gallbladder cancer. Magnetic resonance imaging also has been shown to be highly sensitive in the diagnosis of both gallstones and common duct stones when T2-weighted images are obtained.

TREATMENT

Nonoperative Therapy

The nonsurgical options for the treatment of gallstone disease include oral dissolution therapy with the bile acids, such as ursodeoxycholic acid; contact dissolution therapy with organic solvents (methyl tert-butyl ether); and extracorporeal shock wave biliary lithotripsy. These treatments are rarely used today. Oral dissolution therapy is indicated in symptomatic patients with cholesterol gallstones and a functioning gallbladder. Oral bile acids are only effective in the dissolution of cholesterol gallstones and, therefore, are not indicated if stones are radiopaque or if calcifications can be detected on CT scan. In carefully selected series, complete stone dissolution can be achieved in 40% of patients; however, the recurrence rate is 50% within 5 years if therapy is stopped. Contact dissolution with organic solvents requires cannulation of the gallbladder with direct infusion of the agent into the gallbladder. Again, only cholesterol gallstones are amenable to contact dissolution, and the recurrence rate is similar to that of oral dissolution therapy. Extracorporeal shock wave lithotripsy was originally thought to be a promising nonoperative alternative for the management of symptomatic gallstones. Extracorporeal shock wave lithotripsy is a reasonable therapy for patients with single stones 0.5 to 2 cm in diameter, which have a lower recurrence rate of about 20%. Again, only a small percentage of patients with stones fit these criteria. Moreover, extracorporeal shock wave biliary lithotripsy has never been approved for gallstone dissolution by the U.S. Food and Drug Administration. Finally, the widespread application of laparoscopic cholecystectomy has greatly limited the role of all nonoperative techniques to a very select group of patients.

Operative Therapy

The operative management of gallstones has been the standard of care over the past 140 years. Cholecystectomy is the most common gastrointestinal operation performed in the United States. Since the introduction of laparoscopic cholecystectomy, the number of cholecystectomies performed in the United States has increased from approximately 500,000 per year to 750,000 per year. John Stough Bobb of Indianapolis is credited with performing the first operation on the biliary tract. In 1867, Bobb explored a 32-year-old woman with a large abdominal mass and discovered a massive gallbladder hydrops. A cholecystotomy was made, the gallstones removed, and the gallbladder sutured closed. Fifteen years later, in 1882, Carl Langenbuch of Berlin is credited with performing the first cholecystectomy in a 43-year-old man with a 16-year history of biliary colic. In the late 1980s, German and French surgeons described the first laparoscopic cholecystectomies. Currently, more than 90% of cholecystectomies in the United States are performed laparoscopically.

Laparoscopic Cholecystectomy. Symptomatic cholelithiasis is the main indication for laparoscopic cholecystectomy. As experience with advanced laparoscopy has increased, however, many surgeons will attempt a laparoscopic cholecystectomy in situations of complicated gallstone disease. Contraindications to laparoscopic cholecystectomy include the inability of the patient to withstand a general anesthetic, severe bleeding disorders, and end-stage liver disease. In addition, patients with severe chronic obstructive pulmonary disease or congestive heart failure may not tolerate the pneumoperitoneum required for performing laparoscopic surgery. The technical difficulty of laparoscopic cholecystectomy is increased in several clinical settings. Laparoscopic cholecystectomy can be performed safely in acute cholecystitis albeit with a higher conversion rate and operative time than in the elective setting. Morbid obesity, once thought to be a relative contraindication to the laparoscopic approach, is not associated with a higher conversion rate. Longer trocars and instruments and an increase in intra-abdominal pressure may be helpful in these patients. Prior upper abdominal surgery may increase the difficulty of or preclude laparoscopic cholecystectomy. Elective laparoscopic cholecystectomy also has been completed safely in patients with well-compensated cirrhosis (Child's class A and B), although difficulty retracting the firm liver and increased bleeding from collaterals have been noted.

Patients undergoing laparoscopic cholecystectomy are prepared and draped in a similar fashion to open cholecystectomy. Conversion to an open operation is necessary in up to 3% of patients undergoing elective cholecystectomy and up to 25% of patients undergoing laparoscopic cholecystectomy for acute cholecystitis. A Foley catheter and orogastric tube are inserted to avoid inadvertent injury and improve exposure. Either an open or closed technique can be used to establish a pneumoperitoneum. With the open technique, a small incision is made at the umbilicus, and a blunt cannula (Hasson cannula) is inserted into the peritoneal cavity and anchored to the fascia. In the closed technique a Veress needle is inserted into the peritoneal cavity through a supraumbilical incision and used for insufflation. An 11-mm trocar is inserted through the supraumbilical incision once a pneumoperitoneum is established. A 30-degree laparoscope is then inserted through the umbilical port, and an examination of the peritoneal cavity is performed. An 11-mm operating port is placed subxiphoid, and two additional 5-mm trocars are positioned subcostally in the right upper quadrant in the midclavicular and anterior axillary lines. Single port cholecystectomy is currently under development and may become the procedure of choice in the future.

The two 5-mm ports are used for grasping the gallbladder and exposing the gallbladder and cystic duct (Fig. 60.6). The

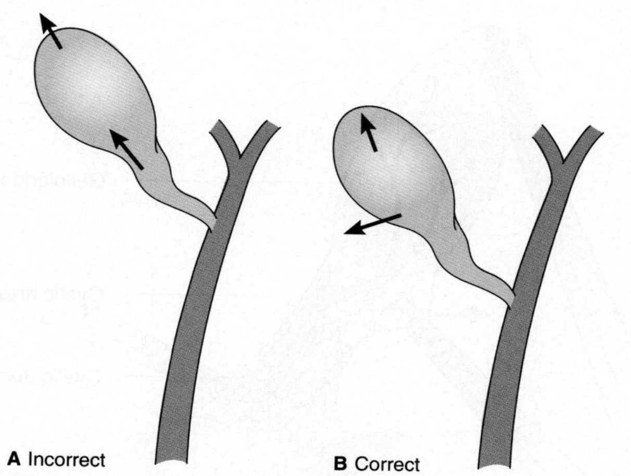

FIGURE 60.7. Incorrect (A) and correct (B) methods of retracting the gallbladder. Incorrect retraction brings the cystic and common ducts into alignment and makes them appear as one.

medial 5-mm cannula is used to grasp the gallbladder infundibulum and retract it laterally to further expose the triangle of Calot. Traction on the fundus should be upward toward the patient's head, and traction on the Hartmann pouch laterally to the right. This combination "disaligns" the common duct and cystic duct so that they appear as distinct structures. Incorrect traction aligns the ducts so that they appear as a continuous structure and as a consequence the chance of biliary injury is increased (Fig. 60.7). The junction of the gallbladder and cystic duct is identified by stripping the peritoneum off the gallbladder neck and removing any tissue surrounding the gallbladder neck and proximal cystic duct. This dissection is continued until the triangle of Calot is cleared of all fatty and lymphatic tissue and the gallbladder infundibulum is elevated off of the liver bed (Fig. 60.8). Visualization of this "critical view" is important in preventing injury to the bile ducts. At this point two structures (cystic artery and cystic duct) should be seen entering the gallbladder. Performance of a cholangiogram may be a factor in avoiding

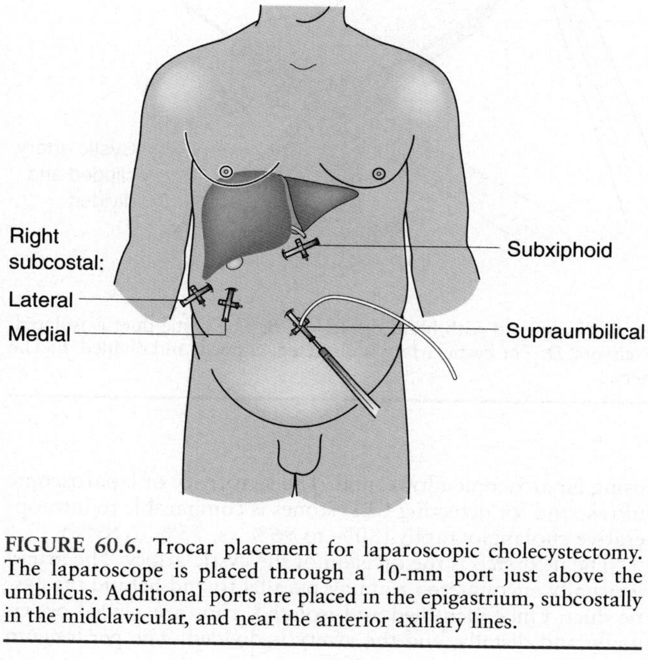

FIGURE 60.6. Trocar placement for laparoscopic cholecystectomy. The laparoscope is placed through a 10-mm port just above the umbilicus. Additional ports are placed in the epigastrium, subcostally in the midclavicular, and near the anterior axillary lines.

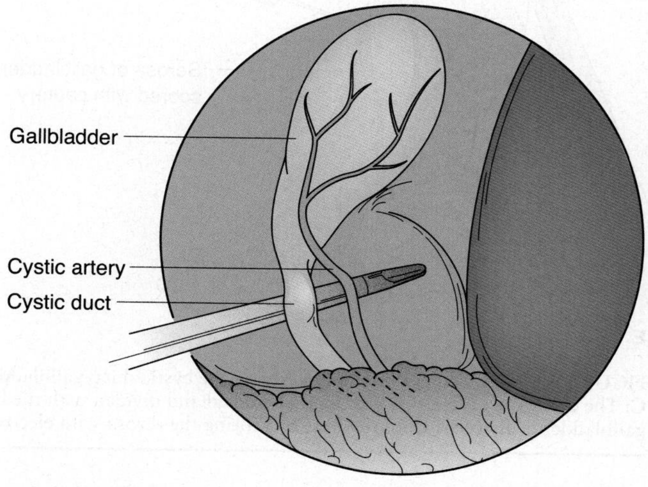

FIGURE 60.8. The "critical view" of safety. The triangle of Calot is dissected free of all tissue except for the cystic duct and artery, and the base of the liver bed is exposed. When this view is achieved, the two structures entering the gallbladder can only be the cystic duct and artery. Visualization of the common bile duct is not necessary. (After Strasberg SM, Hertl M, Soper NJ. An analysis of the problem of biliary injury during laparoscopic cholecystectomy. *J Am Coll Surg* 1995;180:101.)

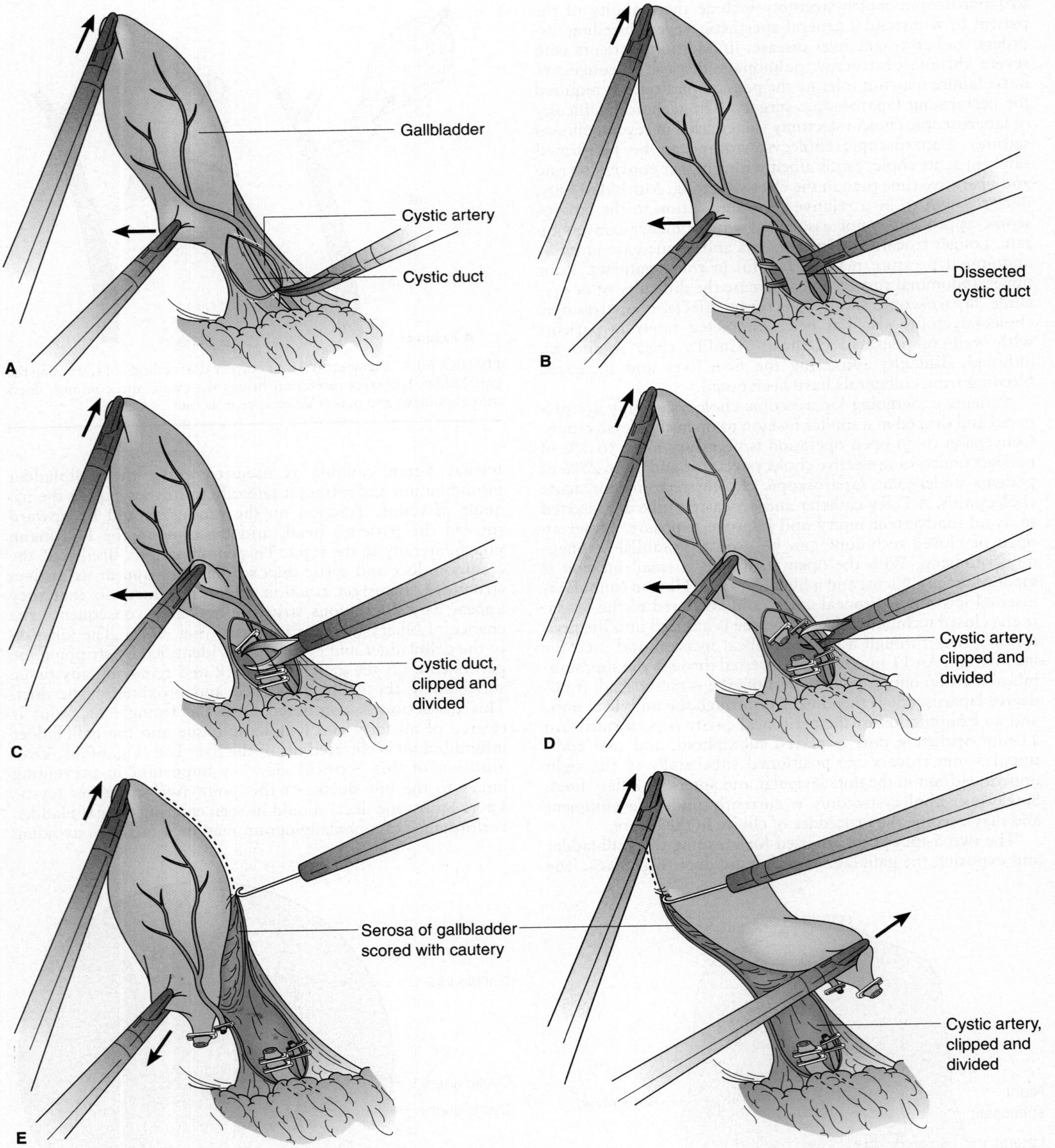

FIGURE 60.9. **A:** The peritoneum overlying the cystic duct–gallbladder junction is opened with blunt dissection. **B:** The cystic duct is isolated. **C:** The cystic duct is clipped proximal and distal and divided with the hook scissors. **D:** The cystic artery is dissected, clipped, and divided. **E:** The gallbladder is dissected from the liver by scoring the serosa with electrocautery.

biliary injury.[13] Once the cystic duct is identified, an intraoperative cholangiogram may be performed by placing a ligating clip proximally on the cystic duct, incising the anterior surface of the duct, and passing a cholangiogram catheter into the cystic duct. Once the cholangiogram is completed, two clips are placed distally on the cystic duct, which is then divided (Fig. 60.9). Alternatively, the CBD may be evaluated for stones using laparoscopic ultrasound. The sensitivity of laparoscopic ultrasound for detecting CBD stones is comparable to intraoperative cholangiography (80% to 96% vs. 75% to 99%).

The next step is the division of the cystic artery. The artery is usually encountered running parallel to and behind the cystic duct. Once identified and isolated, clips are placed proximally and distally, and the artery is divided. The peritoneum overlying the gallbladder is placed on tension using the two grasping forceps, the peritoneum and adventitia between the gallbladder and liver are divided with the cautery, and the gallbladder is dissected out of the gallbladder fossa (Fig. 60.9). Prior to removing the gallbladder from the liver, the operative field is carefully searched for hemostasis and adequate placement of the cystic duct and artery clips is confirmed. The gallbladder is then dissected off the liver and is usually removed through the umbilical port. The fascial defect and skin incision may need to be enlarged to remove the gallbladder and contained gallstones. If the gallbladder has been entered during the dissection or if it is acutely inflamed or gangrenous, the gallbladder should be placed in a plastic specimen retrieval bag prior to removing it from the peritoneal cavity.[14,15]

Elective laparoscopic cholecystectomy can be safely performed as an outpatient procedure.[16] Among patients selected for outpatient management, 77% to 97% of patients can be successfully discharged the same day. Factors contributing to overnight admission include uncontrolled pain, nausea and vomiting, operative duration greater than 60 minutes, and cases completed late in the day.

Routine operative cholangiography has been advocated to avoid ductal injury. However, opinion on the subject is sharply divided. Biliary injuries occur less frequently in the hands of surgeons who perform operative cholangiography routinely. However, in about 50% of ductal injuries, a cholangiogram fails to prevent the injury although abnormal anatomy is present (i.e., cholangiograms are often incorrectly interpreted). The indications for intraoperative cholangiography, when it is performed selectively, are known choledocholithiasis, a history of jaundice, a history of pancreatitis, a large cystic duct and small gallstones, any abnormality in preoperative liver function tests, and dilated biliary ducts on preoperative sonography. Provided these indications are carefully followed, selective cholangiography may be as effective in detecting clinically relevant stones as routine cholangiography.

Serious complications of laparoscopic cholecystectomy are rare, the mortality rate being less than 0.3%. As cholecystectomy rates have risen, however, the total number of deaths has not decreased.[17] The single greatest problem in laparoscopic cholecystectomy is biliary injury. The incidence of major bile duct injury following laparoscopic cholecystectomy is between 0.3% and 0.6%; but if all bile leaks are considered, the injury rate in these reports ranges from 0.6% to 1.5%, which is three to four times the injury rate at open surgery.[18] Major vascular injuries to the hepatic arteries, especially the right hepatic artery, may occur in association with biliary injuries and sometimes lead to intraoperative blood loss. Isolated vascular injuries to hepatic vessels are rare. Although the increase in cholecystectomy rates means that the total number of deaths from cholecystectomy has not decreased, an individual patient's risk for death is smaller.

Spillage of stones into the peritoneal cavity during laparoscopic cholecystectomy occurs in 10% or more of cases. Leaving stones in the peritoneal cavity may not be innocuous.[19] Intra-abdominal abscess, subcutaneous abscess, and later discharge of stones through the abdominal wall or through the lung and trachea have all been described. Every attempt should be made to remove spilled stones by picking and irrigating them out. Clearance is usually quite successful with the use of retractors to lift the liver and the 30-degree laparoscope, which allows the depths of the recess between liver and kidney to be visualized. Laparoscopic ultrasonography may be useful to detect stones. Large stones or massive spills should be cleaned up by laparotomy if necessary. If concern exists that stones have been left behind, the patient should be informed.

As in open cholecystectomy, a gallbladder containing an unsuspected cancer is excised 1 to 3 times per 1,000 laparoscopic cholecystectomies. Therefore, a good practice is to open the gallbladder and inspect it and obtain frozen sections if a suspect lesion is observed. If cancer is suspected, the gallbladder should be extracted in an impermeable bag. If a cancer is discovered, further surgery may be indicated.

Open Cholecystectomy. Open cholecystectomy can be performed through either an upper midline or right subcostal (Kocher) incision. Identification and division of the cystic duct and artery initially limit bleeding from the gallbladder for the remainder of the dissection. With lateral traction on the gallbladder neck, the peritoneum overlying the triangle of Calot is incised, and the cystic duct is identified and ligated distally. A cholangiogram is performed at this time if indicated. The cystic duct is then ligated proximally and divided. Similarly, the cystic artery is ligated and divided after carefully tracing it onto the gallbladder. If the anatomy cannot be clearly identified, the gallbladder should be dissected from the fundus downward toward the gallbladder neck, making the ductal and vascular anatomy easier to identify. The gallbladder is dissected out of the gallbladder bed by incising the overlying peritoneum with cautery.

CLINICAL MANIFESTATIONS

Chronic Calculous Cholecystitis

Pathogenesis. The term *chronic cholecystitis* implies an ongoing or recurrent inflammatory process involving the gallbladder. In most patients (more than 90%), gallstones are the causative factor and lead to recurrent episodes of cystic duct obstruction manifest as biliary pain or colic. Over time, these recurrent attacks can lead to scarring and a nonfunctioning gallbladder. Histopathologically, chronic cholecystitis is characterized by an increase in subepithelial and subserosal fibrosis and a mononuclear cell infiltrate.

Clinical Presentation. The primary symptom associated with chronic cholecystitis or symptomatic cholelithiasis is pain, often labeled *biliary colic*. The pain is usually located in the right upper quadrant and/or epigastrium and frequently radiates to the right upper back, to the right scapula, or between the scapulae (as noted in the previous discussion of symptomatic gallstones). Other symptoms such as nausea and vomiting often accompany each episode (60% to 70% of cases). The physical examination is usually completely normal in patients with chronic cholecystitis, particularly if they are pain-free. During an episode of biliary colic, mild right upper quadrant tenderness may be present. Laboratory values such as serum bilirubin, transaminases, and alkaline phosphatase usually are normal in patients with uncomplicated gallstones.

Diagnosis. The diagnosis of chronic calculous cholecystitis requires two findings: abdominal pain consistent with biliary colic and the presence of gallstones. The presence of symptoms (usually pain) attributable to the gallbladder is necessary to consider any treatment for gallstones. Patients without symptoms (approximately two thirds of patients with gallstones) develop symptoms at a low rate and complications of gallstones at an even lower rate (as noted in the previous discussion of natural history). In most cases treatment is not necessary in these asymptomatic patients. Ultrasound is sensitive (95% to 98%) for documenting the presence of gallstones and also provides additional anatomic information, including the presence of polyps, the diameter of the CBD, and any hepatic parenchymal abnormalities. Gallstones are occasionally identified on abdominal radiographs (15%) or CT scans (50%) because gallstones contain enough calcium to be visualized.

5 **Management.** The treatment of choice for patients with symptomatic gallstones is elective laparoscopic cholecystectomy. The mortality of laparoscopic cholecystectomy is less than 0.3%, with cardiovascular complications being the most

frequent cause of death. The most significant complication following laparoscopic cholecystectomy is injury to the biliary tract. Overall, complications occur in fewer than 10% of patients. Conversion to an open cholecystectomy is necessary in less than 3% of patients undergoing laparoscopic cholecystectomy for chronic cholecystitis. Conversion rates are increased in elderly, obese, and male patients.

The long-term results of laparoscopic cholecystectomy in appropriately selected patients with chronic cholecystitis are excellent. More than 90% of patients with typical biliary pain and gallstones are symptom-free following cholecystectomy. For patients with atypical symptoms or painless dyspepsia (fatty food intolerance, flatulence, belching, or bloating), the percentage of patients experiencing relief of symptoms decreases.

Acute Calculous Cholecystitis

Pathophysiology. Acute cholecystitis is the most common complication of gallstones, occurring in 15% to 20% of patients with symptomatic disease. As in biliary colic, acute cholecystitis results from a stone impaction at the gallbladder–cystic duct junction (Fig. 60.10). The extent of inflammation and the progression of acute cholecystitis are related to the duration and degree of obstruction. In the most severe cases (5% to 18%), this process can lead to ischemia and necrosis of the gallbladder wall. More frequently, the gallstone is dislodged, and the inflammation gradually resolves. Acute cholecystitis is primarily an inflammation and not an infectious process, with bacterial infection appearing as a secondary event. Approximately 50% of patients with acute cholecystitis will have positive bile cultures, with *Escherichia coli* being the most common organism.

Clinical Presentation. Patients with acute cholecystitis typically present with right upper quadrant pain that is similar to that of biliary colic. In acute cholecystitis, however, the pain is usually unremitting, may last several days, and is often associated with nausea, emesis, anorexia, and fever. On physical examination, patients with acute cholecystitis usually have a low-grade fever and exhibit localized right upper quadrant tenderness and guarding, which distinguish the episode from simple biliary colic. The presence of Murphy's sign, an inspiratory arrest during deep palpation of the right upper quadrant, is the classic physical finding of acute cholecystitis. A palpable right upper quadrant mass is appreciated in one third of patients and usually represents omentum that has migrated to the area around the gallbladder in response to the inflammation. Severe jaundice is rare, but mild jaundice may be present—up to 6 mg/dL. Severe jaundice suggests the presence of CBD stones, cholangitis, or obstruction of the common hepatic duct by severe pericholecystic inflammation resulting from impaction of a large stone in the Hartmann pouch, which mechanically obstructs the bile duct (Mirizzi syndrome). Acute cholecystitis may coexist with choledocholithiasis or its complications (acute cholangitis and gallstone pancreatitis). The coexistence of two of these conditions often explains an unusual or atypical clinical presentation.

Laboratory evaluation can show a mild leukocytosis (white blood cell count [WBC] 12,000 to 15,000 cells/mm^3). However, many patients have a normal WBC count. A white cell count greater than 20,000 should suggest further complications of cholecystitis, such as gangrene, perforation, or cholangitis. Mild elevations in serum bilirubin (<4 mg/dL), alkaline phosphatase, the transaminases, and amylase may also be seen with acute cholecystitis.

Diagnosis. Ultrasound is the most useful radiologic examination in the patient with suspected cholecystitis. First, in the patient without known gallstones, ultrasound is a sensitive test for establishing the presence or absence of gallstones. Additional findings suggestive of acute cholecystitis include thickening of the gallbladder wall (>4 mm) and pericholecystic fluid. Focal tenderness directly over the gallbladder (sonographic Murphy's sign) also is suggestive of acute cholecystitis. Ultrasound has a sensitivity and specificity of 85% and 95%, respectively, for diagnosing acute cholecystitis.

Radionuclide scanning is used less frequently for the diagnosis of acute cholecystitis but may provide additional information in the atypical case. Nonfilling of the gallbladder with the radiotracer ^{99}Tc-HIDA indicates an obstructed cystic duct, and in the right clinical setting is highly sensitive (95%) and specific (95%) for acute cholecystitis. Computed tomography (Fig. 60.11) occasionally is performed in evaluating the patient with abdominal pain and acute illness. CT may demonstrate evidence of acute cholecystitis, including gallbladder wall thickening, pericholecystic fluid and edema, gallstones, and air in the gallbladder or gallbladder wall (emphysematous cholecystitis), although it is less sensitive for these conditions than ultrasonography.

Management. Once the diagnosis of acute cholecystitis is made, the patient should be given nothing by mouth, and

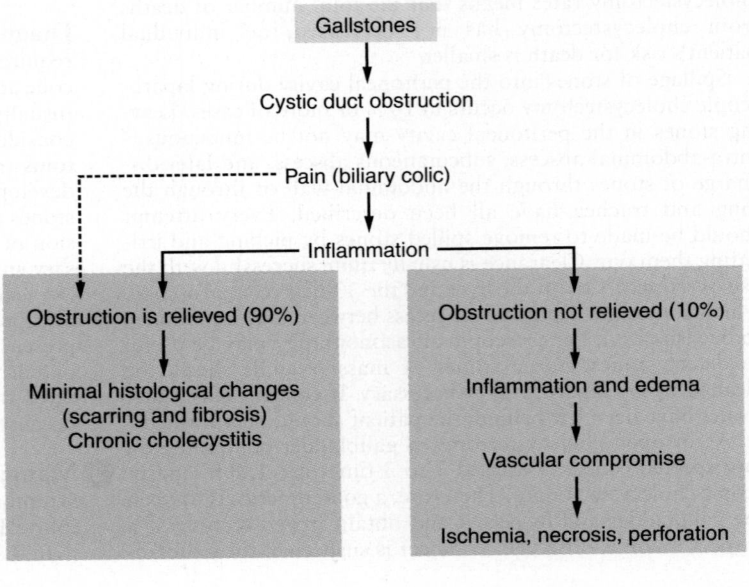

FIGURE 60.10. Pathophysiology of acute cholecystitis.

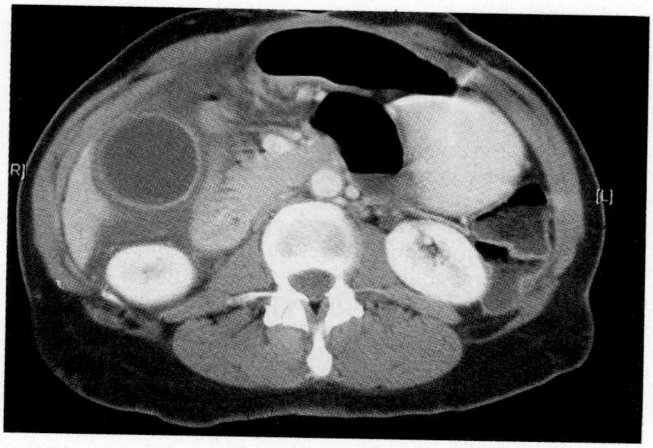

FIGURE 60.11. Computed tomography of a patient with acute cholecystitis showing gallbladder wall thickening and pericholecystic fluid.

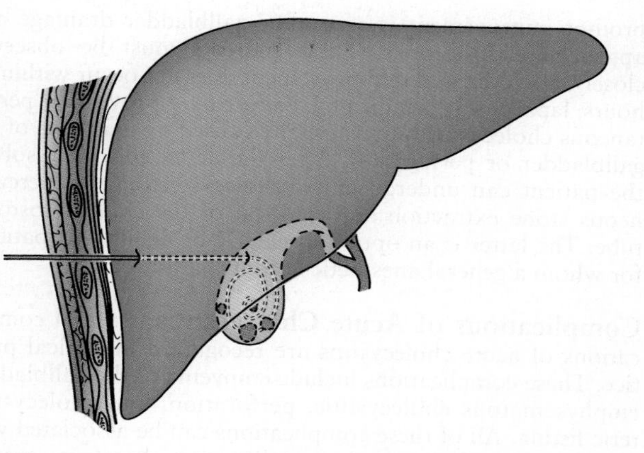

FIGURE 60.12. Schematic demonstration of the technique of percutaneous placement of a pigtail catheter into the gallbladder.

intravenous hydration should begin. A nasogastric tube is placed if persistent nausea and vomiting or abdominal distention are present. In almost all cases, broad-spectrum antibiotics, such as a broad-spectrum penicillin, should be started and maintained into the immediate postoperative period. Parenteral analgesia also should be administered. Unfortunately, narcotics increase biliary pressure, whereas nonsteroidal analgesics, which inhibit prostaglandin synthesis, reduce gallbladder mucin production and, therefore, reduce pressure and pain.

The treatment of choice for acute cholecystitis is cholecystectomy. Open cholecystectomy had been the standard treatment for acute cholecystitis for many years. Initially, acute cholecystitis was felt to be a contraindication to laparoscopic cholecystectomy. As experience has increased, however, laparoscopic cholecystectomy clearly can be performed
6 safely in the setting of acute cholecystitis. In prospective randomized trials, the morbidity rate, length of hospital stay, and time to return to work all have been lower in patients undergoing laparoscopic cholecystectomy than open cholecystectomy.[20] However, the conversion rate in the setting of acute cholecystitis (10% to 25%) is higher than with chronic cholecystitis.

The timing of cholecystectomy for acute cholecystitis has been studied for several decades. In the distant past, delayed cholecystectomy was preferred in the setting of acute cholecystitis. Patients were initially managed nonoperatively and discharged home after their symptoms resolved. Elective cholecystectomy was then performed 6 weeks later after the acute inflammation had resolved. Several prospective randomized trials have shown that early laparoscopic cholecystectomy (within 3 days of symptom onset) can be accomplished with a similar morbidity and mortality rate as delayed cholecystectomy. Representative results are documented in Table 60.4.[21,22] No significant differences were observed in the conversion rate to open cholecystectomy among patients undergoing early cholecystectomy versus those managed with delayed surgery. Hospital stay, and therefore cost, however, were significantly reduced in the trials in the early laparoscopic cholecystectomy group. In addition, approximately 20% of patients in the delayed surgery arms failed initial medical therapy and required operation during the initial admission or before the end of the planned cooling-off period.

Laparoscopic cholecystectomy should be performed within 24 to 72 hours of diagnosis. Early conversion to an open procedure should be considered if dissection is difficult or clear progress cannot be made by the laparoscopic technique. In certain high-risk patients whose medical conditions preclude cholecystectomy, a cholecystostomy can be performed for acute cholecystitis. Although previously performed operatively and under local anesthesia, percutaneous drainage techniques can usually be accomplished (Fig. 60.12). In most cases,

PANCREAS/LIVER

TABLE 60.4 **RESULTS**

RANDOMIZED PROSPECTIVE TRIALS OF EARLY VERSUS DELAYED LAPAROSCOPIC CHOLECYSTECTOMY FOR ACUTE CHOLECYSTITIS

	QUEEN MARY HOSPITAL[20]		PRINCE OF WALES HOSPITAL[21]	
	EARLY	LATE	EARLY	LATE
Number of patients	45	41	53	46
Operative time	135 min	105 min	123 min	106 min
Conversion	11%	23%	21%	24%
Morbidity	13%	29%	21%	24%
Total LOS	6 d	11 d	7.6 d	11.6 d
Recurrent symptoms	—	36%	—	17%

LOS, length of stay.

prompt improvement is seen after gallbladder drainage and appropriate antibiotics. These patients must be observed closely, however, and if improvement does not occur within 24 hours, laparotomy is indicated. Failure to improve after percutaneous cholecystostomy is usually caused by gangrene of the gallbladder or perforation. After the acute episode resolves, the patient can undergo either cholecystectomy or percutaneous stone extraction and removal of the cholecystostomy tube. The latter is an option in elderly or debilitated patients for whom a general anesthetic is contraindicated.[23]

Complications of Acute Cholecystitis. Several complications of acute cholecystitis are recognized in clinical practice. These complications include empyema of the gallbladder, emphysematous cholecystitis, perforation, and cholecystenteric fistula. All of these complications can be associated with significant morbidity and mortality and, therefore, require prompt surgical intervention.

Empyema. Gallbladder empyema represents an advanced stage of cholecystitis with bacterial invasion of the gallbladder and actual pus in the lumen. Patients present with severe right upper quadrant pain, high-grade fever, rigors, and significant leukocytosis. Sepsis including cardiovascular collapse may be seen. Treatment consists of broad-spectrum antibiotics, including anaerobic coverage, and emergent cholecystectomy or cholecystostomy; however, cholecystostomy may not be adequate to relieve sepsis in patients with empyema of the gallbladder.

Emphysematous Cholecystitis. Emphysematous cholecystitis develops more commonly in males and patients with diabetes mellitus. Severe right upper quadrant pain and generalized sepsis are frequently present. Abdominal films or CT scans may demonstrate air within the gallbladder wall or lumen. Prompt antibiotic therapy to cover the common biliary pathogens including *E. coli*, *Enterococcus*, *Klebsiella*, and *Clostridia* species and emergency cholecystectomy are appropriate treatments.

Gangrene/Perforation. Gangrene of the gallbladder occurs when the wall becomes ischemic and leads to perforation. Gallbladder perforation can be categorized as being either localized or free. The incidence of perforation in acute cholecystitis is approximately 10%. Localized perforation generally results in the formation of a pericholecystic abscess as the omentum walls off the perforation and limits it to the right upper quadrant. Free perforation is less frequent (1% of cases) and occurs if the omentum is unable to wall off the inflammatory process. Free perforation results in the spilling of bile into the peritoneal cavity and a generalized peritonitis. Perforation should be suspected if the patient's clinical course deteriorates. Evidence for perforation includes an increase in pain and tenderness, fever and chills, elevation in white blood cell count, and hypotension. These patients require aggressive fluid resuscitation, antibiotics, and emergent operative exploration. Cholecystostomy usually will not be adequate therapy for patients with gangrene or perforation of the gallbladder.

Cholecystenteric Fistula. In 1% to 2% of patients with acute cholecystitis, the gallbladder will perforate into an adjacent hollow viscus. The duodenum (79%) and the hepatic flexure of the colon (17%) are the most common sites. Generally, after the fistula forms, the episode of acute cholecystitis resolves as the gallbladder spontaneously decompresses. If a large gallstone passes from the gallbladder into the small intestine, a mechanical bowel obstruction may result, which is termed *gallstone ileus*. Gallstone ileus occurs in 10% to 15% of patients with a cholecystenteric fistula. Patients with gallstone ileus present with signs and symptoms of intestinal obstruction—nausea, vomiting, and abdominal pain. The pain may be episodic and recurrent as the impacted stone temporarily impacts in the gut lumen and then dislodges and moves distally (tumbling obstruction). A history of gallstone-related symptoms (right upper quadrant pain) may only be present in 50% of these patients. Abdominal films will demonstrate small-bowel distention and air-fluid levels and may give additional clues to the source of the obstruction (pneumobilia or a calcified gallstone distant from the gallbladder). The site of obstruction is most frequently in the narrowest part of the small intestine (ileum) or large intestine (sigmoid colon).

The initial management of gallstone ileus includes relieving the obstruction. Most frequently, this goal can be achieved by removing the gallstone through an enterotomy (Fig. 60.13). Additional gallstones should be sought as recurrent obstruction

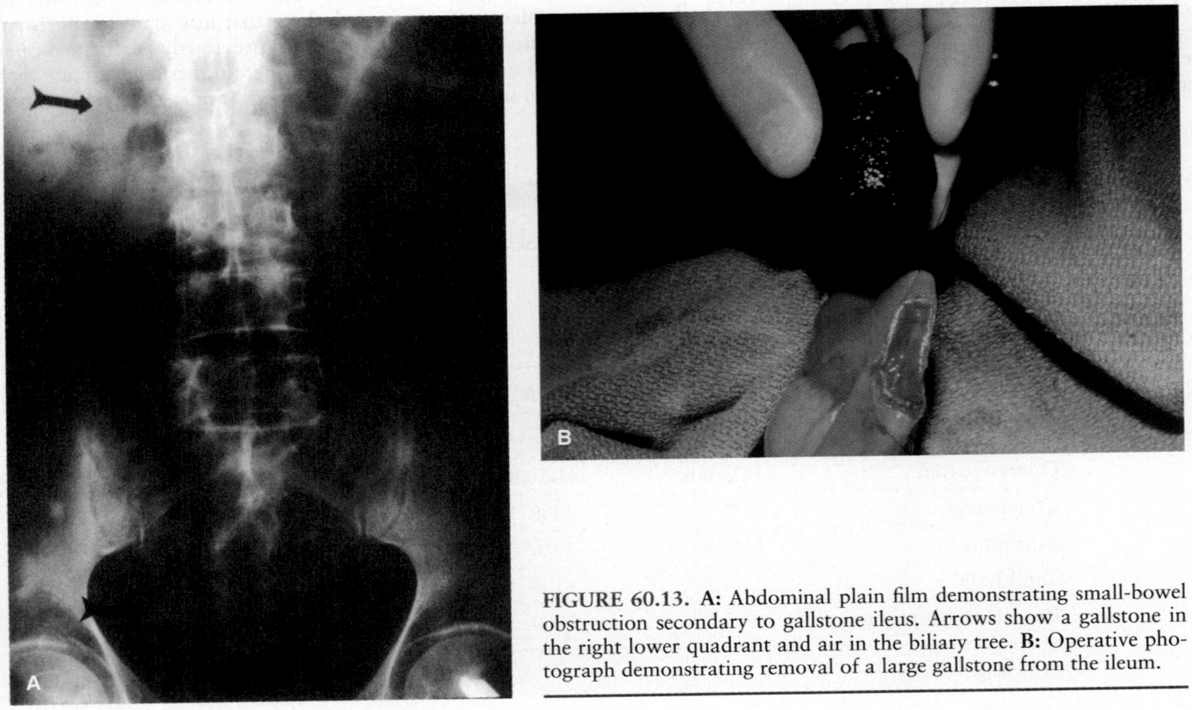

FIGURE 60.13. **A:** Abdominal plain film demonstrating small-bowel obstruction secondary to gallstone ileus. Arrows show a gallstone in the right lower quadrant and air in the biliary tree. **B:** Operative photograph demonstrating removal of a large gallstone from the ileum.

has been reported in up to 10% of patients with gallstone ileus. Takedown of the biliary-enteric fistula and cholecystectomy may be warranted as recurrent cholecystitis and cholangitis are common in patients with a biliary-enteric fistula, and gallbladder cancer has been reported in 15% of these patients. However, in patients with a significant inflammatory process in the right upper quadrant or who are too unstable to withstand a prolonged operative procedure, the fistula can be addressed at a second laparotomy.

Acute Acalculous Cholecystitis

Acute acalculous cholecystitis accounts for 5% to 10% of all patients with acute cholecystitis. The disease often has a more fulminant course than acute calculous cholecystitis and frequently progresses to gangrene, empyema, or perforation. Acute acalculous cholecystitis usually occurs in the critically ill patient following trauma, burns, long-term parenteral nutrition, and major nonbiliary operations such as abdominal aneurysm repair and cardiopulmonary bypass. The etiology of acute acalculous cholecystitis remains unclear, although gallbladder stasis and ischemia have been most often implicated as causative factors. Stasis is common in critically ill patients not being fed enterally and may lead to colonization of the gallbladder with bacteria. Visceral ischemia also is a common denominator in patients with acute acalculous cholecystitis and may explain the high incidence of gallbladder gangrene. Decreased arteriolar and capillary filling is present in acute acalculous cholecystitis in contrast to the dilation of these vessels observed in acute calculous cholecystitis.

The symptoms and signs of acute acalculous cholecystitis are similar to acute calculous cholecystitis with right upper quadrant pain and tenderness, fever, and leukocytosis most frequently present. CT scan and ultrasound findings are similar to calculous cholecystitis and include gallbladder wall thickening and pericholecystic fluid in the absence of gallstones. Cholescintigraphy demonstrates absent gallbladder filling in acute acalculous cholecystitis; however, the false-positive rate (absent gallbladder filling without acute acalculous cholecystitis) may be as high as 40%.

Emergency cholecystectomy is the appropriate treatment once the diagnosis is established or the suspicion is high. The incidence of gangrene, perforation, and empyema exceeds 50%; therefore, cholecystectomy rather than cholecystostomy is usually required in this setting. The mortality rate for acute acalculous cholecystitis remains high (40%) in large part because of the concomitant illnesses in patients who develop this disease.

Chronic Acalculous Cholecystitis

7 A subgroup of patients presenting with typical symptoms of biliary colic (postprandial right upper quadrant pain, fatty food intolerance, and nausea) do not have any evidence of gallstones on ultrasound examination. Further investigations have usually been performed in these patients to exclude any other pathology. This workup often includes an abdominal CT scan, esophagogastroduodenoscopy, or even an endoscopic retrograde cholangiogram. In these patients, the diagnosis of biliary dyskinesia or chronic acalculous cholecystitis should be considered. The cholecystokinin–Tc-HIDA scan has been useful in identifying patients with this disorder. Cholecystokinin (CCK) is infused intravenously after the gallbladder has filled with the ^{99}Tc-labeled radionuclide. Twenty minutes after the administration of CCK, a gallbladder ejection fraction is calculated. An ejection fraction less than 35% at 20 minutes is considered abnormal.

Patients with symptoms of biliary colic and an abnormal gallbladder ejection fraction should be managed with a laparoscopic cholecystectomy. Between 85% and 94% of patients with a low gallbladder ejection fraction and symptoms of biliary colic will be asymptomatic or improved by cholecystectomy. Most of these patients have histopathologic evidence of chronic cholecystitis. Over the past 15 years, the percentage of patients undergoing cholecystectomy for acalculous cholecystitis in the United States has increased from less than 5% to more than 20% of patients having their gallbladder removed. This change parallels the obesity epidemic and may be due to abnormal gallbladder emptying as well as absorption/secretion due to fat within the gallbladder wall (cholecystosteatosis).[24]

Sphincter of Oddi Dysfunction

Sphincter of Oddi dysfunction may be caused by either a structural or functional abnormality involving the sphincter. Fibrosis of the sphincter from gallstone migration, operative or endoscopic trauma, pancreatitis, or other nonspecific inflammatory processes can lead to elevated sphincter pressures. Elevated sphincter pressures also may present in the absence of a structural abnormality, and these cases of sphincter of Oddi dyskinesia or spasm are often associated with more diffuse abnormalities of gastrointestinal motility.[25]

Sphincter of Oddi dysfunction should be suspected in patients with typical episodic biliary-type pain without an obvious organic cause. Approximately 1% of patients undergoing cholecystectomy are estimated to have sphincter of Oddi dysfunction. Numerous diagnostic tests have been used to diagnose sphincter of Oddi dysfunction, but none are sensitive or specific. Elevated serum amylase or transaminases may be present in patients with sphincter of Oddi dysfunction. Ultrasound evidence of sphincter of Oddi dysfunction includes a dilated (>12 mm) CBD, an increase in CBD diameter in response to cholecystokinin, or an increase in pancreatic duct diameter in response to secretin. Delayed emptying of contrast from the CBD after endoscopic retrograde cholangiopancreatography (ERCP) also is indicative of abnormal sphincter function. Endoscopic manometry also has been used to evaluate the sphincter of Oddi, and an elevated basal sphincter pressure (>40 mm Hg) has been correlated with successful response to sphincter ablation.

Both endoscopic sphincterotomy and transduodenal sphincteroplasty with transampullary septotomy have been used to manage patients with sphincter of Oddi dysfunction. Results of both treatments are similar and are more dependent on the presence of objective signs of sphincter dysfunction than on the procedure performed. The endoscopic approach avoids a laparotomy and can be performed safely in expert hands if a temporary pancreatic stent is employed to reduce the risk of pancreatitis when a pancreatic duct sphincterotomy is performed. The surgical approach (transduodenal sphincteroplasty with transampullary septotomy) has the potential advantage that mucosa-to-mucosa apposition can be achieved, minimizing the risk of scarring and restenosis. When objective evidence of sphincter dysfunction is present (elevated transaminases, delayed biliary emptying, dilated CBD, elevated basal sphincter pressure), 60% to 80% of patients will be pain-free or improved following sphincterotomy or sphincteroplasty.[25]

Acute Cholangitis

Acute cholangitis is a bacterial infection of the biliary ductal system, which varies in severity from mild and self-limited to severe and life threatening. The clinical triad of fever, jaundice, and pain associated with cholangitis was first described in 1877 by Charcot. He postulated that stagnant bile associated with obstructive biliary pathology was a significant factor in the pathogenesis of this disease.

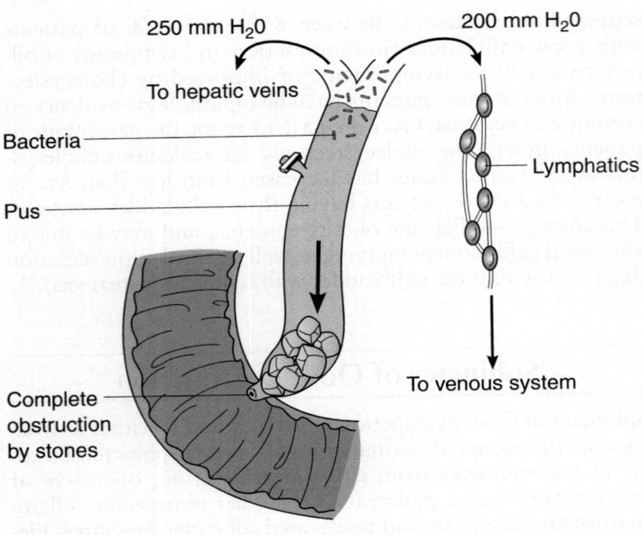

FIGURE 60.14. Cholangitis is caused by the combination of biliary obstruction and bactibilia. Bacteria then reflux into the hepatic veins and perihepatic lymphatics, resulting in systemic bacteremia.

8 **Pathophysiology.** Clinical cholangitis results from a combination of two factors: significant bacterial concentrations in the bile and biliary obstruction. Although cultures of the gallbladder and bile ducts are usually sterile, in the presence of CBD stones or other obstructing pathology the incidence of positive bile duct cultures increases. The most common organisms recovered from the bile in patients with cholangitis include *E. coli, Klebsiella pneumonia*, the enterococci, and *Bacteroides fragilis*.[26] Nevertheless, even in the presence of high biliary bacterial concentrations, clinical cholangitis and bacteremia do not develop unless obstruction causes elevated intraductal pressures.

Normal biliary pressures range from 7 to 14 cm H_2O. In the presence of bactibilia and normal biliary pressures, hepatic vein blood and perihepatic lymph are sterile. In cases of partial or complete biliary obstruction, however, intrabiliary pressures rise to 18 to 29 cm H_2O, and organisms rapidly appear in both the blood and lymph. The fever and chills associated with cholangitis are the result of systemic bacteremia caused by cholangiovenous and cholangiolymphatic reflux (Fig. 60.14).

Etiology. The most common causes of biliary obstruction are choledocholithiasis, benign strictures, biliary enteric anastomotic strictures, and cholangiocarcinoma or periampullary cancer. Prior to 1980, choledocholithiasis was the cause of approximately 80% of the reported cases of cholangitis. In recent years, malignant strictures have become a frequent cause of cholangitis, particularly at tertiary referral centers. Endoscopic cholangiography, percutaneous transhepatic cholangiography, and stent placement via either the endoscopic or percutaneous route are all known to cause bacteremia. These procedures are frequently performed in patients with unresectable malignant obstruction.

Clinical Presentation. Cholangitis may present with a wide spectrum of disease. Patients may have a self-limited illness and never seek attention. At the other end of the spectrum, patients with toxic cholangitis present with a severe illness, including jaundice, fever, abdominal pain, mental obtundation, and hypotension (Reynolds' pentad). Fever is the most common presenting symptom and is often accompanied by chills. Jaundice is a frequent physical finding but may be absent, especially in patients with an indwelling endoprosthesis or biliary stent. Pain is also commonly present but is often mild. Severe pain or marked tenderness should prompt consideration of an alternate diagnosis such as acute cholecystitis. Up to 33% of East Asian patients with choledocholithiasis present with toxic cholangitis characterized by septic shock.[27]

Diagnosis. Although cholangitis is a clinical diagnosis, laboratory tests can support evidence of biliary obstruction. Leukocytosis, hyperbilirubinemia, and elevations of alkaline phosphatase and transaminases all are common in patients with cholangitis. Radiologic studies also are helpful in confirming the diagnosis. CT, ultrasound, and magnetic resonance image scanning can provide noninvasive evidence of biliary ductal dilation, pancreatic masses, and occasionally CBD stones. Cholangiography usually is required prior to or as part of therapy. Both endoscopic and percutaneous transhepatic cholangiography are associated with a 4% to 7% incidence of cholangitis, and systemic antibiotics should be administered prior to these procedures.

Management. The initial treatment of the patient with cholangitis includes antibiotics. Some patients are only mildly ill and can be managed as outpatients with oral antibiotics. Patients with toxic cholangitis may require intensive care unit monitoring and vasopressors to support blood pressure. Most patients will require intravenous fluids and antibiotics. The antibacterial regimen should cover the common pathogens isolated from the biliary tract or be based on current or prior bile cultures.[28]

Most patients with cholangitis respond to antibiotic therapy alone with clinical improvement; however, emergency biliary decompression may be necessary in the 15% of patients who do not respond to antibiotics within 12 to 24 hours or in patients with toxic cholangitis. Biliary decompression may be performed endoscopically or via the percutaneous transhepatic route. The selection of which procedure to perform should be based on the level and nature of the biliary obstruction. In patients with a proximal perihilar obstruction or a biliary-enteric anastomotic stricture, percutaneous drainage may be the preferred route of decompression. Choledocholithiasis and cholangitis associated with periampullary malignancies are best approached endoscopically. Endoscopic biliary drainage may include endoscopic sphincterotomy and stone extraction or simply placement of an endoscopic biliary stent in the hemodynamically unstable patient. In experienced hands, successful endoscopic CBD stone clearance can be achieved in more than 90% of patients.[27] In settings in which either endoscopic or percutaneous biliary drainage is not possible, CBD exploration and placement of a T-tube remains a lifesaving procedure for seriously ill patients with toxic cholangitis. However, the mortality for patients treated surgically is considerably higher than for patients successfully managed endoscopically.

Overall, the mortality rate associated with an episode of cholangitis due to CBD stones is approximately 2% but is higher in patients with toxic cholangitis (5%). Renal failure, hepatic abscess, and malignancy are all associated with higher morbidity and mortality. The success of the initial antibiotic therapy and biliary drainage is significantly lower in patients with malignant biliary obstruction, and these patients frequently require changes in antibiotic therapy and repeat biliary manipulations to adequately decompress the biliary tract.[28] Hepatic abscesses are frequently observed in patients with biliary pathology and should be considered in patients who do not respond to therapy. Patients with cholangitis due to CBD stones should undergo interval laparoscopic cholecystectomy within 6 to 12 weeks because the incidence of recurrent biliary symptoms is significantly higher if the gallbladder is left in situ (6% vs. 25%).[27]

CHOLEDOCHOLITHIASIS

Classification and Etiology

CBD stones can be classified as either primary or secondary. Primary duct stones develop de novo within the bile ducts, whereas secondary stones develop in the gallbladder and subsequently fall into the CBD. In the United States more than 85% of all bile duct stones are secondary. Primary duct stones typically occur in patients with benign biliary strictures, sclerosing cholangitis, choledochal cyst disease, or sphincter of Oddi dysfunction. These conditions are associated with bile stasis, which promotes the overgrowth of bacteria in bile with subsequent deconjugation of bilirubin and the breakdown of biliary lipids, resulting in the formation of brown pigment stones. Secondary bile duct stones have a composition similar to gallbladder stones. Approximately 75% are cholesterol stones, and 25% are black pigment stones. The classification of CBD stones into primary or secondary is of therapeutic importance because primary stones require removal of the stones and a drainage procedure (choledochoenterostomy or sphincteroplasty), whereas secondary stones can be treated by removal of the stones and cholecystectomy.

Clinical Presentation

Common duct stones are often asymptomatic and only discovered during cholangiography at the time of cholecystectomy. CBD stones are present in 8% to 15% of patients with symptomatic gallstones. The incidence varies with age and is less than 5% in younger patients and more than 20% in older patients with gallstones. Patients with symptomatic choledocholithiasis will present with biliary colic, extrahepatic biliary obstruction, cholangitis, or pancreatitis. Clinical features suspicious for biliary obstruction caused by CBD stones include biliary colic, jaundice, lightening of the stools, and darkening of the urine. Typically, the pain and jaundice associated with CBD stones are more intermittent and transient than when the biliary obstruction is caused by a malignancy. In addition, fever and chills may be present in patients with choledocholithiasis and cholangitis. Gallstone pancreatitis can develop from the obstruction of the ampulla of Vater by common duct stones. CBD stones are responsible for up to 50% of all cases of pancreatitis. Most patients with gallstone pancreatitis experience a mild self-limited attack from which they recover within a few days; however, some patients will progress to develop severe pancreatitis with peripancreatic necrosis, infection, or pseudocyst formation.

Predictors of Common Bile Duct Stones

No single clinical variable is completely accurate in predicting the presence of choledocholithiasis. Therefore, the results of a detailed history and physical examination, laboratory evaluations, and diagnostic imaging tests must be taken together when assessing the likelihood that a patient has CBD stones. Serum liver function tests (bilirubin, alkaline phosphatase, and transaminases) can be useful in predicting common duct stones. If any one value of the liver profile is elevated, the risk for CBD stones approaches 20%. With two elevated values the risk increases to nearly 40%, and with three or more elevated values the risk for CBD stones is nearly 50%. However, between 5% and 7% of patients with no liver function abnormalities have CBD stones identified by cholangiography at the
9 time of cholecystectomy. A recent meta-analysis has shown the presence of cholangitis, CBD stones identified on ultrasound, and jaundice to be the strongest indicators of CBD stones.[29] A patient with any one of these indicators has at least 10 times the risk of having CBD stones compared with a patient without the risk factor (Table 60.5).

Diagnostic Studies

Ultrasonography. Ultrasound (US) is very sensitive for the diagnosis of gallstones within the gallbladder. Unfortunately, the sensitivity of US for the detection of CBD stones is only 15% to 30%. Ultrasound can identify CBD dilation, which can suggest choledocholithiasis. If the extrahepatic bile duct diameter is less than 3 mm, CBD stones are exceedingly rare, whereas a diameter greater than 10 mm in a jaundiced patient predicts CBD stones in more than 90% of cases. Ultrasound successfully identifies the presence of CBD stones in only 70% of patients because the distal end of the bile duct is frequently obscured by duodenal or colonic gas.

Magnetic Resonance Imaging. Magnetic resonance cholangiopancreatography (MRCP) is another noninvasive means of imaging the biliary tract (Fig. 60.15). Several studies have shown that MRCP can diagnose CBD stones with a sensitivity

TABLE 60.5 DIAGNOSIS

PREDICTIVE VALUES OF PREOPERATIVE INDICATORS OF COMMON BILE DUCT STONES

INDICATOR	POSITIVE LIKELIHOOD RATIO	NEGATIVE LIKELIHOOD RATIO	SENSITIVITY	SPECIFICITY
Cholangitis	18.3	0.93	0.11	0.99
Common bile duct stones on ultrasound	13.6	0.70	0.38	1.00
Preoperative jaundice	10.1	0.69	0.36	0.97
Elevated bilirubin	4.8	0.77	0.69	0.88
Elevated alkaline phosphatase	2.6	0.65	0.57	0.86
Pancreatitis	2.1	0.96	0.10	0.95
Cholecystitis	1.6	0.94	0.50	0.76
Amylase	1.5	0.99	0.11	0.95

Adapted from Abboud BA, Malet PF, Berlin JA, et al. Predictors of common bile duct stones prior to cholecystectomy: a meta-analysis. *Gastrointest Endosc* 1996;44:450.

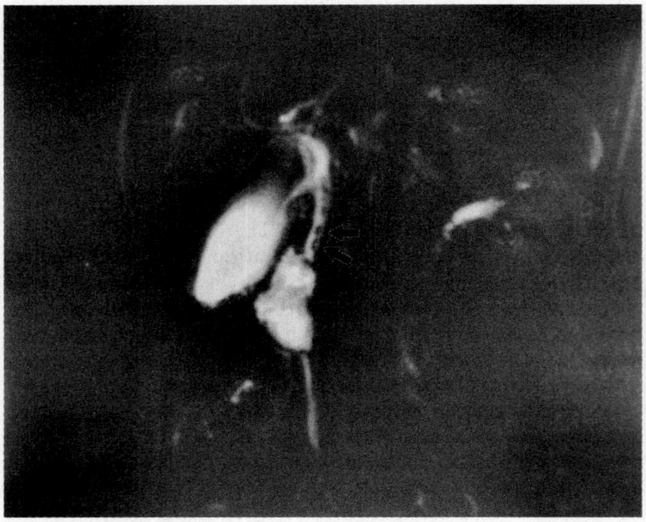

FIGURE 60.15. Magnetic resonance cholangiogram showing common bile duct stones (*arrows*).

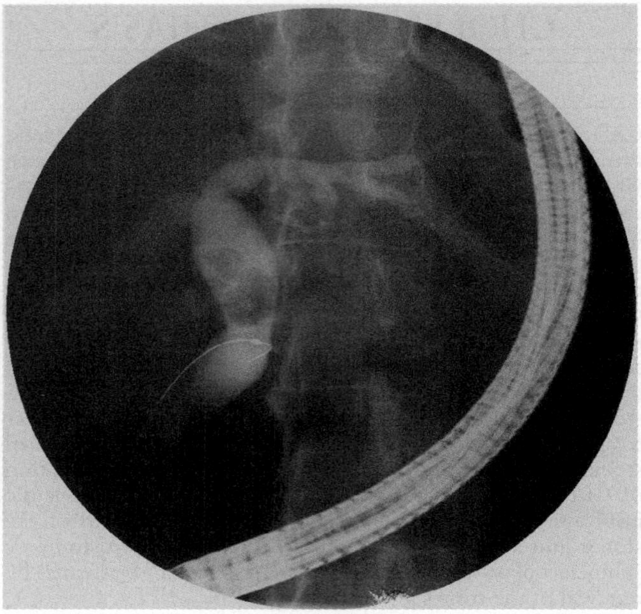

FIGURE 60.16. Endoscopic retrograde cholangiogram showing common bile duct stones.

of 90%, a specificity of 100%, and an overall diagnostic accuracy of 97%. The main advantage of MRCP is that it allows for the direct imaging of the biliary tract without the need for contrast or an invasive procedure. Disadvantages include its relatively high cost and lack of therapeutic capacity. Magnetic resonance cholangiography has been used to screen patients at low and moderate risk of having common duct stones prior to endoscopic cholangiography. A normal magnetic resonance cholangiogram can avoid the need for an invasive endoscopic cholangiogram. MRCP has become more popular as costs have reduced and surgeons have become more skilled with laparoscopic techniques for managing CBD stones.

Endoscopic Ultrasound. Endoscopic ultrasound (EUS) is a semi-invasive test that can be performed with a very low rate of complications (<0.1%).[30] The sensitivity and specificity for the diagnosis of CBD stones by EUS ranges from 92% to 100% and 95% to 100%, respectively. The negative predictive value for EUS is more than 97%.[31] Therefore, when EUS is negative for common duct stones, ERCP or intraoperative cholangiography can be avoided.

Preoperative Cholangiography. Endoscopic cholangiography is the "gold standard" for the diagnosis of CBD stones. Both endoscopic retrograde cholangiography (ERC) and percutaneous transhepatic cholangiography (PTC) techniques can be used to directly visualize the biliary tree. A comparison of endoscopic retrograde cholangiography and percutaneous transhepatic cholangiography techniques is noted in Table 60.6. Endoscopic cholangiography (Fig. 60.16) has the advantage of providing a therapeutic option at the time CBD stones are identified and is therefore the preferred approach for patients with suspected CBD stones. Skilled endoscopists can successfully cannulate the CBD in approximately 90% to 95% of

TABLE 60.6 **TREATMENT**

COMPARISON OF PERCUTANEOUS TRANSHEPATIC CHOLANGIOGRAPHY AND ENDOSCOPIC RETROGRADE CHOLANGIOGRAPHY

CRITERION	TRANSHEPATIC CHOLANGIOGRAPHY	ENDOSCOPIC CHOLANGIOGRAPHY
Success rate	>90% with dilated ducts, 70% with nondilated ducts	80%–90% with either dilated or nondilated ducts
Identification of cause of obstruction	90%–100%	75%–90%
Complications	5% (range, 3%–10%)	5% (range, 2%–7%)
Mortality	0.2%–0.9%	0.1%–0.2%
Expense	Less	More
Skill required	Less	More
Patient selection	Proximal lesions, altered gastroduodenal anatomy, failed endoscopic cholangiography	Distal lesions, pancreatic pathology, coagulopathy, ascites, failed transhepatic cholangiography

patients. Complications of diagnostic cholangiography include pancreatitis and cholangitis and occur in up to 5% of patients. ERC may be unsuccessful in patients with previous gastric surgery (Billroth II reconstruction), periampullary diverticula, or tortuous biliary ducts. Percutaneous transhepatic cholangiography may be used to image the bile ducts if ERC is unsuccessful.

Intraoperative Cholangiography. Intraoperative cholangiography (IOC) also can be successfully accomplished in more than 95% of cases. The cholangiogram should be carefully evaluated for filling defects within the ducts, presence of contrast in the duodenum, and the intrahepatic biliary anatomy. Debate continues over the need to perform routine intraoperative cholangiography at the time of cholecystectomy. Advocates of routine IOC argue that asymptomatic CBD stones can be identified and biliary injuries prevented by performing routine IOC. Critics of this approach suggest that the incidence of retained stones is no greater when cholangiography is performed selectively based on clinical and laboratory criteria. The indications for performing cholangiography during cholecystectomy include (a) a dilated CBD, (b) a wide cystic duct, (c) palpable CBD stones, (d) elevated serum liver function tests or bilirubin, and (e) a history of pancreatitis. If these criteria are strictly followed, approximately 30% of patients will require IOC at the time of cholecystectomy. IOC can identify the size, number, and location of CBD stones in addition to defining biliary anatomy. This information is critical in choosing the most appropriate treatment for CBD stones.

Intraoperative Ultrasonography. Intraoperative ultrasonography also can be used to identify CBD stones at the time of cholecystectomy. In experienced hands, intraoperative ultrasonography has been shown to be comparable to intraoperative cholangiography for the diagnosis of CBD stones. Laparoscopic ultrasonography is performed with a high frequency (7.5- to 10-MHz) probe, and the bile duct is imaged in the transverse and longitudinal planes. The distal bile duct can be visualized in more than 95% of cases.

The choice of radiologic studies used to evaluate a patient with suspected choledocholithiasis should be based on the probability of this diagnosis. Patients at highest risk for choledocholithiasis should undergo endoscopic cholangiography. Patients at intermediate risk may be screened with magnetic resonance cholangiography or endoscopic ultrasound and proceed to laparoscopic cholecystectomy if no stones are identified. Those patients at low risk of harboring common duct stones may be evaluated with intraoperative cholangiography at the time of laparoscopic cholecystectomy with laparoscopic CBD exploration or postoperative endoscopic stone extraction reserved for the few patients with a positive study.[32]

Management

Currently, several options are available to the surgeon for the treatment of CBD stones. In choosing the most appropriate approach for an individual patient, factors such as the local endoscopic expertise, the surgeon's laparoscopic skill, and the patient's clinical condition must be considered. A potential approach to the management of CBD stones is shown in Algorithm 60.1.

10 **Endoscopic.** ERC with endoscopic sphincterotomy permits CBD stones to be removed without the need for conventional surgery. Stones can be successfully removed from the CBD in 85% to 95% of cases. The endoscopic approach is particularly useful for patients prior to cholecystectomy in whom a high suspicion exists for CBD calculi, particularly if laparoscopic

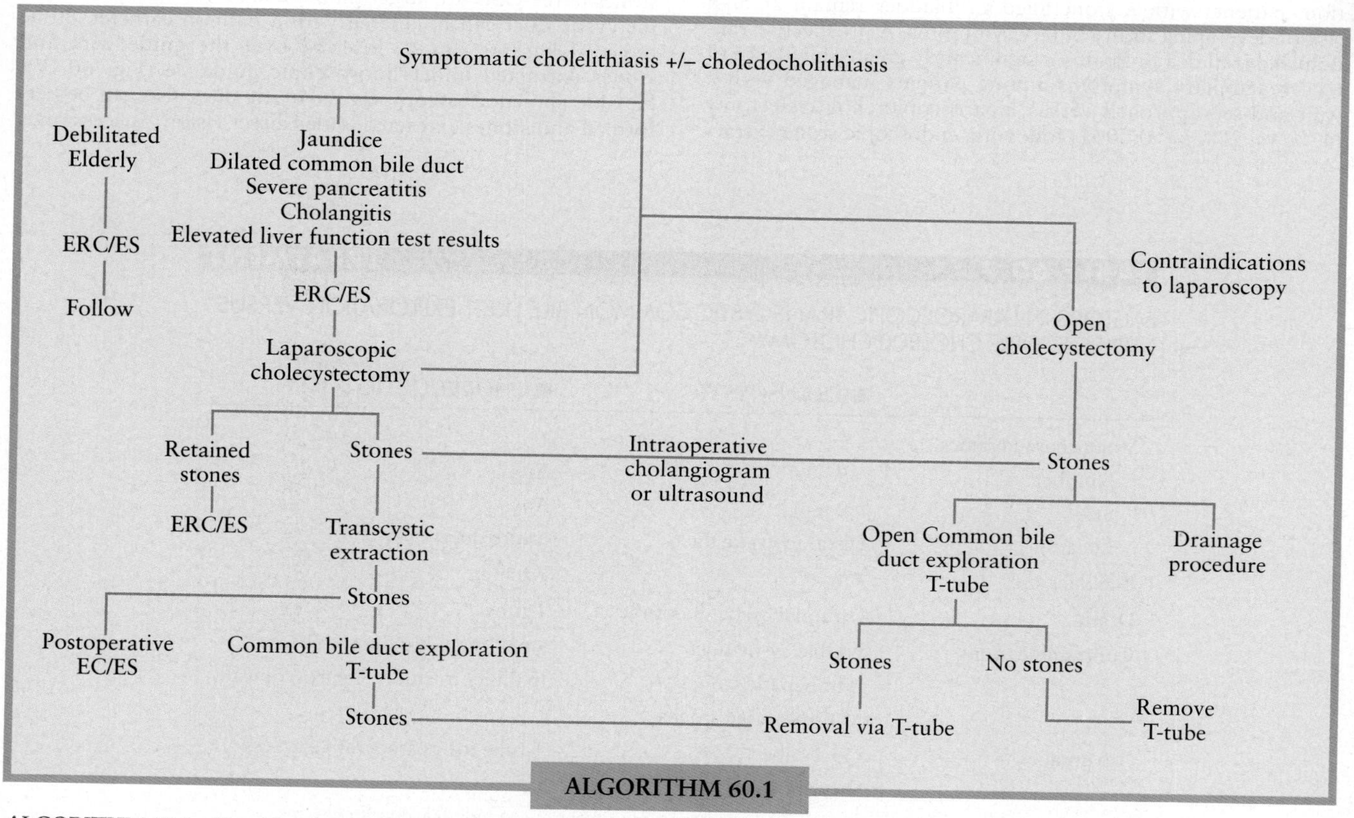

ALGORITHM 60.1. Algorithm for the management of common bile duct stones.

CBD exploration is not available. Endoscopic clearance of stones from the CBD precholecystectomy can avoid the need for an open operation. Furthermore, if endoscopic stone extraction is not possible because of multiple gallstones, intrahepatic stones, large gallstones, impacted stones, duodenal diverticula, prior gastrectomy, or bile duct stricture, this information is known before cholecystectomy, and an open CBD exploration or drainage procedure can be performed. After sphincterotomy, most stones smaller than 1 cm in diameter pass spontaneously. A balloon catheter or stone basket also can be used to retrieve stones if needed. If endoscopic clearance is incomplete, an endoscopic stent can be placed into the CBD to maintain drainage and prevent cholangitis.

Endoscopic sphincterotomy and stone extraction is well tolerated in most patients. Complications occur in 5% to 8% of patients and include cholangitis, pancreatitis, perforation, and bleeding. The overall mortality rate is 0.2% to 0.5%. Complete clearance of all common duct stones is achieved endoscopically in 71% to 75% of patients at the first procedure and in 84% to 95% of patients after multiple endoscopic procedures.[33]

Preoperative ERC plus endoscopic sphincterotomy is the preferred management option for CBD stones in several conditions. In the setting of acute suppurative cholangitis, morbidity and mortality are significantly decreased if preoperative biliary decompression and stone removal are accomplished before cholecystectomy. Patients with severe gallstone pancreatitis or a significant deterioration of their clinical condition also have been shown to benefit from early ERC and stone clearance. Cholecystectomy can then be performed after the pancreatitis has resolved. In patients with a dilated CBD (>8 mm) on ultrasound and jaundice, an ERC also should be performed to rule out a malignancy or biliary stricture that would alter the surgical management. In patients with a high operative risk, ERC plus endoscopic sphincterotomy can be performed to remove CBD stones and the gallbladder left in place.

Following endoscopic sphincterotomy and stone extraction, patients with a stone-filled gallbladder remain at high risk of developing future biliary symptoms. A prospective randomized trial demonstrated a significantly greater incidence of recurrent biliary symptoms among patients managed with a wait-and-see approach versus laparoscopic cholecystectomy (47% vs. 2%, $p < 0.0001$) following endoscopic stone extraction. A large percentage (37%) of patients managed expectantly later required cholecystectomy.[34]

Laparoscopic. Laparoscopic exploration of the CBD for choledocholithiasis enables appropriate patients to undergo complete management of their calculous biliary tract disease with one invasive procedure. This approach is the most cost effective and should become the preferred option as surgeons' laparoscopic skills improve.[35] The laparoscopic approach is ideal for patients with CBD stones identified during intraoperative cholangiography or ultrasound or in patients with suspected choledocholithiasis managed at centers where laparoscopic CBD exploration is routinely performed. Intraoperative cholangiography is accomplished via the cystic duct prior to duct exploration.

The two approaches for laparoscopic bile duct exploration are laparoscopic transcystic common bile duct exploration (LTCBDE) or laparoscopic choledochotomy (Table 60.7). The indications for transcystic duct exploration are filling defects noted on cholangiography (CBD stones), stones less than 9 mm in diameter, stones below the cystic duct entrance to the bile duct, and fewer than six stones. Contraindications to LTCBDE are a small friable cystic duct, more than eight stones in the CBD, common hepatic duct stones, and stones larger than 1 cm. Laparoscopic choledochotomy can be performed if LTCBDE fails or is contraindicated, if stones are present above the cystic duct, or when multiple stones are present. The only contraindication to laparoscopic choledochotomy is a small common duct (<6 mm) that might be narrowed during its closure.

Laparoscopic Transcystic Common Bile Duct Exploration. The technique of LTCBDE involves the blunt dissection of the cystic duct down to its junction with the CBD. A cystic ductotomy is then made and a guide wire inserted into the bile duct. A cholangiocatheter can then be advanced over the guide wire into the bile duct and saline irrigated through the catheter in an attempt to flush small stones out of the bile duct. If the stones in the CBD are larger than the lumen of the cystic duct, the cystic duct can be dilated with a balloon catheter. Stone retrieval baskets can be inserted over the guide wire and stones extracted under fluoroscopic guidance (Fig. 60.17). Flexible choledochoscopy via the cystic duct also can be performed and stones extracted under direct vision. Success rates

TABLE 60.7 **TREATMENT**

FACTORS IN LAPAROSCOPIC TRANSCYSTIC COMMON BILE DUCT EXPLORATION VERSUS LAPAROSCOPIC CHOLEDOCHOTOMY

	■ TRANSCYSTIC	■ CHOLEDOCHOTOMY
Stone characteristics		
Number	<8	Any
Size	>9 mm	Any
Location	Distal to cystic duct	Entire duct
Bile duct size	Any	>6 mm
Drain	Optional cystic duct tube	T-tube
Contraindications	Friable cystic duct Intrahepatic stones Multiple large stones	Small-diameter duct Inability to suture laparoscopically
Advantages	No T-tube Short hospital stay	T-tube for postoperative access

Adapted from Phillips EH, Korman JE. Laparoscopic management of common bile duct stones. In: Cameron JL, ed. *Current Surgical Therapy,* 6th ed. St. Louis, MO: Mosby; 1998.

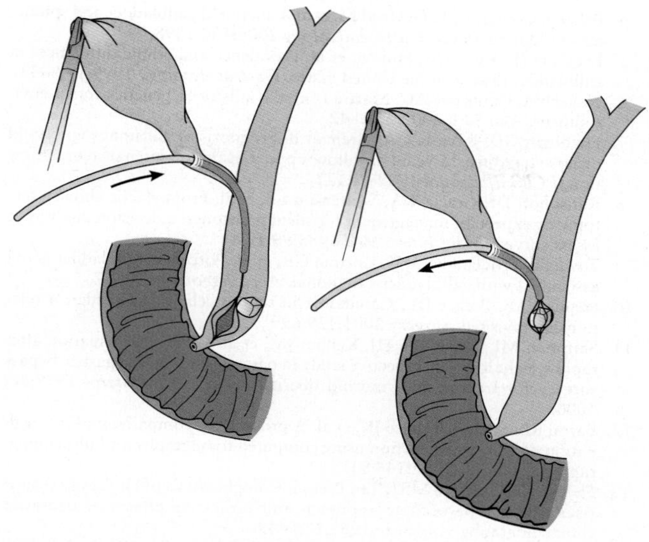

FIGURE 60.17. Laparoscopic transcystic bile duct exploration.

greater than 95% have been reported for bile duct clearance using choledochoscopy. To document stone clearance, a completion cholangiogram should be performed. A cystic duct drainage tube can be left in place if findings on the cholangiogram are equivocal. This tube can be used postoperatively for cholangiography and radiographic treatment of retained stones if necessary.

Laparoscopic Choledochotomy. Laparoscopic choledochotomy is another excellent approach to CBD stones when the CBD diameter is 6 mm or greater. The anterior wall of the CBD is bluntly dissected and a longitudinal choledochotomy made in the anterior wall below the cystic duct. The choledochotomy should be made as long as the diameter of the largest stone. Two stay sutures can be placed in the common duct and used to tent up the anterior wall to facilitate the incision. A larger choledochoscope (3.3 mm, 2.4-mm working channel) can then be placed into the bile duct and stones extracted with baskets or balloon catheters. The choledochotomy is then closed over a T-tube with a 4–0 absorbable suture.

Advantages of laparoscopic choledochotomy over LTCBDE include the ability to remove larger stones (>1 cm), to remove stones from the proximal hepatic ducts, to remove multiple stones, and to use biliary lithotripsy to fragment impacted stones. The disadvantages of laparoscopic choledochotomy are that it requires a T-tube and considerable laparoscopic suturing skill to close the choledochotomy.

Clearance of all CBD stones is achieved in 75% to 95% of patients with laparoscopic CBD exploration.[35] The morbidity and mortality of laparoscopic CBD exploration are similar to laparoscopic cholecystectomy alone. In a prospective randomized trial comparing laparoscopic CBD exploration at the time of laparoscopic cholecystectomy with postoperative endoscopic stone extraction following laparoscopic cholecystectomy, the complication rate and retained stone rate were similar between the two groups. The median hospital stay was significantly shorter for patients managed with the single invasive procedure (1 day vs. 3.5 days).

Open Common Bile Duct Exploration. Open CBD exploration is performed much less frequently with the increased use of endoscopic, percutaneous, and laparoscopic techniques to remove CBD stones. Occasionally, when these methods fail, are not available, or are not possible because of prior surgery, or when open operation is otherwise required, open CBD exploration becomes necessary. The technique will be described briefly because open CBD exploration is not commonly performed in the era of laparoscopic cholecystectomy. The first step is to perform a full Kocher maneuver mobilizing the duodenum so that a hand can be placed behind the head of the pancreas and the distal CBD palpated. Any impacted stones may be milked more proximally. The supraduodenal bile duct is then exposed and two stay sutures placed in the CBD just below the cystic duct. The anterior wall of the bile duct is then elevated with the stay sutures and a longitudinal choledochotomy made. The bile duct then can be explored for stones. Rigid instruments should not be used to extract stones because they can injure the delicate ductal epithelium. A soft rubber irrigating catheter can be used to gently flush out any stones or debris. Balloon-tipped catheters then can be passed proximally and distally into the ducts to retrieve stones. Adequate clearance of the duct should be confirmed visually with flexible choledochoscopy. Remaining stones can be removed by irrigation or the use of instruments such as stone forceps, wire baskets, or balloon catheters. A T-tube should be placed in the bile duct and the choledochotomy closed with 4–0 absorbable suture. Completion cholangiography is performed before closing the abdomen to rule out the presence of retained stones or a bile leak around the T-tube. Postoperatively, a T-tube cholangiogram is performed 3 to 7 days after the exploration. If the cholangiogram is normal, the tube can be clamped and the tube pulled 3 to 6 weeks later. If retained stones are detected, the tract is allowed to mature, and percutaneous extraction can be performed by a radiologist in 4 to 6 weeks. Open CBD exploration can be accomplished with almost no mortality in patients younger than age 60 years but can have a mortality of up to 4% in septic patients.

Drainage Procedures. Patients with an impacted stone at the ampulla that cannot be removed with a CBD exploration or with multiple stones in a nondilated duct may require a transduodenal sphincteroplasty. A sphincteroplasty also is indicated in the presence of an ampullary stenosis or a choledochocele. The first step in a sphincteroplasty is to perform a Kocher maneuver. A small longitudinal duodenotomy is made over the ampulla and two stay sutures placed on each side of the ampulla to elevate it. A small incision is made at the 11-o'clock position in the sphincter taking care to avoid the pancreatic duct, which is usually found at the 5-o'clock position. The sphincterotomy is extended through the sphincter (approximately 1.5 cm) and the impacted stone removed. The bile duct and duodenal mucosa are then reapproximated with interrupted 4–0 absorbable sutures. The duodenotomy should be closed transversely to prevent narrowing of the lumen.

Patients with grossly dilated bile ducts (>2 cm), multiple stones (>5), intrahepatic stones, primary duct stones, or a distal biliary stricture should be considered for a biliary drainage procedure. The two options are a choledochoduodenostomy or a Roux-en-Y choledochojejunostomy. The choledochoduodenostomy can be performed in either a side-to-side or an end-to-side fashion. Advantages of a choledochoduodenostomy are that it can be performed rapidly, it requires only one anastomosis, and the bile duct still can be accessed endoscopically. However, a side-to-side anastomosis leaves the distal CBD in continuity and can lead to the "sump syndrome." In this situation, food debris from the duodenum can enter the distal limb of the duct and obstruct the anastomosis or the pancreatic duct orifice, leading to cholangitis or pancreatitis. Roux-en-Y hepaticojejunostomy or choledochojejunostomy also is an excellent option for biliary drainage. This operation is performed by dividing the hepatic or common duct and doing an end-to-end anastomosis to a 60-cm Roux limb. Development of the sump syndrome is not a concern because a hepaticojejunostomy or choledochojejunostomy is completely diverting.

TABLE 60.8 RESULTS

SUMMARY OF TREATMENT AND OUTCOMES FOR INTRAHEPATIC STONE DISEASE AT THE JOHNS HOPKINS HOSPITAL

Patient, *n*	54
Percutaneous treatment only	26% of patients
Surgical treatment	74% of patients
Postoperative percutaneous treatment	33% of patients
Mean follow-up	60 mo
Successful stone clearance	94% of patients
Symptom-free state	87% of patients
Recurrent stones or stricture	20% of patients

Adapted with permission from Pitt HA, Venbrux AC, Coleman JA, et al. Intrahepatic stones: the transhepatic team approach. *Ann Surg* 1994;219:527.

Intrahepatic Stones

Intrahepatic stones are relatively uncommon in Western countries. These stones are more prevalent in Asia and represent a difficult management problem. Intrahepatic stones are primarily brown pigment stones. They typically occur in association with diseases characterized by prolonged partial bile duct obstruction, such as sclerosing cholangitis, benign and malignant biliary strictures, choledochal cysts, and biliary parasites.

Cholangiography, either endoscopic or percutaneous, is the most valuable technique in the evaluation of patients with intrahepatic stones. The transhepatic percutaneous approach is preferable in most patients because it allows for direct access to the intrahepatic bile ducts for therapeutic interventions. Transhepatic biliary drainage catheters can be inserted and gradually upsized to a 16- to 20-French size. The tract is then allowed to mature for 5 to 6 weeks, and stones are removed by using steerable stone retrieval baskets under fluoroscopic guidance, or with percutaneous choledochoscopy.

Although some patients with intrahepatic stone disease can be managed nonoperatively, many patients will require surgical intervention. A Roux-en-Y hepaticojejunostomy is usually constructed and intraoperative choledochoscopy used to clear the bile ducts of stones. Large-bore transhepatic stents can be placed intraoperatively to provide access to the biliary tree for percutaneous stone extraction or the treatment of strictures postoperatively. Using this approach, a stone clearance rate of greater than 90% can be expected (Table 60.8).[36] Another option for management of intrahepatic stones is the creation of a hepaticocutaneous jejunostomy. This technique involves creating a Roux-en-Y hepaticojejunostomy with a longer than usual Roux limb and extending the Roux limb beyond the anastomosis up to the anterior abdominal wall. The limb is then marked with metal wire or clips, which allows percutaneous access to the biliary system if needed. If the intrahepatic stone disease is isolated to a single lobe or segment of liver and is associated with significant intrahepatic biliary strictures or atrophy, a hepatic resection may be indicated to treat the stone disease.

References

1. National Center for Health Statistics. *Health, United States, 2004 With Chartbook on Trends in the Health of Americans*. Hyattsville, MD: National Center for Health Statistics; 2004.
2. Swartz-Basile DA, Lu D, Basile DP, et al. Leptin regulates gallbladder genes related to absorption and secretion. *Am J Physiol* 2007;293:84.
3. Doty JE, Pitt HA, Kuchenbecker SL, et al. Impaired gallbladder emptying prior to gallstone formation in the prairie dog. *Gastroenterology* 1983;85:168–174.
4. Behar J, Corazziari E, Guelrud M, et al. Functional gallbladder and sphincter of Oddi disorders. *Gastroenterology* 2006;130:1498.
5. Everhart JE, Khare M, Hill M, et al. Prevalence and ethnic differences in gallbladder disease in the United States. *Gastroenterology* 1999;117:632.
6. Nakeeb A, Comuzzie AG, Martin L, et al. Gallstones: genetics versus environment. *Ann Surg* 2002;235:842.
7. Friedman GD, Raviola CA, Fireman B. Prognosis of gallstones with mild or no symptoms: 25 years of follow-up in a health maintenance organization. *J Clin Epidemiol* 1989;42:127.
8. Ransohoff DF, Gracie WA, Wolfenson LB, et al. Prophylactic cholecystectomy or expectant management for silent gallstones: a decision analysis to assess survival. *Ann Intern Med* 1983;99:199.
9. Towfigh S, McFadden DW, Cortina GR, et al. Porcelain gallbladder is not associated with gallbladder carcinoma. *Am Surgeon* 2001;67:7.
10. Stephen AE, Berger DL. Carcinoma in the porcelain gallbladder: a relationship revisited. *Surgery* 2001;129:699.
11. Shiffman ML, Sugerman HJ, Kellum JM, et al. Gallstone formation after rapid weight loss: a prospective study in patients undergoing gastric bypass surgery for treatment of morbid obesity. *Am J Gastroenterol* 1999;86:1000.
12. Baron RL, Stanley RJ, Lee JK, et al. A prospective comparison of the evaluation of biliary obstruction using computed tomography and ultrasonography. *Radiology* 1982;145:91.
13. Fletcher DR, Hobbs MST, Tan P, et al. Complications of cholecystectomy: risks of the laparoscopic approach and protective effects of operative cholangiography. *Ann Surg* 1999;229:449.
14. Cameron JL. *Atlas of Surgery*, Vol 2. Philadelphia, PA: BC Decker, Inc.; 1994.
15. Curet M, Zucker K. Laparoscopic surgery of the biliary tract and liver. In: Zuidema G, ed. *Shackelford's Surgery of the Alimentary Tract*. Philadelphia, PA: WB Saunders; 1996;196–218.
16. Calland J, Tanaka K, Foley E, et al. Outpatient laparoscopic cholecystectomy: patient outcomes after implementation of a clinical pathway. *Ann Surg* 2001;233:704.
17. Steiner CA, Bass EB, Talamini MA, et al. Surgical rates and operative mortality for open and laparoscopic cholecystectomy in Maryland. *N Engl J Med* 1994;330:403.
18. Strasberg SM, Hertl M, Soper NJ. An analysis of the problem of biliary injury during laparoscopic cholecystectomy. *J Am Coll Surg* 1995;180:101.
19. Leslie KA, Rankin RN, Duff JH. Lost gallstones during laparoscopic cholecystectomy: are they really benign? *Can J Surg* 1994;37:240.
20. Lo CM, Liu CL, Fan ST, et al. Prospective randomized study of early versus delayed laparoscopic cholecystectomy for acute cholecystitis. *Ann Surg* 1998;227:461.
21. Kiviluoto T, Siren J, Luukonen P, et al. Randomized trial of laparoscopic versus open cholecystectomy for acute and gangrenous cholecystitis. *Lancet* 1998;351:321.
22. Lai P, Kwong K, Leung K, et al. Randomized trial of early versus delayed laparoscopic cholecystectomy for acute cholecystitis. *Br J Surg* 1998;85:764.
23. Tsuyuguchi T, Takada T, Kawarada Y, et al. Techniques of biliary drainage for acute cholecystitis: Tokyo guidelines. *J Hepatobiliary Pancreat Surg* 2007;14:46–51.
24. Al-Azzawi HA, Nakeeb A, Saxena R, et al. Cholecystosteatosis: an explanation for increased cholecystectomy rates. *J Gastrointest Surg* 2007;11:835.
25. Tzovaras G, Rowlands B. Diagnosis and treatment of sphincter of Oddi dysfunction. *Br J Surg* 1998;85:588.
26. Thompson JE, Pitt HA, Doty JE, et al. Broad spectrum penicillin as an adequate therapy for acute cholangitis. *Surg Gynecol Obstet* 1990;171:275.
27. Poon RT, Liu CL, Lo CM. Management of gallstone cholangitis in the era of laparoscopic cholecystectomy. *Arch Surg* 2001;136:11.
28. Nagino M, Takada T, Kawarada Y, et al. Methods and timing of biliary drainage for acute cholangitis: Tokyo guidelines. *J Hepatobiliary Pancreat Surg* 2007;14(1):68–77.
29. Abboud BA, Malet PF, Berlin JA, et al. Predictors of common bile duct stones prior to cholecystectomy: a meta-analysis. *Gastrointest Endosc* 1996;44:450.
30. Rosch T, Dittler HJ, Fockens P, et al. Major complications of endoscopic ultrasonography: results of a survey of 42,105 cases. *Gastrointest Endosc* 1993;39:341.
31. Vilgrain V, Palazzo L. Choledocholithiasis: role of US and endoscopic ultrasound. *Abdom Imaging* 2001;26:7.
32. Liu T, Consorti E, Kawashima A, et al. Patient evaluation and management with selective use of magnetic resonance cholangiography and endoscopic retrograde cholangiopancreatography before laparoscopic cholecystectomy. *Ann Surg* 2001;234:33.
33. Freeman M, Nelson D, Sherman S, et al. Complications of endoscopic biliary sphincterotomy. *N Engl J Med* 1996;335:909.
34. Boerma D, Rauws W, Keulemans Y, et al. Wait-and-see policy or laparoscopic cholecystectomy after endoscopic cholecystectomy for bile-duct stones: a randomized trial. *Lancet* 2002;360:761.
35. Rhodes M, Sussman L, Cohen L, et al. Randomized trial of laparoscopic exploration of common bile duct versus postoperative endoscopic retrograde cholangiography for common bile duct stones. *Lancet* 1998;351:159.
36. Pitt HA, Venbrux AC, Coleman J, et al. Intrahepatic stones: the transhepatic team approach. *Ann Surg* 1994;219:527.

CHAPTER 61 ■ BILIARY INJURIES AND STRICTURES AND SCLEROSING CHOLANGITIS

KEITH D. LILLEMOE

KEY POINTS

1. Most bile duct injuries or strictures currently occur in association with laparoscopic cholecystectomy, with an overall incidence of 0.3% to 0.7%.
2. Recognition of a bile duct injury during laparoscopic cholecystectomy is uncommon (<30% of cases), but if recognized, repair as either an end-to-end duct-to-duct anastomosis in very selected cases or hepaticojejunostomy should be performed.
3. Cholangiography, usually performed by a percutaneous transhepatic route, should be performed in all cases to define the proximal biliary anatomy needed for reconstruction and to allow placement of biliary catheters to control the ongoing bile leak.
4. Patients with biliary injuries most commonly present in the early postoperative course, usually with bile leakage. Despite recognition of an ongoing bile leak, urgent return to the operating room should be avoided.
5. The repair of a bile duct injury recognized in the postoperative period requires a hepaticojejunostomy in almost all cases and should be performed with transanastomotic biliary stents.
6. A successful result following repair of a bile duct injury can be expected in 80% to 90% of patients. Return to a normal quality of life is also expected. In the modern era, death associated with either bile duct injury or the operative repair is uncommon, occurring in less than 2% of patients.
7. Percutaneous or balloon dilatation of biliary strictures can lead to successful outcomes in selective patients, although the long-term results generally favor surgical reconstruction.
8. Primary sclerosing cholangitis is an autoimmune disease characterized by intrahepatic and extrahepatic inflammatory strictures of the bile ducts. Patients are at risk for the development of cholangiocarcinoma and/or end-stage liver disease. There is no known specific effective medical therapy for primary sclerosing cholangitis. Primary sclerosing cholangitis has become one of the most common indications for liver transplantation.
9. Bile duct strictures associated with alcoholic chronic pancreatitis are best managed by biliary bypass.

Biliary injuries and strictures are among the most difficult challenges that a surgeon faces. Although numerous technologic developments have facilitated diagnosis and management, bile duct injuries and strictures remain a significant clinical problem. If they go unrecognized or are managed improperly, life-threatening early complications such as sepsis and multisystem organ failure or late implications of biliary cirrhosis, portal hypertension, and cholangitis can develop. To avoid these complications, virtually every patient with a bile duct stricture should undergo evaluation and treatment with the goal of relieving the obstruction to bile flow and its associated hepatic injury. Finally, the occurrence of a major bile duct injury during an elective cholecystectomy remains one of the most common indications for charges of medical practice in the United States.

Benign bile duct strictures can have numerous causes (Table 61.1). Most biliary strictures occur after primary operations on the gallbladder or biliary tree. With the introduction of laparoscopic cholecystectomy, bile duct injuries and associated strictures have been seen with increased frequency. Operative injury to the bile ducts can also occur during nonbiliary operations on the gallbladder or biliary tree or as a result of external penetrating or blunt abdominal trauma. Inflammatory conditions and fibrosis caused by chronic pancreatitis, gallstones in the gallbladder or the bile duct, stenosis of the sphincter of Oddi, or biliary tract infections can also cause benign bile duct strictures. Finally, primary sclerosing cholangitis, a rare disease of unknown cause, can result in multiple strictures of the intrahepatic and extrahepatic bile ducts. This chapter focuses primarily on postoperative bile duct strictures and primary sclerosing cholangitis.

POSTOPERATIVE BILE DUCT STRICTURES

Pathogenesis

Most benign bile duct strictures result from operations in or near the right upper quadrant. More than 80% of strictures occur after injury to the bile ducts during cholecystectomy. The exact incidence of bile duct injury is unknown because
1 many cases may go unreported in the literature. Data suggest that the incidence of bile duct injury during open cholecystectomy is 1 in 500 to 1,000 cases. The incidence of bile duct injury during laparoscopic cholecystectomy is clearly higher. Although a wide range in the incidence of injury can be found in reported series, the most accurate data most likely come from surveys encompassing thousands of patients. These reports reflect the results from a large number of surgeons in both community and teaching hospitals. The results of such series suggest an incidence of bile duct injury during laparoscopic cholecystectomy ranging from 0.3% to 0.7%.[1] Furthermore, the incidence of bile duct injury associated with laparoscopic cholecystectomy does not appear to have diminished in more recent surveys, suggesting that the previously observed increase is not simply the result of a learning curve associated

TABLE 61.1 **ETIOLOGY**

CAUSES OF BENIGN BILE DUCT STRICTURES

POSTOPERATIVE STRICTURES
Injury at Primary Biliary Operations
■ Laparoscopic cholecystectomy
■ Open cholecystectomy
■ Common bile duct exploration
Injury at Other Operative Procedures
■ Gastrectomy
■ Hepatic resection
■ Portacaval shunt
Stricture of a biliary-enteric anastomosis
Blunt or penetrating trauma
STRICTURES CAUSED BY INFLAMMATORY CONDITIONS
Chronic pancreatitis
Cholelithiasis and choledocholithiasis
Primary sclerosing cholangitis
Stenosis of the sphincter of Oddi
Duodenal ulcer
Crohn disease
Viral infections
Toxic drugs

with the laparoscopic technique. Finally, due to the high frequency of laparoscopic cholecystectomy, it is estimated that one in every two or three surgeons will create a bile duct injury during his or her career.

A number of factors are associated with bile duct injury during either open or laparoscopic cholecystectomy, including acute or chronic inflammation, inadequate exposure, patient obesity, and failure to identify structures before clamping, ligating, or dividing them. More specific causes of bile duct injury also exist. Bleeding from the cystic or hepatic arteries can lead to bile duct injury during attempts to gain hemostasis. The generous application of Ligaclips at either open or laparoscopic cholecystectomy to hilar areas not well visualized can result in placing a clip on or across a bile duct, with resultant injury (Fig. 61.1). Failure to recognize congenital anatomic anomalies of the bile ducts, such as insertion of the right hepatic duct into the cystic duct or a long common wall between the cystic duct and the common bile duct, can also lead to injury (Fig. 61.2).

A number of technical factors are associated with laparoscopic cholecystectomy that can also increase the risk of bile duct injury compared with the open procedure. These factors include the use of an end-viewing laparoscope, which alters the surgeon's perspective of the operative field. Excessive cephalad retraction of the gallbladder fundus can cause the cystic duct and common bile duct to become aligned in the same plane. This distortion often results in the classic laparoscopic injury, in which the common bile duct is mistaken for the cystic duct and clipped and divided (Fig. 61.3).[2] The role of intraoperative cholangiography (IOC) in preventing bile duct injury during laparoscopic cholecystectomy is controversial. Individual series have failed to demonstrate that either performing routine or selective IOC affects the incidence of bile duct injury. However, a retrospective nationwide cohort analysis of Medicare patients undergoing laparoscopic cholecystectomy between 1992 and 1999 demonstrated that common bile duct injury occurred in 0.39% of patients in which IOC was performed versus 0.58% in patients not undergoing IOC (unadjusted relative risk, 1.49; 95% confidence interval

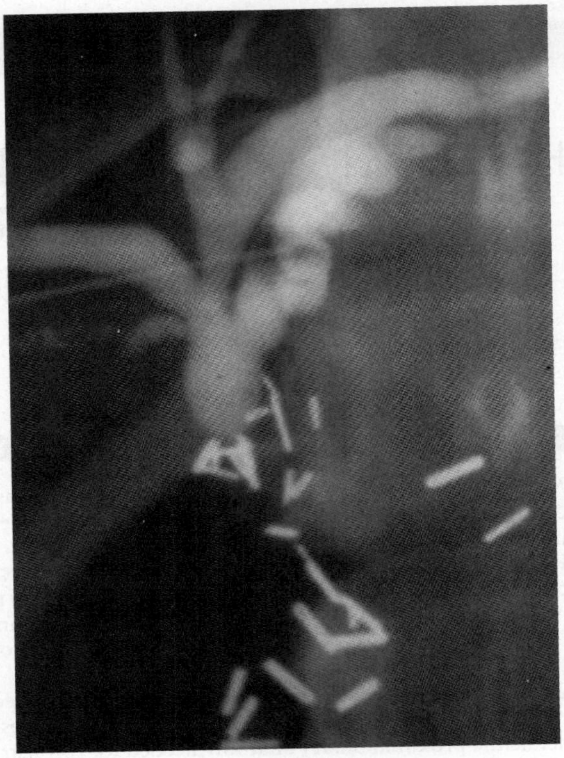

FIGURE 61.1. Percutaneous transhepatic cholangiogram in a patient with a bile duct stricture secondary to iatrogenic injury during cholecystectomy. Numerous surgical clips can be seen in the area of the stricture. (Reproduced with permission from Lillemoe KD, Pitt HA, Cameron JL. Postoperative bile duct strictures. *Surg Clin North Am* 1990;70:1356.)

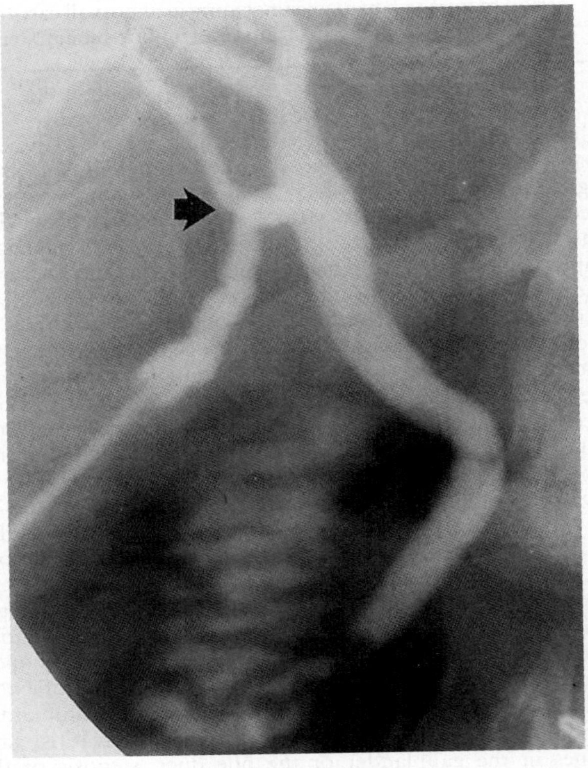

FIGURE 61.2. Operative cholangiogram demonstrating a right lobe segmental bile duct entering the cystic duct (*arrow*). Division of the cystic duct proximal to this insertion can result in a bile leak or obstruction of bile flow from a significant segment of the liver.

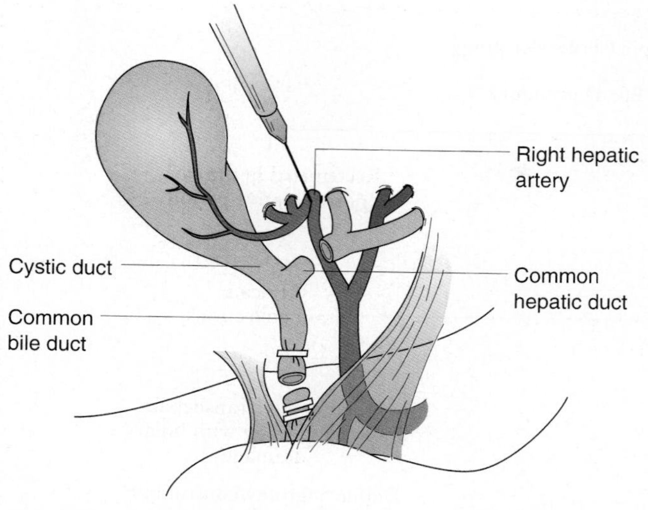

FIGURE 61.3. Classic laparoscopic bile duct injury. The common bile duct is mistaken for the cystic duct and transected. A variable extent of the extrahepatic biliary tree is resected with the gallbladder. The right hepatic artery, in background, is also often injured. (Adapted from Branum G, Schmidt C, Baillie J, et al. Management of major biliary complications after laparoscopic cholecystectomy. *Ann Surg* 1993;217:532.)

1.42–1.57).[3] Furthermore, the proper interpretation of IOC can minimize the extent of injury. Nevertheless, only 27% of surgeons in the United States perform IOC routinely.[4] Finally, ample evidence exists to support the conclusion that the experience of the surgeon in performing laparoscopic cholecystectomy can be correlated with the risk of bile duct injury.

In recent years there has been a growing understanding of surgeon cognitive factors associated with bile duct injury during laparoscopic cholecystectomy. An analysis examining 252 biliary injuries during laparoscopic cholecystectomy using human error factor and cognitive science techniques found that 97% of injuries were caused by visual-perceptual illusion or inadequate visualization.[5] Further work from the same group has determined a major explanation for the surgeon's frequent inability to recognize bile duct injury. These bile duct injuries appear to be associated with confirmation bias, which is a propensity to seek cues to confirm a belief and to discount cues that might discount the belief. Although cognitive factors are important for the understanding of the psychological issues associated with bile duct injuries, surgeons must continue to have the appropriate corrective mechanisms in place to minimize the chance of these injuries, including knowledge of anatomy, typical mechanisms of injury, and an appropriate level of suspicion and logic. An example of such a corrective mechanism is the operative technique of laparoscopic cholecystectomy, which defines the "critical view of safety," which helps prevent misidentification and injury of the major bile ducts.[6]

The importance of ischemia of the bile duct in the formation of postoperative strictures has been emphasized. Injury to the hepatic artery at the time of biliary injury during laparoscopic cholecystectomy has been recognized at an increased incidence, as high as 50%, when investigated at the time of presentation.[7] The presence of an arterial injury, however, does not appear to affect either early or late outcomes. A more clinically important cause of ischemia can be unnecessary dissection around the bile duct during cholecystectomy or bile duct anastomosis, which can divide or injure the major arteries of the bile duct that run in the 3-o'clock and 9-o'clock positions.

Another important factor contributing to the formation of biliary strictures is the intense connective tissue response with fibrosis and scarring that can occur after bile duct injury. Experimental studies of bile duct ligation in a canine model have demonstrated immediate and sustained elevation of bile duct pressure and progressive increase in bile duct diameter. Histologic changes at 1 month after ligation have shown that the bile duct wall is thickened, with a reduction of mucosal folds and loss of surface microvilli, associated with a well-defined epithelial degeneration. Biochemical analysis of connective tissue response to ligation showed that collagen synthesis and prolene hydroxylase activity is increased within 2 weeks in the obstructed bile duct and is sustained throughout the period of observation. Finally, a marked local inflammatory response can develop in the adjacent tissue in association with bile leakage, which occurs with many bile duct injuries. This inflammation can be further intensified in the face of infection. This inflammation results in fibrosis and scarring in the periductal tissue, further contributing to stricture formation. These factors can be of major importance in bile duct injuries during laparoscopic cholecystectomy, which are frequently associated with bile leaks.

After cholecystectomy and common bile duct exploration, the two most common operations associated with bile duct injury are gastrectomy and hepatic resection. The most common situation resulting in bile duct injury during gastrectomy involves dissection of the pyloric region and the first portion of the duodenum in the face of inflammation from peptic ulcer disease. The injury occurs during mobilization of the duodenum either for creation of a Billroth I gastroduodenostomy or for closure of the duodenal stump. Biliary injury during liver resection is most likely to occur during dissection of the hepatic hilum.

In addition to iatrogenic bile duct injury occurring during cholecystectomy or other operations, bile duct strictures can also occur at biliary anastomoses. Such strictures can occur at a biliary-enteric anastomosis performed for reconstruction after resection for benign or malignant disease of the pancreaticobiliary system, or after end-to-end bile duct anastomosis performed for hepatic transplantation or for repair of traumatic injury. Ischemia of the anastomosis caused by excessive skeletonization of the duct in preparation for the anastomosis is an important factor in many such strictures.

Unfortunately, the recurrence of bile duct strictures after an initial attempt at repair is not uncommon and can also account for a number of anastomotic strictures.[8,9] A number of other factors have been evaluated in patients who have a recurrent bile duct stricture, including the location of the stricture, the length of follow-up, the influence of previous operations, the type of operation performed, the type of sutures used, and the use and duration of postoperative stenting.[8] Previous attempts at repair, performance of a procedure other than choledochojejunostomy or hepaticojejunostomy, and stricture location higher in the biliary tree appear to be associated with a higher incidence of recurrent stricture. Finally, long-term follow-up of a bile duct anastomosis is important because strictures can develop years after the original anastomosis.

Clinical Presentation

Most patients with biliary injuries present early after their initial operation (Algorithm 61.1). After open cholecystectomy, only approximately 10% of postoperative strictures are actually suspected within the first week, but nearly 70% are diagnosed within the first 6 months, and more than 80% are diagnosed within 1 year of surgery. In series reporting bile duct injuries during laparoscopic cholecystectomy, the injury is usually recognized either during the procedure (25% to 30%) or, more commonly, in the early postoperative period.

2

Patients suspected of having a postoperative bile duct injury within days to weeks of initial operation usually present in one of two ways. One presentation is the progressive elevation of

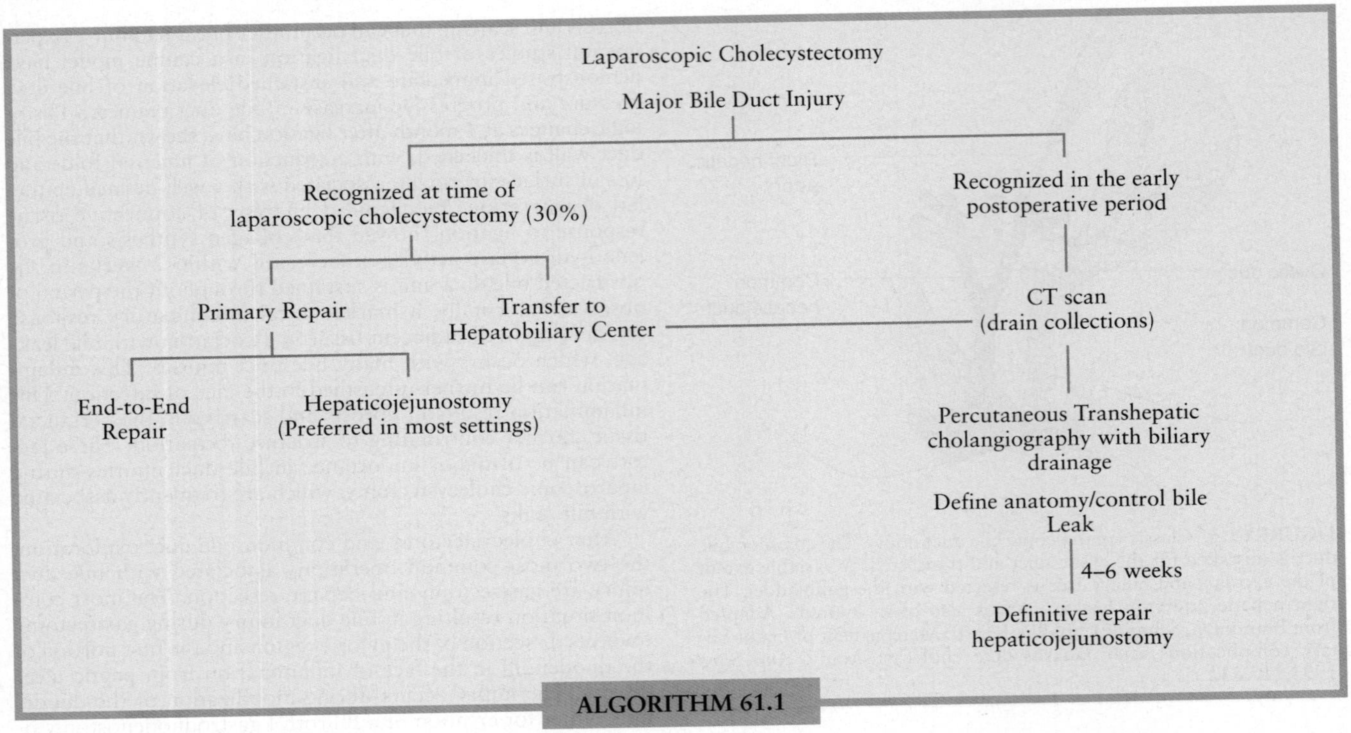

ALGORITHM 61.1. Algorithm for diagnosis and management of bile duct injury associated with laparoscopic cholecystectomy.

liver function test results, particularly total bilirubin and alkaline phosphatase levels. These changes can often be seen as early as the second or third postoperative day. The second mode of early presentation is with leakage of bile from the injured bile duct. This presentation appears to occur most often in patients presenting with bile duct injuries after laparoscopic cholecystectomy. Bilious drainage from operatively placed drains or through the wound after cholecystectomy is abnormal and represents some form of biliary injury. In patients without drains (including patients in whom the drains have been removed), the bile can leak freely into the peritoneal cavity or it can loculate as a collection. Free accumulation of bile into the peritoneal cavity results in either biliary ascites or bile peritonitis. Similarly, a loculated bile collection can result in sterile biloma (Fig. 61.4) or in an infected subhepatic or subdiaphragmatic abscess.

Patients with postoperative bile duct strictures who present months to years after the initial operation frequently have evidence of cholangitis. The episodes of cholangitis are often mild and respond to antibiotic therapy. Repetitive episodes usually occur before the definitive diagnosis. Less commonly, patients may present with painless jaundice and no evidence of sepsis. Finally, patients with markedly delayed diagnoses may present with advanced biliary cirrhosis and its complications.

Laboratory Investigation

Liver function tests usually show evidence of cholestasis. In patients with bile leakage, the bilirubin can be normal or minimally elevated because of absorption from the peritoneal cavity. When elevated, serum bilirubin usually ranges from 2 to 6 mg/dL, unless secondary biliary cirrhosis has developed. Serum alkaline phosphatase is usually elevated. Serum aminotransferase levels can be normal or minimally elevated except during episodes of cholangitis. If advanced liver disease exists, hepatic synthetic function can be impaired, with lowered serum albumin and a prolongation of prothrombin time. Serum electrolytes and complete blood count are typically normal unless there is associated biliary sepsis.

Radiologic Examination

The imaging techniques of abdominal ultrasound and computed tomography (CT) play an important initial role in the evaluation of patients with benign postoperative biliary strictures. In patients who present in the early postoperative period with evidence of a bile leak or biliary sepsis, these studies are useful to rule out the presence of intra-abdominal collections

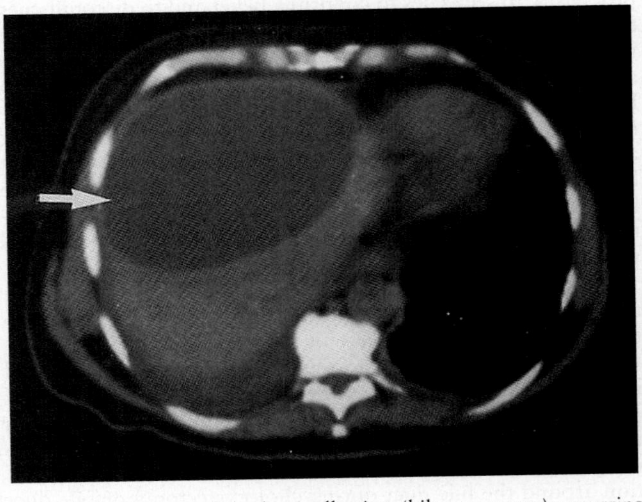

FIGURE 61.4. Large bile duct collection (biloma; *arrow*) occurring after bile duct injury. (Reproduced with permission from Lillemoe KD, Pitt HA, Cameron JL. Post-operative bile duct strictures. *Surg Clin North Am* 1990;70:1362.)

that might require drainage (Fig. 61.4). CT and ultrasound are also important in the initial evaluation of the patient presenting with a bile duct stricture months to years after initial operation. Both studies can confirm biliary obstruction by demonstrating a dilated biliary tree. CT is especially useful in identifying the level of obstruction of the extrahepatic bile duct.

In patients suspected of having early postoperative bile duct injury, a radionucleotide biliary scan can confirm bile leakage. In patients with postoperative external bile fistula, injection of water-soluble contrast media through the drainage tract (sinography) can often define the site of leakage and the anatomy of the biliary tree.

3 The "gold standard" for evaluation of patients with bile duct strictures is cholangiography. Percutaneous transhepatic cholangiography (PTC) is usually more valuable than endoscopic retrograde cholangiography (ERC) in patients with major bile duct injuries following laparoscopic cholecystectomy. PTC is more useful in that it defines the anatomy of the proximal biliary tree that is to be used in the surgical reconstruction (Fig. 61.5). Furthermore, PTC can be followed by placement of percutaneous transhepatic catheters, which can be useful in decompressing the biliary system either to treat or prevent cholangitis and to control an ongoing bile leak. These catheters can also be of assistance in surgical reconstruction and provide access to the biliary tree for nonoperative dilation. ERC is less useful than PTC in major bile duct transections during laparoscopic cholecystectomy because the discontinuity of the extrahepatic bile duct usually prevents adequate filling of the proximal biliary tree (Fig. 61.6). Often, ERC can demonstrate a normal-sized distal bile duct up to the site of the stricture without visualization of the proximal biliary system (Fig. 61.7). This finding is frequently the case in patients with injury during laparoscopic cholecystectomy, when the distal bile duct is often clipped and divided. The development of magnetic resonance cholangiopancreatography has provided a noninvasive technique that provides excellent delineation of the biliary anatomy. The quality of these images has led some surgeons to advocate this technique as the initial step in the evaluation of patients with suspected bile duct injuries and may eliminate the need for a diagnostic ERC in many patients.

Preoperative Management

The preoperative management of a patient with a postoperative bile duct stricture depends primarily on the timing of the presentation. Patients presenting in the early postoperative period can be septic with either cholangitis or intra-abdominal bile collections. Sepsis must be controlled first with broad-spectrum parenteral antibiotics, percutaneous biliary drainage, and percutaneous or operative drainage of biliary leaks. Once sepsis is controlled, there is no hurry in proceeding with surgical reconstruction of the bile duct stricture. The combination of proximal biliary decompression and external drainage allows most biliary fistulas to be controlled or even to close. The patient can then be discharged home to allow several weeks to elapse for resolution of the inflammation in the periportal region and recovery of overall health.

4 The management of a suspected bile duct injury after laparoscopic cholecystectomy presenting with a bile leak deserves special mention. Often, when bile leakage is suspected, the surgeon believes that urgent surgical exploration is necessary. Unfortunately, at laparotomy, the marked inflammation associated with bile spillage and the small decompressed biliary tree that appears retracted high into the porta hepatis make recognition of the injury and repair virtually impossible.

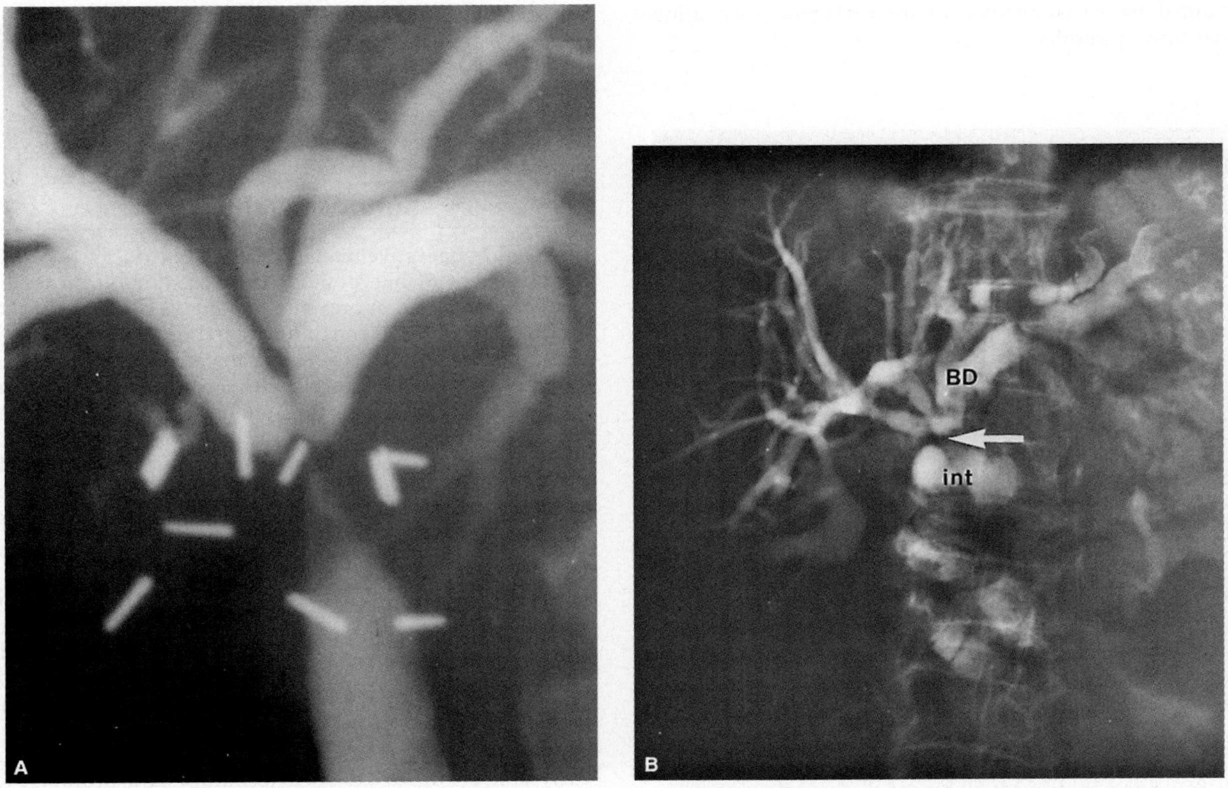

FIGURE 61.5. **A:** Percutaneous transhepatic cholangiogram demonstrating bile duct stricture at hepatic duct bifurcation with proximal duct dilatation. **B:** Percutaneous transhepatic cholangiogram demonstrating stricture (*arrow*) at a hepaticojejunostomy anastomosis. BD, bile duct; int, intestine.

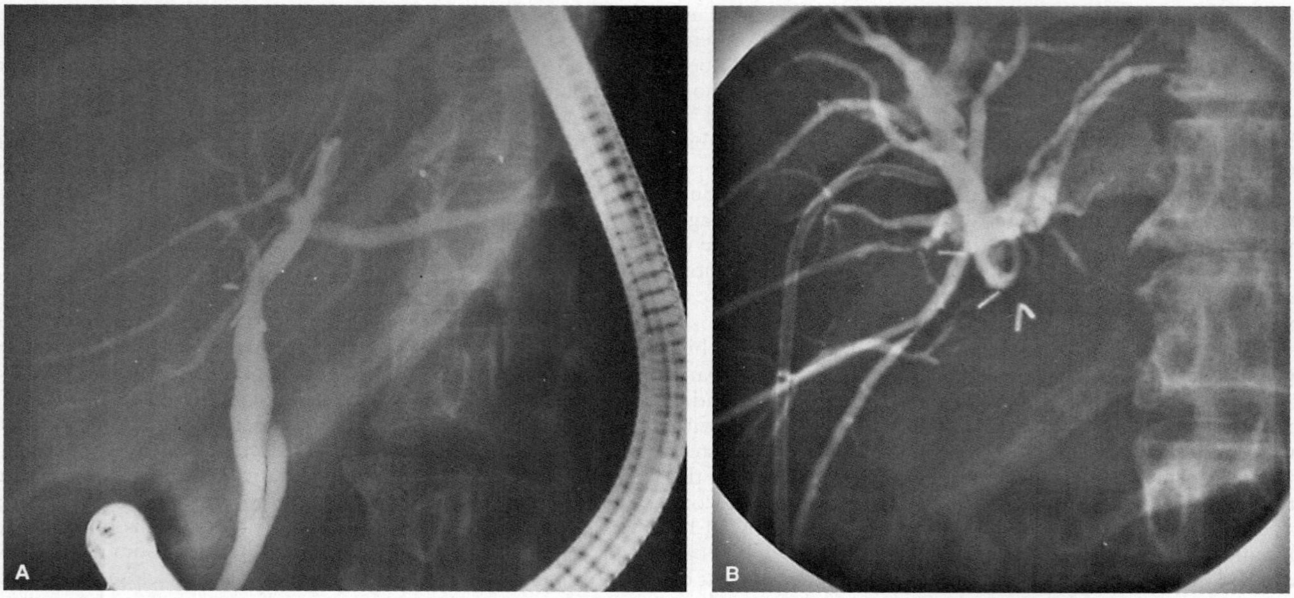

FIGURE 61.6. **A:** Endoscopic retrograde cholangiogram showing a relatively normal biliary tree in a patient with a postoperative bile collection (see Fig. 61.5). **B:** Percutaneous transhepatic cholangiogram of same patient, showing entire right hepatic posterior lobe segment obstructed as the result of ligation of the segmental duct. The patient had an unrecognized anatomic variant similar to that shown in Figure 61.2.

In such cases, every attempt should be made to define the biliary anatomy by preoperative cholangiography and to control the bile leak with percutaneous biliary drainage. In many cases, early operative intervention is not required because the bile collections or ascites can either be drained percutaneously or simply is absorbed from the peritoneal cavity. Delayed reconstruction, aided by percutaneous biliary catheters, then allows optimal surgical results.[10]

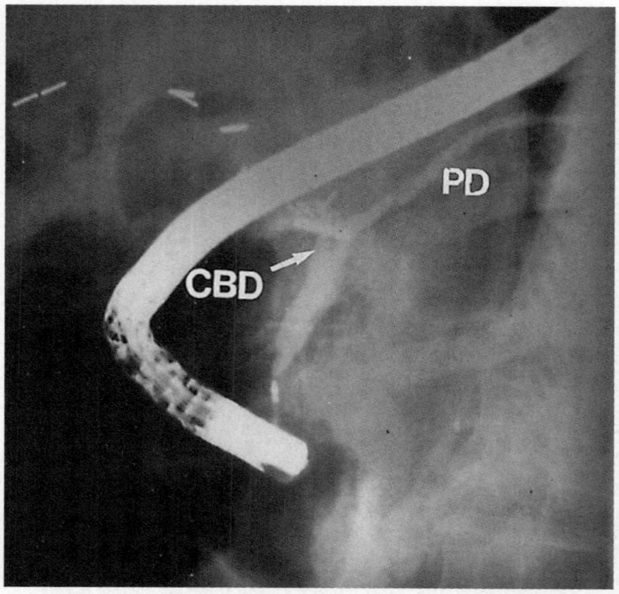

FIGURE 61.7. Endoscopic retrograde pancreaticocholangiogram showing filling of a normal pancreatic duct (PD). The common bile duct (CBD), however, does not fill beyond the large clip that appears to be placed across the duct. (Reproduced with permission from Lillemoe KD, Pitt HA, Cameron JL. Postoperative bile duct strictures. *Surg Clin North Am* 1990;70:1363.)

In patients who present with a biliary stricture remote from the initial operation, symptoms of cholangitis can necessitate urgent cholangiography and biliary decompression. Biliary drainage is best accomplished by the transhepatic method, although successful endoscopic stent placement can also be accomplished. Parenteral antibiotics and biliary drainage should be continued until sepsis is controlled. In patients who present with jaundice but without cholangitis, cholangiography should be performed to define the anatomy. Preoperative biliary decompression in patients without cholangitis has not been demonstrated to improve outcome.

Surgical Management

The goal of operative management of bile duct stricture is the establishment of bile flow into the proximal gastrointestinal tract in a manner that prevents cholangitis, sludge or stone formation, restricture, and biliary cirrhosis. This goal is best accomplished with a tension-free anastomosis between healthy tissues. A number of surgical alternatives exist for primary repair of bile duct strictures, including end-to-end repair, Roux-en-Y hepaticojejunostomy or choledochojejunostomy, choledochoduodenostomy, and mucosal grafting. The choice of repair depends on a number of factors, including the extent and location of the strictures, the experience of the surgeon, and the timing of the repair.

Immediate Repair of Intraoperative Bile Duct Injury. In many cases, initial proper management of bile duct injury recognized at the time of cholecystectomy can avoid the development of a bile duct stricture. Unfortunately, recognition of a bile duct injury is uncommon during either open or laparoscopic cholecystectomy. If bile leakage is observed or atypical anatomy is encountered during laparoscopic cholecystectomy, early conversion to an open technique and prompt cholangiography are imperative. If a segmental or accessory duct less than 3 mm has been injured and cholangiography demonstrates segmental or subsegmental drainage of the injured ductal system, simple ligation of the injured duct is adequate. If the injured duct is 4 mm or larger, however, it is likely to drain multiple hepatic segments or the entire right or left lobe and thus requires operative repair.

If the injury involves the common hepatic duct or the common bile duct, repair should also be carried out at the time of injury. The aims of any repair should be to maintain ductal length and not to sacrifice tissue as well as to effect a repair that will not result in postoperative bile leakage. To accomplish these goals, all repairs at the time of initial operation should involve some sort of external drainage. If the injured segment of the bile duct is short (<1 cm) and the two ends can be opposed without tension, an end-to-end anastomosis can be performed with placement of a T-tube through a separate choledochotomy either above or below the anastomosis (Fig. 61.8A). Generous mobilization of the duodenum out of the retroperitoneum (Kocher maneuver) can be useful to help approximate the injured ends of the bile duct. An end-to-end repair, however, should be avoided if the ductal injury is near the hepatic duct bifurcation.

For proximal injuries or if the injured segment of the bile duct is greater than 1 cm in length, an end-to-end bile duct anastomosis should be avoided because of the excessive tension that usually exists in these situations. In these circumstances, the distal bile duct should be oversewn, and the proximal bile duct should be débrided of injured tissue and anastomosed in an end-to-side fashion to a Roux-en-Y jejunal limb. The use of

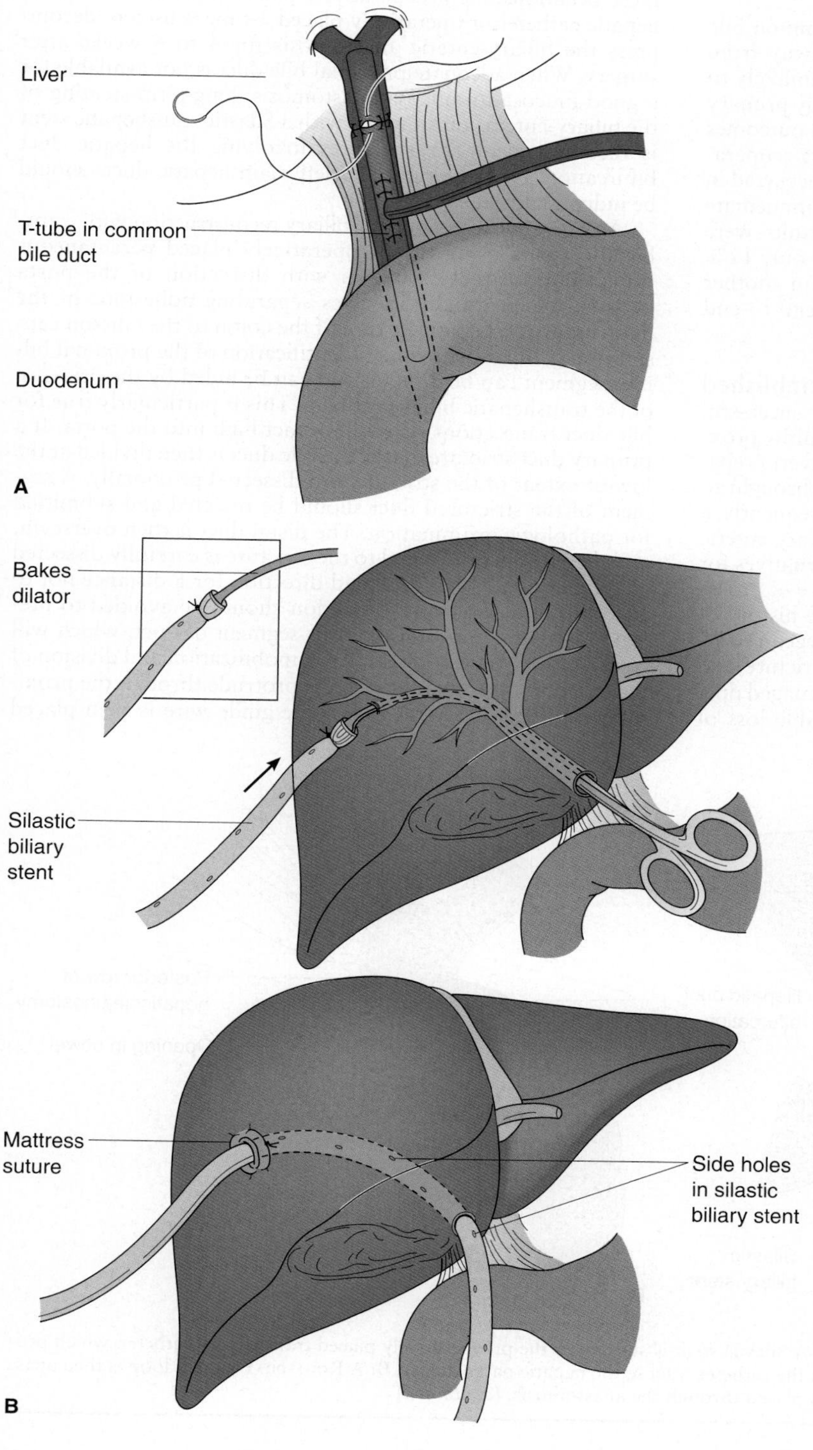

FIGURE 61.8. All biliary anastomoses performed for the reconstruction of acute bile duct injury should have external drainage. **A:** If the injured segment of bile duct is short (<1 cm) and the two ends can be opposed without tension, an end-to-end anastomosis can be performed with placement of a T-tube through a separate choledochotomy either above or below the anastomosis. The T-tube should not be brought out directly through the anastomosis. **B:** With more proximal injuries or if the segment of injured bile duct is greater than 1 cm, an end-to-end bile duct anastomosis should be avoided and a Roux-en-Y hepaticojejunostomy should be constructed. A transanastomotic stent can be placed retrograde through the transected duct and exited to the hepatic parenchyma to allow postoperative external drainage. (Adapted from Cameron JL. Resection of benign bile duct stricture with reconstruction utilizing Silastic transhepatic biliary stents and hepaticojejunostomy. In: *Atlas of Surgery,* vol 1. Ontario: BC Decker; 1990;47.)

a Roux-en-Y jejunal limb is preferable to anastomosis to the duodenum because, in the latter case, an anastomotic leak results in a duodenal fistula. A transanastomotic Silastic stent can be placed retrograde through the transected duct and exiting the hepatic parenchyma (Fig. 61.8B) to allow for postoperative external drainage.

Unfortunately, most bile duct injuries during laparoscopic cholecystectomy occur in the hands of surgeons who are not experienced in performing complex biliary reconstruction. In such settings, the surgeon should consider *not* repairing the injury and not risk further worsening the situation. The biliary tree should be drained via a retrograde catheter to facilitate cholangiography, but the bile duct should not be ligated. The subhepatic space should be well drained to control the biliary leak. Prompt transfer to a tertiary hepatobiliary center should then be made.

The long-term results of immediate repair of common bile duct injuries are uncertain. Most injuries occur away from major centers, and therefore even the successes are unlikely to be reported in the literature. In a Swedish report, early primary repair with end-to-end anastomosis resulted in good outcomes in only 22% of patients. Anastomotic leak requiring reoperation occurred in 32% of patients, and late stricture occurred in another 37% of patients. In patients undergoing immediate repair with a biliary-enteric anastomosis, good results were seen in 54% of patients, with strictures occurring in only 12% of patients. Similar poor late results were observed in another series in which 29 of 36 patients with primary end-to-end repair had postoperative strictures within 4 years.

Elective Repair of Bile Duct Injuries and Established Strictures. Several principles are associated with successful repair of a biliary injury or stricture: exposure of healthy proximal bile ducts that provide drainage of the entire liver; preparation of a suitable segment of intestine that can be brought to the area of the stricture without tension, most frequently a Roux-en-Y jejunal limb; and creation of a direct biliary-enteric mucosal-to-mucosal anastomosis. A number of alternatives for elective repair of bile duct strictures exist. The choice of procedure is dictated by the location of the stricture, the history of previous unsuccessful attempts at repair, and the surgeon's personal preference. Simple excision of a bile duct stricture and end-to-end bile duct anastomosis or repair of the damaged duct can rarely be accomplished because of the invariable loss of duct length as a result of fibrosis associated with the injury. Similarly, anastomosis of the proximal bile duct to the duodenum as a choledochoduodenostomy is not suitable for most postcholecystectomy strictures because an adequate length of bile duct for creating a tension-free anastomosis to the duodenum usually cannot be obtained. Thus, in almost all cases, hepaticojejunostomy constructed to a Roux-en-Y limb of jejunum is the preferred procedure.

5

Many surgeons believe that a transanastomotic stent is helpful in almost all cases. In the early postoperative period, a stent is used to decompress the biliary tree and provide access for cholangiography. If the injury involves the common bile duct or the common hepatic duct at least 2 cm distal to the hepatic duct bifurcation, and adequate proximal bile duct mucosa can be defined, the use of long-term biliary stents is not necessary. In these situations, the preoperatively placed percutaneous transhepatic catheter or operatively placed T-tube is used to decompress the biliary-enteric anastomosis for 4 to 6 weeks after surgery. When adequate proximal bile duct is not available for a good mucosa-to-mucosa anastomosis, long-term stenting of the biliary-enteric anastomosis with a Silastic transhepatic stent is recommended. For strictures involving the hepatic duct bifurcation, both the right and left main hepatic ducts should be individually stented.

An operative technique for biliary reconstruction with transhepatic stents using the preoperatively placed percutaneous transhepatic catheters begins with dissection of the porta hepatis, which usually involves separating adhesions of the duodenum and hepatic flexure of the colon to the Glisson capsule and gallbladder fossa.[11] Identification of the proximal biliary segment can be difficult and can be aided by the presence of the transhepatic biliary catheter. This is particularly true for bile duct transections that will retract high into the porta. If a primary duct stricture exists, the bile duct is then divided at the lowest extent of the stricture and dissected proximally. A segment of the strictured duct should be resected and submitted for pathologic examination. The distal duct is then oversewn, and the bile duct proximal to the stricture is carefully dissected circumferentially in a cephalad direction for a distance not to exceed 5 mm. Excessive dissection should be avoided to prevent vascular compromise of this segment of duct, which will be used for the anastomosis. After mobilization and division of the bile duct, the biliary catheters protrude through the proximal end (Fig. 61.9A). A radiologic guide wire is then placed

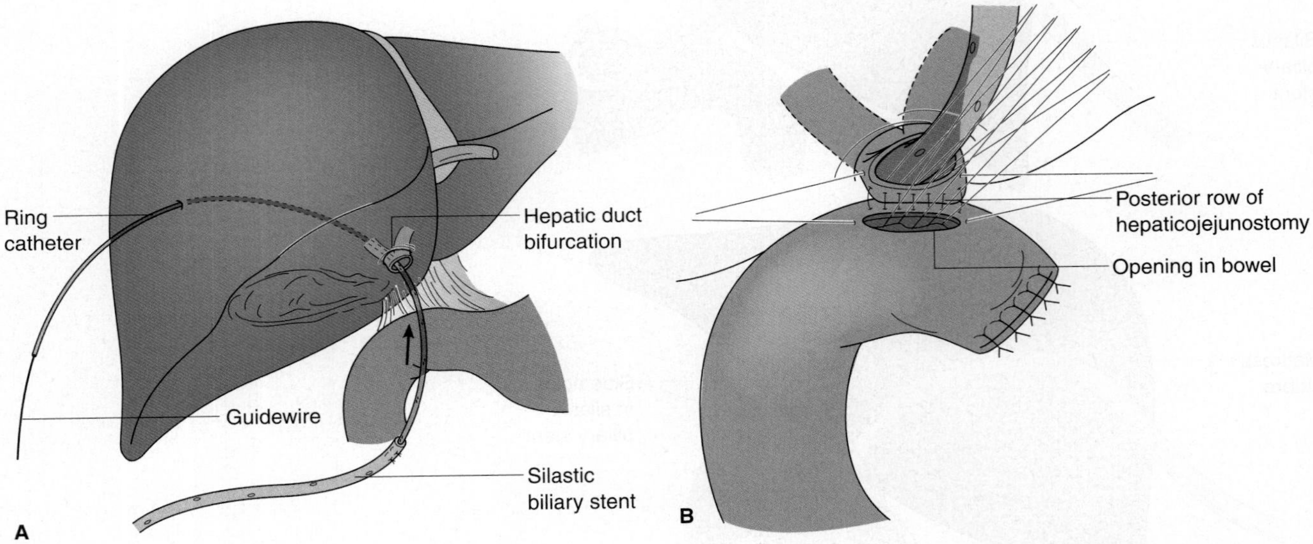

FIGURE 61.9. Technique of biliary reconstruction. **A:** A Silastic stent is sutured to the preoperatively placed transhepatic catheter, which protrudes through the transected hepatic duct and through the catheter tract in the hepatic parenchyma. **B:** A Roux-en-Y jejunal loop is then anastomosed to the hepatic duct and (**C**) the Silastic stent is placed through the anastomosis. (*continued*)

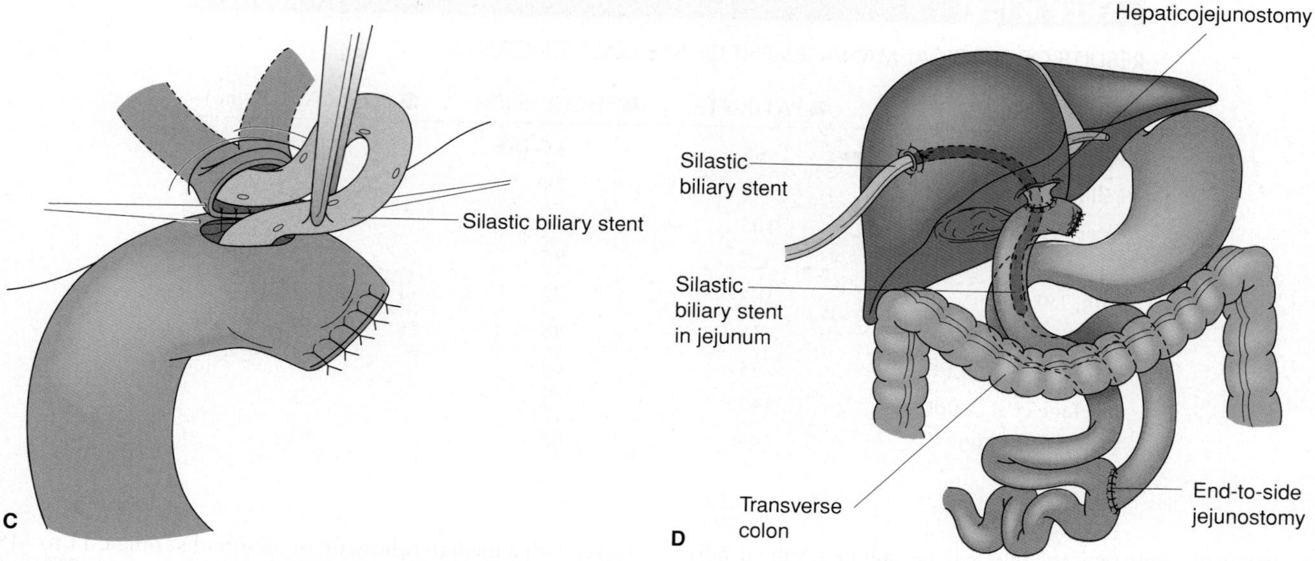

FIGURE 61.9. (*Continued*) D: A completed Roux-en-Y hepaticojejunostomy with a transanastomotic stent. (Adapted from Cameron JL. Resection of benign bile duct stricture with reconstruction utilizing silastic transhepatic biliary stents and hepaticojejunostomy. In: *Atlas of Surgery,* vol 1. Ontario: BC Decker; 1990:45, 55, 57.)

through these catheters. The preoperatively placed catheter can then be exchanged over the wire for a properly sized Silastic stent. These stents are 70 cm long and range from 12 French to 22 French. Multiple side holes are present along 40% of the length of the stent. These side holes are left to reside within the intrahepatic biliary tree and the portion of the Roux-en-Y jejunal limb used for the biliary anastomosis. The end of the stent without the side holes exits through the hepatic parenchyma and is brought out through a stab wound in the upper anterior abdomen. After stent placement, a Roux-en-Y jejunal limb is prepared, and the anastomosis is then performed as an end-to-side hepaticojejunostomy (Fig. 61.9B–D).

An alternative technique has been described for management of bile duct strictures involving the bifurcation and one or both of the hepatic ducts in which a side-to-side anastomosis of the left hepatic duct to the Roux-en-Y limb is constructed. A long opening along the anterior surface of the left hepatic duct is anastomosed to the side of the Roux-en-Y limb. Because it is possible to dissect the anterior surface of the left hepatic duct high up into the hepatic parenchyma, this procedure permits anastomosis to normal mucosa, even though there can be fibrosis and stricture at the bifurcation of the ducts and in the distal portion of the hepatic duct. This technique can avoid the need for postoperative stenting.

Surgical Outcome

Morbidity and Mortality. Repairs of bile duct strictures are performed primarily in major medical centers by experienced surgeons, yet these operations are still associated with significant morbidity and mortality. In 1982, a review of 38 series published since 1900 that included more than 7,643 procedures performed on 5,586 patients reported an overall operative mortality rate of 8.3%.[12] More recently the incidence of operative mortality has decreased markedly with improved technology and a multidisciplinary approach as well as improved surgical experience. A recent series of 200 consecutive patients managed at the Johns Hopkins Hospital reported three deaths in patients who did not undergo an attempt at repair who were referred with sepsis secondary to an uncontrolled biliary leak, for a mortality rate of 1.5%. Definitive surgical reconstruction was performed in 175 patients with a perioperative mortality of only 1.7%.[13] In this series the timing of repair, the mode of presentation, previous attempts of repair, and the level of injury did not influence outcome. Chronic liver disease can be an important factor for operative mortality and morbidity with advanced biliary cirrhosis and portal hypertension leading to mortality rates approaching 30%. Fortunately in the modern era, such advanced disease is uncommon. In most series postoperative morbidity rates are in the range of 20% to 40%. In the recent Hopkins series, complications occurred in 41% of patients. Most of the complications were minor and could be managed with either interventional radiology techniques or conservative management. No patient required reoperation for postoperative complications. The median length of stay in this series was 8 days.

Long-term Results. Historically, excellent long-term results were achieved in 70% to 90% of patients who underwent repair of bile duct strictures (Table 61.2). The definition of satisfactory results in most series requires that patients have no symptoms, jaundice, or cholangitis. Length of follow-up is important in analyzing final results because recurrent strictures can occur up to 20 years after the initial procedure (Fig. 61.10).[8,9] Approximately two thirds of restrictures are evident within 2 years, and 90% are seen within 7 years. The percentage of patients with good results is inversely related to the number of previous repairs. Other factors that favor a good outcome include young age at the time of stricture repair, use of a Roux-en-Y biliary-enteric anastomosis, absence of infection and hepatic fibrosis, and use of transhepatic stents.

As illustrated earlier, in the era before laparoscopic cholecystectomy, excellent long-term results were obtainable in tertiary care centers specializing in the management of these problems. Questions had arisen as to whether the excellent results of bile duct strictures after open cholecystectomy could be directly transferred to patients sustaining laparoscopic bile duct injuries. Some researchers had suggested that the mechanism of bile duct injury during laparoscopic cholecystectomy, the complex nature of many of these injuries, and the frequent association of significant inflammation and fibrosis secondary

TABLE 61.2 **RESULTS**

RESULTS OF SURGICAL MANAGEMENT OF BILE DUCT STRICTURES

INVESTIGATORS	PATIENTS	SUCCESS (%)	FOLLOW-UP (mo)
Pitt et al., 1982[8]	66	86	60
Pelligrini et al., 1984[9]	60	78	102
Genest, 1986	105	82	60
Innes, 1988	22	95	72
Pain, 1988	163	72	133
Pitt et al., 1989[27]	25	88	57
David et al., 1993[28]	35	83	50
Lillemoe et al., 2000[15]	142	91	58
Walsh et al., 2007[17]	144	89	67

to sustained, unrecognized bile leakage might result in poor long-term results. Furthermore, the high percentage of these patients who have undergone unsuccessful operations, often performed by the primary laparoscopic surgeon, might also lead to a poor long-term outcome. Evidence for the latter hypothesis was provided by a review of the records of 85 patients who underwent a total of 112 biliary repairs.[14] Four factors determined the success or failure of treatment in this series. These factors included performance of preoperative cholangiography, the choice of surgical repair, details of the operative repair, and experience of the surgeon performing the repair. The importance of preoperative delineation of anatomy was clear, in that 96% of procedures in which cholangiograms were not obtained before repair were unsuccessful, and 69% of repairs were not successful when the cholangiographic data were incomplete. When cholangiographic data were complete, the initial repair was successful in 84% of patients. The type of repair was also of significance in influencing outcome. A primary end-to-end ductal repair over a T-tube was unsuccessful in all patients in whom a complete transection of the bile duct had taken place, whereas 63% of Roux-en-Y hepaticojejunostomies were successful. Attempts at repair by the primary surgeon were successful only in 17% of cases, and in no case was a secondary repair by the primary surgeon successful. In those cases in which the first repair was performed by a tertiary care biliary surgeon, a 94% success rate was obtained.

The outcome of management of 142 patients with major bile duct injuries treated during the 1990s has been reported.[15] Laparoscopic cholecystectomy was the initial operation in 75% of these patients, and 41% had undergone a previous attempt or attempts at surgical repair before referral. In this series with a median follow-up of 58 months (range, 11 to 119 months), a successful outcome was obtained in 91% of patients. In this series the level of injury, clinical presentation, history of prior repair, and length of biliary stenting did not influence outcome. Comparable results have been reported from other high-volume hepatobiliary centers.[16,17] These results suggest that surgical reconstruction of major bile duct injuries after laparoscopic cholecystectomy can still result in excellent long-term results.

6

Despite the overall success of biliary reconstruction, there is a small subset of patients with major bile duct injuries in whom standard repair techniques appear to be inadequate. Factors such as delay in diagnosis, complex injuries above the hepatic confluence, associated vascular injuries, and liver atrophy can all negatively affect the outcomes of standard reconstruction. In this select population excellent results have been observed with major hepatectomy.[18] Finally, in rare cases with failure of all standard surgical techniques of reconstruction with resultant end-stage liver disease, liver transplantation may offer the opportunity for survival.[19]

Although large series from tertiary referral centers have reported excellent long-term results, the overall impact of bile duct injuries on society is significant in terms of health care costs, disability, and even mortality. In an analysis of patients undergoing laparoscopic cholecystectomy from the U.S. Medicare database, Flum et al. demonstrated that the adjusted hazard ratio for death during the follow-up period was significantly higher (2.79, 95% confidence level 2.71–2.88) for patients with a bile duct injury than in those patients without a bile duct injury.[20] The hazard increased with advancing age and comorbidities and decreased with the experience of the

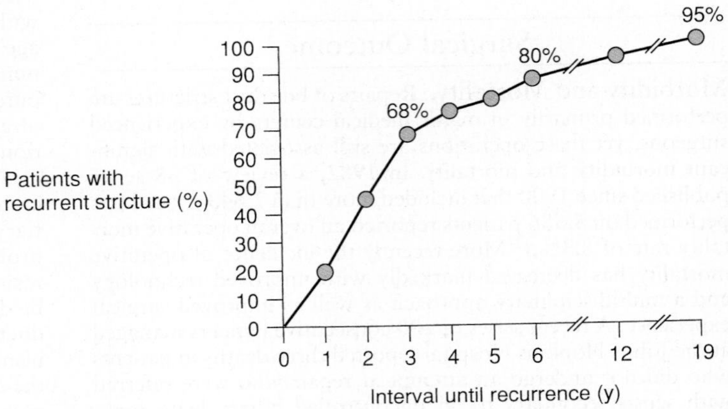

FIGURE 61.10. The cumulative percentage of recurrent strictures with respect to the time from the initial repair until the next repair. (Adapted from Pitt HA, Miyamoto T, Parapatis SK, et al. Factors influencing outcome in patients with postoperative biliary strictures. *Am J Surg* 1982;144:14.)

repairing surgeon. The adjusted hazard of death during follow-up was 11% greater if the repairing surgeon was the same as the injuring surgeon. These data certainly further support the referral of most patients with bile duct injuries to centers with greater experience in the management of the injuries.

Finally, although the overall success of the surgical management of laparoscopic bile duct injuries associated with laparoscopic cholecystectomy is excellent, there is an impression that patients may have an impaired quality of life even after successful repair of their bile duct injury. Quality-of-life assessments after laparoscopic cholecystectomy bile duct injury have been addressed in several recent reports.[21,22] These results have generally reported either comparable or mildly diminished quality of life compared with matched controls. Interestingly, in one study, patients who reported pursuing a law suit following their injury had significantly worse quality-of-life scores in all domains when compared to those who did not entertain legal action.[21]

Nonoperative Management

Operative management of bile duct strictures is technically difficult and continues to be associated with significant postoperative morbidity and mortality. Moreover, in all series, recurrent strictures develop in a proportion of patients. These factors, in addition to technical advances in the fields of therapeutic radiology and endoscopy, have led to the development of nonoperative techniques for management of bile duct strictures. The optimal method for management using these techniques is dependent on the presence and anatomy of biliary-enteric continuity.

Percutaneous Balloon Dilation. The management of benign bile duct strictures using the percutaneous transhepatic route is indicated primarily in patients with a failed prior biliary enteric anastomosis to a jejunal limb. The procedure in many cases can be performed with a combination of local anesthesia and intravenous sedation. In this technique, access to the proximal biliary tree is gained and the stricture is traversed with a guide wire under fluoroscopic guidance. At this point, the stricture is dilated using angioplasty-type balloon catheters, chosen on the basis of the location of the stricture and the diameter of the normal duct (Fig. 61.11). After the procedure, a transhepatic stent is left in place across the stricture to allow access to the biliary tree for follow-up cholangiography, repeat dilation, and maintenance of a lumen during the healing process. In most series, numerous dilations are required.

The results from a number of series have been encouraging (Table 61.3). In a multicenter review of bile duct strictures treated in the open cholecystectomy era, 3-year follow-up showed a 67% patency rate for anastomotic and a 76% patency rate for iatrogenic primary bile duct strictures, yielding an overall 70% success rate.[23] A report of 51 patients with bile duct strictures after laparoscopic cholecystectomy managed with percutaneous dilation showed a success rate of 58% with a mean follow-up of 76 months.[24]

Complications of balloon dilation are frequent. Cholangitis, hemobilia, and bile leaks can occur in up to 20% of patients. Bleeding, usually from the hepatic parenchyma, has been reported, with transfusions often necessary. Sepsis due to cholangitis can occur despite antibiotic prophylaxis. Sepsis and significant bleeding seldom occur in patients dilated by a T-tube tract, suggesting that much of the morbidity is the result of traversing the hepatic parenchyma by the large percutaneously placed catheters.

Endoscopic Balloon Dilation

Endoscopic balloon dilation is technically possible only in patients with primary bile duct strictures or with strictures at a prior primary end-to-end repair or choledochoduodenal anastomosis. This technique begins with ERC and endoscopic sphincterotomy. The stricture is traversed retrograde with an atraumatic guide wire, and sequential balloon dilation is used. Reevaluation with cholangiography is performed every 3 to 6 months. Redilation is performed as necessary. In most cases, an endoprosthesis is left in place after dilation for at least 12 months.

The reported experience with endoscopic dilation of benign bile duct strictures is shown in Table 61.4. The largest experience comes from the group in The Netherlands who recently reported their experience in 110 patients.[25] The mean number of stents placed was two, the mean duration of stenting was 11 months, and stent-related complications occurred in 33% of patients with one death. Twenty percent of patients were eventually referred for surgery. The overall reported success rate was 74% with a mean follow-up of 7.6 years. A similar experience was reported in the United States.[26] In this series, 18 of 25 strictures were postoperative. Strictures were located at the cystic duct junction in 17 patients and in the distal bile duct in the remaining eight patients. Of 25 patients, 22 (88%) had significant clinical benefit from the therapy. Only two complications occurred in this series—one case each of pancreatitis and cholangitis.

Comparative Data

Comparison of results of nonoperative dilation with those of surgery have been difficult. Few centers have significant experience with both operative and nonoperative management. Furthermore, the definition of a successful procedure, the reporting of complications, and the length of follow-up have not been consistent in the literature. There are no prospective randomized studies to compare these techniques; however, two retrospective comparative studies exist. In the first study, a retrospective review of the results at the Johns Hopkins Hospital between 1979 and 1987 compared percutaneous balloon dilation and surgery in 43 patients with benign postoperative bile duct strictures.[27] Twenty-five patients underwent surgical repair with Roux-en-Y hepaticojejunostomy with postoperative transhepatic stenting for a mean of 13 ± 1.3 months. Twenty patients had percutaneous balloon dilation, a mean of 3.9 times, and were stented transhepatically for a mean of 13.3 ± 2 months. Three patients were managed with both surgery and balloon dilation. The two groups were similar with respect to multiple parameters that might have influenced outcome, including age, sex, associated medical problems, and presentation with either obstructive jaundice or biliary fistulas. No patients died after any of the procedures. Procedure-related morbidity occurred in 20% of surgical patients and in 35% of the patients undergoing balloon dilation. For both groups, a successful outcome was defined as no evidence of cholangitis or jaundice requiring another procedure more than 12 months from the onset of treatment. A failed treatment was defined as the need for crossover to the other treatment modality, either operation or dilation, or late death from liver failure, biliary sepsis, or portal hypertension. A successful repair was achieved in 89% of the surgical patients and in only 52% of the balloon dilation patients (Fig. 61.12). The overall late mortality rate in this series was 10%. One late death occurred in the surgical group, whereas three late deaths followed balloon dilation (4% vs. 15%, respectively). No deaths, however, were attributed to liver failure, biliary sepsis, or portal hypertension associated with the bile duct stricture.

To define further the relative benefits of the two procedures, total hospital stay and total procedural costs were determined. As expected, initial hospitalization was longer for surgery than for balloon dilation. When rehospitalization for further dilation, complications, or recurrences was considered, total hospital stay did not differ significantly between the two

TABLE 61.3 **RESULTS**

RESULTS OF TRANSHEPATIC BALLOON DILATION OF BILE DUCT STRICTURES

■ INVESTIGATORS	■ PATIENTS	■ SUCCESS (%)	■ FOLLOW-UP (mo)
Mueller et al., 1986[23]	61	70	36
Williams, 1987	64	78	28
Moore, 1987	18	83	33
Pitt et al., 1989[27]	20	55	59
Citron et al., 1991	28	93	38
Misra et al., 2004[24]	51	58	76

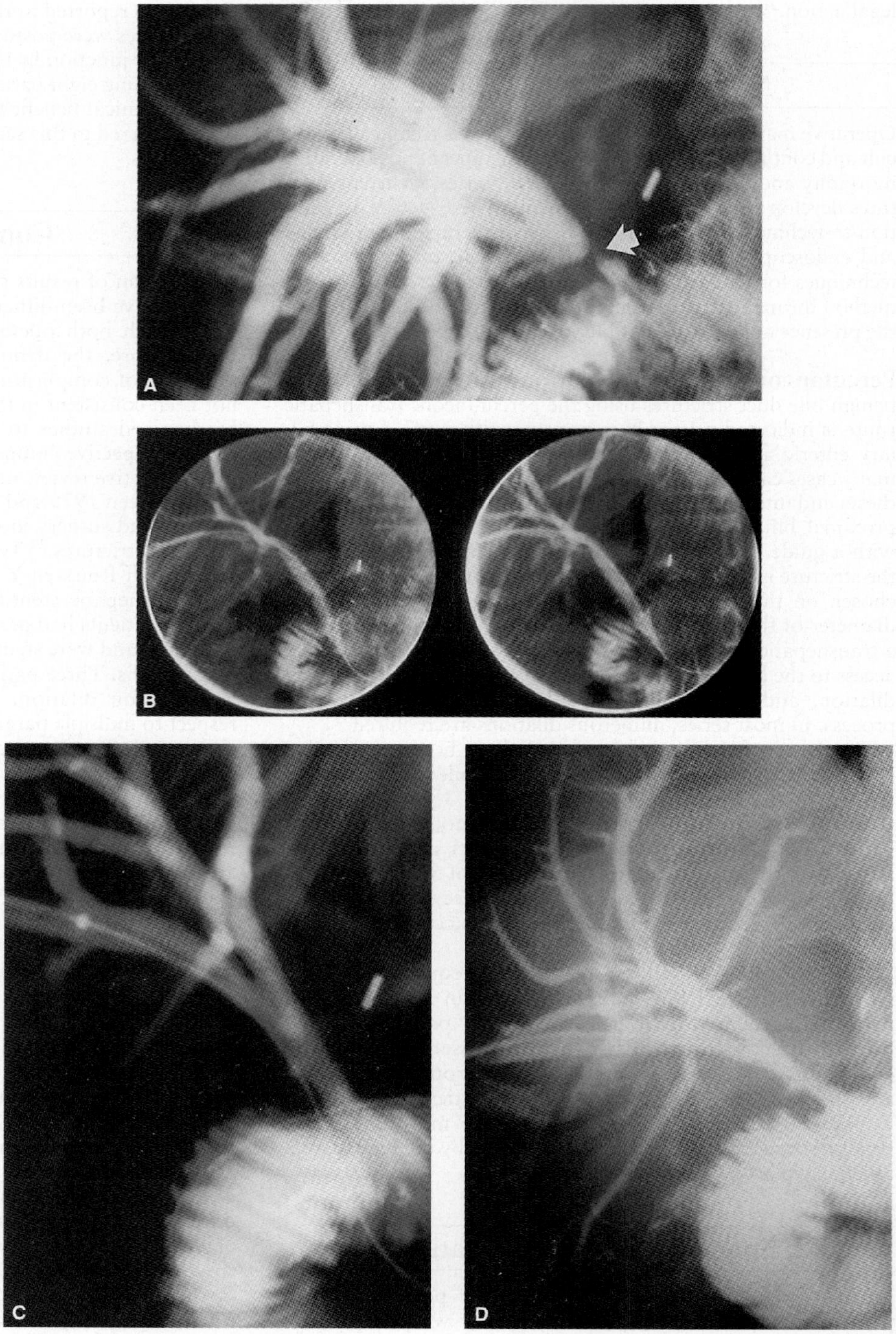

FIGURE 61.11. A: Transhepatic cholangiogram demonstrating stricture (*arrow*) at a previous choledochojejunostomy. **B:** Progressive dilation of the strictured anastomosis with an angioplasty balloon catheter. **C:** Postdilation stenting of the anastomotic stricture for prolonged periods. **D:** Subsequent cholangiogram demonstrating resolution of the anastomotic stricture. (Reproduced with permission from Pitt HA, Kaufman SL, Coleman J, et al. Benign postoperative biliary strictures: operate or dilate? *Ann Surg* 1989;210:417.)

TABLE 61.4 **RESULTS**

RESULTS OF ENDOSCOPIC BALLOON DILATATION OF BILE DUCT STRICTURES

INVESTIGATORS	PATIENTS	SUCCESS (%)	FOLLOW-UP (mo)
Foutsch, 1985	9	55	6
Geenen et al., 1989[26]	25	88	48
David et al., 1993[28]	46	83	48
De Reuver et al., 2007[25]	110	74	91

groups. Cost data paralleled hospitalization data and did not 7 differ significantly between the groups. Thus, the authors concluded that until properly designed, randomized, prospective, controlled trials can be performed, surgical repair for benign postoperative strictures appears to be associated with fewer problems and a greater success rate.

In the second comparative study, the group from The Netherlands compared endoscopic versus surgical treatment of benign bile duct strictures.[28] Thirty-five patients were treated surgically, and 66 were treated by endoscopic stenting. Patient characteristics, initial injury, previous repairs, and the level of obstruction were comparable in both groups. Surgical therapy consisted of Roux-en-Y hepaticojejunostomy, and endoscopic therapy consisted of placement of an endoprosthesis with trimonthly elective exchange for 1 year. Successful stent placement was accomplished in 94% of patients managed endoscopically. Six of the 66 endoscopic patients, however, underwent surgical reconstruction either for failed stent placement or for other reasons. Early complications occurred more frequently in the surgically treated group (26% vs. 8%; $p < 0.03$). However, the only procedure-related death occurred in a patient in whom severe pancreatitis developed after endoscopic stent placement. Late complications, which included primarily episodes of cholangitis, occurred only in the endoscopic group (27%). The overall complication rates, therefore, were similar at 26% for surgical patients and 35% for endoscopic patients. The mean follow-up and definition of success were similar to those in the aforementioned study. After surgery, excellent results were observed in 83% of patients, with a recurrent stricture developing in six patients at a mean of 40 months after the initial operation. After endoscopic stenting, excellent results were observed in 72% of patients, with restricture developing in 18% of patients at a mean of 3 months after stent removal. The investigators concluded that endoscopic stenting should be considered for the initial attempt at definitive management in suitable patients in the hope of avoiding reoperation.

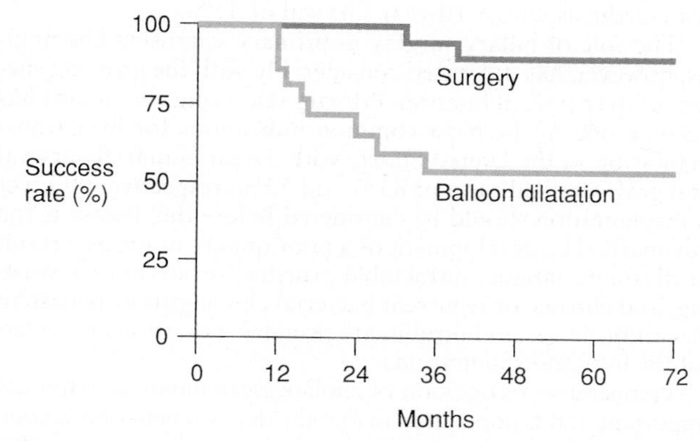

FIGURE 61.12. Actuarial success rates over 72 months for surgery (89%) and balloon dilation (52%). The difference is statistically significant ($p < 0.01$). (Adapted from Pitt HA, Kaufman SL, Coleman J, et al. Benign postoperative biliary strictures: operate or dilate? *Ann Surg* 1989;210:417.)

PRIMARY SCLEROSING CHOLANGITIS

8 Primary sclerosing cholangitis is an idiopathic disease characterized by intrahepatic and extrahepatic inflammatory strictures of the bile ducts that cannot be attributed to other specific causes. The cause of primary sclerosing cholangitis is unknown. Many experts consider primary sclerosing cholangitis to be an autoimmune reaction because it is associated with other autoimmune diseases, such as ulcerative colitis, retroperitoneal fibrosis, and Riedel thyroiditis (Table 61.5). It is likely that a number of causes, including viral or bacterial infections, toxic drug reactions, and congenital anomalies, can all result in the same end-stage injury that is recognized as primary sclerosing cholangitis.

The usual clinical presentation of patients with primary sclerosing cholangitis involves intermittent jaundice, which begins insidiously in the fourth or fifth decade of life. Right upper quadrant pain, pruritus, fever, weight loss, and fatigue can also occur. The disease is characterized by cyclic remissions and exacerbations. Despite the nomenclature, acute

TABLE 61.5

DISEASES ASSOCIATED WITH PRIMARY SCLEROSING CHOLANGITIS

DISEASE	FREQUENCY (%)
Ulcerative colitis	40–60
Pancreatitis	12–25
Diabetes mellitus	5–10
Retroperitoneal fibrosis	Rare
Riedel thyroiditis	Rare
Crohn disease	Rare
Histiocytosis X	Rare
Sicca complex	Rare
Rheumatoid arthritis	Rare
Hypertrophic osteoarthropathy	Rare
Sarcoidosis	Rare
Angioimmunoblastic lymphadenopathy	Rare
Acquired immunodeficiency syndrome	Rare

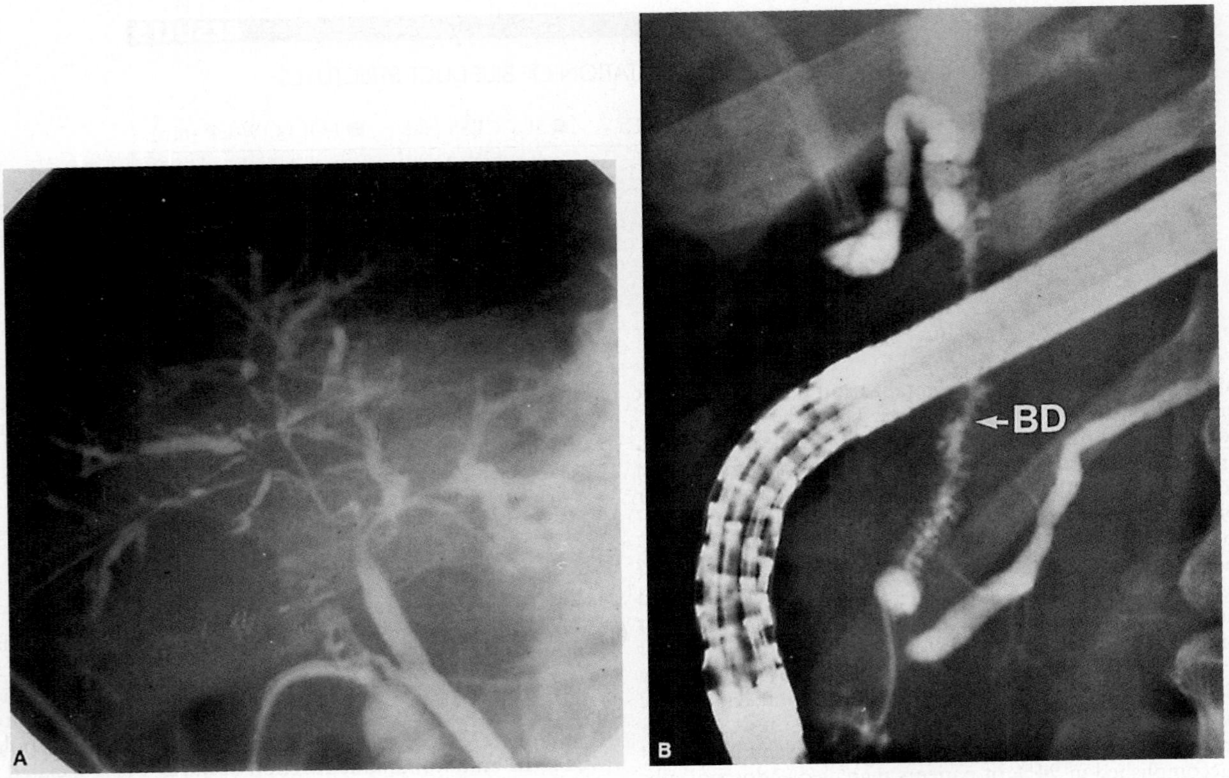

FIGURE 61.13. **A:** Cholangiogram of a patient with primary sclerosing cholangitis. Multiple irregular strictures and dilatation (beading) of intrahepatic bile ducts can be seen. **B:** Endoscopic retrograde cholangiogram showing extensive involvement of extrahepatic bile duct (BD) with primary sclerosing cholangitis. (B reproduced with permission from Lillemoe KD, Pitt HA, Cameron JL. Primary sclerosing cholangitis. *Surg Clin North Am* 1990;70:1390.)

cholangitis is uncommon without previous biliary manipulation or surgery. The diagnosis is suggested by clinical presentation associated with cholestatic liver function test abnormalities. The levels of bilirubin often fluctuate with respect to the remissions and exacerbations of the disease and the extent of hepatic injury. Alkaline phosphatase is usually elevated out of proportion to the serum bilirubin, and is a more persistent finding. The diagnosis, however, usually is confirmed by cholangiography, which reveals multiple dilatations and strictures (beading) of the intrahepatic and extrahepatic bile ducts (Fig. 61.13). Magnetic resonance cholangiopancreatography (MRCP) has become the preferred procedure as it is noninvasive. ERC, however, remains an important tool for both diagnostic and therapeutic procedures. An important distinction must be made as cholangiocarcinoma must be considered in the differential diagnosis of a dominant stricture. Furthermore, cholangiocarcinoma may develop after presentation in up to 30% of patients with primary sclerosing cholangitis. Therefore, endoscopic brushings and biopsies are frequently required. The disease should be followed closely by cholangiography and liver biopsy to provide appropriate management before the development of biliary cirrhosis.

No known specific medical therapy is effective for primary sclerosing cholangitis. The most encouraging results, from a prospective, randomized, placebo-controlled trial, suggest that ursodeoxycholic acid significantly improves serum liver function tests and liver histologic appearance. Unfortunately, there were no significant differences in clinical outcome between the two groups at up to 6 years of follow-up.[29] Nonoperative dilation therapy by the endoscopic route has been used for dominant strictures with favorable results.[30]

An aggressive surgical approach is advocated for selected symptomatic patients with primary sclerosing cholangitis because of the lack of effective medical therapy. One surgical approach, in patients with a dominant stricture at the hepatic duct bifurcation, uses resection of the bifurcation and long-term transhepatic stenting with Silastic stents. This mode of therapy was recently reported in 77 patients with resection of the hepatic duct bifurcation, with hepatic lobectomy performed in another four patients.[31] The perioperative complication rate was 39% and 30-day mortality was 3.9%. Bilirubin improved and 57% of patients had no primary sclerosing cholangitis–related readmissions. At median follow-up of 10.5 years, the 5- and 10-year survival rates were 76.4% and 52.7%, respectively. Cholangiocarcinoma did not develop in any patients and only seven required liver transplant. Over the same period, liver transplant was performed in 49 patients with cirrhosis with a 10-year survival of 57%.

The role of biliary surgery in primary sclerosing cholangitis, however, has decreased considerably with the growing success of liver transplantation. Primary sclerosing cholangitis has become one of the most common indications for liver transplantation in the United States, with 5-year actuarial survival and graft survival rates of 85% and 72%, respectively.[32] Liver transplantation should be considered before the disease is too advanced. The development of a poor quality of life as a result of disabling fatigue, intractable pruritus, severe muscle wasting, and chronic or recurrent bacterial cholangitis or persistent elevations in serum bilirubin are primary indications for referral for liver transplantation.

Preoperative recognition of cholangiocarcinoma is extremely important in this population in that the development of this complication significantly worsens the result after liver transplantation. The presence of known malignancy results in patients being refused transplantation. The microscopic identification of intrahepatic cholangiocarcinoma in the absence of lymph node involvement, often demonstrated in the explanted liver specimen, however, does not usually portend a poor prognosis.

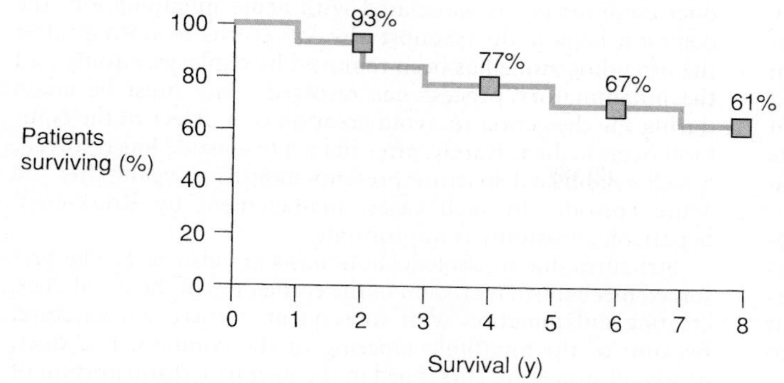

FIGURE 61.14. Actuarial survival rates among 31 noncirrhotic patients with primary sclerosing cholangitis who underwent resection of the hepatic bifurcation and long-term transhepatic stenting. (Reproduced with permission from Lillemoe KD, Pitt HA, Cameron JL. Primary sclerosing cholangitis. *Surg Clin North Am* 1990;70:1397.)

Patients with primary sclerosing cholangitis have a significantly higher rate of development of nonanastomotic biliary strictures after liver transplantation, with histologic features on posttransplantation biopsy consistent with recurrence of the disease. Other causes of stricture, such as hepatic artery thrombosis, preservation-related ischemia, cytomegalovirus infection, and chronic ductopenic rejection, can cause similar lesions. Recurrent primary sclerosing cholangitis usually does not have an aggressive course.

Resection of the hepatic duct bifurcation and long-term transanastomotic stenting in selected patients can preclude or delay the need for hepatic transplantation. Moreover, this operation does not eliminate or influence the results of hepatic transplantation. Resection of the hepatic bifurcation and long-term transhepatic stenting can be recommended for selected patients with primary sclerosing cholangitis with severe strictures at or distal to the hepatic duct bifurcation but without established biliary cirrhosis. In patients with biliary cirrhosis, hepatic transplantation is recommended.

BILE DUCT STRICTURES SECONDARY TO CHRONIC PANCREATITIS

Chronic pancreatitis is an uncommon cause of benign bile duct strictures, resulting in less than 10% of such cases. Transient partial obstruction of the distal common bile duct caused by inflammation and edema frequently occurs in patients with acute pancreatitis. With chronic pancreatitis, however, the clinical problem is distal bile duct obstruction caused by inflammation and parenchymal fibrosis of the gland. These strictures classically involve the entire intrapancreatic segment of the common bile duct and are associated with dilatation of the entire proximal biliary tree (Fig. 61.14). In most cases, the cause of the chronic pancreatitis is alcoholism. Often, advanced disease is present in that the incidence of pancreatic calcification, diabetes, and malabsorption is increased at the time of presentation with jaundice compared with patients with chronic pancreatitis without jaundice. Common bile duct strictures have been reported to occur in 3% to 29% of patients with chronic alcoholic pancreatitis. In a review of a number of clinical series, the overall incidence of common bile duct strictures in patients with chronic pancreatitis was 5.7%.[33] The exact incidence of common bile duct strictures is not known, however, because cholangiography is not routinely performed in patients with chronic pancreatitis.

The clinical presentation of patients with common bile duct strictures secondary to chronic pancreatitis is variable. Some patients have no symptoms, with the diagnosis of bile duct strictures suggested only by abnormal liver function test results. The serum alkaline phosphatase appears to be the most sensitive laboratory finding and is elevated in more than 80% of patients. Abdominal pain with or without jaundice is another common presentation. In some cases, the abdominal pain can be difficult to distinguish from the pain associated with chronic pancreatitis. Failure to recognize and address a bile duct stricture, however, can lead to ultimate failure of operative procedures performed for chronic pain in patients with chronic pancreatitis. Finally, the development of jaundice in patients with chronic pancreatitis must be differentiated from underlying periampullary malignancy.

The definitive evaluation of patients with a bile duct stricture caused by chronic pancreatitis is cholangiography. Either MRCP or endoscopic retrograde cholangiopancreatography (ERCP) is the preferred diagnostic procedure as they both can demonstrate both biliary and pancreatic ductal anatomy, which is essential in optimal surgical management of chronic pancreatitis. ERCP with stenting allows decompression of the obstructed biliary tree if necessary for cholangitis or severe jaundice. A long (usually 2- to 4-cm), smooth, gradual tapering of the common bile duct is most compatible with a benign stricture due to chronic pancreatitis (Fig. 61.15).

The indications for surgical management of common bile duct strictures due to chronic pancreatitis are clear in patients

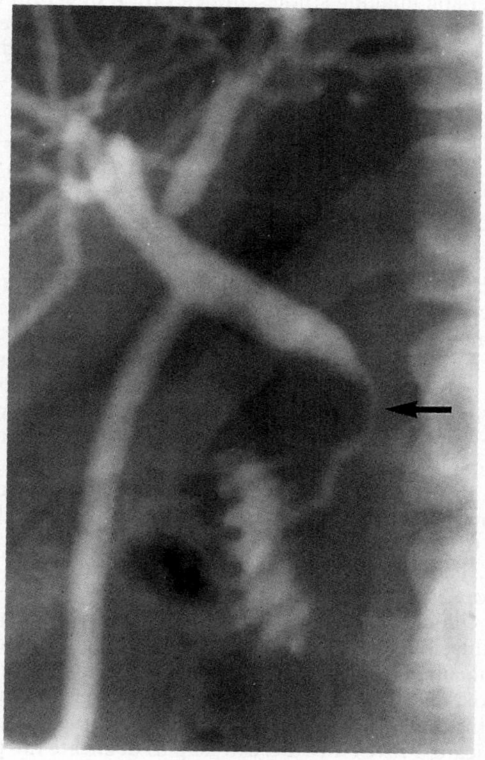

FIGURE 61.15. Cholangiogram of a patient with a long distal common bile duct stricture (*arrow*) caused by chronic pancreatitis.

with significant pain, jaundice, or cholangitis. Controversy exists, however, concerning the necessity of biliary decompression in patients with an asymptomatic elevation of serum 9 alkaline phosphatase. In general, biliary bypass is indicated because changes from obstructive biliary cirrhosis have been observed in liver biopsy specimens obtained from patients with long-standing, functionally significant biliary obstruction due to chronic pancreatitis.[34,35]

Choledochoduodenostomy and Roux-en-Y choledochojejunostomy are acceptable methods of biliary bypass in patients with bile duct strictures caused by chronic pancreatitis. Choledochoduodenostomy is preferred by many surgeons because it does not divert bile from the duodenum, is technically easier to perform, and leaves the jejunum intact for any associated procedures required for decompression of an obstructed gastrointestinal tract or pancreatic duct. Finally, in patients in whom periampullary malignancy cannot be completely ruled out by the clinical course or imaging studies, or in patients with significant chronic pain thought secondary to proximal pancreatic duct disease, pancreaticoduodenectomy offers an excellent treatment option. The results of surgical management of distal bile duct structures due to chronic pancreatitis are usually excellent, with a low rate of perioperative complications and excellent long-term results.

Transduodenal sphincteroplasty is not recommended for the management of common bile duct strictures caused by chronic pancreatitis because the stricture is too long to be managed adequately by this technique. Similarly, endoscopic sphincterotomy has no role in the management of biliary obstruction due to chronic pancreatitis. Limited experience has been reported with balloon dilation of distal bile duct strictures secondary to pancreatitis, with little long-term follow-up.

Over the last decade another variant of chronic pancreatitis has been recognized as a cause of distal bile duct stricture—autoimmune pancreatitis.[36] This process is characterized by a lymphoplasmacytic infiltrate and is associated with secretion of large amounts of immunoglobulin (Ig) 4. The condition can mimic pancreatic cancer and is diagnosed by characteristic imaging studies and elevation of serum Ig4 levels. Treatment is with corticosteroids with surgical resection or bypass reserved for unresponsive cases or when a diagnostic dilemma remains.

MISCELLANEOUS CAUSES OF BILE DUCT STRICTURES

Benign strictures of the bile duct can result from the chronic inflammation associated with gallstones in either the gallbladder or common bile duct. This cause of bile duct strictures is uncommon and is a rare complication of gallstone disease. Bile duct strictures caused by cholelithiasis are usually associated with a narrowing at the level of the common hepatic duct caused by a stone impacted in the infundibulum of the gallbladder. The narrowing can be caused by two means. First, simple compression can occur from a large stone lying adjacent to the common hepatic duct. Second, chronic or acute inflammation arising from the gallbladder or cystic duct can extend to the contiguous bile duct, resulting in stricture formation. The biliary obstruction associated with either of these conditions is known as *Mirizzi syndrome*.

The clinical presentation of a bile duct stricture caused by cholelithiasis is often associated with acute cholecystitis and hyperbilirubinemia. In some long-standing cases, these findings exist in the face of chronic gallbladder symptoms. If hyperbilirubinemia is present and urgent cholecystectomy is not indicated, ERCP or PTC can help to delineate the preoperative biliary anatomy. Most cases that are associated with acute cholecystitis, however, are recognized at the time of cholecystectomy and operative cholangiography. When the duct compression is associated with acute inflammation, the common hepatic duct almost always returns to normal after the offending stone has been removed by cholecystectomy and the inflammatory process has resolved. Care must be taken during the dissection to avoid creation of a defect in the common hepatic duct. Rarely, after the acute episode has resolved, a well-established stricture presents months to years after the acute episode. In such cases, management by Roux-en-Y hepaticojejunostomy is appropriate.

Strictures due to choledocholithiasis are also rare. The presumed mechanism is erosion of the epithelium of the distal duct, creating inflammation with subsequent fibrosis and stricture. Because of the anatomic tapering of the common bile duct, nearly all stones are entrapped in the intrapancreatic portion of the duct and are often difficult to remove by the supraduodenal route.

Excessive intraoperative manipulation at the time of bile duct exploration with forceps, scoops, and catheters can often create additional trauma to an already friable distal duct. After the stone has been removed, the distal bile duct should be gently sized with a soft rubber catheter to be sure that no stricture exists. If a stricture persists after stone removal, it may not be recognized until the time of postoperative T-tube cholangiography. If recognized in the postoperative period, time should be allowed for resolution of inflammation before considering stricture repair. If a distal bile duct stricture does persist, a biliary-enteric anastomosis with either Roux-en-Y choledochojejunostomy or a choledochoduodenostomy is indicated. If the proximal duct is adequately dilated (>2 cm in diameter) to allow a large choledochoduodenal anastomosis, this procedure is usually preferable because of its technical ease and excellent results.

Stenosis of the sphincter of Oddi, or papillitis, is a benign intrinsic obstruction of the outlet of the common bile duct, usually associated with inflammation, fibrosis, or muscular hypertrophy. Sphincter stenosis can result in any of three clinical conditions: (a) common bile duct obstruction due to fibrotic stenosis of the papilla, (b) recurrent pancreatitis, or (c) recurrent right upper quadrant pain without jaundice or pancreatitis. The pathogenesis of the inflammation of sphincter stenosis is unclear. In many cases, it is thought to result from the trauma of the passage of multiple small stones from the common duct through the ampulla. This trauma results in inflammation, scarring, and stricture formation. Many patients with papillary stenosis have no gallstones. Other potential mechanisms include primary sphincter motility disorders and congenital anomalies. The clinical presentation is usually either jaundice or cholangitis. In some cases, an impacted common bile duct stone may be present. The diagnosis can be supported with either PTC or ERC. This condition can be managed by sphincterotomy performed either endoscopically or operatively. If a cholecystectomy was performed previously, endoscopic papillotomy is the initial procedure of choice.

Cholangiohepatitis is an unusual infection of the biliary tree frequently associated with *Clonorchis sinensis* and other parasites. These infections are most commonly seen in natives of Asia. Most patients present with recurrent episodes of cholangitis. Cholangiography can demonstrate multiple strictures of both the intrahepatic and extrahepatic biliary tree, with the bile ducts filled with sludge and stones (Fig. 61.16). Surgical management consists of cholecystectomy and improved biliary drainage with either Roux-en-Y choledochojejunostomy or choledochoduodenostomy. Access to the biliary tree for postoperative management of intrahepatic stones or sludge should be maintained with either transhepatic biliary stents or a choledochojejunocutaneous or subcutaneous fistula. No specific medical management is available for this condition.

Finally, rare causes of benign intrahepatic and extrahepatic bile duct strictures have been reported secondary to intrahepatic arterial infusion of 5-fluorouracil used in the treatment of hepatic metastases of colorectal carcinoma. The clinical picture

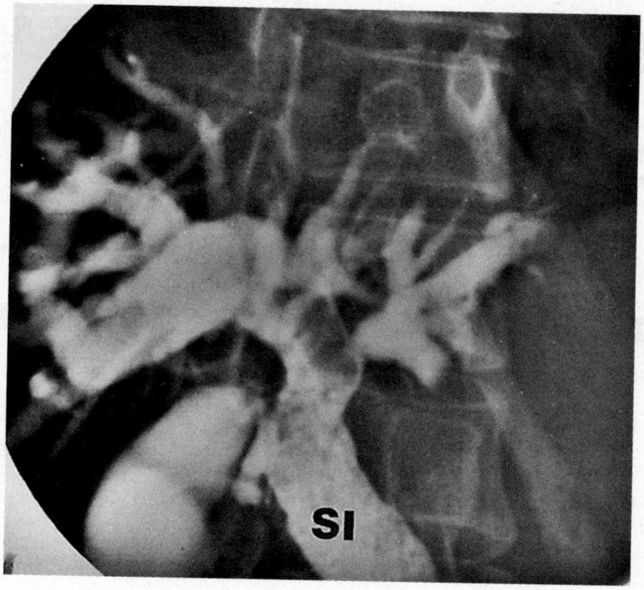

FIGURE 61.16. Cholangiogram of a patient with cholangiohepatitis with diffuse bile duct dilatation. The biliary tree is filled with sludge (SI) and stones.

closely resembles primary sclerosing cholangitis but usually can be managed by simple discontinuation of infusion and, in some cases, percutaneous transhepatic drainage. Surgery should be reserved for patients with persistent evidence of biliary obstruction. A similar cholangiographic appearance has been reported in patients with acquired immunodeficiency syndrome. The pathogenesis of this injury is believed to be viral and related to cytomegalovirus infection. No experience in the surgical management of this condition has been reported.

References

1. Hall JG, Pappas TN. Current management of biliary strictures. *J Gastrointest Surg* 2004;8:1098.
2. Branum G, Schmitt C, Baillie J, et al. Management of major biliary complications after laparoscopic cholecystectomy. *Ann Surg* 1993;17:532.
3. Flum DR, Dellinger EP, Cheadle A, et al. Intraoperative cholangiography and risk of common bile duct injury during laparoscopic cholecystectomy. *JAMA* 2003;289:1639.
4. Massaruch NN, Devlin A, Elrod JA, et al. Surgeon knowledge, behavior and opinions regarding intraoperative cholangiography. *J Am Coll Surg* 2008; 207:821.
5. Way LW, Stewart L, Gantert W, et al. Causes and prevention of laparoscopic bile duct injuries: analysis of 252 cases from a human factors and cognitive psychology perspective. *Ann Surg* 2003;273:460.
6. Strasberg SM, Hertl M, Soper NJ. An analysis of the problem of biliary injury during laparoscopic cholecystectomy. *J Am Coll Surg* 1995;180: 101.
7. Alves A, Farges O, Nicolet J, et al. Incidence and consequence of an hepatic artery injury in patients with postcholecystectomy bile duct strictures. *Ann Surg* 2003;230:93.
8. Pitt HA, Miyamoto T, Parapatis SK, et al. Factors influencing outcome in patients with postoperative biliary strictures. *Am J Surg* 1982;144:14.
9. Pellegrini CA, Thomas MJ, Way LW. Recurrent biliary stricture: patterns of recurrent and outcome of surgical therapy. *Am J Surg* 1984;147:175.
10. Lillemoe KD, Martin SA, Cameron JL, et al. Major bile duct injuries during laparoscopic cholecystectomy: follow-up after combined surgical and radiologic management. *Ann Surg* 1977;225:459–471.
11. Lillemoe KD. Treatment of laparoscopic bile duct injuries. *Curr Tech Gen Surg* 1997;6:1.
12. Warren KW, Christophi C, Armendari ZR. The evolution and current perspectives of the treatment of benign bile duct strictures: a review. *Surg Gastroenterol* 1982;1:141.
13. Sicklick JK, Camp MS, Lillemoe KD, et al. Surgical management of bile duct injuries sustained during laparoscopic cholecystectomy: perioperative results in 200 patients. *Ann Surg* 2005;241:786.
14. Stewart L, Way LW. Bile duct injuries during laparoscopic cholecystectomy. *Arch Surg* 1995;130:1123.
15. Lillemoe KD, Melton GB, Cameron JL, et al. Postoperative bile duct strictures: management and outcome in the 1990s. *Ann Surg* 2000;232:430.
16. Murr MM, Gigot JI, Nagorney DM, et al. Long-term results of biliary reconstruction after laparoscopic bile duct injuries. *Arch Surg* 1999;134: 604.
17. Walsh RM, Henderson JM, Voglt DP, et al. Long-term outcome of biliary reconstruction for bile duct injuries from laparoscopic cholecystectomies. *Surgery* 2007;142:450.
18. Laurent A, Sanvanet A, Farges O, et al. Major hepatectomy for the treatment of complex bile duct injury. *Ann Surg* 2008;248:77.
19. de Santibanes E, Ardilles V, Gadano A, et al. Liver transplantation: the last measure in the treatment of bile duct injuries. *World J Surg* 2008;32:1714.
20. Flum DR, Cheadle A, Prela C, et al. Bild duct injury during cholecystectomy and survival in Medicare beneficiaries. *JAMA* 2003;290:2168.
21. Melton GB, Lillemoe KD, Cameron JL, et al. Major bile duct injuries associated with laparoscopic cholecystectomy: effect on quality of life. *Ann Surg* 2002;235:888.
22. Horgan AM, Hoti E, Winter DC, et al. Quality of life after iatrogenic bile duct injury: a case control study. *Ann Surg* 2009;249:292.
23. Mueller PR, van Sonnenberg E, Ferrucci JT Jr, et al. Biliary stricture dilatation: multicenter review of clinical management in 73 patients. *Radiology* 1986;160:17.
24. Misra S, Melton GB, Geschwind JF, et al. Percutaneous management of bile duct strictures and injuries associated with laparoscopic cholecystectomy: a decade of experience. *J Am Coll Surg* 2004;198:218.
25. de Reuver P, Rauws EA, Vermenlen M, et al. Endoscopic treatment of postsurgical bile duct injuries: long term outcomes and predictors of success. *Gut* 2007;56:1599.
26. Geenen DJ, Geenen JE, Hogan WJ, et al. Endoscopic therapy for benign bile duct strictures. *Gastrointest Endosc* 1989;35:367.
27. Pitt HA, Kaufman SL, Coleman J, et al. Benign postoperative biliary strictures: operate or dilate? *Ann Surg* 1989;210:417.
28. David PHP, Tanka AKF, Rauws EAJ, et al. Benign biliary strictures: surgery or endoscopy? *Ann Surg* 1993;217:237.
29. Lindor KD. Ursodiol for primary sclerosing cholangitis. Mayo Primary Sclerosing Cholangitis-Ursodeoxycholic Acid Study Group. *N Engl J Med* 1997;336:691.
30. Gluck M, Cantone NR, Brandabur JJ, et al. A 20-year experience with endoscopic therapy for primary sclerosing cholangitis. *J Clin Gastroenterol* 2008;42:1032.
31. Pawlik TM, Olbrecht VA, Pitt HA, et al. Primary sclerosing cholangitis: role of extrahepatic biliary resection. *J Am Coll Surg* 2008;206:822.
32. Gross JA, Shackelton CR, Farmer DG, et al. Orthotopic liver transplantation for primary sclerosing cholangitis: a 12-year single center experience. *Ann Surg* 1997;225:472.
33. Stahl TJ, Allen MO, Ansel M, et al. Partial biliary obstruction caused by chronic pancreatitis: an appraisal of indications for surgical biliary drainage. *Ann Surg* 1988;207:26.
34. Warshaw AL, Schapiro RH, Ferrucci JT Jr, et al. Persistent obstructive jaundice, cholangitis, and biliary cirrhosis due to common bile duct stenosis in chronic pancreatitis. *Gastroenterology* 1976;70:562.
35. Afroudakis A, Kaplowitz N. Liver histopathology in chronic bile duct stenosis due to chronic alcoholic pancreatitis. *Hepatology* 1981;1:65.
36. Chari ST, Smyrk TC, Levy MJ, et al. Diagnosis of autoimmune pancreatitis: the Mayo Clinic experience. *Clin Gastro Hepta* 2006;4:1010.

CHAPTER 62 ■ BILIARY NEOPLASMS

SHARON WEBER, BRETT YAMANE, AND YUMAN FONG

KEY POINTS

1. Surgery remains the only curative option for biliary malignancies.
2. Gallbladder cancer is a rare malignancy with a dismal outlook because of its insidious onset, propensity for local invasion, and rapid disease progression.
3. The association of gallstones with carcinoma is probably related to chronic inflammation.
4. Patients with choledochal cysts have an increased risk of carcinoma developing anywhere in the biliary tree, but the incidence is highest in the gallbladder.
5. The only curative option in patients with gallbladder cancer is complete surgical resection.
6. Nonoperative palliative biliary decompression can be accomplished with percutaneous or endoscopic stenting, depending on the level of obstruction.
7. To date, no chemotherapeutic regimen has consistently shown activity against cholangiocarcinoma.

Tumors arising in the gallbladder and biliary tree are often asymptomatic until late in the course of the disease. Consequently, these tumors commonly present in an advanced,
1 often unresectable, stage. Surgery remains the only curative option for biliary malignancies. Resection of biliary neoplasms, however, often requires radical resections and complex biliary reconstructions that have only recently become safe in routine practice. Surgery also offers effective palliation for these cancers, including biliary bypasses for jaundiced patients with unresectable tumors. Both the late diagnosis and the complex operative techniques required for potentially curative resection contribute to the challenge of these cases. In addition, there are no proven effective options for adjuvant treatment. This chapter reviews the incidence, diagnosis, and therapy of these malignancies as well as the outcome of treatment.

GALLBLADDER CARCINOMA

2 Gallbladder cancer is a rare malignancy with a dismal outlook because of its insidious onset, propensity for local invasion, and rapid disease progression. Overall, most series report a 5-year survival of less than 5%. The extent of surgical resection remains ill defined because of the rarity of this lesion and its poor prognosis.

Incidence

Only 6,000 to 7,000 new cases of gallbladder cancer are diagnosed nationally each year.[1] Attesting to the rarity of this lesion, after routine screening of abdominal ultrasounds in asymptomatic patients in Japan, only 19/194,767 (0.01%) were found to have gallbladder cancer.[2] This tumor occurs more frequently in women (female-to-male ratio = 3:1), and peak incidence is in the seventh decade.[1] There is an increased risk of gallbladder cancer in Native American populations of the United States and Mexico.[3] The increased risk of gallbladder cancer with cholelithiasis is well established; 70% to 90% of all patients with carcinoma also have gallstones. However, less than 0.5% of patients with gallstones are found to have gallbladder cancer.[3] After elective cholecystectomy for gallstones, gallbladder cancer is found incidentally in 1% of
3 patients.[4] The association of gallstones with carcinoma is probably related to chronic inflammation. Larger stones (>3 cm) are associated with a 10-fold increased risk of cancer.[5]

The association of gallbladder cancer with gallstone disease has led some investigators to question whether all patients with gallstones should undergo cholecystectomy. The argument against this approach is that the use of cholecystectomy only for symptomatic patients, thus leaving the gallbladder in place in patients with asymptomatic gallstones, has not led to an increase in the prevalence of gallbladder cancer over time. Also, epidemiologic studies have found that the 20-year risk of developing cancer in patients with gallstones is less than 0.5% for the overall population and 1.5% for high-risk groups.[3] Thus, routine cholecystectomy for asymptomatic gallstones because of concern for gallbladder cancer does not appear to be warranted.

In the past, the finding of a calcified gallbladder wall, called "porcelain gallbladder" (Fig. 62.1), was associated with a high risk of cancer, in some series ranging from 25% to 60%.[6] Thus, the recommendation was for all patients with porcelain gallbladder to undergo open cholecystectomy, even if asymptomatic. Recent series evaluating this issue, however, suggest that the risk of gallbladder cancer in patients with porcelain gallbladder has likely been greatly overestimated.[7,8] In fact, although patients with limited areas of calcification of the wall may have a higher incidence of gallbladder cancer (7%), patients with diffuse calcification of the gallbladder wall, the classic presentation for porcelain gallbladder, do not appear to have an increased risk of gallbladder cancer.[7,8]

4 Patients with choledochal cysts have an increased risk of carcinoma developing anywhere in the biliary tree, but the incidence is highest in the gallbladder. This risk increases
5 with age. Therefore, complete surgical resection is recommended for all patients with choledochal cysts at the time of diagnosis.

Pathology and Staging

More than 80% of gallbladder cancers are adenocarcinomas; there are several histologic subtypes, including papillary, nodular, and tubular. Papillary tumors, which grow predominately into the gallbladder lumen, have an improved prognosis compared with the other subtypes.[9] Poor prognostic signs in

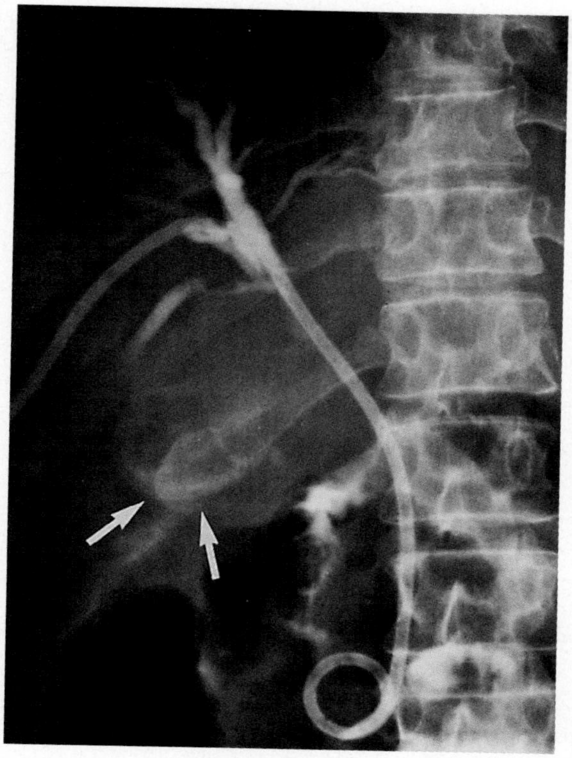

FIGURE 62.1. Unresectable gallbladder cancer demonstrating palliative transhepatic percutaneous stent placed to relieve jaundice. Porcelain gallbladder is present (*arrows*).

gallbladder cancer include grade[9,10] and vascular invasion.[9] The most important prognostic sign may be lymph node status,[11] although 5-year survivors with nodal involvement have been documented.[12] Less than 5% of cases are squamous cell carcinomas, with the remaining 10% being anaplastic lesions.

Gallbladder cancer spreads via the lymphatic and venous drainage. Because of drainage of the cholecystic veins directly into the adjacent liver, these tumors often involve hepatic parenchyma, most often portions of segments IV and V. Lymphatic spread is first to the cystic duct (Calot) node, then to pericholedochal and hilar nodes, and finally to peripancreatic, duodenal, periportal, celiac, and superior mesenteric artery nodes. Nodal disease in the porta hepatis often causes common bile duct obstruction and resultant jaundice, which is the first clinical symptom in 30% of patients. Jaundice may also be caused by tumors arising in the infundibulum, which may spread directly to the cystic duct and common hepatic duct. Although peritoneal metastases are frequent, distant extraperitoneal metastases are not.

Limited information exists regarding the genetic changes in gallbladder cancer. The most widely reported gene abnormalities associated with gallbladder cancer include p53,[13] K-ras,[13,14] and CDKN2 (9p21) mutations.[14,15] The finding that patients with an anomalous pancreaticobiliary junction have a greater frequency of K-ras mutations has led investigators to believe that reflux of pancreatic enzymes into the biliary tree may contribute to the development of cancer.[14] Because of our limited knowledge of the sequence of molecular changes, there are no known detectors of early disease or of risk assessment. Clearly, this is an area that needs improvement, particularly in endemic areas.

The American Joint Committee on Cancer's (AJCC) seventh edition of its tumor, node, metastasis (TNM) staging system (Table 62.1) reflects prognostic characteristics of tumor depth, regional nodal disease, and distant spread. The gallbladder differs histologically from the rest of the gastrointestinal tract in that it lacks a muscularis mucosa and submucosa. The gallbladder wall is composed of (a) a single layer of columnar cells, the mucosa, and lamina propria; (b) a fibromuscular layer; (c) a perimuscular, subserosal layer containing lymphatics and neurovascular structures; and (d) a serosal surface, except where the gallbladder is embedded in the liver.[16] Because lymphatics are present in the subserosal layer only, tumors invading less than the full thickness of the muscular layer have minimal risk of nodal spread. Thus, disease invading into, but not through, the muscular layer of the gallbladder is stage IB disease, whereas invasion into the perimuscular connective tissue is stage II. Stage III disease includes tumors that have perforated the serosa or have directly invaded the liver or other surrounding structures, which are clearly more advanced but still potentially resectable. Lymph node metastasis is now classified as stage IIIB. In line with other pancreaticobiliary malignancies, the stage III grouping refers to locally advanced disease and stage IV indicates metastatic disease.

Clinical Findings and Diagnosis

Most patients are found to have gallbladder cancer during workup or treatment of cholelithiasis or choledocholithiasis. In patients with symptoms, abdominal pain consistent with biliary colic or acute cholecystitis is most common. Patients also present with jaundice, weight loss, anorexia, or an increase in abdominal girth secondary to ascites. Physical findings include right upper quadrant tenderness or a palpable mass, hepatomegaly, and ascites. Laboratory investigation, if abnormal, is most often consistent with biliary obstruction. Because of its nonspecific presentation and the lack of reliable screening tests, gallbladder cancer is not diagnosed preoperatively in more than half the cases.

Imaging evaluation often reveals a thickened gallbladder wall or a mass within or replacing the gallbladder on ultrasound examination. Because polyps and carcinoma can have an echogenicity similar to the gallbladder wall, these lesions are often difficult to distinguish. This is even more difficult when inflammation is present from gallstones. At times, ultrasound can visualize invasion of the liver, adjacent adenopathy, and a dilated biliary tree. The ability of ultrasound to differentiate benign from neoplastic disease is enhanced using endoscopic ultrasound, and may be more specific than computed tomography (CT) or magnetic resonance imaging (MRI).[17,18]

A dynamic contrast-enhanced CT scan may identify a gallbladder mass or invasion into the liver parenchyma or adjacent organs. The classic finding in a patient with gallbladder cancer is asymmetric thickening of the gallbladder wall. The sensitivity and specificity of contrast-enhanced CT in diagnosing neoplastic lesions is close to 90%.[6] Staging of gallbladder carcinoma using CT, however, is limited by poor sensitivity in identifying nodal spread.[19]

In patients who are jaundiced, direct cholangiography may be useful to delineate the extent of biliary involvement as well as to palliate symptoms of biliary obstruction. A mid–bile duct obstruction not caused by gallstones is gallbladder cancer until proved otherwise (Fig. 62.2). More recently, with improvements in MRI technology, magnetic resonance cholangiopancreatography (MRCP) has evolved into a single, noninvasive imaging modality that allows complete assessment of biliary, vascular, hepatic parenchymal, and nodal involvement, as well as involvement of adjacent organs (Fig. 62.3).[20–22]

Surgery

It is clear that the only curative option in patients with gallbladder cancer is complete surgical resection. It is essential for optimal patient care that patients with gallbladder cancer be

TABLE 62.1 **STAGING**

AMERICAN JOINT COMMITTEE ON CANCER 7TH EDITION STAGING SYSTEM FOR GALLBLADDER CARCINOMA

■ STAGE	■ TUMOR	■ NODES	■ METASTASIS
0	Tis	N0	M0
I	T1	N0	M0
II	T2	N0	M0
IIIA	T3	N0	M0
IIIB	T1–3	N1	M0
IVA	T4	N0–1	M0
IVB	Any T	N2	M0
	Any T	Any N	M1

DEFINITION OF TNM

Primary tumor (T)	
TX	Primary tumor cannot be assessed
T0	No evidence of primary tumor
Tis	Carcinoma in situ
T1	Tumor invades lamina propria or muscular layer
T1a	Tumor invades lamina propria
T1b	Tumor invades muscular layer
T2	Tumor invades perimuscular connective tissue; no extension beyond serosa or into liver
T3	Tumor perforates the serosa (visceral peritoneum) and/or directly invades the liver and/or one other adjacent organ or structure, such as the stomach, duodenum, colon, pancreas, omentum, or extrahepatic bile ducts
T4	Tumor invades main portal vein or hepatic artery or invades two or more extrahepatic organs or structures
Regional lymph nodes (N)	
NX	Regional lymph nodes cannot be assessed
N0	No regional lymph node metastases
N1	Nodes confined to the hepatic hilus (including nodes along the common bile duct, hepatic artery, portal vein, and cystic duct
N2	Metastases to celiac, periduodenal, peripancreatic, and/or superior mesenteric artery lymph nodes
Distant metastasis (M)	
M0	No distant metastasis
M1	Distant metastasis

recognized before laparoscopic cholecystectomy is performed, because of the risk of port site seeding and bile spillage, with its potential for subsequent carcinomatosis.[23]

Role of Staging Laparoscopy. Because a large percentage of patients with gallbladder cancer are found to have occult, unresectable disease at the time of surgical exploration, several authors have investigated the use of initial staging laparoscopy for this disease.[24–27] Because gallbladder cancer has such a propensity to spread intra-abdominally, this tumor is ideal for detection of intra-abdominal metastases with laparoscopy. This is demonstrated by the fact that up to 50% of patients are found to have unresectable disease at the time of laparoscopy.[24,28] Patients who are found to have unresectable disease at laparoscopy can begin other forms of systemic therapy earlier and may undergo the procedure as an outpatient. Particularly because patients with unresectable disease have a median survival of only 6 months, the impact on quality of life, including decreased length of stay in the hospital, cannot be overemphasized.

Cholecystectomy with or without Partial Hepatectomy. Gallbladder cancer, if not completely surgically removed, results in rapid local progression and death. In a collected review of 5,836 patients with gallbladder cancer, the overall mean survival was between 2 and 5 months, whereas the 5-year survival was 4%.[3] The 5-year survival of patients undergoing resection with curative intent was 17%. Of the 2,115 patients with unresectable disease, only a single survivor was found at 5 years.[3] Although surgical resection represents the treatment of choice and the only potentially curative therapy available, resection is possible in only 25% of patients at presentation because of the advanced nature of the disease.[3]

There is little doubt that the results of treatment, as well as the scope of operation, are related to depth of tumor penetration (Table 62.2). For tumors limited to the muscular layer of

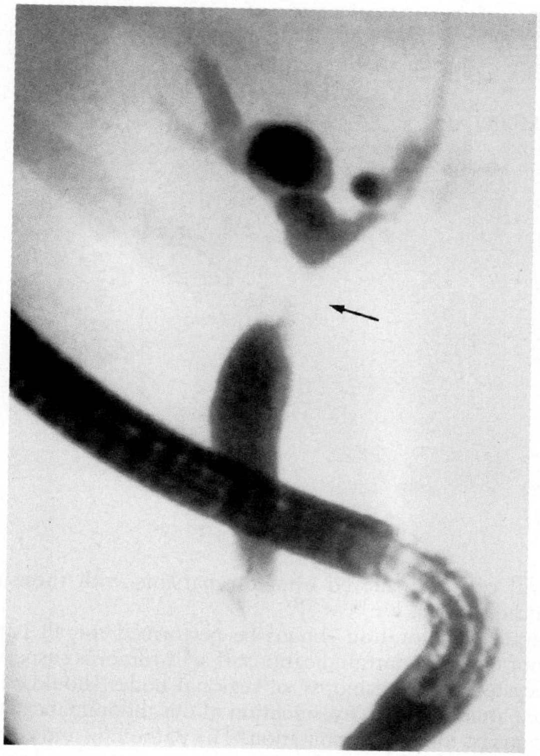

FIGURE 62.2. Endoscopic retrograde cholangiopancreatogram obtained from a patient with gallbladder cancer. Mid–bile duct obstruction (*arrow*) is caused by direct extension of tumor to the cystic and common hepatic duct.

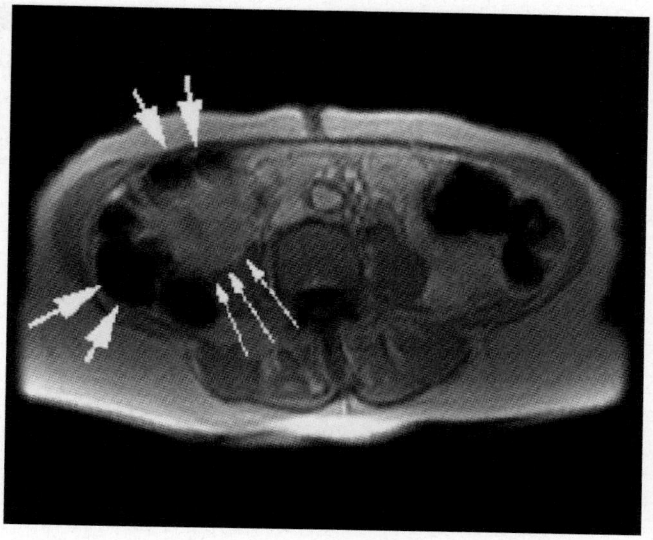

FIGURE 62.3. T_1-weighted magnetic resonance imaging scan of a patient with gallbladder cancer (*small arrows*) with extension into the duodenum and the hepatic flexure of colon (*large arrows*).

the gallbladder (T1), there is near-universal agreement that simple cholecystectomy is adequate.[12,29–31] T1 tumors have not yet invaded the subserosal layer, which contains lymphatics, and therefore lymphadenectomy is not required. Attesting to the fact that early gallbladder carcinoma is completely curable, simple cholecystectomy has resulted in 90% to 100% survival when early cancer is an incidental finding after elective cholecystectomy.[12,32]

Difficulty can arise at the time of surgery in evaluating polypoid lesions of the gallbladder as either benign or early gallbladder cancer. Although it appears that frozen section diagnosis is fairly reliable in distinguishing whether lesions are malignant or benign (95% accurate), the accuracy in correctly assessing depth of invasion is only 70%.[33] Thus, it may be difficult at the time of surgery to determine the extent of resection. Because of this, pursuing a more aggressive resection if the depth of invasion is in doubt is important for adequate tumor clearance.[32]

The extent of surgical resection for T2 or greater tumors is controversial, with recommendations ranging from simple cholecystectomy to radical excision, including hepatectomy. For advanced local disease, some groups have advocated radical

TABLE 62.2 **RESULTS**

FIVE-YEAR SURVIVAL AFTER RESECTION FOR GALLBLADDER CANCER

	■ T1 OR T2 TUMORS		■ T3 OR T4 TUMORS	
■ AUTHOR	■ SIMPLE CHOLECYSTECTOMY (%)	■ RADICAL CHOLECYSTECTOMY OR SEGMENTAL RESECTION (%)	■ SIMPLE CHOLECYSTECTOMY (%)	■ RADICAL CHOLECYSTECTOMY OR SEGMENTAL RESECTION (%)
Wanebo et al., 1982[37]	33	—	3	13
Ouchi et al., 1987[29]	57	100	0	23
Nakamura et al., 1989[34]	—	100	—	15
Donohue et al., 1990[30]	—	—	0	29
Shirai et al., 1992[12]	—	72	—	37
Fong et al., 2000[35]	—	58 (T2)	—	25
Wakai et al., 2001[121]	100[a] (10-year survival, T1b only)	75[a] (10-year survival, T1b only)	—	—
Kai et al., 2007[38]	25	60 (T2)	—	—
Jensen et al., 2009[39]	29	42	—	—

[a]No significant difference.

TABLE 62.3 RESULTS

RESULTS AFTER RADICAL RESECTION FOR GALLBLADDER CANCER

AUTHOR	NUMBER RESECTED	MORTALITY (%)	5-YEAR SURVIVAL (%)
Nakamura et al., 1989[34]	15	0	25
Donohue et al., 1990[30]	42	2	33
Ogura et al., 1991[31]	1,686	5	51
Shirai et al., 1992[12]	40	0	65
Bartlett et al., 1996[11] Fong et al., 2000[35]	102	4	58
Taner et al., 2004[36]	131	2	13
Kai et al., 2007[37]	90	2	40
Jensen et al., 2009[38]	443	—	42

resections, including hepatectomy and pancreatectomy. Whereas it is clear that major hepatic resection can be performed safely with a mortality less than 5% (Table 62.3)[11,12,30–32,34] it has not been universally accepted that more aggressive resections improve survival. To understand the rationale for extensive resections, it is also important to understand the pattern of spread of gallbladder cancer. Direct extension to the adjacent liver parenchyma often occurs first, followed by adjacent organ involvement, including duodenum, colon, and stomach (Fig. 62.2). Lymphatic spread of gallbladder cancer is routine, often involving nodes in the porta hepatis, peripancreatic region, celiac axis, and the aortocaval nodal basins.

Because the gallbladder is not surrounded by serosa where it is attached to the liver in the gallbladder fossa, even T2 tumors (full-thickness invasion of the muscular layer into the perimuscular connective tissue, no extension beyond serosa or into liver) can invade the normal plane of dissection in the gallbladder fossa during simple cholecystectomy. Therefore, T2 tumors cannot be completely removed with cholecystectomy alone, and a radical cholecystectomy, with resection of a 1- to 2-cm rim of normal liver around the gallbladder fossa, is the minimal resection that is required. Many authors, however, have found that segmental resection of segments IVb and V of the liver, which abut the gallbladder fossa, results in a more anatomically controlled dissection with less blood loss.[35] An additional part of the definitive surgical treatment is regional lymphadenectomy, because about half the patients with T2 tumors are found to have nodal spread after resection.[11] Dissection of lymph nodes should include all tissue from the bifurcation of the hepatic ducts to the distal common bile duct. Proponents of this approach advocate liver resection on the basis that it is the only way to obtain an adequate margin on the hepatic side of the gallbladder and resection of the regional nodes allows the best chance for complete tumor clearance. For all of these reasons, simple cholecystectomy is inadequate for T2 or greater tumors. When larger anatomic hepatic resections have been performed in patients with T2 tumors, it has increased the 5-year survival from 25% to 40% after simple cholecystectomy to 70% to 100% after radical resection.[11,29–31,36–40]

For T3 and T4 lesions, there is a high likelihood of intraperitoneal and hematogenous spread and significant morbidity from the radical procedures that are often necessary for excision of local disease. Recent series, however, support an aggressive approach to resection of these large tumors, particularly if no indication of nodal involvement is found (Table 62.3). For T3 and resectable T4 tumors, a minimal resection includes segments 4b and 5, and in many cases an extended right hepatectomy (segments IV, V, VI, VII, and VIII) may be necessary to obtain complete resection. With aggressive resection, long-term survival can be achieved even for patients with these more advanced tumors.[11,12,30,31,34,41]

Surgical exploration should be performed for all patients without medical contraindications. If a T1 tumor is suspected, a cholecystectomy and biopsy of regional nodes should be performed after thorough examination of the abdominal cavity for any signs of tumor dissemination. The pathology and depth of penetration should be confirmed by frozen section, and the procedure terminated if a T1 tumor with negative margins is confirmed. For T2 lesions, either a radical cholecystectomy (wedge resection of the hepatic bed) or a segment IVb and V resection with lymphadenectomy should be performed.[11] For T3 lesions, a segment IVb and V resection or extended right hepatectomy is performed. Finally, for T4 lesions, a more radical excision of the liver, such as extended right hepatectomy, usually must be performed for adequate tumor clearance.

Tumor location may be important in determining the extent of resection. If the tumor arises in the gallbladder infundibulum, the common bile duct is often involved with tumor, either by direct extension or external invasion of the hepatoduodenal ligament. In this case, an extended liver resection and removal of a portion of the common bile duct (CBD) should be performed. Reconstruction is then performed by Roux-en-Y hepaticojejunostomy. Tumor arising in the fundus of the gallbladder, however, can be treated with limited hepatic resection without excision of the CBD. To clear the lymph nodes in the porta hepatis, complete lymphadenectomy should be performed, skeletonizing the CBD, hepatic artery, and portal vein.

Incidentally or Laparoscopically Discovered Gallbladder Cancer. Gallbladder cancer is often discovered during pathologic examination after cholecystectomy for presumed benign gallstone disease. Because of the popularization of laparoscopic cholecystectomy in the past decade, an increasing number of patients with gallbladder cancer are found incidentally. Patients with T2 or greater tumors and no signs of distant disease should be offered radical resection to eradicate all disease. Even if grossly normal, excision of laparoscopic port sites should also be performed because of the well-documented history of port-site seeding.[23,36,42,43]

Patients presenting with gallbladder cancers after a recent cholecystectomy pose additional technical challenges. Often postoperative inflammation occurs in the right upper quadrant that hinders distinction of tumor from normal tissue. Bile spillage at the time of the initial operation may result in carcinomatosis.[44] Determination of ductal or nodal involvement by tumor is always difficult at the time of reoperation. In addition, postoperative fibrosis often encases the right hepatic artery, which crosses behind the bile duct in most patients. Because of this, during a second operation for incidentally discovered gallbladder cancer, an extended right hepatectomy along with excision of the extrahepatic biliary tree and portal lymphadenectomy is often necessary. This resection allows adequate exposure for lymphadenectomy and greater confidence of a negative margin on the bile duct, and also permits biliary reconstruction to only one side of the liver. The disadvantage is that a large portion of normal liver parenchyma is sacrificed, and consequently, transient postoperative liver dysfunction is common. Although it may be more difficult to curatively resect disease in patients with incidentally discovered gallbladder cancer after laparoscopic cholecystectomy, there is no difference in overall survival between patients with incidentally discovered gallbladder cancer who are submitted to curative resection and those patients who undergo initial curative resection.[35]

When a patient presents with T1 gallbladder cancer discovered after simple cholecystectomy, the pathology should be reviewed to determine if the entire gallbladder has been removed and if the cystic duct margin is clear of tumor. If the cystic duct margin is positive, the patient requires bile duct excision. If all margins are negative, no further therapy is warranted. If the tumor is proved to be T2 or greater, the patient should undergo reexcision to attempt complete resection if the extent of disease evaluation is negative. Patients with a known or suspected early gallbladder carcinoma should not undergo laparoscopic cholecystectomy. Rather, open exploration and cholecystectomy should be performed.

Adjuvant Therapy

Adjuvant therapy for gallbladder cancer remains a controversial and unproved consideration. Very few randomized trials have been conducted, and those that have are limited because of the number of patients included. Given the relative rarity of these malignancies in the United States, large-scale, randomized trials are feasible only in the context of a multi-institutional or cooperative group setting.

One recent prospective, randomized phase III trial of adjuvant chemotherapy with 5-fluorouracil and mitomycin C versus surgery alone for patients with pancreaticobiliary malignancies having resection found that in the subset of patients with gallbladder cancer ($n = 112$), the 5-year survival rate was significantly better in the adjuvant group (26%) versus the control group (14%).[46] Similarly, the 5-year disease-free survival rate was 20.3% versus 11.6%, clearly favoring the adjuvantly treated group. This trial suggests that adjuvant chemotherapy may offer benefit for patients with resected gallbladder cancer; however, replication in a larger-scale setting is required before definitive conclusions can be drawn.

Prognosis

The 5-year survival rate for all patients with gallbladder cancer is less than 5% in most series, with a median survival of 6 months. This is primarily because most patients present with unresectable disease. Of those patients undergoing resection, survival is dependent on depth of penetration and nodal status. Nearly 100% survival is reported after simple cholecystectomy for T1 disease, whereas patients with T2 and T3 tumors without nodal disease have a 5-year survival greater than 50%.[11,12,34,36] Node positivity is an ominous finding, with few series reporting 5-year survivors.

Follow-up after Resection for Gallbladder Cancer

The most common sites of recurrence after resection of gallbladder cancer include carcinomatosis, intrahepatic metastases, or nodal recurrence in the retroperitoneum. Jaundice is a common sign, but patients with recurrence may also present with ascites caused by carcinomatosis. For most tumors, local recurrence is found synchronously with diffuse intra-abdominal spread. Therefore, surgical treatment of recurrence has little potential for cure. If recurrent disease is found after resection, prognosis is exceedingly poor, with death occurring secondary to biliary sepsis or liver failure within months of diagnosis.

The main goal of follow-up after resection of gallbladder cancer is to provide palliation for symptomatic recurrences. The main symptoms associated with recurrence requiring palliation are pruritus or cholangitis associated with jaundice, or bowel obstruction associated with carcinomatosis. Additional goals of follow-up are to detect benign complications of surgical treatment such as biliary stricture. When jaundice or cholangitis is the presenting symptom of possible recurrence, a nonsurgical palliative approach using percutaneous transhepatic cholangiogram (PTC) and stenting is usually favored unless a benign postsurgical stricture is suspected. Because of the rapid growth of tumor in patients with recurrence, the hospitalization and recovery time from a surgical bypass is usually not justified for recurrences resulting in biliary obstruction.

6

The routine follow-up of a patient after resection of gallbladder cancer includes office visits every 3 months with physical examination and measurement of liver function tests. Although CA19-9 may be elevated in patients with gallbladder cancer, the sensitivity and specificity are poor[47] and, thus, should not be used for screening patients for recurrence. Because an asymptomatic recurrence of gallbladder cancer has only limited treatment options, overaggressive use of imaging studies is not warranted. Therefore, the use of imaging studies should be individualized.

Issues for the Future

Clearly, improving our ability to recognize early gallbladder cancer in high-risk geographic areas would have an important impact on outcome in these patients. This will likely require improvements in understanding the sequential molecular changes associated with gallbladder cancer. Other improvements in screening programs in high-risk areas, which could result in prophylactic cholecystectomy, would likely be beneficial.[48]

BILE DUCT CARCINOMA

One of the most technically difficult surgical resections occurs in patients with bile duct tumors arising in the hepatic hilus, named Klatskin tumors, or hilar cholangiocarcinoma. Bile duct cancers can arise at other sites, including within the liver (intrahepatic cholangiocarcinoma) and below the biliary bifurcation but above the pancreas (mid–bile duct cholangiocarcinoma). Distal cholangiocarcinoma involves that portion of the bile duct within the pancreas, which requires pancreaticoduodenectomy. The location of the tumor affects prognosis as well as the potential for curative resection.

Resection of biliary neoplasms, particularly hilar cholangiocarcinoma, often requires radical resections and complex biliary reconstructions that have only recently become safe in routine practice. Surgery may also offer effective palliation for these cancers by providing biliary bypass for jaundiced patients with unresectable tumors. Because disease is often diagnosed late in the course and because complex operative techniques are required for potentially curative resection, these tumors represent one of the greatest challenges for definitive treatment. Adding to this is that there are no proved effective options for adjuvant treatment.

Incidence

The overall incidence of hilar cholangiocarcinoma in the United States is 1.0/100,000 per year, although other geographic regions such as Israel and Japan have higher rates.[49] The incidence of intrahepatic cholangiocarcinoma in the United States is approximately 0.7/100,000 with a similar mortality. During the last 30 years, it appears that both the incidence and mortality in the United States are increasing.[50] Most recently, population studies have noted that there has been a trend toward a relative increased incidence of intrahepatic cholangiocarcinoma (ICC) compared to extrahepatic cholangiocarcinoma (ECC).[1,51,52] Using the Surveillance, Epidemiology and End Results-Medicare databases, Welzel et al.[51] noted HCV infection, chronic nonalcoholic liver disease and obesity, and smoking being associated only with ICC and not ECC, possibly explaining the divergent trends in incidence. Cholangiocarcinomas arise slightly more often in males,[9] with a male-to-female ratio of 1.3:1 and an average age of 50 to 70 years.

Known risk factors for this disease include primary sclerosing cholangitis, ulcerative colitis, choledochal cysts, and biliary tract infection, either with *Clonorchis* or in chronic typhoid carriers.[53] Treating patients with cholangiocarcinoma arising from one of these underlying conditions is challenging.[54] Some industrial chemicals (e.g., nitrosamines, dioxin, asbestos, and polychlorinated biphenyls) have also been implicated in the pathogenesis of cholangiocarcinoma.[49] Although there has been some suggestion of an increased risk of cholangiocarcinoma arising after transduodenal sphincteroplasty,[55] it is difficult to determine if this is caused by the surgical intervention or the underlying disease leading to sphincteroplasty.

Pathology and Staging

Similar to gallbladder cancer, bile duct tumors tend to invade locally. More than 95% of these tumors are adenocarcinomas. They are morphologically described as nodular, which is the most common, scirrhous, diffusely infiltrating, or papillary. Histologic subtypes include acinar, ductular, trabecular, alveolar, and papillary. Papillary tumors appear to have an improved outcome. Much less common types of bile duct tumors include cystadenocarcinomas, hemangioendotheliomas, and mucoepidermoid carcinomas. Perineural invasion is clearly a poor prognostic sign.[56]

In patients with intrahepatic cholangiocarcinoma, negative prognostic signs include vascular invasion, multiple tumors, positive margin, large size, and lymph node metastases.[57] These tumors can be either sclerotic, masslike lesions, or cystic lesions.

Historically, cholangiocarcinomas have been classified according to their location in the upper (60%), middle (15%–20%), or lower third (15%–20%) of the bile duct. Middle-third lesions arise between the cystic duct and the superior border of the duodenum. Lower-third lesions are found below the superior border of the duodenum but above the ampulla. The problem with this classification is that the anatomic landmarks are somewhat arbitrary and not clinically useful. Most mid–bile duct malignant obstructions are caused by gallbladder cancer. Even when it is truly a mid–bile duct cholangiocarcinoma, very few of these tumors are amenable to treatment by local excision of the bile duct. A more useful classification is to divide these lesions into upper-half or lower-half tumors, based on the location of the cystic duct as it enters the common duct (in the case of normal anatomy). The usefulness of this classification scheme is that it allows the surgeon to delineate whether a hepatic or pancreatic resection will be required for clearance of tumor. The AJCC TNM staging system (seventh edition) for bile duct cancers is described in Tables 62.4A and B.

Other staging systems have been created that attempt to incorporate clinically important indicators of resectability for hilar cholangiocarcinoma that are defined preoperatively, including hepatic lobe atrophy or portal vein involvement.[58] With the increasing acceptance of major hepatic resection for these tumors, this preoperative staging system attempts to define whether there is ipsilateral involvement alone, because tumors with bilateral extension past the primary biliary radicles are not resectable.

Clinical Findings and Diagnosis

The vast majority of patients with cholangiocarcinoma present with painless jaundice, though mild right upper quadrant pain, pruritus, anorexia, malaise, and weight loss may also be reported. Cholangitis is the presenting symptom in 10% to 30% of patients. Some patients have cancer discovered on evaluation for otherwise asymptomatic elevations of alkaline phosphatase and gamma-glutamyl transferase.

Patients with intrahepatic cholangiocarcinoma are usually asymptomatic. Many patients are found to have a liver tumor present on cross-sectional imaging obtained for other reasons. Many of these patients will present to the surgeon with a biopsy showing adenocarcinoma without a known primary tumor. The standard evaluation in these patients should include tumor markers to rule out an elevated carcinoembryonic antigen (CEA) or α-fetoprotein (AFP); upper and lower endoscopy to evaluate for a gastrointestinal source; CT scan to assess for a primary tumor in the gastrointestinal tract or pancreas; and, in women, a mammogram. If no site of primary disease is found, in most patients, the diagnosis is intrahepatic cholangiocarcinoma.

Various imaging tests are available to assess patients with hilar cholangiocarcinoma. Abdominal ultrasound is noninvasive, easily available, and inexpensive, and thus is commonly used as a first imaging modality. It can establish the level of biliary obstruction and rule out cholelithiasis or choledocholithiasis as the etiology. CT scans frequently reveal dilated intrahepatic biliary ducts with a normal, collapsed gallbladder, and, depending on the level of the tumor, a nondilated or partially dilated extrahepatic biliary tree (Fig. 62.4). In addition, the presence of hilar adenopathy can be assessed. Portal vein patency can be determined with ultrasound or helical CT. In addition, signs of hepatic lobar atrophy should be sought, because this is associated with a high incidence of ipsilateral portal vein involvement by tumor. MRCP offers the potential of evaluating parenchymal, vascular, biliary, and nodal involvement with a single noninvasive examination.[20–22] Frequently, it is possible to visualize the tumor itself with MRI (Figs. 62.5 and 62.6).

In most centers, direct cholangiography is used to evaluate the extent of biliary involvement and provide palliation for jaundice. Endoscopic retrograde cholangiopancreatography (ERCP) has little role to play in high biliary obstruction because opacification of the proximal biliary tree is difficult. ERCP, however, can be effectively used to image more distal lesions. At the time cholangiography is performed, some authors advocate the routine preoperative placement of biliary drainage catheters to aid in intraoperative identification of the bile ducts.[59,60] Others have found a higher incidence of infectious complications[61] and mortality,[62] and a longer hospital stay,[63] after preoperative placement of biliary drainage catheters. The difficulty in making the decision regarding preoperative stenting is that many patients are severely symptomatic because of jaundice and pruritus and require palliation, thus if the operation is delayed, many patients require palliation.

In many cases, it is difficult to obtain pathologic confirmation of cholangiocarcinoma except in very advanced cases, even with the use of biliary brushings and cytology obtained at

TABLE 62.4A **STAGING**

AMERICAN JOINT COMMITTEE ON CANCER, 6TH EDITION, STAGING SYSTEM FOR PERIHILAR BILE DUCT CARCINOMA

STAGE	TUMOR	NODES	METASTASIS
0	Tis	N0	M0
I	T1	N0	M0
II	T2a--b	N0	M0
IIIA	T3	N0	M0
IIIB	T1–3	N1	M0
IVA	T4	N0–1	M0
IVB	Any T	N1–2	M0
	Any T	Any N	M1

Definition of TNM

Primary tumor (T)

TX	Primary tumor cannot be assessed
T0	No evidence of primary tumor
Tis	Carcinoma *in situ*
T1	Tumor confined to bile duct, with extension up to the muscle layer or fibrous tissue
T2a	Tumor invades beyond the wall of the bile duct to surroundng adipose tissue
T2b	Tumor invades adjacent hepatic parenchyma
T3	Tumor invades unilateral branches of the portal vein or hepatic artery
T4	Tumor invades main portal vein or its branches bilaterally; or the common hepatic arter; or the second-order biliary radicals bilaterally; or unilateral second-order biliary radicals with contralateral portal vein or hepatic artery involvement.

Regional lymph nodes (N)

NX	Regional lymph nodes cannot be assessed
N0	No regional lymph node metastasis
N1	Regional lymph node metastasis (including nodes along the cystic duct, common bile duct, hepatic artery and portal vein)
N2	Metastasis to periaortic pericaval, superior mesentary artery, and/or celiac artery lymph nodes

Distant metastasis (M)

M0	No distant metastasis (no pathologic M0; use clinical M to complete stage group)
M1	Distant metastasis

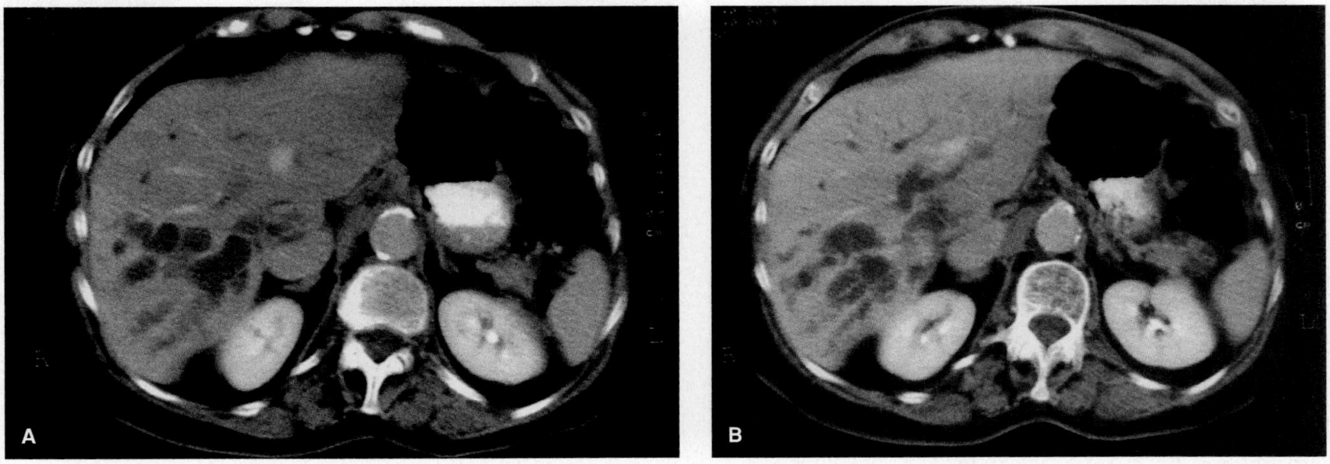

FIGURE 62.4. Computed tomography scan in a patient with hilar cholangiocarcinoma, demonstrating dilated intrahepatic ducts in the right lobe but inability to directly visualize tumor.

TABLE 62.4B **STAGING**

AMERICAN JOINT COMMITTEE ON CANCER, 6TH EDITION, STAGING SYSTEM FOR DISTAL BILE DUCT CARCINOMA

■ STAGE	■ TUMOR	■ NODES	■ METASTASIS
0	Tis	N0	M0
I	T1	N0	M0
II	T2a–b	N0	M0
IIIA	T3	N0	M0
IIIB	T1–3	N1	M0
IVA	T4	N0–1	M0
IVB	Any T	N1–2	M0
	Any T	Any N	M1

DEFINITION OF TNM

Primary tumor (T)

TX	Primary tumor cannot be assessed
T0	No evidence of primary tumor
Tis	Carcinoma *in situ*
T1	Tumor confined to bile duct, with extension up to the muscle layer or fibrous tissue
T2	Tumor invades beyond the wall of the bile duct
T3	Tumor invades gallbladder, pancreas, duodenum, or other adjacent organs without involvement of the celiac axis or the superior mesenteric artery
T4	Tumor involves the celiac axis or the superior mesteteric artery

Regional lymph nodes (N)

NX	Regional lymph nodes cannot be assessed
N0	No regional lymph node metastasis
N1	Regional lymph node metastasis (including nodes along the cystic duct, common bile duct, hepatic artery and portal vein)
N2	Metastasis to periaortic pericaval, superior mesentary artery, and/or celiac artery lymph nodes

Distant metastasis (M)

M0	No distant metastasis (no pathologic M0; use clinical M to complete stage group)
M1	Distant metastasis

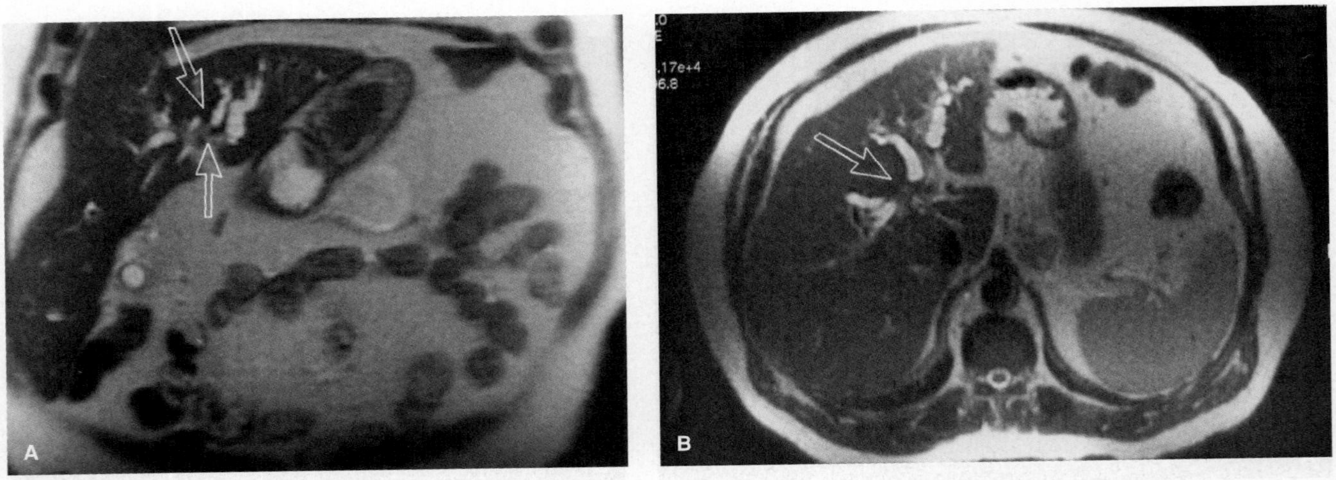

FIGURE 62.5. Coronal (A) and axial (B) magnetic resonance imaging in a patient with hilar cholangiocarcinoma. Dilated intrahepatic ducts are present with a soft tissue density consistent with tumor (*arrows*).

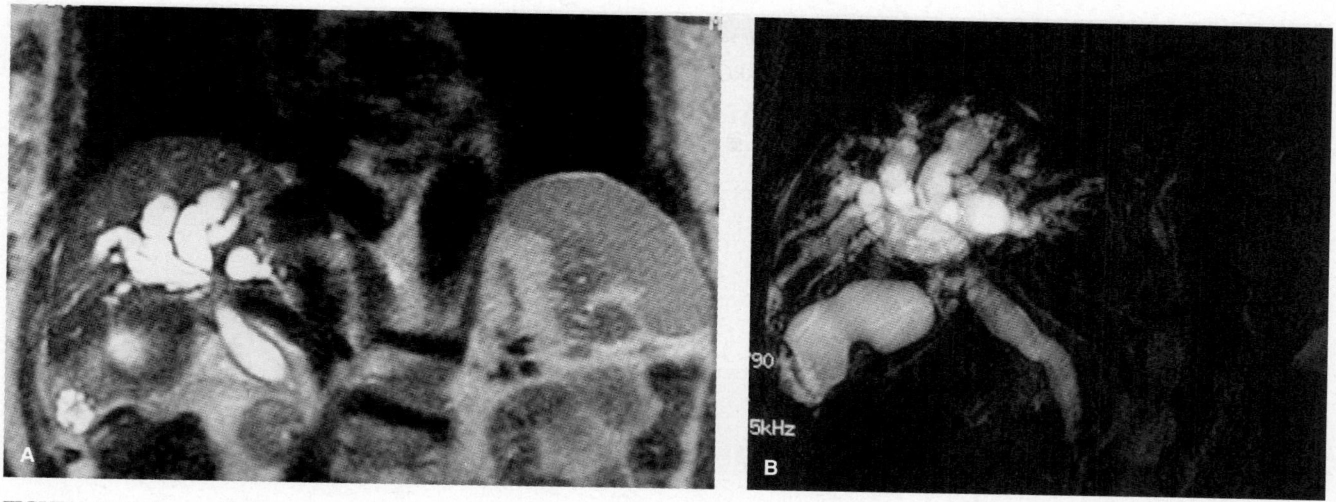

FIGURE 62.6. Coronal (A) magnetic resonance imaging and magnetic resonance cholangiopancreatography (B) in a patient with hilar cholangiocarcinoma, demonstrating dilated intrahepatic ducts narrowing at the area of obstruction.

the time of direct cholangiography. In most cases, patients are offered surgical therapy based on clinical suspicion and radiographic appearance. In patients with intrahepatic cholangiocarcinoma, cross-sectional imaging with CT scan is usually sufficient. Tumors may be masslike or may have cystic areas.

Surgery

Proximal Cholangiocarcinomas. Untreated, most patients with bile duct cancers die within a year of diagnosis.[63,64] Surgical excision is the treatment of choice, with no other potentially curative therapy. The immediate causes of death are most commonly hepatic failure or cholangitis related to tumor growth and inadequate drainage of the biliary tree.[65] Therefore, the objectives of management for patients with cholangiocarcinoma include both complete removal of tumor and adequate biliary drainage. It has become clear over the last three decades that curative treatment for patients with tumors involving the upper half of the bile duct depends on aggressive excision that often requires a major liver resection. Until as recently as one decade ago, treatment of hilar cholangiocarcinomas was associated with mortality as high as 30%.[66–70] Recently, major improvements in the safety of these operations has been demonstrated, and resection of hilar tumors now results in mortality of less than 10%, even when liver resections are required.[66,67,69,71]

Assessment of Resectability and Surgical Procedure. Surgical exploration is often the only means of assessing resectability. Because of the potential morbidity of a laparotomy that has no therapeutic benefit, staging laparoscopy has been advocated to save patients from unnecessary laparotomy. In patients with hilar cholangiocarcinoma, up to 25% will benefit from staging laparoscopy because of detection of occult extrahepatic disease.[24,28] Laparoscopy is a very sensitive means to detect peritoneal metastases or additional intrahepatic disease through the use of laparoscopic ultrasound but is less sensitive in detecting nodal metastases or locally invasive tumors.[24]

Hilar cholangiocarcinoma is considered unresectable because of both local factors and metastatic spread. Clearly, patients with disease outside the liver, including most commonly peritoneal and intrahepatic metastases, are not amenable to curative resection. Local factors that make these tumors unresectable include invasion of the main portal vein or both the right and left portal vein and hepatic arteries and tumor extension into second-order biliary radicals of both right and left hepatic lobes. By contrast, tumors extending into second- or third-order biliary radicles on one side of the liver without vascular involvement can be resected with curative outcome.

The goals of surgical management for cholangiocarcinomas are both eradication of tumor and establishment of adequate biliary drainage. Tumors of the biliary confluence are particularly difficult to treat because symptoms often appear late in the course of disease when the lesion has already involved adjacent structures including the portal vein or adjacent hepatic parenchyma. Complete resection, therefore, requires biliary and hepatic resection and often major vascular reconstruction. It is not surprising, therefore, that in the past the surgical therapy for proximal biliary malignancies consisted mainly of biliary-enteric bypass as palliation for jaundice and cholangitis. The therapeutic approach to hilar cholangiocarcinoma was largely nihilistic, because of difficulty in delineating the extent of disease and the technical challenge of complete resection for such lesions.

Over the last decade, surgical approaches have become more aggressive, as demonstrated by the increasing number of hepatic resections that have been performed for bile duct cancers.[66–70] Recent improvements in ultrasound, CT, MRI, and angiography have greatly facilitated preoperative diagnoses and staging of cholangiocarcinoma. This has allowed improved patient selection and surgical planning. The location and local extension of tumor dictates the extent of resection, with most lesions requiring an extended right or left hepatectomy for complete excision. Caudate resection is often required because of direct extension into caudate biliary radicles or parenchyma.[58,69,70] CBD excision and portal lymphadenectomy are also essential for tumor clearance.

Liver Transplantation for Hilar CCA and the Mayo Protocol. Orthotopic liver transplantation (OLT) was thought to hold promise for patients with hilar CC, because of its ability to achieve adequate margins by complete hepatectomy. Unfortunately, when used as a single treatment modality, results have been poor. Three- and 5-year survival rates have been reported at 25% to 30%.[73–75] Because of this poor outcome, the Mayo Clinic developed a protocol combining neoadjuvant therapy with liver transplant, based on a strategy initially developed by the University of Nebraska. This protocol uses high-dose neoadjuvant 5-fluorouracil and brachytherapy

TABLE 62.5 **RESULTS**

RESULTS AFTER RESECTION FOR HILAR CHOLANGIOCARCINOMA

AUTHOR	N	PERCENT RESECTED	POSTOPERATIVE MORTALITY (%)	5-YEAR SURVIVAL (%)	SURVIVAL (MONTHS) MEAN	SURVIVAL (MONTHS) MEDIAN
Cameron et al., 1990[59]	96	55	2	8		18
Hadjis et al., 1990[70]	131	21	7	12	25	
Altaee et al., 1991[66]	70	21		19		12
Baer et al., 1993[67]	48	44	4	23	34	
McMasters et al., 1997[123]	91	44	0	26		22
Klempnauer et al., 1997[124]	151		10	28		24
Nagino et al., 1999[125]	173	80	10	26		
Nakeeb et al., 2002[126]	72	57		34		
Jarnagin et al., 2001[127]	225	71	10	27		35
Rea et al., 2004[72]	46		9	26		28
Jang et al, 2005[128]	48		0	48		
Konstadoulakis et al., 2008[129]	73	81	7	35		
Yubin et al., 2008[130]	115	100	2	22		40

followed by liver transplantation.[72,76] Inclusion criteria include: (i) locally advanced unresectable disease with either positive intraluminal brush cytology, positive intraluminal biopsy, or CA19-9 ≥100 in the setting of a radiographic malignant stricture; (ii) primary sclerosing cholangitis with resectable disease, and; (iii) absence of medical contraindications for OLT. Since 2003, biliary aneuploidy as demonstrated by digital image analysis (DIA)[77] and fluorescent in situ hybridization have been considered equivalent to cytology.[78] Exclusion criteria include: (i) extrahepatic disease including regional lymph node involvement; (ii) uncontrolled infection; (iii) prior attempt at resection; (iv) prior treatment with radiation or chemotherapy; and (v) previous malignancy within 5 years. In this protocol, patients receive external beam radiotherapy to a target dose of 4,500 cGy with concomitant fluorouracil (5-FU). Following this, transcatheter iridium-192 brachytherapy with a target dose of 2,000 to 3,000 cGy is administered. Thereafter, patients receive oral capecitabine as tolerated until transplantation. It is important that, prior to transplantation, patients undergo a staging laparotomy, at which time biopsy of perihilar lymph nodes as well as any lymph nodes or nodules suspicious for tumor is performed. Only patients with negative staging operations remain eligible for transplantation.[72]

Thus, patients eligible for OLT under this protocol have locally advanced tumors but no pathologic nodal disease. Furthermore, the prolonged course of neoadjuvant therapy, staging laparotomy, and time on the OLT waiting list provides an opportunity to exclude patients demonstrating disease progression. This highly rigorous selection bias in favor of patients with biologically favorable disease is reflected in the early outcomes published from the Mayo group. In a recent review of 71 patients enrolled in this transplant protocol, only 38 underwent transplantation (38%). These patients were compared to 26 patients (of 54 explored, 48%) who underwent successful resection. When compared to those undergoing resection (some with node-positive disease), patients undergoing transplantation were younger ($p < 0.001$) and more likely to have inflammatory bowel disease ($p < 0.03$) and PSC ($p < 0.001$). It is important that only 58% of patients had histologically proven cancer.

In these highly disparate groups, 5-year survival was 82% after transplantation (38 patients) compared to 21% after resection of 26 patients ($p = 0.022$).[72] There were also fewer recurrences in the transplant patients (13% vs. 27%), and recurrences became apparent later after transplantation than after resection (mean 40 months vs. 21 months). Direct comparisons are difficult with this study given the differences between groups. At present, OLT cannot be considered a standard form of therapy for hilar cholangiocarcinoma for patients with resectable disease, but it does offer a potential option for patients with underlying PSC or those with unresectable tumors who fit the rigorous inclusion and exclusion criteria of the protocol.

Prognosis after Resection. Results of major studies on resection of hilar cholangiocarcinoma are summarized in Table 62.5. In patients amenable to curative resection, the median survival is 35 months with a 5-year survival rate of 10% to 30%.[61,68,69,72–80] Surgical resection provides both improved survival and improved quality of life.[79,80] The greatest risk factors for recurrence include the presence of positive margins[79,81] and node-positive tumors.[82]

Prognosis after Resection for Intrahepatic or Distal Cholangiocarcinoma. In patients with intrahepatic cholangiocarcinoma, expected 3-year survival rates as high as 60% have been reported,[24,83] with 5-year survival rates of 30% to 45%.[84] Patients with unresectable disease have a median survival of 12 months.[85,86] Thus, completely resected intrahepatic cholangiocarcinoma appears to have an improved prognosis over proximal (hilar) cholangiocarcinoma.

Most patients with distal cholangiocarcinomas are definitively managed with pancreaticoduodenectomy (Whipple procedure) to obtain adequate clearance of tumor, because of the intrapancreatic location of the distal CBD. Patients with cholangiocarcinomas arising in the distal bile duct have both an increased resectability rate and improved prognosis over those with hilar cholangiocarcinomas.[71] Patients with resectable distal bile duct cancer have a 5-year survival rate of 30% to 50%,[84,87] with a decreased survival if nodes are involved with tumor.[87]

Surgical Treatment of Unresectable Cholangiocarcinoma. For patients with unresectable hilar cholangiocarcinomas, significant improvement in quality of life can occur with surgical bypass. Palliative bypass can be performed in several

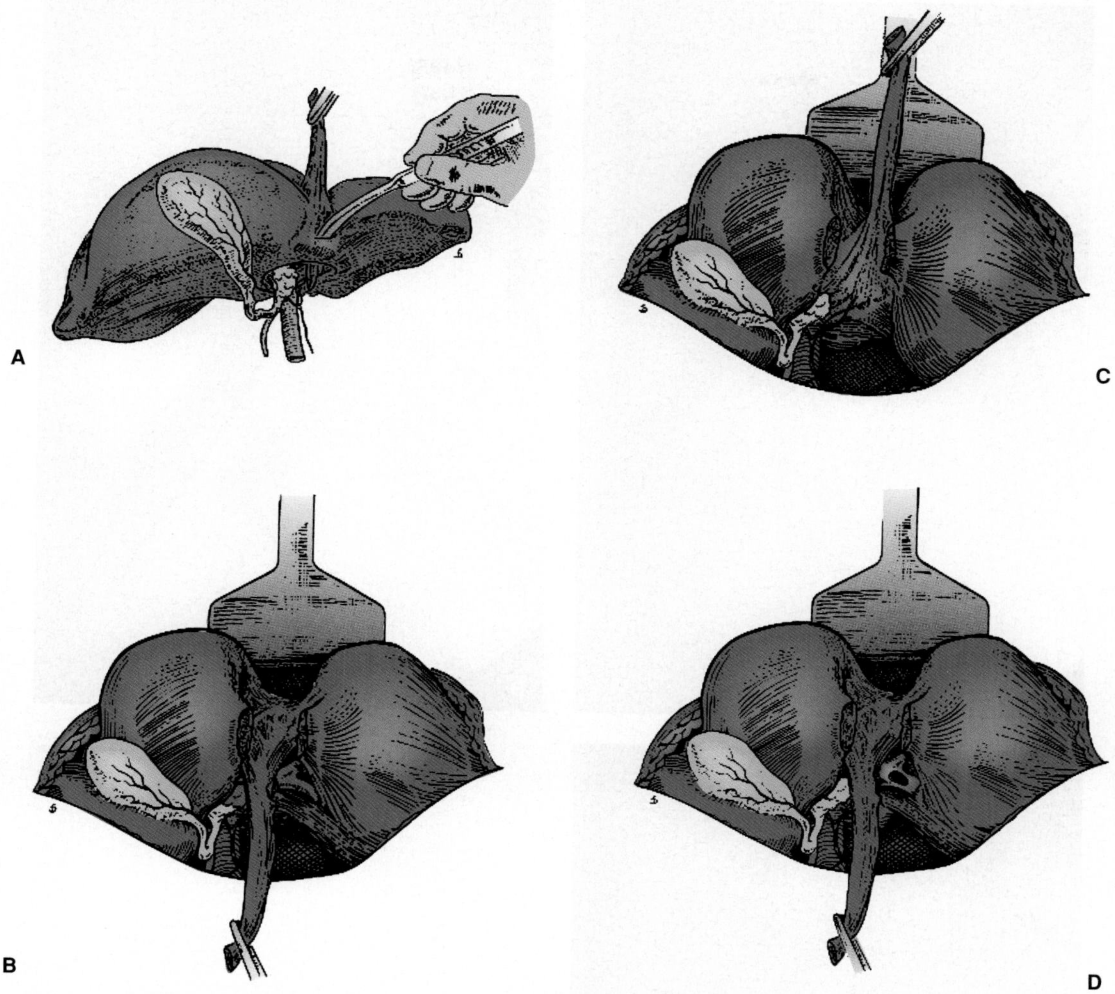

FIGURE 62.7. Surgical approach to segment III duct. **A:** The bridge of tissue present at the base of the liver is divided. **B:** The ligamentum teres is held superiorly to expose the tissue overlying the segment III duct. **C:** The segment III duct is exposed. **D:** The duct is opened in preparation for anastomosis with a Roux-en-Y jejunal limb. (Courtesy of Dr. L. H. Blumgart.)

ways. A partial excision of the left lateral segment and biliary-enteric anastomosis to the left hepatic duct (Longmire procedure) was used commonly in the past, but more recently surgical techniques have become less complicated and do not require hepatic parenchymal transection. One technique involves biliary decompression through the left duct, approached through the round ligament, a segment III bypass (Fig. 62.7). Opening the bridge of tissue just beneath the ligamentum teres allows access to the duct. In this position, a long anastomosis can be performed from the segment III duct to a jejunal limb because of the horizontal course of the duct in this location. Although less commonly used, the right hepatic duct can be approached at the base of the gallbladder fossa. This is technically more difficult and results in a higher rate of late bypass failure.[88]

Nonoperative palliative biliary decompression can be accomplished with percutaneous or endoscopic stenting, depending on the level of obstruction. Proximal lesions are usually approached percutaneously with placement of expandable stents or drainage catheters (Fig. 62.8). Internal stents result in fewer electrolyte abnormalities and improvement in patient comfort, although morbidity and mortality occurs in up to 30% of patients and stent occlusion is common.[89–91] There is a significant risk of cholangitis with external and internal drainage, occurring in more than 90% of patients with metallic expandable internal stents in one series.[90] Bleeding and bile leaks are also frequent complications. More recent techniques (e.g., photodynamic therapy) have been used to palliate patients with biliary obstruction and may hold some promise for the future.[92]

Because patients with unresectable disease have a short median survival, those whose disease is clearly unresectable on preoperative imaging should undergo percutaneous internal or external drainage. In patients who undergo exploratory surgery and whose disease is found to be unresectable, surgical bypass offers fewer episodes of cholangitis, with an improved quality of life. In some series, surgical bypass for patients with unresectable disease is the only biliary drainage procedure ever required by the patient.

In patients with unresectable distal cholangiocarcinomas, palliation can be achieved with surgical bypass, percutaneous biliary drains, or ERCP-placed stents. The simplest and most effective way to relieve jaundice is usually with an ERCP stent. Although surgical bypass offers improved patency and fewer episodes of cholangitis, the morbidity of the procedure is not warranted in patients with these aggressive tumors.

INTRAHEPATIC CHOLANGIOCARCINOMA

Patients with intrahepatic cholangiocarcinoma typically present with single liver lesions. The procedure of choice is anatomically based hepatic resection. Because these tumors

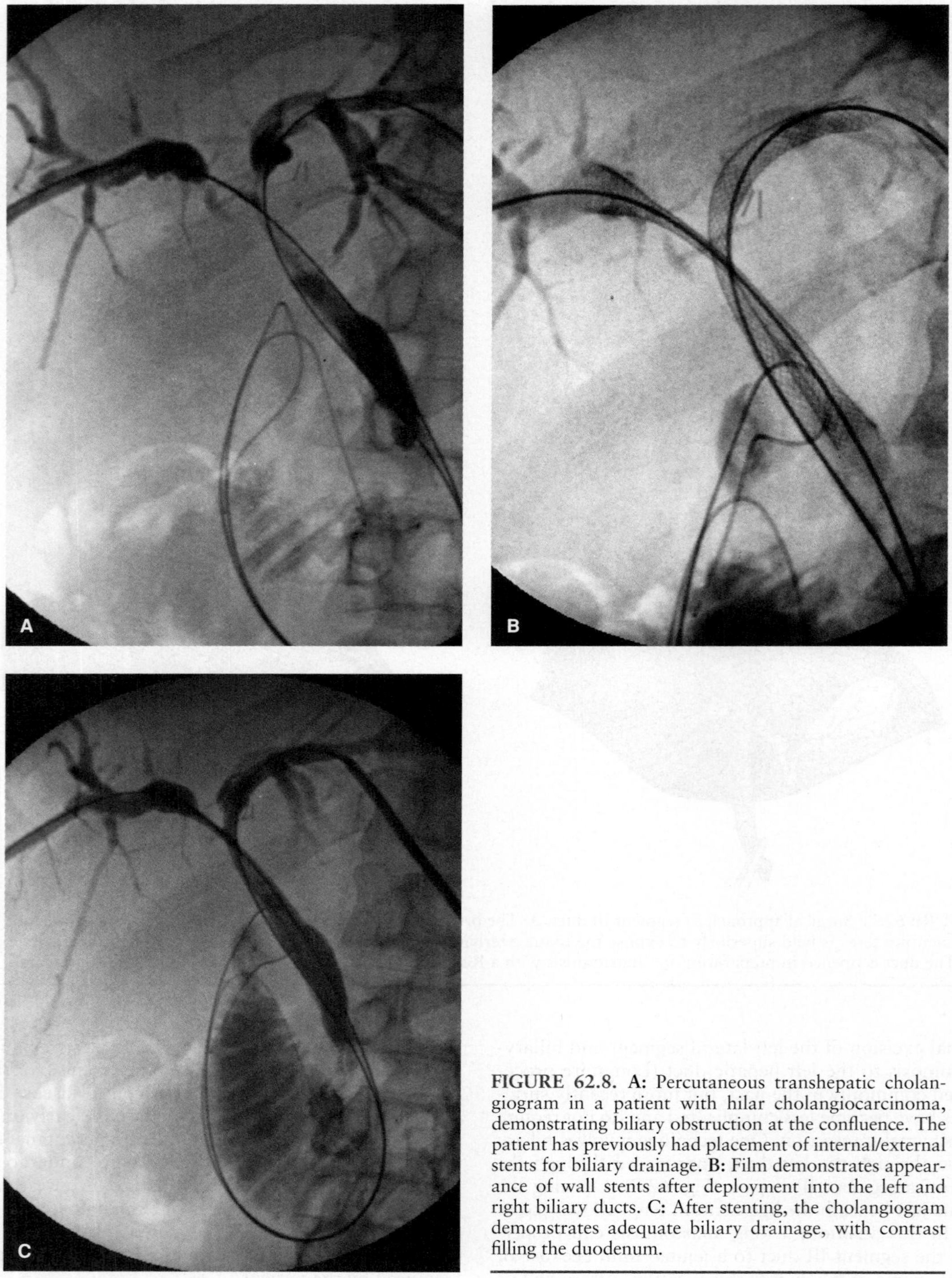

FIGURE 62.8. A: Percutaneous transhepatic cholangiogram in a patient with hilar cholangiocarcinoma, demonstrating biliary obstruction at the confluence. The patient has previously had placement of internal/external stents for biliary drainage. B: Film demonstrates appearance of wall stents after deployment into the left and right biliary ducts. C: After stenting, the cholangiogram demonstrates adequate biliary drainage, with contrast filling the duodenum.

are frequently asymptomatic, there are fewer issues with palliative management.

Adjuvant Therapy

7 To date, no chemotherapeutic regimen has consistently shown activity against cholangiocarcinoma. Many of the issues that pertain to chemotherapy trials in gallbladder cancer are directly relevant to the interpretation of trials for cholangiocarcinomas. Studies performed to date have typically been small, single-institution trials, including patients with both gallbladder and bile duct cancers.[93]

Although 5-fluorouracil (5-FU)–based chemotherapy is often offered to patients with unresectable disease, the likelihood of response is less than 10%. Capecitabine as a single agent may have some modest activity in cholangiocarcinomas.[94] When capecitabine was used in combination with gemcitabine in a recent prospective study,[95] overall survival was 14 months. Gemcitabine and cisplatin combination therapy has also been tested in phase II studies of patients with advanced biliary tract carcinoma.[47,96,97] Results of these studies demonstrated response rates of 27% to 34.5%, and overall survival of 9.7 to 11 months. The use of mitomycin C and doxorubicin (Adriamycin), in combination with 5-FU, has resulted in combined response rates of less than 30%, with higher toxicity than 5-FU alone.[98] There is no proved role for adjuvant chemotherapy in the treatment of cholangiocarcinoma; however, there are recent data to suggest no difference in overall survival (36% vs. 42%, $p = 0.6$) and locoregional recurrence (38% vs. 37%, $p = 0.13$) between patients undergoing RO resections compared with patients with high locoregional recurrence risk who received adjuvant chemoradiation therapy.[99]

In cases of unresectable cholangiocarcinoma, the use of external beam radiation therapy has been explored.[100–103] To date, no study has clearly demonstrated efficacy for this modality. Anecdotal reports of long-term survivors after external beam radiotherapy show that some individuals may benefit from such treatment, but this must be weighed against the potential complications (e.g., duodenal or bile duct stenosis and duodenitis). The most encouraging results involve use of intraoperative[101,104] or interstitial radiation.[90,102,105] Our current practice is to use combined interstitial radiation and external beam radiation in unresectable cases after palliative bypass. In patients whose disease is resected, adjuvant radiotherapy has not been shown to increase quality of life or survival.[106]

Follow-up after Resection of Cholangiocarcinoma

The most likely site of recurrence after resection of a hilar cholangiocarcinoma is locally within the bile duct, regional lymph nodes, or liver. Therapy for recurrence is palliative. Surgical reexcision is usually impossible because of the challenging anatomic location and the radical procedures that are required for resection of the primary tumor. Therefore, the goal of follow-up is diagnosis of symptomatic recurrences to direct palliative therapy and diagnosis of benign complications of surgical treatment (e.g., biliary strictures). The main symptoms of recurrence that demand palliation are pruritus or cholangitis associated with jaundice. For biliary drainage to relieve jaundice or cholangitis, either surgical drainage[90] or drainage by PTC can be effective.[107] Endoscopic drainage has little role in the relief of jaundice in patients who have had Roux-en-Y biliary reconstruction. For limited recurrences, intraluminal brachytherapy[108] or external beam radiotherapy[109] may improve palliation and, potentially, survival.

Routine follow-up consists of office visits every 3 months with physical examination and measurement of liver function tests. Although a rising alkaline phosphatase level is a good indicator of evolving biliary obstruction, patients recovering from liver resection and biliary obstruction can have persistent elevations of alkaline phosphatase. Up to 10% of patients with biliary surgical reconstruction, however, may develop a benign anastomotic stricture. Most patients with recurrence or a benign stricture will present with jaundice or cholangitis. Because there is a low likelihood of effective therapy for recurrences, the routine use of tumor markers is not recommended, although a fair percentage of biliary malignancies will express CEA or CA 19-9. The routine use of imaging studies to follow patients with cholangiocarcinoma after resection should be limited for the same reasons. When patients become symptomatic with jaundice, an abdominal ultrasound should be obtained. Other imaging will usually be dictated by the sonographic findings.

Issues for the Future

The only known curative therapy for intrahepatic and extrahepatic bile duct cancers is surgery. No proven role is seen for adjuvant chemotherapy alone or adjuvant combined chemoradiation, although further studies are needed to fully define the role of these therapies. Continued assessment of new drugs, novel radiosensitizers, and biologic agents is warranted. A better understanding of the molecular pathogenesis and genetics of bile duct cancers may lead to new therapeutic and ultimately preventive strategies for high-risk populations.

BENIGN GALLBLADDER NEOPLASMS

Incidence

Benign tumors of the biliary tract are rare, but have been reported more frequently as imaging modalities (e.g., ultrasound and CT scan) have come into widespread and frequent use. In patients undergoing cholecystectomy, the reported incidence of benign gallbladder tumors is less than 3%.

Pathology

Polyps and Pseudotumors. Benign gallbladder tumors are most frequently polyps or polypoid lesions. The incidence of polyps in asymptomatic patients is about 5%.[2] Cholesterol polyps (cholesterolosis), accounting for half of all gallbladder polypoid lesions,[110] result from epithelium-covered, cholesterol-laden macrophages in the lamina propria. These lesions are likely a result of an error in cholesterol metabolism. They extend from the mucosa on a narrow stalk, grossly appearing as yellow spots on the mucosal surface. Nearly all are multiple, and most are less than 10 mm in size.[6,110,111] When a polyp is pedunculated, it is benign in most cases; alternatively, sessile "polyps" are more often malignant (Fig. 62.9).[111] Inflammatory polyps result from chronic inflammation and extend by a narrow vascularized stalk into the gallbladder lumen. None of these lesions are considered premalignant, although isolated cases of cholesterolosis associated with in situ carcinoma have been reported.[112]

Adenomas. Gallbladder adenomas are found infrequently. They may be tubular or papillary, both arising from the epithelial layer of the gallbladder. Multiple papillary adenomas, or papillomas, are called *papillomatosis*. A direct association between benign adenoma, adenoma containing carcinoma in situ, and invasive carcinoma has been demonstrated; thus

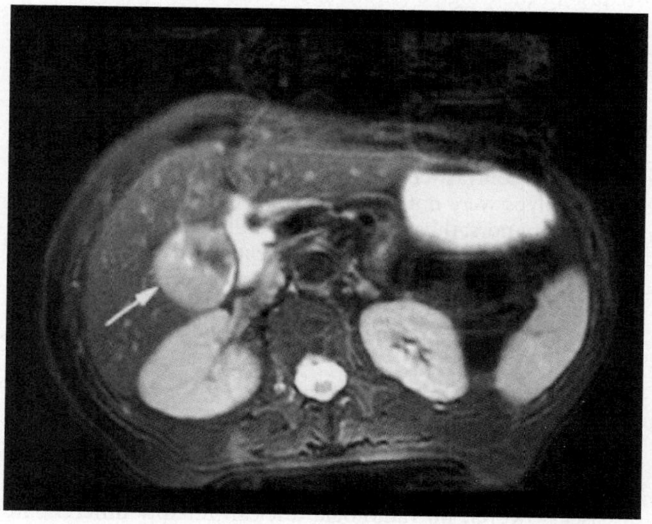

FIGURE 62.9. T_2-weighted magnetic resonance imaging scan showing a sessile polyp within the gallbladder (*arrow*) that was malignant on histologic examination.

these lesions are considered premalignant.[113] Malignant transformation, however, has only rarely been reported, primarily from large adenomas. In one series, all benign adenomas were less than 12 mm in diameter, whereas the adenomas with cancerous foci were greater than 12 mm.[114]

Adenomyomatosis. Adenomyomatosis of the gallbladder is characterized by localized or diffuse hyperplastic extensions of the mucosa into, and often beyond, a hypertrophied gallbladder muscular layer. Hyperplasia occurs at outpouchings of the mucosa of the gallbladder through the wall (Rokitansky-Aschoff sinuses) and through the crypts of Luschka. This can result in focal thickening of the gallbladder wall, resembling gallbladder adenocarcinoma. The etiology is unknown. This lesion may be premalignant, because cases of adenocarcinoma arising in or near adenomyomatosis have been reported,[114,115] but this relationship is unclear.

Other Benign Gallbladder Tumors. Other benign lesions include tumors arising from the tissue of the gallbladder wall, such as leiomyomas, lipomas, hemangiomas, granular cell tumors, and heterotopic tissue, including gastric, pancreatic, or intestinal epithelium.

Clinical Findings

Patients with benign gallbladder tumors typically present with symptoms consistent with choledocholithiasis, including right upper quadrant pain, fatty food intolerance, and nausea. Many benign gallbladder lesions are also discovered incidentally after elective cholecystectomy. Therefore, symptoms caused by benign lesions are difficult to separate from those caused by gallstones. Most lesions, however, are asymptomatic and are discovered incidentally during imaging for other abdominal conditions.

Diagnosis

Diagnosis of benign gallbladder polyps is usually made when an ultrasound study is obtained to evaluate a patient for symptoms consistent with gallstones. On ultrasound, a filling defect that does not change with position is likely a polyp or carcinoma and not a gallstone. Cholesterol polyps are typically small, submucosal, multiple, and hyperechoic on ultrasound because of their high cholesterol content. Other than this typical appearance and the fact that malignant polyps are usually more than 1 cm in size,[6,110,111] it is difficult to differentiate benign from malignant polyps.

Both intravenous contrast-enhanced and unenhanced CT may be important in distinguishing benign from malignant polyps. In a recent series examining 31 polypoid lesions of the gallbladder, contrast-enhanced CT detected all of the lesions. Benign polyps were not visualized with unenhanced CT, unlike neoplastic tumors, thus improving the ability to distinguish these lesions when both enhanced and unenhanced CT scans were obtained.[6] Endoscopic ultrasound has also been used to image these lesions, and may be more accurate than transabdominal ultrasound in differentiating benign from malignant tumors.[17]

Treatment

Large polyps, greater than 10 mm, have the greatest malignant potential.[6,110,111] Without evidence of invasion or metastatic disease, however, no radiologic test can reliably differentiate benign from malignant lesions. Therefore, if large (>1 cm) polyps are present, even in asymptomatic patients without stones, cholecystectomy is warranted.[108] Smaller pedunculated lesions with the gross characteristics of a benign cholesterol polyp may be observed and resected only if symptomatic. Although these lesions have routinely been followed with ultrasound, a recent prospective study suggested that polyps smaller than 1 cm do not progress to carcinoma.[116] Cholecystectomy, however, is still considered the standard of care if there is any increase in size.

BENIGN BILE DUCT NEOPLASMS

Incidence

Benign bile duct tumors, at times clinically resembling hilar cholangiocarcinoma, are less common, occurring in less than 1% of patients.[1]

Pathology

Attesting to the rarity of these lesions, only two cases of benign extrahepatic bile duct disease occurred in 4,200 biliary tract operations in one institution.[117] The most common benign tumors of the extrahepatic biliary tree arise from the glandular epithelium lining the ducts; about two thirds of benign tumors are polyps, adenomatous papilloma, or bile duct adenomas. Most are found in the periampullary region, but they can be distributed throughout the entire biliary tree (Fig. 62.10). Multiple papillomas also have been reported throughout the intrahepatic and extrahepatic biliary tree, termed *multiple biliary papillomatosis*. Although local recurrence and progression to death from obstructive jaundice and cholangitis occur frequently in these rare cases, these tumors have little, if any, malignant potential. Other benign tumors (e.g., cystadenoma, granular cell myoblastoma, leiomyoma, and heterotopic tissue) have also been reported.

One condition that deserves consideration is the case of "malignant masquerade," an inflammatory, fibrotic lesion clinically resembling hilar cholangiocarcinoma, but pathologically consisting only of extensive fibrosis and inflammatory cells without evidence of dysplasia or preneoplastic change.[118–120] In patients being considered for palliative treatment alone with presumed hilar cholangiocarcinoma, it is essential to obtain a tissue diagnosis. It is inappropriate to treat benign lesions by

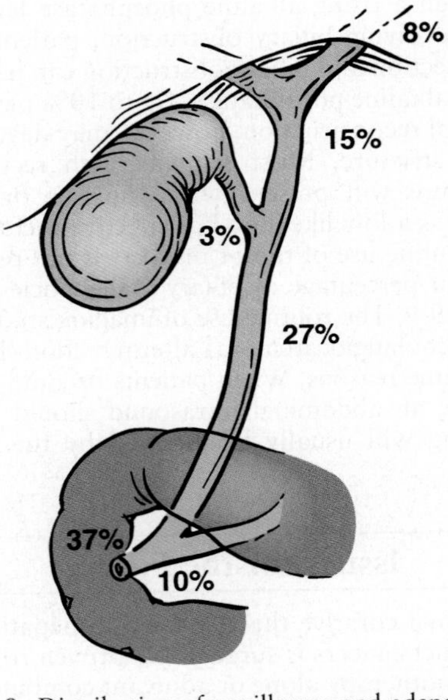

FIGURE 62.10. Distribution of papillomas and adenomas of the biliary tree. The ampulla and common bile duct are the most frequent sites.

percutaneous stenting because of the excellent outcome after resection of these lesions.

Clinical Findings

Biliary obstruction, with resultant jaundice or cholangitis, is frequently the presenting symptom in patients with benign bile duct tumors. Symptoms may also include epigastric pain or nausea. Because these tumors are indolent, symptoms may be intermittent or gradually progressive.

Diagnosis

Because of the presence of jaundice, benign bile duct tumors are usually initially evaluated with ultrasound. Many patients then undergo ERCP or PTC and CT scan. A diagnosis of malignant masquerade should be suspected in patients with mass lesions that resemble hilar cholangiocarcinomas, but without lobar atrophy or portal vein involvement.

Treatment

Resection and reconstruction are performed to relieve jaundice and cholangitis. The preferred reconstruction is a Roux-en-Y choledochojejunostomy to decrease the risk of postoperative biliary stricture or recurrent cholangitis.

References

1. Diehl AK. Epidemiology of gallbladder cancer: a synthesis of recent data. *J Natl Cancer Inst* 1980;65:1209–1213.
2. Okamoto M, Okamoto H, Kitahara F, et al. Ultrasonographic evidence of association of polyps and stones with gallbladder cancer. *Am J Gastroenterol* 1999;94(2):446–450.
3. Piehler JM, Crichlow RW. Primary carcinoma of the gallbladder. *Surg Gynecol Obstet* 1978;147(6):929–942.
4. Anderson JB, Cooper MJ, Williamson RC. Adenocarcinoma of the extrahepatic biliary tree. *Ann R Coll Surg Engl* 1985;67(3):139–143.
5. Diehl AK. Gallstone size and the risk of gallbladder cancer. *JAMA* 1983; 250(17):2323–2326.
6. Shinkai H, Kimura W, Muto T. Surgical indications for small polypoid lesions of the gallbladder. *Am J Surg* 1998;175(2):114–117.
7. Towfigh S, McFadden DW, Cortina GR, et al. Porcelain gallbladder is not associated with gallbladder carcinoma. *Am Surg* 2001;67(1):7–10.
8. Stephen AE, Berger DL. Carcinoma in the porcelain gallbladder: a relationship revisited. *Surgery* 2001;129(6):699–703.
9. Henson DE, Albores-Saavedra J, Corle D. Carcinoma of the gallbladder. Histologic types, stage of disease, grade, and survival rates. *Cancer* 1992; 70(6):1493–1497.
10. Yamamoto M, Nakajo S, Tahara E. Carcinoma of the gallbladder: the correlation between histogenesis and prognosis. *Virchows Arch A Pathol Anat Histopathol* 1989;414(2):83–90.
11. Bartlett DL, Fong Y, Fortner JG, et al. Long-term results after resection for gallbladder cancer. Implications for staging and management. *Ann Surg* 1996;224(5):639–646.
12. Shirai Y, Yoshida K, Tsukada K, et al. Radical surgery for gallbladder carcinoma. Long-term results. *Ann Surg* 1992;216(5):565–568.
13. Wistuba II, Sugio K, Hung J, et al.. Allele-specific mutations involved in the pathogenesis of endemic gallbladder carcinoma in Chile. *Cancer Res* 1995;55(12):2511–2515.
14. Matsubara T, Sakurai Y, Sasayama Y, et al. K-ras point mutations in cancerous and noncancerous biliary epithelium in patients with pancreaticobiliary maljunction. *Cancer* 1996;77(8 suppl):1752–1757.
15. Wistuba II, Albores-Saavedra J. Genetic abnormalities involved in the pathogenesis of gallbladder carcinoma. *J Hepatobiliary Pancreat Surg* 1999;6(3):237–244.
16. Kumar V, Fausto N, Abbas A. eds. *Robbins & Cotran Pathologic Basis of Disease*, 7th ed. Philadelphia: WB Saunders; 2004:89..
17. Sugiyama M, Xie XY, Atomi Y, et al. Differential diagnosis of small polypoid lesions of the gallbladder: the value of endoscopic ultrasonography. *Ann Surg* 1999;229(4):498–504.
18. Mizuguchi M, Kudo S, Fukahori T, et al. Endoscopic ultrasonography for demonstrating loss of multiple-layer pattern of the thickened gallbladder wall in the preoperative diagnosis of gallbladder cancer. *Eur Radiol* 1997;7(8):1323–1327.
19. Ohtani T, Shirai Y, Tsukada K, et al. Spread of gallbladder carcinoma: CT evaluation with pathologic correlation. *Abdom Imaging* 1996;21(3): 195–201.
20. Soto JA, Barish MA, Yucel EK, et al. Magnetic resonance cholangiography: comparison with endoscopic retrograde cholangiopancreatography. *Gastroenterology* 1996;110(2):589–597.
21. Demachi H, Matsui O, Hoshiba K, et al. Dynamic MRI using a surface coil in chronic cholecystitis and gallbladder carcinoma: radiologic and histopathologic correlation. *J Comput Assist Tomogr* 1997;21(4): 643–651.
22. Schwartz LH, Coakley FV, Sun Y, et al. Neoplastic pancreaticobiliary duct obstruction: evaluation with breath-hold MR cholangiopancreatography. *AJR Am J Roentgenol* 1998;170(6):1491–1495.
23. Fong Y, Brennan MF, Turnbull A, et al. Gallbladder cancer discovered during laparoscopic surgery. Potential for iatrogenic tumor dissemination. *Arch Surg* 1993;128(9):1054–1056.
24. Weber SM, DeMatteo RP, Fong Y, et al. Staging laparoscopy in patients with extrahepatic biliary carcinoma. Analysis of 100 patients. *Ann Surg* 2002;235(3):392–399.
25. Barbot DJ, Marks JH, Feld RI, et al. Improved staging of liver tumors using laparoscopic intraoperative ultrasound. *J Surg Oncol* 1997;64: 63–67.
26. Bhargava DK, Sarin S, Verma K, et al. Laparoscopy in carcinoma of the gallbladder. *Gastrointest Endosc* 1983;29(1):21–22.
27. Dagnini G, Marin G, Patella M, et al. Laparoscopy in the diagnosis of primary carcinoma of the gallbladder. A study of 98 cases. *Gastrointest Endosc* 1984;30(5):289–291.
28. Vollmer CM, Drebin JA, Middleton WD, et al. Utility of staging laparoscopy in subsets of peripancreatic and biliary malignancies. *Ann Surg* 2002;235(1):1–7.
29. Ouchi K, Owada Y, Matsuno S, et al. Prognostic factors in the surgical treatment of gallbladder carcinoma. *Surgery* 1987;101(6):731–737.
30. Donohue JH, Nagorney DM, Grant CS, et al. Carcinoma of the gallbladder. Does radical resection improve outcome? *Arch Surg* 1990;125(2): 237–241.
31. Ogura Y, Mizumoto R, Isaji S, et al. Radical operations for carcinoma of the gallbladder: present status in Japan. *World J Surg* 1991;15(3): 337–343.
32. Yamaguchi K, Tsuneyoshi M. Subclinical gallbladder carcinoma. *Am J Surg* 1992;163(4):382–386.
33. Yamaguchi K, Chijiiwa K, Saiki S, et al. Reliability of frozen section diagnosis of gallbladder tumor for detecting carcinoma and depth of its invasion. *J Surg Oncol* 1997;65(2):132–136.
34. Nakamura S, Sakaguchi S, Suzuki S, et al. Aggressive surgery for carcinoma of the gallbladder. *Surgery* 1989;106(3):467–473.
35. Billingsley KG, Jarnagin WR, Fong Y, et al. Segment-oriented hepatic resection in the management of malignant neoplasms of the liver. *J Am Coll Surg* 1998;187(5):471–481.
36. Shirai Y, Yoshida K, Tsukada K, et al. Inapparent carcinoma of the gallbladder. An appraisal of a radical second operation after simple cholecystectomy. *Ann Surg* 1992;215(4):326–331.
37. Wanebo HJ, Castle WN, Fechner RE. Is carcinoma of the gallbladder a curable lesion? *Ann Surg* 1982;195(5):624–631.
38. Kai M, Chijiiwa K, Ohuchida J, et al. A curative resection improves the postoperative survival rate even in patients with advanced gallbladder carcinoma. *J Gastrointest Surg* 2007;11(8):1025–1032.
39. Jensen EH, Abraham A, Habermann EB, et al. A critical analysis of the surgical management of early-stage gallbladder cancer in the United States. *J Gastrointest Surg* 2009;13(4):722–727.
40. Shih SP, Schulick RD, Cameron JL, et al. Gallbladder cancer: the role of laparoscopy and radical resection. *Ann Surg* 2007;245(6):893–901.
41. Chijiiwa K, Tanaka M. Carcinoma of the gallbladder: an appraisal of surgical resection. *Surgery* 1994;115(6):751–756.
42. Drouard F, Delamarre J, Capron JP. Cutaneous seeding of gallbladder cancer after laparoscopic cholecystectomy. *N Engl J Med* 1991;325(18):1316.
43. Pezet D, Fondrinier E, Rotman N, et al. Parietal seeding of carcinoma of the gallbladder after laparoscopic cholecystectomy. *Br J Surg* 1992;79(3): 230.
44. Weiland ST, Mahvi DM, Niederhuber JE, et al. Should suspected early gallbladder cancer be treated laparoscopically? *J Gastrointest Surg* 2002; 6(1):50–56.
45. Fong Y, Jarnagin W, Blumgart LH. Gallbladder cancer: comparison of patients presenting initially for definitive operation with those presenting after prior noncurative intervention. *Ann Surg* 2000;232(4):557–569.
46. Takada T, Amano H, Yasuda H, et al. Is postoperative adjuvant chemotherapy useful for gallbladder carcinoma? A phase III multicenter prospective randomized controlled trial in patients with resected pancreaticobiliary carcinoma. *Cancer* 2002;95(8):1685–1695.
47. Kim HJ, Kim MH, Myung SJ, et al. A new strategy for the application of CA19-9 in the differentiation of pancreaticobiliary cancer: analysis using a receiver operating characteristic curve. *Am J Gastroenterol* 1999;94(7): 1941–1946.
48. Lazcano-Ponce EC, Miquel JF, Munoz N, et al. Epidemiology and molecular pathology of gallbladder cancer. *CA Cancer J Clin* 2001;51(6): 349–364.
49. Pitt HA, Dooley WC, Yeo CJ, et al. Malignancies of the biliary tree. *Curr Probl Surg* 1995;32(1):1–90.
50. Patel T. Increasing incidence and mortality of primary intrahepatic cholangiocarcinoma in the United States. *Hepatology* 2001;33(6):1353–1357.

51. Welzel TM, Graubard BI, El-Serag HB, et al. Risk factors for intrahepatic and extrahepatic cholangiocarcinoma in the United States: a population-based case-control study. *Clin Gastroenterol Hepatol* 2007;5(10):1221–1228.
52. Endo I, Gonen M, Yopp AC, et al. Intrahepatic cholangiocarcinoma: rising frequency, improved survival, and determinants of outcome after resection. *Ann Surg* 2008;248(1):84–96.
53. de Groen PC, Gores GJ, LaRusso NF, et al. Biliary tract cancers. *N Engl J Med* 1999;341(18):1368–1378.
54. Kaya M, de Groen PC, Angulo P, et al. Treatment of cholangiocarcinoma complicating primary sclerosing cholangitis: the Mayo Clinic experience. *Am J Gastroenterol* 2001;96(4):1164–1169.
55. Hakamada K, Sasaki M, Endoh M, et al. Late development of bile duct cancer after sphincteroplasty: a ten- to twenty-two-year follow-up study. *Surgery* 1997;121:488–492.
56. Bhuiya MR, Nimura Y, Kamiya J, et al. Clinicopathologic studies on perineural invasion of bile duct carcinoma. *Ann Surg* 1992;215(4):344–349.
57. Yamamoto M, Takasaki K, Yoshikawa T. Lymph node metastasis in intrahepatic cholangiocarcinoma. *Jpn J Clin Oncol* 1999;29(3):147–150.
58. Burke EC, Jarnagin WR, Hochwald SN, et al. Hilar cholangiocarcinoma: patterns of spread, the importance of hepatic resection for curative operation, and a presurgical clinical staging system. *Ann Surg* 1998;228(3):385–394.
59. Cameron JL, Pitt HA, Zinner MJ, et al. Management of proximal cholangiocarcinomas by surgical resection and radiotherapy. *Am J Surg* 1990;159:91–97; discussion 97–98.
60. Nakayama T, Ikeda A, Okunda K. Percutaneous transhepatic drainage of the biliary tract. *Gastroenterology* 1978;74:554–559.
61. Hochwald SN, Burke EC, Jarnagin WR, et al. Association of preoperative biliary stenting with increased postoperative infectious complications in proximal cholangiocarcinoma. *Arch Surg* 1999;134(3):261–266.
62. McPherson GAD, Benjamin IS, Hodgson HJF, et al. Pre-operative percutaneous transhepatic biliary drainage: the results of a controlled trial. *Br J Surg* 1984;71:371–375.
63. Pitt HA, Gomes AS, Lois JF, et al. Does preoperative percutaneous biliary drainage reduce operative risk or increase hospital cost? *Ann Surg* 1985;201:545–552.
64. Okuda K, Kubo Y, Okazaki N, et al. Clinical aspects of intrahepatic bile duct carcinoma including hilar carcinoma. A study of 57 autopsy proven cases. *Cancer* 1977;39:232–246.
65. Ottow RT, August DA, Sugarbaker PH. Treatment of proximal biliary tract carcinoma: an overview of techniques and results. *Surgery* 1985;97:251–262.
66. Altaee MY, Johnson PJ, Farrant JM, et al. Etiologic and clinical characteristics of peripheral and hilar cholangiocarcinoma. *Cancer* 1991;68:2051–2055.
67. Baer HU, Stain SC, Dennison AR, et al. Improvements in survival by aggressive resections of hilar cholangiocarcinoma. *Ann Surg* 1993;217:20–27.
68. Bengmark S, Ekberg H, Evander A, et al. Major liver resection for hilar cholangiocarcinoma. *Ann Surg* 1988;207:120–125.
69. Bismuth H, Nakache R, Diamond T. Management strategies in resection for hilar cholangiocarcinoma. *Ann Surg* 1992;215:31–38.
70. Hadjis NS, Blenkharn JI, Alexander N, et al. Outcome of radical surgery in hilar cholangiocarcinoma. *Surgery* 1990;107:597–604.
71. Nagorney DM, Donohue JH, Farnell MB, et al. Outcomes after curative resections of cholangiocarcinoma. *Arch Surg* 1993;128:871–879.
72. Rea DJ, Munoz-Juarez M, Farnell MB, et al. Major hepatic resection for hilar cholangiocarcinoma: analysis of 46 patients. *Arch Surg* 2004;139(5):514–523.
73. Meyer CG, Penn I, James L. Liver transplantation for cholangiocarcinoma: results in 207 patients. *Transplantation* 2000;69(8):1633–1637.
74. Brandsaeter B, Isoniemi H, Broome U, et al. Liver transplantation for primary sclerosing cholangitis; predictors and consequences of hepatobiliary malignancy. *J Hepatol* 2004;40(5):815–822.
75. Robles R, Figueras J, Turrion VS, et al. Spanish experience in liver transplantation for hilar and peripheral cholangiocarcinoma. *Ann Surg* 2004;239(2):265–271.
76. Sudan D, DeRoover A, Chinnakotla S, et al. Radiochemotherapy and transplantation allow long-term survival for nonresectable hilar cholangiocarcinoma. *Am J Transplant* 2002;2(8):774–779.
77. Baron TH, Harewood GC, Rumalla A, et al. A prospective comparison of digital image analysis and routine cytology for the identification of malignancy in biliary tract strictures. *Clin Gastroenterol Hepatol* 2004;2(3):214–219.
78. Kipp BR, Stadheim LM, Halling SA, et al. A comparison of routine cytology and fluorescence in situ hybridization for the detection of malignant bile duct strictures. *Am J Gastroenterol* 2004;99(9):1675–1681.
79. Blumgart LH, Hadjis NS, Benjamin IS, et al. Surgical approaches to cholangiocarcinoma at confluence of hepatic ducts. *Lancet* 1984;1:66–69.
82. Reding R, Buard JL, Lebeau G, et al. Surgical management of 552 carcinomas of the extrahepatic bile ducts (gallbladder and periampullary tumors excluded). Results of the French Surgical Association Survey. *Ann Surg* 1991;213:236–241.
83. Lieser MJ, Barry MK, Rowland C, et al. Surgical management of intrahepatic cholangiocarcinoma: a 31-year experience. *J Hepatobiliary Pancreat Surg* 1998;5(1):41–47.
84. Nakeeb A, Pitt HA, Sohn TA, et al. Cholangiocarcinoma: a spectrum of intrahepatic, perihilar, and distal tumors. *Ann Surg* 1996;224:463–475.
85. Weber SM, Jarnagin WR, Klimstra D, et al. Intrahepatic cholangiocarcinoma: resectability, recurrence pattern, and outcomes. *J Am Coll Surg* 2001;193(4):384–391.
86. Berdah SV, Delpero JR, Garcia S, et al. A western surgical experience of peripheral cholangiocarcinoma. *Br J Surg* 1996;83:1517–1521.
87. Fong Y, Blumgart LH, Lin E, et al. Outcome of treatment for distal bile duct cancer. *Br J Surg* 1996;83(12):1712–1715.
88. Jarnagin WR, Burke E, Powers C, et al. Intrahepatic biliary enteric bypass provides effective palliation in selected patients with malignant obstruction at the hepatic duct confluence. *Am J Surg* 1998;175(6):453–460.
89. Glattli A, Stain SC, Baer HU, et al. Unresectable malignant biliary obstruction: treatment by self-expandable biliary endoprostheses. *HPB Surg* 1993;6:175–184.
90. Kuvshinoff BW, Armstrong JG, Fong Y, et al. Palliation of irresectable hilar cholangiocarcinoma with biliary drainage and radiotherapy. *Br J Surg* 1995;82(11):1522–1525.
91. Lee BH, Choe DH, Lee JH, et al. Metallic stents in malignant biliary obstruction: prospective long-term clinical results. *AJR Am J Roentgenol* 1997;168(3):741–745.
92. Rumalla A, Baron TH, Wang KK, et al. Endoscopic application of photodynamic therapy for cholangiocarcinoma. *Gastrointest Endosc* 2001;53(4):500–504.
93. Yee K, Sheppard BC, Domreis J, et al. Cancers of the gallbladder and biliary ducts. *Oncology (Williston Park)* 2002;16(7):939–946, 949.
94. Stemmler J, Heinemann V, Schalhorn A. Capecitabine as second-line treatment for metastatic cholangiocarcinoma: a report of two cases. *Onkologie* 2002;25(2):182–184.
95. Iyer RV, Gibbs J, Kuvshinoff B, et al. A phase II study of gemcitabine and capecitabine in advanced cholangiocarcinoma and carcinoma of the gallbladder: a single-institution prospective study. *Ann Surg Oncol* 2007;14(11):3202–3209.
96. Meyerhardt JA, Zhu AX, Stuart K, et al. Phase-II study of gemcitabine and cisplatin in patients with metastatic biliary and gallbladder cancer. *Dig Dis Sci* 2008;53(2):564–570.
97. Thongprasert S, Napapan S, Charoentum C, et al. Phase II study of gemcitabine and cisplatin as first-line chemotherapy in inoperable biliary tract carcinoma. Ann Oncol 2005;16(2):279–281.
98. Oberfield RA, Rossi RL. The role of chemotherapy in the treatment of bile duct cancer. *World J Surg* 1988;12:105–108.
99. Borghero Y, Crane CH, Szklaruk J, et al. Extrahepatic bile duct adenocarcinoma: patients at high-risk for local recurrence treated with surgery and adjuvant chemoradiation have an equivalent overall survival to patients with standard-risk treated with surgery alone. Ann Surg Oncol 2008;15(11):3147–3156.
100. Cameron JL, Broe P, Zuidema GD. Proximal bile duct tumors. Surgical management with silastic transhepatic biliary stents. *Ann Surg* 1982;196:412–419.
101. Iwasaki Y, Ohto M, Todoroki T, et al. Treatment of carcinoma of the biliary system. *Surg Gynecol Obstet* 1977;144(2):219–224.
102. Fletcher MS, Brinkley D, Dawson JL, et al. Treatment of high bileduct carcinoma by internal radiotherapy with iridium-192 wire. *Lancet* 1981;2:172–174.
103. Kopelson G, Gunderson LL. Primary and adjuvant radiation therapy in gallbladder and extrahepatic biliary tract carcinoma. *J Clin Gastroenterol* 1983;5(1):43–50.
104. Todoroki T, Iwasaki Y, Okamura T, et al. Intraoperative radiotherapy for advanced carcinoma of the biliary system. *Cancer* 1980;46(10):2179–2184.
105. Ikeda H, Kuroda C, Uchida H, et al. Intramural irradiation with iridium-192 wires for extrahepatic bile duct carcinoma. *Nippon Acta Radiologica* 1979;39:1356–1357.
106. Pitt HA, Nakeeb A, Abrams RA, et al. Perihilar cholangiocarcinoma. Postoperative radiotherapy does not improve survival. *Ann Surg* 1995;221:788–798.
107. Polydorou AA, Cairns SR, Dowsett JF, et al. Palliation of proximal malignant biliary obstruction by endoscopic endoprosthesis insertion. *Gut* 1991;32(6):685–689.
108. Aldridge MC, Bismuth H. Gallbladder cancer: the polyp-cancer sequence. *Br J Surg* 1990;77(4):363–364.
109. Shiina T, Mikuriya S, Uno T, et al. Radiotherapy of cholangiocarcinoma: the roles for primary and adjuvant therapies. *Cancer Chemother Pharmacol* 1992;31(suppl):S115–S118.
110. Koga A, Watanabe K, Fukuyama T, et al. Diagnosis and operative indications for polypoid lesions of the gallbladder. *Arch Surg* 1988;123(1):26–29.
111. Furukawa H, Kosuge T, Shimada K, et al. Small polypoid lesions of the gallbladder: differential diagnosis and surgical indications by helical computed tomography. *Arch Surg* 1998;133(7):735–739.
112. Akiyama T, Sahara H, Seto K, et al. Gallbladder cancer associated with cholesterosis. *J Gastroenterol* 1996;31(3):470–474.
113. Kozuka S, Tsubone N, Yasui A, et al. Relation of adenoma to carcinoma in the gallbladder. *Cancer* 1982;50(10):2226–2234.
114. Aldridge MC, Gruffaz F, Castaing D, et al. Adenomyomatosis of the gallbladder. A premalignant lesion? *Surgery* 1991;109(1):107–110.
115. Kurihara K, Mizuseki K, Ninomiya T, et al. Carcinoma of the gallbladder arising in adenomyomatosis. *Acta Pathol Jpn* 1993;43(1–2):82–85.

116. Csendes A, Burgos AM, Csendes P, et al. Late follow-up of polypoid lesions of the gallbladder smaller than 10 mm. *Ann Surg* 2001;234(5): 657–660.
117. Farris KB, Faust BF. Granular cell tumors of biliary ducts. Report of two cases and review of the literature. *Arch Pathol Lab Med* 1979;103(10): 510–512.
118. Hadjis NS, Collier NA, Blumgart LH. Malignant masquerade at the hilum of the liver. *Br J Surg* 1985;72:659–661.
119. Standfield NJ, Salisbury JR, Howard ER. Benign non-traumatic inflammatory strictures of the extrahepatic biliary system. *Br J Surg* 1989;76(8): 849–852.
120. Verbeek PC, Van Leeuwen DJ, de Wit LT, et al. Benign fibrosing disease at the hepatic confluence mimicking Klatskin tumors. *Surgery* 1992;112: 866–871.
121. Wakai T, Shirai Y, Yokoyama N, et al. Early gallbladder carcinoma does not warrant radical resection. *Br J Surg* 2001;88(5):675–678.
122. Taner CB, Nagorney DM, Donohue JH. Surgical treatment of gallbladder cancer. *J Gastrointest Surg* 2004;8(1):83–89.
123. McMasters KM, Tuttle TM, Leach SD, et al. Neoadjuvant chemoradiation for extrahepatic cholangiocarcinoma. *Am J Surg* 1997;174(6):605–608.
124. Klempnauer J, Ridder GJ, von Wasielewski R, et al. Resectional surgery of hilar cholangiocarcinoma: a multivariate analysis of prognostic factors. *J Clin Oncol* 1997;15:947–954.
125. Nagino M, Nimura Y, Kamiya J, et al. Segmental liver resections for hilar cholangiocarcinoma. *Hepatogastroenterology* 1998;45(19):7–13.
126. Nakeeb A, Tran KQ, Black MJ, et al. Improved survival in resected biliary malignancies. *Surgery* 2002;132(4):555–563.
127. Jarnagin WR, Fong Y, DeMatteo RP, et al. Staging, resectability, and outcome in 225 patients with hilar cholangiocarcinoma. *Ann Surg* 2001; 234(4):507–517.
128. Jang JY, Kim SW, Park DJ, et al. Actual long-term outcome of extrahepatic bile duct cancer after surgical resection. *Ann Surg* 2005;241(1):77–84.
129. Konstadoulakis MM, Roayaie S, Gomatos IP, et al. Aggressive surgical resection for hilar cholangiocarcinoma: is it justified? Audit of a single center's experience. *Am J Surg* 2008;196(2):160–169.
130. Yubin L, Chihua F, Zhixiang J, et al. Surgical management and prognostic factors of hilar cholangiocarcinoma: experience with 115 cases in China. *Ann Surg Oncol* 2008;15(8):2113–2119.

CHAPTER 63 COLONIC AND RECTAL ANATOMY AND PHYSIOLOGY

ELIZABETH C. WICK

KEY POINTS

1. The mesorectum is invested by the fascia propria of the rectum.
2. The ileocolic branch of the superior mesenteric artery supplies the right colon and part of the transverse colon.
3. The inferior mesenteric artery supplies part of the transverse colon, sigmoid colon, and rectum.
4. The inguinal lymph nodes drain the lymphatics from the anal canal below the dentate line.
5. The colon has 10^{13} bacteria, which promote mucosal immunity, help digest complex nutrients, and protect against pathogenic organisms.
6. Alterations in the colonic flora have been associated with inflammatory bowel disease and colorectal cancer.
7. Constipation is one of the most common conditions treated by physicians, but only rarely is it due to colonic inertia.
8. During postoperative ileus, the stomach recovers after 1 to 2 days, the small bowel after 1 day, and the colon after 3 days.
9. Thoracic epidural use after colorectal surgery can shorten postoperative ileus.

EMBRYOLOGY OF THE COLON AND RECTUM

The primitive gut is derived from endoderm and begins to form during the third to fourth weeks of gestation. It is divided into three segments: foregut, midgut, and hindgut. The midgut gives rise to the small intestine distal to the ampulla of Vater, the cecum and appendix, the ascending colon, and the right half to two thirds of the transverse colon, all of which receive blood supply from the superior mesenteric artery. During the sixth gestational week, the midgut herniates from the abdominal cavity into the extraembryonic coelom, undergoes a 270-degree counterclockwise rotation around the superior mesenteric artery, and then returns to the abdominal cavity at 10 weeks' gestation. The hindgut gives rise to the distal one third of the transverse colon, descending and sigmoid colon, rectum, and upper portion of the anal canal, all of which receive blood from the inferior mesenteric artery. The terminal end of the hindgut is the endoderm-lined pouch termed the *cloaca*. During development, the cloaca is partitioned by the urorectal septum into the rectum and upper anal canal and urogenital sinus. Ultimately, the distal anal canal arises from canalization of the ectoderm. The pectineal or dentate line marks the junction between tissue derived from endoderm and ectoderm in the anal canal.

ANATOMY OF THE COLON AND RECTUM

On average, the colon is 150 cm long. Characteristics unique to the colon are (a) taeniae coli, (b) haustra, and (c) appendices epiploicae. There are three taeniae (anterior, posterior medial, and posterior lateral), which are condensations of the outer longitudinal muscle layer in the colon. The taeniae originate at the base of the appendix, course along the length of the colon, and then converge at the rectosigmoid junction. The haustra are pockets of colon wall, between the taeniae, that result from the fact that the length of the taeniae is one sixth of the colon length.[1] The epiploicae appendices are fat appendages seen on the colonic serosa. The colon consists of five layers: mucosa, submucosa, circular muscle layer, longitudinal muscle layer, and serosa (Fig. 63.1). Microscopically, the colonic mucosa is a columnar epithelium marked by crypts and goblet cells. Unlike the small intestine, the columnar epithelium of the colon and rectum does not have villi.

The colon begins in the right lower quadrant with the cecum. The cecum extends approximately 6 to 8 cm below the ileocecal valve (where the terminal ileum enters the posteromedial aspect of the cecum) (Fig. 63.2). The cecum is the widest portion of the colon (7.5 to 8.5 cm in diameter) and has the thinnest wall. The appendix originates from the lowest portion of the cecum and can be readily identified by following the converging taeniae. In 85% to 95% of people, the appendix lies posteromedial to the cecum, in line with the terminal ileum, but the position can vary, with the most frequent variants being retrocecal, pelvic, and retroileal.[2] During colonoscopy, visualization of the appendiceal orifice is one of the landmarks required in a complete colonic exam. From the cecum, the right colon ascends to the hepatic flexure (approximately 15 cm). The hepatic flexure is anterior to the inferior pole of the right kidney and overlies the second portion of the duodenum. The hepatic flexure is marked by medial, anterior, and downward angulation of the colon. When the right colon is mobilized during a colectomy, care must be taken to avoid injury to the underlying duodenum. Only the anterior surface of the right colon is invested with peritoneum; laterally, the white line of Toldt marks the extent of the peritoneal covering and serves as an important landmark during surgical mobilization of the colon.

The transverse colon stretches from the hepatic flexure to the splenic flexure and is the longest segment of colon (between 30 and 60 cm). The transverse colon is suspended

COLORECTAL

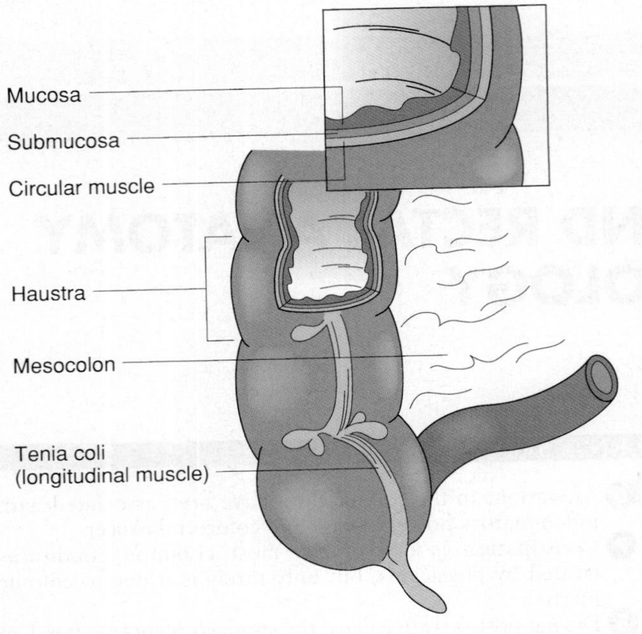

FIGURE 63.1. Layers of the colonic wall.

by the transverse mesocolon and is completely intraperitoneal. It is the most mobile portion of the colon. The greater omentum descends from the greater curve of the stomach in front of the transverse colon and then ascends to attach to the transverse colon on its anterosuperior edge. The splenic flexure is situated high in the left upper quadrant, more cephalad than the hepatic flexure. The flexure lies anterior to the mid-left kidney and abuts the lower pole of the spleen. There are attachments from the colon to the diaphragm and spleen (phrenocolic and splenocolic ligaments) and these must be carefully divided during mobilization of the splenic flexure to avoid splenic injury. The descending colon is approximately 25 cm long and courses from the splenic flexure to its junction with the sigmoid colon at the pelvic brim. It lies anterior to the left kidney and, like the right colon, the anterior, lateral, and medial portions of the descending colon are covered by peritoneum.

The sigmoid colon extends from the pelvic brim to the sacral promontory, where it continues as the rectum and generally measures 30 to 40 cm in length. The rectosigmoid junction is marked by the convergence of the colonic taenia. The sigmoid colon is extremely mobile and has a generous mesentery that extends along the pelvic brim from the iliac fossa across the sacroiliac joint to the second or third sacral segment. Because of its mobile mesentery, the sigmoid colon can twist and cause an obstruction, termed *sigmoid volvulus*. The left ureter runs in the intersigmoid fossa. When the sigmoid colon is being mobilized, the left ureter should be identified to avoid inadvertent injury. Preoperative placement of urinary stents can be useful for locating the ureter intraoperatively in complex, reoperative pelvic surgery.

The rectum, which is 12 to 15 cm long, begins at the level of the sacral promontory and extends to the anorectal ring. The rectum proceeds posterior and caudal along the curvature of the sacrum and coccyx, passing through the levator ani muscles, at which point it turns abruptly caudal and posterior, becoming the anal canal. Anterior to the rectum are the uterine cervix and posterior vaginal wall in women, and the bladder and prostate in men. Posteriorly, the rectum occupies the sacral concavity where the median sacral vessels, presacral veins, and sacral nerves run, all of which are invested in the presacral fascia. The rectum is marked by three curves that correspond to the valves of Houston. The valves are only visible from the lumen and separate the lower third, middle third, and upper third of the rectum, important landmarks when the location of a rectal abnormality is established endoscopically (the lower rectal valve is at 7 to 8 cm from the anal verge, middle rectal valve at 9 to 11 cm, and upper rectal valve at 12 to 13 cm).[3] The anterior and lateral surfaces of the upper third of the rectum are intraperitoneal, whereas only the anterior surface of the middle third of the rectum is intraperitoneal in location. The lower third of the rectum is entirely extraperitoneal. The mesorectum is the term used to describe the areolar tissue surrounding the rectum that contains nerves, lymphatics, and terminal branches of the superior hemorrhoidal branch
❶ of the inferior mesenteric artery. Although it invests the rectum circumferentially, the mesorectum is most prominent posterior to the rectum. It is invested by the fascia propria of

FIGURE 63.2. General anatomic components of the colon.

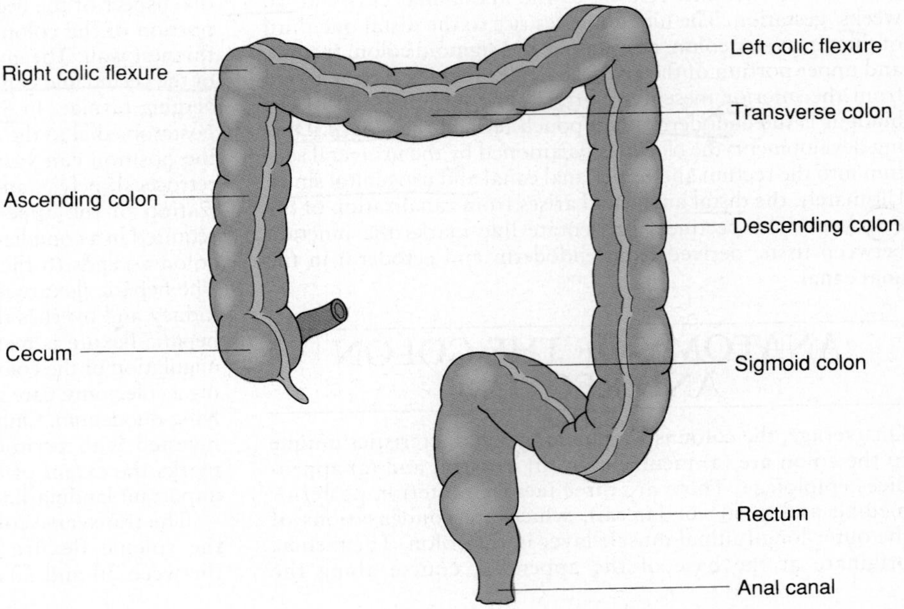

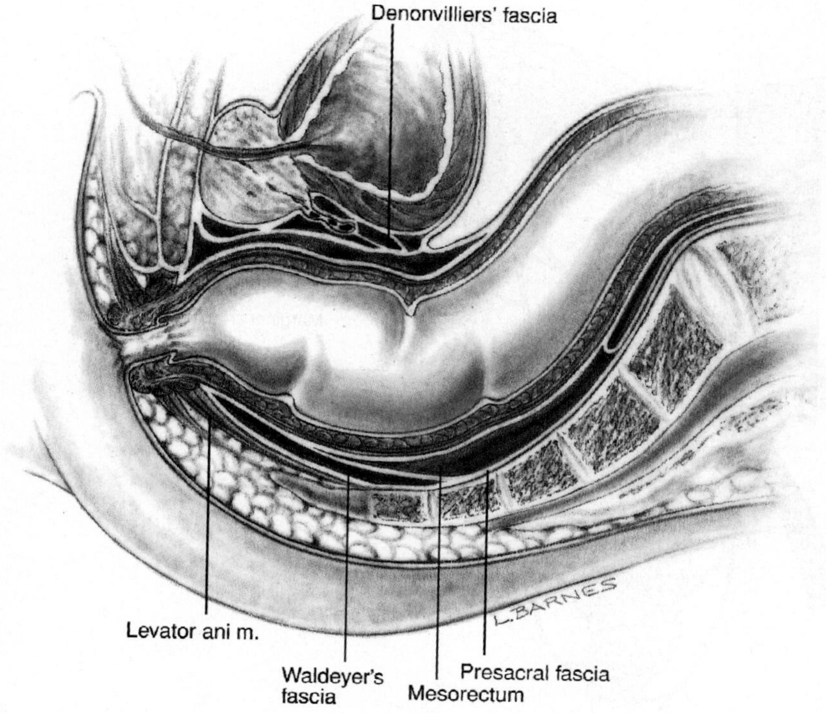

FIGURE 63.3. Fascial relationships of the pelvis. (Reproduced with permission from Fascial relationships of the pelvis. In: Corman ML, ed. *Colon & Rectal Surgery,* 5th ed. Philadelphia, PA: Lippincott Williams & Wilkins; 2004:8, Fig. 1-6.)

the rectum, a continuation of the parietal endopelvic fascia (Fig. 63.3). A total mesorectal excision entails removal of the entire rectum without violating the fascia propria of the rectum. This is accomplished by mobilizing the rectum using the plane between the fascia propria of the rectum and the presacral fascia.

The surgical anal canal begins at the anorectal ring or levator ani muscles and extends to the anal verge. It measures 2 to 4 cm and is usually longer in men than in women. The internal anal sphincter (continuation of the outer longitudinal muscle of the rectal wall) and the external anal sphincter (continuation of the puborectalis muscle) encircle the anal canal and control fecal continence. The dentate line marks the transition between the columnar epithelium of the intestine and the squamous epithelium of the anal canal.

Arterial Blood Supply

The superior mesenteric artery arises from the aorta, runs posterior to the pancreas, and passes anterior to the third
2 portion of the duodenum (Fig. 63.4). In addition to supplying the small bowel through jejunal and ileal branches, the superior mesenteric artery gives rise to the ileocolic, right colic, and middle colic branches that supply the cecum, ascending colon, and proximal transverse colon. The right colic arterial anatomy is particularly variable and can be absent or arise from the ileocolic or the superior mesenteric artery. The middle colic artery has a right and left branch that supply the hepatic flexure and the right portion of the transverse colon, while the left branch supplies the left por-
3 tion of the transverse colon. The inferior mesenteric artery arises from the anterior surface of the aorta, typically 3 to 4 cm above the aortic bifurcation, and supplies the distal transverse colon, descending colon, sigmoid colon, and upper rectum. The inferior mesenteric artery gives rise to the left colic artery and sigmoidal branches, then continues in the sigmoid mesentery, and after crossing the left iliac vessels, is renamed the superior hemorrhoidal artery. The superior hemorrhoidal artery descends behind the rectum and splits into right and left branches in the mesorectum. The middle and inferior hemorrhoidal arteries arise from the hypogastric arteries and supply the distal two thirds of the rectum. The presence of the middle rectal artery, in particular, can be variable. A series of arterial arcades along the mesenteric border of the entire colon, known as the marginal *artery of Drummond,* connect the superior mesenteric and inferior mesenteric arterial systems. The marginal artery may be attenuated or absent at the distal transverse colon/splenic flexure, the delineation between the midgut and hindgut, and thus ischemic colitis most commonly affects this region.

Venous Drainage

The veins that drain the large intestine bear the same terminology and follow a course similar to that of their corresponding arteries (Fig. 63.5). The veins from the right colon and transverse colon, along with the veins draining the small intestine, drain into the superior mesenteric vein. The superior mesenteric vein runs slightly anterior to and to the right of the superior mesenteric artery. The superior mesenteric vein courses beneath the neck of the pancreas, where it joins with the splenic vein to form the portal vein. The inferior mesenteric vein drains blood from the left colon, sigmoid colon, rectum, and superior anal canal. The inferior mesenteric vein ascends over the psoas muscle in a retroperitoneal plane. The vein courses under the body of the pancreas to drain into the splenic vein. During an anterior resection of the rectum, division of the inferior mesenteric vein at the inferior border of the pancreas can provide additional mobility of the left colon to facilitate a coloanal anastomosis. The superior and middle hemorrhoidal veins drain blood from the rectum into the portal system via the inferior mesenteric vein. The inferior hemorrhoidal veins drain blood from the lower rectum and anal canal into the systemic venous circulation via the internal iliac veins. In the setting of portal hypertension,

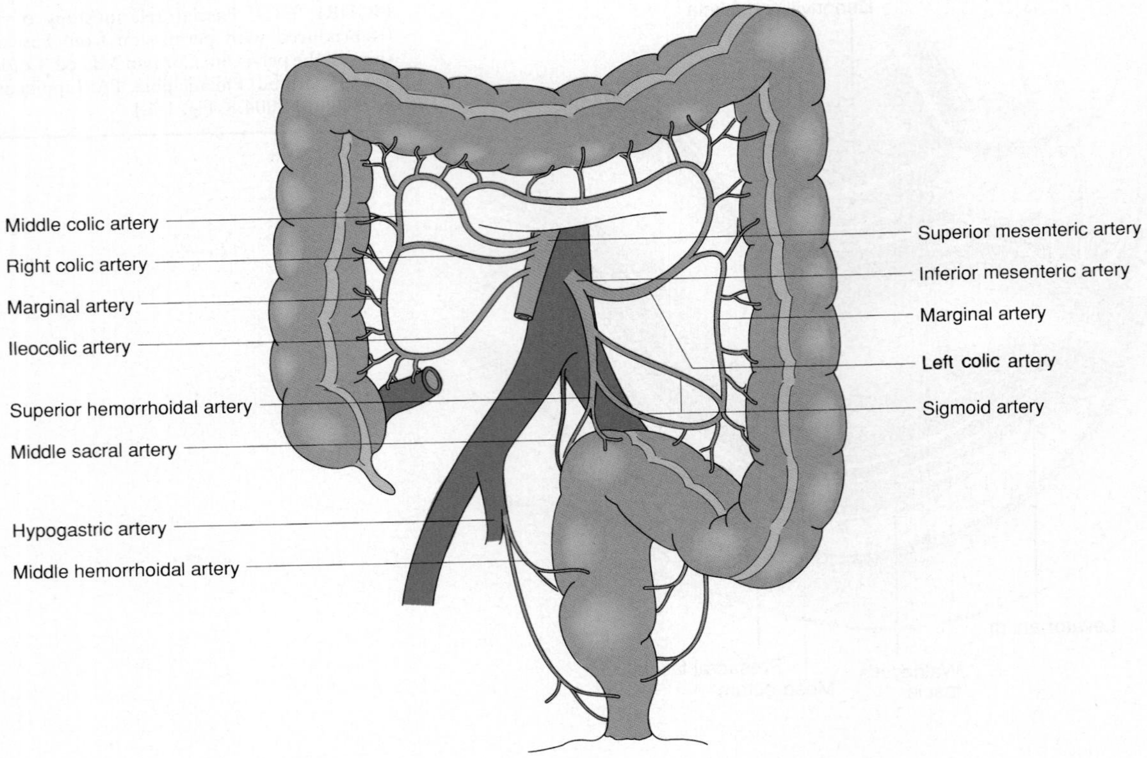

FIGURE 63.4. Arterial blood supply of the colon.

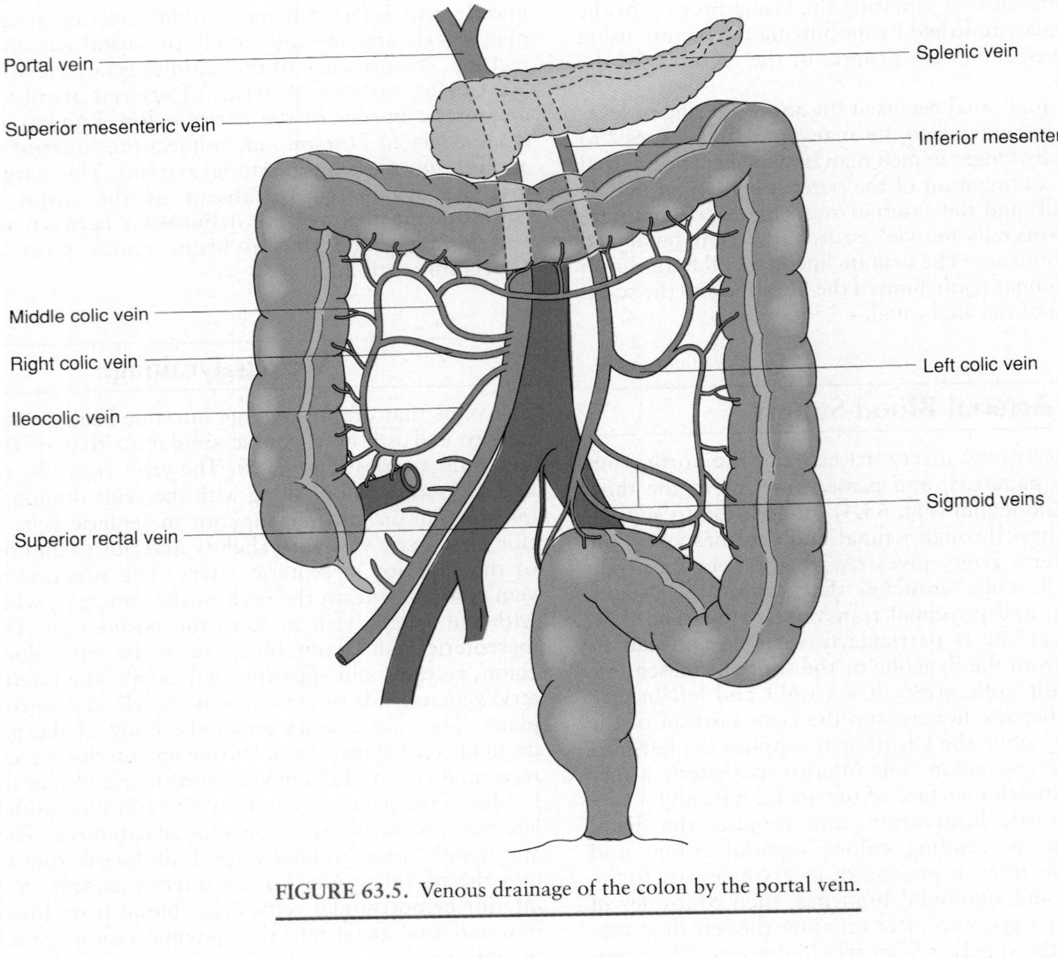

FIGURE 63.5. Venous drainage of the colon by the portal vein.

the superior, middle, and inferior hemorrhoidal veins interact to shunt venous blood from the portal system into the systemic circulation.

Lymphatic Drainage

Lymphatic drainage generally follows the arterial blood supply
4 of the colon and rectum. In the anal canal, lesions above the dentate line drain into the inferior mesenteric lymph nodes. Lesions below the dentate line drain into the internal iliac lymph nodes, but can also drain into the inferior mesenteric lymph nodes.

Neural Components

The colon possesses extrinsic and intrinsic (enteric) neuronal systems. The extrinsic system consists of sympathetic and parasympathetic nerves that inhibit or stimulate colonic peristalsis, respectively. The sympathetic innervation to the right colon originates from the lower thoracic segments of the spinal cord and travels in the thoracic splanchnic nerves to the celiac and superior mesenteric plexuses. Postganglionic fibers emerge from here and course along the superior mesenteric artery and its branches to the right side of the colon. The parasympathetic nerves originate from the right vagus nerve and travel along with the sympathetic nerves to the right side of the colon. The left side of the colon and the rectum receive sympathetic fibers that arise from L1 through L3 segments of the spinal cord. The parasympathetic supply to the left side of the colon and the rectum comes from S2 through S4 spinal cord segments.

The intrinsic, or enteric, nervous system consists of two groups of plexuses that are identified by their location within the colon wall. This system can function independently of the central nervous system and controls motility and exocrine and endocrine functions of the gut, and is involved in intestinal immune regulation and inflammatory responses. The Meissner plexus is located in the submucosa between the muscularis mucosae and the circular muscle of the muscularis propria and is important in secretory control. The myenteric plexus, also known as the *Auerbach plexus*, is located between the inner circular muscle and outer longitudinal muscle layers of the colon and primarily controls intestinal motility.[4]

PHYSIOLOGY

Absorption

The colon absorbs water, sodium, and chloride and secretes potassium and bicarbonate. The physiologic control of colonic water and electrolyte transport requires careful integration of neural, endocrine, and paracrine components. Although colonic epithelium does not actively absorb glucose or amino acids as the small-intestinal epithelium does, the colon does absorb short-chain fatty acids and vitamins that are produced by bacterial breakdown of nonabsorbed sugars and amino acids. These short-chain fatty acids, which include acetate, butyrate, and propionate, are absorbed in a concentration-dependent fashion. They are a major energy substrate for colonic epithelial cells and represent the major fecal anions.[5]

Approximately 1,500 mL of ileal effluent reaches the cecum in a 24-hour period, 90% of which is reabsorbed in the colon; 100 to 150 mL of water remains in stool. The colon has a tremendous capacity that allows it to absorb as much as 5 to 6 L of water within a 24-hour period. When colonic capacity is exceeded, diarrhea results.[6] Normally formed feces consist of 70% water and 30% solid material. Almost half of the solid material is made up of bacteria and the other half is composed of undigested food material and desquamated epithelium. Water absorption in the colon is a passive process that depends primarily on the osmotic gradient established by the active transport of sodium across the colonic epithelium. The composition of ileal effluent and luminal flow rates also play an important role in water absorption. Upsetting the balance of these three factors results in diarrhea. The absorptive capacity is not the same throughout each segment of the colon. Salt and water absorption is greatest in the right colon. Patients undergoing a right hemicolectomy should therefore be counseled preoperatively that they may experience loose bowel movements in the early postoperative period. Patients should also be reassured that this will resolve with time as the remaining colon adapts.

Sodium absorption by the colonic epithelium is an active cellular transport process similar to that seen in small-intestinal and renal epithelial cells.[7] Initially, sodium absorption involves the passive movement of sodium across the apical membrane into the mucosal cell down an electrochemical gradient. To maintain an adequate electrochemical gradient, intracellular sodium is removed from the cell into the interstitial space in exchange for potassium. This is an energy-dependent process that is controlled by Na^+-K^+-adenosine triphosphatase (ATPase). Mineralocorticoids (predominantly aldosterone) and glucocorticoids accelerate sodium absorption and potassium excretion in the colon by increasing Na^+-K^+-ATPase activity.[8] Potassium movement into the colonic lumen is primarily a passive process that depends on the electrochemical gradient generated by the active transport of sodium across colonic epithelial cells. Chloride absorption in the colon is generally thought to be an energy-independent process that is associated with reciprocal exchange for bicarbonate at the luminal border of the mucosal cell.[9]

Colonic Flora

The bacterial flora of the colon is established soon after birth and depends in large part on dietary and environmental fac-
5 tors. The colon is populated by approximately 10^{13} commensal bacteria.[10] The vast majority of the normal colonic flora consists of anaerobic bacteria, with *Bacteroides* species being most prevalent, particularly *B. fragilis*.[11] Aerobic colonic bacteria are mainly coliforms and enterococci, with *Escherichia coli* being the most predominant coliform. The colonic flora is important for (a) digestion and absorption of complex macromolecules, (b) protecting the colon against invasion by noncommensal bacteria, and (c) development of mucosal immunity. Fermentation of carbohydrates generates short-chain fatty acids, including butyrate, which is the primary nutrient for the colonic mucosa. Colonic bacteria also produce certain vitamins, such as vitamin K and B_{12}, which are absorbed by the host. The enterohepatic circulation of bilirubin and bile acids depends on bacterial enzymes produced by fecal flora. The degradation of bile pigments by colonic bacteria gives stool its characteristic brown color. Colonic bacteria also play an important role in preventing infection by controlling the growth of potentially pathogenic bacteria such as *Clostridium difficile*.

Host and colonic flora have a mutualistic relationship; however, disturbances of this coexistence can lead to human disease.[12]
6 Dysregulation of the flora has been implicated in the pathogenesis of inflammatory bowel disease and, to a lesser extent, colorectal cancer. In animal studies, mice with certain immune deficiencies that make them prone to colitis fail to develop colitis when raised under germ-free conditions. Analysis of the microbiota of patients with inflammatory bowel disease revealed markedly different flora compositions in ulcerative colitis, Crohn disease, and healthy control patients. Similarly, certain genetically altered mice

with a propensity to develop colorectal cancer fail to develop tumors in germ-free conditions. Although studies of human flora and colorectal cancer are limited, preliminary studies have raised interest in modulating the colonic flora as a way to treat and/or prevent colitis and other diseases of the colon.

Colonic Motility

Motor activity varies greatly throughout the colon. There are two patterns of colonic motility: segmental contractions, which are single or clustered contractions, and propagated activity, which is either high-amplitude propagated contractions (HAPCs) or low-amplitude propagated contractions (LAPCs). *Segmental contractions* are intermittent contractions of the longitudinal and circular muscles that result in the segmented appearance of the colon.[13] These contractions propel luminal contents in a back-and-forth pattern over short distances, slowing aboral transit and allowing for water reabsorption.[14] *Propagated activity* consists of strong, propulsive contractions of the smooth muscle that involve a long segment of colon.[15] The LAPCs move luminal contents forward at a rate of 0.5 to 1.0 cm/s and typically last for 20 to 30 seconds.[13] HAPCs occur three to four times per day, primarily after awakening, exercise, and after meals.

The orderly progression of colonic luminal contents from cecum to anus requires the coordination of smooth muscle contractions. Calcium-dependent cyclic depolarization and repolarization of the colonic smooth muscle cell membrane generates a basic electrical pattern of slow-wave activity. This activity allows each smooth muscle cell to control its own contraction and to couple with adjacent smooth muscle cells.[16] The extrinsic (autonomic) and intrinsic (enteric) neuronal systems also interact to influence colonic motility.

Defecation

As the fecal mass enters the rectum, the internal anal sphincter relaxes while the external anal sphincter contracts to maintain continence. Distention of the rectum in this setting is the primary stimulus for defecation to begin. At this point, the urge to defecate may be suppressed by conscious contraction of the external anal sphincter. Receptive relaxation of the rectal ampulla accommodates the fecal mass and the urge to defecate passes unless the volume of feces is extremely large or the sphincter mechanism is impaired. If the subject voluntarily accedes to the urge to defecate, a Valsalva maneuver occurs, which increases the intra-abdominal pressure to overcome the resistance of the external anal sphincter. Relaxation of the pelvic muscles causes the pelvic floor to descend and the anorectal angle to straighten. Conscious inhibition of the external anal sphincter then allows passage of the feces. On completion, the pelvic floor returns to its resting position and the anal sphincter muscles return to their resting activity, closing the anal canal. Under normal circumstances, this process occurs once every 24 hours; however, the interval between bowel movements may vary between 8 and 12 hours and 2 to 3 days in normal subjects. The frequency of defecation is influenced by multiple environmental and dietary factors.

DISORDERS OF COLONIC MOTILITY

Constipation

Constipation is common and may affect up to 15% of people, but only a portion of affected individuals seek medical

TABLE 63.1 **DIAGNOSIS**

ROME III CRITERIA FOR THE DIAGNOSIS OF CONSTIPATION

Two or more of the following:
Straining in >25% of bowel movements
Incomplete evacuation of the rectum in >25% of bowel movements
Hard stool consistency in >25% of bowel movements
Three or fewer bowel movements weekly
Manual maneuvers in >25% of bowel movements
Sensation of anorectal obstruction in >25% of bowel movements
Do not meet the criteria for irritable bowel syndrome
Loose stools rarely present without the use of laxatives

From Longstreth GF, Thompson WG, Chey WD, et al. Functional bowel disorders. *Gastroenterology* 2006;130(5):1480–1491.

7 help.[17] Colorectal surgeons, gastroenterologists, gynecologists, and family medicine physicians are frequently called upon to treat constipation.[18] To evaluate constipation, the clinician must ask focused questions about bowel function. Constipation can mean infrequent bowel movements, straining, or hard stools. The Rome criteria were developed to help standardize the diagnosis (Table 63.1). Constipation can be caused by lifestyle choices, side effects of medications taken for other reasons, medical conditions, structural abnormalities of the colon, pelvic floor dysfunction, and colonic inertia (Table 63.2). Evaluation of the constipated patients includes a thorough history, a physical examination including a rectal exam, and evaluation for sources of pelvic floor dysfunction such as rectocele. Colonoscopy may be necessary to eliminate a structural bowel obstruction as the cause of constipation.

After eliminating medication-related or metabolic causes of constipation and in the absence of systemic symptoms, it may be practical to initiate medical therapy before proceeding with radiologic testing for rare conditions such as colonic dysmotility or pelvic floor dysfunction. The goal of first-line medical therapy is to increase stool bulk and physical activity. Fiber intake should be increased to 20 to 30 g/d. To achieve this recommended daily amount, fiber supplementation with either psyllium or methylcellulose is frequently required. At least eight glasses of water should be ingested daily. Fiber and water intake increases stool bulk, and bulky bowel movements stimulate colonic motility. If fiber, water, and exercise do not relieve constipation, then laxatives should be added to the regimen. Laxatives can be divided into different categories by mechanism of action (Table 63.3). Osmotic laxatives are usually the first-line treatment for severe constipation. Long-term use of laxatives, which irritate the colon, should be avoided, however, because they can actually impair colon function. Melanosis coli, a dark discoloration of the colonic mucosa seen on colonoscopy, is a sign of frequent laxative use.

Some patients whose constipation does not respond to standard medical therapy will be found to have slow-transit constipation or pelvic floor dysfunction, both of which require radiologic studies for diagnosis. The most common technique for evaluating colonic transit is a Sitz marker study (Fig. 63.6). To complete this test, all laxatives must be stopped 48 hours before the study. On day 0, a set number of radiopaque markers are ingested; an abdominal radiograph is obtained on day 1 to

TABLE 63.2 **ETIOLOGY**

CAUSES OF CONSTIPATION

LIFESTYLE	
Inadequate fluid intake	
Inadequate fiber intake	
Inactivity	
Laxative abuse	
MEDICATIONS	
Anticholinergics	
Antidepressants	
Antihypertensive medications	
Iron	
Narcotics	
MEDICAL CONDITIONS	
Spinal cord dysfunction	
Multiple sclerosis	
Diabetes mellitus	
Hypothyroidism	
Uremia	
Hypercalcemia	
Electrolyte abnormality	
Depression	
Anorexia	
Sexual abuse	
COLON ABNORMALITY	
Cancer	
Crohn disease	
Chagas disease	
Irradiation	
PELVIC FLOOR DYSFUNCTION	
Nonrelaxing puborectalis	
Anal stenosis	
Rectocele	

From Longstreth GF, Thompson WG, Chey WD, et al. Functional bowel disorders. *Gastroenterology* 2006;130(5):1480–1491.

TABLE 63.3 **TREATMENT**

LAXATIVES

Bulking Agents (Soluble Fiber)	
Psyllium (Konsyl, Metamucil)	
Methylcellulose (Citrucel)	
Calcium polycarbophil (FiberCon)	
Colonic Stimulants/Irritants	
Senna (Senokot and Peri-Colace)	
Cascara	
Bisacodyl (Dulcolax)	
Stool Softeners	
Mineral oil	
Docusate sodium (Colace)	
Osmotic Laxatives	
Lactulose	
Polyethylene glycol (MiraLAX)	
Sodium phosphate (Fleets Phosphosoda)	
Magnesium hydroxide (milk of magnesia)	

document that the markers were ingested, and again on day 5 to determine if the markers have been expelled. Normally, on day 5, more than 80% of the markers should be evacuated. If more than 20% of the markers remain and they are either clustered in the right colon or evenly distributed throughout the colon, the patient has slow-transit constipation. Outlet obstruction is suggested by clustering of the markers in the sigmoid or rectum. Outlet dysfunction can be further evaluated with defecography, a fluoroscopic study of defecation. Slow-transit constipation is best treated with surgery, and obstructed defecation with biofeedback therapy.

Postoperative Ileus

Postoperative ileus is transient impairment of bowel function after an operation. It is most common in patients after

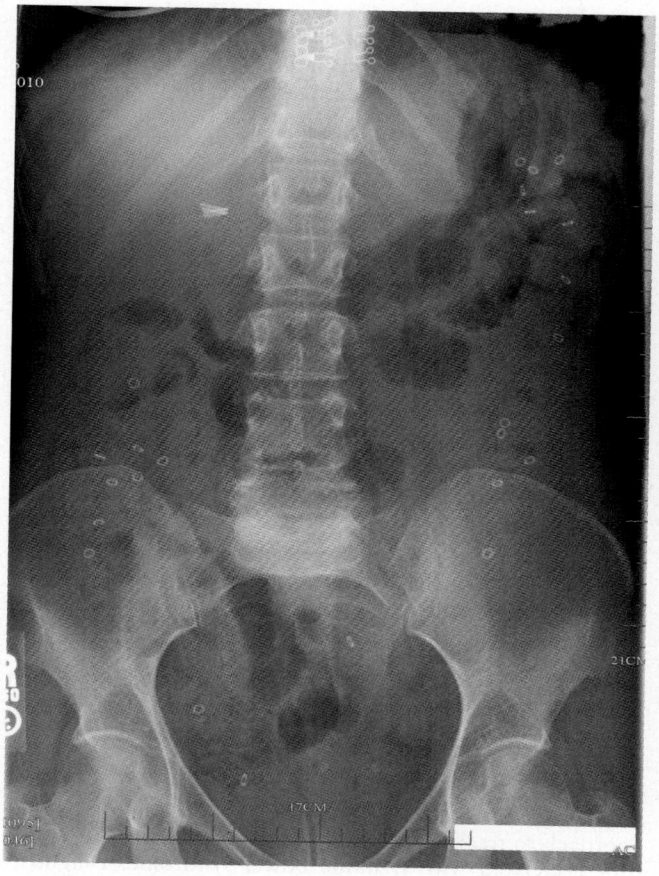

FIGURE 63.6. Sitz marker study demonstrating colonic inertia.

intra-abdominal surgical procedures, particularly colonic operations. Clinically, postoperative ileus is manifested by abdominal distention and delayed passage of flatus and, less
8 frequently, by nausea and vomiting. After an abdominal operation, the colon usually takes 3 to 5 days to recover, whereas the stomach and small bowel resume normal motor function more rapidly (1 to 2 days and 1 day, respectively).[19] In a recent multicenter study, the average length of hospital stay after bowel resection was 6.6 days, with 11.5% of patients requiring a nasogastric tube for ileus.[20] Postoperative ileus is multifactorial. Surgical and anesthetic technique, narcotic use, inactivity, and postoperative infectious complications all have been implicated in prolonged ileus. Bowel manipulation has also been suggested to contribute to the development of ileus.[21] The observation that postoperative ileus is shorter after minimally invasive surgery adds credence to this theory.[22] Use of the anesthetic agent halothane, as well as opioid analgesics, can prolong postoperative ileus.[19] After surgery, systemically administered morphine, in addition to binding to μ opioid receptors in the central nervous system and promoting analgesia, binds to peripheral μ opioid receptors in the colon and causes nonpropulsive electrical activity that can prolong ileus.[23]

Postoperative ileus lengthens hospital stays, and thereby hospital costs. The burgeoning cost of health care has renewed the interest in medications to prevent or shorten postoperative ileus. Research has focused on new pain management strategies that minimize systemic narcotics, and
9 pharmacologic agents to promote intestinal motility. One of the most promising strategies is the use of a thoracic epidural for postoperative analgesia. The thoracic epidural block promotes parasympathetic activity by blunting sympathetic stimulation of the gut. The greatest benefit is seen with epidural infusions of local anesthetic (lidocaine or bupivacaine), as compared to narcotics.[19] Other benefits of using thoracic epidurals in the postoperative period are increased mental acuity and better pain control, both of which promote early mobility, particularly in elderly patients.[24] Currently, alvimopan, an oral medication that blocks the μ opioid receptors in the gastrointestinal tract, is the most studied antidote for ileus. A phase III multicenter study of patients who had a bowel resection or hysterectomy found that alvimopan (12 mg before surgery, then twice a day until discharge) decreased hospital stay by 18 hours as compared to placebo.[25] With an improved understanding of the molecular basis of intestinal motility, we can expect new, targeted medications for decreasing postoperative ileus in the future.

Irritable Bowel Syndrome

Irritable bowel syndrome is defined as abdominal pain that is not associated with an anatomic abnormality and may or may not be associated with alterations in bowel habits. The causes of this disorder are uncertain. Emotional stress and psychiatric illness have been implicated in the pathogenesis of the disorder and may exacerbate symptoms.[26] Physiologic abnormalities have also been demonstrated, as has abnormal colonic motility in response to an ingested meal.[27] Altered myoelectric activity and abnormal gut hormone secretion have also been cited as potential causes.

Because no one, clear cause of irritable bowel syndrome has been demonstrated, no specific treatment regimen has been defined for this disorder. Most patients have asymptomatic periods interrupted by intervals of symptoms. The approach to treatment begins with an evaluation of the factors associated with irritable bowel syndrome. Diagnosis and treatment of an underlying psychiatric problem may resolve the patient's symptoms. A detailed dietary history should also be taken, and factors that contribute to constipation or diarrhea should be adjusted appropriately. If these management strategies are not successful, gradually introducing anticholinergic medications may be helpful. Anticholinergic agents can reduce the rate of myoelectric activity and decrease tonic contractions in the colon, thereby relieving the cramping and bloating that many patients experience. Low doses of tricyclic antidepressants, including imipramine, amitriptyline, and nortriptyline, often decrease or eliminate abdominal symptoms. Constipation is known to be one major side effect of these agents, which may be helpful in patients with irritable bowel syndrome and underlying diarrhea, but a problem in patients with preexisting constipation. The myriad treatment options described for irritable bowel syndrome underscores the poor understanding of this clinical entity.

Colonic Pseudo-obstruction

Colonic pseudo-obstruction, also known as *Ogilvie syndrome*, is massive dilation of the colon without an actual mechanical obstruction. In 1948, Ogilvie described two patients with colonic pseudo-obstruction from malignant infiltration of the celiac plexus that he postulated led to sympathetic inhibition.[28] In the intestine, stimulation of the sympathetic nervous system decreases intestinal motility, whereas activation of the parasympathetic nervous system promotes contractility. Colonic pseudo-obstruction results from an imbalance in the autonomic nervous system of the gastrointestinal tract. Various metabolic conditions, pharmacologic agents, and traumatic factors can alter the balance of the intestinal autonomic nervous system and have been associated with colonic pseudo-obstruction.[29] The most frequent presenting symptoms are abdominal pain and nausea and vomiting. On physical examination, the abdomen is distended and tympanic and may be mildly tender when palpated. Marked colonic distention present on an abdominal radiograph is the hallmark of the condition (Fig. 63.7). Fever and leukocytosis are rare and should raise the concern for perforation.[30] First-line management of colonic pseudo-obstruction is conservative and consists of nasogastric decompression, cessation of oral feedings, correction of fluid and electrolyte imbalances, and avoidance of narcotics and anticholinergics. If abdominal radiographs do not show gas throughout the colon, an abdominal computed tomography scan or a Gastrografin enema should be considered to rule out a mechanical obstruction. With conservative measures, colonic pseudo-obstruction resolves in more than 75% of cases. When the pseudo-obstruction persists for more than 6 days and/or the diameter of the cecum on abdominal radiograph is greater than 12 cm, the risk for cecal perforation increases.[30,31]

Colonic pseudo-obstruction is most commonly seen in elderly patients who may have other significant medical conditions, so when free perforation occurs, it can be associated with significant morbidity and mortality (up to 40% in one study[32]). In patients whose pseudo-obstruction is not responding to conservative therapy but who have no signs of peritonitis, 2.5 mg of neostigmine given intravenously over 2 to 3 minutes has been found to decompress the colon promptly in nearly all patients.[33,34] Neostigmine is a reversible acetylcholinesterase inhibitor that stimulates the intestinal parasympathetic receptors, promoting colonic motility.[35] In a randomized controlled study, the pseudo-obstruction resolved promptly in 10 of 11 patients.[33] If neostigmine fails to decompress the colon, another alternative is decompressive colonoscopy. In one series, 69% of patients had resolution of their pseudo-obstruction after colonoscopy to remove air.[35] Surgery is reserved for patients with obvious peritoneal signs or whose pseudo-obstruction has not improved after all forms of nonsurgical therapy. In

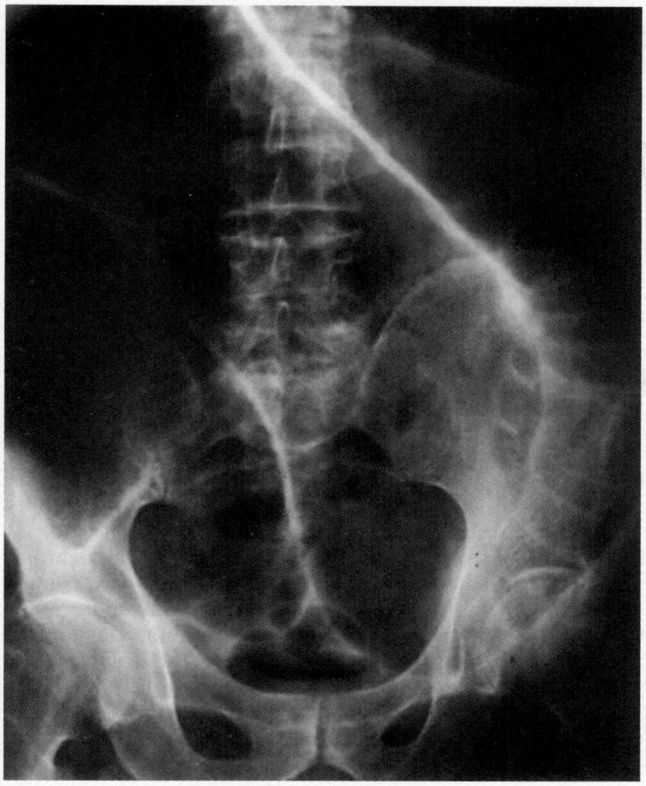

FIGURE 63.7. Pseudo-obstruction of the colon (Ogilvie syndrome).

such patients, when the possibility of cecal perforation is high, a cecostomy can be considered.

References

1. Nivatvongs S, Gordon PH. *Surgical Anatomy.* St. Louis, MO: Quality Medical Publishing; 1992:3–37.
2. Wakely CP. The position of the vermiform appendix as ascertained by an analysis of 10,000 cases. *J Anat* 1933;67(2):277–283.
3. Jorge JM, Habr-Gamma A. *Anatomy and Embryology of the Colon, Rectum and Anus.* New York: Springer; 2007:1–23.
4. Goyal RK, Hirano I. The enteric nervous system. *N Engl J Med* 1996; 334(17):1106–1114.
5. Latella G, Caprilli R. Metabolism of large bowel mucosa in health and disease. *Int J Colorectal Dis* 1991;6(2)127–132.
6. Pemberton JH, Phillips SF. Colonic absorption. *Perspect Colon Rectal Surg* 1988;1:89–103.
7. Grady GF, Duhamel RC, Moore EW. Active transport of sodium by human colon in vitro. *Gastroenterology* 1970;59(4):583–588.
8. Giller J, Phillips SF. Electrolyte absorption and secretion in the human colon. *Am J Dig Dis* 1972;17(11):1003–1011.
9. Powell DW. *Transport in the Large Intestine.* New York: Springer-Verlag; 1978.
10. Hooper LV, Gordon JI. Commensal host-bacterial relationships in the gut. *Science* 2001;292(5519):1115–1118.
11. Dunn DL. Autochthonous microflora of the gastrointestinal tract. *Perspect Colon Rectal Surg* 1989;2:105–119.
12. Rescigno M. The pathogenic role of intestinal flora in IBD and colon cancer. 2008;9(5):395–403.
13. Ritche JA. Movements of segmental constrictions in the human colon. *Gut* 1971;6:251–277.
14. Emmanuel A, Roy A. Small intestine and colon motility. *Medicine* 2007; 35(5):272–276.
15. Herz AF. The passage of food along the human alimentary canal. *Guy's Hosp Rep* 1907;61:389–427.
16. Daniel EE. Electrophysiology of the colon. *Gut* 1975;16:298–329.
17. Higgins PD, Johanson JF. Epidemiology of constipation in North America: a systematic review. *Am J Gastroenterol* 2004;99(4):750–759.
18. Bharucha AE. Constipation. *Best Pract Res Clin Gasterenterol* 2007;21(4): 709–731.
19. Maron DJ, Fry RD. New therapies in the treatment of postoperative ileus after gastrointestinal surgery. *Am J Ther* 2008;15(1):59–65.
20. Delaney CP, Wolff BG, Viscusi ER, et al. Alvimopan, for postoperative ileus following bowel resection: a pooled analysis of phase III studies. *Ann Surg* 2007;245(3):355–363.
21. Delaney CP, Wolff BG, Viscusi ER, et al. Alvimopan, for postoperative ileus following bowel resection: a pooled analysis of phase III studies. *Ann Surg* 2007;245:355–363.
22. Bohm B, Milsom JW, Fazio VW. Postoperative intestinal motility following conventional and laparoscopic intestinal surgery. *Arch Surg* 1995;130(4): 415–419.
23. Frantzides CT, Cowles V, Salaymeh B, et al. Morphine effects on human colonic myoelectric activity in the postoperative period. *Am J Surg* 1992;163(1):144–148; discussion 148–149.
24. Mann C, Pouzeratte Y, Boccara G, et al. Comparison of intravenous or epidural patient-controlled analgesia in the elderly after major abdominal surgery. *Anesthesiology* 2000;92(2):433–441.
25. Wolff BG, Michelassi F, Gerkin TM, et al. Alvimopan, a novel, peripherally acting mu opioid antagonist: results of a multicenter, randomized, double-blind, placebo-controlled, phase III trial of major abdominal surgery and postoperative ileus. *Ann Surg* 2004;240(4):728–734; discussion 734–735.
26. Walker EA, Roy-Byrne PP, Katon WJ. Irritable bowel syndrome and psychiatric illness. *Am J Psychiatry* 1990;147(5):565–572.
27. Munakata J, Naliboff B, Harraf F, et al. Repetitive sigmoid stimulation induces rectal hyperalgesia in patients with irritable bowel syndrome. *Gastroenterology* 1997;112(1):55–63.
28. Olgilvie WH. Large-intestine colic due to sympathetic deprivation: a new clinical syndrome. *Br Med J* 1948;2:671–672.
29. Saunders MD, Cappell MS. Endoscopic management of acute colonic pseudo-obstruction. *Endoscopy* 2005;37(8):760–763.
30. Vanek VW, Al-Salti M. Acute pseudo-obstruction of the colon (Ogilvie's syndrome). An analysis of 400 cases. *Dis Colon Rectum* 1986;29(3):203–210.
31. Johnson CD, Rice RP, Kelvin FM, et al. The radiologic evaluation of gross cecal distension: emphasis on cecal ileus. *AJR Am J Roentgenol* 1985; 145(6):1211–1217.
32. Nanni G, Garbini A, Luchetti P, et al. Ogilvie's syndrome (acute colonic pseudo-obstruction): review of the literature (October 1948 to March 1980) and report of four additional cases. *Dis Colon Rectum* 1982;25(2): 157–166.
33. Ponec RJ, Saunders MD, Kimmey MB. Neostigmine for the treatment of acute colonic pseudo-obstruction. *N Engl J Med* 1999;341(3):137–141.
34. Trevisani GT, Hyman NH, Church JM. Neostigmine: safe and effective treatment for acute colonic pseudo-obstruction. *Dis Colon Rectum* 2000; 43(5):599–603.
35. Saunders MD, Kimmey MB. Systematic review: acute colonic pseudo-obstruction. *Pharmacol Ther* 2005;22(10):917–925.

CHAPTER 64 ■ GASTROINTESTINAL MOTILITY DISORDERS

SANDRA A. TAN AND GEORGE A. SAROSI Jr.

KEY POINTS

1. Ileus is defined as impairment in the aboral passage of intestinal contents secondary to a failure of normal intestinal motility in the absence of an obstructing lesion. Ileus is the most common gastrointestinal motility disorder encountered by surgeons.
2. Irritable bowel syndrome is a chronic gastrointestinal illness characterized by frequent unexplained abdominal pain associated with bloating and disturbance in normal bowel function.
3. Normal esophageal peristalsis interrupted by simultaneous contractions is the hallmark of diffuse esophageal spasm.
4. Diabetic gastroparesis may affect 50% of diabetic patients.
5. Dumping syndrome is a clinically defined spectrum of symptoms observed after gastric surgery thought to be a consequence of accelerated gastric emptying following vagotomy and bypass or destruction of the pylorus.
6. The most common presenting symptom of gallbladder dyskinesia is abdominal pain in the absence of gallstones or other structural cause of right upper quadrant pain.
7. The diagnosis of colonic inertia is established in a chronically constipated patient with markedly prolonged colonic transit time in the absence of anorectal dysfunction.
8. Acute colonic pseudo-obstruction is a clinical syndrome characterized by massive dilation of the colon in the absence of mechanical obstruction. The syndrome generally develops in ill patients hospitalized initially for other significant medical problems.

Orderly progression of a swallowed food bolus from the mouth though the entire digestive system and expulsion of the residual material remaining after digestion is the normal function of gastrointestinal motility. Loss of normal gastrointestinal motor activity causes failure of major gastrointestinal functions, including absorption of nutrients and fluid and secretion of waste products. Although many acute surgical diseases result in secondary failure of gastrointestinal motor function, the majority of diseases causing primary gastrointestinal motor dysfunction are not surgically treated. Because many primary motility disorders can present in a similar fashion to common surgical diseases, and a few primary motility disorders are surgically treated diseases, surgeons must be familiar with gastrointestinal motility disorders. This chapter provides a broad overview of gastrointestinal motility disorders with a focus on the pathophysiology of motility disturbances.

DISORDERS AFFECTING THE ENTIRE DIGESTIVE TRACT

Ileus

1 Ileus is defined as impairment in the aboral passage of intestinal contents secondary to a failure of normal intestinal motility in the absence of an obstructing lesion. Ileus is the most common gastrointestinal motility disorder encountered by surgeons. Broadly defined, there are two major categories of ileus: postoperative ileus and ileus related to metabolic abnormalities, drugs, inflammation, or ischemia (Table 64.1). The most common etiology of ileus is the postsurgical state, as some component of postoperative ileus is associated with essentially all major intra-abdominal procedures and many nonabdominal surgical procedures.[1]

Although the pathophysiology of ileus remains incompletely understood, in recent years the basic mechanisms of postoperative ileus have been elucidated. In the immediate postoperative period, all three functional segments of the gastrointestinal tract, the stomach, small intestine, and colon, display impaired motility characterized by disorganized electrical activity and a lack of coordinated propulsion.[2] Although all segments of the gastrointestinal tract are affected by ileus in the postoperative period, the duration of the dysmotility varies by segment. Small bowel motility normalizes first, often within a few hours.[3] Gastric motility usually returns to normal within 24 to 48 hours, but colonic motility takes 2 to 5 days to normalize, and it is this functional segment that contributes most to the clinical effects of postoperative ileus.[4,5]

The pathophysiologic mechanisms underlying postoperative ileus are multifactorial. Three major contributing factors are spinal and local sympathetic reflexes, local and systemic inflammatory mediators, and exogenous factors including opioid analgesics and electrolyte disturbances. The role of spinal and sympathetic reflexes in ileus has been investigated in animal models, in which interventions such as spinal cord transection or pharmacologic neuronal depletion have been shown to decrease the duration of postoperative ileus.[6] These animal observations have been confirmed in human studies, which demonstrate that interruption of gastrointestinal tract spinal reflexes with epidural local anesthetics significantly reduces the duration of postoperative ileus.[7] Multiple neurotransmitters intrinsic to the enteric nervous system may play a role in regulating gastrointestinal motility in the postoperative period. Nitric oxide, vasoactive intestinal polypeptide (VIP), and substance P reduce intestinal motility and have been linked to postoperative ileus in animal studies.[8,9] In contrast, both motilin and ghrelin promote motility during the resolution of postoperative ileus in both humans and animals.[10,11]

Local inflammation and systemic inflammatory mediators play an important role in postoperative ileus. Animal studies have demonstrated that surgical manipulation results in the accumulation of inflammatory cells in the muscular layer of the small intestine and that the degree of inflammation

TABLE 64.1 ETIOLOGY

CAUSES OF ILEUS

Abdominal surgery
Electrolyte abnormalities
Drugs
Intra-abdominal inflammation
Retroperitoneal trauma or inflammation

correlates with the degree of manipulation. In elegant animal studies, investigators have demonstrated that this infiltrate results in muscular dysfunction and jejunal dysmotility and that the inhibition of leukocyte infiltration reduces ileus.[12] The correlation between intestinal inflammatory cell infiltration and the degree of bowel manipulation may help explain the reduction in postoperative ileus observed with laparoscopic surgical approaches. Elevated serum levels of inflammatory cytokines such as interleukin-1 (IL-1) and IL-6 are seen in the postoperative period and may also be associated with decreased gastrointestinal function.[13]

Opioid analgesics are the mainstay of postoperative pain control and have a powerful influence on gastrointestinal motility through actions on peripheral opioid receptors found throughout the gastrointestinal tract.[14] Opioid analgesics have been shown to directly inhibit gastric, small bowel, and colonic motility, and limited narcotic use reduces postoperative colonic dysmotility in humans.[15,16] Electrolyte abnormalities are common in patients dependent on intravenous fluids for hydration, and one study has linked hypokalemia with prolonged postoperative ileus and demonstrated resolution of ileus with potassium therapy.[17]

Preventing ileus or reducing its duration has enormous potential to reduce health care expenditures and improve patient comfort in the perioperative period. Although no single treatment exists that can eliminate postoperative ileus, there are several interventions that may shorten the duration of this motility disorder. The two most effective interventions are thoracic epidural analgesia with local anesthetics and minimally invasive surgical approaches. Six of eight randomized trials comparing the effects of epidural analgesia to systemic opiates on postoperative ileus demonstrate a statistically significant reduction in the duration of ileus with epidural analgesia, with a typical effect size of 1 to 2 fewer days of ileus.[7] This effect is observed with epidural local anesthetics but not with epidural narcotics. Laparoscopic surgery appears to reduce the duration of postoperative ileus by reducing the amount of bowel manipulation and intraperitoneal inflammatory response. Four of six randomized trials comparing laparoscopic with open colectomy have shown a significant decrease in postoperative ileus with a typical effect size of 24 hours.[7]

Multiple pharmacologic interventions have been studied including promotility agents such as metoclopramide, erythromycin, and cisapride; adrenergic blockade; parasympathomimetic agents; and opiate antagonists. Of these agents, only cisapride, which is no longer available in the United States, and the peripheral opiate antagonist alvimopan (Entereg) have been shown to reduce the duration of postoperative ileus.[18] Nonpharmacologic measures that show promise in reducing postoperative ileus include early enteral feeding, sham feeding, and gum chewing. These interventions have not been proven to have benefit in large randomized trials; however, meta-analysis of small trials suggests that gum chewing can reduce the duration of postoperative ileus after open colectomy by 1 day.[19] Standard interventions such as early ambulation and nasogastric decompression have no effect or prolong postoperative ileus when careful studies are performed, despite being considered standard of care.[20] Multimodality therapy, combining several interventions, shows promise in reducing postoperative ileus, but systematic studies have not yet been performed.

Irritable Bowel Syndrome

2 Irritable bowel syndrome (IBS) is a chronic gastrointestinal illness characterized by frequent unexplained abdominal pain associated with bloating and disturbance in normal bowel function. Although in the strictest sense not a gastrointestinal motility disorder, IBS is associated with many of the symptoms of gastrointestinal motility disorders, and patients with IBS have alterations in gastrointestinal motor function. IBS is a common disorder with an estimated prevalence of 12% in adults in the United States. The peak incidence of the disease is in the second through fifth decades of life, and it is rare in patients older than age 50 years. There is a 2:1 female-to-male predominance.[21] The combination of abdominal pain in association with constipation, diarrhea, or alternating constipation and diarrhea that does not fit the pattern of a conventional gastrointestinal disorder should lead to consideration of the diagnosis of IBS. No single test can diagnose IBS; rather, the condition is diagnosed by the presence of specific symptoms known as the Rome III criteria (Table 64.2) in the absence of other organic diseases.[22]

IBS is characterized by abnormal patterns of small bowel and colon electrical activity known as *discrete clusters of contractions*.[23] Rather than representing a true gastrointestinal motility disorder, these patterns are thought to be an exaggeration of the normal intestinal stress response.[24] Patients with IBS also have increased visceral sensitivity to bowel distention, and are more likely to perceive this distention as a noxious stimulus than normal controls.[25] This combination of heightened sensitivity associated with an exaggerated intestinal motility response to stress is thought to explain the symptoms of IBS. The cause of the heightened sensitivity to visceral stimulation is not clear, but inflammation triggered by infection, the postoperative state, or perhaps food allergies may play a role.[26]

The treatment of IBS is directed at symptomatic control. Importantly for surgeons, patients with IBS appear to have higher rates of common surgical procedures such as cholecystectomy, hysterectomy, and appendectomy than patients without the diagnosis of IBS.[27] The reasons for this observation are not clear. Three possible explanations include the overlap of IBS symptoms with the symptoms of surgically treated diseases, increased health-seeking behavior in IBS patients, and the ability of postsurgical inflammation to create visceral sensitization.

TABLE 64.2 DIAGNOSIS

ROME III DIAGNOSTIC CRITERIA FOR IRRITABLE BOWEL SYNDROME

Recurrent abdominal pain or discomfort at least 3 d per month in the last 3 mo associated with two or more of the following:
Improvement with defecation
Onset is associated with a change in stool frequency
Onset is associated with a change in stool appearance
The criteria must be fulfilled for the last 3 mo with symptom onset at least 6 mo prior to diagnosis

Adapted from Longstreth GF, Thompson WG, Chey WD, et al. Functional bowel disorders. *Gastroenterology* 2006;130:1480–1491.

For these reasons, rigorous attention to surgical indications in patients with IBS symptoms is critical.

Dietary modification and teaching patients to more effectively manage stressful life events that trigger symptoms are the usual starting points of therapy. Psychotherapy, including cognitive-behavioral therapy, has been shown to be beneficial. Management of constipation with fiber therapy and diarrhea with antidiarrheal agents is helpful. Antispasmodic agents may reduce pain symptoms, although they do not appear to affect motility disturbances.[21] Tricyclic antidepressants appear to control motility disturbances in selected patients. This effect is independent from antidepressant actions, as serotonin reuptake inhibitors have not been shown to be effective.[28] Two serotonin axis agents, the serotonin-3 receptor antagonist alosetron and the serotonin-4 agonist tegaserod, have been shown to be beneficial in diarrhea-predominant and constipation-predominant IBS, respectively.[29,30]

DISORDERS AFFECTING SPECIFIC ORGANS

Esophagus

Achalasia. The term *achalasia* is derived from the ancient Greek *chalasis*, or relaxation; thus *achalasis*, failure to relax. This word describes the characteristic motility disorder of achalasia: failure of the lower esophageal sphincter (LES) to relax.[31] Hypermotility of the body of the esophagus is usually the initial response to the functional obstruction of the LES, eventually resulting in hypomotility and aperistalsis. When the esophageal body becomes aperistaltic, the viscus becomes a large pouch in which food remains for days with minimal transit to the stomach. Achalasia is a rare disorder, with an incidence in the Western world of 0.5 to 1.1 per 100,000.[32] Achalasia can occur at any age, and both sexes are equally affected. Symptoms are the hallmarks of the disease; dysphagia is the predominant symptom, with dysphagia for solid food present in more than 50% of patients and dysphagia for liquids present in two thirds of cases. The combination of dysphagia to both liquids and solids is more suggestive of functional disease rather than anatomic obstruction such as a stricture or tumor. The symptoms of dysphagia typically plateau over time, as patients learn to alleviate symptoms and improve esophageal function with postural maneuvers or other strategies that increase intraesophageal pressure and promote esophageal emptying.

Approximately 50% of achalasia patients complain of chest pain. The relationship of pain to esophageal function is unclear as improvement of esophageal emptying does not necessarily ameliorate pain. Regurgitation occurs in 76% of patients and is associated with aspiration of esophageal contents and pulmonary complications in 10%. Heartburn symptoms are noted in roughly 50% of patients. Weight loss usually occurs late in the course of achalasia. The clinical presentation of achalasia is often subtle in early-stage disease but may be dramatic in the decompensated phases of the disease.[33]

A barium swallow study is an appropriate initial test in a patient with suspected achalasia. Abnormal or absent clearance of the barium bolus is seen, particularly in the recumbent position. In achalasia, relaxation of the LES fails to occur with swallowing, causing radiographic findings resembling a "bird's beak." In the late phases of the disease, a dilated esophagus is commonly present. An epiphrenic diverticulum proximal to the LES can be seen in this disease. Its size may vary, and its presence may make diagnostic tests difficult. Esophageal manometry reveals failure of the LES to completely relax in more than 85% of patients with achalasia, often associated with aperistalsis of the esophageal body, and is used as an important confirmatory test in the diagnosis of achalasia.[33] Recent work suggests that high-resolution esophageal manometry may be an even more sensitive test for achalasia than traditional manometry.[34]

The etiology of primary achalasia is not understood; several mechanisms have been postulated including immunologic, infectious, and genetic causes.[35] Dysfunction of inhibitory neurons containing nitric oxide and VIP innervating the LES and proximal portion of the stomach is postulated to be the major mechanism underlying the motor dysfunction of achalasia. Neural degeneration with resultant denervation of the smooth muscle segment of the esophagus has been demonstrated in patients with achalasia.[36] An autoimmune or inflammatory mechanism is suggested by the presence of T lymphocytes infiltrating degenerating nervous fibers.[37] Recent work demonstrates that the lymphocytes infiltrating the LES in achalasia patients are enriched for cytotoxic lymphocytes and that a larger than expected proportion of these lymphocytes target herpes simplex virus (HSV) antigens, suggesting that achalasia may be an autoimmune response to HSV-1 antigens.[38] Patients with achalasia exhibit exaggerated LES contractions in response to acetylcholine and cholecystokinin (CCK), a classic deinnervation response, suggesting that lack of inhibitory neurons is the primary defect.[39] Loss of regulatory inhibition of the sphincter tone results in failure of the LES to relax. Failure of the LES to relax and high resting LES pressure create a functional esophageal obstruction. Over time, this obstruction results in failure of the muscles of the esophageal body with esophageal dilation and aperistalsis. Muscle from the LES in patients with achalasia does not relax compared to muscle from normal individuals.[40]

Restoration of normal motility in the damaged esophagus is not possible and normal peristalsis and LES relaxation are not achievable with any therapeutic modality. All treatment options are targeted at reducing pressure across the LES, which will facilitate esophageal transit by gravity. Reduction of pressure across the LES can be achieved by surgical myotomy, pneumatic dilation, or pharmacologic agents; the choice of treatment depends on the patient's comorbid medical conditions. Because surgical myotomy is the most effective method to provide long-term pressure reduction across the LES, this treatment modality should be offered to patients who are good surgical candidates.[41] Anterior esophageal myotomy is carried out across the esophageal sphincter and should be extended a few centimeters along the anterior gastric wall. Because myotomy destroys the LES in the setting of hypomotility of the esophageal body, inadequate esophageal acid clearance is a potential source of uncontrolled gastroesophageal reflux. Whether an antireflux procedure should be combined with esophageal myotomy remains controversial.[42] Myotomy and fundoplication (Dor, Toupet, or loose Nissen techniques) is usually done laparoscopically through the abdomen. Residual gastroesophageal reflux has been reported in 10% to 40% of patients treated in this way and overall results are satisfactory in 80% to 100% of the patients.

The most effective nonsurgical treatment of achalasia is pneumatic dilation. The goal of this treatment is to "rupture" the LES. This result is obtained with inflation of a balloon across the LES tearing the muscle fibers of the sphincter. The balloons have different sizes (3.0, 3.5, and 4.0 cm), and clinical response is directly proportional to the size of the balloon used for dilation. The procedure can be done on an outpatient basis with minimum discomfort to the patient. With pneumatic dilation, 1-year treatment success rates of greater than 80% are reported, but by 10 years the rate of dysphagia control falls to 61%. Up to 64% of patients require multiple dilations to achieve long-term symptom control.[41] Esophageal perforation is the main complication, with an incidence of about 2%.

Muscle relaxants such as calcium channel blockers or sublingual isosorbide dinitrate can be used before meals or to relieve symptoms. The efficacy of these medications is variable

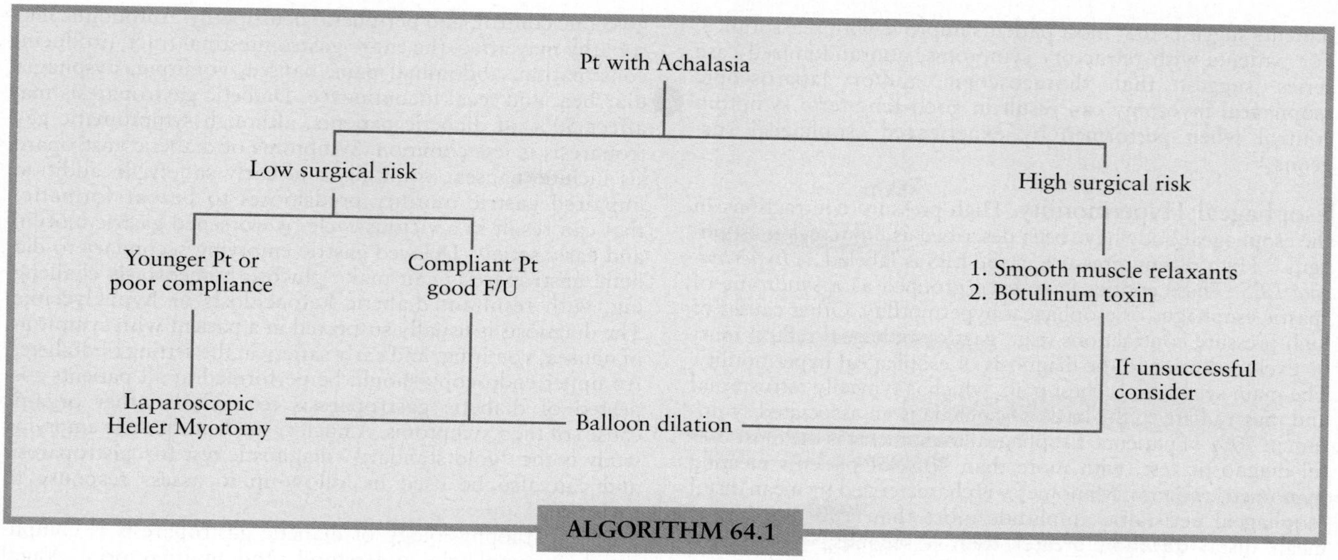

ALGORITHM 64.1. A proposed approach to the patient with achalasia. Pt, patient; F/U, follow-up. (Adapted from Richter JE. Oesophageal motility disorders. *Lancet* 2001;358:823–828.)

and usually decreases with prolonged use.[43] Injection of botulinum toxin into the LES is a relatively new nonsurgical approach for the treatment of achalasia. Botulinum toxin inhibits the release of acetylcholine from nerve terminals, counteracting the effect of loss of the inhibitory neurotransmitters. This treatment has an initial reported efficacy rate of about 80% to 85%. Unfortunately, symptom recurrence occurs in more than 50% of patients within 6 months.[44] Receptor regeneration has been postulated as the main cause of failure after botulinum toxin injection. Some authors reported that myotomy can be more difficult and less effective after botulinum toxin injection.[45] Patient selection is extremely important when considering this type of treatment for achalasia (Algorithm 64.1). Patients with vigorous achalasia and older patients have been reported to have a prolonged response.

Improvement of symptoms is clinically used to evaluate the efficacy of pneumatic dilation or surgical myotomy. Symptom scores are not necessarily correlated with improvement in esophageal emptying; one third of patients have poor esophageal emptying despite symptomatic improvement.[46] Long-term patient follow-up has shown that good esophageal emptying is associated with better long-term results. Manometric or radiologic studies may help to define objective improvement in esophageal body motility and transit through the manipulated LES.

3 Diffuse Esophageal Spasm. Normal esophageal peristalsis interrupted by simultaneous contractions is the hallmark of diffuse esophageal spasm. Roughly 3% to 5% of patients assessed for esophageal motility disorders have diffuse esophageal spasm. Diffuse esophageal spasm can affect patients at any age but is more common in those older than 50 years. The typical symptoms of diffuse esophageal spasm are chest pain and dysphagia. The chest pain of diffuse esophageal spasm is similar to cardiac angina and may respond to nitrites; however, this symptom is usually not related to exertion and is often associated with meals. Intermittent, nonprogressive dysphagia to liquids and solids that can be precipitated by rapid eating, extreme food temperatures, heartburn, and stress is also commonly noted with diffuse esophageal spasm. An association of diffuse esophageal spasm with IBS, urinary disturbances, and sexual dysfunction has been reported.[47] Manometry is the diagnostic test of choice for the diagnosis of diffuse esophageal spasm. The manometric findings are consistent, intermittent simultaneous contractions mixed with normal peristalsis and the presence of simultaneous contractions after 20% or more of wet swallows.[47] Newer work using combined manometry and intraluminal impedance monitoring (MII) shows that patients with diffuse esophageal spasm appear to segregate into two groups, those with effective peristalsis and those without effective peristalsis. Although there are limited data, using MII may play a role in selecting patients with diffuse esophageal spasm who may respond to surgical therapy.[48]

The pathophysiology of diffuse esophageal spasm is unclear, but neural dysfunction has been suggested. Patients with diffuse esophageal spasm are more sensitive to hormonal and cholinergic stimulations, which cause esophageal contractions. Defects in inhibitory neural circuits have been implicated with a possible decrease in nitric oxide synthesis.[49] Gastroesophageal reflux and stress can produce diffuse esophageal spasm, and some patients with diffuse esophageal spasm develop achalasia, suggesting that dysfunction of inhibitory motor circuits may be a common pathogenetic mechanism to both disorders.

Diffuse esophageal spasm is a nonprogressive disorder, and treatment is predominately directed at symptomatic control. Because there are many nonesophageal causes of chest pain, and the relationship between esophageal dysmotility and chest pain can be difficult to confirm, it is critical to exclude these problems before embarking on a course of therapy for dysmotility-induced chest pain. Unrecognized gastroesophageal reflux disease (GERD) can be an important cause of esophageal spasm, so initial therapy should consist of a trial of proton pump inhibitors. If empiric GERD therapy does not improve symptoms, direct treatment of the esophageal motor disorder should be undertaken.[48] Two pharmacologic approaches have been utilized, smooth muscle relaxants such as nitrates and calcium channel blockers, and chronic pain control with antidepressant medication. No randomized trials support the use of nitrates, although uncontrolled studies suggest they help with chest pain symptoms. Three small, randomized trials of calcium channel blockers have shown that despite significant manometric changes, calcium channel blockers were no more effective than placebo in reducing chest pain.[50] Both tricyclic antidepressants and trazodone have shown benefits in symptom relief without improvements in manometric findings in randomized controlled trials.[51] Despite these disappointing results, long-term follow-up of pharmacologically treated patients suggests that most patients improve with reassurance. For patients with refractory symptoms, nonrandomized case series suggest that thoracoscopic and/or laparoscopic esophageal myotomy can result in good long-term symptom control when performed by experienced esophageal surgeons.[52]

Esophageal Hypermotility. High-pressure contractions in the esophageal body have been described as "nutcracker esophagus." High resting pressure in the LES is labeled as *hypertensive LES*. These entities have been grouped as a syndrome of spastic esophagus or esophageal hypermotility. Other causes of high-pressure contractions (e.g., gastroesophageal reflux) must be excluded prior to the diagnosis of esophageal hypermotility. The main symptom is chest pain, which is typically retrosternal and may radiate to the back. Dysphagia is an associated symptom in 50% of patients. Esophageal manometry is the most useful diagnostic test, with more than 40% of patients meeting manometric criteria. Manometry is characterized by mean distal esophageal peristaltic amplitude more than 180 mm Hg or mean distal duration greater than 6 seconds.[53] Treatment options are the same as those for diffuse esophageal spasm, although limited evidence suggests that surgery results in higher failure rates than in diffuse esophageal spasm. Response to treatment is not always predictable.

Esophageal Hypomotility. Low-amplitude peristaltic contractions, simultaneous contractions, or failed contractions in the distal esophagus have been grouped as hypocontracting esophagus or as ineffective esophageal motility. Peristaltic waves with amplitude of less than 30 mm Hg do not provide effective esophageal transport and clearance. Two major groups of patients with esophageal hypomotility exist, those with hypomotility secondary to systemic diseases and those with idiopathic hypomotility. Connective tissue disorders are the most common causes of ineffective esophageal motility, including scleroderma, rheumatoid arthritis, and systemic lupus erythematosus. Up to 80% of patients with scleroderma have esophageal motility disorders, likely secondary to diffuse vasculitis.[54] In the esophagus and gastroesophageal junction, vasculitis affects both smooth muscles and innervation, resulting in low-amplitude peristalsis of the distal esophagus and LES pressures below 10 mm Hg. Other causes of ineffective esophageal motility include autonomic neuropathy, amyloidosis, myxedema, multiple sclerosis, and alcoholism.

Gastroesophageal reflux is present in most patients with ineffective esophageal motility. Acid damage in the distal esophagus may contribute to dysmotility, and diminished esophageal acid clearance is responsible for increased acid exposure with ineffective esophageal motility.[55] The close relationship between esophageal hypomotility and GERD is emphasized by the fact that patients with esophageal hypomotility typically present with reflux symptoms rather than dysphagia.

Many patients with reflux disease have similar manometric findings to patients with primary or secondary esophageal hypomotility. Whether gastroesophageal reflux is the cause or the result of these abnormal manometric findings is a subject of debate. Some patients with esophageal hypomotility in the setting of GERD obtain marked improvement in esophageal contractility with antireflux surgery.[56] There is currently no specific treatment available to improve esophageal contractility, and symptomatic control of the gastroesophageal reflux is the only option for these patients.

Stomach

Diabetic Gastroparesis. Diabetic autonomic neuropathy is one of the major complications of diabetes mellitus and is most common in patients with long-term diabetes, poor glycemic control, and peripheral neuropathy. Autonomic neuropathy may affect the entire gastrointestinal tract, producing constipation, abdominal pain, nausea, vomiting, dysphagia,
4 diarrhea, and fecal incontinence. Diabetic gastroparesis may affect 50% of diabetic patients, although symptomatic gastroparesis is less common. Symptoms of diabetic gastroparesis include nausea, vomiting, and early satiety. In addition, impaired gastric motility predisposes to bezoar formation that can result in a vicious cycle of worsened gastric motility and early satiety. Delayed gastric emptying secondary to diabetic gastroparesis can make glucose homeostasis challenging, with resultant diabetic ketoacidosis or hypoglycemia. The diagnosis is usually suspected in a patient with symptoms of nausea, vomiting, and early satiety in the setting of diabetes. An upper endoscopy should be performed in all patients suspected of diabetic gastroparesis to exclude other organic causes of their symptoms. A nuclear medicine gastric emptying study is the "gold standard" diagnostic test for gastroparesis and can also be used in follow-up to assess response to treatment.

The pathophysiology of diabetic gastroparesis is complicated, incompletely understood, and multifactorial. Vagal nerve dysfunction can cause multiple changes in the normal physiology of gastric emptying. Vagal dysfunction can result in abnormal receptive relaxation of the stomach, decreased gastric antral contractility with failure of the antral pump, and prolonged contraction of the pylorus resulting in pylorospasm.[57] Neuropathy of the gastric enteric nervous system can exacerbate vagal dysfunction and may contribute to gastric myoelectric dysrrythamia.[58] Hyperglycemia itself can disrupt normal gastric motility and delay gastric emptying.[59]

There is no single, specific treatment for diabetic gastroparesis. Aggressive glycemic control may prevent progressive neuropathy. Prokinetic agents such as metoclopramide and domperidone and dopamine antagonists promote gastric tone and improve gastric emptying. In addition, these drugs act as central nervous system–mediated antiemetic agents, reducing symptoms of nausea. The motilin agonist erythromycin has also been shown to be effective in patients with diabetic gastroparesis.[60] Erythromycin use has been limited by long-term tachyphylaxis. Pancreatic transplantation, by restoring glycemic control, has been reported to improve gastric motility as documented by gastric-emptying studies. Gastric electrical pacing using gastric pacemaker leads placed directly on the stomach has shown promise, but remains experimental.[61]

Postsurgical Gastroparesis. Postsurgical gastroparesis is a syndrome characterized by gastric hypomotility in the absence of mechanical obstruction. The incidence of this disorder has been estimated at 2% to 3% after partial gastrectomy and vagotomy.[62] Postsurgical gastroparesis appears to occur more commonly after operations for gastric outlet obstruction and in diabetic patients. Patients with postsurgical gastroparesis develop symptoms of abdominal pain, postprandial nausea, vomiting, and weight loss months after gastric resection. The diagnosis is one of exclusion, and careful evaluation with endoscopy and barium studies is required to exclude mechanical gastric outlet obstruction. A solid-phase gastric emptying study is necessary and is the only abnormal test in 45% of patients with this motility disorder.[63]

The pathogenic mechanism of this syndrome is related to loss of vagal innervation of the stomach, coupled with loss of antral pump function after antrectomy. Underlying gastric motor dysfunction in diabetic patients may also contribute to postsurgical gastroparesis. Treatment of postsurgical gastroparesis consists of prokinetic agents such as metoclopramide and erythromycin or revisional gastric surgery. Most authors recommend a 6- to 12-month trial of medical therapy prior to revisional surgery. Success rates of medical therapy have been disappointing, with response rates in the 20% to 30% range.[63] Surgical therapy is directed at eliminating the gastric reservoir with a near-completion gastrectomy and Roux-en-Y gastrojejunostomy. In selected patient series, symptomatic success rates of 70% to 80% have been reported.[64]

5 **Dumping Syndrome.** Dumping syndrome is a clinically defined spectrum of symptoms observed after gastric surgery thought to be a consequence of accelerated gastric emptying following vagotomy and bypass or destruction of the pylorus. Symptoms occur after the ingestion of food; they are absent in the fasting state. The incidence of dumping syndrome after gastric surgery is variable and depends on the operation performed. Overall, about 10% of patients will have clinically significant symptoms.[65] A diagnosis of dumping is made on clinical grounds and hinges on the presence of typical symptoms in a postoperative patient. Dumping occurs in the postprandial period and is classified into two forms. Early dumping occurs within 30 to 60 minutes of eating and typically presents with both gastrointestinal and vasomotor symptoms. Late dumping occurs 2 to 3 hours after eating and usually presents with only vasomotor symptoms. Gastrointestinal symptoms include postprandial fullness, crampy abdominal pain, nausea, vomiting, and explosive diarrhea. Vasomotor symptoms include diaphoresis, weakness, dizziness, flushing, palpitations, and an intense urge to lie down. In patients with severe dumping symptoms, weight loss and food fear may also be present.

Radioisotopic gastric emptying studies demonstrate rapid gastric emptying. Investigators have suggested a simple provocative test to confirm the diagnosis of dumping. After ingestion of 50 g of oral glucose, a heart rate rise of greater than 10 beats per minute in the first hour is a sensitive predictor of early dumping.[66] Late dumping is confirmed with this test by documenting typical vasomotor symptoms in the postchallenge period.

The pathophysiologies of early and late dumping are different. In early dumping, rapid delivery of hyperosmolar chyme into the small intestine secondary to rapid gastric emptying results in several maladaptive responses. The presence of hyperosmolar proximal small intestinal contents leads to fluid shifts into the intestinal lumen, causing intestinal distention and precipitating gastrointestinal symptoms. Rapid delivery of glucose to the proximal small bowel leads to both peripheral and splanchnic vasodilatation and blood pooling, which results in the vasomotor symptoms of early dumping. In addition, gastrointestinal hormone release is enhanced in patients with early dumping including secretion of enteroglucagon, VIP, peptide YY, pancreatic polypeptide, glucagonlike peptide 1 (GLP-1), and neurotensin.[67,68] Rapid delivery of glucose to the small bowel followed by rapid glucose absorption causes late dumping symptoms by producing an exaggerated serum insulin release. Exaggerated insulin secretion, combined with rapid gastric emptying, results in an excess insulin state 2 to 3 hours after eating with subsequent hypoglycemia and vasomotor symptoms. The cause of the excess insulin secretion is unclear, but the enteric hormone GLP-1 may play a role in late dumping.[69]

Most cases of dumping syndrome fade with time.[70] The initial mainstay therapy for dumping syndrome is dietary modification, which will effectively control dumping symptoms in most patients. An antidumping diet consists of (a) frequent small meals, ideally six or more per day; (b) a diet low in simple sugars with a moderate amount of fat and high in complicated carbohydrates, protein, and fiber; and (c) dry meals with liquid ingestion delayed at least 30 minutes after solid intake. Dietary fiber supplementation has been shown to help with late dumping. Acarbose, a competitive inhibitor of carbohydrate absorption, has also been shown to improve late dumping, although long-term use can cause malabsorption.[68] In patients with severe dumping, or those whose symptoms fail to respond to dietary modification, the next step should be the use of octreotide, the long-acting somatostatin analogue. Octreotide acts to delay intestinal transit time, cause splanchnic vasoconstriction, and suppress the release of a variety of enteral hormones including insulin.[65] For patients with debilitating dumping symptoms that are refractory to dietary modification and octreotide, remedial surgery may be considered. A cautious approach is appropriate, as most cases of dumping will improve with time and no remedial operation has a 100% success rate. Reconstruction of the pylorus and conversion to Roux-en-Y gastrojejunostomy have both been used successfully to correct intractable dumping.[70]

Gallbladder and Biliary Tract

Gallbladder Dyskinesia. The term *biliary dyskinesia* indicates a poorly characterized motility disorder of the gallbladder and the sphincter of Oddi. Gallbladder dyskinesia has been recognized as a cause of biliary symptoms, and may be a manifestation of generalized dysmotility of the gastrointestinal
6 tract.[71] The most common presenting symptom of gallbladder dyskinesia is abdominal pain in the absence of gallstones or other structural cause of right upper quadrant pain. The prevalence of biliary pain without gallstones has been estimated to be 6% to 21% with a 3:1 female-to-male predominance. The diagnosis of gallbladder dyskinesia is usually made by CCK cholescintigraphy obtained after an ultrasound negative for gallstones. During CCK cholescintigraphy, a gallbladder ejection fraction less than 35% is considered diagnostic of the disorder.

Defects in the function and distribution of CCK receptors on cells within the gallbladder wall with resultant abnormal responses to endogenous CCK have been implicated as causes of this disorder. In addition to an intrinsic motility disorder, inflammation and anatomic abnormalities have also been reported. Inflammatory bowel disease is associated with abnormal gallbladder contractility and patients with slow–transit constipation have been reported to have decreased gallbladder ejection fraction.[72,73]

There is no effective medical therapy for this disorder. Laparoscopic cholecystectomy is the major treatment option for patients with gallbladder dyskinesia, with symptomatic improvement noted in 70% to 90% of selected patients. It is unclear if preoperative CCK cholescintigraphy results predict surgical results, although one study suggested that a gallbladder ejection fraction of less than 14% was associated with a higher likelihood of complete symptom relief.[74] Because of the frequent association of gallbladder dyskinesia with other motility disorders of the gastrointestinal tract, symptoms related to gastrointestinal dysmotility may not be relieved; nausea and vomiting are less likely to be relieved than postprandial abdominal pain. Although 81% of the patients with gallstones become asymptomatic after laparoscopic cholecystectomy, only 47% of patients with gallbladder dyskinesia are asymptomatic postoperatively.[75]

Sphincter of Oddi Dysfunction. Sphincter of Oddi dysfunction describes a clinical syndrome arising from abnormalities of sphincter of Oddi contractility. The disorder can be caused by fibrosis and stenosis or by functional obstruction of the pancreaticobiliary junction. Ductal hypertension, hypersensitivity of the papilla, and possible ischemia from spastic contraction have been postulated as causes of pain, pancreatitis, and liver enzyme abnormalities.[76] The disorder can occur at any age and affects women more frequently than men. Although classically diagnosed in patients after cholecystectomy, this disorder can occur in patients with an intact biliary tree. Abdominal pain, usually in the epigastrium or right upper quadrant, is the most common symptom. The pain is often associated with oral intake and use of narcotics and does not respond to acid-reducing or prokinetic medical therapy. Jaundice and fever are uncommon. There are no characteristic findings on physical

TABLE 64.3 **DIAGNOSIS**

ROME III CRITERIA FOR SPHINCTER OF ODDI DYSFUNCTION

Epigastric or right upper quadrant pain and all of the following:
- Pain last for ≥30 min
- Recurrent symptoms occurring at different intervals
- The pain builds up to a steady level
- Pain requires medical attention and affects daily activities
- No evidence of structural abnormalities
- The pain is not relieved by bowel movements, postural change, or antacids

Supportive criteria
- The pain may be associated with nausea and vomiting or back pain or awaken the patient from sleep

Adapted from Behar J, Corazziari E, Guelrud M, et al. Functional gallbladder and sphincter of Oddi dysfunction. *Gastroenterology* 2006;130:1498–1509.

TABLE 64.4 **CLASSIFICATION**

MILWAUKEE CLASSIFICATION: SYMPTOMS

■ BILIARY TYPE	■ DESCRIPTION
I	Patient with biliary-type pain; abnormal AST, ALT, or alkaline phosphatase (two times normal) on two or more occasions; and dilated CBD more than 8 mm diameter at US
II	Patient with biliary-type of pain but only one of two of the above criteria
III	Biliary-type pain only

AST, aspartate aminotransferase; ALT, alanine aminotransferase; US, right upper quadrant ultrasound; CBD, common bile duct. Adapted from Behar J, Corazziari E, Guelrud M, et al. Functional gallbladder and sphincter of Oddi dysfunction. *Gastroenterology* 2006;130:1498–1509.

examination aside from nonspecific abdominal tenderness. Because of the absence of a classic symptom or finding, patients with the diagnosis of sphincter of Oddi dysfunction are sometimes difficult to distinguish from patients with other organic or dysmotility disorders. Rome III criteria for the diagnosis of sphincter of Oddi dysfunction are listed in Table 64.3.[77]

Initial diagnostic tests include complete blood count, liver function tests, and determination of serum amylase and lipase. Imaging studies should begin with ultrasonography to assess for stones and bile duct diameter. All of these tests are most sensitive when performed during active symptoms. Endoscopic retrograde pancreatography (ERCP) is conventionally used to exclude other pathologies that may cause symptoms similar to sphincter of Oddi dysfunction, although with the increased availability and accuracy of magnetic resonance cholangiopancreatography (MRCP), this test should be used before ERCP because it is noninvasive and carries a lower risk of complications. Sphincter of Oddi manometry is considered the "gold standard" for the diagnosis of sphincter of Oddi dysfunction and is the only method available to measure the activity of the sphincter directly. Manometry is usually performed during ERCP with selective cannulation of the pancreatic duct and biliary duct. Although a variety of noninvasive tests have been proposed to evaluate the possible diagnosis of sphincter of Oddi dysfunction, noninvasive testing cannot be recommended for general clinical use due to low sensitivity and specificity.[78] Invasive testing with ERCP and manometry has a high complication rate and is indicated only if definitive therapy is planned in the presence of abnormal results. Because of the difficulty in establishing the diagnosis of sphincter of Oddi dysfunction and predicting the response to therapy, the Milwaukee classification system was developed in an effort to correlate symptoms and diagnostic tests with abnormal manometric findings and predict the response to sphincterotomy (Tables 64.4 and 64.5). Abnormal liver tests in biliary type II disease may predict symptomatic response to endoscopic sphincterotomy.[79]

The aim of therapy for sphincter of Oddi dysfunction is to decrease the resistance to the flow of bile and pancreatic juice. Medical therapy is based on the use of smooth muscle relaxants. Nifedipine has been shown to reduce pain in sphincter of Oddi dysfunction in 75% of the patients in the short term.[80] Long-term outcomes have not been reported. Despite the lack of long-term data, medical approaches should be considered when patients are not severely symptomatic (class II and III sphincter of Oddi dysfunction). Reduction of resistance at the sphincter of Oddi via endoscopic means by stenting or sphincterotomy is the mainstay of therapy for sphincter of Oddi dysfunction.[81] According to the Milwaukee classification, manometry may predict the outcome from sphincter ablation in patients with biliary-type pain. The use of stents in sphincter of Oddi dysfunction is controversial, with a reported high incidence of pancreatitis (38%). Stenting may predict outcome from sphincterotomy when stenting provides resolution of pain for at least 12 weeks. Currently, endoscopic sphincteroplasty is standard therapy for sphincter of Oddi dysfunction, with clinical improvement reported in 55% to 95% of cases.[82] The role of sphincter ablation is evolving; complication rates remain higher than in patients with ductal stones. Surgical

TABLE 64.5 **CLASSIFICATION**

MILWAUKEE CLASSIFICATION: BILIARY SYMPTOMS AND RESPONSE TO TREATMENT

■ PATIENT CHARACTERISTICS	■ ABNORMAL MANOMETRY (%)	■ SPHINCTEROTOMY EFFICACY IF MANOMETRY		■ INDICATION FOR MANOMETRY: PRIOR TO SPHINCTEROTOMY
		■ NORMAL (%)	■ ABNORMAL (%)	
Biliary I	75–95	90–95	90–95	Unnecessary
Biliary II	55–65	35	85	Highly recommended
Biliary III	25–60	<10	55–65	Mandatory

Adapted from Sherman S, Lehman GA. Sphincter of Oddi dysfunction: diagnosis and treatment. *J Pancreas* 2001;2:382–400.

approaches such as transduodenal sphincteroplasty with pancreatic septoplasty have been largely replaced by endoscopic therapy. Patient selection is paramount considering the high complication rate for endoscopic therapy.[82] Evolving manometric techniques are improving our understanding of sphincter of Oddi dysfunction. Patients with abnormal sphincter of Oddi manometry, without gastroparesis or a history of long-term narcotic use, appear to have the best response to endoscopic therapy.

Small Intestine

Chronic Intestinal Pseudo-obstruction. Chronic intestinal pseudo-obstruction is a clinical syndrome caused by ineffective intestinal propulsion and characterized by signs and symptoms of intestinal obstruction in the absence of mechanical cause.[83] The disorder is a rare clinical syndrome, caused by a variety of pathogenic mechanisms. Although sophisticated clinicopathologic classification systems exist for chronic intestinal pseudo-obstruction, important etiologies include visceral myopathies, visceral neuropathies, systemic disorders involving smooth muscle such as systemic sclerosis, developmental abnormalities of the myenteric plexus, and systemic neurodegenerative disorders.[84] Although small intestinal dysmotility is the prominent finding in most cases, the syndrome can involve all portions of the gastrointestinal tract from esophagus to colon.

Patients with intestinal pseudo-obstruction present with variable amounts of abdominal pain, distention, and vomiting. The vomitus often consists of partially digested food and can be feculent in character. Patients with small bowel involvement can develop bacterial overgrowth and may have symptoms of diarrhea and steatorrhea. In patients with significant colonic dysmotility, constipation symptoms may predominate. A family history of similar problems may be present in up to one third of cases, and many patients have a history of abdominal surgery.

On physical examination, patients may exhibit wasting with marked abdominal distention and visible bowel loops against the abdominal wall. Although tenderness is often present, peritonitis is unusual. In most ways it will be impossible to distinguish chronic intestinal pseudo-obstruction from true mechanical bowel obstruction, except for the chronic nature of symptoms and a history of prior episodes with waxing and waning severity. It is imperative for surgeons evaluating patients with chronic intestinal pseudo-obstruction to avoid mistaking this syndrome for mechanical bowel obstruction, because once a patient with chronic intestinal pseudo-obstruction has undergone abdominal surgery, the potential exists for both pseudo-obstruction and adhesive bowel obstruction to coexist. The best way to confirm a suspected diagnosis of chronic intestinal pseudo-obstruction is through barium contrast studies of the entire gastrointestinal tract. The identification of multiple sites of abnormality on such studies in the absence of a clear mechanical transition point is most consistent with the diagnosis. The finding of a single area of dilation isolated to the small intestine should raise suspicion of mechanical small bowel obstruction.

There is no definitive treatment for this motility disorder; no pharmacologic therapy or surgical procedure will correct the underlying motility disorder. Therapy is therefore directed at palliating symptoms and ensuring that patients receive adequate nutrition. A variety of promotility agents have been used. Metoclopramide and domperidone have not been found to be effective.[84] Erythromycin has shown benefit in some patients for up to 1 year, but tachyphylaxis appears to limit its long-term value.[85] Cisapride, although no longer available in the United States, improves symptoms in the majority of patients in noncontrolled trials.[86] Low-dose (50 μg) octreotide may be of benefit in patients with systemic sclerosis, but has not been shown to be useful in other patients with chronic intestinal pseudo-obstruction.[85]

In patients with suspected pseudo-obstruction, avoiding operation is critical because a nontherapeutic operation for bowel obstruction will predispose the patient to adhesive mechanical bowel obstruction in the future. In patients with confirmed chronic intestinal pseudo-obstruction, surgical therapy can be important in palliating specific symptoms of the syndrome such as bloating and malnutrition, or in managing failures of medical management. For patients with localized dysfunctional bowel, bypass or segmental resection of the involved bowel can result in satisfactory long-term results.[87] In patients with diffuse intestinal involvement, venting enterostomy and intravenous access for long-term parenteral nutrition may represent the only surgical options. Small intestinal transplant has been reported in small series with good functional results.[88]

Acquired Jejunoileal Diverticular Disease. Acquired jejunoileal diverticulosis appears to occur as a consequence of a small bowel motility disorder. This rare finding has a prevalence of between 0.1% and 2.3%, depending on whether autopsy or radiologic data are used.[89,90] These lesions are usually found in patients in the seventh decade of life. There is no apparent sex predilection. These acquired lesions are pseudodiverticula whose wall includes only the mucosal and submucosal layers of the bowel. They are found on the mesenteric surface of the bowel and commonly lie within the mesentery. Eighty percent of patients have the diverticula localized to the jejunum; in 15% of patients, lesions are found in the ileum, and 5% have diverticula distributed throughout the small intestine. Eighty percent of patients, particularly those with jejunal diverticula, have multiple lesions.[91]

It has been postulated that these acquired lesions are caused by a motility disturbance of the involved intestine. Poorly coordinated neuromuscular function with ineffective peristalsis and resultant high intraluminal pressures cause protrusion of the mucosa through the muscular layers of the bowel wall at the point that the vasa recta enter the bowel wall. Abnormalities of both intestinal smooth muscle and the myenteric plexus found in patients with jejunoileal diverticulosis support this hypothesis.[92] Mild variants of the same disorders may lead to the development of acquired small bowel diverticulosis. Pseudodiverticula are found in the colon and duodenum in 40% to 50% of patients with jejunoileal diverticulosis, supporting the role of a diffuse intestinal motility disorder in pathogenesis.

The role of surgical therapy in this motility disorder lies in the management of complications and in palliating symptoms secondary to the diverticula. The majority of patients (50% to 60%) have asymptomatic diverticula noted on radiologic study or found incidentally at laparotomy.[90] Because these patients are likely to remain symptom-free, there is no indication for resection in these instances. Twenty to forty percent of patients will present with a nonspecific constellation of chronic abdominal complaints including pain, postprandial bloating, diarrhea, malabsorption, and vitamin B_{12} deficiency.[91] In these patients, symptoms are related to bacterial overgrowth and malabsorption. Most of these patients respond to a regimen of a high-protein, low-residue diet coupled with vitamin B_{12} supplementation and intermittent broad-spectrum antibiotic treatment. Only when this approach fails should resection be contemplated. Ten to fifteen percent of patients will present with acute complications, either bleeding, diverticulitis, or perforation, requiring urgent surgical intervention.[93] In emergent cases, resection of the involved segment of small bowel with anastomosis is the best surgical approach.

Colon

Colonic Inertia. Constipation is a common complaint, affecting up to 20% of the population.[94] Although the overwhelming majority of cases of constipation do not require surgical attention, one disorder, idiopathic slow-transit constipation, is a motility disorder amenable to surgical therapy. Idiopathic slow-transit constipation or colonic inertia (CI) is caused by a variety of pathogenic mechanisms including abnormalities of myenteric plexus formation, disorders of extrinsic enervation of the colon, and disorders of colonic neuromuscular transmission. From a diagnostic and therapeutic standpoint, these disorders may be considered a single syndrome.[95]

7 The diagnosis of colonic inertia is established in a chronically constipated patient with markedly prolonged colonic transit time in the absence of anorectal dysfunction. Patients typically present with complaints of needing regular assistance with bowel movement or of having one bowel movement every 7 days. The normal transit time through the colon can be assessed either with radiopaque markers or by scintigraphic studies. The radiopaque marker study involves the ingestion of a capsule containing 20 or 24 markers. Abdominal radiographs are then taken and analyzed after both 72 and 120 hours of ingestion. CI is defined as retention of at least 20% of the markers in the colon on the fifth day after ingestion. Pancolonic inertia becomes noted if the markers become diffusely scattered throughout the colon.[96] Scintigraphic colonic transit studies are less widely available, but require only 24 hours to obtain accurate segmental transit times.[97] Prior to the diagnosis of CI, tests must be conducted to exclude causes originating from underlying endocrine and/or metabolic diseases. Colonoscopy should be performed to exclude the possibility of a neoplasm.

After establishing a diagnosis of slow colonic transit, anorectal function must be assessed, as disorders of anorectal function will slow colonic transit. Fluoroscopic defecography and anorectal manometry are used to exclude rectocele or rectal intussusception, which is often associated with obstructed defecation. A digital rectal exam can also be a valuable tool to aid a clinician in this diagnosis. Normal findings on these evaluations are required to establish a diagnosis of idiopathic slow-transit constipation.[96,98]

The initial management of chronic constipation is medical, including behavior modification, dietary changes, fiber supplementation (25 g/d), and increased fluid intake to 1.5 to 2 liters daily. The use of psyllium and lactulose has been shown to improve symptoms.[99] Other oral agents, such as senna and milk of magnesia, do help, but the improvement is marginal and outcomes are not statistically significant.[100] The use of low-volume polyethylene glycol electrolyte solution administration does improve clinical outcomes.[101] For some patients, biofeedback has helped with pelvic floor dyssynergia-type constipation.[102] An overview of the management of chronic constipation is illustrated in Algorithm 64.2.

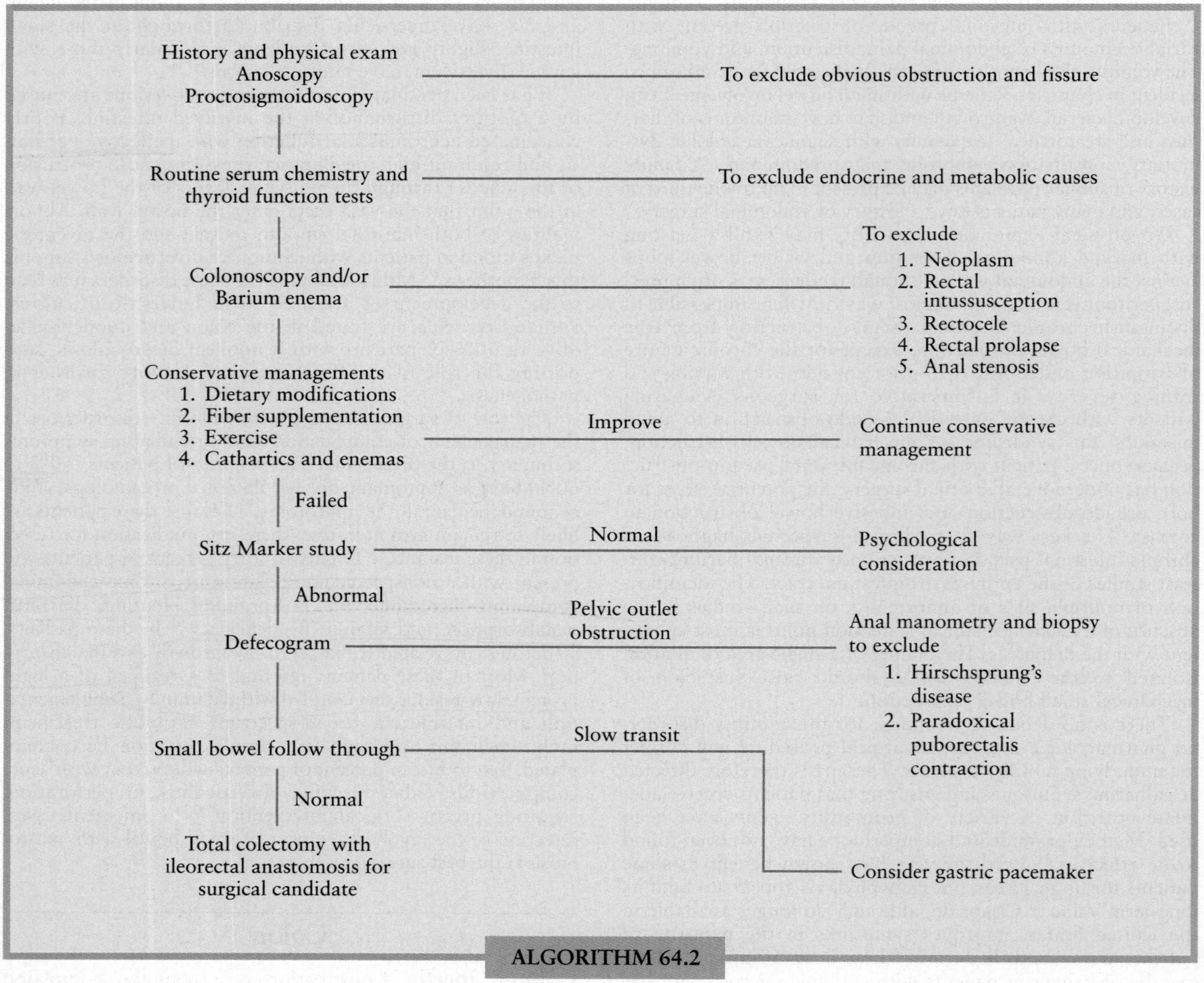

ALGORITHM 64.2. Management of chronic constipation.

TABLE 64.6

SURGICAL OPTIONS FOR CHRONIC CONSTIPATION

SURGICAL OPTION	COMMENTS
Total abdominal colectomy (TAC) with ileorectal (IR) anastomosis	Preferred procedure with over 90% success rate
Subtotal colectomy with ileosigmoid anastomosis	Predisposes to persistent constipation with over 50% conversion to TAC with IR anastomosis
Subtotal colectomy with cecorectal anastomosis	Preserves the ileocecal valve during surgery but can have complications of cecal dilation

In the few patients with intractable constipation found to have isolated colonic inertia, total abdominal colectomy with ileorectal anastomosis results in excellent functional outcomes in 90% of patients. Although subtotal colectomy with ileosigmoid anastomosis and subtotal colectomy with cecorectal anastomosis are available, the results are inferior and often require conversion to total colectomy with ileorectal anastomosis.[96] The key to good results with surgical therapy for constipation is careful preoperative evaluation of colonic function (Table 64.6). In series without complete evaluation, satisfactory outcomes occur in only 67% of patients.[98]

Acute Colonic Pseudo-obstruction (Ogilvie Syndrome).

8 Acute colonic pseudo-obstruction is a clinical syndrome characterized by massive dilation of the colon in the absence of mechanical obstruction. The disorder is characterized by the loss of effective colonic peristalsis and subsequent distention of the proximal colon. This syndrome generally develops in ill patients, hospitalized initially for other significant medical problems, and is also observed in surgical patients after a variety of nongastrointestinal operations.[103] If left untreated, massive colonic dilation can result in ischemia of the right colon and cecum with associated perforation. The overall mortality rate of acute colonic pseudo-obstruction is quite variable, ranging between 0% and 32%, and appears to depend on the underlying cause of the pseudo-obstruction.[104] With the development of ischemia and perforation, mortality rises to 30% to 50%.

The pathophysiology of acute colonic pseudo-obstruction remains unclear. A current hypothesis invokes an imbalance in neural input to the colon distal to the splenic flexure with an excess of sympathetic stimulation and a paucity of parasympathetic input, resulting in a spastic contraction of the distal colon and functional obstruction.[105] Multiple independent circumstantial lines of evidence support this hypothesis, including the finding of colonic dilation in only the right and transverse colon in the majority of cases, the observation that epidural anesthesia improves the condition in a majority of cases, and the effective use of parasympathomimetic agents to treat the syndrome. The role of inhibitory neurotransmitters such as nitric oxide in the pathogenesis of acute colonic pseudo-obstruction has been suggested in vitro, but not yet confirmed in human studies.

Acute colonic pseudo-obstruction should be suspected in a hospitalized patient who develops marked abdominal distention over a period of 1 to 2 days. Obstipation is seen in the majority of patients, but up to 40% of cases will present with diarrhea or passage of flatus. Abdominal discomfort is present in the majority of patients, and tenderness on physical examination raises the concern for bowel ischemia.[103]

Plain films of the abdomen, with the finding of proximal dilation of the colon associated with a decompressed distal colon with some gas in the rectosigmoid region, are highly suggestive of acute colonic pseudo-obstruction. The diagnostic challenge initially is to exclude mechanical colonic obstruction, and early performance of a water-soluble contrast enema is critical if mechanical obstruction cannot be ruled out on clinical grounds. The diameter of the cecum on plain film is important in directing the therapeutic approach to acute colonic pseudo-obstruction. Both animal studies and large retrospective human series suggest that the risk of cecal ischemia and perforation exists with cecal diameters greater than 12 cm and rises dramatically with cecal diameters greater than 14 cm.[103]

For patients with a cecal diameter less than 10 cm, an initial trial of conservative therapy is indicated. Conservative therapy includes correction of electrolyte disorders, avoidance of narcotic and anticholinergic agents, hydration, mobilization, tap-water enemas, and placement of a nasogastric tube.[106] During this course of conservative therapy patients should receive frequent abdominal evaluation and serial abdominal radiographs to assess cecal diameter. Several small cases series suggest that resolution rates of acute colonic pseudo-obstruction approximating 90% can be achieved with a conservative regimen. Roughly 70% of the cases that resolve with conservative therapy do so within 2 days, suggesting that a 48-hour trial in stable patients is warranted.[107] However, postponing colon decompression beyond 4 days increases the mortality rate in patients with acute colonic pseudo-obstruction.[103]

Patients who fail conservative therapy for more than 48 hours should be considered for active intervention with the first-line treatment consisting of intravenous administration of the cholinesterase inhibitor neostigmine. More than five noncontrolled trials and one randomized controlled trial have shown that intravenous neostigmine at a dose of 2 to 2.5 mg given over 3 to 5 minutes results in immediate colonic decompression in 80% to 90% of patients, and sustained colon decompression is achieved in more than 60%.[105,108] Because symptomatic bradycardia is a serious side effect of neostigmine, all patients being treated with the drug require cardiac monitoring. Neostigmine is contraindicated in patients with significant bradycardia. In patients with a contraindication to neostigmine and for those who fail to respond to the drug, decompressive colonoscopy is the next line of therapy. Colonoscopy to the cecum with evacuation of the contents of the proximal colon and placement of a long tube for decompression results in resolution of acute colonic pseudo-obstruction in 70% to 80% of cases. Roughly 40% of cases require multiple colonscopies.[109]

Colonoscopy in this setting is associated with a 2% to 3% perforation rate, and the case fatality rate of acute colonic pseudo-obstruction in patients requiring colonoscopy is up to 30%.[110] In patients who develop findings suggestive of colonic ischemia or those who fail colonoscopic decompression, surgical therapy with either resection or a stoma is necessary, although it is associated with a 30% to 50% mortality rate.[103] Laparoscopic approaches have been reported for stoma creation and may avoid laparotomy in an elderly or frail patient. An algorithm for the management of Ogilvie syndrome is presented in Algorithm 64.3.

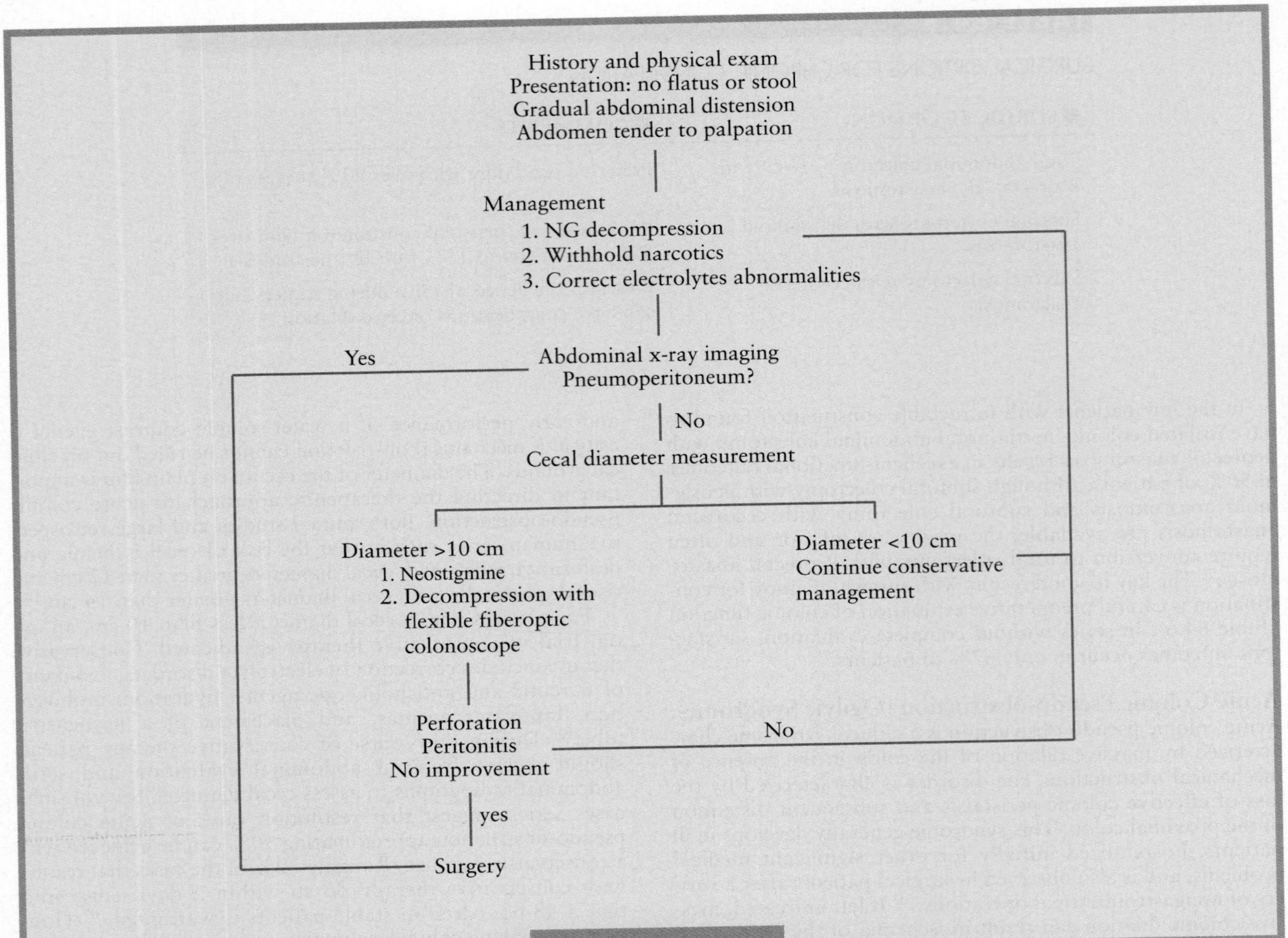

ALGORITHM 64.3

ALGORITHM 64.3. Treatment of Ogilvie syndrome. NG, nasogastric.

References

1. Baig MK, Wexner SD. Postoperative ileus: a review. *Dis Colon Rectum* 2004;47(4):516–526.
2. Livingston EH, Passaro EP Jr. Postoperative ileus. *Dig Dis Sci* 1990;35(1):121–132.
3. Miedema BW, Schillie S, Simmons JW, et al. Small bowel motility and transit after aortic surgery. *J Vasc Surg* 2002;36(1):19–24.
4. Behm B, Stollman N. Postoperative ileus: etiologies and interventions. *Clin Gastroenterol Hepatol* 2003;1(2):71–80.
5. Waldhausen JH, Shaffrey ME, Skenderis BS II, et al. Gastrointestinal myoelectric and clinical patterns of recovery after laparotomy. *Ann Surg* 1990; 211(6):777–784; discussion 785.
6. Holzer P, Lippe IT, Holzer-Petsche U. Inhibition of gastrointestinal transit due to surgical trauma or peritoneal irritation is reduced in capsaicin-treated rats. *Gastroenterology* 1986;91(2):360–363.
7. Holte K, Kehlet H. Postoperative ileus: a preventable event. *Br J Surg* 2000;87(11):1480–1493.
8. De Winter BY, Robberecht P, Boeckxstaens GE, et al. Role of VIP1/PACAP receptors in postoperative ileus in rats. *Br J Pharmacol* 1998;124(6): 1181–1186.
9. Espat NJ, Cheng G, Kelley MC, et al. Vasoactive intestinal peptide and substance P receptor antagonists improve postoperative ileus. *J Surg Res* 1995;58(6):719–723.
10. Rennie JA, Christofides ND, Mitchenere P, et al. Neural and humoral factors in postoperative ileus. *Br J Surg* 1980;67(10):694–698.
11. Trudel L, Tomasetto C, Rio MC, et al. Ghrelin/motilin-related peptide is a potent prokinetic to reverse gastric postoperative ileus in rat. *Am J Physiol Gastrointest Liver Physiol* 2002;282(6):G948–G952.
12. Kalff JC, Schraut WH, Simmons RL, et al. Surgical manipulation of the gut elicits an intestinal muscularis inflammatory response resulting in postsurgical ileus. *Ann Surg* 1998;228(5):652–663.
13. Bellon JM, Manzano L, Larrad A, et al. Endocrine and immune response to injury after open and laparoscopic cholecystectomy. *Int Surg* 1998; 83(1):24–27.
14. Kaufman PN, Krevsky B, Malmud LS, et al. Role of opiate receptors in the regulation of colonic transit. *Gastroenterology* 1988;94(6): 1351–1356.
15. Ferraz AA, Cowles VE, Condon RE, et al. Nonopioid analgesics shorten the duration of postoperative ileus. *Am Surg* 1995;61(12):1079–1083.
16. Yee MK, Evans WD, Facey PE, et al. Gastric emptying and small bowel transit in male volunteers after i. m. ketorolac and morphine. *Br J Anaesth* 1991;67(4):426–431.
17. Lowman RM. The potassium depletion states and postoperative ileus. The role of the potassium ion. *Radiology* 1971;98(3):691–694.
18. Brown TA, McDonald J, Williard W. A prospective, randomized, double-blinded, placebo-controlled trial of cisapride after colorectal surgery. *Am J Surg* 1999;177(5):399–401.
19. Vasquez W, Hernandez AV, Garcia-Sabrido JL. Is gum chewing useful for ileus after elective colorectal surgery? A systematic review and meta-analysis of randomized clinical trials. *J Gastrointest Surg* 2009;13: 649–656.
20. Cheadle WG, Vitale GC, Mackie CR, et al. Prophylactic postoperative nasogastric decompression. A prospective study of its requirement and the influence of cimetidine in 200 patients. *Ann Surg* 1985;202(3): 361–366.
21. Mertz HR. Irritable bowel syndrome. *N Engl J Med* 2003;349(22): 2136–2146.
22. Longstreth GF, Thompson WG, Chey WD, et al. Functional bowel disorders. *Gastroenterology* 2006;130(5):1480–1491.
23. Kellow JE, Gill RC, Wingate DL. Prolonged ambulant recordings of small bowel motility demonstrate abnormalities in the irritable bowel syndrome. *Gastroenterology* 1990;98(5 Pt 1):1208–1218.
24. Kellow JE, Phillips SF, Miller LJ, et al. Dysmotility of the small intestine in irritable bowel syndrome. *Gut* 1988;29(9):1236–1243.

25. Mertz H, Naliboff B, Munakata J, et al. Altered rectal perception is a biological marker of patients with irritable bowel syndrome. *Gastroenterology* 1995;109(1):40–52.
26. Collins SM, Vallance B, Barbara G, et al. Putative inflammatory and immunological mechanisms in functional bowel disorders. *Baillieres Best Pract Res Clin Gastroenterol* 1999;13(3):429–436.
27. Longstreth GF, Yao JF. Irritable bowel syndrome and surgery: a multivariable analysis. *Gastroenterology* 2004;126(7):1665–1673.
28. Jackson JL, O'Malley PG, Tomkins G, et al. Treatment of functional gastrointestinal disorders with antidepressant medications: a meta-analysis. *Am J Med* 2000;108(1):65–72.
29. Camilleri M, Northcutt AR, Kong S, et al. Efficacy and safety of alosetron in women with irritable bowel syndrome: a randomised, placebo-controlled trial. *Lancet* 2000;355(9209):1035–1040.
30. Novick J, Miner P, Krause R, et al. A randomized, double-blind, placebo-controlled trial of tegaserod in female patients suffering from irritable bowel syndrome with constipation. *Aliment Pharmacol Ther* 2002;16(11):1877–1888.
31. Richter JE. Oesophageal motility disorders. *Lancet* 2001;358(9284):823–828.
32. Podas T, Eaden J, Mayberry M, et al. Achalasia: a critical review of epidemiological studies. *Am J Gastroenterol* 1998;93(12):2345–2347.
33. Fisichella PM, Raz D, Palazzo F, et al. Clinical, radiological, and manometric profile in 145 patients with untreated achalasia. *World J Surg* 2008;32(9):1974–1979.
34. Ghosh SK, Pandolfino JE, Rice J, et al. Impaired deglutitive EGJ relaxation in clinical esophageal manometry: a quantitative analysis of 400 patients and 75 controls. *Am J Physiol Gastrointest Liver Physiol* 2007;293(4):G878–G885.
35. Goldblum JR, Whyte RI, Orringer MB, et al. Achalasia. A morphologic study of 42 resected specimens. *Am J Surg Pathol* 1994;18(4):327–337.
36. Cassella RR, Ellis FH Jr, Brown AL Jr. Fine-structure changes in Achalasia of the esophagus. I. Vagus nerves. *Am J Pathol* 1965;46:279–288.
37. Raymond L, Lach B, Shamji FM. Inflammatory aetiology of primary oesophageal achalasia: an immunohistochemical and ultrastructural study of Auerbach's plexus. *Histopathology* 1999;35(5):445–453.
38. Facco M, Brun P, Baesso I, et al. T cells in the myenteric plexus of achalasia patients show a skewed TCR repertoire and react to HSV-1 antigens. *Am J Gastroenterol* 2008;103(7):1598–1609.
39. Clark SB, Rice TW, Tubbs RR, et al. The nature of the myenteric infiltrate in achalasia: an immunohistochemical analysis. *Am J Surg Pathol* 2000;24(8):1153–1158.
40. Misiewicz JJ, Waller SL, Anthony PP, et al. Achalasia of the cardia: pharmacology and histopathology of isolated cardiac sphincteric muscle from patients with and without achalasia. *Q J Med.* 1969;38(149):17–30.
41. Lopushinsky SR, Urbach DR. Pneumatic dilatation and surgical myotomy for achalasia. *JAMA* 2006;296(18):2227–2233.
42. Donahue PE, Horgan S, Liu KJ, et al. Floppy Dor fundoplication after esophagocardiomyotomy for achalasia. *Surgery* 2002;132(4):716–722; discussion 722–723.
43. Lake JM, Wong RK. Review article: the management of achalasia—a comparison of different treatment modalities. *Aliment Pharmacol Ther* 2006;24(6):909–918.
44. Leyden JE, Moss AC, MacMathuna P. Endoscopic pneumatic dilation versus botulinum toxin injection in the management of primary achalasia. *Cochrane Database Syst Rev* 2006;(4):CD005046.
45. Horgan S, Hudda K, Eubanks T, et al. Does botulinum toxin injection make esophagomyotomy a more difficult operation? *Surg Endosc* 1999;13(6):576–579.
46. Tatum RP, Wong JA, Figueredo EJ, et al. Return of esophageal function after treatment for achalasia as determined by impedance-manometry. *J Gastrointest Surg* 2007;11(11):1403–1409.
47. Richter JE, Castell DO. Diffuse esophageal spasm: a reappraisal. *Ann Intern Med* 1984;100(2):242–245.
48. Tutuian R, Castell DO. Review article: oesophageal spasm—diagnosis and management. *Aliment Pharmacol Ther* 2006;23(10):1393–1402.
49. Behar J, Biancani P. Pathogenesis of simultaneous esophageal contractions in patients with motility disorders. *Gastroenterology* 1993;105(1):111–118.
50. Richter JE, Dalton CB, Bradley LA, et al. Oral nifedipine in the treatment of noncardiac chest pain in patients with the nutcracker esophagus. *Gastroenterology* 1987;93(1):21–28.
51. Storr M, Allescher HD, Classen M. Current concepts on pathophysiology, diagnosis and treatment of diffuse oesophageal spasm. *Drugs* 2001;61(5):579–591.
52. Patti MG, Gorodner MV, Galvani C, et al. Spectrum of esophageal motility disorders: implications for diagnosis and treatment. *Arch Surg* 2005;140(5):442–448; discussion 448–449.
53. Spechler SJ, Castell DO. Classification of oesophageal motility abnormalities. *Gut* 2001;49(1):145–151.
54. Bassotti G, Battaglia E, Debernardi V, et al. Esophageal dysfunction in scleroderma: relationship with disease subsets. *Arthritis Rheum* 1997;40(12):2252–2259.
55. Fouad YM, Katz PO, Hatlebakk JG, et al. Ineffective esophageal motility: the most common motility abnormality in patients with GERD-associated respiratory symptoms. *Am J Gastroenterol* 1999;94(6):1464–1467.
56. Rydberg L, Ruth M, Lundell L. Does oesophageal motor function improve with time after successful antireflux surgery? Results of a prospective, randomised clinical study. *Gut* 1997;41(1):82–86.
57. Horowitz M, Edelbroek M, Fraser R, et al. Disordered gastric motor function in diabetes mellitus. Recent insights into prevalence, pathophysiology, clinical relevance, and treatment. *Scand J Gastroenterol* 1991;26(7):673–684.
58. Quigley EM. The pathophysiology of diabetic gastroenteropathy: more vague than vagal. *Gastroenterology* 1997;113(5):1790–1794.
59. Kong MF, Horowitz M. Gastric emptying in diabetes mellitus: relationship to blood-glucose control. *Clin Geriatr Med* 1999;15(2):321–338.
60. Janssens J, Peeters TL, Vantrappen G, et al. Improvement of gastric emptying in diabetic gastroparesis by erythromycin. Preliminary studies. *N Engl J Med* 1990;322(15):1028–1031.
61. Abell T, McCallum R, Hocking M, et al. Gastric electrical stimulation for medically refractory gastroparesis. *Gastroenterology* 2003;125(2):421–428.
62. Eagon JC, Miedema BW, Kelly KA. Postgastrectomy syndromes. *Surg Clin North Am* 1992;72(2):445–465.
63. Pellegrini CA, Broderick WC, Van Dyke D, et al. Diagnosis and treatment of gastric emptying disorders. Clinical usefulness of radionuclide measurements of gastric emptying. *Am J Surg* 1983;145(1):143–151.
64. Eckhauser FE, Conrad M, Knol JA, et al. Safety and long-term durability of completion gastrectomy in 81 patients with postsurgical gastroparesis syndrome. *Am Surg* 1998;64(8):711–716; discussion 716–717.
65. Li-Ling J, Irving M. Therapeutic value of octreotide for patients with severe dumping syndrome—a review of randomised controlled trials. *Postgrad Med J* 2001;77(909):441–442.
66. van der Kleij FG, Vecht J, Lamers CB, et al. Diagnostic value of dumping provocation in patients after gastric surgery. *Scand J Gastroenterol* 1996;31(12):1162–1166.
67. Yamamoto H, Mori T, Tsuchihashi H, et al. A possible role of GLP-1 in the pathophysiology of early dumping syndrome. *Dig Dis Sci* 2005;50(12):2263–2267.
68. Vecht J, Masclee AA, Lamers CB. The dumping syndrome. Current insights into pathophysiology, diagnosis and treatment. *Scand J Gastroenterol Suppl* 1997;223:21–27.
69. Andreasen JJ, Orskov C, Holst JJ. Secretion of glucagon-like peptide-1 and reactive hypoglycemia after partial gastrectomy. *Digestion* 1994;55(4):221–228.
70. Carvajal SH, Mulvihill SJ. Postgastrectomy syndromes: dumping and diarrhea. *Gastroenterol Clin North Am* 1994;23(2):261–279.
71. Moriarty KJ, Dawson AM. Functional abdominal pain: further evidence that whole gut is affected. *Br Med J (Clin Res Ed)* 1982;284(6330):1670–1672.
72. Kamath PS, Gaisano HY, Phillips SF, et al. Abnormal gallbladder motility in irritable bowel syndrome: evidence for target-organ defect. *Am J Physiol* 1991;260(6 Pt 1):G815–G819.
73. Kellow JE, Miller LJ, Phillips SF, et al. Altered sensitivity of the gallbladder to cholecystokinin octapeptide in irritable bowel syndrome. *Am J Physiol* 1987;253(5 Pt 1):G650–G655.
74. Bingener J, Richards ML, Schwesinger WH, et al. Laparoscopic cholecystectomy for biliary dyskinesia: correlation of preoperative cholecystokinin cholescintigraphy results with postoperative outcome. *Surg Endosc* 2004;18(5):802–806.
75. Tabet J, Anvari M. Laparoscopic cholecystectomy for gallbladder dyskinesia: clinical outcome and patient satisfaction. *Surg Laparosc Endosc Percutan Tech* 1999;9(6):382–386.
76. Sherman S, Lehman GA. Sphincter of Oddi dysfunction: diagnosis and treatment. *J Pancreas* 2001;2(6):382–400.
77. Behar J, Corazziari E, Guelrud M, et al. Functional gallbladder and sphincter of Oddi disorders. *Gastroenterology* 2006;130(5):1498–1509.
78. Pereira SP, Gillams A, Sgouros SN, et al. Prospective comparison of secretin-stimulated magnetic resonance cholangiopancreatography with manometry in the diagnosis of sphincter of Oddi dysfunction types II and III. *Gut* 2007;56(6):809–813.
79. Lin OS, Soetikno RM, Young HS. The utility of liver function test abnormalities concomitant with biliary symptoms in predicting a favorable response to endoscopic sphincterotomy in patients with presumed sphincter of Oddi dysfunction. *Am J Gastroenterol* 1998;93(10):1833–1836.
80. Khuroo MS, Zargar SA, Yattoo GN. Efficacy of nifedipine therapy in patients with sphincter of Oddi dysfunction: a prospective, double-blind, randomized, placebo-controlled, cross over trial. *Br J Clin Pharmacol* 1992;33(5):477–485.
81. Rolny P, Geenen JE, Hogan WJ. Post-cholecystectomy patients with "objective signs" of partial bile outflow obstruction: clinical characteristics, sphincter of Oddi manometry findings, and results of therapy. *Gastrointest Endosc* 1993;39(6):778–781.
82. Toouli J, Roberts-Thomson IC, Kellow J, et al. Manometry based randomised trial of endoscopic sphincterotomy for sphincter of Oddi dysfunction. *Gut* 2000; 46(1):98–102.
83. Verne GN, Sninsky CA. Chronic intestinal pseudo-obstruction. *Dig Dis Sci* 1995;13(3):163–181.
84. Schuffler MD. Chronic intestinal pseudo-obstruction. In: Feldman M, Friedman LS, Brandt LJ, eds. *Schleisenger & Fordtran's Gastrointestinal and Liver Disease,* vol 2. Philadelphia, PA: Saunders; 2002:2140–2150.
85. Verne GN, Eaker EY, Hardy E, et al. Effect of octreotide and erythromycin on idiopathic and scleroderma-associated intestinal pseudoobstruction. *Dig Dis Sci* 1995;40(9):1892–1901.
86. Reyntjens A, Verlinden M, Schuermans V. Cisapride in the treatment of chronic intestinal pseudo-obstruction. *Z Gastroenterol* 1990;28(suppl 1):79–84; discussion 92–93.

87. Murr MM, Sarr MG, Camilleri M. The surgeon's role in the treatment of chronic intestinal pseudoobstruction. *Am J Gastroenterol* 1995;90(12): 2147–2151.
88. Iyer K, Kaufman S, Sudan D, et al. Long-term results of intestinal transplantation for pseudo-obstruction in children. *J Pediatr Surg* 2001;36: 174–177.
89. Altemeier WA, Bryant LR, Wulsin JH. The surgical significance of jejunal diverticulosis. *Arch Surg* 1963;86:732–745.
90. Maglinte DD, Chernish SM, DeWeese R, et al. Acquired jejunoileal diverticular disease: subject review. *Radiology* 1986;158(3):577–580.
91. Palder SB, Frey CB. Jejunal diverticulosis. *Arch Surg* 1988;123(7): 889–894.
92. Krishnamurthy S, Kelly MM, Rohrmann CA, et al. Jejunal diverticulosis. A heterogenous disorder caused by a variety of abnormalities of smooth muscle or myenteric plexus. *Gastroenterology* 1983;85(3): 538–547.
93. Kouraklis G, Glinavou A, Mantas D, et al. Clinical implications of small bowel diverticula. *Isr Med Assoc J* 2002;4(6):431–433.
94. Higgins PD, Johanson JF. Epidemiology of constipation in North America: a systematic review. *Am J Gastroenterol* 2004;99(4):750–759.
95. Bassotti G, Iantorno G, Fiorella S, et al. Colonic motility in man: features in normal subjects and in patients with chronic idiopathic constipation. *Am J Gastroenterol* 1999;94(7):1760–1770.
96. Pikarsky AJ, Singh JJ, Weiss EG, et al. Long-term follow-up of patients undergoing colectomy for colonic inertia. *Dis Colon Rectum* 2001;44(2): 179–183.
97. Camilleri M, Zinsmeister AR. Towards a relatively inexpensive, noninvasive, accurate test for colonic motility disorders. *Gastroenterology* 1992; 103(1):36–42.
98. Knowles CH, Scott M, Lunniss PJ. Outcome of colectomy for slow transit constipation. *Ann Surg* 1999;230(5):627–638.
99. Anti M, Pignataro G, Armuzzi A, et al. Water supplementation enhances the effect of high-fiber diet on stool frequency and laxative consumption in adult patients with functional constipation. *Hepatogastroenterology* 1998; 45(21):727–732.
100. Ramkumar D, Rao SS. Efficacy and safety of traditional medical therapies for chronic constipation: systematic review. *Am J Gastroenterol* 2005; 100(4):936–971.
101. Camilleri M, Thompson WG, Fleshman JW, et al. Clinical management of intractable constipation. *Ann Intern Med* 1994;121(7):520–528.
102. Heymen S, Scarlett Y, Jones K, et al. Randomized, controlled trial shows biofeedback to be superior to alternative treatments for patients with pelvic floor dyssynergia-type constipation. *Dis Colon Rectum* 2007;50(4): 428–441.
103. Vanek VW, Al-Salti M. Acute pseudo-obstruction of the colon (Ogilvie's syndrome). An analysis of 400 cases. *Dis Colon Rectum* 1986;29(3): 203–210.
104. Delgado-Aros S, Camilleri M. Pseudo-obstruction in the critically ill. *Best Pract Res Clin Gastroenterol* 2003;17(3):427–444.
105. De Giorgio R, Barbara G, Stanghellini V, et al. Review article: the pharmacological treatment of acute colonic pseudo-obstruction. *Aliment Pharmacol Ther* 2001;15(11):1717–1727.
106. Eisen GM, Baron TH, Dominitz JA, et al. Acute colonic pseudo-obstruction. *Gastrointest Endosc* 2002;56(6):789–792.
107. Sloyer AF, Panella VS, Demas BE, et al. Ogilvie's syndrome. Successful management without colonoscopy. *Dig Dis Sci* 1988;33(11):1391–1396.
108. Ponec RJ, Saunders MD, Kimmey MB. Neostigmine for the treatment of acute colonic pseudo-obstruction. *N Engl J Med* 1999;341(3):137–141.
109. Geller A, Petersen BT, Gostout CJ. Endoscopic decompression for acute colonic pseudo-obstruction. *Gastrointest Endos* 1996;44(2):144–150.
110. Rex DK. Colonoscopy and acute colonic pseudo-obstruction. *Gastrointest Endosc Clin N Am* 1997;7:499–508.

CHAPTER 65 ■ ACUTE GASTROINTESTINAL HEMORRHAGE

LAWRENCE T. KIM AND RICHARD H. TURNAGE

KEY POINTS

1. Eighty percent of patients with an acute gastrointestinal hemorrhage will be bleeding from the esophagus, stomach, or duodenum.
2. The most common cause of acute upper gastrointestinal hemorrhage is peptic ulcer disease, whereas the most common cause of lower gastrointestinal hemorrhage is a colonic diverticulum.
3. The use of nonsteroidal anti-inflammatory drugs, aspirin, and/or Coumadin is an important risk factor for acute gastrointestinal hemorrhage.
4. Approximately 80% of patients suffering an acute gastrointestinal hemorrhage will stop bleeding spontaneously; those who do not or those who rebleed are at particularly high risk to suffer an in-hospital complication, require operative control of their hemorrhage, or die.
5. Esophagastroduodenoscopy (EGD) is an important early diagnostic test in patients suspected to have an acute upper gastrointestinal bleed.
6. Endoscopic therapy, such as thermal coagulation, is effective in controlling bleeding in as many as 90% of patients with bleeding gastric or duodenal ulcers.
7. The operative management of patients with bleeding peptic ulcers is used for those patients in whom endoscopic means are unsuccessful.
8. Endoscopic techniques (e.g., sclerotherapy or banding) will effectively stop acute variceal bleeding in as many as 90% of cases).
9. Localization of the site of bleeding is a crucial step in the successful operative management of patients with lower gastrointestinal hemorrhage.

(1) Acute gastrointestinal (GI) hemorrhage is categorized as upper or lower depending on the location of the bleeding relative to the ligament of Treitz. Upper GI (UGI) hemorrhage (i.e., bleeding from the esophagus, stomach, or duodenum) accounts for about 80% of cases of acute GI blood loss, with most of the remainder coming from the colon. The small intestine is the site of hemorrhage in about 1% to 5% of cases.[1,2] The incidence of UGI bleeding is estimated to be about 37 to 150 episodes per 100,000 individuals depending on the population sampled,[3–5] whereas the incidence of lower GI (LGI) bleeding is about 20 cases per 100,000 individuals.[6] Overall, GI hemorrhage accounts for roughly 300,000 hospitalizations and 30,000 deaths annually in the United States.[7]

The differential diagnosis of overt UGI and LGI hemorrhage and the relative frequency of the most common causes of GI bleeding are shown in Tables 65.1 and 65.2 and Figure 65.1A, B, respectively. The most common causes of acute UGI hemorrhage (2) are peptic ulcer disease (31% to 58%), gastritis and mucosal erosions (9% to 30%), and gastroesophageal varices (3% to 23%),[1,3,8] whereas diverticulosis (24% to 47%), colitis (6% to 26%), neoplasms (9% to 17%), and angiodysplasia (2% to 12%) account for most instances of LGI hemorrhage.[1,6,9–12]

PATIENT CHARACTERISTICS

Patients who suffer significant GI hemorrhage are more commonly older and male than are those individuals without GI bleeding. Furthermore, these individuals are more likely to use alcohol, tobacco, aspirin, nonsteroidal anti-inflammatory drugs

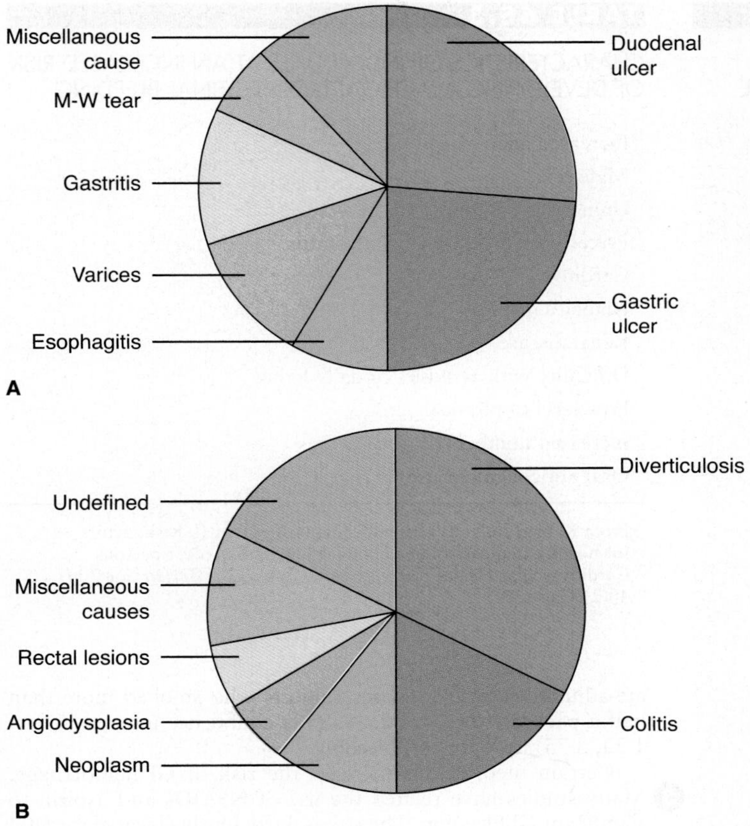

FIGURE 65.1. **A:** The relative frequency of the most common causes of upper gastrointestinal (UGI) hemorrhage in the United States. These data represent the percentage of patients with each of these causes of UGI hemorrhage for 482 patients in a survey of the members of the American College of Gastroenterology published by Peura et al. in 1997.[1] These data are very similar to that reported by Vreeburg in a multi-institutional study of 951 patients sustaining a UGI hemorrhage in the hospitals in and surrounding Amsterdam.[3] **B:** The relative frequency of the most common causes of lower gastrointestinal hemorrhage. These data, reported by Lingenfelser and Ell,[6] are the percentage of patients with each of these causes of lower GI hemorrhage in 912 patients collected in five studies from Europe, the Orient, and the United States.[1,9–12]

TABLE 65.1

DIFFERENTIAL DIAGNOSIS OF ACUTE UPPER GASTROINTESTINAL HEMORRHAGE BY ANATOMIC SITE

Esophagus
- Esophagitis
  - Reflux
  - Infectious (fungal, viral)
- Esophageal varices
- Neoplasms

Stomach
- Peptic ulcer disease
  - Gastric ulcer
- Gastroesophageal varices
  - Portal gastropathy
- Gastric antral vascular ectasia ("watermelon stomach")
- Dieulafoy ulcer
- Arteriovenous malformation
- Neoplasms
  - Gastrointestinal stromal tumors (leiomyoma, leiomyosarcoma)
  - Lymphoma
  - Adenocarcinoma
  - Carcinoid tumors
- Mallory-Weiss tear
- Stress gastritis

Duodenum
- Peptic ulcer disease
  - Duodenal ulcer
- Arteriovenous malformation
- Neoplasms
  - Duodenal adenocarcinoma
  - Pancreatic adenocarcinoma
  - Carcinoid tumors
  - Dieulafoy ulcers
  - Aortoduodenal fistula
  - Diverticula

Hepatopancreatic-biliary
- Hemobilia
- Pancreatitis-induced pseudoaneurysm

TABLE 65.2

DIFFERENTIAL DIAGNOSIS OF ACUTE LOWER GASTROINTESTINAL HEMORRHAGE BY ANATOMIC SITE

Small Intestine
NSAID-induced ulcers
Diverticula
Meckel diverticula
Pseudodiverticula
Neoplasms
Lymphoma
GI stromal tumors (leiomyoma, leiomyosarcoma)
Adenocarcinoma
Carcinoid tumor
Inflammation
Crohn disease
Radiation enteritis
Ischemic enteritis
Infectious enteritis
Arteriovenous malformations
Aortoenteric fistula
Colon and Rectum
Diverticulosis
Colitis
Crohn disease
Ulcerative colitis
Radiation colitis
Infectious colitis
Ischemic colitis
Neoplasms
Adenocarcinoma
GI stromal tumors (leiomyoma, leiomyosarcoma)
Lymphoma
Carcinoid tumors
Arteriovenous malformation
Iatrogenic
Polypectomy sites
Benign rectal diseases
Hemorrhoids
Rectal ulcers

GI, gastrointestinal; NSAID, nonsteroidal anti-inflammatory drug.

(NSAIDs), and anticoagulants.[1,13] Predictors of risk for acute GI bleeding are shown in Table 65.3. Both upper and lower GI hemorrhage are more common in elderly than in younger individuals, with the average age being approximately 60 to 70 years.[1,3]

Coexisting chronic illnesses are common in patients suffering either an upper or lower GI hemorrhage. Various studies have suggested a correlation between GI bleeding and correlates of poor health such as the use of multiple medications, reduced levels of physical activity, and inability to complete basic self-care tasks.[13,14] Cardiovascular disease,[13] hepatic disease, and renal disease[15] are particular risk factors for acute GI bleeding. The presence of these chronic illnesses, as well as chronic obstructive pulmonary disease and cirrhosis, also greatly increases the risk of rebleeding after endoscopic control.[16] Tobacco is also associated with higher rates of significant GI hemorrhage. A prospective cohort study of 5,888 men and women found that the multivariate-adjusted hazard ratio for subjects who smoked more than half a pack per day was 2.14 (95% confidence interval [CI] = 1.22, 3.75) for upper GI bleeding.[13]

TABLE 65.3

CHARACTERISTICS OF INDIVIDUALS AT AN INCREASED RISK OF DEVELOPING ACUTE GASTROINTESTINAL BLEEDING

Increased age
Male sex
Unmarried (vs. married)
Perceived fair or poor health status
Cardiovascular disease
Diabetes mellitus
Renal disease
Difficulty with activities of daily living
Low level of physical activity
Increased numbers of medications
Oral anticoagulant use

From Kaplan RC, Heckbert SR, Koepsell TD, et al. Risk factors for hospitalized gastrointestinal bleeding among older persons. Cardiovascular Health Study Investigators. *J Am Geriatr Soc* 2001; 49(2):126–133.

Certain medications increase the risk of GI hemorrhage. **3** Many studies have related the use of NSAIDs and aspirin to significant GI bleeding. The risk is particularly elevated for UGI bleeding, but NSAIDs increase the risk of LGI hemorrhage as well. In Vreeburg's review of 951 patients with UGI hemorrhage, 41% used NSAIDs or aspirin.[3] Van Leerdam reported that more than half of the patients bleeding from ulcers were actively taking NSAIDs or aminosalicylic acid (ASA).[17] Mellemkjaer et al. found that the observed to expected ratio of UGI hemorrhage in a cohort of 156,138 users of NSAIDs was 4.1 (95% CI = 3.8, 4.5).[18] Other medications known to increase the risk of GI hemorrhage include spironolactone[19] and the selective serotonin reuptake inhibitors (SSRIs).[20,21]

The use of anticoagulants is also an important risk factor for acute GI bleeding. Coumadin is a particularly common cause. Kaplan et al. found that the age- and sex-adjusted hazard ratio for GI bleeding in patients taking oral anticoagulants was 2.59 (95% CI = 1.71, 3.93).[13] Vreeburg et al. reported that 17% of their patients with UGI hemorrhage were taking Coumadin and the international normal ratio (INR) was greater than 4 in more than half of these patients.[3] Because Coumadin metabolism can be affected by so many interfering substances, inadvertent Coumadin toxicity is a common problem, often presenting with GI hemorrhage. The use of antiplatelet agents such as clopidogrel and ticlopidine can also lead to GI hemorrhage.

CLINICAL PRESENTATION

Usually patients with overt GI bleeding present to the hospital after observing the passage of blood from the GI tract as hematemesis, melena, or hematochezia. Hematemesis is the vomiting of blood. Melena is a black, tarry stool resulting from the degradation of blood by enteric bacteria. It may occur with the loss of as little as 50 to 200 mL of blood.[22,23] Bleeding from the small intestine or right colon may also appear black if it has remained in the GI tract for more than 12 to 14 hours.[24] Hematochezia is the passage of bright red blood from the rectum and is usually indicative of a lower GI source, although massive UGI hemorrhage may also cause hematochezia. Patients with acute GI bleeding may present with the hemodynamic consequences of hemorrhage including light-headedness, dizziness, orthostatic syncope or near syncope, shortness of breath, and palpitations from tachycardia.

The medical history and physical examination provide important clues of the etiology of the patient's hemorrhage and the potential risk to the patient's life. The occurrence of melena after several days of worsening epigastric or upper abdominal pain suggests peptic ulcer disease, whereas hematemesis or melena following vomiting or retching strongly suggests a Mallory-Weiss tear. Massive, painless upper GI hemorrhage in a patient with cirrhosis suggests bleeding from gastroesophageal varices, although other etiologies including peptic ulcer disease or a Mallory-Weiss tear must also be considered. The medical history should elicit the presence of risk factors for GI hemorrhage alluded to in the previous paragraphs and listed in Table 65.3.

A systematic physical examination will document the magnitude of bleeding and the patient's ability to compensate for the blood loss. Massive hemorrhage is associated with signs and symptoms of hypovolemic shock, including cool, clammy, mottled skin, tachycardia, tachypnea, flat jugular veins, oliguria, and perhaps hypotension. These responses may be altered by advanced age, concomitant medical problems, and particular medications. Physical examination should also document evidence of cirrhosis and portal hypertension (i.e., ascites, spider angiomas, hepatosplenomegaly, palmar erythema, and large hemorrhoidal veins). A rectal examination may demonstrate bright red blood or melena.

PROGNOSTIC FACTORS

4 Most patients (about 80%) suffering GI hemorrhage will stop bleeding spontaneously; those who don't, or those who rebleed, are at particularly high risk to suffer an in-hospital complication, require operative control of their hemorrhage, or die. Several classification systems have been developed to separate low-risk from high-risk patients with acute upper and lower GI hemorrhage. These systems have also been used to stratify those patients who may be safely managed as outpatients from those requiring in-hospital care.[25] The BLEED classification system addresses both upper and lower GI hemorrhage and consists of the following parameters: ongoing bleeding, low systolic blood pressure, elevated prothrombin time, erratic mental status, and unstable comorbid disease. Patients with at least one BLEED criterion are more likely to suffer in-hospital complications from UGI bleeding (31% vs. 4%) or lower GI bleeding (38% vs. 12%) than are patients who lack these criteria.[26]

Prognostic systems for UGI hemorrhage have been more widely adopted than those for LGI hemorrhage. One widely used system is the Rockall score for assessing the risk of death and rebleeding in patients with UGI hemorrhage (Table 65.4). Using this model, Rockall et al. found that rebleeding occurred in less than 5% of patients and mortality was very low (0% to 0.2%) in patients with scores of 0 to 2. In contrast, one fourth to nearly one half of patients with a Rockall score of 5 to 8+ rebled; the mortality rates for these patients were 11% to 41%. In this study, rebleeding significantly affected the likelihood of death, particularly for patients with intermediate scores of 3 or 4 and 5 to 7 in which there was a three- to fivefold increase in mortality rates.[27]

The Rockall classification has been widely accepted as accurate and, importantly, has been externally validated.[28–31] However, the full classification scheme requires endoscopic assessment. An alternative scoring system based on clear and readily available clinical indices has been proposed, called the Glasgow-Blatchford bleeding score (GBS, Table 65.5). This scoring system has been subjected to a multi-institutional trial and found to be more accurate than the Rockall system.[32] These authors suggested that patients with a score of 0 can be safely managed as outpatients.

TABLE 65.4

ROCKALL RISK SCORING SYSTEM AND RATES OF REBLEEDING AND MORTALITY

	■ SCORE			
Variable	0	1	2	3
Age	<60 y	60–79 y	≥80 y	
Shock	"No shock" Systolic blood pressure ≥100 Heart rate <100	"Tachycardia" Systolic blood pressure ≥100 Heart rate ≥100	"Hypotension" Systolic blood pressure <100	
Comorbidity	None	None	Cardiac failure Ischemic heart disease Any major comorbidity	Renal failure Liver failure Disseminated malignancy
Diagnosis	Mallory-Weiss tear No lesion identified No stigmata of recent hemorrhage	All other diagnosis	Malignancy of the upper gastrointestinal tract	
Major stigmata of recent hemorrhage	None or dark spot only		Blood in upper gastrointestinal tract Adherent clot Visible or spurting vessel	

Score	0	1	2	3	4	5	6	7	8+
Percent mortality	0	0	0.2	2.9	5.3	10.8	17.3	27	41

From Rockall TA, Logan RF, Devlin HB, et al. Risk assessment after acute upper gastrointestinal haemorrhage [see comments]. *Gut* 1996;38(3):316–321.

TABLE 65.5

GLASGOW-BLATCHFORD BLEEDING SCORE (GBS)

	■ SCORE VALUE
Blood Urea (mmol/L)	
<6.5	0
6.5–7.9	2
8.0–9.9	3
10.0–25.0	4
>25.0	6
Hemoglobin for Men (g/L)	
≥130	0
120–129	1
100–119	3
<100	6
Hemoglobin for Women (g/L)	
≥120	0
100–119	1
<100	6

	■ SCORE VALUE
Systolic Blood Pressure (mm Hg)	
100–109	1
90–99	2
<90	3
Other Markers	
Pulse <100	0
Pulse ≥100/min	1
Presentation with melena	1
Presentation with syncope	2
Hepatic disease[a]	2
Cardiac failure[b]	2
Absence of melena, syncope, hepatic disease, or cardiac disease	0

[a]Known history, or clinical and laboratory evidence, of chronic or acute liver disease.
[b]Known history, or clinical and echocardiographic evidence, of cardiac failure.
Adapted from Stanley AJ, Ashley D, Dalton HR, et al. Outpatient management of patients with low-risk upper-gastrointestinal haemorrhage: multicentre validation and prospective evaluation. *Lancet* 2009;373(9657):42–47.

INITIAL EVALUATION AND RESUSCITATION

Upon presentation, patients with GI bleeding should have placement of two large-bore intravenous lines in peripheral veins and intravascular volume resuscitation begun with an isotonic saline solution. Most patients stop bleeding spontaneously, and crystalloid volume resuscitation is all that is required. Blood should be drawn for type and cross match, complete blood count with platelet count, electrolyte determination, liver function tests, and coagulation profiles. It is important to emphasize that on presentation, the hematocrit or hemoglobin level may not accurately reflect the magnitude of acute blood loss. Estimates of the severity of hemorrhage must be based on clinical parameters.

The massively bleeding patient should receive packed red blood cells to restore intravascular volume and oxygen-carrying capacity. The decision to transfuse blood or blood products depends on the individual needs of the patient and the cause of the bleeding. The risks of the blood products (i.e., infection and allergic reactions) must be weighed against the risks of withholding transfusion (i.e., anemia, decreased oxygen-carrying capacity, coagulopathy). In general, blood products are used early in the management of patients with limited cardiac and pulmonary reserve who are unable to withstand or compensate for an acute reduction in their systemic oxygen delivery and those with lesions that are at particularly high risk for continued or recurrent hemorrhage (e.g., gastroesophageal varices).

Careful hemodynamic monitoring of these potentially critically ill patients is vital to successful management. Patients who are actively bleeding and those who have recently sustained significant hemorrhage should be admitted to an intensive care unit for close monitoring of hemodynamic parameters and evidence of continued or recurring hemorrhage. The presence of significant underlying illnesses, such as cardiac, renal, hepatic, or pulmonary insufficiency, may necessitate invasive cardiac monitoring with cardiac and arterial catheters. The information gained from these devices allows cardiac performance to be optimized during intravascular volume replacement. Central venous catheterization should be performed only after initial volume resuscitation through peripheral sites. The placement of a urinary catheter and frequent monitoring of heart rate, blood pressure, gastric aspirate, urine output, and mental status are the minimum necessary to monitor patients who have suffered GI hemorrhage. The importance of prompt, adequate resuscitation and diligent observation cannot be overemphasized as the cornerstone for managing these potentially mortally ill patients.

DIAGNOSTIC APPROACH

After the restoration of circulating blood volume, the next step is to identify the source of bleeding so definitive therapy may be instituted. If the patient presents with hematemesis, localization of the bleeding to the esophagus, stomach, or duodenum is
5 relatively straightforward and esophagogastroduodenoscopy (EGD) should be performed promptly to identify the source of bleeding. When blood or coffee-ground guaiac-positive material is present in the gastric aspirate, EGD should be utilized to define the site of bleeding. Bright red blood per rectum strongly suggests a lower GI source of bleeding unless the patient is hemodynamically unstable, in which case the hemorrhage may originate from a source proximal to the ligament of Treitz. A generalized approach for evaluating patients with acute upper and lower GI hemorrhage is presented in Algorithm 65.1.

Gastric Aspiration

In the absence of hematemesis, aspiration of gastric fluid after the placement of a nasogastric tube has been used to distinguish between an upper and lower GI source of bleeding. Two studies with more than 700 patients found that the presence of blood in the gastric aspirate was a good indicator of a UGI source; however, its absence was unreliable in predicting the presence or absence of a UGI source.[33,34] In one study of 220 patients with a UGI source of bleeding, the sensitivity, specificity, and accuracy

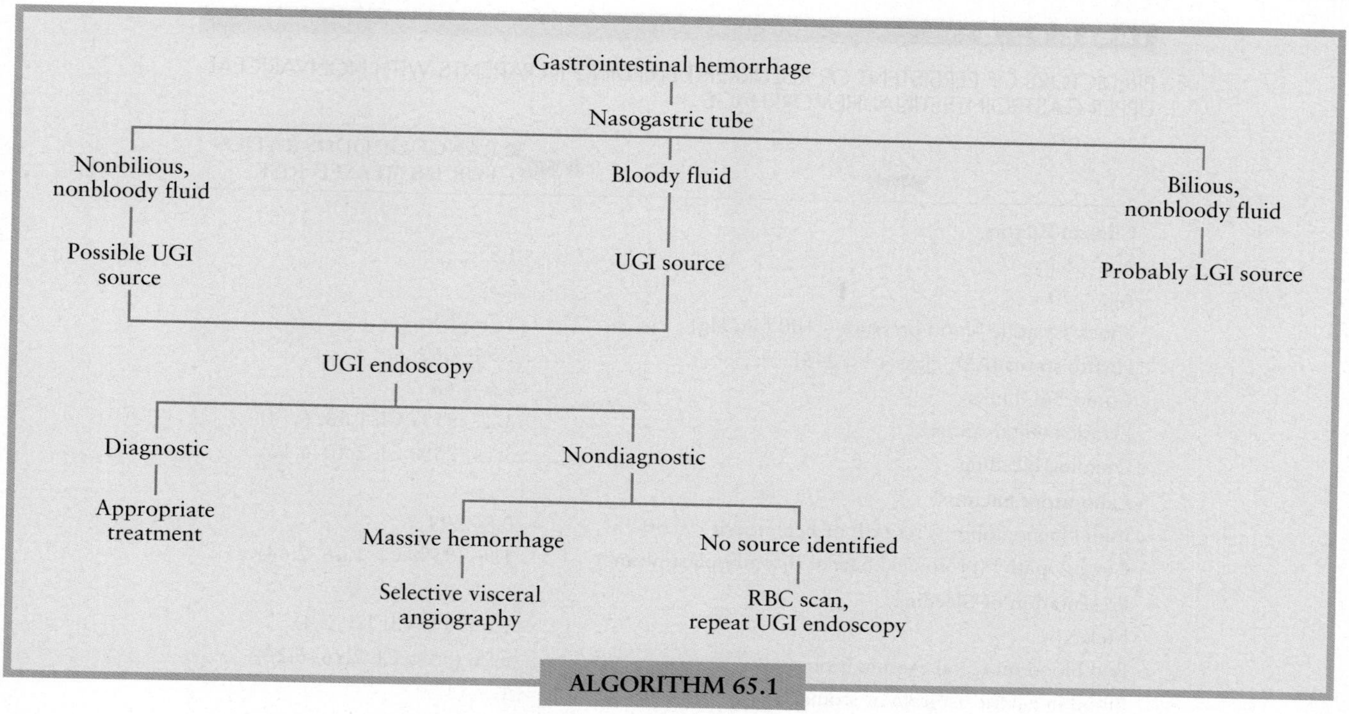

ALGORITHM 65.1. Diagnostic steps in the evaluation of gastrointestinal hemorrhage.

of the nasogastric aspirate were 42% (95% CI = 32, 51), 91% (95% CI = 83, 95), and 66% (95% CI = 59, 72), respectively.[34] Despite the potential for inaccuracy, all patients with acute GI hemorrhage should have a nasogastric tube placed as the initial diagnostic modality since it is inexpensive and safe. While a clear aspirate does not rule out an upper GI source of bleeding, aspiration of blood confirms it.

Endoscopy

Esophagogastroduodenoscopy. EGD will identify the site of bleeding in about 95% of cases of UGI bleeding and is the initial diagnostic study for patients suspected of bleeding from the esophagus, stomach, or duodenum.[35,36] The sensitivity of the procedure is significantly enhanced when performed within the first 24 hours of presentation.[3] A systematic review of the literature found that early endoscopy (i.e., performed within 24 hours of admission) was associated with a decreased transfusion requirement and decreased length of stay.[37] A prospective randomized trial found that early endoscopy allowed the triaging of 46% of patients to outpatient care without any adverse effects.[38] Previous consensus guidelines and several cohort studies have related various endoscopic stigmata of recent or active hemorrhage to a heightened risk of rebleeding or continued bleeding.[39–45] Laine and Peterson[39] analyzed data from 37 prospective trials in which patients with bleeding ulcers did not receive endoscopic therapy; they found that the rate of further bleeding was less than 5% for those patients with a clean ulcer base and increased to 10% for patients with a flat red spot, 22% for those with an adherent clot, 43% for those with a nonbleeding visible vessel, and 55% for those with active bleeding. Endoscopic features predictive of persistent or recurrent bleeding and mortality are shown in Tables 65.6 through 65.8. In addition to these ulcer-specific factors, endoscopy allows identification of lesions with a high risk of continued hemorrhage and mortality (i.e., gastroesophageal varices) and those with a low risk of continued bleeding, such as a Mallory-Weiss tear. The efficacy of endoscopy-based modalities to control UGI hemorrhage is discussed in subsequent sections.

Colonoscopy. Although the efficacy of colonoscopy in determining the cause of occult GI bleeding is undisputed, its role in the evaluation of patients with acute lower GI bleeding is less well agreed upon. The procedure is best suited for patients who are actively bleeding at the time of the study, but not massively bleeding. Colonic gavage with a polyethylene glycol solution will clear the lumen of clot and stool, providing adequate visualization of the mucosa. Others have reported good visualization of the mucosa even in the absence of mechanical bowel preparation.[46]

A meta-analysis examined the role of colonoscopy as the primary diagnostic modality for patients with acute lower GI bleeding and found that 69% (range, 48% to 90%) of urgent colonoscopies identified a source or a presumptive source of bleeding.[47] Even in the setting of unprepped bowel, urgent colonoscopy has been shown to identify bleeding colon and distal ileal lesions in 82 of 85 patients (97%).[46] Stigmata of recent hemorrhage for lower GI bleeding are similar to those of UGI lesions and include an actively bleeding site, a nonbleeding visible vessel, and an adherent clot; these findings have been associated with continued hemorrhage and the need for urgent colectomy.[9,48] Jensen et al. reported that 25% to 50% of patients with *any* of these three factors continued to bleed, or rebled, and required urgent colectomy.[49] Others have found colonoscopy to be less accurate in the diagnosis of lower GI bleeding. For example, Al Qahtani et al. reported a series of 136 patients in which colonoscopy identified only 45% of the sources of lower GI bleeding.[50]

Enteroscopy. For those patients who present with hematochezia in whom the initial EGD and colonoscopy is nondiagnostic, repeating these studies before evaluating the small intestine is warranted given the very small frequency in which the bleeding originates from the small intestine (1%). Repeating the EGD and colonoscopy when the patient is better resuscitated will often detect lesions such as ulcers or vascular ectasias that were obscured by blood at the initial endoscopy or the vasoconstriction of the GI mucosa that accompanies hemorrhagic shock.

Endoscopy of the small bowel with an enteroscope or a pediatric colonoscope will allow inspection of the proximal 60 cm of

TABLE 65.6

PREDICTORS OF PERSISTENT OR RECURRENT BLEEDING IN PATIENTS WITH NONVARICEAL UPPER GASTROINTESTINAL HEMORRHAGE

	RANGE OF ODDS RATIOS FOR INCREASED RISK
Clinical Factors	
Age >65 y	1.3
Age >70 y	2.30
Shock (systolic blood pressure <100 mm Hg)	1.2–3.65
Health status (ASA class 1 vs. 2–5)	1.94–7.63
Comorbid illness	1.6–7.63
Erratic mental status	3.21 (95% CI: 1.53, 6.74)
Ongoing bleeding	3.14 (95% CI: 2.40–4.12)
Laboratory Factors	
Initial hemoglobin <10 g/dL or hematocrit <0.30	0.8–2.99
Coagulopathy (prolonged partial thromboplastin time)	1.96 (95% CI: 1.46, 2.64)
Presentation of Bleeding	
Melena	1.6 (95% CI: 1.1, 2.4)
Red blood on rectal examination	3.76 (95% CI: 2.26, 6.26)
Blood in gastric aspirate or stomach	1.1–11.5
Hematemesis	1.2–5.7
Endoscopic Factors	
Active bleeding on endoscopy	2.5–6.48
Endoscopic high-risk stigmata	1.91–4.81
Clot	1.72–1.9
Ulcer size ≥2 cm	2.29–3.54
Diagnosis of gastric or duodenal ulcer	2.7 (95% CI: 1.2, 4.9)
Ulcer location	
High on lesser curvature	2.79
Superior wall	13.9
Posterior wall	9.2

ASA, American Society of Anesthesiologists.
From Barkun A, Bardou M, Marshall JK, Nonvariceal Upper GI Bleeding Consensus Conference Group. Consensus recommendations for managing patients with nonvariceal upper gastrointestinal bleeding [see comment]. *Ann Intern Med* 2003;139(10):843–857.

the jejunum[51] and the use of a long video-enteroscope may allow visualization of 100 to 150 cm of intestine beyond the ligament of Treitz.[52] Jensen et al., in an experience with more than 200 patients with obscure sources of GI bleeding, reported success in identifying the etiology in 79% of instances using enteroscopy.[53] In their experience, vascular ectasias and postbulbar ulcers were the most common causes of obscure GI bleeding.

Intraoperative enteroscopy using a combination of push enteroscopes per os and per rectum or via enterotomy can allow examination of the entire small bowel. While the endoscopist manipulates the scope, the surgeon manually advances the bowel over the endoscope. After the bowel is telescoped onto the endoscope, it is slowly withdrawn while the endoscopist examines the mucosal lumen and the surgeon watches the transilluminated bowel wall. While this technique can be effective, it is limited by its invasive nature.[54]

Double-balloon Enteroscopy. This technique utilizes a long enteroscope and a long overtube. Both the overtube and the enteroscope have balloons at the end. When the balloon of the enteroscope is inflated, it "grabs" the mucosal surface and allows advancement of the overtube, whose balloon is deflated. The overtube balloon is then inflated while the enteroscope balloon is deflated. The enteroscope is then advanced while the inflated overtube balloon grips the mucosa. Using these alternate inflation–deflation cycles, long-distance advancement of the enteroscope has been achieved.[2] In one U.S. multicenter study, the average distance achieved was 360 cm with a diagnosis made in 43% of cases.[55] In some cases lesions may be seen that are missed by other techniques.[56]

Wireless Capsule Endoscopy. Imaging of the small intestine is also now possible with a wireless capsule endoscope consisting of a battery, light source, imaging-capturing system, and transmitter. This capsule endoscope is 11 × 30 mm and is moved solely by peristalsis. This system captures and sends up to two images per second for about 8 hours to an ultra-high-frequency band radiotelemetry unit worn by the patient. The location of the capsule is suggested by the strength of the signal. Several studies have shown high diagnostic yields using this technique and found it to be superior to push enteroscopy in patients with obscure GI bleeding (reviewed in reference 2). One difficulty with this technique is the very large amount of data to be reviewed. For an 8-hour study, 57,600 images are generated. Even at high frame rates, manual review of the images is difficult and time consuming at best. Software is

TABLE 65.7

PREDICTORS OF MORTALITY IN PATIENTS WITH NONVARICEAL UPPER GASTROINTESTINAL HEMORRHAGE

	■ RANGE OF ODDS RATIOS FOR INCREASED RISK
Clinical Factors	
Age 60–69 y	3.5 (95% CI: 1.5, 4.7)
Age ≥70 y	4.5–12.7
Age >80 y	5.7 (95% CI: 2.9, 10.2)
Shock (systolic blood pressure <100 mm Hg)	1.18–6.4
Health status (ASA class 1 vs. 2–5)	2.6–9.52
Comorbid illness	1.19–12.1
Continued or rebleeding	5.29–76.23
Sepsis	5.4 (95% CI: 1.5, 19.6)
Presentation of bleeding	
Red blood on rectal examination	2.95 (95% CI: 1.29, 6.76)
Blood in gastric aspirate or stomach	0.43–18.9
Hematemesis	2.0 (95% CI: 1.1, 3.5)
Onset of bleeding while hospitalized for other causes	2.77 (95% CI: 1.64, 4.66)
Laboratory Factors	
Elevated blood urea nitrogen level	5.5–18
Elevated serum creatinine level	14.8 (95% CI: 2.6, 83.5)
Elevated serum aminotransferase levels	4.2–20.2

ASA, American Society of Anesthesiologists.
From Barkun A, Bardou M, Marshall JK, Nonvariceal Upper GI Bleeding Consensus Conference Group. Consensus recommendations for managing patients with nonvariceal upper gastrointestinal bleeding [see comment]. *Ann Intern Med* 2003;139(10):843–857.

available to limit the examiner's review time, but its accuracy is not currently known.

Selective Visceral Arteriography

Selective visceral arteriography is primarily useful in patients with upper or lower GI bleeding in whom endoscopy cannot be performed or has been unsuccessful in determining the site of ongoing rapid hemorrhage. Successful angiographic identification of the source of bleeding occurs in 27% to 86% of instances and depends primarily on the presence of active arterial bleeding at the time of the study[50,57,58] (Fig. 65.2). The extravasation of contrast may be detected if the patient is bleeding at rates greater than 0.5 to 1 mL/min[59]; this correlates clinically with the requirement for continuous volume infusion to maintain hemodynamic stability. Pennoyer et al., however, were unable to identify any clinical parameter (including tachycardia, number of transfusions, or orthostatic hypotension) that could increase the diagnostic yield of selective angiography, including scintigraphy demonstrating ongoing

TABLE 65.8

FORREST CLASSIFICATION OF ENDOSCOPIC APPEARANCE OF BLEEDING ULCERS

Ia	Spurting bleeding
Ib	Nonspurting, active bleeding
IIa	Visible vessel
IIb	Nonbleeding ulcer with overlying clot
IIc	Ulcer with hematin-covered (black) base
III	Clean ulcer base

From Laporte JR, Ibanez L, Vidal X, et al. Upper gastrointestinal bleeding associated with the use of NSAIDs: newer versus older agents. *Drug Safety* 2004;27(6):411–420.

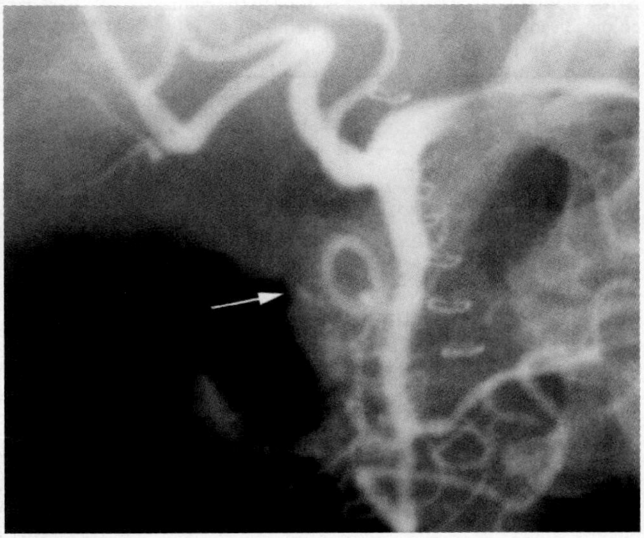

FIGURE 65.2. Selective celiac arteriography with injection into the common hepatic artery in a patient bleeding from a duodenal diverticulum. Extravasation of contrast from a branch of the gastroduodenal artery can be seen (*arrow*).

bleeding.[60] Several groups have used heparin, vasodilators, or thrombolytics to improve the diagnostic yield of arteriography in patients with nondiagnostic studies. Mernagh et al. found that the administration of heparin intravenously for 24 hours increased the diagnostic yield of visceral angiography from 33% (6 of 18) to 67% (12 of 18).[61] Others have found that the intra-arterial infusion of a vasodilator, heparin, and/or urokinase (a thrombolytic) failed to identify the source of bleeding in five of seven patients.[62] It should be noted that these provocative techniques are not commonly employed.

One major advantage of visceral arteriography is its therapeutic potential. Transcatheter embolization of bleeding vessels was first reported in the early 1970s.[63,64] Modern instruments allow superselective catheterization of terminal vessels, leading to satisfactory embolization with less risk for ischemic complications. Further discussion of therapeutic use can be found later.

Abdominal Scintigraphy

Abdominal scintigraphy with ^{99m}technetium (Tc)-labeled red blood cells (RBCs) lacks the spatial resolution and diagnostic precision of angiography and endoscopy; however, it is of most value in detecting intermittently bleeding lesions or those with very low rates of hemorrhage, such as vascular malformations. Abdominal scintigraphy utilizing ^{99m}Tc-RBCs has been shown to detect bleeding rates as low as 0.04 to 0.1 mL/min.[65,66] In a review of seven retrospective studies with nearly 400 patients, the median diagnostic accuracy of scintigraphy was 82% (range, 52% to 95%); in this review, ^{99m}Tc-RBCs were incorrect in 5% to 48% of instances (median 18%).[58] Suzman et al. summarized 20 retrospective studies containing 804 positive studies and reported a false-positive rate of 19%.[67] Precise localization of the site of bleeding may be complicated by the rapid distribution of isotope throughout the intestine by peristalsis or by accumulation in the right colon. More recent techniques of cine-scintigraphy may improve the diagnostic accuracy[68] (Fig 65.3). One area where radionuclide scanning has a clear role is in the diagnosis of Meckel diverticulum. ^{99}Tc-pertechnate is secreted by ectopic gastric mucosa in Meckel diverticula.[69] This study should be considered early in the evaluation of young individuals with lower GI bleeding.

Computed Tomography Scanning

Computed tomography (CT) scanning has been used to detect GI bleeding using a variety of specialized techniques.[70–73] Usually these techniques have been applied in cases of obscure bleeding where standard techniques such as endoscopy have failed. In general, however, these have not been sufficiently sensitive for the fine mucosal imaging necessary in evaluating GI hemorrhage. Research continues, however, using newer multidetector CT scanning combined with oral and intravenous contrast.[74–77] In the future, this may become a more available and useful technique.

COMMON CAUSES OF GASTROINTESTINAL HEMORRHAGE AND TREATMENT

Upper Gastrointestinal Hemorrhage

Peptic Ulcer Disease. Peptic ulcer disease is the most common cause of acute upper GI hemorrhage, accounting for nearly 40% of cases in most series, although this proportion may be decreasing.[78] About 15% to 20% of patients with peptic ulcer disease experience bleeding during the course of their disease, and as many as 20% of these patients will have bleeding as the initial manifestation. Hemorrhage is the principal cause of death from peptic ulcer disease and has replaced intractable pain as the most frequent indication for surgery. Complications of peptic ulcer disease occur more commonly in older patients who often have medical problems that profoundly influence their risk of morbidity and mortality.

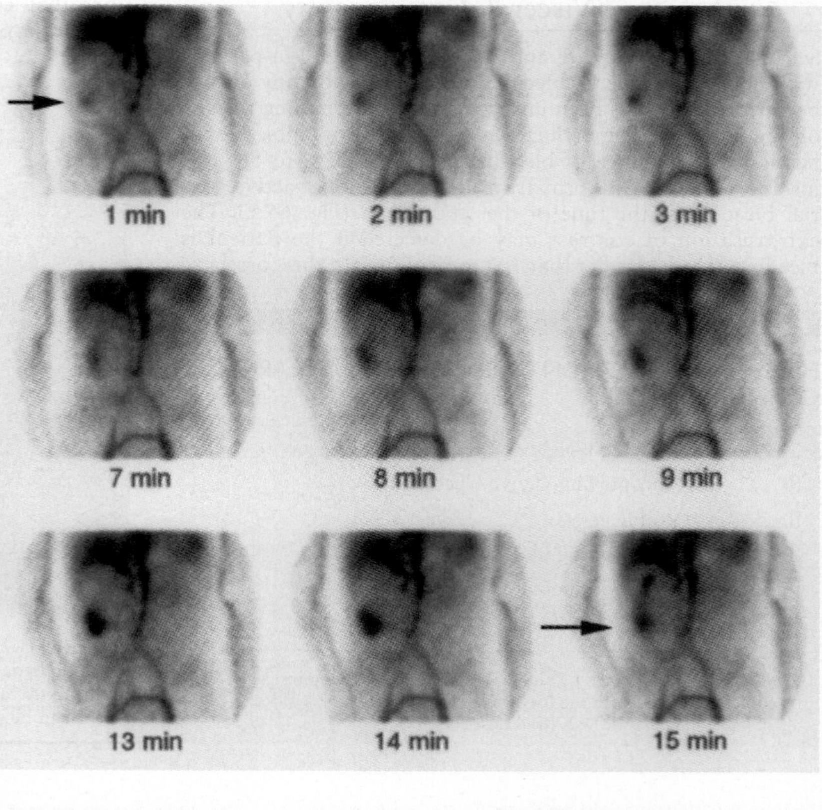

FIGURE 65.3. Cine-^{99m}Tc erythrocyte scintigraphy showing extravasation of isotope in the right colon. Only a small portion of the image set is shown. Arrows point to accumulation of isotope in the right colon. Bleeding was due to delayed hemorrhage following endoscopic polypectomy.

Duodenal ulcers occur slightly more frequently than gastric ulcers. Penetration of the ulcer through the posterior wall of the duodenal bulb is associated with erosion into the gastroduodenal artery or one of its branches, resulting in brisk hemorrhage. Patients may present with hematemesis of bright red blood and clots or with melena alone. Between 80% and 90% of patients stop bleeding spontaneously during the initial stages of therapy with volume resuscitation and gastric lavage.

In general, patients with gastric ulcers tend to be older and have coexisting medical problems that increase morbidity and mortality compared with duodenal ulcers. Bleeding may occur from any site in the stomach, although ulcers located at the incisura are most common. At this site, involvement of the branches of the left gastric artery may result in brisk, if not torrential, hemorrhage. The clinical presentation of patients bleeding from gastric ulcers is similar to that of duodenal ulcers, with hematemesis, melena, and hematochezia.

An important risk factor for the development of GI hemorrhage and gastroduodenal ulcer formation is the use of NSAIDs. NSAID use has been associated with a continuum of mucosal injury ranging from small acute mucosal hemorrhages to large chronic ulcers. It has been estimated that 10% to 15% of regular NSAID users have chronic gastric ulcers.[79] Symptoms correlate poorly with the degree of mucosal injury since as many as 20% of ulcers penetrating the muscularis are asymptomatic.[80] Case-control and cohort studies have suggested that NSAIDs are associated with a relative risk of GI hemorrhage and ulceration ranging from about 2 to 9.1.[81] Ketorolac, in particular, has been associated with a high risk of GI bleeding (relative risk approaches 25).[82,83] The risk of NSAID-associated complications is highest in patients with a history of upper GI bleeding, the elderly, or those patients taking oral anticoagulants[84] or corticosteroids. Patients with a prior history of peptic ulcer disease also appear to be at increased risk of NSAID-associated GI hemorrhage and tend to have a significantly worse outcome when compared to individuals not using NSAIDs.[85,86]

The tremendous frequency with which NSAIDs are used by the elderly underscores the magnitude of this problem. Individuals with a history of NSAID-induced hemorrhage may benefit from the prostaglandin E_1 analogue, misoprostol, which has been shown to prevent NSAID-induced gastric erosions and ulcers.[87] Histamine (H_2)-receptor blockers (ranitidine and cimetidine) are effective in preventing NSAID-induced duodenal ulcers, but appear to have little effect on the occurrence of gastric lesions.[80,88,89] Proton pump inhibitors (PPIs) have also been shown to be protective in patients on NSAIDs, with greater efficacy than H_2 blockers.[90] NSAIDs are also associated with lower GI bleeding, including lesions not generally considered related to NSAID use, such as diverticulosis.[91–93] Selective cyclooxygenase-2 (COX-2) inhibitors have been marketed as being safer than nonselective NSAIDs, although some of these have now been withdrawn from the U.S. market for other safety concerns. It appears that these selective inhibitors cause fewer upper GI problems overall than traditional NSAIDs, the main benefit being fewer uncomplicated ulcers. But there is no decrease in complicated events, including clinically significant bleeding episodes.[94] Selective COX-2 inhibitors do not appear to result in an improvement in lower GI bleeding events.[95]

Medical Treatment. Once bleeding from the upper GI tract is confirmed, treatment with a PPI should be initiated. Acute use of a PPI has been shown in several studies to decrease rebleeding.[43,96–99] Although the Scottish Intercollegiate Guidelines Network (SIGN) recommended withholding PPI therapy until after endoscopy,[100,101] in our opinion the balance of evidence would suggest no harm and perhaps a benefit from early PPI use. An 80-mg intravenous bolus of omeprazole or pantoprazole followed by an infusion at 8 mg/h produces the most reliable acid suppression.[102] All patients should be tested for *Helicobacter pylori* infection and treated if found. Treatment of the infection significantly reduces the recurrence of hemorrhage when compared to no treatment or chronic antisecretory treatment alone.[103,104] Interestingly, *H. pylori* infection may be less common in patients with bleeding ulcers than in those with nonbleeding ulcers.[105]

Endoscopic Treatment. The endoscopic appearance of a bleeding ulcer has important prognostic and therefore therapeutic implications, as alluded to in Tables 65.6 and 65.7. A modification of the system employed by Forrest et al.[106] is shown in Table 65.8. In this system category I findings are indicative of active bleeding, while category II findings provide evidence of recent hemorrhage. In general, only actively bleeding ulcers (i.e., Forrest category I lesions) are treated endoscopically.

6 A variety of endoscopic techniques are available to arrest hemorrhage from bleeding ulcers. The precise method of treatment is less important than the correct selection of patients and the experience of the endoscopist. Mechanical ligation of bleeding vessels can be achieved with endoscopic ligation (banding) or endoscopic clipping or Endoloop ligation.[107–109] Heater probes and monopolar and bipolar electrocoagulation probes also can effectively control upper GI hemorrhage. Monopolar probes apply high-frequency electrical current to the tissue, resulting in localized heating to 100°C and sealing of the bleeding vessel by coagulation necrosis of the surrounding tissue and vessel wall. Multipolar electrocoagulation (BICAP) probes consist of three equally spaced pairs of bipolar microelectrodes. This orientation of electrodes allows coagulation of tissue from tangential approaches and eliminates some of the disadvantages of the monopolar probe, such as the unpredictable depth of thermal injury, adherence of tissue, and clot dislodgement. Direct thermal coagulation of a bleeding point can also be produced by applying a heater probe, consisting of an aluminum tip coated with Teflon. The tip is rapidly heated to 250°C by an inner coil. The tip can be irrigated with a water jet to prevent accumulation of debris and clot. Heat conducted from the probe produces tissue coagulation to a depth of 1 to 5 mm.

Injection of epinephrine to induce vasoconstriction has been used successfully to control acutely bleeding ulcers, particularly as an adjunct to electrocautery or mechanical hemostasis with clips. A meta-analysis of 15 studies concluded that injection alone was inferior to either clips alone or clips plus injection.[110] This study showed no difference between clips and thermocoagulation.

The injection of sclerosants has been well described as a method of treating esophageal varices and has recently been popular for controlling nonvariceal bleeding. Sodium morrhuate and ethanolamine oleate are most commonly used to treat esophageal varices, whereas ethanol and polidocanol are most commonly used for nonvariceal sites. These agents act by thrombosing bleeding vessels and causing necrosis and subsequent fibrosis of surrounding tissue. Clinical experience with sclerosants has been similar to that obtained with electrocoagulation. In one large multicenter study of 332 actively bleeding patients or patients with stigmata of recent hemorrhage who underwent injection of 98% alcohol around the lesions, less than 1% continued to bleed, 6% rebled, and only 3% required emergency operative intervention.[111]

A meta-analysis of 25 randomized trials of endoscopic therapy for bleeding ulcers concluded that endoscopic treatment methods have a beneficial effect on survival by reducing the rate of recurrent hemorrhage. This analysis suggested that endoscopic therapy results in a relative reduction of 69% in recurrent bleeding, 62% in emergent surgery, and 30% in mortality rate, with the greatest benefit seen in actively bleeding ulcers and ulcers with nonbleeding visible vessels.[112] The effectiveness of early aggressive endoscopic diagnosis and treatment is further supported by a report of 562 patients bleeding from a variety of causes, of whom only 2.5% required emergency operations to control hemorrhage.[113]

7 **Operative Treatment.** The successful use of endoscopic therapies has relegated operative procedures to a rescue role for those cases in which endoscopy is unsuccessful in arresting hemorrhage. Numerous studies have attempted to identify those patients at greatest risk of continued or recurrent bleeding. Of the many factors examined, those associated with the highest risk of rebleeding included patients in hypovolemic shock during the initial endoscopy, ulcers greater than 2 cm in diameter, and endoscopic stigmata of recent or ongoing hemorrhage (Forrest type I and II lesions).[114] Many studies have demonstrated the ability of endoscopy to identify those patients at greatest risk of rebleeding. In one review, the presence of active bleeding was associated with a 90% to 100% chance of continued or recurrent hemorrhage. A nonbleeding visible vessel had a 40% to 50% chance, adherent clot 20% to 30%, oozing without visible vessel 10%, flat spot 5% to 10%, and clean-based ulcer 1% to 2%.[115] Even in those patients who rebleed following initial endoscopic therapy, two thirds may be successfully retreated endoscopically, thus avoiding operative intervention.[79] Factors that must be considered in decisions regarding the timing of operative intervention include the magnitude of the initial (or recurrent) hemorrhage, the physiologic ability of the patient to withstand continued or recurrent hemorrhage, and the likelihood of recurrent or continued hemorrhage. It is generally accepted that elderly patients and those with significant concurrent medical problems should undergo operative intervention earlier during the course of the hemorrhage since these individuals will poorly tolerate continued bleeding, recurrent hypotension, and repeated transfusions.

The type of operation depends on the pathology encountered. For bleeding gastric ulcers, the operation of choice depends on the patient's condition and location of the ulcer. For favorably located ulcers, excision of the ulcer with closure of the gastrotomy will suffice. If the ulcer is unfavorably located, for example, near the gastroesophageal junction, simple undersewing of the bleeding ulcer may adequately control bleeding.[116] If a gastric ulcer is left in situ, follow-up endoscopy is necessary 4 to 8 weeks later to either confirm healing or obtain tissue to rule out malignancy. Extensive gastric resections such as antrectomy or subtotal or total gastrectomy are generally not performed in these unstable patients.

For patients bleeding from duodenal ulcers, truncal vagotomy, pyloroplasty, and oversewing of the bleeding vessel is the most widely used operation. Direct ligation of the bleeding vessel through the duodenotomy should incorporate the gastroduodenal artery proximal and distal to the ulcer as well as the transverse pancreatic artery.

Angiographic Embolization. Relatively little has been written about the use of transcatheter embolization for peptic ulcer disease. In general, angiographic embolization is used after failure of endoscopic treatment in patients who cannot or will not undergo surgery. One recent large review (including nonulcer upper GI indications) showed a high technical success rate (i.e., localization of bleeding and deployment of the embolic agent) but a clinical success rate of only 51%.[117] Significant ischemic complications can occur also. While this technique has utility in select patients, it should not be considered a routine treatment option for bleeding peptic ulcers.

Stress Gastritis

Although studies in the 1960s and 1970s demonstrated acute erosions of the gastric mucosa in as many as 60% to 100% of critically ill patients, the incidence has markedly decreased over the past four decades. Factors postulated to have been important in this phenomenon include (a) the widespread use of prophylactic gastric alkalinization, (b) improvements in the ability to detect and treat sepsis, (c) improvements in the ability to monitor and correct hemodynamic instability, and (d) the ability to provide adequate nutritional support of critically ill patients.

In general, stress gastritis is characterized by the appearance of multiple superficial gastric ulcerations within 12 to 14 hours of an acute injury. These lesions, initially localized to the fundus and body of the stomach, later involve the entire gastric surface. Patients at greatest risk include those with sepsis, major burns, or severe trauma. Critically ill patients with a coagulopathy and respiratory insufficiency appear to be at highest risk of developing stress gastritis.[118,119] In this setting, the disease appears to represent the gastric component of the multiorgan failure syndrome.

The pathogenesis of this disease is discussed in detail in Chapter 44. The primary defect is in the protective processes that maintain the integrity of the gastric mucosal barrier. Although some gastric acid secretion is required for the development of stress gastritis, it is clear that the hypersecretion of acid is not the cause of mucosal injury. Altered gastric mucosal blood flow and impaired clearance of hydrogen ions from the mucosa appear to be of particular importance. Stress gastritis should be differentiated from the deep, often solitary ulcerations occurring in patients with severe central nervous system lesions (Cushing ulcers). Generally, hemorrhage is the only symptom that patients with stress gastritis experience. Overt bleeding is often heralded by the appearance of flecks of blood in the gastric aspirate. The superficial nature of the lesions makes perforation unlikely.

Prophylactic therapy is directed toward preventing hemorrhage, primarily by neutralizing gastric acid, augmenting mucosal defenses, and removing or preventing physiologic stress. Antacids, H_2-receptor antagonists, and sucralfate have all been used successfully to prevent stress gastritis. Alkalinization of the gastric contents is associated with oral and fecal flora colonization of the stomach and has raised concerns about an increased risk of nosocomial pneumonia. This concern has prompted the use of sucralfate as a preferred prophylactic agent instead of antacids or cimetidine.[120] However, a prospective, randomized trial of 1,200 critically ill patients receiving either ranitidine or sucralfate for stress ulcer prophylaxis found that those patients receiving ranitidine had a lower bleeding rate (1.7%) than the sucralfate group (3.8%). There was no difference in mortality or incidence of ventilator-assisted pneumonia.[121]

The success of these prophylactic measures has led to a dearth of recent experience in managing patients bleeding from stress gastritis. Based on early reports, attention to blood replacement, intravascular volume restoration, and correction of coagulation defects are associated with the cessation of hemorrhage in nearly 80% of cases and as such are the principal means of initial treatment. A variety of nonoperative techniques have been employed with variable success in arresting hemorrhage from stress gastritis including endoscopic and embolization techniques and the selective catheterization of the left gastric artery with continuous infusion of vasopressin.[122]

Based on these same early experiences, very few patients bleeding from erosive gastritis require operative intervention to arrest hemorrhage. A variety of surgical treatment options have been reported including vagotomy and pyloroplasty with oversewing of bleeding sites, vagotomy and hemigastrectomy, total gastrectomy, and gastric devascularization. The dilemma facing the surgeon is that these critically ill patients poorly tolerate extensive procedures, yet lesser operations often fail to control hemorrhage. Regardless of the operation performed, mortality risk depends on the underlying illness, particularly in the presence of multiple organ failure. Mortality rates between 30% and 60% are commonly quoted, with as many as one fourth of the deaths resulting from continued hemorrhage. Rebleeding rates ranging from 25% to 61% have been reported. The combination of vagotomy, hemigastrectomy, and oversewing of bleeding points has been touted as more successful in these patients; however, rebleeding rates of 11% to 44% and operative mortality rates ranging from 33% to 63% have been associated with this procedure.[123] More extensive operations, such as near-total gastrectomy or total gastrectomy, are associated with significant mortality, although they successfully stop hemorrhage.

Gastroesophageal Varices

Cirrhosis is a leading cause of death in the United States and variceal hemorrhage is a common mode of death for these patients. About 30% of people with cirrhosis develop gastroesophageal varices, and of these individuals, about 30% bleed as a result, usually within 1 to 2 years of diagnosis. Gastroesophageal varices are a significant cause of UGI hemorrhage, accounting for about 20% of such cases. Patients with bleeding gastroesophageal varices tend to have much higher rebleeding rates, transfusion requirements, lengths of hospitalization, and risk of death than do patients bleeding from nonvariceal causes.[113,124,125]

Although the basic tenets of resuscitation for massive variceal hemorrhage are similar to those for any cause of massive bleeding, intravenous volume resuscitation should be particularly judicious. The hyperaldosteronemic state of cirrhosis promotes sodium and water retention with aggravation of ascites and peripheral edema. Accurate blood replacement is imperative since overtransfusion may worsen portal hypertension and exacerbate hemorrhage. Invasive cardiac monitoring with Swan-Ganz catheterization may be particularly useful for guiding volume replacement. Coagulation deficits should be aggressively corrected by administering fresh frozen plasma. Thrombocytopenia, secondary to hypersplenism or dilution, should be treated promptly with pooled platelet transfusions. Sedatives are best avoided or used sparingly because cirrhosis impairs the liver's ability to metabolize many of these drugs. Adequate prophylaxis for delirium tremens should be administered to alcoholics.

As with other sources of upper GI hemorrhage, early endoscopy is imperative for successful diagnosis and therapy. The identification of varices alone is not adequate to incriminate them as the source of the hemorrhage since up to half of patients with cirrhosis bleed from a source other than varices. Furthermore, endoscopy may identify factors associated with a heightened risk of variceal hemorrhage such as the size and number of varices and the presence of red, blue, or other colored spots on the varix. The presence of gastric and duodenal varices and portal hypertensive changes in the gastric mucosa (portal gastropathy) will influence therapeutic decisions and prognosis.

Although vasopressin has commonly been used in the management of variceal hemorrhage, recent reports suggest the superiority of somatostatin or its synthetic analogue, octreotide. It is thought that octreotide causes splanchnic arteriolar vasoconstriction and reduces variceal and azygous vein flow with limited direct effects on portal pressure.[126] Meta-analyses have shown that the infusion of somatostatin is more effective and safer than vasopressin in the pharmacologic control of variceal hemorrhage.[127,128] Other studies have shown that somatostatin or octreotide can improve the results of sclerotherapy or endoscopic variceal ligation.[129–131] In addition to the enhanced efficacy in controlling hemorrhage, the use of octreotide eliminates the cardiac risks of vasopressin infusion (i.e., coronary artery vasoconstriction, myocardial ischemia, and infarction). Although neither somatostatin nor vasopressin plus nitroglycerin definitively treats the bleeding esophageal varices, these modalities may provide initial control of hemorrhage, reducing transfusion requirements and providing time for resuscitation before definitive treatment.

Another temporizing method used for massively bleeding patients is balloon tamponade using a Sengstaken-Blakemore tube or a Minnesota tube. These devices consist of a gastric tube with esophageal and gastric balloons. In the case of a Minnesota tube, a proximal esophageal lumen allows for the aspiration of swallowed secretions. Inflation of the gastric (and, if required, esophageal) balloons tamponade the bleeding varices, controlling hemorrhage in more than 80% of cases. Hemorrhage recurs in 25% to 50% of patients upon deflation of the balloons, thus limiting this technique to a temporizing role.[132] The greatest value of these tubes is for arresting massive hemorrhage that has been unresponsive to other measures, allowing time for resuscitation and angiographic definition of the portal system before definitive treatment.

When used inappropriately, these tubes can be associated with significant morbidity and mortality. Complications occur in 4% to 9% of patients, with the most frequent being aspiration pneumonitis. Measures to prevent pulmonary complications include endotracheal intubation before tube insertion and the placement of an esophageal tube to remove swallowed salivary secretions. Other significant complications include esophageal rupture or necrosis and airway occlusion during the attempted removal of an incompletely deflated gastric balloon.

Endoscopic sclerotherapy, endoscopic clipping, and endoscopic variceal ligation (banding) have become the most widely used modalities for the initial definitive control of bleeding esophageal varices. Several studies have confirmed that these
8 techniques arrest acute variceal hemorrhage in 90% to 95% of patients. In general, a patient bleeding from esophageal varices should undergo urgent sclerotherapy or banding of the varices at the time of the first emergency endoscopy. A single treatment controls variceal bleeding in more than 70% of patients, and a second treatment increases the rate of control to 90% to 95%. Continued or recurrent hemorrhage after endoscopic treatment requires temporary control with balloon tamponade and somatostatin, usually followed by emergency portal decompression either with transjugular intrahepatic portosystemic shunting (TIPS) or with surgery.[133,134] Following an initial episode of variceal hemorrhage, several options are available for the prevention of further hemorrhage. These options and the operative management of bleeding esophageal varices is discussed in detail in Chapter 58.

Mallory-Weiss Tears

The Mallory-Weiss syndrome is acute UGI hemorrhage that occurs after retching or vomiting due to a mucosal tear in the gastric cardia. Mallory and Weiss postulated that violent emesis against an unrelaxed cardia was the mechanism of injury. They were able to produce similar mucosal tears in cadavers by forcing gastric contents against an occluded gastroesophageal junction.[135] The typical patient who develops the syndrome is an alcoholic who begins to retch and vomit after an alcohol binge, although this syndrome may also be found in nonalcoholics with bouts of emesis. Initially, the vomitus consists of gastric contents without blood and subsequently the patient develops hematemesis and/or melena. Overall, these lesions occur in 5% to 10% of patients who present with upper GI bleeding.[113,124,125]

The initial management of these patients is similar to that of patients bleeding from other sources of upper GI hemorrhage and includes volume resuscitation, gastric lavage, and decompression. Most patients with Mallory-Weiss tears stop bleeding spontaneously, either before treatment or after these early measures. Once bleeding has stopped, rebleeding is rare.

In patients who continue to bleed despite these maneuvers, nonoperative and operative therapeutic options are available. Nonoperative management, consisting of endoscopic electrocoagulation, banding, or injection therapy, has been successfully applied to these lesions.[136] In cases not amenable to endoscopic therapy, operative management consists of oversewing the laceration through an anterior longitudinal gastrotomy in the middle third of the stomach.

LOWER GASTROINTESTINAL HEMORRHAGE

Although the passage of maroon or bright red blood per rectum may occur in the presence of a massive upper GI hemorrhage, this finding most commonly indicates a source distal to the ligament of Treitz. The absence of blood in bilious nasogastric lavage fluid further supports a distal location of hemorrhage. Although numerous potential causes of lower GI hemorrhage are possible (see Table 65.2), colonic diverticulosis and colitis are by far the most common. Small-bowel sources and other colonic pathology such as colon cancer are relatively unusual causes of acute GI hemorrhage.

Diagnostic Approach

9 The most important question to answer when presented with a patient with lower GI hemorrhage is not, "What is bleeding?" but rather, "Where is the bleeding?" The common causes of colonic hemorrhage are mucosal in nature, not palpable, and not visible from the serosal surface of the bowel. Therefore, it is imperative that the surgeon make every effort to localize the source of bleeding preoperatively since it is usually impossible to locate the bleeding source intraoperatively. Tagged RBC scanning and/or angiography should be obtained as early as possible after presentation.

After determination that the source is likely from a lower GI source, it is important to first exclude anorectal causes of hemorrhage, such as hemorrhoidal bleeding, by inspection and anoscopy. The authors' approach is then to obtain a tagged RBC scan as soon as practical, or in occasional cases of massive hemorrhage, to proceed directly to angiography. If the tagged RBC scan localizes a bleeding site, then one may continue supportive care to determine if bleeding will stop spontaneously as it will in the majority of cases. If bleeding continues, then the patient may proceed to either surgical excision of the bleeding site or angiography with embolization. If the tagged RBC scan does not demonstrate bleeding, then it is probable that bleeding has stopped. One may then proceed to colonoscopy after adequate mechanical bowel preparation. In the authors' experience, colonoscopy in an actively bleeding patient with an unprepped colon is seldom satisfactory. If the bleeding is rapid enough to warrant emergency surgery, bleeding can usually be demonstrated by one of these modalities. It should be the very rare patient who will need to proceed to surgery for lower GI hemorrhage with failed preoperative localization. In these cases a careful search for small-bowel bleeding sources, possibly including intraoperative small-bowel endoscopy, should be performed. If this still does not demonstrate a source and the blood appears confined to the colon, a total abdominal colectomy should be performed. However, the surgeon should be aware of a significant failure rate even after this radical surgery.

Colonic Diverticulosis

In Western society, the prevalence of colonic diverticula increases with age such that about 60% of people in their seventh decade of life are affected and the incidence increases roughly 1% per year. Only about 20% of patients with diverticulosis have symptoms attributable to these lesions and less than 5% experience hemorrhage.[137] Hemorrhage from diverticular disease is most often massive, associated with hematochezia and varying degrees of hemorrhagic shock. Classically, patients present with a sudden occurrence of mild lower abdominal discomfort, rectal urgency, and the subsequent passage of a large maroon or melanic stool. Because the colon can contain large volumes of blood, neither the volume nor the frequency of bloody stools is a reliable guide to the rate of hemorrhage. Despite the massive nature of hemorrhage, most patients with diverticular disease stop bleeding spontaneously. In one series, 76% of patients initially stopped bleeding spontaneously, though 38% of these rebled. Of those who rebled, less than one fourth required surgery.[138]

Bleeding associated with diverticular disease comes from a perforated vasa recta located at the neck or apex of a diverticulum. The vasa recta penetrates the colonic wall from the serosa to the submucosa through obliquely oriented connective tissue septa. Protrusion of colonic mucosa through this connective tissue plane causes apposition of the diverticulum and the vasa recta (Fig. 65.4). Ulceration of the mucosa within the neck of the diverticulum and disruption of the arterial wall produces hemorrhage into the lumen of the bowel. Although diverticular disease is more prevalent in the left colon, right-sided lesions account for half or more episodes of bleeding.[138,139]

The massive nature of the bleeding caused by colonic diverticula limits the diagnostic usefulness of colonoscopy. Rarely is a bleeding vessel seen within a diverticulum, and the presence of blood or clot within a diverticulum is of no diagnostic benefit. Selective mesenteric arteriography may demonstrate the luminal extravasation of contrast; however, in one study of patients bleeding from diverticulosis, angiographic localization was effective in less than 20% of patients.[140] Failure to visualize a bleeding point is usually due to cessation of active bleeding at the time of angiography.

Given the relatively low risk of recurrent hemorrhage, patients who stop bleeding should be treated expectantly. About 10% of patients bleeding from colonic diverticula continue to bleed and ultimately require operative intervention. Embolization of bleeding vessels in the colon has been reported to be safe and effective in the majority of patients; however, there is a definite risk of ischemic complications.[141–144] The rapid nature of the hemorrhage and the difficulty in defining the site of bleeding through the endoscope have largely thwarted endoscopic attempts at control of diverticular hemorrhage.

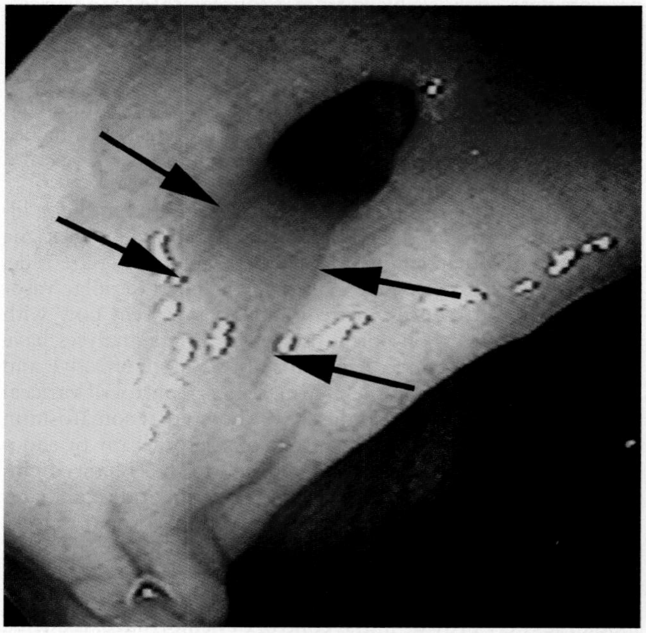

FIGURE 65.4. Colonoscopic view of a colonic diverticulum. A vasa rectum is seen entering the diverticulum and forming one of the walls.

Patients who continue to bleed from diverticular disease should undergo resection of the colon segment that contains the site of bleeding. Even after successful localization of a bleeding source, the least extensive operation that can usually be contemplated is a hemicolectomy or wide segmental colectomy. Tagged red blood cell scanning, while sensitive, cannot pinpoint a bleeding site with great accuracy. Although angiography usually gives more precise localization, correlation between the vascular pattern and the anatomic location is sufficiently imprecise to warrant at least a segmental resection. Lastly, measurement with colonoscopy is notoriously misleading, with even experienced endoscopists making erroneous estimations about the precise site of a lesion.

Although a subtotal colectomy for nonlocalized ongoing colonic hemorrhage may occasionally be necessary, it should be performed only after exhaustive attempts to localize the site of bleeding. Subtotal colectomy is associated with greater perioperative morbidity rates than segmental resection and postoperative diarrhea may present a significant problem to elderly patients. However, if the patient continues to bleed massively from the colon and all attempts at preoperative and intraoperative localization are unsuccessful, subtotal colectomy with ileoproctostomy may be required.

Colonic Angiodysplasia

Sometimes called vascular ectasias or arteriovenous malformations, these lesions are believed to arise from the age-related degeneration of previously normal intestinal submucosal veins and overlying mucosal capillaries. Angiodysplasia is located most frequently in the cecum and ascending colon, although it may be found more distally in 20% to 30% of cases. Multiple lesions may be present in as many as 40% to 75% of cases.[145] Microscopically, angiodysplasia consists of dilated, thin-walled vessels that appear to be ectatic veins and venules localized within the submucosa. A dilated submucosal vein is often found and occasionally an enlarged artery. Angiodysplasia is generally thought to be an acquired lesion associated with aging, but the exact etiology is unknown.

The prevalence of colonic angiodysplasia in the general population appears to be less than 1%.[146] These lesions may present with hematochezia, melena, occult blood loss, or iron deficiency anemia. Bleeding lesions are most commonly found in the right colon. As compared to diverticular bleeding, episodes of hemorrhage from vascular ectasias are usually less severe and are somewhat more likely to recur. After the initial episode of hemorrhage, the majority of patients will stop bleeding spontaneously.[147]

Vascular ectasias may be diagnosed by either colonoscopy or by selective mesenteric angiography. Colonoscopy has been reported to have a sensitivity of 80% in demonstrating vascular ectasias.[148] However, colonoscopic diagnosis of these lesions in actively bleeding patients may be confounded by the presence of other incidental lesions including traumatic and suction artifacts produced during the examination. In addition, after significant bleeding and hypovolemia, the shunting of blood flow away from the intestinal mucosa may obscure these lesions in inadequately resuscitated patients. Colonoscopy can be used effectively to treat vascular ectasias, either by coagulation or possibly injection of sclerosants.[149,150]

Selective mesenteric angiography may also demonstrate these lesions and complement colonoscopy, particularly in patients who are massively bleeding or in whom colonoscopy was unrevealing or incomplete. Characteristic angiographic findings include a densely opacified and slowly emptying, dilated, tortuous vein (found in 90% of patients); a vascular tuft (seen in 66% to 75% of patients); and an early-filling vein (usually a segmental vein in the cecum or right colon, although at times, it may be the ileocolic vein).

The natural history of these lesions was revealed by the clinical course of 101 patients with colonic vascular ectasias.[148] Of the 15 asymptomatic individuals without a history of bleeding, none bled during a period of follow-up to 68 months (mean, 23 months). For 31 patients with overt bleeding or anemia who were treated only with blood transfusion, the rebleeding rate at 1 and 3 years was 26% and 46%, respectively. This study suggests that the risk of bleeding for incidentally discovered lesions is minimal, whereas the risk of recurrent hemorrhage for most symptomatic patients is substantial and may increase with time.

Medical treatment of vascular ectasias has been used, although there is currently no proven effective medical therapy. Hormone treatment using high-dose estrogens and progesterone has been used since the 1950s, but convincing proof of efficacy is lacking. Indeed, most evidence would suggest no antibleeding effect of hormonal treatment.[151] More recently, the antiangiogenic drug thalidomide has been suggested as a treatment option.[152,153]

Patients bleeding from colonic vascular ectasias can be treated endoscopically. Nonrandomized investigations with vascular ectasias managed with monopolar electrocoagulation, endoscopic injection sclerotherapy, contact probes, and lasers have been published with good results. All methods appear to be effective for treating bleeding vascular ectasias and all are associated with procedure-related morbidity rates of 2% to 10%. Perforation has been reported in all of these experiences with rates of 2% to 3%.

Patients bleeding from vascular ectasias in whom endoscopic hemostatic methods are unsuccessful or unavailable can be treated with resection of the colon following preoperative localization of the bleeding site. For the usual patient bleeding from a vascular ectasia in the cecum or ascending colon, a right colectomy with ileotransverse colostomy is the treatment of choice. The value of preoperative localization of the bleeding site cannot be overstated, and every effort should be made to determine the site of hemorrhage prior to laparotomy.

Ischemic Colitis

Ischemic colitis is a common cause of lower gastrointestinal hemorrhage, especially in the elderly. Bleeding is a common presenting manifestation of ischemic colitis, occurring in approximately one half to three fourths of patients, but it is usually not massive.[154,155] Although ischemic colitis may occur with occlusion of a major artery (such as ligation of the inferior mesenteric artery during abdominal aortic aneurysm repair), in most cases it results from impaired local microvascular perfusion of the colonic wall. It occurs most commonly in the elderly, who often have significant medical comorbidities. Renal failure requiring hemodialysis, hypertension, cardiovascular disease, vasoactive medications, and a variety of other risk factors have been associated with the disease.[156] In many cases a specific initiating event cannot be identified. Any segment of the colon may be involved. Profound ischemia may lead to full-thickness necrosis, peritonitis, and perforation. Lesser degrees of ischemia may result in vague abdominal pain, diarrhea, and mild to moderate bleeding. Life-threatening hemorrhage is uncommon.

Ischemic colitis can be diagnosed with colonoscopy, in which case the mucosa may vary from edematous to hemorrhagic and necrotic in appearance. Angiography is usually not helpful in these cases, as it rarely demonstrates major vessel occlusion.[155] Most patients will recover uneventfully with supportive care alone. When operative management is required, it is often necessitated by peritonitis or other signs of full-thickness necrosis. In these critically ill patients the mortality rate is relatively high due to the critical nature of these patients' preexisting comorbid conditions.

UNUSUAL CAUSES OF ACUTE GASTROINTESTINAL HEMORRHAGE

As outlined in Tables 65.1 and 65.2, a wide variety of other pathologic processes may present with acute GI hemorrhage. Although these lesions generally comprise a relatively small percentage of the total number of cases of overt GI hemorrhage, they can present vexing problems to the clinician faced with a bleeding patient in whom the usual etiologies have been excluded. There are a number of case reports in the literature of extremely rare causes of GI bleeding that will not be discussed here. The following lesions occur commonly enough that a clinician is likely to encounter them in his or her practice.

Dieulafoy Vascular Malformation

Dieulafoy vascular malformation is an unusual cause of recurrent hematemesis, in which bleeding originates from an unusually large (1- to 3-mm-diameter) artery running through the gastric submucosa for variable distances. Erosion of the gastric mucosa overlying the vessel results in necrosis of the arterial wall and brisk hemorrhage. The size of the mucosal defect is usually small (2 to 5 mm) and without evidence of chronic inflammation. These lesions may rarely occur in other anatomic locations such as the colon.[157–159]

Painless hematemesis and melena are typical. Recurrent bleeding with spontaneous cessation is also common. In a collective review of 101 cases, the mean age of the patients was 52 years, and the lesion occurred twice as frequently in men as women. There was no significant association with alcohol abuse or antecedent symptoms.[160]

The diagnosis is most frequently made endoscopically by demonstrating arterial bleeding from a pinpoint mucosal defect. Occasionally, a small arterial vessel may be seen protruding from the gastric mucosa. Characteristically, the lesions are located within 6 cm of the esophagogastric junction along the lesser curvature, although they may occur in other sites as well.

Most patients can be managed endoscopically by injection of epinephrine, sclerotherapy, banding, clipping, or coagulation.[161–163] A subset of patients will require retreatment or surgical excision for control of hemorrhage. After cessation of hemorrhage, few patients rebleed from these lesions, even when treated only by endoscopic methods.[164]

Gastric Antral Vascular Ectasia

Sometimes abbreviated as GAVE syndrome, this entity is also known as "watermelon stomach" because of its characteristic endoscopic appearance. Longitudinal erosions are seen in the antrum radiating from the pylorus. It usually causes chronic blood loss and not acute hemorrhage. The etiology is not known, but there is a prominent association with connective tissue disorders. It can usually be treated by endoscopic argon coagulation but occasionally antrectomy is necessary.[165]

Angiodysplasia of the Stomach and Small Intestine

Angiodysplastic lesions may occur throughout the GI tract. Similar to colonic lesions, they appear as minute, flat, or slightly raised red lesions with round or stellate shapes. The margins are characteristically sharp with a pale mucosal halo surrounding the lesion. The lesions are frequently multiple and are found most commonly in the stomach and duodenum, although esophageal and small-intestinal involvement has also been described.

In general, these lesions may be diagnosed by endoscopy, although their minute size and sessile nature may complicate their detection. The lesions may be readily mistaken for submucosal hemorrhage associated with acute gastritis or trauma artifact from a nasogastric tube or the endoscope. These lesions may be demonstrated arteriographically since they have many of the features described for colonic vascular ectasia.

Endoscopic injection of sclerosants, electrocoagulation, and laser photocoagulation have all been used to treat gastroduodenal angiodysplasia with good results. The multiplicity of lesions often necessitates several courses of therapy to eliminate recurring hemorrhage. Surgical resection of the gastric or intestinal wall containing the lesion and oversewing of the bleeding lesion have been reported to successfully control hemorrhage.

Aortoenteric Fistula

Although communication between the aorta and the intestine may occur as a result of aneurysmal disease or infectious aortitis (*primary aortoenteric fistula*), most of those encountered currently are due to the erosion of an aortic vascular prosthesis through the wall of the distal duodenum (*secondary aortoenteric fistula*). The incidence of aortoenteric fistula following aortic reconstructive surgery is about 1%, with most of these fistulas arising from the proximal graft anastomosis. Secondary aortoenteric fistulas are believed to develop after prolonged contact of a prosthetic graft with a fixed segment of intestine. Ultimately, erosion of the graft through the bowel wall results in a low-grade infection around the graft; involvement of the infection with the suture line leads to dehiscence of the anastomosis and massive hemorrhage.

The interval between aortic reconstructive surgery and the onset of GI hemorrhage may range from a few days to many years; the median interval is about 3 years.[166] Most patients have an initial episode of GI bleeding (i.e., herald bleed) that is followed in hours, days, or weeks by catastrophic hemorrhage. Patients may also complain of back or abdominal pain and less commonly have fever or signs of sepsis from infection of the graft.

The diagnosis of an aortoenteric fistula must be considered in any patient with an aortic prosthesis or an abdominal aortic aneurysm who presents with GI hemorrhage. Endoscopy should be urgently performed following resuscitation to disclose evidence of an aortoenteric fistula or another cause of bleeding (e.g., peptic ulcer disease with stigmata of recent hemorrhage). If endoscopy fails to demonstrate an aortoenteric fistula or another convincing source of bleeding and the patient is not massively bleeding, computed tomography may be helpful in detecting perigraft infection or other evidence of an aortoenteric fistula. In patients who are actively bleeding, exploratory laparotomy with exposure of the proximal graft should be undertaken. Identification of an aortoenteric fistula or erosion requires resection of the graft with extra-anatomic bypass and repair of the duodenal wall. The operative management of aortoduodenal fistulas is considered in greater detail in Chapter 88.

Meckel Diverticulum

Bleeding from a Meckel diverticulum is a common cause of lower GI hemorrhage in children but is rare in older adults. Meckel diverticula are present in approximately 2% of the population. The lifetime risk of a complication from a Meckel diverticulum is about 4%.[167] About 25% of patients with symptomatic Meckel diverticula present with hemorrhage.[168]

In a series of 17 patients who bled from Meckel diverticula, 11 experienced frank hemorrhage, while six had chronic occult blood loss. The incidence of GI hemorrhage is greatest in the first decade of life and steadily decreases from that point. In one series, no patient older than 40 years of age, and only one patient older than 31 years, bled from a Meckel diverticulum,[168] although it has been reported in the very elderly.[169] The pathogenesis of this bleeding involves the occurrence of ectopic gastric mucosa with peptic ulceration of adjacent bowel wall. Although these lesions may be demonstrated by enteroclysis, abdominal scintigraphy following the intravenous injection of ^{99}technetium-pertechnetate demonstrates the ectopic gastric mucosa within the diverticulum, suggesting the correct diagnosis. Treatment consists of resecting the diverticulum with a cuff of adjacent bowel. Diverticulectomy alone will be associated with persistence of the ulcer and the possibility of recurrent hemorrhage.

Small-Intestinal Diverticulum

Diverticular disease of the small intestine is another uncommon cause of either upper GI hemorrhage (duodenal) or lower GI hemorrhage (jejunoileal diverticula).[170] The pathogenesis is similar to that of colonic diverticula with erosion of a vasa recta through the diverticular wall and the acute onset of massive hemorrhage. Depending on the location of the diverticulum, patients may present with either hematemesis, melena, or hematochezia. Hemorrhage from this source can be a vexing diagnostic problem because jejunoileal lesions are beyond the reach of the gastroscope and bleeding from duodenal diverticula may be difficult to discern. Mesenteric angiography or intraoperative enteroscopy may localize the site of hemorrhage in actively bleeding patients. Segmental resection of the involved intestine is the treatment of choice.

Hemorrhage Following Endoscopic Procedures

Significant hemorrhage can occur following endoscopic biopsy, sphincterotomy, and other traumatic procedures. Fortunately, these complications are uncommon. Colonoscopy may rarely cause clinically significant bleeding (0.1% to 0.2%).[171] Biopsy of lesions increases the risk up to 10-fold. Usually this is minor and self-limited and may occur up to 12 days after the procedure.[172] The bleeding site can be confirmed by tagged red cell scanning, arteriography, or colonoscopy. Arteriography and colonoscopy can be used therapeutically as described previously. Endoscopically placed bands such as those used for esophageal varices have also been reported to be successful in arresting hemorrhage.[90] Surgical treatment is rarely required.

Hemorrhage following endoscopic biliary sphincterotomy occurs in approximately 2% of patients.[173–175] Mild immediate bleeding is common and is usually self-limited. Late hemorrhage usually occurs within 48 hours of the procedure but can occur many days after sphincterotomy.[176] More severe hemorrhage can usually be controlled by epinephrine injection,[176,177] making the need for operative treatment uncommon.

References

1. Peura DA, Lanza FL, Gostout CJ, et al. The American College of Gastroenterology Bleeding Registry: preliminary findings [see comment]. *Am J Gastroenterol* 1997;92(6):924–928.
2. Raju GS, Gerson L, Das A, et al. American Gastroenterological Association (AGA) Institute technical review on obscure gastrointestinal bleeding. *Gastroenterology* 2007;133(5):1697–1717.
3. Vreeburg EM, Snel P, de Bruijne JW, et al. Acute upper gastrointestinal bleeding in the Amsterdam area: incidence, diagnosis, and clinical outcome. *Am J Gastroenterol* 1997;92(2):236–243.
4. Cutler JA, Mendeloff AI. Upper gastrointestinal bleeding. Nature and magnitude of the problem in the U.S. *Dig Dis Sci* 1981;26(7 suppl): 90S–96S.
5. Yavorski RT, Wong RK, Maydonovitch C, et al. Analysis of 3,294 cases of upper gastrointestinal bleeding in military medical facilities. *Am J Gastroenterol* 1995;90(4):568–573.
6. Lingenfelser T, Ell C. Lower intestinal bleeding [review]. *Best Pract Res Clin Gastroenterol* 2001;15(1):135–153.
7. Cappell MS, Friedel D. Initial management of acute upper gastrointestinal bleeding: from initial evaluation up to gastrointestinal endoscopy. *Med Clin North Am* 2008;92(3):491–509, xi.
8. Rockall TA, Logan RF, Devlin HB, et al. Incidence of and mortality from acute upper gastrointestinal haemorrhage in the United Kingdom. Steering Committee and members of the National Audit of Acute Upper Gastrointestinal Haemorrhage [see comments]. *BMJ* 1995;311(6999):222–226.
9. Richter JM, Christensen MR, Kaplan LM, et al. Effectiveness of current technology in the diagnosis and management of lower gastrointestinal hemorrhage [see comment]. *Gastrointest Endosc* 1995;41(2):93–98.
10. Bramley PN, Masson JW, McKnight G, et al. The role of an open-access bleeding unit in the management of colonic haemorrhage. A 2-year prospective study. *Scand J Gastroenterol* 1996;31(8):764–769.
11. Longstreth GF. Epidemiology and outcome of patients hospitalized with acute lower gastrointestinal hemorrhage: a population-based study [see comment]. *Am J Gastroenterol* 1997;92(3):419–424.
12. Kok KY, Kum CK, Goh PM. Colonoscopic evaluation of severe hematochezia in an Oriental population [see comment]. *Endoscopy* 1998;30(8): 675–680.
13. Kaplan RC, Heckbert SR, Koepsell TD, et al. Risk factors for hospitalized gastrointestinal bleeding among older persons. Cardiovascular Health Study Investigators. *J Am Geriatr Soc* 2001;49(2):126–133.
14. Pahor M, Guralnik JM, Salive ME, et al. Disability and severe gastrointestinal hemorrhage. A prospective study of community-dwelling older persons. *J Am Geriatr Soc* 1994;42(8):816–825.
15. Fiaccadori E, Maggiore U, Clima B, et al. Incidence, risk factors, and prognosis of gastrointestinal hemorrhage complicating acute renal failure. *Kidney Int* 2001;59(4):1510–1519.
16. Cheng HC, Chuang SA, Kao YH, et al. Increased risk of rebleeding of peptic ulcer bleeding in patients with comorbid illness receiving omeprazole infusion. *Hepatogastroenterology* 2003;50(54):2270–2273.
17. van Leerdam ME, Vreeburg EM, Rauws EA, et al. Acute upper GI bleeding: did anything change? Time trend analysis of incidence and outcome of acute upper GI bleeding between 1993/1994 and 2000. *Am J Gastroenterol* 2003;98(7):1494–1499.
18. Mellemkjaer L, Blot WJ, Sorensen HT, et al. Upper gastrointestinal bleeding among users of NSAIDs: a population-based cohort study in Denmark. *Br J Clin Pharmacol* 2002;53(2):173–181.
19. Verhamme K, Mosis G, Dieleman J, et al. Spironolactone and risk of upper gastrointestinal events: population based case-control study. *BMJ* 2006; 333(7563):330.
20. de Abajo FJ, Rodriguez LA, Montero D. Association between selective serotonin reuptake inhibitors and upper gastrointestinal bleeding: population based case-control study. *BMJ* 1999;319(7217):1106–1109.
21. Dalton SO, Johansen C, Mellemkjaer L, et al. Use of selective serotonin reuptake inhibitors and risk of upper gastrointestinal tract bleeding: a population-based cohort study. *Arch Intern Med* 2003;163(1):59–64.
22. Daniel WA Jr, Egan S. The quantity of blood required to produce a tarry stool. *JAMA* 1939;113:2232.
23. Schiff L, Stevens RJ, Shapiro N, et al. Observations on the oral administration of citrated blood in man. II. The effect on the stools. *Am J Med Sci* 1942;203(3):409–412.
24. Hilsman JH. The color of blood-containing feces following the instillation of citrated blood at various levels of the small intestine. *Gastroenterology* 1999;15:131–134.
25. Longstreth GF, Feitelberg SP. Outpatient care of selected patients with acute non-variceal upper gastrointestinal haemorrhage [see comments]. *Lancet* 1995;345(8942):108–111.
26. Kollef MH, O'Brien JD, Zuckerman GR, et al. BLEED: a classification tool to predict outcomes in patients with acute upper and lower gastrointestinal hemorrhage [see comments]. *Crit Care Med* 1997;25(7):1125–1132.
27. Rockall TA, Logan RF, Devlin HB, et al. Risk assessment after acute upper gastrointestinal haemorrhage [see comments]. *Gut* 1996;38(3): 316–321.
28. Sanders DS, Carter MJ, Goodchap RJ, et al. Prospective validation of the Rockall risk scoring system for upper GI hemorrhage in subgroups of patients with varices and peptic ulcers. *Am J Gastroenterol* 2002;97(3): 630–635.
29. Rockall TA, Logan RF, Devlin HB, et al. Selection of patients for early discharge or outpatient care after acute upper gastrointestinal haemorrhage. National Audit of Acute Upper Gastrointestinal Haemorrhage [see comments]. *Lancet* 1996;347(9009):1138–1140.
30. Camellini L, Merighi A, Pagnini C, et al. Comparison of three different risk scoring systems in non-variceal upper gastrointestinal bleeding [see comment]. *Dig Liver Dis* 2004;36(4):271–277.
31. Vreeburg EM, Terwee CB, Snel P, et al. Validation of the Rockall risk scoring system in upper gastrointestinal bleeding. *Gut* 1999;44(3):331–335.

32. Stanley AJ, Ashley D, Dalton HR, et al. Outpatient management of patients with low-risk upper-gastrointestinal haemorrhage: multicentre validation and prospective evaluation. *Lancet* 2009;373(9657):42–47.
33. Aljebreen AM, Fallone CA, Barkun AN. Nasogastric aspirate predicts high-risk endoscopic lesions in patients with acute upper-GI bleeding [see comment]. *Gastrointest Endosc* 2004;59(2):172–178.
34. Witting MD, Magder L, Heins AE, et al. Usefulness and validity of diagnostic nasogastric aspiration in patients without hematemesis. *Ann Emerg Med* 2004;43(4):525–532.
35. Kovacs TO, Jensen DM. Endoscopic control of gastroduodenal hemorrhage [review]. *Annu Rev Med* 1987;38:267–277.
36. Chung YF, Wong WK, Soo KC. Diagnostic failures in endoscopy for acute upper gastrointestinal haemorrhage. *Br J Surg* 2000;87(5):614–617.
37. Spiegel BM, Vakil NB, Ofman JJ. Endoscopy for acute nonvariceal upper gastrointestinal tract hemorrhage: is sooner better? A systematic review [review]. *Arch Intern Med* 2001;161(11):1393–1404.
38. Lee JG, Turnipseed S, Romano PS, et al. Endoscopy-based triage significantly reduces hospitalization rates and costs of treating upper GI bleeding: a randomized controlled trial. *Gastrointest Endosc* 1999;50(6): 755–761.
39. Laine L, Peterson WL. Bleeding peptic ulcer [review]. *N Engl J Med* 1994; 331(11):717–727.
40. Consensus conference: therapeutic endoscopy and bleeding ulcers [review]. *JAMA* 1989;262(10):1369–1372.
41. Hsu PI, Lin XZ, Chan SH, et al. Bleeding peptic ulcer–risk factors for rebleeding and sequential changes in endoscopic findings. *Gut* 1994;35(6): 746–749.
42. Villanueva C, Balanzo J, Espinos JC, et al. Prediction of therapeutic failure in patients with bleeding peptic ulcer treated with endoscopic injection. *Dig Dis Sci* 1993;38(11):2062–2070.
43. Barkun A, Bardou M, Marshall JK, Nonvariceal Upper GI Bleeding Consensus Conference Group. Consensus recommendations for managing patients with nonvariceal upper gastrointestinal bleeding [see comment]. *Ann Intern Med* 2003;139(10):843–857.
44. Chung IK, Kim EJ, Lee MS, et al. Endoscopic factors predisposing to rebleeding following endoscopic hemostasis in bleeding peptic ulcers. *Endoscopy* 2001;33(11):969–975.
45. Terdiman JP, Ostroff JW. Risk of persistent or recurrent and intractable upper gastrointestinal bleeding in the era of therapeutic endoscopy. *Am J Gastroenterol* 1997;92(10):1805–1811.
46. Chaudhry V, Hyser MJ, Gracias VH. Colonoscopy: the initial test for acute lower gastrointestinal bleeding. *Am Surg* 1998;64(8):723–728.
47. Zuckerman GR, Prakash C. Acute lower intestinal bleeding. Part II: etiology, therapy, and outcomes [review]. *Gastrointest Endosc* 1999;49(2): 228–238.
48. Foutch PG. Diverticular bleeding: are nonsteroidal anti-inflammatory drugs risk factors for hemorrhage and can colonoscopy predict outcome for patients? [see comment]. *Am J Gastroenterol* 1995;90(10):1779–1784.
49. Jensen DM, Machicado GA, Jutabha R, et al. Urgent colonoscopy for the diagnosis and treatment of severe diverticular hemorrhage [see comment]. *N Engl J Med* 2000;342(2):78–82.
50. Al Qahtani AR, Satin R, Stern J, et al. Investigative modalities for massive lower gastrointestinal bleeding. *World J Surg* 2002;26(5):620–625.
51. Rossini FP, Pennazio M. Small-bowel endoscopy [review]. *Endoscopy* 2000;32(2):138–145.
52. Kovacs TO, Jensen DM. Recent advances in the endoscopic diagnosis and therapy of upper gastrointestinal, small intestinal, and colonic bleeding [review]. *Med Clin North Am* 2002;86(6):1319–1356.
53. Jensen DM, Kovacs TO, Jutabha R. Gastrointestinal bleeding (GIB) of obscure origin in an era of managed care and push enteroscopy. *Gastrointest Endosc* 1997;45:AB92.
54. Jakobs R, Hartmann D, Benz C, et al. Diagnosis of obscure gastrointestinal bleeding by intra-operative enteroscopy in 81 consecutive patients. *World J Gastroenterol* 2006;12(2):313–316.
55. Mehdizadeh S, Ross A, Gerson L, et al. What is the learning curve associated with double-balloon enteroscopy? Technical details and early experience in 6 U.S. tertiary care centers. *Gastrointest Endosc* 2006;64(5): 740–750.
56. Ross A, Mehdizadeh S, Tokar J, et al. Double balloon enteroscopy detects small bowel mass lesions missed by capsule endoscopy. *Dig Dis Sci* 2008; 53(8):2140–2143.
57. Zuckerman GR, Prakash C. Acute lower intestinal bleeding: part I: clinical presentation and diagnosis [review]. *Gastrointest Endosc* 1998;48(6): 606–617.
58. Vernava AM 3rd, Moore BA, Longo WE, et al. Lower gastrointestinal bleeding [review]. *Dis Colon Rectum* 1997;40(7):846–858.
59. Nusbaum M, Baum S. Radiographic demonstration of unknown sites of GI bleeding. *Surg Forum* 1963;14:374.
60. Pennoyer WP, Vignati PV, Cohen JL. Mesenteric angiography for lower gastrointestinal hemorrhage: are there predictors for a positive study? *Dis Colon Rectum* 1997;40(9):1014–1018.
61. Mernagh JR, O'Donovan N, Somers S, et al. Use of heparin in the investigation of obscure gastrointestinal bleeding. *Can Assoc Radiol J* 2001; 52(4):232–235.
62. Bloomfeld RS, Smith TP, Schneider AM, et al. Provocative angiography in patients with gastrointestinal hemorrhage of obscure origin. *Am J Gastroenterol* 2000;95(10):2807–2812.
63. Rosch J, Dotter CT, Brown MJ. Selective arterial embolization. A new method for control of acute gastrointestinal bleeding. *Radiology* 1972; 102(2):303–306.
64. Bookstein JJ, Chlosta EM, Foley D, et al. Transcatheter hemostasis of gastrointestinal bleeding using modified autogenous clot. *Radiology* 1974; 113(2):277–285.
65. Smith R, Copely DJ, Bolen FH. 99mTc RBC scintigraphy: correlation of gastrointestinal bleeding rates with scintigraphic findings. *AJR Am J Roentgenol* 1987;148(5):869–874.
66. Thorne DA, Datz FL, Remley K, et al. Bleeding rates necessary for detecting acute gastrointestinal bleeding with technetium-99m-labeled red blood cells in an experimental model. *J Nucl Med* 1987;28(4):514–520.
67. Suzman MS, Talmor M, Jennis R, et al. Accurate localization and surgical management of active lower gastrointestinal hemorrhage with technetium-labeled erythrocyte scintigraphy [see comments]. *Ann Surg* 1996;224(1): 29–36.
68. Maurer AH, Rodman MS, Vitti RA, et al. Gastrointestinal bleeding: improved localization with cine scintigraphy [see comments]. *Radiology* 1992;185(1):187–192.
69. Singh PR, Russell CD, Dubovsky EV, et al. Technique of scanning for Meckel's diverticulum. *Clin Nucl Med* 1978;3(5):188–192.
70. Yamaguchi T, Yoshikawa K. Enhanced CT for initial localization of active lower gastrointestinal bleeding. *Abdom Imaging* 2003;28(5):634–636.
71. Ernst O, Bulois P, Saint-Drenant S, et al. Helical CT in acute lower gastrointestinal bleeding. *Eur Radiol* 2003;13(1):114–147.
72. Tew K, Davies RP, Jadun CK, et al. MDCT of acute lower gastrointestinal bleeding. *AJR Am J Roentgenol* 2004;182(2):427–430.
73. Mindelzun RE, Beaulieu CF. Using biphasic CT to reveal gastrointestinal arteriovenous malformations. *AJR Am J Roentgenol* 1997;168(2): 437–438.
74. Huprich JE, Fletcher JG, Alexander JA, et al. Obscure gastrointestinal bleeding: evaluation with 64-section multiphase CT enterography–initial experience. *Radiology* 2008;246(2):562–571.
75. Yoon W, Jeong YY, Shin SS, et al. Acute massive gastrointestinal bleeding: detection and localization with arterial phase multi-detector row helical CT. *Radiology* 2006;239(1):160–167.
76. Paulsen SR, Huprich JE, Hara AK. CT enterography: noninvasive evaluation of Crohn's disease and obscure gastrointestinal bleed. *Radiol Clin North Am* 2007;45(2):303–315.
77. Zink SI, Ohki SK, Stein B, et al. Noninvasive evaluation of active lower gastrointestinal bleeding: comparison between contrast-enhanced MDCT and 99mTc-labeled RBC scintigraphy. *AJR Am J Roentgenol* 2008;191(4): 1107–1114.
78. Boonpongmanee S, Fleischer DE, Pezzullo JC, et al. The frequency of peptic ulcer as a cause of upper-GI bleeding is exaggerated. *Gastrointest Endosc* 2004;59(7):788–794.
79. Hirschowitz BI, Lanas A. NSAID association with gastrointestinal bleeding and peptic ulcer [review]. *Agents Actions Suppl* 1991;35:93–101.
80. Ehsanullah RS, Page MC, Tildesley G, et al. Prevention of gastroduodenal damage induced by non-steroidal anti-inflammatory drugs: controlled trial of ranitidine. *BMJ* 1988;297(6655):1017–1021.
81. Strom BL, Taragin MI, Carson JL. Gastrointestinal bleeding from the non-steroidal anti-inflammatory drugs [review]. *Agents Actions Suppl* 1990;29: 27–38.
82. Garcia RL, Cattaruzzi C, Troncon MG, et al. Risk of hospitalization for upper gastrointestinal tract bleeding associated with ketorolac, other non-steroidal anti-inflammatory drugs, calcium antagonists, and other antihypertensive drugs. *Arch Intern Med* 1998;158(1):33–39.
83. Laporte JR, Ibanez L, Vidal X, et al. Upper gastrointestinal bleeding associated with the use of NSAIDs: newer versus older agents. *Drug Saf* 2004; 27(6):411–420.
84. Shorr RI, Ray WA, Daugherty JR, et al. Concurrent use of nonsteroidal anti-inflammatory drugs and oral anticoagulants places elderly persons at high risk for hemorrhagic peptic ulcer disease. *Arch Intern Med* 1993; 153(14):1665–1670.
85. Armstrong CP, Blower AL. Non-steroidal anti-inflammatory drugs and life threatening complications of peptic ulceration. *Gut* 1987;28(5):527–532.
86. Klein WA, Krevsky B, Klepper L, et al. Nonsteroidal antiinflammatory drugs and upper gastrointestinal hemorrhage in an urban hospital. *Dig Dis Sci* 1993;38(11):2049–2055.
87. Lanza FL, Fakouhi D, Rubin A, et al. A double-blind placebo-controlled comparison of the efficacy and safety of 50, 100, and 200 micrograms of misoprostol QID in the prevention of ibuprofen-induced gastric and duodenal mucosal lesions and symptoms. *Am J Gastroenterol* 1989;84(6): 633–636.
88. Robinson MG, Griffin JWJ, Bowers J, et al. Effect of ranitidine on gastroduodenal mucosal damage induced by nonsteroidal antiinflammatory drugs. *Dig Dis Sci* 1989;34(3):424–428.
89. Roth SH, Bennett RE, Mitchell CS, et al. Cimetidine therapy in nonsteroidal anti-inflammatory drug gastropathy. Double-blind long-term evaluation. *Arch Intern Med* 1987;147(10):1798–1801.
90. Pfaffenbach B, Adamek RJ, Wegener M. Endoscopic band ligation for treatment of post-polypectomy bleeding. *Z Gastroenterol* 1996;34(4): 241–242.
91. Wilcox CM, Alexander LN, Cotsonis GA, et al. Nonsteroidal antiinflammatory drugs are associated with both upper and lower gastrointestinal bleeding. *Dig Dis Sci* 1997;42(5):990–997.
92. Lanas A, Sekar MC, Hirschowitz BI. Objective evidence of aspirin use in both ulcer and nonulcer upper and lower gastrointestinal bleeding. *Gastroenterology* 1992;103(3):862–869.
93. Holt S, Rigoglioso V, Sidhu M, et al. Nonsteroidal antiinflammatory drugs and lower gastrointestinal bleeding. *Dig Dis Sci* 1993;38(9):1619–1623.

94. Laine L, Curtis SP, Cryer B, et al. Assessment of upper gastrointestinal safety of etoricoxib and diclofenac in patients with osteoarthritis and rheumatoid arthritis in the Multinational Etoricoxib and Diclofenac Arthritis Long-term (MEDAL) programme: a randomised comparison. *Lancet* 2007;369(9560):465–473.
95. Laine L, Curtis SP, Langman M, et al. Lower gastrointestinal events in a double-blind trial of the cyclo-oxygenase-2 selective inhibitor etoricoxib and the traditional nonsteroidal anti-inflammatory drug diclofenac. *Gastroenterology* 2008;135(5):1517–1525.
96. Barkun A, Sabbah S, Enns R, et al.; RUGBE Investigators. The Canadian Registry on Nonvariceal Upper Gastrointestinal Bleeding and Endoscopy (RUGBE): endoscopic hemostasis and proton pump inhibition are associated with improved outcomes in a real-life setting [see comment]. *Am J Gastroenterol* 2004;99(7):1238–1246.
97. Lau JY, Leung WK, Wu JC, et al. Omeprazole before endoscopy in patients with gastrointestinal bleeding. *N Engl J Med* 2007;356(16):1631–1640.
98. Chan FK. Proton-pump inhibitors in peptic ulcer disease. *Lancet* 2008; 372(9645):1198–1200.
99. Leontiadis GI, Sharma VK, Howden CW. Proton pump inhibitor therapy for peptic ulcer bleeding: Cochrane collaboration meta-analysis of randomized controlled trials. *Mayo Clin Proc* 2007;82(3):286–296.
100. Management of acute upper and lower gastrointestinal bleeding: a national clinical guideline. Available at: http://www.sign.ac.uk/pdf/sign105.pdf. Accessed 2009.
101. Palmer K, Nairn M. Management of acute gastrointestinal blood loss: summary of SIGN guidelines. *BMJ* 2008;337:a1832.
102. Dore MP, Graham DY. Ulcers and gastritis [review]. *Endoscopy* 2004; 36(1):42–47.
103. Laine LA. Helicobacter pylori and complicated ulcer disease [review]. *Am J Med* 1996;100(5A):52S–77S.
104. Vergara M, Casellas F, Saperas E, et al. Helicobacter pylori eradication prevents recurrence from peptic ulcer haemorrhage. *Eur J Gastroenterol Hepatol* 2000;12(7):733–737.
105. Pilotto A, Leandro G, Di Mario F, et al. Role of Helicobacter pylori infection on upper gastrointestinal bleeding in the elderly: a case-control study. *Dig Dis Sci* 1997;42(3):586–591.
106. Forrest JA, Finlayson ND, Shearman DJ. Endoscopy in gastrointestinal bleeding. *Lancet* 1974;2(7877):394–397.
107. Raju GS, Gajula L. Endoclips for GI endoscopy [review]. *Gastrointest Endosc* 2004;59(2):267–279.
108. Naga MI, Okasha HH, Foda AR, et al. Detachable Endoloop vs. elastic band ligation for bleeding esophageal varices. *Gastrointest Endosc* 2004; 59(7):804–809.
109. Cappell MS, Friedel D. Acute nonvariceal upper gastrointestinal bleeding: endoscopic diagnosis and therapy. *Med Clin North Am* 2008;92(3): 511–550, vii–viii.
110. Sung JJ, Tsoi KK, Lai LH, et al. Endoscopic clipping versus injection and thermo-coagulation in the treatment of non-variceal upper gastrointestinal bleeding: a meta-analysis. *Gut* 2007;56(10):1364–1373.
111. Asaki S. Endoscopic haemostasis by local absolute alcohol injection for UGI tract bleeding: a multicentre study. In: Okabe H, Honda T, Ohshiba S, eds. *Endoscopic Surgery*. New York: Elsevier; 1999:105.
112. Sacks HS, Chalmers TC, Blum AL, et al. Endoscopic hemostasis. An effective therapy for bleeding peptic ulcers. *JAMA* 1990;264(4):494–499.
113. Sugawa C, Steffes CP, Nakamura R, et al. Upper GI bleeding in an urban hospital. Etiology, recurrence, and prognosis. *Ann Surg* 1990;212(4): 521–526.
114. Lau JY, Sung JJ, Lam YH, et al. Endoscopic retreatment compared with surgery in patients with recurrent bleeding after initial endoscopic control of bleeding ulcers [see comments]. *N Engl J Med* 1999;340(10):751–756.
115. Gupta PK, Fleischer DE. Nonvariceal upper gastrointestinal bleeding [review]. *Med Clin North Am* 1993;77(5):973–992.
116. Teenan RP, Murray WR. Late outcome of undersewing alone for gastric ulcer haemorrhage. *Br J Surg* 1990;77(7):811–812.
117. Poultsides GA, Kim CJ, Orlando R 3rd, et al. Angiographic embolization for gastroduodenal hemorrhage: safety, efficacy, and predictors of outcome. *Arch Surg* 2008;143(5):457–461.
118. Schuster DP, Rowley H, Feinstein S, et al. Prospective evaluation of the risk of upper gastrointestinal bleeding after admission to a medical intensive care unit. *Am J Med* 1984;76(4):623–630.
119. Cook DJ, Fuller HD, Guyatt GH, et al. Risk factors for gastrointestinal bleeding in critically ill patients. Canadian Critical Care Trials Group [see comments]. *N Engl J Med* 1994;330(6):377–381.
120. Driks MR, Craven DE, Celli BR, et al. Nosocomial pneumonia in intubated patients given sucralfate as compared with antacids or histamine type 2 blockers. The role of gastric colonization. *N Engl J Med* 1987; 317(22):1376–1382.
121. Cook D, Guyatt G, Marshall J, et al. A comparison of sucralfate and ranitidine for the prevention of upper gastrointestinal bleeding in patients requiring mechanical ventilation. Canadian Critical Care Trials Group [see comments]. *N Engl J Med* 1998;338(12):791–797.
122. Athanasoulis CA. Therapeutic applications of angiography (first of two parts) [review]. *N Engl J Med* 1980;302(20):1117–1125.
123. Robert A, Kauffman GL Jr. Stress ulcers, erosions and gastric mucosal injury. In: Sleisenger MH, Fordtran JS, eds. *GI Disease: Pathophysiology, Diagnosis, Management*, 4th ed. Philadelphia, PA: WB Saunders; 1999:772.
124. Silverstein FE, Gilbert DA, Tedesco FJ, et al. The national ASGE survey on upper gastrointestinal bleeding. II. Clinical prognostic factors. *Gastrointest Endosc* 1981;27(2):80–93.
125. Wilcox CM, Clark WS. Causes and outcome of upper and lower gastrointestinal bleeding: the Grady Hospital experience. *South Med J* 1999;92(1): 44–50.
126. Jenkins SA, Baxter JN, Critchley M, et al. Randomised trial of octreotide for long term management of cirrhosis after variceal haemorrhage. *BMJ* 1997;315(7119):1338–1341.
127. Imperiale TF, Teran JC, McCullough AJ. A meta-analysis of somatostatin versus vasopressin in the management of acute esophageal variceal hemorrhage. *Gastroenterology* 1995;109(4):1289–1294.
128. Burroughs AK. Octreotide in variceal bleeding. *Gut* 1994;35(3 suppl): S23–S27.
129. Avgerinos A, Nevens F, Raptis S, et al. Early administration of somatostatin and efficacy of sclerotherapy in acute oesophageal variceal bleeds: the European Acute Bleeding Oesophageal Variceal Episodes (ABOVE) randomised trial [see comments]. *Lancet* 1997;350(9090):1495–1499.
130. Besson I, Ingrand P, Person B, et al. Sclerotherapy with or without octreotide for acute variceal bleeding. *N Engl J Med* 1995;333(9): 555–560.
131. Sung JJ, Chung SC, Yung MY, et al. Prospective randomised study of effect of octreotide on rebleeding from oesophageal varices after endoscopic ligation [see comments]. *Lancet* 1995;346(8991–8992):1666–1669.
132. Hermann RE, Traul D. Experience with the Sengstaken-Blakemore tube for bleeding esophageal varices. *Surg Gynecol Obstet* 1970;130(5):879–885.
133. Monescillo A, Martinez-Lagares F, Ruiz-del-Arbol L, et al. Influence of portal hypertension and its early decompression by TIPS placement on the outcome of variceal bleeding. *Hepatology* 2004;40(4):793–801.
134. Orloff MJ, Orloff MS, Orloff SL, et al. Three decades of experience with emergency portacaval shunt for acutely bleeding esophageal varices in 400 unselected patients with cirrhosis of the liver [see comments]. *J Am Coll Surg* 1995;180(3):257–272.
135. Mallory GK, Weiss S. Hemorrhages from lacerations of the cardiac orifice of the stomach due to vomiting. *Am J Med Sci* 1929;178:506–515.
136. Park CH, Min SW, Sohn YH, et al. A prospective, randomized trial of endoscopic band ligation vs. epinephrine injection for actively bleeding Mallory-Weiss syndrome. *Gastrointest Endosc* 2004;60(1):22–27.
137. McGuire HH Jr, Haynes BW Jr. Massive hemorrhage for diverticulosis of the colon: guidelines for therapy based on bleeding patterns observed in fifty cases. *Ann Surg* 1972;175(6):847–855.
138. McGuire HH Jr. Bleeding colonic diverticula. A reappraisal of natural history and management. *Ann Surg* 1994;220(5):653–656.
139. Casarella WJ, Kanter IE, Seaman WB. Right-sided colonic diverticula as a cause of acute rectal hemorrhage. *N Engl J Med* 1972;286(9):450–453.
140. Boley SJ, DiBiase A, Brandt LJ, et al. Lower intestinal bleeding in the elderly. *Am J Surg* 1979;137(1):57–64.
141. Nicholson AA, Ettles DF, Hartley JE, et al. Transcatheter coil embolotherapy: a safe and effective option for major colonic haemorrhage [see comments]. *Gut* 1998;43(1):79–84.
142. Kuo WT, Lee DE, Saad WE, et al. Superselective microcoil embolization for the treatment of lower gastrointestinal hemorrhage. *J Vasc Interv Radiol* 2003;14(12):1503–1509.
143. Gady JS, Reynolds H, Blum A. Selective arterial embolization for control of lower gastrointestinal bleeding: recommendations for a clinical management pathway. *Curr Surg* 2003;60(3):344–347.
144. Gordon RL, Ahl KL, Kerlan RK, et al. Selective arterial embolization for the control of lower gastrointestinal bleeding. *Am J Surg* 1997;174(1):24–28.
145. Foutch PG. Angiodysplasia of the gastrointestinal tract [see comments] [review]. *Am J Gastroenterol* 1993;88(6):807–818.
146. Foutch PG, Rex DK, Lieberman DA. Prevalence and natural history of colonic angiodysplasia among healthy asymptomatic people. *Am J Gastroenterol* 1995;90(4):564–567.
147. Sharma R, Gorbien MJ. Angiodysplasia and lower gastrointestinal tract bleeding in elderly patients [review]. *Arch Intern Med* 1995;155(8): 807–812.
148. Richter JM, Hedberg SE, et al. Angiodysplasia. Clinical presentation and colonoscopic diagnosis. *Dig Dis Sci* 1984;29(6):481–485.
149. Gupta N, Longo WE, Vernava AM. Angiodysplasia of the lower gastrointestinal tract: an entity readily diagnosed by colonoscopy and primarily managed nonoperatively. *Dis Colon Rectum* 1995;38(9):979–982.
150. Bemvenuti GA, Julich MM. Ethanolamine injection for sclerotherapy of angiodysplasia of the colon. *Endoscopy* 1998;30(6):564–559.
151. Junquera F, Feu F, Papo M, et al. A multicenter, randomized, clinical trial of hormonal therapy in the prevention of rebleeding from gastrointestinal angiodysplasia [see comment]. *Gastroenterology* 2001;121(5):1073–1079.
152. Bauditz J, Lochs H. Angiogenesis and vascular malformations: antiangiogenic drugs for treatment of gastrointestinal bleeding. *World J Gastroenterol* 2007;13(45):5979–5984.
153. Dabak V, Kuriakose P, Kamboj G, et al. A pilot study of thalidomide in recurrent GI bleeding due to angiodysplasias. *Dig Dis Sci* 2008;53(6): 1632–1635.
154. Medina C, Vilaseca J, Videla S, et al. Outcome of patients with ischemic colitis: review of fifty-three cases. *Dis Colon Rectum* 2004;47(2):180–184.
155. Scharff JR, Longo WE, Vartanian SM, et al. Ischemic colitis: spectrum of disease and outcome. *Surgery* 2003;134(4):624–629.
156. Green BT, Tendler DA. Ischemic colitis: a clinical review. *South Med J* 2005;98(2):217–222.
157. Chaer RA, Helton WS. Dieulafoy's disease [review]. *J Am Coll Surg* 2003;196(2):290–296.

158. Lee YT, Walmsley RS, Leong RW, et al. Dieulafoy's lesion [review]. *Gastrointest Endosc* 2003;58(2):236–243.
159. Gimeno-Garcia AZ, Parra-Blanco A, Nicolas-Perez D, et al. Management of colonic Dieulafoy lesions with endoscopic mechanical techniques: report of two cases. *Dis Colon Rectum* 2004;47(9):1539–1543.
160. Veldhuyzen van Zanten SJ, Bartelsman JF, Schipper ME, et al. Recurrent massive haematemesis from Dieulafoy vascular malformations–a review of 101 cases. *Gut* 1986;27(2):213–222.
161. Baettig B, Haecki W, Lammer F, et al. Dieulafoy's disease: endoscopic treatment and follow up. *Gut* 1993;34(10):1418–1421.
162. Park CH, Sohn YH, Lee WS, et al. The usefulness of endoscopic hemoclipping for bleeding Dieulafoy lesions. *Endoscopy* 2003;35(5):388–392.
163. Cheng CL, Liu NJ, Lee CS, et al. Endoscopic management of Dieulafoy lesions in acute nonvariceal upper gastrointestinal bleeding. *Dig Dis Sci* 2004;49(7–8):1139–1144.
164. Romaozinho JM, Pontes JM, Lerias C, et al. Dieulafoy's lesion: management and long-term outcome. *Endoscopy* 2004;36(5):416–420.
165. Novitsky YW, Kercher KW, Czerniach DR, et al. Watermelon stomach: pathophysiology, diagnosis, and management [review]. *J Gastrointest Surg* 2003;7(5):652–661.
166. Nagy SW, Marshall JB. Aortoenteric fistulas. Recognizing a potentially catastrophic cause of gastrointestinal bleeding [review]. *Postgrad Med* 1921;93(8):211–222.
167. Yahchouchy EK, Marano AF, Etienne JC, et al. Meckel's diverticulum [review]. *J Am Coll Surg* 2001;192(5):658–662.
168. Mackey WC, Dineen P. A fifty year experience with Meckel's diverticulum. *Surg Gynecol Obstet* 1983;156(1):56–64.
169. Lichtstein DM, Herskowitz B. Massive gastrointestinal bleeding from Meckel's diverticulum in a 91-year-old man. *South Med J* 1998;91(8):753–754.
170. El-Haddawi F, Civil ID. Acquired jejuno-ileal diverticular disease: a diagnostic and management challenge. *ANZ J Surg* 2003;73(8):584–589.
171. Rabeneck L, Paszat LF, Hilsden RJ, et al. Bleeding and perforation after outpatient colonoscopy and their risk factors in usual clinical practice. *Gastroenterology* 2008;135(6):1899–1906.
172. Gibbs DH, Opelka FG, Beck DE, et al. Postpolypectomy colonic hemorrhage. *Dis Colon Rectum* 1996;39(7):806–810.
173. Halme L, Doepel M, von Numers H, et al. Complications of diagnostic and therapeutic ERCP. *Ann Chir Gynaecol* 1999;88(2):127–131.
174. Freeman ML, Nelson DB, Sherman S, et al. Complications of endoscopic biliary sphincterotomy [see comments]. *N Engl J Med* 1996;335(13): 909–918.
175. Gholson CF, Favrot D, Vickers B, et al. Delayed hemorrhage following endoscopic retrograde sphincterotomy for choledocholithiasis. *Dig Dis Sci* 1996;41(5):831–834.
176. Vasconez C, Llach J, Bordas JM, et al. Injection treatment of hemorrhage induced by endoscopic sphincterotomy [see comments]. *Endoscopy* 1998;30(1):37–39.
177. Leung JW, Chan FK, Sung JJ, et al. Endoscopic sphincterotomy-induced hemorrhage: a study of risk factors and the role of epinephrine injection. *Gastrointest Endosc* 1995;42(6):550–554.

CHAPTER 66 ■ ULCERATIVE COLITIS

EMILY FINLAYSON

KEY POINTS

1. Ulcerative colitis is a disease largely limited to the mucosa and submucosa of the colorectum. This process is continuous, beginning at the rectum, and extending proximally for variable distances.
2. The acute indications for surgical intervention are bleeding, fulminant disease, and toxic megacolon. Failure of medical management, dysplasia, and cancer are indications for elective surgery.
3. The intestinal manifestations of ulcerative colitis are cured by removal of the colon and rectum.
4. Current surgical options include proctocolectomy with end ileostomy and proctocolectomy with ileal pouch–anal anastomosis.
5. Although operative and late complications after ileal pouch–anal reconstruction are not uncommon, patient satisfaction and quality-of-life scores after surgery are high.

Ulcerative colitis is an idiopathic inflammatory bowel disease (IBD) that affects the mucosa of the colon and rectum. The disease presents with equal frequency in males and females, with onset predominantly in the second to fourth decades. Diarrhea and gastrointestinal bleeding are the hallmark clinical features. Medical treatment temporarily improves symptoms and allows periods of remission. However, 10% to 35% of patients with chronic ulcerative colitis will eventually require surgical intervention for medically refractory symptoms or complications of the disease.[1,2]

EPIDEMIOLOGY

In North America, the incidence of ulcerative colitis is approximately 2.2 to 14.3 cases per 100,000 person-years.[3–6] Rates of disease are highest in northern Europe, the United Kingdom, and North America. The incidence of disease appears to be rising in Asia, Africa, and South America.[7] Although ulcerative colitis typically begins in the teen years or early adulthood, a second and perhaps a third peak of incidence are noted. Secondary peaks of disease activity occur in the 40- to 60-year age range, with a smaller third peak after the age of 70 years. Some studies reveal gender-related differences in late-onset disease, with men more likely than women to be diagnosed later in life.[8]

Etiology and Risk Factors for Ulcerative Colitis

Despite more than five decades of investigation, the underlying biologic mechanisms of the disease process are poorly understood. Many risk factors have been examined without conclusive results. Although diet, oral contraceptive use, breast-feeding, measles infection/vaccination, and other infections have all been implicated, the evidence connecting these factors to ulcerative colitis is weak. Other risk factors, however, have been shown more convincingly to have an association with the disease.

Cigarette Smoking. For more than 20 years, a decreased incidence of ulcerative colitis has been noted in individuals who smoke.[9] In 1989, meta-analytical studies revealed that smokers were 40% as likely as nonsmokers to develop ulcerative colitis.[10] In addition, primary sclerosing cholangitis and pouchitis are both decreased in those who smoke, suggesting a systemic protective effect.[11,12] The mechanisms underlying this protective effect are unclear. Former smokers also appear to be at increased risk of developing ulcerative colitis.[13] Smoking has been associated with a less severe disease course of ulcerative colitis. Active smokers are half as likely to be hospitalized as nonsmokers. Former smokers are 50% more likely to be hospitalized and twice as likely as current smokers or those who have never smoked to require colectomy.[14] One French study revealed that patients with ulcerative colitis who ceased smoking had more active disease, more hospitalizations, and greater need for immunosuppressants that those who continued to smoke.[15]

Appendectomy. Large meta-analyses reveal a protective effect of nearly 70% of appendectomy for the development of ulcerative colitis.[16] Population-based studies in the Netherlands, Sweden,[17] and Denmark[18,19] have documented varying rates of development of chronic ulcerative colitis among patients who have undergone appendectomy. In the Dutch study, the cohorts were followed for 5 million person-years and observed for a subsequent diagnosis of ulcerative colitis. Patients who had undergone appendectomy had only three-quarters the incidence of ulcerative colitis compared with controls. The Danish study, however, revealed only a 13% decreased likelihood for the development of ulcerative colitis.

Like smoking, appendectomy may also influence the course of ulcerative colitis. Results from two studies from Japan and Australia suggest this possibility. In the Japanese study, patients who developed ulcerative colitis after appendectomy were less likely to develop recurrent symptoms than colitis patients with an intact appendix.[20] In the Australian study, ulcerative colitis patients who had undergone appendectomy prior to the diagnosis were significantly less likely to subsequently require colectomy.[21]

Genetics. Inflammatory bowel disease has been shown to cluster within families, implicating genetics in determining susceptibility. Twin studies reveal a concordance rate of 10% in monozygotic twins and 3% in dizygotic twins.[22] Population-based studies report that 5% to 10% of those affected have a positive family history.[23] Population-based studies have demonstrated a 10-fold increased risk for developing ulcerative colitis among relatives of patients with the disease.[24]

Genome-wide scans have been used to type genetic markers in families containing more than one member with ulcerative colitis and to identify shared chromosomal regions. These genetic linkage studies have revealed that the IBD2 locus (12q13) may be associated with ulcerative colitis. Unfortunately, several important genes in this region, including the $\beta 7$ integrin family and signal transducer and activator of transcription 6, have not been found to correlate with this disease.[25] The most intensively studied region has been the chromosome 6 region (IBD3), especially regions associated with major histocompatibility complex class II genes. Meta-analysis combining results from 29 studies reveal positive associations to DR2, DR9, and DRB1*0103.[26]

Although there is mounting evidence that genetic factors play a role in the development of ulcerative colitis, their major role is likely one of making the individual genetically susceptible to other inciting events. Recent evidence suggests that IBD results when the interaction of gut microorganisms, the host epithelium, and the host immune system create an environment of dysregulated immunity.[27] The molecular pathways of these interactions, however, are still debated.

PATHOLOGY

Macroscopic Appearance

1 Ulcerative colitis is a disease largely limited to the mucosa and submucosa of the colon and rectum. The rectum is nearly always involved, and the disease generally presents in a continuous fashion from this point proximally. The proximal extent of disease and the severity vary. When the entire colon is involved, termed *pancolitis*, a phenomenon called *backwash ileitis* may occur, characterized by a dilated, mildly inflamed terminal ileum. The typical presentation may be less clear if a patient develops toxic megacolon initially. In this case, the colon may be diffusely thickened, gangrenous, and perforated. The resultant full-thickness disease may appear similar to Crohn colitis, both macroscopically and microscopically.

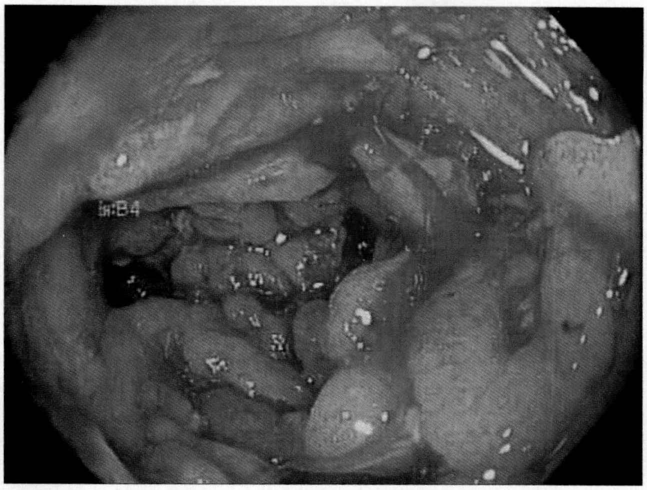

FIGURE 66.1. Pseudopolyps (colonoscopic photo). (Courtesy of Peter Higgins, MD, University of Michigan, Ann Arbor, MI.)

Gross inspection of the colon reveals confluence of numerous ulcers with areas of heaped up, regenerating mucosa, called *pseudopolyps* (Fig. 66.1). This process is continuous, beginning at the rectum, and extending proximally for variable distances. Superficial fissures, consisting of linear coalescence of ulcerating lesions, are seen. In contrast to Crohn disease, ulcerative colitis is not transmural, and therefore tends to lack features of thickening and fibrosis. The loss of the mucosa eventually leads to the loss of the normally visualized endoscopic vascular pattern (Fig. 66.2).

Microscopic Appearance

Early in the inflammatory process, the disease involves acute inflammatory cells, predominantly neutrophils, infiltrating into the crypts of Lieberkühn at the base of the mucosa to form crypt abscesses (Fig. 66.3). As the process continues, crypt abscesses coalesce, and superficial desquamation of overlying epithelium leads to the formation of ulcers. Cryptitis undermines the adjacent mucosa, which becomes edematous. If this inflammation is severe, the muscularis propria may undergo myocytolysis, resulting in hyperemia and wall thinning during severe attacks. Granulation tissue is formed as the ulcerated areas heal, which extends to, but rarely through, the submucosa.

CLINICAL FEATURES/COURSE

Ulcerative colitis is typically characterized by bloody diarrhea. The majority of patients present with a mild attack of predominantly distal disease (80%), while a minority of patients (20%) develop pancolitis.[28] In 10% to 20% of patients, an initial attack will rapidly progress to fulminant colitis, characterized by frequent, bloody bowel movements; fever; and abdominal tenderness.

The signs and symptoms correlate with the severity, duration, and location of disease. Patients with proctitis most often present with urgency, frequency, tenesmus, and bloody, mucoid diarrhea. The abdominal examination is usually unremarkable. On proctoscopy, the rectal mucosa appears inflamed and friable.

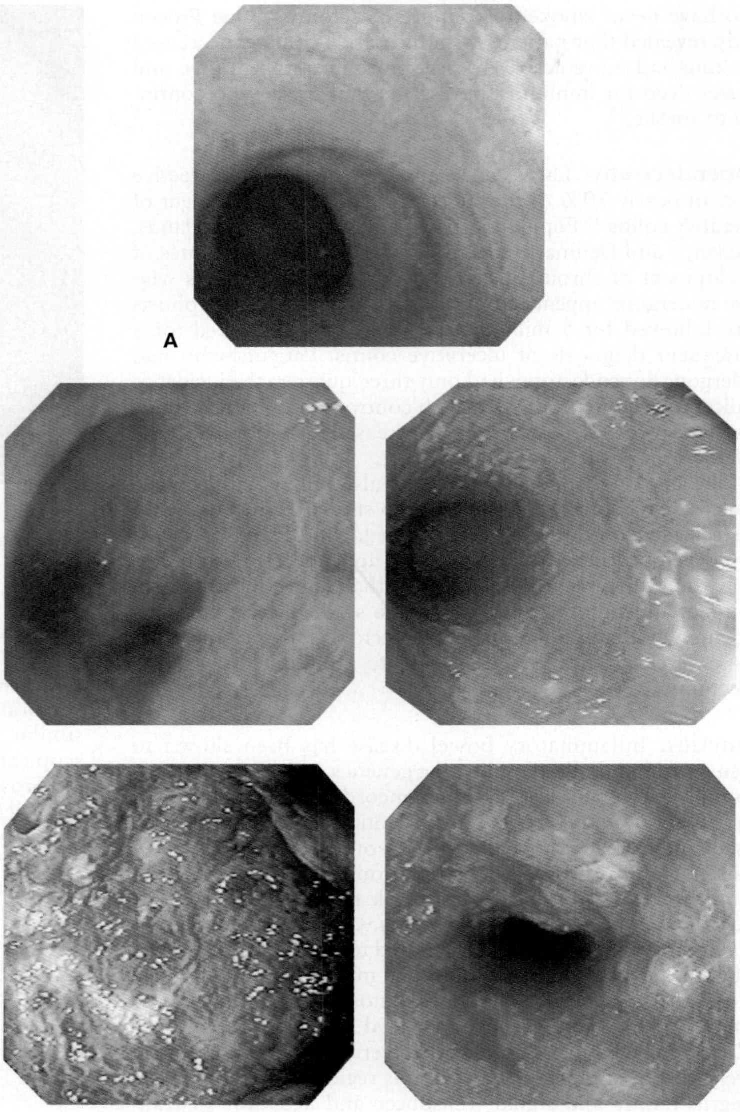

FIGURE 66.2. A: Loss of normal vascular pattern (colonoscopic photo). B: Contact bleeding. C: Granularity. D: Ulceration and friability. E: Colonic stricture. (Reproduced with permission from Corman ML. *Colon and Rectal Surgery,* 5th ed. Philadelphia, PA: Lippincott Williams & Wilkins; 2005.)

In patients with pancolitis, anemia, fatigue, and anorexia may be present. These patients may exhibit weight loss due to decreased oral intake during attacks, increased metabolism, and protein loss during chronic or recurrent episodes. Patients with chronic colitis have loss of mucosal folds and haustra.

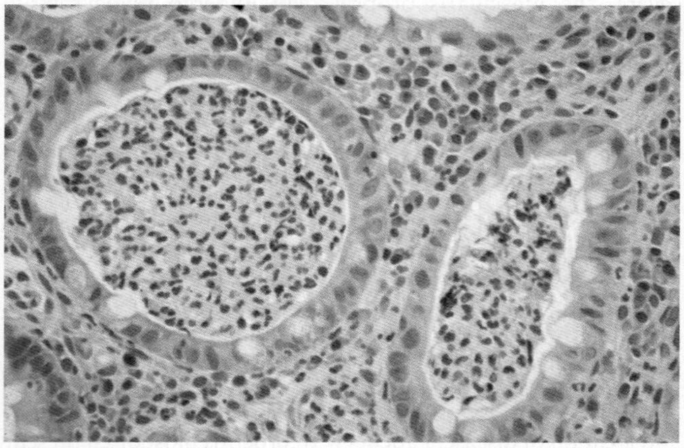

FIGURE 66.3. Histograph of crypt abscess. (Courtesy of Henry Appelman, University of Michigan, Ann Arbor, MI.)

The walls of the colon undergo fibrosis and shortening, leading to a "lead pipe" appearance on contrast radiography (Fig. 66.4). With the loss of functional mucosa, the colon may be unable to absorb fluid, leading to diarrhea.

Extraintestinal manifestations involve dermatologic, ocular, articular, and hepatic tissues (Table 66.1). These manifestations complicate 25% to 30% of cases.[29] With treatment, dermatologic and ocular manifestations may resolve. Unfortunately, hepatic and articular manifestations do not resolve, and primary sclerosing cholangitis may require liver transplantation for management.

Of dermatologic manifestations, erythema nodosum and pyoderma gangrenosum are the most common. Erythema nodosum, found in approximately 9% of patients with ulcerative colitis,[30] is a rash consisting of tender, symmetric, raised erythematous papules, predominantly found on the extensor surfaces of the arms and legs (Fig. 66.5A). Skin disease commonly parallels the activity, but not the severity or extent of bowel disease. Occasionally, the appearance of erythema nodosum precedes the diagnosis of IBD. The uncommon condition of pyoderma gangrenosum is associated with IBD in 50% of cases.[31] Pyoderma gangrenosum begins as an erythematous plaque, papule, or bleb, usually in the pretibial region, but may progress to an ulcerated, necrotizing, tender wound with ill-defined, purple-red margins (Fig. 66.5B). In both diseases, treatment of the underlying bowel disease process is key to management.

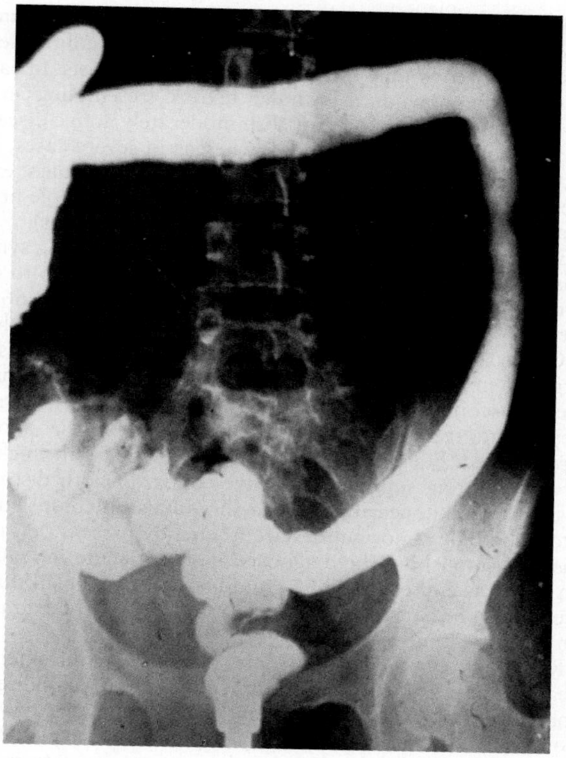

FIGURE 66.4. Lead-pipe colon radiograph. (Reproduced with permission from Corman ML. *Colon and Rectal Surgery*, 5th ed. Philadelphia, PA: Lippincott Williams & Wilkins; 2005, color plate.)

TABLE 66.1 **DIAGNOSIS**

EXTRAINTESTINAL MANIFESTATIONS OF ULCERATIVE COLITIS

DERMATOLOGIC
Pyoderma gangrenosum
Erythema nodosum
Clubbing
OCULAR
Iritis
Uveitis
Scleritis
RHEUMATOLOGIC
Ankylosing spondylitis
Sacroiliitis
Peripheral arthritis
HEPATOBILIARY
Sclerosing cholangitis
Fatty liver
Cirrhosis
VASCULAR
Thromboembolism
Coagulopathy

The ocular manifestations of ulcerative colitis are commonly episcleritis, and less commonly, but more seriously, iritis and uveitis. Episcleritis is characterized by the development of eye redness without visual disturbance, whereas scleritis and iritis/uveitis may be associated with blindness if left untreated. Episcleritis is associated with pain or tenderness to palpation, but is not associated with loss of vision, photophobia, or loss of a normal pupillary response to light. Episcleritis may be confused with conjunctivitis; however, the latter is not associated with discomfort. Scleritis is a more severe ocular disorder, which may result in impaired vision. Scleritis differs from episcleritis in that with episcleritis the sclera remain white, as opposed to pink in scleritis. Scleritis may lead to retinal detachment or optic nerve swelling.[32] Uveitis and iritis are often associated with joint and skin extraintestinal manifestations. The inflammation includes the iris, ciliary body, and, posteriorly, the vitreous, choroids, or retina. These complications are characterized by the acute onset of painful eyes, blurred vision, and headache, and may herald the diagnosis of ulcerative colitis. Slit-lamp examination establishes the diagnosis. Treatment of uveitis typically involves cycloplegics and topical steroids, but may require systemic steroids and immunosuppression.

The musculoskeletal manifestations of ulcerative colitis are the most common extraintestinal complications.[33] The arthritic

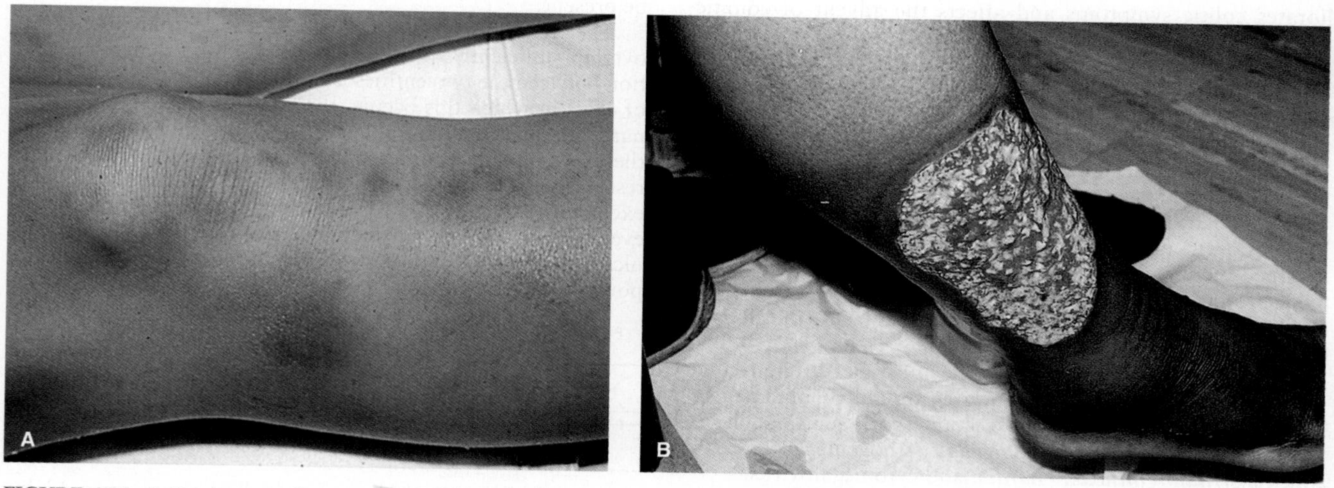

FIGURE 66.5. **A:** Erythema nodosum. **B:** Pyoderma gangrenosum. (A reproduced with permission from Goodheart HP. *A Photoguide of Common Skin Disorders: Diagnosis and Management*. Baltimore, MD: Lippincott Williams & Wilkins; 1999.)

component is believed to be associated with loss of intestinal integrity associated with colitis, and the release of bacteria, lipopolysaccharide, and cytokines. A generalized inflammatory response is manifested as arthritic discomfort. Acute synovitis may occur in up to 20% of patients, reported as sudden joint pain with effusion and tenderness, usually associated with increased disease activity.[33] Medical therapy targeted at improving mucosal integrity or altering bacterial flora relieves symptoms.

Ankylosing spondylitis occurs in a small percentage of patients with ulcerative colitis (3% to 5%), with the highest-risk patients possessing the human leukocyte antigen (HLA) B27 haplotype.[33] Unfortunately, sacroiliitis/spondylitis does not bear a relationship to clinically active bowel disease and thus may progress unnoticed. On examination, these patients have tenderness of the sacroiliac joint and loss of truncal motion and, later, will have decreased chest expansion with cervical fusion. In longstanding disease, pain may dissipate as the spinal ligaments or joints ossify. Neither medical nor surgical therapy has an effect on these manifestations, and thus treatment is geared toward slowing disability and minimizing deformity.

Asymptomatic abnormalities of hepatic enzymes are the most common manifestation of hepatobiliary disturbances in ulcerative colitis. At least 50% of patients have fatty infiltration of the liver, with cirrhosis present in 3% to 5%.[34] Although fatty liver may reverse with treatment of primary disease, cirrhosis will not.

The most severe extraintestinal manifestation of ulcerative colitis is primary sclerosing cholangitis (PSC). This chronic cholestatic syndrome is characterized by fibrosing obliteration of the bile ducts. Best diagnosed by endoscopic retrograde cholangiopancreatography or magnetic resonance cholangiopancreatography, primary sclerosing cholangitis demonstrates beadlike extrahepatic and intrahepatic bile ducts. Epidemiologic studies have shown that nearly 70% of patients with primary sclerosing cholangitis have ulcerative colitis, whereas the incidence of primary sclerosing cholangitis in patients with ulcerative colitis is only 2% to 7%.[35,36] In patients with ulcerative colitis, the relative risk of development of cholangiocarcinoma also is 31 times greater than in PSC patients without ulcerative colitis.[37] In general, primary sclerosing cholangitis is a chronic, progressive disease with the rate of progression being variable. Current medical treatment involves the use of ursodeoxycholic acid and endoscopic dilation of the bile duct strictures until liver failure necessitates transplantation. Currently, the only known curative treatment for primary sclerosing cholangitis is orthotopic liver transplantation. Whether the addition of immunosuppression to maintain the transplanted organ ameliorates colitic symptoms and affects the advent of colonic malignant degeneration is not clear.[38,39]

DIAGNOSIS

The diagnosis of ulcerative colitis requires a combination of history and endoscopic/radiologic findings. Diarrhea, often with blood or mucus, is a dominant symptom. Urgency of bowel movements may be disabling, with tenesmus due to an inflamed rectum. If the disease is more severe, associated systemic symptoms, including fever, arthritis, skin manifestations, and weight loss, may ensue. On a chronic basis, the disease causes fatigue and malaise.

At first presentation, the disease must be differentiated from infectious causes. Stool cultures should be obtained to rule out common infectious colonic pathogens, such as *Campylobacter, Salmonella, Shigella*, pathogenic *Escherichia coli, Clostridium difficile, Giardia*, and cytomegalovirus.

Colonoscopy with ileal intubation or flexible sigmoidoscopy should be the next invasive test. Biopsies of abnormal and quiescent areas are of key importance, with the locations of the biopsies carefully documented. Because the rectum is involved in 90% to 95% of cases with ulcerative colitis, flexible sigmoidoscopy may establish the initial diagnosis. In early cases, findings include a granular texture, resembling small bowel, and mucosal friability. With moderately active disease, spontaneous hemorrhage occurs, whereas in severe cases, the mucosa is ulcerated with copious bleeding and a purulent exudate. Over time, the mucosa regenerates, with multiple areas of raised granulation tissue and mucosa (pseudopolyps).

Examination at initial presentation of accompanying symptoms and histologic examination of biopsies may help to differentiate ulcerative colitis from Crohn disease (Table 66.2). Distinguishing features include the clinical presentation, which for Crohn disease may include cramping abdominal pain, suggestive of small-bowel involvement. At colonoscopy, the presence of discontinuous disease or "skip areas" suggests Crohn disease, and, if possible, ileal intubation with biopsies should be performed. Edema of the interhaustral septa with thickening and blunting suggests ulcerative colitis. In both diseases, grossly normal-appearing mucosa should also be biopsied, as histopathologic abnormalities are frequently present that may assist in establishing the diagnosis. If severe acute inflammation exists, a limited flexible sigmoidoscopy may be all that is necessary to initiate treatment, as a more aggressive examination may result in colonic perforation.

Radiologic examination is helpful to determine the extent of disease and to distinguish ulcerative colitis from Crohn disease. In patients presenting with fulminant colitis, a dilated transverse colon, with a diameter of 5 to 7 cm, is often visible on plain film. Mild cases of ulcerative colitis may be seen on air contrast barium enema with spiculation and collar button ulcers. When contrast studies are used to visualize longstanding ulcerative colitis, the loss of haustra with a flat mucosa and narrowed caliber (lead-pipe colon; see Fig. 66.4) may be seen. Additionally, in Crohn disease, the small bowel is often involved and should be investigated with a small bowel follow-through, video-capsule endoscopy, or computed tomography enterography.

Expression of antibodies may help differentiate the two disease processes. The expression of perinuclear antineutrophil cytoplasmic antibodies versus antibodies to the cell wall of mannan polysaccharide (anti-*Saccharomyces cerevisiae* antibodies [ASCAs]) segregates the diseases in that antineutrophil cytoplasmic antibodies correlate with ulcerative colitis, whereas ASCA is a marker for Crohn disease. Unfortunately, neither antibody is sensitive enough to serve as a sole screening test because up to 64% of patients with Crohn disease have ASCAs.[40] Nevertheless, these antibodies are part of the Prometheus IBD First Step panel, which helps to determine whether a patient may have IBD and which type of disease may be present.

The presentation of ulcerative colitis and Crohn disease may overlap sufficiently in the initial presentation that discrimination between the two entities is not possible. In the 8% to 10% of cases in which this occurs, the colitis is labeled "indeterminate." Because the natural history and surgical management of these two diseases is different, diagnosis is paramount. Prior to restorative proctocolectomy, every attempt should be made to exclude the diagnosis of Crohn disease. Several studies, however, have found similar functional results among patients with ulcerative colitis and those with indeterminate colitis after ileal pouch–anal anastomosis.[41]

MEDICAL MANAGEMENT

Aminosalicylic Acid Compounds

Aminosalicylates are the primary medical treatment modality for mild to moderate ulcerative colitis, used to both induce remission and prevent relapse. Sulfasalazine, composed of

TABLE 66.2 DIAGNOSIS

CLINICOPATHOLOGIC FEATURES OF ULCERATIVE COLITIS VERSUS CROHN DISEASE

MANIFESTATION	ULCERATIVE COLITIS	CROHN DISEASE
Transmural inflammation	Seldom	Common
Granulomas	Seldom	>50%
Fissuring	Rare	Common
Fibrosis	Rare	Common
Submucosal inflammation	Rare	Common
Crypt abscesses	Common	Uncommon
Small-bowel involvement	Rare (backwash ileitis)	Common
Anatomic location	Continuous	Skip
Rectal involvement	Common	May be spared
Bleeding	Common	Absent
Fistulas	Rare	Common
Perianal disease	Rare	Common
Ulcers	Rare	Common
Surrounding mucosa	Pseudopolyps	Relatively normal
Cobblestoning of mucosa	None	Longstanding disease
Mucosal friability	Common	Uncommon
Vascular pattern	Absent	Normal
Fat wrapping	Rare	Common

5-aminosalicylic acid (ASA) linked to sulfapyridine by a diazo-bond, was the first compound in this family to be identified. The active component is 5-ASA, and formulations have been created to release the active moiety at different pH levels. Mesalamine (Asacol) is released at pH greater than 7; for Pentasa, controlled release begins in the duodenum. Rowasa is released at pH greater than 6, thus facilitating distal ileal and colonic exposure. The former is most effective in treating patients with proximal small bowel disease, whereas Rowasa is the preferred medication for ileocolonic disease. Rowasa may be delivered as suppositories or enemas to treat distal colonic disease. Colonic bacteria contain azo-reductase enzymes that are able to split sulfasalazine to liberate 5-ASA in the colon, where it is believed to act topically.

Steroids

Corticosteroids continue to play a major role in the induction of remission in patients with moderate to severe ulcerative colitis or for patients who have failed aminosalicylate treatment. The use of corticosteroids is designed to control symptoms and achieve remission, not to maintain long-term remission. Steroid therapy is followed by a taper to minimize the medical complications of long-term steroid use. In severe cases, prednisone, 40 to 60 mg/d, is used to induce remission. If a hospitalized patient exhibits acute worsening of symptoms (e.g., escalating bloody diarrhea), intravenous steroids, in a dose equivalent to 300 mg of hydrocortisone or 60 mg of methylprednisolone, should be administered.

Budesonide is often effective and has the advantage of producing fewer systemic effects. Budesonide is believed to have greater potency due to high affinity for the glucocorticoid receptor and low systemic bioavailability due to extensive first-pass hepatic metabolism.[42] Budesonide capsules delay the release of the active component until the ileum and ascending colon, where the pH is greater than 5.5.

Immunomodulators

The purine antimetabolites, azathioprine and its metabolite, 6-mercaptopurine, may also be used to achieve steroid-sparing remission. These agents are used to facilitate a remission induced by cyclosporine. These agents act via inhibition of purine biosynthesis, nucleotide interconversions, DNA and RNA synthesis, and chromosomal replication.[43] A prolonged interval of 3 to 6 months may be necessary for these agents to demonstrate their full suppressive potential. Approximately 60% of patients achieve long-term remission with these agents.[44] Measurement of the activity of thiopurine methyltransferase, as well as 6-thioguanine levels, allows for dose adjustment. Toxicities induced by this family of drugs include bone marrow suppression, especially leukopenia, which is dose dependent. Additionally, liver toxicity and allergic reactions, manifested as a combination of fever, rash, myalgias, or arthralgias, may limit utilization. Pancreatitis occurs as another manifestation of hypersensitivity in 2% of patients.[45]

Cyclosporine therapy for refractory colitis is effective in 40% of patients who have failed steroids alone.[46,47] Cyclosporine is a lipophilic peptide with inhibitory effects on both the cellular and humoral immune systems. Cyclosporine down-regulates the cellular immune response by blocking the production of interleukin (IL)-2 by T-helper lymphocytes. Molecularly, cyclosporine binds to cyclophilin, and this complex binds to and inhibits calcineurin, a cytoplasmic phosphatase enzyme involved in the activation of T cells.[48] Cyclosporine also indirectly inhibits B-cell function by interfering with the production of activation factors and interferon-γ by T-helper cells.[49]

The dose of cyclosporine recommended to induce remission is 4 mg/kg per day. Patients with hypocholesterolemia, hypokalemia, or hypomagnesemia must have a reduced dose of 2 mg/kg to avoid the risk of seizures. Long-term therapy is avoided because of the associated side effects of hypertension, renal insufficiency, paresthesias, and seizures. After induction of remission with cyclosporine, patients may be transitioned to either salicylates or to an antimetabolite, such as azathioprine, or 6-mercaptopurine. However, long-term follow-up in these patients fails to demonstrate a decreased incidence of colectomy, with 60% to 80% of these patients requiring operation within 1 year.[50] This delay, however, may allow an elective operation instead of an emergency procedure.

Another calcineurin inhibitor, tacrolimus, a member of the macrolide antibiotic family, may be useful adjunctive therapy for steroid-refractory ulcerative colitis. Tacrolimus has improved absorption compared to cyclosporine. The fact that tacrolimus is a member of the macrolide antibiotic family accounts for its additional promotility effect.[51]

Biologic Agents

Anti–Tumor Necrosis Factor. Recently, anti–tumor necrosis factor (TNF) therapy (infliximab) has been approved for treatment of severe, refractory ulcerative colitis. In a large, multicenter randomized trial, patients with moderate to severe ulcerative colitis who received infliximab therapy were more likely than controls to be in clinical remission at 54 weeks (45% vs. 20%).[52] There appears to be no significant difference in response rates between patients who received 5-mg/kg and 10-mg/kg dosing regimens.

Treatment Algorithms. With many effective agents available to treat ulcerative colitis, there are several options for induction and maintenance of remission. Treatment strategy algorithms have been developed by consensus panels based on up-to-date information on medical therapies[53] (Algorithm 66.1). Patients with mild ulcerative colitis generally begin therapy with oral aminosalicylates. Progression to moderate disease is generally treated with a steroid taper. Patients who become steroid dependent should be started on biologic or immunomodulator therapy. Options for patients unresponsive to steroid therapy and with severe disease include treatment with cyclosporine, infliximab, or surgical resection.

TABLE 66.3 INDICATIONS/CONTRAINDICATIONS

INDICATIONS FOR URGENT SURGERY IN ULCERATIVE COLITIS
Acute severe colitis (70%)
Toxic colonic dilatation (20%)
Perforation (<10%)
Hemorrhage (<5%)

Adapted from Nicholls RJ. Review article: ulcerative colitis—surgical indications and treatment. *Aliment Pharmacol Ther* 2002;16(suppl 4): 25–28.

INDICATIONS FOR SURGICAL INTERVENTION

2 The acute indications for surgical intervention are fulminant disease, toxic megacolon, and hemorrhage (Table 66.3). Failure of medical management, dysplasia, and cancer are indications for elective surgery.

Surgical Emergencies

Acute, severe (fulminant) colitis is the most common indication for acute surgical intervention. Severe colitis is defined as the passage of more than six bloody stools per day with a temperature higher than 37.5°C, tachycardia, hemoglobin less than 75% of normal, and an increased sedimentation rate. Affected patients are hospitalized, resuscitated, and placed on intravenous steroids. Fulminant or severe colitis may be precipitated by superimposed infectious colitis and the latter diagnosis should be ruled out in all patients presenting with severe colitis. Fever, defecation more than 8 to 10 times per 24-hour period, frequent bloody movements, hypoalbuminemia, and abdominal tenderness are findings concerning for failure of

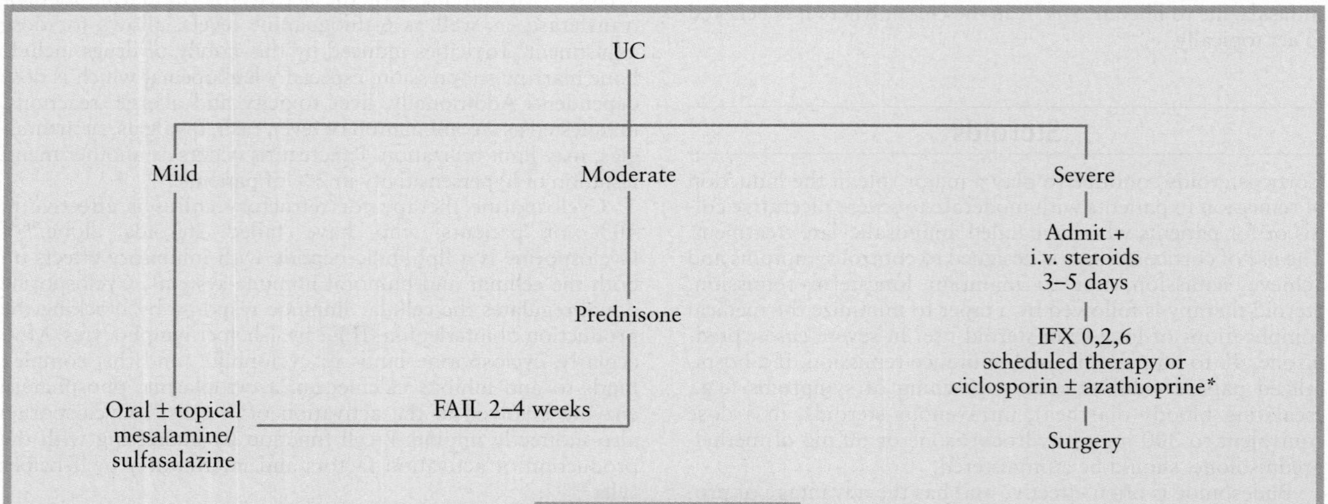

ALGORITHM 66.1

ALGORITHM 66.1. Treatment paradigm for remission induction in ulcerative colitis. (Reproduced with permission from Panaccione R, Rutgeers P, Sandborn WJ, et al. Review article: treatment algorithms to maximize remission and minimize corticosteroid dependence in patients with inflammatory bowel disease. *Aliment Pharmacol Ther* 2008;28:647–688.)

medical management. Barium enema, narcotics, anticholinergic drugs, and antidiarrheal agents should be avoided because these agents may precipitate toxic megacolon. Patients who show no signs of improvement in the first 48 to 96 hours or have an incomplete response after 7 days of medical treatment are likely to fail medical therapy.[54]

Toxic megacolon is the most feared presentation of ulcerative colitis and is characterized by severe systemic signs of illness—fever, abdominal pain and tenderness, tachycardia, leukocytosis—and dilation of the colon (greater than 6 cm transverse colon on abdominal radiograph). Perforation may be present without radiologic evidence in 25% of patients. With either toxic megacolon or severe colitis, perforation is a possible sequela that has historically been associated with a high mortality rate. Recent advances in medical and surgical intervention, however, have decreased mortality rates to less than 3%.[55]

Hemorrhage is an unusual indication for surgery in ulcerative colitis. Most often, bleeding is controlled with medical treatment of the disease. Even with distal disease, total abdominal colectomy is often sufficient to arrest hemorrhage as the fecal stream is diverted. Rectal stump bleeding can be controlled with systemic or topical steroids. In severe cases, hemostasis can be achieved with intrarectal tamponade with epinephrine-soaked gauze. Proctectomy should be a last resort as it complicates later surgical reconstruction.

Emergency Procedures for Ulcerative Colitis. Total abdominal colectomy with end ileostomy is the most common and safest procedure for patients who require emergency intervention for ulcerative colitis. This procedure is rapid, removes the greatest source of the patient's symptoms, and allows withdrawal of steroids postoperatively. The rectum is preserved to minimize the extent of surgery in a systemically ill patient and to facilitate future pelvic procedures (i.e., the creation of a pelvic reservoir). However, this approach may mandate a second procedure (completion proctectomy or pouch formation) and perhaps a third procedure (ileostomy closure). Formerly, blowhole colostomy and ileostomy had been advocated for management of toxic megacolon, in which a dilated, edematous, thin-walled colon might lead to intraoperative spillage with subsequent septic complications. With improved medical management and earlier surgical intervention, fewer patients have advanced disease and perforation at the time of surgery, and therefore this procedure is rarely used.

There are several strategies for securing the rectal stump after subtotal colectomy to prevent "rectal stump blowout." The rectal stump may be managed by either suturing or stapling the proximal end. If the stump is very friable, it may be left with enough sigmoid to create a mucous fistula to the anterior abdominal wall. If the end will not reach the skin, it may be brought through the fascia and sutured in the subcutaneous space. A third option is to place a large catheter intra-anally to stent the sphincters open, facilitating dependent drainage.

Elective Surgery for Ulcerative Colitis

The most common indication for elective proctocolectomy is intractability. These patients often have longstanding colitis and have failed aggressive outpatient medical regimens with significant side effects due to medications.

While biopsy-proven cancer is an absolute indication for proctocolectomy, management of dysplasia is more controversial. In patients with high-grade dysplasia or a dysplasia-associated lesion or mass (DALM), the risk of synchronous cancer is over 40% and surgical resection is warranted.[56] Management of low-grade dysplasia is not as straightforward. Small prospective studies have found a wide range of rates of progression to high-grade dysplasia or cancer, with some studies failing to document an increased risk for cancer.[57,58] A meta-analysis, however, that included over 500 patients found a ninefold increase in the risk of developing cancer.[59] One potential source of confusion is in the histologic diagnosis of dysplasia. Even among experts, there is interobserver variability as high as 60% in the classification of dysplasia.[60]

Cancer prophylaxis is sometimes a motive for elective colectomy. Most investigators believe that oncogenesis is related to the severity and duration of disease. Although the risk is low during the first 8 to 10 years of ulcerative colitis, cancer incidence increases at a rate of 1% to 2% per year following this interval.[61–63] Malignancy may be present in up to 18% of patients with an intact colon having sustained 30 years of disease,[64] and reflects an increase in relative risk of 2.6- to 5.4-fold relative to the general population. Cancers develop in the flat mucosa, not in inflammatory regions. Surveillance colonoscopy is essential. Notably, at the first colonoscopy for surveillance, approximately 10% of patients will already have dysplasia,[56] with a rate of 3% for the development of dysplasia at subsequent follow-up colonoscopy if the first colonoscopy is unrevealing.[65] Current recommendations for surveillance colonoscopy include a minimum of 18 biopsies to have a 95% sensitivity to detect any type of dysplasia, and most studies recommend four biopsies from at least nine sites, with at least four sites in the rectosigmoid.[66]

Procedure Options for Elective Surgery. The advantages, disadvantages, indications, and contraindications for elective surgical options for ulcerative colitis are summarized in Table 66.4.

4 **Total Proctocolectomy with End Ileostomy.** For years, total proctocolectomy with end ileostomy was the operative "gold standard" for ulcerative colitis. This procedure is one of the earliest for ulcerative colitis, and is still considered the standard against which other procedures must be compared. This operation has several advantages. With removal of the entire colon and rectum, cancer risk is eliminated. With an end ileostomy, patients do not experience the urgency and frequency associated with ileoanal pouch. It remains the operation of choice for patients with sphincter dysfunction. An intersphincteric perineal dissection results in a smaller perineal wound than that traditionally created for an abdominoperineal dissection and results in better wound healing rates. Stoma-related complications such as hernia, stenosis, and skin excoriation, however, are not uncommon.

Colectomy with Ileorectal Anastomosis. In this procedure, the entire abdominal colon is removed, and the ileum is anastomosed to the rectum at approximately the level of the sacral promontory. The postoperative leak rate is very low, around 2%,[67] and the procedure is technically easy to perform with either a hand-sewn or stapled anastomosis. The procedure spares the anus. Bowel movements are more numerous and looser than before the operation, but with the addition of bulking agents or antidiarrheal agents, the number of movements may be minimized. The morbidity associated with a pelvic dissection is avoided.

Unfortunately, for most patients with ulcerative colitis, this procedure is not an optimal long-term solution because the disease always involves the rectum and the possibility of neoplastic degeneration mandates surveillance. Indeed, the incidence of carcinoma in the rectal stump at 20 years is approximately 5% to 17%.[68] At least 10% of patients require subsequent proctectomy for refractory proctitis, and another 10% require proctectomy for poor function. This procedure is a compromise for patients with minimal rectal disease who want intermediate-term preservation of parasympathetic nerve function with continence.

Kock Pouch. The Kock pouch is designed to create a reservoir formed from the ileum with a valve that prevents spontaneous

TABLE 66.4 **INDICATIONS/CONTRAINDICATIONS**

ADVANTAGES/DISADVANTAGES AND INDICATIONS/CONTRAINDICATIONS FOR ELECTIVE SURGICAL OPTIONS FOR ULCERATIVE COLITIS

■ PROCEDURE	■ ADVANTAGE	■ DISADVANTAGE	■ CONTRAINDICATIONS
Total proctocolectomy/ ileostomy	Single operation	Permanent ileostomy	
Kock pouch	Continent abdominal reconstruction	Often requires multiple surgical revisions	Crohn disease
Total abdominal colectomy/ ileorectal anastomosis	Single operation, preserves native continence	May require subsequent proctectomy for inflammation or cancer	Active proctitis
Total proctocolectomy/ileal pouch–anal anastomosis	Removes nearly all disease with continent reconstruction	Risk of anastomotic leak, cuffitis, pouchitis, frequent bowel movements/leakage; risk of malignant degeneration in pouch and rectal cuff	Crohn disease, incontinence, distal rectal cancer

emptying. A catheter is inserted through the valve into the reservoir, allowing ileal contents to be emptied by the patient. This construction is created so that motivated patients who did not wish to maintain a permanent, spontaneously emptying ileostomy would be able to intubate the pouch. The nipple valve forms the major source for either a successful or an unsuccessful pouch. The pouch is created from two to three limbs of ileum to form a reservoir, whereas the valve is formed by a portion of the efferent limb intussuscepted into the pouch. This procedure is now rarely performed because of the greater than 50% need for revision due to valve failure and incompetence, technical difficulties with intubation, and fistula formation and because of the advent of the restorative proctocolectomy.

Restorative Proctocolectomy. Parks et al.[69] and Utsonomiya et al.[70] independently reported the development of a technique that adapted Kock's ileal pouch and, instead of connecting the pouch to the abdominal wall, anastomosed it to the anus. This type of reconstruction avoids a permanent ileostomy, and the route of evacuation is sustained. This technique is now commonly referred to as the ileal pouch–anal anastomosis, restorative proctocolectomy, or pelvic pouch.[71]

This procedure has increased in utilization over the past 25 years and is now the most commonly used operation in the elective management of ulcerative colitis.[72] Contraindications include Crohn disease, fulminant colitis, low rectal neoplasia, and incontinence. Relative contraindications include obesity because a thick mesentery will preclude mobilization of the bowel into the distal pelvis. A patient with an android-shaped pelvis or a tall patient may have a similar limitation in pouch creation.

The restorative proctocolectomy is usually performed in two stages: (a) total or completion proctocolectomy, pouch formation and pouch–anal anastomosis, and diverting loop ileostomy, and (b) closure of loop ileostomy. The procedure may be performed with laparoscopic assistance. The colon and rectum are resected and the distal rectum is divided, leaving a short rectal cuff. The small bowel mesentery is then mobilized, and an estimate that a created pouch will reach into the anastomosis is made by grasping the most dependent portion of the pouch and measuring that it will reach 3 to 6 cm beyond the bony symphysis pubis.

If the pouch does not reach the rectal cuff, a number of maneuvers may increase length. The small-bowel mesentery may be mobilized to the third part of the duodenum. Peritoneal windows may be made over the vessels releasing tension to the apical portion of the pouch. These windows may be repeated on both sides of the mesentery. Transillumination will identify vascular arcades that must be preserved, but will also identify vessels that may be ligated to increased length. Application of a vessel clamp with either palpation or Doppler confirmation of adequate blood flow prior to ligation is recommended.

Multiple pouch constructions have been described. Although initially the S- and W-pouches were favored for their increased reservoir capacity and longer length, the J-pouch is now the most popular construction, probably due to the ease of construction, fit into the pelvis, reservoir capacity, and easy emptying. The J-pouch is constructed by stapling two 15- to 20-cm limbs of ileum together, via an enterotomy created at the apex of the J-pouch (Fig. 66.6A). To complete the common wall, another firing of the GIA stapler is necessary, with the distal pouch accordioned onto the forks of the stapler. Other constructions include the S-pouch and W-pouch (Fig. 66.6B,C). An ileoanal anastomosis may be performed by double stapling or, following mucosectomy, via a hand-sewn anastomosis. Stapling preserves the anal transition zone, and this preservation seems to enhance function by retaining neorectal sensation and continence.[73] However, this approach does retain a small area of rectum that has the potential for the development of neoplasia, and therefore some investigators have favored mucosectomy. To facilitate mucosectomy, the perineal operator uses a retractor to expose the dentate line. Dilute epinephrine is injected submucosally to raise the mucosa and to prevent bleeding. A needle-tip cautery is helpful to precisely excise the mucosa for a length of several centimeters. The pouch is then lowered into the pelvis and pulled down endoanally for a hand-sewn anastomosis with absorbable sutures.

Postoperative Complications

The most common early postoperative complications are small-bowel obstruction and sepsis. Small-bowel obstruction complicates 11% to 26% of ileal pouch procedures.[74,75] Creation of a loop ileostomy increases this risk significantly.[76] Analysis of a series of 1,005 patients revealed that 25% of patients had small-bowel obstruction, with two thirds of the patients having the temporary loop ileostomy as the cause.[77] Of this 25%, 7.5% had early obstructions and 18% had later obstructions. Overall, of the 254 patients with a small-bowel obstruction, 28% required reoperation. The most common site of obstruction was at the ileostomy,[78] which has led some surgeons to perform the procedure without ileostomy. Others have implemented the use of Seprafilm (Genzyme Corporation, Cambridge, MA; modified sodium hyaluronic acid and

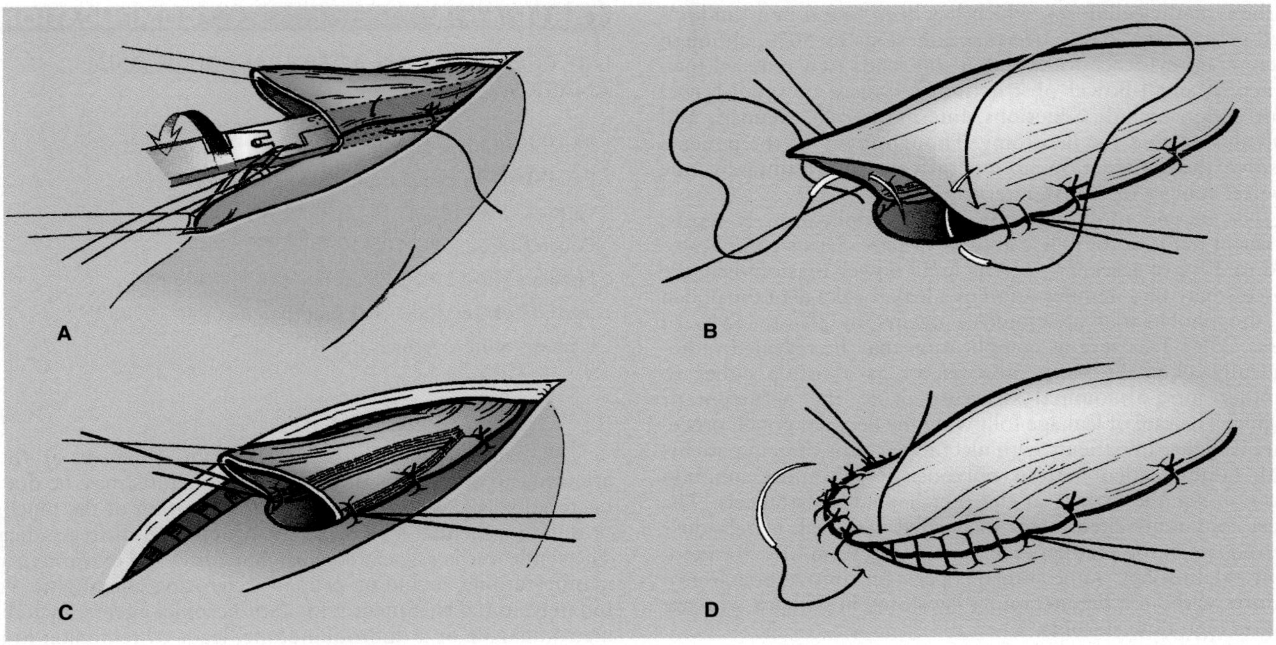

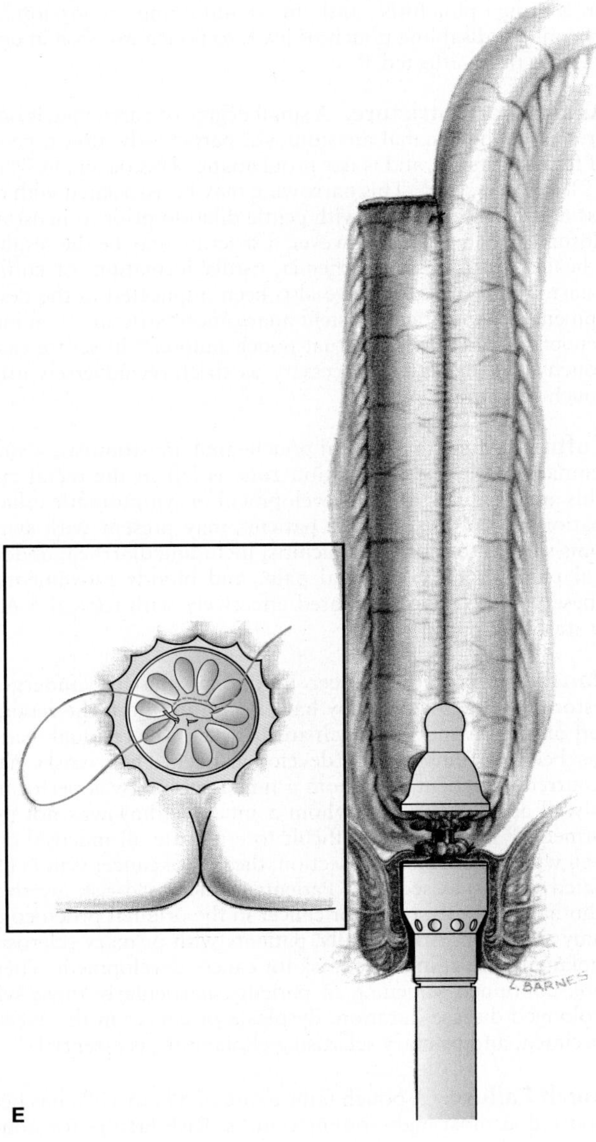

FIGURE 66.6. Ileal pouch construction. **A:** An electrocautery is used to create an enterotomy at the apex of the 15-cm loop of terminal ileum. **B:** The forks of an intestinal anastomosing stapler are pressed into the intestinal limbs, and the instrument is fired. **C:** This is repeated once or twice while the limbs are telescoped onto the stapler, until a 15-cm side-to-side anastomosis is completed. **D:** The apical enterotomy is closed with a simple pursestring stitch. **E:** The stapled construction of the J-pouch. (E reproduced with permission from Corman ML. *Colon and Rectal Surgery*, 5th ed. Philadelphia, PA: Lippincott Williams & Wilkins; 2005:1418.)

COLORECTAL

carboxymethylcellulose), which has been found in a randomized prospective trial to decrease adhesions by 50%, although there is no evidence to date that this leads to a reduced incidence of small-bowel obstruction.[79] Causes of small-bowel obstruction include adhesions, internal hernia, stenosis, and volvulus around the ileostomy. Though many of the patients resolve the obstruction nonoperatively, approximately one quarter require operative intervention.[80]

The second most common early complication is sepsis, either in the form of pelvic abscess or leak. Sepsis complicates 3% to 37% of cases.[74,77,81–83] As in all bowel anastomoses, the abscess may be a manifestation of a leak. Leakage of the pouch or the pouch–anal anastomosis occurs in 2% to 15% of cases.[77,84,85] This serious complication may be revealed radiologically, clinically as an abscess, or as a fistula either to another intra-abdominal structure or to the perineum or vagina. The rate of leakage following the ileoanal pouch procedure is higher in patients with ulcerative colitis than in patients with familial adenomatous polyposis.[84] The most common location for the leak is at the pouch–anal anastomosis. The most commonly cited factor associated with leak is high-dose steroid use in the preoperative period (ingestion of >40 mg of daily prednisone). Some surgeons perform routine pouch procedures without a defunctioning ileostomy in patients who are not on high-dose steroids.[86]

A loop ileostomy does not prevent leakage at the pouch–anal anastomosis, but it may decrease the morbidity associated with the leak. If a leak occurs, it may be adequately managed with diversion and drainage while allowing time for healing. However, the most common cause of eventual pouch excision is an anastomotic leak, usually due to poor long-term functional results. In one series, 58 patients required pouch excision: 39% due to a leak from the ileoanal anastomosis and 12% due to leak from the pouch. Others have reported an association of leak with pouch failure in up to 24% of patients requiring pouch excision.[87]

Fistula is another manifestation of anastomotic leak, which may develop from the pouch or ileoanal anastomosis and extend to another organ, such as the perineum or vagina. Fistula may occur in the early postoperative period, but may also present months or years later. Pouch fistulas occur with a frequency of 2.8% to 12%.[74,77,78,83,86] Fistulas are complex to manage, and regardless of whether a local or abdominal technique is used, only half of attempted repairs will be successful.[88] Contributing factors include pouch ischemia, anastomotic leak, vaginal inclusion in the anastomotic suture line, cryptoglandular infection, and Crohn disease. Abscess drainage, prolonged diversion with loop ileostomy, antibiotics, and local therapy may lead to fistula closure. Variable success has been noted with seton placement, fibrin glue instillation, Surgisis plug placement, ileoanal flaps, and vaginal flaps.[88]

Long-term Sequelae

A summary of the long-term sequelae after ileal pouch–anal anastomosis is listed in Table 66.5.

Pouchitis. Pouchitis is a nonspecific inflammation in the pouch associated with increased stool frequency, urgency, incontinence, bleeding, crampy abdominal pain, malaise, and a low-grade fever. This condition is unique to patients with an ileal pouch and is increased in patients who undergo a pouch procedure for inflammatory bowel disease.[89] Pouchitis occurs in 30% to 50% of these patients.[90] The cumulative probability of suffering a second episode of pouchitis after an initial attack within 2 years of a restorative proctocolectomy is 64%. After a single episode, however, only 15% experience chronic symptoms.[91] On pouchoscopy, the mucosa is inflamed and friable with ulceration and discharge. Mucosal biopsies with histologic analysis must confirm the diagnosis.

TABLE 66.5 COMPLICATIONS

LATE COMPLICATIONS AFTER ILEAL POUCH–ANAL ANASTOMOSIS

Pouchitis (30%–50%)[91]
Small-bowel obstruction (11%–26%)[75,74]
Cuffitis (5%–14%)[97,98]
Pouch failure (5%–10%)[87,97,101,102]
Fistula (3%–12%)[74,77,78,83,86]
Sexual dysfunction—male and female (5%–20%)[104,105]
Cancer—cuff or pouch (rare)[99,100]

The cause of pouchitis is unknown. In most of those affected, no etiology is documented. Pouchitis may be due to bacterial stasis, with toxins causing ulceration of the mucosa, or due to ischemia, leading to the production of free radicals. The syndrome is associated with pancolitis and extraintestinal manifestations, including primary sclerosing cholangitis. Fortunately, initial treatment with antimicrobial agents, including metronidazole or a fluoroquinolone, leads to remission in the majority of cases. In refractory cases, a 5-ASA compound is added. Newer data suggest that probiotics may be beneficial in preventing pouchitis and in maintaining remission.[92,93] Chronic or disabling pouchitis leads to pouch excision in up to 12% of those affected.[94]

Anastomotic Stricture. A small degree of narrowing is often present at the ileoanal anastomosis, particularly after a period of fecal diversion, and is not problematic. This occurs in 7% to 15% of cases.[74,77,95] This narrowing may be associated with disuse and usually resolves with gentle dilation prior to ileostomy closure. In some cases, however, a stricture may be the result of a healed leak, tension, ischemia, fistula formation, or cuffitis. Anastomotic strictures have also been implicated in the development of pouchitis. Persistent anastomotic stricture is an independent predictor of eventual pouch failure.[96] In severe cases, pouch revision may be necessary as strictures adversely affect pouch emptying.

Cuffitis. After stapled ileal pouch–anal anastomosis, a small remnant of the anal transition zone is left in the rectal cuff. This area is at risk for the development of symptomatic inflammation or "cuffitis." These patients may present with symptoms similar to those of pouchitis, including diarrhea, abdominal pain, urgency, perianal pain, and bloody movements.[97] These patients may be treated effectively with topical 5-ASA or steroid suppositories.[98]

Cancer. Reports of cancer in patients having undergone restorative proctocolectomy have been rare. Both the retained cuff of rectum and the pouch are at risk.[99] The residual rectum has been documented to develop cancer. These cases have occurred in patients in whom a mucosectomy was performed as well as in patients in whom a mucosectomy was not performed.[100] Because it is difficult to eradicate all mucosal cells even with a meticulous dissection, the risk of cancer is not eliminated with mucosectomy. Patients at increased risk are those who had either dysplasia or cancer in the original proctocolectomy specimen. Additionally, patients with primary sclerosing cholangitis are at increased risk for cancer development. Therefore, continued screening of patients, particularly those with prolonged disease duration, dysplasia or cancer in the excised specimen, and primary sclerosing cholangitis, is essential.

Pouch Failure. A pouch failure rate of 5% to 10% has been reported at most high-volume centers. Risk factors for pouch failure include (a) patient and disease factors—comorbidity, Crohn disease, and prior anal pathology; (b) operative factors—hand-sewn anastomosis, tension on the ileoanal anastomosis, and use of an ileostomy; and (c) postoperative factors—anastomotic separation, pelvic sepsis, and fistula.[87,97,101,102] Although the development of Crohn disease in the ileoanal pouch has often been implicated in pouch failure, treatment with infliximab can result in acceptable pouch function in up to 67% of patients.[103]

Sexual Dysfunction. Patients undergoing proctectomy are at risk for injury to the parasympathetic nerve trunks. The morbidity from this injury includes difficulty with bladder emptying, and in men, impotence and retrograde ejaculation. These symptoms may be transient or permanent and are reported to occur in 1% to 20% of patients.[104,105]

Women may also suffer from dyspareunia (7% to 30%) and leakage during intercourse (2%).[104,105] There is increasing evidence that fertility following restorative proctocolectomy is substantially reduced, likely secondary to pelvic adhesions.[106] A 2006 meta-analysis study found a threefold increase in infertility among women who had undergone ileal pouch–anal anastomosis compared to women with colitis who were managed medically.[106]

Quality of Life. Quality of life incorporates physical and functional outcomes as well as psychosocial factors that contribute to the well-being of patients. Most patients who have had an operative procedure to manage their disease have high 5 satisfaction scores. Although pelvic pouch patients may experience operative complications and have imperfect functional results (i.e., frequent bowel movements and seepage of stool), 95% of patients report satisfaction with postoperative outcomes.[107–110]

References

1. Langholz E, Munckholm P, Davidsen M, et al. Course of ulcerative colitis: analysis of changes in disease activity over years. *Gastroenterology* 1994; 107:3–11.
2. Vind I, Riis L, Jess T, et al. Increasing incidences of inflammatory bowel disease and decreasing surgery rates in Copenhagen City and County, 2003–2005: a population-based study from the Danish Crohn colitis database. *Am J Gastroenterol* 2006;101(6):1274–1282.
3. Stowe SP, Redmond SR, Stormont JM, et al. An epidemiologic study of inflammatory bowel disease in Rochester, New York. Hospital incidence. *Gastroenterology* 1990;98(1):104–110.
4. Loftus EV Jr, Silverstein MD, Sandborn WJ, et al. Ulcerative colitis in Olmsted County, Minnesota, 1940–1993: incidence, prevalence, and survival. *Gut* 2000;46(3):336–343.
5. Bernstein CN, Blanchard JF, Rawsthorne P, et al. Epidemiology of Crohn's disease and ulcerative colitis in a central Canadian province: a population-based study. *Am J Epidemiol* 1999;149(10):916–924.
6. Langholz E, Munkholm P, Nielsen OH, et al. Incidence and prevalence of ulcerative colitis in Copenhagen county from 1962 to 1987. *Scand J Gastroenterol* 1991;26(12):1247–1256.
7. Sood A, Midha V. Epidemiology of inflammatory bowel disease in Asia. *Indian J Gastroenterol* 2007;26(6):285–289.
8. Stonnington CM, Phillips SF, Melton LJ III, et al. Chronic ulcerative colitis: incidence and prevalence in a community. *Gut* 1987;28(4):402–409.
9. Harries AD, Jones L, Heatley RV, et al. Smoking habits and inflammatory bowel disease: effect on nutrition. *Br Med J (Clin Res Ed)* 1982;284(6323): 1161.
10. Calkins BM. A meta-analysis of the role of smoking in inflammatory bowel disease. *Dig Dis Sci* 1989;34(12):1841–1854.
11. Loftus EV Jr, Sandborn WJ, Tremaine WJ, et al. Primary sclerosing cholangitis is associated with nonsmoking: a case-control study. *Gastroenterology* 1996;110(5):1496–1502.
12. van Erpecum KJ, Smits SJ, van de Meeberg PC, et al. Risk of primary sclerosing cholangitis is associated with nonsmoking behavior. *Gastroenterology* 1996;110(5):1503–1506.
13. Boyko EJ, Koepsell TD, Perera DR, et al. Risk of ulcerative colitis among former and current cigarette smokers. *N Engl J Med* 1987;316(12): 707–710.
14. Boyko EJ, Perera DR, Koepsell TD, et al. Effects of cigarette smoking on the clinical course of ulcerative colitis. *Scand J Gastroenterol* 1988;23(9): 1147–1152.
15. Beaugerie L, Massot N, Carbonnel F, et al. Impact of cessation of smoking on the course of ulcerative colitis. *Am J Gastroenterol* 2001;96(7): 2113–2116.
16. Koutroubakis IE, Vlachonikolis IG, Kouroumalis EA. Role of appendicitis and appendectomy in the pathogenesis of ulcerative colitis: a critical review. *Inflamm Bowel Dis* 2002;8(4):277–286.
17. Andersson RE, Olaison G, Tysk C, et al. Appendectomy and protection against ulcerative colitis. *N Engl J Med* 2001;344(11):808–814.
18. Frisch M, Biggar RJ. Appendectomy and protection against ulcerative colitis. *N Engl J Med* 2001;345(3):222–223.
19. Frisch M, Johansen C, Mellemkjaer L, et al. Appendectomy and subsequent risk of inflammatory bowel diseases. *Surgery* 2001;130(1):36–43.
20. Naganuma M, Iizuka B, Torii A, et al. Appendectomy protects against the development of ulcerative colitis and reduces its recurrence: results of a multicenter case-controlled study in Japan. *Am J Gastroenterol* 2001; 96(4):1123–1126.
21. Radford-Smith GL, Edwards JE, Purdie DM, et al. Protective role of appendicectomy on onset and severity of ulcerative colitis and Crohn's disease. *Gut* 2002;51(6):808–813.
22. Watts DA, Satsangi J. The genetic jigsaw of inflammatory bowel disease. *Gut* 2002;50(suppl 3):III31–III36.
23. Farmer RG, Michener WM, Mortimer EA. Studies of family history among patients with inflammatory bowel disease. *Clin Gastroenterol* 1980;9(2):271–277.
24. Orholm M, Munkholm P, Langholz E, et al. Familial occurrence of inflammatory bowel disease. *N Engl J Med* 1991;324(2):84–88.
25. Satsangi J, Parkes M, Louis E, et al. Two stage genome-wide search in inflammatory bowel disease provides evidence for susceptibility loci on chromosomes 3, 7 and 12. *Nat Genet* 1996;14(2):199–202.
26. Stokkers PC, Reitsma PH, Tytgat GN, et al. HLA-DR and -DQ phenotypes in inflammatory bowel disease: a meta-analysis. *Gut* 1999;45(3):395–401.
27. Shih DQ, Targan SR. Immunopathogenesis of inflammatory bowel disease. *World J Gastroenterol* 2008;14(3):390–400.
28. Holtmann MH, Galle PR. Current concept of pathophysiological understanding and natural course of ulcerative colitis. *Langenbecks Arch Surg* 2004;389(5):341–349.
29. Bernstein CN. Extraintestinal manifestations of inflammatory bowel disease. *Curr Gastroenterol Rep* 2001;3(6):477–483.
30. Apgar JT. Newer aspects of inflammatory bowel disease and its cutaneous manifestations: a selective review. *Semin Dermatol* 1991;10(3):138–147.
31. Danzi T. Extraintestinal manifestation of idiopathic inflammatory bowel disease. *Arch Intern Med* 1988;148:297–302.
32. Mintz R, Feller ER, Bahr RL, et al. Ocular manifestations of inflammatory bowel disease. *Inflamm Bowel Dis* 2004;10(2):135–139.
33. Levine JB, Lukawski-Trubish D. Extraintestinal considerations in inflammatory bowel disease. *Gastroenterol Clin North Am* 1995;24(3):633–646.
34. Raj V, Lichtenstein DR. Hepatobiliary manifestations of inflammatory bowel disease. *Gastroenterol Clin North Am* 1999;28(2):491–513.
35. Olsson R, Danielsson A, Jarnerot G, et al. Prevalence of primary sclerosing cholangitis in patients with ulcerative colitis. *Gastroenterology* 1991; 100(5 Pt 1):1319–1323.
36. Wiesner RH, Grambsch PM, Dickson ER, et al. Primary sclerosing cholangitis: natural history, prognostic factors and survival analysis. *Hepatology* 1989;10(4):430–436.
37. Mir-Madjlessi SH, Farmer RG, Sivak MV Jr. Bile duct carcinoma in patients with ulcerative colitis. Relationship to sclerosing cholangitis: report of six cases and review of the literature. *Dig Dis Sci* 1987;32(2): 145–154.
38. MacLean AR, Lilly L, Cohen Z, et al. Outcome of patients undergoing liver transplantation for primary sclerosing cholangitis. *Dis Colon Rectum* 2003;46(8):1124–1128.
39. Kelly DM, Emre S, Guy SR, et al. Liver transplant recipients are not at increased risk for nonlymphoid solid organ tumors. *Cancer* 1998;83(6): 1237–1243.
40. Nakamura RM, Matsutani M, Barry M. Advances in clinical laboratory tests for inflammatory bowel disease. *Clin Chim Acta* 2003;335(1–2): 9–20.
41. Dayton MT, Larsen KR, Christiansen DD. Equivalent function, quality of life, and pouch survival rates after ileal pouch-anal anastomosis for indeterminate and ulcerative colitis. *Ann Surg* 2002;236(1):43–48.
42. Thalen A, Brattsand R, Andersson PH. Development of glucocorticosteroids with enhanced ratio between topical and systemic effects. *Acta Derm Venereol Suppl (Stockh)* 1989;151:11–19, 47–52.
43. Lennard L. The clinical pharmacology of 6-mercaptopurine. *Eur J Clin Pharmacol* 1992;43(4):329–339.
44. Hawthorne AB, Logan RF, Hawkey CJ, et al. Randomised controlled trial of azathioprine withdrawal in ulcerative colitis. *BMJ* 1992;305(6844): 20–22.
45. Present DH, Meltzer SJ, Krumholz MP, et al. 6-Mercaptopurine in the management of inflammatory bowel disease: short- and long-term toxicity. *Ann Intern Med* 1989;111(8):641–649.
46. Lichtiger S, Present DH. Preliminary report: cyclosporin in treatment of severe active ulcerative colitis. *Lancet* 1990;336(8706):16–19.
47. Lichtiger S, Present DH, Kornbluth A, et al. Cyclosporine in severe ulcerative colitis refractory to steroid therapy. *N Engl J Med* 1994;330(26): 1841–1845.
48. Liu J, Farmer JD Jr, Lane WS, et al. Calcineurin is a common target of cyclophilin-cyclosporin A and FKBP-FK506 complexes. *Cell* 1991;66(4): 807–815.

49. Reed JC, Prystowsky MB, Nowell PC. Regulation of gene expression in lectin-stimulated or lymphokine-stimulated T lymphocytes. Effects of cyclosporine. *Transplantation* 1988;46(2)(suppl):85S–89S.
50. Hyde GM, Thillainayagam AV, Jewell DP. Intravenous cyclosporin as rescue therapy in severe ulcerative colitis: time for a reappraisal? *Eur J Gastroenterol Hepatol* 1998;10(5):411–413.
51. Loftus CG, Egan LJ, Sandborn WJ. Cyclosporine, tacrolimus, and mycophenolate mofetil in the treatment of inflammatory bowel disease. *Gastroenterol Clin North Am* 2004;33(2):141–169, vii.
52. Rutgeerts P, Sandborn WJ, Feagan BG, et al. Infliximab for induction and maintenance therapy for ulcerative colitis. *N Engl J Med* 2005;353(23): 2462–2476.
53. Panaccione R, Rutgeers P, Sandborn WJ, et al. Review article: treatment algorithms to maximize remission and minimize corticosteroid dependence in patients with inflammatory bowel disease. *Aliment Pharmacol Ther* 2008;28:647–688.
54. Travis SP, Farrant JM, Ricketts C, et al. Predicting outcome in severe ulcerative colitis. *Gut* 1996;38:905–910.
55. Hawley PR. Emergency surgery for ulcerative colitis. *World J Surg* 1988; 12(2):169–173.
56. Bernstein CN, Shanahan F, Weinstein WM. Are we telling the truth about surveillance colonoscopy in ulcerative colitis? *Lancet* 1994;343:71–74.
57. Lim CH, Dixon MF, Vail A, et al. Ten year follow up of ulcerative colitis patients with and without low grade dysplasia. *Gut* 2003;52(8):1127–1132.
58. Berfits R, Ljung T, Jaramillo E, et al. Low-grade dysplasia in extensive, long-standing inflammatory bowel disease: a follow-up study. *Dis Colon Rectum* 2002;45(5):615–620.
59. Thomas T, Abrams KA, Robinson RJ, et al. Meta-analysis: cancer risk of low-grade dysplasia in chronic ulcerative colitis. *Aliment Pharmacol Ther* 2007;25(6):657–668.
60. Odze RD, Goldblum J, Noffsinger A, et al. Interobserver variability in the diagnosis of ulcerative colitis-associated dysplasia by telepathology. *Mod Pathol* 2002;15:379–386.
61. Collins RH Jr, Feldman M, Fordtran JS. Colon cancer, dysplasia, and surveillance in patients with ulcerative colitis. A critical review. *N Engl J Med* 1987;316(26):1654–1658.
62. Ekbom A, Helmick C, Zack M, et al. Ulcerative colitis and colorectal cancer. A population-based study. *N Engl J Med* 1990;323(18):1228–1233.
63. Ekbom A. Risk of cancer in ulcerative colitis. *J Gastrointest Surg* 1998; 2(4):312–313.
64. Eaden JA, Abrams KR, Mayberry JF. The risk of colorectal cancer in ulcerative colitis: a meta-analysis. *Gut* 2001;48(4):526–535.
65. Connell WR, Lennard-Jones JE, Williams CB, et al. Factors affecting the outcome of endoscopic surveillance for cancer in ulcerative colitis. *Gastroenterology* 1994;107(4):934–944.
66. Bernstein CN. Ulcerative colitis with low-grade dysplasia. *Gastroenterology* 2004;127(3):950–956.
67. Oakley JR, Jagelman DG, Fazio VW, et al. Complications and quality of life after ileorectal anastomosis for ulcerative colitis. *Am J Surg* 1985; 149(1):23–30.
68. Baker WN, Glass RE, Ritchie JK, et al. Cancer of the rectum following colectomy and ileorectal anastomosis for ulcerative colitis. *Br J Surg* 1978; 65(12):862–868.
69. Parks AG, Nicholls RJ, Belliveau P. Proctocolectomy with ileal reservoir and anal anastomosis. *Br J Surg* 1980;67(8):533–538.
70. Utsunomiya J, Iwama T, Imajo M, et al. Total colectomy, mucosal proctectomy, and ileoanal anastomosis. *Dis Colon Rectum* 1980;23(7):459–466.
71. Martin LW, LeCoultre C, Schubert WK. Total colectomy and mucosal proctectomy with preservation of continence in ulcerative colitis. *Ann Surg* 1977;186(4):477–480.
72. Melville DM, Ritchie JK, Nicholls RJ, et al. Surgery for ulcerative colitis in the era of the pouch: the St Mark's Hospital experience. *Gut* 1994;35(8): 1076–1080.
73. Sugerman HJ, Newsome HH. Stapled ileoanal anastomosis without a temporary ileostomy. *Am J Surg* 1994;167(1):58–65; discussion 65–66.
74. Fleshman JW, Cohen Z, McLeod RS, et al. The ileal reservoir and ileoanal anastomosis procedure. Factors affecting technical and functional outcome. *Dis Colon Rectum* 1988;31(1):10–16.
75. Wexner SD, Rosen L, Lowry A, et al. Practice parameters for the treatment of mucosal ulcerative colitis—supporting documentation. The Standards Practice Task Force. The American Society of Colon and Rectal Surgeons. *Dis Colon Rectum* 1997;40(11):1277–1285.
76. Sagar PM, Lewis W, Holdsworth PJ, et al. One-stage restorative proctocolectomy without temporary defunctioning ileostomy. *Dis Colon Rectum* 1992;35(6):582–588.
77. Fazio VW, Ziv Y, Church JM, et al. Ileal pouch-anal anastomoses complications and function in 1005 patients. *Ann Surg* 1995;222(2): 120–127.
78. Marcello PW, Roberts PL, Schoetz DJ Jr, et al. Obstruction after ileal pouch-anal anastomosis: a preventable complication? *Dis Colon Rectum* 1993;36(12):1105–1111.
79. Becker JM, Dayton MT, Fazio VW, et al. Prevention of postoperative abdominal adhesions by a sodium hyaluronate-based bioresorbable membrane: a prospective, randomized, double-blind multicenter study. *J Am Coll Surg* 1996;183(4):297–306.
80. Senapati A, Nicholls RJ, Ritchie JK, et al. Temporary loop ileostomy for restorative proctocolectomy. *Br J Surg* 1993;80(5):628–630.
81. Mikkola K, Luukkonen P, Jarvinen HJ. Long-term results of restorative proctocolectomy for ulcerative colitis. *Int J Colorectal Dis* 1995;10(1): 10–14.
82. Tan HT, Connolly AB, Morton D, et al. Results of restorative proctocolectomy in the elderly. *Int J Colorectal Dis* 1997;12(6):319–322.
83. Blumberg D, Opelka FG, Hicks TC, et al. Restorative proctocolectomy: Ochsner Clinic experience. *South Med J* 2001;94(5):467–471.
84. Heuschen UA, Hinz U, Allemeyer EH, et al. Risk factors for ileoanal J pouch-related septic complications in ulcerative colitis and familial adenomatous polyposis. *Ann Surg* 2002;235(2):207–216.
85. Heuschen UA, Allemeyer EH, Hinz U, et al. Outcome after septic complications in J pouch procedures. *Br J Surg* 2002;89(2):194–200.
86. Wexner SD, Wong WD, Rothenberger DA, et al. The ileoanal reservoir. *Am J Surg* 1990;159(1):178–183; discussion 183–185.
87. Gemlo BT, Wong WD, Rothenberger DA, et al. Ileal pouch-anal anastomosis. Patterns of failure. *Arch Surg* 1992;127(7):784–786; discussion 787.
88. Shah NS, Remzi F, Massmann A, et al. Management and treatment outcome of pouch-vaginal fistulas following restorative proctocolectomy. *Dis Colon Rectum* 2003;46(7):911–917.
89. Dozois RR, Kelly KA, Welling DR, et al. Ileal pouch-anal anastomosis: comparison of results in familial adenomatous polyposis and chronic ulcerative colitis. *Ann Surg* 1989;210(3):268–271; discussion 272–273.
90. McLeod RS. Surgery for inflammatory bowel diseases. *Dig Dis* 2003; 21(2):168–179.
91. Stocchi L, Pemberton JH. Pouch and pouchitis. *Gastroenterol Clin North Am* 2001;30(1):223–421.
92. Gionchetti P, Amadini C, Rizzello F, et al. Probiotics for the treatment of postoperative complications following intestinal surgery. *Best Pract Res Clin Gastroenterol* 2003;17(5):821–831.
93. Gionchetti P, Rizzello F, Helwig U, et al. Prophylaxis of pouchitis onset with probiotic therapy: a double-blind, placebo-controlled trial. *Gastroenterology* 2003;124(5):1202–1209.
94. Yantiss RK, Sapp HL, Farraye FA, et al. Histologic predictors of pouchitis in patients with chronic ulcerative colitis. *Am J Surg Pathol* 2004;28(8): 999–1006.
95. Kelly KA. Anal sphincter-saving operations for chronic ulcerative colitis. *Am J Surg* 1992;163(1):5–11.
96. Fazio VW, Tekkis PP, Remzi F, et al. Quantification of risk for pouch failure after ileal pouch anal anastomosis surgery. *Ann Surg* 2003:238(4): 605–614; discussion 614–617.
97. Lavery IC, Sirimarco MT, Ziv Y, et al. Anal canal inflammation after ileal pouch-anal anastomosis. The need for treatment. *Dis Colon Rectum* 1995;38(8):803–806.
98. Shen B, Lashner BA, Bennett AE, et al. Treatment of rectal cuff inflammation (cuffitis) in patients with ulcerative colitis following restorative proctocolectomy and ileal pouch-anal anastomosis. *Am J Gastroenterol* 2004; 99(8):1527–1531.
99. Koh PK, Doumit J, Downs-Kelly E, et al. Ileo-anal J-pouch cancer: an unusual case in an unusual location. *Tech Coloproctol* 2008;12:341–345.
100. Laureti S, Ugolini F, D'Errico A, et al. Adenocarcinoma below ileoanal anastomosis for ulcerative colitis: report of a case and review of the literature. *Dis Colon Rectum* 2002;45(3):418–421.
101. MacRae HM, McLeod RS, Cohen Z, et al. Risk factors for pelvic pouch failure. *Dis Colon Rectum* 1997;40(3):257–262.
102. Lepisto A, Luukkonen P, Jarvinen HJ. Cumulative failure rate of ileal pouch-anal anastomosis and quality of life after failure. *Dis Colon Rectum* 2002;45(10):1289–1294.
103. Colombel JF, Ricart E, Loftus EV Jr, et al. Management of Crohn's disease of the ileoanal pouch with infliximab. *Am J Gastroenterol* 2003:98(10): 2239–2244.
104. Damgaard B, Wettergren A, Kirkegaard P. Social and sexual function following ileal pouch-anal anastomosis. *Dis Colon Rectum* 1995;38(3): 286–289.
105. Hueting WE, Gooszen HG, van Laarhoven CJH. Sexual function and continence after ileo pouch anal anastomosis: a comparison between a meta-analysis and a questionnaire study. *Int J Colorectal Dis* 2004;19: 215–218.
106. Waljee A, Waljee J, Morris AM, et al. Threefold increased risk of infertility: a meta-analysis of infertility after ileal pouch anal anastomosis in ulcerative colitis. *Gut* 2006;55(11):1575–1580.
107. McLeod RS, Baxter NN. Quality of life of patients with inflammatory bowel disease after surgery. *World J Surg* 1998;22(4):375–381.
108. Berndtsson I, Lindholm E, Oresland T, et al. Long-term outcome after ileal pouch-anal anastomosis: function and health-related quality of life. *Dis Colon Rectum* 2007:50(10):1545–1552.
109. Pemberton JH, Phillips SF, Ready RR, et al. Quality of life after Brooke ileostomy and ileal pouch-anal anastomosis. Comparison of performance status. *Ann Surg* 1989;209(5):620–626; discussion 626–628.
110. Kohler LW, Pemberton JH, Zinsmeister AR, et al. Quality of life after proctocolectomy. A comparison of Brooke ileostomy, Kock pouch, and ileal pouch-anal anastomosis. *Gastroenterology* 1991;101(3):679–684.
111. Tulchinsky H, Dotan I, Alper A. Comprehensive pouch clinic concept for follow-up of patients after ileal pouch anal anastomosis: report of 3 year experience in a tertiary referral center. *Inflamm Bowel Dis* 2008;14: 1125–1132.

CHAPTER 67 ■ COLONIC POLYPS AND POLYPOSIS SYNDROMES

C. RICHARD BOLAND AND ROBERT S. BRESALIER

KEY POINTS

1. Colorectal neoplasia develops through multistep carcinogenesis that involves the gradual accumulation of genetic and epigenetic alterations in the genome. This process usually requires the presence of some form of genomic or epigenetic instability, and neoplasms may require several decades to evolve from their earliest stages to fully advanced disease.
2. Colorectal carcinoma usually evolves gradually from colorectal adenomas in clinically identifiable stages; removal of adenomas reduces the incidence of colorectal carcinoma.
3. Genetic and familial factors play an important role in the genesis of both the sporadic (common) and syndromic forms of colorectal neoplasia, such as familial adenomatous polyposis and Lynch syndrome.
4. The genetic basis of familial adenomatous polyposis and hereditary nonpolyposis colorectal cancer (called Lynch syndrome) have been identified, which facilitates the early identification and diagnosis of affected individuals.
5. A wide range of clinical heterogeneity is present in the familial colorectal cancer syndromes, and attenuated forms of familial adenomatous polyposis and Lynch syndrome can be subtle and a challenge to the clinician.

COLORECTAL POLYPS

The gastrointestinal tract accounts for more neoplastic disease than any other organ system in the body. In North America, neoplasms of the colon and rectum have attracted the greatest interest because of their relatively high incidence, and because appropriate intervention can dramatically modify the morbidity and mortality associated with them. The adenoma is the most common precursor of colorectal cancer, and early removal of adenomatous polyps can interrupt the natural history of the disease and prevent death.

Colorectal cancers can develop through one of at least three molecular pathways, and each variety appears to have some unique clinical and pathologic features. The adenoma–carcinoma sequence is virtually canonical at this time and describes the common pathway taken by neoplasms that have "chromosomal instability." It has subsequently been proposed that "serrated" polyps may be precursors of colon cancers with the microsatellite instability (MSI) phenotype. These polyps are a pathologic hybrid, showing features of both hyperplastic and adenomatous polyps. It is becoming increasingly important to understand the clinical behavior of colorectal neoplasms in the context of the genetic and molecular bases of these lesions.

Classification of Colorectal Polyps

The term *polyp* (from the Greek *polypous*, "morbid excrescence") refers to a macroscopic protrusion of the colonic mucosa into the bowel lumen. This can result from abnormal growth of the mucosa or from a submucosal process that causes the mucosa to protrude into the lumen. Mucosal polyps can be *sessile*, protruding directly from the colonic wall, or *pedunculated*, extending from the mucosa through a fibrovascular stalk.

Mucosal polyps in the colon can be categorized as *neoplastic*, with malignant potential, and *nonneoplastic*, with no malignant potential (Table 67.1). Neoplastic polyps include benign adenomatous polyps that may evolve to carcinoma, adenomatous polyps that contain foci of intramucosal carcinoma (carcinoma in situ), and adenomatous polyps in which carcinoma has penetrated the muscularis mucosae (invasive carcinoma). A serrated polyp contains adenomatous features admixed with features of a hyperplastic polyp. A serrated polyp appears to originate in a manner unique from typical adenomas, but is also a premalignant lesion. Sometimes a polyp is found in which carcinoma has completely obliterated the adenomatous tissue from which it arose (polypoid carcinoma).

Nonneoplastic mucosal polyps include hyperplastic polyps, juvenile polyps, Peutz-Jeghers hamartomas, and a variety of inflammatory polyps, including those associated with inflammatory bowel disease. Any submucosal lesion can expand to push the mucosa into the bowel lumen and thus appear as a polypoid lesion. Examples include lipomas, leiomyomas, colitis cystica profunda, pneumatosis cystoides intestinalis, lymphoid aggregates, primary or secondary lymphomas, carcinoid tumors, and other metastatic neoplasms.

Neoplastic Mucosal Polyps. Most colorectal cancers arise in preexisting adenomatous polyps. Neoplastic mucosal epithelium evolves through a series of progressive, cumulative molecular and cellular steps that lead to altered proliferation, cellular accumulation, and glandular disarray. In some instances, the polyp also achieves the ability to invade and metastasize through the adenoma-to-carcinoma sequence.

(1) Several lines of evidence support the assumption that colorectal adenocarcinomas arise from adenomatous polyps. The descriptive epidemiology of colonic adenomas parallels that of carcinomas, but the benign lesions occur earlier. Adenomas are rare in geographic regions with a low prevalence of colon cancer, and the distribution of adenomas in the colon parallels that of carcinomas. Adenomas often occur in anatomic proximity to colon cancers, and cancer risk is proportional to the number of adenomas present synchronously or metachronously in a patient. Cancer is often present in polyps removed endoscopically or surgically, and the risk for cancer is proportional to the degree of dysplasia or atypia in the polyp.

TABLE 67.1 CLASSIFICATION

CLASSIFICATION OF COLORECTAL POLYPS

MUCOSAL POLYPS	
Neoplastic	
Benign	
Adenomatous polyps	
Tubular adenoma	
Tubulovillous adenoma	
Villous adenoma	
Serrated polyp	
Malignant	
Carcinoma in situ	
Invasive carcinoma	
Polypoid carcinoma	
Nonneoplastic	
Hyperplastic polyps	
Juvenile polyps	
Peutz-Jeghers polyps	
Inflammatory polyps	
Normal epithelium	
SUBMUCOSAL POLYPS	
Lipomas	
Leiomyomas	
Colitis cystica profunda	
Pneumatosis cystoides intestinalis	
Lymphoid aggregates	
Lymphoma (primary or secondary)	
Carcinoids	
Metastatic neoplasms	

Conversely, histologically evident residual adenomatous tissue may be found surrounding carcinomas. Most important, results from several studies indicate that the systematic removal of adenomatous polyps during screening proctosigmoidoscopy or surveillance colonoscopy decreases the risk for the development of colorectal cancers and death from this disease.

Pathogenesis

Molecular Biology. Genetic changes that lead to the development of adenomas (and carcinomas) can be loosely organized into three major classes: alterations in proto-oncogenes, loss of tumor-suppressor gene activity, and abnormalities of genes involved in DNA repair (Fig. 67.1). Several different mechanisms are involved in altering these genes. Typically, oncogenes become overactive by mutation, rearrangement, or amplification. Tumor-suppressor genes become inactivated by mutation or deletion or silenced through promoter methylation. Tumor-suppressor genes require inactivation of both
2 copies of alleles, making this process more complex. It is now clear, however, that the development of adenoma and carcinoma is always associated with the progressive accumulation of genetic changes, and this process is termed *multistep carcinogenesis*.[1]

In familial adenomatous polyposis (FAP), Lynch syndrome (previously called hereditary nonpolyposis colorectal cancer [HNPCC]), and other familial syndromes, the first genetic alteration is inherited in the germline. Environmental factors are then required for the additional genetic mutations that lead to malignant transformation. The clinical phenotype for the inherited predispositions to gastrointestinal cancer is initially normal; such individuals might be thought of as having an exceptional susceptibility to environmental stress. The germline mutation provides the first "hit," which greatly increases the likelihood of neoplasia and the likelihood that the disease will occur at a
3 young age.[2] FAP and Lynch syndrome account for about 4% of all colorectal cancers, but it is estimated that as many as 30% of colorectal cancers occur in the context of a positive family history.

"Sporadic" polyps and cancers are associated with multiple somatic mutations, all of which are caused by spontaneous decay of DNA, exogenous insults, or are accidents that occur during the replication of DNA. Adenomas and cancers that develop arise through genomic instability, a process that increases the likelihood that epithelial cells will acquire the number of mutations needed to attain a neoplastic state.[3] Destabilization of the genome is a prerequisite to carcinogenesis. This most commonly involves chromosomal instability, which is manifested as widespread chromosomal deletions, duplications, and rearrangements that produce aneuploidy. Alternatively, increased rates of mutations, often in tandemly repeated DNA sequences known as *microsatellites* (microsatellite instability) or a form of epigenetic instability called the CpG island methylator phenotype (CIMP), in which genes are inappropriately silenced by promoter methylation,[4] are mechanisms that can lead to progressive multistep carcinogenesis. Genomic (or epigenetic) instability generates a large number of random alterations, which are largely deleterious, and leads to the demise of the affected cell. However, occasional genetic alterations enhance growth and survival, and the successive accumulation of those changes will eventually facilitate the evolution of the neoplastic cell.

Cellular proto-oncogenes are a group of evolutionarily conserved genes that play a role in signal transduction and the normal regulation of cell growth. They function by being turned on when growth is stimulated and then turned off when sufficient growth has been achieved. Inappropriate activation of these genes, usually through mutation or rearrangement of the promoter sequences, leads to abnormal transmission of growth regulatory signals, which produce excessive cellular proliferation. Mutations of the K-*ras* oncogene, for example, can be found in about half of sporadic colorectal neoplasms, and this accelerates the growth potential of the early adenoma. Only 9% of small adenomas have *K-ras* mutations, whereas 58% of adenomas greater than 1 cm have a mutated *K-ras* gene. *K-ras* mutations are more common in pedunculated than flat adenomas. However, by themselves, *K-ras* mutations are not sufficient either for the neoplastic phenotype or for tumor progression. A combination of altered growth signals is required for an epithelial cell to achieve autonomous growth. The excessive growth then increases the likelihood that additional genetic alterations will occur.

The tumor-suppressor gene *APC* on chromosome 5q is critical to the evolution of the colorectal adenoma. Allelic losses of chromosome 5q occur early during carcinogenesis in the colon, and may be the initial step in the evolution of colorectal neoplasia.[5] A combination of mutation of one allele and loss of the other allele of *APC* (usually by partial chromosomal deletion or promoter methylation) commonly occurs in colorectal adenomas. *APC* acts as the "gatekeeper" of colonic epithelial proliferation, and inactivation of this gene will lead to net cellular proliferation and initiation of neoplasia in the colon.[6] The protein produced by the *APC* gene plays a central role in regulating the intracellular concentrations of the transcription factor, β-catenin. β-Catenin is highly expressed in cells at the base of the colonic crypt, where it stimulates proliferation.[7] As the cell commits to terminal differentiation, the *APC* gene is expressed, which downregulates β-catenin by phosphorylation, targeting it for degradation.

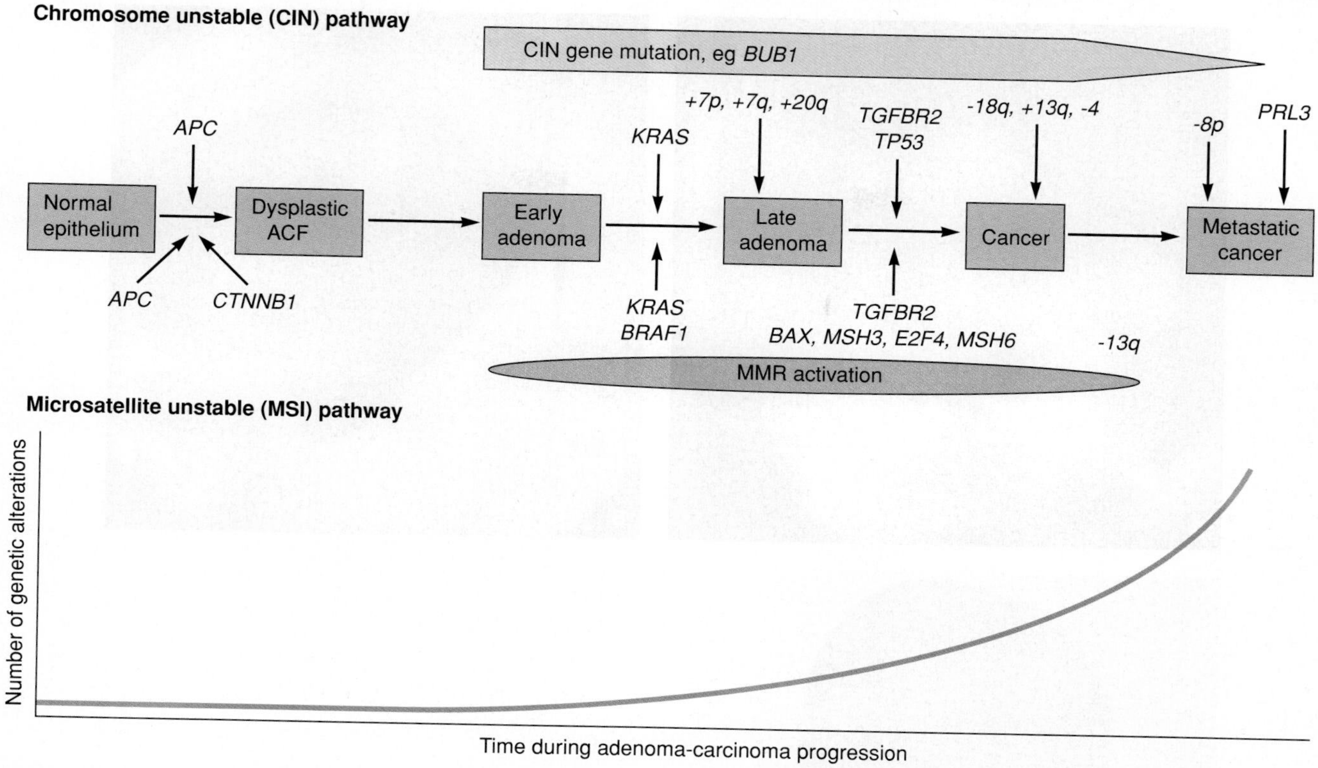

FIGURE 67.1. Proposed sequence of molecular genetic events in the evolution of colon cancer. Carcinomas arise from an accumulation of events whose sequence has been defined for two of the carcinogenesis pathways. As illustrated here, tumors progress through the adenoma-to-carcinoma sequence along pathways marked by chromosomal instability (CIN) or microsatellite instability (MSI). At least one more pathway, characterized by promoter methylation of tumor-suppressor genes, serrated polyps, and cancers with variable degrees of microsatellite instability, is incompletely understood, and not shown here. ACF, aberrant crypt focus; TGF, transforming growth factor. (After Grady WM. Genomic instability and colon cancer. *Cancer Metastasis Rev* 2004;23:11.)

Other genetic changes occur later in the adenoma-to-carcinoma sequence. Stepwise tumor progression is associated, in more than 75% of cases, with loss of one or more tumor-suppressor genes located on chromosome 18q. Several candidate genes are present in this location, and loss of chromosome 18 in the tumor is associated with a poor prognosis. Loss of the *SMAD 4* gene on 18q probably contributes the most to the progressively aggressive nature of neoplasms that advance through the pathway of chromosomal instability. Deletions of chromosome 17p involve the *p53* tumor-suppressor gene, and the p53 protein normally prevents cells with damaged DNA from progressing from the G1 to the S phase in the cell cycle. Inactivation of the *p53* gene mediates the conversion from adenoma to carcinoma.[8]

Alterations in genes that mediate DNA mismatch repair during replication cause Lynch syndrome, which historically was called HNPCC.[9] The genes responsible for Lynch syndrome are *MSH2*, *MLH1*, *MSH6*, and *PMS2*. In the hereditary disease, germline mutations inactivate one copy of the gene, and the other allele is inactivated by one of several "somatic" events that occurs locally in an individual colonic epithelial cell. This creates an inability to repair DNA mismatches and results in a diffuse mutational signature in the tumor called microsatellite instability, or MSI. This defect leads to the mutational inactivation of several key genes important for maintaining normal cellular behavior. The transforming growth factor-β receptor II (TGF-βRII), for example, is mutated in 85% of MSI colorectal cancers. This inactivates the receptor, renders the cell unresponsive to TGF-β, and permits it to escape normal growth regulation. The MSI multistep carcinogenesis pathway to tumor development is seen in about 15% of all colorectal cancers,[10] and progression from adenoma to carcinoma occurs in a shorter time period than occurs the chromosomal instability pathway seen in most colorectal cancers, which is thought to require a period of at least 10 to 20 years. MSI colorectal neoplasms appear to account for two clinical observations. First, the MSI pathway may account for the occurrence of cancers 1 or 2 years after a negative colonoscopic examination. Second, it may account for the relatively small number of adenomatous polyps found with MSI, since they may evolve into cancer in a shorter timeframe than usually occurs.

Histopathology and Malignant Potential

Adenomatous polyps are characterized according to their physical features, size, glandular structure, and degree of dysplasia, which all have important implications for clinical management. Polyps may be sessile, with a broad-based attachment to the colonic wall, or pedunculated, attached to the colonic wall by way of a fibrovascular stalk (Fig. 67.2). Whether a polyp is sessile or pedunculated typically determines whether the endoscopist can remove the polyp completely by snare polypectomy. Diminutive polyps that measure 5 mm or less in diameter are not likely to contain high-grade dysplasia or invasive carcinoma. Malignant potential increases with polyp size in all histologic groups of adenoma.

Adenomas are classified histologically according to their glandular structure. Aberrant (dysplastic) crypts and microadenomas may be the earliest lesions detected in the flat mucosa of patients at risk. These enlarge and progress to macroscopic adenomatous polyps. Tubular adenomas are characterized by a complex network of branching adenomatous glands, whereas villous adenomas contain fronds or folds of mucosa that have

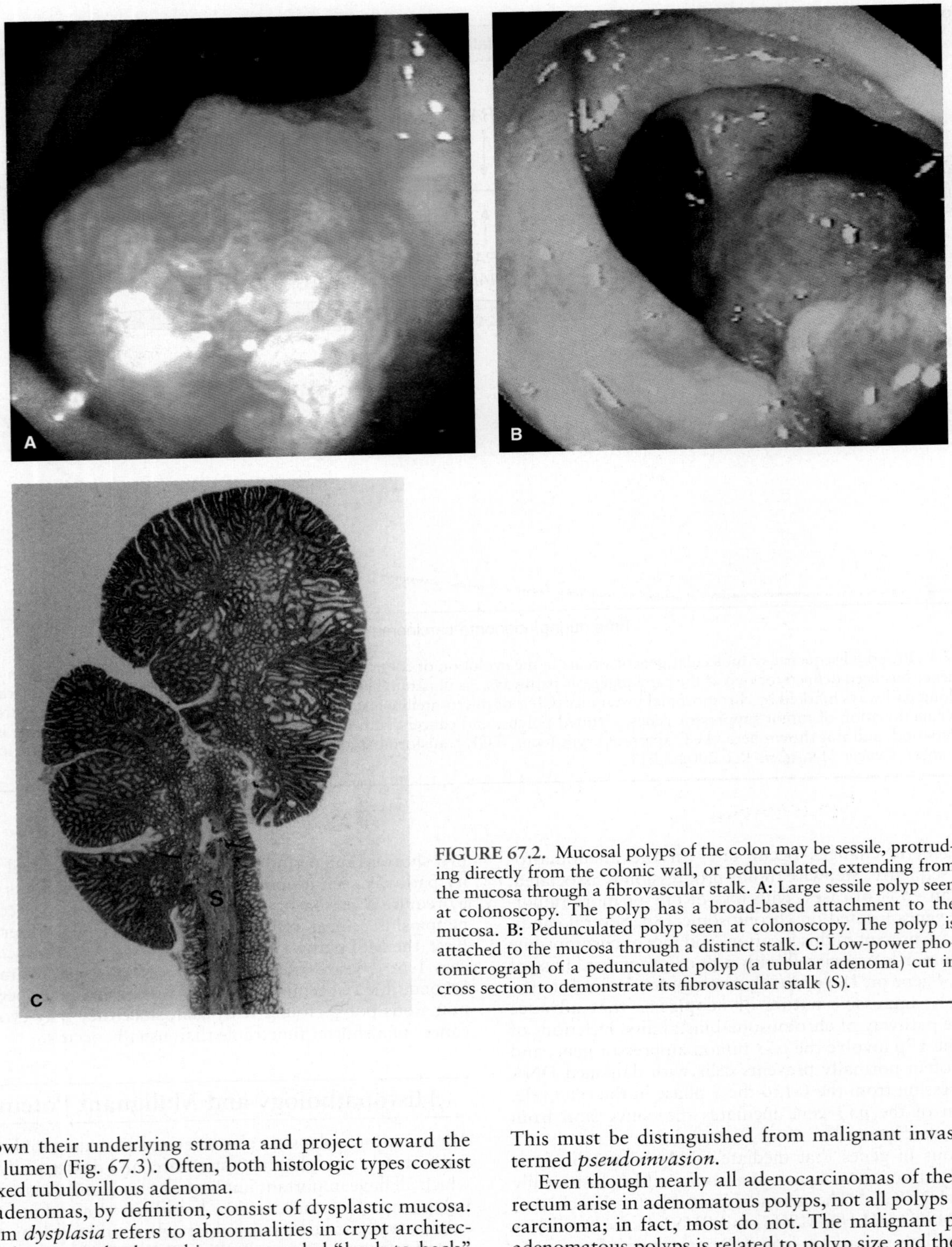

FIGURE 67.2. Mucosal polyps of the colon may be sessile, protruding directly from the colonic wall, or pedunculated, extending from the mucosa through a fibrovascular stalk. **A:** Large sessile polyp seen at colonoscopy. The polyp has a broad-based attachment to the mucosa. **B:** Pedunculated polyp seen at colonoscopy. The polyp is attached to the mucosa through a distinct stalk. **C:** Low-power photomicrograph of a pedunculated polyp (a tubular adenoma) cut in cross section to demonstrate its fibrovascular stalk (S).

overgrown their underlying stroma and project toward the colonic lumen (Fig. 67.3). Often, both histologic types coexist in a mixed tubulovillous adenoma.

All adenomas, by definition, consist of dysplastic mucosa. The term *dysplasia* refers to abnormalities in crypt architecture (such as irregular branching or crowded "back-to-back" glands) and cytologic detail (enlarged, pleomorphic, and hyperchromatic nuclei with multiple mitoses and pseudostratification; Fig. 67.4). Dysplasia may be mild, moderate, or severe, depending on the degree to which these characteristics are present. Severe, or high-grade, dysplasia represents carcinoma in situ when the basement membrane is intact. Extension into the lamina propria denotes intramucosal carcinoma. Invasion into the muscularis mucosae defines invasive carcinoma and the malignant polyp. The degree of dysplasia usually correlates with polyp size and the extent of villous architecture. Occasionally, nonmalignant adenomatous mucosa can be displaced below the muscularis mucosae, probably due to trauma associated with colonic motility. This must be distinguished from malignant invasion and is termed *pseudoinvasion*.

Even though nearly all adenocarcinomas of the colon and rectum arise in adenomatous polyps, not all polyps evolve into carcinoma; in fact, most do not. The malignant potential of adenomatous polyps is related to polyp size and the histologic characteristics. Large polyps and those with predominantly villous architecture are more likely to contain coincident carcinoma (Fig. 67.5). These features are interdependent, however, because large polyps are more likely to be villous and dysplastic. Adenomas that measure 0.5 cm or less are most often tubular adenomas and rarely contain severe dysplasia or carcinoma (<0.5% in autopsy series). Likewise, only 1% to 2% of adenomatous polyps smaller than 1 cm contain carcinoma, but autopsy studies suggest that as many as 40% of adenomas greater than 2 cm contain cancer. Data derived from the examination of colonoscopic polypectomy specimens indicate similar trends but suggest a lower incidence of cancer-containing polyps.

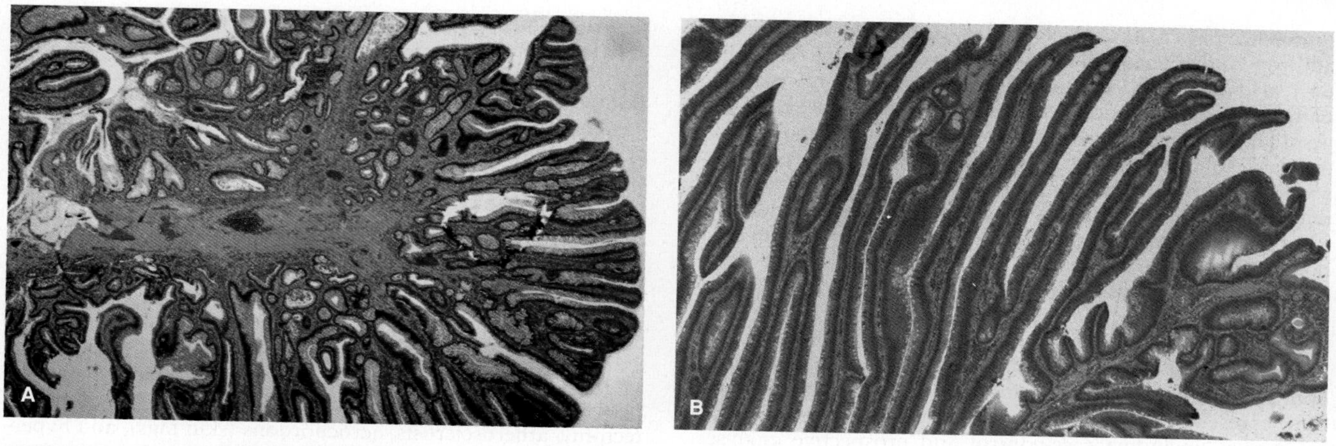

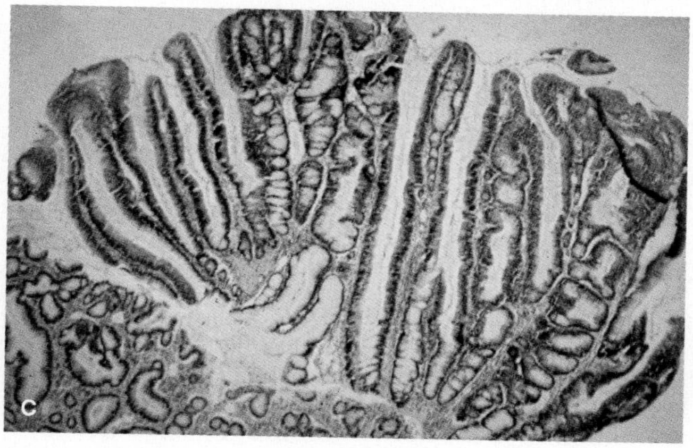

FIGURE 67.3. Histology of adenomatous polyps. **A:** Tubular adenomas are characterized by a complex network of branching adenomatous glands (see also C). **B:** Villous adenomas consist of glands that extend straight down from the surface to the base as fingerlike projections; this pattern may be suggested by the gross appearance of these polyps. **C:** Tubulovillous adenoma.

Epidemiology

Prevalence. The descriptive epidemiology of adenomatous polyps of the colon and rectum parallels that of colorectal carcinoma with relation to geographic distribution, age, prevalence, and genetic susceptibility. Like colorectal cancer, adenomas are common in Western countries such as the United States, but their prevalence traditionally has been low in parts of Asia, South America, and sub-Saharan Africa. Epidemiologic patterns for both adenomas and carcinomas are shifting with the acquisition of a "Western" lifestyle in many areas. Estimates of adenoma prevalence in the United States vary depending on the mode of data collection. Data from older studies were collected from autopsies and sometimes grouped all polyps together, whereas more recent studies have examined adenoma prevalence in the context of endoscopic screening. Studies using colonoscopy suggest an adenoma prevalence in patients without symptoms who are older than 50 years that ranges between 20% and 40%.

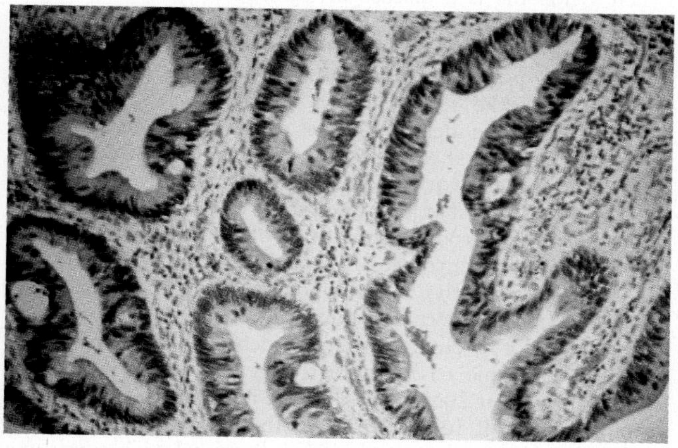

FIGURE 67.4. Moderate dysplasia. Dysplastic mucosa is characterized by crowded, irregular glands and cells with enlarged, hyperchromatic nuclei of varied size and shape that do not line up uniformly on the basement membrane (pseudopalisading). Adenomas are composed of dysplastic mucosa in which the degree of atypia may vary. These changes precede the development of invasive carcinoma.

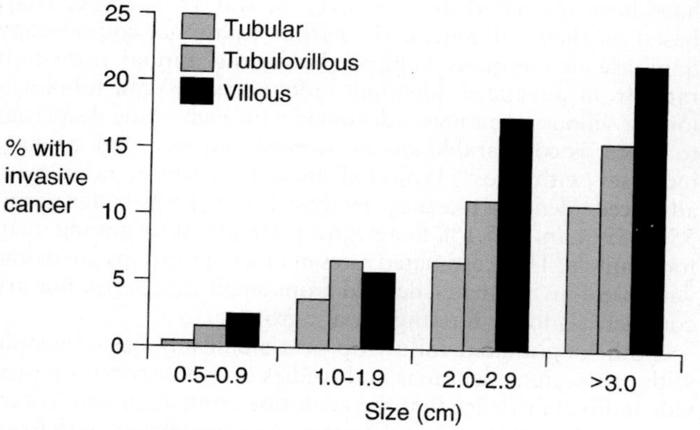

FIGURE 67.5. The relation of adenoma size and histology to malignant potential based on an analysis of 7,000 endoscopically removed polyps. The incidence of polyp-associated carcinoma determined from examination of polypectomy specimens is lower than that derived from early autopsy studies. (Data derived from Shinya H, Wolff WI. Morphology, anatomic distribution, and cancer potential of colonic polyps. *Ann Surg* 1979;1990:675.)

Prevalence rates from autopsy studies are 50% higher. Based on autopsy studies, one half to two thirds of people older than 65 years have colonic adenomas. Adenoma prevalence increases with age in all populations. Age-associated prevalence rates suggest that adenomas precede carcinomas in a given population by at least 5 to 10 years; it may be much longer, as polyps do not produce symptoms and, unlike cancers, dating the onset can only be estimated. Advancing age also correlates with multiplicity of polyps, polyp size, and higher degrees of dysplasia. In addition, 30% to 50% of patients with one adenoma have a synchronous adenoma elsewhere in the colon.[11]

Heredity. Heredity plays a role not only in FAP and Lynch syndrome but also in the development of sporadic adenomas. Sporadic (nonsyndromic) adenomatous polyps and colon cancers represent more than 95% of colorectal neoplasms. Clinical studies, including case-control and prospective analyses, indicate a two- to threefold increased risk for colon cancer among first-degree relatives of patients with a history of colonic adenoma or carcinoma.[12] The relative risk increases when there are more affected relatives and when adenomas and carcinomas occur in young relatives.[13] The impact of family history becomes prognostically insignificant in patients whose polyps are discovered after age 60. In most families, it is not possible to separate the impact of commonly shared genes from the impact of shared environmental exposures.

Anatomic Distribution. Autopsy series and colonoscopic examination of patients who do not have symptoms suggest that although adenomas are uniformly distributed throughout the colon, the distribution of clinically important larger adenomas is more similar to that of carcinomas, with a left-sided predominance.

Natural History. Adenomas are common in people older than 50 years, and although most carcinomas arise in adenomatous polyps, relatively few adenomas progress to carcinoma. Little precise information is available on what percentage of adenomas evolve to carcinomas. In Norway, an example of a high-risk Western population, it has been estimated that colorectal adenomas are present in 29% of the population older than 35 years. The conversion rate from adenoma to carcinoma in this group (based on cancer incidence from multiple tumor registries) has been calculated to be 0.25% per year. In other words, the risk that a colorectal cancer will develop in a polyp-bearing person within 10 years is 2.5%. The annual conversion rates to invasive cancer for people with adenomas larger than 1 cm, villous components, and severe dysplasia have been estimated to be 3%, 17%, and 37%, respectively, based on these inferences. Data from a national colonoscopy database in Germany suggested that the annual transition rates from advanced adenoma (adenomas ≥1 cm, tubulovillous or villous adenomas, adenomas with high-grade dysplasia) to cancer is comparable among women and men, but strongly increases with age.[14] Projected annual transition rates from advanced adenoma to cancer increased from 2.6% in age group 55 to 59 years to 5.1% in age group 80 and older among men, for example. These estimated rates in older age groups are in line with previous estimates derived from small case series but are considerably lower for younger age groups.

Both longitudinal follow-up of a small number of people with unresected adenomas and studies of age distribution provide indirect evidence that the evolution from adenoma to carcinoma takes at least 5 to 10 years. Age prevalence data from the National Polyp Study, for example, suggest that it may take as long as 5 to 10 years for normal-appearing mucosa to develop into a macroscopically visible adenomatous polyp, and an additional 3 to 5 years for invasive carcinoma to develop, in most instances. Case-control studies also support that the development of adenomas in the colon and the evolution to carcinoma occur slowly. Several studies have estimated that a significant protective effect of screening sigmoidoscopy may last at least 10 years.[15]

Associated Disease States. A number of clinical situations have been associated with a greater than average risk for adenoma development, but the evidence in most cases is tenuous. Although adenomas and carcinomas develop frequently in patients who have undergone urinary diversion by way of ureterosigmoidoscopy, this is largely of historical interest. Nonetheless, patients who have undergone this procedure require periodic colonoscopic surveillance for adenoma and carcinoma development. An increased prevalence of colonic adenomas and carcinomas has been reported in patients with acromegaly, and patients with elevated gastrin levels have been reported to be at risk for neoplasia. Alleged associations between colorectal adenomas and a history of prior cholecystectomy, atherosclerosis, acrochordons (skin tags), and hyperplastic polyps remain unproven.

Clinical Features

Adenomatous polyps of the colon and rectum are highly prevalent in Western societies, but most patients with colonic adenomas do not have symptoms directly referable to these lesions. Overt bleeding manifesting as hematochezia may occur with larger polyps, which may be evident when the polyps are located distally in the rectum. Adenomas typically lose less than 1 mL of blood daily unless they are 2 cm or larger in size. Although colorectal polyps are the most common lesions detected in patients without symptoms undergoing colonoscopy because of the presence of fecal occult blood, the polyps are probably not responsible for the bleeding. Very large colonic polyps may be associated with obstructive symptoms, such as lower abdominal cramping or alterations in bowel habits, but this is unusual. Secretory diarrhea with accompanying hypokalemia and hypochlorhydria has been associated with very large villous adenomas of the distal colon and rectum. This is a rare syndrome, and the search for secretagogues such as vasoactive intestinal polypeptide or prostaglandins in patients with polyps and diarrhea is infrequently productive.

Adenomas Associated with Lynch Syndrome and Its Variants

Lynch syndrome is a disease of autosomal dominant inheritance in which cancers arise in discrete adenomas, but polyposis (i.e., dozens or hundreds of polyps) does not occur. Initial case findings used the Amsterdam criteria, but these are not required to make the diagnosis of Lynch syndrome. The Amsterdam criteria identify families who have at least three relatives with colorectal cancer, one of whom is a first-degree relative of the other two; colorectal cancer must involve at least two generations; and at least one cancer case must occur before 50 years of age. Broader definitions of Lynch syndrome take into account the occurrence of extracolonic tumors and smaller kindreds.[16] Currently, the diagnosis of Lynch syndrome is made by finding a germline mutation in the DNA mismatch repair gene, not by clinical criteria. Adenomas and carcinomas in Lynch syndrome arise at an early age (adenomas may occur in patients in their 20s and 30s, with a mean age for carcinoma development of 40 to 45 years) and the polyps are often proximal in location and multiple. Women with Lynch syndrome are prone to cancers of the female genital tract (endometrium and ovary) in addition to colorectal neoplasms. The frequency of Lynch syndrome in the general population is difficult to determine, but Lynch syndrome accounts for about 3% to 4% of all colorectal cancer cases; this suggests that Lynch syndrome may occur in about 2 to 5 per 1,000 of the population.

Turcot syndrome is a term of historical significance, in which there is a concurrence of primary brain tumors and multiple colorectal adenomas or cancer in young people. With the advent of accurate genetic characterization, these families may be categorized as either FAP or Lynch syndrome, as brain tumors are an occasional complication of both diseases.[17]

Diagnosis

Most colorectal adenomas are asymptomatic and often are detected in the setting of an evaluation for unrelated colonic symptoms or occult blood in the stool. Similarly, adenomatous polyps frequently are detected when patients without symptoms are screened for colorectal neoplasia. Nevertheless, data strongly suggest that the detection and removal of adenomatous polyps are important in reducing colorectal cancer–related mortality.

4 In 2008, a joint guideline on screening and surveillance for early detection of colorectal cancer and adenomatous polyps was issued by the American Cancer Society (ACS), the U.S. Multi-Society Task Force on Colorectal Cancer (USMTF), and the American College of Radiology (ACR).[18] This update of previous guidelines is notable in that it grouped screening tests into those that primarily detect cancer (annual fecal occult blood tests [FOBTs] including those that are guaiac based or immunochemical, and stool DNA tests, interval not specified) and those that can detect early cancer and adenomatous polyps (flexible sigmoidoscopy every 5 years, colonoscopy every 10 years, double-contrast barium enema every 5 years, or computed tomography [CT] colonography every 5 years). In November 2008, the U.S. Preventative Services Task Force (USPSTF) also issued updated guidelines (Table 67.2).[19] Based on a targeted evidence-based review and a decision analytic modeling analysis, the USPSTF recommended screening of average-risk individuals age 50 to 75 years with high-sensitivity FOBTs annually, sigmoidoscopy every 5 years plus FOBTs every 3 years, or colonoscopy every 10 years. Notably, the USPSTF indicated that while the benefits of screening outweigh the potential harms for 50- to 75-year-olds, the likelihood that detection and early intervention will yield a mortality benefit declines after age 75 because of the long average time between adenoma development and cancer diagnosis. Routine screening was therefore not recommended for adults age 76 to 85 years, and screening was not recommended at all in adults older than 85 years of age. These guidelines also indicated that for all populations there is insufficient evidence to assess the benefits and harms of screening with CT colonography or fecal DNA testing.

Fecal Occult Blood Tests. Screening studies from both Europe and the United States indicate that a polyp is detected in about 30% of patients without symptoms who are 50 years of age or older and undergo colonoscopy for follow-up of a positive fecal occult blood test result. Blood loss from polyps is related to polyp size, and positive fecal occult blood test results are related to polyp size and proximity to the rectum. In one study in which rehydrated Hemoccult slides were used (rehydration results in greater sensitivity but also increases the number of false-positive findings), only 15% of polyps smaller than 1 cm were associated with a positive Hemoccult test result, whereas 80% of polyps larger than 2 cm were associated with a positive result. In another study, standard testing with Hemoccult cards detected 17% of adenomas smaller than 1 cm and 42% of adenomas larger than 1 cm. A prospective randomized study of fecal occult blood tests in which rehydrated Hemoccult cards were used indicated that annual testing reduces colorectal cancer–related deaths by 33% through 18 years of follow-up.[20] This study, in addition to two European trials, has also demonstrated a 15% to 21% reduction in colon cancer–related death from biennial fecal occult blood testing.[21] Thus, unless one rigorously performs the fecal occult blood test on an annual basis, the reduction in colorectal cancer mortality will be disappointing.

Methods that may decrease the false-positive FOBT rates while maintaining or increasing sensitivity currently are being refined and compared for efficiency with Hemoccult-type slide tests. Fecal immunochemical tests (FITs) are designed to detect human globin and are not affected by diet or drugs. Strategies that use an immunochemical-based FOBT have been shown to be cost-effective when used for colorectal cancer screening in Asia. Quantitative immunochemical FOBT has been shown to

TABLE 67.2 **CLASSIFICATION**

GUIDELINES FOR SCREENING AVERAGE-RISK INDIVIDUALS FOR COLORECTAL CANCER

■ SCREENING TOOL	■ U.S. PREVENTIVE SERVICES TASK FORCE[a]	■ AMERICAN CANCER SOCIETY, U.S. MULTI-SOCIETY TASK FORCE, AMERICAN COLLEGE OF RADIOLOGY JOINT GUIDELINES[b]
High-sensitivity FOBT (guaiac based or immunochemical)	Recommended annually as an option	Recommended annually as an option
Flexible sigmoidoscopy + high-sensitivity FOBT q3y	Recommended q5y as an option	Recommended q5y as an option
Colonoscopy	Recommended q10y as an option	Recommended q10y as an option
Double-contrast barium enema	Not recommended as an option	Recommended q5y
Computed tomography colonography	Not recommended as an option	Recommended q5y
Stool DNA testing	Not recommended	Recommended (interval uncertain)

FOBT, fecal occult blood test.
[a]U.S. Preventive Services Task Force. Screening for colorectal cancer: US Preventative Services Task Force recommendation statement. *Ann Int Med* 2008;149:627–637. The U.S. Preventative Services Task Force recommends screening for adults age 50 to 75 years. Screening for adults age 76 to 85 is not routinely recommended, and for adults older than 85 years screening is not recommended.
[b]Levin B, Lieberman DA, McFarland B, et al. Screening and surveillance for the early detection of colorectal cancer and adenomatous polyps 2008: a joint guideline from the American Cancer Society, the US Multi-Society Task Force on Colorectal Cancer, and the American College of Radiology. *CA Cancer J Clin* 2008;58:130–160. Testing options are divided into those that detect adenomatous polyps and cancer (flexible sigmoidoscopy, colonoscopy, double-contrast barium enema, computed tomography colonography) and those that primarily detect cancer (FOBT, stool DNA testing).

have good sensitivity and specificity for detection of clinically significant neoplasia in recent studies of asymptomatic and symptomatic individuals, but test performance in prospective screening programs has been less well studied. Fecal immunochemical tests have, however, been included in recent screening guidelines (see earlier).

Results from the National Polyp Study strongly indicate that the removal of index polyps detected by fecal occult blood testing and other methods, together with subsequent colonoscopic surveillance, results in a very substantial reduction in colorectal cancer mortality; in fact, the reduction may be as high as 76% to 90% (see later).[22]

Sigmoidoscopy. The benefit of sigmoidoscopy in interrupting the adenoma-to-carcinoma sequence is suggested by a number of studies. Investigators compared the use of rigid sigmoidoscopy in 261 members of the Kaiser Permanente Medical Care Program who died of cancer of the rectum or distal colon versus that in 868 matched controls.[15] Only 8.8% of those with cancer had undergone screening sigmoidoscopy, compared with 24.2% of controls. The impact of sigmoidoscopy was limited to the development of fatal colon cancer within reach of the sigmoidoscope and was long-standing (at least 10 years). Other investigators determined the long-term risk of colorectal cancer development after rigid sigmoidoscopy and polypectomy in 1,618 patients with rectosigmoid adenomas. The overall risk for subsequent rectal cancer in these patients was similar to that in the general population, but subject analysis revealed that risk depended on histologic type, size, and number of adenomas removed.[23] The 60-cm flexible sigmoidoscope has supplanted the rigid scope because it causes less discomfort to the patient, visualizes 2.5 times more surface area, and detects two to three times more adenomas. Flexible sigmoidoscopy can be mastered by paramedical personnel and has been successfully used in screening programs by nurse practitioners. Randomized controlled trials are now under way to measure the effect of screening with flexible sigmoidoscopy on colorectal cancer mortality. The Prostate, Lung, Colon, and Ovarian Cancer Screening Trial (PLCO) has enrolled 155,000 individuals in a recent prospective randomized trial that compares flexible sigmoidoscopy to a usual-care control group. Follow-up is planned through 2015 with cancer-related mortality as the major endpoint. Recent joint guidelines from the American Cancer Society, the U.S. Multi-Society Task Force on Colorectal Cancer, and the American College of Radiology include flexible sigmoidoscopy every 5 years as a screening option, while the USPSTF guidelines include flexible sigmoidoscopy every 5 years in conjunction with high-sensitivity FOBT every 3 years.

Colonoscopy, Barium Enema, Computed Tomography Colonography, and Stool DNA Testing. Colonoscopy may well be the most effective tool for screening for colorectal neoplasia (and especially adenomas), but data from prospective randomized trials are lacking. The National Polyp Study of polypectomy and surveillance strongly suggested a reduction in colorectal cancer mortality as a result of removing adenomatous polyps compared to historic reference populations. A Canadian population-based study compared the risk of developing colorectal cancer after a negative colonoscopy in all Ontario residents with a history of a complete negative colonoscopy with controls consisting of the Ontario population without a history of colonoscopy.[24] In the negative colonoscopy cohort, the relative risk of distal colorectal cancer was significantly lower than the control group in each of the 14 years of follow-up, while the relative risk for proximal colorectal cancer was significantly lower mainly during the last 7 years of follow-up. A second Canadian case-control study demonstrated that complete colonoscopy was also associated with fewer deaths from left-sided colorectal cancer, but not from right-sided cancer. These findings are of interest in light of arguments that colonoscopy is preferable to sigmoidoscopy, because there may be a substantial incidence of proximal colonic cancers and advanced adenomas beyond the reach of the sigmoidoscope. Some of these individuals may not have distal findings on sigmoidoscopy that would trigger a subsequent colonoscopy. Two trials[25,26] suggested that approximately 50% of individuals with advanced proximal neoplasms (adenoma >1 cm; adenoma with villous features or dysplasia; cancer) have no distal neoplasms. Fewer than 2% of those who did not have distal neoplasms, however, had an advanced proximal lesion. A decision analysis commissioned by the USPSTF supports colonoscopy every 10 years as a screening option measured in life-years gained, and the joint guidelines authored by the ACS, USMTF, and ACR suggest colonoscopy as a means of preventing colorectal cancer through adenoma detection and removal.

High-contrast endoscopy using dye or stain solutions combined with colonoscopy (chromoendoscopy) or high-resolution optical methods (e.g., narrow-band imaging, laser confocal endoscopy) has been suggested as a means of identifying lesions in high-risk groups or as an adjunct to colonoscopy where flat lesions (so-called "flat adenomas") are suspected. Recent evidence suggests that flat or depressed neoplasms are more common than previously appreciated and carry a high relative risk of containing in situ or invasive carcinoma.[27]

Air-contrast barium enema (ACBE) has been included as an option in a variety of screening guidelines. No studies, however, have directly addressed the effectiveness of barium enema for colon cancer screening, and especially for detection of adenomas. Several studies have indicated that the sensitivity of ACBE is less than that of colonoscopy, especially for detecting lesions less than 1 cm. A recent population-based study suggested that if a cancer is present, there is approximately a one in five chance that it will be missed by ACBE.

CT colonography, or "virtual" colonoscopy, involves the use of helical CT to generate high-resolution images of the abdomen and pelvis. CT colonography has the potential advantage of being a rapid and safe method of providing full structural evaluation of the entire colon. Two trials provide evidence that CT colonography may be a valid alternative for primary colon cancer screening. The National CT Colonography Trial[28] directed by the American College of Radiology Imaging Network (ACRIN) was a multicenter study that employed CT colonography and same-day colonoscopy using a standard matching protocol in 2,600 asymptomatic individuals. Per patient sensitivity of CT colonography for adenomas greater than 10 mm was 90% with a negative predictive value of 99%. A second trial[29] compared CT colonography and optical colonoscopy in parallel screening cohorts and demonstrated similar rates of detection of advanced neoplasia in both groups. Several key issues need to be addressed as the use of CT colonography becomes more widespread, principal among which is determination of the acceptable size cut-off of a lesion detected by CT colonography that will necessitate a follow-up colonoscopy.

A great deal of knowledge has been accumulated recently about genetic alterations that occur during colon carcinogenesis (discussed earlier). A molecular approach to colorectal cancer screening is therefore attractive since it targets biologic changes that are fundamental to the neoplastic process. Fecal DNA testing relies on the detection of genetic alterations in DNA shed into the stool from neoplastic lesions. While small studies utilizing specimens from patients with known lesions have been promising, larger prospective trials using fecal DNA marker panels have been, to date, disappointing, especially in detecting adenomas. A recently published study[30] compared stool DNA and FOBT for detection of "screen-relevant neoplasia" (curable stage cancer, high-grade dysplasia, or adenomas >1 cm). This blinded, multicenter, cross-sectional study used two different methodologies for detecting alterations in stool DNA, a 23-marker panel and a new test targeting three broadly informative markers (point mutations on *K-ras*, a

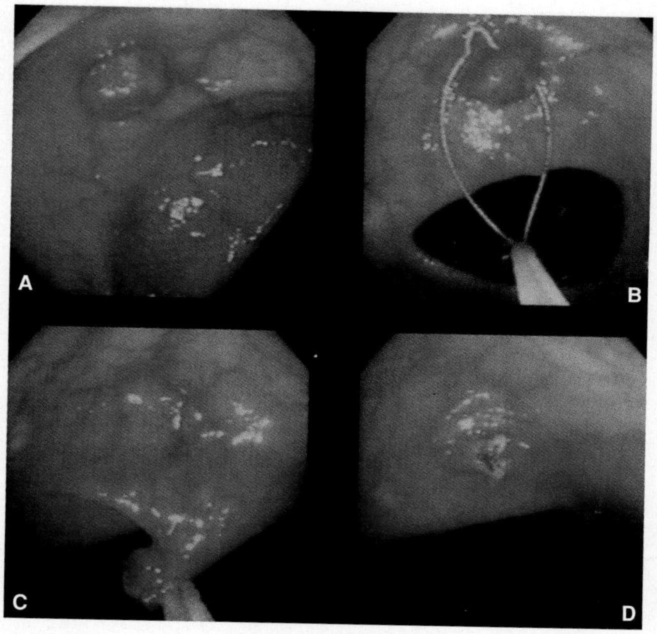

FIGURE 67.6. Endoscopic snare polypectomy. **A:** A small colonic polyp. **B:** The polypectomy snare is placed around the polyp. **C:** The snare is closed around the base of the polyp, and the head of the polyp is gently pulled away from the wall and into the lumen. Current is applied to cut the stalk and cauterize the site. **D:** The site after completion of polypectomy.

scanned mutation cluster region of *APC*, and methylated vimentin). While the multipanel test provided no improvement over FOBT (Hemoccult Sensa) for detection of screen-relevant neoplasms, the newer test showed promise by detecting significantly more neoplasms than FOBT.

Management of Adenomas

Index Polypectomy. Once detected, adenomas should be completely removed, preferably by endoscopic snare polypectomy (Fig. 67.6). Polypectomy is relatively safe and easily performed when adenomas are small or pedunculated but is more difficult when polyps are large or sessile. Potential complications include bleeding and perforation of the polypectomy site. Large sessile villous adenomas (>2 cm) have a great potential for malignant degeneration. If such lesions cannot be completely removed by snare polypectomy, and when there is uncertainty about the polypectomy margin in the case of pathologically advanced lesions, segmental surgical resection may be necessary. Diminutive polyps, on the other hand, carry little malignant potential. If they are too small for snare polypectomy, ablation with a hot biopsy forceps is a reasonable approach. Because 30% to 50% of patients with one adenoma have a synchronous adenoma elsewhere in the colon, the entire colon should be "cleared" by colonoscopy in polyp-bearing patients.

Follow-up. Much of our current practice has come from information gained through the National Polyp Study (NPS), first organized in 1978. Additional metachronous adenomas are likely to develop in patients who have had adenomas removed. Colonoscopic surveillance studies have provided estimates of the frequency and time course of recurrence in these patients. Data from the NPS suggested a recurrence rate of 32% to 42% by 3 years after index polypectomy. A prospective colonoscopic analysis also demonstrated a cumulative recurrence rate at 3 years of 42%. Most adenomas detected at this 3-year interval were small tubular adenomas. Age above 60 years, multiple adenomas at index polypectomy, and large size of the index adenoma predicted polyp recurrence in the NPS, but only multiplicity predicted recurrence of polyps with advanced pathologic features (i.e., >1 cm, high-grade dysplasia, or invasive cancer) at follow-up. The 3-year recurrence rate in patients with a known history of adenoma (42%) was higher than the incidence rate of adenoma appearance de novo during this period in patients who had no adenomas detected on index colonoscopy (16%).[22]

The high recurrence rate of adenomas after index polypectomy supports the use of postpolypectomy surveillance in patients with known histories of adenoma. Colonoscopy is the preferred means of follow-up in these patients. Air-contrast barium enemas are inadequate for surveillance exams; they will miss a substantial number of large lesions and most small polyps. Barium enema will likely be supplanted by the use of CT colonography, as discussed earlier. Colonoscopy is the most accurate means of evaluating the colonic mucosa, and most importantly, allows biopsy and removal of polyps.

Data from the NPS indicate that colonoscopy need not be repeated at intervals shorter than 3 years in patients whose index polyp demonstrates no evidence of high-grade dysplasia or carcinoma. Although patients undergoing postpolypectomy surveillance at both 1 and 3 years after index polypectomy had a greater number of polyps detected in this study than did those undergoing colonoscopy at 3 years only, the percentage of patients whose adenomas had advanced pathologic features was similarly low in both groups (3.3%). Subsequent studies have confirmed the low incidence of recurrent advanced adenomas 3 to 5 years after polypectomy. One recent study examined the relative risk for advanced neoplasia within 5.5 years of a baseline colonoscopy.[31] There was a strong association between the results of baseline screening colonoscopy and the rate of serious incident lesions during surveillance. This study confirmed that patients with one or two small tubular adenomas represent a low-risk group compared with other patients with colorectal neoplasia.

Table 67.3 lists the 2008 ACS/USMTF/ACR guidelines for screening, surveillance, and early detection of colorectal adenomas and cancer for individuals at increased risk or at high risk of disease. These guidelines suggest that those whose index lesion consists of one or two small tubular adenomas with low-grade dysplasia should have a follow-up colonoscopy 5 to 10 years after the initial polypectomy. The precise timing within this interval should be based on clinical factors (prior findings, family history, patient and physician preferences). In those with a large (>1 cm) adenoma, multiple (3 to 10) adenomas, or adenomas with high-grade dysplasia or villous change, colonoscopy should be repeated within 3 years after the initial polypectomy. Although the risk for recurrence of advanced adenomas at this follow-up interval is greater in patients with high-risk adenomas than those with low-risk adenomas, the incremental risk is small.[32] If the exam is normal or shows only one or two small tubular adenomas with low-grade dysplasia, then the interval for the subsequent exam should be 5 years. Patients with more than 10 adenomas on a single examination should have a follow-up colonoscopy less than 3 years after the initial polypectomy and the presence of an underlying familial syndrome should be considered. Patients with sessile adenomas that are removed piecemeal should have follow-up colonoscopy in 2 to 6 months to verify complete removal.

Management of Malignant Polyps

Endoscopic polypectomy is adequate treatment for an adenomatous polyp containing cancer if it can be demonstrated that the cancer is confined to the head of the polyp (i.e., carcinoma

TABLE 67.3

GUIDELINES FOR THE SURVEILLANCE OF ADENOMAS IN PEOPLE AT INCREASED OR HIGH RISK FOR COLORECTAL CANCER

RISK CATEGORY	AGE TO BEGIN SURVEILLANCE	RECOMMENDATION	COMMENT
Increased Risk: Patients with History of Adenomas at Prior Colonoscopy			
Patients with one or two small tubular adenomas with low-grade dysplasia	5–10 y after initial polypectomy	Colonoscopy	Precise timing based on clinical factors, patient and physician preferences
Patients with 3–10 adenomas or one adenoma >1 cm or any adenoma with villous features or high-grade dysplasia	3 y after initial polypectomy	Colonoscopy	If follow-up exam is normal or shows one or two small tubular adenomas, subsequent exam at 5 y
Patients with >10 adenomas on a single examination	<3 y after initial polypectomy	Colonoscopy	Consider familial CRC syndrome
Patients with sessile adenomas that are removed piecemeal	2–6 mo to verify complete removal	Colonoscopy	Surveillance individualized based on endoscopist's judgment
Increased Risk: Patients with Family History			
CRC or adenomatous polyps in a first-degree relative before age 60 years or in two or more first-degree relatives at any age	Age 40 or 10 y before the youngest case in the immediate family	Colonoscopy	Every 5 y
Either CRC or adenomatous polyps in a first-degree relative age ≥60 y or in two second-degree relatives with CRC	Age 40 y	Screening options at intervals recommended for average-risk individuals	Screening should begin at an earlier age, but individuals may be screened with any recommended form of testing
High Risk			
Genetic diagnosis of FAP or suspected FAP without genetic testing evidence	Age 10–12 y	Annual FSIG to determine if the individual is expressing the genetic abnormality and counseling to consider genetic testing	If the genetic test is positive, colectomy should be planned
Genetic or clinical diagnosis of Lynch syndrome, or individuals at increased risk of Lynch syndrome	Age 20–25 y or 10 y before the youngest case in the immediate family	Colonoscopy every 1–2 y and counseling to consider genetic testing for inherited DNA MMR	Genetic testing for Lynch syndrome should be offered to first-degree relatives of persons with a known gene mutation. It should also be offered when the family mutation is not known but one of the first three of the modified Bethesda criteria is present.

CRC, colorectal cancer; FAP, familial adenomatous polyposis; FSIG, flexible sigmoidoscopy; MMR, mismatch repair. Derived from Levin B, Lieberman DA, McFarland B, et al. Screening and surveillance for the early detection of colorectal cancer and adenomatous polyps 2008: a joint guideline from the American Cancer Society, the Multi-Society Task Force on colorectal cancer and the American College of Radiology. *CA Cancer J Clin* 2008;58:130–160.

in situ or intramucosal carcinoma; Fig. 67.7). The adequacy of simple polypectomy has been controversial in cases in which malignant cells have invaded the polyp stalk (Fig. 67.8), but most studies indicate that polypectomy is adequate treatment provided that a margin of more than 2 mm is present, the cancer is not poorly differentiated, and no vascular or lymphatic invasion is noted. The presence of cancer at or near the margin is significantly associated with an adverse outcome, even in the absence of other unfavorable parameters. On the other hand, in the absence of unfavorable histology and with a negative margin, the incidence of residual cancer is low (<1%). These criteria are more difficult to assess in sessile polyps. If an adequate margin cannot be demonstrated or negative histologic parameters are present, surgery is recommended to treat the possibility of regional lymph node metastases.

Primary Prevention of Adenoma Recurrence

Primary prevention relates to the ability to identify genetic, environmental, and biologic factors that cause cancer, and to alter their effects. Laboratory, clinical, and epidemiologic evidence suggests that the regular use of nonsteroidal anti-inflammatory drugs (NSAIDs), including aspirin, is associated with a decreased risk for the development of colorectal cancer. Four recently published trials have demonstrated a reduction in adenoma recurrence in chemoprevention trials involving aspirin.[33,34] Given biologic plausibility, preclinical in vitro and animal data, and data on adenoma regression in patients with FAP, three large randomized trials, which in total studied over 6,000 patients, were undertaken to examine the effect of

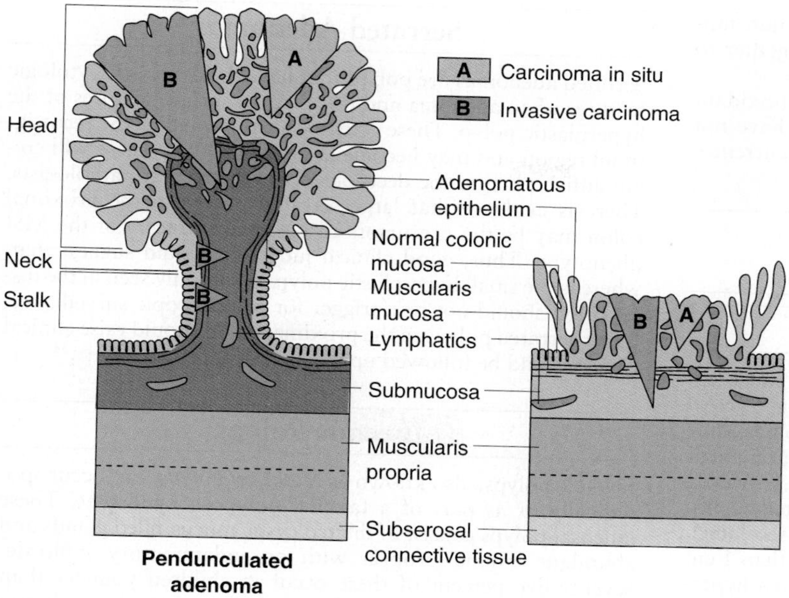

FIGURE 67.7. Diagram representation of cancer-containing polyps. Pedunculated adenoma is described on the left and a sessile adenoma on the right. In carcinoma in situ, malignant cells are confined to the mucosa. These lesions are adequately treated by endoscopic polypectomy. Polypectomy is adequate treatment for invasive carcinoma only if the margin is sufficient (2 mm), the carcinoma is not poorly differentiated, and no evidence of venous or lymphatic invasion is found. (After Haggitt RC, Glotzbach RE, Soffen EE, et al. Prognostic factors in colorectal carcinomas arising in adenomas: implications for lesions removed by endoscopic polypectomy. *Gastroenterology* 1985;89:328.)

cyclooxygenase-2 (COX-2)–selective inhibitors on new adenoma formation in individuals with a history of sporadic adenomas. All of these trials demonstrated a highly significant reduction in new adenoma formation in those taking a COX-2–selective inhibitor (celecoxib, rofecoxib) compared to placebo over 3 years. In the Adenoma Prevention with Celecoxib (APC) trial,[35] for example, use of celecoxib was associated with a dose-dependent 33% to 45% reduction in the development of new adenomas overall by 3 years, with a 57% to 66% reduction in the number of patients developing advanced adenomas. Unfortunately, adverse thrombotic cardiovascular events were associated with COX-2 inhibition in at least two of these trials. Recent data suggest that increased cardiovascular risk may be associated with most NSAIDs, and not just COX-2 inhibitors.

Other agents currently undergoing study for chemoprevention of colorectal neoplasia include the ornithine decarboxylase inhibitor difluoromethylornithine (DFMO), the bile acid ursodiol, the 3-hydroxy-3-methylglutaryl-coenzyme A (HMG-CoA) reductase inhibitors such as pravastatin and lovastatin, epidermal growth factor receptor (EGFR) inhibitors, and matrix metalloproteinase (MMP) inhibitors. The combination of DFMO and the NSAID sulindac were studied in a randomized placebo-controlled trial to assess their efficacy in preventing sporadic adenoma recurrence in 375 subjects. Use of this regimen was associated with a 70% reduction in new adenomas at 3 years compared to placebo.[36] Larger studies are needed to confirm this result and to fully assess toxicity of this combination. A population-based case-control study of individuals with colorectal cancer and matched controls demonstrated a 47% relative reduction of colorectal cancer associated with statin use, but further investigation is needed to assess the overall benefits of this group of agents.

Supplemental calcium reduces proliferative activity in the mucosa of experimental animals and patients at high risk for the development of colorectal cancer. A large body of observational and laboratory studies suggests a role for dietary calcium supplementation in chemoprevention. A prospective, double-blind, placebo-controlled trial showed that supplemental calcium (3,000 mg of calcium carbonate per day, equivalent to 1,200 mg of elemental calcium) reduced the incidence and number of recurrent adenomas in subjects chosen for a recent history of such lesions. The protective effect of calcium supplementation on the risk of colorectal adenoma recurrence extended up to 5 years after cessation of active treatment, even in the absence of continued supplementation.[37] Analysis of

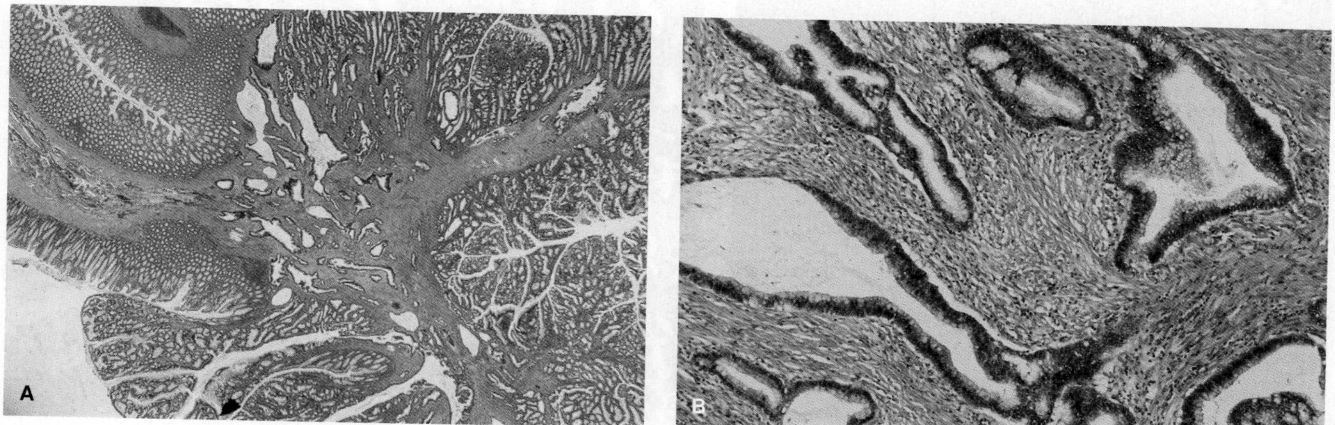

FIGURE 67.8. Invasive carcinoma in the stalk of an adenomatous polyp. **A:** Low-power view. Malignant glands can be seen invading fibrovascular stalk. **B:** High-power magnification of malignant glands in stalk. Nuclei are large, hyperpigmented, and crowded.

serum vitamin D status in subjects suggested that calcium supplementation and vitamin D status appear to act together to reduce the risk of adenoma recurrence.

Trials of supplemental dietary fiber, as well as antioxidant vitamins such as β-carotene and vitamins C and E, have not convincingly demonstrated any effect on adenoma recurrence.

NONNEOPLASTIC MUCOSAL POLYPS

Hyperplastic Polyps

Hyperplastic polyps are small, usually sessile lesions most frequently encountered in the distal colon and rectum (Fig. 67.9A). Although grossly indistinguishable from small adenomas, they carry no significant potential for malignant degeneration particularly when located in the distal colon or rectum. However, hyperplastic polyps must be distinguished from serrated adenomas, which carry significant malignant potential (see later). Macroscopically, these polyps are almost always less than 1 cm in size, and most are in the distal colon. In fact, when hyperplastic polyps are found proximal to the rectosigmoid region, one must consider the possibility of a serrated adenoma. Microscopically, hyperplastic polyps are characterized by a saw-toothed epithelial pattern representing micropapillary luminal infoldings of columnar absorptive cells and mature, frequently hyperdistended goblet cells (Fig. 67.9B). Elongation and subsequent infolding of the epithelium may be caused by an expanded, but otherwise normally located, replication zone in the crypt. The cytologic atypia found in adenomatous polyps is not seen in these lesions.

Hyperplastic polyps are common age-related lesions found in about one third of the population older than 50 years. Although they often coexist with adenomas in polyp-bearing patients, no convincing evidence has been found that hyperplastic polyps per se are harbingers of adenoma development. Because hyperplastic polyps are asymptomatic and carry no malignant potential, no specific treatment is required for these lesions. If a hyperplastic polyp is the only lesion detected on index flexible sigmoidoscopy or colonoscopy, no further evaluation is indicated.

Serrated Adenomas

Serrated adenomas are polyps that have the dysplastic cytologic features of an adenoma and the serrated surface features of the hyperplastic polyp. These often occur proximal to the rectosigmoid region and may become larger than 1 cm. These will create difficult diagnostic decisions for even the best pathologists. There is evidence that large serrated polyps in the proximal colon may be the precursors to colorectal cancers of the MSI phenotype. Thus, good clinical judgment would suggest that, whereas the small hyperplastic polyps commonly seen in the distal colon should not be a trigger for colonoscopic surveillance, larger serrated polyps in the proximal colon should raise clinical concerns and be followed up like an advanced adenoma.[38]

Juvenile Polyps

Juvenile polyps, also known as *retention polyps,* can occur sporadically or as part of a familial polyposis syndrome. These mucosal polyps consist of dilated cystic mucus-filled glands and abundant lamina propria with an inflammatory infiltrate. Seventy-five percent of these occur in children younger than 10 years of age, often appearing as single pedunculated cherry-red polyps with a smooth surface and contour. The exact prevalence of such lesions has not been determined, but they are thought to be acquired lesions detectable in about 2% of children who do not have symptoms. Juvenile polyps often present in the form of hematochezia because they are highly vascularized lesions. Rectal prolapse and autoamputation may occur with distal lesions, whereas intussusception may be precipitated by proximal juvenile polyps found in the context of familial syndromes. Individually, these polyps have no malignant potential, but symptomatic polyps should be removed to prevent further complications. Juvenile polyposis, on the other hand, is associated with an increased risk for the early development of cancer.

Inflammatory Polyps

Inflammatory mucosal polyps are common in the setting of idiopathic inflammatory bowel disease. Marked inflammation

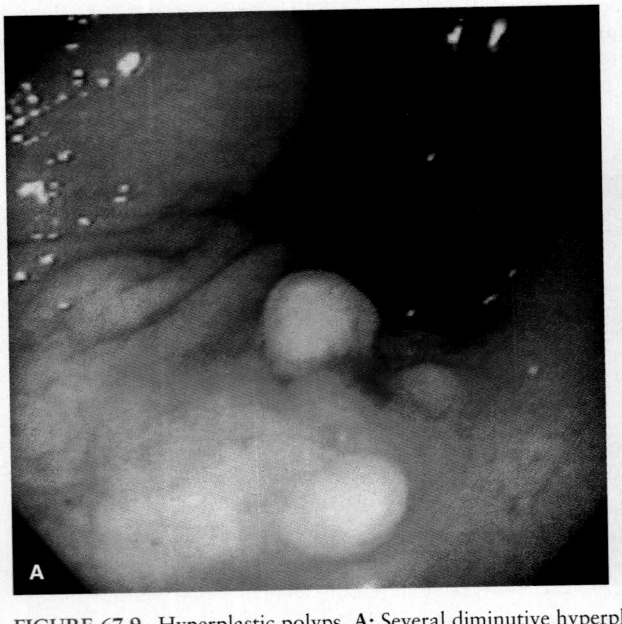

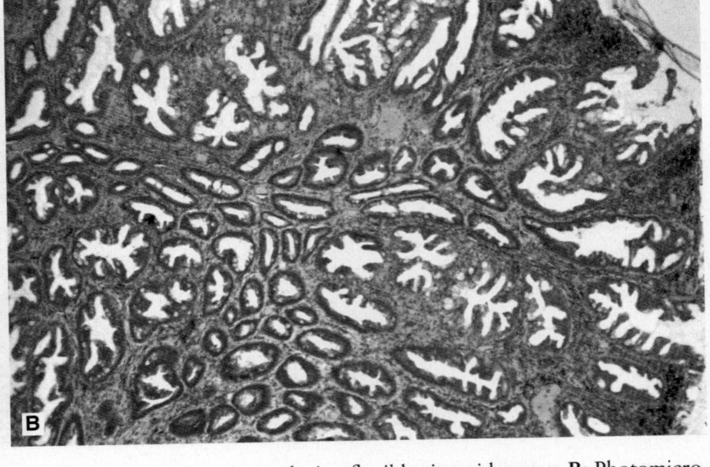

FIGURE 67.9. Hyperplastic polyps. **A:** Several diminutive hyperplastic polyps seen in the rectum during flexible sigmoidoscopy. **B:** Photomicrograph of a hyperplastic polyp, characterized by elongated glands with papillary infoldings that have a typical serrated epithelial pattern.

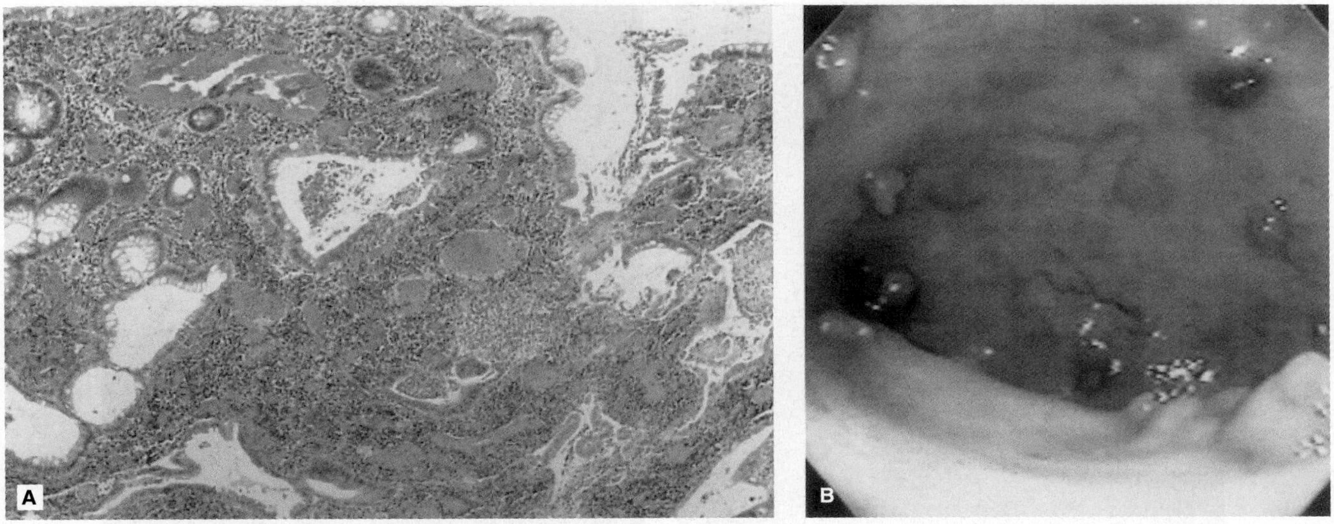

FIGURE 67.10. Inflammatory polyps. **A:** Severe mucosal inflammation with infiltrates and granulation tissue shown here microscopically can appear clinically with a polypoid configuration. **B:** Resolution of inflammation can leave exuberant polyps covered by normal epithelium, which are called pseudopolyps, a misnomer. These are truly polyps, but are not neoplastic.

and ulceration coexist with granulation tissue in a distorted mucosal architecture that appears polypoid because of confluent areas of ulceration, leaving behind islands of intact epithelium (Fig. 67.10A). Subsequent healing leads to the appearance of polypoid, nonneoplastic excrescences covered by normal colonic epithelium, so-called pseudopolyps (Fig. 67.10B). They need not be removed and are important largely because they make it difficult to recognize subtle, early neoplastic lesions in these high-risk patients. Severe chronic inflammation of any kind, including a variety of infectious diseases (tuberculosis, amebiasis, schistosomiasis, amebic colitis), may result in inflammatory polyps that resemble those found in idiopathic inflammatory bowel disease.

Submucosal Polyps

Submucosal masses can expand to push the colonic mucosa into the bowel lumen and thus appear as polypoid lesions. Many submucosal lesions (e.g., lipomas, leiomyomas) are clinically asymptomatic and must be differentiated from neoplastic lesions. Others are malignant lesions that require early detection, such as lymphomas and metastatic tumors. Many submucosal lesions are not detected on endoscopic mucosal biopsy because standard biopsy forceps do not reach beyond the mucosa. If a submucosal lesion is suspected, multiple biopsy specimens of the same site sometimes provide tissue for diagnosis.

Lipomas are benign fatty tumors that occur throughout the gastrointestinal tract but are most commonly found in the cecum near the ileocecal valve (Fig. 67.11). They appear endoscopically as soft, smooth polyps that are pliable and deformable. The overlying mucosa is intact but may be light yellow in appearance. These are benign lesions that have little clinical significance and are commonly seen in obese patients.

Isolated *lymphoid nodules* consisting of benign lymphoid tissue may appear as sessile smooth polyps of various sizes, with a predilection for the distal colon and rectum. These are usually asymptomatic. Diffuse nodular lymphoid hyperplasia also occurs in children as an incidental finding. The nodules must be distinguished from primary or secondary lymphoma of the large intestine, which may present as mucosal nodularity resembling the pseudopolyposis of inflammatory bowel disease or even polyposis (Fig. 67.12). Flow cytometry of the lymphocytes in the lesion will be helpful; benign polyposis is polyclonal, whereas lymphomas are monoclonal and may overexpress cyclin D.

Pneumatosis cystoides intestinalis consists of multiple air-filled cysts within the submucosa. This may be an incidental finding in patients with chronic obstructive pulmonary disease, scleroderma, or asymptomatic pneumoperitoneum secondary to recent surgery or instrumentation, in which air or colonic gas diffuses into the cysts. These sometimes resolve with administration of oxygen. A far more virulent form of pneumatosis is associated with fulminant mucosal inflammation, ischemia, or necrotizing enterocolitis in children. These cysts are thought to result from mucosal invasion by gas-producing bacteria.

Colitis cystica profunda is a rare condition in which the intestinal wall is thickened by submucosal mucus-filled cysts of various sizes and an accumulation of fibroblasts in the lamina propria. It can present as an ulcerating or mass lesion in the rectosigmoid in association with the solitary rectal ulcer syndrome. Although the pathogenesis of this condition is unknown, it may result from the downward displacement of colonic glands during trauma or chronic inflammation followed by healing. The appearance of aberrant submucosal glandular epithelium and acellular mucous lakes must be distinguished from a colloid carcinoma, because this lesion has no malignant potential.

Carcinoid tumors of the rectum appear as isolated, small, yellow-gray submucosal nodules. These are often incidental findings during sigmoidoscopy. Most are smaller than 1 cm, have little malignant potential, and are amenable to local excision. Lesions larger than 2 cm are more likely to be malignant but seldom give rise to metastases. These lesions should be treated aggressively with complete excision. Rectal carcinoid tumors are usually asymptomatic but may present with hematochezia. They are not associated with the carcinoid syndrome. Carcinoid tumors in the proximal colon may be locally invasive or metastasize to the liver, liberating vasoactive peptides into the systemic circulation and producing the carcinoid syndrome.

Other lesions that can present as submucosal polyps include *metastatic tumors*, such as malignant melanoma, and benign lesions, such as *leiomyomas*, *fibromas*, *lymphangiomas*, *hemangiomas*, and *endometriosis*.

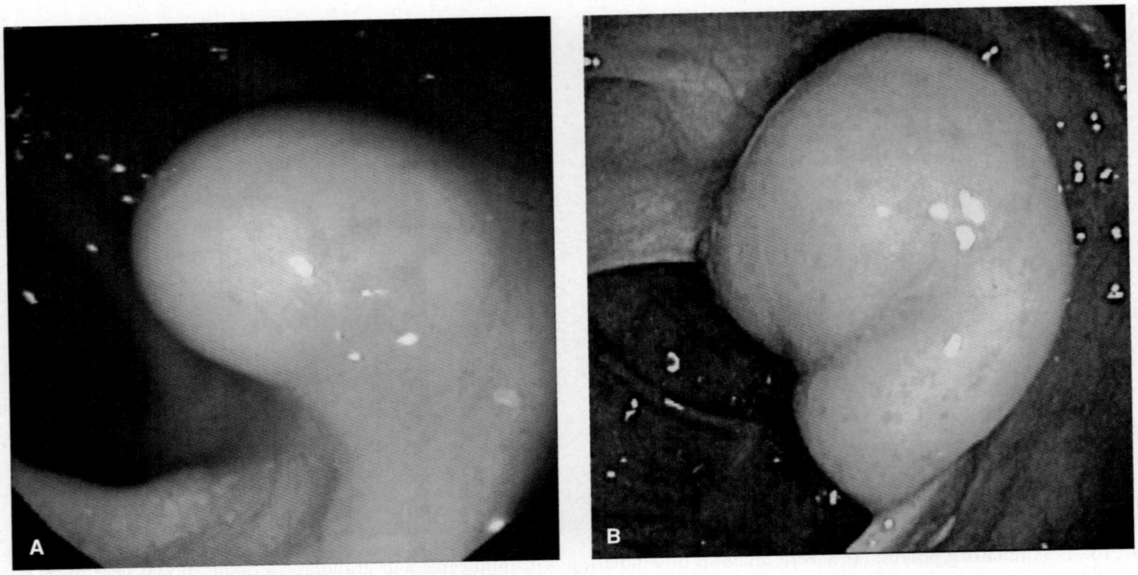

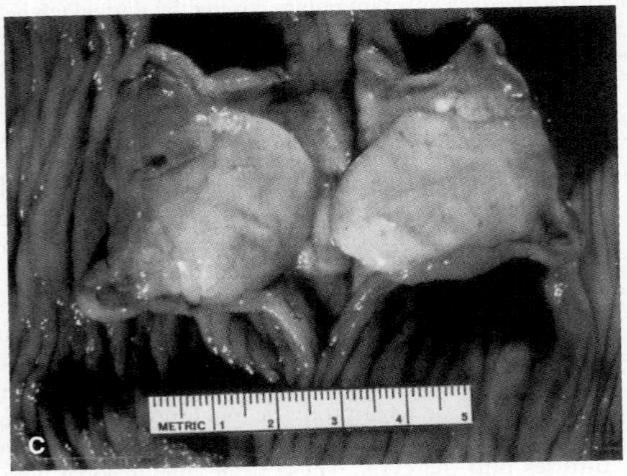

FIGURE 67.11. Submucosal lipomas. **A:** Lipoma seen at colonoscopy. Submucosal fatty tissue causes the mucosa to protrude into the lumen; such protrusion appears as a polyp. Overlying mucosa is smooth. **B:** Lipomatous infiltration of ileocecal valve seen at colonoscopy. **C:** Colectomy specimen showing a large submucosal lipoma cut in cross section.

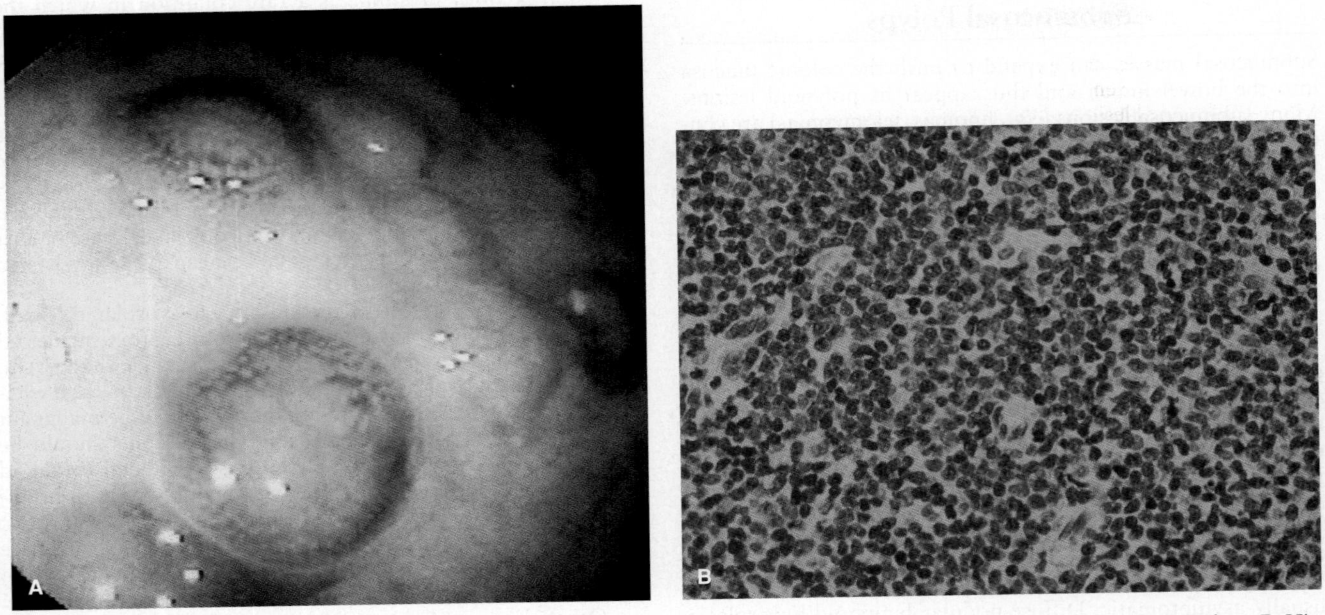

FIGURE 67.12. Lymphomatous polyposis of the colon. **A:** Colonoscopic view of B-cell lymphoma presenting as multiple colonic polyps. **B:** Histology of lymphoma is one of the polyps.

GASTROINTESTINAL POLYPOSIS SYNDROMES

Gastrointestinal polyposis indicates the presence of a systemic process that promotes the development of multiple polyps throughout the gastrointestinal tract. In some instances, the polyps are located predominantly in the colon; however, in others, polyps may be found in the stomach, small intestine, colon, and rectum. The classification of the polyposis syndromes has traditionally been based on the histologic characteristics of the polyps, but gradually an awareness of the genetic basis for the most important of these syndromes has permitted more precise diagnosis and rational approaches to treatment.

Familial Adenomatous Polyposis

FAP is an autosomal dominant, genetic disease characterized by the development of multiple adenomatous polyps throughout the colon and rectum (Fig. 67.13). The polyps first appear in adolescence, with the median age of onset being about 16 years. The number of polyps in each patient is variable, and they increase in number and size with advancing age. The genetic basis for this disease is a germline mutation in the *APC* gene located on chromosome 5q. In part, the age of onset, number of polyps, and age at which cancer develops are determined by the location of the mutation in the *APC* gene (Fig. 67.14). More than 5,000 polyps can develop in patients with specific *APC* mutations, and cancer develops in these patients at a mean age of 35 years. Other mutations in the *APC* gene can give rise to attenuated forms of the disease in which only a few (i.e., 20 to 100) polyps are likely, and the median age for cancer development may be in the 50s or 60s. Additional factors not related to the mutation on the *APC* gene, some genetic and some environmental, also modify the clinical characteristics of the disease.[39,40]

Gastrointestinal Features. Polyps in the stomach and small intestine develop in about 90% of patients with FAP. The gastric polyps consist of fundic gland polyps, which are not premalignant lesions. These may appear to be dysplastic, but in the Western world (North America and Europe), gastric cancer occurs in fewer than 1% of FAP patients. Gastric cancer is a bigger diagnostic problem in FAP in Japan and Korea, however.

Small-intestinal neoplasia is not rare in FAP and principally occurs in the periampullary region of the duodenum. Duodenal adenomatous polyps, which typically appear later than the colonic lesions, may be multiple but tend not to carpet the proximal small intestine. The ampulla of Vater is a particular target for neoplastic development. With time, carcinoma develops in up to 5% to 10% of these patients, so that duodenal surveillance is required. Spigelman has developed a classification system that can be used to determine optimal surveillance for duodenal neoplasia, which is based on the number, size, and histologic features of the duodenal polyps (Table 67.4).

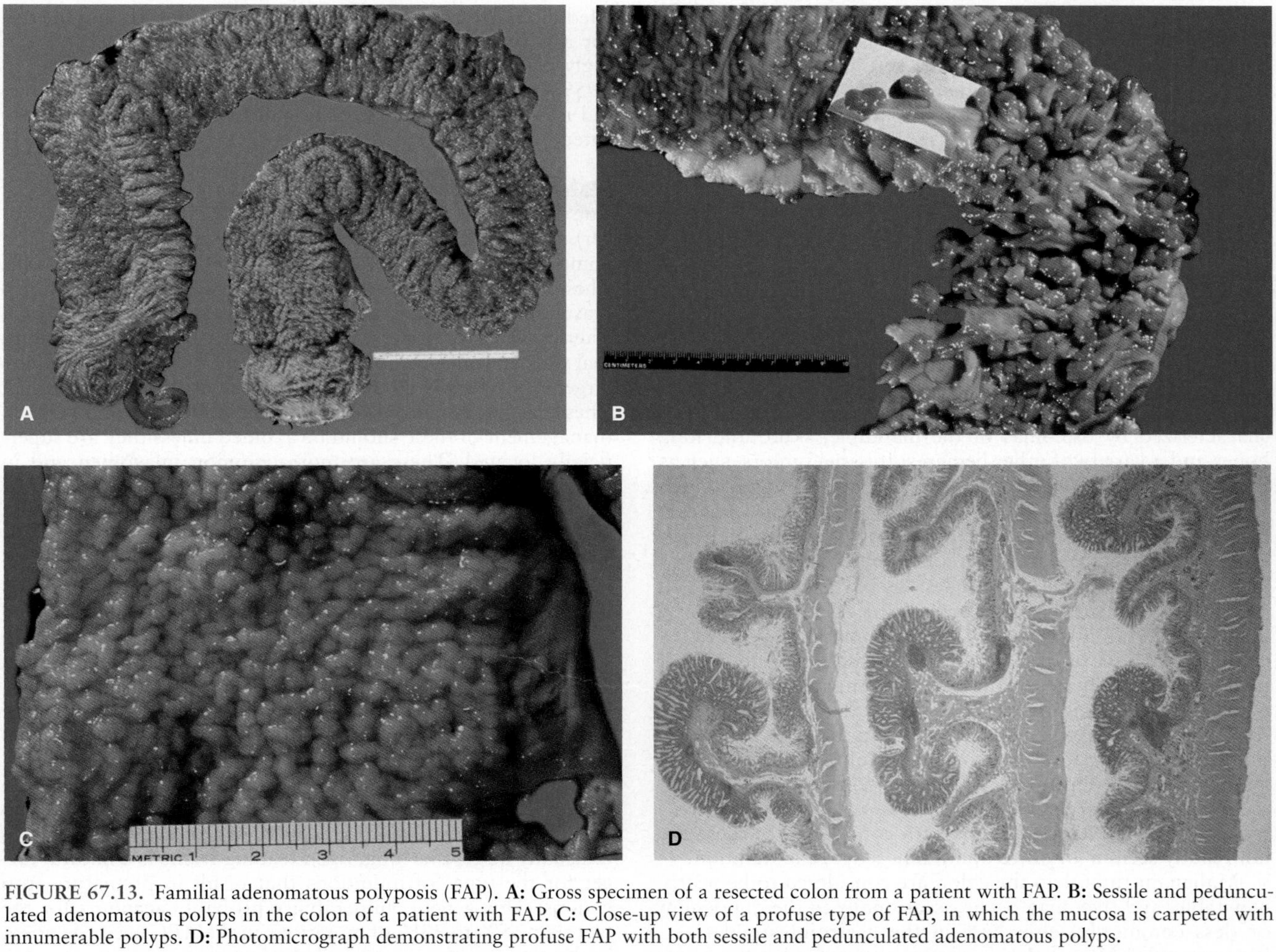

FIGURE 67.13. Familial adenomatous polyposis (FAP). **A:** Gross specimen of a resected colon from a patient with FAP. **B:** Sessile and pedunculated adenomatous polyps in the colon of a patient with FAP. **C:** Close-up view of a profuse type of FAP, in which the mucosa is carpeted with innumerable polyps. **D:** Photomicrograph demonstrating profuse FAP with both sessile and pedunculated adenomatous polyps.

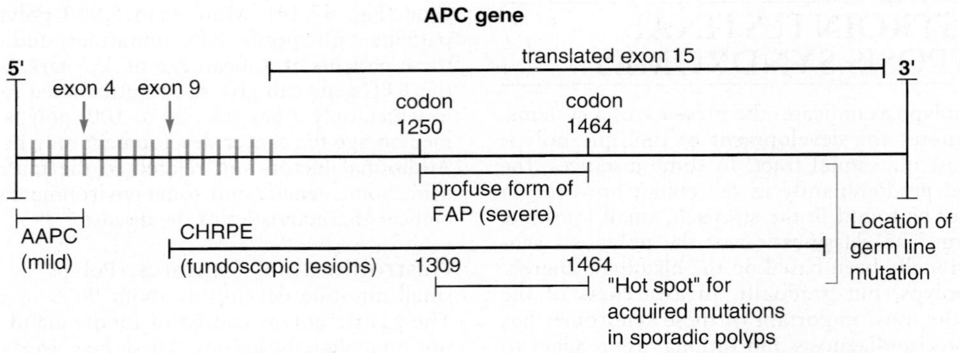

FIGURE 67.14. This scheme of the *APC* (adenomatous polyposis coli) gene illustrates the genotype-phenotype correlations. Most mutations of *APC* result in premature stop codons; therefore, the site of the mutation usually indicates the relative length of the mutant protein product. Mutations at the 5′ end of the gene produce "attenuated" FAP, a milder form of the disease. The retinal lesions (congenital hypertrophy of retinal pigmented epithelium [CHRPE]) occur when the mutations are between exons 9 and 15. The portion of the *APC* gene that binds to other cytoskeletal elements in the cell is represented at the 3′ end of the 15th exon. Mutations in a hot spot immediately downstream from the β-catenin–binding site (between codons 1250 and 1464) result in a more virulent, profuse form of familial adenomatous polyposis. This site is also the location of most of the acquired mutations in sporadic colorectal neoplasms.

Adenomas and carcinomas occur in the jejunum and ileum, but these are rare. Polyps in the terminal ileum may represent lymphoid aggregates rather than adenomas and should be biopsied for diagnostic purposes.

Classically, it has been stated that the natural history of FAP is for cancer to develop at a median age of about 40 years. As mentioned, the development of cancer is variable and is based in part on the location of the germline mutation in the *APC* gene. Colon cancer is rather unusual before 30 years of age, and cancer may not develop in patients with the attenuated form of FAP until they are in their 50s or 60s. Cancer occurring in the teenage years has been reported as a result of a patient who had both FAP and Lynch syndrome.[41] Thus, the treatment of these patients relies increasingly on a genetic characterization of the disease.

Extraintestinal Features. Traditionally, patients with manifestations of FAP together with extraintestinal manifestations were considered to have Gardner syndrome. It is now appreciated that families with FAP all have extraintestinal manifestations and that no distinction can be made between families with Gardner syndrome and those with FAP.[42] FAP is characterized by osteomas of the mandible, skull, and long bones and a variety of other benign soft tissue tumors, such as fibromas, lipomas (Fig. 67.15), and sebaceous cysts, which should not be confused with the sebaceous adenomas and carcinomas seen in the Muir-Torre syndrome variant of Lynch syndrome. Osteomas are commonly found in the skull and may be multiple. Some of these lesions have been reported to regress and later reappear. Osteomas may also be found in the mandible, and radiographs of the mouth may reveal impacted or supernumerary teeth. Congenital hypertrophy of the retinal pigmented epithelium (CHRPE) is present in some families with FAP, depending on the location of the mutation in the *APC* gene. CHRPE lesions may be seen in the general population but are small and usually single. Multiple, bilateral, and large CHRPE lesions are essentially diagnostic of FAP. It will require a slit lamp examination and knowledgeable ophthalmologist to make this diagnosis with confidence, as these are not readily seen in an office ophthalmoscopic examination.

Malignant tumors in the colon are considered to be nearly inevitable, and they may occur occasionally in the duodenum or (less commonly) elsewhere in the gastrointestinal tract. Patients with FAP are also at increased risk for brain tumors (particularly medulloblastomas), thyroid tumors, adrenal tumors, and malignant tumors of the hepatobiliary tree. The occurrence of a malignant brain tumor in conjunction with intestinal polyposis was traditionally referred to as *Turcot syndrome*, although this is not a distinctive disease process. Medulloblastomas are a rare complication of FAP, and the risk for this tumor is increased 99-fold in FAP families. Interestingly, one of the index families initially reported by Turcot in 1959 (and several others characterized as Turcot syndrome) did not have FAP, but actually had Lynch syndrome complicated by astrocytomas.[17]

Desmoid Tumors. Desmoid tumors are currently the major cause of mortality and morbidity in FAP (after colorectal cancer) and develop in 10% to 15% of such patients, often as a complication of laparotomy, but sometimes spontaneously. These are benign but aggressive tumors of mesenteric fibroblasts that can envelop and obstruct the gastrointestinal tract, arteries, veins, or ureters. They frequently occur in the abdominal wall. In some instances, desmoid tumors can become quite large, may virtually fill the abdominal cavity, and can be lethal. These can be visualized on CT of the abdomen, and surgical management of these should be avoided unless they are superficially located. These are more common in women and in those with a positive family history of desmoid tumors.

Genetic Basis. FAP occurs when a germline mutation in the *APC* gene inactivates the function of the *APC* gene product. In most instances, the genetic lesion creates a premature stop codon in the *APC* gene, which in turn leads, to nonsense-mediated decay of the mRNA or the translation of a truncated, nonfunctional APC protein. The *APC* gene encodes a large protein (311 kd) that binds to other intracellular proteins—namely, the catenins and E-cadherin.[5] Depending on the location of the premature stop codon, the mutant protein is of variable length. The *APC* gene encodes 2843 codons (i.e., one for each amino acid) and is broken into 15 translated exons. The structure of the *APC* gene is unique in that the 15th exon makes up about 75% of the coding sequences of the gene. Because it is unusually large, this long, open reading frame is a natural target for the types of mutations that result in premature stop codons. This genetic vulnerability probably accounts for the fact that 25% to 33% of mutations in the *APC* occur de novo, in the absence of a prior family history.

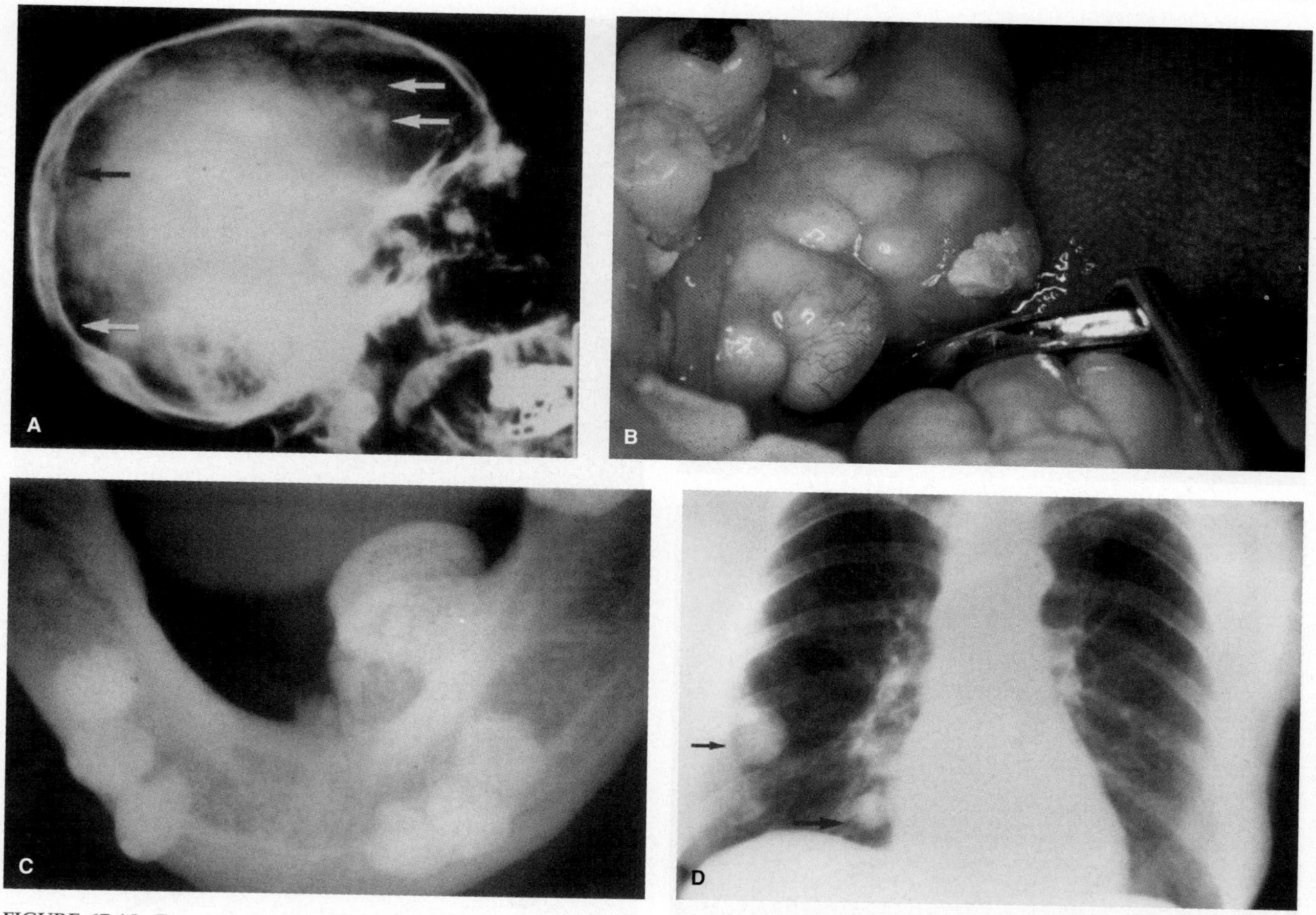

FIGURE 67.15. Extraintestinal manifestations of familial adenomatous polyposis (FAP). **A:** Skull film demonstrating osteomas of the calvarium (*arrows*). **B:** Photograph of the mandible demonstrating protuberant mandibular osteomas. **C:** Mandibular radiograph demonstrating a large osteoma of the mandible. **D:** Chest radiograph demonstrating multiple fibromas (*arrows*) in a patient with FAP.

The location of the germline mutation is of some clinical significance (Fig. 67.16). For example, mutations that occur at the 5′ end of the gene, particularly in the first three exons, result in a clinically mild or "attenuated" form of FAP, in which the number of polyps is smaller and the onset of disease about 10 years later, with cancer developing in the sixth or seventh decade.[43] This occurs because the *APC* gene has a ribosomal reentry site downstream of the mutation, which permits the cell to bypass and ignore the premature stop codon. To complicate the situation, family members with the same mutation may have variable manifestations of the disease. Indeed, some members who inherit this mutation have few polyps and no cancer, yet can pass an increased risk for cancer to their progeny.

In contrast, mutations that occur in the "mutation cluster region" of the 15th exon, in a segment between codons 1250 and 1464, are associated with a particularly virulent form of the disease, in which the number of polyps is greater than 5,000 and the average age for the development of colorectal cancer is significantly earlier (median age, 34 years). Also, mutations at the extreme 3′ end of the gene are also associated with a milder phenotype, with fewer polyps, and later onset of cancer.

In families who have FAP with CHRPE lesions, the mutations are almost always in exons 9 to 15 and rarely in families whose mutations are in the first eight exons. Thus, knowledge of the location of the germline mutation can be useful in predicting the clinical manifestations and guide therapy.

5 **Diagnosis.** The clinical diagnosis of FAP is usually obvious clinically, but the availability of a genetic diagnosis has changed the approach to this disease. Currently, optimal practice is to obtain a germline diagnosis in an individual who is definitely affected, in order to characterize and counsel the family. A mutation in *APC* can be found in most (~90%) of these individuals using commercially available diagnostic laboratories. This will assist in the early and definitive identification of family members who carry the disease-causing mutation and will alleviate anxiety for those who do not. The risk to inherit the mutated gene from an affected parent is 50%, and there is no gender preference. A genetic diagnosis is particularly useful in the attenuated forms of FAP, where the diagnosis is not obvious, and this can help select those family members who need additional surveillance and reassure those who do not.

In some instances, the phenotype indicates FAP, but no mutation can be found in the *APC* gene. In this instance, the relatives at risk should undergo surveillance sigmoidoscopy on an annual basis beginning in their middle teens. If a single adenoma appears in a teenager at risk, the disease is strongly suspected, and the individual should be managed as if he or she is a mutation carrier. Almost no other disease produces multiple adenomatous polyps in young patients.

About 25% of patients have FAP that is not present in either parent. This can represent the autosomal recessive form of the disease (*MYH*-associated polyposis; see later), misattribution

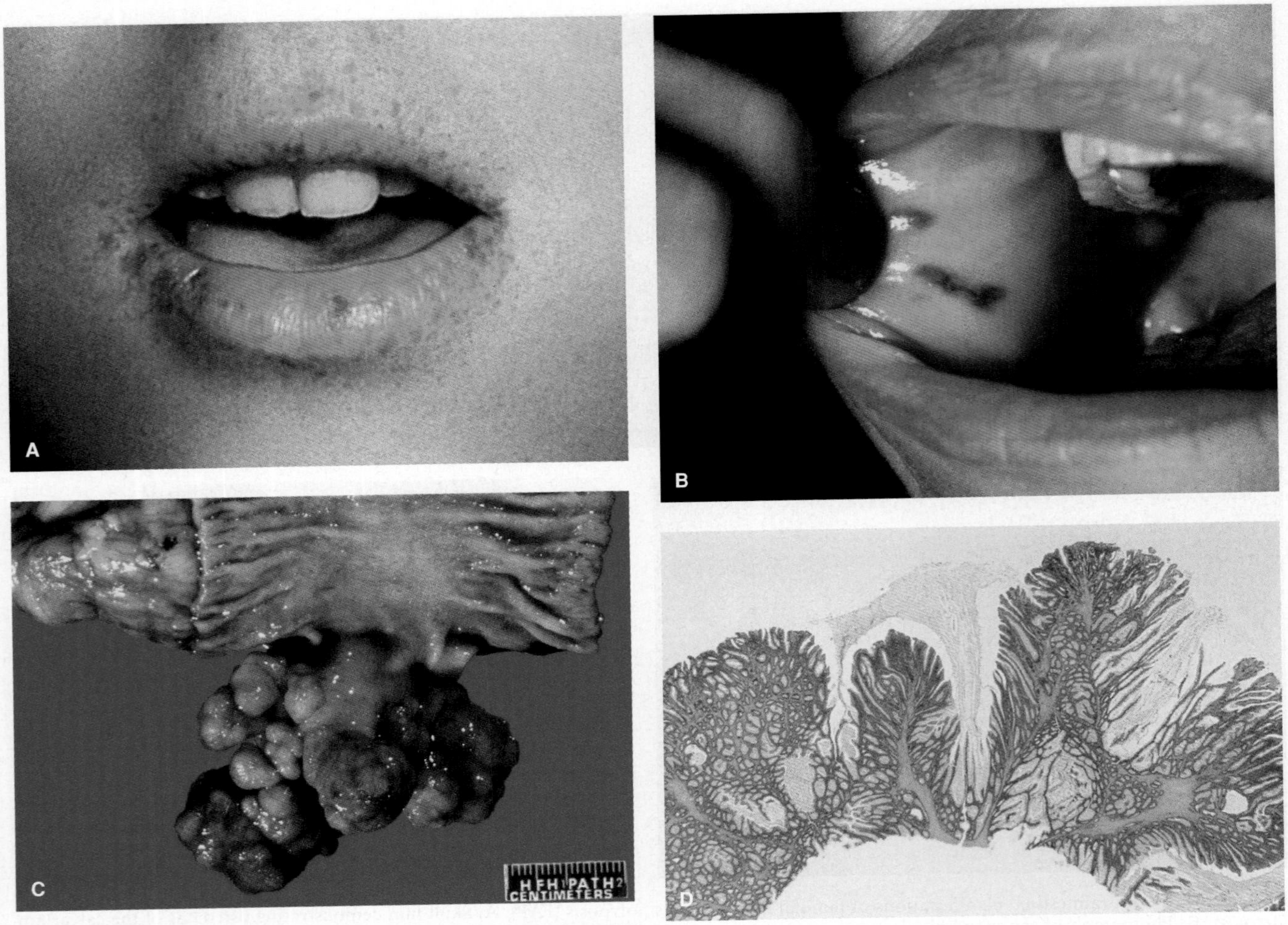

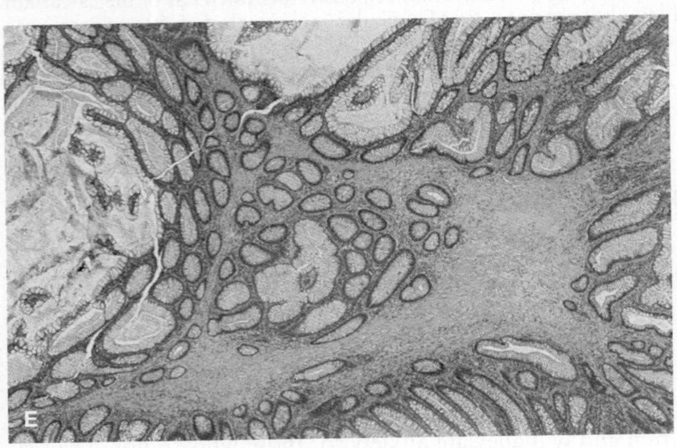

FIGURE 67.16. Peutz-Jeghers syndrome. **A:** Perioral hyperpigmentation. **B:** Hyperpigmented buccal mucosa. **C:** Gross specimen of a Peutz-Jeghers polyp illustrating a large multilobular lesion. **D:** Low-power photomicrograph of a Peutz-Jeghers polyp of the colon revealing smooth muscle stroma covered by nonneoplastic colonic epithelium. **E:** Photomicrograph of the Peutz-Jeghers polyp at higher power indicates that the stroma contains arborizing bands of smooth muscle.

of paternity, or phenotypic variation in which a parent actually has a milder form of the disease.

Genetic testing is an essential part of the clinical management of the hereditary cancer, but it can be a challenge. The genetic results are sometimes ambiguous and difficult for the physician to interpret.[44] Additionally, some patients mistake the germline test as a test for cancer. Issues of guilt and denial are prominent in genetic disorders. It is strongly recommended that physicians enlist the involvement of genetic counselors when performing genetic testing and counseling in such patients.

Management. Surgery is the only reasonable management option in FAP, and the clinical decision involves the selection and timing of the operation. The diagnosis of FAP is often made in adolescence, but the development of cancer may not be anticipated for 20 to 30 years after the first polyp appears, depending on the location of the mutation in the *APC* gene. When a child is found to have a germline mutation in *APC*, sigmoidoscopy should begin in the early teenage years, particularly if the mutation is in the "mutation cluster region" or the family's phenotype is known to be associated with thousands of polyps. Ideally, one would like a patient to reach adulthood prior to the colectomy, as the pelvis is larger and the individual is better able to cope with the disease psychologically.

The safest surgical approach is a total proctocolectomy with an ileoanal pouch anastomosis. No rectal mucosa should be left behind, since it is at risk for the development of neoplasia.

Even with careful endoscopic surveillance of the rectal segment, invasive carcinomas may develop.

The fact that small adenomatous polyps of the rectum can spontaneously regress visibly after a subtotal colectomy and ileorectal anastomosis underscores the reversible nature of the benign adenoma. Additionally, it has been found that adenomas can regress in FAP in response to treatment with sulindac (Clinoril). Several reports have confirmed that even large numbers of polyps regress in patients on 150 to 200 mg of sulindac twice per day.[45] Unfortunately, the polyps reappear when the drug is stopped, and development of cancer despite treatment with sulindac has been reported. Medical treatment is therefore not a safe or reliable first-line treatment for FAP, but it may be of some benefit in patients who delay operative intervention. Although no data are available to support this approach, sulindac may be a useful adjunct in patients with milder forms of FAP (i.e., smaller numbers of polyps with relative rectal sparing) and in circumstances in which residual rectal tissue must be left behind. Sulindac is not effective in the management of upper gastrointestinal tract neoplasia.

Management of Extracolonic Disease. In addition to the risks for colorectal neoplasia, patients with FAP are at risk for the development of osteomas, lipomas, fibromas, and a variety of other lesions. Although these mesenchymal tumors can degenerate into sarcomas, this is a sufficiently rare event that prophylactic surveillance and surgery are not indicated. Likewise, the CHRPE lesions do not require therapy. Gastric carcinoma is distinctly uncommon in North American populations, and it is not necessary to provide endoscopic surveillance of the stomach. The risk for gastric cancer in FAP is 0.5%.

The two major management issues after removal of the colon and rectum are periampullary neoplasia and desmoid tumors. One or more adenomas are found in the duodenum in 90% of patients with FAP, usually close to the ampulla of Vater. These lesions should be excised for biopsy and destroyed by electrocautery, laser, or other ablative approaches. Subsequent examination of the upper gastrointestinal tract is guided by the Spigelman criteria (Table 67.4).

TABLE 67.4

SPIGELMAN'S CLASSIFICATION FOR MANAGEMENT OF DUODENAL ADENOMAS IN INDIVIDUALS WITH FAP

	POINTS		
	1	2	3
A. Duodenal Disease Grading			
Polyp number	1–4	5–20	>20
Polyp size (mm)	1–4	5–20	>20
Histology	Tubular adenoma	Tubulovillous	Villous
Dysplasia	Mild	Moderate	Severe
B. Recommended Upper GI Surveillance in FAP			
Spigelman stage	Interval to EGD		
Stage 0 (0 points)	5 y		
Stage I (1–4 points)	5 y		
Stage II (5–6 points)	3 y		
Stage III (7–8 points)	1–2 y		
Stage IV (9–12 points)	EUS or surgery		

EGD, esophagogastroduodenoscopy; EUS, endoscopic ultrasound; FAP, familial adenomatous polyposis; GI, gastrointestinal.

Complex neoplasms, including adenomas with varying degrees of dysplasia, may require individualized management, including the use of biliary stents while extensive ablative therapy of the periampullary region is performed. Surgical approaches may be required for advanced neoplasms (i.e., carcinoma in situ or invasive carcinoma), but therapeutic endoscopy remains the first option. Duodenotomy with local surgical excision is an option for these lesions; rarely, a Whipple procedure is required for invasive lesions in this region.

Desmoid tumors are aggressive benign tumors of fibroblasts that can cause multiple clinical complications; they are a significant cause of morbidity and mortality in FAP. They typically grow slowly and can surround or compress vascular structures, nerves, or the abdominal viscera. They are more commonly seen in women and may be hormonally responsive, so estrogen administration (oral contraceptives or hormone replacement therapy) should be avoided in these patients. Surgical management is generally avoided unless simple local excision of an abdominal wall lesion is possible, and postoperative recurrences are common. Radiotherapy has been used to control the growth of some of these but is generally reserved for superficial lesions of the abdominal wall. No medical approach to this disease has been uniformly successful. A combination of sulindac plus tamoxifen may be tried for intra-abdominal tumors and has been successful in some patients. Cytotoxic chemotherapy with doxorubicin was successful in a patient whose tumor was refractory to other treatment. Anecdotally, some of these lesions may have *c-kit* mutations and are responsive to imatinib (Gleevec).

Familial Adenomatous Polyposis Variants.

A number of names, especially *Gardner syndrome,* have been attached to variations of FAP to emphasize the presence of particular extracolonic findings. As mentioned, Gardner syndrome is the same entity as FAP. A few families with prominent sebaceous cysts were historically said to have Oldfield syndrome, and families with brain tumors were said to have Turcot syndrome. All these syndromes represent the variable expression of germline mutations in the *APC* gene and are largely of historical interest. The current mode of classifying FAP families is based on the *APC* gene mutation.

MYH-Associated Polyposis

An autosomal recessive form of polyposis has been linked to inheritance of germline mutations in the base excision repair gene *MYH*, a DNA glycolase.[46] This should be considered when multiple adenomatous polyps occur in siblings or in a person who has no vertical family history of polyposis and there is no detectable germline mutation in the *APC* gene. These patients have a relatively mild (attenuated) form of adenomatous polyposis and will develop 20 to 500 adenomas, and the polyposis is typically detected in patients 35 to 65 years old. These patients are at very high risk for colorectal cancer, and the disease may present with cancer. The extraintestinal manifestations of FAP, such as duodenal adenomas or CHRPE lesions, occasionally occur but are less common in this condition. The pathogenesis of this disease is that the germline mutations in *MYH* permit an excess number of acquired mutations in the *APC* gene to occur in the colon; these mutations are typically G:C → T:A transversions, which is a consequence of losing the DNA base excision repair system. More than 1.3% of the Caucasian population carries single Y179C, G396D, and E480X (previously designated Y165C, G382D, and E466X, respectively, but changed due to renumbering of the coding sequence) mutations, and these carriers have a slight increase in colon cancer risk.[47] Many reference laboratories are currently testing for the three commonest *MYH* mutations on DNA sent from patients with a diagnosis of FAP if there is no detectable germline mutation (or deletion) in *APC*.

TABLE 67.5

GENETIC ALTERATIONS IN COLONIC POLYPOSIS SYNDROMES

■ POLYPOSIS SYNDROME	■ CHROMOSOME	■ GENE
Familial adenomatous polyposis (FAP)	5q21 1p35	*APC* (dominant) *MYH* (recessive)
Peutz-Jeghers syndrome	19p13.3	LKB1/STK11
Juvenile polyposis coli	18q21.1	SMAD4/MADH4 BMPR1A ENG
Bannayan-Riley-Ruvalcaba syndrome	10q23	PTEN
Cowden disease	10q23	PTEN
Hereditary mixed polyposis	6q, 15q	unknown

ENG, Endoglin.

Peutz-Jeghers Syndrome

Peutz-Jeghers syndrome is an autosomal dominant familial syndrome associated with multiple gastrointestinal polyps and characteristic skin pigmentation. The gene responsible for this disease is on chromosome 19p3.3 and encodes a serine/threonine kinase called *LKB1* or *STK11* (Table 67.5); carriers of the gene are highly predisposed to a number of early-onset cancers.

Gastrointestinal Features. The gastrointestinal polyps in Peutz-Jeghers syndrome are nonneoplastic hamartomas consisting of a supportive framework of smooth muscle tissue covered by somewhat hyperplastic epithelium (Fig. 67.16). These are histologically distinct from juvenile polyps and show no inflammatory cell infiltrate. Polyps may be found in the stomach, small intestine, or colon, and in each instance they have a distinctive appearance. Peutz-Jeghers polyps can usually be identified as such by the pathologist, and the characteristic cutaneous pigmentation makes this syndrome readily recognizable.

Skin Lesions. The cutaneous manifestations of Peutz-Jeghers syndrome may be found early in life and consist of dark, macular lesions on the mouth (both on the skin and in the buccal mucosa), nose, lips, hands, feet, genitalia, and anus. These lesions tend to become less obvious by the time of puberty. Unlike ordinary freckles, the cutaneous lesions of Peutz-Jeghers syndrome are present from birth. Moreover, ordinary freckles typically do not extend beyond the vermilion border of the lips, nor is the buccal mucosa involved, as it is in Peutz-Jeghers syndrome.

Clinical Complications. The principal complication of Peutz-Jeghers syndrome is intestinal obstruction, which may develop in infancy or childhood. This complication is most prominent in the small intestine because of its narrower diameter. Gastrointestinal bleeding may also be seen in this disease.

Cancer in the small intestine or colon can occur in Peutz-Jeghers syndrome; however, this is an uncommon complication.[48] It is thought that neoplasia may arise from foci of adenomatous epithelium found in some Peutz-Jeghers polyps. The risk for cancer is such that prophylactic surgery is not recommended.

Patients with Peutz-Jeghers syndrome are at increased risk for cancers within and outside the gastrointestinal tract. Cancer developed in about half of the patients in one large study at a median age of about 50 years. At risk are the stomach, small intestine, colorectum, gonads, breasts, pancreas, and biliary tree. Ovarian cysts and sex cord tumors are seen in 5% to 12% of female patients, and boys are at risk for endocrinologically active Sertoli cell testicular tumors that may produce feminizing features before puberty. No internal organ is individually at sufficiently high risk for cancer that a specific screening regimen or prophylactic surgery is indicated. The clinician should be aware of these risks, however, and should be particularly alert to gonadal tumors (which are otherwise rare) and breast cancer (for which screening should start at an early age and bilateral disease should be suspected).

Management. The management of Peutz-Jeghers syndrome is limited to the removal of polyps; endoscopic techniques should be used when possible. Surgery may be required for intussusception caused by small-intestinal polyps. The risk for neoplastic development should be kept in mind, but these patients are not candidates for prophylactic removal of any section of the gastrointestinal tract. As mentioned earlier, gonadal neoplasms and breast cancer are potential complications that may require surgery.

Juvenile Polyposis

Juvenile polyps are pathologically characteristic lesions that can be solitary or part of a polyposis syndrome. Juvenile polyps are most commonly solitary lesions found in the rectum during childhood. The lesions may be large and are made up of an edematous, mildly inflamed lamina propria covered by normal colonic epithelium (Fig. 67.17). If multiple polyps are found, a familial juvenile polyposis syndrome should be suspected. Three different syndromic presentations have been reported; it is not known, however, whether these are truly distinctive syndromes. They may consist of familial juvenile polyposis limited to the colon, familial juvenile polyposis throughout the gastrointestinal tract, and familial juvenile polyposis limited to the stomach. The genetic basis of this syndrome is not understood, but germline mutations in the *SMAD4* (also called the *MADH4* gene) and *BMPR1A* genes each account for about 20% of juvenile polyposis cases in which the genetic cause can be found.[49,50] Both these genes are involved in the TGF-β signaling pathway. Curiously, germline mutations in

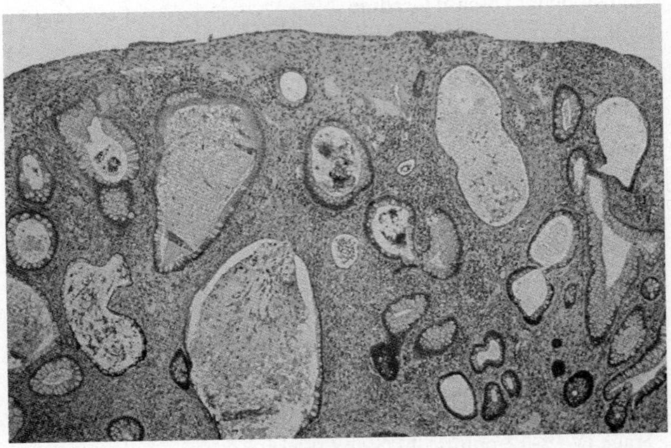

FIGURE 67.17. Photomicrograph of a juvenile polyp reveals an attenuated surface epithelium overlying an edematous lamina propria with fluid- and mucus-filled cystic structures.

these same genes can cause hereditary hemorrhagic telangiectasia. Although alterations in the *PTEN* gene had initially been linked to juvenile polyposis, germline mutations in this gene are only found in the rare Bannayan-Riley-Ruvalcaba variant, a childhood disorder characterized by macrocephaly, intestinal polyps, and unique pigmented macules of the penis[51]; this disorder shares features with Cowden syndrome, which is also caused by *PTEN* mutations.[52] Juvenile polyposis is a topic in need of additional clarification at the genetic and clinical levels.

The manifestations of juvenile polyposis can vary but are largely limited to bleeding, intussusception, obstruction, and the passage of autoamputated lesions. In some children, a life-threatening protein-losing enteropathy may develop that requires surgical resection of the affected segment of intestine. Patients with familial juvenile polyposis are at increased risk for the development of colorectal cancer and require careful surveillance.

Other Familial Polyposis Syndromes

A variety of other rare syndromes may give rise to multiple gastrointestinal polyps. Cowden syndrome consists of multiple gastrointestinal hamartomas and may be complicated by multiple lesions of the face that arise from follicular epithelium and are pathologically trichilemmomas.[53] The diagnosis of Cowden syndrome should be considered for patients with multiple trichilemmomas. Gastrointestinal polyps, which are usually asymptomatic, may develop in these patients. The polyps may include hamartomas, hyperplastic polyps, and ganglioneuromas of the colon. Glycogenic acanthosis of the esophagus may also occur and usually is found incidentally as multiple, diminutive, flat polyps of the esophagus. These patients are at increased risk for the development of breast cancer, uterine cancer, and thyroid neoplasms. No specific therapy need be directed toward the gastrointestinal tract. Germline mutations of the *PTEN* gene can be identified in most families with Cowden syndrome.[54]

Other diseases, such as neurofibromatosis (von Recklinghausen syndrome) and the basal cell nevus syndrome, may be associated with multiple gastrointestinal polyps; however, symptomatic complications of these polyps are uncommon. Bannayan-Riley-Ruvalcaba syndrome is a generalized hamartoma syndrome inherited in an autosomal dominant manner that is characterized by ileal and colonic polyps and lingual lesions. Other characteristics include ocular abnormalities, delayed motor development, lipid storage myopathy, and Hashimoto disease. This disease is most often linked to germline mutations in the *PTEN* gene.

NONFAMILIAL GASTROINTESTINAL POLYPOSIS SYNDROMES

Multiple gastrointestinal polyps are occasionally seen in nonfamilial syndromes. The Cronkhite-Canada syndrome is an acquired, nonfamilial syndrome characterized by cutaneous lesions (Fig. 67.18), chronic diarrhea, protein-losing enteropathy, and gastrointestinal polyps. The enteropathy may produce progressive inanition that can result in death. The diarrhea is attributable to diffuse mucosal injury of the small intestine but may be complicated by bacterial overgrowth. Gastrointestinal polyps are present in most patients and occur in the stomach, small intestine, colon, and rectum. These polyps are pathologically similar to juvenile retention-type polyps. The lamina propria is edematous and contains an inflammatory infiltrate. As has been reported in juvenile polyps, the lesions in this syndrome may contain adenomatous epithelium, and occasionally

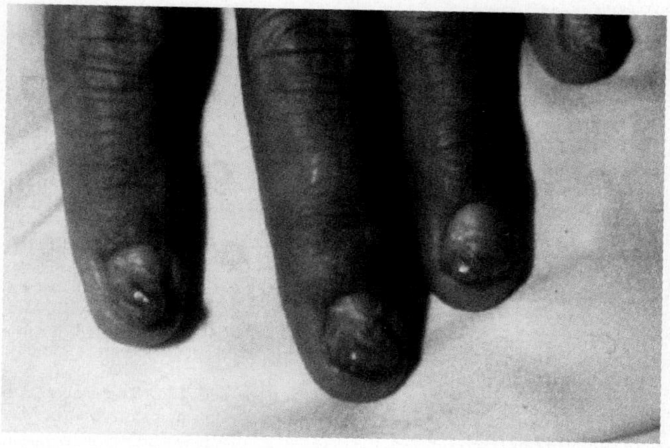

FIGURE 67.18. Cronkhite-Canada syndrome. Onycholysis and hyperpigmentation are characteristic cutaneous manifestations of Cronkhite-Canada syndrome, a nonfamilial, poorly understood, and acquired condition in which multiple juvenile, inflammatory-type gastrointestinal polyps and characteristic cutaneous features are found.

carcinomas have complicated this disease. A variety of medical and surgical measures have been used as treatment, and primary attention should be drawn to the treatment of the diarrhea and maintenance of the nutritional status. The cutaneous lesions consist of onycholysis, alopecia, and hyperpigmentation. Multiple therapeutic approaches have been tried, including broad-spectrum antibiotics, steroids, antihistamines, and extended bowel rest with parenteral nutritional support. Each approach has had occasional success, but none is uniformly effective. Curiously, the cutaneous features may resolve despite persistence of the gastrointestinal polyps.

Other acquired lesions that may present with multiple gastrointestinal polyps include inflammatory pseudopolyps in the setting of inflammatory bowel disease, lymphoma, pneumatosis cystoides intestinalis, and multiple lipomas or hyperplastic polyps. None of these syndromes requires specific surgical treatment.

References

1. Vogelstein B, Kinzler KW. Cancer genes and the pathways they control. *Nat Med* 2004;10:789–799.
2. Kinzler KW, Vogelstein B. Lessons from hereditary colorectal cancer. *Cell* 1996;87:159–170.
3. Boland CR, Ricciardiello L. How many mutations does it take to make a tumor? *Proc Natl Acad Sci U S A* 1999;96:14675–14677.
4. Herman JG, Baylin SB. Gene silencing in cancer in association with promoter hypermethylation. *N Engl J Med* 2003;349:2042–2054.
5. Powell SM, Zilz N, Beazer-Barclay Y, et al. APC mutations occur early during colorectal tumorigenesis. *Nature* 1992;359:235–237.
6. Kinzler KW, Vogelstein B. Cancer-susceptibility genes. Gatekeepers and caretakers. *Nature* 1997;386:761, 763.
7. Su LK, Vogelstein B, Kinzler KW. Association of the APC tumor suppressor protein with catenins. *Science* 1993;262:1734–1737.
8. Boland CR, Sato J, Appelman HD, et al. Microallelotyping defines the sequence and tempo of allelic losses at tumour suppressor gene loci during colorectal cancer progression. *Nat Med* 1995;1:902–909.
9. Boland CR. Evolution of the nomenclature for the hereditary colorectal cancer syndromes. *Fam Cancer* 2005;4:211–218.
10. Umar A, Boland CR, Terdiman JP, et al. Revised Bethesda guidelines for hereditary nonpolyposis colorectal cancer (Lynch syndrome) and microsatellite instability. *J Natl Cancer Inst* 2004;96:261–268.
11. O'brien MJ, Winawer SJ, Zauber AG, et al. The National Polyp Study. Patient and polyp characteristics associated with high-grade dysplasia in colorectal adenomas. *Gastroenterology* 1990;98:371–379.
12. Fuchs CS, Giovannucci EL, Colditz GA, et al. A prospective study of family history and the risk of colorectal cancer. *N Engl J Med* 1994;331:1669–1674.
13. Winawer SJ, Zauber AG, Gerdes H, et al. Risk of colorectal cancer in the families of patients with adenomatous polyps. National Polyp Study Workgroup. *N Engl J Med* 1996;334:82–87.

14. Brenner H, Hoffmeister M, Stegmaier C, et al. Risk of progression of advanced adenomas to colorectal cancer by age and sex: estimates based on 840,149 screening colonoscopies. *Gut* 2009;56:1585–1589.
15. Selby JV, Friedman GD, Quesenberry CP Jr, et al. A case-control study of screening sigmoidoscopy and mortality from colorectal cancer. *N Engl J Med* 1992;326:653–657.
16. Boland CR, Thibodeau SN, Hamilton SR, et al. A National Cancer Institute Workshop on Microsatellite Instability for cancer detection and familial predisposition: development of international criteria for the determination of microsatellite instability in colorectal cancer. *Cancer Res* 1998;58: 5248–5257.
17. Hamilton SR, Liu B, Parsons RE, et al. The molecular basis of Turcot's syndrome. *N Engl J Med* 1995;332:839–847.
18. Levin B, Lieberman DA, Mcfarland B, et al. Screening and surveillance for the early detection of colorectal cancer and adenomatous polyps, 2008: a joint guideline from the American Cancer Society, the US Multi-Society Task Force on Colorectal Cancer, and the American College of Radiology. *CA Cancer J Clin* 2008;58:130–160.
19. U.S. Preventative Services Task Force. Screening for colorectal cancer: U.S. Preventative Services Task Force recommendation statement. *Ann Int Med* 2008;149:627–637.
20. Mandel JS, Bond JH, Church TR, et al. Reducing mortality from colorectal cancer by screening for fecal occult blood. Minnesota Colon Cancer Control Study. *N Engl J Med* 1993;328:1365–1371.
21. Mandel JS. Screening of patients at average risk for colon cancer. *Med Clin North Am* 2005;89:43–59, vii.
22. Winawer SJ, Zauber AG, Ho MN, et al. Prevention of colorectal cancer by colonoscopic polypectomy. The National Polyp Study Workgroup. *N Engl J Med* 1993;329:1977–1981.
23. Atkin WS, Morson BC, Cuzick J. Long-term risk of colorectal cancer after excision of rectosigmoid adenomas. *N Engl J Med* 1992;326:658–662.
24. Lakoff J, Paszat LF, Saskin R, et al. Risk of developing proximal versus distal colorectal cancer after a negative colonoscopy: a population based study. *Clin Gastroenterol Hepatol* 2008;6:1117–1121.
25. Imperiale TF, Wagner DR, Lin CY, et al. Risk of advanced proximal neoplasms in asymptomatic adults according to the distal colorectal findings. *N Engl J Med* 2000;343:169–174.
26. Lieberman DA, Weiss DG, Bond JH, et al. Use of colonoscopy to screen asymptomatic adults for colorectal cancer. Veterans Affairs Cooperative Study Group 380. *N Engl J Med* 2000;343:162–168.
27. Soetikno RM, Kaltenbach T, Rouse RV, et al. Prevalence of nonpolypoid (flat and depressed) colorectal neoplasms in asymptomatic and symptomatic adults. *JAMA* 2008;299:1027–1035.
28. Johnson DJ, Chen M-H, Toledano AY, et al. Accuracy of CT colonography for detection of large adenomas and cancer. *N Engl J Med* 2008;359: 1207–1217.
29. Kim D, Pickhardt PJ, Taylor AJ, et al. CT colonography versus colonoscopy for the detection of advanced neoplasia. *N Engl J Med* 2007; 357:1403–1412.
30. Ahlquist DA, Sargent DJ, Loprinzi CL, et al. Stool DNA and occult blood testing for screen detection of colorectal neoplasia. *Ann Int Med* 2008; 149:441–450.
31. Lieberman DA, Weiss DG, Harford WV, et al. Five year colon surveillance after screening colonoscopy. *Gastroenterology* 2007;133:1077–1085.
32. Laiyermo AO, Murphy G, Albert PS, et al. Postpolypectomy colonoscopy surveillance guidelines: predictive accuracy for advanced adenomas at 4 years. *Ann Int Med* 2008;148:419–426.
33. Logan RF, Grainge MJ, Shepherd VC, et al. Aspirin and folic acid for prevention of recurrent colorectal adenomas. *Gastroenterology* 2008;134:29–38.
34. Baron JA, Cole BF, Sandler RS, et al. A randomized trial of aspirin to prevent colorectal adenomas. *N Engl J Med* 2003;348:891–899.
35. Bertagnolli MM, Eagle CJ, Zauber AG, et al. Celecoxib for the prevention of sporadic colorectal adenomas. *N Engl J Med* 2006;355:873–884.
36. Meyskins FL, McLaren CE, Pelot D, et al. Difluoromethylornithine plus sulindac for the prevention of sporadic colorectal adenomas: a randomized placebo-controlled, double-blind trial. *Cancer Prev Res* 2008;1:9–11.
37. Grau M, Baron JA, Sandler RS, et al. Prolonged effect of calcium supplementation on risk of colorectal adenomas in a randomized trial. *J Natl Cancer Inst* 2007;99:129–136.
38. O'Brien MJ, Yang S, Huang CS, et al. The serrated poly pathway to colorectal carcinoma. *Diagn Histopathol* 2008;14:78–93.
39. Powell SM, Petersen GM, Krush AJ, et al. Molecular diagnosis of familial adenomatous polyposis. *N Engl J Med* 1993;329:1982–1987.
40. Giardiello FM, Krush AJ, Petersen GM, et al. Phenotypic variability of familial adenomatous polyposis in 11 unrelated families with identical APC gene mutation. *Gastroenterology* 1994;106:1542–1547.
41. Scheenstra R, Rijcken FE, Koornstra JJ, et al. Rapidly progressive adenomatous polyposis in a patient with germline mutations in both the APC and MLH1 genes: the worst of two worlds. *Gut* 2003;52:898–899.
42. Giardiello FM, Petersen GM, Piantadosi S, et al. APC gene mutations and extraintestinal phenotype of familial adenomatous polyposis. *Gut* 1997; 40:521–525.
43. Giardiello FM, Brensinger JD, Luce MC, et al. Phenotypic expression of disease in families that have mutations in the 5′ region of the adenomatous polyposis coli gene. *Ann Intern Med* 1997;126:514–519.
44. Giardiello FM, Brensinger JD, Petersen GM, et al. The use and interpretation of commercial APC gene testing for familial adenomatous polyposis. *N Engl J Med* 1997;336:823–827.
45. Giardiello FM, Hamilton SR, Krush AJ, et al. Treatment of colonic and rectal adenomas with sulindac in familial adenomatous polyposis. *N Engl J Med* 1993;328:1313–1316.
46. Sieber OM, Lipton L, Crabtree M, et al. Multiple colorectal adenomas, classic adenomatous polyposis, and germ-line mutations in MYH. *N Engl J Med* 2003;348:791–799.
47. Wang L, Baudhuin LM, Boardman LA, et al. MYH mutations in patients with attenuated and classic polyposis and with young-onset colorectal cancer without polyps. *Gastroenterology* 2004;127:9–16.
48. Giardiello FM, Welsh SB, Hamilton SR, et al. Increased risk of cancer in the Peutz-Jeghers syndrome. *N Engl J Med* 1987;316:1511–1514.
49. Howe JR, Sayed MG, Ahmed AF, et al. The prevalence of MADH4 and BMPR1A mutations in juvenile polyposis and absence of BMPR2, BMPR1B, and ACVR1 mutations. *J Med Genet* 2004;41:484–491.
50. Howe JR, Shellnut J, Wagner B, et al. Common deletion of SMAD4 in juvenile polyposis is a mutational hotspot. *Am J Hum Genet* 2002;70: 1357–1362.
51. Marsh DJ, Coulon V, Lunetta KL, et al. Mutation spectrum and genotype-phenotype analyses in Cowden disease and Bannayan-Zonana syndrome, two hamartoma syndromes with germline PTEN mutation. *Hum Mol Genet* 1998;7:507–515.
52. Chi SG, Kim HJ, Park BJ, et al. Mutational abrogation of the PTEN/MMAC1 gene in gastrointestinal polyps in patients with Cowden disease. *Gastroenterology* 1998;115:1084–1089.
53. Marra G, Armelao F, Vecchio FM, et al. Cowden's disease with extensive gastrointestinal polyposis. *J Clin Gastroenterol* 1994;18:42–47.
54. Eng C. PTEN: one gene, many syndromes. *Hum Mutat* 2003;22:183–198.

CHAPTER 68 ■ COLORECTAL CANCER

ARDEN MORRIS

KEY POINTS

1. Epidemiologic studies have suggested that 15% of colorectal cancers occur in a dominantly inherited pattern. The two best-described familial colorectal cancer syndromes are familial adenomatous polyposis (FAP) and hereditary nonpolyposis colorectal cancer (HNPCC). Currently, it is estimated that 5% of all colorectal cancers occur in persons affected with one of these two syndromes.
2. Mutations in three distinct types of genes are known to contribute to colorectal cancer formation: oncogenes, tumor-suppressor genes, and DNA mismatch repair genes. The former two mechanisms, comprising the loss of heterozygosity or chromosomal instability pathway, account for about 85% of colon and rectal tumors. Mutations in mismatch repair genes, termed the replication error or microsatellite instability pathway, account for about 15% of large bowel tumors.
3. The incidence of invasive malignancy differs markedly for the three histologic subtypes of colon polyps, being lowest in adenomatous polyps, intermediate in tubulovillous adenomas, and highest in villous lesions. Polyp size is directly correlated with the presence of dysplasia or malignancy.

4. The most important prognostic factor in colorectal cancer is dissemination to nearby lymph nodes or distant organs.
5. The surgical goals in the resection of a primary colorectal cancer are to achieve an en bloc resection that encompasses an adequate amount of normal colon proximal and distal to the tumor, to obtain adequate lateral margins if the tumor is adherent to contiguous structures, and to remove the regional lymph node basin.
6. The liver is the most frequent site of blood-borne metastases from primary colorectal cancers.

Adenocarcinoma of the large intestine is the fourth most common malignancy in the United States, with an estimated incidence of 146,970 new cases in 2009.[1] Colorectal cancer is second only to lung cancer as a cause of cancer-related deaths. In 2009, an estimated 49,920 persons died of colorectal cancer in the United States. If diagnosed in its early stages, however, colorectal cancer is one of the most curable malignancies. Most early-stage colorectal cancer is curable by surgical treatment. Because of the potential for surgical cure of early-stage or localized disease, identification of populations at risk and screening of asymptomatic patients are important considerations. For regional disease, controlled clinical trials have demonstrated that a multidisciplinary approach can reduce cancer-specific mortality substantially[2] (Fig. 68.1). For recurrent disease, various therapeutic approaches are reviewed. Other colorectal tumors distinct from adenocarcinoma, such as lymphomas, sarcomas, gastrointestinal stromal tumors, and carcinoid tumors, are discussed at the end of the chapter.

EPIDEMIOLOGY

Incidence and Mortality

Worldwide, colorectal cancer is the third most common cancer in men and the fourth most common cancer in women. An important feature of colorectal cancer is the wide variation in incidence (as much as 30-fold) noted between population groups according to geographic region (Fig. 68.2). Although industrialized countries such as those in Northern and Western Europe have the highest incidence rates, these trends are stable or actually decreasing. In contrast, the incidence of colorectal cancer is increasing notably among economically transitioning areas, such as Eastern Europe, most of Asia, and several parts of South America.[3] These geographic differences cannot be attributed solely to genetic factors for several reasons. First, populations migrating from low- to high-incidence regions can experience an increase in the incidence of colorectal cancer within a single generation.[4–6] Second, even among nonmigrants, incidence rates can change with in-country lifestyle trends. In some parts of Japan, a highly industrialized country, the incidence of new colorectal cancers among men has increased by more than 90%, concurrent with Westernization of the regional diet.[3] These data provide indirect evidence that environmental factors, including diet and lifestyle, are involved in the pathogenesis of this disease—thus, its incidence may be reducible.

In the United States, the incidence of colorectal cancer overall has been in decline since 1992, with a current lifetime incidence risk of just over 5%.[1] This phenomenon is largely attributed to improvements in screening, during which precancerous polyps are detected and removed. The declining incidence of

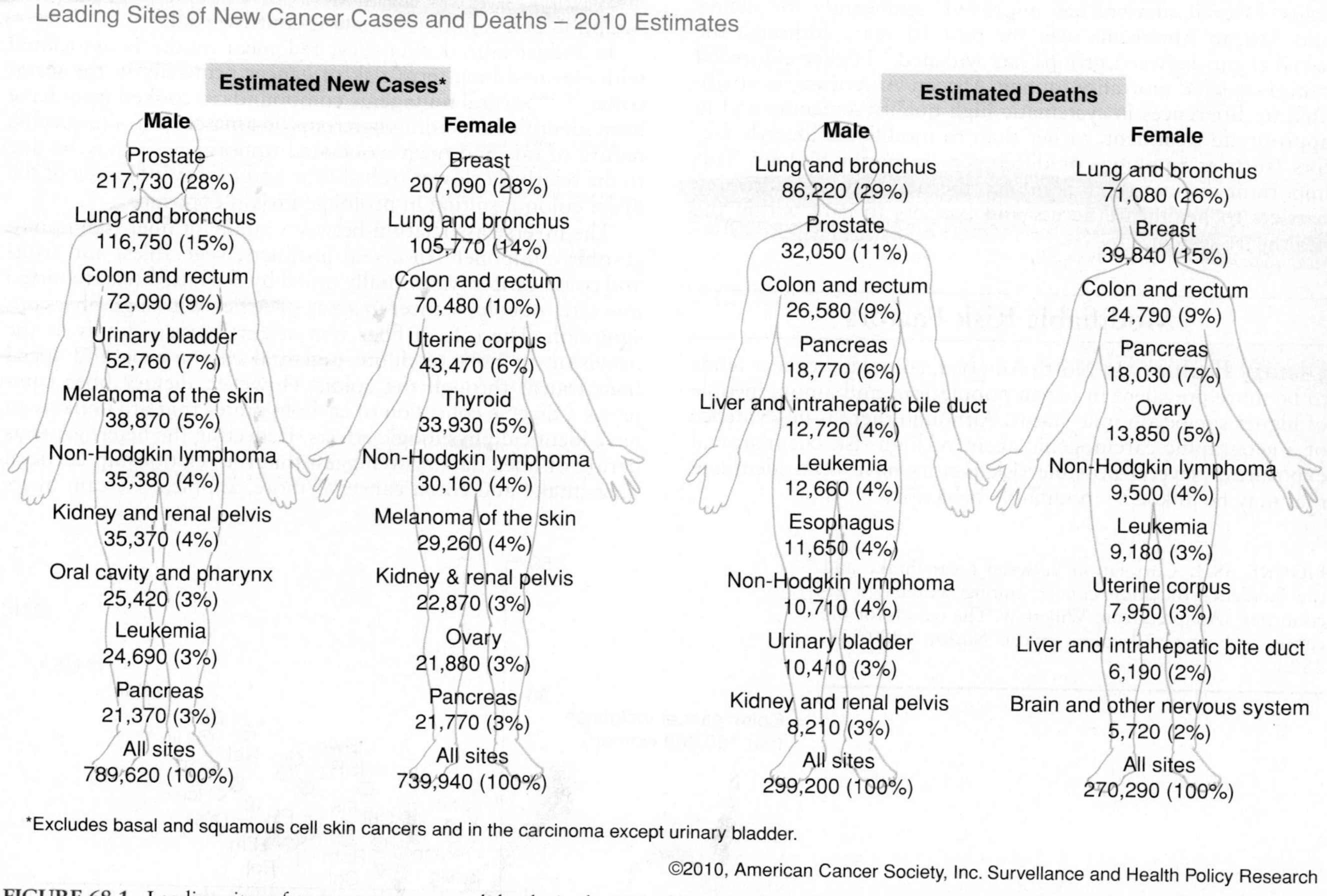

Leading Sites of New Cancer Cases and Deaths – 2010 Estimates
Estimated New Cases*
Male
Prostate
217,730 (28%)
Lung and bronchus
116,750 (15%)
Colon and rectum
72,090 (9%)
Urinary bladder
52,760 (7%)
Melanoma of the skin
38,870 (5%)
Non-Hodgkin lymphoma
35,380 (4%)
Kidney and renal pelvis
35,370 (4%)
Oral cavity and pharynx
25,420 (3%)
Leukemia
24,690 (3%)
Pancreas
21,370 (3%)
All sites
789,620 (100%)
Female
Breast
207,090 (28%)
Lung and bronchus
105,770 (14%)
Colon and rectum
70,480 (10%)
Uterine corpus
43,470 (6%)
Thyroid
33,930 (5%)
Non-Hodgkin lymphoma
30,160 (4%)
Melanoma of the skin
29,260 (4%)
Kidney & renal pelvis
22,870 (3%)
Ovary
21,880 (3%)
Pancreas
21,770 (3%)
All sites
739,940 (100%)
Estimated Deaths
Male
Lung and bronchus
86,220 (29%)
Prostate
32,050 (11%)
Colon and rectum
26,580 (9%)
Pancreas
18,770 (6%)
Liver and intrahepatic bile duct
12,720 (4%)
Leukemia
12,660 (4%)
Esophagus
11,650 (4%)
Non-Hodgkin lymphoma
10,710 (4%)
Urinary bladder
10,410 (3%)
Kidney and renal pelvis
8,210 (3%)
All sites
299,200 (100%)
Female
Lung and bronchus
71,080 (26%)
Breast
39,840 (15%)
Colon and rectum
24,790 (9%)
Pancreas
18,030 (7%)
Ovary
13,850 (5%)
Non-Hodgkin lymphoma
9,500 (4%)
Leukemia
9,180 (3%)
Uterine corpus
7,950 (3%)
Liver and intrahepatic bite duct
6,190 (2%)
Brain and other nervous system
5,720 (2%)
All sites
270,290 (100%)
*Excludes basal and squamous cell skin cancers and in the carcinoma except urinary bladder.
©2010, American Cancer Society, Inc. Surveillance and Health Policy Research

FIGURE 68.1. Leading sites of new cancer cases and deaths in the United States, 2005. (American Cancer Society. *Cancer Facts & Figures 2010.* Atlanta: American Cancer Society; 2010.

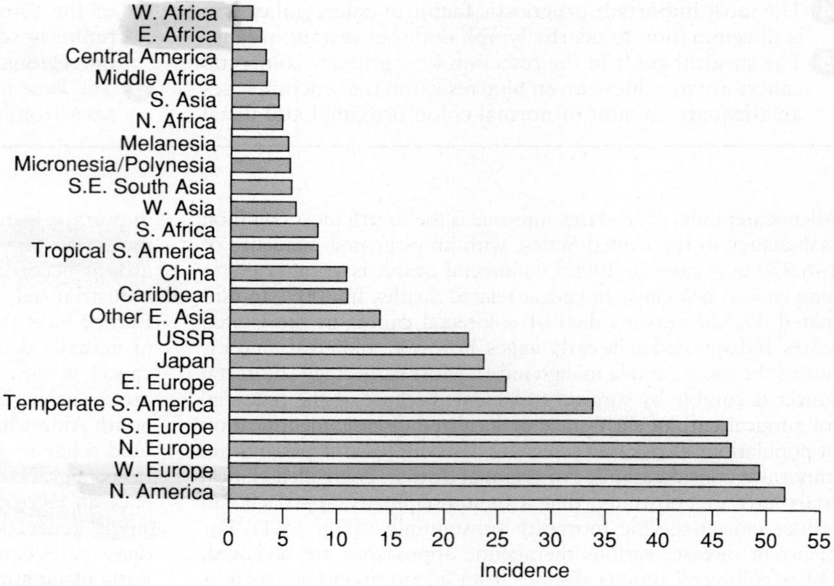

FIGURE 68.2. Incidence of colorectal cancer per 100,000 persons in 23 geographic regions during 1980. (Adapted from Parkin DM, Laara E, Muir CS. Estimates of the worldwide frequency of sixteen major cancers in 1980. *Int J Cancer* 1988;41:184.)

colorectal cancer has been slower among African Americans compared with whites. Among African American men, the colorectal cancer incidence rate is 21% higher than among white men. Among African American women, the incidence rate is 26% higher than among white women. In contrast, among Hispanic men and women the incidence rate is about 25% lower than among their white counterparts.

In 2005, the overall survival rate of colorectal cancer was 66% among whites compared with 55% among African Americans. Overall survival has improved significantly for whites and African Americans over the past 10 years, although the survival gap between groups has widened.[7] Higher colorectal cancer–specific mortality among African Americans is attributed to differences in systematic high-quality screening and in appropriate treatment, rather than to modifiable lifestyle factors (such as smoking) or differences in tumor biology. This important distinction underscores the necessity of addressing barriers to healthcare access and barriers to care within the healthcare system.

Modifiable Risk Factors

Dietary Factors. In North America, colorectal cancer tends to be more prevalent in urban populations and among people of higher socioeconomic status. Although there is no evidence of a geographic carcinogenic agent or high-risk occupational exposures,[8] several possible risk factors have been identified that may be linked to modifiable behaviors.

Epidemiologic studies suggest that dietary factors play causative and protective roles in the development of large-bowel cancers.[9] Red meat and fat intake have the most consistently direct association, and fiber intake has the most consistently inverse association with colorectal cancer (Fig. 68.3). For example, in comparisons between countries, the associations between per capita consumption of total fat, saturated fat, and cholesterol and the national incidence rates of colon cancer are strongly positive.[10] However, whether the responsible mechanism is interaction with bile acids or simply excess fuel consumption and resultant obesity is controversial.[9,11]

In industrialized countries, red meat intake is associated with elevated long-term risk of cancer primarily in the distal colon.[12–14] Several mutagenic compounds in cooked meat have been identified including heterocyclic amines. The site-specific nature of fat- and meat-associated tumorigenesis may be due to the relatively slower transit time and narrowed lumen of the distal colon resulting in prolonged toxin exposure.

The inverse association between intake of fiber (the nondigestible component of cereal products, vegetables, and fruit) and colon cancer was initially noted by Burkitt,[15] who reported low rates of colon cancer in areas of Africa with high fiber consumption. The role of fiber was originally seen simply as the provision of bulk to dilute potential carcinogens and speed their transit through the colon. However, dietary fiber comprises a diverse collection of carbohydrates that are unlikely to have identical physiologic effects. Reflecting the heterogeneous nature of fiber, data now suggest that the relationship between fiber intake and colon cancer is more complex. Certain fibers

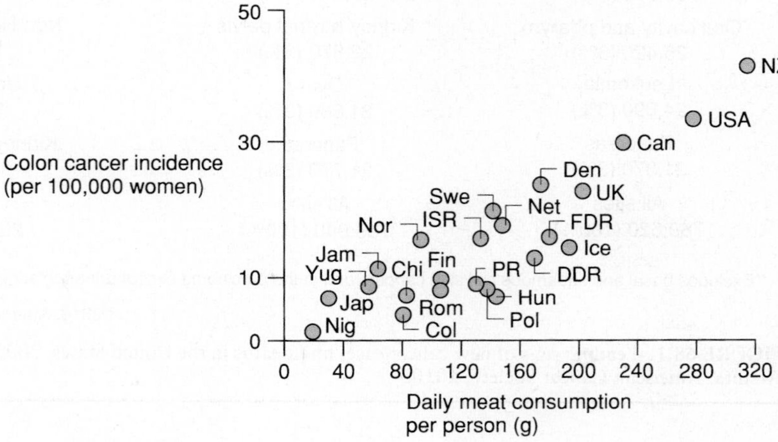

FIGURE 68.3. Correlation between meat intake and the incidence of colon cancer among women in 23 countries. (Adapted from Willett W. The search for the causes of breast and colon cancer. *Nature* 1989;338:389.)

can bind mutagens, reducing their contact with colonic epithelium; others can favorably change the fecal pH or participate in other complex interactions.

Although the protective role of fiber is incompletely defined, recent evidence indicates a potential 20% to 50% risk reduction, particularly noted among frequent consumers of dark green vegetables.[9,11,12] Preliminary data suggest that micronutrients such as folate, methionine, vitamin D, and calcium may provide protection against oxidative stress at the cellular level. Whether the protective effect of leafy green vegetables is due primarily to mechanical effects of fiber or to a chemoprotective effect of micronutrients remains unknown.

Alcohol Consumption. A positive dose response effect of alcohol on colorectal cancer formation has been extensively demonstrated. Beer apparently plays a more important role in mucosal neoplasm formation than wine or spirits.[16] Although the mechanism of mutagenesis has not been determined, the metabolite acetaldehyde is generally considered the culprit. Acetaldehyde may contribute to free radical formation and proliferative growth of mucosal polyps. Folate and calcium appear to have a protective effect, possibly by competing with aldehyde for binding sites at the mucosal surface. These hypotheses are supported by decreased colorectal cancer rates seen among heavy drinkers who consume large quantities of dietary folate, for example in leafy greens, coupled with higher colorectal cancer rates among drinkers with a low intake of leafy green vegetables.

Smoking. After much dissent in the literature, a recent meta-analysis[17] of 106 observational studies has demonstrated 18% higher odds of developing colorectal cancers (CRC) among ever-smokers compared with never-smokers. Risk was significant only among persons who smoked more than 30 years and was dose dependent. The association between cigarette smoking and cancer mortality was even stronger. That is, ever-smokers were 25% more likely to die of colon cancer causes than never-smokers. For unknown reasons, risk was markedly higher for cancers in the rectum compared with those in the colon.

Exercise and Obesity. The cancer prevention benefits of regular exercise have been increasingly recognized for colon (not rectal) cancer. Although the mechanism of action remains unclear, exercise is thought to reduce inflammation and potentially contribute to reduced free radicals. In a pooled analysis of 19 studies, men and women who averaged more than 4 hours per week of moderate exercise demonstrated a 22% and 29% reduction in CRC incidence, respectively.[18] In addition, regular exercise reduces obesity, which is also associated with colorectal cancer incidence. Obesity may contribute to colon cancer formation via fat metabolism pathways or hyperinsulinemia. Notably, central obesity (waist circumference) has an even more robust association with increased colorectal cancer incidence than body mass index.[19,20]

Clinical Risk Factors

Familial Cancer Syndromes. Although up to 30% of persons diagnosed with colorectal cancer have some family history, the vast majority of colorectal cancer cases have no apparent familial association and therefore are considered sporadic. Epidemiologic studies have suggested that at least 15% of all colorectal cancers occur in a dominantly inherited pattern, and that an inherited susceptibility to polyps and cancer could account for up to 90% of the total number of colorectal cancers in the population.[21,22] The two best-described familial colorectal cancer syndromes are familial adenomatous polyposis (FAP) and hereditary nonpolyposis colon cancer (HNPCC). Currently, it is estimated that 5% of all colorectal cancers occur in persons affected with one of these two syndromes (Table 68.1).

TABLE 68.1 **ETIOLOGY**

CLINICAL RISK FACTORS FOR COLORECTAL CANCER

■ GENETIC
POLYPOSIS SYNDROMES
Familial polyposis coli
Gardner syndrome
Turcot syndrome (central nervous system tumors)
Oldfield syndrome (sebaceous cysts)
Peutz-Jeghers syndrome (hamartomas)
NONPOLYPOSIS SYNDROMES
Lynch syndrome I
Lynch syndrome II (associated extracolonic cancers)
PREEXISTING DISEASE
Ulcerative colitis
Crohn disease
Prior colorectal cancer
Neoplastic polyps
Pelvic irradiation
Breast or genital tract cancer
GENERAL
Age >40 years
Family history of colorectal cancer

FAP is an autosomal, dominantly inherited disease caused by mutations in the *APC* gene. In affected subjects, hundreds to thousands of adenomatous polyps typically develop throughout the colon and rectum, each of which has the potential to progress to an invasive cancer. The average age for the diagnosis of colorectal cancer is 42 years, markedly earlier than the average age of 63 years in sporadic cases. Cancer develops in virtually all affected persons by age 55. Polyps are also found in other regions of the gastrointestinal tract in patients with FAP, especially the duodenum and stomach. Duodenal and periampullary polyps in particular are at increased risk of malignant transformation.[23,24] Additionally, several extraintestinal manifestations of FAP have been described, including congenital hypertrophy of the retinal pigment epithelium (CHRPE), osteomas, and desmoid tumors. This and other polyposis syndromes are discussed in more detail in Chapter 67.

HNPCC kindreds were first described in 1913 by Aldred Warthin, a pathologist at the University of Michigan. One kindred, referred to as family G, has been followed extensively through the years and represents a classic example of the HNPCC syndrome.[25,26] A more systematic collection of families and analysis of their pedigrees was performed by Henry Lynch et al. at Creighton University. Although colorectal cancers in this syndrome derive from adenomatous polyps, an associated polyposis phenotype is absent. Thus, the syndrome was given the nonpolyposis designation. Two phenotypic variants of HNPCC have been described: Lynch syndromes I and II. Lynch syndrome I families manifest only colon cancer. Lynch syndrome II families manifest colon cancer in addition to several others, including endometrial, ovarian, gastric, small-bowel, liver and biliary tract, upper urologic tract, and central nervous system cancers. The median age for the development of either colorectal or endometrial cancer in HNPCC patients is 39 to 46 years.[27] HNPCC occurs in about 1 to 2/1,000 individuals, and its penetrance is estimated at 70% to 90% for colon cancer. An unusual clinical variant of HNPCC is the Muir-Torre syndrome, in which affected members have sebaceous tumors (both benign and malignant) and keratoacanthomas in addition to the spectrum of tumors found in Lynch syndrome II.

The clinical criteria necessary for identifying a family as an HNPCC kindred were established initially by an international collaborative conference in Amsterdam in 1990. The Amsterdam criteria are based on exclusion of FAP and a 3-2-1 rule: (i) at least *three* relatives with histologically verified colorectal cancer, with at least one being a first-degree relative of the other two; (ii) at least *two* successive generations affected; and (iii) diagnosis of colorectal cancer in *one* of the relatives before the age of 50 years.[28] With further study of HNPCC kindreds, the Amsterdam criteria were revised as Amsterdam II, to include at least three relatives with HNPCC-associated cancers in lieu of colorectal cancers only.[29] However, a proportion of individuals at risk for HNPCC still do not satisfy the Amsterdam II criteria.[30] To better guide recommendations for genetic evaluation, the Bethesda criteria were developed and recently revised as an alternative system for identifying HNPCC kindreds (Table 68.2).[31,32] Although these criteria schemes provide acceptable capture of patients, test characteristics and ease of use differ. The tumors of patients in families who satisfy Amsterdam II or the revised Bethesda criteria should be tested for microsatellite instability. A positive result includes presence of at least two of five mismatch repair proteins (mononucleotide markers BAT25, BAT26, D2S123, D5S346, D17S250), and indicates further germline analysis for MSH2/MLH1 germline repair gene abnormalities.[33]

Currently, about 40% of familial clusters of colorectal cancer do not have discernable microsatellite instability in their tumors or germline mutations.[34] It is plausible that several predisposing hereditary defects will be identified in the future. Therefore, obtaining a thorough family history is mandatory in the workup of any patient with cancer, especially those with onset at a young age or with multiple tumors.

The easy availability of genetic testing by many commercial laboratories has been problematic, as most physicians are not prepared to interpret the results or to counsel patients regarding their cancer risk and treatment. In a study of patients undergoing genetic testing for familial polyposis by a commercial company, it was found that only 19% of patients received genetic counseling before the test, and in 32% of cases, the physician ordering the test misinterpreted the results.[35] Although most problems with misinterpretation are encountered with negative results, the interpretation of a positive result also can be difficult. It must be emphasized that a negative result can provide reassurance only if the predisposing mutation in the family is already known. Otherwise, a negative result may mean that the mutation was missed, that it occurred in a promoter or intronic sequence not evaluated, or that a cancer predisposition still exists because of a mutation in another known or unknown disease gene.[36] In the case of a positive result, one must be sure that the mutation does in fact confer a cancer risk and that it is not merely a benign polymorphism. Therefore, when identified, patients suspected of having an inherited cancer syndrome should be offered counseling by a cancer geneticist or experienced genetic counselor, both before the test is ordered and after the results are known.

Inflammatory Bowel Disease. A strong association exists between inflammatory bowel disease (IBD) and bowel cancer. For patients with ulcerative colitis, the incidence of malignancy is proportional to the extent of colonic involvement, age at onset, and severity and duration of disease. The duration of inflammatory bowel disease is a critical factor in predicting the likelihood of adenocarcinoma. Cancer develops in about 3% of patients during the first 10 years after the onset of colitis and in an additional 20% during each of the next two decades. The cure rate in patients with ulcerative colitis who are treated for cancer is similar to that in noncolitic patients treated for cancer.[37]

Patients with Crohn disease are also at increased risk for colon cancer in addition to small-bowel cancer. The risk for malignancy is lower than that reported for ulcerative colitis. Like the cancers associated with ulcerative colitis, the cancers associated with Crohn disease tend to occur at an earlier age than those in patients without inflammatory bowel disease.

Carcinogenesis in IBD has been garnering attention recently as a novel model of inflammation-induced cancer.[38] A key molecule in this process is NF-κB, a molecule required for expressing proinflammatory cytokines such as reactive nitrogen and oxygen species, which in turn are likely to stimulate growth of neoplastic epithelium or dysplasia. In chronically inflamed or colitic patients, dysplasia is believed to progress from inflammation, to low-grade, to indefinite, to high-grade dysplasia. The lesions are often flat and therefore may be more difficult to detect by colonoscopy or other traditional diagnostic methods.

Polyps. Traditionally, colorectal polyps have been divided into two broad categories: neoplastic and nonneoplastic. Nonneoplastic polyps included hyperplastic, inflammatory, juvenile, and hamartomatous polyps, none of which were considered precursors to colorectal cancer. Neoplastic polyps were adenomas and had the potential to develop into malignant cancers. The incidence of colorectal malignancy is two to five times higher in patients with adenomatous polyps than in those without them. Carcinoma is twice as likely to develop in patients with multiple polyps as in patients with a single polyp. Evidence suggests the existence of a common inherited susceptibility toward both sporadic colonic adenomatous polyps and colorectal cancer.[21]

Adenoma histology can be classified as tubular (75%–100% tubular components), tubulovillous (25%–75% villous components), or villous (75%–100% villous components). Tubular adenomas, or adenomatous polyps, are the most common type and constitute about 75% of neoplastic polyps[39] (Table 68.3). Tubulovillous adenomas account for 15% and purely villous adenomas for 10% of neoplastic polyps. All adenomas contain some degree of dysplasia or cellular atypia, which can be graded from mild to severe. Carcinoma in situ and severe dysplasia have been grouped together under the classification of high-grade dysplasia. In contrast to invasive carcinoma, carcinoma in situ has not invaded the muscularis mucosa (Fig.
3 68.4). The incidence of invasive malignancy differs markedly for the three histologic subtypes. In general, malignancies are

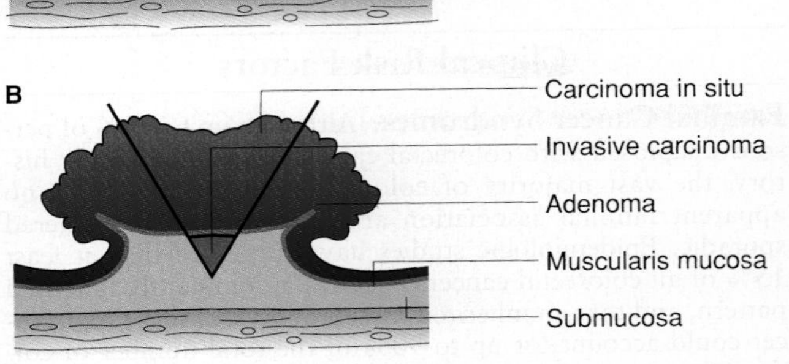

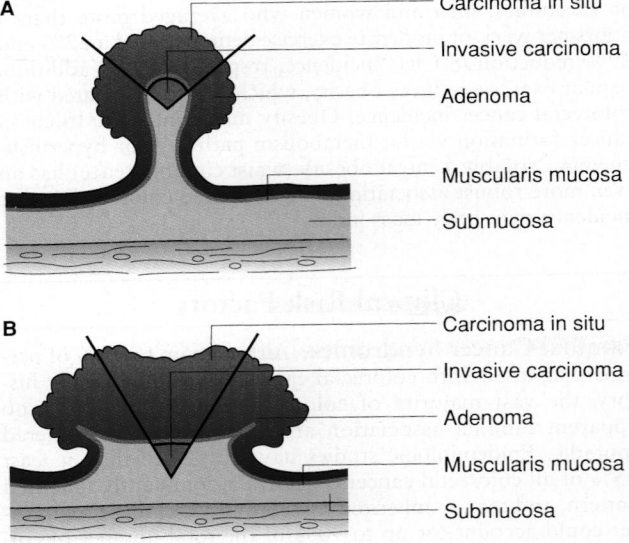

FIGURE 68.4. Anatomic distinction between carcinoma in situ and invasive malignancy in a pedunculated (**A**) and a sessile (**B**) adenomatous polyp. Carcinoma in situ is characterized by the absence of invasion into the muscularis mucosae.

TABLE 68.2

COMPARISON OF CLINICAL CRITERIA FOR HEREDITARY NONPOLYPOSIS COLORECTAL CANCER (HNPCC)[a]

	■ CRITERIA	■ SENSITIVITY[109]	■ SPECIFICITY[109]	■ STRENGTHS	■ WEAKNESSES
AMSTERDAM[28]	Three relatives with colorectal cancer, meeting all of the following criteria: (i) one of whom is a first-degree relative of the other two; (ii) colorectal cancer in at least two generations; (iii) one or more colorectal cancer cases diagnosed before age 50 years	61%	67%	Easy to remember and apply; good specificity	Limited sensitivity
AMSTERDAM II[29]	Three relatives with HNPCC-associated cancer,[b] meeting all of the following criteria: (i) one of whom is a first-degree relative of the other two; (ii) colorectal cancer in at least two generations; (iii) one or more colorectal cancer cases diagnosed before age 50 years	78%	61%	Easy to remember and, apply; good specificity	Improved but limited sensitivity
BETHESDA GUIDELINES[31]	Meeting any of the following criteria:[c] (i) subjects with cancer in families that fulfill Amsterdam criteria; (ii) subjects with two HNPCC-related cancers; (iii) subjects with colorectal cancer and a first-degree relative with HNPCC-related cancer and/or colorectal adenoma; one of the cancers diagnosed at age <45 years and the adenoma diagnosed at age <40 years	94%	49%	Increased sensitivity	Complexity in the clinical setting
REVISED BETHESDA GUIDELINES[32]	Meeting any of the following criteria: (i) colorectal cancer diagnosed in a patient younger than age 50 years; (ii) presence of synchronous or metachronous HNPCC-associated tumors, regardless of age; (iii) colorectal cancer with microsatellite instability high histology in a patient younger than age 60 years; (iv) colorectal cancer in one or more first-degree relatives with an HNPCC-related tumor, with one of the cancers diagnosed at age younger than 50 years; or (v) colorectal cancer diagnosed in two or more first- or second-degree relatives with HNPCC-associated tumors, regardless of age			Easier to apply in the clinical setting	Due to recent development, limited data regarding test

[a]After exclusion of familial adenomatous polyposis.
[b]HNPCC-associated cancers are colorectal, endometrial, ovarian, stomach, small intestine, biliary tract, ureter, renal pelvis, and brain cancers, and sebaceous gland adenomas and keratoacanthomas in Muir-Torre syndrome.
[c]Four additional original Bethesda criteria did not increase the sensitivity, but their inclusion decreased the specificity to 25%: (iv) Subjects with colorectal cancer or endometrial cancer at age <45 years; (v) subjects with right-sided colorectal cancer with an undifferentiated histopathologic pattern diagnosed at age <45 years; (vi) subjects with signet-ring cell type colorectal cancer diagnosed at age <45 years; (vii) subjects with adenomas diagnosed at age <40 years.

TABLE 68.3

NEOPLASTIC COLORECTAL POLYPS

■ TYPE	■ HISTOLOGIC FEATURES	■ INCIDENCE (%)	■ INVASIVE MALIGNANCY (%)
Adenomatous (tabular adenoma)	Branching tubules embedded in lamina propria	75	5
Villous (villous adenoma)	Finger-like projections of epithelium over lamina propria	10	40
Intermediate (tubulovillous adenoma)	Mixture of adenomatous and villous patterns	15	22

seen in 5% of adenomatous polyps, in 22% of tubulovillous adenomas, and in 40% of villous lesions. Although villous lesions are much less common, they are more likely to harbor a malignancy.

Polyp size is also directly correlated with the presence of dysplasia or malignancy.[40] Polyps of size greater than 10 mm have long been considered high risk, harboring invasive carcinoma in about 3% of cases. Polyps of size less than 5 mm are considered to be diminutive, with 0 to 0.05% frequency of carcinoma based on extremely large cohort studies.[41,42] Polyps of size 6 to 9 mm may harbor dysplasia or malignancy, but there is no definitive agreement regarding the benefit-to-risk ratio associated with their removal. Recent reviews have demonstrated 3% of such polyps to have severe dysplasia, but only 0.05% to 0.15% contain invasive cancer.[42,43]

An additional histologic family of neoplastic polyps, the serrated polyps, have been recognized more recently.[44] Serrated polyps include hyperplastic-like polyps, mixed polyps (part hyperplastic, part dysplastic), and serrated adenomas. The serrated polyps appear to be susceptible to or initiated by inactivation of MLH1 by methylation, which in turn is thought to initiate rapid acquisition of microsatellite DNA instability. In contrast to most hyperplastic polyps, which are seen in the distal colon, the serrated hyperplastic-like polyps are found in the proximal colon. Other clinical features include higher prevalence among women and older patients, rapid growth, and large size at diagnosis, all of which are also associated with proximal colon cancer. Although this alternative pathway to colorectal cancer is not universally accepted, supportive data include (i) the frequency of sporadic MSI high cancers but paucity of MSI high adenomatous polyps (except in HNPCC), (ii) loss of expression of MLH1 but not MSH2 among both serrated polyps and sporadic MSI high cancers, and (iii) the natural history of hyperplastic polyposis and associated prevalence of right-sided colon cancer.[44–47]

ETIOLOGY

Mutagenesis

Carcinogenesis in the colon and rectum has been described in terms of an initiation–promotion model based on experimental observations in laboratory animals. According to this simplified model, the first step involves initiating factors that directly interact with cellular DNA to induce mutations in the genome. Afterward, the process is driven by promotional factors, which are not mutagenic by themselves but enhance cellular proliferation of previously mutated cells. One can enhance or reduce tumorigenesis in experimental animals both by maneuvers that modify the generation of a mutagen (or carcinogen) and by those that alter promotional factors long after the administration of an initiating agent.

As described previously, the human diet contains a myriad of naturally occurring mutagens or substances that can be metabolized into mutagens. A wide range of such substances are generated from interactions between the diet, microbial flora, and colonic mucosal enzymes. In addition, protective mechanisms are present throughout the mucosa to detoxify these compounds. The action of carcinogens on DNA appears not to be an entirely random process. Mutagens typically alkylate DNA at specific carbon residues and cause nucleotide misreading during the next cycle of DNA replication. A mutation commonly seen early in colonic carcinogenesis results in activation of the ras protooncogene, one of several genetic events presumed to occur during malignant transformation.[48] The activation of ras may be involved in the initiation or promotion of carcinogenesis. Because of the ubiquitous presence of mutagens in the gut, many strategies that aim to reduce colon cancer attempt to interfere with the interaction between mutagens and the target colonic cells.

In animal studies, for example, the role of fat in the pathogenesis of colon cancer appears to be that of a promotional factor. With increasing fat intake, total fecal bile acid increases significantly. Available data suggest that bile acids stimulate the generation of reactive oxygen metabolites that enhance the conversion of unsaturated fatty acids to compounds that promote cellular proliferation. Theoretically, this would facilitate the emergence of a mutated clone of neoplastic cells. Enhanced proliferation of these transformed cells can either compress the time required for carcinogenesis or, perhaps, make the process more efficient. An extension of this concept is the observation that increased dietary calcium has been associated with a decreased risk for colorectal cancer. Experimental data demonstrate that an increase in dietary calcium tends to inhibit colonic proliferative indices, potentially by binding bile acid salts.

Molecular Genetics

The molecular genetic events that lead to colorectal cancer have served as a paradigm for the multiple-step process of tumorigenesis. This concept arose from frequently clinical and pathologic observations of an orderly progression of cellular transformation from normal colonic or rectal epithelium to small adenoma, then to large adenoma, and finally to carcinoma. Identification of these distinct stages has allowed scientists to elucidate the genetic alterations that may be responsible for the progression of the neoplastic process. Coincident with this line of investigation was the discovery of the genetic basis of several familial cancer syndromes in which colorectal cancer is a prominent feature of the phenotype. Taken together, the evidence

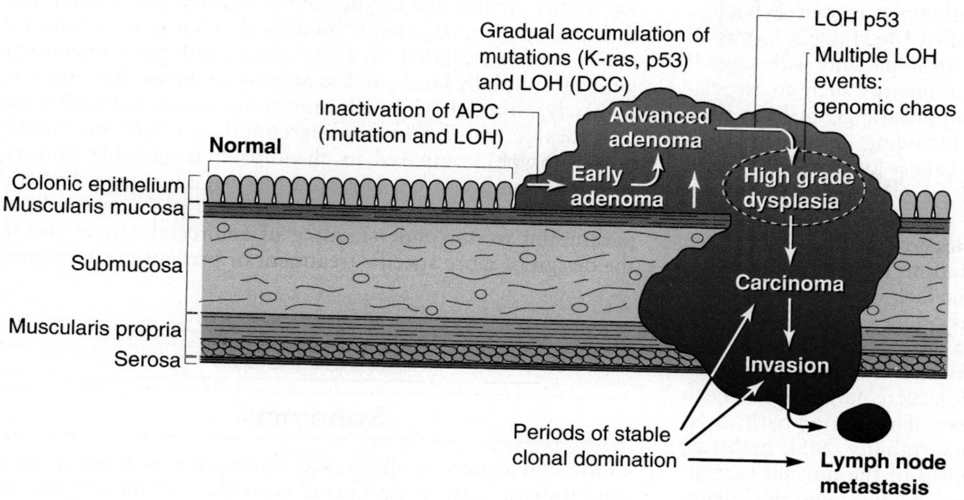

FIGURE 68.5. Model of genetic events mediating neoplastic progression in the colon. LOH, loss of heterozygosity.

suggests that colorectal cancers result from a series of genetic alterations leading to progressive disordering of the normal mechanisms that control cellular growth and differentiation (Fig. 68.5). It must be noted that not every colorectal tumor will acquire each of the mutations described. Furthermore, other genetic events are likely necessary for cancer formation, and each tumor may have a unique genetic profile. Although simplistic, the current model of multiple-step tumorigenesis facilitates
2 understanding the complex molecular genetics of cancer. Within this paradigm, mutations in three distinct types of genes are known to contribute to colorectal cancer formation: oncogenes, tumor-suppressor genes, and DNA mismatch repair genes. The former two gene mutations, comprising the loss of heterozygosity or chromosomal instability pathway, account for about 85% of colon and rectal tumors. Mutations in mismatch repair genes, termed the replication error or microsatellite instability pathway, account for about 15% of large-bowel tumors. Whereas more than half of these mutations are acquired, the remaining ones appear to be inherited.

In colon cancer, the most important genetic alteration is a mutation of the K-ras protooncogene, which is associated with poorer prognosis.[49] The ras protooncogenes are a family of normal genes (N-ras, H-ras, and K-ras) that are highly conserved in nature and encode the production of guanosine triphosphate–binding proteins (G proteins), which are important for signal transduction. G proteins are involved in the transduction of proliferative signals induced by growth factors or factors involved in cell differentiation. The product of a mutated ras gene is an abnormal G protein that becomes constitutively activated and continuously stimulates autonomous cell growth. Experimentally, transfection of normal fibroblasts by mutated ras genes confers neoplastic properties to those cells.

About half of colorectal carcinomas and a similar percentage of adenomas larger than 1 cm in diameter have been found to have the ras gene mutation.[48,50] By contrast, fewer than 10% of adenomas smaller than 1 cm have this mutation. The ras gene mutation may be the initiating event in some colorectal carcinomas or, alternatively, may promote the clonal expansion of a mutated cell population. It appears that the ras gene mutation alone is not responsible for tumorigenesis. Other molecular events are required in addition to ras gene mutations.

The concept of tumor-suppressor genes arose from several observations. Cytogenetic studies demonstrated that tumor cells often have losses of specific chromosomal regions and suggested that loss of a particular gene or genes could contribute to tumor formation and progression. Conversely, experimental evidence documented that replacement of specific chromosomes or portions of chromosomes in tumor cells could result in inhibition of growth. It was thus deduced that genes exist that function to keep cellular growth and proliferation in check, and that their loss results in unregulated growth and neoplastic transformation. One such tumor-suppressor gene associated with colon cancer is the *APC* (adenomatous polyposis coli) gene, mutations in which result in the familial cancer syndrome, familial adenomatous polyposis (FAP). In persons affected with FAP, hundreds to thousands of colorectal adenomatous polyps develop, all of which have the potential to progress to a cancer. The lifetime risk for the development of colon cancer is virtually 100%.[51] When linkage analysis was performed in families with FAP, *APC* was mapped to chromosome 5q21 and was subsequently cloned by several groups.[52,53] The APC gene encodes a large protein of 2,843 amino acids that contains several functional domains. A key function of the protein is to bind and thereby decrease intracellular levels of β-catenin. Mutations of *APC* that result in loss of this binding function lead to an increase in free β-catenin, which then activates the expression of other genes involved in cellular growth.[54,55]

Mutations of *APC* are also commonly found in sporadic cases of colorectal cancer. Approximately 70% of all sporadic cases of colorectal cancer have such mutations. Among those cancers in which *APC* is not mutated, a number have mutations in β-catenin that disrupt its ability to bind to the APC protein, and as such, they are phenotypically similar to those in which *APC* is mutated.[55,56] Mutations in *APC* appear to be an early or initiating event in sporadic colorectal cancer, as mutations in the gene have been identified in aberrant crypt foci, one of the earliest events in the neoplastic proliferation of colonic mucosa.[57]

Mutation or loss of the p53 tumor-suppressor gene, located on chromosome 17p, is another common genetic event in colorectal cancer. Although *p53* mutations have been found in 75% of sporadic colorectal cancers, they are seen infrequently in earlier lesions, which suggests that inactivation of *p53* is an important event in the transition from adenoma to carcinoma. The *p53* gene codes for a 393-amino acid phosphoprotein that has the ability to bind to DNA in a sequence-specific manner. When bound to DNA, the p53 protein can activate the expression of certain genes that are presumed to participate in growth inhibition. Mutations that disrupt this ability to bind DNA result in a decrease in the expression of growth-inhibitory genes and an increase in cellular proliferation.[58] Germline mutations in *p53* are responsible for the Li-Fraumeni syndrome. It is interesting that colorectal cancer is not a prominent feature of the phenotype.

Chromosome 18q21 appears to have an important role in the development of colorectal cancer, as allelic loss of this region is observed in many cases. The clinical importance of such a loss is controversial; one report has identified 18q21 allelic loss as an independent negative prognostic factor in patients with stage II tumors, whereas others have failed to identify such an association.[59,60] Several candidate tumor-suppressor genes have been identified on chromosome 18q21, including deleted in colon cancer (*DCC*), deleted in pancreatic cancer locus 4 (DPC4) and mad-related (smad2) genes. The role of these genes and others in the 18q21 region in colorectal tumorigenesis is not well defined. Investigation has been hampered by the inability to identify a significant number of mutations in any of these genes in sporadic colon cancers and by the lack of any familial syndromes in which germline mutations can be identified.

Similar to the suppressor pathway described previously and characterized by mutations in oncogenes and tumor-suppressor genes, a second and distinct molecular pathway has been implicated in colorectal tumorigenesis. This second pathway is called the mutator or microsatellite instability (MSI) pathway. The MSI pathway involves disruption of the normal surveillance for and repair of DNA damage. Maintaining the fidelity of the genome during DNA replication and cell division is of paramount importance for the normal growth and development of an organism. Ordinarily, cells have numerous mechanisms that constantly survey DNA for damage or replication errors and, if present, repair them. In this manner, the integrity of the genome is ensured and the accumulation and propagation of mutations is minimized. If these survey and repair mechanisms are defective, genetic instability and accelerated rates of mutation follow. If such mutations result in the activation of oncogenes or the inactivation of tumor-suppressor genes, affected cells gain a growth advantage.

In the early 1990s, several investigators observed that a subset of colorectal tumors have widespread instability in microsatellite repeats in tumor DNA and that such instability is present in the tumors of many patients affected by familial nonpolyposis colorectal cancer (HNPCC).[61–63] Simultaneously, bacterial and yeast geneticists described a set of DNA repair enzymes, termed DNA mismatch repair enzymes, that function to excise and repair nucleotide base mismatches that occur during DNA replication. The connection between DNA mismatch repair enzymes and HNPCC was solidified when it was found that tumor cells from patients with HNPCC lack DNA mismatch repair activity in vitro.[64] Subsequently, the first human mismatch repair homologue, hMSH2, was cloned and was found to be mutated in many patients with HNPCC.[65,66] Soon thereafter, a second human homologue of a mismatch repair enzyme, hMLH1, was cloned and demonstrated to be altered in a subset of patients with HNPCC who had normal hMSH2.[67,68]

It is now understood that DNA mismatch repair in the eukaryotic cell requires the participation of at least four other enzymes: hPMS1, hPMS2, hMSH6 (formerly called GTBP), and hMSH3.[69] Together, these enzymes form two complexes that perform the many aspects of the DNA mismatch repair process. Single base pair insertions or errors are recognized by a MSH2-MSH6 heteroduplex, which then binds a MLH1-PMS2 heteroduplex to initiate DNA excision. Similarly, larger DNA insertion or deletion loops are recognized by a MSH2-MSH3 heteroduplex, which again binds a MLH1-PMS2 heteroduplex and initiates DNA excision.[70,71] It follows that hMSH2 or hMLH1 mutator phenotypes result in the highest microsatellite instability and account for more than 60% of the mutations found in HNPCC kindreds. In addition to the germline inactivation of mismatch repair genes seen in HNPCC, spontaneous development of MSI high tumors results from hypermethylation of the promoter region of *MLH1*.

Delineation of the molecular genetic alterations responsible for colorectal tumor development has defined much of our current understanding of the multiple-step process of tumorigenesis. Yet despite these discoveries, an even greater number of questions remain to be answered. For example, among individuals who carry mutations in the APC gene, there is a wide variability in the phenotype; those affected with mutations that preserve the β-catenin binding domain may manifest a much more attenuated, or even absent, polyposis phenotype with substantially later and less aggressive tumor presentation. Similarly, although MSI high tumors are associated with some unfavorable features (poor differentiation, larger size, mucinous subtype) compared to chromosomal unstable tumors, MSI high status confers a marked survival advantage. The elucidation of interacting transformational pathways will be paramount to our understanding of colorectal cancer and to the design of more specific treatment or prevention strategies.

DIAGNOSIS

Symptoms

Colorectal cancer is diagnosed during the evaluation of a symptomatic patient or during screening or surveillance of asymptomatic patients. The symptoms of colorectal cancer tend to be nonspecific, such as vague intermittent abdominal pain, weight loss, sensation of bloating, bleeding per rectum, and at more advanced stages nausea and vomiting. Bleeding may present as melena, which is more commonly associated with right-sided colon cancers, or as gross red blood, associated with left-sided colon and rectal cancers. Lesser amounts of bleeding may be detected on a fecal occult blood test. Patients with chronic blood loss may develop iron deficiency anemia, resulting in fatigue and even cardiac symptoms.

Malignant obstruction can result in crampy abdominal pain with nausea and vomiting. In the presence of obstruction, a perforation may develop either at the site of the tumor or through the proximal uninvolved intestine. With rectal tumors, compromise of the rectal reservoir can cause a change in bowel habits, such as constipation, decreased stool caliber, or even overflow diarrhea with changes in continence. With locally advanced rectal cancers, symptoms of tenesmus, urgency, and perineal pain can occur.

Screening

Screening and Diagnostic Tests. Screening refers to testing that is applied to an asymptomatic group without prior disease to identify those at greater risk for disease. Screening tests should demonstrate simplicity, accuracy and reliability, safety, cost-effectiveness, and good compliance. A broad range of screening and diagnostic studies can be used in the evaluation of a suspected large-bowel cancer. The least expensive and potentially most informative study for rectal tumors is a thorough digital examination geared toward localization of distal rectal and anal neoplasms. An appropriate digital exam should include sensitivity to patient privacy and discomfort, proper positioning, alerting the patient before palpating, noting landmarks (puborectalis muscle and coccyx posteriorly, bilateral ischial tuberosities, prostate anteriorly in men). The examiner should attempt to palpate the levator muscles and complete prostate and note presence of anatomic abnormalities and masses, as well as sphincter function with squeeze and push efforts. The recorded findings should not rely on a clock orientation, which changes depending on positioning. Instead, right, left, anterior, and posterior orientation should be used.

The fecal occult blood test (FOBT) is the most commonly used screening test for colorectal cancer. Stool samples are placed on guaiac-impregnated paper slides that change color in the presence of peroxidase activity from hemoglobin. Patients are instructed to test two samples from three consecutive bowel movements. Several factors affect the utility of this test. First, not all colonic cancers or polyps are associated with

TABLE 68.4

COMPARISON OF TRADITIONAL COLORECTAL CANCER SCREENING TEST CHARACTERISTICS

	UNREHYDRATED	FLEXIBLE		DOUBLE-CONTRAST
	FOBT[61,110]	SIGMOID-OSCOPY[82,111]	COLONOSCOPY[86,111]	BARIUM ENEMA[112–114]
ACCURACY				
Sensitivity	33%–40%	70%	97.5%	70%–85%
Specificity	97%		100%	86%–97%
COST, 2000 $US[115,116]	$3.50	$400	$695	$296
CONSEQUENCES[80,117,118]	Negligible	Perforation = 0 to 0.011%	Hemorrhage = 0.15 to 4% Perforation = 0.2 to 3% Mortality = 0.006%	Negligible
COMPLIANCE	60%–86%	47%–74%	28%–38%	
EFFECTIVENESS (reduction in CRC mortality)[116]	18%–55%	34%–66%	64%–90%	33%–47%

FOBT, fecal occult blood test, unrehydrated; CRC, colorectal cancer.

bleeding, and even in those that are, bleeding is often intermittent in nature. Second, patients must be instructed to remain on diets low in peroxidase (no red meat or horseradish) before testing to avoid false-positive results. Third, certain medications, such as iron, cimetidine, antacids, and ascorbic acid, may interfere with the peroxidase reaction and lead to a false-negative result. The experience with annual, nonrehydrated fecal occult blood testing in asymptomatic populations has shown that about 2.5% of tested patients have positive results. Among these, only 10% to 15% have colorectal cancer.[72] Thus, a positive screening FOBT would necessarily lead to a more specific diagnostic test, colonoscopy, which would lead in turn to the opportunity for biopsy or polypectomy. After 18 years of follow-up, the Minnesota Colon Cancer Control Study[73] determined that, even with 50% to 75% compliance, annual FOBT use decreased the incidence of colorectal cancer by about 20%. Table 68.4 compares test characteristics of FOBT and other traditional screening and diagnostic examinations described in the paragraphs that follow.

Rigid sigmoidoscopy with a 25-cm instrument is comparatively inexpensive but is limited by the length of intestine that can be examined and by patient compliance. Flexible fiberoptic sigmoidoscopy has gained more acceptance. Instruments measuring 35 and 65 cm are available, and an examination of the sigmoid colon and rectum can usually be performed after cleansing enemas have been administered. Patient comfort is much higher than with rigid sigmoidoscopy. In addition, the ability to perform this test adequately without a total bowel cathartic and without sedation have a positive influence on patient compliance. Because of the risk of retained methane gas, electrocautery-assisted biopsy is unsafe.

Colonoscopy with the 180-cm fiberoptic instrument is the most widely used diagnostic study to evaluate the colon, and use has increased substantially in recent years.[74] For some time, direct evidence of an association between colonoscopy and decreased colorectal cancer deaths after colonoscopy was lacking. However, recent case-matched, population-based data indicate a colonoscopy-associated 20% reduction in deaths from left-sided colon cancers.[75] Others have reported that diagnosis of advanced neoplasms decreased by more than 20% when colonoscopic screening increased threefold in the general population.[76]

A valuable aspect of this procedure is the ability not only to obtain mucosal biopsy specimens but to perform polypectomies. That is, colonoscopy provides both diagnostic and therapeutic benefit, making it the accepted criterion standard for assessing other screening and diagnostic tests. Data from the National Polyp Study[77] indicate a lower rate of cancer among patients who have undergone colonoscopic polypectomy. Thus, colonoscopy is the only screening test that can potentially prevent cancer development. Unfortunately, colonoscopy is also the only cancer screening test with an associated mortality rate. The incidence of severe complications that require surgical intervention (e.g., hemorrhage, perforation) is 0.1% to 0.3%.

The barium enema is an historic study for the diagnosis of colonic polyps and cancers. The double-contrast technique in which air insufflation is used is superior to the standard single-contrast barium enema to detect early polyps or cancers. The classic apple core defect has been described for colonic cancers (Fig. 68.6). Colonoscopy has largely supplanted use of barium enema, but the exam is still useful in the setting of strictures or adhesions that cannot be negotiated with a flexible scope. Another advantage of barium enema over colonoscopy is the routine visualization of the right side of the colon, which is not possible in 5% to 10% of colonoscopic examinations.

Two emerging screening tests are virtual colonoscopy or computed tomography (CT) colonography and stool DNA (sDNA) screening. CT colonography was introduced in 1994[78] and has gradually captured public appeal due to its potential to improve patient comfort, minimize risk, and eradicate the need for sedation. After air insufflation of the prepared colon, thin-cut axial images are gathered by a high-speed helical CT scanner; both prone and supine scans are obtained in minutes. Based on both image sets, the two-dimensional axial images are reconstituted into three-dimensional replications of the entire colon (Fig. 68.7). Another advantage of this technique is good visualization of the entire colon, including antegrade and retrograde views of haustral folds that sometimes elude the traditional colonoscopist.

It must be noted that CT colonography is not diagnostic; that is, patients with positive findings must undergo a traditional colonoscopy for biopsy or polypectomy. Among high-risk patients, per-patient sensitivity and specificity as high as 92% and 94%, respectively, for patients with polyps or lesions greater than 6 mm have been reported from a single center.[79] An early multicenter trial examined high-risk patients in nine different institutions and reported a combined sensitivity of

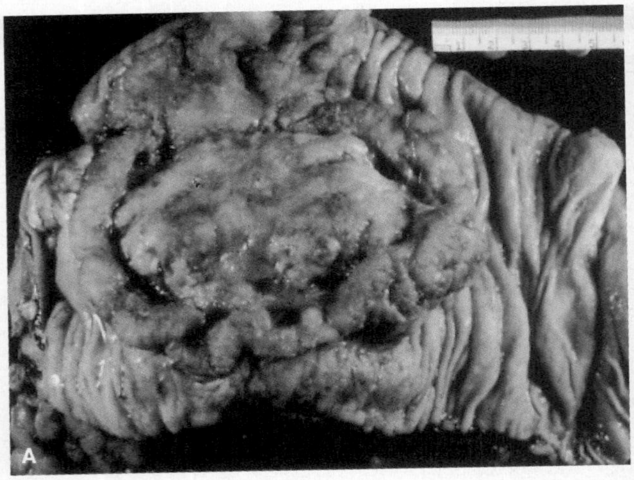

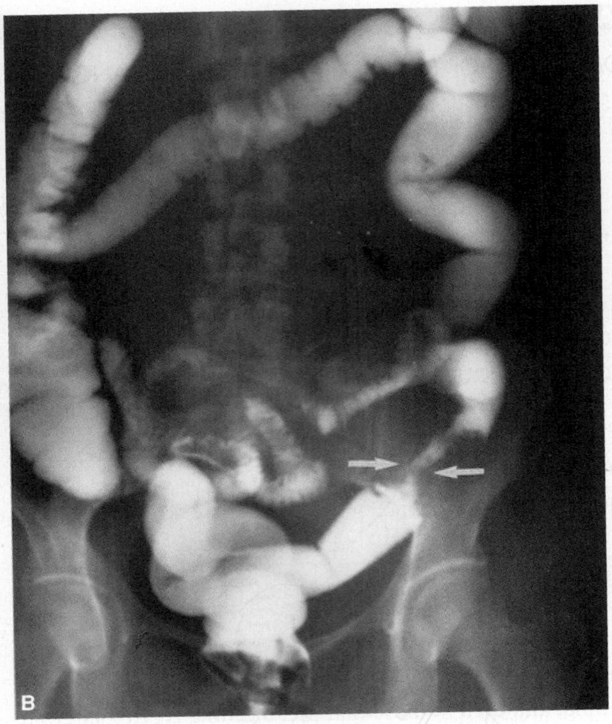

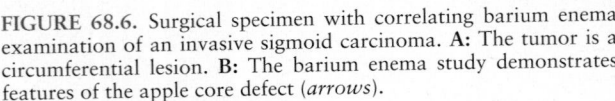

FIGURE 68.6. Surgical specimen with correlating barium enema examination of an invasive sigmoid carcinoma. **A:** The tumor is a circumferential lesion. **B:** The barium enema study demonstrates features of the apple core defect (*arrows*).

only 39% for lesions greater than 6 mm with high interobserver variation.[80] This study has been criticized for its reliance on older technology and high interobserver variation. Such issues may more accurately reflect broadscale generalizability or alternatively may simply indicate a need for methodical credentialing prior to institutional adoption of this technique.

As a rule, test accuracy improves as lesions increase in size, but screening test accuracy declines with decreasing prevalence of disease. It follows that CT colonography test characteristics are less positive among the average-risk population. Table 68.5 demonstrates the range of CT colonography test characteristics based on more recent studies.[81–84] Sensitivity and specificity vary by lesion size and technique, but per patient specificity and negative predictive value is consistently robust even for lesions less than 10 mm. A strong negative-predictive value indicates that a negative test result reliably reflects a lesion-free state; that is, patients with a negative test result may safely forego invasive conventional colonoscopy. False-negative and false-positive results in CT colonography are due primarily to retained stool, which can be minimized by a full bowel cathartic. Stool tagging techniques can also help to distinguish small lesions from fecaliths that adhere to the mucosa despite repositioning.[85]

Stool DNA screening refers to PCR-analysis of sloughed mucosal cells in stool, seeking genetic alterations associated with colorectal cancer. Despite technically challenging contaminants, stool is a useful medium for development of such tests because it reflects mucosal cells from the entire colon. Although the sequence of genetic changes in colorectal cancer is well documented, screening for any of these markers individually may be a painstaking process with no better accuracy than the well-entrenched fecal occult blood test. Conversely, a screening method for some optimal combination of genetic markers can be very useful. Among specimens from known cancer patients, early feasibility studies demonstrated 71% to 91% sensitivity and greater than 93% specificity searching for a combination of K-ras, p53, APC, BAT-26, and long-segment DNA indicating extinguished apoptosis.[86,87] A recent multicenter cohort study of more than 4,400 average-risk patients compared fecal DNA screening to FOBT, using follow-up colonoscopy as a standard.[88] Sensitivity for invasive cancer was 51.6% versus 12.9%, respectively; specificity was 94.4% versus 95.2%, respectively. A newer version of sDNA with purported better test characteristics has become commercially available recently. Concerns about cost-effectiveness relative to FOBT[89,90] may require updating pending greater experience with use and better data-appropriate frequency.

Screening Regimen and Surveillance Recommendations. The previous section described goals and characteristics of screening tests. Screening regimens, that is the periodic application of these tests, should be undertaken for diseases that are serious, prevalent, and curable with early diagnosis. Colorectal cancer is clearly a serious health issue, resulting in approximately 50,000 deaths per year. The increased prevalence among those older than 60 years of age justifies recommendations to begin screening at age 50 years for average-risk individuals. Last, effective treatment is available and earlier stage at diagnosis is associated with better outcome, implying that screening that results in early diagnosis and initiation of treatment confers a survival benefit.

Screening for colorectal cancer begins with risk stratification to determine the appropriate timing of initiation and follow-up. Table 68.6 delineates different risk categories, including average risk, moderate risk, and high risk. For average-risk individuals, no one strategy currently dominates the others in combined cost-effectiveness, patient safety, and compliance.[91] Therefore, the U.S. Multisociety Task Force on Colorectal Cancer (USMSTF) has endorsed various cost-effective screening regimens for asymptomatic, average-risk individuals beginning at age 50 years.[92] Updated recommendations from the USMSTF for average-risk patients have separated tests into polyp and cancer screening tests (structural tests) and cancer screening tests (stool tests), with a strong emphasis on cancer prevention through use of the former (Table 68.7).

Flexible sigmoidoscopy with insertion to 40 cm or the splenic flexure is the simplest structural examination and can be performed in a clinic setting after only a partial bowel preparation with enemas. Approximately 70% of all large-bowel polyps and cancers should be within reach of a flexible sigmoidoscope. Positive flexible sigmoidoscopy must be followed by full colonoscopy. A study of 3,121 veterans demonstrated that

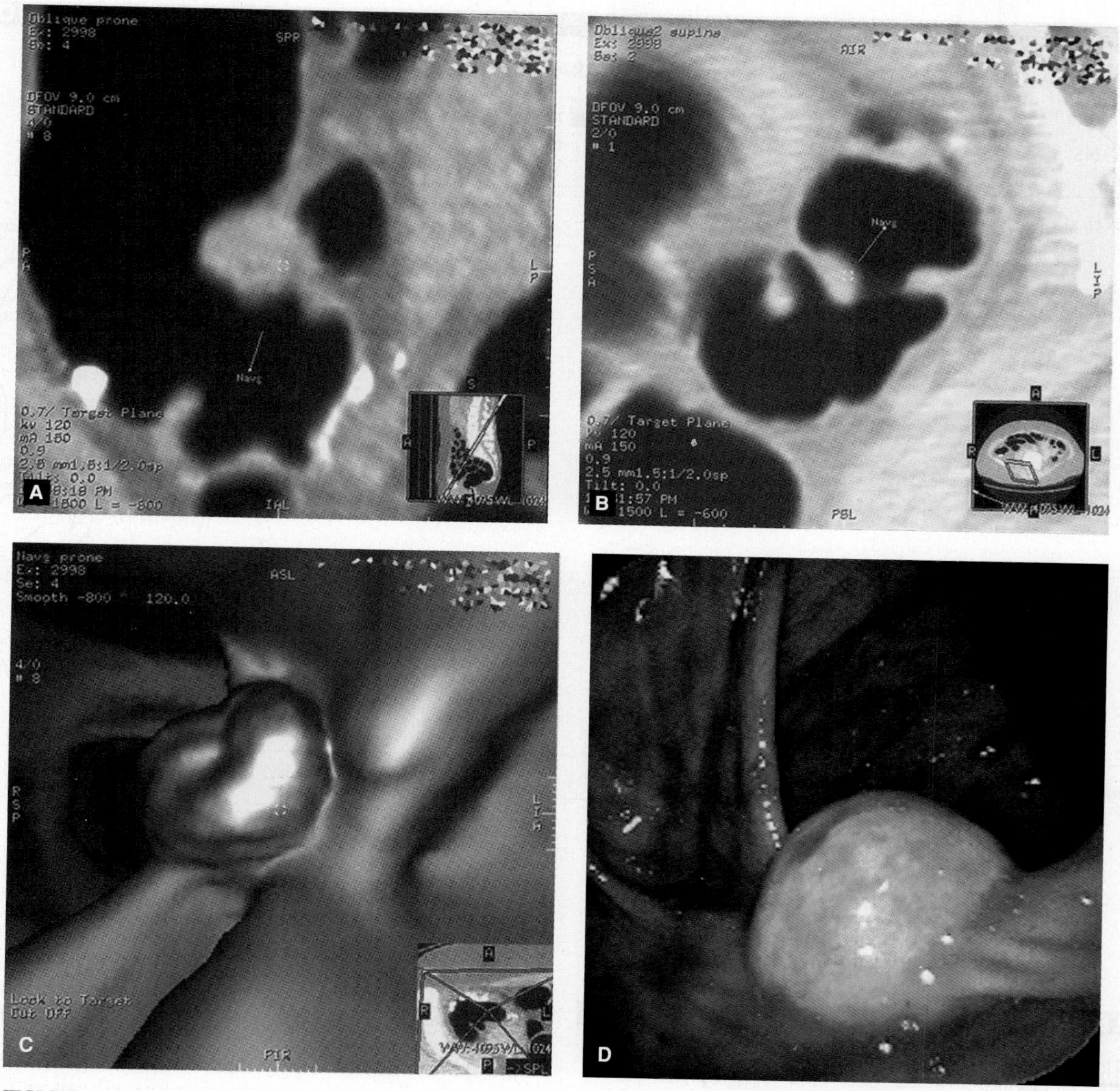

FIGURE 68.7. Prominent ileocecal valve with an associated tumor. **A:** Identified on two-dimensional axial computed tomography image, sagittal view. **B:** Identified on two-dimensional axial computed tomography image, coronal view. **C:** Identified on reconstituted three-dimensional virtual colonoscopy image. **D:** As pictured on colonoscopy performed for biopsy.

flexible sigmoidoscopy, followed by full colonoscopy if a distal polyp was found, would identify 70% to 80% of patients with proximal neoplasia.[93] A recent randomized trial comparing flexible sigmoidoscopy to FOBT found that the tests were equally likely to identify cancers (4 per 1,000 and 3.5 per 1,000 screening exams, respectively), but that flexible sigmoidoscopy was threefold more likely to identify advanced polyps (size ±10 mm, villous features, or high-grade dysplasia).[94] Current recommendations for average-risk individuals include flexible sigmoidoscopy once every 5 years, alone or paired with annual FOBT.

Studies of colonoscopic screening efficacy have been limited by an inability to distinguish screening from diagnostic indications.[75,76] In the classic National Polyp Study, patients who underwent colonoscopy and subsequent removal of benign polyps were followed with periodic colonoscopy for an average duration of 6 years.[77] A 90% decrease in colorectal cancer in patients participating in the National Polyp Study was noted in comparison with a general population registry. The USMSTF recommends colonoscopic screening every 10 years, the estimated time for transformation from an adenoma to invasive malignancy. Recent changes in Medicare coverage to include screening colonoscopy have encouraged the use of this modality.[95]

Double-contrast barium enema (DCBE) is used less commonly but remains an option among screening regimens. The DCBE provides a structural examination of the entire colon and is associated with less than 0.0001% complication rate. The accuracy of this exam is markedly poorer than conventional colonoscopy, and therefore recommended examination intervals have been shortened to every 5 years.

Data regarding the efficacy of CT colonography was recently deemed sufficient to include it as a recommended screening regimen at 5-year intervals.[92] Because of persistent questions regarding test characteristics in specific subpopulations, such as the elderly, the Center for Medicare and Medicaid Services has declined to cover CT colonography as a screening regimen. As data with respect to safety, cost, and standardization of techniques disseminate, this issue is likely to be revisited.[96]

The annual or biennial fecal occult blood test remains the only purely screening regimen that has been shown to directly

TABLE 68.5

COMPUTED TOMOGRAPHY (CT) COLONOGRAPHY TEST CHARACTERISTICS[a]

LESIONS ≥6 mm	SENSITIVITY	SPECIFICITY	POSITIVE-PREDICTIVE VALUE	NEGATIVE-PREDICTIVE VALUE	COMMENTS
Johnson et al., 2008[81]	78%	88%	40%	98%	Multicenter (n = 15), prospective, blinded study High- and average-risk patients (n = 2531) Pre-procedural stool tagging Three-dimensional reconstituted images Multidetector-row CT scanners (>16 rows)
Pineau et al., 2003[84]	84%	83%		95%	Prospective, blinded study High- and average-risk patients (n = 205)
Pickhardt et al., 2003[83]	88.7%	79.6%			Multicenter (n = 3), prospective, blinded study Average-risk patients (n = 1233) Pre-procedural stool tagging Three-dimensional reconstituted images

[a]As compared with subsequent optical colonoscopy.

TABLE 68.6

RISK STRATIFICATION FOR COLORECTAL CANCER SCREENING

Average Risk for Colorectal Cancer (must fulfill all criteria below)
Age 50 years or older
No personal history of polyps or colorectal cancer
No first-degree relatives with polyps or colorectal cancer
Fewer than two second-degree relatives with colorectal cancer
Moderate Risk for Colorectal Cancer (any criteria below)
First-degree relative with colorectal cancer or polyp at age younger than 60 years
First-degree relative with colorectal cancer or polyp at age 60 years or older
Two or more second-degree relatives with colorectal cancer
Increased Risk for Colorectal Cancer (any criteria below)
Gene carrier or at risk for familial adenomatous polyposis
Gene carrier or at risk for hereditary nonpolyposis colorectal cancer
Surveillance (any criteria below)
Personal history of colorectal polyps
Personal history of colorectal cancer
Personal history of inflammatory bowel disease

reduce colorectal cancer mortality. The results of four separate trials comprising more than 400,000 persons with follow-up from 8 to 18 years are summarized in Table 68.8.[73,97–100] Based on intention to treat (screen), annual FOBT was associated with a 33% decrease in colorectal cancer mortality. With exclusion of the noncompliant patients from the Minnesota study, the observable reduction in colorectal cancer mortality would approximate 50%. Clearly, improving compliance with screening can have a major impact on colorectal cancer mortality. Eliminating dietary restrictions may improve patient compliance, as with the newer guaiac-based fecal immunochemical tests.[101] Updated recommendations for the fecal occult blood testing regimen among average-risk adults from the USMSTF includes (i) annual, unrehydrated FOBT with dietary restriction or fecal immunochemical test without restriction, (ii) testing of two samples from three consecutive bowel movements, and (iii) following a positive screening test result with diagnostic colonoscopy.

Currently, about 60% of Americans older than age 50 years have undergone any colorectal cancer screening.[102] It is hoped that choosing a screening regimen based on patient and provider preferences and resources will enhance screening compliance. Although colorectal cancer mortality is decreased with screening, it is unclear whether the overall mortality of the screened populations is different from that of the control groups. Mortality may be shifted to other causes (e.g., cardiovascular deaths) in the screened population. Cost-effective analyses[91] indicate that all of the recommended colorectal cancer screening strategies cost between $10,000 and $25,000 per year of life saved, that is, substantially less than the cost for other currently recommended screening measures (i.e., mammography).

Patients with known disease or a personal history of polyps or cancer are in a separate surveillance category. Surveillance is defined as routine collection of data from a population known

TABLE 68.7

GUIDELINES FOR COLORECTAL CANCER SCREENING[a]

	INDIVIDUALS AT AVERAGE RISK, AGE >50 YEARS	
TEST[b]	**INTERVAL**	**COMMENT**
TESTS THAT DETECT ADENOMATOUS POLYPS OR CANCER (STRUCTURAL TESTS)		
Flexible sigmoidoscopy[b]	Every 5 years	Insertion to 40 cm or splenic flexure. Complete or partial bowel preparation required. Sedation is not usually used.
Colonoscopy	Every 10 years	Complete or partial bowel preparation required. Conscious sedation is used. Risks include perforation and bleeding.
Double-contrast barium enema[b]	Every 5 years	Complete bowel preparation required. Sedation is not usually used.
Computed tomography colonography[b]	Every 5 years	Complete bowel preparation required. Sedation is not usually used.
TEST[b]	**INTERVAL**	**COMMENT**
TESTS THAT PRIMARILY DETECT CANCER (STOOL TESTS)		
Fecal occult blood test	Annually	No rehydration. Two or three specimens should be collected at home to complete testing. Patients must commit to periodic testing; One-time testing is likely to be ineffective.
Fecal immunochemical test	Annually	Two or three specimens should be collected at home to complete testing. Patients must commit to periodic testing; One-time testing is likely to be ineffective.
Stool DNA test	Uncertain	An adequate sample (30 gm) is necessary and requires special packaging.
	INDIVIDUALS AT MODERATE RISK	
RISK	**INITIATE SCREENING**	**COMMENTS**
First-degree relative with colorectal cancer or polyp at age ≥60 years *or* two or more second-degree relatives with colorectal cancer	Age 40 years	Same screening regimens and intervals as average risk
First-degree relative with colorectal cancer or polyp at age <60 years *or* two or more first-degree relatives with colorectal cancer	Age 40 years or 10 years younger than youngest family member at the time of diagnosis, whichever comes first	Colonoscopy every 5 years
	INDIVIDUALS AT INCREASED RISK, COLONOSCOPY ONLY	
FAMILIAL RISK RESULT	**INITIATE SURVEILLANCE**	**INTERVAL IF NORMAL COLONOSCOPY**
Familial adenomatous polyposis; consider genetic counseling and testing; colectomy if genetic testing is positive.	Age 10–12 years	Annual sigmoidoscopy, stopping at age 40 years if normal
Attenuated adenomatous polyposis coli	Late teens	Annual colonoscopy, no stopping at age 40 years
Hereditary nonpolyposis colon cancer	Age 20–25 years or 10 years younger than earliest family diagnosis	Biennial colonoscopy to age 40 years, then annual

[a]Endorsed by the American Cancer Society, American College of Gastroenterology, American Society of Colon and Rectal Surgeons, American Society for Gastrointestinal Endoscopy, Oncology Nursing Society, and Society of American Gastrointestinal Endoscopic Surgeons.
[b]Diagnostic evaluation with colonoscopy should be performed for any patients with either positive findings on this screening examination or symptoms suggestive of colorectal cancer or polyps.

COLORECTAL

TABLE 68.8

SUMMARY OF PROSPECTIVE RANDOMIZED TRIALS OF FECAL OCCULT BLOOD TESTING

STUDY	NO. OF PATIENTS	RANDOMIZED GROUPS	TYPE OF FOBT	CANCERS		RR OF CRC	DEATH WITH SCREENING (95% CI)
				FOLLOW-UP PERIOD (Y)	DETECTED BY FOBT (%)	DUKES A CANCERS (%)	
Mandel et al.[76,96]	46,551	Annual biennial control	Rehydrated	18	Annual 50	Annual 33	Annual 0.67 (0.51–0.89)
					Biennial 39	Biennial 29	Biennial 0.79 (0.62–0.97)
Minnesota, U.S.						Control 25	
Hardcastle et al.[97]	152,850	Biennial control	Unhydrated	7.5 (median)	27	Screen 21	0.85 (0.74–0.98)
						Control 12	
Nottingham, U.K.							
Kronburg et al.[98]	140,000	Biennial control	Unhydrated	10	25	Screen 23	0.82 (0.68–0.99)
						Control 12	
Funen, Denmark	63,308	Two screens, 16–22 mo. apart	Rehydrated	8.2 (median)	28	Screen 26	0.88 (0.69–1.12)
Kewenter et al.[99]							
Gothenburg, Sweden		Control				Control 9	

FOBT, fecal occult blood testing; CRC, colorectal cancer; CI, confidence interval; RR, relative risk.

TABLE 68.9

GUIDELINES FOR COLORECTAL CANCER ENDOSCOPIC SURVEILLANCE[a]

PERSONAL HISTORY RISK	INITIATE SURVEILLANCE	INTERVAL
Following resection of single <1 cm adenoma	5–10 years post-polypectomy	If first colonoscopy is normal, resume average-risk recommendations.
Following resection of 3–10 adenomas, or ≥1 cm adenoma, or polyp with villous features or high-grade dysplasia	3 years post-polypectomy	If first surveillance colonoscopy is normal, repeat at 5 years.
Following resection of >10 adenomas	<3 years post-polypectomy	Consider evaluation for familial syndrome.
Following piecemeal removal of sessile adenoma	2–6 months post-polypectomy	Individualize.
Following curative resection for colorectal cancer	Within 3–6 months if preoperative clearing was not performed. Within 1 year postoperatively following clearance of synchronous disease.	If normal, repeat in 3 years, then if normal every 5 years.
Inflammatory bowel disease	Within 8 years of diagnosis	Survey for dysplasia every 1–2 years.

[a]Endorsed by the American Cancer Society, American College of Gastroenterology, American Society of Colon and Rectal Surgeons, American Society for Gastrointestinal Endoscopy, Oncology Nursing Society, and Society of American Gastrointestinal Endoscopic Surgeons.

to be at high risk for disease. For the purposes of colorectal cancer, this includes patients with inflammatory bowel disease or a personal history of polyps or cancer. The USMSTF Surveillance Guidelines[92,103,104] recommend periodic endoscopy as outlined in Table 68.9.

STAGING

Pathology

Of all large-bowel cancers, 90% to 95% are adenocarcinomas, with the remaining histologic types being squamous cell carcinomas, adenosquamous carcinomas, lymphomas, sarcomas, and carcinoid tumors. Most colonic adenocarcinomas are moderately differentiated or well-differentiated tumors. About 20% of adenocarcinomas are poorly differentiated or undifferentiated, and these are associated with a poorer prognosis. Another commonly described characteristic of adenocarcinomas is the relative amount of mucin that is produced. Ten percent to 20% of tumors are described as mucinous or colloid carcinomas based on the abundant production of mucin. These tumors are associated with a poorer 5-year survival rate in comparison with nonmucinous tumors. Other histologic features associated with a poorer prognosis include blood vessel invasion, lymphatic vessel invasion, and the absence of a lymphocytic response to the tumor.

Staging Classification

Since Dukes' original description, various staging systems based on tumor penetration through the bowel wall have been described. The standard system for staging at this time is the American Joint Committee on Cancer and the International Union Against Cancer (AJCC/UICC) staging system based on the extent of the primary tumor (T), regional node involvement (N), and metastasis (M). The TNM system is correlated with the historical Dukes and modified Astler-Coller stages in Table 68.10. The TNM method is subjected to continuous, data-driven quality improvement reviews. In contrast to the modified Astler-Coller system, the TNM system includes carcinoma in situ (Tis) and stratifies according to number of positive nodes (Fig. 68.8).

Stage 0 represents Tis tumors that do not metastasize, stage I includes T1 and T2 tumors, stage II includes T3 and T4 tumors, and stage III includes any tumors with nodal involvement (N1–N3). Stage IV includes any cancer with distant metastases.

In 2002, the TNM staging system for colorectal cancer was updated to better reflect the impact of depth of penetration and number of involved lymph nodes.[105] National Cancer Database evidence of significantly different survival times among more than 50,000 patients with node-positive cancer led to expansion into subcategories A, B, and C, as displayed in Table 68.10. The prognostic validity of this subclassification has been demonstrated using the SEER national cancer registry. The AJCC 6th edition revised TNM system revealed 5-year colon cancer survival rates of 93.2% for stage I, 84.7% for stage IIA, 72.2% for stage IIB, 83.4% for stage IIIA, 64.1% for stage IIIB, 44.3% for stage IIIC, and 8.1% for stage IV.[106]

Survival of stage IIIA is notably better than that of stage IIB. Two immediate hypotheses may explain this prognostic discrepancy. First, the poorer survival rate among stage IIB patients may reflect the lack of clear recommendations for adjuvant treatment of these patients.[107] Second, an accurate staging system is predicated on adequate node examination. A minimum number of 12 lymph nodes examined has been associated with improved survival[108] and by inference with adequacy of examination. Although there is some controversy regarding the mechanism whereby survival is improved, the 12 lymph node rule—that is, examination of at least 12 lymph nodes in a colon cancer surgical specimen—has been adopted as a surveillance measure of quality of care.[109,110]

NATURAL HISTORY

4 The natural progression of colorectal cancer comprises three processes: local invasion, lymphatic spread, and hematogenous spread. Early studies by Dukes led to the theory of an orderly progression from local tumor invasion to subsequent lymphatic and hematogenous spread after the tumor had penetrated the intestinal wall. Later data have shown that tumors that do not invade through the intestinal wall can progress to lymphatic metastases or distant disease nonetheless. Thus, even patients who undergo curative resection of apparently localized colorectal cancers may harbor blood-borne metastases.

TABLE 68.10

STAGING OF COLORECTAL CANCER[a]

■ STAGE	■ DESCRIPTION
TUMOR-NODE-METASTASIS (TNM) SYSTEM	
Primary Tumor	
TX	Primary tumor cannot be assessed
T0	No evidence of tumor in resected specimen (prior polypectomy or fulguration)
Tis	Carcinoma in situ
T1	Invades into submucosa
T2	Invades into muscularis propria
T3/T4	Depends on whether serosa is present
Serosa Present	
T3	Invades through muscularis propria into subserosa; invades serosa (but not through); invades pericolic fat within the leaves of the mesentery
T4	Invades through serosa into free peritoneal cavity or through serosa into a contiguous organ
NP Serosa (distal two thirds of rectum, posterior left or right colon)	
T3	Invades through muscularis propria
T4	Invades other organs (vagina, prostate, ureter, kidney)
Regional Lymph Node Involvement	
NX	Nodes cannot be assessed (e.g., local excision only)
N0	No regional node metastases
N1	1–3 positive nodes
N2	4 or more positive nodes
N3	Central nodes positive
Distant Metastasis	
MX	Presence of distant metastases cannot be assessed
M0	No distant metastases
M1	Distant metastases present

Stage		**Description**	
0	Tis	N0	M0
I	T1,2	N0	M0
IIA	T3	N0	M0
IIB	T4	N0	M0
IIIA	T1,2	N1	M0
IIIB	T3,4	N1	M0
IIIC	Any T	N2	M0
IV	Any T	Any N	M1

DUKES STAGING SYSTEM CORRELATED WITH TNM SYSTEM	
Dukes A	T1, N0, M0 (stage I)
	T2, N0, M0 (stage I)
Dukes B	T3, N0, M0 (stage II)
	T4, N0, M0 (stage II)
Dukes C	T (any), N1, M0; T (any), N2, M0 (stage III)
Dukes D	T (any), N (any), M1 (stage IV)

MODIFIED ASTLER-COLLER (MAC) SYSTEM CORRELATED WITH TNM SYSTEM	
MAC A	T1, N0, M0 (stage I)
MAC B1	T2, N0, M0 (stage I)
MAC B2	T3, N0, M0 (stage II)
MAC B3	T4, N0, M0 (stage II)
MAC C1	T2, N1, M0; T2, N2, M0 (stage III)
MAC C2	T3, N1, M0; T3, N2, M0 (stage III)
	T4, N1, M0; T4, N2, M0 (stage III)
MAC C3	T4, N1, M0; T4, N2, M0 (stage III)

[a]In all pathologic staging systems, particularly those applied to rectal cancer, the abbreviations m and g may be used; m denotes microscopic transmural penetration; g or m + g denotes transmural penetration visible on gross inspection and confirmed microscopically.

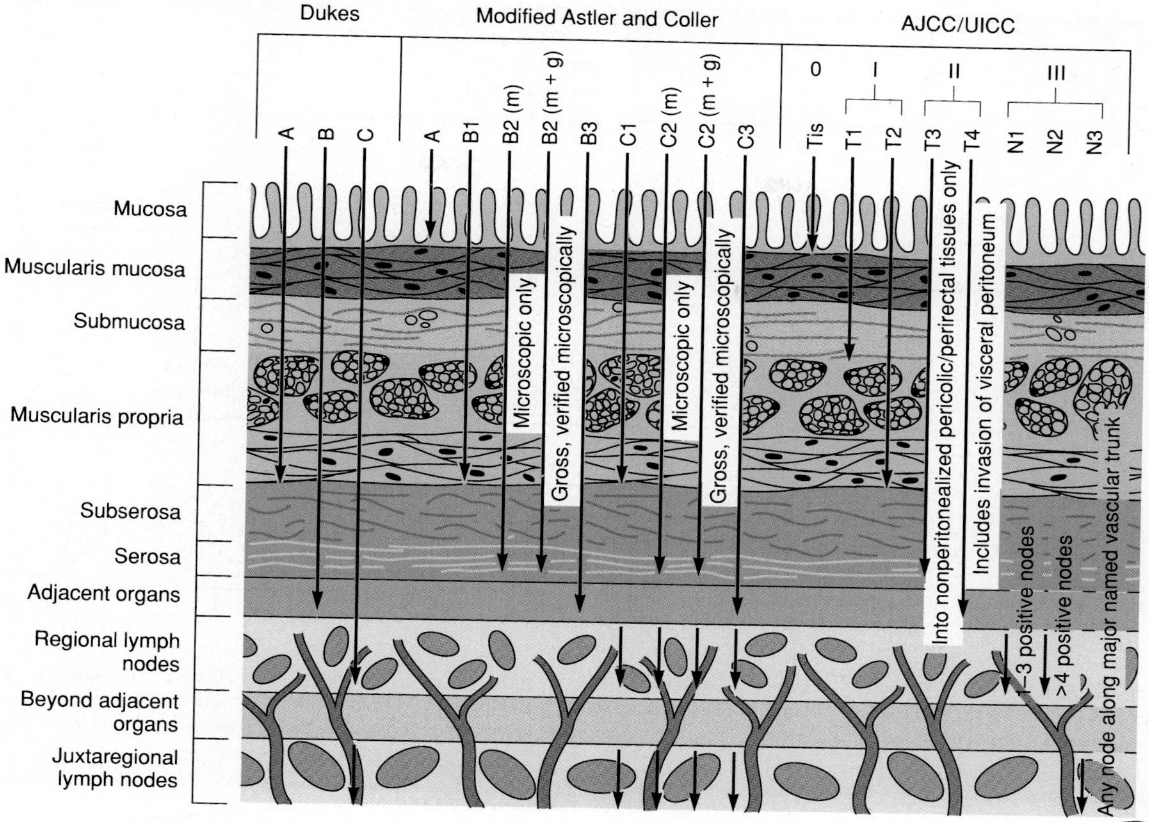

FIGURE 68.8. Schematic description of the staging systems with respect to depth of invasion.

Therapies designed to reduce the development of recurrent disease after surgical resection are discussed in later sections of this chapter.

Often local growth of an adenocarcinoma is characterized by intramural expansion of the tumor into the bowel lumen. Subsequent lateral invasion into the intestinal wall usually progresses in a transverse direction rather than longitudinally and thereby leads to circumferential involvement of the intestine. Although the incidence of lymphatic metastasis increases with extent of local invasion through the intestinal wall, 10% to 20% of patients with cancer limited to the submucosa are found to have positive lymph nodes.

The liver is the most common site of hematogenous spread of colorectal cancer; liver metastasis occurs in about half of all cases eventually.[111] The liver is the first capillary network exposed to tumor emboli traveling through the portal system and represents the major site of venous drainage of the colon and upper rectum. The liver can be the sole site of tumor metastasis, as evidenced by the successful resection of liver metastases for cure in selected patients. By contrast, the lower rectum has a dual drainage system, draining into the portal system and the vena cava by way of the middle and inferior hemorrhoidal veins, respectively. Isolated lung metastases can develop from lower rectal tumors when tumor emboli travel through the systemic venous drainage system. The lung is the second most common site of metastasis from colorectal tumors. Tumor involvement of other sites in the absence of liver and lung metastases is unusual. In certain circumstances, isolated bone metastases to the sacrum or vertebral bodies can arise when tumor emboli travel through portal-vertebral venous communications known as the Batson plexus.

Another potential mode of spread is by intraluminal or extraluminal exfoliation of tumor cells with subsequent implantation. Tumor implantation may occur during surgical resection; spillage of tumor cells can cause recurrences in bowel anastomoses, abdominal incisions, or other intra-abdominal sites. When tumors penetrate the intestinal wall, shed tumor cells can be implanted intraperitoneally and cause peritoneal carcinomatosis.

A summary of the natural history of patients who present with colorectal cancer is depicted in Algorithm 68.1.[111] For every 100 patients initially evaluated, 30 have clinically evident distant spread, and the remaining 70 undergo resection for localized disease. Among these 70 patients, 45 are cured and disease recurs in the remainder. Extrapolation of these figures to the approximately 150,000 patients in whom colorectal cancer is diagnosed each year in the United States implies that 67,500 patients can be cured with surgical resection alone; disease recurs in the remaining 82,500 patients after resection, or they have disseminated tumor at the time of diagnosis.

TREATMENT

Primary Colorectal Tumors

Neoplastic Polyps. Endoscopic polypectomy is the standard approach for the treatment of advanced polyps (size ≥10 mm, villous features, or presence of high-grade dysplasia) unless it is medically contraindicated. Most pedunculated polyps can be removed with a snare endoscopically. Frequently sessile lesions can be removed piecemeal, but several sessions may be required. A resected lesion with a malignant focus presents a dilemma regarding whether to subject the patient to the risks of colectomy. Lesions that are (i) low grade, (ii) without mucosal penetration, (iii) with resection margin greater than 2 mm, and (iv) without lymphovascular invasion should be considered a malignancy in situ that is exceedingly unlikely to metastasize and therefore does not require further surgery.[112–115] If the lesion penetrates the muscularis mucosa, it is an invasive cancer and surgical resection should be strongly considered.

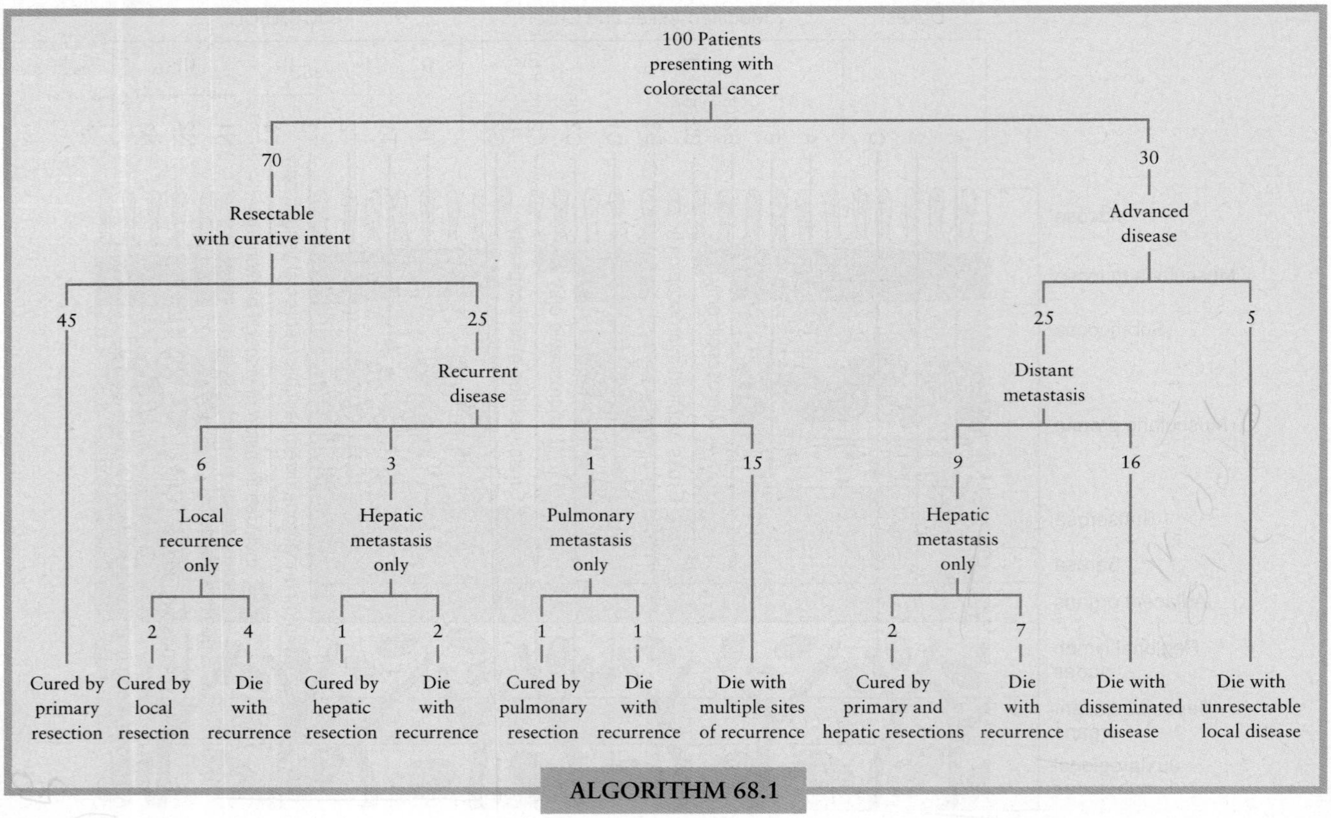

ALGORITHM 68.1. The natural history of colorectal cancer.

Occasionally, colectomy with resection of paracolonic lymph nodes is performed without evidence of residual disease or nodal metastases and the patient goes on to develop widespread metastases. Such a scenario likely reflects aggressive tumor biology refractory to the local control provided by resection.

Large villous tumors of the rectum can pose a therapeutic challenge. Total excision is required to assess the presence of invasive cancer accurately and prevent recurrence, which is estimated to occur in up to 40% of cases. A full-thickness transanal excision with sphincteric muscle and mucosal approximation is preferred and can be facilitated by transanal microscopic endosurgery techniques. However, other approaches, such as low anterior resection, coloanal procedures, or abdominoperineal resection, may have to be used to excise extensive benign rectal lesions totally.

Invasive Colorectal Cancers

Surgery. Surgical options for colorectal cancer depend on the location of the primary tumor. These surgical procedures are summarized in Table 68.11.

Before surgical resection, evaluation for metastatic disease is important. A careful physical examination determines the presence of hepatomegaly, ascites, or adenopathy. Except in the case of an obstructing lesion, a preoperative CT scan has become *de rigueur*. For rectal tumors, the distance of the tumor from the anal verge and its mobility are important in assessing resectability and the type of operation required. Rectal ultrasonography or magnetic resonance imaging are excellent methods for preoperative assessment of local invasion, sphincter involvement, and the presence of enlarged lymph nodes within the mesorectum (Fig. 68.9). Laboratory studies should include a complete blood cell count; a comprehensive metabolic panel to assess nutritional status, serum liver enzymes, and renal function; and a carcinoembryonic antigen (CEA) assay. Determination of a baseline CEA level can be useful in subsequent follow-up of the patient as well as assessment of potential metastases. The presence of metastatic disease may alter the planned surgical procedure and lead to preliminary treatment with chemotherapy or to a more extensive resection. In the unobstructed patient, a full colonoscopy or double-contrast barium enema should be performed to rule out the presence of synchronous colorectal cancers.

5 The surgical goals in the resection of a primary colorectal cancer are to achieve an en bloc resection that encompasses an adequate amount of normal colon proximal and distal to the

TABLE 68.11 **TREATMENT**

SURGICAL OPTIONS FOR COLORECTAL CANCER

INTRAPERITONEAL COLON AND UPPER THIRD OF THE RECTUM
Resection and anastomosis
MIDDLE THIRD OF THE RECTUM
Abdominoperineal resection
Low anterior resection
Abdominosacral resection
Coloanal resection
Local excision or fulguration
Primary radiation therapy
LOWER THIRD OF THE RECTUM
Abdominoperineal resection
Local excision or fulguration
Primary radiation therapy

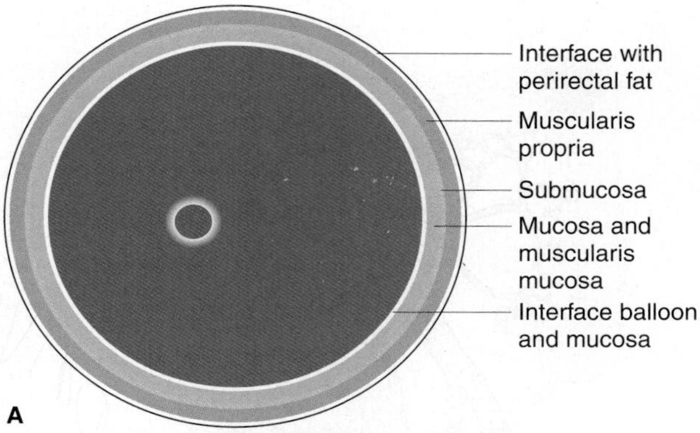

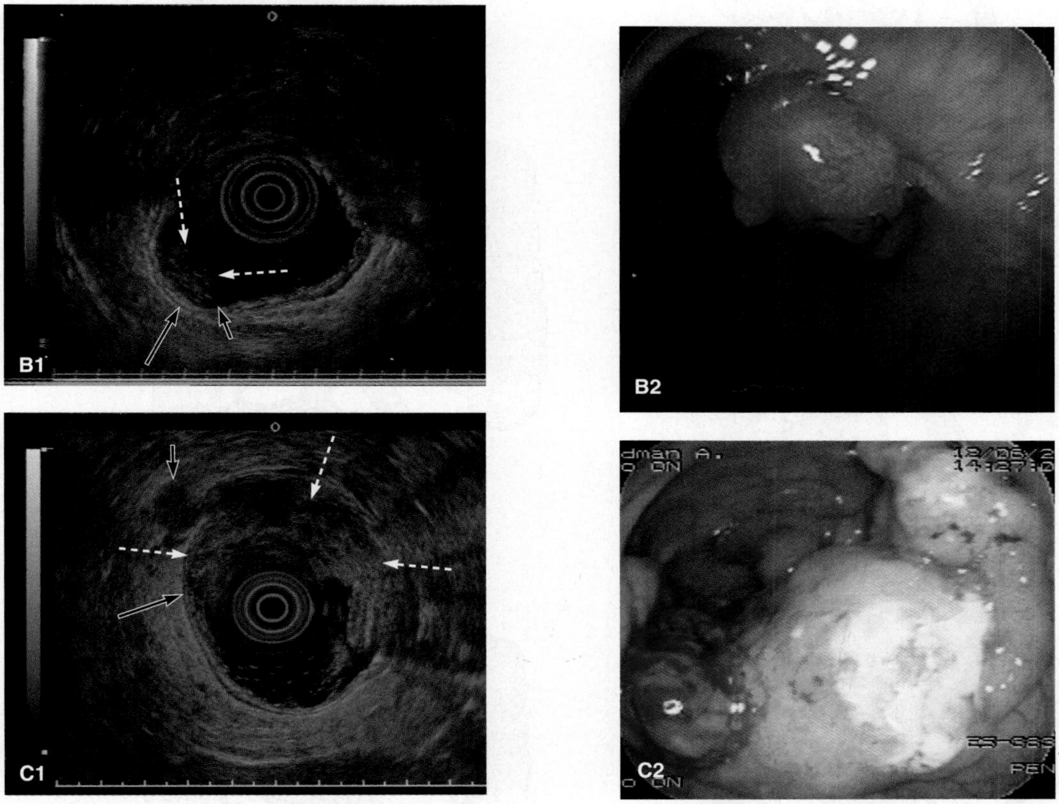

FIGURE 68.9. Endoscopic ultrasound for rectal cancer staging; "u" denotes ultrasound staging. **A:** Schematic view of wall structures. **B1:** Stage uT1N0 rectal tumor; invasion of the submucosa (*short arrow*); no invasion of the muscularis propria (*long arrow*). **B2:** Colonoscopic image of the tumor. **C1:** Stage uT3N1 tumor; invasion through the muscularis propria (*long arrow*) and with nearby lymph node (*short arrow*). **C2:** Colonoscopic image of the same tumor; note the hemicircumferential growth.

tumor, to obtain adequate lateral margins if the tumor is adherent to contiguous structures, and to remove regional lymph nodes. Accomplishment of these goals optimizes the chance of preventing locoregional recurrence of the disease. The extent of bowel resection has been the subject of numerous debates. In pathologic studies, tumor rarely extends intramurally more than 2 cm beyond the area of gross involvement. Traditionally, 5 cm of normal large intestine proximal and distal to the tumor has been advocated as a margin that is adequate to encompass intramural spread completely. The actual margin of intestine removed is often determined by the extent of the lymphadenectomy. The draining lymph nodes to be removed as part of a curative resection include nodes along the named feeding artery (Fig. 68.10). In the event that the tumor is between named arteries, intraoperative judgment should address whether both basins must be removed. Extensive resections of bowel along with more central or retroperitoneal lymph nodes are not indicated because they add minimal oncologic benefit and substantially increase operative complications. At the time of surgical resection, the abdominal viscera, particularly the liver and peritoneal surfaces, should be thoroughly investigated. If evidence of disseminated disease is apparent, a less extensive resection of the primary lesion for palliation to avoid complications of obstruction or bleeding may be indicated.

Intraperitoneal Colon and Upper Third of the Rectum. The surgical resection of cancers in different sites in the colorectum requires attention to specific anatomic details. Resection plus primary anastomosis is the surgical procedure of choice for cancers of the colon and upper and middle third of the rectum. While use of mechanical bowel preparations is in decline, oral antibiotics should be considered preoperatively to reduce infectious complications. The choice of anastomotic technique (i.e., stapling vs. hand sewing) depends on the surgeon's preference.

Tumors of the cecum and ascending colon should be resected by a right hemicolectomy. Ligation of the ileocolic, right colic, and right branches from the middle colic artery is required (Fig. 68.10). For tumors in the hepatic flexure, an extension of a right hemicolectomy is performed with ligation of the middle colic artery near its origin. Care must be taken during the mobilization of the ascending colon and hepatic flexure because the right ureter and testicular or ovarian vessels, inferior vena cava, superior mesenteric vein, and duodenum are all in proximity.

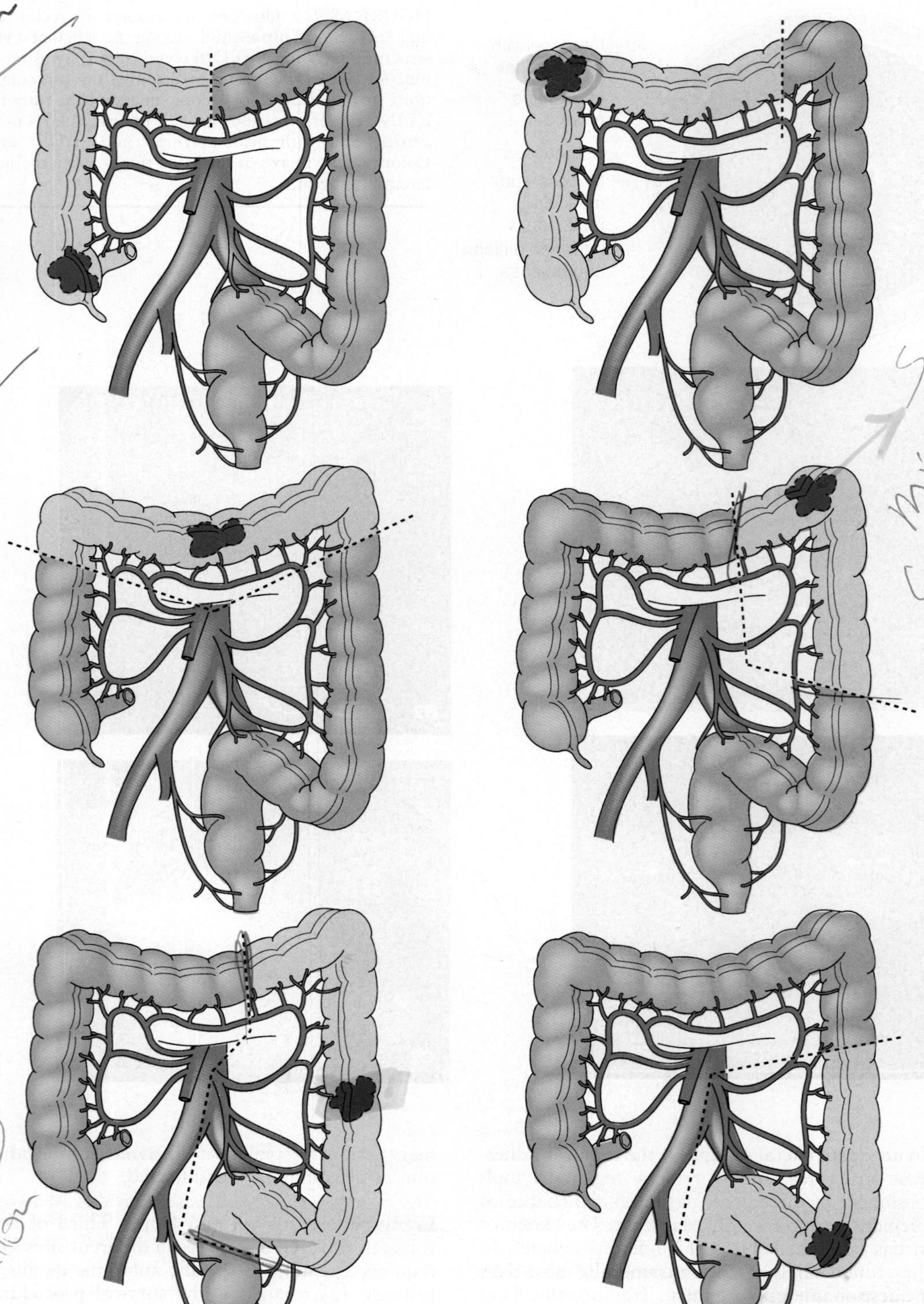

FIGURE 68.10. Segmental resections for cancers of the colon and upper third of the rectum.

For lesions of the transverse colon, a transverse colectomy is accomplished by proximal ligation of the middle colic artery (Fig. 68.10). Cancer of the splenic flexure can be treated with a segmental resection in which the middle transverse colon is anastomosed to the middle descending colon. For this procedure, the left colic artery is divided and the middle colic artery is preserved. Mobilization of the splenic flexure requires care to avoid injury to the spleen.

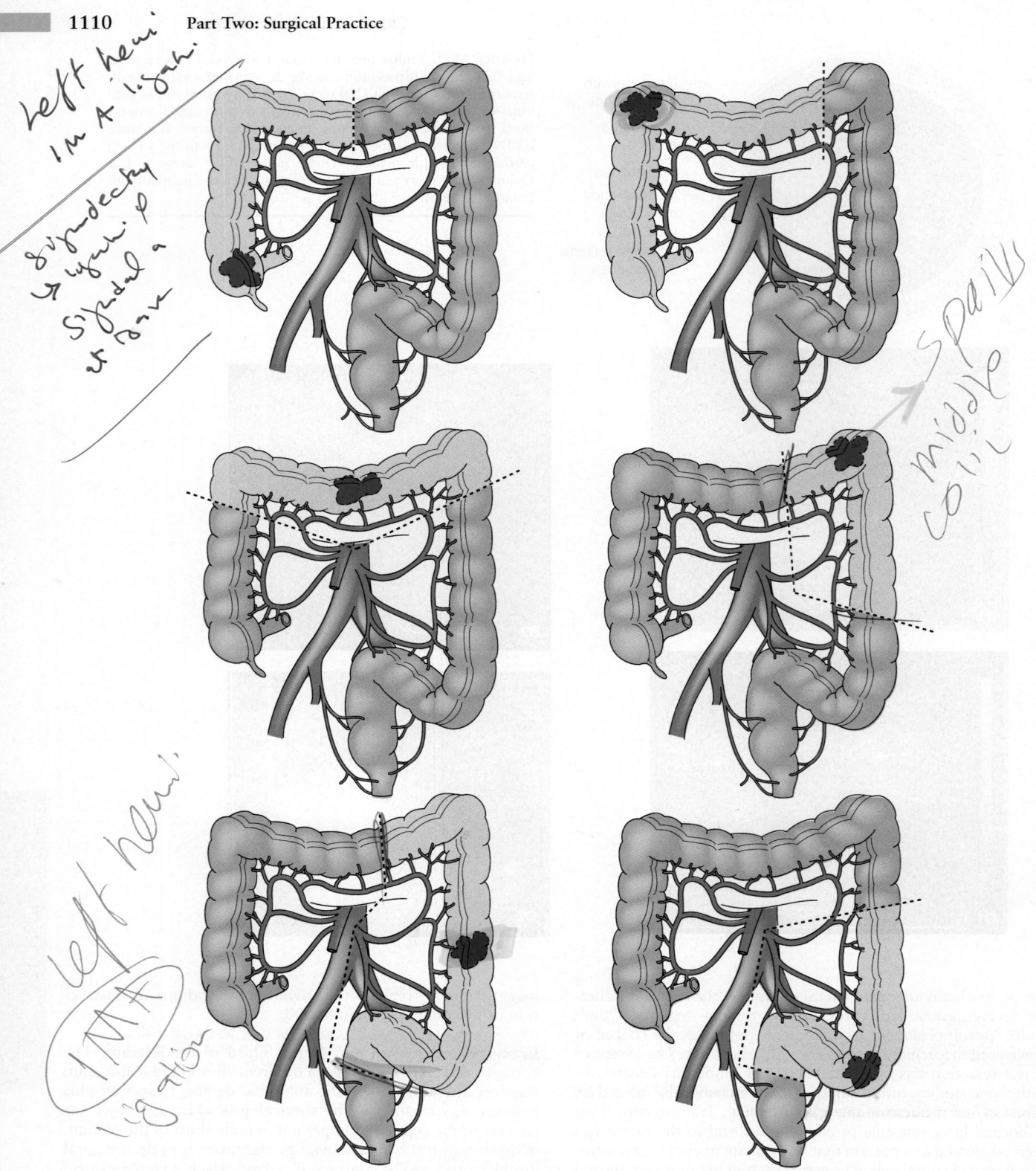

A left hemicolectomy with removal of intestine from the middle transverse to the distal sigmoid colon can be used for tumors of the descending colon (Fig. 68.10). High ligation of the inferior mesenteric artery is necessary in this operation. For cancers of the sigmoid colon, a segmental resection can be

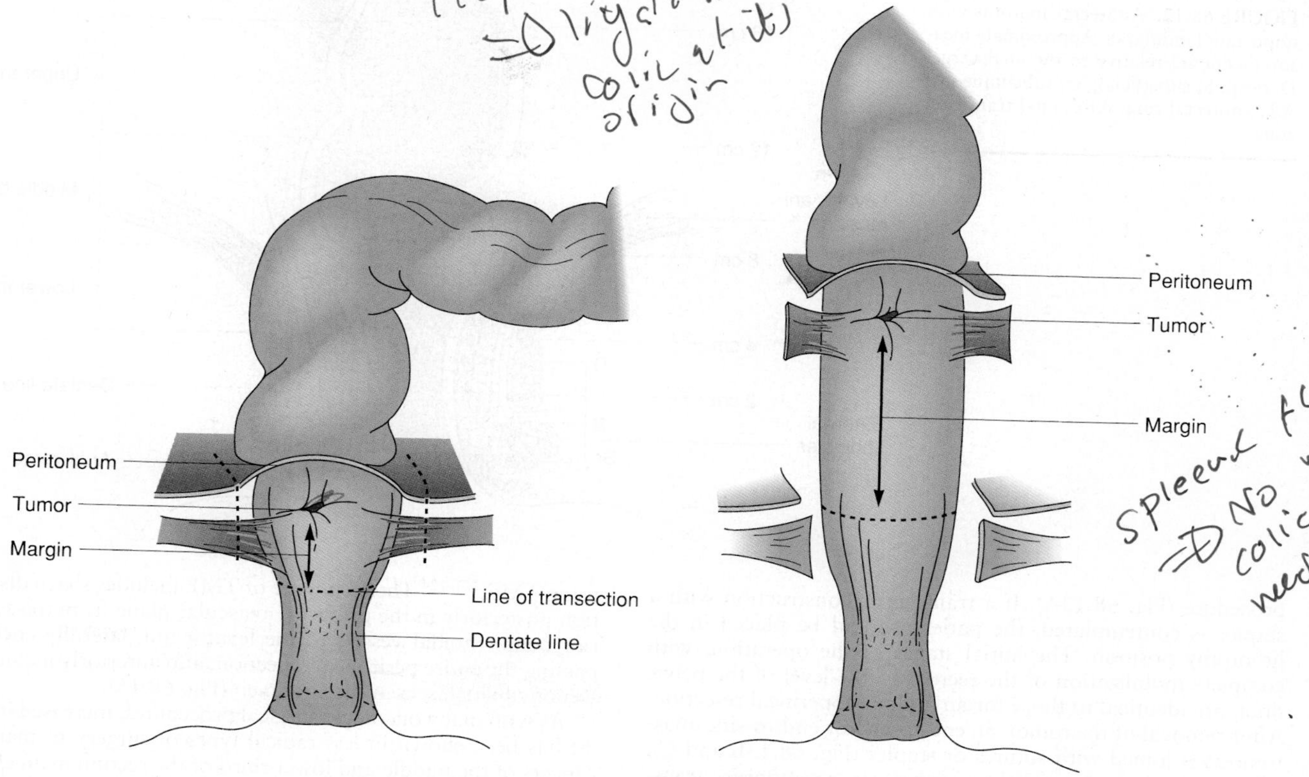

FIGURE 68.11. Extent of surgery in abdominoperineal resection.

performed with ligation of the sigmoid artery near its origin. Rectosigmoid cancers and tumors confined to the upper third of the rectum are removed by an anterior resection. The upper third of the rectum is about 12 to 16 cm from the anal verge and is located above the peritoneal reflection ending proximally where the tenia flare (Fig. 68.11). The pelvic peritoneum is incised circumferentially around the rectum, and the intestine is sharply mobilized from the presacral fascia. Laterally, the middle hemorrhoidal vessels are ligated. Anteriorly, the rectum is mobilized from the seminal vesicles and prostate or the vagina. The mesenteric vessels are divided at the origin of the sigmoid artery or higher, at the origin of the inferior mesenteric artery, if further mobilization of the splenic flexure is required to obtain a tension-free anastomosis.

Laparoscopic and hand-assisted laparoscopic techniques have been widely adopted for resection of colon and upper rectal cancers. Although the operative steps and surgical principles are identical, laparoscopic resection for colorectal cancer was met initially with skepticism. Critics questioned potential for port-site metastases, possible inadequacy of resection, compromise of patient safety, and increased cost and time investment for questionable gain. The Clinical Outcomes and Surgical Therapy (COST) Study Group[116] and others[117] have reported no difference in perioperative complications, cancer recurrence, or overall survival at 3-year follow-up. A large cohort study from the National Cancer Database recently compared overall survival after laparoscopic and open colon cancer resection.[118] After case mix adjustment, overall survival was improved for patients who underwent laparoscopic resection of stage I and II but not stage III colon cancer.

Middle and Lower Third of the Rectum. Cancers located in the lower third of the rectum, between the anorectal ring and 7 to 8 cm from the anal verge, are reliably treated by abdominoperineal resection. The procedure involves wide excision of the rectum to include the lateral attachments and pelvic mesocolon and establishment of a colostomy. The extent of surgery for an abdominoperineal resection is illustrated in Figure 68.13. With the patient in a modified lithotomy position, the abdominal and perineal procedures can be performed simultaneously by two teams or sequentially by one team. Alternatively, the abdominal procedure can be completed with the patient in the supine position, and the perineal portion completed afterward, with the patient turned in the lateral position. On opening of the abdomen, evidence of intra-abdominal spread is ascertained. The discovery of extensive disseminated disease may eliminate the need for an abdominoperineal resection because a local excision or fulguration to preserve anal function may be more appropriate for palliation. If an abdominoperineal resection is performed, ligation of the superior rectal artery at its origin, along with the superior rectal vein, is required. Occasionally, if extensive nodal disease is present, higher arterial ligation may be necessary. The rectum is mobilized in a fashion similar to that described for an anterior resection, but the dissection is carried down to the pelvic floor muscles, which are excised en bloc with the anus. An end-sigmoid colostomy is brought out through the rectus sheath. Efforts to exclude small intestine from a future radiation field by use of the omentum should be considered. Primary closure of the perineal wound over drains often can be accomplished, but a greater than 50% wound infection rate is to be expected. Use of gracilis or other muscle flaps at the time of perineal wound closure should be considered in patients who have undergone neoadjuvant radiation.

Middle and Lower Third of the Rectum. Cancer of the middle third of the rectum, between 8 and 12 cm from the anal verge (Fig. 68.14), can be managed by various techniques. For these tumors, abdominoperineal resection does not yield results superior to those of other procedures that spare the anal sphincter. Therefore, an effort should be made to maintain intestinal continuity. Low anterior resection is a commonly used technique that involves resection of the middle rectum with primary anastomosis. The introduction of the end-to-end anastomosis stapler has increased the use of this sphincter-saving

FIGURE 68.12. Anorectal anatomy with important landmarks. Approximate measurements are relative to the anal verge. D, deep; S, superficial; Sc, subcutaneous; AR, anorectal ring; ATZ, anal transition zone.

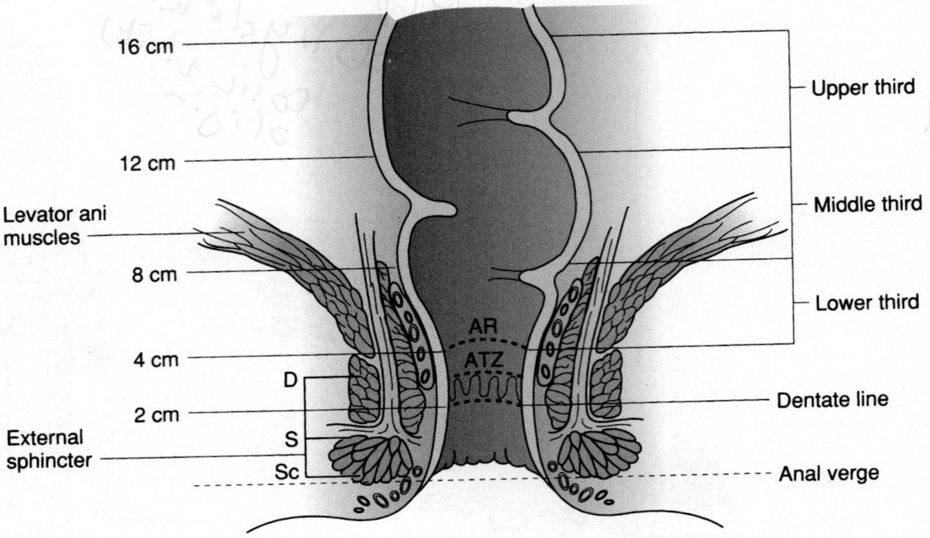

procedure (Fig. 68.13A). If a transanal reconstruction with a stapler is contemplated, the patient should be placed in the lithotomy position. The initial stages of the operation, with complete mobilization of the rectum to the level of the pelvic floor, are identical to those for an abdominoperineal resection. After removal of the tumor, an end-to-end or end-to-side anastomosis is joined with sutures or staples (Fig. 68.13B and C). After ascertaining an airtight anastomosis, a temporary transverse colostomy or loop ileostomy is recommended for patients in whom preoperative radiation was used, the anastomosis is up to 4 cm from the anal verge, or the integrity of the anastomosis is a concern.

Other sphincter-saving approaches have been described for middle rectal cancers.[119] Coloanal anastomosis involves restoring bowel continuity by bringing the colon to the level of the anus and dentate line (Fig. 68.13D). A straight coloanal anastomosis commonly results in stool frequency, urgency, and incontinence for the first year postoperatively. These symptoms can be tempered by a side-to-end anastomosis or a formation of a colonic J-pouch (Fig. 68.13E). Creation of an adequate but not overlarge reservoir is an important technical point to avoid future difficulty with evacuation.

A controversy in sphincter-saving procedures for rectal tumors concerns the length of an adequate distal mucosal margin. The traditional dictum of 5 cm for a margin is not evidence based. Only 2.5% of patients have intramural spread beyond 2 cm from the palpable tumor—and these patients usually have dissemination of tumor despite aggressive local therapy. No correlation has been found between local recurrence and extent of the distal margin when it is greater than 2 cm. Ideally, a surgical margin of 3 cm, measured on the fresh specimen, should be achieved. If the end-to-end anastomosis stapler is used, then a margin of 2 cm plus the additional "doughnut" specimen obtained by the stapler should be adequate. The segment of rectum located between the tumor and the pelvic floor, determined preoperatively, can be lengthened as much as 4 cm after the rectum is mobilized from its pelvic attachments (Fig. 68.14). If in the surgeon's judgment an adequate margin cannot be obtained, then abdominoperineal resection should be performed.

Radial margins are more relevant than longitudinal margins for local control of mid to low rectal cancers. The practical importance of lateral spread is demonstrated by results of total mesorectal excision (TME) en bloc with the rectal specimen. By means of TME, the Basingstoke group initially reported a dramatic reduction in local recurrence from the norm of 30% to 40% to 3.7% over a 4-year follow-up period.[120] Subsequent studies consistently showed a decline in local recurrence of 15% to 40% using conventional techniques to 4% to 11% using TME.[121–124] The technique of TME includes sharp dissection posteriorly in the presacral avascular plane from the superior hemorrhoidal vessels to the levator ani, laterally encompassing the entire peritoneal reflection, and anteriorly including Denonvilliers fascia in the specimen (Fig. 68.15).

As with many oncologic surgical procedures, increased interest has been shown in less radical types of surgery to manage cancers of the middle and lower third of the rectum in an effort to preserve the anal sphincters and avoid an abdominoperineal resection. Initially, these local procedures, such as excision, ablation, and irradiation, were reserved for patients with advanced disease or with medical contraindications to radical surgery. However, for selected patients with low rectal cancers, local excision is an acceptable treatment option that is associated with rates of local recurrence and survival similar to those seen after radical surgery. A multicenter, prospective study was undertaken to address this question.[125] To be eligible, patients had to have an adenocarcinoma of the rectum that was 10 cm or less from the dentate line and 4 cm or less in diameter, and that involved 40% or less of the rectal lumen. All patients registered underwent local excision of their tumor. Those determined to have T1 tumors with negative surgical margins received no further treatment, and those with T2 tumors underwent postoperative radiation and chemotherapy. The 6-year disease-free survival rates were 83% and 87%, respectively, and the overall survival rates were 71% and 85%, respectively, for T1 and T2 tumors. Two of 59 patients with T1 tumors and 7 of 51 patients with T2 tumors experienced an isolated local recurrence and underwent salvage abdominoperineal resection. Four of these died of recurrent local or distal disease.[125] A case-control study from the Minnesota group examining transanal excision versus radical surgery without adjuvant therapy found a significantly higher local recurrence rate of 47% versus 6%, respectively.[126] More important, T2 patients undergoing local versus radical initial excision experienced a respective 5-year survival difference of 65% versus 81% among patients with T2 tumors, in spite of salvage abdominoperineal resection. Detailed prospective data to better understand 3-year survival and other outcomes of preoperative chemoradiotherapy followed by transanal excision of uT2N0 rectal tumors are currently being collected through the American College of Surgeons Oncology Group protocol Z6041.[127]

Other forms of local treatment for low rectal cancers are reserved for patients who are not candidates for abdominoperineal resection or local excision. Ablation by transanal electric fulguration of the tumor in multiple stages has been reported to be an acceptable treatment in patients who are poor surgical candidates; however, this procedure cannot be used for

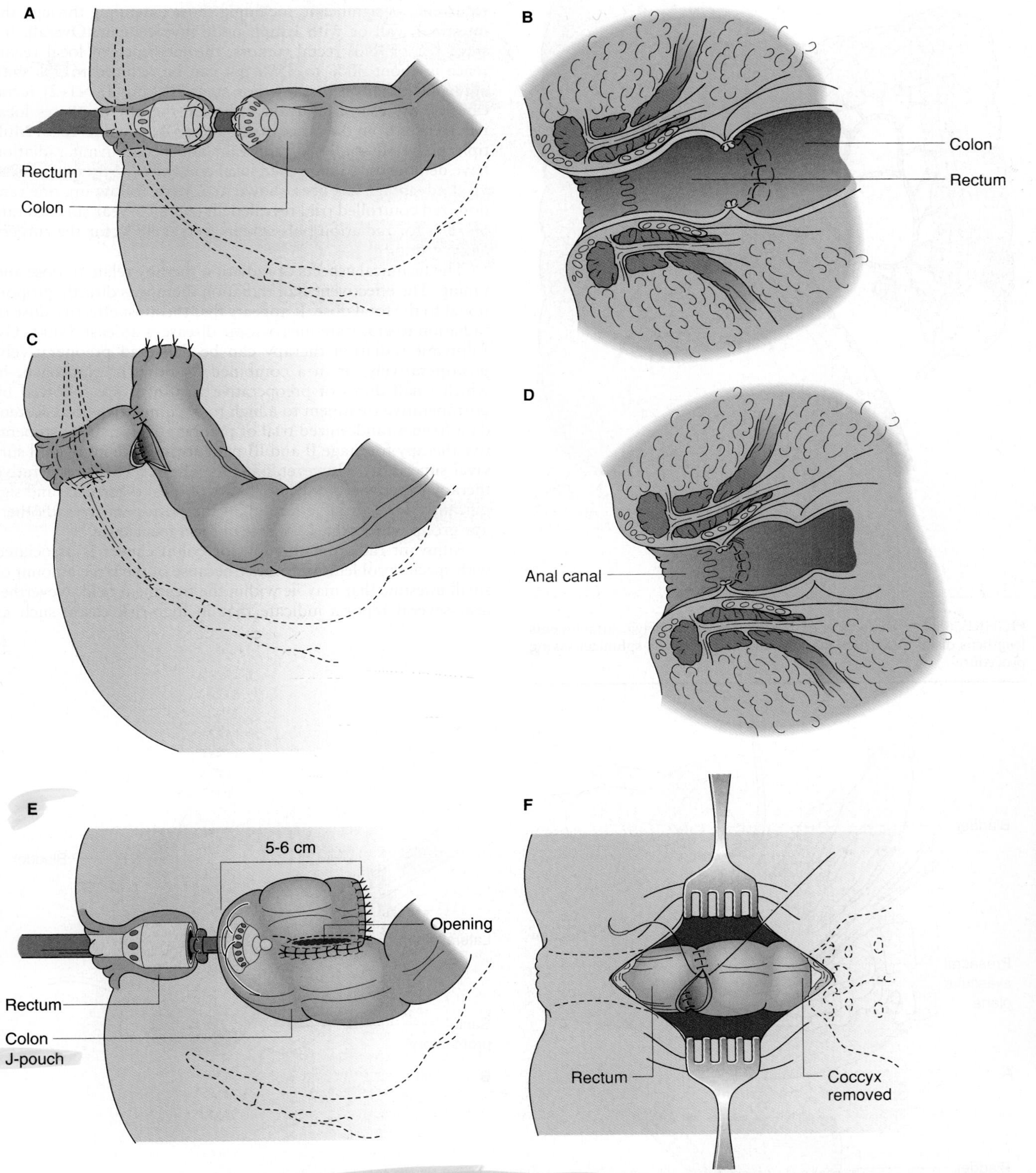

FIGURE 68.13. Techniques for low anterior resections. **A:** End-to-end stapler. **B:** Single layer with sutures. **C:** Side-to-end anastomosis. **D:** Pull-through. **E:** Colon J-pouch (5- to 6-cm pouch). **F:** Transsacral resection.

circumferential tumors.[128] Endocavitary irradiation as a primary curative therapy for early cancers has been reported with some success. The neodymium:yttrium-aluminum garnet laser has been found to be effective in palliating obstructive or bleeding lesions of locally advanced colorectal tumors.

Adjuvant Radiation Therapy

Radiation therapy combined with surgical resection for colorectal cancer has been demonstrated to reduce the incidence of local tumor recurrence. In general, the use of radiation therapy

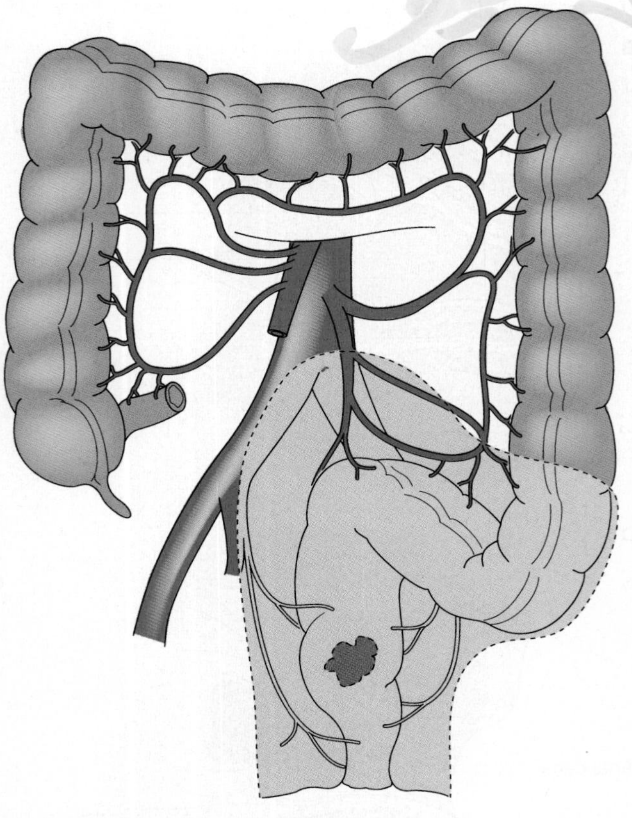

FIGURE 68.14. Dissection of the rectum from pelvic attachments lengthens distal tumor-free margins and may permit a sphincter-saving procedure.

has been limited to rectal tumors in which the incidence of local recurrence is significant, including those extending through the intestinal wall or with lymph node involvement. Overall, for stage IIA (T3N0) rectal tumors, the incidence of local recurrence is about 30% to 35% but can be reduced to 5% with adjuvant radiation therapy. For stage III (any T, N1–2) rectal cancers, the use of adjuvant radiation therapy decreases local recurrences from the range of 45% to 65% down to 10%. Multiple phase III studies of adjuvant and neoadjuvant radiation have demonstrated improved local control.[129] Although no survival advantage has been shown at 2 years follow-up, one randomized controlled trial revealed an overall 5-year survival rate of 58% for radiation plus surgery versus 48% for the surgery alone group.[130]

The technical aspects of radiation therapy relate to dose and timing. The effectiveness of radiation therapy is directly proportional to the total dose. It appears that the most effective dose of radiation to eradicate microscopic disease is at least 5,000 cGy. Adjuvant radiation therapy can be delivered preoperatively, postoperatively, or in a combined "sandwich" approach, in which small doses of preoperative treatment are followed by postoperative treatment to a high total cumulative dose. Recent data from a randomized trial of preoperative versus postoperative therapy for Stage II and III patients indicate no overall survival superiority. However, patients who received preoperative therapy experienced only a 6% rate of local recurrence and significantly fewer toxic effects than the postoperative radiotherapy group who had a 12% rate of local recurrence.[131]

Adjuvant radiation therapy for colon cancer is associated with special problems of toxicity because of the large amount of small intestine that may lie within the treatment field. Nevertheless, several reports indicate that in high-risk cases, such as

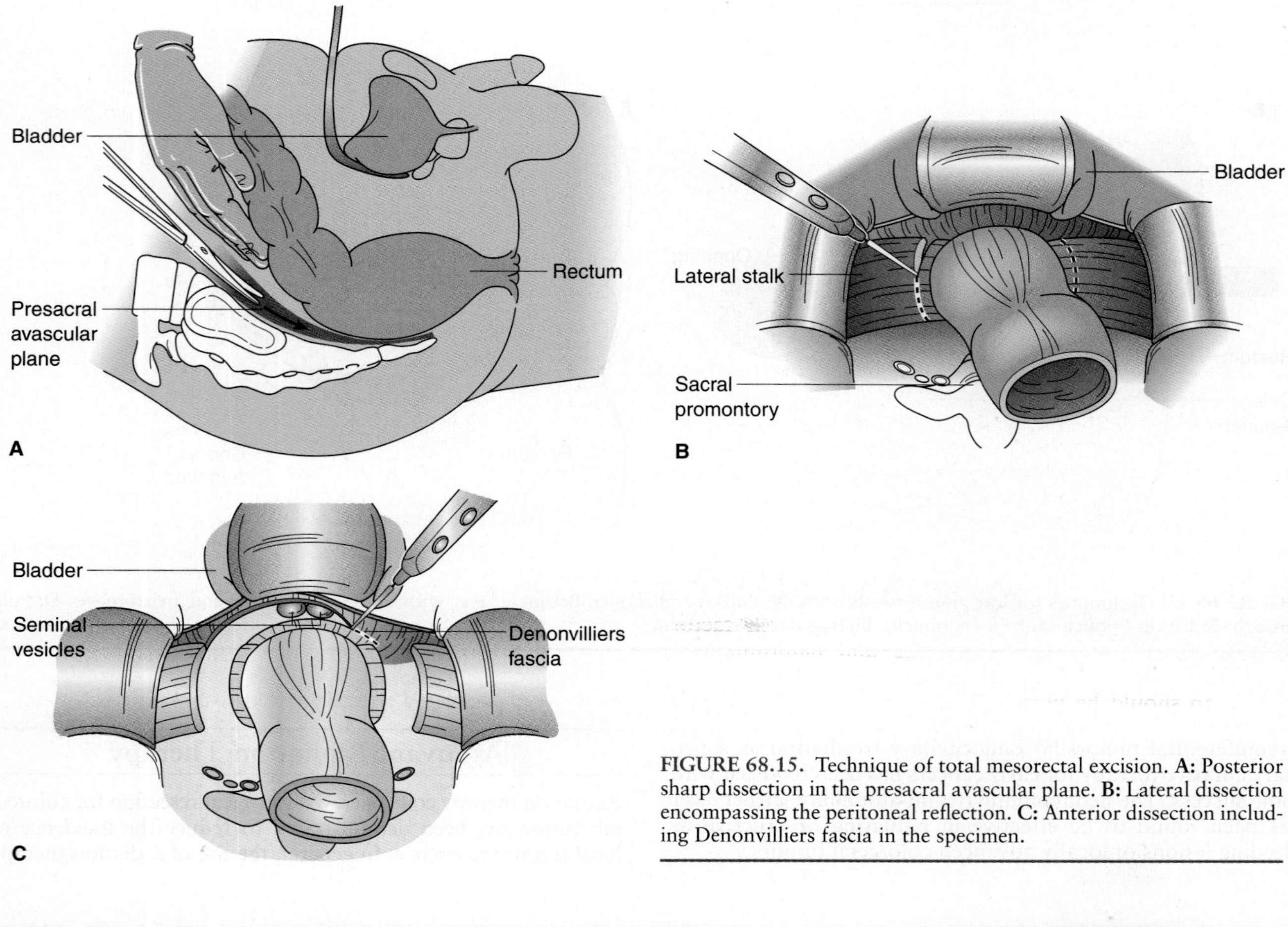

FIGURE 68.15. Technique of total mesorectal excision. **A:** Posterior sharp dissection in the presacral avascular plane. **B:** Lateral dissection encompassing the peritoneal reflection. **C:** Anterior dissection including Denonvilliers fascia in the specimen.

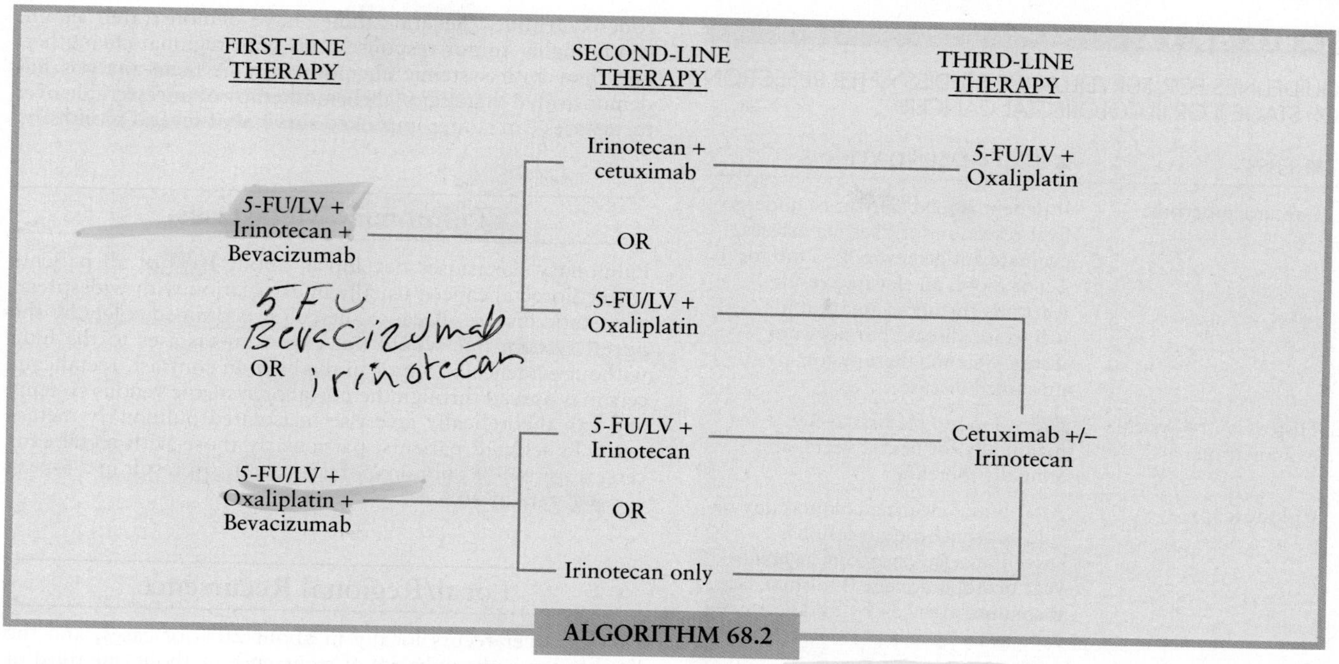

ALGORITHM 68.2. An algorithm for intensive combined, targeted chemotherapy for metastatic colorectal cancer. (Adapted from Goldberg RM, Carrato A. Accomplishments in 2007 in the treatment of advanced colorectal cancer. *Gastrointest Cancer Res* 2008;2(3 suppl):S19–S24.)

tumors involving adjacent viscera or perforated lesions, adjuvant radiation therapy can decrease local and regional recurrences.

Adjuvant Chemotherapy

Even if local tumor control is adequate, patients with colorectal cancer die of disseminated disease. In about 25% of patients with stage II tumors, and 50% of those with stage III tumors, the growth of micrometastatic disease present at the time of primary tumor resection eventually causes death. Several randomized, prospective studies have demonstrated adjuvant systemic chemotherapy benefit to certain subgroups of patients.

The National Comprehensive Cancer Network (NCCN; http://www.nccn.org/index.asp) is a consortium of major cancer centers in the United States that have established practice guidelines for various cancers based on the best evidence available. For node-negative colon cancers, adjuvant chemotherapy may be considered for high-risk lesions (i.e., T4, grade 3–4, lymphovascular invasion, bowel perforation, or bowel obstruction).[132] For the 60% of colorectal cancers diagnosed at stage III or IV, adjuvant chemotherapy is recommended. The standard chemotherapy regimen has traditionally been 5-fluorouracil (5-FU) or its oral equivalent, capecitabine, and leucovorin, for an overall survival benefit of 15% to 20%.

More recently, the addition of oxaliplatin and irinotecan chemotherapeutic agents have substantially improved median survival times of metastatic colorectal cancer. In addition, the survival benefits of regimens that include these agents are further improved by use of new targeted biologic agents including bevacizumab, an anti–vascular endothelial growth factor monoclonal antibody, and cetuximab and panitumumab, anti–epidermal growth factor receptor monoclonal antibodies. Cetuximab should be used as the biologic agent only after ascertaining unmutated, wild-type *K-RAS*.[133] The novel use of these combined agents aggressively and in continuum has led to a paradigm shift in the understanding of metastatic colorectal cancer.[133,134]

Newer recommendations include first-line treatment of unresectable metastatic disease (absent other contraindications to surgery) aggressively with two cytotoxic agents and one biologic agent (Algorithm 68.2). The goal is to shrink the tumor until it may be surgically resected. Even if resection is not achieved, with individually targeted therapies that maximize dosing and minimize toxicities, metastatic colorectal cancer may begin to share more characteristics with chronic disease than an acute terminal illness.

In colon cancer, local recurrence is infrequent; in rectal cancer, the use of adjuvant chemotherapy combined with radiation has proved effective in improving local control and increasing the survival rate. In rectal cancer, it is almost as important to prevent local failure and ensuing symptoms as it is to prevent death from distant metastasis. As noted in the previous section, radiation therapy is routinely recommended for patients with stage IIA (T3, N0) or III (any T, N1–2) rectal cancers. In addition, the NCCN guidelines recommend adjuvant chemotherapy (either 5-FU or oxaliplatin plus fluorouracil and leucovorin [FOLFOX]) for these stages of rectal cancer.

Treatment of Recurrent Colorectal Cancer

A subset of patients with recurrent colorectal cancer can be cured, so that a comprehensive follow-up program in patients who have undergone resection of their primary tumor is appropriate (Table 68.12). Fifty percent of cancers that recur do so within 18 months after surgery, and more than 80% of recurrences are evident by 3 years. Therefore, careful follow-up is important during the 3-year period after primary tumor resection. Besides identifying recurrences, a careful follow-up program also identifies the 5% of patients in whom a metachronous primary tumor of the large intestine develops.

The CEA assay is a sensitive serologic test in the diagnosis of recurrent colorectal cancer. CEA is a glycoprotein that was originally described as a tumor-specific antigen derived from neoplasms of the gastrointestinal tract. It is now known that CEA is not tumor specific because its concentration can be elevated in various malignancies from different sites and in some benign conditions. CEA is an oncofetal antigen that is also

TABLE 68.12

GUIDELINES FOR SURVEILLANCE STUDIES AFTER RESECTION OF STAGE II OR III COLORECTAL CANCER[a]

■ TEST	■ RECOMMENDATIONS
Carcinoembryonic	If patient is medically fit to undergo liver resection for liver metastases, evaluate antigen every 2–3 mo for 2 y or more; an elevated result warrants further evaluation for metastatic disease but does not justify systemic therapy for presumed disease
History and physical examination	Every 3–6 mo for first 2–3 y, biannually for next 2 years, and annually thereafter
Colonoscopy	After initial clearing colonoscopy to rule out synchronous lesions, surveillance colonoscopy at first year postoperatively. If normal, thereafter, every 3–5 y to detect new cancers and polyps
Computed tomography	Individualized
Chest roentgenography	Individualized

[a]Endorsed by the American Society of Clinical Oncology.

expressed by early embryonic or fetal cells. CEA is not useful as a screening or diagnostic test but is useful as a tumor marker. The CEA concentration is elevated in more than 90% of patients with disseminated colorectal cancer and in about 20% of patients with localized disease. Serum levels usually are elevated in proportion to the mass of the tumor present and often correlate with response to therapy. CEA measurement provides useful information when elevated levels fall to normal after curative resection. In about two thirds of patients with recurrent disease, an increased CEA level is the first indicator of tumor recurrence; therefore, serial CEA testing, combined with regular physical examinations, is one of the most useful means for detecting recurrent colorectal cancer. In fact, the CEA determination, along with the history and physical examination, is the only surveillance test recommended for patients after curative resection of stage II or III disease. The NCCN guidelines recommend CEA testing along with history and physical examinations every 3 months for 2 years, then every 6 months for a total of 5 years. Colonoscopy is recommended 1 year after resection and then every 2–3 years thereafter if negative.

Hepatic Metastases

6 The liver is the most frequent site of blood-borne metastases from primary colorectal cancers. In a subgroup of patients, the liver is the only site of recurrent disease, and surgical excision of the metastases is the only curative option for these patients. Overall, surgical resection is associated with a 5-year survival rate of 25% to 30%.[135] Patients eligible for hepatic resection of metastatic disease are those who have no evidence of extrahepatic tumor, no medical contraindications to surgery, and a limited number of lesions that are amenable to resection with negative surgical margins.

Patients who have unresectable hepatic metastases that appear to be confined to that organ have been treated with regional chemotherapy through the hepatic artery (e.g., fluorodeoxyuridine). Several studies have demonstrated significantly higher tumor response rates with regional chemotherapy than with systemic chemotherapy. A meta-analysis has demonstrated that regional chemotherapy of unresectable liver metastases can confer improved survival of several months.

Pulmonary Metastases

Pulmonary metastases develop in about 10% of all patients with colorectal cancer, usually in association with widespread metastatic disease. Because the colon is drained solely by the portal system, one would not expect metastases to the lung without evidence of tumor in the liver. In contrast, rectal cancers may spread through the portal or systemic venous systems and can theoretically give rise to isolated pulmonary metastases. In selected patients, particularly those with rectal cancers, resection of pulmonary recurrences can result in a 5-year survival rate of 20%.[136]

Local/Regional Recurrence

Colon cancer recurs locally in about 20% of cases, and the local lesion is the only site of recurrence in about one third of these cases. If the recurrent tumor is isolated to the suture line, resection of such recurrence can be curative. Locoregional failure occurs in 30% to 65% of patients with transmural or node-positive rectal cancers. Often, pelvic recurrences of rectal cancer after a low anterior or abdominoperineal resection are diffuse and associated with disseminated disease. If pelvic recurrences are localized, they should be resected if negative surgical margins can be achieved. Surgical procedures necessary to accomplish this include en bloc partial sacrectomy or total pelvic exenteration.

Disseminated Disease

Recurrent colorectal cancer is not usually localized to one site that is amenable to surgical resection. More commonly, colorectal cancer recurs in multiple sites. In these cases, systemic therapy may be considered. No studies have clearly documented that systemic therapies for disseminated colorectal cancer improve the survival rate; however, systemic treatment is commonly used for palliation.

The current management of disseminated colorectal cancer uses various active agents, both in combination and as single agents: 5-FU/leucovorin, irinotecan, oxaliplatin, and capecitabine and bevacizumab. The choice of therapy is based upon the performance status of the patient (i.e., whether the patient can tolerate or not tolerate intensive therapy), prior therapies, and patient preference. Patients with poor performance characteristics should receive supportive care only.

Other Colorectal Tumors

Carcinoid Tumors. Carcinoid tumors are neoplasms derived from cells that are capable of synthesizing a wide variety of hormones. Two recent reviews of the Surveillance Epidemiology and End Results database have updated our knowledge of carcinoid tumors.[137,138] In the first study analyzing over 11,000 incident cases between 1973 and 1997, most gastrointestinal tract carcinoids occurred in the ileum, not the appendix as previously thought. The incidence of carcinoid tumors appears to have increased by about 6%.[137] However, it was not possible to discern whether the incidence increase actually represented improvements in diagnosis. In the second study of

TABLE 68.13

STAGING OF CARCINOID TUMORS

STAGE	DESCRIPTION			
TUMOR-NODE-METASTASIS (TNM) SYSTEM				
Primary Tumor				
TX	Primary tumor cannot be assessed			
T0	No evidence of tumor in resected specimen (prior polypectomy or fulguration)			
T1	≤1 cm and any depth of invasion			
	>1 and ≤4 cm and invades up to or including the muscularis propria			
T2	>1 and ≤4 cm and invades beyond the muscularis propria			
	>4 cm and invades up to or including the muscularis propria			
T3	>4 cm and invades beyond the muscularis propria			
Regional Lymph Node Involvement				
NX	Nodes cannot be assessed (e.g., local excision only)			
N0	No regional node metastases			
N1	Positive regional node metastases			
Distant Metastasis				
MX	Presence of distant metastases cannot be assessed			
M0	No distant metastases			
M1	Distant metastases present			
Stage	**Description**			**5-Year Survival Rates**[b]
I	T1	N0	M0	97%
II	T1,2	N1	M0	69%
	T2	Any N		
III	T3	Any N	M0	21%
IV	Any T	Any N	M1	17%

[a]In all pathologic staging systems, particularly those applied to rectal cancer, the abbreviations m and g may be used; m denotes microscopic transmural penetration; g or m + g denotes transmural penetration visible on gross inspection and confirmed microscopically.

[b]Kern KA, Pass HI, Roth JA. Surgical treatment of pulmonary metastases. In: Rosenberg SA, ed. *Surgical Treatment of Metastatic Cancer*. Vol 69. Philadelphia: JB Lippincott; 1987.

incident cases from 1973 to 2004, prognostic variables were assessed and a staging scheme was devised as a tool for more accurate prognostication (Table 68.13).[138] The authors found that tumor size continued to be an important prognostic factor. About 60% of rectal carcinoids present as asymptomatic submucosal nodules measuring less than 2 cm in diameter. Transanal local excision suffices for definitive therapy because small tumors rarely metastasize. More radical excisions of larger rectal lesions may be required for local control; however, the results of radical excisions for large rectal carcinoids are poor because these tumors are more prone to metastasize. In contrast to rectal carcinoids, colon carcinoids should be treated by standard curative operation. Among carcinoid tumors of the colon less than 2 cm in size, 22% have metastasized to regional lymph nodes, while 79% of those greater than 2 cm have positive nodes.[139]

Lymphomas. Colorectal lymphomas are rare and account for fewer than 0.5% of all colorectal malignancies. The documentation of widespread dissemination of lymphoma in most cases underscores the concept that lymphoma of the gastrointestinal tract is a systemic disease in which tumor cells are present in other organ sites. Because this disease is highly responsive to chemotherapy and radiation, surgery is not the primary mode of therapy. If the clinical workup reveals a focal site of disease in the large intestine, surgical resection may be considered. Usually, for localized, low-grade colorectal lymphomas, radiation therapy is considered first-line therapy. For intermediate- and high-grade lymphomas, chemotherapy combined with radiation therapy should be the primary treatment modality. Surgery for colorectal lymphomas has been primarily for diagnostic and staging purposes and for the management of treatment-related complications (i.e., perforation or bleeding).

Sarcomas. Colorectal sarcomas are extremely rare and account for less than 0.1% of all large-bowel malignancies. The most common histologic sarcoma subtype is leiomyosarcoma. With these tumors, the most significant prognostic indicator is the tumor grade. Patients with high-grade tumors do poorly. These tumors usually metastasize to the liver and peritoneal surfaces. If the tumors are clinically localized at initial presentation, a radical en bloc excision should be performed to obtain a margin of uninvolved normal tissue. Because of the rarity of this tumor, no studies have addressed whether adjuvant radiation therapy or chemotherapy is beneficial.

Gastrointestinal Stromal Tumors. Gastrointestinal stromal tumors (GISTs) were previously often mislabelled as sarcoma. GISTs originate from the pluripotential interstitial cells of Cajal, the gastrointestinal pacemaker cell, and can occur anywhere in the gut. These are submucosal, slow-growing tumors that can reach immense sizes before becoming symptomatic.

Frozen section histology is often consistent with a spindle cell appearance; immunohistochemical staining nearly always reveals positive kit receptor. The metastatic potential is assessed by size and field mitotic index. These mesenchymal tumors spread hematogenously, generally recurring locally in the peritoneum or in the liver. The mainstay of treatment is complete surgical resection. GISTs are not responsive to traditional chemotherapy or to radiation. For metastatic disease, a tyrosine kinase inhibitor, imatinib mesylate, is effective at controlling tumor growth and spread.

References

1. Jemal A, Siegel R, Ward E, et al. Cancer statistics, 2009. *CA Cancer J Clin* 2009;59(4):225–249.
2. American Cancer Society. *Cancer Facts & Figures 2010*. Atlanta: American Cancer Society; 2010.
3. Center MM, Jemal A, Ward E. International trends in colorectal cancer incidence rates. *Cancer Epidemiol Biomarkers Prev* 2009;18(6):1688–1694.
4. Lee J, Demissie K, Lu SE, et al. Cancer incidence among Korean-American immigrants in the United States and native Koreans in South Korea. *Cancer Control* 2007;14(1):78–85.
5. Shimizu H, Mack TM, Ross RK, et al. Cancer of the gastrointestinal tract among Japanese and white immigrants in Los Angeles County. *J Natl Cancer Inst* 1987;78(2):223–228.
6. McMichael AJ, McCall MG, Hartshorne JM, et al. Patterns of gastrointestinal cancer in European migrants to Australia: the role of dietary change. *Int J Cancer* 1980;25(4):431–437.
7. DeLancey JO, Thun MJ, Jemal A, et al. Recent trends in Black-White disparities in cancer mortality. *Cancer Epidemiol Biomarkers Prev* 2008; 17(11):2908–2912.
8. Nyren O, Bergstrom R, Nystrom L, et al. Smoking and colorectal cancer: a 20-year follow-up study of Swedish construction workers. *J Natl Cancer Inst* 1996;88(18):1302–1307.
9. Giovannucci E. Modifiable risk factors for colon cancer. *Gastroenterol Clin North Am* 2002;31:925–943.
10. Willett WC, MacMahon B. Diet and cancer—an overview (second of two parts). *N Engl J Med* 1984;310(11):697–703.
11. Forte A, De Sanctis R, Leonetti G, et al. Dietary chemoprevention of colorectal cancer. *Ann Ital Chir* 2008;79(4):261–267.
12. Satia-Abouta J, Galanko JA, Martin CF, et al. Food groups and colon cancer risk in African-Americans and Caucasians. *Int J Cancer* 2004;109(5): 728–736.
13. Chao A, Thun MJ, Connell CJ, et al. Meat consumption and risk of colorectal cancer. *JAMA* 2005;293(2):172–182.
14. Larsson SC, Rafter J, Holmberg L, et al. Red meat consumption and risk of cancers in the proximal colon, distal colon, and rectum: The Swedish Mammography Cohort. *Int J Cancer* 2005;113(5):829–834.
15. Burkitt DP. Epidemiology of cancer of the colon and rectum, 1971. *Dis Colon Rectum* 1993;36(11):1071–1082.
16. Benedetti A, Parent ME, Siemiatycki J. Lifetime consumption of alcoholic beverages and risk of 13 types of cancer in men: results from a case-control study in Montreal. *Cancer Detect Prev* 2009;32:352–362.
17. Botteri E, Iodice S, Bagnardi V, et al. Smoking and colorectal cancer: a meta-analysis. *JAMA* 2008;300:2765–2778.
18. Samad AK, Taylor RS, Marshall T, et al. A meta-analysis of the association of physical activity with reduced risk of colorectal cancer. *Colorectal Dis* 2005;7(3):204–213.
19. Frezza EE, Wachtel MS, Chiriva-Internati M. Influence of obesity on the risk of developing colon cancer. *Gut* 2006;55(2):285–291.
20. Moore LL, Bradlee ML, Singer MR, et al. BMI and waist circumference as predictors of lifetime colon cancer risk in Framingham Study adults. *Int J Obes Relat Metab Disord* 2004;28(4):559–567.
21. Cannon-Albright LA, Skolnick MH, Bishop DT, et al. Common inheritance of susceptibility to colonic adenomatous polyps and associated colorectal cancers. *N Engl J Med* 1988;319(9):533–537.
22. Houlston RS, Collins A, Slack J, et al. Dominant genes for colorectal cancer are not rare. *Ann Hum Genet* 1992;56 (pt 2):99–103.
23. Offerhaus GJ, Giardiello FM, Krush AJ, et al. The risk of upper gastrointestinal cancer in familial adenomatous polyposis. *Gastroenterology* 1992; 102(6):1980–1982.
24. Tonelli F, Nardi F, Bechi P, et al. Extracolonic polyps in familial polyposis coli and Gardner's syndrome. *Dis Colon Rectum* 1985;28(9):664–668.
25. Classics in oncology. Heredity with reference to carcinoma as shown by the study of the cases examined in the pathological laboratory of the University of Michigan, 1895–1913. By Aldred Scott Warthin. 1913. *CA Cancer J Clin* 1985;35(6):348–359.
26. Lynch HT, Krush AJ. Cancer family "G" revisited: 1895–1970. *Cancer* 1971;27(6):1505–1511.
27. Watson P, Lynch HT. Extracolonic cancer in hereditary nonpolyposis colorectal cancer. *Cancer* 1993;71(3):677–685.
28. Vasen HF, Mecklin JP, Khan PM, et al. The International Collaborative Group on Hereditary Non-Polyposis Colorectal Cancer (ICG-HNPCC). *Dis Colon Rectum* 1991;34(5):424–425.
29. Vasen HF, Watson P, Mecklin JP, et al. New clinical criteria for hereditary nonpolyposis colorectal cancer (HNPCC, Lynch syndrome) proposed by the International Collaborative group on HNPCC. *Gastroenterology* 1999;116(6):1453–1456.
30. Lubbe SJ, Webb EL, Chandler IP, et al. Implications of familial colorectal cancer risk profiles and microsatellite instability status. *J Clin Oncol* 2009; 27(13):2238–2244.
31. Rodriguez-Bigas MA, Boland CR, Hamilton SR, et al. A National Cancer Institute Workshop on Hereditary Nonpolyposis Colorectal Cancer Syndrome: meeting highlights and Bethesda guidelines. *J Natl Cancer Inst* 1997; 89(23):1758–1762.
32. Umar A, Boland CR, Terdiman JP, et al. Revised Bethesda Guidelines for hereditary nonpolyposis colorectal cancer (Lynch syndrome) and microsatellite instability. New clinical criteria for hereditary nonpolyposis colorectal cancer (HNPCC, Lynch syndrome) proposed by the International Collaborative group on HNPCC. *J Natl Cancer Inst* 2004;96(4):261–268.
33. Raptis S, Mrkonjic M, Green RC, et al. MLH1 -93G>A promoter polymorphism and the risk of microsatellite-unstable colorectal cancer. *J Natl Cancer Inst* 2007;99(6):463–474.
34. Lindor NM, Rabe K, Petersen GM, et al. Lower cancer incidence in Amsterdam-I criteria families without mismatch repair deficiency: familial colorectal cancer type X. *JAMA* 2005;293(16):1979–1985.
35. Giardiello FM, Brensinger JD, Petersen GM, et al. The use and interpretation of commercial APC gene testing for familial adenomatous polyposis. *N Engl J Med* 1997;336(12):823–827.
36. Ponder B. Genetic testing for cancer risk. *Science* 1997;278(5340): 1050–1054.
37. Gyde SN, Prior P, Thompson H, et al. Survival of patients with colorectal cancer complicating ulcerative colitis. *Gut* 1984;25(3):228–231.
38. Huang EH, Park JC, Appelman H, et al. Induction of inflammatory bowel disease accelerates adenoma formation in Min +/- mice. *Surgery* 2006; 139(6):782–788.
39. Muto T, Bussey HJ, Morson BC. The evolution of cancer of the colon and rectum. *Cancer* 1975;36(6):2251–2270.
41. Nusko G, Mansmann U, Altendorf-Hofmann A, et al. Risk of invasive carcinoma in colorectal adenomas assessed by size and site. *Int J Colorectal Dis* 1997;12(5):267–271.
42. Church JM. Clinical significance of small colorectal polyps. *Dis Colon Rectum* 2004;47(4):481–485.
43. Aldridge AJ, Simson JN. Histological assessment of colorectal adenomas by size. Are polyps less than 10 mm in size clinically important? *Eur J Surg* 2001;167(10):777–781.
44. Jass JR, Young J, Leggett BA. Hyperplastic polyps and DNA microsatellite unstable cancers of the colorectum. *Histopathology* 2000;37(4):295–301.
45. Goldstein NS, Bhanot P, Odish E, et al. Hyperplastic-like colon polyps that preceded microsatellite-unstable adenocarcinomas. *Am J Clin Pathol* 2003;119(6):778–796.
46. Wynter CV, Walsh MD, Higuchi T, et al. Methylation patterns define two types of hyperplastic polyp associated with colorectal cancer. *Gut* 2004; 53(4):573–580.
47. Hyman NH, Anderson P, Blasyk H. Hyperplastic polyposis and the risk of colorectal cancer. *Dis Colon Rectum* 2004;47(12):2101–2104.
48. Bos JL, Fearon ER, Hamilton SR, et al. Prevalence of ras gene mutations in human colorectal cancers. *Nature* 1987;327(6120):293–297.
49. Conlin A, Smith G, Carey FA, et al. The prognostic significance of K-ras, p53, and APC mutations in colorectal carcinoma. *Gut* 2005;54(9): 1283–1286.
50. Fearon ER, Vogelstein B. A genetic model for colorectal tumorigenesis. *Cell* 1990;61(5):759–767.
51. Arvanitis ML, Jagelman DG, Fazio VW, et al. Mortality in patients with familial adenomatous polyposis. *Dis Colon Rectum* 1990;33(8):639–642.
52. Kinzler KW, Nilbert MC, Su LK, et al. Identification of FAP locus genes from chromosome 5q21. *Science* 1991;253(5020):661–665.
53. Groden J, Thliveris A, Samowitz W, et al. Identification and characterization of the familial adenomatous polyposis coli gene. *Cell* 1991;66(3):589–600.
54. Korinek V, Barker N, Morin PJ, et al. Constitutive transcriptional activation by a beta-catenin-Tcf complex in APC-/- colon carcinoma. *Science* 1997;275(5307):1784–1787.
55. Morin PJ, Sparks AB, Korinek V, et al. Activation of beta-catenin-Tcf signaling in colon cancer by mutations in beta-catenin or APC. *Science* 1997;275(5307):1787–1790.
56. Powell SM, Zilz N, Beazer-Barclay Y, et al. APC mutations occur early during colorectal tumorigenesis. *Nature* 1992;359(6392):235–237.
57. Smith AJ, Stern HS, Penner M, et al. Somatic APC and K-ras codon 12 mutations in aberrant crypt foci from human colons. *Cancer Res* 1994; 54(21):5527–5530.
58. Vogelstein B, Kinzler KW. p53 function and dysfunction. *Cell* 1992;70(4): 523–526.
59. Jen J, Kim H, Piantadosi S, et al. Allelic loss of chromosome 18q and prognosis in colorectal cancer. *N Engl J Med* 1994;331(4):213–221.
60. Carethers JM, Hawn MT, Greenson JK, et al. Prognostic significance of allelic lost at chromosome 18q21 for stage II colorectal cancer. *Gastroenterology* 1998;114(6):1188–1195.
61. Thibodeau SN, Bren G, Schaid D. Microsatellite instability in cancer of the proximal colon. *Science* 1993;260(5109):816–819.
62. Ionov Y, Peinado MA, Malkhosyan S, et al. Ubiquitous somatic mutations in simple repeated sequences reveal a new mechanism for colonic carcinogenesis. *Nature* 1993;363(6429):558–561.

63. Aaltonen LA, Peltomaki P, Leach FS, et al. Clues to the pathogenesis of familial colorectal cancer. *Science* 1993;260(5109):812–816.
64. Parsons R, Li GM, Longley MJ, et al. Hypermutability and mismatch repair deficiency in RER+ tumor cells. *Cell* 1993;75(6):1227–1236.
65. Leach FS, Nicolaides NC, Papadopoulos N, et al. Mutations of a mutS homolog in hereditary nonpolyposis colorectal cancer. *Cell* 1993;75(6):1215–1225.
66. Fishel R, Lescoe MK, Rao MR, et al. The human mutator gene homolog MSH2 and its association with hereditary nonpolyposis colon cancer. *Cell* 1993;75(5):1027–1038.
67. Papadopoulos N, Nicolaides NC, Wei YF, et al. Mutation of a mutL homolog in hereditary colon cancer. *Science* 1994;263(5153):1625–1629.
68. Bronner CE, Baker SM, Morrison PT, et al. Mutation in the DNA mismatch repair gene homologue hMLH1 is associated with hereditary nonpolyposis colon cancer. *Nature* 1994;368(6468):258–261.
69. Kolodner R. Biochemistry and genetics of eukaryotic mismatch repair. *Genes Dev* 1996;10(12):1433–1442.
70. Marsischky GT, Filosi N, Kane MF, et al. Redundancy of *Saccharomyces cerevisiae* MSH3 and MSH6 in MSH2-dependent mismatch repair. *Genes Dev* 1996;10(4):407–420.
71. Umar A, Risinger JI, Glaab WE, et al. Functional overlap in mismatch repair by human MSH3 and MSH6. *Genetics* 1998;148(4):1637–1646.
72. Hardcastle JD, Armitage NC, Chamberlain J, et al. Fecal occult blood screening for colorectal cancer in the general population. Results of a controlled trial. *Cancer* 1986;58(2):397–403.
73. Mandel JS, Church TR, Bond JH, et al. The effect of fecal occult-blood screening on the incidence of colorectal cancer. *N Engl J Med* 2000;343(22):1603–1607.
74. Gross CP, Andersen MS, Krumholz HM, et al. Relation between Medicare screening reimbursement and stage at diagnosis for older patients with colon cancer. *JAMA* 2006;296(23):2815–2822.
75. Baxter NN, Goldwasser MA, Paszat LF, et al. Association of colonoscopy and death from colorectal cancer. *Ann Intern Med* 2009;150(1):1–8.
76. Harewood GC, Lieberman DA. Colonoscopy practice patterns since introduction of medicare coverage for average-risk screening. *Clin Gastroenterol Hepatol* 2004;2(1):72–77.
77. Winawer SJ, Zauber AG, Ho MN, et al. Prevention of colorectal cancer by colonoscopic polypectomy. The National Polyp Study Workgroup. *N Engl J Med* 1993;329(27):1977–1981.
78. Vining D, Gelfand D, Bechtold R, et al. Technical feasibility of colon imaging with helical CT and virtual reality [Abstract]. *AJR Am J Roentgenol* 1994;162(suppl):104.
79. Fenlon HM, Nunes DP, Schroy PC III, et al. A comparison of virtual and conventional colonoscopy for the detection of colorectal polyps. *N Engl J Med* 1999;341(20):1496–1503.
80. Cotton PB, Durkalski VL, Pineau BC, et al. Computed tomographic colonography (virtual colonoscopy): a multicenter comparison with standard colonoscopy for detection of colorectal neoplasia. *JAMA* 2004;291(14):1713–1719.
81. Johnson CD, Chen MH, Toledano AY, et al. Accuracy of CT colonography for detection of large adenomas and cancers. *N Engl J Med* 2008;359(12):1207–1217.
82. Kim DH, Pickhardt PJ, Taylor AJ, et al. CT colonography versus colonoscopy for the detection of advanced neoplasia. *N Engl J Med* 2007;357(14):1403–1412.
83. Pickhardt PJ, Choi JR, Hwang I, et al. Computed tomographic virtual colonoscopy to screen for colorectal neoplasia in asymptomatic adults. *N Engl J Med* 2003;349(23):2191–2200.
84. Pineau BC, Paskett ED, Chen GJ, et al. Virtual colonoscopy using oral contrast compared with colonoscopy for the detection of patients with colorectal polyps. *Gastroenterology* 2003;125(2):304–310.
85. Iannaccone R, Laghi A, Catalano C, et al. Computed tomographic colonography without cathartic preparation for the detection of colorectal polyps. *Gastroenterology* 2004;127:1300–1311.
86. Ahlquist DA, Skoletsky JE, Boynton KA, et al. Colorectal cancer screening by detection of altered human DNA in stool: feasibility of a multitarget assay panel. *Gastroenterology* 2000;119(5):1219–1227.
87. Dong SM, Traverso G, Johnson C, et al. Detecting colorectal cancer in stool with the use of multiple genetic targets. *J Natl Cancer Inst* 2001;93(11):858–865.
88. Imperiale TF, Ransohoff DF, Itzkowitz SH, et al. Fecal DNA versus fecal occult blood for colorectal-cancer screening in an average-risk population. *N Engl J Med* 2004;351(26):2704–2714.
89. Song K, Fendrick AM, Ladabaum U. Fecal DNA testing compared with conventional colorectal cancer screening methods: a decision analysis. *Gastroenterology* 2004;126(5):1270–1279.
90. Zauber AG, Lansdorp-Vogelaar I, Wilschut J, et al. *Cost-Effectiveness of DNA Stool Testing to Screen for Colorectal Cancer: Report to AHRQ and CMS from the Cancer Intervention and Surveillance Modeling Network (CISNET) for MISCAN and SimCRC Models*. Rockville, MD: Agency for Health Care Quality and Research; 2007.
91. Pignone M, Saha S, Hoerger T, et al. Cost-effectiveness analyses of colorectal cancer screening: a systematic review for the U.S. Preventive Services Task Force. *Ann Intern Med* 2002;137(2):96–104.
92. Levin B, Lieberman DA, McFarland B, et al. Screening and surveillance for the early detection of colorectal cancer and adenomatous polyps, 2008: a joint guideline from the American Cancer Society, the US Multi-Society Task Force on Colorectal Cancer, and the American College of Radiology. *CA Cancer J Clin* 2008;58(3):130–160.
93. Lieberman DA, Weiss DG, Bond JH, et al. Use of colonoscopy to screen asymptomatic adults for colorectal cancer. Veterans Affairs Cooperative Study Group 380. *N Engl J Med* 2000;343(3):162–168.
94. Segnan N, Senore C, Andreoni B, et al; SCORE2 Working Group-Italy. Randomized trial of different screening strategies for colorectal cancer: patient response and detection rates. *J Natl Cancer Inst* 2005;97(5):347–357.
95. Morris AM. Medicare policy and colorectal cancer screening: will changing access change outcomes? *JAMA* 2006;296(23):2855–2856.
96. Dhruva SS, Phurrough SE, Salive ME, et al. CMS's landmark decision on CT colonography—examining the relevant data. *N Engl J Med* 2009;360(26):2699–2701.
97. Mandel JS, Bond JH, Church TR, et al. Reducing mortality from colorectal cancer by screening for fecal occult blood. Minnesota Colon Cancer Control Study. *N Engl J Med* 1993;328(19):1365–1371.
98. Hardcastle JD, Chamberlain JO, Robinson MH, et al. Randomised controlled trial of faecal-occult-blood screening for colorectal cancer. *Lancet* 1996;348(9040):1472–1477.
99. Kronborg O, Fenger C, Olsen J, et al. Randomised study of screening for colorectal cancer with faecal-occult-blood test. *Lancet* 1996;348(9040):1467–1471.
100. Kewenter J, Brevinge H, Engaras B, et al. Results of screening, rescreening, and follow-up in a prospective randomized study for detection of colorectal cancer by fecal occult blood testing. Results for 68,308 subjects. *Scand J Gastroenterol* 1994;29(5):468–473.
101. Young G, St John J, Winawer S, et al. Choice of fecal occult blood tests for colorectal cancer screening: recommendations based on performance characteristics in population studies. A WHO and OMED Report. *Am J Gastroenterol* 2002;97:2499–2507.
102. Centers for Disease Control and Prevention (CDC). Use of colorectal cancer tests—United States, 2002, 2004, and 2006. *MMWR Morb Mortal Wkly Rep* 2008;57:253–258.
103. Winawer SJ, Zauber AG, Fletcher RH, et al. Guidelines for colonoscopy surveillance after polypectomy: a consensus update by the US Multi-Society Task Force on Colorectal Cancer and the American Cancer Society. *CA Cancer J Clin* 2006;56(3):143–159; quiz 184–185.
104. Rex DK, Kahi CJ, Levin B, et al. Guidelines for colonoscopy surveillance after cancer resection: a consensus update by the American Cancer Society and US Multi-Society Task Force on Colorectal Cancer. *CA Cancer J Clin* 2006;56(3):160–167; quiz 185–186.
105. Greene F, Page D, Fleming I, eds. *AJCC Cancer Staging Manual,* 6th ed. New York, NY: Springer; 2002.
106. O'Connell J, Maggard M, Ko C. Colon cancer survival rates with the new American Joint Committee on Cancer sixth edition staging. *J Natl Cancer Inst* 2004;96(19):1420–1425.
107. Benson Ar, Schrag D, Somerfield M, et al. American Society of Clinical Oncology recommendations on adjuvant chemotherapy for stage II colon cancer. *J Clin Oncol* 2004;22(16):3408–3419.
108. Chang GJ, Rodriguez-Bigas MA, Skibber JM, et al. Lymph node evaluation and survival after curative resection of colon cancer: systematic review. *J Natl Cancer Inst* 2007;99(6):433–441.
109. Wong SL, Ji H, Hollenbeck BK, et al. Hospital lymph node examination rates and survival after resection for colon cancer. *JAMA* 2007;298(18):2149–2154.
110. Wang J, Kulaylat M, Rockette H, et al. Should total number of lymph nodes be used as a quality of care measure for stage III colon cancer? *Ann Surg* 2009;249(4):559–563.
111. August DA, Ottow RT, Sugarbaker PH. Clinical perspective of human colorectal cancer metastasis. *Cancer Metastasis Rev* 1984;3(4):303–324.
112. Haggitt RC, Glotzbach RE, Soffer EE, et al. Prognostic factors in colorectal carcinomas arising in adenomas: implications for lesions removed by endoscopic polypectomy. *Gastroenterology* 1985;89(2):328–336.
113. Williams CB, Saunders BP, Talbot IC. Endoscopic management of polypoid early colon cancer. *World J Surg* 2000;24(9):1047–1051.
114. Whitlow C, Gathright JB Jr, Hebert SJ, et al. Long-term survival after treatment of malignant colonic polyps. *Dis Colon Rectum* 1997;40(8):929–934.
115. Seitz U, Bohnacker S, Seewald S, et al. Is endoscopic polypectomy an adequate therapy for malignant colorectal adenomas? Presentation of 114 patients and review of the literature. *Dis Colon Rectum* 2004;47(11):1789—1796; discussion 1796–1787.
116. Statistics for 2004. website http://www.cancer.org. Accessed January, 2005.
117. Bonjer HJ, Hop WC, Nelson H, et al. Laparoscopically assisted vs open colectomy for colon cancer: a meta-analysis. *Arch Surg* 2007;142(3):298–303.
118. Bilimoria KY, Bentrem DJ, Nelson H, et al. Use and outcomes of laparoscopic-assisted colectomy for cancer in the United States. *Arch Surg* 2008;143(9):832–839; discussion 839–840.
119. Yeatman TJ, Bland KI. Sphincter-saving procedures for distal carcinoma of the rectum. *Ann Surg* 1989;209(1):1–18.
120. Heald RJ, Ryall RD. Recurrence and survival after total mesorectal excision for rectal cancer. *Lancet* 1986;1(8496):1479–1482.
121. Bulow S, Christensen IJ, Harling H, et al. Recurrence and survival after mesorectal excision for rectal cancer. *Br J Surg* 2003;90(8):974–980.
122. Heald RJ, Moran BJ, Ryall RD, et al. Rectal cancer: the Basingstoke experience of total mesorectal excision, 1978–1997. *Arch Surg* 1998;133(8):894–899.
123. Wibe A, Moller B, Norstein J, et al. A national strategic change in treatment policy for rectal cancer—implementation of total mesorectal excision as routine treatment in Norway. A national audit. *Dis Colon Rectum* 2002;45(7):857–866.

124. Martling A, Holm T, Rutqvist LE, et al. Impact of a surgical training programme on rectal cancer outcomes in Stockholm. *Br J Surg* 2005;92(2):225–229.
125. Steele GD Jr, Herndon JE, Bleday R, et al. Sphincter-sparing treatment for distal rectal adenocarcinoma. *Ann Surg Oncol* 1999;6(5):433–441.
126. Mellgren A, Sirivongs P, Rothenberger DA, et al. Is local excision adequate therapy for early rectal cancer? *Dis Colon Rectum* 2000;43(8):1064–1071; discussion 1071–1064.
127. Ota DM, Nelson H. Local excision of rectal cancer revisited: ACOSOG protocol Z6041. *Ann Surg Oncol* 2007;14(2):271.
128. Madden JL, Kandalaft SI. Electrocoagulation as a primary curative method in the treatment of carcinoma of the rectum. *Surg Gynecol Obstet* 1983;157(2):164–179.
129. Colorectal Cancer Collaborative Group. Adjuvant radiotherapy for rectal cancer: a systematic overview of 8,507 patients from 22 randomised trials. *Lancet* 2001;358(9290):1291–1304.
130. Improved survival with preoperative radiotherapy in resectable rectal cancer. Swedish Rectal Cancer Trial. *N Engl J Med* 1997;336(14):980–987.
131. Sauer R, Becker H, Hohenberger W, et al. Preoperative versus postoperative chemoradiotherapy for rectal cancer. *N Engl J Med* 2004;351(17):1731–1740.
132. Benson AB III, Schrag D, Somerfield MR, et al. American Society of Clinical Oncology recommendations on adjuvant chemotherapy for stage II colon cancer. *J Clin Oncol* 2004;22(16):3408–3419.
133. Tol J, Koopman M, Cats A, et al. Chemotherapy, bevacizumab, and cetuximab in metastatic colorectal cancer. *N Engl J Med* 2009;360(6):563–572.
134. Goldberg RM, Carrato A. Accomplishments in 2007 in the treatment of advanced colorectal cancer. *Gastrointest Cancer Res* 2008;2(3 suppl):S19–S24.
135. Resection of the liver for colorectal carcinoma metastases: a multi-institutional study of indications for resection. Registry of Hepatic Metastases. *Surgery* 1988;103(3):278–288.
136. Kern KA, Pass HI, Roth JA. Surgical treatment of pulmonary metastases. In: Rosenberg SA, ed. *Surgical Treatment of Metastatic Cancer*, Vol 69. Philadelphia: JB Lippincott; 1987.
137. Maggard MA, O'Connell JB, Ko CY. Updated population-based review of carcinoid tumors. *Ann Surg* 2004;240(1):117–122.
138. Landry CS, Brock G, Scoggins CR, et al. Proposed staging system for colon carcinoid tumors based on an analysis of 2,459 patients. *J Am Coll Surg* 2008;207(6):874–881.
139. Stinner B, Kisker O, Zielke A, et al. Surgical management for carcinoid tumors of small bowel, appendix, colon, and rectum. *World J Surg* 1996;20(2):183–188.

CHAPTER 69 ■ DIVERTICULAR DISEASE

LAUREN KOSINSKI, KIRK LUDWIG, AND MARY OTTERSON

KEY POINTS

1. Diverticulosis and its complications are common in Western societies.
2. Sigmoid and left colon involvement predominate in non-Asian industrialized nations; the rectum is spared.
3. Lack of dietary fiber, colonic anatomy, and disordered colonic motility are likely contributors to the development of diverticulosis.
4. Computed tomography imaging markedly improves diagnostic accuracy and treatment planning.
5. Early, judicious use of contrast enema studies or colonoscopy can safely help distinguish diverticular stricture from cancer.
6. Antibiotic therapy, bowel rest, and percutaneous drainage of diverticular abscesses can often convert surgical emergencies into elective operations.
7. Bowel resection with primary anastomosis and temporary, diverting loop stoma is favored in acute cases when possible; single-stage operations are preferred for elective cases.

Diverticular disease is one of the most common problems treated by surgeons, and management strategies have evolved significantly in the last 10 years. A short time ago, virtually all cases of acute diverticulitis were treated as surgical emergencies. Patients routinely underwent staged procedures and were taken to the operating room for sigmoid colectomy and temporary end-colostomy within hours of admission. Surgical and radiologic innovations have introduced less invasive options for managing even complex disease. Surgery, when necessary, is often performed electively or semielectively.

Key among recent major shifts in the diagnosis and management of diverticular disease are (a) strategies for converting diverticular surgical emergencies into single-stage, elective operations with avoidance of a colostomy; (b) utilization of computed tomography (CT) imaging for diagnosis and CT-guided percutaneous drainage of diverticular abscesses; (c) reconsideration of indications for elective surgery; and (d) emergence of laparoscopic surgical techniques as state-of-the-art approaches for diverticular disease.

CLASSIFICATION

1 Diverticulosis refers to the presence, whether symptomatic or asymptomatic, of colonic diverticula. In common medical usage, this refers to the presence of pseudodiverticula, a very common acquired condition in Western societies, in which mucosa and submucosa have herniated through the circular layer of the muscularis propria. True diverticula are rare. Diverticular disease refers to the broad range of symptoms and findings associated with diverticulosis and includes diverticulitis, an inflammatory process. Inflammation can be acute or chronic. Acute inflammation can present with a pericolonic phlegmon, colon perforation leading to focal abscess formation, or generalized purulent or fecal peritonitis. Acute and chronic inflammation can cause fistulas between the involved bowel segment and the bladder, vagina, or skin. With chronic inflammation, a colonic stricture can develop, resulting in altered bowel habit or even obstruction.

Anatomy

Colonic diverticula are pulsion diverticula that occur in predictable sites on the bowel wall. Likewise, the pattern of segmental involvement of the colon and its progression are pre-
2 dictable. The sigmoid colon is at highest risk and is affected in 95% of patients. Involvement is isolated to the sigmoid colon in 30% to 60% of cases. Total colonic involvement occurs in 7% to 10% of cases.[1] The rectum is almost always spared. This segmental pattern of involvement is not observed in Asia, where 70% of pseudodiverticula are isolated to the right colon and cecum. The reason for this discrepancy is not known. Right colon pseudodiverticula are more likely to be solitary and tend to originate near the ileocecal valve.[2–4] When true colonic diverticula develop, they

TABLE 69.1

INCIDENCE OF DIVERTICULOSIS IN WESTERN SOCIETY

■ AGE	■ ≤25 y	■ ≤45 y	■ >60 y	■ >80 y
INCIDENCE	1%–2%	33%	40%	60%

are also more likely to be right sided; however, they are still much less common than pseudodiverticula of the right colon.

INCIDENCE

Diverticulosis is rare in nonindustrialized, less affluent societies. The French surgeon Alexis Littre is credited with first describing diverticulosis in 1700, but it wasn't until the mid-1800s that there were reports in the medical literature about the disease process and its treatment.[5] The prevalence of diverticulosis increased after the industrial revolution and through this century. Even before 1940, it was recognized infrequently; retrospective reviews of colon radiographs and pathologic specimens record an incidence of 5% to 10%.[6] An incidence of 46% in people 51 years of age and older was reported by Hughes from postmortem studies in 200 cadavers (Table 69.1).[7] Incidence as a function of gender varies by study, some studies citing an increased incidence among men and others finding a higher incidence among women. It may be that the spectrum of complications and the age at which they develop are gender specific. The majority of people with diverticulosis remain asymptomatic; only 15% to 30% will go on to develop symptomatic disease.[8] Of these, only 30% will require operative treatment.[9] In the United States in 1998, 2.2 million cases of diverticular disease were treated at an estimated cost of $2 billion.[10]

ETIOLOGY

3 Neither the etiology of diverticulosis nor factors causing progression to symptomatic disease have been rigorously defined, but lack of dietary fiber, colonic dysmotility, and colonic structural abnormalities and age-related changes have all been implicated.

Structural/Anatomic Factors

In the colon, the outer, longitudinal layer of the muscularis propria is condensed in three longitudinal bands called the taeniae coli. One of these runs along the mesenteric aspect of the colon; the other two are antimesenteric in location (Fig. 69.1). Mesenteric blood vessels encircle the colon and penetrate the circular muscle in the intertaenial areas between the mesenteric taenia and the two antimesenteric taeniae. Pseudodiverticula develop at areas where these vessels pass through muscle.[11] Postmortem studies of the colon wall showed thinning of the circular muscle associated with early diverticula. Gaps in the circular muscle were observed with larger diverticula.[7]

In contrast to typical pseudodiverticula, giant colonic diverticula almost always arise from the antimesenteric border of the colon. They are assumed to be a complication of ordinary colonic diverticulosis, possibly developing after inflammatory narrowing of the neck of a pseudodiverticulum causes a ball-valve mechanism that entraps gas in the diverticulum, causing it to enlarge[12] (Fig. 69.2).

The observation of colonic diverticula in young patients with connective tissue disorders such as Marfan disease and Ehlers-Danlos syndrome raises the question of whether connective tissue genetic derangements play a role in diverticulosis development.[13,14] Ordinary senescent connective tissue

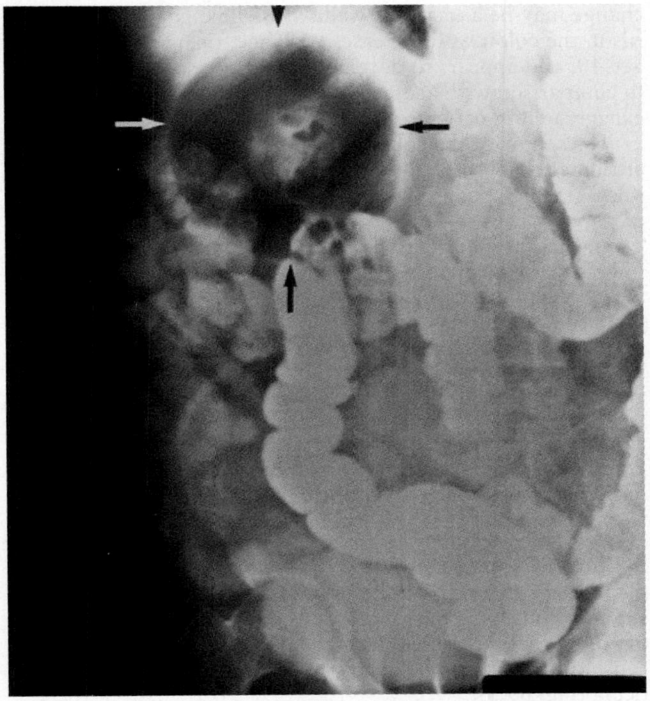

FIGURE 69.2. Postevacuation film of barium enema, demonstrating a giant colonic diverticulum (*arrows*) partially filled with barium. (Reproduced with permission from McNutt R, Schmitt D, Schulte W. Giant colonic diverticula. *Dis Colon* 1988;31:625.)

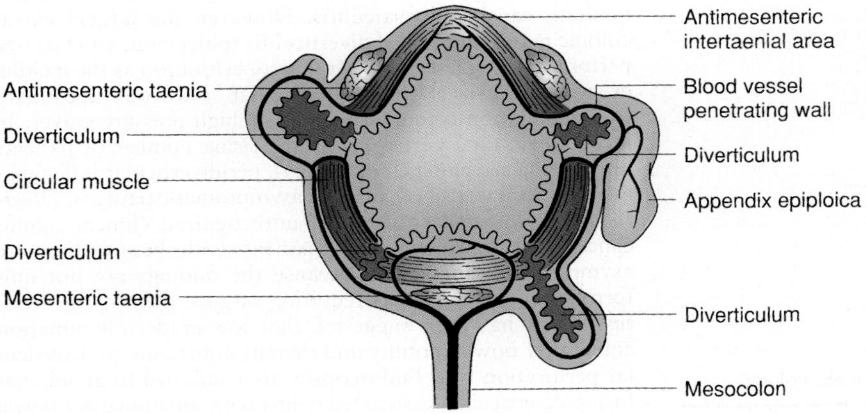

FIGURE 69.1. Cross section of the colon illustrating the relation of diverticula to the blood vessels penetrating the circular muscle layer, the taeniae, and the appendices epiploicae.

COLORECTAL

change may be a factor as well. Cross-linkage of collagen fibrils in the colon wall increases with age, rising markedly after age 40, and appears to decrease compliance of the colon wall. In comparison with age-matched controls, this cross-linkage is exaggerated in patients with diverticulosis.[15]

Thickening of the colon wall in diverticulosis was originally attributed to muscle hypertrophy.[11,16] This was disproven by histologic studies, but increased elastin deposition in the taeniae coli of patients with uncomplicated diverticulosis has been shown. The taeniae are shortened as a result, causing the circular muscle to be accordioned in the two intertaenial zones, the same areas where pseudodiverticula more commonly form.[17] The functional significance of this is not known, but it has been speculated that muscle contractions may be stronger in these areas.

Motility Factors

Four unusual colonic motility patterns have been observed in the setting of diverticulosis: segmentation, high-pressure waves, slow wave motility pattern, and disorganized propulsive activity.

Segmentation. Painter et al. used cineradiography and manometry to study colonic motility and reported that when simultaneous haustral contractions occur in the same segment of colon, high pressure is generated in the intervening bowel, causing ballooning of the colon wall and distention of diverticula (Fig. 69.3).[18]

High-pressure Waves. High-pressure waves are independent of normal peristalsis and have an amplitude of 10 mm Hg in normal patients but have higher amplitude (up to 90 mm Hg) and longer duration in patients with diverticulosis.[19]

Slow Wave Motility Pattern. The normal slow wave pattern in the colon is altered in diverticular disease.[20,21]

Disorganized Propulsive Activity. High-amplitude propulsive contractions occurred more frequently and were more likely to be disorganized in patients with diverticular disease than normal subjects. Retropulsive contractions occurred more frequently in segments of colon with diverticulosis.[22]

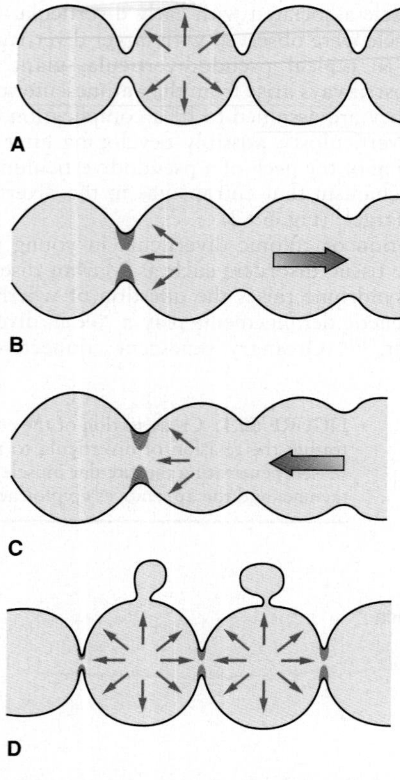

FIGURE 69.3. The role of segmentation in colonic physiology.

Other Factors

Other neurologic and chemical mediators of colonic motility may play a role in pseudodiverticula genesis. Vasoactive intestinal peptide levels are increased in the bowel wall of patients with diverticulosis.[23] Age-related vagal attrition has been postulated to contribute to colonic smooth muscle dysmotility.[24] Alterations of serotonin expression and function are noted after resolution of acute diverticulitis and may contribute to lasting symptoms.[25]

Diet

Decreased dietary fiber is the most consistent factor associated with the high incidence of diverticulosis in Western populations. Painter and Burkitt first elucidated this connection after noting the striking disparity in incidence between British society and sub-Saharan populations. They measured colon transit time and stool weights in over 1,000 individuals in the United Kingdom and sub-Saharan Africa. The rise in incidence of diverticular disease coincident with the rise in refined food products in diets in the West was also noted.[26] Painter and Burkitt also reported improvement of diverticular disease symptoms in patients who increased dietary fiber and recrudescence of symptoms once fiber intake decreased again.[27] There is now a rising incidence of diverticulosis among previously low-risk populations in concert with changes to a Western-style diet as a consequence of economic development or immigration. Japanese immigrants to the United States acquire diverticulosis risk comparable to other Westerners, although the right-sided predominance of diverticulosis seen among Asians persists.[5,28] The exact protective mechanism of stool bulk is not understood.

While the focus on dietary fiber has emphasized insoluble fiber, soluble fiber may also be relevant. Soluble fiber is processed by intestinal flora, which may in turn affect diverticulosis.[28,29] Finally, despite the long-held admonition to avoid eating nuts and seeds, there is no evidence to support this recommendation.[30]

Pathogenesis of Diverticulitis

The process by which a subset of people with diverticulosis develop diverticulitis has yet to be explained. Overwhelming inflammatory changes that develop with perforation or other complications of diverticulitis likely obscure subtle histologic details that might explain the pathogenesis of the disease. Traditionally, it has been postulated that mechanical obstruction by food or fecal material of a diverticulum leads to bacterial proliferation, gas, and toxin production in the occluded diverticulum, causing diverticulitis. However, the largely extracolonic manifestations of diverticulitis (phlegmon, abscess, free perforation) suggest micro- or macroperforation as the inciting event, possibly as a kind of diverticular "blow-out" secondary to segmentation-type contractions or high-pressure waves. In recent years (and perhaps with the rising number of patients undergoing screening colonoscopy), peridiverticular inflammation has been identified, often in asymptomatic patients. *Diverticulitis-associated colitis* is of unrecognized clinical significance, partly because so many patients with these findings are asymptomatic and partly because the findings are not uniformly evident in patients requiring surgical therapy for diverticulitis. It has been suggested that low-grade inflammation could alter bowel motility and thereby contribute to diverticular perforation risk. Endoscopists are cautioned to avoid confusing diverticulitis-associated colitis with inflammatory bowel disease. Probiotics and nonsteroidal anti-inflammatory medications are being explored as potentially protective agents.[28,31,32]

DIAGNOSIS

Noninflammatory Diverticular Disease

Most patients with diverticulosis noted on barium study, colonoscopy, or abdominal CT scan are asymptomatic. In patients who have vague, crampy, left lower quadrant pain in the absence of fever, leukocytosis, or CT findings of focal inflammation, other causes of pain must also be considered. Additional symptoms reported may include nausea, flatulence, bloating, and change of bowel habit. The differential diagnosis includes colonic adenocarcinoma, constipation, inflammatory bowel disease, and irritable bowel syndrome. There are no peritoneal signs on examination, the rectal examination is unrevealing, and proctoscopy shows no inflammation. Postinflammatory neurogenic alteration has been postulated as a cause of visceral hypersensitivity.[33–35] Nonspecific, mild mucosal inflammation and muscle spasm may also contribute. There is considerable overlap with irritable bowel syndrome. In addition to high-fiber modification of the diet and bulk-forming agents such as psyllium or flaxseed, anticholinergics, analgesics, and antibiotics can be prescribed to manage symptoms.

Hemorrhagic Diverticular Disease. Like bleeding from colonic angiodysplasia, diverticular hemorrhage is classically asymptomatic until presentation with lower gastrointestinal hemorrhage that can be massive. This differs from hemorrhage from inflammatory bowel disease or ischemic colitis where there are typically symptoms before bleeding begins. A foregut source of bleeding must be excluded by nasoenteric recovery of bilious, nonbloody aspirate or upper endoscopy. Likewise, an anorectal source of bleeding must be excluded by examination. Localization of lower gastrointestinal hemorrhage of any cause is necessary to help guide appropriate colon resection should that be required. Although most cases of diverticular hemorrhage are self-limited, recurrence or failure of bleeding to stop spontaneously determines the need for resection. Colonoscopy, tagged red blood cell scan, or, if bleeding is brisk enough, angiography is used to localize bleeding (Fig. 69.4).

Giant Colonic Diverticula. Symptoms and signs of giant colonic diverticula may be noninflammatory (pain, bloating, nausea, vomiting, diarrhea, abdominal tenderness and mass) or inflammatory, resulting from perforation (pain, leukocytosis, fever, localized or generalized peritonitis).[12]

Inflammatory Diverticular Disease

The constellation of inflammatory signs and symptoms corresponds to the spectrum of inflammatory complications of diverticular disease. The Hinchey classification[36] categorized the severity of acute diverticulitis and has been modified to reflect refinements of diagnosis enabled by improved CT scan quality (Table 69.2).[37] The modified classification also includes manifestations of chronic inflammation such as fistula formation and stricture/obstruction.

Symptoms of acute diverticulitis include steady, left lower quadrant abdominal pain; fever; change in bowel habits (constipation or diarrhea); anorexia; nausea; vomiting; bloating; and urinary tract symptoms such as urinary frequency or retention. Examination will reveal left lower quadrant tenderness that may be appreciable only with deep palpation in stage 0 inflammation. In stage I or II inflammation, focal peritoneal

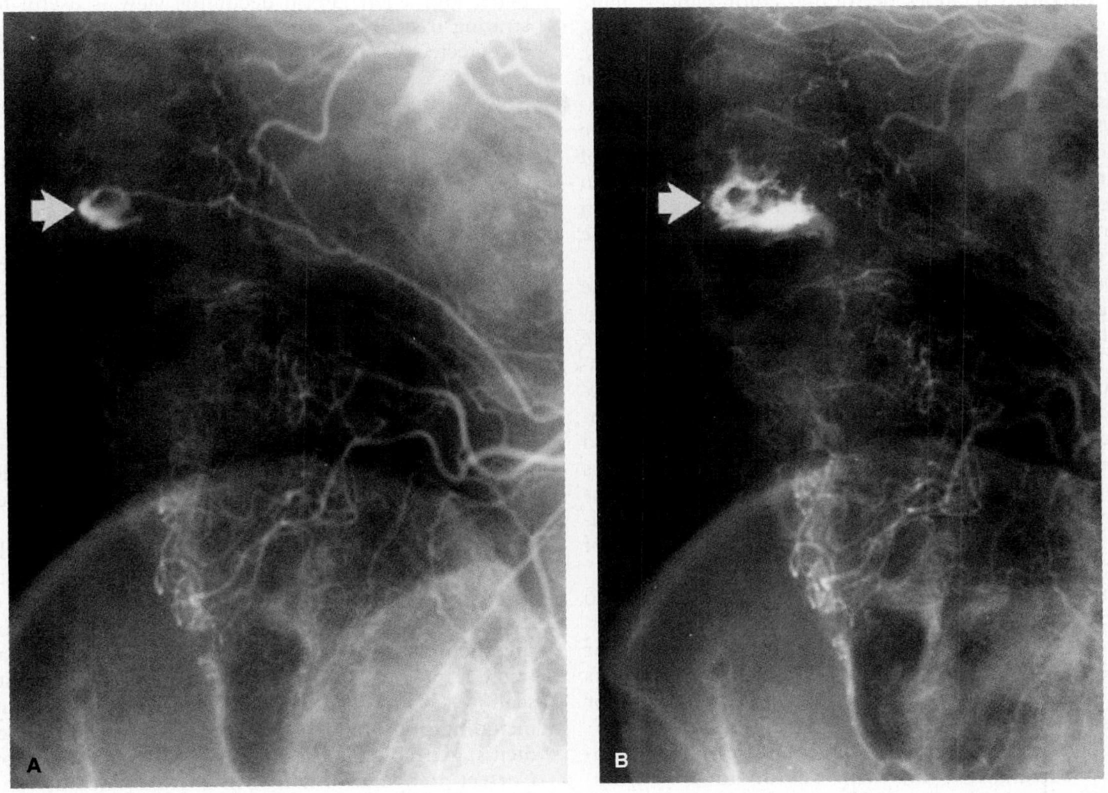

FIGURE 69.4. Superior mesenteric arteriogram from a patient with bleeding from a right colon diverticulum. **A:** Early radiograph with contrast material outlining the diverticulum (*arrow*). **B:** Late radiograph demonstrating overflow of contrast material into the colonic lumen.

COLORECTAL

TABLE 69.2 **CLASSIFICATION**

MODIFIED HINCHEY CLASSIFICATION

■ HINCHEY CLASSIFICATION	■ MODIFIED HINCHEY CLASSIFICATION	■ COMMENTS
	0 Mild clinical diverticulitis	Left lower quadrant pain, elevated white blood cells, fever, no confirmation by imaging or surgery
I Pericolic abscess or phlegmon	Ia Confined pericolic inflammation—phlegmon	
II Pelvic, intra-abdominal, or retroperitoneal abscess	II Pelvic, distant intra-abdominal, or retroperitoneal abscess	
III Generalized purulent peritonitis	III Generalized purulent peritonitis	No open communication with bowel lumen
IV Generalized fecal peritonitis	IV Fecal peritonitis Fistula colovesical/colovaginal/coloenteric/colocutaneous	Free perforation, open communication with bowel lumen
Obstruction	Large- and/or small-bowel obstruction	

signs in the left lower quadrant are likely, and there may be a tender mass. Digital rectal examination may also reveal pelvic tenderness or a tender mass in the cul-de-sac. Generalized peritoneal signs would be expected for stage III or IV inflammation. Dehydration with earlier stages or evolving sepsis with later stages may cause tachycardia and hypotension. Leukocytosis is more likely with advancing stage of inflammation. The differential diagnosis includes perforated colon cancer, acute appendicitis, perforated peptic ulcer, acute ischemic colitis, pancreatitis, and flare of Crohn disease or ulcerative colitis. Normal serum amylase and lipase help exclude a diagnosis of pancreatitis. Imaging studies and endoscopy help to distinguish diverticulitis from the other diagnoses. However, active inflammation or contained perforation may limit the utility of rectal contrast CT, barium enema studies, and endoscopy in the acute setting. Distinguishing perforated colon cancer from diverticular disease can be especially challenging, even in the operating room.

Diverticular fistula formation represents internal drainage of an abscess (or external drainage in the case of colocutaneous fistulas). Approximately half of diverticular fistulas are colovesical fistulas. Women with colovesical or colovaginal fistulas have usually had a hysterectomy.[38,39] Urinary tract infection symptoms, pneumaturia, and fecaluria are common complaints. Recurrent urinary tract infection in elderly men should raise concern for the presence of a colovesical fistula, which is often secondary to diverticular disease. Passage of feces or flatus from the vagina is a characteristic symptom of a colovaginal fistula. Colocutaneous fistulas are a rare complication of diverticular disease.

Thirteen percent of large-bowel obstructions are due to diverticular disease. The concurrent incidence of colon carcinoma in 7% of patients with symptomatic sigmoid diverticular disease confounds diagnosis and treatment.[40] CT scan is not as reliable for distinguishing these diagnoses as colonoscopy or contrast enema studies.

Right-sided diverticulitis frequently is confused with appendicitis, and misdiagnosis is common. The duration of symptoms is usually longer than appendicitis. Patients are usually older than those with appendicitis (late 30s or 40s) but younger than patients with typical left-sided diverticulosis (over 50 years of age).[41,42]

Imaging and Diagnostic Studies for Diverticular Disease

Plain Radiographs. While seldom useful in the diagnosis of uncomplicated diverticulitis, a three-way abdominal series that includes an upright chest radiograph, an abdominal flat plate, and a left lateral decubitus view is useful for demonstrating free air. An ileus pattern or soft tissue mass may also be detected.[43,44]

4 **Computed Tomography Scan.** CT scanning has revolutionized the diagnosis of acute diverticulitis and, sometimes, by way of percutaneous abscess drainage, its treatment. The accuracy of CT scans in the acute setting is central to the trend toward converting what formerly were surgical emergencies into elective, often single-stage operations. Intravenous and water-soluble oral and rectal enteric contrast should be administered. Water-soluble contrast is used to avoid barium peritonitis that may result if barium leaks from a perforated diverticulum into the peritoneal cavity.

A CT scan can reveal the presence and extent of diverticulosis, but its real strength is characterizing extracolonic inflammatory change. Signs of inflammation include colon wall thickening, pericolic fat stranding, or phlegmon formation. Pericolic abscess size and location can be detected (Fig. 69.5). Perforation is evidenced by free air; contained perforation may be identified by loculated extraluminal pericolic air. CT more accurately demonstrates diverticular abscesses and severity of inflammation than contrast enema studies.[45] Air in the bladder or contrast in the vagina may indicate the presence of a fistula (Fig. 69.6).

Rao et al. reported a misdiagnosis rate of up to 67% for diverticulitis in patients with abdominal pain managed without CT imaging.[46] An alternate diagnosis is suggested by CT scan in 45% to 58% of cases when diverticulitis is not found, including small-bowel obstruction, acute cholecystitis, appendicitis, gynecologic disease, and primary epiploic appengitis.[47] Correct preoperative diagnosis of right-sided diverticulitis has also been enhanced by CT scanning.

Not only is CT useful for improving diagnostic accuracy, but also findings can predict failure of medical management or risk of secondary complications following medical management.

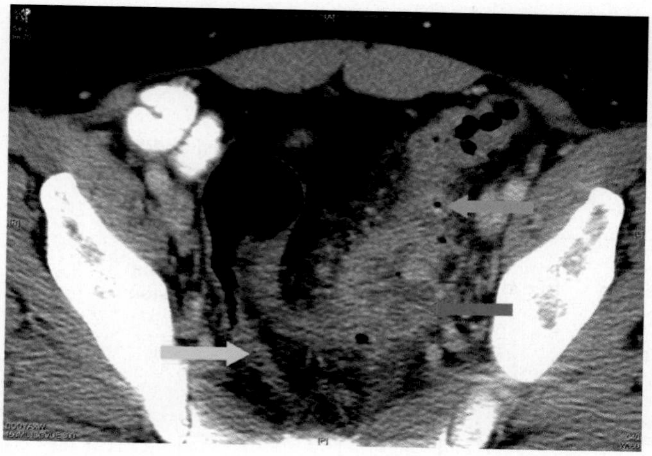

FIGURE 69.5. Sigmoid diverticulitis with pericolic abscess.

Ambrosetti et al. reported on 423 patients with acute diverticulitis on CT scan, categorizing them as having either moderate disease or severe disease. Criteria for moderate disease included localized wall thickening or inflammation of pericolic fat (modified Hinchey stage Ia; see Table 69.2). Severe disease included the presence of extraluminal air or contrast (contained perforation) or abscess (modified Hinchey stages Ib and II). Of the 42 patients who failed nonoperative management, 32 had severe disease. Twenty percent of those patients who were initially successfully managed nonoperatively developed secondary complications such as fistulas (median follow-up 46 months). They concluded that the presence of severe disease at the index episode predicted failure of nonoperative management and that there is a high risk of secondary complications after initial nonoperative management.[48]

Ultrasound. Abdominal ultrasound has been emphasized in the European literature and is attractive as a strategy for limiting radiation exposure. However, its diagnostic limitations (user dependence, interference from overlying bowel gas, and decreased accuracy in obese patients) have precluded its widespread adoption in the United States. In skilled hands, it may have a role in image-guided percutaneous drainage of abscesses.[49]

Contrast Enema Study (Barium Enema). Contrast enemas have been the "gold standard" test for the presence and anatomic distribution of diverticula (Fig. 69.7). For reasons cited earlier, CT scan has supplanted contrast enemas in the

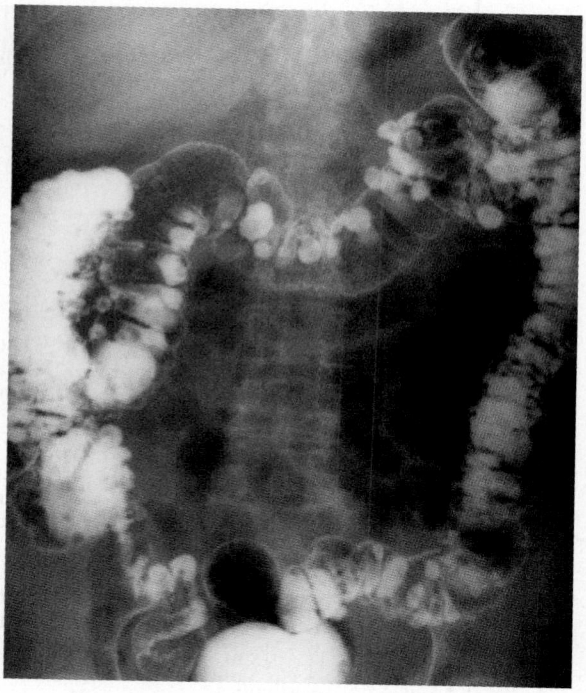

FIGURE 69.7. Barium enema showing multiple diverticula of the colon.

5 acute setting. However, they are better than CT for helping distinguish colon cancer from diverticular obstruction, and contrast can also traverse narrowed areas of the colon impassable by an endoscope. While caution must be used in the acute setting to avoid perforation, these studies can be performed safely. Caveats are that contrast must be administered gently, water-soluble contrast should be used, and a single contrast study is performed in unprepared bowel to avoid the increased risk of perforation and fecal contamination with the administration of air. In chronic diverticular disease, the contrast enema can demonstrate stricture, angulation, and segmentation-type contractions. It can also be useful for the evaluation of fistulas.

Endoscopy. Like contrast enema studies, colonoscopy or flexible sigmoidoscopy can be used judiciously in the acute setting. It is particularly helpful in distinguishing malignancy from diverticular disease and can therefore help guide early management of acute presentations when malignancy as the cause of symptoms is being considered.

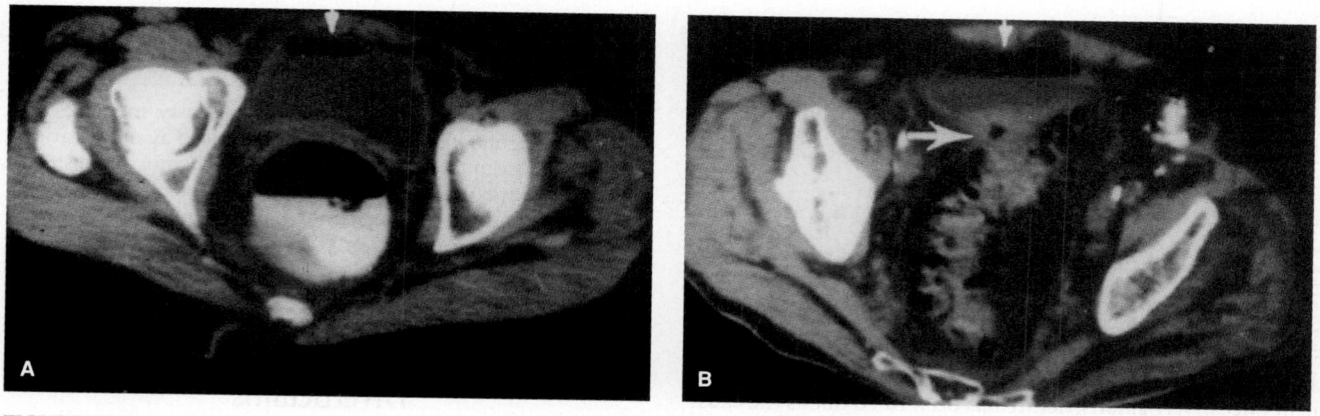

FIGURE 69.6. **A:** Computed tomography scan demonstrating air in the urinary bladder (*arrow*) in the presence of a colovesical fistula secondary to diverticulitis. **B:** Air in the urinary bladder (*small arrow*) in association with a paravesical inflammatory mass (*large arrow*). (Reproduced with permission from Sarr MG, Fishman EK, Goldman SM. Enterovesical fistula. *Surg Gynecol Obstet* 1987;164:2.)

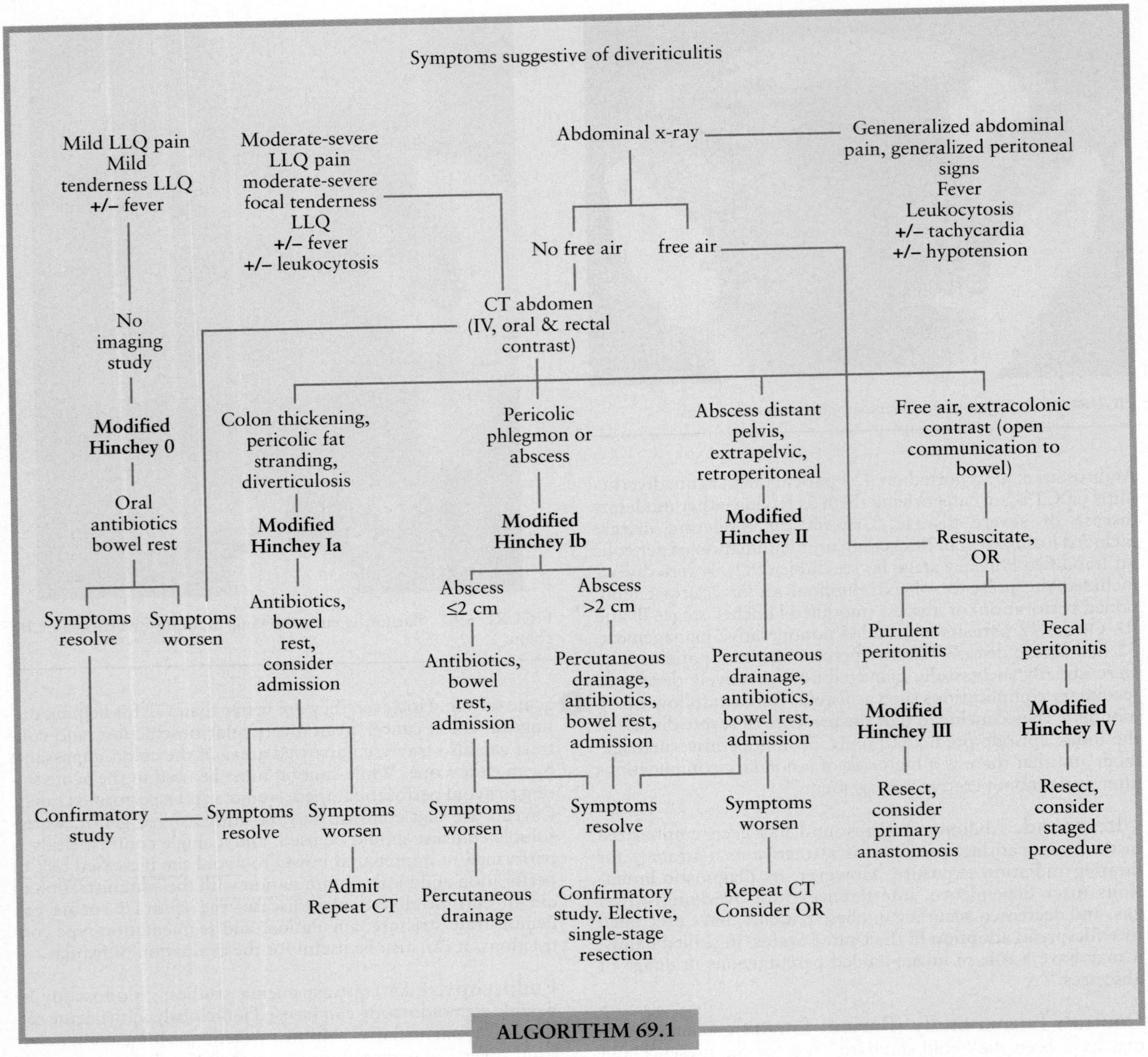

ALGORITHM 69.1.

Cystoscopy. Cystoscopy can help diagnose colovesical fistulas. Although the fistula tract is usually difficult to see, focal hyperemia and inflammation may be noted. Symptoms of a colovesical fistula and air in the uninstrumented bladder on CT scan are usually sufficient for diagnosis.

TREATMENT

Symptomatic Diverticulosis

Fiber supplements and increased dietary fiber (goal 25 to 30 g/d) constitute the cornerstone of symptomatic diverticulosis treatment once diverticular stricture has been ruled out as the cause of symptoms. Stricture is an indication for elective segmental colectomy, typically a sigmoid colectomy to remove the area of stricture and the most dense region of diverticula.

Hemorrhagic Diverticular Disease

Diverticular hemorrhage stops spontaneously in more than 90% of patients; of these, 75% will not bleed again.[50] Patients who have a second episode of diverticular hemorrhage should undergo hemicolectomy of the involved portion of colon[51] after localizing the site of hemorrhage endoscopically with a tagged red blood cell scan or with angiography, because these patients are likely to bleed again. If the site of bleeding cannot be determined definitively as left or right sided, a subtotal colectomy is the procedure of choice.[52]

Diverticulitis

The treatment of diverticulitis typically parallels the Hinchey classification[36]:

- **Stage I,** *confined pericolic abscess*: antibiotics and bowel rest
- **Stage II,** *pelvic or retroperitoneal abscess*: percutaneous abscess drainage
- **Stage III,** *purulent peritonitis*: resuscitation and urgent operation
- **Stage IV,** *feculent peritonitis*: resuscitation and urgent operation

Stage I diverticulitis is mild when patients can tolerate a diet, have no systemic symptoms (no fever, tachycardia, hypotension), and have no substantial peritoneal signs. The CT scan shows either minor pericolic fat stranding or wall thickening in the presence of diverticulosis. Outpatient management is usually appropriate for these patients. Broad-spectrum oral antibiotics are prescribed for 7 to 10 days, and patients start a clear liquid diet, advancing to a solid diet as symptoms resolve. If this is a first episode of presumed diverticulitis, an elective confirmatory study with either barium enema or colonoscopy is planned after inflammation has subsided. Progression of symptoms on this regimen warrants hospital admission and repeat CT scan may be necessary. The vast majority (70% to 100%) of patients with uncomplicated diverticulitis will recover without operative intervention. Although nearly a third will relapse, long-term fiber supplementation appears to reduce this risk.[1]

6 Severe stage I inflammation is indicated by intolerance of diet, possible nausea and vomiting, fever, chills, and peritoneal signs on examination, which are often focal. The CT scan may show a phlegmon or contained pericolic abscess. These patients are admitted to the hospital for parenteral broad-spectrum antibiotics. They are placed on bowel rest, intravenous fluids are administered, and if nausea and vomiting are major symptoms, a nasogastric tube may be placed. Analgesia is provided but limited to enable evaluation of symptom progression. In addition, since narcotics are known to cause strong, nonpropulsive sigmoid colon contractions, their use in patients with diverticulitis should be minimized. Small (<2 cm) pericolic abscesses may resolve with intravenous antibiotics; larger contained abscesses will likely require percutaneous drainage with CT (or possibly ultrasound) guidance.[1,53] If a smaller abscess is treated initially with antibiotics only but symptoms fail to improve, percutaneous drainage should be considered. Progression of symptoms despite percutaneous drainage of an abscess usually indicates the need for surgery. Historically, 10% to 25% of patients requiring hospitalization for treatment of diverticulitis will not improve or will worsen with medical management alone; overall, 30% of hospitalized patients will require an operation. Those patients who recover from an initial episode of complicated diverticulitis (contained perforation or abscess) should be considered for single-stage, elective segmental colectomy after the resolution of acute inflammation.[54] As will be discussed further, minimally invasive surgical techniques are increasingly being used with good outcomes in these patients.

7 Patients who fail nonoperative management of diverticulitis or who present with purulent or feculent peritonitis require operative treatment. The goal of surgery in these patients—especially if they are toxic, developing multisystem organ failure, or hemodynamically unstable—is to resect the perforation and make a stoma. This defines a Hartmann procedure, in which the offending segment of colon is resected, a proximal stoma is constructed, and the distal colon and/or rectum are closed and left in the pelvis. The distal remaining segment of colon and rectum are referred to as a Hartmann pouch. This approach was favored for many years because it is quick and simple and there is no chance of anastomotic leak. However, 30% to 50% of patients treated in this way never undergo reversal of the stoma, and when they do, the complication rate is high (major complications in 5% to 25%, anastomotic leak in 2% to 30%).[55,56]

Despite these problems, this is still the procedure of choice in unstable patients. However, in the more stable patient who requires an urgent operation because of generalized diverticular peritonitis on presentation or failure of nonoperative management, the goal should be resection with primary anastomosis and creation of a diverting stoma, usually a loop ileostomy. The anastomotic leak rate in patients with free diverticular perforation who undergo a single-stage operation acutely is 13%.[57] While diverting ileostomy or colostomy upstream from a primary anastomosis does not prevent an anastomotic leak, it lessens the consequences of a leak by diverting the fecal stream from the area, preventing potentially devastating gross fecal soilage through the defect.

Obstruction

Complete obstruction from diverticular disease is unusual. Partial obstruction resulting from edema, spasm, and inflammation is more common. The differential diagnosis includes cancer and inflammatory bowel disease. Medical treatment and elective resection are usually successful. Rarely is the placement of a colonic stent necessary, but it may be used to allow for bowel preparation before a single-stage resection with primary anastomosis. A diverting stoma may be necessary to relieve obstruction and enable completion of the workup and treatment before definitive resection. If perforation has resulted from obstruction, even when the distinction between obstructive cancer and diverticular obstruction cannot be made, the perforated segment should be resected and diverting end-colostomy performed. If this is a right-sided process in a relatively stable patient, primary anastomosis and diverting loop ileostomy can be considered.

Fistula

The presence of a fistula usually obviates the need for an emergency operation because the abscess has in effect spontaneously drained internally. A single-stage operation should be planned. The bladder side of a colovesical fistula is usually disrupted bluntly at the time of colon resection. No repair of the bladder is needed unless there is a visibly patent opening at the transected fistula tract site. A urinary drainage catheter is left in place for 7 to 10 days after surgery.[38] A cystogram can be done to verify closure of the tract opening and can facilitate discharge without an indwelling catheter following laparoscopic resection, which is often earlier than after open procedures. It is not necessary to leave a pelvic drain at the time of resection. Likewise, fistula tract openings to the vaginal cuff do not require closure. At most, omentum can be draped into the pelvis to separate the fresh colorectal anastomosis from the opening on the vagina.

Giant Colonic Diverticulum

Treatment is surgical resection of the involved segment of colon. Planned electively, a single-stage operation is indicated. Once perforated, the decision process parallels common diverticulitis, preference being given to resection with primary anastomosis and diverting loop stoma in the stable patient.

MANAGEMENT

Operative Strategies

The most important advance in the surgical management of diverticular disease besides trying to convert staged, emergency operations into elective, single-stage operations is the introduction of minimally invasive surgical techniques. No matter what the approach, certain challenges face the surgeon operating for diverticular disease. Inflammation distorts the anatomic planes. Dense fibrosis and adhesions impede sharp dissection and make it difficult to get good traction and countertraction that enable dissection. Inflammatory adhesions interfere with visualization and sometimes even palpation of anatomic structures.

Key concepts apply to both laparoscopic and open procedures. The goal is not to remove every diverticulum but rather to resect the area of inflammation or complication. The proximal resection line should be at soft, pliable bowel. The distal resection line must be at the top of the rectum demarcated by splaying of the bunched longitudinal muscle fibers (taenia coli) into the continuous longitudinal, outer layer of the rectal muscularis propria. The point of transection is almost never below the anterior pelvic peritoneal reflection. The splenic flexure should almost always be mobilized to facilitate creation of a tension-free colorectal anastomosis. The anastomotic site itself must be free from diverticula, which can be difficult in the patient with dense, pandiverticulosis. Manual, pinch dissection (or "finger fracture") techniques are used to separate structures and divide areas of fibrosis and thick adhesions. Dissection commences away from the focus of inflammation, usually proximal to it. The left ureter should be identified as early as possible and before transecting major vessels or the colon. In the setting of severe inflammation in the left lower quadrant or pelvis, it can be very helpful to mobilize and divide the proximal bowel as an initial operative maneuver. Likewise, when dense inflammation makes the standard, lateral-to-medial mobilization of the sigmoid difficult, a medial-to-lateral approach can sometimes provide access to less inflamed tissues. While typically not needed, when a preoperative CT scan shows dense inflammation in proximity to the left ureter, placement of ureteral stents can help with ureteral identification and protection during dissection. Whether using open or laparoscopic techniques, an elective operation should be deferred for 4 to 6 weeks after the last episode of inflammation so that acute inflammatory changes do not interfere with either the dissection or the construction of a safe colorectal anastomosis.[58]

There is growing experience with laparoscopic resection of even complicated diverticular disease. A meta-analysis comparing laparoscopic to open diverticulitis resections concluded that the laparoscopic patients had lower infection rates (overall and wound); decreased pulmonary, gastrointestinal, and cardiovascular complications; and a shorter time to recovery of bowel function and hospital discharge. Although studies in the meta-analysis included acute and chronic indications for surgery and complicated as well as uncomplicated diverticulitis in both groups, the authors cautioned that the retrospective nature of the reviewed studies introduced selection bias.[59] When laparoscopic resections for diverticular disease are performed early (2 to 16 days after hospital admission), the conversion rates are higher than when surgery is delayed (more than 6 weeks).[60] Hand-assisted minimally invasive operations may offer significant benefit compared to pure laparoscopic surgery for diverticular disease, showing lower conversion rates, shorter operative times, and no compromise of the speedy recovery associated with fully laparoscopic operations.[61]

Elective Surgery

Several observations form the basis of recommendations for elective resection following episodes of diverticulitis. Forty percent of diverticulitis patients admitted to the hospital will develop a complication, 23% following a single episode and 58% following two episodes. Thirty to 45% of patients hospitalized for diverticulitis will have another flare, usually within 5 years (90%). Among patients hospitalized a second time, only 10% remain symptom-free.[62–64] Mortality doubles with a second flare. The classic indications for elective resection include two or more episodes of *documented* diverticulitis, a single episode of complicated diverticulitis (modified Hinchey stage Ib or II), one documented episode in an immunocompromised patient, one documented episode in a young patient (40 to 50 years old), and an inability to exclude cancer as the cause of the signs and symptoms.

Practice parameters outlined by the American Society of Colon and Rectal Surgeons note that most patients who present with complicated diverticulitis do so at their first episode, so operating on patients with uncomplicated episodes of diverticulitis may not reduce the risk of emergency surgery and mortality. "The age and medical condition of the patient, the frequency and severity of the attack(s), and whether there are persistent symptoms after the acute episode" may be better determinants of recommendation for elective resection.[1] Complications develop often enough after successful medical management of complicated diverticulitis to warrant recommending elective resection.[48] Kaiser et al. reported that 41% of patients treated with percutaneous drainage of a diverticular abscess will later develop severe sepsis.[37]

It has been noted that the incidence of diverticular disease has steadily increased among young people, from 12% in 1969[65] to 20% in 1998[66] to 54% in a study of young and obese American patients in 2006.[67] Traditionally, elective colon resection was recommended for young people (age younger than 50 years) after one documented episode of uncomplicated diverticulitis. This recommendation was based on the belief that diverticular disease is more virulent in young patients. However, data are conflicting in this regard. There have been reports of young patients', increased risk of complicated disease at presentation, increased frequency of recurrences (in the same time period as older patients, not as a function of longevity), and higher risk of needing emergency surgery and colostomy. Recommendation for elective resection following a single episode of uncomplicated diverticulitis in patients younger than 50 years of age was motivated by an interest in avoiding a colostomy and avoiding major morbidity and mortality. In view of conflicting data and adoption of technical strategies for avoiding end-colostomies in all patients, Nelson et al. have suggested following the same guidelines that are used for older patients.[54,68–74]

Immunocompromised patients are more likely to fail medical management and must be watched closely since the manifestations of failure may be more subtle than in immunocompetent patients. Transplant patients, those on steroids or chemotherapy, diabetics, and dialysis patients are at risk. Elective resection in anticipation of transplant is also considered in some patients with diverticular disease. Interestingly, human immunodeficiency virus (HIV)-positive patients with normal CD4 counts appear to behave as if they were immunologically normal with respect to the incidence of diverticulitis and its clinical course. Since HIV infection has principally been an illness of younger people, most studies of diverticulitis have not included a large number of HIV-positive patients.[75] That may change as longevity improves with current antiretroviral regimens.

SUMMARY

Diverticular disease is common and includes a spectrum of presentations and anatomic locations, favoring the left colon in Western societies. The etiology is likely multifactorial, with a low-residue diet being a common factor. The CT scan has dramatically improved diagnostic accuracy and helped with treatment planning. Treatment often parallels the Hinchey stage, particularly the modified Hinchey classification. Surgical treatment has evolved to favor medical management and image-guided percutaneous drainage of abscesses when feasible to convert surgical-emergency staged procedures into either single-stage procedures or procedures with primary anastomosis and diverting loop stoma. The distinction of complicated diverticular disease and colon cancer can be difficult, but early contrast enema studies or colonoscopy can be safely performed and are the most helpful diagnostic procedures in this setting. The indications for elective resection following successful medical management of diverticular disease are being reconsidered, and it is becoming clear that elective sigmoid resection for diverticular disease should be offered to avoid recurrent symptoms, not primarily to avoid free perforation and the need for an emergent colostomy. Minimally invasive surgery is state of the art, and the hand-assisted techniques are particularly useful for elective diverticular disease resections.

References

1. Rafferty J, et al. Practice parameters for sigmoid diverticulitis. *Dis Colon Rectum* 2006;49(7):939–944.
2. Nakada I, et al. Diverticular disease of the colon at a regional general hospital in Japan. *Dis Colon Rectum* 1995;38(7):755–759.
3. Sugihara K, et al. Diverticular disease of the colon in Japan. A review of 615 cases. *Dis Colon Rectum* 1984;27(8):531–537.
4. Chia JG, et al. Trends of diverticular disease of the large bowel in a newly developed country. *Dis Colon Rectum* 1991;34(6):498–501.
5. Martel J, Raskin JB. History, incidence, and epidemiology of diverticulosis. *J Clin Gastroenterol* 2008;42(10):1125–1127.
6. Spriggs EI, Marxer OA. Intestinal diverticula. *Q J Med* 1925;19:1.
7. Hughes LE. Postmortem survey of diverticular disease of the colon. I. Diverticulosis and diverticulitis. *Gut* 1969;10(5):336–344.
8. Horner JL. Natural history of diverticulosis of the colon. *Am J Dig Dis* 1958;3(5):343–350.
9. Minardi AJ Jr, et al. Diverticulitis in the young patient. *Am Surg* 2001; 67(5):458–461.
10. Sandler RS, et al. The burden of selected digestive diseases in the United States. *Gastroenterology* 2002;122(5):1500–1511.
11. Slack WW. The anatomy, pathology, and some clinical features of diverticulitis of the colon. *Br J Surg* 1962;50:185–190.
12. Gallagher JJ, Welch JP. Giant diverticular of the sigmoid colon: a review of differential diagnosis and operative management. *Arch Surg* 1979;114(9): 1079–1083.
13. Beighton PH, Murdoch JL, Votteler T. Gastrointestinal complications of the Ehlers-Danlos syndrome. *Gut* 1969;10(12):1004–1008.
14. Cook JM. Spontaneous perforation of the colon: report of two cases in a family exhibiting Marfan's stigmata. *Ohio State Med J* 1968;64:73.
15. Wess L, et al. Cross linking of collagen is increased in colonic diverticulosis. *Gut* 1995;37(1):91–94.
16. Morson BC. The muscle abnormality in diverticular disease of the colon. *Proc R Soc Med* 1963;56:798–800.
17. Whiteway J, Morson BC. Elastosis in diverticular disease of the sigmoid colon. *Gut* 1985;26(3):258–266.
18. Painter NS, et al. Segmentation and the localization of intraluminal pressures in the human colon, with special reference to the pathogenesis of colonic diverticula. *Gastroenterology* 1965;49:169–177.
19. Painter NS. The aetiology of diverticulosis of the colon with special reference to the action of certain drugs on the behaviour of the colon. *Ann R Coll Surg Engl* 1964;34:98–119.
20. Taylor I, Duthie HL, Bran tablets and diverticular disease. *Br Med J* 1976; 1(6016):988–990.
21. Snape WJ Jr, et al. Evidence that abnormal myoelectrical activity produces colonic motor dysfunction in the irritable bowel syndrome. *Gastroenterology* 1977;72(3):383–387.
22. Bassotti G, et al. Twenty-four hour recordings of colonic motility in patients with diverticular disease: evidence for abnormal motility and propulsive activity. *Dis Colon Rectum* 2001;44(12):1814–1820.
23. Milner P, et al. Vasoactive intestinal polypeptide levels in sigmoid colon in idiopathic constipation and diverticular disease. *Gastroenterology* 1990; 99(3):666–675.
24. Yun AJ, Bazar KA, Lee PY. A new mechanism for diverticular diseases: aging-related vagal withdrawal. *Med Hypotheses* 2005;64(2):252–225.
25. Costedio MM, et al. Serotonin signaling in diverticular disease. *J Gastrointest Surg* 2008;12(8):1439–1445.
26. Painter NS, Burkitt DP. Diverticular disease of the colon: a deficiency disease of Western civilization. *Br Med J* 1971;2(5759):450–454.
27. Painter NS, Burkitt DP, Diverticular disease of the colon, a 20th century problem. *Clin Gastroenterol* 1975;4(1):3–21.
28. Korzenik JR. Diverticulitis: new frontiers for an old country: risk factors and pathogenesis. *J Clin Gastroenterol* 2008;42(10):1128–1129.
29. Korzenik JR. Case closed? Diverticulitis: epidemiology and fiber. *J Clin Gastroenterol* 2006;40(suppl 3):S112–S116.
30. Strate LL, et al. Nut, corn, and popcorn consumption and the incidence of diverticular disease. *JAMA* 2008;300(8):907–914.
31. Floch MH, Bina I. The natural history of diverticulitis: fact and theory. *J Clin Gastroenterol* 2004;38(5 suppl):S2–S7.
32. West AB. The pathology of diverticulitis. *J Clin Gastroenterol* 2008; 42(10):1137–1138.
33. Simpson J, Scholefield JH, Spiller RC. Origin of symptoms in diverticular disease. *Br J Surg* 2003;90(8):899–908.
34. Stead RH. Nerve remodelling during intestinal inflammation. *Ann N Y Acad Sci* 1992;664:443–455.
35. Brewer DB, et al. Axonal damage in Crohn's disease is frequent, but non-specific. *J Pathol* 1990;161(4):301–311.
36. Hinchey EJ, Schaal PG, Richards GK. Treatment of perforated diverticular disease of the colon. *Adv Surg* 1978;12:85–109.
37. Kaiser AM, et al. The management of complicated diverticulitis and the role of computed tomography. *Am J Gastroenterol* 2005;100(4):910–917.
38. Woods RJ, et al. Internal fistulas in diverticular disease. *Dis Colon Rectum* 1988;31(8):591–596.
39. Grissom R. Snyder TE. Colovaginal fistula secondary to diverticular disease. *Dis Colon Rectum* 1991;34(11):1043–1049.
40. Chintapalli KN, et al. Pericolic mesenteric lymph nodes: an aid in distinguishing diverticulitis from cancer of the colon. *AJR Am J Roentgenol* 1997; 169(5):1253–1255.
41. Graham SM, Ballantyne GH. Cecal diverticulitis. A review of the American experience. *Dis Colon Rectum* 1987;30(10):821–826.
42. Gouge TH, et al. Management of diverticulitis of the ascending colon. 10 years' experience. *Am J Surg* 1983;145(3):387–391.
43. Hayward MW, et al. A pilot evaluation of radiography of the acute abdomen. *Clin Radiol* 1984;35(4):289–291.
44. Field S, et al. The erect abdominal radiograph in the acute abdomen: should its routine use be abandoned? *Br Med J (Clin Res Ed)* 1985; 290(6486):1934–1936.
45. Ambrosetti P, et al. Acute left colonic diverticulitis–compared performance of computed tomography and water-soluble contrast enema: prospective evaluation of 420 patients. *Dis Colon Rectum* 2000;43(10):1363–1367.
46. Rao PM, et al. Helical CT with only colonic contrast material for diagnosing diverticulitis: prospective evaluation of 150 patients. *AJR Am J Roentgenol* 1998;170(6):1445–1449.
47. Rao PM, Rhea JT, Novelline RA. Helical CT of appendicitis and diverticulitis. *Radiol Clin North Am* 1999;37(5):895–910.
48. Ambrosetti P, et al. Computed tomography in acute left colonic diverticulitis. *Br J Surg* 1997;84(4):532–534.
49. Sudakoff GS, Lundeen SJ, Otterson MF. Transrectal and transvaginal sonographic intervention of infected pelvic fluid collections: a complete approach. *Ultrasound Q* 2005;21(3):175–185.
50. Lewis M. Bleeding colonic diverticula. *J Clin Gastroenterol* 2008;42(10): 1156–1158.
51. McGuire HH Jr. Bleeding colonic diverticula. A reappraisal of natural history and management. *Ann Surg* 1994;220(5):653–656.
52. Drapanas T, et al. Emergency subtotal colectomy: preferred approach to management of massively bleeding diverticular disease. *Ann Surg* 1973; 177(5):519–526.
53. Ambrosetti P, et al. Long-term outcome of mesocolic and pelvic diverticular abscesses of the left colon: a prospective study of 73 cases. *Dis Colon Rectum* 2005;48(4):787–791.
54. Chautems RC, et al. Long-term follow-up after first acute episode of sigmoid diverticulitis: is surgery mandatory?: a prospective study of 118 patients. *Dis Colon Rectum* 2002;45(7):962–966.
55. Aydin HN, et al. Hartmann's reversal is associated with high postoperative adverse events. *Dis Colon Rectum* 2005;48(11):2117–2126.
56. Constantinides VA, et al. Operative strategies for diverticular peritonitis: a decision analysis between primary resection and anastomosis versus Hartmann's procedures. *Ann Surg* 2007;245(1):94–103.
57. Salem L, Flum DR. Primary anastomosis or Hartmann's procedure for patients with diverticular peritonitis? A systematic review. *Dis Colon Rectum* 2004;47(11):1953–1964.
58. Reissfelder C, Buhr HJ, Ritz JP. What is the optimal time of surgical intervention after an acute attack of sigmoid diverticulitis: early or late elective laparoscopic resection? *Dis Colon Rectum* 2006;49(12):1842–1848.
59. Purkayastha S, et al. Laparoscopic vs. open surgery for diverticular disease: a meta-analysis of nonrandomized studies. *Dis Colon Rectum* 2006; 49(4):446–463.
60. Zingg U, et al. Early vs. delayed elective laparoscopic-assisted colectomy in sigmoid diverticulitis: timing of surgery in relation to the acute attack. *Dis Colon Rectum* 2007;50(11):1911–1917.
61. Lee SW, et al. Laparoscopic vs. hand-assisted laparoscopic sigmoidectomy for diverticulitis. *Dis Colon Rectum* 2006;49(4):464–469.
62. Parks TG. Natural history of diverticular disease of the colon. *Clin Gastroenterol* 1975;4(1):53–69.
63. Farmakis N, Tudor RG, Keighley MR. The 5-year natural history of complicated diverticular disease. *Br J Surg* 1994;81(5):733–735.
64. Makela J, et al. Natural history of diverticular disease: when to operate? *Dis Colon Rectum* 1998;41(12):1523–1528.
65. Parks TG. Natural history of diverticular disease of the colon. A review of 521 cases. *Br Med J* 1969;4(5684):639–642.

66. Makela J, Kiviniemi H, Laitinen S. Prevalence of perforated sigmoid diverticulitis is increasing. *Dis Colon Rectum* 2002;45(7):955–961.
67. Zaidi E, Daly B. CT and clinical features of acute diverticulitis in an urban U.S. population: rising frequency in young, obese adults. *AJR Am J Roentgenol* 2006;187(3):689–694.
68. Pautrat K, et al. Acute diverticulitis in very young patients: a frequent surgical management. *Dis Colon Rectum* 2007;50(4):472–477.
69. Nelson RS, Velasco A, Mukesh BN. Management of diverticulitis in younger patients. *Dis Colon Rectum* 2006;49(9):1341–1145.
70. Spivak H, et al. Acute colonic diverticulitis in the young. *Dis Colon Rectum* 1997;40(5):570–574.
71. Guzzo J, Hyman N. Diverticulitis in young patients: is resection after a single attack always warranted? *Dis Colon Rectum* 2004;47(7):1187–1190; discussion 1190–1191.
72. Vignati PV, Welch JP, Cohen JL. Long-term management of diverticulitis in young patients. *Dis Colon Rectum* 1995;38(6):627–629.
73. Anaya DA, Flum DR, Risk of emergency colectomy and colostomy in patients with diverticular disease. *Arch Surg* 2005;140(7):681–685.
74. West SD, et al. Diverticulitis in the younger patient. *Am J Surg* 2003;186(6): 743–746.
75. Sachar DB. Diverticulitis in immunosuppressed patients. *J Clin Gastroenterol* 2008;42(10):1154–1155.

CHAPTER 70 ■ ANORECTAL DISORDERS

BARD C. COSMAN, ARDEN M. MORRIS, SANTHAT NIVATVONGS, AND ROBERT D. MADOFF

KEY POINTS

1. The most common manifestation of hemorrhoids is painless, bright red rectal bleeding associated with bowel movements.
2. A high-fiber diet with fiber supplements reduces symptoms of hemorrhoids and is ideal for first- and second-degree hemorrhoids.
3. Rubber band ligation is suitable for symptomatic first- and second- and some third-degree internal hemorrhoids that do not respond to bulk-forming agents.
4. Hemorrhoidectomy is required in only a few patients with symptomatic hemorrhoids. It should be considered when the hemorrhoids are mixed internal and external, are severely prolapsed through the anus, or are complicated by associated pathology, such as ulceration, fissures, fistulas, large hypertrophied anal papillae, or extensive skin tags.
5. Rectal prolapse is a rectal intussusception that extends beyond the anal verge. Fit patients are best treated with transabdominal rectopexy. Patients with significant medical comorbidities are best treated using a perineal approach.
6. Anal fissure is an ischemic ulcer in the lower portion of the anal canal; its treatment, both medical and surgical, involves relaxing the internal anal sphincter.
7. Infection of the anal glands is the origin of perianal abscesses.
8. Anal fistula is a chronic form of perianal abscess, spontaneously or surgically drained, in which the tract persists, with an internal opening at the dentate line and an external opening on the perianal skin.
9. Anal condylomata acuminata are caused by human papillomavirus, as are anal intraepithelial neoplasia and anal cancers.
10. Palpable lesions of the anal canal are not hemorrhoids and may be cancers; examination under anesthesia and biopsy allow for correct diagnosis.

ANATOMY AND PHYSIOLOGY

The Rectum

The rectum, the terminal portion of the large bowel, extends from the level of the sacral promontory to the level of the levator ani muscle and is approximately 15 cm in length. The rectum differs from the colon in that the outer, longitudinal muscular layer is continuous, as opposed to condensing into the three taeniae of the colon. The rectum has two or three lateral curves that form submucosal folds in the lumen, known as the *valves of Houston*. The posterior aspect of the rectum is devoid of peritoneum and adjoins the mesorectum, which is immediately anterior to the presacral fascia. The presacral fascia is a strong, endopelvic fascia that covers the entire anterior surface of the sacrum and also covers the underlying vessels and nerves. At about the level of S4, the presacral fascia runs anteriorly and inferiorly and attaches to the rectum, an area known as the *rectosacral fascia* or *Waldeyer ring* (Fig. 70.1).[1] This fascia must be incised for full mobilization of the rectum during abdominoperineal resection or extended low anterior resection. Peritoneum covers the upper two thirds of the rectum anteriorly and the upper one third of the rectum laterally; the lower third of the rectum is entirely devoid of peritoneum. The level of the anterior peritoneal reflection is variable, but most often is 6 to 8 cm from the anal verge. The extraperitoneal portion of the rectum is surrounded by endopelvic fascia. On the anterior surface, this is called the *Denonvilliers fascia* and lies just posterior to the vagina in females and the seminal vesicles in males.

The Anal Canal and Sphincters

The anal canal, about 4 cm in length, is the transitional organ that extends from the rectum, as it passes through the levator ani or pelvic floor, traverses the anal verge, and extends to the hair-bearing skin of the anal margin. The muscular wall of the anal canal, continuous with the circular smooth muscular layer of the rectum, is thickened and forms the internal anal sphincter. The anal canal is wrapped by the striated external anal sphincter muscle inferiorly. The puborectalis muscle loops around the anorectal junction posteriorly, forming a U-shaped sling that originates on the posterior pubic bones. Although there is functional continuity between the puborectalis and external sphincter, magnetic resonance imaging studies indicate that the deepest portion of the external anal sphincter is separated from the puborectalis by a layer of fat.[2] The elliptical external sphincter muscle extends from the coccyx, where its origin is called the *anococcygeal ligament,* to the perineal body, encircling the anal canal (Fig. 70.2).

At the upper portion of the anal canal, called the *anorectal ring*, the internal sphincter is discretely palpable, and the puborectalis muscle can be palpated digitally. From the level of the anorectal ring distally and between the internal and external sphincter muscles, the longitudinal muscle coat of the rectum

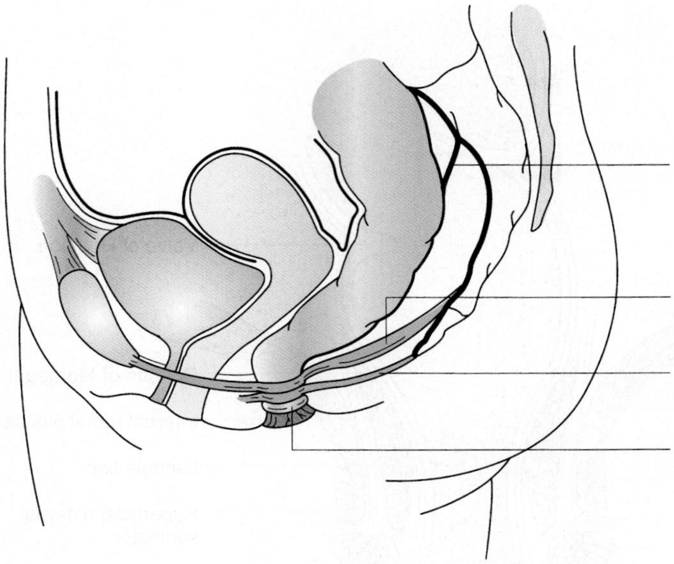

FIGURE 70.1. Fascial attachments of the rectum.

is joined by fibers of the levator ani and puborectalis to form the conjoined longitudinal muscle (Fig. 70.3). These muscle fibers traverse the external sphincter to insert in the skin of the anal verge as the *corrugator cutis ani*, which causes wrinkling of the anal verge. This mixed smooth/striated longitudinal anal muscle may play a significant role in anal function, unifying or coordinating the two sphincters.[3]

At about the midpoint of the anal canal, roughly 2 cm from the anal verge, there is an undulating demarcation called the *dentate* or *pectinate line*, meaning toothed or comblike line. Longitudinal folds of the mucosa above the dentate line are known as the *columns of Morgagni.* For a distance of about 1 cm above the dentate line, the epithelial lining may be columnar, transitional, or stratified squamous epithelium; this area is referred to as the *transitional* or *cloacogenic zone*. The internal hemorrhoidal vascular plexus lies deep to the mucosa at this location. The area above the transitional zone is lined by columnar epithelium, and the area below the dentate line is lined by squamous epithelium (Fig. 70.3).

The 'surgical' anal canal extends from the anorectal ring to the anal verge. The term *anoderm* describes the skin of the anal verge: non–hair-bearing skin distal to the dentate line, but proximal to the hair-bearing skin of the anal margin. The perianal skin (anal margin) extends from the lateral border of the anal verge, where normal hair-bearing skin starts, to 5 to 6 cm from the anal verge.

Pelvic Floor Muscles

The pelvic floor consists of the levator ani muscle and the coccygeus muscle. The levator ani is a broad, thin muscle that forms the floor of the pelvic cavity and is innervated by the fourth sacral nerve and the pudendal nerve. This muscle has two distinct parts, iliococcygeus and pubococcygeus, and regions of the pubococcygeus are further named puborectalis, pubovaginalis, and puboprostaticus.

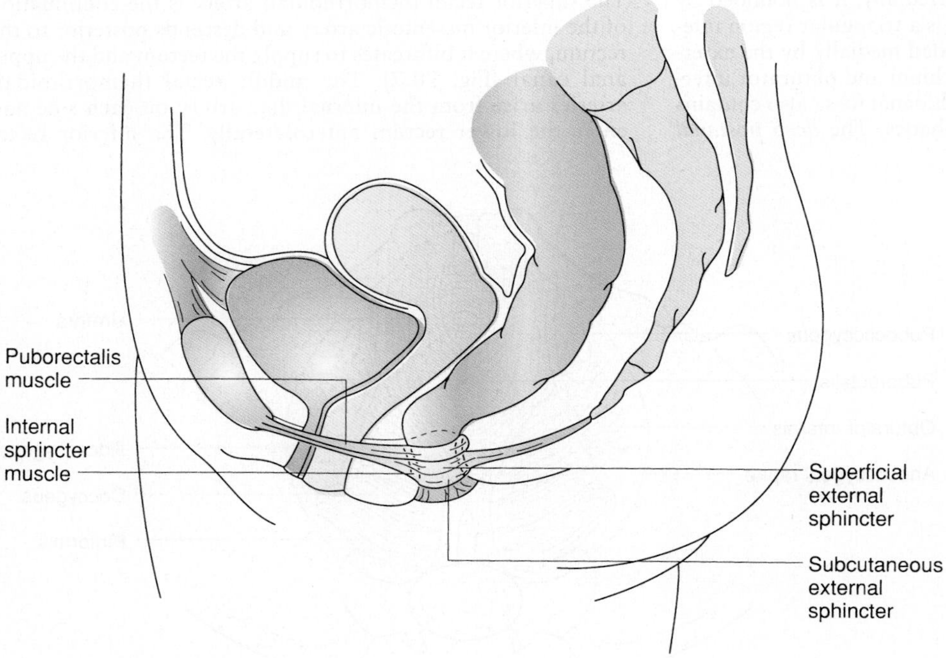

FIGURE 70.2. Arrangement of the external sphincter muscles.

FIGURE 70.3. Anatomy of the anal canal.

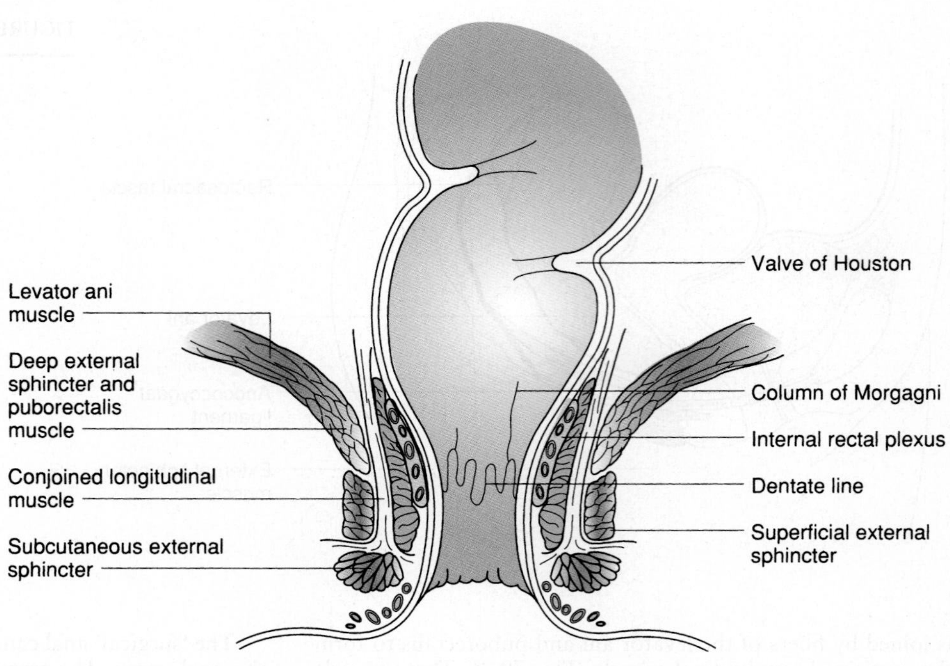

The levator ani arises from the body of the pubis, the ischial spine, and the tendinous arch of the obturator fascia that runs between them, and it inserts on the last two segments of the sacrum, the coccyx, and the *anococcygeal raphe*, which is a decussation with fibers from the opposite site (Fig. 70.4). In the standing position, the puborectalis contraction creates an anorectal angle of nearly 90 degrees, while the levator ani supports the viscera. During defecation, the puborectalis relaxes, straightening the anorectal angle and creating a straight path for evacuation.

Perianal and Perirectal Spaces

Surrounding the anorectum are several potential spaces that are normally filled with areolar tissues and fat, but which can harbor abscesses. The *perianal space* immediately surrounds the anus. Laterally, the perianal space is continuous with the subcutaneous fat of the buttocks. Medially, it is bounded by the anal verge. The *ischioanal fossa* is a triangular region inferior to the levator ani muscle, bounded medially by the external sphincter and laterally by the ischium and obturator internus (Fig. 70.5). The fatty, areolar ischioanal fossa also contains the inferior rectal vessels and lymphatics. The *deep postanal space* (of Courtney) connects the ischioanal space on each side posteriorly and lies between the levator ani muscle superiorly and the anococcygeal ligament inferiorly (Fig. 70.6). The deep postanal space is an important pathway in the formation of abscess; spread from one ischioanal fossa to the other may result in a *horseshoe abscess*, the 'horseshoe' being open anteriorly, where there is no communication between the ischioanal fossae. The *intersphincteric space* lies between the internal and external sphincters. It is continuous with the perianal space below and extends above into the supralevator space. The *supralevator spaces* are situated on each side of the rectum above the levator ani muscle (Fig. 70.5). The supralevator spaces communicate posteriorly and may allow spread of infection cephalad into the retroperitoneum (Fig. 70.6).

Arterial Supply of the Rectum and Anal Canal

The superior rectal (hemorrhoidal) artery is the continuation of the inferior mesenteric artery and descends posterior to the rectum, where it bifurcates to supply the rectum and the upper anal canal (Fig. 70.7). The middle rectal (hemorrhoidal) arteries arise from the internal iliac artery on each side and enter the lower rectum anterolaterally. The inferior rectal

FIGURE 70.4. Muscles of the pelvic floor.

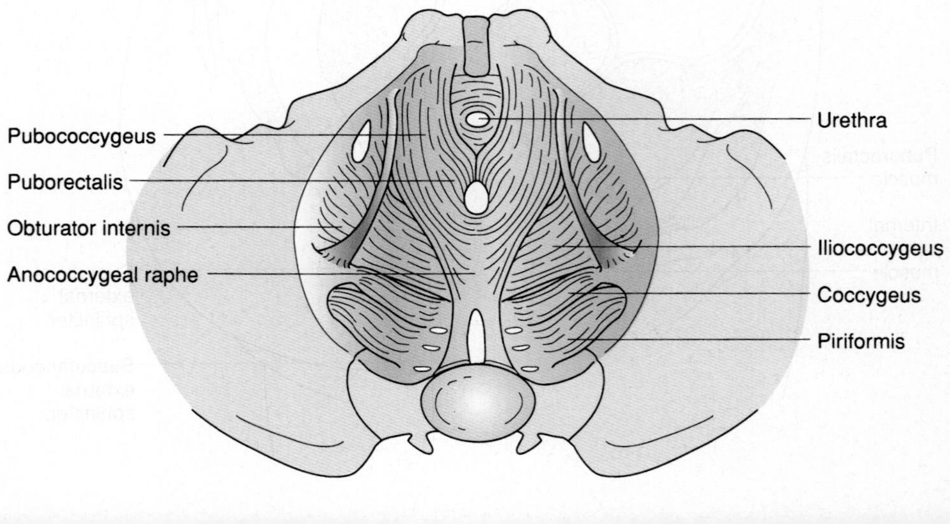

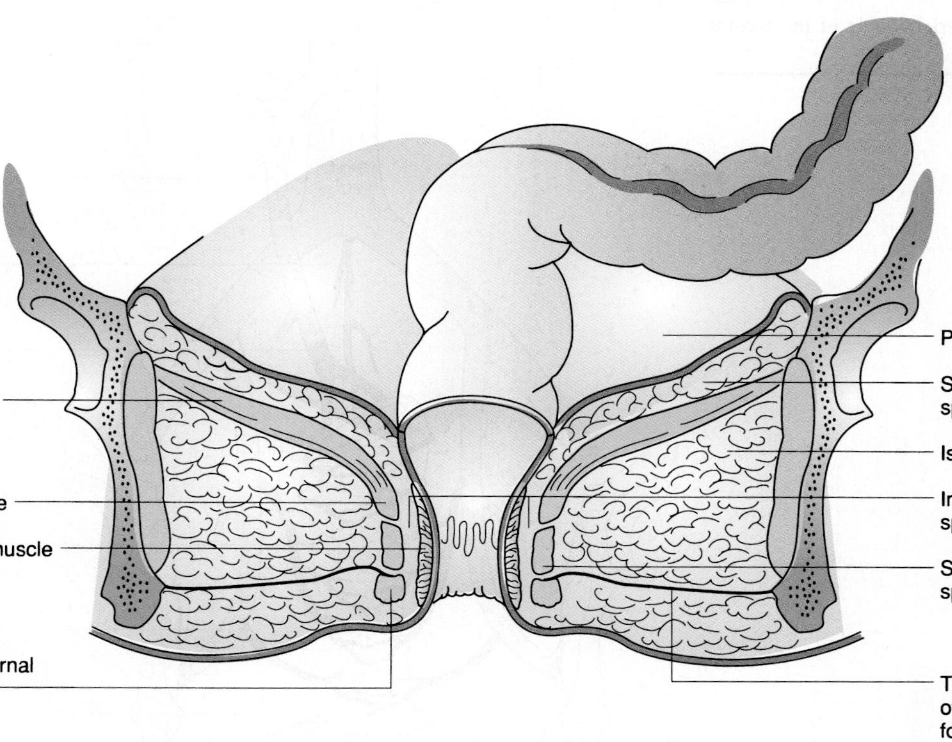

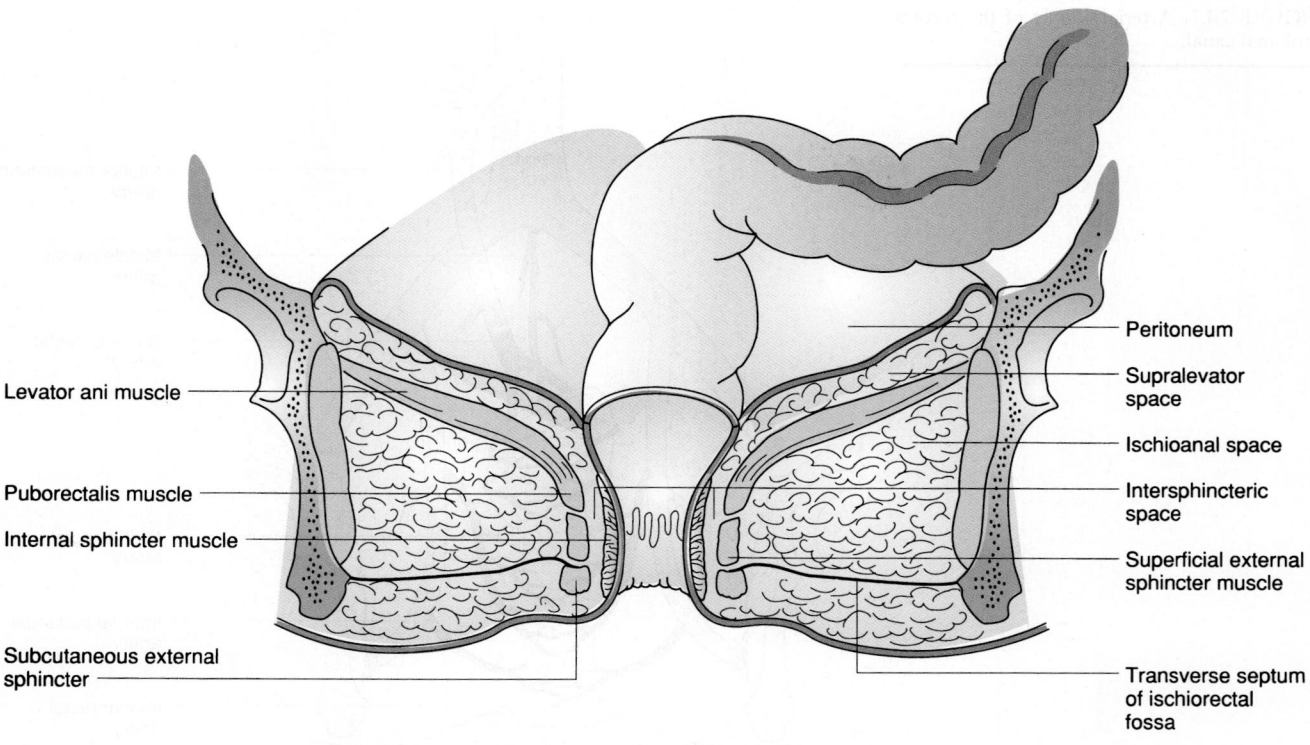

FIGURE 70.5. Anatomy of the perianorectal spaces (anteroposterior view).

(hemorrhoidal) arteries arise from the internal pudendal artery, a branch of the internal iliac artery, and traverse the ischioanal fossa on each side to supply the anal sphincter muscles. There are abundant intramural anastomoses between the superior, middle, and inferior rectal arteries, making rectal ischemia exceedingly rare, even after substantial devascularization.

Venous Drainage of the Rectum and Anal Canal

Venous return from the rectum and anal canal joins both portal and systemic systems (Fig. 70.8). The superior rectal (hemorrhoidal) vein drains the rectum and upper anal canal into the portal system via the inferior mesenteric vein. The middle rectal (hemorrhoidal) veins drain the lower rectum and the upper anal canal into the internal iliac veins. The inferior rectal (hemorrhoidal) veins drain the lower anal canal into the internal pudendal veins, which join the internal iliac veins. Each vein follows the correspondingly named artery. Portal-systemic shunts may thus occur in the rectum as they do in the esophagus, and bleeding rectal varices—not the same as hemorrhoids, and located in the rectum rather than the anus—may result.

Lymphatic Drainage of the Rectum and Anal Canal

Lymph from the upper and middle rectum ascends adjacent to the superior rectal artery to inferior mesenteric lymph nodes.

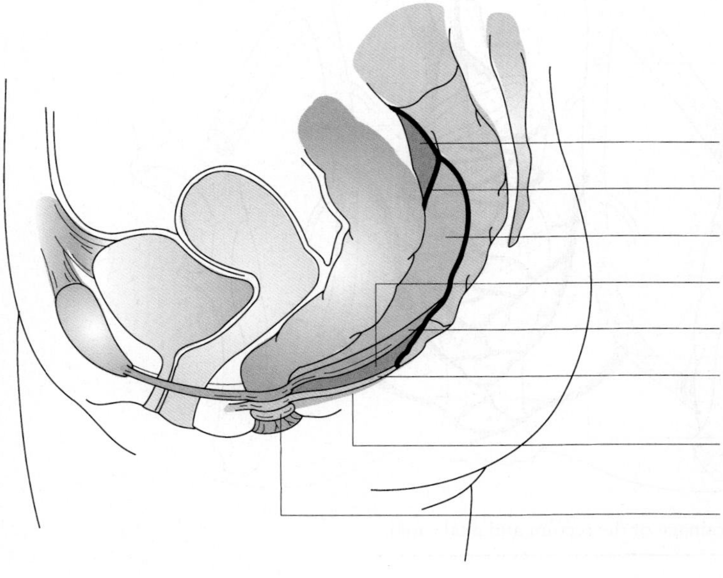

FIGURE 70.6. Anatomy of the perianorectal spaces (lateral view).

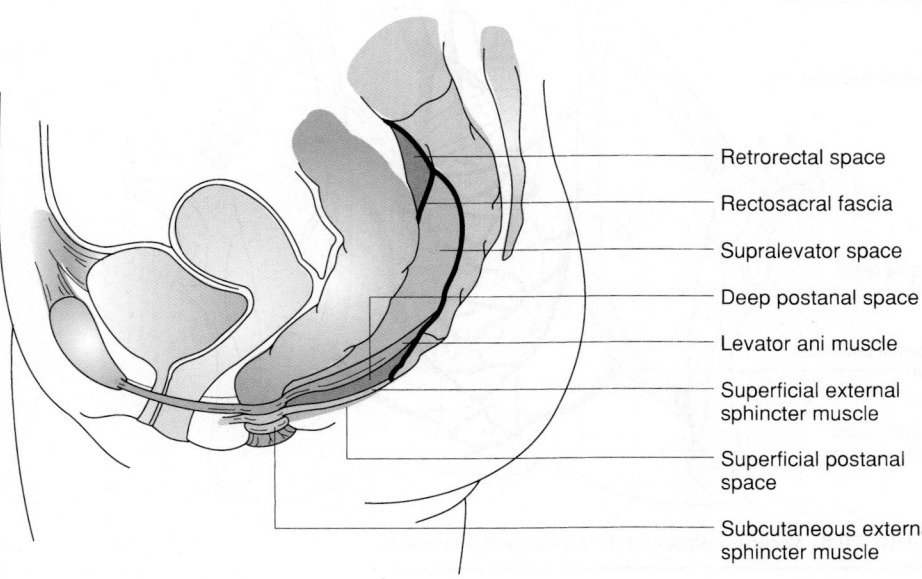

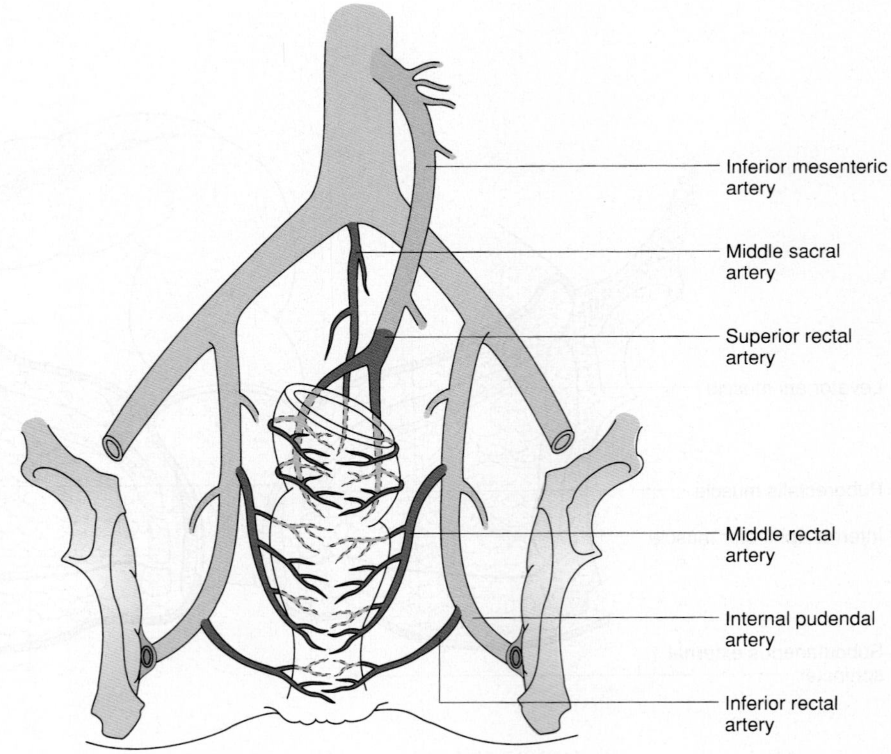

FIGURE 70.7. Arterial supply of the rectum and anal canal.

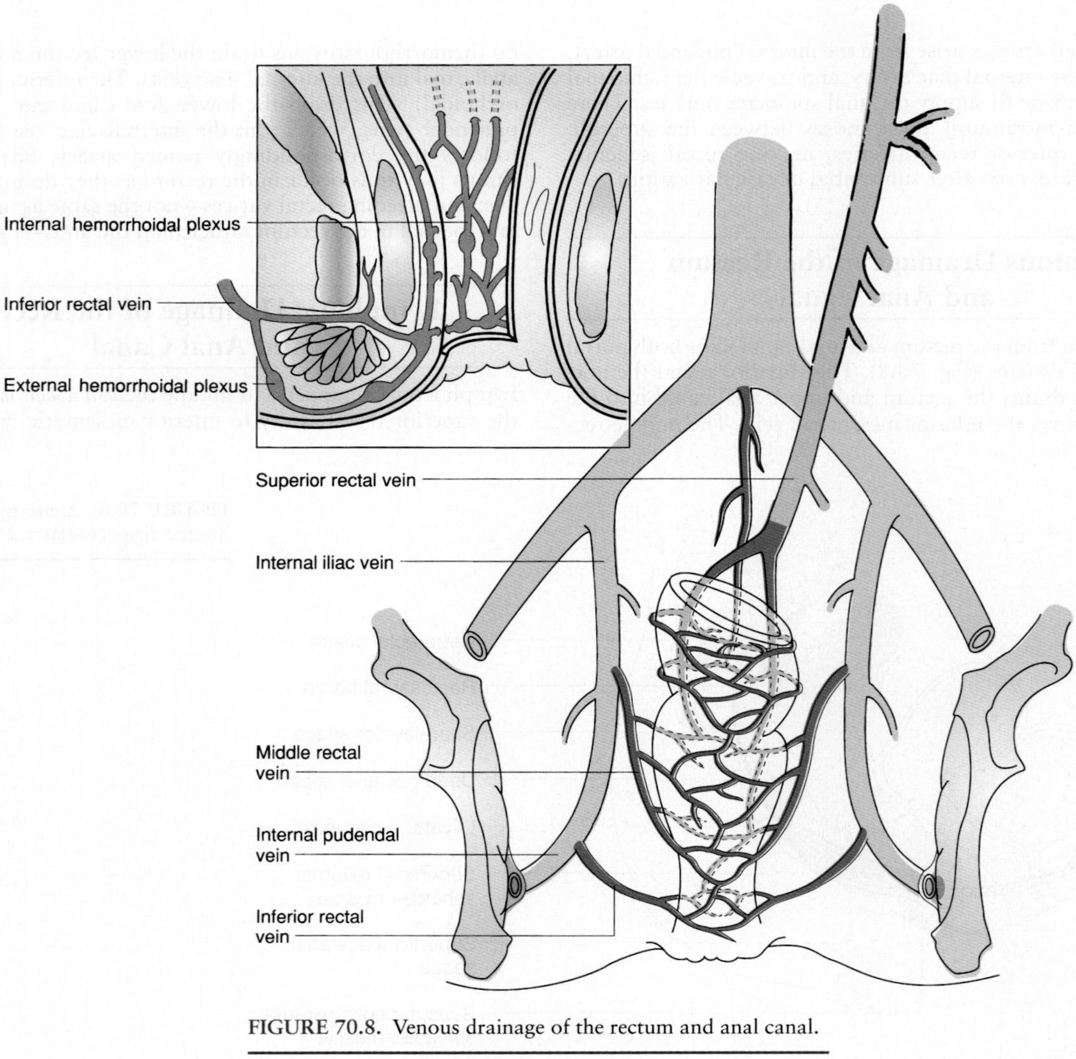

FIGURE 70.8. Venous drainage of the rectum and anal canal.

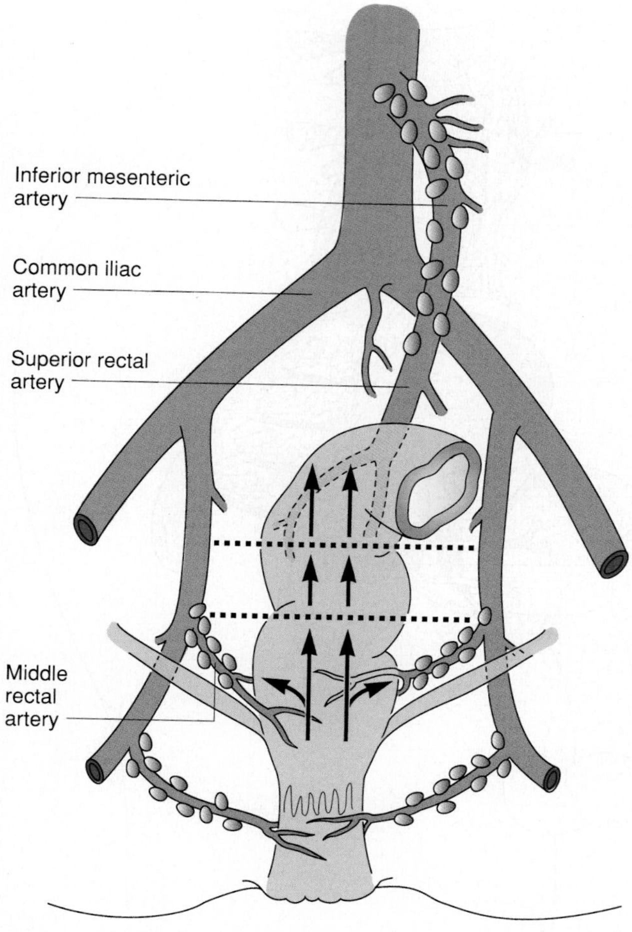

FIGURE 70.9. Lymphatic drainage of the rectum.

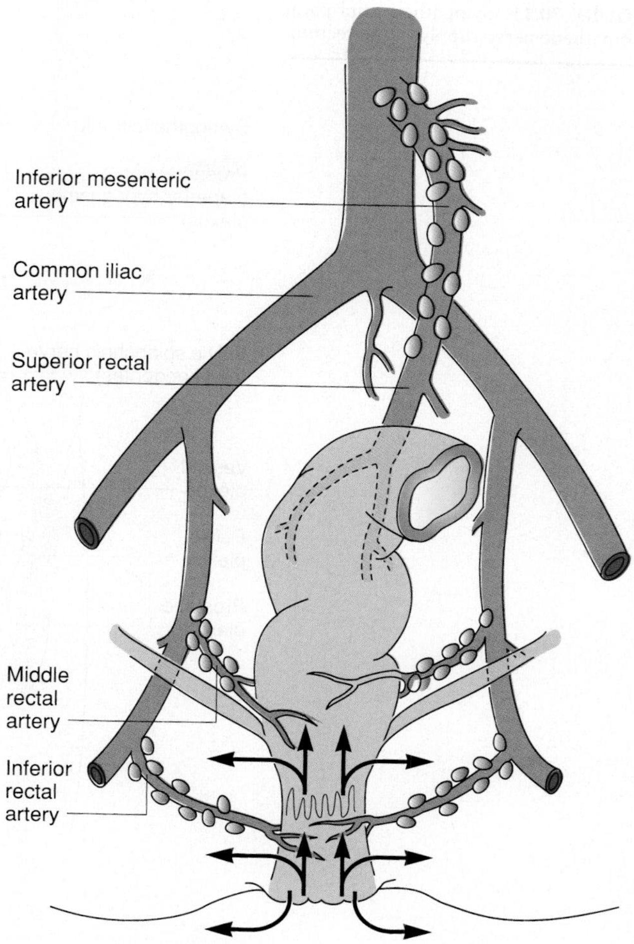

FIGURE 70.10. Lymphatic drainage of the anal canal.

The lower rectum drains likewise to inferior mesenteric nodes, but also laterally to internal iliac nodes (Fig. 70.9). Lymphatics from the anal canal above the dentate line may drain to inferior mesenteric nodes, or laterally, to internal iliac nodes. Lymph from the anus below the dentate line usually drains to inguinal nodes, although it can also drain to inferior mesenteric or internal iliac nodes if obstruction occurs in the primary drainage (Fig. 70.10). Lymphatic drainage of the perianal skin is entirely to the inguinal nodes.

Nerve Supply of the Rectum and Urogenital Organs

Sympathetic and parasympathetic nerves of the autonomic system supply the anus and rectum and also supply the adjacent urogenital organs. Nerve trunks close to the rectum are prone to injury during rectal mobilization unless specific precautions are taken.

Sympathetic fibers to the rectum are derived from the first three lumbar segments of the spinal cord. Sympathetic fibers pass through ganglionated sympathetic chains before forming the preaortic plexus. Preaortic fibers extend below the bifurcation of the aorta to form the hypogastric plexus or the presacral nerve (Fig. 70.11). The plexus thus formed divides into left and right branches, which are joined by the parasympathetic nerves.

The pelvic parasympathetic nerve supply is from pelvic splanchnic nerves (nervi erigentes), which originate from the second, third, and fourth sacral nerve roots. These nerves, joined by sympathetic fibers, form the pelvic plexus. The pelvic plexus is encased in the lateral attachments of the rectum, just superior to the levator ani (Fig. 70.11). From the pelvic plexuses, both types of autonomic nerve fibers distribute to urinary and genital organs.

In women, sympathetic fibers from the hypogastric plexus are directed toward the uterosacral ligament, close to the rectum. In men, fibers from the hypogastric plexus pass immediately adjacent to the anterolateral wall of the rectum in the retroperitoneal tissue.

The pelvic plexus gives rise to the periprostatic plexus, an important subdivision that is essential to sexual function in men. Both parasympathetic and sympathetic systems are involved in sexual function. Parasympathetic activity leads to erection, and a complex coordination between sympathetic, parasympathetic, and somatic systems produces ejaculation. Depending on which nerves are damaged during proctectomy, deficiencies may include incomplete erection, lack of ejaculation, retrograde ejaculation, or total impotence.[4] In women, the consequences of pelvic nerve injuries are poorly understood, but better definition of sexual-dysfunction states will likely lead to a similar list of postoperative complications.[5]

The pudendal nerve arises from the sacral plexus (S2–S4). Leaving the pelvis through the greater sciatic foramen, it reenters via the lesser sciatic foramen and travels in the pudendal canal in the lateral wall of the ischioanal fossa. Its branches include the inferior rectal (anal) nerve, perineal nerve, and dorsal nerves of the penis or clitoris. The pudendal nerve is anatomically protected from injury during mobilization of the rectum. Since sensory stimuli from the penis and clitoris are pudendally mediated, they are preserved after proctectomy.

FIGURE 70.11. Sympathetic and parasympathetic nerve supply of the rectum.

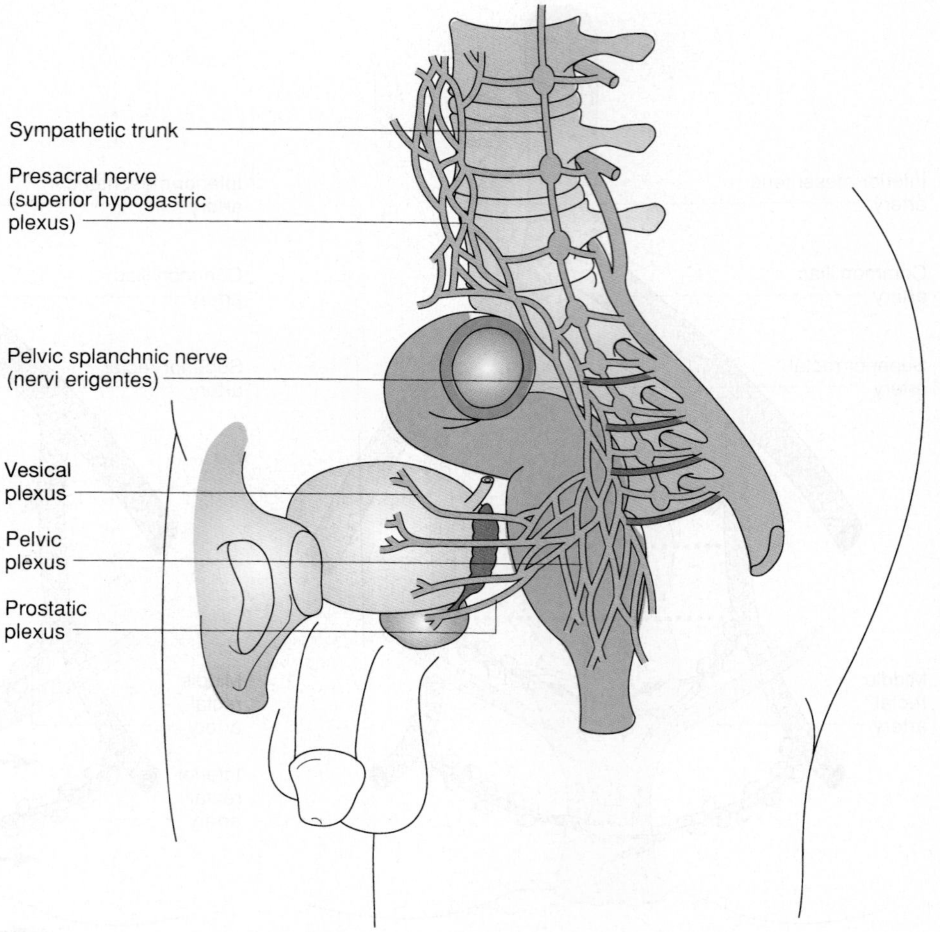

Nerve Supply of the Anal Canal

Motor Innervation. Both sympathetic and parasympathetic nerves supply the internal anal sphincter, which maintains tonic contraction until the complex and coordinated process of defecation allows it to relax. The external sphincter is supplied by the inferior rectal (anal) branch of the pudendal nerve and the perineal branch of the fourth sacral nerve.

Sensory Innervation. The sensory supply of the anal canal comes from the inferior rectal nerve, a branch of the pudendal nerve. The epithelium of the anal canal is profusely innervated with sensory nerve endings, especially at and just distal to the dentate line. Painful sensations in the anal canal can be felt up to 1.5 cm proximal to the dentate line, a fact one must keep in mind when treating internal hemorrhoids in the unanesthetized patient. Such treatment relies on the lack of somatic sensation above the dentate line, so one should test for sensation before banding, injecting, or coagulating in that area.

Physiology of the Anorectum

Sensation of the Anorectum. Complete anal continence cannot be achieved unless the subject can sense material in the rectum and can discriminate the contents by type (gas or feces). The receptors responsible for appreciation of rectal fullness and impending evacuation lie outside the anorectum, probably within the levator ani muscle. The anal canal epithelium is rich with sensory nerve endings, but although this sensitive area helps one discriminate between flatus and stool, it is not a critical factor in preserving anal continence.

Mechanism of Anal Continence. Stool can accumulate in the rectum for hours or days before triggering the urge to defecate. The ability of the rectum to retain stool is called reservoir continence. Continence is partly created by the puborectalis muscle, which functions as a sling, pulling the anal canal forward and creating an anorectal angle of 80 to 90 degrees. This angle, maintained by the continuous tonic activity of the puborectal muscle, is effective in preventing stool from entering the anal canal. Within the anal canal, the hemorrhoidal pillars contribute to continence by functioning as submucosal anal cushions, accounting for about 15% of anal resting pressure.[6]

The autonomically innervated internal anal sphincter is not subject to voluntary control. Under normal circumstances, tonic contraction of this muscle maintains approximately 55% of the anal canal resting pressure in a "high-pressure zone." The somatically innervated external sphincter contributes about 30% to resting anal pressure, and it accounts for all of the increase in pressure during voluntary contraction (squeeze pressure). The high resting pressure in the anal canal acts to preserve continence, preventing leakage of stool and gas.

When the rectum is distended, pressure receptors in the puborectalis stimulate the rectoanal inhibitory reflex. This reflex causes internal anal sphincter relaxation and external anal sphincter contraction, allowing the sensory epithelium of the anal canal to 'sample' anal canal contents without leakage. This allows discrimination of the nature of the material. If rectal distention is maintained—that is, defecation is deferred—the rectal vault relaxes, decreasing the rectal pressure in an *accommodation response*. Incontinence may occur with an abrupt and marked distention of the rectum that inhibits external sphincter contraction. Although volitional contraction

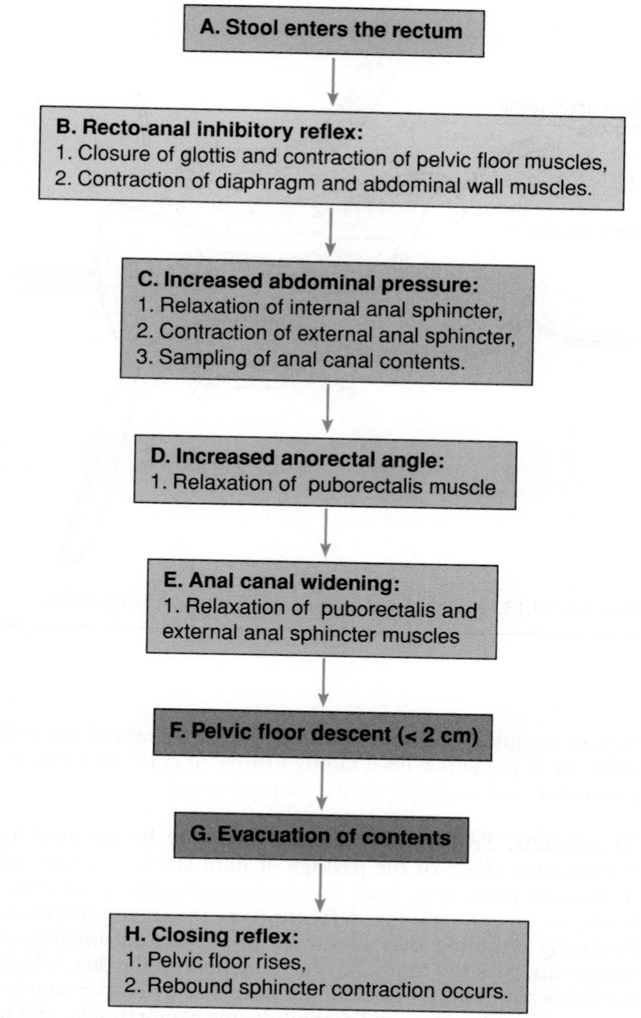
A. Stool enters the rectum
B. Recto-anal inhibitory reflex:
1. Closure of glottis and contraction of pelvic floor muscles,
2. Contraction of diaphragm and abdominal wall muscles.
C. Increased abdominal pressure:
1. Relaxation of internal anal sphincter,
2. Contraction of external anal sphincter,
3. Sampling of anal canal contents.
D. Increased anorectal angle:
1. Relaxation of puborectalis muscle
E. Anal canal widening:
1. Relaxation of puborectalis and external anal sphincter muscles
F. Pelvic floor descent (< 2 cm)
G. Evacuation of contents
H. Closing reflex:
1. Pelvic floor rises,
2. Rebound sphincter contraction occurs.

FIGURE 70.12. Mechanics of defecation.

of the external sphincter can be sustained only for short periods, it is the most important mechanism of voluntary continence and the last line of defense in the continence system.

Mechanism of Defecation. Defecation is a complex process that involves both reflex response and voluntary action (Fig. 70.12). When the anal canal is deemed to have solid contents and a decision to defecate is made, the subject assumes a squatting or sitting position to help straighten the anorectal angle and performs a Valsalva maneuver. With the glottis closed, there is contraction of diaphragm, abdominal wall muscles, and pelvic floor muscles, all increasing abdominal pressure. The puborectalis relaxes, resulting in further straightening of the anorectal angle, and the pelvic floor descends slightly. The external anal sphincter is relaxed, and the anus and rectum are evacuated. On completion of evacuation, the pelvic floor rises and sphincters contract once more in a closing reflex. The external sphincter is contracted voluntarily, and the normal postural tone of the internal sphincter and puborectalis is restored.

BENIGN ANORECTAL DISEASE

Hemorrhoids

In the upper anal canal, superior to the dentate line, the anal (hemorrhoidal) cushions are composed of three submucosal pillars of sinusoids within connective tissue, commonly at the left lateral, right anterior, and right posterior positions. The pathologic term *hemorrhoid* is used to describe the downward displacement of the cushion along with dilation of the contained sinusoids and sometimes bleeding from the arterial, venous, or sinusoidal portions.[7] Thus, hemorrhoids develop when the supporting tissues of the anal cushion deteriorate, or as a result of excessive downward pressure, as in prolonged straining at stool or pregnancy.

TABLE 70.1 CLASSIFICATION

GRADING OF INTERNAL HEMORRHOIDS

■ DEGREE	■ DESCRIPTION
First	Hemorrhoids bleed but do not prolapse
Second	Hemorrhoids prolapse on straining but reduce spontaneously
Third	Hemorrhoids prolapse and require manual reduction
Fourth	Prolapsed hemorrhoids cannot be manually reduced

Classification. *External hemorrhoids* are defined by their original location below the dentate line, i.e., they must be covered with squamous epithelium. Most external hemorrhoids are the external concomitants of internal hemorrhoids, so apart from thrombosis, there is practically no such thing as an independent external hemorrhoid problem. *Thrombosed external hemorrhoids* are intravascular clots in the sinusoids or venules of the external hemorrhoids. *Internal hemorrhoids* are the anal cushions defined by their original internal location—above the dentate line, thus covered with the epithelium of the transitional zone—that are prolapsing and/or bleeding.[8] For practical purposes, internal hemorrhoids are graded according to the degree of prolapse (Table 70.1).

Clinical Manifestations. Popular wisdom notwithstanding, the common complaints of burning, itching, swelling, and pain usually are not from internal hemorrhoids but result from other distinct conditions such as pruritus ani, anal abrasion, anal fissure, thrombosed external hemorrhoids, or prolapsed
1 anal papilla. The most common manifestations of internal hemorrhoids are painless, bright red rectal bleeding associated with bowel movements, and prolapse of tissue with defecation. Symptoms are aggravated by, but never the cause of, constipation and diarrhea. With significant hemorrhoids, the patient commonly describes blood dripping into the toilet bowl. A feeling of incomplete evacuation is also common. In chronic prolapse, exposed transitional mucosa often causes perianal skin irritation and mucous staining on underclothes. Congestion of external hemorrhoids can cause discomfort, and the related skin tags can be a hygiene problem. Except in the presence of obvious thrombosis, pain is rarely an early symptom of hemorrhoidal disease, and other diagnoses, most commonly anal fissure, should be sought and excluded.

Examination. Because many benign and malignant pathologic conditions are initially misdiagnosed as hemorrhoids, a thorough examination is critical for accurate diagnosis (Table 70.2). Although the examination can be performed in prone jackknife position, the left lateral or Sims position is usually less stressful and embarrassing to patients. The physician's discretion, sensitivity, and communication with the patient, for example warning the patient of pressure to the perineum or anus, makes effective examination more likely.

Anal skin tags, an external fistula opening, perianal excoriation from anal discharge, and anal fissure can be easily detected.

TABLE 70.2

THE COMPLETE DIGITAL RECTAL EXAMINATION

PREPARATION
Enema
Left lateral decubitus position
Lighting, gloves, lubrication, anoscope
VISUALIZATION
Distract the buttocks
Inspect for:
Soiling
Excoriation or abrasion
Scarring
Patulous anus, deformity or flattening of folds
Fissure
External fistula opening
Anal wink reflex
Prolapse through anus with strain
External hemorrhoids
PALPATION
Slow insertion of gloved, lubricated finger
Pain with exam
Palpable sphincter defect
Perineal body scarring
Anal stenosis
Relaxed or increased tone
Prostate abnormalities (men) or anterior rectocele (women)
Gross blood present
Muscle function: squeeze
Adequate
Accessory muscle use
Strain
Adequate
Puborectalis relaxation
Prolapsing tissue
Other organ prolapsed

The most accurate method of diagnosis for prolapsing hemorrhoids is to observe the patient straining on a commode.

Internal hemorrhoids are soft and usually cannot be palpated. Digital examination may detect anal stenosis or an anal scar. The anal sphincter tone and sphincter squeeze can be subjectively evaluated. A mass in the anal canal can be detected, and, in male patients, the prostate can and should be carefully examined.

After visual inspection and digital examination, anoscopy can be performed. Anoscopy should not be done in patients with acutely painful conditions such as fissure or perianal abscess; it can be deferred until the painful pathology has resolved. Inserting the anoscope reduces any hemorrhoidal prolapse, so anoscopy in a patient with symptomatic hemorrhoids typically shows only mucosal redundancy above the dentate line. Anoscopy may detect other lesions such as warts or a hypertrophic anal papilla.

Proctoscopy or flexible sigmoidoscopy should be used in all cases in which bleeding is present, to rule out polyps, carcinoma, and inflammatory bowel disease, which can have symptoms identical to hemorrhoidal complaints. Even in young patients, and even if the rectal bleeding is 'obviously' from hemorrhoids, a sigmoidoscopy has minimal risk and is a key component of complete examination. In patients 50 years of age and older, or in patients with a family history of colorectal cancer, a complete colonoscopy should be performed.

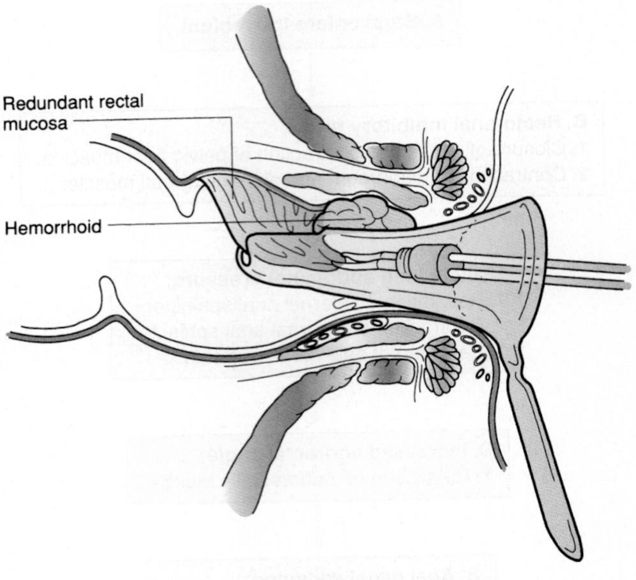

FIGURE 70.13. Rubber band ligation of an internal hemorrhoid.

Treatment. Prolapse of anal cushions may be initiated by the shearing effect of the passage of hard stool, by excessive downward pressure as with constipation, pregnancy, or childbirth, or by precipitous defecation as in urgent diarrhea. Reducing straining may eliminate prolapse and ameliorate symptoms, thus the rationale of adding fiber to the diet, which 2 produces soft, bulky stool. A high-fiber diet with fiber supplements is ideal for first- and second-degree hemorrhoids, and it is an important adjunct to surgical treatment.

3 **Rubber Band Ligation.** Rubber band ligation is suitable for symptomatic first-, second-, and some third-degree internal hemorrhoids that do not respond to fiber supplementation. The procedure is performed in the office through an anoscope, and bowel preparation is not needed. The band should be placed on the upper anal canal or distal rectal mucosa, after pinching to test for somatic sensation (Fig. 70.13). Ligation of up to three hemorrhoids at one setting has good results, and additional ligation can be performed 4 to 6 weeks later.

Rubber band ligation may be painless, but some patients may experience discomfort, aching, or an uncomfortable sense of rectal fullness. Warm sitz baths may help, and an appropriate analgesic should be prescribed. Immediate severe or progressive pain indicates a misplaced band too close to the dentate line and requires immediate removal of the rubber band with a pointed (no. 11) blade or band cutter. Delayed anal pain, urinary retention, and fever suggest infection, which while very rare can be life threatening. Prompt and aggressive treatment includes antibiotics and examination in the operating room, with drainage and débridement as necessary. A large retrospective review indicated a cumulative success rate of 80% for symptomatic relief of all grades of internal hemorrhoids, with a 30% recurrence rate after the first banding episode. Postbanding complication rates were 2.8% for bleeding, 1.5% for thrombosis, and 0.09% for bacteremia.[9]

Sclerotherapy. Sclerotherapy with various substances (phenol, olive oil, sodium tetradecyl sulfate) can be performed in the office setting for first- or second-degree hemorrhoids in conjunction with banding, or for bleeding hemorrhoids that are too small to band. Using an anoscope, a narrow-gauge needle is used to inject 1 to 2 mL of sclerosant in the submucosal space just proximal to the hemorrhoidal bundle.

Infrared Photocoagulation and Electrosurgery. Infrared photocoagulation coagulates tissue protein or evaporates water in the cells, depending on the intensity and duration of application. As in sclerotherapy, an infrared probe is applied just proximal to the internal hemorrhoids through an anoscope. Infrared photocoagulation results for first- and second-degree hemorrhoids are comparable with those of rubber band ligation. Pain and complications are infrequent. An electrocautery unit works as well.

4 **Hemorrhoidectomy.** Hemorrhoidectomy should be considered when the hemorrhoids are mixed internal and external, are severely prolapsed through the anus, or are complicated by associated pathology, such as ulceration, fissures, fistulas, large hypertrophied anal papillae, or extensive skin tags. In many cases, hemorrhoidectomy can be performed using local anesthesia with monitored sedation. In obese individuals, general or spinal anesthesia may be easier. The patient is placed in the prone jackknife position with buttocks taped apart for visualization. An elliptical excision starts at the anoderm, includes external and internal hemorrhoidal components, and ends at the anorectal ring. One to three quadrants are most typically addressed, starting with the largest. It is important to spare all possible anoderm to avoid anal stricture. The mucosa and submucosa are dissected off of the underlying internal sphincter muscle (Fig. 70.14). Excessive bleeding indicates that the hemorrhoidal plexus is being violated, suggesting the dissection is too superficial. Alternatively, excising too deeply damages the internal sphincter fibers. Unless there is an associated anal stenosis or chronic anal fissure, internal sphincterotomy is never performed. The entire wound is closed with running absorbable suture and dressed with ointment, a fluff dressing to the perineum, and mesh shorts.

Urinary retention is a common complication of hemorrhoidectomy, and it can be minimized by restricting intravenous fluids during and after the procedure. Warm sitz baths can be started the next morning, and patients may use a gentle laxative as necessary.

Stapled Anopexy. The Longo stapled anopexy, known as PPH (Procedure for Prolapse and Hemorrhoids) is a significant innovation in the treatment for prolapsing internal hemorrhoids. Instead of removing columns of hemorrhoidal tissue, this operation removes a sleeve of the distalmost rectal mucosa and submucosa, elevating the anal canal and fixing it in place (hence *anopexy*) and radically reducing the redundancy of the mucosa. The conceptual advantage is that the incision is all proximal to the dentate line, so it should hurt much less than a standard hemorrhoidectomy. The PPH procedure is done by placing a purse-string suture in the submucosa 4 to 5 cm proximal to the dentate line (Fig. 70.15). The purse string is tightened as the specially designed circular stapler is inserted into the rectum. After the anvil passes proximal to the purse string, the suture ends are pulled through channels in the stapler to use as stay sutures and manipulate the redundant rectal mucosa. The stapler is closed and fired, and pressure is held to aid in hemostasis. In female patients, one must ascertain before firing that no vaginal tissue is caught in the staple line. After stapler withdrawal, additional sutures are often required to assist with hemostasis.

A randomized trial comparing the PPH procedure with rubber band ligation found significantly increased pain and morbidity using the stapler but significantly increased recurrent bleeding with banding.[10] A systematic review of 15 randomized trials of stapled anopexy compared to excisional hemorrhoidectomy demonstrated significantly shorter operative time (weighted mean difference, −13 minutes), return to work (−4 days), and significantly decreased pain.[11] At 6 months postoperatively, odds of recurrent symptoms using this technique were calculated at 3.64 compared with conventional excision. A report of 1-year follow-up from a randomized trial of the stapled technique versus conventional hemorrhoidectomy reported similar significant short-term benefits.[12]

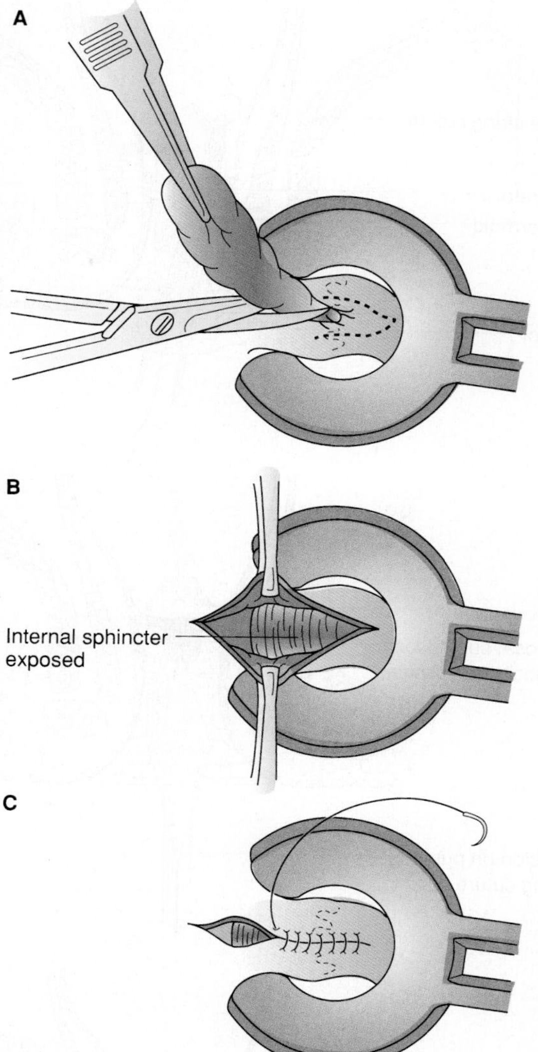

FIGURE 70.14. Technique of interanal closed hemorrhoidectomy. **A:** Exposure of hemorrhoid with elliptic excision starting at perianal skin and extending to anorectal ring. **B:** Submucosal hemorrhoidal plexus dissected from the internal sphincter, anoderm, and mucosa. **C:** Wound closed with a running suture.

Management of Special Hemorrhoid Situations

Thrombosed External Hemorrhoids. Thrombosis is a fairly common complication of hemorrhoidal disease, often appearing as an independent problem, apparently unrelated to internal hemorrhoids. The reason for the acute thrombosis is usually unknown. There is an abrupt onset of anal mass and pain that peaks within 48 hours. Usually, the pain then recedes, leaving a subcutaneous lump. Sometimes the skin overlying the clot becomes necrotic, leading to bleeding and eventual extrusion of the clot. Treatment is aimed at relief of pain, prevention of recurrent thrombosis, and (though this is of secondary importance) prevention of residual skin tags. If the patient presents with severe pain, the thrombosis should be excised in the office or emergency room. This can usually be done under local anesthesia, and the wound is left open without packing. The pain of

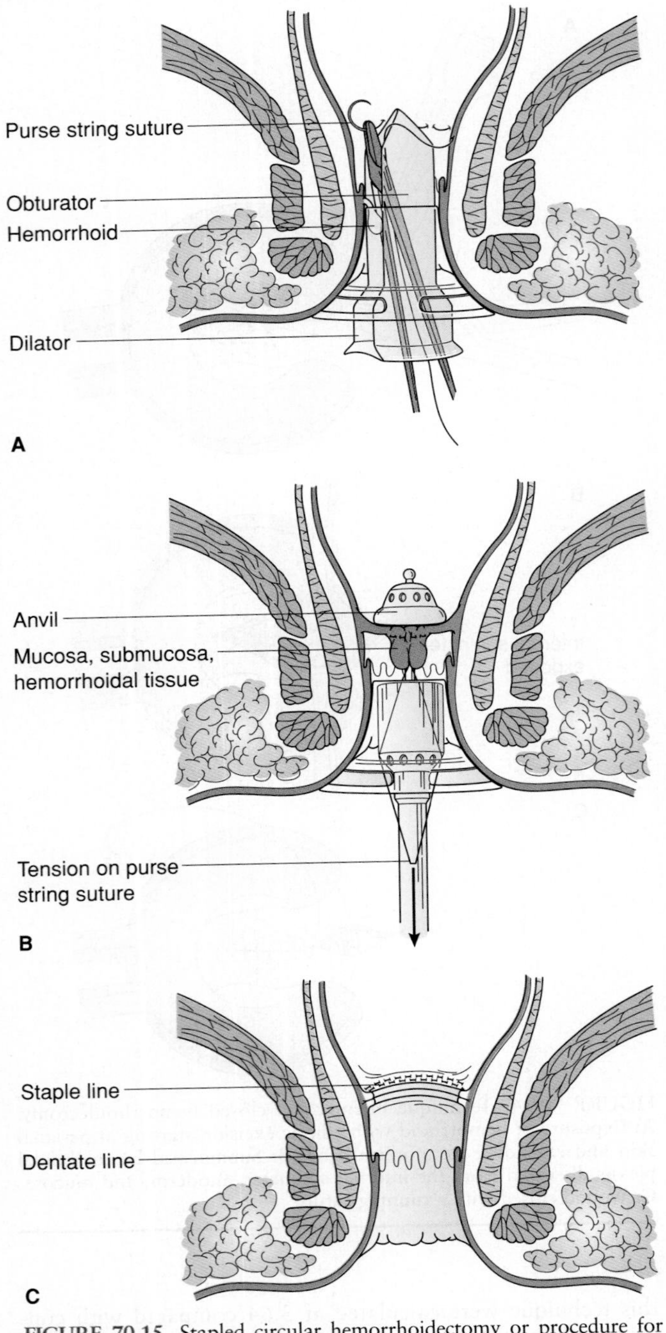

FIGURE 70.15. Stapled circular hemorrhoidectomy or procedure for prolapsing hemorrhoids. **A:** A purse-string suture is placed in the rectal mucosa proximal to hemorrhoids. **B:** The stapler anvil is placed proximal to the purse string, and the purse string is tied down to draw hemorrhoidal tissue into the staple line. **C:** The stapler is fired and removed, excising a sleeve of distal rectal tissue and creating a stapled anastomosis.

incision is usually eclipsed by the relief of pain from the thrombosis, so patients often experience dramatic relief. However, if the pain is already subsiding and the clot resolving, patients may be managed expectantly with warm sitz baths for comfort and fiber supplementation to bulk and soften stool. Patients must be warned of a relatively high recurrence rate of acute thrombosis: 6% after excision and 25% after expectant treatment.[13]

Incarcerated Hemorrhoids. Incarceration indicates irreducibly prolapsed, fourth-degree hemorrhoids. This is the one situation in which internal hemorrhoids cause pain. The diagnosis is obvious on examination: edematous internal hemorrhoids protrude from the anus, usually with large external components as well. Pain is usually severe and urinary retention is common. Untreated, incarceration may progress to strangulation with mucosal necrosis. Treatment is urgent or emergency hemorrhoidectomy. As in other hemorrhoid procedures, antibiotics are not indicated.

Hemorrhoids in Pregnancy and Postpartum. Hemorrhoids can occur as the result of downward pressure from a gravid uterus or from prolonged labor and may be exacerbated by hormonal changes. For thrombosed external hemorrhoids, symptomatic internal hemorrhoids, or incarcerated hemorrhoids, standard treatment can be performed safely and should not be withheld. Left lateral decubitus position is usually recommended in the third trimester.

Bleeding Rectal Varices from Portal Hypertension. The incidence of hemorrhoidal disease of the anus in portal hypertension is no greater than in the normal population. Although uncommon, bleeding from rectal varices in patients with portal hypertension can be life threatening and may initially simulate hemorrhoidal bleeding. Transanal suture of the bleeding vessel should incorporate mucosa, submucosa, and muscular wall of the rectum. This should be done in the operating room, ideally after correcting any coagulopathy. Rubber band ligation and hemorrhoidectomy should not be done on the bleeding portal hypertensive patient, because they create more bleeding opportunities and do not address the source of bleeding. Local control of rectal and anal varices may be achieved by using the PPH anopexy as a devascularization procedure,[14] but definitive control of varices requires reduction of elevated portal pressures by transjugular intrahepatic portosystemic shunting (TIPS) or liver transplantation.

Hemorrhoids in Inflammatory Bowel Disease. Hemorrhoidal problems in inflammatory bowel disease are uncommon. Most anal problems are either inflammatory (anal fistula, atypical fissure, etc.) or the result of diarrhea causing perianal irritation, rather than the result of hemorrhoids themselves. Treating the primary disease symptomatically usually suffices to control secondary anal symptoms. Rubber band ligation, hemorrhoidectomy, and stapled anopexy should almost never be done on the inflammatory bowel disease patient.

Rectal Prolapse

5 Rectal prolapse (procidentia) is an uncommon condition in which the rectum intussuscepts into itself and prolapses through the anal canal. Although the diagnosis is usually obvious, one may have to distinguish early rectal prolapse from severely prolapsed hemorrhoids. Full-thickness rectal prolapse displays concentric circular folds, whereas mucosal prolapse displays radially oriented folds. Rectal prolapse has a female-to-male ratio of at least 5:1. Perhaps associated with dysfunctional bowel habits or with constipating psychotropic medications, rectal prolapse is seen disproportionately among patients with dementia, mental retardation, and schizophrenia.

Pathophysiology.

The cause of rectal intussusception and prolapse is not understood. Intussusception usually starts in the anterior rectum. Many patients with rectal prolapse have a history of constipation and straining or, less commonly, chronic diarrhea. Studies of anorectal function and defecation dynamics reveal that these patients have impaired resting and voluntary sphincter activity, decreased functional rectal capacity, impaired continence, and puborectalis dyssynergy (inappropriate contraction) during defecation. Loss of continence is caused by reduced sphincter tone due to mechanical stretching

TABLE 70.3 **ETIOLOGY**

ANATOMIC DEFECTS OR ABNORMALITIES IN PATIENTS WITH CHRONIC RECTAL PROLAPSE

- Abnormally deep rectovaginal or rectovesical pouch
- Lax and atonic musculature of the pelvic floor
- Lack of normal fixation of the rectum and an elongated mesorectum
- Unusually redundant sigmoid colon
- Lax and atonic anal sphincter

by the prolapsed bowel, traction injury to the pudendal nerves, and loss of normal sensation.

Anatomic Abnormalities. Several anatomic defects or abnormalities are consistently demonstrated in patients with chronic rectal prolapse (Table 70.3). These defects are seen concurrently with long-standing prolapse, making the distinction between cause and effect difficult.

Solitary rectal ulcer syndrome is a vexing condition associated with occult or overt prolapse, in which there is bleeding, tenesmus, and an anterior rectal ulcer that may appear proliferative, like a polyp or cancer.

Evaluation. Physical examination reveals a patulous anus with decreased sphincter tone. When the prolapse itself is not obvious, it is best demonstrated by asking the patient to strain while seated on a commode. Anoscopy or rigid proctoscopy may demonstrate associated conditions, such as anterior rectal erythema or ulceration. Anal manometry documents baseline function preoperatively but does not help predict the outcome of surgery. Cinedefecography confirms the diagnosis of intussusception when in doubt (Fig. 70.16) and it can detect other anatomic and functional abnormalities such as nonrelaxing puborectalis muscle or enterocele. Colonoscopy is indicated to evaluate bleeding and to rule out a cancer or polyp as the lead point for intussusception, a rare but not unheard of condition.

Treatment. Acute prolapse should be reduced with steady manual pressure to prevent incarceration and strangulation. Reduction of an edematous, incarcerated prolapse can be facilitated by application of granulated table sugar. Operations generally suspend or remove the intussuscepting rectum. Methods of repair are abdominal and perineal, the former represented by rectopexy (open or laparoscopic, with or without a concomitant sigmoid resection) and the latter represented by the Altemeier perineal proctectomy and Delorme plication. Abdominal operations generally have recurrence rates less than 10% and are used in fit patients. Transperineal operations have recurrence rates of 15% to 20% (or more in some series) and are most appropriate in patients at high risk for complications of abdominal surgery. Perineal operations are often recommended to young men in an effort to avoid sexual dysfunction following a pelvic dissection, but few comparative data are available. Female sexual function is poorly described following either abdominal or perineal repairs.

Transabdominal rectopexy involves a full mobilization of the rectum to the level of the pelvic floor musculature with suture fixation of the mesorectum to the presacral fascia below the sacral promontory (Fig. 70.17). The recurrence rate has been reported to be 6% to 9% with up to 10-year follow-up.[15] Suture rectopexy is associated with symptomatic constipation in about 50% of cases.[16] About 50% of rectal prolapse patients with fecal incontinence improve after prolapse repair. Because return of continence may take 6 to 12 months, any operation to treat incontinence should be deferred for a year after a successful prolapse repair.

A multicenter cohort study of abdominal approaches to prolapse repair found pooled 5- and 10-year recurrence rates of 7% and 29%, respectively. No recurrence difference was identified based on performance of mobilization, resection, or rectopexy; that is, mobilization-only had the same recurrence rate as mobilization-resection-rectopexy, nor was there a difference in recurrence between suture and mesh rectopexy or between laparoscopic and open approaches.[17] These findings support the notion that prolapse is probably alleviated by formation of presacral adhesions during the postoperative period.

Perineal rectosigmoidectomy (Altemeier operation) is a transanal approach in which the prolapsed rectum and redundant sigmoid colon are excised endorectally, analogous to vaginal hysterectomy. The operation is performed with the patient in the lithotomy (Fig. 70.18) or prone jackknife position. Patients tolerate this operation well, with minimal postoperative pain. A levatorplasty (anterior, posterior, or both) can be performed via the same incision and may help recreate the anorectal angle. Several series report a recurrence rate of about 16% with a relatively short-term follow-up.[18] Major long-term complications include recurrence, fecal urgency due to the smaller sigmoid reservoir after rectal excision, tenesmus, and anastomotic stricture—in other words, the complications of any anterior rectal resection.

The Delorme procedure is another transperineal approach. This is used for rectal near-prolapse (internal intussusception) or for overt prolapse. With the patient in the prone position, the redundant submucosa is stripped circumferentially using electrocautery, continuing proximally until it is taut. The submucosal tube is then transected and the proximal end anastomosed to the dentate line. The denuded rectal wall is incorporated into the suture line with reefing bites to eliminate dead space (Fig. 70.19). Like perineal rectosigmoidectomy, this procedure causes little pain, but it has a high recurrence rate.

A reasonable approach to the problem of rectal prolapse is to use a perineal operation for older, sicker patients and an abdominal approach for younger, healthier ones. The uncertain

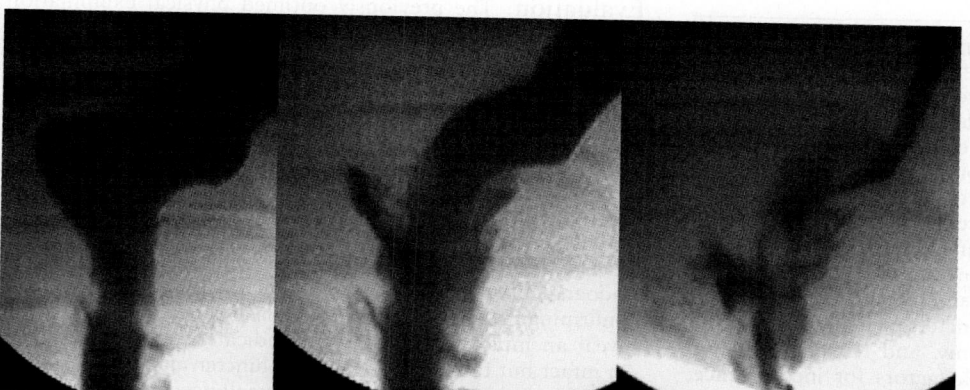

FIGURE 70.16. Cinedefecography demonstrating internal rectal prolapse, or intussusception. (Figure courtesy of Susan Congilosi Parker, M.D.)

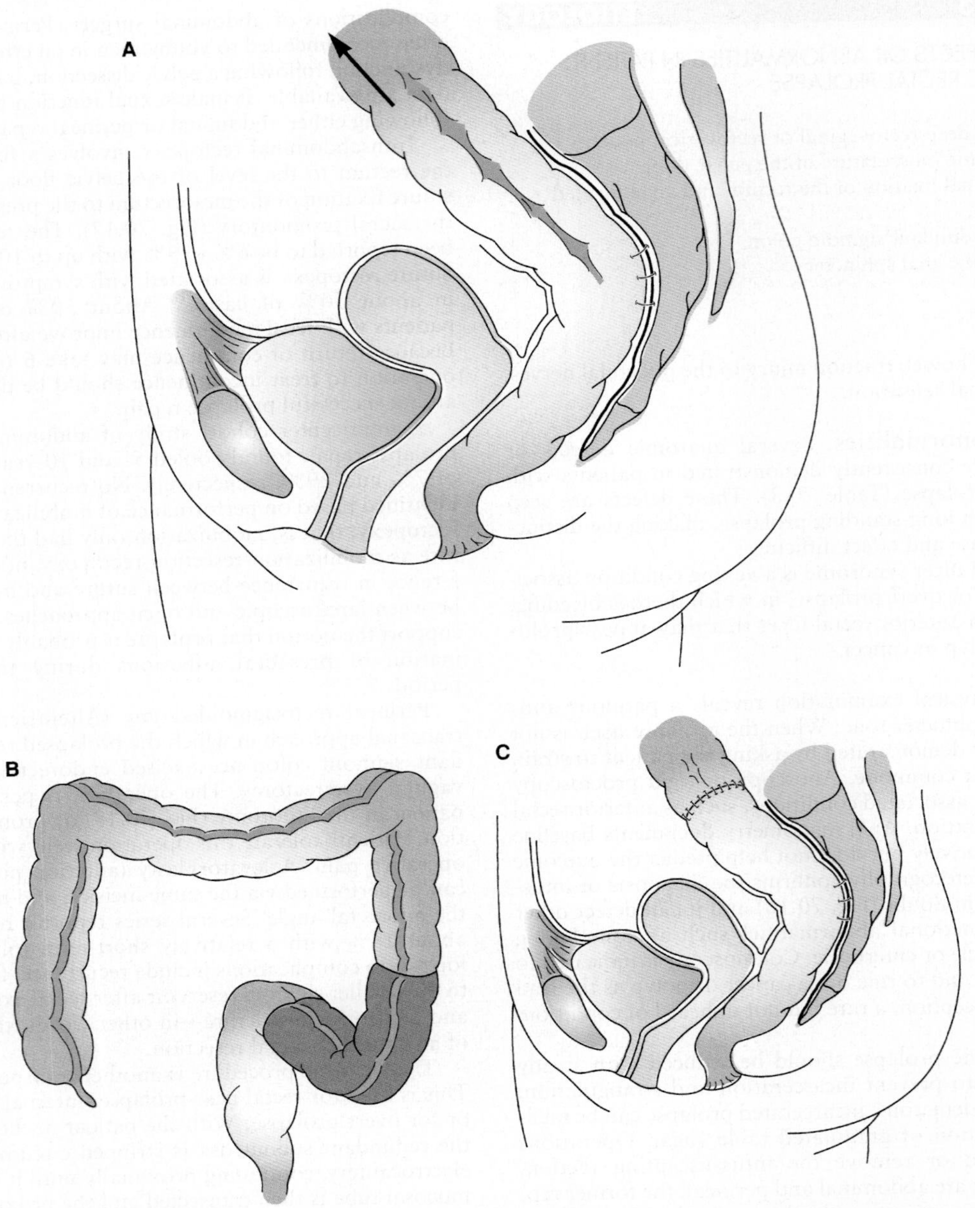

FIGURE 70.17. Transabdominal rectopexy. After full mobilization of the rectum, the endorectal fascia and peritoneum on each side is sutured to presacral fascia, below the promontory of the sacrum.

nature of functional results (constipation, incontinence) should be shared with patients in preoperative discussion.

Anal Incontinence

Definition and Etiology. *Anal incontinence* describes a spectrum of functional impairment that ranges from involuntary passage of flatus to involuntary passage of formed stool. Almost any loss or disturbance of normal anatomy or function—postresection loss of reservoir function, rectal inflammation, and so on—may result in anal incontinence. Disturbance of anorectal sensation may prevent awareness of stool and lead to leakage. A bolus of diarrheal stool emptying rapidly into the rectum may overcome anal continence, even in healthy people. Common mechanical injuries to the sphincters include obstetric tear, fistulotomy, internal sphincterotomy, and trauma. Age and female sex are the two major risk factors for incontinence; these have an important but poorly understood interaction. Incontinence may not manifest for two or more decades after obstetric injury.

Evaluation. The previously outlined physical examination (Table 70.2) can help to differentiate the presence of a neurologic or muscular problem. For example, a patulous or lax anus may indicate neurogenic dysfunction of the sphincter muscles. A scar or defect in the anal region may indicate old surgical injury, and a thin perineal body suggests an obstetric sphincter injury.

In addition to history and physical examination, several anatomic and physiologic tests can be done. The most useful of these, endoanal ultrasonography, provides a circumferential anatomic image of the internal and external sphincter. Endoanal ultrasound can clarify and map sphincter defects, confirming the need for sphincteroplasty, and conversely it can reveal an intact sphincter, contraindicating sphincteroplasty. An intact but thinned portion of sphincter may be due to denervation, which is suggested by a prolonged pudendal nerve

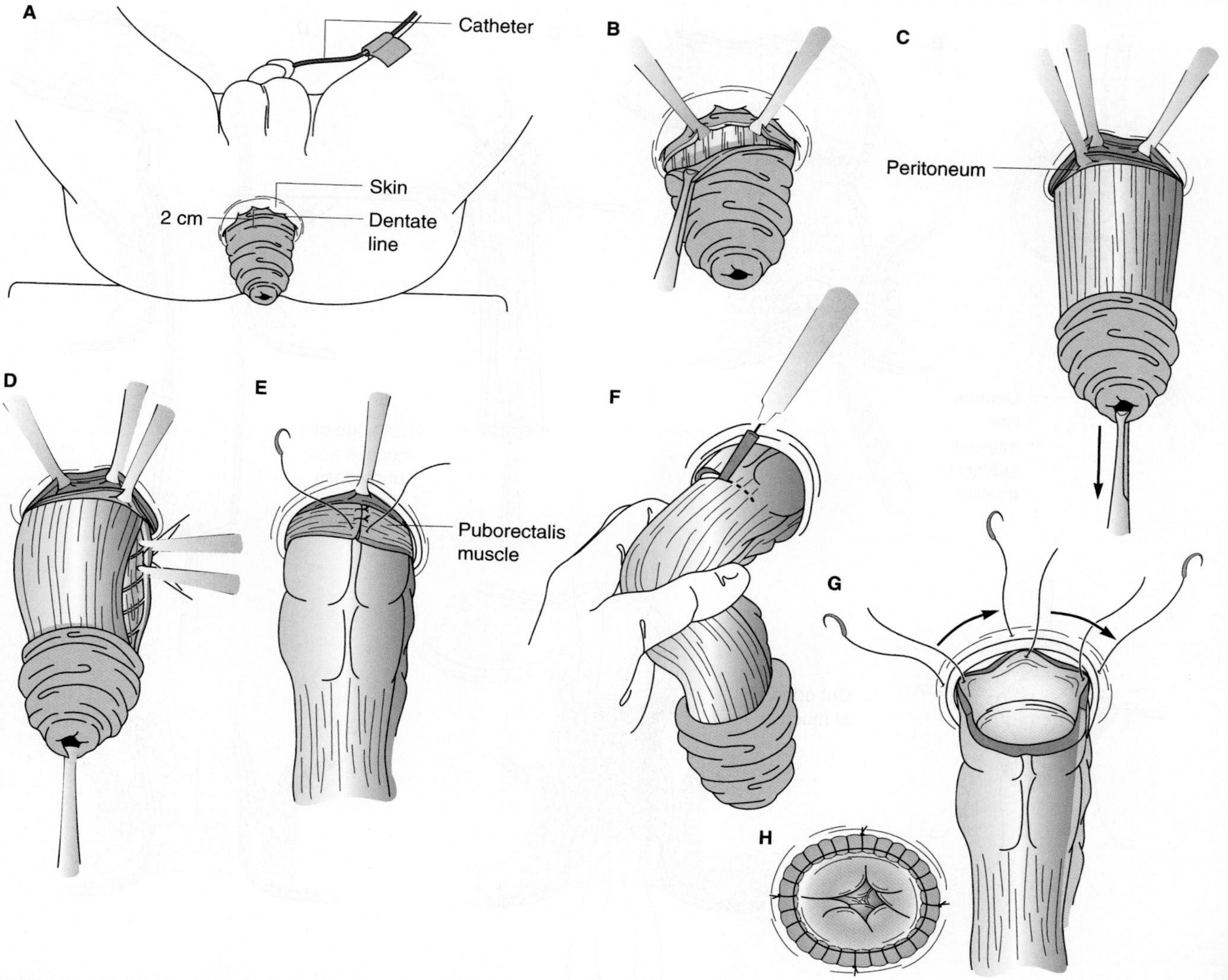

FIGURE 70.18. Perineal rectosigmoidectomy. The patient is placed in the lithotomy position with both legs in gynecologic stirrups. **A** and **B:** A circular incision is made on the prolapsed rectum 2 cm proximal to the dentate line. **C:** The peritoneal attachment is dissected from the anterior rectal wall, thus opening into the peritoneal cavity. **D:** The mesorectum or mesosigmoid is clamped and divided laterally and posteriorly. **E:** This is followed by approximation of the puborectalis. **F:** The anterior wall of the protruding rectum is cut 1 cm distal to the anal verge. **G:** Stay sutures of 3-0 synthetic absorbable material are placed in four quadrants. **H:** Anastomosis with running stitches.

terminal motor latency. Anal manometry establishes baseline resting and squeeze pressures, although results do not correlate well with operative outcomes. Defecography can aid operative planning by identifying previously unrecognized disorders such as rectocele or internal intussusception. None of these tests by itself correlates with incontinence, and fully continent control subjects may also have sphincter defects and manometric abnormalities, so treatment is still geared to the patient's symptoms.

The clinical evaluation of anal incontinence ideally includes an assessment of symptom severity and quality of life. With the same degree of objective incontinence, patients' subjective experience can be surprisingly different. For example, one patient may be housebound because of fear of minor soiling, whereas another patient may make little change in her or his daily activities despite occasional episodes of complete incontinence. Because anal incontinence is more a quality of life problem than a health risk, the patient ultimately determines the need for intervention. Although a formal, validated assessment of quality of life and symptom severity is not necessary, it can help by establishing a baseline score for later comparison. Several validated severity and quality of life scores are available.[19]

Management. One of the key early steps in incontinence treatment is medical regulation of bowel habits, with the goal of decreasing bowel movements to once a day or every other day. Sometimes this simple intervention resolves chronic, difficult symptoms. A high-fiber diet and the use of fiber supplements lead to bulkier stools, which are easier to sense and to control. Antidiarrheal drugs such as loperamide, diphenoxylate, and bile acid binders make stool harder and less frequent, thus easier for the marginal or damaged sphincter to handle.

Biofeedback physical therapy can be used to regain anorectal sensation and to retrain coordinated contraction/relaxation of the pelvic floor and sphincter muscles. Biofeedback training can help up to 85% of patients with anal incontinence, though some of this effect is likely due to the associated counseling and dietary management.[20,21] Most systems include a balloon catheter and pressure transducer. While the patient watches the manometry tracings, the balloon is inflated, and the patient is coached to contract the external sphincter muscle, elevating

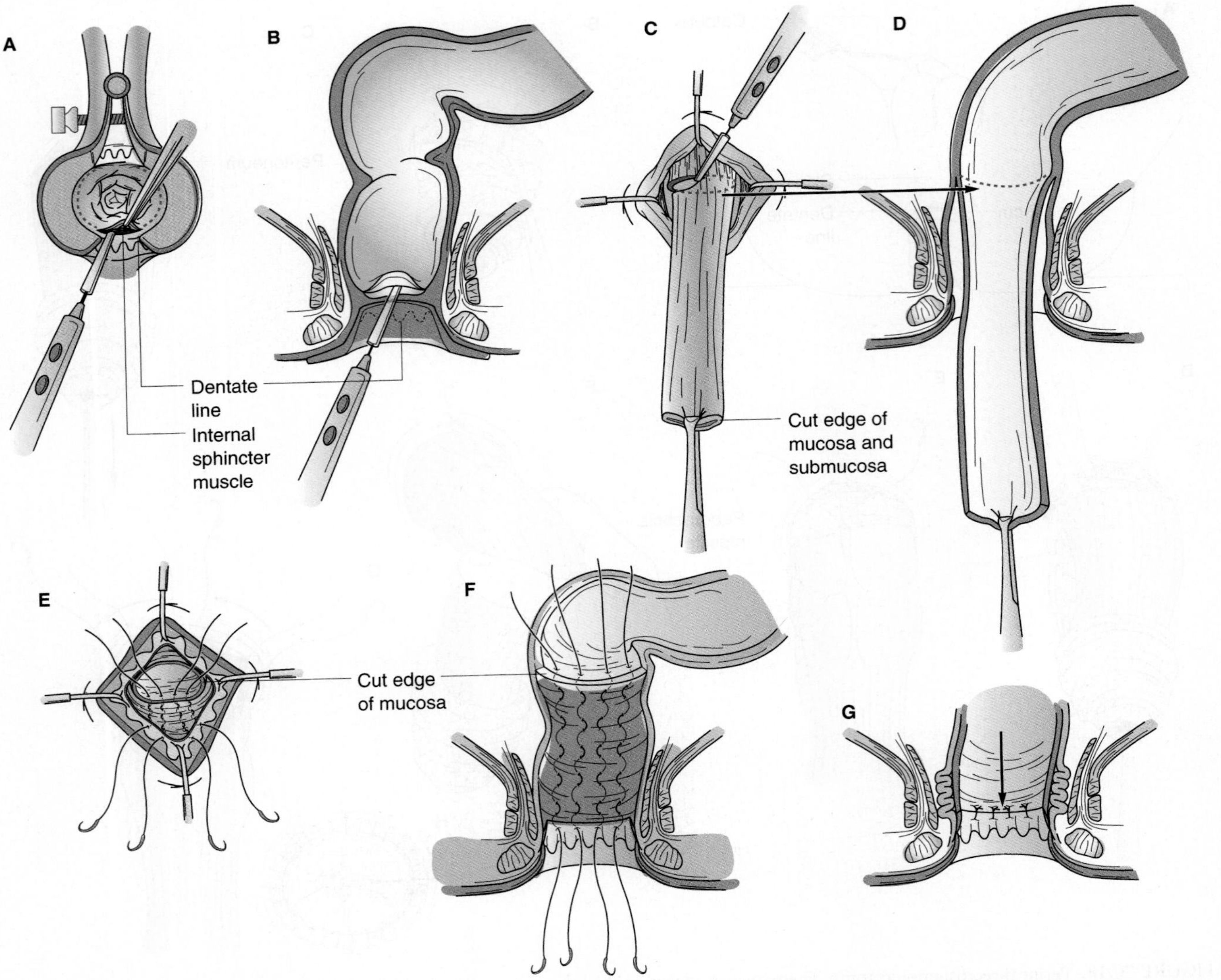

FIGURE 70.19. Modified Delorme procedure. Patient is placed in the prone position. A and B: With a Pratt speculum used for exposure, a circumferential incision is made 1 cm proximal to the dentate line. The submucosa is dissected from the underlying internal sphincter. At the level of the anorectal ring, the Pratt speculum is replaced by Gelpi retractors placed at a right angle to the dentate line. C and D: Proximal to the anorectal ring, the dissection continues in the mucosal plane until the mucosa resists being pulled down. The mucosal tube is then cut. E and F: With 3-0 synthetic absorbable sutures, the mucosa at the upper cut end is brought down to the mucosa at the lower cut end, taking along the denuded anorectal wall. Eight such sutures are placed all around. G: At completion of the anastomosis, the anorectum is plicated.

the tracing. It may take several biofeedback sessions before the patient is aware of the sensation of a full rectum and can contract the sphincter effectively.

Operation is reserved for refractory incontinence. Sphincteroplasty is most suitable for incontinence from obstetric injury or injury after previous anorectal surgery, if there has been preoperative documentation of a sphincter defect. A curved incision is made over the sphincter disruption, parallel to the anal verge. The sphincters are mobilized laterally to allow an overlapping plication with mattress suture, and after plication the anus should still permit digitation (Fig. 70.20). Simultaneous levatorplasty can help support the repair and lengthen the anal canal, but it may contribute to postoperative dyspareunia. Overlapping sphincteroplasty yields short-term improvement in about 85% of patients, but only 40% maintain continence over a 10-year period.[22] Risk of functional failure increased with patient age.

Another sphincter substitute is the artificial anal sphincter (Acticon Neosphincter, American Medical Systems, Minnetonka, MN; Fig. 70.21), the only such device approved by the U.S. Food and Drug Administration (FDA). With a pump in the labium majus or scrotum, a retropubic reservoir, and an inflatable silicone cuff around the upper anal canal, the artificial sphincter can provide satisfactory continence for many patients who have failed or are not amenable to more conventional therapy[23,24] Reoperation is required in about half of patients, primarily because of infection, and this usually necessitates removal of the device. Cuff implantation can be technically difficult due to the common history of multiple previous operations, and success rates are best in the hands of surgeons who are highly experienced with the technique.

Sacral nerve stimulation (SNS) is a novel intervention for anal incontinence that has the advantage of avoiding surgery in the anal region altogether. A quadripolar lead is implanted using a percutaneous technique, most commonly in one of the S3 foramina. The procedure is usually performed under monitored local anesthesia. The patient undergoes a period of test stimulation to assess the effect of stimulation; if continence is significantly improved, a pulse generator is implanted in the buttock at a second operation. The exact mechanism of action

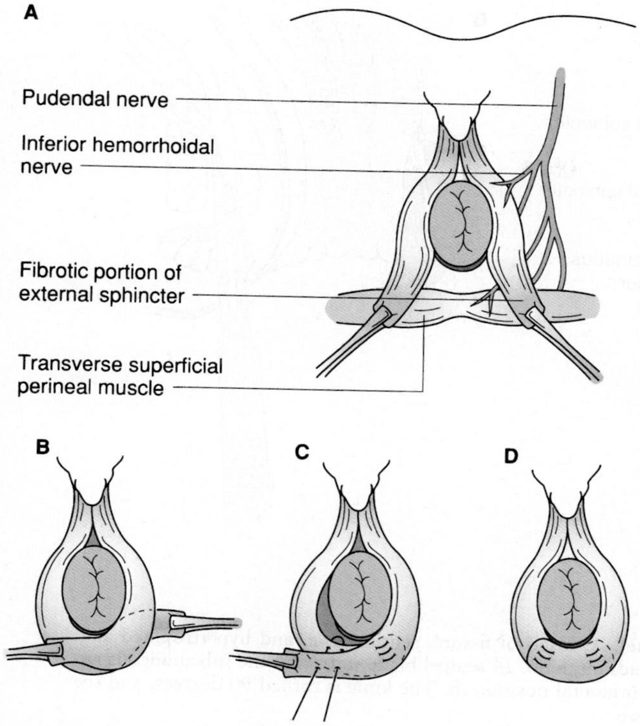

FIGURE 70.20. Overlapping anal sphincteroplasty.

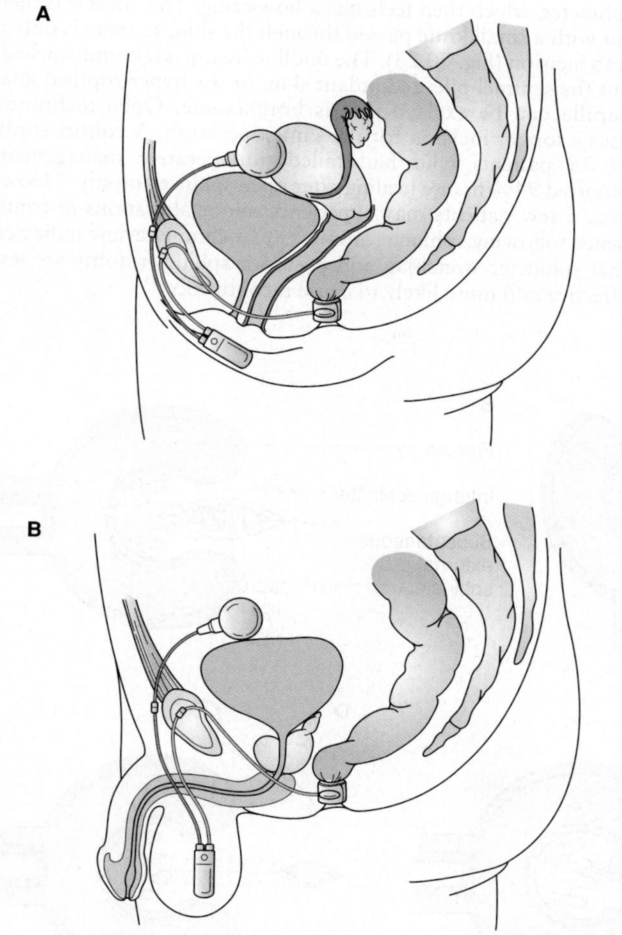

FIGURE 70.21. Implanted silicone neosphincter. **A:** Female. **B:** Male.

for SNS is uncertain. Impressive results have been reported for incontinent patients with and without sphincter defects, and associated morbidity is low.[25] However, at the time of this writing, the FDA has not yet approved SNS for treatment of anal incontinence in the United States.

For patients with refractory and incapacitating anal incontinence, a permanent end-sigmoid colostomy remains a relatively simple and low-risk solution that is generally associated with high patient satisfaction and an improved quality of life.

Anal Fissure

6 **Definition.** Anal fissure is an ulcer in the lower anal canal. Fissures are acute or chronic, primary or secondary. A primary fissure arises without association to other local or systemic disease, whereas a secondary fissure may be due to Crohn disease or ulcerative colitis. Atypical anal ulcers, especially those off the midline, may be due to HIV, anal cancer, tuberculosis, syphilis, or hematologic malignancy.

Pathophysiology. Studies show that resting anal pressure (internal sphincter tone) in patients with anal fissure is significantly higher than normal, whereas squeeze pressure (external sphincter contraction) is normal. Doppler flowmetry has shown anal canal perfusion to be poorest posteriorly, with reduced anodermal blood flow at fissure sites, suggesting that chronic nonhealing fissures are caused and maintained by ischemia. Reduction of anal pressure by sphincterotomy improves anodermal blood flow, resulting in fissure healing.[26]

Clinical Manifestations. Anal pain, particularly during and after bowel movement, is the most prominent symptom, followed by bleeding with defecation. Anal fissure pain can be severe and incapacitating. Constipation is a common association, both as a precipitating event and as a result of deferring painful defecation.

Diagnosis. Although pain and bleeding are typical of anal fissure, the diagnosis is confirmed by examination. When performed gently, inspection by spreading the buttocks will reveal the fissure in most cases. In general, digital and anoscopic examinations are deferred when a fissure is diagnosed because they are too painful. In men, almost all fissures are located in the posterior midline, whereas 10% of fissures in women are in the anterior midline. The *sentinel pile*, a protruding tag at the distal end of the fissure, is often the presenting complaint (a 'painful hemorrhoid'), and patients with anal fissures frequently have an associated hypertrophic anal papilla at the dentate line.

Management. Initial treatment of acute anal fissure is pain relief, with warm sitz baths to relax the anal canal. Application of topical anesthetic gel or ointment directly to the fissure before bowel movement is sometimes helpful. Bulking and softening the stool with fiber supplementation and increased water intake (8–10 glasses/day) is the mainstay of therapy. Acute anal fissures should heal within 6 weeks.

For chronic anal fissure, a reasonable first treatment is the application of 0.2% nitroglycerine or 2% diltiazem ointment directly to the fissure. Both medications reduce anal resting pressure and increase anodermal blood flow. Patients should be warned of possible associated headaches with nitroglycerine; the standard commercially available nitroglycerine ointment is 2%, too strong for topical perianal use, so it must be diluted. Fissure resolution after 6 weeks of topical treatment has been reported at 50% to 75%, but up to half of these will recur. Botulinum toxin A injection into the internal sphincter is another approach to reduce internal anal sphincter hypertonicity,

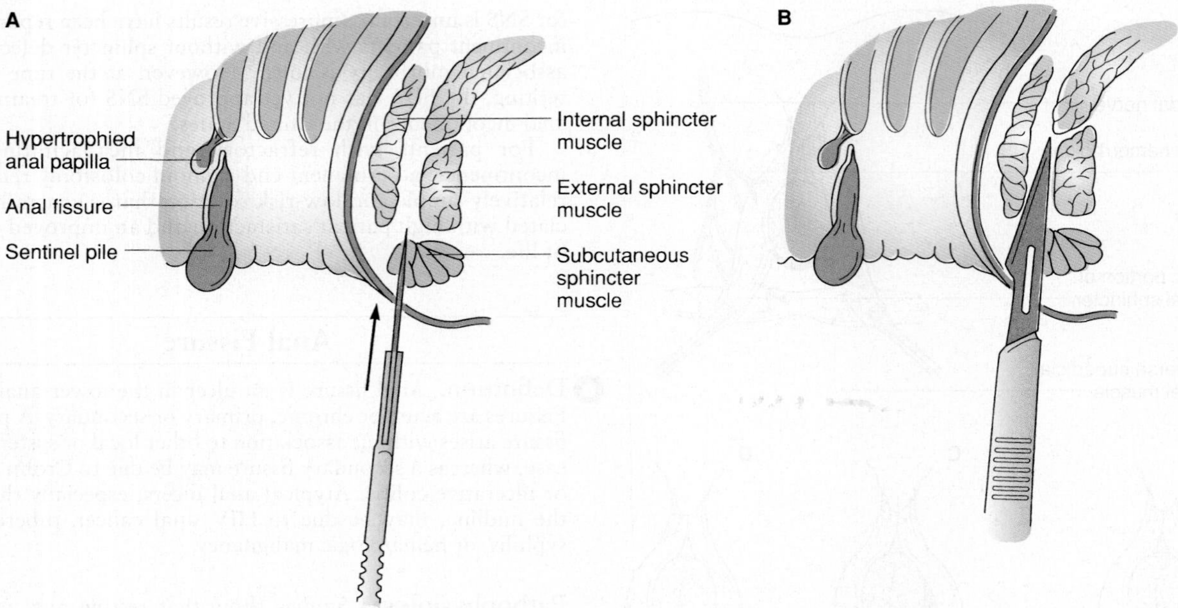

FIGURE 70.22. Lateral internal sphincterotomy (closed technique). A: Triad of fissure, sentinel pile, and hypertrophied anal papilla. With an anal speculum used for exposure of the lateral quadrant, a no. 11 scalpel blade stabs into the subcutaneous tissue from the anal verge to the dentate line, with the knife in the horizontal position. B: The knife is turned 90 degrees, and the internal sphincter muscle is cut while the anal canal is stretched open.

although technique, dose, and success rates have varied significantly. A cohort study of patients treated with botulinum toxin for fissure demonstrated 42% recurrence at a median of 42 months.[27] Potential ill effects of botulinum injection include transitory incontinence (up to 3 months), hematoma, thrombosis, and infection.

Lateral internal sphincterotomy, under local, spinal, or general anesthesia, is the next step for the unhealed chronic anal fissure refractory to medical therapy (Fig. 70.22).[28] Lateral internal sphincterotomy is also indicated in patients whose pain is too severe to tolerate a trial of medical therapy. This is an outpatient procedure that can be performed under local, regional, or general anesthesia. In the closed method of sphincterotomy, a speculum is opened gradually wider, stretching the internal sphincter, which then feels like a bowstring. This muscle is then cut with a small knife passed through the skin, so there is only a stab incision (Fig. 70.23). The midline fissure is left undisturbed, but the sentinel pile, redundant skin, or the hypertrophied anal papilla can be excised if it is bothersome. Open technique uses a longer incision for the same operation. A cohort study of 35 patients who had failed nonoperative management reported 94% fissure healing after open sphincterotomy.[29] However, a few patients may experience minor alterations in continence following sphincterotomy.[30] A Cochrane review indicated that sphincter stretching and posterior sphincterotomy are less effective and more likely to cause incontinence.[31]

FIGURE 70.23. Lateral internal sphincterotomy (open method). A: The fissure in the midline is left alone. B: With a speculum used to expose the left lateral quadrant, an incision is made through the subcutaneous tissue to expose both the subcutaneous external sphincter and the internal sphincter. C: The internal sphincter is incised to its full thickness; care is taken not to cut the external sphincter. D: The wound is closed.

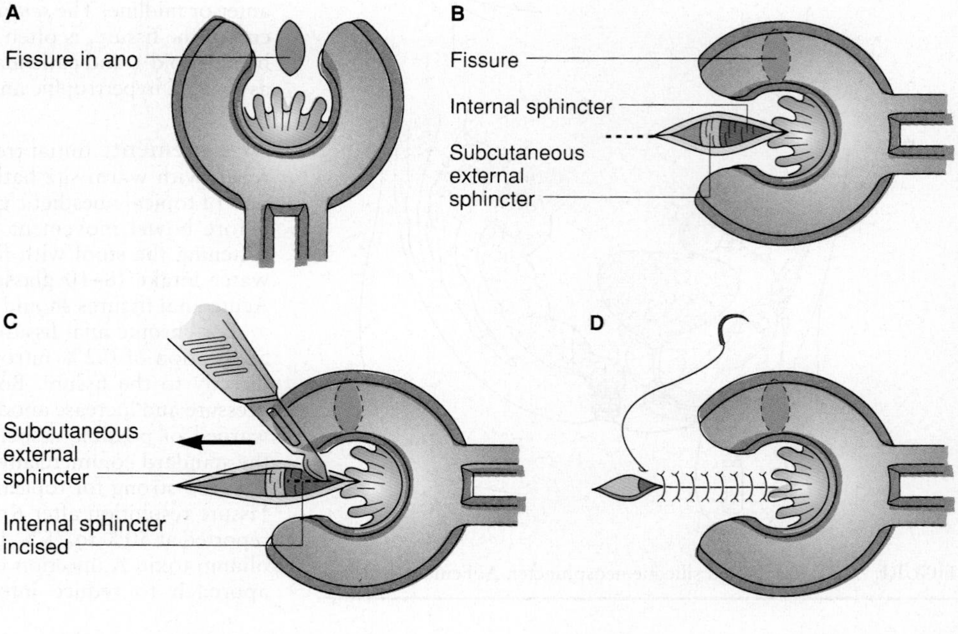

Secondary Anal Fissure. Fissures or ulcers that develop as a result of underlying disease tend to be larger and deeper than primary fissures, and they are less likely located in the posterior midline. Pain is rarely as severe as the pain of primary fissure, and muscle-relaxing therapies (topical medications and sphincterotomy) do not help. A nonmidline or otherwise atypical fissure should be biopsied.

Neutropenic fissures occur in patients with leukemia, aplastic anemia, agranulocytosis, and similar diseases. The fissure may follow a bout of diarrhea or constipation at a time when the patient is neutropenic. This type of fissure is often very painful and may have a necrotic base. Treatment is symptomatic only, and the ulcer should heal when neutropenia resolves.

ANORECTAL ABSCESSES

Pathogenesis

7 In the wall of the anal canal, four to ten anal glands open directly into the anal crypts at the dentate line. Infection of the anal glands, presumably incited by a blocked duct or orifice, is the origin of perianal abscesses. Because the anal glands lie between the internal and external sphincter muscles, an intersphincteric abscess forms first. The infection may then spread to the spaces discussed previously (Fig. 70.24). Abscess locations, in order of frequency, are perianal, ischioanal, intersphincteric, and supralevator.

Clinical Manifestations

The initial symptom of most anorectal abscesses is severe anal pain, aggravated by activity. Swelling is usually prominent, and skin changes become obvious as the abscess nears the surface. Some patients develop urinary retention.

Management

Like all abscesses, the anorectal abscess must be drained as soon as possible. Antibiotics do not help and should be avoided, except in immunosuppressed or immune-deficient patients, in whom antibiotics should be considered. Packing is generally discouraged as painful and impractical.

Perianal abscesses are the most superficial and the easiest to treat. They are usually small and can be drained under local anesthesia. An elliptical or cruciate incision is made on the most prominent part of the skin and subcutaneous tissue overlying the abscess cavity. Redundant skin edges are excised to prevent premature closure of the abscess. No packing should be necessary.

An ischioanal abscess causes a diffuse swelling of the ischioanal fossa, and drainage can be done wherever the abscess is most superficial. Bilateral ischioanal or horseshoe abscess has its origin in the deep postanal space, with spread to both ischioanal spaces. A horseshoe abscess should be drained through the deep postanal space, avoiding division of muscle. A longitudinal incision is made in the skin between the tip of the coccyx and the anus to expose the anococcygeal ligament. The anococcygeal ligament is incised along its fibers, and the deep postanal space is entered. After the abscess cavity is drained and irrigated, a counterincision is made on one or both limbs of the ischioanal space.

Unlike perianal and ischioanal abscesses, there is no external swelling or induration in the perianal area in intersphincteric abscesses. The diagnosis is suspected when there is severe anorectal pain and no evident pathology. Focal tenderness is present when careful, systematic circumanal palpation is performed. Most intersphincteric abscesses are located posteriorly. Intersphincteric abscesses are drained through the anal canal by incising the mucosa and cutting through the internal sphincter muscle.

Supralevator abscess is uncommon and difficult to diagnose. Because it is adjacent to the abdominal cavity, a supralevator abscess can mimic an acute abdomen. Digital examination reveals an indurated or bulging tender mass on either side of the lower rectum or posteriorly above the level of the anorectal ring. The supralevator abscess may arise by extension of an intersphincteric abscess, by extension of an ischioanal abscess, or from intra-abdominal processes such as diverticular, appendiceal, and Crohn disease abscesses. If the abscess is from upward extension of an intersphincteric abscess, it should be drained into the rectum. If such an abscess is drained through the ischioanal fossa, a complicated suprasphincteric fistula can be formed. If the supralevator abscess arises from the upward extension of an ischioanal abscess, it should be drained through the ischioanal fossa.

ANAL FISTULA

8 Anal fistula (fistula in ano) results when an anorectal abscess that is spontaneously or surgically drained does not heal completely, becoming instead an inflammatory tract with an internal opening in the anal crypt at the dentate line and an external opening on the skin. Every abscess becomes a fistula the

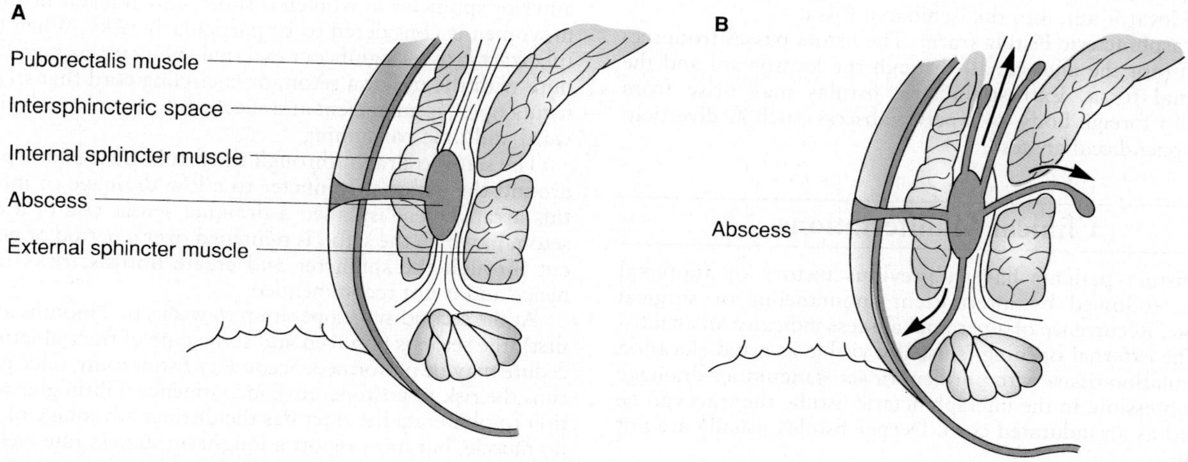

FIGURE 70.24. Pathways of infection start in the intersphincteric space (A) and then spread to perianal spaces, forming perianal abscesses (B).

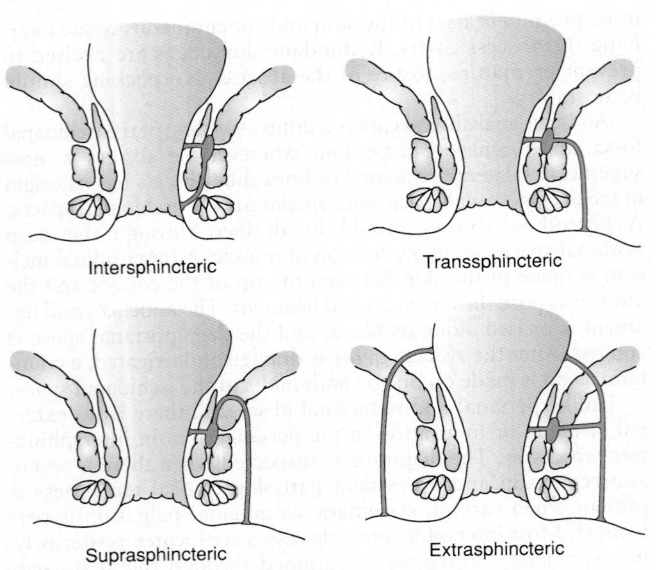

FIGURE 70.25. The four main anatomic types of fistula.

moment it is drained, because of the addition of an external opening, but about half of these fistulas disappear over a 2-month period. If the external opening (incision and drainage site) is still open after 60 days, one may assume it is a chronic anal fistula and will never heal without an operation.

Classification

The four subtypes of anal fistula are named for the relation of the fistula to the sphincter muscles (Fig. 70.25).[32]

Intersphincteric Fistula (most common). The fistulous tract is in the intersphincteric plane. The external opening is in the perianal skin, close to the anal verge. A drained perianal abscess is an intersphincteric fistula.

Transsphincteric Fistula (fairly common). The fistulous tract starts in the intersphincteric plane, then traverses the external sphincter, with the external opening over the ischioanal fossa. Horseshoe fistulas are also in this category. A drained ischioanal abscess is a transsphincteric fistula.

Suprasphincteric Fistula (rare). The fistula typically starts in the intersphincteric plane and then passes upward to a point above the puborectalis muscle. The tract passes laterally over this muscle and downward between the puborectalis muscle and the levator ani, into the ischioanal fossa.

Extrasphincteric Fistula (rare). The fistula passes from rectal wall (not the anal canal) through the levator ani and the ischioanal fossa. Extrasphincteric fistulas may arise from trauma, a foreign body, or a pelvic abscess, such as diverticular or appendiceal abscess.

Clinical Manifestations

Most fistula patients have a previous history of anorectal abscess, followed by intermittent spontaneous or surgical drainage. Recurrence of a perianal abscess indicates an anal fistula. The external opening is usually visible as a red elevation of granulation tissue with purulent or serosanguinous drainage on compression. In the intersphincteric fistula, the tract can be palpated as an indurated cord. Deeper fistulas usually are not palpable.

Anoscopy is done in the operating room to identify the internal opening. Proctoscopy or flexible sigmoidoscopy is usually performed to rule out other lesions and inflammatory bowel disease. A fistula probe can be introduced into the fistulous tract to determine its direction, although it is not always possible to pass the probe through the internal opening. Occasionally the internal fistula opening or fistula pathway may be hard to discern based on physical examination. Injection of the external opening with hydrogen peroxide while performing endoanal ultrasound can demonstrate the tract, effectively creating a fistula map, and can also help to identify an unrecognized internal opening at the time of surgery. Buchanan et al.[33] studied a cohort of 108 patients with recurrent fistulae using digital examination, endoanal ultrasound, and MRI on each patient. Digital examination correctly identified 61% of tracks, compared with 81% of tracks by endoanal ultrasound and 90% by MRI.

Several disorders must be considered in the differential diagnosis of anal fistula. A pilonidal sinus with perianal extension is the closest mimic of anal fistula, although at operation it is obvious that the tract goes the wrong way, away from the anus instead of toward it. Hidradenitis suppurativa usually displays multiple perianal skin openings with surrounding leather-like skin. Infected perianal cysts are multiple and superficial, without a palpable tract. Inflammatory bowel disease fistulas are often in some way atypical, with multiple tracts or unusually superficial or deep tracts. Low rectal and anal canal carcinomas may rarely present as a fistula in the perineum. So as not to miss inflammatory bowel disease and cancers, fistula patients should be considered for flexible endoscopy.

Management

The principles of fistula surgery include unroofing the fistula, eliminating the internal opening, and establishing adequate drainage. Failure to open the entire tract generally leads to recurrence. In most fistulas, the treatment of choice involves opening the entire fistulous tract over a fistula probe. Granulation tissue is curetted out, and the edges of the wound can be marsupialized to facilitate healing. Fistulectomy, the excision of the fistulous tract, has no advantage over fistulotomy, the laying open of the tract. For horseshoe fistula, radical unroofing would result in a large wound and is not necessary. Incision of the deep postanal space combined with counterincision and curettage of the lateral tracts is generally recommended.

Any sphincter muscle division carries with it a risk of impaired continence. Individuals at particular risk include those with compromised continence to begin with, previous sphincter injury, and underlying diarrheal states such as ulcerative colitis or Crohn disease. High fistulas, those involving large amounts of external anal sphincter, are not suitable for treatment by fistulotomy due to the risk of incontinence. The anterior sphincter in women is short, and anterior fistulotomy in women is considered to be particularly risky. When the fistula tract crosses significant external sphincter, a staged procedure with the use of a seton, or encircling cord that stents the fistula open, is an ancient and successful treatment, albeit awkward and time-consuming.

The seton is drawn through the fistula tract and kept loose around the external sphincter to allow drainage of infection; this arrangement is called a draining seton. Use of a cutting seton, in which the seton is tightened over a period of weeks to cut through the sphincter and create fibrosis, risks incontinence and is not recommended.

At the second-stage operation (6 weeks to 3 months after the first), the seton is removed and some type of tract-ablating procedure may be performed. Secondary fistulotomy, once popular, runs the risk of postoperative incontinence. Fibrin glue application to obliterate the tract has the distinct advantage of cutting no muscle, but most report a long-term success rate well under 50%. Fibrin glue can be reapplied and has shown a small success rate among patients with complex fistulae among whom fistulotomy would likely result in incontinence.[34]

The goal of fibrin glue is the formation of a collagen matrix for eventual healing, and that goal is reached more directly by the new biologic fistula plugs made of porcine or bovine collagen. This plug is drawn through the fistula tract and sutured in place. Reported success rates to date have been highly variable.[35]

Endoanal advancement flap is another interventional option for patients who fail less invasive therapy. A U-shaped flap of mucosa and circular muscle is created, encompassing the internal opening near the distal edge. The flap is advanced, and the distal strip with the internal opening is excised. The internal opening is closed with absorbable sutures, and the flap is affixed with sutures to cover this repair.

Anal Fistula Associated with Crohn Disease

Fistulas associated with Crohn disease are often asymptomatic. They may resemble ordinary, cryptoglandular fistulas in that there is an indurated external opening in the skin that exudes pus, and a palpable tract passing toward the anal canal. On the other hand, these fistulas may be complex with multiple tracts, and they may disobey any rule laid down for the expected anatomy of typical fistulas.

The most important part of treatment is adequate and aggressive medical therapy, including medications for active Crohn disease. Metronidazole and ciprofloxacin have been found to be useful in some patients, probably for their anti-inflammatory rather than their antibiotic properties. Methotrexate and azathioprine have had minimal success. Infliximab, a monoclonal antibody directed against tumor necrosis factor, has shown promising efficacy for Crohn disease fistulas. In a placebo-controlled trial of patients with fistulizing Crohn disease in which 90% of patients also had perianal disease, 62% experienced at least 50% reduction in the number of draining fistulas compared with 26% of the placebo group.[36] Nearly half of patients treated with infliximab experienced complete closure of all fistulas with short- to mid-term follow-up.

Aggressive surgical intervention in complex Crohn disease fistulas is discouraged because of extremely poor healing among these patients. The basic principle is to drain any abscess and lay open superficial tracks. Division of any significant quantity of sphincter muscle should be avoided, as these patients are prone to development of additional fistulae and are also at increased risk for incontinence due to diarrhea from their underlying Crohn disease. Long-term indwelling setons are often the best alternative in this patient population.

TABLE 70.4 **ETIOLOGY**

CAUSES OF RECTOVAGINAL FISTULA

Congenital maldevelopment
Trauma
Obstetric
Operative
Blunt and penetrating injury
Foreign body
Infection of anal canal or vaginal septum
Pelvic irradiation
Neoplasm

Rectovaginal Fistula

A rectovaginal fistula is a communication between the anterior wall of the anal canal or rectum and the posterior wall of the vagina. There are many possible causes (Table 70.4), but obstetric injury accounts for most. A rectovaginal fistula is referred to as low if a repair can be done from a perineal approach and high if repair can be accomplished only transabdominally (Fig. 70.26). Simple or complex classification is based on location, size, and cause (Table 70.5).

Clinical Manifestations. Symptoms of rectovaginal fistulas depend on location, size, and cause. In low or small fistulas, the most common complaint is passage of gas per vagina. In large fistulas, symptoms include vaginal discharge with fecal odor, passage of flatus and stool per vagina, and painful vaginitis.

Diagnosis. Diagnosis is made by physical examination. In low fistula, digital examination of the anal canal reveals scar and a defect in the anterior wall. Bimanual examination with one finger in the rectum and a finger of the other hand in the

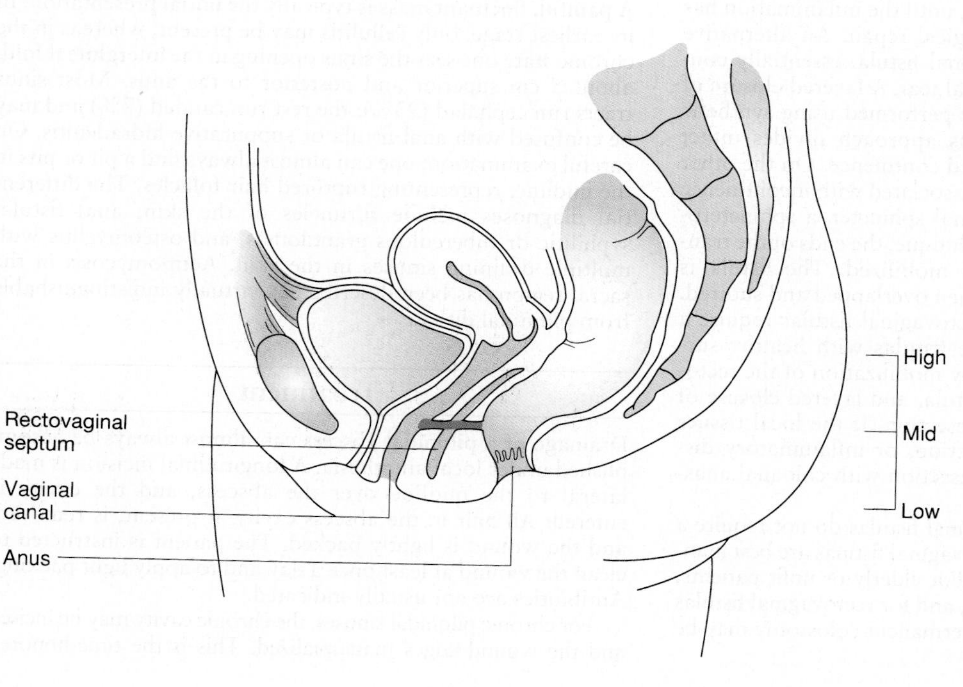

FIGURE 70.26. Rectovaginal fistula classified by location. Fistulas are low when located at or just cephalad to the dentate line, high when near the cervix, and mid when located in between.

TABLE 70.5 CLASSIFICATION

CLASSIFICATION OF RECTOVAGINAL FISTULA

CHARACTERISTIC	SIMPLE	COMPLEX
Location	Low to midvaginal septum	High vaginal septum
Size	2.5 cm or less in diameter	2.5 cm or more in diameter
Cause	Traumatic or infectious cause	Inflammatory bowel disease, irradiation, neoplastic cause

vagina is also helpful. Anoscopy can also detect the opening in the anal canal. Middle and high fistulas require proctoscopy. If the fistula cannot be seen, a tampon is placed in the vaginal canal and 100 mL of dilute methylene blue is instilled into the anorectum. The tampon is then removed and checked for blue staining. Barium enema is usually not helpful but may be indicated in certain patients with inflammatory bowel disease or previous irradiation.

Management. Spontaneous or nonoperative healing of a rectovaginal fistula depends primarily on its cause and, to a lesser extent, on its size. About one half of small rectovaginal fistulas secondary to obstetric trauma heal spontaneously. Fistulas caused by Crohn disease or irradiation rarely heal spontaneously.

For a low, simple fistula and some mid-rectovaginal fistulas, endorectal advancement of an anorectal flap technique gives good results. The rectal flap, which consists of mucosa, submucosa, internal sphincter, and the circular muscle of the lower rectum, is outlined lateral and distal to the fistula. The flap is based at least 4 cm cephalad to the fistula, and the base should be twice the length of the flap to ensure adequate blood supply. After the flap is raised, the underlying fistula and the excess flap are excised. The cut edges of the internal sphincter and the circular muscle of the lower rectum are approximated, obliterating that portion of the fistula tract. The opening in the vagina is left open for drainage. The anorectal flap is then advanced over the repaired area and sutured (Fig. 70.27).

The results of endorectal advancement flap for treatment of simple rectovaginal fistula are good, with 83% of treated patients achieving primary healing of the fistula.[37] It is important to wait, usually 3 to 6 months, until the inflammation has subsided before considering a surgical repair. An alternative repair is to lay open the rectovaginal fistula, essentially converting it to a fourth-degree perineal tear. A layered closure of the anal and vaginal defect can be performed using synthetic absorbable sutures. However, this approach divides intact sphincter muscle and risks impaired continence. On the other hand, if the rectovaginal fistula is associated with incontinence resulting from injury to the external sphincter, a sphincteroplasty is also performed. In this technique, the ends of the transected muscle are identified and mobilized. The fistula is excised, and the muscle ends are then overlapped and sutured.

High fistulas and some mid-rectovaginal fistulas require a transabdominal approach. Simple fistulas with healthy surrounding tissues can be repaired by mobilization of the rectovaginal septum, division of the fistula, and layered closure of the rectal defect without bowel resection. If the local tissues are damaged by irradiation, infection, or inflammatory diseases, an extended low anterior resection with coloanal anastomosis should be performed.

Although most simple rectovaginal fistulas do not require a diverting colostomy, complex rectovaginal fistulas are best managed by a preliminary colostomy. For elderly or unfit patients, for most radiation-induced fistulas, and for rectovaginal fistulas associated with Crohn disease, a permanent colostomy may be prudent.

PILONIDAL SINUS

Pilonidal sinus is an acquired condition, beginning with rupture into the dermis of a hair follicle in the sacrococcygeal region. Why this happens at that location more than other locations, and what predisposes certain people (male sex, second or third decade of life, hirsute habitus, Mediterranean skin type) to develop pilonidal sinus is unclear. Although traditionally conceived as a solitary condition, pilonidal sinus is part of the *acne inversa* tetrad (hidradenitis suppurativa, acne conglobata, dissecting scalp perifolliculitis, and pilonidal sinus), and thus may be the most common manifestation of an incompletely penetrant syndrome. Acne inversa lesions indistinguishable from pilonidal sinus, but in other predictable locations such as the axillae, vulva, scrotum, and so on, are termed *hidradenitis suppurativa*, perhaps reflecting artificial distinctions between treating specialties rather than distinct disease processes. Pilonidal-like lesions have also been reported in unusual locations such as the umbilicus, healed amputation stumps, and interdigital clefts.

Clinical Manifestations

Pilonidal sinus typically begins as an acute abscess at the sacrococcygeal area that drains spontaneously or is drained surgically, leaving a nonhealing sinus with chronic drainage.

Diagnosis

A painful, fluctuant mass is typically the initial presentation. In its earliest stage, only cellulitis may be present, whereas in the chronic state one sees the sinus opening in the intergluteal fold, about 5 cm superior and posterior to the anus. Most sinus tracts run cephalad (93%); the rest run caudad (7%) and may be confused with anal fistula or suppurative hidradenitis. On careful examination, one can almost always find a pit or pits in the midline, representing ruptured hair follicles. The differential diagnoses include furuncles of the skin, anal fistula, syphilitic or tuberculous granulomas, and osteomyelitis with multiple draining sinuses in the skin. Actinomycosis in the sacral region has been described as virtually indistinguishable from pilonidal disease.

Treatment

Drainage of a pilonidal abscess can almost always be accomplished under local anesthesia. A longitudinal incision is made lateral to the midline over the abscess, and the cavity is entered. All hair in the abscess cavity, if present, is removed, and the wound is lightly packed. The patient is instructed to clean the wound at least once a day and to apply light packing. Antibiotics are not usually indicated.

For chronic pilonidal sinuses, the chronic cavity may be incised and the wound edges marsupialized. This is the time-honored

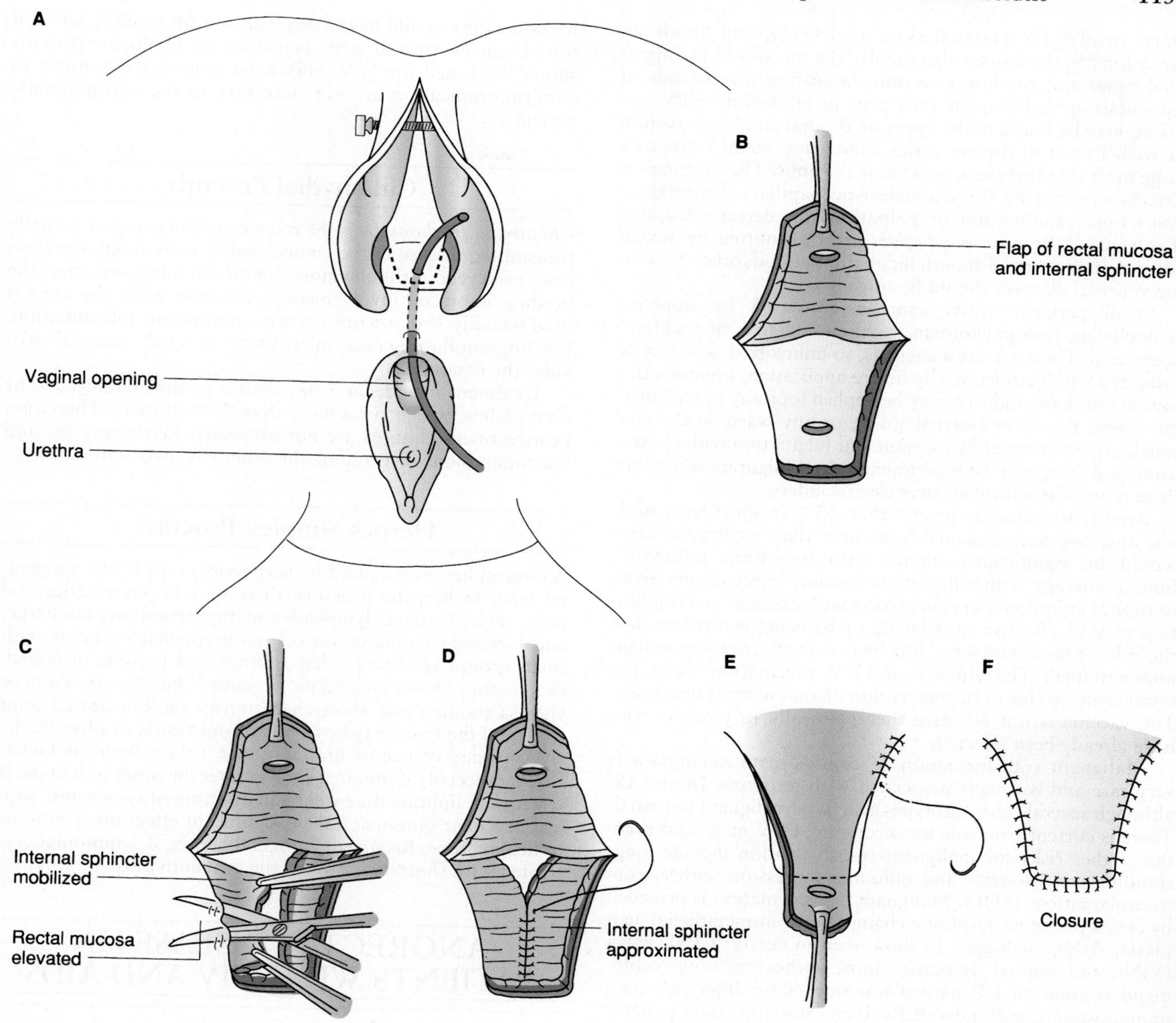

FIGURE 70.27. Endorectal advancement of anorectal flap. **A:** Exposure is gained by an anal speculum, and the fistula is identified. Outline of endorectal flap, extending proximally to 7 cm from the anal verge. **B:** The full-thickness flap is created to include the internal sphincter muscle. **C:** Lateral mobilization is made on each side in the submucosal plane. **D:** Anorectal wall on each side is approximated. **E and F:** The endorectal flap is pulled down to cover the wound and sutured. The fistula is excised. The aperture in the vagina is not sutured but is left open for drainage.

method, and healing is fairly reliable but sometimes prolonged. An alternative is to excise the sinus and perform a local flap repair.[38] Excellent results have been reported from specialty centers using this approach.

A third approach is the Bascom technique, which involves opening the main tract lateral to the midline. The sinus tracts to the midline pits are probed and laid open. Granulation tissue in the cavity is curetted and the wound packed. Healing is reported to be faster than for conventional excision, with the wound completely closed within 4 weeks in most cases.[39] Nonhealing or prolonged healing are problems with all conventional techniques, and there is a substantial corpus of literature on flap procedures for reclosing pilonidal wounds. The Bascom cleft-lift operation is also reported to work for failures of other techniques.[40]

Postoperative Care

Because of the high rate of nonhealing and prolonged healing in this area, much thought has been given to postoperative care, usually described as a critical feature of pilonidal care. However, general principles of open wound care seem to apply here as elsewhere: keeping the wound bed moist and the edges dry, gently debriding devitalized tissue and exudates, and removing foreign bodies.

SEXUALLY TRANSMITTED DISEASES OF THE ANORECTUM

The anus is part of the anogenital tract from the viewpoint of infectious diseases, which are substantially the same as those of the external genitalia.

Anal Condylomata Acuminata

9 Anal condylomata acuminata (warts) are caused by human papilloma viruses (HPV) of various subtypes. In most patients,

warts involve the perianal skin, anal verge, and anoderm. Occasionally, the lesions also involve the mucosa of the upper anal canal and the lower rectum, indicating that islands of squamous epithelium, the only type of epithelium HPV can infect, may be found in the upper anal canal and lower rectum as well. Extent of disease varies from a few small warts to a large mass that threatens to occlude the anus. The diagnosis is usually obvious by the characteristic papillary appearance. Anoscopic examination or palpation can detect intra-anal involvement. Because most cases are transmitted by sexual contact after a 1- to 3-month incubation period, other coexisting venereal diseases should be considered.

Small perianal warts can be destroyed by applying podophyllin, podophyllotoxin, bichloracetic acid, or trichloroacetic acid. These are caustic agents, so uninvolved skin may be protected with petroleum jelly before application. Imiquimod, a topical interferon inducer, may be applied topically to anal margin warts. Extensive external warts, or any warts in the anal canal, are best treated by excision and fulguration with electrocautery. A laser may be used to excise and fulgurate warts, but there is no clear advantage over electrocautery.

Recurrence rates are greater than 65% in short-term studies, and one may reasonably assume that recurrence rates would be significantly higher with long-term follow-up. Immunotherapy with autogenous vaccine, injected interferon, or topical imiquimod in conjunction with excision and fulguration may be effective in delaying or reducing recurrence, but the role of these measures and their cost-effectiveness remain undetermined. The efficacy of HPV vaccination using the tetravalent vaccine in the prevention of anal warts is unknown. The vaccine is not effective therapeutically in patients who have already been infected.

Malignant transformation of condylomata acuminata is very rare and is usually associated with serotypes 16 and 18, although several other serotypes also have malignant potential. There is currently no role for serotyping HPV in clinical practice. Other risks for malignant transformation include long-standing condylomata and immunosuppression, either from transplantation or HIV. Malignant transformation is preceded by development of dysplastic changes (anal intraepithelial neoplasia, AIN), analogous to those seen in cervix (CIN), vulva (VIN), and vaginal dysplasia. Some authorities now recommend routine anal Papanicolaou smears for high risk (i.e., immunosuppressed) individuals. Using this approach, patients found to have high-grade dysplasia (AIN 2–3) undergo high-definition anal microscopy using a colposcope, with focal ablation of areas of high-grade dysplasia. Although several centers have reported encouraging results using this approach, proof of its efficacy in controlled trials is currently lacking.

When malignant transformation occurs, it is almost always to squamous carcinoma rather than adenocarcinoma. Malignancies are treated by location, with Nigro-type chemoradiation for anal canal lesions and surgical excision for anal margin lesions.

Gonococcal Proctitis

Patients with gonococcal proctitis are usually asymptomatic but may have mild anal burning, pain, discharge, or bleeding in the acute phase. Proctoscopy reveals inflamed anorectal mucosa with purulent discharge at the dentate line. In the chronic phase, the anus and rectum may appear normal. Diagnosis is confirmed by observing *Neisseria gonorrheae* on stained smears of the discharge, and by culture. In the United States, gonococcal antimicrobial resistance continues to evolve, and coinfection with *Chlamydia trachomatis* is found in up to 45% of gonorrhea cases.

The recommended treatment is a single injection of ceftriaxone plus a 7-day course of oral doxycycline, which is added for possible coexisting chlamydial infection. All patients treated for gonorrhea should have a serologic test for syphilis, which if found can be treated with penicillin G. High-risk patients should be tested for HIV. Follow-up gonococcal cultures to confirm eradication are not necessary in the asymptomatic patient.

Chlamydial Proctitis

Chlamydia trachomatis is the most common cause of sexually transmitted disease in the United States, with about 4 million cases each year. Although most chlamydial infections affect the urethra, anorectal involvement is common when the anus is used sexually. Proctoscopy reveals a nonspecific inflammation, but immunofluorescence microscopy of swab material provides the diagnosis.

Treatment includes a 7-day course of oral tetracycline or doxycycline, which cures more than 95% of cases. Therefore, posttreatment cultures are not necessary. Erythromycins and fluoroquinolones are among the other effective antibiotics.

Herpes Simplex Proctitis

Anorectal herpes is caused by herpesvirus type II, the anogenital type. In herpetic proctitis, there may be severe anorectal pain, fever, inguinal lymphadenopathy, tenesmus, discharge, and bleeding. Examination reveals erythematous areas with small groups of vesicles that rupture and become ulcerated. Proctoscopy shows nonspecific proctitis,[41] but Papanicolaou or Giemsa staining may show characteristic multinucleated giant cells, and the virus may be isolated from vesicle or ulcer fluid.

A 10-day course of oral acyclovir, valacyclovir, or famciclovir, especially if initiated shortly after the onset of lesions, is effective in limiting the extent and duration of symptoms. Topical acyclovir ointment has no significant effect on symptoms or healing time. Recurrent anorectal herpes, if symptomatic, is treated with shorter courses of the oral antivirals.

ANORECTAL DISEASES IN PATIENTS WITH HIV AND AIDS

Kaposi Sarcoma

Kaposi sarcoma (KS), associated with the herpesvirus HHV-8, is still one of the most common malignancies in AIDS patients. Because it thrives with low CD4 counts, the significance of KS is waning in the era of highly active antiretroviral therapy (HAART). Most colorectal KS is asymptomatic, but bleeding and obstruction may rarely occur; likewise, most KS of the anal verge and anal margin skin is asymptomatic. Treatment is directed at the HIV infection, and KS-specific treatment, if needed, is usually by radiation, chemotherapy, or other ablative measures.

Cytomegalovirus

Symptomatic cytomegalovirus (CMV) proctocolitis occurs in profoundly immunosuppressed AIDS patients. Like KS, CMV is waning in significance because of HAART. Symptoms of CMV proctocolitis include diarrhea, fever, abdominal pain, and weight loss. Proctoscopy may reveal sharply demarcated shallow ulcers with fibrinous exudate, and biopsy gives an accurate diagnosis. Treatment is directed at the HIV infection and the CMV infection. Because proctitis represents systemic infection, CMV is treated by oral or intravenous antivirals, depending on the severity of disease. When surgical complications such as perforation occur, they are usually intra-abdominal, not anorectal.

Lymphoma

Lymphomas occur at higher incidence in patients with HIV. Non-Hodgkin lymphoma was an original AIDS-defining diagnosis in the pre-HAART era, associated with low CD4 counts, whereas Hodgkin lymphoma occurs most commonly in patients with CD4 counts of 300 to 400. Anorectal lymphoma is usually extraluminal, sometimes presenting as perianal ulcer. Any atypical feature of a perianal ulcer in an HIV-positive patient should trigger a biopsy.

Anal Ulcers

Idiopathic anal ulcers were common among HIV-positive patients pre-HAART, and they are still found in AIDS patients with low CD4 counts. Most ulcers are in the posterior midline of the anal canal, straddling the dentate line and thus proximal to site of a typical anal fissure. They can be erosive, dissecting submucosally or intersphincterically, and creating painful areas of acute and chronic inflammation.[42]

Examination of the anus and rectum under anesthesia is usually necessary. Biopsies should be taken and sent for viral, bacterial, and mycobacterial culture, dark-field examination for syphilis, and histopathologic examination to rule out CMV, lymphoma, and squamous cell cancer. About half of HIV-associated ulcers are specific, caused by syphilis, tuberculosis, HSV, cytomegalovirus, and other infections, and about half are nonspecific or idiopathic. Treatment of the latter has been empiric, using metronidazole and/or intralesional steroid injection; treating the HIV infection and raising the CD4 count addresses the underlying problem. Thalidomide has been reported to be effective treatment for HIV-associated aphthous ulcerations, and it might have a role in treating refractory anal ulcerations as well.[43]

Anal Intraepithelial Neoplasia

HPV's role in AIN and anal cancers closely parallels its role in the genesis of cervical carcinoma, a more closely studied process. Oncogenic HPV strains such as 16 and 18 have a higher propensity to initiate the development of carcinoma.[44] These two well-studied serotypes also have a predilection for the less stable epithelium of the upper anal canal (transitional zone) rather than the modified skin of the lower anal canal (anoderm), but they can still be identified in the anal margin skin.

Anal carcinoma and its precursor lesion, anal intraepithelial neoplasia (AIN), both occur at markedly increased incidence in HIV-positive patients and in people with risk factors for HIV. This 'epidemic within the epidemic' is caused by oncogenic strains of HPV and indirectly facilitated by HAART, which has allowed patients to live long enough to develop these lesions. High CD4 counts are not protective. As HIV has become a chronic, manageable condition, anal carcinoma has become more common, necessitating the development of screening and surveillance regimens.[45]

AIN can be detected using cytologic (Papanicolaou) smears, and positive findings can be followed by high-resolution anoscopy, using a colposcope and vital staining. In one prevalence study, AIN was present in 80% of HIV-positive men, and half of the AIN was high-grade (AIN II or III) (Fig. 70.28).[46] Low-grade AIN, like the condyloma it often accompanies, rarely undergoes malignant transformation and can be observed, or it can be ablated if symptomatic. High-grade AIN is the premalignant counterpart of anal squamous carcinoma, identical to carcinoma in situ and Bowen disease. Although the rate of malignant transformation is unknown, one can estimate that it is relatively low to date: Based on prevalence studies, roughly half of the 1,200,000 Americans living with HIV can be presumed to have high-grade AIN, and roughly half of the 5,000 new cases of anal canal cancer per year occur in HIV-positive patients. Thus about 2,500 cases arise annually in an at-risk population of about 600,000—about 0.4% per year. However, based on the analogy to CIN and cervical cancer, progression from high-grade AIN to anal cancer would be expected to take many years, and the incidence of anal cancer in HIV-positive patients may rise sharply with further years of observation on HAART therapy.

Many authors have recommended ablation of detectable lesions, and infrared coagulation is the currently favored ablative technique.[47] High-grade AIN is often very extensive and difficult to detect, so it may be very difficult to ablate completely; multiple treatments and persistence/recurrence are commonplace. Although all authors agree on aggressive treatment of invasive anal cancer (see later), there are many suggested strategies for managing high-grade AIN, from simple surveillance to aggressive ablation of all detectable lesions.[48,49]

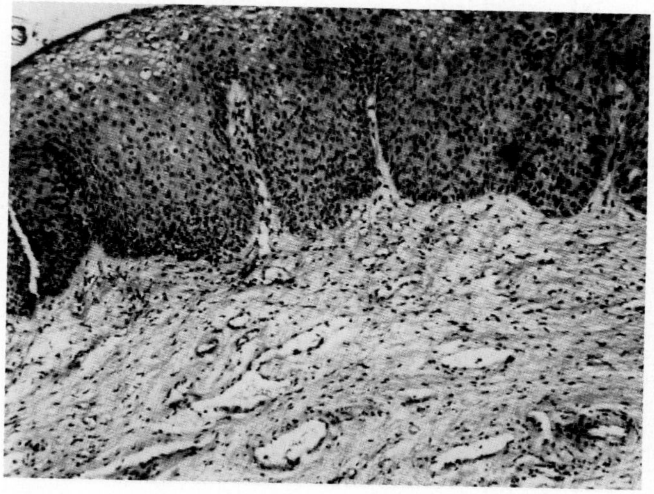

FIGURE 70.28. High-grade anal intraepithelial neoplasia (Bowen disease, carcinoma in situ). Atypical epithelial cells involve the full thickness of the epidermis.

ANAL CANCER

Anal cancers—malignancies of the anal canal and the skin of the anal margin—are uncommon, and the literature is limited by nonuniform terminology and classification. The World Health Organization and the American Joint Committee on Cancer have developed standard terminology for neoplasms of the anal region.

Anal Intraepithelial Neoplasia in the HIV-negative Population

In the HIV-negative population, high-grade AIN (also called Bowen disease) is rare, slow growing, and can occur in any age group but is more prevalent in older women.[50] Immunosuppressed patients, especially those with solid organ transplants, are also a high-risk group for AIN. AIN may appear as a discrete scaly or crusted plaque; it may be pigmented; and it may be difficult to delineate. Biopsy of any atypical anal lesion is mandatory (Fig. 70.28). Once AIN has been detected, one may consider mapping the extent of nonvisible involvement by taking multiple biopsies, but there is no evidence that this practice improves patient outcomes. Once a patient has or has had AIN, lifetime surveillance is essential. Recurrences are reported as late

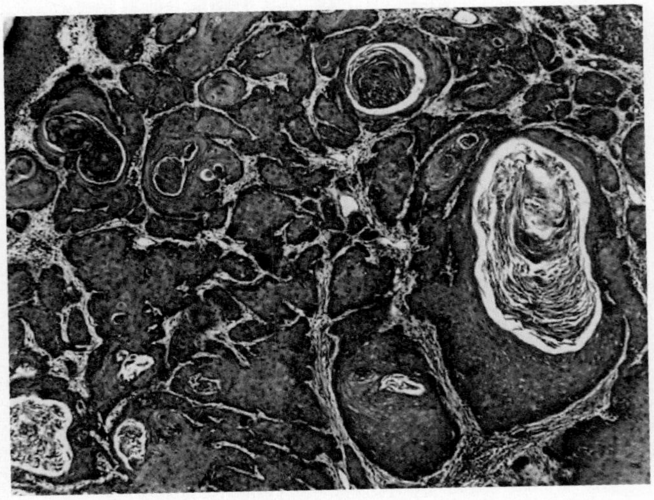

FIGURE 70.29. Photomicrograph of squamous cell carcinoma of the perianal skin. Note the presence of keratin.

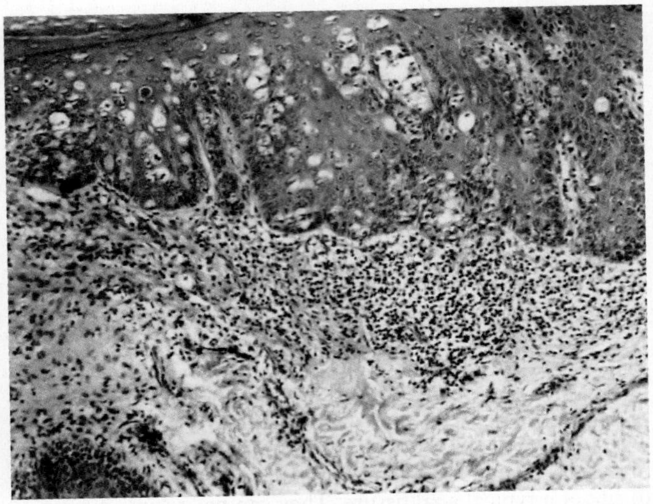

FIGURE 70.30. Perianal Paget disease. Paget cells are above the basal layer.

as 9 years postoperatively; this is not surprising, because surgical intervention does not cure viral infection. Just as in the HIV-positive population, the value of colposcopy (high-resolution anoscopy) for surveillance is debated, and physical examination may be sufficient for detection of new, changed, or suspicious lesions. High-grade AIN in the HIV-negative population probably has a lower rate of malignant transformation than the same lesion in the HIV-positive population.

Squamous Cell Carcinoma

Squamous cell carcinomas of the anal margin resemble those occurring in skin elsewhere. They grow slowly and have rolled, everted edges and central ulceration. Any chronic unhealed or indurated ulceration in the perianal area should be biopsied, looking for squamous cell carcinoma (Fig. 70.29). Lymphatic spread from squamous carcinomas of the perianal area is mainly to inguinal lymph nodes. Despite their superficial location, most lesions are diagnosed late, with half of cases identified more than 22 months after the onset of symptoms; carcinoma is often discovered at a late stage (T3), measuring 5 cm or more. The importance of biopsying atypical 'fissures' and 'external hemorrhoids' cannot be overemphasized.

Wide local excision is the treatment for anal margin squamous cell carcinoma but only in properly selected cases. For microinvasive carcinoma and for cancers that do not invade muscle, local excision should be curative. For large, muscle-invasive (T4), or anal canal-invasive lesions, chemoradiation should be considered, as in anal canal cancer treatment. Abdominoperineal resection is rarely needed for anal margin cancer, though it may be used for patients with extensive lesions who cannot tolerate chemoradiation, or in patients with anal sphincter involvement and incontinence. Size of the carcinoma determines staging and prognosis, as of course do lymph node and distant-metastasis status. Five- and ten-year survival rates for T_1 lesions are both 100%, compared with roughly 60% and 40% for T_2 lesions.

Paget Disease

This intraepithelial adenocarcinoma was initially described in the breast. Extramammary Paget disease can be found in the anogenital region. Most authors agree that Paget cells are of glandular, probably apocrine, origin, from the adnexal organs of the skin.[51] Perianal Paget disease starts out as a benign in situ neoplasm, and it may eventually become invasive as an adenocarcinoma.

Paget disease occurs in the elderly, with an average age of 68.[52] It appears as a slowly spreading pruritic and erythematous, sometimes sharply demarcated perianal rash that may ooze or scale. Because of its gross similarity to other conditions such as idiopathic pruritus ani and AIN, the diagnosis of perianal Paget disease is made by biopsy (Fig. 70.30) and is often delayed. In almost one third of the cases, the lesion involves the entire circumference of the perianal skin.

True Paget disease of the perianal skin must be distinguished from downward intraepidermal spread of a signet-ring cell adenocarcinoma of the rectum, which it resembles histologically. A complete colonoscopy with thorough examination of the rectum and anal canal should be performed. Synchronous visceral carcinomas have been found in up to 50% of patients.[53]

In the absence of invasive carcinoma, wide excision with a microscopically clear margin is the treatment of choice. Because clinically invisible Paget disease may extend beyond the gross margin of the lesion, mapping the extent of involvement by obtaining biopsies in four quadrants at the dentate line, anal verge, and anal margin can assist with planning and establish a baseline for future surveillance. If extensive wide local excision is needed, reconstruction can be performed with large advancement or rotation flaps.[54]

If there is a concomitant rectal adenocarcinoma, then treatment follows rectal cancer protocols, with the possible addition of inguinal lymph node dissection. Because diagnosis is delayed by an average of 4 years from onset of symptoms, about 25% of patients with invasive adenocarcinoma in Paget disease already have distant metastasis. Likely sites of metastasis are the same as those of any distal rectal adenocarcinoma.

Verrucous Carcinoma/Giant Condyloma

An overlapping group of entities is called *giant condyloma acuminatum*, *Buschke-Löwenstein tumor*, and verrucous carcinoma, although the term verrucous carcinoma is also used more broadly to describe a histologic subtype of squamous carcinoma. The giant condyloma is typically a large (>8 cm), slow-growing, symptomatic, warty growth with a soft feel and cauliflower-like appearance. It may arise in the anal margin skin or the anal canal and may be grossly and microscopically indistinguishable from very extensive condylomata acuminata.

Although it may be histologically bland, the lesion's behavior is clinically malignant.

These lesions may relentlessly expand and invade the ischioanal fossa, perirectal tissues, and even the pelvic cavity. Sinuses and fistula tracts may form and create complex lesional anatomy. Verrucous carcinomas rarely metastasize, but they do recur locally.

Treatment is wide local excision, which may even include abdominoperineal resection (APR), if the lesion involves the anal sphincters. Multimodality treatment may be considered.[55]

Basal Cell Carcinoma

Basal cell carcinoma, elsewhere a lesion of sun-exposed skin, occurs rarely on the anal margin. It is usually superficial and rarely metastasizes. Treatment is wide local excision followed by surveillance, because local recurrence is a significant concern.[56]

Anal Canal Neoplasms

Squamous Cell or Epidermoid Carcinoma. Squamous cell carcinoma of the anal canal has an incidence of about 5,000 cases per year in the United States, but this number increases every year with the HIV epidemic. Anal canal cancer differs in treatment and prognosis from anal margin cancer. Squamous cell or epidermoid cancer of the anal canal has various microscopic appearances, including large cell keratinizing (squamous), large cell nonkeratinizing (transitional), and basaloid. The term *cloacogenic carcinoma* has been used for the basaloid and large cell nonkeratinizing (transitional) form of epidermoid carcinoma. Most squamous cell carcinomas of the anal canal above the dentate line are nonkeratinizing (Fig. 70.31).

10 The presentation of epidermoid anal canal carcinoma is commonly a long history of anal problems misinterpreted as pruritus ani, hemorrhoids, or anal fissure, but now characterized by an indurated anal mass. Digital examination of the anal canal should demonstrate all but the smallest anal canal cancers, and the reader is reminded that a palpable 'hemorrhoid' requires biopsy—true internal hemorrhoids are not palpable. Anoscopy confirms digital findings and allows for biopsy.

Once anal canal cancer is diagnosed, colonoscopy is commonly done, but it is not strictly required as there is no association between epidermoid anal canal cancer and colorectal cancer. However, patients are often elderly, may have bled, or simply are due for colorectal cancer screening, so diagnostic colonoscopy is often indicated on its own merits. Computed tomography of the abdomen and pelvis is indicated for staging. Endoanal ultrasonography may be useful in evaluating depth of invasion (not part of anal canal cancer staging) and detecting perirectal lymph node metastasis. Enlarged or suspicious groin lymph nodes should be biopsied, either by excision or fine-needle aspiration, because reactive lymphadenopathy is common. Staging is detailed in Table 70.6.

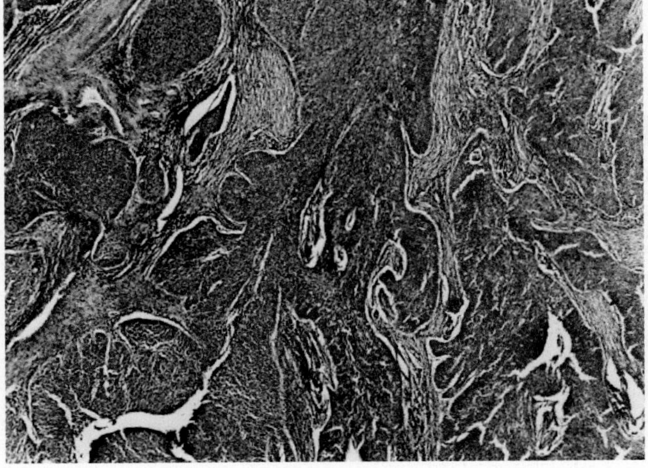

FIGURE 70.31. Squamous cell carcinoma of the anal canal. Note the absence of keratin.

Anal canal lymphatic pathways vary, and the pattern of spread depends on the location of the lesion. About 40% of lymph node metastases are in lymph nodes less than 5 mm in diameter,[57] suggesting a potential role for sentinel node biopsy in this condition.

Inguinal metastasis (stage III) is found in 15% to 20% of patients at the time of diagnosis and becomes apparent later in an additional 10% to 25%.[58] Screening of high-risk groups, such as patients with high-grade AIN (especially in the context of immunosuppression), should decrease the stage at which anal cancers are found. Alertness on the part of surgeons, when evaluating any patient for an atypical 'fissure' or 'hemorrhoid,' is another key defense against advanced disease. When anal cancer is less than 2 cm in diameter (T1), only 3% of patients are found to have lymph node metastasis, and the vast majority of these are curable. Although distant metastasis is uncommon at presentation, subsequent metastasis occurs frequently: 40% of the roughly 700 anal cancer-related deaths per year in the United States occur from disease outside the pelvis.

Treatment for all stages of anal canal cancer is by chemoradiation: The combination of 5-fluorouracil, mitomycin C, and pelvic radiation therapy was pioneered by Nigro in 1972.[59] Abdominoperineal resection had been standard treatment up to that point, but now the surgeon's role is to diagnose the lesion initially by biopsy, then reevaluate the scar 6 to 8 weeks after completion of chemoradiation to rule out persistent disease. Subsequent to Nigro's initial reports, prospective randomized trials established the most effective combination of chemoradiation for local control, avoidance of colostomy, and overall survival.[60] A typical modified Nigro regimen is summarized in Table 70.7; chemotherapy research continues, in the hope of replacing mitomycin C with a less toxic agent.[61] Late adverse effects associated with radiation of the anal region include proctitis, diarrhea, incontinence, anal ulcers, and stenosis, leading to permanent colostomy in about 10% of patients.

Abdominoperineal resection continues to play a role for persistent or recurrent anal canal cancer. All studies of salvage abdominoperineal resection show better survival in recurrent than persistent disease, reflecting the natural history of the two types of lesion. Perineal wound problems are common from this operation, which always takes place in an irradiated field.[62] As patients who undergo chemoradiation for anal cancer have a higher perineal wound complication rate following abdominoperineal resection than do those undergoing chemoradiation for rectal cancer,[63] primary reconstruction with a rectus abdominis myocutaneous flap should be considered.[64]

Adenocarcinoma. Adenocarcinomas of the anus are rare, constituting 3% to 9% of all anal carcinomas.[65] The World Health Organization classifies these malignancies into rectal type, anal gland type, and anorectal fistula type.

Rectal Type. Rectal-type adenocarcinoma arises within the upper anal canal; histology is the same as rectal adenocarcinoma. It is impossible to distinguish this lesion from adenocarcinoma of the lower rectum.

Anal Gland Type. The anal gland ducts are lined by columnar epithelium with mucin-secreting (goblet) cells, from which mucoepidermoid carcinomas can arise. The characteristic feature of anal gland cancer is extramucosal adenocarcinoma without involvement of the anal canal surface epithelium, except where the lesion has spread locally.

TABLE 70.6 **STAGING AND CLASSIFICATION**

AMERICAN JOINT COMMITTEE ON CANCER STAGING CLASSIFICATION FOR SQUAMOUS CELL CARCINOMA OF THE ANAL CANAL

PRIMARY TUMOR (T)	
Tx:	Primary tumor cannot be assessed
T0:	No evidence of primary tumor
Tis:	Carcinoma in situ
T1:	Tumor 2 cm or less in greatest dimension
T2:	Tumor more than 2 cm but not more than 5 cm in greatest dimension
T3:	Tumor more than 5 cm in greatest dimension
T4:	Tumor of any size invades adjacent organ(s), e.g., vagina, urethra, bladder (involvement of sphincter muscle alone is not classified as T4)
REGIONAL LYMPH NODES (N)	
Nx:	Regional lymph nodes cannot be assessed
N0:	No regional lymph node metastasis
N1:	Metastasis in perirectal lymph node(s)
N2:	Metastasis in unilateral internal iliac and/or inguinal lymph nodes
N3:	Metastasis in perirectal and inguinal lymph nodes and/or bilateral internal iliac and/or inguinal lymph nodes
DISTANT METASTASIS (M)	
Mx:	Distant metastasis cannot be assessed
M0:	No distant metastasis
M1:	Distant metastasis
STAGE GROUPING	
Stage 0	Tis, N0, M0
Stage I	T1, N0, M0
Stage II	T2, N0, M0
	T3, N0, M0
Stage IIIA	T1, N1, M0
	T2, N1, M0
	T3, N1, M0
	T4, N0, M0
Stage IIIB	T4, N1, M0
	Any T, N2, M0
	Any T, N3, M0
Stage IV	Any T, Any N, M

TABLE 70.7 **TREATMENT**

MODIFIED NIGRO REGIMEN FOR SQUAMOUS CELL CARCINOMA OF THE ANAL CANAL

■ TREATMENT	■ DOSE	■ SCHEDULE
External radiation	50 Gy, to the primary carcinoma and 35–45 Gy to pelvic inguinal nodes	Start day 1 (2 Gy/d, 5 d/wk for 5 wk)
Systemic chemotherapy	Fluorouracil, 1,000 mg/m^2/24 h as a continuous infusion for 4 d	Start day 1; repeat 4-d infusion starting day 28
Mitomycin C	10–15 mg/m^2 as intravenous bolus	Day 1 only

Anorectal Fistula Type. Mucinous adenocarcinoma may arise within long-standing anorectal fistula tracts. Some authors believe that they originate in the anal glands and ducts, suggesting that the distinction between anal gland–type and anorectal fistula–type adenocarcinoma may be artificial.

Rectal-type adenocarcinoma of the anal canal is treated according to rectal cancer protocols, with local or radical excision depending on depth of invasion, as determined by endoluminal ultrasound or MRI. Abdominoperineal resection is the definitive treatment for most anal canal adenocarcinoma. Although chemoradiation is definitive treatment for epidermoid anal canal cancer, adenocarcinomas of the anal canal are less responsive to nonsurgical therapy.[66]

Melanoma. Melanoma accounts for less than 1% of anal canal malignancies. However, the anal canal is the third most common site for melanoma, after skin and eyes. The female-to-male ratio is approximately 2:1, and the average age at presentation is 63 years.

One should suspect melanoma when one sees a deeply pigmented 'hemorrhoid' causing symptoms. However, most anal melanomas are lightly pigmented or frankly amelanotic, so they are often misdiagnosed as polyps or squamous cell carcinomas. Examination under anesthesia and incisional or excisional biopsy allows for correct diagnosis.

Anal canal melanomas spread submucosally into the rectum but rarely invade adjacent organs, possibly because most patients die before this can occur. Lymphatic spread to mesenteric nodes is seen in about one third of patients at the time of diagnosis; spread to inguinal nodes is less common. Wide hematogenous spread, especially to liver and lung, is common, accounting for most deaths.

Anal canal melanomas do not respond to chemotherapy, radiotherapy, or immunotherapy. While surgery is the only option, it is almost never curative, and abdominoperineal resection confers no survival benefit compared with wide local excision.[67] Sometimes wide local excision involves destroying the anal sphincters, so it must be accompanied by diverting colostomy; when the tumor is large, abdominoperineal resection may be the best option for obtaining local control. Sentinel node excision, a staple of cutaneous melanoma surgery, has not been explored in this population.

References

1. Crapp AR, Cuthbertson AM. William Waldeyer and the rectosacral fascia. *Surg Gynecol Obstet* 1974;138:252–256.
2. Kashyap P, Bates N. Magnetic resonance imaging anatomy of the anal canal. *Australas Radiol* 2004;48:443–449.
3. Macchi V, Porzionato A, Stecco C, et al. Histo-topographic study of the longitudinal anal muscle. *Clin Anat* 2008;21:447–452.
4. Bauer JJ, Gelernt IM, Salky B, et al. Sexual dysfunction following proctocolectomy for benign disease of the colon and rectum. *Ann Surg* 1983;197: 363–367.
5. Izanec J, Nagle D. Impact of proctectomy on continence and sexual function in women. *Am J Gastroenterol* 2006;101(12 suppl):S618–S624.
6. Lestar B, Penninckx F, Kerremans R. The composition of anal basal pressure. An in vivo and in vitro study in man. *Int J Colorectal Dis* 1989;4: 118–122.
7. Loder PB, Kamm MA, Nicholls RJ, et al. Haemorrhoids: pathology, pathophysiology and aetiology. *Br J Surg* 1994;81:946–954.
8. Bernstein WC. What are hemorrhoids and what is their relationship to the portal venous system? *Dis Colon Rectum* 1983;26:829–834.
9. Iyer VS, Shrier I, Gordon PH. Long-term outcome of rubber band ligation for symptomatic primary and recurrent internal hemorrhoids. *Dis Colon Rectum* 2004;47:1364–1370.
10. Peng BC, Jayne DG, Ho YH. Randomized trial of rubber band ligation vs. stapled hemorrhoidectomy for prolapsed piles. *Dis Colon Rectum* 2003; 46:291–297.
11. Nisar PJ, Acheson AG, Neal KR, et al. Stapled hemorrhoidopexy compared with conventional hemorrhoidectomy: systematic review of randomized, controlled trials. *Dis Colon Rectum* 2004;47:1837–1845.
12. Senagore AJ, Singer M, Abcarian H, et al. A prospective, randomized, controlled multicenter trial comparing stapled hemorrhoidopexy and Ferguson hemorrhoidectomy: perioperative and one-year results. *Dis Colon Rectum* 2004;47:1824–1836.
13. Greenspon J, Williams SB, Young HA, et al. Thrombosed external hemorrhoids: outcome after conservative or surgical management. *Dis Colon Rectum* 2004;47:1493–1498.
14. Kaul AK, Skaife PG. Circumferential stapled procedure for bleeding anorectal varices is an effective treatment—experience in nine patients. *Colorectal Dis* 2009;11(4):420–423.
15. Kim DS, Tsang CB, Wong WD. Complete rectal prolapse: evolution of management and results. *Dis Colon Rectum* 1999;42:460–469.
16. Huber FT, Stein H, Siewert JR. Functional results after treatment of rectal prolapse with rectopexy and sigmoid resection. *World J Surg* 1995;19: 138–143.
17. Raftopoulos Y, Senagore AJ, Di Giuro G, et al. Recurrence rates after abdominal surgery for complete rectal prolapse: a multicenter pooled analysis of 643 individual patient data. *Dis Colon Rectum* 2005;48: 1200–1206.
18. Agachan F, Reissman P, Pfeifer J, et al. Comparison of three perineal procedures for the treatment of rectal prolapse. *South Med J* 1997;90:925–932.
19. Baxter NN, Rothenberger DA, Lowry AC. Measuring fecal incontinence. *Dis Colon Rectum* 2003;46:1591–1605.
20. Byrne CM, Solomon MJ, Young JM, et al. Biofeedback for fecal incontinence: short-term outcomes of 513 consecutive patients and predictors of successful treatment. *Dis Colon Rectum* 2007;50:417–427.
21. Norton C. Fecal incontinence and biofeedback therapy. *Gastroenterol Clin North Am* 2008;37:587–604.
22. Bravo Gutierrez A, Madoff RD, Lowry AC, et al. Long-term results of anterior sphincteroplasty. *Dis Colon Rectum* 2004;47:727–731.
23. Wong WD, Congliosi SM, Spencer MP, et al. The safety and efficacy of the artificial bowel sphincter for fecal incontinence: results from a multicenter cohort study. *Dis Colon Rectum* 2002;45:1139–1153.
24. Parker SC, Spencer MP, Madoff RD, et al. Artificial bowel sphincter: long-term experience at a single institution. *Dis Colon Rectum* 2003;46: 722–729.
25. Matzel KE, Lux P, Heuer S, et al. Sacral nerve stimulation for faecal incontinence: long-term outcome. *Colorectal Dis* 2009;11(6):636–641.
26. Schouten WR, Briel JW, Auwerda JJ, et al. Ischaemic nature of anal fissure. *Br J Surg* 1996;83:63–65.
27. Minguez M, Herreros B, Espi A, et al. Long-term follow-up (42 months) of chronic anal fissure after healing with botulinum toxin. *Gastroenterology* 2002;123:112–117.
28. García-Granero E, Sanahuja A, García-Botello SA. The ideal lateral internal sphincterotomy: clinical and endosonographic evaluation following open and closed internal anal sphincterotomy. *Colorectal Dis* 2009;11(5): 502–507.
29. Hyman N. Incontinence after lateral internal sphincterotomy: a prospective study and quality of life assessment. *Dis Colon Rectum* 2004;47: 35–38.
30. Garcia-Aguilar J, Belmonte C, Wong WD. Open vs. closed sphincterotomy for chronic anal fissure: long-term results. *Dis Colon Rectum* 1996;39: 440–443.
31. Nelson R. Non surgical therapy for anal fissure. *Cochrane Database Syst Rev* 2006 Oct 18;(4):CD003431.
32. Parks AG, Gordon PH, Hardcastle JD. A classification of anal fistula. *Br J Surg* 1976;63:1–12.
33. Buchanan GN, Halligan S, Bartram CI, et al. Clinical examination, endosonography, and MR imaging in preoperative assessment of fistula in ano: comparison with outcome-based reference standard. *Radiology* 2004; 233:674–681.
34. Lindsey I, Smilgin-Humphreys MM, Cunningham C, et al. A randomized, controlled trial of fibrin glue vs. conventional treatment for anal fistula. *Dis Colon Rectum* 2002;45:1608–1615.
35. Thekkinkattil D, Botterill I, Ambrose NS, et al. Efficacy of the anal fistula plug in complex anorectal fistulae. *Colorectal Dis* 2009;11(6):584–587.
36. Present DH, Rutgeerts P, Targan S, et al. Infliximab for the treatment of fistulas in patients with Crohn's disease. *N Engl J Med* 1999;340: 1398–1405.
37. Lowry AC, Thorson AG, Rothenberger DA, et al. Repair of simple rectovaginal fistulas. Influence of previous repairs. *Dis Colon Rectum* 1988;31: 676–678.
38. Bessa SS. Results of the lateral advancing flap operation (modified Karydakis procedure) for the management of pilonidal sinus disease. *Dis Colon Rectum* 2007;50:1935–1940.
39. Bascom, J. Pilonidal disease: long-term results of follicle removal. *Dis Colon Rectum* 1983;26:800–807.
40. Bascom J, Bascom T. Utility of the cleft lift procedure in refractory pilonidal disease. *Am J Surg* 2007;193(5):606–609.
41. Milsom J. Herpes simplex infections of the anorectum. *Semin Colon Rectal Surg* 1992;3:222–226.
42. Bernstein M. Benign human immunodeficiency virus/acquired immune deficiency syndrome-specific anorectal conditions. *Semin Colon Rectal Surg* 1998;9:94–98.
43. Kerr AR, Ship JA. Management strategies for HIV-associated aphthous stomatitis. *Am J Clin Dermatol* 2003;4:669–680.
44. Saclarides T, Klem D. Genetic alterations and virology of anal cancer. *Semin Colon Rectal Surg* 1995;6:131–134.
45. Surawicz C, Kiviat N. A rational approach to anal intraepithelial neoplasia. *Semin Colon Rectal Surg* 1998;9:99–106.
46. Palefsky JM, Holly EA, Efirdc JT, et al. Anal intraepithelial neoplasia in the highly active antiretroviral therapy era among HIV-positive men who have sex with men. *AIDS* 2005;19:1407–1414.

47. Goldstone SE, Kawalek AZ, Huyett JW. Infrared coagulator: a useful tool for treating anal squamous intraepithelial lesions. *Dis Colon Rectum* 2005;48:1042–1054.
48. Devaraj B, Cosman BC. Expectant management of anal squamous dysplasia in patients with HIV. *Dis Colon Rectum* 2006;49:36–40.
49. Pineda CE, Welton ML. Controversies in the management of anal high-grade squamous intraepithelial lesions. *Minerva Chir* 2008;63:389–399.
50. Sarmiento JM, Wolff BG, Burgart LJ, et al. Perianal Bowen's disease: associated tumors, human papillomavirus, surgery, and other controversies. *Dis Colon Rectum* 1997;40:912–918.
51. Regauer S. Extramammary Paget's disease—a proliferation of adnexal origin? *Histopathology* 2006;48:723–729.
52. Sarmiento JM, Wolff BG, Burgart LJ, et al. Paget's disease of the perianal region—an aggressive disease? *Dis Colon Rectum* 1997;40:1187–1194.
53. Beck DE. Paget's disease and Bowen's disease of the anus. *Semin Colon Rectal Surg.* 1995;6:143–149.
54. Hassan I, Horgan AF, Nivatvongs S. V-Y island flaps for repair of large perianal defects. *Am J Surg* 2001;181:363–365.
55. De Toma G, Cavallaro G, Bitonti A, et al. Surgical management of perianal giant condyloma acuminatum (Buschke-Löwenstein tumor). Report of three cases. *Eur Surg Res* 2006;38:418–422.
56. Paterson CA, Young-Fadok TM, Dozois RR. Basal cell carcinoma of the perianal region: 20-year experience. *Dis Colon Rectum* 1999;42:1200–1202.
57. Wade DS, Herrera L, Castillo NB, et al., Metastases to the lymph nodes in epidermoid carcinoma of the anal canal studied by a clearing technique. *Surg Gynecol Obstet* 1989;169:238–242.
58. Boman BM, Moertel CG, O'Connell MJ, et al. Carcinoma of the anal canal. A clinical and pathologic study of 188 cases. *Cancer* 1984;54:114–125.
59. Nigro ND. An evaluation of combined therapy for squamous cell cancer of the anal canal. *Dis Colon Rectum* 1984;27:763–766.
60. Flam M, John M, Pajak TF, et al. Role of mitomycin in combination with fluorouracil and radiotherapy, and of salvage chemoradiation in the definitive nonsurgical treatment of epidermoid carcinoma of the anal canal: results of a phase III randomised intergroup study. *J Clin Oncol* 1996;14:2527–2529.
61. Ajani JA, Winter KA, Gunderson LL, et al. Fluorouracil, mitomycin, and radiotherapy vs fluorouracil, cisplatin, and radiotherapy for carcinoma of the anal canal: a randomized controlled trial. *JAMA* 2008;299:1914–1921.
62. Stewart D, Yan Y, Kodner IJ, et al. Salvage surgery after failed chemoradiation for anal canal cancer: should the paradigm be changed for high-risk tumors? *J Gastrointest Surg* 2007;11:1744–1751.
63. Christian CK, Kwaan MR, Betensky RA, et al. Risk factors for perineal wound complications following abdominoperineal resection. *Dis Colon Rectum* 2005;48:43–48.
64. Tei TM, Stolzenburg T, Buntzen S, et al. Use of transpelvic rectus abdominis musculocutaneous flap for anal cancer salvage surgery. *Br J Surg* 2003;90:575–580.
65. Tarazi R, Nelson R. Adenocarcinoma of the Anus. *Semin Colon Rectal Surg.* 1995;6:169–173.
66. Papagikos M, Crane CH, Skibber J, et al. Chemoradiation for adenocarcinoma of the anus. *Int J Radiat Oncol Biol Phys* 2003;55:669–678.
67. Pessaux P, Pocard M, Elias D, et al. Surgical management of primary anorectal melanoma. *Br J Surg* 2004;91:1183–1187.

CHAPTER 71 ■ ABDOMINAL WALL HERNIAS

ROBERT J. FITZGIBBONS Jr., SAMUEL CEMAJ, AND THOMAS H. QUINN

KEY POINTS

1. Surgeons have traditionally been taught the anatomy of the abdominal wall from an outside to inside perspective. However, with the increasing use of intra-abdominal or preperitoneal approaches to abdominal wall reconstruction, a better understanding of the anatomy from the inside to the outside perspective is important.
2. Type I collagen is responsible for tensile strength, while type III collagen is less mature and is most important in the early phases of wound healing. A decreased ratio of type I to type III collagens can be detected in fascial and skin specimens obtained from patients with hernias.
3. Inguinal hernias constitute approximately 75% of abdominal wall hernias, with femoral hernia accounting for 5%. Incisional, umbilical, and epigastric hernias account for 15% and miscellaneous hernias make up the other 5%.
4. Watchful waiting is an acceptable alternative to routine repair for male inguinal hernia patients with minimal symptoms. This does not apply to females because of the higher risk of a hernia accident.
5. The performance of a "tension-free" inguinal hernia repair dramatically reduces the risk of recurrent hernia tc a rate generally reported to be less than 2%.
6. The most popular laparoscopic techniques for repair of an inguinal hernia are the transabdominal preperitoneal repair and the totally extraperitoneal laparoscopic repair.
7. Historical recurrence rates of 30% to 40% following ventral hernia repair have been dramatically reduced by modern tension-free repairs.
8. A recent major prospective, randomized, multicenter trial showed that laparoscopic repair was associated with a significantly increased risk of recurrent hernia than open repair (10.1% vs. 4.9%).
9. The frequency of at least some long-term groin pain may be as high as 50% at 1 year following inguinal hernia repair with moderate to severe pain in up to 10% of patients.
10. Ischemic orchitis occurs in about 1% of primary hernia repairs but is more common following repair of a recurrent hernia.

One of the most frequently performed operations by general surgeons worldwide is the repair of an abdominal wall hernia. According to the National Center for Health Statistics, in the United States in the year 2003, the number of hernia repairs by type was 770,000 inguinal, 175,000 umbilical, 105,000 incisional, 30,000 femoral, and 80,000 miscellaneous (epigastric, spigelian, etc.), for a total cost of approximately $2.5 billion, assuming a conservative estimate of a base cost of $2,000 to $2,500 per procedure.[1] In the past, most training programs relegated the repair of abdominal hernias to the junior members of the surgical team with little regard for results.[2] However, in the modern era of heightened emphasis on accountability to our patients, this is changing rapidly. Interest by the academic community in the science behind hernia repair as well as an explosion in device development by industry has resulted in significant changes in many surgeons' practices. This chapter describes these recent changes in the approach to hernia repair.

ANATOMY OF THE ABDOMINAL WALL AND GROIN

The anatomy of the abdominal wall and the inguinal region are presented, first from the viewpoint of the surgeon using open techniques and subsequently from the perspective of the surgeon utilizing the laparoscope. Anatomic terms for which synonyms and eponyms are commonly used are listed in Table 71.1. Specific anatomic nomenclature can now be found in *Terminologia Anatomica,* the successor to *Nomina Anatomica.*

The abdominal wall spans the gap between the lower ribs and the pelvis; the lowest ribs, pelvic brim, and lumbar spine comprise its only skeletal support. The muscular and aponeurotic structures that provide much of the integrity of the wall must not only compress and contain abdominal viscera but also contribute to the support and movement of the spine and pelvis.

The sheets of relatively thin muscles and aponeuroses that make up the abdominal wall would, individually, seem to predispose to visceral eventration. However, the laminar layout of these sheets over most of the wall precludes this in most cases. The most common sites of hernia formation are found between laminations, where only peritoneum and fascia are found between the viscera and skin. These weak areas are most important to the hernia surgeon and are described in detail in the subsequent sections dealing with the anterior and posterolateral abdominal wall and the inguinal region.

Anterior Abdominal Wall

Superficial Fascia, Vessels, and Nerves. The anterior abdominal wall does not consist solely of muscle and aponeurosis; it can also be the repository for copious amounts of adipose tissue (panniculus adiposus) in its superficial fascial layer, often called *Camper fascia.* This layer, which is continuous inferiorly with the outer layer of fascia covering the perineum and genitalia, also contains the dartos muscle fibers of the scrotum. The major blood vessels of the superficial fatty layer are the superficial epigastric vessels and superficial circumflex iliac vessels, which are tributaries of the femoral vessels. The superficial fascia is also replete with lymphatic vessels that drain into the inguinal lymph nodes inferior to the umbilicus. The lymphatic structures cross the inguinal ligament, so that they are potentially placed in the surgical field during open herniorrhaphy.

TABLE 71.1

ANATOMIC TERMS WITH COMMON SYNONYMS AND EPONYMS

FASCIAL STRUCTURES/SPACES
Fatty layer of superficial fascia; panniculus adiposus; Camper fascia
Investing fascia of external abdominal oblique; fascia innominata
Membranous layer of superficial fascia; Scarpa fascia
Retroinguinal space; space of Bogros
Retropubic space; space of Retzius
LIGAMENTOUS STRUCTURES
Iliopectineal ligament; iliopectineal arch
Iliopubic tract; Thompson ligament (band)
Inguinal ligament; Poupart ligament
Lacunar ligament; Gimbernat ligament
Pectineal ligament; Cooper ligament
APONEUROSIS-DERIVED STRUCTURES
Arcuate line; semicircular line; linea semicirculars; line of Douglas
Falx inguinalis (often incorrectly referred to as *conjoined tendon*)
Reflected inguinal ligament; reflex ligament; Colles ligament
Semilunar line; linea semilunaris; Spigelius line

A second fascial layer in the superficial abdominal wall is the deep fascia of Scarpa. Although most commonly considered a distinct anatomic layer, Scarpa fascia actually consists of compressed fibrous components of the superficial fascia.[3] The deeper fibrous tissue of the superficial fascia forms the fundiform ligament of the penis (suspensory ligament of the female clitoris), continues onto the penis and scrotum, and ultimately fuses with the superficial fascia of the perineum.

The superficial fascia also fuses with the layer of fascia (fascia innominata) investing the external abdominal oblique muscle. This fascia is bound inferiorly to the inguinal ligament and pubis before continuing onto the thigh, where it blends with the fascia lata to seal the space beneath and inferior to the inguinal ligament, which is the inferior portion of the myopectineal orifice (Fig. 71.1). This portion of the inguinal region includes the Hesselbach (inguinal) triangle superiorly and therefore constitutes the weakest aspect of the groin.

The skin of the anterior abdominal wall is segmentally innervated in the familiar dermatome pattern. The nerve branches to this area are derived from the anterior and lateral cutaneous branches of the ventral rami of the 7th to 12th intercostal nerves and from the ventral rami of the first and second lumbar nerves. Disruption of one of these nerves is rarely noted by the postoperative patient because the dermatome fields overlap significantly. The anterior and lateral cutaneous branches reach the subcutaneous layer by coursing between the flat lateral muscles and by piercing the sheath of the rectus abdominis.

Anterior Musculature and Ligaments. The division of the wall into anterior and posterior segments is somewhat artificial because the anterior muscles, with the exception of the rectus abdominis, arise posteriorly and also form part of the posterior wall.

The three muscles of the lateral aspect of the anterior abdominal wall (Fig. 71.2) are composed of a variable amount of muscle with a large aponeurosis. The aponeurosis is the tendon of insertion for the lateral muscles, and it also forms the sheath of the rectus abdominis. The midline decussation of the three aponeuroses forms the linea alba. Fibrous tissue layers are of great importance to the hernia surgeon because of their ability to support sutures. *Fascia* and *aponeurosis* are terms commonly used to describe these fibrous structures but are often confused and used interchangeably. In this chapter, an aponeurosis is defined as the non–muscle-fiber-containing portion of a muscle usually present at insertion points. Muscle fibers are said to "give way" to the corresponding aponeurosis. Fascia, on the other hand, is the fibrous tissue that lines or envelops muscles.

External Abdominal Oblique Muscle and Associated Ligaments. The external abdominal oblique muscle (Figs. 71.2 and 71.3A, B) is the most superficial of the three lateral abdominal muscles. The external abdominal oblique arises from the posterior aspects of the lower eight ribs and interdigitates with both the serratus anterior and the latissimus dorsi at its origin. The direction of the muscle fibers varies from nearly horizontal in its upper portion to oblique in the middle and lower portions. The mostly horizontal fibers, which originate posteriorly, insert onto the anterior portion of the iliac

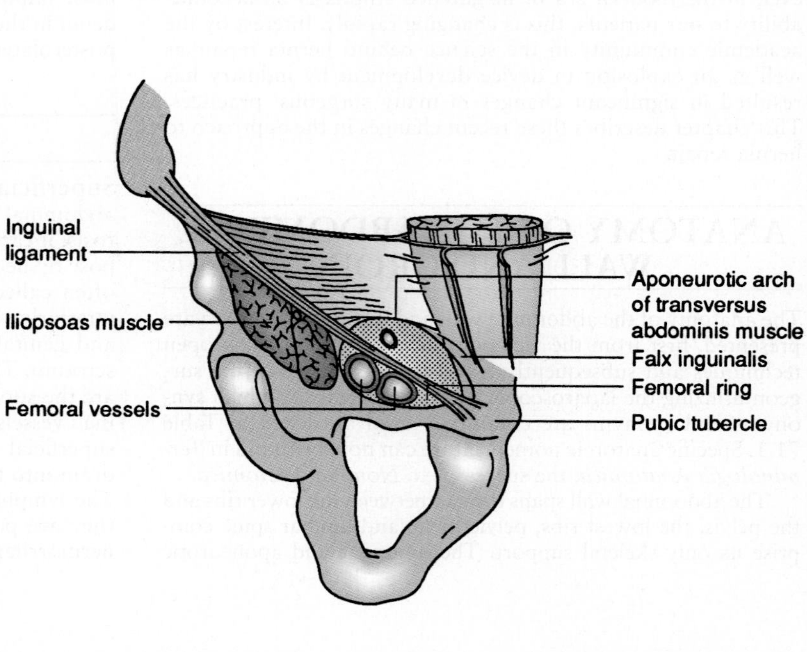

FIGURE 71.1. The myopectineal orifice. Superior to the inguinal ligament, this area includes the inguinal (Hesselbach) triangle. Inferior to the ligament, the orifice transmits the iliopsoas muscle, the femoral nerve and vessels, and the femoral canal and sheath. (Reproduced with permission from Wantz GE. *Atlas of Hernia Surgery*. New York: Raven Press; 1991:4.)

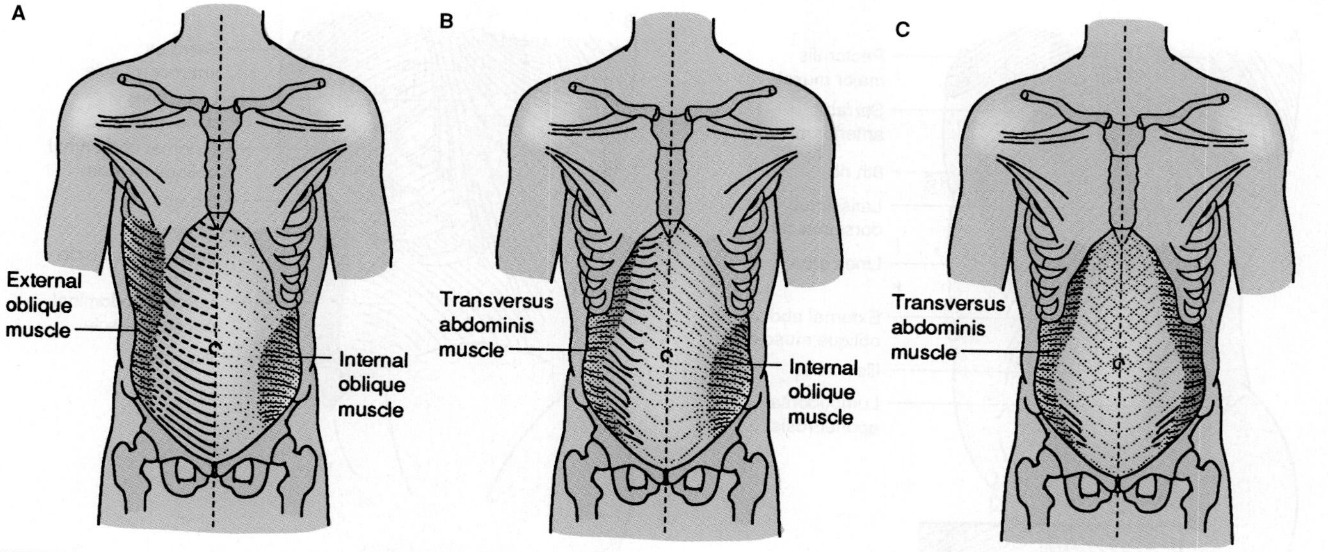

FIGURE 71.2. Pattern of crossing of the aponeurotic fascicles of the abdominal wall musculature. **A:** Fascicles from the right external oblique and anterior lamina of the left internal oblique. **B:** Fascicles from the right transversus abdominis and posterior lamina of the left internal oblique. **C:** Fascicles between the right and left transversus abdominis muscles.

crest. The obliquely arranged anteroinferior fibers of insertion fold on themselves to form the inguinal ligament. The remaining portion of the aponeurosis inserts into the linea alba after contributing to the anterior portion of the rectus abdominis sheath. Some fibers cross the linea alba to reinforce further the anterior rectus sheath of the opposite side.

The more medial fibers of the aponeurosis of the external oblique divide into a medial and a lateral crus to form the external or superficial inguinal ring. The spermatic cord (or round ligament) and branches of the ilioinguinal and genitofemoral nerves pass through this opening. The *inguinal ligament* (Fig. 71.4) is worthy of special consideration because of its important role as both a landmark and an integral component of many groin hernia repairs. The inguinal ligament is formed by obliquely oriented anteroinferior aponeurotic fibers of the external abdominal oblique. The ligament is formed when the aponeurosis folds beneath itself. Its lateral attachment is to the anterior superior iliac crest; its medial insertion is primarily on the pubic tubercle.

The medial insertion of the inguinal ligament in most persons is dual. One portion runs along the superior surface of the pubic tubercle and symphysis to form (or at least reinforce) the superior pubic ligament. The other portion is fan shaped and spans the distance between the inguinal ligament proper and the pectineal line of the pubis. This fan-shaped portion of the ligament is called the *lacunar ligament* (Fig. 71.4). It blends laterally with the pectineal (Cooper) ligament.

Internal Abdominal Oblique Muscle and Aponeurosis. The middle layer of the lateral abdominal group is the internal abdominal oblique muscle (Figs. 71.2 and 71.3B, C). This muscle primarily arises from the iliac fascia along the iliac crest and forms a band of iliac fascia fused with the inguinal ligament. The uppermost fibers course obliquely toward the distal ends of the lower three or four ("floating") ribs. The muscle fibers of the internal oblique fan out following the shape of the iliac crest, so that the lowermost fibers are directed inferiorly. These fibers arch over the round ligament, or spermatic cord. Some of the lower muscle bundles in the male join fibers of the transversus abdominis to form the cremaster muscle. The aponeurosis of the internal oblique (Fig. 71.5A) above the level of the umbilicus splits to envelop the rectus abdominis, re-forming in the midline to join and interweave with the fibers of the linea alba. Below the level of the umbilicus (Fig. 71.5B), the aponeurosis does not split but rather runs anterior to the rectus muscle, continues medially as a single sheet, joins the anterior rectus sheath, and finally contributes to the linea alba. The aponeurotic portion of the internal oblique is widest at the level of the umbilicus.

Transversus Abdominis Muscle and Aponeurosis. The transversus abdominis muscle (Figs. 71.2 and 71.3C) arises from the fascia along the iliac crest and inguinal ligament and from the lower six costal cartilages and ribs, where it interdigitates with the lateral diaphragmatic fibers. The muscle bundles of the transversus abdominis for the most part run horizontally. The lower medial fibers, however, may continue in a more inferomedial course toward the site of insertion on the crest and pecten of the pubis.

The aponeurosis of the transversus abdominis joins the posterior lamina of the internal abdominal oblique, forming above the umbilicus a portion of the posterior rectus sheath. Below the umbilicus, the transversus abdominis aponeurosis is a component of the anterior rectus sheath. The gradual termination of aponeurotic tissue on the posterior aspect of the rectus abdominis forms the arcuate line (of Douglas) (Fig. 71.6). The medial aponeurotic fibers of the transversus abdominis insert on the pecten pubis and the crest of the pubis to form the falx inguinalis. These fibers infrequently are joined by a portion of the internal oblique aponeurosis; only then is a true conjoined tendon formed.[4]

The arch formed by the termination of the aponeurotic fibers of the transversus abdominis is called the *aponeurotic arch* (Fig. 71.6). The area beneath the arch varies. A high arch may be a predisposing factor in direct inguinal hernia. Contraction of the transversus abdominis causes the arch to move down toward the inguinal ligament in a kind of shutter mechanism, which reinforces the weakest area of the groin when intra-abdominal pressure is raised.

Rectus Abdominis. The rectus abdominis (Figs. 71.3D and 71.5) forms the central and anchoring muscle mass of the anterior abdomen. The rectus muscle arises from the fifth to the seventh costal cartilages and inserts on the pubic symphysis and pubic crest. Each rectus muscle is segmented by tendinous intersections at the levels of the xiphoid process and the

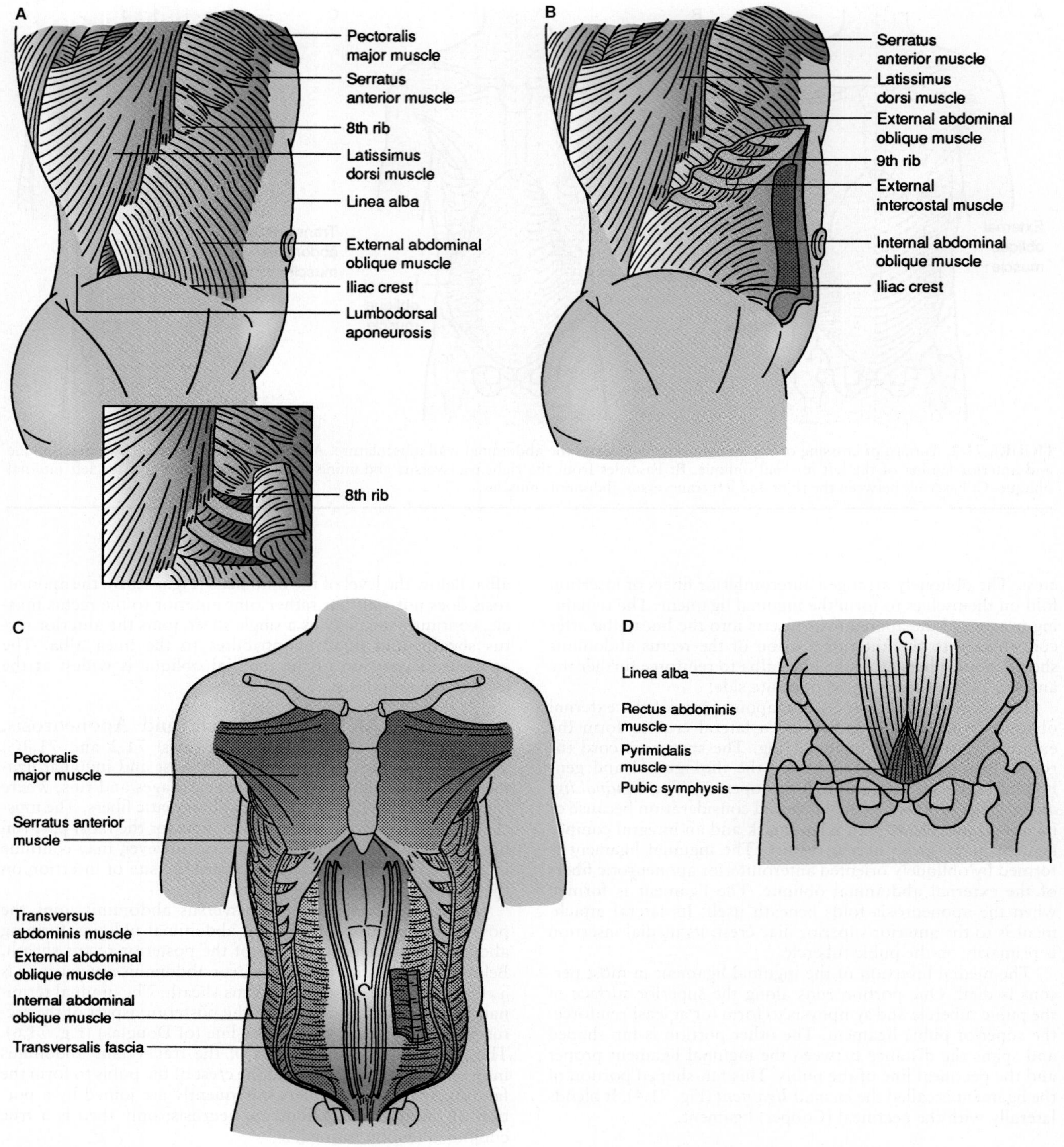

FIGURE 71.3. **A:** External oblique muscle and aponeurosis. **B:** Internal oblique muscle and aponeurosis. **C:** Transversus abdominis muscle and aponeurosis. **D:** Lower rectus abdominis and pyramidalis muscle. The linea alba is formed by the intermeshed fibers of the aponeuroses of the lateral muscle layers; it is tensed by the pyramidalis, which inserts into it.

umbilicus and at a point midway between these two. The principal blood supply reaches the muscle from the superior and inferior epigastric arteries (Fig. 71.5), which anastomose just superior to the umbilicus. Other vessels are anterior branches of the intercostal arteries; these reach the muscle by entering the lateral aspect of the rectus sheath. The innervation of the muscle is from the 7th to the 12th intercostal nerves, which laterally pierce the aponeurotic sheath of the muscle. The lateral edge of the muscle is demarcated by a slight depression in the aponeurotic fibers coursing toward the muscle; this depression is the *semilunar line.*

The small pyramidalis muscle (Fig. 71.3D) accompanies the rectus abdominis at its origin in a minority of people. The pyramidalis arises from the pubic symphysis. It lies within the rectus

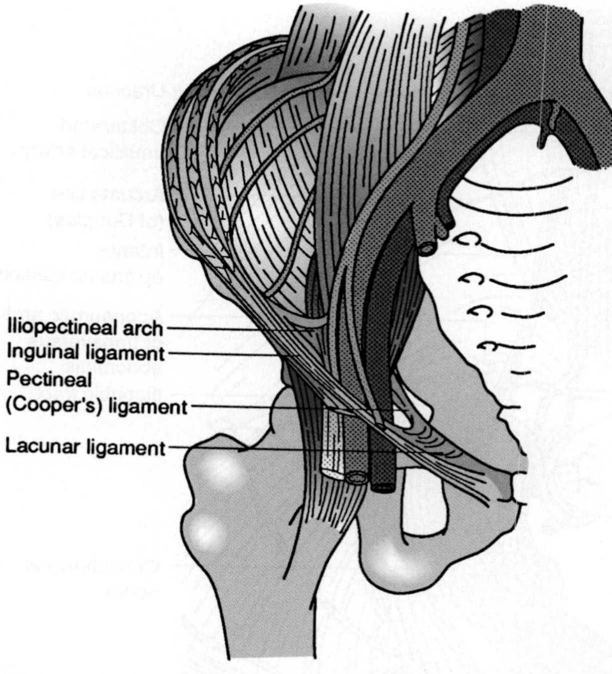

FIGURE 71.4. Ligamentous structures of the inguinal region. The iliopubic tract is not seen in this view because it is obscured by the inguinal ligament. The lacunar ligament is the expanded medial end of the inguinal ligament; on the pecten pubis, it blends with the inguinal (Cooper) ligament.

sheath and tapers to attach to the linea alba, the conjunction of the two rectus sheaths and the major site of insertion of three aponeuroses from all three lateral muscle layers.

Rectus Sheath. Although the components of the rectus sheath individually have been discussed in relation to the three lateral abdominal muscles, it should also be considered as a distinct entity. Three features of the rectus muscle and its sheath can be observed even topographically in well-muscled or very thin subjects:

1. The semilunar line is a slight depression in the aponeurotic fibers corresponding to the lateral edge of the rectus muscle. It marks the site of initial lateral insertion of the aponeurotic tendons of the lateral abdominal muscles.
2. The tendinous inscriptions divide each muscle into three parts.[5] These are the basis of the expression "six pack," popularized by bodybuilders.
3. The linea alba is the midline confluence of the aponeuroses of the rectus muscles and also the internal and external oblique muscles.

The composition of the rectus sheath varies depending on the level sampled. The anterior sheath superior to the umbilicus is composed of the aponeurosis of the external abdominal oblique and the anterior lamina of the internal abdominal oblique. The transversalis aponeurosis does not participate in the formation of the anterior sheath at this level. At a variable level inferior to the umbilicus, the anterior sheath is a composite of all the aponeurotic layers.

The posterior sheath of the rectus muscle superior to the umbilicus is a lamination of the posterior lamina of the aponeurosis of the internal abdominal oblique and the transversus abdominis aponeurosis. The external abdominal oblique does not participate in the formation of the posterior portion of the rectus sheath. At a highly variable site inferior to the umbilicus, all the aponeurotic tendons pass anteriorly to form the anterior rectus sheath. The fibers of the posterior sheath are seen to attenuate gradually. The aponeurotic fibers do not end abruptly at the arcuate line. This transfer of connective tissue away from the posterior rectus sheath causes the arcuate line (of Douglas) to form on the posterior surface of the muscle (Fig. 71.6). The tissue covering the deep surface of the rectus muscle inferior to the arcuate line is primarily the transversalis fascia.

Some have questioned this traditional scheme of rectus sheath composition, contending that each of the aponeurotic layers superior to the umbilicus is actually bifid, with both contributing to the anterior and posterior sheaths.[6] The fibers of the posterior sheath are seen to attenuate gradually. The concept of rectus sheath composition favored by most is shown in Figure 71.7.[7]

Innervation and Blood Supply of the Anterior Abdominal Wall. The innervation of the anterior wall muscles is multiple. The lower intercostal and upper lumbar nerves (T7 to T12, L1, L2) contribute most of the innervation to the lateral muscles and to the rectus abdominis and overlying skin. The nerves pass anteriorly in a plane between the internal abdominal oblique and the transversus abdominis, eventually piercing the lateral aspect of the rectus sheath to innervate the muscle therein. The external oblique muscle receives branches of the intercostal nerves, which penetrate the internal oblique. The anterior ends of the nerves form part of the cutaneous innervation of the abdominal wall. The first lumbar nerve

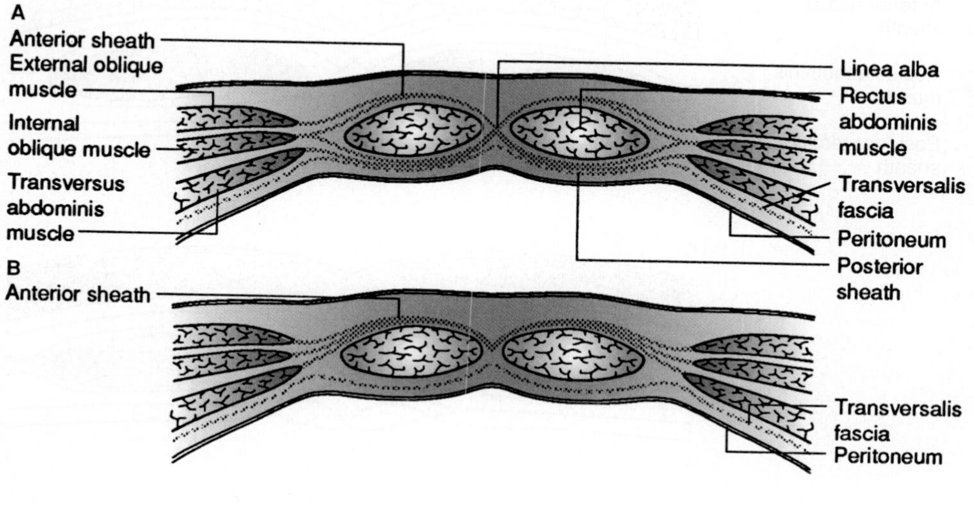

FIGURE 71.5. **A:** Immediately superior to the umbilicus, the rectus sheath consists of anterior and posterior components. The anterior sheath is composed of the aponeuroses of the external and internal abdominal oblique muscles, and the posterior sheath consists of the posterior aponeurotic lamina of the internal oblique and the aponeurosis of the transversus abdominis muscle. **B:** The rectus sheath inferior to the arcuate line (of Douglas) consists of an anterior portion made up of fibers from all aponeurotic layers; the posterior portion at this point comprises only transversalis fascia covered internally by peritoneum.

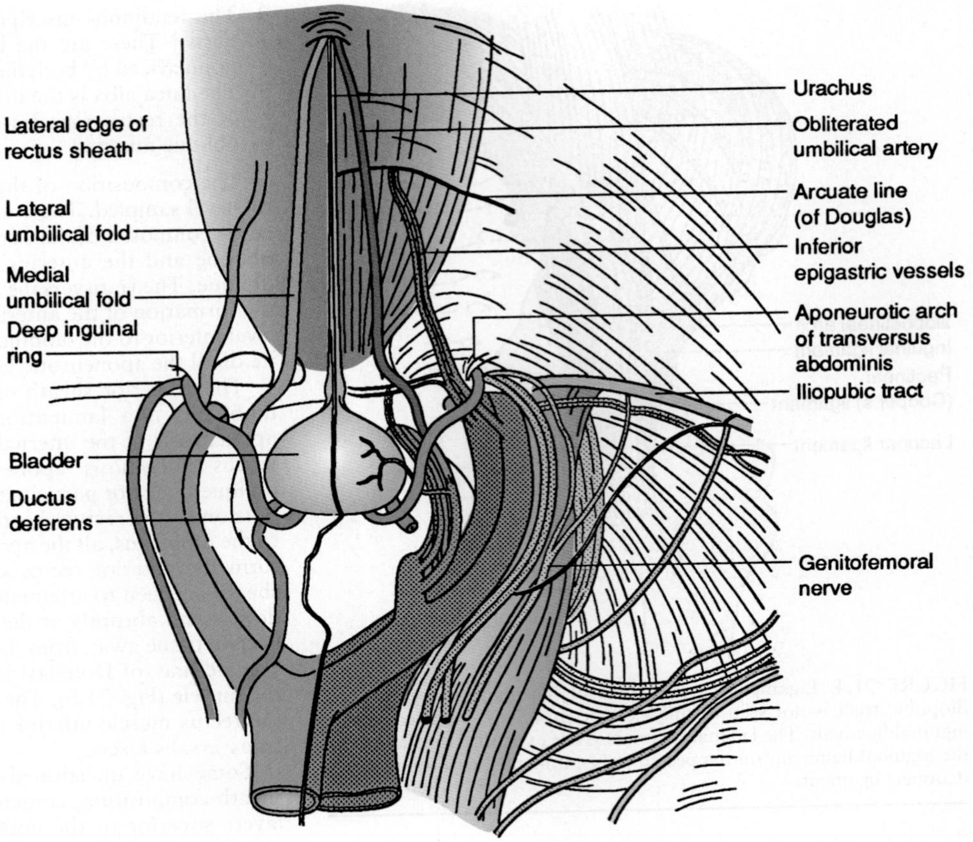

FIGURE 71.6. The deep inguinal region, pelvis, and anterior abdominal wall from the viewpoint of a surgeon using a laparoscopic technique. The anterior wall folds upward approximately at the iliopubic tract in this illustration.

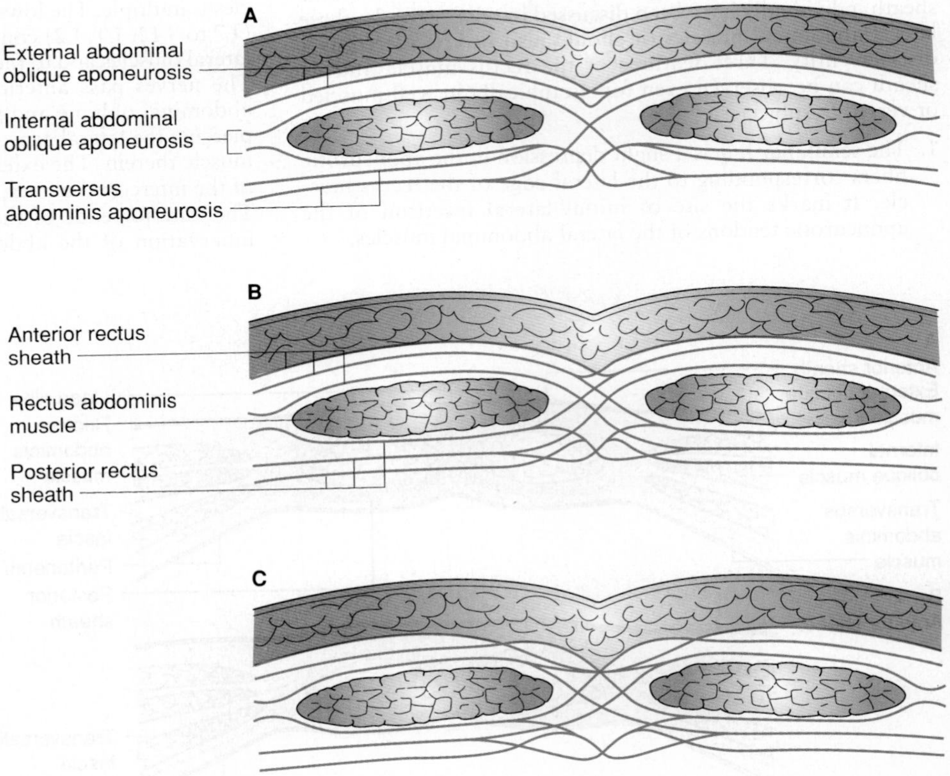

FIGURE 71.7. Patterns of midline decussation of the aponeuroses. A: Single anterior and posterior lines of decussation. B: Single anterior and triple posterior lines of decussation. C: Triple anterior and posterior lines of decussation. (Adapted from Askar O. Surgical anatomy of the aponeurotic expansions of the anterior abdominal wall. *Ann R Coll Surg Engl* 1977;59:313.)

divides into the ilioinguinal and iliohypogastric nerves. These may divide within the psoas major muscle or between the internal oblique and transversus abdominis muscles. The ilioinguinal nerve may communicate with the iliohypogastric nerve before innervating the internal oblique. The ilioinguinal nerve then passes through the external inguinal ring to run with the spermatic cord, whereas the iliohypogastric nerve pierces the external oblique to innervate the skin above the pubis. The cremaster muscle fibers, which are derived from the internal oblique muscle, are innervated by the genitofemoral nerve (L1, L2).

The blood supply of the lateral muscles of the anterior wall is primarily from the lower three or four intercostal arteries, the deep circumflex iliac artery, and the lumbar arteries. The rectus abdominis has a complicated blood supply derived from the superior epigastric artery (a terminal branch of the internal thoracic, or internal mammary, artery), the inferior epigastric artery (a branch of the external iliac artery), and the lower intercostal arteries. The latter arteries enter the sides of the muscle after traveling between the oblique muscles. The superior and inferior epigastric arteries enter the rectus sheath and anastomose near the umbilicus.

Posterolateral (Lumbar) Abdominal Wall

The posterolateral or lumbar portion of the abdominal wall (Fig. 71.8) often is overlooked in discussions of abdominal hernia, perhaps because of the much more common occurrence of groin and femoral hernias. The configuration of the muscle layers in the lumbar area also predisposes to hernia formation. For the purposes of this discussion, the lumbar portion of the abdominal wall is defined as the area bounded superiorly by the 12th rib, inferiorly by the iliac crest, and medially by the erector spinae group. Eight muscles arrayed in three layers constitute the posterolateral or lumbar portion of the abdominal wall.

The most superficial layer is composed of the external abdominal oblique muscle, which arises from the posteroinferior portion of the lower ribs and inserts in part along the posterior iliac crest. Closely associated with the external oblique in this area is the latissimus dorsi, which arises from the posterior iliac crest, the spinous processes of the sacrum and lumbar vertebrae, and the lumbodorsal fascia. The muscle courses obliquely toward its insertion on the medial aspect of the intertubercular groove of the humerus. The triangular space formed by the two muscles just described and the iliac crest is called the *inferior lumbar (Petit) triangle* (Fig. 71.8A).

The middle layer of lumbar abdominal muscles consists of the erector spinae, the internal abdominal oblique, and the extremely thin insignificant serratus posterior inferior. The erector spinae forms a significant portion of the abdominal wall in the lumbar region, with fibers extending nearly the length of the spinal column. The internal abdominal oblique muscle forms the remainder of the layer. The serratus posterior inferior arises from the lumbodorsal fascia and inserts on the lower four ribs. The middle layer of lumbar muscle is associated with the superior lumbar triangle, a more common site of hernia than the inferior lumbar triangle described previously. The superior triangle (Fig. 71.8B) is formed superiorly by the 12th rib, the serratus posterior inferior, and the superior lumbocostal ligament; inferiorly by the upper border of the internal abdominal oblique; and medially by the erector spinae.

The deep layer of the lumbar abdominal wall includes three muscles: the quadratus lumborum, the psoas major, and the transversus abdominis. The quadratus lumborum primarily arises from the posterior iliac crest and inserts on the 12th rib. The psoas major arises from vertebrae T12 through L5 and passes beneath the inguinal ligament to insert on the lesser trochanter of the femur.

Deep Inguinal Region

Laparoscopic View

1 **Deep Aspect of the Anterior Abdominal Wall, Peritoneal Folds, and Associated Structures.** If one creates a space in the abdominal cavity by distending it with gas, an excellent view of the anterior wall can be obtained. The umbilical peritoneal folds (Fig. 71.9) in most subjects are very prominent and provide easily identified landmarks. The folds (ligaments) primarily exist because the peritoneum covers underlying structures.

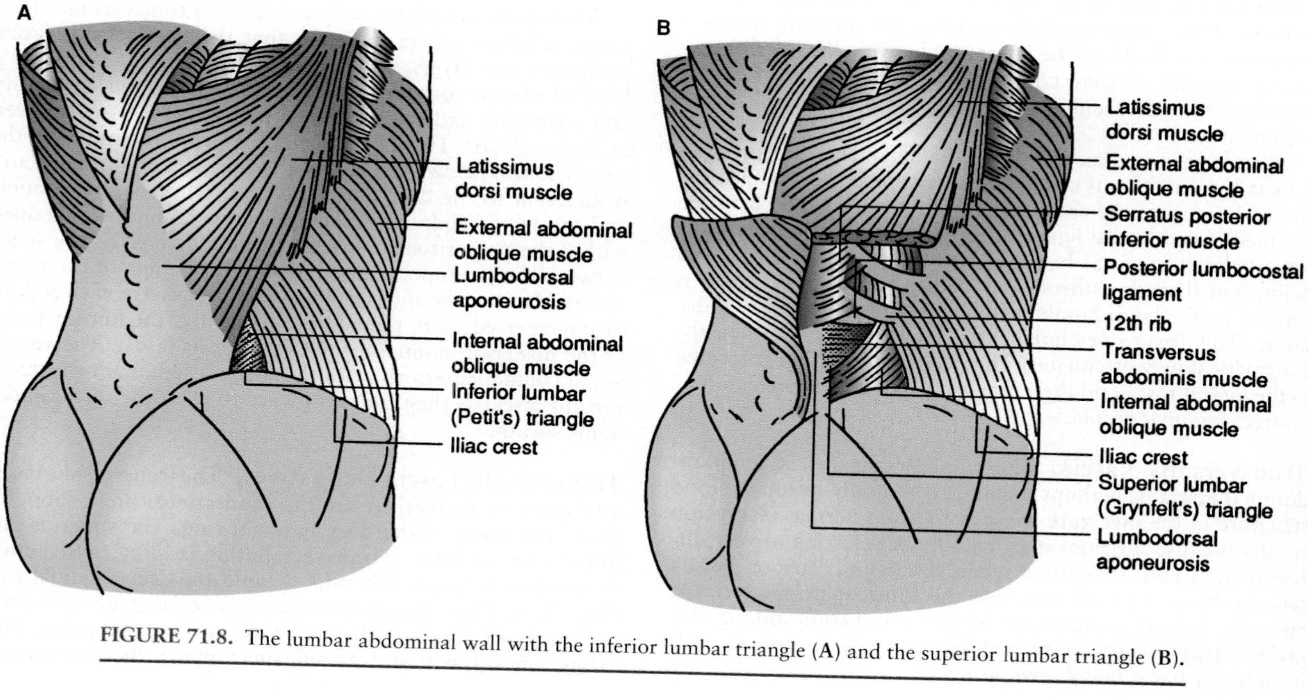

FIGURE 71.8. The lumbar abdominal wall with the inferior lumbar triangle (A) and the superior lumbar triangle (B).

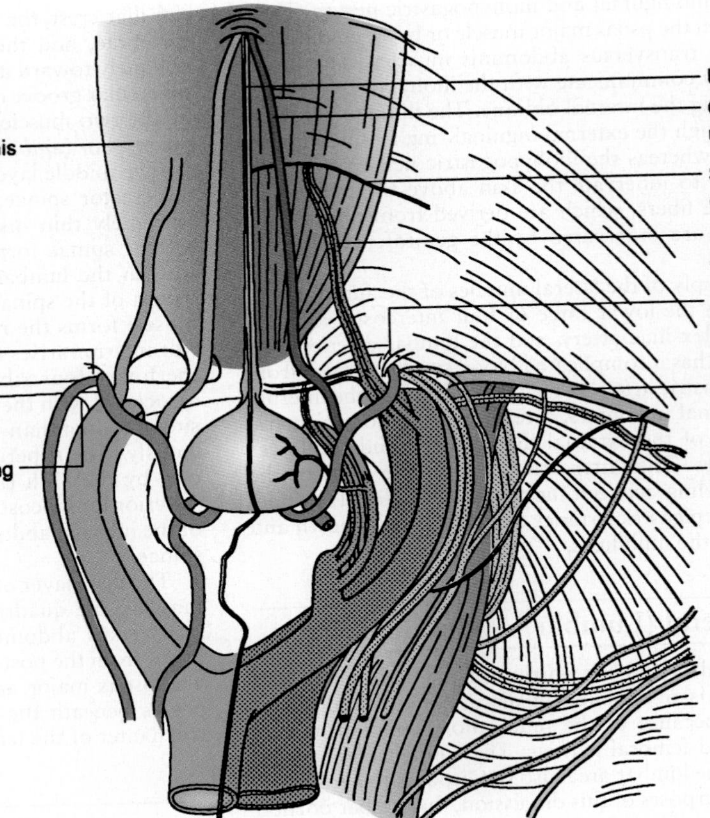

FIGURE 71.9. The deep inguinal region and the anterior abdominal wall seen from within the abdomen. The urachus, the obliterated portion of the umbilical artery, and the inferior epigastric vessels are covered by peritoneal folds, respectively called the median, medial, and lateral umbilical folds.

The single median umbilical fold extends from the umbilicus to the urinary bladder and covers the urachus, the fibrous remnant of the fetal allantois. The urachus may be patent for a short distance in adults or may open into the umbilical scar in newborns. The medial umbilical fold is formed by the underlying obliterated portion of the fetal umbilical artery. This normally cordlike structure, like the urachus, may be patent for a portion of its length. Indeed, the proximal, patent portion of the artery normally supplies the superior vesicular arteries to the bladder. The lateral fold covers the inferior epigastric arteries as they course toward the posterior rectus sheath, which they enter approximately at the level of the arcuate line.

Between the median and the medial ligaments, a depression is usually found that is called the *supravesical fossa*. This is the site of hernias of the same name. The fossa formed between the medial and lateral ligaments is the medial fossa; this is the site of direct inguinal hernias. The lateral fossa is less well delineated than the others. The medial border of the fossa is formed by the lateral umbilical ligament and the rectus abdominis. This fossa does not have a lateral border; rather, the concavity slowly attenuates. The deep inguinal ring is located in the lateral fossa and therefore is the site of the congenital or indirect inguinal hernia.

Transversalis Fascia. The transversalis fascia (endoabdominal fascia) is perhaps the most commonly misunderstood structure in the literature devoted to groin hernia. Confusion results because surgeons may actually be referring to very different anatomic structures when discussing various hernia repairs; however, each may use the same anatomic term or eponym. Indeed, perhaps the biggest reservation among surgeons intent on performing a Shouldice repair is a precise definition of what is being sewn to what.

The transversalis fascia proper is a continuous sheet that extends throughout the extraperitoneal space. The term *transversalis fascia* generally is defined as the deep or endoabdominal fascia covering the internal surface of the transversus abdominis, the iliacus, the psoas muscles, and the obturator internus and portions of the periosteum. One variant of this convention is the use of terms specific to the muscle covered by the fascia (e.g., iliac fascia).

Most authors feel that only one layer of transversalis fascia exists, whereas others maintain that the transversalis fascia comprises two layers, or laminae.[8] The posterior lamina is a layer of fibrous connective tissue that widely varies in density and continuity and is interspersed with adipose tissue, as seen in Figure 71.10. This layer is often referred to simply as the *preperitoneal fascia*. The anterior lamina is more uniform and is adherent to the deep surface of the transversus abdominis and the rectus abdominis. The posterior lamina is contained within the preperitoneal space, which is defined as the space between the peritoneum and the anterior lamina of the transversalis fascia. The inferior epigastric vessels are enclosed by, or interspersed with, the adipose tissue and the fibrous tissue of the posterior lamina of the transversalis fascia. The vessels are in contact anteriorly with the anterior lamina of the transversalis fascia as they course upward to enter the rectus abdominis sheath.

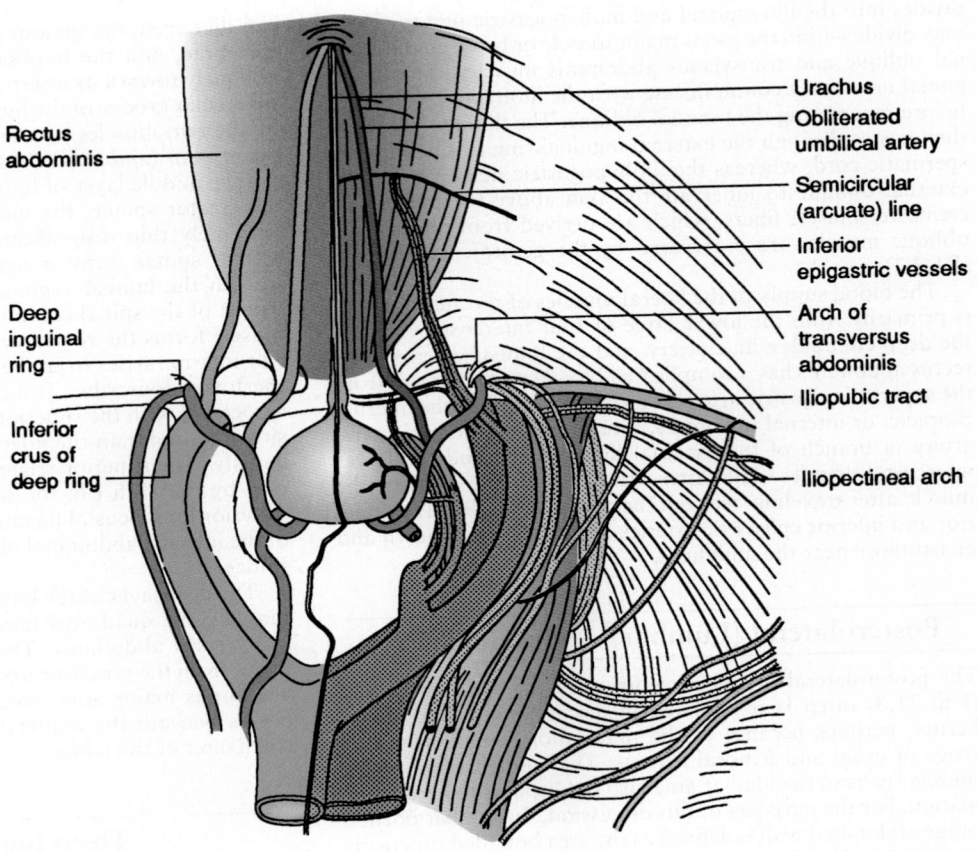

Transversalis Fascia Derivatives. The transversalis fascia analogues or derivatives are the iliopectineal arch, iliopubic tract, and crura of the deep inguinal ring. The superior and inferior crura form a transversalis fascia sling, a structure shaped like a "monk's hood," around the deep inguinal ring (Fig. 71.9). The transversalis fascia also contributes the internal spermatic fascia to the spermatic cord at this point. This "sling" has functional significance; when the transversus

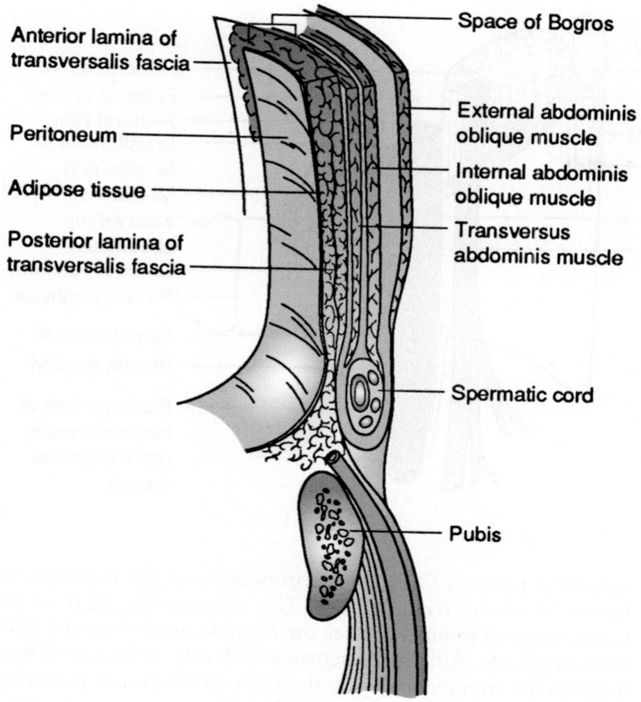

FIGURE 71.10. A parasagittal section through the layers of the anterior abdominal wall and groin. Observe that the transversalis fascia is depicted as a bilaminar structure.

abdominis contracts, the crura of the ring are pulled upward and laterally, which results in a valvular action that helps to prevent the indirect formation of a hernia.

The iliopubic tract (Figs. 71.9 and 71.11) has become an increasingly important landmark for surgeons as the use of laparoscopic technology has increased.[9,10] The iliopubic tract is the thickened band of transversalis fascia formed at the zone of transition between the deep surfaces of the iliac and transversus abdominis muscles. The structure courses parallel to the more superficially located inguinal ligament, is attached to the iliac crest laterally, and inserts on the pubic tubercle medially. The tract forms along its course a portion of the inferior crus of the deep inguinal ring and then contributes to the anterior and medial walls of the femoral sheath. The tract fuses with the inguinal ligament to form a component of the inferior wall of the inguinal canal. At its insertion on the pubic tubercle, it curves backward slightly to blend with the Cooper pectineal ligament. The pectineal ligament actually is a condensation of periosteum and is not a true analogue of the transversalis fascia, but it is reinforced by fibers from the iliopubic tract and inguinal ligament.

The iliopubic tract contains not only fibrous connective tissue but also some elastic fibers.[11] In one series, the iliopubic tract was a substantial structure, suitable for use in hernia repairs, in 42% of the specimens examined. The tract, whether substantial or not, can be used as a readily identified landmark.

The iliopubic tract has particular significance because of its importance as a landmark to the laparoscopic surgeon. Many of the branches of the lumbar plexus run inferior to the tract, and damage to these nerves may be the result of aggressive dissection or the placement of tacks or staples to affix a prosthesis below this structure. The tract is not obviously visible in every patient from a laparoscopic view, but its location should always be immediately known to the surgeon because of its constant relationship to the other landmarks in this area.

The iliopectineal arch (Fig. 71.9) is also a condensation of the transversalis fascia. The iliopectineal arch commences at the medial border of the iliacus muscle, where it is continuous with the iliac fascia, itself a portion of the transversalis (endoabdominal) fascia. The arch separates the vascular compartment containing the femoral vessels from the neuromuscular compartment containing the iliopsoas muscle, femoral nerve, and lateral femoral cutaneous nerve. The iliopectineal arch also contributes to the proximal portion of the femoral sheath, thereby joining the iliopubic tract in the formation of the femoral sheath.

Femoral Sheath, Canal, and Ring. The femoral sheath (Fig. 71.12) is composed primarily of extensions of the transversalis fascia. The sheath is best understood in terms of the

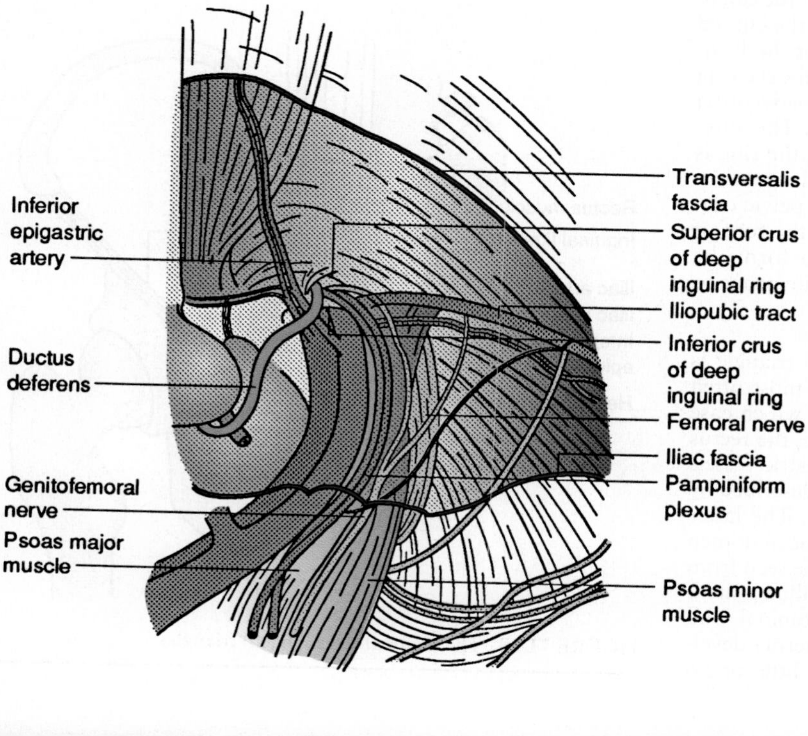

FIGURE 71.11. A schematic representation of the deep inguinal region. The iliopubic tract is shown as a thickening of the transversalis fascia, inferior to which many of the branches of the lumbar plexus exit the pelvis.

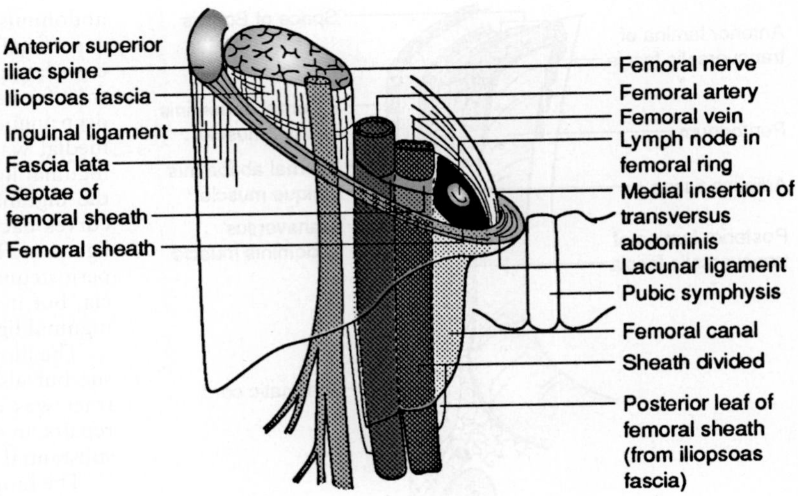

FIGURE 71.12. Schematic view of the femoral sheath, ring, and canal. The transversalis fascia forms the anterior portion of the sheath, and the iliopsoas fascia forms the posterior portion. Septa separate the vessels from each other and the vein from the femoral canal. The femoral ring contains a lymph node. The ring is formed medially by the aponeurosis of the transversus abdominis aponeurosis, anteriorly by the inguinal ligament, posteriorly by the pubic bone, and laterally by the femoral sheath.

structures contained within. As the external iliac artery and vein pass beneath the inguinal ligament to become the femoral vessels, they are covered anteriorly by the transversalis fascia proper. This fascial layer is posteriorly and laterally joined by portions of the iliopsoas fascia, which are themselves continuations of the transversalis fascia. At the inguinal ligament, the iliopsoas fascia forms the iliopectineal arch. This arch divides the vascular compartment (lacuna vasorum), containing the femoral vessels, from the muscular portion (lacuna musculorum), which contains the iliopsoas muscle, femoral nerve, and lateral femoral cutaneous nerve. The vascular lacuna is further divided by septa into compartments for the vessels and the femoral branch of the genitofemoral nerve.

The medial border of the femoral sheath follows the transversus abdominis aponeurosis to its insertion just lateral to that of the lacunar ligament and extends inferiorly to fuse eventually with the medial septum and adventitia of the femoral vein. The resultant cone-shaped cul-de-sac is the femoral canal. The canal normally contains only wisps of connective tissue and small lymphatic nodes. The wider proximal part of the canal, the femoral ring, contains a large node, which is often referred to as the *Cloquet node*.

The femoral ring is the extraperitoneal opening of the canal. The boundaries of the ring are formed medially by the curved edge of the transversus abdominis aponeurosis, not the lacunar ligament, which inserts more medially.[12] Laterally, the ring is bounded by the connective tissue septum and the adventitia that is interposed between it and the femoral vein. The anterior boundary is the inguinal ligament; posteriorly, the ring is reinforced by the iliopubic tract and iliopectineal ligament. The canal is not in direct communication with the pelvic cavity. The transversalis fascia is not a component of the roof of the canal because it is diverted at this point to form the femoral sheath. This weakened area is therefore quite prone to hernia formation, especially in female subjects.

Inguinal (Hesselbach) Triangle. The inguinal triangle is the site of direct inguinal hernias. This triangle is most often described from the anterior aspect (Fig. 71.13), in which case the inguinal ligament forms the base of the triangle, the rectus abdominis the medial border, and the inferior epigastric vessels the superolateral border. The triangle as originally described by Hesselbach had the pectineal ligament as its base. The latter description is quite useful to the surgeon viewing the abdomen from within because the inguinal ligament cannot be seen from this viewpoint. When the inguinal triangle is transilluminated, the thinness and translucency of the area of abdominal wall within the triangle underscores its importance in hernia development and repair. In the most translucent area, little or no muscle is present. Only the peritoneum and the transversalis fascia cover the triangle here. The aponeurotic arch of the transversus abdominis crosses the triangle just below the apex in most people. A high aponeurotic arch affords less reinforcement to the triangle and may therefore predispose a person to the formation of a direct inguinal hernia.

Components of the Spermatic Cord. The spermatic cord (Figs. 71.11 and 71.14) is closely associated with the deep inguinal ring. The spermatic cord is most appropriately described at this point because the deep ring itself is formed by derivatives of transversalis fascia, as is the innermost covering layer of the spermatic cord, the internal spermatic fascia. The middle covering layer is called the *cremasteric fascia* and contains the cremasteric muscle bundles; both are derived from the internal abdominal oblique muscle and fascia. The outermost covering of the spermatic cord is the external spermatic fascia, which is continuous with the investing fascia of the external abdominal oblique muscle.

The tunica vaginalis is initially a component of the cord, but normally it atrophies and closes early in neonatal life. This

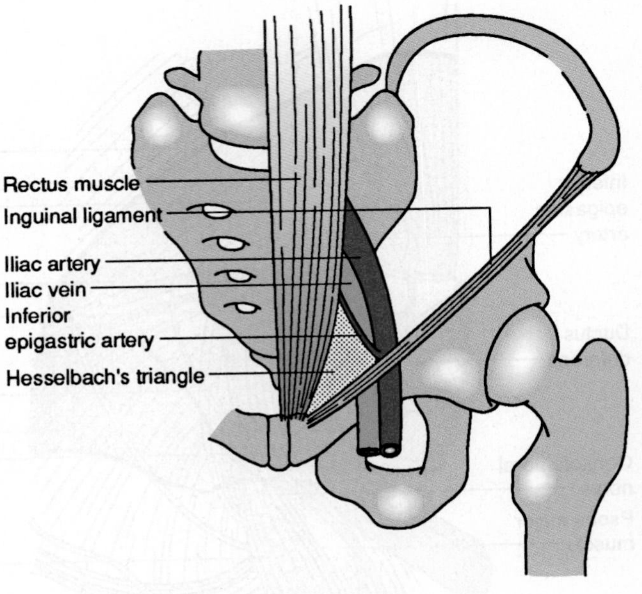

FIGURE 71.13. The inguinal (Hesselbach) triangle.

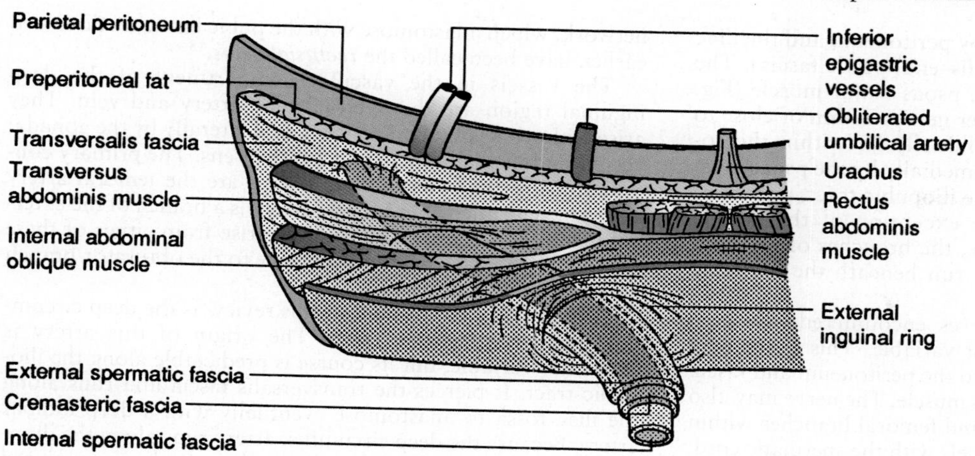

FIGURE 71.14. The component layers covering the contents of the spermatic cord.

structure is an evagination of peritoneum. The testicle descends retroperitoneally in fetal life and is merely in contact with the posterior aspect of the tunica. An indirect congenital hernia enters the patent tunica vaginalis.

The cord structures enclosed by the coverings described earlier are the ductus (vas) deferens, the pampiniform venous plexus, the testicular artery, and the genital branch of the genitofemoral nerve, a branch of the lumbar plexus (Figs. 71.9, 71.11, and 71.15).

Branches of the Lumbar Plexus. The nerves crossing the iliac fossa are some of the most variable in the body. This variability may be the cause of frequent intraoperative injury to the fragile nerves. The lumbar plexus is formed by roots from the 12th thoracic nerve and the first through fourth lumbar nerves. Cutaneous territories innervated by branches of the lumbar plexus are seen in Figure 71.15A. The five terminal branches commonly encountered in laparoscopic herniorrhaphy can be discerned in many people as they course

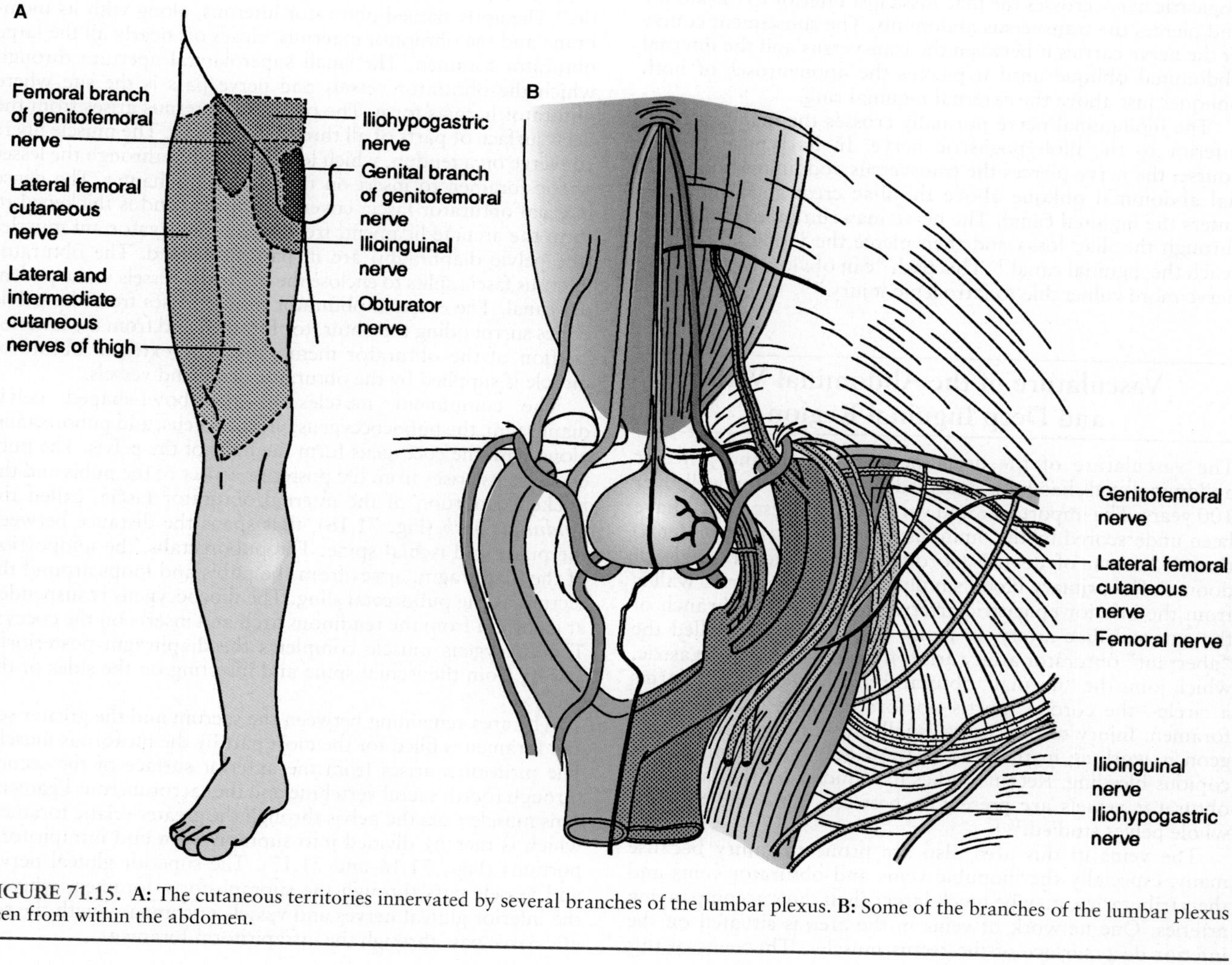

FIGURE 71.15. A: The cutaneous territories innervated by several branches of the lumbar plexus. B: Some of the branches of the lumbar plexus seen from within the abdomen.

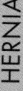

across the iliacus muscle covered by peritoneum and the iliac fascia (a portion of the transversalis–endopelvic fascia). The nerves form within or deep to the psoas major muscle (Fig. 71.15B), often ramifying with other nerves within or close to the muscle. The nerve branches initially lie within the so-called triangle of pain,[13] bordered medially by the psoas muscle, anteriorly and inferiorly by the iliopubic tract, and laterally by the iliac crest. With the exception of the genital branch of the genitofemoral nerve, the branches of the lumbar plexus destined for the thigh run beneath the iliopubic tract.

The most anterior of the nerves encountered, the genitofemoral nerve, is also the most variable. This nerve may occur as a single trunk lying deep to the peritoneum and fascia on the anterior surface of the psoas muscle. The nerve may also divide into its component genital and femoral branches within the muscle. The genital branch travels with the spermatic cord, entering at the deep inguinal ring; it ultimately innervates the cremaster muscle and the lateral scrotum. The femoral branch of the nerve innervates the skin of the proximal midthigh.

The lumbar plexus branch encountered immediately deep to the lateral aspect of the psoas muscle is the large femoral nerve. Although not routinely encountered during laparoscopy, the femoral nerve has been injured in some cases.[14] The lateral femoral cutaneous nerve crosses the iliac fossa under the iliac fascia to run deep to the iliopubic tract and the inguinal ligament, which it pierces to enter the thigh.

The iliohypogastric nerve typically arises with the ilioinguinal by a common trunk from the first lumbar nerve. They may exchange fibers within the muscle, but they usually diverge immediately to form individual nerves. The iliohypogastric nerve crosses the iliac fossa just inferior to the kidney and pierces the transversus abdominis. The subsequent course of the nerve carries it between the transversus and the internal abdominal oblique until it pierces the aponeuroses of both obliques just above the external inguinal ring.

The ilioinguinal nerve normally crosses the iliac fossa just inferior to the iliohypogastric nerve. In its typical further course, the nerve pierces the transversus abdominis and internal abdominal oblique above the iliac crest and eventually enters the inguinal canal. The nerve may run more diagonally through the iliac fossa and then pierce the iliopubic tract to reach the inguinal canal.[15] This path "can obviously render the nerve more vulnerable to iatrogenic injury."[15]

Vasculature of the Abdominal Wall and Deep Inguinal Region

The vasculature of the deep inguinal region and anterior abdominal wall has been analyzed by surgeons for well over 100 years. The importance and variability of these vessels have been underscored by the ominous mnemonics used to refer to them—"crown of death" (*corona mortis*) and "triangle of doom." The primary blood supply to the deep anterior wall is from the inferior epigastric artery. This artery is a branch of the external iliac artery. In many cases, an artery called the "aberrant" obturator artery arises from the inferior epigastric, which joins the "normal" obturator artery and thereby forms a circle—the corona mortis—before entering the obturator foramen. Injury to the circle, usually sustained while the surgeon is working in the area of the Cooper ligament, causes copious bleeding. Recent studies have indicated that aberrant obturator vessels are present in between 60% and 90% of whole pelves studied.[16,17]

The veins in this area also are prone to injury because many, especially the iliopubic veins and obturator veins and their tributaries, may be much larger than their accompanying arteries. One network of veins in the area is situated on the inferior deep surface of the rectus muscles. The veins of this network, which anastomose with the pubic branches discussed earlier, have been called the *rectusial veins.*[18]

The vessels in the vascular compartment of the deep inguinal region are the external iliac artery and vein. They arise within a triangular area bordered laterally by the gonadal vessels and medially by the ductus deferens. The primary continuations of the external iliac vessels are the femoral artery and vein. The inferior epigastric artery is a branch of the external iliac. The obturator artery may arise from either of these arteries as a replacement or accessory to the obturator branch of the internal iliac artery.

A final vessel to consider in this review is the deep circumflex iliac artery (Fig. 71.10). The origin of this artery is extremely variable, but its course is predictable along the iliopubic tract. It pierces the transversalis fascia and runs along the iliac fossa to anastomose eventually with a deep lumbar artery. Because the deep circumflex artery runs along the iliopubic tract, it can inadvertently be stapled or otherwise injured during laparoscopic herniorrhaphy.

Pelvic Floor and Obturator Muscles

The pelvic musculature normally affords remarkable support to the structures within the true pelvis. Although a myoaponeurotic hammocklike sheet forms the pelvic diaphragm, obturator muscles and membrane, and urogenital diaphragm, herniation of fat or viscera through or around any of these layers occurs. The potential for hernia formation is increased because of the openings through which many structures exit or enter the pelvis.

The Latin term *obturator* is translated as "stopper for a bottle." The aptly named obturator internus, along with its membrane and the obturator externus, closes off nearly all the large obturator foramen. The small superolateral aperture through which the obturator vessels and nerve pass is the site where obturator hernias form. The obturator internus arises from the deep surface of parts of all three pelvic bones. The muscle fibers converge on a tendon, which leaves the pelvis through the lesser sciatic foramen to insert on the greater trochanter. The dense internal obturator fascia covers the muscle and is thickened to form the arcuate ligament, from which the levator ani muscles (the pelvic diaphragm) are in part suspended. The obturator internus fascia splits to enclose the pudendal vessels in the pudendal canal. The external obturator muscle arises from the pelvic bones surrounding the obturator foramen and from the anterior portion of the obturator membrane. The external obturator muscle is supplied by the obturator nerve and vessels.

The component muscles of the bowl-shaped pelvic diaphragm, the pubococcygeus, iliococcygeus, and puborectalis, along with the coccygeus form the floor of the pelvis. The pubococcygeus arises from the posterior aspect of the pubis and the thickened portion of the internal obturator fascia, called the *tendinous arch* (Fig. 71.16), that spans the distance between the pubis and ischial spine. The puborectalis, the midportion of the diaphragm, arises from the pubis and loops around the rectum as the puborectal sling. The iliococcygeus is suspended at its origin from the tendinous arch and inserts on the coccyx. The coccygeus muscle completes the diaphragm posteriorly, arising from the ischial spine and inserting on the sides of the coccyx.

The area remaining between the sacrum and the greater sciatic foramen is filled for the most part by the piriformis muscle. The piriformis arises from the anterior surface of the second through fourth sacral vertebrae and the sacrotuberous ligament. This muscle exits the pelvis through the greater sciatic foramen, which is thereby divided into suprapiriform and infrapiriform portions (Figs. 71.16 and 71.17). The superior gluteal nerves and vessels pass through the suprapiriform foramen, whereas the inferior gluteal nerves and vessels in company with the sciatic nerve pass through the infrapiriform foramen.

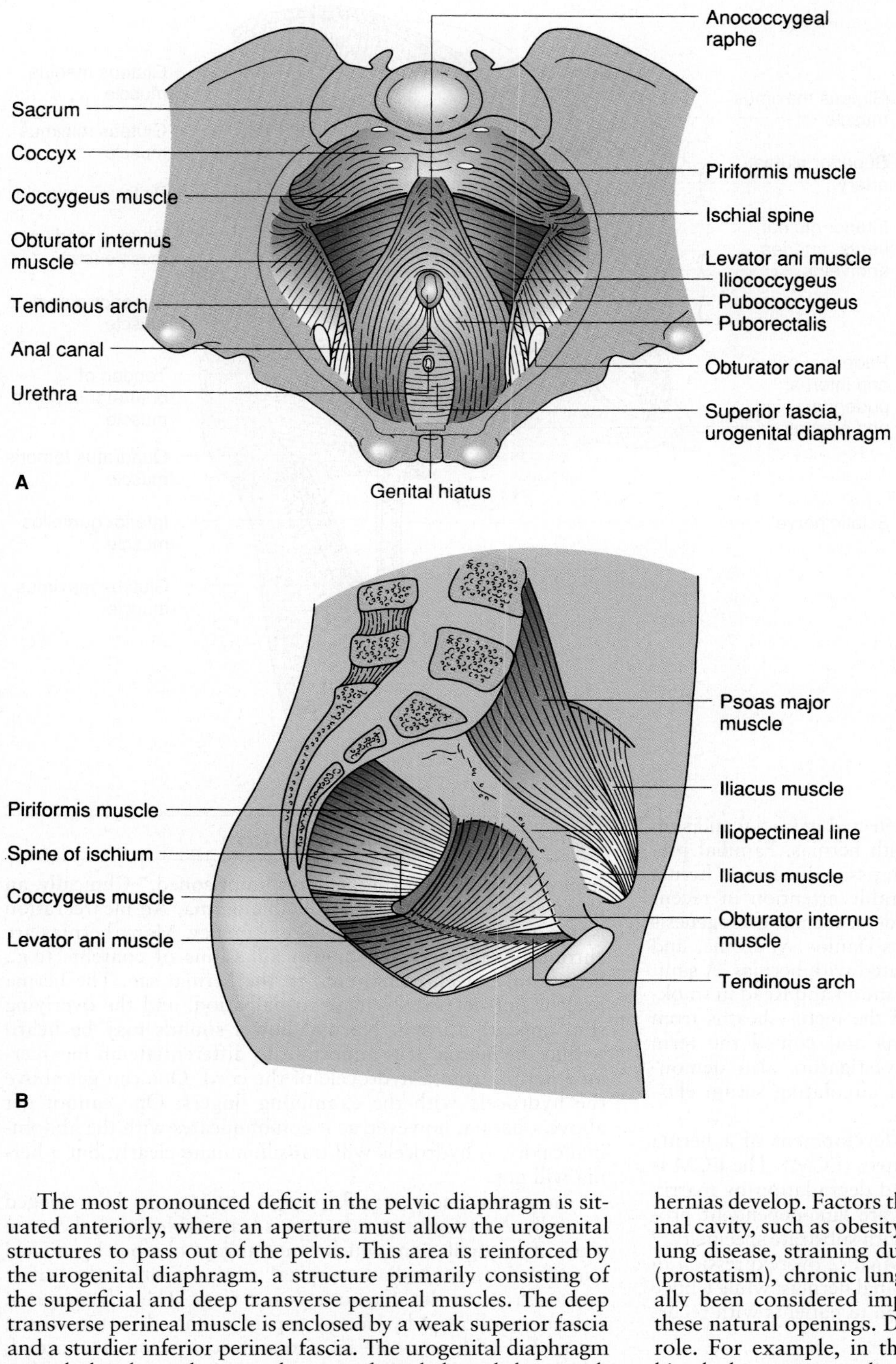

FIGURE 71.16. **A:** The pelvic diaphragm (levator ani and the piriformis) and the urogenital diaphragm viewed from within the pelvis. **B:** Hemisection of the pelvis revealing the levator ani, piriformis, obturator internus, and psoas muscles.

The most pronounced deficit in the pelvic diaphragm is situated anteriorly, where an aperture must allow the urogenital structures to pass out of the pelvis. This area is reinforced by the urogenital diaphragm, a structure primarily consisting of the superficial and deep transverse perineal muscles. The deep transverse perineal muscle is enclosed by a weak superior fascia and a sturdier inferior perineal fascia. The urogenital diaphragm recently has been shown to be more funnel shaped than sandwichlike, as previously depicted in many atlases. The urogenital diaphragm exists only in humans because the human pelvic outlet faces inferiorly, unlike that of quadrupeds.

WHY DO HUMAN BEINGS DEVELOP ABDOMINAL WALL HERNIAS?

The most common hernias develop at sites where the abdominal wall has natural openings such as the internal inguinal ring, the umbilicus, and the esophageal hiatus. Previous surgical entry sites (incisional hernia) are also common areas where hernias develop. Factors that increase the pressure in the abdominal cavity, such as obesity, heavy lifting, coughing with chronic lung disease, straining during a bowel movement or urination (prostatism), chronic lung disease, and ascites, have traditionally been considered important in the etiology, especially at these natural openings. Developmental phenomena also play a role. For example, in the evolution from a quadruped to a biped, the unprotected groin is more vulnerable to changes in intra-abdominal pressure, predisposing to inguinal herniation. The role of heavy lifting, especially a single strenuous event, is an unsettled question and has considerable medical-legal ramifications. There is minimal evidence that vigorous abdominal wall activity is an independent risk factor for abdominal wall hernia development despite the overwhelming opinion to the contrary in the lay literature.[19,20] Indeed, there is not an excessive incidence of hernias in athletes and weightlifters. Nevertheless, there remain some proponents to the theory.[21]

2 Imbalances in collagen, the basic building block of the abdominal wall, are believed to contribute to hernia disease. While type I collagen confers predominantly tensile strength, type III collagen consists of thinner fibers and is regarded as a temporary matrix during tissue remodeling. A decreased ratio

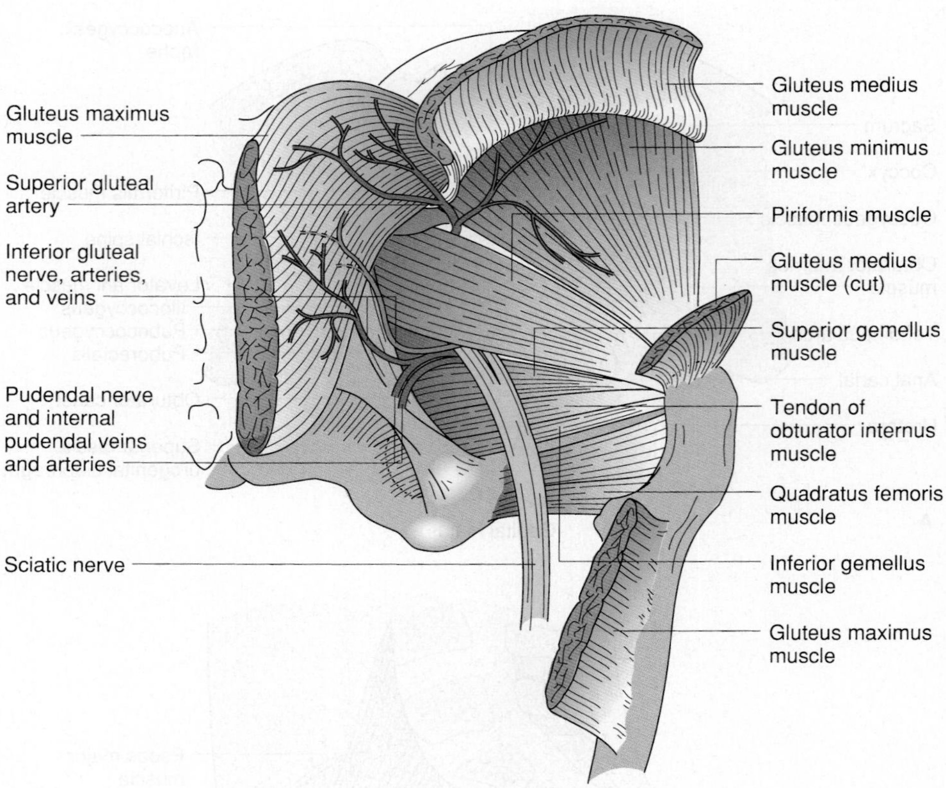

FIGURE 71.17. The gluteal muscles and lateral rotators of the hip. External relations of the sciatic foramen are also evident.

of type I to type III collagens can be detected in fascial and skin specimens obtained from patients with hernias. Familial predisposition and the role of connective tissue diseases in hernia development have received considerable attention in recent years. Various connective tissue disorders, such as osteogenesis imperfecta, Marfan syndrome, Ehlers-Danlos syndrome, and congenital hip dislocation, are associated with hernias. A similar phenomenon was discovered by Cannon and Read in smokers when they performed biopsies of the rectus sheaths from adult smokers with inguinal hernias and coined the term "metastatic emphysema."[22] The investigators also demonstrated significantly greater levels of circulating serum elastolytic activity in patients who smoke.

Recent studies dealing with the development of a hernia have focused on the extracellular matrix (ECM). The ECM is in a dynamic balance of synthesis and degradation by matrix metalloproteinases (MMPs). MMPs are zinc-dependent proteases secreted as latent proenzymes with substrate specificity.[23] Studies by Bellon et al. revealed an MMP-2 overexpression in fibroblasts of patients with direct inguinal hernias, while Klinge et al. detected MMP-13 overexpression in patients with recurrent inguinal hernias.[24,25]

COMPLICATIONS OF HERNIAS

Hernia Accident

For years surgeons have been taught that all hernias should be repaired at diagnosis to prevent a hernia accident, which is defined as a bowel obstruction or incarceration with strangulation, because of the perception that patients presenting with these complications have an unacceptable increase in mortality. This thinking, however, has not stood up when tested in randomized controlled trials. For example, for men with asymptomatic inguinal hernias, randomized controlled trials have shown that a strategy of watchful waiting is safe.[26]

Incarceration

Incarcerated means "trapped" or "imprisoned." Clinically, an incarcerated hernia is an irreducible hernia. An incarceration is not in and of itself a surgical emergency. Many hernias are chronically incarcerated due to adhesions of contents (e.g., omentum, bowel, ovary, etc.) to the hernial sac. The hernia itself is not necessarily tense to palpation, and the overlying skin appears normal. Normal bowel sounds may be heard within the hernia. It is important to differentiate an incarcerated hernia from a hydrocele of the cord. One can get above the hydrocele with the examining fingers. One cannot get above a hernia, however, as it communicates with the abdominal cavity. A hydrocele will transilluminate clearly, but a hernia will not.

An acutely incarcerated, painful hernia must be managed carefully. An attempt at reduction is reasonable unless there are signs of strangulation, which is not always obvious by clinical examination. Immediate surgical exploration is the safest approach when the diagnosis is not clear. The advantage of reduction followed by elective repair is that edematous tissue associated with an acute incarceration can return to normal, which presumably will translate into a better repair with less chance of infection.[27] If an attempt at reduction seems reasonable, the patient is sedated and placed in bed. The Trendelenburg position should facilitate reduction of a groin hernia. An attempt should be made at the initial examination to reduce the hernia. The maneuver of taxis entails grasping the neck of the hernia with the fingers of one hand and then applying intermittent pressure on the most distal part of the hernia with the other hand. Taxis has the effect of elongating the neck of the hernia so that the contents of the hernia may be guided through this area back into the abdominal cavity with a rocking movement. Mere pressure on the most distal part of the hernia causes bulging of the hernial sac around the neck, which can occlude the neck and prevent it from being reduced (Fig. 71.18). The maneuver of taxis should not be performed with excessive

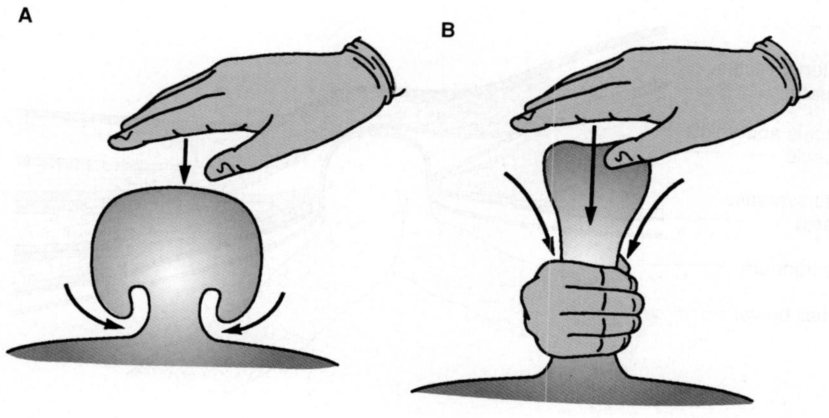

FIGURE 71.18. Reduction of a hernia by taxis. **A:** Applying pressure on the hernia directly occludes the neck. **B:** Elongating the neck of the hernia while applying pressure allows reduction.

pressure or too vigorously. If the hernia is strangulated, gangrenous bowel might be reduced into the abdomen or perforated in the process. One or two gentle attempts should be made at taxis. If they are unsuccessful, this procedure should be abandoned. Rarely, the hernia together with its peritoneal sac and constricting neck may be reduced into the abdomen (reduction en masse). The patient would then have persistent obstruction after reduction of the hernia.

Intestinal Obstruction

One hundred years ago, the most common cause of intestinal obstruction was a hernia. At the present time, hernia is third, after adhesive obstructions and cancer. Hernia is an important cause of obstruction that is not infrequently missed on clinical examination. When a patient with an intestinal obstruction is examined, great emphasis should be placed on adequate exposure of the entire abdominal wall and groin area (from nipples to knees). Proper lighting is essential because previous scars can fade with time and become barely perceptible. The patient with intestinal obstruction as a result of a hernia will have a tense hernia that is irreducible. The abdomen itself will be distended, and high-pitched bowel sounds with frequent rushes will be heard. If the process continues to the complication of strangulation, these signs will disappear. Unlike adhesive small-bowel obstructions, partial small-bowel obstructions secondary to hernia are rare. Most patients will have had vomiting and obstipation.

A plain roentgenogram of the abdomen will reveal the signs of an intestinal obstruction—dilated loops of bowel with air–fluid levels and no bowel gas distal to the obstruction. Frequently on a plain roentgenogram, one can see bowel shadows in the region of the hernia. A lateral view is often useful to demonstrate this feature more clearly. Contrast studies are not usually necessary in this instance. Computed tomography (CT) reliably demonstrates the hernia with characteristic features of obstruction and should be considered if the clinical diagnosis is not certain (Fig. 71.19) because a distal intestinal obstruction secondary to another cause (e.g., adhesions) may result in significant distention of a coincidental nonobstructing hernia of the abdominal wall. Should the examiner focus attention exclusively on the hernia, the real cause of the obstruction may be missed when the hernia is repaired.

The next steps in management include resuscitation followed by urgent surgery. At surgery, an approach directly over the hernia is used. In all patients, the entire gastrointestinal tract must be assessed to eliminate causes of obstruction other than the hernia itself. This is done before the hernia is repaired. The bowel, if viable, is reduced into the abdomen. If difficulty is encountered in reducing the hernia, the neck of the hernia can be widened. In the case of an inguinal hernia, division of the neck with or without ligation and division of the inferior epigastric vessels is safe, and the hernia contents can be reduced into the abdomen. In the case of a femoral hernia, the inguinal ligament can be split anteriorly and the hernia contents reduced into the abdomen. If the bowel is nonviable, then a bowel resection can be performed with anastomosis. The hernia is then repaired.

Strangulation

Strangulation of a hernia is a serious and life-threatening condition in which the hernial contents become ischemic and nonviable. The pathogenesis of this condition involves intra-abdominal contents within the hernia sac. Straining may push more contents into the sac, and the tense sac then causes pressure at the neck. This pressure initially produces venous congestion, resulting in edema. Eventually, the pressure is so great that the arterial supply is obstructed and the contents become gangrenous.

When intestine is involved, in addition to having an irreducible hernia and intestinal obstruction, the patient is toxic, dehydrated, and febrile. Examination of the abdomen reveals the signs of an intestinal obstruction, with distention and increased bowel sounds. Absolute constipation and vomiting are other manifestations. The hernia itself is tense, irreducible, and very tender, and the overlying skin may be discolored with a reddish or bluish tinge. No bowel sounds are heard within the hernia itself. The patient commonly manifests a leukocytosis with a predominance of polymorphonuclear leukocytes. Blood gases may reveal metabolic acidosis.

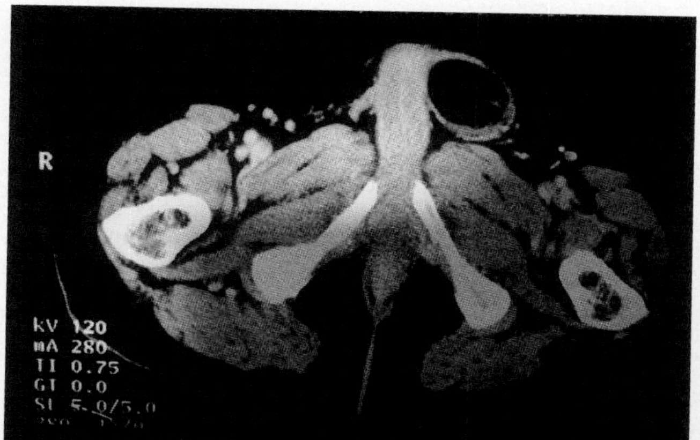

FIGURE 71.19. Computed tomogram showing a left-sided inguinal hernia.

FIGURE 71.20. Richter hernia. Part of the bowel wall herniates through the defect in the abdominal wall.

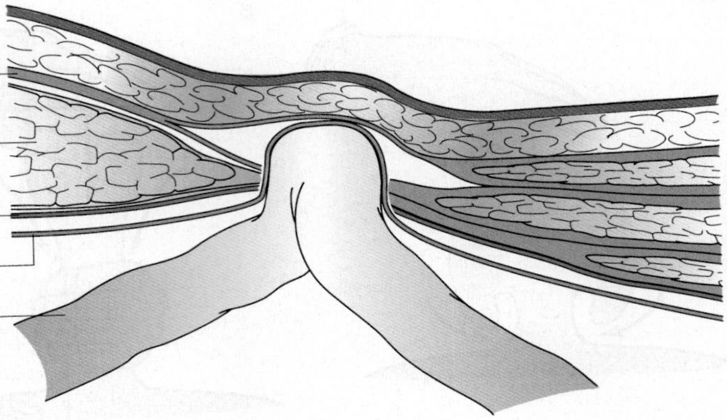

Management of these patients requires urgent attention to detail. No attempt should be made to reduce the hernia. Rapid resuscitation should commence immediately, with nasogastric suction and replacement of fluids and electrolytes. The patient should be given antibiotics. Once the patient is resuscitated, urgent surgery commences to expose the hernia, open the sac, and assess the viability of the bowel. More bowel can be pulled into the hernia so that viable bowel can be transected and the gangrenous portion removed. An end-to-end anastomosis should be performed and the bowel then reduced into the abdominal cavity. The hernia is then repaired.

Richter Hernia

August Gottlob Richter in 1785 described a hernia type that bears his name in which the antimesenteric border of the intestine protrudes into the hernia sac without involving the entire circumference of the intestine, so intestinal obstruction does not occur (Fig. 71.20). The most common site is the femoral ring (36% to 88%), followed by the inguinal canal (12% to 36%) and an abdominal wall incision (4% to 25%). Miscellaneous locations include umbilical, obturator, supravesical, spigelian, triangle of Petit, sacral foramen, Morgagni, internal, and (traumatic) diaphragmatic.[28] The routine use of laparoscopy by general surgeons has resulted in an increased incidence at trocar sites such that most surgeons will repair the fascia for trocar sleeves greater than 5 mm. The surgical treatment is to expose the herniated bowel by opening the sac. The neck of the sac is enlarged to allow delivery of the bowel into the wound. Any areas of gangrene are excised and the bowel wall reconstituted. The hernia is then repaired.

Massive Hernia

Abdominal wall hernias with a large portion of the abdominal contents situated within the sac are said to have "loss of domain" because the contents of the hernia exceed the capacity of the abdominal cavity. Forced reduction of the hernia with replacement of contents into the abdominal cavity and repair of the hernia can increase intra-abdominal tension tremendously, resulting in respiratory insufficiency or abdominal compartment syndrome.[29] In extreme cases, it is impossible to return the contents to the abdomen and repair the hernia defect without resection of intra-abdominal contents, such as colectomy with omentectomy. Complications of repair are common and include respiratory compromise, abdominal compartment syndrome, skin flap necrosis, and wound infection, in addition to the usual surgical complications. Therefore, repair should not be recommended unless there are overwhelming indications such as disabling symptoms, bowel obstruction or strangulation, or extensive skin ulceration caused by the hernia.

Progressive preoperative pneumoperitoneums can be useful in these patients to expand the abdominal cavity by stretching the abdominal wall and the diaphragm.[29] The maneuver involves injecting 500 to 1,500 mL of air every 1 to 3 days for about 3 weeks before the repair. A variety of access techniques have been described including direct puncture with a Veress needle, minilaparotomy with placement of a dialysis-type catheter, and the use of an implantable vascular access device with the catheter placed in the peritoneal cavity.[30] Although theoretically attractive, pneumoperitoneum is not always successful. The injected gas sometimes preferentially enters the hernia sac and distends it with minimal effect on the abdominal cavity. In addition, pneumoperitoneum has been shown to diminish lower extremity venous return. This could translate into a higher risk of thromboembolic complications. Deep venous thrombosis prophylaxis is prudent.

A combination of the techniques described later in this chapter for the repair of ventral hernias is usually required. Large pieces of prosthetic material with or without component separation are useful. A staged procedure has been described in which a large prosthesis is sewed to the circumference of the hernia defect and the skin and subcutaneous tissues closed over it. The prosthesis is purposely placed under some tension to cause "medialization" of the abdominal wall. The patient is returned to the operating room on a scheduled basis and the center portion of the prosthesis is removed and the edges reapproximated. The goal is to eventually be able to close the fascia primarily, usually with an underlay prosthesis.[31]

Prosthetic Materials. The development of a wide variety of materials that can be used for abdominal wall reconstruction now makes it possible to individualize the selection of prostheses so that they can be used in almost all clinical situations. The materials that have the longest track record for routine use in hernia surgery include polypropylene, either monofilament (Marlex, Prolene) or polyfilament (Surgipro); Dacron (Mersilene); and expanded polytetrafluoroethylene (ePTFE) (Gore-Tex). Polypropylene or Dacron work by inciting an intense fibroplastic response to form a strong scar plate interface. Because of this response, they should not be used in situations where contact with intra-abdominal viscera cannot be avoided because of the propensity of these materials to erode into intra-abdominal organs, most commonly intestine, resulting in fistulization. Either a nonmesh material such as ePTFE or a dual-layered prosthesis with a standard plastic mesh on the side facing the abdominal wall with the peritoneal side coated with an adhesion barrier of some type should be used. Recently, a number of dual-sided prosthetics have been introduced with a variety of adhesion barriers (Table 71.2). ePTFE and the adhesion barrier products are effective in decreasing both the amount and tenacity of adhesion, but none can completely eliminate them. Absorbable prostheses such as polyglactin are not durable and almost never result in long-term correction of

TABLE 71.2

PROSTHETIC MATERIALS

NONCOMPOSITE	**COATED PROSTHESIS**
Heavyweight plastic meshes	Polypropylene mesh + coating
Prolene (Ethicon) polypropylene	Glucamesh (Brennen) complex carbohydrate, oat beta glucan (50 g/m^{2}[a])
Marlex (Bard) polypropylene	Sepramesh (Genzyme) carboxymethylcellulose–sodium hyaluronate–polyethylene glycol (102 g/m^{2}[a])
SurgiPro (Covidien) polypropylene	Proceed (Ethicon) polydioxanone–oxidized regenerated cellulose (45 g/m^{2}[a])
Parietex (Covidien) polyester	C-Qur (Atrium) omega-3 fatty acid (50 g/m^{2}[a])
Mersilene (Ethicon) polyester	Polyester mesh + coating
Heavyweight membranes	Parietex composite (Covidien) collagen–polyethylene glycol–glycerol (75 g/m^{2}[a])
Gore-Tex (W L Gore) polyfluorotetraethylene (ePTFE)	**BIOLOGIC PROSTHESIS**
MotifMesh (Proxy Biomedical)	Human dermis
Dual Mesh (W L Gore) ePTFE, one side roughened	AlloDerm (LifeCell)
Dulex (Bard/Davol) ePTFE, one side roughened	AlloMax (Bard/Davol)
Lightweight plastic meshes	FlexHD (MTF)
Ultrapro (Ethicon) polypropylene	Porcine dermis
ProLite (Atrium) polypropylene	Permacol (TSL)
TiMesh (GfE) polypropylene	Collamend (Bard/Davol)
COMPOSITE PROSTHESIS (ePTFE + PLASTIC MESH)	Strattice (LifeCell)
ePTFE + Heavyweight plastic mesh	XenMatrix (Brennan Medical)
Composix EX (Bard/Davol) ePTFE + heavyweight polypropylene	SurgiMend (TEI Biosciences)
Parietex composite (Covidien) polyester–collagen–polyethylene glycol	Porcine small-intestine submucosa
Glycerol	Surgisis (Cook)
ePTFE + lightweight plastic mesh	FortaGen (Organogenesis)
Composix LP (Bard/Davol) ePTFE + lightweight polypropylene	Fetal bovine dermis
	SurgiMend (TEI Biosciences)
	Bovine pericardium
	Tutopatch (Tutogen Medical)
	Veritas (Synovis)

[a]Residual material after coating has absorbed.

an abdominal wall defect but are sometimes useful as a temporary substitute when a nonabsorbable prosthesis is contraindicated (i.e. a grossly infected wound).

The role of the newer biologic prostheses is yet to be determined. Currently available products have been derived from human, porcine, or fetal bovine skin; porcine small intestine submucosa; and bovine pericardium. These materials are processed to remove hair, cells, and cell components as well as other antigens present in the matrix, leaving only the highly organized collagen architecture with the surrounding extracellular ground tissue.[32] These biologic tissue grafts are designed to perform as a surgical prosthesis for soft tissue repair. In general, they possess the physical and mechanical characteristics of a clinically acceptable surgical mesh in that they promote strong tissue in-growth that limits contraction and have sufficient mechanical strength to withstand the physiologic and anatomic stresses of the abdominal wall, at the same time presenting a biologic scaffold to support tissue regeneration.

At the present time best indication for the newer biologic prostheses is contaminated wounds, where a synthetic prosthesis is contraindicated. They are not useful in grossly infected wounds presumably because of the high collagenase content present, which destroys them. A more contentious issue is the routine use for abdominal wall reconstruction. The argument for them is that by remodeling to more normal tissue rather than simply inciting scar tissue as with the plastic meshes, they are more physiologic. It is theorized that this might translate into fewer long-term complications (e.g., postherniorrhaphy wound pain). The argument against them is their expense, as they generally cost 20 to 30 times that of the plastic prostheses. Widespread adoption of these biologic grafts cannot be justified unless there is overwhelming evidence of their superiority. Randomized controlled studies both for inguinal and incisional hernias are now ongoing.

The weight of the polypropylene or polyester meshes, as well as the size of the pores, is a controversial issue currently. As an example, a 7.5 × 15-cm polypropylene mesh (Prolene, Ethicon, Inc.) contains about 80 g/m^2 of polypropylene, while a recently developed polypropylene–poliglecaprone-25 lightweight mesh of the same size (Monocryl, UltraPro, Ethicon, Inc.) contains less than 30 g/m^2 after absorption of the poliglecaprone-25 component. One of the ways of reducing the amount of nonabsorbable material in a mesh is to increase the size of the pores. Many authorities believe that the inflammatory response incited by the small-pore, heavyweight plastic meshes can lead to chronic pain; a sensation of being able to feel the mesh; increased stiffness of the abdominal wall with loss of compliance; and shrinkage, which can lead to recurrence. There is increasing evidence that decreasing the density of polypropylene and increasing the size of the pores reduces this foreign body response, resulting in less long-term pain than normal mesh and at the same time affording the patient a similar recurrence rate.[33–35] This also addresses a theoretical concern about the possible carcinogenic effects of polypropylene, as has been suggested by experimental studies in rats (although there has never been a documented case of a sarcoma developing in a human as a result of an inguinal hernia prosthesis).[36]

GROIN HERNIAS

Hernias are described as inguinal and femoral, the inguinal hernias being further subdivided into direct and indirect hernias (some authorities refer to these as medial and lateral hernias, respectively). Groin hernias may be primary or recurrent. An indirect hernia occurs as a protrusion of abdominal contents through the internal ring, lateral to the inferior epigastric vessels, into the inguinal canal. Indirect inguinal hernias (lateral hernias) are situated within the spermatic cord and therefore may extend into the scrotum. In female patients, the hernia follows the round ligament and may present as a swelling in the labium. A direct hernia (medial hernia) is a protrusion through the triangle of Hesselbach medial to the inferior epigastric vessels. These hernias develop through an area where the endoabdominal fascia is not protected by overlying muscle. Direct hernias do not usually involve the cord, as they tend to protrude forward. However, they occasionally track alongside the cord down the entire length of the inguinal canal and even enter the scrotum. For this reason, the only absolute distinction between a direct and an indirect hernia is the relationship to the inferior epigastric vessels. A femoral hernia protrudes through the femoral canal, which is bordered by the inguinal ligament superiorly, the pubic ramus medially and inferiorly, and the femoral vein laterally. This hernia presents below the inguinal ligament (Fig. 71.21). In a sliding hernia, part of the sac is formed by the viscera, on the left side the sigmoid colon or bladder and on the right side the cecum or bladder (Fig. 71.22).

Epidemiology

3 Inguinal hernias occur in persons of all ages, from the neonate to the elderly. The incidence of inguinal hernias in premature babies is approximately 10%. The lifetime risk of developing a groin hernia is between 15% and 25% in males and less than 5% in females. Right-sided inguinal hernias are more common than left. The male-to-female ratio for inguinal hernias is 7:1, with 8% of groin hernia repairs performed in women. Femoral hernias account for fewer than 10% of all groin hernias; however, 40% present as emergencies, with incarceration or strangulation, and mortality is higher for emergency repair than for elective repair. In men, indirect inguinal hernias outnumber direct by about 2:1, with femoral hernias making up a much smaller proportion. For females, indirect inguinal hernias are most common, followed by femoral hernias, with direct hernias occurring rarely. Emergency operations are required more frequently in females. A study from the Swedish Hernia Registry analyzing 90,648 inguinal hernia operations (88,753 male, 6,895 female) between 1992 and 2003 revealed a higher percentage of emergency operations in women (16.9%) than men (5%), leading to bowel resection in 16.6% and 5.6%, respectively.[37] Femoral recurrences were particularly common in females in whom the diagnosis at the time of the primary repair was direct or indirect (4.6% male, 41.6% female), strongly suggesting a missed hernia at the original procedure. Femoral hernias are also more common in older patients and in those who have previously undergone inguinal hernia repair.

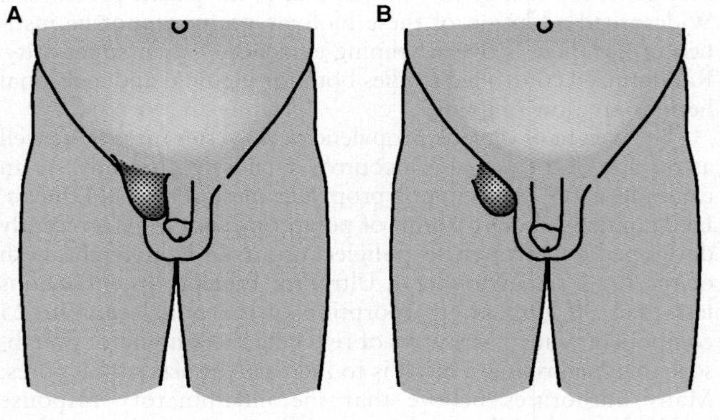

FIGURE 71.21. A: Inguinal hernia. This presents above the inguinal ligament and extends below it. B: Femoral hernia. This presents below the inguinal ligament.

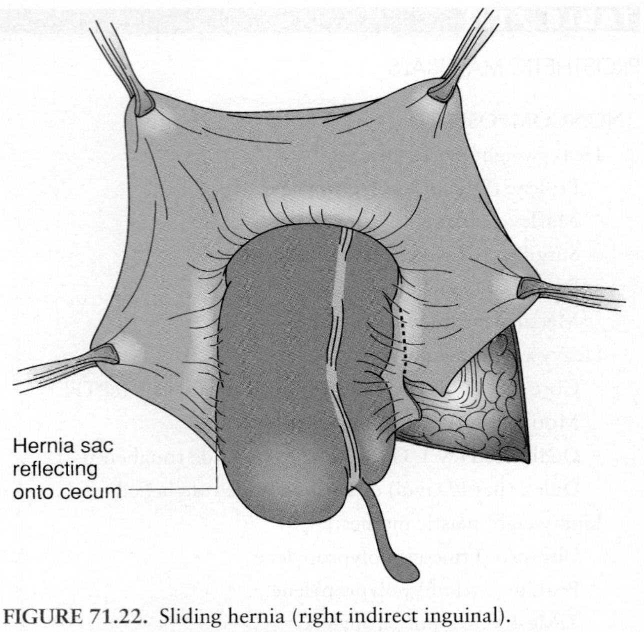

FIGURE 71.22. Sliding hernia (right indirect inguinal).

Classification

The primary purpose of a classification system for any disease is to stratify for severity so that reasonable comparisons can be made between various treatment strategies.[38] However, with the multiplicity of operative techniques and approaches for repair of groin hernias, no one classification system has been accepted by all practitioners. The reason why it is so difficult to develop a classification system that all surgeons can agree on is that in the final analysis, the physical examination represents an important component and no one has been able to eliminate its subjectivity. Nyhus, Gilbert, Schumpelick, Harkins, Casten, Halverson and McVay, Lichtenstein, Bendavid, Stoppa, Alexandre, and Zollinger have developed groin hernia classification systems. The Nyhus system, which is detailed in Table 71.3, is the most widely used.

Clinical Diagnosis

Groin hernias present with a swelling that has a cough impulse. With indirect hernias, the swelling may extend down

TABLE 71.3 CLASSIFICATION

NYHUS CLASSIFICATION OF GROIN HERNIAS

■ TYPE	■ DESCRIPTION
I	Indirect hernia
	Normal-size internal ring
	Typically in infants, children, small adults
II	Indirect hernia
	Dilated internal ring
	Posterior wall intact
	Inferior epigastric vessels not displaced
	Does not extend to the scrotum
III	Posterior wall defect
IIIA	Direct hernia
	Size not taken into account
IIIB	Indirect hernia
	Dilated internal ring encroaching on Hesselbach triangle (massive scrotal, sliding, or pantaloon type)
IIIC	Femoral hernia
IV	Recurrent hernia
IVA	Direct
IVB	Indirect
IVC	Femoral
IVD	Combined

TABLE 71.4 DIAGNOSIS

DIFFERENTIAL DIAGNOSIS OF A GROIN HERNIA

Hydrocele
Encysted hydrocele of the cord
Varicocele
Epididymoorchitis
Torsion of the testis
Undescended testis
Ectopic testis
Testicular tumor
Pseudohernia
Femoral artery aneurysm
Saphena varix
Lipoma of spermatic cord
Inguinal lymphadenopathy
Psoas abscess
Cutaneous lesions (e.g., sebaceous cyst, skin tumor)

into the scrotum. The swelling reduces when the patient lies down. Sometimes, the hernia does not reduce easily and the patient has to reduce it manually. Applying pressure over the midinguinal point (midway between the anterior superior iliac spine and the pubic tubercle and just above the inguinal ligament) with the fingertip will control an indirect hernia and prevent it from protruding when the patient strains. A direct hernia will not be controlled with this maneuver. Similarly, if the scrotum is invaginated with the index finger and the tip of the finger is placed through the external inguinal ring into the canal, and the patient is then asked to strain, an indirect hernia will push against the fingertip, whereas a direct hernia will push against the pulp of the finger. It should be noted that the accuracy of this clinical assessment is questioned by many authorities. A femoral hernia presents as a swelling below the inguinal ligament and just lateral to the pubic tubercle (Fig. 71.21).

Differential Diagnosis

The clinical presentation of a groin hernia, especially when large, is frequently obvious to the examiner. Smaller hernias and recurrent hernias can be confused with a number of different conditions that can be mistaken for a hernia (Table 71.4).

A hydrocele extending into the scrotum or an encysted hydrocele of the cord can involve the groin area. The distinguishing features are that the examining hand can get above a hydrocele but not above a hernia and that a hydrocele transilluminates very clearly. A varicocele does not transilluminate, has the characteristic feel of a "bag of worms," and is more tubelike in conformation. Lesions of the testicle may sometimes mimic a hernia, particularly in inflammatory conditions, such as epididymoorchitis. The distinguishing features are intense pain extending down into the scrotum. The testicle itself is enlarged and tender, as is the epididymis. On rectal examination, the seminal vesicles are tender. This condition may be bilateral. Torsion of the testicle is distinguished by the fact that the testicle is absent from the scrotum and the swelling in the groin feels firm. A sonogram reveals a solid mass in the testicle, which has been pulled up because of the torsion. Testicular tumors, if large enough, may extend up to the groin area, but they have a solid feel and sonography can distinguish them.

Pseudohernia is a condition that occurs in patients with denervation of the abdominal wall musculature (e.g., after polio). The abdominal wall muscles bulge forward on straining and have the appearance of a hernia. An aneurysm of the femoral artery may present as a groin swelling but with an expansile impulse and sometimes a bruit. If thrombosis develops in the aneurysm, pulsation may be lost. In this instance, the aneurysm becomes tender. Femoral aneurysms move from side to side but not up and down. A saphena varix usually presents below the inguinal ligament and represents a varicosity of one of the branches of the long saphenous vein as it emerges from the hiatus. Like a hernia, the varix has a cough impulse and becomes more prominent when the patient is standing. Compression over the femoral hiatus obliterates this lesion. The varix is sometimes associated with varicose veins farther down the lower limb. The overlying skin has an associated bluish discoloration.

A lipoma within the spermatic cord is a very common condition and, from anatomic studies and surgical dissection, is now regarded as a hernia of the extraperitoneal fat.[39] If found at surgery, the lipoma is removed to avoid a persistent bulge in the inguinal region despite a successful hernia repair.

Enlargement of inguinal lymph nodes may also be mistaken for herniation. Inflammatory nodes are usually tender; metastatic lymphadenopathy is usually not tender. If inguinal lymph nodes are replaced by metastasis, a primary lesion should be looked for in the skin in any part of the lower limb. The perineum and anal canal should also be examined. Lymphadenopathy can also be caused by lymphoma, and groin nodes may be the only site. Lymphadenopathy characteristically appears as a well-circumscribed mass below the inguinal ligament that one can get above with the examining hand. Lymph nodes are solid on ultrasonography, and for this reason, it may be difficult to differentiate nodes from a femoral hernia containing omentum.

Surgical Indications. Most standard surgical texts continue to state that all inguinal hernias regardless of symptoms

should be repaired unless specific contraindications are present. This recommendation is based on the presumption that complications of incarceration, obstruction, and strangulation
4 are greater threats than are the risks of operation. This concept is now being challenged for asymptomatic or minimally symptomatic patients. A recent randomized controlled trial comparing a strategy of watchful waiting to routine repair for male inguinal hernia patients with minimal symptoms revealed no difference in quality of life at 2 years and an acceptably low rate of hernia accident.[40] Given the possibility of the development of chronic postherniorrhaphy groin pain in up to 10% of patients undergoing repair, the notion that the presence of an inguinal hernia is an indication for repair can no longer be considered valid.

An alternative to surgical repair is a mechanical device known as a truss. It consists of a belt with a pad that is applied to the groin after spontaneous or manual reduction of a hernia and has been used for centuries. It serves to maintain reduction and possibly prevents enlargement of the hernia. There are insufficient studies to determine how effective trusses actually are and whether they are as good as surgery for the control of symptoms. Most patients find them cumbersome to use and difficult to keep clean. With prolonged usage, atrophy of the spermatic cord has been reported and eventual surgical repair is made more difficult due to fibrosis of the tissues. However, some patients do achieve symptomatic relief.

Treatment

5 Four developments in the latter half of the 20th century significantly decreased morbidity and favorably influenced the recurrence rate to the currently accepted level of less than 2%: (a) the routine use of prosthetic materials, (b) the widespread acceptance of the "tension-free" concept, (c) the realization that the preperitoneal space can be used for hernia repair, and (d) therapeutic laparoscopy. These concepts are discussed in this section; the treatment strategies are divided between an open approach in the conventional anterior space and a preperitoneal approach, either open or laparoscopic.

Open Approach. The simplest Nyhus type I indirect inguinal hernias, which include most inguinal hernias in children, are adequately treated by obliteration of the congenital patent processus vaginalis alone. Since the inguinal floor is otherwise normal, reconstruction is not required. Classically, the hernia sac is dissected from the cord structures, ligated, and removed at its origin at the internal ring, so-called high ligation of the sac, thus the term *herniotomy.* The skin incision starts at the pubic tubercle and is extended laterally. The external oblique aponeurosis is opened in the line of its fibers through the external ring and the lower leaf is freed from the spermatic cord. The spermatic cord is freed from the floor of the inguinal canal and the pubic tubercle. Mobilization of the cord structures is completed by means of blunt dissection, and a Penrose drain is placed around them so that they can be retracted during the procedure.

The genital branch of the genitofemoral nerve and the spermatic vessels are included with the cord. The ilioinguinal and iliohypogastric nerves are usually preserved. The cremasteric fibers are separated, and the hernia sac is dissected from the cord structures to a point proximal to the internal ring. Ligation can be performed at this point (high ligation), followed by division of the neck of the sac. Prior to this the sac can be opened to allow a digital examination of the abdominal cavity and femoral ring. Alternatively, the sac may be simply inverted. The proponents of not opening the sac feel that with this method the patient experiences less pain because the highly innervated peritoneum has not been violated.

The terms *herniorrhaphy* or *hernioplasty* are used when a procedure to reconstruct the inguinal floor is added. For indirect hernias the sac is first dealt with in an identical manner as for a herniotomy. The only exception is large indirect inguinal scrotal hernias where complete removal of the sac might result in too high of an incidence of cord and testicular complications because of the extensive dissection required to completely separate them from the cord. Most authorities believe that these large sacs are best transected at the midpoint of the canal, and the distal sac is left in situ. Direct hernia sacs are almost never removed but instead are dissected from surrounding structures and reduced into the preperitoneal space. Dividing the transversalis fascia circumferentially at the neck (base) of the sac will aid in this reduction in some cases. The defect may be closed primarily at this point to maintain the reduction while a formal repair is being performed. The latter is considered a matter of convenience and adds nothing to the strength of the final outcome. The area of weakness in the posterior wall is then reinforced with the patient's own tissues.

The next step is to reconstruct the inguinal floor. There are two ways to do this. The first is a tissue repair, so named because only the patient's native tissue is used without foreign prosthetic material. The second is the tension-free repair (TFR). This implies the use of a prosthesis to repair the weakened inguinal floor, eliminating the need to reapproximate tissues that were not in apposition naturally. Edoardo Bassini (1844–1924) is considered the father of modern inguinal hernia surgery because in the latter part of the 19th century he introduced the first tissue repair based on solid anatomic principles, which became the "gold standard" for inguinal hernia repair for most of the 20th century. His scientific approach led to the development of several distinct steps essential for the procedure (Table 71.5). Before Bassini's achievements, elective herniorrhaphy was almost never recommended, because the results were so bad.

Today, there are at least 70 named tissue repairs described in the literature.[41] Most are relatively minor modifications of the Bassini, Shouldice, and McVay repairs and therefore, for the purposes of this chapter, only these will be presented. In the Bassini repair, the transversus abdominis aponeurosis together with the transversalis fascia is sutured to the shelving edge of the inguinal ligament with nonabsorbable interrupted sutures (Fig. 71.23). In the Shouldice repair, the transversalis fascia is divided from the internal ring to the pubic tubercle. The musculofascial elements laterally are then sutured to different levels of the inferior flap of the external oblique aponeurosis with four rows of running sutures (Fig. 71.24). Although the suture material originally used for this repair was stainless steel wire, other nonabsorbable materials, such as Prolene, are now used. The McVay repair (Fig. 71.25) addresses both inguinal and femoral hernias. The central attenuated portion of the inguinal floor is excised. The Cooper ligament must be clearly identified. The inguinal floor is then repaired by approximating the transversus abdominis aponeurosis and transversalis fascia to the Cooper ligament between the pubic tubercle and the femoral vein. A so-called transition stitch is then necessary between the transversalis fascia, Cooper ligament, and inguinal ligament to

TABLE 71.5 **TREATMENT**

ESSENTIAL STEPS FOR THE INGUINAL HERNIA REPAIR

1. Complete division of the external oblique aponeurosis and the transversalis fascia
2. Differentiation between indirect and direct defects
3. Isolation of the spermatic cord
4. Ligation and removal of the sac at the deep inguinal ring flush with the peritoneum
5. Oblique reconstruction of the inguinal canal with an anterior and posterior wall and an internal and external ring

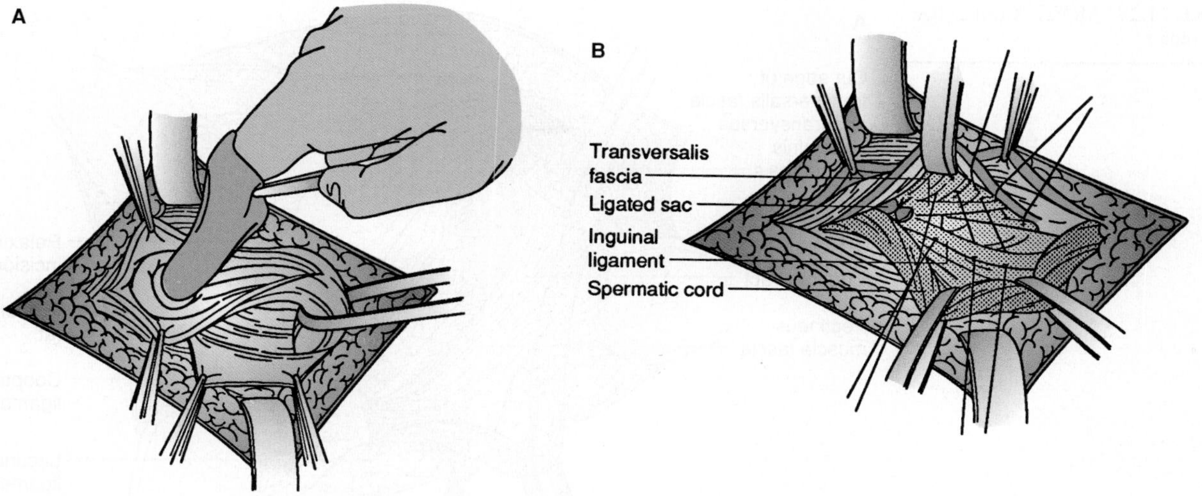

FIGURE 71.23. Bassini repair.

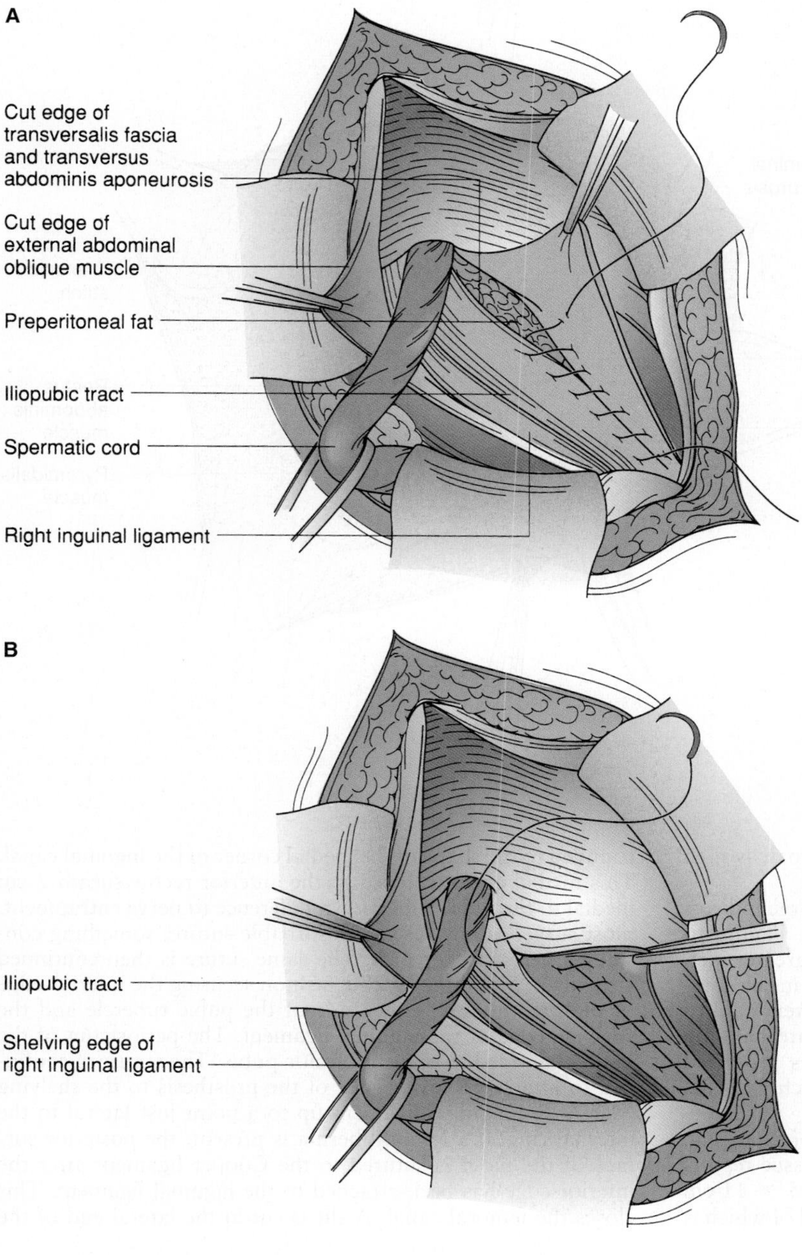

FIGURE 71.24. Shouldice repair.

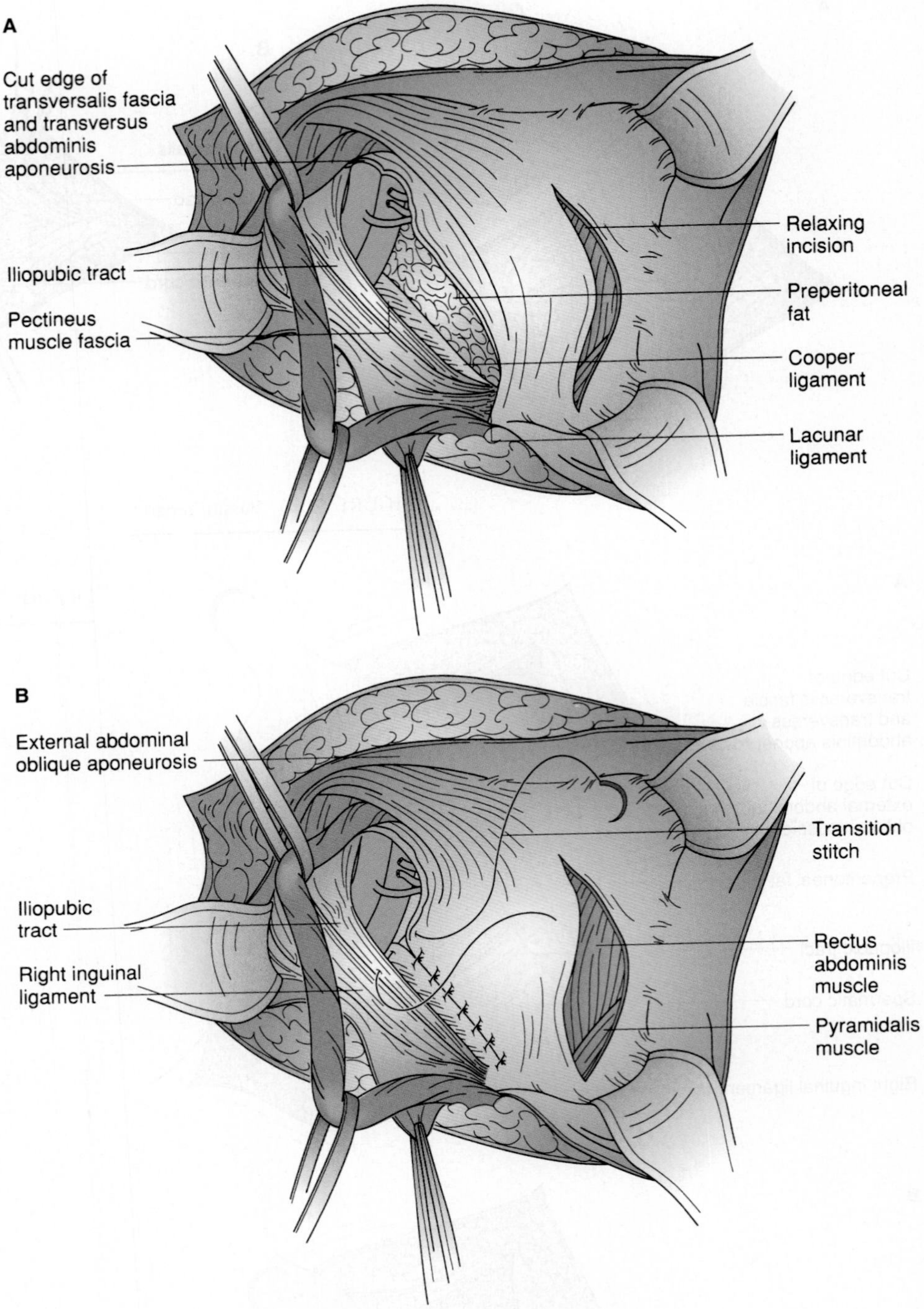

FIGURE 71.25. McVay (Cooper ligament) repair.

bring the repair above the femoral vessels. The repair is then continued laterally along the inguinal ligament.

A relaxing incision is necessary for repairs of large indirect hernias and whenever the McVay repair is used. Failure to make a relaxing incision has been implicated in a greater incidence of recurrence. The relaxing incision is made in the anterior rectus sheath in a vertical direction and is extended 3 to 4 cm above the pubis to a level opposite the internal ring (Fig. 71.25). The resulting defect in the sheath is protected posteriorly by the body of the rectus muscle, which prevents herniation at that site.

The most popular TFR is the Lichtenstein operation (Fig. 71.26).[42] The initial dissection is identical to the tissue repairs described. Once the sac has been dealt with, a 15 × 11-cm sheet of polypropylene mesh is used, the medial end of which is rounded to the shape of the medial corner of the inguinal canal. This medial end is sutured to the anterior rectus sheath 2 cm medial to the pubic tubercle. In deference to nerve entrapment, most surgeons now use an absorbable suture, something considered heresy in the past. The same suture is then continued laterally in a running locking fashion securing the inferior edge of the prosthesis to either side of the pubic tubercle and the shelving edge of the inguinal ligament. The periosteum of the bone is avoided to prevent osteitis pubis. The suture is continued to attach the lower edge of the prosthesis to the shelving edge of the inguinal ligament up to a point just lateral to the internal ring. If a femoral hernia is present, the posterior surface of the mesh is sutured to the Cooper ligament after the inferior edge has been attached to the inguinal ligament. This closes the femoral canal. A slit is cut in the lateral end of the

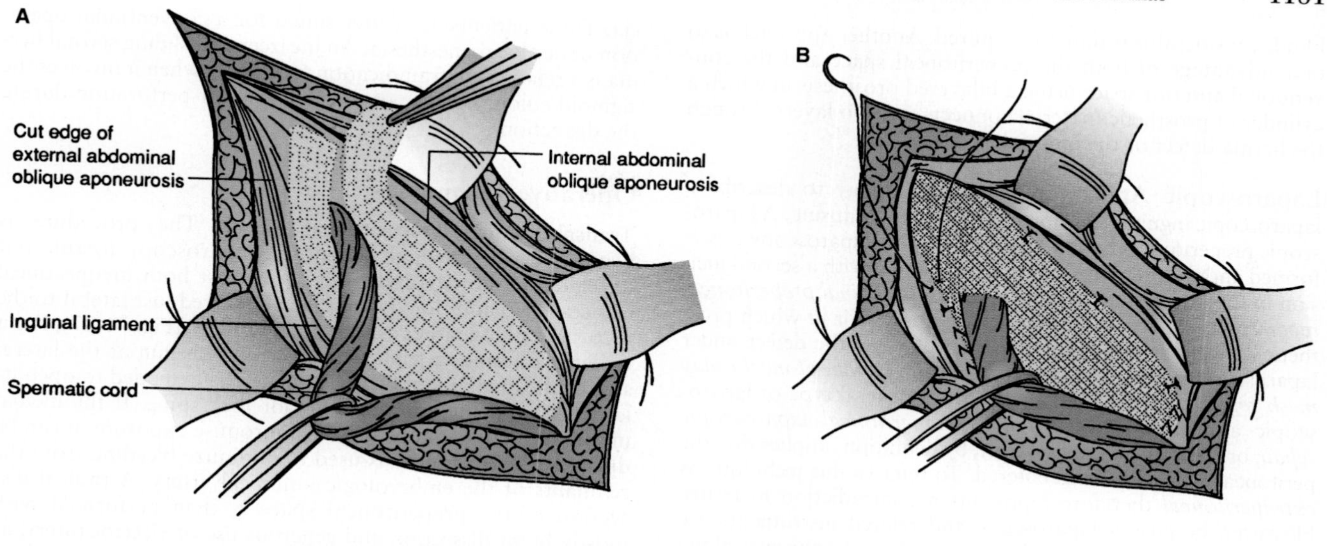

FIGURE 71.26. The Lichtenstein hernioplasty, showing placement of the mesh.

mesh to produce a narrow (one-third width) tail below and a wider (two-thirds width) tail above. The spermatic cord is positioned between the two tails. The wider tail is placed over the narrow one and a so-called shutter valve stitch placed just lateral to the cord including the inferior surface of the superior tail, the inferior surface of the inferior tail, and the inguinal ligament. The tails are then tucked under the external oblique aponeurosis to the level of the anterior superior iliac spine. The external oblique aponeurosis is closed to re-create the external ring. The wound is closed in layers.

A popular modification of the Lichtenstein operation has been termed the plug-and-patch repair. As the name implies, a plug usually constructed from polypropylene is inserted in the defect and secured with interrupted sutures to either the internal ring (for an indirect hernia) or the neck of the defect (for a direct hernia). The patch is then placed over the plug to cover the inguinal floor as in the Lichtenstein. One might argue that this operation is nothing more than a Lichtenstein on top of a plug, and in fact the term "plugstenstein" has been used to describe it. However, the difference with a plug-and-patch repair is that only one or two sutures—or, sometimes, no sutures—are used to secure the flat prosthesis to the underlying inguinal floor. This results in an operation that is fast and very easy to teach.

Femoral hernias can be repaired from a lower approach, in which a vertical incision is made over the femoral triangle in the upper thigh. The hernia is approached from below the inguinal ligament and reduced, and then the defect is closed by suturing the inguinal ligament to the Cooper ligament from below. An alternative is to insert a rolled plug of mesh into the defect and suture the periphery to the inguinal ligament and Cooper ligament.[43] The repair can also be carried out from above via an inguinal approach, as in the McVay repair. The posterior floor of the inguinal canal is dissected out, and the Cooper ligament is repaired after the hernia has been reduced. A third type of femoral hernia repair is the preperitoneal repair. Access to the preperitoneal space is gained through an abdominal incision or laparoscopy. Femoral hernias are more common in women and often present with an acute episode of incarceration, intestinal obstruction, or strangulation, so that emergency surgery is necessary. It can be difficult to reduce the hernia at surgery, and it is not uncommon to have to divide the inguinal ligament to obtain greater freedom to perform this reduction.

Inguinal herniorrhaphy can be performed under local anesthesia. Indeed, throughout the world, local anesthesia has become the standard method of anesthesia for this operation. Its greatest advantage is the virtual elimination of urinary retention when compared to regional or general anesthesia.[44] Hernias in high-risk patients can be safely repaired under local anesthesia.

Preperitoneal Approach. The preperitoneal space is situated between the transversalis fascia and the peritoneum. The final common denominator in all groin hernias is failure of the transversalis fascia to retain the intra-abdominal contents. Repairs performed in this space make the distinction between direct, indirect, and femoral irrelevant because the repair is accomplished behind the defective transversalis fascia, addressing the entire myopectineal orifice.

For a conventional, open operation, the preperitoneal space can be entered via a lower midline incision or a transverse incision placed slightly higher than usual. The rectus muscle is retracted medially and the preperitoneal space entered. A large prosthesis is used that extends far beyond the margins of the myopectineal orifice and envelops the visceral sac. The mesh is held in place by intra-abdominal pressure, which pushes outward toward the undersurface of the transversalis fascia. Because the incision for a preperitoneal hernia repair is away from the groin area and directly accesses the preperitoneal space, dissection of the inguinal canal, spermatic cord, or sensory nerves of the groin is not performed. The complications involving these structures that occur with other hernia repairs are very rare with the preperitoneal repair. If the hernial sac is large, it is amputated or inverted beneath a pursestring suture to smooth the external surface of the visceral sac. The distal peritoneal sac is left in place, undissected, and attached to the cord. With a sliding indirect hernia, the sac is easily dissected away from the cord. Proponents of this technique feel that polyester is better suited than other prostheses because of its pliability. For a bilateral repair, one large chevron-shaped mesh can be used for both sides.

Several newer, less invasive preperitoneal techniques have been developed to place a mesh in the preperitoneal space. For example, in the Kugel procedure, a small incision is made over the deep inguinal ring and the preperitoneal space is developed bluntly followed by the use of a prosthesis with an incorporated reinforcing ring. This ring can be deformed to allow the prosthesis to be introduced into the preperitoneal space and then the ring causes it to spring back to its original shape, providing wide overlap of the myopectineal orifice.[45] The procedure works well in experienced hands but because it is partially blind, considerable training is required. Another approach is to take advantage of both the preperitoneal space and the conventional anterior space using a bilayered prosthesis in which a cylinder of prosthetic material connects the two layers through the hernia defect or the internal ring.[46]

6 **Laparoscopic Approach.** The terminology to describe a laparoscopic inguinal herniorrhaphy can be confusing. A laparoscopic preperitoneal hernia repair, in which a laparoscopy is performed and the preperitoneal space is entered with a second incision in the peritoneum, is called a *transabdominal preperitoneal repair,* or TAPP repair. An inguinal hernia repair in which prosthetic material is placed intraperitoneally over the defect under laparoscopic guidance is referred to as an *intraperitoneal onlay mesh repair,* or IPOM repair. The third general type of laparoscopic approach is the *totally extraperitoneal laparoscopic repair,* or TEP repair. Laparoscopy, by definition, implies that the peritoneal cavity has been entered. To refer to this technique as *extraperitoneal* therefore represents a contradiction in terms. However, because a laparoscope and related instruments are used, it is fitting to discuss the extraperitoneal approach along with the other laparoscopic inguinal herniorrhaphies.

The TAPP and the TEP laparoscopic inguinal herniorrhaphies are the most popular. Both are modeled after the conventional preperitoneal operations. The major difference is that the preperitoneal space is entered through three trocar sites rather than through a large conventional incision. The ensuing radical dissection of the preperitoneal space with placement of a large prosthesis is similar to the conventional preperitoneal operation.

Laparoscopic Versus Conventional Herniorrhaphy. Randomized controlled trials as well as a meta-analysis of pooled data from these trials have shown that on average, patients undergoing laparoscopic herniorrhaphy have less pain initially than open, tension-free herniorrhaphy and return to normal activities sooner.[47] The difference is even greater when the comparison is made to nonprosthetic repairs. However, the potential advantages of laparoscopic herniorrhaphy must be interpreted in light of the disadvantages, which include complications related to the laparoscopy such as bowel perforation or major vascular injury, potential adhesive complications at sites where the peritoneum has been breached or prosthetic material has been placed, the need for a general anesthetic, and increased cost because of the expensive equipment. On the other hand, the conventional operation can be performed under local anesthesia on an outpatient basis, with minimal risk of intra-abdominal injury, and the cost is less.

Patient Selection. Perhaps the most important element in patient selection has nothing to do with the patient but has to do with the surgeon's skill. Laparoscopic inguinal herniorrhaphy is more challenging technically than a conventional open tension-free procedure. Assuming equivalence for recurrence and complication rates between laparoscopic inguinal herniorrhaphy and a tension-free herniorrhaphy for a given surgeon, all adult patients with inguinal hernias who are candidates for general anesthesia can be considered candidates for laparoscopic inguinal hernia repair. Certain hernia types, such as those that are recurrent, bilateral, or otherwise complicated, are particularly suited for the laparoscopic approach.[48] In addition, women may be better served with a laparoscopic operation because the femoral space is addressed, which should eliminate the excessive incidence of femoral recurrence observed with conventional operations such as the Lichtenstein.[37]

Contraindications include intra-abdominal infection and coagulopathy. Relative contraindications include intra-abdominal adhesions from previous surgery, ascites, or previous retropubic space surgery, because of the increased risk for bladder injury. Severe underlying medical illness is also a relative contraindication because of the added risk of general anesthesia. These patients are better suited for a conventional operation under local anesthesia. An incarcerated sliding scrotal hernia is a relative contraindication, especially when it involves the sigmoid colon, because of the high risk for perforation during the dissection.

Operative Techniques

Transabdominal Preperitoneal Repair. The procedure is begun with a thorough diagnostic laparoscopy to rule out unrelated pathology and carefully inspect both myopectineal orifices. Two additional cannulae are placed just lateral to the rectus sheath on either side of the umbilicus (Fig. 71.27). For a unilateral hernia, a transverse incision is begun at the lateral side of the medial umbilical ligament and extended to open its lateral leaf to the anterior superior iliac spine. If the medial umbilical ligament appears to compromise exposure, it can be divided. Electrocautery is used to minimize bleeding from the remnants of the embryologic umbilical artery. A radical dissection of the preperitoneal space is then performed with mostly blunt dissection and generous use of electrocautery, as bleeding in this area is particularly troublesome if it interferes with illumination. The ipsilateral and contralateral pubic tubercles, inferior epigastric vessels, Cooper ligament, and iliopubic tract are identified (Fig. 71.28). The cord structures are mobilized, and the peritoneal flap is dissected several centimeters proximal to the bifurcation of the vas deferens and the internal spermatic vessels. Recurrences have been attributed to inadequate mobilization of the peritoneal flap, which does not allow the prosthesis to lie flat in this area. If small, an indirect sac is mobilized away from the cord structures and reduced. If large, the sac is divided at a convenient point distal to the internal ring and only the proximal portion is mobilized. A direct sac readily reduces during the preperitoneal dissection. An easily visible layer of fatty tissue separates the thinned out transversalis fascia lining the defect and the peritoneum.

A large piece of polypropylene mesh (at least 14×11 cm) is placed in the preperitoneal space to cover the contralateral pubic tubercle medially and extending onto the anterior abdominal wall superiorly at least 2 cm above the hernia defect, to the anterior superior iliac spine laterally, and over the Cooper ligament inferiorly. Most surgeons prefer to fasten the prosthesis with staples, tacks, or glue, but there is increasing evidence that fixation is not necessary when a large prosthesis is used that widely overlaps the entire myopectineal orifice. Staples or tacks are never placed below the iliopubic tract when lateral to the internal spermatic vessel because of the danger of damage to the important nerves in this area. The last step is to cover the prosthesis by closing the peritoneum with sutures, tacks, staples, or glue. The goal is to isolate the prosthesis from the abdominal viscera rather than to always achieve precise approximation of the peritoneal edges. This is because gaps can form if the peritoneum is closed under tension allowing bowel to migrate into the preperitoneal space. A better option is to secure the inferior peritoneal flap to the transversalis fascia above the prosthesis and leave the superior flap alone.

For bilateral inguinal hernias, the same peritoneal incision and preperitoneal dissections are used. The symphysis pubis is completely exposed so that both preperitoneal dissections communicate with each other. This exposure allows the placement of one large prosthesis (at least 25×8 cm) that essentially covers the entire lower pelvis. By not incising the peritoneum between the two medial umbilical ligaments, one avoids the theoretical complication of dividing a patent urachus.

Totally Extraperitoneal Laparoscopic Repair. An incision is made at the umbilicus, as if one were planning to perform open laparoscopy. The rectus sheath is opened on one side and the rectus muscle is retracted laterally. Blunt dissection is then begun in the space between the rectus muscle and the posterior rectus sheath. Once the space is large enough, two additional

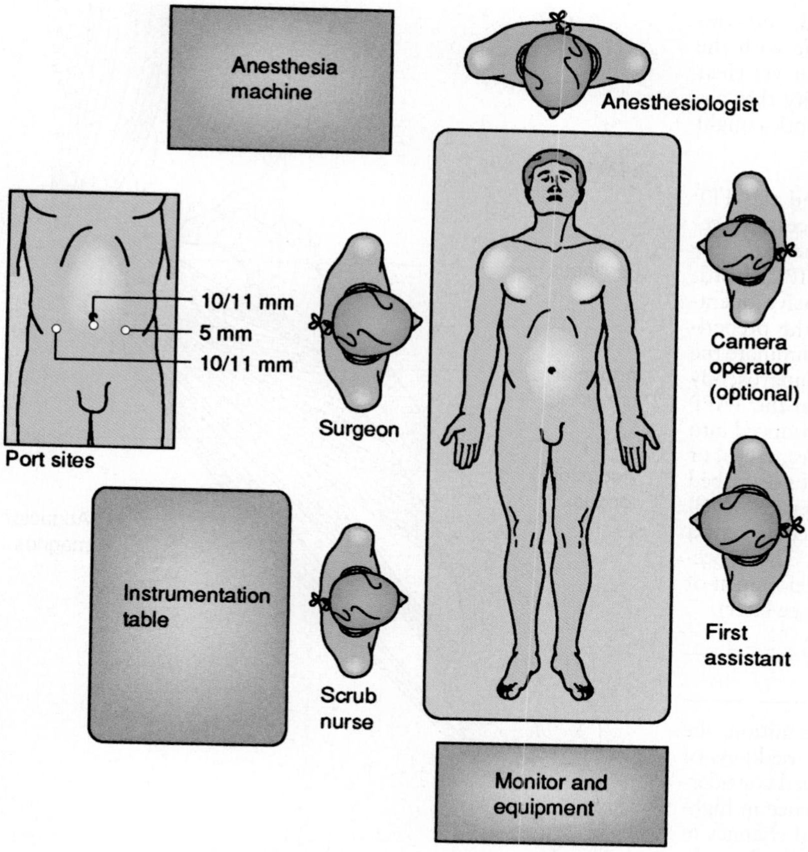

FIGURE 71.27. Typical operative setup and cannula site selection for a transabdominal preperitoneal (TAPP) laparoscopic inguinal herniorrhaphy.

cannulae are placed in the midline, one approximately 5 cm above the symphysis pubis and the other midway between the umbilicus and the symphysis pubis. The dissection of the preperitoneal space is completed under direct vision. The rest of the operation is identical to the TAPP procedure described previously except that peritoneal closure is not necessary. Popular alternatives are to use a water- or air-filled balloon dissector to perform the preperitoneal dissection and to place the two accessory cannulae on either side of the umbilicus, as in the TAPP procedure, instead of in the midline.

The presumed advantages of the TEP procedure are that the inherent complications of entering the peritoneal cavity, such as intra-abdominal organ injury or postoperative bowel obstruction secondary to adhesions or trocar site herniation,

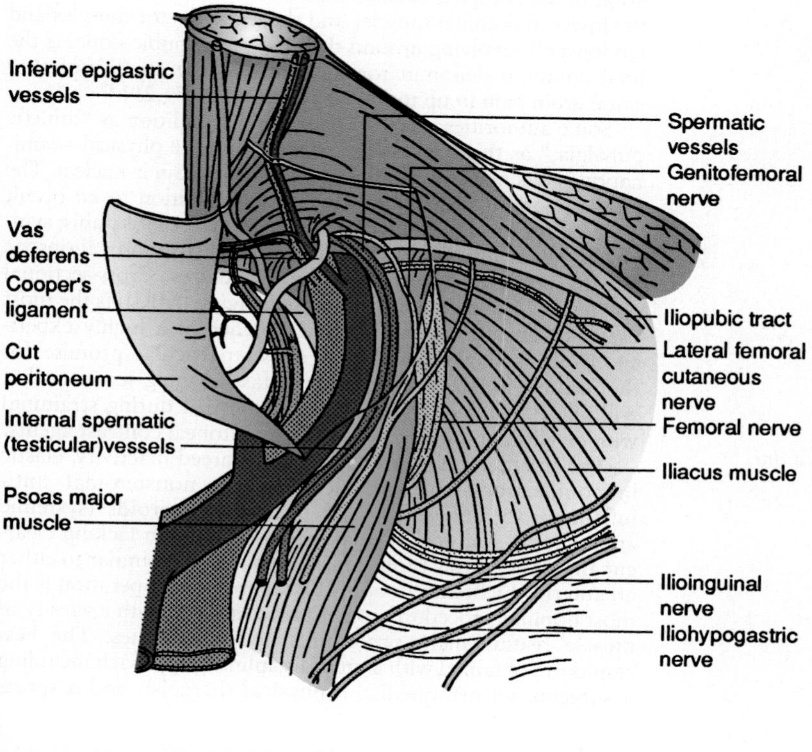

FIGURE 71.28. Important structures that must be identified after a preperitoneal dissection: inferior epigastric vessels, Cooper ligament, spermatic vessels, vas deferens, iliopubic tract, genitofemoral nerve, femoral nerve, lateral femoral cutaneous nerve, ilioinguinal nerve, iliacus muscle, and psoas major muscle.

are avoided. However, the operative space is limited, and considerable experience is required to become familiar with the anatomy from this perspective. In addition, it is not yet clear whether inadvertent breaches in the peritoneal cavity that are difficult to visualize because of the direction of the optics might negate the potential benefits of this approach.

Intraperitoneal Onlay Mesh Repair. The TAPP and the TEP herniorrhaphies are better considered minimal access procedures rather than minimally invasive because of the extensive dissection required in the preperitoneal space. The IPOM procedure was developed to be a truly minimally invasive operation. By placing the prosthesis one layer deep to the preperitoneal space directly onto the peritoneum, one can eliminate the need for a radical preperitoneal dissection. Initial laparoscopy and accessory cannula placement are the same as in the TAPP procedure. A large piece of prosthetic material is introduced into the peritoneal cavity and secured in place with staples, tacks, or sutures. An attempt is made to use the same landmarks described previously for the TAPP procedure. The main concern is development of the complications of intraperitoneal placement of a prosthesis in contact with intra-abdominal organs. The procedure is regaining some popularity because of the development of the adhesion barrier prosthetics for ventral hernia (see later).

SPORTS HERNIA

The term *sports hernia* is confusing because, by definition, the patients do not actually have a hernia but rather a weakness of the posterior inguinal floor. The condition has received considerable attention in the lay press because of its prevalence in high-profile athletes involved in sports who require rapid changes in direction of the hip area such as soccer, football, basketball, track and field, tennis, and hockey. The first step in approaching these patients is to make sure one is not dealing with a cause outside of the groin with referred pain, such as lumbosacral radiculopathic pain, prostatitis, hip disease, and a gastrointestinal cause. The differential diagnosis is listed in Table 71.6. Alteration in the complex balance that must be maintained between the lower abdominal muscles and the leg adductor muscles and tendons, all revolving around the area of the pubic bone, is the final common denominator for many of the conditions that cause groin pain in up to 5% of athletes (Fig. 71.29).[49]

Some authorities prefer to refer to this condition as "athletic pubalgia," as this conveys the concept that the physical examination is inconclusive and the cause of groin pain is unclear. The most important differential diagnoses in addition to an occult groin hernia include adductor tenoperiostitis, osteitis pubis, symphysis syndrome, Gilmore groin (groin disruption), iliopsoas bursitis, stress fractures, or avulsion fractures. Cross-sectional imaging (CT or magnetic resonance imaging [MRI]) is the most useful diagnostic modality in the absence of a highly experienced ultrasonographer.[50] MRI shows particular promise for the future with the development of fast imaging scanners that will allow dynamic imaging (i.e., performed during straining) with or without the addition of intraperitoneal contrast agents.

The treatment is conservative with forced inactivity, elastic immobilization bandages, ice/massage, nonsteroidal anti-inflammatory analgesics, and occasional steroids (systemic and/or local). Surgery is a last resort. Although lacking clear-cut anatomic justification, a mesh hernia repair similar to either an anterior Lichtenstein or a TEP laparoscopic operation is the most popular procedure, sometimes combined with a variety of muscle reattachment procedures and tenotomies. The best results are obtained with a multidisciplinary approach including a surgeon, an orthopedist, a physical therapist, and a sports

TABLE 71.6 DIAGNOSIS

CONDITIONS OTHER THAN A HERNIA ASSOCIATED WITH GROIN PAIN

- Muscle injury
- Adductor strains
- Tendon injury
- Iliopsoas bursitis
- Osteitis pubis
- Pelvic stress fractures
  - Snapping hip syndrome
  - Lumbosacral disorders
  - Connective tissue disease
  - Nerve entrapment
  - Hip disorders
    - Synovitis
    - Avascular necrosis
    - Osteoarthritis
    - Legg-Calvé-Perthes disease
    - Slipped femoral capital epiphysis
    - Osteochondritis dissecans or avascular necrosis of the femoral head
    - Acetabular labral tears
- Prostatitis
- Epididymitis
- Nephrolithiasis
- Urinary tract infection
- Lymphadenitis

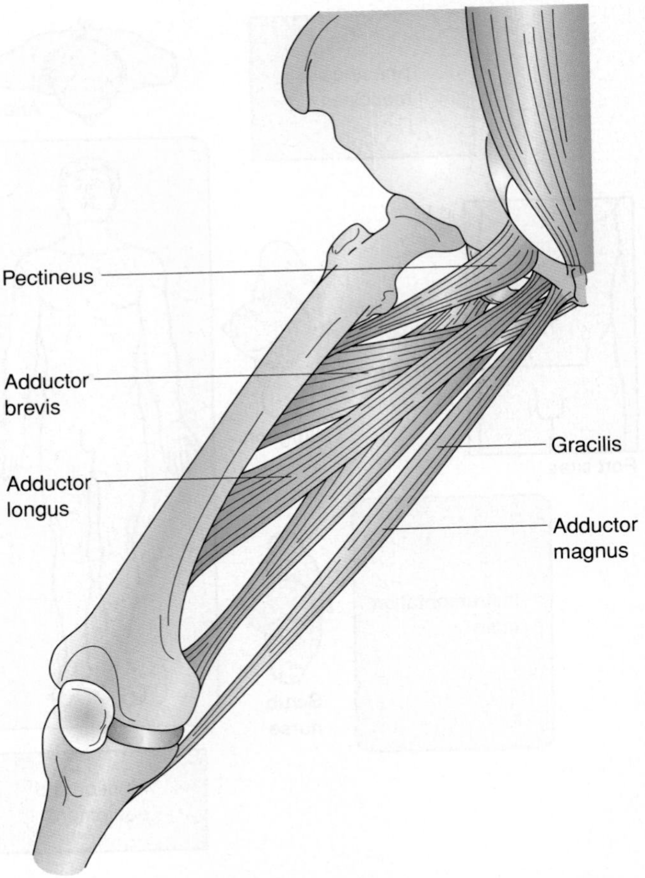

FIGURE 71.29. Complicated arrangement of muscle pulling in different directions that attach to the pubic bone.

TABLE 71.7

VENTRAL ABDOMINAL WALL HERNIAS

Incisional
Umbilical and paraumbilical
Epigastric
Parastomal
Less common variations
Spigelian hernias
Interparietal hernia
Richter hernia
Miscellaneous

medicine physician. Not surprisingly, the results are variable given the lack of objective criteria to recommend operation but can be gratifying in some in this motivated group of patients.

VENTRAL ABDOMINAL WALL HERNIAS

Ventral abdominal wall hernias are best divided into their various subtypes when discussing surgical management because the natural history is different. Results of operations vary depending on the specific hernia. Table 71.7 uses the common terminology familiar to all surgeons for classifying abdominal wall hernias. Table 71.8 is a classification system published by Zollinger that expands upon Table 71.7 by further subdividing ventral hernias based on etiology.[51]

TABLE 71.8

ZOLLINGER CLASSIFICATION OF VENTRAL ABDOMINAL WALL HERNIAS

Congenital
Omphalocele
Gastroschisis
Umbilical (infant)
Acquired
Midline
Diastasis recti
Epigastric
Umbilical
Adult, acquired, paraumbilical
Median
Supravesical
Anterior, posterior lateral
Paramedian
Spigelian
Interparietal
Incisional
Midline
Paramedian
Transverse
Special operative sites
Traumatic
Penetrating, auto-penetrating
Blunt
Focal, minimal injury
Moderate injury
Extensive force or shear
Destructive

UMBILICAL AND PERIUMBILICAL HERNIAS

Umbilical and periumbilical hernias are usually congenital, caused by arrest of the normal spontaneous closure of the umbilical ring through which umbilical blood vessels pass in the developing fetus, which results in a defect in the fascia covered by skin. In infants, the fascial defect varies in size but is most commonly 1 to 2 cm. A large proportion of pediatric umbilical hernias heal spontaneously, and 80% of them close by the time the patient is 2 years old. This is the only abdominal wall defect genetically programmed to close. Persistent umbilical hernias require surgery. In older patients, the onset is usually sudden and the defect is relatively small. There are several syndromes associated with umbilical hernias such as mucopolysaccharide storage diseases, Beckwith-Wiedemann syndrome, and Down syndrome. Predisposing factors for the development of umbilical hernias in adults are multiple pregnancies, obesity, cirrhosis with ascites, and large abdominal tumors, all of which cause an increase in intra-abdominal pressure.[52] The differential diagnosis includes the varicosities that extend radially from the umbilicus in persons with portal hypertension, the so-called caput medusae (Fig. 71.30). The varicosities have a bluish discoloration and fill when the patient is straining. A metastatic deposit of intra-abdominal cancer at the umbilicus may mimic umbilical herniation. Cancer cells reach this area via lymphatics in the falciform ligament. Metastasis presents as a hard nodule, and biopsy is diagnostic. Other periumbilical masses that can be confused with an umbilical

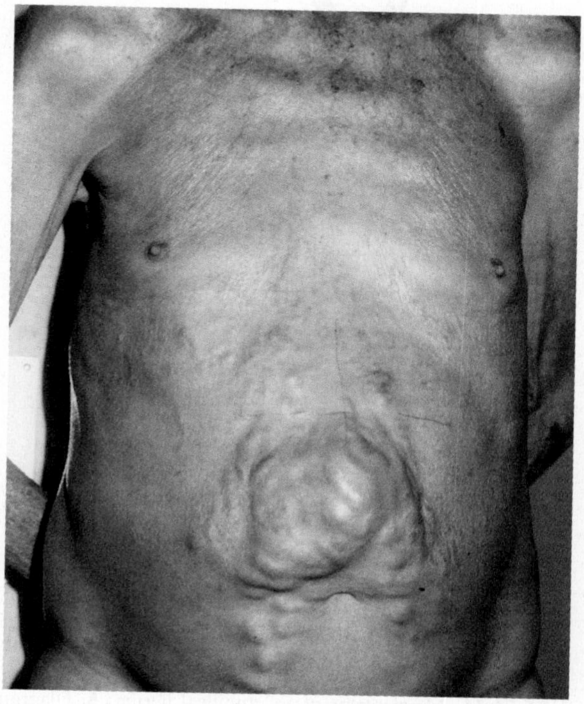

FIGURE 71.30. Caput medusae. Large periumbilical collaterals in a patient with portal hypertension.

HERNIA

hernia include umbilical granulomas, omphalomesenteric duct remnant cysts, and urachal cysts.

The management of umbilical hernias is nonoperative in children up to the age of 2 or 3 years because spontaneous closure is the rule. In those who require surgery, adults or children, the repair depends on the size of the hernia. An infraumbilical semilunar incision is made and the hernia identified. There may or may not be a true peritoneal sac, as smaller hernias usually consist of preperitoneal fat only. If a sac is present, it can be opened and the contents reduced into the abdomen. Alternatively, the hernia can be dissected circumferentially to the fascial opening and reduced without entering the peritoneal cavity. The dissection can be continued beneath the fascias creating a preperitoneal space for the placement of a prosthesis if needed. Several techniques can be used to close the fascial defect. In 1901, James Mayo described the classic overlapping, vest-over-pants (double-breasting or waistcoat) technique, which bears the name of his clinic, in which the upper edge of the linea alba overlaps the lower edge (Fig. 71.31).[53] The operation is losing popularity now because it is generally not consistent with the tension-free concept popular in hernia surgery today.[54] It requires more dissection than other procedures to create the flaps and is therefore more painful. Simple suture herniorrhaphy is the easiest procedure but has the highest recurrence rate and therefore should be used only for small defects. For larger hernias, particularly in adults, the preperitoneal space can be exploited by bluntly dissecting the peritoneum from the undersurface of the posterior rectus sheath for enough distance to be able to place an appropriate prosthesis. If the peritoneum is not entered, a mesh prosthesis is preferred, which is placed in the preperitoneal space and then the fascial edges closed if the defect is small enough. Otherwise, a bridging technique can be used with the fascial edges sewn to the underlying mesh. If the peritoneal cavity is entered, then a composite prosthesis (e.g., ePTFE + polypropylene) or a mesh prosthesis with an adhesion barrier (see prosthetic materials section) can be placed intraperitoneally with the adhesion barrier facing the viscera. A laparoscopic approach for umbilical hernias is a good option for recurrent hernias or hernias with defects larger than 3 cm and, in retrospective reviews, has been shown to decrease operative times and result in faster recovery to normal activities.[52] The technical details are similar to a laparoscopic incisional hernia repair (see incisional hernia section).

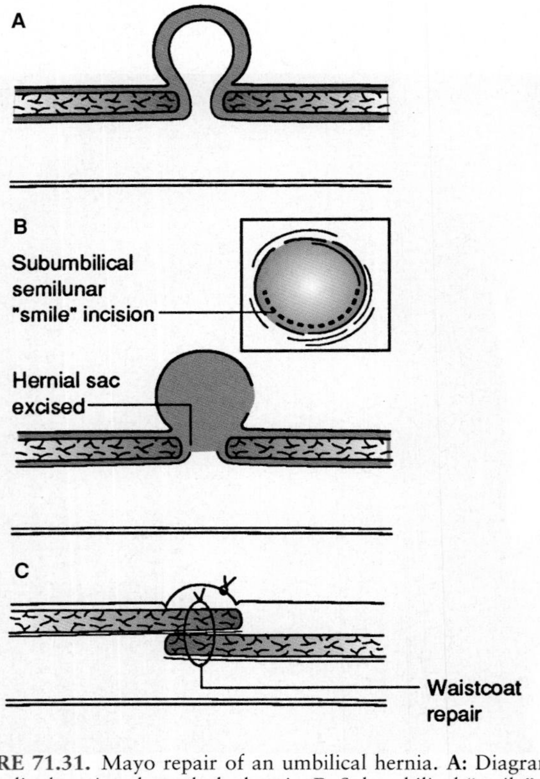

FIGURE 71.31. Mayo repair of an umbilical hernia. **A:** Diagram of longitudinal section through the hernia. **B:** Subumbilical "smile" incision. The hernial sac is excised. **C:** Waistcoat type of closure.

EPIGASTRIC HERNIAS

Epigastric hernias occur through a defect in the linea alba. In the majority of patients, only a single decussation of the fibers of the linea alba is present rather than the usual triple decussation (Fig. 71.7). The incidence of epigastric herniation reported varies from less than 1% to as high as 5%. Epigastric hernias are two to three times more common in men than in women. About 50% of them are asymptomatic. Most are less than 1 cm and contain only incarcerated preperitoneal fat without a peritoneal sac. For this reason, epigastric hernias commonly cannot be visualized with laparoscopy. Patients complain of a painful nodule in the upper midline. Repair by reduction of the preperitoneal fat and simple closure of the defect is curative. These hernias are prone to recur, with rates as high as 10%, which has led many surgeons to routinely include a prosthetic underlay just as in umbilical or incisional hernias.

Left untreated, an epigastric hernia can become large enough for a peritoneal sac to form, into which the intra-abdominal contents can protrude. The sac is usually wide, and serious complications are not common. Twenty percent are multiple, and this needs to be ascertained prior to operation if all the defects are to be addressed, because after anesthesia induction, they can be difficult to identify.

In *diastasis recti,* the two rectus muscles are separated widely. The area of the linea alba is stretched and protrudes like a fin. The condition almost never produces complications and therefore surgical correction is not routinely recommended. However, many patients find the defect unsightly and request treatment. They should be cautioned that many insurance companies consider this a cosmetic defect and will not reimburse. Surgery involves removal of a strip of the weakened linea alba and reapproximation. An alternative is a mesh repair done laparoscopically.

INCISIONAL HERNIAS

Incisional hernias occur as a complication of prior surgery. These hernias can follow any type of abdominal surgery, regardless of the type of incision. More than 2 million laparotomies are performed yearly in the United States, and the reported incidence of incisional hernia varies between 2% and 11%.[55] The highest incidence is with midline incisions (10.5%) and transverse incisions (7.5%), but hernias are well documented following paramedian incisions as well (2.5%).[56] Read and Yoder in a retrospective review found that 17% of incisional hernias are incarcerated or strangulated at presentation.[57] Most of the published literature on treatment options addresses midline defects. The management of nonmidline incisional hernias (i.e., subcostal, transverse, or gridiron incisions) to some extent must be extrapolated.[58] The consequences of unrepaired enlarging symptomatic hernias include loss of abdominal domain; significant biomechanical alterations that affect posture; compromise of activities of daily living, including lifting and straining; and poor cosmetics.

The cumulative incidence of incisional hernias is linear, as they can present after considerable delay following the index operation. Poor surgical technique, rough handling of tissues, use of rapidly degraded absorbable suture materials, closure of

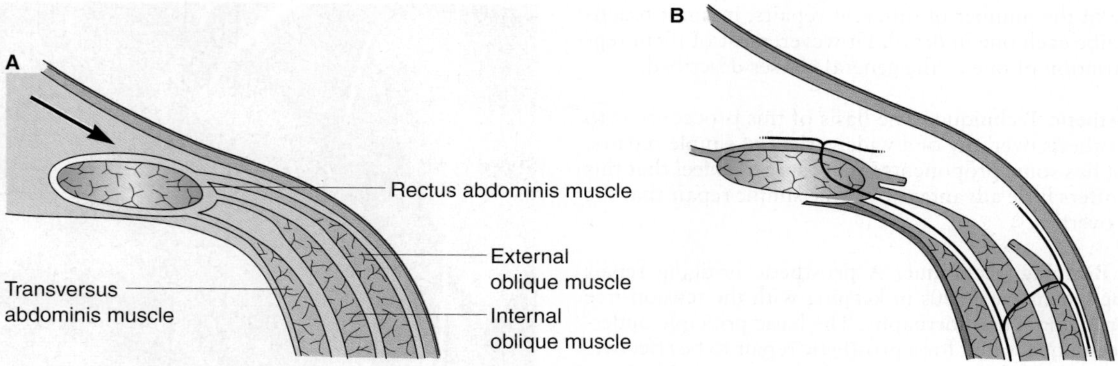

FIGURE 71.32. Component separation technique.

the abdomen under tension, and infection of the wound are technical causes of incisional hernias. Morbid obesity, cigarette smoking, pulmonary disease, debilitation from cancer, chemotherapy, the use of steroids, hypoalbuminemia, and other preexisting comorbid conditions are patient factors that have been incriminated. Patients with an aortic aneurysm or a proven defect in collagen metabolism also exhibit an increased incidence of incisional hernias.[59]

At least some ventral hernias can be prevented by proper abdominal closure after any laparotomy. Sutures should be placed 1 cm away from the edge and 1 cm apart from each other. The length of the suture should be four times the length of the wound to avoid excessive tension.[60] It is now generally agreed that monofilament suture material used in a continuous running fashion is best. Studies have shown that nonabsorbable sutures result in a lower incidence of incisional herniation but at the cost of increased wound pain and chronic suture sinuses when they become infected.[61] These suture sinuses tend to be multiple and take years to eradicate by probing the sinus tracks and removing deep sutures. The development of better monofilament absorbable sutures has caused most surgeons to avoid nonabsorbable closure material.

Treatment

7 **Nonprosthetic Repairs.** Traditionally, the repair of an incisional hernia depended on the size of the hernia. If the defect was solitary and 3 cm or less, primary closure with nonabsorbable suture material was recommended. This concept is now questioned after the publication of a landmark prospective randomized trial by Luijendijk et al. from The Netherlands in the year 2000 and updated in 2004 comparing a prosthetic repair versus primary suture.[62,63] These investigators found a 50% reduction in the recurrence rate when a prosthesis was used, and this even applied to small hernias. For this reason, a simple, nonprosthetic technique should be reserved for only the smallest hernias in patients without risk factors for further recurrence.

A more complex nonprosthetic repair is the component separation technique popularized in the early 1990s by Ramirez et al.[64] The skin and subcutaneous fat are dissected free from the anterior sheath of the rectus abdominis muscle and the aponeurosis of the external oblique muscle. The aponeurosis of the external oblique muscle is transected longitudinally just lateral to the lateral side of the rectus sheath (Fig. 71.32). It is important to extend the incision onto the chest wall at least 5 to 7 cm cranial to the costal margin. The external oblique muscle is separated from the internal oblique muscle, as far laterally as possible. This step is safe because the neurovascular bundle (comprising the intercostal nerves and vessels) lies deep to the internal oblique muscle. The result is that the internal oblique muscle and the rectus abdominis slide medially. When necessary, 2 to 4 cm of additional length can be gained by separating the posterior rectus sheath from the rectus abdominal muscle. Care must be taken not to damage the neurovascular bundle that runs between the internal oblique and transverses abdominis muscle to enter the rectus sheath posterolaterally. The technique can also be used as an adjuvant to the prosthetic repairs described next, but the extensive flap dissection between the two procedures results in an increased incidence of abdominal wall devascularization. A technique that employs a balloon dissector and laparoscopic instruments to lessen the degree of abdominal dissection has been described, but it remains to be seen if it is effective (Fig. 71.32).[65]

Prosthetic Repairs. The concept of prosthetic use is not new as it was proposed by Usher et al. in 1958 for hernia repair using the polypropylene mesh Marlex.[66] Over the ensuing years, lessons have been learned: (a) the use of absorbable mesh leads to a high relapse rate, (b) repetition of a previously inadequate technique frequently fails, (c) a simple inlay technique that bridges the defect has a high failure rate, (d) reinforcement of the entire scar is advisable irrespective of operative findings, and (e) the success of a mesh repair depends on the extent of overlap or underlap.[67]

Numerous techniques for prosthetic incisional hernia repair have been described, which is not surprising since there are so many variables. For example, there are five potential spaces to place a prosthesis (Figs. 71.3 and 71.33).

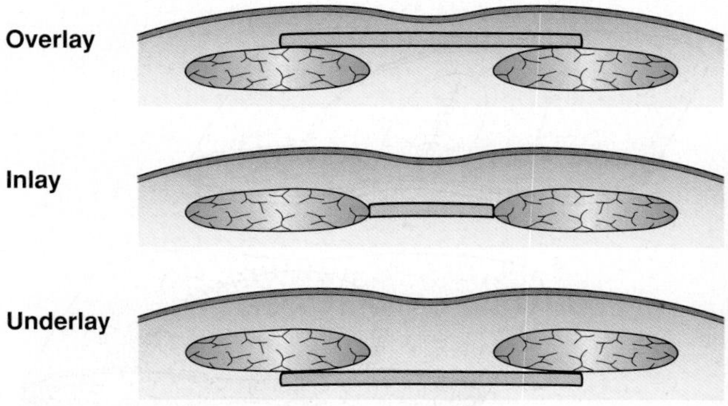

FIGURE 71.33. Potential spaces in the abdominal wall to place prosthetic material: onlay or on top of the anterior abdominal fascia; under the anterior fascia but in front of the muscle (if the mesh bridges that space, it would be an inlay technique; retrorectus space or the underlay technique below the muscle but above the posterior fascia; preperitoneal (important when below the arcuate line); intraperitoneal.

Because of the number of different repairs, it is not practical to describe each one in detail. However, most of them represent a variation of one of the general classes described.

Onlay Prosthetic Technique. The basis of this procedure is to place a prosthesis over any of a wide variety of simple repairs. Although it has some proponents, many surgeons feel that this technique offers little advantage over the simple repair that the prosthesis overlies.[68]

Prosthetic Bridging Technique. A prosthetic bridging repair became popular in the 1990s in keeping with the tension-free concept for inguinal herniorrhaphy. The basic principle underlying this technique is that for a prosthetic repair to be effective, the defect should be bridged. Although this repair is theoretically attractive, it has not been nearly as successful for incisional hernias as for inguinal hernias. The recurrence rate is especially high in obese patients. It is not recommended.

Combined Fascia and Mesh Closure. This group of repairs combines features of the component separation technique with the tension-free concept. By incising the anterior fascia and rotating the medial edge toward the midline in continuity with the posterior fascia, the posterior fascia is effectively lengthened (Fig. 71.34). The posterior fascia is closed primarily, but the anterior fascia is bridged with a prosthesis.

Sublay Prosthetic Technique. The sublay prosthetic repair, sometimes referred to as the retromuscular approach, is characterized by the placement of a large prosthesis in the space between the abdominal muscles and the peritoneum (Fig. 71.17). It was popularized by Velamenta, Stoppa, and Wantz and is particularly suitable for large and multiply

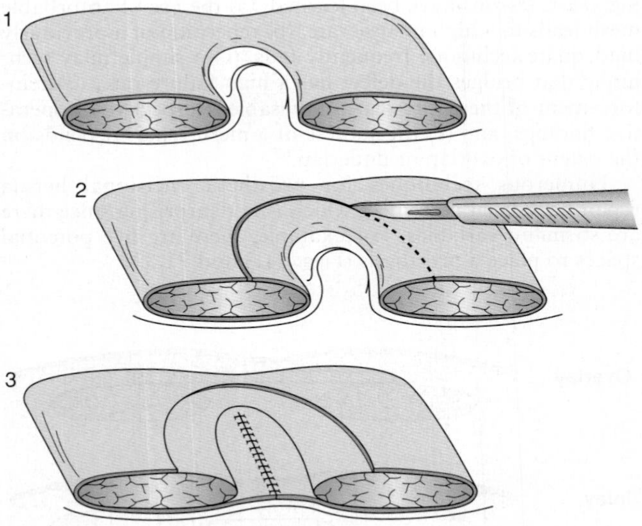

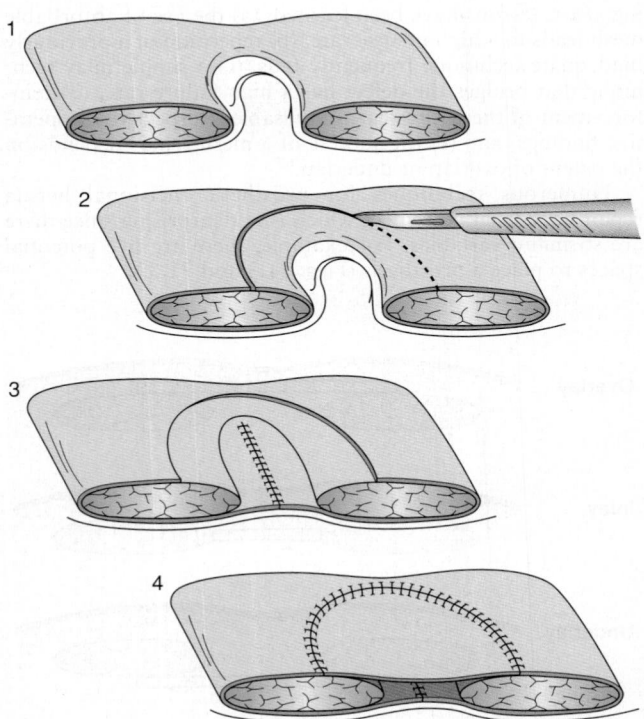

FIGURE 71.34. *1*, Hernia defect with bulging sac. *2*, Anterior fascia is incised longitudinally on either side of the defect. *3*, The anterior fascia is then rotated medially, in effect lengthening the posterior sheath to allow primary closure, isolating the abdominal contents from the anterior fascia. *4*, Prosthetic material is used to bridge the anterior fascia.

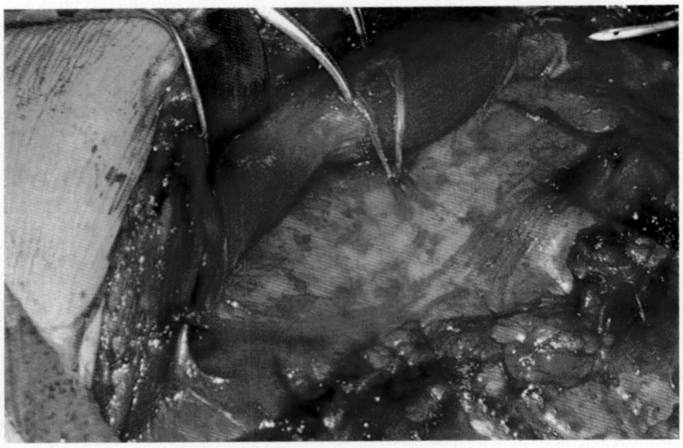

FIGURE 71.35. Perforating blood vessels supplying the rectus muscle.

recurrent hernias when most of the abdominal wall must be reconstructed.[69–71] It is considered the most effective conventional incisional hernia repair and therefore the one against which other procedures must be measured. Its major disadvantage is its need for wide undermining of the abdominal layers with the potential risk of devascularization of the abdominal wall or the creation of a large seroma, which later leads to infection. Suction drains are used by most surgeons, although the literature does not unequivocally support their use.[72]

The procedure is begun by excising the previous scar and dissecting the peritoneal sac of the hernia to the level of the fascia. Occasionally, the sac does not have to be opened and the procedure can be performed totally extraperitoneal. More commonly, the sac is thin and easily disrupted, making entrance into the peritoneal cavity inevitable. The posterior rectus sheath is opened on each edge of the hernia defect and dissected away from the undersurface of the recti to the lateral edge of the rectus sheath, with care being taken to prevent damage to the perforating blood vessels at the lateral side of the sheath (Fig. 71.35). The posterior rectus sheaths are then approximated to each other primarily (unless the peritoneum has not been opened). During this part of the procedure, flaps must be created by dissecting the skin and subcutaneous tissue off of the underlying fascia laterally until enough tension is relieved to allow primary closure of the anterior rectus sheath. It is sometimes necessary to add component separation to further decrease the tension. A large mesh prosthesis (combined with ePTFE or an adhesion barrier if the approximation of the posterior rectus sheath is inadequate) is then placed in this space outside the repaired posterior sheath but beneath the recti. The mesh is secured in this position with several sutures directly to the posterior rectus sheath. An alternative is to use a suture passer to pass the two tails of a suture placed on the lateral side of a prosthesis through the lateral edge of the rectus sheath through separate fascia openings. The suture is then tied in the subcutaneous tissue resulting in a secure anchoring of the prosthesis in the abdominal wall. If the subcutaneous tissue dissection from the anterior rectus sheath has not been too extensive, the sutures cannot be retrieved in the subcutaneous tissue and therefore the suture passer is pushed through the entire thickness of the subcutaneous tissue and then through a small stab incision in the skin. The suture is tied and the knot allowed to retract back into the subcutaneous tissue and the skin is approximated over it. The procedure is completed by reapproximating the anterior rectus sheaths, thus bringing the rectus muscles back to their normal configuration. The best long-term results are obtained when the anterior fascia can be closed bringing the muscles back together because of an improvement in abdominal wall mechanics. However, it is sometimes impossible

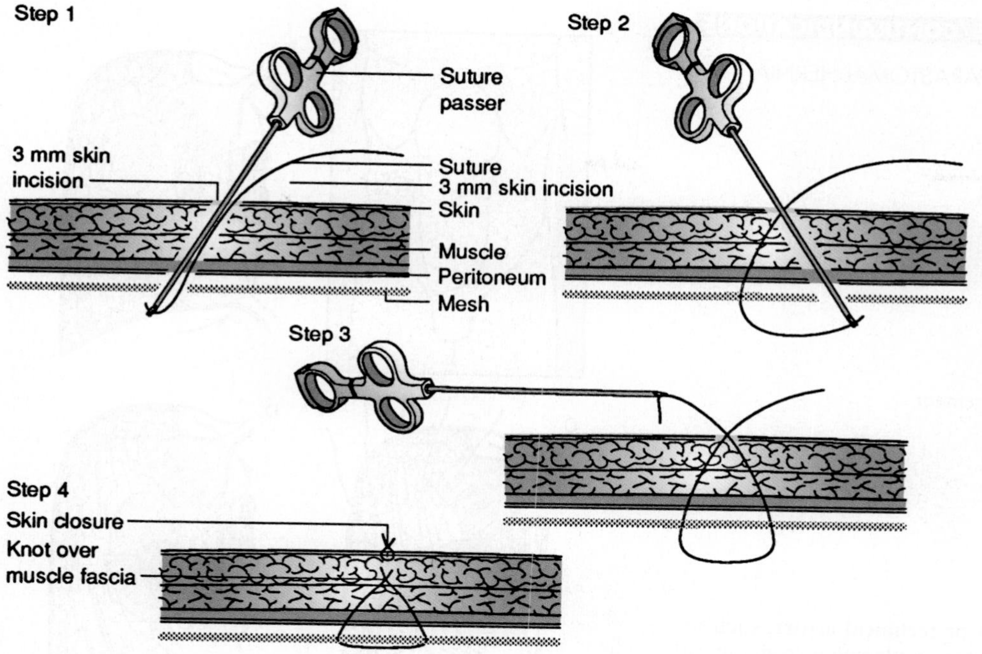

FIGURE 71.36. Fixation of prosthesis to the peritoneal surface of the abdominal wall with use of a suture passer. Step 1: The suture passer device with a heavy nonabsorbable suture is passed through a 3-mm stab incision in the skin at an oblique angle. The device and suture traverse the entire abdominal wall and then the prosthesis. Once the peritoneal cavity is entered, the suture is released and the passer is withdrawn back into the subcutaneous tissue. Step 2: The device is redirected at a different angle through the abdominal wall and prosthesis and the suture is grasped. Step 3: The suture is pulled out of the abdominal cavity so that the two free ends are extracorporeal. Step 4: The suture is tied with the knot resting on the fascia. The skin is then closed.

to achieve this and the gap must be bridged with a prosthesis (Fig. 71.36).

Laparoscopic Ventral Hernia Repair. This operation was developed in the 1990s as a natural extension as surgeons became trained in the laparoscopic method for many commonly performed abdominal procedures. Although smaller hernia defects can be closed primarily, its greatest value is that the "gold standard" sublay technique can be replicated by the intra-abdominal placement of a submuscular prosthesis, eliminating the need for the extensive abdominal wall dissection implicit in the conventional operation. ePTFE has a long track record of safety with contact with intra-abdominal viscera and the development of the adhesion barrier coated mesh prosthesis has made intra-abdominal placement more attractive.

Entrance to the abdominal cavity followed by adhesiolysis can be problematic for a surgeon performing a laparoscopic ventral hernia repair and devastating complications are possible, which is the Achilles heel of this operation. This is because patients with incisional hernias by definition have had previous abdominal surgery and the midline is commonly not usable for initial access because of a previous incision in the area. The surgeon must make an educated guess as to the least likely place for significant adhesions as well as be familiar with alternate access techniques away from the midline. Unrecognized visceral injury can be the consequence if extreme care about entrance and adhesiolysis is not maintained. These injuries commonly go undetected until the patient develops signs of septic shock because it is difficult to differentiate peritoneal signs from ordinary postoperative pain. This accounts for the significant mortality with this complication. Surgeons performing laparoscopic ventral hernia repairs must have the good judgment to abandon the procedure in the face of a hostile abdomen.

Once the abdomen has been safely entered and the adhesiolysis completed, the abdominal contents are reduced from the hernia defect under direct laparoscopic guidance. The number and location of the sites of cannula placement vary depending on the size and location of the hernia. Multiple "swiss cheese defects" are the best indication for the operation because if there is only one or two defects with wide separation of the muscles, the operation is not as effective for two reasons: (a) the prosthesis will tend to balloon out through this defect, simulating a recurrence even though the hernia is technically repaired, and (b) abdominal wall dynamics are addressed more effectively if the muscles can be reapproximated. The muscles can commonly be approximated using a suture passer/trocar site closing device similar to that demonstrated in Figure 71.36. Our group favors conversion to an open, conventional operation in situations where it is not possible to reapproximate the muscles, but this philosophy is not shared by all.

The prosthesis is prepared by placing sutures extracorporeally around its circumference with long tails extending from the nonadhesion barrier side. It is then rolled up and introduced through the largest cannula. After it is unrolled, a suture passer is introduced into the abdomen to grasp each of the suture tails through a single stab incision but separate musculofascial openings in array, which corresponds to the previously placed prosthesis sutures (Fig. 71.36). The sutures can be tied extracorporeally and the knot allowed to retract back into the subcutaneous tissue of the stab incisions. The skin is then closed over them. It is important that the prosthesis be positioned onto the peritoneum so that it widely overlaps the hernia defect (4 to 6 cm, at least). The prosthesis is further secured to the anterior abdominal wall with staples, tacks, or sutures using the suture passer technique.

Complex hernias can be challenging, especially when obesity or a question of loss of domain complicates the problem. An abdominal wall hernia is said to have lost its "right of domain" when so much of the intra-abdominal contents reside outside of the peritoneal cavity in the subcutaneous tissue that there is a question that it can be returned (see section on large hernias). These patients might best be seen in centers with special interest in this area where teams have been assembled to treat complex abdominal wall pathologies.[73]

PARASTOMAL HERNIAS

Parastomal hernias are one of the most common complications of stoma formation. Studies designed with very careful follow-up suggest that a paracolostomy hernia develops in more than 50% of patients followed for longer than 5 years.[74] The rate of herniation with small-bowel stomas is less than for

TABLE 71.9 INDICATIONS/CONTRAINDICATIONS

INDICATIONS FOR REPAIR OF A PARASTOMAL HERNIA

ABSOLUTE	
	Obstruction
	Incarceration with strangulation
RELATIVE	
	Incarceration
	Prolapse
	Stenosis
	Intractable dermatitis
	Difficulty with appliance management
	Large size
	Cosmesis
	Pain

colon stomas. Poor site selection or technical errors, such as making the fascial opening too large or placing a stoma in an incision, account for some of these hernias. Placing a stoma lateral to the rectus sheath is widely touted as a cause, but this is now being challenged. Obesity, malnutrition, advanced age, collagen abnormalities, postoperative sepsis, abdominal distention, constipation, obstructive uropathy, steroid use, and chronic lung disease also contribute. Novel techniques for stomal reconstruction, such as extraperitoneal tunneling, have had little impact.

Fortunately, patients tolerate these hernias well, and life-threatening complications, such as bowel obstruction or strangulation, are rare. Fewer than 20% of patients with parastomal hernias have a complication that mandates repair. Routine repair is therefore not recommended. Table 71.9 lists possible indications. The three general types of stomal hernia repair are fascial repair, stomal relocation, and prosthetic repair. Fascial repair involves a local exploration around the stoma site, with primary closure of the defect. This approach should be considered of historical interest only. Stomal relocation produces better results than simple fascial repair.[74] This approach is especially indicated in patients with other stomal problems, such as skin excoriation or suboptimal stomal construction. The major drawbacks of stomal relocation are the fact that a laparotomy is required, which in and of itself causes more morbidity than some of the other techniques, and it exposes the patient to the risk of three new incisional hernias at (a) the old stoma site, (b) the laparotomy incision site, and (c) the new stoma site.[75]

Whenever possible, a prosthetic repair should be considered as this appears to be the most effective, although few randomized trials have been performed to unequivocally prove this. Options for the location of mesh placement in parastomal hernia repair are as follows:

1. Onlay with the mesh placed anterior to the anterior rectus aponeurosis. A hockey-stick incision is usually performed outside the boundaries of the patient's appliance (Fig. 71.37). The skin and subcutaneous tissue are then undermined to identify the fascial defect, which is closed primarily and reinforced with a prosthetic onlay. The problem with this approach is that the undermining of subcutaneous tissue leads to seroma formation, which sometimes goes on to infection.
2. Inlay with the mesh placed to bridge the defect and sutured to the fascial edges. This alternative has in multiple series been shown to have the highest chance of recurrence and suffers from the seroma problem, as with the onlay.

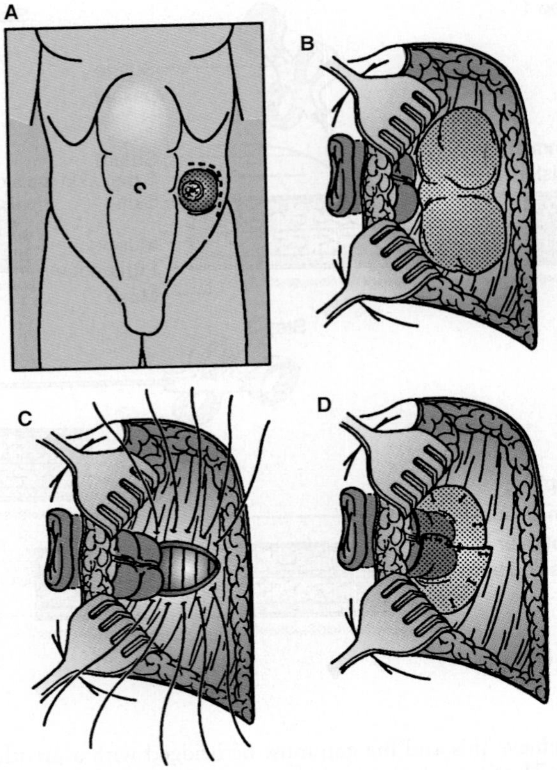

FIGURE 71.37. Repair of a parastomal hernia. **A:** Incision around hernia. **B:** Hernial sac is identified, the contents are reduced, and the peritoneum is closed. **C:** The edges of the fascial defect are reapproximated. **D:** The fascial repair is reinforced with polypropylene mesh, which is wrapped around the subcutaneous portion of the colon and sutured in place. (After Pearl RK. Para-stomal hernias. *World J Surg* 1989;13:569.)

3. Sublay with the mesh placed dorsal to the rectus muscle and anterior to the posterior rectus sheath.
4. Intraperitoneal inlay mesh (IPOM). An intra-abdominal prosthetic repair eliminates the need for the abdominal wall dissection and is therefore becoming increasingly popular. It also enlists the mechanical advantage of placing the prosthesis on the peritoneal side of the abdominal wall.[76] The intra-abdominal approach is particularly suited for laparoscopy, and several techniques have been described.[77]

Janes performed a prospective randomized study using a prophylactic mesh when constructing stomas. He randomized 54 patients to a conventional stoma construction versus the same with the addition of a lightweight, wide-pore prosthesis in a sublay position. He reported that after 5 years, 17 out of 21 patients with the conventional technique had recurred compared to only 2 out of 15 patients in the prophylactic group. There were no fistulas, strictures, or wound infections during the study period.[78]

UNUSUAL HERNIAS

Spigelian Hernia

A Flemish anatomist, Adriaan van der Spieghel, first described the semilunar line, which is the lower limit of the posterior rectus sheath. Also called the spontaneous lateral ventral hernia, a spigelian hernia protrudes through an area of weakness just lateral to the rectus sheath and just below this line (Fig. 71.38). The hernia is usually interparietal, rarely

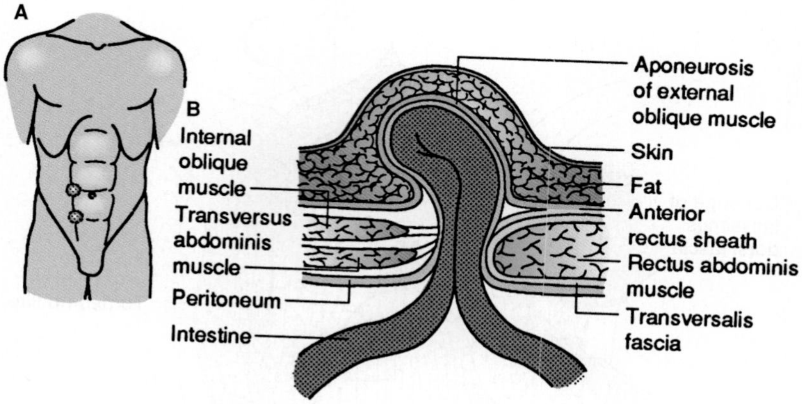

FIGURE 71.38. Spigelian hernia. **A:** Usual site of occurrence. **B:** Transverse section of abdominal wall showing site of defect.

penetrating the external oblique fascia, and therefore can be difficult to appreciate. Most of the time, this hernia appears below the arcuate line. This is an unusual hernia; only 744 cases have been described in the literature. The usual presentation is lower abdominal swelling just lateral to the border of the rectus muscle. Spigelian hernias often occur in elderly female patients. They are usually small, about 1 to 2 cm in diameter, although large hernias up to 14 cm in diameter have been described. Omentum and small or large bowel may enter the sac. Incarceration and strangulation are common complications of this hernia. Because the hernia is deep to the external oblique fascia, the clinical presentation may not be obvious. Pain and tenderness may be the only signs. Plain roentgenograms may show a bowel shadow in this area, and CT can demonstrate the defect well. Treatment is operative repair. A transverse incision is centered over the mass. The external oblique aponeurosis is split to reveal the protrusion. If a large sac is present, it is divided and sutured. The aponeurotic defect is triangular, with its base at or near the lateral border of the rectus muscle. The defect is closed by joining the separated transversus and internal oblique layers. Another option is a laparoscopic repair, done using an intra-abdominal or preperitoneal approach. Recurrence is uncommon.

Lumbar Hernia

The lumbar region is the area bounded inferiorly by the iliac crest and superiorly by the 12th rib, posteriorly by the erector spinae group of muscles, and anteriorly by the edge of the external oblique muscle as it extends from the 12th rib to the iliac crest. The three varieties of lumbar hernia are described in Table 71.10. These hernias require repair if they are large, and because of the size of the defect, synthetic mesh is used. For the inferior lumbar hernia, a rotation flap of fascia lata can be used (Fig. 71.39).

Obturator Hernia

This hernia is the result of abdominal contents protruding through the obturator canal in the pelvis. This canal is the opening in the superior part of the obturator membrane covering the foramen formed by the union of the pubic bone and ischium, through which the obturator nerve, artery, and vein pass from the pelvic cavity into the thigh. A recent history of profound asthenia and weight loss is not unusual, which is most likely due to the loss of the protective fat in the obturator canal.[79] This may account for the fact that women are more often than men afflicted with this hernia because their broader pelvis results in a larger obturator canal. The diagnosis of an obturator hernia is difficult because it is rare and physical examination is rarely helpful because the associated mass is concealed beneath the adductor muscles of the thigh. The main symptom is intermittent pain. The defect is approached transperitoneally; the hernia is reduced and mesh placed over the defect. Depending on the expertise of the responsible surgeon, either a conventional open or laparoscopic operation is reasonable.

Sciatic Hernia

A sciatic hernia is a protrusion of a peritoneal sac through the major or minor sciatic foramen (Fig. 71.40). These very rare hernias present with a swelling on the buttock. The sciatic nerve may be involved. A ureter can become obstructed if it is included with the herniated tissues. The treatment of these

TABLE 71.10

TYPES OF LUMBAR HERNIA

■ TYPE	■ DESCRIPTION
Superior lumbar hernia of Grynfelt	Occurs through a space between the latissimus dorsi, the serratus posterior inferior, and the posterior border of the internal oblique muscle
Inferior lumbar hernia of Petit	Occurs through a defect in the space bounded by the latissimus dorsi posteriorly, the iliac crest inferiorly, and the posterior border of the external oblique anteriorly
Secondary lumbar hernia	Develops as a result of trauma, mostly surgical (e.g., renal surgery), or infection; lumbar hernias were encountered relatively frequently in the past in cases of spinal tuberculosis with paraspinal abscesses

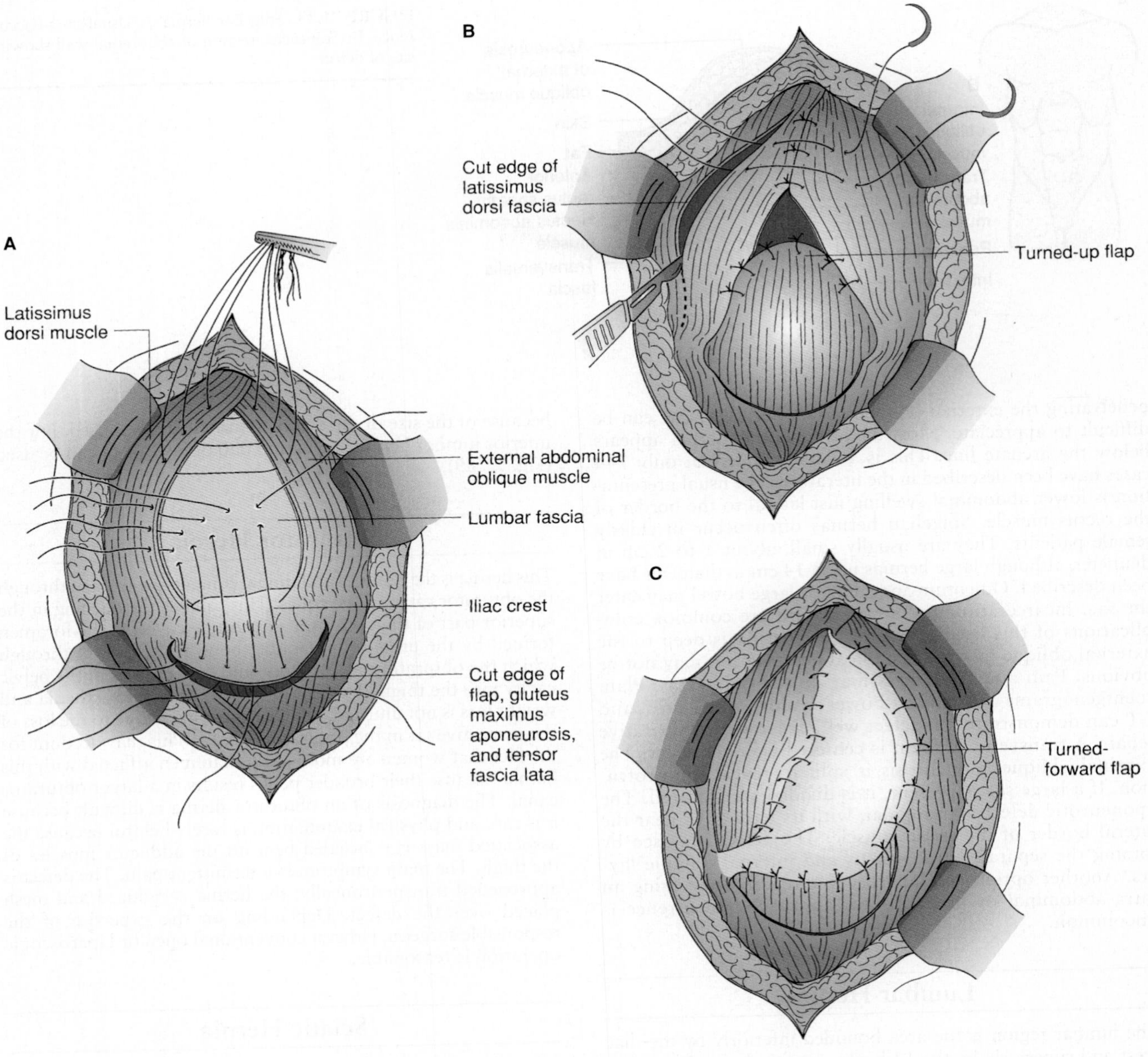

FIGURE 71.39. Technique of repair of inferior lumbar hernia.

hernias is surgical. Both transperitoneal and transgluteal approaches have been described. A combination of the two is sometimes used. The defect usually requires a prosthetic mesh repair.

Supravesical Hernia

This hernia is anterior to the urinary bladder and forms when the integrity of the transversus abdominis muscle and the transversalis fascia fail, both of which insert into the Cooper ligament. The preperitoneal space is continuous with the retropubic space of Retzius, and the hernial sac protrudes into this area. The sac of the hernia is directed laterally, emerges at the lateral border of the rectus muscle, and presents in the inguinal, femoral, or obturator region. It can also be associated with an inguinal, femoral, or obturator hernia. Treatment of this hernia depends on recognizing it at the time of groin exploration and reinforcing the defect.

A second variety of these hernias is known as an internal supravesical hernia. They are classified according to whether they cross in front of, beside, or behind the bladder (Fig. 71.41). Bowel symptoms predominate in patients with these hernias, and urinary tract symptoms develop in up to 30%. The treatment is surgical, and a transperitoneal approach is used through a low midline incision. The hernias can usually be reduced without difficulty. The neck of the sac should be divided and closed.

Interparietal Hernia

This hernia is one in which the hernial sac lies between the layers of the abdominal wall. It may be either *preperitoneal* (between the peritoneum and the transversalis fascia) or *interstitial* (between the muscle layers of the abdominal wall). The majority are inguinal, in which case they are designated *inguinal interstitial* hernias. An *inguinal crural* hernia occurs

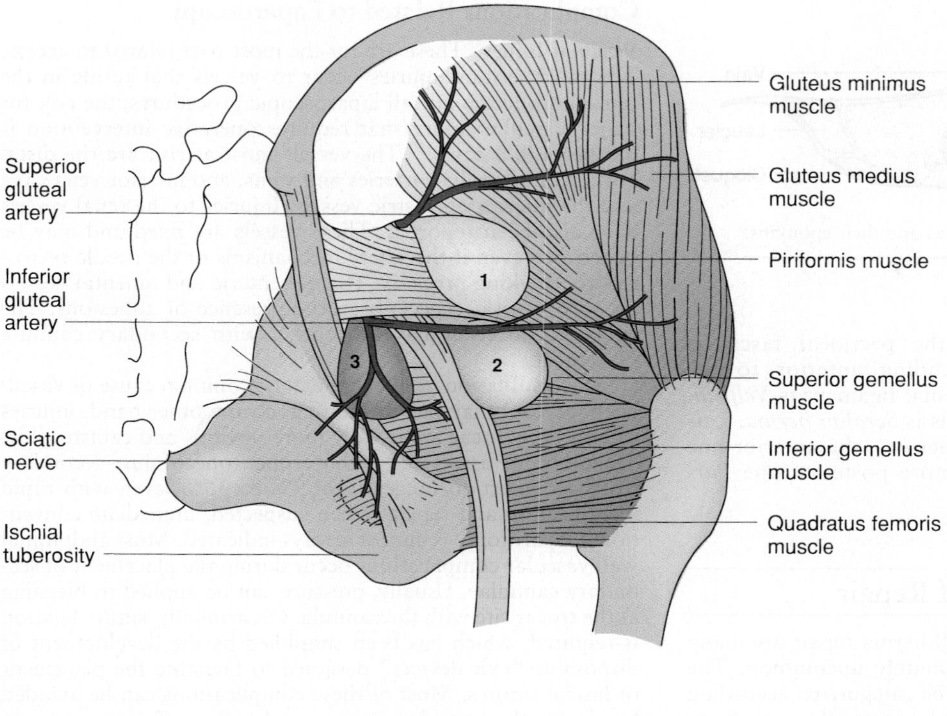

FIGURE 71.40. Sciatic hernia. *1*, Suprapiriform. *2*, Infrapiriform. *3*, Subspinous.

when the sac passes behind the inguinal ligament in the region of the femoral ring.

The cause of these hernias appears to be related to congenital abnormalities; they have been associated with failure of the testis to descend, congenital pouches, and other abnormalities, such as absence of the cremaster and absence of the external abdominal ring.

The diagnosis of these hernias is difficult because no swelling of the abdominal wall is obvious unless the hernia is large. Pain is commonly the only symptom, and it is not unusual for patients to present with intestinal obstruction secondary to incarceration. CT, ultrasonography, and laparoscopy can be helpful in making the diagnosis. Not infrequently, the correct diagnosis is made only at operation. The defect is repaired according to the principles described for inguinal and incisional hernias.

Littre Hernia

Littre hernia is a groin hernia containing a Meckel diverticulum. These hernias sometimes also contain the appendix. If the diverticulum is symptomatic or strangulated, then it is mandatory to resect it at the time of the hernia repair.

Perineal Hernia

These hernias are more common in older female patients and are related to a lax pelvic floor. They are termed *anterior* or *posterior* according to their relationship to the transversus perinei muscle. The anterior hernias usually present as a swelling in the labium or lateral vaginal wall. The posterior hernias present between the rectum and the ischial tuberosity. Surgical repair requires a transperitoneal approach, and, if the opening is large, a prosthetic mesh repair is required.

Perivascular Hernia

These hernias present through defects between the inguinal ligament and the iliopubic bone. They are known by various eponyms according to their position. The hernia protruding through a defect in the lacunar ligament is *Laugier hernia*.

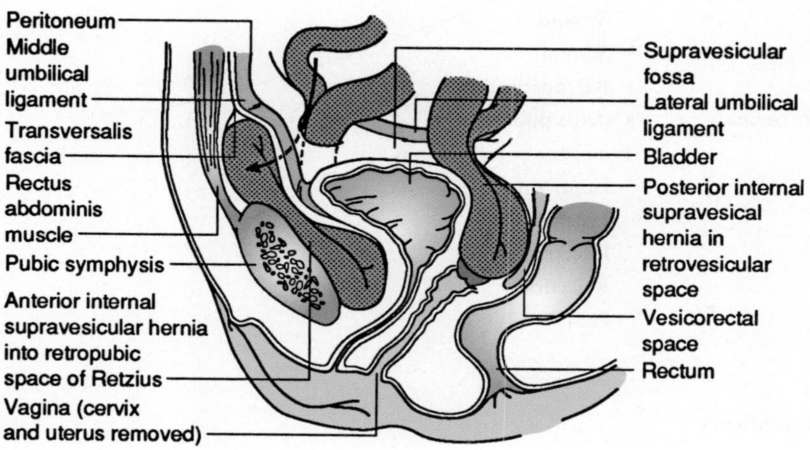

FIGURE 71.41. Internal supravesical hernias. (After Skandalakis JE. Internal and external supravesical hernia. *Am Surg* 1976;42:142.)

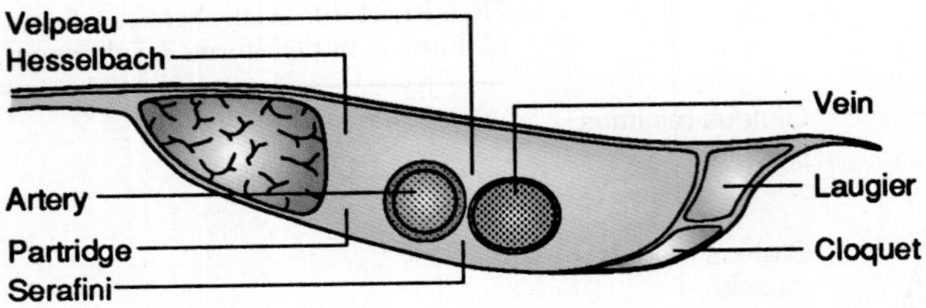

FIGURE 71.42. Perivascular hernias and their eponyms.

The hernia protruding through the pectineal fascia is *Cloquet hernia*. The hernia extending anterior to the femoral vessels but behind the inguinal ligament is *Velpeau hernia*. The hernia behind the vessels is *Serafini hernia*. Lateral to the femoral artery are two hernias, the anterior one being *Hesselbach hernia* and the more posterior one *Partridge hernia* (Fig. 71.42).

Complications of Repair

The complications of abdominal wall hernia repair are many and varied (Table 71.11), but fortunately uncommon. The complications of herniorrhaphy can be categorized according to whether they are related to the laparoscopy, the patient, or the herniorrhaphy. Except for the complications unique to laparoscopy, complications occur at similar rates in both laparoscopic and conventional procedures.

Complications Related to Laparoscopy

Vascular Injury. These are for the most part related to access. The most serious injuries occur to vessels that reside in the retroperitoneum. For all laparoscopic procedures, the risk for major vascular injury that requires operative intervention is 0.9 per 1,000 cases.[80] The vessels most at risk are the distal aorta, common iliac arteries and veins, and inferior vena cava and the inferior epigastric vessels. Injuries to the renal vessels have also been reported. These vessels are fixed and may be penetrated even if the safety mechanisms of the needle or trocar are working properly. The mesenteric and omental vessels are also at risk, especially in the presence of adhesions. The epigastric arteries may be injured with secondary cannula placement.

The insufflation needle is the most common cause of vascular injury but may be self-limiting; on the other hand, injuries caused by a trocar are usually more obvious and catastrophic. The mortality associated with retroperitoneal injury secondary to trocar insertion ranges from 9% to 36%, even with rapid identification and repair. When suspected, immediate conventional laparotomy is almost always indicated. Most abdominal wall vascular complications occur during the placement of secondary cannulae. Usually, pressure can be applied to bleeding at the trocar site with the cannula. Occasionally, suture ligation is required, which has been simplified by the development of disposable "exit devices" designed to facilitate the placement of fascial sutures. Most of these complications can be avoided by placing the secondary trocars under direct vision.

Gas Embolism. This is caused by intravascular insufflation.[81] It is an uncommon complication, unique to the needle insufflation

TABLE 71.11 COMPLICATIONS

COMPLICATIONS OF LAPAROSCOPIC HERNIORRHAPHY

RELATED TO LAPAROSCOPY	RELATED TO HERNIORRHAPHY
Vascular injury	Recurrence
Intra-abdominal	Neurologic
Retroperitoneal	Iliohypogastric
Abdominal wall	Ilioinguinal
Gas embolism	Genitofemoral
Visceral injury	Lateral cutaneous
Bowel perforation	Cord and testicular problems
Bladder perforation	Wound infection
Trocar site complications	Seroma
Hematoma	Hydrocele
Hernia	Hematoma
Wound infection	Wound
Keloid	Scrotal
Bowel obstruction	Retroperitoneal
Trocar or peritoneal closure site hernia	Osteitis pubis
Adhesions	Prosthetic complications
Diaphragmatic dysfunction	Contraction
Hypercapnia	Erosion
RELATED TO PATIENT	Infection
Urinary infection	Rejection
Ileus	Pain
Nausea and vomiting	
Aspiration pneumonia	
Cardiovascular and respiratory insufficiency	

technique. Careful attention to tests confirming proper peritoneal needle placement will keep the incidence of this complication low.

Visceral Injury. Visceral injuries are uncommon, occurring in 1.8 per 1,000 cases of all laparoscopic procedures, but they have a mortality rate of 5%.[80] The most common means of injury is the insufflation needle. Simple repair laparoscopically is usually possible as most are self-limiting. If the injury is caused by a trocar, formal repair of the injury will be needed. The injury can be repaired laparoscopically if the skill of the laparoscopic surgeon is sufficient. Otherwise, laparotomy is mandatory. Quite often, these injuries go unnoticed at the time of insult, so that visceral injury is the most common cause of late morbidity and mortality associated with laparoscopic access. Patients typically present with peritonitis and sepsis 2 days to 1 week after surgery.

Bladder Injury. Bladder injury can be the result of a laparoscopic misadventure or can be directly related to the herniorrhaphy. Laparoscopic peritoneal access can result in a bladder perforation, usually the result of failure to decompress a distended bladder. Less commonly, injury is associated with a congenital bladder abnormality. Bladder injury has not been reported with the open access technique. Injury to the bladder can also occur during secondary suprapubic trocar placement during the course of an operation. When bladder injury occurs, it is usually obvious. After Veress needle insertion, urine is withdrawn into the syringe, or blood and gas are noticed in the urine if the patient is catheterized. In questionable cases, methylene blue dye may be instilled into the bladder to look for leakage. Bladder injury recognized during laparoscopy should be repaired laparoscopically provided the experience of the surgeon is sufficient. This should be followed by bladder drainage for 7 to 10 days.

Bladder injury may present in a delayed fashion with hematuria and lower abdominal discomfort. A retrograde cystogram usually confirms the diagnosis. Small defects may be managed with postoperative decompression via an indwelling catheter for urinary drainage, while larger defects necessitate repair. The bladder is especially prone to injury during preperitoneal herniorrhaphies or when the preperitoneal space has previously been dissected (e.g., previous preperitoneal hernia repair or prostatectomy).[82]

Bowel Obstruction. This problem plagued the developmental stages of laparoscopic inguinal herniorrhaphy for two reasons. First, the importance of closing trocar sites at the fascial level if greater than 5 mm was not appreciated, resulting in the occasional patient with an incarcerated or strangulated ventral hernia at the trocar site, leading to the clinical presentation of a bowel obstruction. There are now several different types of reusable and disposable appliances designed to facilitate trocar site fascial closure, which should minimize the incidence of these hernias (Fig. 71.36). The second is inadequate peritoneal closure over the prosthesis, which allows bowel to migrate into the preperitoneal space, also resulting in intestinal obstruction. Steps taken to avoid tension at the peritoneal closure site (see TAPP technique section) have decreased this problem. Theoretically, the TEP procedure eliminates the possibility of this complication because the abdomen is not entered. However, inadvertent breaches of the peritoneum during a TEP herniorrhaphy are common, especially in patients with thin peritoneum or those who have scar tissue associated with previous lower abdominal surgery. These peritoneal lacerations can be difficult to recognize because they are not in the visual field of the limited working space, and indeed intestinal obstruction has been reported.[83]

Diaphragmatic Dysfunction. Phrenic nerve palsy has been reported with a variety of laparoscopic procedures; it is usually transient but has been known to require a short period of mechanical ventilation. Stretching during the pneumoperitoneum probably causes this complication.

Hypercapnia. This is the result of inadequate compensatory ventilation given the fact that, in the vast majority of laparoscopic procedures, carbon dioxide is used as the insufflating agent.

Complications Related to the Patient

Urinary Retention. The most common predisposing factor for urinary retention after a hernia repair is the use of general or regional anesthesia.[44] It is more common after groin than abdominal wall hernia repairs. Meta-analyses of randomized controlled trials comparing various hernia techniques have not shown a difference in urinary retention rates. Jensen et al. published a review of the literature on urinary retention after inguinal herniorrhaphy from 1966 to 2001. Pooled data from 70 nonrandomized and two randomized studies disclosed that the incidence of urinary retention with local anesthesia was 0.37% (33 in 8,991 patients), with regional anesthesia 2.42% (150 in 6,191 patients), and with general anesthesia 3% (344 in 11,471 patients).[84] The incidence varies widely from as low as 1% to over 20%.[85,86] For example, in a series of laparoscopic inguinal hernia repairs, Koch et al. noted a 22.2% incidence of urinary retention.[87] All cases were done under general anesthesia and postoperative use of narcotics and the administration of postoperative intravenous fluid greater than 500 mL were found to be predictive. Demographic data including age, predisposition to urinary retention, type of procedure (TEP vs. TAPP), surgical time, anesthesia time, use of a Foley catheter intraoperatively, intraoperative fluid restriction, and the development of other complications were not significant risk factors. In addition to overhydration with intravenous fluid and opiates, other studies have found older age and prostatic symptoms to be predictive as predisposing factors.

Intermittent catheterization or temporary placement of an indwelling urinary catheter is usually adequate therapy. Prophylactic use of prazosin after herniorrhaphy may significantly reduce the incidence of urinary retention and the need for catheterization.[88] Phenoxybenzamine hydrochloride, another α-adrenergic blocker, has also been used both prophylactically and therapeutically.

Ileus. Ileus can be seen with either the conventional or the laparoscopic procedure but is more common with the latter. Treatment is symptomatic, and spontaneous resolution is the rule. Nasogastric decompression is occasionally needed.

Complications Related to the Herniorrhaphy

Recurrence. A lower risk for recurrence with the use of prosthetic material for the repair of an inguinal hernia has been clearly proven by meta-analysis.[89] Recurrence rates of 2% or less are now routinely reported from specialty centers performing either laparoscopic or conventional tension-free repairs. Although the recurrence rate for hernia repairs is less than 1% at the Shouldice Clinic, others have not been able to duplicate this outstanding record with this or any of the other nonprosthetic repairs.[90] Complications during the first month after surgery; operation for recurrence; and sutured repairs without mesh, either anterior or preperitoneal techniques, are associated with an increased recurrence rate. A laparoscopic approach is also considered a risk for recurrence because of its higher potential for technical failure, especially in the less experienced. This was felt to be the most likely reason for a higher recurrence rate at 2 years in a Veterans Affairs study for the laparoscopic approach (10%) compared to an open tension-free repair (4% for the Lichtenstein repair).[91]

8

A consistent definition of a recurrent hernia does not exist because of the difficulty in differentiating a lipoma of the cord, a seroma, or an expansile bulge of the internal oblique muscle from a true hernia recurrence. A hernia should not be classified recurrent unless there is a visible bulge or there is unequivocal evidence of a hernia by an imaging modality such as ultrasound, CT, or MRI. This is especially important for patients who present with pain after their hernia repair because their pain is likely due to a preoperative condition or a postinguinal herniorrhaphy pain syndrome and might be exacerbated by further groin surgery. Femoral recurrences are occasionally seen after a Lichtenstein repair because the femoral canal is not routinely closed with the classic technique.

The general principle for managing recurrent hernias depends on the original repair. The logical approach is to perform the herniorrhaphy in the space that has not been dissected. If the patient had a previous conventional repair, then a preperitoneal repair is best chosen. On the other hand, if the index operation was a preperitoneal one, then a repair that is performed in the conventional inguinal space is best. The dissection of the preperitoneal space after a failed herniorrhaphy has been performed there is particularly challenging, with significant risk for vascular, neurologic, and bladder injury.

Several other factors contribute to the poor results obtained in repairing incisional hernias. These include preexisting comorbid conditions, including debilitation from cancer, morbid obesity, the use of steroids, and chemotherapy. Another factor related to recurrence is lateral detachment of the mesh and inadequate mesh fixation caused by mesh distraction.[92] This is more commonly seen in the inlay techniques.[55]

9 **Postherniorrhaphy Groin Pain.** Now that the recurrence rate has been brought down to a minimum using modern hernioplasty techniques, chronic postoperative groin pain syndromes have emerged as the biggest issue facing inguinal hernia surgeons. Poobalan et al. published a critical review of inguinal herniorrhaphy studies between 1987 and 2000.[93] The frequency of at least some long-term groin pain was as high as 53% at 1 year (range, 0% to 53%). On average, moderate or severe postinguinal herniorrhaphy groin pain probably occurs in about 10% of patients. Perhaps the most important single determination for the postherniorrhaphy patient is to decide if the pain is the same or different from that which brought the hernia to the attention of the physician in the first place. There are a variety of conditions that cause groin pain (Table 71.6). CT, ultrasonography, herniography, laparoscopy, and MRI all have their place in the evaluation of these patients. MRI is perhaps the most beneficial because of its ability to differentiate between muscle tear, osteitis pubis, bursitis, and stress fracture. Strain of the adductor muscle complex (adductor longus, brevis, magnus, and gracilis muscles) is commonly overlooked in this group.

True postherniorrhaphy groin pain should be divided into two types: (a) nociceptive pain, which is caused by tissue damage and is further subdivided into somatic and visceral, and (b) neuropathic pain due to direct nerve damage. Somatic pain is the most common and is usually caused by damage to ligaments, tendons, and muscles. Visceral pain refers to that which is related to a specific visceral function such as urination or ejaculation (see dysejaculation syndrome, later). Neuropathic pain is much less common but is important to recognize because surgical treatment is possible if the cause is incorporation of a nerve in staples or suture material. The nerves that are usually involved are the ilioinguinal nerve, the iliohypogastric nerve, both the genital and femoral branches of the genitofemoral nerve, and the lateral cutaneous nerve of the thigh. The former two are especially prone to injury during a conventional herniorrhaphy, whereas the latter are most likely damaged during laparoscopy. A femoral nerve injury is extremely rare and is usually the result of a gross technical misadventure. Pain and/or paraesthesia in their distribution characterize patients' symptoms for the more common nerves. There is significant overlap of these nerves, and therefore it is commonly difficult to sort out exactly which nerve is damaged. Both nociceptive and neuropathic pain is best treated initially with reassurance and conservative treatment with anti-inflammatory medications and local nerve blocks because these will frequently resolve spontaneously. An exception is the patient who complains of severe pain immediately (i.e., in the recovery room). This patient may be best served by immediate reexploration before scar tissue develops. When groin exploration is required, neurectomy and neuroma excision, adhesiolysis, and foreign body removal (i.e., mesh) are options for treatment. The results are often less than satisfying.

Cord and Testicles

Infertility. The cause of infertility can be related to either the vas deferens or the testicle. The incidence of injury to the vas deferens during inguinal herniorrhaphy has been estimated at 0.3% for adults and between 0.8% and 2.0% for children.[94] Injuries to the vas deferens that may present as an obstruction include division, ligation, clipping, stapling, electrocauterization, devascularization, and scarification. In addition, there is evidence that there is a small subset of patients whose inflammatory response to mesh is so severe that vasal obstruction results.[95] Obstruction is not the only reason why an injury to the vas deferens may lead to infertility. For example, traction injuries during normal cord mobilization may damage the muscular layer of the vas deferens, which then interferes with rapid sperm transfer during ejaculation.[96] Sperm antibodies may develop as a result of extravasation of sperm at an injury site, which is why a unilateral injury can also result in infertility.

10 **Ischemic Orchitis.** Damage to the blood supply of the testicle can cause ischemic orchitis and testicular atrophy.[97] Ischemic orchitis occurs in about 1% of primary hernioplasties but is much more common with operations performed for recurrent hernias.[98] It manifests as postoperative inflammation of the testicle developing within 1 to 2 days after surgery. The patient has a painfully enlarged testicle that is hard in consistency and associated with low-grade fever. Pain is severe and may last several weeks. Ischemic orchitis is caused by thrombosis of the veins draining the testicle after extensive dissection of the spermatic cord. It is generally accepted that the incidence can be decreased by division of large inguinal-scrotal sacs leaving the distal sac open in situ rather than excising it.[99] The majority of patients with testicular swelling as an immediate complication of herniorrhaphy recover without testicular atrophy. In one recent report, testicular atrophy developed in 19 patients among 52,583 primary inguinal hernia repairs (0.036%) and 33 patients among 7,169 recurrent inguinal hernia repairs (0.46%).[98] A substantial number of patients who develop testicular atrophy after inguinal herniorrhaphy have no history of a testicular problem at the time of the index operation. The management of a patient with ischemic orchitis is usually conservative with elevation and anti-inflammatory medication. Antibiotics and steroids have been used but their value is unproved.

Miscellaneous. Hydroceles occasionally develop after inguinal herniorrhaphy, but the cause is not known and therefore a preventative measure is not possible. The urologic literature suggests that the practice of leaving the distal aspect of an indirect inguinal sac in situ rather than removing it should be incriminated, but this is not accepted by most experienced hernia surgeons. The treatment is the same as for any other hydrocele. Testicular descent is a complication felt to be related to complete division of the cremasteric muscle, but the occurrence is variable. The cord structures lose their tethering effect, allowing the testicle to descend into the most dependent portion of the scrotum. Due to the elasticity of the scrotum, with time gravity causes the scrotum to elongate. Patients complain their testicle "drops into the toilet" and can be quite unhappy. Few hernia surgeons now routinely completely divide the cremasteric muscle, so it is hoped that this will become a rare phenomena. The dysejaculation syndrome is characterized by searing, burning, painful sensations throughout the groin around the time of ejaculation. The incidence is approximately 0.04%.[98]

Wound Infection. This is a surprisingly rare complication of groin herniorrhaphy (<5%) and the reason for the "protected" status, especially when compared to prosthetic ventral herniorrhaphy, is not known.[99] Most cases of necrotizing facsitis following inguinal hernia repair have been associated either with strangulated bowel or appendicitis in the hernial sac. Necrotizing facsitis has only previously been reported in a few cases following elective hernia repair. On the other hand, the incidence of infection for incisional hernia is much higher, in the range of 10% to 15%, and is probably related to wound ischemia due to the required flap dissection. Other factors leading to infection are preexisting infection or ulceration of the skin over the hernia, obesity, incarcerated or obstructed bowel within the hernia, and perforation of the bowel at the time of hernia repair. Seromas are common when a large prosthesis is required or flap dissection of the subcutaneous layer from the fascia has been extensive. Untreated seromas can become secondarily infected. Suction drains can be useful, but if left in place too long, they also result in infection of the prosthesis. Strategies to prevent and manage seromas are largely based on empiricism and personal opinion, as objective data are nearly absent. It is not always necessary to remove the mesh prosthesis in the presence of infection. A trial of local wound care after opening of the incision and débridement is warranted.

Seromas. Seromas are common with the use of synthetic mesh in laparoscopic hernia repairs and are possibly related to the size of the mesh used. The fluid eventually resorbs spontaneously. Aspiration is performed for symptomatic relief only.

Bleeding. Hemorrhage can occur from the cremasteric, internal spermatic, or inferior epigastric vessels. Conservative treatment with reassurance is preferred for a stable hematoma. Evacuation is rarely required. Injuries to the deep circumflex artery, the corona mortis, or the external iliac vessels may result in a large retroperitoneal hematoma.

Prosthetic Complications. Shrinkage of polypropylene and other meshes should be considered by surgeons when performing prosthetic repairs. Sufficient overlap anticipating a 20% contracture is accepted by most. The decrease in size is felt to be due to scarification of the recipient's tissue. Intestinal obstruction or fistulization is possible by erosion, especially if there is physical contact between intestine and the prosthesis. Intra-abdominal placement of a mesh prosthesis should be avoided in favor of ePTFE or perhaps a biologic prosthesis whenever possible. Rejection because of an allergic response is possible but extremely rare. What patients cite as "rejection" of the mesh is usually the result of infection. Local erosion into the cord structures has also been reported.[100]

References

1. Rutkow IM. Demographic and socioeconomic aspects of hernia repair in the United States in 2003. *Surg Clin North Am* 2003;83(5):1045–51, v–vi.
2. Robson AJ, Wallace CG, Sharma AK, et al. Effects of training and supervision on recurrence rate after inguinal hernia repair. *Br J Surg* 2004;91(6):774–777.
3. Hollingshead HW. The abdominal wall and inguinal region. In: Hollingshead HW, ed. *Anatomy for Surgeons*, vol 2. New York: Hoeber-Harper; 1961:224.
4. Condon RE. Reassessment of groin anatomy during the evolution of preperitoneal hernia repair. *Am J Surg* 1996;172(1):5–8.
5. Milloy FJ, Anson BJ, Mcafee DK. The rectus abdominis muscle and the epigastric arteries. *Surg Gynecol Obstet* 1960;110:293–302.
6. Askar OM. Surgical anatomy of the aponeurotic expansions of the anterior abdominal wall. *Ann R Coll Surg Engl* 1977;59(4):313–321.
7. Cooper A. *The Anatomy and Surgical Treatment of Abdominal Hernia.* Philadelphia, PA: Lee and Blanchard; 1804.
8. Skandalakis PN, Zoras O, Skandalakis JE, et al. Transversalis, endoabdominal, endothoracic fascia: who's who? *Am Surg* 2006;72(1):16–18.
9. Quinn TH, Ryberg A, Annibali R, et al. Anatomy of the anterior abdominal wall and deep inguinal region from the laparoscopic surgeon's perspective. In: Lansafame RJ, ed. *Prevention and Management of Complications in Minimally Invasive Surgery*. New York: Igaku Shoin; 1996:107.
10. Teoh LS, Hingston G, Al-Ali S, et al. The iliopubic tract: an important anatomical landmark in surgery. *J Anat* 1999;194(Pt 1):137–141.
11. Marks SC,Jr, Gilroy AM, Page DW. The clinical anatomy of laparoscopic inguinal hernia repair. *Singapore Med J* 1996;37(5):519–521.
12. Anson BJ, Morgan EH, McVay CB. Surgical anatomy of the inguinal region based upon a study of 500 body-halves. *Surg Gynecol Obstet* 1960; 111:707–725.
13. Annibali R, Quinn TH, Fitzgibbons RJ Jr. Anatomy of the inguinal region from the laparoscopic perspective: critical areas for laparoscopic hernia repair. In: Bendavid R, ed. *Prostheses and Abdominal Wall Hernias*. Austin, TX: Landes; 1994:82.
14. Annibali R, Quinn TH, Fitzgibbons RJ Jr. Avoiding nerve injury during laparoscopic hernia repair: critical areas for staple placement. In: Arregui ME, Nagan R, eds. *Inguinal Hernia: Advances or Controversies?* Oxford, Great Britain: Radcliffe Medical; 1994:41.
15. Brick WG, Colborn GL, Gadacz TR, et al. Crucial anatomic lessons for laparoscopic herniorrhaphy. *Am Surg* 1995;61(2):172–177.
16. Gilroy AM, Hermey DC, DiBenedetto LM, et al. Variability of the obturator vessels. *Clin Anat* 1997;10(5):328–332.
17. Missankov AA, Asvat R, Maoba KI. Variations of the pubic vascular anastomoses in black South Africans. *Acta Anat (Basel)* 1996;155(3):212–214.
18. Bendavid R. The space of Bogros and the deep inguinal venous circulation. *Surg Gynecol Obstet* 1992;174(5):355–358.
19. Read RC. Why do human beings develop groin hernias? In: Fitzgibbons RJ, Greenburg AG, eds. *Nyhus and Condon's Hernia*, 5th ed. Philadelphia, PA: Lippincott Williams & Wilkins; 2002:219–227.
20. Weber A, Garteiz D, Valencia S. Epidemiology of inguinal hernia: a useful aid for adequate surgical decisions. In: Bendavid R, Abrahamson J, Arregui M, et al., eds. *Abdominal Wall Hernia.* New York: Springer; 2001.
21. Sanjay P, Woodward A. Single strenuous event: does it predispose to inguinal herniation? *Hernia* 2007;11(6):493–496.
22. Cannon DJ, Read RC. Metastatic emphysema: a mechanism for acquiring inguinal herniation. *Ann Surg* 1981;194(3):270–278.
23. Jansen PL, Mertens Pr P, Klinge U, et al. The biology of hernia formation. *Surgery* 2004;136(1):1–4.
24. Bellon JM, Bajo A, Ga-Honduvilla N, et al. Fibroblasts from the transversalis fascia of young patients with direct inguinal hernias show constitutive MMP-2 overexpression. *Ann Surg* 2001;233(2):287–291.
25. Klinge U, Zheng H, Si ZY, et al. Synthesis of type I and III collagen, expression of fibronectin and matrix metalloproteinases-1 and -13 in hernial sac of patients with inguinal hernia. *Int J Surg Investig* 1999;1(3):219–227.
26. Turaga K, Fitzgibbons RJ Jr, Puri V. Inguinal hernias: should we repair? *Surg Clin North Am* 2008;88(1):127–138, ix.
27. Harissis HV, Douitsis E, Fatouros M. Incarcerated hernia: to reduce or not to reduce? *Hernia* 2009;13(3):263–266.
28. Boughey JC, Nottingham JM, Walls AC. Richter's hernia in the laparoscopic era: four case reports and review of the literature. *Surg Laparosc Endosc Percutan Tech* 2003;13(1):55–58.
29. Mayagoitia JC, Suarez D, Arenas JC, et al. Preoperative progressive pneumoperitoneum in patients with abdominal-wall hernias. *Hernia* 2006; 10(3):213–217.
30. Fitzgibbons RJ Jr, Filipi CJ, Quinn TH. Inguinal hernias. In: Brunicardi FC, Andersen DK, Billiar TR, et al., eds. *Schwartz's Principles of Surgery*, 8th ed. New York: McGraw-Hill Professional; 2005:1353.
31. Lipman J, Medalie D, Rosen MJ. Staged repair of massive incisional hernias with loss of abdominal domain: a novel approach. *Am J Surg* 2008; 195(1):84–88.
32. Bachman S, Ramshaw B. Prosthetic material in ventral hernia repair: how do I choose? *Surg Clin North Am* 2008;88(1):101–112, ix.
33. Bringman S, Wollert S, Osterberg J, et al. Three-year results of a randomized clinical trial of lightweight or standard polypropylene mesh in Lichtenstein repair of primary inguinal hernia. *Br J Surg* 2006;93(9): 1056–1059.
34. Cobb WS, Kercher KW, Heniford BT. The argument for lightweight polypropylene mesh in hernia repair. *Surg Innov* 2005;12(1):63–69.
35. Conze J, Kingsnorth AN, Flament JB, et al. Randomized clinical trial comparing lightweight composite mesh with polyester or polypropylene mesh for incisional hernia repair. *Br J Surg* 2005;92(12):1488–1493.
36. Klinge U, Klosterhalfen B, Muller M, et al. Foreign body reaction to meshes used for the repair of abdominal wall hernias. *Eur J Surg* 1999; 165(7):665–673.
37. Koch A, Edwards A, Haapaniemi S, et al. Prospective evaluation of 6895 groin hernia repairs in women. *Br J Surg* 2005;92(12):1553–1558.
38. Prasaud P, Cemaj S, Fitzgibbons RJ Jr. Basic features of groin hernia and its repair. In: *Shakelford's Surgery of the Alimentary Tract,* 6th ed. Philadelphia: Saunders; 2006.
39. Nasr AO, Tormey S, Walsh TN. Lipoma of the cord and round ligament: an overlooked diagnosis? *Hernia* 2005;9(3):245–247.
40. Fitzgibbons RJ Jr, Giobbie-Hurder A, Gibbs JO, et al. Watchful waiting vs repair of inguinal hernia in minimally symptomatic men: a randomized clinical trial. *JAMA* 2006;295(3):285–292.
41. Amid PK. Groin hernia repair: open techniques. *World J Surg* 2005;29(8): 1046–1051.

42. Amid PK, Shulman AG, Lichtenstein IL. Open "tension-free" repair of inguinal hernias: the Lichtenstein technique. *Eur J Surg* 1996;162(6): 447–453.
43. Hachisuka T. Femoral hernia repair. *Surg Clin North Am* 2003;83(5): 1189–1205.
44. van Veen RN, Mahabier C, Dawson I, et al. Spinal or local anesthesia in Lichtenstein hernia repair: a randomized controlled trial. *Ann Surg* 2008; 247(3):428–433.
45. Kugel RD. Minimally invasive, nonlaparoscopic, preperitoneal, and sutureless, inguinal herniorrhaphy. *Am J Surg* 1999;178(4):298–302.
46. Gilbert AI, Young J, Graham MF, et al. Combined anterior and posterior inguinal hernia repair: intermediate recurrence rates with three groups of surgeons. *Hernia* 2004;8(3):203–207.
47. Collaboration EH. Laparoscopic compared with open methods of groin hernia repair: systematic review of randomized controlled trials. *Br J Surg* 2000;87(7):860–867.
48. Bisgaard T, Bay-Nielsen M, Kehlet H. Re-recurrence after operation for recurrent inguinal hernia: a nationwide 8-year follow-up study on the role of type of repair. *Ann Surg* 2008;247(4):707–711.
49. Taylor DC, Meyers WC, Moylan JA, et al. Abdominal musculature abnormalities as a cause of groin pain in athletes. Inguinal hernias and pubalgia. *Am J Sports Med* 1991;19(3):239–242.
50. van den Berg JC, de Valois JC, Go PM, et al. Radiological anatomy of the groin region. *Eur Radiol* 2000;10(4):661–670.
51. Zollinger RM Jr. Classification of ventral and groin hernias. In: Fitzgibbons RJ Jr, Greenburg AG, eds. *Nyhus and Condon's Hernia*, 5th ed. Philadelphia, PA: Lippincott Williams & Wilkins; 2002:71.
52. Brandt ML. Pediatric hernias. *Surg Clin North Am* 2008;88(1):27–43, vii–viii.
53. Mayo WJ. An operation for the radical cure of umbilical hernia. *Ann Surg* 1901;34:276–280.
54. Lau H, Patil NG. Umbilical hernia in adults. *Surg Endosc* 2003;17(12): 2016–2020.
55. Shell DH IV, de la Torre J, Andrades P, et al. Open repair of ventral incisional hernias. *Surg Clin North Am* 2008;88(1):61–83, viii.
56. Carlson MA, Ludwig KA, Condon RE. Ventral hernia and other complications of 1,000 midline incisions. *South Med J* 1995;88(4):450–453.
57. Read RC, Yoder G. Recent trends in the management of incisional herniation. *Arch Surg* 1989;124(4):485–488.
58. Moreno-Egea A, Carrillo A, Aguayo JL. Midline versus nonmidline laparoscopic incisional hernioplasty: a comparative study. *Surg Endosc* 2008;22(3):744–749.
59. Franz MG. The biology of hernia formation. *Surg Clin North Am* 2008; 88(1):1–15, vii.
60. Israelsson LA, Jonsson T, Knutsson A. Suture technique and wound healing in midline laparotomy incisions. *Eur J Surg* 1996;162(8):605–609.
61. Hodgson NC, Malthaner RA, Ostbye T. The search for an ideal method of abdominal fascial closure: a meta-analysis. *Ann Surg* 2000;231(3):436–442.
62. Luijendijk RW, Hop WC, van den Tol MP, et al. A comparison of suture repair with mesh repair for incisional hernia. *N Engl J Med* 2000;343(6): 392–398.
63. Burger JW, Luijendijk RW, Hop WC, et al. Long-term follow-up of a randomized controlled trial of suture versus mesh repair of incisional hernia. *Ann Surg* 2004;240(4):578–583; discussion 583–585.
64. Ramirez O, Ruas E, Dellon A. Component separation method for closure of abdominal wall defects: an anatomical and clinical study. *Plast Reconstr Surg* 1990;86:519–526.
65. Rosen MJ, Jin J, McGee MF, et al. Laparoscopic component separation in the single-stage treatment of infected abdominal wall prosthetic removal. *Hernia* 2007;11(5):435–440.
66. Usher FC, Ochsner J, Tuttle LL Jr. Use of Marlex mesh in the repair of incisional hernias. *Am Surg* 1958;24(12):969–974.
67. Klinge U, Conze J, Krones CJ, et al. Incisional hernia: open techniques. *World J Surg* 2005;29(8):1066–1072.
68. Korenkov M, Paul A, Sauerland S, et al. Classification and surgical treatment of incisional hernia. Results of an experts' meeting. *Langenbecks Arch Surg* 2001;386(1):65–73.
69. Temudom T, Siadati M, Sarr MG. Repair of complex giant or recurrent ventral hernias by using tension-free intraparietal prosthetic mesh (Stoppa technique): lessons learned from our initial experience (fifty patients). *Surgery* 1996;120(4):738–743; discussion 743–744.
70. Wantz GE. Incisional hernioplasty with Mersilene. *Surg Gynecol Obstet* 1991;172(2):129–137.
71. Flament JB, Palot JP, Burde A. Treatment of major incisional hernias. *Probl Gen Surg* 1995;12:151.
72. Gurusamy KS, Samraj K. Wound drains after incisional hernia repair. *Cochrane Database Syst Rev* 2007;(1):CD005570.
73. Moreno-Egea A. Multiple prosthesis and tissue repairs: a new technique for very complex cases. *Cir Esp* 2008;83(4):219.
74. Rubin MS, Schoetz DJ Jr, Matthews JB. Parastomal hernia. Is stoma relocation superior to fascial repair? *Arch Surg* 1994;129(4):413–418; discussion 418–419.
75. Israelsson LA. Parastomal hernias. *Surg Clin North Am* 2008;88(1): 113–125, ix.
76. Sugarbaker PH. Peritoneal approach to prosthetic mesh repair of paraostomy hernias. *Ann Surg* 1985;201(3):344–346.
77. Virzi G, Scaravilli F, Ragazzi S, et al. Laparoscopic paracolostomy hernia mesh repair. *Surg Laparosc Endosc Percutan Tech* 2007;17(6):548–550.
78. Janes A, Cengiz Y, Israelsson LA. Preventing parastomal hernia with a prosthetic mesh: a 5-year follow-up of a randomized study. *World J Surg* 2009;33(1):118–121; discussion 122–123.
79. Salameh JR. Primary and unusual abdominal wall hernias. *Surg Clin North Am* 2008;88(1):45–60, viii.
80. Ahmad G, Duffy JM, Phillips K, et al. Laparoscopic entry techniques. *Cochrane Database Syst Rev* 2008;(2):CD006583.
81. Mirski MA, Lele AV, Fitzsimmons L, et al. Diagnosis and treatment of vascular air embolism. *Anesthesiology* 2007;106(1):164–177.
82. Leibl BJ, Schmedt CG, Kraft K, et al. Recurrence after endoscopic transperitoneal hernia repair (TAPP): causes, reparative techniques, and results of the reoperation. *J Am Coll Surg* 2000;190(6):651–655.
83. Rink J, Ali A. Intestinal obstruction after totally extraperitoneal laparoscopic inguinal hernia repair. *JSLS* 2004;8(1):89–92.
84. Jensen P, Mikkelsen T, Kehlet H. Postherniorrhaphy urinary retention–effect of local, regional, and general anesthesia: a review. *Reg Anesth Pain Med* 2002;27(6):612–617.
85. Goldman G, Leviav A, Mazor A, et al. Alpha-adrenergic blocker for posthernioplasty urinary retention. Prevention and treatment. *Arch Surg* 1988;123(1):35–36.
86. Haskell DL, Sunshine B, Heifetz CJ. A study of bladder catheterization with inguinal hernia operations. *Arch Surg* 1974;109(3):378–380.
87. Koch CA, Grinberg GG, Farley DR. Incidence and risk factors for urinary retention after endoscopic hernia repair. *Am J Surg* 2006;191(3):381–385.
88. Gonullu NN, Dulger M, Utkan NZ, et al. Prevention of postherniorrhaphy urinary retention with prazosin. *Am Surg* 1999;65(1):55–58.
89. EU Hernia Trialists Collaboration. Repair of groin hernia with synthetic mesh: meta-analysis of randomized controlled trials. *Ann Surg* 2002; 235(3):322–332.
90. Bendavid R. The Shouldice technique: a canon in hernia repair. *Can J Surg* 1997;40(3):199–205, 207.
91. Neumayer L, Giobbie-Hurder A, Jonasson O, et al. Open mesh versus laparoscopic mesh repair of inguinal hernia. *N Engl J Med* 2004;350(18): 1819–1827.
92. Ziad TA, Varun P, Leblanc K. Mechanisms of ventral hernia recurrence alter mesh repair and a new classification. *J Am College Surg* 2005;201(1): 132–140.
93. Poobalan AS, Bruce J, Smith WC, et al. A review of chronic pain after inguinal herniorrhaphy. *Clin J Pain* 2003;19(1):48–54.
94. Sheynkin YR, Hendin BN, Schlegel PN, et al. Microsurgical repair of iatrogenic injury to the vas deferens. *J Urol* 1998;159(1):139–141.
95. Shin D, Lipshultz LI, Goldstein M, et al. Herniorrhaphy with polypropylene mesh causing inguinal vasal obstruction: a preventable cause of obstructive azoospermia. *Ann Surg* 2005;241(4):553–558.
96. Ceylan H, Karakok M, Guldur E, et al. Temporary stretch of the testicular pedicle may damage the vas deferens and the testis. *J Pediatr Surg* 2003;38(10):1530–1533.
97. Wantz GE. Testicular atrophy and chronic residual neuralgia as risks of inguinal hernioplasty. *Surg Clin North Am* 1993;73(3):571–581.
98. Bendavid R. Complications of groin hernia surgery. *Surg Clin North Am* 1998;78(6):1089–1103.
99. Sanchez-Manuel FJ, Lozano-Garcia J, Seco-Gil JL. Antibiotic prophylaxis for hernia repair. *Cochrane Database Syst Rev* 2007;(3):CD003769.
100. Silich RC, McSherry CK. Spermatic granuloma. An uncommon complication of the tension-free hernia repair. *Surg Endosc* 1996;10(5): 537–539.

CHAPTER 72 ■ ACUTE ABDOMEN AND APPENDIX

JEFFREY B. MATTHEWS AND RICHARD A. HODIN

KEY POINTS

1. Pathologic processes affecting abdominal viscera that produce abdominal pain with characteristic symptoms and signs include obstruction, inflammation, perforation, torsion, and ischemia.
2. Acute abdominal pain in immunosuppressed patients presents a particular diagnostic challenge both in making the diagnosis and due to the unusual infectious causes of abdominal pain that may be present.
3. The cause of acute appendicitis in most patients is luminal obstruction that leads to bacterial overgrowth and increased luminal pressure, leading to obstruction of venous outflow and then arterial inflow, resulting in gangrene and eventual perforation.
4. Ultrasonographic findings of acute appendicitis include demonstration of a so-called target lesion (i.e., a thick-walled, noncompressible, luminal structure in the right lower quadrant with peritoneal fluid and even frank abscess in advanced cases).
5. Computed tomography scanning has become the imaging modality of choice for patients with suspected acute appendicitis. It is highly accurate with sensitivities and specificities reported in the ranges of 95% to 100%.
6. A number of studies suggest that laparoscopic appendectomy is associated with a benefit in regard to shorter hospital stay, narcotic use, and overall recovery, with a perioperative complication rate comparable to open appendectomy.
7. A patient presenting late with appendicitis and an appendiceal mass should undergo initial percutaneous drainage and intravenous antibiotics followed by interval appendectomy in about 8 to 12 weeks.
8. The diagnosis of acute appendicitis in children is difficult, leading to a perforation rate as high as 50%.
9. The diagnosis of acute appendicitis in the elderly is difficult, leading to a perforation rate as high as 50% and higher associated rates of morbidity and mortality.
10. Appendicitis is the most frequent nonobstetric indication for laparotomy during pregnancy and the difficulty in diagnosis leads to a high perforation rate and associated high fetal mortality.
11. Carcinoid tumors less than 1.5 cm are adequately treated by appendectomy, whereas tumors 2 cm in size or greater have metastatic potential and a right hemicolectomy is indicated.

APPROACH TO THE PATIENT WITH ACUTE ABDOMINAL PAIN

Abdominal pain is one of the most frequent reasons for visits to physician offices and hospital emergency rooms and is a leading cause for hospital admission in the United States. Although most patients will be found to suffer from self-limited conditions of little consequence, a subset of patients with acute abdominal pain will harbor serious intra-abdominal or retroperitoneal pathology that requires major surgical or medical intervention. It is this latter population to whom the term "acute abdomen" is commonly applied, although "abdominal emergency" might be more descriptive. The experienced clinician understands that the severity of the pain does not always correlate with the gravity of the situation, nor do all patients with the so-called acute abdomen require surgical intervention. Early diagnosis, and particularly the early distinction of conditions that require urgent operation from those best managed nonsurgically, must be the paramount principle that outweighs all other concerns. Evaluation by a surgical consultant and performance of appropriate radiologic studies must proceed promptly regardless of time of day or disruption of normal routines and schedules.[1] There is considerable interexaminer variability in the evaluation of acute abdominal pain based on the level of experience as well as on specialty (e.g., emergency medicine physician vs. surgeon).[2,3]

In the vast majority of cases, a thorough history and physical examination will reveal the cause of the abdominal pain or at least sufficiently narrow down the possibilities to allow initial treatment decisions to be made.[4] Important features to be elicited include the time and mode of onset of the illness, the location of the pain, the character of the pain, and the presence of associated symptoms and their relation to the pain (Table 72.1). Examination of the patient includes an assessment of general appearance and attitude in bed in addition to the abdominal examination itself (Table 72.2). The ability to group the symptoms and signs of acute abdominal pain and to weigh their relative importance ("pattern recognition") perhaps best distinguishes the novice from the expert diagnostician in this setting. Blood tests may be complementary but are only occasionally of major importance in the initial evaluation. The same is generally true for radiologic studies, although in some circumstances, newer techniques of abdominal imaging do appear to enhance diagnostic accuracy. However, it cannot be overstated that an excessive reliance on tests can lead to unnecessary delay and must be avoided. There is little evidence to support a benefit to decision tools such as computer-based structured checklists or algorithms in the diagnosis of acute abdominal pain.[5] Thus, excessive ordering of tests or complex triage algorithms are unlikely to substitute for a knowledgeable, compassionate surgeon.

Most patients with acute abdominal pain evaluated in the emergency room setting will not require either hospital admission or surgical intervention.[6] The most common causes of abdominal pain requiring admission include acute appendicitis, nonspecific abdominal pain, pain of urologic origin, intestinal obstruction, and biliary tract disease, depending on the population and geographic region considered.[7] With improvements in diagnostic imaging over the past few decades, more patients with acute abdominal pain are able to be assigned a specific diagnosis and there are fewer instances of missed surgical disease.[8]

TABLE 72.1 **DIAGNOSIS**

KEY HISTORICAL FEATURES IN ACUTE ABDOMINAL PAIN

Age
Time and mode of onset of pain
Duration of symptoms
Character of pain
Location of pain and site(s) of radiation
Associated symptoms and their relation to pain
Nausea or anorexia
Vomiting
Diarrhea or constipation
Menstrual history

EMBRYOLOGIC AND PHYSIOLOGIC CONSIDERATIONS

The developing gastrointestinal (GI) tract is divided into three regions based on blood supply and innervation, relationships that are maintained from embryonic to adult life. The foregut consists of the oropharynx, esophagus, stomach, proximal duodenum, pancreas, liver, biliary tract, and spleen. The midgut runs from the distal duodenum (ligament of Treitz) and includes the small intestine, appendix, cecum, ascending colon, and proximal two thirds of the transverse colon. The remainder of the colon and rectum make up the hindgut.

The intestinal tract itself, from the stomach to the distal sigmoid colon (with the exception of the duodenum), is lined by a layer of mesodermally derived visceral peritoneum. The liver, spleen, and gallbladder are largely covered by visceral peritoneum; the pancreas is located within the retroperitoneum. Although continuous with the parietal peritoneum that lines the abdominal cavity, the visceral peritoneum is supplied by autonomic (sympathetic and parasympathetic) nerves. In contrast, the parietal peritoneal layer has an entirely somatic innervation derived from spinal nerves. This difference accounts for the distinct character of the pain associated with irritation or inflammation of the parietal peritoneum (which is generally perceived as sharp, severe, and persistent) compared to painful stimuli involving the visceral peritoneum (perceived as dull, cramping or aching, and poorly localized, and often associated with nausea and/or diaphoresis). The visceral peritoneum and its associated organs are insensitive to touching, pinching, cutting, burning, and electrical stimulation, but the sensation of pain from these sites can be induced by stretching, distention, or vigorous contraction against resistance. Additional painful stimuli to visceral organs include certain chemicals, ischemia, and inflammation. Visceral pain usually indicates the presence of significant intra-abdominal disease but is not in itself an indication for surgical therapy. A transition from visceral to somatic pain implies extension of the underlying disease process to include the parietal peritoneum and often heralds the need for urgent operative intervention (e.g., acute appendicitis, intestinal obstruction with strangulation). However, somatic pain of intra-abdominal origin should not be equated with the invariable need for operation (e.g., acute diverticulitis). In this regard, it is important to distinguish between localized somatic pain and diffuse somatic pain. Although conditions associated with localized peritonitis may require operation, the degree of urgency is far less than in diffuse peritonitis, which almost always indicates a surgical emergency.

The central gut tube is invested with a bilateral nerve supply, accounting for the midline location of the visceral pain originating from these organs. Pain of foregut origin is usually perceived in the epigastrium, midgut pain in the periumbilical region, and hindgut pain in the hypogastrium. In contrast, pain deriving from the bladder, prostate, uterus, ovaries, and fallopian tubes may be localized as pelvic or, occasionally, perineal. Pain originating from the abdominal wall musculature or parietal peritoneum is usually perceived in precise relation to the anatomic location of the stimulus because somatic pain nerve fibers enter the spinal cord ipsilaterally. The anterior and lateral abdominal wall is innervated from vertebral segments T7 to L1, whereas the posterior abdominal wall is from L2 to L5.

In addition to pain of the somatic and visceral categories, a third form of pain related to acute abdominal disorders is referred pain. Referred pain is perceived at a site removed from the anatomic location of the pathology but in a region that shares a common embryonic origin. The most common example is the radiation of pain of biliary origin to the right subscapular region or right shoulder. This phenomenon reflects the fact that the phrenic nerve is derived from the fourth cervical nerve. Thus, irritation of the undersurface of the right hemidiaphragm, such as by an inflamed gallbladder or hepatic abscess, may induce pain or hyperesthesia in the skin distribution of the fourth cervical nerve. Similarly, splenic pathology (e.g., rupture) may be perceived as pain in the left shoulder (Kehr sign). Other examples of referred pain are listed in Table 72.3.

Inflammation of the parietal peritoneum leads to rigidity and tenderness of the overlying muscle groups, a phenomenon of great clinical significance in the diagnosis of acute abdominal pain. These include not only the muscles of the anterior abdominal wall such as the rectus abdominus but also the diaphragm, psoas, quadratus lumborum, erector spinae, pyriformis, and obturator internus. Thus, an inflamed retrocecal appendix overlying the right psoas muscle may produce spasm reflected by the preference of the patient to maintain the right thigh in flexed position; in addition, placing the patient on the

TABLE 72.2 **DIAGNOSIS**

EXAMINATION OF THE PATIENT WITH ACUTE ABDOMINAL PAIN

General observations	
	General appearance
	Attitude in bed
	Vital signs, including temperature
Chest	
	Auscultation
Abdomen	
	Inspection (distention, localized swelling, hernia)
	Percussion (tympany or dullness, tenderness, referred tenderness)
	Palpation (muscle rigidity, tenderness, [rebound pain], hyperesthesia)
	Auscultation
Pelvis	
	Rectal examination (tenderness, presence of stool, occult blood, mass)
	Bimanual examination (cervical motion tenderness, adnexal masses)
	Obturator sign
Back and flanks	
	Percussion (costovertebral angle tenderness)
	Iliopsoas sign

TABLE 72.3

SITES OF REFERRED PAIN

■ SITE	■ ORGAN(S)	■ COMMON EXAMPLES
Right subscapular or shoulder	Diaphragm, gallbladder, liver	Biliary colic, perforated ulcer, pneumoperitoneum
Left subscapular or shoulder	Diaphragm, spleen, stomach, tail of pancreas, splenic flexure	Splenic rupture, pancreatitis
Back	Pancreas, duodenum, aorta	Pancreatitis, ruptured AAA
Coccyx	Uterus, rectum	Uterine colic
Groin or genitalia	Kidney, ureter, iliac arteries	Ureterolithiasis

AAA, abdominal aortic aneurysm.

left side and fully extending the right thigh may produce pain (psoas sign). Similarly, the presence of an inflamed appendix or periappendiceal abscess may be deduced by a positive finding in the so-called obturator test (pain on internal rotation of the right thigh). In contrast, irritation of the deep pelvic peritoneum is generally not associated with any overlying muscle group, accounting for the striking lack of abdominal wall rigidity in cases of pelvic abscess from appendicitis or diverticulitis.

DIFFERENTIAL DIAGNOSIS

The sheer number of conditions that produce acute abdominal pain is overwhelming. However, the differential diagnosis may be narrowed substantially by anatomic considerations and an understanding of the general characteristics of the episode of the pain.

It is useful to subdivide the abdomen into four quadrants and consider the conditions that cause abdominal pain localized to each region (Table 72.4). Pain that does not lateralize in this fashion can be characterized as epigastric, periumbilical, or hypogastric, and a relatively limited differential diagnosis can also be generated for each midline location (Table 72.5). Diffuse abdominal pain (Table 72.6) can be mild and without significant physical findings, as in early acute appendicitis, or it can be severe and associated with generalized abdominal muscle rigidity, as in diffuse peritonitis.

❶ There are a limited number of pathologic processes affecting abdominal viscera that produce abdominal pain, and each is associated with a characteristic evolution of clinical symptoms and signs (Table 72.7). *Obstruction* of a hollow viscus results in a form of pain termed colic, consisting of a deep, nauseating ache that may be cyclical, as in intestinal colic, or steady, as in biliary colic. *Inflammation* can be the result of bacterial infection and generally produces only mild pain until the process becomes transmural, at which point the resultant peritoneal irritation can cause localized somatic pain. *Perforation* or rupture of a hollow viscus or other structure (e.g., an ovarian cyst or a hepatic adenoma) typically results in a pain of sudden onset that builds to maximum intensity over minutes to hours, producing signs of peritoneal irritation that are initially localized but may soon become generalized. *Torsion* may also produce a severe pain of sudden onset, but usually physical findings in the initial phase are limited to the site of torsion and do not generalize. Finally, *ischemia* of a solid or hollow viscus produces a severe pain frequently described as out of proportion to physical findings.

As a first step in differential diagnosis, it is useful to tentatively assign the abdominal pain episode to one of these pathologic processes and to one of the previously mentioned locations. These categories are of course not absolute, because overlapping presentations are seen in a variety of conditions. For example, sigmoid volvulus simultaneously represents torsion and obstruction, whereas acute cholecystitis is initially due to obstruction (of the cystic duct) but then progresses to transmural inflammation. It is not unusual for a pain that is initially due to one process to evolve into another (e.g., intestinal ischemia and infarction developing as a consequence of untreated adhesive obstruction).

EVALUATION OF THE PATIENT WITH ABDOMINAL PAIN

It has been said that the most important diagnostic instrument available to the clinician is a chair, and this is perhaps nowhere more true than in the setting of the evaluation of a patient with acute abdominal pain. While eliciting the history, the clinician should take the opportunity to observe the patient's attitude in bed; the facial expression, particularly during paroxysms of pain; and the contour of the abdomen.[4]

The course of the episode of illness should be retraced, beginning with the exact time and mode of onset of the pain as well as any prodromic events occurring in the hours or days from the point at which the patient was subjectively at baseline health. The location and character of the pain, the direction of radiation of the pain, and changes in intensity or shifts in location over time are elicited. The presence of associated symptoms, in particular anorexia and vomiting, and their relation to the onset and evolution of pain are determined. Nausea and vomiting are usually due either to severe irritation of the peritoneal or mesenteric nerves or to obstruction of a hollow viscus. The character and time of the most recent bowel movement or the occurrence of diarrhea is noted. The relevant past medical history is then documented in detail, with particular attention to prior episodes of similar pain, the presence of major digestive or other systemic disorders, and previous abdominal operations. Current medications are documented. Corticosteroid use or other conditions associated with immunosuppression may diminish the symptoms produced by inflammation and obscure a serious degree of intra-abdominal disease. The presence of familial disorders or concurrent illness in family or other contacts should be noted.

The age of the patient should be taken into account, as the differential diagnosis shifts considerably when dealing with the pediatric versus the geriatric population. In women, a recent menstrual history is obtained and prior pregnancies noted. Gynecologic causes of acute abdominal pain to be considered include Mittelschmerz or ruptured ovarian cyst, pelvic inflammatory disease, ectopic pregnancy, tubo-ovarian abscess (with or without rupture), and ovarian torsion.

TABLE 72.4 **DIAGNOSIS**

PAIN LOCALIZING TO AN ABDOMINAL QUADRANT

RIGHT UPPER QUADRANT PAIN

- Biliary colic/cholecystitis
- Cholangitis
- Hepatic abscess
- Hepatitis (toxic or viral)
- Perihepatitis (Fitzhugh-Curtis syndrome)
- Hepatic congestion
- Budd-Chiari syndrome
- Hepatic tumor (primary or secondary)
- Appendicitis
- Perforated peptic ulcer
- Perinephritis
- Pneumonia (right lower lobe)
- Pulmonary infarction
- Pleuritis
- Myocardial ischemia
- Empyema
- Rib fracture
- Herpes zoster

LEFT UPPER QUADRANT PAIN

- Splenic rupture
- Splenic infarction
- Splenomegaly
- Ruptured splenic artery aneurysm
- Gastritis
- Perforated gastric ulcer (phlegmonous gastritis)
- Jejunal diverticulitis
- Pancreatitis
- Diverticulitis (splenic flexure)
- Perinephritis
- Pneumonia (left lower lobe)
- Pulmonary infarction
- Pleuritis
- Pericarditis
- Myocardial ischemia
- Empyema
- Rib fracture
- Herpes zoster

RIGHT LOWER QUADRANT PAIN

- Appendicitis
- Acute enterocolitis (viral or bacterial)
- Crohn disease (ileitis)
- Foreign body perforation
- Right-sided diverticulitis
- Cecal diverticulitis
- Meckel diverticulitis
- Torsion of appendix epiploica
- Mesenteric adenitis
- Intestinal obstruction
- Perforated peptic ulcer
- Pancreatitis
- Ruptured ovarian cyst (including Mittelschmerz)
- Ovarian torsion
- Endometriosis
- Salpingitis (pelvic inflammatory disease)
- Ectopic pregnancy
- Cholecystitis
- Ruptured iliac artery aneurysm
- Renal or ureteral calculi
- Pyelonephritis
- Psoas abscess
- Seminal vesiculitis
- Rectus sheath hematoma
- Herpes zoster

LEFT LOWER QUADRANT PAIN

- Diverticulitis
- Appendicitis
- Perforated colon cancer
- Intestinal obstruction
- Crohn colitis
- Ischemic colitis
- Ruptured iliac artery aneurysm
- Ruptured ovarian cyst (including Mittelschmerz)
- Ovarian torsion
- Endometriosis
- Salpingitis (pelvic inflammatory disease)
- Ectopic pregnancy
- Renal or ureteral calculi
- Pyelonephritis
- Psoas abscess
- Seminal vesiculitis
- Rectus sheath hematoma
- Herpes zoster

TABLE 72.5 **ETIOLOGY**

CAUSES OF MIDLINE ABDOMINAL PAIN

EPIGASTRIC
- Peptic ulcer
- Pancreatitis
- Gastritis
- Esophagitis
- Mesenteric ischemia
- Appendicitis (early)
- Myocardial ischemia
- Pericarditis
- Cholecystitis

PERIUMBILICAL
- Small-intestinal obstruction
- Appendicitis
- Pancreatitis
- Mesenteric ischemia
- Acute glaucoma

HYPOGASTRIC
- Large-intestinal obstruction
- Intussusception
- Appendicitis
- Diverticulitis
- Enterocolitis
- Ovarian torsion
- Testicular torsion
- Degeneration or torsion of uterine fibroid
- Cystitis

TABLE 72.6 **ETIOLOGY**

CAUSES OF DIFFUSE ABDOMINAL PAIN

- Early appendicitis
- Perforated appendicitis
- Perforated peptic ulcer
- Perforated diverticulitis
- Stercoral perforation of colon
- Peritonitis (primary or secondary)
- Pancreatitis
- Mesenteric adenitis
- Mesenteric ischemia
- Ruptured abdominal aortic aneurysm
- Diabetic coma
- Tuberculous peritonitis
- Food poisoning
- Heavy metal poisoning
- Acute porphyria
- Sickle cell crisis
- Acute leukemia

TABLE 72.7 **ETIOLOGY**

PATHOLOGIC PROCESSES UNDERLYING ABDOMINAL PAIN

■ PROCESS	■ COMMON EXAMPLES
Obstruction	Intestinal colic, renal calculi, biliary colic
Inflammation	Enterocolitis, mesenteric adenitis
Perforation	Perforated peptic ulcer
Torsion	Ovarian torsion, sigmoid volvulus
Ischemia	Mesenteric artery thrombosis, splenic infarction

As indicated previously, the physical examination should begin with inspection of the general appearance, attitude in bed, and facial expression. Unwillingness to change position may indicate underlying peritonitis; conversely, an inability to find a comfortable position may be seen with ureteral colic due to nephrolithiasis. A patient with acute pancreatitis or mesenteric ischemia may prefer to lean forward. Intermittent grimacing may be observed in a patient with intestinal obstruction. Vital signs are measured. The presence of cool, clammy skin or of jaundice may be observed at this time.

Inspection of the abdomen will reveal generalized distention or focal swelling. The presence of a hernia must be specifically excluded by direct examination of all hernial orifices and abdominal incisions. Auscultation of the abdomen may be performed next, although this only rarely provides valuable information. Auscultation of the chest, particularly the basilar regions, may reveal pneumonic consolidation that can simulate an acute abdominal process or may reveal a pleuritic rub. Gentle percussion of the abdomen will help distinguish gaseous distention from ascites; loss of dullness over the liver may indicate free intraperitoneal air, as in perforated duodenal ulcer. Tenderness to percussion, either localized or across the abdomen, suggests focal or diffuse peritonitis. Referred tenderness to percussion (pain perceived away from the site of percussion) is an extremely important finding that is essentially pathognomonic for peritonitis.

Palpation of the abdomen must be gentle. Rough or sudden deep palpation will frighten the patient, cause voluntary guarding, and hamper subsequent attempts to palpate the abdomen. The presence of subtle muscle rigidity (involuntary guarding) or of an intra-abdominal mass is more likely to be detected by a gentle approach. It may be useful to ask the patient to flex the thighs during this phase of the examination. Areas of skin hyperesthesia may be noted during gentle palpation. Elicitation of rebound tenderness rarely provides additional information beyond that obtained by careful percussion and palpation and is not recommended. The psoas and obturator tests may be performed next. In patients with a colostomy or ileostomy, direct examination of the stoma along with digitalization is important. The back is examined with attention to the presence of spinal tenderness or tenderness in the costovertebral angle or flanks.

Examination of the pelvis is extremely important in most patients with abdominal pain. Suprapubic palpation may reveal an enlarged bladder or tenderness indicative of deeper disease. Digital rectal examination may reveal focal tenderness due to a periappendiceal or peridiverticular pelvic abscess. Anterior palpation may reveal the only evidence of pelvic peritonitis, particularly in males. A bimanual vaginoabdominal examination in females will reveal pathology in the pouch of Douglas or involving the uterus, tubes, or ovaries.

Whether it is prudent to administer analgesics to the patient undergoing evaluation for acute abdominal pain has remained a controversial question. Certainly, once the diagnosis is established or a definitive plan of action has been made, it is not justifiable to withhold such treatment. There is a considerable literature to suggest that administration of morphine can provide substantial pain relief without changing important physical signs (in particular, the presence of peritoneal irritation), although there are limited high-quality prospective, randomized data.[9–11]

Laboratory and Radiologic Examination

The common practice of ordering a "routine" panel of tests, even prior to evaluation by a physician, is wasteful of resources and may lead to unnecessary delays in diagnosis and treatment, particularly when normal values lull caregivers into a false sense of security. For example, the white blood cell count is notoriously normal in a substantial fraction of patients with serious intra-abdominal pathology and is frequently elevated in cases of nonsurgical disease.[12] However, a hematocrit and serum electrolytes and blood urea nitrogen may be useful to guide fluid resuscitation. A serum amylase and liver chemistries are usually indicated in patients with upper abdominal pain but only rarely so in lower abdominal pain. Although liberal use of human chorionic gonadotropin testing may avoid a missed tubal pregnancy, its routine use in females with abdominal pain is not likely to be cost-effective. A urinalysis is frequently of value to screen for urologic causes of abdominal pain, but routine urine culture is unnecessary.

Plain radiographs of the abdomen are ordered far in excess of their usefulness in the evaluation of abdominal pain.[13,14] Despite occasional positive findings (e.g., air–fluid levels, a fecalith, gallstones), plain films tend to be relatively nonspecific, complementing what is already obvious on history and examination, and rarely redirect therapeutic thinking. They are most helpful in patients with suspected ureteral calculus or intestinal obstruction. It is important to remember that abdominal films are frequently normal or nondiagnostic in patients with strangulating obstruction. An upright chest film is the least expensive and perhaps best test to identify free intraperitoneal air.

Upper GI series performed with water-soluble contrast is occasionally helpful in detecting ulcer perforation and determining whether such perforation is free or contained. A water-soluble contrast enema may be useful in cases of suspected large bowel obstruction. Intravenous pyelography may be used to identify ureteral stones. All of these studies, however, have been supplanted in many centers by computed tomography (CT), which, although somewhat more expensive, yields considerably more information of practical importance.[15] CT is quite useful in patients with abdominal pain who do not require emergency surgery, particularly in delineating the cause and suggesting a therapeutic strategy in patients with no prior history of abdominal disease.[16] Arteriography may be useful in patients with suspected mesenteric ischemia, although CT angiography and magnetic resonance imaging are increasingly applied to this situation. Ultrasound examination of the right upper quadrant may reveal gallstones, but it is important to remember that ultrasonographic signs of acute cholecystitis may be no more accurate than clinical examination. Ultrasonography for lower abdominal pain may improve diagnostic accuracy beyond clinical impression alone but is highly experience and operator dependent.[17] A guiding principle in ordering radiologic tests is that the result should substantially influence plans for further testing or therapy. Redundant tests should be avoided.

Diagnostic laparoscopy may be appropriate in certain circumstances, especially the evaluation of acute lower abdominal pain in females. This has become a more attractive option as techniques of therapeutic laparoscopy (e.g., appendectomy) have been refined.[18–20] Nevertheless, laparoscopy requires a general anesthetic and should not be used without due consideration.

Conditions Mimicking the Acute Abdomen

A variety of nonsurgical conditions may be associated with acute abdominal pain, including a variety of cardiovascular, respiratory, metabolic, and toxic conditions. For example, myocardial ischemia may produce epigastric pain, nausea, and vomiting that simulate acute cholecystitis; conversely, and perhaps more frequently, acute cholecystitis is mistaken for pain of cardiac origin. Abdominal wall injury, radiculopathy, and rectus sheath hematoma (the latter particularly in patients on anticoagulant therapy) may cause acute abdominal pain. Abdominal pain and vomiting may accompany influenza. Diabetic ketoacidosis and, rarely, blood dyscrasias such as acute porphyria or sickle cell hemolytic crisis may produce severe abdominal pain. Urologic disorders such as pyelonephritis or obstruction of the ureter, renal pelvis, or bladder outlet may be mistaken for intra-abdominal pathology. Urinalysis and renal ultrasound may confirm the diagnosis. Testicular torsion can also be associated with severe abdominal pain.

Abdominal Pain in Special Circumstances

The pediatric population represents a particularly difficult subset in which to evaluate acute abdominal pain. In neonates and infants, congenital causes such as midgut volvulus or pyloric stenosis must be considered, and entities such as intussusception and Meckel diverticulitis are far more common than in adults. It may be impossible to obtain key historical information, and physical examination may be difficult.[21] Evaluation of older children is generally easier. It should be noted that anorexia may be absent in children with appendicitis or other important abdominal pathology. Diarrhea as a manifestation of appendicitis is also frequent and may simulate acute infectious enterocolitis. Abdominal films may be more informative in pediatric than adult patients. In certain instances, it may be appropriate to consider whether child abuse has occurred.

The geriatric population can also present diagnostic difficulty, and if dementia is present, it may be impossible to elicit a meaningful history. In such patients, serious intra-abdominal pathology may present with few or subtle signs, and there may be only minimal tenderness on examination despite diffuse peritonitis. Laboratory values are frequently normal despite the presence of serious pathology in this population.[22] The majority of geriatric patients evaluated in the emergency setting will be found to have significant disease requiring hospitalization.[23]

2 Acute abdominal pain in immunosuppressed patients represents a particular diagnostic challenge, for example, in the setting of organ transplantation, immunosuppressive therapy for autoimmune disorders, chemotherapy, and acquired immunodeficiency syndrome (AIDS). Unusual infectious causes of acute abdominal pain, including cytomegalovirus (CMV), mycobacteria, protozoal species, and fungi, should be considered; these may affect the GI tract, gallbladder, liver, and pancreas. Perforation of the GI tract due to CMV, *Mycobacterium tuberculosis* or *Mycobacterium avium-intracellulare,* lymphoma, or Kaposi sarcoma or associated with corticosteroid use is seen in immunosuppressed patients. Acalculous cholecystitis should be considered in patients with AIDS and is often associated with *Cryptosporidia* or CMV. Splenic abscess due to *Candida* or *Salmonella* may be a cause of left upper quadrant pain. Neutropenic enterocolitis is a common cause of abdominal pain and fever in patients with bone marrow suppression due to chemotherapy. In the transplant population, acute graft-versus-host disease should be considered. Although abdominal pain in immunosuppressed patients is often treated nonoperatively, vigilance must be maintained lest serious surgical pathology be overlooked.

Acute abdominal pain after cardiac or major abdominal vascular surgery merits special mention because of the frequency of serious diagnoses that carry particularly high mortality in this setting. Mesenteric or segmental colonic ischemia is commonly reported, as are acute colitis and cholecystitis (often acalculous). Acute pancreatitis associated with extracorporeal cardiopulmonary bypass occurs in about 2% of cases.[24] Severe acute abdominal pain in hemodialysis patients is most commonly due to mesenteric ischemia.[25]

The diagnosis of abdominal pain in patients with spinal cord injury is particularly challenging. Mortality in this setting is high (about 10%), usually due to delayed diagnosis.[26] Classical signs such as tenderness, guarding, and even fever are unreliable; more helpful are the presence of shoulder pain, abdominal distention, nausea, vomiting, and autonomic dysreflexia.[27]

Finally, evaluation of abdominal pain occurring during pregnancy carries additional considerations.[28] Anatomic relationships may be distorted by the gravid uterus; in particular, the appendix is often displaced upward into the right upper quadrant. Nonsurgical causes of abdominal and pelvic pain are common. Interpretation of blood work should recognize physiologic alterations; leukocytosis is frequently present during normal pregnancy. Although one should not hesitate to obtain radiologic tests when essential, unnecessary exposure to x-rays must be avoided. Ultrasound is a particularly valuable diagnostic modality in these patients. More recently, magnetic resonance imaging has been demonstrated to be useful in the early identification of pregnant patients who are likely to require surgical intervention.[29]

APPENDIX

The clinical entity of appendiceal inflammation followed by perforation, abscess formation, and peritonitis was first described in 1889 by Reginald Fitz.[30] Since that time, appendectomy has remained among the most common abdominal operations and, in fact, is the most common surgical procedure performed on an emergency basis in Western countries. Appendectomy remains the mainstay of treatment, but with the development of modern antibiotics and percutaneous drainage techniques, some cases are best managed nonoperatively. The morbidity and mortality associated with acute appendicitis has diminished over time, although because it usually affects young, healthy people, the overall effect on our workforce remains significant. When not treated appropriately, appendicitis remains a potentially lethal condition. A case in point is that of the famous magician, Harry Houdini, who would occasionally entertain by withstanding punches to the abdomen delivered by members of his audience. Unfortunately, Mr. Houdini once performed this "act" while suffering from an appendiceal abscess, only to die several days later from diffuse peritonitis and sepsis, the abscess having been ruptured from one of the assaults.[31]

Anatomy and Pathophysiology

The appendix is considered a vestigial organ with no known function in human beings. However, examination of the phylogenetic tree reveals that the appendix is absent from a number of carnivores, such as the dog, tiger, and lion, and, surprisingly, there is progressive development of the appendix in apes and as one ascends the primate scale.[32] The appendix contains large amounts of lymphoid aggregates, similar to those within the Peyer patches of gut-associated lymphoid tissue. Lymphoid nodules containing both B and T cells within the lamina propria differentiate the appendix from the adjacent colon.[33] Because of this prominence of lymphoid tissue, some have hypothesized that the appendix may have an immune function similar to that of the thymus or bursa of Fabricius, although no actual function has ever been documented. The appendiceal mucosa produces minimal amounts of fluid and digestive juices, suggesting that it has no important exocrine function. There have been some associations made between the lack of an appendix and various disease states (inflammatory bowel disease), but a causal relationship remains unproved.

The appendix develops as an antimesenteric outpouching from the cecum and is first delineated during the fifth month of gestation. The position of the appendix can vary greatly. In almost two thirds of the population, the appendix is located in a retrocecal position, whereas in others it is located over the pelvic brim, occasionally descending low down in the pelvis. When the appendix occupies an unusual location, the diagnosis of appendicitis may be more difficult and contribute to delays in either presentation and/or diagnosis. The three taeniae coli of the ascending colon meet at the base of the appendix, with the anterior taenia serving as an important landmark. Following the taeniae can be a useful maneuver in identifying a difficult appendix at the time of operation. The appendix can vary in length from 2 to 20 cm, averaging approximately 9 cm. The blood supply of the appendix is from the appendicular artery, which is a branch of the ileocolic. Similarly, the lymphatic drainage follows that of the ileocolic nodes, and these are often hyperplastic in cases of acute appendicitis. The neural innervation of the appendix is derived from the autonomic nervous system. As with other visceral organs, there are no somatic pain fibers within the appendix. As such, early inflammation leads to poorly localizable pain and is referred to the periumbilical region because the autonomic nerves follow the midgut embryologic origin. As inflammation of appendicitis progresses, irritation of the surrounding parietal peritoneum results in the activation of somatic pain fibers and localization of symptoms and signs to the right lower quadrant.

In cross section, the appendix contains the same layers as those of the adjacent colon, including the mucosa, submucosa with prominent lymphoid tissue, circular and longitudinal muscle layers, and overlying serosa. Neurosecretory cells are located within the subepithelial layer and are the presumed source of carcinoid tumors, which are often found within the appendix.

3 The etiology of appendicitis remains somewhat unclear. In most patients, there is probably luminal obstruction that leads to bacterial overgrowth and increased luminal pressure, leading to obstruction of venous outflow and then arterial inflow, resulting in gangrene and eventual perforation. The cause for the luminal obstruction that initiates the process of appendicitis is postulated to involve lymphoid hyperplasia, a condition that is especially common in the teenage years, which correlates with the high incidence of appendicitis in this age group. It is felt that either viral or bacterial infections such as *Shigella*, *Salmonella*, infectious mononucleosis, and so forth can precede the episode of appendicitis, presumably by initiating the lymphoid hyperplasia and subsequent luminal obstruction.

In addition to lymphoid hyperplasia, fecaliths can also lead to appendiceal obstruction and subsequent appendicitis. It is thought that approximately 30% of cases of acute appendicitis in adults are linked to fecaliths. Fecaliths are thought to occur following entrapment of vegetable matter with subsequent mucus deposition and eventual calcification. The "obstructive" model for appendicitis does not appear to explain the etiology in all cases, however, because some patients with appendicitis appear to have a patent lumen by radiologic, gross, and histologic examination. The pathophysiology of these cases remains unclear.

Diagnosis

Early diagnosis remains the most important clinical goal in patients with suspected appendicitis. Although mortality rates in modern series are well under 1%,[34,35] the morbidity of

TABLE 72.8 **DIAGNOSIS**

TYPICAL SEQUENCE OF SYMPTOMS AND SIGNS OF ACUTE APPENDICITIS

Periumbilical pain—vague, visceral, poorly localized
Anorexia, nausea, and/or vomiting
Right lower quadrant pain and tenderness—localized
Fever
Leukocytosis

perforated appendicitis is much higher than in nonperforated cases and is related to increased rates of wound infection, intra-abdominal abscess formation, lengths of hospital stay, and delayed return to full activity.[36]

By a thorough history and physical examination, experienced clinicians can accurately diagnose acute appendicitis in the majority of cases.[4] A typical presentation (Table 72.8) is that of vague periumbilical pain (sometimes located more superiorly in the epigastric region) followed by anorexia, nausea, or even frank vomiting. When vomiting occurs in appendicitis, it is usually of a limited nature, as opposed to patients with viral gastroenteritis, who generally have more severe vomiting. The pain then shifts to the right lower quadrant region as the inflammatory process progresses and involves the localized overlying peritoneum. Eventually, fever ensues and this is followed by the development of leukocytosis. These clinical features are not entirely reliable, however. For example, not all patients will complain of anorexia, so the fact that a given patient expresses hunger should not necessarily deter one from surgical intervention for presumed acute appendicitis. Occasionally, patients will complain of urinary symptoms, perhaps because of some inflammation adjacent to the ureter and/or bladder. Microscopic hematuria is quite common, and the clinician should not mistake the primary problem as residing in the urinary tract. Intestinal function is usually unaffected in appendicitis, but some patients will note diarrhea, perhaps related to the inflammation adjacent to the rectum and/or colon. Appendicitis can also be associated with adynamic ileus, leading to the complaint of constipation.

Physical examination is generally the most reliable indicator of appendicitis. Aside from the young child, very elderly, or otherwise neurologically impaired, patients with appendicitis will have at least some degree of tenderness on palpation of the abdomen. In cases of an appendix located entirely in the pelvis, the tenderness on abdominal examination may be minimal, but on rectal examination the tenderness will be evident as the pelvic peritoneum is manipulated. Pelvic examination with cervical motion will also manipulate the pelvic peritoneum and elicit tenderness when there is an inflamed appendix in that region. Therefore, the finding of cervical motion tenderness does not necessarily indicate gynecologic pathology but rather is a nonspecific sign of inflammation in the pelvis.

Peritoneal irritation can be elicited on physical examination with the findings of percussion and/or rebound tenderness. Any movement including coughing (Dunphy sign) may cause increased pain. The most reliable indicator of peritoneal irritation, however, is involuntary guarding, a reflex contraction of the abdominal wall musculature overlying the inflamed peritoneum. The involuntary nature of this response is less dependent on the individual variation seen in response to external stimuli. Other physical signs (Table 72.9) associated with appendicitis include the occurrence of pain in the right lower quadrant during palpation of the left lower quadrant (Rovsing sign), pain on internal rotation of the hip (obturator sign, suggesting a pelvic appendix), and pain on right hip extension (iliopsoas sign, typical of a retrocecal appendix).

In addition to the history and physical examination, a white blood cell count is usually obtained and in most patients will be elevated, although it may be in the normal range during the early stages. A very high white blood cell count (>20,000 white blood cells per mL) suggests complicated appendicitis with either gangrene or perforation. A urinalysis can also be helpful to rule out pyelonephritis or nephrolithiasis. However, in patients with pyelonephritis, the fever and white blood cell count will generally be much higher than that seen in appendicitis, symptoms of dysuria will be present, and the tenderness is centered more in the flank or costovertebral angle region. Minimal pyuria, frequently seen in elderly women, should not deter one from the correct diagnosis of appendicitis. Although microscopic hematuria is common in appendicitis, gross hematuria is uncommon and may indicate the presence of a kidney stone. As a kidney stone passes down the urinary tract through the distal ureter, pain can often be referred to the right lower quadrant region and occasionally down into the testicle. The pain is quite severe and entirely visceral in nature. Therefore, the signs of peritoneal irritation should not exist in the patient with nephrolithiasis. Other blood tests are generally not helpful nor indicated in the patient with suspected appendicitis.

Plain abdominal radiographs are of little use in the patient with suspected appendicitis. Occasionally, a calcified appendicolith may be evident, but this is a rare event (~17%) and, in any case, does not really establish the diagnosis even if present.[37] Plain abdominal films can show indications of mechanical bowel obstruction or the presence of free intraperitoneal air, but such conditions should rarely be confused with appendicitis.

Given the inherent limitations in establishing the diagnosis of acute appendicitis and a concern that a delay may result in perforation with increased associated morbidity and possible mortality, a false appendectomy rate of approximately 20% has been considered acceptable. Certainly, if the negative appendectomy rate were much higher, one could question the diagnostic acumen and experience of the clinicians involved. On the other hand, in some centers a negative appendectomy rate of less than 10% has been accomplished,[35] and it is likely

TABLE 72.9 **DIAGNOSIS**

SIGNS ON PHYSICAL EXAMINATION SUGGESTIVE OF ACUTE APPENDICITIS

■ SIGN	■ WHAT IT INDICATES	■ DESCRIPTION
Dunphy	Inflammation involving the partial peritoneum	Increased pain with coughing or other movement
Rovsing	Localized peritoneal inflammation in the right lower quadrant	Lower left quadrant palpation induces right lower quadrant pain
Obturator	Pelvic appendicitis	Pain on internal rotation of the right hip
Iliopsoas	Retrocecal appendicitis	Pain on extension of right hip

that the addition of newer imaging modalities to evaluate acute abdominal pain has improved accuracy to the point where the modern standard of care should be substantially better than the historical target of 20%. Clearly, clinical experience and expertise is an important factor in establishing a correct diagnosis. In addition, in-hospital observation has been touted as an excellent way to closely follow patients and quickly intervene for worsening abdominal pain, peritoneal irritation, or fever. Using this approach, White et al.[38] reported a negative appendectomy rate of 6%. Cost-effectiveness of in-hospital observation strategies has not been determined. Of course, with a low negative appendectomy rate, one must ensure that there are few patients who develop perforated appendicitis while being observed in the hospital or after being sent home from an emergency room visit.

4 To improve diagnostic accuracy in patients with suspected appendicitis, other radiologic tests have been used. Ultrasonography has been reported to aid in the diagnosis of acute appendicitis[39,40] by the demonstration of a so-called target lesion (i.e., a thick-walled, noncompressible, luminal structure in the right lower quadrant). In more advanced cases, peritoneal fluid and even a frank abscess may be found. However, a number of large series[41,42] have shown ultrasound to be unreliable, both in terms of sensitivity and specificity, such that it probably should not be used in the routine diagnosis of acute appendicitis. Ultrasound may be helpful if it suggests a diagnosis other than appendicitis, especially gynecologic pathology in women of menstrual age. It must be cautioned, however, that simple cysts of the ovary are common and usually nonpathologic. As such, the presence of an ovarian cyst does not weigh against the diagnosis of acute appendicitis. On the other hand, if ultrasonographic signs of a tubo-ovarian abscess, ovarian torsion, or even rare complications related to uterine fibroids are present, then the diagnosis of appendicitis may be excluded (Fig. 72.1).

5 More recently, abdominal and pelvic CT scan has been used in the setting of suspected acute appendicitis[43,44] and appears to be more accurate than ultrasound.[45] Rao et al.[46] suggested that CT scan can lead to significant cost savings, because a normal study virtually excludes the diagnosis and obviates the need (and costs) of in-hospital observation. CT scan should include thin cuts through the area of the appendix and the use of rectal contrast to distend the cecum and make the adjacent inflammatory changes more evident. The role of CT scan in the diagnosis of appendicitis, however, remains controversial, because in most patients an accurate diagnosis can be reached simply by history and physical examination. In the setting of early acute appendicitis, pathologic changes in the gross appearance of the appendix may be minimal even with direct observation at the time of surgery and may well be missed by all radiologic techniques. One advantage of CT scan, similar to that of ultrasound, may be the detection of pathology other than acute appendicitis.[47]

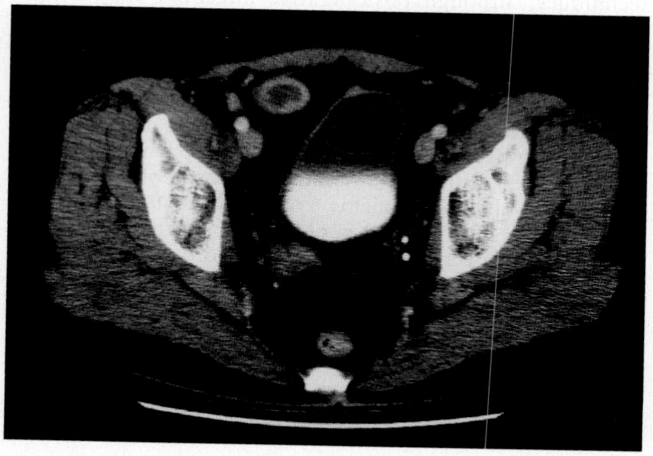

FIGURE 72.1. Acute appendicitis in a 53-year-old woman with fever and right lower quadrant pain and tenderness. Note the thick-walled, fluid-filled appendix with surrounding inflammation. A gangrenous appendix was found at operation.

Barium enema has been used in the past in an attempt to diagnose appendicitis.[48] Failure to fill the appendix has been associated with appendicitis, but up to 20% of normal appendices do not fill and therefore the diagnosis cannot be accurately established using this criterion. Occasionally, in more advanced cases with abscess formation, a mass effect will be seen compressing the adjacent cecum. However, such a finding would probably be better visualized by CT, which also provides the opportunity for percutaneous drainage. On occasion, barium enema can detect a colonic mucosal lesion such as a neoplasm or terminal ileal abnormalities related to Crohn disease, thereby establishing a diagnosis other than appendicitis. Overall, however, barium enema has little role in the modern management of suspected acute appendicitis.

Treatment

The standard treatment for suspected appendicitis is appendectomy via a right lower quadrant incision (Algorithm 72.1). The classical McBurney incision employs an oblique approach, incising each of the three abdominal wall muscle layers lateral to the rectus sheath. Ideally, the incision should follow Langer skin lines to provide an optimal cosmetic result. The aponeurosis overlying the external oblique can be sharply incised, and the remaining muscle layers split by retraction. The peritoneum is opened, the appendix is identified, and its blood supply is then ligated, usually from tip to base. Depending on the degree of surrounding inflammation and the length of time of the illness, mobilization of the appendix may be difficult and may require division of the lateral attachments of the cecum. The appendix itself is usually ligated with an absorbable suture and then inverted into the cecal wall through the use of a pursestring or Z-stitch. Inversion of the appendiceal stump has been advocated to prevent leakage and fistulization, but numerous reports have shown no difference in complication rates between inversion and simple ligation of the appendiceal stump.[49] Following appendectomy, irrigation of the peritoneal cavity should be carried out and then the peritoneum and muscles should be closed in layered fashion, usually with absorbable sutures. The skin incision can generally be safely closed, although in grossly contaminated cases, one may consider delayed primary closure or simply healing by secondary intention. However, based on a large meta-analysis, it appears that there is little if any role for delayed primary closure.[50] Intraperitoneal drains have not proven to be useful even in cases of perforated appendicitis.[51] Although the effectiveness of appendectomy for acute appendicitis is rarely questioned, the supporting evidence is surprisingly meager. Scattered reports have suggested the possibility of nonoperative (antibiotic alone) therapy for selected cases of early acute appendicitis,[52] although this approach remains anathema in classical surgical teaching.

If a normal appendix is found at the time of laparotomy, other causes for the abdominal pain should be sought. The cecum and proximal ascending colon should be examined for right-sided diverticulitis, neoplasms, or other pathology. The terminal ileum should be examined for Crohn disease or acute ileitis, and the ileum should be inspected for at least 2 feet proximal to the ileocecal valve for the presence of a Meckel diverticulum. If Crohn disease is encountered, the appendix may be safely removed as long as the cecum and particularly the base of the appendix are not involved with the inflammatory process. If uncomplicated Crohn inflammation is detected,

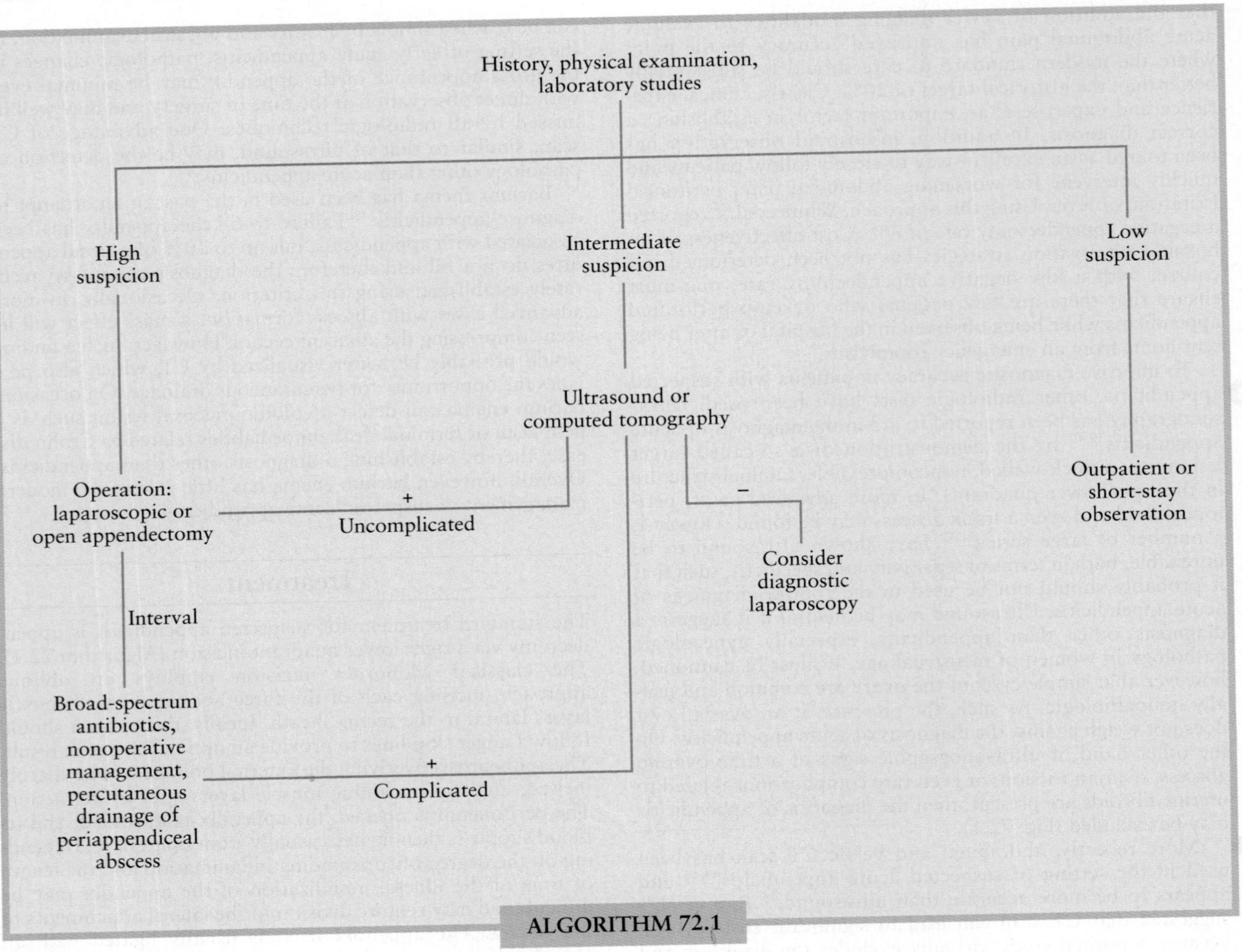

ALGORITHM 72.1. Management of suspected appendicitis.

ileal resection is not indicated, but in the case of a gross perforation or advanced Crohn disease with obstruction, resection should be performed. Occasionally, sigmoid diverticulitis may be mistaken for acute appendicitis, especially when a redundant sigmoid colon reaches the right side of the abdomen. Finally, the fallopian tubes, ovaries, and uterus should be carefully examined in female patients.

Laparoscopy. The role of laparoscopy and laparoscopic appendectomy has expanded greatly in recent years. Many surgeons advocate diagnostic laparoscopy especially for young women. Laparoscopy allows easy visualization of the pelvic organs as well as the appendix and can establish the diagnosis of appendicitis or other processes.[53,54] Laparoscopic appendectomy has gained substantial popularity. Generally, the laparoscope is inserted through a periumbilical incision and then additional trocars are placed, one in the right lower quadrant to grasp the appendix and another on the left side to perform dissection, ligation, and, ultimately, removal of the appendix. Endoscopic stapling devices have simplified transection and closure of the appendiceal stump at its base as well as
6 hemostatic division of the mesoappendix. Numerous series have compared laparoscopic to open appendectomy.[55,56] As in many other minimally invasive procedures, a learning curve clearly exists and may explain the longer operative times in initial reports. With experience, however, operative times for the laparoscopic approach probably equal and may be superior to open appendectomy. Complication rates appear to be low and are probably no different between the laparoscopic and open techniques, although postoperative infections may be less common with laparoscopy. Laparoscopy may also be of benefit in regard to hospital stay and overall recovery. Most reports in the literature indicate that length of stay is significantly shorter using the laparoscopic route, as is narcotic usage and other parameters associated with postoperative morbidity.[57] In a large retrospective series,[35] laparoscopic appendectomy was found to be particularly valuable in cases of gangrenous and/or perforated appendicitis. For simple acute appendicitis, hospital stay and recovery periods were short, regardless of operative approach. However, in the more advanced cases, laparoscopy was associated with shorter hospital stays and faster recovery. Based on a large Cochrane review, the most consistent differences in laparoscopic versus open appendectomy are that laparoscopic appendectomy is associated with a reduction in wound infections (by approximately one half) and intra-abdominal abscesses.[58]

Appendiceal Mass

Some patients with appendicitis will present at a relatively late stage in their illness (greater than about 5 days). Although in

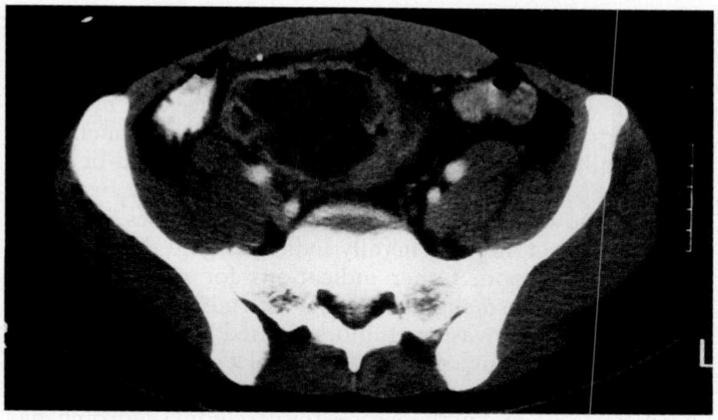

FIGURE 72.2. A 23-year-old man with 2 weeks of right lower quadrant pain, fever, and leukocytosis. Note the large periappendiceal abscess containing gas. The patient was successfully treated with percutaneous drainage and antibiotics.

most cases acute appendicitis progresses to perforation and diffuse peritonitis within the first few days of the illness, virtually forcing the patient to seek medical attention, occasionally an appendiceal perforation is contained by surrounding structures including the omentum and adjacent bowel. Instead of developing diffuse peritonitis, these patients develop a localized inflammatory mass or phlegmon with or without a discrete abscess. The associated pain and other systemic signs are limited by this process, which may explain the delayed presentation. Such patients usually have right lower quadrant abdominal pain, tenderness on examination, and a palpable mass or fullness, although overlying guarding of the abdominal wall musculature may obscure the mass. The key diagnostic feature to be recognized in these patients is the length of time of the illness, because a walled-off appendiceal mass generally requires a minimum of 5 days to form. In such cases, CT scan may establish the diagnosis and allow for percutaneous abscess drainage (Fig. 72.2). In the acute setting, these patients are best treated nonoperatively, because, although the appendix can be removed, there is added risk of injury to adjacent structures, including the small bowel. The overall morbidity in these patients appears to be decreased by the nonoperative approach, with or without percutaneous drainage.[59] Intravenous antibiotics are administered initially, and most of these patients will respond within a 24- to 48-hour period with a decrease in pain and fever. The patients can then be safely discharged on a course of oral antibiotics and a normal diet. The appendiceal inflammation generally subsides within 1 to 2 weeks. Antibiotics should continue for a total of approximately 2 weeks.

7

It should be noted that patients who have undergone percutaneous or open drainage of a periappendiceal abscess rarely develop fistulization from the cecum. Similarly, patients with perforated appendicitis almost always have pus within the peritoneal cavity, rather than actual enteric contents. These observations support the concept that most cases of appendicitis are associated with some obstruction of the lumen of the appendix.

Following the successful nonoperative treatment of an appendiceal mass, consideration should be given to interval appendectomy. A period of approximately 8 to 12 weeks will allow resolution of the inflammatory changes surrounding the appendix. Removal of the appendix after such a time period is generally safe and simple, although in rare circumstances, a significant amount of periappendiceal scar tissue and inflammation will persist. Whether or not to perform an interval appendectomy remains controversial. A number of investigators have examined the incidence of recurrent appendicitis following presentation with an appendiceal mass and successful nonoperative treatment. Based on a recurrence rate of approximately 10% (6-month to 13-year follow-up), Ein and Shandling[60] suggested that interval appendectomy is not indicated in all patients. The incidence of recurrence may be higher in younger patients and therefore the decision to perform the interval appendectomy should probably be individualized by patient age. One must remember, however, especially in the elderly patient, that the original diagnosis of appendicitis may have been mistaken and it is important to rule out a cecal neoplasm in such patients if interval appendectomy is not performed.

More recently, interval laparoscopic appendectomy has been shown to be a safe and simple procedure with a high degree of patient acceptance. The operation can generally be performed on an outpatient basis with minimal morbidity.[61] Laparoscopy, therefore, may have shifted the risk-benefit ratio in favor of interval appendectomy.

Antibiotic Therapy

Patients with acute appendicitis should be treated with perioperative broad-spectrum antibiotics directed against colonic flora, including gram-positive, gram-negative, and anaerobic organisms. Peritoneal cultures are generally not clinically helpful in the selection of the type of antibiotics.[62] The optimal length of antibiotic therapy is not known. In simple cases of acute appendicitis, 24 hours or less is generally sufficient. However, in cases of perforated appendicitis, longer courses of antibiotics are generally used, approximately 5 to 7 days.

Recurrent Appendicitis

Rarely, a patient will present with recurrent episodes of presumed acute appendicitis. At each presentation, spontaneous resolution may occur, with or without the use of antibiotics. Such patients may eventually come to appendectomy, and it is only in retrospect that the previous episodes are recognized to have been due to acute appendicitis. Recurrent appendicitis is occasionally termed *chronic appendicitis*, but this is probably a misnomer because the appendix is almost certainly uninflamed in the interval between episodes. Some patients will present in the outpatient setting for evaluation of chronic or intermittent right lower quadrant pain, raising the question of recurrent and/or chronic appendicitis. This difficult scenario requires clinical expertise to rule out etiologies other than appendicitis and to determine whether surgery is indicated. In general, discrete episodes of right lower quadrant pain, especially associated with fever and/or leukocytosis, are the best indicators of pathology within the appendix, and these patients respond most favorably to appendectomy. In contrast, patients with chronic right lower quadrant pain recurring frequently or even daily, in the absence of associated fever, are unlikely to benefit from appendectomy.

Appendicitis in Special Patient Populations

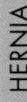

8 **Children.** The diagnosis of acute appendicitis is generally more difficult in young children compared to adults.[21] An accurate history may be difficult to obtain, and some of the signs of appendicitis such as nausea, vomiting, abdominal pain, and tenderness are often seen with other, extra-abdominal processes (e.g., pneumonia, meningitis, otitis media). The difficulty in establishing an accurate diagnosis in children is the presumed reason for a higher perforation rate in this population, reported to be as high as 50%. As such, the use of radiologic studies such as CT scan may be of particular benefit in children with suspected appendicitis. A negative appendectomy rate as low as 4% was reported with the routine use of ultrasound or CT.[63] However, this has not been the experience of all groups, and there is concern about the potential increase

in lifetime risk of cancer in children who have undergone radiation exposure due to a single CT scan.[64]

9 **Elderly Patients.** As in a number of other disease entities, elderly patients tend to present later in their course of appendicitis and clearly have higher associated rates of morbidity and mortality.[65] Perforation rates in elderly patients with appendicitis are quite high (>50%). Elderly patients tend to have less subjective pain, have decreased findings of peritonitis on examination, and may have a delayed leukocytosis. Therefore, the index of suspicion for an intra-abdominal inflammatory/infectious process, including acute appendicitis, must be higher in elderly patients compared to the general population.

Immunocompromised Patients. The patient with an impaired immune system who complains of abdominal pain represents a particularly challenging problem for the clinician.[66] Patients with AIDS or those who have been exposed to high-dose chemotherapy are susceptible to specific disease entities, including CMV-related bowel perforations and typhlitis (neutropenic colitis). Because these disease processes most commonly affect the terminal ileum and cecum, they can often be confused with acute appendicitis. CT scan can be particularly helpful in this setting in order to establish a definitive diagnosis, although in some cases the findings of pericecal inflammation are nonspecific. In general, regardless of the underlying disease process, surgery is indicated in the patient with spreading peritonitis or with systemic signs of sepsis related to an intra-abdominal infection.

10 **Pregnancy.** Appendicitis is the most frequent nonobstetric indication for laparotomy during pregnancy. Pregnant women will often present with abdominal pain, particularly in the lower abdomen, raising the suspicion of appendicitis. A diagnosis can be difficult to establish, especially because abdominal pain, nausea, and vomiting are quite common in early pregnancy. The white blood cell count is slightly elevated in normal pregnancy, adding further difficulties to establishing the diagnosis of appendicitis. In addition, as the uterus enlarges, the anatomic location of the appendix will be shifted upward, and the uterus may cover the appendix, thereby diminishing the signs of peritoneal inflammation. Because of these complicating factors, the perforation rate of appendicitis during pregnancy is probably higher than in the general population.[67,68] Unfortunately, perforated appendicitis is also associated with high fetal mortality (>30%), whereas simple acute appendicitis has a risk of fetal loss in the range of 10% and poses negligible risk to the mother. As such, it is best to be aggressive in recommending surgical exploration in pregnant women with suspected appendicitis, especially because a "negative" appendectomy is well tolerated with minimal morbidity to mother and fetus. Numerous reports have indicated the safety of laparoscopy in the setting of pregnancy.[69] However, in the third trimester, the enlarged uterus may limit the exposure and preclude a laparoscopic approach.

Appendiceal Neoplasms

Approximately 1% of all appendectomy specimens will contain a neoplasm.[70] The most common tumor is the carcinoid. Rare tumors of the appendix include benign and malignant mucoceles, adenocarcinoma, and adenocarcinoids.

Carcinoids. Approximately one third to two thirds of all appendiceal neoplasms are carcinoids, tumors of neural crest origin and derived from enteroendocrine cells. Of all carcinoid tumors within the GI tract, approximately half arise within the appendix. Carcinoid tumors of the appendix are usually found incidentally on pathologic examination of the inflamed appendix. These tumors have a characteristic firm yellow appearance and are often associated with a surrounding desmoplastic reaction. In regard to treatment and prognosis, the key feature
11 is the size of the tumor. Most carcinoids are less than 1.5 cm in diameter, and these tumors are adequately treated by simple appendectomy. The chance of lymphatic or distant metastasis is essentially zero and the prognosis for cure should be excellent. On the other hand, tumors that are 2 cm in size or greater begin to show metastatic potential. In such cases, a formal right hemicolectomy is generally indicated, and the prognosis remains quite good. Other indications for right colectomy include high-grade malignant lesions with a high mitotic index, mesoappendiceal invasion, tumors located at the base of the appendix with positive margins, and goblet cell adenocarcinoid tumors.[71] Rarely, appendiceal carcinoids are associated with liver metastases, and in these cases the carcinoid syndrome may be present. The number and location of liver lesions, as well as the associated symptoms, would dictate treatment in these cases.[72,73]

Mucoceles. Mucoceles of the appendix can be due to both benign and malignant disease, either cystadenomas or cystadenocarcinomas. These tumors obstruct the appendiceal lumen, leading to a large mucin-filled structure, often with calcification in the wall. Such tumors can generally be diagnosed by CT scan.

Appendectomy is curative for benign cystadenomas, even if rupture has occurred with mucinous ascites. However, with rupture of a cystadenocarcinoma, peritoneal tumor implantation can occur, leading to mucin secretion and a condition known as pseudomyxoma peritonei. The presence of mucin-secreting cellular elements in the peritoneal cavity distinguishes this malignant condition from the benign cystadenoma rupture with simple mucinous ascites. There is no effective treatment for pseudomyxoma peritonei, and these patients can develop secondary complications including bowel obstruction and perforation. The neoplastic process tends to be fairly indolent (5-year 50% survival), and repeated debulking procedures may be indicated.[74]

Adenocarcinoma. Adenocarcinoma of the appendix is extremely rare and like other appendiceal neoplasms is generally found unexpectedly at the time of appendectomy. Unfortunately, up to one half of the patients have metastatic disease at the time of diagnosis, usually with peritoneal spread presumably from rupture of the associated inflammatory process. Staging and treatment for appendiceal adenocarcinoma is similar to that for the more common colon carcinoma. Early lesions confined to the mucosa or submucosa (Dukes A) may be treated by simple appendectomy, as long as clear surgical margins are present. Dukes B and C lesions require formal right hemicolectomy, with adjuvant therapy indicated similar to colon carcinoma. Interestingly, appendiceal adenocarcinomas are associated with secondary tumors in up to 35% of patients, most often involving other areas of the GI tract.[75]

References

1. Gill BD, Jenkins JR. Cost-effective evaluation and management of the acute abdomen. *Surg Clin North Am* 1996;76:71.
2. Pines J, Uscher Pines L, Hall A, et al. The interrater variation of ED abdominal examination findings in patients with acute abdominal pain. *Am J Emerg Med* 2005;23(4):483–487.
3. Kharbanda AB, Fishman SJ, Bachur RG. Comparison of pediatric emergency physicians' and surgeons' evaluation and diagnosis of appendicitis. *Acad Emerg Med* 2008;15(2):119–125.
4. Silen W. *Cope's Early Diagnosis of the Acute Abdomen*, 21st ed. New York: Oxford University Press; 2005.
5. Liu JL, Wyatt JC, Deeks JJ, et al. Systematic reviews of clinical decision tools for acute abdominal pain. *Health Technol Assess* 2006;10(47):1–167, iii–iv.
6. Brewer BJ, Golden GT, Hitch DC, et al. Abdominal pain. An analysis of 1000 consecutive cases in a university hospital emergency room. *Am J Surg* 1976;131:219.

7. Hawthorn IE. Abdominal pain as a cause of acute admission to hospital [see comments]. *J Royal Coll Surg Edinb* 1992;37:389.
8. Powers RD, Guertler AT. Abdominal pain in the ED: stability and change over 20 years. *Am J Emerg Med* 1995;13:301.
9. Wolfe JM, Smithline HA, Phipen S, et al. Does morphine change the physical examination in patients with acute appendicitis? *Am J Emerg Med* 2004;22:280.
10. Thomas SH, Silen W, Cheema F, et al. Effects of morphine analgesia on diagnostic accuracy in emergency department patients with abdominal pain: a prospective, randomized trial. *J Am Coll Surg* 2003;196:18.
11. Materola C, Astudillo P, Losada H, et al. Analgesia in patients with acute abdominal pain. *Cochrane Database Syst Rev* 2007;(3):CD005660.
12. Nauta RJ, Magnant C. Observation versus operation for abdominal pain in the right lower quadrant. Roles of the clinical examination and the leukocyte count. *Am J Surg* 1986;151:746.
13. McCook TA, Ravin CE, Rice RP. Abdominal radiography in the emergency department: a prospective analysis. *Ann Emerg Med* 1982; 11:7.
14. Anyanwu AC, Moalypour SM. Are abdominal radiographs still overutilized in the assessment of acute abdominal pain? A district general hospital audit. *J R Coll Surg Edinb* 1998;43:267.
15. Gupta H, Dupuy DE. Advances in imaging of the acute abdomen. *Surg Clin North Am* 1997;77:1245.
16. Siewert B, Raptopoulos V, Mueller MF, et al. Impact of CT on diagnosis and management of acute abdomen in patients initially treated without surgery. *AJR Am J Roentgenol* 1997;168:173.
17. Carrico CW, Fenton LZ, Taylor GA, et al. Impact of sonography on the diagnosis and treatment of acute lower abdominal pain in children and young adults. *AJR Am J Roentgenol* 1999;172:513.
18. Mutter D, Navez B, Gury JF, et al. Value of microlaparoscopy in the diagnosis of right iliac fossa pain. *Am J Surg* 1998;176:370.
19. Memon MA, Fitztgibbons RJ Jr. The role of minimal access surgery in the acute abdomen. *Surg Clin North Am* 1997;77:1333.
20. Chung RS, Diaz JJ, Chari V. Efficacy of routine laparoscopy for the acute abdomen. *Surg Endosc* 1998;12:219.
21. Neblett WW, Pietsch JB, Holcomb GW Jr. Acute abdominal conditions in children and adolescents. *Surg Clin North Am* 1988;68:415.
22. Potts FE, Vukov LF. Utility of fever and leukocytosis in acute surgical abdomens in octogenarians and beyond. *J Gerontol A Biol Sci Med Sci* 1999;54:M55.
23. Marco CA, Schoenfeld CN, Keyl PM, et al. Abdominal pain in geriatric emergency patients: variables associated with adverse outcomes. *Acad Emerg Med* 1998;5:1163.
24. Simic O, Strathausen S, Hess W, et al. Incidence and prognosis of abdominal complications after cardiopulmonary bypass. *Cardiovasc Surg* 1999;7: 419.
25. Bender JS, Ratner LE, Magnuson TH, et al. Acute abdomen in the hemodialysis patient population. *Surgery* 1995;117:494.
26. Sheridan R. Diagnosis of the acute abdomen in the neurologically stable spinal cord-injured patient. A case study. *J Clin Gastroenterol* 1992;15: 325.
27. Bar-On Z, Ohry A. The acute abdomen in spinal cord injury individuals. *Paraplegia* 1995;33:704.
28. Tarraza HM, Moore RD. Gynecologic causes of the acute abdomen and the acute abdomen in pregnancy. *Surg Clin North Am* 1997;77:1371.
29. Oto A, Ernst RD, Ghulmiyyah LM, et al. MR imaging in the triage of pregnant patients with acute abdominal and pelvic pain. *Abdom Imaging* 2009;34:243–250.
30. Fitz R. Perforating inflammation of the vermiform appendix: with special reference to its early diagnosis and treatment. *Trans Assoc Am Physicians* 1886;1:107.
31. Silverman K. *Houdini: The Career of Ehrich Weiss*. New York: HarperCollins; 1996.
32. Scott G. The primate caecum and appendix vermiformis: a comparative study. *J Anat* 1980;131:549.
33. Gray H. *Gray's Anatomy*, 29th ed. Philadelphia, PA: Lea & Febiger; 1973.
34. Styrud J, Eriksson S, Segelman J, et al. Diagnostic accuracy in 2351 patients undergoing appendicectomy for suspected acute appendicitis: a retrospective study 1986–1993. *Dig Surg* 1999;16:39.
35. Nguyen DB, Silen W, Hodin RA. Appendectomy in the pre- and post-laparoscopic eras. *J Gastrointest Surg* 1999;3:67.
36. Hale DA, Molloy M, Pearl RH, et al. Appendectomy: a contemporary appraisal. *Ann Surg* 1997;225:252.
37. Olutola PS. Plain film radiographic diagnosis of acute appendicitis: an evaluation of the signs. *Can Assoc Radiol J* 1988;39:254.
38. White JJ, Santillana M, Haller JA Jr. Intensive in-hospital observation: a safe way to decrease unnecessary appendectomy. *Am Surg* 1975;41: 793.
39. Zielke A, Hasse C, Sitter H, et al. Influence of ultrasound on clinical decision making in acute appendicitis: a prospective study. *Eur J Surg* 1998; 164:201.
40. Ooms HW, Koumans RK, Ho Kang You PJ, et al. Ultrasonography in the diagnosis of acute appendicitis. *Br J Surg* 1991;78:315.
41. Franke C, Bohner H, Yang Q, et al. Ultrasonography for diagnosis of acute appendicitis: results of a prospective multicenter trial. Acute Abdominal Pain Study Group. *World J Surg* 1999;23:141.
42. Wade DS, Marrow SE, Balsara ZN, et al. Accuracy of ultrasound in the diagnosis of acute appendicitis compared with the surgeon's clinical impression. *Arch Surg* 1993;128:1039.
43. Choi YH, Fischer E, Hoda SA, et al. Appendiceal CT in 140 cases. Diagnostic criteria for acute and necrotizing appendicitis. *Clin Imaging* 1998; 22:252.
44. Lane MJ, Katz DS, Ross BA, et al. Unenhanced helical CT for suspected acute appendicitis. *AJR Am J Roentgenol* 1997;168:405.
45. Balthazar EJ, Birnbaum BA, Yee J, et al. Acute appendicitis: CT and US correlation in 100 patients. *Radiology* 1994;190:31.
46. Rao PM, Rhea JT, Novelline RA, et al. Effect of computed tomography of the appendix on treatment of patients and use of hospital resources [see comments]. *N Engl J Med* 1998;338:141.
47. Shaff MI, Tarr RW, Partain CL, et al. Computed tomography and magnetic resonance imaging of the acute abdomen. *Surg Clin North Am* 1988;68: 233.
48. Smith DE, Kirchmer NA, Stewart DR. Use of the barium enema in the diagnosis of acute appendicitis and its complications. *Am J Surg* 1979;138: 829.
49. Street D, Bodai BI, Owens LJ, et al. Simple ligation vs. stump inversion in appendectomy. *Arch Surg* 1988;123:689.
50. Rucinski J, Fabian T, Panagopoulos G, et al. Gangrenous and perforated appendicitis: a meta-analytic study of 2532 patients indicates that the incision should be closed primarily. *Surgery* 2000;127:136.
51. Greenall MJ, Evans M, Pollack AV. Should you drain a perforated appendix? *Br J Surg* 1978;65:880.
52. Mason RJ. Surgery for appendicitis: is it necessary? *Surg Infect (Larchmt)* 2008;9(4):481–488.
53. Tytgat SH, Bakker XR, Butzelaar RM. Laparoscopic evaluation of patients with suspected acute appendicitis. *Surg Endosc* 1998;12:918.
54. Thorell A, Grondal S, Schedvins K, et al. Value of diagnostic laparoscopy in fertile women with suspected appendicitis. *Eur J Surg* 1999;165:751.
55. Chiarugi M, Buccianti P, Celona G, et al. Laparoscopic compared with open appendicectomy for acute appendicitis: a prospective study. *Eur J Surg* 1996;162:385.
56. Chung RS, Rowland DY, Li P, et al. A meta-analysis of randomized controlled trials of laparoscopic versus conventional appendectomy. *Am J Surg* 1999;177:250.
57. Sackier JM. Laparoscopy for acute appendicitis. *Semin Laparosc Surg* 1996;3:185.
58. Sauerland S, Lefering R, Neugebauer EA. Laparoscopic versus open surgery for suspected appendicitis. *Cochrane Database Syst Rev* 2002;(4): CD001546.
59. Brown CV, Abrishami M, Muller M, et al. Appendiceal abscess: immediate operation or percutaneous drainage? *Am Surg* 2003;69:829.
60. Ein S, Schandling B. Is interval appendectomy necessary after rupture of an appendiceal mass? *J Pediatr Surg* 1996;31:849.
61. Nguyen DB, Silen W, Hodin RA. Interval appendectomy in the laparoscopic era. *J Gastrointest Surg* 1999;3:189.
62. Mosdell DM, Morris DM, Fry DE. Peritoneal cultures and antibiotic therapy in pediatric perforated appendicitis. *Am J Surg* 1994;167:313.
63. Kaiser S, Mesas-Burgos C, Söderman E, et al. Appendicitis in children: impact of US and CT on the negative appendectomy rate. *Eur J Pediatr Surg* 2004;14:260.
64. Martin AE, Vollman D, Adler B, et al. CT scans may not reduce the negative appendectomy rate in children. *J Pediatr Surg* 2004;39:886.
65. Horattas MC, Guyton DP, Wu D. A reappraisal of appendicitis in the elderly. *Am J Surg* 1990;160:291.
66. Nylander WA Jr. The acute abdomen in the immunocompromised host. *Surg Clin North Am* 1988;68:457.
67. Tamir IL, Bongard FS, Klein SR. Acute appendicitis in the pregnant patient. *Am J Surg* 1990;60:571.
68. Horowitz MD, Gomez GA, Santiesteban R, et al. Acute appendicitis during pregnancy. Diagnosis and management. *Arch Surg* 1985;120:1362.
69. Nezhat FR, Tazuke S, Nezhat CH, et al. Laparoscopy during pregnancy: a literature review. *J Soc Laparoendosc Surg* 1997;1:17.
70. Connor SJ, Hanna GB, Frizelle FA. Appendiceal tumors: retrospective clinicopathologic analysis of appendiceal tumors from 7970 appendectomies. *Dis Colon Rectum* 1998;41:75.
71. Goede AC, Caplin ME, Winslet MC. Carcinoid tumour of the appendix. *Br J Surg* 2003;90:1317.
72. Moertal CG, Weiland LH, Nagorney DM, et al. Carcinoid tumor of the appendix: treatment and prognosis. *N Engl J Med* 1987;317:1699.
73. Sandor A, Modlin IM. A retrospective analysis of 1570 appendiceal carcinoids. *Am J Gastroenterol* 1998;93:422.
74. Smith JW, Kemeny N, Caldwell C, et al. Pseudomyxoma peritonei of appendiceal origin. The Memorial Sloan-Kettering Cancer Center experience. *Cancer* 1992;70:396.
75. Cortina R, McCormick J, Kolm P, et al. Management and prognosis of adenocarcinoma of the appendix. *Dis Colon Rectum* 1995;38:848.

CHAPTER 73 ■ THE SPLEEN

DOUGLAS L. FRAKER

KEY POINTS

1. The spleen relates to the diaphragm both superiorly and laterally, and it generally spans the 9th, 10th, and 11th ribs along the left mid to posterior axillary line.
2. Accessory spleens are small nodules of splenic tissue that are completely separate from the main body of the spleen. They commonly range in size from 0.5 cm up to 3 to 4 cm.
3. The primary hematologic function of the spleen is removal of senescent erythrocytes or remodeling of abnormal red blood cells, and the recycling of iron by splenic macrophages.
4. The immunologic function of the spleen is to generate an immune response to antigens that are identified and cleared from the blood system.
5. Typically, encapsulated organisms cause the postsplenectomy sepsis-related infection.
6. The spleen is the most common intra-abdominal organ injured by blunt trauma in the United States.
7. The pathophysiology of ITP is development of an IgG antibody to a platelet antigen. In patients who have not achieved a sustained remission with medical therapy, which is most patients with chronic ITP, an elective splenectomy is recommended.
8. Hypersplenism is a physical enlargement of the spleen that can occur due to neoplastic disorders, hematopoietic disorders of the bone marrow, and metabolic or storage disorders. In the neoplastic disorders, the spleen is infiltrated and enlarged by leukemia or lymphoma cells.

The spleen has been a mysterious organ throughout surgical and medical history with a clear understanding and appreciation of its function only in the latter half of the 20th century. The reasons for this paucity of knowledge on the spleen are multifactorial. The spleen has no obvious function that can be discerned from its anatomic structures or features; there are no clear relationships of gross pathology of the spleen to many of the diseases for which it is important; and even in present time it is difficult to obtain a biopsy of the spleen, thereby limiting the amount of tissue available for pathologic study. The diseases (other than trauma) in which the spleen has importance are generally of a hematologic or immunologic nature. Understanding of the normal physiology and subsequent pathophysiology of the spleen is important for surgical decision making regarding when to recommend splenectomy and whether a partial splenectomy is possible. The only surgical procedure for most of the history of medicine applied to the spleen was splenectomy. Current variations on that procedure include laparoscopic splenectomy, partial splenectomy, and other splenic preservation procedures. The history of splenic surgery, the anatomy and physiology, and the disease processes as well as operative techniques involving the spleen will be reviewed.

HISTORY

The spleen has had a colorful history based on the function ascribed to this organ by many of the prominent scientists throughout the ages (Table 73.1).[1] Even the origin of the English term "spleen" is unclear. It is believed to come from the Greek "splen," which may have been derived from the Greek word "splancknon" meaning a viscus or the Greek word "spaw," which means to draw.[1] The dark purple-red color led ancients to believe that the spleen may draw spoiled or bad parts of the blood to itself, which presages one of the major roles of the spleen as a filtration device for senescent red blood cells. In ancient Greece, the spleen was believed to be the source of black bile, which was one of the four cardinal humors related to melancholy.[2] However, ancient authors wrote in the Talmud that the spleen was the seat for laughter and removal of the spleen would limit mirth in that person.[2] The spleen was thought to be a source of discomfort sometimes felt as "a stitch in the side" for athletes and that by removal or ablation of the spleen an individual would run faster. Reports of the earliest procedures on the spleen indicate that runners in ancient Greece may have had their spleens ablated in an effort to improve their performance. This hypothesis was studied in an experimental model almost 2,000 years later at Johns Hopkins in which splenectomized mice versus control mice were evaluated for their ability to run a race and the splenectomized mice were reported to be faster.[2]

During the Renaissance, scientists questioned the functional roles ascribed to the spleen. In the early 16th century, Princelsus rejected the black bile theory and questioned whether the spleen had any meaningful role at all. Zaccarella, one of Princelsus' students, reportedly performed the first splenectomy in 1549 in Palermo, Italy, successfully removing the large spleen of a 24-year-old woman (Table 73.1).[2] This organ was reportedly displayed in the town square after this landmark but unsubstantiated procedure. Versalius during that same era performed splenectomy in mice and other animals and determined that the spleen was not essential to life as there was no clear difference following removal. The first authenticated splenectomy was performed in Germany in 1826 by Carl Frederick Quitterbaum in a patient with secondary hypersplenism due to cirrhosis. This high-risk patient succumbed 6 hours after the procedure. The first successful operation in which the patient survived was performed by Jules Péan in France in 1865 for a large splenic cyst. This patient was operated on for what was thought to be an ovarian cystic mass, but it was found to be arising from the inferior portion of the spleen and required splenectomy for removal. In this early period of splenic surgery, there was much pessimism due to the high operative mortality rate primarily from hemorrhage. A collective series published in 1877 reported 50 splenectomies with 70% mortality. By 1900, Bessel-Hagen reported 360 splenectomies with 40% mortality. An in-depth discussion of the spleen in literature, art, and history was recently published by Morgenstern (3).

The 20th century brought technical advances in terms of hemostasis and blood transfusion as well as an understanding of the pathophysiology of splenic function.[4] The spleen was

TABLE 73.1

HISTORICAL MILESTONES IN SURGERY OF THE SPLEEN

1549	First reported splenectomy by Zaccarella in Italy
1826	First documented splenectomy by Quitterbaum in Germany
1865	First successful splenectomy by Péan in France
1892	First trauma splenectomy by Reigner in Germany
1911	Elective splenectomy for autoimmune hemolytic anemia
1916	Elective splenectomy for immune thrombocytopenia purpura
1952	First report of overwhelming postsplenectomy sepsis
1962	First report of splenic salvage procedure for trauma
1991	Laparoscopic splenectomy

identified as the site of red cell destruction in autoimmune hemolytic anemia by Micheli in 1911. In 1916, Paul Kaznelson, a Czech medical student, postulated that the removal of the spleen in patients with idiopathic thrombocytopenic purpura would be of benefit, and he reported the successful treatment of a patient with that disease by splenectomy. Throughout the 20th century, as understanding of the pathophysiology of hematologic and immune disorders associated with the spleen increased, the roles for splenectomy that are pertinent to modern-day practice became more clear.

EMBRYOLOGY AND ANATOMY

The spleen develops from the mesoderm as an outpouching from the mesogastrium during the 5th week of gestation.[4–6] Natural rotation of the gut during subsequent development places the spleen in its typical position in the left upper quad- 1 rant of the abdomen (Fig. 73.1). In that location, the spleen relates to the diaphragm both superiorly and laterally, and it generally spans the 9th, 10th, and 11th ribs along the left mid to posterior axillary line. The ventral surface of the spleen abuts the greater curvature of the stomach and the tail of the pancreas. The tail of the pancreas touches the splenic capsule in 30% of cases and is 1 cm away in 73% of cases. The inferior pole relates to the left kidney posteriorly and the splenic flexure of the colon anteriorly.

The normal size of the spleen is approximately 13 × 7 × 4 cm.[5] The typical weight of a spleen in a young adult is 150 to 200 g, and this decreases to approximately 100 g in the elderly population (Fig. 73.2).[7,8] If the spleen doubles in size to the range of 300–400 grams, it may project below the costal margin allowing palpation of the spleen tip on abdominal exam on deep inspiration.[9] The splenic weight defining massive splenomegaly has been arbitrarily set at 1,500 g. There is sometimes a significant cleft in the capsule of the spleen that may be confused with splenic disruption on CT scan obtained for trauma.

The vascular anatomy of the spleen is rather straightforward.[10] The splenic artery is one of the three major trunks of the celiac axis, along with the left gastric artery and common hepatic artery (Fig. 73.3). This artery has a characteristic appearance on celiac arteriograms as a serpentine vessel with loops extending both superiorly and inferiorly. There are several small pancreatic branches that supply blood to the body and tail of the pancreas along its length. The first major splenic branch occurs approximately 2 to 3 cm from the hilum, and it is called the superior polar artery. The main artery then divides into three to five segmental branches that enter along the trabecula of the spleen. Additional blood supply to the spleen comes from the left gastroepiploic artery via the short gastric vessels. When the spleen is massively enlarged, it may have direct vessels that are parasitized from the omentum, diaphragm, or the mesentery of the splenic flexure of the colon. The splenic artery generally travels outside the parenchyma of the pancreas just at the superior border although loops that go inferiorly may be completely covered by the posterior surface of the pancreas whereas superior loops may be well away from the pancreatic surface. These curves that are

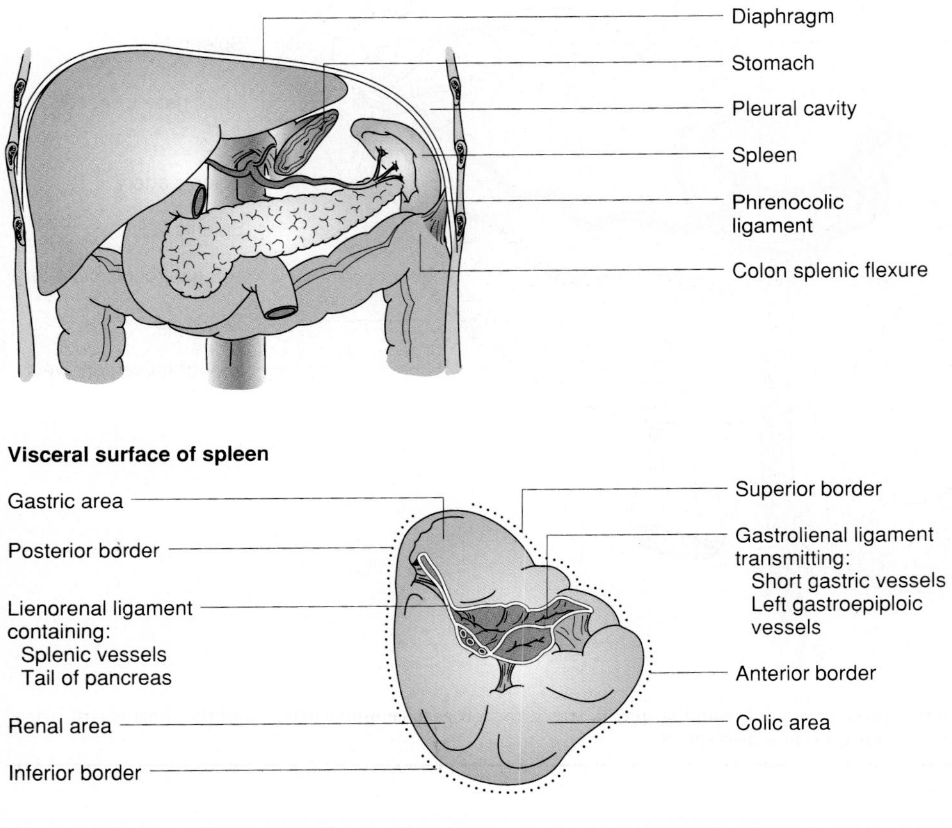

FIGURE 73.1. Anatomic relation of the spleen to the liver, diaphragm, pancreas, colon, and kidney. The stomach is sectioned to illustrate the anatomic relation in situ.

HERNIA

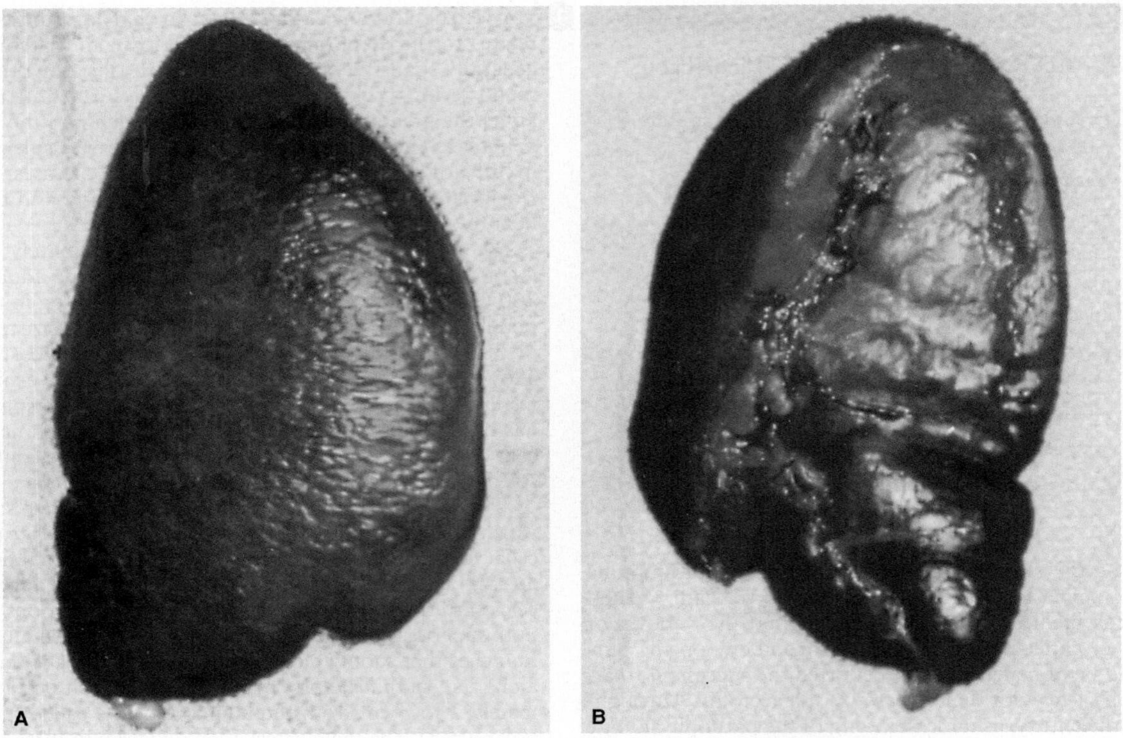

FIGURE 73.2. **A:** The lateral or diaphragmatic surface of the spleen, showing the lobulated edge and the glistening capsule. **B:** The hilar surface of the spleen, showing the ligatures on the cephalad short gastric vessels and the caudal hilar vessels.

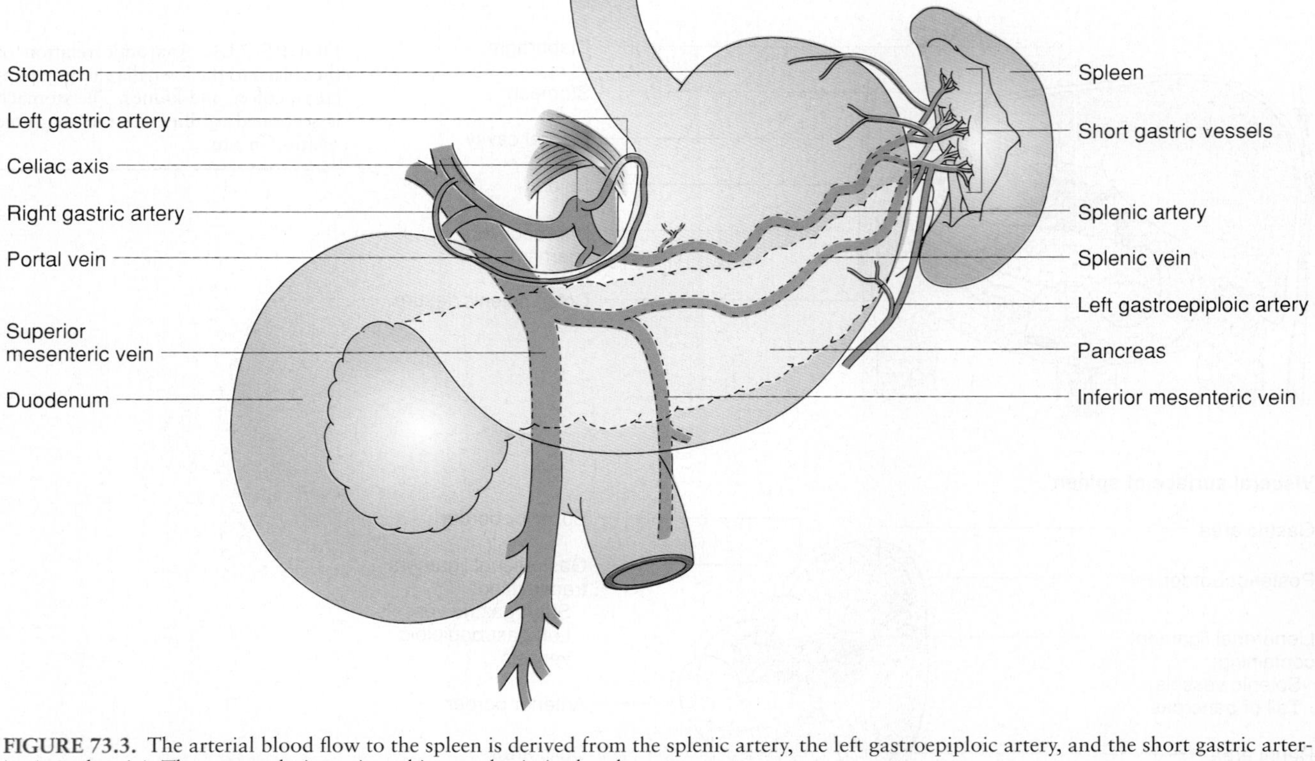

FIGURE 73.3. The arterial blood flow to the spleen is derived from the splenic artery, the left gastroepiploic artery, and the short gastric arteries (vasa brevia). The venous drainage into this portal vein is also shown.

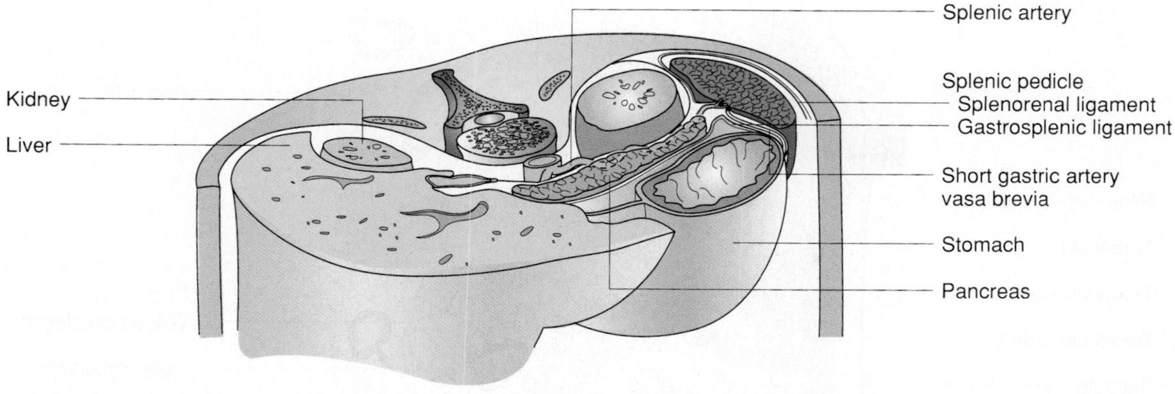

FIGURE 73.4. The relations of the spleen to the abdominal and retroperitoneal viscera are seen in a cross section of the left-facing torso.

exposed along the cranial surface of the pancreas are the optimal location to place a ligature for control of the splenic artery during procedures in which there is significant thrombocytopenia or for enlarged spleens. These are generally areas that have few pancreatic branches and avoid proximity to the splenic vein.

The splenic vein is formed by segmental venous branches that leave the trabecula and coalesce into the main splenic vein in the hilum of the spleen (Fig. 73.3). The splenic vein is intimately associated with the posterior surface of the tail and body of the pancreas from the hilum of the spleen to its junction with the superior mesenteric vein, where they form the portal vein. The inferior mesenteric vein may join the splenic vein directly at several areas along its course or may come together right at the junction of the superior mesenteric vein. There are several pancreatic branches that directly enter the splenic vein. The blood flow to the spleen in the typical adult is estimated to be 200 to 300 mL/minute, or approximately 5% of the cardiac output.[10]

The lymph node drainage generally follows the vasculature. The primary lymph nodes are located in the hilum of the spleen, along the splenic artery at the superior border of the pancreas, and along the short gastric vessels.

There are several ligaments that maintain the spleen in its fixed position in the left upper quadrant (Fig. 73.4).[6] Three of these ligaments are virtually always present (except in the condition of the wandering spleen),[11] and two may be present to variable extents, depending on the individual patient and the disease process. The first ligament that is constant is the splenogastric ligament, which is a left-sided superior extension of the greater omentum along the proximal greater curvature of the stomach. Within this area supplied by the left gastroepiploic vessels are short gastric vessels that branch to the upper pole of the spleen and often provide the upper two thirds of the spleen with alternative blood supply. The second and very important ligament is the splenorenal ligament that runs parallel to the posterolateral border of the spleen and attaches this to the superior pole of the Gerota fascia developing the left kidney. This ligament is divided when mobilizing the spleen during splenectomy and allows reflection of the spleen with or without the tail of the pancreas. The splenocolic ligament is short and may be avascular or have small blood vessels that go from the inferior tip of the spleen to the splenic flexure of the colon. This may be divided by cautery or may have vessels that need to be controlled with ties or clips during mobilization of the splenic flexure of the colon.

Two ligaments that are variably present are the splenoomental attachments and the splenophrenic attachments (Fig. 73.4). The free part of the greater omentum may have variable association with the splenic capsule along the inferior pole. There are often small vessels that can be controlled by electrocautery. This attachment may be absent or may be quite extensive over the lower pole of the spleen. It is this attachment to the omentum that often leads to disruption of the capsule along this inferior pole causing bleeding during other abdominal procedures and may necessitate splenectomy for control after an inadvertent injury. Prior to exerting inferior traction on the omentum during any procedure, the extent of attachments to the lower pole of the spleen should be investigated and if present should be carefully divided prior to further mobilization. There may be direct ligaments connecting the spleen to the diaphragm identified as splenophrenic ligaments. These typically are present to a greater degree when the spleen is diseased or enlarged. They may be avascular or may have branches of vessels parasitized from the diaphragm blood supply.

The anatomy of the spleen itself is segmental, with individual segments fed by arteries and drained by veins that leave via the trabecula.[12] The trabecula are fibrous bands that attach to the splenic capsule. The parenchyma of the spleen between these trabecula is divided into a small area of white pulp surrounding the arteries, a marginal zone, and the larger predominant area of red pulp that constitutes 75% of the splenic parenchyma.[13,14] The capsule of the spleen is quite thin. This consists of a single layer of mesothelium and several layers of fibroelastic tissue. In other mammals but not humans, there may be variable amounts of smooth muscle in the capsule. This smooth muscle allows contraction and mobilization of the circulating blood cells that are stored in the spleen.[15] The trabecular arteries that enter the spleen as continuation of the segmental arterial branches then give off perpendicular branches to form the central arteries (Fig. 73.5). Surrounding these central arteries is the periarterial lymphatic sheath (PALS), which is composed of T lymphocytes as well as follicles with B cells at various stages of development. During antigenic stimulation, this area greatly expands with more mature and secondary follicles. The marginal zone is the border zone between the white pulp and the red pulp; it contains a mixture of lymphatics and macrophages. The structure of the red pulp is made up of splenic cords with an intervening area called splenic sinuses. The splenic cords, also known as the cords of Billroth, are a meshwork of fibroblasts and many mature macrophages. The splenic sinuses are an interconnective meshwork of fairly random red cell spaces that are thin walled and generally filled with many erythrocytes.[14]

Studies on blood flow show two alternative routes to the spleen being fast flow and slow flow.[16] A small proportion of the blood goes through the splenic arteries and returns rapidly to the splenic veins. This fast flow pattern consists of a greater predominance of plasma and few erythrocytes because of streaming and accounts for only 10% of flow. A particularly large portion of the erythrocytes that enter the spleen travels through the highly fenestrated meshwork in the red pulp as part of the filtration process of the spleen. This slow path or slow flow composes up to 90% of the splenic blood flow and relates to the role of the spleen in clearing senescent erythrocytes.

2 Accessory spleens are small nodules of splenic tissue that are completely separate from the main body of the spleen. They commonly range in size from 0.5 cm up to 3 to 4 cm. The incidence of accessory spleens is reported to be between 10% and

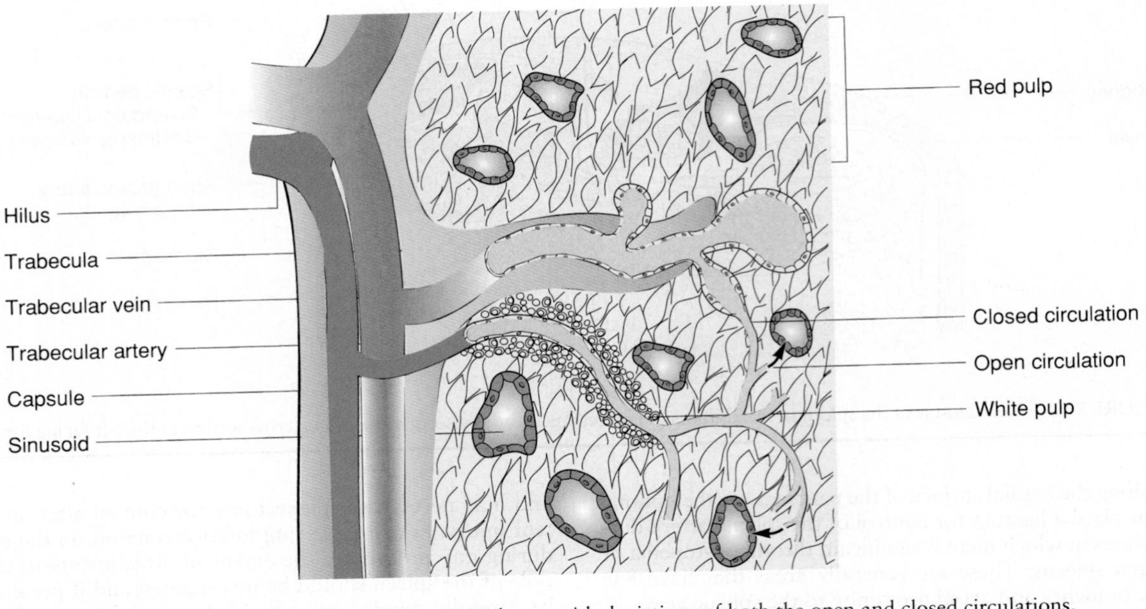

FIGURE 73.5. The splenic microanatomy is shown with depictions of both the open and closed circulations.

20%. The most common location for these small nodules of splenic tissue is in the splenic hilum, the omentum (most commonly between the stomach and transverse colon but also within the greater omentum), and the small bowel mesentery. However, they can occur virtually anywhere in the abdomen including the retroperitoneum behind the spleen and in the pelvis. Accessory spleens are important in disease processes in which a complete removal of all splenic tissue is necessary for long-term cure, such as certain autoimmune disorders. The routine use of laparoscopic splenectomy to treat this disorder highlights the importance of the accessory spleens as they are more difficult to identify during a minimally invasive procedure than during an open operation. However, several reports demonstrate that accessory spleens can be successfully removed laparoscopically, particularly with the aid of a nuclear medicine spleen scan if needed to identify sources of residual tissue.[17]

PHYSIOLOGY

The major functions of the spleen can be divided into two general categories: hematologic functions and immunologic functions (Table 73.2).[14] For hematologic functions, the spleen is primarily related to the destruction or clearance of the circulating blood cell elements as a normal physiologic mechanism. This physiologic filtration function is increased in disease states that produce hypersplenism. The spleen may play a minor role in hematopoiesis and storage of blood cells that can be mobilized for the circulation; the predominantly stored cell type is platelets. In terms of the immunologic functions, the spleen relates to the vascular system in many of the same ways that lymph nodes relate to the lymphatic system. The white pulp and marginal zones are most important for the immunologic functions whereas the red pulp is primarily related to the hematologic functions. However, the macrophages that line or fill the cords in the red pulp are also important in immunosurveillance for intravascular pathogens.

TABLE 73.2

NORMAL FUNCTIONS OF THE SPLEEN

HEMATOLOGIC
Culling or destruction of senescent erythrocytes
Pitting or removal of cytoplasm inclusive in erythrocytes
Reservoir for platelets and granulocytes
Hematopoiesis—as fetus or in conditions with bone marrow destruction
IMMUNOLOGIC
Filtration and trapping of circulatory antigens
Lymphocyte stimulation and proliferation
Antibody production in germinal follicles
Production of opsonin-tuftsin and properdin
Opsonins: tuftsin and properdin

3 The primary hematologic function of the spleen is removal of senescent erythrocytes or remodeling of abnormal red blood cells, and the recycling of iron by splenic macrophages.[14] The average life span of a normal erythrocyte measured on clearance studies in humans is approximately 120 days.[18] The spleen destroys approximately 100 billion erythrocytes daily in the red pulp. The process of removal or phagocytosis of erythrocytes or other blood cells is called culling (Table 73.2). The blood flow patterns of the spleen lead to a hemoconcentrated erythrocyte-laden fluid that enters the sinuses of the red pulp. Here a slow flow through the sinusoid network with adjacent macrophage-filled cords is the environment in which erythrocytes may become trapped and then phagocytized by the macrophages. The precise mechanism by which senescent red cells are identified for destruction in normal physiology is unclear. One hypothesis is that over the course of the life span of an erythrocyte, there is loss of either membrane elements or total membrane material such that the red cells become less compliant and therefore become mechanically trapped in the mesh of the sinusoids. A second hypothesis is that specific cell surface marker molecules may either become more exposed or less available to allow identification of senescent cells targeted for destruction. Pathologic destruction of red cells occurs in diseases such as hereditary spherocytosis or elliptocytosis in which genetic defect creates abnormal red cell pliability limiting its passage through the red pulp. Similarly, in sickle cell anemia, the genetic defect in the hemoglobin alters red cell shape and creates destruction with clogging of the sinusoids. A second pathologic mechanism in which destruction of red cells is increased occurs in disease processes that increase the spleen size and lead to removal of normal red cells because of increased red pulp volume. This condition is called hypersplenism.

The second physiologic process involving circulating erythrocytes is remodeling or pitting, which is partial removal of the cell membrane, typically associated with cytoplasmic inclusions. Erythrocytes with a remnant of the cell nucleus remaining pass more slowly through the splenic red pulp because of their larger size.[14] The nuclear remnant may be trapped passing through a small space in the spleen, and this solid particle that does not allow deformation gets pinched off in the process of pitting. Intracytoplasmic inclusions include Howell-Jolly bodies, which are nuclear remnants; Heinz bodies, which are denatured hemoglobin; and Pappenheimer bodies, which are iron granules.

The destruction of the other circulating cellular elements of the blood (platelets and leukocytes) is typically more pathophysiology of the spleen than normal physiologic function. The disease processes in which these cells are removed are either related to autoantibodies to cell surface elements or to hypersplenism. If either platelets or white blood cells become coated with antibodies, the Fc portion of the immunoglobulin can interact with the Fc receptors on the macrophages in the splenic cords, leading to phagocytosis of these cell types. With splenic enlargement from various causes of hypersplenism, a similar process of destruction can occur even without any autoantibodies or defects in the cells, because of the increase in splenic mass.

The spleen is a potential site for hematopoiesis of all cell types during gestation. In normal humans, there is very little if any production of red cells, granulocytes, or platelets, which is not true in other mammals. In the white pulp of the spleen there are germinal centers with amplification and production of reactive lymphocytes. The cords of the spleen are filled with macrophages, and throughout normal adult life there may be production of lymphocytes and macrophages in the spleen. In certain disease states, the spleen may develop the capacity for erythropoiesis and myelopoiesis. The best example is agnogenic myeloid metaplasia. In this disease, the bone marrow is replaced with fibrotic scar and a portion of the hematopoietic function of the marrow is assumed by the spleen that typically becomes quite enlarged.

The final hematologic function of the spleen is as a reservoir of circulating cellular elements.[15] In humans, the only significant cell type that is stored in the spleen is platelets. It is estimated that 30% of all platelets may reside in the spleen. This function may be more important in other mammals, particularly those with significant smooth muscle lining the capsule of the spleen that allows contracture with expulsion of large numbers of stored cells as a physiologic response to injury.

The immunologic function of the spleen is to generate an
4 immune response to antigens that are identified and cleared from the blood system (Table 73.2). Either opsonized antigens or specific encapsulated microorganisms are important examples of target antigens trapped by the spleen. The spleen is an ideal environment for generation of either a cellular or a humoral immune response. All of the necessary cell types for stimulation of the immune response are present, including phagocytic cells, dendritic cells, T cells, and B cells, which may form germinal follicles to generate specific antibody responses. These interactions primarily occur in the marginal zone in the white pulp, which may become quite enlarged and hypertrophied during antigen stimulation. These cellular components and the structure of the germinal follicles are essentially identical to those found in lymph node tissue, which becomes enlarged in a similar way with antigenic stimulation via microbes or antigens in the lymphatic system.

The spleen is also involved in nonspecific immune responses. It is the site of synthesis of both properdin and tuftsin, which are opsonins. Tuftsin is a small peptide that binds to the surface of granulocytes and promotes phagocytic function by these cells.[19] Properdin can initiate the alternate pathway of complement activation that can be important in destruction of abnormal cells or bacteria that are antibody bound. The spleen is not the only source of these nonspecific immune-enhancing proteins; therefore splenectomy may lead to only a modest alteration in this function.

PATHOPHYSIOLOGY

There are characteristic responses that share many common features under the broad category of hyposplenism and hypersplenism. These features highlight the normal physiologic functions of the spleen and provide guidelines and influence clinical decision making when managing patients after splenectomy or in deciding which patients should undergo splenectomy. By far, the most common cause of hyposplenism is surgical removal.[20] Other causes are an unusual situation of a congenitally small or absent spleen or acquired destruction of splenic tissue as can occur in patients with sickle cell anemia. Hypersplenism is the most frequent indication for elective splenectomy.[21] There are various causes of hypersplenism that are typically neoplastic but may be related to primary blood cell dysfunction or abnormalities, or other condition such as portal hypertension due to cirrhosis or splenic vein thrombosis.

Hyposplenism

Hyposplenism or the changes that occur after a splenectomy are predictable from the known functions of the spleen. There are hematologic changes in the circulating cells from loss of the splenic functions of culling, pitting, and as a reservoir for platelets (Table 73.3). There are changes in the immunologic responses, important primarily in infants or young children, that can lead to overwhelming postsplenectomy sepsis. The two most common nonsurgical causes of hyposplenism are sickle cell anemia and celiac disease.[21]

The changes in circulating blood cells after splenectomy in cases of hyposplenism affect the erythrocytes, leukocytes, and platelets. Over time, the intracytoplasmic inclusions in the red cells that are normally cleared by the spleen accumulate, resulting in the presence of Howell-Jolly bodies, Heinz bodies, and Pappenheimer bodies. Other changes can include target cells with excess red blood cell membrane and increases in the circulating nucleated red blood cells or reticulocytes. As the spleen is the organ of storage for a large proportion of the platelets, a splenectomy often results in thrombocytosis with platelet counts postsplenectomy frequently surpassing 500,000 and sometimes up to one million. This increased platelet count is often transient and may be a reflection that the spleen as a storage organ for platelets may not be a primary area of platelet destruction after the typical half-life of 10 days. The immediate white blood cell response after a splenectomy is leukocytosis, reflecting storage of a large proportion of white blood cells in the spleen.[21] As with thrombocytosis, this effect

TABLE 73.3

RESULTS OF SPLENECTOMY/HYPOSPLENIC CONDITION

HEMATOLOGIC

1. Erythrocytes
   - Howell-Jolly bodies (nuclear fragments)
   - Heinz bodies (hemoglobin deposits)
   - Pappenheimer bodies (iron deposits)
   - Target cells
   - Spur cells (acanthocytes)
2. Platelets
   - Transient thrombocytosis
3. Leukocytes
   - Transient leukocytosis
   - Persistent lymphocytosis
   - Persistent monocytosis

is transient but there may be long-term increases in the proportion of circulating lymphocytes and monocytes after splenectomy. Preserving even a small amount of spleen can preserve splenic clearance of senescent blood cells.[22]

The changes in immune function that occur with hyposplenism or after splenectomy are most importantly manifest by the phenomenon of overwhelming postsplenectomy sepsis.[23,24] This was initially recognized as an important epidemiologic phenomenon in the early 1950s, and multiple studies of splenectomized patients define key features of this increased susceptibility to infection. It is clear that the risk of postsplenectomy sepsis is inversely related to age.[25] The younger the child is, the greater is the impact and risk of developing overwhelming postsplenectomy sepsis.[26] This feature has clinical implications; for example, elective splenectomy should not be generally performed for patients with hereditary erythrocyte syndromes until after 6 to 10 years of age. For adults, there is a 40% to 60% increased risk of sepsis compared to people with normal splenic function. These postsplenectomy septic episodes typically occur within the first 2 years after splenectomy in 80% of the cases. In adults, the reason for the splenectomy also relates to the incidence of sepsis. After splenectomy for trauma, the instance of sepsis in a large series was 1.4% whereas splenectomy for thalassemia was associated with an incidence of 24.8%. Patients with any associated immunodeficiency such as malignancy or patients undergoing chemotherapy for treatment of Hodgkin disease are also at increased risk for sepsis. The mortality rate of postsplenectomy sepsis is 50% to 60% in most series.

5 Typically, encapsulated organisms cause the postsplenectomy sepsis-related infection. These bacteria have special features that allow them to be opsonized and cleared from circulation by the spleen, making them more dangerous in hyposplenic or splenectomized patients. The most common organism causing postsplenectomy sepsis is *Streptococcus pneumoniae*, which accounts for 50% of septic episodes in most series. In decreasing order of frequency, other bacteria associated with postsplenectomy sepsis are *Haemophilus influenza*, *Neisseria meningitidis*, β-hemolytic streptococcus, *Staphylococcus aureus*, *Escherichia coli*, and *Pseudomonas* species.[25] The current recommendations for patients who are having elective splenectomy are to vaccinate susceptible individuals to pneumococcus strains (Table 73.4).[25] This is ideally done 2 weeks before the operation if possible, but should be done at any time preoperatively or even postoperatively if the patient was not vaccinated. Recent studies have shown that administration of vaccine with the first postoperative visit does not lead to beneficial immune stimulation. Waiting for 14 days postoperatively is equivalent to waiting 1 month or longer.[27] Therefore, vaccination at 2 weeks after an unplanned splenectomy is ideal timing. Polyvalent vaccines, including Pneumovax 23, and Pnu-Immune 23, provide protection against virtually all common strains of pneumococcus.[27] For patients who are at particularly high risk because they may be immunosuppressed, there are also polyvalent vaccines against *Neisseria meningitides* and *Haemophilus influenza* type B. Patients younger than the age of 2 years and patients receiving chemotherapy for malignant disease may not be able to generate an immune response to vaccines and should be vaccinated either after age 2 years or when not receiving chemotherapy. Finally, because of the risk of very rapid progression of sepsis in a postsplenectomy state, patients who have had splenectomy for any reason should be given a medic alert bracelet.

TABLE 73.4

GUIDELINES FOR PREVENTION OF POSTSPLENIC SEPSIS

- Vaccinate with polyvalent pneumococcal vaccine at least 10–14 days prior to splenectomy, if possible.
- If splenectomy is urgent, wait until at least 14 days postprocedure to vaccinate
- For high-risk patients (immunosuppressed, children <10 years of age), meningococcal vaccine and *Haemophilus influenza* vaccine
- Antibiotic prophylaxis for children <5 years of age
- Early antibiotic treatment for initial signs of infection
- Medi-Alert bracelet

Two recent studies highlight the incidence of increased relative risk and number of infections after splenectomy. The relative risk for infection within 90 days of a splenectomy was 10.2% compared to 0.6% in the general population. In patients undergoing appendectomy for acute appendicitis, a control group undergoing an abdominal procedure, there was still increased risk of infection in splenectomy of 10.2% compared to patients who had appendectomy of 4.2%.[28] The relative risk of postsplenectomy infection decreased over time with an overall hazard ratio of 4.6-fold between 90 days and 365 days after splenectomy and 2.5-fold for more than 365 days after splenectomy.[28] There is definite evidence that increased use of vaccination decreases this risk of infection. Another large national study from Scotland showed that the overall rate of first severe infection was 7.0 per 100 person-years after splenectomy. In that subgroup of patients who had a severe infection, the rate of subsequent infections was significantly increased, and the second severe infection rate was 44.9 per 100 person-years, and a third episode of severe infection was 109.3 per 100 person-years.[29] This indicates that the patients who had significant postsplenectomy sepsis should be observed very closely and counseled on seeking medical attention for any sign of any infectious process. The increased trend, particularly after blunt splenic trauma and other hematologic diseases, toward splenic preservation by splenorrhaphy or partial splenectomy, is accompanied by an increased risk of infection in these patients comparable to patients who have a complete splenectomy.[30]

A recent survey of practicing surgeons reviewed patterns of use of immunization for splenectomy patients. Virtually all (99.2%) of active surgeons indicated that they do immunize patients they treat with splenectomy.[31] Nearly everyone administered vaccine to pneumococcus; 72.4% of practicing surgeons routinely used a *Haemophilus influenza* type vaccine, 62.8% gave meningococcal vaccination, and 56.7% used all three vaccines. A few practicing surgeons immunized their patients who had splenorrhaphy (15.7%), and a very small proportion immunized patients who had splenic injury but were managed nonoperatively. Current guidelines are that all patients with elective splenectomies should have prophylactic immunization prior to surgery whereas patients who have unexpected splenectomy should have immunization 14 days after the procedure. All patients should get pneumococcal vaccines, and patients at high risk should have vaccination for *H. influenza* and meningococcus.[31,32]

For decades it has been known that patients after splenectomy are susceptible to infections as just described. It has only recently been realized that there are various vascular complications that occur to a greater degree in patients with splenectomy than in a cohort of abdominal surgery patients without splenectomy.[33] These include arterial thrombosis, venous thrombosis, and pulmonary artery hypertension. Data from patients with hereditary spherocytosis who have undergone splenectomy report between a 5.6- and 7.2-fold increase in ischemic heart disease compared to patients who do not have splenectomy. The most marked finding for arterial events occurs in thalassemia in which patients who undergo splenectomy have a 20-fold increase in arterial atherosclerosis of arterial structures. Acute portal venous thrombosis is reported after splenectomy in one series up to 4.8% for various patients.[34] It is clearly more common after splenectomy in patients with cirrhosis and hypersplenism, when the rate of portal vein thrombosis may be 30% to 40%.[35] However, the incidence of venous thrombosis may extend beyond the mesenteric/portal venous system and include deep venous thrombosis in the pelvis and lower extremities as well as subsequent pulmonary embolus to a much greater extent. This

TABLE 73.5

DEFINITION OF HYPERSPLENISM

Decrease in circulating cell count of erythrocytes and/or platelets and/or leukocytes
and
Normal compensatory hematopoietic responses present in bone marrow
and
Correction of cytopenia by splenectomy
with or without
Splenomegaly

also has led to increased evidence of pulmonary arterial hypertension in patients after splenectomy for hematologic diseases.

The pathogenesis of these vascular events after splenectomy is likely multifactorial.[33] They may involve some element of hypercoagulative state due to altered platelet function and number. There may be some disturbances in vascular epithelium related to other blood elements that are altered after splenectomy. There is also evidence that there are changes in lipid profiles after splenectomy that could promote atherosclerosis and thrombosis.[33] Although these vascular events clearly are increased in frequency, they do not occur in an overwhelming number of patients. This phenomenon does mitigate toward using splenectomy conservatively, particularly in high-risk individuals such as patients with thalassemia.

Hypersplenism

Hypersplenism is increased splenic function that is manifested clinically by the decrease in one or more of the circulating blood elements (Table 73.5). The specific criteria for hypersplenism are as follows: (a) documented anemia, thrombocytopenia, or leukopenia; (b) normal compensatory response by the bone marrow to correct the cytopenia; and (c) correction of this cytopenia by splenectomy. Some definitions of hypersplenism may also include splenomegaly among the criteria. If an enlarged spleen is mandatory for hypersplenism, then diseases or disorders of circulating blood cells such as idiopathic thrombocytopenic purpura (ITP) or autoimmune hemolytic anemia would not be included. A second approach to defining hypersplenism is to categorize disorders in which the spleen is normal anatomically and the disease is related to the circulating cells, distinguished from a second category in which the circulating cells are normal and there is a primary anatomic or functional alteration of the spleen (Table 73.6). For either situation the pathophysiology is that the spleen is the site of destruction for one or more circulating blood elements. In cases of a significantly enlarged spleen, additional symptoms can be caused by mass effect from the spleen on adjacent organs. The most important symptom is early satiety and weight loss as the stomach is compressed between the liver and the enlarged spleen. Hypersplenism is the most important indication for elective isolated splenectomy to reverse the cytopenia and often to relieve compressive symptoms from splenomegaly.

TABLE 73.6

CAUSES OF HYPERSPLENISM

I. Primary diseases of blood cells; normal spleen
- A. Congenital
  - i. Erythrocyte abnormalities
    - a. Hereditary spherocytosis
    - b. Hereditary elliptocytosis
    - c. Glucose 6 phosphate dehydrogenase deficiency
    - d. Pyruvate kinase deficiency
  - ii. Hemoglobin abnormalities
    - a. Thalassemia major
    - b. Sickle cell anemia (eventually results in splenic infarction and hyposplenism)
  - iii. Platelet abnormalities
    - a. Wiskott-Aldrich syndrome
- B. Acquired
  - i. Autoimmune hemolytic anemia
  - ii. Autoimmune neutropenia—Felty syndrome
  - iii. Immune thrombocytopenia purpura
  - iv. Thrombotic thrombocytopenia purpura

II. Primary disorders of the spleen
- A. Neoplastic
  - i. Hairy cell leukemia
  - ii. Chronic lymphocytic leukemia
  - iii. Chronic myelogenous leukemia
  - iv. Non-Hodgkin lymphoma
- B. Cellular infiltrative (hematopoiesis)
  - i. Agnogenic myeloid metaplasia
  - ii. Mastocytosis
  - iii. Chediak-Higashi
- C. Metabolic infiltration
  - i. Gaucher disease
  - ii. Sarcoidosis
- D. Vascular
  - i. Splenic vein thrombosis
  - ii. Portal vein hypertension (cirrhosis)

TREATMENT OF DISORDERS OF THE SPLEEN

Splenic Surgery

Until recently, the only pertinent operation involving the spleen was splenectomy. Appreciation of the increased risk of infection in patients who are asplenic or hyposplenic in the late 1960s and the early 1970s led to two new surgical procedures. First, there was an interest in splenic preservation with procedures including splenorrhaphy and other ways to save damaged spleen. Second, procedures for partial splenectomy were developed primarily for elective surgery in which hypersplenism existed but a complete splenectomy was not necessary. The most recent change in surgery of the spleen relates to the advancements in minimally invasive surgery over the past 15 years.[36] Laparoscopic excision is ideal for many splenic operations, and recent reports have used laparoscopic splenectomy for virtually all indications including removal of massive spleens. In most major centers, laparoscopic splenectomy is now the procedure of choice for elective splenectomy.

To better describe and understand operative indications in surgery of the spleen, one could categorize the splenectomy or procedures of the spleen into eight general areas:

1. Trauma or injury to the spleen.
2. Autoimmune/erythrocyte disorders. In this category of disease, there are specific cytopenias related either to antibodies targeting platelets, erythrocytes, or neutrophils, or anemia due to intrinsic structural changes within the erythrocyte. During these procedures, it is typically important to obtain total splenectomy for complete cure.
3. Hypersplenism results in decreased circulating blood cells often including all subtypes of platelets and red blood cells. Hypersplenism may be related to neoplastic infiltration of the spleen or infiltration with lipids and other stored products that leads to a massive spleen. Hypersplenism also may cause symptoms due to the splenic size.

4. Incidental splenectomy. The spleen may be removed as part of a standard operation to remove the distal pancreas most commonly, and also for proximal gastric cancers due to the direct or nodal involvement. Other enlarged tumors of the left upper quadrant and retroperitoneum including sarcoma and adrenal tumor, and left nephrectomy, may require splenectomy because of association with the spleen or its vessels although it is not a primary tumor of the spleen.
5. Iatrogenic splenectomy. This is a category that may be underreported but relates to the splenectomy or splenic preservation procedures due to incidental injury to the spleen during procedures within the general abdominal cavity or specifically, the left upper quadrant.
6. Diagnostic procedures. In some cases, the spleen is removed primarily to make a clinical diagnosis.[37] An example of this is staging laparotomy for Hodgkin disease, though this is now mainly a historical footnote as the treatment of this lymphoma now rarely requires splenectomy to make the diagnosis.
7. Vascular procedures. Splenectomy during vascular procedures includes treatment of patients with splenic vein thrombosis or less commonly splenic artery aneurysms.
8. Miscellaneous procedures. Treatment of simple and neoplastic cysts, echinococcal cysts, and treatment of the wandering spleen when symptomatic as a congenital anomaly.

There were an estimated 22,000 splenectomies performed in the United States in 2005.[21] Two recent reports have been published describing 10-year experiences for all splenectomies done in their respective institutions. The first report is the combined series of 1,280 splenectomies over a 10-year interval from the Barnes Hospital in St. Louis and the Brigham and Women's Hospital in Boston.[37] The second report is a single institution over the identical time period from Vanderbilt University.[38] In the Barnes/Brigham series, there were 1,280 splenectomies and in the Vanderbilt series there were 896 splenectomies (Table 73.7). Dependent on the type of institution and referral patterns, the indications for splenectomy vary to some degree. In the Vanderbilt series most splenectomies were done for trauma, accounting for 41.5% of all operations done in that institution. In the Barnes/Brigham and Women's series, the most common indication was incidental splenectomy in which the spleen was removed as part of an excision of another organ, typically a large tumor in the left upper quadrant of the abdomen. The second most frequent indication for splenectomy was staging laparotomy for Hodgkin disease. This is likely to be different in the ensuing decade as both treatment indications as well as diagnostic techniques have significantly eliminated this practice since 1990. These differences highlight that, in the centers that have a large trauma population, splenectomies are done for that indication whereas in centers with major cancer referral bases, there are alternative indications. If one eliminates the traumatic, incidental, and staging procedures, the most common indication in both series is autoimmune or erythrocyte disorders.

Splenic Trauma

6 The spleen is the most common intra-abdominal organ injured by blunt trauma in the United States, and in many institutions splenectomy remains the most common operative procedure performed on the spleen.[39] The history of splenic surgery mirrors the history of surgery for trauma. In the ancient medical literature, the spleen often herniated through a flank wound and there are reports of either partial splenectomy or total splenectomy of the herniated portions.[40] The first documented splenectomy for penetrating trauma was performed in San Francisco by a British naval surgeon named O'Brien in 1816 when a spleen protruded out the side of a knife wound.[12] In the late 19th century, Theodor Billroth observed during an autopsy of a patient who died of head trauma 5 days earlier that there was minimal blood in the peritoneum from the fracture of the splenic capsule and predicted that these injuries may be managed operatively. Although in the earlier part of the 20th century splenic trauma was uniformly managed by a complete splenectomy, Dr. Campos Christo of Brazil reported partial splenectomy and splenic salvage for both penetrating and blunt trauma in 1962 (Table 73.1).[2,4] This initial report, combined with the ability to obtain repeated cross-sectional imaging, with the understanding of splenic function and with

TABLE 73.7

INDICATIONS FOR SPLENECTOMY IN TWO LARGE SERIES FROM ACADEMIC MEDICAL CENTERS

	BARNES/BRIGHAM AND WOMENS[a]	VANDERBILT[b]
n	1,280	896
Dates	1986–1995	1986–1995
Trauma	167 (13.0%)	372 (41.5%)
Autoimmune/erythrocyte disorders	219 (17.1%)	140 (15.6%)
Hyperplasia	99 (7.7%)	138 (15.4%)
Incidental	336 (26.3%)	110 (12.3%)
Iatrogenic	N.A.	33 (8.1%)
Diagnostic unknown	122 (9.5%)	18 (2.0%)
Diagnostic staging for Hodgkin disease	258 (20.2%)	N.A.
Vascular	74 (5.8%)	21 (2.3%)
Miscellaneous	5 (0.4%)	24 (2.7%)

[a]From Kraus MD, Fleming MD, Vonderheide RH. The spleen as a diagnostic specimen: a review of 10 years' experience at two tertiary care institutions. *Cancer* 2001;91(11):2001–2009.
[b]From Rose AT, Newman MI, Debelak J, et al. The incidence of splenectomy is decreasing: lessons learned from trauma experience. *Am Surg* 2000;66(5):481–486.

TABLE 73.8

SPLEEN INJURY SCALE

GRADE	LACERATION	HEMATOMA
I	<1 cm in depth	Subcapsular <10% of surface
II	1–3 cm in depth not involving a trabecular vessel	Subcapsular 10%–50% of surface area or 5 cm in diameter
III	>3 cm depth or any depth involving a trabecular vessel	Subcapsular >50% of surface area or intraparenchymal
IV	Segmental or hilar vessel involvement	—
V	Shattered spleen or hilar vessel disruption	—

the appreciation for overwhelming postsplenectomy sepsis, has led to the current guidelines for nonoperative management of lower-grade splenic injuries and operative management centered around splenic preservation when possible.[41]

The most common modes of blunt injuries leading to splenic rupture are motor vehicle accidents and bicycle accidents, in which upper abdominal trauma may occur. The signs and symptoms of isolated splenic injury are tenderness in the left upper quadrant of the abdomen. Attention toward the lower lateral left ribs and focal tenderness over ribs 9 through 11 in that region should raise suspicion of possible splenic injury. Approximately 20% of cases of rib fracture can be demonstrated on radiographs. Patients may have referred pain to the left shoulder (the Kehr sign), particularly when placed in the Trendelenburg position with palpation of the upper abdomen. The spleen itself is rarely palpable, but when a left upper quadrant mass is palpable it can represent contained or subcapsular hematoma; this is known as the Ballance sign. Depending on the severity of the injury, patients may have no hemodynamic instability or may be in frank hypovolemic shock. The staging system for splenic trauma is shown in Table 73.8.

The laboratory abnormalities associated with splenic rupture include a decrease in hematocrit and hemoglobin, although initial assessment before volume resuscitation may show normal levels. After a short period of time there is often a leukocytosis of 15,000 to 20,000. Plain abdominal X-ray views may show left rib fractures and displacement or a corrugated appearance along the greater curvature of the stomach due to a hematoma infiltrating the gastrosplenic ligament (Fig. 73.6). Peritoneal lavage can reveal the presence of blood in the abdomen. The most important current tool for diagnosis is the CT scan, particularly in patients who have enough hemodynamic stability to be managed conservatively. Contrast CT scan shows the splenic contour and also demonstrates the amount of extrasplenic blood (Fig. 73.7).[42]

Blunt injuries constitute most splenic trauma, but the spleen is susceptible to penetrating trauma either in the retroperitoneum, lower thoracic region, or upper abdominal area. A 15-year state review of splenic trauma in Pennsylvania reported 10,652 (92%) blunt injuries and 893 (8%) penetrating injuries.[41] The management and diagnosis of penetrating trauma of the thorax and upper abdomen is less of a diagnostic

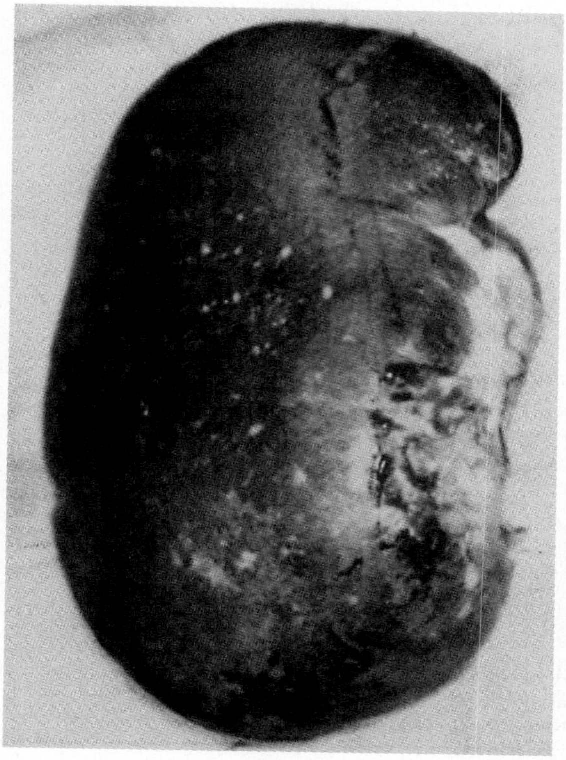

FIGURE 73.6. Abdominal film in a patient with a splenic rupture from blunt trauma with a perisplenic hematoma displacing the greater curvature of the stomach medially. The scalloped appearance is indicative of blood in the gastrosplenic ligament. (Radiograph courtesy of Dr. C. William Schwab.)

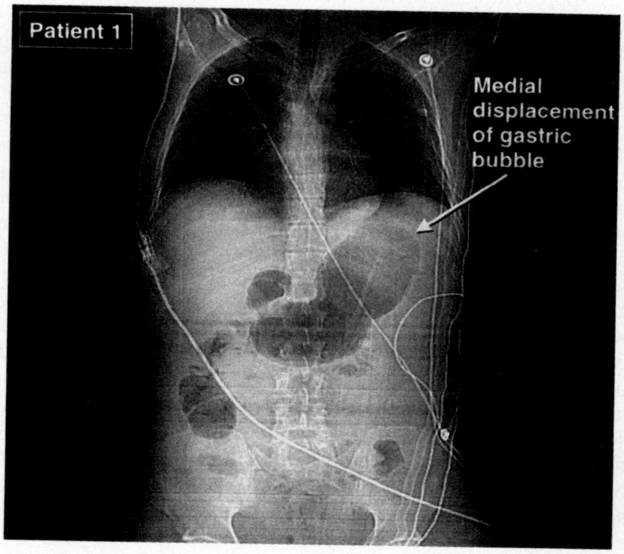

FIGURE 73.7. A contrast CT scan on a patient with splenic rupture near the hilum. There is considerable blood in the perisplenic fossa as well as free blood in the peritoneal cavity around the liver. (Radiograph courtesy of Dr. C. William Schwab.)

dilemma as most of these patients undergo abdominal exploration because of associated injuries. In some series, there are additional injuries in 90% to 100% of patients with penetrating trauma to the spleen and 40% to 60% of patients with associated injuries for blunt trauma.

Management of splenic injuries historically has been a laparotomy with splenectomy. Since Christo introduced the ability to do either partial splenectomy or splenorrhaphy, there has been an increased trend with surgical procedures to try to repair or preserve part if not all of the spleen. The current trend in management is a nonoperative approach with observation by serial CT scans.[43] The presence of peritonitis, associated injuries requiring surgery, the overall injury severity, evidence of hypovolemic shock and ongoing bleeding, and the patient's age are the primary factors that affect decisions regarding nonoperative versus operative management of blunt splenic injuries.[41] When patients have diffuse peritonitis or if patients have hypotension related to hypovolemic shock, urgent laparotomy is indicated (Fig. 73.8). For patients who are hemodynamically stable and do not have other injuries that require surgical management, the recommendation is to attempt nonoperative observation.

The standard nonoperative management protocol includes very close observation in an intensive care unit or a similar monitored environment. Patients have serial abdominal exams as well as serial hemoglobin and hematocrit assessments. Any change in the status of a stable patient is evaluated by CT scan to assess for progressive or ongoing bleeding demonstrated by increased hemoperitoneum or expansion of splenic hematoma. A recent report noted that routine follow-up CT scans did not alter management in patients treated nonoperatively.[44] Only patients with changes in hemodynamic parameters had a change in management. With this conservative management, most patients avoid laparotomy for isolated splenic blunt trauma.[45] If patients are older, have associated injuries, or have ongoing blood loss, a laparotomy is appropriate for blunt splenic trauma.[40,46] The nature of the splenic injury is graded relative to the degree of damage to the splenic parenchyma and the proximity to the splenic hilum and major blood vessels (Table 73.8). The principles of operative management include stopping ongoing hemorrhage while preserving the maximal amount of viable splenic parenchyma. Nonviable or devascularized tissue must be débrided.[47] Partial splenectomy has been used based on the concept of segmental blood supply via the trabecular arteries. Various approaches can be taken to more minor peripheral splenic trauma including primary repair or mesh repair (Fig. 73.9). Multiple materials that are available for hemostasis including microfibrillar collagen, thrombin-soaked Gelfoam, or fibrin glue sealants have been used to obtain control of splenic hemorrhage. The argon beam coagulator is a very useful instrument for capsular tear or avulsions. Of note, all of these techniques that have been applied to the patient suffering from blunt trauma can be similarly applied to patients who have inadvertent trauma to the spleen during operations on the splenic flexure of the colon or the left kidney, adrenal gland, or stomach.

Over the past decade, this increasing trend toward nonsurgical management has expanded the number of patients who were not explored and increased the overall success rate of conservative management. A recent study of more than 625 patients with blunt trauma showed that there was an increase in initial nonoperative management from 61% to 85%.[48] The success rate of nonoperative management increased from 77% to 96% and the splenic salvage rate from 57% to 88%.[48] Part of this may be due to a decreased distribution of more severe splenic injuries and part of it may be due to a trend toward use of embolization of splenic arteries as part of the nonoperative management of blunt trauma.

Since its introduction in 1992 as a potential maneuver to improve the nonoperative management of blunt splenic injury, embolization, with either coils or Gelfoam, of either proximal or distal splenic vessels, has become more common.[49] In a study comparing the outcome of blunt trauma over the past two decades, the use of embolization increased from 2.7% to 22.6%.[48] Most studies provide similar data showing that the overall success rate for nonoperative management is improved with the use of splenic artery embolization, including a

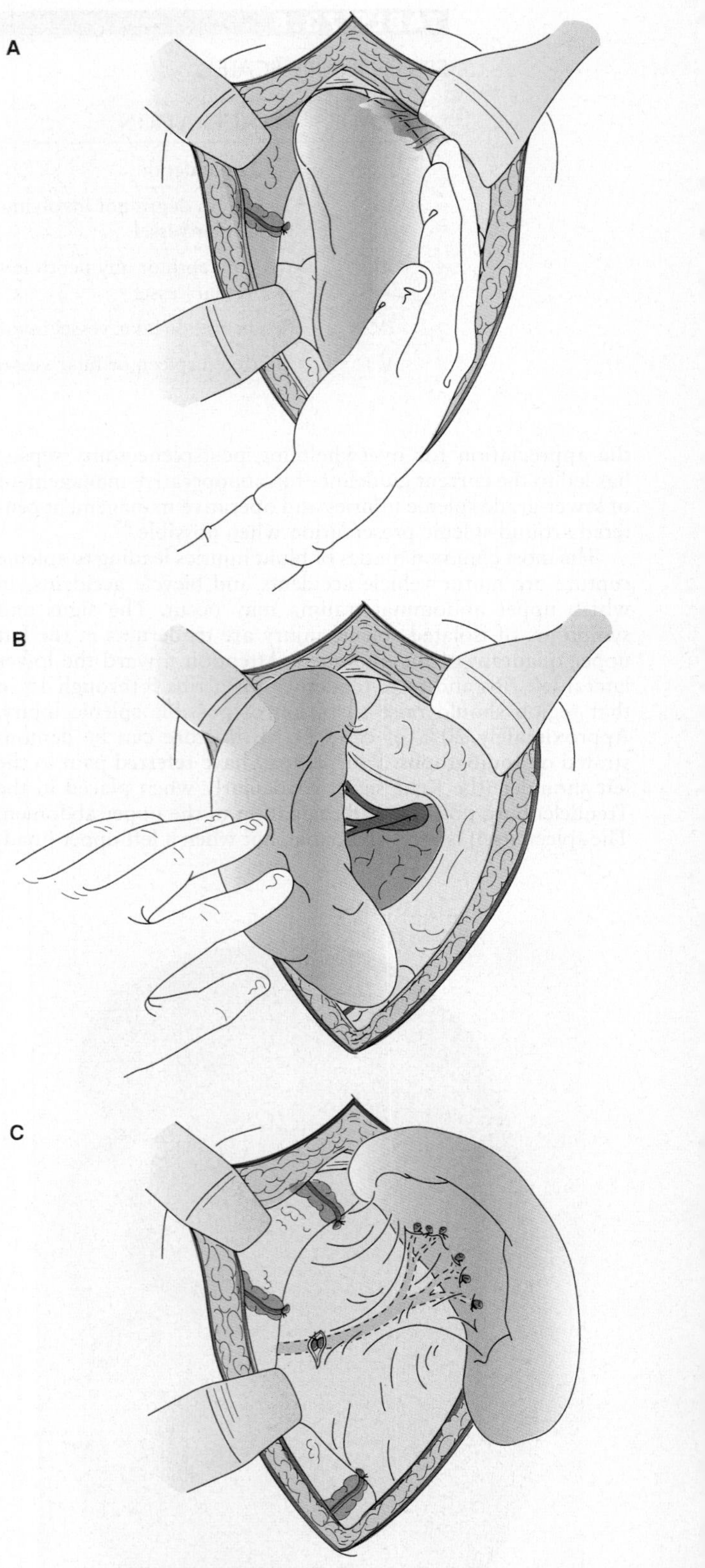

FIGURE 73.8. **A** and **B:** Rapid mobilization of a bleeding spleen can be accomplished in most patients by blunt dissection of the lateral attachments. **C:** The splenic hilum can then be quickly controlled.

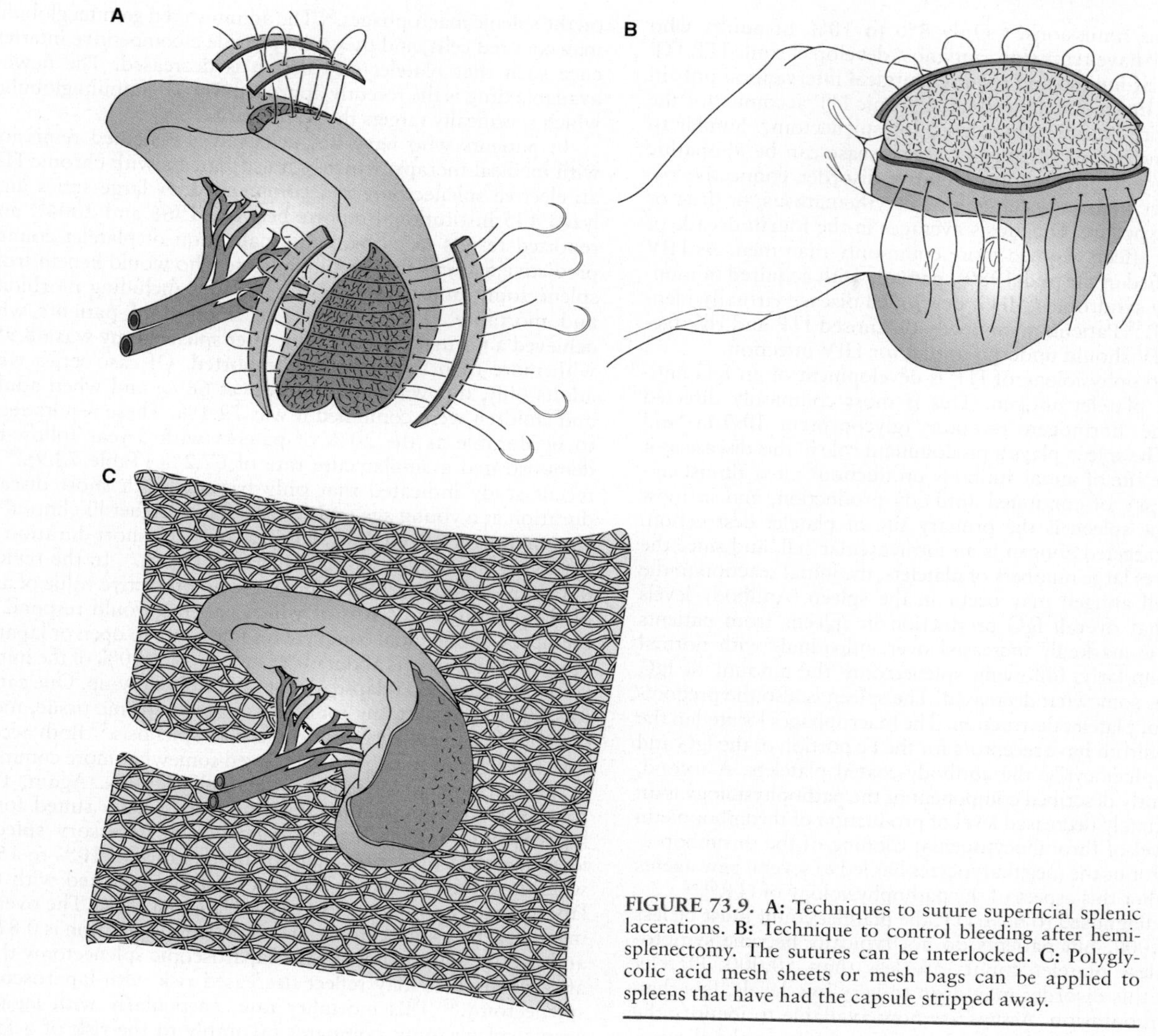

FIGURE 73.9. **A:** Techniques to suture superficial splenic lacerations. **B:** Technique to control bleeding after hemisplenectomy. The sutures can be interlocked. **C:** Polyglycolic acid mesh sheets or mesh bags can be applied to spleens that have had the capsule stripped away.

decreased use of blood products.[50] Some recent studies have stated that embolization may be overused; one reported a failure rate of 27% in patients with embolization who then needed surgical exploration.[51] Again, these comparative studies are not matched in terms of severity of injury or even the techniques used for the splenic artery embolization.

One issue with the nonoperative management of blunt splenic trauma is the risk of delayed rupture. Standard guidelines of conservative management are that patients should have stable hemoglobin for 36 to 48 hours and have resolution of abdominal pain prior to discharge. The delayed rupture rate in a large series of more than 1,900 patients showed that 27 patients were readmitted for splenectomy after discharge.[52] This is a delayed rupture rate of 1.4%.[53] The median time from injury to readmission for splenectomy was 8 days with a range of 3 to 146 days. Similar results were obtained in an institutional study of 450 patients with nonoperative management of blunt splenic injury. In this group, 4% failed with eventual splenectomy due to delayed rupture.[52] Both studies stress that with increased use of nonoperative management, the potential risks of delayed rupture require very specific instructions to patients, emphasizing that re-onset of acute abdominal pain with other signs and symptoms of hypotension requires emergent transportation to the nearest emergency room or hospital facility.

Atraumatic splenic rupture is an unusual occurrence. This spontaneous rupture occurs primarily with enlargement of the spleen due to malignant disorders with either primary or secondary metastases, infectious or inflammatory diseases, or mechanical causes such as pregnancy or peripartum rupture. In a large series of more than 900 patients with atraumatic spontaneous rupture of the spleen, only 6.4% had no pathologic or mechanical causes that were identified.[54]

Autoimmune Disorders

Some splenic disease originates in either autoimmune phenomena or intrinsic diseases within circulating cells that lead to their destruction rather than histology, pathology, or size of the spleen. The most common example of this is immune thrombocytopenic purpura (ITP) in which antibodies to platelet antigens lead to destruction of platelets and thrombocytopenia, with the spleen being the primary source of platelet elimination. Related diseases affecting erythrocytes and neutrophils with specific antibodies and splenic elimination occur less frequently.

Immune Thrombocytopenic Purpura. Immune thrombocytopenic purpura (ITP) is a diagnosis of exclusion once various other causes such as drug-induced thrombocytopenia or evidence of bone marrow failure are eliminated.[55] ITP is a disease characterized by autoimmune destruction of platelets with clinical manifestations of thrombocytopenia such as easy or excess bleeding.[56] ITP occurs as an acute form and a chronic form. Acute ITP generally appears in children younger than 8 years of age following a viral upper respiratory illness. Eighty percent to ninety percent of children with acute ITP have spontaneous remissions.[57] Only 8% to 10% of adults who develop ITP have remission, and most develop chronic ITP. ITP is usually self-limited and requires surgical intervention only in the case of intracranial bleeding. Chronic ITP accounts for the vast majority of cases considered for splenectomy. Similar to autoimmune hemolytic anemia, this disease can be idiopathic or secondary to a lymphoproliferative disorder, connective tissue disorder such as systemic lupus erythematosus, or drug or bacterial exposure. Diagnosis averages in the fourth decade of life, and it affects women more commonly than men. As HIV was identified in the mid-1980s, patients with acquired immunodeficiency syndrome (AIDS) developed disease virtually identical to ITP.[58] Patients with newly diagnosed ITP and risk factors for HIV should undergo testing for HIV infection.

7 The pathophysiology of ITP is development of an IgG antibody to a platelet antigen. This is most commonly directed against the fibrinogen receptor (glycoprotein IIb/IIIa and IR/IX).[59] The spleen plays a predominant role in this disease as it may be the site of initial antibody production[60]; it is almost certainly the site of continued antibody production, and in most patients the spleen is the primary site of platelet destruction. Since the targeted antigen is an intravascular cell, and since the spleen stores large numbers of platelets, the initial reaction to the platelet cell antigen may occur in the spleen. Antibody levels indicate that overall IgG production in spleens from patients with ITP is markedly increased over individuals with normal spleens. Similarly, following splenectomy the amount of IgG antibody is somewhat decreased. The spleen is also the predominant site of platelet destruction. The macrophages located in the cords of Billroth have receptors for the Fc portion of the IgG and bind and phagocytize the antibody-coated platelets. A second, more recently described component of the pathophysiology is an inappropriately decreased level of production of thrombopoietin for the level of thrombocytopenia. Cloning of the thrombopoietin receptor or the megakaryocytes has led to several new agents that can alter this aspect of the pathophysiology of ITP.[61,62]

To be diagnosed to have ITP, the platelet count must be less than 100,000, but patients do not typically become symptomatic unless platelet counts are less than 50,000. Platelet counts in this disorder may drop to very low levels, less than 10,000 on occasion. Assays are now available to identify the IgG antiglobulin on the platelet surface verifying the disease, but more than one third of the patients have no identified antiplatelet antibodies. Bone marrow analysis shows increased megakaryocyte production as compensatory mechanism to the thrombocytopenia. In this disorder, there is usually no splenomegaly and the spleen may be somewhat smaller than typical. Only 2% of patients with ITP have palpable spleens. There is virtually no leukopenia or anemia associated with ITP hypersplenism. Anemia can occur secondary to chronic blood loss. The risk of a fatal hemorrhage in patients with ITP overall is 0.47%/year, and for patients with platelet counts less than 30,000 mortality ranges between 1.6% and 6.9%.[57]

The treatment of ITP includes standard measures to treat any ongoing bleeding, medical therapies designed to increase platelet count, and splenectomy. First-line medical therapy options include platelet transfusion, corticosteroid therapy, gamma-immunoglobulin, and the recently approved Rho(d) immunoglobulin.[63] Platelet transfusions should be limited unless patients are actively bleeding as platelets become rapidly coated with IgG and then sequestered and destroyed in the spleen. High-dose corticosteroid therapy produces an initial response in most patients, but this is usually not sustained. Approximately 75% of patients have an increase in platelet count that is significant within 24 hours of starting high-dose steroids.[64] However, only 15% to 25% of patients with chronic ITP have a sustained remission following steroid therapy. Intravenous IgG immunoglobulin takes between 3 and 5 days to show an effect and generally does not put patients into complete remission. The mechanism of action of immune gamma globulin is believed to be saturation of the Fc receptors on the splenic macrophages.[65] The administered gamma globulin may coat red cells, and they may provide a competitive interference such that platelet destruction is decreased. The newest available drug is the recently approved Rho(d) immunoglobulin, which specifically targets the Fc receptors.

In patients who have not achieved a sustained remission with medical therapy, which is most patients with chronic ITP, an elective splenectomy is recommended. A large series analyzed 135 institutional reports between 1966 and 2004[66] and reported results in terms of normalization of platelet counts, predictive features that would indicate who would benefit from splenectomy, and reported complications including morbidity and mortality (Table 73.9). The fraction of patients who achieved a normal platelet count after splenectomy was 68.9% with more than 5,000 patients reported. Of case series with adults only, this was slightly lower at 66%, and when adults and children were combined it was 72.1%. These results seem to be durable as the 20% of patents with 5-year follow-up demonstrated a similar cure rate of 67.2% (Table 73.9).[66] A recent study indicated that only patients with short disease duration at a young age (<16 years) had a higher likelihood of cure on univariate analysis, whereas only the short duration of disease was a feature in multivariate analysis.[67] In the review of the 135 combined series, there was no predictive value of any of these features in terms of which patients would respond to therapy. Overall initial complete response rate to open or laparoscopic splenectomy is about 60%, and 15% to 20% of the initial responders develop relapse with long-term follow-up. One cause for a failed splenectomy for ITP is residual splenic tissue, most commonly a missed accessory spleen or splenosis.[17] Both accessory spleens and splenosis are believed somewhat more common in the current era of laparoscopic splenectomy. Again, ITP spleens are predominantly small and are ideally suited for a laparoscopic approach. The incidence of accessory spleens identified with open procedures is in the range of 10% to 15% whereas the incidence of accessory spleens reported with the laparoscopic approach is between 5% and 12%.[68] The overall mortality from splenectomy in this patient population is 0.81% and may be slightly lower after laparoscopic splenectomy than after open. This may reflect decreased risk with laparoscopic splenectomy.[69] This mortality rate, particularly with laparoscopic splenectomy, compares favorably to the risk of a fatal hemorrhage in patients who have significant thrombocytopenia with this disease. The overall complication rate was 12%.

Third-line treatment for ITP after splenectomy failure has been accomplished with various new agents. There were initially several studies with rituximab, which is a chimeric humanized monoclonal antibody directing CD20 against B cells.[70–72] It was primarily developed to treat lymphoma, but it has been used in autoimmune disorders and has been tried in phase 2 studies for chronic splenectomy failure ITP. Response rates have been between 25% and 50%. A more promising third-line therapy is agonist agents to stimulate the thrombopoietin receptor on megakaryocytes. There is decreased thrombopoietin production for the degree of thrombocytopenia in ITP. Romiplostim, a fusion protein agonist for thrombopoietin receptor administered by subcutaneous injection, led to response rates of 49% versus 2% for placebo with an overall clinical response of 83%.[59,73] An oral nonpeptide thrombopoietin receptor agonist, eltrombopag, has recently been studied and shows response rates of 59% versus 16% in a placebo-controlled trial.[74,75] Although now proven as effective third-line agents after splenectomy failures, they may be useful as initial therapies for patients who cannot tolerate steroids or patients who are splenectomy candidates who are very high risk for surgery. Future studies will define the role of this new class of compounds and may decrease the incidence and need for splenectomy.

Thrombotic Thrombocytopenia Purpura. Thrombotic thrombocytopenia purpura (TTP), or Moschcowitz syndrome,

TABLE 73.9

RESULTS FROM 135 COMBINED CASE SERIES EVALUATING SPLENECTOMY FOR ITP

CURE RATE		
% of patients with normalized platelet counts		
All reports	68.9%	(3,506/5,086)
Adult series only	66.0%	(1,731/2,623)
Adult pediatric combined	72.1%	(1,785/2,468)
% of patients with normalized platelet counts With 5-year follow-up	67.2%	(779/1,159)
COMPLICATIONS		
Perioperative mortality		
Total	0.81%	51/6,256
Laparotomy	0.96%	48/4,955
Laparoscopy	0.23%	3/1,301
Perioperative complications		
Total	12.0%	406/3,386
Laparotomy	12.9%	318/2,465
Laparoscopy	9.6%	88/921

Adapted from Zarzaur BL, Vashi S, Magnotti LJ, et al. The real risk of splenectomy after discharge home following nonoperative management of blunt splenic injury. *J Trauma* 2009;66:1531–1538.

is a poorly understood much more virulent syndrome than ITP in which thrombocytopenic purpura is only one manifestation. This disease is characterized by widespread occlusion of arterioles and capillaries by hyalin membranes composed of platelets and fibrinogen. The classic pentad of symptoms reflects injury to various organs by this microvascular process. This includes thrombocytopenic purpura, with microvascular disease in the skin, neurologic manifestations due to microvascular disease in the central nervous system, renal failure or hematuria due to microvascular disease in the kidney, microvascular hemolytic anemia due to destruction of red cells traveling to damaged small vessels, and fever. The precise etiology is unknown but may be related to an autoimmune response to a small vessel endothelial cell antigen.

The therapeutic options for this disease include administration of fresh frozen plasma and/or plasmapheresis, high-dose corticosteroids, and antiplatelet drugs.[76] The benefits of plasmapheresis indicate that there is a circulating toxic substance contributing to the etiology, whereas the benefit of administration of fresh frozen plasma indicates lack of some necessary substance yet to be identified. High-dose corticosteroids also have some benefit. Aspirin and dipyridamole block platelet agglutination. A combination of these therapies now leads to significant improvement of symptoms in 70% of patients. For patients failing to respond or patients who relapse, splenectomy has been performed with some success.[77,78] Most of the long-term survivors with TTP have undergone splenectomy, implying that this organ has some major role in the pathophysiology of this disease.[79] The precise mechanism of splenic contribution is unclear. Mortality rates in the past have been as high as 90% to 95% for this disorder but are improving with aggressive treatment plans and a better understanding and diagnosis of this disorder.

Autoimmune Hemolytic Anemia. Autoimmune hemolytic anemia or acquired hemolytic anemia results from antibodies produced to red cell membrane proteins that lead to red cell destruction. This disease is more common in women than men with a ratio of 2:1, and it typically presents in patients older than 50 years of age. Patients present with acute symptoms of anemia, jaundice, and occasional fever. The spleen is enlarged in approximately one half of the patients. Laboratory diagnosis shows a positive direct Coomb test indicating antibodies coating erythrocytes. There is also significant reticulocytosis and increased indirect bilirubin in the serum.

The disease is either idiopathic, in 40% to 50% of the cases in which no identified drug or infectious cause is identified, or secondary to infection or drug. Of the secondary cases, the most common infections are mycoplasmal pneumonia, viral infections, infectious mononucleosis, and AIDS. Neoplastic diseases such as leukemia and lymphoma can also precipitate the syndrome. The major drugs that cause secondary autoimmune hemolytic anemia are penicillin, quinidine, hydralazine, and methyldopa.

Autoimmune hemolytic anemia is also categorized by presence of either cold antibodies or warm antibodies. Warm antibodies are predominantly IgG whereas cold antibodies are predominantly IgM. This distinction is important when considering splenectomy as a treatment. The spleen contains macrophages that bind the Fc portion of IgG. In patients with warm antibody hemolytic anemia, the spleen is the primary source of destruction of the red cells by the red pulp macrophages. However, since the spleen does not contain receptors to bind IgM (the cold antibodies), there is no destruction of the red cells in this form of hemolytic anemia. Rather, IgM either causes complement fixation with destruction of red cells predominantly in the liver, or there is agglutination of red cells in peripheral circulation (such as the distal extremities) leading to peripheral red cell destruction with clinical manifestations similar to the Raynaud phenomenon. Splenectomy for patients with cold antibody or IgM hemolytic anemia is not effective.

The initial treatment of autoimmune hemolytic anemia consists of supportive therapy such as blood transfusions. For patients who have disease secondary to an acute infection such as mycoplasma pneumonia, the disease may be self-limited. For drug-induced hemolytic anemia, the offending agent is removed as quickly as possible. The initial form of treatment is typically high-dose corticosteroids, which cause a beneficial response in 75% of the patients. If patients have drug-induced disease and the offending agent is removed or the acute infection resolves, this may lead to long-term resolution. In idiopathic autoimmune hemolytic anemia, only 25% of patients have sustained remission from corticosteroid therapy. In patients who have relapse after steroid therapy or who are ineligible for steroid therapy and have warm antibodies, a splenectomy has a high likelihood of benefit. Eighty percent of patients have a good response in correcting the anemia by splenectomy.[80] This is almost certainly related to removal of the site of destruction of the erythrocytes but also may be due to decreased production of antibodies.

Autoimmune Neutropenia (Felty Syndrome). Approximately 1% of patients with chronic rheumatoid arthritis develop splenomegaly and neutropenia. This triad of rheumatoid arthritis, neutropenia, and splenomegaly is known as Felty syndrome.[81] High levels of IgG have been identified on the surface of neutrophils with evidence of increased production of granulocytes in the bone marrow. Pathologic analysis of spleens removed in patients with Felty syndrome show a significant but proportional increase in the white pulp of the spleen compared with other conditions of splenomegaly.[82] Microscopically, there is evidence of excess accumulation of neutrophils in the T-cell zone and the white pulp, as well as within the cords and sinuses of the red pulp.

Patients with this disease have recurrent infections due to neutropenia as well as dysfunction of the available neutrophils that are coated with antineutrophil IgG. Recurrent infections as well as chronic leg ulcers are the predominant symptoms. Symptomatic patients should undergo splenectomy, and the vast majority of patients have resolution of their neutropenia within 2 to 3 days.[83] Even patients who do not have a significant increase in neutrophil count should get some benefit because of improved neutrophil function.[84]

Erythrocyte or Platelet Structure Disorders

These diseases are not autoimmune phenomena, but rather, intrinsic cellular defects that lead to a shortened half-life of specific blood components primarily precipitating elimination within the spleen. A normal role of the spleen is to eliminate senescent erythrocytes. If erythrocytes have altered structure, this may lead to more rapid elimination. In other diseases, genetic differences in the hemoglobin may result in changes in splenic clearance of cells, particularly in the hypoxic environment that exists within the splenic sinusoids. The most prevalent example of this is sickle cell anemia. A parallel condition occurs in the platelets in Wiskott-Aldrich syndrome, which is an alteration in a cellular adhesion molecule that leads to increased platelet destruction in the spleen and thus to thrombocytopenia.

Hereditary Spherocytosis. Hereditary spherocytosis, also known as congenital hemolytic jaundice or familial hemolytic anemia, is an autosomal dominant disease and the most common of the congenital hemolytic anemias. It affects 1 in 5,000 individuals.[85] There are various genetic defects in this syndrome that primarily affect spectrin and ankyrin, which alter the binding of the cytoskeleton to the erythrocyte cellular membrane causing decreased cellular plasticity with membrane loss.[86] The normal shape of the erythrocyte is changed from the biconcave disc into a sphere, and the decreased membrane to cell volume ratio causes a lack of deformability, which affects the passage of erythrocytes through channels of the splenic red pulp. Due to this delay in cell transit, there is ATP deprivation resulting in increased cellular destruction. The condition is more frequent in Caucasians than African Americans and is usually noted in childhood or adolescence. Since inheritance is autosomal dominant, patients can be screened and diagnosed at an early age.

The diagnosis is primarily made by evaluation of the red cell smear showing a large number of spherocytes. Spherocytes may also appear during autoimmune hemolytic anemias, but in hereditary spherocytosis the Coombs test is negative and an osmotic fragility test may be performed, which is diagnostic. Also contributing to the diagnosis is a positive family history.

Patients with hereditary spherocytosis have mild to moderate anemia, splenomegaly, and jaundice. The patients may have intermittent flares of disease, which cause significant increased rates of hemolysis causing jaundice. Pigmented gallstones result in 30% to 60% of patients due to the breakdown of hemoglobin and clearance through the liver.[85]

The treatment for hereditary spherocytosis is splenectomy, and this is indicated in virtually all patients.[87] This treatment does not remove the spherocytes, but it relieves all symptoms.[88] The major question involving management of these patients is the timing of splenectomy. Due to the increased incidence of overwhelming postsplenectomy sepsis in very young children, it is usually recommended that patients wait until after the age of at least 4 to 6 years prior to splenectomy. For younger patients who are very symptomatic and require splenectomy, partial splenectomies have been reported to be beneficial in relieving the abdominal symptoms and anemia and may be a useful alternative procedure until patients reach an age at which total splenectomy is safer.[89] Patients after partial splenectomies had regrowth of tissue but in the short term did not have recurrent anemia.[80] Patients should be assessed at the time of scheduling a splenectomy for the presence of gallstones, and a laparoscopic cholecystectomy should be performed if stones are identified.

Hereditary Elliptocytosis. Hereditary elliptocytosis is related to hereditary spherocytosis although the former is not as severe. For patients who are symptomatic, virtually all of the same observations regarding pathophysiology and treatment can be made as for hereditary spherocytosis. This disease is also inherited in an autosomal dominant pattern, and the defect is believed to be in spectrin. The predominant abnormality changes spectrin such that it exists as a dimer instead of a tetramer. This change leads to an alteration in membrane plasticity that creates cells that are more elliptically shaped instead of a biconcave disc.

The signs and symptoms caused in this disease are much more mild than in hereditary spherocytosis in that only 10% of patients have clinical manifestations of anemia, splenomegaly, and in some cases jaundice. The treatment recommendation for symptomatic patients is splenectomy, which may be performed with laparoscopic techniques and also cholecystectomy if gallstones are present.

Hereditary Nonspherocytic Hemolytic Anemia. This is a heterogeneous group of rare hemolytic anemias caused by inherited defects, primarily enzymes involved in glycolysis. These genetic defects may decrease cellular energy production such that during passage through the red pulp of the spleen, these patients may have cells that do not have the ability to produce ATP in a relatively hypoxic environment, leading to increased red cell destruction. The most common subtypes in this group of hemolytic anemias are pyruvate kinase deficiency and glucose 6-phosphate dehydrogenase deficiency (G6PD). Patients present with anemia, jaundice, increased reticulocytes, and sometimes cholelithiasis. Differentiation from spherocytosis and elliptocytosis can be made in that the shape of the cell does not show spherocytes and there is normal osmotic fragility.

The primary treatment for these diseases is blood transfusion. In G6PD deficiency, splenectomy is not usually beneficial though it may reverse some of the symptoms associated with pyruvate kinase deficiency.

Thalassemia. Thalassemia is an autosomal dominant disease with various structural defects in one of the globin chains. The disease is either alpha, beta, gamma, or delta thalassemia depending on which of the globin chains is defective. The vast majority of patients in North America have beta-thalassemia. Thalassemia major, otherwise known as Mediterranean anemia or Cooley anemia, is a homozygous expression of this genetic defect. Thalassemia minor is heterozygous expression; these patients are only mildly symptomatic and are carriers for the more severe form of the disease.

The pathophysiology of thalassemia major or beta-thalassemia is the lack of production of normal beta-chain hemoglobin leading to a surplus of alpha-chain hemoglobin in adults. These excess globin chains precipitate in the cytoplasm and attach to the inner surfaces of cytoplasmic membrane, leading to poor passage of these cells through the splenic sinusoids. This intracellular inclusion then leads to increased destruction and over time causes significant splenomegaly due to this increased clearance of red cells.

The diagnosis is made by identifying microcytic hypochromic anemia with target cells and increase in reticulocytes on the peripheral smear. Protein electrophoresis shows very low levels of hemoglobin A with predominant amounts of the fetal hemoglobin, or hemoglobin F. The clinical symptom of alpha-thalassemia major is severe anemia within the first year of life. Decreased growth rate, enlargement of the head, splenomegaly, and hepatomegaly are the typical clinical findings.[90]

The primary treatment for thalassemia major is frequent transfusions combined with iron chelation therapy. Some patients develop significant splenomegaly due to overload or hypertrophy from excess trapping of red cells.[91] Patients may be referred for splenectomy for symptomatic splenomegaly or for massive and frequent transfusion requirements. One report suggested that episodes of transfusion are decreased from 18 per year down to 4 per year after splenectomy. In general, if there are symptoms of massive splenomegaly, these are resolved by splenectomy. As with other hematologic disorders in children, there has been a recent trend toward partial splenectomy, particularly in children younger than 4 to 5 years of age.[92] This results in symptomatic improvement for 1 to 2 years with recurrent disease due to hypertrophy of the residual splenic remnant.[93]

Although splenectomy may be beneficial in terms of the transfusion requirements and local symptoms, the typical mode of death with this disease is myocardial failure due to hemosiderin accumulation. Splenectomy does not alter this cardiac problem to any great extent. In fact, recent data suggest splenectomy in thalassemia patients increases vascular complications.

Sickle Cell Anemia. Sickle cell anemia is a hereditary hemolytic anemia due to a genetic alteration of a single amino acid in the beta chain. This results in a change from glutamic acid to valine in the sixth amino acid position of the beta chain of the hemoglobin molecule. Because of this substitution, patients who are homozygous for sickle cell defect have a characteristic stiffening or sickling of the red blood cells when the cells become hypoxic.[94] This change in red cell shape leads to blockage in hypoxic areas such as the red pulp of the spleen. There can occasionally be sequestration crises in which a portion of the blood volume gets actively trapped or sequestered to the spleen during the sickle cell crisis. This pattern of red cell shape change in relatively hypoxic areas can lead to tissue infarction with bone pain, hematuria, abdominal pain, or priapism.

Sickle cell anemia occurs almost exclusively in the black population, and the incidence of homozygous disease is approximately 0.5%, though approximately 8% of African Americans are carriers for the sickle cell trait. Patients who have a combination of a sickle cell allele as well as a beta-thalassemia allele manifest a similar disease process.

The clinical signs of the disease usually present during the second 6 months of life. In early infancy the patient is asymptomatic due to the presence of fetal hemoglobin. Patients may have acute crises with abdominal pain and bone pain in conjunction with significant anemia. During acute crises of splenic sequestration, there can be massive enlargement of the spleen and an urgent decompressive splenectomy can be required. Patients who do not need splenectomy for splenic sequestration can be followed as this disease goes through a natural progression of ischemic necrosis of large areas of the spleen with eventual hyposplenism with a shrunken organ by early adolescence. Splenectomy is reserved for the very young patients who have massive splenomegaly during sequestration crises early in life.

Wiskott-Aldrich Syndrome. Wiskott-Aldrich syndrome is an X-linked disease characterized by thrombocytopenia, combined B- and T-cell deficiency, eczema, and a propensity to develop other malignancies. The genetic defect in this disease is related to an abnormal adhesion molecule affecting immune cell interaction as well as platelet adhesion. Thrombocytopenia is the major problem with this rare disease, and most patients present at a young age with manifestations of poor clotting, bloody diarrhea, epistaxis, and petechiae. The platelet counts typically range between 20,000 and 40,000, and the platelets that are present are 25% to 50% of normal platelet volume and dysfunctional. In this disease, the spleen sequesters platelets and partially degrades them releasing "microplatelets" back into the circulation.[95]

Splenectomy in the Wiskott-Aldrich syndrome was initially avoided as there was a very problematic postoperative course characterized by severe and fatal infections due to the underlying immunodeficiency combined with the potential for overwhelming postsplenectomy infection. However, splenectomy does increase the number, size, and function of platelets and can lead to amelioration of the bleeding problems in very symptomatic patients.[95] The combination of splenectomy with antibiotic therapy may be beneficial, particularly in younger patients. The optimal treatment for Wiskott-Aldrich syndrome is an HLA-matched sibling bone marrow transplant.[96] However, splenectomy with antibiotics results in better survival than unmatched bone marrow transplantation. Patients who do not undergo bone marrow transplantation or splenectomy typically do not survive past the age of 5 years. The pathology of spleens removed for Wiskott-Aldrich syndrome show a near complete depletion of white pump supporting the clinical immune deficiency seen in this syndrome.[97]

Hypersplenism

8 Hypersplenism is a physical enlargement of the spleen that can occur due to neoplastic disorders, hematopoietic disorders of the bone marrow, and metabolic or storage disorders. In the neoplastic disorders, the spleen is infiltrated and enlarged by leukemia or lymphoma cells. This often happens in the mid or late course of the disease but can be associated with isolated splenomegaly in which splenectomy is performed not only to treat hypersplenism, but also to make the definitive diagnosis (see Diagnostic Splenectomy section later). Hypersplenism associated with diseases of hematopoiesis related to myeloid metaplasia in which the bone marrow is infiltrated with fibrotic material and the spleen becomes a site of secondary non–bone marrow hematopoiesis. Enlargement can lead to symptoms of hypersplenism due to the massive size of the spleen. Often the benefits of extramedullary hematopoiesis are outweighed by circulating blood cell destruction in this enlarged spleen. Secondary hypersplenism can also occur due to deposition of lipid within the spleen, such as in Gaucher disease, leading to enlargement that can cause pancytopenia. Each of these etiologies of secondary hypersplenism is associated with pancytopenia and mass effect of the spleen causing early satiety and weight loss. These disorders typically lead to spleen size greater than 1,500 g and can produce spleens that fill the entire left side of the abdomen.

Chronic Lymphocytic Leukemia. Chronic lymphocytic leukemia (CLL) is the most common of all chronic leukemias. It predominantly affects males with 2:1 gender predominance and has a peak incidence in the sixth decade of life. This indolent disease presents with fatigue, lymphadenopathy, hepatosplenomegaly,

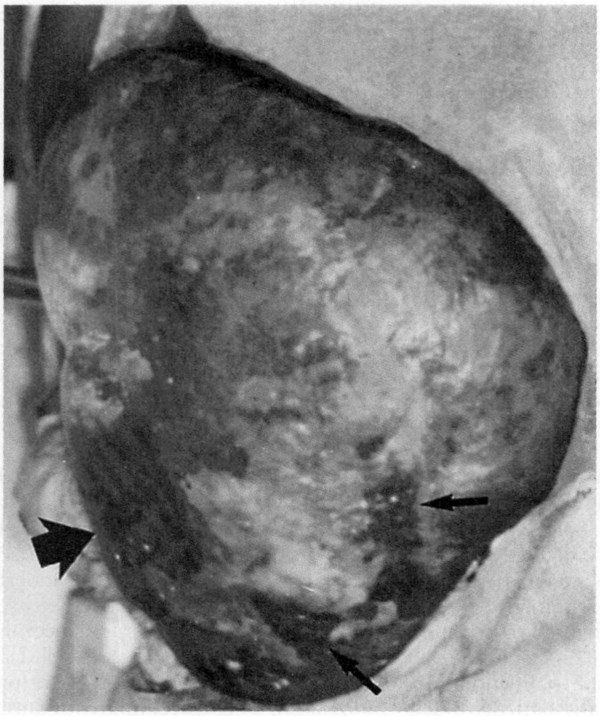

FIGURE 73.10. A massively enlarged, 2.2-kg spleen from a patient with chronic lymphocytic leukemia. Superficial areas of infarction are indicated by *thin arrows* and splenic infarction by the *thick arrow*.

and eventually anemia and thrombocytopenia. Disease progression often occurs over a 5- to 10-year period.

Patients in stage II or greater CLL have splenomegaly and anemia and thrombocytopenia secondary to hypersplenism. Splenomegaly often reaches very large sizes, and patients may have symptoms secondary to the compressive effects of the large spleen on the stomach with early satiety and pain (Fig. 73.10). Treatment for early-stage disease is either observation or treatment with nontoxic doses of alkylating agents such as chlorambucil or cyclophosphamide. A newer agent that is frequently used is fludarabine. Medical therapy is never curative, and eventually the predominant symptoms are due to hypersplenism and splenomegaly. Splenic radiation has been used for patients who are nonoperative candidates.[98] Splenic radiation can decrease the size of the spleen, improving symptoms due to mass effect, but it can have complications of further thrombocytopenia and leukopenia.

Splenectomy is a highly successful treatment for both the pressure effects due to splenomegaly as well as the cytopenias.[99–101] Published reports include 85% resolution of thrombocytopenia and 100% resolution of anemia.[102] The negative feature of splenectomy in this patient population is that they are typically elderly and debilitated from having gone through years of having CLL and prior chemotherapy treatment. In one series in which a prospective comparison was made between splenectomy and fludarabine for later-stage CLL, there was a 9% perioperative mortality in the splenectomy group primarily due to sepsis.[103] However, in this same study, there were highly significant improvements in thrombocytopenia and anemia. The patients who are younger and have larger spleens tend to do better. In this comparative study, patients with Rai stage IV CLL had a 55% survival in the splenectomy arm and a 29% survival in the fludarabine arm. At present, splenectomy is recommended for patients who have failed medical therapy and have anemia with transfusion requirements, thrombocytopenia with bleeding, or compressive symptoms such as splenomegaly.

Chronic Myelogenous Leukemia. Chronic myelogenous leukemia (CML) is a leukemia with a primitive hematopoietic cell as the cell of origin. This precursor cell can differentiate into myeloid cell lines, erythroid cell lines, platelet cell lines, and possibly B lymphoid and T lymphoid cells. CML occurs preferentially in men to women at a 1.5:1 ratio and, like CLL, typically occurs in the sixth decade of life or older. This disease varies from CLL in that it invariably progresses from a chronic stage to an accelerated (blast) stage whereas CLL remains more indolent. The initial chronic phase lasts between 1 and 5 years and is characterized by splenomegaly, constitutional symptoms of fatigue, abdominal fullness, and weight loss.[104] The accelerated phase is apparent with 15% of circulating cells being more immature blast cells. Within 3 to 6 months this generally converts to the terminal blast phase in which the blastic cells fill the bone marrow and the circulating blood at greater than 30% of leukocytes and cause destruction of other organs. Death due to infection or bleeding invariably results after the blast crisis begins.

The diagnosis of CML is made by the leukocytosis with myeloid differentiation and presence of granulocytes filling the bone marrow space. Ninety percent of patients have the classic Philadelphia chromosome, which is a reciprocal translation between chromosomes 9 and 22. On the basis of randomized trials, there is no benefit in terms of delaying the accelerated and blast phases of the disease by doing a splenectomy during the chronic phase of the disease. Certain select patients who have significant hypersplenism or splenomegaly may have symptomatic benefit from splenectomy during the chronic phase.[105,106]

A recent study from M.D. Anderson Cancer Center reports their experience of splenectomy during the accelerated or blast phase of disease.[107] Patients were referred for this procedure with symptoms of splenomegaly in 42% of cases, thrombocytopenia in 30% of cases, to potentially improve administration of chemotherapy by reducing the hypersplenism in 19% of cases and because of symptoms with both hypersplenism and thrombocytopenia in 9% of cases. The perioperative mortality in this series of 55 patients was 2% (one patient death).[93] There was universal benefit of symptoms related to splenomegaly, and there was a marked improvement of platelet count and requirement for platelet transfusions in patients with preoperative thrombocytopenia. The median 6-month transfusion requirement decreased from 21 down to 1 (both platelet and red cell transfusions). The median post-splenectomy survival was 19 months for patients in the accelerated phase and 6.5 months for patients in the blastic phase of their disease. This report concludes that for select patients who have severe transfusion requirements and/or severe symptoms of splenomegaly, there is objective benefit with relatively low morbidity in patients with this later stage of CML.

Non-Hodgkin Lymphoma. Non-Hodgkin lymphoma (NHL) is the most common lymphoma, outnumbering Hodgkin disease by a ratio of almost 6:1 in the United States. Non-Hodgkin lymphoma is a much more heterogeneous disease with a large range of histologic cell types defined by morphology and immunohistochemistry to differentiate subgroups of the disease. The clinical course of these subgroups correlates with the microscopic findings. In general, diffuse or infiltrative non-Hodgkin lymphoma has a worse prognosis than nodular NHL. The diffuse high-grade type occurs most commonly in the younger patient population (age <35 years) or the very elderly. More aggressive non-Hodgkin lymphomas are T-cell lymphomas, whereas the low-grade tumors are usually B-cell. Non-Hodgkin lymphoma presents in approximately one third of cases at extranodal sites, whereas two thirds are limited to lymphadenopathy.[108,109] In general, the disease is more diffuse at the time of presentation, mandating treatment by combination chemotherapy.

In patients dying of NHL, up to 80% have significant splenomegaly due to lymphatic infiltration.[110,111] As is true

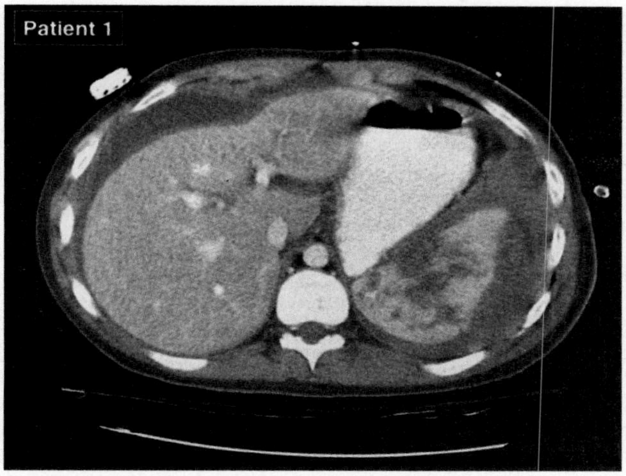

FIGURE 73.11. Spleen from a patient with hairy cell leukemia. Note the whitened anterior edge of the spleen and the white "sugar-coating" spots on the surface.

with other infiltrative neoplastic diseases, symptoms of pancytopenia and splenomegaly are common in patients with NHL. Patients who are operative candidates have significant benefit with up to 80% of patients having decreased transfusion requirements and most patients having relief of gastric oppression and pain symptoms due to splenomegaly.[112] The response of the pancytopenias is somewhat dependent on the bone marrow reserve, which may be altered by prior chemotherapy and/or radiation therapy. There is no test to identify adequate marrow reserve, and the only assessment in that situation is whether a patient has a response following splenectomy.

Hairy Cell Leukemia. Hairy cell leukemia is a low-grade lymphoproliferative disorder with characteristic "hairy" cells due to irregular filament projections from the cell surface visible under light microscopy.[113] This leukemia is a B-lymphocyte tumor that infiltrates the bone marrow and spleen with almost no peripheral lymphadenopathy. There may be enlargement of the liver. The disease is much more common in males than females by a fourfold difference, and the onset of disease is typically in the fifth or sixth decade of life.

The initial symptoms most commonly relate to enlargement of the spleen either by direct effects of splenomegaly or by pancytopenia due to hypersplenism (Fig. 73.11).[114] Patients can have early satiety or upper quadrant pain with a large palpable spleen infiltrated with leukemic cells. The enlarged spleen often causes symptoms related to anemia with a transfusion requirement, bleeding due to thrombocytopenia, and frequent infections due to leukopenia. In the past, hairy cell leukemia was described as the "surgical leukemia" as splenectomy was recommended as the primary treatment, and virtually all patients had resolution of symptoms of splenomegaly. Thus, splenectomy was the standard of care.[115] However, the vast majority of patients relapsed, some as early as 6 to 12 months later, and only 40% to 50% of patients received long-term benefit from the cytopenias due to bone marrow replacement with hairy cell infiltrates.

In 1984, medical therapy led to responses, initially with recombinant alpha-interferon.[116] Newer trials with purine analogues such as pentostatin (2-doxycoformycin) and 2-chlorodoxydenosine provided a beneficial nonsurgical therapy.[117] A randomized trial comparing pentostatin with α-interferon showed a complete response rate of 78% with pentostatin versus 11% with α-interferon, and this has now become a first-line therapy.[118] The 10-year survival rate for pentostatin was 96% and 100% for Cladribine.[119] Five percent to 10% of patients who are resistant to medical therapy should be offered splenectomy as a salvage therapy.

Myelodysplastic Syndrome. Agnogenic myeloid metaplasia (AMM) or myelodysplastic syndrome (MDS) with myeloid metaplasia is a poorly understood disorder characterized by a fibrotic replacement of the bone marrow compartment with extramedullary hematopoiesis and massive splenomegaly.[120] The pathophysiology of the disease is poorly understood but includes a nonclonal proliferation of fibroblasts making a dense fibrous stroma that fills the marrow space and contributes to hepatosplenomegaly and lymphadenopathy. This fibrous proliferation may be under control of secreted growth factors such as transformin growth factor-beta.[121] Other myeloproliferative diseases include polycythemia vera and essential or idiopathic thrombocytosis.

The clinical symptoms and features of MDS relate to anemia and splenomegaly via direct mass effects or hypersplenism.[122] Patients are usually in the fifth decade of life or older. They present with constitutional symptoms including weight loss and fatigue, as well as abdominal fullness and discomfort due to splenomegaly. Splenic infarctions can cause pain. Patients may present with bleeding due to thrombocytopenia. Hepatomegaly is present in 50% to 75% of patients, and splenomegaly is present in virtually all patients. The massively enlarged spleens in MDS are some of the largest spleens by weight in most clinical series.

The combination of massive splenomegaly with increased blood flow via the enlarged spleen and hepatomegaly with fibrosis can lead to relative portal hypertension. Clinical symptoms may be similar to portal hypertension from other causes including varices and ascites. The diagnosis is made by evaluation of peripheral blood smear that shows immature red cells with poikilocytes and tear-shaped cells. There can either be thrombocytopenia or thrombocytosis with platelet counts of greater than one million. Similarly, there may be leukopenia or elevated white cell counts similar to CML. Bone marrow biopsy often produces a hypocellular sample due to the fibrotic replacement of the marrow space.

Treatment is generally targeted to palliate symptoms.[122] Anemia and thrombocytopenia can be treated with transfusions. There is some role for alkylating agents and steroids, and in patients with thrombocytosis, hydroxyurea is of benefit.[123] Splenectomy is indicated for relief of significant symptoms of hypersplenism or splenomegaly.[124] Hypersplenism is manifested by anemia and thrombocytopenia with increasing transfusion requirements. Patients who have significant pain and early satiety with massively enlarged spleens may benefit by removal of mass effect. Finally, MDS is a unique situation in which splenectomy may treat portal hypertension, decreasing variceal bleeding and possibly ascites.[125]

The Mayo Clinic has updated use of splenectomy over the past three decades for patients with myelofibrosis.[126] A total of 314 patients have been treated overall with 91 patients treated during the last 10 years. The primary indications for surgery were mechanical symptoms of compression due to massive splenomegaly in 49%, severe anemia in 25%, portal hypertension in 15%, and thrombocytopenia in 11%. The meaningful improvement in symptoms was observed in 30% to 50% of patients, but the overall complication rate was 28% and there were 6.7% perioperative deaths.[126] Furthermore, there is no clear overall impact on patient survival, disease course, or the intramedullary manifestations of myeloid metaplasia after splenectomy. Given these results, all factors including severity of symptoms and comorbidities must be considered before recommending splenectomy for this hematologic disorder.

Treatment strategies have changed in MDS in the past 5 years. One new therapy is antiangiogenic therapy, and the other is immunosuppressive treatment.[122] There is an increase in neovascularity of the bone marrow in patients with MDS, and vascular endothelial cell growth factor appears to play a prominent role in pathophysiology. Specific antiangiogenic therapy to block vascular endothelial growth factor (VEGF), including the recently reported trial of thalidomide, led to independence from transfusions in a subgroup of patients with MDS. Interest in immunosuppressive therapy in MDS occurred because the subset of these patients with refractory anemia has autoimmune pathophysiology. Young patients or patients with HLA-DR 15 appear to have autoimmune etiology and have responded to immunosuppressive therapy. A new treatment includes JAk2 inhibitors, as the 63% of myelodysplasias patients with a JAK mutation have a much higher incidence of splenomegaly.[127]

Metastatic Disease to the Spleen. The incidence of splenic metastases in autopsy studies of patients succumbing to malignancy ranges between 2.3% and 7.1%.[128] It is rare that splenic metastatic lesions are isolated disease. This can occur in colon cancer and ovarian cancer. In patients who have multiple areas of intra-abdominal malignancies, the most common histologies are breast, lung, colorectal, ovarian, and melanoma. There can rarely be isolated metastasis that may be excised for increase in disease-free survival, particularly for colorectal cancer and melanoma.[129] Techniques to differentiate benign from malignant lesions include fine-needle aspiration biopsy, MRI with gadolinium contrast to assess enhancement patterns, and specific ultrasound techniques.[130]

Metabolic or Infiltrative Diseases. Gaucher disease is an autosomal recessive disorder with a deficiency in the lysosomal hydrolase, α-glucosidase, encoded by chromosome 1. Gaucher disease is the most common lysosomal storage disease. α-Glucosidase typically degrades sphingolipids like glucocerebroside. There is a markedly increased incidence of this disorder in Ashkenazi Jews. There are three types of this disease. Type I, the adult form, composes 99% of cases and is the one in which splenectomy was useful in the past. The defect in the acid α-glucosidase causes an accumulation of undegraded glycolipids that are taken up by the reticuloendothelial cells and result in infiltration of the spleen, liver, and bone marrow. The most common symptoms of this disease relate to hypersplenism as well as direct effects of massive splenomegaly. Thrombocytopenia with bleeding problems or anemia causing fatigue are the most common effects of hypersplenism. Patients also may have such massive spleens that they have early satiety and weight loss due to gastric compression.

The diagnosis can be confirmed by the measurement of acid α-glucosidase activity in peripheral white blood cells or cultured fibroblasts. Now that the genetic abnormality is known, patients can be screened by molecular techniques to identify carriers. Prenatal diagnosis is also available by amniocentesis or chorionic villous sampling.

In the past, treatment has included supportive care with platelet transfusions as well as erythrocyte transfusions. Splenectomy was frequently performed for advanced cases, and in this disease a significant experience with partial splenectomy was developed in the early 1990s.[131–133] The goals of the subtotal splenectomy are partially to prevent the complications of overwhelming postsplenectomy sepsis and to partially protect the liver and bone marrow by leaving a residual splenic fragment for continued deposition of lipid. In this disease, the technique to safely perform partial splenectomy leaves a small residual upper pole fragment vascularized from the short gastric vessels.

Recently, it has been established that enzyme replacement with purified placental acid α-glucosidase is safe with good efficacy. Patients receive enzyme intravenously, 30 to 60 units per kg every other week, and the symptoms and signs are typically reversed. A recombinant α-glucosidase (alglucerase) is now available for therapy, and the role of splenectomy has been displaced by medical management.

INCIDENTAL SPLENECTOMY

In a large series evaluating reasons for splenectomy from Barnes Hospital and Brigham and Women's Hospital, the single most common indication for removing the spleen was incidental during a procedure for nonsplenic pathology.[37,38] This was primarily because removal of an adjacent organ or tumor required removal of the spleen either for completeness of resection or because of removal or ligation of the splenic vasculature. In this large series, more than 26% of the splenectomies performed over a 10-year period were incidental splenectomies (Table 73.7).[37] The actual primary treatments of those various disease entities in adjacent organs are subjects of multiple other chapters within this textbook, but a few comments can be made regarding the reasons for splenectomy and whether it is always appropriate.

The one common indication for an incidental splenectomy is during removal of the distal pancreas. For decades, the standard procedure when a distal pancreatectomy was performed was to include a splenectomy. The reason for splenectomy is that the splenic vein is intimately associated with the undersurface of the pancreas and has many direct branches to the pancreatic parenchyma. The splenic artery generally is superior to the pancreatic border and could be preserved, but because of removal of the splenic vein and for completeness of the resection, an en bloc resection of the distal pancreas and spleen is typically performed. Because of the interest in splenic preservation due to the incidence of postsplenectomy infection, two different approaches have been used to remove the distal pancreas without removing the spleen. The more technically challenging operation is a distal pancreatectomy with preservation of the splenic artery and vein. This can be performed if there is a relatively small amount of invasive tumor or benign neoplasia in which the splenic vein can be dissected away from the pancreatic tissue, tying multiple side branches and then dividing the pancreatic parenchyma leaving the splenic vessels intact. The second spleen-preserving distal pancreatectomy involves ligation of the splenic artery and vein but preservation of short gastric vessels and using those vessels as collateral inflow and outflow to maintain splenic viability. A recent report demonstrated no increased risks of preoperative complications or morbidity with this approach.[134] Removal of the distal pancreas with splenic preservation has also been recently reported as a laparoscopic procedure as well.[135] For patients with tumors that mandate removal of the lymph nodes of the splenic hilum or with direct association of the tumor with splenic parenchyma, it is more appropriate to do an operation based on neoplastic principles and perform a distal pancreatectomy with splenectomy. In other indications, if the anatomy is appropriate and the completeness of tumor resection is not compromised by splenic preservation, it is certainly possible.

Additional procedures in which it is quite common to perform a splenectomy include proximal gastric cancers. The importance of complete nodal dissection in long-term results in gastric resections has been debated for several decades. A report from Japan noted that in 20% of proximal gastric cancers there were positive splenic hilum nodes identified as level X lymph nodes.[136] These authors emphasize the need to perform associated splenectomy for grossly positive nodal disease in the splenic hilum. A long-term retrospective review from Memorial Sloan-Kettering Cancer Center noted that in 23% of gastrectomies in which complete resection of cancer was accomplished, adjacent organs had to be removed, the most common being the spleen.[137] There was long-term survival in this patient population, but it was emphasized that this aggressive surgery should be used only when removal of all gross disease is achieved.[138] A recent randomized study from Korea showed no benefit in doing a splenectomy if splenic hilum nodes were grossly normal.[139]

Other tumors of the left upper quadrant and retroperitoneum that may require splenectomy include large renal cell carcinomas, left adrenal tumors, and retroperitoneal sarcomas that can infiltrate into the spleen. Often splenectomy is useful to provide adequate exposure to cleanly dissect bulky disease posterior to the spleen. Although the asplenic state does make patients susceptible to infections (see previous Hyposplenism), there should be no hesitation to remove the spleen in those settings to achieve the appropriate complete resection.

IATROGENIC SPLENECTOMY

An uncommonly discussed area of spleen surgery is removal or preservation of the iatrogenically traumatized spleen during unrelated abdominal operations. Procedures in which mobilization of the left upper quadrant such as reflection of the spleen and pancreas medially to expose retroperitoneal tissue, left adrenalectomy, and left nephrectomy put the spleen at risk.[140] Simple mobilization of the splenic flexure of the colon can lead to bleeding from the inferior pole of the spleen that can be difficult to control. The ligaments that go directly from the omentum to the capsule of the spleen are the most common cause of iatrogenic splenic trauma as retraction of the omentum for exposure can strip the splenic capsule from the organ. A national database on antireflux procedures of 86,411 patients reported an incidence of iatrogenic splenectomy of 2.3%, which is 1,987 iatrogenic splenectomies for that indication alone.[141]

Probably the best data for the incidence of iatrogenic splenectomy comes from the recently reported series from Vanderbilt, which listed 73 iatrogenic splenectomies over a 10-year period or an average of 7 per year.[38] This constituted 8.1% of all splenectomies performed during that time interval. There are likely more minor or moderate injuries to the spleen during unrelated operations in which the spleen was not removed but was repaired or salvaged. Just as in trauma to the spleen, the techniques of splenorrhaphy can be used to preserve the spleen. A recent report indicates that use of a mesh wrap splenorrhaphy even in the setting of bowel surgery does not lead to an increased incidence of infection.[43] For minor capsular disruption, the use of the argon beam coagulator for surface cautery is a helpful technique.

Two large recent reports have evaluated the incidence and effects of inadvertent splenic injury during colectomy. The Mayo Clinic surveyed 13,897 colectomies and found 59 splenic injuries (0.42%). Most of these occurred during mobilization of the splenic flexure.[142] The 30-day morbidity rate for this subgroup of patients was 34%, and the mortality rate was 17%. There were no clear episodes of sepsis. A second large study from the California Cancer Registry of almost 42,000 patients showed that there was a similar rate of inadvertent splenectomy of 0.58%.[143] This was associated with a distal transverse colon or splenic flexure primary and increased the length of hospital stay by 37.4%. It also increased the probability of perioperative death to 40%.

The primary teaching point regarding iatrogenic injuries is that the best way to preserve the spleen is to not damage it in the first place. This requires caution in mobilizing tissue in and around the spleen as well as visual inspection of the attachments of the spleen prior to blunt mobilization. Whenever possible, the spleen should be preserved to decrease the risk of postsplenectomy sepsis.

DIAGNOSTIC SPLENECTOMY

Splenectomy is sometimes necessary for diagnosis in an otherwise asymptomatic patient. The situation in which splenectomy may be needed to make a diagnosis includes when a mass lesion is identified within the spleen on CT scan, ultrasound, or MRI scan for which a definitive diagnosis cannot be made radiographically. Another example is when patients have either palpable spleens on physical examination or enlarged spleens by scan and otherwise have no clear disorder. Table 73.10 lists the final pathology diagnoses in spleens removed for these two indications over a 10-year period in two major academic medical centers.[37] In that series, a total of 122 diagnostic splenectomies were performed; 52 were for splenic mass, and 41 were for splenomegaly with no other clear diagnosis. An additional 29 were done to further characterize a known hematologic malignancy.

TABLE 73.10

FINAL PATHOLOGIC DIAGNOSES IN 122 SPLEENS REMOVED FOR DIAGNOSTIC PURPOSES

Total number of diagnostic splenectomies	122
Indication-Splenic mass	52
Lymphomas	17
Metastatic cancer	14
Carcinoma	12
Sarcoma	2
Benign	20
Cysts	11
Hamartoma	3
Hemangioma	3
Other	3
Indication-Splenomegaly	41
Lymphoma	24
Benign lymphoid proliferation	5
Benign vascular	4
Granulomatous disease	4
Infarction/hemorrhage	4
Indication-Categorize lymphoma	29
Malignant (successful)	28
Benign	1

Adapted from Thomsen RW, Schoonen WM, Farkas DK, et al. Risk for hospital contact with infection in patients with splenectomy: a population-based cohort study. *Ann Intern Med* 2009;151:546–555.

Of the patients who had an isolated splenic mass, 60% had malignant lesions and 40% had benign lesions (Table 73.10).[37] Most of the malignant lesions were lymphoma, with another large group of metastatic carcinomas including some in which the primary diagnosis had not been made previously. There were two patients with metastatic sarcoma to the spleen. Of the benign diagnoses, more than half were cysts and there were also splenic hamartomas and splenic hemangiomas.

In the diagnosis of an isolated splenic mass, most of these lesions could have been diagnosed by a fine-needle aspiration biopsy. Certain of these lesions such as the cystic lesions or the hemangiomas have a classic appearance on gadolinium-enhanced MRI scan, which can be used to sort out mass lesions without tissue biopsy. Although there may be some hesitation to do fine-needle aspiration biopsies on splenic lesions due to the risk of bleeding, for most mass lesions this would have made the diagnosis, and with the exception of splenic hemangiomas, essentially all of these lesions could be aspirated without any significant consequence.

The second diagnostic indication for splenectomy is unexplained splenomegaly. In this series over 10 years there were 41 cases, or 4 cases per year at these two hospitals in which a massively enlarged spleen was removed purely for diagnosis.[37] Most of these (58%) turned out to be lymphoma. The remaining 42% were split relatively evenly between benign lymphoid proliferation, benign vascular lesions, and granulomatous disease, as well as splenic infarction and hemorrhage. The role of fine-needle aspiration and other percutaneous biopsies for splenomegaly is limited as there is considerable risk of bleeding for this indication, and there would be a very low yield in terms of being able to make that diagnosis by that form of biopsy.

Staging laparotomy for Hodgkin disease is a diagnostic procedure that is infrequently necessary in current practice. A standard practice for pathologic staging between 1960 and 1990 was performance of a staging laparotomy in most patients with Hodgkin disease. The reason to perform this invasive procedure was based on reports that laparotomy altered the clinical stage of disease in approximately 35% of patients. Of these patients, approximately two thirds, or 20% to 25%, were up-staged to a more advanced level by staging laparotomy, and approximately one third, or 10% to 15%, were down-staged to a lower clinical level based on laparotomy results. Since the treatment of Hodgkin disease depended on accurate staging (i.e., early stages were treated differently than more advanced stages), the staging laparotomy was essential in determining the proper therapeutic intervention for patients with Hodgkin disease.

Staging laparotomy was performed via an upper abdominal midline incision.[144] This included exploration of the entire abdomen for any abnormal lymph nodes, including nodes identified by lymphogram. Even if no abnormalities were found, multiple tissues were removed for pathologic assessment (Fig. 73.12). This included removal of the spleen, bilobar hepatic wedge resections, bilobar hepatic core biopsies, and multiple lymph nodes samplings. Lymph nodes were typically removed from the porta hepatis area, the celiac region, the splenic hilum, the periaortic region, and the bowel mesentery. If any iliac lymph nodes were palpated, they were removed as well. The spleen removed during a staging laparotomy for Hodgkin disease was sliced at 3 to 4 mm thicknesses, and any suspicious nodule, particularly in the white pulp, was examined microscopically for the presence of Hodgkin disease.

There are several reasons why the incidence of performing staging laparotomy has decreased over the past two decades.[145] The primary reason is that it no longer alters treatment of Hodgkin disease. The treatment of patients with stages IB, IIB, IIIB, IVB, IIIA, and IVA Hodgkin disease almost always involves systemic chemotherapy. Accurate pathologic staging makes no impact on the treatment outcome or treatment decisions. The only patients who may theoretically benefit from staging laparotomy at present are patients with stage IA or IIA Hodgkin disease who typically may receive treatment with radiation therapy. Even in this subgroup of patients there is a trend toward not performing staging laparotomy. First, many oncologists use combination chemotherapy even for early stage disease. Second, for patients who were treated with radiation therapy alone for stage IA and IIA disease, it has been demonstrated in several recent clinical series that the ultimate outcome is equivalent whether these patients undergo staging laparotomy or whether they are treated initially with radiation therapy.[146,147] The reason is that if these patients recur outside of the radiation field during long-term follow-up, salvage can be obtained with systemic chemotherapy. Third, performance of staging laparotomy is a major abdominal operation with potential for morbidity and the treatment for the Hodgkin disease must be delayed for 4 to 6 weeks. Finally, there are data that patients who survive Hodgkin disease and receive combination chemotherapy are at increased risk for the development of a secondary malignancy that is primarily acute, nonlymphocytic leukemia (ANLL).[148,149] In some series, the risk of developing ANLL is increased up to tenfold in patients who have undergone splenectomy as part of their

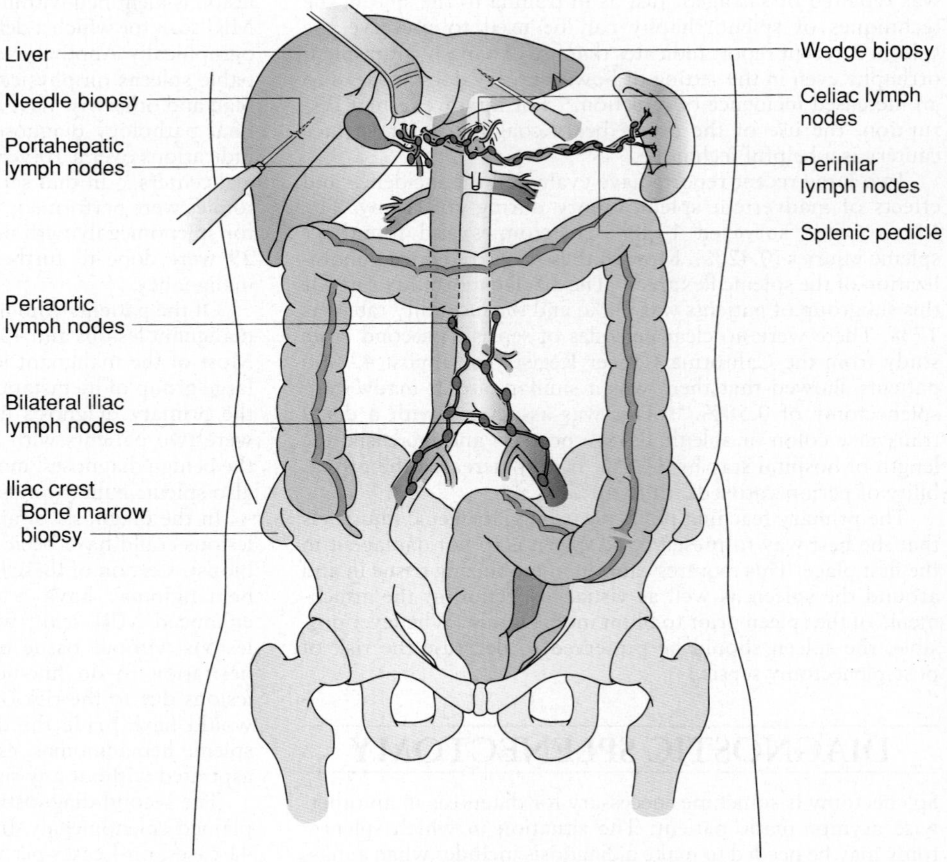

FIGURE 73.12. The tissues to be removed or to undergo biopsy in a staging laparotomy for Hodgkin disease. Splenectomy, liver biopsy, and lymph node sampling in the specific sites are shown. Bone marrow biopsy can be done if necessary.

staging workup for Hodgkin disease compared to patients undergoing similar chemotherapy regimens who did not undergo splenectomy. For all of these reasons, this procedure that also accounted for a large number of the splenectomies performed in major tertiary referral centers and cancer centers is rarely performed now.

VASCULAR DISORDERS OF THE SPLEEN

Vacular problems with the spleen that can require splenectomy include both venous and arterial problems. The most common is splenic vein thrombosis; splenectomy in this setting is typically curative in sinistral portal hypertension. Splenic artery aneurysms are one of the more common visceral aneurysms and also can be an indication for splenectomy.

Splenic Vein Thrombosis

Splenic vein thrombosis is an unusual cause of upper gastrointestinal hemorrhage that can be cured by splenectomy. The pathophysiology of this disease is an isolated thrombosis of the splenic vein as it traverses along the posterior pancreatic body and tail. After thrombosis, splenic venous outflow is diverted to the short gastric vessels as the main collateral venous outflow. This increased flow via the short gastric veins leads to a high pressure with a dilatation of the submucosal venous plexus primarily in the gastric cardia and fundus and development of gastric varices.[150]

The cause of the splenic vein thrombosis does not typically involve any pathology of the spleen, but rather, typically pathology of the pancreas and possibly the stomach. Pancreatitis or pancreatic pseudocyst is the cause of splenic vein thrombosis in more than 50% of patients in most series. Pancreatic carcinoma with direct invasion and infiltration of the splenic vein is the second most common cause. Other unusual causes may be a penetrating gastric ulcer posteriorly or retroperitoneal fibrosis.

The diagnosis is made in patients who have upper gastrointestinal bleeding with only gastric varices on endoscopy. Because there is no portal venous hypertension and no cirrhosis of the liver, there are no esophageal varices. The spleen may or may not be enlarged, but again there are no other signs and symptoms of cirrhosis. Definitive diagnosis in the past has been made by a celiac angiogram, which demonstrates absence of the splenic vein with collateral flow via the gastric veins. MR angiograms/venograms as well as high-resolution ultrasound can also make the diagnosis.

Splenectomy is curative as it removes the blood flow via the splenic artery through this organ. This removes all the excess collateral flow that leads to the venous hypertension, and the associated symptoms resolve. Whenever splenic vein thrombosis is diagnosed, even if the patient has not had an episode of bleeding, elective splenectomy should be performed as a prophylactic measure.

Patients with portal hypertension and cirrhosis or partial vein thrombosis have a complex collection of symptoms that include hypersplenism with splenomegaly, thrombocytopenia, and anemia. However, the operative risk associated with portal vein hypertension is excessive, and splenectomy is virtually never indicated in this setting.

Splenic Artery Aneurysm

Splenic artery aneurysm is uncommon, though it is the second most frequent abdominal artery to undergo aneurysmal changes.[151] Splenic aneurysms occur twice as often in women as in men. Patients can be divided into two distinct groups. First, there are elderly patients whose aneurysms are manifestations of atherosclerosis. Second, some young women have an apparent congenital predisposition to form splenic artery aneurysms. In these women, there is an increased risk of rupture of these aneurysms during pregnancy. Inflammatory processes such as pancreatitis may involve the splenic artery and occasionally lead to aneurysm but more frequently lead to acute bleeding.

Splenic artery aneurysms are typically asymptomatic and may be initially identified as a widened rim of calcification in the left upper quadrant defining the aneurysm boundaries. They may also be discovered as incidental findings on CT scan. If symptomatic, patients experience left upper quadrant pain, nausea, and vomiting. The presence of symptoms suggesting pending aneurysmal rupture indicates urgent splenectomy with ligation of the splenic artery.

When a calcified atherosclerotic splenic artery aneurysm is discovered in a patient older than 60 years of age with no splenomegaly and no symptoms, surgical excision is not indicated and the aneurysm may be followed for evidence of enlargement. In younger patients who have an asymptomatic aneurysm identified, particularly young women of childbearing age, an elective splenectomy is recommended to prevent rupture. Nonsurgical approaches include embolization of the splenic artery in patients who are poor risks for open laparotomy.[152]

MISCELLANEOUS INDICATIONS FOR SPLENECTOMY

Splenectomy is performed relatively infrequently for a miscellaneous collection of indications including splenic cysts, infectious cysts, and splenic abscesses. The wandering spleen is a normal spleen that lacks ligamental attachments to keep it in the left upper quadrant. This can present in various ways from an undiagnosed mass to torsion of the splenic hilum causing acute pain.

Cysts of the Spleen

Splenectomy is performed as described previously often for hematologic malignancies including multiple forms of leukemias and lymphoma, primarily for symptoms of hypersplenism or splenomegaly or as a staging procedure. Splenectomy for primary neoplasms of the spleen is an infrequent indication. These primary neoplastic processes are listed in Table 73.11.

Hemangioma is the most common benign primary neoplasm of the spleen. It is often an incidental finding and may be solitary or multiple. During operation, it can be identified as a more intensely bluish-purple colored lesion when seen from the surface compared to the reddish-purple color of the splenic parenchyma. The hemangiomas can be identified with excellent sensitivity and specificity by MRI characteristics. It is not advised to biopsy a lesion that may be a splenic hemangioma.[153,154] Hemangiomas of the spleen rarely cause symptoms, but massive

TABLE 73.11

PRIMARY NEOPLASMS AND CYSTS OF SPLEEN

Hemangioma
Hemangioendothelioma
Lymphangioma
Pseudotumor
Mycobacterial pseudotumor
Hamartomas
Primary cyst
Echinococcal cyst

hemangiomas can either rupture spontaneously or make the spleen more susceptible to a traumatic rupture. In cases of massive hemangioma with capsular distention and pain, either a splenectomy or partial splenectomy may be helpful.

Hemangioendothelioma is a slightly more aggressive neoplasm than the typical benign hemangioma. Pathologically it is an intermediate benign hemangioma and malignant angiosarcoma. It does not seem to have metastatic potential and generally is an incidental finding. Larger lesions can cause symptoms or be noted for their size and rupture either spontaneously or with minor trauma.

Lymphangiomas also occur in the spleen and are much less common than hemangiomas. They can be multiple or solitary and can be identified by a lighter color and compressibility when seen in surgery.

Two mass lesions that occur in the spleen that are not true neoplasms are hamartomas and inflammatory pseudotumors. Hamartomas are focal developmental abnormalities that occur in spleen and other solid organs such as the liver. Hamartomas contain normal cellular elements and are nonneoplastic but have a random fibrotic organization.[155] The major significance of hamartomas is that they are identified either at laparotomy as incidental findings or they are seen as incidental lesions on CT scans done for other reasons.[156] Inflammatory pseudotumors are described throughout most organs and have also been described in the spleen. These sometimes are quite large with a wide variety of reactive cells. A subcategory of inflammatory pseudotumors of the spleen are related to mycobacterial infection, particularly in HIV-positive patients. There have been reports of primary splenic pregnancy, which is considered the rarest site of ectopic pregnancies.

Cysts of the spleen are almost uniformly unrelated to parasitic infection. They are also relatively common lesions seen across all age groups and may be multifocal. The diagnosis of splenic cysts can be ascertained by ultrasound or CT scan. These benign lesions have no clinical significance unless they reach a large size. The first reported case of a successful elective splenectomy was done for a splenic cyst. This was an enormous cyst at the tip of the spleen and was believed to be an ovarian mass and found to be arising from the spleen at laparotomy (Fig. 73.13). Today a cyst enucleation or partial splenectomy for peripheral cystic lesions that are large and symptomatic would be sufficient. An alternative approach is unroofing the cyst and leaving a portion of the cyst wall in place; this can be done laparoscopically.[157]

The only parasitic cyst involving the spleen is from *Echinococcus granulosus* or a hydatid cyst. The incidence of

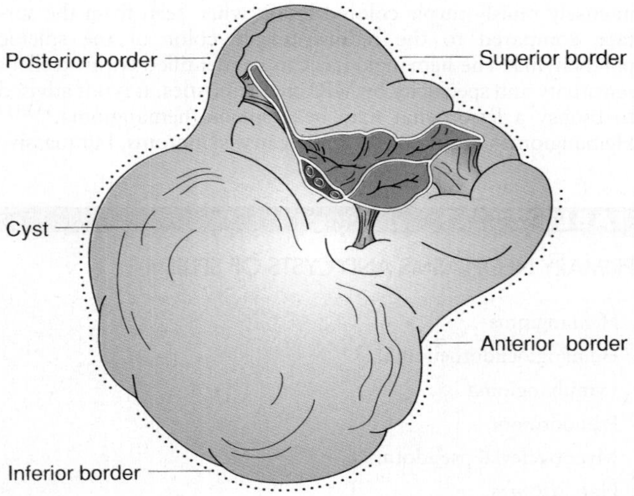

FIGURE 73.13. The visceral surface of a spleen with a true congenital splenic cyst.

echinococcal cyst in the spleen compared to the liver is a ratio of approximately 30:1. However, the spleen is the third most common site of echinococcal cysts behind the liver and lung.[158] Diagnosis should be suspected in patients in areas where echinococcal disease is common such as New Zealand, Australia, and parts of the western United States. The complement fixation test is the most reliable serologic study for this organism. The treatment of echinococcal cysts can include splenectomy. As with echinococcal cysts of the liver, it is of utmost importance not to rupture the cyst and expose the patient to the scoleces. For large and peripheral cysts in which risk of rupture is high, the contents of the cyst should be carefully aspirated and replaced with hypertonic saline.[159] In a recent report from Greece, surgeons preserved 8 of 19 spleens with echinococcal cysts by doing partial splenectomy.[158]

Abscess of the Spleen

Splenic abscess is an uncommon but important disease because it is associated with a significant mortality rate and may be cured by splenectomy.[160] In most series, the mortality rate ranges between 40% and 100%.[161] The typical patient has hematogenous seeding of the spleen by bacteria from a remote source such as endocarditis or from intravenous drug abuse.[162] There may be in some cases direct spread of infection from adjacent intra-abdominal sources. Finally, splenic trauma treated conservatively may eventually result in an infected splenic hematoma. In 80% of cases, there is an additional source of infection in locations other than the spleen, and in only 20% of cases is the splenic abscess the sole source of sepsis identified. Enteric organisms account for two thirds of the splenic abscesses and staphylococcus and streptococcus cause the remainder of the cases.

The patients present with signs and symptoms of sepsis including fever, malaise, and leukocytosis. When the spleen is the sole site of infection, patients have significant left upper quadrant tenderness and guarding. Abdominal X-ray views may show gas in the spleen, and an ultrasound or CT scan with contrast can be diagnostic to show an abscess with reactive rim.

Splenectomy is the treatment of choice for patients who can undergo a laparotomy and who have the splenic abscess as an isolated or prominent component of septic syndrome. If the spleen is the only site of infection, removal of the spleen should be curative and result in the recovery of the patient. If patients have multiple sites of infection or are too sick to undergo laparotomy, percutaneous drainage of splenic abscesses may be attempted, but this is often not successful because of spillage and accumulation of infection in the left upper quadrant of the abdomen.

Ectopic Spleen (Wandering Spleen)

Ectopic spleens, or the so-called wandering spleens, occur because of either extreme laxity or absence of the normal ligaments that attach the spleen to the left upper quadrant. This allows the spleen to drop to the lower abdomen in either the right lower quadrant or left lower quadrant by the force of gravity, though still attached by its vascular pedicle.[163] This condition of a wandering spleen occurs thirteen times more frequently in women than in men. The wandering spleen presents most commonly in adults but can cause symptoms in children.[164] The diagnosis may be made by palpable lower abdominal mass confirmed by CT scan or a nuclear imaging spleen scan finding of splenic tissue. The ectopic spleen creates symptoms typically when there is torsion of the pedicle causing acute ischemia and acute pain. The treatment for a wandering spleen as an incidental finding at laparotomy or if the torsion can be corrected and the spleen appears to be viable is to do a splenopexy, affixing it to its native position in the left upper quadrant. If the spleen is infarcted, a splenectomy must be performed.[165] The wandering spleen is ideally suited for laparoscopic splenectomy as it is generally free from ligaments or attachments to other organs.[166]

SPLENECTOMY

The choices of operations available currently to approach the spleen in an elective manner are open splenectomy, laparoscopic splenectomy, or partial splenectomy. Table 73.12 lists indications for splenectomy and whether a partial splenectomy is indicated. Certain principles apply to all patients undergoing elective splenectomy. First, all patients should receive appropriate preoperative vaccination with Pneumovax and possibly also vaccination against *Haemophilus influenza* and *Neisserian* meningococcus 10–14 days prior to the procedure if possible. Patients must have appropriate blood products ready as often patients are anemic and thrombocytopenic due to hypersplenism.

The operative technique for open splenectomy involves either a midline abdominal incision or a left subcostal incision. For patients with massive splenomegaly, defined as greater than 1,500 g in adults and greater than 1,000 g in children, a long midline incision should be used.[167] The components of the splenectomy include division of the avascular lateral and posterior attachments to mobilize the spleen, ligation of the short gastric vessels separating the upper half of the spleen from the greater curvature of the stomach, and ligation of splenic hilar vessels in a controlled manner to avoid injury to the pancreatic tail. One approach, particularly for small spleens that are mobile, is to initially divide the lateral attachments and place packs in the left upper quadrant to elevate the spleen and then proceed with the vascular dissection (Fig. 73.14), but this should be discouraged particularly in patients who are thrombocytopenic or patients with massive splenomegaly. In this situation,

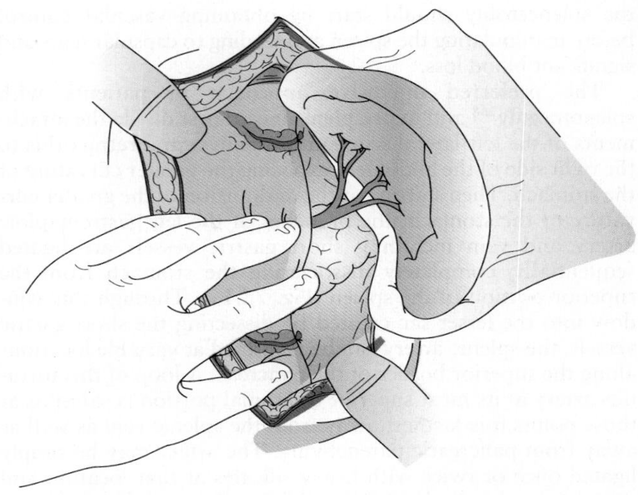

FIGURE 73.14. Lateral mobilization permits the spleen to reach the surface of a midline wound despite the presence of intact hilar vessels.

TABLE 73.12

OPERATIVE INDICATIONS FOR SPLENECTOMY

DISEASE	NEED FOR SPLENECTOMY	PARTIAL SPLENECTOMY
Hereditary spherocytosis	Always	Yes
Hereditary elliptocytosis	Sometimes	Yes
Thalassemia	Sometimes	Yes
Sickle cell anemia	Rarely	No
Wiskott-Aldrich	Sometimes	No
Autoimmune hemolytic anemia	Usually	No
Autoimmune neutropenia	Sometimes	No
Immune thrombocytopenia purpura	Usually	No
Thrombotic thrombocytopenia purpura	Sometimes	No
Hairy cell leukemia	Rarely[a]	No
Chronic lymphocytic leukemia	Sometimes	No
Chronic myelogenous leukemia	Sometimes	No
Non-Hodgkin lymphoma	Sometimes	No
Angiogenic myeloid metaplasia	Sometimes	Yes
Mastocytosis	Rarely	No
Gaucher	Rarely[a]	Yes
Hodgkin disease	Rarely[b]	No
Splenic vein thrombosis	Always	No
Splenic abscess	Usually	No
Splenic cyst	Rarely	Yes
Echinococcal cyst	Always	No

[a]Splenectomy rarely indicated in current practice because of effective medical therapy.
[b]Splenectomy rarely indicated because of change in current therapy.

the splenectomy should start by obtaining vascular control before manipulating the spleen and leading to capsular tears and significant blood loss.

The preferred operative approach in patients with splenomegaly[168] and hypersplenism is to first divide the attachments of the left lateral segment of the liver and retract this to the right side of the abdomen, exposing the greater curvature of the stomach. Then starting at the midportion of the greater curvature of the stomach, the branches of the left gastroepiploic artery and vein including short gastric vessels are ligated sequentially, completely dissociating the stomach from the superior portion of the spleen (Fig. 73.15). Through this window into the lesser sac created by dissecting the short gastric vessels, the splenic artery can be identified at variable locations along the superior border of the pancreas. A loop of this tortuous artery at its most superior or cranial portion is safest as at those points it is farthest away from the splenic vein as well as away from pancreatic parenchyma. The artery may be simply ligated once or twice with heavy silk ties at that location and does not need to be divided. By dividing short gastric arteries as well as ligating the main splenic artery, the vast majority if not all of blood flow into the spleen is controlled prior to even touching the spleen to mobilize it. If capsular disruption occurs, the amount of blood loss then is greatly minimized. Following vascular control, the lateral and posterior attachments are divided and the spleen is elevated to near the level of the abdominal wall musculature ventrally. The splenic hilum can then be dissected, tying vessels in a controlled manner.

For patients with ITP, platelets should not be given until the spleen is either removed or at least until the arterial inflow is controlled, because of clearance of transfused platelets by the spleen in this disease. Similarly, for this disease as well as other diseases in which the spleen is the site of platelet or blood cell destruction, it is important to identify and remove accessory spleens. Most of the accessory spleens occur in the splenic hilum, though they can also occur in the omentum, along the superior border of the pancreas, in the bowel mesentery, and in the pelvis in some situations. The incidence of accessory spleens identified during open splenectomy is between 15% and 30%.

Partial splenectomy can be performed based on the segmental blood supply to the spleen. The spleen is mobilized with good visualization. The inferior segmental arteries are generally ligated, and the artery and veins are ligated as a predemarcation of blood flow to the spleen. The splenic parenchyma is then transected, and the cut surface bleeding can be controlled using materials that induce coagulation or the argon beam coagulator.[169,170]

For the past 5 to 10 years, the standard approach for an elective splenectomy in most large centers has become a laparoscopic approach.[36,171,172] Even patients with massive splenomegaly can now have laparoscopic splenectomy with use of a hand port. In one recent series, there were no conversions in 16 consecutive patients with massive splenomegaly.[173] Another series noted a higher incidence of conversion to an open procedure when the spleen has weighed more than 2,000 g.[174]

The technique of laparoscopic splenectomy begins with the patient either supine with a roll under the hip to prop the left side of the abdomen up approximately 30 degrees, or in the lateral decubitus position. The omental, inferior attachments and the short gastric vessels are divided, often with a powered dissection instrument. It has been reported that careful exposure of the splenic hilum with the direct ligation of the vessels is a much safer technique than division of the hilum with staples without precise vessel dissection.[175] Once the vessels are ligated, the spleen is placed into a large plastic bag and brought to the most convenient port for careful morselization. This can allow removal of the spleen without having to enlarge the port incisions and without fracture and spillage in the abdomen. Laparoscopic resection has extended to include massive splenomegaly[176] and partial splenectomy.[177]

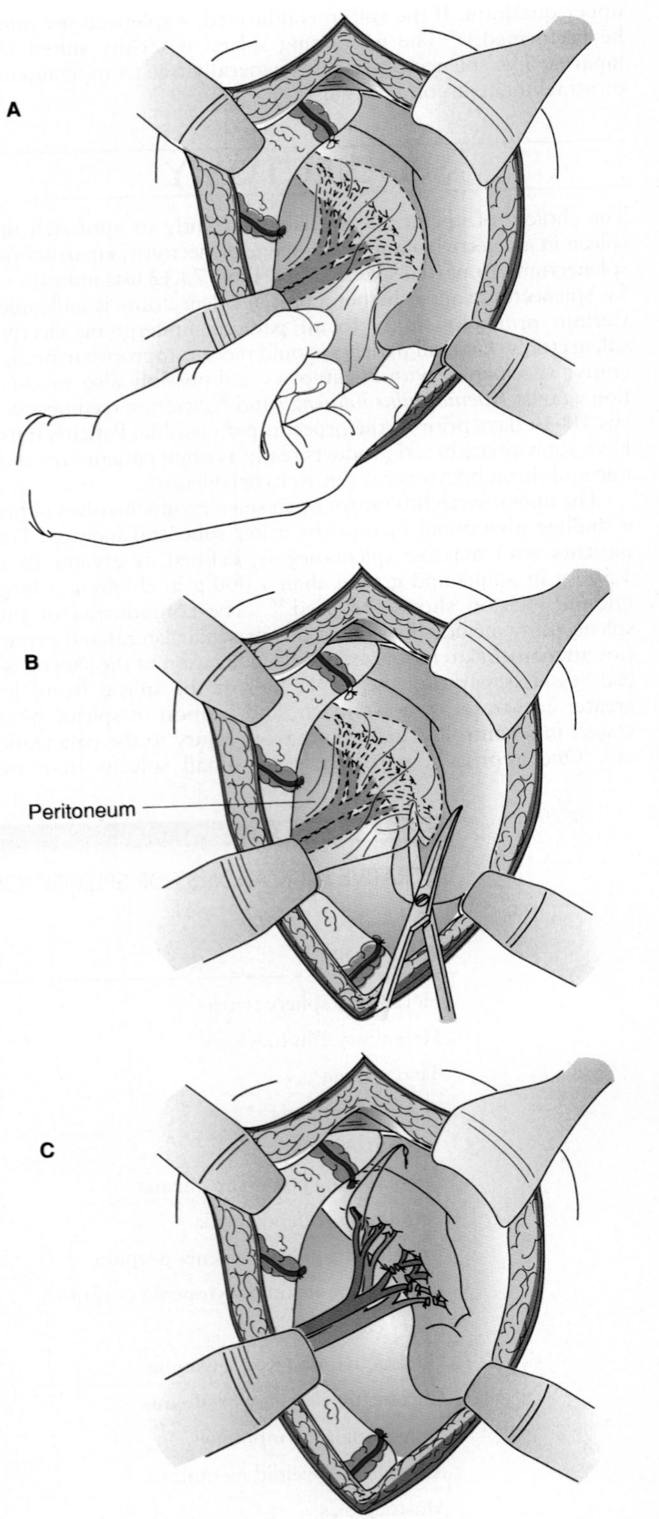

FIGURE 73.15. Technique for elective splenectomy. **A:** The inferior pole is reflected laterally by the assistant's fingers, exposing the lower edge of the hilar peritoneal envelope. **B:** The hilar peritoneum is opened, here shown progressing from inferior to superior. **C:** Individual vessels are identified and suture ligated.

Virtually all indications for splenectomy can be approached laparoscopically.[178] Laparoscopic splenectomy has been reported for removal of the wandering spleen.[179] In this indication it is actually a much easier operation as the spleen is free and the hilum is exposed. Accessory spleens may be identified less frequently and consequently left in place more often with a laparoscopic approach. The use of lymphoscintigrams after failed splenectomy can identify accessory spleens. The removal of accessory spleens can be done laparoscopically as well; adding a hand port for palpation assists in this type of procedure.[180]

Radiofrequency ablation is a new technique added to treatment of splenic disorders.[181,182] Radiofrequency ablation was developed in the mid-1990s primarily to treat liver lesions. There are various commercial products that essentially destroy tissue indiscriminately by heating to 100°C. The largest experience is with either primary or metastatic tumors in the liver, but this has also been used in treatment of bone metastasis, kidney lesions, lung lesions, and breast cancer. Recent reports indicate that radiofrequency ablation probes can be used successfully as a minimally invasive technique to treat splenic disorders such as thalassemia. There also may be a role for radiofrequency ablation to treat trauma to the spleen as a way to control severe injuries.[182]

References

1. McClusky DA 3rd, Skandalakis LJ, Colborn GL, et al. Tribute to a triad: history of splenic anatomy, physiology, and surgery—part 1. *World J Surg* 1999;23(3):311–325.
2. Morgenstern L. A history of splenectomy. In: Hiatt JR, Phillips EH, Morgenstern L, eds. *Surgical diseases of the spleen*. Berlin, Germany: Springer-Verlag; 1997.
3. Morgenstern L. Love in the time of spleen: a personal memoir. *J Am Coll Surg* 2006;202:335–339.
4. McClusky DA 3rd, Skandalakis LJ, Colborn GL, et al. Tribute to a triad: history of splenic anatomy, physiology, and surgery—part 2. *World J Surg* 1999;23(5):514–526.
5. Patterson KD, Drysdale TA, Krieg PA. Embryonic origins of spleen asymmetry. *Development* 2000;127(1):167–175.
6. Brendolan A, Rosado MM, Carsetti R, et al. Development and function of the mammalian spleen. *Bioessays* 2007;29:166–177.
7. Sprogoe-Jakobsen S, Sprogoe-Jakobsen U. The weight of the normal spleen. *Forensic Sci Int* 1997;88(3):215–223.
8. Ravaglia G, Forti P, Biagi F, et al. Splenic function in old age. *Gerontology* 1998;44(2):91–94.
9. Hoefs JC, Wang FW, Lilien DL, et al. A novel, simple method of functional spleen volume calculation by liver-spleen scan. *J Nucl Med* 1999;40(10); 1745–1755.
10. Skandalakis PN, Colborn GL, Skandalakis LJ, et al. The surgical anatomy of the spleen. *Surg Clin N Amer* 1993;73(4):747–768.
11. Desai DC, Hebra A, Davidoff AM, et al. Wandering spleen: a challenging diagnosis. *South Med J* 1997;90(4):439–443.
12. Liu DL, Xia S, Xu W, et al. Anatomy of vasculature of 850 spleen specimens and its application in partial splenectomy. *Surgery* 1996;120(3):574.
13. Kraus MD. Pathology of the spleen. Introduction. *Semin Diagn Pathol* 2003;20(2):83.
14. Mebius RE, Kraal G. Structure and function of the spleen. *Nat Rev Immunol* 2005;5:606–614.
15. Espersen K, Frandsen H, Lorentzen T, et al. The human spleen as an erythrocyte reservoir in diving-related interventions. *J Appl Physiol* 2002; 92(5):2071–2079.
16. Peters AM. Splenic blood flow and blood cell kinetics. *Clin Haematol* 1983;12:421.
17. Phom H, Kumar A, Tripathi M, et al. Comparative evaluation of Tc-99m-heat-denatured RBC and Tc-99m-anti-D IgG opsonized RBC spleen planar and SPECT scintigraphy in the detection of accessory spleen in post-splenectomy patients with chronic idiopathic thrombocytopenic purpura. *Clin Nucl Med* 2004;29(7):403–409.
18. Werre JM, Willekens FL, Bosch FH, et al. The red cell revisited—matters of life and death. *Cell Mol Biol* 2004;50(2):139–145.
19. Zoli G, Corazza GR, D'Amato G, et al. Splenic autotransplantation after splenectomy: tuftsin activity correlates with residual splenic function. *Br J Surg* 1994;81(5):716–718.
20. Feder HM Jr, Pearson HA. Assessment of splenic function in familial asplenia. *NEJM* 1999;341(3):210–212.
21. William BM, Corazza GR. Hyposplenism: a comprehensive review. Part I: Basic concepts and causes. *Hematology* 2007;12(1):1–43.
22. Resende V, Petroianu A. Functions of the splenic remnant after subtotal splenectomy for treatment of severe splenic injuries. *Am J Surg* 2003; 185(4):311–315.
23. Lutwick LI. Life threatening infections in the asplenic or hyposplenic individual. *Curr Clin Top Infect Dis* 2002;22:78–96.
24. Caditi Ali, de Gara C. Complications of splenectomy. *Am J Med* 2008;121: 371–375.
25. Hansen K, Singer DB. Asplenic-hyposplenic overwhelming sepsis: post-splenectomy sepsis revisited. *Pediatr Develop Pathol* 2001;4(2):105–121.
26. Lane PA. The spleen in children. *Curr Opin Pediatr* 1995;7(1):36–41.
27. Shatz DV, Romero-Steiner S, Elie CM, et al. Antibody responses in post-splenectomy trauma patients receiving the 23-valent pneumococcal polysaccharide vaccine at 14 versus 28 days postoperatively. *J Trauma Inj Inf Crit Care* 2002;53(6):1037–1042.
28. Thomsen RW, Schoonen M, Faras DK, et al. Risk for hospital contact with infection in patients with splenectomy. A population based cohort study. *Ann Intern Med* 2009;151:546–555.
29. Kyaw MH, Holmes EM, Toolis F, et al. Evaluation of severe infection and survival after splenectomy. *Am J Med* 2006;119:276.e1–276.e7.
30. Nakae H, Shimazu T, Miyauchi H, et al. Does splenic preservation treatment (embolization, splenorrhaphy, and partial splenectomy) improve immunologic function and long-term prognosis after splenic injury? *J Trauma* 2009;67:567–574.
31. Shatz DV. Vaccination practices among North American trauma surgeons in splenectomy for trauma. *J Trauma* 2002;53(5):950–956.
32. Mourtzoukou EG, Pappas G, Peppas G, et al. Vaccination of asplenic or hyposplenic adults. *Br J Surg* 2008;95:273–280.
33. Crary SE, Buchanan GR. Vascular complications after splenectomy for hematologic disorders. *Blood* 2009;114:2861–2868.
34. Stamou KM, Toutouzas KG, Kekis PB, et al. Prospective study of the incidence and risk factors of postsplenectomy thrombosis of the portal, mesenteric, and splenic veins. *J Arch Surg* 2006;141:663–669.
35. Kawanaka H, Akahoshi T, Kinjo N, et al. Impact of antithrombin III concentrates on portal vein thrombosis after splenectomy in patients with liver cirrhosis and hypersplenism. *Ann Surg* 2010;251:76–83.
36. Singla A, Li Y, Ng SC, et al. Is the growth in laparoscopic surgery reproducible with more complex procedures? *Surgery* 2009;146:367–374.
37. Kraus MD, Fleming MD, Vonderheide RH. The spleen as a diagnostic specimen: a review of 10 years' experience at two tertiary care institutions. *Cancer* 2001;91(11):2001–2009.
38. Rose AT, Newman MI, Debelak J, et al. The incidence of splenectomy is decreasing: lessons learned from trauma experience. *Am Surg* 2000;66(5): 481–486.
39. Peitzman AB, Ford HR, Harbrecht BG, et al. Injury to the spleen. *Curr Probl Surg* 2001;38(12):932–1008.
40. Upadhyaya P. Conservative management of splenic trauma: history and current trends. *Ped Surg Int* 2003;19(9–10):617–627.
41. Harbrecht BG, Zenati MS, Ochoa JB, et al. Evaluation of a 15-year experience with splenic injuries in a state trauma system. *Surgery* 2007;141: 229–238.
42. Gavant ML, Schurr M, Flick PA, et al. Predicting clinical outcome of non-surgical management of blunt splenic injury: using CT to reveal abnormalities of splenic vasculature. *AJR Am J Roentgenol* 1997;168(1): 207–212.
43. Berry MF, Rosato EF, Williams NN. Dexon mesh splenorrhaphy for intra-operative splenic injuries. *Am Surg* 69(2):2003;176–180.
44. Uecker J, Pickett C, Dunn E. The role of follow-up radiographic studies in nonoperative management of spleen trauma. *Am Surg* 2001;67(1):22–25.
45. Konstantakos AK, Barnoski AL, Plaisier BR, et al. Optimizing the management of blunt splenic injury in adults and children. *Surgery* 1999; 126(4):805–812.
46. Gaunt WT, McCarthy MC, Lambert CS, et al. Traditional criteria for observation of splenic trauma should be challenged. *Am Surg* 1999;65(7): 689–691.
47. Khan ZA, Dikki PE. Return of a normal functioning spleen after traumatic splenectomy. *J R Soc Med* 2004;97(8):391–392.
48. Rajani RR, Claridge JA, Yowler CJ, et al. Improved outcome of adult blunt splenic injury: a cohort analysis. *Surgery* 2006;140:625–632.
49. Duchesne JC, Simmons JD, Schmieg RE, et al. Proximal splenic angioembolization does not improve outcomes in treating blunt splenic injuries compared with splenectomy: a cohort analysis. *J Trauma* 2008;65:1346–1353.
50. Wei B, Hemmila MR, Arbabi S, et al. Angioembolization reduces operative intervention for blunt splenic injury. *J Trauma* 2008;64:1472–1477.
51. Smith HE, Biffl WL, Majercik SD, et al. Splenic artery embolization: have we gone too far? *J Trauma* 2006;61:541–546.
52. McCray VW, Davis JW, Lemaster D, et al. Observation for nonoperative management of the spleen: how long is long enough? *J Trauma* 2008;65: 1354–1358.
53. Zarzaur BL, Vashi S, Magnotti LJ, et al. The real risk of splenectomy after discharge home following nonoperative management of blunt splenic injury. *J Trauma* 2009;66:1531–1538.
54. Renzulli P, Hostettler A, Schoepfer AM, et al. Systematic review of atraumatic splenic rupture. *Br J Surg* 2009;96:1114–1121.
55. Cines DB, Bussel JB. How I treat idiopathic thrombocytopenic purpura (ITP). *Blood* 2005;106(7):2244–2251.
56. Morris KT, Horvath KD, Jobe BA, et al. Laparoscopic management of accessory spleens in immune thrombocytopenic purpura. *Surg Endosc* 1999;13(5):520–522.
57. Ballem PJ, Belzberg A, Devine DV, et al. Kinetic studies of the mechanism of thrombocytopenia in patients with human immunodeficiency virus infection. *NEJM* 1992;327(25):1779–1784.

58. Ballem PJ, Belzberg A, Devine DV, et al. Kinetic studies of the mechanism of thrombocytopenia in patients with human immunodeficiency virus infection. *NEJM* 1992;327(25):1779–1984.
59. Cersosimo RJ. Romiplostim in chronic immune thrombocytopenic purpura. *Clin Ther* 2009;31(9):1887–1907.
60. Hoo M, Lv B, He Q, et al. Both splenic CD5(+) B and CD5(–) B cells produce platelet glycoprotein-specific autoantibodies in chronic ITP. *Thromb Res* 2003;110(1):1–5.
61. Bromberg ME. Immune thrombocytopenic purpura—the changing therapeutic landscape. *NEJM* 2006;355:1643–1645.
62. Bussel JB, Kuter DJ, George JN, et al. AMG 531, a thrombopoiesis-stimulating protein, for chronic ITP. *NEJM* 2006;355:1672–1681.
63. Dan K, Gomi S, Kuramoto A, et al. A multicenter prospective study on the treatment of chronic idiopathic thrombocytopenic purpura. *Int J Hematol* 1992;55(3):287–292.
64. Andersen JC. Response of resistant idiopathic thrombocytopenic purpura to pulsed high-dose dexamethasone therapy. *NEJM* 1994;330(22): 1560–1564.
65. Sandler SG. The spleen and splenectomy in immune (idiopathic) thrombocytopenic purpura. *Semin Hematol* 2000;37:10–12.
66. Kojouri K, Vesely SK, Terrell DR, et al. Splenectomy for adult patients with idiopathic thrombocytopenic purpura: a systematic review to assess long-term platelet count responses, prediction of response, and surgical complications. *Blood* 2003;104(9):2623–2634.
67. Tsereteli Z, Smith CD, Branum GD, et al. Are the favorable outcomes of splenectomy predictable in patients with idiopathic thrombocytopenic purpura (ITP)? *Surg Endosc* 2001;15(12):1386–1389.
68. Targarona EM, Espert JJ, Balague C, et al. Residual splenic function after laparoscopic splenectomy: a clinical concern. *Arch Surg* 1998;133(1): 56–60.
69. Sampath S, Meneghetti AT, MacFarlane JK, et al. An 18-year review of open and laparoscopic splenectomy for idiopathic thrombocytopenic purpura. *Am J Surg* 2007;193:580–584.
70. Godeau B, Porcher R, Fain O, et al. Rituximab efficacy and safety in adult splenectomy candidates with chronic immune thrombocytopenic purpura: results of a prospective multicenter phase 2 study. *Blood* 2008;112: 999–1004.
71. Arnold DM, Nazi I, Santos A, et al. Combination immunosuppressant therapy for patients with chronic refractory immune thrombocytopenic purpura. *Blood* 2010;115:29–31.
72. Arnold DM, Dentall F, Crowther MA, et al. Systematic review: efficacy and safety of rituximab for adults with idiopathic thrombocytopenic purpura. *Ann Intern Med* 2007;146:25–33.
73. Kuter DJ, Bussel JB, Lyons RM, et al. Efficacy of romiplostim in patients with chronic immune thrombocytopenic purpura: a double-blind randomized controlled trial. *Lancet* 2008;271:395–403.
74. Bussel JB, Provan D, Shamsi T, et al. Effect of eltrombopag on platelet counts and bleeding during treatment of chronic idiopathic thrombocytopenic purpura: a randomized, double-blind, placebo-controlled trial. *Lancet* 2009;373:641–648.
75. Bussel JB, Cheng G, Saleh MN, et al. Eltrombopag for the treatment of chronic idiopathic thrombocytopenic purpura. *NEJM* 2007;357: 2237–2247.
76. Onundarson PT, Rowe JM, Heal JM, et al. Response to plasma exchange and splenectomy in thrombotic thrombocytopenic purpura. A 10-year experience at a single institution. *Arch Int Med* 1992;152(4):791–796.
77. Wells AD, Majumdar G, Slater NG, et al. Role of splenectomy as a salvage procedure in thrombotic thrombocytopenic purpura. *Br J Surg* 1991; 78(11):1389–1390.
78. Aqui NA, Stein SH, Konkle BA, et al. Role of splenectomy in patients with refractory or relapsed thrombotic thrombocytopenic purpura. *J Clin Apher* 2003;18(2):51–54.
79. Modic M, Cernelc P, Zver. Splenectomy: the last option of immunosuppressive therapy in patients with chronic or relapsing idiopathic thrombotic thrombocytopenic purpura? *Transplant Proc* 2002;34(7): 2953–2954.
80. Rice HE, Oldham KT, Hillery CS, et al. Clinical and hematologic benefits of partial splenectomy for congenital hemolytic anemias in children. *Ann Surg* 2003;237(2):281–288.
81. Balint GP, Balint PV. Felty's syndrome. *Best Pract Res Clin Rheumatol* 2004;18(5):631–645.
82. Van Krieken JH, Breedveld FC, de Velde J. The spleen in Felty's syndrome: a histological, morphometrical, and immunohistochemical study. *Eur J Haematol* 1988;40:58.
83. Blumfelder TM, Logue GL, Shimm DS. Felty's syndrome: effects of splenectomy upon granulocyte count and granulocyte-associated IgG. *Ann Int Med* 1981;94(5):623–628.
84. Logue GL, Huang AT Shimm DS. Failure of splenectomy in Felty's syndrome. The role of antibodies supporting granulocyte lysis by lymphocytes. *NEJM* 1981;304(10):580–583.
85. Perrotta S, Gallagher PG, Mohandaqs N. Hereditary spherocytosis. *Lancet* 2008;372:1411–1426.
86. Eber S, Lux SE. Hereditary spherocytosis—defects in proteins that connect the membrane skeleton to the lipid bilayer. *Semin Hematol* 2004;41(2): 118–141.
87. Bolton-Maggs PH, Stevens RF, Dodd NJ, et al. Guidelines for the diagnosis and management of hereditary spherocytosis. 2004;126(4):455–474.
88. Reliene R, Mariana M, Zanella A, et al. Splenectomy prolongs in vivo survival of erythrocytes differently in spectrin/ankyrin- and band 3-deficient hereditary spherocytosis. *Blood* 2002;2208–2215.
89. Tsereteli Z, Smith CD, Branum GD, et al. Are the favorable outcomes of splenectomy predictable in patients with idiopathic thrombocytopenic purpura (ITP)? *Surg Endosc* 2001;15(12):1386–1389.
90. Olivieri NF, Nathan DG, MacMillan JH, et al. Survival in medically treated patients with homozygous beta-thalassemia. *NEJM* 1994;331(9): 574–578.
91. Pinca A, DiPalma A, Soriani S, et al. Effectiveness of partial splenic embolization as treatment for hypersplenism in thalassemia major: a 7-year follow up. *Eur J Haemat* 1992;49(2):49–52.
92. Idowu O, Hayes-Jordan A. Partial splenectomy in children under 4 years of age with hemoglobinopathy. *J Ped Surg* 1998;33(8):1251–1253.
93. Al-Salem AH, al-Dabbous I, Bhamidibati P. The role of partial splenectomy in children with thalassemia. *Eur J Ped Surg* 1998;8(6):334–338.
94. Levasseur DN, Ryan TM, Reilly MP, et al. A recombinant human hemoglobin with anti-sickling properties greater than fetal hemoglobin. *J Biol Chem* 2004;279(26):27518–27524.
95. Corash L, Shafer B, Blaese RM. Platelet-associated immunoglobulin, platelet size, and the effect of splenectomy in the Wiskott-Aldrich syndrome. *Blood* 1985;65(6):1439–1443.
96. Muller CA, Anderson KD, Blaese RM. Splenectomy and/or bone marrow transplantation in the management of the Wiskott-Aldrich syndrome: long-term follow-up in 62 cases. *Blood* 1993;82:2961.
97. Verni W, Blanzuoli L, Kraus MD, et al. The spleen in the Wiskott-Aldrich syndrome: histopathologic abnormalities of the white pulp correlate with the clinical phenotype of the disease. *Am J Surg Path* 1999;23(2):182–191.
98. Elliott MA, Tefferi A. Splenic irradiation in myelofibrosis with myeloid metaplasia: a review. *Blood Rev* 1999;13(3):163–170.
99. Delpero JR, Houvenaeghel G, Gastaut JA, et al. Splenectomy for hypersplenism in chronic lymphocytic leukemia and malignant non-Hodgkin's lymphoma. *Br J Surg* 1990;77(4):554–559.
100. Thiruvengadam R, Piedmonte M, Barcos M, et al. Splenectomy in advanced chronic lymphocytic leukemia. *Leukemia* 1990;4(11):758–760.
101. Delpero JR, Houvenaeghel G, Gastaut JA, et al. Splenectomy for hypersplenism in chronic lymphocytic leukemia and malignant non-Hodgkin's lymphoma. *Br J Surg* 1990;77:443–449.
102. Neal TF Jr, Tefferi A, Witzig TE, et al. Splenectomy in advanced chronic lymphocytic leukemia: a single institution experience with 50 patients. *Am J Med* 1992;93(4):435–440.
103. Seymour JF, Cusack JD, Lerner SA, et al. Case/control study of the role of splenectomy in chronic lymphocytic leukemia. *J Clin Oncol* 1997;15(1): 52–60.
104. Savage DG, Szydlo RM, Goldman JM. Clinical features at diagnosis in 430 patients with chronic myeloid leukemia seen at a referral centre over a 16-year period. *Br J Haematol* 1997;96(1):111–116.
105. Hester JP, Waddell CC, Coltman CA, et al. Response of chronic myelogenous leukemia patients to COAP-splenectomy: a Southwest Oncology Group Study. *Cancer* 1984;54:1977–1982.
106. The Italian Cooperative Study on Chronic Myeloid Leukemia: results of a prospective randomized trial of early splenectomy in chronic myeloid leukemia. *Cancer* 1984;54:333–338.
107. Bouvet M, Babiera GV, Termuhlen PM, et al. Splenectomy in the accelerated or blastic phase of chronic myelogenous leukemia: a single-institution, 25-year experience. *Surgery* 1997;122(1):20–25.
108. Morel P, Dupriez B, Gosselin B, et al. Role of early splenectomy in malignant lymphomas with prominent splenic involvement (primary lymphomas of the spleen). A study of 59 cases. *Cancer* 1993;71(1):207–215.
109. Nair S, Shukla J, Chandy M. Non-Hodgkin's lymphoma presenting with prominent splenomegaly—clinicopathologic diversity in relationship to immunophenotype. *Acta Oncologica* 1997;36(7):725–727.
110. Lehne G, Hannisdal E, Langholm R, et al. A 10-year experience with splenectomy in patients with malignant non-Hodgkin's lymphoma at the Norwegian Radium Hospital. *Cancer* 1994;74(3):933–939.
111. Tsimberidou AM, Catovsky D, Schlette E, et al. Outcomes in patients with splenic marginal zone lymphoma and marginal zone lymphoma treated with rituximab with or without chemotherapy or chemotherapy alone. *Cancer* 2006;107:125–135.
112. Brodsky J, Abcar A, Styler M. Splenectomy for non-Hodgkin's lymphoma. *Am J Clin Oncol* 1996;19(6):558–561.
113. Grever MR. How I treat hairy cell leukemia. *Blood* 2010;115:21–28.
114. Tallman MS, Hakimian D Peterson L. Massive splenomegaly in hairy cell leukemia. *J Clin Oncol* 1998;16(3):1232–1233.
115. Katz SC, Pachter HL. Indications for splenectomy. *Am Surg* 2006;72: 565–580.
116. Smalley RV, Connors J, Tuttle RL, et al. Splenectomy vs alpha interferon: a randomized study in patients with previously untreated hairy cell leukemia. *Am J Hematol* 1992;41(1):13–18.
117. Saven A, Piro L. Newer purine analogues for the treatment of hairy-cell leukemia. *NEJM* 1994;330(10):691–697.
118. Grever M, Kopecky K, Foucar MK, et al. Randomized comparison of pentostatin versus interferon alpha-2a in previously untreated patients with hairy cell leukemia: an intergroup study. *J Clin Oncol* 1995;13(4): 974–982.
119. Else M, Ruchlemer R, Osuji N, et al. Long remissions in hairy cell leukemia with purine analogs. A report of 219 patients with a median follow-up of 12.5 years. *Cancer* 2005;104:2442–2448.

120. Reilly JT. Pathogenesis of idiopathic myelofibrosis: present status and future directions. *Br J Haematol* 1994;88(1):1–8.
121. Kraus MD, Bartlett NL, Fleming MD, et al. Splenic pathology in myelodysplasia: a report of 13 cases with clinical correlation. *Am J Surg Path* 1998;22(10):1255–1266.
122. Mesa RA. How I treat symptomatic splenomegaly in patients with myelofibrosis. *Blood* 2009;113:5394–5400.
123. Benbassat J, Gion D, Penchas S. The choice between splenectomy and medical treatment in patients with advanced agnogenic myeloid metaplasia. *Am J Hematol* 1990;33(2):128–135.
124. Barosi G, Ambrosetti A, Buratti A, et al. Splenectomy for patients with myelofibrosis with myeloid metaplasia: pretreatment variables and outcome prediction. *Leukemia* 1993;7(2):200–206.
125. Lopez-Guillermo A, Cervantes F, Bruguera M, et al. Liver dysfunction following splenectomy in idiopathic myelofibrosis: a study of 10 patients. *Acta Haematologica* 1991;85(4):184–188.
126. Mesa RA, Nagorney DS, Schwager S, et al. Palliative goals, patient selection, and perioperative platelet management: outcomes and lessons from 3 decades of splenectomy for myelofibrosis with myeloid metaplasia at the Mayo Clinic. *Cancer* 2006;107:361–370.
127. Barosi G, Bergamaschi G, Marchetti M, et al. JAK2 V617 mutational status predicts progression to large splenomegaly and leukemic transformation in primary myelofibrosis. *Blood* 2007;110:4030–4036.
128. Camperat E, Bardier-Dupas A, Camparo P, et al. Splenic metastasis. Clinicopathologic presentation, differential diagnosis, and pathogenesis. *Arch Pathol Lab Med* 2007;131:965–969.
129. Sileri P, D'Ugo S, Benavoli D, et al. Metachronous splenic metastasis from colonic carcinoma five years after surgery: a case report and literature review. *South Med J* 2009;102(7):733–735.
130. Stang A, Keles H, Hentschke S, et al. Differentiation of benign from malignant focal splenic lesions using sulfur hexafluoride-filled microbubble contrast-enhanced pulse-inversion sonography. *AJR Am J Roentgenol* 2009; 193:709–721.
131. Cohen IJ, Katz K, Freud E, et al. Long-term follow-up of partial splenectomy in Gaucher's disease. *Am J Surg* 1992;164(4):345–347.
132. Morgenstern L, Verham R, Weinstein I, et al. Subtotal splenectomy for Gaucher's disease: a follow-up study. *Am Surg* 1993;59(12):860–865.
133. Zer M, Freud E. Subtotal splenectomy in Gaucher's disease: towards a definition of critical splenic mass. *Br J Surg* 1992;79(8):742–744.
134. Rodriguez JR, Madanat MG, Healy BC, et al. Distal pancreatectomy with splenic preservation revisited. *Surgery* 2007;141:619–625.
135. Fermandez-Cruz L, Martinez I, Gilabert R, et al. Laparoscopic distal pancreatectomy combined with preservation of the spleen for cystic neoplasms of the pancreas. *J Gastrointest Surg* 2004;8(4):493–501.
136. Ikeguchi M, Kaibara N. Lymph node metastasis at the splenic hilum in proximal gastric cancer. *Am Surg* 2004;70(7):645–648.
137. Martin RC, Jaques DP, Brennan MF, et al. Extended local resection for advanced gastric cancer: increased survival versus increased morbidity. *Ann Surg* 2002;236(2):159–165.
138. Martin RC, Jaques DP, Brennan MF, et al. Achieving RO resection for locally advanced gastric cancer: is it worth the risk of multiorgan resection? *J Am Coll Surg* 2002;194(5):568–577.
139. Yu W, Choi GS, Chung HY. Randomized clinical trial of splenectomy versus splenic preservation in patients with proximal gastric cancer. *Br J Surg* 2006;93:559–563.
140. Cassar K, Munro A. Iatrogenic splenic injury. *J R Coll Surg Edinb* 2002; 47(6):731–741.
141. Flum DR, Koepsell T, Heagerty P, et al. The nationwide frequency of major adverse outcomes in antireflux surgery and the role of surgeon experience. *J Am Coll Surg* 2002;195(5):611–618.
142. Holubar SD, Wang JK, Wolff BG, et al. Splenic salvage after intraoperative splenic injury during colectomy. *Arch Surg* 2009;144(11):1040–1045.
143. McGory ML, Zingmond DS, Sekeris E, et al. The significance of inadvertent splenectomy during colorectal cancer resection. *Arch Surg* 2007; 142(7):668–674.
144. Muskat PC, Johnson RA, Bowers GJ. Staging laparotomy in Hodgkin's lymphoma. *Am J Surg* 1991;162(6):603–606.
145. Mendenhall NP, Cantor AB, Williams JL, et al. With modern imaging techniques, is staging laparoscopy necessary in pediatric Hodgkin's disease? A Pediatric Oncology Group study. *J Clin Oncol* 1993;11(11):2218–2225.
146. Gospodarowicz MK, Sutcliffe SB, Clark RM, et al. Analysis of supradiaphragmatic clinical stage I and II Hodgkin's disease treated with radiation alone. *Int J Radiat Oncol Biol Phys* 1992;22:859.
147. Wasserman TH, Trenkner DA, Fineberg B, et al. Cure of early stage Hodgkin's disease with subtotal nodal irradiation. *Cancer* 1991;68:1208.
148. Swerdlow AJ, Douglas AJ, Vaughan Hudson G, et al. Risk of second primary cancer after Hodgkin's disease in patients in the British National Lymphoma Investigation: relationships to host factors, histology, and stage of Hodgkin's disease, and splenectomy. *Br J Cancer* 1993;68(5):1006–1011.
149. Linet MS, Yren O, Gridley G, et al. Risk of cancer following splenectomy. *Int J Cancer* 1996;6(5):611–616.
150. Loftus JP, Nagorney DM, Ilstrup D, et al. Sinistra portal hypertension. Splenectomy or expectant management. *Ann Surg* 1993;217(1):35–40.
151. Lambert CJ Jr, Williamson JW. Splenic artery aneurysm. A rare cause of upper gastrointestinal bleeding. *Am Surg* 1990;56(9):543–555.
152. Lambert CJ Jr, Williamson JW. Splenic artery aneurysm. A rare cause of upper gastrointestinal bleeding. *Am Surg* 1990;56(9):543–545.
153. Keagan MT, Freed KS, Parks EK, et al. Imaging-guided percutaneous biopsy of focal splenic lesions: update on safety and effectiveness. *AJR Am J Roentgenol* 1999;172(4):933–937.
154. Lishner M, Lang R, Hamlet E, et al. Fine needle aspiration biopsy in patients with diffusely enlarged spleens. *Acta Cytologica* 1996;40(2):196–198.
155. Lee H, Maeda K. Hamartoma of the spleen. *Arch Pathol Lab Med* 2009;133:147–151.
156. Yu RS, Zhang SZ, Hua JM. Imaging findings of splenic hamartoma. *World J Gastroent* 2004;10(17):13–15.
157. Mackenzie RK, Youngson GG, Mahomed AA. Laparoscopic decapsulation of congenital splenic cysts: a step forward in splenic preservation. *J Ped Surg* 2004;39(1):88–90.
158. Atmatzidis K, Papaziogas B, Mirelis C, et al. Splenectomy versus spleen-preserving surgery for splenic echinococcosis. *Dig Surg* 2003;20(6): 527–531.
159. Manouras AJ, Nikolaou CC, Katergiannakis VA, et al. Spleen-sparing surgical treatment for echinococcosis of the spleen. *Br J Surg* 1997;84:1162.
160. Alonso Cohen MA, Galera MJ, Ruiz M, et al. Splenic abscess. *World J Surg* 1990;14(4):513–516.
161. De Bree E, Tsiftsis D, Christodoulakis M, et al. Splenic abscess: a diagnostic and therapeutic challenge. *Acta Chirurgica Belgica* 1998;98(5):199–202.
162. Robinson SL, Saxe JM, Lucas CE, et al. Splenic abscess associated with endocarditis. *Surgery* 1992;112(4):781–786.
163. Misawa T, Yoshida K, Shiba H, et al. Wandering spleen with chronic torsion. *Surgery* 2008;195:504–505.
164. Flum DR, Koepsell T, Heagerty P, et al. The nationwide frequency of major adverse outcomes in antireflux surgery and the role of surgeon experience. *J Am Coll Surg* 2002;195(5):611–618.
165. Haj M, Bickel A, Weiss M, et al. Laparoscopic splenopexy of a wandering spleen. *J Laparoendosc Adv Surg Tech A* 1999;9(4):357–360.
166. Corcione F, Caiazzo P, Cuccurullo D, et al. Laparoscopic splenectomy for the treatment of wandering spleen. *Surg Endosc* 2004;18(3):554–556.
167. Nelson EW, Mone MC. Splenectomy in high-risk patients with splenomegaly. *Am J Surg* 1999;178(6):581–586.
168. Letoquart JP, LaGamma A, Kunin N, et al. Splenectomy for splenomegaly exceeding 1000 grams: analysis of 47 patients. *Br J Surg* 1993;80(3): 334–335.
169. Petroianu A, da Silva RG, Simal CJ, et al. Late postoperative follow-up of patients submitted to subtotal splenectomy. *Am Surg* 1997;63(8):735–740.
170. Targarona EM, Espert JJ, Balague C, et al. Splenomegaly should not be considered a contraindication for laparoscopic splenectomy. *Ann Surg* 1998;228(1):35–39.
171. Naoum JJ, Silverfein EJ, Zhou W, et al. Concomitant intraoperative splenic artery embolization and laparoscopic splenectomy versus laparoscopic splenectomy: comparison of treatment outcome. *Am J Surg* 2007; 193:713–718.
172. Rescorla F, West KW, Engum SA, et al. Laparoscopic splenic procedures in children experience in 231 children. *Ann Surg* 2007;246:683–688.
173. Borrazzo ED, Daly JM, Morrisey KP, et al. Hand-assistant laparoscopic splenectomy for giant spleen. *Surg Endosc* 2003;17(6):918–920.
174. Terrosu G, Baccarani U, Bresadola V, et al. The impact of splenic weight on laparoscopic splenectomy for splenomegaly. *Surg Endosc* 2002;16(1): 103–107.
175. Machado MA, Makdissi FF, Herman P, et al. Exposure of splenic hilum increases safety of laparoscopic splenectomy. *Surg Laparosc Endosc Percutan Tech* 2004;14(1):23–25.
176. Grahn SW, Alvarez J, Kirkwood K. Trends in laparoscopic splenectomy for massive splenomegaly. *Arch Surg* 2006;141:755–762.
177. Breitenstein S, Scholz T, Schafer M, et al. Laparoscopic partial splenectomy. *J Am Coll Surg* 2007;204:179–181.
178. Tanoue K, Okita K, Akahoshi T, et al. Laparoscopic splenectomy for hematologic diseases. *Surgery* 2002;131:S318–S323.
179. Corcione F, Caiazzo P, Cuccurullo D, et al. Laparoscopic splenectomy for the treatment of wandering spleen. *Surg Endosc* 2004;18(3):554–556.
180. Kaban GK, Czerniach DR, Perugini RA, et al. Use of a laparoscopic hand-assist device for accessory splenectomy. *Surg Endosc* 2004;18(6):1001.
181. Rasekhi AR, Naderifar M, Bagheri MH, et al. Radiofrequency ablation of the spleen in patients with thalassemia intermedia: a pilot study. *AJR Am J Roentgenol* 2009;192:1425–1429.
182. Jiao LR, Tierris I, Ayav A, et al. A new technique for spleen preservation with radiofrequency. *Surgery* 2006;140:464–466.

CHAPTER 74 ■ BREAST DISEASE

TARI A. KING AND MONICA MORROW

KEY POINTS

1. Screening mammography reduces breast cancer mortality by 20% to 30% and increases the likelihood of breast-conserving surgery.
2. Needle biopsy is the preferred method of diagnosing both palpable and nonpalpable breast masses. A benign needle biopsy diagnosis of a clinically or mammographically suspicious mass is an indication for surgical biopsy.
3. The most common causes of pathologic nipple discharge are a solitary papilloma (60%) or duct hyperplasia (15% to 20%), followed by ductal carcinoma in situ in 5% to 20% of patients.
4. If aspiration of a breast cyst yields nonbloody fluid and the mass resolves, no further therapy is needed; whereas if the fluid is bloody, the palpable abnormality does not resolve completely, or the same cyst recurs multiple times, biopsy to exclude malignancy is required.
5. A dominant breast mass should not be dismissed as a cyst unless the diagnosis is confirmed by ultrasonography or aspiration of fluid.
6. Mutations in the susceptibility genes *BRCA1* and *BRCA2* are present in 5% to 10% of women with breast cancer. They should be considered in women diagnosed before age 40 years and those with a family history of two or more relatives in the same bloodline with breast cancer, or in the presence of breast and ovarian cancer, bilateral breast cancer, or male breast cancer in the family.
7. The use of tamoxifen for 5 years in high-risk pre- or postmenopausal women results in an approximately 50% reduction in risk for invasive and noninvasive breast cancer. The use of raloxifene in postmenopausal women for 5 years has a similar effect and fewer side effects.
8. Improvements in local control rates of greater than 10% at 5 years through the use of radiotherapy after lumpectomy or mastectomy are associated with improved breast cancer–specific and overall survival at 15 years.
9. There is no difference in survival for patients with invasive breast cancer treated with mastectomy and those treated with lumpectomy and radiotherapy.
10. For breast-conserving therapy to be successful in the treatment of invasive breast cancer, three conditions must be met. It must be possible to (a) reduce the tumor burden to a microscopic level likely to be controlled by irradiation, (b) safely deliver radiation therapy, and (c) promptly detect local recurrence.
11. Radiation therapy leads to an approximately 75% reduction in local recurrence after breast conservation therapy. Subgroups of women with invasive cancer not requiring radiation, other than women over age 70 with small, estrogen receptor–positive tumors, have not been reproducibly identified.
12. Regardless of the technique of sentinel node biopsy used, a sentinel node will be identified in 95% of breast cancer patients and will predict the status of the remaining axillary nodes in about 90% of cases.
13. Locally advanced breast cancer includes T3 and T4 tumors, those with extensive regional nodal involvement (N2 or N3), and inflammatory breast cancer, and should be treated with a combination of induction chemotherapy, surgery, and postoperative radiation therapy.

ANATOMY

The adult female breast lies between the second and sixth ribs and between the sternal edge and the midaxillary line (Fig. 74.1). Breast tissue frequently extends into the axilla as the axillary tail of Spence. Posteriorly, the upper portion of the breast rests on the fascia of the pectoralis major muscle; inferolaterally, it is bounded by the fascia of the serratus anterior. Bands of fibrous tissue, known as *Cooper ligaments*, extend from the fascia to the fibrous tissue of the dermis and support the breast. The size of the adult female breast varies widely among individuals, and there is considerable discrepancy in breast size between the breasts of an individual woman. This is rarely a sign of breast disease. The breast is composed of skin, subcutaneous tissue, and breast tissue. The breast tissue includes both epithelial parenchymal elements and stroma. The epithelial component comprises about 10% to 15% of the breast mass, with the remainder being stroma. Each breast consists of 15 to 20 lobes of glandular tissue that are supported by a framework of fibrous connective tissue. The space between lobes is filled by adipose tissue. Variations in breast size are accounted for by differences in the amount of adipose tissue in the breast rather than the epithelial elements. Much of the epithelial tissue of the breast is found in the upper outer quadrant, which is why this is the most frequent site of both benign and malignant breast disease.

The lobes of the breast are subdivided into lobules, which are made up of branched tubuloalveolar glands. Each lobe ends in a lactiferous duct, 2 to 4 mm in diameter. Beneath the areola, the lactiferous ducts dilate into lactiferous sinuses and then open through a constricted orifice onto the nipple (Fig. 74.2).

The nipple is located over the fourth intercostal space in the nonpendulous breast and is surrounded by a circular, pigmented areola. Beneath the nipple and areola are bundles of radially arranged smooth muscle fibers that are responsible for the erection of the nipple in response to a variety of stimuli. The nipple and areola contain sebaceous glands and apocrine sweat glands, but no hair follicles. In addition, the tubercles of Morgagni are nodular elevations formed by the

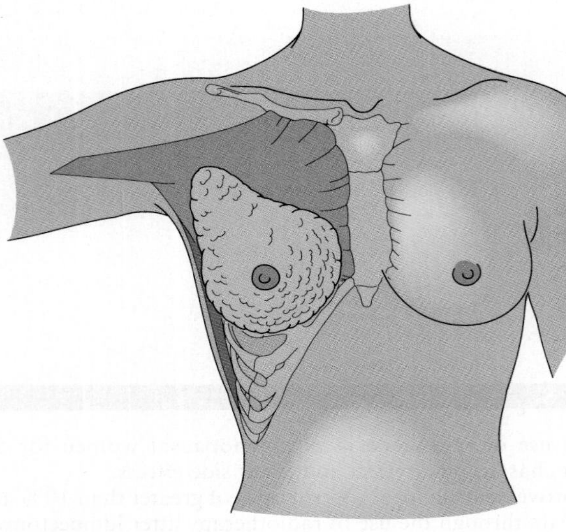

FIGURE 74.1. The adult female breast. The upper and medial portions of the breast rest on the pectoralis major muscle, and the inferolateral portion rests on the serratus anterior.

openings of the Montgomery glands at the periphery of the areola. These glands are capable of secreting milk and are believed to represent an intermediate stage between sweat and mammary glands. The nipple and areolar region, as well as the remainder of the breast, is richly supplied with sensory innervation.

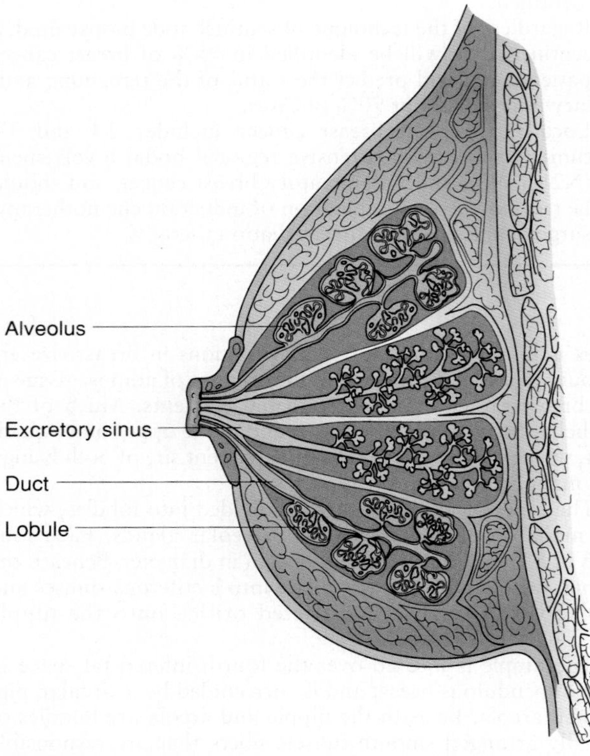

FIGURE 74.2. The breast consists of 15 to 20 lobes of glandular tissue. Within each lobe, the lobules are composed of branched tubuloalveolar glands. Each lobule ends in a lactiferous duct. These ducts dilate into lactiferous sinuses beneath the nipple.

The blood supply of the breast is derived from the internal mammary and lateral thoracic arteries. The medial and central portions of the breast receive their major blood supply from anterior perforating branches of the internal mammary artery, and the upper outer quadrant is primarily supplied by the lateral thoracic artery. In general, the venous drainage of the breast follows the arterial supply.

LYMPHATIC DRAINAGE

The lymphatics of the breast are thin-walled, valveless vessels that drain unidirectionally except when obstructed by inflammatory or neoplastic disease. The superficial subareolar lymphatic plexus drains primarily the skin of the breast and the nipple and areola, in addition to some of the central portion of the gland. This plexus is interconnected with the deep lymphatic plexus, which drains most of the breast parenchyma. Injections of radioactively labeled colloid have demonstrated that about 97% of the lymphatic flow from the breast drains directly into the axillary lymph nodes, with the remaining 3% draining into the internal mammary nodes.[1] All quadrants of the breast drain into the axillary nodes.

The axillary space is bordered by the axillary vein superiorly, the latissimus dorsi laterally, and the serratus anterior medially (Fig. 74.3). The pectoralis major lies anterior to the axillary space, and the subscapularis comprises its posterior wall. Structures of clinical importance within this space include the long thoracic nerve, which innervates the serratus anterior; the thoracodorsal neurovascular bundle, which innervates and supplies blood to the latissimus dorsi; and the intercostobrachial nerves, which are sensory to the upper inner aspect of the arm.

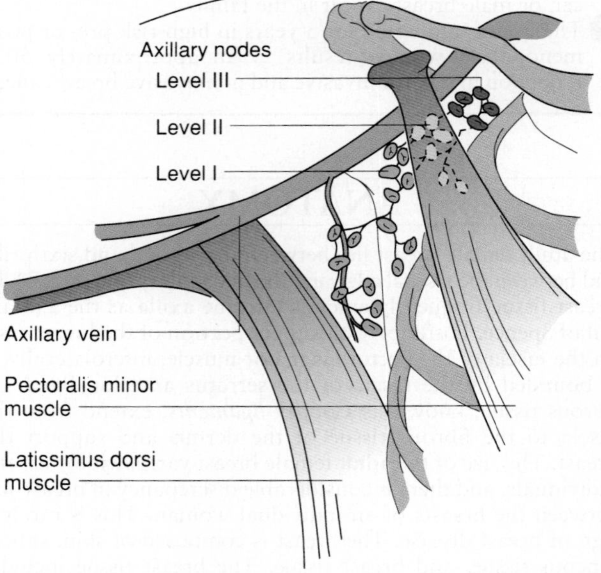

FIGURE 74.3. The axillary lymph nodes are divided into three levels by the pectoralis minor muscle. The level I nodes are inferior and lateral to the pectoralis minor, the level II nodes are below the axillary vein and behind the pectoralis minor, and the level III nodes are medial to the muscle against the chest wall.

The axillary nodes are embedded in fat and are variable in number. Surgeons have traditionally divided the axillary nodes into three levels: level I nodes, inferior and lateral to the pectoralis minor; level II nodes, behind the pectoralis minor and inferior to the axillary vein; and level III nodes, medial to the pectoralis minor and against the chest wall. The interpectoral (or Rotter) nodes are located between the pectoralis major and minor muscles along the lateral pectoral nerve. Involvement of this node group in the absence of axillary metastases is extremely rare,[2] and thus they are of limited clinical significance. The supraclavicular nodes are contiguous with the apex of the axilla. Metastatic involvement of this nodal group in the absence of extensive axillary disease is also uncommon, although direct lymphatic drainage to this node group occurs occasionally.

The internal mammary nodes are located in the first six intercostal spaces within 3 cm of the edge of the sternum. The highest concentration of internal mammary nodes is found in the first three intercostal spaces.[3]

PHYSIOLOGY

Development of the Breast

Breast development is controlled by a large number of hormonal and biochemical factors. In the female, estrogens interact with the primordial breast bud to promote ductal development, whereas in the male, the interaction of androgen with the breast bud results in destruction of the epithelial component. In the female, ductal elongation and branching begin in puberty and are regulated by pituitary growth hormone, which may act through insulinlike growth factor I locally.[4] In addition, the presence of estrogen and progesterone is required to stimulate DNA synthesis. This effect is believed to occur through both receptor-mediated and paracrine pathways.

Changes in breast size and shape begin at puberty and are secondary to growth of both the glandular and stromal elements of the breast. Russo and Russo[5] have described three types of breast lobules related to a woman's parity and menopausal status. The type 1 (or virginal) lobule consists of a cluster of 11 alveolar buds around a terminal duct; it is the predominant lobule in nulliparous and postmenopausal women. Type 2 lobules contain an average of 47 alveolar buds, and type 3 lobules have 80, at which time they are referred to as *ductules* or *alveoli*. In parous women, type 3 lobules predominate, with a peak frequency in the early reproductive years until they begin to decline in the fourth decade of life. Cells within these lobules have been shown to proliferate at different rates, the rate being 10 times higher in type 1 than in type 3 lobules, and three times higher in type 1 than in type 2 lobules. The presence of estrogen receptor-α (ER-α) and the progesterone receptor within these lobules is directly proportional to the rate of cell proliferation.[6] These differences in cell proliferation may explain some of the differences in breast cancer risk observed on the basis of parity and age at first birth (see section on breast cancer risk factors).

The cyclic increases in estrogen and progesterone that occur in the menstrual cycle also influence the gross and microscopic character of the breast. Many women experience increased breast fullness, nodularity, and sensitivity in the premenstrual period. During the follicular phase of the menstrual cycle (days 4 through 14), epithelial proliferation occurs, with epithelial sprouting and an increased mitotic rate. During the luteal phase of the cycle (days 15 through 28), when progestins predominate, proliferation is maximal, with ductal dilation and differentiation of the alveolar epithelial cells to secretory cells. This results in the formation of lipid droplets in the alveolar cells and some intraluminal secretion. With the onset of menstruation, secretory activity regresses secondary to epithelial apoptosis, or programmed cell death.

Pregnancy

Significant ductal, lobular, and alveolar growth occurs during pregnancy as a result of exposure to estrogen, progesterone, growth hormone, prolactin, and placental hormones. Clinically, this is manifested as breast enlargement, with associated dilation of the superficial veins and darkening of the nipple. At delivery, the breast may be three times the size of the nonlactating breast. Microscopically, lobular-alveolar differentiation to type 3 lobules begins in the first trimester, and the stromal elements of the breast are gradually replaced by the proliferating glandular epithelium. During the third trimester, terminal differentiation of the epithelium results in the development of secretory cells that are able to synthesize and secrete milk proteins. Oxytocin induces myoepithelial proliferation and differentiation.[6]

Lactation and Involution

After delivery, the sudden fall in estrogen and progesterone levels results in lactation. Prolactin, in conjunction with growth hormone and insulin, induces the production and secretion of milk. Initially, colostrum, a sticky serous fluid rich in growth factors, is secreted, followed by milk. Milk secretion is regulated by the pituitary production of oxytocin, which is released in response to neural reflexes activated by suckling.

Following weaning, the secretory activity of the lactogenic epithelium gradually decreases. Retained secretory products are removed by phagocytosis, although ruptured alveoli containing milk may be clinically manifested as galactoceles. Atrophy of glandular, ductal, and stromal elements results in a decrease in breast size. Withdrawal of the steroid hormones and growth factors of pregnancy and lactation results in apoptosis of the terminally differentiated secretory cells of the epithelial lumen. As previously noted, however, type 3 lobules persist.

Menopause

After menopause, the breast undergoes regression. Type 1 lobules predominate, as in the breasts of nulliparous women. Overall, involution of the ductal and glandular elements of the breast occurs, and the breast becomes predominantly fat and stroma. With aging, a progressive decrease in the fat content and supporting stroma results in breast shrinkage and loss of contour.

BREAST EXAMINATION

A careful history is the initial step in a breast examination. Regardless of the presenting complaint, baseline information regarding menstrual status and breast cancer risk factors should be obtained. The basic elements of a breast history are listed in Table 74.1. In premenopausal women, knowing the date of the last menstrual period and the regularity of the cycle is useful in evaluating breast nodularity, pain, and cysts. Postmenopausal women should be questioned about the use of hormone replacement therapy, given that many benign breast problems are uncommon after menopause in the absence of exogenous hormones. Specific information about the patient's presenting complaint is then elicited. A breast lump is most often the clinical problem that causes women to

TABLE 74.1 **DIAGNOSIS**

MEDICAL HISTORY OF A BREAST PROBLEM

GENERAL
Age at menarche
Number of pregnancies
Number of live births
Age at first birth
Family history of breast cancer, including affected relative, age of onset, and presence of bilateral disease
History of breast biopsies (and histologic diagnosis, if available)
Premenopausal women
Date of last menstrual period
Length and regularity of cycles
Use of oral contraceptives
Postmenopausal women
Date of menopause
Use of hormone replacement therapy
SPECIFIC
Onset
Duration
Frequency
Severity
Relationship to menstrual cycle or use of hormone replacement therapy

seek treatment and remains the most common presentation of breast carcinoma. Today, many women present for a breast examination after an abnormality has been identified on a screening mammogram. Although the majority of these lesions are not clinically evident, a careful physical examination is an important part of the evaluation of a patient with an abnormal mammogram. Breast pain, a change in the size and shape of the breast, nipple discharge, and changes in the appearance of the skin are infrequent symptoms of carcinoma. The evaluation and management of these conditions are described in the section on clinical breast problems. For any breast complaint, the duration of the symptoms, their persistence over time, and their fluctuation with the menstrual cycle or relationship to exogenous estrogen should be ascertained.

Technique

A woman must be disrobed from the waist up for a complete breast examination. Although attention to modesty is appropriate and a gown or drape should be provided, inspection is an important part of the examination, and subtle abnormalities are best appreciated by comparing the appearance of both breasts. The breast examination should be performed with the patient in both the sitting and supine positions, and care should be taken at all times to be gentle. The steps of a breast examination are illustrated in Figure 74.4.

The breasts are initially inspected while the patient is in the sitting position with the arms relaxed. The size and shape of the breasts should be compared. If a discrepancy in size is noted, determine its chronicity. In many women, the breasts

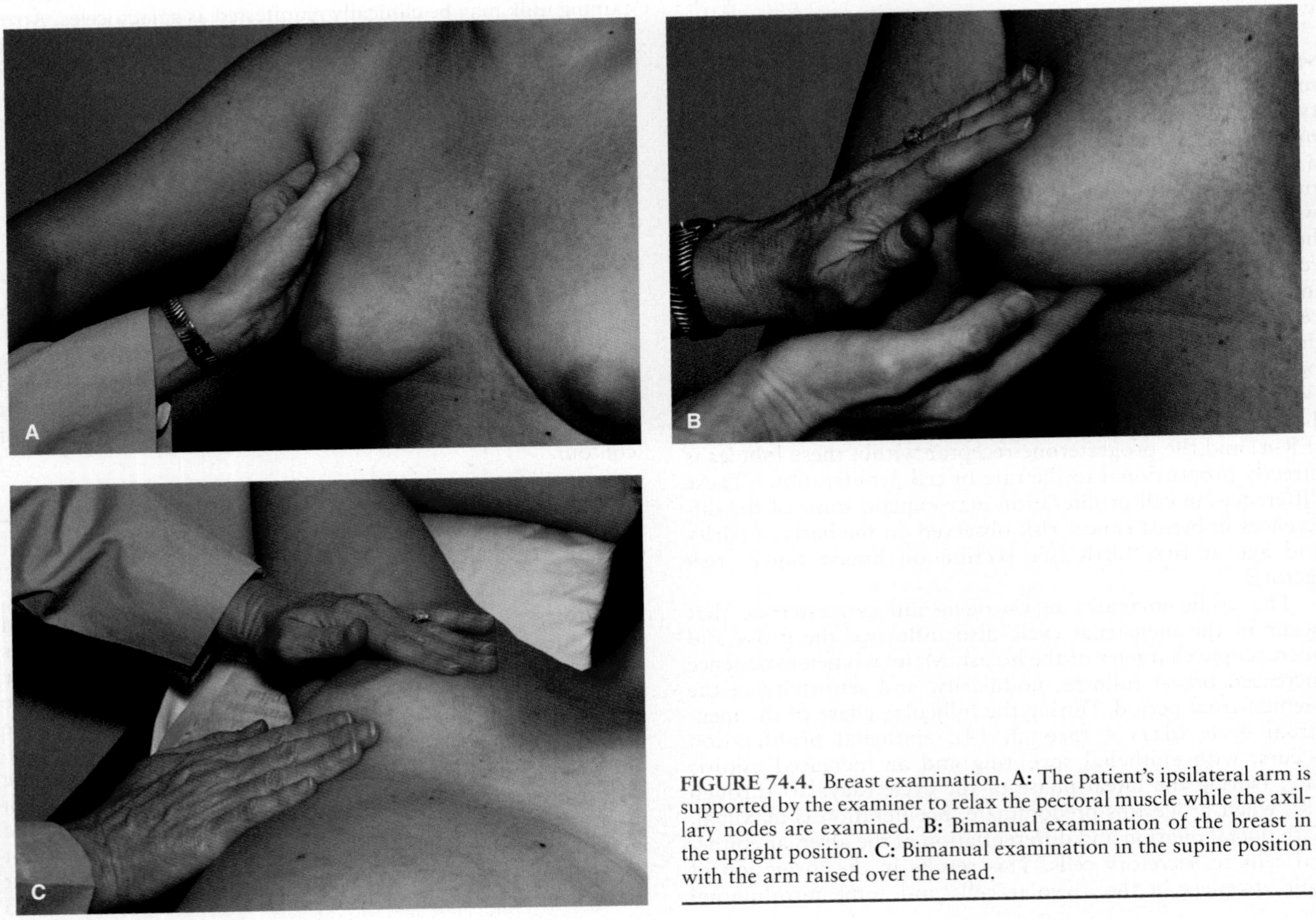

FIGURE 74.4. Breast examination. **A:** The patient's ipsilateral arm is supported by the examiner to relax the pectoral muscle while the axillary nodes are examined. **B:** Bimanual examination of the breast in the upright position. **C:** Bimanual examination in the supine position with the arm raised over the head.

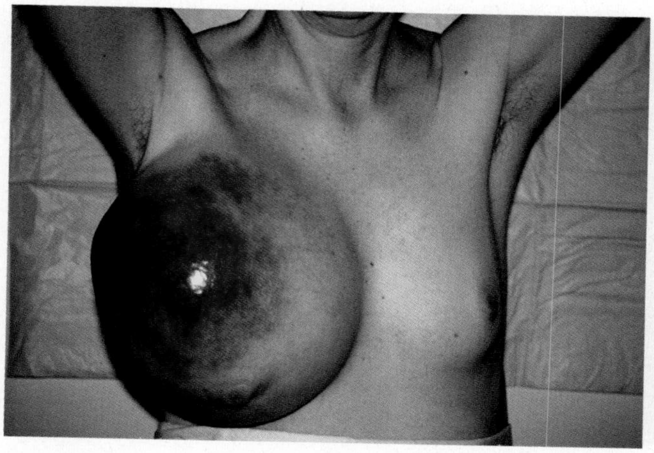

FIGURE 74.5. Breast asymmetry resulting from a benign phyllodes tumor. Skin changes are caused by pressure necrosis.

are not identical in size, and the finding of small discrepancies in size is rarely a sign of malignancy. Differences in breast size of recent onset or progressive in nature, however, may be caused by both benign and malignant tumors and require further evaluation (Fig. 74.5). Alterations in breast shape, in the absence of previous surgery, are of more concern. Superficially located tumors can cause bulges in the breast contour or retraction of the overlying skin. The skin retraction evident with superficial tumors may be caused by direct extension of tumor or fibrosis. Tumors deep within the substance of the breast that involve the fibrous septa (Cooper ligaments) can also cause retraction. Retraction is not itself a prognostic factor except when it is caused by the direct extension of tumor into the skin, and for this reason, it is not a part of the clinical staging of breast cancer.[7] Although retraction is usually a sign of malignancy, benign lesions of the breast, such as granular cell tumors and fat necrosis, also cause retraction. Other benign causes of retraction include surgical biopsy and thrombophlebitis of the thoracoepigastric vein (Mondor disease).

The skin of the breast and the nipples should also be carefully inspected. Edema of the skin of the breast (*peau d'orange*), when present, is usually extensive and readily apparent. Localized edema is frequently most prominent in the lower half of the breast and periareolar region, and is most noticeable when the patient's arms are raised. Erythema is another sign of disease that is evident on inspection. It may be caused by cellulitis or abscess in the breast, but a diagnosis of inflammatory carcinoma should always be considered.

Examination of the nipples should include inspection for symmetry, retraction, and changes in the character of the skin. The new onset of nipple retraction should be regarded with a high index of suspicion, except when it occurs immediately after cessation of breast-feeding. Ulceration and eczematous changes of the nipple may be the first signs of Paget disease.

After inspection with the arms relaxed, ask the patient to raise her arms to allow a more complete inspection of the lower half of the breasts. A final inspection is made with the hands on the hips and the pectoral muscles contracted.

The regional nodes are then examined with the patient upright. Assess the size, character (soft, tender, firm), and number, and note whether the nodes are matted. The axillary nodes are most readily examined with the ipsilateral arm supported to relax the pectoral muscle (Fig. 74.4A). Bimanual examination of the breast is also carried out with the patient upright (Fig. 74.4B).

Complete the breast examination with the patient in the supine position and the ipsilateral arm raised above the head (Fig. 74.4C). Then systematically examine the breast tissue. Whether the examination is performed with a radial or a concentric circular search pattern is unimportant, provided that the entire breast is examined. The examination should extend superiorly to the clavicle, inferiorly to the lower rib cage, medially to the sternal border, and laterally to the midaxillary line.

One of the most difficult aspects of breast examination relates to the nodular, irregular texture of normal breasts in premenopausal women. Normal breasts tend to be most nodular in the upper outer quadrants, where the glandular tissue is concentrated; in the inframammary ridge area; and in the subareolar region. Generalized lumpiness is not a pathologic finding. Comparing the breasts is often helpful in determining whether a questionable area requires further evaluation. When the patient notices a mass that is not evident to the examiner, she should be asked to indicate the area of concern. If uncertainty remains regarding the significance of an area of nodular breast tissue in a premenopausal woman, a repeat examination at a different time during the menstrual cycle may clarify the issue. If a dominant mass is identified, measure it and record its location, mobility, and character in the medical record. The evaluation of a breast mass is discussed in detail in the section on clinical breast problems.

Screening Mammography

A screening mammogram consists of two views of the breast (craniocaudal and mediolateral oblique), which are obtained in asymptomatic women in an effort to detect cancer in a preclinical state, when the likelihood of cure is higher. It is important that screening not be confused with a diagnostic workup, which is performed to evaluate a woman with a clinical breast complaint and is discussed in the section on diagnostic imaging.

1 The ultimate measure of the effectiveness of a screening test is its effect on mortality. Eight randomized clinical trials, beginning with the Health Insurance Plan of New York study in 1963, have compared breast cancer mortality in women undergoing screening mammography at 1- to 2-year intervals with mortality in control populations. A 20% to 30% decrease in mortality has been demonstrated for screened women age 50 and older.[8] The benefit of screening in women ages 40 to 49 has been controversial. Many of the trials were not designed to allow a separate analysis of women in this age group, and mortality benefits were often not apparent until after 8 years or more of follow-up. A meta-analysis of women ages 40 to 49 in the randomized trials, however, suggests a 29% mortality reduction with screening in this age group.[9]

The mortality reduction from screening is achieved by identifying abnormalities that cannot be detected on physical examination. These include microcalcifications and masses smaller than 1 cm in size, the usual clinical limit of detection. In addition to reducing breast cancer mortality, identifying smaller tumors increases the likelihood that a woman will be a candidate for breast-conserving surgery. In one study, only 10% of women with tumors 2 cm or less in size had contraindications to breast conservation, compared with 30% of women with tumors larger than 2 cm but less than 5 cm in size.[10] Current screening recommendations are for annual mammography for women age 40 and older.

Screening mammography is a sensitive but nonspecific test, and only 20% to 30% of mammographically detected abnormalities that are examined further are found to be malignant. Biopsies for clinically occult, benign lesions represent the major induced cost of screening. The positive predictive value

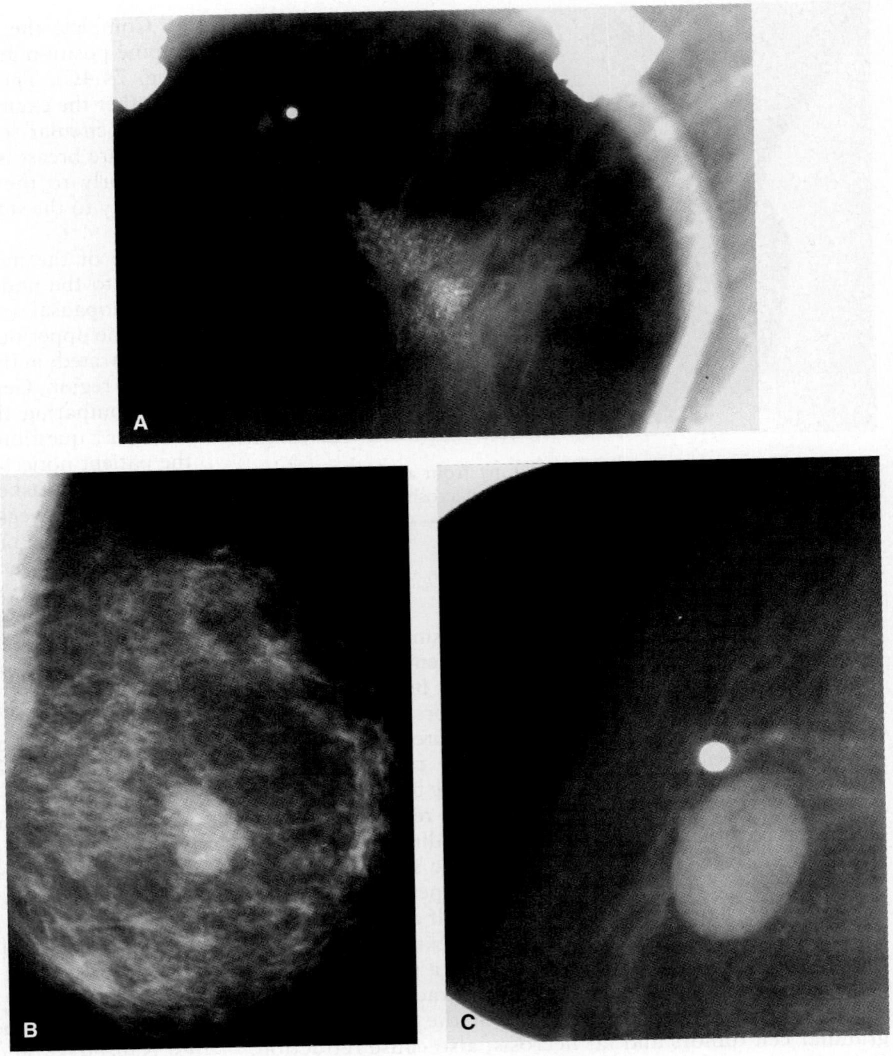

FIGURE 74.6. Mammographic masses. A: Spiculated mass with calcifications. B: Lobulated mass with indistinct posterior margin. C: Well-circumscribed mass.

of a mammographic lesion varies with its appearance. For spiculated or stellate masses, the likelihood of malignancy is 75%; this falls to 20% for lobulated masses with slightly irregular margins and to 5% for well-circumscribed masses (Fig. 74.6). The classification of calcifications has proved to be even more difficult. Calcifications are analyzed based on their size, number, distribution, and morphology; those that are irregular in size and shape, particularly when they have a branching pattern suggestive of a ductal distribution, are most likely to be malignant (Fig. 74.7).

In an effort to standardize the reporting of mammographic abnormalities, the American College of Radiology has created a breast imaging reporting and data system (BI-RADS).[11] The BI-RADS classification is listed in Table 74.2. Category 3 lesions are those with a less than 2% probability of malignancy, and short-interval follow-up usually consists of repeated imaging studies at 6 months. Category 4 lesions range in risk from 2% to 50%, and a decision regarding biopsy is based on the appearance of the lesion and the patient's level of risk.

The BI-RADS also includes a category 0, which is used when analysis is incomplete and additional studies, such as magnification views or ultrasonography, are needed before a final BI-RADS classification can be assigned. In practice, the

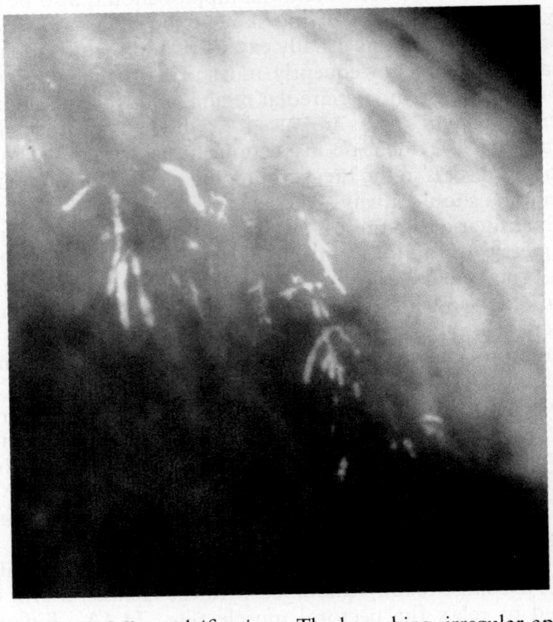

FIGURE 74.7. Microcalcifications. The branching, irregular appearance is classic for ductal carcinoma in situ.

TABLE 74.2 **CLASSIFICATION**

BI-RADS CLASSIFICATION OF MAMMOGRAPHIC ABNORMALITIES

■ CATEGORY	■ ASSESSMENT	■ RECOMMENDATION
1	Negative	Routine screening
2	Benign finding	Routine screening
3	Probably benign finding	Short-interval follow-up
4	Suspicious abnormality	Definite probability of malignancy; consider biopsy
5	Highly suggestive of malignancy	High probability of cancer; appropriate action should be taken

BI-RADS, breast imaging reporting and data system.

majority of abnormalities detected on screening mammography should undergo a diagnostic workup before biopsy. With additional views, the need for biopsy of benign lesions is often avoided, as illustrated in Figure 74.8, where what appears to be a mass lesion resolves with spot compression and magnification views. Sickles[12] reported that of 302 cases of calcifications felt to be equivocal (i.e., BI-RADS category 4) after a screening examination, 61% were shown to be benign on additional views. Even with lesions that are clearly malignant on a screening examination, additional views allow a better definition of the extent of the lesion for treatment planning.

Biopsy Techniques for Lesions Detected on Screening

After a physical examination has confirmed that a mammographically detected abnormality is not clinically evident, a histologic diagnosis can be obtained by needle localization and excision, or an image-guided core biopsy. For many years, needle localization with excision was the "gold standard" for the diagnosis of mammographic abnormalities. Recognition that the majority of mammographic abnormalities are benign, however, has resulted in the replacement of surgical biopsy with image-guided needle biopsy techniques.

Mass lesions can be sampled under ultrasonographic or stereotactic guidance; calcifications generally require stereotactic guidance. A comparison of the results of stereotactic core biopsy and surgical biopsy demonstrates concordance rates of 71% to 99%.[13–15] Based on clinical experience, a number of circumstances in which a benign core biopsy should be followed by a surgical excision have been identified. These are listed in Table 74.3. The finding of atypical ductal hyperplasia on a core biopsy is associated with carcinoma in 18% to 50% of cases, even when large vacuum-assisted biopsy devices are used.[15,24,25] The majority of these are intraductal carcinomas, but approximately one third are invasive

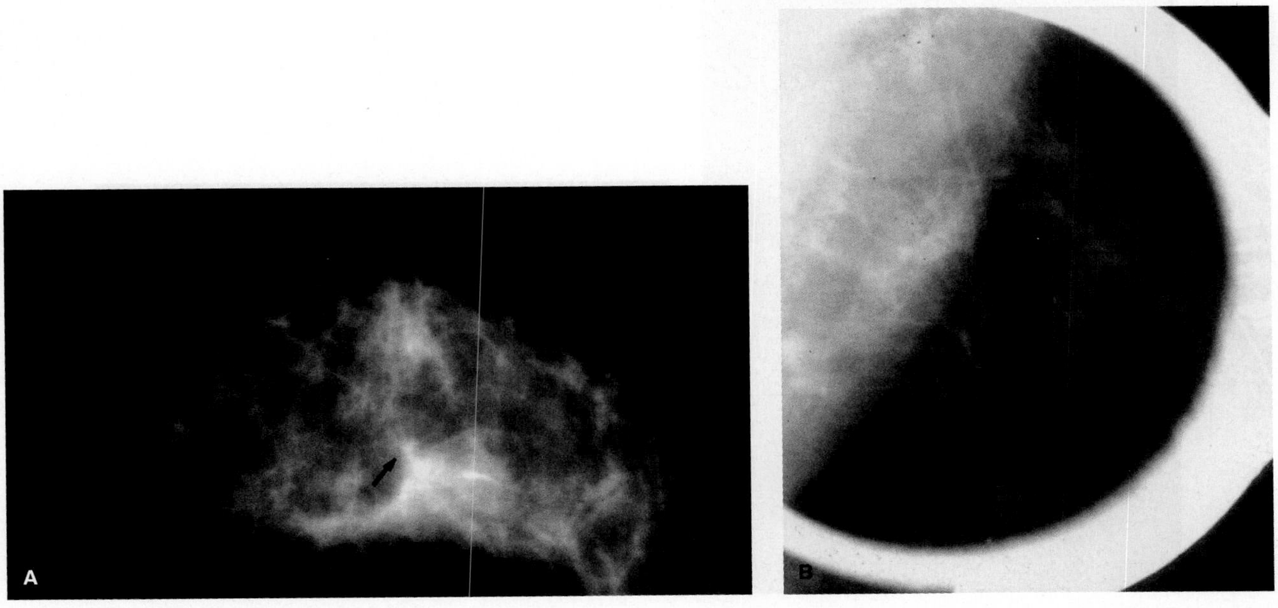

FIGURE 74.8. Workup of abnormal screening mammogram. **A:** Craniocaudal view showing an increased density with a slightly spiculated appearance (*arrow*). **B:** Spot magnification view of the density demonstrating normal breast tissue.

TABLE 74.3 INDICATIONS/CONTRAINDICATIONS

INDICATIONS FOR SURGICAL BIOPSY AFTER CORE BIOPSY

- Atypical ductal hyperplasia
- Atypical lobular hyperplasia[16–18]
- Radial scar
- Lobular carcinoma in situ[16–19]
- Columnar cell hyperplasia with atypia
- Papillary lesions[20–23]
- Lack of concordance between appearance of mammographic lesion and histologic diagnosis
- Nondiagnostic specimen (including absence of calcifications on specimen radiograph when biopsy is performed for calcifications)

lesions. Similarly, radial scar has been found to be associated with coexistent carcinoma in 20% of cases. Lesions suspected of being radial scars are best approached initially with needle localization and excision. Columnar cell lesions with atypia warrant surgical excision due to their frequent association with tubular carcinoma. Approximately 80% of patients with tubular carcinoma have associated columnar cell lesions with atypia.[26,27]

Lack of concordance between the appearance of a mammographic abnormality and the histologic diagnosis obtained with core biopsy is an important indication for surgical biopsy. For example, the finding of a small amount of hyperplasia in a largely fatty specimen would not adequately explain a mass lesion identified on a mammogram. In addition, biopsies that reveal only fat, provide material insufficient for diagnosis, or lack calcifications on specimen radiography (if performed for that indication) must be repeated. An assessment of the cause of an insufficient sample (i.e., superficial location of the lesion, poor targeting, breast too thin after compression) will aid in determining if a repeated core biopsy is appropriate or if surgical excision is needed.

2 For most mammographic abnormalities, core biopsy is a more cost-effective, less morbid diagnostic technique than needle localization and excision, and diagnosis by core biopsy increases the likelihood that local therapy will be completed with a single surgical procedure.[28,29] When needle localization and excision is indicated, the localizing wire should be placed within 1 cm of the lesion, and the incision should be placed over the abnormality (Fig. 74.9). Incisions at the point of wire entry should be used only when the wire has a short course within the breast. Specimen radiography should be performed routinely to document removal of the target abnormality. The clinical approach to a patient with a mammographic abnormality is summarized in Algorithm 74.1.

CLINICAL BREAST PROBLEMS

Most breast complaints that cause a woman to seek medical attention are benign. The purpose of the evaluation of any breast problem is first to determine if it is caused by a benign or malignant condition. If the process is malignant, a prompt diagnosis with sufficient information to plan treatment is the goal. If the process is benign, reassurance and relief of troublesome symptoms are the goals. Clinical breast problems can be divided into the general categories of breast pain, nipple discharge, breast masses, and breast infections. Each is associated with different causes and a different risk for malignancy, and each is considered separately.

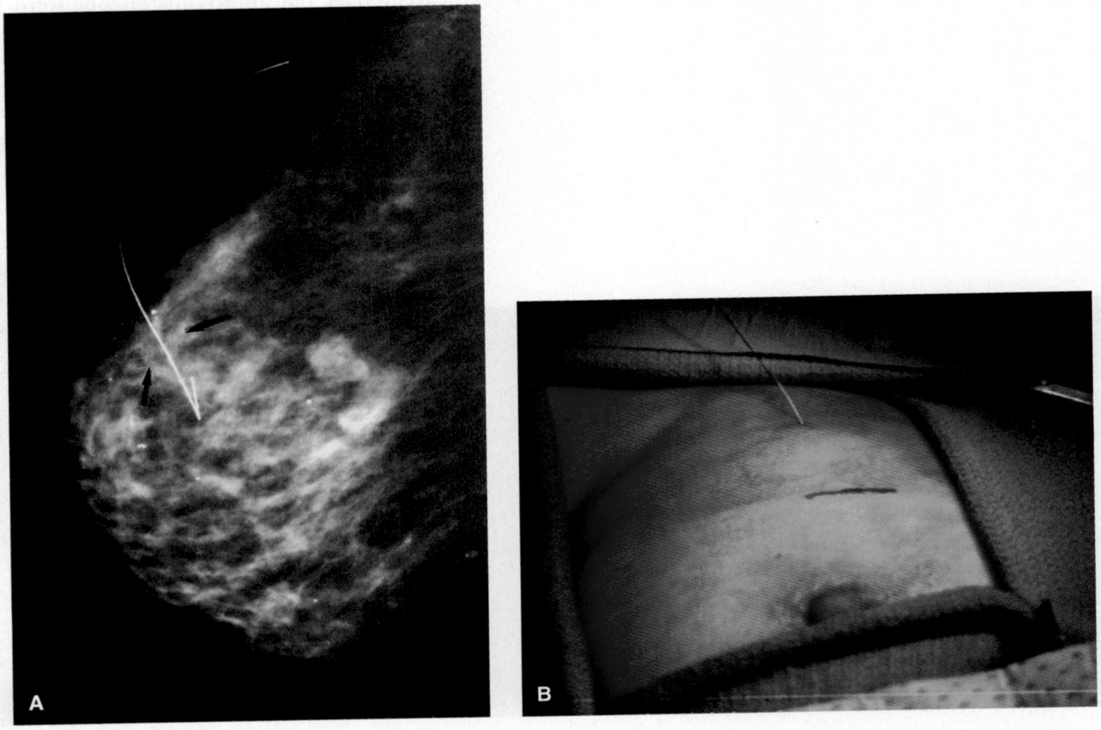

FIGURE 74.9. Incision placement for needle localization biopsy. **A:** The mammogram demonstrates that the lesion (*arrow*) is inferior to the point of wire entry. **B:** Incision placement inferior to wire entry to allow access to the lesion.

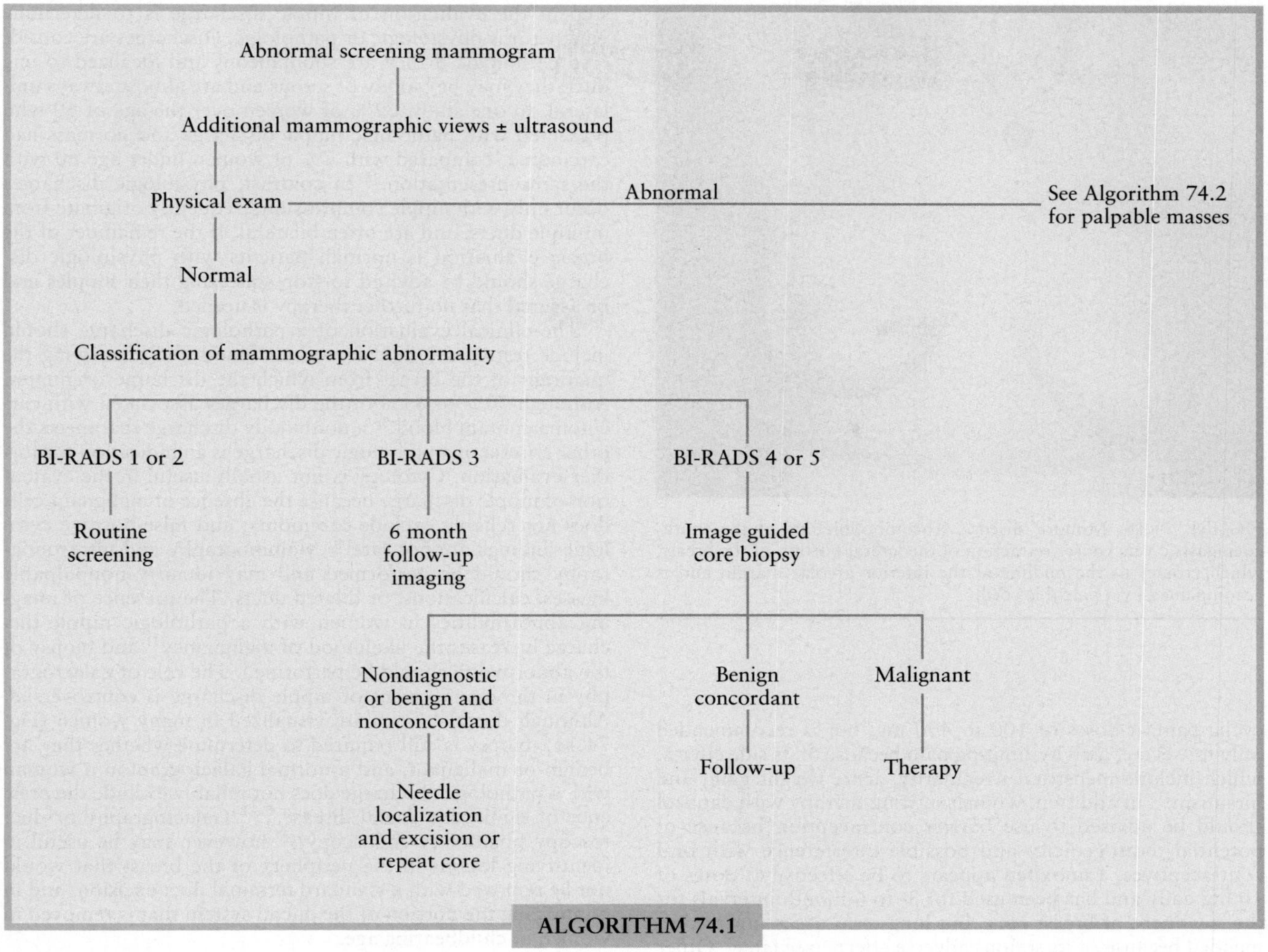

ALGORITHM 74.1. Diagnosis and management of mammographically detected breast lesions. A careful physical examination and a diagnostic imaging workup must be performed before a decision is made about the need for biopsy. *BI-RADS*, breast imaging reporting and data system.

Breast Pain

Breast pain is a common problem that is rarely a presenting sign of breast carcinoma. Breast pain may originate from the breast itself or may be referred from extramammary structures, such as the ribs, the vertebrae, or occasionally the teeth. Clinically, breast pain can be divided into two categories: cyclic and noncyclic. Cyclic breast pain waxes and wanes with the menstrual cycle, is frequently bilateral, and often involves the upper outer quadrants of the breasts with radiation to the axillae or down the arms. It tends to be most severe immediately before the menses, but may persist throughout the month. In contrast, noncyclic pain occurs in postmenopausal women or, in premenopausal women, bears no relationship to the menstrual cycle.

No specific hormonal abnormalities or histologic correlates have been identified in women with breast pain, but the problem is clearly hormonally related because it affects premenopausal women much more frequently than their postmenopausal counterparts. Breast pain is often precipitated by hormonal change, and a history of menstrual irregularity or a new medication should be sought. In the evaluation, it is important to ascertain whether fear of an underlying cancer or the need for pain relief is the patient's primary concern. In almost all cases, fear of cancer predominates. A careful physical examination should be performed to exclude a specific cause of the pain, particularly for focal, noncyclic mastalgia, which is occasionally secondary to the presence of a fibroadenoma or cyst and may be relieved by treatment of the underlying lesion. In women age 35 and older, a mammogram is usually part of the evaluation of breast pain unless one has been obtained within the preceding year. In the vast majority of women with breast pain, examination and mammography demonstrate no evidence of breast disease. In these cases, reassurance that a malignancy is not the cause of the pain and a discussion of the normal physiology of the breast are usually all that is necessary. In the patient with persistent, localized pain, physical examination should be accompanied by imaging studies, including ultrasound, to exclude the presence of carcinoma.

Approximately 5% of patients have disabling breast pain requiring further treatment. Several agents have been tested in randomized controlled trials; these include danazol (an antigonadotropin),[30] bromocriptine (a dopaminergic agonist),[31] and tamoxifen (a selective estrogen receptor [ER] modulator).[32] Danazol, which appears to be more effective than bromocriptine, has a response rate of approximately 50% for

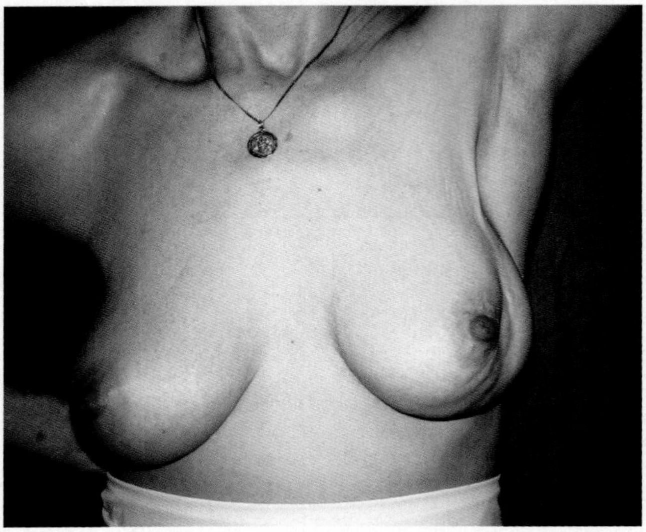

FIGURE 74.10. Mondor disease. Thrombophlebitis of the thoracoepigastric vein causes retraction of the lateral portion of the breast, which crosses to the midline at the inferior areolar margin and is accompanied by a palpable cord.

cyclic pain at doses of 100 to 400 mg, but is recommended only for severe, activity-limiting pain because of its side effects, which include menstrual irregularity, acne, weight gain, and hirsutism.[33] In addition, women starting therapy with danazol should be advised to use barrier contraception because of potential teratogenicity and possible interference with oral contraceptives. Tamoxifen appears to be effective at doses of 10 mg daily and has been used for 3- to 6-month intervals for the treatment of breast pain, but long-term use is not recommended because of its serious adverse effects (see later). Other agents, such as vitamins E and B_6, diuretics, and avoidance of caffeine have failed to demonstrate a reduction in symptoms in controlled clinical trials.[34–36] Evening primrose oil, which contains the long-chain fatty acid γ-linolenic acid, has also been proposed as therapy for cyclic breast pain, but clear evidence of its efficacy is lacking. Surgery should be avoided, even for apparently localized pain, because it rarely results in long-term pain relief.

Mondor disease, or thrombophlebitis of the lateral thoracic or superior thoracoepigastric vein, is an uncommon cause of breast pain that is readily identified clinically by the presence of a tender, subcutaneous cord in the lateral aspect of the breast. Skin retraction may be associated (Fig. 74.10), which raises concern about the presence of carcinoma. Mondor disease may develop secondary to trauma, surgical procedures on the breast, or breast irradiation. In approximately 50% of cases, no predisposing condition can be identified. Mondor disease occurs occasionally in women with a nonpalpable breast cancer,[37] and for this reason, a mammogram should be obtained in women age 35 and older who present with the condition. Mondor disease resolves spontaneously and requires no specific therapy, although anti-inflammatory agents may be used for pain relief.

Nipple Discharge

Evaluation. Nipple discharge is a common complaint, particularly in premenopausal women, and has a benign cause in approximately 95% of women who present with it. The initial step in the evaluation of nipple discharge is to determine whether it is physiologic or pathologic. Discharges are considered pathologic if they are spontaneous and localized to one duct; they may be bloody or serous and are almost always unilateral. In one study, 32% of women over the age of 60 who presented with pathologic nipple discharge and no mass had carcinoma, compared with 7% of women under age 60 with the same presentation.[38] In contrast, physiologic discharges occur only with nipple compression, frequently originate from multiple ducts, and are often bilateral. If the remainder of the breast evaluation is normal, patients with physiologic discharge should be advised to stop squeezing their nipples and be assured that no further therapy is needed.

The clinical evaluation of a pathologic discharge should include testing the fluid for occult blood and identifying the quadrant of the breast from which the discharge originates. Although 70% to 85% of the discharges associated with carcinoma contain blood,[39] a nonbloody discharge that meets the other criteria of a pathologic discharge is an indication for further evaluation. Cytology is not usually useful in the evaluation of nipple discharge because the absence of malignant cells does not reliably exclude carcinoma, and false-positive cytologic findings are not rare.[40] Mammography and ultrasonography should be performed and may identify nonpalpable masses, calcifications, or dilated ducts. The presence of imaging abnormalities in women with a pathologic nipple discharge increases the likelihood of malignancy[41] and biopsy of the abnormality should be performed. The role of galactography in the management of nipple discharge is controversial. Although ductal lesions are visualized in many women (Fig. 74.11), biopsy is still required to determine whether they are benign or malignant, and a normal galactogram in a woman with a pathologic discharge does not reliably exclude the presence of significant ductal disease.[40,42] Galactography or ductoscopy (mammary endoscopy),[43] however, may be useful in identifying lesions in the periphery of the breast that would not be removed with a standard terminal duct excision, and in minimizing the portion of the ductal system that is removed in women of childbearing age.

Galactorrhea, defined as the nonpuerperal discharge of milky fluid from both nipples, is not a sign of primary breast pathology. It should prompt a workup to exclude an underlying endocrine disorder, particularly a variety of amenorrhea syndromes that result in hyperprolactinemia. In addition, it may be secondary to hypothyroidism, pituitary adenoma, or chest trauma (including thoracotomy). A variety of medications, including oral contraceptives, phenothiazines, tricyclic antidepressants, metoclopramide, and reserpine, also cause galactorrhea. Persistent galactorrhea in a patient not taking any of these medications should be evaluated with measurement of the prolactin level. A persistently elevated prolactin level should prompt a search for a pituitary adenoma, but if there is no evidence of an endocrine abnormality, these women may be followed without intervention.

3 **Etiology.** The most common cause of pathologic discharge identified in surgical specimens is a solitary papilloma (about 60% of cases); these lesions are most common in the major subareolar ducts. They consist of an epithelial layer covering a fibrovascular stroma. Peripheral papillomas are a distinctly different clinical entity in which multiple papillomas develop in the peripheral ducts of the breast. These lesions are less likely to produce nipple discharge and tend to present as a palpable or image-detected mass.[44] Duct hyperplasia, typical or atypical, is found in 15% to 20% of women undergoing duct excision for spontaneous nipple discharge, whereas ductal carcinoma in situ is found in 5% to 20%.[39,41] Invasive carcinoma presenting as discharge alone is rare. Ductal ectasia may also cause nipple discharge, which is classically thick and opaque, and varies in color from pale yellow to blue-green. It

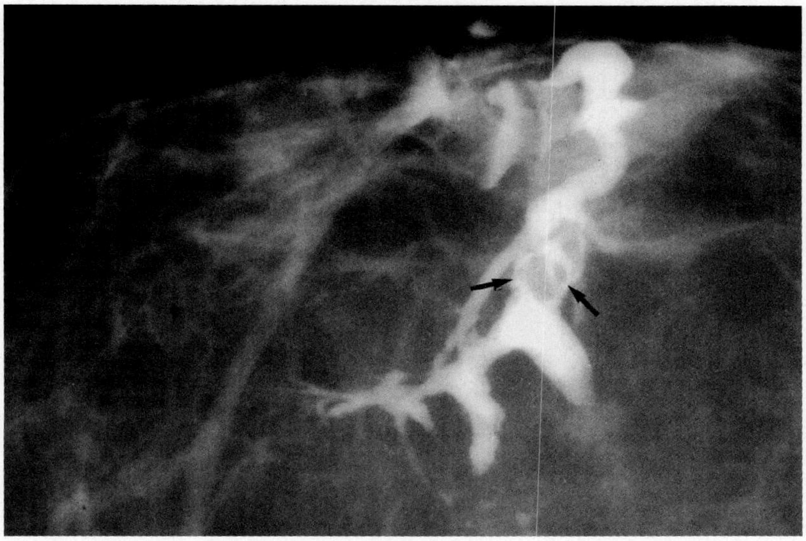

FIGURE 74.11. Ductogram. A large defect (*arrows*) represents an intraductal papilloma.

may be accompanied by periductal mastitis, causing nipple inversion, and mimic carcinoma. The discharge of ductal ectasia is sometimes mistaken for an infectious process, but the ducts are usually sterile.[45]

Management. When a pathologic discharge has been identified, an attempt should be made to localize the source of the discharge within the ductal tree by galactography, or by ductoscopy. If the intraductal lesion is centrally located, terminal duct excision, also called *microdochectomy*, is the appropriate management. If the lesion is peripheral, it is necessary to localize it for excision, either by wire localization of the abnormal area on galactogram, or by ductoscopy immediately preceding the surgical excision. In a woman with clearly pathologic nipple discharge, it is reasonable to proceed with terminal duct excision even if radiologic investigations (including galactography) are normal.[40,42] Exceptions to this rule include women with a single, nonreproducible episode of discharge with normal imaging evaluation, and women with bloody nipple discharge during pregnancy.

Terminal duct excision is carried out through a circumareolar incision that includes a quarter to a third of the circumference of the areola. Duct removal should begin on the dermal surface of the nipple, as ductal disease often occurs in the proximal duct. The dilated duct is visualized after the subareolar space has been entered and excised to a depth of 2 to 3 cm in the breast parenchyma. Identification of the diseased duct can be aided by inserting a lacrimal probe into the discharging ductal orifice, or the instillation of blue dye. If ductoscopy is performed before the duct excision, the outer cannula of the endoscope can be left in place to guide resection of the appropriate segment of the duct. Patients should be warned that some nipple sensation may be lost after the procedure, in addition to the ability to breast-feed.

Breast Masses

Definition. The first step in the evaluation of a woman with a complaint of a breast mass is to verify that a dominant mass is actually present. Dominant masses may be cystic or solid and are characterized by their persistence throughout the menstrual cycle. They may be discrete or poorly defined, but they differ in character from the surrounding breast tissue and the corresponding area in the contralateral breast. Often, what the patient perceives as a breast mass is actually a normal variant of breast tissue. In premenopausal women, the normal glandular tissue of the breast is nodular, and patients often confuse such nodular glandular tissue with a dominant breast mass. Nodularity, particularly when it waxes and wanes during the menstrual cycle, is a physiologic process and not a predictor of breast disease. Morrow et al.[46] reviewed 605 women younger than 40 years of age who were referred for evaluation of a breast mass. Only 36% of the 484 masses detected by patient self-examination and 29% of the 121 masses detected by a primary care provider were confirmed surgically. The differential diagnosis of a palpable breast mass includes macrocyst, fibroadenoma, prominent areas of fibrocystic change, fat necrosis, and carcinoma.

Cysts. Cysts are a common cause of dominant breast masses, with a peak incidence in women in their 40s and perimenopausal years. Cysts are thought to result from cystic lobular involution; acini within the lobule distend to form microcysts, which in turn give rise to macrocysts. Clinically evident macrocysts are estimated to develop in 7% of Western women.

Cysts are usually well demarcated from the surrounding breast tissue, mobile, and firm. It is often difficult to distinguish a cystic from a solid lesion on physical examination, although cysts may fluctuate with the menstrual cycle, whereas solid lesions do not. Cystic lesions in postmenopausal women who are not on hormone replacement therapy are uncommon, and they should be regarded with a higher degree of suspicion than those found in premenopausal women because they may be secondary to ductal obstruction by a malignant lesion.

4 The initial step in the evaluation of a possible cyst is aspiration. If fluid is obtained that is not grossly bloody and the mass resolves completely, no further therapy other than a follow-up examination is needed. However, if the cystic fluid is bloody, the palpable abnormality does not resolve completely, or the same cyst recurs multiple times in a short time period, a biopsy to exclude the presence of a malignant lesion in the cyst wall is required. Cytologic examination of cyst fluid is of little value because intracystic carcinoma is rare and malignant cells are identified in fewer than 1% of cases.[47] The presence of atypical cells, an indication for surgical biopsy, is not uncommon when cyst fluid is examined, and it may pose a dilemma when a patient's cyst has resolved with aspiration, and the examination and mammographic findings are now normal.

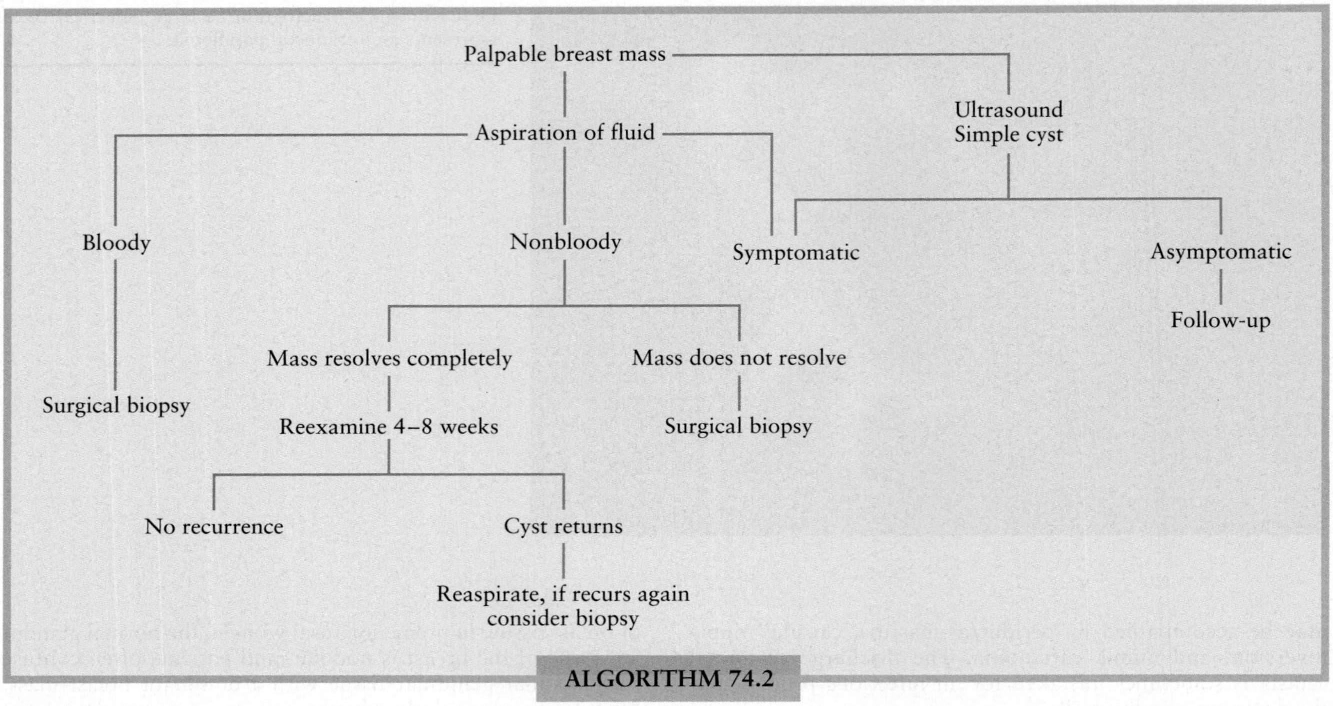

ALGORITHM 74.2. Diagnosis and management of cystic lesions. Bloody fluid on aspiration, failure of the mass to resolve completely, and prompt refilling of the same cyst are indications for surgical biopsy.

Many patients present to the surgeon with a palpable mass and an ultrasonographic examination demonstrating that the mass is a simple cyst. If the cyst is symptomatic or alarming to the patient, it can be aspirated. Otherwise, because the diagnosis has been made, it can be left alone. Nonpalpable lesions that are proved to be simple cysts by ultrasonography do not require aspiration. The management
5 of cystic lesions is summarized in Algorithm 74.2. A dominant breast mass should not be dismissed as a cyst unless the diagnosis is confirmed by ultrasonography or aspiration of fluid.

Solid Masses

Fibroadenomas. Fibroadenomas present most frequently in patients between the ages of 20 and 50 years. Their characteristic clinical presentation is that of a well-defined palpable mass that is rubbery in texture and mobile. Fibroadenomas present as multiple lesions in 10% to 15% of cases. Although they have a characteristic clinical appearance, a clinical diagnosis of fibroadenoma is accurate in only one half to two thirds of cases.[48] In women younger than age 20, however, fibroadenomas account for 75% of breast biopsies.

Fibroadenomas are thought to be the result of a minor aberration in the normal process of lobular development. Hormonal factors appear to be important in their growth, as evidenced by the clinical observation of the involution of fibroadenomas after menopause and their dramatic increase in size during pregnancy. In postmenopausal women receiving estrogen alone, fibroadenomas may increase in size relative to the surrounding breast parenchyma.

Sonographic criteria for the diagnosis of fibroadenoma include a round or oval, well-circumscribed, solid mass with homogeneous, low-level internal echoes and intermediate acoustic attenuation. As many as 30% of fibroadenomas, however, lack these "classic" features.

In rare circumstances, fibroadenomas have been associated with carcinoma. More than 160 cases of associated cancers have been reported in the literature, including ductal carcinoma in situ, and infiltrating lobular and ductal carcinomas. Historically, it has been widely accepted that fibroadenomas do not confer an increased breast cancer risk. However, four population-based retrospective studies have shown a small (relative risk of 1.3 to 1.9) but significant increased risk for breast cancer development that persists over time.[49–52] This slight increase in risk should have no impact on the clinical management of fibroadenomas. Although fibroadenomas can be suspected on the basis of their characteristic clinical presentation, a final diagnosis cannot be made without histologic or cytologic confirmation.

Fibrocystic Disease. *Fibrocystic disease* is a common term that is used to describe a variety of benign breast disorders. It is not a clinically meaningful term because it encompasses a heterogeneous group of processes, some pathologic and some physiologic, with widely varying cancer risks. The cancer risks associated with benign breast disease are discussed in the section on breast cancer risk factors. The term *fibrocystic change* is not a synonym for lumpy breasts and, if used at all, it should be reserved for women in whom a breast biopsy has demonstrated one of the histologic components of fibrocystic change. Frequently, when a breast biopsy is performed for vague areas of nodularity that lack mammographic or ultrasonographic correlates, a fibrocystic process is the diagnosis.

Fat Necrosis. Fat necrosis in the breast may occur secondary to trauma, breast surgery, infection, or radiation therapy, although in approximately 50% of cases, no antecedent cause can be identified. Fat necrosis occurs most commonly in women with pendulous breasts and those who are overweight. It is clinically significant in that on both physical examination and mammography, it may be indistinguishable from carcinoma. The lesions of fat necrosis are typically firm, painless, and poorly defined. Because fat necrosis usually

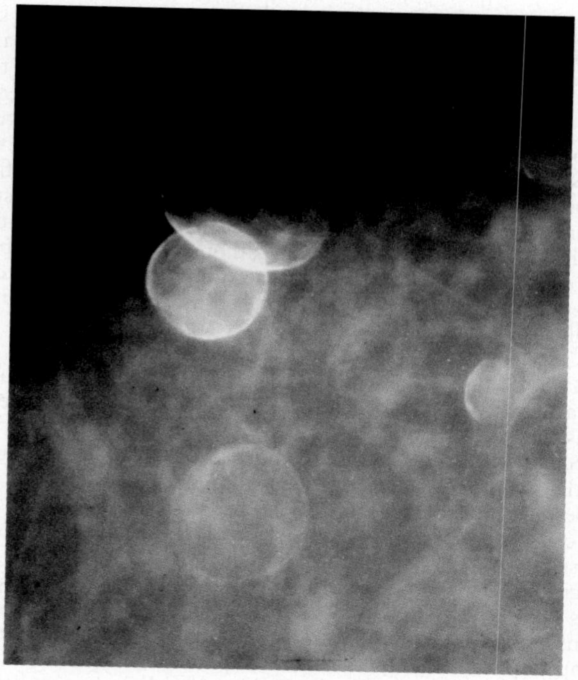

FIGURE 74.12. Oil cysts. The calcified rims of these cysts in a patient with a history of trauma are diagnostic.

occurs in the superficial breast tissue, it may be accompanied by skin thickening, dimpling, or retraction. The mammographic findings of fat necrosis include spiculated masses, microcalcifications, and architectural distortion. Only when the characteristic oil cyst, a circumscribed mass of mixed soft tissue density and fat with a rim that is often calcified, is present can an unequivocal diagnosis of fat necrosis be made radiographically (Fig. 74.12). In the absence of this finding or a clear history of trauma, biopsy is required to exclude the presence of malignancy.

Diagnostic Imaging

Mammography and Ultrasonography. When a clinical abnormality has been identified in a woman over age 40, a diagnostic mammogram should be obtained before a histologic diagnosis is attempted. Imaging studies are used to define the extent of a potential malignancy and to identify nonpalpable masses or associated calcifications elsewhere in the ipsilateral or contralateral breast that might influence definitive therapy. The decision to perform a biopsy, however, is based on the clinical determination that a dominant mass is present, and nonvisualization of a mass on imaging studies should not dissuade the surgeon from performing a breast biopsy. In two reports, between 10% and 22% of patients with palpable breast cancer had tumors that were not visible by mammography.[53,54] Obtaining a diagnostic rather than a screening mammogram ensures that a marker will be placed on the area of palpable concern, so that the clinical and radiographic findings can be correlated. Identifying the site of a lesion also ensures that lesions at the periphery of the breast will be included on the film, which helps to eliminate one cause of false-negative mammograms. A diagnostic mammogram also includes magnification views of the lesion, which are useful in determining the extent of any associated calcifications.

The routine use of ultrasonography for the evaluation of solid palpable masses remains controversial. Studies of high-resolution ultrasonography have demonstrated that the technique is more accurate and sensitive, and has a better negative predictive value than mammography alone.[55] If follow-up of a clinically benign lesion is being considered, ultrasonography is a useful adjunct to mammography, as discussed in the section on the clinical approach to the patient with a solid breast mass. In the patient with a clinically suspect mass who will undergo biopsy regardless of the results of imaging studies, ultrasonography provides a more accurate estimate of lesion size than mammography,[56] and it may also identify satellite lesions not identified on mammography. Ultrasonography is also useful in the woman with a palpable mass that is not clearly delineated on mammography; in such cases, it may help to define the extent of the lesion more completely than physical examination alone.

In women under age 40 presenting with a clinically unworrisome breast mass, the rationale for mammographic imaging is less compelling because carcinoma is uncommon and the density of the breasts often obscures mass lesions. Directed ultrasonography allows the presence of a true mass lesion to be confirmed when the significance of a physical finding is clinically uncertain.[46] The presence of benign characteristics on ultrasonography also supports the use of a follow-up approach. In younger women with clinically suspect masses, mammography should be performed.

Magnetic Resonance Imaging. Magnetic resonance imaging (MRI) of the breast is increasingly being used for clinical breast imaging. Initially it was hoped that MRI would reduce the number of biopsies done for benign breast lesions. However, in a prospective study of 821 breast abnormalities identified mammographically (404 malignant), the sensitivity and specificity of MRI for the diagnosis of carcinoma were 88% and 68%, respectively.[57] These findings indicate that a normal MRI does not obviate the need for biopsy of a lesion that has suspicious clinical or mammographic features.[57] There is great interest in the use of MRI in women with known breast cancer to improve selection for breast-conserving therapy (BCT). In a meta-analysis of 19 studies involving 2,763 breast cancer patients, MRI identified additional disease in 16% of patients, resulting in a mastectomy or wider surgical excision that would not have been done otherwise.[58] It is not clear that these more extensive procedures are beneficial to patients. In one retrospective study, local recurrence rates did not differ between women selected for BCT with and without MRI.[59] A decrease in the need to convert from BCT to mastectomy, or a greater likelihood of obtaining negative margins with a single excision have not been demonstrated in patients selected for BCT with MRI,[60] so the ultimate role of this technology in the patient with cancer remains to be determined.

Other clinical applications of MRI are to detect an implant rupture and to look for a primary breast tumor in patients presenting with axillary adenopathy caused by metastatic tumor from an unknown primary site (see section on occult primary tumor presenting with nodal metastases). MRI also has a role in assessing the response of a tumor to preoperative chemotherapy is also under study. The role of screening MRI in women at very high risk of breast cancer development is discussed in the section on management of the high-risk woman.

Biopsy Techniques for Solid Breast Masses. A variety of biopsy techniques are available to obtain a pathologic diagnosis of clinically evident breast masses. Each has advantages and disadvantages, and no single technique is applicable to all clinical circumstances.

Fine-needle Aspiration Biopsy. Fine-needle aspiration (FNA) cytology has a very high diagnostic accuracy rate in the hands of experienced clinicians and cytopathologists. In a review of 31,340 procedures,[61] its sensitivity ranged from 65% to 98%.

TABLE 74.4 TREATMENT

MANAGEMENT OF BREAST MASSES BASED ON FINE-NEEDLE ASPIRATION (FNA) DIAGNOSIS

■ FNA DIAGNOSIS	■ TREATMENT
Malignant	Definitive therapy
Suspicious	Surgical or core needle biopsy
Atypia	Surgical biopsy
Benign	Possible observation[a]
Nondiagnostic	Repeated FNA or surgical biopsy

[a]See discussion in text on clinical approach to the patient with a solid breast mass.

In most series, false-positive rates are less than 1%, false-negative rates are below 10%, and the incidence of insufficient specimens ranges from 4% to 13%. Small tumor size, fibrotic tumors, and certain histologic tumor types, such as infiltrating lobular, tubular, and cribriform carcinoma, have been associated with a higher likelihood of false-negative results. Most false-negative results are the consequence of sampling errors rather than misinterpretation by the cytopathologist.

The advantages of FNA include its simplicity and quickness, low cost, low morbidity, and availability as an office procedure. Because an unequivocal diagnosis of malignancy by FNA is reliable, treatment options can be discussed with the patient and definitive surgery can be performed without the need for a surgical biopsy. The management of breast lesions on the basis of FNA results is summarized in Table 74.4.

Core Needle Biopsy. Core needle biopsy is another office diagnostic technique that is rapid, inexpensive, and relatively painless. A core needle biopsy differs from FNA in that a core of tissue is obtained for histologic examination, so that a more detailed characterization of the lesion is possible and the adequacy of the specimen can be evaluated at the time of the biopsy. In addition, the material can be evaluated by any surgical pathologist. A core biopsy specimen allows the determination of ER and HER2 status at the time of diagnosis. False-negative results occur when the needle is deflected into the surrounding fat by a hard tumor mass. In practice, the selection of the type of needle biopsy (FNA or core) often depends on the availability of a cytopathologist and the surgeon's level of comfort with a cytologic diagnosis of malignancy without further histologic detail, although core biopsy is preferred in patients who will receive neoadjuvant therapy. The difference between an FNA specimen and a core needle specimen is illustrated in Figure 74.13.

Excisional Biopsy. Excisional biopsy is the complete removal of a breast mass. It is definitive therapy for a benign breast mass and may also serve as a therapeutic lumpectomy if the specimen includes a margin of normal breast tissue around a malignant tumor. The adequacy of an excision cannot be assessed unless the margins of the specimen are inked. The use of orienting sutures in two margins of the specimen makes it possible to identify which margin contains tumor should the excision be incomplete; as a result, less normal breast tissue has to be removed in a repeated excision. In this era of breast-conserving surgery, orientation and inking of excisional breast biopsy specimens should be routine practice.

However, diagnosis by needle biopsy techniques is reliable, more cost-effective than surgical biopsy, and avoids placement of an incision on the breast before definitive local therapy. For the vast majority of breast masses, needle biopsy is the preferred diagnostic technique.

Incisional Biopsy. Incisional biopsy is a diagnostic procedure reserved for masses that are too large to be completely excised. Today, the indications for incisional biopsy are few, because FNA or core needle biopsy can be used to make a diagnosis of breast cancer with less morbidity and at lower cost.

Clinical Approach to the Patient with a Solid Breast Mass. The accuracy of physical examination alone to detect carcinoma is limited because the clinical characteristics of benign and malignant masses are not absolute, and a clinical diagnosis is

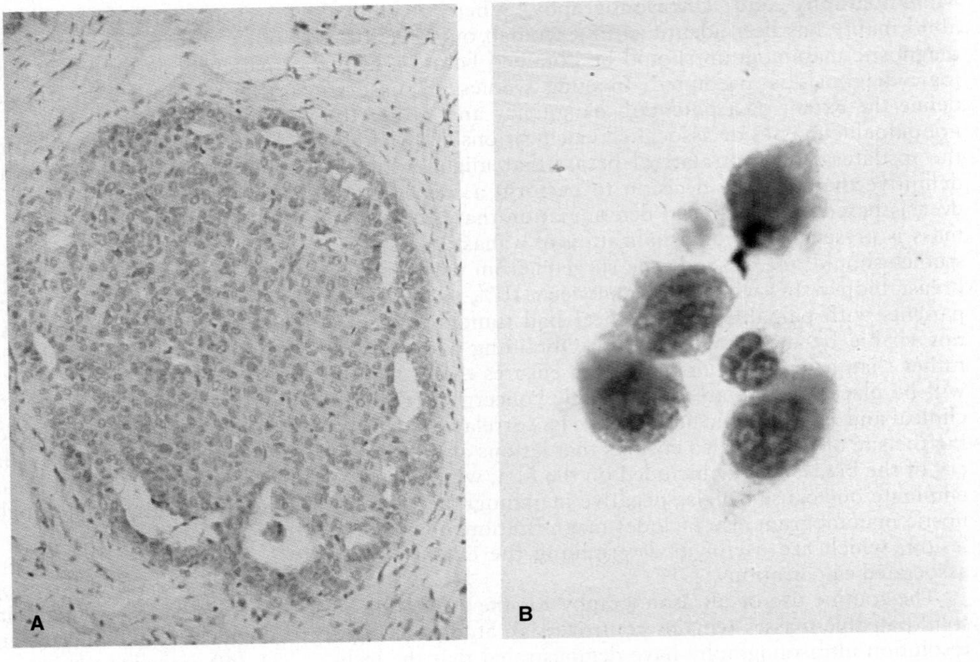

FIGURE 74.13. Comparison of core needle biopsy specimen (A) and fine-needle aspiration specimen (B). Only the core specimen can demonstrate the architectural detail.

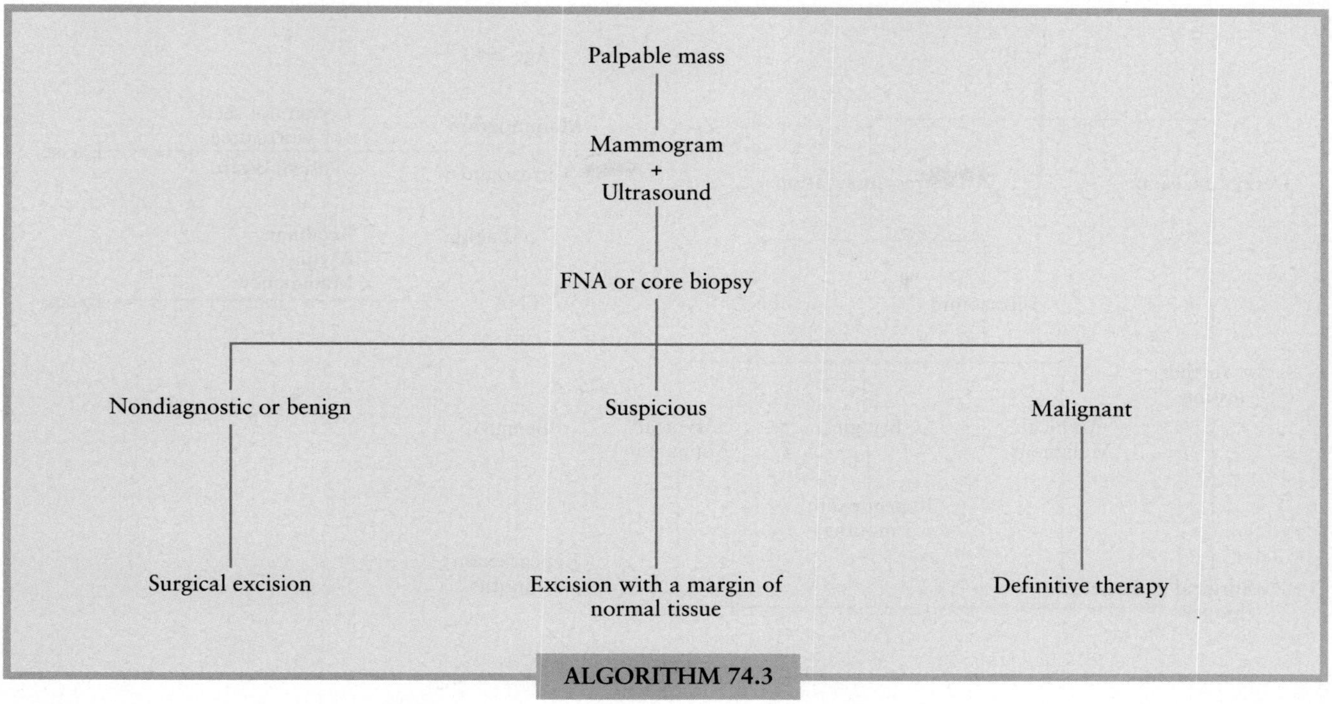

ALGORITHM 74.3. Diagnosis and management of the patient with a clinically indeterminate or suspect solid breast mass. In this circumstance, imaging studies are insufficient to exclude malignancy, and tissue sampling is required.

correct in only 60% to 85% of cases.[62,63] The difficulty of distinguishing benign from malignant lesions is greatest in young women, and the use of other studies to confirm the clinical diagnosis of a benign breast mass is essential before the patient is returned to routine follow-up.

The extent of the workup necessary to exclude the presence of carcinoma varies with the degree of suspicion and the age of the patient. In the patient with a clinically suspect mass, regardless of age, diagnostic mammography and ultrasonography should be performed before a histologic diagnosis is sought. A needle biopsy (either aspiration cytology or core biopsy) is the preferred initial method of making a diagnosis, for the reasons discussed in the preceding section on biopsy technique. If a diagnosis of malignancy is obtained, treatment options are discussed with the patient. If a diagnosis of cancer is not obtained, excisional biopsy is undertaken because of the known false-negative rates of both FNA and core biopsy. This approach is summarized in Algorithm 74.3.

In the woman with a clinically benign mass, management varies somewhat with age (Algorithm 74.4). In women under age 40, the first step is to determine if the patient wants the mass to be excised, regardless of the likelihood of malignancy. If so, imaging studies are not indicated because of the low risk for carcinoma in this age group. For the patient who desires follow-up, ultrasonography and FNA or core biopsy should be performed. If both confirm that the lesion has benign features, clinical follow-up can be undertaken, with regular monitoring of the lesion for a period of 1 to 2 years to confirm that carcinoma is not present. The combination of clinical examination, FNA, and ultrasonography provides an accurate differentiation between benign and malignant lesions in 95% of cases.[64] For this reason, in addition to the low risk for malignancy in this age group, follow-up is a safe approach.

In patients over age 40, mammography and ultrasonography should be obtained before a decision about the need for excision or follow-up is made. If follow-up is chosen, needle biopsy is also performed. If the mass is visualized on mammography and appears benign, and if the needle biopsy is benign, the risk for carcinoma ranges from 0.6% to 3.4%.[65,66] It must be emphasized that if any elements of the "triple test" cannot be evaluated (i.e., lesion not visualized on imaging studies, aspirate contains only blood and fat), these statistics do not apply. A follow-up approach to new breast lesions in women older than age 40 should be undertaken only by clinicians with experience in the management of breast disease, and patients must be advised of the small, but real, possibility of a delay in the diagnosis of breast carcinoma.

Breast Infections

Breast infections can be classified as lactating or nonlactating. Lactating infections are usually caused by *Staphylococcus aureus,* and are most common during the first 4 to 6 weeks of breast-feeding or during weaning. They are caused by the proliferation of bacteria in poorly drained breast segments, and present as cellulitis with fever, pain, redness, and swelling. Antibiotics are the first line of treatment, and breast-feeding should be continued to facilitate drainage of the engorged segment. Tetracycline, chloramphenicol, and ciprofloxacin should be avoided because they enter breast milk. If the infection fails to resolve, an abscess should be considered. When the breast skin is intact, repeated aspiration of the abscess combined with antibiotics is the preferred treatment.[67] When the skin is thinned, a small incision will facilitate drainage.

In nonlactating women, a syndrome characterized by periareolar inflammation, sometimes associated with a purulent nipple discharge, which affects premenopausal women, is the most common form of breast infection. Periareolar abscess and mammary duct fistulas may develop secondary to this

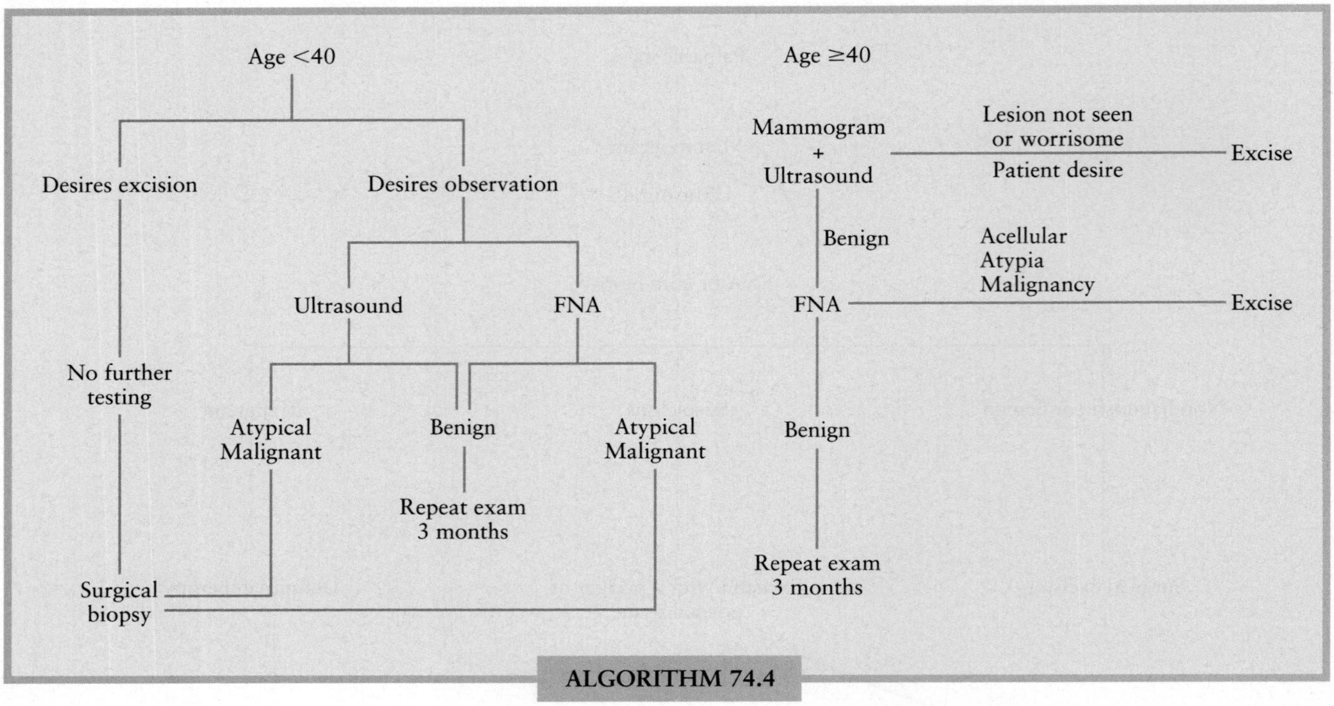

ALGORITHM 74.4. Diagnosis and management of clinically benign breast masses. The use of imaging studies varies according to age because carcinoma is infrequent in women under age 40.

condition, and infection can be troublingly recurrent. Recurrent periareolar abscess is associated with smoking,[68] apparently by promoting squamous metaplasia of the duct lining.[69] Antibiotics that provide coverage for aerobic and anaerobic bacteria should be used in patients with periareolar inflammation without abscess formation. Abscesses can be treated with aspiration. For patients with recurrent episodes of infection, terminal duct excision is indicated.

Peripheral breast abscesses, which are less common than periareolar infections, should be treated with aspiration or incision and drainage. In any patient with a breast infection, particularly in older women, the possibility of an underlying malignancy should be considered. A biopsy should be performed on any apparent "infection" that fails to respond to appropriate antibiotics and drainage to exclude the presence of an underlying carcinoma.

RISK FACTORS FOR BREAST CANCER

Breast cancer is the most common cancer in American women, the second most common cause of cancer death, and a major cause of cancer death in most industrialized nations. Approximately 180,000 cases of breast cancer and 41,000 breast cancer deaths occur annually in American women.[70] Many factors that increase the risk for the development of breast cancer have been identified, and have become clinically important since the demonstration that chemoprevention can protect high-risk women from breast cancer (see section on management of the high-risk woman). Risk can be described as the absolute risk for the development of breast cancer, either over the lifetime (usually to age 90) or within a given time interval (e.g., 2.5% during the next 5 years). Risk may also be expressed as a relative risk (RR), a comparison of the incidence of disease in a population having a particular risk factor with the incidence in a population lacking that risk factor. Understanding the clinical implications of RR requires knowledge of the absolute risk of breast cancer in the index population and, although it is a useful measure for research purposes, it is not particularly useful for the discussion of risk clinically. Risk information is best provided to patients as absolute risk within a given time period.

Age

The most common breast cancer risk factor is age. Half of a woman's lifetime risk for breast cancer development occurs after age 65. Between the ages of 35 and 55, the risk for breast cancer development is only 2.5%, and the risk for breast cancer death is only about one third of that.[71] The incidence of breast cancer across age groups has been fairly stable, although an increase in the number of young women in the population has resulted in an increase in the number of cases in this group, without a change in incidence rate. Breast cancer at a young age is more common in black women than in white women. At age 40, the incidence curves cross, and the disease becomes more common in white women.

Family History

6 There are two distinct types of risk associated with a family history of breast carcinoma. Approximately 20% to 30% of women with breast cancer have a family history of the disease, but only 5% to 10% have an inherited mutation in a breast cancer susceptibility gene.[72,73] Distinguishing between familial and true hereditary breast cancer is important because the associated level of risk varies widely.

The majority of cases of genetic breast cancer are caused by mutations of *BRCA1* and *BRCA2*. Mutations of either of

TABLE 74.5 RESULTS

ESTIMATED LIFETIME CANCER RISKS FOR *BRCA1* AND *BRCA2* MUTATIONS (TO AGE 70)

■ TYPE OF CANCER	■ GENERAL POPULATION (%)	■ *BRCA1* CARRIER (%)	■ *BRCA2* CARRIER (%)
Breast cancer	8.0	40–85	40–85
Contralateral breast cancer	0.5–1/y	40–65	40–65
Male breast cancer	0.1	1–5	5–10
Ovarian cancer	1.4	30–45	10–20

Modified from Isaacs C, Peshkin BN, Lerman C. Evaluation and management of women with a strong family history of breast cancer. In: Harris JR, Lippman ME, Morrow M, et al., eds. *Diseases of the Breast*, 3rd ed. Philadelphia, PA: Lippincott Williams & Wilkins; 2004:316.

these genes carry a lifetime risk for breast cancer development of 37% to 85%,[74,75] a high risk of contralateral breast cancer, and an increased risk for ovarian cancer. Although the risk for ovarian cancer is elevated with mutations of both *BRCA1* and *BRCA2*, it is greater in carriers of the *BRCA1* mutation. In *BRCA2* families, the risk for male breast cancer, prostate cancer, and pancreatic cancer is increased.[76,77] These mutations can be inherited from both maternal and paternal relatives, and are summarized in Table 74.5. The carrier frequency of these mutations varies with the population under study. The frequency of *BRCA1* mutations is between 1 in 500 and 1 in 800, and the frequency of *BRCA2* mutations is lower in the general population. In persons of Ashkenazi Jewish descent, however, two specific mutations of *BRCA1* (185delAG and 5382insC) and one *BRCA2* mutation (6174delT) occur with a background frequency of 2.3%.[74] These are known as *founder mutations*, thought to arise from common ancestry, and have been identified in other ethnic populations in Iceland, France, Russia, Holland, Sweden, and Belgium.

Features of the family history that suggest mutations in *BRCA1* or *BRCA2* include having two or more relatives affected with early-onset breast or ovarian cancer, or both, with involvement of two or more generations in a pattern consistent with autosomal dominant inheritance. This can be through maternal or paternal relatives. A typical pedigree is shown in Figure 74.14. The likelihood of a mutation also varies with ethnic ancestry. For example, in an Ashkenazi Jewish family with two cases of breast cancer and one case of ovarian cancer, the chance of a *BRCA1* mutation is 75%, but in a non-Ashkenazi family with the same history, the probability is only 33%.[78] Models have been developed and validated to assist clinicians in estimating the probability of a mutation.[79]

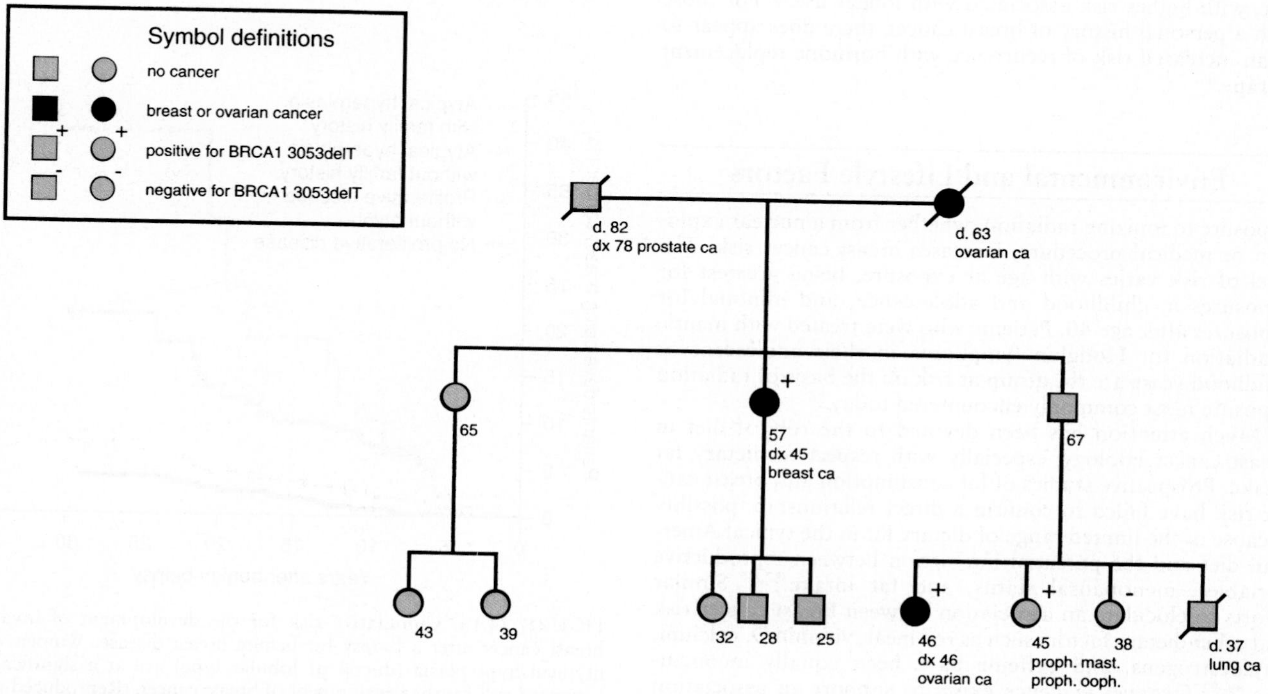

FIGURE 74.14. Pedigree of genetic breast cancer. The family illustrated in the pedigree carries a mutation of the *BRCA1* gene; multiple relatives are affected with breast and ovarian cancer.

Genetic testing for mutations of *BRCA1* and *BRCA2* is now a commercially available option for women with a family history suggestive of a genetic mutation. Genetic testing should always be preceded by a counseling session in which the complexities of genetic testing and the potential emotional and financial ramifications of test results are discussed. The information obtained from testing will be maximized by first testing a family member affected with breast or ovarian cancer, or both. If the affected person does not carry a mutation, testing an unaffected relative is unlikely to be informative.

Other, infrequent genetic breast cancer syndromes include the Li-Fraumeni syndrome, Cowden syndrome, and the Lynch syndromes. The Li-Fraumeni syndrome is associated with mutations in the tumor-suppressor gene *p53*, and is an autosomal dominant condition characterized by soft tissue sarcomas, osteosarcomas, brain tumors, leukemia, adrenocortical malignancies, and early-onset breast cancer.[80]

For the majority of women with a family history of breast cancer that is not associated with an inherited mutation, the level of risk is much lower and rarely exceeds 30%.

Hormonal Factors

Numerous studies have linked breast cancer risk to the lifetime exposure to estrogens, as reflected by age at menarche, menopause and first pregnancy, and postmenopausal obesity.[81] Conversely, women who undergo bilateral oophorectomy before menopause are at decreased risk, with the magnitude of benefit increasing as the age at oophorectomy decreases. In general, hormonal risk factors are associated with a RR in the range of 1.5 to 2.0. Studies of the effect of lactation on breast cancer risk have been inconclusive, but a long duration of lactation appears to reduce risk in premenopausal women.[82]

In healthy women, there is no convincing evidence for an effect of oral contraceptive use on breast cancer risk, despite extensive study,[83] but use of combination postmenopausal hormone replacement therapy (estrogen plus progesterone) appears to be associated with a small increase in breast cancer risk, with higher risk associated with longer use.[84] For those with a personal history of breast cancer, there does appear to be an increased risk of recurrence with hormone replacement therapy.[85]

Environmental and Lifestyle Factors

Exposure to ionizing radiation, whether from a nuclear explosion or medical procedure, increases breast cancer risk. The level of risk varies with age at exposure, being greatest for exposures in childhood and adolescence, and minimal for exposures after age 40. Patients who were treated with mantle irradiation for Hodgkin lymphoma in their adolescent or childhood years are the group at risk on the basis of radiation exposure most commonly encountered today.[86]

Much attention has been devoted to the role of diet in breast cancer etiology, especially with respect to dietary fat intake. Prospective studies of fat consumption and breast cancer risk have failed to confirm a direct relationship, possibly because of the limited range of dietary fat in the typical American diet and the potential interaction between reproductive variables, menopausal status, and fat intake.[87,88] Similar efforts to elucidate an association between breast cancer risk and other dietary factors such as red meat, vitamin D, calcium, phytoestrogens, and caffeine have been equally inconclusive.[89–92] Stronger evidence exists to support an association between alcohol intake and breast cancer risk.[93]

Regular physical exercise appears to provide modest protection against breast cancer, particularly among postmenopausal women.[94,95] There is no evidence of a direct association between active cigarette smoking and breast cancer risk.[93]

TABLE 74.6 CLASSIFICATION

CLASSIFICATION OF BENIGN BREAST DISEASE

NONPROLIFERATIVE: NO INCREASE IN RISK
Cysts: micro or macro
Ductal ectasia
Simple fibroadenoma
Mastitis
Fibrosis
Metaplasia: squamous or apocrine
Mild hyperplasia
PROLIFERATIVE: RR 1.5–2.0
Complex fibroadenoma
Papilloma
Sclerosing adenosis
Hyperplasia: moderate or severe
PROLIFERATIVE WITH ATYPIA: RR 4.5–5.0
Atypical ductal hyperplasia
Atypical lobular hyperplasia

RR, relative risk.

BENIGN BREAST DISEASE

Benign breast lesions are classified as nonproliferative, proliferative, or proliferative with atypia (Table 74.6). Nonproliferative lesions, which are not associated with an increased risk for breast cancer development, account for approximately 70% of palpable breast masses.[96] Proliferative lesions without

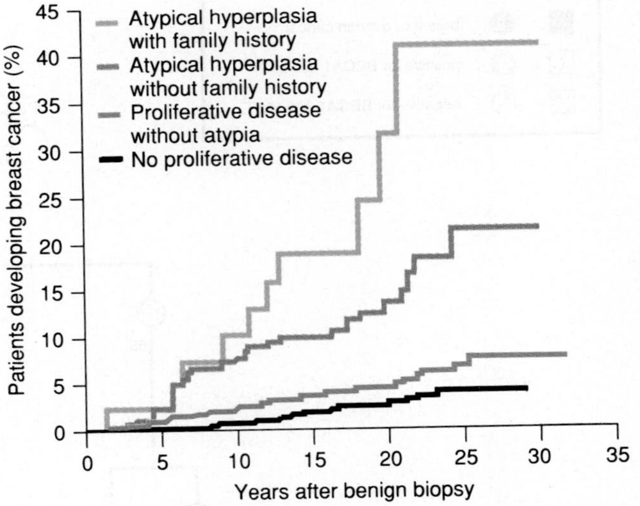

FIGURE 74.15. Cumulative risk for the development of invasive breast cancer after a biopsy for benign breast disease. Women with atypical hyperplasia (ductal or lobular type) are at a significantly increased risk for the development of breast cancer. (Reproduced with permission from Page DL, Dupont WD. Anatomic markers of human premalignancy and risk of breast cancer. *Cancer* 1990;66:1326.)

TABLE 74.7 **RESULTS**

RISK FOR BREAST CANCER DEVELOPMENT AFTER LOBULAR CARCINOMA IN SITU

STUDY	NO. PATIENTS	INVASIVE CANCER (%)	FOLLOW-UP (y)	RELATIVE RISK
Haagensen[98]	287	18	16.3	6.9
Rosen et al.[99]	99	12.5	24	9.0
Andersen[100]	47	26.4	15	12.0
Page et al.[101]	44	23	18	9.0
Salvadori et al.[102]	80	6.3	5	10.3
Ottesen et al.[103]	69	11.6	5	11.0
Bodian et al.[104]	236	26[a]	18	5.4
Fisher et al.[105]	182	33	5	—

[a]Includes intraductal and invasive cancer.

atypia are associated with a small increase in breast cancer risk (RR, 1.5 to 2.0). Proliferative lesions with atypia are uncommon, comprising only 3.6% of palpable breast masses and 7% to 10% of nonpalpable abnormalities. Atypical lesions are associated with a RR of 4.0 to 5.0, which increases to 9.0 when they are found in a woman having a first-degree relative with breast cancer.[96] As illustrated in Figure 74.15, however, breast cancer will have developed at 15 years in only 10% of women with atypical hyperplasia alone.

Lobular Carcinoma In Situ

Lobular carcinoma in situ (LCIS), first described by Foote and Stewart in 1941 as a favorable malignancy,[97] has been accepted as a risk factor for breast cancer since the mid-1980s. This paradigm shift was based on the unique biologic features of LCIS, which include a lack of clinical or radiographic findings, multifocality and bilaterality in up to 50% of cases, and clinical experience demonstrating the risk of subsequent breast cancer to be equal in both breasts, and lower than expected. Although invasive lobular carcinoma is more frequent after LCIS than in the general population, infiltrating ductal carcinoma is the most common histologic tumor type, casting further doubt upon the role of LCIS as a precursor lesion.[98–104] The term *lobular intraepithelial neoplasia* (LIN), with lobular hyperplasia without atypia being described as grade 1 LIN, atypical lobular hyperplasia as grade 2 LIN, and LCIS as grade 3 LIN, was suggested with the intention of clarifying its role as a high-risk lesion rather than a malignancy; however, LCIS remains more commonly used in clinical practice. LCIS occurs predominantly in premenopausal women and is usually identified incidentally with other benign changes in women who undergo biopsy. Women diagnosed with grade 3 LIN or LCIS have a RR for breast cancer development ranging from 5.4 to 12.[98–105] This translates in most studies to a risk for breast cancer development of about 1% per year (Table 74.7), and this risk persists indefinitely.

While historical series suggest that the increased risk of breast cancer is conferred equally to both breasts and subsequent cancers are equally likely to be infiltrating ductal or lobular carcinomas, recent evidence suggests that subsequent cancer is up to three times more likely in the ipsilateral breast, and the observed frequency of infiltrating lobular carcinoma (ILC) following a diagnosis of LCIS (50%) far exceeds the frequency of ILC observed in large series of unselected breast cancer patients (10% to 15%).[106–108] These observations, combined with emerging laboratory evidence suggesting phenotypic and genotypic similarities between coexisting LCIS and invasive lobular cancers,[109,110] have reopened the debate over the malignant potential of LCIS and its possible role as a precursor lesion. To date, there is no direct clinical evidence that LCIS is a precursor lesion, and studies attempting to show an increased risk of local recurrence when LCIS is found in the lumpectomy specimen of patients undergoing breast conservation, particularly when LCIS is at the specimen margin, have failed to demonstrate a relationship between LCIS and local recurrence,[111–116] arguing against its true malignant potential.

The recognition of histologic variants of LCIS, such as pleomorphic LCIS, with molecular profiles suggestive of a more aggressive biology[117] and the broader spectrum of lesions now classified as lobular neoplasia based on immunohistochemical staining for e-cadherin, raises new questions regarding the biology of these lesions and appropriate clinical management.

CLINICAL ASSESSMENT OF RISK

Many factors that increase breast cancer risk have been identified in studies of large populations and are summarized in Table 74.8, but are of uncertain benefit in counseling the individual woman. Several of these have been integrated into a model to allow calculation of risk for an individual woman by Gail et al.[118] These include age, age at menarche, age at first live birth, number of first-degree relatives with breast cancer, number of prior breast biopsies, and whether or not any of the biopsies showed atypical hyperplasia. This model calculates risk over a defined time interval, allows comparison with age-specific incidence figures, and predicts risk accurately in groups of women undergoing annual mammographic screening. It is a useful tool for counseling women who are concerned about their level of risk. It is not an appropriate model, however, for women at risk because of a strong family history of breast cancer, particularly early-onset breast cancer, or those with LCIS. A sample Gail model risk calculation is shown in Figure 74.16. A more appropriate risk model for women with strong family histories, which has not, however, been validated to the same extent as the Gail model, was described by Claus et al.[119] and considers both the age at onset in affected relatives and the history of cancer in second-degree relatives.

TABLE 74.8 **CLASSIFICATION**

MAGNITUDE OF KNOWN BREAST CANCER RISK FACTORS

RELATIVE RISK <2
Early menarche
Late menopause
Nulliparity
Proliferative benign disease
Obesity
Alcohol use
Hormone replacement therapy
RELATIVE RISK 2–4
Age >35 first birth
First-degree relative with breast cancer
Radiation exposure
Prior breast cancer
RELATIVE RISK >4
Gene mutation
Lobular carcinoma in situ
Atypical hyperplasia

MANAGEMENT OF THE HIGH-RISK WOMAN

Counseling women who are at high risk for breast cancer should include a discussion of the options for enhanced surveillance, chemoprevention, and prophylactic surgery. If a woman is at high risk secondary to a strong family history of breast cancer or very early onset of breast or ovarian cancer, genetic counseling should be offered. For patients with known or suspected *BRCA1* or *BRCA2* mutations, most experts suggest aggressive surveillance consisting of an annual mammogram, annual MRI, and clinical breast exam every 4 to 6 months beginning at age 25. For patients with a more moderate family history, annual mammographic screening and clinical breast exam should begin within 10 years of age of breast cancer diagnosis in a first-degree relative or age 40, whichever comes first.

The use of MRI screening for women at high risk is supported by the results of seven clinical trials demonstrating greater sensitivity of MRI as compared with mammography for the detection of breast cancer.[120] Participants in each of these seven studies had either a documented *BRCA1* or *BRCA2* mutation, or a very strong family history of breast cancer. Some of the studies included women with a prior personal history of breast cancer. The cancer detection rate in these studies ranged from 1% to 9% (average 4%). Overall, the studies reported a high sensitivity for MRI, ranging from 71% to 100%, compared with 13% to 40% for mammography. Based on these studies, the American Cancer Society issued guidelines in 2007 recommending annual screening MRI in addition to annual screening mammography in women with a known *BRCA1* or *BRCA2* gene mutation, a lifetime risk of breast cancer exceeding 20%, or a history of mantle radiation for Hodgkin disease before the age of 30.[121]

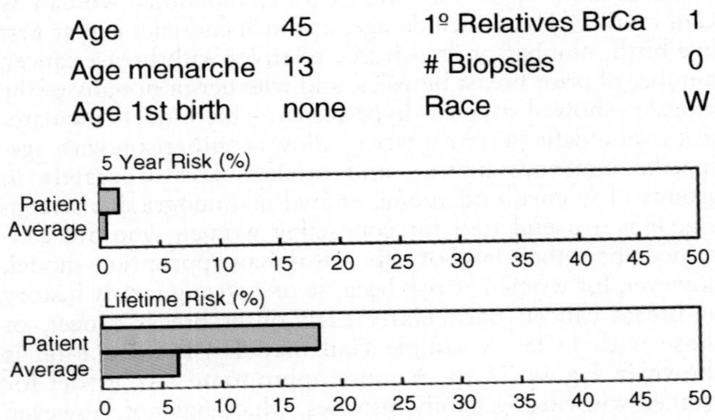

FIGURE 74.16. Breast cancer risk assessment according to the Gail model. This woman's 5-year risk for the development of breast cancer is 1.6%, and her lifetime risk is 18%.

The use of chemopreventive agents for breast cancer risk reduction should be individualized for each patient based on menopausal status, medical history, family history, and a
7 quantified estimate of breast cancer risk. Tamoxifen (Nolvadex) and raloxifene (Evista) are both selective ER modulators (SERMs) that have been shown to reduce the risk of breast cancer. Tamoxifen has been used to treat breast cancer for more than 25 years. Data from treatment trials[122,123] demonstrating that women taking tamoxifen for 5 years had a significantly reduced rate of contralateral breast cancer led to studies of tamoxifen as a chemopreventive agent for women at increased risk of breast cancer. The National Surgical Adjuvant Breast and Bowel Project (NSABP) P-1 prevention trial randomized 13,388 women at increased risk for breast cancer development to tamoxifen or placebo.[105] Risk was defined by the Gail model.[118] Eligible women included those who were age 60 or older, or those between the ages of 35 and 59 years with a predicted 5-year breast cancer risk of 1.66% or more. After a median follow-up of 54.6 months, a 49% reduction in the risk for invasive cancer and a 50% reduction in the risk for noninvasive cancer were found in the tamoxifen group. The reduction occurred only in ER-positive tumors; the occurrence of ER-negative tumors was unchanged. Tamoxifen was of benefit in all age groups, in women at risk on the basis of a family history, and in those eligible for the study on the basis of other risk factors. Women at risk on the basis of LCIS and atypical hyperplasia had particular benefit, with risk reductions of 65% and 86%, respectively.[123] Updated results from the P-1 study based on 7 years of follow-up noted similar reductions in breast cancer incidence.[124] A meta-analysis of five completed tamoxifen prevention trials demonstrated a 38% reduction in breast cancer incidence in populations at varying levels of risk.[125]

The most common side effects of tamoxifen were hot flashes and vaginal discharge. Participants who took tamoxifen had a 2.5 times greater risk for endometrial carcinoma than those in the placebo group, and postmenopausal women carried all of the excess risk. An increased risk for venous thrombosis, including pulmonary embolism, occurs in the postmenopausal women taking tamoxifen. The rate of pulmonary embolism in these women, however, was 1 in 1,000 annually. The presence of these competing risks, particularly in postmenopausal women, led to the search for other acceptable chemopreventive agents. The NSABP Study of Tamoxifen and Raloxifene (known as the STAR or P-2 trial) randomized 19,747 postmenopausal women at increased risk for breast cancer to either tamoxifen 20 mg/d or raloxifene 60 mg/d for 5 years. Raloxifene is a second-generation SERM that reduces the incidence of breast cancer in preclinical models and in clinical trials evaluating its use for the prevention of osteoporosis and heart disease in postmenopausal women.[126] Similar to the P-1 trial, increased risk was defined as a 5-year predicted breast cancer risk of 1.66% as determined by the Gail model or a personal history of LCIS treated by excision alone. After 6 years of follow-up, raloxifene was found to be equivalent to tamoxifen in reducing the incidence of invasive breast cancer (50% reduction) but with fewer side effects (Fig. 74.17).[127] Raloxifene was inferior to tamoxifen in reducing the risk of ductal carcinoma in situ. The reason for this selective effect remains unclear.

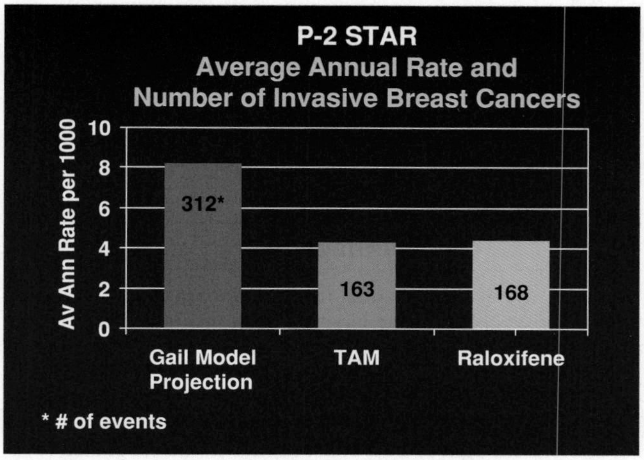

FIGURE 74.17. Both tamoxifen and raloxifene when taken for 5 years in the National Surgical Adjuvant Breast and Bowel Project P-2 (STAR trial) were equally effective at reducing the risk of invasive breast cancer.

The incidence of uterine cancer was lower in the raloxifene arm, with the difference approaching statistical significance, but more than half the women in the STAR trial had previously undergone a hysterectomy, limiting the ability to assess the effect of raloxifene on the uterus. Pulmonary embolism and deep venous thromboses occurred less often in the raloxifene group (RR, 0.70); however, there was an equal number of strokes and transient ischemic attacks. Rates of fracture were virtually identical in the two treatment arms, and there were no statistically significant differences in patient-reported quality-of-life outcomes, although specific symptoms showed significant differences.[128] When counseling postmenopausal women, differences such as the frequency of hot flashes and sexual side effects may be an important factor in determining which drug is most appropriate for an individual patient.

Aromatase inhibitors (AIs) block the conversion of androgens to estrogens by the aromatase enzyme and lower circulating estrogen levels. AIs have proven effective in breast cancer treatment among postmenopausal women with hormone-sensitive tumors, and clinical trial data from three studies show that AIs decrease the incidence of contralateral breast cancers by 37% to 55%.[129–131] Clinical trials assessing the chemopreventive potential of AIs among women at increased risk for breast cancer are currently under way.

Surgical options for women at increased risk for breast cancer include prophylactic mastectomy and prophylactic salpingo-oophorectomy. Both subcutaneous and total (simple) mastectomies have been used for breast cancer prevention; however, neither provides 100% protection. The development of carcinoma in residual breast tissue has been reported after both types of surgery. The efficacy of prophylactic mastectomy in a group of high-risk women was defined in a study of 639 women from the Mayo Clinic, of whom 90% underwent subcutaneous mastectomy and 10% received total mastectomy.[132] At a median of 14 years, prophylactic mastectomy reduced the risk for breast cancer by 90%. Trials in women at risk on the basis of *BRCA1* and *BRCA2* mutations have confirmed a similar efficacy for prophylactic mastectomy in this group. Prophylactic mastectomy is a prevention option that should be undertaken only after a complete risk assessment, consultation with a reconstructive surgeon, and a thorough discussion of management alternatives. Women should be advised of their level of risk and assisted in determining if that level of risk is unacceptable to them, rather than being told to undergo prophylactic surgery. When prophylactic mastectomy is performed, the procedure should be a total mastectomy extended to the same anatomic limits as a therapeutic mastectomy. Patients undergoing prophylactic mastectomy are ideal candidates for a skin-sparing approach to facilitate immediate breast reconstruction (Fig. 74.18). The role of nipple-sparing mastectomy for prophylaxis remains controversial.

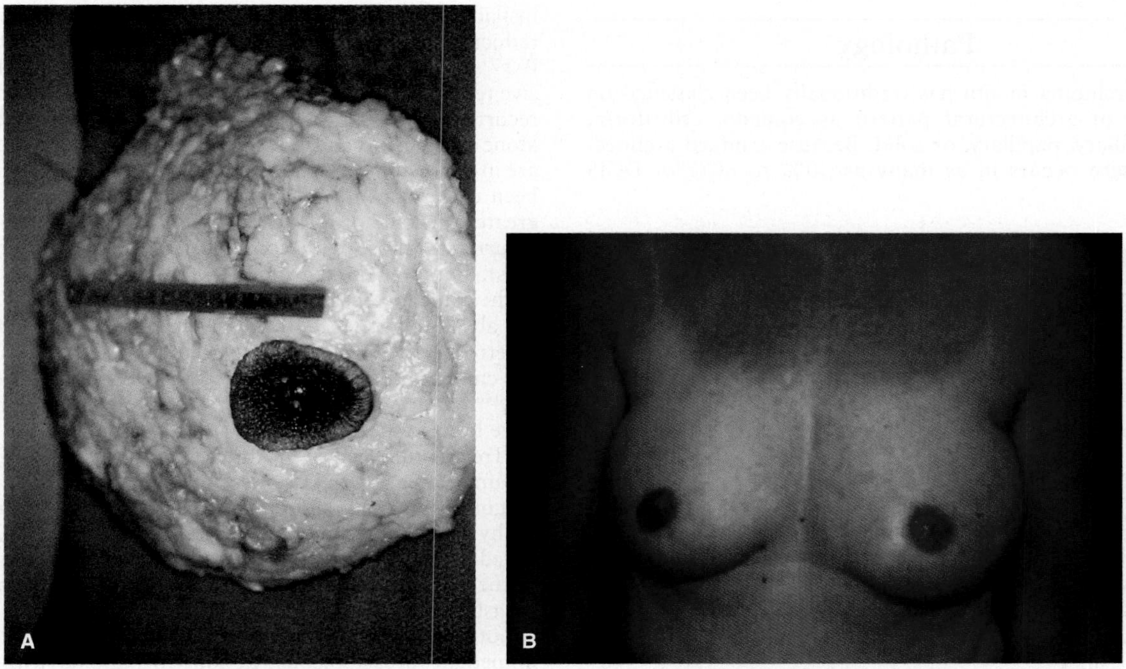

FIGURE 74.18. Skin-sparing mastectomy. **A:** The only skin removed was the nipple–areola complex. **B:** Cosmetic outcome after bilateral skin-sparing mastectomy and transverse rectus abdominis myocutaneous (TRAM) flap reconstruction.

Bilateral salpingo-oophorectomy as a risk reduction strategy is generally limited to women with *BRCA1* and *BRCA2* mutations. In this population prophylactic salpingo-oophorectomy reduces the risk of breast cancer by 50%[133,134] and reduces the risk of ovarian cancer by 98%.

DUCTAL CARCINOMA IN SITU

Ductal carcinoma in situ (DCIS), also known as *intraductal carcinoma,* is a distinct entity from LCIS, the other lesion classified as noninvasive breast cancer, with differences in both clinical presentation and biologic potential. DCIS is characterized by a proliferation of abnormal, presumably malignant epithelial cells that are confined within the basement membrane of the mammary ductal-lobular system (Fig. 74.19).

Presentation

Ductal carcinoma in situ has a variety of clinical presentations: palpable mass, pathologic nipple discharge, or Paget disease of the nipple, all of which are relatively uncommon. The overwhelming majority of palpable breast cancers are invasive carcinoma; fewer than 2% are DCIS. Today, clustered microcalcifications on a mammogram are the most frequent presentation of DCIS, although approximately 10% of nonpalpable masses may also be DCIS. In many reports of biopsies performed for mammographic abnormalities, DCIS accounts for 30% to 50% of the malignancies identified. The number of cases of DCIS between 1975 and 2004 increased by 560% as screening mammography became widely adopted.[135] This increase was observed in both white and black women, and in those over and under 50 years of age, DCIS may also lack both clinical and mammographic findings and be discovered incidentally in a biopsy done for other indications. Of lesions initially diagnosed as DCIS by large-gauge vacuum-assisted core biopsy, 15% to 20% will be found to contain invasive carcinoma when completely excised. Invasive carcinoma is most frequently found in large, high-grade DCIS lesions.[136]

Pathology

Ductal carcinoma in situ has traditionally been classified on the basis of architectural pattern as comedo, cribriform, micropapillary, papillary, or solid. Because a mixed architectural pattern occurs in as many as 30% to 60% of DCIS lesions, however, the utility of this classification system is limited. Newer systems classify DCIS lesions on the basis of nuclear grade and necrosis, and usually recognize three groups of lesions: high, intermediate, and low grade. Multiple systems have been proposed, but their reproducibility and ability to predict the behavior of DCIS remain to be proved.

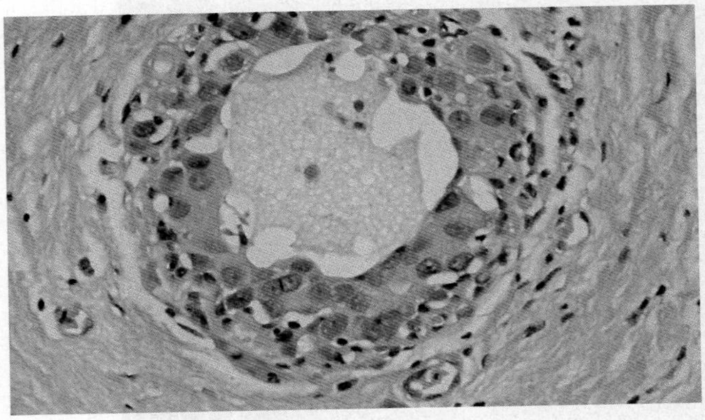

FIGURE 74.19. Photomicrograph of ductal carcinoma in situ. The abnormal cells do not cross the ductal basement membrane. The necrotic debris in the center of the duct is responsible for the calcification visible on mammography.

Management

Mastectomy, excision and irradiation (radiation therapy [RT]), and excision alone have all been proposed as management strategies for DCIS because of uncertainty about the natural history of the disease. Mastectomy is a curative treatment for approximately 98% of patients with DCIS, regardless of lesion size or grade.[137,138] Treatment failure after mastectomy for DCIS is thought to be a consequence of unrecognized invasive carcinoma.

Although mastectomy is an effective treatment for DCIS, it is a radical approach for a lesion that may not progress to invasive carcinoma during a patient's lifetime and is too small to be detected clinically. The use of BCT with excision and RT for invasive carcinoma (see section on local management of stages I and II breast cancer) has stimulated greater interest in the use of this approach for DCIS. No randomized trial has ever compared the treatment of DCIS by mastectomy with treatment by excision and RT. A large number of clinical studies have demonstrated that the local recurrence rate after treatment with excision and RT is 10% to 15% of cases after 10 years,[137–141] and that approximately half of the local recurrences are invasive carcinoma. Deaths from DCIS are rare; 14 breast cancer deaths occurred in 814 patients followed for 8 years after treatment with excision and RT.[140]

Because DCIS is a local problem in the breast and all DCIS does not progress to invasive carcinoma during a patient's lifetime, some authors have suggested that DCIS can be treated by wide excision alone. Four prospective, randomized trials have compared the outcome of excision alone to excision and RT, and the results are summarized in Table 74.9. Despite differences in study design, the trial results are remarkably similar.[142–145] The studies demonstrate that the use of RT reduces ipsilateral breast tumor recurrence by 50% to 60%, and this reduction persists through 12 years of follow-up in the NSABP B-17 study. The use of RT reduces both invasive and noninvasive recurrences; with the use of RT, the annual rate of invasive recurrence is 0.5% to 1.0%. In patients treated with excision alone or excision and RT, approximately 50% of recurrences are invasive and 50% are DCIS. No survival benefit for RT has been observed. In a more detailed pathologic analysis,[145] the greatest benefits of RT were in the patients at highest risk for recurrence (those with comedo necrosis and uncertain margins), but even in the most favorable subgroup (absent or slight comedo necrosis, clear margins), the use of RT reduced the absolute incidence of breast recurrence by 7% at 8 years. A retrospective study has suggested that excision of DCIS with a 1-cm margin of normal breast tissue eliminates the need for RT,[146] but attempts to prospectively duplicate this observation have been unsuccessful.[147]

Treatment selection for the patient with DCIS begins with a careful evaluation of the extent of the DCIS lesion by means of magnification mammography. Standard two-view mammography significantly underestimates the extent of well-differentiated DCIS.[148] If the extent of the DCIS is too large, relative to the patient's breast size, to allow a cosmetically acceptable breast-conserving approach, the patient should be counseled about the options of mastectomy alone or mastectomy with immediate breast reconstruction. In patients with localized DCIS suitable for a breast-conserving approach, the decision regarding the need for RT should be made based on the estimated risk for recurrence and the patient's attitude toward

TABLE 74.9

RESULTS

RESULTS OF RANDOMIZED TRIALS OF RADIOTHERAPY IN DUCTAL CARCINOMA IN SITU

STUDY	PATIENTS (No.)	MEDIAN FOLLOW-UP (Mo)	IBTR (%)	
			E	RT
NSABP B-17[140,141]	813	44	40	17
EORTC 10853[142]	1,010	126	26	15
United Kingdom[143]	1,030	53	14	6
SweDCIS[144]	1,046	96 (mean)	27	12

DCIS, ductal carcinoma in situ; E, excision alone; EORTC, European Organization for Research and Treatment of Cancer; IBTR, ipsilateral breast tumor recurrence; NSABP, National Surgical Adjuvant Breast Project; RT, radiation therapy.

risk. Patients with larger tumors, high-grade lesions, and close margins appear to derive the greatest benefit from RT. It also appears that younger women are at higher risk for recurrence than their older counterparts.[142,149] However, even patients with small, low-grade lesions appear to benefit from RT,[142–145] and it is in this low-risk subgroup that the patient's attitude toward risk becomes important.

Tamoxifen is of benefit in reducing the risk for subsequent invasive carcinoma in patients with DCIS. In NSABP B-24,[149] 1,804 women with DCIS treated by excision and RT were randomized to tamoxifen or placebo for 5 years. Tamoxifen caused a reduction in the incidence of all breast cancer events from 17% to 10.0% ($p = 0.01$). The benefit of tamoxifen was observed in women over and under age 50, and in those with negative and positive margins. A benefit for tamoxifen was also observed whether or not comedo necrosis was present in the tumor. A subset analysis of 676 patients for whom ER status could be determined was performed retrospectively. The benefit of adding tamoxifen to RT in reducing all breast cancer events was 59% in ER-positive women, compared with 37% in the overall patient population. There was little benefit for tamoxifen in ER-negative DCIS, and its use is not warranted in these patients. The UK trial[143] compared treatment with excision alone with excision plus tamoxifen. After a median follow-up of 53 months, there were no differences in the rate of local recurrence between groups. The findings of this study indicate that tamoxifen is not a replacement for RT. The effects of RT and tamoxifen in the NSABP B-17 and B-24 trials[140,149] are illustrated in Figure 74.20. The decision to use RT, tamoxifen, or both in the patient with DCIS will depend on the patient's personal level of risk and attitude toward small benefits from therapeutic intervention, but both should be considered. Identification of markers that predict which women with DCIS will develop an invasive recurrence is a research priority that will greatly improve our ability to tailor treatment to an individual's level of risk.

Axillary nodal involvement in DCIS is rare and presumed to be due to unrecognized invasive carcinoma. In NSABP B-17 and B-24, the axillary recurrence rates, regardless of treatment, were less than 1 per 1,000 patient-years of follow-up.[150] For this reason, axillary staging is not routinely indicated in the patient with a diagnosis of DCIS. Most would agree that sentinel node biopsy should be performed in patients undergoing mastectomy for DCIS since the opportunity for sentinel node biopsy is lost if not performed at the time of mastectomy. In addition, many of these patients have large areas of DCIS where the risk of sampling error after a needle biopsy diagnosis of DCIS is highest.

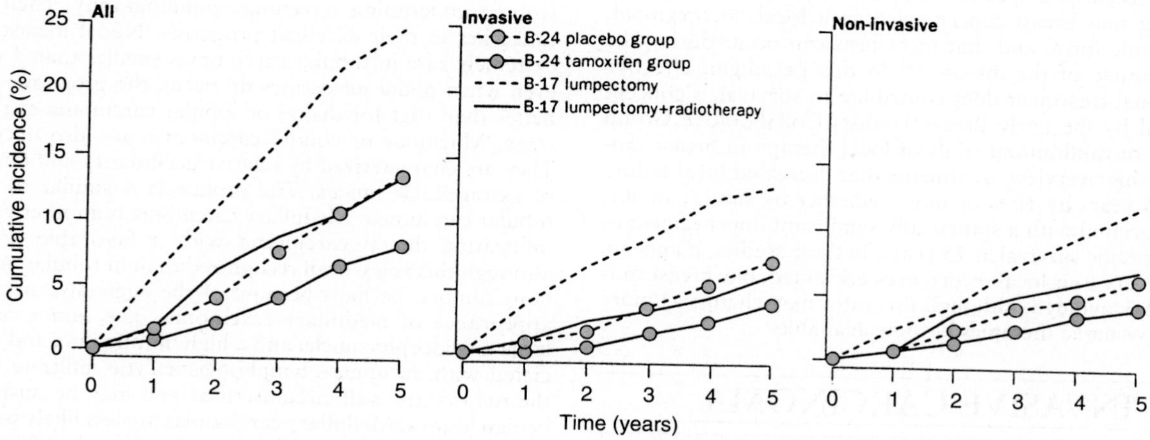

FIGURE 74.20. Benefits of radiation therapy and tamoxifen in ductal carcinoma in situ. The cumulative incidence of breast cancer events in the ipsilateral and contralateral breasts for patients treated in the National Surgical Adjuvant Breast and Bowel Project B-17 and B-24 trials is shown. The reduction in recurrence is greatest for patients receiving radiotherapy and tamoxifen.

BIOLOGY AND NATURAL HISTORY OF BREAST CANCER

Breast cancer is a disease characterized by marked heterogeneity among patients and a long natural history. This is evident in the Middlesex Hospital series, in which Bloom et al.[151] reported the outcome of 250 patients with breast cancer observed without treatment between 1805 and 1933. Patients were generally admitted for advanced disease, with only 2% having stage II disease, 23% having stage III, and 74% having stage IV. Only 39% presented within 1 year of their first symptom. Despite this, 18% of patients receiving no treatment survived 5 years, and 4% survived 10 years. The mortality was constant over time, with approximately 25% of patients who were alive at the beginning of any given year dying during that year. In modern series, patients with varying annual hazards of death can also be identified, and these remain constant for at least 10 years after the diagnosis. For this reason, some have concluded that breast cancer is never cured, and that if death from other causes did not intervene, cancer eventually would recur in all patients. Although this may be true in the abstract, from a practical point of view, failures more than 20 years after treatment are rare, and many patients have a normal life expectancy after breast cancer treatment. The clinical variations in breast cancer are believed to reflect variable genetic changes that result in the disease.

The initial clinical understanding of breast cancer, as articulated by Halsted,[152] was one of orderly disease progression, suggesting that en bloc extirpation of the primary tumor with a wide margin of normal tissue (i.e., the breast) and the draining lymphatics was the most likely strategy to cure breast cancer. Over time, it became clear that the majority of women with breast cancer were not cured by radical mastectomy. Recognition of this fact initially led to larger operations, such as the extended radical mastectomy to remove more of the lymphatic drainage of the breast. When these procedures failed to improve survival, however, a dramatic shift in thinking occurred. In the new disease paradigm, championed by Bernard Fisher,[153] most breast cancer was considered to be systemic at the time of diagnosis, so that the extent of locoregional treatment would have little impact on survival from breast cancer. Acceptance of this concept led to the adoption of the modified radical mastectomy, and subsequently breast-conserving surgery, for the treatment of stages I and II breast cancer, in addition to the widespread use of adjuvant chemotherapy and hormonal therapy.

More recently, a spectrum hypothesis has been advanced suggesting that breast cancer exists in a local, locoregional, and systemic form, and that metastasis can occur during the clinical course of the disease.[154] In this paradigm, effective locoregional treatment does contribute to survival, a concept supported by the Early Breast Trialists Collaborative Group overview of randomized trials of local therapy in breast can-
8 cer.[155] In this overview, treatments that decreased local failure rates at 5 years by 10% or more, whether by surgery or RT, were associated with a statistically significant improvement in disease-specific survival at 15 years. In these studies, it appears that for every four local recurrences prevented, one breast cancer death is avoided, although this ratio may change as more effective systemic therapies become available.

INVASIVE CARCINOMA

Pathology

Invasive carcinomas are defined as those in which tumor cells have crossed the basement membrane and have the biologic capability to metastasize. Any breast lesion that is surgically removed should be considered potentially malignant. Breast biopsy specimens should be oriented in the operating room and inked before sectioning so that the margin status can be assessed. The pathologic evaluation of a breast tumor should routinely include size, histologic type, grade, margin status, hormone receptor, and HER2 status.

Histologic Type

Infiltrating ductal carcinoma is the most common type of breast carcinoma, accounting for 65% to 80% of all cases of breast cancer. Microscopically, infiltrating ductal carcinomas vary widely in appearance and often have features of other histologic subtypes of breast cancer, with areas of lobular, medullary, or tubular differentiation. For prognostic purposes, these mixed tumors are considered to be infiltrating ductal carcinomas.

Infiltrating lobular carcinoma is the second most frequently encountered subtype of invasive carcinoma. Approximately 10% of cancers are classified as lobular. Histologically, lobular cancers grow as a single file of malignant cells that tend to be arranged circumferentially around ducts and lobules. Because of this growth pattern, they are often difficult to recognize on clinical examination and mammography because they may not produce the distinctive mass lesions characteristic of infiltrating ductal carcinomas. Infiltrating lobular carcinoma has been said to have a rate of bilaterality as high as 30% to 50%. When patients with LCIS are excluded from consideration, however, the incidence of contralateral breast cancer in patients with infiltrating lobular carcinoma differs little from that in patients with ductal carcinoma. In one study of 4,748 patients, a contralateral cancer had developed after 5 years in 5.3% of patients with infiltrating lobular cancer, and in 4.0% of those with infiltrating ductal tumors.[156] Thus, the routine use of bilateral mastectomy for patients with tumors of lobular histology cannot be justified. Lobular carcinoma is more likely to metastasize to the intra-abdominal viscera, uterus, ovaries, and peritoneal surfaces than other histologic types of breast carcinoma. Most studies have found no difference in survival between patients with infiltrating ductal and those with lobular carcinoma after stratification for appropriate prognostic factors.

Favorable histologic subtypes of breast carcinoma include pure tubular and mucinous carcinoma. Tubular carcinomas form normal-appearing breast ductules or tubules. At least 75% of a tumor must be tubular to be classified in this subtype. Tubular carcinomas are uncommon, accounting for 2% or fewer of all cancers, although they are more frequent in women undergoing screening mammography. Their significance lies in their excellent prognosis. Nodal metastases are extremely rare in tubular carcinomas smaller than 1 cm, and even when nodal metastases do occur, the prognosis is much better than that for ductal or lobular carcinoma at the same stage. Mucinous or colloid carcinomas are also uncommon. They are characterized by relative acellularity and large pools of extracellular mucus. The prognosis is similar to that for tubular carcinoma. Medullary carcinoma is another variant of infiltrating ductal carcinoma with a favorable prognosis, although this is less well recognized than in tubular and mucinous tumors, perhaps because of the aggressive microscopic appearance of medullary carcinoma. The tumor cells have large pleomorphic nuclei and a high mitotic rate, and are associated with an intense lymphoplasmacytic infiltrate. Grossly, the tumors are well circumscribed and may be mistaken for benign lesions. Medullary carcinomas are less likely to be associated with axillary nodal metastases than ductal or lobular carcinomas of the same size, and survival is also better. Other histologic types of breast cancer account for fewer than 2% of all cancers.

Grading Systems

The grade of a carcinoma is an estimate of differentiation. It may be histologic or nuclear. Nuclear grading is a cytologic assessment of the similarity of tumor nuclei to the nuclei of normal cells. The nuclear grade is usually reported as well differentiated, intermediate, or poorly differentiated. The histologic grade considers not only the cytologic differentiation but also the growth pattern of the carcinoma. The extent of tubule formation, nuclear hyperchromasia, and the mitotic index are assessed. In one of the most widely used systems, the Elston modification of the Scharf-Bloom-Richardson classification, each of these three elements is scored on a scale of 1 to 3, with a resultant classification of grade 1 (score of 3 to 5), grade 2 (score of 6 or 7), or grade 3 (score of 8 or 9).[157] Approximately 19% of the 2,000 cases reviewed by Elston and Ellis[157] were grade 1, 34% were grade 2, and 47% were grade 3. A study of the molecular phenotypes associated with histologic grade demonstrated distinct genetic profiles for grade 1 and grade 3 tumors, but a profile for grade 2 tumors could not be identified. Instead, tumors classified as grade 2 were found to have the genetic profile of grade 1 or grade 3 tumors, calling into question the existence of a grade 2 group as a distinct prognostic group.[158]

Hormone Receptors and HER2

The concept of an estrogen receptor was described by Jensen and Jacobsen in 1962,[159] based on the observation that estrogens tagged with radioactive isotopes are preferentially concentrated in the estrogen target organs of animals (i.e., breast, uterus, vagina) and in human breast cancers. Subsequently, a second hormone receptor, the progesterone receptor (PR), was identified. ERs and PRs belong to a superfamily of nuclear hormone receptors that function as transcription factors when bound to their respective ligands. Approximately 70% of breast carcinomas are hormone receptor positive; well-differentiated tumors and those occurring in older postmenopausal women have the highest rates of receptor positivity. Approximately 60% of patients with ER-positive tumors respond to endocrine therapy, but only 5% to 10% of patients with ER-negative tumors do so, and responses probably result from false-negative receptor results.[160] It is now apparent that there are two receptors for estrogen, ERα (the classic receptor identified by Jensen) and ERβ, identified by Gustaffson's laboratory in 1996.[161] At present, the clinical significance of ERβ in breast cancer management is uncertain. Tumor ERα and PR content is measured by immunohistochemical techniques. Determination of hormone receptor status is a critical part of the pathologic analysis of breast tumors and is used to ascertain whether the patient is a candidate for hormonal therapy (see section on adjuvant systemic therapy).

The HER2 gene, also known as HER2/neu or c-erbB2, is located on chromosome 17q. HER2 is a member of the epidermal growth factor receptor (EGFR) family of transmembrane tyrosine kinases and is normally involved in regulation of cell proliferation. The HER2 gene is a proto-oncogene, a normal gene with the potential to become an oncogene upon molecular alterations, such as mutation, amplification, or overexpression of its protein product. The HER2 protein is overexpressed and/or its gene is amplified in ~20% of invasive breast cancers. HER2 amplification is associated with a more aggressive phenotype and predicts for response to trastuzumab therapy, a recombinant humanized monoclonal antibody specific for the external region of HER2[162] (see section on adjuvant systemic therapy). Immunohistochemistry for membrane-bound HER2 protein is most commonly employed for semiquantitative analysis of staining (0, 1+, 2+, or 3+) followed by fluorescence in situ hybridization (FISH) for confirmation of gene amplification in cases scored as positive (2+ or 3+).[163]

Molecular Subtyping

Over the last decade, advances in DNA microarray technology and sophisticated genomic analyses have led to the development of classification systems of breast cancer based on gene expression profiles. As such, breast cancer is increasingly being recognized as a heterogeneous family of diseases with implications for both tumor biology and treatment. First described in the seminal papers by Perou and Sorlie,[164,165] and subsequently validated by others,[166,167] the intrinsic breast cancer subtypes have been identified as HER2 positive, ER positive luminal A, ER positive luminal B, and basal-like or "triple negative." These intrinsic subtypes, which characterize the primary tumor and remain constant through the metastatic process, have been shown to be prognostic for clinical outcome as well as predictive of response to therapy, and provide important insights into tumor biology.

The basal-like group was named for the higher expression of genes characteristic of normal basal cells of breast epithelium including keratins 5, 14, or 17; HER1 (epidermal growth factor receptor); and smooth muscle actin.[164] Basal-like cancers are generally high-grade, poorly differentiated tumors with a poor prognosis. They are predominantly negative for ER, PR, and HER2, and clinical adoption of this breast tumor classification uses immunohistochemical "triple negativity" as the most practical surrogate for the identification of basal-like tumors. Basal-like tumors are more common in younger women, women of African descent,[168] and carriers of *BRCA1* germline mutations.

Clinical Evaluation and Staging

The extent of the preoperative workup should be guided by the clinical stage of the disease and the patient's symptoms. Patients with DCIS do not require screening for metastatic disease. Bone scans are frequently used as a preoperative screening test for patients with invasive cancer, but in a large review, the incidence of occult bony metastases detected by scanning in patients with stage I or II disease was less than 5%.[169] False-positive results are frequent, especially in older women. In asymptomatic women with stage III disease, 8.3% had bony metastases. The yield of liver screening studies is less than 1%, even for women with stage III disease, and the test is of little benefit in preoperative evaluation. Positron emission tomography (PET) scans are also not indicated in the routine preoperative evaluation of asymptomatic women.

Serum tumor markers have not been shown to be of value preoperatively. Studies of carcinoembryonic antigen, CA15-3, CA27.29, and the shed extracellular domain of erbB2 do not demonstrate sufficient sensitivity or specificity to indicate or exclude the presence of occult metastatic disease.

Staging refers to the grouping of patients according to the extent of their disease. The stage is useful in (a) determining the choice of treatment for an individual patient, (b) estimating prognosis, and (c) comparing the results of different treatment programs. Staging can be based on either clinical or pathologic findings.

Currently, the staging of cancer is determined by the American Joint Committee on Cancer (AJCC). The AJCC system is a clinical and pathologic staging system based on the TNM (tumor, node, metastasis) system.[7]

The clinical stage is based on all the information available before the first definitive treatment is administered. This

STAGING

TABLE 74.10

TUMOR, NODE, METASTASIS (TNM) CLASSIFICATION FOR BREAST CANCER STAGING

TNM DEFINITIONS

Primary Tumor

Tx	Primary tumor cannot be assessed
T0	No evidence of primary tumor
Tis	Carcinoma in situ, ductal or lobular or Paget disease of the nipple with no tumor
T1	Tumor 2 cm or less in greatest dimension
T2	Tumor more than 2 cm but not more than 5 cm in greatest dimension
T3	Tumor more than 5 cm in greatest dimension
T4	Tumor of any size with direct extension to the chest wall (not including pectoralis muscle), skin edema, skin ulceration, satellite skin nodules, or inflammatory carcinoma

Regional Lymph Nodes (pathologic)

Nx	Nodes cannot be assessed
N0	No regional node metastases histologically, no additional examination for isolated tumor cells (ITCs)
N1	Metastasis to one to three axillary nodes or in internal mammary (IM) nodes with microscopic disease detected by sentinel node biopsy, which is not clinically apparent
N2	Metastases in four to nine axillary nodes or in clinically apparent IM nodes in the absence of axillary node metastasis
N3	Metastases in 10 or more axillary nodes, or in infraclavicular nodes, or in IM nodes in the presence of one or more positive axillary nodes; or in more than three axillary nodes with IM metastases, or in supraclavicular nodes

Distant Metastases

Mx	Distant metastasis cannot be assessed
M0	No distant metastasis
M1	Distant metastasis

STAGE GROUPING

Stage 0	Tis	N0	M0
Stage I	TI	N0	M0
Stage IIA	T0	N1	M0
	T1	N1	M0
	T2	N0	M0
Stage IIB	T2	N1	M0
	T3	N0	M0
Stage IIIA	T0	N2	M0
	T1	N2	M0
	T2	N2	M0
	T3	N1	M0
	T3	N2	M0
Stage IIIB	T4	N0	M0
	T4	N1	M0
	T4	N2	M0
Stage IIIC	Any T	N3	M0
Stage IV	Any T	Any N	M1

includes the findings from physical examination, imaging studies, operation, and pathologic examination of the breast or other tissues. The clinical stage is useful in selecting and evaluating therapy.

The pathologic stage (designated pTNM) is based on all the data used for clinical staging in addition to data derived from the pathologic examination of the primary carcinoma and axillary lymph nodes. A tumor cannot be evaluated for pathologic staging (pTX) if excision of the primary carcinoma reveals tumor in any margin of resection by gross pathologic examination. The pathologic stage provides the most precise data to estimate the prognosis and calculate the end result. The current staging system is given in Table 74.10.[7]

Local Management of Stage I and Stage II Breast Cancer

The goal of the local therapy of breast cancer is to eradicate all clinically evident tumor in the breast and axillary lymph nodes. In the breast, this can be accomplished with a total

TABLE 74.11 **RESULTS**

SURVIVAL IN PROSPECTIVE RANDOMIZED TRIALS COMPARING BREAST-CONSERVING THERAPY WITH MASTECTOMY

■ TRIAL	■ FOLLOW-UP (y)	■ OVERALL SURVIVAL ■ BCT (%)	■ OVERALL SURVIVAL ■ MASTECTOMY (%)	■ LOCAL RECURRENCE ■ BCT (%)	■ LOCAL RECURRENCE ■ MASTECTOMY (%)
Institut Gustave-Roussy[170]	15	73	65	9	14
Milan I[171]	20	42	41	7	2
NSABP B-06[172]	20	46	47	14	10
NCI[173]	20	54	58	31	6
EORTC[174]	10	65	66	20	12
Danish[175]	6	79	82	3	4

BCT, breast-conserving therapy; EORTC, European Organization for Research and Treatment of Cancer; NCI, National Cancer Institute; NSABP, National Surgical Adjuvant Breast and Bowel Project.

mastectomy, a total mastectomy with immediate breast reconstruction, or BCT, which consists of removal of the primary tumor with a margin of normal tissue and RT. Six modern prospective, randomized trials have compared mastectomy with BCT and have demonstrated no survival differences, even after long-term follow-up (Table 74.11).[170–175] Mastec-
9 tomy alone has never been compared with mastectomy and reconstruction in a randomized trial, but there is no reason to suspect that reconstruction would decrease survival. In the absence of survival differences, the role of the surgeon is to identify medical contraindications to the procedures and to counsel the patient regarding what is involved in each one.

10 **Breast-conserving Therapy.** For BCT to be successful, three conditions must be met. It must be possible to (a) reduce the tumor burden to a microscopic level likely to be controlled by irradiation, (b) safely deliver radiation therapy, and (c) promptly detect local recurrence. The contraindications to BCT arise logically from these conditions. In 1992, a joint committee of the American College of Surgeons, American College of Radiology, College of American Pathologists, and Society of Surgical Oncology developed guidelines for BCT. These were updated in 2007 and are listed in Table 74.12.[176]

The incidence of the contraindications to BCT in the breast cancer population determines the number of patients who are advised to undergo mastectomy for medical reasons. Morrow et al.[10] reported a study in which a multidisciplinary team of physicians prospectively evaluated 456 patients with DCIS, clinical stage I breast cancer, or clinical stage II breast cancer between 1988 and 1991. Medical contraindications to breast preservation were present in only 26% of the patients, and the incidence and type of contraindications varied significantly by stage, with only 10% of patients with stage I disease having contraindications to BCT.

In an effort to increase the number of patients eligible for breast conservation, the use of neoadjuvant chemotherapy to shrink the primary tumor before surgical therapy has been studied.[177] In a large randomized trial, NSABP protocol B-18, 1,523 patients with tumors of any size were randomized to receive four cycles of doxorubicin (A) and cyclophosphamide (C) either preoperatively or postoperatively.[178] All patients over age 50 received tamoxifen. A reduction in tumor diameter of 50% was noted clinically in 80% of the patients, and in 37%, no tumor could be felt after chemotherapy. However, only one fourth of the patients thought to be complete responders had no tumor identified microscopically after surgery. Significant axillary down-staging also occurred, with pathologically negative nodes in 60% of the neoadjuvant group and in 42% of the postoperative adjuvant group ($p < 0.001$). Despite these impressive response rates, the rate of breast conservation increased by only 8%, from 60% to 68%. In a subsequent study, the addition of docetaxel to AC treatment preoperatively increased the clinical complete response rate from 40.1% to 63.6% ($p < 0.001$) and the pathologic complete response rate from 13.7% to 26.1% ($p < 0.001$).[179] Despite this increase in response rate, the use of BCT did not differ between patients receiving preoperative AC and those receiving AC plus Taxotere. This is probably because of the inability of the physical examination and imaging studies to reliably predict the degree of pathologic response. To date, neoadjuvant therapy has not been shown to improve survival in comparison with therapy given postoperatively.

TABLE 74.12 **INDICATIONS/CONTRAINDICATIONS**

CONTRAINDICATIONS TO BREAST-CONSERVING THERAPY IN INVASIVE CARCINOMA

ABSOLUTE CONTRAINDICATIONS

- Two or more primary tumors in separate quadrants of the breast
- Persistent positive margins after reasonable surgical attempts
- Pregnancy is an absolute contraindication to the use of breast irradiation. When cancer is diagnosed in the third trimester, it may be possible to perform breast-conserving surgery and treat the patient with irradiation after delivery.
- A history of prior therapeutic irradiation to the breast region that would result in re-treatment to an excessively high radiation dose
- Diffuse malignant-appearing microcalcifications

RELATIVE CONTRAINDICATIONS

- A history of scleroderma or active systemic lupus erythematosus
- Large tumor in a small breast that would result in cosmesis unacceptable to the patient. In this circumstance, preoperative chemotherapy should be considered.
- Very large or pendulous breasts if reproducibility of patient setup and adequate dose homogeneity cannot be ensured

In addition to the medical contraindications to BCT discussed earlier, patient desire is another indication for mastectomy. Not all women who are eligible for BCT opt for this therapy. In one study, greater patient involvement in the decision-making process was associated with a significantly higher mastectomy rate than when the surgeon was the primary decision maker.[180]

The amount of breast tissue to be resected in a lumpectomy to minimize the risk for local recurrence while optimizing the cosmetic appearance remains a major issue. There is no consensus on what constitutes an adequate margin for a lumpectomy. The only microscopic margin definition used in randomized trials has been tumor cells not touching ink. There is little convincing evidence that wider margins reduce the risk of local recurrence. Studies have shown that the risk of residual tumor varies with the histology of the primary tumor, being lowest in pure infiltrating ductal carcinoma and highest in infiltrating ductal carcinoma with an extensive intraductal component (EIC); the risk in infiltrating lobular carcinoma falls between the other two.[181] These studies indicate that the ideal balance between cosmesis and local failure is unlikely to be achieved by resecting the same amount of breast tissue in all patients. Magnification mammography is essential to identify the extent of the tissue that must be resected, and it allows large "quadrantectomy"-type resections to be reserved for patients with multifocal disease. With the use of physical examination and magnification mammography, the patients who can undergo breast conservation can be identified with a success rate higher than 95%.[182] The extent of surgical resection is the major determinant of cosmetic outcome, and approximately 90% of patients treated with conservative resection rate their cosmetic outcome as excellent or good (Fig. 74.21).

Local recurrence of tumor in the breast after BCT has been the subject of many studies. Local recurrence may be a consequence of inappropriate patient selection, inadequate surgery or RT, or biologic characteristics of the tumor. The presence of tumor at the margin of resection significantly increases the risk for local recurrence, as does the use of radiation doses to the
11 whole breast of less than 4,500 to 5,000 cGy. Six randomized trials have attempted to identify a subgroup of patients with invasive carcinoma who do not require RT. All have shown a large reduction (average, 75%) in the rate of local recurrence with RT,[183] and RT should be considered a standard part of BCT for invasive carcinoma. This is particularly true since the 2005 overview analysis[111] of trials of local therapy has demonstrated that absolute improvements in local control of more than 10% at 5 years, whether obtained by surgery or radiation therapy, are associated with statistically significant reductions in breast cancer mortality 15 years after diagnosis. Studies are now ongoing to evaluate the efficacy of partial breast irradiation to the quadrant of the tumor on local control. Patient factors, such as young age, have also been associated with an increased risk for local failure after BCT. In contrast, a family history of breast cancer does not increase local failure rates. In women with mutations of *BRCA1* or *BRCA2*, the risk of new second primary cancers is increased in both breasts, but the risk of local failure does not seem to be elevated.[184] A number of tumor factors, such as size and involvement of axillary lymph nodes, that are strong predictors of the risk for distant recurrence are not associated with the risk for recurrence in the breast. Histologic tumor type also is not a risk factor, and studies have shown that recurrence rates after excision of infiltrating lobular carcinoma to negative margins do not differ from those after excision of infiltrating ductal tumors. Most studies also indicate that histologic grade is not predictive of recurrence. Some studies have identified lymphatic invasion at the primary tumor site as a risk factor, but this has also been shown to be a risk factor for local recurrence after mastectomy.

In the past, an EIC, defined as the presence of intraductal carcinoma both within an infiltrating ductal carcinoma and in adjacent grossly normal breast tissue, was thought to be associated with an increased risk for local, but not distant, recurrence. More recent studies indicate that when EIC-positive tumors are excised to negative margins, local failure rates are similar to patients with EIC-negative tumors.[185] The use of adjuvant chemotherapy or tamoxifen in patients who have received breast RT reduces the risk for breast recurrence by approximately 50%. In modern series, local failure rates of 4% to 8% at 10 years are commonly reported in patients receiving RT plus systemic therapy. The information on factors associated with local recurrence suggests that two types of recurrences develop after BCT. One type of recurrence represents a heavy tumor burden in the breast that is not controlled by breast irradiation. This type of recurrence can be minimized by meticulous patient selection and attention to the technical details of surgery and irradiation. The other type of recurrence is a manifestation of a biologically aggressive tumor and represents a first site of metastatic disease. This type of recurrence is similar to the majority of chest wall recurrences after mastectomy.

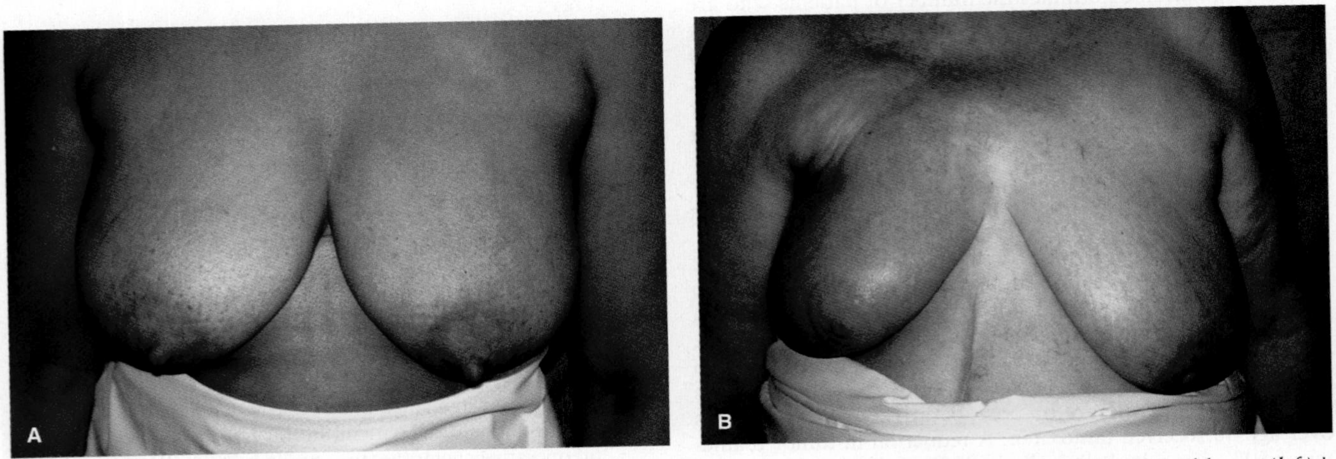

FIGURE 74.21. Cosmetic outcome after breast-conserving therapy with radiation. **A:** Excellent cosmetic outcome. The treated breast (*left*) is identical to the untreated breast. **B:** Fair cosmetic outcome. Significant shrinkage and loss of ptosis is evident in the treated right breast.

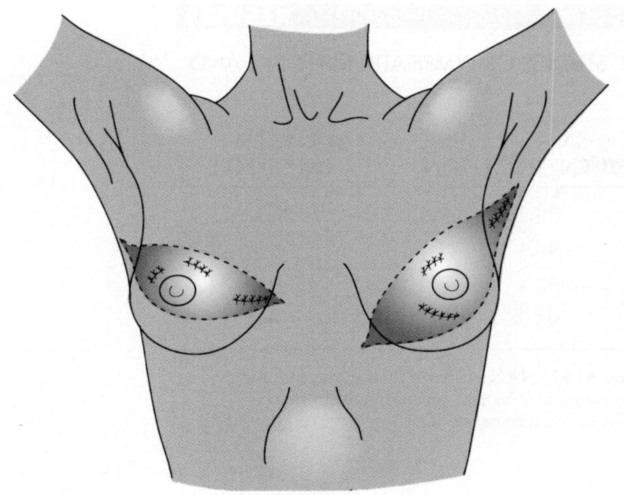

FIGURE 74.22. Incision placement for modified radical mastectomy. The incision should include the nipple–areola complex, biopsy scar, and excess skin of the breast.

Mastectomy. The term *mastectomy* describes the removal of all grossly evident breast tissue. If only the breast is removed, the operation is called *total* or *simple mastectomy*. If the breast and most or all of the axillary lymph nodes are removed, the procedure is termed *modified radical mastectomy*. Mastectomy has traditionally been performed through an elliptical incision that encompasses the nipple–areola complex and the biopsy scar, if an open biopsy has been performed, in addition to the excess skin of the breast (Fig. 74.22). If the skin is needed for reconstruction, it can be preserved and exposure obtained through incision rather than excision, a procedure known as *skin-sparing mastectomy*. Skin flaps are raised in the plane between the subcutaneous fat and the underlying breast tissue. To encompass all the breast tissue, the dissection should extend superiorly to the inferior border of the clavicle, medially to the lateral border of the sternum, inferiorly to the superior extent of the rectus sheath, and laterally to the latissimus dorsi. The fascia overlying the pectoralis major is the deep margin of resection, but it can be preserved when needed to facilitate reconstruction.

Mastectomy is an extremely safe operation. A review of the Surveillance, Epidemiology, and End Results (SEER) from the National Center for Health Statistics data for 10,056 patients treated between 1960 and 1973 reports a 30-day operative mortality of 0.35%.[186] Early postoperative complications include wound infections, which often present as cellulitis and occur in 2% to 14% of cases.[187] Open surgical biopsy before mastectomy (as opposed to a needle biopsy technique) increases the rate of infection. Skin flap necrosis is relatively uncommon today. Factors associated with flap necrosis include vertical incisions, technical error with denuding of the subcutaneous fat from the flap, and closure under tension. Seromas form in 100% of patients and should be considered a side effect and not a complication. Extensive axillary nodal involvement is the strongest predictor of prolonged lymphatic drainage after mastectomy. Seroma formation can be minimized by leaving suction drains in place until their output is less than 30 mL per 24 hours rather than arbitrarily removing them on a predetermined day. Anesthesia of the chest wall is another side effect of mastectomy that patients should be informed of preoperatively.

Mastectomy and Immediate Reconstruction. The techniques of breast reconstruction have evolved dramatically during the past 30 years, and the switch from radical mastectomy to total mastectomy has made immediate reconstruction an option for most women. Tissue expansion followed by removal of the expander and replacement with a permanent implant is the most common form of reconstruction in the United States. The advantage of this technique is that it adds little to the length of surgery or the time of recovery. Disadvantages include the need for a second surgical procedure routinely and the limitations in cosmetic outcome, particularly for women with large or pendulous breasts. These differences, however, are minimized when a bra is worn (Fig. 74.23).

The alternative to implant reconstruction is the use of autologous tissue flaps. Both the transverse rectus abdominis myocutaneous (TRAM) flap and a latissimus dorsi flap have been used for reconstruction. These flaps have the advantage of allowing a more natural look and feel to the breasts than can be achieved with implants (see Fig. 74.18B). The TRAM reconstruction has the added advantage of an abdominoplasty. Both, however, add significant time to the operative procedure, hospitalization, and recovery period, and they may not be suitable for patients with major comorbid conditions. In addition,

ENDOCRINE

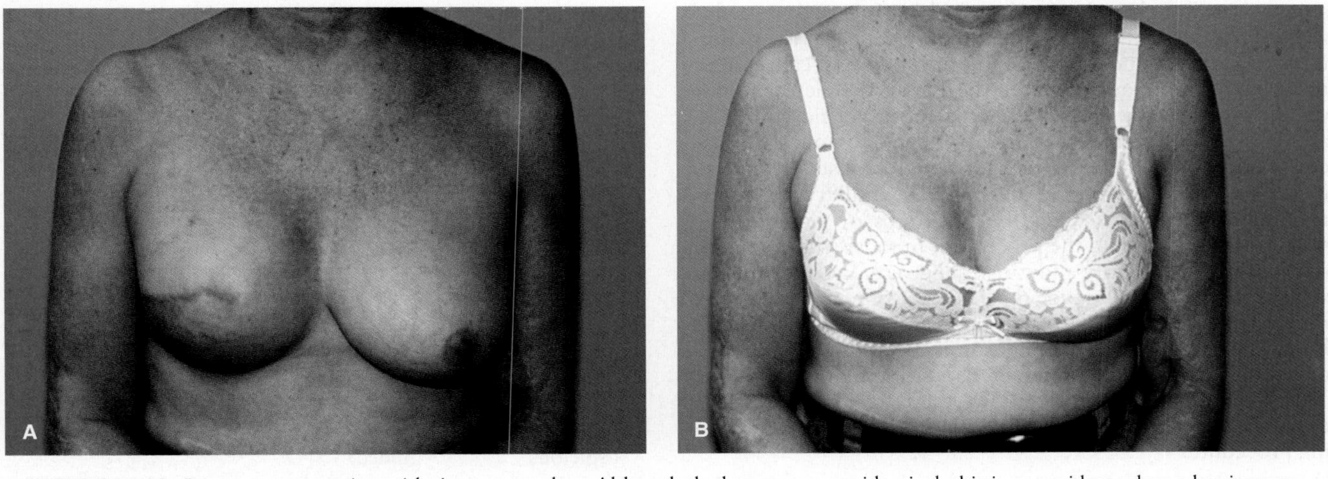

FIGURE 74.23. Breast reconstruction with tissue expanders. Although the breasts are not identical, this is not evident when a bra is worn.

TABLE 74.13 **RESULTS**

RESULTS OF PROSPECTIVE, MULTI-INSTITUTIONAL STUDIES OF LYMPHATIC MAPPING AND SENTINEL NODE BIOPSY

STUDY	NO. PATIENTS	% SN IDENTIFICATION	% FALSE NEGATIVE
ACOSOG Z10[191]	5,237	98.7	N/A
ALMANAC[192]	803	96.1	6.7
NSABP B-32[193]	5,611	97.1	9.8
Sentinella/GIVOM[194]	697	95	16.7

ACOSOG, American College of Surgeons Oncology Group; ALMANAC, Axillary Lymphatic Mapping Against Nodal Axillary Clearance; GIVOM, Gruppo Interdisciplinare Veneto Oncologia Mammaria; NSABP, National Surgical Adjuvant Breast and Bowel Project; SN, sentinel node.

in most women the latissimus flap does not provide enough tissue to create a breast mound, and an implant must be added.

Retrospective studies indicate that immediate reconstruction, even after skin-sparing mastectomy, does not increase the risk of local failure.[188] The detection of local failure also does not appear to be altered by the presence of a reconstruction because the majority of chest wall failures occur in the skin or subcutaneous fat. An important issue is the use of immediate reconstruction in patients who will require postoperative RT. The incidence of implant loss and poor cosmetic outcome is clearly increased in patients who undergo postoperative RT, whereas flap necrosis, fibrosis, and shrinkage can occur in TRAM flaps after radiation. As the indications for postoperative RT have expanded (discussed later), the issue of the optimal method and timing of reconstruction has become a subject of great controversy. Good cosmetic outcomes have been reported after irradiation of both implants and tissue flaps. Alternative approaches include the placement of an expander to allow skin preservation at the time of initial surgery,[189] with a decision to continue with the expander and implant, to switch to a flap reconstruction at the completion of oncologic therapy, or to delay reconstruction until after the completion of irradiation.

Management of the Axillary Nodes

Axillary dissection has been a part of the surgical management of breast cancer since the era of Halsted. Initially, axillary dissection was thought to be therapeutic, but came to be regarded as a staging procedure when it became evident that the majority of women with nodal metastases died of breast cancer after receiving local therapy alone. In the 1990s, the increasing use of adjuvant systemic therapy for node-positive and node-negative breast cancer, the more frequent detection of small cancers associated with a low risk for nodal metastases, and an increased awareness of the morbidity of axillary dissection resulted in attempts to identify subgroups of patients who would not benefit from the procedure. In most studies, tumor size was used to identify a low-risk subgroup. Even for tumors smaller than 5 mm, however, the incidence of nodal metastases ranges from 3% to 12%.[183] For the majority of patients with breast cancer, the axillary nodal status cannot be reliably predicted on the basis of the characteristics of the primary tumor. Today, sentinel node biopsy allows the reliable identification of patients with axillary metastases with a low-morbidity staging procedure.

Sentinel Node Biopsy. A sentinel lymph node (SN) is defined as the first lymph node that receives drainage from a cancer. The procedure of lymphatic mapping can be performed with Lymphazurin blue dye, colloids labeled with radioactive isotopes (usually technetium), or a combination of the two agents. The SN technique was initially developed and validated in studies from single surgeons or institutions where SN biopsy was followed by axillary dissection.[190]

A number of prospective, multi-institutional studies have examined the ability to identify an SN and the accuracy of the SN in predicting the status of the remaining axillary
12 nodes.[191–194] These are summarized in Table 74.13. These studies indicate that regardless of the technique used, surgeons learning the procedure can identify a SN in approximately 95% of patients, which will predict the status of the remaining axillary nodes in about 90% of cases. It is apparent that SN biopsy can be performed in most patients with breast cancer. The management of the axillary lymph nodes is listed in Table 74.14. A randomized comparison has demonstrated that equal numbers of node-positive women are identified with SN biopsy and axillary dissection.[195] The morbidity of SN biopsy is significantly lower than that of axillary dissection, both 6 months and 2 years postoperatively, and the incidence of lymphedema is significantly lower.[181] After SN biopsy alone, isolated axillary recurrence occurs in fewer than 1% of patients, making it the axillary staging procedure of choice for most patients with breast cancer. Sentinel node biopsy also offers the pathologist the opportunity to perform a much more detailed study of the lymph node that is most likely to contain metastases than is possible when an entire axillary specimen containing 15 to 30 nodes is evaluated. With the use of multiple sections or immunohistochemistry, it is possible to identify tumor deposits in approximately 20% of nodes found to be "negative" with routine sectioning and hematoxylin and eosin staining. The prognostic significance of these micrometastases,

TABLE 74.14

APPROACH TO THE AXILLARY NODES

FINDING	APPROACH
Clinically negative	Sentinel node biopsy
Radiographically suspicious	Ultrasound-guided fine-needle aspiration Axillary dissection if positive Sentinel node biopsy if negative
Clinically suspicious	Fine-needle aspiration (image or hand guided) Follow-up management as for radiographically suspicious

however, is uncertain. Prospective clinical trials performed by the American College of Surgeons Oncology Group and the NSABP will determine whether immunohistochemistry of the SN is a useful way to refine our ability to predict the risk for recurrence.

Axillary Dissection. Axillary dissection is indicated in patients found to have metastatic disease in the SN or those with contraindications to SN biopsy. The extent of axillary dissection has been defined on the basis of the number of nodes removed or their anatomic location. As discussed in the section on anatomy, the axilla is divided into three anatomic levels. Removal of the level I and II nodes accurately identifies metastases in 98% of patients because isolated metastases to level III are uncommon. A level I and II dissection is standard practice, with the removal of level III being reserved for patients with evidence of gross nodal involvement. Isolated axillary recurrence after a level I and II dissection is uncommon, occurring in fewer than 3% of patients undergoing BCT. With random node removal, a clear relationship is noted between the number of nodes removed and the incidence of axillary failure.

It has become increasingly apparent that axillary dissection is accompanied by significant morbidity. Major complications, such as injury to the axillary vein and motor nerves of the axilla, are rare, but numbness in the distribution of the intercostobrachial nerve occurs in 70% to 80% of patients unless the nerve is preserved, and 20% to 30% of patients have pain and weakness 1 year after surgery.[195] The risk of lymphedema after axillary surgery persists for the patient's lifetime, and the frequency of lymphedema increases as the time from surgery increases. In a review of reports published in the 1990s,[196] the incidence of lymphedema was found to range from 6% to 30%. The incidence of lymphedema is related to the extent of axillary dissection, being higher when level III is removed than when lesser dissections are performed. The radiation of an axillary field after surgical dissection significantly increases the risk for lymphedema. Beyond these two treatment-related factors, there is little agreement regarding which patient characteristics are associated with an increased risk for lymphedema.

Postmastectomy Radiotherapy

The reasons for irradiating the chest wall and draining lymph node basins after mastectomy are twofold: first, to reduce the risk for locoregional recurrence of tumor, and second, to improve survival by eradicating residual locoregional disease that may be resistant to systemic therapy. The risk for local failure after mastectomy is significant and is clearly related to the presence of axillary node metastases, and large (>5 cm) tumor size. Reported locoregional recurrence rates in randomized trials of mastectomy alone range from 4% to 26%.[197] In patients with negative axillary nodes, local failure rates are usually less than 4%. An overview analysis of 40 trials (19,582 women) of RT after both mastectomy and BCT demonstrated that RT reduces the risk for local recurrence by approximately two thirds.[198] A much smaller decrease in breast cancer mortality was also observed (proportional reduction: 9%) but, in older studies, was offset by a significant increase in late cardiac mortality in women who underwent radiation for left-sided cancers.

Recent studies have examined the use of RT in patients receiving adjuvant systemic therapy and have reported an improvement in survival with the addition of RT in node-positive women. The Early Breast Cancer Trialists' Collaborative Group Overview[155] demonstrated a survival benefit for RT when used for patients with both one to three, and four or more, involved axillary nodes. However, the extent of the axillary dissections performed in some of these studies was limited, resulting in a relatively high rate of axillary recurrences than is observed in many studies in the United States. For this reason, debate continues on the need for RT in women with breast cancers less than 5 cm in size and involvement of one to three axillary nodes. In patients with involvement of four or more nodes, RT is recommended routinely, regardless of tumor size.

PROGNOSTIC FACTORS

The clinical course of breast cancer varies from patient to patient. Prognostic factors can be used to predict the natural history of a tumor, usually in terms of disease-free or overall survival. Prognostic factors must be distinguished from predictive factors, which are associated with response to a particular therapy. Clinically, prognostic factors are used to determine which patients have such a favorable outcome after local therapy that adjuvant systemic therapy is not warranted. Although multiple prognostic factors have been described, those in standard use today include axillary lymph node status, tumor size, histologic subtype (discussed in the section on pathology), nuclear or histologic grade, and ER and PR status. Measurements of proliferation, such as S-phase fraction or Ki67, are more controversial but are used in many institutions. Newer factors under study include cyclins, growth factor receptors, plasminogen activators, and inhibitors and markers of cell death (e.g., BCL-2).

The presence of metastases to the axillary nodes is the single most important prognostic factor in breast cancer. Although clinical studies usually divide patients into groups with negative nodes, one to three positive nodes, and four or more positive nodes, the number of involved nodes indicates the prognosis as a continuous variable. Because patients with node-positive disease are uniformly recognized as requiring adjuvant systemic therapy, most studies have concentrated on prognostic factors in patients with node-negative disease. Tumor size is another strong predictor of outcome.[199,200] Only 10% or less of patients with tumors 1 cm or less in size and negative axillary lymph nodes experience recurrence during long-term follow-up.[199]

Tumor grade has also been shown to predict outcome in breast cancer. However, the availability of multiple grading systems, poor reproducibility among different observers unless specific guidelines are provided, and the failure in the past of many pathologists to include a grade on the pathology report have limited its utility as a prognostic factor. Hormone receptor (ER and PR) status has long been recognized as a predictive factor for response to endocrine manipulations (e.g., tamoxifen or oophorectomy). In addition, studies have demonstrated that ER and PR are prognostic factors that are associated with increases in disease-free survival of about 10% at 5 years.[201] ER and PR levels are strongly correlated with histologic grade and patient age, and inversely correlated with measures of proliferation.

Although many prognostic factors have been examined, relatively few have shown clinical utility. In addition, most studies of prognostic factors have examined one or two factors, making it difficult to predict the outcome of patients with a mixture of favorable and unfavorable prognostic features. Drawing on information from the SEER database, the results of individual clinical trials, and published literature, Ravdin et al.[202] developed a novel computerized system called Adjuvant! that projects patient outcomes at 10 years based on a combination of classic clinicopathologic features. Adjuvant! is an evidence-based tool to facilitate clinical decisions based on the risk of recurrence and the potential benefit from adjuvant therapies. This prognostic tool has been independently validated, and observed outcomes were within 2% for most demographic, pathologic, and treatment-defined subgroups.[203]

The advent of genomic technology for the analysis of human tumor samples has added an additional source of information to aid in determining prognosis and clinical decisions. The intrinsic subsets of breast cancer, as first described by Perou et al.[164] (HER2, luminal A, luminal B, and basal-like), are associated with different relapse-free and overall survival rates, with those in the luminal subgroup having the best prognosis and those in the basal cell group having a significantly worse prognosis.[165,166] Efforts to define more limited sets of genes for prognostic purposes include a 70-gene expression profile first described by van de Vijver et al. in 2002.[204] Commonly referred to as the Amsterdam signature, this expression profile was used to classify 295 patients with breast cancer into a good- or poor-prognosis groups, on the basis of distant relapse and overall survival. Interestingly, women with node-positive and node-negative disease were evenly distributed between the two groups, whereas other recognized poor-prognostic factors (e.g., ER negativity, high histologic grade) were clustered in the poor-prognosis group. The 10-year disease-free survival was 94.5% in the good-prognosis group and 50.6% in the poor-prognosis group. This genomic assay, which requires fresh frozen tumor samples, is now commercially available as MammaPrint and is undergoing clinical validation as part of a multicenter trial.

Another gene-based approach is a 21-gene assay using reverse transcription polymerase chain reaction (RT-PCR) on RNA isolated from paraffin-embedded breast tumors (Oncotype DX). This assay provides individualized risk estimates based on measurements of 16 cancer-related genes and five reference genes. It was originally developed for use in ER-positive, node-negative patients by retrospective analysis of available tumor tissue from 447 patients treated with tamoxifen ± chemotherapy in three clinical trials, and the risk of recurrence at 10 years was quantified (recurrence score [RS]).[205] Independent validation was performed on 668 stage I or II, node-negative, hormone receptor–positive patients treated with tamoxifen from the NSABP B-14 trial.[206] In the validation study, the RS was superior to age, tumor size, and grade in predicting prognosis, and when subdivided into low-risk (RS <18), intermediate-risk (RS 18 to 30), and high-risk (RS >31) groups, the 10-year disease-free survival was 69% for the high-risk group and 93% for the low-risk group. Further analysis of patients from the NSABP B-20 trial demonstrated that patients in the high-risk group experienced a significant benefit from the addition of chemotherapy to tamoxifen, whereas those in the intermediate- and low-risk groups derived little to no benefit from chemotherapy. This 21-gene expression assay has been accepted as a clinical practice tool for appropriately selected patients; however, optimal therapy for patients in the intermediate-risk group remains unclear, and this question is being tested in a prospective trial (TAILORx) where Oncotype DX will be used to select hormone receptor–positive, node-negative patients with an intermediate RS for randomization to hormonal therapy or combined hormonal therapy and chemotherapy. Additional studies have shown that the recurrence score is also prognostic and predictive of the benefit of chemotherapy in node-positive, ER-positive patients.

ADJUVANT SYSTEMIC THERAPY

Adjuvant therapy is defined as the use of cytotoxic chemotherapy or endocrine therapy after the local treatment of breast cancer to eliminate clinically occult micrometastases, thereby preventing recurrence and increasing survival. Initially, adjuvant systemic therapy trials were carried out in patients with node-positive disease, who are at the highest risk of relapse. Subsequently, the recognition that breast cancer death occurs in up to 40% of patients with node-negative breast cancer led to trials of systemic treatment in that group.

The Early Breast Cancer Trialists Collaborative Group has conducted meta-analyses of the major prospective, randomized trials of chemotherapy, with the most recent analysis published in 2005 (Table 74.15).[207] After 15 years of follow-up, this analysis confirmed that adjuvant chemotherapy reduces the proportional risk of death equally in patients with node-positive and node-negative disease. There is a small benefit for anthracycline-based treatment (e.g., doxorubicin) versus Cytoxan, methotrexate, and fluorouracil. The benefit of chemotherapy was greatest in younger women, reducing the odds of death by 29% in those under 40 and by 9% in those ages 60 to 69. A separate meta-analysis of 16 randomized trials comparing taxane (paclitaxel or docetaxel)–containing regimens to non–taxane-containing regimens in the adjuvant setting for women with node-positive and high-risk node-negative disease demonstrates a small added benefit with the use of taxanes for this group of patients.[208] The next Oxford Overview by the Early Breast Cancer Trialists Collaborative Group will also examine this question.

TABLE 74.15 **RESULTS**

OVERVIEW ANALYSIS OF CHEMOTHERAPY, 2005

■ TREATMENT	■ REDUCTION IN ANNUAL ODDS: ■ BREAST CANCER RECURRENCE (% ± SE)	■ BREAST CANCER DEATH (% ± SE)
Any multidrug chemotherapy	33 ± 2	17 ± 2
CMF vs. none, age <50	41 ± 4	34 ± 5
CMF vs. none, age 50–69	19 ± 3	10 ± 3
Anthracycline vs. none, age <50	33 ± 8	26 ± 9
Anthracycline vs. none, age 50–69	21 ± 4	17 ± 5
Anthracycline vs. CMF	11 ± 3	16 ± 3

CMF, Cytoxan, methotrexate, 5-fluorouracil; SE, standard error.
Modified from Stearns V, Davidson NE. Adjuvant chemotherapy and chemoendocrine therapy. In: Harris JR, Lippman ME, Morrow M, et al., eds. *Diseases of the Breast,* 3rd ed. Philadelphia, PA: Lippincott Williams & Wilkins; 2004:895.

The advent of trastuzumab (Herceptin) therapy in the adjuvant management of HER2-positive breast cancer in 2005 was a major breakthrough in the application of targeted therapy to breast cancer. Herceptin is a recombinant humanized monoclonal antibody specific for the external region of the HER2 transmembrane tyrosine kinase. To date, results from five studies, which have randomized 11,650 women with early-stage HER2-positive breast cancer to trastuzumab- versus non–trastuzumab-based adjuvant chemotherapy, have demonstrated that the addition of trastuzumab results in a significant improvement in both disease-free (50%) and overall survival (33%).[209–213] The clinical benefit of trastuzumab appears to be limited to tumors with HER2 amplification. Lapatinib, a next-generation tyrosine kinase inhibitor, which reversibly inhibits both the EGFR (HER1) and HER2 kinases, has been approved for use in the metastatic setting. The role of lapatinib in early-stage disease is being explored both in the adjuvant and neoadjuvant settings.

Adjuvant endocrine therapy is standard therapy for both pre- and postmenopausal women with hormone receptor–positive disease. Tamoxifen is a nonsteroidal agent that exhibits site-specific estrogen agonist and antagonist properties.[214] It was the first drug identified in the class now referred to as SERMs. Tamoxifen acts as an antiestrogen in the breast through competitive blockade of the ER. In bones and lipids, tamoxifen acts as an estrogen agonist, preserving bone density and lowering blood cholesterol. Tamoxifen also acts as an agonist in the uterus, increasing the incidence of endometrial carcinoma (see section on management of the high-risk woman). The most recent Early Breast Cancer Trialists Collaborative Group meta-analysis also included more than 48,000 patients in 56 trials of tamoxifen.[207] The use of tamoxifen for 5 years reduces the annual odds of breast cancer recurrence by 41% and the annual odds of death by 34%. Tamoxifen is beneficial in women of all ages, and 5 years of therapy is superior to shorter durations of treatment. These benefits are limited to patients whose tumors express ER, PR, or both.

Tamoxifen was the cornerstone of endocrine therapy for postmenopausal women with hormone receptor–positive disease until the recent reporting of several adjuvant AI trials. AIs function by inhibiting the peripheral conversion of androgens to estrogen, thereby lowering estrogen levels. Adjuvant AIs have been compared to tamoxifen in a number of study designs including sequential strategies[215] (AI given after 2 to 3 years of tamoxifen), upfront strategies[216] (AI instead of tamoxifen), and extended strategies[217] (AI given after 5 years of tamoxifen). All of these strategies have demonstrated significant recurrence-free survival benefits over tamoxifen alone; however, the superiority of any given strategy remains to be determined. One of these agents, anastrozole, was compared with tamoxifen alone or in combination with anastrozole in a randomized trial of more than 9,000 postmenopausal women (ATAC trial).[216] At 9 years' follow-up, the anastrozole-alone arm showed a 4.8% recurrence-free survival benefit over tamoxifen alone; however, no overall survival benefit has been observed. The tolerability profile of anastrozole is somewhat better than that for tamoxifen, with fewer hot flashes, no endometrial effects, and fewer thromboembolic events. However, arthralgias and myalgias are more commonly reported, and the risk of fracture is increased during the 5 years of treatment.

The overview analysis of randomized trials[207] also demonstrates that combined therapy with chemotherapy and tamoxifen is superior to treatment with either agent alone in both premenopausal and postmenopausal women. In postmenopausal women, however, the benefit from the addition of chemotherapy is modest and must be weighed against the toxicity of the treatment in the context of the patient's overall health. General guidelines for the use of adjuvant therapy are shown in Table 74.16, but final treatment decisions are influenced by the individual attitudes of patients toward possibly small benefits and treatment toxicities. The Oncotype DX assay to predict benefit from therapy is being increasingly used in clinical practice for node-negative, hormone receptor–positive tumors (see discussion under prognostic factors).

TABLE 74.16 **TREATMENT**

RECOMMENDATIONS FOR ADJUVANT THERAPY

■ PATIENT GROUP	■ RECOMMENDED TREATMENT
NODE NEGATIVE, LOW RISK	
Tumor <1 cm	No treatment or endocrine therapy if ER+
Special histologic types 1–2 cm, grade 1, ER+	
NODE NEGATIVE, HIGHER RISK	
ER+	Endocrine therapy OR chemotherapy + endocrine therapy
ER–	Chemotherapy
Any HER2+	Add trastuzumab to chemotherapy
NODE POSITIVE	
ER+	
Premenopausal	Chemotherapy + endocrine therapy
Postmenopausal	Chemotherapy + endocrine therapy OR endocrine therapy alone
ER–	Chemotherapy
Any HER2+	Add trastuzumab to chemotherapy

ER+, estrogen receptor positive; ER–, estrogen receptor negative.

SPECIAL PROBLEMS

Breast Cancer in the Elderly

Approximately 50% of breast cancers in the United States are diagnosed in women age 65 and older. Therapy in the elderly should be based on physiologic, not chronologic, age. Mastectomy can be performed safely in the majority of older women, regardless of age, albeit with a slightly higher mortality (0.39% for all ages, and 0.9% for the subgroup of women age 75 and older).[186] Mastectomy is an excellent means of obtaining local control and may minimize outpatient visits, but many older women prefer BCT if offered this option. This is clearly a lesser operative procedure than a mastectomy, and several studies[218] suggest that local failure rates after BCT with RT are lower in women over age 65 than in their younger counterparts. Radiotherapy is generally well tolerated by older women, but daily visits for RT may be difficult for the elderly patient with limited mobility. In elderly women with tumors under 2 cm in size, the benefit of RT may be marginal, and treatment with wide excision of the tumor and endocrine therapy is an option.[219] When omission of breast irradiation in the treatment of an elderly patient with larger tumors is considered, it is useful to remember that the majority of local failures occur in the first 6 postoperative years. Sentinel node biopsy is a low-morbidity staging technique that is particularly well suited to older women. However, if nodal status will not change the recommendation for systemic therapy (e.g., an ER-positive patient not a candidate for chemotherapy), then the routine performance of sentinel node biopsy adds little to patient management.

In the elderly woman with significant comorbid conditions, tamoxifen has been studied as an alternative to conventional surgical treatment. In a review of seven randomized trials, including more than 1,500 women 70 years of age or older, there was no survival advantage for surgical therapy.[220] Although wide resection with free surgical margins was not uniformly required in these studies, significant improvements in local control were noted in the surgically treated woman. The aromatase inhibitor letrozole has been compared with tamoxifen in a randomized trial of neoadjuvant therapy, with letrozole producing a superior local response. Response rates to primary endocrine therapy are high, but 12 months or more are often needed to achieve the best response. With long-term follow-up, the risk for disease progression may be significant. Because surgical treatment is well tolerated by the majority of older women, there is no reason to routinely substitute primary endocrine therapy. For the elderly woman with a limited life span who is a poor operative risk, however, endocrine therapy represents a viable alternative as a primary therapy.

Breast Cancer in Pregnancy

Breast cancer occurring during pregnancy is relatively uncommon when all cases of breast cancer are considered. If only patients with breast cancer in their childbearing years are evaluated, 7% to 14% are found to be pregnant at diagnosis.[221] If pregnant women are used as a denominator, approximately 2.2 breast cancers per 10,000 pregnancies can be anticipated.

The clinical presentation of breast cancer during pregnancy is the same as in the nonpregnant patient, and a palpable mass is the most common symptom. Mammography is not particularly helpful in the evaluation of breast masses in pregnant women because of the increased density of the breast. Ultrasonography is often useful in distinguishing a true mass from the normal nodularity of pregnancy, but ultimately the decision about the need for biopsy should be made on the basis of the physical examination. Delay in the diagnosis of breast cancer during pregnancy remains a major problem, and most of this delay is physician induced. Core needle biopsy or breast biopsy under local anesthesia is safe at any time during pregnancy and should be performed for any suspicious mass.

The options for the local treatment of breast cancer during pregnancy are limited for the woman who wishes to continue her pregnancy. The use of irradiation during any trimester of pregnancy is contraindicated because of the inability to shield the fetus from internal radiation scatter. If breast cancer is diagnosed in the third trimester, lumpectomy can be performed and radiation delayed until after delivery. The effect of longer delays in radiation to allow breast preservation is unknown and may be detrimental. Immediate reconstruction with tissue flaps is also contraindicated during pregnancy because of the risk to the fetus of a more prolonged anesthesia and increased blood loss, in addition to the inability to obtain symmetry with the postpartum breast. Thus, mastectomy remains the mainstay of the surgical therapy of breast cancer during pregnancy. The safety of radiocolloids and blue dyes used for SN biopsy during pregnancy is unclear,[222] so axillary staging is done with an axillary dissection, although newer modeling studies suggest that the dose of radioactivity used for lymphatic mapping is safe during pregnancy. Therapeutic abortion does not appear to play a role in the treatment of nonmetastatic breast carcinoma. A number of small, nonrandomized studies have failed to show a survival advantage associated with termination of pregnancy. Some patients may opt to terminate a pregnancy because of concerns about the long-term prognosis or the risk for fetal damage, but patients should not be advised that this is of therapeutic benefit.

Breast cancer during pregnancy is often thought to be a particularly aggressive disease with a poor prognosis. Much of the poor prognosis, however, seems to be secondary to advanced disease at the time of diagnosis. These women are generally too young to undergo regular mammographic screening before pregnancy, and even in recent series, more than 60% of patients with pregnancy-associated breast cancer had positive axillary nodes. After correction for age and tumor stage, some studies suggest that survival in women treated during pregnancy is similar to that of nonpregnant patients. Population-based studies in Denmark, Sweden, and the United States indicate, however, that survival decreases significantly when breast cancer is diagnosed during pregnancy or shortly thereafter.[223–225]

Chemotherapy can be given to the pregnant patient with breast cancer but is generally delayed until after the first trimester. Fetal malformation occurs in approximately 20% of patients treated during the first trimester, and this risk falls to about 2% for exposure in the second and third trimesters. Some series, however, have reported low birth weight in as many of 40% of infants exposed to chemotherapy during pregnancy, and the long-term effects of chemotherapy exposure on growth, development, and cancer risk are largely unknown.[226] The decision to treat any woman with chemotherapy during pregnancy depends on her risk for relapse and the woman's desire for treatment after a thorough discussion of the risks and benefits, and these decisions must be resolved on a case-by-case basis. When breast cancer is diagnosed in the third trimester, chemotherapy can usually be delayed until fetal maturity, when delivery can be induced. The effects of longer delays on the efficacy of chemotherapy are unknown. Tamoxifen is contraindicated in pregnant women, and women undergoing chemotherapy or endocrine therapy should not breastfeed.

Male Breast Cancer

Cancer of the male breast is an uncommon disease. Risk factors include Klinefelter syndrome, a family history of breast cancer, mutations of the *BRCA2* gene, hepatic disorders, and radiation exposure. With the exception of the gynecomastia in Klinefelter disease, there is no clear association with gynecomastia. The mean age of patients at presentation with male breast cancer is approximately 10 years older than that of women with the disease.[227] The typical presentation is a mass beneath the nipple–areola complex, with retraction or ulceration of the nipple; nipple discharge is less frequent. Approximately 80% of male breast cancers are hormone receptor positive.

The most common local treatment for male breast carcinoma is mastectomy. Radical mastectomy is no longer the standard therapy, and when the tumor is not fixed to the pectoral muscle, a total mastectomy can be performed. With limited muscle involvement, the portion of the pectoralis adherent to the tumor can be excised. When extensive pectoral muscle invasion is present, radical mastectomy may be necessary, although preoperative chemotherapy, as in female breast cancer, is also an option. BCT for male breast carcinoma is rarely feasible because of the small size of the breast and the central location of most tumors. Several small studies in men with breast cancer support the use of SN biopsy if the axilla is clinically negative; axillary dissection is indicated if nodal metastases are documented preoperatively.[228]

The survival rate of men with breast cancer is similar to that in women with disease of the same stage,[229] and axillary nodal status is the major predictor of outcome. The benefit of adjuvant systemic therapy in male breast cancer has not been evaluated in randomized clinical trials, but the natural history and response to therapy of metastatic breast carcinoma in men is similar to that in postmenopausal women, leading to similar practice in the adjuvant setting. Because most male breast cancers contain hormone receptors, the largest adjuvant experience has been gained with hormonal therapy. The administration of tamoxifen to men with stage II or III disease resulted in a 55% 5-year survival, versus 28% in historical controls who received no systemic treatment.[230] Tamoxifen, however, may not be as well tolerated in men as in women, and frequently causes decreased libido. The use of aromatase inhibitors in men with breast cancer is being explored, but an AI alone is not appropriate. Only 80% of circulating estrogen in men is derived from peripheral aromatization, and inhibition of aromatization activates the hypothalamic-pituitary axis negative feedback loop, resulting in increased androgen production.[231] Therefore, complete estrogen suppression is not achieved with an AI alone, and tamoxifen remains the mainstay of endocrine therapy in men. In general, the use of adjuvant systemic therapy should be based on prognosis and hormone receptor status, and the guidelines for postmenopausal women should be followed. Orchiectomy is an option as second-line hormonal manipulation in men with metastatic disease, with an 80% response rate to castration, in men with receptor-positive cancer.[232]

Occult Primary Tumor Presenting with Nodal Metastases

Breast cancer presenting as metastatic disease in the axillary nodes with no evident tumor in the breast is uncommon, accounting for fewer than 1% of cases in most large series. Metastatic adenocarcinoma in axillary nodes may be secondary to a variety of primary cancers, but in women, breast cancer is by far the most common type. In the patient without historical or clinical evidence suggesting a primary tumor at another site, the radiologic evaluation should be confined to breast imaging and a chest radiograph. Examination of the nodal tissue for hormone receptors and HER2 overexpression helps to confirm a breast primary tumor if the tissue is hormone receptor or HER2 positive, but the breast cannot be excluded as the site of the primary tumor if the nodal tissue does not contain receptors.

Magnetic resonance imaging is often successful in identifying a primary tumor when mammography and ultrasound are normal. Buchanan et al.[233] identified a primary tumor in 26 of 55 (47%) patients presenting with axillary adenopathy in the absence of distant disease. In patients presenting with axillary adenopathy and synchronous distant disease, MRI identified the primary tumor in 12 of 14 (86%) patients. Identification of a primary tumor greatly facilitates BCT and, in this circumstance, the patient can be managed in the same way as any stage II cancer.

Historically, when a primary tumor has not been identified, most women with axillary node metastases secondary to a presumed breast cancer have been treated with mastectomy, and a breast carcinoma was identified during the pathologic evaluation in approximately 65% of these cases. In older reports, the size of the occult tumors varied widely, with lesions as large as 6 cm reported. In more recent studies of patients evaluated with modern imaging techniques, large tumors are uncommon, and this has stimulated interest in breast preservation even when the tumor cannot be identified. In the largest reported series from the Institute Curie, 54 patients received whole breast irradiation (median dose 59 Gy). The 5- and 10-year rates of ipsilateral breast recurrence were 7.5% and 20%, respectively, supporting the idea that this is a reasonable approach.[234] In contrast, studies in which the breast was observed without treatment indicate that evident breast cancers develop in close to 50% of patients within 5 years.[235,236] Additional positive axillary nodes are frequent in this circumstance, so axillary dissection should be performed regardless of the method that is selected for managing the breast. The prognosis for patients with occult primary tumors is similar to that for patients with clinically evident tumors matched for the number of involved nodes, and adjuvant systemic therapy should be administered according to established guidelines for patients with node-positive disease.

Locally Recurrent Breast Carcinoma

Local recurrence in the breast after BCT may be a consequence of inappropriate patient selection, poor surgical or radiotherapeutic technique, or tumor biology. When errors in technique and selection are excluded, local recurrence in the first 2 postoperative years is uncommon. From years 2 to 6, local recurrence develops at a constant rate, usually at or adjacent to the site of the original tumor. After year 6, most local recurrence develops in other quadrants of the breast, which suggests that these are new primary tumors rather than true local failures. This idea is supported by the observation that the risk for late recurrence in other quadrants of the breast, approximately 1% annually, is equal to the risk for development of a new contralateral breast carcinoma.

Most recurrences are in the breast parenchyma, with approximately 5% to 10% developing in the skin as diffuse inflammatory-type recurrences.[237] Before further local therapy, an evaluation to exclude metastatic disease is appropriate because concomitant distant metastases are present in 5% to 10% of cases. In the absence of distant metastases, complete mastectomy has been the mainstay of therapy. Five-year relapse-free survival rates range from 60% to 79% after the procedure, and further chest wall recurrences are uncommon. Small experiences with further attempts at breast preservation by using excision alone or repeated irradiation of small areas of the breast after surgical excision have been reported, but larger numbers of patients and longer follow-up periods are needed to determine the role of these therapies. The role of adjuvant systemic therapy in the management of recurrence is not well defined. In patients who have not received prior systemic therapy, we use the same criteria for treatment that are used for patients with newly diagnosed cancer. Treatment decisions for patients who received adjuvant systemic therapy at the time of diagnosis are made on a case-by-case basis.

Local recurrence after mastectomy develops in a different time frame, and the predictors and outcome are different than for local recurrence after BCT. Approximately 75% of cases of local recurrence after mastectomy develop in the first 3 postoperative years, and about half of these are associated with the development of distant metastases at the time of local recurrence or within a few years. The number of axillary nodes containing metastasis is the best predictor of the risk for chest wall recurrence.

An evaluation for distant metastases is an essential part of the workup of local recurrence after mastectomy. Small, localized recurrences are usually excised, but even with complete excision, RT should be administered to the chest wall because it is safe to assume that all the lymphatics are seeded with tumor. The supraclavicular space is usually included in the radiation field because these nodes are the second most frequent site of locoregional recurrence. The value of treating the axillary space and the internal mammary nodes is uncertain because clinical recurrence at these sites is uncommon. The value of additional systemic therapy for patients who have received postoperative adjuvant therapy is also uncertain.

Paget Disease of the Nipple

Paget disease of the nipple comprises 1% to 3% of all breast cancers. It is characterized by eczematoid changes of the nipple (Fig. 74.24), frequently present for 6 months or more before diagnosis, and often accompanied by itching, erythema, and nipple discharge. Paget disease is diagnosed histologically by the presence of large cells with pale cytoplasm and prominent nucleoli (Paget cells) involving the epidermis of the nipple. In 1874, Sir James Paget reported that this condition is invariably followed by cancer of the breast, usually within 1 year of diagnosis.[238] It is now recognized that the majority of women with Paget disease have an associated infiltrating or intraductal carcinoma, which may manifest as a palpable mass or as mammographic findings.

Paget disease has traditionally been treated with mastectomy. The reasons include the need to sacrifice the nipple–areola complex, the fact that subareolar ducts may be diffusely involved with tumor, and the observation that carcinoma may be found at a considerable distance from the nipple. A limited experience with breast-conserving procedures in the management of Paget disease has been described. Because Paget disease is a noninvasive carcinoma involving the nipple that usually is associated with intraductal or invasive carcinoma in the underlying breast parenchyma, the appropriateness of BCT is determined by the extent of the underlying involvement. A detailed mammographic evaluation (including magnification views of the subareolar region) and histologic evaluation with margin assessment are essential components of this assessment. Further evaluation with breast MRI may be considered in patients with Paget disease and a negative mammographic evaluation.[239] For patients with evidence of diffuse involvement or disease at a distance from the nipple, mastectomy remains the standard therapy. In patients with disease localized to the subareolar area or the nipple–areola complex, BCT can be considered. This treatment requires removal of the entire nipple–areola complex and some of the underlying ductal region. In carefully selected patients, local failure rates with this approach appear to be similar to those reported for other breast carcinomas. Radiotherapy has been increasingly employed as part of BCT for Paget disease, but no randomized trials have been performed because of the rarity of the condition.[240] The prognosis in Paget disease is related to the stage of the disease and appears to be similar to that of women with other types of breast carcinoma. If invasive breast cancer is found, adjuvant systemic therapy should be administered according to the same guidelines used for other patients with invasive cancer.

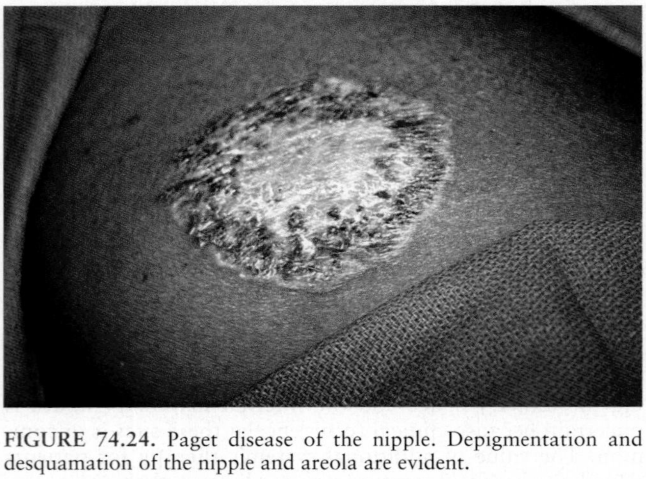

FIGURE 74.24. Paget disease of the nipple. Depigmentation and desquamation of the nipple and areola are evident.

Phyllodes Tumor

The term *phyllodes tumor* denotes a group of lesions of varying malignant potential, ranging from completely benign tumors to fully malignant sarcomas. (The previous name, *cystosarcoma phyllodes*, is now reserved for fully malignant lesions.) A palpable mass is the most common clinical presentation, and rapid growth is often reported. On examination, phyllodes tumors are smooth, rounded, multinodular lesions that may be indistinguishable from fibroadenomas. Skin ulceration can occur with very large tumors, but this is usually caused by pressure necrosis rather than invasion of the skin by malignant cells (see Fig. 74.5). Histologically, phyllodes tumor, like fibroadenoma, is composed of epithelial elements and a connective tissue stroma.

Phyllodes tumors are classified as benign, borderline, or malignant, based on the nature of the tumor margins (pushing or infiltrative) and the presence of cellular atypia, mitotic activity, and overgrowth in the stroma. Which of these criteria is most important is a matter of disagreement, although most experts favor stromal overgrowth. The percentage of phyllodes tumors classified as malignant ranges from 23% to 50%.[241,242] Axillary metastases are reported in fewer than 5% of cases but are a poor prognostic sign when present. Metastases more commonly follow the pattern observed with sarcomas (with the lung as the most common site) and histologically resemble sarcomas. Approximately 20% of benign and malignant phyllodes tumors recur locally if excised with no margin or a margin of a few millimeters of normal breast tissue. Barrio et al.[243] reported that in addition to positive margins, fibroproliferation in the surrounding breast tissue and necrosis were associated with a marked increase in local recurrence rates. A wide excision with a 1- to 2-cm margin of normal breast tissue is appropriate therapy for benign and borderline phyllodes tumors unless they are so large that this is not cosmetically feasible. In the past, many authors advocated mastectomy for the management of malignant phyllodes tumors. Because phyllodes tumors are not multicentric, there is no clear-cut biologic rationale for mastectomy, and the successful treatment of malignant phyllodes tumors with wide excision has been reported.[244] The use of systemic therapy for malignant phyllodes tumors is based on the guidelines for treating sarcomas.

OTHER CANCERS IN THE BREAST

Sarcomas, lymphomas, and melanomas may all present as breast masses and are generally managed as recommended when they develop in other sites. Angiosarcoma is reported to involve the breast more frequently than other sites in the body. The tumors frequently grow rapidly and may be associated with a bluish discoloration of the skin. Bilateral disease is not uncommon. Angiosarcoma has traditionally been treated with mastectomy to clear margins. Axillary metastases are rare, and axillary dissection is not routinely indicated. The prognosis appears to be related to the grade of the lesion. No advantage has been proved for adjuvant RT or chemotherapy. Other sarcomas occur infrequently in the breast. Surgery is the primary therapy, and the decision to perform mastectomy or wide local excision is based on tumor size.

Melanoma arising from the skin of the breast is a more frequent finding in men than women. The diagnosis, treatment, and prognosis of melanoma arising in the breast are the same as for melanoma arising in other parts of the body. Mastectomy is not necessary for treatment of this lesion.

Primary breast lymphomas are rare and account for fewer than 1% of breast malignancies. They are believed to arise from intramammary lymph nodes or periductal and perilobular lymphoid tissue. Bilateral disease is present in as many as 25% of patients. The diagnosis is usually made only after a biopsy, as neither the clinical nor the mammographic appearance of these lesions is diagnostic. Once the diagnosis of lymphoma is established, treatment is with chemotherapy or RT, or both, according to the disease stage and histologic subtype.

LOCALLY ADVANCED BREAST CANCER

13 The designation of *locally advanced breast cancer* includes T3 and T4 tumors, those with extensive regional nodal involvement (N2 or N3), and inflammatory breast cancer (Fig. 74.25).

Historical studies have demonstrated that for inflammatory carcinoma and tumors with evidence of skin involvement, chest wall fixation, or extensive axillary nodal disease, initial surgical therapy is associated with a high rate of locoregional recurrence and very poor 5-year survival, with treatment failure usually occurring within 2 years of diagnosis.[245] For this reason, locally advanced breast cancer is now approached with a combination of chemotherapy, surgery, and RT. Anthracycline-based neoadjuvant chemotherapy results in partial (50% reduction in primary tumor volume) or complete clinical response (no clinically detectable residual tumor) in 60% to 80% of patients.[246] Response rates are further increased by the addition of taxanes to the neoadjuvant protocol, with an increase in clinical complete response (80%–95%), and an increase in pathologic complete response (no residual invasive tumor present on pathologic examination) from 15% to 31%.[247] Newer studies also suggest that the addition of Herceptin in the neoadjuvant setting for HER2-positive tumors may further increase the pathologic complete response rate.[248] Women who experience a pathologic complete response have significantly better long-term survival than those who do not.[249] Although induction chemotherapy is effective in reducing tumor burden and facilitates surgical therapy, no survival advantage has been demonstrated for the use of preoperative, as opposed to postoperative, chemotherapy in randomized trials.

For patients with stage IIIB carcinoma, induction chemotherapy is the standard initial approach. All planned chemotherapy is generally given preoperatively followed by surgery. Depending on the pretreatment stage and extent of residual tumor, chest wall RT may be indicated to reduce the risk of local recurrence. For the patient with stage IIIA carcinoma that is operable by traditional criteria, the initial therapy can be surgery or chemotherapy. If the patient desires breast preservation, chemotherapy can shrink the tumor sufficiently to allow this in some women. If not, mastectomy can be performed, with chemotherapy and RT given postoperatively in the traditional sequence.[250] Women with hormone receptor–positive disease should receive endocrine therapy. Inflammatory breast cancer is a special subtype of locally advanced breast cancer that is characterized by erythema, edema, and peau d'orange, and by diffuse thickening of the breast tissue. This appearance is caused by obstruction of the dermal lymphatics with tumor cells. Inflammatory cancer is always treated with chemotherapy as the initial approach. If all inflammatory skin changes resolve, mastectomy is performed. Radiation to the chest wall is also part of therapy. With modern combined-modality therapy, locoregional control can be maintained in 80% of patients with locally advanced and inflammatory cancer, and 5-year survival rates of 50% to 80% have been reported.[247,249–251] However, 50% of patients eventually die of metastatic disease, which underscores the need for further research in this area.

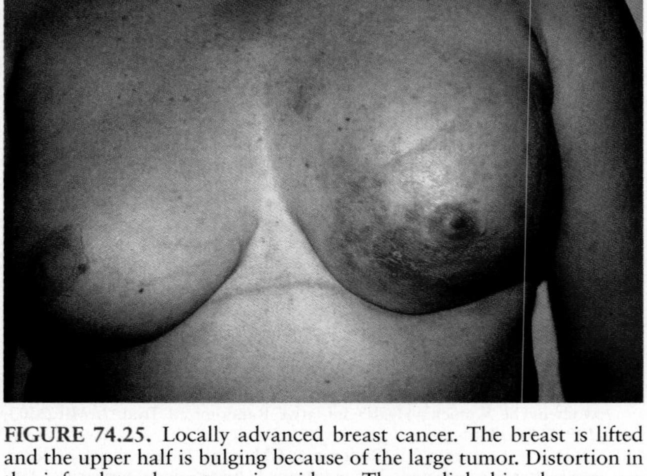

FIGURE 74.25. Locally advanced breast cancer. The breast is lifted and the upper half is bulging because of the large tumor. Distortion in the inferolateral contour is evident. The medial skin changes are caused by dermal tumor satellites.

References

1. Turner-Warwick RT. The lymphatics of the breast. *Br J Surg* 1959;46:574.
2. Cody HS III, Egeli RA, Urban JA. Rotter's node metastases. Therapeutic and prognostic considerations in early breast carcinoma. *Ann Surg* 1984; 199:266–270.
3. Sacre R. Modern thoughts on lymph nodes in breast cancer. *Semin Surg Oncol* 1989;5:118–125.
4. Daniel C, Silberstein, GB. Development of the mammary gland. In: Neville M, Daniel CW, eds. *The Mammary Gland*. New York: Plenum; 1987: 3–10.
5. Russo J, Russo IH. Development of the human breast. In: Russo J, Russo IH, eds. *Encyclopedia of Reproduction*. New York: Academic Press; 1998: 71–76.
6. Dickson RB, Russo J. Biochemical control of breast development. In: Harris JR, Lippman ME, Morrow M, eds. *Diseases of the Breast*. Philadelphia, PA: Lippincott Williams & Wilkins; 2000:303–318.
7. American Joint Committee on Cancer. Breast. In: Edge SB, Byrd DR, Compton CC, et al. *Cancer Staging Manual*, 7th ed. New York: Springer; 2009:345–376.
8. Shapiro S. Screening: assessment of current studies. *Cancer* 1994;74: 231–238.
9. Hendrick RE, Smith RA, Rutledge JH III, et al. Benefit of screening mammography in women aged 40–49: a new meta-analysis of randomized controlled trials. *J Natl Cancer Inst Monogr* 1997;(22):87–92.
10. Morrow M, Bucci C, Rademaker A. Medical contraindications are not a major factor in the underutilization of breast conserving therapy. *J Am Coll Surg* 1998;186:269–274.
11. American College of Radiology. *Breast Imaging Reporting and Data System (BI-RADS)*, 2nd ed. Reston, VA: American College of Radiology; 1995.
12. Sickles EA. Further experience with microfocal spot magnification mammography in the assessment of clustered breast microcalcifications. *Radiology* 1980;137:9–14.
13. Dowlatshahi K, Yaremko, ML, Kluskens LF, et al. Nonpalpable breast lesions: findings of stereotactic needle-core biopsy and fine-needle aspiration cytology. *Radiology* 1991;183:745–750.
14. Parker SH, Burbank F, Jackman RJ, et al. Percutaneous large-core breast biopsy: a multi-institutional study. *Radiology* 1994;193:359–364.
15. Venta L. Image-guided breast biopsy. In: Harris J, Lippman ME, Morrow M, et al. *Diseases of the Breast,* 3rd ed. Philadelphia, PA: Lippincott Williams & Wilkins; 2004:199–219.
16. Margenthaler JA, Duke D, Monsees BS, et al. Correlation between core biopsy and excisional biopsy in breast high-risk lesions. *Am J Surg* 2006; 192(4):534–537.
17. Elsheikh TM, Silverman JF. Follow-up surgical excision is indicated when breast core needle biopsies show atypical lobular hyperplasia or lobular carcinoma in situ: a correlative study of 33 patients with review of the literature. *Am J Surg Pathol* 2005;29(4):534–543.
18. Brem, RF, Lechner, MC, Jackman RJ, et al. Lobular neoplasia at percutaneous breast biopsy: variables associated with carcinoma at surgical excision. *AJR Am J Roentgenol* 2008;190(3):637–641.
19. Liberman L, Sama M, Susnik B, et al. Lobular carcinoma in situ at percutaneous breast biopsy: surgical biopsy findings. *AJR Am J Roentgenol* 1999;173(2):291–299.

20. Philpotts LE, Shaheen NA, Jain KS, et al. Uncommon high-risk lesions of the breast diagnosed at stereotactic core-needle biopsy: clinical importance. *Radiology* 2000;216(3):831–837.
21. Valdes EK, Tartter PI, Genelus-Dominique E, et al. Significance of papillary lesions at percutaneous breast biopsy. *Ann Surg Oncol* 2006;13(4): 480–482.
22. Mercado CL, Hamele-Bena D, Oken SH, et al. Papillary lesions at percutaneous core-needle biopsy. *Radiology* 2006;238(3):801–808.
23. Liberman L, Tornos C, Huzjan R, et al. Is surgical excision warranted after benign, concordant diagnosis of papilloma at percutaneous breast biopsy? *AJR Am J Roentgenol* 2006;186(5):1328–1334.
24. Liberman L, Cohen MA, Dershaw DD, et al. Atypical ductal hyperplasia diagnosed at stereotaxic core biopsy of breast lesions: an indication for surgical biopsy. *AJR Am J Roentgenol* 1995;164:1111–1113.
25. Jackman RJ, Burbank F, Parker SH, et al. Atypical ductal hyperplasia diagnosed at stereotactic breast biopsy: improved reliability with 14-gauge, directional, vacuum-assisted biopsy. *Radiology* 1997;204: 485–488.
26. Abdel-Fatah TM, Powe DG, Hodi Z, et al. High frequency of coexistence of columnar cell lesions, lobular neoplasia, and low grade ductal carcinoma in situ with invasive tubular carcinoma and invasive lobular carcinoma. *Am J Surg Pathol* 2007;31(3):417–426.
27. Brandt SM, Young GQ, Hoda SA. The "Rosen triad": tubular carcinoma, lobular carcinoma in situ, and columnar cell lesions. *Adv Anat Pathol* 2008;15(3):140–146.
28. Golub RM, Bennett CL, Stinson T, et al. Cost minimization study of image-guided core biopsy versus surgical excisional biopsy for women with abnormal mammograms. *J Clin Oncol* 2004;22:2430–2437.
29. Morrow M, Venta L, Stinson T, et al. Prospective comparison of stereotactic core biopsy and surgical excision as diagnostic procedures for breast cancer patients. *Ann Surg* 2001;233:537–541.
30. Mansel RE, Wisbey JR, Hughes LE. Controlled trial of the antigonadotropin danazol in painful nodular benign breast disease. *Lancet* 1982; 1:928–930.
31. Mansel RE, Dogliotti L. European multicentre trial of bromocriptine in cyclical mastalgia. *Lancet* 1990;335:190–193.
32. Fentiman IS, Caleffi M, Hamed H, et al. Dosage and duration of tamoxifen treatment for mastalgia: a controlled trial. *Br J Surg* 1988;75:845–846.
33. Pye JK, Mansel RE, Hughes LE. Clinical experience of drug treatments for mastalgia. *Lancet* 1985;2:373–377.
34. London RS, Sundaram GS, Murphy L, et al. The effect of vitamin E on mammary dysplasia: a double-blind study. *Obstet Gynecol* 1985;65:104–106.
35. Allen SS, Froberg DG. The effect of decreased caffeine consumption on benign proliferative breast disease: a randomized clinical trial. *Surgery* 1987;101:720–730.
36. Smallwood J, Ah-Kye D, Taylor I. Vitamin B_6 in the treatment of premenstrual mastalgia. *Br J Clin Pract* 1986;40:532–533.
37. Catania S, Zurrida S, Veronesi P, et al. Mondor's disease and breast cancer. *Cancer* 1992;69:2267–2270.
38. Seltzer MH, Perloff LJ, Kelley RI, et al. The significance of age in patients with nipple discharge. *Surg Gynecol Obstet* 1970;131:519–522.
39. King TA, Carter KM, Bolton JS, et al. A simple approach to nipple discharge. *Am Surg* 2000;66:960–965.
40. Simmons R, Adamovich T, Brennan M, et al. Nonsurgical evaluation of pathologic nipple discharge. *Ann Surg Oncol* 2003;10:113–116.
41. Cabioglu N, Hunt KK, Singletary SE, et al. Surgical decision making and factors determining a diagnosis of breast carcinoma in women presenting with nipple discharge. *J Am Coll Surg* 2003;196:354–364.
42. Dawes LG, Bowen C, Venta LA, et al. Ductography for nipple discharge: no replacement for ductal excision. *Surgery* 1998;124:685–691.
43. Dietz JR, Crowe JP, Grundfest S, et al. Directed duct excision by using mammary ductoscopy in patients with pathologic nipple discharge. *Surgery* 2002;132:582–587.
44. Schnitt S, Connelly J. Pathology of benign breast disorders. In: Harris J, Lippman ME, Morrow M, eds. *Diseases of the Breast,* 2nd ed. Philadelphia, PA: Lippincott Williams & Wilkins; 2000:75–94.
45. Aitken RJ, Hood J, Going JJ, et al. Bacteriology of mammary duct ectasia. *Br J Surg* 1988;75:1040–1041.
46. Morrow M, Wong S, Venta L. The evaluation of breast masses in women younger than forty years of age. *Surgery* 1998;124:634–640.
47. Cowen PN, Benson EA. Cytological study of fluid from breast cysts. *Br J Surg* 1979;66:209–211.
48. Wilkinson S, Anderson TJ, Rifkind E, et al. Fibroadenoma of the breast: a follow-up of conservative management. *Br J Surg* 1989;76:390–391.
49. Dupont WD, Page DL, Parl FF, et al. Long-term risk of breast cancer in women with fibroadenoma. *N Engl J Med* 1994;331:10–15.
50. Dupont WD, Parl FF, Hartmann WH, et al. Breast cancer risk associated with proliferative breast disease and atypical hyperplasia. *Cancer* 1993;71: 1258–1265.
51. London SJ, Connolly JL, Schnitt SJ, et al. A prospective study of benign breast disease and the risk of breast cancer. *JAMA* 1992;267:941–944.
52. McDivitt RW, Stevens JA, Lee NC, et al. Histologic types of benign breast disease and the risk for breast cancer. The Cancer and Steroid Hormone Study Group. *Cancer* 1992;69:1408–1414.
53. Shelty MK, Shah YP, Sharman RS. Prospective evaluation of the value of combined mammographic and sonographic assessment in patients with palpable abnormalities of the breast. *J Ultrasound Med* 2003;22: 263–268.
54. Morrow M, Schmidt RA, Bucci C. Breast conservation for mammographically occult carcinoma. *Ann Surg* 1998;227:502–506.
55. Lister D, Evans AJ, Burrell HC, et al. The accuracy of breast ultrasound in the evaluation of clinically benign discrete, symptomatic breast lumps. *Clin Radiol* 1998;53:490–492.
56. Yang WT, Lam WW, Cheung H, et al. Sonographic, magnetic resonance imaging, and mammographic assessments of preoperative size of breast cancer. *J Ultrasound Med* 1997;16:791–797.
57. Bluemke DA, Gatsonis CA, Chen MH, et al. Magnetic resonance imaging of the breast prior to biopsy. *JAMA* 2004;292(22):2735–2742.
58. Houssami N, Ciatto S, Macaskill P, et al. Accuracy and surgical impact of magnetic resonance imaging in breast cancer staging: systematic review and meta-analysis in detection of multifocal and multicentric cancer. *J Clin Oncol* 2008;26(19):3248–3258.
59. Solin LJ, Orel SG, Hwang WT, et al. Relationship of breast magnetic resonance imaging to outcome after breast-conservation treatment with radiation for women with early-stage invasive breast carcinoma or ductal carcinoma in situ. *J Clin Oncol* 2008;26(3):386–391.
60. Bleicher RJ, Ciocca RM, Egleston BL, et al. The influence of routine pretreatment MRI on time to treatment, mastectomy rate and positive margins [abstract 227]. *ASCO Breast* 2008.
61. Giard RW, Hermans J. The value of aspiration cytologic examination of the breast. A statistical review of the medical literature. *Cancer* 1992;69: 2104–2110.
62. Shabot MM, Goldberg IM, Schick P, et al. Aspiration cytology is superior to Tru-Cut needle biopsy in establishing the diagnosis of clinically suspicious breast masses. *Ann Surg* 1982;196:122–126.
63. Layfield LJ, Glasgow BJ, Cramer H. Fine-needle aspiration in the management of breast masses. *Pathol Annu* 1989;24(Pt 2):23–62.
64. Greenberg R, Skornick Y, Kaplan O. Management of breast fibroadenomas. *J Gen Intern Med* 1998;13:640–645.
65. Bell DA, Hajdu SI, Urban JA, et al. Role of aspiration cytology in the diagnosis and management of mammary lesions in office practice. *Cancer* 1983;51:1182–1189.
66. Donegan WL. Evaluation of a palpable breast mass. *N Engl J Med* 1992; 327:937–942.
67. Dixon JM. Repeated aspiration of breast abscesses in lactating women. *Br Med J* 1988;297:1517–1518.
68. Bundred NJ, Dover MS, Aluwihare N, et al. Smoking and periductal mastitis. *Br Med J* 1993;307:772–773.
69. Meguid MM, Oler A, Numann PJ, et al. Pathogenesis-based treatment of recurring subareolar breast abscesses. *Surgery* 1995;118:775–782.
70. American Cancer Society. *Breast Cancer Facts & Figures 2007–2008.* Atlanta, GA: American Cancer Society Inc.; 2007.
71. National Center for Health Statistics. *SEER Cancer Statistics Review, 1973–1995.* Bethesda, MD: National Cancer Institute; 1998.
72. Slattery ML, Kerber RA. A comprehensive evaluation of family history and breast cancer risk. The Utah Population Database. *JAMA* 1993;270: 1563–1568.
73. Claus EB, Risch NJ, Thompson WD. Age at onset as an indicator of familial risk of breast cancer. *Am J Epidemiol* 1990;131:961–972.
74. Struewing JP, Hartge P, Wacholder S, et al. The risk of cancer associated with specific mutations of BRCA1 and BRCA2 among Ashkenazi Jews. *N Engl J Med* 1997;336:1401–1408.
75. King MC, Marks JH, Mandell JB. Breast and ovarian cancer risks due to inherited mutations in BRCA1 and BRCA2. *Science* 2003;302: 643–646.
76. Kirchhoff T, Kauff ND, Mitra N, et al. BRCA mutations and risk of prostate cancer in Ashkenazi Jews. *Clin Cancer Res* 2004;10:2918–2921.
77. Hahn SA, Greenhalf B, Ellis I, et al. BRCA2 germline mutations in familial pancreatic carcinoma. *J Natl Cancer Inst* 2003;95:214–221.
78. Shattuck-Eidens D, Oliphant A, McClure M, et al. BRCA1 sequence analysis in women at high risk for susceptibility mutations. Risk factor analysis and implications for genetic testing. *JAMA* 1997;278: 1242–1250.
79. Euhus DM, Smith KC, Robinson L, et al. Pretest prediction of BRCA1 or BRCA2 mutation by risk counselors and the computer model BRCAPRO. *J Natl Cancer Inst* 2002;94:844–851.
80. Hisada M, Garber JE, Fung CY, et al. Multiple primary cancers in families with Li-Fraumeni syndrome. *J Natl Cancer Inst* 1998;90:606–611.
81. Colditz GA. Epidemiology of breast cancer. Findings from the nurses' health study. *Cancer* 1993;71:1480–1489.
82. Newcomb PA, Storer BE, Longnecker MP, et al. Lactation and a reduced risk of premenopausal breast cancer. *N Engl J Med* 1994;330:81–87.
83. Collaborative Group on Hormonal Factors in Breast Cancer. Breast cancer and hormonal contraceptives: collaborative reanalysis of individual data on 53,297 women with breast cancer and 100,239 women without breast cancer from 54 epidemiological studies. *Lancet* 1996;347: 1713–1727.
84. Chlebowski RT, Hendrix SL, Langer RD, et al. Influence of estrogen plus progestin on breast cancer and mammography in healthy postmenopausal women: the Women's Health Initiative Randomized Trial. *JAMA* 2003; 289:3243–3253.
85. Holmberg L, Iversen OE, Rudenstam CM, et al. Increased risk of recurrence after hormone replacement therapy in breast cancer survivors. *J Natl Cancer Inst* 2008;100:475–482.
86. Hancock SL, Tucker MA, Hoppe RT. Breast cancer after treatment of Hodgkin's disease. *J Natl Cancer Inst* 1993;85:25–31.

87. Hunter DJ, Spiegelman D, Adami HO, et al. Cohort studies of fat intake and the risk of breast cancer—a pooled analysis. *N Engl J Med* 1996;334: 356–361.
88. Willett W, Hunter, DJ, Stampfer, MJ, et al. Dietary fat and fiber in relation to risk of breast cancer: an 8 year follow-up. *JAMA* 1992;268:2037–2044.
89. Cho E. Red meat intake and risk of breast cancer among premenopausal women. *Arch Intern Med* 2006;166(20):2253–2259.
90. Lin J. Intakes of calcium and vitamin d and breast cancer risk in women. *Arch Intern Med* 2007;167(10):1050–1059.
91. Ganmaa D. Coffee, tea, caffeine and risk of breast cancer: a 22-year follow-up. *Int J Cancer* 2008;122(9):2071–2076.
92. Verheus M. Plasma phytoestrogens and subsequent breast cancer risk. *J Clin Oncol* 2007;25(6):648–655.
93. Hamajima N, Hirose K, Tajima K, et al. Alcohol, tobacco and breast cancer—collaborative reanalysis of individual data from 53 epidemiological studies, including 58,515 women with breast cancer and 95,067 women without the disease. *Br J Cancer* 2002;87:1234–1245.
94. McTiernan A, Kooperberg C, White E, et al.; Women's Health Initiative Cohort Study. Recreational physical activity and the risk of breast cancer in postmenopausal women: the Women's Health Initiative Cohort Study. *JAMA* 2003;290(10):1331–1336.
95. Patel AV, Callel EE, Bernstein L, et al. Recreational physical activity and risk of postmenopausal breast cancer in a large cohort of US women. *Cancer Causes Control* 2003;14(6):519–529.
96. Dupont WD, Page DL. Risk factors for breast cancer in women with proliferative breast disease. *N Engl J Med* 1985;312:146–151.
97. Foote FW, Stewart FW. Lobular carcinoma in situ. *Am J Pathol* 1941;17(4): 491–495.
98. Haagensen CD. Lobular neoplasia (lobular carcinoma in situ). In: Haagensen CD, Bodian C, Haagensen DE, eds. *Breast Carcinoma: Risk and Detection.* Philadelphia, PA: WB Saunders; 1981:238–291.
99. Rosen P, Kosloff, C, Lieberman PH, et al. Lobular carcinoma in situ of the breast: detailed analysis of 99 patients with average follow-up of 24 years. *Am J Surg Pathol* 1978;2:225–251.
100. Andersen JA. Lobular carcinoma in situ of the breast. An approach to rational treatment. *Cancer* 1977;39:2597–602.
101. Page DL, Kidd TE Jr, Dupont WD, et al. Lobular neoplasia of the breast: higher risk for subsequent invasive cancer predicted by more extensive disease. *Hum Pathol* 1991;22:1232–1239.
102. Salvadori B, Bartoli C, Zurrida S, et al. Risk of invasive cancer in women with lobular carcinoma in situ of the breast. *Eur J Cancer* 1991;27: 35–37.
103. Ottesen GL, Graversen HP, Blichert-Toft M, et al. Lobular carcinoma in situ of the female breast. Short-term results of a prospective nationwide study. The Danish Breast Cancer Cooperative Group. *Am J Surg Pathol* 1993;17: 14–21.
104. Bodian CA, Perzin KH, Lattes R. Lobular neoplasia. Long term risk of breast cancer and relation to other factors. *Cancer* 1996;78:1024–1034.
105. Fisher B, Costantino JP, Wickerham DL, et al. Tamoxifen for prevention of breast cancer: report of the National Surgical Adjuvant Breast and Bowel Project P-1 Study. *J Natl Cancer Inst* 1998;90:1371–1388.
106. Page DL, Schuyler PA, Dupont WD, et al. A typical lobular hyperplasia as a unilateral predictor of breast cancer risk: a retrospective cohort study. *Lancet* 2003;361(9352):125–129.
107. Lakhani SR, Audresch W, Cleton-Jenson JM, et al. The management of lobular carcinoma in situ (LCIS). Is LCIS the same as ductal carcinoma in situ (DCIS)? *Eur J Cancer* 2006;42(14):2205–2211.
108. Fisher ER, Land SR, Fisher B, et al. Pathologic findings from the National Surgical Adjuvant Breast and Bowel Project: twelve-year observations concerning lobular carcinoma in situ. *Cancer* 2004;100:238.
109. Morandi L, Marucci G, Foschini MP, et al. Genetic similarities and differences between lobular in situ neoplasia (LN) and invasive lobular carcinoma of the breast. *Virchows Arch* 2006;449(1):14–23.
110. Aulmann S, Penzel R, Longerich T, et al. Clonality of lobular carcinoma in situ (LCIS) and metachronous invasive breast cancer. *Breast Cancer Res Treat* 2008;107:331–335.
111. Abner AL, Connolly JL, Recht A, et al. The relation between the presence and extent of lobular carcinoma in situ and the risk of local recurrence for patients with infiltrating carcinoma of the breast treated with conservative surgery and radiation therapy. *Cancer* 2000;88(5):1072–1077.
112. Ben-David MA, Kleer CG, Paramagul C, et al. Is lobular carcinoma in situ as a component of breast carcinoma a risk factor for local failure after breast-conserving therapy? Results of a matched pair analysis. *Cancer* 2006;106(1):28–34.
113. Jolly S, Kestin LL, Goldstein NS, et al. The impact of lobular carcinoma in situ in association with invasive breast cancer on the rate of local recurrence in patients with early-stage breast cancer treated with breast-conserving therapy. *Int J Radiat Oncol Biol Phys* 2006;66(2):365–371.
114. Moran M, Haffty BG. Lobular carcinoma in situ as a component of breast cancer: the long-term outcome in patients treated with breast-conservation therapy. *Int J Radiat Oncol Biol Phys* 1998;40(2):353–358.
115. Sasson AR, Fowble B, Hanlon AL, et al. Lobular carcinoma in situ increases the risk of local recurrence in selected patients with stages I and II breast carcinoma treated with conservative surgery and radiation. *Cancer* 2001;91(10):1862–1869.
116. Ciocca RM, Li T, Freedman GM, et al. Presence of lobular carcinoma in situ does not increase local recurrence in patients treated with breast-conserving therapy. *Ann Surg Oncol* 2008;15(8):2263–2271.
117. Middleton LP, Palacios DM, Byrant DR, et al. Pleomorphic lobular carcinoma: morphology, immunohistochemistry, and molecular analysis. *Am J Surg Pathol* 2000;24(12):1650–1656.
118. Gail MH, Brinton LA, Byar DP, et al. Projecting individualized probabilities of developing breast cancer for white females who are being examined annually. *J Natl Cancer Inst* 1989;81:1879–1886.
119. Claus EB, Risch N, Thompson WD. Autosomal dominant inheritance of early-onset breast cancer. Implications for risk prediction. *Cancer* 1994; 73:643–651.
120. Lehman CD. Role of MRI in screening women at high risk for breast cancer. *J Magn Reson Imaging* 2006;24(5):964–970.
121. Saslow D, Boetes C, Burke W, et al.; American Cancer Society Breast Cancer Advisory Group. American Cancer Society guidelines for breast screening with MRI as an adjunct to mammography. *CA Cancer J Clin* 2007; 57(2): 75–89.
122. Cuzick J, Baum M. Tamoxifen and contralateral breast cancer. *Lancet* 1985;2:282.
123. Fisher B, Costantino J, Redmond C, et al. A randomized clinical trial evaluating tamoxifen in the treatment of patients with node negative breast cancer who have estrogen receptor positive tumors. *N Engl J Med* 1989;320:479–484.
124. Fisher B, Costantino JP, Wickerham DL, et al. Tamoxifen for the prevention of breast cancer: current status of the National Surgical Adjuvant Breast and Bowel Project P-1 study. *J Natl Cancer Inst* 2005;97(22): 1652–1662.
125. Cuzick J, Powles T, Veronesi U, et al. Overview of the main outcomes in breast-cancer prevention trials. *Lancet* 2003;361(9354):296–300.
126. Cummings SR, Eckert S, Krueger KA, et al. The effect of raloxifene on risk of breast cancer in postmenopausal women: results from the MORE randomized trial. Multiple outcomes of raloxifene evaluation. *JAMA* 1999; 281:2189–2197.
127. Vogel VG, Costantino JP, Wickerham DL, et al.; National Surgical Adjuvant Breast and Bowel Project (NSABP). Effects of tamoxifen vs raloxifene on the risk of developing invasive breast cancer and other disease outcomes: the NSABP Study of Tamoxifen and Raloxifene (STAR) P-2 trial. *JAMA* 2006;295(23):2727–2741.
128. Land SR, Wickerham DL, Costantino JP, et al. Patient-reported symptoms and quality of life during treatment with tamoxifen or raloxifene for breast cancer prevention: the NSABP Study of Tamoxifen and Raloxifene (STAR) P-2 trial. *JAMA* 2006;295(23):2742–2751.
129. Coombes RC, Hall E, Gibson LJ, et al.; Intergroup Exemestane Study. A randomized trial of exemestane after two to three years of tamoxifen therapy in postmenopausal women with primary breast cancer. *N Engl J Med* 2004;350(11):1081–1092.
130. Goss PE, Ingle JN, Martino S, et al. A randomized trial of letrozole in postmenopausal women after five years of tamoxifen therapy for early-stage breast cancer. *N Engl J Med* 2003;349(19):1793–1802.
131. Baum M, Budzar AU, Cuzick J, et al.; ATAC Trialists' Group. Anastrozole alone or in combination with tamoxifen versus tamoxifen alone for adjuvant treatment of postmenopausal women with early breast cancer: first results of the ATAC randomised trial. *Lancet* 2002;359(9324): 2131–2139.
132. Hartmann LC, Schaid DJ, Woods JE, et al. Efficacy of bilateral prophylactic mastectomy in women with a family history of breast cancer. *N Engl J Med* 1999;340:77–84.
133. Rebbeck TR, Levin AM, Eisen A. Breast cancer risk after bilateral prophylactic oophorectomy in BRCA1 mutation carriers. *J Natl Cancer Inst* 1999;91(17):1475–1479.
134. Rebbeck TR, Lynch HT, Neuhausen SL, et al. Prevention and Observation of Surgical End Points Study Group. Prophylactic oophorectomy in carriers of BRCA1 or BRCA2 mutations. *N Engl J Med* 2002;346(21): 1616–1622.
135. Ries LAG, Melbert D, Krapcho M, et al. *Seer Cancer Statistics Review, 1975–2004.* Bethesda, MD: National Cancer Institute; 2007. Based on November 2006 SEER data submission, posted to the SEER website.
136. Houssami N, Ciatto S, Ellis I, et al. Underestimation of malignancy of breast core-needle biopsy: concepts and precise overall and category-specific estimates. *Cancer* 2007;109(3):487–495.
137. Boyages J, Delaney G, Taylor R. Predictors of local recurrence after treatment of ductal carcinoma in situ: a meta-analysis. *Cancer* 1999;85(3): 616–628.
138. Lee LA, Silverstein MJ, Chung CT, et al. Breast cancer-specific mortality after invasive local recurrence in patients with ductal carcinoma-in-situ of the breast. *Am J Surg* 2006;192(4):416–419.
139. Solin LJ, Kurtz J, Fourquet A, et al. Fifteen-year results of breast-conserving surgery and definitive breast irradiation for the treatment of ductal carcinoma in situ of the breast. *J Clin Oncol* 1996;14:754–763.
140. Fisher B, Dignam J, Wolmark N, et al. Lumpectomy and radiation therapy for the treatment of intraductal breast cancer: findings from National Surgical Adjuvant Breast and Bowel Project B-17. *J Clin Oncol* 1998;16: 441–452.
141. Fisher B, Land S, Mamounas E, et al. Prevention of invasive breast cancer in women with ductal carcinoma in situ: an update of the national surgical adjuvant breast and bowel project experience. *Semin Oncol* 2001;28(4): 400–418.
142. Bijker N, Meijnen P, Peterse JL, et al.; EORTC Breast Cancer Cooperative Group, EORTC Radiotherapy Group. Breast-conserving treatment with or without radiotherapy in ductal carcinoma-in-situ: ten-year results of European Organisation for Research and Treatment of Cancer randomized phase III trial 10853—a study by the EORTC Breast Cancer Cooperative Group and EORTC Radiotherapy Group. *J Clin Oncol* 2006;24(21): 3381–3387.
143. UK Coordinating Committee on Cancer Research Ductal Carcinoma in Situ Working Party. Radiotherapy and tamoxifen in women with

completely excised ductal carcinoma in situ of the breast in the UK, Australia, and New Zealand: randomized controlled trial. *Lancet* 2003;362: 95–102.
144. Holmberg L, Garmo H, Granstrand B, et al. Absolute risk reductions for local recurrence after postoperative radiotherapy after sector resection for ductal carcinoma in situ of the breast. *J Clin Oncol* 2008;26(8): 1247–1252.
145. Fisher ER, Dignam J, Tan-Chiu E, et al. Pathologic findings from the National Surgical Adjuvant Breast Project (NSABP) eight-year update of protocol B-17: intraductal carcinoma. *Cancer* 1999;86:429–438.
146. Silverstein MJ, Lagios MD, Groshen S, et al. The influence of margin width on local control of ductal carcinoma in situ of the breast. *N Engl J Med* 1999;340:1455–1461.
147. Wong JS, Carolyn M, Kaelin CM, et al. Prospective study of wide excision alone for ductal carcinoma in situ (DCIS) of the breast. *J Clin Oncol* 2006;24:1031–1036.
148. Holland R, Hendriks JH, Vebeek AL, et al. Extent, distribution, and mammographic/histological correlations of breast ductal carcinoma in situ. *Lancet* 1990;335:519–522.
149. Fisher B, Dignam J, Wolmark N, et al. Tamoxifen in treatment of intraductal breast cancer: National Surgical Adjuvant Breast and Bowel Project B-24 randomised controlled trial. *Lancet* 1999;353:1993–2000.
150. Julian TB, Land SR, Fourchotte V, et al. Is sentinel node biopsy necessary in conservatively treated DCIS? *Ann Surg Oncol* 2007;14(8): 2202–2208.
151. Bloom HJ, Richardson WW, Harries EJ. Natural history of untreated breast cancer (1805–1933). Comparison of untreated and treated cases according to histological grade of malignancy. *Br Med J* 1962;5299: 213–221.
152. Halsted W. The results of radical operations for the cure of carcinoma of the breast. *Ann Surg* 1907;66:1–19.
153. Fisher B. Laboratory and clinical research in breast cancer—a personal adventure: the David A. Karnofsky memorial lecture. *Cancer Res* 1980;40: 3863–3874.
154. Hellman S. Karnofsky Memorial Lecture. Natural history of small breast cancers. *J Clin Oncol* 1994;12:2229–2234.
155. Clarke M, Collins R, Darby S, et al.; Early Breast Cancer Trialists' Collaborative Group (EBCTCG). Effects of radiotherapy and of differences in the extent of surgery for early breast cancer on local recurrence and 15-year survival: an overview of the randomised trials. *Lancet* 2005;366(9503): 2087–2106.
156. Broet P, de la Rochefordiere A, Scholl SM, et al. Contralateral breast cancer: annual incidence and risk parameters. *J Clin Oncol* 1995;13: 1578–1583.
157. Elston CW, Ellis IO. Pathological prognostic factors in breast cancer. I. The value of histological grade in breast cancer: experience from a large study with long-term follow-up. *Histopathology* 1991;19:403–410.
158. Sotiriou C, Wirapati P, Loi S, et al. Gene expression profiling in breast cancer: understanding the molecular basis of histologic grade to improve prognosis. *J Natl Cancer Inst* 2006;98(4):262–272.
159. Jensen C, Jacobsen HI. Basic guides to the mechanism of estrogen action. *Recent Prog Horm Res* 1962;18:387.
160. McGuire W, Carbone P, Sears M, et al. Estrogen receptors in human breast cancer: an overview. In: McGuire W, Vollmer E, Carbone P, eds. *Estrogen Receptors in Human Breast Cancer*. New York: Raven Press; 1975:1–7.
161. Kuiper G, Enmark E, Pelto-Huikko M, et al. Cloning of a novel receptor expressed in rat prostate and ovary. *Proc Natl Acad Sci U S A* 1996;93: 5925–5930.
162. Burstein HJ. The distinctive nature of HER2-positive breast cancers. *N Engl J Med* 2005;353(16):1652–1654.
163. Carlson RW, Moench SJ, Hammond ME, et al. HER 2 testing in breast cancer: NCCN task force report and recommendations. *J Natl Compr Canc Netw* 2006;4(suppl 3):S1–S22.
164. Perou CM, Sorlie T, Eisen MB, et al. Molecular portraits of human breast tumours. *Nature* 2000;406:747–752.
165. Sørlie T, Wang Y, Xiao C, et al. Distinct molecular mechanisms underlying clinically relevant subtypes of breast cancer: gene expression analyses across three different platforms. *BMC Genomics* 2006;7:127.
166. Sotiriou C, Neo SY, McShane LM, et al. Breast cancer classification and prognosis based on gene expression profiles from a population-based study. *Proc Natl Acad Sci U S A* 2003;100(18):10393–10398.
167. Yu K, Lee CH, Tan PH, Tan P. Conservation of breast cancer molecular subtypes and transcriptional patterns of tumor progression across distinct ethnic populations. *Clin Cancer Res* 2004;10(16):5508–5517.
168. Carey LA, Perou CM, Livasy CA, et al. Race, breast cancer subtypes, and survival in the Carolina Breast Cancer Study. *JAMA* 2006;295(21): 2492–2502.
169. Myers RE, Johnston M, Pritchard K, et al. Baseline staging tests in primary breast cancer: a practice guideline. *CMAJ* 2001;164:1439–1444.
170. Arriagada R, Le MG, Rochard F, et al. Conservative treatment versus mastectomy in early breast cancer: patterns of failure with 15 years of follow-up data. Institut Gustave-Roussy Breast Cancer Group. *J Clin Oncol* 1996; 14:1558–1564.
171. Veronesi U, Cascinelli N, Mariani L, et al. Twenty-year follow-up of a randomized study comparing breast-conserving surgery with radical mastectomy for early breast cancer. *N Engl J Med* 2002;347: 1227–1232.
172. Fisher B, Anderson S, Bryant J, et al. Twenty-year follow-up of a randomized trial comparing total mastectomy, lumpectomy, and lumpectomy plus irradiation for the treatment of invasive breast cancer. *N Engl J Med* 2002;347:1233–1241.
173. Poggi MM, Danforth DN, Sciuto LC, et al. Eighteen-year results in the treatment of early breast carcinoma with mastectomy versus breast conservation therapy: the National Cancer Institute Randomized Trial. *Cancer* 2003;98:697–702.
174. van Dongen JA, Voogd AC, Fentiman IS, et al. Long-term results of a randomized trial comparing breast-conserving therapy with mastectomy: European Organization for Research and Treatment of Cancer 10801 trial. *J Natl Cancer Inst* 2000;92:1143–1150.
175. Blichert-Toft M, Rose C, Andersen JA, et al. Danish randomized trial comparing breast conservation therapy with mastectomy: six years of life-table analysis. Danish Breast Cancer Cooperative Group. *J Natl Cancer Inst Monogr* 1992;(11):19–25.
176. Morrow M, Harris JR. Practice guideline for breast conservation therapy in the management of invasive breast carcinoma. *J Am Coll Surg* 2007; 205:362–376.
177. Bonadonna G, Veronesi U, Brambilla C, et al. Primary chemotherapy to avoid mastectomy in tumors with diameters of three centimeters or more. *J Natl Cancer Inst* 1990;82:1539–1545.
178. Fisher B, Bryant J, Wolmark N, et al. Effect of preoperative chemotherapy on the outcome of women with operable breast cancer. *J Clin Oncol* 1998;16:2672–2685.
179. Bear H, Anderson, S, Brown A, et al. The effect on tumor response of adding sequential preoperative docetaxel to preoperative doxorubicin and cyclophosphamide: preliminary results from National Surgical Adjuvant Breast and Bowel Project B-27. *J Clin Oncol* 2003;22: 4165–4174.
180. Katz SJ, Lantz PM, Janz NK, et al. Patient involvement in surgery treatment decisions for breast cancer. *J Clin Oncol* 2005;23(24):5526–5533.
181. Schmidt-Ullrich RK, Wazer DE, DiPetrillo T, et al. Breast conservation therapy for early stage breast carcinoma with outstanding 10-year locoregional control rates: a case for aggressive therapy to the tumor bearing quadrant. *Int J Radiat Oncol Biol Phys* 1993;27:545–552.
182. Morrow M, Schmidt R, Hassett C. Patient selection for breast conservation therapy with magnification mammography. *Surgery* 1995;118: 621–626.
183. Morrow M, Harris JR. Local management of invasive cancer: breast. In: Harris J, Lippman ME, Morrow M, et al. *Diseases of the Breast*, 3rd ed. Philadelphia, PA: Lippincott Williams & Wilkins; 2004:719–744.
184. Haffty BG, Harrold E, Khan AJ, et al. Outcome of conservatively managed early-onset breast cancer by BRCA1/2 status. *Lancet* 2002;359: 1471–1477.
185. Schnitt SJ, Abner A, Gelman R, et al. The relationship between microscopic margins of resection and the risk of local recurrence in patients with breast cancer treated with breast-conserving surgery and radiation therapy. *Cancer* 1994;74:1746–1751.
186. Schneiderman M, Axtell LM. Deaths among female patients with carcinoma of the breast treated by surgical procedure alone. *Surg Gynecol Obstet* 1979;148:193–196.
187. Platt R, Zucker JR, Zaleznik DF, et al. Prophylaxis against wound infection following herniorrhaphy or breast surgery. *J Infect Dis* 1992;166: 556–560.
188. Chagpar AB. Skin-sparing and nipple-sparing mastectomy: preoperative, intraoperative, and postoperative considerations. *Am Surg* 2004;70: 425–432.
189. Cordiero P, Pusic A, Disa JJ, et al. Irradiation after immediate tissue expander/implant breast reconstruction. *Plast Reconstr Surg* 2004;113: 877–881.
190. Giuliano AE, Kirgan DM, Guenther JM, et al. Lymphatic mapping and sentinel lymphadenectomy for breast cancer. *Ann Surg* 1994;220: 391–398.
191. Posther KE, McCall LM, Blumencranz PW, et al. Sentinel node skills verification and surgeon performance: data from a multicenter clinical trial for early-stage breast cancer. *Ann Surg* 2005;242(4):593–599.
192. Goyal A, Newcombe RG, Chhabra A, et al.; ALMANAC Trialists Group. Factors affecting failed localisation and false-negative rates of sentinel node biopsy in breast cancer—results of the ALMANAC validation phase. *Breast Cancer Res Treat* 2006;99(2):203–208.
193. Krag DN, Anderson SJ, Julian TB, et al.; National Surgical Adjuvant Breast and Bowel Project. Technical outcomes of sentinel-lymph-node resection and conventional axillary-lymph-node dissection in patients with clinically node-negative breast cancer: results from the NSABP B-32 randomised phase III trial. *Lancet Oncol* 2007;8(10):881–888.
194. Zavagno G, De Salvo GL, Scalco G, et al.; GIVOM Trialists. A randomized clinical trial on sentinel lymph node biopsy versus axillary lymph node dissection in breast cancer: results of the Sentinella/GIVOM trial. *Ann Surg* 2008;247(2):207–213.
195. Veronesi U, Paganelli G, Viale G, et al. A randomized comparison of sentinel-node biopsy with routine axillary dissection in breast cancer. *N Engl J Med* 2003;349:546–553.
196. Petrek JA, Heelan MC. Incidence of breast carcinoma-related lymphedema. *Cancer* 1998;83:2776–2781.
197. Morrow M. Postmastectomy radiation therapy: a surgical perspective. *Semin Radiat Oncol* 1999;9:269–274.
198. Early Breast Cancer Trialists' Collaborative Group. Favourable and unfavourable effects on long-term survival of radiotherapy for early

breast cancer: an overview of the randomized trials. *Lancet* 2000;355: 1757–1770.
199. Morrow M, Krontiras H. Who should not receive chemotherapy? Data from American databases and trials. *J Natl Cancer Inst Monogr* 2001;(30): 109–113.
200. Quiet CA, Ferguson DJ, Weichselbaum RR, et al. Natural history of node-positive breast cancer: the curability of small cancers with a limited number of positive nodes. *J Clin Oncol* 1996;14:3105–3111.
201. Clark GM, McGuire WL. Steroid receptors and other prognostic factors in primary breast cancer. *Semin Oncol* 1988;15:20–25.
202. Ravdin PM, Siminoff LA, Davis GJ, et al. Computer program to assist in making decisions about adjuvant therapy for women with early breast cancer. *J Clin Oncol* 2001;19(4):980–991.
203. Olivotto IA, Bajdik CD, Ravdin PM, et al. Population-based validation of the prognostic model ADJUVANT! for early breast cancer. *J Clin Oncol* 2005;23(12):2716–2725.
204. van de Vijver MJ, He YD, van't Veer LJ, et al. A gene-expression signature as a predictor of survival in breast cancer. *N Engl J Med* 2002;347:1999–2009.
205. Paik S, Tang G, Shak S, et al. Gene expression and benefit of chemotherapy in women with node-negative, estrogen receptor-positive breast cancer. *J Clin Oncol* 2006;24(23):3726–3734.
206. Paik S, Shak S, Tang G, et al. A multigene assay to predict recurrence of tamoxifen-treated, node-negative breast cancer. *N Engl J Med* 2004; 351(27):2817–2826.
207. Early Breast Cancer Trialists' Collaborative Group (EBCTCG). Effects of chemotherapy and hormonal therapy for early breast cancer on recurrence and 15-year survival: an overview of the randomised trials. *Lancet* 2005; 365(9472):1687–1717.
208. De Laurentiis M, Cancello G, D'Agostino D, et al. Taxane-based combinations as adjuvant chemotherapy of early breast cancer: a meta-analysis of randomized trials. *J Clin Oncol* 2008;26(1):44–53.
209. Romond EH, Perez EA, Bryant J, et al. Trastuzumab plus adjuvant chemotherapy for operable HER2-positive breast cancer. *N Engl J Med* 2005;353(16):1673–1684.
210. Piccart-Gebhart MJ, Procter M, Leyland-Jones B, et al.; Herceptin Adjuvant (HERA) Trial Study Team. Trastuzumab after adjuvant chemotherapy in HER2-positive breast cancer. *N Engl J Med* 2005;353(16):1659–1672.
211. Perez EA, Romond EH, Suman VJ, et al. NCCTG/NSABP, Updated results of the combined analysis of NCCTG N9831 and NSABP B-31 adjuvant chemotherapy with/without trastuzumab in patients with HER2-positive breast cancer. *J Clin Oncol* 2007;25(suppl 18):512.
212. Smith I, Procter M, Gelber RD, et al.; HERA study team. 2-year follow-up of trastuzumab after adjuvant chemotherapy in HER2-positive breast cancer: a randomised controlled trial. *Lancet* 2007;369(9555):29–36.
213. Joensuu H, Kellokumpu-Lehtinen PL, Bono P; FinHer Study Investigators. Adjuvant docetaxel or vinorelbine with or without trastuzumab for breast cancer. *N Engl J Med* 2006;354(8):809–820.
214. Jordan VC, Morrow M. Tamoxifen, raloxifene, and the prevention of breast cancer. *Endocr Rev* 1999;20:253–278.
215. Coombes RC, Kilburn LS, Snowdon CF, et al.; Intergroup Exemestane Study. Survival and safety of exemestane versus tamoxifen after 2–3 years' tamoxifen treatment (Intergroup Exemestane Study): a randomised controlled trial. *Lancet* 2007;369(9561):559–570.
216. Baum M, Buzdar A, Cuzick J, et al. Anastrozole alone or in combination with tamoxifen versus tamoxifen alone for adjuvant treatment of postmenopausal women with early-stage breast cancer: results of the ATAC (arimidex, tamoxifen alone or in combination) trial efficacy and safety update analyses. *Cancer* 2003;98:1802–1810.
217. Goss PE, Ingle JN, Martino S, et al. Randomized trial of letrozole following tamoxifen as extended adjuvant therapy in receptor-positive breast cancer: updated findings from NCIC CTG MA.17. *J Natl Cancer Inst* 2005;97(17):1262–1271.
218. Veronesi U, Salvadori B, Luini A, et al. Conservative treatment of early breast cancer. Long-term results of 1232 cases treated with quadrantectomy, axillary dissection, and radiotherapy. *Ann Surg* 1990;211:250–259.
219. Hughes KS, Schnaper LA, Berry D, et al.; Cancer and Leukemia Group B; Radiation Therapy Oncology Group; Eastern Cooperative Oncology Group. Lumpectomy plus tamoxifen with or without irradiation in women 70 years of age or older with early breast cancer. *N Engl J Med* 2004; 351(10):971–977.
220. Hind D, Wyld L, Beverley CB, et al. Surgery versus primary endocrine therapy for operable primary breast cancer in elderly women (70 years plus). *Cochrane Database Syst Rev* 2006;(1):CD004272.
221. Rugo HS. Management of breast cancer diagnosed during pregnancy. *Curr Treat Options Oncol* 2003;4:165–173.
222. Mondi MM, Cuenca RE, Ollila DW, et al. Sentinel lymph node biopsy during pregnancy: initial clinical experience. *Ann Surg Oncol* 2007;14(1): 218–221.
223. Kroman N, Wohlfahrt J, Andersen KW, et al. Time since childbirth and prognosis in primary breast cancer: population based study. *Br Med J* 1997;315:851–855.
224. Rosenberg L, Thalib L, Adami HO, et al. Childbirth and breast cancer prognosis. *Int J Cancer* 2004;111:772–776.
225. Whiteman MK, Hillis SD, Curtis KM, et al. Reproductive history and mortality after breast cancer diagnosis. *Obstet Gynecol* 2004;104: 146–154.
226. Ebert U, Loffler H, Kirch W. Cytotoxic therapy and pregnancy. *Pharmacol Ther* 1997;74:207–220.
227. Anderson WF, Althuis MD, Brinton LA, et al. Is male breast cancer similar or different than female breast cancer? *Breast Cancer Res Treat* 2004;83: 77–86.
228. Port ER, Fey JV, Cody HS III, et al. Sentinel lymph node biopsy in patients with male breast carcinoma. *Cancer* 2001;91:319–323.
229. Giordano SH, Cohen DS, Buzdar AU, et al. Breast carcinoma in men: a population-based study. *Cancer* 2004;101:51–57.
230. Ribeiro G, Swindell R. Adjuvant tamoxifen for male breast cancer (MBC). *Br J Cancer* 1992;65:252–254.
231. Mauras N, O'Brien KO, Klein KO, et al. Estrogen suppression in males: metabolic effects. *J Clin Endocrinol Metab* 2000;85(7):2370–2377.
232. Donegan WL, Redlich PN. Breast cancer in men. *Surg Clin North Am* 1996;76:343–363.
233. Buchanan CL, Morris EA, Dorn PL, et al. Utility of breast magnetic resonance imaging in patients with occult primary breast cancer. *Ann Surg Oncol* 2005;12(12):1045–1053.
234. Fourquet A, Melinier M, Campana F. Occult primary cancer with axillary metastases. In: Harris J, Lippman ME, Morrow M, et al., eds. *Diseases of the Breast*, 3rd ed. Philadelphia, PA: Lippincott Williams & Wilkins; 2004:1047–1054.
235. Ellerbroek N, Holmes F, Singletary E, et al. Treatment of patients with isolated axillary nodal metastases from an occult primary carcinoma consistent with breast origin. *Cancer* 1990;66:1461–1467.
236. Merson M, Andreola S, Galimberti V, et al. Breast carcinoma presenting as axillary metastases without evidence of a primary tumor. *Cancer* 1992;70: 504–508.
237. Gage I, Schnitt SJ, Recht A, et al. Skin recurrences after breast-conserving therapy for early-stage breast cancer. *J Clin Oncol* 1998;16:480–486.
238. Paget J. Disease of the mammary areola preceding cancer of the mammary gland. *St Bartholomews Hosp J* 1874;10:79–89.
239. Morrogh M, Morris EA, Liberman L, et al. MRI identifies otherwise occult disease in select patients with Paget disease of the nipple. *J Am Coll Surg* 2008;206(2):316–321.
240. Bijker N, Rutgers EJ, Duchateau L, et al. Breast-conserving therapy for Paget disease of the nipple: a prospective European Organization for Research and Treatment of Cancer study of 61 patients. *Cancer* 2001;91: 472–477.
241. Salvadori B, Cusumano F, Del Bo R, et al. Surgical treatment of phyllodes tumors of the breast. *Cancer* 1989;63:2532–2536.
242. Kessinger A, Foley JF, Lemon HM, et al. Metastatic cystosarcoma phyllodes: a case report and review of the literature. *J Surg Oncol* 1972;4: 131–147.
243. Barrio AV, Clark BD, Goldberg JI, et al. Clinicopathologic features and long-term outcomes of 293 phyllodes tumors of the breast. *Ann Surg Oncol* 2007;14(10):2961–2970.
244. Zissis C, Apostolikas N, Konstantinidou A, et al. The extent of surgery and prognosis of patients with phyllodes tumor of the breast. *Breast Cancer Res Treat* 1998;48:205–210.
245. Haagensen CD, Stout AP. Carcinoma of the breast. II. Criteria of operability. *Ann Surg* 1943;118:859–872.
246. Hortobagyi G, Singletary SE, Strom EA. Locally advanced breast cancer. In: Harris J, Lippman ME, Morrow M, et al., eds. *Diseases of the Breast*, 3rd ed. Philadelphia, PA: Lippincott Williams & Wilkins; 2004: 951–969.
247. Smith IC, Heys SD, Hutcheon AW, et al. Neoadjuvant chemotherapy in breast cancer: significantly enhanced response with docetaxel. *J Clin Oncol* 2002;20:1456–1466.
248. Buzdar AU, Ibrahim NK, Francis D, et al. Significantly higher pathologic complete remission rate after neoadjuvant therapy with trastuzumab, paclitaxel, and epirubicin chemotherapy: results of a randomized trial in human epidermal growth factor receptor 2-positive operable breast cancer. *J Clin Oncol* 2005;23(16):3676–3685.
249. Thomas E, Holmes FA, Smith TL, et al. The use of alternate, non-cross-resistant adjuvant chemotherapy on the basis of pathologic response to a neoadjuvant doxorubicin-based regimen in women with operable breast cancer: long-term results from a prospective randomized trial. *J Clin Oncol* 2004;22:2294–2302.
250. Chen AM, Meric-Bernstam F, Hunt KK, et al. Breast conservation after neoadjuvant chemotherapy: the MD Anderson Cancer Center experience. *J Clin Oncol* 2004;22:2303–2312.
251. Low JA, Berman AW, Steinberg SM, et al. Long-term follow-up for locally advanced and inflammatory breast cancer patients treated with multimodality therapy. *J Clin Oncol* 2004;22:4067–4074.

CHAPTER 75 ■ THYROID GLAND

BARBRA S. MILLER AND PAUL G. GAUGER

KEY POINTS

1. Thyroid follicular tissue in the carotid sheath or the lateral compartments of the neck represents a regional nodal metastasis of an occult thyroid cancer until proven otherwise.
2. The tubercle of Zuckerkandl is an anatomic feature of the thyroid that helps facilitate identification of the recurrent laryngeal nerve and the superior parathyroid gland.
3. Ultrasound is the imaging procedure of choice for nodular thyroid disease, and surgeon-performed ultrasound helps facilitate operative planning.
4. Additional thyroid resection or adjuvant treatment with radioiodine is seldom required for an incidental papillary microcarcinoma found in the surgical specimen.
5. Complete investigation of a follicular/indeterminate lesion by fine-needle aspiration currently requires thyroid resection to differentiate a follicular adenoma from a follicular carcinoma based on the presence of capsular or vascular invasion.
6. Genotype/phenotype correlation using the specific RET proto-oncogene mutation identified in each patient/family can help determine the appropriate age for prophylactic thyroidectomy in patients with hereditary medullary thyroid carcinoma.
7. Extranodal lymphoma of the thyroid or anaplastic thyroid cancer should be considered in the hypothyroid patient who experiences rapid growth of the thyroid.
8. Advantages of total thyroidectomy over thyroid lobectomy for differentiated thyroid carcinoma include (a) removal of multifocal intrathyroidal tumors; (b) facilitation of radioiodine imaging and ablation for residual, regional, or metastatic disease; and (c) use of serum thyroglobulin as a sensitive marker of persistent or recurrent disease.
9. Routine prophylactic lymph node dissection of the central compartment (level VI) in patients with known papillary thyroid cancer may decrease postoperative thyroglobulin levels and prevent the need for future reoperation in the same compartment.

Excellent patient outcomes for surgical treatment of thyroid disorders are obtainable only by a thorough understanding of embryology, anatomy, physiology, and relevant pharmacology. Delicate and deliberate surgical technique and careful attention to detail are necessary to prevent common complications of thyroid resections.

EMBRYOLOGY AND SURGICAL IMPLICATIONS

Developmental Embryology

As the first endocrine gland to develop, the thyroid is mostly derived of endoderm from the ventral embryologic digestive tract. A midline diverticulum arises in the area of the foramen cecum at the base of the tongue at approximately 4 weeks of gestation. The tissue descends as the median thyroid component, which ultimately becomes the isthmus and the majority of each lateral lobe. The foramen cecum ruptures and resorbs during week 6 of gestational age, leaving behind a regressive fibrous tract, which becomes the thyroglossal duct tract (including the portion associated with the central hyoid bone). The distal end associated with the isthmus persists as a recognizable pyramidal lobe in about 30% to 50% of individuals. The lateral thyroid component develops on each side from the caudal pharyngeal endoderm (with contribution from the fourth and fifth branchial pouches), which arises later in development than the median component.[1] The lateral components become increasingly removed from the pharynx, leaving a tapering connection on each side, which eventually detaches. The residual posterolateral projection from the lateral thyroid component toward the pharynx, when present, is known as the tubercle of Zuckerkandl. Because of its branchial pouch origin, the lateral thyroid component is closely associated with the superior parathyroid anlage (from the fourth pouch). The lateral components fuse with the posterior portion of the median component on each side, and accompanying C cells (from neural crest origin) migrate into the superolateral portion of the lobes and eventually secrete calcitonin. The unified thyroid begins to differentiate into thyroid follicles between weeks 8 and 11. Basic glandular function begins on a cellular level by the third month of gestation when iodine trapping occurs and thyroid hormones are first manufactured.

Congenital Abnormalities

An uncommon developmental malformation is the lingual thyroid gland. It represents a failure of the median thyroid component to descend from the foramen cecum. The size of a lingual thyroid can often be decreased by using exogenous thyroid hormone to suppress thyroid-stimulating hormone (TSH) or by ^{131}I ablation. Surgical excision may be required if airway obstruction, obstructive dysphagia, or hemorrhage occurs. Ectopic thyroid tissue can be found in other areas of the central cervical compartment and the mediastinum. These can be sequestered nodules associated with multinodular goiters or they may be
1 embryologic rests of thyroid tissue.[2] Although the concept of *lateral aberrant thyroid* tissue was originally used to describe the findings of follicular tissue in the carotid sheath or the lateral compartments of the neck, it is now generally agreed that this cannot occur as an embryologic abnormality. If thyroid tissue is found in these areas, it represents a regional nodal metastasis of an occult thyroid cancer. Thyroglossal duct cysts occur in the midline of the neck along the path of descent of the median thyroid component. They may occur from the base of the tongue to the low central neck, although most are located just inferior to the hyoid bone. Although they are often discovered during infancy and childhood, it is not uncommon for them to present

in adulthood—discovered either because of mass effect or infection. When examining the patient, elevation of the mass with protrusion of the tongue is very suggestive of a thyroglossal duct cyst. Resection of a thyroglossal duct cyst involves excision of the entire thyroglossal duct including the cyst. The tract courses through the central portion of the hyoid bone and, for that reason, excision of this segment of bone is critical to prevent recurrence (Sistrunk procedure). The epithelial lining usually contains some thyroid cells and, thus, thyroid carcinomas (usually of papillary type) can arise within thyroglossal duct cysts. Excision of the cyst and the thyroglossal duct may be sufficient for small, limited carcinomas less than 1 cm, but if multifocal elements or regional nodal metastases are present or if the tumor is of sufficient size, total thyroidectomy should be performed to facilitate subsequent ^{131}I scanning and therapy.

ANATOMY AND SURGICAL IMPLICATIONS

A normal thyroid gland (in patients from iodine-sufficient regions) weighs between 15 and 20 g. The upper portion of the isthmus typically crosses at or below the level of the cricoid cartilage. The isthmus itself is approximately 1 to 2 cm in transverse and vertical dimensions and the lower margin of the lobe is normally near the fourth or fifth tracheal ring. The lateral lobes lie adjacent to the thyroid cartilage and cricothyroideus muscles as well as the lateral trachea and a portion of the lateral esophagus on each side. The two lobes are roughly conical, approximately 5 cm in craniocaudal and 2 to 3 cm in transverse and anteroposterior dimensions.

Muscular, Fascial, and Airway Relationships

The thyroid lies in the central compartment of the neck bordered by the contents of the carotid sheath on each side. The anterolateral surface is covered by the sternothyroid muscles, which do not completely meet in the midline above the level of the isthmus. Superficial to the sternothyroid muscles are the sternohyoid muscles that meet in the midline raphe marking the most common plane of dissection used to expose the thyroid gland. These muscles are innervated on the inferolateral aspect by the ansa cervicalis (ansa hypoglossi). The thyroid is invested in a thin layer of connective tissue that is an expansion of the pretracheal fascia (often called the "thyroid sheath"). The sheath is not to be confused with the thyroid capsule, which is more integral to the gland itself. The plane defined by this layer is usually easy to develop as the thyroid is mobilized away from surrounding structures. Especially near the superior portion of the thyroid, the sheath defines a coronal plane that, when opened, exposes the potential space between the pharynx/esophagus and the cervical vertebral bodies. The sheath is condensed as the anterior suspensory ligament above the isthmus. The sheath also attaches the posterior surface of the thyroid gland to the tracheal rings. It is condensed posteromedially into the ligament of Berry on each side. The ligament of Berry is a very firm attachment to the trachea near the cricothyroid space, which means that it is often intimately associated with the recurrent laryngeal nerve (RLN) near its insertion. It is in the course of dividing these posterior attachments that the RLN is most vulnerable to iatrogenic injury. The superior parathyroid gland may be found between the sheath and the thyroid capsule, within the sheath, or posterior to the sheath.

Vascular Relationships

The thyroid gland has a very high blood flow index per tissue mass and receives its arterial supply from a paired system of superior thyroid arteries (originating from the external carotid arteries) and inferior thyroid arteries (originating from the thyrocervical trunks). The superior artery courses along the inferior pharyngeal constrictor muscle group and branches near the tip of the superior pole of the thyroid, usually into at least an anterior and posterior branch. The inferior thyroid artery (ITA) courses upward behind the carotid artery and then crosses medially to serve the thyroid lobe. The ITA has multiple branches that course in a plane between the sheath and the capsule of the gland. The relationship of the ITA to the RLN is an important landmark. There is always an intersection (except in the case of a direct/nonrecurrent laryngeal nerve), but the specific relationship (anterior, posterior, or interdigitated) may be variable. Occasionally, an arteria thyroidea ima arises from the aorta or innominate artery and directly serves the inferior portion of the thyroid gland. Venous drainage is by a widely anastomosing system that condenses into three main trunks. The superior thyroid veins course adjacent to the superior thyroid arteries but empty into the internal jugular vein at the level of the carotid bifurcation. Middle thyroid veins are present in more than half of patients and drain laterally to the internal jugular vein. These veins are divided early in the course of mobilizing the thyroid lobe. In tracing a vessel laterally, if it passes anterior to the carotid artery, it is a middle thyroid vein, whereas if it passes deep to the carotid, it is the ITA. The inferior thyroid veins form nearly all of the vascular connections found at the inferior poles of the thyroid lobes. The number and configuration of these veins can be quite variable, but in general they descend along the course of the thyrothymic tract to drain into the ipsilateral innominate or brachiocephalic veins.

Neurologic Relationships

Two nerves have critical importance during thyroidectomy: the RLN (also known as the inferior laryngeal nerve) and the external branch of the superior laryngeal nerve. The right recurrent laryngeal nerve arises from the vagus at the level of the subclavian artery and passes (recurs) around the posterior aspect of the artery before ascending into the central compartment. The nerve takes an oblique course in the central neck and may be 1 to 2 cm lateral to the trachea low in the central neck before traveling toward its entry into the larynx. The left RLN arises from the vagus nerve as it crosses the aortic arch. It passes inferior and medial to the arch and ascends to the larynx in the tracheoesophageal groove along a course that is typically linear and more vertical. The RLN often lies immediately posterolateral to the ligament of Berry, but it is not infrequent that it can be embedded in the fibrous connections of the ligament itself, especially the anterior branch of the nerve if it bifurcates outside the larynx. Pelizzo et al. have described the tubercle of
2 Zuckerkandl as a constant anatomic landmark to facilitate identification of the recurrent laryngeal nerve during thyroid resection.[3] In the standard anatomic relationship, the tubercle of Zuckerkandl lies immediately lateral to and covers the RLN (Fig. 75.1). An uncommon but high-risk anatomic arrangement

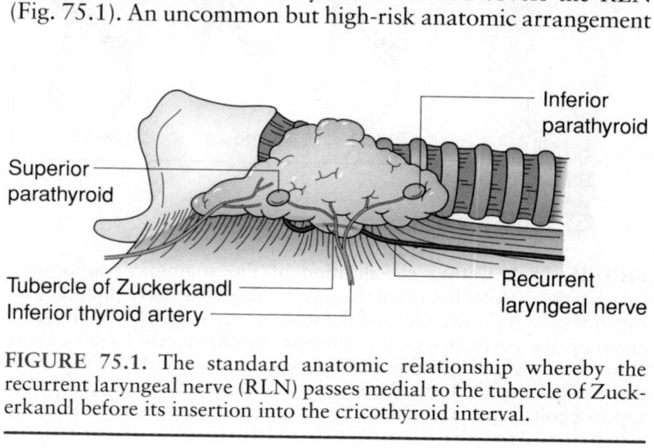

FIGURE 75.1. The standard anatomic relationship whereby the recurrent laryngeal nerve (RLN) passes medial to the tubercle of Zuckerkandl before its insertion into the cricothyroid interval.

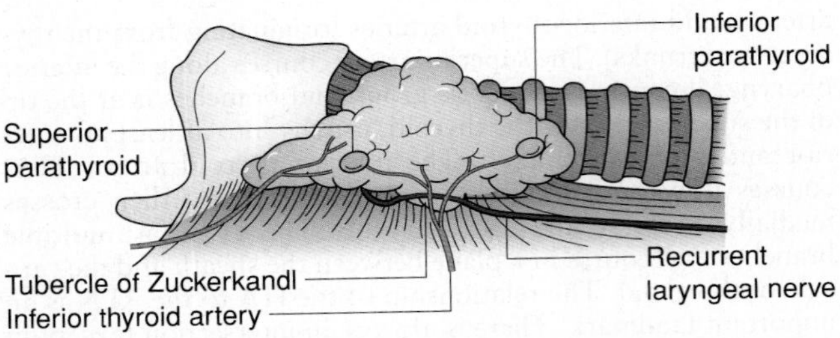

FIGURE 75.2. The uncommon but high-risk anatomic variation where the recurrent laryngeal nerve (RLN) courses lateral to the tubercle of Zuckerkandl, which is often enlarged. The nerve is encountered much earlier in the dissection required for thyroidectomy and is at risk of being misidentified as a vascular structure.

occurs when the RLN is found lateral to the tubercle of Zuckerkandl (Fig. 75.2). If the surgeon is unaware of this possibility (which may exist when the tubercle has undergone nodular enlargement), the nerve is subject to iatrogenic injury.[4] The nerve usually bifurcates extralaryngeally but often at a point less than 0.5 cm from the cricoid cartilage. Up to 58% of recurrent laryngeal nerves will bifurcate proximal to the inferior border of the cricoid cartilage.[5]

It is critical to be aware of the occasional "direct" laryngeal nerve (also called the "nonrecurrent laryngeal nerve"). This anomaly results from abnormal embryonic development of the aortic arch. The anomaly is more common on the right (approximately 0.5% to 0.7%) than on the left (approximately 0.04%).[6] On the right, a direct nerve is the consequence of the formation of the arteria lusoria vascular abnormality, in which the innominate artery is absent and the right common carotid and right subclavian arteries originate directly from the arch. The subclavian artery takes a retroesophageal course. To have a direct nerve on the left side, a number of other anomalies must exist. Specifically, the aortic arch must be right sided (as occurs in situs inversus viscerum), the origin of the left subclavian artery must be abnormally sited on the aortic arch, and the ligamentum arteriosum must be displaced to the right. A "false" nonrecurrent inferior laryngeal nerve has been described as a communicating branch between the cervical sympathetic system and the RLN, which can mimic a nerve that appears to emerge from the region of the vagus nerve as would a direct nerve.[7]

The superior laryngeal nerve arises from the vagus at the nodose ganglion near the base of the skull and descends along the course of the internal carotid artery. At the level of the hyoid bone, it divides into the internal branch (which enters the larynx at the thyrohyoid membrane to provide sensory innervation to the superior larynx) and the external branch (which provides motor innervation to the cricothyroideus muscle). It has a variable course in relation to the inferior pharyngeal constrictor muscle and the branches of the superior thyroid artery. It is this fact that makes the external branch of the superior laryngeal nerve (EBSLN) vulnerable to iatrogenic injury. One classification of the anatomic variations is depicted in Figure 75.3.[8]

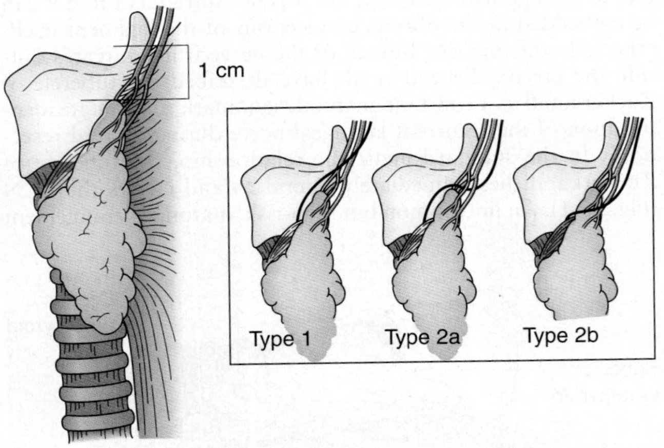

FIGURE 75.3. Cernea classification of the anatomic relationships between the external branch of the superior laryngeal nerve (EBSLN), the superior pole of the thyroid, and the superior thyroid artery. With type 1 anatomy, the nerve crosses the superior thyroid vessels 1 cm or more above the superior thyroid pole. With type 2 anatomy, the nerve crosses the vessels less than 1 cm above (type 2a) or even below (type 2b) the superior pole. Type 2 variants are the most vulnerable to iatrogenic injury.

Lymphatic Relationships

The thyroid gland has intracapsular lymph channels, which provide some communication from lobe to lobe across the isthmus. A rich plexus of lymphatics surrounds the region of the thyroid; consequently, lymph flows in multiple directions from the gland. These factors are important to understand for treatment of thyroid malignancies. Within the anterior suspensory ligament is a small group of midline prelaryngeal lymph nodes known as the Delphian nodes. Along with the pretracheal and paratracheal nodes and those along the recurrent laryngeal nerves, these central compartment lymph nodes are classified as level VI. The upper jugular (level II), midjugular (level III), and lower jugular (level IV) lymph nodes divide the central compartment from the lateral compartment of the neck, whereas the posterior triangle lymph nodes are level V (Fig. 75.4). Thyroid cancers with regional lymph node metastases tend to involve level VI lymph node metastases before involving levels II, III, IV, and ultimately V.[9] Level I (submental) and level VII

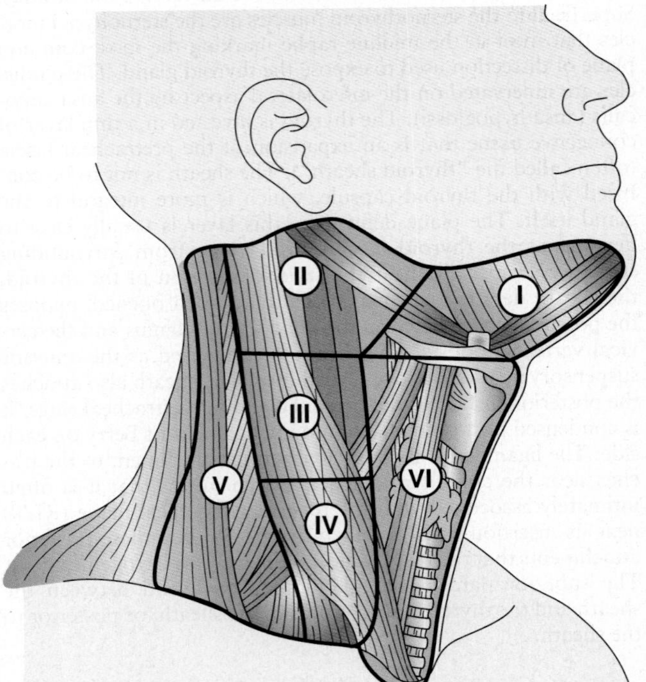

FIGURE 75.4. Classification scheme for regional lymph node basins in the neck.

(superior mediastinal) involvement is less common but can occur. Documented cases of "skip" metastases directly to the lateral compartment with no level VI involvement have been reported.[10]

Parathyroid Relationships

Parathyroid glands in typical locations are encountered during thyroidectomy by virtue of their association with the thyroid gland. Parathyroid glands in ectopic locations will typically not be encountered during thyroidectomy. The superior parathyroid gland is usually located in a relatively constant area largely because of the embryologic association between the lateral thyroid component and the superior parathyroid anlage (both associated with the fourth branchial pouch). The tubercle of Zuckerkandl is anatomically associated with the position of the ipsilateral superior parathyroid gland as well as the recurrent laryngeal nerve. In relation to the point at which the RLN intersects the inferior thyroid artery, a 2-cm circumscribed area on the cranial aspect will often contain the superior parathyroid gland. It may also be found tucked posterior to the inferior thyroid artery or even posteromedial to the superior thyroid pole. Superior parathyroid glands are very rarely found within the thyroid capsule. There is an 80% chance that a superior parathyroid gland will be found in a position similar to its contralateral partner.

The location of the inferior parathyroid gland may be more variable. It may be found on the anterior aspect of the inferior thyroid pole (especially with Hashimoto disease or large multinodular goiter) but is often on the inferolateral aspect. It may also be in the triangular region caudal to the inferior thyroid artery and anterior to the RLN. If it is not in these locations, it is often embedded in fat and thymic tissue within the thyrothymic tract. It may also be located under the thyroid capsule in an intrathyroidal position. The symmetry of inferior parathyroid glands from side to side is approximately 70%.

THYROID PHYSIOLOGY

Production of Thyroid Hormones

The thyroid gland produces thyroxine (T_4), triiodothyronine (T_3), and calcitonin under complicated regulatory mechanisms. Approximately 100 to 150 μg of dietary iodide is required for normal thyroid hormone synthesis to occur. In most developed regions of the world, daily intake from iodine-containing foods is usually far in excess of this requirement. The kidneys excrete the iodide not utilized by the thyroid. The availability of thyroid hormones to all tissues results from hormone production within the thyroid gland (specifically within the follicular cells) and the delivery and metabolism of the hormones in peripheral tissues. The integration of these systems to maintain a euthyroid state is ultimately orchestrated by the anterior pituitary gland through its secretion of thyrotropin (TSH). The active uptake of iodide in the thyroid occurs on the basolateral aspect of the follicular cells and is performed by a Na^+/K^+-adenosine triphosphatase (ATPase)-mediated pump. Both TSH and the circulating concentration of iodide influence this symporter system. TSH acts within the thyroid gland to regulate the synthesis of thyroglobulin (Tg), the active uptake of iodide, its incorporation with tyrosine (an oxidative reaction catalyzed by thyroid peroxidase [TPO]), and the subsequent production of T_4 and T_3 (and their storage bound to Tg in the colloid component of the gland), and ultimately the release of both T_4 and T_3 into the circulation. Hormone release is an active process of micropinocytosis that involves resorption of the bound Tg into the follicular cell where enzymatic degradation releases T_4 and T_3, which is released from the basal portion of the cell into the circulation. T_4 is produced in preference to T_3 in the thyroid gland by a ratio of approximately 13:1 in normal states. T_4 has a relatively weak biologic action, so peripheral conversion to the more active T_3 hormone is required. Most of this takes place in the plasma and liver by type 1 deiodinase enzymes. All of the T_4 in the circulation is derived from the thyroid, whereas less than 20% of T_3 in the circulation is from the thyroid, the majority being produced enzymatically from monodeiodination of T_4 in nonthyroidal sites. In circulation, most thyroid hormone (>99% of both T_4 and T_3) is bound to proteins such as thyroxine-binding globulin (TBG), albumin, and thyroxine-binding prealbumin. Protein-bound thyroid hormones are considered biologically inert because they do not enter cells until they are released from proteins to circulate in the very small free fraction. The half-life of T_4 is approximately 7 days, whereas the half-life of T_3 is much shorter—on the order of 8 to 12 hours.

Action of Thyroid Hormones

Thyroid hormones have many effects on various body tissues. The peripheral conversion from T_4 to T_3 increases the binding affinity of thyroid hormone for the nuclear thyroid receptor protein at least 10-fold. Triiodothyronine acts within the nucleus of peripheral tissues via four T_3 nuclear receptor subtypes to activate T_3-regulated gene transcription. Ultimately, the physiologic actions of thyroid hormone relate to growth, differentiation, calorigenesis, and TSH suppression.

Calcitonin is a 32-amino-acid polypeptide that is physiologically effective in many other species, but in humans it is apparently less important. Although exogenous calcitonin may have a therapeutic effect, endogenous calcitonin secretion rarely results in an impact on serum calcium levels.

RELEVANT LABORATORY TESTS

An understanding of the normal relationship between free T_4 (FT_4) levels and TSH levels is critical for appropriate interpretation of thyroid function tests. Thyroid dysfunction can be determined directly, by measuring FT_4 levels, or indirectly, by measuring TSH. If TSH is to be used as the primary indicator of thyroid dysfunction, an intact hypothalamic–pituitary axis is required. Normally, a log/linear inverse relationship between TSH and FT_4 is defined by the negative feedback inhibition of TSH secretion by circulating thyroxine levels. Therefore, high TSH and low FT_4 levels are indicative of hypothyroidism and, conversely, low TSH and high FT_4 levels are characteristic of hyperthyroidism. It is likely that each individual has a genetically determined FT_4 set point. Early subtle deviation from that set point (via in situ conversion to FT_3 in the pituitary) will cause amplified changes in the TSH value, thus making TSH a very sensitive and clinically useful early indicator of incipient thyroid dysfunction.

Calcitonin

Basal calcitonin levels are generally less than 16 pg/mL for healthy people and for nearly all patients with thyroid disease, other than medullary thyroid carcinoma (MTC). Therefore, calcitonin serves as a very specific tumor marker for MTC. Basal calcitonin levels are useful for diagnosis and observation of these patients.

Free Thyroxine and Free Triiodothyronine

Technically, it is easier to measure the total (free + protein-bound) hormone levels (measured at nanomolar levels) as compared to the very small free hormone concentrations (measured at picomolar ranges). Because T_4 is more tightly protein bound than T_3, it is less bioavailable and, consequently, very difficult to measure directly. Ligand assays performed on automated immunoassay analyzers are fairly common in clinical use and are standardized against known hormone concentrations. Because this method does not rely on physical separation of the free and protein-bound hormone fractions, it is more accurately considered a free hormone estimate. The only reason to measure FT_4 or free triiodothyronine (FT_3) in preference to total thyroxine (TT_4) or total triiodothyronine (TT_3) is to improve the ability to detect thyroid dysfunction in the presence of thyroid hormone–binding abnormalities, which are relatively common. For example, some common drugs such as phenytoin, carbamazepine, furosemide, and aspirin may compete with thyroid hormone for binding to serum proteins.

Thyroglobulin

Serum thyroglobulin is reflective of three factors: the mass of thyroid tissue present; the presence of injury or inflammation of the gland, which allows leakage of Tg; and the degree of stimulation of the TSH receptor. The primary clinical use of Tg measurement is as a tumor marker, which serves as an index of the amount of differentiated thyroid cancer present (assuming that total thyroidectomy has been performed, thereby removing all normal thyroid tissue). Tg is measured in the serum by radioimmunoassay methods or by immunometric assays. The latter is more susceptible to competitive interference by thyroglobulin autoantibodies (TgAbs), which cause an artifactual decrease in the measured levels. In fact, sensitive quantitative TgAb determination is a critical accompaniment to serum Tg measurement, which is common during management of differentiated thyroid carcinoma (DTC). The particular assay utilized must be sensitive enough to detect Tg levels at the lower end of the reference range (1 to 3 μg/L) to be useful in monitoring for recurrence of DTC. It is critical to understand that the TSH level is a major influence on the level of Tg and, consequently, interpretation of any level requires an understanding of whether the patient was hypothyroid or not at the time of measurement.

Thyroid Autoantibodies

Measurement of thyroid peroxidase autoantibodies (TPOAbs) is the most sensitive test for detecting autoimmune thyroid disease. TPOAb is often the first abnormality to appear in Hashimoto disease; however, a significant fraction (up to 12%) of people with no apparent thyroid disorder may also have positive TPOAb titers.

TgAb may be present in approximately 3% to 10% of the general population and are even more common (20%) in patients with differentiated thyroid carcinoma. TgAb measurements are not as useful as TPOAb in evaluation of autoimmune thyroid disease.

Thyroid-stimulating hormone receptor autoantibodies (TRAbs) are heterogeneous and may mimic the action of TSH to cause hyperthyroidism as in Graves disease or, conversely, may block the action of TSH and cause hypothyroidism as occurs in neonates of a mother with thyroid autoantibodies. The specific different types include thyroid-stimulating antibodies (TSAbs), TSH receptor–blocking antibodies (TBAbs), thyroid growth-simulating immunoglobins (TGIs), and thyroid binding inhibiting immunoglobulins (TBIIs).

Thyroid-stimulating Hormone (Thyrotropin)

As the sensitivity and specificity of current TSH assays are quite high, the indirect approach of measuring TSH levels is the most sensitive method for detecting thyroid dysfunction. The inverse relationship between TSH and FT_4 also dictates that small alterations in FT_4 will lead to a larger response in TSH, thus adding further support to this strategy. Modern methods are generally based on immunometric assays and are able to achieve a sensitivity of 0.02 mIU/L or less. At present, the upper limit of the normal range is considered to be approximately 5 mIU/L, but this is likely to be redefined at approximately 2.5 to 3.0 mIU/L in the future. This is because greater than 95% of rigorously screened normal euthyroid volunteers have values in this range, and it is becoming evident that many patients in the interval between these upper limit values progress to develop hypothyroidism, especially if thyroid autoantibodies are present. It is the range of 0.3 to 3.0 mIU/L that is generally considered the target range for TSH when patients are treated with levothyroxine (LT_4) for hypothyroidism because, consequently, most patients then have FT_4 levels in the upper third of the normal reference range.[11]

Total Thyroxine and Total Triiodothyronine

Total hormone assays require an inhibitor to block or displace the hormone from its binding proteins. This factor, along with large sample dilution, allows binding of the hormone to the antibody reagent. Because of the 10-fold lower concentrations of T_3 in the serum, the TT_3 assay requires even greater sensitivity and precision. Because of variability in the quantity and the binding capacity of serum proteins, however, abnormal TT_4 and TT_3 measurements are more commonly caused by these factors instead of true thyroid dysfunction.

THYROID IMAGING TECHNIQUES

It is common for patients to present to the surgeon after having undergone multiple imaging tests. In general, only ultrasonography is routinely useful in evaluation of the patient with a thyroid nodule. In other specific circumstances, various other tests may be useful.

Nuclear Medicine Imaging

Radionuclide imaging is unique when compared with other thyroid imaging techniques in that the image provided depends on the specific functional characteristics of the thyroid tissue; however, it provides little anatomic detail.

Technetium Pertechnetate ^{99m}Tc Scintigraphy. ^{99m}Tc is the radionuclide most commonly available for thyroid imaging. The ^{99m}Tc pertechnetate component is actively trapped by functional thyroid cells in a manner similar to iodine but is not organified or stored in the thyroid. The isotope emits gamma (γ) radiation (the mechanism of scintigraphic imaging) and very small amounts of other types of radiation. Because the thyroid rapidly absorbs the injected ^{99m}Tc pertechnetate, imaging can occur early after administration and an entire study may take only an hour. A normal result demonstrates equal distribution bilaterally. Abnormal results include either concentration of the tracer in the region of a known nodule indicating an area of hyperfunction or, conversely, an area of photopenia (the "cold nodule") indicating a region of hypofunction. Before the era of fine-needle aspiration (FNA) biopsy, this finding increased the concern for potential malignancy.

^{123}Iodine Scintigraphy. Because ^{123}I is trapped and organified by the thyroid gland, it can better indicate the functional characteristics of thyroid tissue. ^{123}I emits x-rays, some β particles, and γ rays. It has a short half-life of about 13 hours. After administration of an oral dose, the thyroid absorbs sufficient isotope to allow imaging by 4 hours. Images are also obtained at 24 hours, and the total fraction of dose retained by the thyroid can then be calculated as the 24-hour radioactive iodine uptake (RAIU).

^{131}Iodine Scintigraphy. ^{131}I concentrates in the thyroid by the same mechanism as ^{123}I, but has a much longer half-life (about 8 days) and emits much more β radiation along with β radiation at a range that is suboptimal for clear image creation. However, because of its long half-life and thorough clearance from background tissues, it remains the isotope of choice for imaging of patients with differentiated thyroid carcinoma. Ultimately, treatment or ablation of residual or metastatic carcinoma (largely by the effect of β irradiation) is accomplished with higher doses of the isotope than required for imaging.

Positron Emission Tomography. ^{18}F fluorodeoxyglucose positron emission tomography (PET) scanning with three-dimensional tomographic reconstruction can be very helpful in imaging thyroid carcinomas, and allows anatomic and functional evaluation. Because of the expense and the inconsistent insurance coverage, usage is currently limited to unusual circumstances such as recurrent thyroid malignancy that is otherwise occult (Fig. 75.5). The sensitivity in thyroid carcinomas is approximately 60% to 70%.[12] PET scanning is so frequently used in the evaluation of other solid malignancies that occult thyroid carcinomas are discovered in 2% to 3%.[13] Incidentally discovered thyroid nodules identified on PET scans can be malignant in 14% to 47% and have a higher incidence of malignancy compared with nodules identified by other imaging modalities.[13,14] Some overlap does occur for standard uptake values of benign and malignant nodules, so each nodule should be carefully evaluated.

^{99m}Tc Sestamibi Scintigraphy. Although ^{99m}Tc sestamibi scintigraphy is commonly used in localization of parathyroid tumors, it has incidentally been noted to concentrate in follicular tumors, most notably those with Hürthle cell cytology. For this reason, it may have a role in localizing persistent disease in patients with Hürthle cell carcinoma. In contrast to radioactive iodine, however, it does not have therapeutic potential in ablating tissue. If a thyroid nodule is incidentally imaged on sestamibi scanning, there is no capability to predict whether it is a benign or malignant tumor.[15]

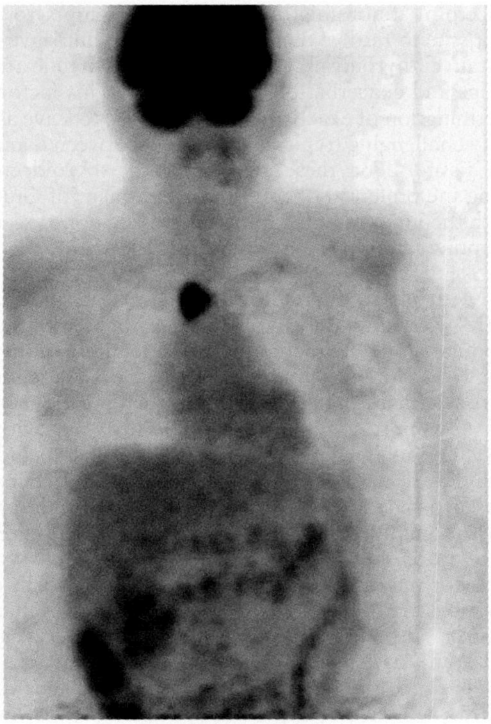

FIGURE 75.5. ^{18}F fluorodeoxyglucose (FDG) positron emission tomography scan of a patient with late recurrence of differentiated thyroid carcinoma in the mediastinum. The tumor is the intensely FDG-avid mass superior to the cardiac activity.

^{111}Indium-Octreotide Scintigraphy. Octreotide scanning (somatostatin receptor scintigraphy) has been occasionally useful in imaging differentiated thyroid carcinoma, especially when radioiodine scintigraphy has failed to do so. It is a useful imaging modality for patients with medullary thyroid cancer. Its therapeutic potential is undefined.

Ultrasonography

3 Ultrasound (US) has become the imaging technique of choice to evaluate the thyroid gland and its surrounding structures. It is best performed using a high-frequency "small parts" probe (7.5 to 15 mHz). It is the most sensitive and specific technique to determine the size, number, and distribution of thyroid nodules. US often detects very small, subtle nodules that are not otherwise clinically evident. Studied prospectively, the prevalence of asymptomatic thyroid nodules (thyroid incidentalomas) detected by ultrasonography is approximately 67%,[16] whereas physical examination identifies thyroid nodules in approximately 5% to 8%. Hyperechoic nodules are often benign, whereas thyroid malignancies, regardless of cell type, are often hypoechoic. Irregular margins between the nodule and surrounding tissues raise concern for malignancy. An anechoic rim around the nodule is referred to as a "halo" sign and is much more likely to be associated with a benign nodule. Larger macrocalcifications with posterior acoustic shadowing are usually indicative of chronicity and are more likely associated with a benign nodule, whereas subtle microcalcifications, which cause a "twinkling" effect when the transducer is moved across the nodule, are correlated with malignancy. In practical terms, selective FNA biopsy should be limited to those nodules greater than 1 cm, those with concerning ultrasound features, or those that have increased in size under serial US measurement. Because US can detect nodules at a preclinical stage, it follows that proper perspective about the significance or insignificance of these nodules must be maintained. As with any imaging technique that depends on individual performance of the test, a user-dependent factor exists. US can be especially useful when performed by the surgeon and allows appropriate preoperative planning. Additionally, it has an important role in the preoperative staging and postoperative follow-up of patients with differentiated thyroid carcinoma. In experienced hands, it is a very sensitive technique for detecting abnormally enlarged lymph nodes or tumor recurrence within the thyroid bed, and for guiding subsequent confirmatory biopsy. It is especially important for identifying sites of recurrent thyroid cancer in those patients with negative radioactive iodine (RAI) scans or dedifferentiated tumors that are no longer iodine avid.

Cross-sectional Imaging

Computed tomography (CT) scans and magnetic resonance imaging (MRI) scans are useful in certain circumstances. In large nodules firmly fixed to contiguous structures or accompanied by new vocal cord paralysis, the concern for an invasive thyroid cancer is raised. CT scan may suggest invasion of the laryngeal or tracheal cartilages, which may modify the operative approach. Large goiters that have an obvious substernal component on physical examination or that are accompanied by an upper airway obstructive component may warrant preoperative CT scan to define the extent of the goiter, not only to help plan the specific operative plan but also to facilitate

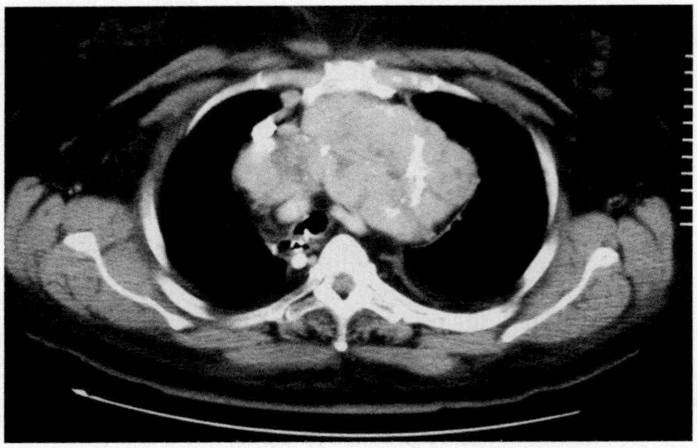

FIGURE 75.6. Example of a multinodular goiter with a large substernal component causing tracheal displacement and compression.

anesthetic evaluation for difficult airway management techniques such as fiberoptic intubation (Fig. 75.6).

FUNCTIONAL DISORDERS AND GENERAL TREATMENT CONSIDERATIONS

Hyperthyroidism

Hyperthyroidism can be caused by diverse pathophysiology, such as Graves disease, toxic multinodular goiter, and solitary toxic adenoma. Typical symptoms are heat intolerance, sweating, palpitations, tremor, hyperphagia, thirst, and sleep disturbances. Elderly patients can present with muscle wasting, atrial fibrillation, angina pectoris, or congestive heart failure. Regardless of specific cause, the need to control hyperthyroidism before operation is critical to prevent thyroid crisis (i.e., thyroid storm). Maximal safety is assured with thionamides combined with beta blockade, but studies suggest that propranolol or metoprolol used without thionamides are as safe and effective.[17,18] Beta blockade alone is not universally accepted because of the occasional occurrence of postoperative thyroid crisis, tachycardia, hyperhidrosis, or anxiety. Doses of beta-blockers must continue through the morning of surgery and should not be stopped abruptly in the postoperative setting.

Graves Disease. Graves disease, which was described by Dr. Robert Graves in the 1830s as a toxic diffuse goiter associated with exophthalmos and palpitations, is an autoimmune disorder with a genetic predisposition and a female predominance (five to seven times greater than males). It is characterized by the presence of TSAbs. These antibodies bind to the TSH receptor on follicular cells and stimulate thyroid hormone release. In addition, the autoimmune disease process may affect the eyes, causing exophthalmos secondary to inflammatory cell infiltration into the extraocular muscles and orbital connective tissue. Graves ophthalmopathy may be the first manifestation of disease, and it covers a wide spectrum from very mild changes in visual acuity or ocular dryness to obvious proptosis. It may be so severe as to require aggressive ophthalmologic treatment in approximately 5% of patients. Aside from the ophthalmopathic findings of proptosis and lid lag on physical examination, patients with Graves disease may have involvement of the pretibial regions, leading to myxedema. Patients with Graves disease usually have a diffuse goiter, which may be smooth or occasionally irregular. The gland is by nature very vascular and may occasionally have an audible bruit overlying it. T_4 and T_3 levels are increased and TSH levels are suppressed. The uptake of RAI generally shows a symmetrically enlarged gland with increased 24-hour RAIU measurements.

Three main treatment modalities for Graves disease are medical therapy, radioactive iodine treatment, and thyroidectomy. Selection of therapy depends on age, disease severity, goiter size, and patient preference. Practice patterns differ dramatically across the world, especially regarding the use of radioiodine (it is less common in Europe and especially Japan compared to the United States). The most common initial treatment involves thionamides and often beta blockade. In a small fraction of patients, antithyroid drugs may be the only therapy necessary, but in general, this strategy is considered an impermanent solution. Although the drugs may theoretically be used long term, they are associated with a small but real risk of life-threatening agranulocytosis. Additionally, a number of less severe side effects make tolerance difficult for many, and the recurrence of thyrotoxicosis can be unpredictable. Ultimately, most patients pursue a permanent or "ablative" therapy such as RAI or surgery. Treatment with RAI is very effective and has not been associated with secondary risk of development of a new malignancy, yet there is still hesitancy to use this treatment in young children. RAI may take up to 6 months to provide definitive results and thus antithyroid medications must continue during this period. In a small percentage of patients, a second treatment may be necessary. Although euthyroidism is the most common result of therapy, the effects are slowly progressive such that over 95% of patients become hypothyroid within 10 years following treatment. RAI therapy has been occasionally associated with exacerbation of Graves ophthalmopathy, although the effect is ameliorated by corticosteroids and the early addition of LT_4 posttreatment.[19–21] Because of this concern, patients with severe ophthalmopathy should consider total thyroidectomy instead of RAI to prevent such an exacerbation; however, ultimate resolution of ophthalmopathy is no more likely with operation.

Surgery for Graves disease has the advantage of rapid correction of the hyperthyroid state. The specific operation has typically been either bilateral subtotal thyroidectomy or total thyroidectomy. Subtotal thyroidectomy attempts to remove enough tissue to resolve the hyperthyroidism but leave enough to maintain euthyroidism. Graves disease is dynamic and, thus, remissions and exacerbations are common. This factor makes the determination of exactly how much tissue to leave as a remnant very challenging (typically estimated between 4 and 8 g of thyroid tissue). For these reasons, total thyroidectomy is becoming the preferred operation for treatment of Graves disease with the intention of eliminating the chance of recurrence but accepting hypothyroidism requiring LT_4 therapy.

Toxic Multinodular Goiter. The term *toxic multinodular goiter* (MNG) refers to thyrotoxicosis that is caused by a multinodular goiter that may be of endemic or nonendemic etiology. H.S. Plummer first distinguished toxic adenomatous goiter from Graves disease. Although the eponym "Plummer disease" now more commonly refers to the patient with a solitary toxic nodule (see later), many clinicians still include toxic MNG under the same historical blanket. Thyrotoxicosis may occur as a progression from euthyroid multinodular goiter that was originally TSH dependent, which then progressed to a state of autonomy whereby it is not suppressible with LT_4. After that, it may progress to a toxic state in which distinct nodular areas are overproducing T_4 and T_3 with resultant TSH suppression. Although the cause is clearly distinct, it is possible that some patients included in this diagnostic category actually have Graves disease with nodular degeneration of their diffuse goiter. Patients with toxic MNG, however, are often easily distinguished from those with Graves disease. The typical patient is female and more than 50 years old with a previous history of multinodular goiter. Thyrotoxicosis may be precipitated in a MNG with or without areas of autonomy when an iodide load is provided (Jod-Basedow phenomenon).

Historically, public health efforts to iodinate salt or flour in an iodine-deficient population have caused this to follow over a period of years. This can occur after exposure to iodinated radiographic contrast media, expectorants, or iodide-containing drugs such as amiodarone.

Hyperthyroidism present in a patient with MNG can involve a wide spectrum of severity such that it is not uncommon for a patient having indications for thyroidectomy, for reasons such as continued nodular growth or substernal extension, to have a suppressed TSH in the absence of major functional symptoms. This subclinical thyrotoxicosis is another potential indication for thyroidectomy because it rarely resolves spontaneously and prolonged hyperthyroidism, even when mild, may have deleterious health effects. Thyroidectomy is a relatively common treatment for toxic MNG, with radioiodine treatment representing a less common alternative because it often requires high doses or repeated treatments because of the large goiter size and low radioiodine uptake. Long-term remissions from antithyroid drug treatment are even less common or predictable than in treatment of Graves disease.[22]

Solitary Toxic Adenoma. Patients with thyrotoxicosis and a dominant thyroid nodule may have a toxic adenoma. Nodules usually grow to at least 2 cm in size before hyperthyroidism is clinically evident. As expected, T_3 or T_4 or both are elevated and TSH is suppressed. Thyroid scintigraphy will demonstrate a single "hot" area corresponding to the known nodule with suppression of the remainder of the thyroid substance. FNA is rarely helpful and the incidence of malignancy within these nodules is negligible. Treatment options include ^{131}I RAI therapy or resection. RAI is effective in controlling the hyperthyroidism, but depending on nodule size, may leave behind a palpable abnormality. In particular, younger patients with sizable nodules may choose operation. The resection is typically a hemithyroidectomy and isthmusectomy. The contralateral lobe is often normal and will maintain normal thyroid hormone production after the hyperthyroidism is remedied.

Hypothyroidism

Primary hypothyroidism can arise from intrinsic thyroid disease, iatrogenic thyroid removal or destruction, and antithyroid drug effects. Secondary hypothyroidism can also occur from failure of thyrotropic function (via TSH) of the pituitary gland because of disease, removal, or destruction of that gland as well. Rarely, tertiary hypothyroidism can occur with destructive disorders of the hypothalamus via decreased production of thyrotropin-releasing hormone. The most common cause of primary hypothyroidism in adult patients is Hashimoto thyroiditis. In large part, hypothyroidism is straightforward to address with exogenous LT_4 therapy, with the exception of the patient with thyroid hormone resistance. As defined by hypothyroidism itself, the role for surgical therapy is limited. A structural thyroid disorder associated with the hypothyroidism, however, may be an indication for thyroidectomy (e.g., goiter).

Thyroiditis

A summary of conditions causing a painful neck mass is delineated in Table 75.1. Inflammatory conditions of the thyroid are a disparate family of conditions that require surgical therapy in the minority of situations. However, they can be quite prevalent in patients undergoing evaluation for thyroid surgery and a thorough understanding is required to avoid diagnostic and therapeutic misadventures.

Hashimoto Thyroiditis. Also known as chronic thyroiditis, autoimmune thyroiditis, and lymphocytic thyroiditis, this condition was described by Hashimoto in 1912 as struma lymphomatosa based on the histologic findings. It affects approximately 10% of the general population and is the most common cause of both goiter and hypothyroidism in the United States. Although it can occur at nearly any age, the peak is from age 30 to 60. Female-to-male preponderance is as high as 9:1. It is clearly an autoimmune condition and there is a moderate genetic predisposition, associated with human leukocyte antigen (HLA)-DR3, -DR5, and -B8. The disease prevalence is increased in iodine-sufficient regions and this may be because immunogenicity of the thyroglobulin molecule increases with the degree of iodination. The histologic changes are characterized by lymphocytic infiltration with fibrosis and germinal centers. Some follicular cells may undergo metaplasia to Hürthle cells. The typical presentation is that of a painless diffuse goiter in a young woman discovered on physical examination associated with or without hypothyroidism. Patients often note a sense of fullness in, or awareness of, the region of the thyroid. When the associated goiter is large, compressive symptoms of dysphagia or dyspnea may occur. The goiter is typically firm and rubbery and slightly "bumpy" with prominent lateral lobes. Nodular disease can and does occur in a gland affected by Hashimoto disease and needs to be investigated with FNA to rule out coexisting malignancy, typically papillary cancer or, rarely, thyroid lymphoma. Some data suggest that Hashimoto disease may actually be a risk factor for papillary thyroid cancer.[23] Thyroid autoantibody titers are elevated, TPOAb primarily and TgAb secondarily. In approximately 5% of patients, a transient phase of hyperthyroidism, termed "Hashitoxicosis," occurs at the onset of disease and the subsequent pattern in thyroid function changes are nearly indistinguishable from that of silent thyroiditis. Many patients are hypothyroid, but they may be euthyroid at the time of presentation. If so, approximately 5% per year will progress to hypothyroidism.[24] For the majority of patients, treatment of Hashimoto thyroiditis is limited to LT_4 therapy in those with hypothyroidism. Surgery is indicated in patients with large goiters, significant compressive symptoms, local symptoms refractory to LT_4 therapy, or the inability to rule out malignancy (typically in the setting of nodules or rapid growth).

Painless or Postpartum Thyroiditis. Sporadic silent (painless) thyroiditis and postpartum thyroiditis are known as destruction-induced thyroiditities and are probably variants of

TABLE 75.1 **DIAGNOSIS**

DIFFERENTIAL DIAGNOSIS OF THE PAINFUL NECK MASS

THYROIDAL CAUSES
Acute thyroiditis
Subacute thyroiditis
Acute thyroid cyst (hemorrhage into cyst or nodule)
Rapidly enlarging thyroid carcinoma
Painful Hashimoto thyroiditis
Radiation thyroiditis
NONTHYROIDAL CAUSES
Infected thyroglossal duct cyst
Infected branchial cleft cyst
Infected cystic hygroma
Cervical adenitis
Globus hystericus (no mass palpable)

Adapted from Farwall AP, Braverman LE. Thyroiditis. In: Randolph GW, ed. *Surgery of the Thyroid and Parathyroid Glands*. Philadelphia, PA: WB Saunders; 2003:49.

ENDOCRINE

the same process, distinguished only by the relationship to pregnancy.[25] Along with subacute thyroiditis, these conditions are characterized by the onset of thyrotoxicosis and a goiter, and low 24-hour RAIU. Even excluding postpartum cases, there is a female predominance by 2:1 and the age range of affected patients is broad. The cause appears to be autoimmune, but the genetic predisposition is low. There is no fever or malaise and the goiter is painless but persistent. Thyroid autoantibody titers are often high, and the erythrocyte sedimentation rate (ESR) is usually normal. Thyroid function is dynamic and follows a pattern similar to that of subacute thyroiditis with the abrupt onset of thyrotoxicosis followed by a period of euthyroidism, then hypothyroidism. Permanent hypothyroidism is fairly common. A 24-hour RAIU is very low (usually $<5\%$), consistent with a thyroid gland that is damaged on the cellular level. At the histologic level, lymphocytic infiltration is present along with destruction of follicular cells. If it is pregnancy associated, it is likely to relapse with future pregnancies. If symptoms of thyrotoxicosis are significant, β-adrenergic–blocking drugs may be used, but antithyroid drugs are not appropriate because the gland is not hyperfunctioning at the follicular cell level. If LT_4 therapy is instituted during the hypothyroid phase for symptomatic relief, it can be withdrawn after 6 to 9 months to determine if recovery has occurred.

Subacute Thyroiditis. Subacute thyroiditis is a common form of thyroiditis that affects women more often than men by a 5:1 ratio and often in the age group of 20 to 60. There are a number of synonymous terms, such as de Quervain thyroiditis, giant cell thyroiditis, pseudogranulomatous thyroiditis, subacute painful thyroiditis, and subacute granulomatous thyroiditis. The cause is not entirely certain, but it appears to be virally related. There may be moderate genetic predisposition. A prodrome consistent with an upper respiratory viral infection is very common. The patient often has fever and malaise and an exquisitely painful and firm goiter that is also transient. The goiter is usually unilaterally dominant, and the patient may have pain that radiates to the ipsilateral ear. Giant cells (which may also be observed on FNA, thus supporting the diagnosis) and granulomas often infiltrate the thyroid. It is common to identify a dynamic picture of thyroid function with subclinical or obvious thyrotoxicosis followed by hypothyroidism, which may occasionally be permanent. Consistent with follicular cell destruction, serum Tg levels may be elevated. Antithyroid antibodies may be present in low titers and the ESR is often high. A 24-hour RAIU is usually quite low ($<5\%$). Management is similar to painless thyroiditis in that beta-blockers may be used, but antithyroid medications are not useful. Salicylates or nonsteroidal anti-inflammatory drugs (NSAIDs) are adequate to control pain in most cases, with the occasional need for oral glucocorticoids. Although the course of disease can be protracted for weeks or months, relapse is rare and management is usually limited to management of symptoms.

Amiodarone-induced Thyrotoxicosis or Thyroiditis. Although the significance of amiodarone-induced thyrotoxicosis or thyroiditis is usually related to the thyrotoxicosis induced by the Jod-Basedow mechanism, increased understanding of the condition has led to the realization that it often includes a component of destructive thyroiditis as well (common in the United States), especially when background iodine deficiency is not a factor.[26] The antiarrhythmic drug amiodarone is 37% iodine by weight and the iodine load can induce thyrotoxicosis. Amiodarone therapy results in thyrotoxicosis in 3% of patients in iodine-sufficient regions and up to 10% of patients in iodine-deficient regions.[27] In addition, the drug inhibits 5′-deiodinase. Medical treatment of the hyperthyroidism is difficult because of both the long half-life of the drug and the decompensation in cardiac function related to underlying heart disease. Two types of amiodarone-induced hyperthyroidism can occur, but distinction between the types can be clinically difficult. Type I is iodine induced and is more common in iodine-deficient areas (type Ia is often associated with preexisting multinodular goiter). In general, amiodarone should be stopped and thionamides may be variably effective. A 24-hour RAIU may be normal or elevated in iodine-deficient areas (allowing that therapeutic possibility), but in iodine-sufficient areas (type Ib is often associated with Graves disease), 24-hour RAIU is decreased. Type II, defined primarily by destructive thyroiditis, usually occurs in iodine-sufficient areas and can be self-limited. Decreased thyroid parenchymal blood flow on color flow Doppler imaging is typical. A 24-hour RAIU is typically very low and serum interleukin-6 may be elevated. Corticosteroids are used therapeutically and, if tolerated, beta-blockers as well. If hyperthyroidism is severe in either type I or II, thyroidectomy may be required to resolve the thyrotoxicosis and allow continuation of amiodarone. Some recommend iopanoic acid before thyroidectomy, which markedly inhibits peripheral conversion of T_4 to T_3. Because of the cardiac decompensation, thyroidectomy may need to be done under local anesthesia and sedation to avoid the risks of general anesthesia.

Acute Thyroiditis. Acute thyroiditis refers to a rare suppurative condition caused by bacterial organisms. It may occur in children or young adults (approximately age 20 to 40 years) with equal sex predisposition and no evidence of genetic predisposition. Patients with acquired immunodeficiency syndrome (AIDS) may be at risk for this condition. A clinical prodrome, usually a viral or bacterial upper respiratory infection, may occur and the patient is often affected by a significant fever and malaise and may have radiating pain to the region of the ipsilateral ear. *Staphylococcus aureus* and *Streptococcus pyogenes* are the most common pathogens. A painful but ultimately transient goiter may be evident, which often is a thyroidal or perithyroidal abscess. The patient usually remains euthyroid and antithyroid antibody titers are normal. ESR may be elevated. If a 24-hour RAIU scan is performed, it is often normal but uptake may be focally decreased in the region of active infection. Bacterial infection of the thyroid may occur via hematologic spread from a distant site or local infiltration from other head and neck infections. If acute thyroiditis is related to a fistulous communication with the pyriform sinus, the condition may recur repeatedly. It is the potential for abscess formation or pyriform sinus fistula that makes this a disease that occasionally requires surgical intervention even if FNA is able to determine the causative organism and if appropriate parenteral antibiotics are instituted.

Riedel Thyroiditis. Also known as Riedel struma or invasive fibrous thyroiditis, this rare disorder affects mainly women (by a ratio of 4:1) and usually occurs between the ages of 30 and 60. The cause is unknown and a genetic predisposition is not apparent. The patient presents with a painless but persistent, and often progressive, goiter. Patients are usually euthyroid at presentation but may eventually become hypothyroid. They may have detectable antithyroid antibody titers and a normal ESR. If obtained, the 24-hour RAIU is often normal or somewhat decreased. Physical examination reveals an exceptionally firm goiter often described as "woody." Most commonly, this is a diffuse, bilobar process. Histologically, the disease is characterized by extensive fibrosis, which may progress to a point of compression of adjacent structures such as the trachea and esophagus. Riedel thyroiditis is often accompanied by other equally mysterious focally sclerotic conditions such as retroperitoneal fibrosis, mediastinal fibrosis, retro-orbital fibrosis, and sclerosing cholangitis.[28] Because of its infiltrative nature, it is important to differentiate Riedel thyroiditis from thyroid carcinoma. FNA is often inadequate and open biopsy may be required. If substantial compression exists, surgery is often required to relieve these symptoms. Extensive resection is often unsafe or impossible, and wedge resections, especially of the isthmus, may be very effective in relieving symptoms. Medical therapy, including corticosteroids, methotrexate, or tamoxifen, may have a positive impact in the chronic setting.[29]

NODULAR THYROID DISEASE AND GENERAL TREATMENT CONSIDERATIONS

Nontoxic Multinodular Goiter

From a world health perspective, endemic goiter is still a significant issue. Endemic goiters are caused by dietary iodine deficiency, which ultimately is also responsible for endemic cretinism—another major world health issue. Goitrogenic substances found in diets may also be contributory. Iodine deficiency in a region is addressed over time by iodination of dietary components (e.g., salt, bread flour, or vegetable oil).

In endemic goiter, T_4 levels may be normal or decreased, whereas T_3 levels are normal or often increased. This reflects an adaptive regulatory mechanism by which the thyroid preferentially shifts production to the more biologically potent T_3. Exogenous thyroxine therapy will induce a decrease in goiter size in roughly 80% of patients treated. Resection may be indicated for large size, increase in size while on T_4, or compression of the trachea, esophagus, or superior vena cava.

In most developed countries, the term *goiter* generically refers to the group of diseases causing thyroid enlargement in patients not affected by iodine deficiency. In common usage, *goiter* typically refers to patients with nodular goiter. Asymptomatic multinodular goiter is common, and if reasonable assurance that the goiter is not harboring a malignancy can be obtained by FNA, thyroidectomy is not usually indicated. Sometimes, because of the number of nodules of significant size (>1 cm), repeated FNA during longitudinal observation becomes impractical. Patients may grow frustrated with the process of multiple FNAs and elect to undergo thyroidectomy to simplify management. Compressive symptoms involving the airway or esophagus are also an indication for thyroidectomy. A multinodular goiter causing subclinical or obvious thyrotoxicosis (toxic multinodular goiter) should also be removed. Total thyroidectomy is the procedure of choice because of the significant chance for recurrent nodular degeneration of the thyroid remnant after subtotal thyroidectomy and the attendant increase in morbidity during reoperation. If a goiter develops in a substernal position, thyroidectomy is warranted because of the inability to monitor continuing growth in the mediastinum. If tracheal compression develops gradually, it may be largely asymptomatic until a critical point of narrowing is reached, which inhibits passage of air in a sudden and catastrophic manner. Because all of the important attachments to the thyroid parenchyma remain in the neck, even very large substernal goiters can be removed through a cervical incision. Less than 5% will require partial sternotomy for full removal.[30]

Solitary or Dominant Thyroid Nodule

Nodular thyroid disease is very common, whereas thyroid malignancy is relatively rare. The prevalence of thyroid nodules is approximately 4% to 7% in the general population; however, thyroid nodules are in fact present in up to 60% of patients undergoing autopsy. In contrast, the population incidence of thyroid cancer has increased from 3.72 to 12.08 cases per 100,000 person-years.[31] This increase is only partially explained by improved surveillance. Appropriately identifying patients with malignancy who require operation while appropriately avoiding operation for the majority of patients with benign, noncompressive nodules can be a difficult task.

When assessing a patient with a solitary thyroid nodule, the physician should first query factors in the history that may indicate the likelihood of benign or malignant disease. A new thyroid nodule that occurs at the extremes of age is more likely to be malignant than one that occurs in the third through seventh decades. The risk of a solitary thyroid nodule in a child under 14 being malignant may be as high as 50%.[32] Patient gender itself does not generally confer risk of malignancy, and the fact that thyroid cancer occurs in a greater number of women than men is related somewhat to the increased prevalence of nodular thyroid disease in women. A new thyroid nodule that occurs after the age of 60, however, is more likely to be malignant in a man than in a woman.

Many factors apparent on physical examination or imaging can also be used to assess the potential for malignant disease in the patient with a thyroid nodule. The consideration that nodular disease is uninodular (e.g., solitary) instead of multinodular has traditionally implied that the former situation is more concerning for malignancy. Especially in the era of thyroid US, this distinction is overemphasized because at least half of nodules considered solitary by clinical examination are ultimately found to be a dominant nodule within a multinodular goiter. It is mostly a practical consideration that the dominant nodule (largest or most apparent) of a multinodular gland is the one that dictates subsequent clinical decision making. The characteristics of a nodule assessed by physical examination (size, firmness, texture) have a limited ability to predict malignancy. Significant fixation to surrounding tissues can heighten the level of concern. Associated lymphadenopathy in the central or lateral cervical compartments is certainly concerning for potential malignancy. Although many patients with benign thyroid disease describe hoarseness or a change in voice, this is often largely subjective and is of limited concern unless accompanied by objective hoarseness and ipsilateral recurrent laryngeal nerve paralysis. Thyroid functional status can be important in two ways. First, if the nodule is truly solitary and the patient is hyperthyroid, it may be a toxic autonomous nodule. If this is confirmed by nuclear scintigraphy, the risk of malignancy in this nodule is negligible. If the patient is chronically hypothyroid (likely from Hashimoto disease), a firm, rapidly enlarging, indistinct nodule raises the possibility of the presence of an extranodal lymphoma or anaplastic thyroid cancer.

A critical question in assessing any patient with a thyroid nodule is whether any history of radiation exposure exists. At least 90% of radiation-associated thyroid cancers are of the papillary type. Typical exposures to radiation in the 1940s and 1950s included external beam irradiation treatment for acne, tinea capitis, external otitis, recurrent tonsillitis, or neonatal thymic enlargement. In the current era, excessive diagnostic radiation or high-dose therapeutic irradiation (e.g., treatment of lymphoma or head and neck malignancies) is responsible for relevant exposures. The association is well documented and there appears to be a linear relationship between the dose of radiation and the risk for thyroid cancer, with even a higher risk among those exposed at a young age.[33] The typical latent period between exposure and clinically evident cancer appears to be in the 3- to 8-year range. It is not clear when, if ever, the risk is no longer present. Cases appear to increase for up to three decades after exposure and then begin to tail off. Another source of radiation exposure to the thyroid gland is nuclear fallout, related to either atomic weapons or nuclear power plant accidents, such as Chernobyl in 1986, which exposed 1.5 million people in southern Belarus and northern Ukraine. This acute γ-radiation exposure is likely the main risk factor, but longer-term exposure to diverse radioisotopes of iodine that secondarily contaminate the regional water and food supplies may also be contributory.

Another critical question to investigate is whether a family history of thyroid cancer or associated conditions exists. The key issue is to uncover a family history of medullary thyroid cancer, which suggests the potential for an inherited syndrome such as familial medullary thyroid carcinoma or multiple endocrine neoplasia type 2. Papillary thyroid cancer, however, may have a familial association as well, either independently or, more commonly, associated with Cowden syndrome or Gardner syndrome (familial adenomatous polyposis).

In most situations, extensive thyroid function testing is not necessary and a TSH is all that is required. After initial clinical assessment, thyroid nodular disease is often assessed by US. Relevant factors include the size of the nodule and other sonographic characteristics previously explained. Also important is whether the nodule is truly solitary or whether there are additional nodules, especially in the contralateral lobe, which may affect the specific surgical recommendations. Although it is not uncommon for patients to undergo thyroid scintigraphy, its utility is actually very limited and should not be routinely used to evaluate thyroid nodules. The only helpful role is to determine the specific nature of a nodule in a patient with hyperthyroidism. The additional diagnostic information provided by knowing the nodule is "cold" or "photopenic" is very limited, especially in the era of US and FNA, which can characterize the potential for malignancy to a much greater degree. Although smaller cysts may resolve with aspiration, recurrence is very likely if the cyst is 4 cm or greater and, consequently, resection should be considered.

FNA is the cornerstone of diagnostic evaluation of the thyroid nodule. It can reliably identify colloid nodules, benign nodular hyperplasia, thyroiditis, papillary thyroid carcinoma (PTC), medullary thyroid carcinoma, and anaplastic thyroid carcinoma. FNA may suggest an extranodal lymphoma, but usually more tissue for diagnosis and flow cytometry is required. FNA can also classify nodules as follicular lesions or Hürthle cell lesions. These lesions are indeterminate and currently require at least partial thyroidectomy (e.g., lobectomy) to determine whether it is a follicular (or Hürthle cell) adenoma or follicular (or Hürthle cell) carcinoma. Determination of malignancy in these lesions can be made only by the demonstration of capsular or vascular invasion. FNA should have a false-positive rate of 0% to 0.5% and a false-negative rate of 0% to 5%. The potential for a nondiagnostic interpretation is directly related to the number of follicular cells recovered for analysis. This is ultimately related to technique and the number of needle passes performed. US guidance can help ensure that the biopsy results are representative of the nodule of interest.

Standard disposable needles ranging in size from 23 to 27 gauge and 10-mL syringes are used. The target nodule is located using ultrasound guidance while multiple passes through the most concerning appearing solid portions of the nodule are made. An average of three separate biopsy maneuvers is reasonable practice. The technique does not rely heavily on aspiration or suction as the name might imply. The ideal sample remains mostly in the needle hub and barrel before expelling it onto a slide or into fixative for cytologic preparation. Current limitations require that decisions based on FNA are contingent on the cytologic appearance. It is likely that in the near future, however, specific molecular markers or gene expression data will be identified that will allow specific testing of FNA specimens to indicate risk of malignancy.

THYROID MALIGNANCY AND GENERAL TREATMENT CONSIDERATIONS

General Considerations

Thyroid cancers exhibit a wide spectrum of behavior, from the inconsequential, occult, well-differentiated thyroid carcinoma to the nearly uniformly fatal undifferentiated anaplastic cancers. Fortunately, at least 98% of thyroid cancers are well differentiated and long-term prognosis is excellent. Although the general treatment strategy for thyroid carcinomas is familiar (surgical resection, staging of disease, appropriate adjuvant treatments, and secondary screening or follow-up), a number of unique points are emphasized below.

Tumor Classification

Differentiated thyroid cancers are of follicular cell origin (papillary thyroid carcinoma and its variants, follicular thyroid carcinoma, and Hürthle cell carcinoma) or parafollicular (C-cell) origin (medullary thyroid carcinoma). There is a spectrum of dedifferentiation that exists between these tumors and undifferentiated cancers such as anaplastic carcinoma. Tumors such as insular or tall cell variants exist along this spectrum. In a general sense, prognosis is directly related to the degree of differentiation. A number of classification systems exist. The American Thyroid Association (ATA), the Armed Forces Institute of Pathology (AFIP), and the World Health Organization (WHO) all consider papillary thyroid cancers (including classic papillary carcinoma, mixed papillary-follicular variants, follicular variants, and follicular thyroid carcinomas [FTC]) as differentiated thyroid cancer. Still, some disagreement exists about the classification of Hürthle cell carcinomas (HCCs). In general, the ATA and WHO consider HCC as a subtype of follicular thyroid carcinoma, although the AFIP does not. Support for considering HCC as a subtype of follicular thyroid carcinoma includes the histologic demonstration of the transition of follicular to Hürthle cells, an intact TSH receptor adenylate cyclase system in Hürthle cells, and the ability of Hürthle cells to produce thyroglobulin and thus maintain Tg positivity on immunohistochemical staining.[34] Other characteristics, however, such as higher oncogene expression in HCC than FTC and the general impression that HCC can display a more aggressive clinical course than FTC cause some to classify HCC tumors outside the FTC family.[35] Medullary thyroid carcinoma is also a differentiated thyroid carcinoma but is of parafollicular cell origin.

Papillary Thyroid Carcinoma. Papillary thyroid carcinoma (PTC) accounts for approximately 80% of thyroid carcinomas. Although it occurs across a wide spectrum of ages from childhood to the elderly, the peak incidence begins in the third and fourth decades of life. It is more common in females than males. It is especially prevalent in iodine-sufficient regions of the world. Papillary carcinoma arises from the follicular cells, is characterized by papillary architecture, and is often associated with calcifications, psammoma bodies, squamous metaplasia, and fibrosis. Cytology is diagnostically important and typical findings include large, overlapping nuclei that are optically clear (known as Orphan Annie nuclei) and intranuclear grooves. As a whole, the prognosis is excellent, especially in those patients with tumors that define a low risk for recurrence. Greater than 30% of PTC is multicentric and found throughout the thyroid. Although multifocality does not signify a worse prognosis, this characteristic, in part, influences the rationale for total thyroidectomy discussed later. The incidence of cervical lymph node metastases varies across series and is influenced by whether lymphadenectomy is performed for prophylactic or therapeutic reasons. In general, it approximates 30% to 40%. Distant metastases occur in 2% to 14% of patients with PTC.[34] At least 70% of PTC can take up radioiodine and thus, RAI scanning is an important part of the treatment strategy.

Variants. A follicular variant of papillary thyroid carcinoma essentially combines the histologic and architectural appearance of follicular tumors with the cytologic features of papillary carcinoma. In terms of treatment and biologic behavior, this variant behaves in the same manner as classic PTC. The dilemma caused by this variant is based on the fact that, in contrast to classic PTC, it is very difficult to diagnose on frozen section analysis. It is often interpreted as a follicular lesion with the final diagnosis deferred until formal histopathology can be completed to identify the atypical features. More aggressive variants of papillary carcinoma include tall cell and columnar types, which also exist along the spectrum of dedifferentiation.

Microcarcinoma. PTCs less than 1 cm in size are considered microcarcinomas (occult or incidental tumors). They may be multifocal and are usually clinically silent until thyroidectomy is performed for another indication. Although they are by definition malignant, this group of tumors requires a different set of considerations based on "nonmalignant" biologic behavior and patient outcome. Prognosis is exceptionally good, with a 0.4%
4 cause-specific mortality rate.[36] If such a solitary microcarcinoma is found after lobectomy, adequate treatment has already been rendered and completion thyroidectomy or radioiodine scanning or both are not typically indicated. Somewhat in contrast, if these microcarcinomas are diagnosed preoperatively, which may be difficult because of their small size, thyroid resection is usually recommended. Some groups, however, have chosen to follow these patients closely with ultrasound. Approximately 70% do not increase in size significantly.[37] Nonetheless, these tumors cannot be completely discounted. Metastases to central neck (level VI) lymph nodes occur, and it is not uncommon for PTC to be diagnosed by biopsy of a lateral compartment lymph node even if the associated primary tumor is not apparent. If these patients are treated with total thyroidectomy, very careful histologic sectioning will be required to find the associated primary tumor, which may be as small as 1 mm.

Follicular Carcinoma.

FTC accounts for approximately 10% to 20% of all thyroid cancers. Again, there is a female-to-male predominance, and the incidence begins to increase in the
5 fifth decade of life. Determination that a follicular lesion/neoplasm is a carcinoma is contingent not only on the specific cellular architecture but also on the findings of vascular and capsular invasion. This determination is rarely able to be made on frozen section and the information is often not available until final histopathology results.[37] FTC is often more advanced at the time of diagnosis compared with PTC. It is more common for FTC to be locally infiltrative of muscles and perithyroidal vascular structures. Because of this difference in stage at diagnosis, the overall 10-year survival for patients with FTC is slightly worse than for those with PTC, but when patients are matched for age and stage with PTC, this difference largely disappears.[38] In contrast to PTC, follicular cancers are usually solitary. Approximately one third of patients with FTC have distant metastases at the time of diagnosis and the pattern is consistent with a mechanism of hematogenous spread, with lung and bone most often being involved. Lymph node involvement is limited to only about 10% of patients. Importantly, at least 80% of FTC will take up radioiodine.

Minimally Invasive Follicular Carcinoma. Follicular neoplasms with demonstrable capsular invasion but no vascular invasion are classified as minimally invasive follicular cancers. These patients have an excellent prognosis, conceptually equivalent to patients with incidental papillary microcarcinomas. If such a tumor is found after hemithyroidectomy, there is no reason for most patients to undergo completion thyroidectomy and radioiodine scanning as would be recommended for true FTC.[39]

Hürthle Cell Carcinoma.

Malignant Hürthle cell neoplasms account for approximately 5% of thyroid carcinomas and, in general, occur in patients slightly older than those with PTC or FTC. Despite their relatively uncommon nature, HCC enters diagnostic consideration frequently because Hürthle cells are frequently present on FNA cytology from thyroid nodules. Patients with Hashimoto disease or colloid nodules commonly demonstrate Hürthle cells; however, it is the nodule that contains almost entirely Hürthle cells that raises concern for HCC. If HCC is suggested by FNA cytology, a diagnostic thyroid lobectomy at the minimum is required to definitively establish the nature of the tumor. Hürthle cell adenomas (neoplasms with no evidence of capsular or vascular invasion) certainly exist, but occasionally a tumor that is otherwise histologically compatible with a Hürthle cell adenoma is found to be associated with lymph node or distant metastases. For these reasons and considering the perspective that HCC may behave more aggressively, many surgeons advocate total thyroidectomy for any Hürthle cell neoplasm.[40] HCC is more prevalent in women than men and is more often associated with lymph node metastases and distant metastases than PTC and FTC in general. Although it is a DTC likely of follicular cell origin, very few HCC tumors take up radioiodine (approximately 10%). For this reason, and taking into consideration the more aggressive nature of HCC, complete surgical resection is especially important in this disease. Therefore, total thyroidectomy is often combined with central compartment lymphadenectomy and perhaps modified radical neck dissection if lateral compartment lymph node involvement is evident.

Medullary Carcinoma.

MTC arises from the parafollicular C cells and accounts for about 5% to 7% of all thyroid malignancies. Approximately 75% occur in a sporadic fashion and 20% to 25% may be familial (multiple endocrine neoplasia [MEN] types 2A and 2B, as well as familial medullary thyroid carcinoma [FMTC]). These are autosomal dominant inherited endocrinopathies related to a group of specific mutations on chromosome 10q11.2 (RET proto-oncogene) (Table 75.2). The familial forms of MTC have different degrees of aggressiveness related to the specific syndrome. Familial MTC has the most indolent course, whereas MEN 2B has the most aggressive course, with MEN 2A intermediate to these. Most sporadic MTC is relatively slow growing and may be quite indolent. Typically, these patients do not present before 30 years of age. A subset of patients with sporadic MTC have a much more aggressive course. This variability in biologic behavior accounts for the overall 10-year survival rate of approximately 50%. Overall, MTC is more aggressive than other DTCs and is more likely to metastasize. At least 50% to 75% of patients with sporadic MTC have nodal metastases already present at the time of diagnosis. To some degree this is correlated with tumor size and contralateral cervical metastases are conceptually systemic disease.[41] Distant metastases may involve the liver, lungs, and bone. FNA can be diagnostic for medullary cancer, especially if the specimen is stained for calcitonin. MTC is unique in that calcitonin is a very specific tumor marker used for diagnosis and to guide subsequent follow-up. Most MTCs also make carcinoembryonic antigen (CEA).

Approximately 20% of patients thought to have sporadic MTC may in fact be index cases of familial MTC. Therefore, any patient with a new diagnosis of MTC should have genetic testing for the RET proto-oncogene mutations associated with MEN 2 and FMTC. Appropriate screening for pheochromocytoma (which would be treated prior to thyroidectomy) and hyperparathyroidism are required.

The treatment strategy for MTC is somewhat distinguished from that of DTC of follicular cell origin. Because of the high likelihood of lymph node metastases and the fact that there is no effective adjuvant therapy (MTC does not take up radioiodine), more extensive initial surgical resection is warranted. With few exceptions, the appropriate operation for MTC is a total thyroidectomy with central compartment lymphadenectomy (level VI). Because intraoperative assessment of lymph node involvement is relatively inaccurate, consideration should be given to ipsilateral modified radical neck dissection as well. Some authors even advocate bilateral modified radical neck dissection initially or very extensive "microdissection."[42] Because of technical issues and an unclear influence on prognosis, this approach has not met with widespread acceptance.

TABLE 75.2 CLASSIFICATION

DISEASE PHENOTYPES RELATED TO MUTATION OF THE RET PROTO-ONCOGENE

PHENOTYPE	GENETIC DEFECT	CLINICAL FEATURES	PREVALENCE (%)
MEN 2A (60%)	Germline mutations in cysteine codons of extracellular and transmembrane domains of RET	Medullary thyroid carcinoma	100
		Pheochromocytoma	10–60
		Hyperparathyroidism	5–20
MEN 2B (5%)	Germline activating mutation in tyrosine kinase domain or RET	Medullary thyroid carcinoma	100
		Pheochromocytoma	50
		Marfanoid habitus	100
		Mucosal neuromas (gut) and ganglioneuromatosis	100
FMTC (35%)	Germline mutations in cysteine codons of extracellular or transmembrane domains of RET	Medullary thyroid carcinoma	100

FMTC, familial medullary thyroid carcinoma; MEN, multiple endocrine neoplasia.

It is common for patients to have persistent hypercalcitoninemia even after an extensive initial operation. Most patients have a subsequent indolent course, although some patients will progress more rapidly. Experience with remedial neck dissections in an attempt to render the patient normocalcemic has generally been disappointing and requires an appropriate search for distant metastases before operation is planned. This may include extensive imaging tests such as CT scanning, ultrasound, somatostatin receptor scintigraphy scanning, selective venous sampling for calcitonin levels, and laparoscopy to investigate for hepatic metastases.[43] For most patients, the strategy of observation by clinical examination, biochemical markers, and imaging tests is adopted with interval reassessment for resectable regional and metastatic disease. When this is detected, especially if it is in a location whereby ongoing growth could cause significant morbidity (e.g., tracheoesophageal groove), resection can be offered. Hepatic resections for diffuse metastatic disease are inadequate, whereas such an operation may be considered for isolated bulky metastatic deposits. Chemotherapy has largely been ineffective, although trials with selective and nonselective tyrosine kinase–inhibiting drugs are ongoing. Progress has been limited by difficulty in establishing the desired degree of RET inhibition. Somatostatin analogues can be helpful in slowing the growth of the tumor in some patients. External beam radiotherapy may be useful for locoregional tumor control, especially in those patients with evidence of locally aggressive tumor behavior[44]; however, this should not be employed until appropriate surgical options are exhausted.

Provocative testing (e.g., pentagastrin or calcium-stimulated calcitonin levels) was until recently a standard screening maneuver to identify patients with heritable forms of MTC. Now, these familial forms of MTC, or at least the risk of developing the manifestations, may be diagnosed with the aid of genetic testing for mutations in the RET proto-oncogene. The best use of such testing is to identify the specific mutation in affected family members, which then guides testing of the progeny. When other kindred members with the mutation are identified, thyroidectomy may be performed before malig-
6 nancy develops. Worldwide cooperation has allowed for genotype/phenotype correlation based on youngest age of diagnosis according to the specific mutation identified. Recommendations for the age of prophylactic thyroidectomy to be performed are based on this information (Table 75.3). The thyroid resection must be absolutely complete because the region of thyroid that remains after a near-total or subtotal thyroidectomy is the region that is most densely populated with C cells. If hyperparathyroidism is present and enlarged parathyroid glands are encountered at operation, they should be removed as well. A subtotal parathyroidectomy or total parathyroidectomy and autotransplantation (similar to that which would be considered for MEN 1) are excessive options for the parathyroid disease encountered in MEN 2A and, instead, resection may be guided by morphologic changes in the parathyroid glands. Children identified to have MEN 2B should undergo thyroidectomy and central compartment lymph node dissection as soon as the diagnosis is made, definitely by 2 years of age, but even by 6 months of age as guided by mutation analysis.[45] If MTC is already evident at the time of diagnosis (as opposed to only C-cell hyperplasia), patients should also undergo ipsilateral neck dissection. There is no consensus about at which age patients confirmed to have FMTC mutation should undergo thyroidectomy, although this decision may be guided by the specifics of the family history.

Anaplastic Carcinoma. Although it formerly accounted for a larger fraction of thyroid malignancies, undifferentiated or anaplastic cancer now accounts for just 1% to 2% of thyroid cancers. Most commonly, this occurs in elderly patients with a long-standing history of a goiter. There is significant evidence to infer that most anaplastic thyroid cancers of the spindle cell or giant cell type arise from transformation of DTC, especially follicular and papillary carcinoma. Anaplastic thyroid carcinoma is one of the most aggressive and rapidly

TABLE 75.3 TREATMENT

AGE OF PROPHYLACTIC THYROIDECTOMY BASED ON GENOTYPE/PHENOTYPE CORRELATION

Level 3 HIGHEST RISK (codons 883, 918, 922)
Total thyroidectomy and CCLND by age 6 mo
Level 2 INTERMEDIATE RISK (codons 611, 618, 620, 634, 804)
Total thyroidectomy ± CCLND by age 5 y
Level 1 LOWEST RISK (codons 609, 768, 790, 791, 804, 891)
Total thyroidectomy individualized by kindred history, calcitonin levels, earliest reported age for genotype.

CCLND, central compartment lymph node dissection.

lethal malignancies known. Nearly all are too far advanced at the time of diagnosis to be adequately treated by currently available therapies. The diagnosis may be made by appropriate clinical suspicion (rapidly growing firm thyroid mass) and FNA. If not, excisional biopsy at operation may be required. If airway compromise is present or impending, operation may include debulking and tracheostomy. Occasionally, a small anaplastic cancer is found that is confined to the thyroid or is minimally invasive to surrounding tissues (e.g., trachea). Especially in a young patient, aggressive resection may be legitimately considered. The long-term prognosis for these patients, however, is usually limited by metastatic disease, which may not be apparent at diagnosis. Adjuvant or primary palliative therapy consisting of chemotherapy and external beam radiotherapy is frequently employed. It is common to see a measurable response early in therapy, but eventual tumor progression is typical. Unfortunately, the overall impact is often very limited, so no single regimen has become a standardized approach. Although doxorubicin, Taxol, and other drugs have been tried, doxorubicin and cisplatin are more frequently used. Radiation therapy is often given in combination with chemotherapy by using a hyperfractionated routine such as two daily fractions, 5 days per week, until a total of 40 Gy is delivered to the cervical compartments and superior mediastinum.[46] Most often, chemotherapy and radiotherapy follow an operation performed for diagnosis or airway protection, but such a regimen may also be used occasionally as neoadjuvant therapy before an attempt at resection is undertaken.

Thyroid Lymphoma. Primary thyroid lymphomas are rare tumors that account for fewer than 5% of thyroid malignancies. The majority are classified as non-Hodgkin lymphomas of B-cell origin. Nearly all arise from within a background of Hashimoto thyroiditis. Most patients present with a rapidly enlarging thyroid mass and compressive symptoms (e.g., dyspnea, dysphagia, choking, pain) and have a history of hypothyroidism (Fig. 75.7A, B). Because the rarity of the diagnosis has limited the number of prospective randomized trials that have evaluated the optimal treatment for thyroid lymphomas, most recommendations are based solely on retrospective case series. Patients with diffuse large B-cell lymphoma are generally treated with combination chemotherapy (cyclophosphamide, doxorubicin, vincristine, and prednisone [CHOP]) followed by radiation therapy for stage IE or IIE disease.[47] In those with pure marginal zone B-cell lymphoma, some have advocated for single-modality therapy (surgery or radiation) given its more indolent behavior, but this still remains controversial and would be limited to those with stage IE nonbulky disease.[48] There are limited reports on the use of immunochemotherapy (rituximab + CHOP) for thyroid non-Hodgkin lymphoma (NHL), but given the central role that this combination has in the general treatment of many extranodal B-cell NHLs, it may be of value to extrapolate those results when considering therapy for thyroid lymphoma.[49] The diagnosis must be firmly established. Modern immunophenotypic analysis often allows this to occur with a small amount of tissue obtained by FNA or core needle sampling. Open biopsy is still occasionally required to establish the diagnosis. Substantial surgical resection is often not required, but there is a subset of patients with significant compressive symptoms from respectable tumors who benefit from palliative total or subtotal thyroidectomy.[50]

7

Metastases to the Thyroid Gland. Isolated metastases from other primary cancers can occur in the thyroid gland, although they are rare. The most common tumor type to do so is renal cell carcinoma, although it can occur from breast, lung, and gastrointestinal carcinomas, as well as melanoma and sarcoma.[51]

ENDOCRINE

Staging of Thyroid Malignancy

A number of patient factors have been investigated to predict risk and prognosis for patients with DTC, such as age, gender, tumor size, involvement of lymph nodes, extrathyroidal invasion, tumor grade or histologic features, and completeness of surgical removal. Although there are differences in these systems, in general, they agree that younger patients with smaller tumors have an excellent prognosis with decreased risk of recurrence and death compared with older patients. One early prognostic staging scheme was the AGES system (*a*ge, histologic *g*rade, *e*xtrathyroidal disease [invasion and distant metastases], and tumor *s*ize).[52] Although useful, the scheme was later modified to exclude histologic tumor grade because there was not uniform agreement on DTC grading by pathologists. Another system is the AMES system (*a*ge, *m*etastases, *e*xtrathyroidal invasion, and tumor *s*ize), which was originally described for patients with DTC.[53] The main criticism of this scheme is that it was defined based on a patient population that included both papillary and follicular thyroid carcinomas, and that there was no accounting for those patients with low-risk versus high-risk FTC. Another

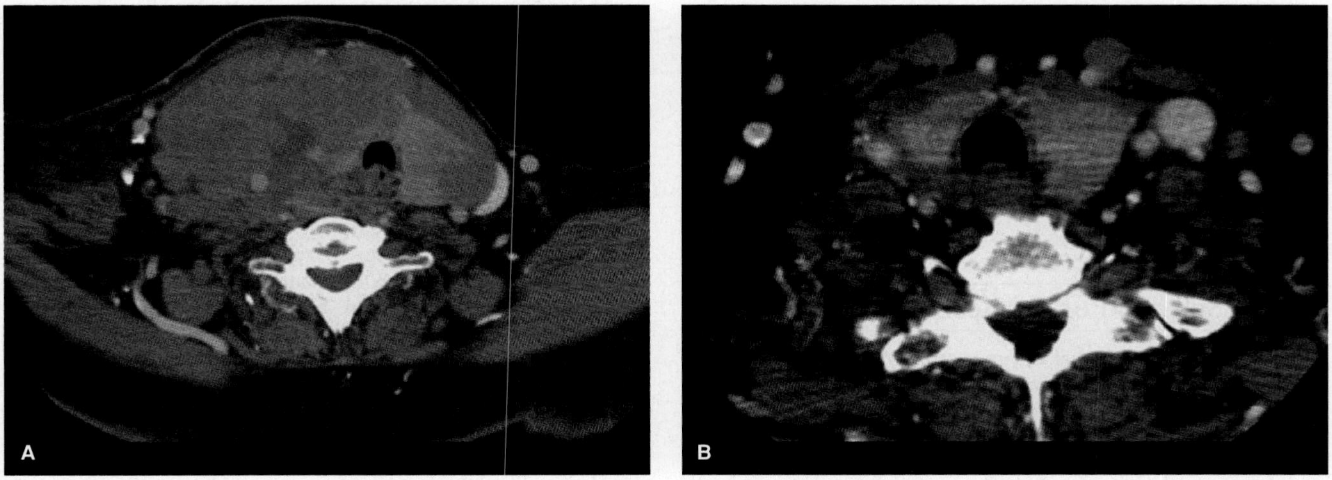

FIGURE 75.7. **A:** Initial computed tomography (CT) scan of patient with thyroid lymphoma. Note encasement of right carotid artery and deviation of trachea by tumor. **B:** Repeat CT scan of patient's neck after receiving chemotherapy.

TABLE 75.4 **STAGING**

TUMOR, NODE, METASTASIS STAGING SYSTEM FOR DIFFERENTIATED THYROID CARCINOMA (PAPILLARY AND FOLLICULAR TYPES)

STAGE	AGE <45 Y	AGE >45 Y
I	T_{any} N_{any} M0	T1 N0 M0
II	T_{any} N_{any} M1	T2 N0 M0
III		T3 N0 M0 or T1–3 N1a M0
IV		T4 N0 M0 or T4a N1a M0 or T1–3 N1b M0
IVB		T4b Any N M0
IVC		T_{any} N_{any} M1

T1, <2 cm; T2, 2–4 cm, >4 cm; T3, >4 cm; T4a, extrathyroidal extension; T4b, invades prevertebral fascia or encases carotid artery or mediastinal vessels.
N0, no nodal involvement; N1, regional nodal metastases; N1a, metastasis to level 6 lymph nodes; N1b, metastasis to unilateral, bilateral, or contralateral cervical or superior mediastinal lymph nodes; M0, no distant metastases; M1, distant metastases.

useful prognostic system is the MACIS scoring system (*m*etastases, *a*ge, *c*ompleteness of resection, extrathyroidal *i*nvasion and distant metastases, and tumor *s*ize). This system calculates a composite score based on these factors, then stratifies prognosis in proportion to these scores (<6.00 is very low risk and >8.00 represents greatly increased risk).[54] The European Organization for Research on Treatment of Cancer (EORTC) based its prognostic scoring system on a multivariate analysis of patients with all types of thyroid malignancies and found that patients with scores of less than 50 had a 5-year survival rate of 95%, whereas those with scores greater than 109 had a 5-year survival rate of 5%.[55] This system has not been universally adopted for use in DTC because the high-risk, poor-prognostic group contained a large fraction of patients with anaplastic thyroid cancer. Although medullary thyroid carcinoma is considered a differentiated cancer, its biologic behavior differs sufficiently from DTC of follicular cell origin such that its inclusion in this staging system also confounds the prognostic ability somewhat. The familiar TNM system (*t*umor size, *n*odal status, distant *m*etastases) is also used to provide prognostic information for patients. When used for thyroid cancer, the TNM system has been modified to account for the risk-reducing influence of low patient age (Table 75.4). This system can provide consistency when comparing patients across different series. This system, like all prognostic scoring systems, still has limited utility in guiding initial treatment decisions (e.g., extent of resection) because the important components are unable to be determined until after resection.

Selection of Surgical Procedure

Although thyroidectomy as a primary treatment for DTC is well accepted to be both effective and safe, some controversy persists about the extent of thyroidectomy necessary for low-risk
8 patients. The advantages of total thyroidectomy for all DTCs of follicular cell origin include (a) removal of multifocal intrathyroidal tumors; (b) use of radioiodine to localize and treat small amounts of residual normal thyroid tissue, and more importantly, regional or distant metastases; and (c) after radioiodine ablation, use of serum thyroglobulin as a sensitive marker of persistent or recurrent disease. If only thyroid lobectomy is performed, radioiodine treatment is usually not optimal because of the increased avidity for RAI of normal thyroid tissue compared to thyroid cancer tissue, and thyroglobulin measurements also lose their utility. After treatment with lobectomy, recurrence develops in the contralateral lobe in about 7% of patients, and half go on to die of thyroid cancer.[34] It has been difficult to demonstrate a survival advantage related to extent of thyroidectomy, but a recent study comparing extent of thyroid surgery in patients with PTC showed that patients with PTC greater than 1 cm who underwent total thyroidectomy had a significantly lower risk of recurrence and lower mortality compared with those undergoing thyroid lobectomy.[56]

Lymphadenectomy

Lymphadenectomy for thyroid cancer has been advocated for patients with clinically positive lymph nodes, or those found to have micrometastases by FNA or frozen section. In general, regional lymph node metastases are found in 30% to 40% of patients, although wider ranges have been reported (20% to 90%).[57–59] A compartment-oriented approach to lymphadenectomy is currently preferred over the previously advocated technique of "berry picking" (removing only grossly positive nodes) if central compartment lymph node dissection and modified radical neck dissection can be performed without significantly
9 increasing morbidity or mortality. Prophylactic central compartment lymph node dissection (CCLND) is an emerging standard in the treatment of papillary thyroid cancer because lymph node involvement is both common and difficult to treat with a remedial operation in the future. Metastatic disease to central compartment lymph nodes can be found in up to 60% of patients with lymph nodes that appear clinically negative. If CCLND is to be added to the routine performance of total thyroidectomy to treat low-risk PTC, it must be assured that the incidence of RLN injury and hypoparathyroidism is not increased, because it can be technically difficult to maintain parathyroid vascularization with a thorough level VI lymphadenectomy. For the first time, in 2006, the American Thyroid Association management guidelines[59] suggested routine CCLND be considered for patients with papillary thyroid cancer and Hürthle cell cancer if it can be done without increasing morbidity. Properly performed CCLND at the initial operation may diminish the higher risk of damage to nerves or parathyroid glands that is associated with reoperation for a local recurrence. Current evidence suggests that prophylactic CCLND in PTC may decrease disease recurrence with limited data to suggest a survival benefit.[60] Residual subclinical disease, as indicated by postoperative serum thyroglobulin levels, can be decreased using this strategy.[61]

Preoperative Ultrasound

In recent years, US has taken on a more important role for preoperative planning, especially in patients with thyroid cancer. The use of palpation alone to rule out metastases to the central or lateral neck lymph nodes is highly unreliable. Preoperative US should be obtained in all patients with thyroid nodules, and particular attention should be paid to evidence of lymphadenopathy accompanied by concerning imaging appearances (lack of a hilar line, microcalcifications, loss of the typical flattened ovoid shape). A number of institutions have reported detection by US of nonpalpable lymph node metastases in 24% to 39% of patients with papillary thyroid cancer diagnosed by FNA.[62–64] Even in patients with palpable lymphadenopathy, US can alter the extent of lymphadenectomy in approximately 40% of patients undergoing initial or reoperative surgery.[63]

Radioiodine Therapy

Radioiodine may be used in two ways after thyroidectomy: low doses are used to demonstrate remaining thyroid tissue or metastatic disease as part of a diagnostic radioiodine scan, whereas higher doses are used for ablation or therapy. The timing of the initial postoperative scan is dictated by the physiology of T_4 and the fact that remnant thyroid tissue or DTC must be stimulated by elevated levels of TSH to take up RAI. Although no precise threshold has been established, a general consensus is held that the TSH should be at least 30 mIU/mL. Traditionally, the rise in TSH level has been achieved by withdrawal of supplemental thyroxine. The half-life of thyroxine is approximately 7 days, so TSH values are significantly elevated 4 to 5 weeks after total thyroidectomy or withdrawal from thyroxine treatment. To minimize the duration of hypothyroid symptoms, patients can be managed with T_3 until 2 weeks prior to scanning, as T_3 has a much shorter half-life (8 to 12 hours) than T_4.

The use of recombinant human TSH (rhTSH) for ^{131}I uptake scans has become more readily accepted for use in patients with thyroid cancer.[65] The use of rhTSH avoids the long withdrawal from thyroid hormone replacement and development of troublesome hypothyroid symptoms that occurs over several weeks. It also allows for the opportunity to follow some patients with rhTSH-stimulated serum thyroglobulin levels without performing ^{131}I whole-body scans, especially as ^{131}I whole-body scans are used less frequently and reliance on high-frequency US for early identification of recurrent tumor is now the more favored modality for long-term surveillance of patients with thyroid cancer.

Radioiodine therapy is a rational therapy for DTC because most tumor cells retain the ability to concentrate radioiodine. Additionally, many studies have shown a decreased rate of recurrence and increased disease-specific and overall survival when ^{131}I is used. In 1997, Mazzaferri reported a threefold decrease in the incidence of distant metastatic disease and local tumor recurrence in tumors treated with radioiodine.[66] In another study, the risk of cancer death was decreased by half (from 16% to 8%) when radioiodine was used after surgery compared with hormone replacement or external radiation alone.[67] Many clinicians agree that radioiodine is beneficial and well tolerated, but this is certainly not a unanimous opinion.

There are no prospective randomized trials with subgroup analysis to shed light on the dilemma of which patients should receive postoperative radioiodine. The argument is further complicated by the fact that because of the multiple staging and prognostic systems used, comparisons across studies can be difficult. Postoperative RAI is commonly used, even for lower-risk cancers, and thyroid remnant ablation is generally accepted as part of the postoperative treatment of patients who have undergone total or near-total thyroid excision for DTC. It is not entirely evident that using postoperative radioiodine to "clear" a whole-body scan will impact the patient's recurrence or survival. Perhaps the most appropriate approach is to select patients for postoperative radioiodine therapy based on individual risk assessment.

Several situations exist wherein it is generally agreed that ^{131}I is not beneficial. If the cancer is undifferentiated and does not concentrate radioiodine, ablative or therapeutic efforts will be futile. Intrathyroidal cancers smaller than 1 cm without evidence of metastatic disease are not treated with radioiodine because of their exceptionally low potential for local or distant recurrence. Finally, if only a lobectomy is performed, radioiodine ablation is possible only 25% of the time because of the volume of residual tissue and its avidity for RAI.

Proponents of ^{131}I therapy advocate that all patients who meet the indications for total thyroidectomy should undergo postoperative radioiodine therapy because it should not be assumed that even negligible amounts of residual thyroid tissue in the neck are tumor-free. Importantly, more than 30% of well-differentiated thyroid cancers will be multifocal, multicentric, or microscopic. In these settings, postoperative remnant thyroid ablation after total thyroidectomy serves to destroy remaining thyroid tissue that may harbor occult microscopic carcinoma. Additionally, it is less confounding to manage and follow a patient without residual thyroid tissue. Without competing normal tissue, visualization of local or distant recurrences on follow-up ^{131}I scanning is possible. If large amounts of thyroid tissue remain after the initial operation, the bright emission of ^{131}I from the residual thyroid will obscure any small areas of local recurrence. Significant residual thyroid tissue will not allow TSH to rise, which can decrease the uptake of ^{131}I during postoperative imaging. Finally, thyroglobulin measurements are the most specific tests for recurrent cancer when no normal thyroid tissue or TgAbs are present and when the Tg level is measured during a period of hypothyroidism—none of which is feasible when a remnant of the thyroid gland remains. It follows, therefore, that only patients with a small cancer (<1 cm) carrying an exceptionally low risk of recurrence should be routinely excluded from consideration of treatment with postoperative radioiodine therapy.

External Beam Radiotherapy

If gross residual disease remains after surgical resection, external radiotherapy may be considered to assist with local tumor control. This is most often a consideration with tumors that invade the tracheoesophageal axis. This occurrence is frequent with poorly differentiated tumors, but it certainly can complicate DTC as well. It has also been considered for patients with extensive lymph node involvement that is characterized by extranodal invasion of metastatic tumor. Bone metastases are rarely treated completely with ^{131}I and, thus, external beam radiotherapy may be effective.[68] Complications include skin erythema and desquamation and tracheoesophageal mucositis.

Thyroid-stimulating Hormone Suppression

Levothyroxine therapy to suppress TSH levels is commonly recommended for patients with differentiated thyroid carcinoma because TSH is considered a trophic factor for these cancers. The efficacy is inferred from uncontrolled retrospective studies. It is important to individualize the degree of suppression in patients, balancing the risk of recurrence with the risks of subclinical hyperthyroidism (e.g., osteoporosis, cardiac arrhythmias). Many physicians will suppress TSH to undetectable levels (<0.1 mIU/L) in high-risk cancers and less severely (TSH 0.1 to 0.5 mIU/L) in low-risk cancers. If a patient has no evidence of recurrence and has extremely low or undetectable thyroglobulin levels 5 to 10 years after treatment, it may be appropriate to lessen the degree of TSH suppression.

New Horizons and Future Directions

Adjunctive treatment of DTC is dependent on the uptake and concentration of radioiodine by cancerous thyroid tissue. Problematically, it has been reported that as many as 30% of advanced DTC will eventually dedifferentiate, and a portion of these cancers will lose the ability to concentrate radioiodine. Molecular testing of thyroid tumors has become available to help characterize thyroid tumors in pre- and postoperative settings. Several well-documented molecular mutations have been identified in various types of thyroid cancer.[69] Translocations of partner genes RET/PTC (1, 2, or 3) are found in up to 40% of papillary carcinomas and are more common in radiation-induced tumors. PAX8-PPARγ translocations can be identified in up to 40% of follicular carcinomas. Mutation of the BRAF gene in papillary carcinomas is estimated to be present in up to 60% of cases. Sorafenib, a multikinase inhibitor that inhibits serine/threonine kinase Raf (BRAF and c-RAF) and RET, c-kit, and receptor tyrosine kinases (platelet-derived growth factor receptor [PDGFr] and vascular endothelial growth factor receptor [VEGFr]), inhibits tumor growth in anaplastic thyroid carcinoma xenografts with BRAF mutations. In an orthotopic mouse model with PTC harboring a RET/PTC1 mutation, tumor volume was reduced by 94%, and those with BRAF mutations saw a 54% reduction in tumor volume.[70] Eventually, preoperative molecular testing of fresh or frozen tissue samples (FNA or surgical specimen) will be used to differentiate benign from malignant thyroid nodules. Molecular profiling of thyroid tumors for pre- or postoperative use is a burgeoning field that will likely become commonplace in the next 5 to 10 years and will likely deliver other signaling pathways that could be used for targeted therapeutics.

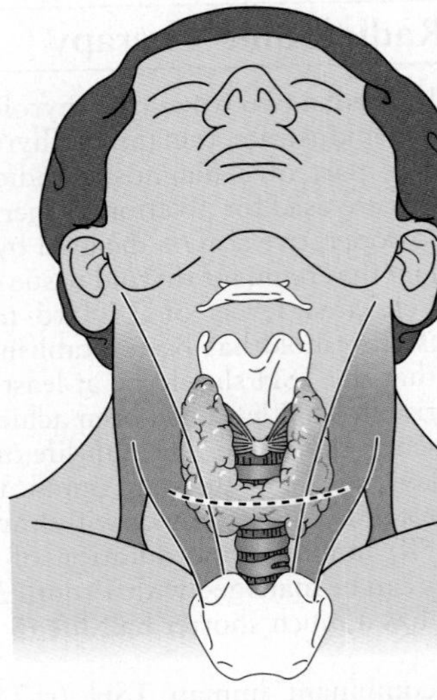

FIGURE 75.8. With the patient's neck extended, the line above indicates the appropriate site of incision for thyroid resection. Camouflage within an existing skin crease is often possible.

THYROID SURGERY

After an inauspicious beginning, thyroid surgery has improved remarkably over the last century. Substantial improvements began with the discovery of anesthesia, antisepsis, and improved hemostasis. With these improvements, Albert Theodor Billroth, Theodor Kocher, and William Halsted were able to make substantial technical contributions and lay the foundation of thyroidectomy as a safe and efficacious operation.

Technique

There is little, if any, place for subtotal lobar resections (e.g., nodulectomy) and only an occasional role for isthmusectomy alone. Total thyroid lobectomy is the total extracapsular removal of the lobe and the isthmus while preserving both parathyroid glands, the recurrent laryngeal nerve, and the external branch of the superior laryngeal nerve. Total thyroidectomy is merely a matter of performing a total thyroid lobectomy on the contralateral side during the same operation. Subtotal thyroidectomy is intentional subtotal lobar resection, either unilaterally or bilaterally, and is rarely indicated. Near-total thyroidectomy involves intentionally leaving a minor amount of thyroid tissue to protect the insertion of the RLN and the superior parathyroid gland. When properly performed, it is essentially interchangeable with total thyroidectomy when considering surgical outcomes. For most thyroid procedures, the patient is placed in a supine position or a semi-Fowler position with the arms tucked to the side. A support is placed transversely under the shoulders to aid in extending the neck. This extension must not be too extreme or a significant amount of postoperative pain may occur in the occipitocervical region. After skin preparation, a curvilinear incision is made approximately one to two fingerbreadths above the clavicular heads and not any higher than the level of the cricoid cartilage (Fig. 75.8). If possible, it should be disguised in an existing skin crease. Subplatysmal skin flaps are raised to the level of the thyroid cartilage above, the sternal notch below, and laterally to the sternocleidomastoid muscles. The midline raphe is opened to expose the anterior trachea and the isthmus. The sternohyoid and sternothyroid are then the separated from the thyroid lobe. It is this maneuver that leads to division of the thyroid sheath layer as the paraesophageal space is entered. The middle thyroid veins are divided and ligated.

If a pyramidal lobe is present, it is mobilized and divided from the fibrous tissue in any remaining thyroglossal duct tract. The anterior suspensory ligament is divided to mobilize the superior aspect of the isthmus.

Thyroid resection should be performed in a logical orderly sequence as follows: (a) exposure of the thyroid gland, (b) capsular dissection of the superior pole of the thyroid with preservation of the external branch of the superior laryngeal nerve, (c) capsular dissection of the inferior pole of the thyroid lobe with preservation of the inferior parathyroid gland, and (d) capsular dissection of the posterolateral aspect of the thyroid gland with preservation of the superior parathyroid gland and the recurrent laryngeal nerve. Unequivocal identification of the recurrent laryngeal nerve occurs early in the operation and involves progressive exposure superiorly as the dissection continues in order to identify and avoid any extralaryngeal RLN branches. Figure 75.9 indicates the plane of dissection relevant to steps (c) and (d).

Dissection of the superior pole of the thyroid must take place in the plane directly adjacent to the thyroid capsule after the largely avascular space between the pole and the cricothyroideus muscle is dissected. To do so more proximally along the superior pole vessels imperils the EBSLN. This nerve is not always identified during thyroidectomy, but it can nearly always be preserved by utilizing this technique. Unequivocal identification of the recurrent laryngeal nerve is mandatory. This is done by many surgeons as direct dissection and exposure in the proximal portion of the RLN before its intersection

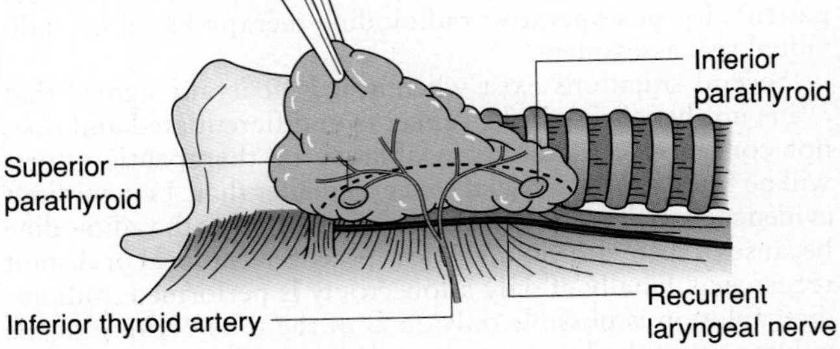

FIGURE 75.9. The capsular dissection necessary to preserve well-vascularized parathyroid tissue and a fully functional recurrent laryngeal nerve begins in the area outlined above.

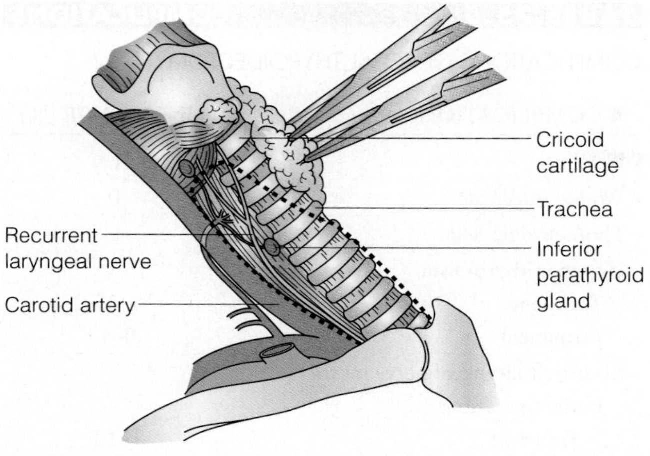

FIGURE 75.10. Boundaries showing high-risk area of central compartment dissection involving the vascular supply to the Superior and inferior parathyroid glands and the recurrent larygeal nerve. (Adapted from Grodski S, Cornford L, Sywak M, et al. Level VI lymph node dissection for papillary thyroid cancer: Surgical technique. *ANZ J Surg.* 2007;77(4):203–208.)

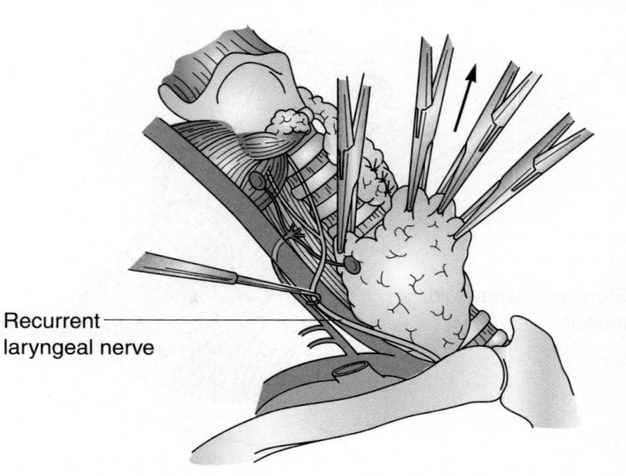

FIGURE 75.12. The recurrent laryngeal nerve is carefully repositioned laterally and medially as needed to dissect all fibrofatty and lymphatic tissue from level VI structures. (Adapted from Grodski S, Cornford L, Sywak M, et al. Level VI lymph node dissection for papillary thyroid cancer: Surgical technique. *ANZ J Surg.* 2007; 77(4):203–208.)

with the ITA and the ligament of Berry. The safety provided by this maneuver, however, is contingent on continuing the exposure more distally along the nerve as it approaches the cricothyroid space, because it is at this point of genu near the ligament of Berry that the nerve is most vulnerable to iatrogenic injury. Another technique of nerve exposure is provided by the close capsular dissection that takes place when the lobe is retracted anteromedially and the terminal branches of the ITA are divided. As the ligament of Berry is divided, the genu of the nerve is identified and protected. Although visual identification of the RLN remains the "gold standard," palpation can aid in the process. The nerve is often easy to palpate as a slightly firm linear structure in the tracheoesophageal groove with the lobe retracted anteromedially. Although helpful in guiding early dissection, this technique cannot supplant visual confirmation.

The ability to routinely preserve well-vascularized parathyroid tissue during thyroidectomy is mandatory for surgeons performing these operations. Normal parathyroid tissue is subtle and may be difficult to identify. It can be distinguished from surrounding fat by a slight brownish color and a fine

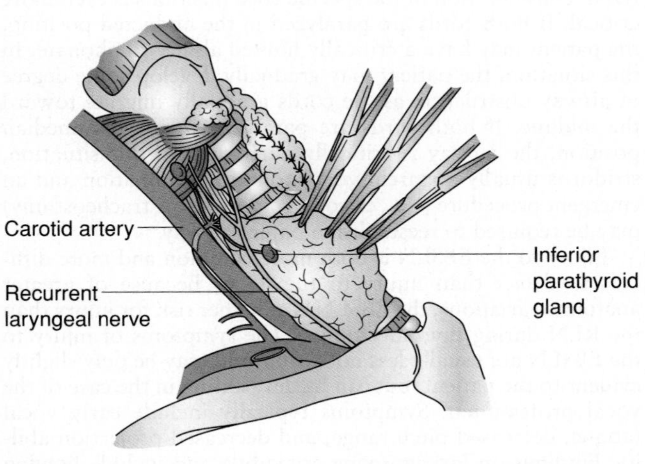

FIGURE 75.11. The recurrent laryngeal nerve is carefully isolated and dissected free from surrounding tissue in level VI. (Adapted from Grodski S, Cornford L, Sywak M, et al. Level VI lymph node dissection for papillary thyroid cancer: Surgical technique. *ANZ J Surg.* 2007; 77(4):203–208.)

capillary vascular pattern that is not present in the adjacent fat or thymus.

The central compartment of the neck contains level VI lymph nodes and is bordered by the hyoid bone above, the innominate artery below, and the carotid arteries laterally. Removal of these lymph nodes is a critical component of an operation to treat medullary thyroid carcinoma or in the case of clinically evident lymphadenopathy. To perform a CCLND, the prelaryngeal (Delphian) lymph node(s) adjacent to the pyramidal lobe is excised. After the ipsilateral thyroid lobe is completely resected, the lateral and medial extent of dissection is defined to mobilize the level VI nodes. The superior parathyroid gland must be carefully preserved on its vascular supply as the inferior parathyroid gland is often embedded in the nodal tissue to be removed and must be autotransplanted (Fig. 75.10). The cervical portion of the RLN is completely exposed in a retrograde direction using gentle dissection to divide the overlying fibrofatty and nodal tissue (Fig. 75.11). It is important to remove the nodes located posterior to the RLN and anterior to the prevertebral fascia in addition to the more easily removed nodes located anterior to the RLN (Fig. 75.12). If the nerve is adequately mobilized, this can usually be accomplished en bloc and the nodes may even be left attached to the inferior pole of the thyroid. The block of nodal tissue is then removed down to the level VII nodes at the superior margin of the innominate vein. In order to accomplish this, the cervical thymus must be removed. If unable to be preserved on a branch of the ITA, the inferior parathyroid is autotransplanted into the adjacent sternocleidomastoid muscle (Fig. 75.13).

Minimally invasive techniques for thyroid surgery have evolved significantly in some centers. Attention to detail and knowledge of anatomy is critical when performing operations through very small incisions or even from an entirely endoscopic approach. Patient selection for these approaches is extremely important for success. In general, patients with known Hashimoto thyroiditis, those who have undergone previous surgery within the central neck, or those with large thyroid nodules having a volume greater than 30 mL are usually not considered candidates for minimally invasive approaches for thyroidectomy. Minimally invasive approaches are most often used for patients with indeterminate thyroid nodules undergoing diagnostic thyroid lobectomy. Although more extensive oncologic procedures including CCLND can be performed with these techniques, the most appropriate indications remain benign thyroid disease.[71]

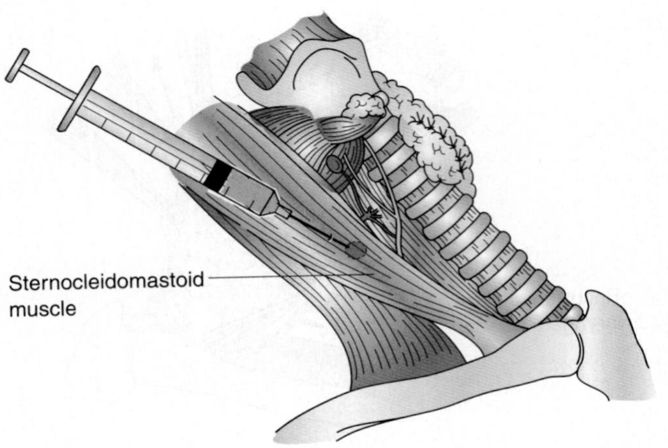

FIGURE 75.13. It is not uncommon for the inferior parathyroid gland(s) to become devascularized during dissection of the central compartment. Devascularized parathyroid tissue should be retrieved, minced into 1-mm pieces, and autotransplanted to the ipsilateral sternocleidomastoid muscle. (Adapted from Grodski S, Cornford L, Sywak M, et al. Level VI lymph node dissection for papillary thyroid cancer: Surgical technique. *ANZ J Surg*. 2007;77(4):203–208.)

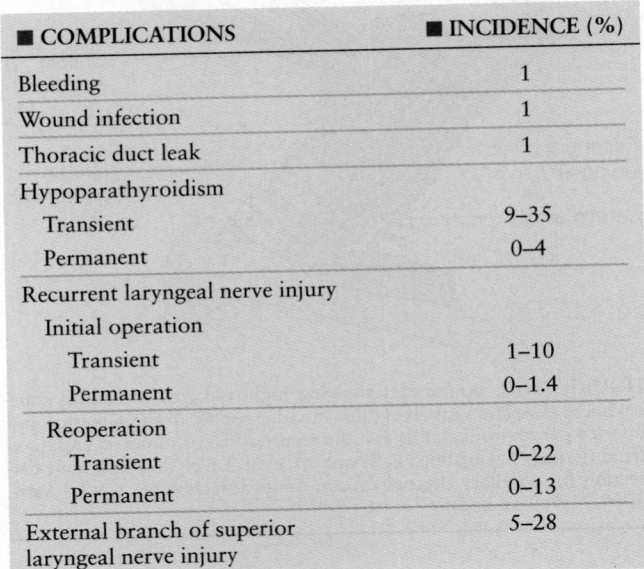

TABLE 75.5 **COMPLICATIONS**

COMPLICATIONS OF TOTAL THYROIDECTOMY

■ COMPLICATIONS	■ INCIDENCE (%)
Bleeding	1
Wound infection	1
Thoracic duct leak	1
Hypoparathyroidism	
Transient	9–35
Permanent	0–4
Recurrent laryngeal nerve injury	
Initial operation	
Transient	1–10
Permanent	0–1.4
Reoperation	
Transient	0–22
Permanent	0–13
External branch of superior laryngeal nerve injury	5–28

Three general techniques have been developed. The largest experience exists for minimally invasive video-assisted thyroidectomy (MIVAT), initially developed by Miccoli et al. The MIVAT procedure uses a 5-mm 30-degree laparoscope to aid visualization of dissection planes, nerves, and parathyroid glands while the procedure is performed through an incision of 2.5 cm or smaller. An electrosurgical device is usually used to ligate and divide vessels. The incision may be less painful and more cosmetically pleasing to patients, but average operating time is slightly longer than conventional thyroid surgery.[72] Slightly different from MIVAT, minimally invasive thyroid surgery (MITS) is done with direct visualization (without video assistance) of critical structures through a small lateral incision (2 to 3 cm). Again, advantages include reduced pain and improved cosmesis with equivalent safety.[73] Largely in Asia, there is an evolving experience with a totally endoscopic approach using multiple 5-mm port sites placed either in the axilla or areola of the nipple to avoid cervical incision and allow dissection with laparoscopic equipment.[74] This places the incision away from the neck in a less noticeable position. Operating time is considerably longer. Morbidity and mortality are not significantly different in experienced hands, but dissemination of this complicated technique has been limited.

Traditional thyroidectomy was developed using standard clamping and tying surgical techniques. Advanced surgical energy instruments for bipolar vessel sealing and ultrasonic scalpels have now been integrated into thyroid resections. The main benefit in thyroidectomy is decreased operative time.[75–77] Most series indicate that complication rates (hematoma, RLN injury, hypoparathyroidism) are comparable to conventional techniques. Heat generation and lateral thermal spread for a particular instrument are critical to understand and may limit safe application near the RLN and parathyroid glands.

Complications

The risk of death or major disability during thyroidectomy should be diminutive. The key outcomes by which to measure the quality of surgical care, especially relevant to total thyroidectomy, include recurrent laryngeal nerve paralysis and hypoparathyroidism (Table 75.5). Although both complications can occur in a self-limited fashion, the persistence or permanence (defined at 6 months after operation) of these complications is a critical measure. For most surgeons, the rate of unintended permanent recurrent laryngeal nerve dysfunction should be no greater than 1% and the rate of permanent hypoparathyroidism should be no greater than 1% to 2%.

Injury to an RLN results in paralysis of the vocal cord it innervates. Depending on the specific branch or combination of branches injured, the cord may remain in a paramedian position (also called cadaveric position) or may remain abducted. If the contralateral cord is able to adduct to the midline or beyond, the patient may have a voice that is not particularly hoarse, but is weak. If the cord is paralyzed in the abducted position, vocal quality is very poor because of the difficulty in approximating the cords during speaking. The patient's cough also has a bovine quality where there is a lack of a sharp, percussive initiation. If both vocal cords are paralyzed, consideration of the specific cord positions is even more critical. If both cords are paralyzed in the abducted position, the patient may have a critically limited ability to phonate. In this situation, the patient may gradually develop some degree of airway obstruction as the cords gradually migrate toward the midline. If both cords are paralyzed in the paramedian position, the airway is critically narrowed. In this situation, stridor is usually apparent very soon after extubation and an emergent procedure (e.g., cricothyroidotomy or tracheostomy) may be required to reestablish a patent airway.

Injury to the EBSLN is both more common and more difficult to detect than injury to the RLN. Because of greater anatomic variations, the EBSLN is at higher risk for injury than the RLN during thyroidectomy.[78] The symptoms of injury to the EBSLN are usually less noticeable and may be only slightly evident to the patient, but can be devastating in the case of the vocal professional. Symptoms typically include early vocal fatigue, decreased pitch range, and decreased projection ability. Findings on laryngoscopy are subtle and include bowing and inferior displacement of the affected vocal cord and rotation of the posterior glottis toward the injured side. Laryngeal videostroboscopy or percutaneous electromyography of the cricothyroideus muscle may be required to detect injury in subtle cases. Because there is no effective treatment for this condition, prevention is extremely important.

Functional monitoring of EBSLN integrity is feasible but somewhat cumbersome and is not routinely employed. If nerve monitoring is employed, the stimulator probe can also be used to demonstrate the location of the EBSLN by observing a motor response in the ipsilateral cricothyroideus muscle. Recurrent laryngeal nerve monitoring is increasingly common in recent thyroid surgery practice. Although the technology has improved to a point that the technique is relatively easy to employ, large studies have failed to detect a major improvement in RLN injury rates (largely related to the low incidence of this complication when thyroidectomy is performed in the proper hands despite the specific technique employed).[79] Even so, RLN monitoring can be very helpful in facilitating nerve identification and protection during a complex reoperation or initial thyroidectomy for very large goiter or aggressive malignancy, even if it will not materially change the chance of injury.[80] Since current technologies are essentially nerve integrity monitors, the information provided (loss of action potential at the vocalis muscle) indicates when an injury has or has not occurred and therefore does not indicate when a nerve is under stress from dissection or traction. Therefore, whether or not RLN monitoring is employed, prevention of injury still requires meticulous and precise surgical technique.

The parathyroid glands are at risk during thyroid resection by virtue of the fact that they are often firmly invested within the thyroid sheath or occasionally even within the thyroid capsule. Inferior parathyroid glands are ultimately supplied by the inferior thyroid artery. Superior parathyroid glands are often served by the inferior thyroid artery but may also have contributions from the superior thyroid artery distribution as well. Ligation of the trunk of the ITA must be avoided to preserve blood supply to the parathyroid glands. Every attempt should be made to mobilize the parathyroid glands away from the thyroid tissue being resected while preserving the blood supply. If the gland appears pale or dark and devascularized, the arterial supply is probably compromised. Such a parathyroid gland is unlikely to survive after the operation and should be immediately autotransplanted. This may be done by mincing the gland into 1-mm pieces and inserting or injecting the pieces into well-vascularized skeletal muscle (e.g., sternocleidomastoid or pectoralis).[81] Even during thyroid lobectomy, meticulous technique must be used to preserve parathyroid viability, even though permanent, or even temporary, hypoparathyroidism is unlikely. With total thyroidectomy, careful dissection is even more critical. Temporary hypoparathyroidism is relatively common and is due to mild devascularization or venous congestion of parathyroid glands during mobilization. Approximately 20% to 40% of patients will have mild temporary hypocalcemia beginning about 12 to 36 hours after operation. If symptomatic, it can be treated with oral calcium or occasionally vitamin D supplements (e.g., calcitriol). Severe symptomatic hypocalcemia can be treated with intravenous calcium gluconate. Temporary hypoparathyroidism complicating thyroidectomy usually resolves over days to weeks, although occasionally it may take months to do so. Hypoparathyroidism that persists longer than 6 months is usually destined to be permanent. The transient hypocalcemia after total thyroidectomy may be worse in the patient with Graves disease because of the increased bone turnover observed with hyperthyroidism; however, recovery is expected and the incidence of permanent hypoparathyroidism should be no higher than in euthyroid patients.

Regardless of the specific extent or technique of thyroidectomy, these complications can largely be avoided or ameliorated by delicate and deliberate surgical technique. A thorough understanding of the function and anatomy, both normal and abnormal, of the thyroid gland, and of the rationale behind various treatment options, is critical to ensure the best outcomes for our patients.

ACKNOWLEDGMENTS

The authors would like to acknowledge the efforts of Jana Mitchell for her administrative assistance with this chapter. The authors have nothing to disclose.

References

1. Gauger P, Delbridge LW, Thompson NW, et al. Incidence and importance of the tubercle of Zuckerkandl in thyroid surgery. *Eur J Surg* 2001;167: 249–254.
2. Sackett W, Reeve TS, Barraclough B, et al. Thyrothymic thyroid rests: incidence and relationship to the thyroid gland. *J Am Coll Surg* 2002;195: 635–640.
3. Pelizzo M, Toniato A, Gemo G. Zuckerkandl's tuberculum: an arrow pointing to the recurrent laryngeal nerve (constant anatomical landmark). *J Am Coll Surg* 1998;187:333–336.
4. Bliss R, Gauger PG, Delbridge LW. Surgeon's approach to the thyroid gland: surgical anatomy and the importance of technique. *World J Surg* 2000;2:891–897.
5. Katz A. Extralaryngeal division of the recurrent laryngeal nerve. *Am J Surg* 1986;152:407–410.
6. Henry J, Audiffret J, Denizot A, et al. The nonrecurrent inferior laryngeal nerve: review of 33 cases, including two on he left side. *Surgery* 1988;104: 977–984.
7. Raffaelli M, Iacobone M, Henry JF. The "false" nonrecurrent inferior laryngeal nerve. *Surgery* 2000;128:1082–1087.
8. Cernea C, Ferraz AR, Nishio S, et al. Surgical anatomy of the external branch of the superior laryngeal nerve. *Head Neck* 1992;14: 380–383.
9. Kupferman ME, Patterson M, Mandel SJ, et al. Patterns of lateral neck metastases in papillary thyroid carcinoma. *Arch Otolaryngol Head Neck Surg* 2004;130:857–860.
10. Machens A, Holzhausen JJ, Dralle H. Skip metastases in thyroid cancer leaping the central lymph node compartment. *Arch Surg* 2004;139: 43–45.
11. Baskin HJ, Cobin RH, Duick DS, et al.; American Association of Clinical Endocrinologists. American Association of Clinical Endocrinologists medical guidelines for clinical practice for the evaluation and treatment of hyperthyroidism and hypothyroidism. *Endocr Pract* 2002; 8:457–569.
12. Scanga DR, Martin WH, Delbeke D. Value of FDG PET imaging in the management of patients with thyroid, neuroendocrine, and neural crest tumors. *Clin Nuc Med* 2004;29:86–90.
13. Davis P, Perrier ND, Adler L, et al. Incidental thyroid carcinoma identified by positron emission tomography scanning obtained for metastatic evaluation. *Am Surg* 2001;67:582–584.
14. Katz SC, Shaha A. PET-associated incidental neoplasms of the thyroid. *J Am Coll Surg* 2008;27:259–264.
15. Boi F, Lai ML, Deias C, et al. The usefulness of 99mTc-SestaMIBI scan in the diagnostic evaluation of thyroid nodules with oncocytic cytology. *Eur J Endocrinol* 2003;149:493–498.
16. Tan G, Gharib H. Thyroid incidentalomas: management approaches to nonpalpable nodules discovered incidentally on thyroid imaging. *Ann Intern Med* 1997;126:226–231.
17. Lennquist S, Jortso E, Anderberg B, et al. Beta blockers compared with antithyroid drugs as preoperative treatment in hyperthyroidism: drug tolerance complications, and postoperative thyroid function. *Surgery* 1985; 98:1141–1146.
18. Alderberth A, Stenstrom G, Hasselgren P. The selective beta 1 blocking agent metoprolol compared with antithyroid drug and thyroxine as preoperative treatment of patients with hyperthyroidism. Results from a prospective randomized study. *Ann Surg* 1987;205:182–188.
19. Tallstedt L, Lundell G, Blomgren H, et al. Does early administration of thyroxine reduce the development of Graves' ophthalmopathy after radioiodine treatment? *Eur J Endocrinol* 1994;130:494–497.
20. Tallstedt L, Lundell G, Torring O, et al. Occurrence of ophthalmopathy after treatment for Graves' hyperthyroidism. The Thyroid Study Group. *N Engl J Med* 1992;326:1733–1738.
21. Bartalena L, Marcocci C, Bogazzi F, et al. Use of corticosteroids to prevent progression of Graves' ophthalmopathy after radioiodine therapy for hyperthyroidism. *N Engl J Med* 1989;321:1349–1352.
22. van Soestbergen M, van der Vijver J, Graafland A. Recurrence of hyperthyroidism in multinodular goiter after long-term drug therapy: a comparison with Graves' disease. *J Endocrinol Invest* 1992;15: 797–800.
23. Repplinger D, Bargren A, Zhang YW, et al. Is Hashimoto's thyroiditis a risk factor for papillary thyroid cancer. *J Surg Res* 2008;150:49–52.
24. Tunbridge W, Brewis M, French JM, et al. Natural history of autoimmune thyroiditis. *Br Med J Clin Res* 1981;282:258–262.
25. Smallridge R, DeKeyser FM, VanHerle AJ, et al. Thyroid iodine content and serum thyroglobulin: cues to the natural history of destruction-induced thyroiditis. *J Clin Endocrinol Metab* 1986;62:1213–1219.

26. Bartalena L, Grasso L, Brogioni S, et al. Serum interleukin-6 in amiodarone-induced thyrotoxicosis. *J Clin Endocrinol Metab* 1994;78:423–427.
27. Harjai K, Licata AA. Effects of amiodarone on thyroid function. *Ann Intern Med* 1997;126:63–73.
28. Violaris N, Windle-Taylor PC. Idiopathic fibrosis of the upper aero-digestive tract. *J Laryngol Otol* 1989;103:333–334.
29. Few J, Thompson NW, Angelos P, et al. Riedel's thyroiditis: treatment with tamoxifen. *Surgery* 1996;120:998–999.
30. White ML, Doherty GM, Gauger PG. Evidence-based management of substernal goiter. *World J Surg* 2008;32:1285–1300.
31. Enewold L, Zhu K, Ron E, et al. Rising thyroid cancer incidence in the United States by demographic and tumor characteristics. *Cancer Epidemiol Biomarkers Prev* 2009;18:784–791.
32. Harness J, Thompson NW, Nishiyama RH. Childhood thyroid carcinoma. *Arch Surg* 1971;102:278–284.
33. DeGroot L, Kaplan EL, McCormick M, et al. Natural history, treatment, and course of papillary thyroid carcinoma. *J Clin Endocrinol Metab* 1990;71:414–424.
34. Kebebew E, Clark OH. Differentiated thyroid cancer: "complete" rational approach. *World J Surg* 2000;24:942–951.
35. Jossart G, Clark OH. Well-differentiated thyroid cancer. *Curr Probl Surg* 1994;31:933–1012.
36. Ito Y, Tomoda C, Uruno T, et al. Papillary microcarcinoma of the thyroid: how should it be treated? *World J Surg* 2004;28:1115–1121.
37. Chen H, Nocol TL, Udelsman R. Follicular lesions of the thyroid. Does frozen section evaluation alter operative management? *Ann Surg* 1995;222:101–106.
38. Emerick G, Duh QY, Siperstein AE, et al. Diagnosis, treatment, and outcome of follicular thyroid carcinoma. *Cancer* 1993;72:3287–3295.
39. van Heerden J, Hay ID, Goellner JR, et al. Follicular thyroid carcinoma with capsular invasion alone: a non-threatening malignancy. *Surgery* 1992;112:1130–1138.
40. Thompson N, Nishiyama RH, Harness JK. Thyroid carcinoma: current controversies. *Curr Probl Surg* 1978;15:1–67.
41. Moley JF, DeBenedetti MK. Patterns of nodal metastases in palpable medullary thyroid carcinoma. Recommendations for extent of node dissection. *Ann Surg* 1999;229:880–887.
42. Tisell L, Hansson G, Jansson S, et al. Reoperation in the treatment of asymptomatic metastasizing medullary carcinoma of the thyroid. *Surgery* 1986;99:60–66.
43. Tung WS, Vessely TM, Moley JF. Laparoscopic detection of hepatic metastases in patients with residual or recurrent medullary thyroid cancer. *Surgery* 1995;118:1024–1029.
44. Fersht N, Vini L, A'Hern R, et al. The role of radiotherapy in the management of elevated calcitonin after surgery for medullary thyroid cancer. *Thyroid* 2001;11:1161–1168.
45. Skinner M, DeBenedetti MK, Moley JR, et al. Medullary thyroid carcinoma in children with multiple endocrine neoplasia types 2A and 2B. *J Pediatr Surg* 1996;31:177–181.
46. Crevoisier R, Baudin E, Bachlot A, et al. Combined treatment of anaplastic thyroid carcinoma with surgery, chemotherapy, and hyperfractionated accelerated external radiotherapy. *Int J Radiat Oncol Biol Phys* 2004;60:1137–1143.
47. Mack LA, Pasieka JL. An evidence-based approach to the treatment of thyroid lymphoma. *World J Surg* 2007;31:978–986.
48. Green LD, Mack L, Pasieka JL. Anaplastic thyroid cancer and primary thyroid lymphoma: a review of these rare thyroid malignancies. *J Surg Oncol* 2006;94:725–736.
49. Dai CW, Zhang GS, Pei MF, et al. Thyroid diffuse large B cell lymphoma (DLBCL) following thyroid medullary cancer: long-term complete remission with R-CHOP therapy. *Ann Hematol* 2009;88:701–702.
50. Sippel R, Gauger PG, Angelos P, et al. Palliative thyroidectomy for malignant lymphoma of the thyroid. *Ann Surg Oncol* 2002;9:907–911.
51. Mirallie E, Rigaud J, Mathonnet M, et al. Management and prognosis of metastases to the thyroid gland. *J Am Coll Surg* 2005;200:203–207.
52. Hay I, Grant CS, Taylor WF, et al. Ipsilateral lobectomy versus bilateral lobar resection in papillary thyroid carcinoma: a retrospective analysis of surgical outcome using a novel prognostic scoring system. *Surgery* 1987;102:1088–1095.
53. Cady B, Rossi R. An expanded view of risk-group definition in differentiated thyroid carcinoma. *Surgery* 1988;104:947–953.
54. Hay I, Bergstralh EJ, Goellner JR, et al. Predicting outcome in papillary thyroid carcinoma: development of a reliable prognostic scoring system in a cohort of 1779 patients surgically treated at one institution during 1940 through 1989. *Surgery* 1993;114:1050–1057.
55. Byar D, Green SB, Dor P, et al. A prognostic index for thyroid carcinoma: a study of the E.O.R.T.C. thyroid cancer cooperative group. *Eur J Cancer* 1979;15:1033–1041.
56. Bilimoria K, Bentrem DJ, Ko CY, et al. Extent of surgery affects survival for papillary thyroid cancer. *Ann Surg* 2007;246(3):375–384.
57. Grebe S, Hay ID. Thyroid cancer nodal metastasis: biologic significance and therapeutic considerations. *Surg Oncol Clin N Am* 1996;5:43–63.
58. Loh K, Greenspan FS, Gee L, et al. Pathological tumor-node-metastasis (pTNM) staging for papillary and follicular thyroid carcinomas: a retrospective analysis of 700 patients. *J Clin Endocrinol Metab* 1997;82:3553–3562.
59. Cooper D, Doherty GM, Haugen BR, et al. Management guidelines for patients with thyroid nodules and differentiated thyroid cancer. *Thyroid* 2006;16(2):109–142.
60. White ML, Gauger PG, Doherty GM. Central lymph node dissection in differentiated thyroid cancer. *World J Surg* 2007;31:895–904.
61. Sywak M, Cornford L, Roach P, et al. Routine ipsilateral level VI lymphadenectomy reduces postoperative thyroglobulin levels in papillary thyroid cancer. *Surgery* 2006;140:1000–1007.
62. Stulak JM, Grant CS, Farley DR, et al. Value of preoperative ultrasonography in the surgical management of initial and reoperative papillary thyroid cancer. *Arch Surg* 2006;141(5):494–496.
63. Kouvaraki MA, Shapiro SE, Fornage BD, et al. Role of preoperative ultrasonography in the surgical management of patients with thyroid cancer. *Surgery* 2003;134(6):946–955.
64. Solorzano CC, Carneiro DM, Ramirez M, et al. Surgeon-performed ultrasound in the management of thyroid malignancy. *Am Surg* 2004;70(7):580–582.
65. Mazzaferri EL, Kloos RT. Using recombinant human TSH in the management of well-differentiated thyroid cancer: current strategies and future directions. *Thyroid* 2000;10(9):767–778.
66. Mazzaferri E. Thyroid remnant 131 I ablation for papillary and follicular thyroid carcinoma. *Thyroid* 1997;7:265–271.
67. Mazzaferri EL, Jhiang SM, Long-term impact of initial surgical and medical therapy on papillary and follicular thyroid cancer. *Am J Med* 1994;97:418–428.
68. Brierley J, Tsang RW. External-beam radiation therapy in the treatment of differentiated thyroid cancer. *Semin Surg Oncol* 1999;16:42–49.
69. Hunt J. Molecular testing in solid tumors. *Arch Pathol Lab Med* 2008;132:164–167.
70. Henderson Y, Soon-Hyun A, Kang Y, et al. Sorafenib potently inhibits papillary thyroid carcinomas harboring RET/PTC1 rearrangement. *Clin Cancer Res* 2008;14(15):4908–4914.
71. Miccoli P, Minuto MN, Ugolini C, et al. Minimally invasive video-assisted thyroidectomy for benign thyroid disease: an evidence-based review. *World J Surg* 2008;32:1333–1340.
72. Miccoli P, Berti P, Raffaelli G, et al. Comparison between minimally invasive video-assisted thyroidectomy and conventional thyroidectomy: a prospective randomized study. *Surgery* 2001;130:1039–1043.
73. Alvarado R, McMullen T, Sidhu SB, et al. Minimally invasive thyroid surgery for single nodules: an evidence-based review of the lateral mini-incision technique. *World J Surg* 2008;32:1341–1348.
74. Jeryong K, Jinsun L, Hyegyong K, et al. Total endoscopic thyroidectomy with bilateral breast areola and ipsilateral axillary (BBIA) approach. *World J Surg* 2008;32:2488–2493.
75. Franko J, Kish KJ, Pezzi CM, et al. Safely increasing the efficiency of thyroidectomy using a new bipolar electrosealing device (LigaSure) versus conventional clamp-and-tie technique. *Am Surg* 2006;72:132–136.
76. Siperstein A, Berber E, Morkoyun E. The use of the harmonic scalpel vs. conventional knot tying for vessel ligation in thyroid surgery. *Arch Surg* 2002;137:137–142.
77. Cardon C, Fajardo R, Ramirez J. A randomized, prospective, parallel group study comparing the harmonic scalpel to electrocautery in thyroidectomy. *Surgery* 2005;137:337–3341.
78. Teitelbaum B, Wenig BL. Superior laryngeal nerve injury from thyroid surgery. *Head Neck* 1995;17:36–340.
79. Dralle H, Sekulla C, Haerting J, et al. Risk factors of paralysis and functional outcome after recurrent laryngeal nerve monitoring in thyroid surgery. *Surgery* 2004;136:1310–1322.
80. Yarbrough D, Thompson GB, Kasperbauer JL, et al. Intraoperative electromyographic monitoring of the recurrent laryngeal nerve in reoperative thyroid and parathyroid surgery. *Surgery* 2004;136:1107–1115.
81. Gauger P, Reeve TS, Wilkinson M, et al. Routine parathyroid autotransplantation during total thyroidectomy: the influence of technique. *Eur J Surg* 2000;166:605–609.

CHAPTER 76 ■ PARATHYROID GLANDS

GERARD M. DOHERTY

ENDOCRINE

KEY POINTS

1. The normal parathyroid glands are flat, ovoid, and red-brown to yellow. Their dimensions are 5 to 7 mm × 3 to 4 mm × 0.5 to 2 mm, and they weigh between 30 and 50 mg each.
2. Parathyroid hormone is the single most important hormonal regulator of calcium and phosphate metabolism in humans with direct effects on the skeleton and kidney and indirect effects on the intestine, mediated through vitamin D.
3. The demonstration of an elevated plasma parathyroid hormone concentration alone does not establish the diagnosis of hyperparathyroidism; with a simultaneous elevated serum calcium level, this finding is virtually diagnostic.
4. A large proportion of patients with the diagnosis of hyperparathyroidism are minimally symptomatic or asymptomatic and the appropriate treatment for these patients remains controversial.
5. It is routinely possible to identify abnormal parathyroid glands prior to operation for most patients, allowing the surgeon to know where to start the exploration; intraoperative parathyroid hormone measurement can be used to confirm removal of all hyperfunctioning parathyroid tissue, that is, when to stop the operation.

ANATOMY

Typically, a person has four parathyroid glands—two superior
1 and two inferior (Fig. 76.1).[1] The normal parathyroid glands are flat, ovoid, and red-brown to yellow. They measure 5 to 7 mm × 3 to 4 mm × 0.5 to 2 mm and weigh between 30 and 50 mg each. The lower glands are usually larger than the upper glands. The superior glands are most often embedded in the fat on the upper posterior surface of the thyroid lobe near the site where the recurrent laryngeal nerve enters the larynx. The inferior glands are usually more ventral and lie close to or within the portion of the thymus gland that extends from the inferior pole of the thyroid gland into the chest. Although this anatomy is fairly consistent, substantial variations from the usual can occur, and it is essential that the surgeon have a thorough understanding of these anatomic variations.

Variations in parathyroid gland anatomy are primarily caused by differences in patterns of embryogenesis. During the fourth and fifth weeks of fetal development, a series of four pharyngeal pouches develop (Fig. 76.2). The superior parathyroid gland arises from the fourth pharyngeal pouch in conjunction with the lateral thyroid, and the inferior gland arises from the third pouch along with the thymus. The derivatives of each pouch then migrate together so that the superior parathyroid gland usually remains in close association with the upper pole of the thyroid, although it may occasionally be loosely attached by a long vascular pedicle, migrating caudad along the esophagus into the posterior mediastinum. Occasionally, a gland may be totally embedded in the thyroid parenchyma. The inferior parathyroid gland descends with the thymus, but this migration is extremely variable. Inferior glands can be found anywhere from the pharynx to the mediastinum. Regardless of their location, they usually adhere to the thymus or are within the thyrothymic ligament. Supernumerary glands can be identified in up to 15% of patients, most often in association with the thymus. Autopsy studies suggest that four parathyroid glands are virtually always present.

The arterial supply to both the superior and inferior parathyroid glands is usually from the inferior thyroid artery, although it may arise from the superior thyroid or thyroidea ima arteries or from the rich anastomosis of vessels supplying the larynx, trachea, and esophagus. A mediastinal parathyroid gland that descended during embryonic development usually receives its blood supply from either the internal mammary artery or small arteries within the thymus; however, an enlarged parathyroid gland that grows into the mediastinum usually carries with it the corresponding branch of the inferior thyroid artery. The inferior, middle, and superior thyroid veins, which drain the parathyroid glands, empty into the internal jugular vein or the innominate vein.

Histologically, the normal adult parathyroid gland is about half parenchyma and half stroma, including fat cells (Fig. 76.3). In children, the gland is almost entirely composed of parenchymal chief cells. Beginning at puberty, adipocytes appear and, with age, occupy an increasing proportion of the gland. Also with increasing age, acidophilic, mitochondria-rich oxyphil cells are present in increasing numbers and are intermixed with the glycogen-laden, polygonal, water-clear cells. The functional significance of the various cell types remains unclear, although the water-clear cells and oxyphil cells are probably derived from the chief cells and secrete parathyroid hormone (PTH).

PHYSIOLOGY

The primary physiologic role of the parathyroid gland is the endocrine regulation of calcium and phosphate metabolism. Average daily exchanges of these ions from the gastrointestinal tract, bone, and kidney are shown in Fig. 76.4.

Calcium

Calcium ion plays a critical role in all biologic systems. It participates in enzymatic reactions and is a mediator in hormone metabolism. Calcium is intimately involved in the physiology of neurotransmission, muscle contraction, and blood coagulation. It is the major cation in bone and teeth. It represents about 2% of the average body weight, and almost all calcium is contained in the skeleton. The normal range of serum calcium is 9 to 10.5 mg/dL (4.5 to 5.2 mEq/L), and the daily variation in a

FIGURE 76.1. Schematic illustration of the location of the superior (A) and inferior (B) parathyroid glands from 503 autopsy studies. The more common locations are indicated by the shaded areas. The numbers represent the percentage of glands found at each location. Typically, the glands were posterolateral to the thyroid and above or below the junction of the inferior thyroid artery with the recurrent laryngeal nerve. (After Akerstrom G, Malmaers J, Bergstrom R. Surgical anatomy of human parathyroid glands. *Surgery* 1984;95:14.)

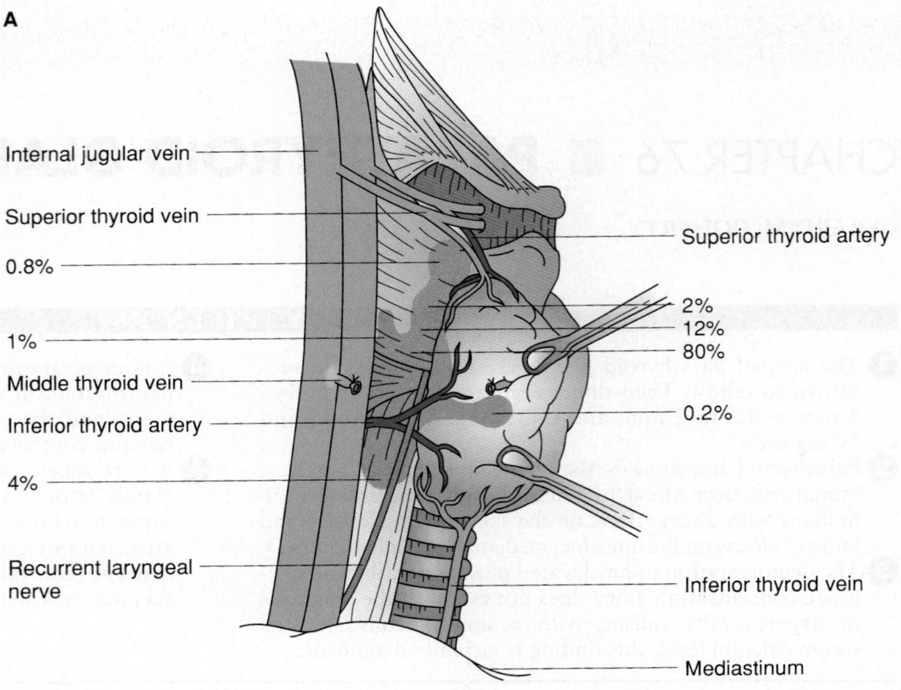

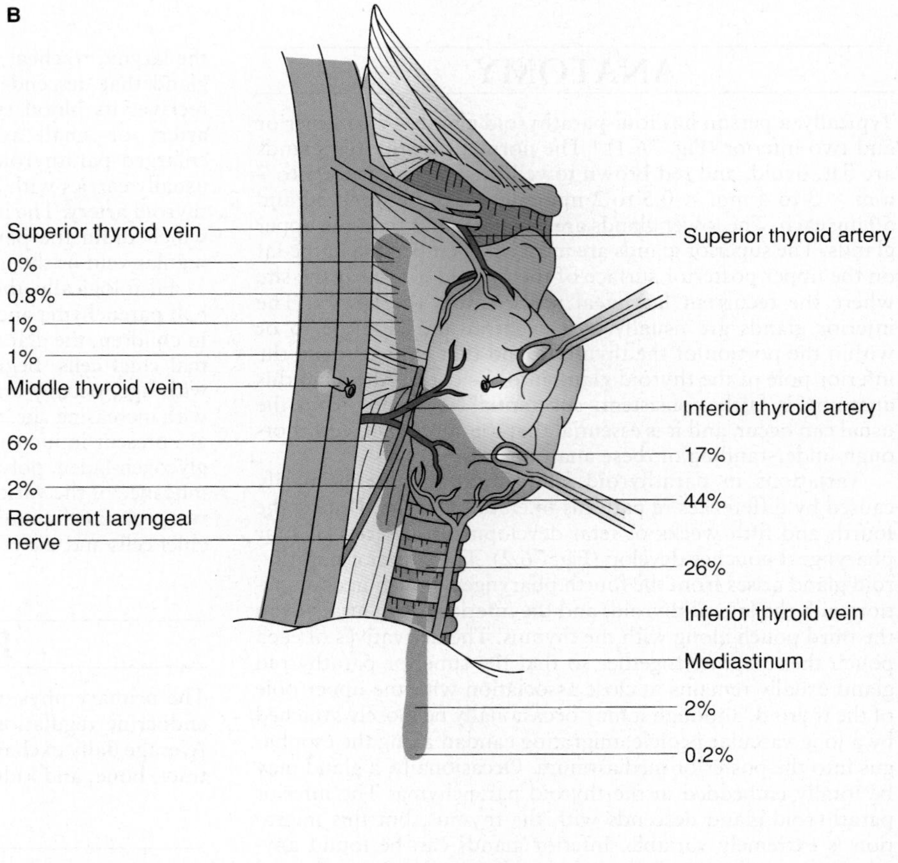

normal person is generally less than 10%. About half of the total serum calcium is in an ionized, biologically active form; 40% is bound to serum protein, mainly albumin, and 10% forms compounds with organic ions, such as citrate. The total serum calcium concentration is a function of the serum protein content, and because hydrogen ion competes with calcium for the same binding sites on albumin, the body fluid pH is important. In general, for every change of 1 g/dL in the serum albumin level, a direct alteration of 0.8 mg/dL occurs in the serum calcium concentration. Almost all the physiologically important activity of calcium is represented by the unbound, or free, fraction.

Calcium is absorbed in its inorganic form from the duodenum and proximal jejunum. The rate of absorption is precisely regulated according to body calcium status. The calcium in the extracellular fluid is constantly being exchanged with that in the intracellular fluid, the exchangeable bone, and the glomerular filtrate. Calcium reabsorption by the kidney is closely related to that of sodium, and about 99% of the filtered load is reabsorbed under normal conditions.

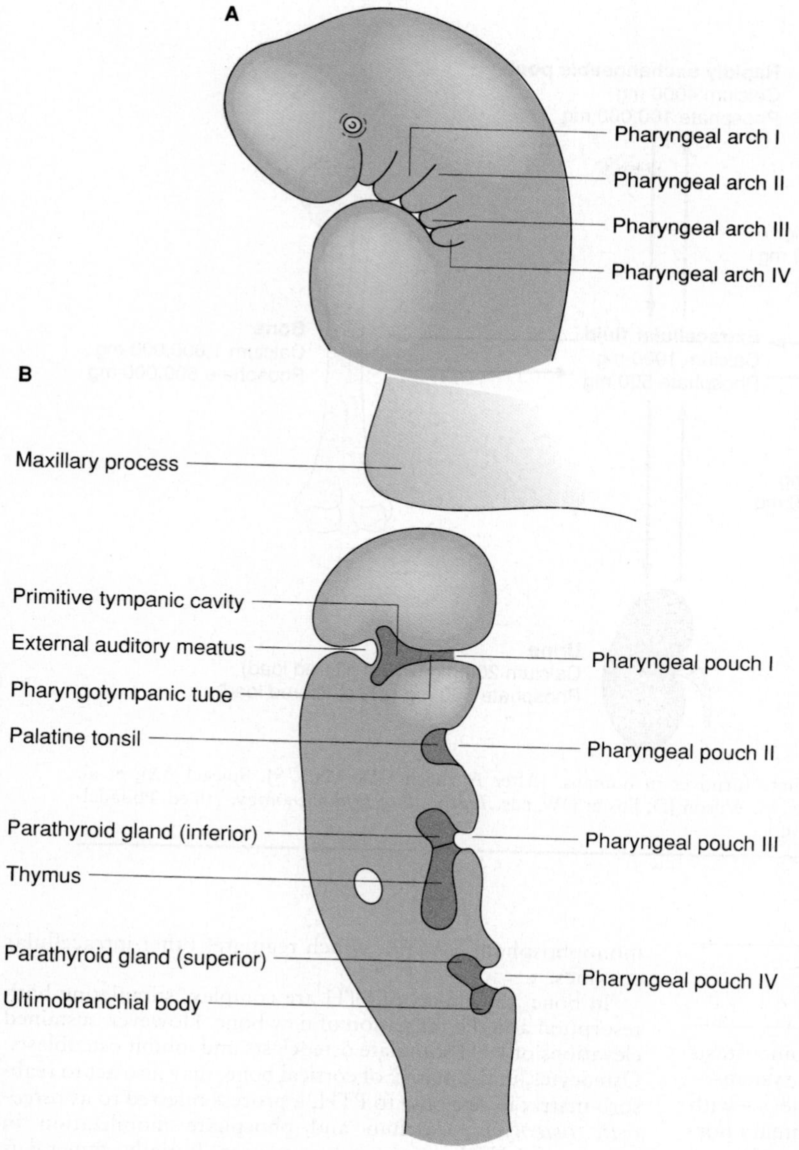

FIGURE 76.2. **A:** Pharyngeal arches in a 5-week embryo. The corresponding pouches extend from within the pharynx into each arch. **B:** Schematic representation of the differentiating epithelium of the respective pharyngeal pouches. (After Langman J. *Medical Embryology and Human Development: Normal and Abnormal*. Baltimore, MD: Williams & Wilkins; 1975:262.)

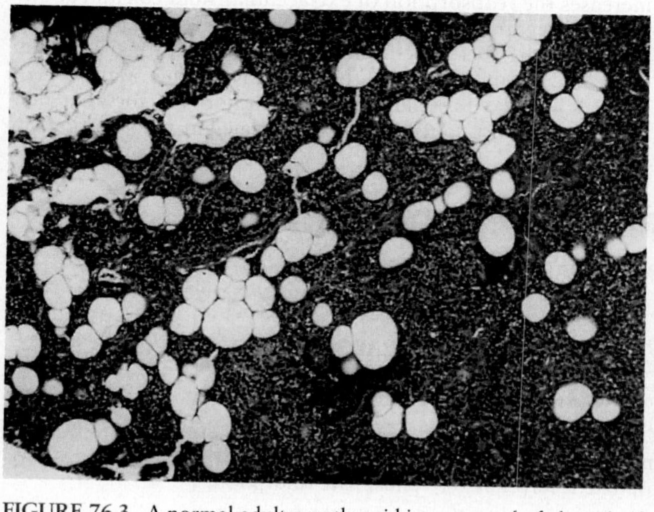

FIGURE 76.3. A normal adult parathyroid is composed of about half parenchyma and half fat (×150).

Phosphate

Phosphate anion is also an integral component of most biologic systems. It is critical to the pathways of glycolysis and is the functional group for a number of high-energy transfer compounds, including adenosine triphosphate. It is also the major anion in crystalline bone. Normal levels of plasma phosphate range from 2.5 to 4.3 mg/dL, and the level varies inversely with the serum level of calcium. The relation is such that the product of plasma calcium and phosphate is relatively constant ranging between 30 and 40 (with calcium and phosphate both expressed in mg/dL). When the product is above this level, the potential for the precipitation of calcium phosphate in body tissues increases.

In contrast to the percentage of calcium absorbed, the percentage of phosphate absorbed from the diet is relatively constant, and excretion usually provides the major mechanisms for regulating phosphate balance (Fig. 76.4). Unlike stores of calcium, the readily exchangeable soft tissue stores of phosphate, such as those in muscle, are large.

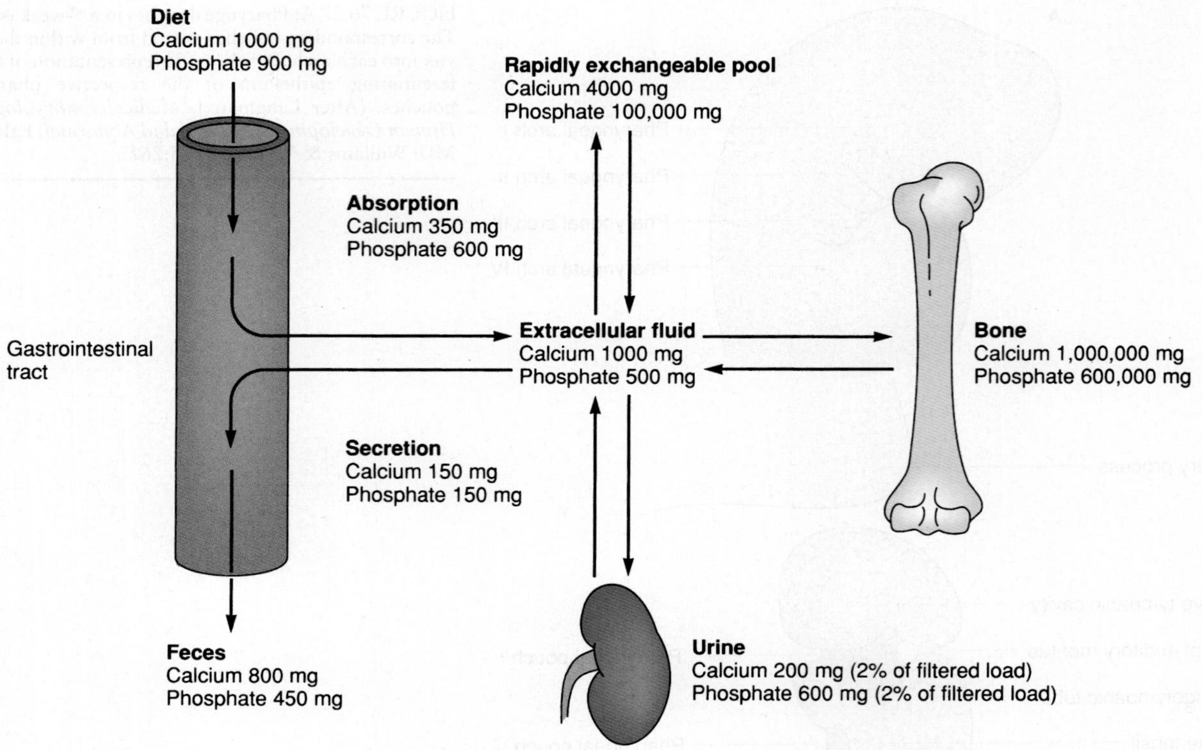

FIGURE 76.4. Average daily calcium and phosphate turnover in humans. (After Aurbach GD, Marx SJ, Spiegel AM, et al. Parathyroid hormone, calcitonin, and the calciferols. In: Wilson JD, Foster DW, eds. *Textbook of Endocrinology*, 7th ed. Philadelphia, PA: WB Saunders; 1985:1144, with permission.)

Regulation of Calcium and Phosphate Metabolism

The maintenance of calcium and phosphate homeostasis depends on major contributions from three organ systems—the gastrointestinal tract, the skeleton, and the kidneys—with minor contributions from the skin and liver.[2] The primary hormonal regulators of this metabolism are PTH, vitamin D, and calcitonin. The actions of each of these hormones in the organs are summarized in Table 76.1.

2 **Parathyroid Hormone.** PTH is the single most important hormonal regulator of calcium and phosphate metabolism in humans. It has direct effects on the skeleton and kidney and indirect effects on the intestine, mediated through vitamin D. In target tissues, PTH binds first to membrane receptors, activating adenyl cyclase to generate cyclic adenosine monophosphate (cAMP), which regulates other intracellular enzymes.

In bone, the effects of PTH are complex, stimulating both resorption and the formation of new bone. However, sustained elevations of PTH stimulate osteoclasts and inhibit osteoblasts. Osteocytes, in the matrix of cortical bone, may also act to reabsorb matrix in response to PTH, a process referred to as *osteocytic osteolysis*. Calcium and phosphate mobilization in response to PTH occurs in two phases. Initially, mineral is mobilized from areas of rapid equilibrium. This phase is followed by a more sustained release mediated by newly synthesized lysosomal and hydrolytic enzymes. In the kidney, PTH increases the reabsorption of extracellular fluid calcium at any given concentration, although excess secretion, because of hypercalcemia, increases the net daily amount of urinary calcium excretion. Reabsorption in the proximal tubule and loop of Henle is linked with sodium transport such that factors that alter sodium transport concomitantly alter calcium reabsorption. In

TABLE 76.1

HORMONAL REGULATION OF CALCIUM AND PHOSPHATE METABOLISM

■ LOCATION	■ PARATHYROID HORMONE	■ VITAMIN D	■ CALCITONIN
Gastrointestinal tract	No direct effect	Stimulates calcium and phosphate absorption	No direct effect
Skeleton	Stimulates calcium and phosphate resorption	Stimulates calcium and phosphate resorption	Inhibits calcium and phosphate resorption
Kidneys	Stimulates calcium resorption	No direct effect	Inhibits calcium and phosphate resorption

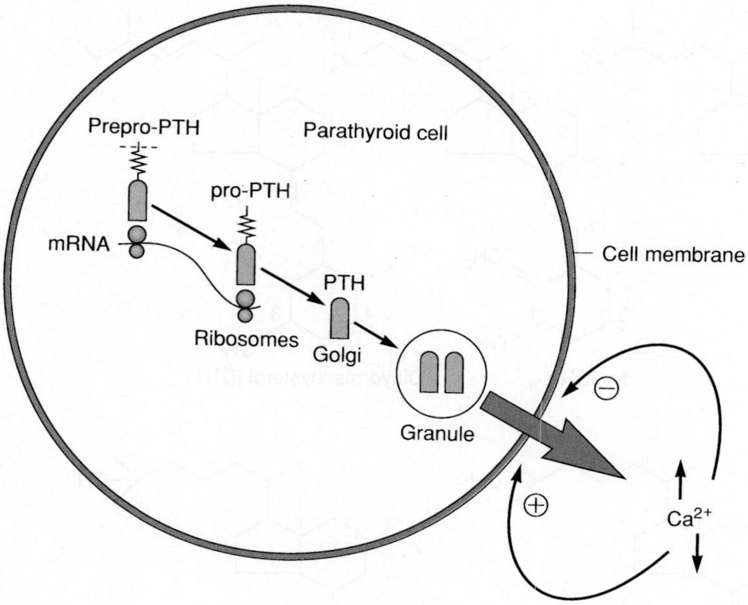

FIGURE 76.5. The parathyroid gland produces a precursor of parathyroid hormone (PTH), prepro-PTH, that is sequentially cleaved to pro-PTH and PTH. PTH secretion is controlled by the extracellular fluid calcium concentration. (After Klee GG, Kao PC, Heath H. Hypercalcemia. *Endocrinol Metab Clin North Am* 1988;17:573.)

contrast, reabsorption in the distal nephron is independent of sodium and directly influenced by PTH. PTH also increases phosphate excretion. This action is accompanied by enhanced bicarbonate secretion. PTH probably has only indirect effects on the gastrointestinal tract, by stimulating the hydroxylation of 25-hydroxyvitamin D to 1,25-dihydroxyvitamin D in the kidney.

PTH is synthesized initially as a precursor, preproPTH, which is sequentially cleaved in the parathyroid gland to proPTH and then to PTH (Fig. 76.5). Secretion of this 84-amino-acid molecule is controlled by a negative feedback loop with extracellular fluid calcium. Most PTH is secreted in this form and then cleaved in the liver into N- and C-terminal fragments. The N-terminus contains most of the biologic activity and is rapidly degraded by the liver, whereas the inactive C-terminus is slowly metabolized by the kidney.

Vitamin D. Vitamin D acts at two major sites. It increases intestinal absorption of calcium and phosphate. In addition, in the skeleton, it promotes mineralization and enhances PTH-mediated mobilization of calcium and phosphate. It probably has no direct effect on the kidney.

Vitamin D_3, or cholecalciferol, is produced normally by the action of sunlight on 7-dehydrocholesterol in the skin (Fig. 76.6). It is then hydroxylated in the liver (25 position) and kidney (1 position) to form the active 1,25-dihydroxyvitamin D_3 (calcitriol). Vitamin D_2 is normally present in yeast and fungi but not in humans. It is the major pharmacologic source of vitamin D. Pharmaceutical preparations include vitamin D_2 (ergocalciferol), 25-hydroxycholecalciferol (calcifediol), and 1,25-dihydroxycholecalciferol (calcitriol). 1-Hydroxycholecalciferol and dihydrotachysterol are synthetic preparations that require only 25-hydroxylation for activity and so are useful for supplementation in patients with renal failure, who lack the 1-hydroxylase.

Calcitonin. Calcitonin is a 32-amino-acid protein produced by the parafollicular C (calcitonin) cells of the thyroid. The C cells are embryologically derived from the neural crest and, in lower animals, are found in the ultimobranchial bodies, which are glandular structures derived from the lowest branchial pouch. In humans, these structures are incorporated into the superior and lateral aspects of the thyroid lobes.

Total thyroidectomy, with removal of all the C cells, is well tolerated. Calcitonin is not essential for the normal control of calcium metabolism in adult humans. It does inhibit bone resorption and can produce hypocalcemia in experimental animals. It also increases urinary calcium and phosphate excretion. These effects are mediated primarily through cAMP. Several secretagogues for calcitonin have been identified, including catecholamines, gastrin, and cholecystokinin, but the most potent appear to be calcium and pentagastrin. Exogenously administered calcitonin can be useful pharmacologically to reduce serum calcium levels.

Mineral Homeostasis. Under normal conditions, serum calcium and phosphate levels vary minimally during the course of the day. Regulation occurs primarily through PTH but also through a series of feedback loops involving vitamin D and calcitonin (Fig. 76.7). A fall in serum ionized calcium increases PTH secretion and stimulates the production of 1,25-dihydroxyvitamin D_3. Conversely, increases in serum calcium inhibit PTH secretion and the formation of active calciferol.

Pathophysiology

Diseases of the parathyroid glands present almost exclusively as disorders of calcium metabolism. Hypercalcemia is the most common manifestation, and in the patient who presents with an elevated serum calcium level, the differential diagnosis can be complex. A thorough understanding of both hypercalcemia and hypocalcemia is essential for the successful treatment of patients undergoing parathyroid surgery. Primary disorders of plasma phosphate are not usually related to surgical disease and are not discussed in detail here.

HYPERCALCEMIA

Hypercalcemia is a relatively common clinical problem.[3,4] In the general population and in hospital outpatients, the incidence is between 0.1% and 0.5%. Most patients in this group have primary hyperparathyroidism. In contrast, hypercalcemia is identified in almost 5% of hospitalized patients, and nearly two thirds of them have a malignancy.

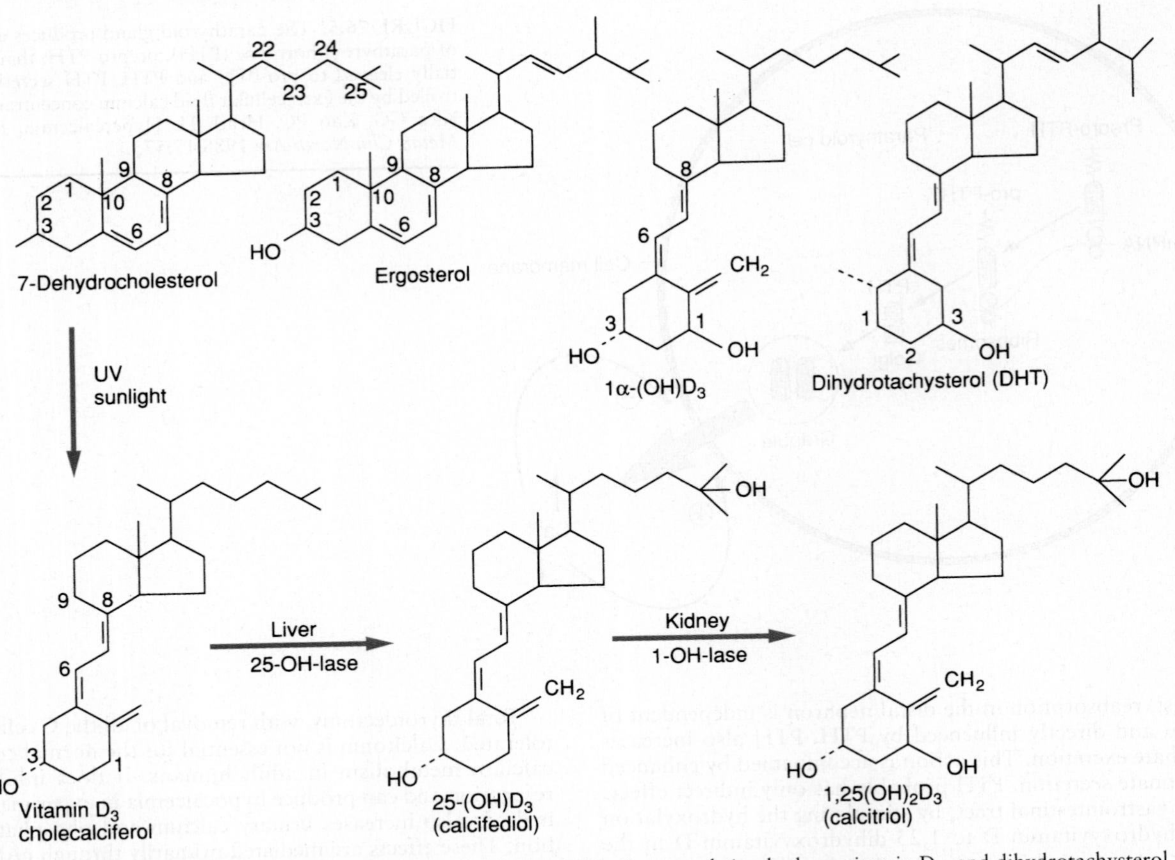

FIGURE 76.6. Schematic illustration of the synthesis of vitamin D_3. Ergosterol, 1-α-hydroxyvitamin D_3, and dihydrotachysterol are synthetic preparations of vitamin D. (After Klee GG, Kao PC, Heath H. Hypercalcemia. *Endocrinol Metab Clin North Am* 1988;17:573.)

Clinical Manifestations

The symptoms of hypercalcemia are varied and nonspecific (Table 76.2). Severity is a function of both the magnitude and rapidity of onset of the hypercalcemia. Many of the manifestations are subtle and are evident only in retrospect, after the patient has been successfully treated for the cause of the elevated calcium. Specific symptoms and diagnostic tests are addressed in more detail in the section on hyperparathyroidism.

Differential Diagnosis

Although the diagnosis of primary hyperparathyroidism can, after appropriate investigation, be established with confidence in most patients, all causes of hypercalcemia must be considered and excluded. The multiple causes of hypercalcemia are listed in Table 76.3.

Etiology

Hyperparathyroidism. The diagnosis of hyperparathyroidism is discussed in detail later. Patients typically have elevated plasma concentrations of calcium and PTH, increased urinary excretion of calcium, and a low plasma concentration of phosphate.

Malignancy. Generally, patients with hypercalcemia and malignancy (humoral hypercalcemia of malignancy) can be classified into two groups.[5–7] Patients with solid tumors, such as lung carcinoma (25% of all cases of humoral hypercalcemia

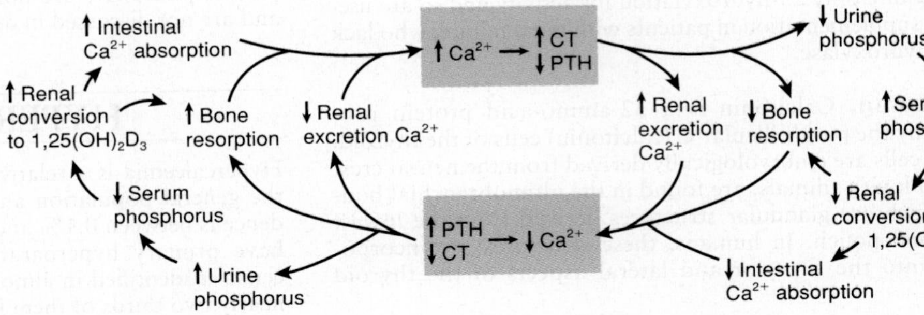

FIGURE 76.7. Feedback loops involved in the regulation of serum calcium and phosphorus. CT, calcitonin; PTH, parathyroid hormone.

TABLE 76.2 **DIAGNOSIS**

CLINICAL FEATURES OF HYPERCALCEMIA

Neurologic ■ Lethargy ■ Confusion ■ Coma ■ Headache ■ Depression ■ Paranoia ■ Muscle weakness ■ Hyporeflexia ■ Incontinence ■ Memory loss ■ Hearing loss ■ Ataxia	Cardiovascular ■ Electrocardiogram changes (short QT interval, widened T wave) ■ Bradycardia ■ Heart block ■ Hypertension Renal ■ Polyuria ■ Uremia ■ Renal colic ■ Nephrocalcinosis
Gastrointestinal ■ Constipation ■ Anorexia ■ Nausea and vomiting ■ Polydipsia ■ Weight loss ■ Pancreatitis ■ Peptic ulcer ■ Abdominal pain	Other ■ Band keratopathy ■ Conjunctivitis ■ Change in vision ■ Pruritus ■ Thrombosis ■ Myalgia

of malignancy); breast carcinoma (20%); squamous cell carcinoma of the head, neck, esophagus, or female genital tract (19%); or renal cell cancer (8%), account for three fourths of all cases. Humoral hypercalcemia of malignancy in this setting generally appears late in the disease, with nearly all patients having known, or readily evident, malignancy. These patients have elevated levels of serum calcium, low levels of serum phosphorus, and elevated levels of urinary cAMP, consistent with increased PTH activity but normal or low serum PTH levels. The hypercalcemia is now known to be caused by PTH-related protein secreted by the tumor, rather than by the bony metastases that many of these patients have because of the advanced nature of their cancers. In the second group, accounting for one fourth of cases, are patients with hematologic malignancies, such as multiple myeloma, certain lymphomas and leukemias, and a subset of the patients with breast cancer. These patients have elevated levels of serum calcium, but in contrast to most patients with solid tumors and humoral hypercalcemia of malignancy, they have elevated levels of serum phosphate and low levels of urinary cAMP. These patients always have lytic bony lesions and histologically demonstrate increased

TABLE 76.3 **ETIOLOGY**

CAUSES OF HYPERCALCEMIA

- ■ Hyperparathyroidism
- ■ Malignancy
- ■ Vitamin A or D intoxication
- ■ Thiazide diuretics
- ■ Hyperthyroidism
- ■ Milk–alkali syndrome
- ■ Sarcoidosis and other granulomatous diseases
- ■ Familial hypocalciuric hypercalcemia
- ■ Immobilization
- ■ Paget disease
- ■ Lithium therapy
- ■ Addisonian crisis
- ■ Idiopathic hypercalcemia of infancy

osteoclast bone resorption adjacent to tumor cells. This osteoclast-activating activity is an effect of cytokines, mainly interleukin-1β and tumor necrosis factor-β (lymphotoxin). These cytokines promote local net bone resorption and thus produce hypercalcemia and hyperphosphatemia.

Vitamin D and Vitamin A Intoxication. When administered in excess, vitamins A and D can produce hypercalcemia. Affected patients tend to have normal or elevated serum phosphate levels associated with a low PTH level. Metastatic calcification may occur.

Thiazide Diuretics. Thiazides may increase serum calcium levels to a mild degree, primarily through hemoconcentration and decreased renal excretion. Serum phosphate may also be depressed. It often takes several weeks for the hypercalcemia to resolve after the medication is discontinued.

Hyperthyroidism. Hyperthyroidism is associated with increased bone resorption. Often, the plasma PTH is low, and a history of other thyrotoxic symptoms can be elicited. The hypercalcemia usually resolves as the patient becomes euthyroid.

Milk–Alkali Syndrome. Typically, the milk–alkali syndrome occurs in patients with peptic ulcers who consume large quantities of milk and absorbable antacids. Usually, some degree of renal failure is present. PTH levels are low. This syndrome has become much less common with the increased use of nonabsorbable antacids, histamine 2–receptor antagonists, and proton pump inhibitors as therapy for peptic ulcer disease.

Sarcoidosis and Other Granulomatous Diseases. These syndromes are associated with hypersensitivity to vitamin D. The granulomas can convert inactive vitamin D to its active form. Patients have elevated plasma globulins and low PTH levels. The administration of large doses of corticosteroids for 10 days usually reduces the hypercalcemia. Biopsy of lymph nodes or the liver may confirm the diagnosis.

Familial Hypocalciuric Hypercalcemia. This disease is an asymptomatic, autosomal dominant condition characterized by mild to moderate hypercalcemia, hypocalciuria, and normal or only slightly elevated PTH levels. It develops in people heterozygous for a mutation in the calcium-sensing receptor.[8,9] The mutation causes an increase in the set point for extracellular calcium concentration, so that the "normal" calcium level is higher in these people than in the normal population. No treatment is necessary, although people with this disease should receive genetic counseling. Neonatal severe hyperparathyroidism, which can be fatal, develops in children homozygous for mutations in this receptor. Treatment for neonates with this disease is controversial, but they appear to benefit from early surgical management.

Immobilization. Immobilization produces hypercalcemia by increasing the ratio of bone resorption to bone formation. These patients can usually be distinguished by history, although on laboratory evaluation they have elevated serum levels of calcium and phosphate and a decreased serum concentration of PTH. Often, hypercalciuria is present, which may lead to the development of renal stones. Treatment is early mobilization and forced diuresis.

Other Causes. A variety of other diseases may produce hypercalcemia. For example, Paget disease (osteitis deformans) typically causes mild elevations in serum calcium. Paget disease can be diagnosed on the basis of the characteristic radiographic lesion. Adrenal insufficiency may be associated with hypercalcemia, although the symptoms are typically those of the primary abnormality. Lithium therapy appears to produce hypercalcemia by altering the parathyroid set point for inhibition by calcium and, over long courses of therapy, may also be associated with hyperparathyroidism. Idiopathic hypercalcemia of infancy is a rare disorder that is probably the result of hypersensitivity to vitamin D. It occurs in infants with mental retardation and is satisfactorily treated with glucocorticoids. Other causes include aluminum-induced renal osteomalacia and a host of analytic errors related to improper specimen collection with prolonged tourniquet times, tube contamination, and instrument drift.

Medical Treatment

Although the choice of therapy is tailored to the cause of the hypercalcemia, several general measures can prove effective.[4,10,11]

For the patient with mild hypercalcemia, a trial of a decrease in dietary calcium is indicated. A reduction in intake of milk and other dairy products is suggested, along with discontinuation of thiazide diuretics and vitamin D preparations. Mobilization prevents bone demineralization.

Patients with more marked hypercalcemia or severe symptoms should be admitted to the hospital for treatment, with careful observation and monitoring. In the patient with severe hyperparathyroidism, although the definitive therapy is surgical, it is unwise to proceed with neck exploration until the calcium has been reduced to near-normal levels. The mainstay of therapy is intravenous hydration, preferably with normal saline solution in sufficient quantities to maintain the urine output above 100 mL/h. These patients are often dehydrated before therapy, and fluid can be administered intravenously at a rate of 200 mL/h. Caution must be exercised in older patients, whose cardiac reserve may be marginal. This therapy exploits the parallel handling of calcium and sodium by the kidneys. The diuretic furosemide also increases sodium and calcium excretion but should not be used until the patient is well hydrated.

The endpoints of therapy are a decrease in the serum calcium level and a reduction of symptoms. Diuresis with saline solution is usually effective when the hypercalcemia results from hyperparathyroidism or a benign cause. In contrast, the hypercalcemia of malignancy may produce severe symptoms associated with extremely high serum calcium levels that are difficult to control. In this setting, a variety of other measures may be considered (Table 76.4). Some of the agents used to treat hypercalcemia cause significant toxicity, and close patient monitoring is required during treatment. Calcitonin is a fairly weak hypocalcemic agent, but it acts rapidly and is associated with less toxicity than many of the other drugs.[11] Salmon calcitonin is the most potent preparation. Treatment with glucocorticoids is particularly efficacious in patients with sarcoidosis and other granulomatous diseases. Plicamycin has proved useful in patients with hypercalcemia of malignancy, but it causes a cumulative toxicity (thrombocytopenia, hepatotoxicity, and nephrotoxicity). Bisphosphonates inhibit osteoclast activity directly. These agents are administered orally or parenterally and are particularly efficacious, although long-term use may be associated with significant osteomalacia.[5,12] Prostaglandin synthetase inhibitors were initially considered useful, but their efficacy has proved to be limited. Intravenous phosphates and chelating agents have largely been abandoned because of their severe toxicity; however, oral phosphates may be beneficial in patients requiring prolonged therapy.

HYPOCALCEMIA

Hypocalcemia can occur as a consequence of various acquired and hereditary diseases.[13,14] Generally, these disorders produce a deficiency or defect in the action of either PTH or vitamin D. It is most commonly a significant clinical problem after neck operation for thyroid disease. Chronic vitamin D deficiency is associated with compensatory PTH excess. The end result is rickets in children or osteomalacia in adults.

TABLE 76.4 **TREATMENT**

TREATMENT OF HYPERCALCEMIA

Therapy of Primary Disease
- Tumor resection (hypercalcemia of malignancy)
- Parathyroidectomy (primary hyperparathyroidism)

Expansion of Extracellular Volume
- Infusion of saline solution
- Enhancement of urinary calcium excretion
- Extracellular volume expansion
- Loop diuretics (furosemide and ethacrynic acid)

Inhibition of Bone Resorption
- Calcitonin
- Glucocorticoids
- Plicamycin (mithramycin)
- Bisphosphonates
- Gallium nitrate

Reduction of Intestinal Calcium Absorption
- Low-calcium diet
- Glucocorticoids

Other Treatments
- Dialysis
- Mobilization
- Oral phosphate
- Estrogens or progestogens (postmenopausal women with primary hyperparathyroidism)
- Chloroquine (sarcoidosis)

Modified from Attie MF. Treatment of hypercalcemia. *Endocrinol Metab Clin North Am* 1989;18:802.

Clinical Features

The major signs and symptoms of hypocalcemia are a direct consequence of the reduction in plasma levels of ionized calcium, which increases neuromuscular excitability (Table 76.5).

TABLE 76.5 **DIAGNOSIS**

CLINICAL FEATURES OF HYPOCALCEMIA

Neurologic
- Circumoral paresthesia
- Light-headedness
- Depression
- Anxiety
- Confusion
- Chvostek sign
- Trousseau sign
- Irritability
- Laryngeal spasm
- Seizures

Musculoskeletal
- Tetany
- Cramps
- Involuntary twitching
- Osteomalacia

Cardiovascular
- Electrocardiogram changes (prolonged QT interval, T-wave peaking)
- Arrhythmia
- Tachycardia, hypotension

Other Features
- Lenticular cataracts

TABLE 76.6 **ETIOLOGY**

CAUSES OF HYPOCALCEMIA

- Hypoparathyroidism
- Vitamin D deficiency
- Pseudohypoparathyroidism
- Hypomagnesemia
- Malabsorption
- Pancreatitis
- Hypoalbuminemia
- Chelation of calcium
- Osteoblastic metastases
- Toxic shock syndrome
- Hyperphosphatemia

The earliest clinical manifestations are numbness and tingling in the circumoral area, fingers, and toes. Mental symptoms are also common. Patients become anxious, depressed, and occasionally confused. Tetany may develop, characterized by carpopedal spasm, tonic–clonic convulsions, and laryngeal stridor. The magnitude of symptoms at any given plasma concentration of ionized calcium varies from patient to patient. On physical examination, contraction of the facial muscles is elicited by tapping anterior to the ear, over the facial nerve (Chvostek sign), although this sign may be present in 10% of normal patients. Trousseau sign is elicited by occluding blood flow to the forearm for 3 minutes. The development of carpal spasm indicates hypocalcemia, although the test is unpleasant and clinically impractical.

Etiology

Some of the causes of hypocalcemia are listed in Table 76.6. The most common cause of hypocalcemia by far is excision of or damage to the parathyroid glands during thyroid surgery.

Postoperative Hypoparathyroidism. Postoperative hypoparathyroidism commonly develops after total thyroidectomy.[14–16] Most patients undergoing operation on the thyroid experience some alteration in serum calcium, although they often are asymptomatic; the low calcium probably represents contusion or temporary alteration of the blood supply to the parathyroid glands. The hypocalcemia is usually transient and is not treated unless significant symptoms develop. Occasionally, in hyperparathyroid patients who have parathyroidectomy and significant bone disease, a marked skeletal deposition of calcium and symptomatic hypocalcemia occurs, so-called *bone hunger*. The plasma calcium usually reaches its nadir at 48 to 72 hours after surgery and then slowly returns to normal within several days. These patients may require calcium and vitamin D therapy for weeks or months after parathyroidectomy.

Idiopathic Hypoparathyroidism. A less common form of hypoparathyroidism is idiopathic lack of function. It occurs both sporadically and in families. In some cases, it develops as part of a polyglandular disorder and is thought to have an autoimmune basis. DiGeorge syndrome is a group of congenital disorders involving the branchial pouches that produces partial or complete agenesis of the thymus and parathyroid glands. Hypoparathyroidism can also develop in newborns as a result of prenatal suppression of the fetal parathyroid glands as a consequence of maternal hypercalcemia.[17] It is also common in otherwise normal but premature infants.

Vitamin D Deficiency. Vitamin D deficiency can occur as a result of dietary deficiency or lack of sun exposure. Likewise, renal disease produces a decrease in the 1-hydroxylase activity necessary for the formation of active vitamin D. The result is a decrease in calcium absorption and an increased secretion of PTH by the stimulated parathyroid glands. Osteomalacia, abnormal fractures, and the deformities of rickets may result.

Pseudohypoparathyroidism. Pseudohypoparathyroidism is a familial disease characterized by a rotund appearance, shortening of the extremities, and sometimes mental deficiency. The defect is not in PTH secretion; in fact, most patients have elevated plasma levels of PTH with evidence of increased bone resorption. Rather, the kidney is unresponsive to the hormone, and as a consequence, hypocalcemia and hyperphosphatemia develop. The deficit appears to be in the renal adenyl cyclase system.

Hypomagnesemia. This unusual deficit may result from chronic alcoholism, malabsorption, parenteral nutrition, or increased renal clearance during therapy with aminoglycosides. The deficit appears to block the physical response to PTH in addition to its release from the parathyroid gland.

Other Causes. In short-gut syndrome, after extensive small-bowel resection or bypass, or after some forms of bariatric surgery, vitamin D and calcium may be absorbed in insufficient quantities. In pancreatitis, the massive soft tissue destruction and saponification that occur with hemorrhagic disease may sequester significant amounts of calcium in the retroperitoneum. Some undefined systemic factor also appears to contribute to hypocalcemia in these patients. Hypoalbuminemia causes a reduction in the total plasma calcium level, although the level of ionized calcium remains within the normal range and patients are asymptomatic. Circulatory substances, such as the citrate used to anticoagulate banked blood and radiographic contrast media, may bind to calcium. In patients with osteoblastic metastases, particularly associated with prostate carcinoma, hypocalcemia has been attributed to increased calcium flux into the lesions. Toxic shock syndrome is sometimes associated with hypocalcemia, but the mechanism has not been defined. Acute hyperphosphatemia, as a consequence of exogenous administration of phosphate or during the cytolytic chemotherapy of highly responsive tumors (e.g., Burkitt lymphoma and acute lymphoblastic leukemia), may produce symptomatic hypocalcemia associated with soft tissue calcification.

Treatment

The treatment of hypocalcemia is summarized in Table 76.7. For acute symptomatic hypocalcemia, calcium should be administered intravenously. Calcium gluconate is less irritating to the veins than calcium chloride, and the calcium release is slower, without a risk for overcorrection. Usually, 20 to 30 mL of 10% solution is infused over a 15- to 20-minute period, and then 50 to 100 mL is administered over the next 12 hours in adults. A practical guide after an initial bolus dose includes 60 mL of 10% calcium gluconate in a 500-mL bag of dextrose 5% in water, infused at 1 mL/kg per hour, and adjusted every 4 hours based on the serum level of calcium and patient symptoms. Bicarbonate precipitates any calcium infused through the same intravenous line. Serum magnesium should always be measured, and hypomagnesemia should be corrected if present. In patients with convulsions from advanced tetany, diphenylhydantoin therapy is useful, but symptoms should never be allowed to progress to this point.

Long-term therapy is gauged on the basis of symptoms. In the postoperative patient, the continued stimulus of mild hypocalcemia to any remaining parathyroid gland tissue may prove useful. Concomitant therapy with calcium and vitamin D is effective in a timely fashion. A starting dose of 2 g of oral calcium carbonate per day in divided doses is usually well

TABLE 76.7 TREATMENT

TREATMENT OF HYPOCALCEMIA

■ SYMPTOM OR GOAL	■ TREATMENT
Symptomatic hypocalcemia	Oral calcium carbonate or intravenous calcium gluconate, and possibly vitamin D supplements to increase the efficiency of absorption of oral supplements
Symptomatic tetany	Intravenous calcium gluconate
Correction of hypomagnesemia	Intravenous magnesium chloride
Vitamin D supplementation	Ergocalciferol, calcifediol (liver disease), calcitriol (renal disease)
Long-term therapy	Calcium carbonate; low-phosphate, low-oxalate diet; parathyroid grafting (immunosuppressed or cryopreserved autograft)

tolerated. Vitamin D can be administered as calcitriol, an active synthetic vitamin D analogue. Most adults respond to a dose of 0.5 to 1.0 μg/d; reduced doses may be necessary for patients with renal dysfunction.

HYPERPARATHYROIDISM

Definitions

Parathyroid neoplasms are rarely identified by physical enlargement but rather are sought because of the peripheral effects of excess hormone. Primary hyperparathyroidism develops spontaneously, without apparent cause but possibly in response to exogenous stimuli. When the normal control of serum calcium is disturbed and the autonomous production of PTH is increased, the state is referred to as *primary hyperparathyroidism*. This category includes both benign single- and multiple-gland enlargements and the much rarer parathyroid carcinoma. In some cases, the disease is familial. In contrast, *secondary hyperparathyroidism* occurs when a defect in mineral homeostasis leads to a compensatory increase in parathyroid function. This occurs most commonly in response to renal disease but may also develop as a consequence of the hypocalcemia associated with some diseases of the gastrointestinal tract, bones, or other endocrine organs. Occasionally, with prolonged secondary stimulation, the hyperfunctioning glands are no longer physiologically responsive to an increase in ionized calcium. This uncommon (affecting about 2% of patients after renal transplantation), relatively autonomous state, referred to as *tertiary hyperparathyroidism*, develops most commonly after renal transplantation when the renal defect in calcium homeostasis is corrected.

Incidence

The advent in the 1970s of the widespread assessment of serum calcium as part of automated multichannel analysis has considerably altered our understanding of hyperparathyroidism. Before that time, primary hyperparathyroidism was thought to be a relatively rare condition. Most patients presented with symptoms of disease, usually renal stones or bony manifestations. Currently, most patients are asymptomatic or have only vague symptoms or signs that can be related to hyperparathyroidism.[18,19] Occasionally, patients recognize that they had symptoms only after their well-being improves following parathyroidectomy. Incidence varies with both age and gender (Table 76.8), but hyperparathyroidism is believed to develop in about 50 to 100 people per 100,000 in the general population, with approximately 50,000 new cases occurring annually in the United States.[20,21] Marked variations have been noted worldwide; the reasons for these differences remain unclear.

Etiology

The cause of primary hyperparathyroidism is not known. Although the sequence of progression from secondary to tertiary disease in response to chronic stimulation has a logical appeal, it is difficult to draw parallels with primary disease. Most patients with primary hyperparathyroidism have disease of a single rather than of multiple glands, which is not what might be predicted if an external stimulus were part of the pathophysiology. Hyperparathyroidism is most common in postmenopausal women, the population group with the highest incidence of osteoporosis and the most significant alterations in calcium and phosphate metabolism. Loss of renal function with aging is associated with elevations in PTH and decreases in phosphate clearance. It has been suggested but not demonstrated that a renal calcium leak, if sufficient, might result in a chronic calcium deficit stimulating the parathyroid glands.

Genetic studies of parathyroid adenomas have described an oncogene (*PRAD1*) that may be one step in the path to neoplasia in these tumors. Overexpression of the normal *PRAD1* gene, also known as *cyclin D1*, allows progression of the cell cycle from the G1 phase to the S phase, thus promoting cellular growth and division. *PRAD1* is overexpressed in 20% to 40% of parathyroid adenomas; further research may reveal

TABLE 76.8

AGE-SPECIFIC AND GENDER-SPECIFIC INCIDENCE OF PRIMARY HYPERPARATHYROIDISM

	■ NEW CASES PER 100,000	
■ AGE (y)	■ MEN	■ WOMEN
<39	5	8
40–50	26	104
>60	92	189
Total	18	56

After Heath H III, Hodgson SF, Kennedy MA. Primary hyperthyroidism: incidence, morbidity, and potential economic impact in a community. *N Engl J Med* 1980;302:189.

other genetic alterations that contribute to the neoplastic growth. The *MEN1* tumor-suppressor gene has also been implicated in the molecular pathogenesis of sporadic hyperparathyroidism. About 15% to 20% of sporadic parathyroid adenomas have either somatic mutation or biallelic deletion of the *MEN1* gene.[22]

Hyperparathyroidism occurs in several familial forms. It is a major component of the multiple endocrine neoplasia (MEN) syndromes types 1 and 2A. The parathyroid disease of MEN-1 syndrome is multiple parathyroid adenomas that appear with increasing frequency over the patient's lifetime.[23] In other families, hyperparathyroidism is inherited in an autosomal dominant fashion without other manifestations of MEN-1 or MEN-2; some have osseous abnormalities (tumor–jaw syndrome) and some apparently have isolated disease.

Pathology

Single-gland Versus Multiple-gland Disease. Microscopically, the cell most commonly involved in primary hyperparathyroidism is the chief cell. Less frequently, the oxyphil cell is the predominant cell type. Diseased glands typically have an increase in the proportion of stromal cells and a reduction in the proportion of stromal fat. Single diseased glands, or adenomas, have been classically described with a predominance of chief cells centering in a single focus, with a compressed rim of surrounding normal tissue (Fig. 76.8). In contrast, parathyroid hyperplasia has been characterized as a diffuse proliferation of clear cells in multiple glands, with little remaining normal tissue (Fig. 76.9). These criteria have proved totally unreliable. Although pathologic studies can usually distinguish parathyroid glands from other tissue, they may not prove useful beyond this capacity. Intraoperative decisions frequently depend on recognizing disease of one or more parathyroid glands, and in this regard, the histologic description of adenoma or hyperplasia is generally unreliable in primary hyperparathyroidism.[24]

Patients with multiple-gland disease may have one gland that appears to be an adenoma and another that appears diffusely involved or even histologically normal with gross enlargement. The most reliable index of abnormality is the determination of glandular enlargement by visual inspection. The incidence of single- and multiple-gland enlargement as judged by visual inspection in 66 consecutive patients with hyperparathyroidism is shown in Table 76.9. The visual assessment and judgment of the experienced surgeon have proved to

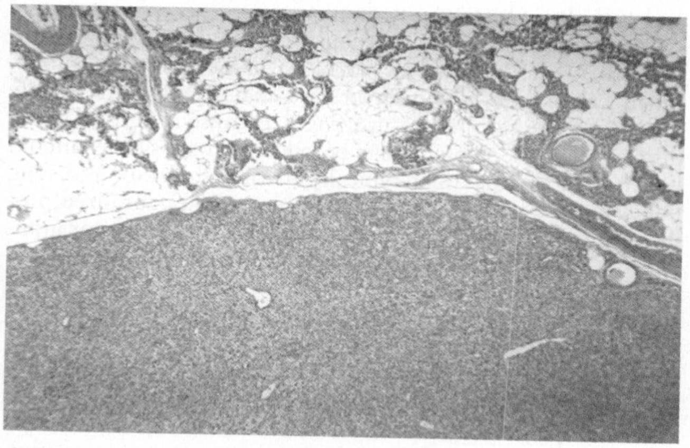

FIGURE 76.8. Parathyroid adenoma. The tumor consists of sheets of neoplastic chief cells and is separated from normal parenchyma by a thin capsule. (Reproduced with permission from Rubin E, Farber JL. *Pathology*, 3rd ed. Philadelphia, PA: Lippincott Williams & Wilkins; 1999.)

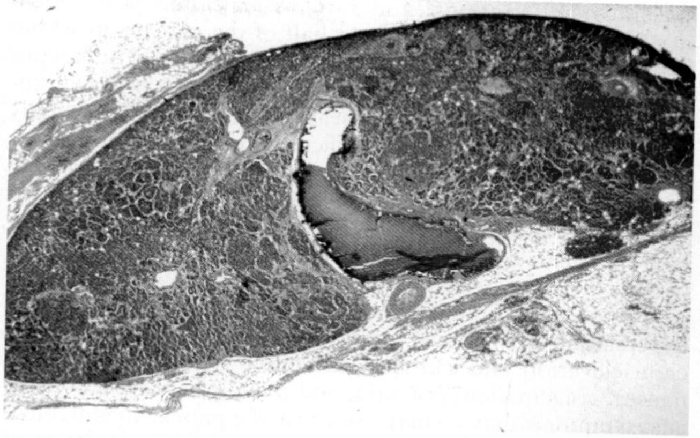

FIGURE 76.9. Primary parathyroid hyperplasia. The normal adipose tissue of the gland has been replaced by sheets and trabeculae of hyperplastic chief cells. (Reproduced with permission from Rubin E, Farber JL. *Pathology*, 3rd ed. Philadelphia, PA: Lippincott Williams & Wilkins; 1999.)

be an effective basis for intraoperative decisions. This approach requires that all four parathyroid glands be evaluated at the time of operation. However, the recent ability to rapidly measure PTH during operation has provided a method to assess gland function rather than size. This experience indicates that there may be more enlarged glands than there are hyperfunctioning glands.[25]

Carcinoma. Parathyroid carcinoma is a rare entity, and the histologic diagnosis can be exceedingly difficult. The surgeon may suspect the diagnosis when dense invasion and scarring are encountered, although this may also be secondary to some other inflammatory disease in the neck. Pathologic criteria include marked mitotic activity, dense fibrous stroma, and evidence of local invasion into the capsule or surrounding vessels.[26] Malignant-appearing tumors, however, may pursue an apparently benign clinical course; the converse is less frequently true. The only reliable criteria of malignancy are metastases, most commonly to the lymph nodes, lung, or liver, and true local invasion.

Systemic Effects

The use of automated technology for determining serum calcium has changed not only the estimated incidence of hyperparathyroidism but also the usual mode of presentation. Before screening, three fourths of patients presented with renal disease, particularly nephrolithiasis; one third to one half had

TABLE 76.9

GLAND ENLARGEMENT IN 66 CONSECUTIVE PATIENTS WITH PRIMARY HYPERPARATHYROIDISM

PATHOLOGY	PATIENT, *n*	PERCENTAGE
Adenoma	50	76%
Double adenoma	4	6%
Hyperplasia	12	18%

From Lowney JK, Weber B, Johnson S, et al. Minimal incision parathyroidectomy: cure, cosmesis, and cost. *World J Surg* 2000;24: 1442–1445.

ENDOCRINE

skeletal manifestations; and rare patients had both. Most recent series suggest that at least half of the patients in whom hyperparathyroidism is diagnosed do not have renal or osseous disease and many are minimally symptomatic or asymptomatic. Manifestations of the disease are protean but generally nonspecific, and they may be difficult to elicit in the history. A significant proportion of patients present without a readily quantifiable index of disease severity. This finding has created some controversy about the need for surgery in the asymptomatic patient and particularly for the elderly or high-risk patient.[21,27]

The earliest complaints are often the vague symptoms of hypercalcemia. These vary with the magnitude of plasma calcium elevation and can include muscle weakness, anorexia, nausea, constipation, polyuria, and polydipsia. These nonspecific symptoms may or may not cause the patient to seek medical attention. Some symptomatic patients have evidence of chronic disease involving the kidney or skeleton. Usually, only one of these systems is significantly involved in any individual patient. The treatment of hyperparathyroidism is designed to eliminate or halt the progression of the complications of the disease. Symptomatic patients can be divided into two groups. Members of the first group have renal manifestations, a slower onset of symptoms, and generally lower serum calcium concentrations. Patients in the second group have a more rapid onset of symptoms, higher serum calcium levels, and significant bone disease. No recognizable histologic or physiologic characteristics distinguish patients with renal disease from those with bone disease.

Renal Manifestations. Renal complications develop because the hypercalcemia leads to an increase in urinary calcium excretion and because PTH increases the excretion of phosphate and produces urinary alkalosis. Both these events predispose to stone formation. Urinary stones can be treated surgically or with lithotripsy, and subsequent definitive treatment of the hyperparathyroidism reduces the rate of re-formation. Of patients who present for the first time with renal colic, 5% to 10% are found to have primary hyperparathyroidism. Nephrocalcinosis (Fig. 76.10) is calcification of the renal parenchyma and occurs in 5% to 10% of patients with hyperparathyroidism. It causes more significant renal damage than nephrolithiasis does. In general, the more severe the renal damage, the less likely it is that nephrocalcinosis will regress after parathyroidectomy.

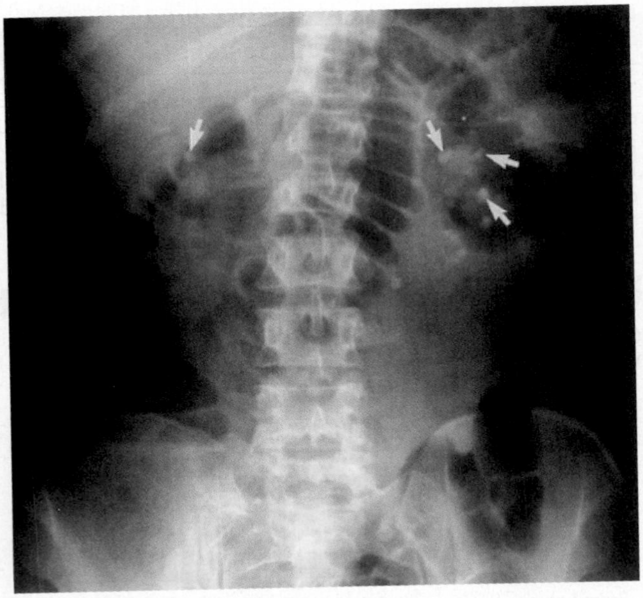

FIGURE 76.10. Abdominal film demonstrating nephrocalcinosis, or diffuse calcification of the renal parenchyma (*arrows*).

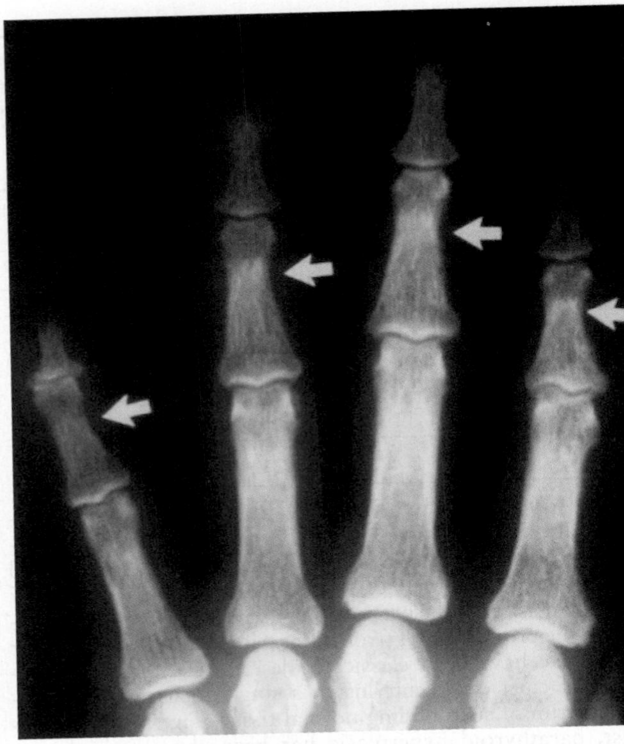

FIGURE 76.11. Magnification radiograph of the fingers in hyperparathyroidism. Subperiosteal cortical resorption (*arrows*) typically is most visible on the radial aspect of the middle phalanges.

The incidence of hypertension in hyperparathyroidism increases with the degree of renal impairment. Hypertension may be a significant cause of the morbidity associated with hyperparathyroidism, but although a decrease in blood pressure has been demonstrated in some patients after parathyroidectomy, the correlation between the two conditions is not clear.

Skeletal Manifestations. Parathyroid bone disease in its most classic and severe form, osteitis fibrosa cystica, is seldom encountered; however, 5% to 15% of patients with parathyroid bone disease present with significant symptoms of skeletal disease. Most commonly, these symptoms include bone pain and pathologic fractures.

Bone changes are often demonstrable on detailed plain radiographs of the hands (Fig. 76.11). Characteristically, subperiosteal resorption is evident on the radial aspect of the middle phalanx of the second or third finger. Because of tufting of the distal phalanges, clubbing may be evident on physical examination. Other findings that typically involve the skull and long bones include bone cysts, "brown" tumors (i.e., localized proliferations of osteoclasts), and diffuse demineralization or granularity. More subtle bone loss can be detected by iliac crest bone biopsy or dual-energy x-ray absorptiometry scan. The risk of bone fracture increases with increasing severity of bone loss.

Gastrointestinal Manifestations. Hypercalcemia is clearly associated with nonspecific gastrointestinal complaints, including nausea, vomiting, constipation, and anorexia, but attempts to demonstrate a definite relation between hyperparathyroidism and either peptic ulcer disease or pancreatitis remain unconvincing. Hypercalcemia stimulates gastric acid secretion experimentally and clinically, and has been associated with pancreatitis. Therefore, a theoretic rationale for the complex of hyperparathyroidism and gastrointestinal symptoms does exist.

Neuromuscular Manifestations. Neurologic and muscular complaints are those of hypercalcemia in general. Fatigability and proximal muscle weakness are among the most debilitating manifestations. Atrophy of type II muscle fibers, consistent with a neuropathic and not a myopathic cause, has been demonstrated. Sensory complaints include dysesthesia, a reduced vibratory sense, and stocking–glove sensory deficits.

Psychological Manifestations. The emotional disturbances of hyperparathyroidism are often subtle and difficult to quantify. As with other forms of hypercalcemia, they range from depression or anxiety to psychosis and coma. Patients undergoing parathyroidectomy frequently experience a sense of well-being and relief from fatigue and dullness postoperatively, even if they may have had no noticeable complaints preoperatively.

Other Manifestations. A variety of signs and symptoms of soft tissue calcification have been described. Nonspecific arthralgia, particularly involving the proximal interphalangeal joints of the hands, is characteristic. The incidence of chondrocalcinosis is increased. Pruritus, vascular and cardiac calcification, and band keratopathy of the cornea have all been noted. Some reports have suggested an increased risk of malignancy and coronary artery disease, but the effects remain unsubstantiated, and it is not clear if the mortality risk is modifiable by correction of hyperparathyroidism.[28–30]

Physical Findings. Except in patients with the classic deformities of advanced bone disease, the physical examination is seldom helpful. Diseased parathyroid glands are infrequently palpable, except in patients with parathyroid carcinoma. A mass in the anterior neck in a patient with primary hyperparathyroidism is most commonly a thyroid nodule.

Laboratory Findings. Tests for calcium, PTH, phosphate, bicarbonate, and magnesium, in addition to other laboratory tests, are useful to establish the diagnosis of hyperparathyroidism.

Calcium. Hypercalcemia is the single most important diagnostic finding; however, particularly in early or mild cases, serial analysis may show fluctuations in and out of the normal range. Coexistent hypoalbuminemia and acidosis may produce an apparently normal total serum level of calcium, even though the ionized fraction is actually elevated. Serum concentrations of ionized calcium may be helpful in the patient with intermittent or mild hypercalcemia.

Parathyroid Hormone. PTH measurement is an important method for establishing the diagnosis of hyperparathyroidism. Because of the heterogeneity of the various circulating forms of PTH, measurement of C-terminal or N-terminal fragments give conflicting and confusing results. Intact hormone assays and
3 whole molecule assays are the most dependable. The demonstration of an elevated plasma PTH concentration alone does not establish the diagnosis of hyperparathyroidism. With a simultaneous elevated serum calcium level, this finding is virtually diagnostic (Fig. 76.12).

Phosphate. PTH increases renal phosphate excretion and, in about half of patients, produces hypophosphatemia. In the presence of renal disease, however, the serum phosphate levels may be normal or significantly elevated.

Bicarbonate. PTH also increases bicarbonate excretion, so that a hyperchloremic metabolic acidosis may develop. It has been suggested that the finding of an elevated serum chloride-to-phosphate ratio may be helpful in the differential diagnosis of hypercalcemia. A ratio greater than 30 is considered highly suggestive of hyperparathyroidism.

Magnesium. Hypomagnesemia develops in 5% to 10% of patients with hyperparathyroidism. After parathyroidectomy, if both hypocalcemia and hypomagnesemia are present, it may be difficult to correct the calcium until the serum magnesium has been corrected.

Other Diagnostic Tests. A variety of special diagnostic tests for hyperparathyroidism are available. None is more specific than the measurement of serum concentrations of calcium and PTH, although they may be useful in equivocal cases. For example, the 24-hour urinary calcium excretion is usually elevated, but may be normal, in patients with hyperparathyroidism, although the finding is not specific for this disease. This test is helpful in identifying patients with familial hypercalcemic hypocalciuria, in whom the rate of urinary calcium excretion is low. Measurements of tubular reabsorption of phosphate below 30% suggest primary hyperparathyroidism. Urinary cAMP is generated

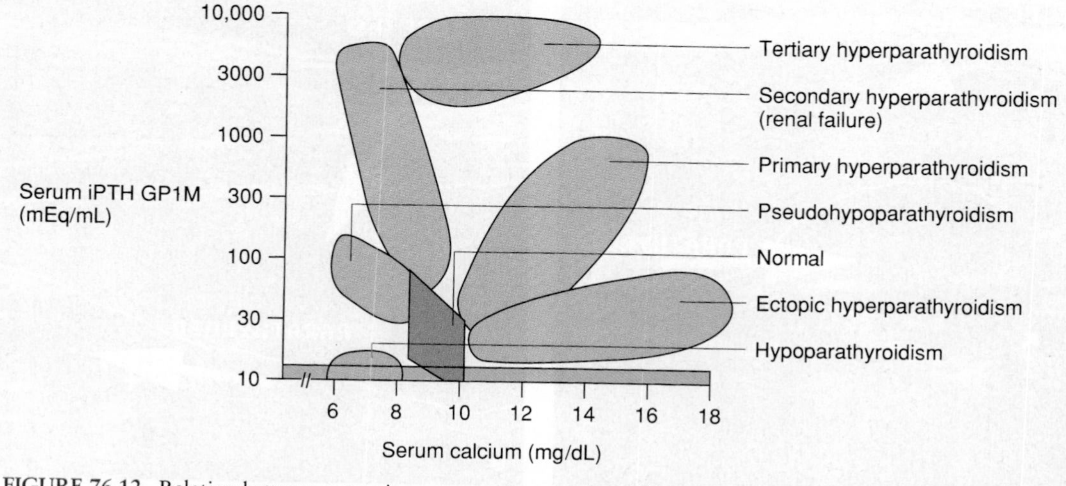

FIGURE 76.12. Relation between serum immunoreactive parathyroid hormone and serum calcium in patients with hypoparathyroidism, pseudohypoparathyroidism, ectopic hyperparathyroidism, and primary, secondary, and tertiary hyperparathyroidism. GP1M, guinea pig antiserum 1M. (After Clark OH, Way LW. Thyroid and parathyroid. In: Way LW, ed. *Current Surgical Diagnosis and Treatment*, 8th ed. Norwalk, CT: Appleton & Lange; 1989:249.)

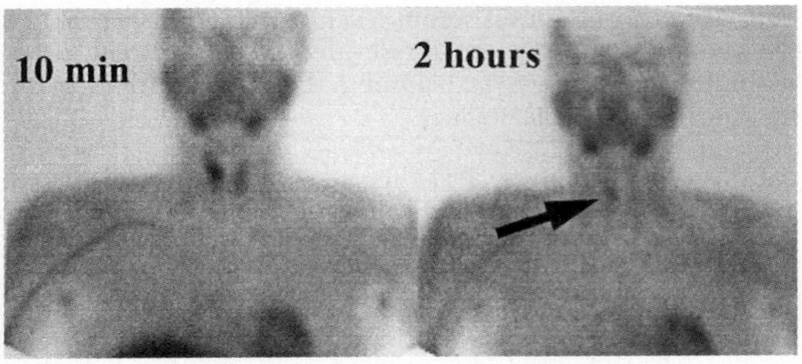

FIGURE 76.13. ^{99m}Technetium sestamibi scan of a patient with a parathyroid adenoma. The radionuclide is present in both thyroid and parathyroid tissue on the 10-minute film; however, by 2 hours, the radionuclide has washed out of the thyroid and remains only in the right-sided parathyroid gland. This scan shows a 794-mg right upper parathyroid adenoma (*arrow*).

specifically as a consequence of PTH activation of renal tubular adenyl cyclase. Increased urinary concentrations are identified in most patients with primary hyperparathyroidism. These measurements are rarely necessary because of the reliability of the intact PTH measurement.

Localization with Imaging Techniques. In order to try to simplify the operative approach to hyperparathyroidism, an attempt is usually made to localize enlarged glands preoperatively. In the hands of an experienced surgeon, the cure rate for hyperparathyroidism at the initial operation without preoperative localization exceeds 95% with the conventional full neck exploration. However, technologic developments have led surgeons to pursue alternatives to the full neck exploration. These innovations are increasingly accurate preoperative localization with ^{99m}technetium sestamibi scintigraphy or high-resolution ultrasound, combined with intraoperative intact PTH measurement that allows termination of the operation without visualization of all four parathyroid glands. Surgeons have used these technologies in various combinations to limit the extent of the neck exploration. All of the current alternative strategies, however, depend on a preoperative parathyroid localization study to direct the exploration.

The study most frequently used for imaging previously unoperated patients is ^{99m}technetium sestamibi scintigraphy (Fig. 76.13). Sestamibi scanning can identify the site of abnormal tissue in 75% to 80% of patients but has limitations in patients with small adenomas or multiple-gland disease. Sestamibi was originally developed for cardiac imaging. The use of a single nuclide with a short half-life and a high-energy profile has advantages in lateral, oblique, and three-dimensional imaging that technetium-thallium scanning, which was formerly used, does not provide.

High-resolution ultrasound examination of the neck is also used for localization of abnormal parathyroid tissue, particularly when it is available for use by the clinician. The current machines scan at high frequencies (10 to 13 MHz) that allow demonstration of small abnormalities in the neck (Fig. 76.14). The examination is best done by a clinician in real time, as that allows the most complete assessment of the neck, rather than scans performed by a technician for later review of still pictures by the physician. The sensitivity of cervical ultrasound for abnormal parathyroid glands is about the same as for sestamibi scanning. Ultrasonography is an operator-dependent technique. It is rapid and relatively inexpensive and can direct fine-needle aspiration for cytologic confirmation and immunoassay for PTH.

In patients with persistent or recurrent hyperparathyroidism, preoperative imaging is important to guide the exploration. High-resolution real-time ultrasonography, computed tomography (CT), magnetic resonance imaging (MRI), and sestamibi scanning all appear to have comparable sensitivities of 50% to 60%. The results of these examinations may be less successful at centers without significant experience in their use.

Computed tomography is more expensive but less operator dependent than ultrasonography. It clearly is superior in identifying deeper structures and for examining the retrosternal mediastinum. MRI is considerably more expensive than CT and has not been shown to be superior. Most surgeons prefer to have results of two or more imaging tests that confirm an abnormality before exploration in the reoperative setting.[31]

Treatment

Indications for Surgery. Generally, the only practical therapeutic option is surgery. Nephrolithiasis, bone disease, and

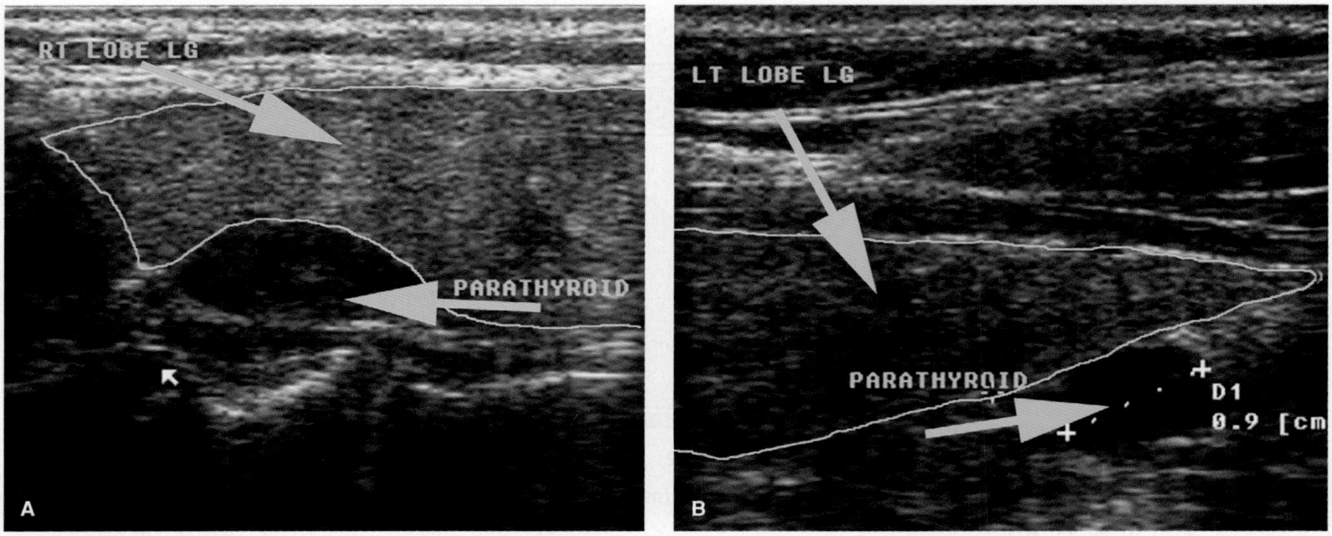

FIGURE 76.14. Ultrasound views of parathyroid adenomas. **A:** Sagittal image of the upper pole of the right lobe of the thyroid gland, demonstrating a hypoechoic parathyroid adenoma posterior to the thyroid parenchyma. **B:** Sagittal image of the lower pole of the left lobe of the thyroid gland with an adjacent hypoechoic parathyroid adenoma measuring 9 mm in greatest dimension.

neuromuscular symptoms all respond well to surgical intervention. In contrast, surgery in patients with renal failure, hypertension, and psychiatric symptoms is not so uniformly successful, although it benefits some patients and is usually indicated in all except those at highest risk. The question of how to manage the large group of patients with apparently asymptomatic disease requires particularly careful consideration.

Management of Asymptomatic Hyperparathyroidism.

4 A large proportion of patients with the diagnosis of hyperparathyroidism are minimally symptomatic or asymptomatic. The appropriate treatment for these patients remains controversial. Although little evidence indicates that irreversible complications, such as renal failure, eventually develop in patients with asymptomatic mild disease, the natural history of the disease remains incompletely defined. Many of the manifestations of this disease may go unrecognized until they are corrected surgically. Still unanswered is the question of how much asymptomatic disease may contribute to generalized osteopenia in this predominantly postmenopausal female population.

One study followed a group of 142 asymptomatic patients without operation.[23] At the end of the 10-year study, more than 20% of the patients had required surgery for an increase in serum calcium to above 11 mg/dL or for specific complications attributable to the disease. Another 20% were lost to or declined follow-up. The remaining patients either died of unrelated causes or had persistent asymptomatic disease. The authors concluded that because of the large percentage (about 40%) of patients who either required operation or were lost to follow-up, they could not reliably recommend conservative management.

A more recent report detailed the 15-year natural history of 116 patients with asymptomatic hyperparathyroidism.[21] Operation was recommended for those in whom symptoms or findings developed, according to the guidelines of the National Institutes of Health Consensus Conference (see later). During the monitoring period, 51% of the patients had operation, and biochemical normalization and increased bone mass were observed in those who underwent surgery. However, the patients who did not undergo operative correction continued to have biochemical abnormalities and the cortical bone mass fell significantly. These data confirm the impression of most clinicians that mild hyperparathyroidism rarely takes a precipitously worsening clinical course; however, the differential bone effects that are evident by 15 years call into question how long such patients can be monitored without correction.

In October 1990, a National Institutes of Health Consensus Development Conference reviewed the available evidence regarding the management of asymptomatic primary hyperparathyroidism.[32] After interval developments, a panel of experts reconvened in 2002 and revisited this issue.[20] The panel agreed that operation is the indicated treatment for all patients with symptoms; however, they recognized a subgroup of patients who have no symptoms attributable to hyperparathyroidism, and their conclusions included several indications for surgical intervention in these asymptomatic patients (Table 76.10).

The panel mandated close (every 6 months) follow-up for those patients not treated by operation. In addition, they recommended surgery for cases in which medical surveillance is neither desirable nor suitable, such as when a patient requests surgery, consistent follow-up is unlikely, coexistent illness complicates management, or a patient is younger than age 50 years.

This remains an area of considerable controversy. The complication rate of operation by an experienced surgeon is very low. Within a short period, the financial cost of medical follow-up exceeds that of treatment by operation. Based on these considerations, most patients should undergo operation, and those who do not must be closely followed.

TABLE 76.10 INDICATIONS/CONTRAINDICATIONS

NATIONAL INSTITUTES OF HEALTH CONSENSUS DEVELOPMENT CONFERENCE'S INDICATIONS FOR SURGICAL INTERVENTION IN PATIENTS WITH ASYMPTOMATIC PRIMARY HYPERPARATHYROIDISM

- Markedly elevated serum calcium (>1.0 mg/dL above normal)
- History of an episode of life-threatening hypercalcemia
- Reduced creatinine clearance
- Presence of one or more kidney stones detected by abdominal radiography
- Markedly elevated 24-h urinary calcium excretion
- Substantially reduced bone mass as determined by direct measurement (dual-energy x-ray absorptiometry T score < −2.5)

ENDOCRINE

Principles of Surgical Correction

Although neck exploration for hyperparathyroidism may be straightforward, it sometimes becomes an arduous procedure requiring considerable patience because of the variability in both the location and the number of diseased glands. Persistent hyperparathyroidism and the necessity for reexploration can usually be avoided by a meticulous initial procedure. Reoperation is predictably more difficult than the initial operation, and the risks for damage to the recurrent laryngeal nerves and hypoparathyroidism are greater during reoperation.

It is essential that the surgeon be confident of the preoperative diagnosis and prospectively discuss the procedure with the patient. The potential complications of damage to either the recurrent laryngeal nerve or the superior laryngeal nerve and the development of hypocalcemia require discussion. Likewise, the possibility of an unsuccessful initial operation must be explained, and the patient should recognize that reexploration, including median sternotomy, may be required. Although alternatives to full neck exploration are often now applied, no patient should be explored by a surgeon who is unfamiliar with the principles and techniques of the conventional full neck exploration.

For a full neck exploration, the patient is placed under general anesthesia with a roll beneath the shoulders and the neck extended. The neck is opened through a transverse incision overlying the thyroid isthmus, and the platysma is similarly divided. Superior and inferior flaps are developed. The strap muscles are separated in the midline and retracted laterally; division is unnecessary. One lobe of the thyroid is chosen and rotated medially. Important landmarks include the tracheoesophageal groove, the recurrent laryngeal nerve, the inferior and superior thyroid arteries, and the middle thyroid vein (Fig. 76.15). In most patients, the nerve lies in the tracheoesophageal groove or just laterally. Occasionally, it may be situated more anteriorly. Uncommonly, it may originate directly from the vagus without passing around the right subclavian artery. Both of these latter variations make the recurrent nerve more susceptible to injury. The external branch of the superior laryngeal nerve, which innervates the cricothyroid muscle, usually lies medial to the superior thyroid vessels and should be carefully preserved.

For a full neck exploration, all four glands should be identified at the initial exploration because of the possibility of multiple-gland disease. Supernumerary glands may be present and should be sought at the initial procedure. Although frozen section has not been helpful in differentiating diseased from normal glands, it is generally reliable for confirming the presence or absence of parathyroid tissue. Small, thin biopsy specimens are sharply incised from the gland, with extreme care

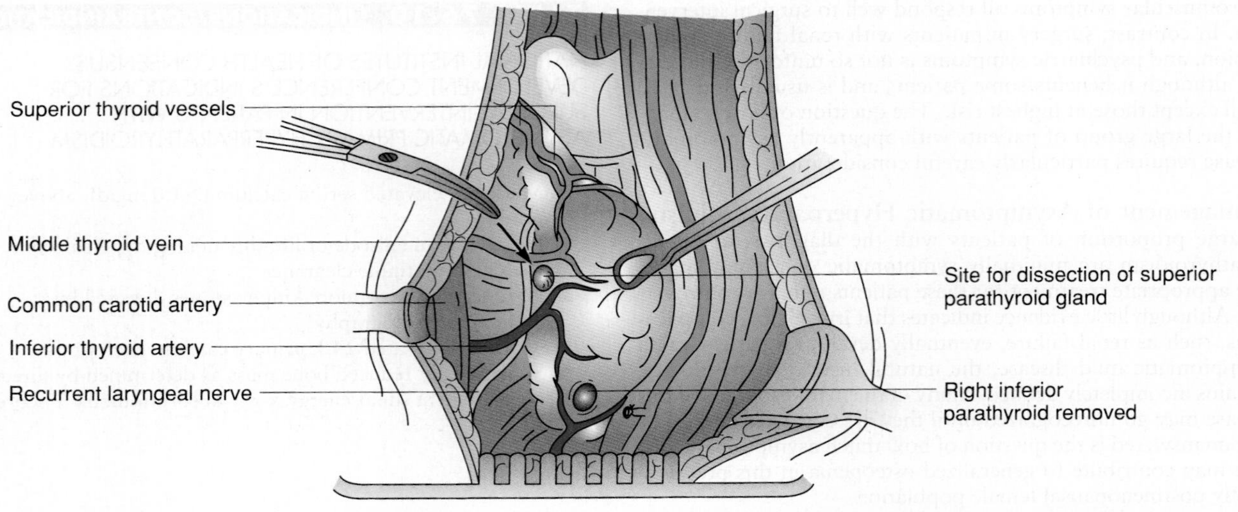

FIGURE 76.15. Lateral view of the right side of the neck after rotation of the thyroid lobe. The important anatomic landmarks are emphasized.

taken to avoid damaging its delicate blood supply. Most surgeons use frozen section selectively to confirm suspected abnormal parathyroid tissue or to document difficult or confusing situations.[33]

The upper glands are usually located far dorsally on the surface of the thyroid lobe at the level of the upper two thirds of the gland. The lower glands are less constant and may be located anywhere from well above the thyroid to the anterior mediastinum. The lower glands are most typically in the region where the thyrothymic ligament attaches to the lower pole of the thyroid lobe. If the inferior glands cannot be localized, the thymic pedicle should be carefully examined and mobilized. Because of their common embryologic origin, the inferior gland is frequently associated with the thymic remnant. Parathyroid glands within the mediastinum sometimes can be removed by mobilizing the thymus through the cervical incision. If this technique is unsuccessful in identifying the parathyroid gland, the thyroid lobe on the side of the missing gland is mobilized and palpated. Intraoperative ultrasonographic examination may identify an intrathyroidal parathyroid gland. As a last resort, excision of the thyroid lobe may be indicated.

If after meticulous exploration of all these areas three or four parathyroid glands have been identified, none of which is enlarged, most surgeons favor terminating the operation.

Limited Surgical Exploration

5 With the availability of accurate preoperative localization methods, it has become routinely possible to identify abnormal parathyroid glands prior to operation for most patients. This allows the surgeon to know where to start the exploration. Then, intraoperative PTH measurement can be used to confirm removal of all hyperfunctioning parathyroid tissue, that is, when to stop the operation. This strategy of directed, limited neck exploration is applicable to about 75% of initial parathyroid explorations, and has about the same success rate as full neck exploration.[34–36] The preoperative localization can be done by either ^{99m}technetium sestamibi nuclear medicine scan or by high-resolution ultrasound. The intraoperative PTH measurement is first assessed at the outset of the procedure and/or immediately preceding parathyroid gland excision (the pre-excision baseline). Blood samples are obtained at time intervals after parathyroid gland resection. A decrease of the PTH level by 50% from the higher of the incision or pre-excision baseline predicts long-term normocalcemia.[37] Other investigators use more sensitive criteria for the detection of multigland disease, including reduction of the PTH level into the normal range and kinetic assessments of the rate of PTH decrease.[38] This increase in sensitivity comes with the cost of decreased specificity, however. Blood samples can be obtained either centrally or peripherally.[39]

The limited nature of this operative approach also makes it easier to perform this operation under regional or local anesthesia in an ambulatory setting. However, because of the possibility of multiple-gland disease or inaccurate preoperative localization, all surgeons undertaking this approach should also be skilled in the full neck exploration for hyperparathyroidism.[40–42]

Extent of Resection. The operative procedure performed has been based on the number of enlarged glands identified at full neck exploration; however, with the use of intraoperative PTH monitoring, it has become clear that not all enlarged parathyroid glands are hyperfunctioning.[43] In contrast, nearly all hyperfunctioning glands are enlarged and hypercellular. The full neck exploration experience has demonstrated that removing all enlarged glands is a highly successful approach to curing hyperparathyroidism, and in the absence of PTH monitoring, this remains an accepted approach. Typically, single-gland disease has been treated by simple excision, whereas any combination of two- or three-gland enlargement is treated by resecting the diseased tissue and leaving the normal glands in place. The question of whether two- or three-gland enlargement implies the presence of disease in all glands (hyperplasia) has not been resolved. If one gland is large and the remaining three are normal in size, resection of the single parathyroid cures virtually all patients. Of 76 patients with two- or three-gland disease treated by excising the large glands and leaving the normal glands, only eight (10.5%) had recurrent hypercalcemia, which tended to be mild (follow-up of 12 to 140 months postoperatively). This approach seems satisfactory in most patients.[44]

Treating patients with four-gland disease has been more difficult. In many of these patients, the disease occurs as a component of one of the familial syndromes, particularly MEN-1. Patients with four-gland parathyroid disease can be treated by subtotal parathyroidectomy (removing three and a half glands) or by total parathyroidectomy with autotransplantation of some parathyroid tissue into the nondominant forearm. Both operations depend on meticulous identification of all parathyroid tissue for adequate results. The putative advantage of the subtotal parathyroidectomy is that it leaves the remaining parathyroid tissue with its native blood supply. Total parathyroidectomy with autograft has the advantage of removing all the abnormal parathyroid tissue from the neck and placing it in a site where reoperation for recurrent hyperparathyroidism is simpler.

The reported incidence of recurrent hypercalcemia after subtotal parathyroidectomy for nonfamilial parathyroid hyperplasia is 0% to 16%; the incidence of permanent hypoparathyroidism is 4% to 5%. Total parathyroidectomy with autograft is associated with a similar risk for permanent hypoparathyroidism in the sporadic setting (5%) and a higher reported risk for recurrent hypercalcemia (20%). Reoperation for recurrent hypercalcemia is greatly simplified by the approach of total parathyroidectomy with autotransplantation. Thus, given the current data, sporadic parathyroid hyperplasia can be acceptably treated by either operation. In patients with MEN-1, the disease is not the same as sporadic hyperplasia. Rather, defects in the *MEN1* gene cause multiple parathyroid adenomas that arise independently over the life of the patient.[23] The operative results reflect this independent capability of all parathyroid tissue in these patients to become neoplastic. The hypercalcemia recurrence rate is 26% to 36% with long-term follow-up after subtotal parathyroidectomy, and similar after total parathyroidectomy with autograft. However, the incidence of permanent hypoparathyroidism after autograft in MEN-1 is also significant (reported as high as 46%). While both approaches are currently accepted, most experienced centers now advocate subtotal parathyroidectomy as the initial operation in MEN-1 hyperparathyroidism, and anticipate that recurrent disease is likely, manageable, and less problematic than permanent hypocalcemia.[45–48]

Technique of Parathyroid Autotransplantation. The parathyroid gland is sliced into 15 to 20 pieces and autografted into a forearm muscle bed. The sites are marked with silk sutures. This location permits easy subsequent access under local anesthesia if recurrent hypercalcemia develops. Function of the autograft is documented by (a) normocalcemia, with the autograft as the only source of PTH; (b) by measuring higher concentrations of hormone in the antecubital vein draining the graft bed than in the corresponding vein in the opposite arm; or (c) "transient parathyroidectomy," by placing a venous occlusive tourniquet on the arm above the graft and measuring changes over several minutes in the PTH levels drawn from the contralateral arm.[49] Lack of function is unusual outside of the MEN-1 patients; hypoparathyroidism develops in about 5% of patients. Glands can also be cryopreserved in dimethyl sulfoxide and serum. If in the postoperative period it becomes clear that the patient is aparathyroid, the cryopreserved tissue can be reimplanted under local anesthesia.

Special Situations

Persistent or Recurrent Hyperparathyroidism. Persistent hyperparathyroidism occurs in fewer than 5% of patients after exploration by an experienced surgeon. Most commonly, it is the result of a single diseased gland remaining in the neck or the mediastinum. Recurrent disease develops after an interval of normocalcemia and may be the result of regrowth of diseased tissue, implantation from a tumor broken at the initial procedure, or recurrent parathyroid carcinoma.

In the evaluation of these patients, it is essential to document that the initial diagnosis was correct. Familial hypocalciuric hypercalcemia should be excluded by measuring urinary calcium excretion.

Reviewing the original operative notes and pathology reports may provide clues to the position of missed glands. The locations of parathyroid tumors not found at the initial operation but identified on subsequent exploration in one large series are shown in Fig. 76.16.

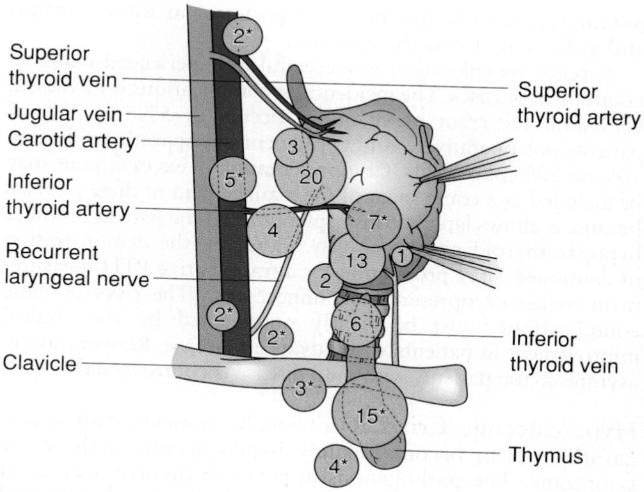

FIGURE 76.16. Location of parathyroid tumors missed on initial exploration but identified on subsequent operation. (After Jaskowiak N, Norton JA, Alexander HR, et al. A prospective trial evaluating a standard approach to reoperation for missed parathyroid adenoma. *Ann Surg* 1996;224:308–320.)

It is generally agreed that localization studies do have a place in the management of recurrent disease. Noninvasive methods are used first, and if these are unsuccessful in identifying the diseased gland, selective angiography and venous sampling for PTH are used. The utility of the techniques vary across institutions, dependent on local experience, expertise, and preference. Selective angiography localizes 50% to 80% of parathyroid glands that cannot be detected by any other modality. Venous sampling may also be helpful in some patients, although interpretation can be complicated by the collateralization that occurs postoperatively. Because it provides no direct image but indicates the side and level of the neck where the hyperfunctioning tissue is located, it may help to direct the evaluation of imaging studies and the exploration to one or the other side of the neck. Both these invasive radiographic techniques require considerable expertise. Transient cortical blindness, transverse myelitis, and cerebrovascular accidents have all been reported as complications of arteriography. Angiographic ablation of mediastinal parathyroid tissue with large doses of ionic contrast has been successful in selected patients. This technique may be used in some patients with mediastinal parathyroid adenomas who are at increased surgical risk and who have other functional parathyroid tissue remaining.[50]

Surgical reexploration can be a difficult procedure. The neck should almost always be reexplored first. If the thymic remnant has not already been removed, it should be excised at this time. Two adjunctive techniques, intraoperative ultrasonography to locate glands and intraoperative measurement of PTH to document the adequacy of resection, may be useful in patients undergoing operation for persistent disease.[31]

If the gland is not identified in the neck by means of the maneuvers described, the mediastinum is examined; most surgeons do this only if there is imaging evidence of disease in the mediastinum, rather than unguided exploration. Median sternotomy and exploration are necessary in only 1% to 2% of patients with hyperparathyroidism. Successful transcervical mediastinal exploration is sometimes possible with use of the Cooper thymectomy retractor, a substernal retractor that permits more extensive mediastinal exploration and thymectomy through a cervical incision.[51] Any remaining thymic tissue is first isolated and examined. Inferior parathyroid glands most commonly migrate into the anterior mediastinum. If the results of this exploration are negative, the area posterior and lateral to the trachea is then explored. The location of superior parathyroid glands may be as far posterior as the esophagus and as far superior as the pharynx.

Surgical reexploration is successful in experienced hands in about 80% of cases. The incidence of complications is increased. Unilateral recurrent nerve injury occurs in 5% to 10% of patients postoperatively, and permanent hypoparathyroidism in 10% to 20% of patients. Cryopreservation of excised tissue may be included as a component of the management of these patients because it allows later autotransplantation if the patient becomes hypoparathyroid postoperatively. However, the demonstration of continued PTH production by intraoperative PTH measurement makes cryopreservation unnecessary. The risks of these complications must be clearly outweighed by the clinical improvement in patients with advanced disease. Reoperation in asymptomatic patients with mild disease is controversial.

Hypercalcemic Crisis. Occasionally, patients with hyperparathyroidism become acutely hypercalcemic with severe symptoms. The pathogenesis appears to involve a cycle of uncontrolled PTH secretion followed by hypercalcemia and secondary polyuria, dehydration, and reduced renal function, which exacerbate the hypercalcemia. Serum calcium concentrations may reach 16 to 20 mg/dL, and the syndrome is manifested by rapidly developing muscle weakness, nausea and vomiting, lethargy, fatigue, and even coma. Ultrasonography, sestamibi scan, or CT scan may help to identify the enlarged gland to allow expedient correction.

Definitive treatment involves resecting the diseased parathyroid tissue, which is almost always curative. Generally, however, it is safer to lower the serum calcium level before operation.

Hyperparathyroidism in Pregnancy. Hyperparathyroidism in pregnancy is a rare disorder that not only causes hypercalcemia in the mother but also is associated with increased morbidity and mortality rates in the fetus. Even the newborn is at risk for the development of tetany. The risk for fetal complications is higher if the hyperparathyroidism is left untreated. The mother should undergo operation in the second trimester.[17,52,53]

Neonatal Hyperparathyroidism. Neonatal hyperparathyroidism occurs in infants who are homozygous for a mutation of the calcium-sensing receptor and is characterized by hypotonia, poor feeding, constipation, and respiratory distress. Each parent of these children is affected by familial hypocalciuric hypercalcemia. The 1-year survival rate in children with symptoms is less than 50%, and patients without symptoms appear to have significant bone disease. Total parathyroidectomy with autotransplantation is the treatment of choice.[54]

Secondary Hyperparathyroidism. Secondary hyperparathyroidism develops as a consequence of chronic renal failure. Phosphate retention and hyperphosphatemia reduce the serum calcium levels. This effect is aggravated by the reduction in 1-hydroxylase activity in the kidney, necessary for the activation of vitamin D_3. The secondary increase in PTH levels to compensate for the hypocalcemic effects is exacerbated by aluminum accumulation in bone. Aluminum, present both in the dialysate fluid and in phosphate-binding medications, contributes to the osteomalacia (renal osteodystrophy) that develops in all these patients after several years of dialysis. Therapy includes controlling the hyperphosphatemia with dietary restriction and phosphate-binding gels, calcium supplementation orally and in the dialysate bath, correction of acidosis, administration of vitamin D sterol, and reduction in aluminum intake in both the dialysate and the diet. Therapy should be initiated carefully because metastatic soft tissue calcification can occur. Indications for surgical therapy include persistent, symptomatic hypercalcemia that cannot be controlled medically, particularly in prospective renal transplant patients; bone pain and abnormal fractures; ectopic calcification; and intractable pruritus. Subtotal parathyroidectomy and total parathyroidectomy with heterotopic autotransplantation both appear to be acceptable options, although reexploration for recurrent disease is less complicated after total parathyroidectomy with autotransplantation. Parathyroidectomy can enhance aluminum deposition, so any excess should be corrected preoperatively through chelation.

Parathyroid Carcinoma. Parathyroid carcinoma is a rare condition, accounting for less than 1% of all cases of hyperparathyroidism. Histologic criteria remain controversial, and the diagnosis is securely made only on the basis of local invasion or distant metastases. In comparison to patients with benign disease, these patients tend to be somewhat younger and more symptomatic. In contrast to the marked female predominance in benign disease, the male-to-female ratio in carcinoma is equal. Serum calcium, PTH, and alkaline phosphatase levels are relatively more elevated, and patients often have an elevated level of human chorionic gonadotropin. Patients may have manifestations of both renal and bone disease. The affected gland is palpable in almost half of patients.

Initial treatment should include radical resection of the involved gland, ipsilateral thyroid lobe, and regional lymph nodes. Neither chemotherapy nor radiation therapy has shown any benefit. If the disease recurs, resection should be attempted because without treatment these patients usually succumb to uncontrolled hypercalcemia. The long-term prognosis is poor, and the opportunity for survival depends on complete initial resection.[26,55,56]

MULTIPLE ENDOCRINE NEOPLASIA

Although these familial disorders are typically characterized by a predisposition to the development of tumors of multiple endocrine organs, the parathyroid is characteristically involved in two of them. The disorders are all inherited in an autosomal dominant fashion, and the tumors tend to be multicentric. The tumors can be benign or malignant and can occur metachronously or synchronously. MEN-1 is characterized by the concurrence of parathyroid hyperplasia, pancreatic islet cell tumors, and pituitary adenomas. MEN-2A consists of medullary thyroid carcinoma (MTC), pheochromocytoma, and parathyroid hyperplasia. MEN-2B includes MTC, pheochromocytoma, mucosal neuromas, and a distinctive marfanoid habitus. Together these syndromes encompass much of the spectrum of endocrine neoplasia.

Pathogenesis

The genetic abnormality in MEN-1 has been identified and described in detail.[57,58] As a tumor-suppressor gene, the first mutation is inherited and becomes unmasked only when a second mutation, in some cases a deletion, develops in susceptible tissues. The resulting complete loss of the tumor suppressor allows neoplasia to develop. The occurrence of multiple second mutations explains the characteristic multicentric involvement of these diseases. Direct genetic testing is now available for some families with known mutations.

Mutations of the *RET* proto-oncogene are the cause of MEN-2A.[59,60] Genetic testing is now available to identify affected family members and provide the opportunity for early treatment of MTC in affected persons.

Clinical Features and Management of Multiple Endocrine Neoplasia Type 1

Characteristically, MEN-1 presents in the third and fourth decades, without any gender predilection.[61] The syndrome is expressed with nearly complete penetrance, and autopsy studies suggest that all three organs are affected in more than 90% of patients. The phenotype varies, however; more than 90% of patients have hyperparathyroidism, but evidence of islet cell neoplasms (30% to 80%) and pituitary tumors (15% to 50%) is less common. The cause of death in carriers of the MEN-1 mutation is related to MEN-1 in about 45% of patients and often caused by malignant islet cell or carcinoid tumors.[62]

Parathyroid Disease. Hypercalcemia secondary to hyperparathyroidism is usually the first biochemical abnormality detected in MEN-1 and represents the best screening opportunity for members of affected kindreds until direct genetic screening is available in a specific family. Many of these patients are asymptomatic and have relatively mild hypercalcemia. When symptoms do develop, they typically involve the urinary tract rather than the skeleton.

Typically, the patients have four-gland disease, which may be particularly difficult to manage. The disease is characterized by metachronous development of multiple parathyroid adenomas. There is no curative operation; the two accepted approaches (subtotal parathyroidectomy and total parathyroidectomy with autograft) each have faults (see earlier). Over time, the subtotal parathyroidectomy approach is becoming the preferred choice by most surgeons.

Pancreatic Tumors. In patients with pancreatic tumors, multicentric and diffuse hyperplasia of the pancreatic islets may occur in areas distant from any grossly evident tumor. The management of these tumors is controversial because although some patients have aggressive, malignant tumors, many patients have a fairly benign course. No reliable criteria are available to detect malignant tumors. Tumor size is often cited as a useful marker of prognosis, but substantial overlap has been noted between the sizes of primary benign and malignant tumors (Fig. 76.17).[63] Because of the difficulty in identifying the more aggressive subset, some authors have chosen a liberal policy of early operation to try to prevent metastasis and death. Pancreatic tumors are typically multicentric and frequently malignant. Somatostatin receptor scintigraphy can be a useful imaging technique to demonstrate the extent of tumor (Fig. 76.18).[64]

Gastrinoma is the most common functional tumor in MEN-1; typically, a severe ulcer diathesis (Zollinger-Ellison syndrome) develops that is associated with secretory diarrhea. Serum gastrin levels are usually markedly elevated (>1,000 pg/mL); when levels are equivocal (250 to 1,000 pg/mL), provocative testing with secretin (2 m/kg) may be useful. An absolute serum gastrin increase of 200 pg/mL is diagnostic. The primary tumors are often in the submucosa of the duodenal wall.

Biochemical cure of these gastrinomas is almost never possible, which is different than patients with sporadic gastrinomas, although exploration can reduce the need for antisecretory medications and may reduce the risk for liver metastasis. Histamine 2–receptor antagonists or proton pump inhibitors are effective in controlling acid secretion, although very high doses may be necessary; the malignant disease is often indolent. Total gastrectomy is no longer ever necessary to eliminate acid secretion.

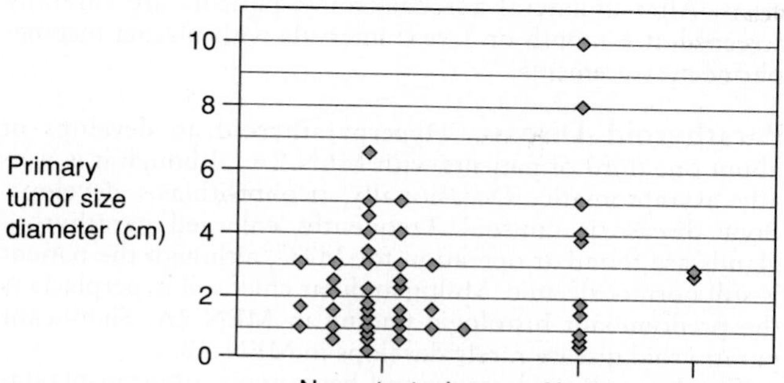

FIGURE 76.17. Scatter plot of largest primary tumor size versus metastatic status in 43 patients with pancreatic islet cell tumors associated with multiple endocrine neoplasia type 1. Each point represents a single patient. Tumor size is not correlated with the presence of liver or lymph node metastases. (Reproduced with permission from Lowney JK, Frisella MM, Lairmore TC, et al. Islet cell tumor metastasis in multiple endocrine neoplasia type I: correlation with primary tumor size. *Surgery* 1998;124:1043–1049.)

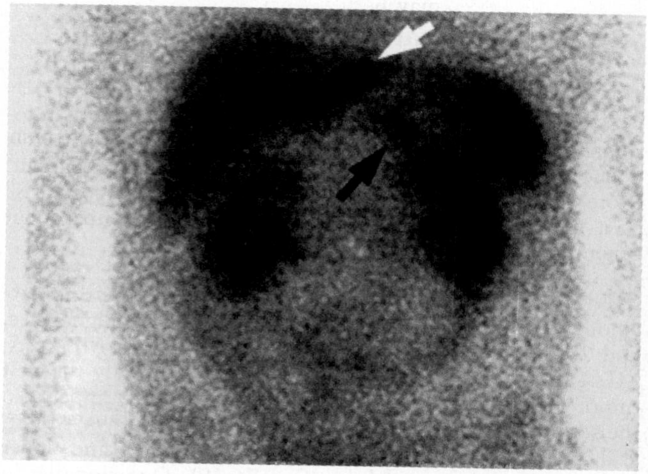

FIGURE 76.18. Somatostatin receptor scintigraphy in a patient with multiple endocrine neoplasia type 1. This scintiscan detected an otherwise unrecognized metastasis to the left lateral segment of the liver (*white arrow*), which was resected along with the small primary tumor (*black arrow*).

Insulinoma is the next most common functional pancreatic neoplasm in MEN-1. Patients present with a history of sweating, dizziness, confusion, and syncope, consistent with neuroglycopenia; these symptoms are relieved by consuming carbohydrates. The diagnosis is verified by documenting fasting hypoglycemia associated with inappropriately elevated plasma insulin levels. Preoperative tumor localization is usually achieved by a combination of CT and arteriography. Calcium is injected into various pancreatic arteries and plasma insulin levels in the hepatic vein plasma are measured to detect a gradient after the injection of specific pancreatic arteries localizing the area of the pancreas containing the functional tumor.

Because the available medical therapy for insulinoma is limited, patients are treated operatively. Lesions in the tail of the gland can be enucleated if they are small; however, distal pancreatectomy carries little morbidity. Tumors of the head can usually be enucleated, so that pancreaticoduodenectomy can be avoided. In patients with malignant disease, metastases may respond to streptozocin; diazoxide, verapamil, or octreotide, may successfully reduce insulin secretion and control symptoms. A diet of complex carbohydrates can also help stabilize serum glucose levels in the hyperinsulinemic patient.

Nonfunctional tumors are the most common pancreas lesions in MEN-1. Their management is specific to their size and risk of malignancy.

Pituitary Adenomas. Prolactin-secreting tumors occur most commonly in this setting, although Cushing disease or acromegaly develops in an occasional patient. Symptoms may result from compression of the optic chiasm, which produces bitemporal hemianopsia, or from prolactin excess, which produces amenorrhea and galactorrhea in female patients and hypogonadism in male patients.

Bromocriptine inhibits prolactin secretion and shrinks many prolactinomas. Refractory tumors and those producing other hormones can be managed by pituitary ablation or radiation.

Other Tumors. MEN-1 is associated much less frequently with adrenocortical tumors and benign thyroid adenomas. Lipomas and carcinoid tumors may also occur.

ENDOCRINE

Clinical Features and Management of Multiple Endocrine Neoplasia Type 2

Like MEN-1, the MEN-2 syndromes are inherited in an autosomal dominant fashion with complete penetrance but variable phenotype. Bilateral MTC occurs in every affected patient. More frequently than the other syndromes, MEN-2B can arise as a new mutation that can be transmitted to subsequent generations.

Medullary Thyroid Carcinoma. Medullary thyroid carcinoma accounts for about 10% of all thyroid malignancies, and 20% of cases occur in the familial setting of MEN-2A, MEN-2B, or familial non-MEN MTC. It is usually the first tumor that develops in these patients and typically appears in the second or third decade. Tumors are virtually always bilateral and develop in multiple areas of the middle and upper portions of the thyroid lobe (Fig. 76.19). Occasionally, in young people, a diffuse proliferation of parafollicular C cells, termed *C-cell hyperplasia*, is present without frankly invasive carcinoma. This finding is highly suggestive of one of the familial MTC syndromes. Patients typically present with a neck mass and may have hoarseness, dysphagia, or palpable cervical adenopathy. MTC may produce a variety of hormones, including calcitonin, adrenocorticotropic hormone, prostaglandin, and serotonin. The hypercalcitoninemia is often asymptomatic, although severe diarrhea can develop.

By detecting minimal elevations of plasma calcitonin, it is possible to diagnose MTC at a clinically occult stage. Basal plasma calcitonin levels in normal subjects are in the range of 30 to 100 pg/mL. An increase to levels of 150 to 200 pg/mL occurs, however, after the administration of the potent secretagogues calcium and pentagastrin. The plasma calcitonin levels of patients with MTC show striking increases (>1,000 pg/mL) after provocative testing, so that they can be identified readily. Patients with occult disease may have only minimally elevated basal calcitonin levels that increase in response to secretagogues. The combined infusion of calcium and pentagastrin was the most effective screening test for familial MTC before genetic testing became available. By means of provocative testing in kindred members at risk for disease, MTC was diagnosed at a preclinical stage, and a greater percentage of these patients were cured by surgical therapy. With genetic testing now available, prophylactic thyroidectomy to prevent the development of MTC is possible for all affected people.

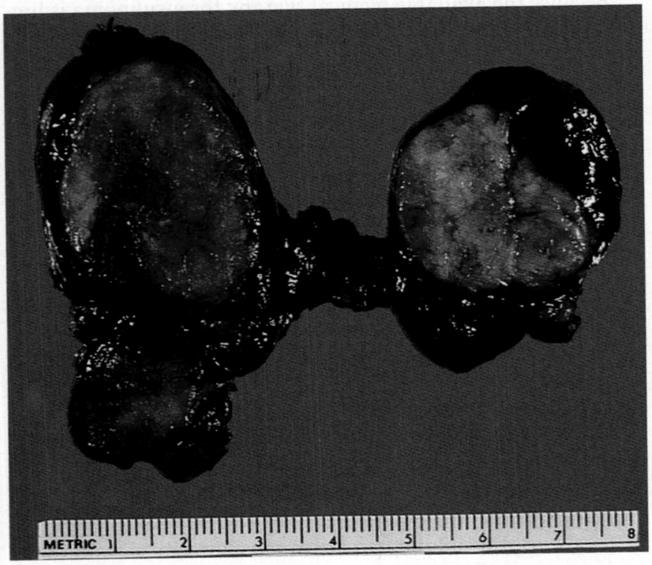

FIGURE 76.19. Medullary thyroid carcinoma. Coronal section of a total thyroid resection shows bilateral involvement by a firm, pale tumor. (Reproduced with permission from Rubin E, Farber JL. *Pathology*, 3rd ed. Philadelphia, PA: Lippincott Williams & Wilkins; 1999.)

Postoperatively, the presence of residual MTC can be readily detected by provocative testing. Meticulous reoperation in patients with recurrent or persistently elevated plasma calcitonin levels postoperatively, including mediastinal dissection on occasion, can normalize elevated plasma calcitonin levels and apparently cure many of them.[65] For the patient with unresectable metastases, few therapeutic options are available. Neither radiation nor chemotherapy is of significant benefit.

The clinical course of patients with the MEN-2 syndromes is determined primarily by the status of their MTC. In the setting of MEN-2A, the tumors are often indolent and survival prolonged, even in the presence of metastatic disease. By contrast, the tumors in patients with MEN-2B occur at an earlier age and are generally more aggressive neoplasms. Patients may succumb to the disease at a young age. As a consequence of this aggressiveness, the size of kindreds with the disease is typically small, and usually only a few generations are affected.

Pheochromocytoma. Pheochromocytomas are usually detected during the initial screening or follow-up of patients in whom MTC has already been diagnosed. They typically appear in the second or third decade of life, and about 80% are bilateral. Usually, pheochromocytomas are benign but multicentric, and they almost always arise in the adrenal medulla. In patients with MEN-2A or MEN-2B, hyperplasia of the adrenal medulla may develop first, grossly characterized by thickening of the medullary tissue in both adrenal glands.

Pheochromocytomas can be asymptomatic, but most commonly, patients have pounding frontal headaches, episodic diaphoresis, palpitations, or anxiety. Hypertension also occurs and is often episodic.

The diagnosis is made by measuring the plasma concentration of metanephrines. Patients with MEN-2A or MEN-2B and MTC should be evaluated for pheochromocytoma before they undergo thyroidectomy. If a patient is found to have both lesions, adrenalectomy should be performed first, followed by neck exploration. The abdomen is explored through a bilateral subcostal incision or, more typically, with a laparoscope.[66] Bilateral pheochromocytomas are treated by bilateral adrenalectomy. In patients with MEN-2A or MEN-2B and a unilateral pheochromocytoma, only the diseased adrenal gland is removed. In about 30% of patients treated in this manner, a tumor eventually develops in the opposite gland. In the remaining patients, this approach avoids the need for glucocorticoid and mineralocorticoid replacement and the risk for addisonian crisis. After unilateral adrenalectomy, patients are carefully screened at 6-month or 1-year intervals with plasma metanephrine measurements.

Parathyroid Disease. Hyperparathyroidism develops in about one third of patients with MEN-2A, although it is usually asymptomatic. Occasionally, nephrolithiasis develops. Bone disease is unusual. Frequently, enlarged parathyroid glands are found at operation for MTC, although the patient is still normocalcemic. Multiglandular chief cell hyperplasia is the predominant histologic finding in MEN-2A. Significant parathyroid disease rarely develops in MEN-2B.

Total parathyroidectomy and heterotopic autotransplantation are performed in hypercalcemic patients with MEN-2A. In normocalcemic patients with MEN-2A undergoing thyroidectomy for MTC, total parathyroidectomy and heterotopic autotransplantation are performed in one session to ensure that the complete thyroidectomy does not compromise the parathyroid blood supply and to avoid reoperation in the neck for subsequent hyperparathyroidism. Evidence suggests that these patients are more easily treated, with a lower incidence of recurrent hyperparathyroidism, than patients with MEN-1.

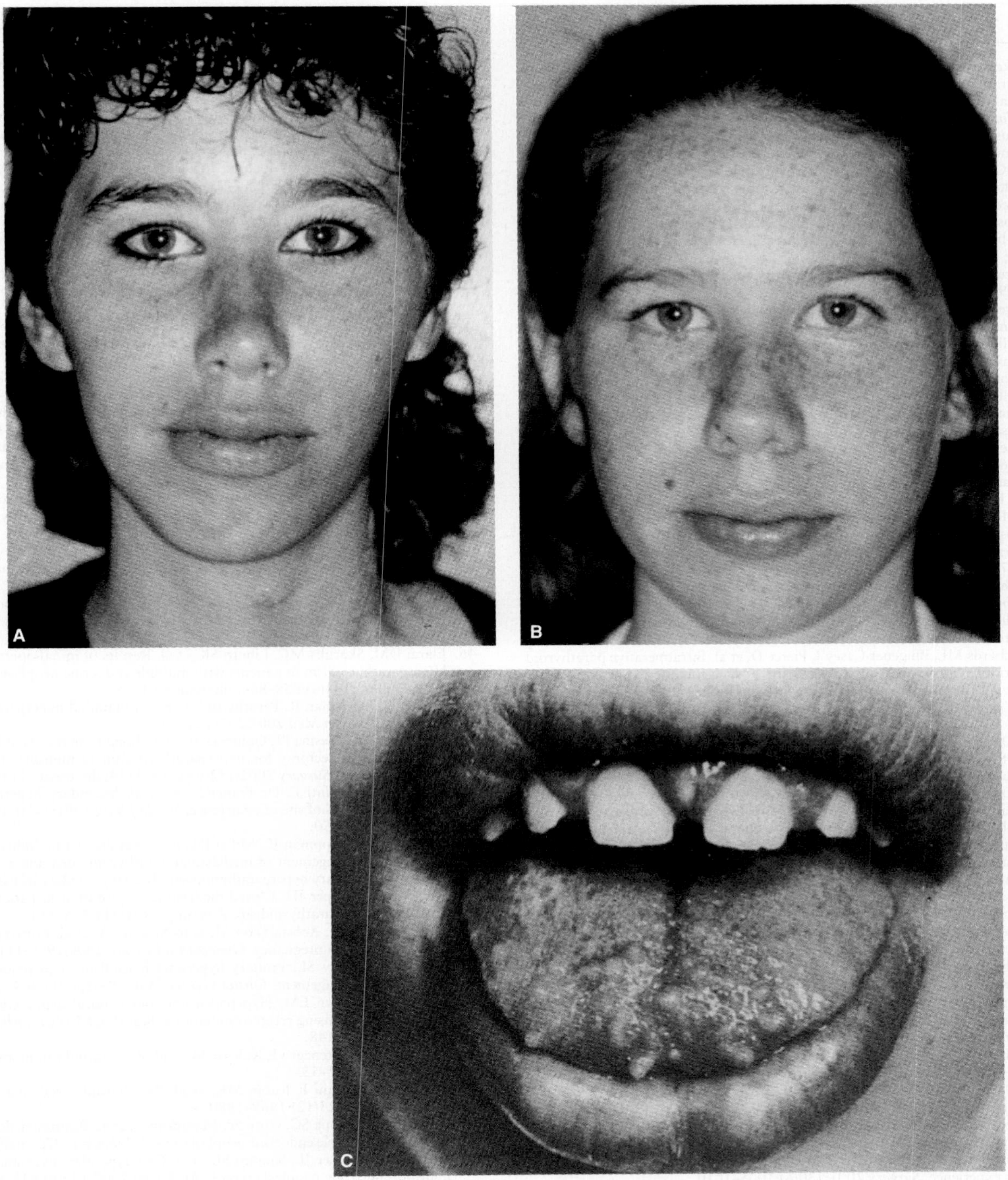

FIGURE 76.20. **A, B:** Characteristic appearance of patients with multiple endocrine neoplasia type 2B (MEN-2B), including thick lips. **C:** Multiple mucosal neuromas on the tongue of a patient with MEN-2B. (Reproduced with permission from Norton JA, Froome LC, Farrell FE, et al. Multiple endocrine neoplasia type 2b: the most aggressive form of medullary thyroid carcinoma. *Surg Clin North Am* 1979;59:109.)

Nonendocrine Manifestations of Multiple Endocrine Neoplasia Type 2B

In addition to MTC and pheochromocytoma, marked abnormalities of the nervous and musculoskeletal systems develop in patients with MEN-2B. The classic phenotype is characterized by thick lips and a thin, marfanoid habitus (Fig. 76.20A, B). The incidence of associated skeletal abnormalities is high; these include kyphosis, pectus excavatum, pes planus or cavus, and congenital dislocation of the hip. Diffuse autonomic nervous hypertrophy is another feature. Mucosal neuromas appear on the tongue (Fig. 76.20C), eyelids, lips, and pharynx. Slit-lamp examination may reveal hypertrophied corneal nerves. Ganglioneuromatosis develops in the submucosal and myenteric plexuses of the gastrointestinal tract. Constipation is common, and radiographic findings may suggest megacolon or Hirschsprung disease.

References

1. Akerstrom G, Malmaeus J, Bergstrom R. Surgical anatomy of human parathyroid glands. *Surgery* 1984;95:14.
2. Mallette LE. Regulation of blood calcium in humans. *Endocrinol Metab Clin North Am* 1989;18:601–610.
3. Nussbaum SR. Pathophysiology and management of severe hypercalcemia. *Endocrinol Metab Clin North Am* 1993;22:343–362.
4. LeGrand SB, Leskuski D, Zama I. Narrative review: furosemide for hypercalcemia: an unproven yet common practice [see comment]. *Ann Intern Med* 2008;149(4):259–263.
5. Ross JR, Saunders Y, Edmonds PM, et al. A systematic review of the role of bisphosphonates in metastatic disease. *Health Technol Assess (Winchester, England)* 2004;8(4):1–176.
6. Strewler GJ, Nissenson RA. Hypercalcemia in malignancy. *West J Med* 1990;153:635–640.
7. Strewler GJ, Nissenson RA. Peptide mediators of hypercalcemia in malignancy. *Annu Rev Med* 1990;41:35–44.
8. Pollak MR, Brown EM, Chou Y-HW, et al. Mutations in the human Ca-sensing receptor gene cause familial hypocalciuric hypercalcemia and neonatal severe hyperparathyroidism. *Cell* 1993;75:1297–1303.
9. Pollak MR, Chou Y-HW, Marx SJ, et al. Familial hypocalciuric hypercalcemia and neonatal severe hyperparathyroidism: effects of mutant gene dosage on phenotype. *J Clin Invest* 1994;93:1108–1112.
10. Bilezikian JP. Management of acute hypercalcemia. *N Engl J Med* 1992; 326:1196–1203.
11. Martinez-Zapata MJ, Roque M, Alonso-Coello P, et al. Calcitonin for metastatic bone pain [update of Cochrane Database Syst Rev. 2003;(3):CD003223; PMID: 12917954]. *Cochrane Database Syst Rev* 2006;(3):CD003223.
12. Ross JR, Saunders Y, Edmonds PM, et al. Systematic review of role of bisphosphonates on skeletal morbidity in metastatic cancer. *BMJ* 2003; 327(7413):469.
13. Tohme MF, Bilezikian JP. Hypocalcemic emergencies. *Endocrinol Metab Clin North Am* 1993;22:363–375.
14. Pallotti F, Seregni E, Ferrari L, et al. Diagnostic and therapeutic aspects of iatrogenic hypoparathyroidism. *Tumori* 2003;89(5):547–549.
15. Richards ML, Bingener-Casey J, Pierce D, et al. Intraoperative parathyroid hormone assay: an accurate predictor of symptomatic hypocalcemia following thyroidectomy [see comment]. *Arch Surg* 2003;138(6):632–635; discussion 635–636.
16. Lo CY. Postthyroidectomy hypocalcemia [comment]. *J Am Coll Surg* 2003;196(3):497–498.
17. Ip P. Neonatal convulsion revealing maternal hyperparathyroidism: an unusual case of late neonatal hypoparathyroidism. *Arch Gynecol Obstet* 2003;268(3):227–229.
18. Heath H. Clinical spectrum of primary hyperparathyroidism: evolution with changes in medical practice and technology. *J Bone Miner Res* 1991; 6(suppl 2):S63–S70.
19. Heath H, Hodgson SF, Kennedy MA. Primary hyperparathyroidism: incidence, morbidity and potential economic impact in a community. *N Engl J Med* 1980;302:189–193.
20. Bilezikian JP, Potts JT Jr, Fuleihan Gel H, et al. Summary statement from a workshop on asymptomatic primary hyperparathyroidism: a perspective for the 21st century. *J Clin Endocrinol Metab* 2002;87(12):5353–5361.
21. Rubin MR, Bilezikian JP, McMahon DJ, et al. The natural history of primary hyperparathyroidism with or without parathyroid surgery after 15 years. *J Clin Endocrinol Metab* 2008;93(9):3462–3470.
22. Arnold A, Shattuck TM, Mallya SM, et al. Molecular pathogenesis of primary hyperparathyroidism. *J Bone Miner Res* 2002;17(suppl 2):N30–N36.
23. Doherty GM, Lairmore TC, DeBenedetti MK. Multiple endocrine neoplasia type 1 parathyroid adenoma development over time. *World J Surg* 2004;28(11):1139–1142.
24. Johnson SJ, Sheffield EA, McNicol AM. Best practice no 183. Examination of parathyroid gland specimens. *J Clin Pathol* 2005;58(4):338–342.
25. Gauger PG, Agarwal G, England BG, et al. Intraoperative parathyroid hormone monitoring fails to detect double parathyroid adenomas: a 2-institution experience. *Surgery* 2001;130(6):1005–1010.
26. DeLellis RA. Parathyroid carcinoma: an overview. *Adv Anat Pathol* 2005;12(2):53–61.
27. Bilezikian JP, Khan AA, Potts JT Jr. Guidelines for the management of asymptomatic primary hyperparathyroidism: summary statement from the third international workshop. *J Clin Endocrinol Metab* 2009;94(2): 335–339.
28. Hedback G, Oden A, Tisell L-E. The influence of surgery on the risk of death in patients with primary hyperparathyroidism. *World J Surg* 1991; 15:399–407.
29. Hedback G, Tisell L-E, Bengtsson B-A, et al. Premature death in patients operated on for primary hyperparathyroidism. *World J Surg* 1990;14: 829–836.
30. Hagstrom E, Hellman P, Larsson TE, et al. Plasma parathyroid hormone and the risk of cardiovascular mortality in the community. *Circulation* 2009;119(21):2765–2771.
31. Udelsman R, Donovan PI. Remedial parathyroid surgery: changing trends in 130 consecutive cases [see comment]. *Ann Surg* 2006;244(3):471–479.
32. Potts JT Jr, Ackerman IP, Barker CF, et al. Diagnosis and management of asymptomatic primary hyperparathyroidism: consensus development conference statement. *Ann Intern Med* 1991;114:593–597.
33. Oertli D, Richter M, Kraenzlin M, et al. Parathyroidectomy in primary hyperparathyroidism: preoperative localization and routine biopsy of unaltered glands are not necessary. *Surgery* 1995;117:392–396.
34. Carty S, Worsey M, Virji M, et al. Concise parathyroidectomy: the impact of preoperative SPECT ^{99m}Tc sestamibi scanning and intraoperative quick parathormone assay. *Surgery* 1997;122:1107–1116.
35. Udelsman R, Pasieka JL, Sturgeon C, et al. Surgery for asymptomatic primary hyperparathyroidism: proceedings of the third international workshop. *J Clin Endocrinol Metab* 2009;94(2):366–372.
36. Carling T, Udelsman R. Focused approach to parathyroidectomy. *World J Surg* 2008;32(7):1512–1517.
37. Carneiro DM, Solorzano CC, Nader MC, et al. Comparison of intraoperative iPTH assay (QPTH) criteria in guiding parathyroidectomy: which criterion is the most accurate? *Surgery* 2003;134(6):973–979; discussion 979–981.
38. Gauger PG, Mullan MH, Thompson NW, et al. An alternative analysis of intraoperative parathyroid hormone data may improve the ability to detect multiglandular disease. *Arch Surg* 2004;139(2):164–169.
39. Woodrum DT, Saunders BD, England BG, et al. The influence of sample site on intraoperative PTH monitoring during parathyroidectomy. *Surgery* 2004;136(6):1169–1175.
40. Irvin GL III, Sfakianakis G, Yeung L, et al. Ambulatory parathyroidectomy for primary hyperparathyroidism. *Arch Surg* 1996;131(10):1074–1078.
41. Lowney JK, Weber B, Johnson S, et al. Minimal incision parathyroidectomy: cure, cosmesis, and cost. *World J Surg* 2000;24(11):1442–1445.
42. Carling T, Donovan P, Rinder C, et al. Minimally invasive parathyroidectomy using cervical block: reasons for conversion to general anesthesia. *Arch Surg* 2006;141(4):401–404; discussion 404.
43. Clerici T, Brandle M, Lange J, et al. Impact of intraoperative parathyroid hormone monitoring on the prediction of multiglandular parathyroid disease. *World J Surg* 2004;28(2):187–192.
44. Wells SA, Leight GS, Hensley M, et al. Hyperparathyroidism associated with the enlargement of two or three parathyroid glands. *Ann Surg* 1985; 202:533–538.
45. Marx SJ, Simonds WF, Agarwal SK, et al. Hyperparathyroidism in hereditary syndromes: special expressions and special managements. *J Bone Miner Res* 2002;17(suppl 2):N37–N43.
46. Elaraj DM, Skarulis MC, Libutti SK, et al. Results of initial operation for hyperparathyroidism in patients with multiple endocrine neoplasia type 1. *Surgery* 2003;134(6):858–864; discussion 64–65.
47. Carling T, Udelsman R. Parathyroid surgery in familial hyperparathyroid disorders. *J Intern Med* 2005;257(1):27–37.
48. Arnalsteen LC, Alesina PF, Quiereux JL, et al. Long-term results of less than total parathyroidectomy for hyperparathyroidism in multiple endocrine neoplasia type 1. *Surgery* 2002;132(6):1119–1124; discussion 1124–1125.
49. Casanova D, Sarfati E, De Francisco A, et al. Secondary hyperparathyroidism: diagnosis of site of recurrence. *World J Surg* 1991;15(4):546–549; discussion 549–550.
50. Doherty GM, Doppman JL, Miller DL, et al. Results of a multidisciplinary strategy for management of mediastinal parathyroid adenoma as a cause of persistent primary hyperparathyroidism. *Ann Surg* 1992;215(2):101–106.
51. Wells SA Jr, Cooper JD. Closed mediastinal exploration in patients with persistent hyperparathyroidism. *Ann Surg* 1991;214:555–561.
52. Amaya Garcia M, Acosta Feria M, Soto Moreno A, et al. Primary hyperparathyroidism in pregnancy. *Gynecol Endocrinol* 2004;19(2):111–114.
53. Schnatz PF, Curry SL. Primary hyperparathyroidism in pregnancy: evidence-based management. *Obstet Gynecol Surv* 2002;57(6):365–376.
54. Egbuna OI, Brown EM. Hypercalcaemic and hypocalcaemic conditions due to calcium-sensing receptor mutations. *Best Pract Res Clin Rheumatol* 2008;22(1):129–148.
55. Cordeiro A, Montenegro F, Kulcsar M, et al. Parathyroid carcinoma. *Am J Surg* 1998;175:52–55.
56. Marcocci C, Cetani F, Rubin MR, et al. Parathyroid carcinoma. *J Bone Miner Res* 2008;23(12):1869–1880.
57. Chandrasekharappa SC, Guru Sc, Manickam P, et al. Positional cloning of the gene for multiple endocrine neoplasia-type 1. *Science* 1997;276:404–407.
58. Kouvaraki MA, Lee JE, Shapiro SE, et al. Genotype-phenotype analysis in multiple endocrine neoplasia type 1. *Arch Surg* 2002;137(6):641–647.
59. Mulligan LM, Kwok JBJ, Healey CS, et al. Germ-line mutation of the RET proto-oncogene in multiple endocrine neoplasia type 2A. *Nature* 1993; 363:458–460.
60. Donis-Keller H, Dou S, Chi D, et al. Mutations in the RET proto-oncogene are associated with MEN 2A and FMTC. *Hum Mol Genet* 1993;2: 851–856.
61. Doherty GM. Multiple endocrine neoplasia type 1. *J Surg Oncol* 2005; 89(3):143–150.
62. Doherty GM, Olson JA, Frisella MM, et al. Lethality of multiple endocrine neoplasia type I. *World J Surg* 1998;22(6):581–586; discussion 586–587.
63. Lowney JK, Frisella MM, Lairmore TC, et al. Islet cell tumor metastasis in multiple endocrine neoplasia type I: correlation with primary tumor size. *Surgery* 1998;124:1043–1049.
64. Yim JH, Siegel BA, DeBenedetti MK, et al. Prospective study of the utility of somatostatin-receptor scintigraphy in the evaluation of patients with multiple endocrine neoplasia type 1. *Surgery* 1998;124(6):1037–1042.
65. Quayle FJ, Moley JF. Medullary thyroid carcinoma: including MEN 2A and MEN 2B syndromes. *J Surg Oncol* 2005;89(3):122–129.
66. Brunt LM, Lairmore TC, Doherty GM, et al. Adrenalectomy for familial pheochromocytoma in the laparoscopic era. *Ann Surg* 2002;235(5):713–720.

CHAPTER 77 ■ ADRENAL GLAND

JOHN A. OLSON, Jr., AND RANDALL P. SCHERI

KEY POINTS

1. Adrenocortical steroid hormones, glucocorticoids, mineralocorticoids, and androgenic steroids are all synthetic derivatives of cholesterol that are either extracted from plasma or synthesized intracellularly.
2. Catecholamines of the adrenal medulla include epinephrine, norepinephrine, and dopamine, the vasoactive synthetic derivatives of the amino acid tyrosine.
3. Cushing syndrome is adrenocorticotropic hormone dependent in 80% to 90% of cases, most often because of an ACTH-secreting pituitary adenoma, though ectopic ACTH-producing nonendocrine tumors (mostly non–small cell lung cancer and bronchial carcinoids) represent 10% to 20% of cases of ACTH-dependent Cushing syndrome; the remainder have a primary adrenal cause of hypercortisolism.
4. An aldosterone-producing adrenal adenoma (Conn syndrome) is the source of primary hyperaldosteronism in 60% to 70% of cases whereas idiopathic bilateral adrenal hyperplasia causes most of the remaining cases of primary hyperaldosteronism; adrenocortical carcinoma is a rare cause of primary hyperaldosteronism.
5. Surgical removal by laparoscopic adrenalectomy of an aldosterone-secreting adenoma results in durable improvement of hypertension and hypokalemia in 70% to 90% of patients; management of idiopathic adrenal hyperplasia is medical, because fewer than 20% to 30% of patients with this disease are cured by adrenalectomy.
6. The congenital adrenal hyperplasias are autosomal recessive conditions resulting from inherited defects of one or several of the enzymes necessary for cortisol biosynthesis leading to ACTH overproduction and secondary hyperplasia of the adrenal cortex with shunting of cortisol precursors into adrenal androgen pathways; peripheral conversion of the excess adrenal androgens to testosterone causes virilization of the patient.
7. Adrenocortical carcinoma has an estimated incidence of 0.5 to 2 cases per million per year and is very aggressive (most patients present with locoregionally advanced or distant disease); hormone overproduction syndromes are frequent including hypercortisolism, hyperaldosteronism, or virilization.
8. The *rule of tens* is a useful way to characterize pheochromocytoma: Tumors are bilateral in 10% of cases, extra-adrenal in 10%, familial in 10%, multicentric in 10%, and malignant in 10%, and occur in children in 10% of cases; determination of plasma-fractionated metanephrines is the best test for diagnosis of pheochromocytoma.
9. Unsuspected adrenal masses are detected by computed tomography in 0.6% to 1.9% of healthy patients; the goal of evaluation is to distinguish and remove those adrenal masses that are functioning or likely to be malignant versus those that are neither and can be observed.

ANATOMY

The adrenal glands are bilateral, retroperitoneal, endocrine organs located adjacent to the superior pole of each kidney. These glands appear grossly as flat, triangular structures each weighing approximately 4 g. Each adrenal gland is composed of two distinct endocrine organs, the cortex and medulla. The outer adrenal cortex is bright yellow and nodular, whereas the adrenal medulla is red-brown and is sandwiched between the thin layers of the cortex. The adrenals are embedded in retroperitoneal perinephric fat but can be identified as distinct structures by their golden brown, nodular appearance. The right adrenal gland abuts the inferior vena cava medially and lies in close proximity to the diaphragmatic crus posteriorly and the liver anteriorly. The left adrenal gland resides between the kidney and aorta, immediately deep to the tail of the pancreas and spleen.

Embryologically, fetal and definitive adrenal cortices arise from coelomic mesoderm near the urogenital ridge during the fourth to sixth weeks of gestation. Postnatally, the fetal cortex involutes, leaving only the definitive cortex to differentiate into the three adult zonae, the glomerulosa, fasciculata, and reticularis. The adrenal medulla develops from the neural crest during the fifth gestational week and migrates along paraaortic and paravertebral routes to join the developing cortex. Ectopic adrenal cortex and medulla may be found anywhere along their respective paths of embryologic migration. Most neural crest tissue regresses; however, extraadrenal neural crest derivatives may be found along the retroperitoneum and at the aortic bifurcation (organ of Zuckerkandl).

The adrenal cortex is composed of three distinct zones. The outer zona glomerulosa, located just beneath the fibrous gland capsule, is the site of mineralocorticoid production. The middle zona fasciculata, composed of linear arrays of large, foamy cells with lipid inclusions, is the predominant site of glucocorticoid and adrenal sex steroid biosynthesis. The inner zona reticularis is the primary location of synthesis of adrenal androgens. Both the zona fasciculata and zona reticularis respond to stimulation by adrenocorticotropic hormone (ACTH). The adrenal medulla is smaller than the cortex. Cells of the adrenal medulla appear as homogeneous sheets, with large, irregular, atypical-looking nuclei. The cytoplasm of these cells has numerous secretory granules containing catecholamines, neuron-specific enolase, and chromogranin. Catecholamines in these granules precipitate chromium salts, which is the basis for the term *chromaffin cells*.

The adrenal glands have an extensive vascular supply derived from branches of the inferior phrenic artery superiorly, the aorta medially, and the renal artery inferiorly. Venous return from the right adrenal gland empties directly into the inferior vena cava through a wide but short central vein. Venous drainage from the left adrenal gland empties into a smaller vein that shares a common trunk with the left phrenic vein. Together they join the left renal vein (Fig. 77.1).

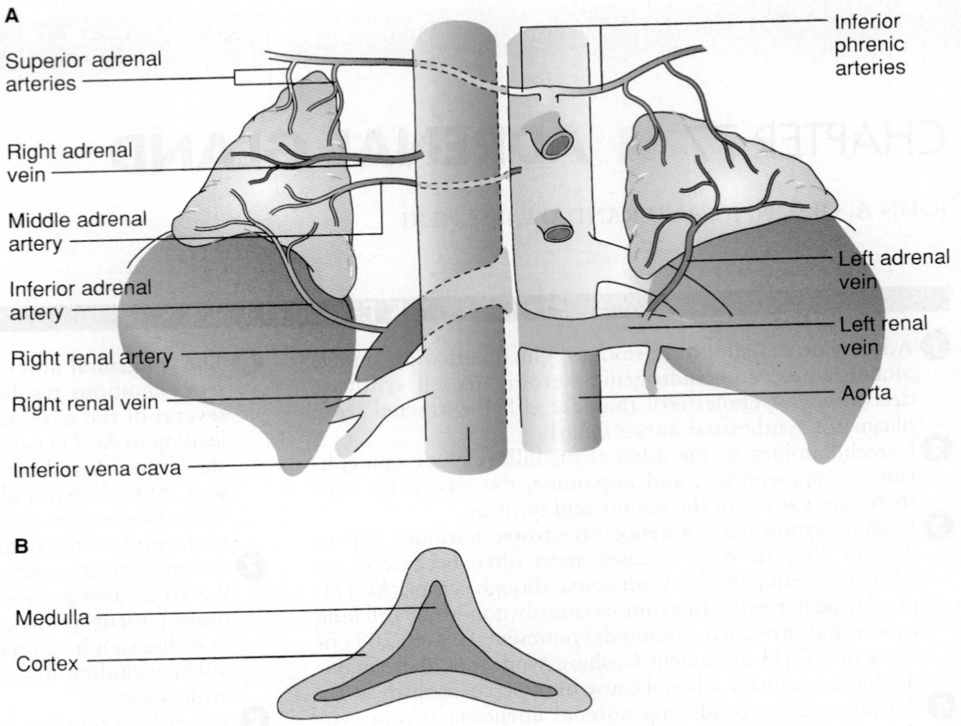

FIGURE 77.1. **A:** Arterial (*dark shaded*) and venous (*light shaded*) anatomy of the adrenal glands. **B:** Schematic showing outer adrenal cortex (*light shaded*) and inner adrenal medulla (*dark shaded*).

BIOCHEMISTRY AND PHYSIOLOGY

Adrenal Cortex

1 Adrenocortical steroid hormones, glucocorticoids, mineralocorticoids, and androgenic steroids are all synthetic derivatives of cholesterol that are either extracted from plasma or synthesized intracellularly (Fig. 77.2). In mitochondria of cells in the adrenal cortex, cholesterol is converted by desmolase (CYP11A1) to delta-5-pregnenolone, the common parent compound for all adrenal cortex steroids. Pregnenolone is then shunted to the three biosynthetic pathways, each compartmentalized within the adrenal according to synthetic capabilities within each zone. In the zonae fasciculata and reticularis,

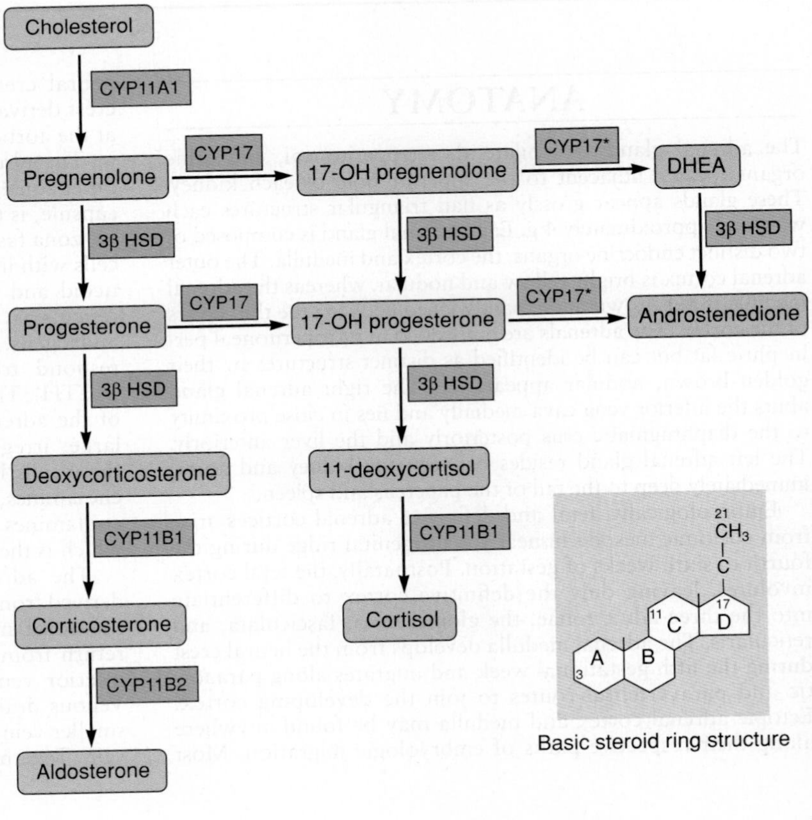

FIGURE 77.2. Steroid biosynthetic pathways in the adrenal cortex. Steroids and precursors are shown in *square boxes*. Enzymes are shown in *stippled boxes*. Enzyme gene symbol designations are as follows: CYP11A1, desmolase; CYP17, 17α hydroxylase >>?(±17,20 lyase*); 3β HSD, 3β hydroxysteroid dehydrogenase; CYP21A2, 21 hydroxylase; CYP11B1, 11β hydroxylase; CYP11 B2, aldosterone synthase. **Inset:** Basic steroid ring structure. The four basic carbon rings are designated A, B, C, and D. Individual carbons at sites of steroidogenic enzyme activity are designated numerically.

pregnenolone is either converted to progesterone by 3-beta-hydroxysteroid dehydrogenase or is oxidized at position 17 by 17-alpha hydroxylase (CYP17) to form 17-hydroxypregnenolone. In the zona fasciculata, progesterone is hydroxylated by CYP17 at position 17 to form 17-hydroxyprogesterone. Subsequently, 17-hydroxyprogesterone is sequentially hydroxylated at the 21 position by 21-beta hydroxylase (CYP21A2) and at position 11 by 11-beta hydroxylase (CYP11B1) to form cortisol. In the zona reticularis, the androgenic steroids dehydroepiandrosterone (DHEA) and androstenedione are made from 17-hydroxypregnenolone and 17-hydroxyprogesterone, respectively. Collectively, the glucocorticoid and androgenic steroids are known as *17-hydroxy corticosteroids* and *17-hydroxy ketosteroids*. In the zona glomerulosa, progesterone is not hydroxylated at the 17 position owing to the lack of enzyme at this location. Instead aldosterone is made from progesterone by a sequential series of hydroxylation steps at position 21 by CYP21A2, position 11 by CYP11B1, and position 18 by aldosterone synthase (CYP11B2 and P450c11as). The zona glomerulosa is well suited to aldosterone biosynthesis because of the relative lack of 17-hydroxylase and the exclusive expression of aldosterone synthase, required for the conversion of corticosterone to aldosterone.

Cortisol. Cortisol is the predominant glucocorticoid in humans. Production and release of cortisol is tightly regulated by a complex feedback relationship between the hypothalamus, corticotrophs of the anterior pituitary, and cells of the adrenal cortex zonae fasciculata and reticularis. This endocrine system is called the *hypothalamic-pituitary-adrenal (HPA) axis*. Communication within the HPA axis is mediated by synthesis and secretion of corticotrophin-releasing hormone (CRH) by the hypothalamus and ACTH production by corticotrophs of the anterior pituitary (Fig. 77.3). ACTH is a cleavage product of a precursor polypeptide, proopiomelanocortin (POMC) that is built of 241 amino acid residues within corticotroph cells of the anterior and intermediate lobes of the pituitary. Several derivatives of POMC are important biologically active substances, including ACTH. Under stimulation of hypothalamic CRH, POMC can be cleaved into ACTH and β-lipotropic hormone in the anterior lobe. ACTH acts directly on the adrenal to regulate cortisol production by cells within the zonae fasciculata and reticularis. Feedback loops involving cortisol, hypothalamic CRH, and pituitary ACTH keep the concentration of cortisol in plasma within a narrow range of 10 to 15 μg/dL. Typical daily production of cortisol in humans ranges between 10 to 30 mg and can increase to as high as 300 mg per day under conditions of maximal stress.

In circulation, cortisol is protein bound to transcortin and albumin with a small percentage of free cortisol available to target tissues. The half-life of cortisol in circulation is 90 minutes. Cortisol is metabolized in the liver to the inactive metabolites dihydrocortisol and tetrahydrocortisol, which become conjugated to glucuronidase and excreted in the urine. These urinary metabolites, collectively known as *17-hydroxycorticosteroids*, as well as free cortisol, can be measured in the urine.

Cortisol binds to specific intracellular cytoplasmic receptors, causing translocation of activated receptor-ligand complexes to the nucleus. Biologic effects result from transcriptional activation of genes and may be grouped into intermediary metabolism, immunomodulation, and regulation of intravascular volume (Table 77.1). Important effects of cortisol on intermediary metabolism center on raising blood glucose directly and indirectly by providing substrate for gluconeogenesis by the liver. These effects include (a) stimulation of glucagon and inhibition of insulin-stimulated glucose uptake by cells; (b) decrease in peripheral protein synthesis and increase in proteolysis, thus delivering gluconeogenic amino acids to the liver; and (c) stimulation of peripheral lipolysis. In effect, cortisol acts anabolically in vital organs to preserve glucose supply and catabolically in peripheral tissues to mobilize gluconeogenic substrates. Cortisol also possesses profound anti-inflammatory and immunosuppressive activities. Impairment of cellular immunity is due to

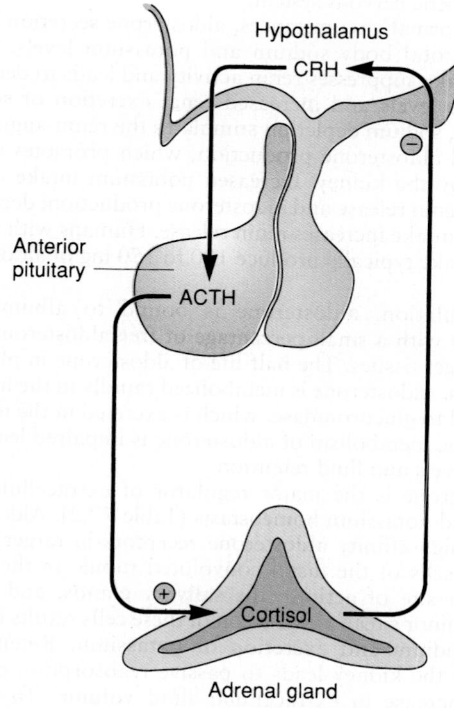

FIGURE 77.3. Schematic of hypothalamic-pituitary-adrenal axis for cortisol. Regulatory feedback relationships are designated with *arrows*.

TABLE 77.1

SYSTEMIC EFFECTS OF CORTISOL

■ FUNCTION	■ NORMAL AMOUNTS	■ EXCESSIVE AMOUNTS
Metabolic		
Protein	Proteolysis	Muscle wasting
Glucose	Gluconeogenesis	Hyperglycemia
Fat	Low-use peripheral lipolysis	Limb thinness
	Central lipogenesis	Truncal obesity
Gastrointestinal	Mucosal cells	Ulceration
	Prostaglandin	Pancreatitis (?)
Cardiovascular	Chronotropic, inotropic	Hypertension
	Vascular resistance	
Renal	Sodium resorption	Hypertension
Bone	Osteoblastic development	Osteoporosis
Inflammatory and immune	Circulating cells	Infection
	Soluble mediators	
	Antigen processing	
Wound healing	Fibroblasts	Striae
	Epithelial cell	Dehiscence

FIGURE 77.4. Regulatory relationships of renin, the angiotensins, and their sites of production and enzymatic conversion.

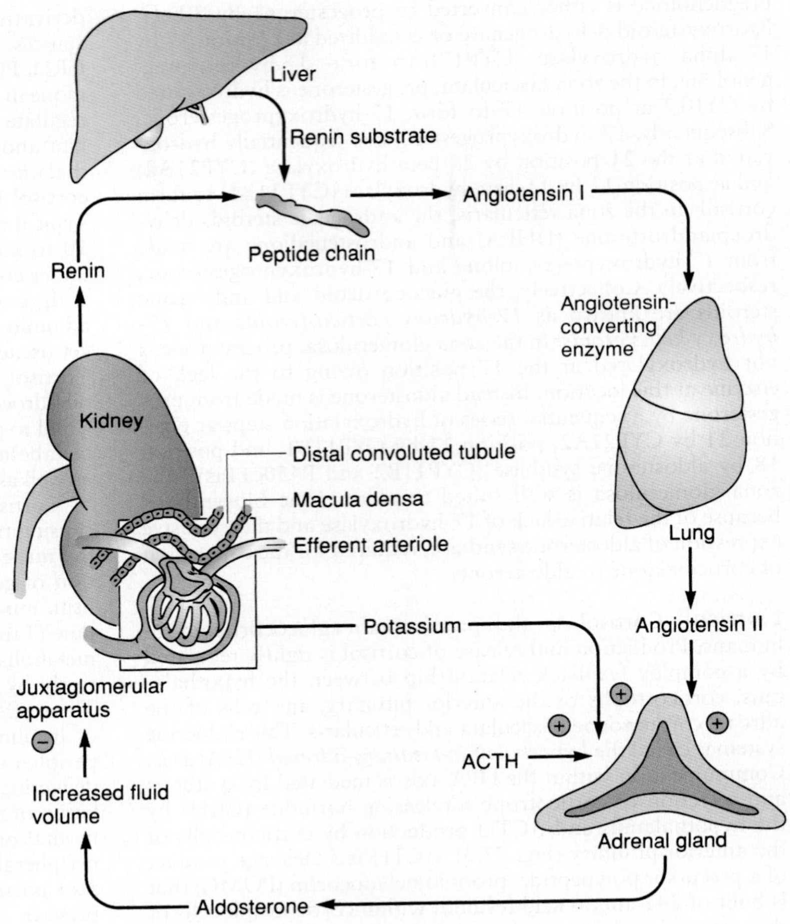

inhibition of interleukin production, impairment of monocyte and neutrophil chemotaxis despite raised leukocyte counts, and reduction of T-cell activation. Humoral immunity is inhibited by inhibition of T-cell stimulation of B cells and by direct inhibition of B-cell proliferation and activation. These immunomodulatory effects may also underlie the impairment of normal wound healing seen in states of cortisol excess. Cortisol also regulates intravascular volume through renal retention of sodium and maintains blood pressure through inotropic and chronotropic effects on the heart as well as by increasing peripheral vascular resistance. In bone, glucocorticoids promote osteopenia by inhibition of bone formation by osteoblasts.

Aldosterone. Aldosterone is the principle mineralocorticoid in humans. Aldosterone secretion by the cells of the adrenal zona glomerulosa is regulated by the renin-angiotensin system and by plasma potassium (Fig. 77.4). Aldosterone is also regulated to a lesser degree by ACTH and plasma sodium concentration. Juxtaglomerular myoepithelial cells lining afferent arterioles of the kidney sense renal blood flow and pressure, and they secrete renin in response to decreased perfusion. Renin enzymatically activates angiotensinogen to the inactive decapeptide precursor, angiotensin I. Angiotensin I is converted to angiotensin II by angiotensin-converting enzyme in the lung. Angiotensin II has three major effects: (a) arteriolar vasoconstriction; (b) renal sodium retention; and (c) increased aldosterone biosynthesis, each of which results in sodium retention and potassium excretion by the kidney. These effects work together to maintain arterial blood pressure as well as blood volume. Physiologic conditions that stimulate the renin-angiotensin cascade and aldosterone release include dehydration, upright posture, and hemorrhage. Inhibitory factors include volume repletion. Postural changes in renin-angiotensin and aldosterone are mediated by the sympathetic nervous system.

Under normal circumstances, aldosterone secretion is controlled by total body sodium and potassium levels. Excess sodium intake suppresses renin activity and leads to decreased aldosterone levels and increased renal excretion of sodium. Conversely, sodium depletion stimulates the renin-angiotensin system and aldosterone production, which promotes sodium retention by the kidney. Increased potassium intake directly decreases renin release and aldosterone production; decreasing potassium intake increases renin release. Humans with normal sodium intake typically produce 100 to 150 mg of aldosterone per day.

In circulation, aldosterone is bound to albumin and transcortin with a small percentage of free aldosterone available to target tissues. The half-life of aldosterone in plasma is 15 minutes. Aldosterone is metabolized rapidly in the liver and conjugated to glucuronidase, which is excreted in the urine. In liver failure, metabolism of aldosterone is impaired leading to elevated levels and fluid retention.

Aldosterone is the major regulator of extracellular fluid volume and potassium homeostasis (Table 77.2). Aldosterone binds to high-affinity aldosterone receptors in target tissues, including cells of the distal convoluted tubule in the kidney (the major site of action), the salivary glands, and colonic mucosa (minor sites). Stimulation of these cells results in retention of sodium and excretion of potassium. Retention of sodium in the kidney leads to passive reabsorption of water and an increase in extracellular fluid volume. To balance aldosterone-mediated retention of positively charged sodium ions, the kidney epithelium releases intracellular potassium into the distal convoluted tubule for excretion in the urine.

TABLE 77.2

EFFECTS OF ALDOSTERONE SECRETION

■ TUBULAR ACTION	■ NORMAL AMOUNTS	■ EXCESSIVE AMOUNTS
Increased resorption of sodium	Protects against low-volume states	Hypertension Positive sodium balance Hyporeninemia
Decreased resorption of potassium	Protects against hyperkalemia	Hypokalemia Metabolic alkalosis Hyperglycemia Nocturia, polyuria Muscle weakness

Hydrogen ion is also released causing acidification of the urine.

Adrenal Androgens. Adrenal C-19 androgenic steroids, which include DHEA and delta-4 androstenedione, are synthesized in cells of the zona reticularis. These steroids promote secondary sexual characteristics in men and virilization in women. DHEA is the major adrenal androgen, while androstenedione is relatively minor. Both are relatively weak androgens and exert their effects on target tissue after local tissue conversion to testosterone. Unlike gonadal androgens, adrenal androgens are regulated by ACTH, not gonadotropins, and can therefore be inhibited by glucocorticoid administration.

Adrenal Medulla

2 Catecholamines of the adrenal medulla include epinephrine, norepinephrine, and dopamine. These vasoactive hormones are synthetic derivatives of the amino acid tyrosine (Fig. 77.5). The biosynthetic pathway that converts tyrosine to active catecholamines involves four sequential enzymatic reactions: (a) Tyrosine is converted to L-dihydroxyphenylalanine (dopa) by tyrosine hydroxylase; (b) dopa is converted to dopamine by aromatic-L-amino acid decarboxylase; (c) dopamine is converted to norepinephrine by dopamine beta hydroxylase; and (d) norepinephrine is converted to epinephrine by phenylethanolamine-N-methyltransferase (PNMT). Epinephrine is the major (80%) catecholamine stored in the adrenal medulla, followed by norepinephrine (20%) and dopamine (<1%). Tissue expression of the enzyme PNMT is limited to cells of either the adrenal medulla or organ of Zuckerkandl, located near the aortic bifurcation; thus most extraadrenal pheochromocytomas produce norepinephrine, rather than epinephrine.

A complex regulatory network governs synthesis and secretion of catecholamines. Factors that increase catecholamine release include splanchnic nerve stimulation, stress, and glucocorticoids. The metabolic milieu within the adrenal medulla also greatly influences catecholamine synthesis by regulating enzymatic activity: Glucocorticoids, phospholipids, cyclic adenosine monophosphate, adenosine triphosphate, protein kinase, and magnesium increase activity of PNMT and decrease catecholamine negative feedback. Catecholamines are stored and secreted from granules within cells of the medulla in association with the matrix protein chromogranin. Chromogranin A is measurable in the blood, and its measurement may support the biochemical testing for pheochromocytoma, as well as other functional neuroendocrine tumors.

Catecholamines act on target tissues through membrane-bound receptors. Pharmacologic distinction of adrenergic receptors is made based on their relative responsiveness to natural and artificial bioamines. Alpha-adrenergic receptors show the highest affinity for norepinephrine, less for epinephrine, and least for isoproterenol. Beta-adrenergic receptors are most responsive to isoproterenol and least to norepinephrine. In addition, specific antagonists recognize each receptor class: Alpha-receptors are antagonized by phentolamine and phenoxybenzamine, and beta-receptors are blocked by propranolol and related compounds. Beta-adrenergic receptor subtypes include beta-1, which is present in cardiac muscle, adipose tissue, and small intestine, and beta-2 receptors, which are found in vascular, tracheal, and uterine smooth muscle, skeletal

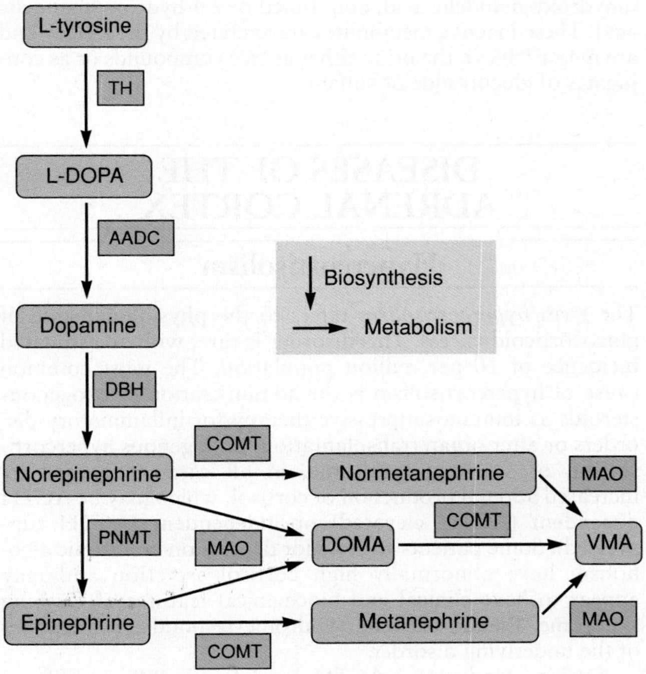

FIGURE 77.5. Catecholamine biosynthetic and metabolism pathways. Precursors, catecholamines, and metabolites are shown in *square boxes*. Enzymes are shown in *stippled boxes*. Enzyme gene symbol designations are as follows: TH, tyrosine hydroxylase; AADC, aromatic-L-amino acid decarboxylase; DBH, dopamine β hydroxylase; PNMT, phenylethanolamine-N-methyltransferase; COMT, catechol-O-methyl-transferase; MAO, monoamine oxidase; VMA, 3-methoxy-4-hydroxy-mandelic acid.

TABLE 77.3

CATECHOLAMINE EFFECTS

■ RECEPTOR CLASS	■ NORMAL AMOUNTS	■ EXCESSIVE AMOUNTS
β_1	Chronotropic, inotropic	Tachycardia
	Sweat glands	Sweating
	Decreased glucose use	Hyperglycemia
β_2	Smooth muscle relaxation	Hypotension
α_1	Smooth muscle contraction	Hypertension
	Gluconeogenesis	
	Glycogenolysis	Hyperglycemia
	Suppressed insulin effects	
α_2	Smooth muscle contraction[a]	Pallor

[a]Platelet aggregation.

muscle, and liver. Alpha-adrenergic receptors are similarly subdivided: Alpha-1 receptors mediate vasoconstriction whereas alpha-2 receptors modulate presynaptic norepinephrine release and platelet aggregation (Table 77.3).

Metabolism of catecholamines occurs through three mechanisms: by specific uptake by sympathetic neurons, by nonspecific uptake and degradation by peripheral tissues, and by excretion in the urine. Catecholamines are metabolized in liver and kidney by two enzymes, monoamine oxidase and catechol-O-methyltransferase (Fig. 77.5). In these tissues, monoamine oxidase and catechol-O-methyltransferase convert epinephrine or norepinephrine to normetanephrine, metanephrine, 3,4-dihydroxy-mandelic acid, and 3-methoxy-4-hydroxy-mandelic acid. These inactive metabolites are excreted by the kidney and are measurable in the urine either as free compounds or as conjugates of glucuronide or sulfate.

DISEASES OF THE ADRENAL CORTEX

Hypercortisolism

The term *hypercortisolism* refers to the physiologic state of glucocorticoid excess. This disorder is rare, with an estimated incidence of 10 per million population. The most common cause of hypercortisolism is the administration of exogenous steroids as immunosuppressive therapy for inflammatory disorders or after organ transplantation. Endogenous hypercortisolism, or Cushing syndrome, in all cases is caused by increased adrenal production of cortisol, which may be ACTH dependent (ACTH elevated) or independent (ACTH suppressed). Some patients with major depression or chronic alcoholism have abnormally high cortisol secretion and may appear to have clinical and biochemical features of Cushing syndrome. Pseudo-Cushing syndrome responds to treatment of the underlying disorder.

3 Cushing syndrome is ACTH dependent in 80% to 90% of cases. Such ACTH-dependent hypercortisolism is most often (80%–90% of cases) caused by an ACTH-secreting pituitary adenoma (termed *Cushing disease*). Ectopic ACTH-producing nonendocrine tumors (mostly non–small cell lung cancer and bronchial carcinoids) represent 10% to 20% of cases of ACTH-dependent Cushing syndrome. All causes of ACTH-dependent Cushing syndrome involve bilateral adrenal hyperplasia in response to ACTH stimulation.

4 Of patients with endogenous Cushing syndrome, 10% to 25% have ACTH-independent disease caused by a primary adrenal cause. A solitary adrenal adenoma is present in 80% to 90% of these patients and is often associated with atrophy of both adjacent and contralateral adrenocortical tissue. Nodular cortical hyperplasia of both glands causes the remaining cases of primary adrenal Cushing syndrome. Although nodular hyperplasia represents a diffuse process, one or more distinct nodules may simulate adenomas. Rarely tumors secrete CRH ectopically, leading to ACTH-independent (though ACTH is elevated) Cushing syndrome with secondary adrenal hypertrophy.

Signs and Symptoms. Clinical features of cortisol excess are listed in Table 77.1. Truncal obesity (*orange on toothpicks*), accumulation of fat around the head and neck (*moon facies* and *buffalo hump*), and muscle wasting are present in most patients. Patients often have purple striae and purpura on the abdomen and extremities. Hirsutism may be present in women. High blood pressure is common and is usually moderate, although malignant hypertension has been observed. Muscle weakness and bone pain, particularly backache, are also common. Weakness is caused partly by proximal muscle wasting but also by hypokalemia. Osteoporosis is common, and pathologic fractures are observed in advanced cases. Neurologic symptoms, including headache, emotional lability, depression, and even psychosis may be observed. Glucose intolerance is common but can often be managed by alterations in diet alone. The serum potassium level may be low secondary to the weak mineralocorticoid properties of cortisol. Autonomous glucocorticoid production without specific signs and symptoms of Cushing syndrome is termed *subclinical Cushing syndrome.* This condition is being diagnosed with increased frequency because of the detection of adrenal incidentalomas by routine CT. A substantial percentage of incidentalomas are hormonally active, with 5% to 20% of the tumors producing glucocorticoids. The estimated prevalence of subclinical hypercortisolism is 77 cases per 100,000 persons, substantially higher than classic Cushing syndrome. Depending on the amounts of glucocorticoids secreted by the tumor, the clinical spectrum ranges from slightly attenuated diurnal cortisol rhythm to atrophy of the contralateral adrenal gland. Patients with subclinical Cushing syndrome lack the classical stigmata of hypercortisolism but have a high prevalence of obesity, hypertension, and type 2 diabetes.

Diagnosis. The investigation of suspected Cushing syndrome should answer two questions: (a) Does the patient have hypercortisolism? (b) If the answer is yes, then what is the cause? It is worthwhile to emphasize that the diagnosis of Cushing syndrome is biochemical. Radiologic investigations should not be undertaken until Cushing syndrome has been confirmed and its likely etiology characterized biochemically.

Hypercortisolism insensitive to suppression by administration of exogenous glucocorticoid is the sine qua non of Cushing syndrome. The low-dose dexamethasone suppression test is the best test in patients with suspected Cushing syndrome. For this test, 1 mg of dexamethasone is administered orally at 11 p.m. and plasma cortisol is obtained at 8 a.m. the following day. Normal individuals suppress cortisol to less than 5 μg/dL. Patients with Cushing syndrome fail to suppress less than 5 μg/dL. False-positive test results occur in 10% to 15% of cases with the overnight test and occur especially in patients with obesity or alcoholism or in those taking estrogens or phenytoin. Measurement of free cortisol (not metabolites) in three consecutive 24-hour collections of urine is also a good screening test for Cushing syndrome. Collections should include concurrent creatinine measurement to evaluate the completeness of the collection. A 24-hour urinary free cortisol level greater than 100 μg is diagnostic of Cushing syndrome. This test may be less sensitive than the low-dose dexamethasone suppression test in mild hypercortisolism. Plasma cortisol levels can normally vary considerably

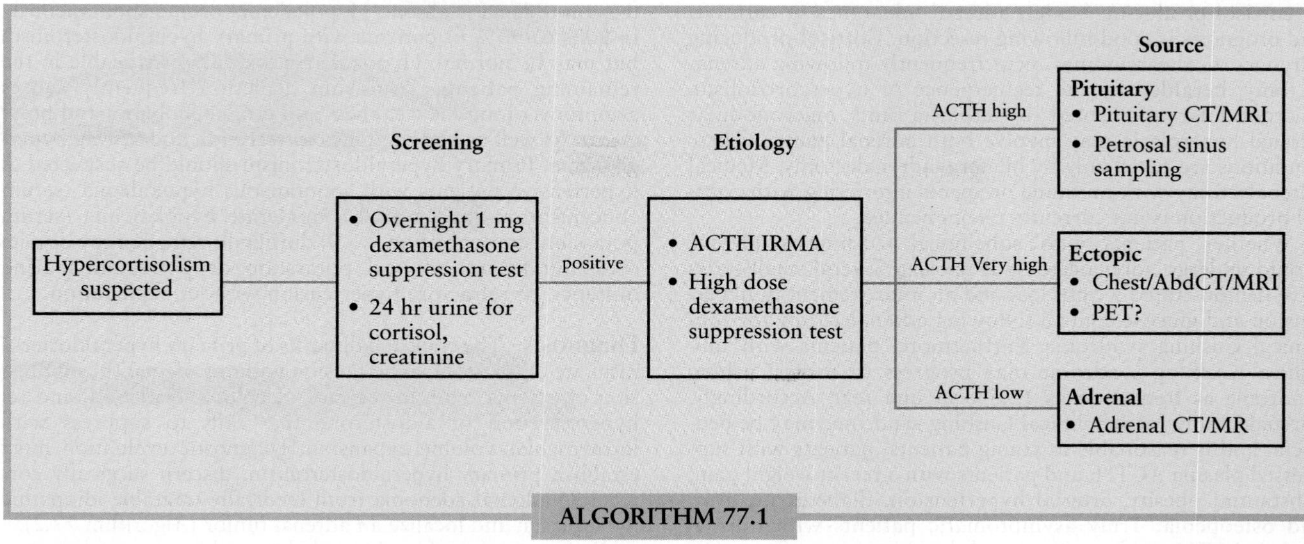

ALGORITHM 77.1. Diagnosis of hypercortisolism. ACTH, adrenocorticotropic hormone; IRMA, immunoradiometric assay; CT, computed tomography; MRI, magnetic resonance imaging; PET, positron emission tomography.

during a 24-hour period, so a single random plasma cortisol level is not helpful in establishing a diagnosis of Cushing syndrome.

Once the presence of hypercortisolism is established, the next task is to determine ACTH-dependent (pituitary or ectopic source) from ACTH-independent (primary adrenal) causes. Measurement of basal ACTH by immunoradiometric assay is the best test to make this distinction. Plasma ACTH levels are normally between 10 and 100 pg. Suppression of the absolute level of ACTH less than 5 pg per mL is nearly diagnostic of adrenocortical neoplasms, which secrete high levels of cortisol and inhibit ACTH release by the pituitary. Patients with pituitary neoplasms and secondary bilateral adrenocortical hyperplasia have ACTH levels that may range from the upper limits of normal (15 pg per mL) to 500 pg per mL. The highest plasma levels of ACTH (>1,000 pg per mL) are in patients with ACTH-producing nonendocrine tumors such as non-small cell lung cancer.

Although 80% to 90% of patients with ACTH-dependent Cushing syndrome have Cushing disease, a high-dose dexamethasone suppression test may be required to exclude ectopic ACTH syndrome. Hypercortisolism caused by ACTH-secreting pituitary adenomas is suppressed at least partially by high dexamethasone, whereas hypercortisolism caused by adrenal tumors and ectopic ACTH-producing tumors is not suppressed. For this test 2 mg dexamethasone is administered orally every 6 hours for 2 days, and a 24-hour urine collection for free cortisol is taken during the second day. About 90% of patients with pituitary source Cushing disease have a 50% reduction in urine free cortisol. The specificity of the test can be improved to 100% for diagnosing pituitary disease if more than 90% suppression in urinary free cortisol is used.

Biochemical testing of suspected Cushing syndrome is followed by radiologic studies. Pituitary adenomas are best imaged with gadolinium-enhanced MRI of the sella turcica, which has a sensitivity approaching 100%, although small pituitary microadenomas may be missed. Patients with ACTH-independent Cushing syndrome require thin-section CT or MRI of the adrenal, which identifies adrenal abnormalities with more than 95% sensitivity. CT or MRI of the chest may identify a source of ectopic ACTH and should be undertaken in patients with elevated ACTH and hypercortisolism that cannot be suppressed by high-dose dexamethasone.

Despite the accuracy of biochemical testing and radiographic localization, a pituitary versus ectopic source of ACTH sometimes cannot be determined. Bilateral inferior petrosal sinus sampling is the best test to settle this issue. Simultaneous bilateral petrosal sinus and peripheral blood samples are obtained before and after peripheral intravenous injection of 1 μg per kg CRH. An inferior petrosal sinus to peripheral plasma ACTH ratio of 2.0 at basal stimulated or of 3.0 after CRH administration is 100% sensitive and specific for pituitary adenoma. Comparison of right and left inferior petrosal sinus ratios may also lateralize the adenoma.

The laboratory approach to the diagnosis of Cushing syndrome is summarized in Algorithm 77.1. A careful history and physical examination form the basis for suspecting this condition. A low-dose dexamethasone suppression test and/or urinary free cortisol measurement provide initial evidence for the diagnosis. Plasma ACTH determination and the high-dose dexamethasone suppression test are then used to identify the underlying cause of excess cortisol production by the adrenal cortex. Imaging studies support the cause of Cushing syndrome suggested by biochemical testing and localize the site for subsequent treatment.

Treatment. ACTH-dependent Cushing syndrome is best treated by removing the source of ACTH excess. In the case of Cushing disease, transsphenoidal resection of the pituitary microadenoma is successful in 80% or more of cases. If a microadenoma is not found, then hemihypophysectomy may be performed with the understanding that fertility may be impaired. Pituitary irradiation is a good treatment option when fertility is desired, when a tumor is not found or is unresectable, or cure is not achieved by transsphenoidal resection of a tumor. Debulking of unresectable primary lesions or recurrences with or without bilateral adrenalectomy may provide palliation in some patients. Treatment of ectopic ACTH syndrome involves removal of the primary lesion. Medical adrenalectomy with metyrapone, aminoglutethimide, and mitotane has been used to suppress production of corticosteroid in inoperable cases for both pituitary and ectopic sources of ACTH. Bilateral adrenalectomy is a good option for patients intolerant of mitotane.

ACTH-independent Cushing syndrome is best treated by removal of the adrenal tumor and affected gland. Small lesions, less than 6 cm in diameter, may be resected laparoscopically. Lesions larger than 6 cm or those suspected of being carcinoma require an anterior open approach. Resection of cortisol-producing benign adrenal adenomas is curative, and prognosis is good following resection. Cortisol-producing adrenocortical carcinomas recur frequently following adrenalectomy, heralded by the reemergence of hypercortisolism. Micronodular pigmented hyperplasia and macronodular adrenal hyperplasia may involve both adrenal glands. These conditions are cured only by bilateral adrenalectomy. Medical adrenalectomy with mitotane or agents interfering with cortisol production is not currently recommended.

Whether patients with subclinical Cushing syndrome should undergo adrenalectomy is unclear. Several small series have demonstrated weight loss and an improvement in hypertension and glucose control following adrenalectomy for subclinical Cushing syndrome. Furthermore, patients with subclinical Cushing syndrome may progress to overt Cushing syndrome as frequently as 12.5% at one year. Accordingly, adrenalectomy for subclinical Cushing syndrome may be beneficial and is reasonable in young patients, patients with suppressed plasma ACTH, and patients with a recent weight gain, substantial obesity, arterial hypertension, diabetes mellitus, and osteopenia. Truly asymptomatic patients with normal plasma ACTH concentrations and the elderly or unfit may be observed. Demonstration of the benefits of surgery versus conservative treatment in patients with subclinical Cushing syndrome will require a randomized prospective trial.

All patients who undergo adrenalectomy for Cushing syndrome require perioperative and postoperative glucocorticoid replacement, since the contralateral gland is suppressed. Replacement therapy with hydrocortisone, 12 mg/m^2 per day, may be required as long as 2 years postoperatively. Adequacy of replacement is monitored clinically. The duration of replacement therapy is guided by normalization of the ACTH stimulation test.

Hyperaldosteronism

Hyperaldosteronism is a syndrome of hypertension and hypokalemia caused by autonomous adrenal secretion of the mineralocorticoid aldosterone. Hyperaldosteronism may be primary, as a result of an adrenal neoplasm with suppressed plasma renin, or may be secondary, as a result of elevated plasma renin. Primary hyperaldosteronism is twice as common in women as in men, and it usually occurs between the ages of 30 and 50 years. Screening of hypertensive patients with plasma aldosterone and plasma renin activity (PRA) has suggested that primary hyperaldosteronism may be the underlying cause of up to 15% of cases of essential hypertension.

5 An aldosterone-producing adrenal adenoma (Conn syndrome) is the source of primary hyperaldosteronism in 60% to 70% of cases. Idiopathic bilateral adrenal hyperplasia causes the remaining cases of primary hyperaldosteronism. Adrenocortical carcinoma is a rare cause of primary hyperaldosteronism. Autosomal dominant glucocorticoid-suppressible hyperaldosteronism is a rare cause of hyperaldosteronism resulting from the fusion of the ACTH-responsive 11-beta hydroxylase gene promoter to the aldosterone synthase gene in cells of the adrenal cortex.

Secondary hyperaldosteronism is a physiologic response of the renin-angiotensin system to decreased renal perfusion due to renal artery stenosis, cirrhosis, congestive heart failure, and normal pregnancy. The adrenal cortex functions normally and secretes aldosterone in response to the elevated plasma renin and angiotensin caused by these conditions. Secondary hyperaldosteronism responds to treatment of the underlying cause.

Signs and Symptoms. Clinical manifestations of primary hyperaldosteronism are attributable to hypersecretion of aldosterone by the adrenal gland (Table 77.2). Aldosterone-mediated retention of sodium and excretion of potassium and hydrogen ion by the kidney causes moderate diastolic hypertension. Edema is absent. Hypokalemia occurs spontaneously in 80% to 90% of patients with primary hyperaldosteronism but may be normal. Hypokalemia is easily provocable in the remaining patients. Potassium depletion frequently causes symptoms of muscle weakness and fatigue, polyuria and polydipsia, as well as impaired insulin secretion and fasting hyperglycemia. Primary hyperaldosteronism should be suspected in hypertensive patients with spontaneous hypokalemia (serum concentration <3.5 mEq/L), moderate hypokalemia (serum potassium concentration <3.0) during diuretic therapy despite concomitant use of oral potassium or potassium-sparing diuretics, or refractory hypertension without explanation.

Diagnosis. The clinical hallmarks of primary hyperaldosteronism are (a) diastolic hypertension without edema; (b) suppression of plasma renin in the face of volume depletion; and (c) hypersecretion of aldosterone that fails to suppress with intravascular volume expansion. Diagnostic evaluation must establish primary hyperaldosteronism, discern surgically correctable adrenal adenoma from medically treatable idiopathic hyperplasia, and localize an adrenal tumor (Algorithm 77.2).

Demonstration of an elevated plasma aldosterone concentration (PAC) in the setting of suppressed PRA is the best test to establish primary hyperaldosteronism. The ratio in normal subjects and patients with essential hypertension is 4 to 10 compared with more than 30 in most patients with primary hyperaldosteronism. A PAC of greater than 20 ng/dL and a PAC/PRA ratio of greater than 30 are diagnostic for aldosteronoma with almost 90% sensitivity. A serum potassium value less than 3.5 mEq/L and urinary potassium excretion greater than 30 mEq per day also support a diagnosis of primary hyperaldosteronism. Before biochemical evaluation, patients need to be potassium repleted and have an adequate sodium intake. Medications including ACE inhibitors and spironolactone should be withheld for at least 4 weeks before study.

An elevated PAC/PRA ratio alone does not establish the diagnosis of primary hyperaldosteronism, which must be confirmed by demonstrating inappropriate aldosterone secretion with salt loading. This involves a 24-hour urine collection for sodium and aldosterone after 3 days of a high-sodium diet. The 24-hour urinary excretion of aldosterone should be greater than 14 μg per 24 hours after a high-salt diet for patients with primary hyperaldosteronism. An intravenous saline infusion test or captopril challenge test is also a reliable method to confirm primary hyperaldosteronism. These tests are not usually required.

After the diagnosis of primary hyperaldosteronism is made, distinction must be made between an aldosteronoma and idiopathic adrenal hyperplasia. The first test measures aldosterone in blood collected at 8 a.m. from a patient who has been supine overnight. Laboratory studies are repeated 4 hours later after the patient has been upright. Aldosterone secretion in patients with an aldosteronoma is unaffected by postural changes (<20 ng/dL), whereas, in patients with idiopathic adrenal hyperplasia, plasma aldosterone levels are elevated 33% (>20 ng/dL) or more by postural changes.

High-resolution adrenal computed tomography (CT) is the best test for localization of an adrenal tumor (Fig. 77.6). CT will detect an aldosterone-producing adenoma in 90% of cases overall. The presence of a unilateral adenoma greater than 1 cm on CT and supportive biochemical evidence of an aldosteronoma are generally all that is needed to make the diagnosis in most patients younger than 40 years of age. Magnetic resonance imaging (MRI) is less effective and more costly but may be useful during pregnancy or in situations in which intravenous contrast medium injection is undesirable. Scintigraphy with [6-beta](131I)-iodo-methyl-19-norcholesterol (NP-59) identifies functional tumors and discriminates aldosteronoma from adrenal hyperplasia with an overall accuracy of approximately 75%, but requires a tumor of sufficient size (>1 cm) for imaging to be dependable.

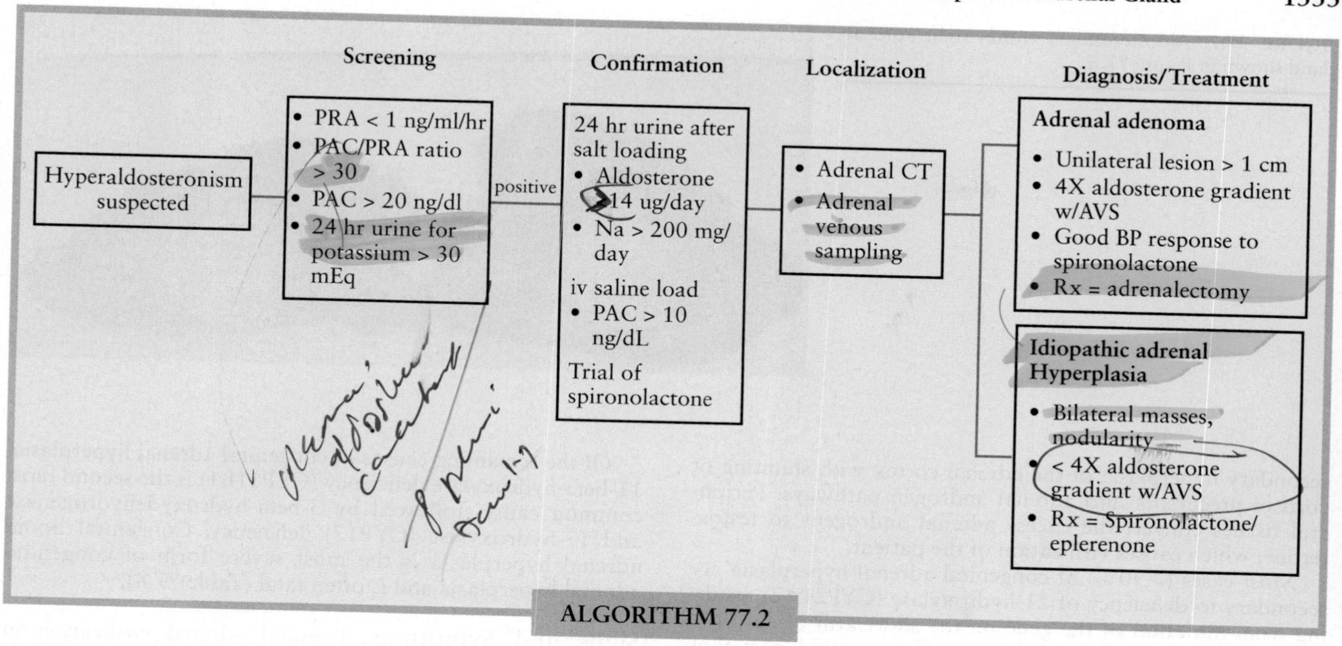

ALGORITHM 77.2. Diagnosis and management of hyperaldosteronism. PRA, plasma renin activity; PAC, plasma aldosterone concentration; CT, computed tomography; AVS, bilateral adrenal venous sampling.

Adrenal vein sampling to lateralize the source of aldosterone production is useful in patients with hyperaldosteronism when there is no adrenal abnormality on CT or MRI or when both adrenal glands are abnormal but asymmetric. Furthermore, patients older than 40 years, in whom the possibility of a nonfunctioning adenoma is statistically higher, may benefit from routine sampling. Percutaneous transfemoral cannulation of both adrenal veins is performed and intravenous ACTH (50 μ/h) is administered. Simultaneous adrenal vein blood samples for aldosterone and cortisol are taken before and after ACTH injection, and their ratios are determined. The PAC is markedly higher (at least fourfold) on the side of an adenoma, whereas there is little or no left-right gradient present in cases of bilateral adrenal hyperplasia. A 10-fold gradient of cortisol in adrenal veins to a peripheral sample ensures adequate adrenal vein cannulation. This study is greater than 90% accurate and has been shown to alter management in 30% to 50% of patients, even in those with an apparent unilateral adenoma. This test is technically difficult and may be unsuccessful in 25% of patients. Emerging data suggest that adrenal vein sampling may be superior to CT in differentiating the source of aldosterone production in patients with hyperaldosteronism.

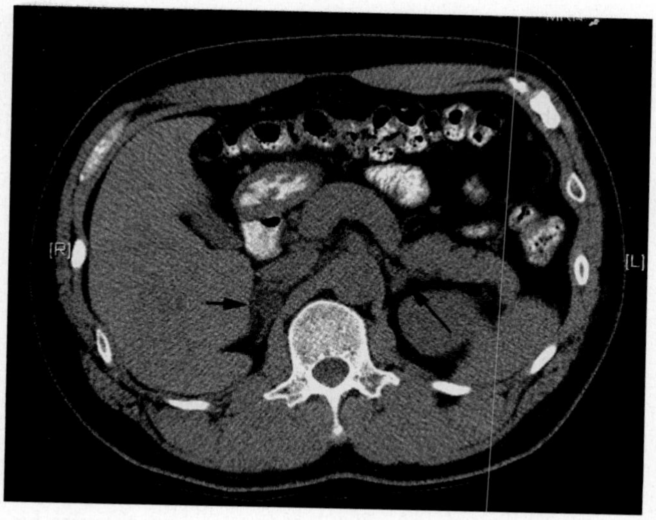

FIGURE 77.6. Computed tomography scan of right adrenal aldosteronoma. *Short arrow* shows aldosteronoma. *Long arrow* shows normal contralateral adrenal gland.

6 **Treatment.** Surgical removal of an aldosterone-secreting adenoma (Fig. 77.7) results in durable improvement of hypertension and hypokalemia in 70% to 90% of patients. Laparoscopic adrenalectomy is the preferred approach to remove these tumors. Morbidity and mortality following these procedures are almost negligible. Preoperative spironolactone or eplerenone and potassium are given to replenish potassium stores and correct alkalosis before anesthesia. Preoperatively, a significant fall in blood pressure with aldosterone receptor antagonists predicts a successful outcome after adrenalectomy. Response to adrenalectomy is also influenced by the duration and severity of hypertension and by the presence of histologic changes in the kidney. Age greater than 50 years, male sex, and the presence of multiple nodules within the adrenal is also associated with a poor response to surgery.

7 Management of idiopathic adrenal hyperplasia is medical because fewer than 20% to 30% of patients with this disease are cured by adrenalectomy. Idiopathic adrenal hyperplasia is treated with spironolactone or with the newer aldosterone antagonist eplerenone. Other potassium-sparing diuretics may be used including triamterene and amiloride. Treatment of glucocorticoid-suppressible hyperaldosteronism includes dexamethasone 0.5 to 1.0 mg daily. Glucocorticoids are used in small doses to avoid Cushing syndrome.

Congenital Adrenal Hyperplasia

8 The congenital adrenal hyperplasia syndromes are autosomal recessive conditions resulting from inherited defects of one or several of the enzymes necessary for cortisol biosynthesis (Fig. 77.8). Cortisol deficiency leads to ACTH overproduction and

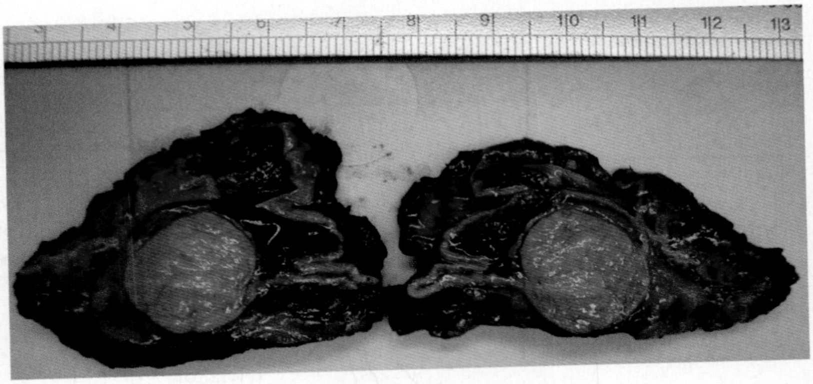

FIGURE 77.7. Aldosteronoma within right adrenal gland shown in Figure 77.6.

secondary hyperplasia of the adrenal cortex with shunting of cortisol precursors into adrenal androgen pathways. Peripheral tissues convert the excess adrenal androgens to testosterone, which causes virilization of the patient.

Most cases (>90%) of congenital adrenal hyperplasia are secondary to deficiency of 21-hydroxylase (CYP21A2) resulting from mutation of the gene on the short arm of chromosome 6. Two forms of this deficiency are recognized: partial or complete. The complete form is characterized by androgen excess at birth, with virilization, hypovolemia, hyponatremia, hyperkalemia, and hyperpigmentation. The partial form is characterized by virilization only and may present in adolescence or adulthood.

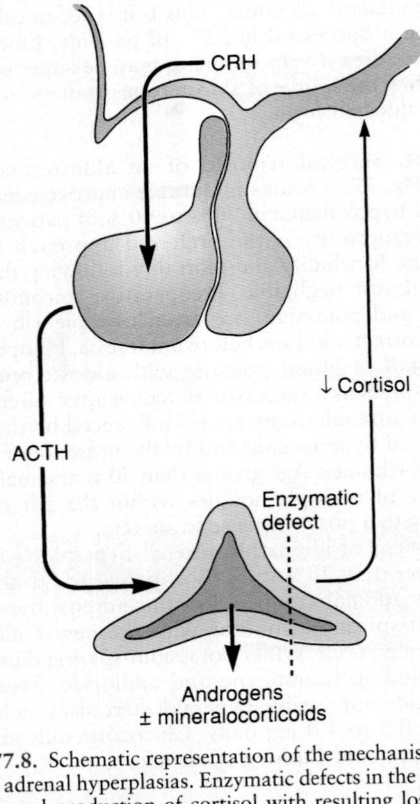

FIGURE 77.8. Schematic representation of the mechanism underlying congenital adrenal hyperplasias. Enzymatic defects in the adrenal gland prevent normal production of cortisol with resulting loss of negative feedback to the hypothalamus and pituitary. Chronic adrenocorticotropic hormone stimulation of the adrenal gland shunts steroid precursors through androgenic and mineralocorticoid pathways, leading to the overproduction of androgens and mineralocorticoids. The most common deficiencies are CYP21A2 (21-hydroxylase), CYP11B1 (11β-hydroxylase), and 3-β-HSD (3-β-hydroxysteroid dehydrogenase).

Of the remaining causes of congenital adrenal hyperplasia, 11-beta-hydroxylase deficiency (CYP11B1) is the second most common cause, followed by 3-beta-hydroxydehydrogenase and 17-hydroxylase (CYP17) deficiency. Congenital lipoid adrenal hyperplasia is the most severe form of congenital adrenal hyperplasia and is often fatal (Table 77.4).

Signs and Symptoms. Prenatal adrenal virilization in females produces ambiguous external genitalia (female pseudohermaphrodism). The ovaries, fallopian tubes, and uterus develop normally, and patients are fertile. Postnatal congenital adrenal hyperplasia causes virilization of females and precocious puberty of males. Females develop hirsutism, polycystic ovaries, and irregular menses. Male patients exhibit secondary sexual characteristics by age 2 or 3 years. Fertility is often impaired. Both sexes experience rapid somatic growth and short stature. Virilization, salt wasting, and hyperpigmentation are variably present with the non–21-hydroxylase forms of congenital adrenal hyperplasias.

Diagnosis. Elevated plasma 17-hydroxyprogesterone is the most characteristic abnormality found in 21-hydroxylase deficiency. Both plasma cortisol and 24-hour free urinary cortisol excretion are variably reduced. Diagnosis of other forms of the disease involves demonstration of elevated levels of enzyme substrate: corticosterone and 11-deoxycortisol for 11-beta hydroxylase; dehydroepiandrosterone and 17 delta-5 hydroxypregnenolone for 3-beta hydroxydehydrogenase; and deoxycorticosterone and corticosterone for 17 beta-hydroxylase deficiency (Table 77.4).

Treatment. The treatment of 21-hydroxylase deficiency is glucocorticoid and mineralocorticoid replacement. Clinical management is often complicated by inadequately treated hyperandrogenism or iatrogenic hypercortisolism, or both. New treatment approaches under investigation include combination therapy to block androgen action and inhibit estrogen production, and bilateral adrenalectomy in the most severely affected patients. Female patients with ambiguous genitalia may require surgical correction as infants. Treatment of congenital adrenal hyperplasias caused by other enzyme deficiencies includes steroid and electrolyte replacement and surgical correction of the external genitalia in affected female infants.

Virilizing and Feminizing Adrenal Tumors

Excess production of adrenal androgens by an adrenal adenoma or carcinoma can produce virilizing features either alone or more commonly in addition to Cushing syndrome. Development of an adrenal virilizing tumor in women causes hirsutism and masculinization. Males with these tumors may present late with signs and symptoms of tumor enlargement or distant metastases develop. Virilizing tumors secrete androgen

TABLE 77.4

CONGENITAL ADRENAL HYPERPLASIA SYNDROMES

■ DISEASE	■ 21-HYDROXYLASE DEFICIENCY	■ 11β-HYDROXYLASE DEFICIENCY	■ ALDOSTERONE SYNTHASE DEFICIENCY	■ 17α-HYDROXYLASE DEFICIENCY	■ 3β-HYDROXYSTEROID DEHYDROGENASE DEFICIENCY	■ LIPOID HYPERPLASIA
Defective gene	*CYP21*	*CYP11B1*	*CYP11 B2*	*CYP17*	*HSD3 B2*	*STAR*
Ambiguous genitalia	Females	Females	No	Males	Males	Males
Addisonian crisis	Present	Rare	Salt wasting only	Absent	Present	Present
Incidence (general population)	1:10–18,000	1:100,000	Rare	Rare	Rare	Rare
HORMONES						
Glucocorticoids	Reduced	Reduced	Normal	Corticosterone normal	Reduced	Reduced
Mineralocorticoids	Reduced	Elevated	Reduced	Elevated	Reduced	Reduced
Androgens	Elevated	Elevated	Normal	Reduced	Reduced (males) Elevated (females)	Reduced
Estrogens	Reduced (females)	Reduced in females	Normal	Reduced	Reduced	Reduced
PHYSIOLOGY						
Blood pressure	Reduced	Elevated	Reduced	Elevated	Reduced	Reduced
Na balance	Reduced	Elevated	Reduced	Elevated	Reduced	Reduced
K balance	Elevated	Reduced	Elevated	Reduced	Elevated	Elevated
Acidosis	Present	Absent	Present	Absent	Present	Present
Elevated metabolites	17-OHP	DOC, 11-deoxycortisol	Corticosterone ± 18-hydroxy-corticosterone	DOC corticosterone	DHEA, $17\Delta^5$ preg	None

OHP, hydroxyprogesterone; DOC, deoxycorticosterone; DHEA, dehydroepiandrostenedione.
(Modified with permission from White PC, Speiser PW. Congenital adrenal hyperplasia due to 21-hydroxylase deficiency. *Endocr Rev.* 2000;21:245–291.)

precursor, dehydroepiandrosterone, which can be measured either directly in plasma or in urine as a 17-ketosteroid. Feminizing adrenal neoplasms are extremely rare. Abdominal CT is subsequently used to localize the lesion. Resection of tumor and involved adrenal gland is the primary treatment for patients with adrenal virilizing tumors. Tumor recurrence is heralded by return of virilization or by detection of increased 17-ketosteroids in the urine. Tumor debulking or inhibition of steroidogenesis with aminoglutethimide or mitotane may be useful in controlling signs and symptoms in patients with metastatic disease.

Adrenocortical Carcinoma

9 Adrenocortical carcinoma is a rare malignancy with an estimated incidence of 0.5 to 2 cases per million per year. Presentation peaks in the first and fifth decades of life. The prevalence is higher in females than in males (1.4 to 2:1). The cause of adrenocortical carcinoma is unknown, although somatic mutations in P53 and inheritance of this tumor in patients with germline mutations in P53 (Li Fraumeni syndrome) implicate this tumor suppressor gene in its pathogenesis.

10 **Signs and Symptoms.** Adrenocortical carcinoma is a very aggressive malignancy, and most patients (up to 75%) present with locoregionally advanced or distant disease. Syndromes of adrenal hormone overproduction are frequent (up to 60%) and may include hypercortisolism, hyperaldosteronism, or virilization. Patients with rapidly progressive Cushing syndrome or mixed presentations with signs of both Cushing syndrome and virilization should be suspected of having adrenocortical carcinoma. Nonfunctioning adrenocortical carcinomas present most commonly as abdominal pain or mass with vague symptoms of nausea, weight loss, and fatigue.

Diagnosis. Patients with suspected adrenocortical carcinoma should have biochemical testing to identify hormone overproduction followed by staging investigations including cross-sectional imaging and bone scans. Contrast-enhanced CT of the abdomen and chest is important to preoperatively diagnose local tumor invasion and metastatic lesions as well as to confirm a functioning contralateral kidney (Fig. 77.9). In the absence of distant metastases or local invasion, preoperative distinction between large adenomas and carcinomas can be difficult, although large (>6 cm) adrenal masses that extend to nearby structures on CT scanning should be approached as carcinomas. Biopsy of adrenal lesions suspected of being adrenocortical carcinoma is unnecessary and should be avoided. The risk of seeding and the inability of histologic examination to distinguish between adenoma and carcinoma make biopsy useless and potentially harmful. Biopsy of extraadrenal lesions may be performed to confirm metastatic disease.

A definitive diagnosis of adrenocortical carcinoma requires pathologic demonstration of tumor invasion to adjacent organs or spread to lymph nodes or distant sites. Practically, any adrenal neoplasm larger than 6 cm or weighing more than 100 g should be considered malignant. Histologic features of tumor necrosis, hemorrhage, and local invasion are gross pathologic evidence of carcinoma, while cells with large, hyperchromatic nuclei and more than 20 mitoses per high-power field suggest malignancy.

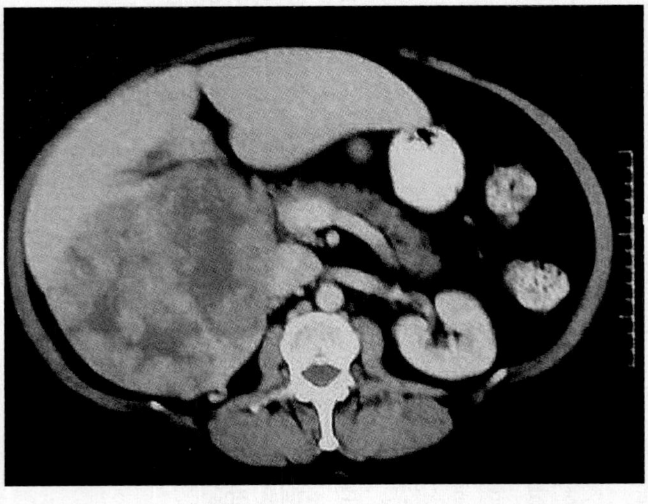

FIGURE 77.9. Computed tomography scan of right adrenocortical carcinoma showing invasion of liver and inferior vena cava. Note that a contralateral kidney is present and functioning.

Treatment. Surgical resection is the mainstay of treatment for all stages of adrenocortical carcinoma. Complete resection of locally confined tumor is the only chance for cure from adrenocortical carcinoma. However, distant or local spread is evident in 65% of cases at presentation. and a few patients are resectable with curative intent. Recurrence rates after surgery range from 38% to 85%, depending on stage at presentation (Table 77.5).

Many patients with adrenocortical carcinoma present with metastatic disease, involving the lung, lymph nodes, liver, or bone. Resection or surgical debulking of locally advanced or metastatic lesions may provide symptomatic relief for select patients, especially those with low-grade, slow-growing, hormonally productive cancers. Symptomatic recurrent or metastatic disease is best treated by resection when feasible.

Chemotherapy for adrenocortical carcinoma usually includes mitotane, although no controlled studies have established its efficacy in this disease. Partial responses to mitotane occur in less than a third of patients, and survival is unchanged. Adjuvant chemotherapy with mitotane after complete resection

TABLE 77.5 STAGING

AMERICAN JOINT COMMITTEE ON CANCER STAGING OF ADRENOCORTICAL CARCINOMA, WITH 5-YEAR SURVIVAL RATES

STAGE	CRITERIA	
Tumor		
T1	Tumor <5 cm, no invasion	
T2	Tumor >5 cm, no invasion	
T3	Tumor with invasion to fat	
T4	Tumor with organ invasion	
Lymph nodes		
N0	No lymph node metastasis	
N1	Lymph node metastasis present	
Metastasis		
M0	No distant metastasis	
M1	Distant metastasis present	
Stage Group	**TNM**	**5-Year Survival Rate**
I	T1 (<5 cm) N0M0	30%–45%
II	T2 (>5 cm) N0M0	12%–57%
III	T1–2, N1, M0 T3N0M0	5%–18%
IV	Any T, any N, M1 T3–4N1M0	0

for adrenocortical carcinoma is unproven and toxic so that many oncologists reserve its use for recurrent, unresectable, or metastatic disease. Cisplatin in combination with mitotane or doxorubicin and 5-fluoruracil has been applied in metastatic disease with partial responses noted.

The prognosis of adrenocortical carcinoma is poor. Median survival following diagnosis for all patients is approximately 18 months. Overall survival following resection for all stages of adrenocortical cancer is 15% to 47% at 5 years. Stage-specific 5-year survival is 30% to 45% for stage I, 12% to 57% for stage II, 5% to 18% for stage III, and 0 for stage IV disease.

DISEASES OF THE ADRENAL MEDULLA

Pheochromocytoma

Pheochromocytomas are functional adrenal tumors that arise from neuroectodermal cells of the adrenal medulla or in certain extraadrenal sites. These tumors are uncommon, occurring in 0.005% to 0.1% of persons, but occur with increased frequency in hypertensive populations (0.2% incidence) and in heritable endocrine tumor syndromes. The peak incidence of pheochromocytoma occurs during the fourth and fifth decades
11 of life, and men and women are affected about equally. The *rule of tens* is a useful way to characterize pheochromocytoma: Tumors are bilateral in 10% of cases, extraadrenal in 10%, familial in 10%, multicentric in 10%, and malignant in 10%, and occur in children in 10% of cases.

Approximately 10% of pheochromocytomas are extraadrenal, although most (98%) are still located within the abdomen. Extraadrenal pheochromocytomas can occur at any site in the abdomen where chromaffin tissue is located and have been found in the paravertebral ganglia, the organ of Zuckerkandl, and the urinary bladder. Clues to the presence of extraadrenal pheochromocytoma are predominance of norepinephrine because extraadrenal sites lack the enzyme necessary to convert norepinephrine to epinephrine.

Familial pheochromocytoma is a component of two autosomal dominant syndromes: von Hippel-Lindau syndrome and multiple endocrine neoplasia II (MEN2). Patients with von Hippel-Lindau syndrome have pheochromocytoma (usually bilateral), retinal angiomas, cerebellar hemangioblastoma, epididymal cystadenoma, renal and pancreatic cysts, and renal cell carcinoma. Patients with MEN2A develop pheochromocytoma (usually bilateral), medullary carcinoma of the thyroid (MTC), and primary parathyroid hyperplasia. Patients with MEN2B develop pheochromocytoma (usually bilateral), MTC, mucosal neuromas, and intestinal ganglioneuromatosis, and have a characteristic marfanoid body habitus. Pheochromocytoma also occurs in neurofibromatosis type 1 and familial paraganglioma. The frequency of pheochromocytoma in these disorders is 10% to 20% in von Hippel-Lindau syndrome, 50% in MEN2, and 0.1% to 5.7% with neurofibromatosis type 1.

In some families, patients with pheochromocytomas have no other clinical abnormalities, suggesting the existence of a separate disease limited to the formation of adrenal medullary tumors. In a study of three generations of an affected kindred, a novel mutation was found in the von Hippel-Lindau gene even though there were no other clinical manifestations of this disorder. Patients with bilateral pheochromocytoma, young patients with pheochromocytoma, and patients with paraganglioma should be screened for MEN2 and von Hippel-Lindau syndrome.

The etiology and pathogenesis of pheochromocytoma is unknown. A genetic component seems certain because pheochromocytoma occurs not only as a part of familial syndromes but also as an isolated disorder because of mutation in the RET gene or the MEN2 gene. Familial pheochromocytoma as well as sporadic pheochromocytoma occurs also with mutations in the succinate dehydrogenase complex, subunit B, iron sulfur protein (SDHB). Either germline or somatic mutations in the SDHD gene are another cause of pheochromocytoma.

Signs and Symptoms. Symptoms of pheochromocytoma are attributable to the effects of excessive circulating catecholamines on target tissues (Table 77.3). The classic triad of symptoms in patients with a pheochromocytoma is episodic headache, sweating, and tachycardia. Hypertension is common with pheochromocytoma and is sustained in roughly half of patients, is paroxysmal in one third, and is absent in one fifth. Orthostatic hypotension results from diminished plasma volume and blunted autonomic reflexes. Other symptoms include palpitations, anxiety, and tremulousness. Cardiovascular sequelae include myocardial infarction, cardiac dysrhythmias, and stroke. Gastrointestinal motility is also impaired. Asymptomatic patients with functioning tumors are rare, and nonfunctioning tumors are distinctly uncommon. Sudden death has been reported in patients with pheochromocytoma who have undergone surgical procedures or childbirth.

Diagnosis. Elevation of catecholamines and their metabolites in either urine or blood is essential for the diagnosis of pheochromocytoma. Either a 24-hour urine collection for catecholamines and their metabolites (metanephrines) or plasma-fractionated metanephrines can be used to make the diagnosis. Urine catecholamines/metanephrines is the most reliable test with a sensitivity and specificity of 98%. Plasma fractionated metanephrines is similarly sensitive (99%), but lacks specificity (85%). Accordingly, plasma-fractionated metanephrines should be reserved for patients with a high pretest probability for pheochromocytoma—adrenal incidentalomas, classic symptoms, family history of genetic syndromes associated with pheochromocytoma (MEN, etc.)—whereas urine catecholamines/metanephrines is useful as a screening tests for patients who are less likely to have a pheochromocytoma. Measurement of plasma catecholamines is not as useful in distinguishing patients with pheochromocytoma from those with essential hypertension. Measurement of plasma chromogranin A is nonspecific and a poor diagnostic but potentially helpful confirmatory test.

Many medications alter or interfere with measurement of either plasma or urine catecholamines. Such medications should be discontinued to ensure accurate testing. These drugs include acetaminophen, labetalol, clonidine withdrawal, tricyclic antidepressants, antipsychotics, and ethanol. To control blood pressure, other antihypertensives such as calcium channel blockers may be substituted.

In normotensive or mildly hypertensive patients with elevated plasma catecholamine levels (1,000–2,000 pg/mL), a clonidine suppression test may be used to distinguish from pheochromocytoma. An oral 0.3-mg dose of clonidine suppresses centrally mediated release of catecholamines to less than 500 pg/mL within 2 to 3 hours but does not affect release of catecholamines by a pheochromocytoma.

Biochemical confirmation of the diagnosis should be followed by radiologic evaluation to locate the tumor. Pheochromocytomas are best imaged with CT or MRI. Contrast-enhanced CT readily detects tumors 1 cm and larger and has sensitivity of 87% to 100% for pheochromocytoma (Fig. 77.10A). MRI is similarly sensitive, and a T2-weighted image brightness three times greater than liver is highly specific for pheochromocytoma (Fig. 77.10B and C). MRI is useful in suspected malignant pheochromocytoma to evaluate for inferior vena cava thrombus or liver invasion.

Functional nuclear imaging with iodine-131-metaiodobenzylguanidine (131-I MIBG) is a useful adjunct to cross-sectional imaging for pheochromocytoma (Fig. 77.10D). MIBG resembles norepinephrine and is taken up by adrenergic tissues including pheochromocytoma. An MIBG scan can detect

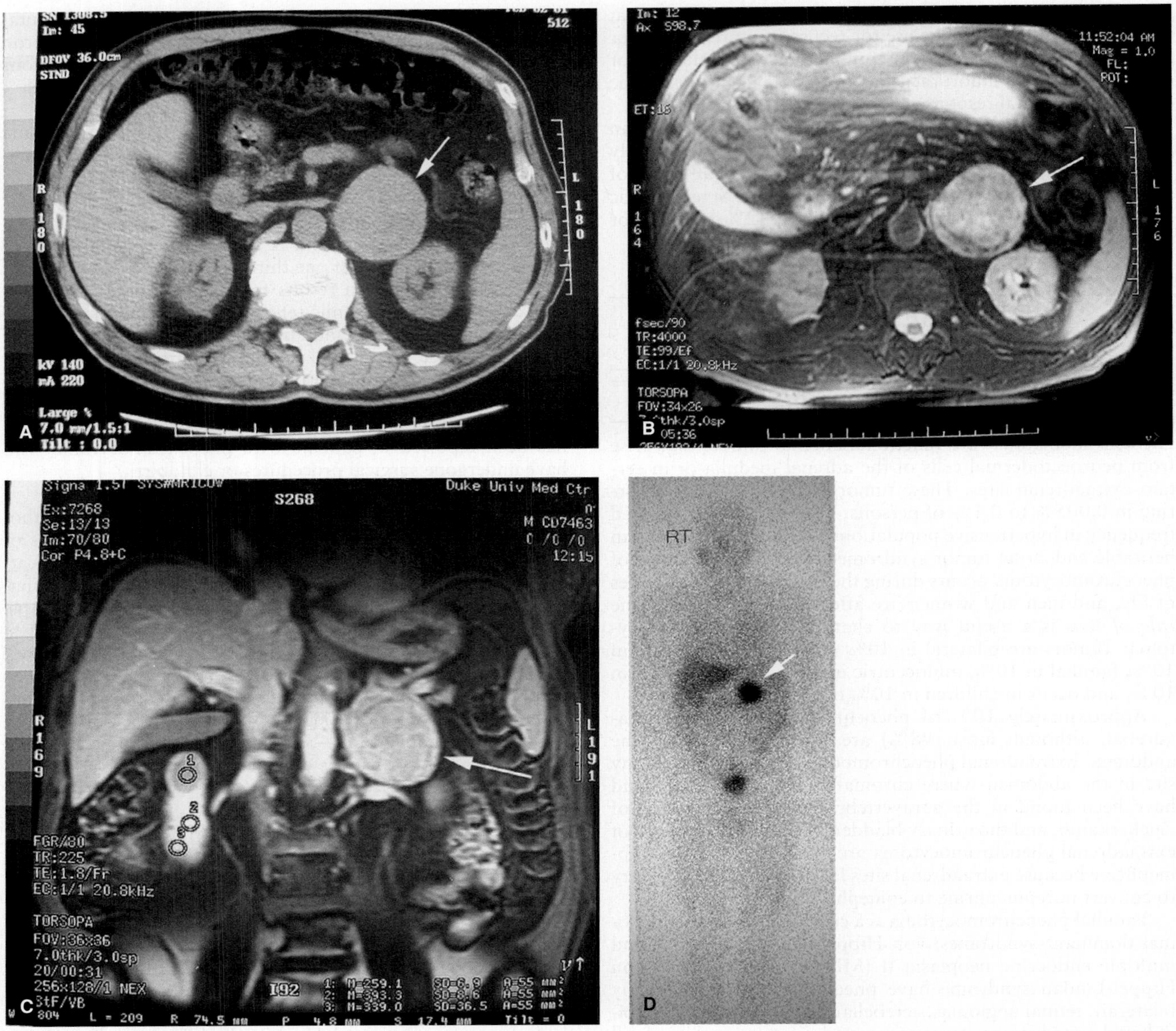

FIGURE 77.10. Imaging of pheochromocytoma (*arrows*). **A:** Computed tomography scan shows well-circumscribed left adrenal mass. **B:** T2-weighted magnetic resonance imaging shows the mass to be heterogeneously bright consistent with pheochromocytoma. **C** and **D:** Coronal contrast-enhanced MRI and near-simultaneous ^{131}I-metaiodobenzylguanine (^{131}I-MIBG) scanning show location of the pheochromocytoma and relationship to surrounding structures.

tumors not detected by CT or MRI or multiple tumors when CT or MRI is positive. Multi-institutional experience with this technique has demonstrated an overall sensitivity of 77% to 87% and a specificity of 96% to 100%. This test is usually not necessary for sporadic pheochromocytoma unless urinary or plasma catecholamines and metabolites are marginally elevated, or if malignant or extraadrenal pheochromocytoma is suspected. 131-I MIBG scanning is also useful to screen patients with metastatic pheochromocytoma for high-dose 131-I MIBG therapy. 111-In-pentetreotide scintigraphy may also identify pheochromocytoma and can be used therapeutically as with 131-I MIBG.

Treatment. Surgical resection is the only cure for pheochromocytoma. When the diagnosis of pheochromocytoma has been established and localization studies are completed, preoperative preparation of the patient centers on blood pressure control. Usually 1 to 3 weeks before operation, alpha-adrenergic blockade is performed first with phenoxybenzamine, starting at 10 mg twice a day and increasing by 10 to 20 mg per day, until blood pressure normalizes. Side effects of alpha blockade include postural hypotension, reflex tachycardia, nasal congestion, and an inability to ejaculate. Preoperative alpha blockade also reverses the relative hypovolemia that is usually present in patients with pheochromocytoma and also prevents severe blood pressure swings during intraoperative manipulation of the tumor. Metyrapone added preoperatively to phenoxybenzamine can achieve a greater degree of sympathetic blockade.

Beta-adrenergic blockade with propranolol added after alpha blockade can manage patients who develop tachycardia or who have inducible cardiac arrhythmias or ischemia. Propranolol may enhance pressor response to endogenous norepinephrine and thus should not be given until adequate alpha blockade has been established. Propranolol can also produce profound bradycardia, myocardial depression, and congestive heart failure. Newer drug regimens to manage hypertension in pheochromocytoma include selective alpha-1-adrenergic antagonists (terazosin and doxazosin) and calcium channel blockers (nifedipine and nicardipine).

Patients with pheochromocytoma can be expected to have blood pressure volatility and high intravascular volume requirements during and immediately after surgery. Elderly patients or those with a history of heart disease may require pulmonary catheter insertion and arterial line placement for careful monitoring of blood pressure and arterial pH. Anesthetic agents may trigger the release of catecholamines from pheochromocytomas. The anesthetic plane is now considered more important than the choice of agent, and both enflurane and isoflurane have been used successfully. Magnesium administration during surgery is an effective way to control blood pressure in patients with pheochromocytoma. Intraoperative hypertension is best treated with a sodium nitroprusside drip, and cardiac arrhythmias are best managed with short-acting beta-blockers (esmolol) or lidocaine.

Formerly, an anterior approach through either a midline or bilateral subcostal incision was used exclusively to resect pheochromocytomas. Today, CT, MRI, and nuclear scans permit preoperative localization of tumor in 95% or more of cases, so that the surgical approach may be more directed using a laparoscopic approach. Regardless of approach, important common principles include minimal handling of the tumor, early isolation and ligation of the adrenal vein, and avoidance of capsular rupture. Recurrence following resection of benign pheochromocytoma is infrequent, and its presence indicates malignancy.

Recurrent, malignant pheochromocytoma can include locally advanced disease or metastasis to bone, liver, lymph nodes, lungs, and the central nervous system. Treatment of malignant pheochromocytoma involves resection of metastases when feasible and medical control of hypertension. Radiation therapy may be helpful to ameliorate pain from bony metastases. Ablative therapy with 131-I MIBG may also produce partial responses and palliation of hormonal symptoms. Radiofrequency ablation of hepatic and bone metastases can be effective in selected patients. Combination chemotherapy with cyclophosphamide, vincristine, and dacarbazine can also be effective. Overall 5-year survival for patients with malignant pheochromocytoma ranges from 36% to 60%.

Metastasis to the Adrenal Glands

The adrenal glands are frequent sites for metastases from many cancers. Carcinoma of the lung and breast account for most adrenal metastases; however, virtually any cancer including melanoma, lymphoma, and kidney and ovarian carcinoma can spread to the adrenals. Autopsy series of patients with carcinoma show that the adrenal glands are involved in more than 25% of cases. Among cancer patients, 50% to 75% of newly discovered adrenal masses represent metastases. Usually, either a primary site is obvious or widespread disease is apparent. Biopsy of adrenal masses in patients with a history of carcinoma may be performed after pheochromocytoma is excluded. Resection of isolated adrenal metastases in select patients with long disease-free intervals from lung cancer, renal cell carcinoma, and melanoma can be considered, although subsequent extraadrenal disease usually develops. Median survival after complete resection of isolated adrenal metastases from various tumors ranges from 13 to 60 months with actuarial 2- and 5-year survival of 40% to 50% and 20%, respectively.

Incidental Adrenal Mass

Clinically inapparent adrenal masses (also called *adrenal incidentalomas*) have become commonplace over the past 20 years with the increased use of abdominal imaging such as CT and MRI. The estimated prevalence of incidental adrenal neoplasms varies by population studied and method of detection. Unsuspected adrenal masses are detected by CT in 0.6% to 1.9% of healthy patients, a figure that is somewhat lower than the estimated prevalence of up to 8.7% based on unselected autopsy data. Patients with a prior history of malignancy have a prevalence of adrenal masses of up to 4.4%. Adrenal masses increase in frequency with advancing age, ranging from 3% in midlife to 10% in the elderly. The combination of an aging population and increased application of abdominal imaging promises to create a significant public health challenge.

Over the past 10 years, increased awareness of morbidity associated with subclinical hormone overproduction, as well as the increased availability of minimally invasive laparoscopic adrenalectomy, has resulted in a lower threshold for treatment of adrenal masses. The goal of evaluation is to distinguish and remove those adrenal masses that are functioning or likely to be malignant versus those that are neither and may be observed.

Expectations of the yield for the workup of adrenal masses may be informed by epidemiologic reports and reports of pathologic findings in resected incidentalomas. Epidemiologic data indicate that up to 6.5% of incidentalomas are pheochromocytoma, 7% produce aldosterone, 0.035% produce cortisol, and 0.06% are carcinoma. A recent review of 44 reports describing more than 3,000 such cases reported that 41% were cortical adenomas, 19% were metastases from other primary cancers, 10% were adrenocortical carcinomas, and 8% were pheochromocytomas, with the remainder including myelolipomas and cysts.

Diagnosis. The evaluation of incidental adrenal masses, previously considered controversial, can now be standardized. Two simple questions must be answered: Is it functional? Is it malignant? The diagnostic approach should proceed to answer these questions sequentially (Table 77.6). Current opinion is that all asymptomatic patients with adrenal masses should be screened for pheochromocytoma, hypercortisolism, and hyperaldosteronism (Algorithm 77.3).

All patients require a complete history and physical examination, biochemical evaluation of pertinent hormones, and select imaging studies. Attention must be paid to episodes of hypertension, tachycardia, and anxiety that suggest pheochromocytoma. Physical findings such as muscle wasting, purple striae, hirsutism, and gynecomastia may suggest either Cushing syndrome or a virilizing tumor. Secondary metastases from underlying malignancy must be considered and evaluated with appropriate history, physical examination, and select tests including mammograms in women and chest radiography in all patients, especially smokers.

Biochemical testing should routinely exclude pheochromocytoma, hypercortisolism, and hyperaldosteronism. Pheochromocytoma is evaluated either by 24-hour urine collection for catecholamines, metanephrines, and 3-methoxy-4-hydroxymandelic acid, or by plasma-fractionated metanephrines. Subclinical or clinically apparent Cushing syndrome is best evaluated with the overnight 1-mg dexamethasone suppression test. Hyperaldosteronism is best assessed by concurrent measurement of serum or plasma aldosterone and PRA.

Imaging studies usually include cross-sectional imaging with either CT or MRI. CT is the best test for identifying and characterizing most adrenal masses. Using a fast scanner and 1-m scanning intervals, both adrenal glands can be identified in 97% to 99% of patients and lesions as small as 5 mm can be readily identified. Currently, attenuation values expressed in Hounsfield units (HU) have better performance than size or other criteria to differentiate adenomas from adrenal malignancy and nonadenomas such as pheochromocytoma. Adenomas are usually lipid rich and have attenuation values less than 18 HU on unenhanced CT, a threshold with high sensitivity and specificity (85%–95% and 93%–100%, respectively).

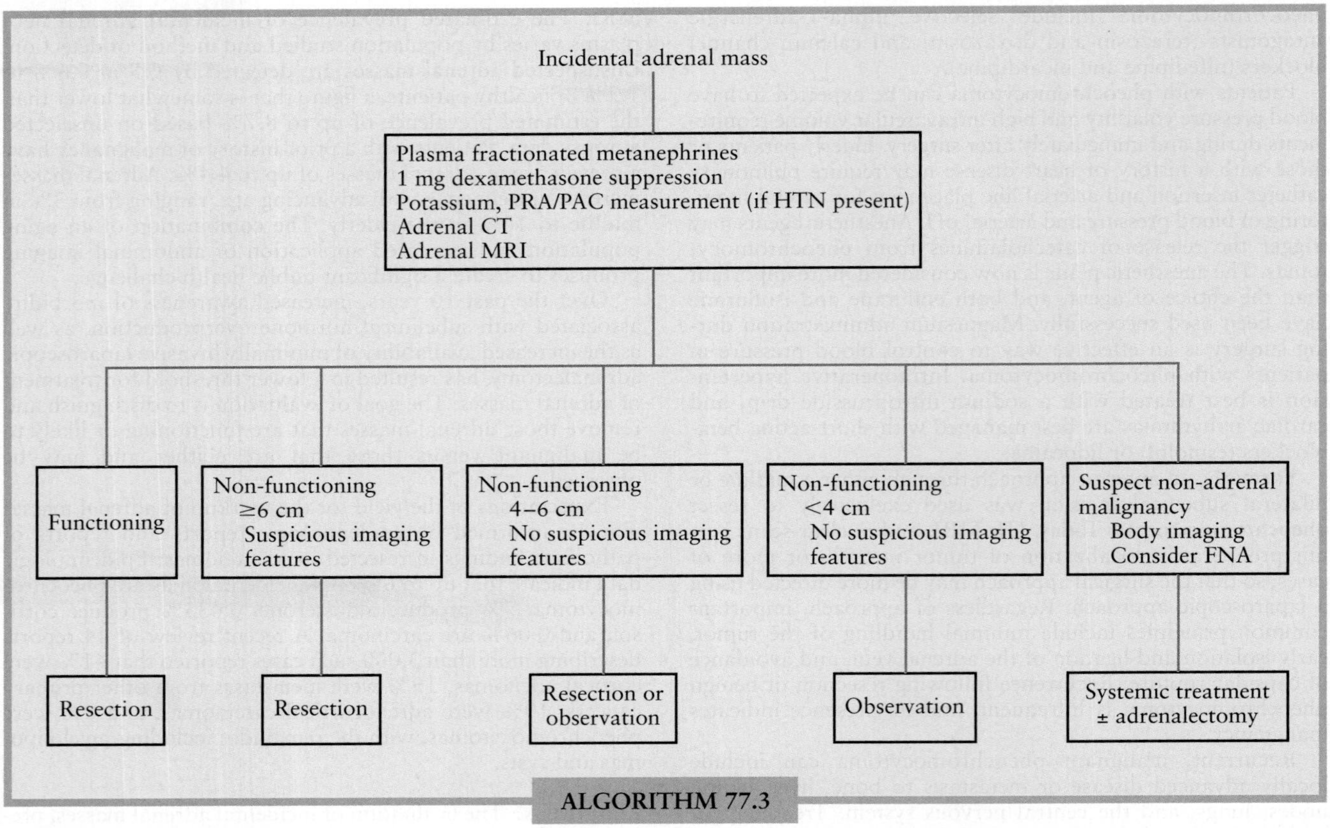

ALGORITHM 77.3. Diagnosis and management of the incidental adrenal mass. PRA, plasma renin activity; PAC, plasma aldosterone concentration; HTN, hypertension; CT, computed tomography; MRI, magnetic resonance imaging; FNA, fine-needle aspiration.

Generally, further workup is unnecessary when an adrenal lesion has an attenuation of less than 10 HU, suggesting lipid-rich adrenal adenoma. A notable exception is lipid-poor adenoma, which has higher HU density. In these cases, rapid washout of intravenous contrast suggests an adenoma. Using a 10- to 15-minute delayed enhanced CT, a washout value of 50% to 60% of the initial enhancement is used to distinguish adenoma from nonadenoma.

MRI can differentiate adenomas, metastases and pheochromocytomas, although the best MRI technique for evaluating adrenal masses is complex and controversial. Adenomas usually show a loss in signal intensity on chemical shift MRI

TABLE 77.6 **DIAGNOSIS**

SUMMARY OF TESTS FOR EVALUATION OF INCIDENTAL ADRENAL MASS

■ QUESTION	■ BEST TEST	■ ALTERNATIVE TEST	■ DIAGNOSIS
Is it functioning?	Plasma fractionated metanephrines	24-h urine for catecholamines, metanephrines, VMA	Pheochromocytoma
	- mg dexamethasone suppression test	24-h urine for cortisol	Hypercortisolism
	Serum potassium	24-h urine for potassium	Hyperaldosteronism
	Plasma renin/plasma aldosterone ratio		
Is it malignant?	Computed tomography	Magnetic resonance imaging	Cortical adenoma
			Adrenocortical
			Carcinoma
			Pheochromocytoma
			Myelolipoma
			Cyst
	Fine-needle aspiration		Metastasis

because of high lipid content. Malignant masses tend to be bright on T2-weighted images because of higher fluid content. Secondary metastases to the adrenal are hypointense to liver on T1-weighted images and are brighter than liver on T2-weighted images. Metastases also typically show strong contrast enhancement. Pheochromocytomas most often have low lipid content and high water content, giving low T1 signal intensities and very bright T2 signal intensities. Comparison of the adrenal mass to liver and spleen intensities on various sequences adds to specificity and sensitivity of the test.

Masses that appear cystic may be aspirated under CT guidance. Fine-needle aspiration biopsy may be of value in patients with known extraadrenal malignancy; however, it is not indicated in the evaluation of primary adrenal neoplasms and is contraindicated if pheochromocytoma is suspected.

Treatment. Resection is indicated for all functioning adrenal incidentalomas and those suspected of harboring primary adrenal cancer. Size cutoff for resecting adrenal incidentalomas has drifted to include smaller and smaller lesions. The prevalence of primary adrenal carcinoma in adrenal incidentalomas is related to mass size. The risk of primary adrenal carcinoma is less than 2% in lesions smaller than 4 cm whereas the incidence rises to 25% for lesions larger than 6 cm. Lesions larger than 6 cm and smaller lesions with suspicious criteria on imaging should be resected. Lesions smaller than 4 cm with benign imaging characteristics should be followed. For lesions between 4 and 6 cm, either resection or observation is acceptable. Decisions should not be based on size alone, but also on imaging characteristics including CT attenuation values. Resection of secondary adrenal malignancy is not generally recommended except for highly select patients.

Adrenal Insufficiency

Adrenal insufficiency reflects inadequate glucocorticoid and mineralocorticoid production by the adrenals, either secondary to suppression of the HPA axis or by destruction or removal of the adrenal glands. The most common causes of primary adrenal insufficiency are autoimmune adrenalitis, infection, and gland replacement with metastatic disease. Chronic exogenous steroid use with HPA suppression and surgical resection of adrenal glands are important causes of secondary adrenal insufficiency.

Clinical signs and symptoms usually do not become manifest until at least 90% of the gland is destroyed. Adrenal insufficiency usually occurs gradually unless the patient experiences stress, which may precipitate acute crisis.

Signs and Symptoms. Acute adrenal insufficiency usually manifests as shock in a patient with undiagnosed chronic adrenal insufficiency who has been subjected to physiologic stress. Similarly, patients with established adrenal insufficiency caused by exogenous steroid use may experience crisis if they do not increase glucocorticoid replacement during times of stress or illness. Symptoms of adrenal insufficiency reflect glucocorticoid and mineralocorticoid deficiencies. Signs and symptoms of acute insufficiency include fever, nausea, vomiting, refractory hypotension, and lethargy (Table 77.7). Acute adrenal insufficiency is a medical emergency and should be suspected in stressed patients with a history of either adrenal insufficiency or exogenous steroid use. Chronic adrenal insufficiency presents more subtly, with fatigue, weight loss, anorexia, nausea and vomiting, abdominal pain, and diarrhea.

Diagnosis. Laboratory findings of adrenal insufficiency include hyponatremia, hyperkalemia, azotemia, and fasting or reactive hypoglycemia. Hypercalcemia may also be present. The rapid ACTH stimulation test is the best test for both acute and chronic adrenal insufficiency. Synthetic ACTH (250 μg) is administered intravenously, and plasma cortisol levels are measured 30 and 60 minutes later. Normal peak cortisol response should exceed 20 μg/dL. Measurement of ACTH by immunoradiometric assay (IRMA) is then used to distinguish primary from secondary and tertiary adrenal insufficiency. High plasma concentration of ACTH (>200 pg/dL) and low plasma cortisol (<10 mg/dL) are diagnostic of primary adrenal insufficiency. Low levels of plasma ACTH indicate secondary (pituitary) or tertiary (hypothalamic) adrenal insufficiency.

TABLE 77.7 **DIAGNOSIS**

SYMPTOMS AND SIGNS OF ACUTE ADRENAL INSUFFICIENCY

SYMPTOMS
- Lethargy
- Confusion or disorientation
- Nausea and vomiting
- Abdominal pain

SIGNS
- Hypotension
- Hyponatremia, hyperkalemia, azotemia,
- Hypoglycemia
- Fever
- Anemia

Treatment. Acute adrenal insufficiency is based on clinical suspicion before laboratory confirmation is available. Intravenous volume replacement with isotonic fluids and immediate intravenous steroid replacement therapy with 4 mg dexamethasone is essential. A rapid ACTH stimulation test is then performed to establish the diagnosis of adrenal insufficiency after resuscitation and corticosteroid replacement. Hydrocortisone acetate is detected in laboratory measurement for cortisol so dexamethasone should be used for replacement of glucocorticoid function until ACTH testing is complete. Thereafter, 100 mg of hydrocortisone is administered intravenously every 6 to 8 hours and is tapered to standard replacement doses as the patient's condition stabilizes. Mineralocorticoid replacement is not required until oral intake resumes. Chronic adrenal insufficiency requires both corticosteroid and mineralocorticoid replacement. Usual daily dosing is 12 mg/m^2 of hydrocortisone and 0.05 to 0.10 mg fludrocortisone.

Patients who have known adrenal insufficiency or who have received supraphysiologic doses of corticosteroid for at least 1 week in the year preceding surgery should receive perioperative stress-dose corticosteroids. Administration of 100 mg hydrocortisone the morning of major surgery followed by 100 mg of hydrocortisone every 8 hours during the perioperative 24 hours is usually more than sufficient. Steroids can be rapidly tapered to replacement levels as the patient's condition permits.

ADRENALECTOMY

Surgical approaches to the adrenal glands include the laparoscopic approach, the anterior transabdominal approach, and less commonly, the combined thoracoabdominal approach or posterior retroperitoneal approach. Either adrenal gland can be removed using any of these approaches. The choice of approach depends on the suspected pathology, the size of the adrenal lesion, and the expertise of the surgeon. Small benign-appearing tumors that are localized with confidence by imaging studies are resected using a laparoscopic or posterior approach. Posterior retroperitoneal adrenalectomy, once the most common method of adrenalectomy, is less commonly used since most lesions amenable to this approach can be removed laparoscopically. Large adrenal masses and those that may harbor malignancy should be resected using an anterior approach to adequately explore the entire abdomen and gain sufficient exposure for safe resection. Very large adrenocortical carcinomas may require a thoracoabdominal approach for en bloc resection with involved adjacent structures. Recently, a retroperitoneal laparoscopic approach has been advocated as an alternative method for small tumors, particularly for patients with prior abdominal surgery.

Laparoscopic Adrenalectomy

Laparoscopic adrenalectomy is now the preferred approach to most small, benign adrenal lesions including functioning and nonfunctioning adenomas and pheochromocytomas. Enthusiasm for the laparoscopic approach is based on the expectation of decreased postoperative pain, faster rehabilitation, and fewer complications. Numerous studies have shown the efficacy and safety of this procedure for tumors up to 6 cm. Larger lesions can be approached by experienced surgeons in select circumstances. It is important that expertise in open adrenalectomy is absolutely necessary for the laparoscopic surgeon to convert to an open procedure and promptly rectify any intraoperative laparoscopic complications.

Laparoscopic adrenalectomy begins with induction of general anesthesia, placement of a urinary catheter and orogastric tube, and positioning of the patient in the lateral decubitus position with the affected side up. Exposure is facilitated by extension of the operating table at the patient's waist. A total of three or four intraperitoneal ports (one camera, one retractor particularly for the right side, and two working ports) are placed at least 5 cm apart in a transverse line from the lateral edge of the rectus sheath to the midaxillary line between the costal margin and iliac crest (Fig. 77.11A). Four-quadrant exploration of the peritoneal cavity is first performed with the videoscope through the medialmost port, and the videoscope is then transferred to the middle port. A retractor is placed

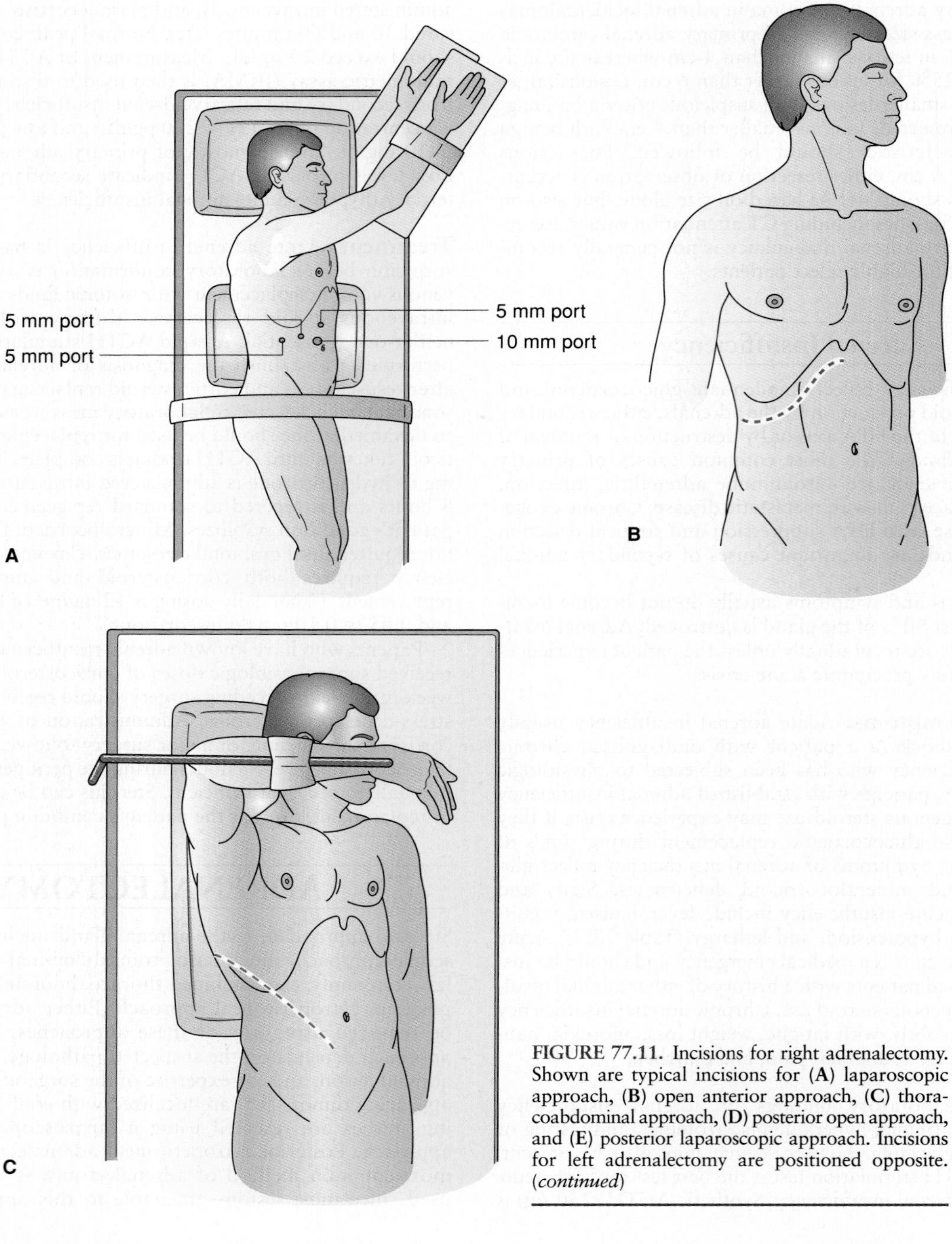

FIGURE 77.11. Incisions for right adrenalectomy. Shown are typical incisions for (A) laparoscopic approach, (B) open anterior approach, (C) thoracoabdominal approach, (D) posterior open approach, and (E) posterior laparoscopic approach. Incisions for left adrenalectomy are positioned opposite. (*continued*)

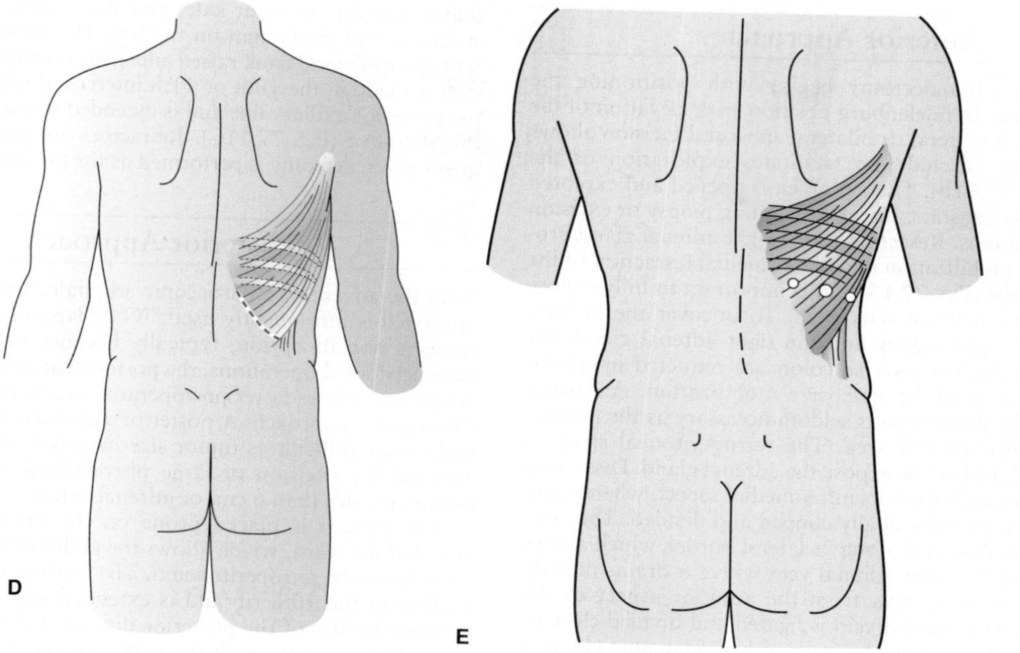

FIGURE 77.11. (*Continued*)

through the medialmost port to retract the viscera medially. Operating instruments are alternately placed within the abdomen through the lateral ports.

Laparoscopic adrenalectomy proceeds similar to the open anterior approach. Right adrenalectomy begins with mobilization of the liver to open the retroperitoneum and allow retraction of the right lobe anteriorly and medially using the most medial port. The adrenal gland is then identified posterolateral to the inferior vena cava and superior to the kidney. Dissection usually begins by developing the plane between right adrenal and inferior vena cava using careful blunt dissection, with small vessels sequentially coagulated using electrosurgical or harmonic energy. The right adrenal vein is identified, carefully dissected, and then doubly clipped and divided (Fig. 77.12A). Dissection then continues circumferentially around the gland with additional small vessels coagulated or clipped. The adrenal gland subsequently is placed in a bag and removed through an expanded port.

Left adrenalectomy is performed with mirror-image patient and port site orientation as right adrenalectomy. After port placement, dissection begins with mobilization of the splenic flexure of the colon and spleen from the left retroperitoneum. Subsequent medial retraction of the spleen, tail of the pancreas, and stomach is accomplished with the fan or similar retractor if necessary. Often after full mobilization, no retractor is necessary, and thus only three ports are needed. The left adrenal gland is identified in perinephric fat at the superior renal pole. Intraoperative laparoscopic ultrasound can be useful for this on the left side, particularly in Cushing syndrome with the associated increased truncal fat. Once identified, left adrenal gland dissection proceeds circumferentially around the gland, with identification, ligation, and division of the left adrenal vein at the inferiormost aspect of the dissection (Fig. 77.12B). Care is needed to identify and avoid the inferior phrenic vein, which courses along the medial aspect of the left adrenal gland. Following circumferential dissection, the gland is removed.

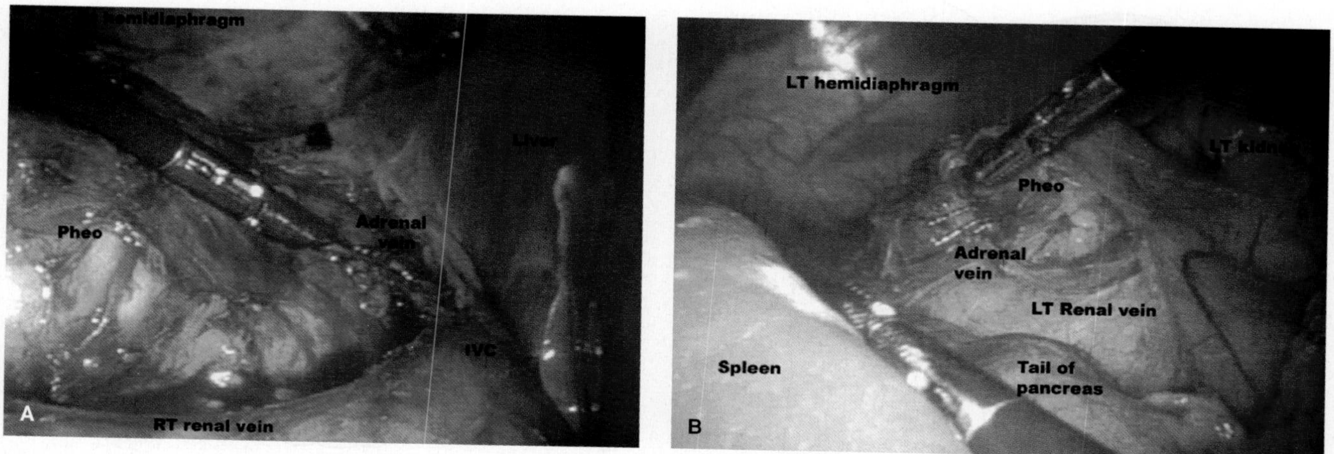

FIGURE 77.12. Laparoscopic adrenalectomy. Shown are intraoperative views of exposed right (A) and left (B) adrenal pheochromocytomas (pheo) in a patient with multiple endocrine neoplasia (MEN)-2 A. Note clips on each adrenal vein. IVC, inferior vena cava.

ENDOCRINE

Anterior Approach

Anterior open adrenalectomy begins with positioning the patient in reverse Trendelenburg position with elevation of the right flank. An ipsilateral or bilateral subcostal incision allows access to either adrenal and facilitates exploration of the abdomen (Fig. 77.11B). The abdomen is opened and explored for evidence of metastatic disease, including biopsy or excision of suspicious lesions. Resection of the right adrenal gland proceeds with full mobilization and anteromedial retraction of the right hepatic lobe (Fig. 77.13A). It is important to fully expose the retrohepatic inferior vena cava. To uncover the inferior vena cava, the right kidney and the right adrenal gland, the hepatic flexure, and transverse colon are retracted inferiorly, usually without need for extensive mobilization. A Kocher maneuver of the duodenum is seldom necessary as the adrenal gland is superior to this area. The retroperitoneal space is entered behind the liver to expose the adrenal gland. Dissection of the gland proceeds from its inferomedial aspect, where small feeding arteries are individually clipped and divided. The vena cava is carefully dissected along its lateral border, which allows identification of the right adrenal vein where it drains directly into the inferior vena cava from the anterior aspect of the adrenal gland. The adrenal vein is ligated and divided close to the vena cava. If necessary because of hemodynamic changes during an operation for a pheochromocytoma, the adrenal vein is identified and ligated early to avoid catecholamine surges and blood pressure fluctuations during manipulation of the gland. Once the adrenal vein is ligated, arterial feeding vessels are clipped and divided sequentially, beginning at the superolateral aspect of the gland and continuing medially.

Resection of the left adrenal gland requires mobilization of the spleen, tail of pancreas, and left colon. The left colon is freed from its peritoneal attachments and is reflected inferiorly. The spleen is then delivered from the left upper quadrant medially, and the splenocolic ligament is divided. The spleen, stomach, and pancreatic tail are retracted medially en bloc to expose the left kidney and adrenal (Fig. 77.13B). The left adrenal vein is ligated and divided at its junction with the left renal vein. The gland is dissected, and the arterial vessels are ligated and divided sequentially, beginning at the superolateral aspect of the gland and continuing medially.

Thoracoabdominal Approach

The thoracoabdominal approach is used for large adrenal lesions with invasion of surrounding structures including the liver and diaphragm on the right side, and the spleen, pancreatic tail, stomach, and diaphragm on the left. The patient is positioned with the ipsilateral flank raised and arm extended cephalad. Incision is made in the 10th or 11th intercostal space beginning at the posterior axillary line and is extended toward the midline of the abdomen (Fig. 77.11C). Retractors are placed, and subsequent adrenalectomy is performed as for the anterior approach.

Posterior Approach

With the advent of laparoscopic adrenalectomy, the posterior approach is infrequently used. When laparoscopic adrenalectomy is not an option, typically because of extensive prior transperitoneal operations, the posterior approach is better tolerated and allows faster postoperative recovery compared with the anterior approach. A posterior approach becomes increasingly more difficult as tumor size increases and is not recommended for excision of large pheochromocytomas, adrenal tumors greater than 6 cm, or adrenal carcinoma.

The patient is placed prone on the operating table and flexed at the waist, which allows the abdominal contents to fall away from the retroperitoneum. The incision is made from the midline at the 10th rib and is extended inferolaterally to the superior border of the posterior iliac crest (Fig. 77.11D). Dissection proceeds through the subcutaneous fat and latissimus dorsi muscle to the lumbodorsal fascia. This fascia is incised longitudinally, and the underlying sacrospinalis muscle. The sacrospinalis muscle is retracted medially, and the 12th rib and vascular bundle are resected as far medially as possible. The 12th intercostal nerve is preserved and gently retracted superiorly. The retroperitoneum is entered and the diaphragm is bluntly elevated from the Gerota fascia, the pleura are separated from the diaphragm, and the diaphragm is then divided. The Gerota fascia is incised, and the kidney is retracted inferiorly to expose the adrenal gland. The arterial blood supply is controlled first by clipping and ligating numerous arterial vessels, which course posteriorly. The adrenal vein, located deep to the arteries, is ligated as it is encountered. On the right, the adrenal vein exits from the anterior aspect of the gland and courses to the inferior vena cava. Once the adrenal vein is divided, the gland is then freed circumferentially from its lateral to medial aspect. The inferior border of the gland is dissected last to maintain attachment to the kidney and allow inferior retraction of the gland. The procedure is completed by repair of the diaphragm and any incidental pleural defects, reapproximation of the lumbodorsal fascia, and closure of the skin.

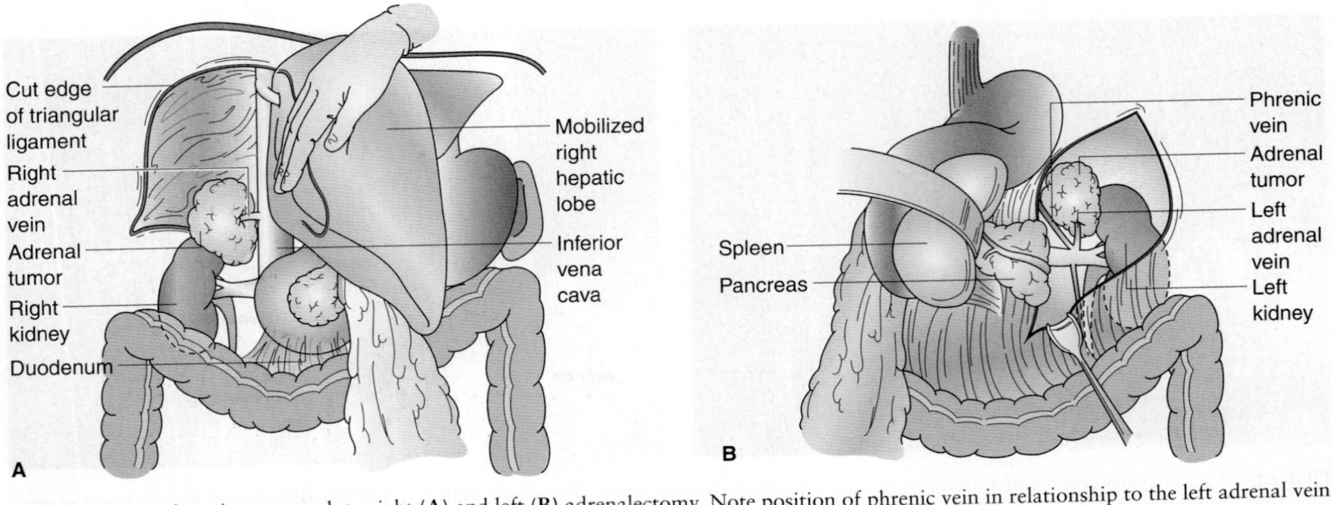

FIGURE 77.13. Anterior approach to right (**A**) and left (**B**) adrenalectomy. Note position of phrenic vein in relationship to the left adrenal vein and tumor.

Posterior Retroperitoneal Laparoscopic Adrenalectomy

Posterior retroperitoneal laparoscopic adrenalectomy, also known as posterior retroperitoneoscopic adrenalectomy, maintains the advantages of a laparoscopic approach while avoiding the abdominal cavity. This approach is ideal for patients with prior abdominal surgery or for bilateral adrenalectomy as both adrenal glands can be removed without repositioning the patient.

Posterior retroperitoneal laparoscopic adrenalectomy begins with placing the patient in the prone jackknife position on a spinal table allowing the abdominal contents to hang forward. The hips and knees are positioned at 90-degree angles to the spine and femur and carefully padded. The first port is placed just below the tip of the 12th rib; after the incision is made, the retroperitoneal space is entered sharply, a space is created bluntly with the index finger, and a blunt 10-mm trocar is placed. A second medial 10-mm trocar is placed along the paraspinous muscle at a 45-degree angle toward the adrenal gland. A lateral 5-mm port is placed 5 cm lateral to the first port in a similar fashion (Fig 77.11E). Pneumoretroperitoneum to 20 to 24 mm Hg is created with CO_2 to create an adequate working space. The videoscope is transferred from the initial middle port to the medial port to complete the dissection. The retroperitoneal space beneath the diaphragm is created bluntly and sharply. The superior border of the kidney is immediately identified, and the Gerota fascia is entered. The upper pole of the kidney is retracted caudally, and the tissue superior to the kidney that contains the adrenal gland is completely separated from the kidney. The medial dissection is then begun by carefully bluntly dissecting medial to the adrenal gland, identifying the adrenal vein, and dividing it between clips. Identification of the adrenal vein, particularly on the right side, is easier than with the transabdominal laparoscopic approach. Dissection is completed circumferentially around the gland using electrosurgical or harmonic energy to coagulate any small vessels. Once the gland is completely free, it is placed in a bag and removed through the middle port.

Bibliography

Bravo EL, Tagle R. Pheochromocytoma: state-of-the-art and future prospects. *Endocr Rev* 2003;24:539–553.

Brunt LM, Lairmore TC, Doherty GM, et al. Adrenalectomy for familial pheochromocytoma in the laparoscopic era. *Ann Surg* 2002;235:713–720.

Findling JW, Raff H. Diagnosis and differential diagnosis of Cushing syndrome. *Endocrinol Metab Clin North Am* 2001;30:729–747.

Harrison LE, Gaudin PB, Brennan MF. Pathologic features of prognostic significance for adrenocortical carcinoma after curative resection. *Arch Surg* 1999;134:181–185.

Kalady MF, McKinlay R, Olson JA Jr, et al. Laparoscopic adrenalectomy for pheochromocytoma. A comparison to aldosteronoma and incidentaloma. *Surg Endosc* 2004;18:621–625.

Lenders JW, Pacak K, Walther MM, et al. Biochemical diagnosis of pheochromocytoma: which test is best? *JAMA* 2002;287:1427–1434.

Magill SB, Raff H, Shaker JL, et al. Comparison of adrenal vein sampling and computed tomography in the differentiation of primary aldosteronism. *J Clin Endocrinol Metab* 2001;86:1066–1071.

Mansmann G, Lau J, Balk E, et al. The clinically inapparent adrenal mass: update in diagnosis and management. *Endocr Rev* 2004;25:309–340.

Mulatero P, Stowasser M, Loh KC, et al Increased diagnosis of primary aldosteronism, including surgically correctable forms, in centers from five continents. *J Clin Endocrinol Metab* 2004;89:1045–1050.

Ng L, Libertino JM. Adrenocortical carcinoma: diagnosis, evaluation and treatment. *J Urol* 2003;169:5–11.

NIH state-of-the-science statement on management of the clinically inapparent adrenal mass ("incidentaloma"). *NIH Consens State Sci Statements* 2002;19:1–25.

OMIM Online Mendelian Inheritance in Man [database online] #202300. Baltimore, MD: Johns Hopkins; 2005. Available at: http:// www.ncbi.nlm.nih.gov/entrez/dispomim.cgi?id5202300. Accessed June 9, 2005.

OMIM Online Mendelian Inheritance in Man [database online] #171300. Baltimore, MD: Johns Hopkins; 2005. Available at: http:// www.ncbi.nlm.nih.gov/entrez/dispomim.cgi?id5171300). Accessed June 9, 2005.

Orth DN. Adrenal insufficiency. *Curr Ther Endocrinol Metab* 1994;5:124–130.

Pacak K, Linehan WM, Eisenhofer G, et al. Recent advances in genetics, diagnosis, localization, and treatment of pheochromocytoma. *Ann Intern Med* 2001;134:315–329.

Perrier ND, Kennamer DL, Bao R, et al. Posterior retroperitoneoscopic adrenalectomy, preferred technique for removal of benign tumors and isolated metastases. *Ann Surg* 2008;248:666–673.

Reincke M. Subclinical Cushing syndrome. *Endocrinol Metab Clin North Am* 2000;29:43–56.

Shen WT, Sturgeon C, Duh QY. From incidentaloma to adrenocortical carcinoma: the surgical management of adrenal tumors. *J Surg Oncol* 2005;89: 186–192.

Sippel RS, Chen H. Subclinical Cushing's syndrome in adrenal incidentalomas. *Surg Clin North Am* 2004;84:875–885.

Speiser PW, White PC. Congenital adrenal hyperplasia. *N Engl J Med* 2003;349: 776–788.

Stojadinovic A, Ghossein RA, Hoos A, et al. Adrenocortical carcinoma: clinical, morphologic, and molecular characterization. *J Clin Oncol* 2002;20:941–950.

Werbel SS, Ober KP. Acute adrenal insufficiency. *Endocrinol Metab Clin North Am* 1993;22:303–328.

White PC, Speiser PW. Congenital adrenal hyperplasia due to 21-hydroxylase deficiency. *Endocr Rev* 2000;21:245–291.

Young WF Jr. Minireview: primary aldosteronism–changing concepts in diagnosis and treatment. *Endocrinology* 2003;144:2208–2213.

ENDOCRINE

CHAPTER 78 ■ PITUITARY GLAND

WILLIAM F. CHANDLER, ARIEL L. BARKAN, AND RICARDO V. LLOYD

KEY POINTS

1. The hypothalamus of the brain is the principal integrating organ for regulating the internal environment of the body, and the pituitary is its major link with the organs outside the nervous system.
2. The adenohypophysis constitutes 80% of the gland and contains the pars distalis, pars tuberalis, and remnant of the pars intermedia.
3. The neurohypophysis, or posterior pituitary, is small and is virtually an extension of the hypothalamus of the brain.
4. Magnetic resonance imaging has evolved as the first choice for diagnostic imaging of the pituitary and is often the only test needed for a therapeutic decision to be made.
5. The findings of Cushing syndrome often include central obesity, hypertension, hirsutism, fatigue, easy bruising, striae, moonlike facies, dorsal fat pad, and often depression or other mental changes. The cause of hypercortisolism is an adrenocorticotropic hormone (ACTH)-secreting pituitary adenoma (Cushing disease) in up to 80% of cases; the remainder are caused by an adrenocortical tumor or an endocrine tumor that secretes ACTH or corticotropin-releasing hormone.
6. The three goals of surgery for nonfunctioning macroadenomas are establishment of a diagnosis, decompression of surrounding structures, and gross total removal of tumor tissue, if possible.
7. The goals of treatment of adenomas secreting growth hormone are to lower the circulating growth hormone and insulinlike growth factor-1 (IGF-1) levels to a normal range and to reduce the size of the mass lesion that is causing compression-related symptoms.

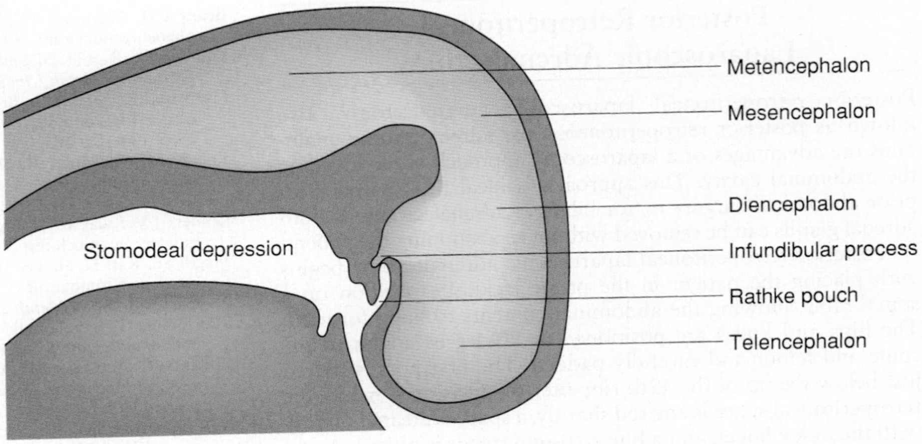

FIGURE 78.1. Diagram of a 4-week-old embryo illustrating how the Rathke pouch meets the infundibular process to form the anterior and posterior lobes, respectively, of the pituitary gland.

1 The pituitary gland, or hypophysis, is a remarkably complex way station in the connection between the brain and a wide range of organs throughout the body. The hypothalamus of the brain is the principal integrating organ for regulating the internal environment of the body, and the pituitary is its major link with the organs outside the nervous system. The pituitary has been called the "master gland"; even with advances in modern neuroendocrinology, it remains worthy of that description.

EMBRYOLOGY, ANATOMY, AND PHYSIOLOGY

By the fourth week of gestation, an evagination develops in the roof of the stomodeal depression that is lined by ectodermal cells of the cavity destined to become the pharynx (Fig. 78.1). This structure is known as the *Rathke pouch*. At the same time, a depression develops in the floor of the diencephalon; this is called the *infundibular process*. It too is lined with ectodermal cells. These are cells of the future diencephalic portion of the brain and, therefore, are more similar to the cells of central nervous system tissue. During a period of weeks, the two structures grow to meet each other—the infundibular process forming the neurohypophysis (pars neuralis) and the Rathke pouch forming the adenohypophysis (pars distalis). In lower animals, an intermediary lobe (pars intermedia) also forms, but in humans this is present only as a minor cleft. As the adenohypophysis enlarges, its upper portion (pars tuberalis) partially surrounds the stalk connecting the pituitary to the brain. Eventually, the connection between the adenohypophysis and the oral cavity disappears, but occasionally ectopic remnants of nonfunctioning pituitary cells, known as *pharyngeal pituitary tissue*, are left along its path.

In an adult, the dimensions of the hypophysis are 6 × 9 × 12 mm, and it weighs about 0.6 g. It enlarges during preg-
2 nancy and weighs up to 1 g in multiparous women. The adenohypophysis constitutes 80% of the gland and contains the pars distalis, pars tuberalis, and remnant of the pars intermedia. The pars distalis is the major functional portion of the adenohypophysis, and in this chapter, it is considered synonymous with
3 the adenohypophysis, or anterior pituitary. The neurohypophysis, or posterior pituitary, is small and is virtually an extension of the hypothalamus of the brain.

The combined neurohypophysis and adenohypophysis are connected to the base of the brain by a common stalk (Fig. 78.2A). The stalk blends into the median eminence of the hypothalamus and serves to transport both hormone-rich portal blood to the adenohypophysis and nerve fibers to the neurohypophysis. The optic chiasm lies directly above the pituitary, just anterior to the stalk; thus, it is vulnerable to compression by a pituitary tumor. The supraoptic and paraventricular nuclei of the hypothalamus are depicted in Figure 78.2A because they are the principal locations of cell bodies with axons directed toward the neurohypophysis.

The median eminence is where hormonal contributions from axons originating in various nuclei of the hypothalamus enter blood destined for the adenohypophysis (Fig. 78.2B). Blood reaches this region primarily through the superior hypophyseal artery and flows into gomitoli, which are small capillary plexuses within the median eminence through which hormones enter the blood. The blood then travels through the portal system to the adenohypophysis, where the hormones modulate the activity of secretory cells. These cells, in turn, secrete hormones into the general circulation to stimulate end organs. This system comprises the hormones listed in Table 78.1. Each of these hormonal combinations constitutes a feedback system in which the brain (hypothalamus) senses the level of end-organ hormone output and, in turn, positively or negatively adjusts the secretion of the various hypothalamic hormones into the portal system.

The neurohypophysis differs significantly from the adenohypophysis in that it does not receive controlling hormones by means of the portal system but rather by direct transport through nerve fibers. The principal input into the neurohypophysis is via the supraoptic–hypophyseal tract, which arises from cells within the supraoptic and paraventricular nuclei. The tuberohypophyseal tract, which originates from the central and posterior portions of the hypothalamus, also contributes input to the neurohypophysis. These tracts carry both antidiuretic hormone (ADH; vasopressin) and oxytocin. ADH is secreted into the general circulation and causes the kidneys to reabsorb free water. Elevated levels of ADH (syndrome of inappropriate ADH secretion) cause water retention and hyponatremia, and inadequate levels of ADH (diabetes insipidus) cause dehydration and hypernatremia. Interestingly, surgical loss of the neurohypophysis does not usually result in diabetes insipidus because the stalk itself can still secrete ADH into the circulation. The feedback mechanism to the brain for release of ADH is mainly serum osmolarity, with hyperosmolar conditions causing the release of ADH and retention of water. Blood volume also affects the release of ADH; thus, hemorrhage causes water retention. Oxytocin functions only during pregnancy and causes both uterine contractions and milk letdown within the breasts.

The gross surgical anatomy of the pituitary is also critical to the surgeon because the pituitary is closely surrounded by a number of important structures. Figure 78.3A illustrates the coronal cross section of the anatomy of the pituitary as viewed from the front. The pituitary sits within the bony confines of the sella turcica ("Turkish saddle") and is bordered laterally by the cavernous sinuses (venous), inferiorly and anteriorly by the sphenoid sinus (air), posteriorly by the dorsum sellae, and superiorly by the membranous diaphragma sellae. The cavernous

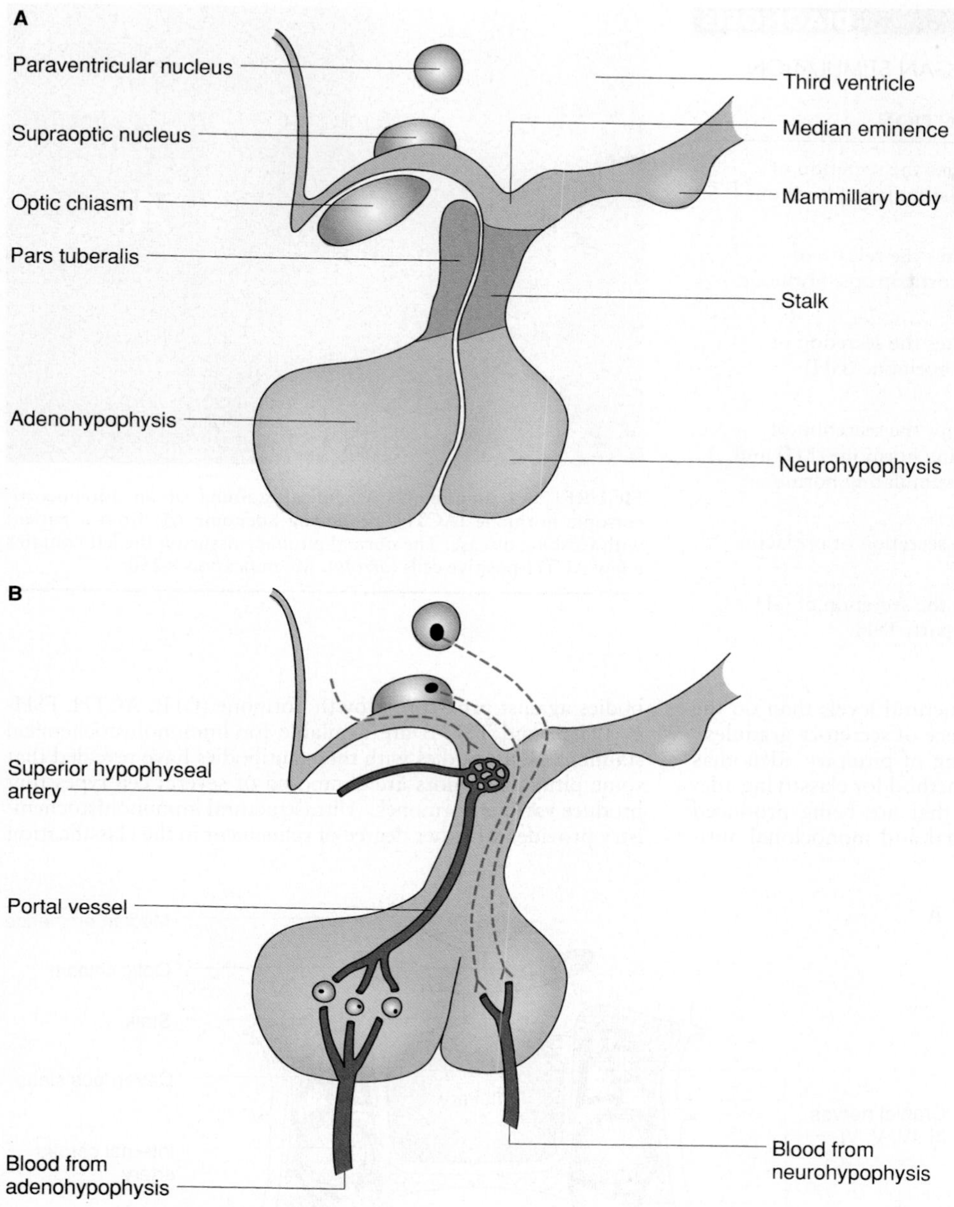

FIGURE 78.2. **A:** Schematic diagram of the pituitary and floor of the third ventricle as seen in a midline sagittal view. Anterior is to the left. **B:** Physiology of hormone release. The adenohypophysis receives releasing hormones through a portal venous system, and the neurohypophysis receives hormones directly from hypothalamic nuclei by means of neurons.

sinuses each contain the siphon region of the internal carotid artery and portions of cranial nerves III, IV, V, and VI, all within a venous plexus. The optic chiasm lies 10 to 15 mm above the diaphragma sellae. Directly below the anterior and inferior portions of the sella is the aerated sphenoid sinus. This is sufficiently large in 97% of patients to allow a transnasal, transsphenoidal surgical approach to the pituitary (Fig. 78.3B).

METHODS OF CELL ANALYSIS

Pituitary adenomas have been classified historically as acidophilic, basophilic, and chromophobic. Adenomas may show a variable staining pattern with conventional hematoxylin and eosin dyes, so it is difficult to classify adenomas based on these stains. For example, prolactinomas and sparsely granulated growth hormone adenomas may be acidophilic or chromophobic after hematoxylin and eosin staining (Table 78.2). Immunohistochemistry, ultrastructural studies, and in situ hybridization analyses for specific hormones are the most reliable methods of classifying pituitary adenomas today.

Other conventional stains that help in the analysis of pituitary adenomas include the reticulin stain, which helps to distinguish between pituitary hyperplasia and adenomas. The normal reticulin pattern is retained in hyperplasia and is similar to normal pituitary tissue, but it becomes disrupted in neoplasia. The periodic acid–Schiff reaction stains carbohydrates in adrenocorticotropic hormone (ACTH)-, thyroid-stimulating hormone (TSH)-, follicle-stimulating hormone (FSH)-, and luteinizing hormone (LH)-producing tumors.

The ultrastructural analysis of pituitary adenomas provides a great deal of information about size and type of secretory granules, cellular synthetic activity, and unique features of specific adenoma subtypes. For example, misplaced exocytosis occurs in prolactin-producing tumors, type I microfilaments are present in ACTH-producing tumors, and abundant mitochondria are characteristic of oncocytic null cell adenomas. The unique honeycomb pattern of the Golgi complex is a distinct morphologic feature of FSH/LH-producing adenomas in women.[1] Because of the pleomorphism and variations in size that are typical of secretory granules, the classification of adenomas is more reliably based on immunohistochemical findings

TABLE 78.1 DIAGNOSIS

HORMONES INVOLVED IN END-ORGAN STIMULATION

■ HORMONE	■ FUNCTION
Thyrotropin-releasing hormone (TRH)	Stimulates the secretion of thyroid-stimulating hormone (TSH)
Corticotropin-releasing hormone (CRH)	Stimulates the release of adrenocorticotropic hormone (ACTH)
Growth hormone–releasing hormone (GHRH)	Stimulates the secretion of growth hormone (GH)
Gonadotropin-releasing hormone (GnRH)	Stimulates the secretion of luteinizing hormone (LH) and follicle-stimulating hormone (FSH)
Prolactin-inhibitory factor (dopamine)	Inhibits secretion of prolactin
Somatostatin	Inhibits the secretion of GH and, in part, TSH

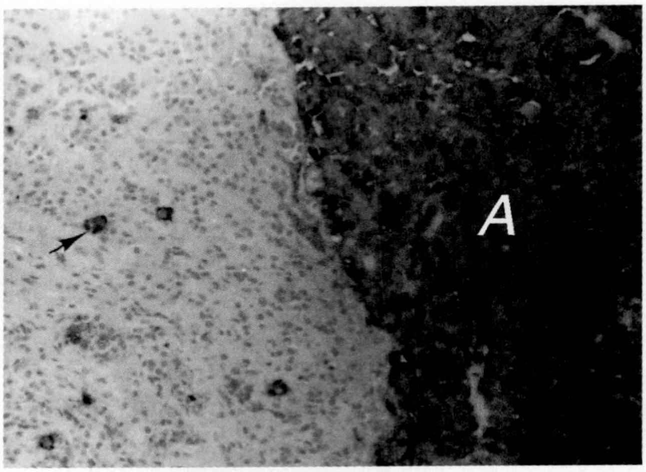

FIGURE 78.4. Immunohistochemical staining of an adrenocorticotropic hormone (ACTH)-producing adenoma (*A*) from a patient with Cushing disease. The normal pituitary tissue on the left contains a few ACTH-positive cells (*arrow*). Magnification ×250.

at the light microscopic and ultrastructural levels than on the ultrastructural morphologic appearance of secretory granules.

The immunohistochemical staining of pituitary adenomas with specific antibodies is a reliable method for classifying adenomas according to the hormones that are being produced (Fig. 78.4). Highly purified polyclonal and monoclonal antibodies against prolactin, growth hormone (GH), ACTH, FSH-β, LH-β, and TSH-β are available for immunohistochemical staining. Many studies with these antibodies have revealed that some pituitary tumors are composed of several cell types that produce various hormones.[1] Ultrastructural immunohistochemistry provides a further degree of refinement in the classification

FIGURE 78.3. **A:** Midpituitary coronal view of parasellar region. The sphenoid sinus is below and the cavernous sinuses are lateral. **B:** Midsagittal view of pituitary and surrounding bony structures. Note the approach for transsphenoidal surgery. Anterior is to the left.

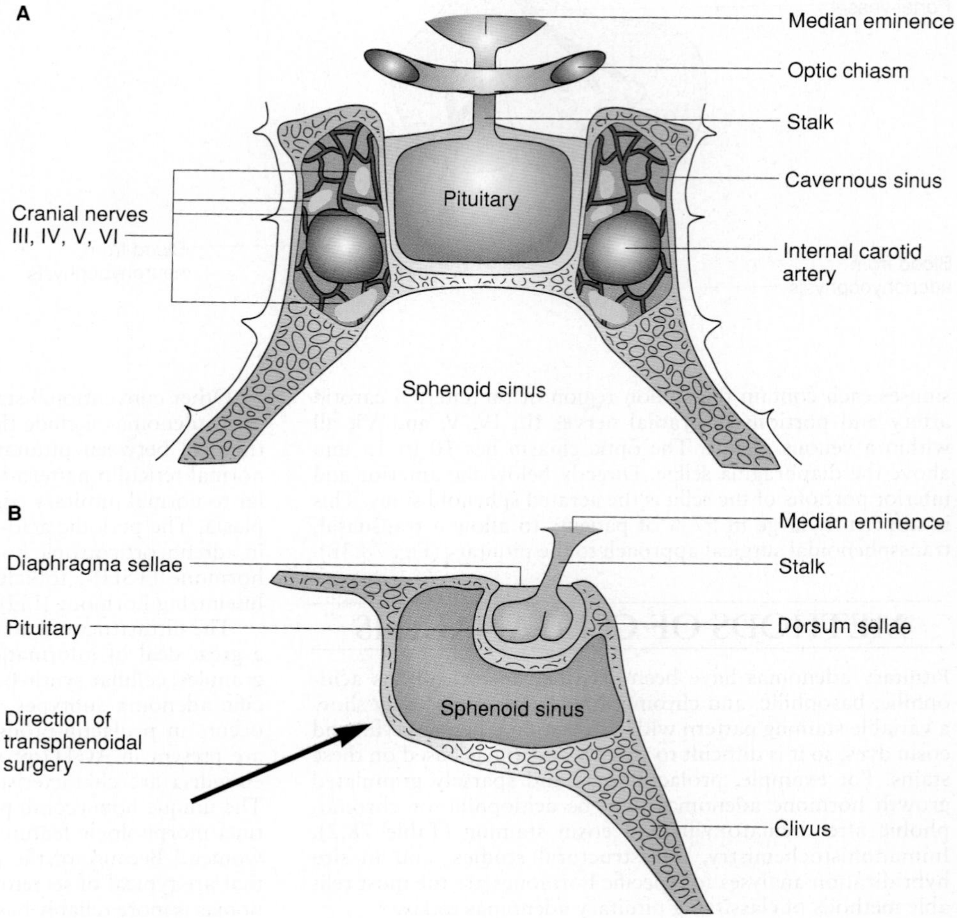

TABLE 78.2

FUNCTIONAL PITUITARY ADENOMAS: PATHOLOGIC FINDINGS

ADENOMA TYPE	INCIDENCE (%)	STAINING[a]	IMMUNOREACTIVITY	ULTRASTRUCTURE
PRL secreting				
Sparsely granulated	28	C	PRL	Few SG 150–500 nm Misplaced exocytosis
Densely granulated	1	A	PRL	SG 400–1,200 nm
GH secreting				
Sparsely granulated	5	C-A	GH	SG 300–600 nm Fibrous bodies
Densely granulated	5	A	GH	SG 100–250 nm
Mixed GH cell–PRL cell	5	A-C	GH, PRL	Variable pattern
Mixed GH cell–PRL cell	1	A	GH, PRL	SG 150–450 nm and 350–1,000 nm
ACTH secreting	10	B	ACTH	SG 250–700 nm Prominent type I microfilaments
Gonadotrope cell	7–10	C-B	FSH, LH	SG 50–150 nm Distinct female pattern of honeycomb, Golgi region
Thyrotrope cell	1	C-B	TSH	SG 50–250 nm

[a]Conventional hematoxylin and eosin staining: A, acidophil; B, basophil; C, chromophobe
ACTH, adrenocorticotropic hormone; FSH, follicle-stimulating hormone; GH, growth hormone; LH, luteinizing hormone; PRL, prolactin; SG, secretory granules; TSH, thyroid-stimulating hormone.

and study of adenomas, because the exact site of hormone storage in secretory granules and the subcellular sites of production and processing in the rough endoplasmic reticulum and Golgi regions can be visualized with this technique.

Some adenomas may not store specific hormones, so immunohistochemical staining may be weak or absent. Messenger ribonucleic acid (mRNA) is usually present in the cytoplasm of adenomas. The localization of mRNA for specific protein hormones is becoming more widely used in the study and classification of pituitary adenomas. In situ hybridization studies have shown that many GH-producing adenomas in patients with acromegaly also express prolactin mRNA.[2] Recent studies with microRNAs using polymerase chain reaction methods have demonstrated the importance of specific microRNA in pituitary tumor development.[3] In situ and Northern hybridization studies have contributed to the understanding of adenoma subtypes. Null cell adenomas, which constitute up to 15% of pituitary neoplasms, commonly express the mRNA for gonadotropic hormones.

IMAGING OF THE PITUITARY AND PARASELLAR REGION

Modern, computerized imaging technology now provides remarkably detailed multiplanar images of the pituitary and
4 parasellar structures. Magnetic resonance imaging (MRI) has evolved as the first choice for diagnostic imaging and is often the only test needed to make a therapeutic decision. With the intravenous infusion of a paramagnetic substance (e.g., gadolinium), MRI demonstrates intrasellar tumors as small as 5 mm and shows the growth pattern of larger tumors. It reveals the extent of suprasellar and sphenoid sinus extension, in addition to lateral extension into the cavernous sinuses (Fig. 78.5). Cysts and hemorrhages can be differentiated, as can blood flowing within an aneurysm.

Computed tomography (CT) also has a place in pituitary imaging and, if MRI is unavailable, may well suffice as the only mode of imaging. CT shows calcification better than MRI and, thus, is often helpful in imaging a craniopharyngioma. CT, even with intravenous contrast, cannot differentiate an aneurysm, so MRI or angiography must be performed if this is suspected.

Plain skull radiographs are not needed if the diagnosis has been reached by CT or MRI, but they remain a way to identify incidental lesions. A pituitary macroadenoma (>10 mm) causes enlargement of the sella turcica, which can easily be observed on a plain lateral skull radiograph. If this finding is noted on a radiograph performed for any reason (e.g., trauma), a more detailed study (e.g., MRI or CT) should be obtained.

Angiography is performed only if an aneurysm is suspected or if a lesion is so large that occlusion or compression of one or both internal carotid arteries is in question.

CLINICAL AND ENDOCRINE EVALUATION

General Clinical Signs and Symptoms

Patients with pituitary lesions may present with symptoms and signs related to a mass effect on the pituitary and its surrounding structures, hypersecretion of hormones by the lesion itself, or a combination of both. Tumors or other mass lesions are generally larger than 1 cm before they produce symptoms related to compression. As a lesion enlarges, it may cause a loss of pituitary function, usually manifested by a decrease in hormone secretion from the adenohypophysis. This may result in a loss of TSH and subsequent hypothyroidism. A decrease in ACTH results in low serum cortisol levels, and a decrease in

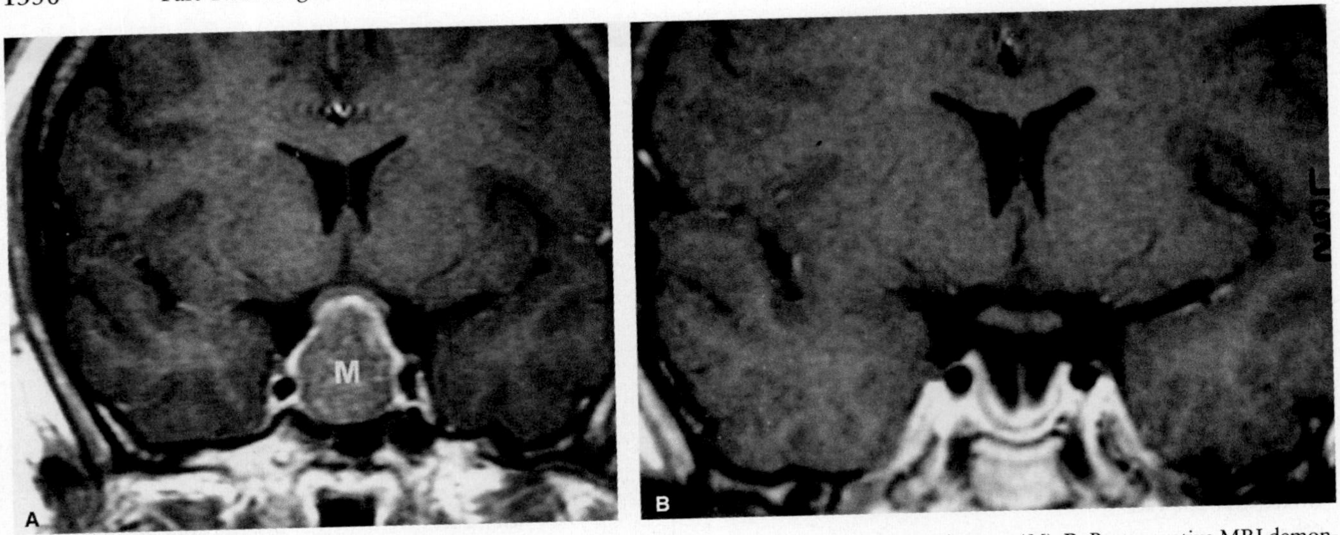

FIGURE 78.5. **A:** Midpituitary coronal magnetic resonance imaging (MRI) shows a pituitary macroadenoma (*M*). **B:** Postoperative MRI demonstrates gross total resection of tumor with cerebrospinal fluid in the sella.

LH and FSH causes amenorrhea in women and hypogonadism in men. A decline in GH is noted only in children with a loss of normal growth progress.

The one exception to this pattern is that generalized pituitary compression may cause a rise in prolactin levels because the secretion of prolactin-inhibitory factor (dopamine) from the hypothalamus or its delivery to the lactotropes may be compromised by the compression. Generalized compression from within the sella rarely results in a loss of ADH from the neurohypophysis and subsequent diabetes insipidus. Lesions that originate in the region of the pituitary stalk, however, often present with early signs of diabetes insipidus. Symptoms related to a loss of pituitary function are usually insidious in onset, except for those of sudden hemorrhage within the sella, or so-called pituitary apoplexy. Such hemorrhages are usually associated with a pituitary adenoma.

When mass lesions in the region of the pituitary enlarge, they may compress or invade nearby structures and cause symptoms unrelated to endocrine function. As tumors or other lesions grow laterally from the sella, they encounter the various contents of the cavernous sinuses. These include the third, fourth, first two divisions of the fifth, and sixth cranial nerves, in addition to the internal carotid artery. Compression of cranial nerves III, IV, or VI causes diplopia, and compression of cranial nerve V causes ipsilateral facial numbness. Invasion or constriction of the carotid artery may cause occlusion of this vessel, which in rare cases results in cerebral infarction. Upward growth of a tumor, which is relatively unrestricted, is much more common and often results in compression of the optic chiasm and loss of vision, typically a bitemporal hemianopsia. Extensive upward intracranial growth may compress the hypothalamus or the third ventricle and cause hydrocephalus. Rarely, intracranial extension results in cortical irritation and associated seizures. Downward growth of tumors into the sphenoid sinus is common but causes no clinical symptoms or signs.

The syndromes associated with hypersecretion of pituitary hormones include Cushing disease (ACTH), acromegaly (GH), hyperprolactinemia (prolactin), and Nelson syndrome (ACTH after adrenalectomy). Rare cases of TSH-secreting adenomas have been documented. Traditionally, pituitary adenomas have been divided into nonfunctioning and functioning tumors, but it has become clear through immunohistochemical studies that many nonfunctioning tumors are in fact endocrinologically active. Although secreted hormones may not cause clinical symptoms or signs, they may serve as a marker for the presence of a tumor before and after treatment.

General Endocrine Evaluation

The extent of the endocrine evaluation of a patient with a pituitary lesion depends on the urgency of the situation (e.g., impaired vision) and whether a hypersecretory state is suspected. If time permits, a careful evaluation of the endocrine status is warranted, including testing of pituitary reserve. Although this is most critical after treatment, it is ideal to obtain a complete pretreatment evaluation for comparison. A pituitary endocrine evaluation should include baseline values for prolactin, GH, insulinlike growth factor-1 (IGF-1), LH, FSH, testosterone, morning cortisol, ACTH, electrolytes, and glucose. Thyroid function tests, including TSH and free thyroxine (T_4), should be performed. Because baseline values may not reflect the ability of the pituitary to respond to stress, it is sometimes necessary to test the reserve capacity of the pituitary. The most efficient way to do this is to administer insulin to induce hypoglycemia. Provided the patient has no contraindication to transient hypoglycemia (i.e., ischemic heart disease, cerebrovascular disease, or seizure disorder), insulin is given in a dose of 0.10 to 0.15 IU/kg, such that the serum glucose falls below 40 mg/dL. In the patient with normal pituitary function, transient hypoglycemia causes a rise in cortisol to above 20 μg/dL and a rise in GH to above 10 μg/L. In patients with compromised ACTH or GH production, a response is not noted.

If urgent surgical decompression is indicated, the previously mentioned baseline values are obtained, and the patient is prepared for surgery with sufficient hydrocortisone to cover the possibility of inadequate cortisol response to stress. Careful postoperative evaluation is then carried out to determine if long-term replacement therapy is needed. If the patient receives postoperative radiation therapy, the status of the pituitary should be checked periodically during the following years because pituitary function may slowly decline after radiation exposure.

If diabetes insipidus is suspected, urine and serum osmolality and serum sodium should be assessed, and fluid intake and output should be carefully evaluated.

Cushing Disease

Although the diagnosis of hypercortisolism (Cushing syndrome) is often determined after physical examination by an astute physician, sometimes the physical manifestations are not obvious. Often, the precise cause of hypercortisolism is difficult to ascertain, even with detailed endocrine testing and imaging. The findings of Cushing syndrome often include central obesity, hypertension, hirsutism, fatigue, thin skin, easy bruising, striae, moonlike facies, dorsal fat pad, and depression or other mental changes. Less common abnormalities include headache, osteoporosis, diabetes mellitus, galactorrhea, and amenorrhea. Often, a patient presents without the classic cushingoid appearance and complains only of severe fatigue or depression.

The cause of hypercortisolism is an ACTH-secreting pituitary adenoma (Cushing disease) in up to 80% of cases; the remainder are caused by an adrenocortical tumor or an endocrine tumor that secretes ACTH or corticotropin-releasing hormone. Pituitary-dependent hypercortisolism is much more common in women (80%), and an ectopic cause is more common in men (80%). Thus, if an adult man presents with a rapid onset of Cushing syndrome, particularly with weight loss, hypertension, edema, or hypokalemia, an ectopic neoplasm must be strongly considered. Increased cortisol levels can occur in patients with primary depression, alcoholism, obesity, or drugs such as estrogens and phenytoin.

Because imaging studies are nondiagnostic in up to 60% of patients with pituitary disorders, the diagnosis is often based completely on the results of endocrine testing.[4] Multiple measurements of cortisol and ACTH to evaluate the diurnal pattern are important but often misleading. They are mainly of value when clearly elevated. Urinary free cortisol excretion over 24 hours is an extremely important measurement, but it may also be elevated in cases of depression or alcoholism. Undetectable plasma or urinary cortisol in a patient with clinically florid Cushing syndrome is unequivocal evidence of exogenous steroid therapy ("iatrogenic Cushing syndrome"). When the result of the overnight dexamethasone screening test (1 mg at 11:00 PM) is an 8:00 AM serum cortisol level below 1.8 μg/dL, hypercortisolism is rarely present. The recent development of the salivary cortisol assay permits spot measurement of the free circulating cortisol concentration. Elevated salivary cortisol at 11:00 PM appears to provide strong evidence in favor of endogenous hypercortisolism. The differential diagnosis starts with measurements of plasma cortisol and ACTH: undetectable ACTH in a patient with clinical Cushing syndrome and elevated cortisol establishes the diagnosis of a cortisol-producing adrenal tumor. Plasma ACTH above 200 pg/mL and certainly above 500 pg/mL strongly suggests an ectopic source of ACTH. Most patients with Cushing disease have ACTH within the normal or slightly elevated range. The overlap with the cases of ectopic ACTH secretion, however, is significant and poses the greatest diagnostic difficulty. Generally, the cortisol level of patients with a pituitary cause of hypercortisolism is not suppressed with the low-dose dexamethasone test (0.5 mg given every 6 hours for 2 days), but is with the higher dose (2 mg given every 6 hours for 2 days). The cortisol level of patients with adrenal or ectopic disorders classically is not suppressed with either dose. There are exceptions with both of these tests (Algorithm 78.1).

When metyrapone is given, a rise in serum 11-deoxycortisol (or urinary 17-hydroxycorticosteroids) follows in normal patients or those with Cushing disease, but not in those with adrenal tumors of ectopic ACTH secretion. A positive response, however, does not absolutely rule out an adrenal or ectopic source of hypercortisolism. The most specific differential diagnostic test to distinguish an ectopic ACTH source from Cushing disease is the measurement of ACTH levels in both inferior petrosal sinuses by transfemoral catheterization, along with simultaneous measurement of peripheral blood levels. This should be done prior to and 2 to 10 minutes after an intravenous bolus of corticotropin-releasing hormone. This provides convincing evidence for the existence of an ACTH-secreting pituitary tumor.[5] Inferior petrosal sinus sampling should be carried out in every case of suspected Cushing disease when MRI results are not *definitive* for a tumor. If the results of standard endocrine testing are conclusive for hypercortisolism and indicate a pituitary source and if MRI clearly shows a tumor, then invasive petrosal sinus sampling is not necessary before surgery.

Nelson Syndrome

In 1958, Nelson et al. identified a syndrome of progressive hyperpigmentation, visual field loss, and amenorrhea associated with elevated ACTH levels related to an ACTH-secreting pituitary adenoma in a patient who had undergone bilateral adrenalectomy for hypercortisolism.[6] This syndrome today generally represents a missed diagnosis of Cushing disease that has been treated with adrenalectomy. Often these tumors are aggressive or occasionally malignant.

Acromegaly

Like Cushing syndrome, acromegaly can be diagnosed clinically when patients present with advanced stages of the disease. The enlargement of the facial features and extremities may be subtle, and the presenting symptoms may be nonspecific headaches, fatigue, arthralgias, decreased libido, or amenorrhea. Patients often have hypertension, diabetes mellitus, and an early onset of atherosclerotic cardiovascular disease. It is critical that this disease be diagnosed and treated because the associated mortality rate is 50% above normal per decade beyond the age of 40 years. With rare exceptions, the cause of acromegaly is a GH-secreting pituitary adenoma. Like other functioning adenomas, the tumors may be either small or large and invasive. Patients with larger tumors may present with visual loss. Rarely, elevated GH levels are secondary to the production of GH-releasing hormone by an ectopic tumor.

The endocrine diagnosis now rests largely on serum levels of IGF-1, also known as *somatomedin C.* Even though 90% of patients with acromegaly have GH levels higher than 10 ng/mL, and although GH in a resting, nonstressed patient is normally below 5 ng/mL, both normal patients and patients with acromegaly may have levels below 5 ng/mL.[7] IGF-1, which mediates the effect of GH on peripheral tissues, should be measured in *all* circumstances in which acromegaly is suspected (Algorithm 78.2).

Hyperprolactinemia

Because 60% to 70% of prolactin-secreting pituitary adenomas are microadenomas, most patients present with endocrine symptoms rather than local mass effects. Hyperprolactinemia in women usually causes amenorrhea and often galactorrhea; thus, young women have a reason to seek medical evaluation while the tumor is still at an early stage. Because men do not have these early warning signs, they almost invariably present with macroadenomas associated with loss of libido, infertility, or loss of vision. The finding of amenorrhea or galactorrhea together with an elevated prolactin level does not always indicate the presence of a pituitary tumor. Table 78.3 lists other possible causes of hyperprolactinemia. Most important among these are renal failure, hypothyroidism, and the use of various drugs. Compression of the pituitary stalk by any type of mass lesion results in an increased secretion of prolactin. If the prolactin level is above 200 ng/mL, a pituitary tumor is almost invariably the cause, but microadenomas are often associated with prolactin levels below 100 ng/mL. The size of pituitary adenomas correlates with the degree of prolactin elevation; levels may reach thousands of nanograms per milliliter. No reliable provocative tests are available to differentiate prolactinomas from other causes of hyperprolactinemia, so the diagnosis relies on ruling out other causes and imaging the adenoma (Algorithm 78.3).

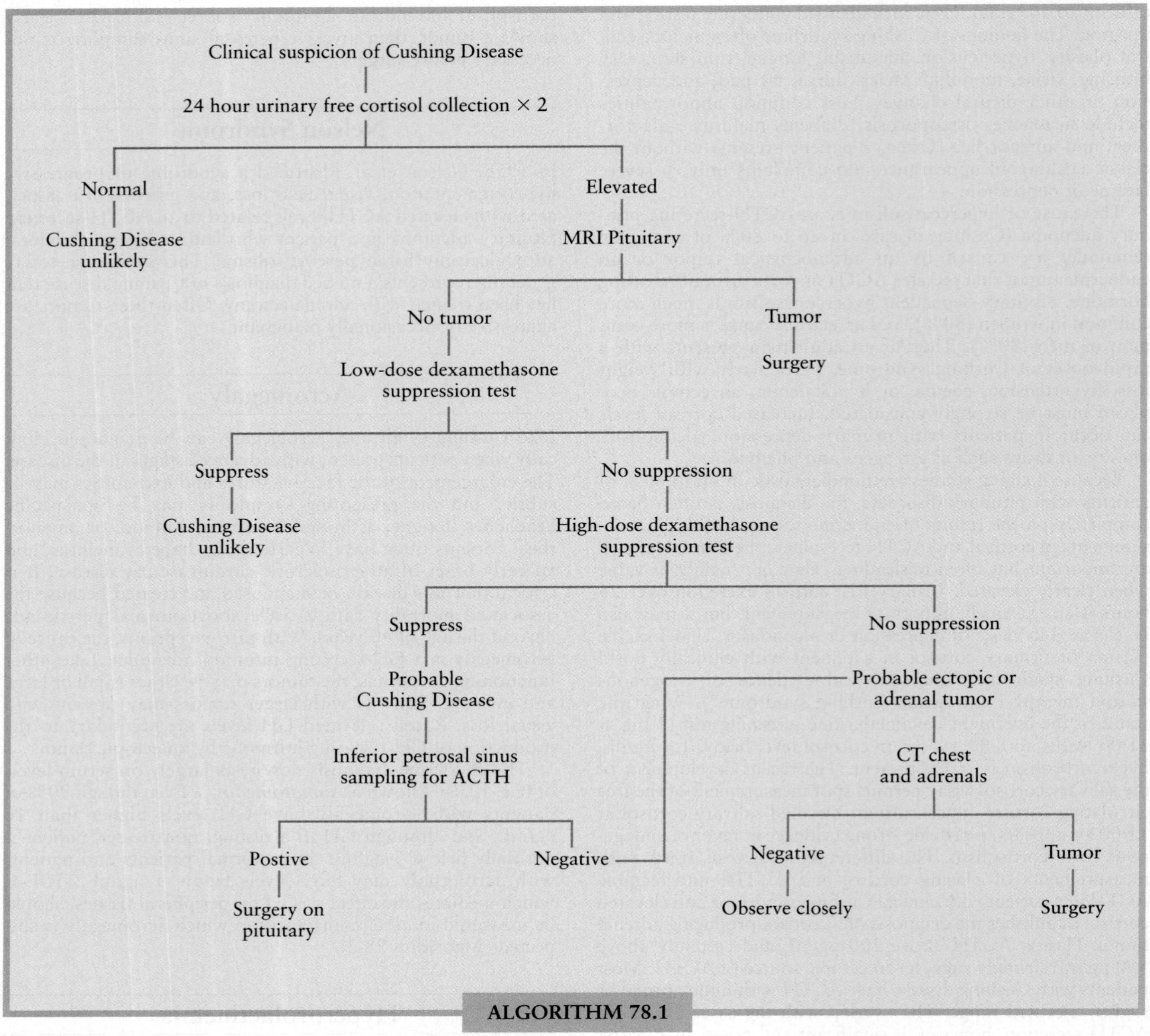

ALGORITHM 78.1. Workup and treatment of Cushing disease.

Currently, prolactin is measured by immunoradiometric (IRMA) or immunoluminometric (ILMA) assays, both employing two-site technology. These assays offer rapid and accurate measurement, but suffer from the pitfall of the so-called "hook effect." At very high prolactin concentrations the assay may report falsely normal or only slightly elevated values. Thus, in any patient having a large pituitary mass (usually >4 cm) that has the potential for being a pituitary adenoma, prolactin needs to be measured in a 1:1,000 diluted sample. Failure to do so may lead to an erroneous diagnosis of a nonfunctioning adenoma and inappropriate surgery instead of medical treatment with a dopamine agonist.

DIFFERENTIAL DIAGNOSIS

Table 78.4 lists the possible lesions that may occur within the sella or in the parasellar region. Pituitary adenomas head the list, because they are the most common lesion in this region and constitute 8% to 10% of all intracranial tumors. In the report of the Central Brain Tumor Registry of the United States (CBTRUS) for 2000–2004, pituitary tumors are the most common intracranial tumor in the 20- to 34-year age group and the second most common tumor in the 34- to 44-year age group.[8] They are 30% more common in the black population.

Occasionally, they are cystic and confused with other lesions. Craniopharyngiomas are the next most common tumor, and although more often suprasellar in location, they may be exclusively intrasellar. They are more common in children, but up to one third occur in adults. They are usually cystic and are calcified in 70% of children and 40% of adults. Meningiomas are also more commonly suprasellar and enhance strongly on CT and MRI. Germinomas, or so-called ectopic pinealomas, generally involve the pituitary stalk and often cause diabetes insipidus. If a patient presents with diabetes insipidus, the lesion is likely something other than a pituitary adenoma. Metastatic malignancies, commonly from lung and breast primary tumors, may be found in the pituitary, with

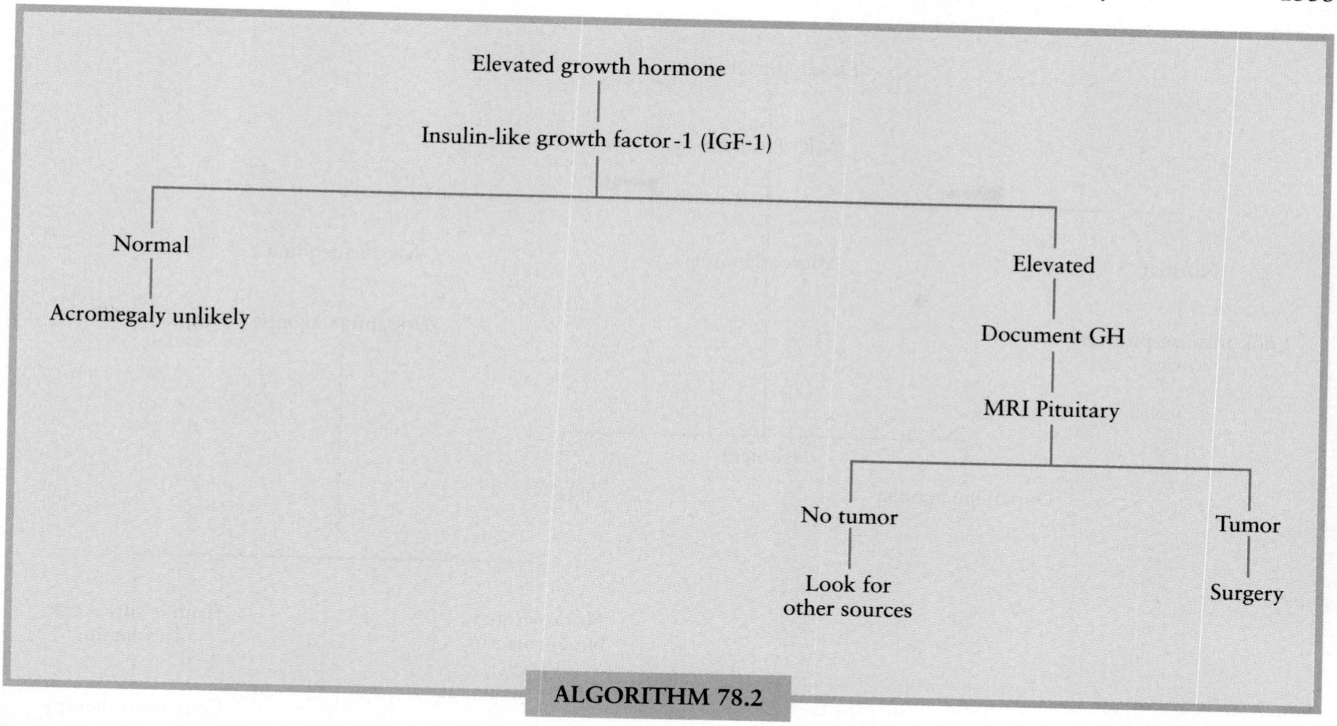

ALGORITHM 78.2. Workup and treatment of acromegaly.

TABLE 78.3 **ETIOLOGY**

CAUSES OF HYPERPROLACTINEMIA

Pituitary disease
Prolactinoma
Growth hormone–secreting adenoma
Pituitary stalk section (any concomitant structural lesion)
Empty sella syndrome
Hypothalamic disease
Tumors
Sarcoidosis
Radiation
Primary hypothyroidism (severe)
Chronic renal failure
Hepatic disease
Drugs
Phenothiazines
Metoclopramide
Tricyclic antidepressants
Estrogen
Opiates
Reserpine
Verapamil
Others
Pregnancy
Stress

70% residing in the posterior pituitary. Optic nerve gliomas and hypothalamic gliomas may occasionally be confused with pituitary adenomas, as can the rare granular cell tumor (choristoma). Dermoids and epidermoids may occur within the sella, and fifth nerve neuromas may compress the sella.

Rathke cysts are benign congenital remnants that develop within the sella and can cause a loss of pituitary function by local compression. These can be confused on imaging studies with cystic adenomas or craniopharyngiomas, and biopsy and surgical decompression is required if the cyst is enlarging or causing symptoms.

Inflammatory and granulomatous processes include bacterial abscesses within the sella and hypophysitis. Sarcoidosis may involve the pituitary or its stalk, as can the granulomas associated with Langerhans granulomatosis (histiocytosis X). Hamartomas may involve the pituitary stalk and hypothalamus and are impossible to differentiate from invasive gliomas on imaging studies.

Aneurysms, usually from the internal carotid arteries but occasionally from the basilar artery, may appear within the sella and must be ruled out preoperatively with MRI or angiography.

The empty-sella syndrome is generally just an anatomic variation that rarely causes symptoms. If a patient with headaches or head trauma undergoes skull radiography or CT, an enlarged sella may be found. With high-resolution MRI, usually the elongated stalk reaches the sellar floor, so that a cystic lesion can be ruled out. A contrast cisternogram may be used to visualize cerebrospinal fluid within the sella if necessary.

Pituitary apoplexy occurs symptomatically only rarely but may cause a profound and emergent situation. Infarction and hemorrhage, usually in a preexisting pituitary adenoma, cause a sudden intrasellar expansion with severe headache and a rapid loss of pituitary function, resulting in hypotension. A sudden loss of vision and other cranial nerve palsies may also develop. Treatment in severe cases involves the administration of steroids and surgical decompression of the sella. Smaller hemorrhages may be managed medically with hormone replacement and serial imaging.

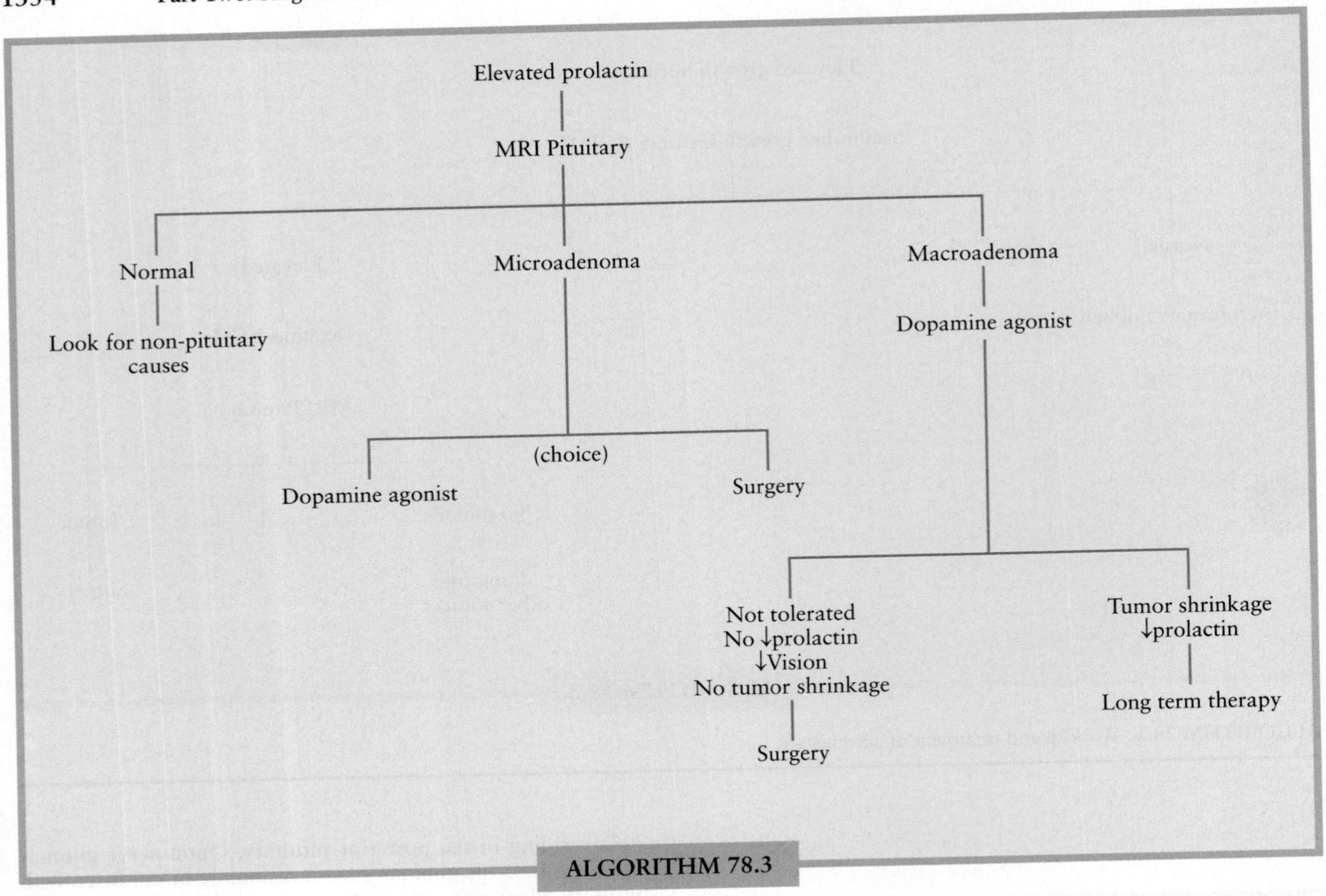

ALGORITHM 78.3. Diagnostic tests and treatment for hyperprolactinemia.

TREATMENT AND RESULTS

The treatment of primary pituitary adenomas is generally surgical, although there are certain exceptions. Even with modern imaging techniques, the unequivocal diagnosis of an adenoma is not reached until tissue is obtained. As shown in Table 78.4, the list of possible parasellar lesions is extensive. Along with surgical removal or decompression of pituitary adenomas, additional treatment in the form of radiation or medical therapy is often indicated. In addition to treatment directed at the primary lesion, it is critical to assess pituitary function thoroughly before and after treatment to decide whether hormone replacement is indicated.

More than 95% of pituitary adenomas can be approached by the transsphenoidal route, usually through a transnasal approach to the sphenoid sinus using the three-dimensional operating microscope. Some pituitary surgeons choose to use the two-dimensional endoscope during part or all of the surgery. Once the sphenoid sinus is entered, the anterior wall of the sella is carefully drilled away, and the dura surrounding the pituitary is identified. The dura is opened, and if a macroadenoma is present, the tumor is usually identified directly beneath the dura. If a microadenoma is present, the surgeon must carefully dissect around and often through the pituitary to identify the small tumor. In selected cases, it is helpful to use a frameless stereotactic system to define the anatomy of the sella and to localize a small tumor. This requires that either preoperative or intraoperative CT or MRI be entered into one of several commercially available frameless stereotactic systems.[9] This three-dimensional precise localizing system adds to the safety of the transsphenoidal approach and reduces the chance of injury to surrounding structures, such as the carotid arteries or the cavernous sinuses.

Contraindications to the transsphenoidal approach, and therefore indications for a craniotomy, include massive suprasellar extension, extensive lateral intracranial extension, and the rare dumbbell-shaped tumor with a tight construction at the level of the diaphragma sellae. If a craniotomy is necessary, a right subfrontal approach to the optic nerve and chiasm is required; the tumor is removed in a piecemeal fashion with use of the operating microscope and microinstruments.

NONFUNCTIONING ADENOMAS

Because patients with nonfunctioning adenomas usually present with the effects of a mass lesion, these tumors are rarely microadenomas. Although their location can be either exclusively intrasellar or extensively suprasellar, almost all of these tumors are currently approached via the transsphenoidal route.

6 The three goals of surgery for nonfunctioning macroadenomas are establishment of a diagnosis, decompression of surrounding structures, and gross total removal of tumor tissue, if possible. The first goal is usually accomplished easily, and although most tumors turn out to be adenomas, surprise findings are not unusual. Decompression is also usually accomplished readily because most tumors are soft and easily removed. Fewer than 5% of adenomas are so fibrous that decompression is difficult. Evidence of adequate decompression is the consistent finding that 75% to 80% of patients with visual field loss show recovery after transsphenoidal tumor removal.[10] The third goal, total tumor resection, is much more

TABLE 78.4 **DIAGNOSIS**

DIFFERENTIAL DIAGNOSIS OF INTRASELLAR AND PARASELLAR LESIONS

Tumors
Pituitary adenoma
Craniopharyngioma
Meningioma
Lymphoma
Germinoma
Chordoma
Granular cell tumor (choristoma)
Neuroma (arising from cranial nerve V)
Metastatic
Optic nerve glioma
Epidermoid
Dermoid
Infundibuloma
Hypothalamic glioma
Cysts
Rathke cleft cyst
Pituitary cyst
Inflammatory and granulomatous lesions
Bacterial abscess
Sarcoidosis
Eosinophilic granuloma (histiocytosis X)
Tuberculosis
Mycoses
Granulomatous hypophysitis
Aneurysm
Hamartoma
Empty sella syndrome
Pituitary apoplexy

difficult to accomplish with macroadenomas. Most macroadenomas (88% to 94%) invade at least the dura mater, and many grossly invade surrounding structures. Such invasion makes complete surgical resection impossible and, therefore, these patients need to be followed indefinitely with high-quality imaging to monitor tumor progression or recurrence. Whereas it was once common practice to administer postoperative radiation to all macroadenomas, most neurosurgeons are now content to watch for progression with high-resolution imaging and reserve local radiation for progression or recurrence.[11] Currently, no medical treatment is available for nonfunctional adenomas.

CUSHING DISEASE

Once it has been established that the cause of a patient's hypercortisolism is a pituitary lesion, the treatment of choice is transsphenoidal exploration of the pituitary. Only 40% of such patients have positive results on imaging studies and, therefore, careful and systematic exploration of the sellar contents by an experienced pituitary surgeon is required in many cases.[4] Microadenomas secreting ACTH may be very small and are often located deep within the gland itself. If a tumor is not evident when the dura is opened and all surfaces of the pituitary are examined, then incisions must be made into the gland and an internal exploration carried out. These microadenomas are usually located in one of the lateral aspects of the pituitary gland, and the initial choice of which side to explore can be guided by lateralization in the preoperative petrosal sinus sampling for ACTH levels. If no tumor is identified, then a decision must be made regarding whether to resect all or a portion of the gland. If the endocrine evidence is convincing for a pituitary origin and the patient has no desire to have children, then total hypophysectomy is warranted. If petrosal sinus sampling clearly indicates laterality of the ACTH secretion, then an appropriate hemiresection of the gland is carried out. Macroadenomas are treated with maximal tumor resection, but endocrine remission is, of course, more difficult to accomplish in these situations. Obviously, patients with adrenal or ectopic lesions are treated by resection of tumors in these locations. Microadenomas are the source of ACTH secretion in about 75% of patients.[4,12,13] The postoperative remission rate in these patients is 88% to 96%, and the long-term recurrence rate appears to be no more than 5%. Therefore, selective microsurgical tumor resection in patients with microadenomas is clearly the current treatment of choice. Postoperative plasma cortisol concentrations below 1 μg/dL are a very good predictor of surgical cure, although even in these cases recurrence of Cushing disease occurs in up to 25% of patients within 5 years.[14] If cortisol levels are not in this subnormal range and just in the normal range, a long-term cure is unlikely and the chance of recurrence goes up.

Some 10% to 20% of patients who undergo exploration have macroadenomas, and postoperative remission rates in these patients have been reported to be from 33% to 61%.[4,12,13,15,16] Most of them require postoperative radiation therapy, which leads to remission in some of the surgical failures. Those whose tumors fail to remit after both surgery and radiation require either a surgical adrenalectomy or medical suppression of adrenal function. In a small percentage of patients who have undergone adrenalectomy, the pituitary tumors continue to grow and secrete ACTH (Nelson syndrome).

ACROMEGALY

Like Cushing disease, acromegaly is a condition that ultimately threatens life. For this reason, it must be treated aggressively, even at the expense of normal pituitary function. During the past two decades, a variety of medical, surgical, and radiation therapies have evolved that have proved effective in lowering GH levels. No single treatment is uniformly effective, and 7 often a combination of treatments is necessary. The goals of treatment are to lower the circulating GH and IGF-1 levels to a normal range and to reduce the size of the mass lesion that is causing compression-related symptoms.

Only 20% to 34% of GH-secreting tumors are microadenomas, however, so that microsurgical tumor resection is less effective than in Cushing disease. When a microadenoma is selectively removed transsphenoidally, endocrine remission may be expected in 80% to 88% of cases. When a macroadenoma is resected, immediate postoperative remission is reported in 30% to 68% of cases.[17] Remission rates are inversely related to preoperative GH levels and the size and invasiveness of tumors.

Radiation therapy has proved moderately effective in conjunction with partial surgical resection. Proton beam heavy-particle therapy was reported in 510 patients, 428 of whom had been observed for 1 to 20 years.[18] Analysis of these patients revealed a progressive fall in GH levels beginning immediately after treatment and continuing for up to 20 years. After 2 years, 47.5% of patients had GH levels below 10 ng/mL; at 4, 10, and 20 years, the rates were 65%, 87.5%, and 97.5%, respectively. A GH level below 5 ng/mL is achieved in

75% of patients at 10 years and 92.5% of patients at 20 years. Conventional radiation therapy provides comparable results (10-year posttreatment levels below 10 ng/mL in 81% and below 5 ng/mL in 69%). A recent review of our own patients, however, showed that after an average follow-up of 6.8 years, normalization of IGF-1 levels was attained in only 2 of 36 patients who received radiation (45 to 50 Gy) after surgical failure.[19] The remaining 34 patients had persistently elevated IGF-1 levels (219 ± 26% of upper normal limit) despite plasma GH levels averaging 4.6 ± 1.1 μg/L. Normalization of IGF-1 is usually achieved in up to 80% of patients within 5 years after conventional radiation, but the long delay requires medical therapy.[20] A report by Landolt et al. suggests that stereotactic radiosurgery may be more effective than fractionated radiotherapy for persistent acromegaly after failed surgical treatment, but there is currently no conclusive evidence that focused radiosurgery is more effective than fractionated radiotherapy.[21]

Bromocriptine, a dopamine-receptor agonist, lowered GH levels in 71% of 126 patients.[22] GH levels below 10 ng/mL, however, were achieved in only 14% of patients in this study. Bromocriptine does not appear to be an effective primary treatment for acromegaly, but may help to control GH and IGF-1 levels as an adjuvant therapy. Cabergoline offers an advantage of longer action and lower incidence of side effects, but only rarely normalizes IGF-1 on its own.

Somatostatin analogues, octreotide (Sandostatin LAR), and lanreotide (Somatuline Depot) have been demonstrated to reduce GH and IGF-1 levels significantly in most patients and may provide tumor shrinkage, but GH levels rise again after cessation of the drug. A GH-receptor blocker, pegvisomant, has proved useful in lowering IGF-1 levels in patients whose disease cannot be controlled by surgery or somatostatin analogues. Because this drug works peripherally, there is still concern that the pituitary tumor may grow and enlarge during this treatment, although recent data suggest that this may not be the case.

Given the variety of treatment modalities, a rational therapeutic approach is to resect tumors surgically when possible and to provide medical and radiation therapy to those patients in whom a remission cannot be achieved. The recurrence rate of GH-secreting tumors appears to be only 4% after successful surgery and less than 1% after radiation.[21]

PROLACTINOMAS

Prolactin-secreting adenomas are the most common functioning pituitary tumors but remain somewhat controversial with regard to treatment. The controversy exists because, unlike ACTH- or GH-secreting adenomas, prolactinomas can be treated medically with dopamine agonists, with excellent results. The treatment options include medical therapy, usually with a dopamine agonist; transsphenoidal surgical resection; radiation therapy; or, in some cases, no treatment. Because treatment considerations depend on tumor size, the treatments are discussed on that basis.

Macroadenomas

The goal in treating a patient with a large, prolactin-secreting adenoma is to decompress the optic pathways if they are involved and to reduce the prolactin levels to normal concentrations. Surgery is effective in improving vision in 80% of cases, but vision also usually improves in patients treated with dopamine agonists. The success of surgery in reducing prolactin levels to normal has generally been disappointing. The uniform finding of various investigators has been that the likelihood of surgical normalization of prolactin levels is greatly reduced if the initial concentration is above 200 ng/mL or if the macroadenoma is larger than 10 mm.

The administration of dopamine agonists to patients with macroadenomas reduces prolactin levels significantly in almost all instances, and reductions to normal ranges have been reported in more than 46%.[23] In 90% of patients, the size of the tumor is decreased to some degree and, in many, the reduction is dramatic. With rare exceptions, however, the tumor returns to its original size once bromocriptine or cabergoline is stopped. It is recognized that up to 25% of patients with macroadenomas experience an increase in tumor size during pregnancy, whereas this is true in fewer than 1% of patients with microadenomas.[23]

In most instances patients with macroprolactinomas are treated initially with a dopamine agonist and surgery is reserved for the rare situation in which the patient is not responsive to this medication. Occasionally, patients with prolactinomas present with significant hemorrhage within the tumor and require surgical debulking of the hemorrhage and surrounding tumor.

Microadenomas

Primary medical treatment with a dopamine agonist is safe and effective and is currently the treatment of choice for most patients with a prolactin-secreting microadenoma. As in macroadenomas, long-term continued therapy is indicated because prolactin levels rapidly rise with cessation of dopamine agonists in most patients. Pregnancy is of less risk to the patient with a microadenoma because tumor expansion and visual loss are rare.

The surgical treatment of prolactin-secreting microadenomas results in postoperative remission in a much higher percentage of patients. Two large series reported remission in 77%[24] and 72%[25] of patients. In the latter report, 88% of patients with preoperative prolactin levels below 100 ng/mL were in remission, as opposed to only 50% in those who had preoperative prolactin levels above 100 ng/mL. The incidence of new postoperative hypogonadism was only 1%. The recurrence rate in patients initially in remission after microsurgical tumor removal, however, has been disappointing compared with the rates after removal of other functioning tumors. Recurrences have uniformly been found to be higher in patients with postoperative prolactin levels in the upper end of the normal range. Recurrence rates of 17% to 50% during 5 years have been reported. Radiation therapy does not play a role in the treatment of microadenomas unless they recur in an aggressive manner.

References

1. Kovacs K, Horvath E. Tumors of the pituitary gland. In: Hartmann WH, ed. *Atlas of Tumor Pathology*, Series 2, fascicle 21. Washington, DC: Armed Forces Institute of Pathology; 1986:192.
2. Lloyd RV, Cano M, Chandler WF, et al. Human growth hormone- and prolactin-secreting pituitary adenomas analyzed by in situ hybridization. *Am J Pathol* 1989;134:605.
3. Zatelli MC, degli Uberti EC. MicroRNAs and possible role in pituitary adenoma. *Semin Reprod Med* 2008:26;453–460.
4. Chandler WF, Schteingart DE, Lloyd RV, et al. Surgical treatment of Cushing's disease. *J Neurosurg* 1987;66:204.
5. Oldfield EH, Chrousos GP, Schulte HM, et al. Preoperative lateralization of ACTH-secreting pituitary microadenomas by bilateral and simultaneous inferior petrosal venous sinus sampling. *N Engl J Med* 1985;312: 100–103.
6. Nelson DH, Meakin JW, Dealy JB, et al. ACTH-producing tumor of the pituitary gland. *N Engl J Med* 1958;259:161.
7. Dimaraki EV, Jaffe CA, DeMott-Friberg R, et al. Acromegaly with apparently normal GH secretion: implications for diagnosis and follow-up. *J Clin Endocrinol Metab* 2002;87:3537–3542.
8. Central Brain Tumor Registry of the United States. *Statistical report: primary brain tumors in the United States, 2000–2004*. Hinsdale, IL: Central Brain Tumor Registry of the United States; 2008.

9. Fox WC, Wawrzyniak S, Chandler WF. Intraoperative acquisition of three-dimensional imaging for frameless stereotactic guidance during transsphenoidal pituitary surgery using the Arcadis Orbic System. *J Neurosurg* 2008;108:746–750.
10. Ebersold MJ, Quast LM, Laws ER, et al. Long-term results in transsphenoidal removal of nonfunctioning pituitary adenomas. *J Neurosurg* 1986; 64:713.
11. Park P, Chandler WF, Barkan AL, et al. The role of radiation therapy after surgical resection of nonfunctional pituitary macroadenomas. *Neurosurgery* 2004;55:100–107.
12. Boggan JE, Tyrrell JB, Wilson CB. Transsphenoidal microsurgical management of Cushing's disease. *J Neurosurg* 1983;59:195.
13. Hardy J. Cushing's disease: 50 years later. *Can J Neurol Sci* 1982;9:375.
14. Patil CG, Prevedello DM, Lad SP, et al. Late recurrences of Cushing's disease after initial successful transsphenoidal surgery. *J Clin Endocrinol Metab* 2008;93:358–362.
15. Kuwayama A, Kageyama N. Current management of Cushing's disease: part II. *Contemp Neurosurg* 1985;7:1.
16. Salassa RM, Laws ER, Carpenter PC, et al. Cushing's disease: 50 years later. *Trans Am Clin Climatol Assoc* 1982;94:122.
17. Tindall GT, Tindall SC. Transsphenoidal surgery for acromegaly: long-term results in 50 patients. In: Black PM, Zervas NT, Ridgeway EC, et al., eds. *Secretory Tumors of the Pituitary Gland.* New York: Raven Press; 1984:175.
18. Kliman B, Kjellberg RN, Swisher B, et al. Proton beam therapy of acromegaly: a 20-year experience. In: Black PM, Zervas NT, Ridgeway EC, et al., eds. *Secretory Tumors of the Pituitary Gland.* New York: Raven Press; 1984:191.
19. Barkan AL, Halasz I, Dornfeld KJ, et al. Pituitary irradiation is ineffective in normalizing plasma insulin-like growth factor I in patients with acromegaly. *J Clin Endocrinol Metab* 1997;82:3187–3191.
20. Barrande G, Pittino-Lungo M, Coste J, et al. Hormonal and metabolic effects of radiotherapy in acromegaly: long-term results in 128 patients followed in a single center. *J Clin Endocrinol Metab* 2000;85:3779–3785.
21. Landolt AM, Haller D, Lomas N, et al. Stereotactic radiosurgery for recurrent surgically treated acromegaly: comparison with fractionated radiotherapy. *J Neurosurg* 1998;88:1002–1008.
22. Besser GM, Wass JAH. The medical management of acromegaly. In: Black PM, Zervas NT, Ridgeway EC, et al., eds. *Secretory Tumors of the Pituitary Gland.* New York: Raven Press; 1984:155.
23. Thorner MO, Evans WS, Vance ML. Medical management of prolactinomas: I. In: Black PM, Servas NT, Ridgeway EC, et al., eds. *Secretory Tumors of the Pituitary Gland.* New York: Raven Press; 1984:53.
24. Hardy J. Transsphenoidal microsurgery of prolactinomas. In: Black PM, Zervas NT, Ridgeway EC, et al., eds. *Secretory Tumors of the Pituitary Gland.* New York: Raven Press; 1984:73.
25. Randall RV, Laws ER, Abboud CF, et al. Transsphenoidal microsurgical treatment of prolactin-producing pituitary adenomas. *Mayo Clin Proc* 1983;58:108.

CHAPTER 79 ■ LUNG NEOPLASMS

ANDREW C. CHANG AND JULES LIN

KEY POINTS

1. Lung cancer remains the leading cause of cancer-related death in the United States.
2. Resection remains the mainstay in the treatment of lung cancer, yet only about 20% of all patients diagnosed with lung cancer are considered resectable (stages I to IIIA). Video-assisted thoracoscopic surgery/robotic approaches have changed the landscape for operation, although the principles of oncologic resection remain unchanged.
3. Advances in molecular biology including genomic and proteomic techniques constitute promising methodologies for the diagnosis and patient-tailored management of non-small cell lung cancer (NSCLC), but to date these strategies have not been validated for broad clinical implementation.
4. Updated staging criteria for NSCLC are available that stratify patient survival based on outcomes data collected worldwide.
5. Common sites of distant metastases are bone, liver, bone marrow, and the central nervous system; therefore, the metastatic evaluation includes a bone scan and computed tomogram of the chest, abdomen, and brain.
6. Taken as a whole, neoadjuvant therapy trials have demonstrated the feasibility of induction chemotherapy and radiation followed by resection for the treatment of selected stage IIIA NSCLC. Most studies show improved rates of resectability and survival in comparison with the historical experience for surgical resection or radiation alone.
7. In addition to new chemotherapeutic agents, new radiation techniques, such as hyperfractionated or accelerated schedules, also merit further exploration in neoadjuvant trials with concurrent chemotherapy.
8. Generally, a solitary lesion is more likely to be a metastasis if the primary tumor was a sarcoma or a melanoma. If the primary tumor originated in the head, neck, or breast, it is more likely to be a new primary lung cancer.

Although population estimates of both the incidence and mortality of lung cancer have begun to decline, lung cancer was second only to heart disease among all causes of mortality reported for 2005. Lung cancer is second in cancer prevalence only to prostate cancer among men and breast cancer among
1 women. With 215,020 new cases and 161,840 deaths projected for 2008, lung cancer remains the leading cause of cancer-related death in both sexes in the United States. Although annual mortality rates due to lung cancer are decreasing among men, lung cancer–related deaths among women continued to increase by 0.2% per year from 1995 to 2004.[1] There is also significant regional variation in both lung cancer incidence and mortality. Among men, lung cancer mortality has decreased from 1996 through 2005 in over 80% of the 50 states and the District of Columbia, whereas among women over the same period, mortality decreased in only three states (California, New Jersey, and Texas) and has increased in 13 other states, primarily in the Midwest and South.[2]

The best predictor of survival for patients with lung
2 cancer is still tumor stage. Resection remains the mainstay in the treatment of lung cancer, yet only approximately 20% of all patients diagnosed with lung cancer are considered resectable (stages I to IIIA). Even among patients who have undergone complete curative resection for early-stage disease, as determined using pathologic tumor–node–metastasis (TNM) criteria, a substantial number will have recurrence of their cancer.[3]

Clinical trials continue to demonstrate that adjuvant chemotherapy can improve survival over surgery alone for early-stage lung cancer,[4–6] but it remains to be seen whether earlier tumor detection by modalities such as screening chest computed tomography (CT) will impact overall survival.[7,8] In addition, as understanding of the molecular changes occurring in lung cancer evolves, new strategies that allow for early detection and classification of lung cancer will provide valuable information for the treatment of patients.

HISTORY

Ferdinand Sauerbruch, whose interests included the physiology of pneumothorax and who is considered one of the pioneers of thoracic surgery, reported the first successful lobectomy for lung carcinoma in 1920. At that time, it was believed that only total pneumonectomy would provide a cure for lung cancer. Although this was neither the first pulmonary resection nor pneumonectomy, Dr. Evarts A. Graham performed the first successful single-stage pneumonectomy for a left upper lobe bronchogenic carcinoma in 1933,[9] establishing the modern era of thoracic surgery for lung cancer. Ultimately, Dr. Graham succumbed to lung cancer in 1957 and was outlived by his patient, Dr. James L. Gilmore, who had continued to smoke.[10]

EPIDEMIOLOGY

Recently, population studies have demonstrated a continued decline in lung cancer incidence among men (83.5 cases per 100,000) and stabilization of disease incidence among women (49.2 per 100,000) as of 2001. African American men continue to have the greatest incidence of lung cancer, in excess of nearly 50% (124.5 per 100,000) over the cases reported for all men.[11] The decline in incidence as well as mortality may be due in part to public health efforts to promote smoking cessation.[12] In a follow-up to the Seven Countries Study of smoking-related mortality, follow-up analysis of the initial cohorts studied from Europe, the United States, and Japan confirmed that cigarette smoking increased the risk for death due to lung cancer with a hazard ratio of 4.2 per pack of cigarettes smoked. Furthermore, the death rates due to lung cancer decreased to that of never-smokers after 10 years of smoking cessation.[13] Exposure to environmental "second-hand" cigarette smoke can also contribute to an increased risk of lung cancer.[14] The European Prospective Investigation into Cancer and Nutrition (EPIC), a recent nested case-control study of a cohort of 123,479 EPIC enrollees, demonstrated that former smokers and subjects with environmental smoke exposure were at greater risk for developing lung cancer over a median follow-up period of 7 years.[15]

PATHOLOGIC CLASSIFICATION

Uniform classification of lung cancer is important both to provide consistent treatment for patients and to allow standardization in reports of epidemiologic, clinical, and basic scientific studies. Currently, the classification is largely histologic and is based on light microscopy findings determined from specimens obtained by resection or needle biopsy, permitting its wide application by surgical pathology laboratories where more advanced techniques might not be readily available. Nevertheless, immunohistochemical and electron microscopy analyses are important, particularly in the diagnosis of neuroendocrine tumors or in distinguishing between primary bronchogenic adenocarcinoma and metastatic lesions. The most recent revision of the World Health Organization (WHO) classification (Table 79.1) was published in 2004[16] but is largely unchanged from the previous revision in 1999.[17] Guidelines for defining preinvasive lesions such as squamous dysplasia and carcinoma in situ are provided. Recognition and definition of the heterogeneity among adenocarcinomas is reflected in the subclassification of this group, including more restrictive definitions for bronchioloalveolar carcinoma (BAC). Definitions for the spectrum of neuroendocrine tumors, ranging from typical and atypical carcinoid to small cell lung cancer (SCLC) and large cell neuroendocrine carcinomas, are provided.

TABLE 79.1 **CLASSIFICATION**

WORLD HEALTH ORGANIZATION HISTOLOGIC CLASSIFICATION OF LUNG TUMORS

1. Squamous cell carcinoma	
Variants:	1.1 Papillary
	1.2 Clear cell
	1.3 Small cell
	1.4 Basaloid
2. Small cell carcinoma	
Variant:	2.1 Combined small cell carcinoma
3. Adenocarcinoma	
3.1 Acinar adenocarcinoma	
3.2 Papillary adenocarcinoma	
3.3 Bronchioloalveolar carcinoma	
3.4 Solid adenocarcinoma with mucin	
3.5 Adenocarcinoma with mixed subtypes	
Variants: Fetal, mucinous ("colloid"), mucinous cystadenocarcinoma, signet ring, clear cell	
4. Large cell carcinoma	
Variants:	4.1 Large cell neuroendocrine carcinoma
	4.2 Others
5. Adenosquamous carcinoma	
6. Carcinoma with pleomorphic, sarcomatoid, or sarcomatous elements	
7. Carcinoid	
7.1 Typical	
7.2 Atypical	
8. Carcinoma of salivary gland type	
8.1 Mucoepidermoid carcinoma	
8.2 Adenoid cystic carcinoma	
8.3 Epithelial-myoepithelial	
9. Unclassified	

Adapted from *World Health Organization Classification of Tumors, Pathology and Genetics of Tumours of the Lung, Pleura, Thymus and Heart*. Lyon, France: IARC Press; 2004.

TUMOR BIOLOGY

Genetic alterations in several regulatory pathways including apoptosis, the cell cycle, and mitogenic signaling have been identified in tumors of patients with non–small cell lung cancer (NSCLC). Chromosomal loss of heterozygosity (LOH) or allelic gain appears to occur more frequently among patients with adenocarcinoma and history of tobacco exposure than among patients without any smoking history. Mutations among the Ras oncogenes, particularly K-ras, are characterized by the accumulation of DNA adducts within these genes, predominantly among patients with a history of tobacco use.[18] This has been attributed to the exposure to tobacco carcinogens such as benzo[a] pyrene (BaP); its activated form, benzo[a]pyrene diol epoxide (BPDE); and N-nitrosamines. These genes encode guanosine triphosphate (GTP)-binding proteins that participate in cellular signal transduction; their mutation results in constant Ras activation. Another family of oncogenes, Myc, encoding several transcription factors, is activated by gene amplification, primarily in SCLC.[18]

The tumor-suppressor gene p53 is the most frequently mutated gene in human cancer. Among patients with a history of tobacco use, mutations within p53 were identified in over 50% of patients with NSCLC, particularly squamous cell carcinoma (SCC) and non-BAC adenocarcinoma.[19,20] Among patients with stage I tumors, those with mutations, particularly truncating, structural, or those that abolished DNA contact, demonstrated significantly worse actuarial survival in comparison with patients who had wild-type p53. In contrast, those patients with missense mutations did not demonstrate significantly different survival than those with wild-type p53. In patients with more-advanced-stage tumors, mutations in p53 did not identify patients at risk for worse outcomes, suggesting that the effects of p53 mutation may be diluted by the accumulation of mutations at loci important in the later stages of tumorigenesis.[19] Interestingly, investigators have also identified p53 protein expression, determined by immunohistochemical analysis, as a predictor of poor outcome in patients with stage I NSCLC.[21] Furthermore, p53 expression is also associated with tumors more likely to demonstrate distant metastases.[22] Although mutational analyses were not reported in these immunohistochemical studies, these findings may be concordant, since it is possible that p53 mutations may result in greater steady-state levels of p53 protein, allowing for increased detection by immunohistochemistry.[23]

Epigenetic mechanisms of gene regulation also appear to participate in tumorigenesis of lung cancer. In particular, gene promoter inactivation by hypermethylation may be an important mechanism in the inactivation of tumor-suppressor genes such as $p16^{INK4a}$ (p16), an inhibitory regulator in the cyclin D–retinoblastoma cell cycle pathway. In patients with premalignant lesions such as squamous dysplasia and carcinoma in situ, both allelic loss and hypermethylation of p16 have been identified, with associated decreases in p16 protein expression,[24] suggesting that loss of p16 may be an important early event in NSCLC tumorigenesis.[25]

3 Investigators have attempted to identify genome-wide molecular events occurring in lung cancer and to relate these changes to tumor classification, patient prognosis, or even response to therapy. Microarray analyses, encompassing a multitude of methodologic approaches, have the potential to provide the investigator with an abundance of data describing changes in gene or protein expression.[26] Several groups have demonstrated that large-scale gene expression studies can identify patterns of expression distinguishing squamous cell carcinoma, adenocarcinoma, and small cell lung cancer.[27,28] Furthermore, within groups of patients with bronchogenic adenocarcinoma, tumor heterogeneity can be identified, distinguishing not only tumor grade and differentiation but also patient outcomes.[28–31] These studies, although largely retrospective, demonstrate the potential for gene and protein expression "profiles" to be utilized as diagnostic and prognostic tools in the treatment of lung cancer. Before these techniques can be broadly applied, even in prospective clinical trials, issues of reproducibility between institutions and across analytic platforms must be addressed.[32] Distinguishing those genes that appear to be involved causally in lung cancer tumorigenesis from those genes that are regulated secondarily is critical for our understanding of this disease and for the identification of potential targets for therapeutic intervention.

Historically, clinical trials demonstrated that only 10% to 19% of patients with chemotherapy-refractory advanced NSCLC responded to treatment with the tyrosine kinase inhibitor gefitinib. Furthermore, the addition of gefitinib to standard chemotherapy yielded no demonstrable benefit.[33] As proof of concept for targeted molecular therapy, two groups demonstrated that tumors obtained from patients who exhibited rapid and dramatic tumor response to gefitinib were more likely to have mutations in the epidermal growth factor receptor (EGFR).[33,34] In contrast, gefitinib-insensitive tumors did not contain similar mutations. Supporting this finding, retrospective analyses of patients with NSCLC indicated that patients with adenocarcinoma of bronchioloalveolar subtype and "never-smokers," defined as patients with a less than 100-cigarette lifetime smoking history, were more likely to respond to treatment with gefitinib,[35] and mutational analysis of these gefitinib-sensitive tumors contained similar somatic mutations.[36] These data represent an exciting potential application of gene expression studies for use in determining patient prognosis and in the clinical management of lung cancer in preventing over- or undertreatment of patients.

NON–SMALL CELL LUNG CANCER

4 The diagnosis of lung cancer should be directed by the presumed stage of disease at patient presentation. Accurate and reproducible TNM staging of lung cancer allows clinicians to provide consistent treatment of lung cancer and provides the basis for uniform reporting of clinical research across institutions and study groups. In 1997, revisions in the International System for Staging Lung Cancer (Table 79.2) were adopted by the American Joint Committee on Cancer (AJCC) and the Union Internationale Contre le Cancer (UICC), based on 5,319 cases of lung cancer.[3] Changes for the seventh edition of the TNM classification of malignant tumours for NSCLC staging[37] were proposed by the International Association for the Study of Lung Cancer (IASLC). The revisions arise from evaluation of 67,725 cases of NSCLC with broad geographic diversity including subjects from Asia, Australia, Europe, and North America.[37,38] The revisions address both T[39] and M[40] designations (Table 79.3), with no changes suggested for the current nodal classification schema (Table 79.4).[41] Stratification of patient survival, particularly among subjects with pathologic stage IB and IIA cancers, was more distinct with application of the seventh edition criteria (Table 79.5).

Guidelines for surveillance of the incidentally detected subcentimeter nodule (<8 to 10 mm) or larger solitary pulmonary nodule (8 to 10 mm or larger) have been published by the Fleischner Society for Thoracic Imaging and Diagnosis,[42] the American College of Chest Physicians,[43] and others[44] and are incorporated in a suggested algorithm (Algorithm 79.1) for evaluation of these common incidental chest findings. As with any algorithm, assessment of patient risk factors (pretest probability) for cancer[43] as well as comorbidities[42] should be taken into consideration before following these guidelines in one's practice.

The aims of the initial evaluation of a patient with NSCLC are to determine whether distant metastatic disease is present and to assess the extent of intrathoracic disease. A multidisciplinary approach, involving input from pulmonary medicine, chest radiology, oncology, and thoracic surgery, should be undertaken in the selection of the most suitable testing for any individual patient. One general algorithm for patient evaluation and decision making is shown in Algorithm 79.2. A thorough history and physical examination, combined with a plain chest radiograph and baseline laboratory data (complete blood cell count and measurement of serum sodium, calcium, alkaline phosphatase, and lactate dehydrogenase levels), can
5 suggest the presence of metastatic disease. Common metastatic sites include the brain, supraclavicular nodes, contralateral lung, bones, liver, and adrenal glands. Abnormal findings are then investigated further with chest CT and fluorodeoxyglucose positron emission tomography (FDG-PET) body scans. If necessary, needle aspiration biopsy or open biopsy can be performed to determine the extent of disease.

If the initial clinical evaluation does not suggest the presence of distant disease, the extent of further evaluation by various scans is controversial. Some physicians always perform a complete metastatic workup with CT of the chest and abdomen, CT or magnetic resonance imaging (MRI) of the brain, and FDG-PET scan. CT of the chest and upper abdomen has become standard, as much to evaluate the extent of the primary tumor and the status of the mediastinal lymph nodes as to detect metastases in the ipsilateral or contralateral lung, liver, or adrenals. Additional scans in asymptomatic patients may detect the 5% to 10% of metastases that are occult, but these scans are not clearly cost-effective in patients with clinical stage I or II tumors.

Patients presenting with suspected NSCLC and a pleural effusion should undergo thoracentesis, followed by thoracoscopy should initial cytology specimens be nondiagnostic. Those patients presenting with metastatic (stage IV) disease involving a solitary distant site should obtain tissue confirmation at the site of metastasis, if technically feasible. If noninvasive testing demonstrates multiple metastases (e.g., multiple liver, brain, or bone lesions), then diagnosis of the primary lesion might provide the most efficient means of diagnosis, followed by the initiation of palliative chemotherapy.[45] In patients who are suitable candidates for operation, who have a suspicious solitary pulmonary nodule that is of indeterminate origin despite appropriate evaluation, excisional biopsy and subsequent lobectomy of resectable lung cancer should be pursued.[46]

Recent multi-institutional studies have indicated a benefit for a combined modality approach in the treatment of stage IIIA NSCLC, consisting of neoadjuvant chemotherapy and radiation followed by resection (Intergroup0139/RTOG9309). Therefore, tissue confirmation of mediastinal nodal involvement has implications not only for the staging but also the management of patients who are otherwise candidates for resection of locoregionally advanced NSCLC. Regional lymph node involvement (N) has been defined as follows: N0 = no lymph node metastasis; N1 = metastasis to lymph nodes in the peribronchial or the ipsilateral hilar region or both, including direct extension;

TABLE 79.2 **CLASSIFICATION**

TNM CLASSIFICATION FOR STAGING SYSTEM OF NON–SMALL CELL LUNG CANCER (6TH EDITION)

■ STAGE	■ TNM STATUS
IA	T1 N0 M0
IB	T2 N0 M0
IIA	T1 N1 M0
IIB	T2 N1 M0
	T3 N0 M0
IIIA	T3 N1 M0
	T1–3 N2 M0
IIIB	T4 Any N M0
	Any T N3 M0
IV	Any T any N M1

TNM DEFINITIONS

T	TX	Positive malignant cells, but primary tumor not visualized by imaging or bronchoscopy
	T0	No evidence of primary tumor
	Tis	Carcinoma in situ
	T1	Tumor ≤3 cm, surrounded by lung or visceral pleura, without bronchoscopic evidence of invasion more proximal than the lobar bronchus[a]
	T2	Tumor with any of the following features of size or extent:
		>3 cm in greatest dimension
		Involves main bronchus, ≥2 cm distal to the carina
		Invades the visceral pleura
		Associated with atelectasis or obstructive pneumonitis that extends to the hilar region but does not involve the entire lung
	T3	Tumor of any size that directly invades any of the following: chest wall (including superior sulcus tumors), diaphragm, mediastinal pleura, or parietal pericardium; tumor in the main bronchus <2 cm distal to the carina, but without involvement of the carina; or associated atelectasis or obstructive pneumonitis of the entire lung
	T4	Tumor of any size that invades any of the following: mediastinum, heart, great vessels, trachea, esophagus, vertebral body, or carina; or tumor with a malignant pleural or pericardial effusion, or with satellite tumor nodule(s) within the ipsilateral primary tumor lobe of the lung[b]
N	NX	Regional lymph nodes cannot be assessed
	N0	No regional lymph node metastasis
	N1	Metastasis to ipsilateral peribronchial and/or ipsilateral hilar lymph nodes, and involvement of intrapulmonary nodes by direct extension of the primary tumor
	N2	Metastasis to ipsilateral mediastinal and/or subcarinal lymph node(s)
	N3	Metastasis to contralateral mediastinal, contralateral hilar, ipsilateral or contralateral scalene, or supraclavicular lymph node(s)
M	MX	Presence of distant metastasis cannot be assessed
	M0	No distant metastasis
	M1	Distant metastasis present (including metastatic tumor nodule[s] in the ipsilateral nonprimary tumor lobe of the lung)

[a]The uncommon superficial tumor of any size with its invasive component limited to the bronchial wall that may extend proximal to the main bronchus is classified as T1.
[b]Most pleural effusions associated with lung cancer are caused by tumor. There are, however, some few patients in whom the pleural fluid (more than one specimen) is negative for tumor on cytopathologic examination and in whom the fluid is nonbloody and is not an exudate. In cases in which these elements and clinical judgment dictate that the effusion is not related to the tumor, the patient should be staged T1, T2, or T3, with effusion excluded as a staging element. Pericardial effusion is classified according to the same rules.

N2 = metastasis to ipsilateral mediastinal lymph nodes and subcarinal lymph nodes; and N3 = metastasis to contralateral mediastinal lymph nodes, contralateral hilar lymph nodes, and ipsilateral or contralateral scalene or supraclavicular lymph nodes (Table 79.4).[47]

Chest CT provides only anatomic clues for tumor involvement of mediastinal lymph nodes (enlargement >10 mm), as demonstrated in a recent meta-analysis of over 3,400 evaluable patients, with a pooled sensitivity of 57% and specificity of only 82%. This meta-analysis also demonstrated that FDG-PET scanning appears to provide increased sensitivity of 84% and specificity of 89% in over 1,100 patients studied for the detection of mediastinal malignancy.[48] Several single-institution prospective studies have also indicated the superior diagnostic accuracy of FDG-PET imaging.[49–51] A recent multi-institutional trial involving 271 patients confirmed these findings. Although

TABLE 79.3

DESCRIPTORS, PROPOSED T AND M CATEGORIES, AND PROPOSED STAGE GROUPINGS

6TH EDITION T/M DESCRIPTOR		PROPOSED T/M	N0	N1	N2	N3
T1	(≤2 cm)	T1a	IA	IIA	IIIA	IIIB
T1	(>2–3 cm)	T1b	IA	IIA	IIIA	IIIB
T2	(≤5 cm)	T2a	IB	IIA	IIIA	IIIB
T2	(>5–7 cm)	T2b	IIA	IIB	IIIA	IIIB
T2	(>7 cm)	T3	IIB	IIIA	IIIA	IIIB
T3	Invasion		IIB	IIIA	IIIA	IIIB
T4	(same lobe nodules)		IIB	IIIA	IIIA	IIIB
T4	(extension)	T4	IIIA	IIIA	IIIB	IIIB
M1	(ipsilateral lung)		IIIA	IIIA	IIIB	IIIB
T4	(pleural effusion)	M1a	IV	IV	IV	IV
M1	(contralateral lung)		IV	IV	IV	IV
M1	(distant)	M1b	IV	IV	IV	IV

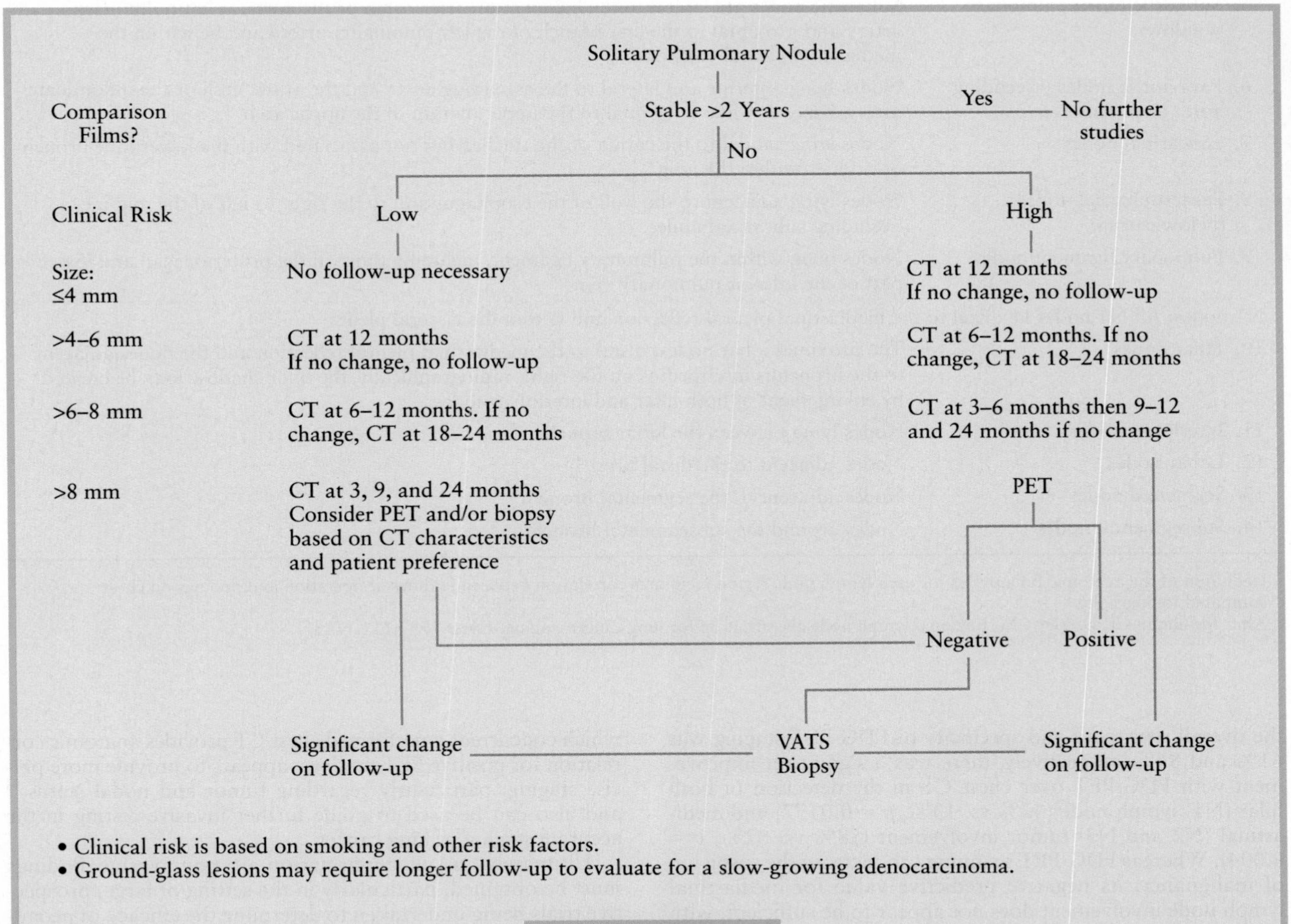

ALGORITHM 79.1

ALGORITHM 79.1. Management of the incidental solitary pulmonary nodule. (Partially based on MacMahon H, Austin JHM, Gamsu G, et al. Guidelines for management of small pulmonary nodules detected on CT scans: a statement from the Fleischner Society. *Radiology* 2005;237: 395–400.)

TABLE 79.4 **CLASSIFICATION**

THE MOUNTAIN-DRESLER LYMPH NODE MAP

NODAL STATION	ANATOMIC LANDMARKS
N2 nodes: All N2 nodes lie within the mediastinal pleural envelope	
1. Highest mediastinal nodes	Nodes lying above a horizontal line at the upper rim of the brachiocephalic (left innominate) vein where it ascends to the left, crossing in front of the trachea at its midline
2. Upper paratracheal nodes	Nodes lying above a horizontal line drawn tangential to the upper margin of the aortic arch and below the inferior boundary of No. 1 nodes
3. Prevascular and retrotracheal nodes	Prevascular and retrotracheal nodes may be designated 3A (anterior to the vessels) and 3P (prevertebral); midline nodes are considered to be ipsilateral.
4. Lower paratracheal nodes	The lower paratracheal nodes on the right lie to the right of the midline of the trachea between a horizontal line drawn tangential to the upper margin of the aortic arch and a line extending across the right main bronchus at the upper margin of the upper lobe bronchus, and contained within the mediastinal pleural envelope; the lower paratracheal nodes on the left lie to the left of the midline of the trachea between a horizontal line drawn tangential to the upper margin to the aortic arch and a line extending across the left main bronchus at the level of the upper margin of the left upper lobe bronchus, medial to the ligamentum arteriosum and contained within the mediastinal pleural envelope.
	Researchers may want to designate the lower paratracheal nodes as No. 4s (superior) and No. 4i (inferior) subsets for study purposes; the No. 4s nodes may be defined by a horizontal line extending across the trachea and drawn tangential to the cephalic border of the azygos vein; the No. 4i nodes may be defined by the lower boundary of No. 4s and the lower boundary of No. 4 as described above.
5. Subaortic (aortopulmonary window)	Subaortic nodes are lateral to the ligamentum arteriosum or the aorta or left pulmonary artery and proximal to the first branch of the left pulmonary artery and lie within the mediastinal pleural envelope.
6. Para-aortic nodes (ascending aorta or phrenic)	Nodes lying anterior and lateral to the ascending aorta and the aortic arch or the innominate artery, beneath a line tangential to the upper margin of the aortic arch
7. Subcarinal nodes	Nodes lying caudal to the carina of the trachea but not associated with the lower lobe bronchi or arteries within the lung
8. Paraesophageal nodes (below carina)	Nodes lying adjacent to the wall of the esophagus and to the right or left of the midline, excluding subcarinal nodes
9. Pulmonary ligament nodes	Nodes lying within the pulmonary ligament, including those in the posterior wall and lower part of the inferior pulmonary vein
N1 nodes: All N1 nodes lie distal to the mediastinal pleural reflection and within the visceral pleura	
10. Hilar nodes	The proximal lobar nodes, distal to the mediastinal pleural reflection and the nodes adjacent to the bronchus intermedius on the right; radiographically, the hilar shadow may be created by enlargement of both hilar and interlobar nodes.
11. Interlobar nodes	Nodes lying between the lobar bronchi
12. Lobar nodes	Nodes adjacent to the distal bronchi
13. Segmental nodes	Nodes adjacent to the segmental bronchi
14. Subsegmental nodes	Nodes around the subsegmental bronchi

Definition of the anatomic boundaries for each lymph node region facilitates correlation between findings at operation and findings on chest computed tomography.
After Mountain CF, Dresler CM. Regional lymph node classification for lung cancer staging. *Chest* 1997;111:1718.

the overall sensitivity and specificity of FDG-PET staging was 61% and 84%, respectively, there was a significant improvement with FDG-PET over chest CT in the detection of both hilar (N1) lymph node (42% vs. 13%, $p = 0.0177$) and mediastinal (N2 and N3) tumor involvement (58% vs. 32%, $p = 0.004$). Whereas FDG-PET scanning can increase the suspicion of malignancy, its negative predictive value for mediastinal lymph node involvement does not appear to be sufficient, with a false-negative rate reported as high as 13%.[52] PET evaluation of the solitary pulmonary nodule also appears to be somewhat insensitive, with a negative predictive value for benign lesions of only 57%, indicating a false-negative rate of 47%. Reliance on this modality could lead to delayed treatment for resectable early-stage (IA) NSCLC.[53] Integrated CT-PET imaging, in which concurrently performed chest CT provides anatomic correlation for positive PET findings, appears to provide more precise staging, particularly regarding tumor and nodal status,[54] and also can be used to guide further invasive testing in the accurate staging of lung cancer.

Ultimately, tissue confirmation of noninvasive findings must be obtained, particularly in the setting of large, prospective trials being undertaken to determine the efficacy of neoadjuvant and adjuvant therapy.[55] Noninvasive techniques for clinical staging, particularly chest CT, have a reported false-negative rate of approximately 10% to 15%. FDG-PET scan also has a reported false-positive rate of as high as 50%.[49] Clinical staging of NSCLC, particularly mediastinal lymph node involvement, can be accomplished by needle aspiration

TABLE 79.5 **RESULTS**

IASLC LUNG CANCER STAGING PROJECT: OVERALL 5-YEAR SURVIVAL BY CLINICAL AND SURGICAL 6TH AND PROPOSED 7TH EDITION TNM STAGE

	■ CLINICAL STAGE				■ SURGICAL STAGE			
	■ 6TH ED. TNM		■ PROPOSED 7TH ED. TNM		■ 6TH ED. TNM		■ PROPOSED 7TH ED. TNM	
■ STAGE	■ NO. PATIENTS	■ PATIENTS SURVIVING (%)	■ NO. PATIENTS	■ PATIENTS SURVIVING (%)	■ NO. PATIENTS	■ PATIENTS SURVIVING (%)	■ NO. PATIENTS	■ PATIENTS SURVIVING (%)
IA	831	50	831	50	3,666	73	3,666	73
IB	1,842	40	1,284	43	4,426	54	3,100	58
IIA	25	24	483	36	562	48	2,579	46
IIB	2,151	25	2,248	25	2,982	38	2,252	36
IIIA	3,005	18	3,175	19	3,091	25	3,792	24
IIIB	1,224	8	758	7	1,042	19	297	9
IV	2,458	2	2,757	2	183	21	266	13
TOTAL	11,536				15,952			

IASLC, International Association for the Study of Lung Cancer.
Adapted from Goldwstraw P, Crowley J, Chansky K, et al. The IASLC Lung Cancer Staging Project: proposals for the revision of the TNM stage groupings in the forthcoming (seventh) edition of the TNM Classification of malignant tumours. *J Thorac Oncol* 2007;2:706–714.

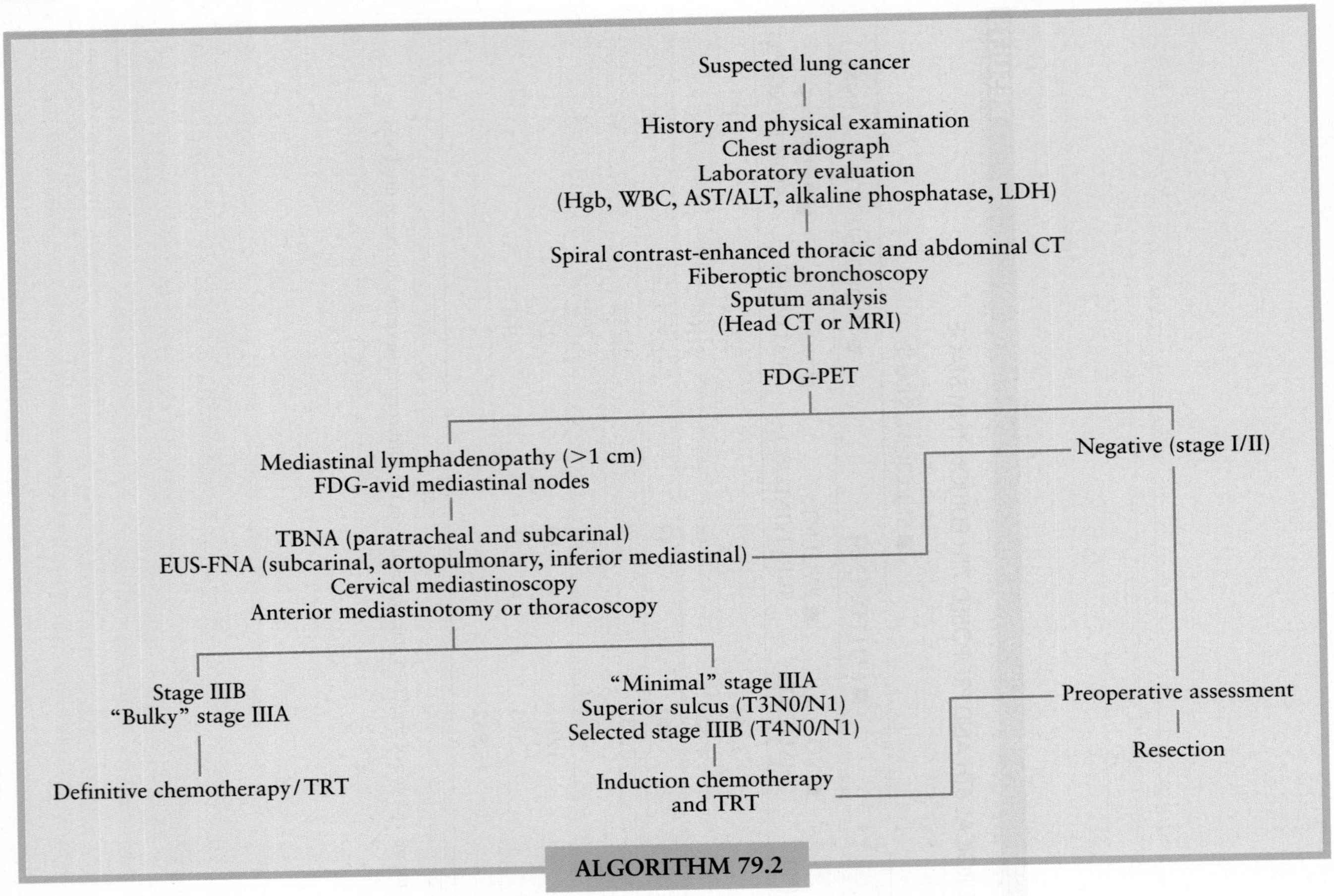

ALGORITHM 79.2. Evaluation of the patient who presents with a pulmonary mass.

techniques from several approaches: transbronchial (TBNA) with or without endobronchial ultrasound (EBUS) guidance, transthoracic, or transesophageal. Transesophageal endoscopic ultrasound with fine-needle aspiration (EUS-FNA) appears to be particularly useful for sampling of posterior mediastinal nodes such as the subcarinal, periesophageal, or aortopulmonary window stations, particularly in patients with mediastinal lymphadenopathy in these regions. Diagnostic yield is improved with practitioner experience, sampling needle size, and on-site cytology examination to determine adequacy of the obtained samples.

Cervical mediastinoscopy remains the "gold standard" for tissue diagnosis of mediastinal lymphadenopathy, with procedural sensitivity greater than 90% and specificity of 100%.[56] A recent retrospective review of a single institutional experience with routine mediastinoscopy, including 1,745 patients with known or suspected lung cancer, demonstrated overall sensitivity of 85%, with most false-negative results due to lymph node involvement in regions inaccessible to standard mediastinoscopic technique; morbidity of 0.6%; and perioperative mortality of 0.05%. Furthermore, of the patients found to have N2 or N3 disease at mediastinoscopy, only 6.6% (28/422) subsequently underwent resection, including several patients treated on neoadjuvant protocol.[57] For patients with clinically suspicious aortopulmonary lymph node involvement (stations 5 and 6), an area that is generally not accessible by standard mediastinoscopy, anterior mediastinotomy, extended cervical mediastinoscopy, or, as of more recently, thoracoscopy can be performed.

One recent goal in the diagnosis of lung cancer has been the early detection of tumors arising in asymptomatic high-prevalence populations (e.g., older patients with a history of tobacco use). Whether such efforts actually alter the natural history of disease remains controversial.[7,8,58,59] While newer modalities of noninvasive imaging, such as FDG-PET imaging, have improved the accuracy of staging for lung cancer,[52] these techniques still rely on factors such as tumor cell volume, tumor density, and metabolic activity. Current staging procedures do not detect all lymph node or distant hematogenous metastases.

Risk Assessment

Having established that resection is feasible, a significant number of patients with lung cancer cannot undergo operation due to associated comorbidity that increases operative mortality and postoperative morbidity. Age alone should not preclude patients with resectable disease from operation.[60] In a population with a high prevalence of prior or continuing tobacco use that has a greater predisposition to atherosclerotic cardiovascular disease, preoperative cardiovascular risk assessment with further noninvasive cardiac testing or coronary angiography, if indicated, should be considered.[61]

Preoperative spirometry, particularly the forced expiratory volume in 1 second (FEV_1), as an assessment of patients' suitability for pulmonary resection is essential. Measurement of the diffusing capacity of the lung for carbon monoxide (DLCO) provides complementary data to standard spirometry, particularly for patients with evidence of interstitial lung disease or exertional dyspnea. Generally, if a patient demonstrates a FEV_1 greater than 2 L (>60% predicted) or DLCO greater than 50% predicted, further evaluation of pulmonary capacity prior to resection, including pneumonectomy, is not necessary.[62,63] Patients with limited pulmonary reserve, including those with a FEV_1 less than 1.2 L (40% predicted) or DLCO 35% to 40% predicted, are at higher risk for significant morbidity or mortality following anatomic resection and should undergo further evaluation.[64]

Preoperative room-air arterial blood gas testing can identify patients at greater risk for perioperative complications or death. In particular, patients with an arterial oxygen concentration less than 60 mm Hg, partial pressure of arterial carbon dioxide ($PaCO_2$) greater than 45 mm Hg, or oxygen saturation less than 90% may be at greater risk for pulmonary resection. Quantitative perfusion scanning allows the assessment of predicted postoperative (ppo) lung function in patients with marginal pulmonary function and can be calculated as follows: $ppoFEV_1$ (% predicted) = preoperative FEV_1 (% predicted) × (1 − fraction of total number of anatomic segments to be resected). Patients with a $ppoFEV_1$ less than 0.8 L, or 35% to 40% predicted, are likely at substantially increased risk for perioperative death or complication.[65,66]

If available, further testing with formal cardiopulmonary exercise testing (CPET) in order to calculate maximal oxygen consumption (VO_{2max}) may allow further risk stratification in marginal patients. In several series, patients with a VO_{2max} less than 10 to 15 mL/min per kg were at very high risk for postoperative complications, whereas those with a VO_{2max} greater than 20 mL/min per kg underwent operation without complication or death.[66] These findings were corroborated by a recent cooperative group study (CALGB 9238) conducted to determine whether pulmonary resection could be accomplished safely in patients with peak exercise oxygen capacity greater than 15 mL/min per kg, regardless of FEV_1. In this prospective study of 346 patients who underwent thoracotomy for NSCLC, there were 86 subjects whose peak exercise oxygen capacity was less than the threshold of less than 15 mL/min per kg, or 60% of predicted. This group experienced significantly more cardiorespiratory complications, respiratory failure, or death than the remaining subjects whose peak exercise oxygen capacity was greater than 15 mL/min per kg. From these data, the authors concluded that patients with peak exercise oxygen capacity greater than 15 mL/min per kg, even if the FEV_1 and/or DLCO were less than 70% predicted, could undergo pulmonary resection with curative intent.[67]

Informal exercise testing, particularly stair climbing, may also aid the clinician in determining a patient's suitability for resection. Patients who are able to climb five flights of stairs will likely tolerate pneumonectomy, whereas those who cannot climb a single flight will likely not tolerate pulmonary resection. Furthermore, oxygen desaturation greater than 4% during exercise testing may also be an indicator for increased risk of perioperative complication. Careful preoperative physiologic assessment will allow the clinician to identify patients at increased risk for perioperative complication or death and allow such patients to make an informed decision regarding operation.[68] Measures to minimize postoperative complications, including aggressive efforts to encourage smoking cessation, pre- and postoperative chest physiotherapy, incentive spirometry, early extubation and mobilization, and the use of postoperative thoracic epidural analgesia, are important for all patients undergoing pulmonary resection, especially those with marginal pulmonary function (Algorithm 79.3).

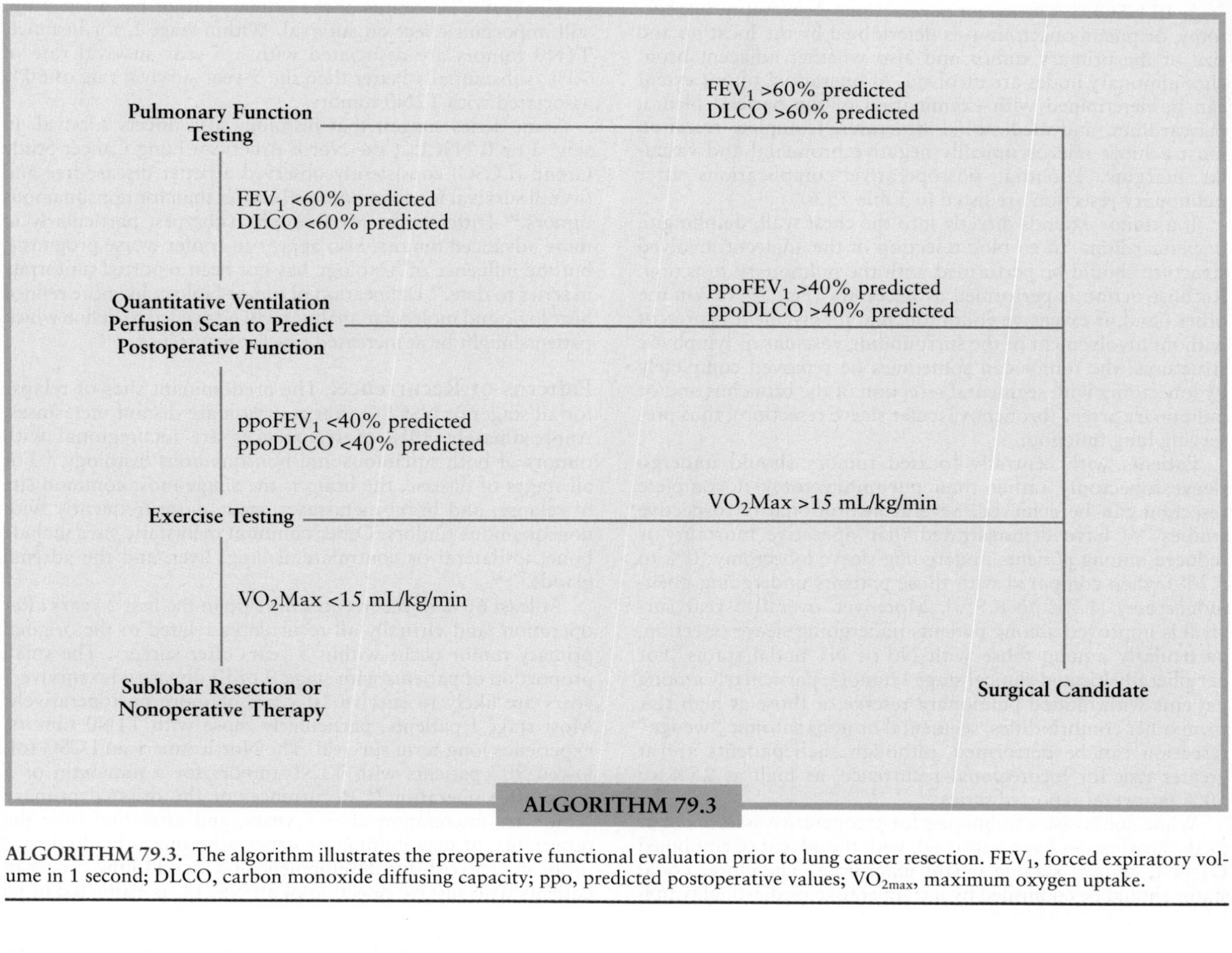

ALGORITHM 79.3

ALGORITHM 79.3. The algorithm illustrates the preoperative functional evaluation prior to lung cancer resection. FEV_1, forced expiratory volume in 1 second; DLCO, carbon monoxide diffusing capacity; ppo, predicted postoperative values; VO_{2max}, maximum oxygen uptake.

TABLE 79.6 **COMPLICATIONS**

POSTOPERATIVE COMPLICATIONS AFTER PULMONARY RESECTION[a]

■ COMPLICATION	■ INCIDENCE (%)
Atrial arrhythmia	2.9–14.4
Prolonged air leak	4–7.6
Pneumonia	1–2.5
Subcutaneous emphysema	0.8–1.1
Myocardial infarction	0.4–0.9
Recurrent laryngeal nerve injury	0.4–0.7
Bronchopleural fistula	0.3–0.5
Respiratory failure	0.1–5.5
Hemorrhage	0–1.5
Empyema	0–1.1
Mortality	0.7–1.4

[a]Includes thoracoscopic and open series.
Based on Berry MF, et al. Complications of thoracoscopic pulmonary resection. *Semin Thorac Cardiovasc Surg* 2007;19:350–354.

Treatment

Pulmonary resection, with definitive tumor staging, remains the mainstay of treatment for stage I, stage II, and selected stage III NSCLC. The extent of resection—lobectomy, bilobectomy, or pneumonectomy—is determined by the location and size of the primary tumor and also whether adjacent bronchopulmonary nodes are involved. At operation, tumor extent can be determined with examination of the parietal pleura, pericardium, and mediastinal structures. Complete resection must achieve microscopically negative bronchial and vascular margins. Potential postoperative complications after pulmonary resection are listed in Table 79.6.

If a tumor extends directly into the chest wall, diaphragm, or pericardium, an en bloc resection of the adjacent involved structure should be performed with the pulmonary resection. Reconstruction is performed as necessary (Fig. 79.1). On the other hand, if extensive endobronchial involvement is present without involvement of the surrounding vascular or lymphatic structures, the tumor can sometimes be removed completely by lobectomy with segmental resection of the bronchus and/or pulmonary artery (bronchovascular sleeve resection), thus preserving lung function.

Patients with centrally located tumors should undergo sleeve lobectomy rather than pneumonectomy if complete resection can be achieved. Several institutional retrospective studies[69–73] have demonstrated that operative mortality is reduced among patients undergoing sleeve lobectomy (0% to 5.2%) when compared with those patients undergoing pneumonectomy (1.7% to 8.9%). Moreover, overall 5-year survival is improved among patients undergoing sleeve resection, particularly among those with N0 or N1 nodal status. For peripherally located clinical stage I tumors, particularly among patients with limited pulmonary reserve or those at high risk from other comorbidities, segmental or nonanatomic "wedge" resection can be performed, although such patients are at greater risk for locoregional recurrence, as high as 25% to 50% in several reported series.[74–77]

While noninvasive techniques for preoperative assessment of mediastinal nodes have improved, with the advent of combined CT-PET, clinical staging is still inaccurate. Therefore, nodal status should be confirmed by intraoperative mediastinal lymph node sampling or mediastinal lymph node dissection. Accurate pathologic staging not only provides prognostic information but is also important in the decision on whether to proceed with adjuvant chemotherapy. Systematic sampling should include, for right-sided resections, at least one subcarinal, right paratracheal, and tracheobronchial angle lymph node each, and for left-sided resections, at least one subcarinal and para-aortic or aortopulmonary lymph node each, using standard nomenclature and numbering as depicted in Table 79.4. Several groups advocate complete mediastinal lymph node dissection, with en bloc removal of the nodal packets from the same levels as in systematic sampling.[78] Complete mediastinal lymph node dissection does not appear to confer increased perioperative morbidity,[79] but whether mediastinal lymph node dissection rather than sampling confers a survival advantage among patients undergoing major pulmonary resection remains controversial, and is one of the questions addressed in a recently completed multicenter clinical trial, Z0030, conducted by the American College of Surgeons Oncology Group (ACOSOG).

Survival

The long-term survival after resection for NSCLC is linked to the pathologic stage of disease. The overall 5-year survival rates are shown in Table 79.5. They range from 60% to 70% for stage I tumors, from 40% to 50% for stage II tumors, and from 15% to 30% for stage IIIA tumors. Nodal involvement has the strongest adverse influence on survival. Large peripheral tumors that extend directly into the chest wall without nodal involvement (T3N0) are associated with a 5-year survival rate of 40% after complete resection, whereas involvement of mediastinal nodes is associated with only a 20% survival rate. The status of the primary tumor has a lesser but still important effect on survival. Within stage I, for instance, T1N0 tumors are associated with a 5-year survival rate of 70%, substantially better than the 5-year survival rate of 60% associated with T2N0 tumors.

Some series suggest that histology also affects survival. In stage I or II NSCLC, the North American Lung Cancer Study Group (LCSG) consistently observed a better disease-free and overall survival for squamous cell cancer than for nonsquamous tumors.[80] Different adenocarcinoma subtypes, particularly in more advanced tumors, also appear to confer worse prognosis, but the influence of histology has not been reported uniformly in series to date.[81] Delineation of tumor biology by more refined histologic and molecular analyses will be needed to define which patients might be at increased risk for recurrence.

Patterns of Recurrence. The predominant sites of relapse for all stages of NSCLC after resection are distant metastases. Approximately 30% of recurrences are locoregional with tumors of both squamous and nonsquamous histology.[76] For all stages of disease, the brain is the single most common site of relapse, and brain metastases occur more frequently with nonsquamous tumors. Other common metastatic sites include bone, ipsilateral or contralateral lung, liver, and the adrenal glands.[76,82]

At least 60% of recurrences develop in the first 2 years after operation, and virtually all recurrences related to the original primary tumor occur within 5 years after surgery. The small proportion of patients with stage II or III disease who survive 5 years are likely to survive 10 years or more postoperatively. Most stage I patients, particularly those with T1N0 tumors, experience long-term survival. The North American LCSG followed 907 patients with T1N0 tumors for a minimum of 5 years after operation.[82] Recurrences of the original primary tumor are uncommon after 5 years, and after that time the occurrence of new pulmonary cancers becomes the dominant problem. The risk for development of a second lung cancer in patients who survive resection of an NSCLC is estimated to be

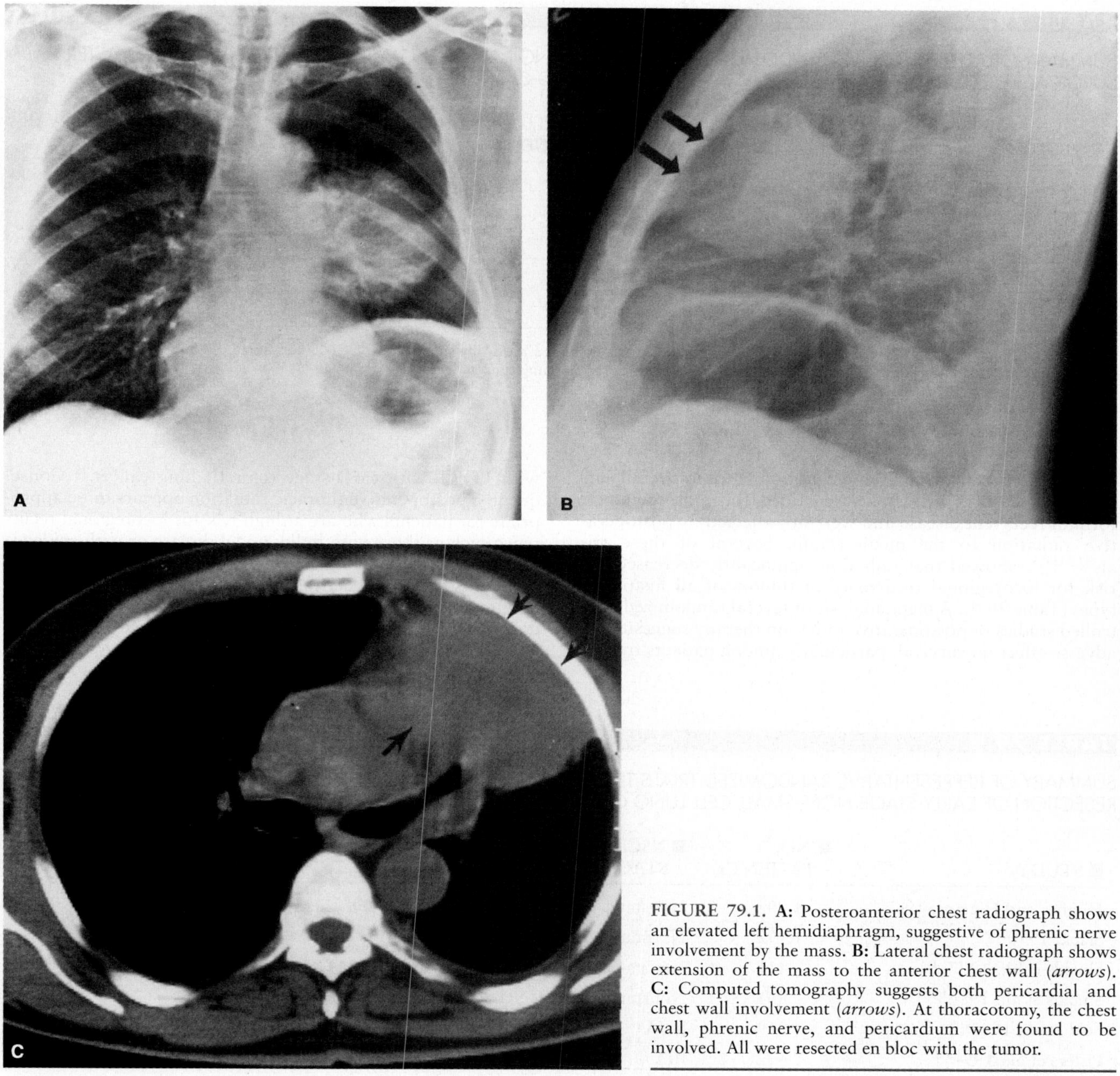

FIGURE 79.1. **A:** Posteroanterior chest radiograph shows an elevated left hemidiaphragm, suggestive of phrenic nerve involvement by the mass. **B:** Lateral chest radiograph shows extension of the mass to the anterior chest wall (*arrows*). **C:** Computed tomography suggests both pericardial and chest wall involvement (*arrows*). At thoracotomy, the chest wall, phrenic nerve, and pericardium were found to be involved. All were resected en bloc with the tumor.

2% to 3% per patient per year,[83] with a second lung cancer developing rarely in never-smokers at the time of initial resection and at rates of 1.8% per patient-year in former smokers and 2.7% per patient-year in current smokers.[84] Patients also face a consistent risk for the development of new, nonpulmonary primary cancers during the first 5 years after operation and thereafter. New, nonpulmonary malignancies develop in a wide variety of sites, but breast, colon, and prostate cancers are the most common.[76]

These data underscore the importance of long-term follow-up after resection of early-stage NSCLC. Traditionally, most thoracic oncologists recommend oncologic surveillance for their lung cancer patients in coordination with a primary or referring physician every 3 to 4 months during the first 2 years after operation, then every 6 months the following 2 years and annually thereafter. Although there is no single modality to detect recurrence, follow-up should include a combination of history, physical examination, serial chest radiographs, and low-dose spiral chest CT. While the cost-effectiveness of this approach is unproven,[85] cost decision analysis suggests that inclusion of annual surveillance chest CT could be beneficial, depending on factors such as patient age, cost of chest CT, rate of false-positive findings, and annual risk of a second primary lung cancer.[86]

Adjuvant Therapy for Non–Small Cell Lung Cancer.

The risk for recurrent disease, even after resection of early-stage NSCLC, has led to efforts to improve overall survival rates through the use of adjuvant therapy, even though no specific method is available to identify which patients will relapse. Various types of adjuvant therapy have been tested, including immunotherapy,[87–89] radiation, chemotherapy, and combined chemotherapy and radiation.

Radiation has been evaluated extensively as adjuvant therapy. Although early retrospective series suggested that postoperative radiation therapy (PORT) potentially improved overall survival,[90–92] subsequent relatively small randomized trials comparing adjuvant radiation with no further treatment

TABLE 79.7 **RESULTS**

SUMMARY OF REPRESENTATIVE RANDOMIZED TRIALS COMPARING RADIATION WITH NO FURTHER TREATMENT AFTER SURGICAL RESECTION OF EARLY-STAGE NON–SMALL CELL LUNG CANCER

STUDY	NO. PATIENTS	NSCLC STAGE[a]	RADIATION DOSE (Gy)	OVERALL SURVIVAL DIFFERENCE
Van Houtte et al., 1980[97]	224	I, II	60	NS
LCSG, 1986[96]	210	II, IIIA	50	NS
Lafitte et al., 1996[95]	132	IB	45–60	NS
MRC, 1996[94]	308	II, IIIA	40 (15 fractions)	NS
Mayer et al., 1997[93]	155	IA–IIIA	50–56	NS

LCSG, Lung Cancer Study Group; MRC, Medical Research Council; NS, not statistically significant; NSCLC, non–small cell lung cancer.
[a]The stages are listed according to the 1997 international system for staging lung cancer.

failed to demonstrate any significant difference in overall survival.[93–97] Distant metastases remained the most common form of recurrent disease and were not affected by postoperative radiation to the mediastinum. Several of these trials[93,94,96,97] showed that radiation significantly decreased the risk for locoregional recurrence in tumors of all histologic types (Table 79.7). A meta-analysis of several randomized controlled studies of postoperative radiation therapy suggested an adverse effect on survival, particularly among patients treated with PORT with early-stage (I or II) lung cancer.[98] Consequently, postoperative thoracic radiation appears to be appropriate for patients who are at high risk for locoregional recurrence such as those with bulky nodal disease or with evidence of residual tumor at surgical margins.

Because distant metastases are the predominant mode of relapse after resection of early-stage NSCLC, multiple randomized trials (Table 79.8) have been performed to determine if postoperative adjuvant chemotherapy improves survival.

TABLE 79.8 **RESULTS**

SUMMARY OF REPRESENTATIVE RANDOMIZED TRIALS TESTING THE BENEFIT OF ADJUVANT CHEMOTHERAPY AFTER RESECTION OF EARLY-STAGE NON–SMALL CELL LUNG CANCER

STUDY	NO. PATIENTS	NSCLC STAGES[a]	CHEMOTHERAPY AGENTS	OVERALL SURVIVAL DIFFERENCE
Hughes and Higgins, 1962[99]	1,002	Not stated	HN2 vs. no Rx	NS
Slack, 1970[100]	1,192	Not stated	HN2 vs. no Rx	NS
Shields et al., 1977[101]	417	Not stated	Cytoxan vs. Cytoxan + MTX	NS
Shields et al., 1982[102]	865	Not stated	CCNU + hydroxyurea vs. no Rx	NS
Feld et al., 1993[109]	269	I–IIA	CAP vs. no Rx	NS
Pisters et al., 1994[118]	72	IIIA	VP + RT vs. RT	NS
Dautzenberg et al., 1995[214]	267	I–IIIA	COPAC, RT vs. RT	NS
Wada et al., 1996[104]	323	I–IIIA	VP, UFT vs. UFT vs. no Rx	$p = 0.053$
Keller et al., 2000[110]	488	II, IIIA	EP + RT vs. RT	NS
Scagliotti et al., 2003[215]	1209	I–IIIA	MVP vs. no Rx	NS
IALT, 2004[4,106]	1867	I–IIIA	CDDP based ± RT vs. RT vs. no Rx	Overall, NS; DFS, $p = 0.02$
Nakagawa et al., 2005[105]	332	I	UFT vs. no Rx	Overall, NS; T1N0, $p = 0.036$
Winton et al., 2004[5,107]	482	IB–II	CDDP, Vnb vs. no Rx	Overall, $p = 0.011$; DFS, $p = 0.0003$
Strauss et al., 2008[108]	344	IB	Carboplatin, paclitaxel vs. no Rx	NS
ANITA, 2006[6]	840	I–IIIA	CDDP, Vnb vs. no Rx	Overall, $p = 0.017$

[a]The stages are listed according to the 1997 international system for staging lung cancer.[3]
ANITA, Adjuvant Navelbine International Trialist Association; CAP, cyclophosphamide, doxorubicin, cisplatin; CCNU, J-12-chlorethyl)-3-cyclohexyl-J nitrosourea; CDDP, cisplatin; COPAC, cyclophosphamide, doxorubicin, cisplatin, vincristine, lomustine; Cytoxan, cyclophosphamide; DFS, disease-free survival; EP, etoposide, cisplatin; HN2, nitrogen mustard; IALT, International Adjuvant Lung Cancer Trial; M, mitomycin C; MTX, methotrexate; NS, not significant; no Rx, no adjuvant treatment; RT, radiation; UFT, tegafur plus uracil; Vnb, vinorelbine; VP, vindesine, cisplatin.

Early trials evaluated agents, including nitrogen mustards, Cytoxan, methotrexate, and nitrosourea, now known to have no activity in NSCLC.[99–102] More recently, several studies have demonstrated that cisplatinum-based chemotherapy regimens appear to provide a modest survival benefit. A meta-analysis of 9,387 patients entered into 52 randomized clinical trials showed a 5% survival benefit at 5 years for adjuvant cisplatin-based chemotherapy in comparison with surgery alone. Trials comparing adjuvant radiation with radiation plus chemotherapy showed an absolute survival benefit of 4% at 2 years in favor of combined-modality treatment.[103]

Recent trials of adjuvant chemotherapy in patients with completely resected NSCLC appear to indicate a therapeutic benefit. Initial studies from the West Japan Study Group indicated that postoperative treatment with uracil-tegafur (UFT), a well-tolerated oral analogue of fluorouracil, confers a survival advantage.[104] Although a recent randomized phase III trial from this same group failed to demonstrate a survival advantage among patients with resected stage I adenocarcinoma or squamous cell carcinoma, subset analysis of patients with pT1N0M0 tumors indicated a significant improvement in overall survival.[105] The prolonged low-dose administration of fluorouracil, generally not considered to be an active drug against NSCLC, used in this trial appeared to have a significant antitumor effect.

The International Adjuvant Lung Cancer Trial evaluated the effect of cisplatin-based adjuvant chemotherapy on survival after complete resection of non–small cell lung cancer. A total of 1,867 patients with resected stage I, II, or III NSCLC were randomized to receive cisplatin-based chemotherapy, cisplatin-based chemotherapy and radiation, radiation alone, or no adjuvant treatment. Individual institutions administered additional chemotherapeutic agents at their discretion ("open-choice design"), with nearly half of the treated patients receiving cisplatin (100 mg/m^2) and etoposide for three or four cycles. The total dose delivered of cisplatin was greater than 240 mg/m^2 for 73.8% of treated patients. Additional agents used were vinorelbine, vinblastine, or vindesine. Cisplatin dosing varied from 80 to 120 mg/m^2 per cycle, for a total expected dose of 300 to 400 mg/m^2. Statistically significant benefits were observed for both overall (absolute difference, 4.1%) and disease-free (absolute difference, 5.1%) survival at 5 years for patients treated with cisplatin-based chemotherapy, with or without adjuvant radiation.[4] Planned radiotherapy did not appear to provide any added benefit. In subgroup analysis, the benefits of cisplatin-based adjuvant chemotherapy appeared to confer the greatest benefit upon patients with stage III NSCLC. In longer-term follow-up, disease-free survival hazard ratio remained improved at 0.88 (95% confidence interval [CI], 0.78–0.98; p = 0.02) for patients receiving adjuvant therapy at 7 years following operation, but the previously observed improvement in overall survival was no longer statistically significant with a hazard ratio of 0.91 (95% CI, 0.81–1.02; p = 0.10).[106]

Several subsequent studies support the use of adjuvant chemotherapy, particularly in stage II and III lung cancer. In the National Cancer Institute of Canada-Clinical Trials Group (JBR.10), adjuvant treatment with vinorelbine and cisplatin resulted in prolonged overall and disease-free survival for patients with resected stage IB or II (excluding T3N0M0) NSCLC.[5] These survival differences were demonstrated despite poor patient compliance, with only 50% of patients completing their prescribed regimen of adjuvant therapy.[107] In a phase III trial in which 840 patients with completely resected stage IB, II, and IIIA NSCLC were randomized to observation or adjuvant vinorelbine and cisplatinum, the Adjuvant Navelbine International Trialist Association (ANITA) reported that risk-adjusted overall mortality was reduced significantly in subjects assigned to chemotherapy, with a hazard ratio of 0.80 (95% CI, 0.66–0.96; p = 0.017).[6] Again, only 50% of patients receiving treatment completed the planned regimen.

The Cancer and Leukemia Group B (CALGB) 9633 trial reported 344 patients undergoing pulmonary resection for T2N0M0 (stage IB) NSCLC, randomized either to adjuvant therapy with paclitaxel and carboplatin or observation. With a median follow-up of 74 months, no statistical difference in overall survival was observed between treatment groups, with a hazard ratio of 0.83 (95% CI, 0.64–1.08; p = 0.12) for patients receiving adjuvant therapy. Unplanned subgroup analysis indicated a significant survival benefit for patients with larger tumors (>4 cm), but as a group, adjuvant chemotherapy for stage IB NSCLC is not considered standard of care currently.[108]

Notably, several of these trials have shown that approximately half of all patients actually received the planned dose of chemotherapy.[109,110] It remains to be determined whether patients undergoing minimally invasive approaches to pulmonary resection can tolerate adjuvant chemotherapy better than similar patients recovering from open operations. In a recent report by Petersen et al., thoracoscopic lobectomy was found to improve the delivery of adjuvant chemotherapy.[111] In a series of 100 patients, 43 underwent thoracotomy and 57 had pulmonary resection performed by thoracoscopy. Those undergoing thoracoscopic resection were found to have a higher compliance rate. Chemotherapy doses were delayed in significantly fewer patients in the thoracoscopic group (18% versus 58%). Chemotherapy doses were reduced in 26% in the thoracoscopy group versus 49% in the thoracotomy group, which was also significant. In addition, a significantly higher percentage of patients received 75% or more of the planned regimen. There was no significant difference in the time to initiation of chemotherapy or toxicity.

Treatment of Stage III Disease

Stage III NSCLC indicates locoregionally advanced disease that encompasses several anatomic subsets that vary considerably in the likelihood that resection will provide durable oncologic benefit. Stage IIIB is generally considered unresectable. There is no role for resection for patients with T4 (stage IIIB) disease due to malignant pleural or pericardial effusion, infiltration of the heart or vertebra, or contralateral or supraclavicular nodal metastases (N3). However, several small series from specialized centers have demonstrated that surgery can be considered for selected patients with invasion of mediastinal structures such as the superior vena cava, left atrium, carina, or aorta, with consideration for induction chemoradiation, in order to "downstage" such tumors.[112,113] These series indicate that complete resection is essential in order to obtain survival benefit from this approach.

Stage IIIA includes patients with extrapulmonary disease involving the ipsilateral hemithorax (i.e., T3N1 and T1–3N2). The management of patients with stage IIIA disease due to mediastinal nodal involvement (N2) continues to evolve, and is discussed in the following sections.

Role of Resection. The most controversial and complex part of the treatment of stage IIIA NSCLC is the management of patients with N2 disease. Reported 5-year survival rates after resection for N2 disease are usually 20% to 30% but range from zero to 40%. This variation reflects the extent of mediastinal nodal involvement, the T status of the primary tumor, and the ability to perform a complete resection. With respect to mediastinal nodal involvement, adverse prognostic factors include the presence of extracapsular nodal disease, multiple levels of involved lymph nodes, and superior mediastinal nodal metastases.[114,115]

Historically, several series presented an inappropriately optimistic view of the benefit of resection for N2 disease because they focused on highly selected patients. The experience reported by Martini and Flehinger[116] from Memorial Sloan-Kettering Cancer Center places resection for N2 disease in perspective because it examines the outcome of treatment of all patients with N2 disease, not just a small subset. From 1974 to 1981, a total of 1,598 patients with NSCLC, of whom 706 had mediastinal nodal metastases, were seen by the thoracic service. Only 151 patients, or 21% of all patients with N2 disease, had technically complete resections of the primary tumor and all accessible mediastinal lymph nodes. The overall survival of these 151 patients was 29% at 5 years. Moreover, 33 of these 151 patients who had "clinical" N2 disease (mediastinal nodal involvement extensive enough to be visible on chest radiography or bronchoscopy) had only an 8% survival rate at 3 years. Thus, only 16.7% of all patients potentially benefited in the long term from resection. Overall survival was also influenced by the T status of the primary tumor; patients with T2 or T3 tumors fared significantly worse than those with T1 tumors. Based on these and other data, most surgeons consider for resection only those patients who have a T1 or T2 primary tumor and single-level intranodal N2 disease.

Rationale for Neoadjuvant Therapy. Although some patients with "minimal" N2 disease survive for long periods of time after resection, most have more extensive nodal involvement and do not benefit from surgery as their primary treatment. Until the 1980s, the standard treatment for such patients was radiation. The reported survival rates after radiation are harder to interpret than those after resection because most series include a mixture of stage IIIA and IIIB patients and do not define the precise extent of nodal involvement. Sequential trials by the Radiation Therapy Oncology Group (RTOG) showed that high-dose, continuous radiation yields the best chance of local control.[117] Many attempts have been made to intensify radiation dose without increasing radiation side effects, either by altering radiation fractionation schemes or by using three-dimensional conformal treatment planning. On the whole, these efforts have led to minimal improvements in both local control and survival because most patients relapse in distant sites, just as they do after resection. For this reason, postoperative chemotherapy has been used as adjuvant therapy to surgery and radiation therapy in patients with N2 disease, although no benefit in survival has been shown.[118] The poor long-term survival and the risk for distant metastatic disease prompted an investigation of neoadjuvant multimodality therapy for stage III NSCLC.

Two small randomized clinical trials further challenged the concept of resection as the primary treatment for any patient with N2 disease. Rosell et al.[119,120] randomized 60 patients with stage IIIA NSCLC (16 of whom did not have N2 disease) to undergo resection or to receive three cycles of cisplatin-based chemotherapy followed by resection. The median survival of the patients who received preoperative chemotherapy was significantly longer (26 vs. 8 months) than the survival of patients who underwent only resection. A study of similar design from the M. D. Anderson Cancer Center corroborated these results.[121,122] Both trials were stopped early because of highly significant differences between the two study arms. These two studies suggest that it is appropriate to consider all patients with N2 disease diagnosed at mediastinoscopy for induction chemotherapy. Unfortunately, because pretreatment mediastinoscopy was not mandated in either trial, some patients who did not have N2 disease were included. The results of these trials are not universally accepted because of the small numbers of patients enrolled, the lack of systematic pretreatment staging, and the unusually poor survival of the patients in the control (surgery-only) arms.

Early Trials of Neoadjuvant Therapy. The concept of preoperative therapy followed by resection (neoadjuvant therapy) dates back to 1955, when Bromley and Szur[123] used radiation (at an average dose of 47 Gy) to treat 66 patients before resection. At operation, no viable tumor was found in 29 of 62 (47%) patients, but 10 patients died of complications in the first month, and only two patients survived to 5 years after operation. At the time, the natural history of NSCLC was not well understood, the methods of staging before resection not very accurate, and the risk for distant metastases not fully recognized. Effective chemotherapy did not exist and it was hoped that an approach that increased resectability might lead to better long-term survival. Thus, early neoadjuvant trials focused on the use of preoperative radiation.

Several subsequent studies further explored this approach.[124] All these trials were flawed by a lack of pretreatment staging, by the use of widely varying amounts of radiation, and by excessively long intervals between irradiation and resection. Nonetheless, it became apparent that aggressive local treatment did not improve long-term survival, even though radiation could sterilize tumor in a significant number of patients. The development of distant metastases in 50% to 80% of patients during or shortly after treatment underscored the need for systemic therapy in stage III NSCLC.

Recent Trials of Neoadjuvant Therapy. Because of a better understanding of the natural history of early-stage lung cancer and the revision of the international staging system in 1986, recent trials have defined more uniform patient populations, so that it has been easier to interpret trial results. Although many different treatment regimens have been used in neoadjuvant trials, they can be grouped into three major categories: (a) chemoradiation without resection, (b) chemotherapy followed by resection, and (c) chemoradiation followed by resection.

Trials of Chemoradiation without Resection. These trials cannot be equated with trials of neoadjuvant therapy that include resection because patients entered into nonsurgical trials are staged clinically without the benefit of mediastinoscopy. Therefore, nonsurgical trials include a mix of patients with stage IIIA and IIIB cancers, and they might even include some patients with earlier-stage disease who were thought erroneously to have stage III disease because of benign mediastinal adenopathy diagnosed only by CT.

With the acceptance of chemotherapy and radiation as standard treatment, attention has focused recently on the optimal means to deliver both modalities. A study suggests that concurrent treatment is superior to sequential chemoradiotherapy. Furuse et al.[125] randomized 314 patients with stage III NSCLC to MVP (cisplatin, 80 mg/m^2 on day 1; mitomycin, 8 mg/m^2 on days 1 and 29; and vindesine on days 1, 8, 29, and 36) with concurrent split-course radiation or to MVP followed by standard radiation. Patients who received concurrent treatment had a significantly better response and survival.

The results of several phase III randomized trials comparing radiation alone with either sequential or concurrent chemotherapy and radiation are shown in Table 79.9. These trials confirm the feasibility of combined-modality treatment and overall have shown that patients receiving chemoradiation have a better survival than those receiving either standard fractionated or hyperfractionated radiation alone. In most studies, the addition of chemotherapy improved median survival from between 9 and 10 months to 14 months and 5-year survival from 5% to between 15% and 20%. The somewhat variable results among these trials are related to several factors, including differences in total radiation dose and method of administration (split vs. continuous course); differences in chemotherapy dose, especially with respect to cisplatin; and differences in patient selection based on staging criteria.

Trials of Neoadjuvant Therapy with Resection. These trials have used two different treatment strategies: induction chemotherapy alone or concurrent chemoradiation before resection. The rationale for chemotherapy alone as induction treatment is that it potentially allows the use of a more intense dose and the use of some drugs, such as mitomycin, that cannot be administered in conjunction with radiation. Proponents of this approach also believe that chemotherapy is as effective as induction treatment as is combined chemoradiation, and that separating the two modalities allows irradiation to be

TABLE 79.9 **RESULTS**

RESULTS OF PHASE III TRIALS COMPARING RADIOTHERAPY ALONE WITH CHEMORADIOTHERAPY FOR STAGE III NON–SMALL CELL LUNG CANCER

INVESTIGATORS	NO. PATIENTS	CT	RT (Gy)	GROUP	MEDIAN SURVIVAL (mo)	SURVIVAL AT 2 Y (%)	*p*
TRIALS SHOWING NO ADVANTAGE							
Trovo et al., 1990[216]	111	CAMP	45 (seq)	CT-RT	11.7	17[a]	ND
				RT	10.0	19[a]	
Morton et al., 1991[217]	114	MACC	60 (seq)	CT-RT	10.6	21	>0.2
				RT	10.4	16	
Le Chevalier et al., 1991[218]	353	VCPC	65 (seq)	CT-RT	12.0	21	0.08
				RT	10.0	14	
Blanke et al., 1995[219]	214	CDDP	60–65 (con)	CT-RT	10.0	18	0.35
				RT	10.7	13	
TRIALS IN FAVOR OF COMBINED THERAPY							
Schaake-Koning et al., 1992[220]	331	CDDP	55 (con)	CT daily-RT	—	26	0.01
				CT wkly-RT	—	19	ND
				RT	—	13	
Jeremic et al., 1995[221]	169	Carbo	64.8 (con)	CT (wkly)-HXFRT	18.0	23[b]	0.003
		+VP-16		CT (other wk)-HXFRT	13.0	16	ND
				HXFRT	8.0	6.6	
Dillman et al., 1996[222]	155	CDDP	60 (seq)	CT-RT	13.7	26	0.01
		+Vbl		RT	9.6	13	
Sause et al., 2000[223]	458	CDDP	60 (seq)	CT-RT	13.2	32	0.04
		+Vbl		HFXRT (69.6 Gy)	12.0	24	ND
				RT	11.4	21	

CAMP, cyclophosphamide, doxorubicin, methotrexate, procarbazine; CDDP, cisplatin; con, concurrent; CT, chemotherapy; HFXRT, hyperfractionated radiation therapy; MACC, methotrexate, doxorubicin, cyclophosphamide, lomustine; ND, no difference; RT, radiotherapy; seq, sequential; VCPC, vindesine, cyclophosphamide, cisplatin, lomustine; Vbl, vinblastine; VP-16, etoposide.
[a]From survival curve.
[b]Survival at 3 years.

used postoperatively, when a higher total dose can be given. Proponents of concurrent preoperative chemoradiation believe that this approach provides adequate systemic treatment of micrometastatic disease and more effective control of bulky primary and mediastinal tumors.

Neoadjuvant Trials of Chemotherapy Alone before Resection. One of the best-known early trials to demonstrate the feasibility of combining induction chemotherapy with subsequent pulmonary resection in patients with stage III NSCLC was developed by Martini et al.[126] at Memorial Sloan-Kettering Cancer Center. In 1984, they initiated a trial of high-dose, cisplatin-based (120 mg/m^2) chemotherapy followed by resection for patients with clinical N2 disease. Vindesine or vinblastine and subsequently mitomycin were added to form the so-called "MVP" regimen. Postoperative radiation was given to patients who had persistent mediastinal nodal tumor at thoracotomy, and all patients received two additional cycles of chemotherapy postoperatively. In 136 patients treated from 1984 to 1991, the major response rate to induction chemotherapy was 77% (105/136), and the complete resection rate was 65% (89/136). A complete pathologic response was noted in 19 patients (21%) at the time of resection. The overall survival at 5 years was 17% and the median survival was 19 months: a distinct improvement over the historical survival for this group of patients. Seven treatment-related deaths (5%) occurred in this study, five of which were postoperative.

A phase II trial, reported by the CALGB in 1995, of induction chemotherapy enrolled 74 patients, treated with two cycles of cisplatin (100 mg/m^2 on days 1 and 29) and vinblastine (5 mg/m^2 per week) without mitomycin followed by resection for patients with mediastinoscopy-proven stage IIIA N2 disease.[127] In addition, two cycles of chemotherapy and 59.4 Gy of radiation were given postoperatively. Sixty-three patients (85%) had either an objective response or stable disease after induction therapy and underwent thoracotomy, with an operative mortality rate of 3.2%. Twenty-three patients (37% of thoracotomies, 31% of all patients) had a complete resection, with 3-year survival of 46%. The overall 3-year survival was 23%. The lower resectability rate in this trial than in the study performed at Memorial Sloan-Kettering potentially reflects both the multi-institutional nature of this trial and the use of a less intensive chemotherapy regimen (primarily because of the omission of mitomycin). However, the overall long-term survival appears similar for the two trials.

Trials of Induction Chemoradiation Followed by Resection. The second approach to combined-modality therapy and resection for stage III NSCLC has been to combine chemotherapy and radiation preoperatively (Table 79.10).

TABLE 79.10 **RESULTS**

RESULTS OF REPRESENTATIVE NEOADJUVANT TRIALS FOR STAGE III NON–SMALL CELL LUNG CANCER: INDUCTION CHEMORADIOTHERAPY FOLLOWED BY RESECTION

STUDY	NO. PATIENTS	CHEMOTHERAPY	RADIOTHERAPY (Gy)	SURVIVAL MEDIAN (mo)	SURVIVAL OVERALL (%)
Rush-Presbyterian, Faber et al., 1989[130]	IIIA: 85 (including 19 N0)	CDDP (60 mg/m^2) + 5-FU ± VP-16 × 4	40(S), 20 fractions	21.7	40 (3 y)
LCSG, Weiden et al., 1991[129]	IIIA, IIIB: 85	CDDP (75 mg/m^2) + 5-FU × 2	30(C), 5 fractions	13	22 (2 y)[a]
CALGB, Strauss et al., 1992[131]	IIIA: 41 (including 8 N0–1)	CDDP (100 mg/m^2) + Vbl + 5-FU × 2	30(C), 15 fractions	15.5	30 (2 y)[a]
SWOG, Albain et al., 1995[132]	IIIA, IIIB: 126	CDDP (50 mg/m^2 days 1 and 8) + VP-16 × 2	45(C), 30 fractions	13 (IIIA) 17 (IIIB)	37 (2 y) (IIIA) 39 (2 y) (IIIB)
M.D. Anderson, Taylor et al., 2004[137]	IIIA: 107 (including 21 N1)	CDDP-based or carboplatin/paclitaxel	None	31	33 (5 y)
		CDDP + Vbl	Daily, 60–63 (C)	27	30 (5 y)
		CDDP + VP-16	69.6 (H)		
North American Intergroup, Albain et al., 2003[224]	Resection: 201 patients	CDDP (50 mg/m^2) + VP-16 × 4; 2 cycles consolidation	45 (C)	22.0 (OS), 13.4 (PFS)	3 y: 37 (OS) 27 (PFS)
	No surgery: 191	CDDP (55 mg/m^2) + VP-16	61 (C)	22.3 (OS)	3 y: 34 (OS)
	(264 patients eligible)		45, twice daily	11.8 (PFS)	19 (PFS)
German Lung Cancer Cooperative Group, Thomas et al., 2008[139]	131 resected[b]	Carboplatin + vindesine		32.4 (OS)	3 y: 48 (OS)
	CT			19.6 (PFS)	36 (PFS)
	CRT surgery (260 patients eligible)			33 (OS)	3 y: 45 (OS)
	141 resected[b]	CDDP (55 mg/m^2) + VP-16		21.3 (PFS)	37 (PFS)
	CT surgery		54, daily		
	PORT				

5-FU, 5-fluorouracil; (C), continuous course; CALGB, Cancer and Leukemia Group B; CDDP, cisplatin; (H), hyperfractionated; LCSG, Lung Cancer Study Group; OS, overall survival; PFS, progression-free survival; PORT, postoperative radiation therapy; RTOG, Radiation Therapy Oncology Group; (S), split course; SWOG, Southwest Oncology Group; Vbl, vinblastine; VP-16, etoposide.
[a]From survival curve.
[b]Survival data for patients found to be resectable at thoracotomy.

This strategy aims to control micrometastatic disease while utilizing the synergism of concurrent radiation and chemotherapy to reduce tumor bulk in the primary site and mediastinum. In one of the first trials of this type, performed by the North American LCSG, 39 patients with stage III NSCLC received three cycles of chemotherapy with cyclophosphamide, doxorubicin, and cisplatin (CAP) and 1,500 cGy of radiation in 300-cGy fractions given concurrently with cycles 2 and 3 of the chemotherapy. The overall response rate to induction therapy was 51% (20/39), and 33% (13/39) of patients had a complete resection at thoracotomy. However, the overall 2-year survival was only 8%, with a median survival of 11 months. No treatment-related deaths occurred.[128]

The LCSG subsequently performed another phase II induction trial of cisplatin, 5-fluorouracil, and partially concurrent low-dose radiation (3,000 cGy in 15 fractions) in 85 patients with stage IIIA N2 or stage IIIB NSCLC.[129] Although the cisplatin dose in this trial was higher than in the previous study (75 instead of 60 mg/m^2 per dose), the overall response rate and complete resection rates were similar (56% and 34%). The median survival was 13 months. Four of 54 patients (7%) died postoperatively.

Faber et al.[130] at Rush-Presbyterian performed two sequential phase II neoadjuvant trials of 5-fluorouracil and low-dose cisplatin (60 mg/m^2) plus 4,000 cGy of split-course radiation administered concurrently with the four cycles of induction chemotherapy. The second group of 74 patients also received etoposide in addition to the cisplatin and 5-fluorouraci1. Of the 130 patients entered into these trials, 85 were candidates for surgery after induction therapy, and 62 (73%) underwent thoracotomy. The complete resection rate was 68% (58/85), and the overall survival rate was 40% at 3 years, with a median survival of 22 months. The induction therapy was associated with significant toxicity, but only one treatment-related death occurred. The operative mortality rate was 5% (3/62). The excellent results of these trials may reflect the inclusion of some patients who did not have N2 disease but were considered at that time to have stage III NSCLC by virtue of T3 (chest wall) N0 tumor status.

A neoadjuvant trial of similar design was performed by the CALGB in which high-dose cisplatin (100 mg/m^2), vinblastine, and 5-fluorouracil were given with 3,000 cGy of continuous radiation in 15 fractions to patients with stage IIIA disease.[131] The overall response rate was 51% (21/41), and the complete resection rate was 61% (25/41). The median survival was 15.5 months. Significant toxicity occurred, and treatment-related mortality was high at 15% (6/41).

The largest reported phase II neoadjuvant trial of concurrent chemotherapy and radiation was a multi-institutional study performed by the Southwest Oncology Group.[132] Both stage IIIA and stage IIIB patients were entered, although notably, pathologic documentation of the initial tumor stage, usually by mediastinoscopy, was required. The induction regimen included two cycles of cisplatin (50 mg/m^2 on days 1 and 8) and etoposide with 4,500 cGy of concurrent radiation in 25 fractions. All patients underwent thoracotomy unless their disease progressed. The objective response rate to induction therapy in the 126 eligible patients was 59%. The resectability rates were 85% for the IIIA N2 group and 80% for the IIIB group. Nearly two thirds of the patients had no viable tumor or only minimal residual foci of tumor in their surgical specimens. The 3-year survival rate was 27% for the IIIA group and 24% for the IIIB group, with median survival of 13 and 17 months, respectively. The best predictor of survival after surgery was the absence of tumor in the mediastinal nodes at surgery (3-year survival of 44%). The majority of recurrences were distant, and the brain was the single most common site. The operative mortality rate was 6%, and the overall treatment-related mortality was 10%. An important finding of SWOG 8805 was that survival was the same for patients with stage IIIB NSCLC by virtue of T4 tumor status and patients with stage IIIA N2 disease. Patients with N3 disease had a poor overall survival. Importantly, the long-term follow-up of this study showed that the survival rates at 3 years were sustained at 6 years.[133]

Important differences between the Southwest Oncology Group trial and earlier neoadjuvant trials were the careful documentation of pretreatment stage, the use of a higher dose of continuous radiation (4,500 cGy rather than 3,000 cGy of continuous or 4,000 cGy of split-course radiation), and the fully concurrent manner in which the chemotherapy and radiation were administered. Early attempts to intensify this therapeutic approach by increasing or accelerating the radiation were associated with unacceptable toxicity. Two small single-institution trials illustrate this problem. Yashar et al.[134] treated 36 patients who had stage IIIA N2 disease with two cycles of cisplatin (25 mg/m^2 per day for 4 days) and etoposide and 55 Gy of concurrent radiation. All patients underwent exploratory thoracotomy, and 31 (86%) underwent resection, 27 with pneumonectomy. Although the overall 3-year survival rate was 34%, two operative deaths (5.6%) occurred, six patients required prolonged intubation because of postoperative acute respiratory distress syndrome (ARDS), and a bronchial stump leak developed in three patients.

In the second study, Fowler et al.[135] treated 13 patients who had stage IIIA N2 disease with two cycles of cisplatin (20 mg/m^2 per day for 4 days), 5-fluorouracil, and etoposide and 60 Gy of concurrent radiation in 30 fractions. Six patients then underwent lobectomy, and seven patients underwent pneumonectomy. The complication rate was unacceptably high; ARDS developed in one of the lobectomy patients and in five of the seven pneumonectomy patients, and was fatal in two patients. Bronchial stump leaks developed in three pneumonectomy patients, of whom one died. The trial was closed prematurely after 13 patients had been accrued because of the excessive morbidity and mortality. An additional 27 patients who received the same induction therapy but did not undergo thoracotomy tolerated the treatment without major problems.

Two additional trials have tested concurrent induction chemoradiation in stage III NSCLC. Milstein et al.[136] conducted a phase II trial in which 36 patients (10 with T3N0 or T3Nl disease and 11 with IIIB disease) received two cycles of cisplatin (25 mg/m^2) and etoposide plus concurrent radiation to 50 Gy during 28 sessions. Twenty-four patients (21 with IIIA and three with IIIB disease) underwent thoracotomy, with complete resection in 20 (86%). Three of the 21 IIIA patients had complete tumor sterilization. The overall survival at 2 years was 39% (57% for resectable patients and 15% for unresectable patients), and the median survival was 15 months. One death from sepsis occurred during the induction treatment, and two postoperative deaths resulted from ARDS and bronchopleural fistula. This attempt to intensify induction chemoradiation by increasing the dose of radiation was not successful.

One study from the University of Texas M. D. Anderson Cancer Center addresses the question of whether radiation augments the benefit of induction chemotherapy before resection.[137] This retrospective review identified 107 patients who underwent resection for stage IIIA disease. Patients had been treated with induction chemotherapy (55 patients) with cisplatin (100 mg/m^2) or carboplatin/Taxol; concurrent chemoradiation (15 patients) with cisplatin (75 mg/m^2) and vinblastine plus daily radiation to 60 to 63 Gy; or concurrent chemoradiation (37 patients) with cisplatin (50 mg/m^2) and etoposide plus hyperfractionated radiation to 69.6 Gy. Postoperatively, 35 patients treated with induction chemotherapy received adjuvant radiation therapy.

A North America Intergroup clinical trial sought to determine whether neoadjuvant therapy including resection is superior to nonsurgical treatment with chemotherapy and higher-dose radiation in patients with stage IIIA NSCLC. In the Intergroup 0139/RTOG 9309 trial,[138] patients with proven pN2, stage IIIA NSCLC were randomized to receive neoadjuvant chemotherapy with concurrent thoracic radiation therapy (TRT) followed by operation or continuation with definitive TRT.

Of 429 patients accrued over 92 months, 392 patients were considered eligible and were treated with cisplatin (50 mg/m^2) on days 1 and 8 and etoposide (50 mg/m^2) on days 1 through 5 every 3 weeks for two cycles, as well as 45 Gy TRT. Patients randomized to resection (n = 201) underwent operation 4 to 6 weeks later. Patients randomized to definitive radiation (n = 191) continued without break to a total of 61 Gy. Following operation or completion of TRT, consolidation with two cycles of cisplatin and etoposide was given. Of note, less than two thirds of patients undergoing operation received consolidation treatment, compared with over 75% of patients receiving chemoradiation only. There was no mortality in either group during induction chemoradiation. Surgical mortality was 7%, with 12 of 14 deaths occurring in patients undergoing pneumonectomy.

Progression-free survival (PFS) was improved from a median of 11.8 months to 13.4 months, and 3-year PFS from 19% to 27% with the addition of surgery. There appeared to be improved local control with the addition of surgery, with local failure occurring in only 5% of surgically treated patients compared with 16% in the nonsurgical group, although this was not statistically significant. However, no statistically significant differences were seen in overall survival, with 3-year survival of 34% and 37% for the chemoradiation alone and chemoradiation and surgery groups, respectively. Survival for patients undergoing complete resection in this study has not yet been published. This study indicated that carefully selected patients with N2-positive stage IIIA NSCLC can be treated with multimodality therapy including resection.

The role of surgery for patients whose tumors appear to require pneumonectomy remains controversial as well. In the recently published German Lung Cancer Study Group trial, patients were randomized to induction chemotherapy (cisplatin and etoposide) followed by chemoradiation (concurrent carboplatin and vindesine) followed by resection, or induction chemotherapy followed by surgery alone. Of 524 patients deemed eligible, randomized, and started on treatment, 296 underwent operation and 272 underwent tumor resection. In an intention-to-treat analysis of patients eligible and randomized to different arms of this study, no differences in progression-free or overall survival were observed between the treatment groups. Patients receiving preoperative chemoradiation were more likely to achieve complete resection among those with resectable tumors (98/131 vs. 84/141, $p = 0.008$), and were more likely to have evidence for mediastinal downstaging and pathologic response, but again with no significant difference observed in progression-free or overall survival. Of 104 patients who required pneumonectomy, including 39 right sided, for resection, mortality was slightly greater among patients treated with preoperative chemoradiation (7/50 vs. 3/54), but this was not statistically significant.[139] Parenchymal-preserving bronchoplastic techniques also can be considered for those patients who might otherwise require pneumonectomy.[140] Whether such technically challenging approaches can be undertaken in the setting of recent radiation therapy remains to be established.

Stimulated by the promising results of the Southwest Oncology Group 8805 trial for patients with T4 disease, Grunenwald et al.[113] performed a phase II trial of similar design for stage IIIB T4 NSCLC. The induction regimen consisted of cisplatin (100 mg/m^2), 5-fluorouracil, and vinblastine with 45 Gy of concurrent hyperfractionated (twice daily) radiation. Of 25 patients enrolled, 16 were subsequently eligible for surgery, and 12 had complete resection. No induction treatment–related or operative deaths occurred. This study confirms that complete resection after induction therapy is feasible in a significant number of stage IIIB T4 tumors, a subset of stage IIIB tumors previously considered inoperable under any circumstances.

6 Current Status of Neoadjuvant Therapy and Resection. Taken as a whole, neoadjuvant therapy trials have demonstrated the feasibility of induction chemotherapy and resection for the treatment of stage III NSCLC. Most studies show improved rates of resectability and survival in comparison with the historical experience for resection or radiation alone. The optimal treatment approach to these locally advanced tumors has not yet been fully defined, especially because neoadjuvant trials vary with respect to eligibility criteria, inclusion of both stage IIIA and stage IIIB tumors, accuracy of pretreatment staging, and type of induction regimens. Moreover, the response, resectability, and survival rates are not uniformly reported. In some cases, instead of reporting results as a percentage of the total number of patients entered into the study, the authors report resectability rates as a percentage of the patients with a radiographic response, and only the survival rates of patients who underwent resection are emphasized.

The potential toxicity of neoadjuvant regimens should not be overlooked. Induction regimens in which high-dose cisplatin ($\geq$100 mg/m^2) or radiation doses of 4,000 to 4,500 cGy are used have been well tolerated, but radiation doses of 5,500 cGy or higher have been associated with an excessive risk for postoperative ARDS and bronchial stump leak. Good response rates have been achieved with chemotherapeutic agents including paclitaxel, docetaxel, gemcitabine, and carboplatin, and they are better tolerated by patients. Determining the contribution of these agents in combined-modality therapy will require further trials, especially as the major form of relapse continues to be distant metastatic disease.

7 Future Directions. In addition to new chemotherapeutic agents, new radiation techniques, such as hyperfractionated or accelerated schedules, also merit further exploration in neoadjuvant trials with concurrent chemotherapy. Adelstein et al.,[141] from the Cleveland Clinic, conducted a study in which 45 patients with stage IIIA or IIIB NSCLC received induction cisplatin, paclitaxel, and 30 Gy of accelerated hyperfractionated radiation therapy (1.5-Gy fraction twice daily). Surgery was then performed approximately 4 weeks after induction. The overall response rate was 54%. Forty patients (89%) proceeded to surgery, and 32 patients (71%) underwent complete resection. Five complete pathologic remissions were seen. Fourteen patients overall were downstaged. Patients received a consolidation dose of chemotherapy and additional radiation to a total of 60 to 63 Gy. The 2-year relapse-free survival rate was 47%, and the 2-year survival rate was 65%. No apparent therapy-related deaths occurred, but the toxicity was high, with 89% of patients experiencing significant mucositis and 20% experiencing esophagitis of grade 3 or worse. Three-dimensional conformal therapy permits higher radiation dosing (>70 Gy) of the tumor while sparing surrounding normal lung in order to provide improved local control.[142,143]

The management of stage III NSCLC is complex and still evolving. Many trials indicate that resectability and survival rates are probably improved with the use of combined-modality therapy than with radiation or resection alone. Regimens incorporating high-dose cisplatin with or without moderate-dose radiation have achieved the best results with acceptable levels of toxicity. Careful patient management leads to complete resection, and the operative risk is comparable with that of standard pulmonary resection. Importantly, combined-modality treatment requires close collaboration among medical oncologists, radiation oncologists, surgeons, pulmonologists, and anesthesiologists. In the future, three key areas warrant further investigation: (a) the optimal combination and sequence of newer, less toxic chemotherapeutic agents and a variety of new radiation techniques; (b) whether concurrent chemoradiation is superior to chemotherapy alone as preoperative induction therapy; and (c) the identification of the molecular features that dictate tumor response to different chemotherapeutic agents, allowing a more individualized selection of induction treatment regimens, which may lead to improved long-term outcomes.

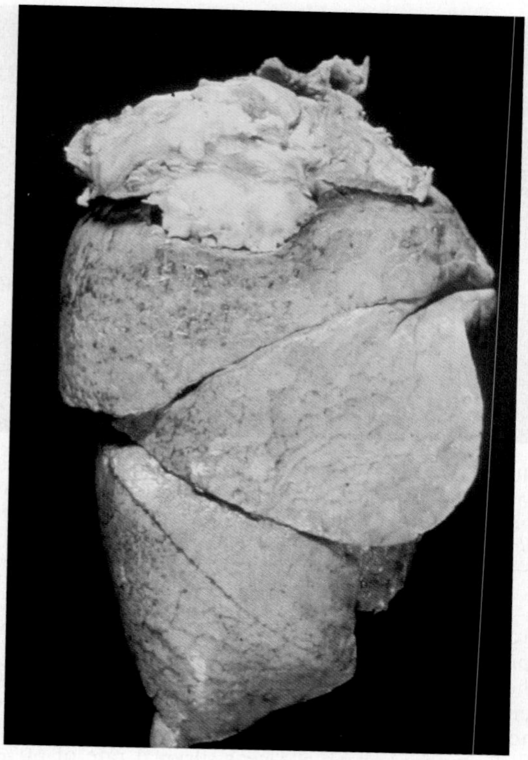

FIGURE 79.2. Gross figure of a squamous cell carcinoma showing a superior sulcus tumor (*Pancoast tumor*) arising from apex of the right lung. (Reproduced with permission from Cagle PT. *Color Atlas and Text of Pulmonary Pathology*. Philadelphia, PA: Lippincott Williams & Wilkins; 2005.)

Superior Sulcus Tumors. Tumors of the superior sulcus (Fig. 79.2), described in detail by H. K. Pancoast in 1932,[144] represent an uncommon (3%) and challenging subset of NSCLC. Tumors frequently involve the brachial plexus, subclavian vessels, or spine and typically fall into two categories: T3N0–1 (stage IIB or IIIA) or T4N0–1 (stage IIIB).[145] Until the 1950s, these tumors were felt to be almost universally fatal, with no benefit provided by resection. In 1961, Shaw and Paulson demonstrated that preoperative thoracic radiation followed by resection was potentially curative.[146] For the subsequent 30 to 35 years, reports demonstrated 5-year survival of approximately of 25% to 30%. In a single-institutional experience spanning 24 years, during which 225 patients underwent thoracotomy at Memorial Sloan-Kettering Cancer Center, 5-year survival for patients undergoing resection for stage IIB, IIIA, and IIIB superior sulcus tumors was 46%, 0%, and 13%, respectively.[147] In this retrospective study, the mode of preoperative therapy, with radiation and/or chemotherapy, or adjuvant therapy did not appear to affect survival, which was influenced only by completeness of resection and tumor and nodal status in a multivariate analysis. As in other retrospective series, locoregional recurrence was the most common form of relapse, occurring in 40% of patients.[148]

Spurred by reports of the apparent success of neoadjuvant chemotherapy and thoracic radiation in achieving improved local control and survival for patients with locoregionally advanced NSCLC, the Southwestern Oncology Group coordinated a phase II trial, the first prospective, multicenter trial (SWOG 9416/Intergroup 0160) for superior sulcus tumors.[149] Of 111 patients eligible, including 31 patients with T4 disease, 102 completed induction chemoradiation and 95 were eligible for operation. Patients with mediastinal lymph node metastases (N2) were excluded from this trial. Of the 88 patients who underwent thoracotomy, over 90% had a complete resection, with 65% of patients demonstrating complete pathologic response (R0) or minimal residual disease (R1). Overall treatment mortality was 4.5%, including an operative mortality of 2.4%. Of note, intracranial and other distant metastases were more common (22% each) than locally recurrent disease only (11%). Overall 2- and 5-year survival was 55% and 41% for all patients enrolled, and 70% and 53% for patients with a complete response, respectively.

NEUROENDOCRINE TUMORS

Neuroendocrine tumors of the lung include a varied group of lesions ranging from tumors with low-grade malignant potential (typical carcinoid) to SCLC, which is among the most rapidly growing and aggressive of human tumors. Between those two extremes, atypical carcinoid and large cell neuroendocrine carcinoma have been defined.[150]

Typical and Atypical Carcinoid Tumors

Carcinoid tumors, which are neoplasms with a low-grade malignant potential, account for about 2% of lung tumors in the United States. They arise from neuroendocrine stem cells of the bronchial epithelium and are classified as either typical or atypical. Histologically, typical carcinoids consist of uniform polygonal cells with round nuclei and fine granular chromatin (Fig. 79.3). Mitotic figures are rare. Atypical carcinoids show increased mitotic activity, nuclear pleomorphism, areas of disorganized architecture, and tumor necrosis[151] (Fig. 79.4).

Carcinoid tumors occur equally in both sexes and at a median age of 55 years. Half of patients present with pulmonary symptoms, including hemoptysis, dyspnea, and recurrent or persistent pneumonitis, because 40% of lesions are centrally located in the main or lobar bronchi (Figs. 79.5 and 79.6). The lesions may be diagnosed by bronchoscopy, appearing as pink or purple friable endobronchial masses covered by intact epithelium. In the other half of patients, carcinoid tumors are diagnosed when radiologic abnormalities are detected on a chest roentgenogram as part of a routine examination.[152]

Lymph node metastases occur in approximately 10% to 15% of patients at diagnosis but are more frequent in atypical carcinoids. The carcinoid syndrome is associated with bronchial carcinoids in only 2% of cases, usually in patients

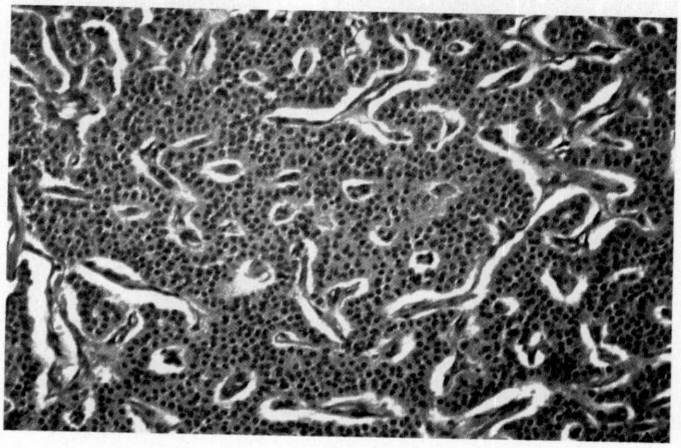

FIGURE 79.3. Typical carcinoid tumor of the lung. A microscopic view shows ribbons of tumor cells embedded in a vascular stroma. (Reproduced with permission from Rubin E, Farber JL. *Pathology*, 3rd ed. Philadelphia, PA: Lippincott Williams & Wilkins; 1999.)

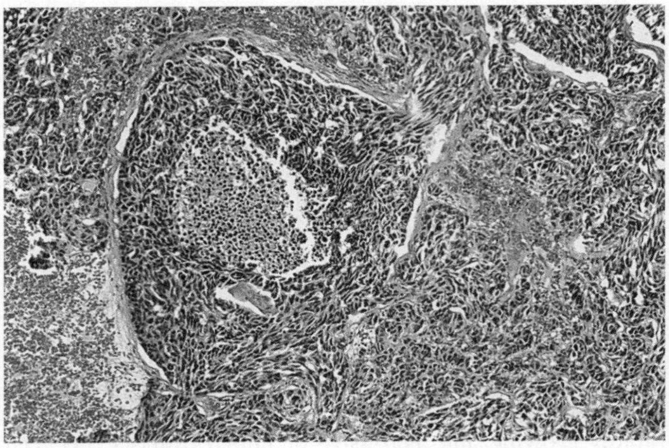

FIGURE 79.4. Atypical carcinoid tumor of the lung. A cellular tumor shows central necrosis and a disorganized architecture. (Reproduced with permission from Rubin E, Farber JL. *Pathology*, 3rd ed. Philadelphia, PA: Lippincott Williams & Wilkins; 1999.)

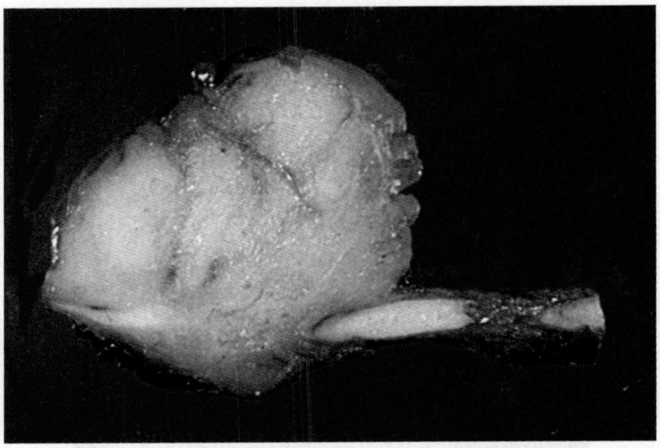

FIGURE 79.6. Gross figure of a resected carcinoid tumor cut in cross section to show invasion through the bronchial cartilage. (Reproduced with permission from Cagle PT. *Color Atlas and Text of Pulmonary Pathology*. Philadelphia, PA: Lippincott Williams & Wilkins; 2005.)

with metastatic disease, particularly of the liver. The most common sites of metastases are lung, bone, liver, adrenals, and brain.[152]

The standard treatment for bronchial carcinoid is complete resection, regardless of the presence of nodal involvement, with mediastinal lymph node sampling or dissection.[153] Lobectomy is required in about 50% of patients. Lesser resection (segmentectomy, sleeve resection) is adequate for complete resection in about 20% of patients. Endoscopic resection is invariably associated with local recurrence and should be used only as a palliative maneuver in patients whose general medical condition precludes thoracotomy and pulmonary resection.[152]

The long-term survival rate after resection exceeds 90% in patients with typical carcinoids, even when hilar or mediastinal nodal metastases are present. In contrast, patients with atypical carcinoids have a 5-year survival rate of 60% after complete resection. The outcome is more closely linked to histology than to tumor size, location, or nodal involvement. Recurrence is more frequent with tumors larger than 3 cm and in patients who present with lymph node metastases.[152]

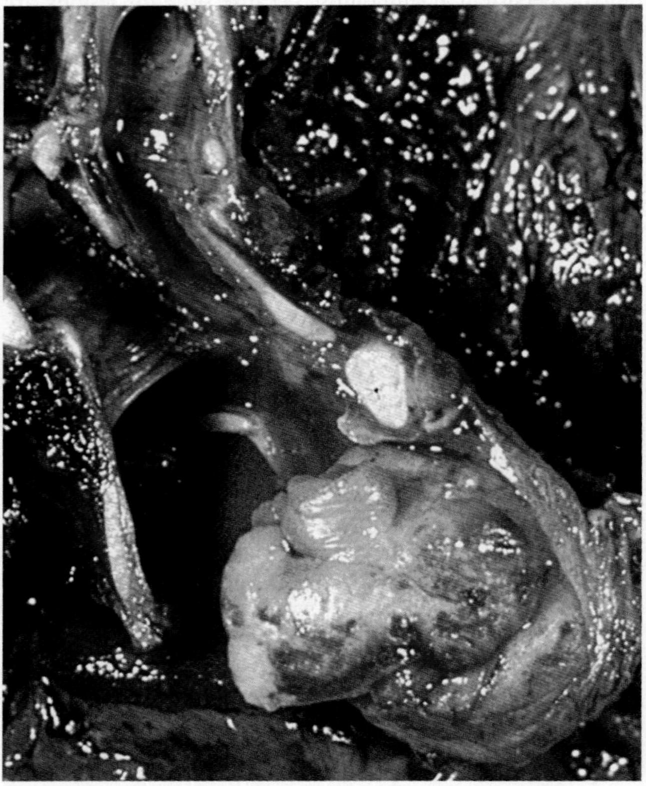

FIGURE 79.5. Gross figure of a carcinoid tumor protruding into the bronchial lumen. (Reproduced with permission from Cagle PT. *Color Atlas and Text of Pulmonary Pathology*. Philadelphia, PA: Lippincott Williams & Wilkins; 2005.)

Large Cell Neuroendocrine Carcinomas

Large cell neuroendocrine carcinoma is characterized by the microscopic features of neuroendocrine tumors, but the tumor cells are large, have a high mitotic rate, and frequently show necrosis[150,151] (Fig. 79.7). According to Travis et al.,[154,155] large cell neuroendocrine carcinomas are related to smoking, as is SCLC, and are high-grade tumors with 5- and 10-year survival

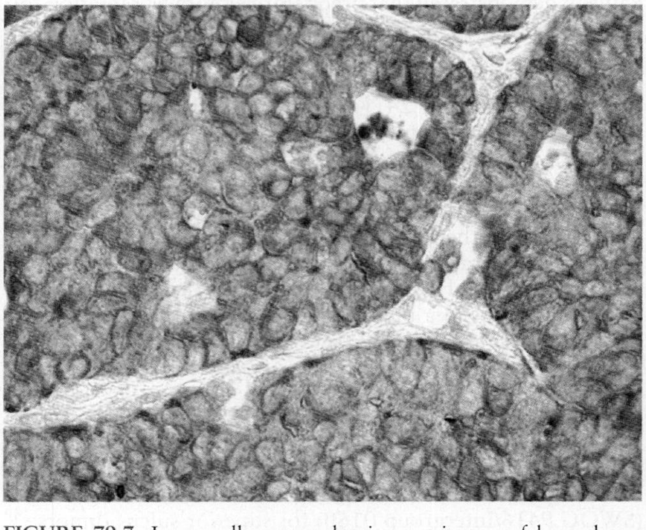

FIGURE 79.7. Large cell neuroendocrine carcinoma of lung shows positive immunostaining with synaptophysin antibody. (Reproduced with permission from Cagle PT. *Color Atlas and Text of Pulmonary Pathology*. Philadelphia, PA: Lippincott Williams & Wilkins; 2005.)

rates of 27% and 9%, respectively, despite complete resection. Few data are available concerning adjuvant therapy. For the time being, the management of large cell neuroendocrine carcinoma is identical to that of NSCLC.[156]

Small Cell Lung Cancer

Small cell carcinoma of the lung has the most aggressive clinical course of any type of pulmonary tumor and is often widely disseminated by the time of diagnosis. In contrast to non–small cell tumors, these lesions are notably responsive to chemotherapy and are rarely within the domain of the surgeon. The staging system for SCLC was developed by the Veterans Administration Lung Cancer Staging Group and divides patients into those with limited and those with extensive disease. This distinction was first based on what could be encompassed by a tolerable radiation portal. After clarification by the International Association for the Study of Lung Cancer, limited disease includes patients with tumors confined to one hemithorax and regional lymph nodes (hilar, ipsilateral, and contralateral mediastinal nodes, and ipsilateral and contralateral supraclavicular nodes) as well as patients with ipsilateral pleural effusion, regardless of whether the cytology is positive or negative. On the other hand, both pericardial and bilateral pulmonary involvement are considered extensive disease.[157]

Common sites of distant metastases are bone, liver, bone marrow, and the central nervous system, and therefore the metastatic evaluation includes a bone scan and CT of the chest, abdomen, and brain. Some oncologists also perform bone marrow biopsies, but because the marrow is the sole site of extensive disease in fewer than 5% of patients, biopsies are usually judged unnecessary. After the staging process, approximately 30% to 40% of patients are found to have limited disease.

For patients with limited disease, response rates of 85% to 90% and complete response rates of 50% to 60% can be expected with the combination of etoposide and cisplatin and radiation therapy.[158] The median survival is 18 to 24 months, and the 2-year survival rates are 40% to 50% (5% more than before the use of radiation therapy).[159,160] In extensive SCLC treated with chemotherapy, response rates reach 75% to 85%, although complete response is seen in only 15% to 25% of patients. The median survival is between 7 and 11 months, with a 2-year survival near zero. The prognosis in SCLC depends primarily on the anatomic extent of disease, but after a review of prognostic variables in its 2,580-patient SCLC database, the Southwest Oncology Group determined that the two-stage system should be extended into a four-stage system, with serum lactate dehydrogenase level, age, and pleural effusion used as additional staging criteria.[161]

The small numbers of patients with SCLC seen by the surgeon represent fewer than 10% of all patients with SCLC. They have peripheral tumors with no nodal involvement or only hilar nodal involvement, which would be classified as T1–2 N0–1 tumors in the NSCLC staging system. In the past, such tumors were often diagnosed at exploratory thoracotomy for an asymptomatic coin lesion, but with the increasing use of diagnostic percutaneous needle aspiration, more patients with early-stage SCLC are now identified preoperatively. Such patients should be evaluated in conjunction with a medical oncologist, and resection should be considered after distant disease has been excluded by a complete metastatic evaluation. For such cases, it has been suggested that the TNM classification be used in future trials and studies.[162]

Retrospective series have demonstrated a 5-year survival rate of 30% to 50% after resection of T1 N0 or T2 N0 SCLC.[162–164] Because of the propensity for small cell cancers to disseminate, adjuvant chemotherapy has traditionally been given to patients after resection, even though, by virtue of the small numbers of patients available, no prospective randomized trials have demonstrated whether this is of benefit.[164] Relapse at the primary site, which is a problem for most patients with limited-stage SCLC, is distinctly uncommon after complete resection of these early tumors.[165] Radiation therapy to the chest has been suggested after surgically complete resection, but because insufficient information is available in the literature and local relapse is uncommon, it cannot be considered a standard treatment.[163,164]

Because the role of resection in patients with mediastinal nodal involvement (N2 disease) is questionable, mediastinoscopy should be considered mandatory to exclude mediastinal nodal disease.[166] This should ideally be performed separately from thoracotomy because it can be difficult for the pathologist to diagnose small cell cancer on a frozen section. The intraoperative management of SCLC is not significantly different from that of NSCLC, and an incomplete resection does not benefit the patient.

The addition of resection after a response to induction chemotherapy has been proposed by some surgeons to cure a small number of patients with limited SCLC without mediastinal involvement.[167] To date, the LCSG has performed the only prospective randomized trial evaluating the role of surgery in limited SCLC.[168] All patients enrolled in that study received chemotherapy, and those in whom at least a partial response was achieved were randomized to undergo or not undergo surgery. Because the survival rate was the same in both groups, this trial did not support the addition of pulmonary resection to the multimodality treatment of SCLC. Finally, the occurrence of a second primary lung carcinoma after treatment for SCLC has been reported in the few patients with prolonged survival. It should not be assumed that the new tumor is of small cell histology, and these patients should be evaluated for the possibility of resection.[169] The average risk for the development of a second lung cancer in patients who survive SCLC is approximately 6% per patient per year.[83]

BRONCHIAL GLAND CARCINOMAS

Bronchial gland carcinomas are rare primary tumors of the lung. They constitute about 1% of all lung neoplasms and 2% of the tumors for which resection is performed. These tumors are also called primary salivary gland–type tumors of the lung because the tracheal and bronchial airway submucosa and the salivary glands contain serous and mucous glands that are histologically similar.[170] Often, they are called bronchial adenomas, but this term is misleading because they are malignant. Care must be taken to separate these primary tumors from metastases of primitive salivary gland tumors.[171] This group of carcinomas includes adenoid cystic carcinoma, mucoepidermoid carcinoma, and the even rarer mixed tumor (pleomorphic adenoma). The only truly benign tumors are mucous gland adenomas.

The symptomatology of these tumors is determined essentially by their location and size.[171] Peripheral tumors, which are less frequent, are asymptomatic, generally presenting as a nodule on routine chest radiography. Proximally located tumors present with symptoms of bronchial irritation and obstruction, including cough, shortness of breath, hemoptysis, recurrent infection, wheezing, and stridor. Sometimes, patients have constitutional symptoms, such as weight loss and pain. On chest radiography, the nodule may be seen with pneumonia or atelectasis. Because of the slow growth of these tumors, signs and symptoms may develop over a period of years. Incompletely obstructing tumors frequently masquerade as asthma for prolonged periods of time. Smoking does not seem to be a risk factor for these tumors.

Peripheral tumors are diagnosed by percutaneous needle aspiration biopsy or at the time of thoracotomy. Tumors in major airways are diagnosed by bronchoscopy. Other studies, such as CT, are rarely required to make the diagnosis but may be of value in planning therapy. Because most of these tumors do not metastasize, complete excision, with preservation of as much pulmonary tissue as possible, is the goal. Whenever possible, sleeve resections of main bronchi are performed to preserve pulmonary tissue.

Adenoid Cystic Carcinoma

Adenoid cystic carcinomas are slowly growing malignant tumors that arise from the submucosal glands of the trachea and main bronchi (Fig. 79.8). They have also been called cylindromas, adenoid cystic basal cell carcinomas, adenomyoepitheliomas, and pseudoadenomatous basal cell carcinomas. Adenoid cystic carcinomas behave much like the major and minor salivary gland tumors of the same name, to which they are microscopically identical. An important aspect of their clinical behavior is that they tend to spread in the submucosal plane along the perineural lymphatics, well beyond the obvious endoluminal component of the tumor (Fig. 79.9). In a small biopsy specimen, it can be difficult to distinguish adenoid cystic carcinoma from a conventional adenocarcinoma. Immunohistochemical stains may help the pathologist differentiate the two by showing the presence of the myoepithelial cell immunophenotype in adenoid cystic carcinoma.[171]

Whenever possible, total excision by tracheal resection or tracheobronchial resection is the treatment of choice.[172–175] This is not always possible because of the extensive submucosal spread of tumor. In such cases, palliative resection may be necessary. Postoperative radiation is indicated because these tumors are radiation sensitive.

When no resection is feasible because of the extent of the lesion, a palliative treatment option is endoscopic laser removal followed by radiation (brachytherapy, external beam irradiation, or both). When complete resection is possible, the prognosis is excellent. However, because of the slow-growing nature of the tumor and its responsiveness to radiation, prolonged survival is possible even with incomplete resection or palliative measures. Patients frequently live 10 years or more with persistent disease, including pulmonary metastases. In such cases, repeated efforts at palliation are indicated.

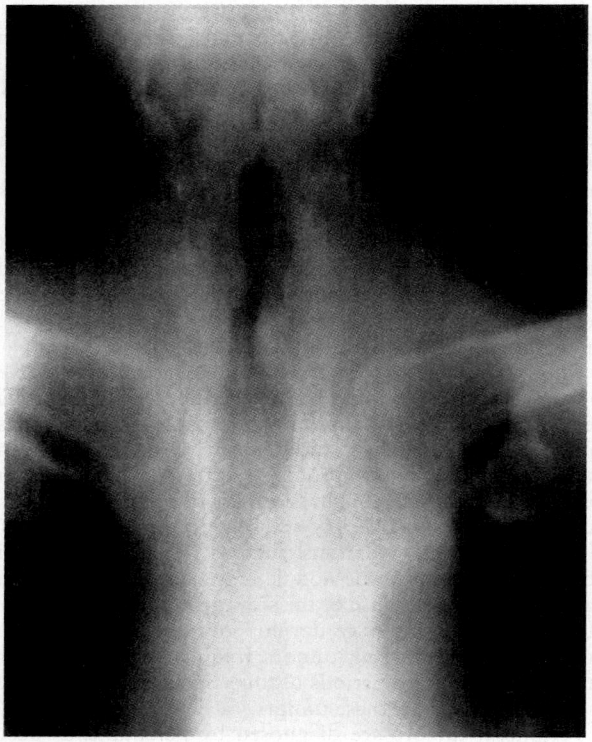

FIGURE 79.8. Tracheogram demonstrating airway obstruction by an adenoid cystic carcinoma of the upper trachea.

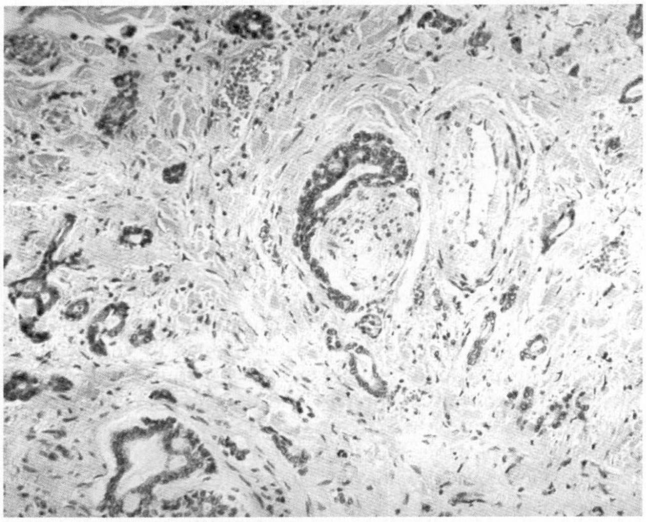

FIGURE 79.9. Adenoid cystic carcinoma. A photomicrograph shows perineural infiltration by the tumor. (Reproduced with permission from Rubin E, Farber JL. *Pathology*, 3rd ed. Philadelphia, PA: Lippincott Williams & Wilkins; 1999.)

Mucoepidermoid Carcinoma

Mucoepidermoid carcinomas may be of low- or high-grade malignancy and have the same microscopic appearance as mucoepidermoid tumors of salivary gland origin. These tumors also arise in the glandular submucosa, presenting as submucosal lesions. The distinction between low-grade and high-grade tumor is based on mitotic activity, cellular necrosis, and nuclear pleomorphism.[170]

The principles of treatment of mucoepidermoid tumors are similar to those of carcinoid tumors. The more malignant variety must be treated as bronchogenic carcinoma. Some authors even think that adenosquamous carcinoma is the same entity as mucoepidermoid carcinoma, but arising in the periphery of the lung.[170] The outlook for these tumors depends on the grade of malignancy and the stage of the disease. High-grade tumors have the same prognosis as bronchogenic carcinoma. Complete resection is the mainstay of treatment. Mucoepidermoid tumors are too rare to permit an evaluation of combined-modality therapy for more aggressive, high-grade tumors.[170]

Mucous Gland Adenoma

Mucous gland adenomas are rare submucosal tumors that arise from mucous glands. They are also known as bronchial cysts and papillary cystadenomas. Because of their totally benign behavior, they can usually be treated by endoscopic excision. Thoracotomy and resection are indicated only if the distal lung has been destroyed by chronic infection or if endoscopic removal is technically contraindicated or incomplete.

OTHER MALIGNANT TUMORS OF THE LUNG

The lung is composed of epithelial, mesodermal, and endodermal cells, and malignant tumors may arise from any of these cells. This group represents fewer than 1% of all primary lung cancers and is usually subdivided into lymphoid tumors, soft tissue sarcomas, mixed epithelial/mesenchymal tumors, and ectopic tissue tumors.[176,177] Primary pulmonary lymphomas usually are excised for confirmatory diagnosis. Sarcomas arising from soft tissue or large vessels are treated in a similar fashion to sarcomas occurring elsewhere. Treatment of the other rare tumors, including pulmonary blastomas, primary melanomas of the bronchus, and malignant teratomas, primarily involves complete resection. Radiation and chemotherapy do not have well-defined roles in the treatment of any of these tumors but are occasionally used in particular situations.

RESECTION OF PULMONARY METASTASES

Historical Background

The first report of the resection of a pulmonary metastasis performed as a separate procedure is attributed to Divis in 1926. In North America, the most quoted case of lobectomy for a metastatic carcinoma was that performed by Barney and Churchill in 1939.[178] Their patient underwent nephrectomy for an adenocarcinoma and was known to have a pulmonary mass. After the renal resection, the pulmonary tumor did not respond to radiation treatment and increased in size. Following exploration and resection of the pulmonary lesion, the patient survived disease-free for more than 20 years.

From 1940 to the mid-1960s, pulmonary metastasectomy was performed infrequently and only in highly selected patients. A total of 169 pulmonary metastasis resections were performed on 165 patients at the Mayo Clinic from 1941 to 1959.[179] This large number of operations may reflect the high volume of cases seen at the Mayo Clinic rather than the common use of resection at that time. The first principles of pulmonary resection for metastatic disease included complete removal of the primary disease, no evidence of recurrence or metastatic disease other than the lung lesion, and the patient is in good general condition. Multiple lesions were not considered a contraindication to resection (Fig. 79.10), but it was thought that bilateral disease indicated a poor prognosis and should not be resected. Surgeons were already convinced that the resection should be as conservative of lung function as possible.

Since then, experience from several institutions suggests that more liberal indications for pulmonary metastasectomy are appropriate.[180] A striking example was the treatment of metastatic osteogenic sarcoma at Memorial Sloan-Kettering Cancer Center. From 1940 to 1965, only five such patients were treated surgically. During the same period, only 24 of 145 patients (17%) survived 5 years after resection of their primary tumors, and 118 of these patients (81%) died of pulmonary metastases. This experience prompted a more aggressive approach to the management of pulmonary metastases. Starting in 1965, a consecutive series of 22 patients with osteogenic sarcoma underwent pulmonary metastasectomy. Patients were considered for operation even if they had bilateral metastases or required multiple thoracotomies to remove all gross tumor. A total of 59 thoracotomies were performed in these 22 patients, with an overall 5-year survival rate of 32%. The dramatic improvement in survival in comparison with the historical experience strongly supported the aggressive use of pulmonary metastasectomy in these patients.[181]

During the past 30 years, resection has become a widely accepted treatment for certain pulmonary metastases; however, some of the criteria for patient selection remain controversial. In addition, advances in chemotherapy have changed the indications for resection. With some cancers, pulmonary metastasectomy is performed to prolong life expectancy, whereas with others, it serves mainly to restage disease or to provide adjuvant treatment after initial chemotherapy. The role of pulmonary metastasectomy will undoubtedly continue to evolve as improvements in systemic treatment are made.

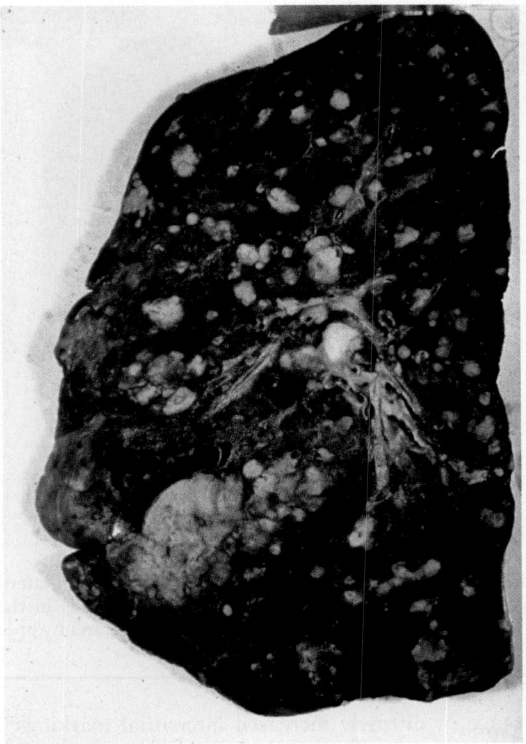

FIGURE 79.10. Metastatic carcinoma of the lung. A section through the lung shows numerous nodules of metastatic carcinoma, corresponding to "cannon ball" metastases seen radiologically. (Reproduced with permission from Rubin E, Farber JL. *Pathology*, 3rd ed. Philadelphia, PA: Lippincott Williams & Wilkins; 1999.)

Clinical Presentation and Diagnosis

Metastases are asymptomatic 85% of the time and are usually detected on a routine chest radiograph. Patients who undergo resection of a primary tumor with a known tendency to metastasize to the lung should have a chest radiograph as part of their routine follow-up care. On a chest radiograph, metastases usually present as well-circumscribed, spherical solid masses with well-defined borders (Fig. 79.11). Cavitation is occasionally seen in large lesions with central necrosis, mostly squamous cell cancers. The distribution of lung metastases is predominantly subpleural or in the outer third of lung fields.[182]

Metastases to the lung usually arise in the pulmonary parenchyma. Endobronchial metastases are uncommon but occur most typically with renal cell, colon, and breast cancers. Even with endobronchial metastases, half of patients are asymptomatic.[183] More often, endobronchial disease represents an extension of contiguous parenchymal disease. The extent of endobronchial tumor can affect the approach to resection. For these reasons, bronchoscopy should be performed before thoracotomy, especially if centrally located metastases are present.

Hilar or mediastinal nodal involvement sometimes accompanies pulmonary metastases. Several retrospective series have indicated that metastatic nodal involvement is a poor prognostic indicator, independent of disease-free interval or number of nodules.[184,185] However, the determinants of nodal involvement and the prognostic and therapeutic implications remain poorly understood. Lymphangitic spread can occur with or without concomitant pulmonary nodules. This happens most frequently in breast cancer and produces a characteristic radiographic

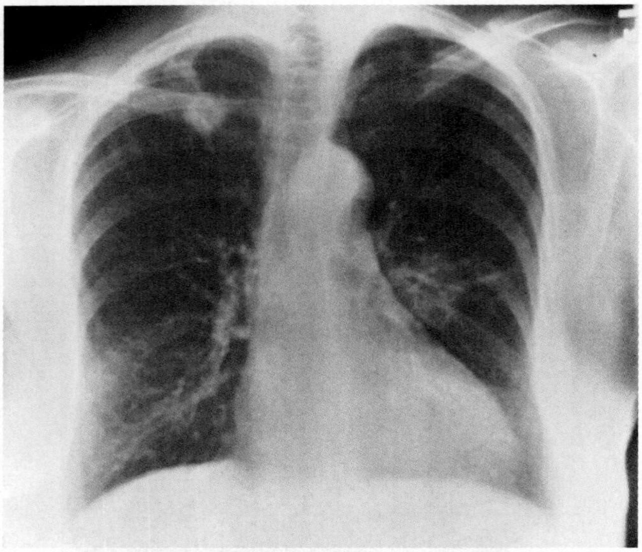

FIGURE 79.11. Chest radiograph of a patient with bilateral pulmonary metastases from endometrial cancer. The mass in the right upper lobe is well circumscribed and has the radiographic appearance typical of a metastasis.

appearance of diffusely increased interstitial markings and a clinical presentation of severe dyspnea that is out of proportion to the radiographic findings.

When pulmonary metastases are thought to be present on a chest radiograph, CT should be performed to determine their number, location, size, and potential resectability. Plain chest radiographs detect only lesions at least 9 mm in size. New lesions of this size seen on a chest radiograph in a patient already treated for a malignancy have a 90% chance of being malignant.[186] Even though CT can identify lesions as small as 3 mm, it often underestimates the number of pulmonary metastases (Fig. 79.12). When radiologic and surgical findings are correlated, only 75% of malignant nodules are detected by CT. Fifteen percent of CT studies overestimate the number of lung metastases for an accurate radiologic assessment of 61%.[187,188] FDG-PET scan appears to have a role as well in the preoperative evaluation of resectable pulmonary metastases, enhancing the detection of extrathoracic or mediastinal involvement that might preclude complete resection.[189]

Patients who present with multiple pulmonary nodules in the setting of a previously treated malignancy rarely pose a diagnostic dilemma. Patients who present with solitary pulmonary
8 nodules are more problematic. Generally, a solitary lesion is more likely to be a metastasis if the primary tumor was a sarcoma or a melanoma. If the primary tumor originated in the head, neck, or breast, it is more likely to be a new primary lung cancer.[190] It has an equal chance of being a metastasis or a new primary tumor if the initial tumor was of gastrointestinal or genitourinary origin. Percutaneous fine-needle aspiration biopsy usually yields a tissue diagnosis, but the necessity of a biopsy in the case of a solitary lesion is questionable. If the patient fits the criteria for resection, a biopsy of the lesion is best performed as an excisional biopsy. Because the findings on needle biopsy do not alter the recommendations for excision of a solitary lesion, this procedure should be undertaken only if the patient is not an operative candidate, if an alternative method of treatment is indicated, or if the patient requests that the diagnosis be established before consenting to operation.

Criteria for Resection

The disease-free interval, number of metastatic nodules, and tumor doubling time all have been used as criteria for the resection of pulmonary metastases. Each of these remains controversial with respect to its effect on long-term outcome.[191] The disease-free interval is defined as the time from resection of the primary tumor to the diagnosis of metastases. The length of the disease-free interval is thought to be of prognostic significance and varies greatly among published reports from 7 months to 5 years.[192]

The number of metastatic nodules resected has also been considered predictive of survival. In sarcomas, some have reported that the presence of four nodules is a significant breakpoint in survival; however, the significance of the number of nodules varies among reported series. Most consider the completeness of resection the best predictor of survival.[193] Obviously, when a shower of numerous, tiny (1- to 2-mm) lesions is encountered, complete resection is not possible.

Tumor doubling time is a measure of the aggressiveness of tumor growth. The prognostic importance of tumor doubling time, however, is questioned because various doubling times, from 20 to 136 days, have been found to be significant in different studies.[192] Many do not consider this a criterion for resection. The disease-free interval, number of metastatic nodules, and tumor doubling time in fact reflect the intrinsic tumor biology.

In 1991, the International Registry of Lung Metastases was established. Five thousand two hundred six cases of pulmonary metastases were analyzed retrospectively with regard to prognostic variables.[187] Multivariate analysis showed a better prognosis for patients with germ cell tumors, a disease-free interval of 36 months or more, a single metastasis, and complete resection. A simple system of classification into prognostic groups was designed (Table 79.11).

Several guidelines must be met before a patient is considered for resection of pulmonary metastases: (a) control of the primary tumor, (b) absence of extrathoracic metastases, (c) a general medical condition that permits thoracotomy, (d) pulmonary function that allows complete resection of all metastases, and (e) lack of a more effective systemic treatment. Resection should be undertaken only if complete resection is considered technically feasible.[194]

If the metastatic lesion is found at the same time as a recurrence at the primary site, the recurrent primary tumor should be treated before the metastatic disease is treated to prevent further seeding of the metastatic site. When the primary tumor and the metastasis are diagnosed simultaneously, lung resection may precede operation for the primary disease if it is doubtful whether the pulmonary disease can be completely resected and immediate subsequent resection of the primary tumor is planned.

When a patient meets the criteria for resection of one or more pulmonary metastases, the natural history of the tumor and whether effective systemic therapy is available must be considered. Experience in breast cancer, testicular cancer, and osteogenic sarcoma illustrate this point.[195] In contrast to metastatic sarcoma, which is usually confined to the lungs, metastatic breast cancer to the lungs signals the development of widely disseminated disease. Although effective systemic therapy is available, patients with a solitary metastatic lesion, long disease-free interval following treatment for the primary breast cancer, and good performance status appear to have longer median and 5-year survival following pulmonary resection.[196,197]

The advent of effective chemotherapy has altered the management of pulmonary metastases of germ cell cancer and rendered an incurable disease curable. Platinum-based chemotherapy is now the primary form of treatment.[198] Resection is reserved for patients who have a complete serologic response (normal levels of ß-human chorionic gonadotropin and α-fetoprotein) with residual pulmonary lesions, evidence of persistent intrathoracic disease with elevated markers despite a full course of chemotherapy, or lesions that do not respond or that progress with chemotherapy.[199] Approximately one third of the resected pulmonary lesions contain viable tumor,

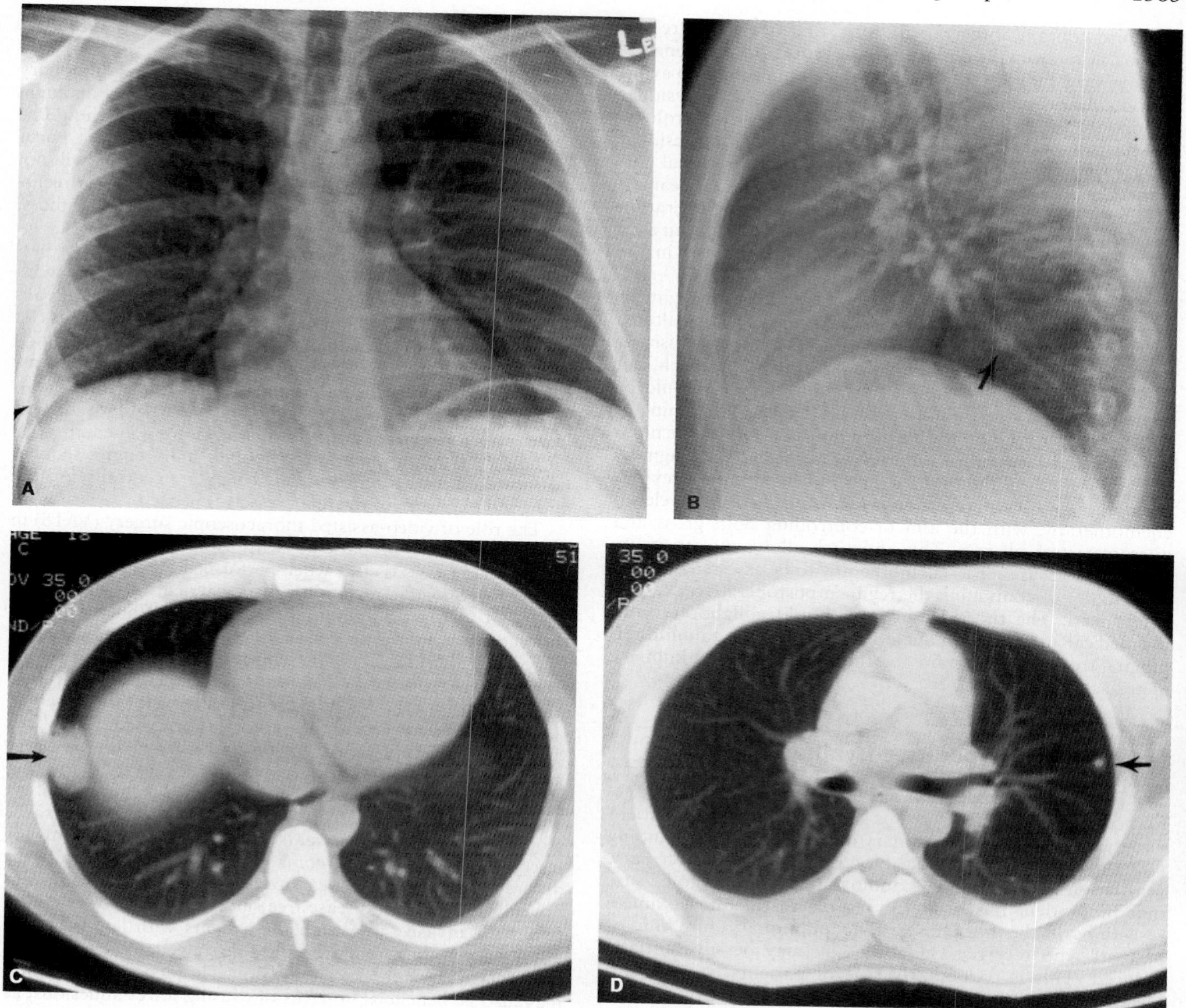

FIGURE 79.12. Imaging studies from a patient with metastatic embryonal rhabdomyosarcoma. Chest radiographs show a mass in the right lower lobe (*arrow,* **A**) that is best seen on the lateral view (*arrow,* **B**). Computed tomography (CT) confirmed the presence of this mass (*arrow,* **C**) and showed an additional nodule in the left upper lobe (*arrow,* **D**). At surgical exploration, however, multiple bilateral pulmonary metastases were found that measured less than 5 mm and therefore could not be seen on CT.

TABLE 79.11 **RESULTS**

SURVIVAL BY PROGNOSTIC GROUP: THE INTERNATIONAL REGISTRY OF LUNG METASTASES

■ GROUPS		■ MEDIAN SURVIVAL (mo)
I	Resectable, no risk factor (DFI ≥36 mo and single metastasis)	61
II	Resectable, one risk factor (DFI >36 mo and multiple metastases)	34
III	Resectable, two risk factors (DFI >36 mo and multiple metastases)	24
IV	Unresectable	14

DFI, disease-free interval.
From Pastorino U, Buyse M, Friendel G, et al. Long-term results of lung metastasectomy: prognostic analyses based on 5206 cases. *J Thorac Cardiovasc Surg* 1997;11:34–49.

one third contain fibrosis or necrosis, and one third are teratomas. A teratoma is removed to prevent it from degenerating to a more malignant form of germ cell tumor and to avoid the potential complications of local tumor growth. Residual tumors are found mostly in patients with positive serology, and the prognosis is usually not as good as when no residual disease is present.[200] In addition, the presence of residual pulmonary disease, as opposed to mediastinal disease, appears to portend a worse survival. Patients who are fit for operation can derive significant long-term survival, even though surgical thoracic metastasectomy has a strictly adjuvant role in the treatment of malignant germ cell tumors.[201]

The development of more effective chemotherapy regimens for sarcomas, especially osteogenic sarcomas, has also altered the management of pulmonary metastases in this disease. Resection is part of a multimodality treatment approach, but the manner in which chemotherapy and resection should be combined is less clear than in germ cell cancer. The timing of an operation in relation to chemotherapy depends on the number, size, and location of pulmonary metastases at diagnosis and on whether the patient has received any previous chemotherapy. Often, resection is performed between cycles of chemotherapy, with the aim of controlling both gross and micrometastatic disease. This approach allows the sensitivity of the patient's tumor to chemotherapy to be assessed, and the advisability of continuing the regimen postoperatively can be determined. The thoracic surgeon should collaborate with the medical and radiation oncologists in planning a multidisciplinary treatment program for the patient with pulmonary metastases of sarcoma.

Preoperative Evaluation

The preoperative evaluation of the patient undergoing resection of pulmonary metastases is similar to that of the patient undergoing removal of a primary lung cancer. Tests including pulmonary function, arterial blood gases, and, if necessary, ventilation-perfusion lung scanning are performed to be sure that the patient has sufficient reserve to tolerate complete resection of the metastases. The pulmonary function of patients who received chemotherapy may be substantially reduced. This is particularly true of patients treated with bleomycin and mitomycin, which can markedly diminish the diffusion capacity and, occasionally and unpredictably, cause an acute respiratory distress type of syndrome postoperatively. Maintaining patients on 35% or less inspired oxygen intraoperatively is thought to help prevent this complication. Like patients with primary lung cancers, these patients should stop smoking. Patients who smoke actively up to the time of operation are at risk for postoperative atelectasis or pneumonia.

It is also important to assess the patient's general medical condition and cardiovascular status. Older patients may have underlying coronary artery disease that requires preoperative treatment and additional perioperative monitoring. The cardiac function of patients who previously received chemotherapy, especially doxorubicin, may be impaired. A preoperative radionuclide scan or echocardiogram should be performed to determine the left ventricular ejection fraction and assess whether intraoperative hemodynamic monitoring is necessary. Other drugs, such as cisplatin, can impair renal or neurologic function and may influence perioperative management.

If a patient has recently undergone chemotherapy, the timing of surgery should be planned after consultation with the medical oncologist, so that the operation is not performed when the patient is neutropenic or thrombocytopenic. Resumption of chemotherapy postoperatively should also be a joint decision between the surgeon and medical oncologist so that it does not compromise wound healing.

Surgical Technique

Two principles guide the approach to resecting pulmonary metastatic lesions: complete resection of disease and maximal sparing of functioning lung tissue. Wedge resections should be performed whenever possible. A lobectomy or even a pneumonectomy may be performed when wedge resection will not provide a complete resection. This may be necessary for recurrences (completion pneumonectomy), centrally located tumors, or multiple metastases.[202,203]

Unilateral disease is approached by a standard anterolateral or posterolateral thoracotomy incision. Patients with bilateral pulmonary metastases should have a simultaneous resection of the bilateral lesions if technically feasible. This can be accomplished by a median sternotomy or a clamshell incision (bilateral anterior thoracotomy with or without transverse sternotomy). A clamshell incision provides better exposure to the posterior aspects of the lungs, particularly the left lower lobe, which is difficult to access by a median sternotomy.[204] Bilateral pulmonary nodules may require sequential posterolateral thoracotomies if they are centrally located and good exposure of the hilar vessels is needed.

The role of video-assisted thoracoscopic surgery (VATS) in the management of patients with isolated suspected pulmonary metastasis is clear when performed for diagnostic purposes. VATS wedge resection can be carried out with a high degree of success and minimal morbidity.[205] While the use of thoracoscopy in the resection of pulmonary metastases is increasing, its use remains controversial. In a series of 318 patients reported by Petersen et al. undergoing resection of metastatic melanoma, 40 patients underwent thoracoscopic resection.[206] According to the authors, thoracoscopy has been their preferred approach to metastasectomy in the past few years; they use chest CT for preoperative localization and ring clamp or digital palpation for intraoperative confirmation.

Gossot et al. compared 31 patients undergoing thoracoscopic resection to 29 patients undergoing thoracotomy for resection of metastatic sarcoma.[207] They found no significant difference in 1-, 3-, or 5-year survival. There was also no significant difference in disease-free survival. They recommend a minimally invasive approach for patients with less than two pulmonary nodules that are amenable to wedge resection with no mediastinal or chest wall invasion. Thoracoscopic resection may also be beneficial in terms of causing fewer adhesions, as Briccoli et al. have shown that 35% of patients undergoing metastasectomy for sarcoma will require a repeat resection, resulting in acceptable survival rates as long as pulmonary function is maintained.[208]

Results

Resection remains the mainstay of treatment for pulmonary metastases from many solid tumors that cannot be treated effectively with chemotherapy. These include melanoma, colon, renal cell, head and neck, and endometrial cancers. The histologic subtypes of the pulmonary metastases in the International Registry of Lung Metastases are listed in Table 79.12.[187]

Globally, the actuarial survival after complete metastasectomy is 36% at 5 years and 26% at 10 years (median survival of 35 months).[187] The experience at Memorial Sloan-Kettering Cancer Center in the resection of pulmonary metastases from renal cell carcinoma, head and neck tumors, colorectal cancers, testicular germ cell tumors, and soft tissue sarcoma are summarized (Table 79.13). These results again demonstrate that complete resection of metastatic disease is associated with prolonged survival in carefully selected patients. Furthermore, patients who are persistently free of disease at the primary tumor location but who have recurrent resectable

TABLE 79.12 CLASSIFICATION

HISTOLOGIC SUBTYPES FROM THE INTERNATIONAL REGISTRY OF LUNG METASTASES

HISTOLOGIC GROUPS	NO. PATIENTS (%)	SUBTYPES
Carcinoma	2,260 (47)	Breast
		Lung
		Bowel
		Kidney
		Uterus
		Head and neck
Sarcoma	2,173 (45)	Osteosarcoma
		Other bone sarcomas
		Histiocytoma
		Leiomyosarcoma
		Synovial sarcoma
		Other soft tissue sarcoma
Other types	328 (8)	Wilms tumor
		Teratoma
		Embryonal carcinoma
		Other germ cell tumor
		Melanoma

From Pastorino U, Buyse M, Friedel G, et al. Long-term results of lung metastasectomy: prognostic analyses based on 5206 cases. *J Thorac Cardiovasc Surg* 1997;113:37–49.

metastatic disease of the lung also benefit from repeated surgery.[209] Mortality rates of pulmonary metastasectomy do not differ from those of thoracic surgery performed for lung cancers, varying between 0.6% and 2%.[180,199,210] The surgical removal of pulmonary metastases is widely accepted, but its role has changed as more effective chemotherapy has become available for some cancers. It is important that the surgeon understand the indications for operation, the potential side effects of initial chemotherapy, and the ways in which resection should be integrated into the overall treatment plan for these patients.

BENIGN TUMORS OF THE LUNG

Benign tumors of the lung are rare neoplasms. Few series are found in the literature, but in a 10-year surgical review (1958 to 1968) from the Mayo Clinic, 130 patients were found to have benign tumors.[211] Like malignant tumors, benign tumors arising from epithelial, mesodermal, or endodermal cell lines can develop in the lung. They may present as endobronchial lesions but more commonly as peripheral nodules.[212] Endobronchial tumors present with signs and symptoms related to airway obstruction or bleeding. Tumors arising in peripheral airways or within pulmonary parenchyma usually present as asymptomatic solitary pulmonary nodules. Types of benign lung tumors are listed in Table 79.14.

Hamartoma

The most frequent benign tumors are hamartomas, which represent 75% of benign lesions. They show a predilection for

LUNG

TABLE 79.13 RESULTS

RESULTS OF PULMONARY RESECTIONS FOR METASTASES AT MEMORIAL SLOAN-KETTERING CANCER CENTER

	NO. PATIENTS	SURVIVAL (5 y, %)
Renal cell carcinoma (1980–1993)[225]		
Solitary metastasis	50	54
Head and neck cancer (1966–1995)[210]		
Squamous cell	41	34
Glandular tumors	36	64
Overall	83	50
Colorectal cancer (1965–1988)[226]		
Overall	144	44
Soft tissue sarcoma (1982–1997)[227,a]		
Complete resection	161	46
Incomplete resection	52	23
No resection	473	17
Unknown	33	
Overall	719	25
Testicular germ cell tumors		
1967–1995[199]		
1967–1974	22	41
1975–1984	69	65
1984–1995	66	82
Overall	157	68

[a]Survival at 3 years.

TABLE 79.14 CLASSIFICATION

BENIGN TUMORS OF THE LUNG

Epithelial
Polyps
Papilloma
Mucous gland adenoma
Mesenchymal
Vessel
Sclerosing hemangioma
Lymphangioma
Nerve
Granular cell tumor
Neurilemoma
Neurofibroma
Muscle
Leiomyoma
Miscellaneous
Hamartoma
Teratoma
Clear cell (sugar) tumor
Others
Lipoma
Chondroma
Fibroma
Inflammatory pseudotumors
Plasma cell granuloma
Pulmonary hyalinizing granuloma

men.[213] A hamartoma consists of an abnormal arrangement of normal cells. In the lung, the most frequent component is cartilage. A hamartoma usually presents as a solitary pulmonary nodule with an extremely slow growth pattern. Classically, the radiographic appearance is that of a well-circumscribed nodule that may contain popcorn calcification. If previous chest radiographs are available, these tumors are found to have been present for many years. Their growth pattern is variable but generally slow. These lesions can be diagnosed by CT if appropriate calcification is demonstrated. Needle aspiration is frequently diagnostic of a cartilaginous benign lesion.

Controversy exists regarding whether these lesions should be excised for pathologic diagnosis. Certainly, they do not require excision unless they are proximally located and cause symptoms related to endobronchial obstruction or unless carcinoma cannot be ruled out. If transthoracic needle aspiration biopsy confirms the presence of a hamartoma, many surgeons elect to follow patients with annual chest radiography rather than surgical excision. Occasionally, significant growth during follow-up necessitates excision.

Other Benign Tumors

Other benign tumors may present as endobronchial lesions (commonly fibromas, lipomas, chondromas, and granular cell myoblastomas). These tumors may be removed endoscopically, but frequently they also require surgical excision when the diagnosis is in doubt or when endoscopic excision has been incomplete. Peripheral tumors often are removed for diagnosis.

References

1. Jemal A, Siegel R, Ward E, et al. Cancer statistics, 2008. *CA Cancer J Clin* 2008;58:71–96.
2. Jemal A, Thun MJ, Ries LAG, et al. Annual report to the nation on the status of cancer, 1975–2005, featuring trends in lung cancer, tobacco use, and tobacco control. *J Natl Cancer Inst* 2008;100(23):1672–1694.
3. Mountain C. Revisions in the International System for Staging Lung Cancer. *Chest* 1997;111:1710–1717.
4. Arriagada R, Bergman B, Dunant A, et al. Cisplatin-based adjuvant chemotherapy in patients with completely resected non-small-cell lung cancer. *N Engl J Med* 2004;350:351–360.
5. Winton T, Livingston R, Johnson D, et al. Vinorelbine plus cisplatin vs. observation in resected non-small-cell lung cancer. *N Engl J Med* 2005; 352:2589–2597.
6. Douillard J-Y, Rosell R, De Lena M, et al. Adjuvant vinorelbine plus cisplatin versus observation in patients with completely resected stage IB-IIIA non-small-cell lung cancer (Adjuvant Navelbine International Trialist Association [ANITA]): a randomised controlled trial. *Lancet Oncol* 2006; 7:719–727.
7. Miller YE. Minimizing unintended consequences of detecting lung nodules by computed tomography. *Am J Respir Crit Care Med* 2008;178:891–892.
8. The International Early Lung Cancer Action Program Investigators. Survival of patients with stage I lung cancer detected on CT screening. *N Engl J Med* 2006;355:1763–1771.
9. Graham EA, Singer JJ. Successful removal of an entire lung for carcinoma of the bronchus. *JAMA* 1933;101:1371–1374.
10. Warren WH. Historical facets of thoracic surgery emphasizing lung cancer. In: Gruhn JG, Rosen ST, eds. *Lung Cancer: The Evolution of Concepts.* New York: Field and Wood Medical Publishers, Inc.; 1989:73–106.
11. Jemal A, Clegg LX, Ward E, et al. Annual report to the nation on the status of cancer, 1975–2001, with a special feature regarding survival. *Cancer* 2004;101:3–27.
12. DeLancey JOL, Thun MJ, Jemal A, et al. Recent trends in black-white disparities in cancer mortality. *Cancer Epidemiol Biomarkers Prev* 2008;17: 2908–2912.
13. Jacobs DR Jr, Adachi H, Mulder I, et al. Cigarette smoking and mortality risk: twenty-five-year follow-up of the Seven Countries Study. *Arch Intern Med* 1999;159:733–740.
14. Vineis P, Alavanja M, Buffler P, et al. Tobacco and cancer: recent epidemiological evidence. *J Natl Cancer Inst* 2004;96:99–106.
15. Vineis P, Airoldi L, Veglia P, et al. Environmental tobacco smoke and risk of respiratory cancer and chronic obstructive pulmonary disease in former smokers and never smokers in the EPIC prospective study. *BMJ* 2005;330: 277.
16. Travis WD, Brambilla E, Müller-Hermelink HK, et al., eds. *World Health Organization Classification of Tumors, Pathology and Genetics of Tumours of the Lung, Pleura, Thymus and Heart.* Lyon, France: IARC Press; 2004.
17. Brambilla E, Travis WD, Colby TV, et al. The new World Health Organization classification of lung tumours. *Eur Respir J* 2001;18:1059–1068.
18. Sanchez-Cespedes M. Dissecting the genetic alterations involved in lung carcinogenesis. *Lung Cancer* 2003;40:111–121.
19. Ahrendt SA, Hu Y, Buta M, et al. p53 mutations and survival in stage I non-small-cell lung cancer: results of a prospective study. *J Natl Cancer Inst* 2003;95:961–970.
20. Ahrendt SA, Chow JT, Yang SC, et al. Alcohol consumption and cigarette smoking increase the frequency of p53 mutations in non-small cell lung cancer. *Cancer Res* 2000;60:3155–3159.
21. D'Amico TA, Aloia TA, Moore M-BH, et al. Molecular biologic substaging of stage I lung cancer according to gender and histology. *Ann Thorac Surg* 2000;69:882–886.
22. D'Amico TA, Aloia TA, Moore M-BH, et al. Predicting the sites of metastases from lung cancer using molecular biologic markers. *Ann Thorac Surg* 2001;72:1144–1148.
23. Carbone DP, Mitsudomi T, Chiba H, et al. p53 Immunostaining positivity is associated with reduced survival and is imperfectly correlated with gene mutations in resected non-small cell lung cancer: a preliminary report of LCSG 871. *Chest* 1994;106:377S–381S.
24. Belinsky SA, Nikula KJ, Palmisano WA, et al. Aberrant methylation of p16INK4a is an early event in lung cancer and a potential biomarker for early diagnosis. *Proc Natl Acad Sci U S A* 1998;95:11891–11896.
25. Esteller M, Corn PG, Baylin SB, et al. A gene hypermethylation profile of human cancer. *Cancer Res* 2001;61:3225–3229.
26. Meyerson M, Franklin W, Kelley M. Molecular classification and molecular genetics of human lung cancers. *Semin Oncol* 2004;31:4–19.
27. Garber ME, Troyanskaya OG, Schluens K, et al. Diversity of gene expression in adenocarcinoma of the lung. *Proc Natl Acad Sci U S A* 2001;98: 13784–13789.
28. Bhattacharjee A, Richards WG, Staunton J, et al. Classification of human lung carcinomas by mRNA expression profiling reveals distinct adenocarcinoma subclasses. *Proc Natl Acad Sci U S A* 2001;98:13790–13795.
29. Beer DG, Kardia SL, Huang CC, et al. Gene-expression profiles predict survival of patients with lung adenocarcinoma. *Nat Med* 2002;8:816–824.
30. Motoi N, Szoke J, Riely GJ, et al. Lung adenocarcinoma: modification of the 2004 WHO mixed subtype to include the major histologic subtype suggests correlations between papillary and micropapillary adenocarcinoma

subtypes, EGFR mutations and gene expression analysis. *Am J Surg Pathol* 2008;32:810–827.
31. Shedden K, Taylor JMG, Enkemann SA, et al. Gene expression-based survival prediction in lung adenocarcinoma: a multi-site, blinded validation study. *Nat Med* 2008;14:822–827.
32. Parmigiani G, Garrett-Mayer ES, Anbazhagan R, et al. A cross-study comparison of gene expression studies for the molecular classification of lung cancer. *Clin Cancer Res* 2004;10:2922–2927.
33. Lynch TJ, Bell DW, Sordella R, et al. Activating mutations in the epidermal growth factor receptor underlying responsiveness of non-small-cell lung cancer to gefitinib. *N Engl J Med* 2004;350:2129–2139.
34. Paez JG, Janne PA, Lee JC, et al. EGFR mutations in lung cancer: correlation with clinical response to gefitinib therapy. *Science* 2004;304: 1497–1500.
35. Miller VA, Kris MG, Shah N, et al. Bronchioloalveolar pathologic subtype and smoking history predict sensitivity to gefitinib in advanced non-small-cell lung cancer. *J Clin Oncol* 2004;22:1103–1109.
36. Pao W, Miller V, Zakowski M, et al. EGF receptor gene mutations are common in lung cancers from "never smokers" and are associated with sensitivity of tumors to gefitinib and erlotinib. *Proc Natl Acad Sci U S A* 2004;101:13306–13311.
37. Goldstraw P, Crowley J, Chansky K, et al. The IASLC Lung Cancer Staging Project: proposals for the revision of the TNM stage groupings in the forthcoming (seventh) edition of the TNM Classification of malignant tumours. *J Thorac Oncol* 2007;2:706–714.
38. Groome PA, Bolejack V, Crowley JJ, et al. The IASLC Lung Cancer Staging Project: validation of the proposals for revision of the T, N, and M descriptors and consequent stage groupings in the forthcoming (seventh) edition of the TNM classification of malignant tumours. *J Thorac Oncol* 2007;2:694–705.
39. Rami-Porta R, Ball D, Crowley J, et al. The IASLC Lung Cancer Staging Project: proposals for the revision of the T descriptors in the forthcoming (seventh) edition of the TNM classification for lung cancer. *J Thorac Oncol* 2007;2:593–602.
40. Postmus PE, Brambilla E, Chansky K, et al. The IASLC Lung Cancer Staging Project: proposals for revision of the M descriptors in the forthcoming (seventh) edition of the TNM classification of lung cancer. *J Thorac Oncol* 2007;2:686–693.
41. Rusch VW, Crowley J, Giroux DJ, et al. The IASLC Lung Cancer Staging Project: proposals for the revision of the N descriptors in the forthcoming seventh edition of the TNM classification for lung cancer. *J Thorac Oncol* 2007;2:603–612.
42. MacMahon H, Austin JHM, Gamsu G, et al. Guidelines for management of small pulmonary nodules detected on CT scans: a statement from the Fleischner Society. *Radiology* 2005;237:395–400.
43. Gould MK, Fletcher J, Iannettoni MD, et al. Evaluation of patients with pulmonary nodules: when is it lung cancer?: ACCP evidence-based clinical practice guidelines (2nd edition). *Chest* 2007;132:108S–130S.
44. Ost D, Fein AM, Feinsilver SH. The solitary pulmonary nodule. *N Engl J Med* 2003;348:2535–2542.
45. Postmus PE, Rocmans P, Asamura H, et al. Consensus report IASLC workshop Bruges, September 2002: pretreatment minimal staging for non-small cell lung cancer. *Lung Cancer* 2003;42:3–6.
46. Rivera MP, Mehta AC. Initial diagnosis of lung cancer: ACCP evidence-based clinical practice guidelines (2nd edition). *Chest* 2007;132: 131S–148S.
47. Mountain C, Dresler C. Regional lymph node classification for lung cancer staging. *Chest* 1997;111:1718–1723.
48. Silvestri GA, Gould MK, Margolis ML, et al. Noninvasive staging of non-small cell lung cancer: ACCP evidenced-based clinical practice guidelines (2nd edition). *Chest* 2007;132:178S–201S.
49. Gonzalez-Stawinski GV, Lemaire A, Merchant F, et al. A comparative analysis of positron emission tomography and mediastinoscopy in staging non-small cell lung cancer. *J Thorac Cardiovasc Surg* 2003;126: 1900–1904.
50. Kernstine KH, McLaughlin KA, Menda Y, et al. Can FDG-PET reduce the need for mediastinoscopy in potentially resectable nonsmall cell lung cancer? *Ann Thorac Surg* 2002;73:394–402.
51. Vesselle H, Pugsley JM, Vallieres E, et al. The impact of fluorodeoxyglucose F 18 positron-emission tomography on the surgical staging of non-small cell lung cancer. *J Thorac Cardiovasc Surg* 2002; 124:511–519.
52. Reed CE, Harpole DH, Posther KE, et al. Results of the American College of Surgeons Oncology Group Z0050 trial: the utility of positron emission tomography in staging potentially operable non-small cell lung cancer. *J Thorac Cardiovasc Surg* 2003;126:1943–1951.
53. Kozower BD, Meyers BF, Reed CE, et al. Does positron emission tomography prevent nontherapeutic pulmonary resections for clinical stage IA lung cancer? *Ann Thorac Surg* 2008;85:1166–1170.
54. Cerfolio RJ, Ojha B, Bryant AS, et al. The accuracy of integrated PET-CT compared with dedicated pet alone for the staging of patients with nonsmall cell lung cancer. *Ann Thorac Surg* 2004;78:1017–1023.
55. Krasna MJ, Reed CE, Nugent WC, et al. Lung cancer staging and treatment in multidisciplinary trials: cancer and leukemia group B cooperative group approach. *Ann Thorac Surg* 1999;68:201–207.
56. Detterbeck FC, Jantz MA, Wallace M, et al. Invasive mediastinal staging of lung cancer: ACCP evidence-based clinical practice guidelines (2nd edition). *Chest* 2007;132:202S–220S.
57. Hammoud ZT, Anderson RC, Meyers BF, et al. The current role of mediastinoscopy in the evaluation of thoracic disease. *J Thorac Cardiovasc Surg* 1999;118:894–899.
58. Henschke CI, McCauley DI, Yankelevitz DF, et al. Early Lung Cancer Action Project: overall design and findings from baseline screening. *Lancet* 1999;354:99–105.
59. Swensen SJ, Jett JR, Sloan JA, et al. Screening for lung cancer with low-dose spiral computed tomography. *Am J Respir Crit Care Med* 2002;165: 508–513.
60. Burfeind WR Jr, Tong BC, O'Branski E, et al. Quality of life outcomes are equivalent after lobectomy in the elderly. *J Thorac Cardiovasc Surg* 2008; 136:597–604.
61. Eagle KA, Berger PB, Calkins H, et al. ACC/AHA guideline update for pPerioperative cardiovascular evaluation for noncardiac surgery–executive summary: a report of the American College of Cardiology/American Heart Association Task Force on Practice Guidelines (committee to update the 1996 guidelines on perioperative cardiovascular evaluation for noncardiac surgery). *Circulation* 2002;105:1257–1267.
62. Miller JI, Grossman GD, Hatcher CR. Pulmonary function test criteria for operability and pulmonary resection. *Surg Gynecol Obstet* 1981;153: 893–895.
63. Datta D, Lahiri B. Preoperative evaluation of patients undergoing lung resection surgery. *Chest* 2003;123:2096–2103.
64. Pate P, Tenholder MF, Griffin JP, et al. Preoperative assessment of the high-risk patient for lung resection. *Ann Thorac Surg* 1996;61:1494–1500.
65. Cerfolio RJ, Allen MS, Trastek VF, et al. Lung resection in patients with compromised pulmonary function. *Ann Thorac Surg* 1996;62:348–351.
66. Burke JR, Duarte IG, Thourani VH, et al. Preoperative risk assessment for marginal patients requiring pulmonary resection. *Ann Thorac Surg* 2003; 76:1767–1773.
67. Loewen GM, Watson D, Kohman L, et al. Preoperative exercise Vo2 measurement for lung resection candidates: results of Cancer and Leukemia Group B Protocol 9238. *J Thorac Oncol* 2007;2:619–625.
68. Beckles MA, Spiro SG, Colice GL, et al. The physiologic evaluation of patients with lung cancer being considered for resectional surgery. *Chest* 2003;123:105S–114S.
69. Deslauriers J, Gregoire J, Jacques LF, et al. Sleeve lobectomy versus pneumonectomy for lung cancer: a comparative analysis of survival and sites or recurrences. *Ann Thorac Surg* 2004;77:1152–1156.
70. Gaissert H, Mathisen D, Moncure A, et al. Survival and function after sleeve lobectomy for lung cancer. *J Thorac Cardiovasc Surg* 1996;111: 948–953.
71. Okada M, Yamagishi H, Satake S, et al. Survival related to lymph node involvement in lung cancer after sleeve lobectomy compared with pneumonectomy. *J Thorac Cardiovasc Surg* 2000;119:814–819.
72. Suen H-C, Meyers BF, Guthrie T, et al. Favorable results after sleeve lobectomy or bronchoplasty for bronchial malignancies. *Ann Thorac Surg* 1999;67:1557–1562.
73. Yoshino I, Yokoyama H, Yano T, et al. Comparison of the surgical results of lobectomy with bronchoplasty and pneumonectomy for lung cancer. *J Surg Oncol* 1997;64:32–35.
74. Ginsberg RJ, Rubinstein LV. Randomized trial of lobectomy versus limited resection for T1 N0 non-small cell lung cancer. *Ann Thorac Surg* 1995;60: 615–622.
75. Landreneau R, Sugarbaker D, Mack M, et al. Wedge resection versus lobectomy for stage I (T1 N0 M0) non-small-cell lung cancer. *J Thorac Cardiovasc Surg* 1997;113:691–700.
76. Martini N, Bains MS, Burt ME, et al. Incidence of local recurrence and second primary tumors in resected stage I lung cancer. *J Thorac Cardiovasc Surg* 1995;109:120–129.
77. Yano T, Yokoyama H, Yoshino I, et al. Results of a limited resection for compromised or poor-risk patients with clinical stage I non-small cell carcinoma of the lung. *J Am Coll Surg* 1995;181:33–37.
78. Keller SM, Adak S, Wagner H, et al. Mediastinal lymph node dissection improves survival in patients with stages II and IIIa non-small cell lung cancer. Eastern Cooperative Oncology Group. *Ann Thorac Surg* 2000;70: 358–365.
79. Allen MS, Darling GE, Pechet TTV, et al. Morbidity and mortality of major pulmonary resections in patients with early-stage lung cancer: initial results of the randomized, prospective ACOSOG Z0030 trial. *Ann Thorac Surg* 2006;81:1013–1020.
80. Feld R, Rubinstein LV, Weisenberger TH. Sites of recurrence in resected stage I non-small-cell lung cancer: a guide for future studies. *J Clin Oncol* 1984;2:1352–1358.
81. Hirsch FR, Spreafico A, Novello S, et al. The prognostic and predictive role of histology in advanced non-small cell lung cancer: a literature review. *J Thorac Oncol* 2008;3:1468–1481.
82. Thomas P, Rubinstein L. Cancer recurrence after resection: T1 N0 non-small cell lung cancer. Lung Cancer Study Group. *Ann Thorac Surg* 1990; 49:242–246.
83. Johnson BE. Second lung cancers in patients after treatment for an initial lung cancer. *J Natl Cancer Inst* 1998;90:1335–1345.
84. Rice D, Kim H-W, Sabichi A, et al. The risk of second primary tumors after resection of stage I nonsmall cell lung cancer. *Ann Thorac Surg* 2003;76: 1001–1008.
85. Virgo KS, Naunheim KS, McKirgan LW, et al. Cost of patient follow-up after potentially curative lung cancer treatment. *J Thorac Cardiovasc Surg* 1996;112:356–363.

86. Kent MS, Korn P, Port JL, et al. Cost effectiveness of chest computed tomography after lung cancer resection: a decision analysis model. *Ann Thorac Surg* 2005;80:1215–1223.
87. Gail MH. A placebo-controlled randomized double-blind study of adjuvant intrapleural BCG in patients with resected T1N0, T1N1, or T2N0 squamous cell carcinoma, adenocarcinoma, or large cell carcinoma of the lung. LCSG Protocol 771. *Chest* 1994;106:287S–292S.
88. Ludwig Lung Cancer Study Group. Adverse effect of intrapleural Corynebacterium parvum as adjuvant therapy in resected stage I and II non-small cell carcinoma of the lung. *J Thorac Cardiovasc Surg* 1985;89: 842–847.
89. Ratto GB, Zino P, Mirabelli S, et al. A randomized trial of adoptive immunotherapy with tumor-infiltrating lymphocytes and interleukin-2 versus standard therapy in the postoperative treatment of resected nonsmall cell lung carcinoma. *Cancer* 1996;78:244–251.
90. Green N, Kurohara SS, George FW III, et al. Postresection irradiation for primary lung cancer: the impact of surgical adjuvant thoracic radiation therapy for patients with nonsmall cell lung carcinoma with ipsilateral mediastinal lymph node involvement. *Radiology* 1975;116:405–407.
91. Kirsh M, Rotman H, Argenta L, et al. Carcinoma of the lung: results of treatment over ten years. *Ann Thorac Surg* 1976;21:371–377.
92. Sawyer TE, Bonner JA, Gould PM, et al. The impact of surgical adjuvant thoracic radiation therapy for patients with nonsmall cell lung carcinoma with ipsilateral mediastinal lymph node involvement. *Cancer* 1997;80: 1399–1408.
93. Mayer R, Smolle-Juettner FM, Szolar D, et al. Postoperative radiotherapy in radically resected non-small cell lung cancer. *Chest* 1997;112:954–959.
94. Stephens RJ, Girling DJ, Bleehen NM, et al. The role of post-operative radiotherapy in non-small-cell lung cancer: a multicentre randomised trial in patients with pathologically staged T1–2, N1–2, M0 disease. Medical Research Council Lung Cancer Working Party. *Br J Cancer* 1996;74: 632–639.
95. Lafitte JJ, Ribet ME, Prevost BM, et al. Postresection irradiation for T2 N0 M0 non-small cell carcinoma: a prospective, randomized study. *Ann Thorac Surg* 1996;62:830–834.
96. The Lung Cancer Study Group. Effects of postoperative mediastinal radiation on completely resected stage II and stage III epidermoid cancer of the lung. *N Engl J Med* 1986;315:1377–1381.
97. Van Houtte P, Rocmans P, Smets P, et al. Postoperative radiation therapy in lung caner: a controlled trial after resection of curative design. *Int J Rad Oncol Biol Phys* 1980;6:983–986.
98. PORT Meta-analysis Trialist Group. Postoperative radiotherapy in non-small-cell lung cancer: systematic review and meta-analysis of individual patient data from nine randomised controlled trials. *Lancet* 1998;352: 257–263.
99. Hughes FA, Higgins G. Veterans Administration Surgical Adjuvant Lung Cancer Chemotherapy Study: present status. *J Thorac Cardiovasc Surg* 1962;44:295–304.
100. Slack NH. Bronchogenic carcinoma: nitrogen mustard as a surgical adjuvant and factors influencing survival. University surgical adjuvant lung project. *Cancer* 1970;25:987–1002.
101. Shields TW, Humphrey EW, Eastridge CE, et al. Adjuvant cancer chemotherapy after resection of carcinoma of the lung. *Cancer* 1977;40: 2057–2062.
102. Shields TW, Higgins GA Jr, Humphrey EW, et al. Prolonged intermittent adjuvant chemotherapy with CCNU and hydroxyurea after resection of carcinoma of the lung. *Cancer* 1982;50:1713–1721.
103. Non-small Cell Lung Cancer Collaborative Group. Chemotherapy in non-small cell lung cancer: a meta-analysis using updated data on individual patients from 52 randomised clinical trials. *BMJ* 1995;311:899–909.
104. Wada H, Hitomi S, Teramatsu T. Adjuvant chemotherapy after complete resection in non-small-cell lung cancer. West Japan Study Group for Lung Cancer Surgery. *J Clin Oncol* 1996;14:1048–1054.
105. Nakagawa M, Tanaka F, Tsubota N, et al. A randomized phase III trial of adjuvant chemotherapy with UFT for completely resected pathological stage I non-small-cell lung cancer: the West Japan Study Group for Lung Cancer Surgery (WJSG)–the 4th study. *Ann Oncol* 2005;16:75–80.
106. Wakelee H, Chhatwani L. Adjuvant chemotherapy for resected non-small cell lung cancer. *Semin Thorac Cardiovasc Surg* 2008;20:198–203.
107. Alam N, Shepherd FA, Winton T, et al. Compliance with post-operative adjuvant chemotherapy in non-small cell lung cancer: an analysis of National Cancer Institute of Canada and intergroup trial JBR.10 and a review of the literature. *Lung Cancer* 2005;47:385–394.
108. Strauss GM, Herndon JE II, Maddaus MA, et al. Adjuvant paclitaxel plus carboplatin compared with observation in stage IB non-small-cell lung cancer: CALGB 9633 with the Cancer and Leukemia Group B, Radiation Therapy Oncology Group, and North Central Cancer Treatment Group study groups. *J Clin Oncol* 2008;26:5043–5051.
109. Feld R, Rubinstein L, Thomas PA. Adjuvant chemotherapy with cyclophosphamide, doxorubicin, and cisplatin in patients with completely resected stage I non-small-cell lung cancer. The Lung Cancer Study Group. *J Natl Cancer Inst* 1993;85:299–306.
110. Keller SM, Adak S, Wagner H, et al. A randomized trial of postoperative adjuvant therapy in patients with completely resected stage II or IIIA non-small-cell lung cancer. *N Engl J Med* 2000;343:1217–1222.
111. Petersen RP, Pham D, Burfeind WR, et al. Thoracoscopic lobectomy facilitates the delivery of chemotherapy after resection for lung cancer. *Ann Thorac Surg* 2007;83:1245–1249.
112. Rendina EA, Venuta F, De Giacomo T, et al. Induction chemotherapy for T4 centrally located non-small cell lung cancer. *J Thorac Cardiovasc Surg* 1999;117:225–233.
113. Grunenwald DH, Andre F, Le Pechoux C, et al. Benefit of surgery after chemoradiotherapy in stage IIIB (T4 and/or N3) non-small cell lung cancer. *J Thorac Cardiovasc Surg* 2001;122:796–802.
114. Okada M, Tsubota N, Yoshimura M, et al. Prognosis of completely resected pN2 non-small cell lung carcinomas: what is the significant node that affects survival? *J Thorac Cardiovasc Surg* 1999;118:270–275.
115. Sagawa M, Sakurada A, Fujimura S, et al. Five-year survivors with resected pN2 nonsmall cell lung carcinoma. *Cancer* 1999;85:864–868.
116. Martini N, Flehinger BJ. The role of surgery in N2 lung cancer. *Surg Clin North Am* 1987;67:1037–1049.
117. Perez CA, Pajak TF, Rubin P, et al. Long-term observations of the patterns of failure in patients with unresectable non-oat cell carcinoma of the lung treated with definitive radiotherapy. Report by the Radiation Therapy Oncology Group. *Cancer* 1987;59:1874–1881.
118. Pisters KM, Kris MG, Gralla RJ, et al. Randomized trial comparing post-operative chemotherapy with vindesine and cisplatin plus thoracic irradiation with irradiation alone in stage III (N2) non-small cell lung cancer. *J Surg Oncol* 1994;56:236–241.
119. Rosell R, Gomez-Codina J, Camps C, et al. A randomized trial comparing preoperative chemotherapy plus surgery with surgery alone in patients with non-small-cell lung cancer. *N Engl J Med* 1994;330:153–158.
120. Rosell R, Gomez-Codina J, Camps C, et al. Preresectional chemotherapy in stage IIIA non-small-cell lung cancer: a 7-year assessment of a randomized controlled trial. *Lung Cancer* 1999;26:7–14.
121. Roth J, Fossella F, Komaki R, et al. A randomized trial comparing perioperative chemotherapy and surgery with surgery alone in resectable stage IIIA non-small-cell lung cancer. *J Natl Cancer Inst* 1994;86:673–680.
122. Roth JA, Atkinson EN, Fossella F, et al. Long-term follow-up of patients enrolled in a randomized trial comparing perioperative chemotherapy and surgery with surgery alone in resectable stage IIIA non-small-cell lung cancer. *Lung Cancer* 1998;21:1–6.
123. Bromley LL, Szur L. Combined radiotherapy and resection for carcinoma of the bronchus; experiences with 66 patients. *Lancet* 1955;269:937–941.
124. Payne DG. Is preoperative or postoperative radiation therapy indicated in non-small cell cancer of the lung? *Lung Cancer* 1994;10:S205–S212.
125. Furuse K, Fukuoka M, Kawahara M, et al. Phase III study of concurrent versus sequential thoracic radiotherapy in combination with mitomycin, vindesine, and cisplatin in unresectable stage III non-small-cell lung cancer. *J Clin Oncol* 1999;17:2692–2699.
126. Martini N, Kris M, Flehinger B, et al. Preoperative chemotherapy for stage IIIa (N2) lung cancer: the Sloan- Kettering experience with 136 patients. *Ann Thorac Surg* 1993;55:1365–1373.
127. Sugarbaker DJ, Herndon J, Kohman LJ, et al. Results of cancer and leukemia group B protocol 8935: a multiinstitutional phase II trimodality trial for stage IIIa (N2) non-small-cell lung cancer. *J Thorac Cardiovasc Surg* 1995;109:473–485.
128. Eagan RT, Ruud C, Lee RE, et al. Pilot study of induction therapy with cyclophosphamide, doxorubicin, and cisplatin (CAP) and chest irradiation prior to thoracotomy in initially inoperable stage III M0 non-small cell lung cancer. *Cancer Treat Rep* 1987;71:895–900.
129. Weiden P, Piantadosi S. Preoperative chemotherapy (cisplatin and fluorouracil) and radiation therapy in stage III non-small-cell lung cancer: a phase II study of the Lung Cancer Study Group. *J Natl Cancer Inst* 1991; 83:266–273.
130. Faber L, Kittle C, Warren W, et al. Preoperative chemotherapy and irradiation for stage III non-small cell lung cancer. *Ann Thorac Surg* 1989;47: 669–675.
131. Strauss G, Herndon J, Sherman D, et al. Neoadjuvant chemotherapy and radiotherapy followed by surgery in stage IIIA non-small-cell carcinoma of the lung: report of a Cancer and Leukemia Group B phase II study. *J Clin Oncol* 1992;10:1237–1244.
132. Albain KS, Rusch VW, Crowley JJ, et al. Concurrent cisplatin/etoposide plus chest radiotherapy followed by surgery for stages IIIA (N2) and IIIB non-small-cell lung cancer: mature results of Southwest Oncology Group phase II study 8805. *J Clin Oncol* 1995;13:1880–1892.
133. Albain K, Rusch V, Crowley J, et al. Long-term survival after concurrent cisplatin/etoposide (PE) plus chest radiotherapy (RT) followed by surgery in bulky, stages IIIA(N2) and IIIB non-small cell lung cancer (NSCLC): 6-year outcomes from Southwest Oncology Group Study 8805. *Proc Am Soc Clin Oncol* 1999;18:467a.
134. Yashar J, Weitberg A, Glicksman A, et al. Preoperative chemotherapy and radiation therapy for stage IIIa carcinoma of the lung. *Ann Thorac Surg* 1992;53:445–448.
135. Fowler W, Langer C, Curran W Jr, et al. Postoperative complications after combined neoadjuvant treatment of lung cancer. *Ann Thorac Surg* 1993;55:986–989.
136. Milstein D, Kuten A, Saute M, et al. Preoperative concurrent chemoradiotherapy for unresectable stage III nonsmall cell lung cancer. *Int J Rad Oncol Biol Phys* 1996;34:1125–1132.
137. Taylor NA, Liao ZX, Cox JD, et al. Equivalent outcome of patients with clinical stage IIIA non-small-cell lung cancer treated with concurrent chemoradiation compared with induction chemotherapy followed by surgical resection. *Int J Rad Oncol Biol Phys* 2004;58:204–212.
138. Albain KS, Swann RS, Rusch VW, et al. Radiotherapy plus chemotherapy with or without surgical resection for stage III non-small-cell lung cancer: a phase III randomised controlled trial. *Lancet* 2009;374:379–386.

139. Thomas M, Rübe C, Hoffknecht P, et al. Effect of preoperative chemoradiation in addition to preoperative chemotherapy: a randomised trial in stage III non-small-cell lung cancer. *Lancet Oncol* 2008;9:636–648.
140. Burfeind WR Jr, D'Amico TA, Toloza EM, et al. Low morbidity and mortality for bronchoplastic procedures with and without induction therapy. *Ann Thorac Surg* 2005;80:418–421.
141. Adelstein DJ, Rice TW, Rybicki LA, et al. Accelerated hyperfractionated radiation, concurrent paclitaxel/cisplatin chemotherapy and surgery for stage III non-small cell lung cancer. *Lung Cancer* 2002;36:167–174.
142. Weil MD, Roach I, Mack, et al. 3D conformal radiotherapy in the sagittal plane for centrally located thoracic tumors. *Med Dosim* 1995;20:11–14.
143. Hayman JA, Martel MK, Ten Haken RK, et al. Dose escalation in non-small-cell lung cancer using three-dimensional conformal radiation therapy: update of a phase I trial. *J Clin Oncol* 2001;19:127–136.
144. Pancoast H. Superior pulmonary sulcus tumor: tumor characterized by pain, Horner's syndrome, destruction of bone and atrophy of hand muscles. *JAMA* 1932;99:1391–1396.
145. Vallieres E, Kraut M, Thomas C. Pancoast (superior sulcus) neoplasms. *Curr Prob Cancer* 2003;27:81–104.
146. Shaw R, Paulson D, Kee JJ. Treatment of the superior sulcus tumor by irradiation followed by resection. *Ann Surg* 1961;154:29–40.
147. Rusch V, Parekh K, Leon L, et al. Factors determining outcome after surgical resection of T3 and T4 lung cancers of the superior sulcus. *J Thorac Cardiovasc Surg* 2000;119:1147–1153.
148. Detterbeck FC. Pancoast (superior sulcus) tumors. *Ann Thorac Surg* 1997;63:1810–1818.
149. Rusch V, Giroux D, Kraut M, et al. Induction chemoradiation and surgical resection for non-small cell lung carcinomas of the superior sulcus: initial results of Southwest Oncology Group Trial 9416 (Intergroup Trial 0160). *J Thorac Cardiovasc Surg* 2001;121:472–483.
150. Travis WD, Linnoila RI, Tsokos MG, et al. Neuroendocrine tumors of the lung with proposed criteria for large-cell neuroendocrine carcinoma. An ultrastructural, immunohistochemical, and flow cytometric study of 35 cases. *Am J Surg Pathol* 1991;15:529–553.
151. Vuitch F, Sekido Y, Fong K, et al. Neuroendocrine tumors of the lung. Pathology and molecular biology. *Chest Surg Clin N Am* 1997;7:21–47.
152. McCaughan B, Martini N, Bains M. Bronchial carcinoids. Review of 124 cases. *J Thorac Cardiovasc Surg* 1985;89:8–17.
153. Martini N, Zaman MB, Bains MS, et al. Treatment and prognosis in bronchial carcinoids involving regional lymph nodes. *J Thorac Cardiovasc Surg* 1994;107:1–7.
154. Jiang S-X, Kameya T, Shoji M, et al. Large cell neuroendocrine carcinoma of the lung: a histologic and immunohistochemical study of 22 cases. *Am J Surg Pathol* 1998;22:526–537.
155. Travis WD, Rush W, Flieder DB, et al. Survival analysis of 200 pulmonary neuroendocrine tumors with clarification of criteria for atypical carcinoid and its separation from typical carcinoid. *Am J Surg Pathol* 1998;22:934–944.
156. Zacharias J, Nicholson AG, Ladas GP, et al. Large cell neuroendocrine carcinoma and large cell carcinomas with neuroendocrine morphology of the lung: prognosis after complete resection and systematic nodal dissection. *Ann Thorac Surg* 2003;75:348–352.
157. Stahel RA, Ginsberg R, Havemann K, et al. Staging and prognostic factors in small cell lung cancer: a consensus report. *Lung Cancer* 1989;5:119–126.
158. Shepherd FA. The role of chemotherapy in the treatment of small cell lung cancer. *Chest Surg Clin N Am* 1997;7:113–133.
159. Pignon JP, Arriagada R, Ihde DC, et al. A meta-analysis of thoracic radiotherapy for small-cell lung cancer. *N Engl J Med* 1992;327:1618–1624.
160. Warde P, Payne D. Does thoracic irradiation improve survival and local control in limited- stage small-cell carcinoma of the lung? A meta-analysis. *J Clin Oncol* 1992;10:890–895.
161. Albain K, Crowley J, LeBlanc M, et al. Determinants of improved outcome in small-cell lung cancer: an analysis of the 2580-patient Southwest Oncology Group data base. *J Clin Oncol* 1990;8:1563–1574.
162. Inoue M, Miyoshi S, Yasumitsu T, et al. Surgical results for small cell lung cancer based on the new TNM staging system. *Ann Thorac Surg* 2000;70:1615–1619.
163. Kreisman H, Wolkove N, Quoix E. Small cell lung cancer presenting as a solitary pulmonary nodule. *Chest* 1992;101:225–231.
164. Brock MV, Hooker CM, Syphard JE, et al. Surgical resection of limited disease small cell lung cancer in the new era of platinum chemotherapy: its time has come. *J Thorac Cardiovasc Surg* 2005;129:64–72.
165. Shepherd F, Evans W, Feld R, et al. Adjuvant chemotherapy following surgical resection for small-cell carcinoma of the lung. *J Clin Oncol* 1988;6:832–838.
166. Shah S, Thompson J, Goldstraw P. Results of operation without adjuvant therapy in the treatment of small cell lung cancer. *Ann Thorac Surg* 1992;54:498–501.
167. Shepherd F, Ginsberg R, Patterson G, et al. Is there ever a role for salvage operations in limited small-cell lung cancer? *J Thorac Cardiovasc Surg* 1991;101:196–200.
168. Lad T, Piantadosi S, Thomas P, et al. A prospective randomized trial to determine the benefit of surgical resection of residual disease following response of small cell lung cancer to combination chemotherapy. *Chest* 1994;106:320S–323S.
169. Inoue H, Iwasaki M, Ogawa J, et al. Surgical resection of a second primary lung carcinoma in a survivor of small cell carcinoma. *Ann Thorac Surg* 1993;56:1160–1161.
170. Heitmiller R, Mathisen D, Ferry J, et al. Mucoepidermoid lung tumors. *Ann Thorac Surg* 1989;47:394–399.
171. Moran CA. Primary salivary gland-type tumors of the lung. *Semin Diagn Pathol* 1995;12:106–122.
172. Webb BD, Walsh GL, Roberts DB, et al. Primary tracheal malignant neoplasms: the University of Texas MD Anderson Cancer Center experience. *J Am Coll Surg* 2006;202:237–246.
173. Gaissert HA, Grillo HC, Shadmehr MB, et al. Long-term survival after resection of primary adenoid cystic and squamous cell carcinoma of the trachea and carina. *Ann Thorac Surg* 2004;78:1889–1897.
174. Maziak DE, Todd TRJ, Keshavjee SH, et al. Adenoid cystic carcinoma of the airway: thirty-two-year experience. *J Thorac Cardiovasc Surg* 1996;112:1522–1532.
175. Chin H, DeMeester T, Chin R, et al. Endobronchial adenoid cystic carcinoma. *Chest* 1991;100:1464–1465.
176. Miller DL, Allen MS. Rare pulmonary neoplasms. *Mayo Clin Proc* 1993;68:492–498.
177. Berho M, Moran CA, Suster S. Malignant mixed epithelial/mesenchymal neoplasms of the lung. *Semin Diagn Pathol* 1995;12:123–139.
178. Barney JD, Churchill ED. Adenocarcinoma of the kidney with metastases to the lung cured by nephrectomy and lobectomy. *J Urol* 1939;42:269–276.
179. Clagett OT, Woolner LB. Surgical treatment of solitary metastatic pulmonary lesion. *Med Clin North Am* 1964;48:939–943.
180. Mountain C, McMurtrey M, Hermes K. Surgery for pulmonary metastasis: a 20-year experience. *Ann Thorac Surg* 1984;38:323–330.
181. Martini N, Huvos A, Mike V, et al. Multiple pulmonary resections in the treatment of osteogenic sarcoma. *Ann Thorac Surg* 1971;12:271–280.
182. Crow J, Slavin G, Kreel L. Pulmonary metastasis: a pathologic and radiologic study. *Cancer* 1981;47:2595–2602.
183. Heitmiller R, Marasco W, Hruban R, et al. Endobronchial metastasis. *J Thorac Cardiovasc Surg* 1993;106:537–542.
184. Loehe F, Kobinger S, Hatz RA, et al. Value of systematic mediastinal lymph node dissection during pulmonary metastasectomy. *Ann Thorac Surg* 2001;72:225–229.
185. Ercan S, Nichols FC III, Trastek VF, et al. Prognostic significance of lymph node metastasis found during pulmonary metastasectomy for extrapulmonary carcinoma. *Ann Thorac Surg* 2004;77:1786–1791.
186. Johnson H Jr, Fantone J, Flye MW. Histological evaluation of the nodules resected in the treatment of pulmonary metastatic disease. *J Surg Oncol* 1982;21:1–4.
187. Pastorino U, Buyse M, Friedel G, et al. Long-term results of lung metastasectomy: prognostic analyses based on 5206 cases. *J Thorac Cardiovasc Surg* 1997;113:37–49.
188. McCormack P, Ginsberg K, Bains M, et al. Accuracy of lung imaging in metastases with implications for the role of thoracoscopy. *Ann Thorac Surg* 1993;56:863–865.
189. Pastorino U, Veronesi G, Landoni C, et al. Fluorodeoxyglucose positron emission tomography improves preoperative staging of resectable lung metastasis. *J Thorac Cardiovasc Surg* 2003;126:1906–1910.
190. Deleyiannis F, Thomas D. Risk of lung cancer among patients with head and neck cancer. *Otolaryngol Head Neck Surg* 1997;116:630–636.
191. Robert JH, Ambrogi V, Mermillod B, et al. Factors influencing long-term survival after lung metastasectomy. *Ann Thorac Surg* 1997;63:777–784.
192. Rusch V. Pulmonary metastasectomy. Current indications. *Chest* 1995;107:322S–331S.
193. Girard P, Baldeyrou P, Le Chevalier T, et al. Surgery for pulmonary metastases. Who are the 10-year survivors? *Cancer* 1994;74:2791–2797.
194. McCormack P. Surgical resection of pulmonary metastases. *Semin Surg Oncol* 1990;6:297–302.
195. La Quaglia MP. Osteosarcoma. Specific tumor management and results. *Chest Surg Clin N Am* 1998;8:77–95.
196. Singletary SE, Walsh G, Vauthey J-N, et al. A role for curative surgery in the treatment of selected patients with metastatic breast cancer. *Oncologist* 2003;8:241–251.
197. Friedel G, Pastorino U, Ginsberg RJ, et al. Results of lung metastasectomy from breast cancer: prognostic criteria on the basis of 467 cases of the international registry of lung metastases. *Eur J Cardiothorac Surg* 2002;22:335–344.
198. Feldman DR, Bosl GJ, Sheinfeld J, et al. Medical treatment of advanced testicular cancer. *JAMA* 2008;299:672–684.
199. Liu D, Abolhoda A, Burt ME, et al. Pulmonary metastasectomy for testicular germ cell tumors: a 28-year experience. *Ann Thorac Surg* 1998;66:1709–1714.
200. Kesler KA, Rieger KM, Hammoud ZT, et al. A 25-year single institution experience with surgery for primary mediastinal nonseminomatous germ cell tumors. *Ann Thorac Surg* 2008;85:371–378.
201. Kesler KA, Wilson JL, Cosgrove JA, et al. Surgical salvage therapy for malignant intrathoracic metastases from nonseminomatous germ cell cancer of testicular origin: analysis of a single-institution experience. *J Thorac Cardiovasc Surg* 2005;130:408–415.
202. Putnam J Jr, Suell D, Natarajan G, et al. Extended resection of pulmonary metastases: is the risk justified? *Ann Thorac Surg* 1993;55:1440–1446.
203. Koong HN, Pastorino U, Ginsberg RJ. Is there a role for pneumonectomy in pulmonary metastases? *Ann Thorac Surg* 1999;68:2039–2043.
204. Bains M, Ginsberg R, Jones W II, et al. The clamshell incision: an improved approach to bilateral pulmonary and mediastinal tumor. *Ann Thorac Surg* 1994;58:30–32.

205. Liu H, Lin P, Hsieh M, et al. Application of thoracoscopy for lung metastases. *Chest* 1995;107:266–268.
206. Petersen RP, Hanish SI, Haney JC, et al. Improved survival with pulmonary metastasectomy: an analysis of 1720 patients with pulmonary metastatic melanoma. *J Thorac Cardiovasc Surg* 2007;133:104–110.
207. Gossot D, Radu C, Girard P, et al. Resection of pulmonary metastases from sarcoma: can some patients benefit from a less invasive approach? *Ann Thorac Surg* 2009;87:238–243.
208. Briccoli A, Rocca M, Salone M, et al. Resection of recurrent pulmonary metastases in patients with osteosarcoma. *Cancer* 2005;104:1721–1725.
209. Kandioler D, Kromer E, Tuchler H, et al. Long-term results after repeated surgical removal of pulmonary metastases. *Ann Thorac Surg* 1998;65: 909–912.
210. Liu D, Labow DM, Dang N, et al. Pulmonary metastasectomy for head and neck cancers. *Ann Surg Oncol* 1999;6:572–578.
211. Arrigoni M, Woolner L, Bernatz P, et al. Benign tumors of the lung. A ten-year surgical experience. *J Thorac Cardiovasc Surg* 1970;60:589–599.
212. Oldham HN Jr. Benign tumors of the lung and bronchus. *Surg Clin North Am* 1980;60:825–834.
213. Hansen C, Holtveg H, Francis D, et al. Pulmonary hamartoma. *J Thorac Cardiovasc Surg* 1992;104:674–678.
214. Dautzenberg B, Chastang C, Arriagada R, et al. Adjuvant radiotherapy versus combined sequential chemotherapy followed by radiotherapy in the treatment of resected nonsmall cell lung carcinoma. A randomized trial of 267 patients. GETCB (Groupe d'Etude et de Traitement des Cancers Bronchiques). *Cancer* 1995;76:779–786.
215. Scagliotti GV, Fossati R, Torri V, et al. Randomized study of adjuvant chemotherapy for completely resected stage I, II, or IIIa non-small-cell lung cancer. *J Natl Cancer Inst* 2003;95:1453–1461.
216. Trovo MG, Minatel E, Veronesi A, et al. Combined radiotherapy and chemotherapy versus radiotherapy alone in locally advanced epidermoid bronchogenic carcinoma. A randomized study. *Cancer* 1990;65:400–404.
217. Morton RF, Jett JR, McGinnis WL, et al. Thoracic radiation therapy alone compared with combined chemoradiotherapy for locally unresectable non-small cell lung cancer. A randomized, phase III trial. *Ann Int Med* 1991; 115:681–686.
218. Le Chevalier T, Arriagada R, Quoix E, et al. Radiotherapy alone versus combined chemotherapy and radiotherapy in nonresectable non-small-cell lung cancer: first analysis of a randomized trial in 353 patients. *J Natl Cancer Inst* 1991;83:417–423.
219. Blanke C, Ansari R, Mantravadi R, et al. Phase III trial of thoracic irradiation with or without cisplatin for locally advanced unresectable non-small-cell lung cancer: a Hoosier Oncology Group protocol. *J Clin Oncol* 1995;13:1425–1429.
220. Schaake-Koning C, van den Bogaert W, Dalesio O, et al. Effects of concomitant cisplatin and radiotherapy on inoperable non-small-cell lung cancer. *N Engl J Med* 1992;326:524–530.
221. Jeremic B, Shibamoto Y, Acimovic L, et al. Randomized trial of hyperfractionated radiation therapy with or without concurrent chemotherapy for stage III non-small-cell lung cancer. *J Clin Oncol* 1995;13:452–458.
222. Dillman R, Herndon J, Seagren S, et al. Improved survival in stage III non-small-cell lung cancer: seven-year follow-up of cancer and leukemia group B (CALGB) 8433 trial. *J Natl Cancer Inst* 1996;88:1210–1215.
223. Sause W, Kolesar P, Taylor S, IV, et al. Final results of phase III trial in regionally advanced unresectable non-small cell lung cancer: Radiation Therapy Oncology Group, Eastern Cooperative Oncology Group, and Southwest Oncology Group. *Chest* 2000;117:358–364.
224. Albain KS, Scott CB, Rusch VR, et al. PL-4 phase III study of concurrent chemotherapy and full course radiotherapy (CT/RT) versus CT/RT induction followed by surgical resection for stage IIIA(pN2) non-small cell lung cancer (NSCLC): first outcome analysis of North American Intergroup trial 0139 (RTOG 93–09). *Lung Cancer* 2003;41:S4.
225. Kavolius J, Mastorakos D, Pavlovich C, et al. Resection of metastatic renal cell carcinoma. *J Clin Oncol* 1998;16:2261–2266.
226. McCormack PM, Burt ME, Bains MS, et al. Lung resection for colorectal metastases. 10-year results. *Arch Surg* 1992;127:1403–1406.
227. Billingsley KG, Burt ME, Jara E, et al. Pulmonary metastases from soft tissue sarcoma: analysis of patterns of diseases and postmetastasis survival. *Ann Surg* 1999;229:602–610.

CHAPTER 80 ■ CHEST WALL, PLEURA, MEDIASTINUM, AND NONNEOPLASTIC LUNG DISEASE

RISHINDRA M. REDDY

KEY POINTS

1. Surgical intervention for chest wall tumors depends on the type of lesion and goals of surgery (resection vs. diagnosis). Reconstruction varies depending on the size of the defect and location on the chest wall.
2. Thoracic outlet syndrome may be arterial, venous, or neurogenic. Neurogenic TOS is the most difficult to diagnose, and surgery for this should be performed in high-volume centers.
3. The primary treatment for a lung abscess is antibiotic therapy.
4. Hemoptysis can be life threatening from suffocation due to a low volume of blood in the lungs, *not* from blood volume loss requiring transfusion.
5. Primary spontaneous pneumothoraces will recur in only 30% of patients after initial treatment. When they recur, the treatment should include a thoracoscopic evaluation and possible pleurodesis.
6. Transudative pleural effusions should be treated medically, whereas exudative effusions may need more intervention. One quarter of pleural effusions in a community hospital are due to malignancy.
7. Empyema is a part of a spectrum of disease that may be treated early on with drainage alone, but may require débridement and decortication in more advanced cases.
8. Complications of tracheostomies are usually due to improper placement of the tracheostomy on the trachea (below the third ring, risking a tracheoinnominate fistula) or to the use of high pressures in the cuff of the tracheostomy (causing ischemia and long-term stenosis).
9. Mediastinitis is life threatening and warrants immediate evaluation, antibiotic therapy, and surgical drainage.

This chapter is meant as a resource for the general surgery community and general surgery trainees with regard to pathology in the chest. It will cover a wide variety of topics including most noncardiac congenital disease processes in the thorax. The outline for this chapter is from the Thoracic Surgery Director's Association curriculum for the topics mentioned in the title. The full curriculum can be accessed at www.tsda.org.

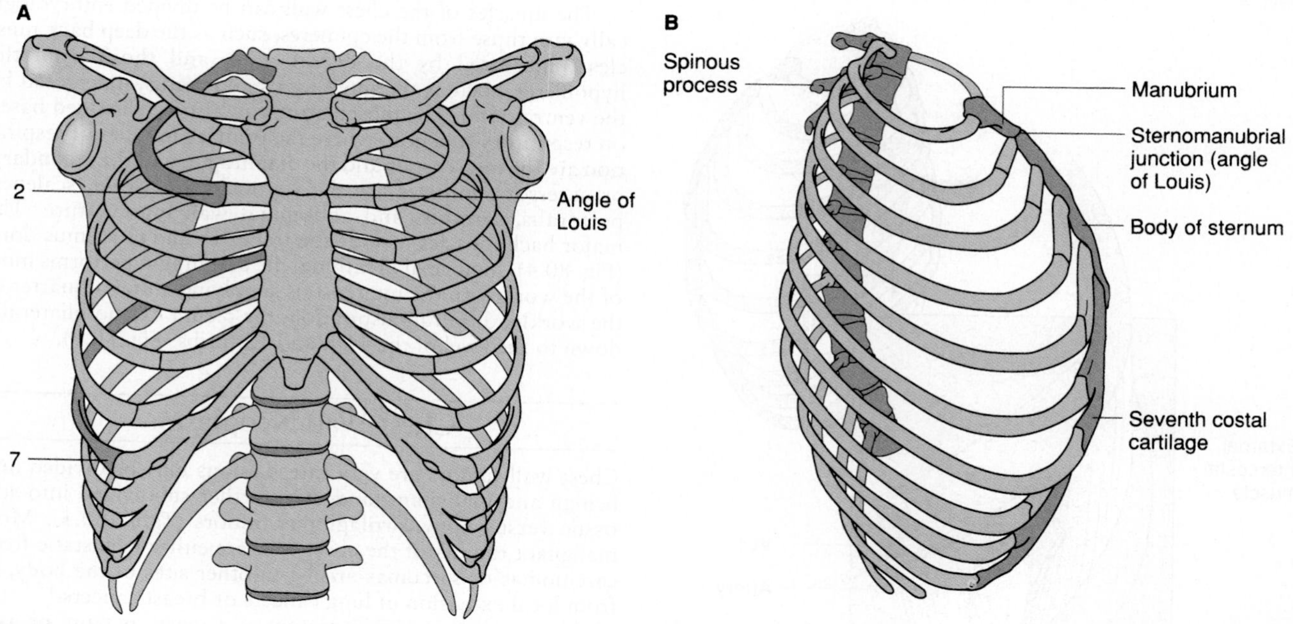

FIGURE 80.1. Skeletal support of the thorax. Anterior (A) and lateral (B) views. Note the anterior cartilaginous component of the upper 10 ribs, the fused costal cartilages of ribs 7 through 10, the location of the sternomanubrial junction (angle of Louis) at the level of the second rib, and the oblique course of the ribs laterally from posterior to anterior.

CHEST WALL

Chest Wall Anatomy

The chest wall is the musculoskeletal structure that contains and protects the structures of the upper trunk or thorax. There are two openings to the thorax: the superior aperture, or the thoracic inlet, and the inferior aperture, which leads to the abdominal cavity. The head and arms connect to the intrathoracic structures via the inlet, whereas the diaphragm separates the thoracic and abdominal cavities at the inferior aperture. The inferior vena cava, esophagus, and aorta all travel to the abdomen through the diaphragm at levels T8, T10, and T12, respectively.

The sternum, commonly known as the breast bone, is composed of three parts: the manubrium, the body, and the xiphoid. The manubrium attaches to the clavicles and the first costal cartilages. The sternal angle where the manubrium and body connect is called the angle of Louis and is an important landmark. The second ribs attach to the sternum at this angle, and they allow one to count the ribs from this point down, as the first ribs are not palpable. The body of the sternum contains articular facets for ribs 2 to 7 and connects to the cartilaginous xiphoid inferiorly. The xiphoid may be bifid and will eventually ossify in older adults (Fig. 80.1).

The ribs are split into two groups; the upper seven pairs are the true ribs, with articulations to the sternum, while the lower five pairs are the false ribs. Ribs 8, 9, and 10 connect to each other and the upper ribs via their costal cartilage. Ribs 11 and 12 are called floating ribs as they have no anterior connection. Rib 1 is unique in its shape as it is flat, short, and extremely curved. Ribs 2 through 10 have a more standard configuration with the head containing articular facets for the vertebrae. After the neck the tubercle contains the facet for the vertebral transverse process. The costal groove along the inferior portion of the shaft houses the intercostal bundle, consisting of the nerve, artery, and vein (Fig. 80.2). Because of this inferior placement, most chest wall procedures such as thoracostomy tube placement or thoracentesis should be aimed at the superior aspect of the rib to avoid injury to this bundle.

There are three intercostal muscles: the external intercostal, the internal intercostal, and the innermost intercostal muscle. The intercostal bundle lies just external to the innermost intercostal layer (Fig. 80.3). On the inner aspect of the chest wall, the internal thoracic (mammary) artery and vein runs between the innermost intercostal muscle and the transversus thoracis muscles, which connect the ribs to the lower half of the sternal body. The intercostal arteries have two sources, one posterior and one anterior. The posterior arteries almost all arise from the descending thoracic aorta, while the anterior arteries branch off the internal thoracic artery. The intercostal nerve is a branch off the ventral ramus after it joins the sympathetic trunk. The intercostal veins follow the arteries and posteriorly drain into the azygos and hemiazygos veins. Lymphatic drainage from the posterior chest wall drains into the thoracic duct on the left and into the right lymphatic duct on the right.

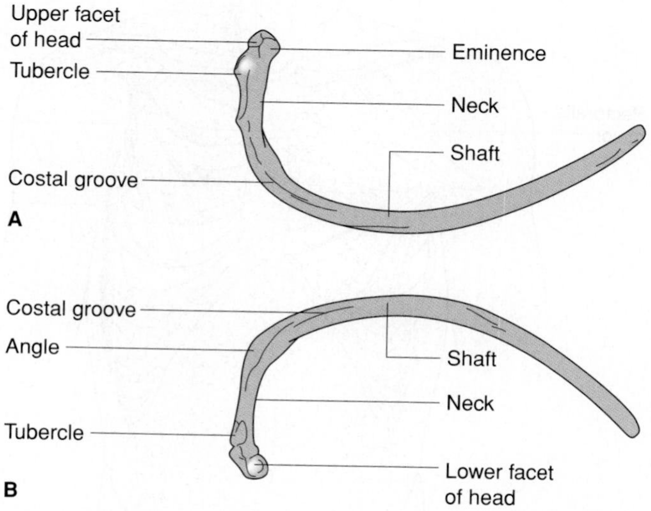

FIGURE 80.2. Anatomy of ribs 2 to 10 as viewed from above (A) and below (B).

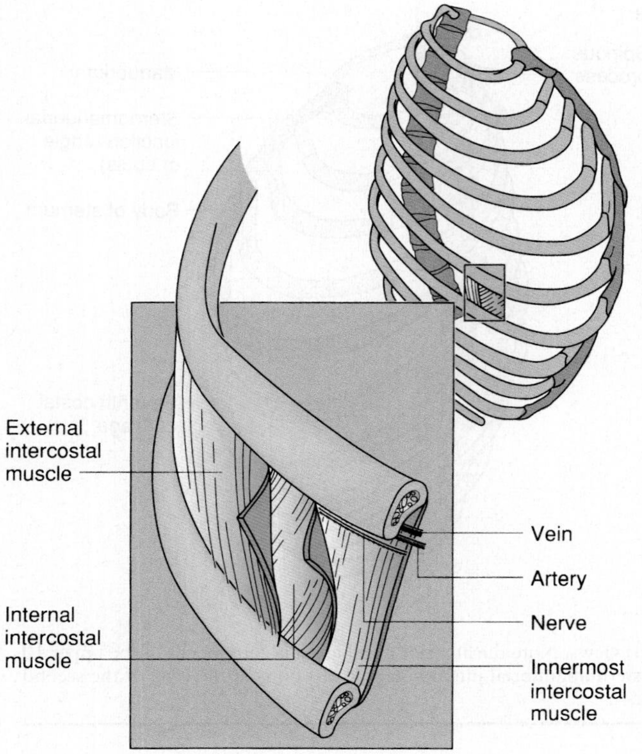

FIGURE 80.3. Anatomy of the intercostal space. The major intercostal muscles are the external and internal. The neurovascular bundle courses in the costal groove along the inferior aspect of the rib.

The muscles of the chest wall can be divided embryologically into those from the epimeres, such as the deep back muscles, innervated by the dorsal rami, and those from the hypomeres, such as the intercostals and rectus, innervated by the ventral rami. The musculature can also be classified based on respiratory function, where the primary muscles of respiration are the intercostals and the diaphragm, and the secondary, or accessory, muscles are the sternocleidomastoid, scalenes, pectoralis, serratus, and abdominal wall musculature. The major back muscles include the trapezius and latissimus dorsi (Fig. 80.4). In normal breathing, the diaphragm performs most of the work with the intercostals supplying about a quarter of the workload. In full inspiration, the pleura extend bilaterally down to the level of the 11th and 12th ribs (Fig. 80.5).

Chest Wall Neoplasms

Chest wall tumors are very rare. Lesions may be divided into benign and malignant, and then further subdivided into soft tissue versus bony/cartilaginous tumors (Table 80.1). Most malignant tumors of the chest wall are either metastatic from carcinomas or sarcomas arising in other sites of the body, or from local extension of lung cancers or breast cancers.[1]

Almost all lesions will present as a mass, as pain, or as a combination of both. Occasionally they will be asymptomatic and be identified on imaging for cancer surveillance or other reasons.[2] Fever can occasionally be a presenting symptom in the setting of a systemic neoplastic process. Evaluation of these lesions includes a thorough history and physical and appropriate imaging, which may begin with plain radiographs, but should include three-dimensional imaging such as a CT scan and/or MRI. This will allow for evaluation of the depth of the lesion, the relationship of the lesion to nerve and vascular structures, and the pulmonary fields for possible

FIGURE 80.4. Thoracic musculature. Anterior (**A**) and posterior (**B**) views.

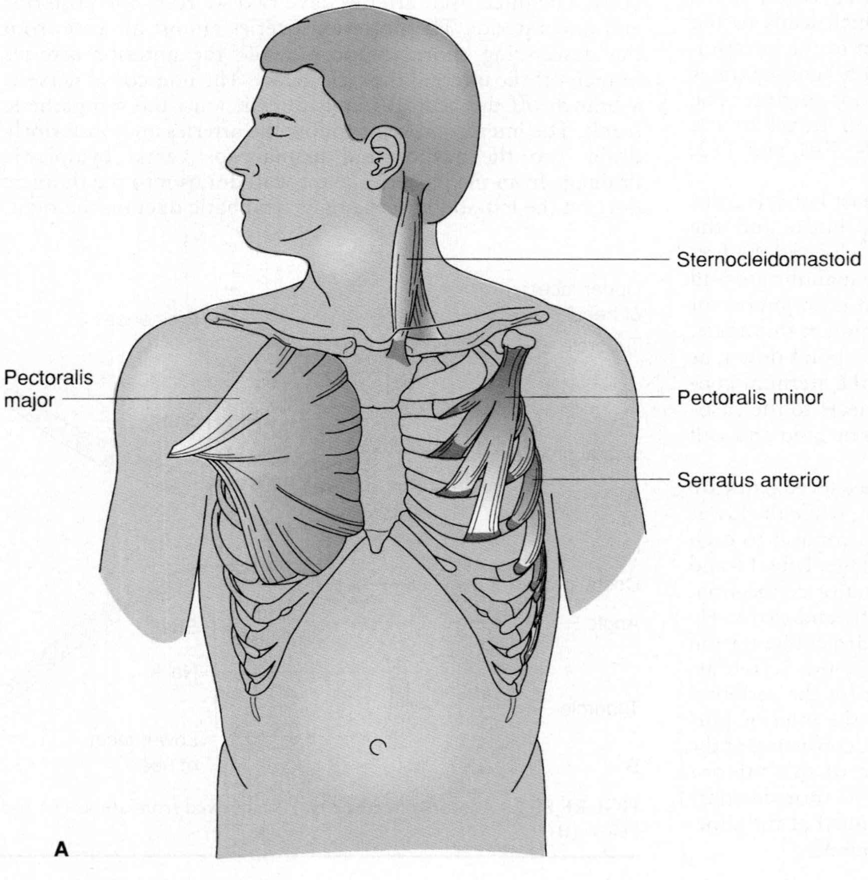

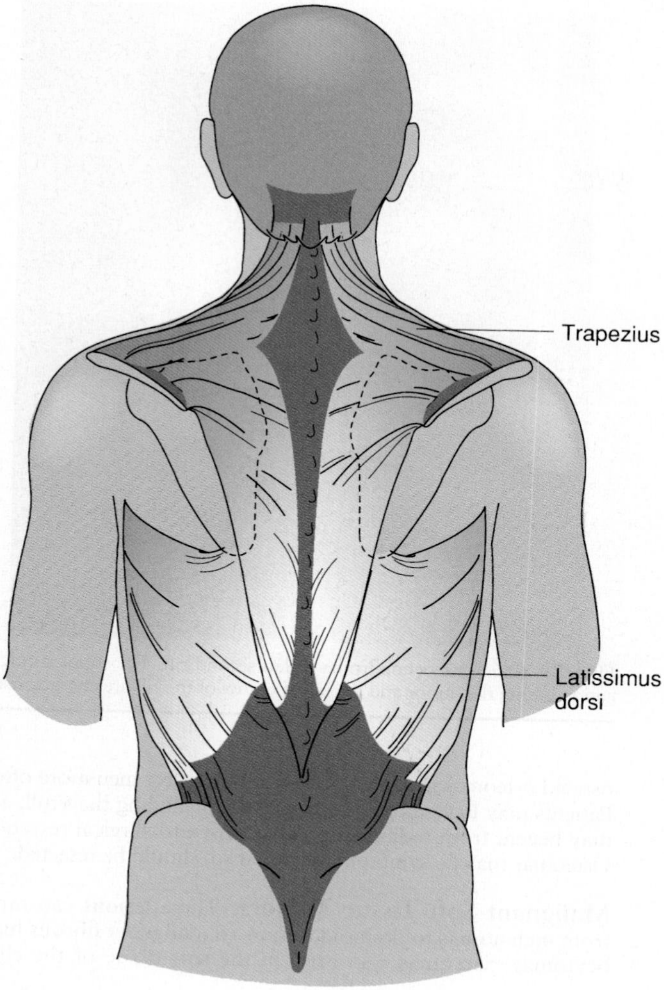

FIGURE 80.4. (*Continued*)

metastases. Depending on the situation, PET scans may also be useful.[1] Prior films may help ascertain the rate of growth of the lesion.[3]

Surgical intervention depends on the type of lesion and the goal of surgery. Tumors that are suspected metastases may require only a needle or an incisional biopsy to confirm the diagnosis. Lesions that are possible primary tumors, whether benign or malignant, require excisional biopsies. Some low-grade malignant tumors may be underdiagnosed and considered benign if the entire specimen is not removed and examined. If a tumor is proven to be a primary malignant lesion, wide excision is required, with margins up to 4 cm.[3]

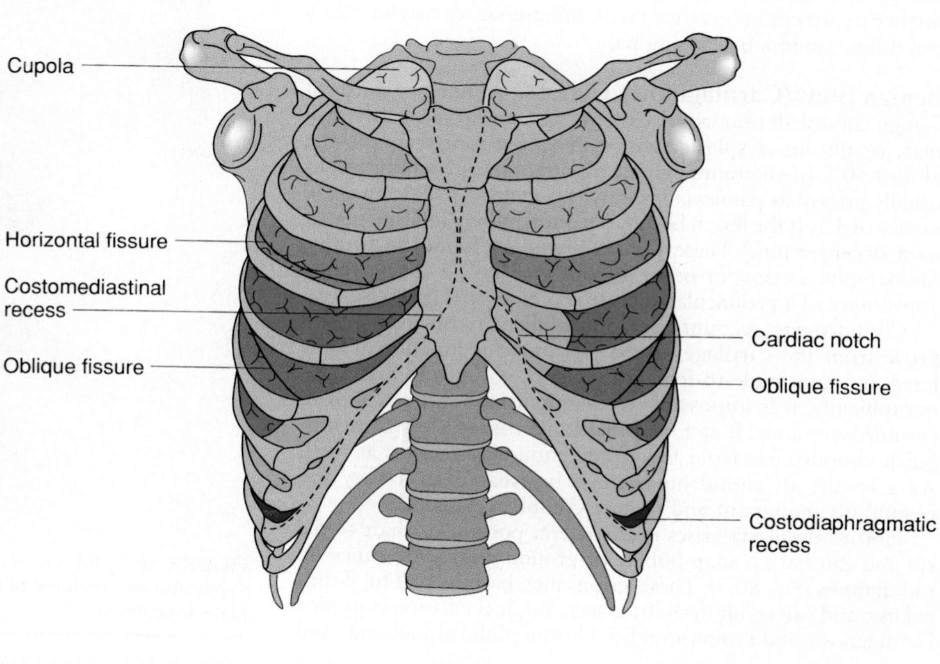

FIGURE 80.5. Topographic relations of the pleura to the chest wall. Laterally, the pleura extends to the level of the 11th to 12th ribs. The anterior reflection of the mediastinal and costal pleurae forms the costomediastinal recess, whereas the reflections of the costal and diaphragmatic pleurae form the costodiaphragmatic recess.

TABLE 80.1

CHEST WALL TUMOR CLASSIFICATION

■ Benign tumors
Soft tissue tumors
Lipomas
Fibromas
Hemangiomas
Neurofibromas
Granulomas
Inflammatory tumor
Tuberculoma
Bony/Cartilagenous tumors
Osteochondromas
Chondromas
Fibrous dysplasia
Eosinophilc granuloma
Osteoid osteomas
Osteomyelitis
Chondro/Osteoblastomas
■ Malignant tumors
Soft tissue tumors
Melanomas and other cutaneous cancers
Sarcomas
Desmoid tumors/low-grade fibrosarcomas
Lymphoma
Malignant fibrous histiocytoma
Bony/Cartilagenous tumors
Chondrosarcomas
Osteogenic sarcomas
Ewing's sarcomas
Solitary plasmocytoma
Lymphoma
■ Metastatic tumors
Breast cancer
Lung cancer
Mediastinal tumors
Mesothelioma
Other sarcomas or carcinomas

Benign Soft Tissue Tumors. These tumors include lipomas, fibromas, hemangiomas, and neurofibromas, among others. These can be removed by excisional biopsy and require no further treatment unless they recur. Inflammatory osteomyelitis can mimic tumors by causing pain.

Benign Bony/Cartilaginous Tumors. About two thirds of benign chest wall tumors are either osteochondromas, chondromas, or fibrous dysplasia, with osteochondromas composing almost 50% of all nonmalignant rib tumors. Osteochondromas usually present as painless masses with a male-to-female predominance of 3:1. If the lesion becomes painful, it may indicate malignant degeneration.[3] These tumors are often found on routine radiographic exams for other reasons and have a characteristic appearance of a pedunculated bony prominence (Fig. 80.6).

Chondromas account for 15% of benign rib lesions and grow from the cartilage at the sternocostal junction.[1] They have an equal male-to-female incidence. Clinically and radiographically, it is impossible to distinguish chondromas from chondrosarcomas. It can be difficult microscopically to distinguish chondromas from low-grade chondrosarcomas as well. As a result, all chondromas must be treated as if they are potentially malignant and require complete excision.[3]

Fibrous dysplasia arises in the lateral portion or shaft of the rib and can have a soap bubble or ground-glass appearance on radiographs (Fig. 80.7). These lesions may become painful if they enlarge and can result in rib fractures. Surgical excision is needed for diagnosis and symptom relief.[4] Eosinophilic granulomas and

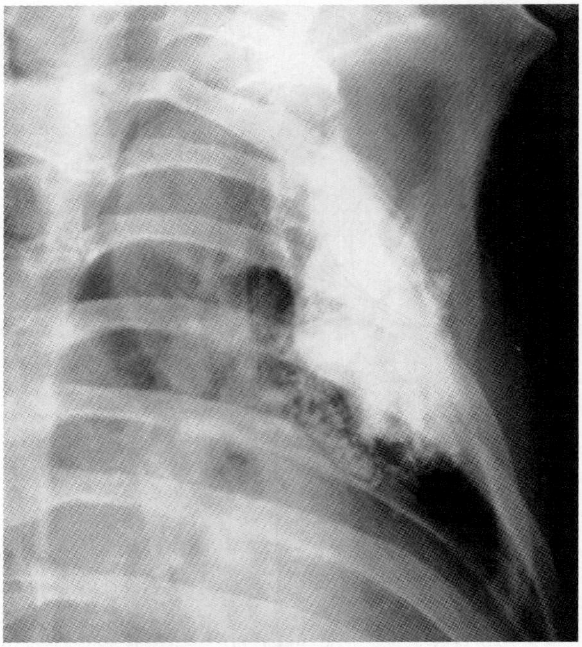

FIGURE 80.6. Osteochondroma of left second rib. The stippled calcification within the tumor and the intact cortex of the rib are characteristic.

osteoid osteomas are rare conditions that affect men more often. Patients may have multiple granulomas, including the skull, and may benefit from radiotherapy as opposed to surgical resection. Osteomas may be symptomatic and if so, should be resected.

Malignant Soft Tissue Tumors. These lesions can range from melanomas to desmoid tumors to malignant fibrous histiocytomas. Sarcomas also arise in the soft tissue of the chest

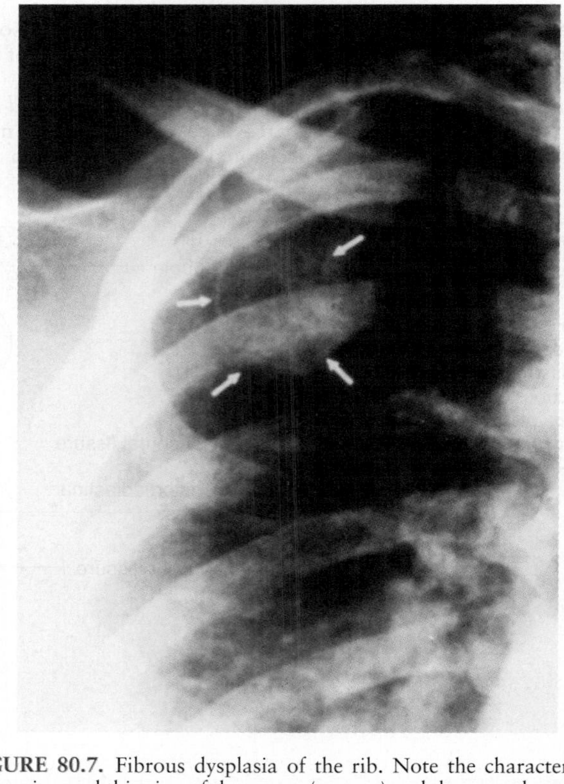

FIGURE 80.7. Fibrous dysplasia of the rib. Note the characteristic expansion and thinning of the cortex (*arrows*) and the central ground-glass appearance.

wall, but they compose less than 10% of all sarcomas.[2] Desmoid tumors are borderline lesions between a benign and malignant classification and are sometimes considered low-grade fibrosarcomas.[1] Almost half of all desmoids occur in the chest wall and shoulder where they can encapsulate the brachial plexus. They require wide local excision and have a high rate of recurrence. If they encircle vital structures, they can be treated with radiotherapy after surgical excision.

Malignant fibrous histiocytoma (MFH) is the most common primary chest wall tumor. These tumors are more frequent in men (2:1 ratio) and generally occur in those older than 50 years of age. They are slow growing, painless, and spread along the fascial planes or between muscle fibers. MFH are unresponsive to other forms of therapy and require wide local excision. Because of the lesion's propensity for fascial plane infiltration, there is a high rate of recurrence following resection, and patients who have undergone resection have a 5-year survival of less than 40%.[3] Rhabdomyosarcoma is the second most common soft tissue lesion of the chest wall and usually occurs in children and younger adults. It grows rapidly from the striated muscle but is usually painless. It is treated with wide excision followed by radiation and chemotherapy with a reported 70% survival at 5 years.[3] A recent review of soft tissue sarcomas in the chest wall suggested that tumor size greater or less than 5 cm correlates with overall prognosis. Also, patients with low-grade tumors had a 100% 5-year survival rate versus a 69.2% survival in those with high-grade tumors. There was a trend toward improved survival in patients who received a complete resection versus those left with residual disease, but it did not achieve statistical significance due to small sample size.[2]

Malignant Bony/Cartilagenous Tumors. Chondrosarcomas are the most common primary malignant bony tumors, accounting for 20% to 30% of lesions. These are well-differentiated tumors and on microscopic examination may be difficult to distinguish from their benign counterparts. Local recurrence can occur after excision, and if untreated, distant metastases can develop.[3] Osteogenic sarcomas are more common in the limbs but also occur in the ribs. Radiographs depict a characteristic sunburst pattern. These tend to grow quickly and often have metastases at the time of initial presentation. Patient evaluation should include a CT scan and bone scan to check for the presence of metastatic disease. Surgery with adjuvant chemotherapy is the treatment of choice for local disease.[5] Ewing sarcomas constitute 5% to 10% of chest wall tumors. They occur in children and younger adults with a male-to-female ratio of 1.6:1. Symptoms include pain, fever, and fatigue. Radiographs show a large soft tissue mass with bony destruction. Patients often present with metastatic disease, and ultimately three quarters of patients will develop metastases. Multimodality treatment is the key to treatment. Survival may be less than 30% at 5 years in patients with metastatic disease.[6]

Solitary plasmocytoma is a rare tumor of the plasma cells and can be part of a systemic disease in multiple myeloma. Lesions can be painful and usually occur in men older than 50 years of age. X-ray findings show cortical destruction of the rib (Fig. 80.8). In the setting of systemic disease, only a needle biopsy may be needed, but if the lesion is small and symptomatic, resection can be offered. For larger lesions, radiotherapy is the primary treatment.[1]

Metastatic Tumors. As discussed before, metastatic lesions can arise from various other cancers, and treatment depends on the primary histology, time to recurrence, and goals of intervention. For isolated metastases with a long interval before recurrence, surgical resection may be warranted. Each case should be individualized and discussed within a multidisciplinary team.

Chest Wall Reconstruction

Chest wall defects can result from cancer, radiation, trauma, or infection.[7] The goals of repair are to protect the thoracic

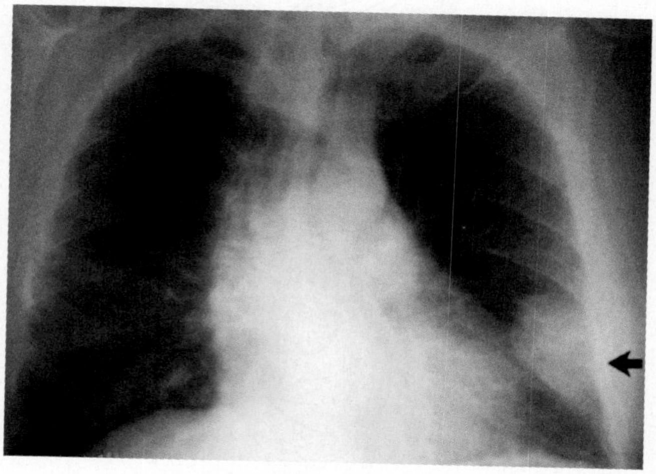

FIGURE 80.8. Plasmacytoma of the left seventh rib, showing characteristic cortical destruction and relatively large soft tissue component projecting into the chest.

1 cavity, minimize complications of respiration due to a flail chest, and to provide cosmetic coverage as needed. Surgical repair involves chest wall stabilization and soft tissue coverage. Stabilization depends on the size and the location of the defect. Often, if the defect is small enough, no stabilization is needed. In larger defects, or when the patient has an intrinsic lung disease limiting the ability to breathe, stabilization using prosthetic materials is warranted. Soft tissue coverage of the defect can vary from mobilization of soft tissue edges, to muscle/omental pedicled flaps, to free muscle flaps.[8]

Size and location generally determine the need for chest wall stabilization. Defects less than 5 cm anywhere in the chest wall or defects less than 10 cm in the posterior chest wall that are anterior to the scapula do not usually need stabilization.[7,9] An alternative criteria is to use the number of ribs resected, and to avoid stabilization when a portion of three ribs or fewer have been removed.[10] Techniques for closure of the defect include utilizing absorbable Vicryl mesh, used in the setting of infection or if small defects are present. This approach does not provide any stabilization. More definitive repairs use polytetrafluoroethylene (PTFE) or a polypropylene methylmethacrylate (PPM) sandwich mesh. PTFE is a flexible, soft material, whereas the PPM sandwich mesh resembles a hardened piece of plaster between two portions of woven mesh. Different surgeons prefer different approaches, but some of the benefits cited for the PTFE repair include greater stretch and the ability to create a watertight seal.[7] The PPM sandwich repair, on the other hand, allows the ability to mold the prosthetic and provides a firmer stabilization (Fig. 80.9).[9] Mortality rates from chest wall reconstruction in the setting of cancer resections have been reported at 4% in multiple series.[7,9,10]

Flap coverage of the soft tissue defect will almost always require the assistance of a plastic surgeon, and he or she should be involved preoperatively in the planning of a chest wall resection and reconstruction. The decision-making process for which flap to use depends on the location of the defect, the size of the defect, the corresponding size of the flap, and its vascular source. The pectoralis major flap is the most common in the upper chest/neck region. Its blood source can be from the thoracoacromial artery or from intercostal perforators from the internal thoracic arteries (Fig. 80.10). The latissimus dorsi flap is also commonly used for large, ipsilateral defects. Its blood source is from the thoracodorsal artery or from perforators from the posterior intercostal vessels. It has a large arc of rotation from the thoracodorsal pedicle and can cover a wide area of the chest wall (Fig. 80.11). Also commonly used are rectus abdominal muscle flaps in either a vertical (VRAM) or transverse (TRAM) orientation (Fig. 80.12). External obliques can

LUNG

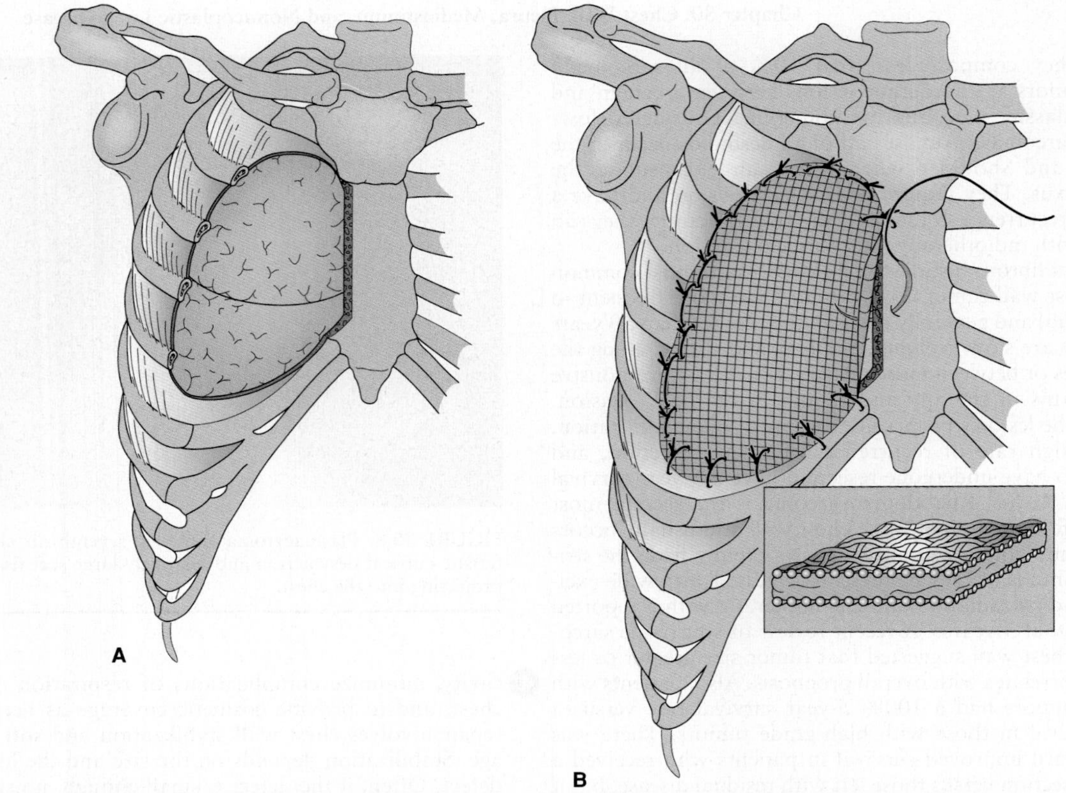

FIGURE 80.9. Marlex methylmethacrylate sandwich technique for chest wall reconstruction. **A:** Upper anterior chest wall defect resulting from resection of ribs two to five and a portion of sternum. **B:** Marlex methylmethacrylate prosthesis being sutured in place. Heavy, nonabsorbable sutures either encircling the ribs or passed through the sternum are used to anchor the prosthesis in place. **Insert:** Detail of prosthesis showing sandwich of hardened methylmethacrylate between two sheets of Marlex.

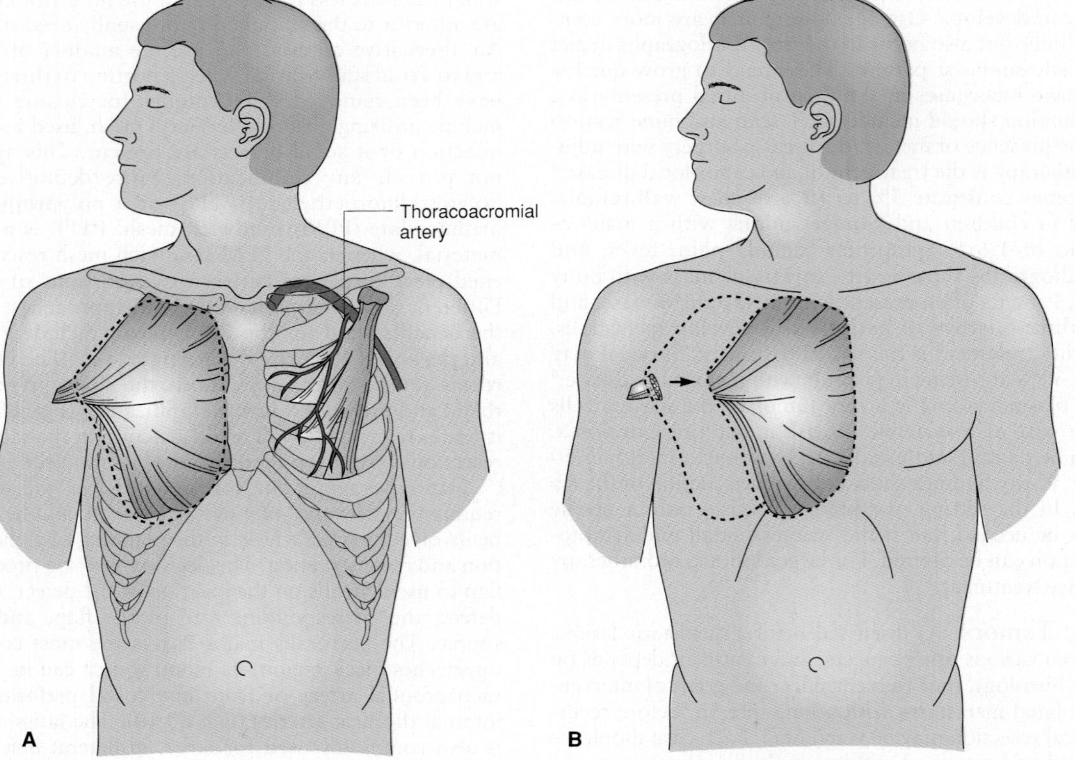

FIGURE 80.10. Pectoralis major muscle rotation flap. **A:** Mobilization of the flap by detaching the clavicular, sternal, and chest wall origins as well as the insertion of the muscle on the greater tubercle of the humerus. The dominant blood supply, the thoracoacromial artery, which arises from the axillary artery medial to the proximal border of the pectoralis minor muscle, is shown on the left side where the pectoralis major muscle has been removed. **B:** Medial transposition of the muscle flap, preserving the thoracoacromial neurovascular bundle.

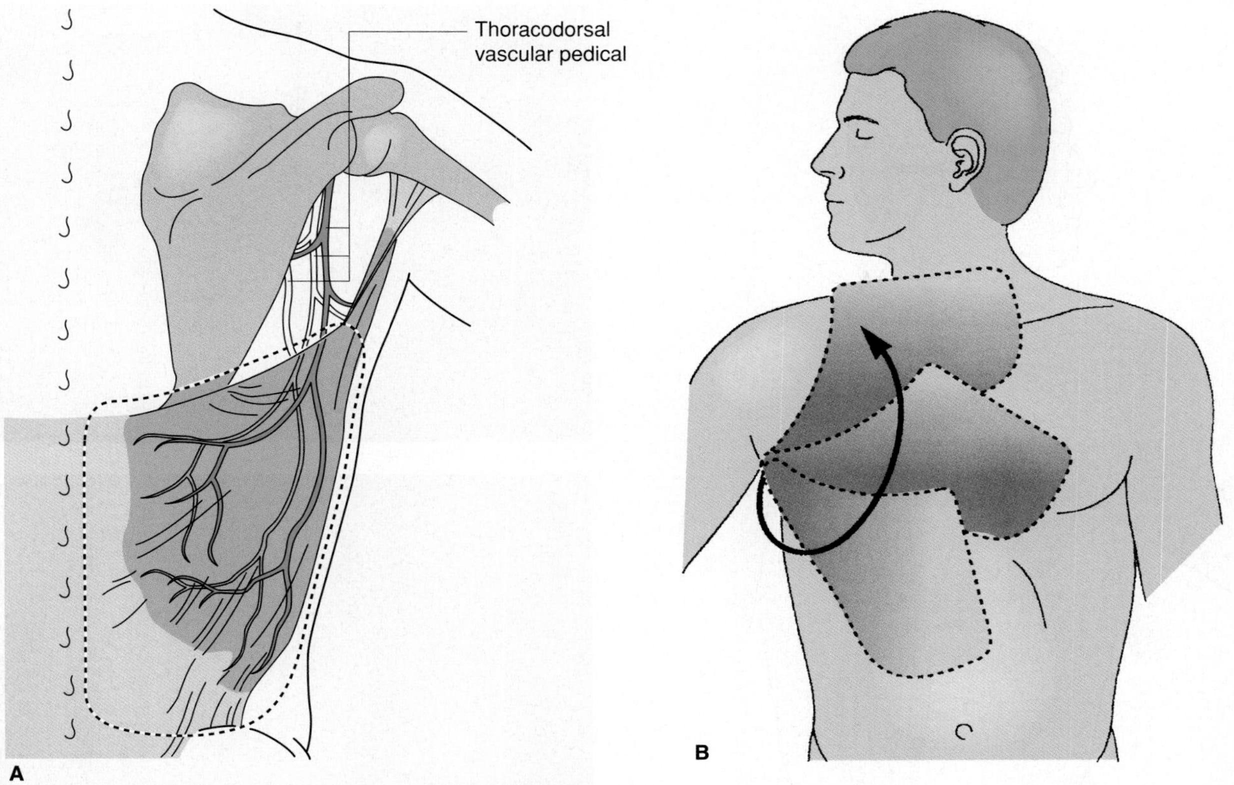

FIGURE 80.11. Latissimus dorsi muscle rotation flap for chest wall reconstruction. A: Posterior view showing detachment of the origins of the muscle. The dominant blood supply, the thoracodorsal artery, is preserved. B: Anterior view showing the extent to which the mobilized muscle reaches.

be used on the lower anterior chest wall, and the trapezius can be used in the midback.[11] Omental flaps are extremely useful and versatile. They can be used to cover large defects or to fill cavities, such as the pleural space in the setting of a bronchopleural fistula and empyema. The omentum can be taken off the right or left gastroepiploic artery, but using the right arterial source allows a greater arc of rotation than from the left. The limitations of this flap are that it requires a laparotomy, although laparoscopic techniques have been described,[12] and that the size of the omentum can be variable and difficult to assess preoperatively (Fig. 80.13).[11]

Chest Wall Congenital Abnormalities and Thoracic Outlet Syndrome

Pectus Excavatum and Pectus Carinatum. Chest wall deformities occur in 1/1,000 live births. They are five times more common in men than women, and pectus excavatum is five times more common than pectus carinatum. Up to 6% of people with these deformities will also have a connective tissue disorder. Scoliosis is frequently seen in this population.[13] Pectus excavatum appears as a sternal depression that can be off midline approximately 50% of the time. Pectus carinatum is the opposite, with a sternal protrusion, often described as a "pigeon chest" deformity. Less common deformities include sternal clefts, which are incomplete fusions of the sternum, and Poland syndrome, where there is an absence of a pectoralis muscle and underlying bony support in the chest wall.

Pectus excavatum is the most common of these deformities, and the techniques for surgical correction have been evolving, including the Ravitch and Nuss procedures. Despite this, less than 15% of patients undergo surgery.[14] Most patients present as children with notable deformities. People can be physiologically asymptomatic but can also present with fatigue, limited stamina, and cardiopulmonary limitations. The workup includes pulmonary function testing, echocardiography, and CT scans. The use of CT scans has been debated in children as the radiation exposure poses a risk. Some advocate that CT scans are needed to show the three-dimensional aspect of the defect and can better reflect the right heart compression. The pectus severity index (Haller index) can be calculated by dividing the inner thorax width by the depth measured from the posterior aspect of the sternum to the anterior aspect of the spine (Fig. 80.14). Normal values are 2 to 2.2, and repair is recommended only when the index is at least greater than 3.1.[13,15] The age of the patient at which repair should be performed is also somewhat controversial, as some surgeons advocate waiting until after the age of 10 years, but many series have reported on many patients treated at a much younger age with good outcomes.[14] There is a growing experience with treating adults also, as some patients seek repair at a later age (Fig. 80.15).[16,17]

The most commonly used open repair was first described by Dr. Ravitch and is based on removing sections of the deformed cartilage from around the sternum laterally at the ribs, while preserving the perichondrium. Many advocate using a stabilizing bar for a minimum of 6 months, usually placed in an intrathoracic position, to minimize the occurrence of flail chest and to allow the sternum to heal in an anterior position. An essential part of the procedure is a transverse sternal wedge resection through the anterior table to allow the inferior aspect of sternum to bend forward.[13,17] Incisions may be in a vertical midline over the lower half of the sternum or in an inframammary position (Fig. 80.16). Recurrences occur in 5% to 10% of patients, with recurrence more common in patients with connective tissue disorders.

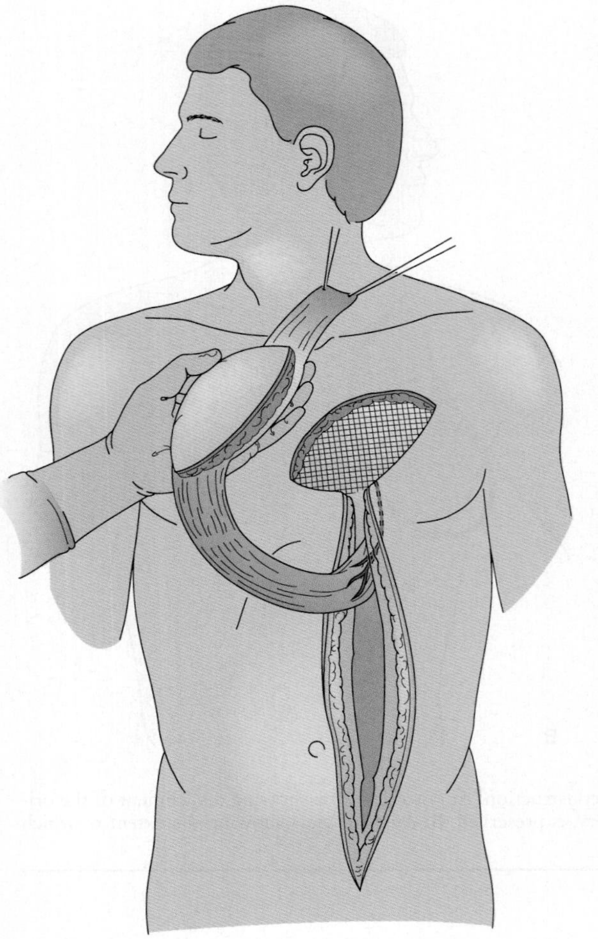

FIGURE 80.12. Rectus abdominis muscle rotation flap. Shown is the mobilization of the rectus abdominis muscle, which is based on the superior epigastric artery (the continuation of the internal thoracic artery), and rotation of the muscle and overlying skin to fill an anterior chest wall defect.

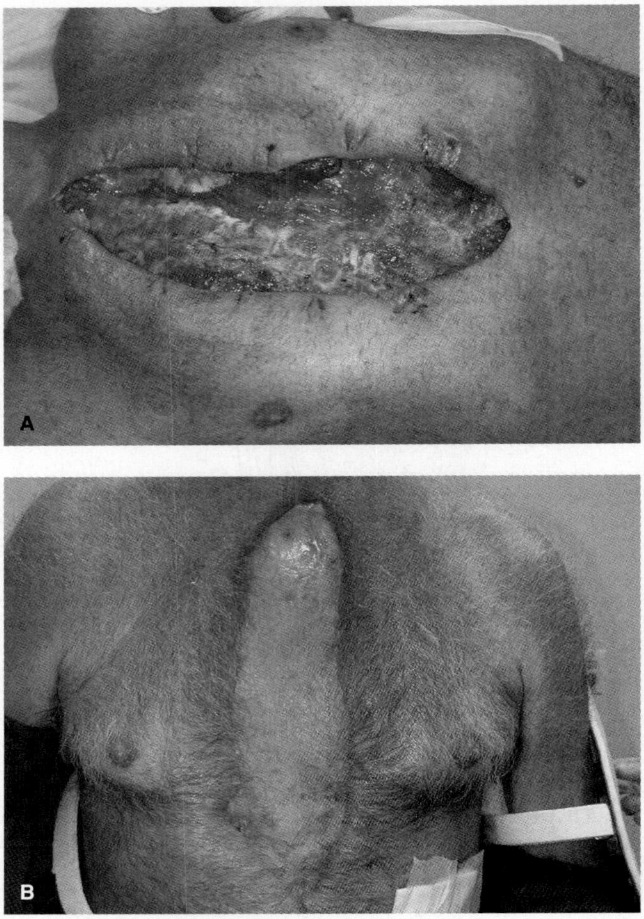

FIGURE 80.13. The omentum can be used to cover large defects. Shown is an open sternal wound after débridement with failed prior muscle flap (**A**). Wound 6 months after omental flap placement (**B**). (Reproduced with permission from Ghazi B, Carlson G, Losken A. Use of the greater omentum for reconstruction of infected sternotomy wounds: a prognostic indicator. *Ann Plast Surg* 2008;60(2):169–173.)

Since the 1990s, the Nuss procedure, which uses a minimally invasive approach, has been described and performed. The Nuss procedure uses one or two stabilization bars, secured to the ribs laterally in multiple points of fixation. It routinely employs thoracoscopy, either unilateral or bilateral. Skin incisions are limited to small lateral locations at the site of the bar insertion and thoracoscopic port sites. In both the Ravitch and Nuss procedures, the stabilization bars stay in for at least 6 months.[18] As the Nuss procedure has grown in popularity, many modifications have been made, including precise shaping of the bars and increased bar stabilization with wire fixation around the ribs to minimize bar displacement.[19]

Pectus carinatum doesn't have the same cardiac compression concerns as pectus excavatum, but the chest is held in an enlarged position, limiting normal respiration mechanics. Patients can have increased residual lung volumes, and their respiratory physiology can mimic emphysema physiology. This can result in breathing difficulties and limited stamina.[17] The Ravitch procedure is most commonly performed to remove the deformed cartilage. Special attention is placed on the transverse sternal osteotomy, to depress the sternum and align it with the anterior ribs (Fig. 80.17).[13]

Sternal Clefts. Sternal clefts are much rarer than either pectus deformity. They result from the failure of the sternum to fuse in the midline. They can vary from minor defects with the upper half of the sternum separated, to complete dissociation and thoracic ectopia cordis (the heart being outside the chest wall). Upper sternal defects have a U- or V-shaped appearance and usually extend to the fourth intercostal space (Fig. 80.18). Repair of these defects can be easily performed by incision, complete sternotomy, oblique chondrotomies of the sternal halves, and closure. Complete sternal clefts are associated with diastasis recti and an opening between the peritoneal and pericardial cavities. Inferior clefts are associated with the pentalogy of Cantrell, a constellation of defects that include: supraumbilical abdominal wall defect, lower sternal cleft, defect in the anterior diaphragm, defect in the associated pericardium, and congenital cardiac defects, often tetrology of Fallot. With the increased use of prenatal ultrasound, most cases are diagnosed early and are being appropriately referred to specialists prior to birth.[20]

Poland Syndrome. Poland syndrome is the clinical absence of a pectoralis muscle and underlying bony support in the chest wall, and it occurs in 1/30,000 live births. It is usually a right-sided, unilateral defect. Patients commonly have associated limb abnormalities and may also present with renal and spinal lesions (Fig. 80.19). Clinical symptoms may be absent, though lung herniation can occur, requiring a more urgent repair. The surgical approach is usually multidisciplinary and ideally is deferred until after the patient has stopped growing. Repairs

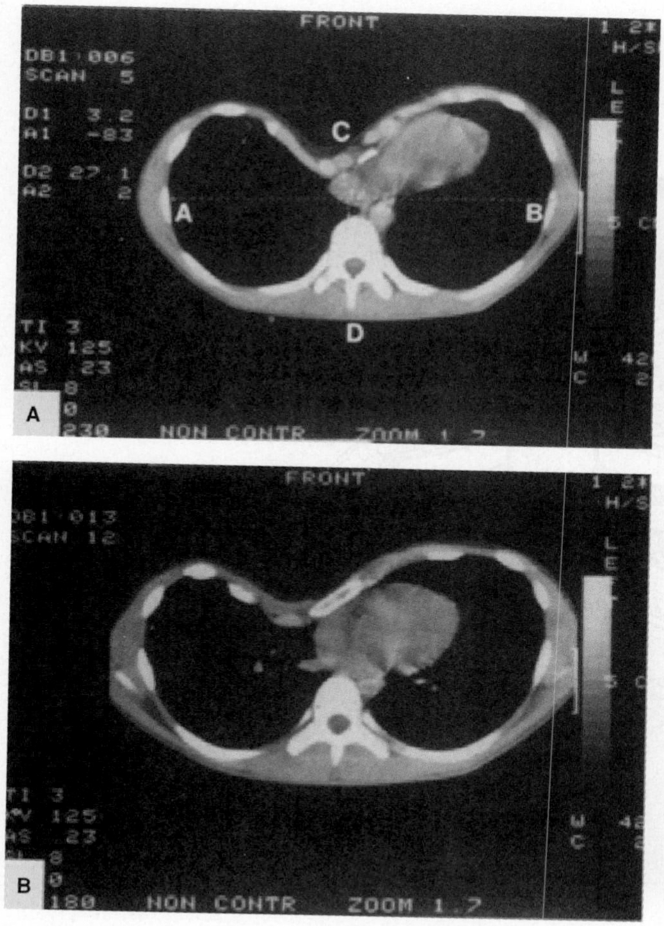

FIGURE 80.14. Chest CT of pectus excavatum. CT image at xiphoid with A-B (transverse diameter) and C-D (anterior-posterior diameter) indicated for the calculation of the pectus severity index A-B/C-D (**A**). CT image demonstrating angulation of the sternum to the right in the severe defect (**B**). (Reproduced with permission from Haller JA Jr, et al. Evolving management of pectus excavatum based on a single institutional experience of 664 patients. *Ann Surg* 1989;209(5):578–582.)

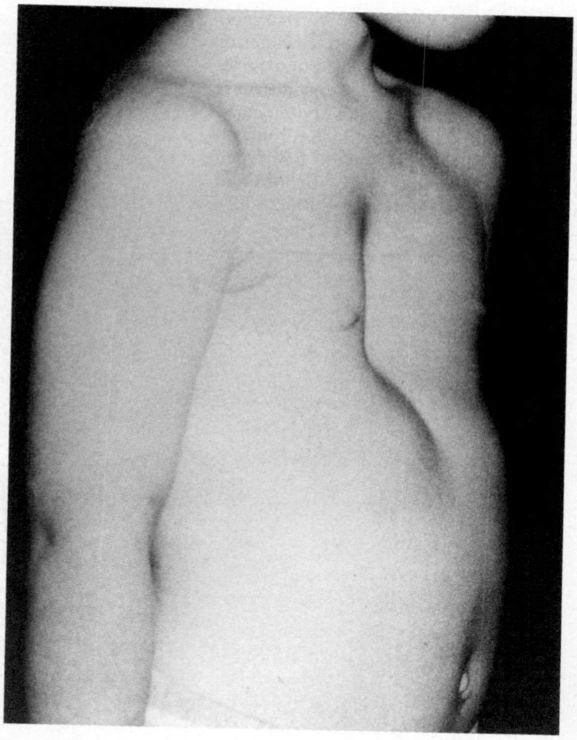

FIGURE 80.15. Photograph of a 4.5-year-old girl with a symmetric pectus excavatum deformity. Note that the depression extends to the sternal notch. (Adapted with permission from Shamberger RC. Chest wall deformities. In: Shields TW, ed. *General Thoracic Surgery*, 4th ed. Baltimore: Williams & Wilkins; 1994:529–557.)

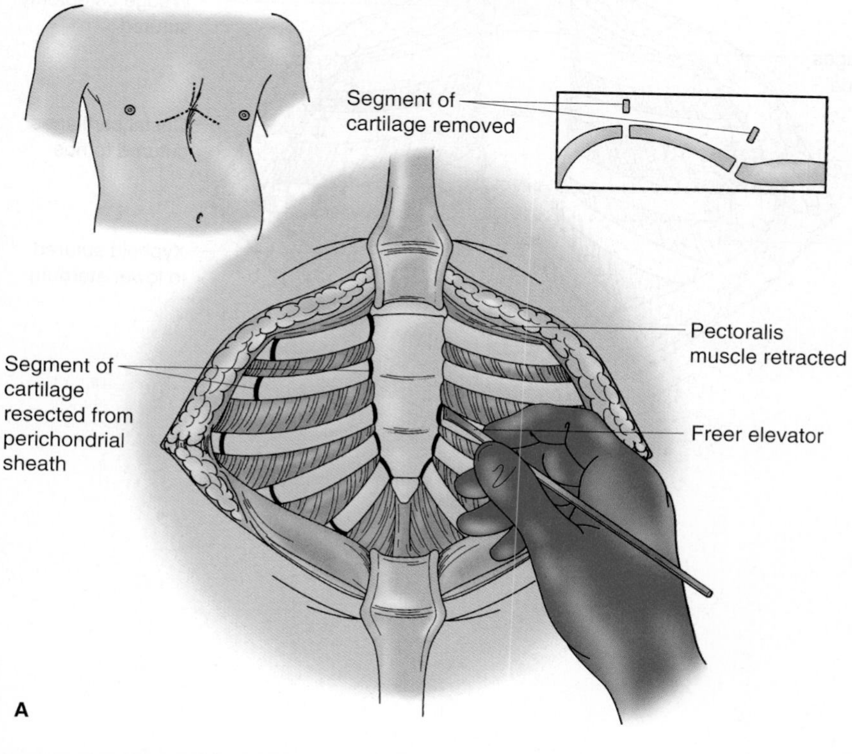

FIGURE 80.16. A chevron incision is made with flaps elevated. The perichondrium on the deformed cartilage is removed (**A**). (*continued*)

FIGURE 80.16. (*Continued*) A transverse wedge osteotomy is made across the anterior table of the sternum. The lower sternum is elevated to the desired level (**B**). A metal strut is placed posterior to the sternum and attached to the ribs with fine wire (**C**). (Reproduced with permission from Fonkalsrud EW. Open repair of pectus excavatum with minimal cartilage resection. *Ann Surg* 2004;240(2): 231–235.)

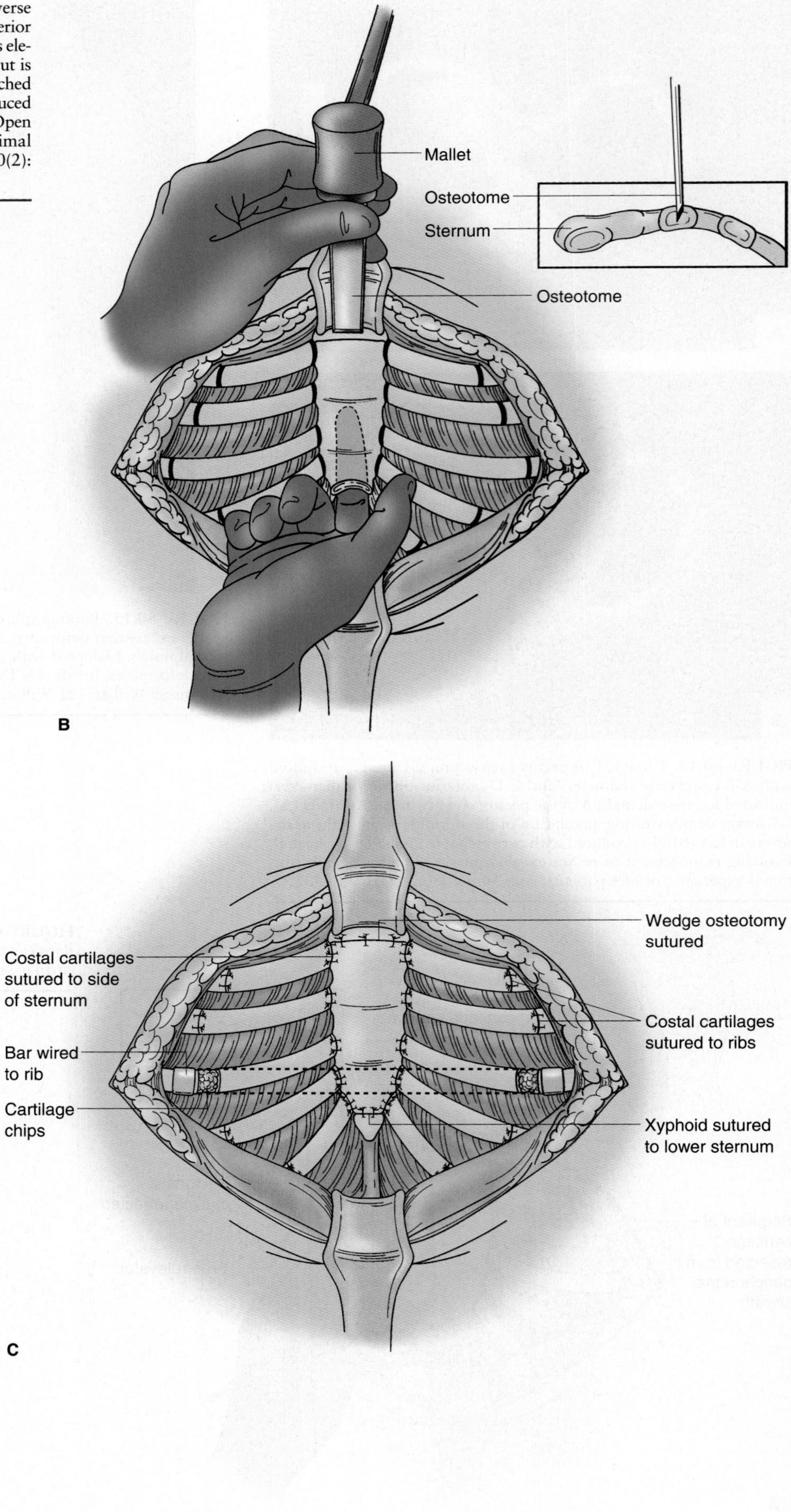

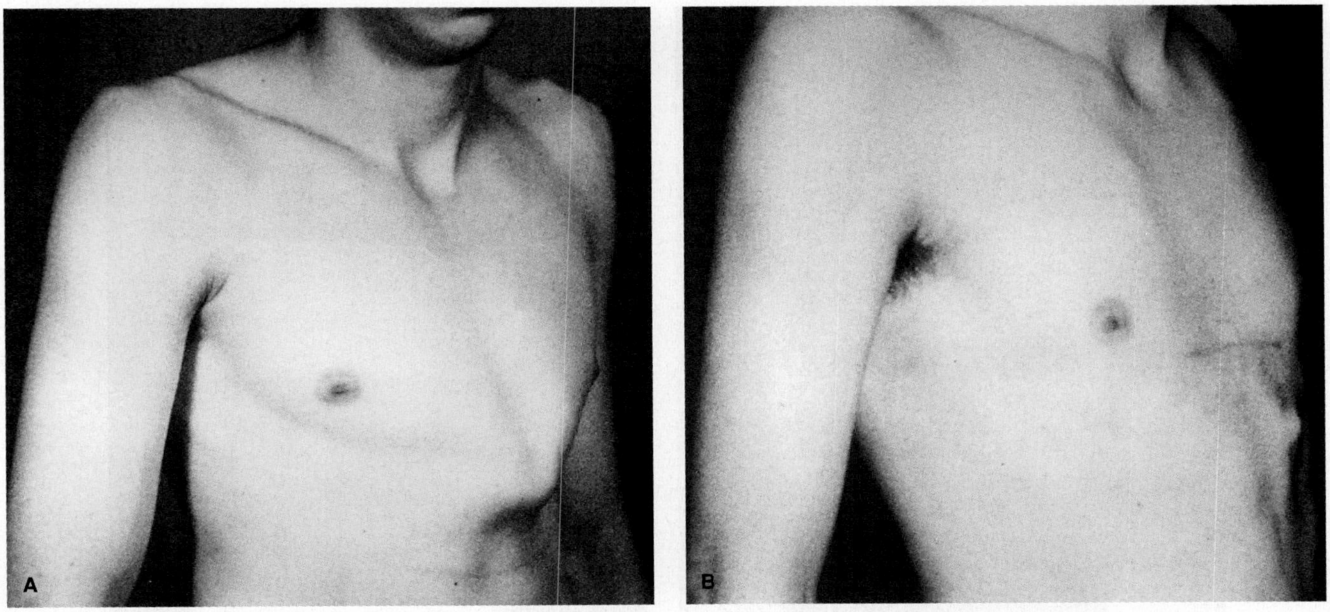

FIGURE 80.17. Photograph of (**A**) symmetric chondrogladiolar pectus carinatum in a 19-year-old man. Postoperative photograph (**B**) shows correction of the protruding sternum and costal cartilages. (Adapted with permission from Shamberger RC. Chest wall deformities. In: Shields TW, ed. *General Thoracic Surgery*, 4th ed. Baltimore: Williams & Wilkins; 1994:529–557.)

typically use mesh placement over the defect, and/or muscle flap placement.[21]

Thoracic Outlet Syndrome (TOS).

The thoracic outlet in TOS refers to the area described at the beginning of this chapter as the thoracic inlet, the correct anatomic term for the region of the first rib and the middle and anterior scalene muscles. Through these structures, the brachial plexus, subclavian artery, and subclavian vein travel to the upper limbs (Fig. 80.20). Because of the close proximity in this area, these conduits may be subjected to abnormal compression by inflammation around the muscles or abnormal bony structures such as cervical ribs, causing pain, thrombosis, and other symptoms that are described as TOS. TOS can be divided into arterial, venous, or neurogenic diseases, or a combination, depending on the symptoms and clinical findings. Vascular TOS is easier to document with vascular imaging. Neurogenic TOS is more difficult to diagnose. Unfortunately for neurogenic TOS, there is no gold standard diagnostic test to confirm the syndrome. As a result there has been significant controversy over the diagno-

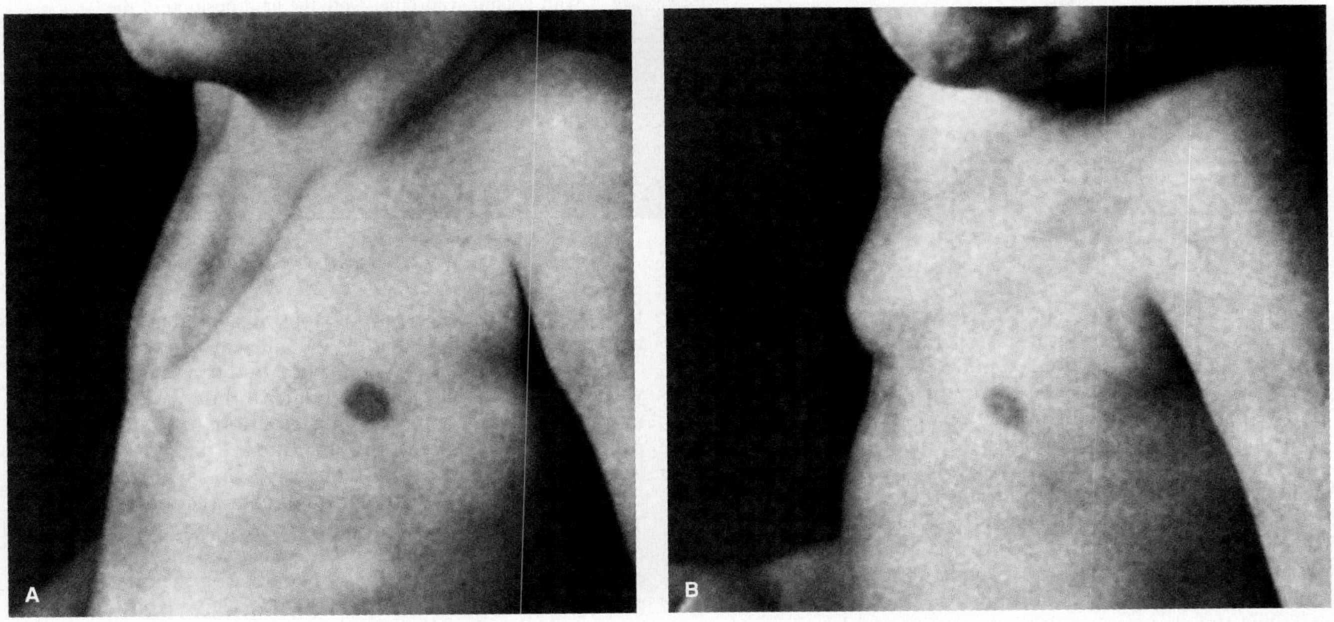

FIGURE 80.18. Cleft sternum at rest (**A**) and during forced expiration (**B**). Superior clefts of the sternum are variously V- or U-shaped. The appearance of the child as he cries explains the term ectopia cordis, although the heart is actually not misplaced. In the newborn, defects of this kind can be corrected by direct apposition of the sternal halves. In this child, closure of the defect was made possible by sliding chondrotomies on either side. (Reproduced with permission from Sabiston DC Jr. The surgical management of congenital bifid sternum with a partial ectopia cordis. *J Thorac Surg* 1958;35:118.)

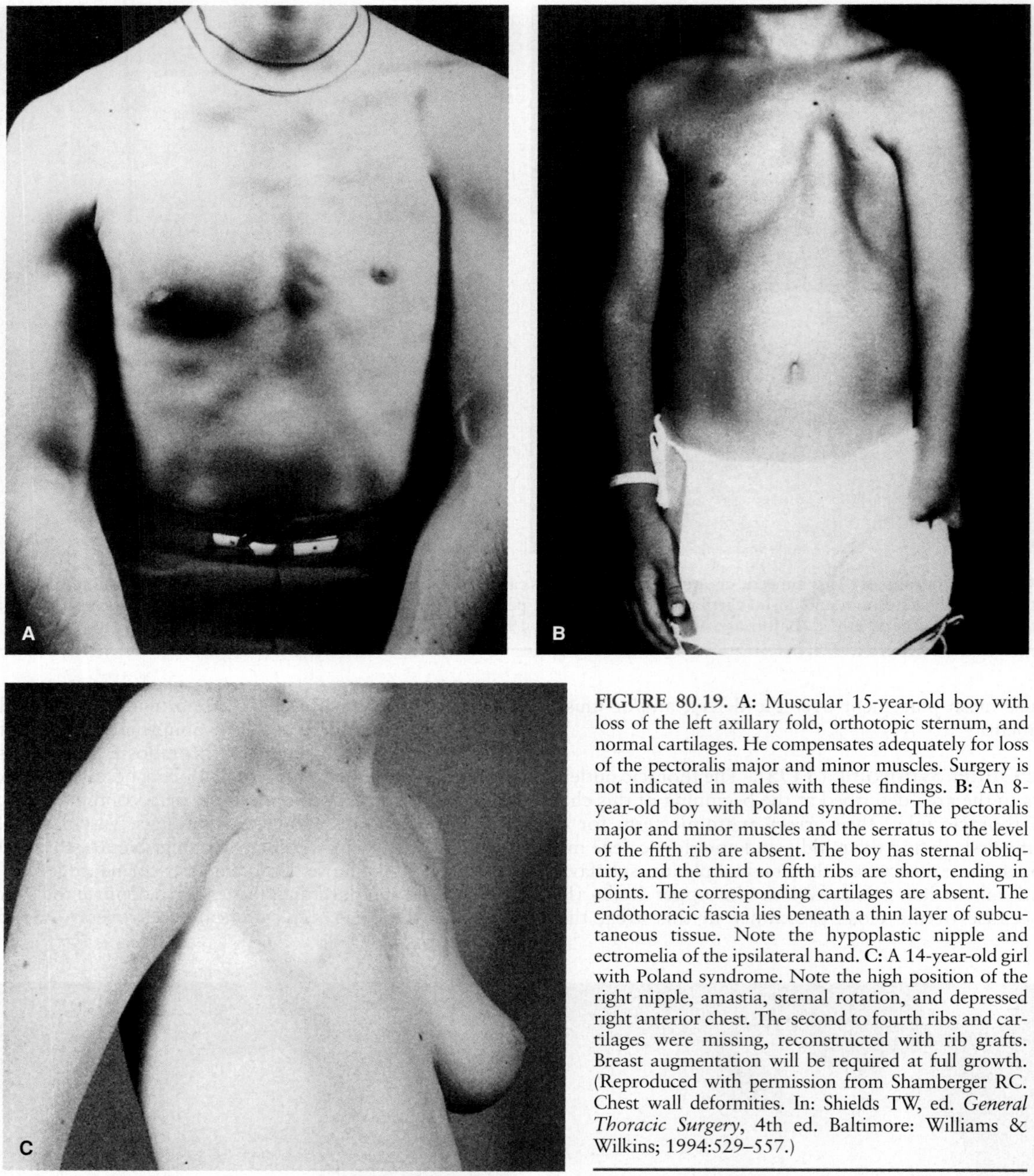

FIGURE 80.19. **A:** Muscular 15-year-old boy with loss of the left axillary fold, orthotopic sternum, and normal cartilages. He compensates adequately for loss of the pectoralis major and minor muscles. Surgery is not indicated in males with these findings. **B:** An 8-year-old boy with Poland syndrome. The pectoralis major and minor muscles and the serratus to the level of the fifth rib are absent. The boy has sternal obliquity, and the third to fifth ribs are short, ending in points. The corresponding cartilages are absent. The endothoracic fascia lies beneath a thin layer of subcutaneous tissue. Note the hypoplastic nipple and ectromelia of the ipsilateral hand. **C:** A 14-year-old girl with Poland syndrome. Note the high position of the right nipple, amastia, sternal rotation, and depressed right anterior chest. The second to fourth ribs and cartilages were missing, reconstructed with rib grafts. Breast augmentation will be required at full growth. (Reproduced with permission from Shamberger RC. Chest wall deformities. In: Shields TW, ed. *General Thoracic Surgery*, 4th ed. Baltimore: Williams & Wilkins; 1994:529–557.)

sis and the indications for surgical treatment, especially in light of the potential for significant postoperative complications.[22,23]

Vascular TOS can be divided into venous disease and arterial disease. Venous disease results in thrombosis of the subclavian vein and is also called Paget-Schroetter syndrome. This syndrome usually presents in men who use their upper bodies and dominant arm for work. Symptoms may present as pain, swelling, and cyanotic discoloration.[22] Contrast venography is the best test to make the diagnosis, and the radiologist should be instructed to perform positional maneuvers with the patient's arm to replicate narrowing that occurs with arm movement.[23] Arterial TOS accounts for about 5% of all cases of TOS[24] and also may result from repetitive and strenuous use. Patients will present with arm fatigue and may even have evidence of ischemia in their distal digits. Patient evaluation includes pulse exam with the arm relaxed and elevated, bruit exam for poststenotic dilatation, and blood pressure readings in both arms. Duplex scanning and angiography will often confirm the diagnosis. Decompression of the scalene muscles and any abnormal bony structures will alleviate these symptoms.[22]

Neurogenic TOS presents with limb pain, numbness, or weakness. Symptoms may be bilateral, but are usually worse in the dominant arm. The distribution may not follow a peripheral nerve pattern, thus making the diagnosis confusing, but also ruling out more distal compression syndromes such as carpal tunnel in the wrist or cubital compression at the elbow. The physical exam should be focused on duplicating the patient's symptoms. The Adson maneuver may detect artery compression and is performed by palpating the affected radial pulse and having the patient take a deep inspiration while turning the head away from the affected arm (Fig. 80.21). The test is positive if the pulse disappears, but a positive result can also be seen in asymptomatic people without TOS. Another test requires the patient to elevate the arms in a "surrender" position and open and close their hands repeatedly. Most people with neurogenic TOS will be fatigued within a minute and be

ORIENTATION

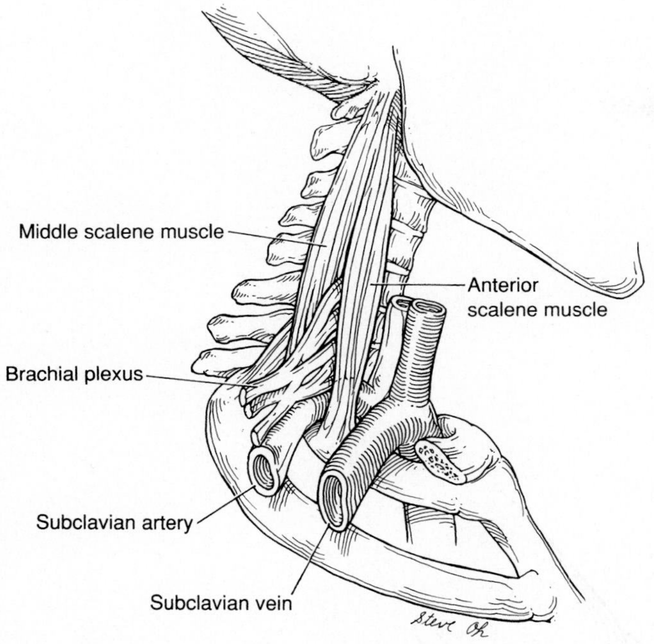

FIGURE 80.20. Important structures in the thoracic outlet. (Reproduced with permission from Scott-Conner CE, Dawson DL, Shirazi MK, et al. *Operative Anatomy*, 3rd ed. Philadelphia: Lippincott Williams & Wilkins; 2008:Fig. "Orientation" in Chapter 29)

unable to continue (Fig. 80.22). Plain radiographs may show bony abnormalities, but no other imaging will help diagnose neurogenic TOS. Physical rehabilitation is the first step to treat patients with neurogenic TOS, and over a third of patients may get a significant improvement in their symptoms. If there is no significant improvement in symptoms, then surgical intervention is suggested.[23]

The surgical approach for TOS was traditionally a transaxillary first-rib resection (Fig. 80.23). In recent years, a supra-

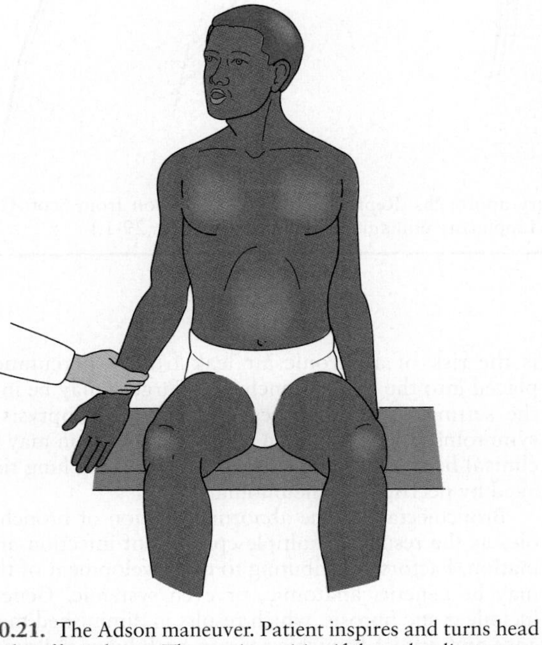

FIGURE 80.21. The Adson maneuver. Patient inspires and turns head away from the affected arm. The test is positive if the pulse disappears.

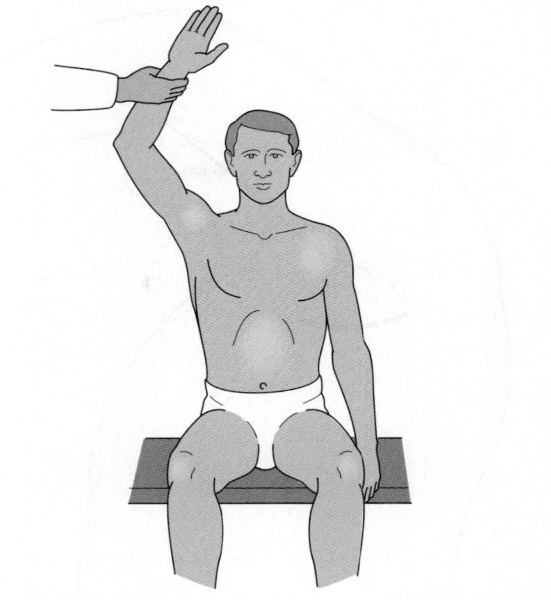

FIGURE 80.22. Surrender position with opening and closing of hand. Early fatigue is seen in neurogenic TOS.

clavicular approach has become increasingly popular as it gives better exposure to the scalene muscles and any cervical ribs. In either approach, the first rib is exposed and the anterior and middle scalene muscles are removed from their attachments to the rib. Once this is performed, the first rib is removed (Fig. 80.24). Special attention must be paid to the phrenic nerve laying along the anterior scalene and the axillary branches off the brachial plexus. Small drains may be placed in the apex of the thorax if the pleural space is entered.[23,25] The supraclavicular approach also gives access to perform a cervical sympathectomy if indicated for symptoms consistent with sympathetic overactivity. In patients with arterial aneurysms, reconstruction with synthetic grafts or autologous conduits such as an external iliac artery can be performed. For patients with venous TOS, care should be taken to perform a circumferential venolysis and to remove the medial aspect of the first rib.[25]

Postoperative complications include pneumothorax, lymphatic leaks (especially on the left side where the thoracic duct enters the operative field), phrenic nerve palsy, and traction injury to the brachial plexus.[24] Patients should have good pain control and may need muscle relaxants to minimize muscle spasm. There should be limited restrictions to the operated extremity to maximize movement and minimize the risk of developing a frozen shoulder. Rehabilitation should be restarted as soon as possible after surgery.[23,25] Up to 12.5% of patients may not get any symptom relief after the surgery, and long-term physical rehabilitation is recommended.[24] Patients with combined symptoms of venous and neurogenic TOS have worse outcomes when compared to patients with only venous disease. A higher percentage of patients had persistent pain in the neurogenic group as might be expected.[26] The treatment of this disease process requires a significant investment into the preoperative and postoperative care of these patients and should be done only in centers with a high volume and expertise in this syndrome.

NONNEOPLASTIC LUNG DISEASE

Lung Abscess and Bronchiectasis

Complications from pulmonary infections that require surgery are not common relative to the frequency of pneumonias in

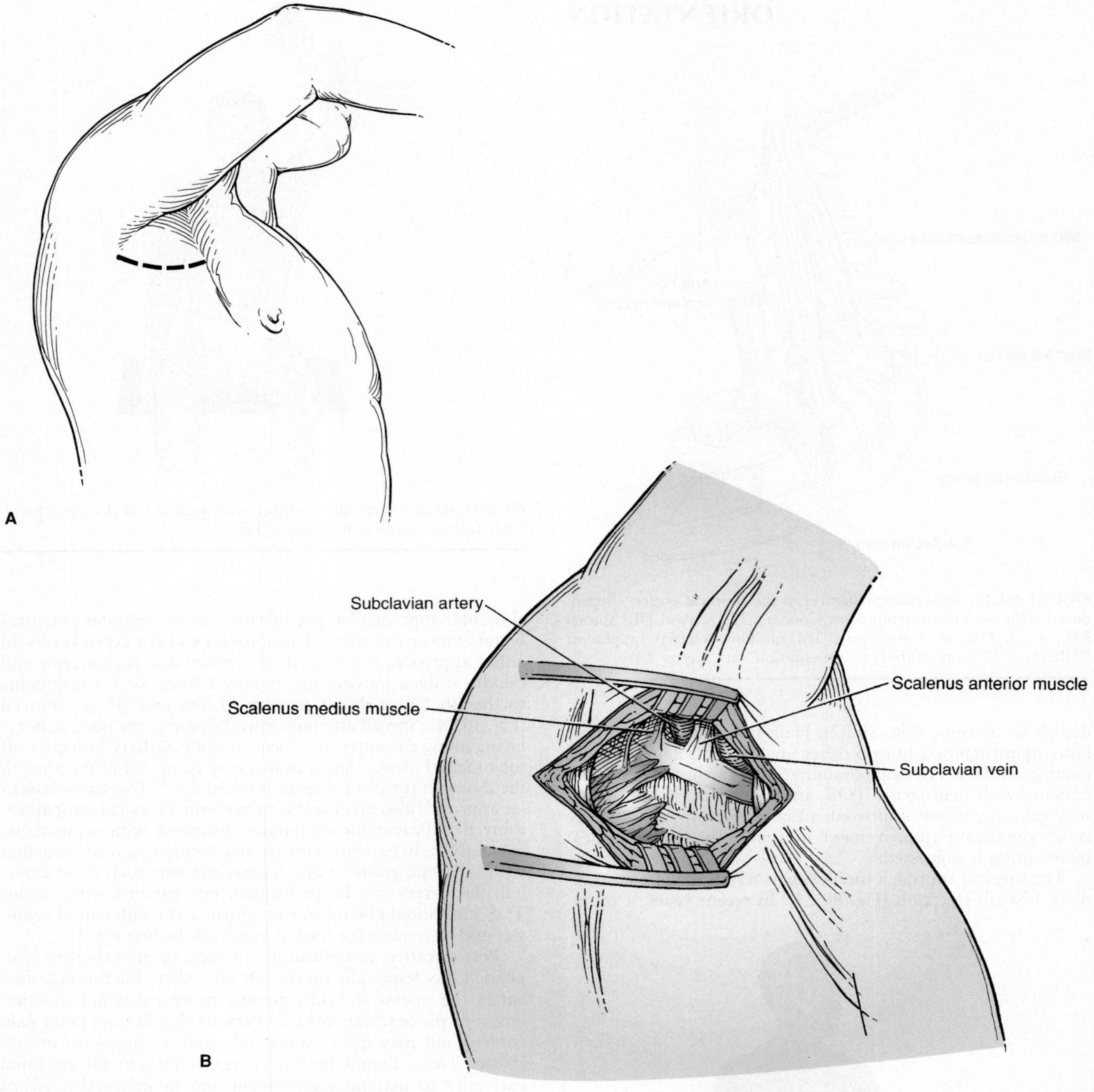

FIGURE 80.23. Position of the patient and skin incision for transaxillary approach. (Reproduced with permission from Scott-Conner CE, Dawson DL, Shirazi MK, et al. *Operative Anatomy*, 3rd ed. Philadelphia: Lippincott Williams & Wilkins; 2008:Fig. 29-1.)

both the inpatient and outpatient community. However, in some patients, treatment of lung abscesses and bronchiectasis may include surgical intervention. Lung abscesses can result from aspiration or occur after necrotizing pneumonia. Patients may present with chest pain and fever. Routine use of antibiotics for pneumonias has dramatically reduced the rate of lung abscess sequelae. In more than 80% of cases, a pathogen can be found, and in immunocompromised patients, there are usually multiple organisms involved including *Pseudomonas*
3 *aeruginosa* and *Haemophilus* species. The primary treatment for lung abscesses is medical with antibiotics. If a patient is clinically not improving with medical therapy alone, a guided drainage tube may be placed. A complication of this approach is the risk of a chronic air leak from a percutaneous tube placed into the lung parenchyma. Surgery may be indicated in the setting of large abscesses causing hemoptysis or other symptoms (Algorithm 80.1). Surgical resection may also be of clinical benefit in some patients by removing lung tissue damaged by necrotizing pneumonia.[27]

Bronchiectasis is the abnormal dilation of bronchi/bronchioles as the result of multiple episodes of infection and inflammation. Factors contributing to the development of this disease may be genetic, anatomic, or even systemic. Genetic causes include cystic fibrosis, which results in diminished mucus clearance and diffuse bronchiectasis in both lungs.[28] Primary ciliary dyskinesia is an autosomal recessive syndrome resulting in

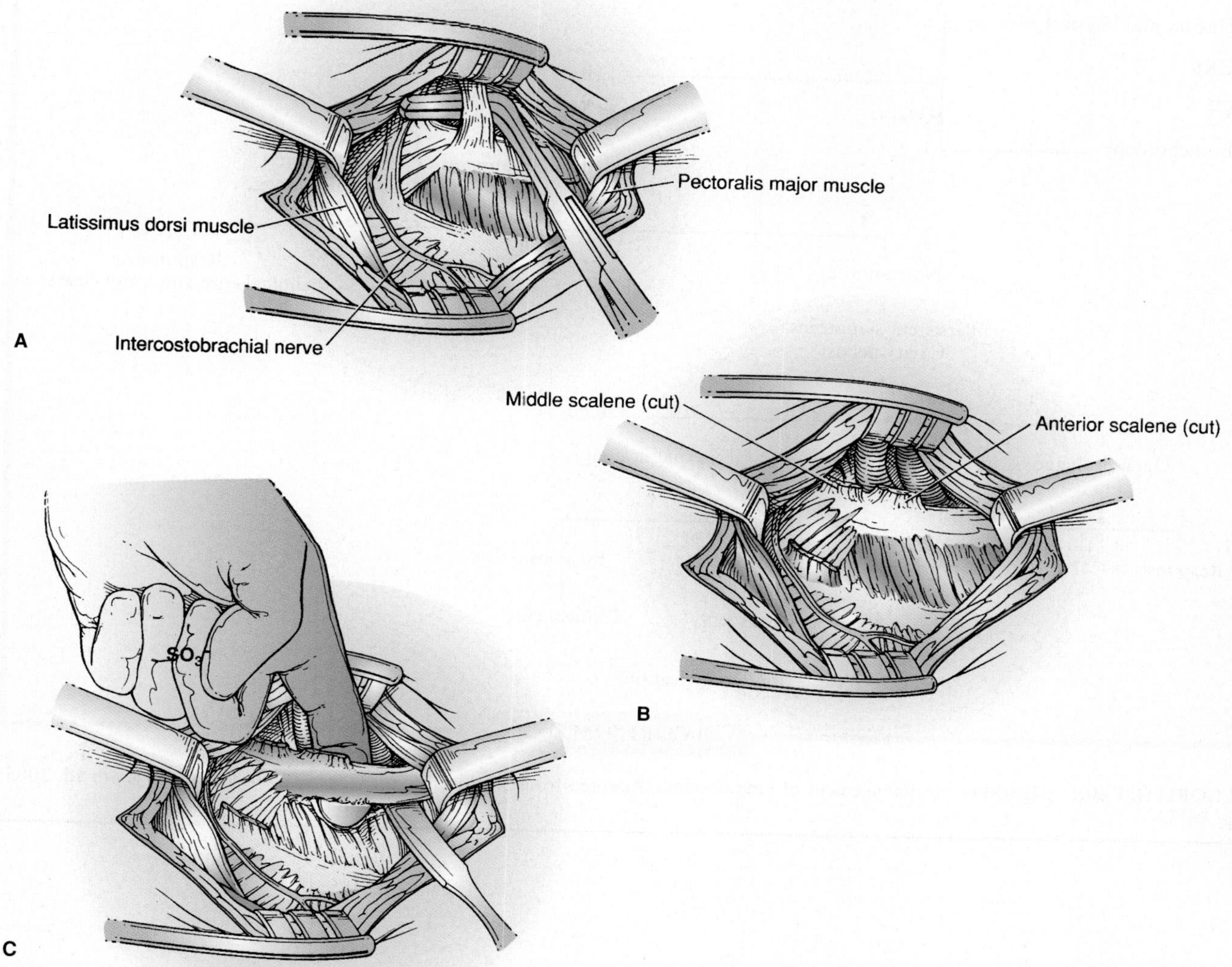

FIGURE 80.24. Division of the scalene muscles and the first rib. (Reproduced with permission from Scott-Conner CE, Dawson DL, Shirazi MK, et al. *Operative Anatomy*, 3rd ed. Philadelphia: Lippincott Williams & Wilkins; 2008:Fig. 29-2.)

abnormal cilia that cannot clear secretions leading to multiple infections. Individuals with alpha1-antitrypsin deficiency can also develop bronchiectasis. Anatomic causes include postsurgical changes or acquired diseases such as chronic obstructive pulmonary disease (COPD) that lead to an increased risk of infection, again by the inability to clear secretions. Autoimmune diseases such as rheumatoid arthritis and inflammatory bowel disease have been associated with increased rates of bronchiectasis.[28,29] Infectious causes include allergic bronchopulmonary aspergillosis and nontuberculous *Mycobacterium* infections. Reflux disease is also being studied as a potential contributor. Most often the etiology of the disease is idiopathic.[28]

There are estimated to be 110,000 patients in the United States being treated for non–cystic fibrosis bronchiectasis each year. The diagnosis is increasingly being made as a result of an increasing number of chest CT scans being performed for other nonrelated reasons. Patients can present with respiratory symptoms such as dyspnea, hemoptysis, or pleuritic pain, or alternatively may present only with systemic changes such as fatigue and weight loss.[28] Almost all patients will have a chronic cough with or without sputum production.[29] Pulmonary function tests may demonstrate moderate to severe airflow obstruction.[28] A chest CT scan is the optimal test to diagnose bronchiectasis (Fig. 80.25), and once the diagnosis is made, the search for an etiology should begin, including obtaining sputum cultures and blood tests for autoimmune markers such as rheumatoid factor.[29]

The treatment of the disease includes antibiotic therapy to control infection, the treatment of underlying diseases if they exist, reducing inflammation, improving secretion clearance, and surgery to remove focally damaged areas or transplantation if needed for more diffuse, severe disease. Antibiotic therapy includes inhaled tobramycin and gentamicin.[29] Macrolide antibiotics have been increasingly studied for their nonantibiotic effects. Erythromycin and clarithromycin have anti-inflammatory benefits. They disrupt the biofilm produced in *Pseudomonas* infections resulting in decreased sputum volume and improved symptoms.[30] Secretion removal is also essential to improving symptoms. Besides the standard treatments of percussive therapy and postural drainage, the use of nebulized

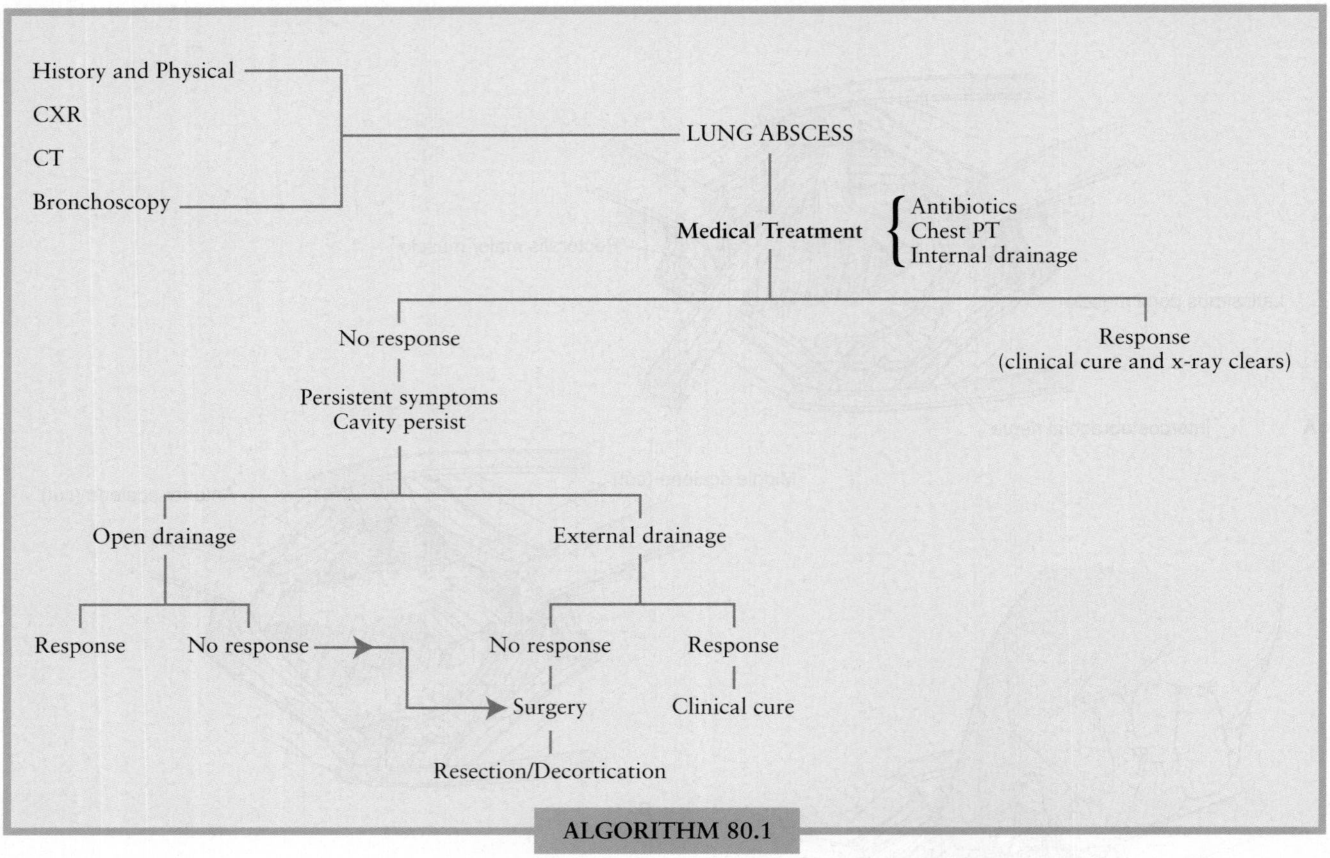

ALGORITHM 80.1. Algorithm for management of lung abscess. (Adapted from Shields TW, ed. *General Thoracic Surgery*, 6th ed. 2005: Fig. 86-7.)

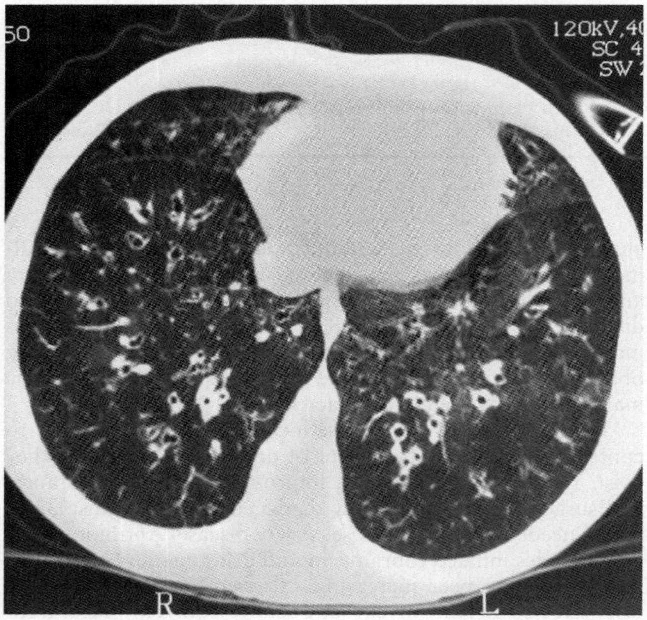

FIGURE 80.25. CT scan of bronchiectatic lungs. (Reproduced with permission from Shields TW, ed. *General Thoracic Surgery*, 6th ed. 2005:Fig. 86-2.)

acetylcysteine[29] or hypertonic saline[30] have been shown to improve mucus clearance.

Surgical intervention may occur at many stages of the disease process. Bronchoscopy can be useful to clear secretions or to manage hemoptysis. If the bronchiectasis is localized to a single lobe, resection can eliminate the disease and the source of chronic infection. If a patient has a genetic disease such as cystic fibrosis, a double lung transplant may be the best treatment if the patient's symptoms are severe enough.[29] Pulmonary tuberculosis can have similar indications for surgical intervention when it results in bronchiectasis or hemoptysis.[31] The rise of more multi–drug-resistant tuberculosis strains has led to the increasing need for surgical intervention.[32]

Hemoptysis

Hemoptysis is often used to describe any blood streaking associated with cough. True hemoptysis may be only a few drops
4 of blood, and it requires investigation. Massive hemoptysis is acutely life threatening, not from blood or volume loss, but rather from suffocation secondary to blood in the airway. The immediate goals when this is encountered are airway control, improved oxygenation, and resuscitation if needed. Intubation may or may not be necessary, depending on the volume of blood in the airway and the patient's ability to cough.[33] If the bleed is able to be lateralized, the patient should be placed

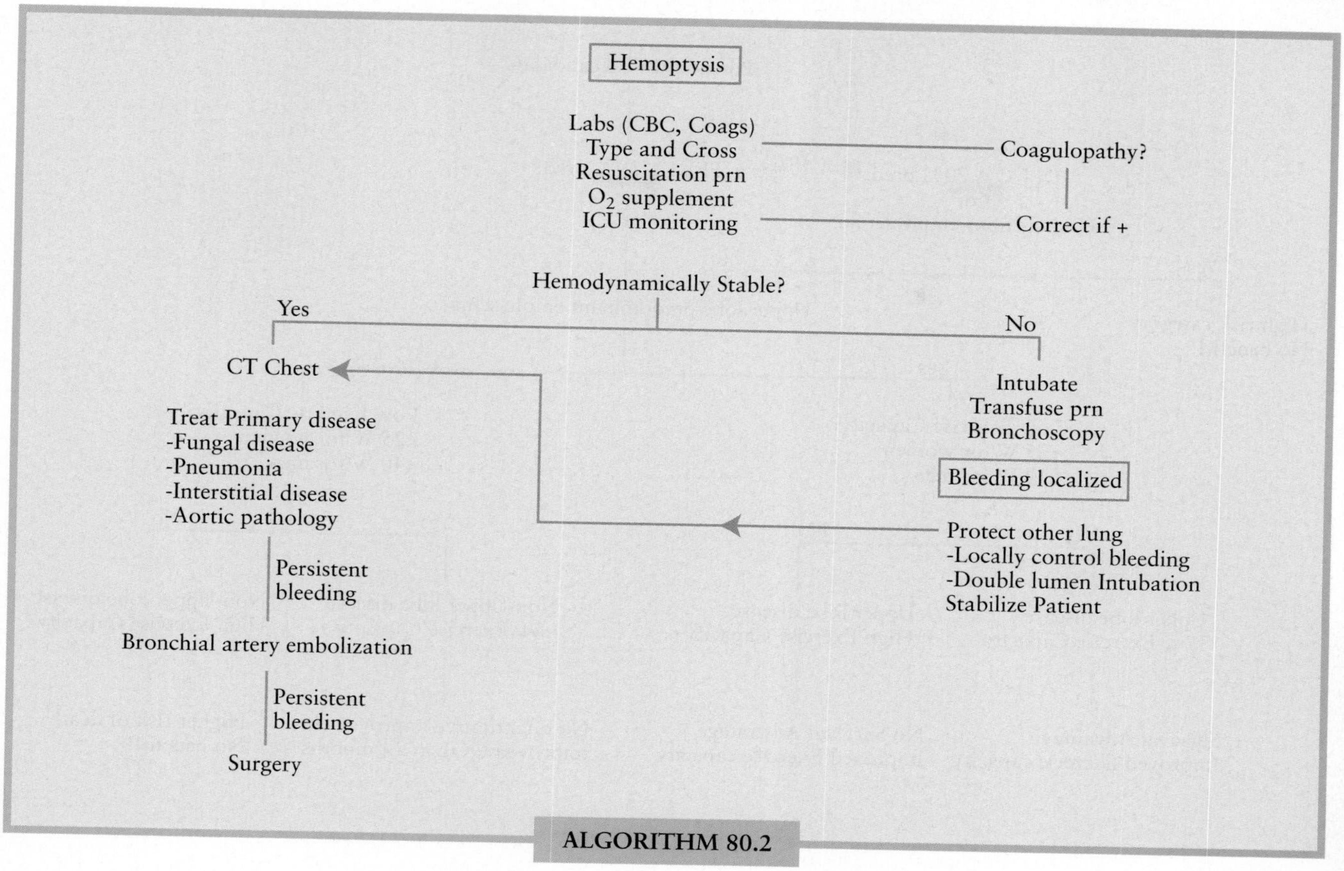

ALGORITHM 80.2. Hemoptysis management. (Adapted from Jean-Baptiste E. *Crit Care Med* 2000;28(5):1642–1647.)

in a lateral decubitus position with the bleeding side in the dependant position. The causes of hemoptysis include cancer, infections/bronchiectasis, vascular injuries, vasculitides, and coagulopathies.[34]

In patients with hemoptysis, any coagulopathy should be corrected. Early bronchoscopy is essential, and the goals are to lateralize the side of bleeding and identify the site and cause of the bleeding. Flexible bronchoscopy may be done, but rigid bronchoscopy is the best approach to maintain airway control, in particular in the setting of large-volume hemoptysis. Initial treatment may include topical therapy such as cold saline lavage, bronchial tamponade, and intubation of the contralateral good lung. Double lumen endotracheal tubes may also be useful to isolate and protect the uninvolved lung from blood from the contralateral side obstructing its lumen.[33] If a patient is stable, a chest CT scan is useful to identify tumors or other potential sources of bleeding.[34]

Once a patient is stabilized and appropriate diagnostic tests performed, the treatment of continued bleeding includes the use of interventional radiology and bronchial artery embolization (BAE).[35] First introduced in 1973, BAE is the best nonsurgical treatment of massive hemoptysis, with a success rate of up to 98% within 24 hours.[34] Surgery is reserved to treat the underlying condition once the patient has been stabilized and bleeding controlled by other methods. Emergent surgery to treat bleeding may have a mortality rate as high as 38%[35] and increase to 59% in the setting of malignancy.[34] Depending on the patient's baseline lung function, a lobectomy, let alone a pneumonectomy, may not be tolerated. A risk assessment of the benefits of surgery must be performed. In the setting of a vascular etiology of the hemoptysis such as a ruptured aortic aneurysm, surgical repair is essential and should not be delayed once the patient is hemodynamically stable and the airway is controlled.[34] A detailed algorithm in the assessment and treatment of hemoptysis is shown in Algorithm 80.2.

COPD and Lung-Volume Reduction

Chronic obstructive pulmonary disease (COPD) includes a broad group of diseases that result in airflow obstruction and hyperinflation. Medical therapy involves smoking cessation, bronchodilator treatment, steroids, home oxygen, and antibiotics as needed. Despite improvements in the medical management of this condition, patients continue to suffer severe limitations due to their breathing and exercise capacity. As a result, surgical interventions have continued to play a role in trying to ameliorate symptoms and improving survival in these patients.[36,37]

There is a more than 50-year history in the literature recording various surgical approaches to help treat COPD. Interest has diminished, however, because of the high mortality associated with surgical intervention in this patient population. In the 1990s, a renewed interest in lung-volume reduction surgery (LVRS) was observed following reports that this procedure was associated with a low published mortality rate and a significant improvement in forced expiratory volume in 1 s (FEV1) seen on pulmonary function testing. There was a national increase in interest in the procedure, as many centers began offering it. Despite continued publication of low mortality rates, evaluation of Medicare data in 1996 showed a mortality of 23% in surgically treated patients at 12 months, and Medicare reimbursement for the procedure stopped. This led to the development of the National Emphysema Treatment

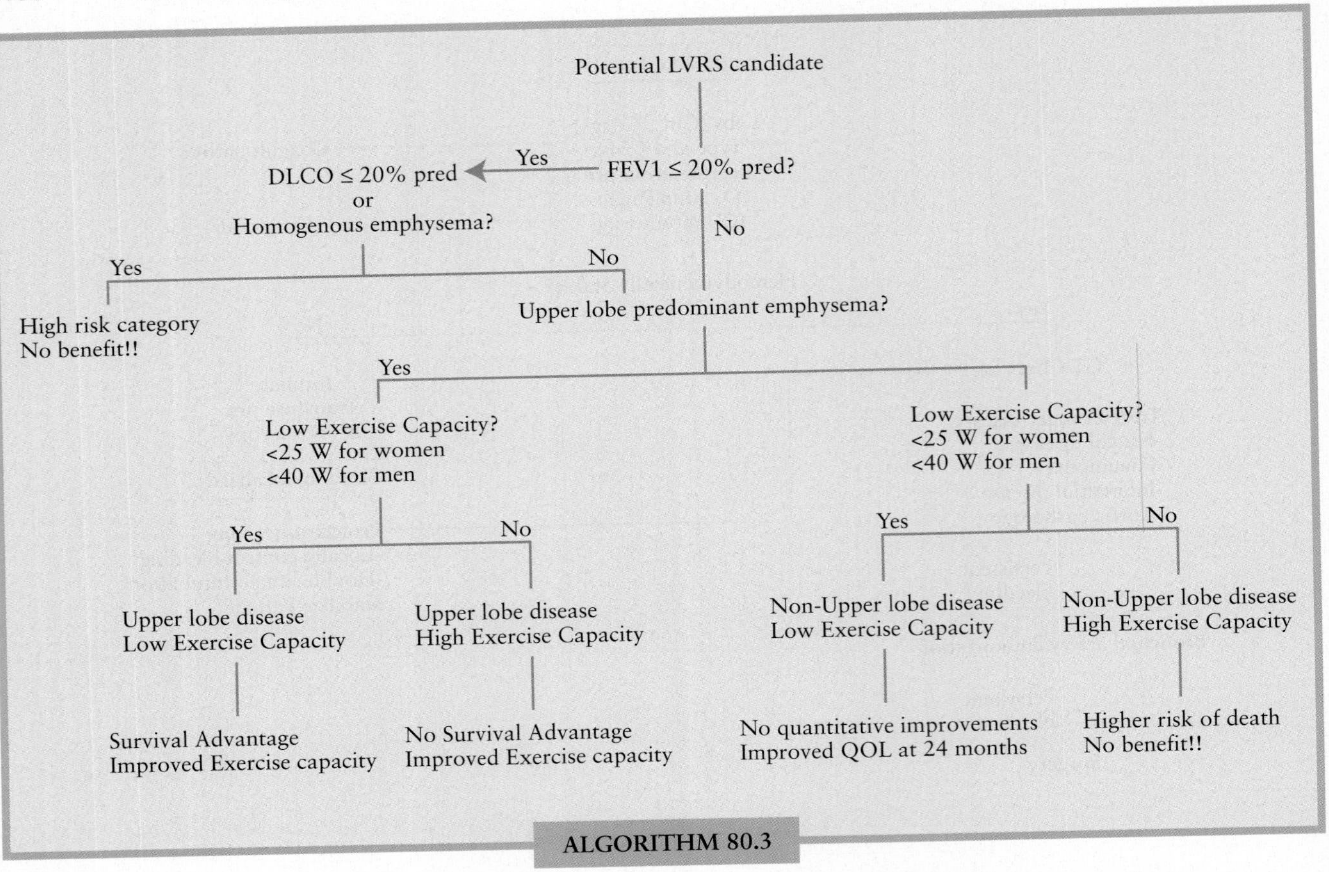

ALGORITHM 80.3. LVRS candidate workup. (Adapted from Martinez FJ, Chang A. *Semin Respir Crit Care Med* 2005;26(2):167–191.)

Trial (NETT), a prospective randomized trial to evaluate the outcomes of lung-volume reduction surgery compared to optimal medical treatment.[36]

The goal of the NETT study was to evaluate short- and long-term survival, lung function, exercise capacity, and quality of life. Centers used both median sternotomy and bilateral video-assisted thoracoscopic surgery (VATS) approaches to perform the operative procedure. Interim analysis identified a high-risk subgroup with a higher mortality. These patients had low FEV1 (less than 20% predicted) and either a homogenous pattern of emphysema in both upper and lower lungs or a low carbon monoxide diffusing capacity (DLCO) (less than 20% predicted). The mortality at 30 days was 16%, and the risk was felt to be prohibitive. As the study continued, two preoperative factors appeared to be associated with decreased mortality: dominant upper-lobe emphysema and having a higher preoperative exercise capacity. Using these factors, patients were divided into four subgroups. Patients with upper-lobe disease and a low exercise capacity, defined as achieving less than the 40th percentile on exercise testing, 25 Watts for women and 40 Watts for men, showed a survival advantage and improved exercise capacity after surgery. Patients with upper-lobe disease and high exercise capacity, achieving more than the 40th percentile cutoff, showed no survival advantage but did have improved long-term exercise capacity. Patients with non–upper-lobe disease and low exercise capacity had no survival or exercise improvements but did note an improved quality of life at 24 months. The remaining patients with non–upper-lobe disease and high exercise capacity had a higher risk of death and no significant improvement in exercise capacity or quality of life. The 30-day mortality in the non–high-risk subgroup was 5.5%. Long-term follow-up showed the same results in all subgroups except in the non–upper-lobe disease and low exercise capacity group. The quality of life improvement had disappeared by 3 years (Algorithm 80.3).[36] This subgroup analysis has allowed surgeons to better counsel patients as to the benefits of LVRS, based on which group they fall in.

When the different surgical approaches were evaluated, there was no difference in mortality or benefit from sternotomy versus video-assisted thoracoscopic (VATS) approaches. Sternotomy patients had a longer hospital stay and higher costs noted at 6 months. The cost effectiveness of LVRS was also evaluated. The mean cost for LVRS was much higher at 1 year than for the medical therapy group, $71,515 versus $23,371, respectively.[38] In the subgroup with upper-lobe disease and low exercise capacity, at 2 years of follow-up, there was a cost of $98,000 per quality-adjusted life-year (QALY). This was predicted to fall to $21,000 at 10 years. In comparison, coronary artery bypass graft surgery has a cost of $64,000 per QALY.[38,39]

A new technique aimed to provide the same benefit of LVRS but without the surgical risk is the placement of one-way endobronchial valves. These are designed to allow air to escape the hyperinflated apical regions and not allow air to re-enter. Endobronchial stents have been designed to cross bronchioles into hyperinflated regions of the lung and allow decompression. Other approaches being tested include the bronchoscopic introduction of biologic substances such as trypsin or thrombin into hyperinflated regions of the lung with the goal of causing local scarring and reduce the hyperinflation.[38] Other surgical procedures in the treatment of COPD include bullectomy in selected patients and lung transplants in patients with end-stage disease.[37]

Tracheobronchial Foreign Body (TFB) Aspiration

TFB aspiration occurs most often in children, but up to 20% of cases have been reported in adults. Risk factors in adults include older age, as elderly patients have a higher incidence of neurologic disease and an impaired cough reflex. Symptoms usually involve an episode of choking, followed by a protracted cough. Fever, dyspnea, and wheezing can also be present.[40] Chest x-ray view may aid in the diagnosis if the aspirated TFB is radiopaque or if there is associated air trapping, atelectasis, or pneumonia; however, the TFB is visible less than a quarter of the time as most foods are not radiopaque.[41] Chest CT scans are a more sensitive imaging modality but not necessarily more specific. Bronchoscopy should be performed if TFB aspiration is suspected. Removal of the TFB can usually be accomplished by flexible bronchoscopy but may require rigid bronchoscopy in difficult cases.[40,41]

Pneumothorax

Pneumothoraces are classified as spontaneous, primary or secondary, traumatic, or iatrogenic. Primary spontaneous pneumothoraces occur in patients with no known lung disease, whereas secondary spontaneous ones occur in patients with underlying lung pathology thought to predispose those patients to a pneumothorax. Iatrogenic pneumothoraces may occur in either the postsurgical or postprocedural setting, typically following central line placement or thoracentesis.[42] Traumatic pneumothoraces are covered elsewhere in this text.

5 Primary spontaneous pneumothoraces occur more frequently in men than in women, with an incidence of 7 to 18 cases per 100,000 people for men, compared to an incidence rate of 1 to 6 cases per 100,000 people in women. Most cases occur in males younger than 30 years of age, and they rarely occur in people older than the age of 40 years. Even though many patients with primary pneumothoraces do not have apparent lung disease, almost all are found to have subpleural bullae, the pathophysiology of which is unknown.[42] Most bullae are apical in location.[43] Patient symptoms can range from minimal to severe and usually include pleuritic pain, dyspnea, or both. Tachycardia may also be present, and if a person is tachycardic and hypotensive, a tension pneumothorax must be high on the differential and appropriate needle decompression considered. A tension pneumothorax occurs when air entering the pleural cavity cannot escape and the air compresses the vena cava and even the heart, resulting in hemodynamic instability (Fig. 80.26). Urgent needle decompression followed by chest tube placement is the preferred treatment. Most spontaneous pneumothoraces occur while patients are at rest.[42,44]

Observation is often the treatment of a stable, small pneumothorax, defined as being less than 3 cm from the apex. For a larger pneumothorax, chest tube placement is the standard treatment, though some advocate a trial of aspiration. Most patients will have a complete resolution of their pneumothorax and not need further treatment. In the group of patients who have a persistent air leak from the initial pneumothorax, or the 30% who have a recurrent pneumothorax, usually within 2 years, further treatment is warranted. This involves some form of pleurodesis, chemical or mechanical, either via a chest tube (talc infusion), or during a thoracoscopic evaluation where apparent blebs can also be resected (Algorithm 80.4).[43,44]

Secondary spontaneous pneumothoraces can occur due to various lung diseases, but COPD is the most common.[45] Although primary pneumothoraces can be mild clinical events, secondary ones are much more concerning because of the baseline lung disease and poor pulmonary reserve. Observation has no role in this patient population, who should undergo definitive treatment to prevent a recurrence during the first event. Here a thoracoscopic approach may be more effective in establishing an adequate pleurodesis and allow the evaluation for sources of air leaks.[44] Iatrogenic pneumothoraces can result from transthoracic needle lung biopsies, central line placement, thoracentesis, transbronchial lung biopsies, pleural biopsies, and positive-pressure ventilation. Patients with underlying lung disease are at a higher risk of developing a pneumothorax after these procedures. Treatment should follow the same paradigm as for spontaneous pneumothoraces. Patients with a small, asymptomatic, stable pneumothorax and no underlying lung

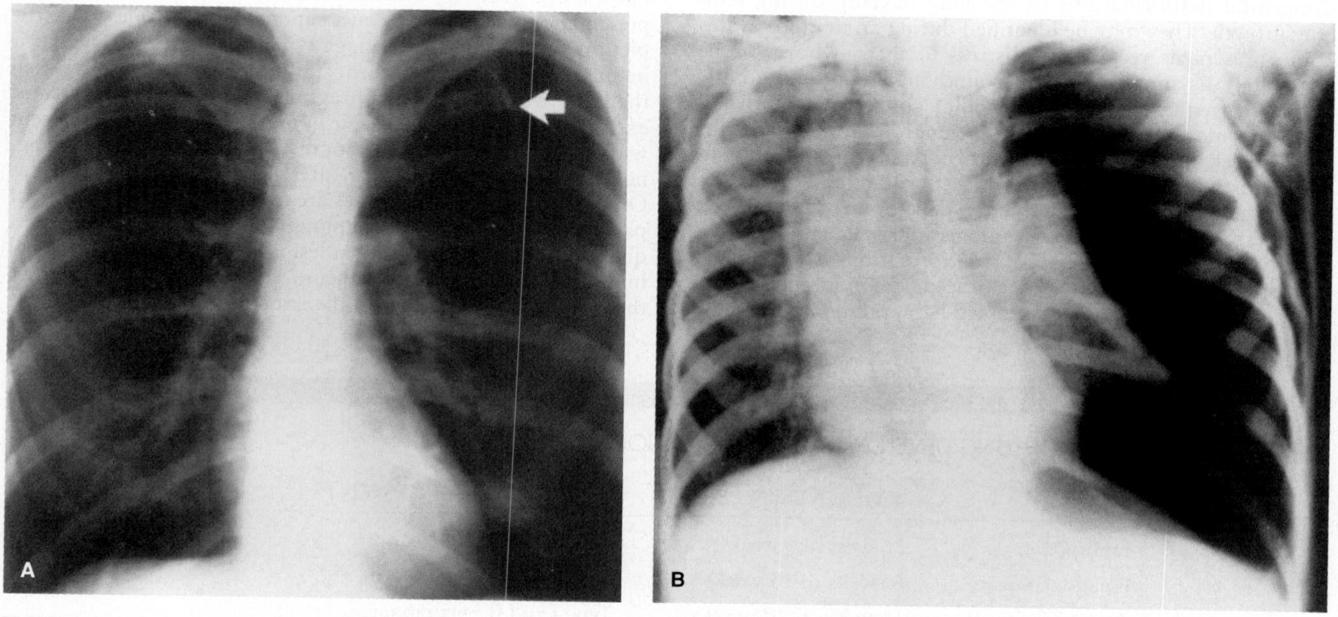

FIGURE 80.26. **A:** A 40% left-sided spontaneous pneumothorax (*arrow*). **B:** Progression of simple pneumothorax to a tension pneumothorax, showing the characteristic radiographic findings—virtual collapse of the entire involved lung, shift of the mediastinum to the contralateral side, and compression of the contralateral lung. Subcutaneous air dissecting along the left chest wall is also evident.

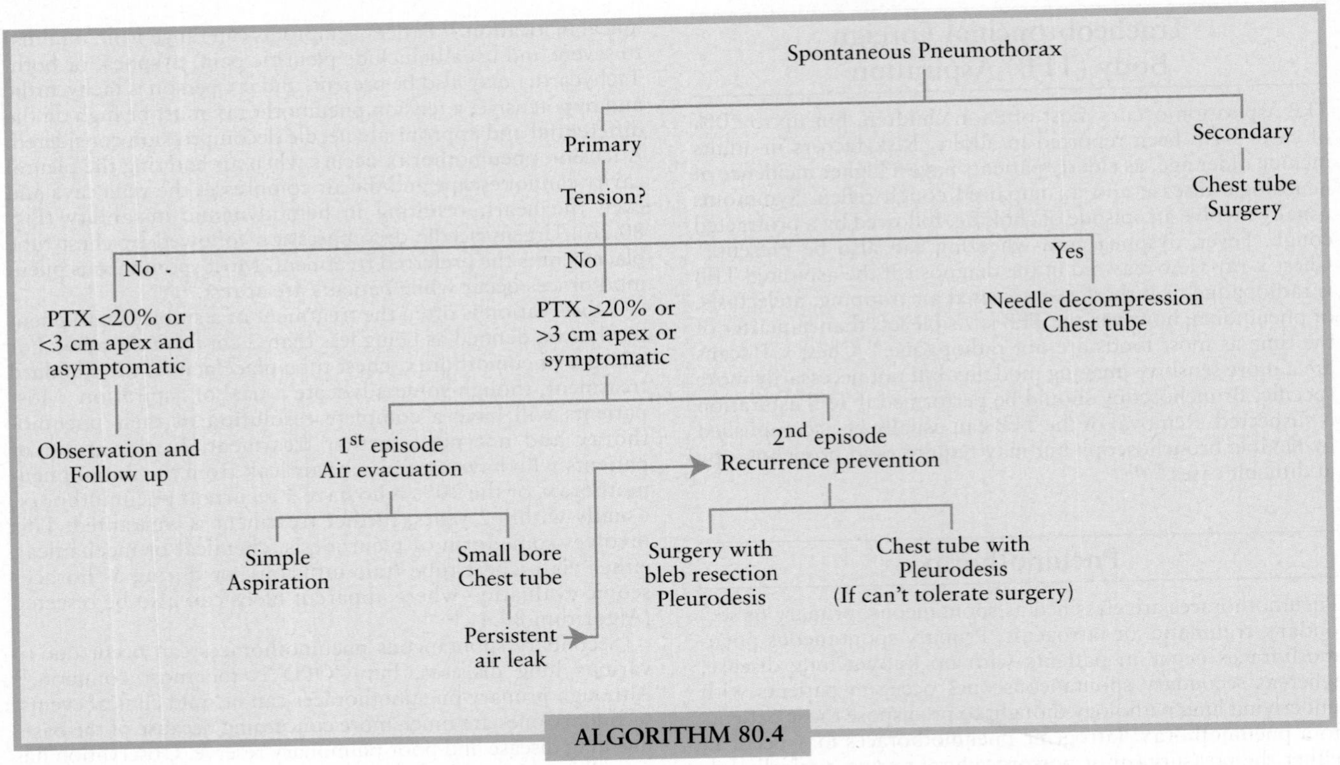

ALGORITHM 80.4. Algorithm to treat pneumothorax. (Adapted from Baumann MH, Noppen M. *Respirology* 2004;9(2):157–164.)

disease may be safely observed, although all others should undergo placement of a chest tube.[44] Some studies have suggested immediate aspiration of air after a CT-guided lung biopsy resulting in a pneumothorax, with an 85% success rate in avoiding the need for chest tube placement.[43]

Congenital Lung Disease

Congenital malformations of the lung develop during fetal lung growth. They may be identified during an in utero evaluation, present as respiratory distress in the newborn, or be completely asymptomatic and found in patients as adults. They can frequently occur with other congenital malformations and may be life threatening. Lung development begins during week 3 from the foregut. It progresses through birth to approximately 2 years of age when alveolar development is complete. The five stages of lung development have been divided into the embryonic, pseudoglandular, acinar, saccular, and alveolar stages (Table 80.2). Malformations may occur at each step and lead to different pathologic conditions.[46] Four separate conditions will be discussed here; pulmonary sequestration, lobar emphysema, congenital cystic adenomatoid malformation (CCAM), and bronchogenic cysts.[47]

Pulmonary Sequestrations. Pulmonary sequestrations are defined as pieces of parenchymal lung separated from the respiratory tree, with the sequestration receiving its blood supply from an anomalous artery arising from the aorta rather than having the blood supply arising from the pulmonary artery. Sequestrations have been further subdivided into extralobar and intralobar lesions, with very distinct anatomic alterations and clinical presentations. Extralobar sequestrations reside outside of the true pleural space. Venous drainage is usually into the azygos or hemiazygos veins. They are most often on the left side between the left lower lobe and diaphragm (Fig. 80.27). Up to 80% of extralobar sequestrations occur in males. Most patients present with dyspnea in the first 6 months of life. They may be diagnosed by fetal ultrasound or after birth by chest x-ray view. Other congenital abnormalities are found in up to two thirds of patients, with congenital diaphragmatic hernias present in a quarter of patients.[46] Intralobar lesions reside within the normal lung and within the normal pleura. They are almost always in the lower lobes and occur in the left side just over 50% of the

TABLE 80.2

PHASES OF LUNG DEVELOPMENT CLASSIFICATION

■ PHASE	■ GESTATION PERIOD	■ MAJOR DEVELOPMENTS
Embryonic	26 days to 6 weeks	5 lobar bronchi
Pseudoglandular	6 weeks to 16 weeks	Cartilage rings, cilia form
Acinar/Canalicular	16 weeks to 28 weeks	Type I and II pneumoncytes
Saccular	28 weeks to 34 weeks	Distal airspace development
Alveolar	34 weeks to 2 years	Alveoli proliferate from 20 to 600 million

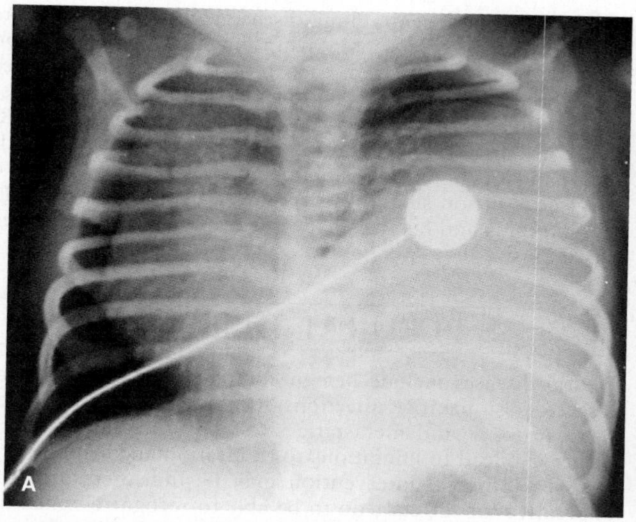

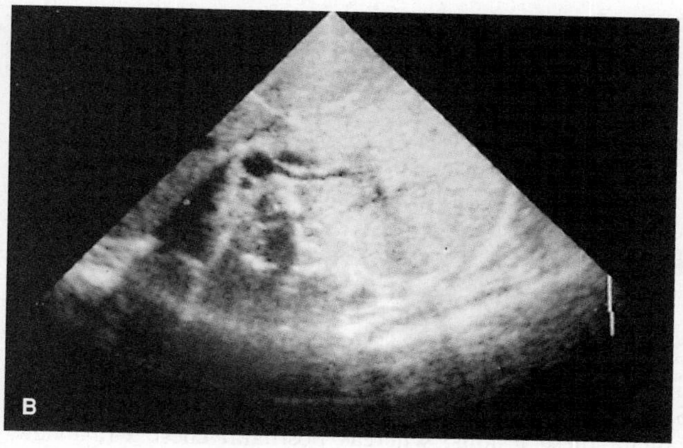

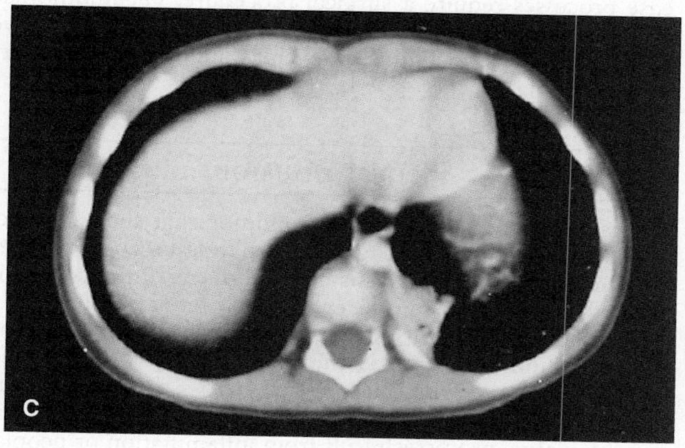

FIGURE 80.27. **A:** Abnormal radiograph of the chest of a newborn with respiratory distress (**A**). Ultrasound identified the anomalous vessel coursing through the diaphragm and entering the sequestration (**B**). This computed tomographic scan clearly demonstrates the anomalous artery arising from the thoracic aorta and entering the sequestered lung (**C**). (Reproduced with permission from Shields TW, ed. *General Thoracic Surgery*, 6th ed. 2005:Fig. 80-15.)

time. Venous drainage is usually through the pulmonary vein. It is suggested that intralobar sequestration may be an acquired disease, caused by repeated episodes of inflammation that lead to bronchiole narrowing and scarring. Ultimately the "lobe" becomes isolated and may develop new feeding blood vessels from collateral arteries in the inferior pulmonary ligament. A complete assessment of a sequestered lesion must be performed prior to resection and should include assessment of any potential airway or gut connection, determining the vascular supply of the sequestration, and determining if there are any other congenital malformations.[46]

Congenital Lobar Emphysema. Lobar emphysema is the cause of half of the episodes of newborn respiratory distress that are due to structural anomalies. Two thirds of the cases occur in males. Distention of the distal lung occurs from obstruction of the airway, either from an intrinsic cause, such as meconium or torsion, or an extrinsic cause, such as obstructing lymph nodes. In up to half of the cases, no cause can be found. Almost all cases occur in the upper lobes, with almost equal distribution between sides. Half of the lesions will present in newborns, and the remaining 50% will reveal themselves by 6 months. Chest x-ray studies are diagnostic (Fig. 80.28).[46] Surgical resection may not be immediately necessary and may be delayed until the child has grown or until he or she develops a failure to thrive. Even after surgical resection, patients may have bronchomalacia and a tendency toward bronchospasm.[48]

Congenital Cystic Adenomatoid Malformation. CCAM lesions are the second most common cause (25%) of newborn respiratory distress, secondary to structural problems. Children will present either at birth or in early childhood with recurrent respiratory infections. The anomalies are due to an overgrowth of bronchioles, likely during the acinar phase of fetal lung development. Lesions can occur on either side and usually are isolated to one lower lobe. The classification system by Stocker (Table 80.3) organizes these lesions based on pathologic

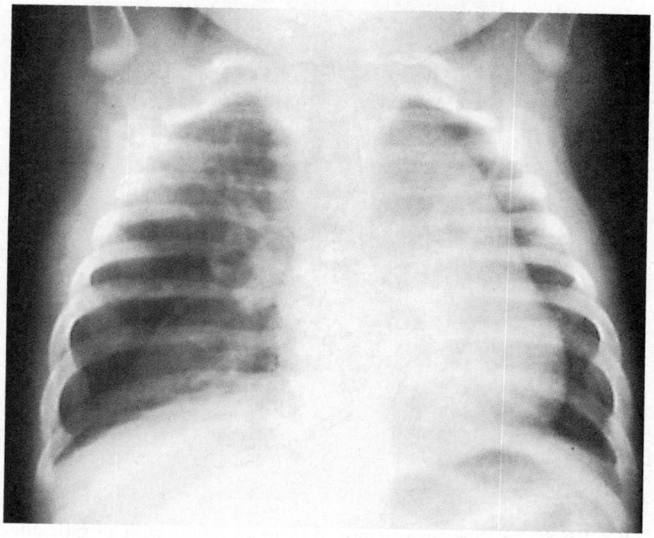

FIGURE 80.28. Radiograph of a newborn with lobar emphysema involving the right middle lobe. Note the compressed right lower lobe and mediastinal shift. (Reproduced with permission from Shields TW, ed. *General Thoracic Surgery*, 6th ed. 2005:Fig. 80-6.)

TABLE 80.3

THE STOCKER CLASSIFICATION OF CCAM

- Type I
  75% of lesions
  Few large cysts
  Parenchymal compression
- Type II
  Numerous, <1 cm cysts
  Associated with other congenital anomalies
  Worse prognosis
- Type III
  Rarest type
  Cysts are solid and smaller (few mm in diameter)

appearance and clinical outcome. Prenatal MRI best serves to evaluate these lesions, whereas postnatal chest x-ray view and/or chest CT scan can be used to differentiate CCAMs from other lesions.[46] Even though lesions may be small and asymptomatic, these lesions possess the potential for malignant transformation and should be resected (Fig. 80.29).[48]

Bronchogenic Cysts. Bronchogenic cysts are formed from primitive foregut tissue present in the airway. They can present as single or multiple cysts in a wide variety of locations in the thorax. They usually present in young children who develop symptoms such as stridor due to airway obstruction or compression caused by the cysts.[47] Alternatively, cysts located within the lung parenchyma can become infected and present as an abscess. Therapeutic aspiration may be temporizing, but ultimately surgery is needed.[49] Resection may have a mortality of up to 14%, but untreated lesions have a 100% mortality.[47]

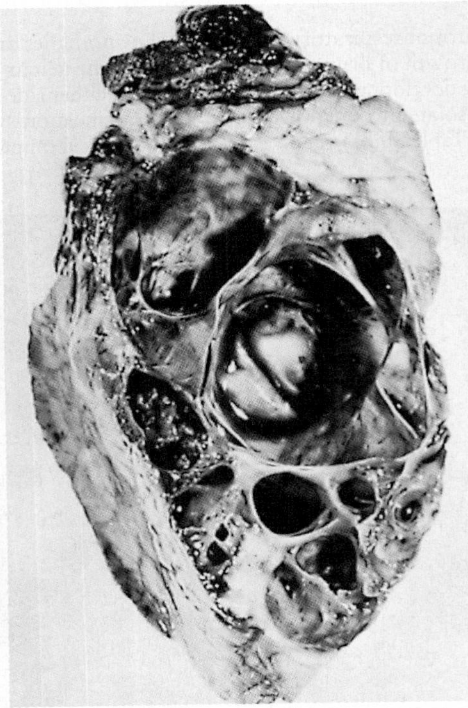

FIGURE 80.29. Specimen removed from an infant with a cystic adenomatoid malformation. Microscopically, there was marked proliferation of terminal bronchioles, and cartilage was lacking (Reproduced with permission from Shields TW, ed. *General Thoracic Surgery*, 6th ed. 2005:Fig. 80-24.)

Most cases of congenital lung disease will present in the first 6 months of life. The main symptom is usually respiratory distress, but once children reach 1 year in age, chronic infections become the most common symptom. Diagnostic tests begin with chest x-ray views but can include ultrasound, MRI, CT scans, angiography, and bronchoscopy, depending on the lesion and location.[50] Decision making regarding the timing of surgical resection should incorporate the patient's acuity due to symptoms and his or her overall ability to tolerate surgery based on size.

PLEURAL DISEASE

Pleural diseases include benign complications from systemic disease, postoperative infections, local infections, and cancers from primary and metastatic sites. Diseases involving the pleura can lead to limitations to respiration and symptoms of dyspnea. Surgical intervention may be indicated, and it is imperative for the surgeon to be able to recognize which disease processes require a surgical procedure. Pneumothoraces are discussed earlier in this chapter, and here we will cover pleural effusions, including empyemas and malignant pleural mesotheliomas.

Pleural Effusions

Pleural effusions are a common condition that elicit a surgical consult for potential drainage and even thoracoscopic intervention to assist in the diagnosis and treatment of the condition. The essential first step in the evaluation of a new effusion is to determine if it is a transudative or exudative process. A transudative fluid collection is the result of a poorly balanced hydrostatic and/or osmotic pressure across the pleural membrane resulting in increased serum leak across the pleural barrier. Exudative processes result from inflammation or neoplastic processes that cause increased capillary leak at the pleural membrane. Because of the leaky membrane, larger proteins can enter the pleural fluid resulting in higher protein and lactate dehydrogenase (LDH) levels in the exudative fluid compared to the transudative fluid (Table 80.4).[51] One of the tests used most often to make the diagnosis is the Light criteria, where the serum and pleural fluid protein and LDH levels are measured (Table 80.5). If one or more of the criteria are met, then the fluid is considered exudative.[52] Other tests have been evaluated, including measuring cholesterol ratios and the albumin gradient, but the Light criteria is still the best overall test.[51]

Transudative effusions are most often caused by congestive heart failure. Even if a patient has no other symptoms of heart failure, in the setting of a transudative effusion, a complete cardiac workup should be considered. Other causes include cirrhosis, which may or may not be associated with ascites. Isolated right- and left-sided effusions due to liver disease have been described. Effusions can be seen in more than 20% of patients with nephrotic syndrome, and so all patients with new effusions should be evaluated for the presence of proteinuria. Rarer causes include retroperitoneal urine leaks or cerebrospinal fluid leaks.[52] 6 Surgical interventions, such as chest tube placement, should be avoided in these disease settings, as patients will continue to drain fluid from their chest until the primary cause is treated. Aspiration of fluid may help temporarily while systemic treatment is instituted but should only be done as part of a larger treatment plan.

Exudative effusions have several etiologies, but malignancy is the number one cause.[52] Approximately a quarter of pleural effusions in a community hospital setting have been attributed to cancer. The malignancies that cause the effusions are, in order of decreasing frequency, lung cancer, breast cancer, and hematologic cancers such as lymphoma. Other malignancies, such as ovarian cancer, can also cause effusions.[53] The next most

TABLE 80.4 DIAGNOSIS

DIFFERENTIAL DIAGNOSIS OF PLEURAL EFFUSIONS

Transudative pleural effusions	Collagen vascular diseases
Congestive heart failure	Rheumatoid pleuritis
Pericardial disease	Systemic lupus erythematosus
Cirrhosis	Drug-induced lupus erythematosus
Nephrotic syndrome	Immunoblastic lymphadenopathy
Peritoneal dialysis	Sjögren syndrome
Superior vena cava obstruction	Wegener granulomatosis
Myxedema	Churg-Strauss syndrome
Pulmonary emboli	Postcardiac injury syndrome
Sarcoidosis	Asbestos exposure
Urinothorax	Sarcoidosis
EXUDATIVE PLEURAL EFFUSIONS	Uremia
Neoplastic diseases	Meigs syndrome
Metastatic disease	Yellow nail syndrome
Mesothelioma	Drug-induced pleural disease
Infectious diseases	Nitrofurantoin
Bacterial infections	Dantrolene
Tuberculosis	Methysergide
Fungal infections	Bromocriptine
Viral infections	Procarbazine
Parasitic infections	Amiodarone
Pulmonary embolization	Trapped lung
Gastrointestinal disease	Radiotherapy
Esophageal perforation	Electric burns
Pancreatic disease	Urinary tract obstruction
Intra-abdominal abscess	Iatrogenic injury
Diaphragmatic hernia	Ovarian hyperstimulation syndrome
Postabdominal surgery	Chylothorax
Endoscopic variceal sclerotherapy	Hemothorax

common causes of exudative effusions are infections, including pneumonias causing parapneumonic effusions, tuberculosis (TB), and fungal infections. Although rarer in the United States, TB is still a common etiology worldwide. If someone is suspected of having pleural TB, the pleural fluid should be evaluated for adenosine deaminase (ADA) and gamma-interferon levels, which if low will rule out the diagnosis of TB. If other infections are suspected, the pleural fluid should be cultured. Pancreatitis may also cause an exudate, and elevated serum amylase levels will support the diagnosis. Autoimmune processes, such as rheumatoid disease and lupus, can also cause effusions. Chylothorax presents after problems with thoracic duct lymph drainage in the chest lead to an accumulation of lymphatic fluid in one or both thoraces. The thoracic duct collects lymph from the cisterna chyli, the plexus of lymphatics in the upper abdomen, and travels anterior to the spine and just posterolateral to the aorta. It follows behind the aorta and enters the left neck where it empties into the confluence of the left internal jugular and subclavian veins (Fig. 80.30). Chylous leaks are due primarily to thoracic duct injury from trauma, surgery, or lymphomas resulting in obstructed lymphatics. Pleural triglyceride and cholesterol levels will be elevated, and the fluid will have a milky color. Treatment for persistent chylothoraces include thoracic duct ligation by surgery or by embolization of the site of leak in the interventional suite.[52]

TABLE 80.5

CRITERIA FOR EXUDATIVE EFFUSIONS BASED ON RATIO OF PLEURAL FLUID PROTEIN AND LDH CONCENTRATIONS TO SERUM CONCENTRATION

Protein/serum protein >0.5
LDH/serum LDH >0.6
Pleural LDH 1.67 times normal serum LDH

LDH, lactate dehydrogenase.

The management of malignant pleural effusions includes various options, but critical to the decision-making process is the knowledge of the median life expectancy in that patient due to the underlying malignancy. Chest tube drainage may be therapeutic and diagnostic, allowing fluid drainage and alleviation of symptoms of dyspnea. It will also allow determination of whether the underlying lung is able to expand. If not, it is described as a "trapped lung" and although the fluid may be gone, a persistent pneumothorax appears on chest x-ray views as the lung cannot expand and fill the thorax. In these settings, an indwelling pleural drainage catheter may be the best option to intermittently drain accumulating fluid. Decortication is not recommended, as most patients with malignancy in this setting have a limited life expectancy and the success rate is low

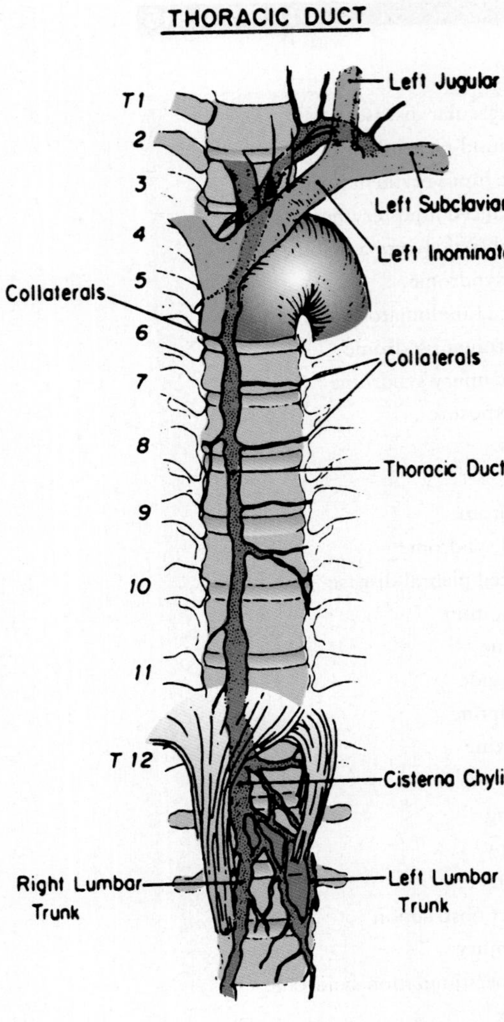

FIGURE 80.30. Schematic drawing of the most usual pattern and course of the thoracic duct. The single duct that enters the chest through the aortic hiatus between T12 and T10 is a relatively consistent finding and the usual site for surgical ligation.

compared to decortication in the setting of an empyema. VATS exploration may also be used to remove loculated fluid collections and to evaluate for lung re-expansion after the procedure. If the lung re-expands, further treatment includes pleurodesis, using talc, doxycycline, or bleomycin. These medications will cause an inflammatory reaction between the parietal and visceral pleura resulting in the lung being "stuck" in an expanded state. Mechanical pleurodesis can also be performed by mechanical débridement of the pleura via VATS. Chemical pleurodesis may be performed via VATS or through an existing thoracostomy tube. The goal of treatment in the setting of a malignant pleural effusion is palliation.[53]

Empyema. 7 Empyemas are defined as frank pus in the thoracic cavity. This represents part of the continuum of disease that begins with simple parapneumonic effusion, where exudative fluid is not infected and not loculated. As the disease progresses, fluid becomes loculated with fibrinous septations and becomes infected, leading to pus and ultimately the development of a fibrinous peel. Up to half of pneumonias have an associated effusion, but less than 5% of cases lead to an empyema.[54] Other causes include surgical thoracotomies and/or other infections from nearby organs, such as esophageal injuries. Pleural infections have been categorized into three overlapping stages. The first is the exudative stage, where the fluid is thin, sterile, has a lower white blood cell (WBC) count and LDH levels, and the glucose level is still greater than 40 mg/dL (Table 80.6). Treatment usually involves addressing the underlying etiology, such as a pneumonia. The second stage is the fibrinopurulent stage, where the fluid becomes infected and fibrin deposits accumulate on the pleura. The LDH and WBC count increase, and the glucose and pH levels drop. The fluid becomes thick and purulent, and the lung is often unable to expand. Chest tube drainage alone at this stage may not be effective to remove the fluid. The third stage is the organizing stage, and a thick pleural peel is created by migrating fibroblasts. At this point, a formal débridement and decortication is required to allow the lung to return to full function.[54]

Organisms causing empyemas have shifted from predominately *S. pneumoniae* in the preantibiotic era, to anaerobic organisms in up to three quarters of empyemas in the current era. Imaging to evaluate the presence of an empyema begins with a simple chest x-ray view but requires a chest CT to show potential loculations. After the institution of antibiotic therapy, surgical intervention depends on the stage of the disease but may require a VATS exploration or even a thoracotomy to débride the thorax effectively and to decorticate the pleural peel off the lung to allow re-expansion.[54] Postpneumonectomy empyemas are an especially difficult problem as there is no lung tissue to occupy the empty thorax. Risk factors in this setting include right pneumonectomies (vs. left), the need for postoperative ventilation, lower starting hemotocrit levels, and poor preoperative pulmonary function test results.[55,56] Treatments of these empyemas are particularly difficult and may include an Eloesser flap or the Clagett procedure, which allow for the creation of an open wound that permits packing and granulation tissue to form in the empyema cavity.[57]

Mesothelioma. Malignant pleural mesothelioma (MPM) is a cancer of the serosal pleura, related to the exposure to asbestos. Multiple hypotheses have been formed regarding how asbestos causes mesothelioma and include the idea that asbestos fibers are inhaled deeply into the lung and penetrate the parenchymal surface, causing irritation of the pleura and repeated episodes of inflammation, ultimately leading to cancer. Other potential mechanisms include asbestos interfering with mitosis, inducing free-radical production, and induction of proto-oncogene kinases by asbestos fibers.[58] Exposure to asbestos usually occurs decades prior to presentation with mesothelioma and has been seen in miners exposed to asbestos dust, industrial workers such as plumbers and carpenters who used asbestos products, and even in 20% of patients with no

TABLE 80.6

DIAGNOSTIC CRITERIA FOR PLEURAL FLUID IN EMPYEMA

■ STAGE	■ FLUID/PEEL	■ WBC	■ LDH (cells/mm^3)	■ pH (IU)	■ BACTERIA
Exudative	Thin/elastic	<1000	<500	>7.3	Absent
Fibrinopurulent	Purulent/inelastic	>5000	>1000	<7.1	Present
Organizing	Thick/rigid peel	Varies	Varies	<7.1	Varies

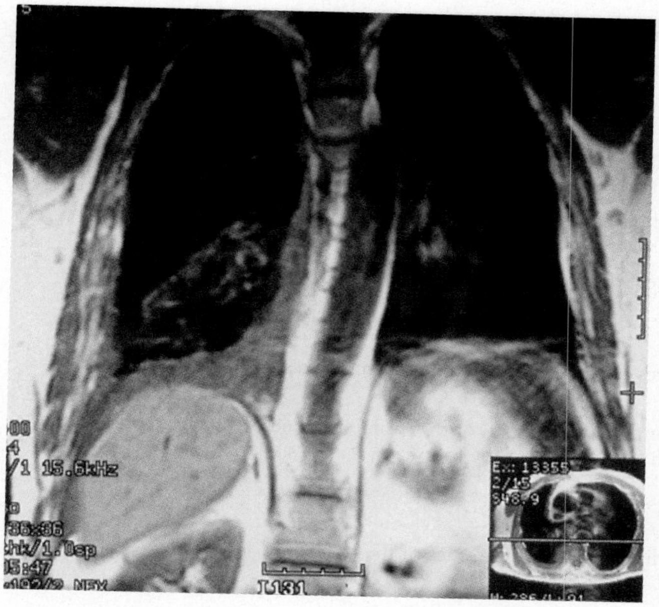

FIGURE 80.31. Magnetic resonance imaging of the patient in Figure 80.25 shows a large amount of tumor within the pleural space and into the diaphragmatic sulcus with no evidence of extension outside the hemithorax. (Reproduced with permission from Flores RM, Sugarbaker DJ. Malignant mesothelioma of the pleural space. *Ann Thorac Surg* 2000;70:306.)

known exposure but living in industrial countries. Mesothelioma is a relatively rare malignancy, with less than 5,000 cases in the United States per year.[59]

Patients with mesothelioma may present with dyspnea or chest pain. Often, patients are asymptomatic and the diagnosis is made after abnormalities are seen on a chest x-ray view performed for another reason. Radiographs may show unilateral effusions and a loss of volume on the affected side, as the lung capacity is diminished due to disease. As the disease progresses, patients may have weight loss, worsening pain, and night sweats. Median survival may be as little as 1 year from the time of diagnosis.[60] Diagnostic studies include a chest CT scan or MRI to show the extent of pleural thickening (Fig. 80.31). Lymphadenopathy or signs of local spread through the diaphragm or chest wall can also be seen with three-dimensional imaging. The pathologic diagnosis almost always requires a tissue biopsy. Cytologic examination of pleural fluid from a thoracentesis cannot differentiate between mesothelioma cells and other potential lung cancers. CT-guided biopsy of pleural thickening can often give the diagnosis, but ultimately a VATS approach or limited thoracotomy may be needed to obtain a diagnosis. If the patient is being considered for surgical resection, a limited thoracotomy in the site of a potential later incision is optimal to limit seeding of the tumor.[60]

Mesotheliomas can be categorized into epithelial, sarcomatoid, and mixed histologies. Patients with epithelial histology do better than those with a sarcomatoid histology.[60] There are various staging systems for mesothelioma, including the Butchart system, the revised Brigham and Women's Hospital system, and the TNM-based system by the International Mesothelioma Interest Group (IMIG) (Table 80.7).[60,61] The IMIG system allows for better reproducibility of the interpretation of local and regional lymph node spread. Laparoscopy may be useful to evaluate the patient for transdiaphragmatic spread of the tumor, differentiating between T3 and T4 tumors.[61]

Treatment for mesothelioma may include chemotherapy, radiation therapy, and surgery. Surgical treatment ranges from a pleurodesis for palliation in the setting of effusions and unresectable disease, to pleurectomy/decortication for limited disease, and to the most aggressive treatment of an extrapleural pneumonectomy (EPP), with the goal of complete tumor resection. Less than a third of patients are candidates for any surgical intervention. Preoperative workup for an EPP should include a cardiac evaluation, and optimal surgical candidates have pulmonary function tests with an FEV1 of greater than 2 L/s and an age younger than 70 years.[61] Surgery involves an en bloc removal of the lung, pleura, pericardium, and diaphragm with reconstruction of the pericardium and diaphragm. Pleurectomy and decortication is reserved for very early-stage disease and involves removal of the pleura only with preservation of the lung parenchyma. Multimodality approaches have shown better results, with neoadjuvant chemotherapy and adjuvant radiation therapy.[62] Chemotherapy for advanced disease includes pemetrexed and cisplatin or the combination of gemcitabine and cisplatin. Both have shown similar levels of palliation. Radiotherapy may also be used but is limited by the large field requiring treatment and the risks of pneumonitis and esophagitis.[58] It is best used in combination with EPP for local control after surgery or to treat local painful areas.[61] Because of the few cases per year, most patients who are considered for surgery should be referred to high-volume centers where surgeons and other clinicians are comfortable treating this disease.

TRACHEA

The trachea is a well-known structure to general surgeons who may perform tracheostomies and bronchoscopies as part of their clinical practice. A thorough knowledge of the anatomy and vascular supply is essential to minimize complications such as postintubation tracheal stenosis and tracheoinnominate fistulas after tracheostomies.

Anatomy

The trachea is the connection from the cricoid cartilage to the carina that allows ventilation and mucous clearance from the lungs. It is oval, with C-shaped cartilaginous rings creating the anterior and lateral borders. A soft tissue membrane forms the posterior wall to complete the oval shape. In the average male, the anterior-posterior dimension is 1.8 cm, whereas the lateral aspect is 2.3 cm. Tracheal length reaches almost 12 cm with almost two rings per centimeter. Trachea in women are 10% to 20% smaller. In children, the shape is more circular, but becomes gradually more ovoid as they age. There is a significant amount of flexibility in the normal trachea, and remodeling can occur in chronic disease states such as emphysema. The inner lining consists of ciliated pseudostratified columnar epithelium with goblet and mucous cells interspersed. At the carina, the right and left mainstem bronchi split off. The right side is characterized by the quick take-off of the right upper lobe bronchus, with the bronchus intermedius continuing into the middle- and lower-lobe bronchi. The left side has a longer mainstem bronchus with a split into the upper and lower lobes.[63] The blood supply begins with the inferior thyroid artery supplying the cervical trachea through three tracheoesophageal branches. The lower trachea is supplied by bronchial arteries arising off the aorta. As the arteries approach the trachea, they further split to supply separate segments. Even within segments, they will branch into anterior and posterior transverse intercartilaginous arteries (Fig. 80.32). Because of this segmental blood supply, there should be minimal circumferential dissection around the trachea to limit impairment of the blood supply and healing in tracheal/bronchial surgery.

Surgical Airways

The most common tracheal procedure is a tracheostomy. Over the last 20 years, there has been an increasing use of percutaneous

STAGING

TABLE 80.7

THE NEW INTERNATIONAL STAGING SYSTEM (IMIG)

T–TUMOR		
T1	1a	Tumor limited to the ipsilateral parietal pleura, including mediastinal and diaphragmatic pleura; noninvolvement of the visceral pleura
	1b	Tumor involving the ipsilateral parietal pleura, including mediastinal and diaphragmatic pleura; scattered foci of tumor also involving the visceral pleura
T2		Tumor involving each of the ipsilateral pleural surfaces (parietal, mediastinal, diaphragmatic, and visceral pleura) with at least one of the following features:
		Involvement of diaphragmatic muscle
		Confluent visceral pleural tumor (including the fissures) or extension of tumor from visceral pleura into the underlying pulmonary parenchyma
T3		Locally advanced but potentially resectable tumor; tumor involving all of the ipsilateral pleural surfaces (parietal, mediastinal, diaphragmatic, and visceral pleura) with at least one of the following features:
		Involvement of the endothoracic fascia
		Extension into the mediastinal fat
		Solitary, completely resectable focus of tumor extending into the soft tissues of the chest wall
		Nontransmural involvement of the pericardium
T4		Locally advanced technically unresectable tumor; tumor involving all of the ipsilateral pleural surfaces (parietal, mediastinal, diaphragmatic, and visceral) with at least one of the following features:
		Diffuse extension or multifocal masses of tumor in the chest wall, with or without associated rib destruction
		Direct transdiaphragmatic extension of tumor to the peritoneum
		Direct extension of tumor to the contralateral pleura
		Direct extension of tumor to one or more mediastinal organs
		Direct extension of tumor into the spine
		Tumor extending through to the internal surface of the pericardium with or without pericardial effusion; or tumor involving the myocardium
N–LYMPH NODES		
NX		Regional lymph nodes cannot be assessed
N0		No regional lymph node metastases
N1		Metastases in the ipsilateral bronchopulmonary or hilar lymph nodes
N2		Metastases in the subcarinal or ipsilateral mediastinal lymph nodes, including the ipsilateral internal mammary nodes
N3		Metastases in the contralateral mediastinal, contralateral internal mammary, ipsilateral or contralateral supraclavicular lymph nodes
M–METASTASES		
MX		Presence of distant metastases cannot be assessed
M0		No distant metastasis
M1		Distant metastasis present
STAGE		**DESCRIPTION**
I		
Ia		T1aN0M0
Ib		T1bN0M0
II		T2N0M0
III		Any T3M0
		Any N1M0
		Any N2M0
IV		Any T4
		Any N3
		Any M1

Adapted with permission from Rusch VW. A proposed new international TNM staging system for malignant pleural mesothelioma. From the International Mesothelioma Interest Group. *Chest* 1995;108:1122–1128.

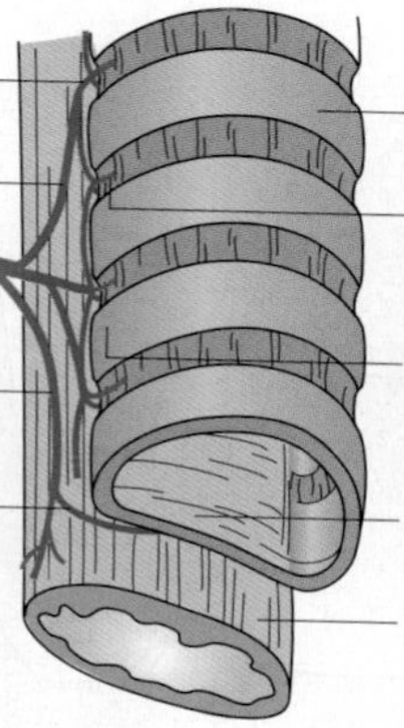

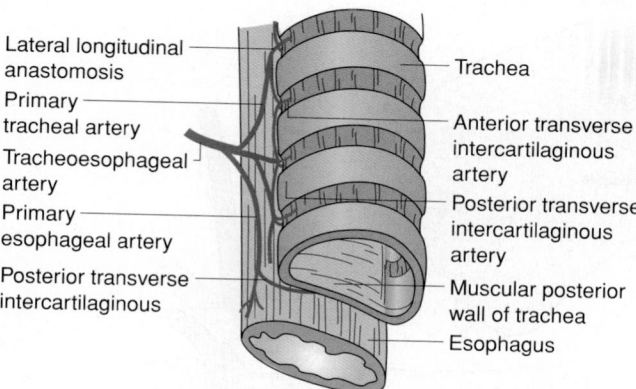

FIGURE 80.32. Semischematic view of the tracheal microscopical blood supply. Transverse intercartilaginous arteries derived from the lateral longitudinal anastomosis penetrate the soft tissues between each cartilage to supply a rich vascular network beneath the endotracheal mucosa. (Adapted from Salassa JR, Pearson BW, Payne WS, et al. Gross and microscopical blood supply of the trachea. *Ann Thorac Surg* 1977;24:100–107.)

tracheostomy. For patients who are intubated, the indication for and timing of tracheostomy depends on a multitude of factors, of which there is very little consensus in the medical literature. The goal of a tracheostomy is to limit the risk of laryngeal stenosis caused by prolonged endotracheal intubation, to improve pulmonary toilet, and to improve oral hygiene. Generally, tracheostomy should be considered after a patient has been intubated for more than 7 days, without clear expectation for immediate extubation.[64] Ideally, patients should be on minimal ventilator settings, but tracheostomy may be performed in patients with elevated oxygen (FiO_2 of up to 60%) and ventilatory (positive end-expiratory pressure [PEEP] less than 10) requirements. Patients requiring more support are at high risk of decompensating if they lose their airways, even if just for a moment, and the decision to perform a tracheostomy should be carefully considered in this setting.[65]

Tracheostomies are performed with the neck extended. A 2- to 3-cm incision is made approximately 2 cm above the sternal notch. Dissection is carried down through the platysma, and the strap muscles are divided longitudinally. Exposure of the trachea and the second and third rings may require elevation of the thyroid. Lateral traction sutures may be placed around the second or third rings. A vertical incision is made between rings two and four and gradually dilated. A tracheostomy tube is placed under direct vision.[64,66] Percutaneous tracheostomy placement is based on the Seldinger technique. A needle is placed percutaneously into the trachea at the estimated level of the second or third rings with bronchoscopic visualization. A guidewire is placed into the airway and serial dilations performed, until a tracheostomy tube is able to be advanced over the wire.[65] Cricothyroidotomy should be performed only in the emergent setting. The cricothyroid membrane is palpated below the superior thyroid notch. A transverse incision is made to the lateral borders of the thyroid cartilage. Rapid dilation is followed by tube insertion.[64]

8 Complications can vary depending on the technique. For open tracheostomy, they include damage to the carotid artery, internal jugular vein, posterior tracheal wall/anterior esophagus, and apex of the lung.[65] Also reported are fires due to the use of electrocautery in the setting of nitrous oxide and oxygen.[64] In percutaneous tracheostomies, complications include pneumothorax, mediastinal emphysema, paratracheal insertion, tracheoesophageal fistula, and airway loss.[65,67] Common complications include local hemorrhage and infection. Major late complications include tracheal stenosis and tracheoinnominate fistulas. Fistulas result from erosion of the tracheostomy tube into the innominate artery. Improper placement of the tracheostomy into rings lower than the third ring place patients at higher risk for this complication. A sentinel bleed may be the initial presentation. Pressure on the fistula with immediate repair or ligation of the vessel is required (Fig. 80.33).[68] Postintubation stenosis is usually due to necrosis caused by high-pressure cuffs resulting in impaired blood flow to the segmental area of the trachea. This leads to the long-term loss of cartilage and narrowing of the airway. The use of low-pressure cuffs has reduced the incidence of this complication but not eliminated it. Bronchoscopy and dilation may alleviate symptoms, but resection of the stenotic area may be needed (Fig. 80.34).[66]

Tracheal Tumors

Benign lesions of the trachea are less common than malignant ones. They include papillomas, chondromas, hamartomas, fibromas, and hemangiomas. Papillomas are associated with the human papilloma virus and can degenerate into malignant lesions, thus requiring resection. Chondromas arise from the cartilage and may recur after resection. Hamartomas are composed of cartilage and epithelial and lymphatic tissue. Recurrence is rare after resection. Fibromas can be resected via bronchoscopy. Hemangiomas are the most common pediatric tracheal mass. They may regress without treatment and can be observed if not causing obstructive symptoms. Biopsy is generally avoided due to bleeding risk. Surgery may be required if lesions persist.[69]

Although more common than benign lesions, malignant tracheal tumors are very rare with only 600 to 700 cases in the United States per year. Lesions may be primary tracheal lesions, tumors from adjacent organs growing into the trachea, or metastatic lesions.[70] Primary tumors are most commonly squamous cell carcinomas or adenoid cystic carcinomas in the trachea, followed by carcinoids in the bronchi.[70,71] Adjacent tumors may arise in the lung, esophagus, thyroid, or mediastinum. The most common cancers that cause tracheal metastases include renal cell cancers, sarcomas, breast cancers, and colon cancers.[70] Patients will present with stridor and wheezing and have often been recently diagnosed with adult-onset asthma and treated with inhalers and even steroids without alleviation of symptoms. Hemoptysis may also occur, though it is more common in lung cancer than in tracheal disease.[71] Patients should undergo imaging such as a neck and chest CT scan to assist in making the proper diagnosis. Bronchoscopy with a flexible or rigid endoscope is essential to aid in the evaluation of the extent of disease and to control the airway if necessary. Treatment includes tracheal resection for primary tumors if possible. For metastatic disease, palliative treatment includes endoluminal resection and/or radiotherapy.[71] Endoluminal treatments include mechanical core out, YAG-laser treatment, photodynamic therapy (PDT), cryotherapy, or brachytherapy. Stenting also may play a role to maintain airway patency, either for a temporary period during radiation treatment or in the setting of end-stage disease (Algorithm 80.5).[70]

Tracheomalacia and Airway Stents

Tracheomalacia occurs when the trachea loses its rigid form and the posterior membranous wall approaches the anterior wall, causing luminal narrowing and obstruction leading to dyspnea. Patients have a characteristic seal-like cough. Chest CT scans may demonstrate this condition, and pulmonary function testing in these patients will show reduced FEV1, forced vital capacity (FVC), and peak expiratory flow rates. Bronchoscopy is the best diagnostic test and reveals real-time airway collapse with expiration. Etiologies include congenital tracheomalacia, extrinsic compression, postintubation stenosis and inflammation, relapsing polychondritis, and chronic obstructive pulmonary disease.[72] Surgical intervention may

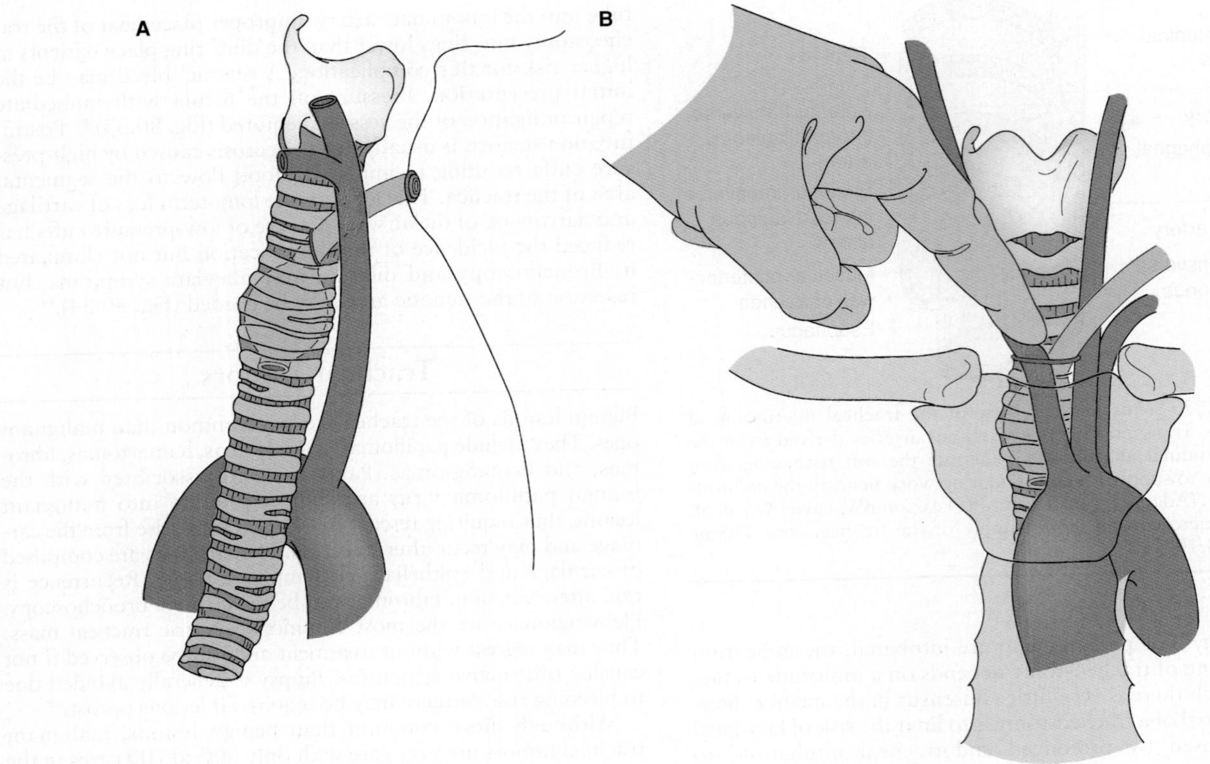

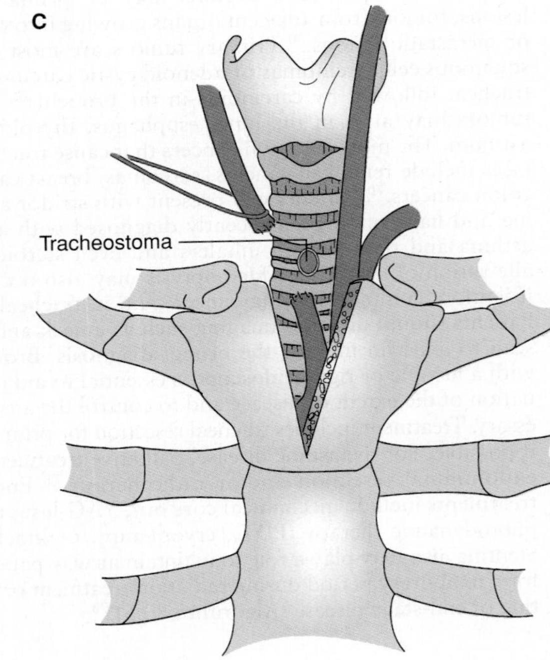

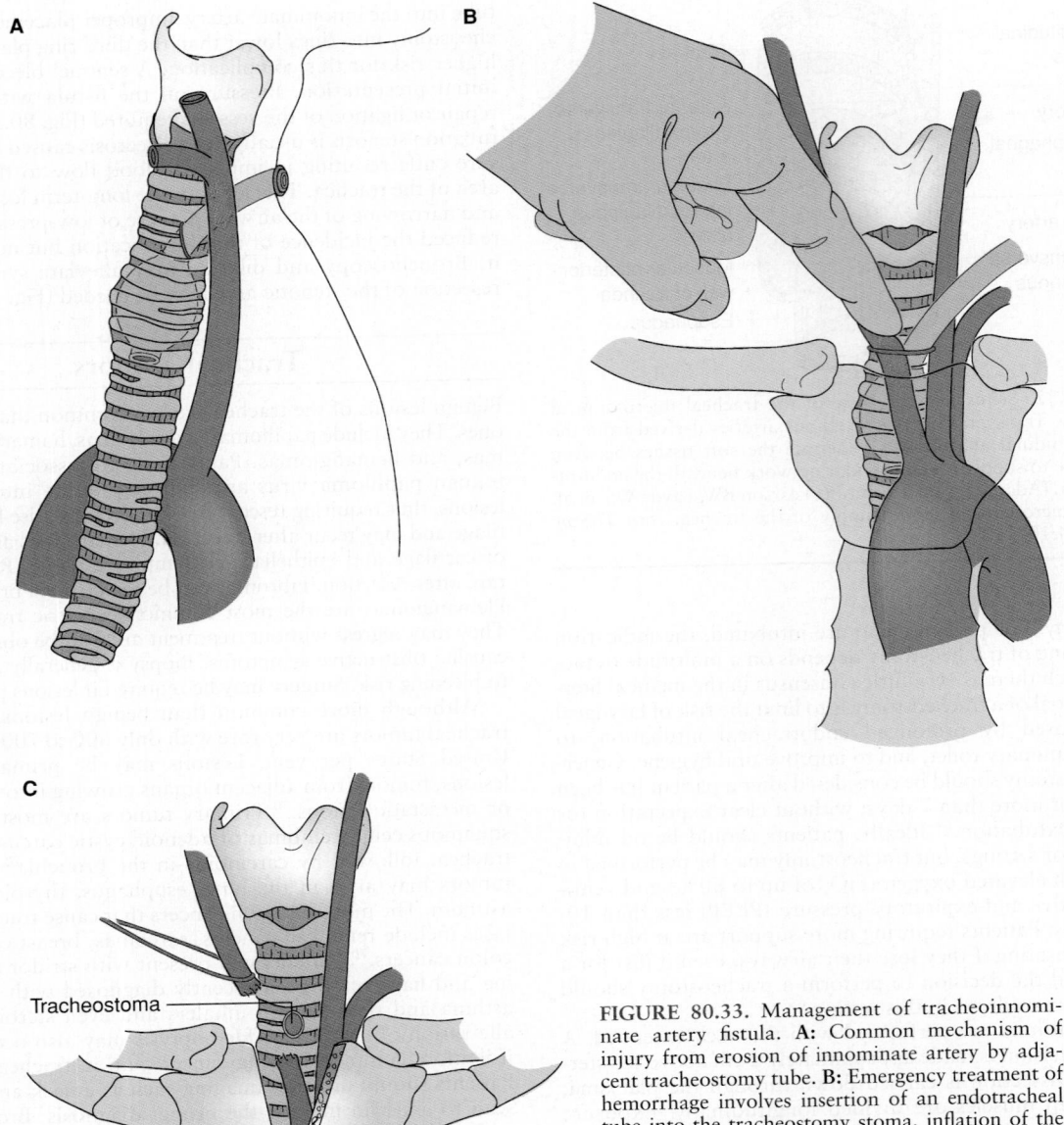

FIGURE 80.33. Management of tracheoinnominate artery fistula. **A:** Common mechanism of injury from erosion of innominate artery by adjacent tracheostomy tube. **B:** Emergency treatment of hemorrhage involves insertion of an endotracheal tube into the tracheostomy stoma, inflation of the cuff, and downward and outward pressure on the fistula by the finger inserted through the tracheostomy incision to further tamponade the bleeding. **C:** Through a partial upper sternal split, the segment of involved innominate artery is resected and the oversewn ends covered with adjacent mediastinal fat or muscle. Tracheal resection is usually not necessary. A new tracheostomy tube may have to be inserted higher in the trachea or, if possible, the tracheostomy tube removed and the stoma covered with a sternohyoid muscle flap.

include resection for localized involvement, tracheoplasty, or stenting.[72,73] Airway stents can be divided into two groups, silicone and metal, with each type having distinct advantages (Table 80.8). Silicone stents require rigid bronchoscopy to place, have a narrower inner lumen, and are more easily displaced. Advantages to the use of silicone stents are that they are easily adjustable or removable, they do not develop tissue ingrowth, and they are nonreactive to the endoluminal lining. Metal stents can be placed by flexible bronchoscopy and conform to the trachea better. They are permanent and difficult to adjust. Placement requires fluoroscopy, and granulation tissue often grows in between metal struts making subsequent removal difficult.[70] Newer stents being developed include covered metal stents that prevent tumor ingrowth along the stent, but unfortunately still allow granulation tissue to grow in at the ends.[74] In addition to being useful in the setting of tracheal stenosis, they can also play an essential role in palliating post-transplant bronchial stenosis.[75]

MEDIASTINUM

The mediastinum contains several important structures and may be involved in different disease processes. Mediastinal

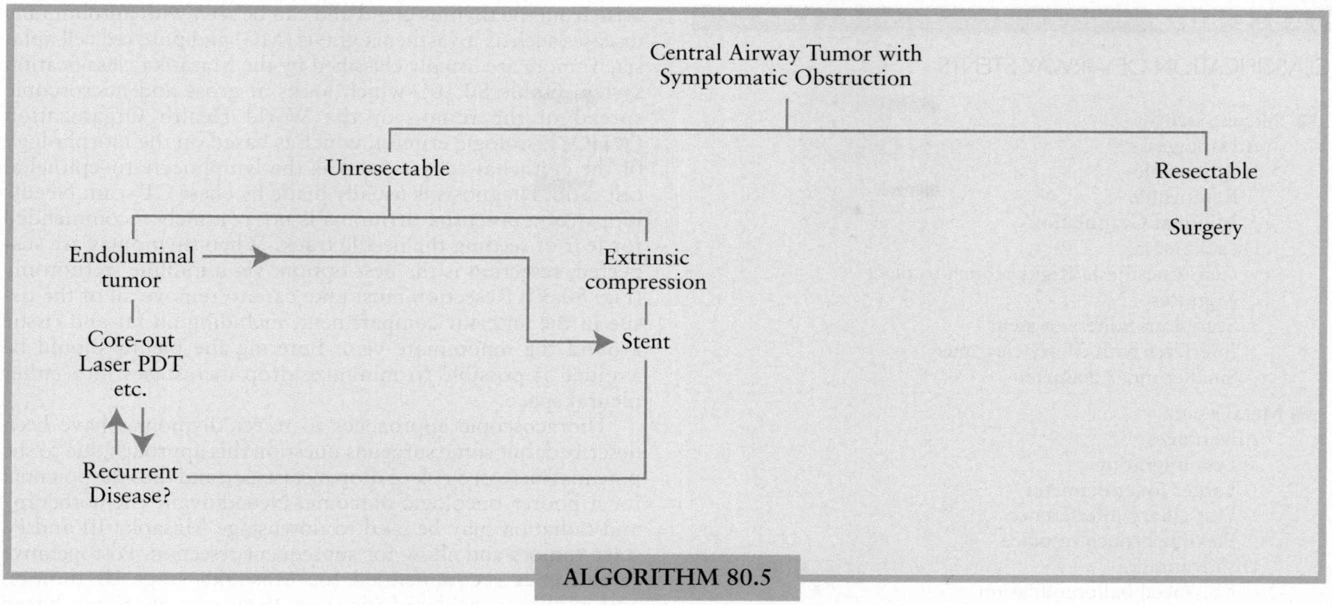

ALGORITHM 80.5. Algorithm for management of tracheal masses. (Adapted from Wood DE. *Surg Clin North Am* 2002;82(3):621–642).

infections are not as common as they were in the past, but when they present, they are life-threatening situations. The mediastinum is divided into several compartments, including the superior, anterior, middle, and posterior regions. Sometimes the lower three compartments are extended superiorly and only three are described (Fig. 80.35). The anterior mediastinum includes the fat and lymph nodes posterior to the sternum but anterior to the pericardium. The middle compartment includes the pericardium, heart, aorta, and trachea. The posterior compartment includes the esophagus, sympathetic chain, and vertebral column (Fig. 80.36). Most lesions are found in asymptomatic patients, but presenting symptoms include dyspnea and chest pain. Symptoms may be local, related to compression on mediastinal structures, or systemic, caused by the release of cytokines or inflammatory factors, such as in lymphomas or thymomas with myasthenia gravis. Imaging begins with plain radiographs, but CT scans are essential. MRI scans may be helpful to evaluate

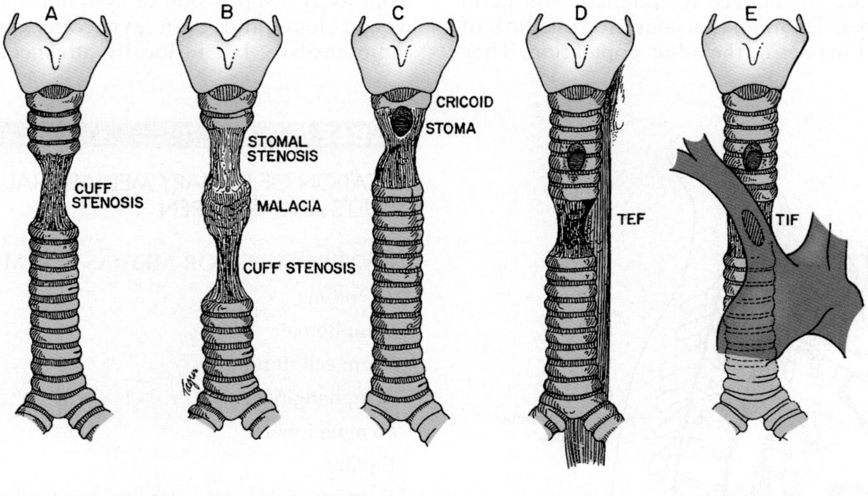

FIGURE 80.34. Diagrams of principal postintubation tracheal lesions. **A:** Cuff stenosis from the cuff of an endotracheal tube. **B:** Cuff stenosis from the cuff of a tracheostomy tube, usually lower in the trachea than that from an endotracheal tube. Stomal stenosis also occurs at the site of the tracheostomy itself. Malacia may occur either at the level of the cuff or in the segment between the stoma and the cuff stenosis. **C:** Cuff stenosis at the site of a high tracheostomy stoma, which has eroded into the lower margin of the cricoid cartilage. In older patients, this may erode back farther into the subglottic larynx, producing a laryngotracheal stenosis. A stoma placed in the cricothyroid membrane will, by definition, produce an intralaryngeal stenosis. **D:** Tracheoesophageal fistula (TEF) produced by pressure of the cuff against the "party wall," often abetted by an indwelling firm nasogastric tube. **E:** One type of tracheoinnominate fistula (TIF) as the result of a high-pressure cuff erosion. The more common type, but also rare, is that seen with a low-placed tracheostomy stoma, which rests against the innominate artery itself. (Reproduced with permission from Grillo HC. Surgical treatment of postintubation tracheal injuries. *J Thorac Cardiovasc Surg* 1979;78:860–875.)

TABLE 80.8

CLASSIFICATION OF AIRWAY STENTS

- Silicone stents
  - Advantages
    - Adjustable
    - Removable
    - Minimal Granulation
  - Disadvantages
    - Gen. Anesthesia/Rigid bronch to place
    - Migrates
    - Secretions adhere to stent
    - Interferes with ciliary clearance
    - Smaller inner diameter
- Metal stents
  - Advantages
    - Less migration
    - Larger inner diameter
    - Less ciliary interference
    - Flexible bronch to place
  - Disadvantages
    - May need balloon dilation
    - Difficult to remove
    - Granulation and tumor ingrowth in the stent
    - Radial force may lead to necrosis/fistula

vascular or spinal involvement. PET scans are increasingly used as they may further aid in staging. Biopsy and/or surgical resection is required to confirm the diagnosis in almost all patients.[76]

Anterior Mediastinum

The anterior mediastinum can contain various tumors (Table 80.9). Most common are thymomas, lymphomas, and germ cell tumors, in that order. Thymomas account for one fifth of all anterior mediastinal masses in the adult population. They arise from the thymus gland and can be seen with autoimmune diseases such as myasthenia gravis (MG) and pure red cell aplasia. Tumors are usually classified by the Masaoka classification system (Table 80.10), which looks at gross and microscopic spread of the tumor, or the World Health Organization (WHO) histologic criteria, which is based on the morphology of the epithelial cells as well as the lymphocyte-to–epithelial cell ratio. Diagnosis is usually made by chest CT scan. Needle biopsy of a potential thymoma is not routinely recommended for fear of seeding the needle track. When thymomas are suspected, resection is the best option, via a midline sternotomy (Fig. 80.37) Resection must take care to remove all of the tissue in the anterior compartment, including all fat and tissue around the innominate vein. Entering the pleura should be avoided if possible to minimize drop metastases into either pleural space.

Thoracoscopic approaches to resect thymomas have been described, but some surgeons question this approach due to the potential increased risk of drop metastases, and thus the potential for a poorer oncologic outcome. Neoadjuvant chemotherapy and radiation may be used to downstage Masaoka III and IV stage tumors and allow for subsequent resection. Postoperative radiation is recommended for Masoaka stage III tumors, and may be considered for stage II disease. Platinum-based chemotherapy is typically used in the unresectable setting.[77] Patients with MG present with diplopia, ptosis, fatigue, and weakness. One-third to one half of patients with thymomas have MG, but only 10% of patients with MG have thymomas. Anti–acetylcholine receptor antibody levels may be measured to evaluate for MG in patients with suspected thymomas.[78] Thymic carcinomas and thymic carcinoids are other tumor types that can also arise from the thymus.

Germ cell tumors can present as benign teratomas, seminomas, and embryonal tumors, which include nonseminomatous germ cell tumors and malignant teratomas. Benign teratomas have a good prognosis, and resection is the best treatment. Seminomas constitute up to half of mediastinal germ cell malignant tumors. Patients may have symptoms from local compression or systemic symptoms such as fever, weight loss, and even gynecomastia. These tumors are radiosensitive, but in locally advanced disease, chemother-

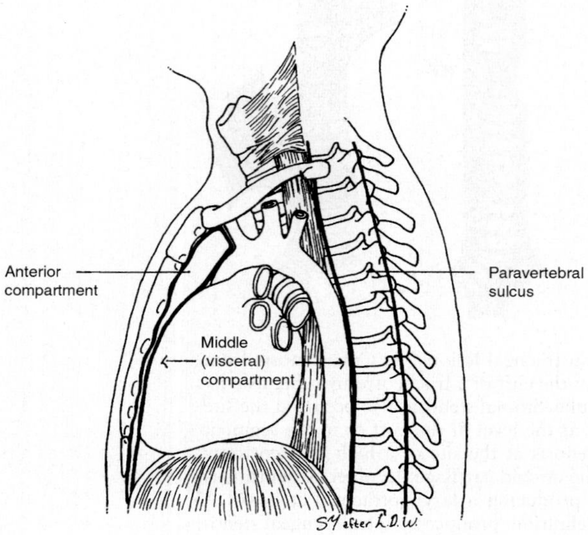

FIGURE 80.35. The mediastinal subdivisions. Note that the paravertebral sulcus encompasses the posterior compartment. (Reproduced with permission from Shields TW, ed. *General Thoracic Surgery*, 6th ed. 2005:Fig. 154–1.)

TABLE 80.9

LOCATION OF PRIMARY MEDIASTINAL MASSES IN ADULTS AND CHILDREN

ANTEROSUPERIOR MEDIASTINUM
Thymoma
Lymphoma
Germ cell tumor
Lymphangioma
Hemangioma
Lipoma
Carcinoma
Thyroid adenoma
Parathyroid adenoma
MIDDLE MEDIASTINUM
Pericardial cyst
Bronchogenic cyst
Lymphoma
POSTERIOR MEDIASTINUM
Neurogenic tumor
Enteric cyst

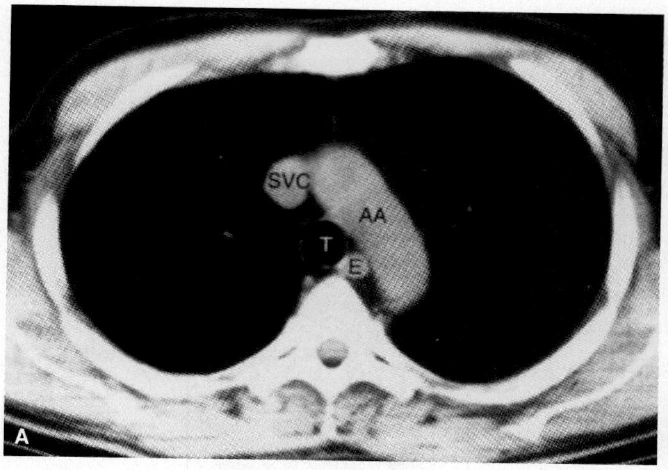

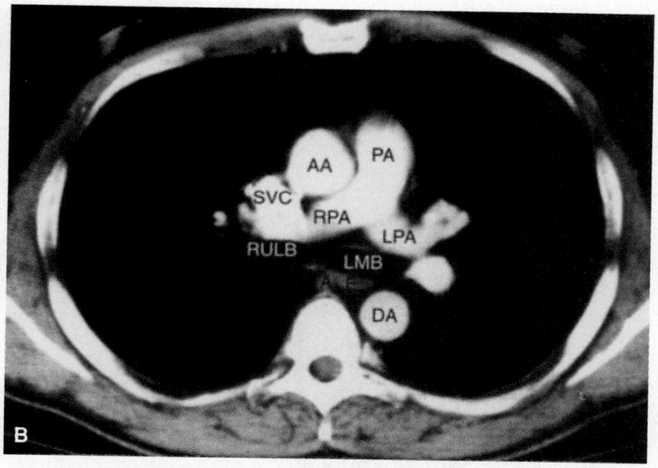

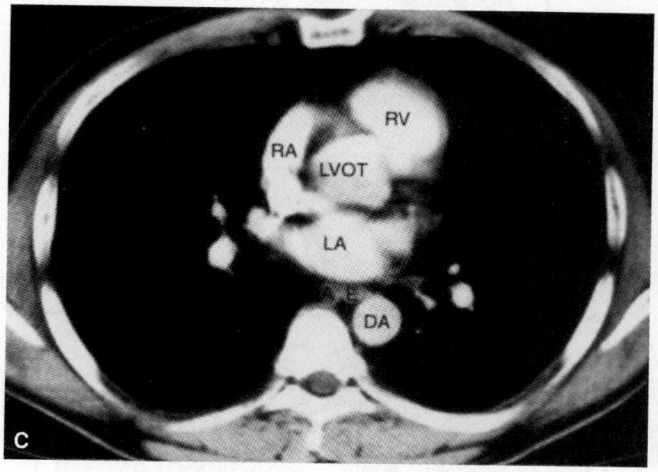

FIGURE 80.36. Normal mediastinal anatomy as shown with computed tomography scans. **A:** Scan at level of the aortic arch and midtrachea. T, trachea; E, esophagus; AA, aortic arch; SVC, superior vena cava. **B:** Scan at level of carina. RULB, right upper-lobe bronchus; LMB, left mainstem bronchus; AA, ascending aorta; DA, descending aorta; A, azygos vein; E, esophagus; SVC, superior vena cava; PA, main pulmonary artery; LPA and RPA, left and right pulmonary arteries. **C:** Scan at the level of the left atrium. LA, left atrium; RA, right atrium; LVOT, left ventricular outflow tract; RV, right ventricle; A, azygos vein; E, esophagus; DA, descending aorta.

apy with later surgical resection is the favored treatment. Nonseminomatous tumors include a wide variety of histologic malignancies. They usually occur in young men and are often symptomatic (Fig. 80.38). Elevated alpha-fetal protein(AFP) and beta-human chorionic gonadotropin (β-hCG) levels are seen with these tumors and should be measured. Chemotherapy is the best treatment, but patients have a poorer prognosis when compared to those with seminomas. Lymphomas in the mediastinum are usually part of a wider spectrum of disease. Two thirds of cases are Hodgkin disease. Most patients present with symptoms of fevers, night sweats, and even weight loss. Treatment is always chemotherapy based, and surgery in the form of a biopsy is used only to help make the diagnosis.[78]

TABLE 80.10

MASAOKA STAGING SYSTEM FOR THYMOMA

■ STAGE	■ DEFINITION
I	Macroscopically, completely encapsulated; microscopically, no capsular invasion
IIA	Macroscopic invasion in surrounding fatty tissues or mediastinal pleura
IIB	Microscopic invasion into the capsule
III	Macroscopic invasion into a neighboring organ, such as pericardium, great vessels, or lung
IVA	Pleural or pericardial dissemination
IVB	Hematogenous or lymphogenous metastases

Adapted from Masaoka A, Monden Y, Nakahara K, et al. Follow-up study of thymomas with special references to their clinical stages. *Cancer* 1981;48:2485, with permission.

Middle and Posterior Mediastinum

Middle mediastinal masses include esophageal and bronchogenic cysts, pericardial cysts, lymphangiomas, and lymphomas (Fig. 80.39). For cystic lesions, surgical resection is the best treatment option. Posterior lesions include neurogenic tumors, which may be benign or malignant. Almost 95% of tumors come from the sympathetic chain or intercostal nerve rami. Up to two thirds of these tumors are benign nerve sheath tumors and are usually discovered incidentally. An MRI scan may be used to evaluate intraspinal extension.[78]

Pediatric Mediastinum

The presentation of mediastinal masses in the pediatric population varies from what is observed in adults. The rate of malignancy is slightly lower in children, and while thymomas are the most common adult masses seen, neurogenic tumors are more common in children (Table 80.11). Just over half of all mediastinal tumors arise in the posterior compartment.[79] Anterior masses may include the normal thymus in a young

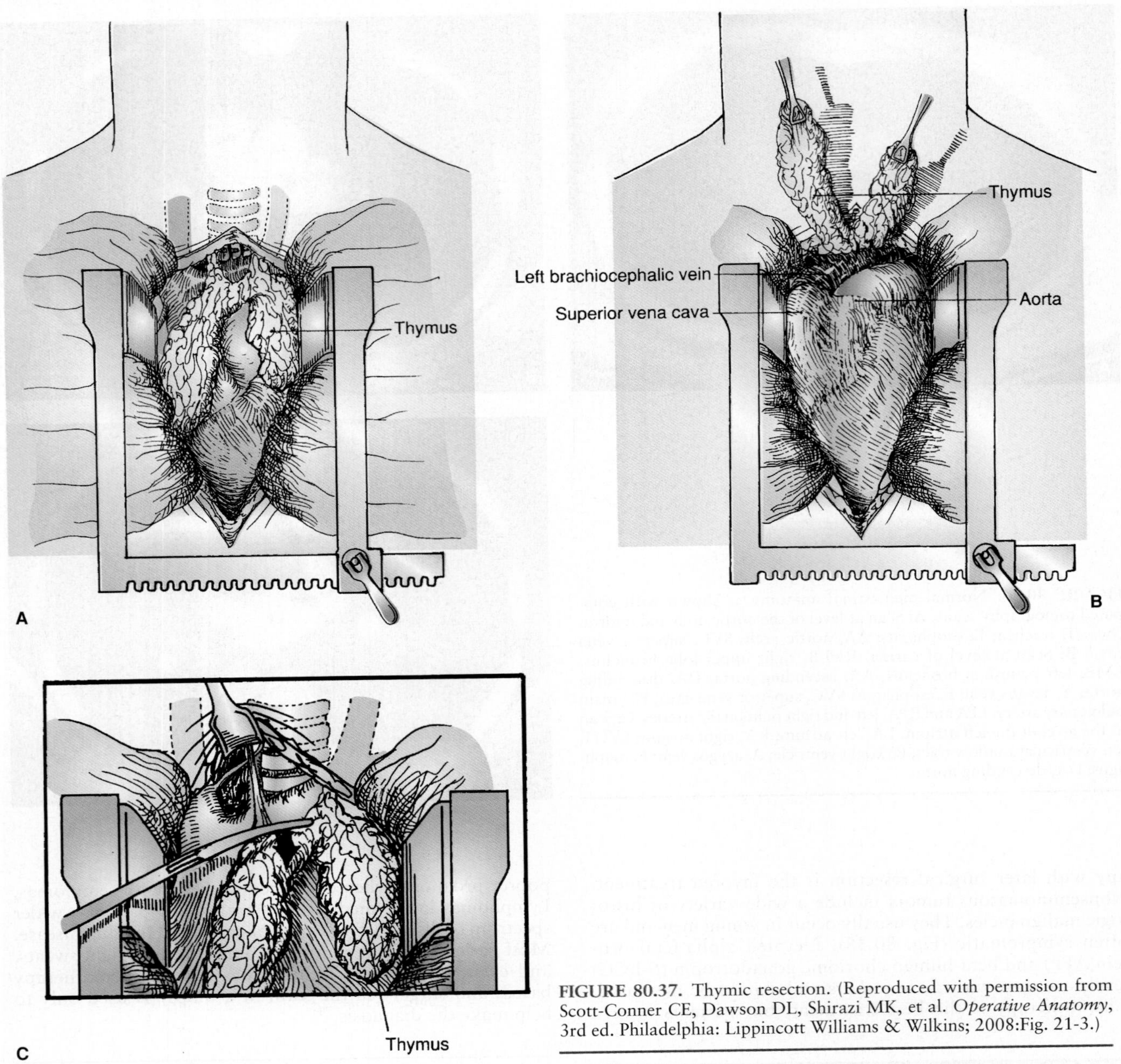

FIGURE 80.37. Thymic resection. (Reproduced with permission from Scott-Conner CE, Dawson DL, Shirazi MK, et al. *Operative Anatomy*, 3rd ed. Philadelphia: Lippincott Williams & Wilkins; 2008:Fig. 21-3.)

TABLE 80.11

MEDIASTINAL TUMORS IN CHILDREN

■ TYPE OF TUMOR	■ INCIDENCE REPORTED IN SERIES (%)
Neurogenic	35
Lymphoma	25
Germ cell	11
Primary malignancy	2
Cysts	25

From Davis RD Jr, Oldham HN Jr, Sabiston DC Jr. The mediastinum. In: Sabiston DC Jr, Spencer FC, eds. *Surgery of the Chest*, 5th ed. Philadelphia: WB Saunders; 1990:507.

child. Teratomas are the most common germ cell tumor seen.[79] Vascular anomalies may be seen in children and include hemangiomas and cystic hygromas.[80] Middle compartment tumors are usually foregut cysts, as in the adult population. Posterior tumors are most often malignant neurogenic tumors, compared to more benign pathology in adults.[79]

Mediastinitis

9 Mediastinal inflammation can arise from different sources, but it is most often infectious in nature. Acute mediastinitis is life threatening and usually results from a perforated esophagus, postcardiac procedure, or trauma. Oral infections can also result in organisms traveling through the neck into the mediastinum along fascial planes. These infections can travel as quickly as necrotizing fasciitis in other parts of the body. A wide variety of organisms can cause mediastinitis. Patients will have

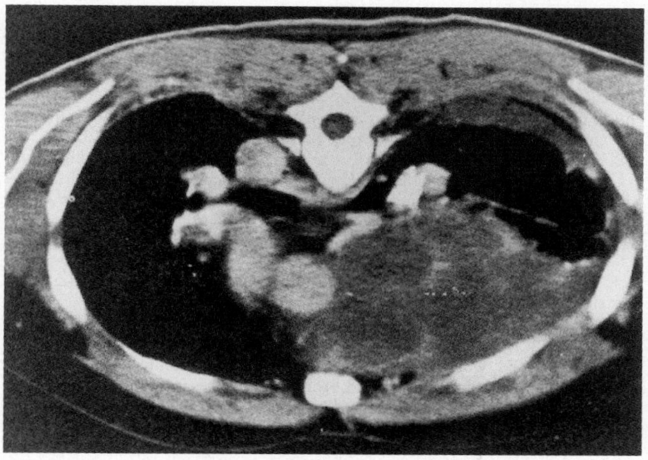

FIGURE 80.38. Computed tomography scan of a malignant nonseminomatous germ cell tumor of the anterior mediastinum reveals the inhomogeneous anterior mediastinal mass in contrast to the homogeneous density of a seminoma. Pleural effusion is also demonstrated in the right hemithorax. (Reproduced with permission from Shields TW. Primary lesions of the mediastinum and their investigation and treatment. In: Shields TW, ed. *General Thoracic Surgery*. Baltimore: Williams & Wilkins; 1994:1724–1769.)

chest pain, dyspnea, and fevers. Radiographic films may show pneumomediastinum or pneumothoraces. If an esophageal perforation is suspected, an esophagogram should be performed. Treatment is broad-spectrum antibiotics and surgical drainage via a cervical incision and/or thoracotomy. Quick débridement and drainage are key to patient survival. Minimally invasive approaches to the chest may be adequate, but surgeons should have a low threshold to perform a posterolateral thoracotomy, which may give the best exposure and opportunity to débride the chest. Sternal infections after cardiac surgery can also be a serious problem requiring drainage and débridement. Ultimate repair of the defect following débridement may involve muscle or omental flaps for sternal reconstruction.

Chronic mediastinitis is a separate entity from acute mediastinitis and may arise from infectious sources or autoimmune disorders. Patients may be asymptomatic until a mass effect is seen on their mediastinal organs. CT scans are the best imaging modality to diagnose this condition, and surgery is reserved only for diagnosis or in the end stages of the disease to relieve compression on other organs. Sclerosing mediastinitis may be seen in patients with retroperitoneal fibrosis.[81]

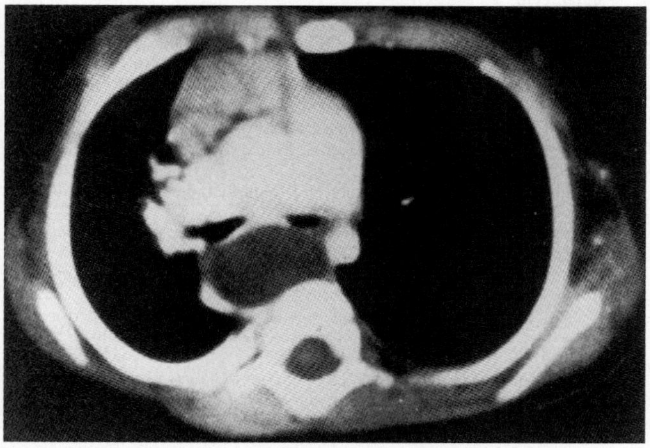

FIGURE 80.39. Computed tomography scan reveals a bronchogenic cyst located in the subcranial area with compression of the left mainstem bronchus with hyperinflation of the left lung and a mediastinal shift to the right. (Reproduced with permission from Shields TW. Primary lesions of the mediastinum and their investigation and treatment. In: Shields TW, ed. *General Thoracic Surgery*. Baltimore: Williams & Wilkins; 1994:1764–1769).

Superior Vena Cava (SVC) Syndrome

Superior vena cava syndrome is a rare condition seen when a mediastinal mass compresses the SVC, resulting in facial and upper body edema. Only 15,000 cases per year are seen in the United States. Patients may present with cough, dyspnea, or even stridor from upper airway edema. When patients start to have symptoms, collateral venous drainage develops to drain into the azygos vein or inferior vena cava. This process usually takes weeks. Malignant tumors are the most common cause, but venous thrombosis and nonmalignant lesions cause up to one third of cases. CT scans are the best diagnostic test. Treatment is based on supportive care and addressing the underlying condition causing the obstruction. If a malignant tumor is causing the obstruction, chemotherapy or radiotherapy may shrink the tumor and lessen symptoms. Surgical resection with SVC reconstruction may be used in specific tumors such as locally advanced thymomas. Angioplasty and stenting may be of benefit but is usually palliative.[82] Although it is often felt to be an emergency, most cases of SVC syndrome have a slowly progressive course. When a patient develops symptoms, supportive care, including possible intubation, will allow time for collateral venous drainage to develop and symptoms to improve without other interventions. Although the median survival is typically 6 months or less in patients with SVC syndrome from malignant obstruction, some have seen long-term survivors when the primary tumors have responded to appropriate treatment.[83] When patients present with severe symptoms, it is a mistake to rush to surgical intervention without a long-term plan. Symptoms should be managed and the etiology discovered and treated appropriately.

References

1. Incarbone M, Pastorino U. Surgical treatment of chest wall tumors. *World J Surg* 2001;25(2):218–230.
2. Gross JL, Younes RN, Haddad FJ, et al. Soft-tissue sarcomas of the chest wall: prognostic factors. *Chest* 2005;127(3):902–908.
3. Pairolero PC. Chest wall tumors. In: Sellke FW, del Nido PJ, Swanson SJ, eds. *Sabiston and Spencer: Surgery of the Chest*, 7th ed. Philadelphia: Elsevier Saunders; 2005:395.
4. Anderson BO, Burt ME. Chest wall neoplasms and their management. *Ann Thorac Surg* 1994;58(6):1774–1781.
5. Douglas YL, Meuzelaar KL, van der Lei B, et al. Osteosarcoma of the sternum. *Eur J Surg Oncol* 1997;23(1):90.
6. Gladish G, Sabloff B, Munden R, et al. Primary thoracic sarcomas. *Radiographics* 2002;22(3):621.
7. Deschamps C, Tirnaksiz BM, Darbandi R, et al. Early and long-term results of prosthetic chest wall reconstruction. *J Thorac Cardiovasc Surg* 1999;117(3):588–591; discussion 591–592.
8. Graeber GM. Chest wall resection and reconstruction. *Semin Thorac Cardiovasc Surg* 1999;11(3):251–263.
9. Weyant MJ, Bains MS, Venkatraman E, et al. Results of chest wall resection and reconstruction with and without rigid prosthesis. *Ann Thorac Surg* 2006;81(1):279–285.
10. Chang RR, Mehrara BJ, Hu QY, et al. Reconstruction of complex oncologic chest wall defects: a 10-year experience. *Ann Plast Surg* 2004;52(5):471–479; discussion 479.
11. Skoracki RJ, Chang DW. Reconstruction of the chest wall and thorax. *J Surg Oncol* 2006;94(6):455–465.
12. Acarturk T, Swartz W, Luketich J, et al. Laparoscopically harvested omental flap for chest wall and intrathoracic reconstruction. *Ann Plast Surg* 2004;53(3):210.
13. Lopushinsky SR, Fecteau AH. Pectus deformities: a review of open surgery in the modern era. *Semin Pediatr Surg* 2008;17(3):201–208.
14. Fonkalsrud EW, Dunn JC, Atkinson JB. Repair of pectus excavatum deformities: 30 years of experience with 375 patients. *Ann Surg* 2000;231(3):443–448.

15. Kelly RE Jr. Pectus excavatum: historical background, clinical picture, preoperative evaluation and criteria for operation. *Semin Pediatr Surg* 2008; 17(3):181–193.
16. Mansour KA, Thourani VH, Odessey EA, et al. Thirty-year experience with repair of pectus deformities in adults. *Ann Thorac Surg* 2003;76(2): 391–5; discussion 395.
17. Jaroszewski DE, Fonkalsrud EW. Repair of pectus chest deformities in 320 adult patients: 21 year experience. *Ann Thorac Surg* 2007;84(2):429–433.
18. Nuss D. Minimally invasive surgical repair of pectus excavatum. *Semin Pediatr Surg* 2008;17(3):209–217.
19. Park HJ, Lee SY, Lee CS, et al. The Nuss procedure for pectus excavatum: evolution of techniques and early results on 322 patients. *Ann Thorac Surg* 2004;77(1):289–295.
20. Engum SA. Embryology, sternal clefts, ectopia cordis, and Cantrell's pentalogy. *Semin Pediatr Surg* 2008;17(3):154–160.
21. Moir CR, Johnson CH. Poland's syndrome. *Semin Pediatr Surg* 2008; 17(3):161–166.
22. Mackinnon SE, Novak CB. Thoracic outlet syndrome. *Curr Probl Surg* 2002;39(11):1070–1145.
23. Thompson RW, Petrinec D. Surgical treatment of thoracic outlet compression syndromes: diagnostic considerations and transaxillary first rib resection. *Ann Vasc Surg* 1997;11(3):315–323.
24. Maxey TS, Reece TB, Ellman PI, et al. Safety and efficacy of the supraclavicular approach to thoracic outlet decompression. *Ann Thorac Surg* 2003;76(2):396–399; discussion 399–400.
25. Thompson RW, Petrinec D, Toursarkissian B. Surgical treatment of thoracic outlet compression syndromes: II. Supraclavicular exploration and vascular reconstruction. *Ann Vasc Surg* 1997;11(4):442–451.
26. Divi V, Proctor MC, Axelrod DA, et al. Thoracic outlet decompression for subclavian vein thrombosis: experience in 71 patients. *Arch Surg* 2005; 140(1):54–57.
27. Mansharamani NG, Koziel H. Chronic lung sepsis: lung abscess, bronchiectasis, and empyema. *Curr Opin Pulm Med* 2003;9(3):181–185.
28. O'Donnell AE. Bronchiectasis. *Chest* 2008;134(4):815–823.
29. Barker AF. Bronchiectasis. *N Engl J Med* 2002;346(18):1383–1393.
30. Ilowite J, Spiegler P, Chawla S. Bronchiectasis: new findings in the pathogenesis and treatment of this disease. *Curr Opin Infect Dis* 2008;21(2): 163–167.
31. Naidoo R. Surgery for pulmonary tuberculosis. *Curr Opin Pulm Med* 2008;14(3):254–259.
32. Souilamas R, Riquet M, Barthes FP, et al. Surgical treatment of active and sequelar forms of pulmonary tuberculosis. *Ann Thorac Surg* 2001;71(2): 443–447.
33. Cahill BC, Ingbar DH. Massive hemoptysis. assessment and management. *Clin Chest Med* 1994;15(1):147–167.
34. Jean-Baptiste E. Clinical assessment and management of massive hemoptysis. *Crit Care Med* 2000;28(5):1642–1647.
35. Shigemura N, Wan IY, Yu SC, et al. Multidisciplinary management of life-threatening massive hemoptysis: a 10-year experience. *Ann Thorac Surg* 2009;87(3):849–853.
36. Edwards M, Hazelrigg S, Naunheim K. The national emphysema treatment trial: summary and update. *Thorac Surg Clin* 2009;19(2):169.
37. Martinez FJ, Chang A. Surgical therapy for chronic obstructive pulmonary disease. *Semin Respir Crit Care Med* 2005;26(2):167–191.
38. Shah AA, D'Amico TA. Lung volume reduction surgery for the management of refractory dyspnea in chronic obstructive pulmonary disease. *Curr Opin Support Palliat Care* 2009;3(2):107–111.
39. Trow TK. Lung-volume reduction surgery for severe emphysema: appraisal of its current status. *Curr Opin Pulm Med* 2004;10(2): 128–132.
40. Swanson KL, Edell ES. Tracheobronchial foreign bodies. *Chest Surg Clin N Am* 2001;11(4):861–872.
41. Boyd M, Chatterjee A, Chiles C, et al. Tracheobronchial foreign body aspiration in adults. *South Med J* 2009;102(2):171–174.
42. Sahn SA, Heffner JE. Spontaneous pneumothorax. *N Engl J Med* 2000; 342(12):868–874.
43. Rahman NM, Davies RJ, Gleeson FV. Pleural interventions: management of acute and chronic pneumothorax. *Semin Respir Crit Care Med* 2008; 29(4):427–440.
44. Baumann MH, Noppen M. Pneumothorax. *Respirology* 2004;9(2): 157–164.
45. Shen KR, Cerfolio R. Decision making in the management of secondary spontaneous pneumothorax in patients with severe emphysema. *Thorac Surg Clin* 2009;19(2):233.
46. Mendeloff EN. Sequestrations, congenital cystic adenomatoid malformations, and congenital lobar emphysema. *Semin Thorac Cardiovasc Surg* 2004;16(3):209–214.
47. Horak E, Bodner J, Gassner I, et al. Congenital cystic lung disease: diagnostic and therapeutic considerations. *Clin Pediatr (Phila)* 2003;42(3): 251–261.
48. Schwartz DS, Reyes-Mugica M, Keller MS. Imaging of surgical diseases of the newborn chest. Intrapleural mass lesions. *Radiol Clin North Am* 1999; 37(6):1067–1078, v.
49. Evrard V, Ceulemans J, Coosemans W, et al. Congenital parenchymatous malformations of the lung. *World J Surg* 1999;23(11):1123–1132.
50. Takeda S, Miyoshi S, Inoue M, et al. Clinical spectrum of congenital cystic disease of the lung in children. *Eur J Cardiothorac Surg* 1999;15(1): 11–17.
51. Heffner J. Discriminating between transudates and exudates. *Clin Chest Med* 2006;27(2):241.
52. Light RW. The undiagnosed pleural effusion. *Clin Chest Med* 2006;27(2): 309–319.
53. Putnam J Jr. Malignant pleural effusions. *Surg Clin North Am* 2002;82(4): 867.
54. de Hoyos A, Sundaresan S. Thoracic empyema. *Surg Clin North Am* 2002;82(3):643–671, viii.
55. Wright CD, Wain JC, Mathisen DJ, et al. Postpneumonectomy bronchopleural fistula after sutured bronchial closure: incidence, risk factors, and management. *J Thorac Cardiovasc Surg*1996;112(5):1367–1371.
56. Deschamps C, Bernard A, Nichols FC III, et al. Empyema and bronchopleural fistula after pneumonectomy: factors affecting incidence. *Ann Thorac Surg* 2001;72(1):243–247; discussion 248.
57. Vallieres E. Management of empyema after lung resections (pneumonectomy/lobectomy). *Chest Surg Clin N Am* 2002;12(3):571–585.
58. Robinson BW, Musk AW, Lake RA. Malignant mesothelioma. *Lancet* 2005;366(9483):397–408.
59. Robinson BW, Lake RA. Advances in malignant mesothelioma. *N Engl J Med* 2005;353(15):1591–1603.
60. Pistolesi M, Rusthoven J. Malignant pleural mesothelioma: update, current management, and newer therapeutic strategies. *Chest* 2004;126(4): 1318–1329.
61. Singhal S, Kaiser LR. Malignant mesothelioma: options for management. *Surg Clin North Am* 2002;82(4):797–831.
62. van Ruth S, Baas P, Zoetmulder FA. Surgical treatment of malignant pleural mesothelioma: a review. *Chest* 2003;123(2):551–561.
63. Minnich D, Mathisen D. Anatomy of the trachea, carina, and bronchi. *Thorac Surg Clin* 2007;17(4):571.
64. Walts PA, Murthy SC, DeCamp MM. Techniques of surgical tracheostomy. *Clin Chest Med* 2003;24(3):413–422.
65. Angel L, Simpson C. Comparison of surgical and percutaneous dilational tracheostomy. *Clin Chest Med* 2003;24(3):423.
66. Wain JC. Postintubation tracheal stenosis. *Chest Surg Clin N Am* 2003; 13(2):231–246.
67. Fellerkopman D. Acute complications of artificial airways. *Clin Chest Med* 2003;24(3):445.
68. Mathisen DJ. Surgery of the trachea. *Curr Probl Surg* 1998;35(6):453.
69. Mathisen DJ. Tracheal tumors. *Chest Surg Clin N Am* 1996;6(4):875.
70. Wood DE. Management of malignant tracheobronchial obstruction. *Surg Clin North Am* 2002;82(3):621–642.
71. Gaissert H. Primary tracheal tumors. *Chest Surg Clin N Am* 2003;13(2):247.
72. Wright CD. Tracheomalacia. *Chest Surg Clin N Am* 2003;13(2):349–357, viii.
73. Jaquiss RD. Management of pediatric tracheal stenosis and tracheomalacia. *Semin Thorac Cardiovasc Surg* 2004;16(3):220–224.
74. Chin CS, Litle V, Yun J, et al. Airway stents. *Ann Thorac Surg* 2008;85(2): S792–S796.
75. Mulligan MS. Endoscopic management of airway complications after lung transplantation. *Chest Surg Clin N Am* 2001;11(4):907–915.
76. Date H. Diagnostic strategies for mediastinal tumors and cysts. *Thorac Surg Clin* 2009;19(1):29–35, vi.
77. Tomaszek S, Wigle DA, Keshavjee S, et al. Thymomas: review of current clinical practice. *Ann Thorac Surg* 2009;87(6):1973–1980.
78. Duwe BV, Sterman DH, Musani AI. Tumors of the mediastinum. *Chest* 2005;128(4):2893–2909.
79. Wright CD. Mediastinal tumors and cysts in the pediatric population. *Thorac Surg Clin* 2009;19(1):47–61, vi.
80. Jaggers J, Balsara K. Mediastinal masses in children. *Semin Thorac Cardiovasc Surg* 2004;16(3):201–208.
81. Athanassiadi KA. Infections of the mediastinum. *Thorac Surg Clin* 2009; 19(1):37–45, vi.
82. Wilson LD, Detterbeck FC, Yahalom J. Clinical practice. Superior vena cava syndrome with malignant causes. *N Engl J Med* 2007;356(18): 1862–1869.
83. Yu JB, Wilson LD, Detterbeck FC. Superior vena cava syndrome—a proposed classification system and algorithm for management. *J Thorac Oncol* 2008;3(8):811–814.

CHAPTER 81 CONGENITAL HEART DISEASE

JENNIFER C. HIRSCH, ERIC J. DEVANEY, RICHARD G. OHYE, AND EDWARD L. BOVE

KEY POINTS

1. The first successful treatment of a congenital lesion was the closure of a patent ductus arteriosus (PDA) by Gross and Hubbard in 1938. Prostaglandin inhibitors, such as indomethacin and ibuprofen, can be used to induce closure of a PDA in the premature newborn with a success rate of 80%. When this is not successful, surgical closure may be necessary in small infants. Coil occlusion can be performed in older children presenting with a PDA.
2. An atrial septal defect (ASD) is a hole in the atrial septum. ASDs are the third most common congenital heart defect, occurring in 1 out of 1,000 live births and representing 10% of congenital heart defects. ASDs cause right heart volume overload and can lead to pulmonary vascular obstructive disease later in life. The majority of ASDs are now closed with a device in the catheterization laboratory.
3. Ventricular septal defects (VSDs) are the most common congenital heart defect (with the exception of bicuspid aortic valve, which occurs in about 1.3% of the population). VSDs cause left heart volume overload.
4. Over 50% of children with trisomy 21 have a congenital heart defect. The most common heart defect in this patient population is an atrioventricular septal defect. All infants with trisomy 21 should have an echocardiogram to rule out congenital heart disease.
5. Tetralogy of Fallot (TOF) is the most common cyanotic congenital heart defect. It occurs in 0.6 per 1,000 live births and has a prevalence of about 5% among all patients with congenital heart disease. The pathologic anatomy is frequently described as having four components: ventricular septal defect, overriding aorta, pulmonary stenosis, and right ventricular hypertrophy.
6. Transposition of the great arteries is a congenital cardiac anomaly in which the aorta arises from the right ventricle and the pulmonary artery originates from the left ventricle (ventriculoarterial discordance). It is the most common congenital heart defect presenting with cyanosis in the first week of life. This malformation accounts for approximately 10% of all congenital cardiovascular malformations in infants.
7. Upper extremity hypertension with diminished femoral pulses are hallmark clinical findings in patients with aortic coarctation.
8. Coronary arteriovenous fistula is the most common major coronary anomaly.

HISTORY

Cardiac surgery, as a specialty, is notable for the rapid technical advances that have been made during the past few decades. Much of the original interest was focused on attempts to treat congenital heart defects associated with cyanosis and early mortality. **1** The first successful treatment of a congenital lesion was the closure of a patent ductus arteriosus (PDA) by Gross and Hubbard in 1938.[1] The description of the subclavian artery–to–pulmonary artery (PA) shunt by Blalock and Taussig in 1945[2] introduced the palliation of many complex cyanotic lesions—most notably, tetralogy of Fallot (TOF). The 1950s represented the decade of greatest advances, which laid the foundation for the field of cardiac surgery. Lewis and Taufic in 1952[3] performed the first open closure of an atrial septal defect (ASD) by using surface hypothermia and inflow occlusion. In 1953, Gibbon[4] performed the first repair of an ASD with the use of a pump oxygenator that became the model for modern cardiopulmonary bypass. Next, Warden et al.[5] used controlled cross-circulation with an adult as the oxygenator during intracardiac repairs. Building on the work of Gibbon, Kirklin et al.[6] then published the first series of eight intracardiac operations performed at the Mayo Clinic with the use of cardiopulmonary bypass. With these landmark efforts focused on congenital heart disease, the field of cardiac surgery was established.

ATRIAL SEPTAL DEFECT

Cardiac septation occurs between the third and sixth weeks of fetal development. The septum primum, which arises from the roof of the common atrium and descends inferiorly, initially divides the common atrium. The ostium primum is the opening below the inferior edge of the septum primum, which is obliterated as the septum primum fuses with the endocardial cushions. The ostium secundum forms in the midportion of the septum primum prior to closure of the ostium primum. The septum secundum also arises from the roof of the atrium and descends along the right side of the septum primum and covers the ostium secundum. This creates a flap valve whereby blood from the inferior vena cava may preferentially stream beneath the edge of the septum secundum and through the ostium secundum into the left atrium. After birth, the increase in left atrial pressure usually closes this pathway.

2 An ASD is a hole in the atrial septum (Fig. 81.1). ASDs are the third most common congenital heart defect, occurring in 1 out of 1,000 live births and representing 10% of congenital heart defects.[7] The most common ASD is the secundum defect, which occurs when the ostium secundum is too large for complete coverage by the septum secundum. Ostium secundum defects account for about 80% of ASDs. An ostium primum ASD, representing 10% of ASDs, occurs from failure of fusion of the septum primum with the endocardial cushions. The ostium primum defect is discussed later in the section on atrioventricular septal defects (AVSDs). A third type of ASD is the sinus venosus defect, seen in about 10% of cases. Sinus venosus ASDs are caused by abnormal fusion of the venous pathways with the atrium and are characterized by defects high in the atrial septum near the orifice of the superior vena cava or, less commonly, low in the atrial septum near the inferior vena cava. Sinus venosus defects are frequently associated with partial anomalous pulmonary venous connection, usually with the right upper pulmonary vein draining into the superior vena

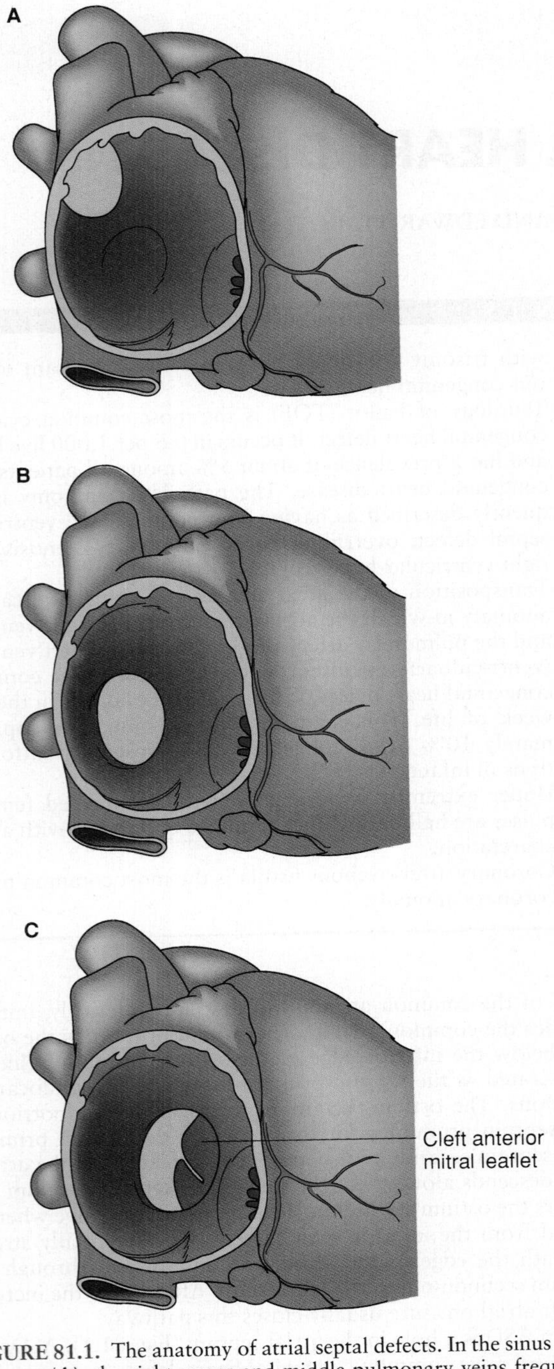

FIGURE 81.1. The anatomy of atrial septal defects. In the sinus venosus type (A), the right upper and middle pulmonary veins frequently drain to the superior vena cava or right atrium. B: Secundum defects generally occur as isolated lesions. C: Primum defects are part of a more complex lesion and are best considered as incomplete atrioventricular septal defects.

cava near the cavoatrial junction. The rarest type of ASD is the unroofed coronary sinus septal defect. This occurs when there is loss of the common wall between the coronary sinus and the left atrium adjacent to the atrial septum. This unroofing of the coronary sinus leads to a communication between the right and left atria at the site of the coronary sinus.

Failure of postnatal fusion of the septum secundum to the septum primum results in a persistent slitlike communication known as a patent foramen ovale (PFO). PFOs are extremely common in the general population, and autopsy studies have demonstrated a prevalence of 27%.[8] PFOs are generally considered separate from other ASDs due to the absence of significant shunting, but they remain important clinically due to the occurrence of paradoxical embolization. A paradoxical embolus is a blood clot arising from a systemic vein that would normally pass to the lungs, but in the presence of a septal defect, may instead cross into the systemic circulation.

ASDs lead to increased pulmonary blood flow (PBF) secondary to left-to-right shunting. Shunting at the atrial level is determined by the size of the defect and by the relative ventricular compliance (i.e., blood preferentially fills the more compliant ventricle). At birth, both chambers are equally compliant, but as pulmonary vascular resistance (PVR) falls, the right ventricle remodels and becomes more compliant. Shunting across the atrial septum causes a volume load on the right heart. A volume load is created by additional venous return to a chamber during diastole.

The volume overload from an ASD is usually well tolerated, and patients are frequently asymptomatic. Symptoms tend to develop when the ratio of pulmonary to systemic blood flow (Q_p/Q_s) exceeds two. The most common symptoms are fatigue, shortness of breath, exercise intolerance, and recurrent respiratory infections. Older patients with untreated ASDs tend to develop atrial dysrhythmias, and adults may develop congestive heart failure (CHF) and right ventricular dysfunction. Pulmonary vascular obstructive disease may occur rarely as a late complication of an untreated ASD. Paradoxical embolization is also an important potential complication of an ASD.

The classic physical findings in patients with ASDs include fixed splitting of the second heart sound and a systolic ejection murmur at the left upper sternal border due to relative pulmonary stenosis (PS) (increased flow across a normal pulmonary valve). A diastolic flow murmur across the tricuspid valve is occasionally audible. A prominent right ventricular lift and increased intensity of the pulmonary component of the second heart sound may occur with pulmonary hypertension. Chest radiography shows cardiomegaly, with enlargement of the right atrium, right ventricle, and pulmonary artery. Electrocardiography frequently demonstrates right axis deviation and an incomplete right bundle branch block. When right bundle branch block occurs with a leftward or superior axis, the diagnosis of AVSD should be considered. Echocardiography confirms the diagnosis of ASD and defines the anatomy. Cardiac catheterization is important in selected cases to assess PVR in older patients, but it is used more frequently with therapeutic intent for device closure of ASDs.

Due to the long-term complications associated with ASDs, repair is recommended for all patients with symptomatic defects and in asymptomatic patients in whom the Q_p/Q_s is greater than 1.5. Repair is usually performed in children prior to school age. Closure of ASDs may be performed surgically or using a device deployed in the cardiac catheterization laboratory.

Surgical repair is usually recommended for large secundum defects and for most other types of ASDs. The heart is exposed by median sternotomy. Other surgical approaches have been proposed, including minimally invasive techniques, but there are technical drawbacks associated with each of the alternative approaches. In most cases, a limited midline incision with a partial lower sternal split provides adequate exposure and a cosmetically acceptable scar. The heart is carefully inspected for anomalies of systemic and pulmonary venous return.

Cardiopulmonary bypass is required with cooling to between 32°C and 35°C. The superior and inferior vena cava are separately cannulated for venous drainage, and the arterial cannula is placed in the ascending aorta. Following aortic clamping and arrest of the heart with cardioplegia, the atrial septum is exposed through a right atriotomy. Small secundum defects or PFOs may sometimes be closed primarily by suturing the edge of the septum primum to the edge of the septum secundum. More commonly, larger defects are closed using a patch (polytetrafluoroethylene or autologous pericardium) and a running polypropylene suture. When anomalous pulmonary venous drainage is present, a baffle is created to redirect the flow across the ASD. In all cases, care is taken to de-air the left atrium to avoid the complication of air embolization. Surgical closure of an ASD can be accomplished with a mortality approaching zero and minimal morbidity.[9] Common postoperative complications include atrial arrhythmias and postpericardiotomy syndrome.

The first transcatheter device closure of an ASD was performed in 1976.[10] A number of devices are currently available for percutaneous closure of secundum ASDs.[11] The contemporary success rate for device deployment is 96% with complete closure at 24 hours of 99% or greater.[12,13] The presence of a deficient rim is the most common reason for failed implantation.[13] Device closure has the advantages of fewer complications and a shorter hospitalization. Device closure of small to moderate secundum ASDs and PFOs has now become the standard of care at most large centers. Surgical closure remains the procedure of choice for large or multiple defects, insufficient rims, sinus venous–type defects, and primum ASDs.

The long-term survival for patients undergoing ASD repair in childhood is normal.[14,15] The major long-term complication following surgical closure of ASD is the development of supraventricular arrhythmias, although the risk is lowered when the ASD is closed in childhood.[15,16] The persistence of this risk despite relief of right-sided volume overload is thought to be related to incomplete atrial remodeling or due to the presence of the atriotomy scar. Longer follow-up will be required to determine whether device closure alters the risk of atrial dysrhythmias.

Occasionally, adults will present with a newly diagnosed ASD. Many studies have confirmed that ASD closure in adults over the age of 40 increases survival and limits the development of heart failure.[17,18] When the Q_p/Q_s is less than 1.5 and the ratio of pulmonary to systemic vascular resistance (R_p/R_s) is greater than 0.7, significant pulmonary vascular obstructive disease is usually present. A PVR in excess of 10 to 12 Woods units/m^2 represents a contraindication to ASD closure.

VENTRICULAR SEPTAL DEFECT

Ventricular septation is a complex process that requires accurate development and alignment of a number of structures including the muscular interventricular septum, the atrioventricular (AV) septum (arising from the endocardial cushions), and the infundibular septum (which divides the outflow tracts of the right and left ventricles). The membranous septum is a fibrous portion of the ventricular septum that is adjacent to the central fibrous body (where the mitral, tricuspid, and aortic valve annuli make contact).

3 Ventricular septal defects (VSDs) are the most common congenital heart anomalies (with the exception of bicuspid aortic valve, which occurs in about 1.3% of the population). VSDs are present in about 4 of 1,000 live births and represent about 40% of congenital heart defects.[7] VSDs are classified based on their location in the ventricular septum (Fig. 81.2).

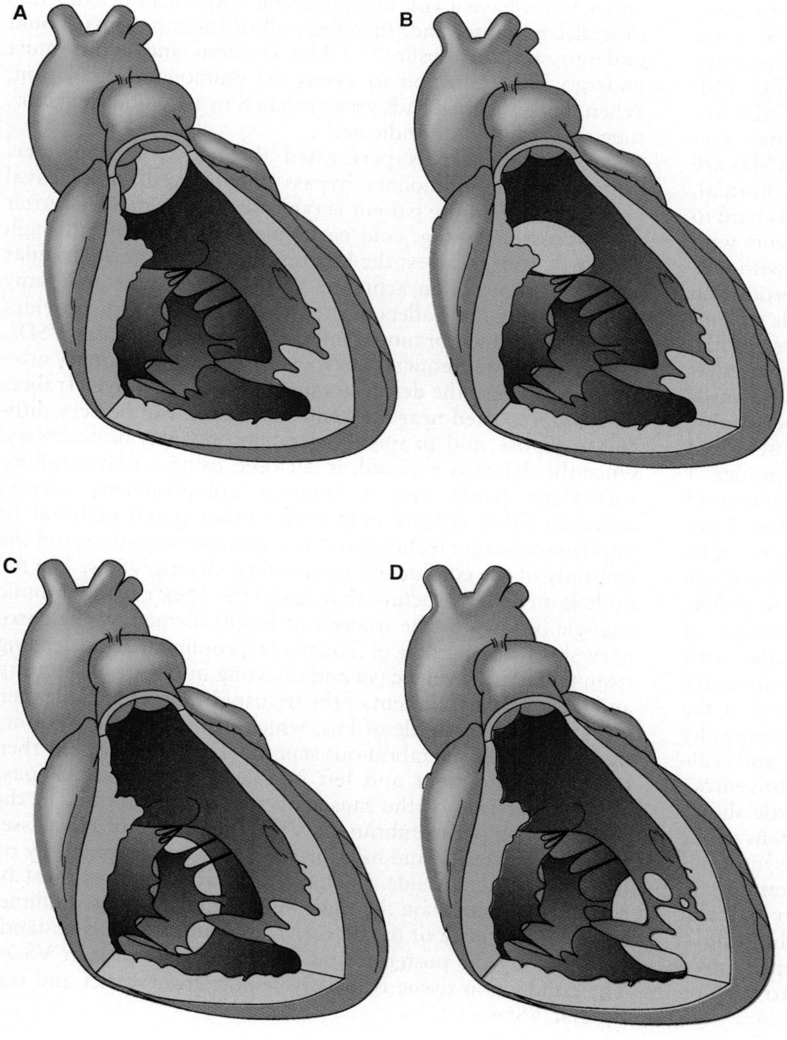

FIGURE 81.2. The anatomy of ventricular septal defects (VSDs) as seen through the right ventricle. A: Outlet, or subarterial, VSDs are generally bordered superiorly by the pulmonary valve annulus. B: Perimembranous VSDs are most common, extending from the membranous septum into the infundibular septum. C: Inlet defects are located predominantly beneath the septal leaflet of the tricuspid valve. D: Muscular VSDs are situated away from the valves, toward the cardiac apex.

The most common defects are perimembranous (80%), which are located in the area of the membranous septum. Inlet defects (5%) are located beneath the septal leaflet of the tricuspid valve and are sometimes called AV canal-type defects. Defects located high in the ventricular septum are outlet defects (10%). Outlet VSDs are typically adjacent to both the pulmonary and aortic valves. Outlet defects are also known by several other names, including supracristal, infundibular, or doubly committed subarterial. Outlet defects are more common in the Asian population. Trabecular (or muscular) VSDs (5%) are completely bordered by muscle. Trabecular VSDs are frequently multiple and may be associated with perimembranous or outlet defects. The size of VSDs varies. By definition, a VSD is nonrestrictive when its size (or the cumulative size of multiple defects) is greater than or equal to the size of the aortic annulus.

A VSD causes increased PBF due to left-to-right shunting primarily during systole. This creates a volume load on the left heart (the left atrium and ventricle receive the increased venous return during diastole). The right ventricle is not volume loaded (blood is ejected from the left ventricle [LV] through the VSD and directly into the pulmonary circulation); however, it does experience a pressure load. The volume of shunt flow is determined by the size of the defect and by the ratio of pulmonary to systemic vascular resistance. After birth the PVR is still high and shunting across a VSD is sometimes minimal. Over the first several weeks of life, shunting tends to increase as the PVR normally falls. Therefore, a patient with a large VSD may be asymptomatic at birth and develop severe CHF symptoms over the first 6 weeks of life.

The natural history for patients with isolated VSDs is highly variable. Most VSDs are restrictive and tend to close spontaneously during the first year of life. Large VSDs are nonrestrictive, resulting in right ventricular and pulmonary pressures that are systemic or nearly systemic, and high PBF with Q_p/Q_s ratios greater than 2.5 to 3. Moderate VSDs are restrictive, with pulmonary pressures that are one-half systemic (or less) and Q_p/Q_s ratios of 1.5 to 2.5. Small VSDs are highly restrictive; right ventricular pressures remain normal, and the Q_p/Q_s is less than 1.5. Patients with large VSDs tend to develop symptoms of CHF by 2 months of age. Patients with smaller VSDs may remain asymptomatic. In patients with outlet VSDs, prolapse of the aortic valve may occur, producing aortic insufficiency.[19] Untreated, excessive PBF leads to pulmonary vascular obstructive disease by the second year of life. The histologic changes associated with pulmonary vascular obstructive disease have been classified by Heath and Edwards based on severity.[20] Grade 1 consists of medial hypertrophy; grade 2 reflects intimal proliferation; grade 3 is characterized by intimal fibrosis and vascular occlusion; and grades 4 through 6 describe progressive vessel dilatation, angiomatoid malformation, and necrotizing arteritis. Grades 1 and 2 are considered reversible, whereas the latter stages are irreversible.

Signs of heart failure in infants with large VSDs include tachypnea, hepatomegaly, poor feeding, and failure to thrive. On physical examination, there is a holosystolic murmur at the left sternal border. Usually, the murmur is louder with smaller defects. The precordium is active. The pulmonary component of the second heart sound is accentuated in the presence of pulmonary hypertension. Chest radiography shows increased pulmonary vascular markings and cardiomegaly. Electrocardiography is significant for right ventricular hypertrophy. Patients with small VSDs have little shunting and are usually asymptomatic, having only a pansystolic murmur. Patients with moderate VSDs manifest symptoms and signs that are proportional to the degree of shunting. In patients who have developed significant pulmonary vascular obstructive disease, the volume of left-to-right shunting is decreased, and the murmur may disappear. Eisenmenger physiology results when the shunt flow reverses to right to left, creating cyanosis.

The diagnosis of VSD is confirmed by echocardiography, which accurately defines the anatomy and excludes the presence of associated defects. Cardiac catheterization is used selectively in older children and adults in whom elevated PVR is suspected. PVR is calculated by the following formula:

$$PVR = (PA_{mean} - LA)/Q_p$$

where PA_{mean} is the mean pulmonary artery pressure and LA is the left atrial pressure. The units of resistance by this formula-tion (using pressures in millimeters of mercury and pulmonary flow in liters per minute) are Woods units (which can be expressed in dynes/s per cm^5 by multiplying by 80). In the pediatric population, vascular resistance is frequently calculated using the cardiac output indexed to the body surface area (in square meters) with the resulting indexed resistance units of Woods units/m^2. PVR may be fixed or reactive, and, at the time of cardiac catheterization, response to nitric oxide or 100% fraction of inspired oxygen (FiO_2) may be assessed.

The management of a patient with a VSD depends on the size of the defect, the type of defect, the shunt volume, and the PVR. In general, patients with large defects who have intractable CHF or failure to thrive should undergo early surgical repair. If the congestive symptoms can be moderated by medical therapy, then surgery may be deferred until 6 months of age. Patients with moderate VSDs may be safely followed. If closure has not occurred by school age, then surgical closure is indicated. Small VSDs with a Q_p/Q_s ratio of less than 1.5 do not require closure unless there is evidence of left-sided chamber enlargement. There is a small long-term risk of endocarditis for these patients, but this can be minimized with the appropriate use of prophylactic antibiotics.[21] Patients with outlet VSDs have a risk of developing aortic insufficiency due to leaflet prolapse, and, therefore, all of these patients should undergo surgical closure.[22] Older children and adults must undergo catheterization to assess the pulmonary circulation. When there is a fixed PVR greater than 8 to 10 Woods units/m^2, then surgery is contraindicated.

Surgical closure is performed through a median sternotomy. Cardiopulmonary bypass is employed with bicaval cannulation, and the patient is typically cooled to 32°C. After aortic cross-clamping, cold cardioplegia is delivered through the aortic root to arrest the heart. Exposure of the ventricular septum is most often achieved by making a right atriotomy and retracting the leaflets of the tricuspid valve. This provides access to perimembranous, inlet, and most trabecular VSDs. Outlet VSDs are frequently best exposed via a pulmonary arteriotomy because the defect lies just beneath the valve. Trabecular VSDs located near the ventricular apex can be very difficult to expose, and an apical ventriculotomy may be necessary. Once the defect is exposed, it is closed using a polytetrafluoroethylene patch and a running polypropylene suture, although other centers may prefer other patch material or interrupted suture technique. It is important to understand the anatomy of the conduction tissue when closing VSDs. The AV node is an atrial structure that lies at the apex of an anatomic triangle (known as the triangle of Koch) formed by the coronary sinus, the tendon of Todaro (a prominent band leading from the inferior vena cava and inserting in the atrial septum), and the septal attachment of the tricuspid valve. The node then gives rise to the bundle of His, which penetrates the AV junction beneath the membranous septum. The bundle of His then bifurcates into right and left bundle branches, which pass along either side of the muscular ventricular septum. In the presence of a perimembranous VSD, the bundle of His passes along the posterior and inferior rim of the defect, generally on the left ventricular side. In this critical area, sutures must be placed superficially on the right ventricular side a few millimeters from the edge of the defect. The bundle of His also tends to run along the posterior and inferior margin of inlet VSDs. The conduction tissue is usually remote from outlet and trabecular VSDs.

PA banding is a palliative maneuver that is used to protect the pulmonary circulation from excessive blood flow. PA banding is currently performed only in patients who are felt to be poor candidates for VSD closure, either due to associated illness or due to anatomic complexity, such as multiple trabecular VSDs ("Swiss cheese" septum). Banding is performed without the need for cardiopulmonary bypass. A band is placed around the main PA and tightened to achieve a distal PA pressure of about one-half systemic. The band is secured to the adventitia of the PA to prevent its migration. Distal migration may result in narrowing and poor growth of one or both branch pulmonary arteries, whereas proximal migration can cause deformity of the pulmonary valve. Later, when the patient is a candidate for VSD closure, the band must be removed. Repair of the main PA at the band site is also usually necessary and can typically be accomplished by scar resection and primary closure or patch repair.

Surgical closure of a VSD is associated with a mortality of about 1%.[23] Potential complications include injury to the conduction tissue and injury to the tricuspid or aortic valves. Transient heart block may result from tissue swelling or injury from retraction, but permanent heart block occurs in less than 1% of cases. When heart block develops after surgery, patients are usually observed for a period of 7 to 10 days prior to permanent pacemaker implantation. Closure of perimembranous and inlet VSDs may result in distortion of the tricuspid valve, which may cause significant regurgitation. Aortic valve injury may occur as a result of inaccurate suturing, especially in perimembranous and outlet defects. A residual VSD is seen in about 5% of cases, and reoperation is indicated when significant shunting persists (Q_p/Q_s ratio >1.5). The Q_p/Q_s ratio can be calculated by measuring oxygen saturations and using the following formula derived from the Fick equation:

$$Q_p/Q_s = (Ao - SVC)/(PV - PA)$$

where Ao is the aortic (or systemic) saturation, SVC is the saturation in the superior vena cava, PV is the saturation in the pulmonary veins (which is usually estimated to be 95% to 100%), and PA is the saturation in the pulmonary arteries. Intraoperative echocardiography is used routinely to identify residual defects, which can then be repaired before the patient leaves the operating room.

Recently, transcatheter devices have been developed to allow closure of some VSDs in the cardiac catheterization laboratory or by perventricular deployment without the use of cardiopulmonary bypass.[24,25] Device closure is optimal for large muscular defects with sufficient rims for securing the device. These defects are often difficult to visualize and close surgically. Perventricular closure allows the use of VSD device closure in smaller infants with symptomatic muscular VSDs with excellent results without the challenges of transvenous access in this population.[25] The use of devices for perimembranous VSDs remains limited by the risk of damage to the conduction system or impingement on the function of the tricuspid or aortic valves. A recent series demonstrated a 22% rate of complete heart block, which is prohibitively high in comparison to the surgical rate of complete heart block of less than 1%.[26]

ATRIOVENTRICULAR SEPTAL DEFECT

Defects in the embryologic development of the endocardial cushions may result in a variety of morphologic abnormalities in the AV valves and the atrial and ventricular septa. These anomalies range from ostium primum ASD to complete AVSD (or AV canal defect), with a spectrum of intermediate forms. PDA and TOF are occasionally seen in association with these defects. A high percentage of patients with abnormalities of the AV structures have trisomy 21 (Down syndrome). All infants with trisomy 21 should have an echocardiogram to rule out congenital heart disease given a prevalence of 50%.

TABLE 81.1

RASTELLI CLASSIFICATION OF ATRIOSEPTAL VENTRICULAR DEFECTS

■ TYPE	■ DESCRIPTION
A	The anterior bridging leaflet is divided and attached to the septum by multiple chordae.
B	The anterior bridging leaflet is attached to a papillary muscle in the right ventricle.
C	The anterior bridging leaflet is free-floating, with no attachments except to the valve annulus.

Complete AVSD is an anomaly characterized by a common AV orifice, rather than separate mitral and tricuspid orifices, and a deficiency of endocardial cushion tissue, which results in a primum ASD and an inlet type of VSD. Complete AVSDs were subclassified by Rastelli et al.[27] into three types according to the morphology of the anterior leaflet of the common AV valve (Table 81.1). Incomplete AVSDs are variants in which there is partial fusion of the AV valves, resulting in separate right and left AV valve orifices. The ostium primum ASD is a type of incomplete AVSD in which the VSD component is absent.

When both left and right AV valves equally share the common AV valve orifice, the AVSD is termed *balanced*. Occasionally, the orifice may favor the right AV valve (right dominance) or the left AV valve (left dominance). In marked right dominance, the left AV valve and LV are hypoplastic, and frequently coexist with other left-sided abnormalities, including aortic stenosis, hypoplasia of the aorta, and coarctation. Conversely, marked left dominance results in a deficient right AV valve with associated hypoplasia of the right ventricle, pulmonary stenosis or atresia, and TOF. Patients with severe imbalance require staged single-ventricle reconstruction.

The conduction tissue is displaced in an ASVD and is at risk during surgical repair. The AV node is located posteriorly and inferiorly of its normal position toward the coronary sinus in what has been termed the *nodal triangle*. This triangle is bounded by the coronary sinus, the posterior attachment of the inferior bridging leaflet, and the rim of the ASD. The bundle of His courses anteriorly and superiorly to run along the leftward aspect of the crest of the VSD, giving off the left bundle branch and continuing as the right bundle branch.

A number of other cardiac anomalies are associated with AVSDs including a PDA (10%) and TOF (10%).[28] Important abnormalities of the left AV valve include single papillary muscle (parachute mitral valve) (2% to 6%) and double orifice mitral valve (8% to 14%).[29] A persistent left superior vena cava with or without an unroofed coronary sinus is encountered in 3% of patients with an AVSD. DORV (2%) significantly complicates or may even preclude complete surgical correction.[28] Left ventricular outflow tract obstruction from subaortic stenosis or redundant AV valve tissue occurs in 4% to 7%.[30,31]

Patients with an incomplete AVSD generally present in a similar fashion as a patient with a large secundum ASD. Patients with a complete AVSD with both atrial and ventricular level shunting generally present early in infancy with signs and symptoms of CHF. In addition, moderate or severe left AV valve regurgitation occurs in approximately 10% of patients with an AVSD, worsening the clinical picture. On physical examination, the precordium is hyperactive, often with a prominent thrill. Auscultatory findings include a systolic murmur along the left sternal border, a high-pitched murmur at the apex from left AV valve regurgitation, and a middiastolic flow murmur across the common AV valve. In the presence of elevated PVR, there may be a split first heart sound. Significant cardiomegaly and pulmonary overcirculation are found on the chest radiograph. Electrocardiography (ECG) reveals biventricular hypertrophy, atrial enlargement, prolonged PR interval, leftward axis, and counterclockwise frontal plane loop. Doppler/echocardiography is diagnostic, defining the atrial and ventricular level shunting, valvular anatomy, and any associated anomalies. Cardiac catheterization should be performed for patients older than 1 year of age, for patients with signs or symptoms of increased PVR, or in some cases to further evaluate other associated major cardiac anomalies. If the PVR is high, it is important to remeasure it while the child is breathing 100% oxygen with and without nitric oxide. If the pulmonary resistance falls, it implies that much of the elevated resistance is dynamic and can be managed in the perioperative period by ventilatory manipulation, supplemental oxygen, and nitric oxide. More recently, sildenafil has been shown to decrease elevation in PVR in children with CHF.[32] Markedly elevated pulmonary resistance (>10 Woods units/m^2) that does not respond to oxygen administration is generally considered a contraindication to repair.

Operative treatment is almost always necessary as soon as symptoms are observed to prevent further clinical deterioration. Even in the absence of symptoms, operation is best performed before 6 months of age. PA banding, which permits delaying the repair until the child is larger, is no longer used today except in select complex or single-ventricle cases, extremely low birth weight or prematurity, and very poor clinical condition. This approach exposes the child to the risks of two operations, and the overall mortality exceeds that of primary repair in infancy.

Correcting AVSDs requires patch closure of both septal defects, with any necessary valve reconstruction. Separate atrial and ventricular patches or a single patch for both chambers can be used.[33] During closure of the ventricular defect, the surgeon must carefully avoid injury to the conduction system, which passes along the posterior and inferior rim of the ventricular septum.

The short- and long-term success of the operation is highly dependent on the status of the PVR and the surgeon's ability to maintain competence of the mitral valve. Although earlier reports recommend that the cleft in the left AV valve should not be closed and the valve treated as a trileaflet structure, most surgeons now believe that closure of the cleft is an important mechanism in preventing postoperative left AV valve regurgitation. Significant AV valve regurgitation at the conclusion of surgery, severe dysplasia of the left AV valve, and failure to close the cleft of the left AV valve have been identified as important risk factors for reoperation.[34] Significant postoperative left AV valve regurgitation is also a risk factor for operative and long-term mortality.[30,34] The cleft should not be completely closed in the presence of a single papillary muscle to avoid causing left AV valve stenosis. In the case of a double-orifice valve, the bridging tissue should not be divided to create a single opening in the valve.

Operative mortality is related largely to associated cardiac anomalies and left AV valve regurgitation. Mortality for repair of uncomplicated incomplete AVSDs ranges from 0% to 0.6%, and the addition of left AV valve regurgitation increases mortality to 4% to 6%.[30,35] For complete AVSDs, the mortality without left AV valve regurgitation is approximately 5%, compared with 13% when significant degrees of regurgitation are present.[30]

The majority of reoperations after repair of AVSD are due to left AV valve regurgitation or subaortic stenosis with reoperation rates at 5 years of 11% and 10%, respectively.[36] Significant postoperative AV valve regurgitation occurs in 10% to 15% of patients, necessitating reoperation for valve repair or replacement in 7% to 12%.[34,37,38] Long-term survival is excellent with rates at 1, 3, and 5 years of 98%, 95%, and 95%, respectively.[36]

TETRALOGY OF FALLOT

5 TOF is the most common cyanotic congenital heart defect. It occurs in 0.6 per 1,000 live births and has a prevalence of about 5% among all patients with congenital heart disease.[7] The pathologic anatomy is frequently described as having four components: VSD, overriding aorta, PS, and right ventricular hypertrophy (Fig. 81.3). Embryologically, the anatomy of TOF is thought to result from a single defect: anterior malalignment of the infundibular septum.[39] The infundibular septum normally separates the primitive outflow tracts and fuses with the ventricular septum. Anterior malalignment of the infundibular septum creates a VSD due to failure of fusion with the ventricular septum and also displaces the aorta over the VSD and right ventricle. Infundibular malalignment also crowds the right ventricular outflow tract, causing PS and, secondarily, right ventricular hypertrophy. Prominent muscle bands also extend from the septal insertion of the infundibular septum to the right ventricular free wall and contribute to the obstruction of the right ventricular outflow tract. The pulmonary valve is usually stenotic and is bicuspid in 58% of cases.[40] Pulmonary atresia occurs in about 7% of cases of TOF. The branch pulmonary arteries in TOF may exhibit mild diffuse hypoplasia or discrete stenosis (most frequently of the left PA at the site of ductal insertion). Coronary artery anomalies are frequently present. The origin of the left anterior descending from the right coronary artery, which occurs in 5% of cases, is clinically important because the vessel crosses the right ventricular infundibulum and is vulnerable to injury at the time of surgery. A right aortic arch is present in 25% of patients with TOF. Associated defects include ASD, complete AVSD, PDA, or multiple VSDs.

Patients with TOF develop cyanosis due to right-to-left shunting across the VSD. The degree of cyanosis depends on the severity of obstruction of the right ventricular outflow tract. Frequently, cyanosis is mild at birth and may remain undetected for weeks or months. Neonates with severe infundibular obstruction or pulmonary atresia will develop symptoms shortly after birth and will require a prostaglandin infusion to maintain ductal patency to ensure adequate PBF. In other patients, the right ventricular outflow tract obstruction

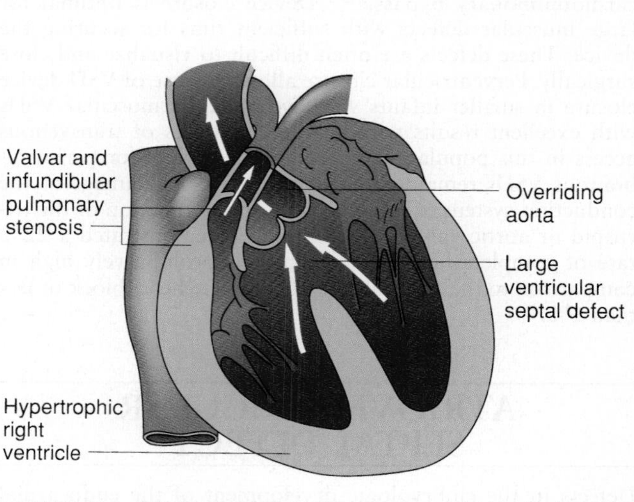

FIGURE 81.3. The four anatomic features of tetralogy of Fallot. The primary morphologic abnormality, anterior and superior displacement of the infundibular septum, results in a malalignment ventricular septal defect, overriding of the aortic valve, and obstruction of the right ventricular outflow. Right ventricular hypertrophy is a secondary occurrence.

is minor, and the predominant physiology is that of a large VSD with left-to-right shunting and CHF.

The occurrence of intermittent cyanotic spells is a well-known feature of TOF. The etiology of spelling is still controversial but is clearly related to a transient imbalance between pulmonary and systemic blood flow. A spell may be triggered by hypovolemia or peripheral vasodilation (e.g., after a bath or vigorous physical exertion). Spells may occur in neonates, but are most frequently reported in infants between the ages of 3 and 18 months. Most spells resolve spontaneously within a few minutes, but some spells may be fatal. Older children have been observed to spontaneously squat to terminate spells. The squatting position is thought to increase systemic vascular resistance, which thereby favors PBF.

Cyanosis is the most frequent physical finding in tetralogy. Auscultation reveals a normal first heart sound and a single second heart sound. A systolic ejection murmur is present at the left upper sternal border. Older children may develop clubbing of the fingers and toes. Chest radiography typically demonstrates a boot-shaped heart due to elevation of the cardiac apex from right ventricular hypertrophy. Pulmonary vascular markings are usually reduced. A right aortic arch may be present. An ECG shows right ventricular hypertrophy. Echocardiography is definitive, and catheterization is not necessary in most cases.

The medical management of TOF is directed toward the treatment and prevention of cyanotic spells. The immediate treatment of the spelling patient includes administration of oxygen, narcotics for sedation, and correction of acidosis. Transfusion is indicated for anemic infants. α-Agonists are useful for increasing systemic vascular resistance (which favors PBF). Some centers have used beta-blockers as a form of long-term therapy to suppress the incidence of spells.

All patients with TOF should undergo surgical repair. Asymptomatic patients should be repaired electively between 4 and 6 months of age. Early repair is indicated for neonates with severe cyanosis and for infants who have had a documented spell or worsening cyanosis.

Classically, the repair of TOF was accomplished in two stages. During the first stage, PBF was augmented by creating a connection (or shunt) between a systemic artery and the PA. At the second stage, the shunt was taken down, and a complete repair was performed. The first shunt procedure was the Blalock-Taussig shunt, in which the subclavian artery was mobilized and divided distally, and an end-to-side anastomosis was created between the inferiorly deflected subclavian and the ipsilateral PA. Other shunt operations were subsequently developed and involved connections between the ascending aorta and right PA (Waterston shunt) or between the descending aorta and left PA (Potts shunt). The modified Blalock-Taussig shunt is the most common type of shunt used today and consists of an interposition graft (polytetrafluoroethylene) between the innominate or subclavian artery and the ipsilateral PA. Creation of a shunt may be accomplished with or without the use of cardiopulmonary bypass.

Currently, one-stage repair of TOF is preferred by most centers. Initial palliation with a shunt is still indicated for some patients who are at high risk for early complete repair, such as those with multiple congenital anomalies, severe concurrent illness, intracranial hemorrhage, or an anomalous coronary artery crossing a hypoplastic infundibulum. In the absence of these risk factors, complete repair in the symptomatic neonate can be performed with lower mortality and reoperation rate compared to staged palliation.[41,42]

Complete repair of TOF is performed using a median sternotomy and cardiopulmonary bypass with bicaval venous cannulation. By a transatrial approach, the right ventricular outflow tract can be examined through the tricuspid valve. Muscle bundles obstructing the right ventricular outflow tract are divided or rarely resected. The VSD is closed with a patch. Pulmonary valvotomy is performed, when indicated, via a vertical incision in the main PA. When the pulmonary valve annulus or infundibulum is severely hypoplastic, a transannular outflow tract patch may be necessary to relieve the obstruction. When an anomalous coronary artery crosses the infundibulum, a transannular incision may be contraindicated. In these cases, and in patients with pulmonary atresia, placement of a conduit (cryopreserved homograft, valved xenograft, or bioprosthetic heterograft) between the right ventricle (via a separate ventriculotomy) and main PA will be necessary. Patients who have a transannular patch develop pulmonary insufficiency as a consequence. This is surprisingly well tolerated in most infants and children, as long as the tricuspid valve is competent. As these patients grow older, some will develop right ventricular failure due to chronic pulmonary insufficiency, and pulmonary valve implantation may be necessary, often in the second or third decade of life.[43,44]

The early mortality following repair of TOF is between 1% and 5%.[40,45] The results are worse for patients with TOF and pulmonary atresia. Long-term complications include recurrent obstruction of the right ventricular outflow tract and development of right ventricular dysfunction due to chronic pulmonary insufficiency. Actuarial survival at 20 years is 86% with excellent functional status.[46]

DOUBLE-OUTLET RIGHT VENTRICLE

Double-outlet ventricle includes a variety of malformations in which, by 50% or more, both great arteries arise from one ventricle. Although double-outlet LVs occur, a far more common anomaly is the double-outlet right ventricle (DORV). A VSD is usually present in DORV, in addition to other defects, including discordant ventriculoarterial connections, valvar or subvalvar stenosis of the PA and aortic outflow, and single ventricle.

The physiologic consequences of DORV vary depending on the associated defects. The three most critical factors determining the net effects on the circulation are the size of the VSD, the presence or absence of PS, and the presence and degree of left-sided obstruction. As a result, DORV may clinically resemble an isolated VSD, TOF, or transposition of the great arteries.

The size and location of the VSD are important considerations in planning operative management. The VSD may be primarily directed toward the aorta, toward the PA, equally toward both arteries (doubly committed), or remote from both great vessels (noncommitted). The location of the VSD affects the direction of flow of oxygenated blood and thus affects the degree of cyanosis. VSDs in DORV seldom close spontaneously. This is fortunate, as closure would result in severe hemodynamic decompensation or death.

If the VSD is large, nonrestrictive, and committed to the aorta, it can be closed with a tunnel-like patch that directs left ventricular flow into the aorta. A restrictive VSD must be enlarged to avoid creating subaortic stenosis. For patients with DORV and PS, repair requires right ventricular outflow tract reconstruction with a patch or a valved allograft conduit, in addition to patch closure of the VSD.

DORV with transposition-type physiology (malposed great vessels with the VSD committed to the PA), also known as a Taussig-Bing anomaly, may be treated by a variety of methods, depending on the specific anatomic details. The preferred approach would be to perform an arterial switch operation, thus making the VSD committed to the aorta, and baffling the left ventricular outflow from the VSD to this neoaorta. Another preferred approach, which depends on a favorable orientation of the two great vessels and VSD, would be an intraventricular tunnel from the VSD to the aorta. A third approach utilizes the Damus-Kaye-Stanzel operation (DKS).

During the DKS, the proximal PA is anastomosed end to side into the aorta. The VSD is baffled to both semilunar valves, which both connect to the aorta. An extracardiac conduit is then placed to reconstruct right ventricle–to–PA continuity. This approach may also be useful when the VSD is doubly committed or noncommitted, so that making a direct connection to either single great vessel is problematic.

The current results for correction of DORV with subaortic VSD are excellent, with a 15-year survival, including hospital mortality, of 96%.[47,48] Mortality for the more complex repairs tends to be slightly higher. Hospital mortality for an arterial switch operation with VSD closure for DORV ranges from 3.7% to 14.3%.[49,50]

TRANSPOSITION OF THE GREAT ARTERIES

6 Transposition of the great arteries (TGA) is a congenital cardiac anomaly in which the aorta arises from the right ventricle and the PA originates from the LV (ventriculoarterial discordance; Fig. 81.4). Looping refers to the right or left looping of the primitive heart tube during fetal development, which determines whether the atria and ventricles are concordant (right atrium attaches to right ventricle and left atrium attaches to LV) or discordant. Levo-TGA (l-TGA) is associated with AV discordance (right atrium attaches to LV and left atrium attaches to right ventricle), and is also termed *congenitally corrected TGA*. l-TGA is a rare variant of TGA and is beyond the scope of this chapter, which will focus on dextro-TGA (d-TGA). The defect can be subdivided into d-TGA with intact ventricular septum (IVS) (55% to 60%) and d-TGA with VSD (40% to 45%), one third of which are hemodynamically insignificant. Pulmonic stenosis (PS), causing significant left ventricular outflow tract obstruction, occurs rarely with an IVS and in approximately 10% of d-TGA/VSD.[51]

d-TGA is a relatively common cardiac anomaly and is the most common form of congenital heart disease presenting as cyanosis in the first week of life. The malformation accounts for approximately 10% of all congenital cardiovascular malformations in infants.[52] The degree of cyanosis depends on the amount of mixing between the pulmonary and systemic circulations. In d-TGA, oxygenated pulmonary venous blood is returned to the lungs and desaturated systemic blood is returned to the body. Because the two circulations exist in parallel, some mixing between them must occur to allow oxygenated blood to reach the systemic circulation and the desaturated blood to reach the lungs. Mixing may occur at a number of levels, most commonly at the atrial level through an ASD or a PFO. Generally, two levels of mixing are necessary to maintain adequate systemic oxygen delivery with a VSD or PDA serving as an additional site for cardiac mixing. In d-TGA, there can be no fixed shunt in one direction without an equal amount of blood passing in the other direction; otherwise, one circulation would eventually empty into the other. Therefore, the amount of desaturated blood reaching the lungs (effective PBF) must equal the amount of saturated blood reaching the aorta (effective systemic blood flow). Clinical characteristics are dependent on the degree of mixing and the amount of PBF. These factors relate to the specific anatomic subtype of d-TGA. Neonates with d-TGA with IVS (or small VSD) have mixing limited to the atrial level and PDA. The ASD may be restrictive and the PDA generally will close over the first days to week of life. As the degree of mixing decreases, the patient becomes increasingly cyanotic and will eventually suffer cardiovascular collapse. Fortunately, the majority of these neonates will manifest cyanosis early in life, which is recognized by a nurse or physician within the first hour in 56% and in the first day in 92%.[53] In d-TGA with a large VSD, there is additional opportunity for mixing and increased PBF. The neonate with d-TGA/VSD may only manifest mild cyanosis, which may be initially overlooked. However, generally within 2 to 6 weeks signs and symptoms of CHF will emerge. Tachypnea and tachycardia become prominent, whereas cyanosis may remain mild. Auscultatory findings are consistent with CHF with increased PBF, including a pansystolic murmur, third heart sound, middiastolic rumble, gallop, and narrowly split second heart sound with increased pulmonary component. Neonates with d-TGA and significant PS present with severe cyanosis at birth. Lesser degrees of PS will result in varying levels of cyanosis. The ECG is normal at birth, demonstrating the typical pattern of right ventricular dominance. Although the classic chest radiographic appearance of an egg-shaped heart with a narrow superior mediastinum may be seen, this finding is often obscured by an enlarged thymic shadow. The abnormal ventriculoarterial connection is clearly seen on echocardiography, which demonstrates that the posterior great vessel arising from the LV is a PA that bifurcates soon after its origin. The anterior great vessel is the aorta and arises from the right ventricle. Associated lesions, including VSD, left ventricular outflow tract obstruction, and coarctation, may also be diagnosed. Although used less frequently, cardiac catheterization may be helpful to confirm the basic anatomy, discern associated lesions, define the coronary anatomy, and improve cardiac mixing by means of balloon atrial septostomy.

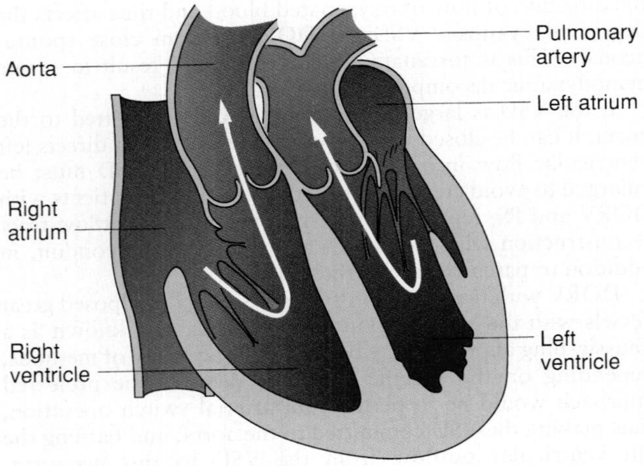

FIGURE 81.4. Anatomy of the most common type of transposition of the great arteries. The location of the ascending aorta is usually anterior to and to the right of the pulmonary artery.

The infant with d-TGA and severe cyanosis requires prompt diagnosis and treatment to improve mixing and increase the arterial oxygen saturation. The first intervention to improve mixing in a cyanotic newborn suspected of having d-TGA is to ensure ductal patency by beginning an infusion of prostaglandin E_1 (PGE_1). In the presence of a restrictive ASD, a balloon atrial septostomy, a technique developed by William Rashkind[54] in 1966, is performed. The procedure involves inserting a balloon-tipped catheter across the foramen ovale into the left atrium. Inflation and forcible withdrawal of the catheter tears the septum primum and enlarges the ASD. Mixing generally increases immediately, with a substantial increase in arterial oxygen saturation.

Without intervention, d-TGA is universally fatal. Untreated, 30% of neonates will die in the first week of life, 50% by the first month, 70% within 6 months, and 90% by 1 year.[55] The definitive surgical treatment of patients with d-TGA has changed dramatically in the past decade with the advent of the arterial switch operation. Before this procedure, repair of d-TGA was generally delayed until patients were at least 6 months of age. Historically, palliative procedures were often

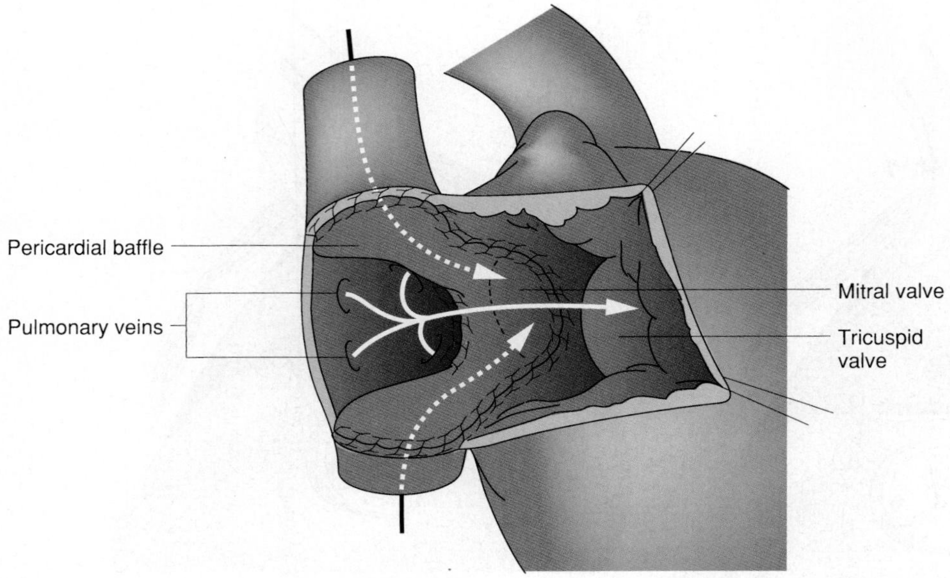

FIGURE 81.5. The Mustard operation for transposition of the great arteries. In this procedure, the atrial septum is excised and replaced with a pericardial baffle, so that pulmonary venous blood is redirected over the baffle to the tricuspid valve. Superior and inferior vena caval blood then drains to the mitral valve.

necessary to improve the systemic saturation or protect the pulmonary vascular bed before definitive repair. If balloon atrial septostomy failed to enlarge the ASD adequately, a Blalock-Hanlon septectomy was performed. Rarely used today, this operation is a method of surgically enlarging the ASD without cardiopulmonary bypass. In patients with large VSDs, significant CHF and pulmonary hypertension are present early in life. Historically, the main PA was banded to reduce distal PA pressure and prevent the development of pulmonary vascular occlusive disease. Changes of pulmonary vascular disease may develop in about 25% of patients with hemodynamically large VSDs by 3 months of age; therefore, early reduction of PA pressure was essential. In those cases of transposition with severe left ventricular outflow tract obstruction, total pulmonary flow is reduced and systemic-to-PA shunting was undertaken until definitive repair could be accomplished.

Historically, definitive repair was achieved by redirecting venous inflow at the atrial level. First successfully performed by Senning[56] in 1959, the operation was further modified by Mustard[57] in 1964 (Fig. 81.5). In both techniques, the atrial septum is repositioned such that superior and inferior vena caval blood is rerouted to the mitral valve and then to the LV and PA. Pulmonary venous blood is redirected to the tricuspid valve and right ventricle. The right ventricle then ejects the oxygenated blood to the systemic circulation. The Mustard operation uses a large patch of pericardium or prosthetic material to create the intra-atrial baffle. In the Senning procedure, the patient's atrial tissue is used, and little or no foreign material is necessary. Although physiologic repair at the atrial level is associated with a low operative mortality rate (<5%), even in infants, a number of late problems have occurred. Obstruction to vena caval inflow, particularly at the junction of the superior vena cava and the right atrium, still occurs in about 5% of patients and may be more common when the procedure is performed in an infant. Additionally, pulmonary venous obstruction may develop and is often difficult to repair. Perhaps because of the complex atrial suture lines, atrial dysrhythmias are common and occur in more than half of patients observed on a long-term basis. In addition, pacemakers may be necessary for troubling bradyarrhythmias in as many as 10% of these patients.

The most serious long-term complication of repair by either the Senning or Mustard technique has been right ventricular dysfunction. Right ventricular failure with an enlarged, poorly contractile chamber and secondary tricuspid regurgitation has been found in a significant number of these patients in long-term follow-up studies. The true incidence of significant right ventricular failure in these cases remains difficult to define and is clearly influenced by an earlier era of operation with different methods of myocardial protection and surgical technique. The fact that many of these infants underwent definitive repair after many months of significant cyanosis may also have influenced right ventricular function.

The long-term complications of atrial repair prompted a reexamination of direct arterial repair for transposing the great arteries. The "arterial switch" operation, first successfully performed by Jatene in 1975, has become the optimal surgical procedure for infants with this condition.[58] Current techniques have reduced the operative mortality to levels comparable with those of atrial repair. Additionally, because the operation is performed early in life, this approach has virtually eliminated the interim morbidity and mortality associated with postponement of surgery until at least 6 months of age. The operative technique involves transection of both great vessels and direct reanastomosis to reestablish ventriculoarterial concordance (Fig. 81.6). Additionally, the coronary arteries are removed from the anterior aorta and relocated to the posterior great vessel (neoaorta). The extensive experience gained with this procedure has confirmed that any variant of coronary artery anatomy can be successfully repaired. Certain coronary anatomy variants were previously felt to be associated with higher risk; however, this concern has been neutralized in recent series.[59,60] Many patients with d-TGA have an IVS, and left ventricular pressure falls early in life as PVR decreases. In this situation, it is essential that the arterial repair be performed within the first 1 to 2 weeks of life, while the LV is still able to meet systemic workloads. In patients presenting later, the LV can be retrained with a preliminary PA banding and an aorticopulmonary shunt, if necessary, followed by the definitive arterial repair. Although patients with large VSDs do not require early repair because they maintain systemic left ventricular pressures, experience has indicated that, even in this subgroup, the operation is best performed within the first month of life, before secondary complications such as pulmonary hypertension, CHF, or infection develop.

Patients with fixed left ventricular outflow tract obstruction are not candidates for the arterial repair because correction would result in systemic ventricular outflow tract obstruction. Most of these patients also have large VSDs. Palliation early in life with systemic-to-PA shunting is an option, with definitive repair postponed until somatic growth results in cyanosis as

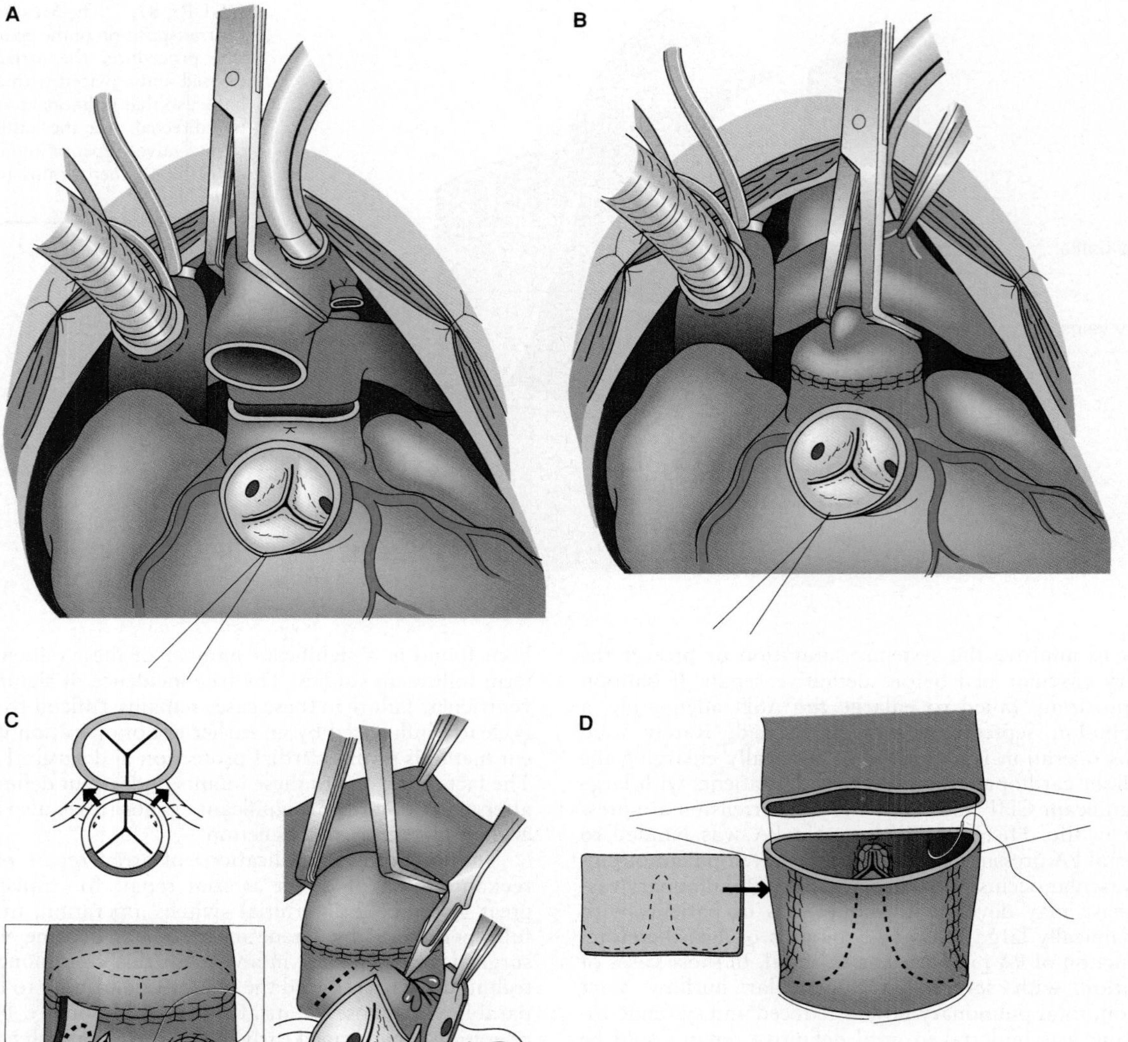

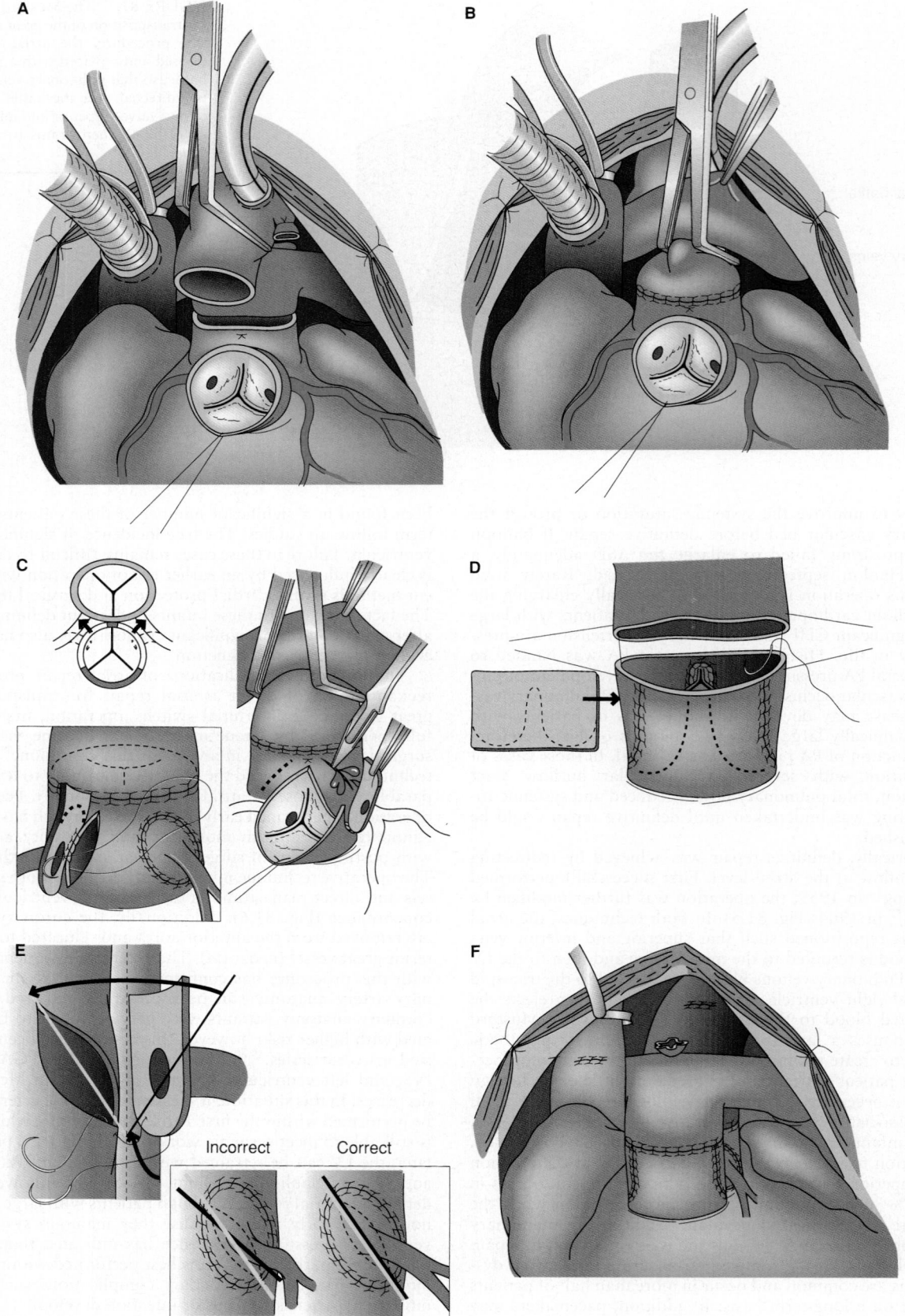

FIGURE 81.6. Arterial switch procedure for transposition of the great arteries. A: Division of aorta and pulmonary artery. B: LeCompte maneuver; posterior translocation of the aorta. C: Mobilization of the coronary arteries. D: Placement of pantaloon-shaped pericardial patch. E: Proper alignment of the coronary arteries on the neoaorta. F: Completed repair.

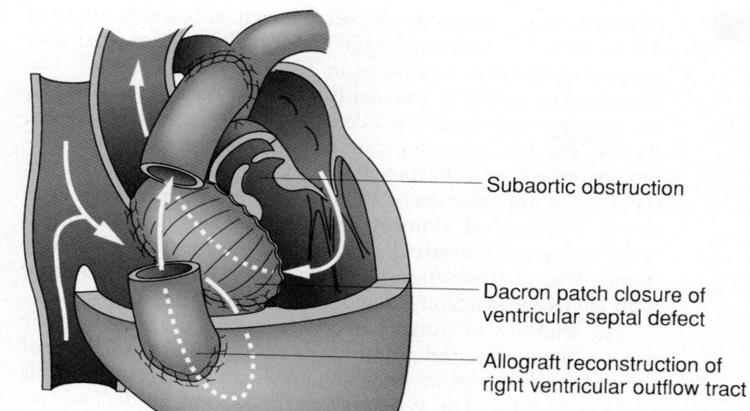

FIGURE 81.7. The Rastelli procedure for transposition of the great arteries with ventricular septal defect and pulmonary stenosis. A prosthetic patch placed within the right ventricle directs left ventricular blood through the defect to the aorta. The main pulmonary artery is ligated, and right ventricular blood then passes through a conduit to the distal pulmonary arteries.

the shunt is outgrown. At that time, the Rastelli procedure is performed, in which left ventricular blood is redirected through the VSD and to the anterior aorta by placement of an intraventricular patch (Fig. 81.7). The PA is ligated, and right ventricle–to–distal PA continuity is reestablished with a valved conduit. An increasing number of experienced centers currently recommend early complete repair in the neonatal period using a Rastelli procedure. Early repair eliminates the interim morbidity and mortality associated with a systemic-to-PA shunt and chronic cyanosis.

Current hospital survival for the arterial switch operation ranges from approximately 90% to 98%.[51,59–62] In earlier eras, d-TGA/IVS had a lower operative mortality than d-TGA/VSD; however, recent studies have neutralized this difference.[59,60] Complex d-TGA including d-TGA/VSD/PS and d-TGA/VSD with aortic arch hypoplasia are independent predictors of increased operative mortality.[63,64] Coronary artery anatomy does not affect mortality.[59] Long-term survival at 5 to 10 years and 15 years ranges from 87% to 93% and 86% to 88%, respectively.[60–62] The most common cause for reintervention is supravalvar pulmonic stenosis, occurring in 3.9% to 16%.[61,62] Late follow-up of arterial switch operation patients has led to increased concern regarding coronary artery patency and neoaortic root dilation.[65]

TRUNCUS ARTERIOSUS

Truncus arteriosus is a rare anomaly that accounts for 0.4% to 4% of all cases of congenital heart disease.[66–68] A single arterial vessel arises from the heart, overriding the ventricular septum and giving rise to the systemic, coronary, and pulmonary circulations. Two classification schemes have been proposed: one by Collett and Edwards[69] in 1949 and the other by Van Praagh and Van Praagh[70] in 1965 (Fig. 81.8). The Collett and Edwards classification focused on the origin of the pulmonary arteries from the common arterial trunk (Table 81.2). The system offered by Van Praagh and Van Praagh, a somewhat more surgically oriented scheme, is based on the presence or absence of a VSD, the degree of formation of the aorticopulmonary septum, and the status of the aortic arch (Table 81.3).

Persistent truncus arteriosus is the result of failed development of the aorticopulmonary septum and subpulmonary infundibulum (conal septum). Normal septation leads to the development of both pulmonary and systemic outflow tracts, division of the semilunar valves, and formation of the aorta and pulmonary arteries. Failure of septation results in a VSD (absence of the infundibular septum), a single semilunar valve, and a single arterial trunk. Most cases are associated with a

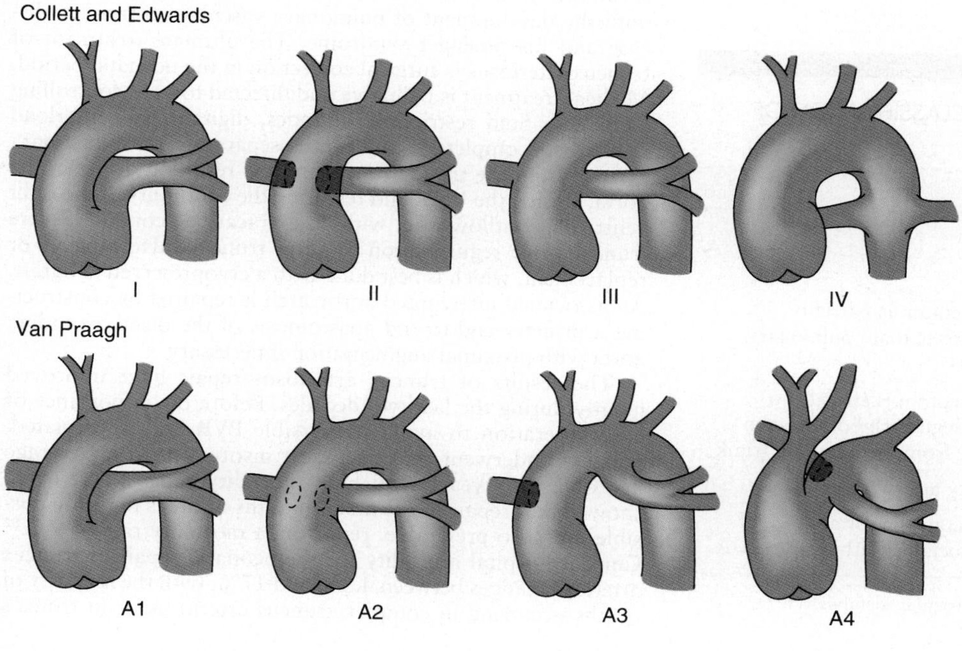

FIGURE 81.8. Truncus arteriosus: classification schemes as described by Collett and Edwards[69] and by Van Praagh and Van Praagh.[70] (Adapted from Hernanz-Schulman M, Fellows KE. Persistent truncus arteriosus: pathologic, diagnostic, and therapeutic considerations. *Semin Roentgenol* 1985;20:121.)

TABLE 81.2

COLLETT AND EDWARDS CLASSIFICATION OF TRUNCUS ARTERIOSUS

■ TYPE	■ DESCRIPTION
I	Common arterial trunk gives rise to a main pulmonary artery and the aorta.
II	Right and left pulmonary arteries arise directly and in close proximity from the posterior wall of the truncus.
III	Right and left pulmonary arteries arise from more widely separated orifices on the posterior truncal wall.
IV	Branch pulmonary arteries are absent. Pulmonary blood flow is derived from aorticopulmonary collaterals.

VSD reminiscent of the VSD associated with TOF. However, in this anomaly, the superior margin of the defect is formed by the truncal valve. The truncal valve leaflets are generally dysmorphic, and their motion may be restricted. Leaflet number is highly variable, with about 65% tricuspid, 22% quadricuspid, 9% bicuspid, and rarely unicuspid or pentacuspid.[71] As a result of these abnormally developed valve leaflets, a moderate or greater degree of truncal insufficiency is present in 20% to 26% of patients.[72,73] Mild stenosis is common; however, significant stenosis is present in only 4% to 7%.[72,73] Significant obstruction is predicted by gradients of more than 30 mm Hg in the presence of a normal cardiac output.[74] The PAs are usually of normal size and most often arise from the left posterolateral aspect of the truncal artery, often in close proximity to the truncal valve and ostium of the left coronary artery.

Other cardiac anomalies are common, with a PFO usually present. A true ASD is found in 9% to 20%, a persistent left superior vena cava in 4% to 9%, and mild tricuspid valve stenosis in 6%.[28,75] An interrupted aortic arch, most commonly type B, is present in association with truncus arteriosus (Van Praagh type A4/B4) in approximately 10% to 20%.[76,77] The arch is rightward, generally with mirror-image branching, in 21% to 36%.[75,77] Aberrant origins of the brachiocephalic vessels are reported, most commonly an aberrant right subclavian artery in 4% to 10%.[75,78] Coronary ostial abnormalities are of particular surgical significance and occur in 37% to 49% of cases.[79] The left coronary artery is frequently noted to have a high origin, not uncommonly near the takeoff of the pulmonary arteries. Rarely, the left coronary can originate from the main pulmonary trunk or a branch PA.[78] Extracardiac anomalies are reported in approximately 28% of patients with truncus arteriosus.[72] Described abnormalities include skeletal, genitourinary, and gastrointestinal deformities. As mentioned earlier, monoallelic microdeletion of chromosome 22q11 is common, with DiGeorge syndrome diagnosed in at least 11%.[72]

The anatomy of truncus arteriosus results in the obligatory mixing of systemic and pulmonary venous blood at the level of the VSD and truncal valve, which produces arterial saturations of 85% to 90%. The systemic arterial saturation depends on the volume of pulmonary blood flow, which in turn is determined by the PVR. As the PVR begins to fall, excessive pulmonary circulation ensues and leads to pulmonary congestion and signs and symptoms of CHF. This nonrestrictive left-to-right shunt may cause early development of irreversible pulmonary vascular obstructive disease.

The presence of truncal valve abnormalities poses further hemodynamic burdens. Truncal valve regurgitation leads to ventricular dilatation and low diastolic coronary perfusion pressures that can result in myocardial ischemia. Truncal valve stenosis promotes ventricular hypertrophy, increases the myocardial oxygen demand, and limits coronary and systemic perfusion, especially with the large volume of runoff into the pulmonary vascular bed.

Neonates with truncus arteriosus present with signs of CHF and collapsing peripheral pulses. Chest radiography shows marked cardiomegaly; pulmonary plethora, often with minimal thymus shadow; and a right aortic arch. The ECG most often depicts biventricular hypertrophy. Echocardiography is the diagnostic procedure of choice and can demonstrate the truncal vessel, the structure and function of the truncal valve, associated lesions such as interrupted aortic arch, and often the pulmonary arterial anatomy. Cardiac catheterization is not performed unless the anatomy is unclear, further information is needed about the status of the truncal valve, or the status of the pulmonary vasculature is unclear (i.e., infants older than 3 months at diagnosis).

The natural history of patients born with truncus arteriosus is early demise. Approximately 40% of infants are dead within 1 month, 70% by 3 months, and 90% by 1 year.[80] Early death is caused by CHF. Survivors may do well for a period of time until the development of pulmonary vascular obstructive disease and Eisenmenger syndrome. The ultimate treatment of truncus arteriosus is surgical correction in the neonatal period. Medical treatment is palliative and directed toward controlling CHF with fluid restriction, diuretics, digitalis, and afterload reduction. Complete repair entails separating the pulmonary arteries from the truncus, repairing the resulting defect in the aorta, closing the VSD, and restoring the continuity of the right ventricular outflow tract with an extracardiac conduit. Severe truncal valve regurgitation requires truncal valve repair[81] or replacement, which is best done with a cryopreserved allograft. An associated interrupted aortic arch is repaired by constructing a primary end-to-end anastomosis of the distal ascending aorta with proximal augmentation if necessary.

The results of truncus arteriosus repair have improved greatly during the last two decades. Before the importance of early operation to avoid irreversible PVR was appreciated, patients underwent repair at most institutions at an average age of 2 to 5 years with high mortality rates. Ebert et al. showed that repair in the first 6 months of life is not only possible, but also preferable, reporting a mortality rate of 9%.[82] Current hospital mortality for the neonatal repair of truncus arteriosus ranges between 4.3% and 17%, with the majority of deaths occurring in complex truncus arteriosus or in truncus

TABLE 81.3

VAN PRAAGH AND VAN PRAAGH CLASSIFICATION OF TRUNCUS ARTERIOSUS

■ TYPE	■ DESCRIPTION
A	With a VSD
B	Without a VSD
1	The aorticopulmonary septum is partially developed (partially separate main pulmonary artery).
2	The aorticopulmonary septum is absent (no main pulmonary artery segment); both branch pulmonary arteries arise from the common trunk.
3	Either branch pulmonary artery is absent.
4	Hypoplasia, coarctation, atresia, or absence of the aortic isthmus is associated with a large PDA.

PDA, patent ductus arteriosus; VSD, ventricular septal defect.

arteriosus with associated severe truncal valve regurgitation.[72–74,83–85] Risk factors for poor outcome identified in various studies include significant truncal regurgitation, need for truncal valve replacement, birth weight less than 2.5 kg, presence of interrupted aortic arch or coronary artery anomalies, pulmonary reconstruction with a technique other than valved heterograft or allograft, and age older than 100 days.[72–74,83–87] Other recent studies have demonstrated that interrupted aortic arch has been neutralized as a risk factor.[74,84]

AORTIC STENOSIS

Aortic stenosis (AS) refers to a form of left ventricular outflow tract obstruction that may occur at the valvar (70%), subvalvar (25%), or supravalvar (5%) level (Fig. 81.9). Aortic stenosis occurs in about 4% of patients with congenital heart disease.[7] The severity of AS may be graded by echocardiography or catheterization. Classification by echocardiography peak instantaneous pressure gradient is mild (<40 mm Hg), moderate (40 to 70 mm Hg), and severe (>70 mm Hg). Classification by catheterization peak-to-peak pressure gradient is mild (<30 mm Hg), moderate (30 to 50 mm Hg), and severe (>50 mm Hg).

Valvar AS occurs secondary to maldevelopment of the aortic valve. Most commonly, a bicuspid valve is present, although tricuspid and unicuspid valves are also represented. In valvar AS, the leaflets are thickened and frequently dysmorphic, and there is a variable degree of leaflet fusion along the commissures. The aortic annulus may be hypoplastic. In 20% of cases, valvar AS is associated with other cardiac defects, most commonly coarctation of the aorta, PDA, VSD, or mitral stenosis. Males with valvar AS outnumber females by a ratio of 4:1. There is a wide spectrum of clinical presentation of valvar AS, but patients tend to present in one of two groups: younger patients (neonates and infants) with severe AS develop symptoms of rapidly progressive CHF, whereas older patients, with less severe obstruction at birth, have a more indolent course.

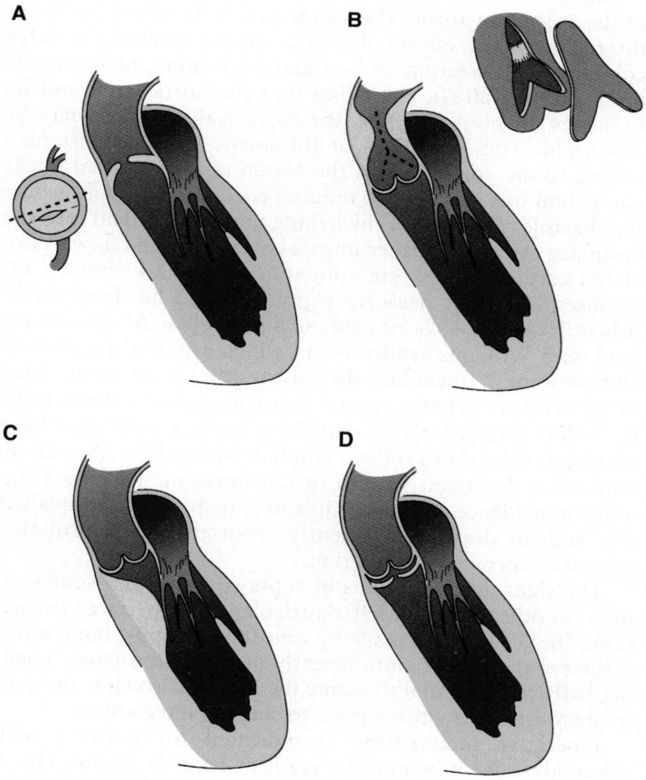

FIGURE 81.9. Anatomy of the types of congenital aortic stenosis. **A:** Valvar aortic stenosis. **B:** Supravalvar aortic stenosis and its repair (*inset*). **C:** Diffuse (tunnel) subvalvar aortic stenosis. **D:** Discrete subvalvar aortic stenosis.

Severe AS is usually well tolerated during fetal development. Although left ventricular output and antegrade flow across the aortic valve are decreased, the right ventricle compensates with increased output, and systemic perfusion is maintained by flow across the ductus. After birth, there is increased venous return to the left heart, and this exacerbates the pressure load created by the stenotic aortic valve, leading to left ventricular dysfunction. As the ductus closes during postnatal life, systemic malperfusion may develop with resulting hypotension, acidosis, and oliguria. Coronary perfusion is also impaired due to the combination of systemic hypotension and elevated left ventricular end-diastolic pressure. Patients with critical AS typically exhibit severe left ventricular dysfunction. These patients show signs of distress soon after birth. On examination, there is impaired distal perfusion with poor capillary refill and diminished, thready pulses. A systolic ejection murmur may be absent if the cardiac output is severely diminished. Differential cyanosis may be observed due to perfusion of the lower body with desaturated blood shunting through the ductus. The ECG shows left ventricular hypertrophy, and the chest radiograph displays cardiomegaly and pulmonary congestion. Echocardiography establishes the diagnosis.

Fetal echocardiography has allowed for early diagnosis of critical aortic stenosis. For some, this may predict the progression to hypoplastic left heart syndrome or may result in irreversible left ventricular dysfunction. A few centers in the United States have been able to successfully balloon dilate the aortic valve in utero to promote left ventricular growth and preserve function in select cases.[88–90]

The neonate or infant with critical AS represents a true emergency. Endotracheal intubation and inotropic support are routine. Ductal patency is maintained with prostaglandins, and acidosis is corrected. All patients with critical AS require some form of urgent intervention. The approach is determined by the valve morphology and by the presence of associated defects. In its most extreme form, critical AS may be associated with underdeveloped left-sided cardiac chambers and therefore may represent a form of hypoplastic left heart syndrome. In these cases, single-ventricle palliation must be undertaken. For patients with adequate left-sided chambers, relief of AS may be achieved by one of the following three approaches: percutaneous balloon valvuloplasty, surgical valvotomy, or aortic valve replacement. Balloon valvuloplasty is generally considered the procedure of choice when the aortic valve annulus is adequate and there are no associated cardiac defects. Alternatively, surgical valvotomy may be accomplished by closed or open techniques. The closed approach is performed using cardiopulmonary bypass, but without aortic cross-clamping. Dilators of increasing size are passed through a ventriculotomy in the left ventricular apex and advanced across the aortic valve. Some centers prefer open surgical valvotomy, which allows a precise valvotomy under direct vision, although aortic cross-clamping with cardioplegia is necessary and results are similar to transventricular dilation. In all cases, the goal of therapy is to relieve stenosis without creating excessive aortic insufficiency. Dramatic clinical improvement is expected following balloon or surgical valvotomy, and early survivals of greater than 80% have been reported regardless of approach.[91,92] The incidence of aortic insufficiency is slightly higher following balloon valvotomy. In most cases, however, stenosis will recur and repeat valvotomy or aortic valve replacement will eventually be required. Aortic valve replacement is problematic in the neonate due to small patient size. In these cases, many consider the best valve replacement to be a pulmonary autograft

(Ross procedure)[93] with enlargement of the aortic annulus (Konno aortoventriculoplasty).[94] The Ross-Konno procedure has been used successfully for neonates with critical AS in whom the aortic annulus is hypoplastic and for selected patients in whom valvuloplasty was unsuccessful. Survival following the Ross-Konno procedure in infants has been shown to be excellent.[95] Growth of the pulmonary autograft has been documented, thereby making it an ideal valve replacement for children. Unfortunately, as part of the Ross procedure, the pulmonary valve must be replaced using a cryopreserved homograft that does not grow, and homograft replacement must be anticipated at intervals as the patient grows.

In contrast to infants with critical AS, older children with valvar AS usually present with less severe stenosis (mild or moderate), and most are asymptomatic. Symptoms of angina, syncope, and CHF are not commonly reported. Congenital valvar AS is a progressive lesion, however, and survival is dependent on the severity of stenosis and the rate of its progression. Sudden cardiac death is the most common cause of mortality. Endocarditis occurs in less than 1% of patients. The diagnosis of valvar AS in older children can frequently be made on physical exam. There is a classic systolic crescendo-decrescendo murmur at the upper sternal border, which radiates to the neck. An ejection click is often present. A visible apical impulse is suggestive of significant left ventricular hypertrophy. In severe cases, the pulse may be weak and delayed (pulsus tardus et parvus). The ECG shows left ventricular hypertrophy. The chest radiograph is usually normal. Echocardiography accurately defines the level of stenosis and its severity. Using Doppler techniques, the pressure gradient across the stenotic valve may be estimated using a simplified form of Bernoulli's equation, $P = 4V^2$, where P is the pressure gradient and V is the peak flow velocity. Cardiac catheterization is generally reserved for therapeutic intervention.

All patients with severe valvar AS should undergo intervention, as should all symptomatic patients with moderate stenosis. Asymptomatic patients with mild or moderate stenosis are generally observed. As described previously for critical AS, the techniques used to relieve AS in older patients include percutaneous balloon valvuloplasty, surgical valvulotomy, and valve replacement. Balloon valvuloplasty is usually performed as the primary intervention, and is associated with a success rate of nearly 90% and a mortality of less than 1%.[96] Open surgical valvotomy is an alternative approach with similar results.[97] For valves that are severely dysplastic, develop restenosis after intervention, or become insufficient as a result of prior intervention, valve replacement may be necessary. For older children, there are more options for valve replacement. The choices include mechanical prostheses, bioprosthetic valves, and tissue substitutes, such as porcine xenografts, cryopreserved human allografts, and pulmonary autografts (Ross procedure). The mechanical valves are the most durable, but require chronic anticoagulation. The bioprosthetic and tissue valves do not require long-term anticoagulation, but tend to deteriorate over time (with the exception of the pulmonary autograft). The pulmonary autograft has the potential advantage of growth but the homograft used to replace the pulmonary valve will require replacement. Selection of the appropriate replacement valve is a complex decision that requires input from all involved parties.

Subvalvar AS occurs below the level of the aortic valve and may be discrete (80%) or diffuse (20%). Discrete (or membranous) subaortic stenosis is rarely seen in infants and tends to progress over time. This lesion consists of a crescentic or circumferential fibrous or fibromuscular membrane that protrudes into the left ventricular outflow tract. The pathogenesis of discrete subaortic stenosis is unknown, but it is thought to be an acquired lesion that develops secondary to a congenital abnormality of the left ventricular outflow tract in which abnormal flow patterns lead to endocardial injury with resultant fibrosis. Although the aortic valve leaflets are usually normal in discrete subaortic stenosis, the turbulent flow created by the obstruction can cause leaflet thickening and progressive aortic insufficiency. Diffuse subaortic stenosis is a more severe form that creates a long, tunnel-like obstruction. Diffuse subaortic stenosis should be distinguished from hypertrophic cardiomyopathy. Both forms of subaortic stenosis are associated with a high risk of endocarditis. The clinical findings in subvalvar AS are similar to those for valvar stenosis.

Intervention for discrete subvalvar stenosis is usually undertaken when the gradient exceeds 30 to 50 mm Hg or when aortic insufficiency is present. In these patients, resection of the membrane is readily performed by a transaortic approach. To reduce the incidence of restenosis, we advocate concurrent performance of a septal myomectomy to alter the geometry of the left ventricular outflow tract.[98] Operative mortality approaches zero. The recurrence rate of discrete stenosis following membrane resection and myomectomy has been reported to be as low as 4%.[99] Complications associated with membrane resection can include heart block, VSD, or damage to the aortic or mitral valve leaflets.

The indications for operative intervention in diffuse subaortic stenosis are similar to those for valvar stenosis. When diffuse subaortic stenosis is associated with hypoplasia of the aortic annulus, repair is best achieved with a Konno aortoventriculoplasty, whereby an incision is carried across the aortic annulus and subjacent ventricular septum, the opening patched, and an aortic valve implanted. Patients with an adequate aortic annulus may undergo a septoplasty (modified Konno), in which the septal incision is confined to the immediate subvalvar area and a patch is used to widen the left ventricular outflow tract without replacing the aortic valve. Despite the technical complexity of repair for diffuse subaortic stenosis, excellent results have been reported with high survival and freedom from reoperation.[100]

Supravalvar AS is characterized by thickening of the wall of the ascending aorta. The lesion may be localized (80%) to the region of the sinotubular ridge (at the level of the valve commissures), creating an hourglass deformity, or it may be more diffuse (20%), extending into the aortic arch and its branches. In both varieties, the aortic valve leaflets may be abnormal. The free edges of the aortic valve leaflets may adhere to the aortic wall in the region of intraluminal thickening, and this may lead to reduced coronary blood flow during diastole. Aortic wall thickening may also extend into the coronary ostia and further impair coronary blood flow. Associated cardiac lesions are common, particularly branch PA stenoses. A genetic basis for supravalvar AS has been established.[101] About 50% of cases of supravalvar AS are associated with Williams syndrome, in which a partial deletion of chromosome 7 (including the elastin gene) leads to the triad of supravalvar stenosis, mental retardation, and a characteristic "elfin" facies. Isolated mutations in the elastin gene have also been shown to produce familial supravalvar AS with an autosomal dominant pattern of transmission. There is a significant incidence of endocarditis in patients with supravalvar AS. Sudden death is frequently reported and is probably related to coronary obstruction.

The signs and symptoms of supravalvar AS are similar to those in other forms of left ventricular outflow tract obstruction. The diagnosis is made by echocardiography, but cardiac catheterization (and more recently magnetic resonance imaging [MRI]) is essential to define the aortic, coronary, and pulmonary arterial anatomy prior to surgical intervention.

Operative intervention is indicated for patients with supravalvar AS in whom the gradient exceeds 50 mm Hg. A number of operations have been proposed for the treatment of localized supravalvar stenosis. The classic repair involves a longitudinal incision across the obstruction in the ascending aorta, which is extended into the noncoronary sinus. The thickened, hypertrophic ridge is resected by endarterectomy and the aortotomy is augmented with an elliptical patch. A variation of this repair involves creation of an inverted-Y aortotomy with one limb of the Y extended into the noncoronary sinus and the other into the right coronary sinus. A Y-shaped patch is then used to augment the aortotomy. Finally, the Brom repair is performed by transection of the ascending aorta beyond the supravalvar ridge. Separate incisions are then made through the supravalvar ridge into each sinus of Valsalva. Triangular patches are placed to augment each of these incisions, thereby relieving the supravalvar obstruction. Reconnection of the aortic root to the ascending aorta completes the repair. The repair of the diffuse type of supravalvar stenosis is performed under circulatory arrest with extensive patching of the ascending aorta, transverse arch, and involved arch arteries. Branch pulmonary stenoses are best managed using transcatheter techniques.

The results of surgery for localized supravalvar AS are generally good with low operative mortality and excellent long-term survival.[102–104] The diffuse form is more difficult to treat, and recurrence is more likely. Overall results are much worse when severe bilateral PA stenoses are present.

COARCTATION OF THE AORTA

Coarctation of the aorta is a narrowing of the proximal descending thoracic aorta distal to the origin of the left subclavian artery, near the insertion of the ductus arteriosus (or ligamentum arteriosum). The severity of luminal narrowing and the length of the aorta affected are variable. Coarctation is thought to occur as a result of ectopic tissue from the ductus arteriosus, which migrates into the wall of the adjacent aorta. After birth, as the ductus closes, the ectopic tissue in the aorta also constricts. Frequently, a posterior shelf of tissue is present at the point of most severe obstruction. The aortic obstruction caused by coarctation creates a pressure load on the LV.

The incidence of coarctation is about 0.5 per 1,000 live births, and its prevalence is 5% of congenital heart defects.[7] Coarctation is commonly associated with other heart defects including bicuspid aortic valve (in more than 50% of cases), PDA, and VSD. Other left-sided obstructive lesions may also be present, such as aortic arch hypoplasia, AS, mitral stenosis, and left ventricular hypoplasia. Coarctation is also recognized to occur in association with Turner syndrome.

Patients with severe coarctation present in the newborn period. Aortic obstruction is so significant that perfusion of the lower body is dependent on flow from the ductus arteriosus. Spontaneous ductal closure typically worsens the aortic obstruction and may lead to malperfusion of tissues distal to the coarctation. The pressure load on the LV may precipitate CHF. Patients may develop shock with severe acidosis, oliguria, and diminished distal pulses. Infants with severe coarctation will generally not survive without intervention.

7 Older children with coarctation are usually asymptomatic. The diagnosis is commonly made on the basis of hypertension in the upper extremities with decreased pulses in the lower extremities. Noninvasive blood pressure measurements in all four extremities help to quantify the severity of aortic obstruction. These older patients tend to develop extensive collateral arteries that bypass the obstruction. Life expectancy for these patients is limited due to the development of heart failure later in life. Other long-term complications of coarctation include chronic hypertension, endocarditis (frequently involving a bicuspid aortic valve), endarteritis (in the poststenotic area of the aorta at the site of the jet of turbulent flow), aortic dissection, aortic aneurysm, and intracranial hemorrhage (from Berry aneurysms, which occur more commonly in patients with coarctation).[105]

The diagnosis of coarctation can usually be made clinically. The infant with significant coarctation is frequently asymptomatic at birth, but following closure of the ductus develops signs of heart failure such as irritability, tachypnea, and poor feeding. Lower extremity pulses are absent, and upper extremity pulses may be weak. Chest radiography shows cardiomegaly and pulmonary venous congestion. There is a left ventricular strain pattern on the ECG. Echocardiography is usually diagnostic, demonstrating narrowing of the aorta at the coarctation site with a loss of pulsatility in the descending aorta.

In older children and adults with coarctation, there is usually a pressure gradient between the arms and legs, which can be demonstrated by measuring cuff pressures in all four extremities. On chest radiography, rib notching may be evident, secondary to erosion of the inferior rib borders from the development of large intercostal collateral vessels. Echocardiography usually confirms the diagnosis. Anatomic details may also be clarified with computed tomography (CT) and MRI. Cardiac catheterization is usually not necessary.

Generally, all patients with coarctation should undergo surgical repair. For neonates, the acute medical management includes initiation of PGE_1 for the purpose of reopening the ductus; this maneuver partially relieves the aortic obstruction and augments perfusion of the lower body due to improved antegrade flow across the arch, as well as right-to-left flow across the ductus. Prostaglandins are usually effective for reopening the ductus when initiated within 7 to 10 days of life, but are less successful thereafter.

Surgical repair of coarctation is usually performed through a left posterolateral thoracotomy via the third or fourth intercostal space. Neonates with an associated hypoplastic aortic arch may require sternotomy for extended arch augmentation with either primary extended end-to-end repair or patch augmentation. For repair via thoracotomy, the descending thoracic aorta, ductus (or ligamentum), transverse aortic arch, and brachiocephalic vessels are mobilized. Care is taken to preserve the vagus nerve and its recurrent laryngeal branch. The preferred surgical approach to coarctation in infants and children is a resection with end-to-end anastomosis or extended end-to-end repair if there is associated mild distal arch hypoplasia.[106] In older children and adults, it may not be possible to perform a resection with primary repair without creating excessive tension on the anastomosis, which may lead to hemorrhage or scarring with recurrent coarctation. An alternative strategy is necessary in these cases. Patch aortoplasty may be performed in children in whom further growth is anticipated.[107,108] The subclavian flap repair augments the narrowed aorta using native arterial tissue. Blood flow to the left arm is maintained by collateral vessels, although long-term studies have demonstrated a slight discrepancy in limb length in some patients. Prosthetic patch material may also be used. By avoiding circumferential prosthetic material, growth potential of the native aorta is preserved. The disadvantage of patch repair is a high risk of aneurysm formation. In adults, in whom growth is no longer a concern, resection of the coarctation may be performed with subsequent placement of a prosthetic interposition graft (either Dacron or polytetrafluoroethylene).

One of the principal concerns during coarctation repair is interruption of distal aortic blood flow, especially to the spinal cord. The anterior spinal artery is fed by major radicular branches from intercostal arteries. In patients without well-formed collaterals, ischemia of the spinal cord may be precipitated by aortic cross-clamping, and paraplegia may result. Protective measures include induction of mild hypothermia, maintenance of a high proximal aortic pressure, and minimization of cross-clamp time. In older patients, distal aortic perfusion may be maintained by the technique of left heart bypass, in which oxygenated blood is taken from the left atrium and delivered to the femoral artery or distal aorta using a centrifugal pump.[109] This is usually not necessary due to the presence of significant collaterals. Overall, the incidence of paraplegia following coarctation repair is less than 1%.[110]

Following repair, patients may develop severe hypertension. This can be managed using intravenous beta-blockers (e.g., esmolol). Uncontrolled hypertension can lead to the complication of mesenteric arteritis. Hypertension usually resolves within days to weeks after repair, although older children and adults may require lifelong antihypertensive therapy. Repair of coarctation during infancy is thought to minimize the risk of late hypertension.[111]

Transcatheter intervention for primary therapy of discrete coarctation in young children and adolescents remains controversial. Technical success rates range from 80% to 98%, with reintervention rates of 10% to 20%.[112–114] Placement of a stent has been associated with higher success rates and lower restenosis rates[114]; however, the long-term outcome of stents in this population remains unknown, and stents are not an ideal option in younger children. There is no evidence to date, therefore, that demonstrates superiority or equivalence of catheter intervention compared to surgery. In addition, there is a high complication rate of 5% to 11.7%, including recurrent coarctation, need for multiple interventions, injury to the femoral vasculature (for access), aortic dissection, and aneurysm formation.[113,115–117] On the other hand, balloon angioplasty is widely accepted for the treatment of recurrent coarctation following surgery, in which the success rate is on the order of 90% with low recurrence rates.[118–120]

The early mortality following repair of coarctation in neonates is 2% to 10%, whereas the risk in older children and adults is about 1%.[106,121] The incidence of recurrent coarctation following resection and end-to-end repair is about 4% to 8%.[106,122,123] The long-term survival following repair of coarctation is determined by the presence of associated defects and the persistence of hypertension.

PATENT DUCTUS ARTERIOSUS

The ductus arteriosus is a normal fetal vascular structure that allows blood from the right ventricle to bypass the high-resistance pulmonary vascular bed and pass directly to the systemic circulation. The ductus communicates between the main PA (or proximal left PA) and the proximal descending thoracic aorta. Histologically, the media of the ductus contains a predominance of smooth muscle cells, whereas the media of the aorta and PA contain well-developed elastic fibers. Vasocontrol of the ductus is mediated by two important mechanisms: oxygen tension and prostaglandin levels. During fetal development, low oxygen tension and high levels of circulating prostaglandin maintain ductal patency. During the final trimester, the ductus becomes less sensitive to prostaglandins and more sensitive to the effects of oxygen tension. Following birth, the rise in oxygen tension and a fall in prostaglandins (which were previously supplied principally by the placenta) lead to ductal closure, which is usually complete by 12 to 24 hours. After closure, the ductus becomes a fibrous cord known as the ligamentum arteriosum. Failure of closure of the ductus leads to the condition called patent ductus arteriosus. PDA occurs in about 1 out of 1,200 live births and accounts for 7% of congenital heart defects.[7] The incidence is much higher in premature infants (>20%).[124] This elevated incidence is thought to be related to immaturity of the ductal wall resulting in impaired sensitivity to oxygen tension.

PDA may occur as an isolated defect, or it may occur in association with a number of other anomalies. Patency of the ductus arteriosus is desirable in a number of defects in which there is either inadequate PBF (such as pulmonary atresia) or inadequate systemic blood flow (as in severe coarctation of the aorta). The discovery that extrinsic delivery of prostaglandins can maintain ductal patency has played a critical role in improving the survival of these patients.[125]

The physiologic manifestation of PDA is shunting of blood across the ductus. The shunt volume is determined by the size of the ductus and by the ratio of pulmonary to systemic vascular resistance. At birth, the PVR drops dramatically and continues to decline over the first several weeks of life. As a result, shunting across a PDA is from left to right. Excessive PBF can lead to CHF. In extreme cases, hypotension and systemic malperfusion may result. Patients with a large PDA who survive infancy tend to develop pulmonary vascular obstructive disease. Eisenmenger physiology results when the PVR exceeds the systemic vascular resistance, producing a reversal of shunting across the ductus to right to left. This leads to cyanosis and, eventually, right ventricular failure. Small PDAs may persist to adulthood without producing any symptoms or physiologic derangement. Endocarditis and endarteritis have been reported as long-term complications of PDA.[126]

In patients with PDA, symptoms are proportional to the shunt volume and the presence of associated defects. Left-to-right shunting produces volume overload of the left heart. Infants with CHF demonstrate symptoms of tachypnea, tachycardia, and poor feeding. Older children may present with recurrent respiratory infections, fatigue, and failure to thrive. Physical findings include a widened pulse pressure and a continuous "machinery" murmur heard best along the left upper sternal border. Chest radiography shows increased pulmonary vascular markings and left heart enlargement. Left ventricular hypertrophy and left atrial enlargement may be evident on the ECG. Echocardiography is the diagnostic method of choice. Diagnostic cardiac catheterization is performed only in older patients with suspected pulmonary hypertension to evaluate for pulmonary vascular obstructive disease. More frequently, catheterization is utilized for transcatheter occlusion of the ductus in selected cases.

PDA closure is performed for all symptomatic patients. Closure is also recommended for asymptomatic patients due to the risk of heart failure, pulmonary hypertension, and endocarditis. Closure of the ductus may be accomplished by one of three approaches: pharmacologic, surgical, and endovascular. Indomethacin and ibuprofen, which are cyclooxygenase inhibitors, stimulate PDA closure in premature infants.[127,128] Both are rarely effective in full-term infants. Due to improved side effect profile of gastrointestinal bleeding and renal dysfunction, ibuprofen is the current drug of choice.[128] The dosing regimen is 10 mg/kg intravenously, followed by 5 mg/kg intravenously at 24-hour intervals for a total of three doses. This is effective in about 70% to 80% of premature babies.[128,129] Due to their side effects, indomethacin and ibuprofen are contraindicated in patients with sepsis, renal insufficiency, intracranial hemorrhage, or bleeding disorders. Failure of ibuprofen after two complete courses results in referral for surgical closure.

The surgical approach to PDA is through a left posterolateral thoracotomy via the third or fourth intercostal space. The pleura is incised over the proximal descending thoracic aorta. This allows medial retraction of the vagus nerve. The recurrent laryngeal nerve curves behind the ductus and should be protected throughout the procedure. Dissection is then performed to demonstrate the pertinent anatomy. In many cases, the ductus is the largest vascular structure present, and it must not be confused with the aorta. Ductal tissue is extremely friable, so direct manipulation is minimized. In premature infants, the ductus is controlled with a single surgical clip; this procedure is commonly performed in the neonatal intensive care unit, thereby avoiding problems associated with patient transfer.[130,131] In older patients, occlusion of the ductus is achieved with simple silk ligature, or, preferably, by division between ligatures to minimize recurrence.

Thoracoscopic techniques have been developed to perform PDA ligation.[132] This approach has the potential benefits of decreased pain and quicker recovery. Disadvantages include a substantial learning curve and increased operating time.

A number of endovascular devices have been developed for the purpose of transcatheter occlusion of the PDA.[133–135] This approach is very successful in older infants, children, and adults with small and moderate-sized PDAs and has become the treatment of choice at many centers. Surgical therapy is reserved for PDAs having a large diameter or very short length.

Rarely, an adult will present with a significant PDA. These patients must be carefully evaluated for the presence of pulmonary vascular obstructive disease prior to ductal closure. If the patient is not a candidate for device closure, surgical closure can be problematic. Calcification of the ductal wall is common in adults, making ligation hazardous. In some cases, cardiopulmonary bypass may be required with closure of the ductus from within the PA.[136,137]

Closure of the ductus by surgical or transcatheter techniques is achieved with a mortality that approaches zero.[130] Potential complications include pneumothorax, phrenic nerve injury, recurrent laryngeal nerve injury, and chylothorax (from injury to the thoracic duct). Long-term survival should be normal following PDA ligation in most patients. Survival in premature infants depends primarily on the extent of prematurity with its attendant complications.

VASCULAR RINGS

Vascular rings comprise a spectrum of vascular anomalies of the aortic arch, pulmonary artery, and brachiocephalic vessels. The clinically significant manifestation of these lesions is a varying degree of tracheoesophageal compression. These vascular anomalies can be divided into complete vascular rings and partial vascular rings. Incomplete vascular rings include aberrant right subclavian artery, innominate artery compression, and pulmonary artery sling. The incidence of clinically significant vascular rings is 1% to 2% of all congenital heart defects.[7]

Vascular rings and pulmonary slings have been described in conjunction with other cardiac defects, including tetralogy of Fallot, atrial septal defect, branch pulmonary artery stenosis, coarctation, atrioventricular septal defect, ventricular septal defect, interrupted aortic arch, and aortopulmonary window. Significant associated cardiac anomalies occur in 11% to 20% of patients with a vascular ring.[138,139] A right aortic arch is generally associated with a greater incidence of coexisting anomalies.

By the end of the fourth week of embryonic development, the six aortic or branchial arches have formed between the dorsal aortae and ventral roots. Subsequent involution and migration of the arches results in the anatomically normal or abnormal development of the aorta and its branches. The majority of the first, second, and fifth arches regress. The third arch forms the common carotid artery and proximal internal carotid artery. The right fourth arch forms the proximal right subclavian artery. The left fourth arch contributes to the portion of the aortic arch from the left carotid to left subclavian arteries. The proximal portion of the right sixth arch becomes the proximal portion of the right pulmonary artery, while the distal segment involutes. Similarly, the proximal left sixth arch contributes to the proximal left pulmonary artery, and the distal sixth arch becomes the ductus arteriosus.

Children with a complete vascular ring generally present within the first weeks to months of life. Typically, children with a double aortic arch present earlier in life than those with a right arch and retroesophageal left ligamentum. In the younger age group, respiratory symptoms predominate, as liquids are generally well tolerated. Respiratory symptoms may include stridor, nonproductive cough, apnea, or frequent respiratory infections. The cough is classically described as a "seal bark" or "brassy." These symptoms may mimic asthma, respiratory infection, or reflux, and children with vascular rings are often initially misdiagnosed. With the transition to solid food, dysphagia becomes more apparent.

The presentation of a patient with an incomplete vascular ring is variable. Children with innominate artery compression usually present within the first 1 to 2 years of life with respiratory symptoms. Aberrant right subclavian artery is the most common arch abnormality, occurring in approximately 0.5% to 1% of the population, and it rarely causes symptoms. Classically, when symptoms do occur, they present in the seventh and eighth decades, as the aberrant vessel becomes ectatic and calcified, causing *dysphagia lusoria* due to impingement of the artery on the posterior esophagus.

Children with pulmonary artery slings generally present with respiratory symptoms within the first few weeks to months of life. As with complete rings, respiratory symptoms may include stridor, nonproductive cough, apnea, or frequent respiratory infections and may mimic other conditions, leading to misdiagnosis. Pulmonary artery slings are associated with complete tracheal rings in 30% to 40% of patients, leading to focal or diffuse tracheal stenosis.

The methods for diagnosing a vascular ring are variable, due to the variability in presentation and the spectrum of diagnostic tests available. A child with a presumptive diagnosis of asthma or tracheomalacia may be referred to a pulmonologist and a diagnosis of vascular ring made or suspected initially by chest radiograph and bronchoscopy. In some situations, the diagnosis is made by echocardiography during evaluation for concurrent cardiac defects. Regardless, the diagnosis generally begins with a chest radiograph. Complementary studies may include barium esophagogram, CT, MRI, and bronchoscopy. CT, MRI, and bronchoscopy are important modalities to define the tracheal anatomy in a patient with a pulmonary artery sling. Echocardiography may be diagnostic, and may be used to rule out other cardiac anomalies. Tracheograms and cardiac catheterizations, which have been used extensively in the past, are rarely currently indicated.

A double aortic arch occurs when the distal portion of the right dorsal aorta fails to regress. The two arches form a complete ring, encircling the trachea and esophagus. The right arch is dominant in the majority of the cases, followed by left dominant, with codominant arches being the least common. The left and right carotid and subclavian arteries generally arise from their respective arches. The ligamentum arteriosum and descending aorta usually remain on the left.

The approach to repair of a double aortic arch is via a left posterolateral thoracotomy. The pleura is incised, after identifying the vagus and phrenic nerves. The ligamentum or ductus arteriosum is divided while preserving the recurrent laryngeal nerve. The nondominant arch is then divided between two vascular clamps at the point where brachiocephalic flow is optimally preserved. If there is concern regarding the location for division, the arches can be temporarily occluded at various points while monitoring pulse and blood pressure in each limb. If there is an atretic segment, the division is done at the point of the atresia. Dissection around the esophagus and trachea in the regions of the ligamentum/ductus and nondominant arch allows for retraction of the vascular structures and lysis of any residual obstructing adhesions.

The surgical approach for a right aortic arch with retroesophageal left ligamentum arteriosum is the same as for a double arch. The ligamentum is divided and any adhesions around the esophagus and trachea are lysed. Rarely, the Kommerell diverticulum has been reported to cause compression even after division of the ligamentum. As such, it may be prudent to resect or suspend the diverticulum posteriorly.

In innominate artery compression syndrome, the aortic arch and ligamentum are in their normal leftward position. However, the innominate artery arises partially or totally to the left of midline. As the artery courses from left to right anterior to the trachea, it causes tracheal compression. The symptoms of innominate artery compression may be mild to severe. With mild symptoms and minimal tracheal compression on bronchoscopy, children can be observed expectantly as the symptoms may resolve with growth. Indications for surgery include apnea, severe respiratory distress, significant stridor, and recurrent respiratory tract infection. Several approaches for the correction of innominate artery compression syndrome have been described. These include simple division, division with reimplantation into the right side of the ascending aorta, and suspension to the overlying sternum.

An aberrant right subclavian artery occurs when there is regression of the right fourth arch between the right common carotid and right subclavian arteries. The right subclavian then arises from the leftward descending aorta, laying posterior to the esophagus as it crosses from left to right. Although the artery can compress the esophagus posteriorly, it is rarely the cause of symptoms in children. Surgical treatment involves simple division via a left posterolateral thoracotomy. Rarely, reimplantation or grafting from the right carotid or aortic arch may be necessary.

Normally, the right and left sixth aortic arches contribute to the proximal portions of their respective pulmonary arteries. If the proximal left sixth arch involutes and the bud from the left lung migrates rightward to meet the right pulmonary artery, a pulmonary artery sling is formed. Pulmonary artery slings are associated with complete tracheal rings and tracheal stenosis in 30% to 40% of patients.

Initial attempts at the repair of a pulmonary artery sling involved reimplantation after division of the left pulmonary artery (LPA) and translocation of the trachea without cardiopulmonary bypass. These early reports had a high incidence of LPA thrombosis. This has led some authors to advocate division of the trachea and translocation of the LPA. This approach would seem sensible if the trachea were being divided in the course of tracheal reconstruction. However, currently most authors advocate the reimplantation of the LPA, which has resulted in excellent results. The procedure is done via a median sternotomy on cardiopulmonary bypass to ensure optimal visualization of the repair. Aortic cross-clamping is not necessary. The LPA is divided off of the right pulmonary artery, translocated anterior to the trachea, and reimplanted into the main pulmonary artery.

Any necessary reconstruction of the trachea is done concurrently with bronchoscopic assistance. Many techniques for tracheal reconstruction have been described, the most common of which are resection with primary reanastomosis and sliding tracheoplasty for short-segment stenosis, and rib cartilage or pericardial patch for long areas of narrowing.[140]

Over 95% of vascular rings without concurrent cardiac defects can be performed through a left thoracotomy. A right thoracotomy is indicated for the rare cases where there is a right ligamentum arteriosum. In addition, a double aortic arch with an atretic segment proximal to the right carotid artery is more easily divided through a right thoracotomy. The approach to these anomalies is the same as for a left-sided ring division, with the caveat that the right recurrent laryngeal nerve will loop around the right ligamentum.

Repair of vascular rings has been described using video-assisted thoracoscopic surgery (VATS) both with and without robotic assistance. Candidates for thoracoscopic division are limited to those patients requiring only the division of non-patent vascular structures. In general, VATS is used for patients greater than 15 kg due to current size limitations of the instruments.[141]

Mortality for the repair of a vascular ring is 0% to 4%, with improved survival occurring in more recent series.[138,139,142] The majority of deaths are related to other cardiac defects or respiratory infection and failure. Backer et al. reported a series of 16 patients repaired utilizing LPA division and reimplantation for pulmonary artery sling, all of whom also required tracheal reconstruction. There were no operative mortalities and one late death due to respiratory complications.[140] The major source of morbidity, as well as mortality, in this and other series is related to the tracheal reconstruction.

CORONARY ARTERY ANOMALIES

Coronary artery anomalies occur in 0.3% to 1.3% of the population.[143,144] They can be classified as minor, secondary, or major based on their clinical significance.[145] Minor defects have no functional significance and are usually detected as incidental findings at cardiac catheterization. Secondary defects have no intrinsic significance, but alter surgical management when they are present. An example of a secondary defect is an anomalous origin of the left anterior descending artery from the right coronary artery that crosses the hypoplastic infundibulum in a patient with TOF. The presence of this vessel may prevent the safe performance of a transannular incision and thereby mandate the use of a conduit. Major defects are the most important form of coronary anomaly, because they exert an intrinsically adverse effect on the myocardium. Major anomalies can be subdivided based on anatomy: coronary arteriovenous fistula, anomalous pulmonary origin of a coronary artery, anomalous aortic origin of a coronary artery, myocardial bridging, or coronary artery aneurysm.

8 Coronary arteriovenous fistula is the most common major coronary anomaly. An abnormal connection exists between a coronary artery (usually the right) and another vascular structure (usually one of the right heart chambers). Most fistulas are isolated and solitary. The fistula leads to left-to-right shunting, which can produce CHF. Other symptoms include angina, endocarditis, myocardial infarction, arrhythmia, and sudden death. The diagnosis is suggested by echocardiography and confirmed by catheterization. All symptomatic fistulas should be occluded, either surgically or by transcatheter techniques. In some cases, coronary bypass grafting may be necessary when distal flow is compromised by fistula occlusion. Treatment of asymptomatic fistulas is controversial, but occlusion should probably be undertaken when significant left-to-right shunting is present.

The second most common major coronary anomaly is origin of a coronary artery from the PA. The most common manifestation is the anomalous left coronary artery arising from the pulmonary artery (ALCAPA). The right coronary (or both coronaries) may also arise anomalously from the PA, but only in very rare cases. ALCAPA is usually well tolerated during fetal development, but after birth, the pulmonary systolic pressure usually drops (following ductal closure and decline in PVR) and the anomalous coronary is perfused with desaturated blood at low pressure. Collateral vessels develop between the normal right coronary artery and the abnormal left coronary, but the benefit is negated due to the development of coronary steal, whereby the collateral blood shunts left to right by retrograde flow in the anomalous coronary into the low-pressure PA. Most patients will present between 6 weeks and 3 months of life. Typical symptoms include irritability, difficulty in feeding, and other signs of CHF. Untreated, ALCAPA is nearly always fatal. Rarely, patients will survive to adulthood and present with symptoms of angina or sudden death. On examination, patients with ALCAPA frequently have a holosystolic murmur of ischemic mitral regurgitation. The pulmonary component of the second heart sound may be pronounced due to pulmonary hypertension. Chest radiography is significant for cardiomegaly and pulmonary edema. Electrocardiographic evidence of ischemia and infarction is usually present. Echocardiography is usually diagnostic and is useful for assessing the severity of left ventricular dysfunction and ischemic mitral regurgitation, which are commonly present. Catheterization is occasionally necessary to clarify the anatomy, but this technique is used less frequently due to the risk of inducing life-threatening arrhythmias.

Surgical repair is indicated for all patients with ALCAPA. Historically, the initial surgical approach involved ligation of the proximal left coronary artery. This served to eliminate coronary steal and allow perfusion of the left coronary system by collaterals from the right. Despite the ease of simple ligation, most centers have abandoned this approach in favor of establishment of a two-coronary system, which offers better long-term freedom from ischemia. In older patients, this may be achieved by proximal ligation of the left coronary artery in conjunction with coronary artery bypass, ideally with a left internal mammary graft. Coronary bypass is technically difficult in neonates, and a number of alternative operations have been devised to create a direct connection between the aorta and the anomalous coronary artery. Most commonly, this can be achieved by removing the origin of the left coronary artery (along with a button of adjacent PA) and reimplanting the vessel directly into the side of the aorta. Another approach involves creation of a side-to-side connection between the aorta and PA with placement of an intrapulmonary baffle to direct flow from this connection to the anomalous left coronary ostium. With improved coronary transfer techniques learned from the arterial switch operation, direct reimplantation of the anomalous coronary artery is always feasible and preferred. Survival following surgical repair of ALCAPA has improved over the years.[146] Recent reports have suggested an operative mortality of 6% or less.[147,148] Ventricular function tends to normalize after surgery.[149] In most patients, mitral valve function also improves,[147,149] but for patients with severe mitral regurgitation, concurrent mitral valve repair may rarely be indicated.

Anomalous aortic origins of the coronary arteries are usually minor defects, but a potentially dangerous abnormality exists when the left main coronary artery arises from the right coronary sinus and passes between the PA and aorta. This defect has been associated with cardiac symptoms and sudden death, as has the origin of the right coronary artery from the left coronary sinus (usually when the right coronary is dominant).[150,151] The etiology of ischemia in both defects is thought to be related to the acute angle of origin and slitlike orifice of the anomalous vessel often with an intramural course and the extrinsic compression created by the opposing walls of the aorta and PA. These defects usually present in older patients. Symptomatic patients are treated surgically by unroofing the coronary ostia into the aorta or by coronary artery bypass.

Myocardial bridging occurs when a segment of an epicardial coronary artery (usually the left anterior descending) takes an intramyocardial course over a short segment. Although this is a common incidental finding at cardiac catheterization, this defect has been associated in some cases with myocardial ischemia. Treatment involves dividing the muscle bridge to free the coronary, coronary bypass beyond the bridge, or transcatheter stenting.

Coronary aneurysms occur rarely, usually in conjunction with an inflammatory condition such as Kawasaki syndrome, polyarteritis nodosa, Takayasu arteritis, or syphilis. Coronary aneurysms may thrombose or lead to distal coronary stenosis or embolization. Rupture occurs uncommonly. Treatment ranges from antiplatelet therapy to coronary bypass grafting.

UNIVENTRICULAR HEART

In the univentricular heart, only one ventricular chamber is connected to the atria. To be classified as a ventricle, a chamber must receive at least half of an inlet valve. In the most common form of univentricular heart, both the mitral and tricuspid valves connect to a morphologic LV (double-inlet LV), which ejects blood through a hypoplastic outlet chamber and then, due to malposition of the great arteries, to the aorta. The outlet chamber is not considered to be a ventricle, regardless of its size, because it does not receive an inlet valve. Similarly, the intracardiac communication is not termed a VSD, but a bulboventricular foramen. Univentricular hearts are frequently associated with malpositions of the great vessels and varying degrees of obstruction to PBF. In double-inlet LV, the aorta is usually anterior and to the left of the PA.

The presentation of infants with univentricular heart is variable, depending on the amount of PBF.[152] When the pulmonary flow is excessive, cyanosis may be mild, and the dominant feature is CHF. Associated PS decreases the PBF, and the degree of cyanosis is increased. Associated lesions may further complicate the picture, such as coarctation, subaortic stenosis, or a restrictive ASD. Patients with moderate PS may achieve a well-balanced circulation with acceptable systemic oxygenation and normal PA pressure. These patients may be symptom-free well into adolescence. Most patients, however, require intervention early in life to reduce excessive PBF or to increase it in the presence of significant PS. Pulmonary vascular obstructive disease develops early when PBF is excessive. With the possible exception of patients in whom the pulmonary and systemic blood flow is well balanced, the prognosis for patients with unoperated univentricular hearts is poor, with more than half dying early of CHF or dysrhythmias.

In the presence of excessive PBF and pulmonary hypertension, operation should be performed early in life to control PBF and prevent the development of pulmonary vascular occlusive disease. Options include PA banding or division of the main PA in conjunction with a controlled aortopulmonary shunt. PA banding is a less complicated procedure; however, it is often difficult to adjust the pulmonary flow accurately, and too proximal or too distal a band can lead to distortion of the pulmonary valve or branch pulmonary arteries, which further complicates later operations. Simple division of the PA with placement of a modified Blalock-Taussig shunt can be undertaken in the presence of an adequate bulboventricular foramen providing unobstructed flow to the aorta. This option avoids the problems associated with a PA band, and more accurately controls the PBF. Another similar technique is division of the main PA, side-to-side anastomosis of the proximal PA with the native aorta, and placement of a modified Blalock-Taussig shunt (modified Damus-Kaye-Stanzel procedure). It is not uncommon for the bulboventricular foramen to decrease in size over time due to progressive ventricular hypertrophy. Maintaining continuity from both the outlet chamber and the LV eliminates the possibility of subaortic obstruction, which can occur when the systemic blood flow depends entirely on egress through a bulboventricular foramen. In infants who are well balanced and can be safely managed medically until the age of 4 to 6 months, a hemi-Fontan or bidirectional Glenn, in which the superior vena caval flow is directed into the pulmonary arteries, can be used to increase the effective PBF. This procedure maximizes pulmonary flow without causing a volume overload to the single ventricle. It is most commonly used as part of an interim stage to a complete atriopulmonary connection or Fontan procedure.

The ultimate goal of surgical correction in patients with a univentricular heart is the total diversion of all vena caval blood directly into the pulmonary arteries. The Fontan procedure was first successfully performed in a patient with tricuspid atresia, but has since evolved as an excellent way to establish physiologic repair for patients with more complex forms of univentricular heart.[153] The superior vena caval blood returns directly via an end-to-side anastomosis with the PA (bidirectional Glenn) or through a right atrial–PA connection (hemi-Fontan). The inferior vena caval flow is directed to the PA with an intra-atrial baffle (lateral tunnel technique, Fig. 81.10) or an extracardiac conduit. All oxygenated pulmonary venous flow empties into the ventricular chamber through the

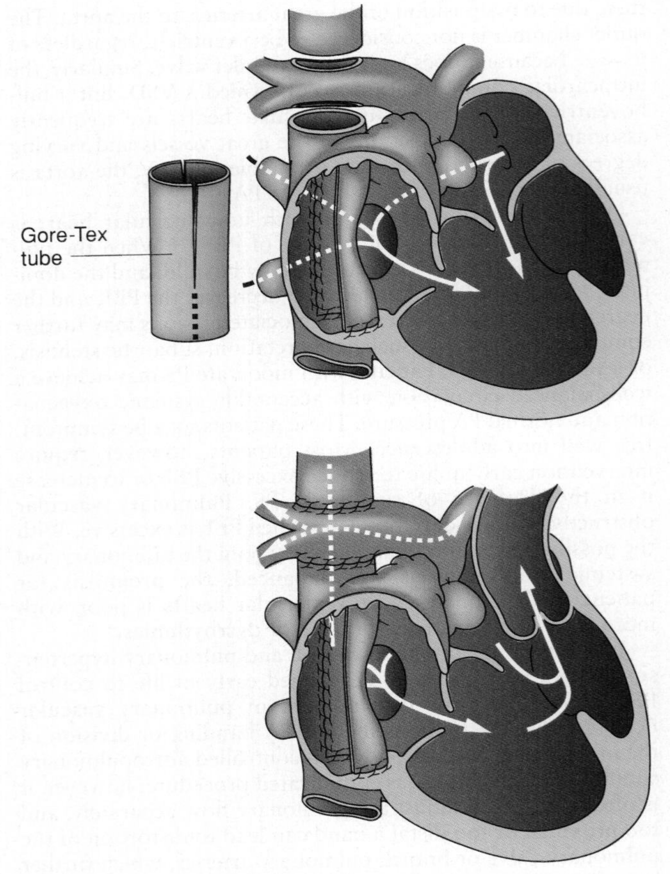

FIGURE 81.10. Total cavopulmonary connection for univentricular heart. The internal orifices of the superior and inferior venae cavae are connected in the right atrium with a patch cut of polytetrafluoroethylene. The superior vena cava is divided just above its junction with the right atrium, and both ends are anastomosed to the right pulmonary artery. The main pulmonary artery is ligated.

AV valves to be ejected to the systemic circulation, while superior and inferior vena caval blood flows directly to the lungs to acquire oxygen prior to returning to the heart. For the Fontan procedure to be performed with a low operative mortality and an acceptable functional result, certain criteria must be met. Normal PA pressure (<20 mm Hg) and PVR (<2 Woods units/m^2) are the most important prerequisites. Additionally, it is essential that ventricular function and AV valve function be normal. Many of the criteria originally proposed, including normal cardiac rhythm, right atrial hypertrophy, normal systemic venous return, and age older than 4 years, are of little or no importance in the current era. Although the Fontan procedure cannot be considered a truly corrective operation, it offers benefits that cannot be equaled by any of the other palliative procedures. The major advantages include restoration of normal systemic oxygen saturation and reduction of ventricular volume overload.

Ventricular septation procedures have also been successfully performed in patients with univentricular hearts. The subset of patients with a double-inlet LV, anterior and leftward aorta, nonrestrictive outlet foramen, and mild or no PS are best suited for septation. This anatomy allows placement of a relatively direct and straight prosthetic patch in the ventricle that separates the pulmonary and systemic circulations. The septation procedure has been associated with a relatively high morbidity, primarily related to complete heart block, so that its overall effectiveness is reduced. Few centers have continued to apply this procedure in carefully selected patients.

The current results for the Fontan are excellent, with hospital mortality ranging from 2% to 9%.[154–158] The condition of survivors is generally good and most attain a functional status of New York Heart Association class I or II. The long-term results have been reported with a 93% to 97% 5-year survival and a 91% 10-year survival.[156,157] Although long-term results are encouraging, late complications may be seen. Continued surveillance for arrhythmias, CHF, protein-losing enteropathy, and hepatic dysfunction remains important.

HYPOPLASTIC LEFT-HEART SYNDROME

Hypoplastic left-heart syndrome (HLHS) refers to a constellation of congenital cardiac anomalies characterized by marked hypoplasia or absence of the LV and severe hypoplasia of the ascending aorta. The systemic circulation is dependent on the right ventricle via a PDA and there is obligatory mixing of pulmonary and systemic venous blood in the right atrium. There is associated aortic valve stenosis or atresia, and mitral valve stenosis or atresia. The descending aorta is essentially a continuation of the ductus arteriosus, and the ascending aorta and aortic arch are a diminutive branch from this vessel. Initial management includes a prostaglandin infusion to maintain ductal patency and correction of metabolic acidosis. The patient may require intubation and ventilator adjustment to reduce supplemental oxygen and maintain a partial pressure of carbon dioxide (PCO_2) of about 40 mm Hg to avoid excessive pulmonary flow.

Treatment options for this problem include cardiac transplantation and staged reconstructive surgery. Transplantation for HLHS is generally performed with the same techniques that are standard for transplantation in older children and adults. However, it is necessary to have a generous amount of donor aortic arch that can be used to augment the hypoplastic recipient arch. Results of transplantation in neonates have been excellent in centers with extensive experience in this area, and a 2-year survival as high as 70% has been reported.[159] In the context of improving results for staged reconstruction, risks of immunosuppression, and limited donor availability, competing risk analysis favors staged repair, and most centers pursue this option as primary therapy for HLHS.[160] Transplantation is generally reserved for very high-risk patients, such as those with depressed right ventricular function or severe tricuspid regurgitation.

The first successful palliation of HLHS was reported by Norwood et al. on a series of infants operated on between 1979 and 1981.[161] This procedure has been technically refined over the years, but three essential components remain: atrial septectomy, anastomosis of the proximal PA to the aorta with homograft augmentation of the aortic arch, and aortopulmonary shunt or right ventricle–PA conduit (Fig. 81.11). As described previously for the univentricular heart, subsequent reconstructive management of HLHS includes an interim hemi-Fontan procedure or bidirectional Glenn anastomosis at 4 to 6 months of age, followed by a Fontan procedure at about 18 to 24 months.

Universally fatal only two decades ago, tremendous strides have been made in improving the outcomes for patients with HLHS. Of the three stages, the highest-risk stage of the repair remains the Norwood operation. During the 1990s, the hospital survival for the Norwood procedure across the United States was approximately 40%.[162] Currently, select centers have reported hospital survivals of 90% or greater.[163–167] Reported survivals for the hemi-Fontan and Fontan procedures have also been excellent at 98% for both operations.[155,157,168]

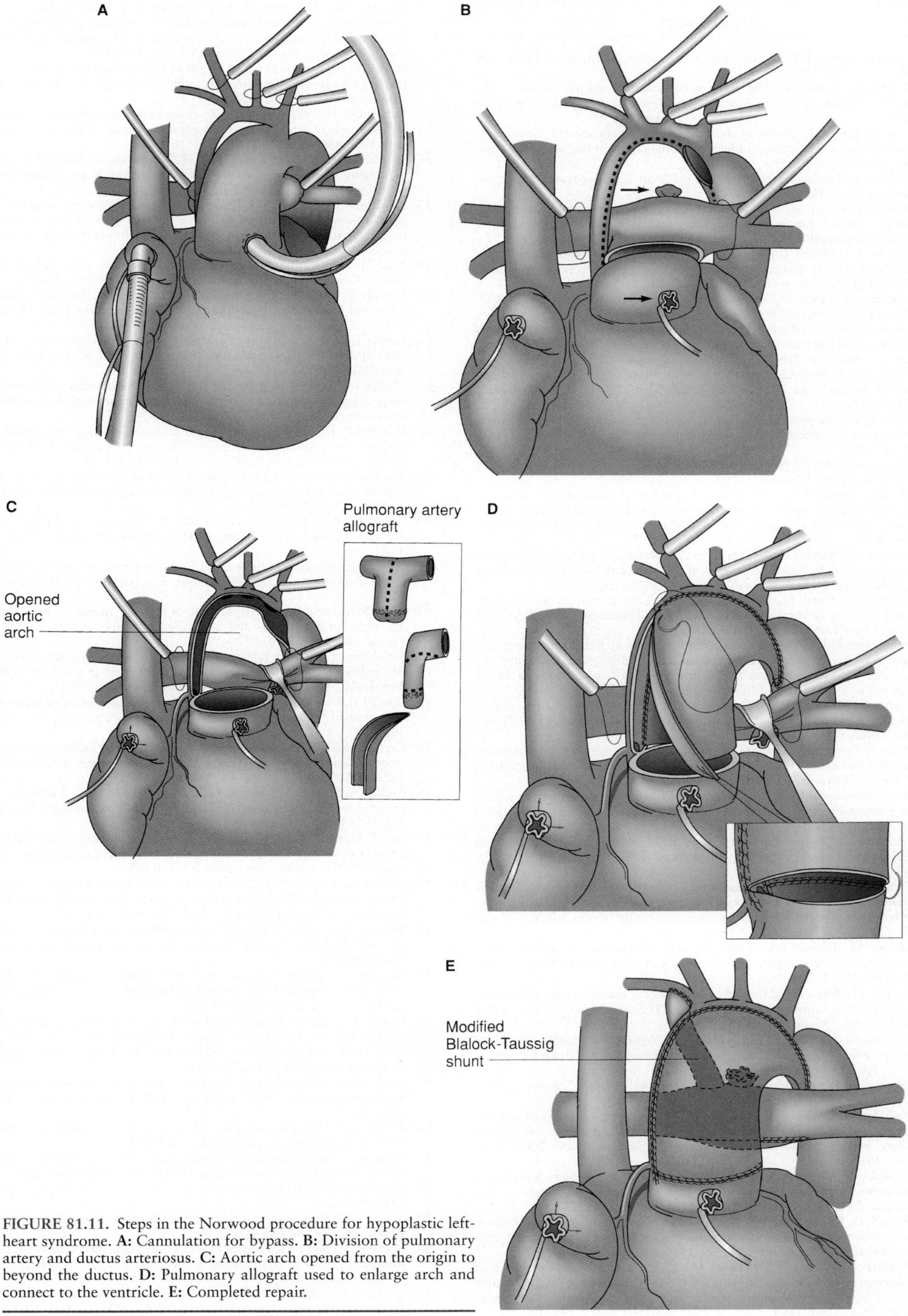

FIGURE 81.11. Steps in the Norwood procedure for hypoplastic left-heart syndrome. **A:** Cannulation for bypass. **B:** Division of pulmonary artery and ductus arteriosus. **C:** Aortic arch opened from the origin to beyond the ductus. **D:** Pulmonary allograft used to enlarge arch and connect to the ventricle. **E:** Completed repair.

References

1. Gross R, Hubbard J. Surgical ligation of a patent ductus arteriosus. *JAMA* 1939;112:729–731.
2. Blalock A, Taussig H. The surgical treatment of malformations of the heart in which there is pulmonary stenosis or atresia. *JAMA* 1945;128: 189.
3. Lewis F, Taufic M. Closure of atrial septal defects with the aid of hypothermia: experimental accomplishments and the report of one successful case. *Surgery* 1953;33:53–59.
4. Gibbon J. Application of a mechanical heart-lung apparatus to cardiac surgery. *Minn Med* 1954;37:171.
5. Warden E, Cohen M, Read C. Controlled cross-circulation for open intracardiac surgery: physiologic studies and results of creation and closure of ventricular septal defects. *J Thorac Surg* 1954;28:331–343.
6. Kirklin J, DuShane J, Patrick R. Intracardiac surgery with the aid of a mechanical pump-oxygenator system (Gibbon type): report of eight cases. *Proc Staff Meet Mayo Clin* 1955;30:201–206.
7. Hoffman JI, Kaplan S. The incidence of congenital heart disease. *J Am Coll Cardiol* 2002;39(12):1890–900.
8. Hagen PT, Scholz DG, Edwards WD. Incidence and size of patent foramen ovale during the first 10 decades of life: an autopsy study of 965 normal hearts. *Mayo Clin Proc* 1984;59(1):17–20.
9. Hopkins RA, Bert AA, Buchholz B, et al. Surgical patch closure of atrial septal defects. *Ann Thorac Surg* 2004;77(6):2144–2149; author reply 2149–2150.
10. King TD, Thompson SL, Steiner C, et al. Secundum atrial septal defect. Nonoperative closure during cardiac catheterization. *JAMA* 1976; 235(23): 2506–2509.
11. O'Laughlin MP. Catheter closure of secundum atrial septal defects. *Tex Heart Inst J* 1997;24(4):287–292.
12. Du ZD, Koenig P, Cao QL, et al. Comparison of transcatheter closure of secundum atrial septal defect using the Amplatzer septal occluder associated with deficient versus sufficient rims. *Am J Cardiol* 2002;90(8): 865–869.
13. Everett AD, Jennings J, Sibinga E, et al. Community use of the Amplatzer atrial septal defect occluder: results of the multicenter MAGIC Atrial Septal Defect Study. *Pediatr Cardiol* 2008;30(3):240–247.
14. Murphy JG, Gersh BJ, McGoon MD, et al. Long-term outcome after surgical repair of isolated atrial septal defect. Follow-up at 27 to 32 years. *N Engl J Med* 1990;323(24):1645–1650.
15. Roos-Hesselink JW, Meijboom FJ, Spitaels SE, et al. Excellent survival and low incidence of arrhythmias, stroke and heart failure long-term after surgical ASD closure at young age. A prospective follow-up study of 21–33 years. *Eur Heart J* 2003;24(2):190–197.
16. Gatzoulis MA, Freeman MA, Siu SC, et al. Atrial arrhythmia after surgical closure of atrial septal defects in adults. *N Engl J Med* 1999;340(11): 839–846.
17. Attie F, Rosas M, Granados N, et al. Surgical treatment for secundum atrial septal defects in patients >40 years old. A randomized clinical trial. *J Am Coll Cardiol* 2001;38(7):2035–2042.
18. Konstantinides S, Geibel A, Olschewski M, et al. A comparison of surgical and medical therapy for atrial septal defect in adults. *N Engl J Med* 1995; 333(8):469–473.
19. Momma K, Toyama K, Takao A, et al. Natural history of subarterial infundibular ventricular septal defect. *Am Heart J* 1984;108(5): 1312–1317.
20. Heath D, Edwards JE. The pathology of hypertensive pulmonary vascular disease; a description of six grades of structural changes in the pulmonary arteries with special reference to congenital cardiac septal defects. *Circulation* 1958;18(4 Part 1):533–547.
21. Dajani AS, Taubert KA, Wilson W, et al. Prevention of bacterial endocarditis. Recommendations by the American Heart Association. *Circulation* 1997;96(1):358–366.
22. Backer CL, Idriss FS, Zales VR, et al. Surgical management of the conal (supracristal) ventricular septal defect. *J Thorac Cardiovasc Surg* 1991; 102(2):288–295; discussion 295–296.
23. Mavroudis C, Backer CL, Jacobs JP. Ventricular septal defect. In: Mavroudis C, Backer CL, eds. *Pediatric Cardiac Surgery*, 3rd ed. Philadelphia, PA: Mosby; 2003 298–320.
24. Hijazi ZM. Device closure of ventricular septal defects. *Catheter Cardiovasc Interv* 2003;60(1):107–114.
25. Crossland DS, Wilkinson JL, Cochrane AD, et al. Initial results of primary device closure of large muscular ventricular septal defects in early infancy using perventricular access. *Catheter Cardiovasc Interv* 2008;72(3): 386–391.
26. Predescu D, Chaturvedi RR, Friedberg MK, et al. Complete heart block associated with device closure of perimembranous ventricular septal defects. *J Thorac Cardiovasc Surg* 2008;136(5):1223–1228.
27. Rastelli G, Kirklin JW, Titus JL. Anatomic observations on complete form of persistent common atrioventricular canal with special reference to atrioventricular valves. *Mayo Clin Proc* 1966;41(5):296–308.
28. Bharati S, Kirklin JW, McAllister HA Jr, et al. The surgical anatomy of common atrioventricular orifice associated with tetralogy of Fallot, double outlet right ventricle and complete regular transposition. *Circulation* 1980;61(6):1142–1149.
29. Draulans-Noe HA, Wenink AC, Quaegebeur J. Single papillary muscle ("parachute valve") and double-orifice left ventricle in atrioventricular septal defect convergence of chordal attachment: surgical anatomy and results of surgery. *Pediatr Cardiol* 1990;11(1):29–35.
30. Studer M, Blackstone EH, Kirklin JW, et al. Determinants of early and late results of repair of atrioventricular septal (canal) defects. *J Thorac Cardiovasc Surg* 1982;84(4):523–542.
31. Piccoli GP, Ho SY, Wilkinson JL, et al. Left-sided obstructive lesions in atrioventricular septal defects: an anatomic study. *J Thorac Cardiovasc Surg* 1982;83(3):453–460.
32. Schulze-Neick I, Hartenstein P, Li J, et al. Intravenous sildenafil is a potent pulmonary vasodilator in children with congenital heart disease. *Circulation* 2003;108(suppl 1):II167–II173.
33. Weintraub RG, Brawn WJ, Venables AW, et al. Two-patch repair of complete atrioventricular septal defect in the first year of life. Results and sequential assessment of atrioventricular valve function. *J Thorac Cardiovasc Surg* 1990;99(2):320–326.
34. Puga FJ. Reoperation after repair of atrioventricular canal defects. *Semin Thorac Cardiovasc Surg Pediatr Card Surg Annu* 1998;1:123–128.
35. Stewart S, Alexson C, Manning J. Partial atrioventricular canal defect: the early and late results of operation. *Ann Thorac Surg* 1987;43(5):527–529.
36. Suzuki T, Bove EL, Devaney EJ, et al. Results of definitive repair of complete atrioventricular septal defect in neonates and infants. *Ann Thorac Surg* 2008;86(2):596–602.
37. Minich LL, Tani LY, Pagotto LT, et al. Size of ventricular structures influences surgical outcome in Down syndrome infants with atrioventricular septal defect. *Am J Cardiol* 1998;81(8):1062–1065.
38. Hanley FL, Fenton KN, Jonas RA, et al. Surgical repair of complete atrioventricular canal defects in infancy. Twenty-year trends. *J Thorac Cardiovasc Surg* 1993;106(3):387–394; discussion 394–397.
39. Van Praagh R, Van Praagh S, Nebesar RA, et al. Tetralogy of Fallot: underdevelopment of the pulmonary infundibulum and its sequelae. *Am J Cardiol* 1970;26(1):25–33.
40. Hirsch JC, Bove EL. Tetralogy of Fallot. In: Mavroudis C, Backer CL, eds. *Pediatric Cardiac Surgery*, 3rd ed. Philadelphia, PA: Mosby; 2003 383–397.
41. Hirsch JC, Mosca RS, Bove EL. Complete repair of tetralogy of Fallot in the neonate: results in the modern era. *Ann Surg* 2000;232(4):508–514.
42. Tamesberger MI, Lechner E, Mair R, et al. Early primary repair of tetralogy of Fallot in neonates and infants less than four months of age. *Ann Thorac Surg* 2008;86(6):1928–1935.
43. de Ruijter FT, Weenink I, Hitchcock FJ, et al. Right ventricular dysfunction and pulmonary valve replacement after correction of tetralogy of Fallot. *Ann Thorac Surg* 2002;73(6):1794–1800; discussion 1800.
44. Discigil B, Dearani JA, Puga FJ, et al. Late pulmonary valve replacement after repair of tetralogy of Fallot. *Thorac Cardiovasc Surg* 2001;121(2): 344–351.
45. Karl TR, Sano S, Pornviliwan S, et al. Tetralogy of Fallot: favorable outcome of nonneonatal transatrial, transpulmonary repair. *Ann Thorac Surg* 1992;54(5):903–907.
46. Bacha EA, Scheule AM, Zurakowski D, et al. Long-term results after early primary repair of tetralogy of Fallot. *J Thorac Cardiovasc Surg* 2001; 122(1):154–161.
47. Belli E, Serraf A, Lacour-Gayet F, et al. Biventricular repair for double-outlet right ventricle. Results and long-term follow-up. *Circulation* 1998;98 (suppl 19):II360–II365; discussion II365–II367.
48. Kirklin JW, Pacifico AD, Blackstone EH, et al. Current risks and protocols for operations for double-outlet right ventricle. Derivation from an 18 year experience. *J Thorac Cardiovasc Surg* 1986;92(5):913–930.
49. Walters HI, Pacifico A. Double outlet ventricles. In: Mavroudis C, Backer CL, eds. *Pediatric Cardiac Surgery*, 3rd ed. Philadelphia, PA: Mosby; 2003:408–441.
50. Musumeci F, Shumway S, Lincoln C, et al. Surgical treatment for double-outlet right ventricle at the Brompton Hospital, 1973 to 1986. *J Thorac Cardiovasc Surg* 1988;96(2):278–287.
51. Kirklin J. Complete transposition of the great arteries. In: Kirklin J, ed. *Cardiac Surgery*. New York: Churchill Livingston; 1993:1383–1467.
52. Fyler D. Report of the New England regional infant cardiac program. *Pediatrics* 1980;65(2 Pt 2):375–461.
53. Levin DL, Paul MH, Muster AJ, et al. d-Transposition of the great vessels in the neonate. A clinical diagnosis. *Arch Intern Med* 1977;137(10): 1421–1425.
54. Rashkind WJ. Historical aspects of surgery for congenital heart disease. *J Thorac Cardiovasc Surg* 1982;84(4):619–625.
55. Liebman J. Natural history of transposition of the great arteries: anatomy and birth and death characteristics. *Circulation* 1969;40:237–262.
56. Senning A. Surgical correction of transposition of the great vessels. *Surgery* 1959;45:966.
57. Mustard W. Successful two stage correction of transposition of the great vessels. *Surgery* 1964;55:469.
58. Jatene AD, Fontes VF, Paulista PP, et al. Successful anatomic correction of transposition of the great vessels. A preliminary report. *Arq Bras Cardiol* 1975;28(4):461–464.
59. Qamar ZA, Goldberg CS, Devaney EJ, et al. Current risk factors and outcomes for the arterial switch operation. *Ann Thorac Surg* 2007;84(3): 871–878; discussion 878–879.

60. Brown JW, Park HJ, Turrentine MW. Arterial switch operation: factors impacting survival in the current era. *Ann Thorac Surg* 2001;71(6): 1978–1984.
61. Haas F, Wottke M, Poppert H, et al. Long-term survival and functional follow-up in patients after the arterial switch operation. *Ann Thorac Surg* 1999;68(5):1692–1697.
62. Losay J, Touchot A, Serraf A, et al. Late outcome after arterial switch operation for transposition of the great arteries. *Circulation* 2001;104(12) (suppl 1):I121–I126.
63. Gottlieb D, Schwartz ML, Bischoff K, et al. Predictors of outcome of arterial switch operation for complex D-transposition. *Ann Thorac Surg* 2008;85(5):1698–1702; discussion 1702–1703.
64. Blume ED, Altmann K, Mayer JE, et al. Evolution of risk factors influencing early mortality of the arterial switch operation. *J Am Coll Cardiol* 1999;33(6):1702–1709.
65. Schwartz ML, Gauvreau K, del Nido P, et al. Long-term predictors of aortic root dilation and aortic regurgitation after arterial switch operation. *Circulation* 2004;110(11)(suppl 1):II128–II132.
66. Rowe R, Freedom R, Mehrizi A. *The Neonate with Congenital Heart Disease*. Philadelphia, PA: WB Saunders; 1981.
67. Calder L, Van Praagh R, Van Praagh S, et al. Truncus arteriosus communis. Clinical, angiocardiographic, and pathologic findings in 100 patients. *Am Heart J* 1976;92(1):23–38.
68. Tandon R, Hauck AJ, Nadas AS. Persistent truncus arteriosus. A clinical, hemodynamic, and autopsy study of nineteen cases. *Circulation* 1963;28: 1050–1060.
69. Collett R, Edwards J. Persistent truncus arteriosus: a classification according to anatomic type. *Surg Clin North Am* 1949;29:1245.
70. Van Praagh R, Van Praagh S. The anatomy of common aorticopulmonary trunk (truncus arteriosus communis) and its embryologic implications: a study of 57 necropsy cases. *Am J Cardiol* 1965;16:406.
71. Fuglestad SJ, Puga FJ, Danielson GK, et al. Surgical pathology of the truncal valve: a study of 12 cases. *Am J Cardiovasc Pathol* 1988;2(1): 39–47.
72. Urban AE, Sinzobahamvya N, Brecher AM, et al. Truncus arteriosus: ten-year experience with homograft repair in neonates and infants. *Ann Thorac Surg* 1998;66(6 suppl):S183–S188.
73. Lacour-Gayet F, Serraf A, Komiya T, et al. Truncus arteriosus repair: influence of techniques of right ventricular outflow tract reconstruction. *J Thorac Cardiovasc Surg* 1996;111(4):849–856.
74. Bove EL, Lupinetti FM, Pridjian AK, et al. Results of a policy of primary repair of truncus arteriosus in the neonate. *J Thorac Cardiovasc Surg* 1993;105(6):1057–1065; discussion 1065–1065.
75. Marcelletti C, McGoon DC, Danielson GK, et al. Early and late results of surgical repair of truncus arteriosus. *Circulation* 1977;55(4):636–641.
76. Nath PH, Zollikofer C, Castaneda-Zuniga W, et al. Persistent truncus arteriosus associated with interruption of the aortic arch. *Br J Radiol* 1980; 53(633):853–859.
77. Butto F, Lucas RV Jr, Edwards JE. Persistent truncus arteriosus: pathologic anatomy in 54 cases. *Pediatr Cardiol* 1986;7(2):95–101.
78. Bharati S, McAllister HA Jr, Rosenquist GC, et al. The surgical anatomy of truncus arteriosus communis. *J Thorac Cardiovasc Surg* 1974;67(4): 501–510.
79. Shrivastava S, Edwards JE. Coronary arterial origin in persistent truncus arteriosus. *Circulation* 1977;55(3):551–554.
80. Kirklin J, Barrat-Boyes B. *Cardiac Surgery*. New York: John Wiley & Sons; 1993.
81. Backer CL. Techniques for repairing the aortic and truncal valves. *Cardiol Young* 2005;15(suppl 1):125–131.
82. Ebert PA, Turley K, Stanger P, et al. Surgical treatment of truncus arteriosus in the first 6 months of life. *Ann Surg* 1984;200(4):451–456.
83. Brown JW, Ruzmetov M, Okada Y, et al. Truncus arteriosus repair: outcomes, risk factors, reoperation and management. *Eur J Cardiothorac Surg* 2001;20(2):221–227.
84. Thompson LD, McElhinney DB, Reddy M, et al. Neonatal repair of truncus arteriosus: continuing improvement in outcomes. *Ann Thorac Surg* 2001;72(2):391–395.
85. Konstantinov IE, Karamlou T, Blackstone EH, et al. Truncus arteriosus associated with interrupted aortic arch in 50 neonates: a Congenital Heart Surgeons Society study. *Ann Thorac Surg* 2006;81(1):214–222.
86. Hanley FL, Heinemann MK, Jonas RA, et al. Repair of truncus arteriosus in the neonate. *J Thorac Cardiovasc Surg* 1993;105(6):1047–1056.
87. Rajasinghe HA, McElhinney DB, Reddy VM, et al. Long-term follow-up of truncus arteriosus repaired in infancy: a twenty-year experience. *J Thorac Cardiovasc Surg* 1997;113(5):869–878; discussion 878–879.
88. Selamet Tierney ES, Wald RM, McElhinney DB, et al. Changes in left heart hemodynamics after technically successful in-utero aortic valvuloplasty. *Ultrasound Obstet Gynecol* 2007;30(5):715–720.
89. Makikallio K, McElhinney DB, Levine JC, et al. Fetal aortic valve stenosis and the evolution of hypoplastic left heart syndrome: patient selection for fetal intervention. *Circulation* 2006;113(11):1401–1405.
90. Tworetzky W, Wilkins-Haug L, Jennings RW, et al. Balloon dilation of severe aortic stenosis in the fetus: potential for prevention of hypoplastic left heart syndrome: candidate selection, technique, and results of successful intervention. *Circulation* 2004;110(15):2125–2131.
91. McCrindle BW, Blackstone EH, Williams WG, et al. Are outcomes of surgical versus transcatheter balloon valvotomy equivalent in neonatal critical aortic stenosis? *Circulation* 2001;104(12)(suppl 1):I152–I158.
92. Cowley CG, Dietrich M, Mosca RS, et al. Balloon valvuloplasty versus transventricular dilation for neonatal critical aortic stenosis. *Am J Cardiol* 2001;87(9):1125–1127, A10.
93. Ross DN. Replacement of aortic and mitral valves with a pulmonary autograft. *Lancet* 1967;2(7523):956–958.
94. Konno S, Imai Y, Iida Y, et al. A new method for prosthetic valve replacement in congenital aortic stenosis associated with hypoplasia of the aortic valve ring. *J Thorac Cardiovasc Surg* 1975;70(5):909–917.
95. Ohye RG, Gomez CA, Ohye BJ, et al. The Ross/Konno procedure in neonates and infants: intermediate-term survival and autograft function. *Ann Thorac Surg* 2001;72(3):823–830.
96. Moore P, Egito E, Mowrey H, et al. Midterm results of balloon dilation of congenital aortic stenosis: predictors of success. *J Am Coll Cardiol* 1996; 27(5):1257–1263.
97. Chartrand CC, Saro-Servando E, Vobecky JS. Long-term results of surgical valvuloplasty for congenital valvar aortic stenosis in children. *Ann Thorac Surg* 1999;68(4):1356–1359; discussion 1359–1360.
98. Lupinetti FM, Pridjian AK, Callow LB, et al. Optimum treatment of discrete subaortic stenosis. *Ann Thorac Surg* 1992;54(3):467–470; discussion 470–471.
99. Rayburn ST, Netherland DE, Heath BJ. Discrete membranous subaortic stenosis: improved results after resection and myectomy. *Ann Thorac Surg* 1997;64(1):105–109.
100. Jahangiri M, Nicholson IA, del Nido PJ, et al. Surgical management of complex and tunnel-like subaortic stenosis. *Eur J Cardiothorac Surg* 2000; 17(6):637–642.
101. Chowdhury T, Reardon W. Elastin mutation and cardiac disease. *Pediatr Cardiol* 1999;20(2):103–107.
102. McElhinney DB, Petrossian E, Tworetzky W, et al. Issues and outcomes in the management of supravalvar aortic stenosis. *Ann Thorac Surg* 2000; 69(2):562–567.
103. Stamm C, Kreutzer C, Zurakowski D, et al. Forty-one years of surgical experience with congenital supravalvular aortic stenosis. *J Thorac Cardiovasc Surg* 1999;118(5):874–885.
104. Brown JW, Ruzmetov M, Vijay P, et al. Surgical repair of congenital supravalvular aortic stenosis in children. *Eur J Cardiothorac Surg* 2002; 21(1):50–56.
105. Reifenstein GH, Levine SA, Gross RE. Coarctation of the aorta. A review of 104 autopsied cases of the "adult type," 2 years of age or older. *Am Heart J* 1947;33(2):146–168.
106. Backer CL, Mavroudis C, Zias EA, et al. Repair of coarctation with resection and extended end-to-end anastomosis. *Ann Thorac Surg* 1998;66(4): 1365–1370; discussion 1370–1371.
107. Backer CL, Paape K, Zales VR, et al. Coarctation of the aorta. Repair with polytetrafluoroethylene patch aortoplasty. *Circulation* 1995;92(9 suppl): II132–II136.
108. del Nido PJ, Williams WG, Wilson GJ, et al. Synthetic patch angioplasty for repair of coarctation of the aorta: experience with aneurysm formation. *Circulation* 1986;74(3 Pt 2):I32–I326.
109. Wong CH, Watson B, Smith J, et al. The use of left heart bypass in adult and recurrent coarctation repair. *Eur J Cardiothorac Surg* 2001;20(6): 1199–1201.
110. Brewer LA III, Fosburg RG, Mulder GA, et al. Spinal cord complications following surgery for coarctation of the aorta. A study of 66 cases. *J Thorac Cardiovasc Surg* 1972;64(3):368–381.
111. Seirafi PA, Warner KG, Geggel RL, et al. Repair of coarctation of the aorta during infancy minimizes the risk of late hypertension. *Ann Thorac Surg* 1998;66(4):1378–1382.
112. Hornung TS, Benson LN, McLaughlin PR. Interventions for aortic coarctation. *Cardiol Rev* 2002;10(3):139–148.
113. Karl TR. Surgery is the best treatment for primary coarctation in the majority of cases. *J Cardiovasc Med (Hagerstown)* 2007;8(1):50–56.
114. Golden AB, Hellenbrand WE. Coarctation of the aorta: stenting in children and adults. *Catheter Cardiovasc Interv* 2007;69(2):289–299.
115. Tynan M, Finley JP, Fontes V, et al. Balloon angioplasty for the treatment of native coarctation: results of Valvuloplasty and Angioplasty of Congenital Anomalies Registry. *Am J Cardiol* 1990;65(11):790–792.
116. Ovaert C, McCrindle BW, Nykanen D, et al. Balloon angioplasty of native coarctation: clinical outcomes and predictors of success. *J Am Coll Cardiol* 2000;35(4):988–996.
117. Cooper RS, Ritter SB, Rothe WB, et al. Angioplasty for coarctation of the aorta: long-term results. *Circulation* 1987;75(3):600–604.
118. Hellenbrand WE, Allen HD, Golinko RJ, et al. Balloon angioplasty for aortic recoarctation: results of Valvuloplasty and Angioplasty of Congenital Anomalies Registry. *Am J Cardiol* 1990;65(11):793–797.
119. Hijazi ZM, Fahey JT, Kleinman CS, et al. Balloon angioplasty for recurrent coarctation of aorta. Immediate and long-term results. *Circulation* 1991;84(3):1150–1156.
120. Yetman AT, Nykanen D, McCrindle BW, et al. Balloon angioplasty of recurrent coarctation: a 12-year review. *J Am Coll Cardiol* 1997;30(3): 811–816.
121. van Heurn LW, Wong CM, Spiegelhalter DJ, et al. Surgical treatment of aortic coarctation in infants younger than three months: 1985 to 1990. Success of extended end-to-end arch aortoplasty. *J Thorac Cardiovasc Surg* 1994;107(1):74–85; discussion 85–86.
122. Presbitero P, Demarie D, Villani M, et al. Long term results (15–30 years) of surgical repair of aortic coarctation. *Br Heart J* 1987;57(5): 462–467.

123. Wright GE, Nowak CA, Goldberg CS, et al. Extended resection and end-to-end anastomosis for aortic coarctation in infants: results of a tailored surgical approach. *Ann Thorac Surg* 2005;80(4):1453–1459.
124. Siassi B, Blanco C, Cabal LA, et al. Incidence and clinical features of patent ductus arteriosus in low-birthweight infants: a prospective analysis of 150 consecutively born infants. *Pediatrics* 1976;57(3):347–351.
125. Elliott RB, Starling MB, Neutze JM. Medical manipulation of the ductus arteriosus. *Lancet* 1975;1(7899):140–142.
126. Campbell M. Natural history of persistent ductus arteriosus. *Br Heart J* 1968;30(1):4–13.
127. Heymann MA, Rudolph AM, Silverman NH. Closure of the ductus arteriosus in premature infants by inhibition of prostaglandin synthesis. *N Engl J Med* 1976;295(10):530–533.
128. Sekar KC, Corff KE. Treatment of patent ductus arteriosus: indomethacin or ibuprofen? *J Perinatol* 2008;28(suppl 1):S60–S62.
129. Gersony WM, Peckham GJ, Ellison RC, et al. Effects of indomethacin in premature infants with patent ductus arteriosus: results of a national collaborative study. *J Pediatr* 1983;102(6):895–906.
130. Coster DD, Gorton ME, Grooters RK, et al. Surgical closure of the patent ductus arteriosus in the neonatal intensive care unit. *Ann Thorac Surg* 1989;48(3):386–389.
131. Taylor RL, Grover FL, Harman PK, et al. Operative closure of patent ductus arteriosus in premature infants in the neonatal intensive care unit. *Am J Surg* 1986;152(6):704–708.
132. Burke RP, Jacobs JP, Cheng W, et al. Video-assisted thoracoscopic surgery for patent ductus arteriosus in low birth weight neonates and infants. *Pediatrics* 1999;104(2 Pt 1):227–230.
133. Cowley CG, Lloyd TR. Interventional cardiac catheterization advances in nonsurgical approaches to congenital heart disease. *Curr Opin Pediatr* 1999;11(5):425–432.
134. Goyal VS, Fulwani MC, Ramakantan R, et al. Follow-up after coil closure of patent ductus arteriosus. *Am J Cardiol* 1999;83(3):463–466, A10.
135. Patel HT, Cao QL, Rhodes J, et al. Long-term outcome of transcatheter coil closure of small to large patent ductus arteriosus. *Catheter Cardiovasc Interv* 1999;47(4):457–461.
136. Omari BO, Shapiro S, Ginzton L, et al. Closure of short, wide patent ductus arteriosus with cardiopulmonary bypass and balloon occlusion. *Ann Thorac Surg* 1998;66(1):277–278.
137. Goncalves-Estella A, Perez-Villoria J, Gonzalez-Reoyo F, et al. Closure of a complicated ductus arteriosus through the transpulmonary route using hypothermia. Surgical considerations in one case. *J Thorac Cardiovasc Surg* 1975;69(5):698–702.
138. Backer CL, Mavroudis C, Rigsby CK, et al. Trends in vascular ring surgery. *J Thorac Cardiovasc Surg* 2005;129(6):1339–1347.
139. Woods RK, Sharp RJ, Holcomb GW III, et al. Vascular anomalies and tracheoesophageal compression: a single institution's 25-year experience. *Ann Thorac Surg* 2001;72(2):434–438; discussion 438–439.
140. Backer CL, Mavroudis C, Dunham ME, et al. Pulmonary artery sling: results with median sternotomy, cardiopulmonary bypass, and reimplantation. *Ann Thorac Surg* 1999; 67(6):1738–1744; discussion 1744–1745.
141. Koontz CS, Bhatia A, Forbess J, et al. Video-assisted thoracoscopic division of vascular rings in pediatric patients. *Am Surg* 2005;71(4):289–291.
142. Alsenaidi K, Gurofsky R, Karamlou T, et al. Management and outcomes of double aortic arch in 81 patients. *Pediatrics* 2006;118(5):e1336–e1341.
143. Alexander RW, Griffith GC. Anomalies of the coronary arteries and their clinical significance. *Circulation* 1956;14(5):800–805.
144. Yamanaka O, Hobbs RE. Coronary artery anomalies in 126,595 patients undergoing coronary arteriography. *Cathet Cardiovasc Diagn* 1990;21(1):28–40.
145. Dodge-Khatami A, Mavroudis C, Backer CL. Congenital Heart Surgery Nomenclature and Database Project: anomalies of the coronary arteries. *Ann Thorac Surg* 2000;69(4 suppl):S270–S297.
146. Dodge-Khatami A, Mavroudis C, Backer CL. Anomalous origin of the left coronary artery from the pulmonary artery: collective review of surgical therapy. *Ann Thorac Surg* 2002;74(3):946–955.
147. Huddleston CB, Balzer DT, Mendeloff EN. Repair of anomalous left main coronary artery arising from the pulmonary artery in infants: long-term impact on the mitral valve. *Ann Thorac Surg* 2001;71(6):1985–1988; discussion 1988–1989.
148. Ando M, Mee RB, Duncan BW, et al. Creation of a dual-coronary system for anomalous origin of the left coronary artery from the pulmonary artery utilizing the trapdoor flap method. *Eur J Cardiothorac Surg* 2002;22(4):576–581.
149. Schwartz ML, Jonas RA, Colan SD. Anomalous origin of left coronary artery from pulmonary artery: recovery of left ventricular function after dual coronary repair. *J Am Coll Cardiol* 1997;30(2):547–553.
150. Basso C, Maron BJ, Corrado D, et al. Clinical profile of congenital coronary artery anomalies with origin from the wrong aortic sinus leading to sudden death in young competitive athletes. *J Am Coll Cardiol* 2000; 35(6):1493–1501.
151. Frommelt PC, Frommelt MA. Congenital coronary artery anomalies. *Pediatr Clin North Am* 2004;51(5):1273–1288.
152. Hawkins JA, Thorne JK, Boucek MM, et al. Early and late results in pulmonary atresia and intact ventricular septum. *J Thorac Cardiovasc Surg* 1990;100(4):492–497.
153. Fontan F, Fernandez G, Costa F, et al. The size of the pulmonary arteries and the results of the Fontan operation. *J Thorac Cardiovasc Surg* 1989;98(5 Pt 1):711–719; discussion 719–724.
154. Cetta F, Feldt RH, O'Leary PW, et al. Improved early morbidity and mortality after Fontan operation: the Mayo Clinic experience, 1987 to 1992. *J Am Coll Cardiol* 1996;28(2):480–486.
155. Bove EL. Current status of staged reconstruction for hypoplastic left heart syndrome. *Pediatr Cardiol* 1998;19(4):308–315.
156. Stamm C, Friehs I, Mayer JE Jr, et al. Long-term results of the lateral tunnel Fontan operation. *J Thorac Cardiovasc Surg* 2001;121(1):28–41.
157. Hirsch JC, Goldberg C, Bove EL, et al. Fontan operation in the current era: a 15-year single institution experience. *Ann Surg* 2008;248(3):402–410.
158. Hirsch JC, Ohye RG, Devaney EJ, et al. The lateral tunnel Fontan procedure for hypoplastic left heart syndrome: results of 100 consecutive patients. *Pediatr Cardiol* 2007;28(6):426–432.
159. Bailey LL, Gundry SR, Razzouk AJ, et al. Bless the babies: one hundred fifteen late survivors of heart transplantation during the first year of life. The Loma Linda University Pediatric Heart Transplant Group. *J Thorac Cardiovasc Surg* 1993;105(5):805–814; discussion 814–815.
160. Jenkins PC, Flanagan MF, Sargent JD, et al. A comparison of treatment strategies for hypoplastic left heart syndrome using decision analysis. *J Am Coll Cardiol* 2001;38(4):1181–1187.
161. Norwood WI, Lang P, Casteneda AR, et al. Experience with operations for hypoplastic left heart syndrome. *J Thorac Cardiovasc Surg* 1981;82(4):511–519.
162. Gutgesell HP, Gibson J. Management of hypoplastic left heart syndrome in the 1990s. *Am J Cardiol* 2002;89(7):842–846.
163. Azakie A, Martinez D, Sapru A, et al. Impact of right ventricle to pulmonary artery conduit on outcome of the modified Norwood procedure. *Ann Thorac Surg* 2004;77(5):1727–1733.
164. Mair R, Tulzer G, Sames E, et al. Right ventricular to pulmonary artery conduit instead of modified Blalock-Taussig shunt improves postoperative hemodynamics in newborns after the Norwood operation. *J Thorac Cardiovasc Surg* 2003;126(5):1378–1384.
165. Pizarro C, Malec E, Maher KO, et al. Right ventricle to pulmonary artery conduit improves outcome after stage I Norwood for hypoplastic left heart syndrome. *Circulation* 2003;108(Suppl 1):II155–II160.
166. Sano S, Ishino K, Kawada M, et al. Right ventricle-pulmonary artery shunt in first-stage palliation of hypoplastic left heart syndrome. *J Thorac Cardiovasc Surg* 2003;126(2):504–509; discussion 509–510.
167. Hirsch JC, Gurney JG, Donohue JE, et al. Hospital mortality for Norwood and arterial switch operations as a function of institutional volume. *Pediatr Cardiol* 2008;29(4):713–717.
168. Douglas WI, Goldberg CS, Mosca RS, et al. Hemi-Fontan procedure for hypoplastic left heart syndrome: outcome and suitability for Fontan. *Ann Thorac Surg* 1999;68(4):1361–1367; discussion 1368.

CHAPTER 82 ■ VALVULAR HEART DISEASE AND CARDIAC TUMORS

TOMISLAV MIHALJEVIC, CRAIG M. JARRETT, AND A. MARC GILLINOV

KEY POINTS

1. The most common cause of aortic stenosis is degenerative calcific disease, followed by congenital aortic stenosis due to bicuspid valve anatomy.
2. Two-dimensional echocardiography with Doppler allows precise real-time analysis of valvular anatomy and function, and is the study of choice for the diagnosis and management of valvular lesions.
3. The current indication for cardiac catheterization in patients with valvular heart disease is limited to preoperative evaluation of coronary artery disease.
4. There is no effective medical therapy for patients with severe aortic stenosis. Mechanical relief of the obstruction to blood flow is the only effective treatment.
5. The most common causes of aortic regurgitation include bicuspid valve disease, rheumatic fever, and endocarditis.
6. Mitral stenosis is almost exclusively caused by rheumatic fever.
7. The most common cause of mitral regurgitation is degenerative mitral valve disease. Other causes include rheumatic valve disease, endocarditis, certain drugs, and collagen vascular diseases.
8. The most common cardiac tumors are secondary tumors, which usually originate from the lung in men and from the breast in women.

VALVULAR HEART DISEASE

Valvular Anatomy

The basic structural framework of all heart valves is provided by the fibrous cardiac skeleton (Fig. 82.1). The skeleton is a collection of dense connective tissue in the shape of four interconnected rings in the plane between the atria and the ventricles. The interconnecting areas include the right fibrous trigone, which is between the aortic and tricuspid rings and contiguous with the membranous septum, and the left trigone and fibrous continuity, which are between the aortic and mitral rings and form the posterior wall of the left ventricular (LV) outflow tract. The cardiac skeleton maintains the integrity of the valve orifices and provides points of attachment for the valve leaflets. It also serves as a partition by electrically isolating the atria and ventricles except at the atrioventricular bundle, which passes through the right fibrous trigone near the septal leaflet of the tricuspid valve.

The normal aortic valve (AV) consists of three semilunar leaflets or cusps projecting outward and upward into the lumen of the ascending aorta (Fig. 82.2). The space between the free edge of each leaflet and the points of attachment to the aorta comprise the sinuses of Valsalva. Since the coronary arteries arise from two of the three sinuses, the sinuses and the respective leaflets are named the right coronary, left coronary, and noncoronary (or posterior) sinuses and leaflets.

The properties of the AV ensure minimal obstruction to flow when open and minimal flow reversal when closed. Opening and closing of the valve are passive, as it functions only in response to pressure differences between the left ventricle and aorta during the cardiac cycle. The pressure generated from ventricular contraction forces the valve open, and the subsequent recoil of blood from the aorta fills the sinuses of Valsalva and forces the leaflets closed.

There are two structures in close proximity to the AV and, therefore, susceptible to injury during AV surgery (Fig. 82.2). First, the anterior leaflet of the mitral valve (MV) is positioned under the commissure between the left and noncoronary leaflets. Second, the left bundle of His is positioned under the commissure between the right and noncoronary leaflets.

In contrast to the simplistic anatomy and passive opening and closing mechanism of the AV, the anatomy and active valve mechanism of the MV are more complex. Indeed, proper functioning of the MV depends on the organized interaction of all components of the MV apparatus, which consists of the leaflets, annulus, LV papillary muscles, and chordae tendineae.

The normal MV consists of two leaflets: the anterior and posterior leaflets. The anterior leaflet is semicircular in shape, extends from the anteromedial aspect of the mitral annulus, and encompasses approximately one third of the annular circumference. The posterior leaflet is rectangular in shape, extends from the posterolateral aspect of the mitral annulus, and encompasses approximately two thirds of the annular circumference. The leaflets are separated from one another at the annulus by the posteromedial and anterolateral commissures. Both leaflets are divided by clefts into three scallops, named laterally to medially A1, A2, and A3, and P1, P2, and P3, and together comprise an average cross-sectional area of 5 to 11 cm^2.

The mitral annulus is formed anteriorly by the confluence of the right, left, and intervalvular fibrous trigones and posteriorly by a fibrous band. Since the anterior aspect of the mitral annulus is composed of the fibrous trigones, it has limited flexibility. Conversely, the posterior aspect of the annulus, which is not surrounded by any rigid structures, has more flexibility. This increased flexibility of the posterior aspect relative to the anterior aspect has important implications during the cardiac cycle. In systole the mitral annulus contracts (primarily the posterior aspect) and adopts an elliptical shape (shortening occurs perpendicular to the line of leaflet coaptation), and in diastole it relaxes and adopts a circular shape.[1,2] This dynamic motion of the annulus provides

FIGURE 82.1. Schematic diagram of the fibrous cardiac skeleton.

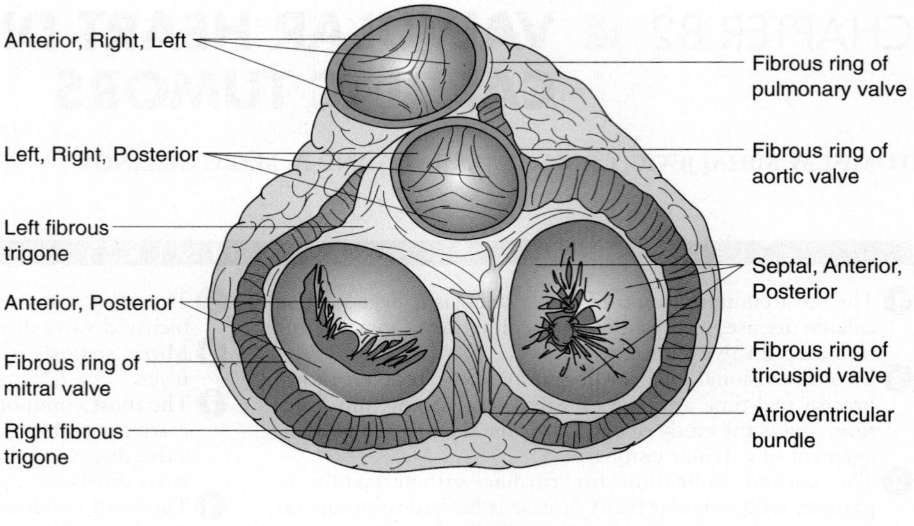

increased leaflet coaptation during systole and increased orifice area during diastole.

Two papillary muscles arise directly from the ventricular wall: the anterolateral and posteromedial papillary muscles. Importantly, the anterolateral papillary muscle usually is supplied by two coronary arteries, the left anterior descending artery and branches of the circumflex artery. On the other hand, the posteromedial papillary muscle is usually supplied by a single coronary artery, either from the right coronary or the circumflex artery, which makes it twice as likely to rupture from ischemia and infarction as the anterolateral papillary muscle. The papillary muscles play an important role in the proper function of the MV. MV closure and appropriate leaflet coaptation are permitted by end-diastolic and early systolic lengthening of the papillary muscles.[3]

Chordae tendineae attach the leaflets to the papillary muscles or directly to the ventricular wall and can be categorized based on the attachments. Primary chordae attach to the leaflets at the free edge to ensure proper coaptation without prolapse or flail. The secondary chordae attach along the line of coaptation and are more prominent on the anterior leaflet. Tertiary chordae arise directly from the ventricle or trabeculae carneae and are only present on the posterior leaflet. Lastly, commissural chordae attach to both leaflets and arise from either papillary muscle.

The structures in close proximity to the MV and, therefore, susceptible to injury during MV surgery include the AV, the atrioventricular node, and the circumflex coronary artery (Fig. 82.3).

FIGURE 82.2. Schematic diagram of the relationship of the aortic valve to the underlying structures.

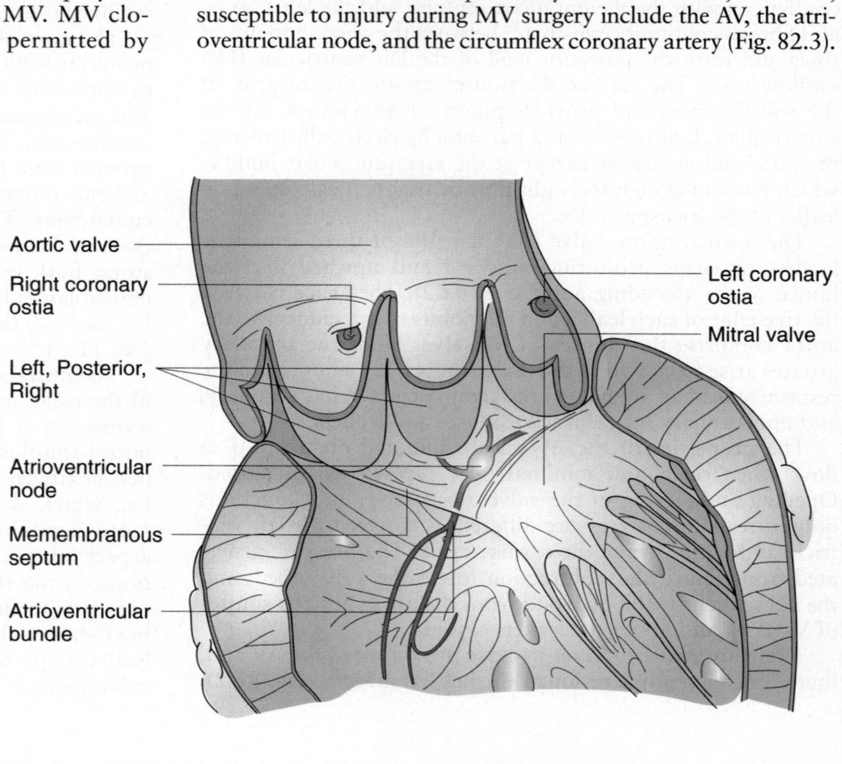

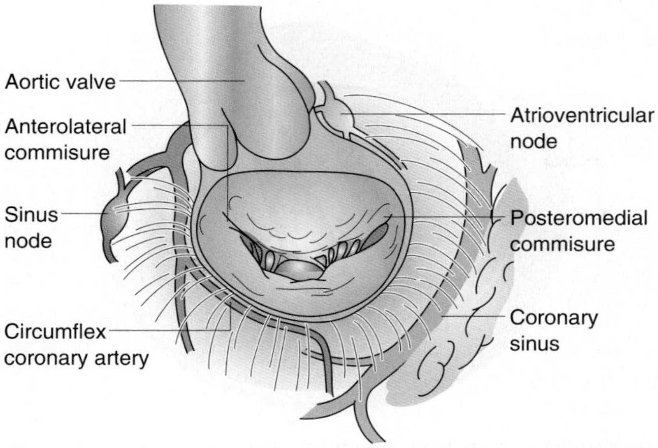

FIGURE 82.3. Schematic diagram of the relationship of the mitral valve to the underlying structures.

AORTIC STENOSIS

Prevalence and Etiology

1 Aortic stenosis (AS) is the most prevalent valvular heart disease in developed countries. The most common cause of AS is degenerative calcific disease, followed by congenital AS due to bicuspid valve anatomy. Rheumatic AS is becoming exceedingly uncommon in developed countries due to efficient prevention of rheumatic heart disease.

Degenerative Calcific Aortic Stenosis. The most frequent cause of AS is degenerative calcification of the AV. The prevalence of degenerative AS in persons older than 65 years, which is the most commonly affected age group, is 2%.[4] The degenerative process that leads to stiffening of the aortic leaflets is the result of proliferative and inflammatory changes with lipid accumulation and infiltration of macrophages and T lymphocytes.[4–9] Fibrosis and calcification initially affect the base of the leaflets, but ultimately progress to immobilization of the leaflets due to large calcific deposits that can extend deep into the annulus. These deposits may also extend onto the ventricular surface of the anterior leaflet of the MV, as well as into the wall of the ascending aorta. The risk factors for the development of calcific AS are similar to those for atherosclerosis and include elevated serum levels of low-density lipoprotein (LDL) cholesterol, diabetes, smoking, and hypertension.[10,11]

Bicuspid Aortic Stenosis. Calcification of bicuspid AVs, which are present in approximately 2% of the general population, represents the most common form of congenital AS. In patients with bicuspid AVs, the left and right coronary cusps are usually fused, while the noncoronary cusp is freestanding. Gradual calcification of the bicuspid valve results in AS with typical onset of symptoms in the fifth or sixth decade of life, in contrast to degenerative AS, which causes symptoms in elderly individuals. Bicuspid AS is frequently associated with degenerative changes in the wall of the ascending aorta with resultant dilatation or aneurysm formation.

Rheumatic Aortic Stenosis. Introduction of effective antibiotic therapy has resulted in a decline in the prevalence of rheumatic fever and rheumatic valve disease. Rheumatic AS is caused by inflammation and thickening of the AV leaflets, producing a mixture of AS and regurgitation. Rheumatic AS is rarely an isolated disease, and usually occurs in conjunction with MV stenosis.[12]

Pathophysiology

Regardless of the etiology of AS, the pathophysiologic consequences are similar. Narrowing of the AV to one quarter of its normal area of 3.0 to 4.0 cm^2 produces a significant pressure gradient between the left ventricle and aorta. There is a resultant increase in LV workload and compensatory LV hypertrophy.

Even though this hypertrophy is an appropriate response to the increased afterload, there are numerous harmful effects. First, the increased wall thickness makes the ventricle stiff and less compliant. This leads to diastolic dysfunction and increased wall tension. In addition to diastolic dysfunction, systolic dysfunction, typically occurring later in the course of the disease, can develop from chronic ischemia. All of the following contribute to increased myocardial oxygen demand: increased LV muscle mass, increased wall tension, increased systolic ventricular pressure, and increased systolic ejection time. There is also decreased coronary artery perfusion, which occurs during diastole, due to increased wall tension, increased diastolic ventricular pressure, and decreased diastolic aortic pressure.[13,14] The subsequent ischemia of the subendocardium due to increased oxygen demand and decreased perfusion leads to cell death and fibrosis. Chronically, this ischemia results in systolic dysfunction.

Diagnosis

Symptoms. The most common symptoms of AS are angina pectoris, syncope, and heart failure.[15] Angina pectoris occurs in 30% to 50% of patients with severe AS. It is a reflection of myocardial ischemia caused by increased metabolic demands and decreased coronary perfusion. Coronary artery disease, which affects more than 70% of elderly patients with degenerative AV disease, causes further deterioration of myocardial perfusion and lowers the threshold for angina.

Syncope is most commonly due to reduced cerebral perfusion that occurs during exertion. Reduced cerebral perfusion is a result of decreased mean arterial pressure from peripheral vasodilation in the presence of a fixed cardiac output. Approximately 15% of patients present with syncope and only 50% of these survive for 3 years.

Congestive heart failure in patients with severe AS is typically a sign of advanced and longstanding disease. It is marked by shortness of breath and dyspnea with exertion, and results from ongoing LV outflow obstruction. Heart failure is a consequence of the aforementioned diastolic and systolic dysfunction from decreased compliance and ischemia, respectively. In addition, as the left ventricle becomes less compliant, atrial systole becomes more important for maintaining cardiac output and the onset of atrial fibrillation may result in worsening of congestive heart failure.

Some patients with severe AS may develop serious gastrointestinal bleeding secondary to angiodysplasias, occurring predominantly in the right colon, and also in the small bowel and stomach. These result from shear stress–induced platelet aggregation with reduction in high-molecular-weight multimers of von Willebrand factor.

Signs. Signs of AS include a loud systolic ejection murmur that radiates to the neck and is often accompanied by a thrill. "Pulsus parvus et tardus" describes a weak and prolonged arterial pulse characteristic of advanced AS. The weak pulse is a reflection of a narrowed pulse pressure, while the slow rise in pulse reflects a prolonged ejection of blood volume through a stenotic valve.[16]

TABLE 82.1 **DIAGNOSIS**

CLASSIFICATION OF AORTIC STENOSIS SEVERITY

■ INDICATOR	■ MILD	■ MODERATE	■ SEVERE
Jet velocity (m/s)	<3.0	3.0–4.0	>4.0
Mean gradient (mm Hg)	<25	25–40	>40
Valve area (cm^2)	>1.5	1.0–1.5	<1.0
Valve area index (cm^2/m^2)			<0.6

Adapted from Bonow RO, Carabello BA, Chatterjee K, et al. 2008 focused update incorporated into the ACC/AHA 2006 guidelines for the management of patients with valvular heart disease. *J Am Coll Cardiol* 2008;52(13):e1–e142.

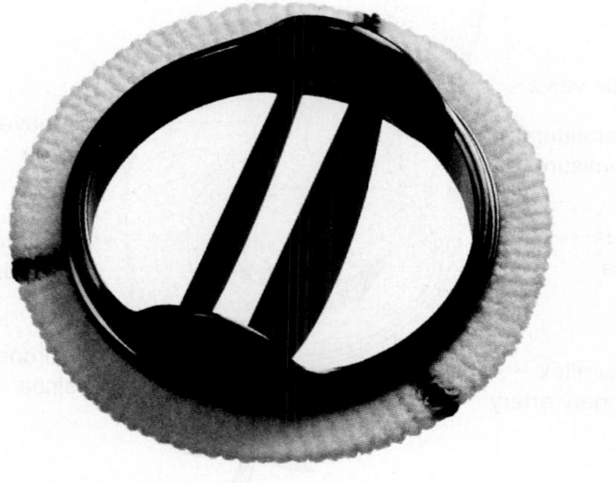

FIGURE 82.5. St. Jude Medical Regent Valve.

Electrocardiogram and Imaging. The electrocardiogram typically shows signs of LV hypertrophy, which is found in the majority of patients with AS. Echocardiography represents the
2 "gold standard" modality for the diagnosis of AS. Two-dimensional (2D) echocardiography with Doppler allows precise real-time analysis of ventricular and valvular anatomy and function. The most important objective of echocardiography is correct assessment of the severity of AS using Doppler echocardiography to calculate jet velocity, mean transvalvular pressure gradient, and valve orifice area (Table 82.1). It is also used to assess valve thickening and calcification, as well as reduced leaflet motion. Distinction between bicuspid and tricuspid valves is often possible, particularly when the amount of calcification is small.

Two-dimensional echocardiography is also invaluable in detecting associated MV disease and in assessing LV hypertrophy, systolic function, and diastolic performance. Ejection fraction is used to measure LV systolic function. However, a severe decrease in ejection fraction can falsely lower estimates of severity of AS due to low-pressure gradients. Stress echocardiography with dobutamine administration may be required to properly assess the severity of valvular disease and to distinguish it from primary contractile dysfunction with lack of contractile reserve.[17]

Cardiac catheterization with direct measurement of the pressure gradients across the AV to calculate the severity of stenosis has been replaced by less invasive echocardiography.
3 The current indication for cardiac catheterization is limited to preoperative evaluation of coronary artery disease.

Natural History

The natural history of AS is marked by a prolonged latent period with few symptoms and minimal morbidity. Even patients with moderately severe AS have a slow decrease in AV area, generally by approximately 0.1 cm^2 per year.[18,19] The natural history of severe AS correlates well with the onset and severity of symptoms. Life expectancy of patients with severe, untreated AS and angina is approximately 5 years. Patients presenting with syncope have life expectancies of 3 years. Presence of congestive heart failure in patients with severe, untreated AS is associated with a worse prognosis, with the time of death occurring less than 2 years from the onset of symptoms (Fig. 82.4).[20]

Treatment

4 There is no effective medical therapy for patients with severe AS. Diuretics and digitalis may improve the symptoms of congestive heart failure. Mechanical relief of AS is accomplished by surgical AV replacement (AVR), percutaneous AVR, or percutaneous balloon aortic valvotomy.

Surgical Aortic Valve Replacement. The primary indication for surgery is the presence of symptoms in patients with severe AS. AVR is also indicated in patients with severe AS and reduced LV function and in patients with moderate to severe AS who also require coronary, other valve, or aortic surgery.[17] Recent studies suggest that AVR may also be beneficial in patients with asymptomatic severe AS and severe LV hypertrophy.[21]

Choice of valve prosthesis for AVR is primarily influenced by the patient's age. Mechanical prostheses are made of carbon, require lifelong anticoagulation, and are very durable (Fig. 82.5). Mechanical prostheses are therefore indicated in patients younger than 65 years old. Stented biologic prostheses

FIGURE 82.4. Natural history of aortic stenosis without operative treatment. Onset of symptoms identifies patients at high risk of death over the next 2 to 5 years.

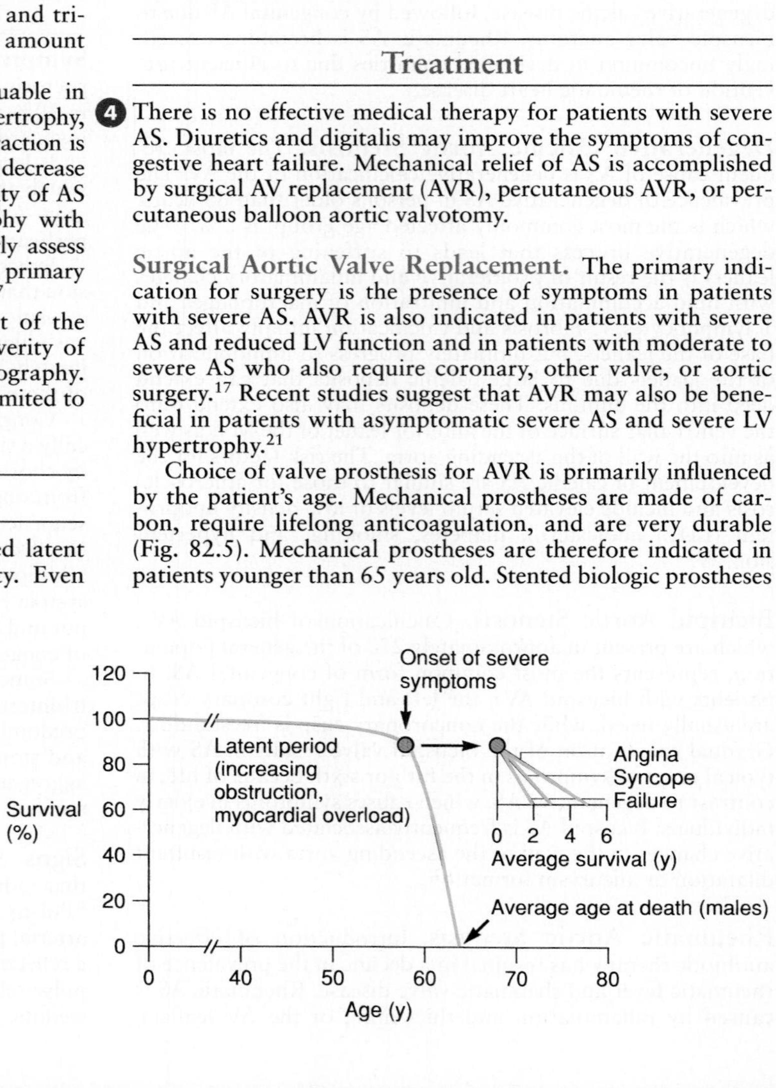

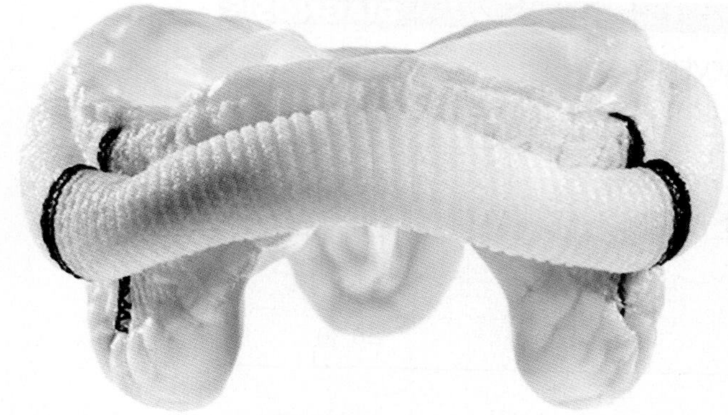

FIGURE 82.6. St. Jude Medical Epic Valve.

are most commonly made of bovine pericardium or porcine valve leaflets, do not require anticoagulation, and have a limited durability of approximately 15 years (Fig. 82.6). Biologic prostheses are used in elderly patients (older than 65 years) and in younger patients in whom long-term anticoagulation with warfarin is contraindicated (bleeding diathesis, peptic ulcer disease, etc.).

Percutaneous Aortic Valve Replacement. Percutaneous AVR is a novel form of AVR that uses a bioprosthesis sutured to a balloon-expandable stainless steel or nitinol stent (Fig. 82.7). The prosthesis is introduced through the femoral artery retrogradely into the aorta and placed at the midpart of the native stenotic AV by balloon inflation. The radial forces of the stent push the native AV aside to increase the valve orifice area. In patients with severe peripheral vascular disease, the retrograde arterial approach cannot be used. In these patients, similar prostheses can be inserted directly into the beating heart through the LV apex (transapical approach). Safety and efficacy of percutaneous AVR in high-risk and inoperable patients is currently being evaluated in clinical trials.

Percutaneous Balloon Aortic Valvotomy. Percutaneous balloon aortic valvotomy (PBAV) is a procedure in which a balloon is placed across a stenotic AV and inflated in order to decrease the degree of valve narrowing. This procedure is a valuable tool for treatment of AS in children and young adults. Rapid development of restenosis and clinical deterioration limits its application in the treatment of adults to those with severe AS who are not candidates for conventional surgical AVR.

AORTIC REGURGITATION

Prevalence and Etiology

Aortic regurgitation (AR) results from the improper coaptation of the AV leaflets due to either intrinsic leaflet abnormalities or aortic root distortion. The most common causes of AR include bicuspid valve disease, rheumatic fever, and endocarditis. Regurgitant bicuspid AVs are often partly calcified, which results in limited opening and closing of the valve and a mixture of AR and AS. Rheumatic fever causes inflammation and fibrosis of the leaflets, while endocarditis causes destruction of leaflets. In addition, AR can occur as a secondary phenomenon of aortic root enlargement due to Marfan syndrome, anuloaortic ectasia, or aortic dissection. Most of these causes produce chronic AR with a slow increase in LV size. Some lesions, in particular acute aortic dissection and endocarditis, cause acute AR with a sudden decrease in cardiac output.

Pathophysiology

In patients with AR, inappropriate coaptation of the aortic leaflets causes diastolic reflux of blood from the aorta into the left ventricular with a consequent increase in LV end-diastolic volume and pressure. In chronic AR, compensatory mechanisms of the left ventricular result in dilatation and hypertrophy. LV hypertrophy and dilatation ultimately result in a decrease in LV function and heart failure.

Diagnosis

Symptoms. Chronic AR is usually well tolerated and patients with even severe AR often remain asymptomatic for years. Initial symptoms of severe AR include fatigue, shortness of breath, and dyspnea on exertion. Advanced AR is marked by the onset of congestive heart failure, syncope, and angina. Acute onset of severe AR, such as in cases of aortic dissection or endocarditis-induced valve destruction, causes a sudden increase in LV end-diastolic volume and pressure with subsequent cardiogenic shock and pulmonary edema.

Signs. Lateral displacement of the point of maximum impulse is seen in chronic AR due to LV dilation and hypertrophy. The classic auscultatory findings of AR are best heard at the right sternal border of the second intercostal space and include a high-pitched, blowing holodiastolic decrescendo murmur; an S_3 heart sound; and a systolic ejection murmur.

VASCULAR

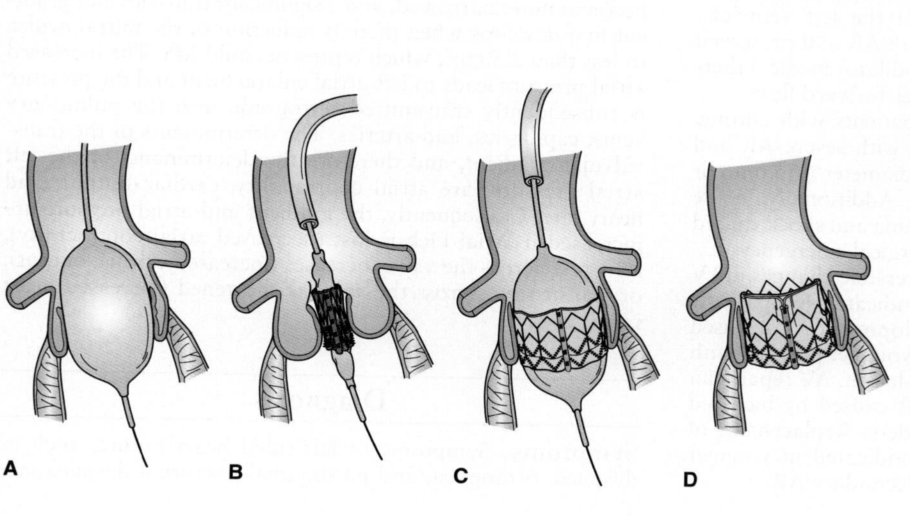

FIGURE 82.7. Schematic diagram of percutaneous aortic valve replacement. **A:** Balloon valvuloplasty. **B:** Balloon catheter with valve in the native diseased valve. **C:** Balloon inflation to secure the valve. **D:** Valve in place.

TABLE 82.2

CLASSIFICATION OF AORTIC REGURGITATION SEVERITY

■ INDICATOR	■ MILD	■ MODERATE	■ SEVERE
Angiographic grade	1+	2+	3–4+
Jet width	<25% LVOT	25%–65% LVOT	>65% LVOT
Regurgitant volume (mL/beat)	<30	30–59	≥60
Regurgitant fraction (%)	<30	30–49	≥50
Regurgitant orifice area (cm^2)	<0.10	0.10–0.29	≥0.30

LVOT, left ventricular outflow tract.
Adapted from Bonow RO, Carabello BA, Chatterjee K, et al. 2008 focused update incorporated into the ACC/AHA 2006 guidelines for the management of patients with valvular heart disease. *J Am Coll Cardiol* 2008;52(13):e1–e142.

Additionally, the widened pulse pressure leads to a number of interesting findings, such as bounding pulses (water-hammer pulse), Quincke pulse (pulse in fingernail bed), De Musset sign (rhythmic bobbing of the head), Duroziez sign (systolic and diastolic murmurs heard over the femoral artery when it is gradually compressed), and Muller sign (pulsations of the uvula).[16]

Imaging. Echocardiography represents the diagnostic "gold standard" for patients with AR. It allows assessment of the valvular and aortic anatomy, the severity of regurgitation, and the size and function of the left ventricle. Assessment of the severity of AS is determined by color Doppler jet width, regurgitant volume, regurgitant fraction, and regurgitant orifice area (Table 82.2). The role of coronary angiography is reduced to the preoperative diagnosis of coronary artery disease.

Natural History

The natural history of AR is strongly dependent on the presence of symptoms and LV dysfunction at the time of presentation. Asymptomatic patients with normal LV function develop symptoms and/or LV dysfunction at 6% per year. Asymptomatic patients with LV dysfunction at presentation develop cardiac symptoms at 25% per year. Lastly, the mortality rate of symptomatic patients is 10% per year.[17]

Treatment

Management of patients with AR depends on the severity of symptoms and the size and function of the left ventricle. Asymptomatic patients with chronic severe AR and preserved LV size and function are treated with vasodilator medical therapy, which reduces afterload and improves forward flow.

Surgery is indicated in symptomatic patients with chronic severe AR and in asymptomatic patients with severe AR and evidence of LV dilatation (end-systolic LV diameter >55 mm) or dysfunction (ejection fraction <50%). Additionally, acute severe AR with consequent pulmonary edema and shock caused by endocarditis or aortic dissection is a surgical emergency.

AVR should be performed before irreversible changes in LV function occur. Mechanical valves are indicated for patients younger than 65 years of age. Stented bioprostheses are used for AVR in patients older than 65 and in younger patients with contraindications to long-term anticoagulation. AV repair can be performed in patients with severe AR caused by bicuspid valve disease or connective tissue disorders. Replacement of the ascending aorta with AV repair is indicated in younger patients with aortic root dilatation and secondary AR.

MITRAL STENOSIS

Prevalence and Etiology

6 Mitral stenosis (MS) is predominantly caused by rheumatic fever. The steady rate of decline of rheumatic fever in developed countries has resulted in a similar decline in the prevalence of MS. Other far less common causes of MS include severe annular and leaflet calcification, congenital malformations, malignant carcinoid, left atrial myxoma, left atrial thrombus, and endocarditis. A definitive history of rheumatic fever can only be obtained in 50% to 60% of cases and women are affected more often than men by a 2:1 ratio.[22,23] Rheumatic fever commonly occurs in childhood or adolescence and can lead to a postinfective pancarditis, affecting to various degrees the valves, endocardium, myocardium, and pericardium. In MS due to rheumatic fever, there is leaflet thickening and calcification, chordal shortening and fusion, and commissural fusion, which all lead to a smaller, funnel-shaped mitral orifice. This deformation can also prevent complete closure of the valve, which is evidenced by concomitant regurgitation in about half of patients with MS.

Pathophysiology

The cross-sectional area of the normal MV is 4 to 5 cm^2. Normally, there is a trivial diastolic pressure gradient present to move blood across the MV from the left atrium into the left ventricle. An increasing gradient is required as the MV becomes more narrowed, and a significant transvalvular gradient first develops when there is reduction of the mitral orifice to less than 2.5 cm^2, which represents mild MS. The increased atrial pressure leads to left atrial enlargement and the pressure is subsequently transmitted retrograde into the pulmonary veins, capillaries, and arteries. The determinants of the transvalvular gradient, and therefore the determinants of the left atrial pressure, are atrial contractility, cardiac output, and heart rate. Consequently, the gradient and atrial pressure are increased if atrial kick is lost (decreased atrial contractility), flow rate across the valve increases (increased cardiac output), or transit time across the valve is shortened (increased heart rate).

Diagnosis

Symptoms. Symptoms of left-sided heart failure, such as dyspnea, orthopnea, and paroxysmal nocturnal dyspnea, are the primary indicators of MS and are typically triggered by exertion, stress, infection, pregnancy, or the abrupt onset of atrial fibrillation. The increased heart rate and cardiac output that can occur under these circumstances, and the mechanical obstruction inherent to MS, lead to an increased transvalvular gradient and left atrial pressure. The ensuing pulmonary congestion results in dyspnea. Likewise, the loss of atrial kick with atrial fibrillation increases the gradient and atrial pressure. Patients with atrial fibrillation may also present with palpitations or systemic embolization.

Patients infrequently present with hoarseness, dysphagia, hemoptysis, and symptoms of right-heart failure. Hoarseness and dysphagia may result if left atrial enlargement is sufficient to compress surrounding structures. Hemoptysis may occur from significant pulmonary venous hypertension. Symptoms of right-sided heart failure arise when right ventricular function is impaired due to an increased afterload from the stenotic MV and secondary pulmonary hypertension. Still, other patients may present without symptoms but have an abnormal physical examination.

Signs. The left ventricle is typically not enlarged; thus, the point of maximum impulse is not displaced. The typical auscultatory findings of MS are best heard at the apex and include a low-pitched, rumbling mid-diastolic murmur; an accentuated first heart sound; and an opening snap. These findings may be absent with a heavily calcified immobile valve, severe pulmonary hypertension, or low cardiac output. Physical findings of pulmonary hypertension, such as a loud pulmonic component of the second heart sound (P_2), a right ventricular heave, distended neck veins, hepatomegaly, ascites, and peripheral edema, can also be observed with MS.[16]

Imaging. Echocardiography is the principal tool used in the diagnosis of MS. It is used to assess the morphologic characteristics of the valve apparatus, which include leaflet mobility, flexibility, and thickness; presence of calcifications and subvalvular fusion; and appearance of the commissures. Additionally, Doppler echocardiography is utilized to determine the hemodynamic severity by measurement of the mean transvalvular pressure gradient, pulmonary artery systolic pressure, and valve area (Table 82.3). This morphology and severity information is fundamental in determining the timing and type of intervention to be used.[17]

The enlarged left atrium gives rise to characteristic findings on the chest radiograph, which includes displacement of the left main-stem bronchus superiorly and displacement of the esophagus posteriorly. Additionally, calcification of the mitral leaflets and enlarged pulmonary arteries with cephalization of pulmonary blood flow can be seen.

TABLE 82.3 **DIAGNOSIS**

CLASSIFICATION OF MITRAL STENOSIS SEVERITY

INDICATOR	MILD	MODERATE	SEVERE
Mean gradient (mm Hg)	<5	5–10	>10
Pulmonary artery systolic pressure (mm Hg)	<30	30–50	>50
Valve area (cm^2)	>1.5	1.0–1.5	<1.0

Adapted from Bonow RO, Carabello BA, Chatterjee K, et al. 2008 focused update incorporated into the ACC/AHA 2006 guidelines for the management of patients with valvular heart disease. *J Am Coll Cardiol* 2008;52(13):e1–e142.

Similar to the diagnosis of other valvular heart disease, cardiac catheterization with direct pressure measurement has largely been replaced by echocardiography.

Natural History

The natural history of MS is that of a continuous decline usually consisting of a slow, stable course followed by a progressive acceleration. The latent period from rheumatic fever to the onset of symptoms is typically 20 to 40 years, with another decade before symptoms become disabling. Depending on the symptoms at presentation, the overall 10-year survival of untreated patients presenting with MS is 50% to 60%. Once disabling symptoms occur, the 10-year survival is a bleak 0% to 15%.[22–25] Mortality in untreated patients is due to pulmonary and systemic congestion, systemic embolism, pulmonary embolism, and infection.[24,26]

Treatment

For the asymptomatic patient with mild MS in sinus rhythm, prophylaxis against rheumatic fever is the only therapy indicated. A yearly history, physical examination, chest radiograph, and electrocardiogram should be obtained; serial echocardiograms are only warranted in patients with severe MS or when there is a change in symptoms.[17]

Mechanical relief is considered in symptomatic patients with moderate to severe MS. In symptomatic patients with mild MS, further exercise testing or dobutamine stress testing is useful to determine whether or not mechanical relief is warranted. Patients with a significant elevation of mean transmitral gradient (>15 mm Hg), pulmonary artery systolic pressure (>60 mm Hg), or pulmonary artery wedge pressure (>25 mm Hg) during provocative testing have hemodynamically significant MS and should be considered for mechanical relief.[17] The options for mechanical relief of MS include percutaneous balloon mitral valvotomy, open mitral commissurotomy, and MV replacement.

Percutaneous Balloon Mitral Valvotomy. Percutaneous balloon mitral valvuloplasty (PBMV), where one or more large balloons are inflated across the MV by a catheter-based approach, is the treatment of choice for select patients with MS.[17] Patients with pliable, noncalcified valves and minimal fusion of the subvalvular apparatus are the best candidates for PBMV. Contraindications to this procedure include the presence of a left atrial thrombus, moderate to severe MR, heavy annular or leaflet calcification, and severe subvalvular distortion.

Procedural mortality of PBMV is 1% to 2% in large series. Rare risks of the procedure include MR, iatrogenic creation of an atrial septal defect, perforation of the left ventricle, embolic events, and myocardial infarction.[27–31] Overall, 80% to 95% of patients have a successful initial outcome with a doubling of the MV area and a 50% to 60% reduction in the transvalvular gradient.

Open Mitral Commissurotomy. Open mitral commissurotomy (OMC) permits direct inspection of the MV apparatus and allows debridement of calcium deposits, division of the commissures, and splitting of fused chordae tendineae under direct vision. Additionally, the left atrial appendage can be surgically oversewn from within the left atrium, reducing the risk of postoperative embolization. The contraindications to OMC are similar to those of PBMV.

The operative mortality of OMC is less than 2%,[32,33] and complication rates are similar to those of PBMV.[34,35] Short- and long-term hemodynamic results and symptomatic results are similar between PBMV and OMC in younger patients with less severe valve pathology (lower Wilkins scores).[34] More favorable results are seen with OMC in older patients with subvalvular fusion, leaflet calcification, and less valve flexibility (higher Wilkins scores).[35]

Mitral Valve Replacement. MV replacement (MVR) is necessary in symptomatic patients with moderate to severe MS when there is a significant amount of calcification or subvalvular fusion, since PBMV and OMC are less likely to be successful. MVR is also necessary in symptomatic patients with moderate to severe MS and concomitant moderate to severe MR.[17] The choice of valve prosthesis for MVR is determined in a similar manner as choosing the prosthesis for AVR. Biologic prostheses are used in the elderly and those in whom long-term warfarin is contraindicated. Regardless of the prosthesis used, it is well established that preservation of the papillary muscle attachments to the annulus plays an important roll in the maintenance of LV function.[36–40]

The operative mortality of MVR is 5% to 6% and freedom from reoperation at 15 years is 50% to 75%.[41]

MITRAL REGURGITATION

Prevalence and Etiology

Since competency of the MV is dependent on the entire MV apparatus, dysfunction of any one of the components can lead
7 to mitral regurgitation (MR). The most common overall cause of MR is degenerative MV disease. Other causes of MR include rheumatic valve disease, endocarditis, certain drugs, and collagen vascular disease. In some cases, functional MR develops as a result of dilatation of the left ventricular from cardiomyopathy or severe ischemic heart disease. Lastly, rupture of a papillary muscle from myocardial infarction or endocarditis, or rupture of a chord can lead to the onset of acute, severe MR.

Pathophysiology

MR is caused by deficient coaptation of the MV leaflets, which results in blood flow from the left ventricle into the left atrium during systole. Regardless of etiology, the pathophysiology of chronic MR is similar. MR results in gradual enlargement of the left atrium as a result of volume overload. Decrease in the functional stroke volume causes an increase in LV size with a subsequent decrease in LV function.

On the other hand, the pathologic process that takes place in acute MR is quite different. Sudden volume overload results in an increase in LV preload and a decrease in forward stroke volume, since compensatory LV eccentric hypertrophy has not had time to develop. Similarly, acute volume overload of the left atrium results in an increase in left atrial pressure and pulmonary congestion.

Diagnosis

Symptoms. Symptoms of chronic MR include fatigue, dyspnea on exertion, and shortness of breath. More advanced stages of disease are characterized by the development of heart failure. Acute, severe MR is characterized by acute pulmonary edema and cardiogenic shock.

Signs. The point of maximum impulse is typically laterally displaced. The classic auscultatory findings of MR are best heard at the apex and include a high-pitched, blowing, holosystolic murmur radiating to the axilla; a diminished S_1; and an S_3.

Imaging. Echocardiography is used to assess the severity of MR, morphology of the MV, and size and function of the left ventricular and atrium. Assessment of the severity of MR is determined by the jet area/left atrial area, regurgitant volume, regurgitant fraction, and regurgitant orifice area (Table 82.4). Additionally, magnetic resonance imaging allows accurate measurements of the severity of regurgitation and quantification of regurgitant volumes, along with assessment of LV size and function.

Natural History

Patients with mild to moderate MR usually remain asymptomatic with little or no hemodynamic compromise for many years. In patients with severe MR caused by flail leaflets, mortality is 6% to 7% per year, and 90% of patients die or require an MV operation within 10 years.[42]

Treatment

Medical therapy is indicated in asymptomatic patients with mild to moderate chronic MR and preserved LV function.

Surgery is indicated in symptomatic patients with severe MR as well as in asymptomatic patients with severe MR and LV dysfunction. MV repair is the preferred surgical therapy for most patients with MR, since it preserves the native valve and avoids the need for anticoagulation, which is required in the majority of patients who undergo valve replacement.[43] Preservation of the MV and chordae preserves LV function and improves survival. Success rates of MV repair depend on the etiology of regurgitation. Durable MV repair can be accomplished

TABLE 82.4 DIAGNOSIS

CLASSIFICATION OF MITRAL REGURGITATION SEVERITY

INDICATOR	MILD	MODERATE	SEVERE
Angiographic grade	1+	2+	3–4+
Jet size			Wall-impinging jet of any size
Jet area/left atrial area (%)	<20	20–40	>40
Regurgitant volume (mL/beat)	<30	30–59	≥60
Regurgitant fraction (%)	<30	30–49	≥50
Regurgitant orifice area (cm^2)	<0.20	0.20–0.39	≥0.40

Adapted from Bonow RO, Carabello BA, Chatterjee K, et al. 2008 focused update incorporated into the ACC/AHA 2006 guidelines for the management of patients with valvular heart disease. *J Am Coll Cardiol* 2008;52(13):e1–e142.

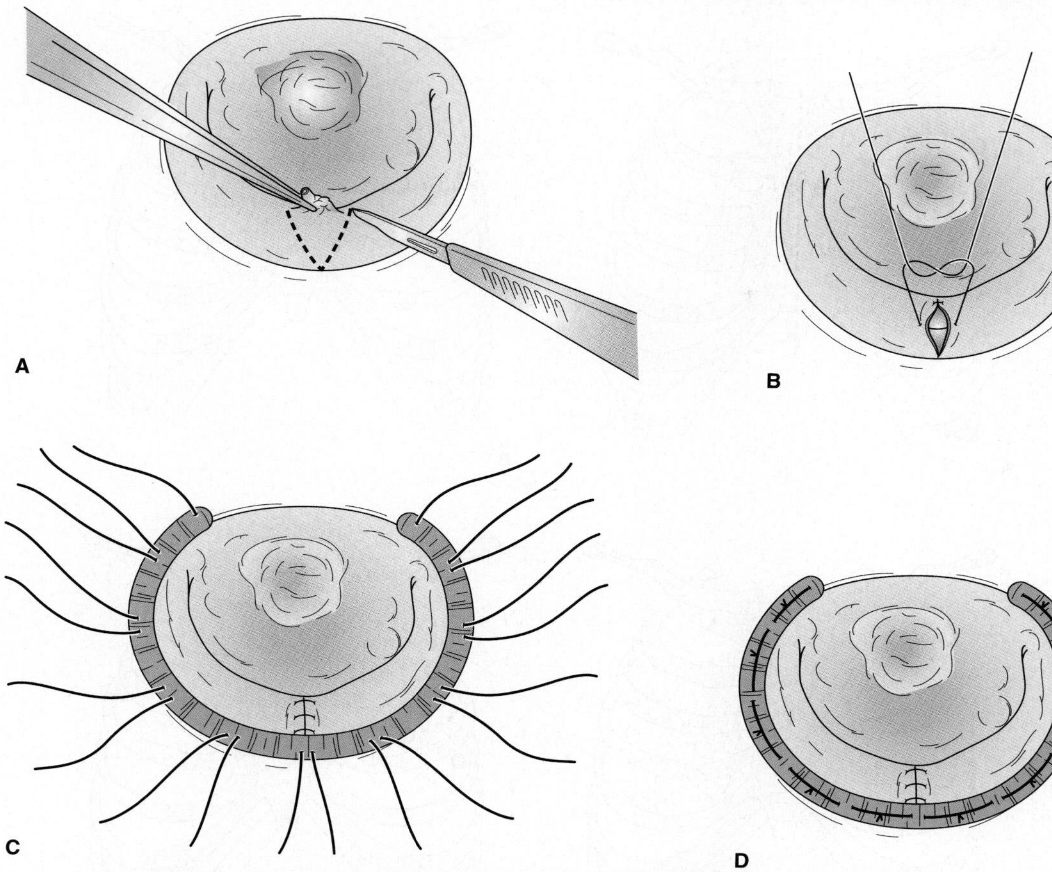

FIGURE 82.8. Schematic diagram of posterior mitral valve repair and insertion of annuloplasty ring.

in more than 90% of patients with degenerative MV disease. Standard techniques for MV repair include resection of the prolapsed portion of the MV leaflet, leaflet reconstruction, and insertion of an annuloplasty ring (Fig. 82.8).

Mortality of isolated MV repair is less than 1%, with greater than 90% freedom from reoperation at 10 years. Functional MR is usually repaired with the use of an undersized annuloplasty ring to reduce the diameter of the mitral annulus and restore valve competency. MV repair is also the preferred surgical therapy in patients with MV endocarditis. Resection of all infected valve tissue is the mainstay of valvular reconstruction in patients with endocarditis. This is followed by leaflet reconstruction, commonly with the use of an autologous pericardial patch and an annuloplasty (Fig. 82.9).

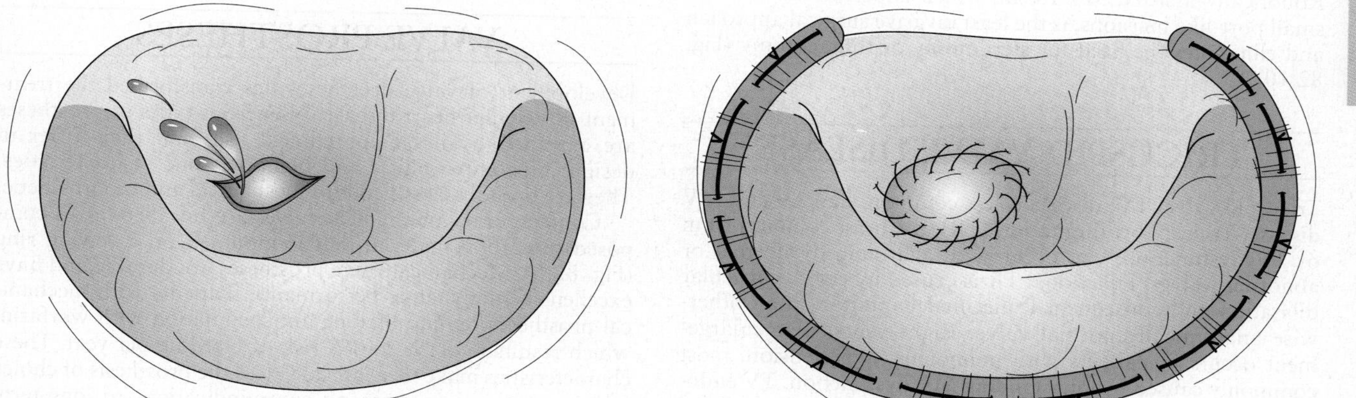

FIGURE 82.9. Schematic diagram of mitral valve repair with autologous pericardial patch and insertion of an annuloplasty ring.

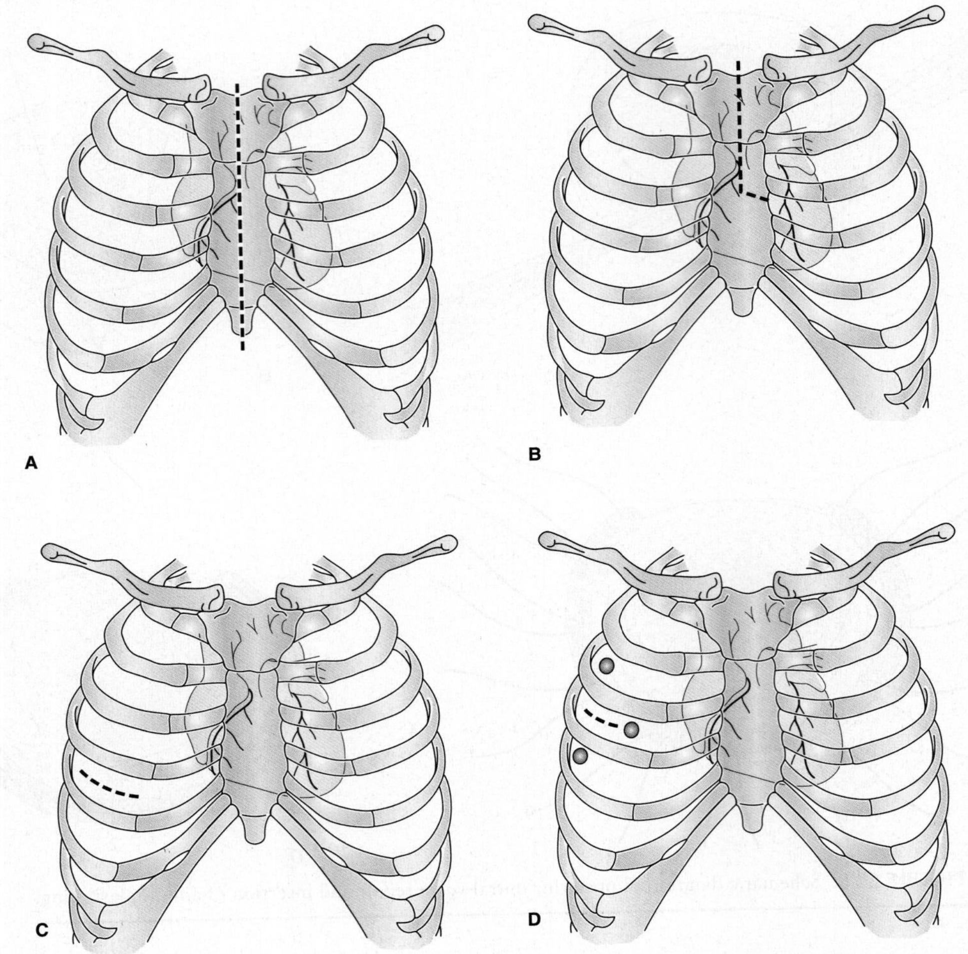

FIGURE 82.10. Surgicalapproaches to the mitral valve. **A:** Full sternotomy. **B:** Partial sternotomy. **C:** Limited right anterolateral mini-thoracotomy. **D:** Robotically assisted.

MVR is indicated for patients in whom adequate MV repair cannot be accomplished. Mechanical valve replacements are indicated in patients younger than 65 years of age and stented bioprostheses are indicated in the elderly.

Isolated MV repair and replacement are most commonly performed through a full sternotomy. Minimally invasive approaches, which include the partial upper and lower sternotomy and limited right thoracotomy, decrease the degree of surgical trauma and blood loss and allow faster recovery. Robotically assisted MV repair, which is performed through small port-like incisions, is the least invasive surgical approach and eliminates the need for sternotomy or thoracotomy (Fig. 82.10).[44]

TRICUSPID VALVE DISEASE

Tricuspid valve (TV) disease is less common than AV and MV disease. Tricuspid regurgitation (TR), the most common form of TV dysfunction, can occur with anatomically normal or abnormal valves. Functional TR is caused by right ventricular dilatation and consequent leaflet malcoaptation in an otherwise anatomically normal valve. Right ventricular enlargement occurs in patients with pulmonary hypertension, most commonly caused by longstanding MV dysfunction. TV endocarditis most commonly occurs in intravenous drug users and causes TR by destruction of the leaflets.

Echocardiography is used to assess the degree of TR, anatomy of the TV, right ventricular function, and pulmonary pressures.

Mild to moderate degrees of TR often resolve spontaneously once the MV disease causing the pulmonary hypertension is corrected. Severe functional TR is corrected by reduction in the diameter of the tricuspid annulus, most commonly using an annuloplasty ring. Severe endocarditis requires complete resection of infected valve tissue, followed by TV replacement with a bioprosthesis. In active drug users, insertion of a valve prosthesis may be delayed by several months to decrease the risk of recurrent endocarditis.

VALVE PROSTHESES

Development of valve prostheses has transformed the treatment of valvular heart disease. Numerous types of prostheses are currently available for clinical use, and they differ in design, biocompatibility, and hemodynamic characteristics. They are broadly classified into mechanical and bioprosthetic.

Contemporary mechanical valves are bileaflet valves composed of carbon material that is mounted on a sewing ring (Fig. 82.5). Mechanical valve prostheses are durable and have excellent hemodynamic performance. Patients with mechanical prostheses require lifelong anticoagulation with warfarin, which results in a 1% to 3% risk of bleeding per year. These characteristics make mechanical valves the prosthesis of choice for younger patients with no contraindications to long-term anticoagulation.[17]

Biologic prostheses are composed of valve leaflets created from bovine pericardium or porcine valve leaflets mounted on a sewing ring (Fig. 82.6). Biologic prostheses have slightly inferior hemodynamic characteristics when compared with mechanical prostheses and a limited durability of 10 to 15 years. However, bioprostheses are not thrombogenic and therefore do not require anticoagulation. Bioprostheses are generally indicated in older individuals and younger patients who have contraindications to long-term anticoagulation. There has been an increased use of bioprostheses in younger individuals due to recent improvements in design of the prostheses, expected increases in valve durability, and decreased risk of reoperations.

Aortic homografts are cryopreserved allografts that are composed of AVs and ascending aortas. Homografts are not thrombogenic, have excellent hemodynamic characteristics, and have high resistance to infection. Homografts are indicated in patients with AV endocarditis. Their use for primary AVR is limited due to the complexity of the operation and limited durability (10 years).

CARDIAC TUMORS

Cardiac tumors can be located in the epicardium, myocardium, endocardium, or any combination of the three. In general, tumors that involve the parietal pericardium are not classified as cardiac tumors.

Tumors of the heart are classified as either primary or secondary. Primary tumors arise in the heart and are either benign or malignant. Secondary tumors are metastases from primary tumors arising elsewhere and hence are always malignant. Primary tumors are rare, with an autopsy incidence of less than
8 0.1%.[45] Secondary tumors are observed more commonly, with a postmortem incidence of about 1%.[46]

Cardiac tumors present with variable symptoms. Symptoms are frequently determined by the intracardiac location of the tumor. Intracavitary tumors can obstruct blood flow, causing signs and symptoms that mimic those of valvular heart disease. Intracavitary tumors can also cause embolic events, resulting in symptoms related to the site of embolization. Intramyocardial tumors can trigger cardiac rhythm disturbances, including sudden death.[47] Cardiac tumors can also cause systemic symptoms mimicking collagen vascular disease, malignancy, or infective endocarditis.[47]

BENIGN PRIMARY CARDIAC TUMORS

Myxomas

Definition, Incidence, and Prevalence. Myxomas are the most common primary cardiac tumors. They are benign. Although myxomas have been reported in both genders and in all age groups, they most often occur in women in the third to sixth decades of life. Myxomas are usually sporadic, but at least 7% occur as part of an autosomal dominant syndrome.

Morphology. Arising from the endocardium, myxomas usually extend into a cardiac chamber. They are generally polypoid, pedunculated lesions with a smooth surface that may be covered with thrombus (Fig. 82.11A). The tumors range in size from 1 to 15 cm, but are most commonly about 5 cm.[48–51] Myxomas are thought to arise from pluripotent mesenchymal cells. Histologically, myxomas consist of a matrix of acid mucopolysaccharide (Fig. 82.11B).[45] Myxomas most commonly occur in the atria. Approximately 75% arise in the left atrium, and 15% to 20% arise in the right atrium.[50] The remainder of myxomas are located in the ventricles.

Clinical Characteristics. Many patients with myxomas are asymptomatic. The myxoma may be detected by routine

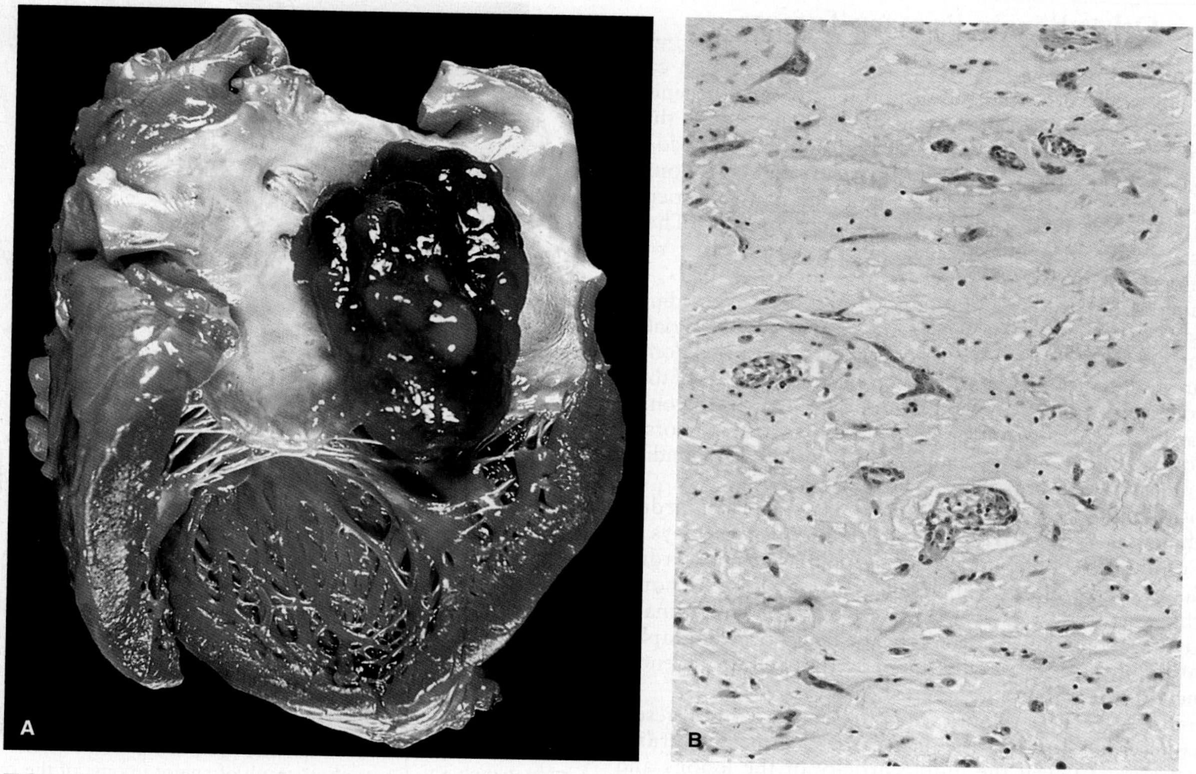

FIGURE 82.11. Left atrial myxoma. **A:** Gross photograph showing large pedunculated lesion arising from the left atrium and extending into the mitral valve orifice. **B:** Microscopic appearance, with abundant acid mucopolysaccharide, scattered collections of myxoma cells, and abnormal vascular formations (*arrow*). (Reproduced with permission from Kumar V, Abbas AK, Fausto N. *Robbins and Cotran Pathologic Basis of Disease*, 7th ed. Philadelphia: Elsevier; 2005.)

VASCULAR

screening echocardiography performed for other indications. Asymptomatic myxomas should be excised in order to prevent emboli, valvular dysfunction, or constitutional symptoms.

Patients with myxomas can have a variety of symptoms. In the sporadic form, classic findings include emboli, congestive heart failure caused by obstruction of cardiac blood flow, and constitutional symptoms. These sequelae are related to the location, size, and mobility of the tumor. Because most myxomas arise in the left atrium, systemic embolization is common, occurring in 30% to 50% of cases.[52–54]

Myxomas also can display signs and symptoms related to cardiac obstruction. Typically, the findings are related to the tumor's ability to impede filling of the ventricles; in such instances, signs and symptoms may mimic those of mitral or tricuspid valve stenosis. Constitutional symptoms include fever, malaise, rash, weight loss, and myalgia.

Diagnosis. Echocardiography is the imaging modality of choice for diagnosis of myxomas. In cases of diagnostic uncertainty, magnetic resonance imaging (MRI) and computed tomography (CT) may be helpful. Final diagnosis is confirmed by pathologic examination.

Management. Surgical resection is the mainstay of treatment. Great care must be taken to minimize manipulation of the heart before cross-clamping the aorta to reduce the risk of intraoperative tumor embolization. A variety of approaches are available for resection of left atrial tumors. In the absence of other cardiac disease, a minimally invasive or robotically assisted operation can be employed to speed postoperative recovery. The tumor is resected en bloc. Tumors that arise from a relatively well-defined pedicle can be excised without full-thickness excision of a button of atrial wall. The results of surgical excision are good with a low risk of morbidity and mortality (0% to 3%).[55–57]

Other Benign Primary Tumors

Rhabdomyoma. Rhabdomyoma is the most common cardiac tumor in children and the second most common benign cardiac tumor overall.[50] Most occur in children younger than 1 year of age. Rhabdomyoma is a benign tumor composed of cardiac myocytes. About one half of patients with rhabdomyoma have tuberous sclerosis, and about one half of patients with tuberous sclerosis develop rhabdomyomas.[58] These tumors occur sporadically or in conjunction with other rare congenital heart malformations.

Rhabdomyomas usually are found deep in the myocardium; they may extend into the cardiac chambers. They are of variable size, ranging from 1 mm to several centimeters. Most rhabdomyomas are multicentric and involve both ventricles. Because of their morphologic appearance and multicentric nature, rhabdomyomas are classified as hamartomas rather than as true tumors.[59] Pathologically, they are distinguishable from the surrounding myocardium by their firm, gray, nodular characteristics.[60]

Most children with rhabdomyomas display cardiac arrhythmias or obstructive symptoms in the first few days or weeks of life. Rhabdomyomas causing significant intracardiac obstruction to blood flow can result in death within 24 hours of birth; patients with less severe disease may be asymptomatic for years. The diagnosis is usually made by echocardiography. One of the curiosities of this tumor is the well-documented tendency for these tumors to regress.[61,62]

In most cases these tumors are not resected. Surgical resection is reserved for masses that cause significant cardiac obstruction.[63,64] Given the multicentricity of the lesions and their limited growth potential, the operative approach is conservative debulking, with the goal being relief of outflow obstruction with preservation of electrical conduction and myocardial and valvular function.

Lipomas. Lipomas are encapsulated masses of adipose tissue that usually arise from the myocardium or pericardium.[50] They are usually small but can grow to be massive. Lipomas involving the pericardium may be mistaken for pericardial cysts and may be associated with pericardial effusions. Although most of these tumors are identified after death, they can be diagnosed by echocardiography and MRI. Most cardiac lipomas can be observed. However, lipomas causing obstructive symptoms or arrhythmias should be resected.

Papillary Fibroelastoma. Papillary fibroelastomas are the most common tumors affecting cardiac valves.[65,66] They usually involve the valves of the left side of the heart, and typically occur in adult patients.[67] Although papillary fibroelastomas usually are asymptomatic, when symptoms occur, they are most frequently related to embolization. The tumors are identified by echocardiography. Surgical excision is advised, even in asymptomatic patients.[65,68,69] When resection is performed, a minimally invasive surgical approach is generally possible.

MALIGNANT PRIMARY CARDIAC TUMORS

Angiosarcoma

Most malignant cardiac tumors are metastases from other malignancies.[51] Almost all primary malignant tumors of the heart are sarcomas[70]; angiosarcoma is the most common malignant primary cardiac tumor.[50] Angiosarcomas are usually solitary, large bulky masses that originate in the right atrium (Fig. 82.12). They may extend into the right atrial cavity, causing valvular obstruction, right-sided heart failure, or

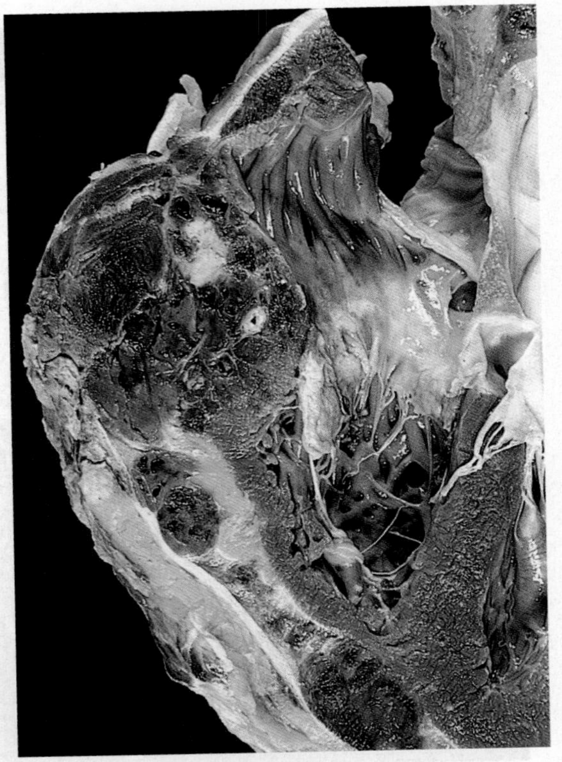

FIGURE 82.12. Gross photograph of angiosarcoma of the right ventricle. (Reproduced with permission from Kumar V, Abbas AK, Fausto N. *Robbins and Cotran Pathologic Basis of Disease*, 7th ed. Philadelphia: Elsevier; 2005.)

hemorrhagic pericardial effusion with tamponade.[70] Most of these tumors metastasize, most commonly to the lung, liver, or brain.[71] Angiosarcomas are very aggressive, and survival after diagnosis ranges from 3 to 15 months.[59] Given their rapid growth and poor prognosis, surgical resection is rarely successful.

Rhabdomyosarcoma

Rhabdomyosarcoma is the second most common cardiac sarcoma. Like angiosarcoma, it is more common in men.[72–74] Unlike angiosarcoma, rhabdomyosarcoma does not have a predilection for a particular cardiac chamber.[50] It may occur at multiple sites and extend into the pericardium. Patients may have cardiac obstructive or constitutional symptoms. Prognosis is poor, and surgical resection is usually ineffective.

SECONDARY CARDIAC TUMORS: METASTASES TO THE HEART

Metastatic tumors to the heart, or secondary tumors, are much more common than are primary cardiac tumors. Secondary tumors are usually carcinomas rather than sarcomas because of the relative frequency of these cancers.[70] Hematogenous spread is the most common mode of metastasis, but lymphatic spread and direct extension also occur.

Symptoms occur most commonly in patients with pericardial metastases rather than intramural or intracavitary involvement. The symptoms associated with metastases are congestive heart failure and arrhythmias. Metastases to the heart should be suspected in patients with known neoplasms who develop congestive heart failure.

Carcinoma of the lung and breast may directly invade the parietal and visceral pericardium, causing myocardial restriction and pericardial effusion.[70] Melanoma commonly metastasizes to the myocardium, as do leukemia and lymphoma. The treatment of metastatic tumors depends on the tumor type and symptoms. Given the late stage at which cardiac metastases occur and the poor prognosis, few of these patients are candidates for cardiac surgical intervention. Lymphoma and leukemia may respond to chemotherapy or radiotherapy. Symptomatic malignant pericardial effusions may be drained by creation of a pericardial window, temporarily relieving symptoms.

References

1. Tsakiris AG, Von Bernuth G, Rastelli GC, et al. Size and motion of the mitral valve annulus in anesthetized intact dogs. *J Appl Physiol* 1971;30(5):611–618.
2. Ormiston JA, Shah PM, Tei C, et al. Size and motion of the mitral valve annulus in man. I. A two-dimensional echocardiographic method and findings in normal subjects. *Circulation* 1981;64(1):113–120.
3. Marzilli M, Sabbah HN, Stein PD. Mitral regurgitation in ventricular premature contractions. The role of the papillary muscle. *Chest* 1980;77(6):736–740.
4. Otto CM, Lind BK, Kitzman DW, et al. Association of aortic-valve sclerosis with cardiovascular mortality and morbidity in the elderly. *N Engl J Med* 1999;341(3):142–147.
5. Ghaisas NK, Foley JB, O'Briain DS, et al. Adhesion molecules in nonrheumatic aortic valve disease: endothelial expression, serum levels and effects of valve replacement. *J Am Coll Cardiol* 2000;36(7):2257–2262.
6. O'Brien KD, Shavelle DM, Caulfield MT, et al. Association of angiotensin-converting enzyme with low-density lipoprotein in aortic valvular lesions and in human plasma. *Circulation* 2002;106(17):2224–2230.
7. Olsson M, Thyberg J, Nilsson J. Presence of oxidized low density lipoprotein in nonrheumatic stenotic aortic valves. *Arterioscler Thromb Vasc Biol* 1999;19(5):1218–1222.
8. Galante A, Pietroiusti A, Vellini M, et al. C-reactive protein is increased in patients with degenerative aortic valvular stenosis. *J Am Coll Cardiol* 2001;38(4):1078–1082.
9. Rajamannan NM, Gersh B, Bonow RO. Calcific aortic stenosis: from bench to the bedside–emerging clinical and cellular concepts. *Heart* 2003;89(7):801–805.
10. Mohler III ER, Gannon F, Reynolds C, et al. Bone formation and inflammation in cardiac valves. *Circulation* 2001;103(11):1522–1528.
11. Rajamannan NM, Subramaniam M, Rickard D, et al. Human aortic valve calcification is associated with an osteoblast phenotype. *Circulation* 2003;107(17):2181–2184.
12. Alpert JS. Aortic stenosis: a new face for an old disease. *Arch Intern Med* 2003;163(15):1769–1770.
13. Bache RJ, Vrobel TR, Ring WS. Regional myocardial blood flow during exercise in dogs with chronic left ventricular hypertrophy. *Circ Res* 1981;48(1):76–87.
14. Marcus ML, Doty DB, Hiratzka LF. Decreased coronary reserve. A mechanism for angina pectoris in patients with aortic stenosis and normal coronary arteries. *N Engl J Med* 1982;307(22):1362–1366.
15. Carabello BA. Evaluation and management of patients with aortic stenosis. *Circulation* 2002;105(15):1746–1750.
16. Swartz MH. *Textbook of Physical Diagnosis: History and Examination*, 4th ed. Philadelphia: W.B. Saunders Company; Philadelphia, PA: 2001.
17. Bonow RO, Carabello BA, Chatterjee K, et al. 2008 focused update incorporated into the ACC/AHA 2006 guidelines for the management of patients with valvular heart disease: a report of the American College of Cardiology/American Heart Association Task Force on Practice Guidelines (Writing Committee to revise the 1998 guidelines for the management of patients with valvular heart disease). Endorsed by the Society of Cardiovascular Anesthesiologists, Society for Cardiovascular Angiography and Interventions, and Society of Thoracic Surgeons. *J Am Coll Cardiol* 2008;52(13):e1–e142.
18. Faggiano P, Aurigemma GP, Rusconi C, et al. Progression of valvular aortic stenosis in adults: literature review and clinical implications. *Am Heart J* 1996;132(2 Pt 1):408–417.
19. Wagner S, Selzer A. Patterns of progression of aortic stenosis: a longitudinal hemodynamic study. *Circulation* 1982;65(4):709–712.
20. Ross Jr J, Braunwald E. Aortic stenosis. *Circulation* 1968;38(suppl 1):61–67.
21. Mihaljevic T, Nowicki ER, Rajeswaran J, et al. Survival after valve replacement for aortic stenosis: implications for decision making. *J Thorac Cardiovasc Surg* 2008;135(6):1270–1278; discussion 1278–1279.
22. Rowe JC, Bland EF, Sprague HB, et al. The course of mitral stenosis without surgery: ten and twenty year perspectives. *Ann Intern Med* 1960;52:741–749.
23. Wood P. An appreciation of mitral stenosis. *Br Med J* 1954;1:1051–1063.
24. Olesen KH. The natural history of 271 patients with mitral stenosis under medical treatment. *Br Heart J* 1962;24:349–357.
25. Selzer A, Cohn KE. Natural history of mitral stenosis: a review. *Circulation* 1972;45(4):878–890.
26. Roberts WC, Perloff JK. Mitral valvular disease. A clinicopathologic survey of the conditions causing the mitral valve to function abnormally. *Ann Intern Med* 1972;77(6):939–975.
27. Cohen DJ, Kuntz RE, Gordon SPF, et al. Predictors of long-term outcome after percutaneous balloon mitral valvuloplasty. *N Engl J Med* 1992;327(19):1329–1335.
28. Feldman T. Hemodynamic results, clinical outcome, and complications of Inoue balloon mitral valvotomy. *Cathet Cardiovasc Diagn* 1994(suppl 2):2–7.
29. Davis K. Multicenter experience with balloon mitral commissurotomy: NHLBI balloon valvuloplasty registry report on immediate and 30-day follow-up results. *Circulation* 1992;85(2):448–461.
30. Dean LS. Complications and mortality of percutaneous balloon mitral commissurotomy: a report from the National Heart, Lung, and Blood Institute Balloon Valvuloplasty Registry. *Circulation* 1992;85(6):2014–2024.
31. Palacios IF, Sanchez PL, Harrell LC, et al. Which patients benefit from percutaneous mitral balloon valvuloplasty? Prevalvuloplasty and postvalvuloplasty variables that predict long-term outcome. *Circulation* 2002;105(12):1465–1471.
32. Gross RI, Cunningham JN Jr, Snively SL. Long-term results of open radical mitral commissurotomy: ten year follow-up study of 202 patients. *Am J Cardiol* 1981;47(4):821–825.
33. Halseth WL, Elliott DP, Walker EL, et al. Open mitral commissurotomy. A modern re-evaluation. *J Thorac Cardiovasc Surg* 1980;80(6):842–848.
34. Farhat MB, Ayari M, Maatouk F, et al. Percutaneous balloon versus surgical closed and open mitral commissurotomy: seven-year follow-up results of a randomized trial. *Circulation* 1998;97(3):245–250.
35. Cotrufo M, Renzulli A, Ismeno G, et al. Percutaneous mitral commissurotomy versus open mitral commissurotomy: a comparative study. *Eur J Cardiothorac Surg* 1999;15(5):646–652.
36. David TE, Uden DE, Strauss HD. The importance of the mitral apparatus in left ventricular function after correction of mitral regurgitation. *Circulation* 1983;68(3 Pt 2):II76–II82.
37. David TE, Burns RJ, Bacchus CM. Mitral valve replacement for mitral regurgitation with and without preservation of chordae tendineae. *J Thorac Cardiovasc Surg* 1984;88(5 Pt 1):718–725.
38. Hennein HA, Swain J, McIntosh CL, et al. Comparative assessment of chordal preservation versus chordal resection during mitral valve replacement. *J Thorac Cardiovasc Surg* 1990;99(5):828–837.
39. Rozich JD, Carabello BA, Usher BW, et al. Mitral valve replacement with and without chordal preservation in patients with chronic mitral regurgitation: mechanisms for differences in postoperative ejection performance. *Circulation* 1992;86(6):1718–1726.

40. Horskotte D, Schulte HD, Bircks W, et al. The effect of chordal preservation on late outcome after mitral valve replacement: a randomized study. *J Heart Valve Dis* 1993;2(2):150–158.
41. Hammermeister K, Sethi GK, Henderson WG, et al. Outcomes 15 years after valve replacement with a mechanical versus a bioprosthetic valve: final report of the Veterans Affairs randomized trial. *J Am Coll Cardiol* 2000;36(4):1152–1158.
42. Ling LH, Enriquez-Sarano M, Seward JB, et al. Clinical outcome of mitral regurgitation due to flail leaflet. *N Engl J Med* 1996;335(19):1417–1423.
43. Enriquez-Sarano M, Schaff HV, Orszulak TA, et al. Valve repair improves the outcome of surgery for mitral regurgitation: a multivariate analysis. *Circulation* 1995;91(4):1022–1028.
44. Chitwood WR Jr, Rodriguez E, Chu MW, et al. Robotic mitral valve repairs in 300 patients: a single-center experience. *J Thorac Cardiovasc Surg* 2008;136(2):436–441.
45. Reynen K. Frequency of primary tumors of the heart. *Am J Cardiol* 1996;77(1):107.
46. Lam KY, Dickens P, Chan AC. Tumors of the heart. A 20-year experience with a review of 12,485 consecutive autopsies. *Arch Pathol Lab Med* 1993;117(10):1027–1031.
47. Shapiro LM. Cardiac tumours: diagnosis and management. *Heart* 2001;85(2):218–222.
48. Goodwin JF. Diagnosis of left atrial myxoma. *Lancet* 1963;1(7279):464–468.
49. Hall RJ, Cooley DA, McAllister HA. Neoplastic heart disease. In: Hurst JW, ed. *The Heart, Arteries, and Veins*, 7th ed. New York: McGraw-Hill; 1990:1382–1403.
50. McAllister HA, Fenoglio JJ. Tumors of the cardiovascular system, fascicle 15. In: Hartman WH, Cowan W. *Atlas of Tumor Pathology*, 2nd ed. Washington, DC: Armed Forces Institute of Pathology; 1978:1–20.
51. Prichard RW. Tumors of the heart; review of the subject and report of 150 cases. *AMA Arch Pathol* 1951;51(1):98–128.
52. Bortolotti U, Maraglino G, Rubino M, et al. Surgical excision of intracardiac myxomas: a 20-year follow-up. *Ann Thorac Surg* 1990;49(3): 449–453.
53. Fyke FE III, Seqard JB, Edwards WD, et al. Primary cardiac tumors: experience with 30 consecutive patients since the introduction of two-dimensional echocardiography. *J Am Coll Cardiol* 1985;5(6):1465–1473.
54. Goodwin JF. The spectrum of cardiac tumors. *Am J Cardiol* 1968;21(3):307–314.
55. Fang BR, Chiang CW, Hung JS, et al. Cardiac myxoma–clinical experience in 24 patients. *Int J Cardiol* 1990;29(3):335–341.
56. Hanson EC, Gill CC, Razavi M, et al. The surgical treatment of atrial myxomas. Clinical experience and late results in 33 patients. *J Thorac Cardiovasc Surg* 1985;89(2):298–303.
57. St John Sutton MG, Mercier LA, Giuliani ER, et al. Atrial myxomas: a review of clinical experience in 40 patients. *Mayo Clin Proc* 1980;55(6): 371–376.
58. Corno A, de Simone G, Catena G, et al. Cardiac rhabdomyoma: surgical treatment in the neonate. *J Thorac Cardiovasc Surg* 1984;87(5):725–731.
59. Brizard C, Latremouille C, Jebara VA, et al. Cardiac hemangiomas. *Ann Thorac Surg* 1993;56(2):390–394.
60. Choi JY, Bae EJ, Noh CI, et al. Cardiac rhabdomyoma in childhood tuberous sclerosis. *Cardiol Young* 1995;5(02):166–171.
61. Alkalay AL, Ferry DA, Lin B, et al. Spontaneous regression of cardiac rhabdomyoma in tuberous sclerosis. *Clin Pediatr (Phila)* 1987;26(10):532–535.
62. Beghetti M, Gow RM, Haney I, et al. Pediatric primary benign cardiac tumors: a 15-year review. *Am Heart J* 1997;134(6):1107–1114.
63. Gutierrez de Loma J, Villagra F, Perez de Leon J, et al. Rhabdomyoma of the heart: surgical treatment. *J Cardiovasc Surg (Torino)* 1982;23(2):149–154.
64. Foster ED, Spooner EW, Farina MA, et al. Cardiac rhabdomyoma in the neonate: surgical management. *Ann Thorac Surg* 1984;37(3):249–253.
65. Edwards FH, Hale D, Cohen A, et al. Primary cardiac valve tumors. *Ann Thorac Surg* 1991;52(5):1127–1131.
66. Ryan PE Jr, Obeid AI, Parker FB Jr. Primary cardiac valve tumors. *J Heart Valve Dis* 1995;4(3):222–226.
67. Darvishian F, Farmer P. Papillary fibroelastoma of the heart: report of two cases and review of the literature. *Ann Clin Lab Sci* 2001;31(3):291–296.
68. Gallo R, Kumar N, Prabhakar G, et al. Papillary fibroelastoma of mitral valve chorda. *Ann Thorac Surg* 1993;55(6):1576–1577.
69. Topol EJ, Biern RO, Reitz BA. Cardiac papillary fibroelastoma and stroke. Echocardiographic diagnosis and guide to excision. *Am J Med* 1986;80(1):129–132.
70. Roberts WC. Primary and secondary neoplasms of the heart. *Am J Cardiol* 1997;80(5):671–682.
71. Thomas CR Jr, Johnson GW Jr, Stoddard MF, et al. Primary malignant cardiac tumors: update 1992. *Med Pediatr Oncol* 1992;20(6):519–531.
72. Hajar R, Roberts WC, Folger GM Jr. Embryonal botryoid rhabdomyosarcoma of the mitral valve. *Am J Cardiol* 1986;57(4):376.
73. Hui KS, Green LK, Schmidt WA. Primary cardiac rhabdomyosarcoma: definition of a rare entity. *Am J Cardiovasc Pathol* 1988;2(1):19–29.
74. Shirani J, Roberts WC. Clinical, electrocardiographic and morphologic features of massive fatty deposits ("lipomatous hypertrophy") in the atrial septum. *J Am Coll Cardiol* 1993;22(1):226–238.

CHAPTER 83 ■ ISCHEMIC HEART DISEASE

JONATHAN W. HAFT

KEY POINTS

1. Because of its unique physiology, the heart is particularly susceptible to ischemic injury.
2. Atherosclerotic plaques cause ischemia from chronic flow limitations or from unstable plaque rupture.
3. Patients with coronary artery disease will present with either chronic stable angina or an acute coronary syndrome, which consists of unstable angina, a non–ST-segment myocardial infarction, or an ST-segment myocardial infarction.
4. Several well-described complications from myocardial infarctions must be anticipated and recognized early.
5. Medical treatment of coronary artery disease includes lifestyle modifications and medications to slow the progression and stabilize atherosclerotic plaques.
6. Percutaneous intervention (PCI) of coronary lesions has improved dramatically in recent years to include drug-eluting intracoronary stents.
7. Coronary artery bypass grafting (CABG) involves creation of alternative conduits from the systemic circulation to the epicardial coronary arteries.
8. The left internal mammary artery is the superior conduit for CABG.
9. CABG remains superior to both medical treatment and PCI for patients with left main or three-vessel disease or for patients with two-vessel disease involving the left anterior descending artery associated with left ventricular dysfunction.

CORONARY ANATOMY AND PHYSIOLOGY

The right and left coronary arteries originate from the aorta just above the aortic valve cusps (Fig. 83.1). The orifices of the two arteries within the sinuses of Valsalva designate the right and left coronary cusps. The third aortic valve cusp is referred to as the noncoronary cusp. The coronary circulation is traditionally divided into three major territories: the left anterior descending (LAD) and the circumflex territories originate from the left coronary artery, and the right coronary territory usually comes from the right coronary artery.

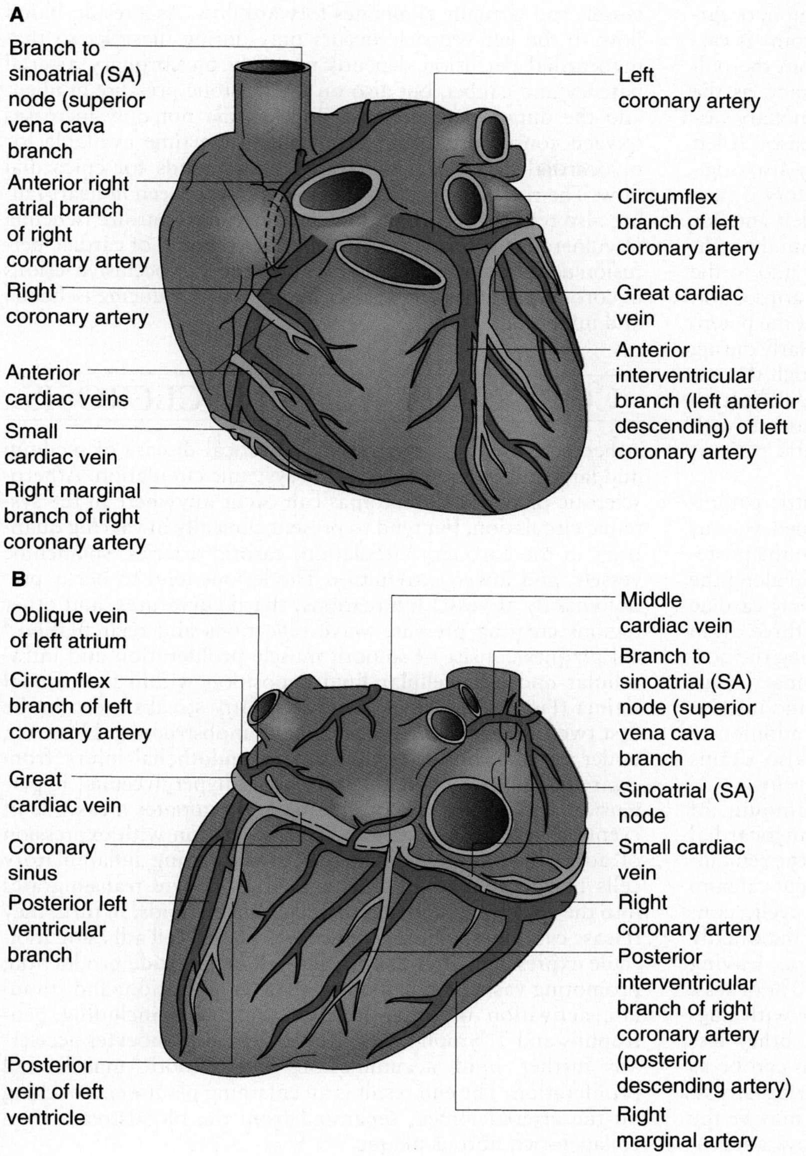

FIGURE 83.1. Anatomy of the cardiac circulation. **A:** Anterior view. **B:** Posterior view.

The origin of the left coronary artery is referred to as the left main and travels posterolaterally to the left behind the pulmonary artery, where it divides into two main branches, the LAD and the circumflex coronary artery. The length of the left main coronary artery is variable, but rarely exceeds 2 cm. Unusually, the left main is absent, where the circumflex and LAD originate from the aorta via two separate ostia.

The LAD coronary artery emerges from behind the pulmonary artery and travels inferiorly within the interventricular groove to the cardiac apex, sometimes wrapping around it onto the posterior interventricular groove. The LAD gives off two different types of branches: diagonals and septals, both of which are highly variable in size and number. The diagonals take off at acute angles and perfuse the anterolateral surface of the left ventricle. Septal branches, the first of which is typically quite prominent, emerge at a right angle from the LAD and supply the interventricular septum. The LAD is the most prominent of the three coronary territories described, and carries approximately 50% of left ventricular myocardial blood flow, supplying the anterior, anterolateral, septal, and apical walls.

The circumflex coronary artery continues from the left main coronary and travels within the posterior atrioventricular groove. Branches from the circumflex are called obtuse marginal arteries, and also vary greatly in size and number. In 80% to 90% of people, the terminal branch of the circumflex supplies the posterolateral wall of the left ventricle. In the remaining 10% to 20%, the circumflex continues to the posterior interventricular septum and terminates as the posterior descending artery (PDA). This is referred to as a left dominant heart, where the left main coronary artery is supplying the posterior interventricular septum. Some patients will have a third branch of the left main referred to as the ramus intermedius, or intermediate branch. If present, this vessel is typically large, and supplies much of the anterolateral wall of the left ventricle.

The right coronary artery originates from the anterior right sinus of Valsalva and descends in the right atrioventricular groove. One or more acute marginal branches feed the right ventricular free wall. In 80% to 90% of patients, the right coronary artery continues to the posterior interventricular septum and supplies the PDA and often a variable-sized right posterolateral artery. This is referred to as a right dominant heart. Near the origin of the posterior descending branch, a small characteristic vessel can be seen supplying the atrioventricular node. This branch can become important in acute right coronary artery occlusions, resulting in life-threatening heart block and bradycardia. A small proximal branch of the right coronary artery supplies the sinus node on the anterolateral surface of the superior vena cava.

Anomalous origin of the coronary arteries is common, occurring in 0.3% to 1% of the population, and their anatomy is varied and complex. Rarely, the left coronary arises from the pulmonary artery. This pathology is diagnosed in infancy, as the myocardium becomes profoundly ischemic when pulmonary vascular resistance falls and myocardial perfusion decreases. If left uncorrected, it is universally fatal. The coronaries may also originate from atypical aortic root sinuses, and their trajectory is variable. The most worrisome problem occurs when the left anterior descending or left main coronary artery originates from the right sinus of Valsalva. When the LAD travels posteriorly and to the left, it courses between the pulmonary artery and the aortic root. This trajectory is described as "malignant" because of the potential for compression between the great vessels, particularly during accentuated wall stress, such as with exercise. Although there is little evidence, it is generally accepted that a revascularization strategy should be considered in symptomatic patients with "malignant" coronary anomalies or in asymptomatic patients with demonstrable ischemia on noninvasive testing.[1]

Venous anatomy is more predictable, and very little pathology within this system is encountered. Three named venous branches can be identified: the middle cardiac vein in the posterior interventricular groove, the posterior cardiac vein along the obtuse margin of the heart, and the great (or anterior) cardiac vein along the anterior interventricular groove. All three drain into one confluence known as the coronary sinus along the posterior atrioventricular groove (Fig. 83.1). The coronary sinus empties posteriorly into the right atrium between the inferior vena cava and the annulus of the tricuspid valve. In addition to these identifiable named veins, the myocardium also drains directly into all chambers of the heart via thebesian veins.

1 Myocardial work consumes an enormous amount of energy substrate. In fact, only 10% to 20% of myocardial energy requirements are related to basal functions; the remainder is utilized during the continuous energy-dependent calcium mobilization and myofilament cross-linking from cyclic contraction and relaxation. Even at rest, the heart maximally extracts oxygen delivered from the bloodstream, leaving venous saturation in the coronary sinus typically 20% or less. Thus, increased energy requirements must be met with augmentation in blood oxygen delivery. Contrarily, other less oxygen-dependent tissues, where venous saturation can be as high as 80%, can extract additional oxygen during stress. When insufficient supply of oxygen is available, as may be the case with extreme consumption or limited blood flow, anaerobic metabolism cannot generate enough energy substrate to perform myocardial contraction.[2] As a result, cardiac function deteriorates immediately and can be observed clinically essentially within heartbeats. Increases in cardiac oxygen consumption must be met with proportional increases in myocardial blood flow.

The heart and its coronary circulation have a unique capacity to dramatically increase blood flow, and thus oxygen delivery, during periods of increased needs.[3] While basal coronary blood flow is approximately 10 mL/kg, this value can increase up to sixfold with exercise by autoregulatory mechanisms and feedback loops. Specifically, adenosine accumulates from the breakdown of the energy substrate adenosine triphosphate (ATP). Vasodilatory receptors within the media of coronary arteries are particularly avid for adenosine, increasing blood flow to myocardial regions with increased energy consumption. In addition, increased myocardial activity activates nitric oxide synthase within coronary endothelial cells, producing the powerful vasodilator nitric oxide. By immediately altering the vessel diameter and thus changing the resistance properties of epicardial vessels, these two short-acting mediators can rapidly alter coronary flow rates to meet changing energy requirements.

In addition to the high metabolic requirements of the heart and its dependence on responsive changes in blood flow, the coronary circulation is further uniquely challenged. During systole, increased cavitary pressure compresses intramyocardial vessels and virtually eliminates forward flow. As a result, blood flow to the left ventricle occurs only during diastole, so that myocardial perfusion depends not only on coronary arterial patency and caliber, but also on the diastolic pressure gradient and the duration of diastole. Tachycardia not only increases oxygen consumption, but also reduces the time available for myocardial perfusion, increasing the demands for epicardial flow. The rise in ventricular diastolic pressure seen in heart failure also reduces perfusion pressure and can jeopardize ischemia in vulnerable territories. With an understanding of cardiac perfusion needs and mechanics, it is apparent why occlusive lesions in coronary arteries can restrict blood flow, producing ischemia and infarction.

CORONARY ATHEROSCLEROSIS

Atherosclerosis is a progressive multifocal disease of medium and large muscular arteries of the systemic circulation. Atherosclerotic plaques or atheromas can occur anywhere in the systemic circulation, but tend to present clinically in varying quantities in the coronary circulation, carotid arteries, splanchnic vessels, and lower extremities. The lesions tend to occur predominantly at vessel bifurcations, sharp curvatures, and other regions creating pressure wave reflections and recirculation.[4] All plaques consist of smooth muscle proliferation and intracellular and extracellular lipid deposition within the arterial intima (Fig. 83.2). The predecessor "fatty streaks" seen in the first two decades of life are small and unobstructing. However, under certain clinical circumstances, endothelial injury from cigarette smoke, hypercholesterolemia, hyperglycemia, hypertension, or other causes of inflammation initiates a cascade of events. These include endothelial dysfunction with expression of adhesion molecules, which bind circulating inflammatory cells like monocytes. The activated monocyte transmigrates into the vessel wall and ingests accumulated lipids. In turn, they release cytokines, which enhance endothelial cell adhesion molecule expression; alter endothelial cell nitric oxide production, promoting vasoconstriction and platelet activation; and stimulate activation of other inflammatory cells including neutrophils and T lymphocytes. The activated monocytes accelerate further lipid accumulation and smooth muscle cell proliferation. The end result is an enlarging plaque encroaching on the arterial lumen, separated from the bloodstream by a collagen-rich fibrous plaque.

Within the coronary circulation, atherosclerotic stenotic lesions are generally restricted to the proximal regions of the large epicardial coronary arteries. In particular, stenosis found in the LAD and circumflex vessels are frequently isolated, short, and in the proximal segments. The right coronary artery, however, develops diffuse obstructions, although
2 rarely extending into the posterior descending or intramural branches. For reasons that are unclear, atherosclerosis is rarely found within intramyocardial segments of the coronary arteries. Symptoms from these atherosclerotic plaques can occur from a variety of proposed mechanisms. First, the lesion can cause flow limitations, particularly when the luminal cross-sectional area is reduced by at least 75%. With this degree of obstruction, the vasodilatory reserve required during increased myocardial demand is restricted, resulting in transient myocardial ischemia until demand returns to baseline, also known as exertional angina. The atherosclerotic plaque also causes coronary ischemia when the lesion becomes unstable. The fibrous plaque can fracture or rupture, exposing the bloodstream to the highly thrombogenic internal plaque contents. This can lead to complete epicardial thrombosis, the presumed mechanism of ST-segment elevation myocardial infarction (STEMI). Additionally, subtotal plaque disruption can cause vasoconstriction, platelet activation, and embolization, resulting in ischemia without total occlusion of the epicardial vessel. This is the presumed mechanism of

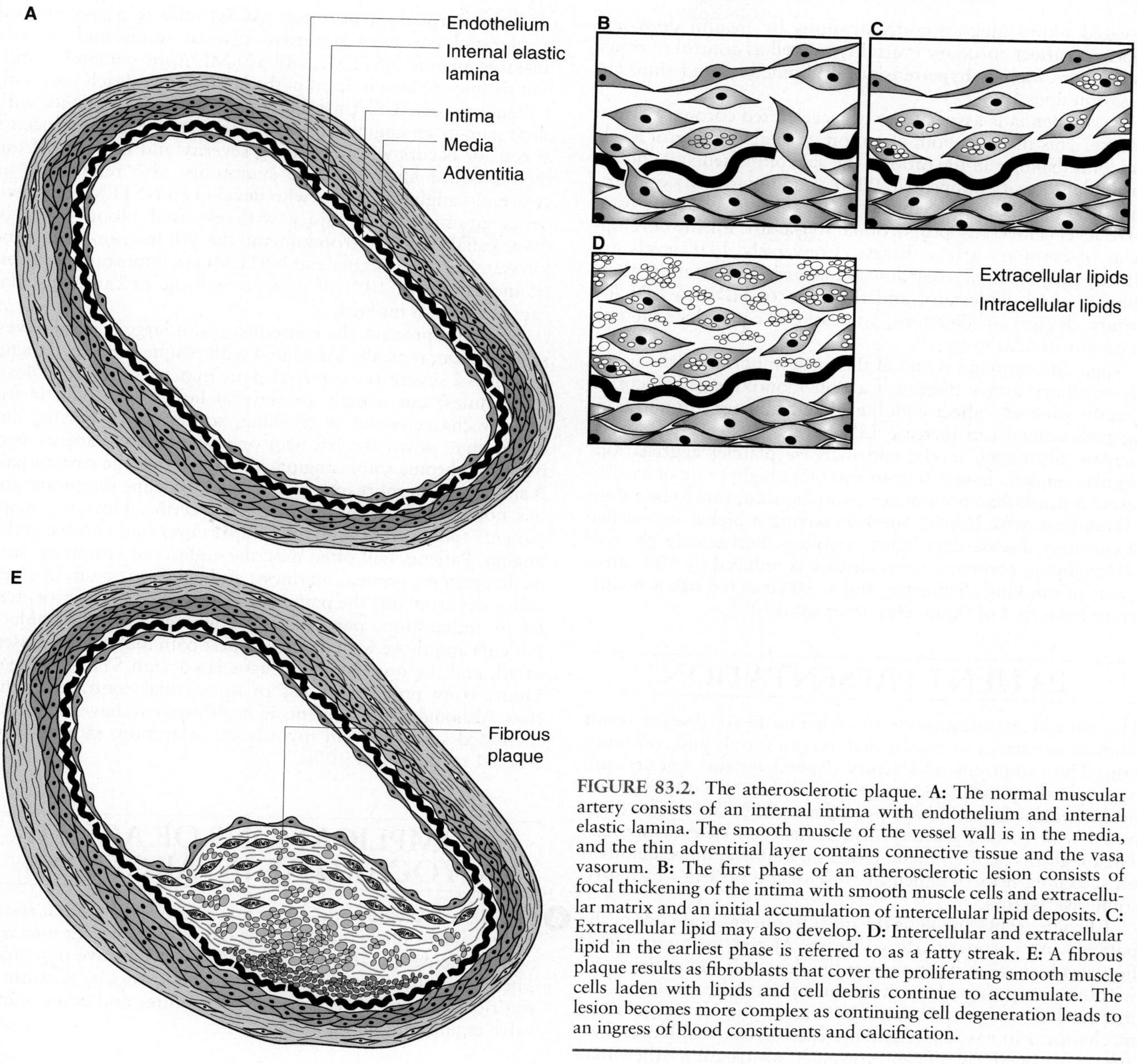

FIGURE 83.2. The atherosclerotic plaque. **A:** The normal muscular artery consists of an internal intima with endothelium and internal elastic lamina. The smooth muscle of the vessel wall is in the media, and the thin adventitial layer contains connective tissue and the vasa vasorum. **B:** The first phase of an atherosclerotic lesion consists of focal thickening of the intima with smooth muscle cells and extracellular matrix and an initial accumulation of intercellular lipid deposits. **C:** Extracellular lipid may also develop. **D:** Intercellular and extracellular lipid in the earliest phase is referred to as a fatty streak. **E:** A fibrous plaque results as fibroblasts that cover the proliferating smooth muscle cells laden with lipids and cell debris continue to accumulate. The lesion becomes more complex as continuing cell degeneration leads to an ingress of blood constituents and calcification.

unstable angina and non–ST-segment elevation myocardial infarction (NSTEMI). Some plaques are more prone to rupture than others, and the composition of the fibrous cap may be an identifiable feature of an unstable lesion. Activation of inflammatory cells may increase the activity of matrix metalloproteinases, which degrade components of the fibrous cap. Some theorize that certain stressors can stimulate activation of these inflammatory cells, such as acute infections, extreme cold, and even emotional distress.[5] The inflammatory component of coronary artery disease has been demonstrated by the strong relationship between C-reactive protein and the incidence of acute myocardial infarctions.[6]

Although the characteristics, locations, and severity of lesions in each person can vary, a number of established risk factors appear to predispose to atherosclerosis. These include advanced age, family history, male sex, hypertension, diabetes mellitus, dyslipidemia, and cigarette smoking. Recognizing the presence of these risk factors can help identify patients at risk of coronary atherosclerosis. In addition, some of these risk factors are modifiable, and simple interventions can reduce their risk of future cardiac events.

Hypertension is strongly associated with the development of atherosclerotic heart disease and the risk of death from cardiovascular causes. Although the mechanism is uncertain, it has been suggested that an increase in shear stress at particular vessel locations may injure the vascular endothelium, predisposing to lipid deposition and plaque development. Systolic hypertension appears to be more predictive than diastolic hypertension, particularly in elderly patients. Numerous interventions can control hypertension, but the most effective appears to be lifestyle modifications including reduction in dietary sodium, exercise, and weight loss. Several classes of medications are used for blood pressure control, and each is variably efficacious in different populations of patients.[7] Unequivocally, reduction in elevated systolic blood pressure reduces the risk of death from cardiovascular disease, and in particular of atherosclerotic coronary artery disease.

Patients with diabetes are two to four times more likely to have coronary artery disease, and even more so when they are insulin dependent and in diabetic women. In addition, patients with diabetes and coronary disease have worse outcomes than age-matched nondiabetics. Unfortunately, rigorous control of elevated blood glucose concentrations by insulin does not appear to affect coronary mortality as well as control of other risk factors such as hypertension, dyslipidemia, and smoking cessation does.[8]

Dyslipidemia is associated with accelerated coronary artery disease. This includes both elevation of total cholesterol levels and an imbalance in the ratio of the subcomponents of cholesterol: high-density lipoprotein (HDL) and low-density lipoprotein (LDL).[9] HDL levels appear to be protective, as the total HDL level is inversely proportional to the risk for the development of coronary artery disease. Conversely, LDL levels are directly proportional to cardiovascular risk. Importantly, alteration in total cholesterol and the ratio of HDL to LDL by dietary changes, medications, and exercise can reduce the risk of cardiovascular events.[10]

Cigarette smoking is one of the most important risk factors for coronary artery disease. Carbon monoxide and nicotine directly adversely affect endothelial cell function. In addition, cigarette smoke can increase LDL levels, reduce HDL levels, increase fibrinogen levels, and increase platelet aggregation. Regular smokers have a four to five times higher rate of cardiovascular death than nonsmokers, and there appears to be a dose relationship, with heavier smokers having a higher prevalence of coronary disease than lighter smokers. Fortunately, the risk of developing coronary artery disease is reduced by 50% after 1 year of smoking abstinence, and at 10 years the risk is no different from that of those who never smoked.[11]

PATIENT PRESENTATION

The clinical manifestations of ischemic heart disease result from an imbalance of myocardial oxygen supply and consumption. The symptoms and acuity depend on the severity and nature of the patient's occlusive lesions, but also on his or her other medical comorbidities. As many as 25% of patients diagnosed with coronary artery disease have no clear symptoms. The diagnosis is often made based on abnormalities identified on screening tests obtained because of the presence of worrisome risk factors.

3 Chronic stable angina is the most frequent complaint of the patient with coronary artery disease. At rest, coronary blood flow is adequate to meet myocardial demand, and patients are without symptoms. However, during exercise or stress, as myocardial oxygen demand increases, the autoregulatory mechanisms to vasodilate and increase myocardial blood flow are constrained. Significant coronary obstructing atheromas become flow limiting, resulting in an imbalance of oxygen demand and supply. Chest pain develops rapidly and builds up quickly, typically described as tightness, squeezing, constricting, or aching. It is usually midsternal and radiates to the left shoulder, arm, jaw, or neck. The classically described Levine sign with a clenched fist over the sternum is a common finding. Some patients, however, will describe symptoms that are collectively referred to as "anginal equivalents." These include dyspnea, diaphoresis, nausea, abdominal pain, heartburn, and dizziness or presyncope. Although the differential diagnoses of these "atypical" symptoms are broad, they should prompt the clinician to think of coronary disease, particularly if risk factors predominate. Interestingly, women are more likely to describe atypical symptoms, resulting in late or missed diagnosis of coronary atherosclerosis. Although the clinical manifestations of angina are variable, the pathognomonic feature of chronic stable angina is that the symptoms occur predictably with exertion and are always relieved with rest. Symptoms of patients with coronary atherosclerosis can be categorized according to the Canadian Heart Association Classification scheme. Class I patients have no symptoms, class II patients have angina with significant exertion, class III patients describe angina with mild exertion, and class IV patients have angina at rest.

Acute coronary syndromes (ACSs) refer to a spectrum of accelerated coronary occlusive disease states and include unstable angina, NSTEMI, and STEMI. Approximately 1 million people are hospitalized in the United States each year with a diagnosis of ACS. Unstable angina refers to patients with chest pain or an anginal equivalent that is new in onset, occurs at rest, or occurs with increasing severity and frequency from their baseline chronic stable symptoms, also referred to as crescendo angina. Patients who develop an NSTEMI have evidence of myocardial injury with elevated blood levels of myocardial enzymes (troponin and the MB fraction of creatine kinase). Unstable angina and NSTEMI are important prognostic indicators, as 10% of patients will die of cardiovascular causes within 6 months.

STEMI represents the consequences of large epicardial vessel occlusion, typically associated with plaque rupture. Patients describe a severe retrosternal pain that persists for at least 30 minutes, but usually for several hours. The pain is frequently characterized as crushing, squeezing, or boring, and can radiate down the left arm or into the jaw. Patients with previous chronic stable angina will report that the current pain is similar to but more intense than their baseline symptoms and has not resolved with rest or nitroglycerine. However, many patients that present with an STEMI never had chronic stable angina. Patients will often describe additional symptoms such as diaphoresis, nausea, dizziness, and epigastric pain. In emergency departments, the pain is often mistaken for gastroenteritis or indigestion, particularly in women. Often in elderly patients and those with diabetes, chest pain may not be present at all, and the only symptom associated with STEMI is heart failure from progressive loss of myocardial contractile function. Although improvements in health systems have drastically increased survival from myocardial infarction, mortality for STEMI remains near 10%.

COMPLICATIONS OF ACUTE MYOCARDIAL INFARCTIONS

4 STEMIs can create widespread myocyte necrosis, often resulting in catastrophic complications that require urgent intervention. Anticipation and early diagnosis can improve outcomes. These complications include cardiogenic shock, postinfarct ventricular septal defect, free wall rupture, and acute mitral valve regurgitation (Table 83.1).

Cardiogenic Shock

Cardiogenic shock is a state in which cardiac output is insufficient to meet metabolic demands, despite adequate intravascular filling pressures. Between 5% and 10% of patients with acute myocardial infarctions develop cardiogenic shock. A large proportion of these patients progress to shock not upon arrival, but more than 24 hours after initial presentation.[12] Overall mortality is approximately 60%, with very little improvement over recent decades. Treatments include fluids and inotropic agents to optimize myocardial contraction. Insertion of an intra-aortic balloon counterpulsation pump (IABP) can improve coronary perfusion by diastolic augmentation of perfusion pressure. This can have a profound impact by improving contractile function of peri-infarct territories. Although there is significant afterload reduction afforded by the IABP, cardiac output typically increases by only 15% to 20%. Emergent salvage revascularization can reduce mortality, with sustained benefits seen over long-term follow-up.[13] When shock persists despite using these aggressive strategies, consideration must be made regarding the patient's candidacy for mechanical circulatory support using ventricular assist devices or extracorporeal membrane oxygenation.[14] While

TABLE 83.1

COMPLICATIONS OF ACUTE MYOCARDIAL INFARCTIONS

■ COMPLICATION	■ DIAGNOSIS	■ TREATMENT
Cardiogenic shock	Echocardiography, pulmonary artery catheter	Inotropes, intra-aortic balloon pump, VAD
Ventricular septal defect	Echocardiography, cardiac catheterization	Surgical ventricular septal defect repair
Papillary muscle rupture	Echocardiography	Surgical valve replacement
Ventricular free wall rupture	Echocardiography, ventriculography	Emergent repair of ventricular defect

these options may only be available in selected regional medical centers, durable long-term survival can be obtained in a highly selected patient population.[15]

Postinfarction Ventricular Septal Defect

A postinfarction ventricular septal defect (VSD) is an infrequent complication occurring after fewer than 1% of acute myocardial infarctions. The infarct is most commonly in the LAD territory, with the defect in the distal septum. Alternatively, a postinfarct VSD can form from acute right coronary occlusion, with the infarct predominantly in the posterobasilar septum. They typically present 5 to 10 days following initial presentation, but can occur earlier, particularly if late thrombolytic therapy was administered. The diagnosis should be considered in a patient in whom cardiogenic shock with refractory hypotension and pulmonary edema develops suddenly following a myocardial infarction. On physical examination, an unmistakable holosystolic murmur can be heard over the entire precordium. The diagnosis is confirmed with echocardiography using Doppler techniques to demonstrate flow across the interventricular septum. Right heart catheterization will reveal a step-up in oxygen saturation from the right atrium to the pulmonary artery. Medical therapy involves stabilization to optimize cardiac output and end-organ perfusion. Refractory hypotension is typical, excluding the use of afterload reducing agents. Intra-aortic balloon counterpulsation can occasionally be helpful for afterload reduction and to optimize coronary perfusion. Emergent surgical intervention is required if there is any hope of survival. Infarcted muscle is débrided, and the defect is typically closed using prosthetic material. For surgical candidates, survival rates of approximately 50% can be expected.[16]

Papillary Muscle Rupture

Severe regurgitation of the mitral valve can occur after acute myocardial infarctions, with a frequency of less than 1%. The mechanism is related to infarction of the tip or trunk of one of the papillary muscles, with resultant disruption of the mitral subvalvar apparatus and failed leaflet coaptation. Posteroinferior MIs lead to this complication two to three times more frequently than anterior infarctions, presumably because there is more collateral blood flow to the anterolateral papillary muscle compared to the posteriomedial. While chronic mitral regurgitation can be well tolerated through adaptive changes in the left atrium and pulmonary vascular bed, severe acute mitral regurgitation results in immediate heart failure, as the small left atrium offers little compliance for the massive volume overload. Papillary muscle rupture develops typically between the third and fifth days following myocardial infarction, when infarcted myocardium is at its weakest. However, it can present within the first 24 hours. Patients will describe acute-onset dyspnea, pulmonary edema, and possibly signs of cardiogenic shock. The diagnosis should be suspected in any patient after myocardial infarction with a new holosystolic murmur heard at the apex, associated with dyspnea and hypotension. Bedside surface echocardiography typically demonstrates the mitral regurgitation, and the flail leaflet may be seen. For more definitive imaging, transesophageal echocardiography (TEE) can be performed. Not only will the mitral valve pathology be clearly seen, but also alternative diagnoses such as a postinfarct VSD can be excluded. In addition to the treatments typically employed for myocardial infarctions, immediate medical therapy of ruptured papillary muscles involves afterload reduction when tolerated, with infusions of nitroglycerine or nitroprusside. If cardiac output cannot be maintained, intra-aortic balloon counterpulsation can be helpful. Definitive therapy involves prompt surgical correction. Although mortality rates are generally high, there are no survivors without surgical correction.[17] If coronary angiography demonstrated occlusive epicardial lesions in territories other than the acute infarction, simultaneous coronary bypass grafting can be performed. Under most circumstances, the diseased mitral valve is excised and replaced. Because the ventricular cavity is typically small, the valve is usually replaced with a low-profile mechanical prosthesis to avoid left ventricular outflow obstruction from the protruding struts of stented bioprosthetic valves.

Ventricular Free Wall Rupture

Ventricular free wall rupture after myocardial infarction is infrequently encountered clinically, likely because of the exceedingly high mortality. The actual incidence is unknown, but may represent up to 30% of all deaths after acute myocardial infarctions. Like postinfarct VSD and papillary muscle ruptures, they tend to occur between the third and sixth days after infarction, when the myocardium is at its weakest. Free wall ruptures can present in essentially one of two ways: (a) a simple full-thickness tear with catastrophic hemorrhage and death from tamponade or (b) a complex serpiginous tear, partially contained. The latter is more likely to require surgical intervention, often presenting weeks from the initial infarction with symptoms of delayed cardiac tamponade. In rare cases, it is completely contained and may go unrecognized until a pseudoaneurysm develops, which is often diagnosed at a later date. Patients with free wall rupture will typically present with cardiogenic shock and may have features suggesting tamponade. Echocardiography will demonstrate a large pericardial effusion, frequently with echo-dense clot or ventricular wall defects. Urgent surgical intervention is required, often without coronary angiography or other time-consuming diagnostic tests. Once the pericardium is opened and cardiac tamponade is relieved, hemodynamic stability is often

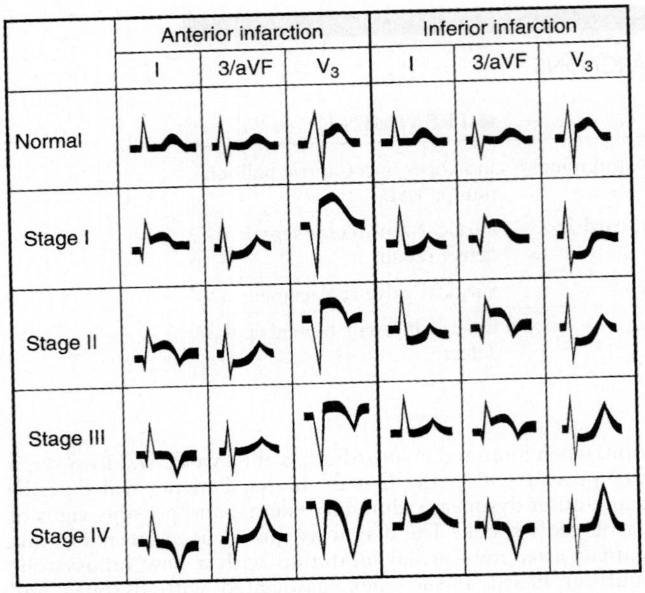
Anterior infarction
Inferior infarction
I
3/aVF
V3
I
3/aVF
V3
Normal
Stage I
Stage II
Stage III
Stage IV

FIGURE 83.3. The electrocardiogram in an acute myocardial infarction.

achieved. The site of hemorrhage is identified by the necrotic-appearing myocardium and adherent thrombus. The defect can be closed with large mattress sutures reinforced with Teflon felt strips. Care must be taken while tying the suture, as the necrotic muscle is weak and friable. Some have advocated covering the defect with a large Teflon felt patch using biologic adhesives, avoiding sutures altogether.[18] Whatever the technique, outcomes are likely determined by the hemodynamic status of the patient prior to arrival in the operating room and the quality of the remaining viable myocardium.

DIAGNOSIS

The initial diagnostic tool for patients presenting with chest pain is the resting electrocardiogram (ECG). Although the majority of patients with chronic stable angina will have a normal ECG pattern, evidence of previous myocardial infarctions may be identified, either with the presence of Q waves or conduction abnormalities. Patients with an acute myocardial infarction may demonstrate ST-segment elevation (Fig. 83.3), prompting urgent intervention. Occasionally, more subtle ECG findings may provide clues that the chest pain is ischemic in etiology. Although nonspecific, these changes may include mild ST-segment depression or T-wave inversions.

During a myocardial infarction, the dying myocytes release enzymes specific to cardiac muscle into the bloodstream. These enzymes can be detected from laboratory analysis and are pathognomonic of myocardial infarction. The MB fraction of creatine kinase is cardiac specific and rises within 8 to 24 hours of infarction and returns to baseline within 2 days. Cardiac troponin has even greater specificity and serum levels rise faster than creatine kinase, improving both the speed and accuracy in the laboratory diagnosis of an acute myocardial infarction in the absence of clear ECG changes.[19]

For asymptomatic patients, or those with chronic stable angina, the most widely used diagnostic test to evaluate for coronary artery disease is exercise electrocardiography, or a "stress test." Using standardized protocols, patients are exercised on a treadmill while the 12-lead ECG is continuously recorded. Alternatively, for those patients unable to walk, a bicycle ergometer may be used. Testing is continued until patient symptoms are noted or until the development of significant downward-sloping ST-segment depression, suggesting myocardial ischemia (Fig. 83.4). The diagnostic accuracy of exercise stress ECG testing can be enhanced with myocardial perfusion imaging. Several radioactive tracers are used clinically, the most frequent of which is thallium-201. Because of its similarities to potassium ions, it is taken up preferentially by viable cardiac myocytes. Its distribution within the myocardium is proportional to the rate of perfusion. During stress, regions of underperfused myocardium will take up less thallium, resulting in a visible defect. Following a period of rest and reperfusion, thallium uptake normalizes, demonstrating a "reversible defect."

In some cases, patients are unable to exercise because of additional physical or psychological limitations. Pharmacologic agents can substitute for exercise by increasing myocardial oxygen demand (dobutamine) or by directly vasodilating coronary arteries (adenosine or dipyridamole), thus demonstrating regions with fixed restrictions in myocardial blood flow. Echocardiography can be used as an alternative to nuclear perfusion imaging to improve the accuracy of exercise ECG testing. Regional changes in wall motion will be observed during myocardial ischemia, followed by restoration of normal myocardial contraction after rest or discontinuation of dobutamine. Echocardiography can also identify valvular abnormalities or other conditions that may influence treatment choices.

Coronary angiography, also known as cardiac catheterization, is the definitive tool for diagnosing coronary atherosclerotic

FIGURE 83.4. Electrocardiogram during an exercise test showing precordial leads V_1 through V_6. **A:** During exercise, depression of the ST segment and ischemia are seen in leads V_4 through V_6. **B:** These resolve after exercise is stopped.

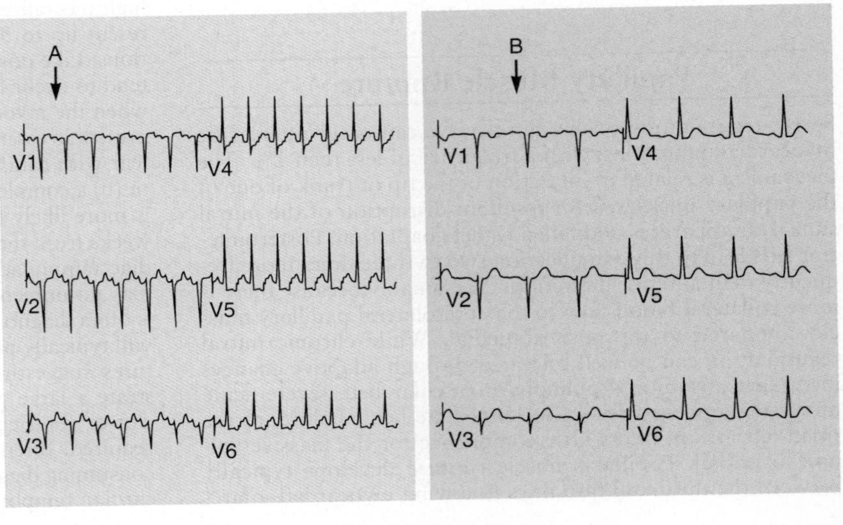

disease. Indications include symptomatic patients with typical angina refractory to medical treatments, patients with significant ischemia on exercise or pharmacologic stress testing, patients with an STEMI, or patients with an NSTEMI and persistent pain despite medical treatment. Patients with valvular heart disease who are scheduled to undergo surgical correction should also undergo coronary angiography to identify coexisting coronary occlusions, which can be addressed at the time of the valve surgery. After percutaneous access is obtained in the femoral, brachial, or radial arteries, preformed catheters of varying sizes are advanced fluoroscopically to selectively engage the ostia of the left and right coronary arteries. Radio-opaque contrast is injected with imaging of the opacified coronary artery. Standardized views are obtained of both the right and left coronary systems to provide different projections to clearly define the vascular anatomy and to quantify the severity of occlusive lesions (Fig. 83.5). Automated computer analysis systems can calculate area reduction, improving interobserver consistency. Additionally, catheters can be inserted across the aortic valve into the left ventricular cavity, providing information about ventricular pressure throughout the cardiac cycle. Contrast injection for ventriculography can illustrate ventricular systolic function, cavity size, and the presence of left-sided valvular abnormalities. New microtipped pressure sensors can be advanced across coronary lesions and document a clinically significant drop in perfusion pressure, either at rest or after provocation with vasodilating agents.[20] In addition, intravascular ultrasound imaging sensors can now be loaded onto tiny catheters and advanced into the left main coronary artery, helping to clarify the significance of lesions that may appear equivocal in severity on standard angiography.[21]

Newer imaging techniques using high-resolution multislice computed tomography (CT) scanning with three-dimensional reconstruction and magnetic resonance imaging are increasingly being utilized. These noninvasive approaches have the potential to improve the safety and convenience of coronary imaging;

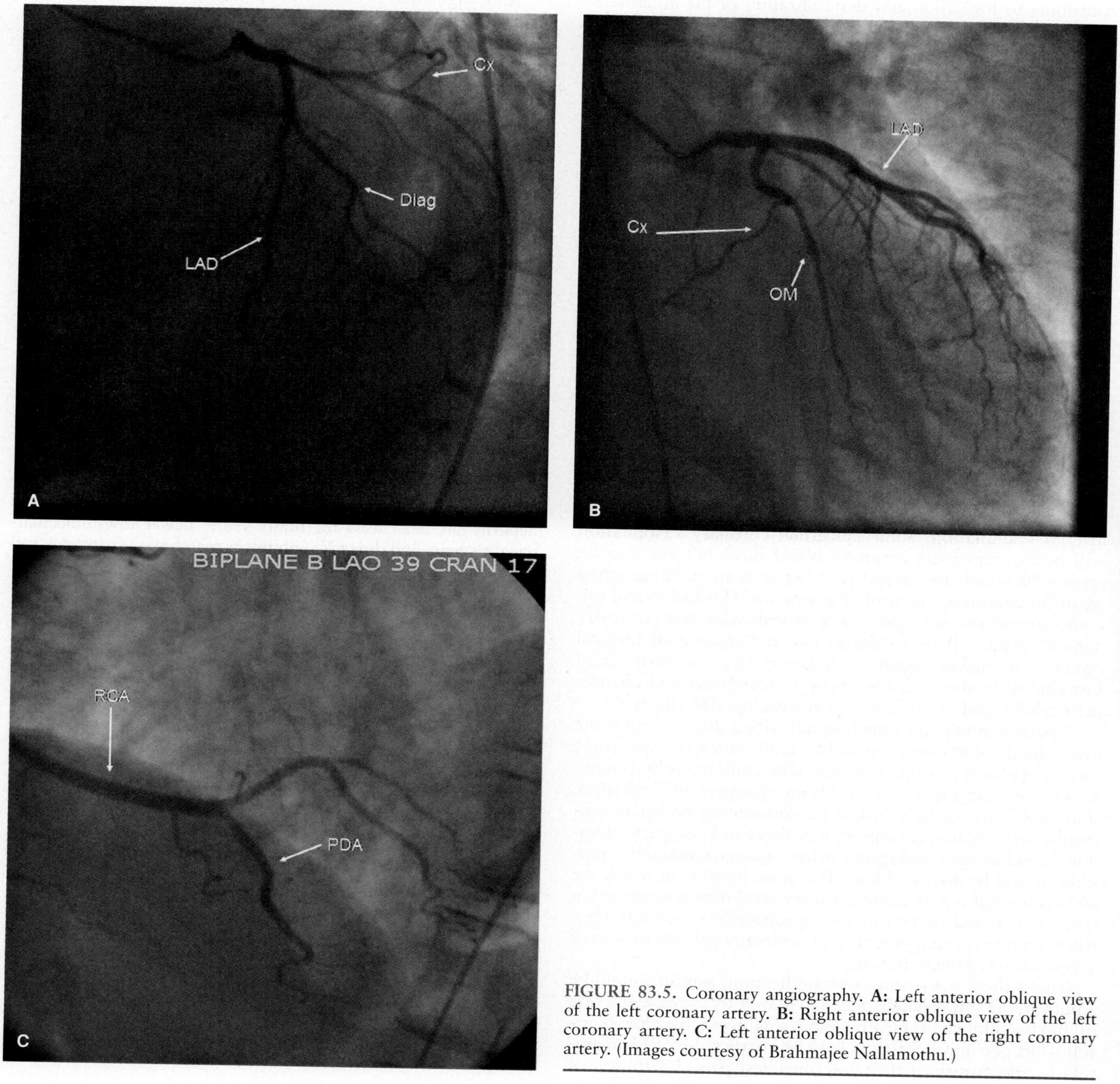

FIGURE 83.5. Coronary angiography. **A:** Left anterior oblique view of the left coronary artery. **B:** Right anterior oblique view of the left coronary artery. **C:** Left anterior oblique view of the right coronary artery. (Images courtesy of Brahmajee Nallamothu.)

VASCULAR

however, resolution remains inferior to standard coronary angiography. These techniques are often used as screening tests and are frequently followed up with traditional angiography.[22]

MEDICAL TREATMENT

5 Medical therapy of coronary artery disease is designed to slow the rate of progression of coronary artery atherosclerosis, to reduce the rate of complications from these lesions, and to control symptoms. Treatments are aimed at slowing plaque growth, reducing risk of plaque rupture, and reducing myocardial oxygen consumption. While advances in pharmacologic agents have improved the treatment of atherosclerosis and reduced mortality, lifestyle modification remains the most important intervention and the most difficult to achieve. These lifestyle modifications include cessation of cigarette smoking, weight loss, dietary control of diabetes, salt restriction, reduction in the consumption of foods high in cholesterol and fat, and exercise.

Medical therapy begins with controlling risk factors that contribute to formation and destabilization of the atherosclerotic plaque. Medical treatment alone is often satisfactory for many patients with coronary artery disease affecting only one or two epicardial vessel territories. Statins can decrease cholesterol levels and improve the ratio of low- to high-density lipoproteins and have been demonstrated to reduce rates of myocardial infarction and death.[23] Statins also appear to reduce macrophage accumulation within atheromatous plaques, matrix metalloprotease activity, and collagen degradation. Angiotensin-converting enzyme (ACE) inhibitors have been shown to reduce mortality and myocardial infarction in patients with coronary artery disease.[24] Aspirin inhibits cyclooxygenase-1 (COX-1) activity and thromboxane production, irreversibly inhibiting platelet aggregation by inhibiting platelet activity, and should be prescribed to all patients unless significant contraindications exist. Aspirin has been shown to reduce death and myocardial infarctions in patients with significant coronary artery disease. By binding the catecholamine-mediated B1 receptor on cardiac myocytes, beta-blocking agents reduce myocardial oxygen consumption by reducing heart rate and contractility, and increase perfusion by extending diastolic perfusion time. Beta-blockers are effective at controlling angina[26] and, in selected patients, reduce cardiovascular mortality.[27] Nitrates also reduce myocardial oxygen demand by decreasing cardiac preload via venodilation and by reducing afterload via arterial vasodilation. Some epicardial coronary vasodilation will occur, improving coronary blood flow. Nitrates can be given sublingually for immediate relief or as an oral long-acting agent for continuous control of symptoms. Headaches and tolerance are notable side effects. For patients who have refractory angina despite all revascularization and traditional medical options, a newer agent, ranolazine, has recently been introduced. It alters cardiac myocyte membrane ion channel permeability and can relieve angina with few side effects.[28]

A patient admitted to the hospital with a diagnosis of acute myocardial infarction or possible acute coronary syndrome should be placed in an environment with continuous ECG monitoring and the capacity to perform emergent defibrillation, since these patients are at risk of life-threatening malignant ventricular arrhythmias. Patients with evidence of ST-segment elevation should undergo emergent cardiac catheterization when possible, as will be discussed later. For those patients in which the ECG is normal but an acute coronary syndrome is suspected, a stress test should be performed expeditiously to identify their risk for future coronary events and to identify patients in need of urgent cardiac catheterization.

Unless there is a strong contraindication, aspirin should be administered immediately, ideally chewed to increase the rate of bioavailability. Typically, aspirin is given by emergency transport personnel. Patients may be instructed by 911 operators to take aspirin if they describe chest pain. Institution of oxygen therapy is important to maximizing oxygen delivery, particularly for patients in whom hypoxemic respiratory dysfunction is also present. Intravenous nitroglycerine as a continuous infusion is typically effective at controlling symptoms of pain, which is essential in reducing unnecessary myocardial strain. Small randomized trials have suggested that nitroglycerine can reduce hospital mortality, although this has not been validated in larger trials.[29] When necessary, narcotics should be added, as unrelenting pain not only increases myocardial oxygen consumption, but also may contribute to plaque instability. Beta-blocking agents can reduce myocardial oxygen consumption but can also exacerbate heart failure, particularly in the setting of severely decreased systolic ventricular function. They should be considered cautiously in hemodynamically stable patients. ACE inhibitors reduce mortality after acute myocardial infarctions, particularly those with decreased ventricular function.[30] Benefits are not just restricted to the afterload reduction effects. Some evidence suggests they have a role in alteration of the myocardial intercellular matrix and scar formation.[31]

Anticoagulation is among the most important interventions in patients presenting with an acute myocardial infarction. In recent years, patients with myocardial infarctions were placed on newer antiplatelet glycoprotein (Gp) IIb/IIIa inhibitors, which affect adenosine diphosphate (ADP)-mediated platelet adhesion. Thienopyridines are a newer class of antiplatelet agents that act by binding to the ADP receptors on the platelet surface and inhibiting the GpIIb/IIIa pathway. Specific agents include clopidogrel (Plavix) and ticlopidine (Ticlid). There is strong evidence that the addition of clopidogrel to aspirin reduces death, myocardial infarction, and stroke in the setting of ACS.[32] Clopidogrel is irreversible and has a long half-life, resulting in bleeding complications, particularly if surgery is required. Surgical intervention should ideally be delayed for 3 to 5 days.[33] Abciximab (ReoPro) is a murine antibody that binds directly to the GpIIb/IIIa receptor on platelet surfaces, preventing fibrinogen binding and activation. The half-life is short, and platelet activity generally returns to normal within 24 hours. Eptifibatide (Integrilin) is a synthetic antagonist of the GpIIa/IIIb receptor and has a half-life of 3 to 4 hours. The benefit of these agents in patients with ACS treated medically is unclear, but they have become routine in the setting of percutaneous treatment of coronary stenoses. Unless contraindications exist, inhibition of the coagulation cascade is also recommended for patients with acute myocardial infarctions. Although standard unfractionated heparin has been used for many years, newer low-molecular-weight agents and direct Xa inhibitors may have advantages and are used with increasing frequency.[34,35]

With STEMI, significant myocardium is at risk, potentially resulting in either cardiogenic shock or ventricular arrhythmias. Emergency recanalization of acutely occluded vessels can salvage cardiac function and save lives. Various fibrinolytic drugs, which convert plasminogen to plasmin, can be given emergently and restore flow in vessels obstructed by acute thrombus. A number of clinical trials were performed in the 1980s using streptokinase and demonstrated reduced survival when it was given within 12 hours.[36] Newer agents are now available including tissue plasminogen inhibitor (tPA) and reteplase, which are faster in onset and may further improve outcomes, although they are more costly.

The main drawbacks of fibrinolytic therapy are bleeding complications and failure of recanalization. Systemic intravenous thrombolytic therapy unquestionably decreases morbidity and mortality after MI and continues to be used in 40% to 50% of eligible patients. The earlier the treatment, the greater the impact, with the greatest benefit accruing in patients treated within 1 to 2 hours after the onset of symptoms.

In 1977, Dr. Andreas Gruentzig performed the first percutaneous intervention with balloon angioplasty on a stenotic lesion in the LAD. This pioneer laid the foundation for a revolution in the treatment of coronary artery disease worldwide.

Percutaneous treatment of acute STEMI is now standard practice in centers in which this therapy is available, with outcomes that are superior to pharmacologic reperfusion.[37] Although percutaneous intervention may be better than fibrinolysis, the treatment requires numerous experienced personnel and highly technologic equipment, which is not always available in every facility. Complex interhospital and intrahospital systems are now in place to improve the efficiency and application of this treatment strategy, and guidelines have defined minimum "door to balloon" times to salvage myocardium at risk.[38]

PERCUTANEOUS CORONARY INTERVENTIONS

6 Since the inception of percutaneous transcoronary balloon angioplasty (PTCA), catheter-directed treatment of coronary artery disease has evolved into one of the most commonly performed procedures worldwide. Advances in technology have improved outcomes and expanded the indications, particularly for the acutely ischemic heart. Using the same techniques described for cardiac catheterization, small, highly flexible and steerable guide wires can be advanced through the lumen of epicardial coronary arteries. Over this guide wire, balloon-tipped catheters can be advanced and centered across discrete stenotic lesions and inflated to 4 to 10 atmospheric pressures, stretching and dilating the affected vessel (Fig. 83.6). Typically, the vessel tears or cracks at the junction of the plaque and the normal vessel wall. Acute thrombosis or coronary dissection could result in immediate closure of the vessel, often necessitating emergent surgical coronary bypass grafting in approximately 5% of cases. Restenosis is common, occurring in nearly 40% to 50% of patients, either from mechanical elastic recoil or progressive neointimal hyperplasia.

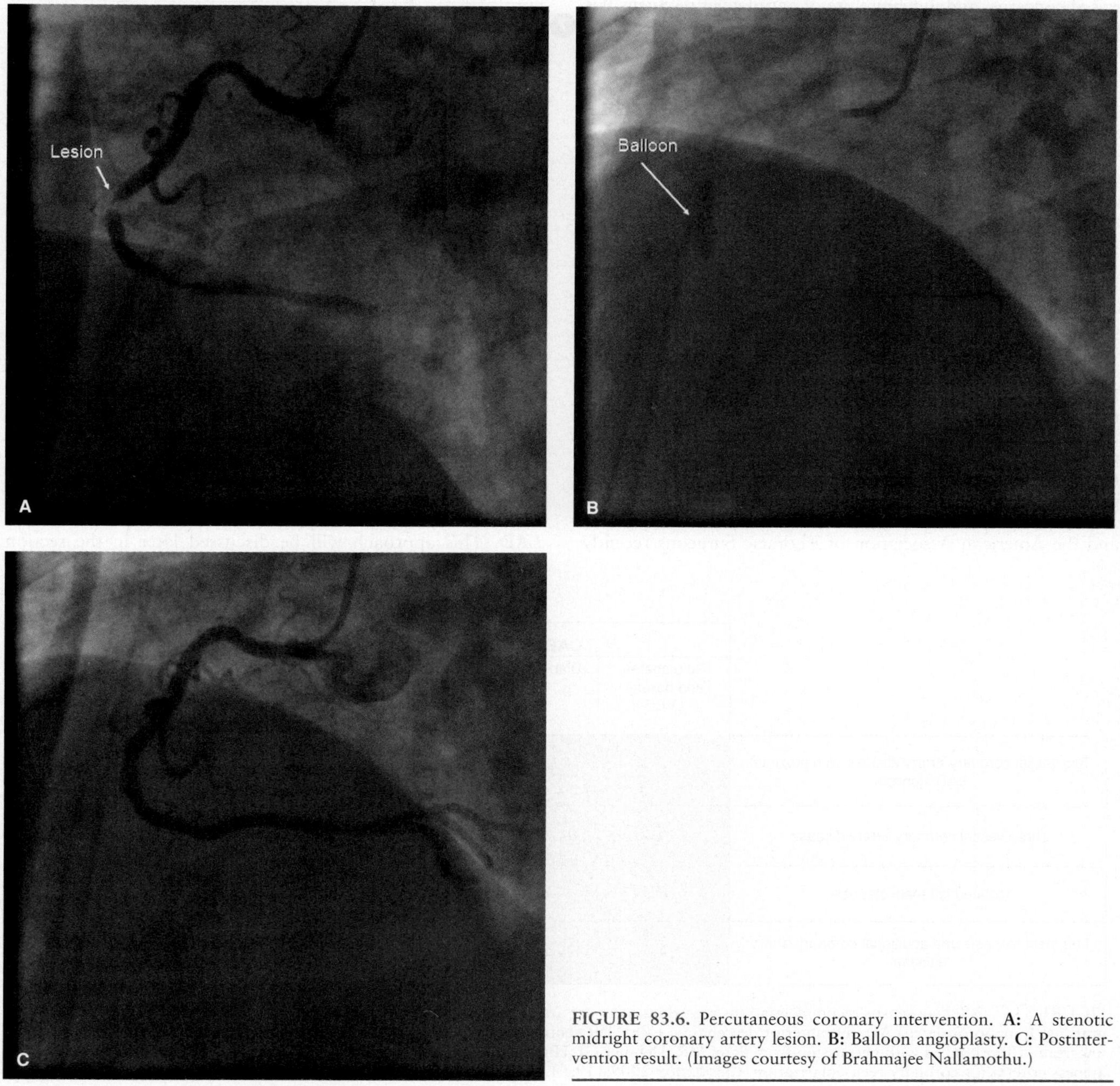

FIGURE 83.6. Percutaneous coronary intervention. **A:** A stenotic midright coronary artery lesion. **B:** Balloon angioplasty. **C:** Postintervention result. (Images courtesy of Brahmajee Nallamothu.)

The addition of stents, nitinol scaffolding devices, has nearly eliminated acute vessel occlusion, and the need for salvage surgical revascularization is below 1%. In addition, stents have greatly reduced restenosis rates down to nearly 20% and are used in nearly 90% of percutaneous procedures in the United States. The stents are delivered crimped onto a deflated balloon. With balloon inflation, the stent expands, restoring the vessel lumen to its anatomic dimensions. The stent prevents elastic recoil and coronary dissection, improving immediate outcomes, but the problem of neointimal hyperplasia remains, resulting in the persistent rates of restenosis. Stents have been improved even further by impregnating antiproliferative drugs onto the scaffolds. Sirolimus and paclitaxel are immunosuppressants that act by different mechanisms. Paclitaxel is a mitotic inhibitor, which retards microtubule breakdown. Sirolimus binds intracellularly to FK-binding protein and inhibits interleukin-2 (IL-2) production via the target of rapamycin pathway. Both sirolimus- and paclitaxel-eluting stents have further reduced the rate of target vessel restenosis and the need for repeat interventions.[39] However, reports of late stent thrombosis have raised concerns, and indefinite use of antiplatelet regimens has been recommended.[40]

CORONARY BYPASS GRAFTING

Indications

Coronary artery bypass grafting (CABG) is one of the most common and most studied surgical procedures performed in the United States. As one might expect, CABG consumes more resources than any other single cardiovascular procedure. Dozens of multicenter, prospective, randomized trials have been performed comparing the surgical treatment of coronary artery disease to both medical and percutaneous options. Some of these landmark studies will be discussed in detail later in the chapter, as proper understanding of these trials is important in determining appropriate treatment strategies for individual patients. In summary, these studies consistently demonstrate that CABG continues to be the best revascularization strategy, reducing rate of both myocardial infarctions and the need for repeat revascularization in patients with a broad degree of occlusive disease. A task force made up of numerous medical societies including the American College of Cardiology, the American Heart Association, the Society of Thoracic Surgeons, and the American Association of Thoracic Surgeons recently published guidelines on the indications for coronary artery revascularization and made recommendations regarding the mode of revascularization.[41] The group considered a number of variables, including clinical symptoms and mode of presentation, the degree of ischemia determined by noninvasive imaging, and the severity of coronary disease based on angiographic imaging. In summary, patients are more likely to benefit from surgical revascularization if they have worse symptoms, more severe myocardial ischemia, and more extensive coronary artery occlusions. The recommendations are summarized in Figure 83.7, where recommendations are categorized as "appropriate," "uncertain," and "inappropriate." Interestingly, these guidelines have not changed markedly over the last several decades, despite vast improvements in both medical treatment and percutaneous technology. Today, CABG remains the best mode of cardiac revascularization in symptomatic patients.

Standard Technique

7 The basic principles in coronary bypass grafting are to restore normal unimpeded perfusion of ischemic myocardial territories by providing alternative routes for blood flow. Previous approaches to surgically revascularize the myocardium included creation of intramyocardial tunnels and arterialization of the coronary sinus. However, it was the aortocoronary bypass pioneered by a surgeon named Rene Favaloro at the Cleveland Clinic in the late 1960s that revolutionized the treatment of coronary atherosclerosis. The technique has evolved considerably over the decades, and there remains significant variability in how this complex procedure is conducted even today.

The heart is typically exposed via a median sternotomy. This incision allows exposure of the anterior surface of the heart, as well as the great vessels, for initiation of cardiopulmonary bypass. Except for the severely hypertrophic heart, the entire epicardial surface can be exposed with manipulation and traction on the left ventricle. Alternatively, a left lateral thoracotomy can be used. This limits visualization to the obtuse margin of the heart but can be advantageous, particularly if the patient has previously had a median sternotomy with dense adhesions hazarding catastrophic injury during sternal reentry. Another alternative has been a limited left anterior thoracotomy, which exposes only a small portion of the anterior wall of the left ventricle, usually limited to revascularization of the LAD. This approach will be discussed later in the section

	CABG			PCI		
	No diabetes and normal LVEF	Diabetes	Depressed LVEF	No diabetes and normal LVEF	Diabetes	Depressed LVEF
Two vessel coronary artery disease with proximal LAD stenosis	A	A	A	A	A	A
Three vessel coronary artery disease	A	A	A	U	U	U
Isolated left main stenosis	A	A	A	I	I	I
Left main stenosis and additional coronary artery disease	A	A	A	I	I	I

FIGURE 83.7. 2009 consensus recommendations regarding coronary artery revascularization. A, appropriate; CABG, coronary artery bypass grafting; I, inappropriate; LAD, left anterior descending; LVEF, left ventricular ejection fraction; PCI, percutaneous coronary intervention; U, uncertain. (Reproduced with permission from Patel MR, Dehmer GJ, Hirshfeld JW, et al. ACCF/SCAI/STS/AATS/AHA/ASNC 2009 appropriateness criteria for coronary revascularization. *Circulation* 2009;119:1330–1353.)

describing minimally invasive approaches to surgical revascularization.

The key to constructing a durable and reproducible anastomosis to small diseased epicardial vessels is creation of a quiet and bloodless surgical field. The advent of cardiopulmonary bypass (CPB) using extracorporeal circulation along with cardiac standstill using cardioplegia has allowed precisely this environment. The epicardial vessels are motionless and can be brought directly into the surgical field. Epicardial blood flow is eliminated, allowing direct visualization of the lumen without arterial control, avoiding potential clamp or snare injury to the fragile vessels.

After anticoagulation with 300 IU/kg of heparin is confirmed with an activated clotting time (ACT), the patient is cannulated in the distal ascending aorta. Patients may have significant atherosclerotic disease, and the cannulation site should be carefully inspected for mobile lesions using transesophageal echocardiography and manual palpation. Some centers advocate epiaortic ultrasonic imaging for more accurate visualization. After insertion, the cannula is manually deaired and connected to the arterial limb of the CPB circuit (Fig. 83.8). Venous drainage is accomplished with a cannula in the right atrium, typically in the atrial appendage. Bleeding from the cannulation sites is controlled by pursestring sutures around the cannulas. Bypass is initiated by venous drainage into a reservoir, emptying the heart of venous return. Blood is pumped into a membrane oxygenator and returned into the aortic cannula, typically at a blood flow rate of 2.4 L/min per m^2 of body surface area. With full flow, ventilation of the patient can be discontinued, further improving visualization and minimizing motion in the surgical field. The extracorporeal blood is cooled, creating mild hypothermia, varying from 28°C to 32°C. Systemic cooling minimizes end-organ injury from relative hypotension or hypoperfusion from nonpulsatile blood flow.

After adequate cardiopulmonary bypass is confirmed, the heart is arrested by applying a clamp across the midascending aorta, proximal to the aortic cannulation site. This clamp isolates the native coronary vessels from the remainder of the systemic circulation. Cardioplegia is then delivered to the myocardium via a needle or catheter in the aortic root. There are a variety of cardioplegia solutions commercially available, but the most important components are dilute blood, cold temperature (8°C to 15°C), potassium at 15 to 30 mM/L, citrate for calcium binding, dextrose for myocardial substrate, and pH buffers. The cold temperature and potassium maintain the heart in diastolic arrest, reducing myocardial oxygen consumption. Cardioplegia is typically delivered intermittently, approximately every 15 to 20 minutes, to provide adequate oxygen and nutrient delivery and to minimize myocardial activity. Additionally, some surgeons utilize cardioplegia delivered in a retrograde fashion via a specially designed balloon-tipped catheter inserted into the coronary sinus. Protocols relying entirely upon antegrade delivery of cardioplegia hazard incomplete myocardial protection, particularly in territories of severe coronary artery stenosis or total occlusions. In addition, an incompetent aortic valve will limit cardioplegia delivery down the coronaries, and leaking into the left ventricle will result in significant ventricular distention. Furthermore, antegrade cardioplegia

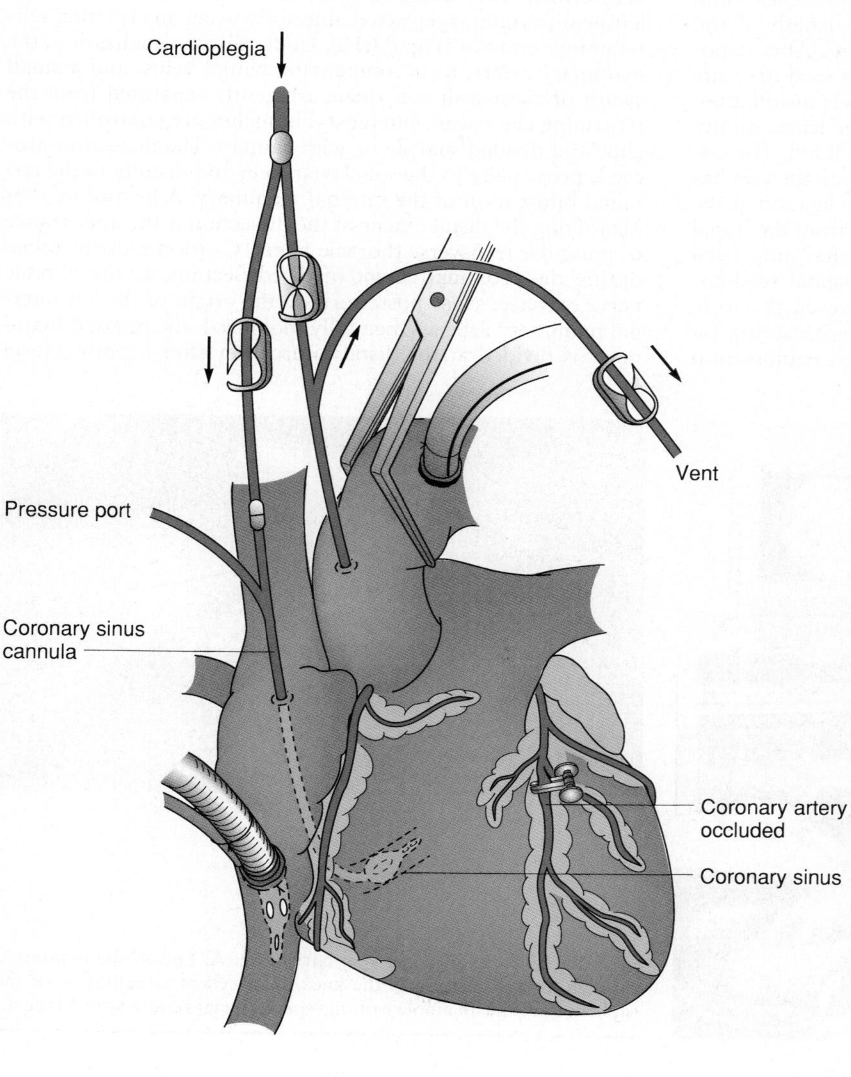

FIGURE 83.8. Instrumentation for cardiopulmonary bypass.

can be delivered under supraphysiologic pressures from the extracorporeal mechanical blood pumps. This can result in epicardial vessel injury and embolization of atheromatous debris, particularly in the reoperative setting in which old vein grafts often contain mobile and highly friable lesions. The use of retrograde cardioplegia can overcome these limitations, and some evidence suggests outcomes can be improved.

Conduits used for coronary bypass grafting are variable. The oldest and most frequently chosen conduit is the greater saphenous vein because of its availability, accessibility, reasonable size match, the facility with which vascular anastomoses can be created, and the avoidance of morbidity in harvesting the vein. The adequacy and size of the vein can be assessed preoperatively using ultrasound techniques. Generally, a conduit of 2 to 4 mm in diameter is considered suitable. Alternative veins, such as the lesser saphenous vein and cephalic vein, are infrequently used for coronary bypass grafting because patency rates have been reported to be low. The greater saphenous vein can be exposed with a single long incision, beginning at the ankle, midway between the medial malleolus and the anterior tibial tendon. It is important to handle the vein gently and avoid electrocautery directly on the vein to minimize traumatic or thermal injury to the endothelial cells. The side branches are carefully ligated, and the vein is preserved in a solution of cold heparinized blood, often with vasodilating agents such as papaverine and nitroglycerine. If dissection is minimized and hemostasis is meticulously ensured, the incidence of infection and wound healing complications is generally low. Patients will complain of pain along the length of the incision, but this typically resolves after several weeks.

In more recent years, minimally invasive approaches using endoscopic techniques can harvest the entire length of the greater saphenous vein with three small incisions. After exposure of the vessel at the knee, a blunt dissector is used to create a tissue plane, which is then expanded with CO_2 insufflation. Direct visualization with magnifying endoscopic lenses allows identification and ligation of side branches (Fig. 83.9). The dissection proceeds both proximally and distally, until the vein has been fully mobilized. Small stab incisions allow ligation at the groin and the ankle, and extraction of the vein from the initial incision. This technique has reduced pain, has improved patient satisfaction, and appears to reduce hospital readmission from wound healing complications. However, the technique is more time consuming, which can be aggravating for the impatient surgeon. In addition, the disposable equipment is expensive, increasing the costs by approximately $500 to $1,000, depending on the manufacturer and negotiated contract pricing. More importantly, a recent nonrandomized report described the use of endoscopic vein harvesting as an independent predictor of vein graft occlusion, hospital readmission for major cardiac adverse event, and mortality, as compared to open saphenous vein harvesting techniques.[42] This study was in contrast to the previous smaller randomized trials but raises concerns about the use of this strategy. Proponents of endoscopic vein harvesting argue that the observational trial did not describe the operator's previous experience using minimally invasive harvesting and suggest that many centers remained on the early part of their learning curve. In addition, newer technology now allows for safer delivery of bipolar electrocautery, minimizing the potential for heat transmission and endothelial injury. In addition, many centers are now administering low doses of heparin before initiating the dissection to reduce the likelihood of in situ thrombus during manipulation of the vein. It is likely that the debate regarding minimally invasive saphenous vein harvesting will continue in the near future.

Arterial conduits for coronary bypass grafting have been increasingly utilized because of early neointimal hyperplasia and late accelerated atherosclerosis seen in saphenous vein
8 grafts. The most important of these arterial conduits is the left internal mammary artery, which originates from the left subclavian artery and descends caudally behind the chest wall, just lateral to the sternal edge. It gives off intercostal branches until it terminates distally as the bifurcation into the superior epigastric and musculophrenic arteries. The artery is typically mobilized as a pedicle, left intact at its origin from the subclavian artery. After completion of the median sternotomy, the left hemisternum is retracted anteriorly using an elevating self-retaining retractor (Fig. 83.10). Under direct visualization, the mammary artery, its accompanying paired veins, and a small swath of chest-wall soft tissue are gently separated from the remaining chest wall. Intercostal branches are controlled with clips and divided sharply or with cautery. The dissection proceeds proximally to the subclavian vein and distally to the terminal bifurcation of the internal mammary. A helpful marker identifying the distal extent of the dissection is the appearance of muscular transverse thoracic fibers. Caution must be taken during the proximal extent of the dissection, as the phrenic nerve traverses close posteriorly to the origin of the left internal mammary artery. Once fully mobilized, the internal mammary is divided at the distal bifurcation after heparinization

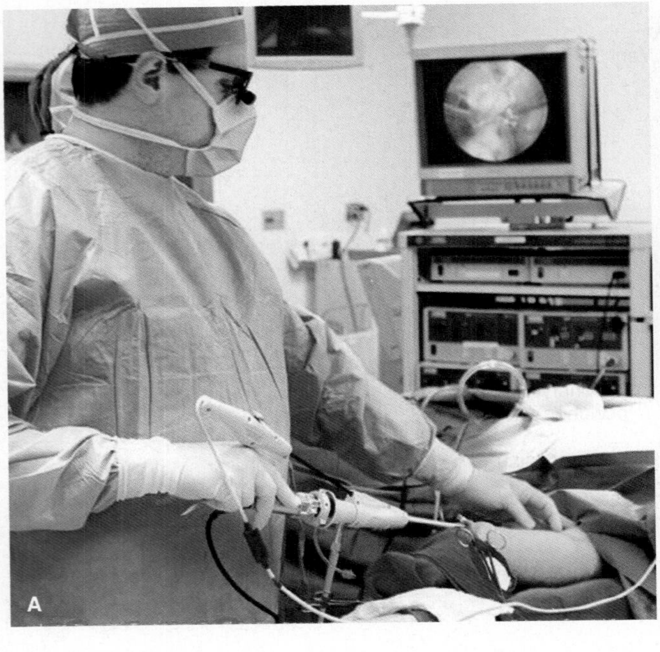

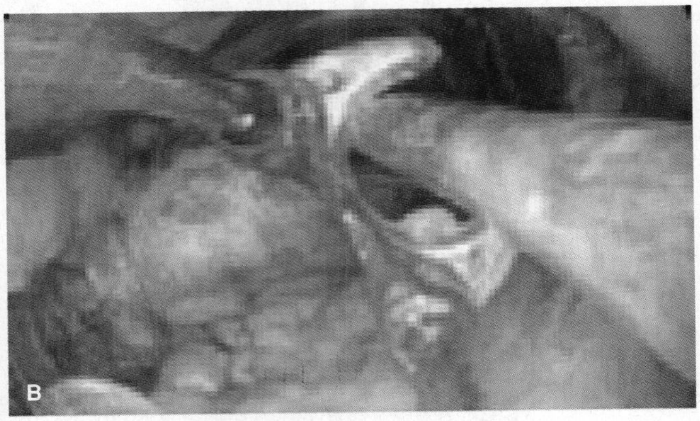

FIGURE 83.9. Endoscopic vein harvesting. **A:** Endoscope is inserted through a small incision in the knee. **B:** Excellent visualization of the saphenous vein with ample working space. (Images courtesy of Maquet.)

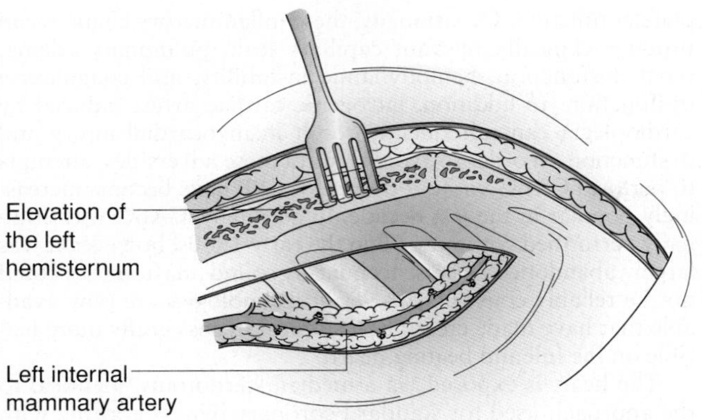

FIGURE 83.10. Elevation of the left hemisternum for visualization of the left internal mammary artery.

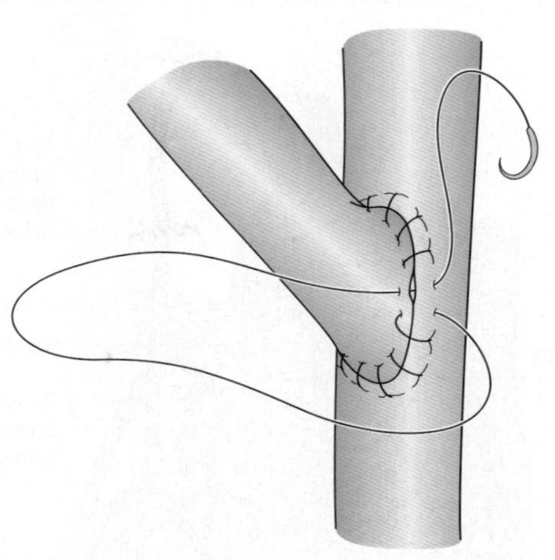

FIGURE 83.11. Distal coronary anastomosis with saphenous vein conduit. Excellent visualization in a quiet bloodless field is required to achieve a hemostatic and unobstructed graft.

and soaked in a solution of vasodilating agents to overcome spasm from manipulation.

Other arterial conduits are also increasingly utilized, such as the right internal mammary artery, the radial artery, the gastroepiploic artery, and the inferior epigastric artery. The internal mammary artery tends to be spared of atherosclerotic disease, and its patency rates are excellent many years following bypass surgery. As such, many surgeons routinely harvest both internal mammary arteries to take advantage of this biologic privilege. However, utilization of both internal mammary arteries can devascularize the sternum and increase the risk of postoperative sternal wound infections, particularly in obese diabetics.[43] The radial artery can be harvested safely in the majority of patients, as a complete palmar arch allows collateral flow to the hand from the ulnar artery. Preoperative ultrasound in addition to a bedside Allen test can reliably identify patients in which hand ischemia precludes radial artery use. Although the radial artery is more resistant to late occlusions typical in saphenous vein grafts, it tends to be prone to spasm from competitive flow originating from subcritically stenosed native coronary vessels. Radial arteries should only be used on coronary targets with at least 70% proximal stenoses. The inferior epigastric artery has been used as an arterial conduit, but limitations in length and the need for an abdominal incision have diminished enthusiasm. The right gastroepiploic artery can be used, since it has more than adequate length after mobilization off of the greater curve of the stomach. It is left on its pedicle from the gastroduodenal artery and tunneled through a hole in the diaphragm. It is most frequently used to revascularize the posterior descending coronary branch, but will easily reach posterolateral branches as well. Patency has generally been reported to be excellent, but its widespread use is restricted by the additional morbidity of laparotomy and risks of intra-abdominal complications.

Once conduits have been harvested, cardiopulmonary bypass has been instituted, and cardioplegia infusion has resulted in adequate diastolic arrest, the heart is manipulated to expose the epicardial vessels of interest. Occasionally, the coronary arteries are in fact not on the epicardial surface but run within the epicardial fat or deep within the myocardium. This is common for intermediate branches and the LAD. Careful dissection is often required. If the midportion of the LAD cannot be found, the vessel can be opened at the apex and a small coronary probe can be inserted proximally and palpated to better localize the vessel. Care must be taken to ensure the target has been properly identified. Even the most seasoned cardiac surgeons have mistakenly anastomosed grafts to epicardial veins. Once the target vessel is properly located, an appropriate site for anastomotic construction should be identified. It is important to have a thorough understanding of the angiographic location of significant obstructions to ensure the graft is bypassing all significant lesions. The anastomotic site should ideally be relatively spared of atherosclerotic disease, although in patients with advanced diabetes this is not always possible. The vessel is dissected using a #64 sharp scalpel and opened vertically in the midline. This maneuver is among the most essential and challenging, and requires precision and experience. Eccentric incisions, inadvertent incisions in the posterior wall, or incisions in friable plaques can result in stenotic or leaky constructions. The arteriotomy is extended using fine Potts scissors 3 to 4 mm in length. The conduit is beveled to the appropriate length and the anastomosis is created with a continuous running polypropylene suture, usually size 7–0 or 8–0 (Fig. 83.11). Absolute technical precision is crucial, and skills required for these distal coronary anastomoses take practice and experience. A motionless and dry surgical field, 2.5 to 3.5 magnifying loupes, experienced assistance, and a steady hand are essential. Some surgeons use gentle insufflation of CO_2 to clear the field of obscuring blood and to distend the coronary artery to improve visualization of the toe and heal. After completion of the anastomosis, saphenous vein grafts or free arterial grafts can be hand injected with cold saline to visualize patency of the vessel and competence of the construction. Pedicled arterial grafts can be opened, and flow down the target will be easily visualized.

The proximal ends of the grafts are usually connected to the ascending aorta. The grafts are cut to the appropriate length. This maneuver also requires experience, as a short graft will create tension, potentially impinging upon the distal anastomosis, and an excessively long graft may kink. The graft is distended to prevent twisting, and the aortic root is filled by infusing antegrade cardioplegia to help determine optimal graft length. One must take into account the change in geometry as the heart fills after weaning from cardiopulmonary bypass. In general, the conduits should take a straight trajectory toward their target (Fig. 83.12). An aortotomy is created using a specially designed punch of 4 or 5 mm diameter. The grafts are beveled, and the proximal anastomosis is created with continuous running 5–0 or 6–0 polypropylene. Alternatively, the aortic cross-clamp can be removed after completion of all of the distal coronary anastomoses, and a side-biting partial aortic clamp can be placed. This technique can reduce total cardioplegia time but may increase risk of atheroembolic complications from additional aortic manipulation.

After completion of all distal and proximal anastomoses and the aortic cross-clamp has been removed, the temperature

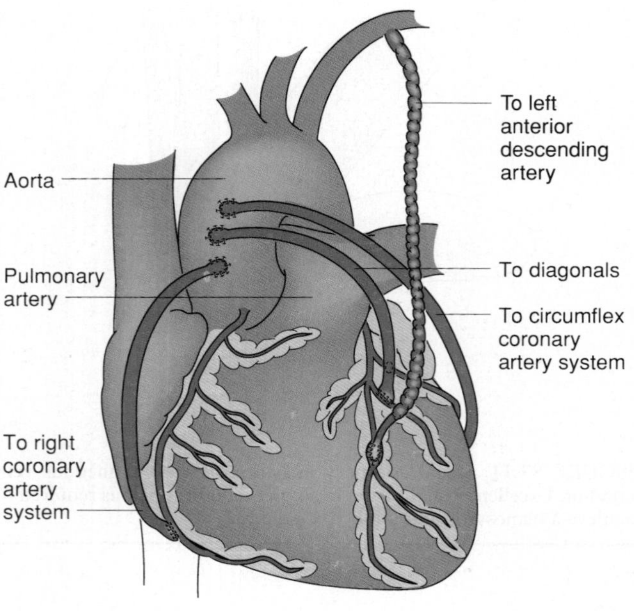

FIGURE 83.12. Bypass grafts take gentle curving but a direct approach to the coronary targets. The pericardium is typically left open to avoid kinking.

of extracorporeal circulation is warmed. Ventricular fibrillation often occurs but can easily be defibrillated with a single internal shock. Ventilation of the lungs is resumed, and CPB flow is gradually reduced. Careful inspection of myocardial contractility and volume is required during weaning, as transient dysfunction often occurs. It is important to avoid distention of ventricular chambers, which causes unnecessary increased myocardial strain. A period of empty beating reperfusion is often helpful, particularly if the aortic cross-clamp period was prolonged or if the heart was severely ischemic preoperatively. Temporary sinus node or atrioventricular node conduction abnormalities are common, and it is standard to place temporary pacemaker leads on the ventricle, although permanent conduction abnormalities are very rare. Suture lines should be inspected for hemostasis, and cannulas for cardiopulmonary bypass are removed. Although not essential for routine CABG, pulmonary artery catheters and transesophageal echocardiography are helpful in weaning from CPB. Excessive pulmonary artery pressures or new regional wall motion abnormalities can suggest perfusion abnormalities and should prompt careful inspection of the bypass grafts. Once satisfactory hemodynamics are achieved, protamine is administered to reverse the anticoagulation of heparin. A notch in the pericardium to the left of the pulmonary artery must be created to allow unhindered passage of the pedicled left internal mammary artery to its distal target. The pericardium is typically left open after coronary bypass grafting to avoid graft kinking or compression; however, mediastinal and thymic fat can be carefully placed over the aorta and proximal anastomoses to protect them from future sternal reentry. Drains are left within the mediastinum to collect shed blood, and the sternum is closed with steel wires, cables, or plates.

Off-pump Technique

While the use of cardiopulmonary bypass was essential in allowing safe and reproducible coronary anastomoses, it is now well understood that extracorporeal circulation incites a powerful inflammatory response, activating neutrophils and monocytes to release cytokines and inhibiting the clotting cascade and platelet function. Occasionally, these inflammatory changes can produce clinically relevant capillary leak, pulmonary edema, renal dysfunction, hemodynamic instability, and coagulation dysfunction. In addition, iatrogenic cardiac arrest induced by cardioplegia can infrequently result in myocardial injury and dysfunction. In order to avoid some of these adversities, attempts to perform CABG without the use of CPB have become increasingly popular in the last decade. Interestingly, CABG was originally performed without CPB in the early 1960s; however, it was largely abandoned because technically sound anastomoses could not be reliably constructed. Newer technologies are now available that have made creation of surgical bypass grafts more feasible on the full and beating heart.

The heart is exposed via a median sternotomy, identical to the approach used for standard coronary bypass grafting with cardiopulmonary bypass. Additional sutures are placed deep within the posterior pericardium, which can be used to facilitate retraction of the heart anteriorly and rightward, exposing the anterior, anterolateral, and obtuse marginal surfaces. Typically, the vessel with the most severe occlusion is grafted first, since occlusion of the vessel will result in the least myocardial ischemia and revascularization of this territory may collateralize other regions and improve tolerance to alternate vessel occlusion. For saphenous vein and free arterial grafts, the proximal anastomoses are performed first to allow immediate revascularization of ischemic territories following completion of the distal anastomoses. A dose of heparin is administered, typically 150 IU/kg, and adequate anticoagulation is confirmed with an ACT. A partial occlusion clamp is placed on the ascending aorta for control. Alternatively, newer sealing systems allow clampless control of the ascending aorta during construction of the proximal anastomoses, and sutureless connectors are available that can variably create satisfactory graft–aorta constructs. Once the proximal connections are complete, the grafts are carefully cut to the appropriate length after identification of the anticipated sites of the distal targets.

Of the potential epicardial vessels, the LAD is the easiest to expose, since it lies anteriorly. Gentle retraction on the pericardial sutures, occasionally along with a pad placed behind the heart, will usually expose the vessel adequately. The diagonal branches are exposed with slightly further rightward retraction. The obtuse marginal vessels can be exposed with the help of a suction device placed on the apex of the heart and slowly and gently retracting the apex anteriorly and rightward. This maneuver must be performed carefully, as cardiac chamber and/or outflow tracts can become compressed. The anesthesiologist must be alerted to and familiar with these maneuvers, as temporary vasoactive infusions may be required. Exposure of the right coronary artery and its branches is often the most challenging. The right ventricle can become compressed with retraction superiorly. The suction apparatus placed on the acute margin can facilitate exposure, as can stiff retraction of the right-sided pericardial edges.

Once the epicardial vessel of interest is identified, a U-shaped epicardial suction stabilizing device is applied around the vessel (Fig. 83.13). This device can reduce myocardial motion in a small region of interest, maintaining reasonable contractility. Silastic tapes loaded on blunt needles are carefully encircled around the proximal and distal portions of the coronary artery and gently retracted for blood flow control. A variable degree of ischemia may be seen on the electrocardiogram and transesophageal echocardiogram. The vessel is dissected and opened in the same way as is done for on-pump techniques. If ischemia is pronounced, small shunts can be inserted in the arteriotomy and the silastic snares released to reestablish some distal flow. Continuous insufflation of CO_2 can reduce obscuring blood from the field. The anastomosis is constructed, and competency is assessed. Electrocardiographic normalization should be seen immediately, confirming graft patency. Once all the grafts are complete, protamine is given to reverse the anticoagulation effect of heparin. Hemostasis is confirmed and closure proceeds routinely.

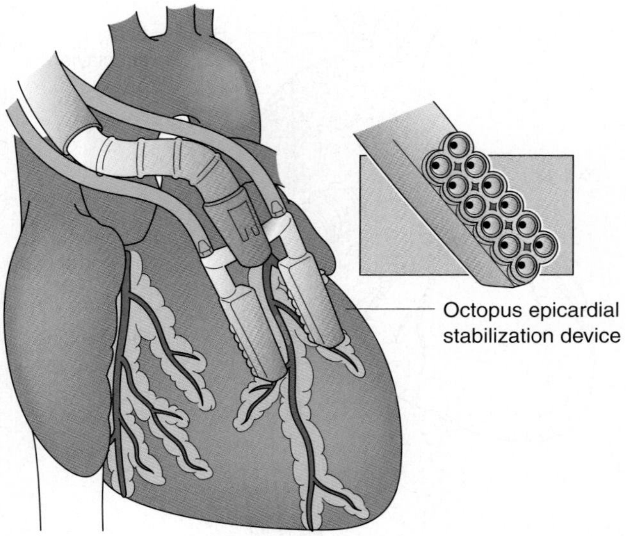

FIGURE 83.13. Suction-stabilizing devices allow isolation and immobilization of epicardial coronary targets.

Despite early enthusiasm for off-pump coronary bypass surgery, concerns regarding long-term patency of bypass grafts have prompted investigation into its true benefits and general application. A large multicenter randomized trial recently published investigated short- and midterm outcomes of patients undergoing either standard coronary bypass surgery with cardiopulmonary bypass or off-pump bypass.[44] Over 2,000 patients referred for coronary bypass grafting were randomly assigned to undergo standard versus off-pump CABG. All patients were felt to be suitable candidates for both approaches, and all surgeons had previously completed a median of 50 off-pump procedures to ensure competency. The primary endpoints were morbidity and mortality at 30 days and 1 year, and secondary endpoints were graft patency and neuropsychologic testing. Thirty-day mortality was similar in both groups (1.6% vs. 1.2% in off-pump vs. on-pump, respectively; $p = 0.47$), as was the rate of perioperative stroke (1.3% vs. 0.7%; $p = 0.28$). However, at 1 year, there was a higher rate of cardiac death in the off-pump group (2.7% vs. 1.3%; $p = 0.03$). At 1 year, 65% of patients underwent routine cardiac catheterization, revealing a significantly reduced rate of graft patency in the off-pump group (82.6% vs. 87.8%; $p < 0.01$), particularly for saphenous vein grafts (76.6% vs. 83.8%; $p < 0.01$). Neuropsychologic testing was performed to attempt to quantify benefits from eliminating proposed neurocognitive dysfunction attributed to cardiopulmonary bypass. Fifty-four percent of randomized patients completed neuropsychologic testing at baseline and at 1 year, and interestingly, there were no significant differences observed from baseline to 1 year between off-pump and on-pump strategies. In summary, this important and well-conducted study showed no advantages and potential disadvantages of off-pump surgical revascularization in this selected cohort of patients. While there are valid criticisms of this study, these data certainly suggest that routine use of off-pump CABG is not superior, and perhaps should be reserved to selected populations. This author uses off-pump techniques for patients with a heavily calcified or atheromatous ascending aorta or those with severe renal or hepatic dysfunction.

In addition to off-pump CABG, a variety of "minimally invasive" approaches have been conceptualized. The minimally invasive direct coronary bypass (MIDCAB) involves creating a small left anterior thoracotomy. After entering the chest in the fourth intercostal space and resecting a portion of the fourth costal cartilage, a portion of the left internal mammary artery is mobilized under direct vision. Using off-pump techniques and stabilizing equipment, the internal mammary artery is anastomosed to the LAD using conventional open instruments. Although experiences at selected single centers have described satisfactory patency and reduced cost, complications, and postoperative length of stay,[45] the MIDCAB has not achieved widespread application. Technical considerations and exposure have raised concerns about graft patency, and in the era of increased percutaneous intervention, very few patients are referred with isolated single-vessel disease. Some groups have advocated for a hybrid approach, in which the LAD is surgically grafted using the MIDCAB approach and the right coronary and circumflex branches are treated percutaneously.[46] Robotic systems, such as the da Vinci (Intuitive Surgical, Sunnydale, CA), benefit from high-definition three-dimensional video visualization and precise remotely controlled instruments with 6- or 7-degree freedom of motion. They have been increasingly used in noncardiac surgery, particularly in gynecology and urologic specialties. Some centers have begun using robotic technology to harvest the internal mammary artery along its entire length, followed by a MIDCAB, also known as robotically assisted CABG (RASCAB).[47] Others have gone one step further, performing complete coronary revascularization using robotic instruments: the totally endoscopic coronary artery bypass (TECAB).[48,49] The procedure has been performed with or without cardiopulmonary bypass and cardiac arrest. Although in selected centers the procedure appears feasible, the widespread utilization of minimally invasive coronary artery bypass remains in question because of concerns regarding patency, particularly in light of recent evidence regarding off-pump surgery in general. Despite changes in technology, there has been little growth in minimally invasive coronary artery bypass procedures.

POSTOPERATIVE CARE

Most patients after undergoing coronary bypass grafting require very little physician intervention, particularly if the operation was conducted according to the preoperative plan. The use of clinical care pathways is now routine, and they have been demonstrated to reduce morbidity, cost, and length of hospital stay. However, complications can occur, which must be anticipated for early recognition and treatment.

Patients after cardiac surgery are routinely admitted to the intensive care setting. Most centers delay extubation until systemic warming is complete, typically within 4 to 6 hours. This also gives ample opportunity to ensure adequate hemostasis and hemodynamic stability. Many centers routinely use pulmonary artery catheters, or Swan-Ganz catheters, for assessment of intracardiac filling pressures as well as calculation of cardiac output. Cardiac output (CO) can be calculated in one of two ways: thermodilution or the modified Fick technique. Using thermodilution, room temperature saline of a known quantity is injected briskly into the right atrium. As the saline mixes with blood traveling through the right ventricle, blood is cooled. The blood temperature is then recorded in the pulmonary artery over time. A curve is generated, denoting the change in temperature from baseline, and the area under this curve is inversely proportional to the cardiac output (e.g., the higher the cardiac output, the lower the impact the small saline aliquot has on blood temperature). Clinicians should be aware that severe tricuspid regurgitation can interfere with the validity of the thermodilution technique, typically underestimating forward flow. The Fick technique relies on the principle of mass balance proposed by Adolph Fick in 1870. Oxygen consumption (VO_2) must equal the difference in oxygen content of arterial and venous blood times the cardiac output. Assumptions can be made about oxygen consumption at rest, and arterial and venous oxygen content (CaO_2 and CVO_2) can be calculated by the hemoglobin concentration and oxyhemoglobin saturation:

$$CO = VO_2/(CaO_2 - CVO_2)$$

Goals for hemodynamic stability generally include maintenance of a mean arterial pressure between 65 and 75 mm Hg and a cardiac index of at least 2 L/min per m^2. Outcomes should be individualized, as a chronically hypertensive patient may require a higher arterial pressure to maintain satisfactory tissue perfusion, and a postoperative patient with bleeding from a tenuous aortic suture line may benefit from a more restrictive blood pressure approach. Hypotension is quite common following cardiac surgery and is often related to hypovolemia, as well as vasodilation from systemic warming and an inflammatory response from extracorporeal circulation with activation of vasodilatory mediators. Intravascular hypovolemia is extremely common in the immediate perioperative period. Causes are multifactorial and include capillary leak from inflammation, venodilation from warming, unrecognized and unreplaced blood loss, and excessive diuresis, particularly if osmotic diuretics such as mannitol are given during cardiopulmonary bypass. Patients may require 2 to 3 liters of fluid in the first several hours after surgery. Those with ventricular hypertrophy and diastolic dysfunction may require additional fluid to maintain cardiac output. Although not essential, the pulmonary artery catheter can be instrumental in guiding fluid resuscitation. While colloids, such as albumin and hetastarch, can reduce the total volume required to maintain stability, there are no prospective randomized data clearly demonstrating its superiority with regard to outcome benefits.

Vasoconstrictors are used to treat hypotension, but should only be initiated if the patient has been adequately fluid resuscitated and myocardial function and cardiac output is preserved. α-Agonists, such as Neo-Synephrine, will increase vascular tone without increasing contractility or heart rate and do not exacerbate dysrhythmias. Similarly, vasopressin has no effect on cardiac function, but uniquely will not increase pulmonary vascular resistance, as there are no vasopressin receptors in the pulmonary vascular bed. Additionally, vasopressin preferentially constricts efferent renal arterioles rather than afferent arterioles, resulting in maintained glomerular filtration and urine output. Norepinephrine, epinephrine, and dopamine are also frequently used to counteract a vasodilatory state. These catecholamines are also inotropic agents, which can be useful if myocardial function is depressed. However, they all increase heart rate and myocardial oxygen consumption and can be arrhythmogenic.

Myocardial dysfunction can occur from stunning after cardioplegic arrest, particularly if the cross-clamp period was long. This can be problematic if systolic function is severely depressed preoperatively. Inadequate myocardial protection from insufficient cardioplegia can also result in catastrophic and unrecoverable postoperative heart failure. Unless the heart is acutely ischemic at the time of surgery, it is unusual to expect immediate improvement in contractility after surgical revascularization. In fact, the acutely ischemic heart often tolerates cardiopulmonary bypass and cardioplegia poorly. Contractility can be globally severely depressed after emergent coronary bypass grafting in the setting of a sizable STEMI, especially if the patient was in preoperative shock. If cardiac dysfunction and low cardiac output are detected intraoperatively, careful assessment of bypass graft position and patency should be undertaken. This is especially true if new wall motion abnormalities are regional.

Once surgical problems have been corrected, efforts are made to optimize myocardial contractility. Inotropic agents will improve cardiac function and can be easily titrated to the desired effect. Catecholamines, such as dopamine, epinephrine, and dobutamine, are frequently used. All of these agents, through their effects on β receptors, will increase heart rate, predispose to arrhythmias, and increase myocardial oxygen consumption. Nonetheless, these agents are generally safe, particularly at low doses. Phosphodiesterase inhibitors, such as milrinone, also improve contractility and have less effect on heart rate or myocardial contractility. These agents are also vasodilators, and should be used with caution in patients who are hypotensive. Both catecholamines and phosphodiesterase inhibitors exert their inotropic effects by increasing cytosolic calcium. For these agents to be effective, there must be adequate calcium stores. Infusion of supplemental calcium often potentiates the effect of both classes of drugs. Likewise, acidosis decreases the effectiveness of inotropic agents, and normalization of blood pH, either by replacement of sodium bicarbonate or hyperventilation, can have an immediate effect on myocardial function.

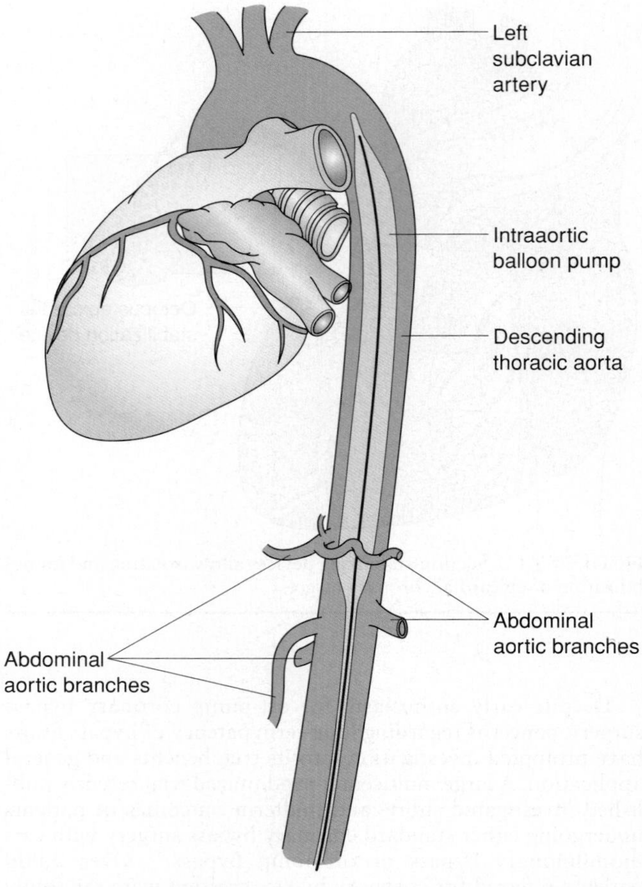

FIGURE 83.14. Intra-aortic balloon pump positioned within the descending thoracic aorta. The device must be positioned to not occlude the left subclavian artery or the abdominal aortic branches. (Images courtesy of Datascope Corporation.)

When postoperative ventricular dysfunction is entirely related to myocardial stunning, inotropes should be weaned within the first 24 hours. However, if postoperative cardiogenic shock is severe and refractory to high-dose inotropic infusions, insertion of an intra-aortic balloon pump should be considered. Positioned within the thoracic aorta (Fig. 83.14), balloon pump actuation is timed with the patient's electrocardiogram or arterial pressure tracing. Inflation occurs during diastole, augmenting coronary perfusion, and deflates during systole, reducing afterload and increasing cardiac output. Insertion of a ventricular assist device may be beneficial; however, many of these patients subsequently require heart transplantation, so careful patient selection is essential.

Postoperative bleeding is infrequent but can occur, especially when patients are taking irreversible platelet inhibitors. Output from mediastinal chest drains is monitored closely, and markers of coagulation are assessed. Coagulopathy should be corrected with appropriate blood component transfusions. Retransfusion of shed blood is generally avoided, as it may exacerbate coagulopathy. Return to the operating room should be considered if drainage exceeds 600 to 800 mL in 4 to 5 hours, without signs of slowing.

Inhibitors of plasminogen can be helpful in reducing postoperative coagulopathy and bleeding complications. There are three agents in this class of drug: ε-aminocaproic acid (Amicar, Xanodyne Pharmaceuticals, New Port, KY), tranexamic acid, and aprotinin (Trasylol, Bayer Leverkusen, Germany). The first two agents are synthetic binders of plasminogen or plasmin. Aprotinin is a naturally occurring serine protease inhibitor that can inhibit plasminogen, as well as many other proteases. Although meta-analysis suggested that aprotinin was superior to the other agents,[50] concerns regarding the safety of aprotinin have been raised, suggesting a higher incidence of renal failure[51] and even mortality.[52] A subsequent prospective randomized trial concluded that aprotinin was independently associated with a higher rate of death,[53] and as such its approval has been halted by the U.S. Food and Drug Administration.

There has recently been great enthusiasm for using a blood conservation strategy. Transfusion of as little as a single unit of packed red cells is independently associated with increased morbidity after coronary bypass surgery.[54] Efforts to minimize hemodilution using retrograde priming and hemofiltration can be very effective at reducing transfusion rates, but the most important adjunct to reduce blood usage is reduced transfusion triggers. Evidence exists that hemoglobin concentrations as low as 7 g/dL can be safe and are very well tolerated in intensive care unit patients.[55]

Cardiac tamponade is an infrequent but feared complication that can be fatal and is often difficult to diagnose. The classic scenario is a patient with initially high chest drainage that suddenly ceases. The patient then insidiously develops oliguria, followed by low cardiac output and refractory hypotension. Signs such as bulging neck veins, elevated central venous pressure, pulsus paradoxus, and widened mediastinal silhouette on chest radiography may be variably present. Echocardiography can establish the diagnosis by demonstrating a pericardial effusion with right atrial and right ventricular compression. However, it is important to note that echocardiography cannot rule out the diagnosis. Timely diagnosis usually requires experience and a low index of suspicion. Treatment involves immediate return to the operating room, where removal of the obstructing fluid and clot results in immediate relief of constriction and normalization of hemodynamic parameters. When tamponade occurs late, it may be treatable with percutaneous drains if the pericardial fluid content is thin and without significant clot burden.

Atrial fibrillation is extremely common following CABG, with a frequency of 25% to 30%. Its occurrence is higher for older patients and those with lung disease, and after combined CABG and valve surgery, decreased ventricular function, prolonged aortic cross-clamp period, and more severe hypothermia. Interestingly, the rate of atrial fibrillation does not appear to be reduced after off-pump CABG.[56] It most frequently occurs between the second and fourth postoperative day, and can be precipitated by electrolyte imbalances, particularly hypokalemia or hypomagnesemia. If the rate is excessively high or the patient has significant ventricular hypertrophy, atrial fibrillation can result in hemodynamic compromise producing hypotension and oliguria. The most frequently used treatment for postoperative atrial fibrillation is amiodarone. It can achieve adequate rate control after an intravenous load of 150 mg in the majority of patients, with minimal effect on blood pressure or contractility. As a class III antiarrhythmic, amiodarone is also very effective at facilitating conversion to sinus rhythm. When given preoperatively, amiodarone can also reduce the rate of postoperative atrial fibrillation, although bradycardia is more common in protocols that use higher doses.[57] Beta-blocking agents are also effective at achieving rate control, and when given routinely preoperatively and reinitiated immediately after surgery, they have reduced the occurrence of atrial fibrillation.[58] Diltiazem is immediately effective at controlling rapid atrial fibrillation, and is typically given as a 5- to 10-mg load, followed by a continuous infusion of 5 to 10 mg/h. Although it is associated with hypotension, its short half-life makes this complication quite manageable. For atrial fibrillation with rapid ventricular response refractory to amiodarone, beta-blockers, and diltiazem, it may be reasonable to add digoxin. This drug should be used with caution, because it is proarrhythmic. Drug concentrations should be followed and potassium levels maintained aggressively. If rapid ventricular response results in significant hemodynamic instability, electrical cardioversion should be performed. Cardioversion may also be considered if atrial fibrillation persists after 24 to 36 hours because of the risk of clot formation within the left atrial appendage. Cardioversion should not be performed if atrial fibrillation has been present for more than 48 hours. If atrial fibrillation is persistent, anticoagulation must be considered and weighed against the potential for postoperative bleeding complications. The vast majority of patients who develop atrial fibrillation after CABG will revert to sinus rhythm, and the complication rate is generally low. However, atrial fibrillation does increase the length of stay and cost of hospitalization, so efforts to reduce its incidence are necessary.

Deep sternal wound infection involving the bone occurs in approximately 0.5% to 1% of patients. Independent risk factors are obesity, diabetes, immunosuppression, use of both internal mammary arteries, chronic lung disease, and malnutrition. The most frequent organism is *Staphylococcus aureus*, although gram negatives can be seen in diabetics and immunosuppressed patients. Helpful preventative strategies include decontamination of nasal *Staphylococcus* species with mupirocin, preoperative Hibiclens wash, and tight postoperative glucose control. The diagnosis is established with sternal wound drainage and palpable sternal instability. Systemic antibiotics should be initiated and the patient returned to the operating room expeditiously for sternal débridement. Delay could result in mediastinitis with sepsis and shock. Under most circumstances, the chest wall is reconstructed with myocutaneous flaps based on the pectoralis and rectus abdominus muscles.

RESULTS OF CORONARY BYPASS GRAFTING

Overall, the mortality rate following coronary bypass grafting is between 2% and 3%. This number has been progressively declining despite rising median age and worsening severity of disease (Fig. 83.15). Improved outcomes can be attributed to advances in surgical technique, anesthetic approaches, preoperative timing and patient selection, sophistication of intensive care systems, and superior pharmacology, including antiplatelet agents, beta-blockers, and statins. Increased competition, both between cardiac surgeons and with percutaneous interventionalists, and public reporting of data have undoubtedly improved efficiency and contributed significantly to better outcomes. Major morbidity is estimated to be 10% to 12%. Risk of stroke is approximately 1% to 2%, renal failure requiring renal replacement therapy is 0.5% to 1%, deep sternal wound infection is 0.5% to 1%, and need for urgent reoperation is 3% to 5%. Overall median length of hospital stay is approximately 6 days.

The Society of Thoracic Surgeons (STS) maintains a voluntary registry for cardiac surgery outcomes. Participation throughout the United States is extremely high, and the database is generally considered an excellent representation of cardiac surgery outcomes. Overall, coronary bypass procedures have increased in volume, although at a slower pace in recent years, presumably as a result of expanded medical and percutaneous treatments. In 2008, 163,000 isolated coronary bypass procedures were submitted to the STS database. With over 1.4 million individual cases embedded in the dataset, enormous information can be obtained regarding risk factors for mortality and morbidity. Independent predictors of death are listed in Table 83.2 and include coronary reoperation, preoperative shock, dialysis dependence, immunosuppressed state, advanced age, diabetes mellitus, nonwhite race, female

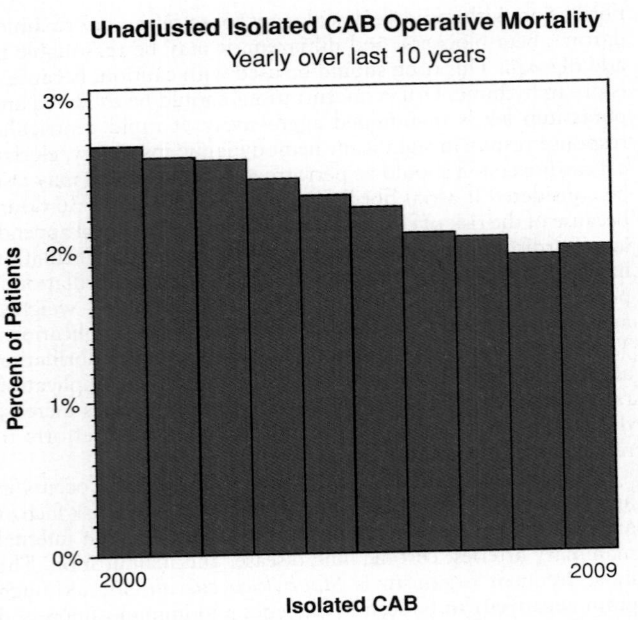

FIGURE 83.15. Unadjusted isolated coronary artery bypass operative mortality: 2000–2009. (This graph is reprinted from the Society of Thoracic Surgeons adult cardiac database 4th 2009 harvest report executive summary. http://www.sts.org/documents/pdf/ndb2010/20094thHarvestExecutiveSummary.pdf. © The Society of Thoracic Surgeons. Used with permission. All rights reserved.)

gender, previous stroke, advanced heart failure symptoms, peripheral vascular disease, and chronic lung disease. While the presence of these predictors are not contraindications for coronary bypass grafting, these prognostic tools are helpful both in balancing potential benefits from predicted risks and in correctly informing patients, families, and referring physicians. There are two well-described predictive models that can be used to estimate risk of death following coronary bypass surgery. Each model has been created using large voluntary registry data, one from the Society of Thoracic Surgeons, and one created from the European registry from 128 hospitals across eight countries. Both models incorporate features related to the patients, the nature of their clinical presentation, and the planned operative intervention. Although far from perfect, both models can be very helpful in determining patient selection and preoperative optimization and in tailoring the therapy to the unique clinical circumstances.

TABLE 83.2

INDEPENDENT PREDICTORS OF MORTALITY FOLLOWING CORONARY BYPASS PROCEDURES

■ VARIABLE	■ ODDS RATIO
Age	1.05 (1.05, 1.05)
African American race	1.34 (1.23, 1.45)
Chronic lung disease	1.41 (1.35, 1.48)
Diet controlled diabetes	1.15 (1.09, 1.21)
Insulin requiring diabetes	1.50 (1.42, 1.58)
First reoperation	2.76 (2.72, 2.91)
Immunosuppression	1.75 (1.1.57, 1.95)
Renal failure	1.88 (1.80, 1.96)
Shock	2.04 (1.90, 2.19)
Male gender	0.84 (0.80, 0.89)
NYHA class IV symptoms	1.15 (1.10, 1.20)

Another risk factor for death after coronary bypass grafting that is not included in either stratification model is incomplete revascularization. Incomplete revascularization refers to failure to construct a bypass graft to a territory natively perfused by a vessel with at least a 50% proximal stenosis. Under most circumstances, the revascularization is incomplete because target vessels were unsuitable for bypassing because they were small, inaccessible, or too heavily diseased. The differences observed are typically not apparent in 30-day survival but manifest as a reduced long-term prognosis. Although the angiographic appearance of potential coronary targets may suggest unsuitability, interpretation of vessel quality is extremely subjective and very difficult to quantify, which is why it has not been incorporated into the two large risk creation models. Nonetheless, the quality of the bypass targets should be considered when weighing the options for treatment of advanced coronary artery disease.

The purpose of coronary bypass surgery is to create unimpeded blood flow to ischemic myocardial territories. While short- and long-term mortality may reflect the adequacy of revascularization, bypass graft patency is a more precise assessment of the technical success of the operation. Patency rates are typically reported based on clinical trials in which routine angiography is performed at regular intervals, excluding biases from studies in which angiography is only performed in symptomatic patients. Saphenous vein grafts are hampered by a higher early graft loss, as much as 20% in the first year. Mechanisms include technical anastomotic problems, graft kinking, inadequate epicardial run-off, vein graft endothelial dysfunction from injury or chronic stasis, competitive flow from relatively unobstructed native coronary flow, and early development of neointimal hyperplasia. Late vein graft occlusion develops at a rate of approximately 5% per year from progressive native vessel disease and the development of accelerated vein graft atherosclerosis. Patency at 10 years is generally 40% to 50%. It remains to be seen if these outcomes improve with advances in statin and antiplatelet agents. As described previously, the internal mammary artery is generally spared of both atherosclerotic disease and early development of neointimal hyperplasia. Not surprisingly, its patency is vastly superior,[59] although these outcomes may be biased by the fact that the left internal mammary artery is typically placed on the LAD. The higher outflow of this target results in greater flow rates, reducing the risk of stagnation from limited run-off. In addition, its anterior location make it less likely to kink. Patency at 1 year is approximately 95%, and there is very little attrition over time, with 85% to 90% patency at 10 years. In fact, the use of the internal mammary artery is an independent predictor of long-term survival, presumably because of better graft outcomes.[60] The radial artery is generally intermediate to saphenous vein grafts and the internal mammary artery. Patency rates have been described as 90% at 1 year and 80% to 90% at 5 years. The radial artery is particularly prone to spasm from competitive flow, resulting in a patent but dysfunctional graft, referred to as a string sign. The radial artery should be avoided when stenotic lesions are less than 70%.

COMPARATIVE TRIALS

With the advent of coronary bypass surgery in the late 1960s, questions arose as to which patients are appropriate to offer this highly invasive and costly treatment. Three landmark randomized trials were constructed comparing CABG with
9 medical treatment for a variety of patient populations. The Veterans Administration Cooperative Study,[61] the European Coronary Surgery Study,[62] and the Coronary Artery Surgery Study[63] all demonstrated that CABG improves survival as compared to

medically treated patients, and the benefits of CABG are enhanced by more severe disease, as well as left ventricular dysfunction. Although these trials are now more than 30 years old and medical and surgical treatments have evolved considerably, the principles continue to apply and are repeatedly described in more contemporary series.

Although these clinical trials definitively demonstrated the superiority of CABG over medical therapy for patients with advanced coronary artery disease, the advent and widespread adoption of intracoronary balloon angioplasty raised the possibility that a less invasive approach to revascularization may be as beneficial as the surgical approach. Several multicenter clinical trials were conducted comparing CABG with angioplasty for a variety of patient populations. The most notable of these studies was the Bypass Angioplasty Revascularization Investigation, or BARI trial.[64] A total of 1,829 patients were deemed eligible and were randomized to angioplasty or CABG in 18 centers across the United States and Canada. While there were no differences for in-hospital death or 5-year survival, the rate of repeat revascularization was significantly higher in the percutaneously treated patients. Only 8% of patients in the CABG group required repeat revascularization within the first 5 years, as compared to 54% in the angioplasty group. Although survival analysis was intention to treat, 31% of patients in the angioplasty group underwent subsequent CABG. Importantly, subgroup analysis demonstrated a survival advantage at 5 years for diabetic patients treated with CABG as opposed to angioplasty (80.6% vs. 65.5%; $p = 0.003$). The BARI study demonstrated that surgical revascularization was more durable and resulted in improved survival for diabetic patients with advanced coronary artery disease.

Angioplasty alone carries a restenosis rate of 30% to 40% from at least two mechanisms. One is entirely mechanical, related to elastic recoil, and is seen within weeks of intervention. The other mechanism is related to progressive neointimal hyperplasia, likely occurring as a result of local trauma. Intracoronary stents have reduced the restenosis rate and improved outcomes of percutaneous intervention. In the setting of these advances, several multicenter, prospective, randomized trials were performed, again with the hypothesis that percutaneous intervention would be superior or equivalent to surgical revascularization for patients with advanced coronary artery disease. Among the most prominent of these studies was the SoS, or Surgery or Stent, trial.[65] A total of 988 patients from 53 medical centers in 11 countries were enrolled based on eligibility criteria, including the presence of multivessel coronary artery disease. Patients were randomly assigned to receive either coronary bypass surgery or percutaneous intervention using intracoronary stents. At a median follow-up of 2 years, 20.7% of patients in the stent arm required repeat revascularization, as compared to only 6% in the CABG arm ($p < 0.001$). Surprisingly, there was also a survival advantage seen with surgery (mortality 4.5% vs. 1.6%, stent vs. surgery, respectively; $p = 0.01$). These mortality advantages persisted with a median follow-up of 6 years (10.9% vs. 6.8%; $p = 0.02$).[66] Consistent with previous clinical trials, the survival advantage was even more pronounced for diabetics (17.6% vs. 5.4%). The SoS trial was similar to other randomized trials comparing coronary stents with CABG with respect to superior rates of repeat revascularization. However, SoS was unique in describing a mortality benefit. Some have argued that enrollment criteria were much less stringent in SoS, enrolling sicker patients with more complex anatomic lesions. SoS may therefore better reflect "real world" practice.

Among the biggest limitations of bare metal intracoronary stents is the development of obstructing neointimal hyperplasia resulting in in-stent restenosis, which occurs at a rate of 15% to 30%. Recently, antiproliferative drugs have been incorporated into the platform of stents to inhibit this occlusive process. These drug-eluting stents have been demonstrated in prospective randomized fashion to reduce the rate of repeat revascularization, when compared to bare metal stents. Because of improved outcomes using this new technology, a prospective, multicenter, randomized trial was conducted comparing coronary bypass grafting with a strategy using drug-eluting stents for patients with left main or three-vessel coronary stenosis.[67] Eighty-five centers in the United States and Europe enrolled patients who met these criteria and whose anatomic disease was determined by both the surgeon and interventional cardiologist to be amenable to either strategy. A total of 3,075 patients were enrolled, but only 1,800 patients were randomized, 897 to CABG and 903 to PCI with the Taxus drug-eluting stent (Boston Scientific). The remaining patients were not felt to be good candidates for both procedures, and 1,077 underwent CABG and 198 underwent PCI. Outcomes of these excluded patients were collected into a separate registry. Of the randomized patients, more patients in the PCI arm had major cardiac or cerebrovascular events at 12 months (12.4% vs. 17.8%, CABG vs. PCI, respectively; $p = 0.002$). The majority of these differences were seen in the rate of repeat revascularization (5.9% vs. 13.5%; $p < 0.001$). The authors also created a numerical system to comparatively describe the complexity of the coronary anatomy. This "syntax" score was higher for chronic total occlusions, bifurcation lesions, heavily calcified vessels, and lesions greater than 20 mm in length. The differences in major cardiac or cerebrovascular events between CABG and PCI were even more pronounced in the subgroup of patients with a high "syntax" score (10.9% vs. 23.4%). This study once again demonstrated that despite improved outcomes of percutaneous treatment of coronary artery disease with drug-eluting stents, CABG remains the best therapy for patients with significant left main and three-vessel coronary artery disease. The benefits of CABG are accentuated for patients with more severe and complex disease.

These important randomized trials have consistently demonstrated that surgical coronary artery revascularization is the ideal technique to reduce symptoms, myocardial infarctions, cardiac-related future hospitalizations, and death in patients with advanced coronary artery atherosclerosis. Improvements in nonsurgical therapy, both medical and percutaneous, have prompted recurring investigations into the comparative efficacy of coronary bypass surgery. Surgical treatment continues to successfully compete, largely because of simultaneous advances in surgical technique, intraoperative patient care, and postoperative management. Despite concerns raised every year that CABG will no longer be performed in the future, outcomes remain superior and as a result, volumes continue to rise. It is likely that surgical revascularization of the ischemic heart will continue to be the dominant strategy for many years to come.

References

1. Davies JE, Burkhart HM, Dearani JA, et al. Surgical management of anomalous aortic origin of a coronary artery. *Ann Thorac Surg* 2009;88: 844–847.
2. Messer JV, Wagman RJ, Levine HJ, et al. Patterns of myocardial oxygen extraction during rest and exercise. *J Clin Invest* 1962;41:725.
3. Berne RM. The role of adenosine in the regulation of coronary blood flow. *Circ Res* 1980;47:807.
4. Malek AM, Alper SL, Izumo S. Hemodynamic sheer stress and its role in atherosclerosis. *JAMA* 1999;282:2035–2042.
5. Samnegard A, Hulthe J, Silveira A, et al. Gender specific associations between matrix metalloproteinases and inflammatory markers in post myocardial infarction patients. *Atherosclerosis* 2009;202:550–556.
6. Singh SK, Suresh MV, Voleti B, et al. The connection between C-reactive protein and atherosclerosis. *Ann Med* 2008;40:110–120.
7. Psaty BM, Lumley T, Furberg CD, et al. Health outcomes associated with various antihypertensive therapies used as first-line agents: a network meta-analysis. *JAMA* 2003;289:2534–2544.
8. Duckworth W, Abraira C, Moritz T, et al. Glucose control and vascular complications in veterans with type 2 diabetes. *New Engl J Med* 2009;360: 129–139.
9. Expert Panel on Detection, Evaluation, and Treatment of High Blood Cholesterol in Adults. Executive Summary of the Third Report of the National Cholesterol Education Program (NCEP) Expert Panel on Detection, Evaluation, and Treatment of High Blood Cholesterol in Adults (Adult Treatment Panel III). *JAMA* 2001;285:2486–2497.

10. The Lipid Research Clinics Program Primary Prevention Trial. Results II. The relationship of reduction in incidence of coronary heart disease to cholesterol lowering. *JAMA* 1984;251:365–374.
11. Wilson K, Gibson N, Willan A, et al. Effect of smoking cessation on mortality after myocardial infarction: meta-analysis of cohort studies. *Arch Intern Med* 2000;160:939–944.
12. Hasdai D, Topol EJ, Califf RM, et al. Cardiogenic shock complicating acute coronary syndromes. *Lancet* 2000;356:749–756.
13. Hochman JS, Sleeper LA, Webb JG, et al. Early revascularization in acute myocardial infarction complicated by cardiogenic shock. SHOCK Investigators. Should we emergently revascularize occluded coronaries for cardiogenic shock. *N Engl J Med* 1999;341:625–634.
14. Bakhtiary F, Keller H, Dogan S, et al. Venoarterial extracorporeal membrane oxygenation for treatment of cardiogenic shock: clinical experiences in 45 adult patients. *J Thorac Cardiovasc Surg* 2008;135:382–388.
15. Haft JW, Pagani FD, Romano MA, et al. Short- and long-term survival of patients transferred to a tertiary care center on temporary extracorporeal circulatory support. *Ann Thorac Surg* 2009;88:711.
16. Jeppsson A, Liden H, Johnsson P, et al. Surgical repair of post infarction ventricular septal defects: a national experience. *Eur J Thorac Cardiovasc Surg* 2005;27:216–221.
17. Russo A, Suri RM, Grigioni F, et al. Clinical outcome after surgical correction of mitral regurgitation due to papillary muscle rupture. *Circulation* 2008;118:1528–1534.
18. Vohra HA, Chaudhry S, Satur CM, et al. Sutureless off-pump repair of post-infarction left ventricular free wall rupture. *J Cardiothorac Surg* 2006;1:11.
19. Ohman EM, Armstrong PW, Christenson RH, et al., GUSTO IIA Investigators. Cardiac troponin T levels for risk stratification in acute myocardial ischemia. *N Engl J Med* 1996;335:1333–1341.
20. Tonino PA, De Bruyne B, Pijls NH, et al. Fractional flow reserve versus angiography for guiding percutaneous coronary intervention. *N Engl J Med* 2009;360:213–224.
21. Bruining N, de Winter S, Serruys PW. Intravascular ultrasound registration/integration with coronary angiography. *Cardiol Clin* 2009;27: 531–540.
22. Budoff MJ, Achenbach S, Blumenthal RS, et al. Assessment of coronary artery disease by cardiac computed tomography: a scientific statement from the American Heart Association Committee on Cardiovascular Imaging and Intervention, Council on Cardiovascular Radiology and Intervention, and Committee on Cardiac Imaging, Council on Clinical Cardiology. *Circulation* 2006;114:1761–1791.
23. Ross SD, Allen IE, Connelly JE, et al. Clinical outcomes in statin treatment trials: a meta-analysis. *Arch Intern Med* 1999;159:1793–1802.
24. Yusuf S, Sleight P, Pogue J, et al. Effects of an angiotensin-converting enzyme inhibitor, ramipril, on cardiovascular events in high risk patients. *N Engl J Med* 2000;342:145–153.
25. Antiplatelet Trialists' Collaboration. Collaborative overview of randomised trials of antiplatelet therapy—I: prevention of death, myocardial infarction, and stroke by prolonged antiplatelet therapy in various categories of patients. *BMJ* 1994;308:81–106.
26. Ryden L. Efficacy of epanolol versus metoprolol in angina pectoris: report from a Swedish multicentre study of exercise tolerance. *J Intern Med* 1992; 231:7–11.
27. Chobanian AV, Bakris GL, Black HR, et al. The Seventh Report of the Joint National Committee on Prevention, Detection, Evaluation, and Treatment of High Blood Pressure: the JNC 7 report. *JAMA* 2003;289:2560–2572.
28. Chaitman BR, Skettino SL, Parker JO, et al. Anti-ischemic effects and long-term survival during ranolazine monotherapy in patients with chronic severe angina. *J Am Coll Cardiol* 2004;43:1375–1382.
29. Yusuf S, Collins R, MacMahon S, et al. Effect of intravenous nitrates on mortality in acute myocardial infarction: an overview of the randomised trials. *Lancet* 1988;1:1088–1092.
30. Rutherford JD, Pfeffer MA, Moye LA, et al., SAVE Investigators. Effects of captopril on ischemic events after myocardial infarction: results of the Survival and Ventricular Enlargement trial. *Circulation* 1994;90:1731–1738.
31. Beckwith C, Munger MA. Effect of angiotensin-converting enzyme inhibitors on ventricular remodeling and survival following myocardial infarction. *Ann Pharmacother* 1993;27:755–766.
32. Yusuf S, Zhao F, Mehta SR, et al. Effects of clopidogrel in addition to aspirin in patients with acute coronary syndromes without ST-segment elevation. *N Engl J Med* 2001;345:494–502.
33. Mehta RH, Roe MT, Mulgund J, et al. Acute clopidogrel use and outcomes in patients with non-ST-segment elevation acute coronary syndromes undergoing coronary artery bypass surgery. *J Am Coll Cardiol* 2006;48:281–286.
34. Ferguson JJ, Califf RM, Antman EM, et al. Enoxaparin vs unfractionated heparin in high-risk patients with non-ST-segment elevation acute coronary syndromes managed with an intended early invasive strategy: primary results of the SYNERGY randomized trial. *JAMA* 2004;292:45–54.
35. Yusuf S, Mehta SR, Chrolavicius S, et al. Comparison of fondaparinux and enoxaparin in acute coronary syndromes. *N Engl J Med* 2006;354: 1464–1476.
36. Fibrinolytic Therapy Trialists' (FTT) Collaborative Group. Indications for fibrinolytic therapy in suspected acute myocardial infarction: collaborative overview of early mortality and major morbidity results from all randomised trials of more than 1000 patients. *Lancet* 1994;343:311–322.
37. Keeley EC, Boura JA, Grines CL. Primary angioplasty versus intravenous thrombolytic therapy for acute myocardial infarction: a quantitative review of 23 randomised trials. *Lancet* 2003;361:13–20.
38. Bradley EH, Nallamothu BK, Herrin J, et al. National efforts to improve door-to-balloon time: results from the door-to-balloon alliance. *J Am Coll Cardiol* 2009;54:2423–2429.
39. Di Lorenzo E, Sauro R, Varricchio A, et al. Long-term outcome of drug-eluting stents compared with bare metal stents in ST-segment elevation myocardial infarction: results of the paclitaxel- or sirolimus-eluting stent versus bare metal stent in primary angioplasty (PASEO) randomized trial. *Circulation* 2009;120:964–972.
40. van Werkum JW, Heestermans AA, Zomer AC, et al. Predictors of coronary stent thrombosis: the Dutch Stent Thrombosis Registry. *J Am Col Cardiol* 2009;53:1399–1409.
41. Patel MR, Dehmer GJ, Hirshfeld JW, et al. ACCF/SCAI/STS/AATS/AHA/ASNC 2009 appropriateness criteria for coronary revascularization. *Circulation* 2009;119:1330–1353.
42. Lopes RD, Hafley GE, Allen KB, et al. Endoscopic versus open vein-graft harvesting in coronary-artery bypass surgery. *N Engl J Med* 2009;361:235–244.
43. Savage EB, Grab JD, O'Brien SM, et al. Use of both internal thoracic arteries in diabetic patients increases deep sternal wound infection. *Ann Thorac Surg* 2007;83:1002–1006.
44. Shroyer AL, Grover FL, Hattler B, et al. On-pump versus off-pump coronary-artery bypass surgery. *N Engl J Med* 2009;361:1827–1837.
45. Mehran R, Dangas G, Stamou SC, et al. One-year clinical outcome after minimally invasive direct coronary artery bypass. *Circulation* 2000;102: 2799–2802.
46. Zhao DX, Leacche M, Balaguer JM, et al. Routine intraoperative completion angiography after coronary artery bypass grafting and 1-stop hybrid revascularization results from a fully integrated hybrid catheterization laboratory/operating room. *J Am Coll Cardiol* 2009;53:232–241.
47. Ishikawa N, Watanabe G, Iino K, et al. Robotic internal thoracic artery harvesting. *Surg Today* 2007;37:944–946.
48. de Canniere D, Wimmer-Greinecker G, Cichon R, et al. Feasibility, safety, and efficacy of totally endoscopic coronary artery bypass grafting: multicenter European experience. *J Thorac Cardiovasc Surg* 2007;134:710–716.
49. Bonatti J, Schachner T, Bonaros N, et al. Robotic totally endoscopic double-vessel bypass grafting: a further step toward closed-chest surgical treatment of multivessel coronary artery disease. *Heart Surg Forum* 2007;10: E239–E242.
50. Levi M, Cromheecke ME, de Jonge E, et al. Pharmacologic strategies to decrease excessive blood loss in cardiac surgery: a meta-analysis of clinically relevant end points. *Lancet* 1999;354:1940–1947.
51. Mangano DT, Tudor IC, Dietzel C. The risk associated with aprotinin in cardiac surgery. *N Engl J Med* 2006;354:353–365.
52. Mangano DT, Miao Y, Yuylsteke A, et al. Mortality associated with aprotinin during 5 years following coronary artery bypass surgery. *JAMA* 2007;297:471–479.
53. Fergusson DA, Hebert PC, Mazer CD, et al. A comparison of aprotinin and lysine analogues in high risk cardiac surgery. *N Engl J Med* 2008;358: 2319–2331.
54. Koch CG, Li L, Duncan AI, et al. Morbidity and mortality risk associated with red blood cell and blood-component transfusion in isolated coronary artery bypass grafting. *Crit Care Med* 2006;34:1608–1616.
55. Hébert PC, Wells G, Blajchman MA, et al. A multicenter, randomized, controlled clinical trial of transfusion requirements in critical care. *N Engl J Med* 1999;340:409–417.
56. Salamon T, Michler RE, Knott KM, et al. Off-pump coronary artery bypass grafting does not decrease the incidence of atrial fibrillation. *Ann Thorac Surg* 2003;75:505–507.
57. Daoud EG, Strickberger SA, Man KC, et al. Preoperative amiodarone as prophylaxis against atrial fibrillation after heart surgery. *N Engl J Med* 1997;337:1785–1791.
58. Crystal E, Connolly SJ, Sleik K, et al. Interventions on prevention of postoperative atrial fibrillation in patients undergoing heart surgery: a meta-analysis. *Circulation* 2002;106:75–80.
59. Sabik JF, Lytle BW, Blackstone EH, et al. Comparison of saphenous vein and internal thoracic artery graft patency by coronary system. *Ann Thorac Surg* 2005;79:544–551.
60. Loop FD, Lytle BW, Cosgrove DM, et al. Influence of the internal-mammary-artery graft on 10-year survival and other cardiac events. *N Engl J Med* 1986;314:1–6.
61. Detre KM, Takaro T, Hultgren H, et al., and the study participants. Long-term mortality and morbidity results of the Veterans Administration randomized trial of coronary artery bypass surgery. *Circulation* 1985; 72(Suppl V):84–89.
62. Varnauskas E, and the European Coronary Surgery Study Group. Twelve-year follow-up of survival in the randomized European Coronary Surgery Study. *N Engl J Med* 1988;319:332–337.
63. Myers WO, Marshfield WI, Gersh BJ, et al. Medical versus early surgical therapy in patients with triple-vessel disease and mild angina pectoris: a CASS registry study of survival. *Ann Thorac Surg* 1987;44:471–486.
64. Comparison of coronary bypass surgery with angioplasty in patients with multivessel disease. The Bypass Angioplasty Revascularization Investigation (BARI) Investigators. *N Eng J Med* 1996;335:217–225.
65. The SoS Investigators. Coronary artery bypass surgery versus percutaneous coronary intervention with stent implantation in patients with multivessel coronary artery disease: a randomised controlled trial. *Lancet* 2002;360:965–969.
66. Booth J, Clayton T, Pepper J, et al. Randomized, controlled trial of coronary artery bypass surgery versus percutaneous coronary intervention in patients with multivessel coronary artery disease: six-year follow-up from the Stent or Surgery Trial (SoS). *Circulation* 2008;118:381–388.
67. SYNTAX Investigators. Percutaneous coronary intervention versus coronary-artery bypass grafting for severe coronary artery disease. *N Engl J Med* 2009;360:961–972.

CHAPTER 84 ■ MECHANICAL CIRCULATORY SUPPORT FOR CARDIAC FAILURE

SANJEEV AGGARWAL, KEITH D. AARONSON, AND FRANCIS D. PAGANI

KEY POINTS

1. The term "mechanical circulatory support" (MCS) refers to a broad array of cardiac support devices that are distinguished by a number of important features including the location of the pumping chamber of the device, ventricle being supported, and pumping mechanism.
2. Indications for MCS include bridge to recovery, bridge to transplantation, and destination therapy (permanent implantation as an alternative to transplantation).
3. The major types of devices utilized for bridge to recovery are temporary, extracorporeal systems that can be placed utilizing percutaneous techniques.
4. Devices utilized for bridge to transplantation or destination therapy are durable, long-term devices that require major operative implantation and permit patient hospital discharge with untethered "hands free" mobility.
5. Delay in instituting any type of MCS increases the need for biventricular support as opposed to just left ventricular support alone. As the severity of illness and organ dysfunction increases, patients are more likely to require biventricular support and have a decreased survival secondary to the greater degree of organ failure present at implant.
6. Patient selection is the single most crucial factor in determining outcome of patients who receive mechanical circulatory support.
7. Major adverse events following initiation of MCS include stroke, infection, bleeding, right heart failure, and device malfunction.
8. The Interagency Registry of Mechanically Assisted Circulatory Support (INTERMACS) is a National Institutes of Health–funded data registry to study outcomes for patients receiving durable, long-term implantable ventricular assist devices.
9. Major technologic advances in device design for both temporary and long-term durable devices have incorporated continuous flow rotary pumps with axial or centrifugal design.

1 The term "mechanical circulatory support" (MCS) refers to a broad array of cardiac support devices. These devices are distinguished by a number of important features including (a) the location of the pumping chamber of the device, whether located outside the body or inside the body (extracorporeal vs. intracorporeal or "implantable") (Fig. 84.1), (b) the ventricle being supported (left ventricular assist device [LVAD] vs. right ventricular assist device [RVAD] vs. biventricular assist device [BiVAD] vs. total artificial heart [TAH]) (Fig. 84.2), and (c) the pumping mechanism (pulsatile, volume displacement device vs. continuous flow rotary device with axial or centrifugal design) (Algorithm 84.1). Generally, systems designed for short-term use have the pumping chamber located outside the body (extracorporeal or paracorporeal location), while "durable" systems intended for long-term (months to years) use have the pumping system located within the body.

INDICATIONS FOR MECHANICAL CIRCULATORY SUPPORT AND DEVICE SELECTION

The spectrum of MCS therapy is complex due to multiple indications for use and availability of numerous types of MCS
2 devices. Currently, there are three accepted indications for MCS. These treatment paradigms have been developed based on regulatory oversight by the U.S. Food and Drug Administration (FDA) and historical use of the therapy.

"Bridge to recovery" (BTR) refers to the use of MCS in patients who are presenting with acute cardiogenic shock or decompensated heart failure, despite the use of optimal medical therapy including intravenous inotropes and/or vasoconstrictors, with a reasonable expectation that the myocardial injury is reversible and that myocardial function will recover during a short period of temporary MCS (generally days to several weeks). The short-term utilization of MCS for BTR is the most common application of MCS in the United States.[1] Examples of reversible forms of myocardial injury include acute myocardial infarction, viral myocarditis, and postcardiotomy cardiogenic shock with failure to wean from cardiopulmonary bypass (CPB) following open heart cardiac procedures due to ischemic myocardial stunning or inadequate valvular repair or replace-
3 ment. Several types of devices can provide temporary MCS in these circumstances and include an intra-aortic balloon pump (IABP), extracorporeal ventricular assist device (VAD), and extracorporeal membrane oxygenation (ECMO, or preferably referred to as extracorporeal life support [ECLS], which provides both cardiac and pulmonary support). Generally, temporary MCS devices are placed percutaneously to facilitate rapid initiation of cardiac support and, alternatively, ease of removal when cardiac function returns. Some types of extracorporeal VAD systems require major operative procedures with sternotomy for access and placement and are more frequently utilized at the time of postcardiotomy failure to wean while the heart is exposed through sternotomy from the prior open heart procedure.

The second indication for MCS applies to patients presenting with cardiogenic shock or decompensated advanced heart failure refractory to optimal medical management in whom myocardial function is unlikely to recover and the patients are considered candidates for heart transplantation (long-standing ischemic, valvular, or idiopathic cardiomyopathy; severe acute
4 myocardial infarction or myocarditis). Durable MCS devices designed for long-term use that are implantable and permit untethered patient mobility and discharge from the hospital are

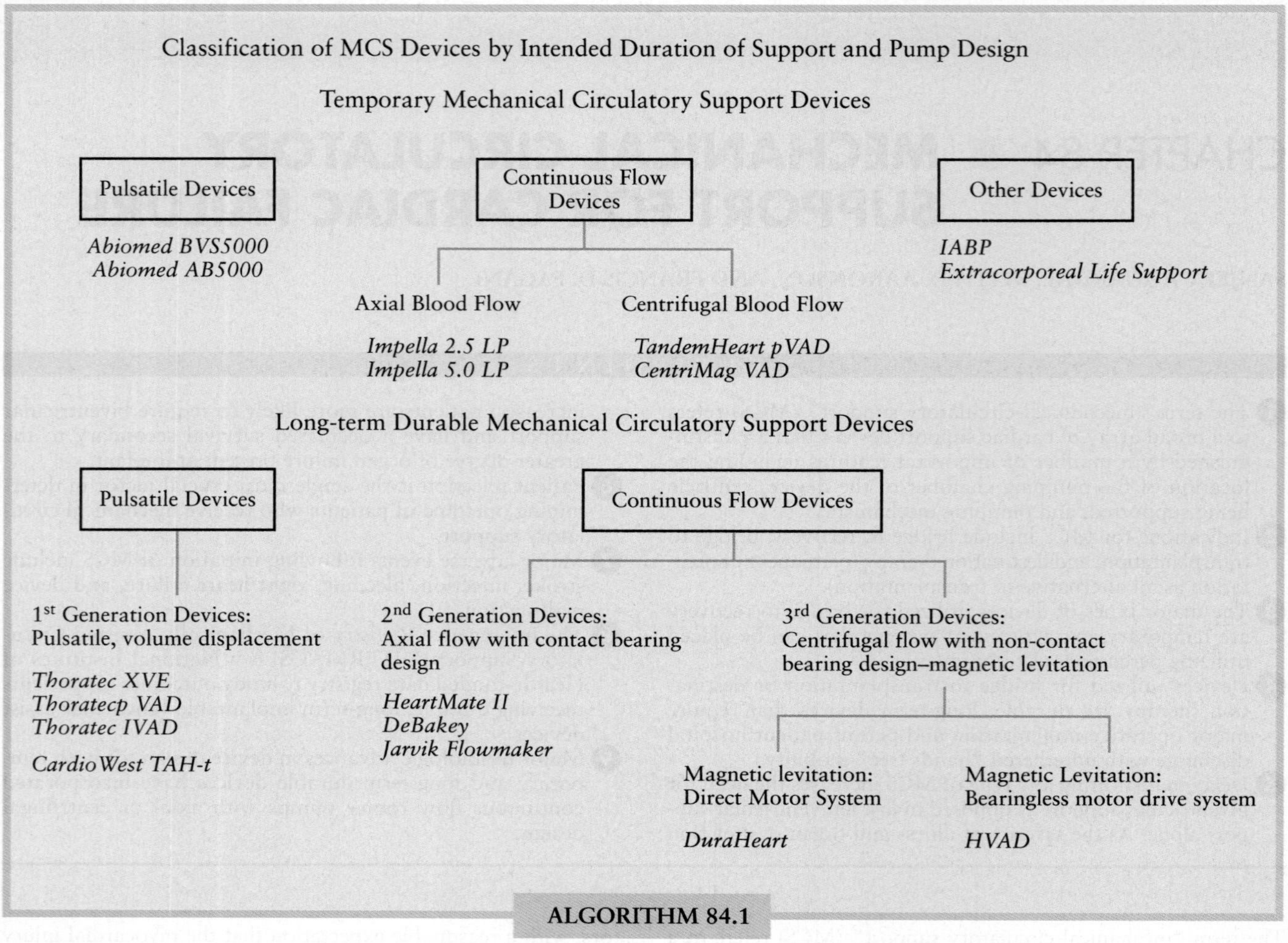

ALGORITHM 84.1. Classification of mechanical circulatory support devices by the pumping mechanism (pulsatile, volume displacement, or continuous flow rotary pumps) (Abiomed BVS 5000, Abiomed AB 5000, Impella 2.5 LP, Impella 5.0 LP, Abiomed Corporation, Danvers, MA; HeartMate XVE, Thoratec pVAD, Thoratec IVAD, HeartMate II, Thoratec Corporation, Pleasanton, CA; CardioWest TAH, Syncardia Systems, Tucson, AZ; Tandem Heart pVAD, Cardiac Assist Corporation, Pittsburgh, PA; CentriMag VAD, Levitronix LLC, Waltham, MA; HeartAssist 5 [DeBakey LVAD], Micromed Cardiovascular Corporation, Houston, TX; Jarvik LVAD, Jarvik Heart Corporation, New York, NY; DuraHeart LVAD, Terumo Heart Corporation, Ann Arbor, MI; HVAD LVAD, HeartWare Corporation, Miami, FL).

appropriate devices for a "bridge to transplantation" (BTT) indication. Implantable pumps require a major operative procedure for placement, including CPB in many instances, and are ideally placed in patients with significant symptoms of heart failure who are dependent on intravenous inotropes but with stable hemodynamics and end-organ function.

The third indication for MCS applies to patients with chronic refractory symptoms of advanced heart failure due to irreversible forms of either nonischemic or ischemic cardiomyopathy and who are not eligible for heart transplantation. The application of MCS in this setting is termed "destination therapy" (DT). Implantable devices with proven long-term reliability permitting untethered "hands free" patient mobility at home are appropriate devices in this clinical situation.[2] Again, these implantable pumps require a major operative procedure for placement and are ideally placed in patients with significant symptoms of heart failure but with stable hemodynamics. The survival, functional, and quality-of-life benefit of MCS for DT for the treatment of chronic advanced heart failure was established in a prospective randomized trial known as REMATCH (Randomized Evaluation of Mechanical Assistance in the Treatment of Congestive Heart Failure).[2] REMATCH evaluated the use of an implantable LVAD compared to optimal medical therapy for refractory chronic advanced heart failure. LVAD therapy halved (relative risk, 0.52; 95% confidence limit, 0.34–0.78) the mortality seen in the control population treated with optimal medical therapy, which was 92% at 2 years. Despite serious adverse events attributable to MCS from infection, bleeding, and device malfunction, LVAD recipients had an improved survival rate and experienced a superior quality of life than the medical therapy group. Currently, patients evaluated for DT must meet specific criteria that include (a) New York Heart Association (NYHA) class IV or stage D heart failure symptoms, (b) a left ventricular ejection fraction of less than 25%, (c) a peak exercise oxygen consumption of less than 14 mL/kg per minute, and (d) significant functional limitations despite the use of maximally tolerated doses of drugs outlined in the recent guidelines for heart failure treatment for at least 60 of 90 days.

The intended use and indication for MCS has significant influences on the appropriate device selection and use. The decision to initiate MCS must include an analysis of the intended use, clinical setting, patient variables and condition, type of MCS devices available, and FDA approval and guidelines for use of the device. The paradigms of BTR, BTT, and DT have become integrated into the way that MCS is currently delivered by clinicians, regulatory agencies, and insurance payers. These paradigms do not consistently describe all clinical situations and

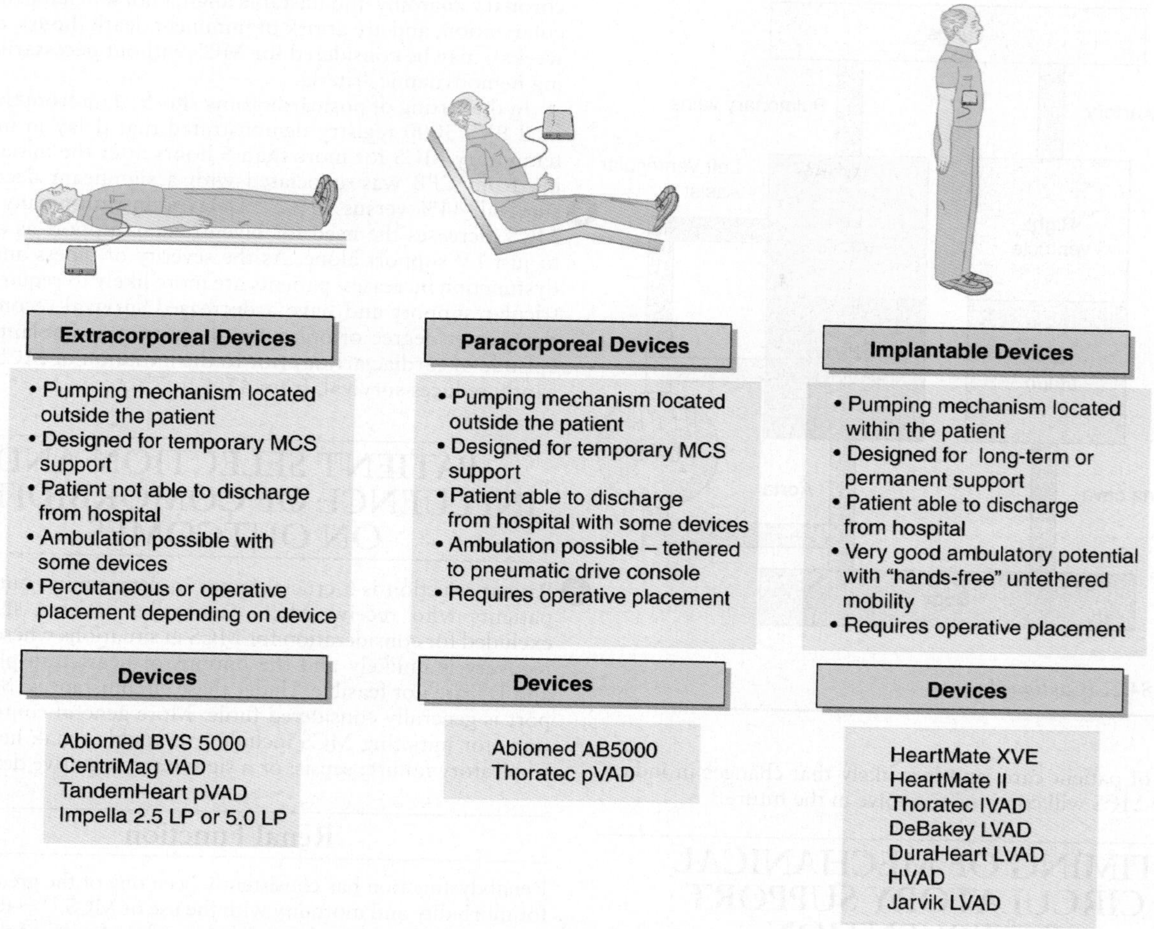
Extracorporeal Devices
• Pumping mechanism located outside the patient
• Designed for temporary MCS support
• Patient not able to discharge from hospital
• Ambulation possible with some devices
• Percutaneous or operative placement depending on device
Devices
Abiomed BVS 5000
CentriMag VAD
TandemHeart pVAD
Impella 2.5 LP or 5.0 LP
Paracorporeal Devices
• Pumping mechanism located outside the patient
• Designed for temporary MCS support
• Patient able to discharge from hospital with some devices
• Ambulation possible – tethered to pneumatic drive console
• Requires operative placement
Devices
Abiomed AB5000
Thoratec pVAD
Implantable Devices
• Pumping mechanism located within the patient
• Designed for long-term or permanent support
• Patient able to discharge from hospital
• Very good ambulatory potential with "hands-free" untethered mobility
• Requires operative placement
Devices
HeartMate XVE
HeartMate II
Thoratec IVAD
DeBakey LVAD
DuraHeart LVAD
HVAD
Jarvik LVAD

FIGURE 84.1. Classification of mechanical circulatory support devices by location of pumping mechanism (extracorporeal, paracorporeal, and implantable).

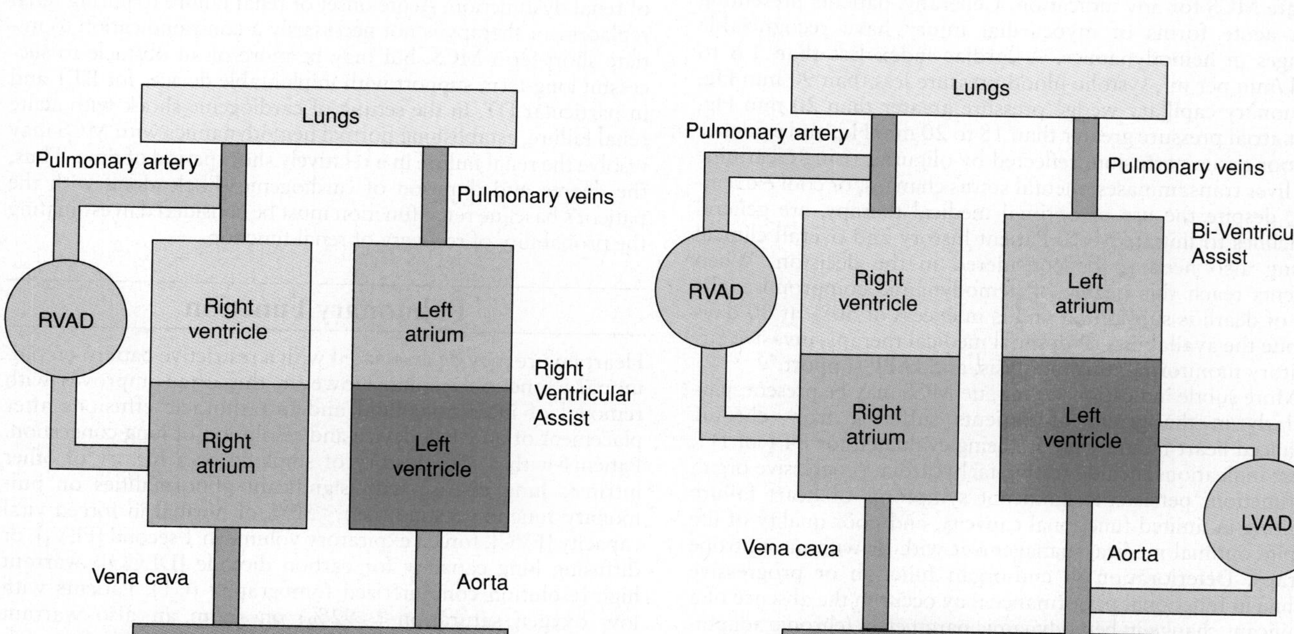

FIGURE 84.2. Classification of mechanical circulatory support devices by the ventricle being assisted (right ventricular assist, left ventricular assist, and biventricular assist). (*continued*)

VASCULAR

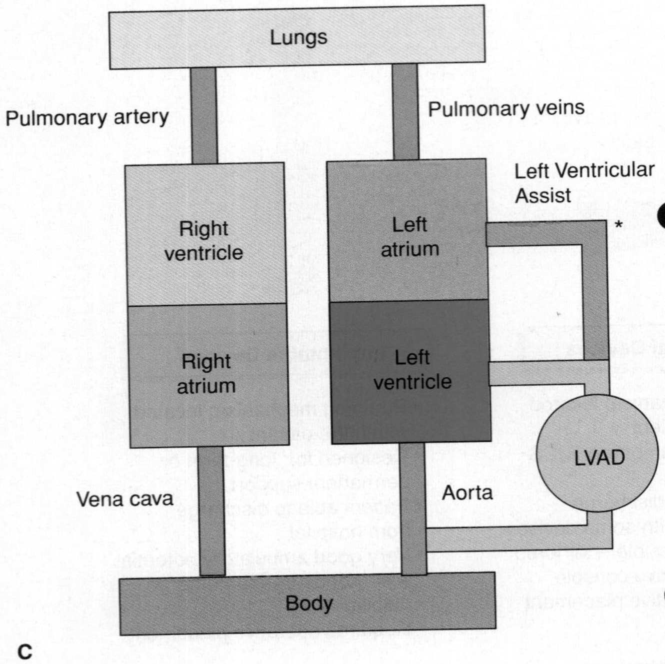

FIGURE 84.2. (*Continued*)

realities of patient care, and it is likely that changes in indications for MCS will continue to evolve in the future.[3]

TIMING OF MECHANICAL CIRCULATORY SUPPORT INTERVENTION

Timing the initiation of MCS is crucial to patient outcome. There are no absolute hemodynamic criteria to meet in order to initiate MCS for any indication. Generally, patients presenting with acute forms of myocardial injury have recognizable changes in hemodynamics. A cardiac index less than 1.8 to 2.2 L/min per m^2, systolic blood pressure less than 90 mm Hg, pulmonary capillary wedge pressure greater than 20 mm Hg, right atrial pressure greater than 18 to 20 mm Hg, and evidence of poor tissue perfusion, reflected by oliguria, rising creatinine and liver transaminases, mental status changes, or cool extremities, despite the use of optimal medical therapy, are general guidelines to initiate MCS. Patient history and overall clinical setting also need to be considered in the decision. When patients reach this degree of hemodynamic compromise, the risk of death is substantial and is in excess of 50% at 30 days despite the availability of optimal medical therapy, invasive circulatory monitoring, thrombolysis, and IABP support.[4,5]

More subtle indications to initiate MCS may be present, particularly in the group of patients suffering from chronic advanced heart failure who are being evaluated for BTT or DT. These indications include resting tachycardia, progressive organ dysfunction, persistent significant symptoms of heart failure resulting in limited functional capacity, and poor quality of life despite optimal medical management with or without inotrope therapy. Deterioration in end-organ function or progressive decline in functional performance may occur in the absence of a significant change in hemodynamic parameters (chronic adaptation to low cardiac output). In addition, patients who do not tolerate optimal medical management for advanced heart failure and experience renal insufficiency or hypotension in the setting of optimal dosages of angiotensin-converting enzyme (ACE) inhibitors or beta-blockers may need evaluation for MCS therapy. Patients who do not tolerate inotrope therapy as a result of refractory ventricular arrhythmias or have life-threatening coronary anatomy and unstable angina not amenable to revascularization, and are at risk of imminent death (hours, days, or weeks), may be considered for MCS without necessarily meeting hemodynamic criteria.

In the setting of postcardiotomy shock, data from the Abiomed BVS 5000 registry demonstrated that delay in initiating temporary MCS for more than 6 hours after the initial weaning from CPB was associated with a significant decrease in
5 survival, 44% versus 14%.[6–8] Delay in instituting any type of MCS increases the need for biventricular support as opposed to just LV support alone. As the severity of illness and organ dysfunction increases, patients are more likely to require biventricular support and have a decreased survival secondary to the greater degree of organ failure present at implant.[9–14] An episode of cardiac arrest prior to the initiation of MCS significantly reduces survival, from 47% to 7%.[6,7]

PATIENT SELECTION AND INFLUENCE OF COMORBIDITIES ON OUTCOMES

6 Patient selection is a crucial factor in determining outcome of patients who receive MCS. Generally, patients should be excluded for consideration for MCS in situations where cardiac recovery is unlikely and the options of heart transplantation and DT are not feasible. Under these circumstances, MCS support is generally considered futile. More general contraindications for initiating MCS include irreversible renal, hepatic, or respiratory failure; sepsis; or a significant cognitive deficit.

Renal Function

Renal dysfunction has consistently been one of the greatest risks for morbidity and mortality with the use of MCS.[15–20] Renal dysfunction is often secondary to decreased perfusion of the kidney in cardiogenic shock, but may also be due to nephrotoxic effects of drugs utilized for heart failure therapy. In patients with shock or advanced heart failure, it is difficult to assess the reversibility of renal dysfunction. Acute onset of renal failure requiring renal replacement therapy is not necessarily a contraindication to initiate short-term MCS, but may be more of an obstacle to successful long-term support with implantable devices for BTT and in particular DT. In the setting of cardiogenic shock with acute renal failure, establishing normal hemodynamics with MCS may resolve the renal failure in a relatively short period of time. Thus, the degree and duration of cardiogenic shock along with the patient's baseline renal function must be considered in estimating the probability of recovery of renal function.

Pulmonary Function

Heart failure may be associated with a restrictive pattern on pulmonary function testing. However, this often improves with removal of interstitial fluid and intrathoracic effusions after placement of an MCS device and resolution of lung congestion. Patients with a long history of smoking or a history of other intrinsic lung disease with significant abnormalities on pulmonary function testing (i.e., <50% of normal in forced vital capacity [FVC], forced expiratory volume in 1 second [FEV_1], or diffusing lung capacity for carbon dioxide [DLCO]) warrant high-resolution computerized tomography (CT). Patients with low oxygen saturation (<92%) on room air also warrant evaluation with echocardiography to rule out a right-to-left shunt from an atrial septal defect or patent foramen ovale (PFO) and, if negative, a spiral CT or nuclear scan to rule out thromboembolic disease. Patients with severe pulmonary disease may have an elevated pulmonary vascular resistance that is fixed (not responsive to pulmonary artery vasodilators). High fixed pulmonary vascular resistance (generally >6 Wood units) represents a contraindication to heart transplantation and thus BTT indication. Perioperative hypoxia as a result of significant underlying lung disease may also contribute to pulmonary vasoconstriction leading to right ventricular (RV) failure following institution of LVAD support. Moderate elevations in pulmonary vascular resistance can be encountered in patients with cardiogenic shock and does not preclude successful use of MCS if reversibility or lowering of the pulmonary vascular resistance is achieved with inotropes or pulmonary vasodilators.

Liver Function

Previous studies have reported that total bilirubin levels and hepatic cellular enzymes more than three times normal are independent risk factors for adverse outcomes.[15–18] The etiology of the hyperbilirubinemia may be multifactorial, including "cardiac congestion" or cirrhosis, cholestatic jaundice, or a combination of etiologies. Abnormal liver function is often associated with abnormal coagulation factors, as well as low serum albumin. Attempts should be made to normalize all measurements of liver function and their cause(s) preoperatively. The presence of portal hypertension with liver cirrhosis is a contraindication to initiating MCS support. A history of significant alcohol use should be reviewed in all potential candidates for MCS therapy, especially those with abnormal liver function. Patients should also be tested for previous infection with hepatitis A, B, or C or other viruses. Ultrasound visualization of the liver is a good screen for patients with significant hepatomegaly to rule out infiltrative disease, mass, or other pathology that may warrant biopsy. Improvement in hepatic congestion and recovery of synthetic functions of the liver can occur with institution of MCS.

Right Ventricular Failure

Patients with advanced heart failure frequently have coexisting RV failure. RV failure may be one of the most prominent causes of mortality or morbidity following initiation of MCS.[10–14,21–23] RV failure in most patients is due to LV failure. Patients with a nonischemic etiology often present with significant RV failure and may have a three- to fourfold increased risk of requiring both LV and RV support. Patients who require BiVAD support have significantly higher preoperative creatinine and total bilirubin levels and a greater need for mechanical ventilation before MCS device insertion as compared to patients requiring LVAD support only. The institution of BiVAD support adversely influences survival for both short-term and long-term MCS devices as a consequence of worse preoperative organ function.[10–14,21–23] RV failure is a prominent factor leading to renal dysfunction after LVAD implantation, as right atrial pressures greater than 20 mm Hg lead to changes in glomerular filtration from cortical to medullary nephrons, with secondary reduction in urine output and resistance to diuretic therapy.[24] Preoperative optimization of RV function with a goal right atrial pressure ideally less than 15 mm Hg is important for reducing the need for postoperative RV support. The higher the left atrial or wedge pressure at the time of device implantation, the greater is the benefit to the RV and pulmonary artery pressure when the LV is totally unloaded and left atrial pressure falls. However, the recovery of the right ventricle may lag for several days as total decompression of the left ventricle allows a significant shift of the interventricular septum toward the left ventricle, with further distention and dysfunction of the right ventricle.[25–27]

Coagulation Parameters

Coagulopathy is a significant risk factor and a common abnormality noted in patients with refractory heart failure. An abnormal international normalized ratio (INR) in the absence of warfarin use is of added concern, as it may reflect chronically high right atrial pressures, leading to hepatic congestion and, ultimately, to hepatic fibrosis and cirrhosis. Prolonged abnormal INR and low platelet count combined with use of anticoagulation or antiplatelet therapy are associated with significant perioperative bleeding, requiring multiple transfusions, leading to increased pulmonary vascular resistance, RV failure, decline in renal function, hemodynamic instability, and multiple organ failure.[28] In addition, patients with severe heart failure commonly have a nutritional basis for abnormal coagulation due to depletion of several specific coagulation factors, such as factor VII. The minimum preoperative screen for coagulation abnormalities should include prothrombin time (PT), partial thromboplastin time (PTT), INR, platelet count, platelet aggregation studies, and possibly a heparin-induced thrombocytopenia (HIT) assay. The presence or development of HIT is associated with a high risk of bleeding as well as thrombosis of MCS devices.[29]

Nutrition

Nutrition is an important contributor to overall outcome with MCS. A low serum albumin (<3.3 mg/dL) was the prominent risk factor for mortality and was associated with a relative increase in risk of 6.6-fold in the study by Lietz et al.,[30,31] who evaluated outcomes with LVAD therapy for DT. Significant nutritional deficiency is often associated with poor wound healing and an increased risk of infection and impaired T-lymphocyte cell function, as manifest by cutaneous skin test anergy. Body habitus is a marker of nutrition and an important consideration in patient selection and is reliably defined by body mass index (BMI). Patients whose BMI is either less than 22 or greater than 36 are at risk for perioperative complications, but outcomes are more adversely impacted by cachexia than obesity.[32–34] Cachexia is often due to poor appetite due to elevated tumor necrosis factor (TNF) and other cytokines, limitations in exertion and work of breathing, and early satiety in those with significant hepatomegaly.[35] Cessation of calorie intake for as little as 24 hours may be associated with a 50% reduction in production of critical proteins needed for wound repair. Delay in instituting MCS therapy may be warranted for several weeks when feasible to allow improvement in nutritional status, either by ingestion of various oral nutritional supplements or enteral feedings using a small feeding tube, preferentially with nocturnal feeding in those unable to consume adequate calories during the day. Early, aggressive caloric supplementation in the postoperative period is also critical to preventing or reversing malnutrition.

OTHER IMPORTANT MEDICAL CONSIDERATIONS IN INSTITUTING MECHANICAL CIRCULATORY SUPPORT

Valvular Heart Disease

Abnormalities of the cardiac valves have important adverse consequences in patients being considered for MCS and may require repair or replacement in order to initiate successful MCS or achieve weaning from support. Mild to moderate aortic stenosis in the absence of insufficiency is not a contraindication to placement of a VAD. Severe aortic stenosis should be corrected prior to placement of a VAD, preferably with a bioprosthetic valve, to facilitate future weaning or optimize native heart function in the event of device failure. The presence of even mild to moderate aortic insufficiency can have a significant impact on the effectiveness of MCS therapy. In cases where LV assistance is initiated with left atrial to aortic cannulation, aortic insufficiency will result in LV distention in the presence of significant LV dysfunction. LV distention adversely affects subendocardial blood flow and can prevent weaning from MCS. In cases where MCS support is initiated with devices that require LV apical to aortic cannulation, reductions in LV pressure elicited by MCS increase the pressure gradient across the aortic valve and increase the degree of aortic insufficiency. Blood pumped into the aorta by the LVAD will flow backward across the incompetent aortic valve (aortic insufficiency), decreasing net forward flow and compromising end-organ perfusion. Mild to moderate aortic insufficiency may become more severe with initiation of MCS from an LVAD because the elevated LV end-diastolic pressure will be significantly reduced by emptying of the LV cavity by the device and the aortic root pressure will be elevated above baseline because of device flow. The presence of significant aortic insufficiency can be confirmed by echocardiography. Patients with a mechanical valve prosthesis in the aortic valve position should have the mechanical valve replaced with a bioprosthetic valve prior to institution of LV assistance. During complete unloading of the left ventricle by a VAD, the aortic valve may not open and the mechanical valve may be prone to thrombus formation.

Patients with significant mitral stenosis at the time of initiation of device support may require correction of the valvular problem before implantation of a device depending on device selection and site of cannulation. In the setting of significant mitral stenosis, LV filling is impaired. VADs that utilize apical ventriculotomy for cannula placement for ventricular drainage may experience limitations in device filling due to mitral stenosis. This problem can be circumvented by either choosing a device that can utilize left atrial drainage or by correcting the underlying valvular pathology (mitral valve repair or replacement with a bioprosthetic valve). Mitral regurgitation does not have an impact on the filling of a VAD. In situations where weaning from MCS may be feasible, correction of the mitral pathology, either stenosis or regurgitation, is necessary in order to optimize ventricular function.

Adequate RV function is extremely important to maintain LVAD flow in the early postoperative period. Severe tricuspid regurgitation can significantly impair the forward flow of blood from the right ventricle, particularly in situations of high pulmonary vascular resistance. Severe tricuspid regurgitation contributes to elevated central venous pressure, hepatic congestion, and renal dysfunction. Severe tricuspid regurgitation may be present preoperatively in the setting of volume overload and biventricular failure or may develop following institution of LVAD support as a consequence of RV dilation from leftward shift of the interventricular septum.[25–27] If severe tricuspid regurgitation is present during the initiation of LVAD support, tricuspid valve repair should be performed to improve RV performance.

Coronary Artery Disease

Patients with significant obstructive coronary artery disease or patients with postcardiotomy shock following failed coronary bypass operations may experience angina during MCS. Generally, coronary artery disease does not have adverse hemodynamic consequences during the period of MCS. However, the presence of obstructive coronary disease with ongoing ischemia may limit the degree of myocardial recovery and impact the ability to wean from temporary MCS.

Perioperative ischemia of the right ventricle may be of hemodynamic significance during institution of LVAD support. RV ischemia causing myocardial stunning or infarction that occurs during or soon after implantation of an LVAD can elicit RV failure, resulting in decreased flow to the LVAD. In patients who have had coronary bypass surgery and are candidates for MCS, patent bypass grafts, particularly to the right coronary artery or left anterior descending coronary artery, should be preserved in order to reduce the risk of perioperative RV failure and arrhythmias. In selected situations it may be important to perform a coronary artery bypass to the right coronary artery or left anterior descending coronary artery systems to optimize RV function in the perioperative period if significant obstructive coronary lesions amenable to bypass are present in the distribution of these arteries.

Arrhythmias

Atrial and ventricular arrhythmias are common in patients with cardiogenic shock and underlying ischemic or idiopathic cardiomyopathies. These arrhythmias generally persist in the immediate postoperative period and subsequently resolve with time as the hemodynamic condition of the patient improves and inotrope therapy is weaned. Some patients will have persistent arrhythmias due to their underlying pathology (i.e., giant cell myocarditis). Severe ventricular arrhythmias have traditionally been thought to be a contraindication to univentricular support. However, recent experience has revealed that the hemodynamic consequences in patients in whom these arrhythmias develop in the late postoperative period are generally not life-threatening.[36–38] In the absence of pulmonary hypertension and elevated pulmonary vascular resistance in the postoperative period, patients maintain adequate LVAD flows during ventricular fibrillation. This situation is analogous to a Fontan (systemic vein to pulmonary artery) circulation. In the early perioperative period, some patients with refractory ventricular arrhythmias may require biventricular support until the pulmonary vasculature resistance drops and a Fontan circulation is tolerated. The addition of RV support for hemodynamic compromise due to refractory ventricular arrhythmia is unusual. In situations where weaning from MCS is feasible or planned, elimination of the ventricular arrhythmias with antiarrhythmic therapy is essential.

Intracardiac Shunts

Intracardiac shunts, such as a patent foramen ovale or atrial septal defect, should be closed at the time of implantation of an LVAD to prevent right-to-left shunting. These anomalies should be identified prior to surgery using transesophageal echocardiogram.[39] During the initiation of LV assistance, left atrial pressure is reduced compared to right atrial pressure. This gradient causes shunting of deoxygenated blood from the right atrium into the left, resulting in significant systemic hypoxemia.

PATIENT OUTCOMES AND MAJOR ADVERSE EVENTS FOLLOWING INITIATION OF MECHANICAL CIRCULATORY SUPPORT

Survival, as well as the occurrence of significant adverse events following the initiation of MCS therapy, is dependent on the clinical presentation, indication for MCS therapy, and type of device utilized. Generally, adverse outcomes are associated with a greater acuity and severity of illness and are generally higher when temporary MCS devices are utilized in the 7 emergent situation. Bleeding, stroke and thromboembolism, infection, and RV failure are the most frequent complications that occur in the early postoperative period following initiation of MCS. Major adverse events most common in the late postoperative period include infection and device failure.

Bleeding

Bleeding is a frequent, early complication in patients supported by MCS and generally requires reoperation in the early postoperative period. Risk factors for bleeding include preoperative hepatic congestion and failure, poor preoperative nutritional status, prolonged CPB times, extensive surgical dissection, reoperative surgery, multiple cannulation sites, decreased platelet function, and induction of fibrinolysis as a result of contact with biomaterial surfaces during CPB and MCS devices. In the early experience of MCS, about 50% of patients required reoperation for bleeding. The rate still remains significant even with the incorporation of new device technology.

Right Ventricular Failure (see Right Ventricular Failure under Patient Selection and Influence of Comorbidities on Outcomes)

RV failure occurs in approximately 7% to 20% of patients supported by LV assistance alone. The etiology of RV failure is multifactorial and includes pathologies within the pulmonary vascular bed and/or right ventricle. Factors contributing to RV failure include impaired RV function as a result of intraoperative air embolism, myocardial stunning as a result of poor intraoperative myocardial protection, ischemia and infarction from coronary artery disease, arrhythmias, volume loading, and alteration of RV septal geometry induced by LV unloading. Several studies have demonstrated that factors, such as elevated central venous pressure, reduced RV stroke work index, low preoperative pulmonary artery pressures, transpulmonary gradient greater than 16 mm Hg, acute decrease in pulmonary artery pressures equal to or greater than 10 mm Hg at the onset of LVAD support, degree of preoperative pulmonary edema, increased need for perioperative transfusions, increasing degree of renal and hepatic dysfunction, female gender, nonischemic etiology, and preoperative temporary MCS support, all increase the need for RV MCS following LVAD implantation.[12–14,23,40,41] Acute unloading of the left ventricle by MCS may cause the septum to shift leftward, increasing RV volume loading and reducing its function.[25–27] The negative consequences of this phenomenon may be offset by the reduction in pulmonary artery pressures and RV afterload caused by device-mediated LV decompression.[25–27] Hemodynamic stability can be attained with isolated mechanical LV support in approximately 90% of patients, even in those patients with substantial RV dysfunction, if there is effective replacement of left-sided heart function and aggressive treatment of pulmonary hypertension. More recently, the improved perioperative management of elevated pulmonary vascular resistance including the use of inhaled nitric oxide, a specific, potent pulmonary vasodilator, in combination with milrinone, isoproterenol, or dobutamine has significantly reduced the need for placement of a RVAD.[42–44] In patients with marked elevation of central venous pressure, multiorgan failure, or severe RV dysfunction with low pulmonary artery pressures, early biventricular support may be indicated.[12–14,23]

Stroke and Thromboembolism

The occurrence of thromboembolic events following MCS is variable and depends on a number of factors including the type of device, duration of support, location and number of cannulation sites, and presence of prosthetic valves within the heart. Approximately 10% of patients receiving MCS with implantable devices will experience a thromboembolic event or stroke.[45,46] This rate is in the range of 20% for patients on short-term extracorporeal MCS devices. Improvement in the rate of thromboembolic events has come from more aggressive antiplatelet therapy in conjunction with warfarin, improved device design, and more frequent use of LV apical as compared to left atrial cannulation. In patients supported for short durations only, anticoagulation is usually achieved with heparin and antiplatelet therapy. Longer-term support usually requires transition to warfarin and antiplatelet therapy for most, but not all, devices.

Infection

Infections can be device related (i.e., device endocarditis, percutaneous lead or cannula site infection, pocket infection [infection external to an implanted device]) or non–device related (i.e., pneumonia, urinary tract infection). The incidence of early nosocomial non–device-related or device-related infections in patients undergoing MCS is approximately 30% to 40% in many series and is related to the acuity of illness in this population of patients.[46–54] Patients with persistent or recurrent sepsis and those patients with device-related infections tend to have a higher mortality than patients without these complications. In patients on long-term MCS, infection remains the single most significant obstacle to successful outcome. Infection was the most common cause of mortality during LVAD support seen in the REMATCH trial, with infection contributing to 41% of deaths.[3] Within 3 months after implantation, the probability of infection with the device was 28%. Most of these late infections began in the percutaneous tube (driveline) tract and pocket of the device. However, clinical experience has revealed that VAD infection rates can be minimized with attention to infection control guidelines, optimal implantation techniques, meticulous wound care, and the utilization of new continuous flow rotary pump technology.[46,55,56]

Risk factors for development of infection that are present before device insertion include preoperative infection at remote sites (not in the area of implantation), malnutrition, prolonged hospitalization, immobilization, broad-spectrum antibiotic therapy, immunosuppressive medications (i.e., steroids), mechanical ventilation, and the presence of central venous catheters. The percutaneous lead of the device can be a portal of entry for bacterial and fungal pathogens. Intracorporeal device infections can occur within the pumps themselves and on their outer surfaces, which are generally caused by biofilm-forming bacteria and fungi (e.g., *Staphylococcus* species). Device-related infections can sometimes be successfully treated with antibiotic suppression and device exchange or removal. Infections involving the preperitoneal pocket (subfascial space created for device placement) surrounding implantable VADs require more aggressive treatment, including open drainage, débridement, and rerouting of the percutaneous lead through a fresh exit site. However, patients who are device dependent and awaiting transplantation generally cannot tolerate device removal as a therapeutic option to eradicate the infection. Antibiotic suppression and transplantation remain the only chance for cure of device-related infections in these instances. These infections do not generally preclude heart transplantation, and transplant outcomes and survival are generally not significantly affected in this situation.[50,56]

Device Malfunction

As with any mechanical device, malfunction is an anticipated occurrence. The types and severity of device malfunctions vary with each of the devices. Many devices have built-in backup systems that, in the event of catastrophic device failure, provide support to the patient. Also, most patients supported by a VAD have enough residual LV function to help sustain them until corrective measures can be taken. New technology incorporating continuous flow rotary pump design presents new challenges to device malfunction. These devices do not contain valves to direct the flow of blood, and stoppage of the pump is associated with significant regurgitation of blood through the device, resulting in significant LV distention. This phenomenon is similar to the development of acute aortic insufficiency. Fortunately, the reported frequency of this event is low.[46] Device malfunctions in total artificial hearts are more problematic as there is no native heart to provide hemodynamic support in the event of a total device failure. Stringent quality control measures in fabrication and testing and very low mechanical failure rates are therefore even more essential with total artificial hearts.

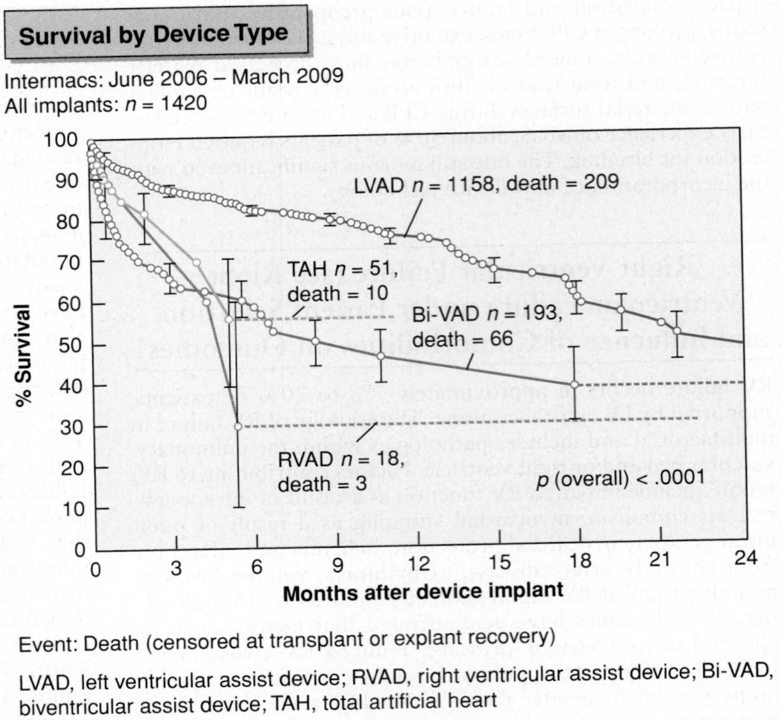

FIGURE 84.3. Survival analysis for patients on mechanical circulatory support by Interagency Registry for Mechanically Assisted Circulatory Support (INTERMACS) profile and entered into the INTERMACS registry from June 2006 through December 2009. (Figure adapted from the INTERMACS Registry website: http://www.uab.edu/ctsresearch/intermacs/presentations.htm and previously presented at the International Society of Heart and Lung Transplantation, 28th Meeting and Scientific Sessions, April 2008. Reproduced with permission.)[59]

Interagency Registry for Mechanically Assisted Circulatory Support

8 The Interagency Registry for Mechanically Assisted Circulatory Support (INTERMACS) database, funded by the U.S. National Heart, Lung and Blood Institute (NHLBI), is a registry for patients who receive implantable or "durable" VAD devices that are approved by the FDA.[57–60] The INTERMACS registry represents one of the largest available data repositories for the study of VAD outcomes intended for BTT or DT. The most recent published data analysis of MCS outcomes for VAD therapy reviews the nearly 3 years of data entry into the registry and largely represents outcomes from patients undergoing implantation with the first generation of pulsatile, volume displacement technology, such as the HeartMate XVE (Thoratec Corporation, Pleasanton, California), Thoratec pVAD (Thoratec Corporation, Pleasanton, California), Thoratec IVAD (Thoratec Corporation, Pleasanton, California), and Novacor LVAD (World Heart Corporation, Oakland, California), and second-generation technology with continuous flow rotary pumps.[57–60] Survival with LVAD support alone at 2 years was approximately 50% and was significantly worse for those patients requiring BiVAD support or support with a TAH[57–60] (Figs. 84.3 and 84.4 and Table 84.1). Patients undergoing implantation of an MCS device in the

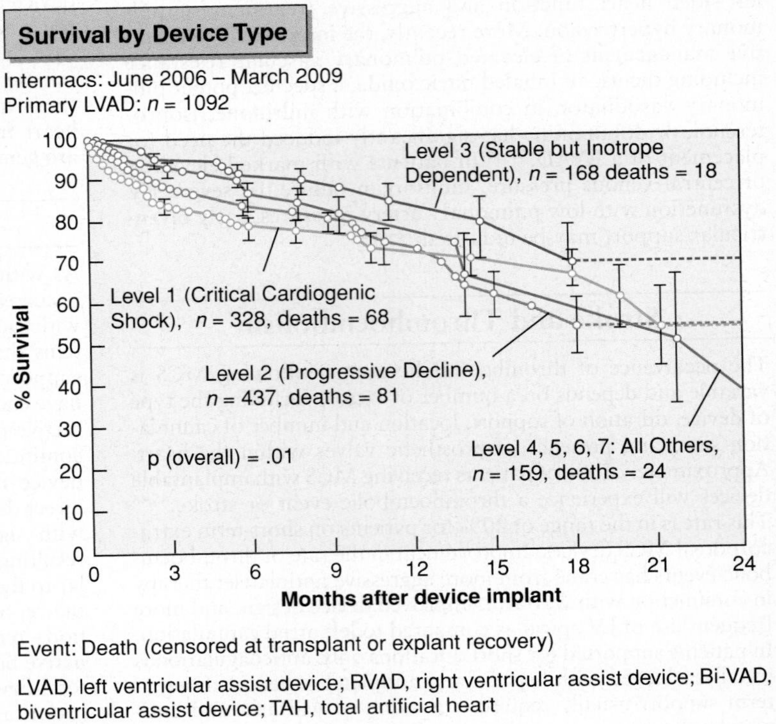

FIGURE 84.4. Survival analysis for patients on mechanical circulatory support by INTERMACS Profile and entered into the INTERMACS Registry from June 2006 through December 2009. (Figure adapted from the INTERMACS Registry Web site: http://www.uab.edu/ctsresearch/intermacs/presentations.htm and previously presented at the International Society of Heart and Lung Transplantation, 28th Meeting and Scientific Sessions, April 2008. Reproduced with permission.)[5]

TABLE 84.1

DESCRIPTION OF INTERMACS PROFILES DESCRIBING DEGREE OF HEART FAILURE SYMPTOMS AND HEMODYNAMIC STATUS AT THE TIME OF MECHANICAL CIRCULATORY SUPPORT IMPLANTATION AND INCLUDING THE TIME FRAME FOR INTERVENTION[57]

■ INTERMACS PROFILE DESCRIPTIONS	■ TIME FRAME FOR INTERVENTION
Profile 1: Critical cardiogenic shock Patients with life-threatening hypotension despite rapidly escalating inotropic support, critical organ hypoperfusion, often confirmed by worsening acidosis and/or lactate levels. *"Crash or burn."*	Definitive intervention needed within hours.
Profile 2: Progressive decline Patient with declining function despite intravenous inotropic support, may be manifest by worsening renal function, nutritional deprivation, inability to restore volume balance. "Sliding on inotropes." Also describes declining status in patients unable to tolerate inotropic therapy.	Definitive intervention needed within few days.
Profile 3: Stable bu inotrope dependent Patient with stable blood pressure, organ function, nutrition, and symptoms on continuous intravenous inotropic support (or a temporary circulatory support device or both), but demonstrating repeated failure to wean from support due to recurrent symptomatic hypotension or renal dysfunction. *"Dependent stability."*	Definitive intervention elective over a period of weeks to few months.
Profile 4: Resting symptoms Patient can be stabilized close to normal volume status but experience daily symptoms of congestion at rest or during ADL. Doses of diuretics generally fluctuate at very high levels. More intensive management and surveillance strategies should be considered, which may in some cases reveal poor compliance that would compromise outcomes with any therapy. Some patients may shuffle between 4 and 5.	Definitive intervention elective over period of weeks to few months.
Profile 5: Exertion intolerant Comfortable at rest and with ADL but unable to engage in any other activity, living predominantly within the house. Patients are comfortable at rest without congestive symptoms, but may have underlying refractory elevated volume status, often with renal dysfunction. If underlying nutritional status and organ function are marginal, patient may be more at risk with INTERMACS 4, and require definitive intervention.	Variable urgency, depends upon maintenance of nutrition, organ function, and activity.
Profile 6: Exertion limited Patient without evidence of fluid overload is comfortable at rest, and with ADLs and minor activities outside the home but fatigues after the first few minutes of any meaningful activity. Attribution to cardiac limitation requires careful measurement of peak oxygen consumption, in some cases with hemodynamic monitoring to confirm severity of cardiac impairment. *"Walking wounded."*	Variable, depends upon maintenance of nutrition, organ function, and activity level.
Profile 7: Advanced NYHA III A placeholder for more precise specification in future, this level included patients who are without current or recent episodes of unstable fluid balance, living comfortably with meaningful activity limited to mild physical exertion.	Transplantation or circulatory support may not currently be indicated.
Modifiers for Profiles	**Possible Profiles to Modify**
TCS: Temporary Circulatory Support can modify only patients in hospital (other devices would be INTERMACS devices). Includes IABP, ECMO, TandemHeart, Levitronix, BVS 5000 or AB5000, Impella	1, 2, 3 in hospital.
A-Arrhythmia: can modify any profile. Recurrent ventricular tachyarrhythmias that have recently contributed substantially to clinical compromise. This includes frequent ICD shock or requirement for external defibrillator, usually more than twice weekly.	Any profile.
FF: Frequent Flyer can modify only outpatients, designating a patient requiring frequent emergency visits or hospitalizations for diuretics, ultrafiltration, or temporary intravenous vasoactive therapy.	3 if at home, 4, 5, 6. A frequent flyer would rarely be profile 7.

INTERMACS, Interagency Registry for Mechanically Assisted Circulatory Support.
From Stevenson LW, Pagani FD, Young JB, et al. INTERMACS profiles of advanced heart failure: the current picture. *J Heart Lung Transplant* 2009;28:535–541.

presence of critical cardiogenic shock (i.e., INTERMACS level 1) had worse outcomes compared to device implantation in patients with more stable forms of advanced heart failure (INTERMACS levels 2 through 7)[57–60] (Figs. 84.3 and 84.4 and Table 84.1). These observations highlight the importance of proper patient selection and timing of initiation of MCS therapy on outcomes. Patients with significant organ dysfunction at the time of MCS device implant, accompanied by a greater degree of hemodynamic compromise, have a significantly higher risk of requiring BiVAD support, higher risk of major adverse events, and significantly higher risk of death during VAD support.

Since May 2008, following FDA approval of the HeartMate II LVAD, an increasing number of patients entered into the INTERMACS registry have received MCS device support with the new generation of continuous flow rotary pump technology. Subsequent reports from the INTERMACS registry will highlight outcomes from new continuous flow rotary pump technology and offer unique insight with comparison to older technology for BTT indications.

WEANING PATIENTS FROM MECHANICAL CIRCULATORY SUPPORT

Weaning from Short-term Mechanical Circulatory Support

A number of factors are considered when weaning patients from MCS. The first consideration is an assessment of pathologic abnormalities of the heart, such as valvular disease or severe coronary disease, that have not been addressed and corrected. If the underlying pathology that has caused the patient to require MCS is not corrected, then the chances of weaning from MCS will be negligible. Cardiac tamponade must also be excluded. Bleeding is a major early complication of MCS and reoperation for cardiac tamponade and bleeding is frequent. Transesophageal echocardiogram may not reliably identify cardiac tamponade in the early postoperative period. Thus, a high index of suspicion and low threshold for reoperation is critical to rule out tamponade. Volume status, preload and afterload, cardiac rhythm, and degree of inotropic support should be optimized for weaning. Noncardiac causes can contribute to failure to wean from MCS. Pulmonary edema, elevated pulmonary vascular resistance, acute respiratory distress syndrome (ARDS), and pneumonia may hinder RV function.

Once a patient's status has been optimized, weaning from MCS with the use of transesophageal echocardiogram is ideal. As device flows are reduced, transesophageal echocardiogram provides information on ventricular filling and performance and valve function. If patients can maintain satisfactory hemodynamics with reduction of pump flow, they can be considered for weaning. In the setting of biventricular support, it is important that device flows on the right side be reduced prior to turning down left-sided device flows to prevent pulmonary edema in the event of inadequate LV function. As device flows are reduced, native heart function will begin to support the circulation. If hemodynamics are unsatisfactory during the weaning trial, the patient will require continued support and subsequent weaning trials. When weaning from MCS is not possible, patients should be evaluated for heart transplantation and bridged to a long-term MCS device if feasible.

Weaning from Long-term Mechanical Circulatory Support

Anecdotal observations from the cumulative experience with long-term MCS for BTT and recent small clinical studies have demonstrated that long-term MCS, associated with sustained mechanical unloading of the left ventricle, can improve myocardial function in those patients thought to have irreversible, dilated, end-stage nonischemic cardiomyopathies.[61–63] Several studies have demonstrated that long-term MCS can restore ventricular geometry; improve myocyte function, orientation, and size; reduce myocyte apoptosis; reduce myocardial cytokine gene and protein expression; reverse abnormal neurohormonal patterns associated with advanced heart failure; and improve myocardial mitochondrial function.[61–63] These observations have led clinicians to consider MCS alone, or in conjunction with other future possible therapies (novel medications, gene therapy, myocyte or stem cell implantation), as a potential modality to reverse end-stage cardiomyopathy.

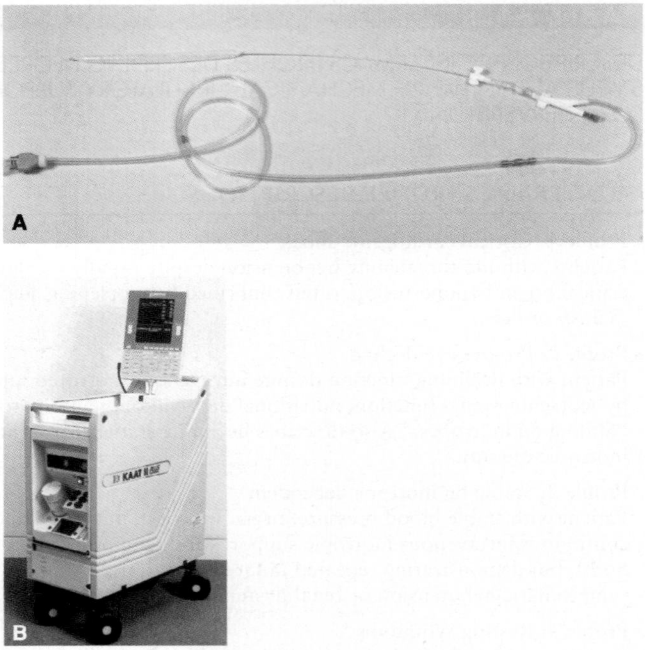

FIGURE 84.5. Intra-aortic balloon pump. **A:** Catheter-mounted balloon is positioned within the thoracic aorta through a percutaneous insertion in the groin. **B:** Console for the intra-aortic balloon pump.

Whether these observations hold under future rigorous experimental scrutiny remains unknown at this time.

MECHANICAL CIRCULATORY SUPPORT DEVICES

There are two broad categories of MCS devices separated by the intent of the duration to support patients and their ability to discharge patients safely to home.

Devices Intended for Short-term Mechanical Circulatory Support

Intra-aortic Balloon Pump. The most frequent MCS device in utilization today is the IABP (Figs. 84.5 and 84.6).

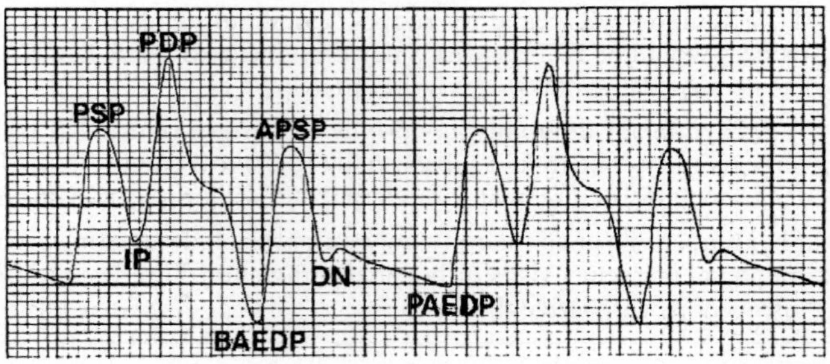

FIGURE 84.6. Aortic pressure tracing during intra-aortic balloon pump support. Balloon counterpulsation is occurring after every other heartbeat (1:2 counterpulsation). With correct timing, balloon inflation (IP) begins immediately after aortic valve closure, signaled by the dicrotic notch (DN). Compared with unassisted ejection, the pump augments diastolic blood flow by increasing peak aortic pressure during diastole (PDP). Balloon deflation before systole decreases ventricular afterload, with lower aortic end-diastolic pressure (balloon aortic end-diastolic pressure [BAEDP] vs. patient aortic end-diastolic pressure [PAEDP]) and lower peak systolic pressure (assisted peak systolic pressure [APSP] vs. peak systolic pressure [PSP]). (Courtesy of St. Jude Medical, Inc., Cardiac Assist Division, Minneapolis, MN.)

The first clinical use of the IABP was reported by Kantrowitz et al. in 1968.[64] The IABP can be inserted percutaneously and is positioned within the descending thoracic aorta. The IABP may augment cardiac output by 10% to 25% depending on the balloon size, patient size, degree of aortic compliance, cardiac rhythm, blood pressure, and IABP settings and timing. The concept for the IABP was based on the observation that the area under the arterial pressure trace (time-tension index) was an indirect estimation of the heart's oxygen consumption. Deflation just before ejection effectively decreases afterload and thus the work of the heart during systole. Balloon inflation during diastole increases diastolic pressure and hence coronary perfusion. Cardiac output improves from enhanced myocardial contractility as a result of increased coronary blood flow and reduced afterload and preload. Patients with ischemic cardiomyopathy have the greatest potential in increase in cardiac output from improved cardiac contractility resulting from enhanced coronary perfusion during diastole. Complications from use of the IABP include leg ischemia, balloon rupture, thrombosis within the balloon, sepsis, infection at the insertion site, bleeding, false aneurysm formation, lymph fistula, femoral neuropathy, vessel perforation with hemorrhage, and aortic dissection from catheter passage below the intima. Depending on the extent of peripheral vascular disease, balloon position can occlude major branches of the aorta and elicit ischemia of the tissues supplied by these vessels. Female gender, peripheral vascular disease, diabetes, smoking, advanced age, obesity, and cardiogenic shock are risk factors for the development of leg ischemia. The IABP has several disadvantages. In the best of circumstances, cardiac output is augmented by 25% as compared to LVADs, which can augment cardiac output by three to five times baseline flows. Mobilization and ambulation of the patient is limited while the IABP is being utilized.

Extracorporeal Life Support. ECLS, traditionally referred to as ECMO, is a temporary form of MCS that provides circulatory assistance as well as oxygenation and carbon dioxide removal from blood.[65–67] The ECLS circuit is similar in concept to cardiopulmonary bypass routinely used in the operating room for cardiac procedures. However, with ECLS, safe application for extended periods of time (days) has required certain modifications, particularly the inclusion of membrane or hollow-fiber oxygenators. The first successful use of prolonged ECLS was reported by Hill et al. in 1972.[68] Subsequently, ECLS has been used in an increasing number of indications including neonatal, pediatric, and adult respiratory support; neonatal, pediatric, and adult postcardiotomy support; and as a bridge to a LVAD or heart and lung transplantation.

ECLS supports the circulation by unloading the right ventricle and draining blood from the venous circulation, oxygenating it, and returning it to the arterial circulation. ECLS does not unload the left ventricle, although LV preload is reduced by decreasing pulmonary venous return. In patients with severe LV dysfunction, the use of an IABP helps reduce LV afterload during systole and improves myocardial contractility. The use of the IABP and inotrope therapy can maintain sufficient cardiac contractility to prevent stasis within the ventricle where clot formation is possible.[69] If LV function is so severely reduced that there is no ejection, an atrial septostomy can be performed to vent pulmonary venous return. Alternatively, a left-sided vent can be connected to the venous line to relieve LV distention. It is important during ECLS support to maintain some degree of pulmonary blood flow to prevent thrombosis. Additionally, it is important to continue ventilation of the lungs to maintain the oxygen saturation of the blood ejected from the left ventricle above 90%. Poorly oxygenated blood ejected from the left ventricle will perfuse the coronary arteries and add hypoxic damage to the already injured heart. Venovenous ECLS, unlike venoarterial ECLS, maintains flow through the heart. Venoarterial ECLS is used primarily for cardiac or cardiorespiratory support, while venovenous ECLS is used for pulmonary support.

Current ECLS circuits are typically composed of a centrifugal pump with either a hollow fiber or membrane oxygenator, an oxygen blender, a pump console, a heat exchanger, and a pump cart. A roller pump is used by some centers. Cannulation for ECLS is extremely variable and depends on the clinical situation and whether venoarterial or venovenous circuit is desired. Percutaneous cannulation of the femoral vein and artery can be performed in emergent situations where institution of MCS is needed within minutes (acute cardiac and/or respiratory arrest). In less urgent situations, cut-down on the internal jugular and carotid artery or respective femoral vessels can be performed. In cases of postcardiotomy failure in the operating room, venous access can be obtained by insertion of the cannula in the right atrium and arterial outflow obtained by cannulation of the ascending aorta.

Numerous large clinical series have reported successful use of ECLS for cardiac and/or respiratory support in adult, pediatric, and neonatal patients. In the largest series reported to date, Bartlett et al. at the University of Michigan reported on the outcome of 1,000 patients supported with ECLS from 1980 through 1998.[70] Survival to hospital discharge was 88% for 586 cases of neonatal respiratory failure, 70% for 132 cases of respiratory failure in children, and 56% for 146 cases of respiratory failure in adult patients. Venovenous ECLS was the preferred method of respiratory support since 1988. For patients with cardiac failure, 33% of adult patients (31 cases) and 48% of pediatric patients (105 cases) survived to hospital discharge. Survival in adult patients was improved by utilizing ECLS as a bridge to longer-term implantable devices in patients who did not demonstrate early recovery of myocardial function.[71–74] Conversely, the availability of long-term implantable devices has extended the use of ECLS in situations where recovery of myocardial function is unlikely.[71–74]

Tandem Heart pVAD. The Tandem Heart pVAD (Cardiac Assist Technologies, Inc., Pittsburgh, Pennsylvania) is a percutaneous left atrial–to–femoral artery VAD[75] (Figs. 84.7 and 84.8). The pump is a low-speed, continuous flow, centrifugal pump. It is a dual-chamber pump composed of an upper housing and a lower housing assembly. The upper housing provides a conduit for inflow and outflow of blood. The lower housing assembly provides communication with the controller, the means for rotating the impeller of the VAD, and an anticoagulation infusion line integral to the pump to provide a hydrodynamic bearing, cooling of the bearing, and local anticoagulation. The controller is a microprocessor-based electromechanical drive and infusion system that is designed to be operated on AC current or on internal batteries.

Implantation of the device is performed percutaneously through the right femoral vein. A standard Brockenbrough catheter is inserted into the superior vena cava and the interatrial septum is punctured in the fossa ovalis using a Ross needle. The Brockenbrough catheter is then exchanged for a stiff guide wire with a distal soft wire loop identical to the device used for mitral valvuloplasty by the Inoue method. The transseptal puncture site is then dilated to 21 French with a two-stage dilator followed by insertion of a venous inflow cannula, which is sutured to the skin of the thigh. An arterial perfusion catheter of 14 French to 19 French is inserted percutaneously into the right femoral artery or two arterial perfusion catheters of 12 French into both femoral arteries.

In a randomized comparison of IABP with the Tandem Heart pVAD, Thiele et al. reported a more effective improvement in cardiac power index as well as other hemodynamic and metabolic variables with the Tandem Heart pVAD compared to the IABP. However, complications such as severe bleeding and limb ischemia were encountered more frequently after VAD support. Thirty-day mortality was similar between the groups.[75] The Tandem Heart pVAD is FDA approved for temporary MCS for cardiogenic shock in patients refractory to optimal medical therapy and IABP.

CentriMag VAD. The CentriMag VAD (Levitronix LLC, Waltham, Massachusetts) is an extracorporeal system composed

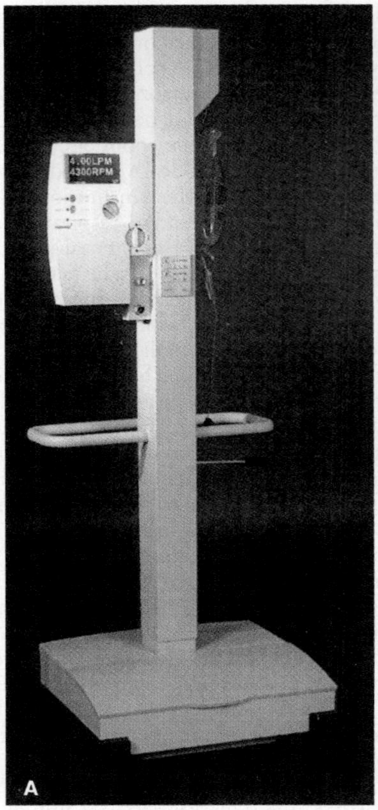

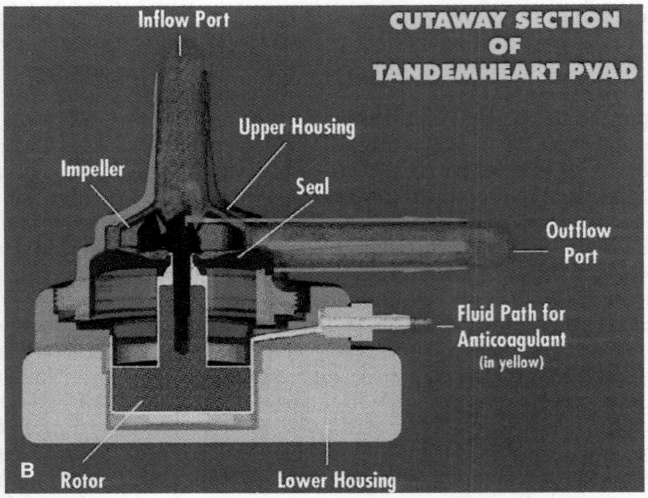

FIGURE 84.7. **A:** The Tandem Heart pVAD centrifugal pump. The Tandem Heart pVAD is an extracorporeal, continuous flow rotary pump providing temporary mechanical circulatory support (left ventricle). The Tandem Heart pVAD utilizes a bearing design in the pump for impeller positioning and rotation. **B:** Electrical control console for the Tandem Heart pVAD centrifugal pump. (Photographs courtesy of Cardiac Assist Corporation, Pittsburgh, PA.)

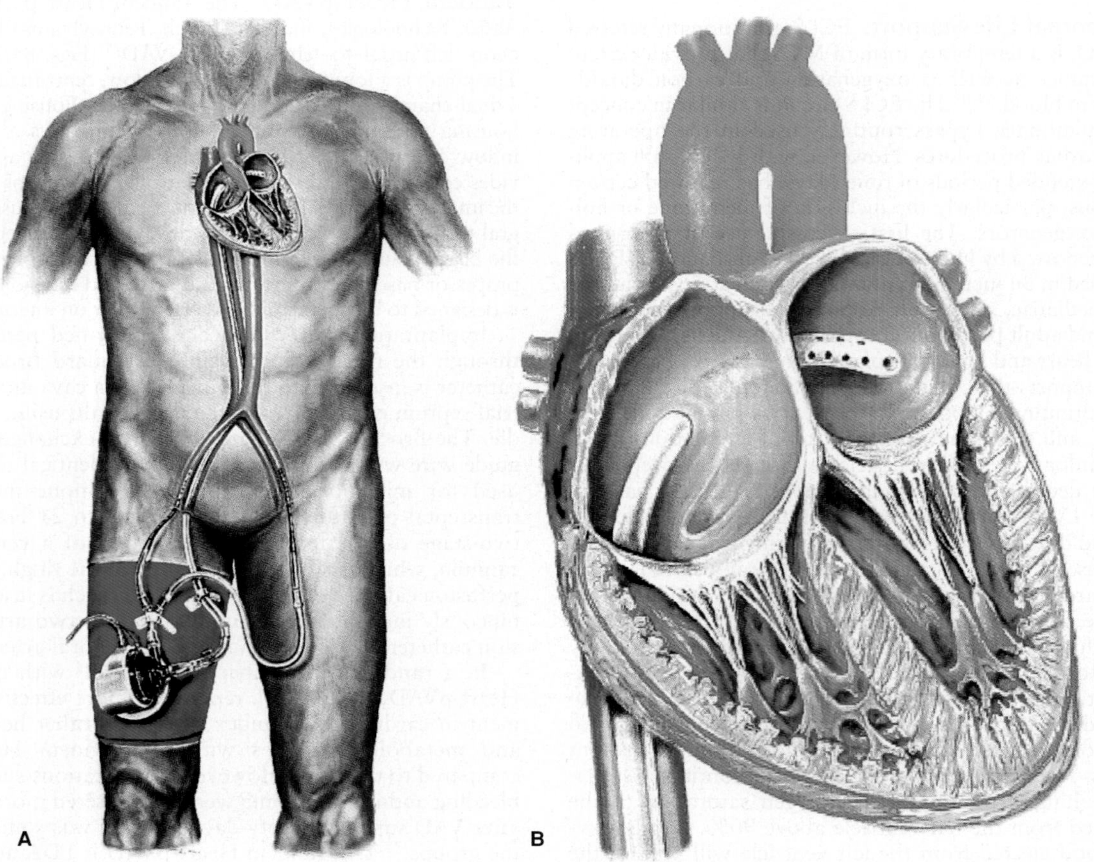

FIGURE 84.8. Schematic representation of the cannulation of the femoral artery and femoral vein with the transseptal placement of the inflow catheter within the left atrium from the femoral vein. The centrifugal pump of the Tandem Heart pVAD is secured to the patient's right thigh. (Photographs courtesy of Cardiac Assist Corporation, Pittsburgh, PA.)

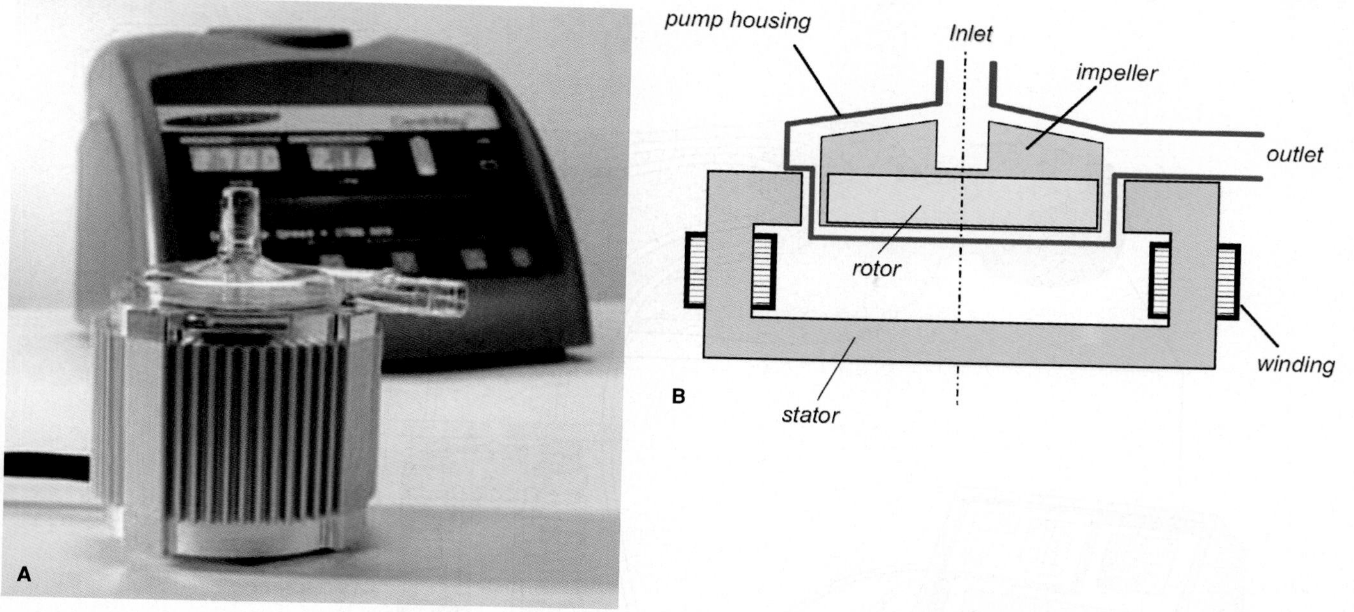

FIGURE 84.9. The CentriMag VAD. The CentriMag VAD is an extracorporeal, continuous flow rotary pump with centrifugal design utilized for temporary mechanical circulatory support. The CentriMag can provide univentricular or biventricular support. **A:** The CentriMag console (background) and pump/motor (foreground). **B:** Schematic representation of the CentriMag pump. The rotor located within the upper pump housing is magnetically coupled to the lower motor housing to produce rotor levitation and spin. (Photograph courtesy of Levitronix LLC, Waltham, MA; copyright IHC 2004.)

of a centrifugal blood pump, a motor, a console, a flow probe, and a circuit[76] (Fig. 84.9). The device is based on a magnetically levitated "bearingless motor" design. The rotor located within the upper pump housing is magnetically coupled to the lower motor housing to produce rotor levitation and spin, which combines the drive, the magnetic bearing, and the rotor function into a single unit. The motor generates the magnetic bearing force that levitates the rotor into the pump housing while also generating the torque necessary to produce the unidirectional flow. This device can produce flows of up to 10 L/min under normal physiologic conditions, with a priming volume of 31 mL. Single-center reports have demonstrated successful use of the CentriMag device as a BTR or bridge to long-term implantable VAD.[76,77]

Impella Recover LP 2.5. The Impella Recover LP 2.5 (Abiomed Corporation, Danvers, Massachusetts) is a catheter-based, impeller-driven, axial flow pump with a maximal flow of 2.5 L/min from the left ventricle to the ascending aorta. The device is positioned across the aortic valve with the inlet port below the valve and outlet port above the aortic valve. The device can be implanted via a percutaneous approach.[78,79] In a prospective randomized clinical trial comparing the Impella Recover LP 2.5 to IABP, cardiac index was significantly increased in patients with the LP 2.5 compared to patients supported with an IABP. Overall mortality at 30 days was similar in both groups.[80] The Impella is also available in a larger model, LP 5.0, that is capable of up to 5 L/min flow. The Impella LP 5.0 can be placed directly into the ascending aorta through the femoral artery or axillary artery.[81]

Extracorporeal Pulsatile Flow Circulatory Support Devices

Abiomed BVS 5000 and AB 5000. The Abiomed BVS 5000 (Abiomed Corporation, Danvers, Massachusetts) is an automated ventricular support device intended to provide complete temporary LV and/or RV support[6–8] (Figs. 84.10 and 84.11). The Abiomed BVS 5000 is FDA approved for short-term MCS as a bridge to recovery in cases of cardiogenic shock due to postcardiotomy failure to wean, acute myocarditis, and myocardial infarction. Positioned externally, this pulsatile

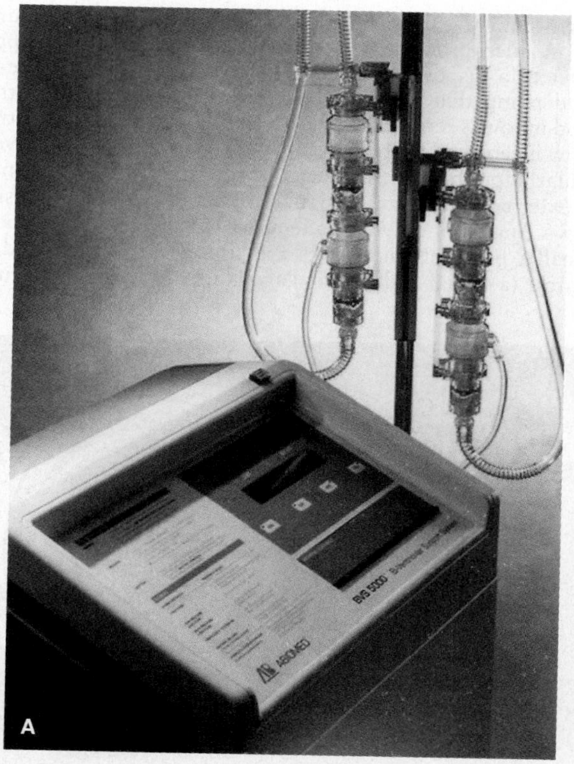

FIGURE 84.10. **A:** The Abiomed BVS 5000 (Abiomed Corporation, Danvers, MA) is an extracorporeal, pulsatile, displacement pump designed for temporary biventricular or univentricular mechanical circulatory support. Shown are the drive console and blood pumps. (*continued*)

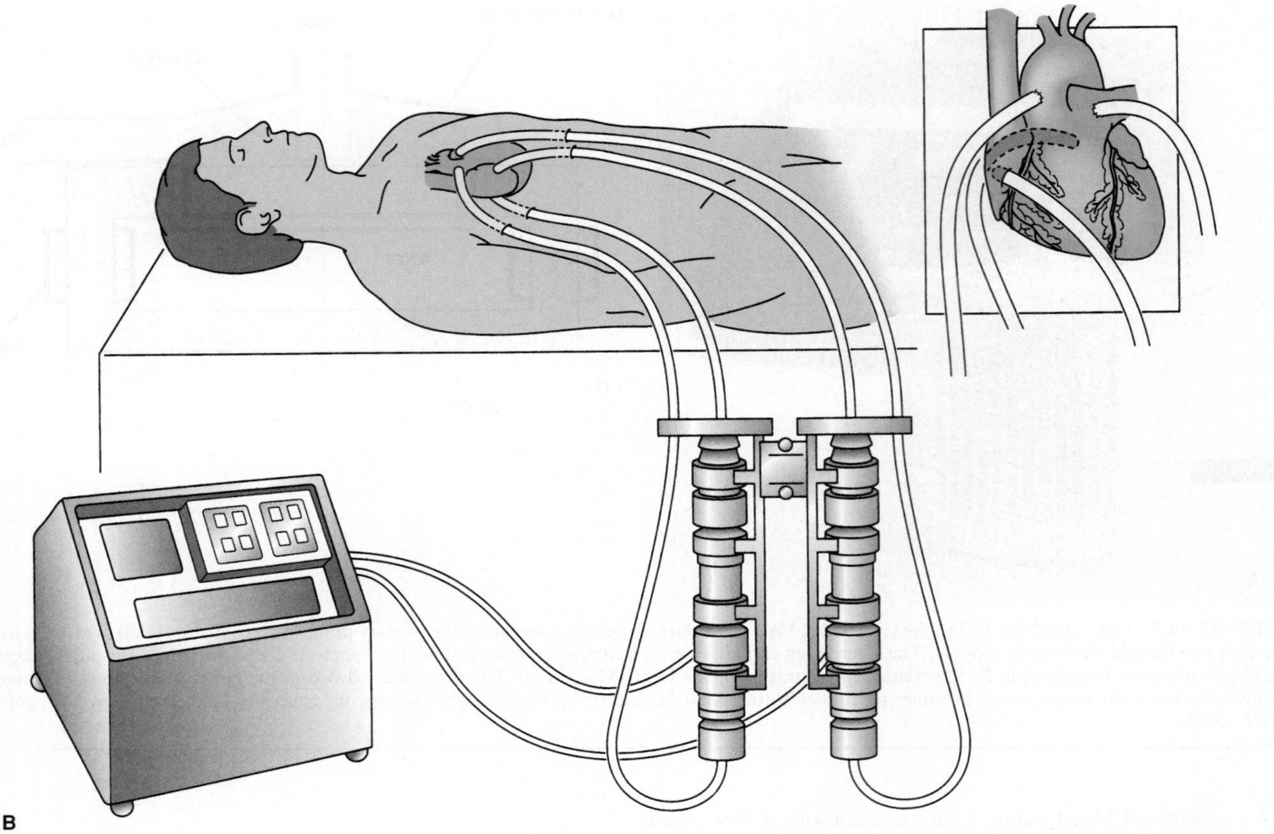

FIGURE 84.10. (*Continued*) **B:** Schematic representation of the Abiomed BVS 5000 with biventricular support configuration (see insert).

system simulates normal physiologic mechanical cardiac function. A microprocessor-based drive console is used to supply power to a disposable, pneumatically driven two-chambered blood pump that supports one side of the heart. Left atrial blood inflow is returned to the ascending aorta and right atrial inflow is returned to the pulmonary artery in the case of biventricular support. Transthoracic cannulas are used to connect the external system to the patient. Each blood pump consists of two Angioflex polyurethane atrioventricularlike chambers. Trileaflet polyurethane valves are strategically positioned to separate (a) atrial and ventricular bladders and (b) ventricular bladders and outflow cannulas. One or two disposable blood pumps are operated by a single BVS console, which automatically adjusts beat rate and systolic-to-diastolic ratio based on compressed air flow into and out of the external system. The blood pump is a dual-chamber device that incorporates an atrial (filling) chamber and a ventricular (pumping) chamber. Unidirectional flow is ensured by two trileaflet polyurethane valves fabricated from Angioflex, a biomaterial. The durations of pump systole and diastole are calculated automatically by the microprocessor to optimize pump filling and maintain a stroke volume of 83 mL. The console drives and adjusts left and right sides independently of each other. In addition to the traditional blood pumps and console, new blood pump designs and console, designated the AB 5000, have recently been introduced and approved by the FDA for short-term circulatory support. These blood pumps are connected to the patient in a paracorporeal configuration to enhance patient mobility (Fig. 84.11).

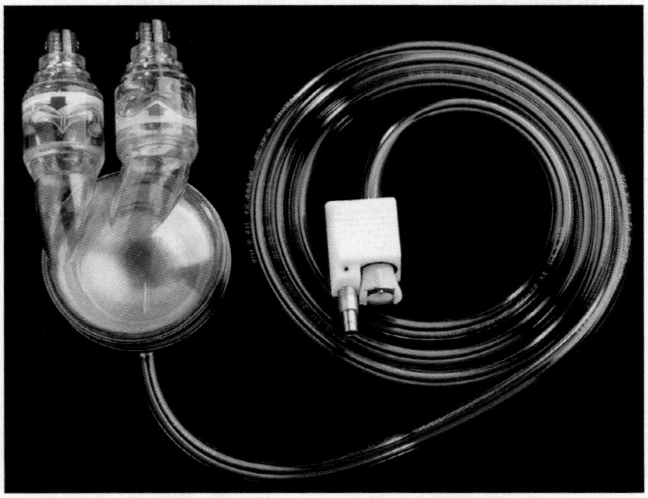

FIGURE 84.11. Abiomed AB 5000 (Abiomed Corporation, Danvers, MA). The AB 5000 is a pneumatically driven, pulsatile, volume displacement blood pump designed for a paracorporeal location.

Implantable Devices Intended for Long-term Mechanical Circulatory Support for Out-of-hospital Use (Bridge to Transplantation and Destination Therapy Indications)

The majority of patients receiving long-term MCS have been supported by devices engineered with pulsatile, volume displacement designs that are represented by the HeartMate VE and XVE (Thoratec Corporation, Pleasanton, California), Thoratec pVAD and IVAD (Thoratec Corporation, Pleasanton, California), or Novacor (World Heart Corporation, Oakland, California).[82–87] These first-generation devices are engineered with an internal reservoir chamber and inflow and outflow valves that permit cyclic filling and emptying of the device with pump actuation elicited by either pneumatic (Thoratec pVAD and

IVAD) or electrical (HeartMate VE and XVE and Novacor) drive systems. The inlet cannula of these devices is generally sewn to the left ventricular apex and the outflow graft sewn to the ascending aorta. Blood entering the left ventricle is diverted to the pump chamber and exits to the ascending aorta. The pump lies in a preperitoneal pocket created by surgical dissection below the diaphragm adjacent to the apex of the left ventricle. A percutaneous cable carrying the power supply to the pump, either pneumatic or electrical, is tunneled from the preperitoneal pocket to an external power source through the abdominal wall in the right upper quadrant.

Extended periods of MCS have highlighted limitations in the design of pulsatile, volume displacement pumps and include a large pump size restricting mobility, requirement for extensive surgical dissection for implant leading to bleeding and infection complications, a large body habitus of the recipient limiting options for device therapy for women, the presence of a large-diameter percutaneous lead for venting air, and audible pump operation. A critical limitation of these devices, particularly the HeartMate VE device and the subsequent later model, the HeartMate XVE, was the high incidence of reoperation for device exchange because of device malfunction.[88] Reports on the HeartMate VE and XVE have
9 demonstrated a greater than 50% rate of device failure at 2 years. To overcome these limitations, newer device designs incorporating continuous flow rotary pump technology with an axial or centrifugal blood path represent the next generation of devices for long-term MCS therapy.[88]

Implantable, Pulsatile, Volume Displacement Mechanical Circulatory Support Devices

HeartMate XVE Left Ventricular Assist Device. The HeartMate XVE is an implantable, pulsatile, volume displacement LVAD designed for long-term MCS[82,83] (Fig. 84.12). The unique feature of this device is that its blood-contacting surfaces of the pump are textured with sintered titanium spheres on the rigid surface and integrally textured polyurethane on the movable surfaces to encourage the deposition of circulating cells with the formation of a biologic layer, obviating the need for anticoagulation with warfarin. The HeartMate blood pump consists of a flexible polyurethane diaphragm within a ridged outer titanium alloy housing. The inflow and outflow conduits of the HeartMate device each contain a 25-mm porcine valve within a titanium cage to ensure unidirectional blood flow. Diaphragm movement and blood ejection depend on an electric motor positioned below the diaphragm. The electric rotary motor within the titanium housing drives a cam up and down (translational movement) causing diaphragm movement. An external vent equalizes the air pressure and permits emergency pneumatic actuation in the event of electrical failure. The drive line is covered with a polyester velour that promotes tissue bonding and anchoring to the skin. The XVE LVAD is powered by two rechargeable batteries. The wearable electrical devices currently available have external backup mechanisms to continue support without the need for reoperation in case of failure of the device. The maximum pump flow is 9.6 L/min for the HeartMate XVE.

Thoratec IVAD. The Thoratec IVAD is a small implantable ventricular assist device (IVAD) based on the Thoratec pVAD[89–93] (Figs. 84.13 and 84.14). The IVAD is a pneumatically driven pulsatile, volume displacement VAD that has a polyurethane blood pumping sac housed within a smooth-contoured, polished titanium alloy outer shell. The IVAD is controlled with the Thoratec TLC-II portable VAD driver, which is a small, briefcase-sized, battery-powered, pneumatic control unit that permits patient discharge from the hospital. A small flexible (9-mm outside diameter) percutaneous pneumatic driveline for each VAD is tunneled out of the body from the LVAD or RVAD in a pre- or intraperitoneal position. The major feature of this small pump is that it can be implanted to provide left, right, or biventricular support.

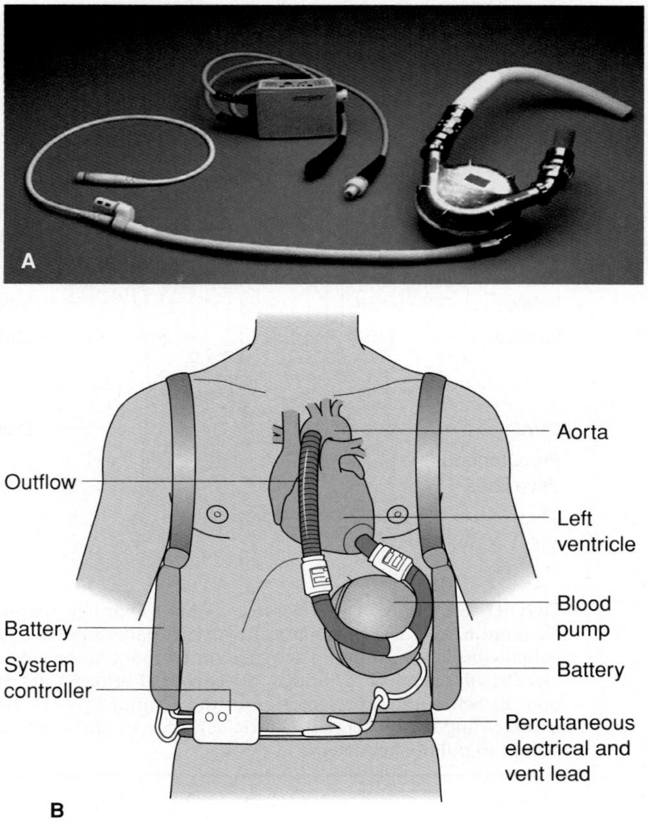

FIGURE 84.12. **A:** The HeartMate XVE (Thoratec Corporation, Pleasanton, CA) is an implantable, electrically driven, pulsatile, volume displacement left ventricular assist device designed for long-term mechanical circulatory support for bridge to transplant or destination therapy. **B:** Schematic representation of the preperitoneal pump placement for left ventricular assist and percutaneous drive line, external controller, and power source (batteries).

Implantable, Continuous Flow Mechanical Circulatory Support Devices (Rotary Pumps with Axial Flow Design). Implantable, continuous flow rotary pumps with axial flow design represent the second generation of implantable VAD technology and have now replaced first-generation, pulsatile devices for long-term MCS indications.[46,94–96] The term "second-generation rotary pump" has largely been used to describe those continuous flow rotary pumps, typically with an "axial" blood flow path, that have an internal rotor within the blood flow path that is suspended by contact bearings. Rotary pumps with axial flow design offer several advantages over pulsatile, volume displacement pumps. These advantages include smaller size, fewer moving parts, durability, absence of valves to direct blood flow, smaller blood-contacting surfaces, and reduced energy requirements. Blood flow is accomplished by the spinning of an internal rotor at high speed that imparts significant kinetic energy to the blood. The spinning of the rotor is accomplished by actuating an electrical current and magnetic field around the rotor that contains internal magnets. Blood flow from the left ventricle to the aorta occurs continuously during the systolic and diastolic phases of the cardiac cycle. Although blood flow is continuous during the cardiac cycle, phasic changes in the flow of blood occur during the cardiac cycle due to changes in ventricular pressure and aortic afterload. These phasic changes in blood flow impart a diminished pulsatility to the aortic waveform. The ability to design smaller pumps using axial flow technology is a result of the elimination of a large blood chamber necessary with pulsatile systems. An additional important feature of these pumps is the lack of need for a compliance chamber. This feature alleviates the problem of internal compensation that is associated with conventional

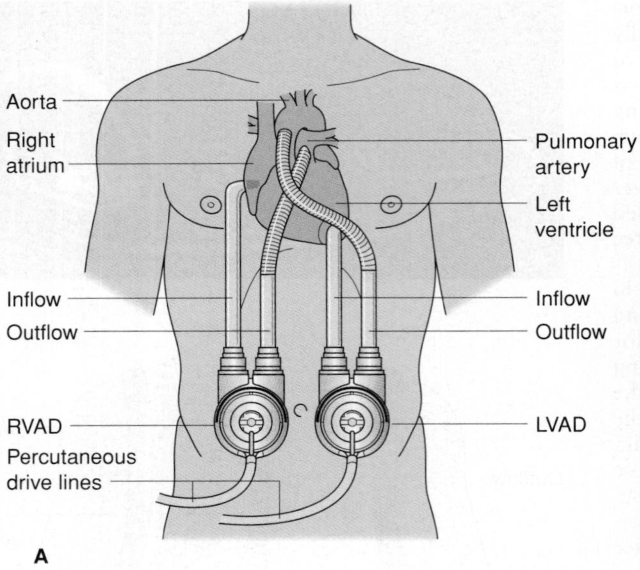

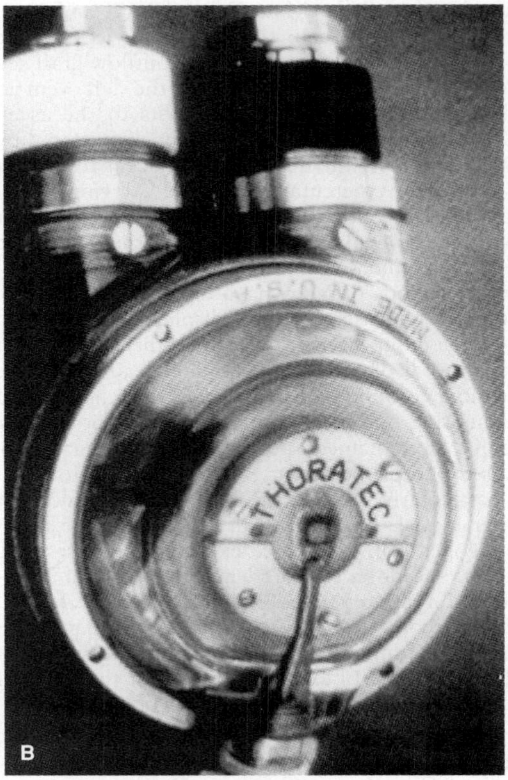

FIGURE 84.13. **A:** The Thoratec pVAD (Thoratec Corporation, Pleasanton, CA) is a pneumatically driven, paracorporeal, pulsatile, volume displacement pump designed for temporary univentricular or biventricular support for bridge to recovery or bridge to transplantation. **B:** Schematic representation of the Thoratec pVAD for biventricular support. LVAD, left ventricular apex to aorta; RVAD, right atrium to pulmonary artery.

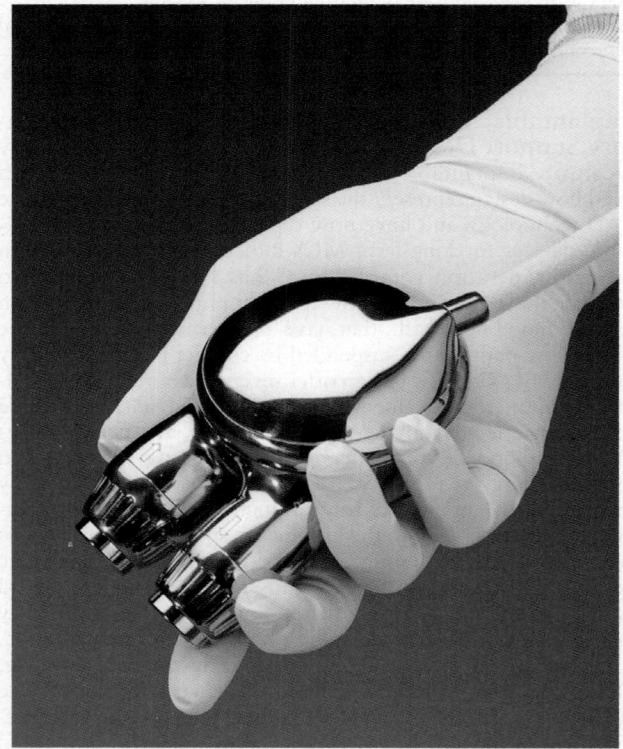

FIGURE 84.14. The Thoratec IVAD (Thoratec Corporation, Pleasanton, CA) is an implantable version of the Thoratec pVAD. The device is designed for longer-term univentricular or biventricular support for bridge to transplantation.

pulsatile pumps that, to date, has significantly hindered total internalization.

Device designs incorporating second-generation rotary pump technology with an axial blood path have accumulated significant human clinical experience and are either currently in late stages of clinical trials in the United States or have been recently been approved by the FDA for BTT. Reports from clinical trials of the second-generation rotary pumps have demonstrated efficacy in providing hemodynamic support, a favorable risk-to-benefit assessment, and improvement in mechanical performance.[46,96] Further, the human experience with second-generation rotary pumps with axial design has established the long-term safety of mechanical circulatory support with minimal pulse pressure.[97,98] Results from clinical studies have demonstrated early improvement followed by long-term stability of renal and hepatic function and no adverse effects on neurocognitive performance.[46] These improvements in device technology with the second-generation of continuous flow rotary pumps with axial design have increased the acceptance of LVAD therapy for long-term MCS indications.

HeartMate II. The HeartMate II is a continuous flow rotary pump with axial design that is representative of the second generation of LVAD technology in clinical use in the United States[46] (Fig. 84.15). The HeartMate II recently completed an FDA evaluation for BTT therapy in the United States in a cohort of 133 patients. To date, over 400 patients have been evaluated with the HeartMate II LVAD for BTT therapy and the device has received approval by the FDA for BTT indication in May 2008. In an extended follow-up report of 280 patients evaluated for BTT therapy with the HeartMate II device, 222 patients (79%) either received a transplant, recovered cardiac function and underwent device explantation, or remained alive with ongoing LVAD support at 18-month follow-up.[99] At 18 months, 157 (55.8%) patients had received a heart transplant, 58 (20.6%) remained alive with ongoing LVAD support, 56 (19.9%) died, 7 (2.5%) recovered cardiac function and underwent device explantation, and 3 (1%) were withdrawn from the study after device explantation and exchange for another type of LVAD. Overall survival

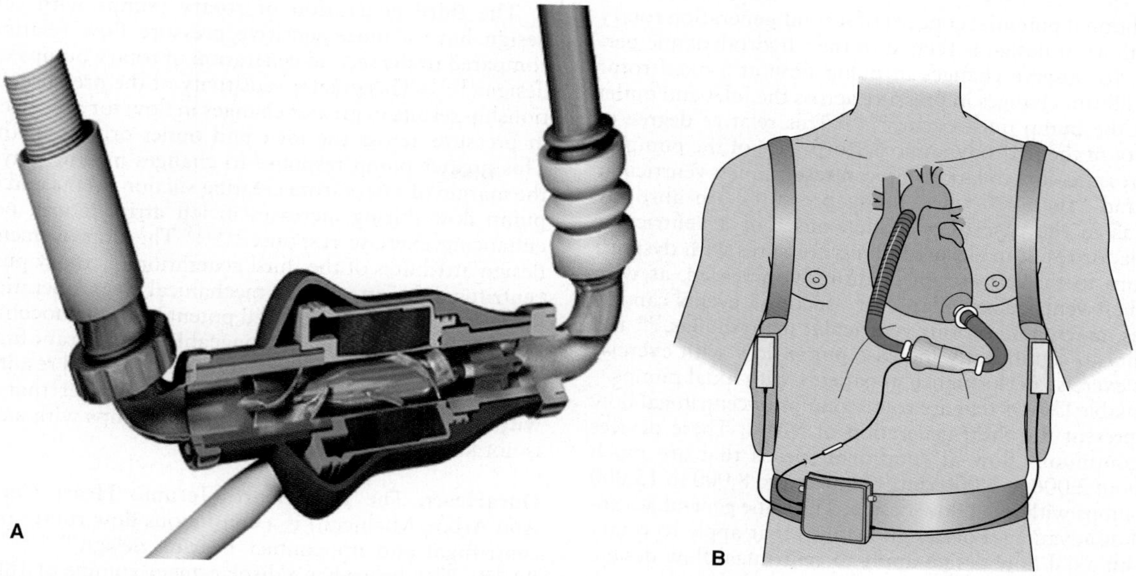

FIGURE 84.15. **A:** The HeartMate II LVAD (Thoratec Corporation, Pleasanton, CA) is an implantable, continuous flow rotary left ventricular assist device with axial design intended for long-term mechanical circulatory support for bridge to transplantation or destination therapy. Schematic drawing shows internal rotor, stators, and bearings and external motor coils. (Drawing courtesy of Thoratec Corporation, Pleasanton, CA.) **B:** Schematic representation of the HeartMate II in the preperitoneal position with associated percutaneous lead, external controller, and power source (batteries).

for the patients who continued on LVAD support was 82% (95% confidence interval [CI]: 77% to 87%) at 6 months, 73% (95% CI: 66% to 80%) at 1 year, and 72% (95% CI: 65% to 79%) at 18 months.

Jarvik 2000. The Jarvik 2000 (Jarvik Heart, Inc., New York, New York) is an implantable, continuous flow rotary pump with axial flow design.[100–102] The unique feature of the Jarvik device is the placement of the pump within the left ventricle to eliminate the inflow cannula along with orientation of the outflow graft to the descending aorta (Fig. 84.16). The Jarvik 2000 pump is inserted through a sewing cuff sewn into the apex of the left ventricle. The outflow orifice of the pump is attached to a Dacron graft for anastomosis to the descending thoracic aorta. The current adult version of the Jarvik 2000 measures 2.5 cm in diameter by 5.5 cm in length, with a weight of 85 g and a displacement volume of 25 mL. The adult pump functions at speeds of 8,000 to 12,000 rpm, achieving blood flow up to 8 L/min. Percutaneous power is delivered from external batteries via a controller unit. Internal electrical wires are brought via the left pleural cavity to the apex of the chest and then subcutaneously across the neck to the base of the skull, where a percutaneous titanium pedestal transmits fine electrical wires through the skin of the scalp. The Jarvik 2000 LVAD is currently in clinical trial.

DeBakey Left Ventricular Assist Device. The DeBakey is an axial flow pump that measures approximately 86 mm long and 25 mm wide (about the size of an AA battery).[95,103–105] It weighs 95 g and has a displacement of 15 cm^3. The pump is designed to produce flows of 5 L/min against 100 mm Hg pressure with a rotor speed of 10,000 rpm with less than 10 W of power. The DeBakey LVAD is currently under investigation in clinical trial.

Implantable, Continuous Flow Mechanical Circulatory Support Devices (Rotary Pumps with Centrifugal Flow Design). Although significant improvements in pump design have occurred with the second generation of rotary pumps with an axial blood flow path, there remain potential concerns with this technology. The presence of contact bearings in the blood path that suspend the rotor represents a potential point of frictional wear resulting in device failure and subsequent need for device exchange.[94,106] The second-generation rotary pumps with axial design still demonstrate the potential for thrombus formation on the device rotor and bearing interface due to the presence of stasis and incomplete "wash" of the bearings.[46,95,107] The presence of stators to suspend and redirect blood flow also represents an obstruction within the blood flow path. Clinical studies have documented the problem with device thrombus requiring device exchange or treatment with thrombolytic therapy, and have also shown a reduced but persistent risk of stroke.[46,107] In addition, this technology still requires long-term antithrombotic therapy and, subsequently, hemorrhagic complications are observed with this therapy.[46,95,96]

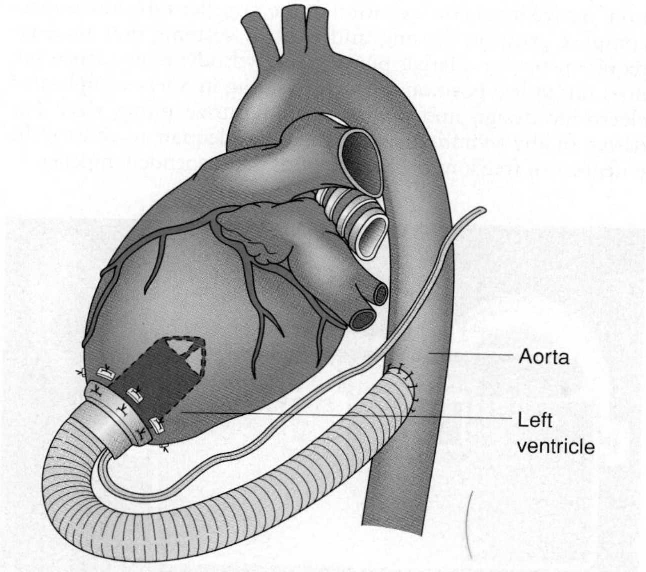

FIGURE 84.16. The Jarvik 2000 (Jarvik Heart Corporation, New York, NY) is an implantable, continuous flow rotary left ventricular assist device with axial design intended for long-term mechanical circulatory support for bridge to transplant or destination therapy. Schematic representation of the placement of the Jarvik 2000 within the left ventricle.

An additional potential concern of second-generation rotary pumps with axial design is related to their hydrodynamic performance. To observe changes in pump flow at a fixed rotor speed, significant changes in pressure across the inlet and outlet orifices of the pump must occur.[108,109] This relative degree of insensitivity of the hydrodynamic performance of the pump or "steep" pressure–flow relationship can result in left ventricular collapse and "suction" when filling pressures are abruptly reduced, as in the case of a sudden onset of a ventricular arrhythmia, or result in elevated filling pressures with dyspnea when return to the left atrium is abruptly increased, as with exercise. Left ventricular collapse or "suction" events can, by themselves, precipitate serious ventricular arrhythmias,[110] and the inability to significantly increase pump flow with exercise may limit exercise performance in patients with axial pumps.

Implantable LVADs that are rotary pumps of centrifugal flow design represent the third generation of VADs. These devices provide continuous flow at rotational speeds that are much slower, about 2,000 to 4,000 rpm, compared to 8,000 to 15,000 rpm for pumps with axial flow design. The same general advantages and disadvantages of design features that apply to rotary pumps with axial flow design apply to centrifugal flow design. The major feature of the third generation of rotary pumps with centrifugal flow design is that the impeller is rotated and levitated in a magnetic field, eliminating the need for bearings and the subsequent problems associated with bearing wear; these pumps have a potential for very long durability[94,106,111] (Fig. 84.17). Impeller rotation to elicit blood flow is achieved through magnetic coupling to the pump motor. Levitation systems utilized in third-generation rotary pumps suspend the moving impeller within the blood field without any mechanical contact, thus eliminating frictional wear and reducing heat generation that would normally take place at the contact surface with a contact bearing design. These levitation forces may be achieved through magnetic or hydrodynamic bearing design. Magnetic forces may be passive without the consumption of power (permanent magnet) or active (induction of magnetic field with electricity) in design.[94,106,111,112] Hydrodynamic levitation depends on fluid forces generated by the rotating impeller to levitate the internal impeller. Pump designs can be further distinguished by the utilization of hydrodynamic levitation only, hydrodynamic levitation working in synergy with magnetic levitation for suspension, or variations of active and/or passive magnetic levitation. Active magnetic levitation of the impeller typically utilizes complex position sensing and control systems that increase requirements for a larger pump size. Hydrodynamic suspension does not utilize position sensors, resulting in a less complicated electronic design and ability to miniaturize pump size. The design of any levitation system must be adequate to control the 6 degrees of freedom of movement of the suspended impeller.

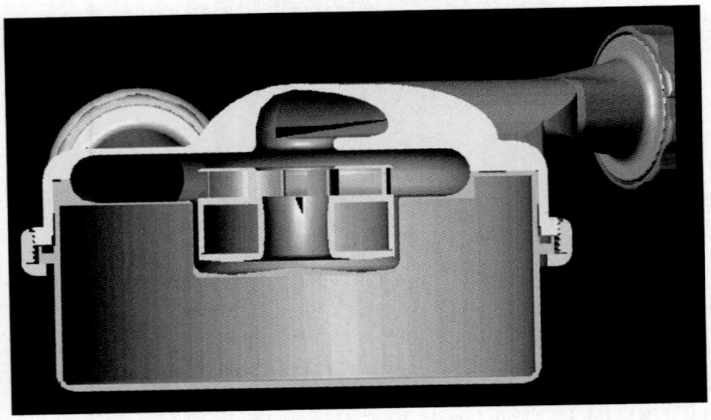

FIGURE 84.17. Schematic representation of a third-generation continuous flow rotary pump utilizing magnetic coupling of the internal impeller for levitation and rotation that obviates the need for bearings in the blood flow path.

The third generation of rotary pumps with centrifugal design have a more sensitive pressure–flow relationship as compared to the second generation of rotary pumps with axial design.[111,113] This greater sensitivity of the pressure–flow relationship results in greater changes in flow for any given change in pressure across the inlet and outlet orifices of the pump. This greater pump response to changes in flow may increase the margin of safety from creating suction events and improves pump flow during increases in left atrial return, potentially enhancing exercise response.[114,115] The improvements in the design attributes of the third generation of rotary pumps with centrifugal design, such as mechanical wear, operation at low flow, and perceived improved potential for hemocompatibility while still maintaining a manageable size warrant further clinical investigation. Whether these attributes will result in significant improvement in clinical outcomes over that observed with the second generation of rotary pumps with axial design is not known at this time.

DuraHeart. The DuraHeart (Terumo Heart Corporation, Ann Arbor, Michigan) is a continuous flow rotary pump with centrifugal and noncontact bearing design[106,112,113,116] (Fig. 84.18). The device has a displacement volume of 180 cm^3 and a weight of 540 g. Its external dimensions are 72 mm in width and 45 mm in height. The pumping unit consists of an upper housing with the levitation system, an impeller, and a bottom housing containing the external drive motor. The device is designed with active magnetic levitation of the impeller along with hydrodynamic bearings to support impeller levitation in case of failure of the magnetic levitation system. The impeller is rotated through magnetic coupling between permanent magnets embedded on the motor side of the impeller and an external drive motor that utilizes a bearing design. Three electromagnets and three position sensors are mounted in the upper housing. Tilting and axial displacements of the impeller are monitored and controlled using a 3-degrees-of-freedom control. The ferromagnetic ring on the opposite side of the impeller is levitated by the electromagnet, and position sensors

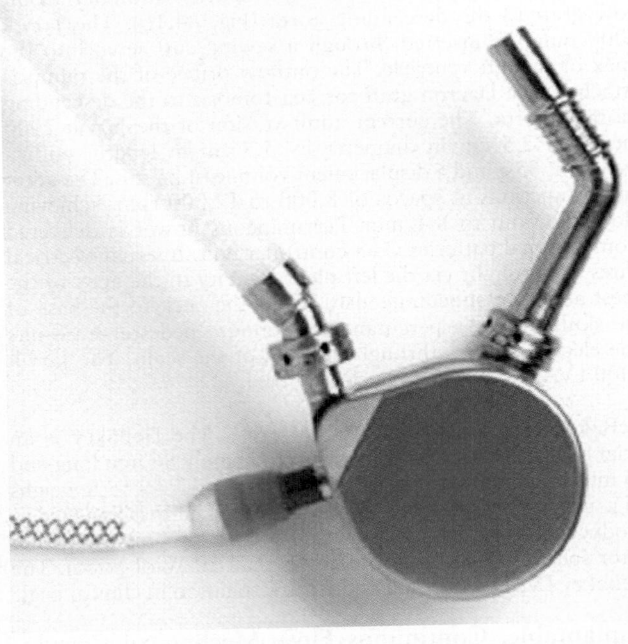

FIGURE 84.18. The DuraHeart (Terumo Heart Corporation, Ann Arbor, MI) is an implantable, continuous flow rotary pump with centrifugal design intended for long-term left ventricular assist for bridge to transplant or destination therapy. The device uses active magnetic coupling of the internal impeller for levitation and rotation. (Photograph courtesy of Terumo Heart Corporation, Ann Arbor, MI.)

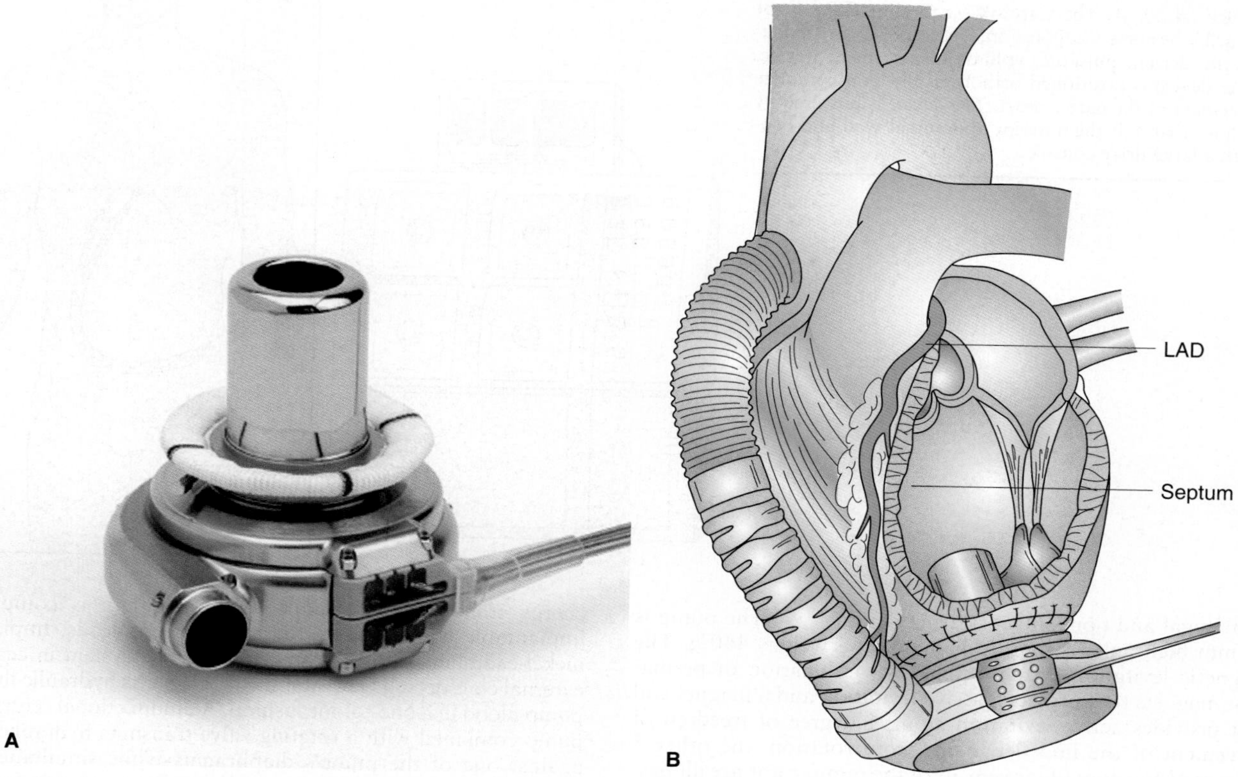

FIGURE 84.19. **A:** The HVAD left ventricular assist device (HeartWare Corporation, Miami, FL) is an implantable, continuous flow rotary pump with centrifugal design. The device incorporates passive magnetic and hydrodynamic forces for impeller levitation and rotation. **B:** Schematic representation of the HVAD with the inlet cannula inserted into the apex of the left ventricle. The outflow cannulas and graft are anastomosed to the ascending aorta. (Photograph courtesy of HeartWare Corporation, Miami, FL.)

control the impeller so that it is always positioned at the center of the blood chamber. Radial impeller movement is passively suspended with a bias flux through the electromagnetic rotor and drive magnet rotor.

Clinical evaluation of the DuraHeart device has recently concluded in Europe and the device is undergoing clinical evaluation in the United States. A preliminary report of the European experience was recently presented at the International Society of Heart and Lung Transplantation in April 2008.[116] Thirty-five patients with advanced heart failure (NYHA class IV, 14 ischemic, 5 females) who were eligible for heart transplantation underwent implantation of the DuraHeart device from January 2004 through September 2007. Median age of the patients was 56 (range, 29 to 73) years. The average duration of device support was 330 ± 220 (17 to 808) days with a cumulative duration of 21 years. Fourteen patients (40%) underwent heart transplantation at 194 ± 146 days. Nineteen patients (54%) were supported for at least 6 months and seven (20%) patients were supported for greater than 1 year. Fourteen patients (40%) remained alive with ongoing device support (330 ± 292 days). Kaplan-Meier survival at 2 years was 78%. There were seven deaths (median time to deaths, 29 days). Six early deaths occurred in the initial 11 patients and 4 were associated with excessive anticoagulation/antiplatelet therapy that resulted in fatal intracerebral hemorrhage or subdural hematoma. After implementing less intensive anticoagulation and antiplatelet therapy comparable to mechanical heart valves, there was no ischemic or hemorrhagic stroke for the last 24 patients. Stroke-free survival for the last 24 patients was 94% at 2 years. Twenty-six patients (86% of 1-month survivors) were discharged home, and the readmission rate was 1.5 patients per year.

HVAD. The HVAD (HeartWare Corporation, Miami, Florida) is a small continuous flow rotary pump with centrifugal and noncontact bearing design. The unique feature of the HVAD is its small design size[117,118] (Fig. 84.19). It has a displacement volume of 45 mL and weighs 145 g with a flow capacity of up to 10 L/min. The device is small enough to place within the pericardial cavity without the need for dissection and creation of a preperitoneal pocket. The impellor of the HVAD is suspended in place by combination of passive magnetic and hydrodynamic bearing systems. The impeller suspension system uses a passive magnetic bearing for radial stiffness. Axial magnetic preload and hydrodynamic bearings on top of each impeller blade provide axial constraint. The magnetic bearing consists of a stack of rare-earth ring magnets near the impeller's inside diameter that repel the magnetic force of a similar stack of magnets inside the center post. The axial alignment of the center-post magnet stack is set to provide an axial force that pushes the impeller toward the forward housing (the assembly with the inflow cannula). Physical contact between the housing and the impeller is prevented by a thin blood film generated by the hydrodynamic bearings.

The HVAD has undergone clinical evaluation in Europe and Australia and is undergoing clinical evaluation in the United States. In a multi-institutional trial in Europe and Australia, 20 patients underwent implantation of the HVAD from March 2006 through September 2007.[117] Mean age of the patients was 46 ± 12 (range, 28 to 68) years. Mean duration of HVAD device support was 167 ± 143 days (range, 13 to 425 days). Range of blood flow provided by the pump was 4.0 to 6.5 L/min. Three patients were successfully transplanted after 426, 349, and 157 days, respectively. One patient was weaned from pump support on postoperative day 266, two patients died on device (postoperative days 13 and 203), and 14 patients remained alive with ongoing device support. Actuarial survival at 1 year was 80%.

Levacor. The Levacor (World Heart Corporation, Oakland, California) device is a continuous flow rotary pump with

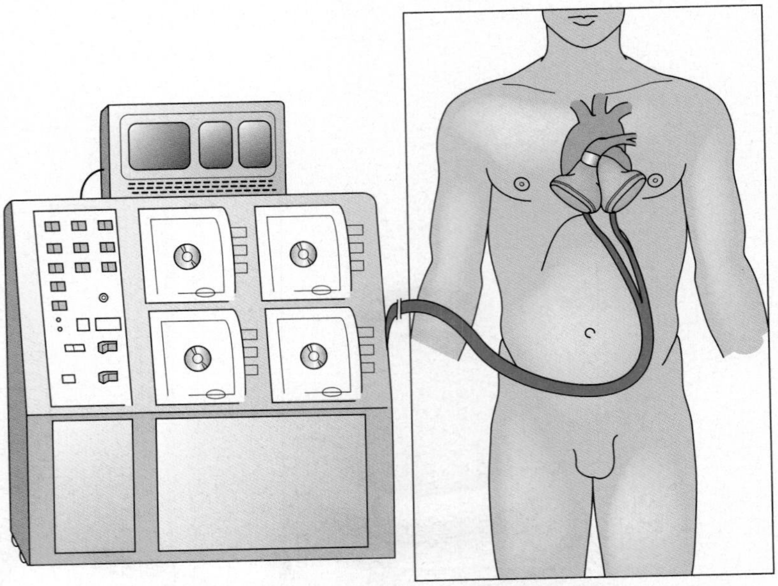

FIGURE 84.20. **A:** The CardioWest total artificial heart (Syncardia Systems Corporation, Tucson, AZ) is a pneumatically driven, pulsatile, volume displacement device. **B:** The device is positioned orthotopically as a complete replacement of the native heart. The device is powered by drivelines that exit the anterior abdominal wall and connect to a large drive console.

centrifugal and noncontact bearing design.[106,119] The pump is 35 mm high and 75 mm in diameter and weighs 440 g. The magnetic levitation system utilizes a combination of permanent magnets that provide passive levitation and a magnet coil that provides active levitation along 1 degree of freedom of movement of the impeller. Aside from rotation, the other 5 degrees of freedom of movement of the pump rotor are all passively controlled except axial movement in the z-direction, which is actively controlled by the coil and electronics. The motor is integrated directly into the pump housing and rotor and no external motor is required for rotation.

Clinical evaluation of the Levacor device has been initiated in Europe and Canada with successful results reported in a BTR protocol.[119] Clinical evaluation in the United States is scheduled for 2010.

Total Artificial Hearts

CardioWest Total Artificial Heart. The CardioWest TAH (SynCardia Systems Corporation, Tucson, Arizona) is a pulsatile, volume displacement, total artificial heart[120–123] (Fig. 84.20). The rigid polyurethane pump contains a flexible polyurethane diaphragm that separates blood and air chambers. Two Medtronic-Hall mechanical valves located at the inflow and outflow orifices ensure unidirectional blood flow. Compressed air from the external drive console moves the diaphragm upward, pressurizing the blood chamber and causing ejection of blood. The pump has a maximum stroke volume of 70 mL and a maximum flow rate of 15 L/min, although the average flow rate is less than 8 L/min. Pump rate, duration of systole, and driving pressure can be adjusted to achieve optimal flow conditions. The TAH is surgically implanted in the mediastinal space after the ventricles have been excised, while the atrial cuffs are retained. The pneumatic drivelines are externalized percutaneously and attached to the drive console. Patients may be ambulatory, but their mobility is frequently restricted by the large drive console. A portable drive console is in clinical trial evaluation. The CardioWest TAH is approved by the FDA for bridge to heart transplant indication. In a recent study, Copeland et al. reported a 79% survival to heart transplantation compared to 46% for the observational arm.[121] One-year posttransplant survival was 86%.

Abiomed Total Replacement Heart. The AbioCor TAH (Abiomed, Inc., Danvers, Massachusetts) is an orthotopically positioned total artificial heart pump.[124] The system uses brushless DC motors that are powered by TETS (transcutaneous energy transmission system), and the system is completely implantable with no need for percutaneous leads. Implanted nickel-cadmium batteries can also drive the system in case the external coils detach. The Abiomed TAH shifts hydraulic fluid to pump blood in a one-to-one fashion. A unidirectional centrifugal pump combined with a rotating valve transmits hydraulic fluid against one of the pump's diaphragms while simultaneously withdrawing fluid from the contralateral side. In this fashion, alternating filling and emptying of the pumps with blood occurs. The system incorporates 24-mL polyether urethane trileaflet valves in both the inlet and outlet orifices. The control schemes of this system demonstrate so-called Starling behavior so that increases in venous return elicit a commensurate increase in left pump output until a maximum output is reached. Optimal pumping rate is made a function of right atrial pressure, inferred from transducer-measured pressure readings within the right hydraulic chamber. Compensation for right and left flow imbalances depends on a flexible, 20-mL hydraulic chamber positioned against the left atrium. This compliance chamber, in continuity with the right pump's hydraulic chamber, exerts negative feedback on right pump filling. As left atrial pressure rises, hydraulic fluid shifts into the right hydraulic chamber, limiting the passive diastolic filling of the right pump's blood chamber. Less blood is then delivered to the left side until left atrial pressure decreases. The AbioCor TAH has received humane device exemption in the United States for clinical use for permanent replacement for patients not eligible for heart transplantation and at imminent risk of death from advanced heart failure.

FUTURE DIRECTIONS

Recent rapid technologic advancements and successful clinical applications of MCS have made the future of this field optimistic, but uncertain. It is possible that long-term MCS will provide a viable alternative to heart transplantation and medical therapy for patients with advanced heart failure. Due to the technologic advancements, it will be difficult to predict what devices will ultimately prove to be the most efficacious. It is likely that a variety of devices will become available for use depending on clinical circumstances and patient characteristics.

References

1. Stevenson LW, Kormos RL, Barr ML, et al. Mechanical cardiac support 2000: current applications and future trial design: June 15 and 16, 2000 Bethesda, Maryland. *Circulation* 2001;103:337–342.

2. Rose EC, Gelijns AC, Moskowitz AJ, et al. Long-term use of a left ventricular assist device for end-stage heart failure. *N Engl J Med* 2001;345: 1435–1443.
3. Felker GM, Rogers JG. Same bridge, new destinations rethinking paradigms for mechanical cardiac support in heart failure. *J Am Coll Cardiol* 2006;47:930–932.
4. Hochman JS, Sleeper LA, Webb JG, et al. Early revascularization in acute myocardial infarction complicated by cardiogenic shock. *N Engl J Med* 1999;341:625–634.
5. Norman JC, Cooley DA, Igo SR, et al. Prognostic indices for survival during postcardiotomy intra-aortic balloon pumping. *J Thorac Cardiovasc Surg* 1977;74:709–720.
6. Guyton RA, Schonberger J, Everts P, et al. Postcardiotomy shock: clinical evaluation of the BVS 5000 biventricular support system. *Ann Thorac Surg* 1993;56:346–356.
7. Jett GK. Postcardiotomy support with ventricular assist devices: selection of recipients. *Semin Thorac Cardiovasc Surg* 1994;6:136–139.
8. Gray LA, Champsaur GG. The BVS 5000 biventricular assist device. The worldwide registry experience. *ASAIO J* 1994;40:M460–M464.
9. Pae WE. Ventricular assist devices and total artificial hearts: A ASAIO-ISHLT registry experience. *Ann Thorac Surg* 1993;55:295–298.
10. Pennington DG, Merjavy JP, Swartz MT, et al. The importance of biventricular failure in patients with postoperative cardiogenic shock. *Ann Thorac Surg* 1985;39:16–26.
11. Farrar DJ, Hill JD, Pennington DG, et al. Preoperative and postoperative comparison of patients with univentricular and biventricular support with the Thoratec ventricular assist device as a bridge to cardiac transplantation. *J Thorac Cardiovasc Surg* 1997;113:202–209.
12. Fitzpatrick JR III, Frederick JR, Hsu VM, et al. Risk score derived from pre-operative data analysis predicts the need for biventricular mechanical circulatory support. *J Heart Lung Transplant* 2008;27:1286–1292.
13. Matthews JC, Koelling TM, Pagani FD, et al. The right ventricular failure risk score: a pre-operative tool for assessing the risk of right ventricular failure in left ventricular assist device candidates. *J Am Coll Cardiol* 2008; 51:2163–2172.
14. Kormos RL, Gasior TA, Kawai A, et al. Transplant candidate's clinical status rather than right ventricular function defines the need for univentricular versus biventricular support. *J Thorac Cardiovasc Surg* 1996;111: 773–783.
15. Reedy JE, Swartz MT, Miller LW, et al. Bridge to transplantation: importance of patient selection. *J Heart Lung Transplant* 1990;9:473–480.
16. Farrar DJ. Preoperative predictors of survival in patients with Thoratec ventricular assist devices as a bridge to transplantation. *J Heart Lung Transplant* 1994;13:93–100.
17. Stevenson LW. Patient selection for mechanical bridging to transplantation. *Ann Thorac Surg* 1996;61:380–387.
18. Aaronson KD, Patel H, Pagani FD. Patient selection for left ventricular assist device therapy. *Ann Thorac Surg* 2003;75(suppl 6):S29–S35.
19. Miller LW. Patient selection for the use of ventricular assist devices as a bridge to transplantation. *Ann Thorac Surg* 2003;75(suppl 6):S66–S71.
20. Rao V, Oz MC, Flannery MA, et al. Revised screening scale to predict survival after insertion of a left ventricular assist device. *J Thorac Cardiovasc Surg* 2003;125:855–862.
21. Tsukui H, Teuteberg JJ, Murali S, et al. Biventricular assist device utilization for patients with morbid congestive heart failure: a justifiable strategy. *Circulation* 2005;112(suppl 9):I-65–I-72.
22. Kavarana MN, Pessin-Minsley MS, Urtecho J, et al. Right ventricular dysfunction and organ failure in left ventricular assist device recipients: a continuing problem. *Ann Thorac Surg* 2002;73:745–753.
23. Ochiai Y, McCarthy PM, Smedira NG, et al. Predictors of severe right ventricular failure after implantable left ventricular assist device insertion: analysis of 245 patients. *Circulation* 2002;106:198–202.
24. Firth JD, Raine AE, Ledingham JG. Raised venous pressure. A direct cause of renal sodium retention in edema. *Lancet* 1988;1:1033–1035.
25. Santamore WP, Gray LA. Left ventricular contributions ot right ventricular systolic function during LVAD support. *Ann Thorac Surg* 1996;61: 350–356.
26. Pavie A, Leger P. Physiology of univentricular versus biventricular support. *Ann Thorac Surg* 1996;61:347–349.
27. Mandarino WA, Winowich S, Gorcsan J, et al. Right ventricular performance and left ventricular assist device filling. *Ann Thorac Surg* 1997;63: 1044–1049.
28. Goldstein DJ, Seldomridge JA, Chen JM, et al. Left ventricular assist device and bleeding: adding insult to injury. *Ann Thorac Surg* 1995;59: 1063–1068.
29. Dewald O, Schmitz DO, Reichart B, et al. Platelet activation markers in patients with heart assist devices. *Artif Organs* 2005;29:292–299.
30. Pasini E. Cachexia in chronic heart failure patients. *Ital Heart J* 2003;4: 232–235.
31. Lietz K, Long JW, Kfoury AG, et al. Outcomes of left ventricular assist device implantation as destination therapy in the post-REMATCH era: implications for patient selection. *Circulation* 2007;116:497–505.
32. Engelman DJ. Impact of body mass index (BMI) and albumin on morbidity and mortality after cardiovascular surgery. *J Thorac Cardiovasc Surg* 1999;118:866–873.
33. Reeves BC, Ascione R, Chamberlain MH, et al. Effect of body mass index on early outcomes in patients undergoing coronary bypass surgery. *J Am Coll Cardiol* 2003;42:668–676.
34. Filippatos GS, Anker SD, Kremastinos DT. Pathophysiology of peripheral muscle wasting in cardiac cachexia. *Curr Opin Clin Nutr Metab Care* 2005;8:249–254.
35. Sharma R, Anker SD. Cytokines, apoptosis, and cachexia: the potential for TNF antagonism. *Int J Cardiol* 2002;85:161–171.
36. Aria H, Swartz MT, Pennington DG, et al. Importance of ventricular arrhythmias in bridge patients with ventricular assist devices. *ASAIO Trans* 1991;37:M427–M428.
37. Oz MC, Rose EA, Slater JP, et al. Malignant ventricular arrhythmias are well tolerated in patients receiving long-term left ventricular devices. *J Am Coll Cardiol* 1994;24:1688–1691.
38. Salzberg SP, Lachat ML, Zünd G, et al. Left ventricular assist device (LVAD) enables survival during 7 h of sustained ventricular fibrillation. *Eur J Cardiothorac Surg* 2004;26:444–446.
39. Shapiro GC, Leibowitz DW, Oz MC, et al. Diagnosis of patent foramen ovale with transesophageal echocardiography in a patient supported with a left ventricular assist device. *J Heart Lung Transplant* 1995;14:594–597.
40. Nakatani S, Thomas JD, Savage RM, et al. Prediction of right ventricular dysfunction after left ventricular assist device implantation. *Circulation* 1996;94(9 Suppl):II-216–II-221.
41. Fukamachi K, McCarthy PM, Smedira NG, et al. Preoperative risk factors for right ventricular failure after implantable left ventricular assist device insertion. *Ann Thorac Surg* 1999:68:2181–2184.
42. Argenziano M, Choudhri AF, Moazami N, et al. Randomized, double-blind trial of inhaled nitric oxide in LVAD recipients with pulmonary hypertension. *Ann Thorac Surg* 1998;65:340–345.
43. Salamonsen RF, Kaye D, Esmore DS. Inhalation of nitric oxide provides selective pulmonary vasodilation, aiding mechanical cardiac assist with the Thoratec left ventricular assist device. *Anaesth Intensive Care* 1994;22: 209–210.
44. Hare JM, Shernan SK, Body SC, et al. Influence of inhaled nitric oxide on systemic flow and ventricular filling pressure in patients receiving mechanical circulatory assistance. *Circulation* 1997;95:2250–2253.
45. Rose EA, Levin HR, Oz MC, et al. Artificial circulatory support with textured interior surfaces: a counterintuitive approach to minimizing thromboembolism. *Circulation* 1994;90(Suppl II):II-87–II-91.
46. Miller LW, Pagani FD, Russell SD, et al. Use of a continuous-flow device in patients awaiting heart transplantation. *N Engl J Med* 2007;357:885–896.
47. Holman WL, Fix RJ, Foley BA, et al. Management of wound and left ventricular assist device pocket infection. *Ann Thorac Surg* 1999;68: 1080–1082.
48. McKellar SH, Allred BD, Marks JD, et al. Treatment of infected left ventricular assist device using antibiotic-impregnated beads. *Ann Thorac Surg* 1999;67:554–555.
49. Arabia FA, Copeland JG, Smith RG, et al. Infections with the CardioWest total artificial heart. *ASAIO J* 1998;44:M336–M339.
50. Argenziano M, Catanese KA, Moazami N, et al. The influence of infection on survival and successful transplantation in patients with left ventricular assist devices. *J Heart Lung Transplant* 1997;16:822–831.
51. Hermann M, Weyand M, Greshake B, et al. Left ventricular assist device infection is associated with increased mortality but is not a contraindication to transplantation. *Circulation* 1997;95:814–817.
52. Fischer SA, Trenholme GM, Costanzo MR, et al. Infectious complications in left ventricular assist device recipients. *Clin Infect Dis* 1997;24:18–23.
53. Holman EL, Murrah CP, Ferguson ER, et al. Infections during extended circulatory support: University of Alabama at Birmingham experience 1989 to 1994. *Ann Thorac Surg* 1996;61:366–371.
54. Gordon SM, Schmitt SK, Jacobs M, et al. Nosocomial bloodstream infections in patients with implantable left ventricular assist devices. *Ann Thorac Surg* 2001;72:725–730.
55. Holman WL, Park SJ, Long JW, et al., for the REMATCH Investigators. Infection in permanent circulatory support: experience from the REMATCH trial. *J Heart Lung Transplant* 2004;23:1359–1365.
56. Poston RS, Husain S, Sorce D, et al. LVAD bloodstream infections: therapeutic rationale for transplantation after LVAD infection. *J Heart Lung Transplant* 2003;22:914–921.
57. Stevenson LW, Pagani FD, Young JB, et al. INTERMACS profiles of advanced heart failure: the current picture. *J Heart Lung Transplant* 2009; 28:535–541.
58. Holman WL, Kormos RL, Naftel DC, et al. Predictors of death and transplant in patients with a mechanical circulatory support device: a multi-institutional study. *J Heart Lung Transplant* 2009;28:44–50.
59. Kirklin JK, Naftel DC, Stevenson LW, et al. INTERMACS database for durable devices for circulatory support: first annual report. *J Heart Lung Transplant* 2008;27:1065–1072.
60. Kirklin JK, Naftel DC, Kormos RL, et al. Second INTERMACS annual report: more than 1000 primary LVAD implants. *J Heart Lung Transplant* 2010;29:1–10.
61. Young JB. Healing the heart with ventricular assist device therapy: mechanisms of cardiac recovery. *Ann Thorac Surg* 2001;71:S210–S219.
62. Burkhoff D, Klotz S, Mancini DM. LVAD-induced reverse remodeling: basic and clinical implications for myocardial recovery. *J Card Fail* 2006; 12:227–239.
63. Birks EJ, Tansley PD, Hardy J, et al. Left ventricular assist device and drug therapy for the reversal of heart failure. *N Engl J Med* 2006;355: 1873–1884.
64. Kantrowitz A, Tjonneland S, Freed PS, et al. Initial clinical experience with intraaortic balloon pumping in cardiogenic shock. *JAMA* 1968;203:135.

65. Muehrcke DD, McCarthy PM, Stewart RW, et al. Extracorporeal membrane oxygenation for postcardiotomy cardiogenic shock. *Ann Thorac Surg* 1996;61:684–691.
66. Smedira NG, Wudel JH, Hlozek CC, et al. Venovenous extracorporeal life support for patients after cardiotomy. *ASAIO J* 1997;43:M444–M446.
67. McGovern GJ, Magovern JA, Benckart DH, et al. Extracorporeal membrane oxygenation-preliminary results in patients with postcardiotomy cardiogenic shock. *Ann Thorac Surg* 1994;57:1462–1467.
68. Hill JD, O'Brien TG, Murray JJ, et al. Extracorporeal oxygenation for acute post-traumatic respiratory failure. *N Eng J Med* 1972;286:629–634.
69. Bavaria JE, Furukawa S, Kreiner G. Effect of circulatory assist devices on stunned myocardium. *Ann Thorac Surg* 1990;49:123–128.
70. Bartlett RH, Roloff DW, Custer JR, et al. Extracorporeal life support: the University of Michigan experience. *JAMA* 2000;283:904–908.
71. Pagani FD, Lynch W, Swaniker F, et al. Extracorporeal life support to left ventricular assist device bridge to heart transplant: a strategy to optimize survival and resource utilization. *Circulation* 1999;100(19):II206–II210.
72. Pagani FD, Aaronson KD, Dyke DB, et al. Assessment of an extracorporeal life support to LVAD bridge to heart transplant strategy. *Ann Thorac Surg* 2000;70:1977–1985.
73. Bowen FW, Carboni AF, O'Hara ML, et al. Application of "double bridge mechanical" resuscitation for profound cardiogenic shock leading to cardiac transplantation. *Ann Thorac Surg* 2001;72:86–90.
74. Smedira NG, Moazomi N, Golding CM, et al. Clinical experience with 202 adults receiving extracorporeal membrane oxygenation for cardiac failure: survival at five years. *J Thorac Cardiovasc Surg* 2001;122:92–102.
75. Thiele H, Sick P, Boudriot E, et al. Randomized comparison of intra-aortic balloon support with a percutaneous left ventricular assist device in patients with revascularized acute myocardial infarction complicated by cardiogenic shock. *Eur Heart J* 2005;26:1276–1283.
76. Haj-Yahia S, Birks EJ, Amrani M, et al. Bridging patients after salvage from bridge to decision directly to transplant by means of prolonged support with the CentriMag short-term centrifugal pump. *J Thorac Cardiovasc Surg* 2009;138:227–230.
77. John R, Liao K, Lietz K, et al. Experience with the Levitronix CentriMag circulatory support system as a bridge to decision in patients with refractory acute cardiogenic shock and multisystem organ failure. *J Thorac Cardiovasc Surg* 2007;134:351–358.
78. Jurmann MJ, Siniawski H, Erb M, et al. Initial experience with miniature axial flow ventricular assist devices for postcardiotomy heart failure. *Ann Thorac Surg* 2004;77(5):1642–1647.
79. Thiele H, Smalling RW, Schuler GC. Percutaneous left ventricular assist devices in acute myocardial infarction complicated by cardiogenic shock. *Eur Heart J* 2007;28:2057–2063.
80. Seyfarth M, Sibbing D, Bauer I, et al. A randomized clinical trial to evaluate the safety and efficacy of a percutaneous left ventricular assist device versus intra-aortic balloon pumping for treatment of cardiogenic shock caused by myocardial infarction. *J Am Coll Cardiol* 2008;52:1584–1588.
81. Sassard T, Scalabre A, Bonnefoy E, et al. The right axillary artery approach for the Impella Recover LP 5.0 microaxial pump. *Ann Thorac Surg* 2008; 85:1468–1470.
82. Frazier O, Rose E, Macmanus Q, et al. Multicenter clinical evaluation of the Heart Mate 1000 IP left ventricular assist device. *Ann Thorac Surg* 1992;53:1080–1090.
83. Frazier OH, Rose EA, Oz MC, et al. Multicenter clinical evaluation of the HeartMate vented electric left ventricular assist system in patients awaiting heart transplantation. *J Thorac Cardiovasc Surg* 2001;122:1186–1195.
84. Slaughter MS, Tsui SS, El-Banayosy A, et al. Results of a multicenter clinical trial with the Thoratec Implantable Ventricular Assist Device. *J Thorac Cardiovasc Surg* 2007;133:1573–1580.
85. Joyce LD, Noon GP, Joyce DL, et al. Mechanical circulatory support—a historical review. *ASAIO J* 2004;50:x–xii.
86. Portner PM, Oyer PE, McGregor CGA, et al. First human use of an electrically-powered implantable ventricular assist system [Abstract]. *Artif Organs* 1985;9:36.
87. Dagenais F, Portner PM, Robbins RC, et al. The Novacor left ventricular assist system: clinical experience from the Novacor registry. *J Card Surg* 2001;16:267–271.
88. Dembitsky WP, Tector AJ, Park S, et al. Left ventricular assist device performance with long-term circulatory support: Lessons from the REMATCH trial. *Ann Thorac Surg* 2004;78:2123–2130.
89. McBride LR, Naunheim KS, Fiore AC, et al. Clinical experience with 111 Thoractec ventricular assist devices. *Ann Thorac Surg* 1999;67: 1233–1238.
90. El-Banayosy A, Korfer R, Arusoglu L, et al. Bridging to cardiac transplantation with the Thoratec ventricular assist device. *Thorac Cardiovasc Surg* 1999;47(suppl 2):307–310.
91. Farrar DJ, Buck KE, Coulter JH, et al. Portable pneumatic biventricular driver for the Thoratec ventricular assist device. *ASAIO J* 1997;43: M631–M634.
92. El-Banayosy A, Arusoglu L, Kizner L, et al. Predictors of survival in patients bridged to transplantation with the Thoratec VAD device: a single-center retrospective study on more than 100 patients. *J Heart Lung Transplant* 2000;19:964–968.
93. Reichenbach SH, Farrar DJ, Hill JD. A versatile intracorporeal ventricular assist device based on the Thoratec VAD system. *Ann Thorac Surg* 2001; 71:S171–S175.
94. Takatani S. Progress of rotary blood pumps: presidential address, International Society for Rotary Blood Pumps 2006, Leuven, Belgium. *Artif Organs* 2007;31:329–344.
95. Goldstein DJ, Zucker M, Arroyo L, et al. Safety and feasibility trial of the MicroMed DeBakey ventricular assist device as a bridge to transplantation. *J Am Coll Cardiol* 2005;45:962–963.
96. Siegenthaler MP, Frazier OH, Beyersdorf F, et al. Mechanical reliability of the Jarvik 2000 Heart. *Ann Thorac Surg* 2006;81:1752–1758.
97. Radovancevic B, Vrtovec B, de Kort E, et al. End-organ function in patients on long-term circulatory support with continuous- or pulsatile-flow assist devices. *J Heart Lung Transplant* 2007;26:815–818.
98. Westaby S, Banning AP, Jarvik R, et al. First permanent implant of the Jarvik 2000 heart. *Lancet* 2000;356:900–903.
99. Pagani FD, Miller LW, Russell SD, et al. Extended mechanical circulatory support with a continuous-flow rotary left ventricular assist device. *J Am Coll Cardiol* 2009;54:312–321.
100. Frazier OH, Myers TJ, Gregoric ID, et al. Initial clinical experience with the Jarvik 2000 implantable axial-flow left ventricular assist system. *Circulation* 2002;105:2855–2860.
101. Westaby S, Frazier OH, Beyersdorf F, et al. The Jarvik 2000 Heart. Clinical validation of the intraventricular position. *Eur J Cardiothorac Surg* 2002;22:228–232.
102. Frazier OH, Myers TJ, Westaby S, et al. Clinical experience with an implantable, intracardiac, continuous flow circulatory support device: physiologic implications and their relationship to patient selection. *Ann Thorac Surg* 2004;77:133–142.
103. Salzberg S, Lachat M, Zünd G, et al. Left ventricular assist device as bridge to heart transplantation – lessons learned with the MicroMed DeBakey axial blood flow pump. *Eur J Cardiothorac Surg* 2003;24:113–118.
104. DeBakey ME. Development of a ventricular assist device. *Artif Organs* 1997;21:1149–1153.
105. DeBakey ME. A miniature implantable axial flow ventricular assist device. *Ann Thorac Surg* 1999;68:637–640.
106. Hoshi H, Shinshi T, Takatani S. Third-generation blood pumps with mechanical noncontact magnetic bearings. *Artif Organs* 2006;30: 324–338.
107. Jahanyar J, Noon GP, Koerner MM, et al. Recurrent device thrombi during mechanical circulatory support with an axial-flow pump is a treatable condition and does not preclude successful long-term support. *J Heart Lung Transplant* 2007;26:200–203.
108. Stepanoff AJ. *Centrifugal and Axial Flow Pumps: Theory, Design, and Application*, 2nd ed. New York: John Wiley and Sons; 1957.
109. Akimoto T, Yamazaki K, Litwak P, et al. Rotary blood pump flow spontaneously increases during exercise under constant pump speed: results of a chronic study. *Artif Organs* 1999;23:797–801.
110. Vollkron M, Voitl P, Ta J, et al. Suction events during left ventricular support and ventricular arrhythmias. *J Heart Lung Transplant* 2007;26: 819–825.
111. Farrar DJ, Bourque K, Dague CP, et al. Design features, developmental status, and experimental results with the HeartMate III centrifugal left ventricular assist system with a magnetically levitated rotor. *ASAIO J* 2007; 53:310–315.
112. Nojiri C, Kijima T, Maekawa J, et al. Development status of Terumo implantable left ventricular assist system. *Artif Organs* 2001;25:411–413.
113. Nishinaka T, Schima H, Roethy W, et al. The DuraHeart VAD, a magnetically levitated centrifugal pump. The University of Vienna bridge to transplant experience. *Circ J* 2006;70:1421–1425.
114. Ayre PJ, Vidakovic SS, Tansley GD, et al. Sensorless flow and head estimation in the VentrAssist rotary blood pump. *Artif Organs* 2000;24: 585–588.
115. Tsukiya T, Akamatsu T, Nishimura K, et al. Use of motor current in flow rate measurement for magnetically suspended centrifugal blood pump. *Artif Organs* 1997;21:396–401.
116. Nojiri C, Fey O, Jaschke F, et al. Long-term circulatory support with the DuraHeart mag-lev centrifugal left ventricular assist system for advanced heart failure patients eligible to transplantation: European experiences. *J Heart Lung Transplant* 2008;27:S245.
117. Wieselthaler GM, Strueber M, O'Driscoll GA, et al. Experience with the novel HeartWare HVAD with hydromagnetically levitated rotor in a multi-institutional trial. *J Heart Lung Transplant* 2008;27:S245.
118. Tuzun E, Roberts K, Cohn WE, et al. In vivo evaluation of the HeartWare centrifugal ventricular assist device. *Texas Heart Inst J* 2007;34:406–411.
119. Pitsis AA, Visouli AN, Vassilikos V, et al. First human implantation of a new rotary blood pump: design of the clinical feasibility study. *Hellenic J Cardiol* 2006;47:368–376.
120. Arabia FA, Copeland JG, Pavie A, et al. Implantation technique for the CardioWest total artificial heart. *Ann Thorac Surg* 1999;68:698–704.
121. Copeland JG, Smith RG, Arabia FA, et al. Cardiac replacement with a total artificial heart as a bridge to transplantation. *N Engl J Med* 2004; 351:859–867.
122. Copeland JG, Smith RG, Arabia FA, et al. Total artificial heart bridge to transplantation: a 9-year experience with 62 patients. *J Heart Lung Transplant* 2004;23:823–831.
123. Copeland JG, Arabia FA, Tsau PH, et al. Total artificial hearts: bridge to transplantation. *Cardiol Clin* 2003;21:101–113.
124. Dowling RD, Gray LA, Etoch SW, et al. The AbioCor implantable replacement heart. *Ann Thorac Surg* 2003;75:93–99.

CHAPTER 85 ■ PERICARDIUM

JULES LIN

KEY POINTS

1. Prompt recognition and treatment of cardiac tamponade can be lifesaving.
2. The echocardiogram is the most useful noninvasive test in evaluating pericardial disease.
3. The electrocardiogram is important in the diagnosis of acute pericarditis and classically shows diffuse ST elevations.
4. The hemodynamic significance of a pericardial effusion depends on the volume and the rate of accumulation.
5. Postoperative tamponade should always be in the differential diagnosis with low cardiac output after cardiac surgery.
6. Distinguishing constrictive pericarditis from restrictive cardiomyopathy can be difficult, but is important since the treatment is significantly different.
7. Metastatic disease is the most common cause of pericardial effusion.

The pericardium supports and protects the heart. The smooth pericardial surface and the small amount of normal pericardial fluid provide a frictionless chamber, which improves cardiac efficiency and serves as a barrier to infection. The pericardium can be susceptible to a variety of disease processes including 1 inflammation, infection, malignancy, and trauma. Changes in compliance and the accumulation of pericardial fluid can impair cardiac function, and its prompt recognition and treatment can be lifesaving.

HISTORY

Hippocrates first described the pericardium in 460 BC. Three hundred years later, Galen described a pericardial effusion and the inflammatory changes associated with pericarditis. Lower first reported pericardial tamponade in humans in 1669. Lancisi and Morgagni described constrictive pericarditis, and Laennec wrote of the "bread and butter" appearance of acute pericarditis in 1819.[1] Kussmaul described the hemodynamic changes known as pulsus paradoxus, and Beck and Griswald performed experimental studies in the 1930s leading to a better understanding of the pathophysiology of pericardial effusion.[2,3] Karanaeff first described relieving the symptoms of tamponade using pericardiocentesis in 1840,[4] and Rehn reported methods to resect the pericardium in 1913.[5]

EMBRYOLOGY AND ANATOMY

The pleuropericardial membranes fuse during the fifth week of gestation, dividing the thoracic cavity into pleural and pericardial spaces and forming the fibrous pericardium.[6] The serous pericardium is a single layer of mesothelial cells that produce and reabsorb pericardial fluid. The serous and fibrous pericardium form the parietal pericardium, which is normally 2 mm in thickness. The visceral pericardium covers the heart and the intrapericardial great vessels. The phrenic nerves are contained in the parietal pericardium, and there is a risk of diaphragmatic paralysis with any operation on the pericardium. The pericardial folds form the oblique sinus, a blind cul-de-sac behind the left atrium, and the transverse sinus between the aorta and pulmonary artery superiorly and the left and right atrium inferiorly (Fig. 85.1). Lymphatic drainage is to the bronchial and tracheal lymph nodes and the thoracic duct. The pericardium normally produces 15 to 50 mL of serous fluid with a protein level lower than plasma.[7]

NORMAL PHYSIOLOGY

Although there are no significant consequences of the congenital absence or surgical resection of the pericardium as long as the defect does not lead to cardiac herniation, the pericardium has some function in the normal patient. The pericardium anchors the heart and prevents torsion and acute distention.[8] The pericardium also contributes to the diastolic coupling of the ventricles along the Starling curve. Mechanoreceptors in the pericardium may also regulate blood pressure and heart rate. The pericardium stretches up to 20% with small changes in pressure but becomes abruptly stiff and resistant with larger volumes. Compliance depends on the rate of fluid accumulation, and the hemodynamic response is also partially dependent on intravascular volume status.

The normal pericardial pressure is less than atmospheric pressure and is the same as the intrapleural pressure. With inspiration, right-sided venous return and preload increase. Blood pools in the lungs and decreases left-sided venous return and aortic blood flow. The arterial pressure normally decreases less than 10 mm Hg with inspiration. The normal jugular waveforms are shown in Figure 85.2. The a wave is the normal atrial contraction. The c wave reflects the bulging of the atrioventricular valve into the atrium during isovolumic ventricular systole. The v wave represents passive atrial filling from the vena cava. The x descent occurs with systolic collapse during ventricular systole and atrial relaxation. The y descent reflects diastolic collapse with opening of the atrioventricular valve and passive ventricular filling. Inspiration decreases intrathoracic pressure and leads to a lower x descent compared to the y descent.

DIAGNOSTIC STUDIES

While the electrocardiogram (ECG) is nonspecific, it can be helpful in suggesting the diagnosis. In acute pericarditis, the ECG classically shows diffuse ST elevations, and a low-voltage QRS is seen with a large pericardial effusion. The chest radiograph in a patient with a pericardial effusion shows an enlarged cardiac silhouette described as a water bottle. Pericardial calcification can

FIGURE 85.1. This drawing illustrates the pericardial attachments of the great vessels and pulmonary veins. The oblique sinus forms a blind cul-de-sac behind the left atrium, and the transverse sinus is a space between the aorta and pulmonary artery superiorly and the left and right atrium inferiorly. (Reproduced with permission from Bradley SM. Pericardium. In: Mulholland MW, Lillemoe KD, eds. *Greenfield's Surgery: Scientific Principles and Practice*, 4th ed. Philadelphia, PA: Lippincott Williams & Wilkins; 2006: 1521.)

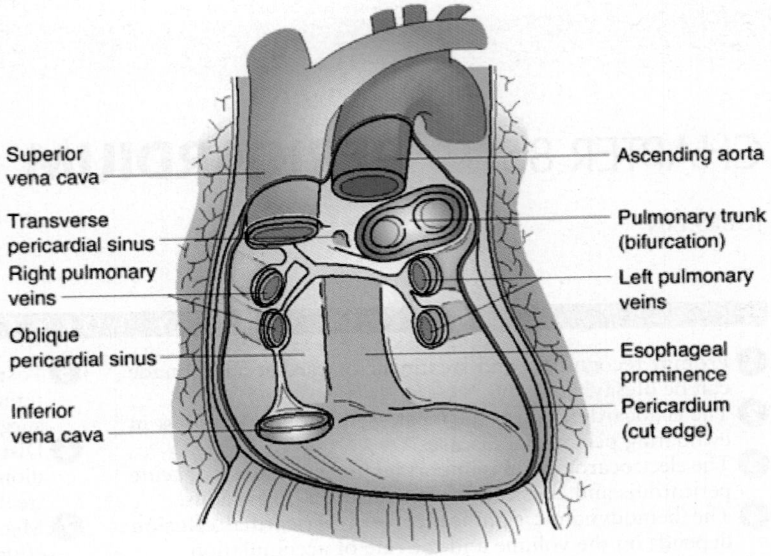

be seen in chronic constrictive pericarditis secondary to tuberculosis.

2 The echocardiogram is the most useful noninvasive test in evaluating pericardial disease. The echocardiogram can identify an effusion, pericardial thickening, or masses. By using Doppler and assessing changes in chamber size, the echocardiogram is useful in assessing hemodynamics and can help differentiate tamponade, constriction, and restriction. It can also be used to help guide procedures such as pericardiocentesis. Computed tomography (CT) and magnetic resonance imaging (MRI) can identify pericardial masses and pericardial thickening or calcification.[9] Cardiac catheterization provides pressure tracings that help to distinguish cardiac tamponade, constriction, and restriction. Endomyocardial biopsy can also be useful in diagnosing restrictive cardiomyopathy.

CONGENITAL ABNORMALITIES

Congenital absence of the pericardium is usually partial, but can be complete. It is most common on the left side and is more frequent in males. Associated congenital cardiac defects include atrial septal defect, a bicuspid aortic valve, and pulmonary malformations. Defects on the right side can lead to cardiac herniation. Patients can present with chest pain, syncope, or death. The electrocardiogram can show a right bundle branch block. The pericardial defect can be appreciated on CT or MRI. The treatment of a partial defect is total pericardiectomy or patch closure with polytetrafluoroethylene or bovine pericardium. Total pericardial absence is usually asymptomatic and is found incidentally.

Pericardial cysts are rare benign cysts that generally measure 1 to 15 cm in size. They are most commonly found at the right cardiophrenic angle and are asymptomatic. Patients may present with mediastinal compression and respiratory symptoms. The differential diagnosis includes a Morgagni hernia, lipoma, mediastinal tumor, or bronchogenic cyst. CT scans are used to confirm the location and relationship to surrounding structures. The cyst is excised if the patient is symptomatic or the diagnosis is unclear.

ACUTE PERICARDITIS

Acute pericarditis is an inflammatory process that has involved the pericardium for less than 2 weeks (Table 85.1). Patients often present with a 3- to 7-day prodrome of low-grade fevers, malaise, and muscle aches. Acute pericarditis occurs in 5% of those who present to the emergency department with nonischemic chest pain[10] and in 1% of those with ST elevation.[11] It is important to distinguish pericarditis from the chest pain of an acute myocardial infarction. Acute pericarditis usually causes sharp, pleuritic pain that can last several days. The pain most commonly radiates to the trapezius ridge and is improved by leaning forward. Patients can present with shortness of breath, a nonproductive cough, and clear lung fields. The differential diagnosis also includes aortic dissection and pneumothorax. On physical examination, a friction rub may be heard and is sometimes intermittent. The classic friction rub has three components during systole, early diastolic filling, and atrial contraction.

3 The electrocardiogram is important in the diagnosis and classically shows diffuse ST elevations without Q waves or T-wave inversion. PR depression can also be seen. There is a four-stage progression in the changes seen on ECG, with diffuse ST elevations followed by normalization of ST segments with flattening of T waves. The ECG then evolves with T-wave inversions prior to normalization of the ECG. Pericarditis and associated myocarditis can cause elevations in creatinine kinase and troponin I.[12] The minimal workup should include an ECG, complete blood count, cultures, chemistry profile, and antibody titers for collagen diseases.

FIGURE 85.2. The jugular venous pulse waveform. (Reproduced with permission from Bradley SM. Pericardium. In: Mulholland MW, Lillemoe KD, eds. *Greenfield's Surgery: Scientific Principles and Practice*, 4th ed. Philadelphia, PA: Lippincott Williams & Wilkins; 2006:1522.)

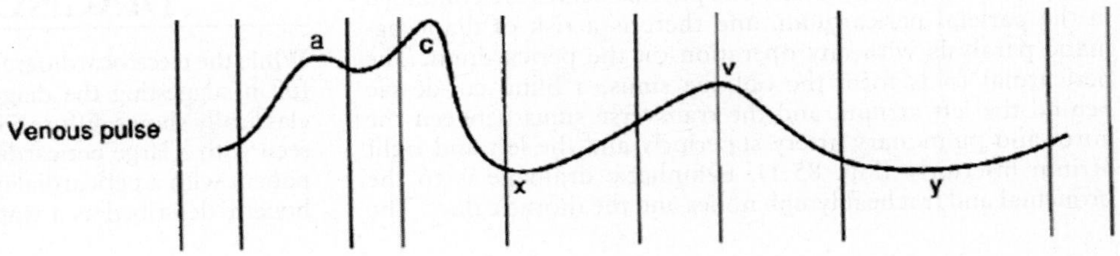

TABLE 85.1 ETIOLOGY

CAUSES OF PERICARDITIS

Idiopathic
Infectious
Neoplastic
Hemopericardium
Blunt and penetrating trauma
Post–cardiac surgery
Aortic dissection
Autoimmune and inflammatory
Connective tissue disorders
Post–myocardial infarction
Medication induced
Miscellaneous
Radiation induced
Hypothyroidism
Uremic

Idiopathic and Viral Pericarditis

Idiopathic causes of pericarditis are the second most common after neoplastic disease. The majority are likely viral, although routine testing is not usually performed. A virus is only identified in 15% to 20% of cases, with the most common being coxsackievirus, echovirus, adenovirus, influenza, and cytomegalovirus. Patients present with chest pain, malaise, and fever and often have an elevated erythrocyte sedimentation rate. The episode is self-limited in 70% to 90% of cases.[10] Initial treatment is with nonsteroidal anti-inflammatory drugs (NSAIDs). There is a 15% to 30% relapse rate, at which point specific causes, such as autoimmune disorders, should be investigated.[10,13] A repeat course of NSAIDs, colchicine, or steroids is generally successful. Pericardiectomy is recommended if the patient is unresponsive to medical treatment or constriction develops.

Acquired Immunodeficiency Syndrome

A pericardial effusion develops in up to 20% of patients with human immunodeficiency virus (HIV) and is usually a poor prognostic sign.[14] This may be partly due to a generalized capillary leak syndrome as well as increased cytokine expression seen in the more advanced stages of HIV. Other contributing factors include tubercular and mycobacterial infections, lymphoma, Kaposi sarcoma, or congestive heart failure. The majority are idiopathic and do not require further therapy if asymptomatic. Symptomatic effusions are drained.

Tuberculous Pericarditis

Tuberculous pericarditis occurs in 1% to 8% of patients.[15] In immunocompromised patients, infection by *Mycobacterium avium* or *Mycobacterium intracellulare* can lead to pericarditis. The incidence of tuberculous pericarditis has decreased, although it continues to be a significant issue in immunocompromised patients, particularly HIV patients in Africa. Patients present with fever, night sweats, cough, dyspnea, and weight loss. While infection usually results from hematogenous spread, it can also extend directly from lymph nodes or through lymphatics. Pericardial changes occur in four stages: fibrinous, effusive, fibrous, and constrictive fibrous. Making the diagnosis from pericardial fluid alone is rare. Pericardial biopsy with acid-fast staining provides the diagnosis 80% to 90% of the time. Treatment includes multidrug antitubercular therapy and pericardiocentesis. Steroids have not been shown to be beneficial for mortality or progression to constriction, but lead to a faster resolution of symptoms and reaccumulation.[16] If patients present with late constriction, pericardiectomy may be required.

Purulent Pericarditis

Bacteria can be introduced into the pericardial space by direct injury, pneumonia, extension from head and neck infections, or hematogenous and lymphatic spread. Patients present with chest pain, fever, and leukocytosis. The most common organisms in adults are staphylococcus, pneumococcus, and streptococcus. Purulent pericarditis can evolve rapidly into tamponade and can be confused with septic shock. Fungal infections are less common, but immunocompromised patients and drug addicts are at greater risk. Pericardial fluid in purulent pericarditis has low glucose, high protein, and elevated lactate dehydrogenase (LDH) and neutrophils. An air-fluid level may be seen on chest radiography with gas-producing organisms. Treatment includes antibiotics and drainage. Surgical drainage may be needed for thick fluid or refractory effusions. The prognosis for purulent pericarditis is poor, with a survival of 30%.[10,17]

Uremic Pericarditis

Fifty percent of patients with untreated renal disease develop pericarditis. The incidence is decreased to approximately 20% in patients on hemodialysis. The exact cause is unknown but is not directly related to the blood urea nitrogen (BUN) or creatinine. Other possible etiologies include hypercalcemia, viral infection, and autoimmune disease. Chest pain is usually less common, and the large effusions accumulate gradually. Treatment includes more intensive dialysis, NSAIDs, and steroids. The fluid is generally bloody and care should be taken in heparinizing these patients for dialysis. If patients develop tamponade or the effusion is unresponsive, pericardiocentesis or surgical drainage is performed.

Vasculitis, Connective Tissue Disease, and Drugs

Pericarditis can result from a variety of vasculitic and connective tissue diseases, including rheumatoid arthritis, Wegener granulomatosis, rheumatic fever, lupus, scleroderma, Reiter syndrome, Behçet disease, dermatomyositis, polyarteritis nodosa, dermatomyositis, sarcoidosis, and amyloidosis. Treatment includes management of the underlying disease process and NSAIDs. Pericardiocentesis is performed if necessary. Several medications can also lead to pericarditis including warfarin, hydralazine, isoniazid, procainamide, phenytoin, dantrolene, cromolyn, and methysergide.

Dressler and Postpericardiotomy Syndrome

Pericarditis can occur following acute myocardial infarction in 3% to 5% of patients.[18] Pericarditis can develop early in the first 1 to 3 days, particularly with transmural infarction. Forty percent of large Q-wave infarctions cause pericardial inflammation, although the incidence is decreasing with the use of thrombolytics and early revascularization. Patients are usually asymptomatic and are found to have a pericardial rub on examination, although they can present with pleuritic chest pain. Treatment is usually with NSAIDs. Steroids can prevent conversion of infracted myocardium to scar, leading to greater thinning and risk of rupture.[19,20]

Patients can also present with pericarditis 1 week to a few months after a myocardial infarction with a friction rub, typical ECG changes, and chest pain, although the incidence has decreased with increased revascularization. Pericardial inflammation is thought to be from an autoimmune reaction to myocardial cells.[20] Similar symptoms can also occur after cardiac surgery, blunt trauma, and pacemaker placement. Patients can develop a pericardial effusion and even tamponade. Treatment includes NSAIDs and colchicine for 2 to 3 weeks and occasionally steroids. The syndrome is usually self-limited.

Radiation-induced Pericarditis

Pericarditis can result from mediastinal and thoracic radiation for cancer, including lymphoma and breast carcinoma, and is related to the dosage delivered. With modern techniques, the incidence is 2%, but can be as high as 20% if the entire pericardium is treated. Patients may develop chest pain and fever.[20] Symptoms are usually self-limited, and tamponade is rare. Delayed symptoms can develop years later and can result in pericardial constriction. Due to the history of malignancy, the etiology can be confused with a malignant effusion. If pericardial constriction develops, the treatment is pericardiectomy, although the mortality is higher than for other etiologies.

PERICARDIAL EFFUSION AND TAMPONADE

Any of the etiologies mentioned previously for pericarditis can also lead to pericardial effusion. Other causes include blunt or penetrating trauma, retrograde bleeding from an aortic dissection, and a transudative effusion from congestive heart failure. Effusions due to a bacterial or fungal infection, HIV, or malignancy have a higher incidence of progressing to tamponade. Twenty percent of large symptomatic effusions of unknown cause are due to an undiagnosed cancer.[21]

Normally there is only a small reserve volume before pericardial fluid causes significant cardiac compression and prevents **4** adequate cardiac filling. The hemodynamic significance of a pericardial effusion depends on the volume and the rate of accumulation. The compensatory adrenergic response to a pericardial effusion leads to tachycardia and increased contractility, and patients on beta-blockers are less likely to compensate. Tamponade usually occurs when filling pressures reach 15 to 20 mm Hg, although tamponade can occur at lower pressures in conditions where blood volume is reduced, including dialysis, with diuretic therapy, and bleeding. Cardiac pressures become elevated and are most closely equalized during inspiration. Tamponade generally affects right heart filling first, which then leads to underfilling of the left heart.[22]

Patients may present with dyspnea, tachycardia, and diaphoresis. The three classic signs of Beck's triad are hypotension, jugular venous distention, and muffled heart sounds, although each may be absent in patients with tamponade.[23] Symptoms can be confused with right heart failure and pulmonary embolus. The jugular waveform changes characteristically with loss of the y descent.[24] Since the total heart volume is fixed in tamponade, blood only enters the heart when blood leaves. The y descent represents opening of the tricuspid valve and is lost since no blood is ejected from the heart. Pulsus paradoxus is also noted with a fall in the systolic blood pressure of greater than 10 mm Hg with inspiration. Pulsus paradoxus is absent in left ventricular dysfunction, atrial septal defect, positive-pressure ventilation, aortic insufficiency, and regional tamponade. The ECG shows variation in the morphology of every other QRS complex, or electrical alternans, due to swinging of the heart in the pericardial effusion (Fig. 85.3). Chest radiography shows an enlarged, rounded cardiac

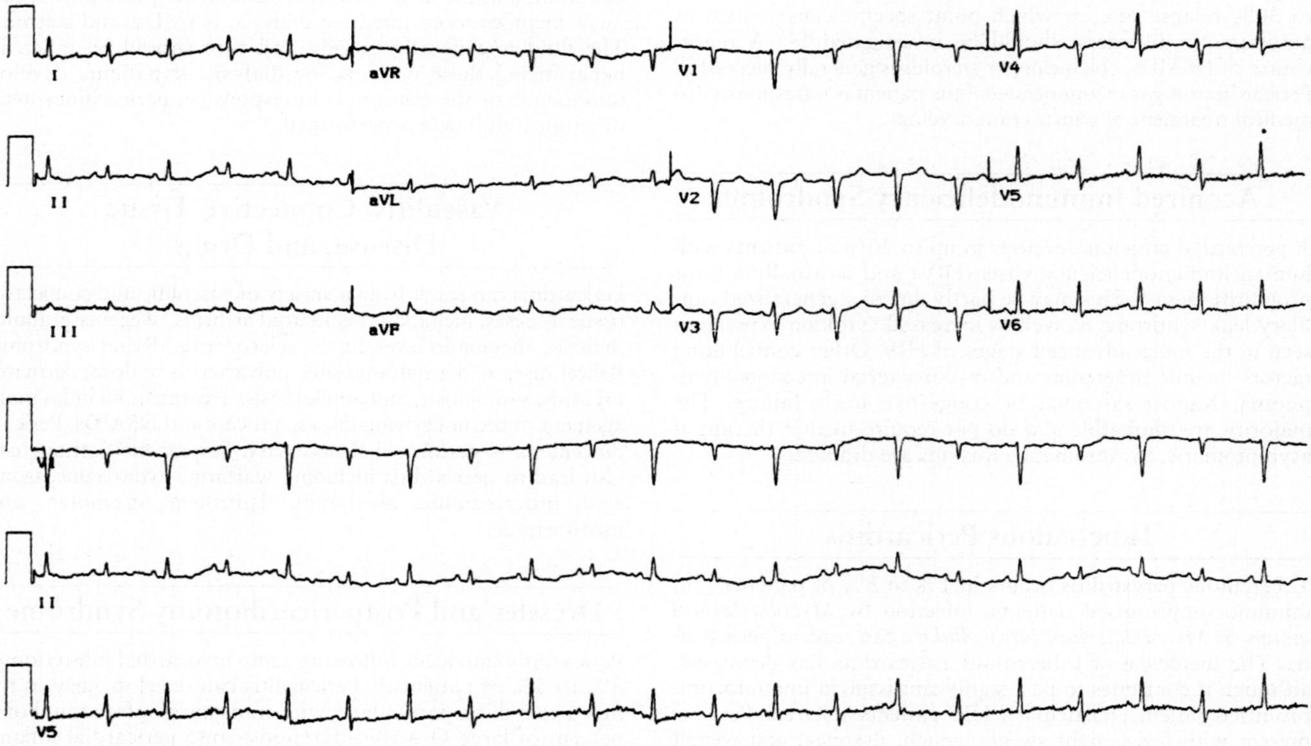

FIGURE 85.3. The 12-lead electrocardiogram shows electrical alternans with variation in the morphology of every other QRS complex in a patient with a large pericardial effusion. (Reproduced with permission from Joffe II, Jacobs LE, Kotler MN. Pericardial tamponade. *Circulation* 1996;94:2667.)

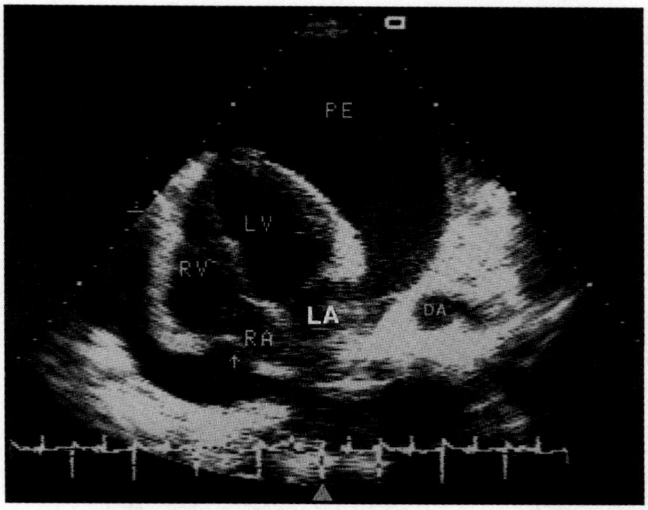

FIGURE 85.4. The echocardiogram shows a large pericardial effusion with diastolic right atrial collapse (*arrow*). (Reproduced with permission from Joffe II, Jacobs LE, Kotler MN. Pericardial tamponade. *Circulation* 1996;94:2667.)

silhouette. The pericardial fat pad sign is seen when the pericardial fat is separated from the heart by the effusion.

Echocardiography is the most useful test in diagnosing pericardial effusion and tamponade. Signs of tamponade include early diastolic right ventricular and right atrial collapse during diastole (Fig. 85.4) and distention of the cava that does not diminish with inspiration. Doppler is useful in evaluating blood flow and shows exaggerated respiratory variation with an increase with inspiration on the right and a decrease on the left side of the heart. Echocardiography is also useful in identifying localized atrial compression, which can lead to tamponade with the other changes described previously.

The approach to a patient with a large pericardial effusion is outlined in Algorithm 85.1. If there are significant hemodynamic changes, emergent pericardiocentesis should b formed. Intravenous fluid and inotropes can tempori hypotension but should not delay pericardiocentesis. effusion is loculated or contains blood clots, open dra may be necessary. There should be a higher suspicion for ponade in situations involving bleeding, bacterial or tube lous pericarditis, or an acute or increasing moderate to la effusion.

Postoperative Cardiac Tamponade

5 Postoperative tamponade should always be in the differentia diagnosis with low cardiac output after cardiac surgery. Patients may have rising filling pressures, hypotension, and decreased urine and cardiac output. Mediastinal chest tube output may increase or abruptly stop. Hypovolemia during the postoperative period can limit the increase in filling pressures. Pulsus paradoxus may also be masked by positive-pressure ventilation. On chest radiography, the cardiac silhouette is enlarged. In the postoperative cardiac patient, the epicardial pacing wires may move farther from the pericardium with increasing tamponade on chest films. Tamponade can result from relatively small amounts of blood with localized atrial compression from blood clots. There should be a low threshold for reexploration, which also provides a definitive diagnosis. Patients can also present with delayed tamponade after being started on anticoagulants.

PERICARDIAL CONSTRICTION

Constriction develops when the heart becomes constrained by a fibrotic pericardium. The process can progress over years, and the most common causes in the developed world are radiation treatment, postsurgical changes, and idiopathic. Tuberculosis was the most common cause before antitubercular drug therapy. Other causes include amyloidosis, scleroderma, sarcoidosis, hemochromatosis, and malignant disease. Patients develop signs and symptoms of right heart failure due to obstruction of the right ventricular outflow tract including hepatomegaly, ascites, and peripheral edema. Patients can also

VASCULAR

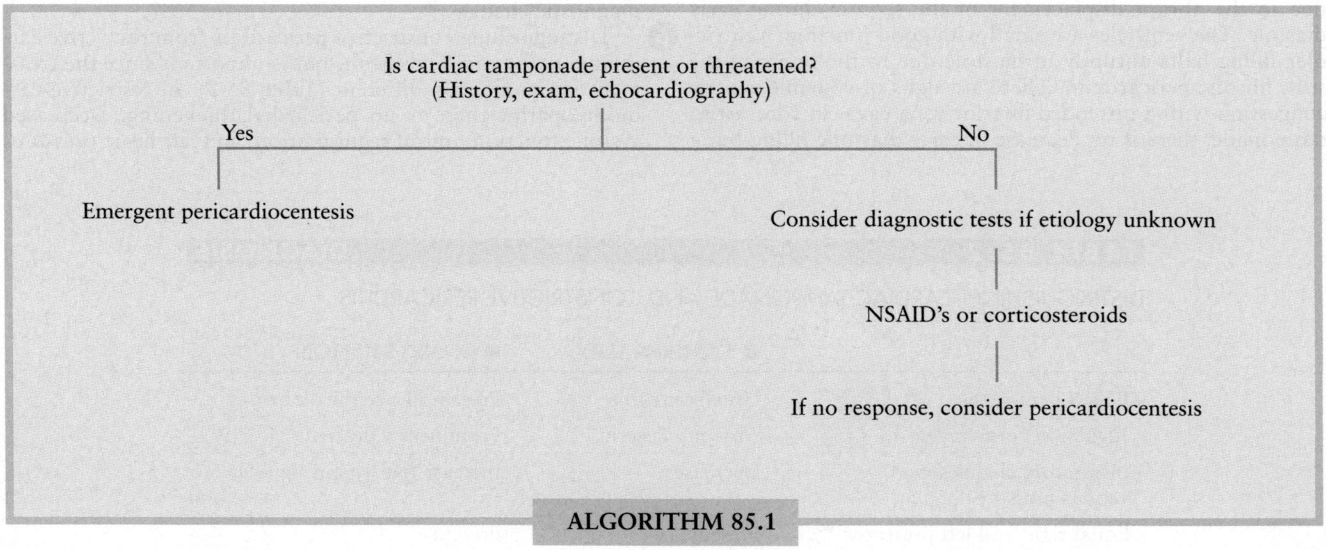

ALGORITHM 85.1. This algorithm outlines the initial approach to a patient with a large pericardial effusion.

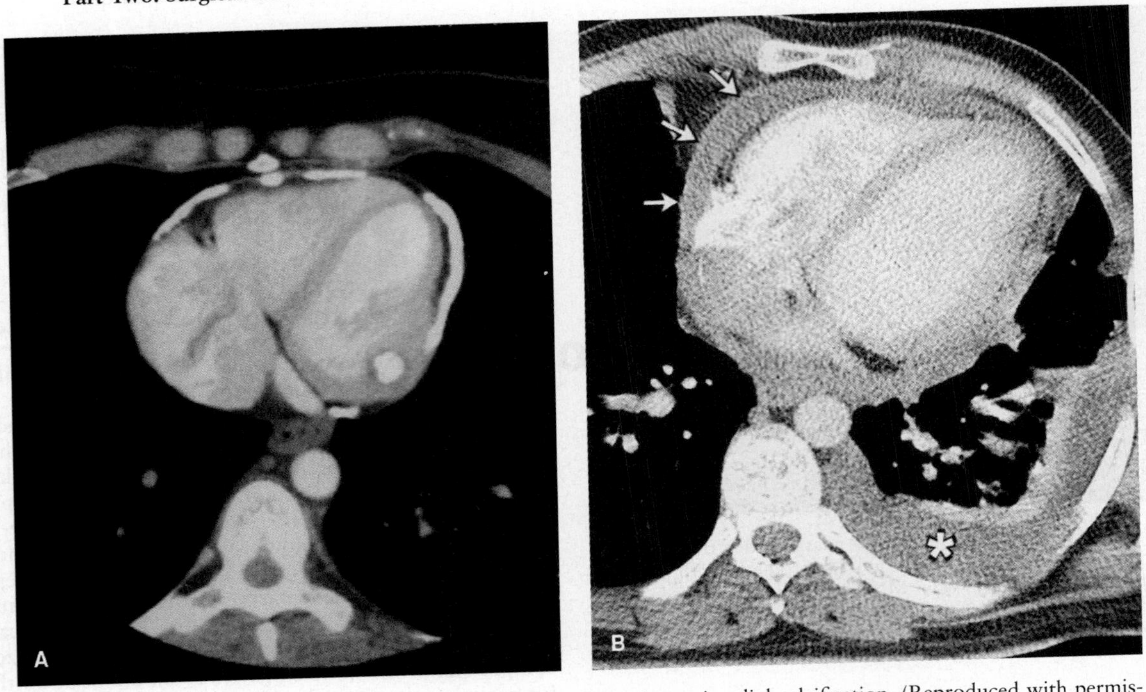

FIGURE 85.5. **A:** Chest computed tomography (CT) shows extensive pericardial calcification. (Reproduced with permission from Cavendish JJ, Linz PE. Constrictive pericarditis from a severely calcified pericardium. *Circulation* 2005; 112:e138.). **B:** Chest CT shows thickening of the pericardium in a patient with constrictive pericarditis. (Reproduced with permission from Tom CW, Oh JK. A case of transient constrictive pericarditis. *Circulation* 2005;111:e364.).

have dyspnea, pleural effusions, fatigue, and weight loss. On physical examination, a pericardial knock, or a loud third heart sound, can be heard, which corresponds to the abrupt cessation of diastolic filling. The Kussmaul sign is increased jugular venous distention with inspiration. Atrial fibrillation or flutter is present in up to 25% of patients, and tricuspid regurgitation is also common.

Pericardial calcification is pathognomonic but is only seen in 40% of cases. Thickened pericardium can be seen on CT or MRI (Fig. 85.5), although the pericardium was normal in thickness in 18% of patients in one series.[25] The normal pericardial thickness is 2 mm on CT and 4 mm on MRI. Echocardiography shows thickened pericardium and a septal bounce due to the abrupt displacement of the septum during early diastole. The ventricles are small with good function. Ventricular filling halts abruptly in diastole due to the limits of the stiff, fibrotic pericardium. There are signs of systemic venous congestion with a distended inferior vena cava. In contrast to tamponade, there is no decrease in early diastolic filling but a sudden decrease in late diastole (Table 85.2).[24] When the myocardium is involved by fibrosis, ventricle dysfunction is present, which is associated with a poorer response to pericardiectomy.

On right heart catheterization, the y descent is deeper and more rapid than normal. The right atrial waveform is M- or W-shaped. The right ventricular tracing is described as the "square root" sign with an early diastolic decrease with a rapid increase and plateau (Fig. 85.6). Pulmonary artery and right ventricular pressures can be moderately elevated, but more severe pulmonary hypertension suggests a different disease process. In addition, hypovolemia can mask these findings, and patients may need to be volume challenged to see the diagnostic changes.[26]

6 Distinguishing constrictive pericarditis from restrictive cardiomyopathy can be difficult, but is important since the treatment is significantly different (Table 85.3). In restrictive cardiomyopathy, there is no pericardial thickening. Decreased systolic function, mitral regurgitation, and left heart pressures

TABLE 85.2 — DIAGNOSIS

DISTINGUISHING CARDIAC TAMPONADE AND CONSTRICTIVE PERICARDITIS

	■ TAMPONADE	■ CONSTRICTION
Pulsus paradoxus	Usually present	Present in one third of cases
Jugular venous waveform	Absent y descent	Prominent y descent (M or W)
Inspiratory changes in venous pressure	Decrease	Increase (Kussmaul sign)
Equal right and left pressures	Present	Present
"Square-root" sign of ventricular pressure	Absent	Present

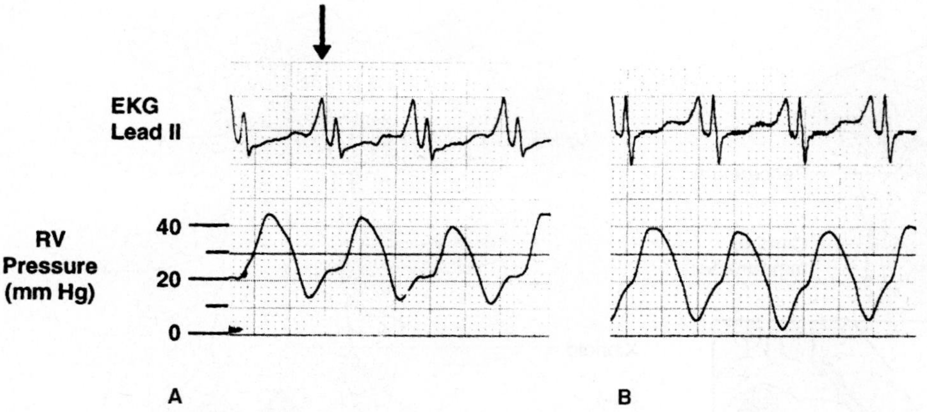

FIGURE 85.6. **A:** The right ventricular (RV) pressure tracing shows elevated RV diastolic pressure with the dip-and-plateau waveform known as the "square-root" sign. The electrocardiogram tracing shows a large P wave indicative of right atrial enlargement. **B:** The postoperative RV tracing shows normalization of the RV waveform. (Reproduced with permission from Correa SD, Amsterdam EA. Constrictive pericarditis. *Circulation* 1998;97:806.)

greater than right are more common in restrictive cardiomyopathy. Early diastolic filling is slower. In addition, left and right ventricular pressures move in the same direction on inspiration rather than in opposite directions.[27]

Constrictive pericarditis is generally progressive, although it can be transient after cardiac surgery and should be observed for several months. Diuretics with fluid and salt restriction help initially, but pericardiectomy is the only definitive treatment. Tachycardia is a compensatory response, and beta-blockers and calcium channel blockers should be avoided.

NEOPLASTIC PERICARDIAL DISEASE

Primary tumors of the pericardium are rare and include benign fibromas, hemangiomas, lipomas, lymphangiomas, leiomyomas, and neurofibromas. Malignant pleural tumors include mesothelioma, teratoma, and fibrosarcoma. Surgical resection is therapeutic and diagnostic. Malignancies can also extend directly
7 from the mediastinum, esophagus, and lung. Metastatic disease is the most common cause of pericardial effusion. Cardiac involvement is found in 5% to 10% of patients dying of cancer, with 85% of those having pericardial involvement. The most common cancers are lung and breast carcinoma, lymphoma, melanoma, and leukemia. Patients often present with tamponade. The diagnosis is made on echocardiography or CT. Cytology of pericardial fluid is negative in 20% to 50% of cases, and pericardial biopsy may be helpful. Palliation includes sclerosing agents such as tetracycline, radiotherapy, intrapericardial chemotherapy, and catheter drainage.

PERICARDIOCENTESIS

Pericardiocentesis can be diagnostic and therapeutic. Ideally, it should be performed in the catheterization lab so the hemodynamic response can be monitored. Normal pericardial fluid is an ultrafiltrate with an LDH 2.4 times serum and protein 0.6 times serum.[28] Uremic fluid is bloody. Rheumatic effusions are high in protein and leukocytes and low in glucose. Cholesterol crystals are seen with myxedema, tuberculosis, and rheumatoid arthritis.

Generally, a 16- to 22-gauge needle is inserted to the left of the xiphoid. The needle is angled at 45 degrees toward the left shoulder (Fig. 85.7). An ECG lead may also be attached to the needle to monitor for an injury current, although

TABLE 85.3 **DIAGNOSIS**

DISTINGUISHING CONSTRICTIVE PERICARDITIS FROM RESTRICTIVE CARDIOMYOPATHY

	■ RESTRICTION	■ CONSTRICTION
Pericardial knock	Absent	Present
Pulsus paradoxus	Absent	Present in one third of cases
Thickened pericardium	Absent	Present
Atrial enlargement	Biatrial	Possibly left atrial
Septal bounce	Absent	Present
Equal right and left pressures	Left 3–5 mm Hg > than right	Present
Filling pressures >25 mm Hg	Present	Uncommon
Pulmonary artery SBP >60 mm Hg	Present	Absent
"Square root" sign of ventricular pressure	Variable	Present
Prominent y descent	Variable	Present

SBP, systolic blood pressure.

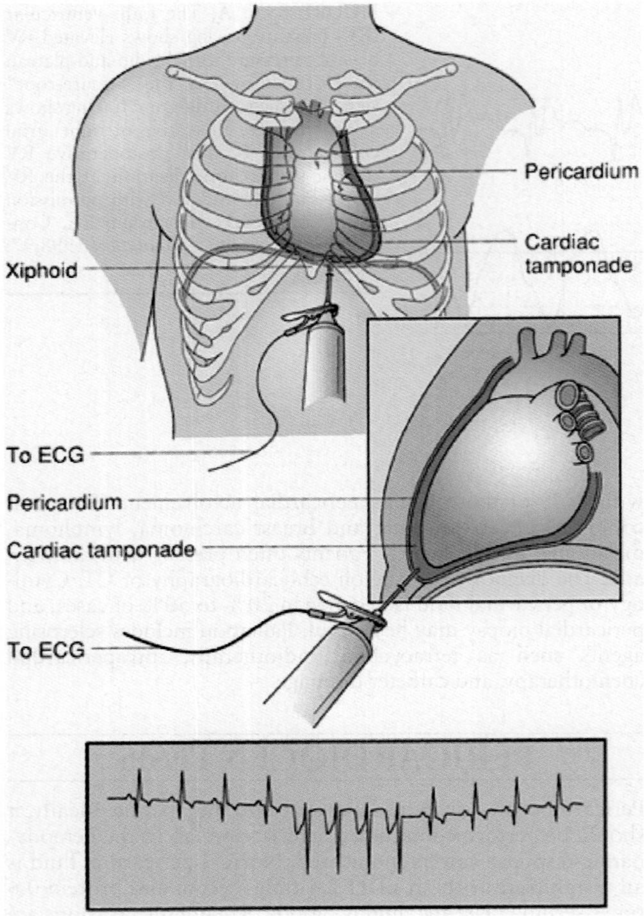

FIGURE 85.7. Pericardiocentesis is performed by inserting a needle to the left of the xiphoid and toward the left shoulder at a 45-degree angle. An electrocardiogram lead may be attached to the needle to monitor for Q waves indicating contact with the epicardium. (Reproduced with permission from Bradley SM. Pericardium. In: Mulholland MW, Lillemoe KD, eds. *Greenfield's Surgery: Scientific Principles and Practice,* 4th ed. Philadelphia, PA: Lippincott Williams & Wilkins; 2006:1526.)

echocardiography is more commonly used for guidance. There is a 97% success rate with a complication rate of 4.7% (Table 85.4).[29] If the effusion is anterior, a parasternal approach is used 1 to 2 cm to the left of the sternum in the fourth or fifth intercostal space. The removal of even a small amount of fluid can lead to significant hemodynamic improvement. For longer-term drainage, a catheter can be placed over a guide wire. Pericardiocentesis may not be effective for purulent or bloody effusions, which may require open drainage.

TABLE 85.4 COMPLICATIONS

POTENTIAL COMPLICATIONS FROM PERICARDIOCENTESIS

Injury to surrounding organs
Liver laceration
Lung (pneumothorax)
Coronary arteries
Myocardium
Arrhythmias
Pulmonary edema from acute left ventricular failure
Recurrence

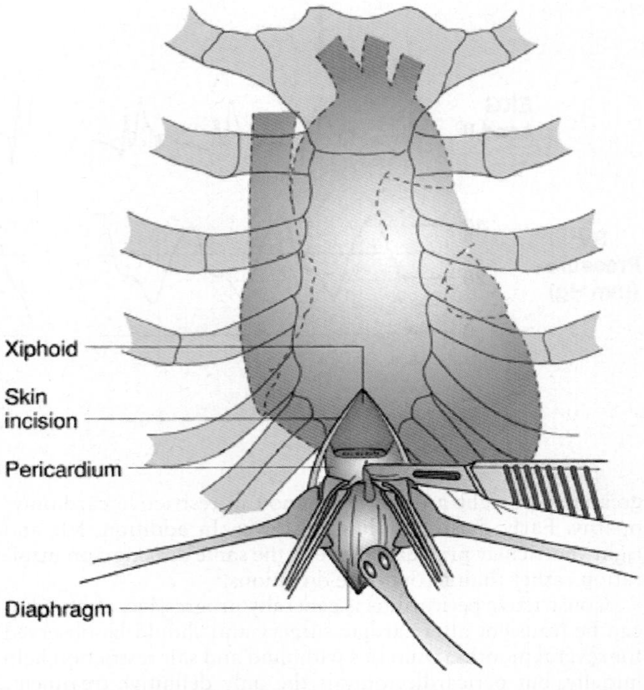

FIGURE 85.8. Open pericardial biopsy or drainage is performed through an upper midline incision. The xiphoid is retracted or removed, providing exposure to the pericardium. (Reproduced with permission from Bradley SM. Pericardium. In: Mulholland MW, Lillemoe KD, eds. *Greenfield's Surgery: Scientific Principles and Practice,* 4th ed. Philadelphia, PA: Lippincott Williams & Wilkins; 2006:1527.)

PERICARDIAL BIOPSY AND SURGICAL DRAINAGE

Pericardial biopsy is useful when pericardiocentesis is nondiagnostic, which is not uncommon in neoplastic and tubercular effusions. This can be approached through a subxiphoid incision, through an anterior thoracotomy, or thoracoscopically (Fig. 85.8). Open drainage may be useful if the fluid is viscous, including bloody or purulent effusions or in patients who have recurrent effusions. Loculated effusions may also require open drainage. The subxiphoid approach is better for purulent effusions to prevent contamination of the pleural space. Chronic or malignant effusions can be drained through a pericardial window into the left pleura. Preinduction pericardiocentesis or intravenous fluids may be necessary for patients to tolerate general anesthesia.

PERICARDIECTOMY

Pericardiectomy is most commonly performed for constrictive pericarditis. It can be performed through a median sternotomy or a left anterior thoracotomy in the fifth intercostal space. Anterior thoracotomy allows removal of the pericardium over the left ventricle with minimal manipulation. Femoral cannulation is used if bypass is necessary. Median sternotomy is the most common approach (Fig. 85.9). Cardiopulmonary bypass increases the risk of bleeding and is used when significant cardiac manipulation is needed or the dissection is difficult. The pericardium over the left ventricle is resected first to avoid pulmonary edema from the right ventricle ejecting against a constricted left ventricle. The pericardium is removed from phrenic nerve to phrenic nerve. Some patients have an immediate improvement in hemodynamics and symptoms, while others do

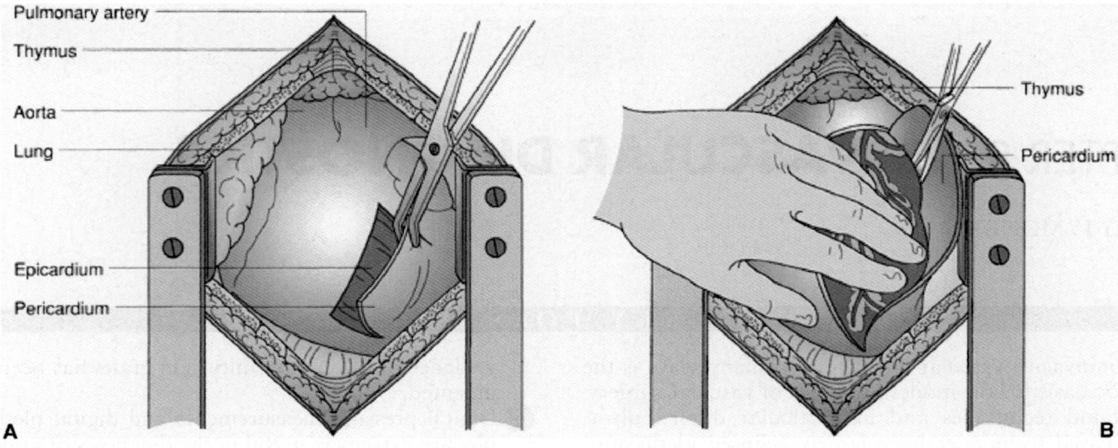

FIGURE 85.9. Pericardiectomy is most commonly approached through a median sternotomy. **A:** The pericardium is incised and the fibrous pericardium dissected from the left ventricle. **B:** The heart is retracted to the right so that the pericardium can be resected from phrenic nerve to phrenic nerve. (Reproduced with permission from Bradley SM. Pericardium. In: Mulholland MW, Lillemoe KD, eds. *Greenfield's Surgery: Scientific Principles and Practice,* 4th ed. Philadelphia, PA: Lippincott Williams & Wilkins; 2006:1527.)

not improve until weeks or months later. A delayed or incomplete response is thought to be due to an incomplete resection of the visceral pericardium or myocardial atrophy and fibrosis. Left ventricular function returned to normal in 40% of patients.

Perioperative mortality has been reported between 5% and 15% and is due to low cardiac output, sepsis, bleeding, and renal or respiratory failure.[30] Seventy percent of mortality is due to low cardiac output. Mortality is directly related to the patient's preoperative status[31] and is 1% for New York Heart Association class I to II, 10% for class III, and 46% for class IV.[32] Five-year survival is 84%, and 99% of late survivors were class I or II. Patients with constriction due to radiotherapy have a higher mortality rate, which may be due to radiation-induced myocardial injury. Other poor prognostic factors are renal failure, advanced age, pulmonary hypertension, hyponatremia, and reduced cardiac output.[30,33]

References

1. Laennec R. *Traite d'Auscultationo oMedicale et des Maladies su Poumon et du Coeur*. Paris, France: Brosson & JS Chaude; 1819.
2. Beck C, Griswald RA. Pericardiectomy in the treatment of the Pick syndrome: experimental and clinical observations. *Arch Surg* 1930;21:1064.
3. Kussmaul A. Ueber schwielige Mediatino-perikarditis und dem Paradoxen Puls. *Berl Klin Wochenschr* 1873;10:433.
4. Karanaeff P. Paracentese des Brustkastens und des Pericardiums. *Med Z* 1840;9:251.
5. Rehn L. Zurexperimentellen pathologic des herzbeutels. *Verh Dtsch Ges Chir* 1913;42:339.
6. Sadler T. *Langman's Medical Embryology*, 7th ed. Baltimore: Williams & Wilkins; 1995.
7. Gibbon A, Segal MB. A study of the composition of pericardial fluid with special reference to the probable mechanism of fluid formation. *J Physiol* 1940;277:635.
8. Spodick DH. Macrophysiology, microphysiology, and anatomy of the pericardium: a synopsis. *Am Heart J* 1992;124:1046–1051.
9. Moncada R, Kotler MN, Churchill RJ, et al. Multimodality approach to pericardial imaging. *Cardiovasc Clin* 1986;17:409–441.
10. Troughton RW, Asher CR, Klein AL. Pericarditis. *Lancet* 2004;363: 717–727.
11. Brady WJ, Perron AD, Martin ML, et al. Cause of ST segment abnormality in ED chest pain patients. *Am J Emerg Med* 2001;19:25–28.
12. Imazio M, Demichelis B, Cecchi E, et al. Cardiac troponin I in acute pericarditis. *J Am Coll Cardiol* 2003;42:2144–2148.
13. Lange RA, Hillis LD. Clinical practice. Acute pericarditis. *N Engl J Med* 2004;351:2195–2202.
14. Heidenreich PA, Eisenberg MJ, Kee LL, et al. Pericardial effusion in AIDS. Incidence and survival. *Circulation* 1995;92:3229–3234.
15. Mayosi BM, Burgess LJ, Doubell AF. Tuberculous pericarditis. *Circulation* 2005;112:3608–3616.
16. Strang JI, Kakaza HH, Gibson DG, et al. Controlled clinical trial of complete open surgical drainage and of prednisolone in treatment of tuberculous pericardial effusion in Transkei. *Lancet* 1988;2:759–764.
17. Sagrista-Sauleda J, Barrabes JA, Permanyer-Miralda G, et al. Purulent pericarditis: review of a 20-year experience in a general hospital. *J Am Coll Cardiol* 1993;22:1661–1665.
18. Dressler W. A post-myocardial infarction syndrome; preliminary report of a complication resembling idiopathic, recurrent, benign pericarditis. *JAMA* 1956;160:1379–1383.
19. Little WC, Freeman GL. Pericardial disease. *Circulation* 2006;113: 1622–1632.
20. Maisch B, Seferovic PM, Ristic AD, et al. Guidelines on the diagnosis and management of pericardial diseases executive summary; the task force on the diagnosis and management of pericardial diseases of the European Society of Cardiology. *Eur Heart J* 2004;25:587–610.
21. Ben-Horin S, Bank I, Guetta V, et al. Large symptomatic pericardial effusion as the presentation of unrecognized cancer: a study in 173 consecutive patients undergoing pericardiocentesis. *Medicine (Baltimore)* 2006;85: 49–53.
22. Ditchey R, Engler R, LeWinter M, et al. The role of the right heart in acute cardiac tamponade in dogs. *Circ Res* 1981;48:701–710.
23. Beck C. Two cardiac compression triads. *JAMA* 1935;104:714.
24. Shabetai R, Fowler NO, Guntheroth WG. The hemodynamics of cardiac tamponade and constrictive pericarditis. *Am J Cardiol* 1970;26:480–489.
25. Talreja DR, Edwards WD, Danielson GK, et al. Constrictive pericarditis in 26 patients with histologically normal pericardial thickness. *Circulation* 2003;108:1852–1857.
26. Abdalla IA, Murray RD, Lee JC, et al. Does rapid volume loading during transesophageal echocardiography differentiate constrictive pericarditis from restrictive cardiomyopathy? *Echocardiography* 2002;19:125–134.
27. Hatle LK, Appleton CP, Popp RL. Differentiation of constrictive pericarditis and restrictive cardiomyopathy by Doppler echocardiography. *Circulation* 1989;79:357–370.
28. Ben-Horin S, Shinfeld A, Kachel E, et al. The composition of normal pericardial fluid and its implications for diagnosing pericardial effusions. *Am J Med* 2005;118:636–640.
29. Tsang TS, Enriquez-Sarano M, Freeman WK, et al. Consecutive 1127 therapeutic echocardiographically guided pericardiocenteses: clinical profile, practice patterns, and outcomes spanning 21 years. *Mayo Clin Proc* 2002; 77:429–436.
30. Ling LH, Oh JK, Schaff HV, et al. Constrictive pericarditis in the modern era: evolving clinical spectrum and impact on outcome after pericardiectomy. *Circulation* 1999;100:1380–1386.
31. Seifert FC, Miller DC, Oesterle SN, et al. Surgical treatment of constrictive pericarditis: analysis of outcome and diagnostic error. *Circulation* 1985; 72:II264–II273.
32. McCaughan BC, Schaff HV, Piehler JM, et al. Early and late results of pericardiectomy for constrictive pericarditis. *J Thorac Cardiovasc Surg* 1985;89:340–350.
33. Bertog SC, Thambidorai SK, Parakh K, et al. Constrictive pericarditis: etiology and cause-specific survival after pericardiectomy. *J Am Coll Cardiol* 2004;43:1445–1452.

CHAPTER 86 ■ VASCULAR DIAGNOSTICS

GREGORY L. MONETA

KEY POINTS

1. The noninvasive vascular laboratory in many ways is the scientific basis for the modern practice of vascular surgery.
2. Ultrasound techniques and in particular duplex ultrasound-based techniques have largely eclipsed plethysmographic techniques in most vascular laboratories.
3. Detecting carotid stenosis involves a combination of spectral analysis, color and grayscale imaging, and, in selected cases, power Doppler.
4. The noninvasive vascular laboratory, in combination with the history and physical examination, has a critical role in providing objective diagnosis of lower extremity arterial occlusive disease in asymptomatic patients, those with intermittent claudication, and those with critical arterial insufficiency.
5. The ankle-brachial index (ABI) is a very useful measure of overall lower extremity perfusion.
6. Arterial duplex scanning provides detailed anatomic and hemodynamic information from the infrarenal aorta to the distal tibial vessels that cannot be determined by indirect testing. The role of duplex ultrasound scanning in the surveillance of lower extremity vein grafts has been well documented.
7. Digital pressure measurements and digital plethysmography are extremely useful in the diagnosis of upper extremity arterial disease and can be as accurate as arteriography in assessing patients with hand ischemia.
8. Duplex ultrasonography can serve as a valuable noninvasive screening test for splanchnic artery stenosis in patients with possible chronic mesenteric ischemia and for follow-up of mesenteric artery reconstructions.
9. Physical examination is not sensitive or specific for the detection of acute deep venous thrombosis (DVT). At a minimum, vascular laboratory duplex ultrasound evaluation for lower extremity DVT should include examination of the common femoral, profunda femoral, femoral, and popliteal veins.
10. Vascular laboratory ultrasound screening of males older than 65 years with a history of cigarette smoking for abdominal aortic aneurysm (AAA) has been shown to be effective in preventing aneurysm-related deaths.

1 The noninvasive vascular laboratory in many ways is the scientific basis for the modern practice of vascular surgery. It provides accurate, safe, and objective evidence of the presence of vascular disease throughout the body and, in many cases, its physiologic significance. There are two broad categories of testing available in the noninvasive vascular laboratory: plethysmographic techniques and ultrasound-based techniques.

PLETHYSMOGRAPHY

Plethysmography is based on the detection of limb volume changes in response to arterial inflow. In addition to volume flow, the technology can be modified to determine digital pressures and produce pulse waveforms. Mercury strain gauge plethysmography, air plethysmography (pulse volume recordings), and photoplethysmography are examples of plethysmographic techniques used clinically.

ULTRASOUND

2 Ultrasound techniques and in particular duplex ultrasound-based techniques have largely eclipsed plethysmographic techniques in most vascular laboratories. Duplex ultrasound was introduced in 1974 and was applied first to the carotid artery. The term "duplex" derives from the fact that the technique combines information from ultrasound-generated images (B mode) and Doppler analysis of blood flow direction and velocity. Duplex ultrasound is used extensively in the modern evaluation of carotid arteries, intra-abdominal arteries, and veins as well as upper and lower extremity arteries and veins. Since its inception, the technique has been advanced by (a) improved B-mode imaging; (b) better low-frequency scan heads, permitting deeper penetration of the ultrasound beam from the skin surface; (3) improvements in online computer-based microprocessor software; and (4) perhaps most importantly, the addition of color flow to the B-mode image.

In essence, color flow is superimposing a real-time color image of blood flow onto a standard grayscale B-mode picture. Returning echoes from stationary tissues generate the B-mode image, while those interacting with moving substances (blood) generate a significant enough phase shift that they can be processed separately and color-coded by operator selection to give information on the direction and velocity of blood flow according to the magnitude and direction of the Doppler frequency shift. It is color flow, combined with the ability of the current generation of duplex scanners to detect very low blood flow velocities (<5 cm/s), that makes duplex scanning practical on a routine basis throughout the body. Color flow dramatically reduces the time required to perform duplex examinations by allowing more rapid identification of vessels to be examined. It appears essential for duplex examination of some vessels such as tibial arteries and veins.

BASICS OF DUPLEX ULTRASOUND

An ultrasonic wave is produced in tissue by placing a vibrating source in contact with the tissue. This vibrating source is the ultrasound transducer. The transducer is contained within the ultrasound scan head. The purpose of the scan head is to steer and focus the sound beam arising from the transducer. These functions are crucial in deriving an ultrasound image from the returning echoes.

The transducer converts electrical energy into vibrational energy and, conversely, turns the vibrational energy of returning echoes into electrical signals that can be analyzed by the software of the duplex machine. The frequency of the vibrations, which determines the wavelength of the resulting sound wave, is determined by the design of the transducer. The relationship between frequency and wavelength is expressed mathematically as follows:

$$\lambda = c/f \quad (86.1)$$

where λ is the wavelength, c is the speed of sound in tissue, and f is the frequency.

The speed of sound in soft tissues averages 1,540 m/s and varies only minimally from this average in the soft tissues insonated in the clinical application of duplex ultrasound. The wavelength of the sound beam as it moves through the tissue is the principal physical determinant of how well the ultrasound beam penetrates the tissue. Because the speed of sound within tissue is, for all practical purposes, constant (1,540 m/s), the ability of ultrasound to penetrate tissue depends on the frequency of the vibrating source (transducer). As noted earlier, transducer frequency is determined by the design of the transducer and is thus controlled by the manufacturer of the duplex device. For examination of the carotid artery, transducer frequencies of 5 to 7.5 MHz provide optimal tissue penetration for clinical purposes.

As noted earlier, the term "duplex" refers to the combination of Doppler and B-mode ("B" stands for "brightness") ultrasound in the same device. Both types of ultrasound require analysis of reflected echoes of the original sound beam initially created by placing the ultrasound transducer in contact with the tissue. The B-mode component of the duplex machine is most concerned with analyzing the strength (intensity) and origin of the reflected echo, while the Doppler component is most concerned with analyzing shifts in frequency of an original sound wave produced by the transducer.

B-mode Ultrasound

As a sound wave passes through tissue, its relative strength at any point as it moves away from the transducer depends on the degree to which the beam has been attenuated, scattered, and reflected up to that point. The strength of the reflected echo depends in part on relative differences in acoustic impedance between two different media. Major differences in acoustic impedance reflect a large proportion of the sound beam back to the transducer, while small differences result in little reflection and continued propagation of the beam through the tissue.

In B-mode ultrasound, the strength of the returning echo is reflected in the brightness of the individual pixels comprising the ultrasound image. This is the ultrasound grayscale and the resulting image is termed a grayscale image. (As we will see later, the primary purpose of the grayscale image in duplex ultrasonography is to aid in properly positioning the Doppler sample volume.)

Very bright pixels represent sites of large differences in acoustic impedance between media, while less dramatic differences are represented by proportionally less bright pixels on the B-mode image. Thus, gallstones, which differ dramatically in acoustic properties from soft tissue, result in strong echoes and proportionally brighter pixels on an ultrasound image, while blood, which differs little from soft tissue in acoustic characteristics, frequently cannot be distinguished from soft tissue in a grayscale image.

Of course, the strength of the reflected echo will also be dependent on the strength of the sound beam at the point of its reflection. Grayscale images do not show the percentage of the beam reflected, but rather represent the absolute strength of the reflected echo arriving back at the transducer. Thus, if the sound beam is very weak at the site of its reflection, even areas of significant differences in acoustic impedance will not result in a bright pixel on the ultrasound image.

In addition to reflection, the strength of the ultrasound beam at any point also depends on the degree to which the beam has been attenuated as it passes through the tissue. Attenuation of a sound wave in tissue depends on both the tissue traversed and the frequency of the wave. The frequency of the wave depends on the frequency of the transducer used to generate the wave (see discussion earlier and Equation 86.1). In any given tissue, sound waves resulting from higher-frequency transducers are attenuated more rapidly than sound waves resulting from lower-frequency transducers. Higher-frequency transducers therefore provide a relatively weak echo to be reflected from a deep structure and thus a comparatively poor B-mode image compared to a lower-frequency transducer.

The linear resolution of an ultrasound image depends on the ability to focus the beam. Sound beams emanating from high-frequency transducers can be more precisely focused than those from low-frequency transducers and thus provide clearer B-mode images of more superficial structures. Because the carotid artery is superficial, higher-frequency transducers can be used to provide much clearer B-mode images than is possible with deeper vessels such as the aorta or iliac arteries.

Doppler Ultrasound

In a continuous wave Doppler, a transducer continually emits vibrations into the tissue. Echoes are therefore continually reflected back to the transducer. A transducer cannot, however, simultaneously generate and receive an echo. A continuous wave Doppler therefore must have separate transmitters and receivers to both generate and receive echoes.

Duplex devices utilize pulse Doppler. A pulse Doppler uses the same transducer to generate and receive echoes. Because the speed of sound is relatively constant in tissue, and with a pulse Doppler it is possible to know when an echo is generated and when it is received, it is possible to tell from what depth in the tissue a reflected echo originated. The sample volume of the duplex device is thus determined by specifying from what depth one wishes the pulse Doppler to receive reflected echoes.

The transducer is gated, based on the total time from original sound wave generation to arrival of the reflected echo back at the transducer, to only receive echoes from the specified depth of the sample volume. The "position" of the sample volume is determined from the B-mode image, and in duplex examination of a blood vessel corresponds to particular points within the lumen of the vessel examined. Because B-mode images and Doppler waveforms cannot be generated simultaneously, the technologist must continually update the B-mode image during the course of the examination to ensure proper placement of the sample volume.

When a sound wave encounters moving reflectors, such as red blood cells within the lumen of an artery or vein, the frequency of the reflected wave changes from that of the original wave generated by the transducer. The magnitude of this frequency shift depends on the velocity of the moving reflector and its angle with the incident sound beam. Because the frequency of the original sound wave is known and the frequency of the received echo can be determined by the software of the duplex machine, the velocity of the moving reflectors (red blood cells) can be calculated provided the angle of the incident sound beam with the moving reflectors is also known. This relationship is reflected in the Doppler equation:

$$f_r - f_o = [(2f_o v)/c]\cos\theta \quad (86.2)$$

where f_r is the received frequency, f_o is the originating frequency, v is the velocity of the reflector, c is the speed of sound in tissue, and θ is the angle of the incident sound beam with the moving reflectors, the so-called Doppler angle.

To solve the Doppler equation for the velocity of the moving reflectors, the Doppler angle must be known. To standardize the results of duplex scanning, it has been traditionally

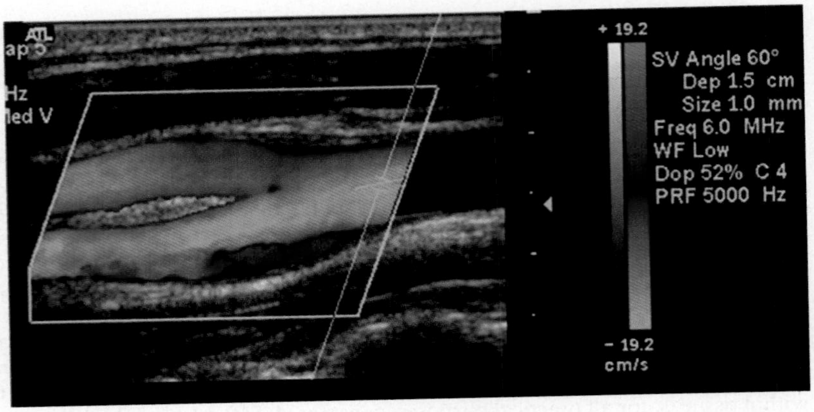

FIGURE 86.1. Color flow image of a normal carotid bifurcation. The color bar on the right of the image indicates that flow toward the probe is blue and away from the probe is red. Note that the black line separating the blue and red on the color bar indicates no Doppler shift. Therefore, when the color on the image goes from red to black to blue, this indicates true flow reversal. The area of reverse flow on the lateral wall of the carotid bulb opposite the flow divider in this image is a normal finding and indicates a carotid bulb free of significant atherosclerosis.

recommended that examinations be conducted as close as possible to a Doppler angle of 60 degrees. At this angle, errors in velocity calculations secondary to misreading of the Doppler angle are small as a percentage of the true velocity. When the Doppler angle approaches 70, these errors become much more significant. Small errors in determining the Doppler angle when the angle of insonation is less than 60 degrees have little overall impact on the calculation of the velocity of the moving red cells. Indeed, Doppler angles from 45 to 60 degrees are acceptable for most clinical studies. Most often an angle of 60 degrees can be easily obtained in carotid artery duplex examinations and, in line with traditional teaching, 60 degrees is chosen whenever possible as the Doppler angle in carotid duplex studies. In examination of other vessels, it may be much more difficult to adhere to a 60-degree angle.

As noted earlier, pulse Doppler both transmits and receives echoes with the same transducer. This dual function places limits on the frequencies that can be displayed in the spectral waveform. The maximum frequency that can be displayed is half the pulse-transmitting frequency or pulse-repetition frequency (PRF), and is known as the Nyquist limit. If frequencies are encountered that exceed the Nyquist limit, they are flipped and appear on the reverse flow side of the spectrum. This is termed "aliasing." If aliasing is encountered, the PRF should be increased to increase the Nyquist limit. The PRF is adjusted by changing the scale displayed on the right side of the spectral waveform or by adjusting the baseline. If aliasing still occurs, the operator should consider switching to a lower-frequency transducer or to the use of a continuous wave Doppler. A continuous wave Doppler is not affected by aliasing.

Color Flow

A color flow image is produced by assigning color to Doppler shifts. Returning echoes that are not Doppler shifted are shown in grayscale. The net result is what appears to be color superimposed on a grayscale image. The hue and intensity of the color are determined by the direction and magnitude of the Doppler shifts. The technologist can adjust the color settings as desired. Varying shades of red and blue are used to distinguish flow away from or toward the transducer. By convention, most technologists assign red to arterial flow and blue to venous flow.

When the Doppler angle is 90 degrees, there is no Doppler shift. When this occurs, the assigned color is black and corresponds to the horizontal black bar serving as the baseline on the color scale that appears on the right side of a color flow image (Fig. 86.1). Aliasing can be readily recognized on a color flow image as a mosaic pattern or as a transition from red to blue or blue to red without an intervening black line. In areas of actual reverse flow, the blue and red colors are separated by a black border. Just as with pulsed Doppler, color aliasing can be reduced by increasing the PRF. This is often quite important, as an extensive mosaic pattern can obscure clear visualization of a stenotic site.

Power Doppler is a variant of color Doppler. Power Doppler, however, assigns no direction of flow to the color image and velocity information is not calculated. Any detected Doppler shift is colorized without consideration of the direction of the Doppler shift or the magnitude of the Doppler shift. It is therefore not subject to aliasing or affected by Doppler angle. Its principal utility lies in the ability to detect blood moving at very low velocity and in outlining the course of tortuous vessels. It can be useful in detecting flow in small distal veins and flow in arteries distal to a very high-grade stenosis.

It is tempting to try and directly estimate the severity of a stenosis from the color flow image. It is generally agreed, however, that such estimates are probably less accurate than measurements of stenosis derived from spectral analysis. Color serves primarily as a guide in locating the vessels and selecting specific sites for examination with the pulse Doppler. The absence of color can indicate extensive mural calcification and difficulty in obtaining a pulse Doppler waveform.

CAROTID AND VERTEBRAL ARTERIES

Historically, the vascular laboratory began with assessing internal carotid artery (ICA) stenosis. Duplex diagnosis of ICA stenosis, and arterial stenoses in general, is based on duplex ultrasound and focuses on three areas, the prestenotic region, the stenosis
3 itself, and the poststenotic region. Detecting carotid stenosis involves a combination of spectral analysis, color and grayscale imaging, and, in selected cases, power Doppler. The primary interest is in the detection of increased flow velocities within the area of suspected stenosis and therefore, in most cases, spectral analysis dominates in the detection of carotid stenosis. The exception is in distinguishing ICA occlusion from a very high-grade stenosis where color flow or power Doppler flow can identify very low flow in the area of the stenosis or distal to the stenosis that may not be detected by pulse Doppler.

In all cases, the pulsed Doppler and color flow findings should be cross-checked for concordance. If there is disagreement between the impression obtained with the color and pulsed Doppler examinations (i.e., color Doppler suggests high-grade stenosis but velocities are only moderately elevated), the findings of both should be reviewed to resolve the discrepancy.

COMMON CAROTID ARTERY WAVEFORMS

In the majority of cases, carotid stenosis or occlusion occurs in the proximal ICA at or just beyond the carotid bifurcation. A

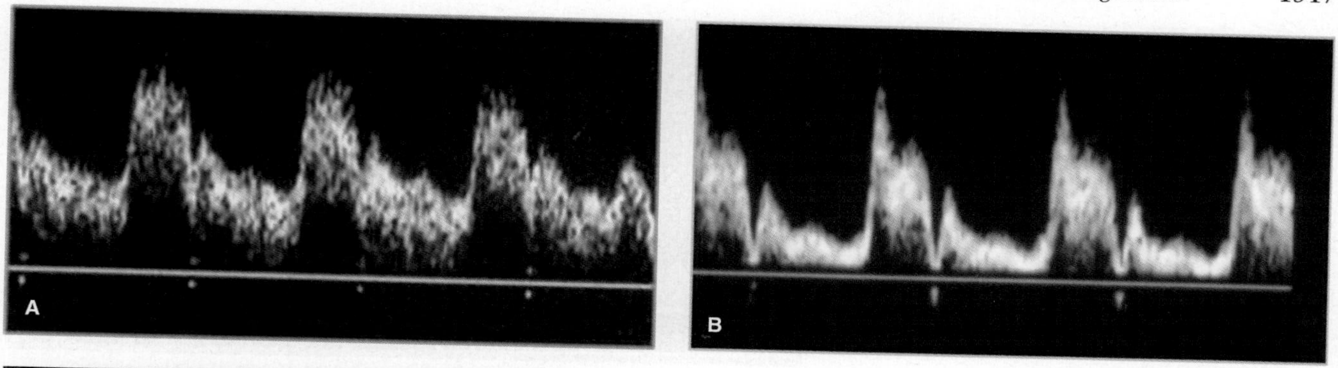

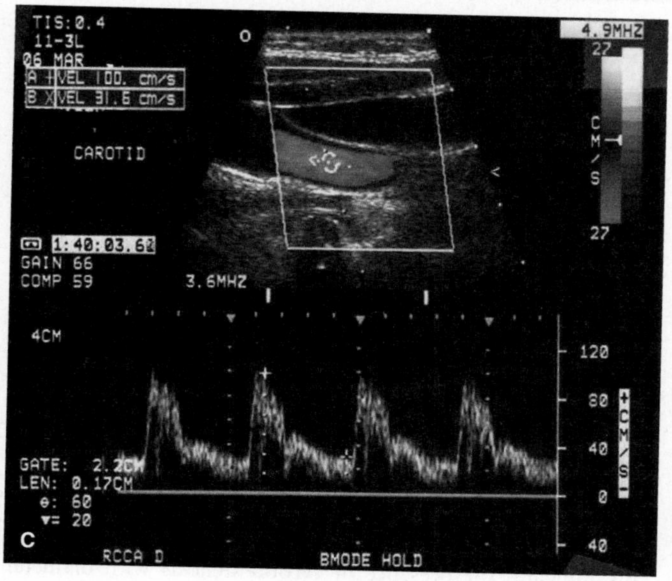

FIGURE 86.2. A normal internal carotid artery (ICA) waveform has low resistance; therefore, flow is relatively high at the end of diastole (A). The external carotid artery (ECA) supplies primarily the scalp and face, a higher-resistance circulation, and therefore end-diastolic flow is lower (B). Normally, 80% of common carotid artery (CCA) flow is directed to the ICA. Normal CCA end-diastolic flow is therefore generally well above baseline (C) and more closely resembles an ICA rather than an ECA waveform.

normal internal carotid artery waveform reflects the low resistance of the cerebral circulation with high flow at the end of the diastolic component of the waveform (Fig. 86.2A). The external carotid artery (ECA) supplies the relatively higher-resistance circulation of the scalp and face and therefore has a low end-diastolic flow component (Fig. 86.2B). The common carotid artery waveform reflects the fact that normally 80% of common carotid artery (CCA) flow is directed to the ICA. CCA end-diastolic flow is therefore generally well above baseline and exceeds ECA diastolic flow (Fig. 86.2C). In the presence of a very high-grade ICA stenosis or ICA occlusion, outflow is primarily through the higher-resistance external carotid circulation. The CCA waveform then takes on the high flow resistance characteristics of an ECA, with flow to zero, or nearly zero, in end diastole[1] (Fig. 86.3). In addition, the peak systolic velocity (PSV) and the overall flow velocity may be substantially lower than normal due to reduced carotid artery flow. By observing these changes in the CCA, one can reliably predict the presence of high-grade stenosis or occlusion of the ICA.

The CCA contralateral to an ICA stenosis or occlusion may demonstrate an increased flow velocity with particular elevation of the velocity at the end of diastole, so-called end-diastolic velocity (EDV). These changes represent a compensatory increase in blood flow volume in the nonobstructed ICA in response to reduced contribution to cerebral perfusion from the opposite carotid artery. This compensatory hemodynamic change can be substantial and stenosis-related flow velocities may be artificially elevated on the side with compensatory high-volume flow.[2]

In the presence of a significant stenosis at the origin of a CCA or the innominate artery, the ipsilateral CCA waveform may be dampened, with low overall PSVs and EDVs and a slower rise to peak systole when compared with the contralateral CCA waveform (Fig. 86.4). The CCA flow changes seen with proximal stenosis are also important in the diagnosis of ICA stenosis because the overall reduction in flow velocity may artificially lower velocities in an ipsilateral ICA stenosis, leading to underestimation of the severity of ICA stenosis. In some cases of proximal CCA or innominate artery stenosis, the ipsilateral CCA waveform may exhibit poststenotic turbulence low in the neck, representing disturbed flow distal to the more proximal stenosis.

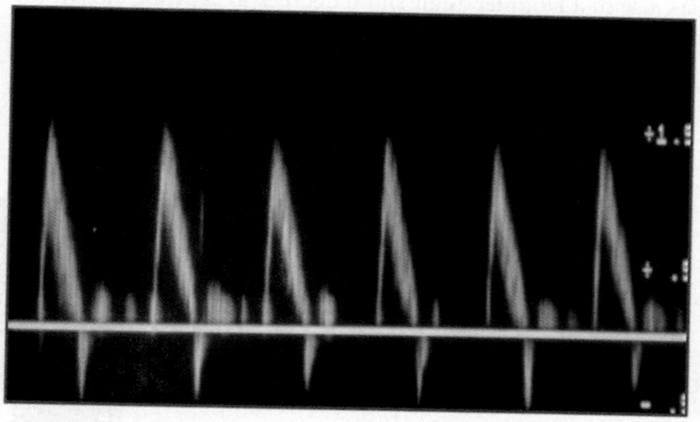

FIGURE 86.3. Common carotid artery waveform from a patient with an internal carotid artery occlusion. There is essentially no end-diastolic flow, indicating that flow in this common carotid artery is now supplying the high-resistance circulation of the external carotid artery.

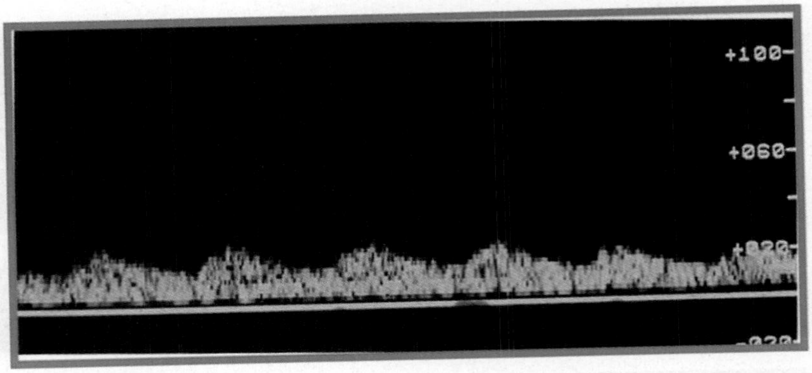

FIGURE 86.4. Common carotid artery (CCA) waveform distal to a more proximal high-grade CCA stenosis. The systolic upstroke is delayed and the amplitude of the waveform depressed, reflecting the presence of the proximal lesion. Diastolic flow is still well above baseline as the ipsilateral internal carotid artery was not significantly narrowed in this patient.

INTERNAL CAROTID ARTERY WAVEFORMS

As noted earlier, the normal ICA spectral waveform is indicative of high flow in a low-resistant circulation. The systolic upstroke is rapid, PSV is less than 125 cm/s, and flow is maintained throughout diastole[3] (Fig. 86.2A). In the absence of plaque there is generally a clear spectral window under the outline of the spectral waveform, as there is little turbulent flow. The presence of color shifts, indicating high-velocity flow, and color mosaics, indicating poststenotic turbulence, aids in selecting potential areas for examination with the pulsed Doppler.

Hemodynamic quantification of the severity of ICA stenosis is primarily achieved by analysis of Doppler spectral waveforms and measurements of peak systolic and end-diastolic velocity or comparison of peak systolic velocities in the ICA to those in the CCA just proximal to the carotid bifurcation, the ICA/CCA ratio. As a stenosis develops, the PSV first becomes elevated. PSV is the principal measure of stenosis severity. EDV lags behind, relatively speaking, as stenosis severity progresses but rises rapidly as the stenosis becomes severe (diameter reductions of ≥60%). Thus, elevation of EDV is a good marker for high-grade stenosis[4] (Fig. 86.5). The ICA/CCA ratio is also a very important measure of stenosis severity.[5] Because it is a ratio, it compensates for abnormally high and low flow states that may skew the PSV and EDV upward or downward.

To accurately measure flow velocity, the sample volume must be placed within the area of greatest stenosis. Color flow imaging has demonstrated that the orientation of the stenotic jet within a stenosis is frequently not along the longitudinal axis of the vessel. This finding has resulted in controversy with regard to the proper technique of obtaining velocity waveforms at sites of stenosis. In areas of mild to moderate stenosis, use of a Doppler angle of 60 degrees to the long axis of the vessel is recommended. However, in areas of more severe stenosis and/or wall abnormalities, the Doppler angle of 60 degrees should be defined by the long axis of the stenotic flow jet, as demonstrated by color flow.

The sample volume size should be kept as small as possible, usually 1.5 mm, to detect discreet changes in flow velocity. This is important as the highest velocities may be localized to a small area in the flow stream that emanate from the stenosis. A large sample volume that incorporates flow from many points within the vessel in the generation of the spectral waveform may give the false impression of disturbed flow, potentially leading to the misdiagnosis of moderate disease in an otherwise normal vessel. In practice, the sonographer, having identified the stenosis, gently moves a small sample volume around until the point of highest velocity is found.

Damping of spectral Doppler waveforms may be seen in the region distal to the carotid stenosis when the lesion is severe enough to be flow reducing. The most common abnormality seen distal to a carotid stenosis is spectral broadening caused by disturbed blood flow or frank turbulence. At best, poststenotic flow disturbance is a qualitative measure of arterial stenosis; nevertheless, its detection is important. With proper gain settings "fill-in" of the Doppler spectral waveform generally indicates the presence of carotid stenosis with diameter reduction of at least 50%. However, this level of disturbed flow occasionally can be seen with nonstenotic disease. Diagnostically, the most significant poststenotic flow disturbance produces a simultaneous forward and reverse spectral Doppler signal, accompanied by poor definition of the upper spectral border. Such disturbed flow implies the presence of severe carotid stenosis. Severely disturbed flow distal to a highly calcified plaque may be the only substantial evidence for the presence of clinically significant stenosis if calcification prevents direct insonation of the stenosis.

Vertebral Artery

On rare occasions, a stenosis may be found in the cervical portion of the vertebral artery associated with cervical osteoarthritis. However, the origin of the vertebral artery from the subclavian artery is by far the most common site of disease in the vertebral artery. The vertebral artery origin lies deep in

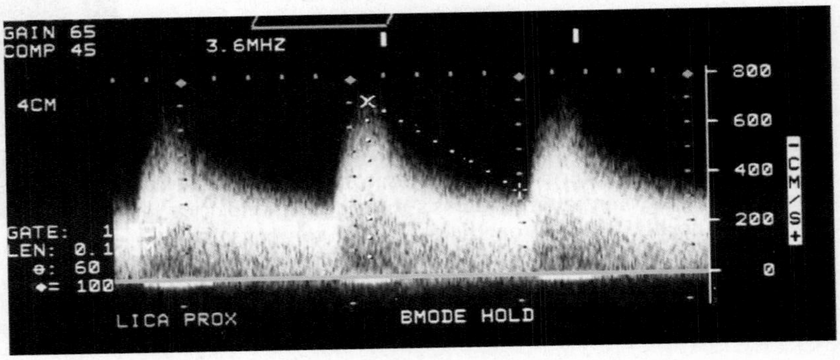

FIGURE 86.5. Internal carotid artery (ICA) waveform from the site of a greater than 80% ICA stenosis. Both peak systolic and end-diastolic velocities are very elevated.

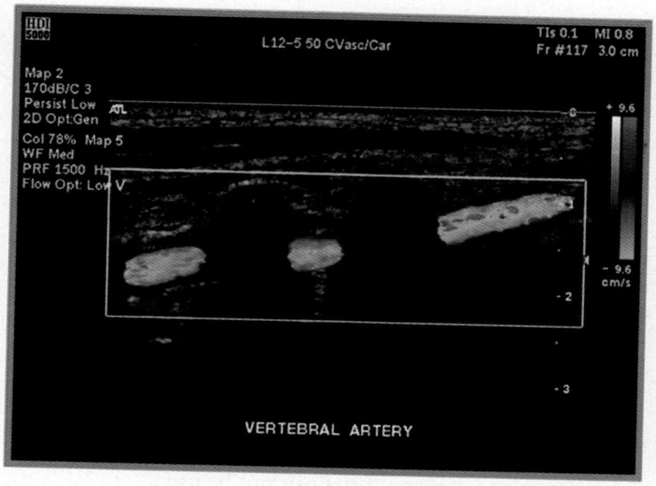

FIGURE 86.6. Color flow image of a vertebral artery. The Doppler cannot penetrate the vertebral bodies; therefore, there is no Doppler shift and no color where the artery passes through the vertebral foramen.

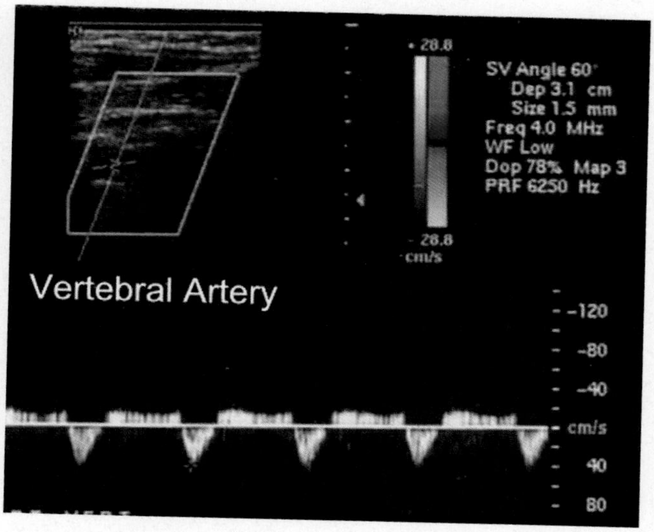

FIGURE 86.7. This patient has reverse flow in the vertebral artery (systolic flow below the baseline), indicating the presence of a high-grade ipsilateral subclavian artery or innominate artery stenosis, so-called subclavian steal syndrome. In the absence of symptoms this finding is of uncertain significance.

the base of the neck and may be difficult to access. Mean vertebral artery diameter is about 4 mm but the vertebral arteries are frequently asymmetric in size, with one, most commonly the left, being larger than the other.

The vertebral artery is most commonly interrogated with ultrasound further distally in the neck, from an anteroposterior window, as it threads through the transverse processes of the cervical spine. The vertebral bodies serve as a reference to ensure the vertebral artery is actually under examination (Fig. 86.6). The artery is usually seen deeper but adjacent to the vertebral vein. Color Doppler is helpful to locate the vessel. A spectral waveform from the vertebral artery in the midneck provides information about direction of flow, waveform shape, and velocity but does not rule out disease at the origin. The normal vertebral artery waveform is similar to that of the ICA with normal PSVs reported to be 20 to 40 cm/s.[6] Velocities up to 80 cm/s are, however, frequently seen without apparent clinical importance and may represent collateral flow through a dominant vertebral artery, or a small but disease-free vertebral artery. Evaluation of disturbed flow distally may help determine which elevated velocities are associated with a vertebral artery stenosis and which are not. Velocity patterns are usually similar in the two vertebral arteries, but systolic and diastolic velocities may differ if vertebral artery diameters are asymmetric. For this reason, if there is concern for stenosis based on an elevated peak systolic velocity in a vertebral artery, recording of vertebral artery diameters is important.

Flow in the vertebral artery flow is normally antegrade with a rapid upstroke and continuous diastolic flow. In cases of anatomic subclavian steal, color flow provides an important initial clue to the diagnosis as flow in the artery will be retrograde in the same direction as the vein (Fig. 86.7). Spectral Doppler must still be used to verify arterial flow and will demonstrate reverse or bidirectional flow in cases of subclavian steal.

External Carotid Artery

The ECA is smaller in diameter than the ICA at the level of the carotid bulb but similar in diameter beyond the bulb. It has little clinical significance in most cases but can serve as an important source of collateral flow to the brain in cases of ICA very high-grade stenosis or occlusion. The ECA may also serve in such cases as a conduit for emboli to the brain, so-called carotid stump syndrome.[7]

The ECA waveform has a sharp upstroke, a prominent dicrotic wave in late systole or early diastole, and velocity that is near or at the zero baseline in end diastole. The PSV of the ECA is normally higher than the ICA. The ECA may adopt the characteristics of the ICA in end diastole as the resistance in the face and scalp decreases with temperature change and/or in the presence of disease.

CLASSIFYING CAROTID STENOSIS

Duplex criteria for quantifying carotid artery stenosis were developed by comparing duplex-derived spectral waveforms and contrast arteriograms. Duplex-derived categories of stenosis are relatively broad. Sensitivities and specificities for spectral analysis of duplex-derived waveforms for detecting an ICA stenosis of greater than 50% to 99% are between 90% and 95%. There are numerous spectral criteria for classifying ICA stenosis. Some focus on categories of stenosis, while others focus on threshold levels of stenosis.

One of the most widely accepted classification schemes for categories for ICA stenosis was developed at the University of Washington under the direction of Dr. Eugene Strandness. These criteria were useful in the study of the natural history of carotid atherosclerosis and in clinical practice. In the University of Washington system, velocity waveform analysis and spectral criteria were used to classify ICA angiographic stenosis as normal; 1% to 15%, 16% to 49%, 50% to 79%, or 80% to 99% stenosis; and occlusion. Prospective validation of these criteria has demonstrated an overall agreement of 82% with contrast angiography. The ability of the criteria to detect carotid disease is 99% sensitive and the ability of the criteria to recognize normal arteries is 84% specific.[3]

Criteria for detecting carotid artery stenosis scanning have undergone reevaluation to remain relevant to current clinical practice. This reevaluation was stimulated by the randomized trials testing the efficacy of carotid endarterectomy (CEA) that took place over the last two decades (Table 86.1).[8–12] These trials have had a profound impact on validating the indications for CEA in patients with carotid bifurcation atherosclerosis. The trials identified significant benefit, in terms of stroke reduction, for CEA in patients with specific levels of ICA

TABLE 86.1

MAJOR RANDOMIZED TRIALS ASSESSING EFFICACY OF CAROTID ENDARTERECTOMY

Symptomatic stenosis
North American Symptomatic Carotid Endarterectomy Trial (NASCET)[8]
European Carotid Surgery Trial (ECST)[9]
Veterans Affairs Cooperative Study 309[10]
Asymptomatic stenosis
Asymptomatic Carotid Atherosclerosis Study (ACAS)[11]
Asymptomatic Carotid Surgery Trial (ACST)[12]

stenosis. In particular, patients with symptomatic ICA stenosis greater than 70% to 99% had dramatic benefit from CEA, while patients with symptomatic ICA stenosis between 50% and 69% and patients with asymptomatic ICA stenosis between 60% and 99% also benefited, albeit to a lesser extent, from CEA.

In the North American trials of CEA, ICA stenosis was calculated from arteriograms by comparing the diameter of the minimal residual lumen to the diameter of the distal cervical ICA.[13] The University of Washington duplex criteria for categories of stenosis preexisted the endarterectomy trials and were developed comparing the diameter of the residual ICA lumen at its narrowest point with an estimate of the diameter of the ICA bulb if it were free of atherosclerosis. Because the bulb has a greater diameter than the distal ICA, the two methods of measurement do not give the same calculated percentage of angiographic stenosis for the same lesion. Calculations of angiographic stenosis using the distal ICA as the reference vessel result in lower calculated stenosis percentages than calculations using the bulb as the reference site. This effect is particularly striking for modest lesions.

In a review of 1,001 internal carotid angiograms, 34% of the ICAs were classified as stenosis of 70% to 99% using the ICA bulb as the reference vessel. In contrast, when the distal cervical ICA was used as the reference site, only 16% of the ICAs were classified as 70% to 99% stenosis.[14] More than 99% of distal ICA-based calculations of stenosis were less than bulb-based calculations. Thus, the duplex stenosis criteria using the bulb as the reference vessel are not and were not directly applicable to the results of the clinical trials.

CURRENT CRITERIA FOR INTERNAL CAROTID ARTERY STENOSIS

Since the randomized CEA trials were completed, additional duplex criteria were developed comparing duplex scans to angiographic ICA stenosis using the distal ICA as the reference vessel in calculating angiographic stenosis. Such criteria are considered more useful by many in selection of patients for carotid intervention because they are directly applicable to the threshold levels of carotid stenosis addressed in the CEA trials.

The initial studies addressing the issue of duplex criteria relevant to the CEA trials were performed at the Oregon Health & Science University (OHSU)[5,15] with subsequent publications from many different institutions, most of which proposed different criteria for the identification of the clinically relevant threshold levels of ICA stenosis.[16–21]

Recognizing that duplex criteria from different centers differed for the threshold levels of angiographic stenosis determined by the CEA trials, a panel of authorities from a variety of medical specialties assembled to review the carotid ultrasound literature. The panel developed a consensus regarding the key components of the carotid ultrasound examination and reasonable criteria for stratification of ICA stenosis.[22]

The consensus committee recommended that all carotid examinations be performed with grayscale imaging, color Doppler, and spectral Doppler. Examinations should be performed by a credentialed vascular technologist in accordance with the standards of one of the accrediting bodies. Doppler waveforms should be measured with an insonation angle as close to 60 degrees as possible but not exceeding 60 degrees, and the sample volumes should be placed within the area of maximal stenosis. The panelists recommended the consistent use of relatively broad diagnostic strata to estimate the degree of ICA stenosis. The panel also concluded that Doppler is relatively inaccurate for subcategorizing ICA stenoses less than 50% and recommended that these lesions be reported under a single category as less than 50% stenosis and that the subcategories for minor degrees of stenosis not be used.

The consensus panel noted that PSV is easy to obtain. However, data suggest that reproducibility of PSV, even among experienced vascular technologists, has sufficient problems that PSVs should not be used as a continuous variable in clinical carotid duplex scanning. Even so, the degree of stenosis estimated by ICA PSV and the degree of narrowing of the ICA lumen seen on grayscale and color Doppler should correlate with PSV as the primary parameters for determining ICA stenosis. Additional parameters such as the ICA/CCA PSV ratio and ICA EDV are secondary parameters and should be employed as internal checks. They are especially useful when ICA PSV may not be representative of the extent of disease. After their discussions the consensus panel recommended criteria, stratifying ICA stenosis into specific categories relevant to the CEA trials (Table 86.2). These criteria have not been subjected to retrospective or prospective evaluation and do not represent the results of any one laboratory or study. They are not meant to serve as a substitute for continuous quality assurance in individual laboratories.

BILATERAL HIGH-GRADE INTERNAL CAROTID ARTERY STENOSIS

Doppler-derived flow velocities from the ICA opposite an ICA occlusion or high-grade stenosis may suggest a higher degree of narrowing than is observed angiographically.[2] This is likely due to compensatory flow. Duplex scan overestimation of stenosis is more common in less severe categories of stenosis than in higher-severity categories.[23]

STENTED CAROTID ARTERIES

Carotid artery stenosis is increasingly treated with an intraluminal stent. However, ultrasound criteria developed for native ICAs are likely not applicable to stented carotid arteries, especially to more modest lesions in the stented arteries. With rare exceptions, the number of patients in studies of stented carotid arteries that have actually had severe in-stent restenosis is small. No study has correlated the degree of stenosis or increase in ICA velocities within a stented carotid artery with clinical symptoms or outcomes. Studies have also not evaluated the effect of the stented carotid artery on the opposite nonstented artery. Currently, it appears that for more modest lesions, higher PSVs (i.e., >125 cm/s) will be needed to identify a greater than 50% stenosis in a stented ICA, whereas criteria to detect high-grade stenosis in native ICAs still work reasonably well to identify high-grade stenosis in stented ICAs.[24]

TABLE 86.2

CONSENSUS PANEL RECOMMENDATIONS FOR CLASSIFICATION OF INTERNAL CAROTID ARTERY STENOSIS

Normal: The ICA PSV is <125 cm/s and there is no visible plaque or intimal thickening. Normal arteries should also have an ICA/CCA PSV ratio of <2.0 and ICA EDV of <40 cm/s.
ICA stenosis <50% is present when the ICA PSV is <125 cm/s and there is visible plaque or intimal thickening. Such arteries should also have an ICA/CCA PSV ratio of <2.0 and an ICA EDV of <40 cm/s.
ICA stenosis of 50%–69% is present when the ICA PSV is 125 cm/s to 230 cm/s and there is visible plaque. Such arteries should also have an ICA/CCA PSV ratio of 2.0–4.0 and an ICA EDV of 40–100 cm/s.
ICA stenosis ≥70%–99% but less than near occlusion is present when the ICA PSV is >230 cm/s and there is visible plaque with lumen narrowing on grayscale and color Doppler imaging. The higher the PSV, the more likely (higher positive predictive value) it is to have severe disease. Such stenoses should also have an ICA/CCA PSV ratio of >4.0 and an ICA EDV of >100 cm/s.
Near occlusion of the ICA: The velocity parameters may not apply. "Preocclusive" lesions may be associated with high, low, or undetectable velocity measurements. The diagnosis of near occlusion is therefore established primarily by demonstration of a markedly narrowed lumen with color Doppler. In some near-occlusive lesions, color Doppler can distinguish between near occlusion and occlusion by demonstrating a thin wisp of color traversing the lesion.
Occlusion: There is no detectable patent lumen on grayscale imaging and no flow with spectral, color, and power Doppler. Near-occlusive lesions may be misdiagnosed as occlusions when only grayscale ultrasound and spectral Doppler are used.

CCA, common carotid artery; ICA, internal carotid artery; EDV, end-diastolic volume; PSV, peak systolic velocity.
From Grant EG, Benson CB, Moneta GL, et al. Carotid artery stenosis: gray-scale and Doppler US diagnosis—Society of Radiologists in Ultrasound Consensus Conference. *Radiology* 2003; 229:340–346.

COMMON CAROTID ARTERY AND EXTERNAL CAROTID ARTERY STENOSIS

Criteria used for classifying disease in the ICA have not been tested for application to the ECA or the CCA. However, as with the ICA, relative degrees of stenosis may be determined by the presence of plaque with B-mode imaging, aberration in color flow on duplex examination, spectral broadening, and increases in PSV. Although not specifically tested, stenosis of more than 50% can be inferred by the presence of a focally increased PSV followed by poststenotic turbulence. As noted earlier, the CCA waveform normally has attributes of the ICA and ECA. The CCA will take on the quality of the "normal" vessel (ICA or ECA) when the other is occluded. If there is a proximal CCA (or innominate artery) high-grade stenosis or occlusion, the ipsilateral CCA Doppler flow quality will be dampened with low PSVs, as compared with the contralateral side. Poststenotic turbulence also may be seen. There are no widely employed validated criteria to give a diameter reduction for stenosis in the CCA or ECA. Stenosis of more than 50% is inferred by a PSV of more than 125 cm/s associated with poststenotic turbulence.

LOWER EXTREMITY ARTERIAL DISEASE

4 The noninvasive vascular laboratory, in combination with the history and physical examination, has a critical role in providing objective diagnosis of lower extremity arterial occlusive disease in asymptomatic patients, those with intermittent claudication, and those with critical arterial insufficiency. Both plethysmographic and ultrasound techniques are used in the evaluation of peripheral arterial disease.

In many patients the clinical history and physical examination is all that is necessary to establish a diagnosis of intermittent claudication (IC). Almost all patients with IC have diminished or absent lower extremity pulses. However, palpation of pulses is subjective and poorly reproducible. Therefore, in almost all cases, the pulse examination in a patient suspected of having arterial disease should be supplemented with objective testing in the noninvasive vascular laboratory. On occasion, a patient will give a history suggesting IC yet have what appear to be normal resting pedal pulses. Exercise testing with postexercise Doppler-measured ankle-brachial systolic blood pressure ratios is crucial to confirm the diagnosis of IC secondary to arterial disease (see later).

Many patients with peripheral arterial disease (PAD) have atypical leg symptoms or are asymptomatic. Such patients have similar increased risk of cardiovascular death as patients with typical IC symptoms. The recognition of these patients has resulted in an increased interest in screening for the presence of PAD in patients with atypical leg symptoms and/or atherosclerotic risk factors.

Patients with exercise-induced lower extremity and/or buttock pain should be asked the location of the pain, its relationship to walking, severity and duration of symptoms, and symptom progression over time. Only exercise-induced muscular pain of the calf, thigh, or buttock, relieved within a few minutes of rest and reproduced by additional walking, can be reliably improved by lower extremity arterial revascularization. There are no data on the response of atypical leg symptoms to revascularization in patients with evidence of PAD.

Ischemic pain is a clinical diagnosis. It is suspected when a patient complains of pain and/or numbness in the forefoot, toes, or instep at rest. In such patients the vascular laboratory can objectively confirm and quantify the magnitude of arterial insufficiency.

PLETHYSMOGRAPHIC TECHNIQUES

Volume Flow

Calf or foot blood flow can be recorded with a mercury-in-silastic strain gauge. Electrical resistance of the mercury column depends on the length of the column and changes in electrical resistance reflecting. Changes in the volume of the extremity, are based on detection of minute changes in the length of the column. However, neither calf nor foot blood flow at rest differs between normal subjects and patients with even rather severe IC.[25] Hyperemic volume flow is often lower in patients with occlusive disease, but such testing can be quite painful for the patient.[26] Measurements of volume flow therefore are not very useful in the evaluation of lower extremity ischemia.

Pulse Volume Recordings

Air plethysmography can be used to display pulse volume waveforms.[27] Pulsed volume recordings are obtained with

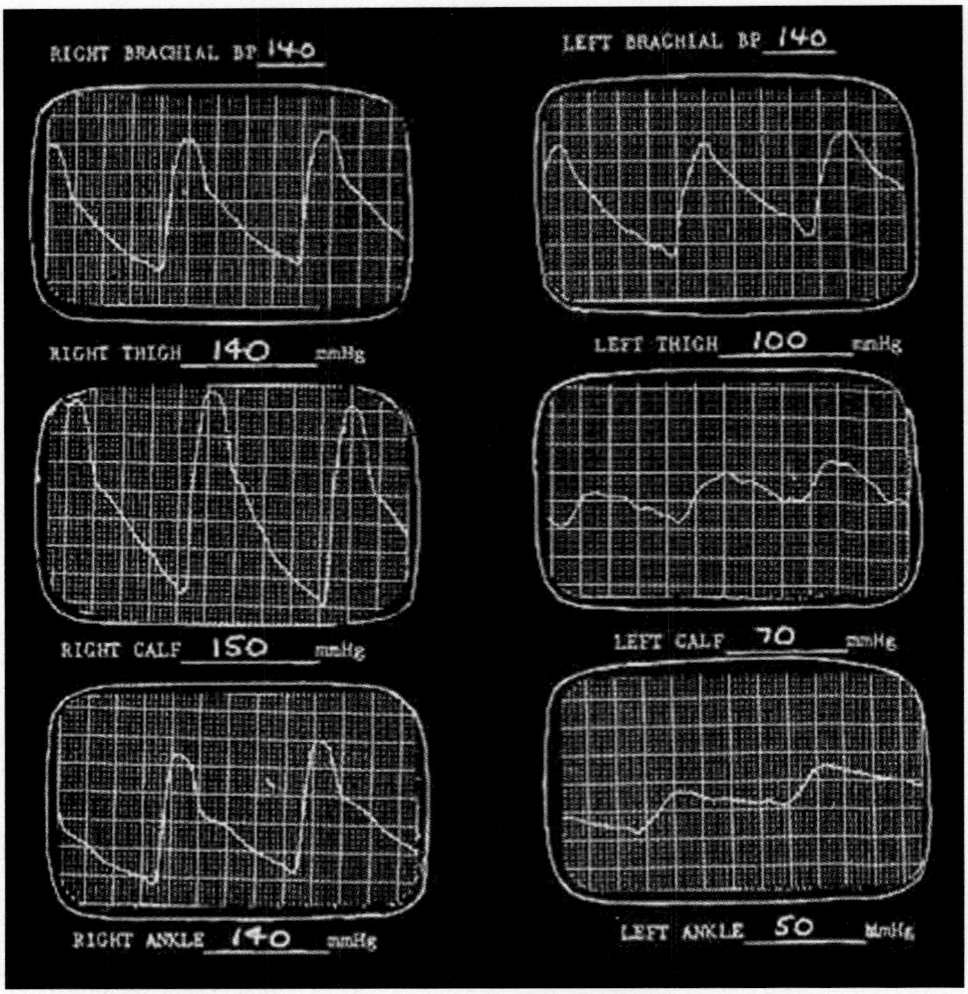

FIGURE 86.8. The pulse volume recordings (PVRs) are normal on the right with rapid upstrokes and a dicrotic notch on the downstroke of the waveform. PVRs on the left are abnormal with loss of amplitude, delay in rise of the waveform, and absence of the dicrotic notch.

partially inflated blood pressure cuffs that detect volume changes sequentially down a limb. Volume changes beneath the cuffs resulting from the pulse wave result in small pressure changes within the cuffs. These changes are displayed as arterial waveforms with the use of appropriate transducers. A normal pulse volume waveform has a sharp systolic upstroke and peak, as well as a prominent dicrotic notch on the downward portion of the curve. With increasing proximal arterial occlusion, the dicrotic notch is lost. The peak of the pulse wave becomes rounded and there is loss of amplitude of the wave as disease is more severe. With even more severe disease there are nearly equal upstroke and downstroke times, and in very severe proximal disease the pulse wave is absent[28] (Fig. 86.8). Evaluation of pulse volume waveforms is qualitative based on the shape of the curve, the presence or absence of the dicrotic notch, and the amplitude of the waveform.[29] Lack of quantitative data limits the utility of pulse volume recordings. More quantitative data for the evaluation of lower extremity arterial disease are available using ultrasound-based techniques.

ULTRASOUND TECHNIQUES

Ankle-Brachial Index

5 The ankle-brachial index (ABI) is a very useful measure of overall lower extremity perfusion. The test is performed with the patient supine and having rested for a few minutes. A pneumatic pressure cuff is placed just above the ankle and inflated to suprasystolic levels. A continuous wave Doppler probe is positioned over the posterior tibial or dorsalis pedal artery distal to the cuff. The cuff is deflated and the pressure reading when the Doppler signal returns is recorded. The sequence is repeated for the other ankle artery and the values compared with the highest brachial artery systolic pressure, also obtained with the Doppler. For clinical purposes, the higher ipsilateral dorsal pedal or posterior tibial pressure is divided by the higher brachial artery systolic pressure, yielding an ABI for that lower extremity. The use of a ratio makes the test relatively independent of day-to-day variations in arterial blood pressure.

A normal ABI is 1.0 to 1.2, with progressively lower values corresponding to worsening arterial disease (Table 86.3). ABIs

TABLE 86.3

CORRELATION BETWEEN ANKLE-BRACHIAL INDEX (ABI) AND CLINICAL SEVERITY OF LOWER EXTREMITY ARTERIAL ISCHEMIA

■ ABI	■ CLINICAL STATUS
>1.3	Abnormal, significant arterial wall calcification
1.1 ± 0.1	Normal
0.6 ± 0.2	Intermittent claudication
0.3 ± 0.1	Ischemic rest pain
0.1 ± 0.1	Impending tissue necrosis

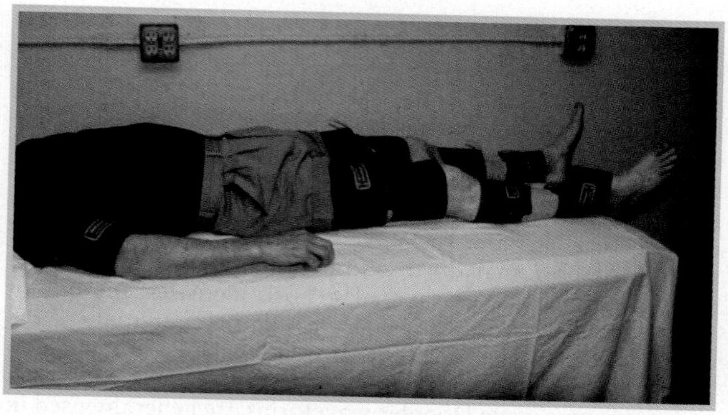

FIGURE 86.9. Placement of blood pressure cuffs for measurement of lower extremity segmental pressures using the four-cuff technique.

below normal indicate relative lower extremity arterial insufficiency and increased risk of cardiovascular death, with the risk increasing with the magnitude of depression of the ABI. This test has several limitations. Significant bilateral subclavian or axillary artery occlusive disease results in a falsely elevated ABI. Calcified tibial arteries that can occur with diabetes or renal failure may be inadequately compressed by the pressure cuff. This also results in a falsely elevated (suprasystolic) ankle pressure. An ABI greater than 1.4 should also be considered abnormal. Such patients have severe arterial disease and are also at increased risk of cardiovascular death. When the ABI may be falsely elevated, qualitative analysis of Doppler-derived analogue or plethysmographic waveforms or measurement of digital systolic pressures is a more appropriate indicator of the arterial status of the lower extremity. Other problems with the ABI include confusion with venous signals when the ankle arterial pressure is low or unmeasurable and relative insensitivity to certain patterns of progression of arterial disease. A tibial artery can occlude without a change in ABI if the remaining tibial vessels remain patent. High-grade stenosis may also progress to occlusion without a change in ABI.

Segmental Limb Pressures

Multiple pneumatic cuffs may be used along the lower extremity to determine the arterial blood pressure at each level (Fig. 86.9). These segmental leg pressures are compared with the higher brachial artery systolic pressure, with other locations in the ipsilateral leg, and with the corresponding levels in the contralateral extremity. Three or four cuffs may be used. In the four-cuff technique cuffs are placed (a) as far proximal on the thigh as possible, (b) immediately above the knee, (c) just below the knee, and (d) just proximal to the ankle. Each cuff width should be 20% greater than the diameter of the limb at the point of application to avoid falsely elevated pressure readings induced by too narrow a cuff.[30] In the thigh, this would generally necessitate a single, wide, thigh cuff. Use of two cuffs above the knee, however, can permit assessment of inflow at or proximal to the common femoral artery with the proximal cuff and permit evaluation for the presence of superficial femoral artery disease with the distal thigh cuff. With two thigh cuffs the most proximal thigh cuff is often too narrow. An artificially elevated pressure in the proximal thigh is then expected. Therefore, the high-thigh index, comparing the proximal thigh pressure to the brachial pressure, is normally about 1.4 with the four-cuff technique and 1.0 to 1.1 with the three-cuff technique.

A hand-held Doppler is used to detect the most prominent Doppler signal at the ankle. Examination proceeds proximal to distal. First, the high-thigh cuff is inflated until the ankle Doppler signal is no longer audible. The cuff is then deflated and the pressure where there is return of the Doppler signal at the ankle is the high-thigh pressure. The above-knee, below-knee, and ankle pressures are similarly determined. If there is no audible ankle Doppler signal, the popliteal artery is insonated with the Doppler to determine high-thigh and above-knee pressures. Comparison of the pressures measured at each location permits an estimation of the location of occlusive lesions (Fig. 86.10).

There are limitations in the interpretation of segmental limb pressures. The high-thigh pressure is subject to particular interpretation difficulties. A diminished high-thigh pressure can reflect an occlusive lesion anywhere at or proximal to the common femoral artery bifurcation. Low high-thigh pressures therefore may reflect a pressure-reducing stenosis in the ipsilateral common or external iliac artery, a common femoral artery lesion, tandem pressure-reducing lesions in the profunda femoris and the proximal superficial femoral artery, or any combination of such lesions. The accuracy of segmental pressures is also affected by mural calcification resulting in artificially elevated pressures. Diminished proximal pressures may also mask gradients that exist further down the leg. Segmental pressures do not allow differentiation between short- and

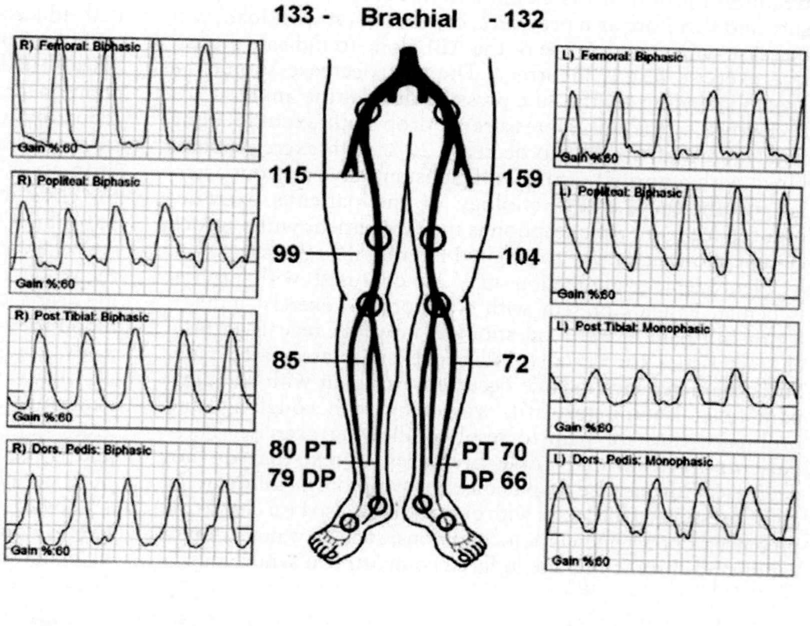

FIGURE 86.10. Segmental pressures indicate the presence of a significant occlusive lesion at or proximal to the common femoral artery bifurcation on the right and a significant superficial femoral artery lesion on the left. See text for explanation.

VASCULAR

long-segment occlusions or between occluded and patent, but highly stenotic, arteries.

Exercise Testing

Doppler-determined pressures can be combined with treadmill exercise testing in patients without a contraindication to exercise. After determination of resting supine ankle pressures and ABIs, the patient walks on a treadmill with a predetermined incline at a predetermined rate. The test continues for 5 minutes or until the patient is forced to stop. The type, time to onset, and location of symptoms are recorded. At completion of the test, the patient is immediately placed supine and absolute ankle pressures and ABIs determined.

In most patients exercise testing serves only to confirm a diagnosis of claudication. It is not required in a patient with classic symptoms of claudication, absent peripheral pulses, and a diminished ABI. In some cases exercise testing can document a physiologic response to revascularization or provide an objective assessment of the potential postoperative physiologic benefit.

Exercise testing is particularly useful in the patient with symptoms of claudication and who has palpable pedal pulses and a normal ABI. Patients with exercise-induced leg pain occurring on the basis of arterial insufficiency will show a decrease in the postexercise ABI. Exercise testing can also be used to document an ischemic response to exercise in patients with PAD and other conditions that may limit their ability to walk. Patients with COPD, arthritis, venous disease, and PAD are often more limited in their walking ability by these coexisting conditions than by their PAD. If the patients cannot complete a treadmill examination, but no ischemic pressure response to exercise occurs, it is highly unlikely their walking ability would be improved by a revascularization procedure.

The precise endpoints and techniques of exercise testing are controversial. Some laboratories exercise patients at low speeds with no inclination of the treadmill, while others utilize various inclines and graded increases in treadmill speed. Both initial and absolute claudication distances can be determined. Initial claudication distance is the point where the patient initially experiences claudication-type pain. The absolute claudication distance is where the patient can no longer continue to walk on the treadmill.

Criteria for a positive exercise test include a decrease in the ankle pressure of 20 mm Hg or 20%, a decrease in the ABI of 0.2 in the symptomatic extremity, or failure of the ankle pressure to return to baseline within 3 minutes of completing the treadmill portion of the examination. Because systemic pressure and therefore arm pressures, depending on workload, will increase with exercise, use of the ABI alone to indicate a positive exercise test is incorrect. The ABI decrease should be accompanied by an absolute pressure drop at the ankle.

Failure of the ankle pressure to drop with exercise along with failure of the ABI to decrease 20% with exercise, combined with a normal resting ABI, substantially rules out arterial insufficiency as the etiology of the patient's exercise-induced leg pain. An exception is the rare patient with buttock claudication secondary to isolated internal iliac disease.

Neurogenic claudication may be confused with arterial ischemia. Patients present with symptoms of exercise-induced leg or calf pain. Careful questioning, however, reveals atypical characteristics for vascular-induced exercise-associated pain. Such characteristics include occurrence of pain with standing, pain relief leaning forward, worsening with coughing, and prolonged time for pain to resolve following exercise. These patients have normal ankle pressures at rest that do not decrease with exercise despite onset of symptoms. Failure of the ankle pressures to decrease with exercise may also be a clue to the presence of other uncommon conditions, such as venous claudication and chronic exercise-induced compartment syndromes.

Doppler Analogue Waveform Analysis

Similar to plethysmographic waveforms, continuous wave Doppler waveforms may also be analyzed qualitatively. Normal lower extremity Doppler waveforms are described as triphasic with a sharp systolic upstroke and an end-systolic reverse flow component followed by low flow forward through diastole. The shape of the waveform changes with increasing severity of proximal obstruction. Initially, the reverse flow component is lost. As proximal stenosis increases, the rate of rise of the systolic upstroke is decreased, the amplitude of the waveform is diminished, and diastolic flow increases relative to systolic flow.

Continuous wave Doppler waveforms are generally used in conjunction with measurement of segmental Doppler pressures similar to the use of pulse volume recordings. Doppler waveform analysis can also be used to assess iliac artery inflow to the common femoral artery. An attenuated common femoral artery waveform indicates proximal disease.

Peripheral Artery Duplex Scanning

6 Arterial duplex scanning provides detailed anatomic and hemodynamic information from the infrarenal aorta to the distal tibial vessels that cannot be determined by indirect testing. Arterial duplex scanning has been prospectively compared with angiography to establish standard criteria for normal and diseased arteries.[31] Sensitivity of duplex examination for detecting the presence of a hemodynamically important lesion (>50%) ranges from 89% at the iliac artery to 68% at the popliteal artery. Overall sensitivities for predicting interruption of patency are 90% for the anterior and posterior tibial arteries and 82% for the peroneal artery. The technique is versatile and does not appear to be influenced by the presence of previous operations or multilevel disease (Fig. 86.11).

Velocity Patterns and Classification of Percent Stenosis

Lower extremity waveforms from normal resting peripheral arteries are triphasic. End-diastolic flow is near zero, reflecting the high end-organ resistance associated with the peripheral circulation. Triphasic waveforms are maintained throughout the length of the lower extremity, but PSV decreases from the iliac to the tibial vessels. There is no significant difference in velocity measurements among the three tibial arteries in normal subjects.

Important changes in the velocity waveforms that signify disease include the absence of an end-systolic reverse flow component and elevation of the peak systolic velocity. A 50% reduction in arterial diameter (equivalent to a cross-sectional surface area reduction of 75%) is associated with a pressure drop across the lesion. The University of Washington criteria for classification of peripheral arterial stenoses is shown in Table 86.4.[32]

A PSV ratio, comparing the velocity within the stenosis to the velocity just proximal to the stenosis, is also useful for grading degree of stenosis. PSV ratios are independent of changes in blood pressure, cardiac output, and vascular compliance. Typically, grading stenoses using the PSV ratio has been found to be highly reproducible.[33,34] Fifty percent stenoses in lower extremity arteries correlate with a PSV ratio from 1.4 to 3.0.[31,35–38] A velocity ratio of 2.0 is a reasonable compromise and is used by many vascular laboratories as indicative of a 50% peripheral arterial stenosis.

Lower extremity duplex scanning can serve as an alternative to contrast arteriography in the preoperative assessment of candidates for arterial intervention. In selected centers,

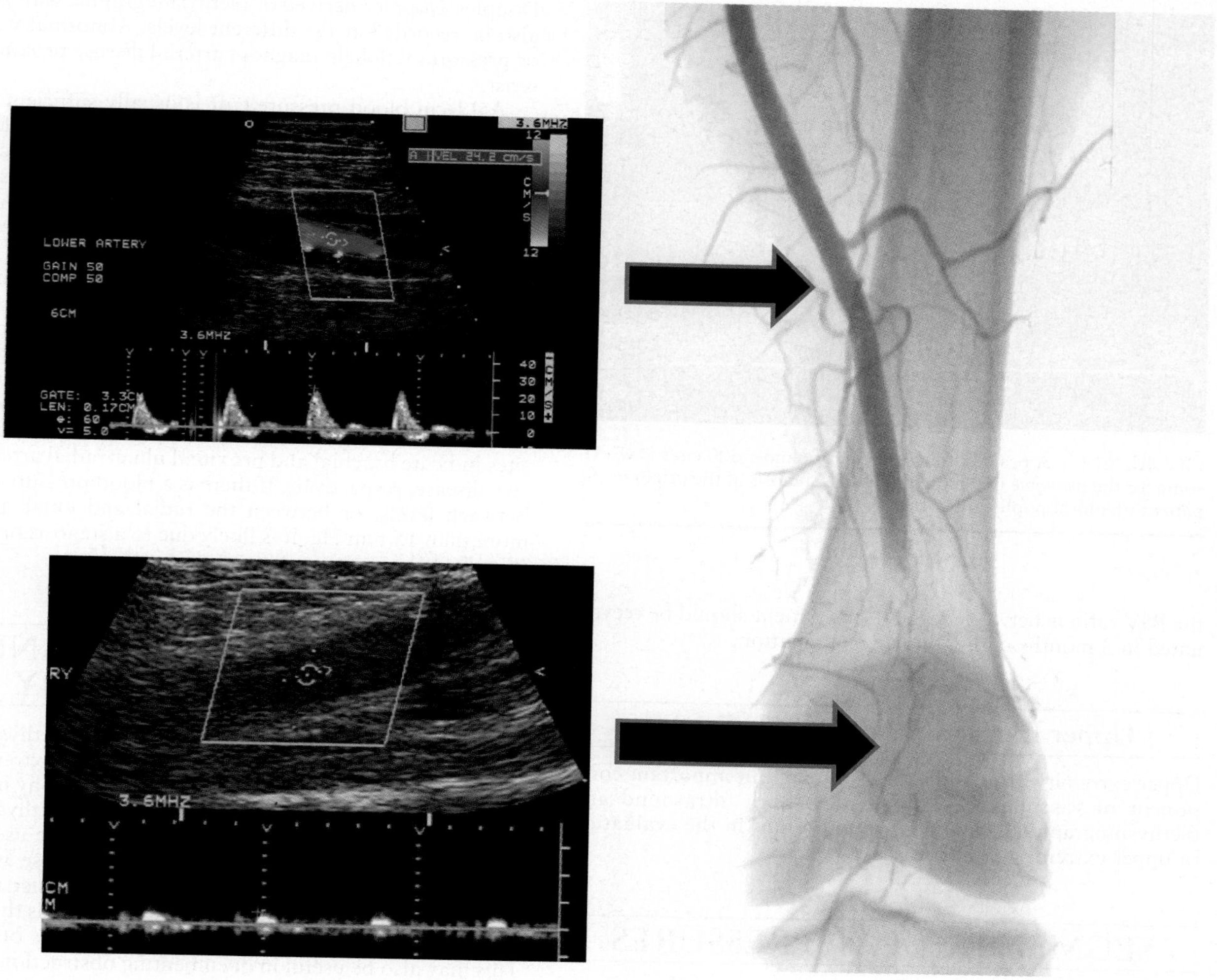

FIGURE 86.11. Duplex waveforms and a corresponding angiogram in a patient with acute lower extremity ischemia. Note the absence of ultrasound-detected flow in the area of the popliteal artery occlusion.

TABLE 86.4

UNIVERSITY OF WASHINGTON DUPLEX CRITERIA FOR DETERMINATION OF STENOSIS IN LOWER EXTREMITY ARTERIES

■ DEGREE OF STENOSIS (%)	■ DUPLEX ULTRASOUND CRITERIA
0	Normal waveform and velocities
1–19	Normal waveform and velocities with spectral broadening
20–49	Marked spectral broadening, 30% increase in PSV
50–99	Marked spectral broadening, 100% increase in PSV
	Loss of reverse-flow component of waveform
Occluded	No detectable flow signal in well-visualized artery

PSV, peak systolic velocity.

successful lower extremity revascularization either by open arterial bypass grafting or with catheter-based techniques has been reported using only arterial duplex in a high percentage of cases.[39–41] The limiting factor with preoperative arterial duplex is the ability to accurately identify the best site for the distal anastomosis of a bypass graft, especially when the distal anastomotic site is below the knee.[42]

The role of duplex ultrasound scanning in the surveillance of lower extremity vein grafts has been well documented (Figs. 86.12 and 86.13). Detection and repair of graft-threatening stenoses detected by duplex scanning appear to improve secondary graft patency.[43–46] Twenty to thirty percent of vein grafts will develop a severe enough stenosis that revision is recommended.[47] Approximately 80% of these graft stenoses develop in the first postoperative year. However, graft-threatening lesions can develop at any time. Surveillance is therefore generally recommended for the life of the graft. A widely utilized protocol for vein graft duplex surveillance is every 3 months for the first year and every 6 months thereafter. The examination involves insonation of the proximal inflow artery, proximal anastomosis, midgraft, distal anastomosis, and distal outflow artery. A PSV ratio of 4, or a PSV above 300 cm/s, indicates a critical graft stenosis, and repair of the lesion by open or catheter-based techniques should be considered.[48] If

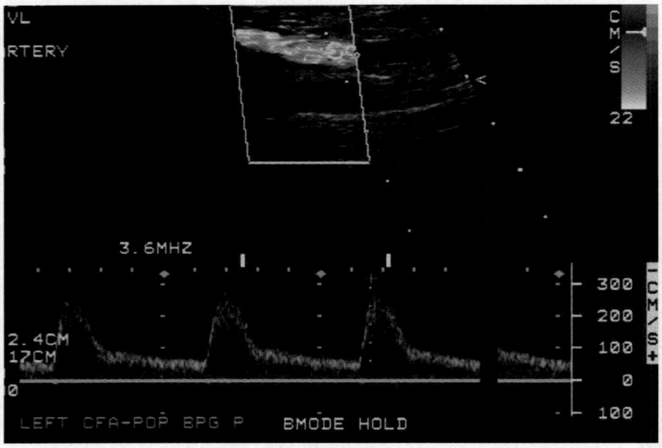

FIGURE 86.12. A peak systolic velocity of almost 300 cm/s is worrisome for the presence of a more than 50% stenosis at the origin of the patient's femoral popliteal bypass.

the PSV ratio is between 2 and 4, the patient should be reevaluated in 3 months with a duplex examination.

Upper Extremity Arterial Evaluation

Upper extremity arterial disease is a small but important component of vascular surgical practice. Both ultrasound and plethysmographic techniques are important in the evaluation of upper extremity arterial disease.

SEGMENTAL ARM PRESSURES

Upper extremity segmental pressures are obtained by measuring blood pressure with pneumatic cuffs above the elbow, below the elbow, and above the wrist while insonating the radial or ulnar artery at the wrist using a continuous wave Doppler. Doppler-derived or plethysmographic waveforms can also be recorded at the different levels. Abnormal waveforms or pressures will help diagnose arterial disease proximal to the wrist.

A 12-cm blood pressure cuff is usually sufficient for measuring the brachial artery pressure, while a 10-cm blood pressure cuff is used at the wrist to measure the systolic pressure from the radial and ulnar arteries. A systolic pressure measurement is taken from the upper arm (brachial artery) and at the wrist (radial and ulnar arteries). Normally, there is not a recordable gradient between any of these sites and a normal wrist/brachial blood pressure ratio is 1.0. If there is a blood pressure difference between the two arms of more than 15 mm Hg, it is likely that there is a stenosis or occlusion somewhere on the side of the lower pressure. Abnormal waveforms and decreased pressures at the above-elbow cuff site indicate axillary, subclavian, or brachiocephalic arterial occlusive disease. Similarly, abnormalities at the below-elbow and above-wrist sites indicate brachial and proximal ulnar/radial arterial occlusive disease, respectively. If there is a blood pressure difference between levels, or between the radial and ulnar arteries, of more than 15 mm Hg, it is likely due to a stenosis or occlusion (Fig. 86.14).

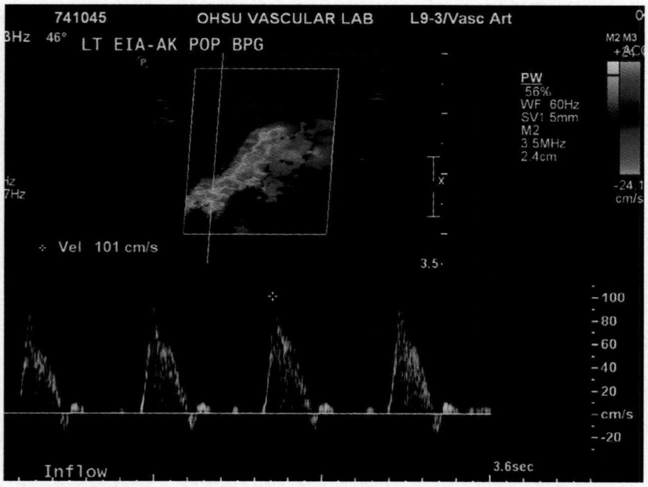

FIGURE 86.13. The peak systolic velocity in this patient's lower extremity bypass graft is normal and the waveform exhibits normal triphasic flow. There is no evidence of stenosis in the graft at this point. The graft must, however, be examined along the entire length of the graft as stenoses can exist distally with normal proximal waveforms and velocity measurements.

DIGITAL PRESSURES AND PLETHYSMOGRAPHY

7 Digital pressure measurements and digital plethysmography are extremely useful in the diagnosis of upper extremity arterial disease and can be as accurate as arteriography in assessing patients with hand ischemia.[49] Either photoplethysmography (PPG) or strain-gauge plethysmography can be used to measure digital blood pressure and to obtain pulse waveforms. PPG is preferred because the equipment is easier to use and more durable. An additional advantage of PPG is that it is possible to record the volume pulses from the tips of the digits. This may also be useful in documenting obstruction within the digit arteries themselves.

The photo cell is attached to the fingertip pulp with double-sided tape or small strain gauges are placed around the fingertip. One-inch (2.5 cm) blood pressure cuffs are placed around the proximal phalanx (Fig. 86.15). Waveforms are recorded using pulse tracings obtained at high speed to evaluate the shape of the waveform. Waveforms are normal if the upstroke time is less than 0.2 seconds (Fig. 86.16A, B). They may or may not have a dicrotic notch. An abnormal obstructive waveform will have a rounded peak, as opposed to the normal notched peak. Upstroke time is prolonged. The amplitude of the waveform is not important. Finger PPG waveforms are not quantitative. The amplitude of the waveform is dependent on the gain setting, not blood flow.

Patients with vasospasm will often have an abnormally shaped waveform termed a "peaked pulse," which is thought to represent abnormal elasticity and rebound of the palmar and digital vessels (Fig. 86.17).

Finger blood pressures are measured by inflating the cuffs placed at the base of the fingers. At reduced chart recorder speed the pulsations are recorded while the blood pressure cuffs are inflated. When digit pulsations are obliterated, the cuff is slowly deflated until the pulsation returns. The pressure reading at this point is recorded and represents the digital artery pressure.

It is extremely important to measure and record finger temperature before performing digital plethysmography and obtaining finger blood pressures. If the finger temperature is less than 28°C to 30°C, false-positive results may be obtained secondary to cold-induced vasospasm. It is recommended that hand and/or whole body warming be performed in patients with low finger temperatures. The technologist should record

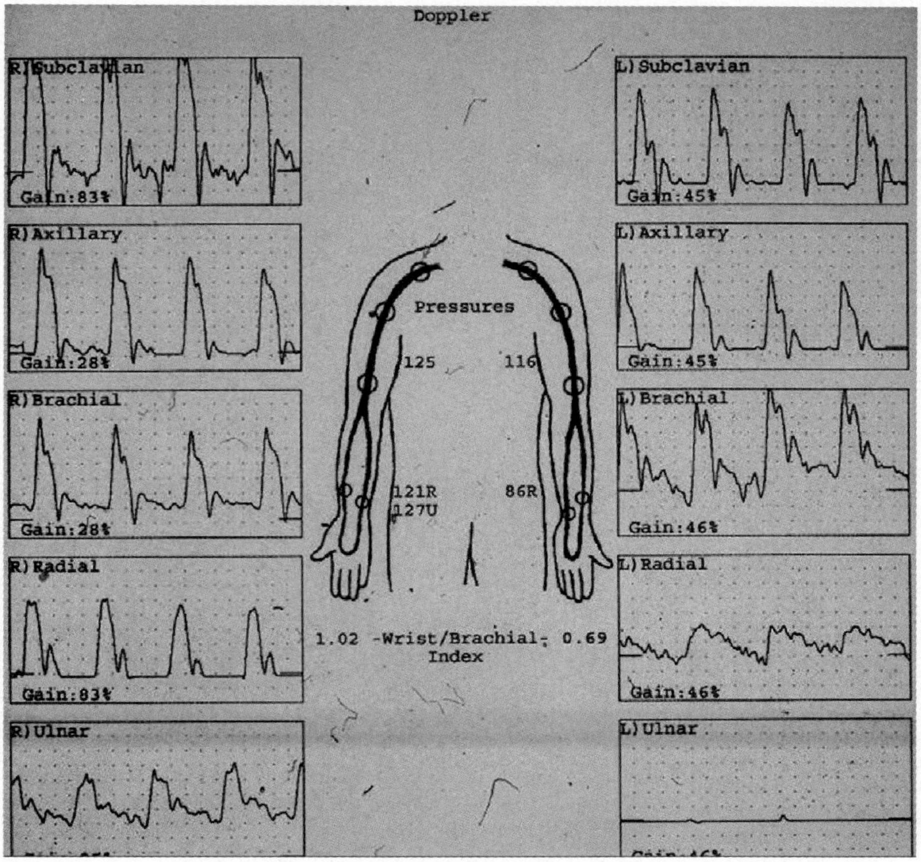

FIGURE 86.14. Upper extremity segmental pressures and Doppler-derived waveforms. Pressures and waveforms are normal on the right but indicate the presence of radial artery occlusive disease and ulnar artery occlusion on the left. The normal axillary and subclavian artery waveforms on the left suggest the absence of significant occlusive disease proximally on the left. The study is compatible with embolization from a left subclavian artery aneurysm.

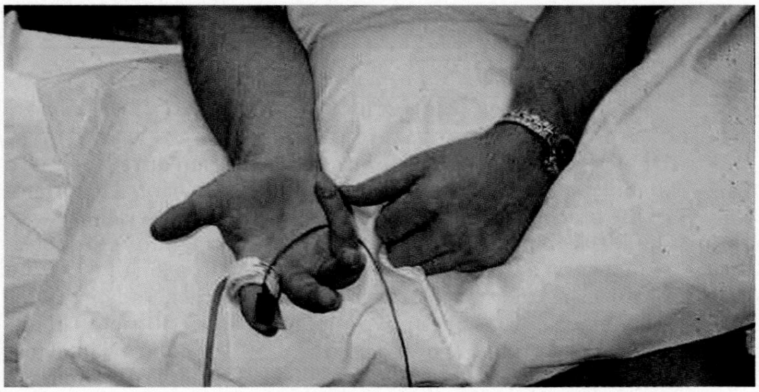

FIGURE 86.15. Digital blood pressure cuff and photoplethysmography sensor for measurement of digital artery blood pressures.

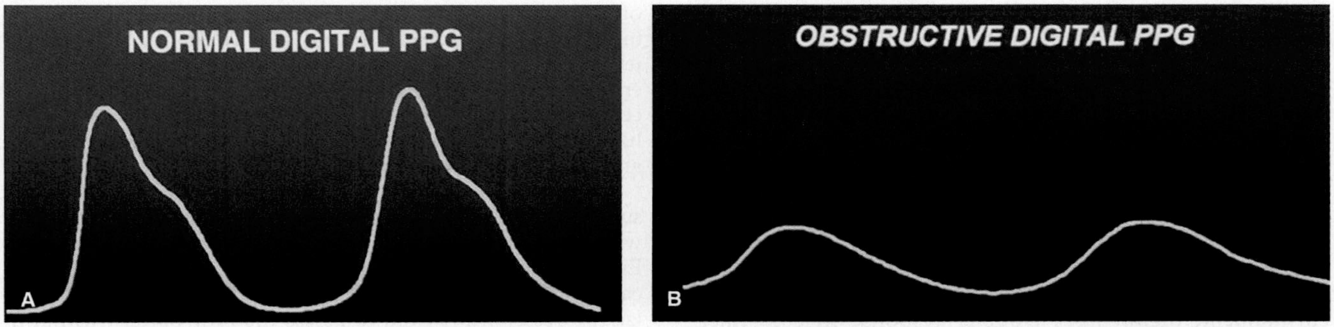

FIGURE 86.16. Normal (**A**) and obstructive (**B**) digital photoplethysmographic (PPG) waveforms. The normal waveform has a rapid upstroke and a sharp apex, while the obstructive waveform demonstrates a delayed upstroke and rounded apex.

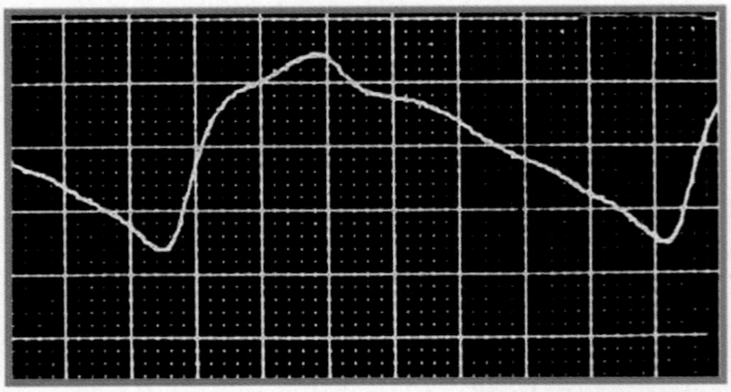

FIGURE 86.17. A so-called peak pulse digital PPG waveform demonstrating a dicrotic notch high on the systolic down-slope of the waveform. This type of waveform can be seen in patients with the purely vasospastic form of Raynaud's syndrome.

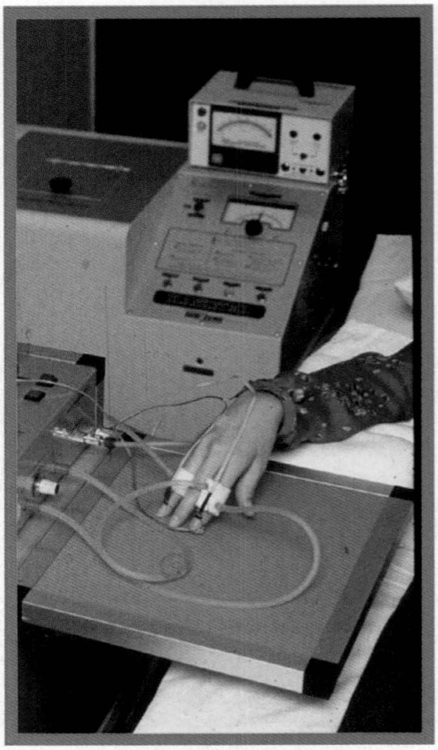

FIGURE 86.18. Device for performance of digital hypothermic challenge or Nielsen test. The cuff on the second finger is used to cool the test finger and measure digital pressure. This allows controlled application of cold to induce a vasospastic response. The fourth finger is the reference finger. Strain gauges on the finger tips are used to measure the digital pressures. See text.

the finger temperatures to ensure the interpreting physician that chances of vasospasm have been minimized.

Digital blood pressure is normally within 20 to 30 mm Hg of brachial pressure. A ratio of finger systolic pressure to brachial systolic pressure of greater than 0.80 is normal but does not necessarily rule out digital artery occlusive disease. It is important to remember that there are occasional patients with very distal digital artery occlusive disease with normal finger pressures since the digital cuff is around the proximal phalanx. Also, occlusive disease in a single digital artery can be missed if the other digital artery in that finger is normally patent.

COLD CHALLENGE TESTING

The simplest cold intolerance test is to measure the digital temperature recovery time after immersion of the hand in ice water for a short time period. Preimmersion digital temperatures must be above 30°C. Hand and body warming may be required prior to immersion.

Using a thermistor probe to measure finger temperatures, the patient's hand is immersed in a container of ice water for 30 to 60 seconds. After the hand is dried, the fingertip pulp temperatures are measured every 5 minutes for 45 minutes, or until the temperature returns to preimmersion levels. Normal individuals will have a recovery time to preimmersion levels of less than 10 minutes. This test is very sensitive for detecting cold-induced vasospasm but is nonspecific, with approximately one half of patients with a positive test having no clinical symptoms of cold sensitivity.[50] Cold immersion testing is also uncomfortable and poorly tolerated by patients with significant Raynaud's syndrome symptoms. Pressures often fall to unrecordable levels in such patients.

A better test for cold sensitivity is the digital hypothermic challenge test as described by Nielsen and Lassen[51] (Fig. 86.18). This test involves placing a finger cuff around the proximal phalanx on the test finger and perfusing the cuff with progressively cooler fluid. The pressure in the test finger is then compared with that in a reference finger that is not cooled. The Nielsen test is interpreted as positive for abnormal cold-induced vasospasm if the test finger pressure is reduced by more than 17% compared with the reference finger.

Other tests for cold-induced vasospasm include thermal entrainment, digital laser Doppler response to cold, thermography, venous occlusion plethysmography, and digital artery caliber measurement. None is widely accepted or employed.[52–54]

UPPER EXTREMITY DUPLEX SCANNING

Duplex scanning of the upper extremity is carried out in a manner similar to arterial examination elsewhere. The origins of the brachial cephalic vessels can be difficult to visualize with duplex scanning. For examination of the origin of the subclavian artery, a 3- or 5-MHz transducer with a small footprint probe using the sternal notch as a window generally gives the best images. A recent study found that 48 of 50 right subclavian artery origins (96%) and 25 of 50 left subclavian artery origins (50%) could be visualized by color duplex scanning.[55]

Criteria for stenosis at the origins of brachial cephalic arteries are slightly different than those used elsewhere. A peak systolic velocity ratio of 2 or more indicates stenosis at the origin of a brachial cephalic artery. Stenosis can also be implied by monophasic flow without actual visualization of a high-velocity jet and by reverse flow in a vertebral artery. Such additional criteria are necessary to assess the origins of the brachiocephalic vessels. If only peak systolic velocity ratios were utilized, there would be higher numbers of both false-positive and false-negative results.[55]

More distally the upper extremity arteries are relatively superficial and fairly constant in location. They are best scanned with a higher-frequency probe such as a 7.5- or 10-MHz probe. Either a sector or linear scan head may be used, but in either case a standoff or mound of acoustical gel is helpful to visualize the vessel clearly and to assess the flow pattern within it. Color facilitates identification of the vessels (Fig. 86.19A, B), and tortuosity of the upper extremity arteries may be more easily seen with color flow imaging.

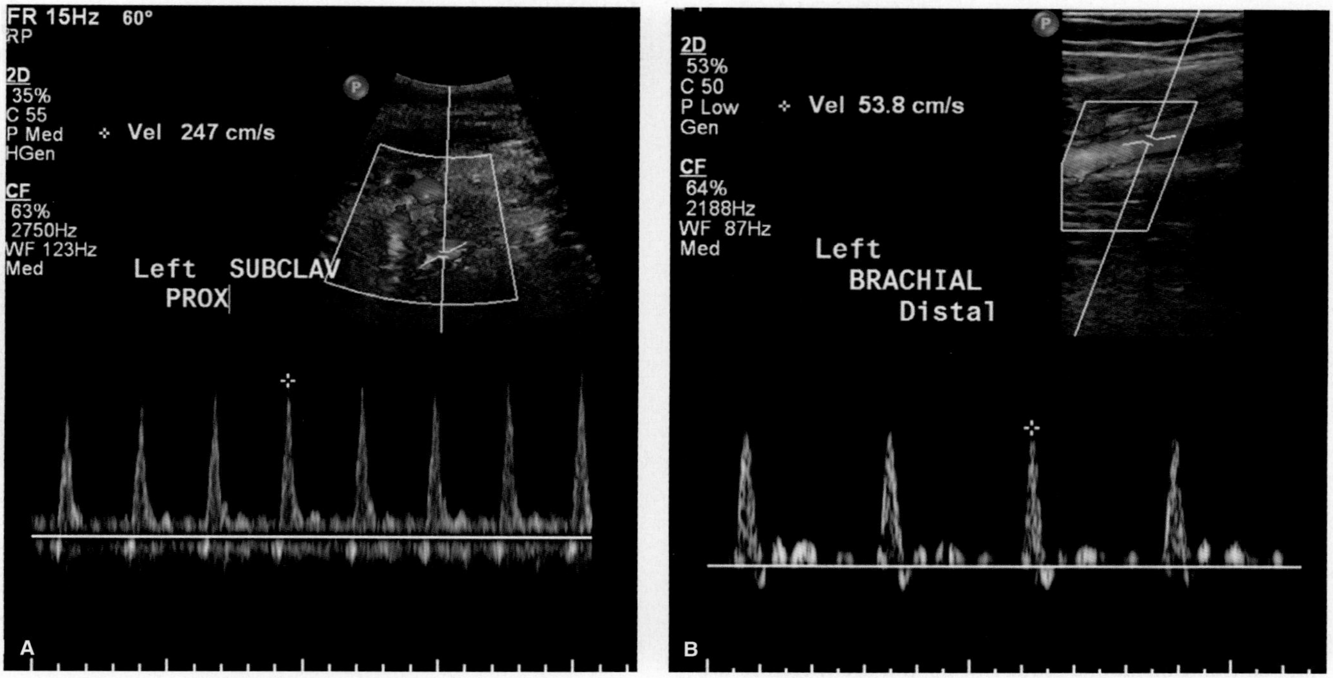

FIGURE 86.19. A peak systolic velocity of almost 250 cm/s (**A**) suggests a moderate to severe stenosis in the proximal subclavian artery. The hemodynamic significance of the lesion can be ascertained by comparing brachial blood pressures in the right and left upper extremities and inspecting distal waveforms. In this case, the ipsilateral brachial artery (**B**) has a normal velocity and a normal triphasic waveform, suggesting that the subclavian lesion is unlikely to be pressure reducing.

The interpretation of duplex findings in the upper extremity beyond the origins of the vessels is similar to the interpretation of B-mode images and Doppler signals gathered in other arterial systems.[56] Normal waveforms in the upper extremity arteries are usually triphasic. As elsewhere in the arterial system, stenoses will produce high-velocity jets, poststenotic turbulence, and dampened distal waveforms. There are, however, at present no specific frequency or velocity criteria with which to gauge the severity of stenoses in the upper extremity arteries. Some general guidelines are listed in Table 86.5. The diagnosis of arterial occlusion is made by imaging the artery and using the pulsed Doppler to show that there is no flow within the lumen.

For patients with unilateral symptoms who may have a surgically correctable lesion such as a subclavian artery aneurysm or stenosis, duplex scanning is quite useful.[57] The duplex evaluation of aneurysms is based on the B-mode image appearance, with the most important feature being the size of the enlarged artery and the presence of intraluminal thrombosis that may serve as a source of distal embolization. Presence or absence of flow within the aneurysm can be determined by the Doppler component.

Duplex scanning may be of use in patients with suspected embolization to identify proximal aneurysms, but the evaluation should also include echocardiography to look for mural thrombi and valvular lesions. While duplex scanning alone cannot be used to make the diagnosis of Takayasu arteritis, it can be a helpful adjunct in following the progression or regression of arterial involvement in response to treatment.[58]

TABLE 86.5

DUPLEX ULTRASOUND CRITERIA FOR EVALUATION OF UPPER EXTREMITY ARTERIAL STENOSIS

■ CONDITION	■ CHARACTERISTICS
Normal	Uniform waveforms; biphasic or triphasic waveforms; clear window beneath systolic peak
<50% diameter reduction	Focal velocity increase; spectral broadening; possibly triphasic or biphasic flow
>50% diameter reduction	Focal velocity increase; loss of triphasic or biphasic velocity waveform; poststenotic flow (color bruit)
Occlusion	No flow detected

VISCERAL ARTERIES

Mesenteric Arteries

8 Duplex ultrasonography can serve as a valuable noninvasive screening test for splanchnic artery stenosis in patients with possible chronic mesenteric ischemia and for follow-up of mesenteric artery reconstructions. Despite the accuracy of duplex detection of mesenteric artery stenoses, angiographic confirmation of high-grade stenoses or occlusion of the splanchnic vessels and appropriate history and physical examination are still required for the diagnosis of chronic mesenteric ischemia. The examination is technically difficult and is best performed by vascular technologists with extensive experience in intra-abdominal ultrasound techniques.

Interpretation of Mesenteric Duplex Ultrasound Studies. In healthy individuals, fasting blood flow velocity waveforms differ in the superior mesentery artery (SMA) versus the celiac artery (CA). Arterial waveforms reflect end-organ vascular resistance. The liver and spleen have relatively

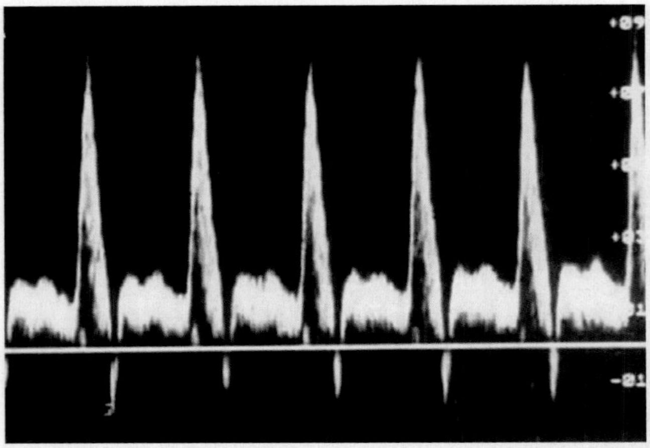

FIGURE 86.20. A normal fasting superior mesenteric artery (SMA) waveform may exhibit reverse flow at the end of systole and relatively low end-diastolic velocity, reflecting relatively high resistance of the intestinal circulation in the fasting state.

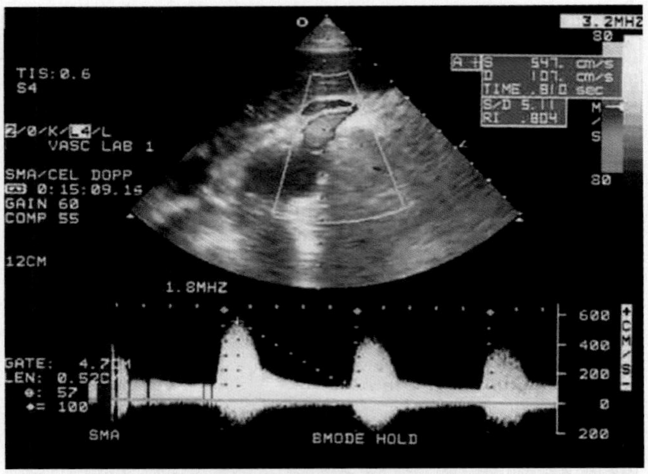

FIGURE 86.22. Color flow image and duplex-derived superior mesenteric artery (SMA) waveform in a patient with possible chronic mesenteric ischemia. A peak systolic velocity of 547 cm/s indicates a high-grade SMA stenosis and is compatible with a clinical picture of chronic mesenteric ischemia.

high constant metabolic requirements and are therefore low-resistance organs. As a result, CA waveforms are generally biphasic, with a peak systolic component, no reversal of end-systolic flow, and a relatively high end-diastolic velocity. The normal fasting SMA velocity waveform is triphasic, reflecting the high vascular resistance of the intestinal tract at rest. There is a peak systolic component, often an end-systolic reverse flow component, and a minimal diastolic flow component[59] (Fig. 86.20).

Changes in Doppler-derived arterial waveforms in response to feeding are also different in the CA and SMA. Because the liver and spleen have basically fixed metabolic demands, there is no significant change in CA velocity waveform after eating. Blood flow in the SMA, however, increases markedly after a meal, reflecting a marked decrease in intestinal arterial resistance. The postprandial waveform changes in the SMA include a near doubling of systolic velocity, tripling of the end-diastolic velocity, and loss of end-systolic reversal of blood flow[60] (Fig. 86.21). These changes are maximal at 45 minutes after ingestion of a test meal and depend on the composition of the meal ingested. Mixed-composition meals produce the greatest flow increase in the SMA when compared with equal caloric meals composed solely of fat, glucose, or protein.[61]

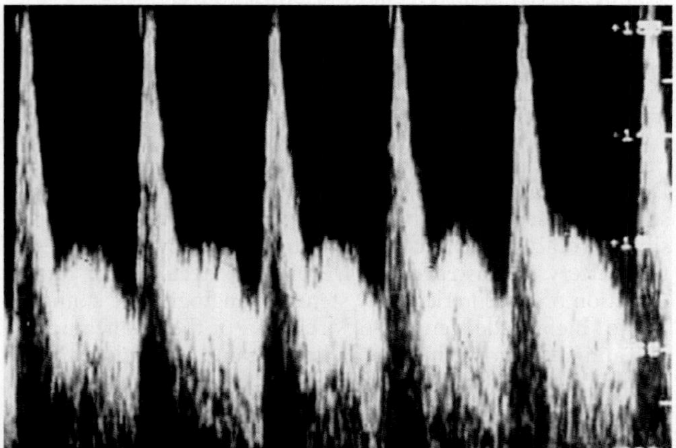

FIGURE 86.21. Postprandial superior mesentery artery (SMA) waveform. There has been, in comparison to Figure 86.20, loss of end-systolic reverse flow and an increase in end-diastolic flow as resistance in the intestinal arterial circulation falls following feeding.

Detection of Splanchnic Arterial Stenosis. Duplex ultrasound can detect hemodynamically significant stenoses in splanchnic vessels. In a blinded prospective study of 100 patients who underwent mesenteric artery duplex scanning and lateral aortography, a PSV in the SMA of 275 cm/s or more indicated an SMA stenosis of 70% or more with a sensitivity of 92%, a specificity of 96%, a positive predictive value of 80%, a negative predictive value of 99%, and an accuracy of 96% (Fig. 86.22). In the same study, a PSV of greater than or equal to 200 cm/s identified an angiographic celiac artery stenosis of 70% or more with a sensitivity of 87%, a specificity of 80%, a positive predictive value of 63%, a negative predictive value of 94%, and an accuracy of 82%.[62]

Other duplex criteria for mesenteric artery stenoses are also in use. An SMA EDV greater than 45 cm/s correlates with an SMA stenosis of 50% or more with a specificity of 92% and a sensitivity of 100%, while a CA EDV of 55 cm/s or greater predicts a CA stenosis of 50% or more with a sensitivity of 93%, specificity of 100%, and accuracy of 95%.[63]

Surgical revascularization of the mesenteric arteries is standard treatment for chronic mesenteric ischemia. Most often bypass grafts are constructed to the superior mesenteric and/or celiac arteries. Mesenteric artery bypass grafts can be followed postoperatively with mesenteric artery duplex scanning (Fig. 86.23). Flow velocities within mesenteric artery bypass grafts vary little with the origin of the graft (supraceliac or infrarenal aorta or a common iliac artery) and remain stable over time. Serially increasing velocities over time in a mesenteric bypass likely suggest the development of a graft or anastomotic stenosis.[64]

Placement of an intraluminal stent is emerging as a viable alternative to surgical bypass in the treatment of mesenteric artery stenosis. Similar to the carotid artery (see earlier), there is reason to suspect duplex criteria developed for stenosis in native mesenteric arteries may not be applicable to stented superior mesenteric arteries. However, to date, only a single study has examined this issue. Mesenteric duplex scans pre- and postplacement of a superior mesenteric artery stent were compared and correlated with pressure gradients measured at

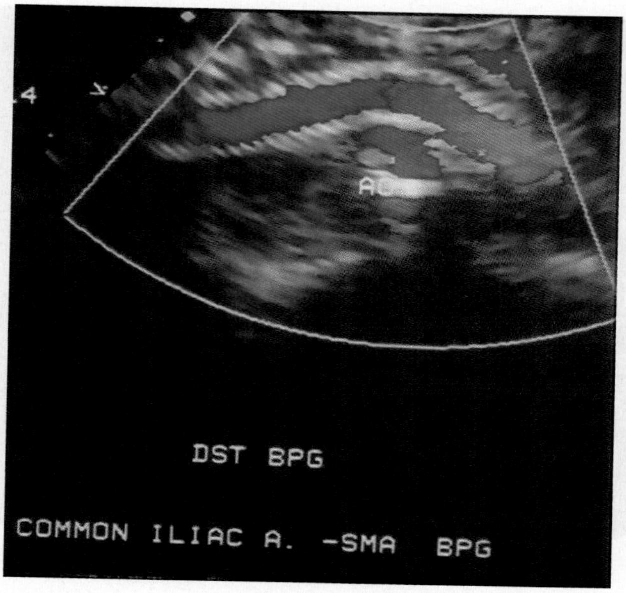

FIGURE 86.23. Color flow image of a common iliac–to–superior mesenteric artery (SMA) bypass graft.

the time of angiography. The data indicate that SMA stenting provides good anatomic results and significantly reduces angiographically measured pressure gradients. Duplex-measured SMA PSVs are reduced after stent placement but, despite good angiographic results, seem to remain in most cases above criteria predicting high-grade native artery SMA stenosis.[65]

Renal Arteries

Indirect Assessment of Renal Artery Stenosis. Indirect methods to assess renal artery stenosis evaluate interlobar arteries. Decreased acceleration times and/or presence of tardus/parvus waveforms (waveforms with delayed or slowed upstrokes) may suggest the presence of a main renal artery stenosis. These techniques are quicker and easier to perform than direct examination of the main renal artery but have not been widely validated. Improved visualization of the main renal arteries with modern duplex scanners has made indirect methods of assessing the main renal artery essentially obsolete. These techniques are even less accurate in patients with bilateral stenoses and are not applicable in patients with a single patent renal artery.

Direct Assessment of Renal Artery Stenosis. Normal renal arteries have a PSV less than 180 cm/s and low-resistance waveforms reflecting the high metabolic demands of the kidney. A ratio of the PSV in the renal artery to that in the aorta (renal-to-aortic ratio [RAR]) of 3.5 or higher indicates a greater than or equal to 60% diameter-reducing renal artery stenosis (84% to 88% sensitivity, 97% to 99% specificity, 94% to 98% positive predictive value)[66] (Fig. 8.24). A PSV of greater than or equal to 200 cm/s has also been suggested to indicate a renal artery stenosis of 60% or more, while a velocity in the renal artery of greater than 185 cm/s has been suggested to indicate a less than 60% renal artery stenosis. Therefore, a renal artery can be considered normal when the PSV is less than 180 cm/s and the RAR is less than 3.5. With a PSV greater than 180 cm/s and a RAR less than 3.5, the renal artery can be considered to have a less than 60% stenosis. RARs of greater than 3.5 indicate a greater than 60% renal artery stenosis regardless of whether the renal artery PSV is less than

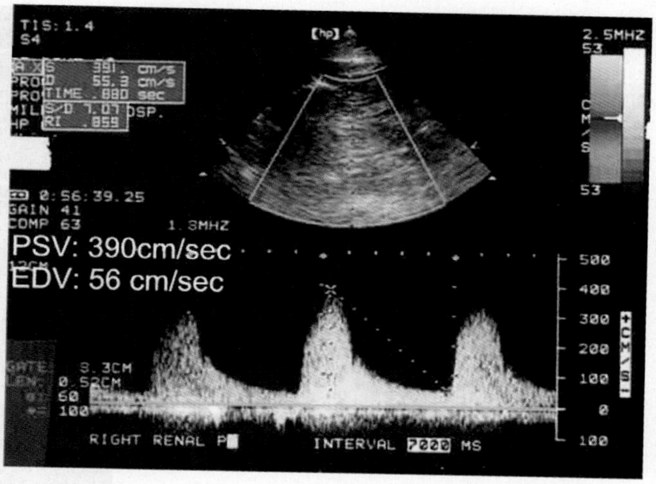

FIGURE 86.24. Renal artery waveform in a patient with severe hypertension. The high peak systolic velocity is compatible with a high-grade stenosis of the right renal artery.

or more than 180 cm/s.[67] When the end-diastolic velocity exceeds 150 cm/s, data suggest a greater than 80% renal artery stenosis.[68] The same criteria have been used to evaluate the patency of renal arterial reconstructions but, similar to stented carotid and mesenteric arteries, may need modification for stented renal arteries.[69]

Predicting Success of Renal Artery Interventions. EDVs tend to be lower in patients with renal insufficiency, indicating decreased diastolic flow and suggesting increased parenchymal resistance to blood flow. Decreased parenchymal diastolic velocities may therefore suggest renal parenchymal disease (Fig. 86.25). Many patients, 20% to 40%, treated with renal artery angioplasty and stenting or open surgical reconstructions do not have postprocedure blood pressure or renal function improvement. An estimate of resistance to flow within the renal parenchyma can be made by comparisons of EDVs and PSVs of renal artery waveforms obtained from renal

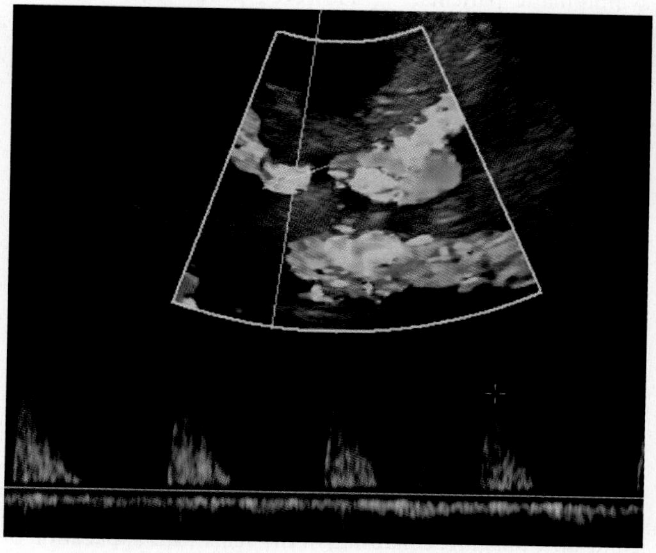

FIGURE 86.25. Low diastolic flow from the parenchyma of this transplanted kidney suggests parenchymal renal disease.

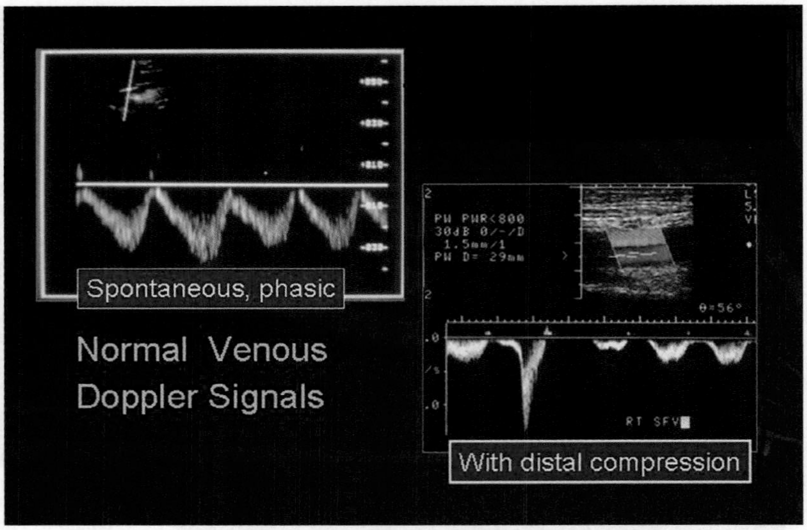

FIGURE 86.26. Venous flow is typically depicted below the baseline. Venous flow in the proximal lower extremity veins should be spontaneous, vary with respiration, and augment with distal compression.

parenchymal arteries. The so-called resistive index (RI) is calculated as follows:

$$RI = [1 - (EDV/PSV)] \times 100$$

In effect, a high resistive index, greater than 0.7, is bad, suggesting renal parenchymal disease, while a low resistive index is good, indicating healthy renal parenchymal tissues. Evaluation of parenchymal resistance has been suggested as a possible preprocedure predictor of clinical success of renal artery interventions.[70]

VENOUS DISEASE

Acute Deep Venous Thrombosis

9 Physical examination is not sensitive or specific for the detection of acute deep venous thrombosis (DVT).[71] Prior to the acceptance and widespread use of venous duplex scanning, impedance plethysmography (IPG) was employed as the initial noninvasive test for patients with suspected acute lower extremity DVT. IPG is a reasonably sensitive (87%) and specific (up to 100%) test for proximal lower extremity DVT in symptomatic patients.[72–74] However, lower sensitivities for proximal DVT (65%) have been reported in studies that exclude clinical outcomes and only report in comparison to venography. IPG may not detect nonocclusive proximal DVT or occlusive proximal DVT present in parallel venous systems, such as duplicated femoral or popliteal veins, and cannot detect DVT isolated to the calf veins.[75,76] While IPG is still sometimes used for clinical situations felt to require serial evaluations of the proximal veins, the limitations noted here make it a substandard examination for routine clinical assessment of lower extremity DVT.[77] Currently, color flow duplex scanning performed by skilled operators provides the most practical and cost-effective method for assessment of DVT of the lower and upper extremity veins as well as for superficial venous thrombosis.

At a minimum, vascular laboratory duplex ultrasound evaluation for lower extremity DVT should include examination of the common femoral, profunda femoral, femoral, and popliteal veins. Venous waveforms from the right and left common femoral veins should always be compared. A normal lower extremity examination will show patency of the veins on color flow imaging, collapsing of the veins with application of pressure by the ultrasound probe, and venous flow patterns in the common femoral and femoral veins that decrease with inspiration and increase with expiration. Flow within a patent vein should also increase with application of compression distal to the site of examination (Fig. 86.26).

The primary ultrasound diagnostic criteria for acute venous thrombosis is failure of the vein to collapse with application of pressure with the ultrasound probe (Fig. 86.27). A continuous flow pattern in one common femoral vein and not the other suggests ipsilateral iliac vein thrombosis or external compression of the ipsilateral iliac vein. Bilateral pulsatile common femoral waveforms suggest volume overload, tricuspid regurgitation, or heart failure.

Not all venous ultrasound examinations for DVT are the same. Some vascular laboratories do not include evaluation of the calf veins as part of their routine evaluation for lower extremity DVT, even in symptomatic patients. This results from outdated perceptions of inaccuracy of calf vein ultrasound evaluation for DVT. Failure to perform a complete initial examination necessitates serial ultrasound examinations or alternative strategies to detect possible extension of venous thrombi initially isolated to the calf veins. Such strategies are inefficient, ineffective for noncompliant patients, and not cost-effective compared to a single stand-alone color flow duplex study of the proximal and calf veins in patients with suspected lower extremity DVT.

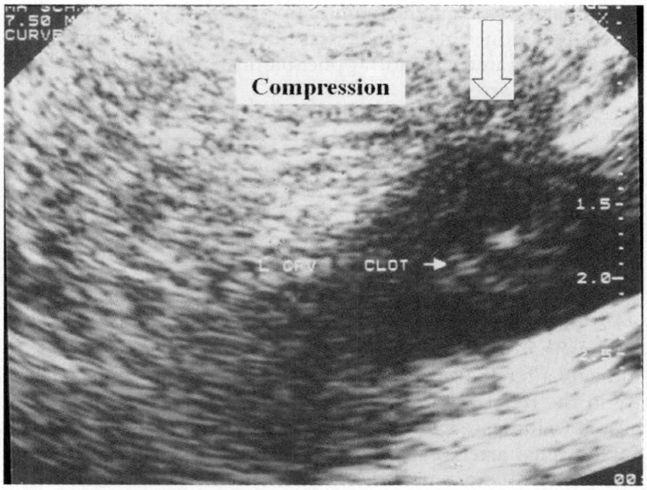

FIGURE 86.27. Failure of the common femoral vein to compress with pressure applied by the ultrasound scanhead indicates the presence of thrombus in the common femoral vein.

Limited ultrasound studies for acute DVT may include compression ultrasound (B-mode imaging only), duplex ultrasound (B-mode imaging and Doppler waveform analysis), and color Doppler alone. The sensitivities and specificities for detecting acute DVT differ among the examinations, and different examinations are appropriate for different veins. Compression ultrasound is typically performed for evaluation of proximal deep veins, specifically the common femoral, femoral, and popliteal veins. A combination of duplex ultrasound and color Doppler is more often used for calf and iliac veins. Color flow alone may be used to assess patency of the calf veins as they are difficult to reliably compress especially in subjects with larger legs.

Many factors will influence which venous segments can be evaluated in an individual examination. These include the presence of morbid obesity, lower extremity edema or tenderness, and the presence of immobilization devices and bandages. Overall, a complete color and Doppler examination has become the standard of care for assessment of lower extremity DVT. It is recommended that whenever possible, a venous duplex examination to exclude the presence of DVT consist of an evaluation of both the proximal and calf veins.

A well-trained technologist can interrogate calf veins in 80% to 98% of cases using a combination of B mode, Doppler waveform analysis, and color Doppler.[78,79] Overall accuracy of venous ultrasonography in comparison to venography has been well established. The weighted mean sensitivity and specificity of venous ultrasonography (including all types) for the diagnosis of symptomatic proximal DVT are 97% and 94%, respectively.[77] As suggested earlier, in technically adequate studies, the sensitivity and specificity of color Doppler to identify isolated calf vein thrombosis exceeds 90%.[79] The high specificity of venous ultrasonography allows treatment for DVT to be initiated without further confirmatory tests, and the high sensitivity in diagnosing proximal DVT makes it possible to withhold treatment if the examination is negative.

Some ultrasound examinations are limited by practical constraints. Inability of the patient to fully cooperate with regard to positioning for the examination and/or intolerance of the pressure of the ultrasound scan head on the skin, or inability of the examiner to obtain a complete examination secondary to bandages, casts, or extremity wounds, may lead to a requirement for serial examinations. An alternative diagnostic procedure, such as catheter-based contrast, magnetic resonance (MR), or computed tomography (CT) venography, may be indicated when a complete ultrasound examination is not possible or if the patient cannot or is unlikely to return for a follow-up examination. Currently, repeat or serial venous ultrasonography is advisable for negative examinations in symptomatic patients highly suspicious for DVT in whom an alternative form of imaging is unavailable or contraindicated.

The diagnosis of pulmonary embolism (PE), like that for DVT, also cannot be established without objective testing. Several studies have evaluated lower extremity venous ultrasound examinations in patients suspected of PE. These studies, often employing ultrasound of only the proximal veins and nuclear medicine–based ventilation-perfusion (V/Q) scanning, unfortunately have little relevance to modern practice where complete proximal and distal vein ultrasound examinations are usually routine, and where CT pulmonary angiography (CTPA) or MR pulmonary angiography (MRPA) have largely supplanted V/Q scanning.

The rationale for venous ultrasonography in patients who present with symptoms of PE is that a diagnosis of DVT may indirectly suggest a diagnosis of PE, making additional investigation to exclude PE unnecessary in some clinical settings. However, ultrasound cannot make a definitive diagnosis of PE. Patients can have DVT and pulmonary symptoms or hemodynamic instability from causes other than PE.

Normal bilateral proximal venous ultrasound scans do not rule out PE. When PE is definitively present, DVT of the proximal lower extremity veins is detectable by compression ultrasound in only 50% of patients.[80] When a PE is objectively diagnosed with no evidence of lower extremity DVT, the PE may have originated from pelvic veins or arm veins, or possibly embolized completely from a lower extremity vein. An objective diagnostic test for PE is therefore indicated in most cases. Currently, in most centers this would be a CT pulmonary angiogram.

Chronic Venous Insufficiency

The presence of venous insufficiency can also be evaluated with either air or photoplethysmography and with duplex scanning.[81] In theory, air plethysmography (APG) can provide an analysis of overall venous hemodynamics including evaluation of the individual components of venous function, reflux, and the efficacy of the calf muscle pump. A flexible chamber is placed on the calf and volume changes are then induced by a series of positional and exercise maneuvers. Measurements derived from these maneuvers are then used to calculate measures of venous reflux (venous filling index [VFI]) and calf muscle pump function (ejection fraction [EF]) as well as a measure of overall venous function, termed the residual volume fraction. Of these values, VFI has the potential for being the most important. A VFI of greater than 2 mL/s indicates abnormal reflux, with values greater than 10 mL/s indicating increased risk of cutaneous changes associated with chronic venous insufficiency. APG, while theoretically interesting, is used only infrequently in clinical practice.

PPG is a variant of plethysmography techniques to assess venous reflux. It detects changes in the blood content of the skin that theoretically reflect venous volume. It consists of a light-emitting diode and a photosensor. The diode transmits light into subcutaneous tissues. Blood attenuates light in proportion to its content in tissue. The PPG machine amplifies the difference between the transmitted and reflected signal and converts it into a waveform. To assess for venous reflux the sensor is typically applied to the medial ankle area (Fig. 86.28). The patient performs a series of plantar and dorsal flexions of

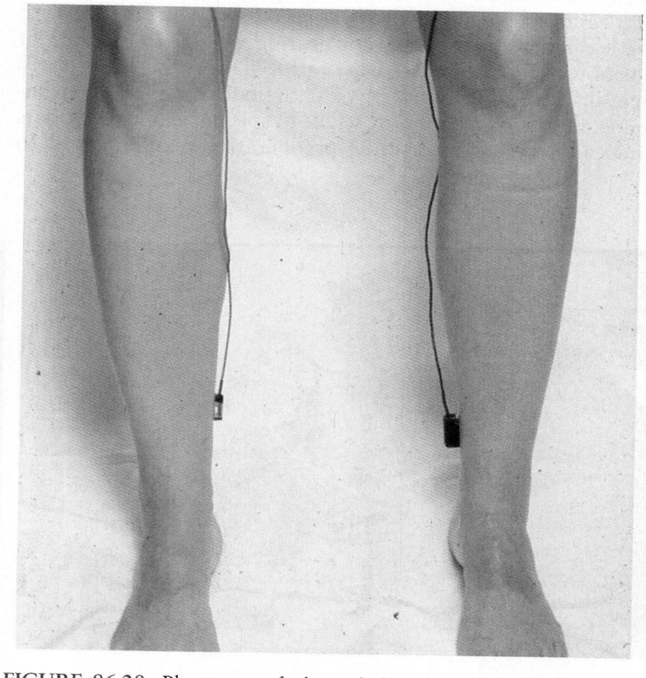

FIGURE 86.28. Placement of photoplethysmographic (PPG) probes for assessment of venous reflux. See text.

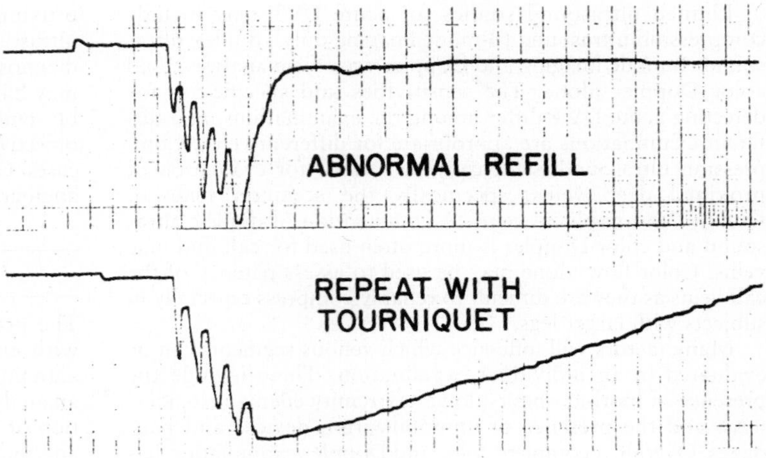

FIGURE 86.29. Venous photoplethysmographic (PPG) waveforms in a patient with superficial venous reflux. The patient is asked to perform 10 dorsal and plantar flexions of the ankle, resulting in emptying the leg of venous blood. In the top panel the veins refill very rapidly, indicating the presence of venous reflux. Refill slows with application of a tourniquet to occlude the superficial veins, indicating this patient likely has only reflux in the superficial venous system and no deep venous reflux.

the foot, decreasing the venous volume of the extremity. The time for the waveform to return to baseline is termed the "venous recovery time" (VRT). A normal venous recovery is 20 seconds or greater. Shorter times indicate the presence of venous reflux. If the VRT returns to normal with the application of a superficial venous tourniquet, then the reflux is confined to the superficial venous system (Fig. 86.29). If the VRT does not correct with a superficial venous tourniquet, deep venous reflux is present. Neither APG nor PPG can provide information about the specific venous segments that are abnormal. That information can be provided by duplex ultrasound.

Duplex ultrasound can provide important physiologic and anatomic information in patients with possible chronic venous insufficiency. Both sites of reflux and of venous obstruction can be determined in deep, superficial, and perforating veins. In patients with valve incompetence, reflux can be stimulated and then detected with duplex using a Valsalva maneuver, manual compression proximal to the transducer, or release of compression distal to the transducer. The examination has been standardized with the patient upright and using deflation of a series of pneumatic cuffs at specific sites on the leg with the leg under examination not bearing weight. In the upright position, reflux stimulated by cuff deflation that lasts more than 0.5 second is indicative of pathologic reflux.[82] The technique allows localization of reflux to specific venous segments and can serve as a valuable preoperative planning tool to target specific venous segments for removal or reconstruction (Fig. 86.30A, B). It has a sensitivity of 82% and specificity of 100% for the identification of competent and incompetent perforating veins. Duplex determination of reflux sites and sites of venous occlusion as a means of assessing overall venous hemodynamics is not established. Currently, duplex assessment of venous reflux provides the basis of planning for the large majority of venous procedures designed to treat the manifestations of superficial venous reflux.

SELECTED MISCELLANEOUS EXAMINATIONS

Evaluation for Abdominal Aortic Aneurysm

10 Vascular laboratory ultrasound screening of males older than 65 years with a history of cigarette smoking for abdominal aortic aneurysm (AAA) has been shown to be effective in preventing aneurysm-related deaths in this cohort.[83] Ultrasound is highly accurate and reproducible in measuring the diameter of infrarenal AAAs (Fig. 86.31). Typically, patients with AAA diameters below accepted threshold levels for repair are followed with serial ultrasound examinations to monitor for enlargement of the aneurysm to a diameter where repair is indicated.

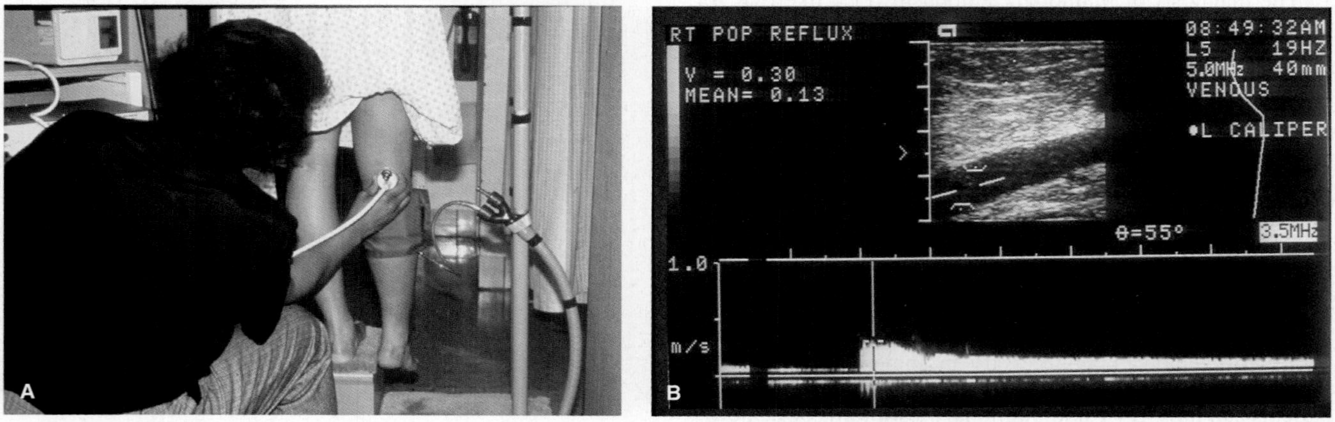

FIGURE 86.30. Technique (A) and popliteal venous waveform (B) with cuff deflation for duplex assessment and localization of venous reflux. Reflux lasting longer than 0.5 to 1 second is abnormal.

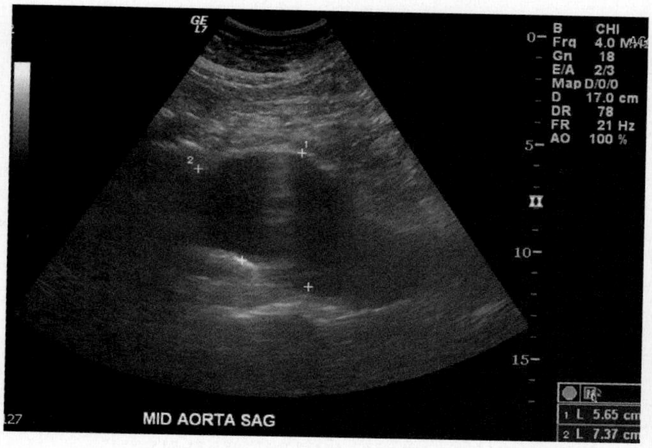

FIGURE 86.31. Ultrasound image of an infrarenal abdominal aortic aneurysm.

Evaluation of Aortic Endografts

Placement of endoluminal stent grafts is now standard therapy for most patients with AAA. With stent grafting of an AAA, the aneurysm is left in situ and blood flow diverted through the stent graft. Some stent grafts eventually leak at proximal or distal attachment sites. AAAs with these so called type I endoleaks are at risk for rupture. In addition, AAAs treated with stent grafts may also occasionally enlarge because of back-pressure in the aneurysm sac from patent lumbar vessels, type II endoleak. Patients whose AAAs enlarge in association with type II endoleaks after endografting are also considered at risk for aneurysm rupture.

Standard monitoring of endoluminal stent grafts is with serial CT scans to detect endoleak and changing sac diameter. However, there are increasing concerns about repeated doses of contrast and radiation exposure associated with serial CT scans. It now appears that many stent grafts can be followed with serial duplex ultrasound examinations. Duplex ultrasound is capable of measuring sac diameter and detecting both type I and II endoleaks. Even if an endoleak cannot be detected by ultrasound, an increase in sac diameter following stent grafting should prompt further investigation. In some centers duplex ultrasound has replaced CT scanning as the preferred method of follow-up of AAA stent grafts.[84,85]

Evaluation and Treatment of Groin Pseudoaneurysms

Pseudoaneurysms can occur as a complication of an arterial puncture in the groin performed for diagnostic or therapeutic angiography. Groin pseudoaneurysms are readily detected with duplex ultrasound (Fig. 86.32). Color flow demonstrates a typical collection of flowing blood usually anterior to the artery from which the pseudoaneurysm originates. The native artery and pseudoaneurysm are connected by a so-called "neck." To-and-fro flow within the neck of the pseudoaneurysm is characteristic and pathognomonic of a pseudoaneurysm arising from an arterial puncture.

Treatment of pseudoaneurysms may be with direct surgical repair or, utilizing the vascular laboratory, direct compression of the pseudoaneurysm until it thromboses using the ultrasound scanhead to both locate the pseudoaneurysm and apply pressure. Alternatively, the pseudoaneurysm is visualized with the ultrasound scanhead and a needle introduced into the body of the pseudoaneurysm for injection of small amounts of thrombin to induce thrombosis of the pseudoaneurysm.[86,87] All of these techniques are effective, but currently direct thrombin injection is favored in most cases as it is relatively noninvasive, less painful, and more effective than prolonged compression alone.

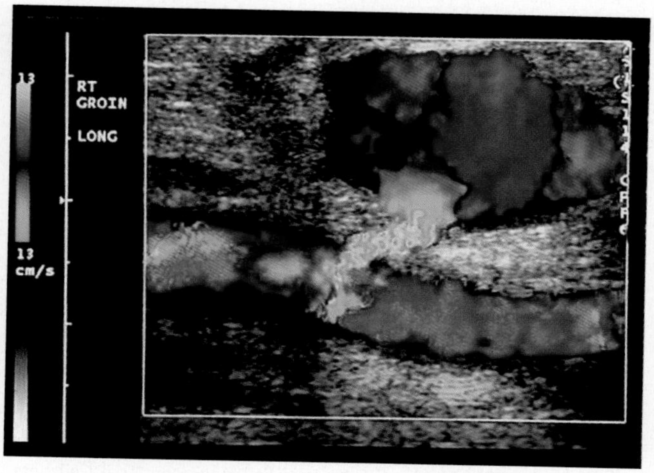

FIGURE 86.32. Color flow image of a groin pseudoaneurysm. See text.

Transcutaneous Oxygen Measurements

Measurements of transcutaneous oxygen ($TCpO_2$) can be performed as an aid in predicting healing of pedal lesions or healing of an amputation at the site where the measurement is taken (Fig. 86.33). In general, a $TCpO_2$ greater than 30 mm Hg indicates that healing is likely, measurements between 20 and 30 mm Hg are equivocal for healing, and measurements below 20 mm Hg indicate that healing is unlikely.[88] Measurements are not influenced by the presence of diabetes, but it has been suggested that the level for predicting healing be increased to 40 mm Hg in patients with diabetes. The test is less accurate in the presence of edema, cellulitis, or hyperkeratosis and in older patients.

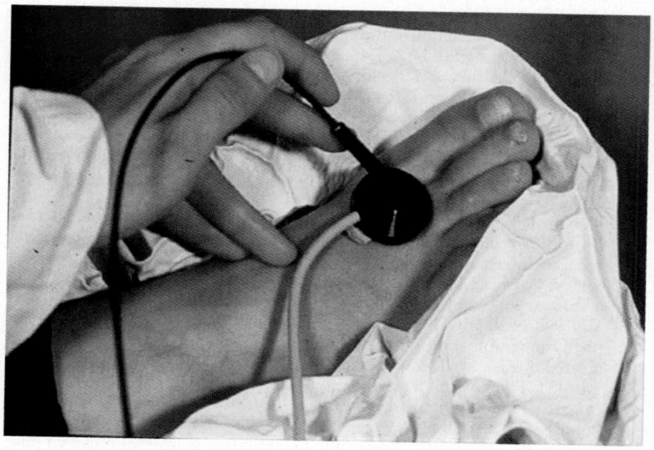

FIGURE 86.33. Device for measuring transcutaneous oxygen pressures.

References

1. Roederer GO, Langlois YE, Chan AT, et al. Ultrasonic duplex scanning of the extracranial carotid arteries: improved accuracy using new features from the carotid artery. *J Cardiovasc Ultrasonography* 1982;1:373–380.
2. Abou-ZamZam AM Jr, Moneta GL, Edwards JM, et al. Is a single preoperative duplex scan sufficient for planning bilateral carotid endarterectomy? *J Vasc Surg* 2000;31:282–288.
3. Strandness DE Jr. *Duplex Scanning in Vascular Disorders*. New York: Raven Press; 1990:92–120.
4. Roederer GO, Langlois YE, Jager KA, et al. A simple spectral parameter for accurate classification of severe carotid artery disease. *Bruit* 1989;3:174–178.
5. Moneta GL, Edwards JM, Chitwood RW, et al. Correlation of North American Symptomatic Carotid Endarterectomy Trial (NASCET): angiographic definition of 70% to 90% internal carotid artery stenosis with duplex scanning. *J Vasc Surg* 1993;17:152–159.
6. Bendick PJ, Glover JL. Hemodynamic evaluation of the vertebral arteries by duplex ultrasound. *Surg Clin North Am* 1990;70:235–244.
7. Kumar SM, Wang JC, Barry MC, et al. Carotid stump syndrome: outcome from surgical management. *Eur J Vasc Endovasc Surg* 2001;21:214–219.
8. North American Symptomatic Carotid Endarterectomy Trial Collaborators. NASCET: beneficial effect of carotid endarterectomy in patients with high-grade carotid stenosis. *N Engl J Med* 1991;325:445–453.
9. European Carotid Surgery Trialists' Collaborative Group (ECST). MRC European Carotid Surgery Trial: interim results for symptomatic patients with severe (70–99%) or with mild (0–29%) carotid stenosis. *Lancet* 1996;347:1591–1593.
10. Mayberg MR, Wilson SE, Yatsu F, et al. Carotid endarterectomy and prevention of cerebral ischemia in symptomatic carotid stenosis: Veterans Affairs Cooperative Studies Program 309 Trialist Group. *JAMA* 1991;266:3289–3294.
11. Executive Committee for Asymptomatic Carotid Atherosclerosis Study. Endarterectomy for asymptomatic carotid artery stenosis. *JAMA* 1995;273:1421–1428.
12. MRC Asymptomatic Carotid Surgery Trial (ACST) Collaborative Group. Prevention of disabling and fatal strokes by successful carotid endarterectomy in patients without recent neurological symptoms: randomized controlled trial. *Lancet* 2004;363:1491–1502.
13. North American Symptomatic Carotid Endarterectomy (NASCET) Steering Committee. North American symptomatic carotid endarterectomy trial: methods, patient characteristics, and progress. *Stroke* 1991;22:711–720.
14. Rothwell PM, Gibson RJ, Slattery J, et al. Equivalence of measurements of carotid stenosis: a comparison of three methods on 1001 angiograms. *Stroke* 1994;25:2435–2439.
15. Moneta GL, Edwards JM, Papanicolaou G, et al. Screening for asymptomatic internal carotid artery stenosis: duplex criteria for discriminating 60% to 99% stenosis. *J Vasc Surg* 1995;21:989–994.
16. AbuRahma AF, Robinson PA, Stickler DL, et al. Proposed new duplex classification for threshold stenoses used in various symptomatic and asymptomatic carotid endarterectomy trials. *Ann Vasc Surg* 1998;12:349–358.
17. Carpenter JP, Lexa FJ, Davis JT. Determination of duplex Doppler ultrasound criteria appropriate to the North American symptomatic carotid endarterectomy trial. *Stroke* 1996;27:695–699.
18. Hood DB, Mattos MA, Mansour A, et al. Prospective evaluation of new duplex criteria to identify 70% internal carotid artery stenosis. *J Vasc Surg* 1996;23:254–261.
19. Carpenter JP, Lexa FJ, Davis JT. Determination of 60% or greater carotid artery stenosis by duplex Doppler ultrasonography. *J Vasc Surg* 1995;22:697–703.
20. Browman MW, Cooperberg PL, Harrison PB, et al. Duplex ultrasonography criteria for internal carotid stenosis of more than 70% diameter: angiographic correlation and receiver operating characteristic curve analysis. *Can Assoc Radiol J* 1995;46:291–295.
21. Neale ML, Chambers JL, Kelly AT, et al. Reappraisal of duplex criteria to assess significant carotid stenosis with special reference to reports from the North American Symptomatic Carotid Endarterectomy Trial and the European Carotid Surgery Trial. *J Vasc Surg* 1994;20:642–649.
22. Grant EG, Benson CB, Moneta GL, et al. Carotid artery stenosis: grayscale and Doppler US diagnosis—Society of Radiologists in Ultrasound Consensus Conference. *Radiology* 2003;229:340–346.
23. Fujitani RM, Mills JL, Wang LM, et al. The effect of unilateral internal carotid arterial occlusion upon contralateral duplex study: criteria for accurate interpretation. *J Vasc Surg* 1992;16:459–467.
24. Setacci C, Chisci E, Setacci F, et al. Grading carotid intra-stent re-stenosis: a six-year follow-up study. *Stroke* 2008;30:1189–1196.
25. Yao JST, Nedham TN, Gourmos C. A comparative study of strain gauge plethysmography and Doppler ultrasound in the assessment of occlusive arterial disease of the lower extremities. *Surgery* 1972;71:4–9.
26. Yao JST, Flinn WR. Plethsymography. In: Kempczinski RF, Yao JST, eds. *Practical Noninvasive Vascular Diagnosis*. Chicago, IL: Yearbook Medical Publishers; 1987:80–94.
27. Darling RC, Raines JK, Brener BF. Quantitative segmental pulse volume recorder: a clinical tool. *Surgery* 1972;72:873–887.
28. Strandness DE. *Peripheral Arterial Disease: A Physiologic Approach*. Boston, MA: Little, Brown; 1969:112–130.
29. Kempczinski RF. Segmental volume plethysmography: the pulse volume recorder. In: Kempczinski RF, Yao JST, eds. *Practical Noninvasive Vascular Diagnosis*. Chicago, IL: Yearbook Medical Publishers; 1987:140–153.
30. Krikendall WM, Burton AC, Epstein FH, et al. Recommendations for human blood pressure determination by sphygmomanometers: report of a subcommittee of the postgraduate education committee, American Heart Association. *Circulation* 1967;36:980–988.
31. Moneta GL, Yeager RA, Antonovic R, et al. Accuracy of lower extremity arterial duplex mapping. *J Vasc Surg* 1992;15:275–284.
32. Jager KA, Ricketts HJ, Strandness DE. Duplex scanning for evaluation of lower limb arterial disease. In: Bernstein EF, ed. *Noninvasive Diagnostic Techniques in Vascular Disease*. St Louis, MO: Mosby; 1985:619–631.
33. Whyman MR, Hoskins PR, Leng GC, et al. Accuracy and reproducibility of duplex ultrasound imaging in a phantom model of femoral artery stenosis. *J Vasc Surg* 1993;17:524–530.
34. Leng GC, Whyman MR, Donnan PT, et al. Accuracy and reproducibility of duplex ultrasonography in grading femoropopliteal stenoses. *J Vasc Surg* 1993;17:510–517.
35. Sacks D, Robinson ML, Marinelli DL, et al. Peripheral arterial Doppler ultrasonography: diagnostic criteria. *J Ultrasound Med* 1992;11:95–103.
36. Jager KA, Phillips DJ, Martin RL, et al. Noninvasive mapping of lower limb arterial lesions. *Ultrasound Med Biol* 1985;11:515–521.
37. Sensier Y, Hartshorne T, Thrush A, et al. A prospective comparison of lower limb colour-coded duplex scanning with arteriography. *Eur J Vasc Endovasc Surg* 1996;11:170–175.
38. de Smet AA, Ermers EJ, Kitslaar PJ. Duplex velocity characteristics of aortoiliac stenoses. *J Vasc Surg* 1996;23:628–636.
39. Elsman BH, Legemate DA, van der Heijden FH, et al. Impact of ultrasonographic duplex scanning on therapeutic decision making in lower-limb arterial disease. *Br J Surg* 1995;82:630–633.
40. Ascher E, Mazzariol F, Hingorani A, et al. The use of duplex ultrasound arterial mapping as an alternative to conventional arteriography for primary and secondary infrapopliteal bypasses. *Am J Surg* 1999;178:162–165.
41. Mazzariol F, Ascher E, Salles-Cunha SX, et al. Values and limitations of duplex ultrasonography as the sole imaging method of preoperative evaluation for popliteal and infrapopliteal bypasses. *Ann Vasc Surg* 1999;13:1–10.
42. Larch E, Minar E, Ahmadi R, et al. Value of color duplex sonography for evaluation of tibioperoneal arteries in patients with femoropopliteal obstruction: a prospective comparison with anterograde intraarterial digital subtraction angiography. *J Vasc Surg* 1997;25:629–636.
43. Landry GJ, Moneta GL, Taylor LM Jr, et al. Patency and characteristics of lower extremity vein grafts requiring multiple revisions. *J Vasc Surg* 2000;32:23–31.
44. Johnson BL, Bandyk DF, Back MR, et al. Intraoperative duplex monitoring of infrainguinal vein bypass procedures. *J Vasc Surg* 2000;31:678–690.
45. Idu MM, Blankenstein JD, de Gier P, et al. Impact of a color-flow duplex surveillance program on infrainguinal vein graft patency: a five-year experience. *J Vasc Surg* 1993;17:42–52; discussion 52–53.
46. Lundell A, Lindblad B, Bergqvist D, et al. Femoropopliteal-crural graft patency is improved by an intensive surveillance program: a prospective randomized study. *J Vasc Surg* 1995;21:26–33; discussion 33–34.
47. Passman MA, Moneta GL, Nehler MR, et al. Do normal early color-flow duplex surveillance examination results of infrainguinal vein grafts preclude the need for late graft revision? *J Vasc Surg* 1995;22:476–481; discussion 482–484.
48. Mills JL Sr, Wixon CL, James DC, et al. The natural history of intermediate and critical vein graft stenosis: recommendations for continued surveillance or repair. *J Vasc Surg* 2001;33:273–278; discussion 278–280.
49. McLafferty RB, Edwards JM, Taylor LM Jr, et al. Diagnosis and long-term clinical outcome in patients presenting with hand ischemia. *J Vasc Surg* 1995;22:361–369.
50. Porter JM, Snider RL, Bardana EJ, et al. The diagnosis and treatment of Raynaud's phenomenon. *Surgery* 1975;77:11–23.
51. Nielsen SL, Lassen NA. Measurement of digital blood pressure after local cooling. *J Appl Physiol* 1977;43:907–910.
52. Lutolf O, Chen D, Zehnder T, et al. Influence of local finger cooling on laser Doppler flux and nailfold capillary blood flow velocity in normal subjects and in patients with Raynaud's phenomenon. *Microvasc Res* 1993;46:374–382.
53. Lafferty K, de Trafford JC, Roberts VC, et al. Raynaud's phenomenon and thermal entrainment: an objective test. *BMJ Clin Res* 1983;286:90–92.
54. Singh S, de Trafford JC, Baskerville PA, et al. Digital artery caliber measurement: a new technique of assessing Raynaud's phenomenon. *Eur J Vasc Surg* 1991;5:199–205.
55. Yurdakul M, Tola M, Uslu OS. Color Doppler ultrasonography in occlusive diseases of the brachiocephalic and proximal subclavian arteries. *J Ultrasound in Med* 2008;27:1065–1070.
56. Strandness DE. *Duplex Scanning in Vascular Disorders*. New York: Raven Press; 1993:159–196.
57. Grosveld WJ, Lawson JA, Eikelboom BC, et al. Clinical and hemodynamic significance of innominate artery lesions evaluated by ultrasonography and digital angiography. *Stroke* 1988;19:958–962.
58. Reed AJ, Fincher RME, Nichols FT. Case report: Takayasu's arteritis in a middle-aged Caucasian woman: clinical course correlated with duplex ultrasonography and angiography. *Am J Med Sci* 1989;298:324–327.
59. Jagar KA, Fortner GS, Thiele BI, et al. Noninvasive diagnosis of intestinal angina. *J Clin Ultrasound* 1984;12:588–591.

60. Gentile AT, Moneta GL, Masser P, et al. Fasting and postprandial superior mesenteric artery duplex scanning in the diagnosis of high-grade superior mesenteric artery stenosis. *Am J Surg* 1995;169:476–479.
61. Moneta GL, Taylor DC, Helton WS, et al. Duplex ultrasound measurement of postprandial intestinal blood flow: effect of meal composition. *Gastroenterology* 1988;95:1294–1301.
62. Moneta GL, Lee RW, Yeager RA, et al. Mesenteric artery duplex scanning: a blinded prospective study. *J Vasc Surg* 1993;17:79–86.
63. Zwolak RM, Fillinger MF, Walsh DB, et al. Mesenteric and celiac duplex scanning: a validation study. *J Vasc Surg* 1998;27:1078–1087.
64. Liem TK, Segall JA, Wei Wei, et al. Duplex scan characteristics of bypass grafts to mesenteric arteries. *J Vasc Surg* 2007;45(5):922–928.
65. Mitchell EL, Chang EY, Landry GJ, et al. Duplex criteria for native superior mesenteric arteries stenosis overestimates stenosis in stented superior mesenteric arteries. *J Vasc Surg* 2009;50:335–340.
66. Taylor DC, Kettler MD, Moneta GL, et al. Duplex ultrasound in the diagnosis of renal artery stenosis: a prospective evaluation. *J Vasc Surg* 1988;7:363–369.
67. Hoffman U, Edwards JM, Carter S, et al. Role of duplex scanning for detection of atherosclerotic renal artery disease. *Kidney Int* 1991;39:1232–1238.
68. Olin JW, Piedmonte MR, Young JR, et al. The utility of duplex ultrasound scanning of the renal arteries for diagnosing significant renal artery stenosis. *Ann Intern Med* 1995;122:833–840.
69. Mohabbat W, Greenerg RK, Mastracci BW, et al. Revised duplex criteria and outcomes for renal stents and stent grafts following endovascular repair of juxtarenal and thoracoabdominal aneurysms. *J Vasc Surg* 2009;49;827–837.
70. Radermacher J, Chavan A, Bleck J, et al. Use of Doppler ultrasonography to predict the outcome of therapy for renal-artery stenosis. *N Engl J Med* 2001;344:410–416.
71. Wells PS, Hirsh J, Anderson DR. Accuracy of clinical assessment of deep-vein thrombosis. *Lancet* 1995;345:1326–1330.
72. Hull R, van Aken WG, Hirsh J, et al. Impedance plethysmography using the occlusive cuff technique in the diagnosis of venous thrombosis. *Circulation* 1976;53:696–700.
73. Hull R, Hirsh J, Sackett DL, et al. Combined use of leg scanning and impedance plethysmography in suspected venous thrombosis: an alternative to venography. *N Engl J Med* 1977;296:1497–1500.
74. Hull R, Taylor DW, Hirsh J, et al. Impedance plethysmography: the relationship between venous filling and sensitivity and specificity for proximal vein thrombosis. *Circulation* 1978;58:898–902.
75. Hull R, Hirsh J, Sackett DL, et al. Replacement of venography in suspected venous thrombosis by impedance plethysmography and ^{125}I-fibrinogen leg scanning: a less invasive approach. *Ann Intern Med* 1981;94:12–15.
76. Anderson DR, Lensing AWA, Wells PS, et al. Limitations of impedance plethysmography in the diagnosis of clinically suspected deep vein thrombosis. *Ann Intern Med* 1993;118:25–30.
77. Kearon C, Julian JA, Math M, et al. Noninvasive diagnosis of deep vein thrombosis. McMaster Diagnostic Imaging Practice Guidelines Initiative. *Ann Intern Med* 1998,128:663–677.
78. Schindler JM, Kaiser M, Gerber A, et al. Color coded duplex sonography in suspected deep vein thrombosis. *Br J Surg* 1991;78:611–613.
79. Rose SC, Zwiebel WJ, Nelson BD, et al. Symptomatic lower extremity deep venous thrombosis: accuracy, limitations, and role of color duplex flow imaging in diagnosis. *Radiology* 1990;175:639–644.
80. Kearon C. Diagnosis of pulmonary embolism. *CMAJ* 2003;168(2):183–194.
81. Welch Hg, Faliakou EC, McLaughlin RL, et al. Comparison of descending phlebography with quantitative photoplethysmography, air plethysmography and duplex quantitative valve closure time in assessing deep venous reflux. *J Vasc Surg* 1989;10:425–432.
82. van Bemmelen PS, Bedford G, Beach K, etal. Quantitative segmental evaluation of venous valvular reflux with duplex ultrasound scanning. *J Vasc Surg* 1989;10:425–431.
83. Fleming C, Whitlock EP, Beil TL, et al. Screening for abdominal aortic aneurysm: a best evidence systematic review for the U.S. preventive services task force. *Ann Intern Med* 2005;142;203–211.
84. Sanford RM, Brown MJ, Fisfwick G, et al. Duplex ultrasound scanning is reliable in the detection of endoleak following endovascular aneurysm repair. *Eur J Vasc Endovasc Surg* 2006;32:537–541.
85. Chaer RA, Gushchin A, Rhee R, et al. Duplex ultrasound as the sole long-term surveillance method post endovascular aneurysm repair: a safe alternative for stable aneurysms. *J Vasc Surg* 2009;49;845–849.
86. Cox GS, Young JR, Gray BR, et al. Ultrasound guided compression repair of postcatheterzation pseudoaneurysms: results of treatment in 100 cases. *J Vasc Surg* 1994;19:683–690.
87. Kang SS, Labropoulos N, Mansour MA, et al. Expanded indications for ultrasound guided thrombin injection of pseudoaneurysms. *J Vasc Surg* 2000;31:289–296.
88. Ballard JL, Eke CC, Bunt TJ, et al. A prospective evaluation of transcutaneous oxygen measurements in the management of diabetic foot problems. *J Vasc Surg* 1995;22;485–492.

CHAPTER 87 ■ ENDOVASCULAR TREATMENT OF DISEASE

MATTHEW J. EAGLETON AND SUNITA D. SRIVASTAVA

VASCULAR

KEY POINTS

1. The treatment of vascular disease has progressed significantly over the past several years with the evolution and application of endovascular procedures.
2. Endovascular treatment of carotid artery stenosis is less invasive and thus may be associated with a lower morbidity and mortality compared with carotid endarterectomy (CEA).
3. In order for carotid artery stenting to gain full acceptance, it must provide clinical outcomes that rival CEA.
4. With the advent of lower-profile sheaths, wires, and stents, percutaneous interventions have become more feasible and often the first-line treatment in the setting of mesenteric occlusive disease.
5. Percutaneous transluminal angioplasty is the treatment of choice for nonorificial atherosclerotic lesions and fibromuscular dysplasia.
6. Results from surgical revascularization and renal interventions are comparable.
7. The most important aspect of aortic endograft placement takes place prior to graft placement in determining whether a patient is indeed a suitable candidate for endograft placement, choosing an appropriate endograft device, and properly determining the size graft to be placed.
8. Postoperative surveillance is extremely important in patients undergoing endovascular abdominal aortic aneurysm repair.
9. Endovascular treatment of aortoiliac occlusive disease has become increasingly prominent over the past several years and has assumed a dominant role in the treatment of this disease.
10. There have been mixed results reported for outcomes of patients treated with percutaneous balloon angioplasty of femoropopliteal artery stenosis.

(1) The treatment of vascular disease has progressed significantly over the past several years with the evolution and application of endovascular procedures. In particular, the endovascular treatments of aortic aneurysm disease and carotid artery stenosis

have received intense scrutiny. Intravascular treatment of disease, however, is not a new concept. In the 1960s, radiologist Charles Dotter pioneered the concept of endovascular therapy.[1] He conceived the idea of using dilators of varying diameters to serially expand stenotic atherosclerotic lesions in the iliac arteries. Since then, the technology has continued to evolve. The development of guide wire–directed catheter technology has allowed physicians to percutaneously access nearly any blood vessel in the body. This combined with the development of the angioplasty balloon revolutionized percutaneous interventions and allowed for the treatment of stenotic lesions through a percutaneous arterial puncture. This procedure has been further enhanced by the development of metallic stents to assist in maintaining long-term patency of percutaneous angioplasty. With advancing technology, more endovascular procedures are being applied to the treatment of peripheral vascular disease. The goal of this chapter is to outline many of the applications of endovascular therapies for the treatment of peripheral vascular disease including technical aspects, complications, and outcomes.

BASIC CONCEPTS

The basic concept of most endovascular procedures is to obtain percutaneous access of a blood vessel and then to gain access across the lesion (either a stenosis or aneurysm) with a guide wire. This allows for endovascular treatment of the disease. Most arterial and venous access is obtained through a percutaneous puncture over the femoral vessels. From this location, most other branches of the arterial tree can be reached. Access from the femoral vessels, however, is not always possible or ideal, and in those instances percutaneous access is generally obtained through an alternate site, such as the brachial artery or the jugular vein. Once blood vessel access is obtained, a guide wire is inserted through the needle and into the artery or vein. Generally, the needle is then removed and a sheath is placed into the vessel over the wire. A sheath is a specialized piece of equipment, with a valve on one end, which allows continuous access to the blood vessel. This allows for continued introduction and removal of a variety of pieces of equipment

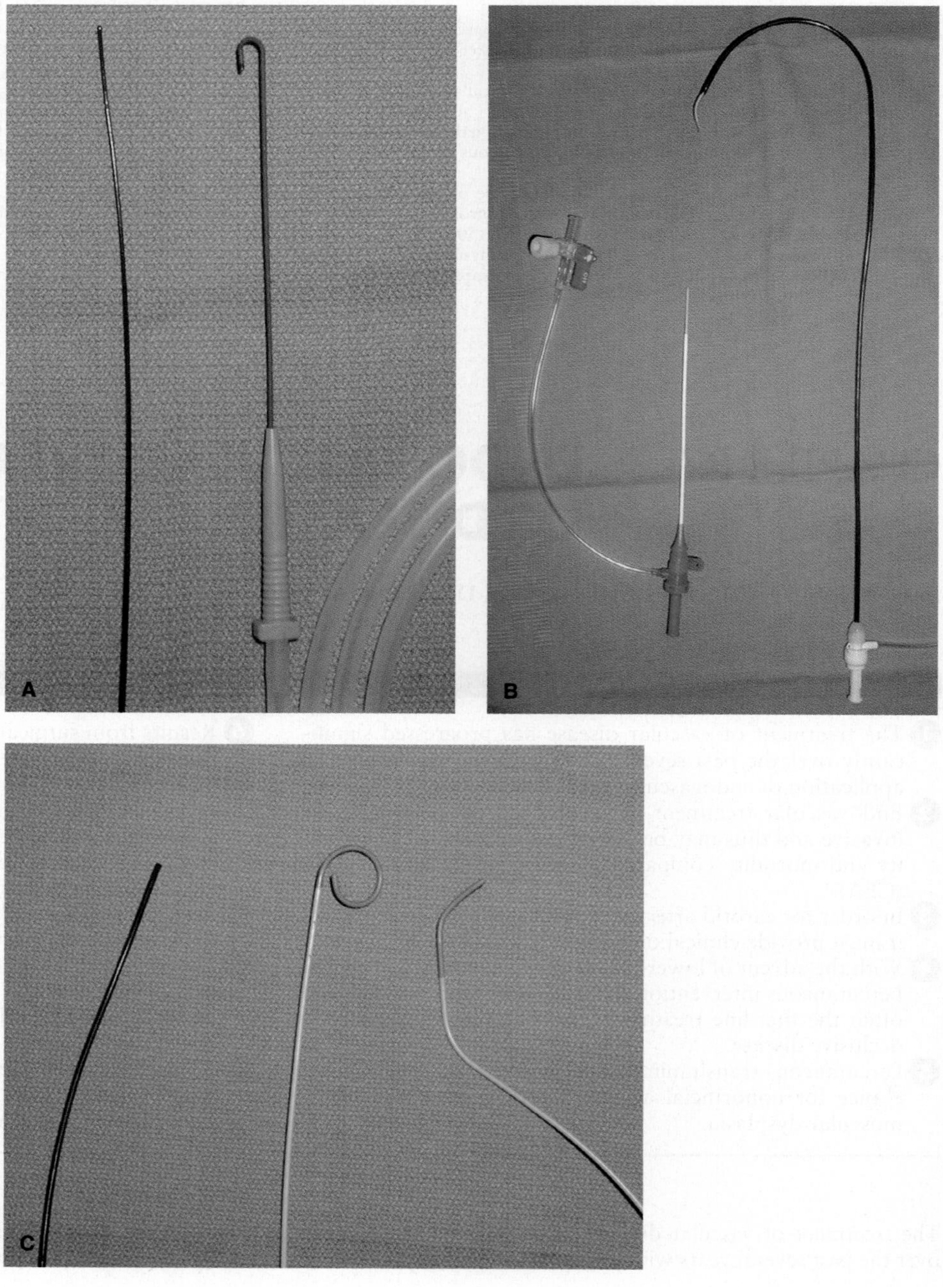

FIGURE 87.1. **A:** An example of two different endovascular wires. The one on the left has a straight tip, and it is coated with a hydrophilic substance, which increases its maneuverability in stenotic lesions. The wire on the right has a J-tip on the end, which allows it to be less traumatic to the arterial wall. **B:** An example of two different types of sheaths. The smaller sheath on the left is representative of the standard access sheath used for many endovascular procedures, whereas the larger one on the right demonstrates a more specialized sheath of a larger size with a preshaped curve. **C:** An example of angiographic catheters. The catheter on the left represents a straight catheter that is hydrophilic coated. It is an end-hole catheter that is used for selective catheterization of vessels. The catheter in the middle is a nonselective catheter that has a "pigtail" shape. It has multiple side holes and is most generally used for nonselective angiography. The catheter on the right is also a selective catheter that has a preformed shape that allows the interventionalist the ability to access vessels in unique anatomic locations.

while protecting the vessel wall from repeated trauma. Sheaths are available in a variety of sizes and a variety of shapes, and the exact sheath used depends on the procedure being performed and the blood vessel being accessed (Fig. 87.1).

The next tool to consider once a secured entry into the blood vessel is obtained is the guide wire, which allows remote access across the lesion. Guide wires are constructed in a variety of sizes; the three most commonly used sizes are 0.035, 0.018, and 0.014 inches in diameter. The length of the guide wire is also important and generally varies from 145 to 300 cm. The guide wire length needs to be long enough to cover the cumulative distance required both inside and outside the patient. This will vary based on lesion location, the type of procedure performed, and the type of other pieces of technology being used. There are several factors that are important in guide wire construction, including the stiffness of the wire, the coating on the wire, and the tip shape (Fig. 87.1). Some of these factors affect the steerability and trackability of the wire. Steerability refers to the ability to direct the intravascular tip of the wire by manipulating the extravascular portion, and trackability refers to the ability of the wire to allow a catheter to follow its course. The tip of the wire may be straight, angled, or J-tipped, and the tip may be stiff or floppy, making it less traumatic. Many wires have a tightly wound inner steel core that confers differing magnitudes of stiffness to the body of the guide wire. A surrounding wrap of lighter, more flexible wire helps prevent fracture and fragmentation while the guide wire is in use. Most guide wires have a hydrophilic coating of either polytetrafluoroethylene or silicone, which decreases the coefficient of friction during catheter exchange or while traversing a stenosis.

Catheters are another vital piece of equipment important in performing endovascular procedures. They are used to perform diagnostic procedures, maintain access across a lesion while a more suitable wire is exchanged, and support devices, such as balloons and stents, that are delivered to the lesion attached to the catheter. Catheters are constructed from a variety of materials including polyurethane, polyethylene, polypropylene, and nylon. Catheters are also available in a variety of diameters (measured in French) and lengths. Catheters constructed from polyethylene have a low coefficient of friction and are pliable with good shape memory. They are useful for selective catheterization. Polyurethane catheters are softer, are more pliable, and follow guide wires more easily but have a higher coefficient of friction. Nylon catheters are stiffer but tolerate higher flow rates. The construction of the catheter affects several important properties, including trackability (the ability of the catheter to follow the direction of the wire), pushability (the ability of force applied on one end of the catheter to induce movement on the other end), crossability (the facility with which a catheter will follow the wire across a lesion), and steerability. The shape of the catheter's head is variable and dictates the catheter's function (Fig. 87.1). Functionally, catheters are classified as selective or nonselective. Nonselective catheters, also known as flush catheters, often have multiple side holes that allow large amounts of contrast to exit in a short period of time. These catheters' head shapes are usually either straight or curved. Selective catheters have only one end hole but are available in a variety of shapes, including straight, angled, reverse curved, and double-curved. The choice of catheter used depends on the type of procedure being performed.

An important tool in endovascular procedures is the angioplasty balloon. This is a balloon mounted on the end of a catheter that has the ability to be inflated and deflated through a port on the extravascular portion of the catheter (Fig. 87.2). The function of the angioplasty balloon is to provide a dilating force on the endoluminal surface of a blood vessel. As with all catheters, angioplasty balloon catheters are constructed with a number of variables, most specific to the balloon itself. Balloons vary in sizes that range from 1.5 to 40 mm, and they are selected with the intent to slightly overdilate the vessel being treated. The length of the balloon is also variable and can range from one to several centimeters in length. Typically, there are radiopaque markers on either end of the balloon that allow for accurate placement at the site of the lesion. The rounded area of the balloon that extends beyond the markers is termed the *shoulder* of the balloon. The length of the shoulders of the balloon varies from balloon type to balloon type. In addition, balloons are constructed of a variety of types of material, which alters the way in which the balloons respond to inflation. Most balloons are constructed of polyethylene, polyethylene terephthalate, or other low-compliance polymers. These allow for a low or noncompliant balloon, which allows the balloon at high inflation pressures to exert more radial force without increasing the balloon diameter. Other balloons, particularly those used in aortic endografting, are more compliant and will continue to change diameter with increases in pressure, thus reducing the radial force applied. Furthermore, specialized balloons have been developed that provide specific functions while performing an angioplasty. One such balloon is a "cutting balloon." This is a balloon that

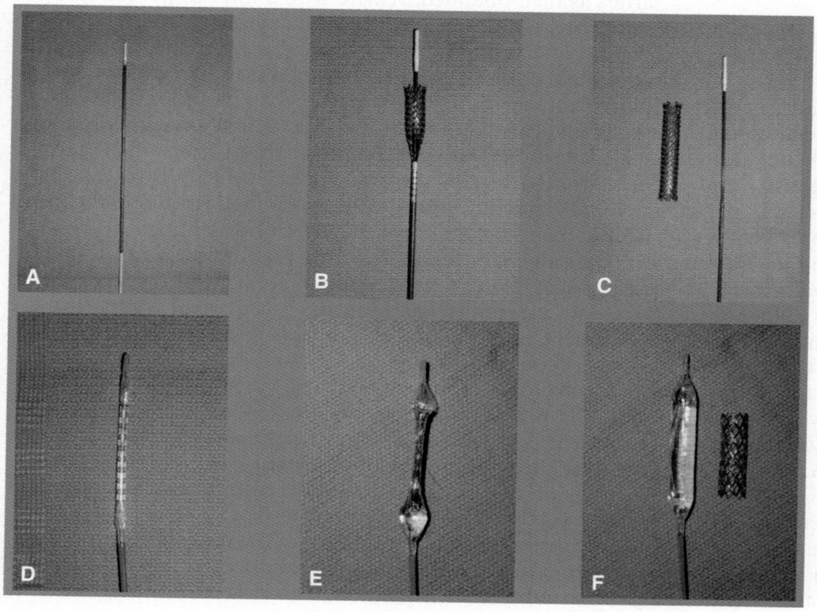

FIGURE 87.2. **A–C:** These pictures depict a self-expanding stent at various stages of deployment. **A:** The stent ensheathed on the catheter prior to deployment. **B:** The stent partially deployed. Note the expansion of the stent in the unsheathed portion. **C:** The self-expanding stent fully deployed. **D–F:** These pictures depict a balloon-expandable stent at various stages of deployment. **D:** The balloon-expandable stent mounted on a catheter prior to deployment and **(E)** at the start of expansion. **F:** A fully expanded balloon-expandable stent adjacent to the inflated balloon used to deploy it.

has strips of metal, or blades, along the length of the balloon that can cut the area of stenosis, assisting in the balloon's ability to dilate the region.

As discussed in more detail later, balloon angioplasty is often supplemented with the placement of an intravascular stent. The evolution of stents has occurred along two fundamental design philosophies: balloon-expandable stents and self-expanding stents (Fig. 87.2). Stents are composed of a variety of metals including steel, nitinol, tantalum, platinum, and various metal alloys. The construction is also variable and includes laser cut, woven, knitted, coiled, or welded. The construction of the stent helps to determine its properties. The ideal stent properties are high radial force, minimal induction of neointimal hyperplasia, longitudinal flexibility, high radiopacity, radial elasticity, ability to conform to the vessel, low profile with high expansion ratio, no foreshortening, durable, and affordable.[2] Balloon-expandable stents are best exemplified by the prototypical Palmaz stent. The basic mechanism is a metal tube (stent) placed around a balloon. The balloon is expanded, thus dilating the metal tube, which then maintains the nominal diameter of the balloon. Most are made of stainless steel alloy, providing greater radial and hoop strength with minimal foreshortening, which allows for exact placement. These same properties, however, allow little flexibility and render the stents susceptible to irreversible deformation when subjected to external compressive forces. The prototype of the self-expanding stents is the Wallstent. These stents function on the principle of elasticity, as the stents self-expand to their nominal diameter when released from a constrained state within the delivery catheter. A stent of a larger nominal diameter than the target vessel is chosen so that it exerts a continuous outward expansile force. The final diameter is the equilibrium that is reached between the elastic recoil of the vessel and the expansile force of the stent. Some general properties of self-expanding stents are that they are flexible, track better than balloon-expandable stents, and have crush resistance. Unfortunately, these stents foreshorten during placement and thus can only be accurately positioned at one end. With improving technology and the development of better alloys (e.g., nitinol, a nickel and titanium alloy), many of the adverse properties of both balloon- and self-expanding stents are overcome and they approach closer the properties of the ideal stent. As discussed in more detail later, the specific choice of stent to use in a given situation depends on the procedure being performed.

CAROTID ARTERY INTERVENTIONS

Stroke occurs in nearly 700,000 patients annually in the United States resulting in an estimated 164,000 deaths and contributing $54 billion in health care costs.[3] Nearly one third of strokes are attributable to carotid artery stenosis, and nearly 200,000 carotid endarterectomies (CEAs) are performed each year in the United States to help prevent this debilitating problem.[4] The value of CEA to reduce the risk of stroke has been proven in a number of randomized, prospective clinical trials. CEA has been documented to reduce the incidence of both stroke and combined stroke and death in symptomatic patients with a stenosis greater than 70%.[5] In the North American Symptomatic Carotid Endarterectomy Trial, life-table estimates of the cumulative risk of any ipsilateral stroke at 2 years were 26% in patients treated with aspirin alone versus 9% in those patients treated with CEA. For major or fatal ipsilateral stroke the estimates were 13.1% and 2.5% for medical versus surgical treatment, respectively. For patients with asymptomatic disease, although the results are not as dramatic, there is a significant decrease in stroke risk with CEA versus medical therapy. The Asymptomatic Carotid Atherosclerosis Study randomized 4,657 patients with greater than 60% stenosis to receive either CEA or medical therapy.[4] The aggregate risk over 5 years for ipsilateral stroke and any perioperative stroke or death was 5.1% for surgical patients and 11.0% for patients treated medically. The results from the Asymptomatic Carotid Surgery Trial were very similar.[6] CEA has also proven durable, with reoperation for recurrent stenosis reported from as low as 1% to as high as 9%.

2 Endovascular treatment of carotid artery stenosis is less invasive and thus may be associated with a lower morbidity and mortality compared with CEA. The underlying indications for treatment of carotid artery stenosis do not change with the application of percutaneous techniques. However, carotid artery stenting must at least demonstrate clinical equipoise with CEA to become an accepted alternative. In the United States, most applications of carotid artery stenting currently are reserved for patients who are characterized as "high risk" for conventional CEA or in patients who are enrolled in ongoing clinical trials. In May 2007, the Centers for Medicare and Medicaid Services (CMS) expanded coverage of carotid angioplasty and stenting to those patients at high risk for carotid endarterectomy with symptomatic high-grade stenosis of 50% to 70% and asymptomatic stenosis of greater than 80%.

Percutaneous treatment of carotid artery stenosis was first described in 1980 by Kerber et al.,[7] at which time they described the application of percutaneous transluminal balloon angioplasty (PTA) of an atherosclerotic lesion. Since that time the procedure has evolved tremendously and now includes the application of either a balloon-expandable or self-expanding stent. Currently, patients are premedicated with aspirin and either ticlopidine or clopidogrel at least 1 day prior to the procedure. Heparin anticoagulation is standard once arterial access has been obtained. The majority of the procedure does not differ significantly from the performance of PTA and stent placement at other sites. Percutaneous arterial access is obtained through a common femoral artery puncture. Brachial artery access is possible, although more difficult, if femoral access is prohibitive. Selective catheterization of the common carotid artery is performed utilizing one of a variety of preformed catheters that best fit the anatomic variability. The common carotid artery is cannulated with a 6- or 7-French introducer sheath or guide catheter. An inability to access the common carotid artery with these devices due to vessel tortuosity or anatomic variation is the principle cause of procedure failure. During advancement of the sheath, distal guide wire access is maintained in the external carotid artery. Guide wire access across the lesion in the internal carotid artery is then obtained. A wire with a filter or net for cerebral protection is advanced to allow for embolic protection prior to carotid intervention. In cases where there is thrombus, ulcerated plaque, or higher risk of embolization with initial wire placement, reversal of flow devices can be utilized. This technique involves placement of a special balloon catheter allowing occlusion of both the common carotid artery and the external carotid artery. A separate 9-French sheath is placed in the femoral vein and reversal of flow through the internal carotid is initiated to facilitate protected carotid stenting.

Typically, the lesion requires predilation with a smaller angioplasty balloon to facilitate placement of the stent. Little outcome variability has been described when comparing the placement of a balloon-expandable versus a self-expanding stent, although most often self-expanding stents are placed due to the balloon-expandable stents' vulnerability to compression.[8] If necessary, the stent is extended from the internal carotid artery into the common carotid artery, effectively "jailing" the external carotid artery ostia.

One of the most catastrophic complications of carotid artery stenting is stroke, which is most often due to atheroemboli or thromboemboli dislodged at the time of the procedure. Unfortunately, unlike in peripheral interventions when a surgical therapy can often be used to correct an interventional

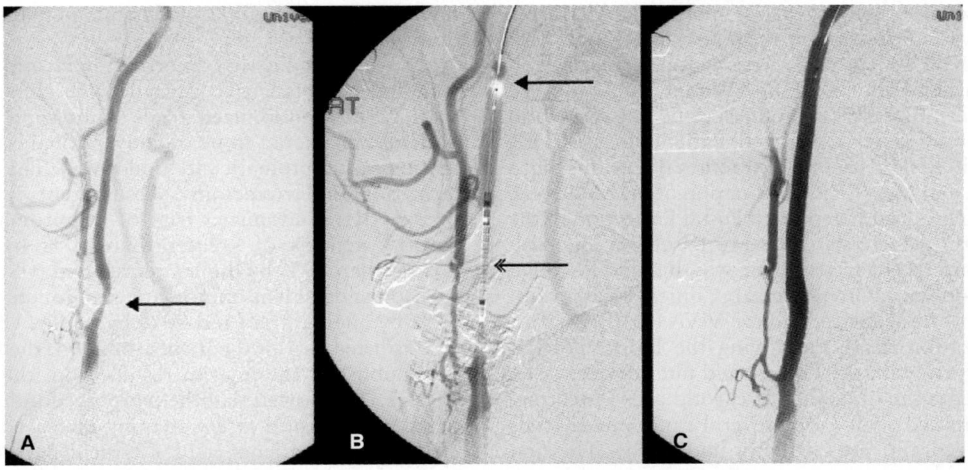

FIGURE 87.3. Angiograms from a patient undergoing a carotid artery stent. **A:** There is an 85% recurrent stenosis within the internal carotid artery (*arrow*). The patient had undergone a carotid endarterectomy 1 year prior. **B:** After wire access was obtained across the lesion, a balloon occlusion protection device was placed prior to angioplasty and stenting. This current angiogram shows placement of a self-expanding stent at the site of the internal carotid narrowing (*top arrow*). The balloon occlusion device can be seen in the distal internal carotid artery (*bottom arrow*). Note the absence of contrast beyond the protection device. After stent deployment and prior to balloon deflation, the contents of the common carotid artery and proximal internal carotid artery will be aspirated and discarded. **C:** After stent deployment, there is resolution of the internal carotid artery narrowing.

complication, it is rare that an operation can correct distal cerebral embolization. To decrease the incidence of these complications, several cerebral protection devices have been developed and are utilized at the time of stent placement. Several series evaluating the efficacy of cerebral protection devices have shown up to an 80% reduction in the rate of acute neurologic events related to embolic complications compared with unprotected procedures.[9–12] There are a number of different types of cerebral protection devices, including distal occlusive balloons, distal filter systems, and proximal protection systems. The distal protection devices must cross the lesion prior to stent placement and before they are opened; thus, some embolization may occur as they cross the lesion. Distal occlusive balloons consist of a 0.014-inch guide wire with the balloon on the distal portion. The balloon is inflated in the extracranial internal carotid artery distal to the lesion occluding blood flow (Fig. 87.3). After placement of the stent, stagnant blood and debris is suctioned from the region before blood flow is resumed by deflating the balloon. Distal filter systems are placed in a similar location, but allow for continuous blood flow through the filter while it traps emboli. Proximal protection systems provide protection by occluding flow in the common carotid artery and external carotid artery. The collateral flow through the circle of Willis then provides a "back-pressure" that prevents distal embolization during the procedure. After stent placement, the blood in the internal carotid artery is then evacuated to prevent embolization of debris when antegrade flow is reestablished.

Carotid artery stent placement complications can be divided into three stages.[13] Stage I complications occur primarily during access of the common carotid artery. Stage II complications occur during positioning of the distal protection device in a straight cervical segment of the internal carotid artery. Stage III complications occur during predilation, stent deployment, and postdilation of the stent. When a neurologic event does occur, one should have an understanding of the cerebral circulation to proceed with neurologic rescue procedures.[14] In patients with a transient ischemic attack (TIA) or minor stroke and a normal angiogram, medical management should ensue. In patients with minor or major strokes and evidence of occlusion of an intracranial vessel, catheter-directed thrombolysis should be initiated and glycoprotein platelet receptor antagonists administered.[13]

3 In order for carotid artery stenting to gain full acceptance, it must provide clinical outcomes that rival CEA. Early studies evaluating carotid stent outcomes were derived from single-institution case series and registries. The first large series reported was by Yadav et al.[15] and included 126 carotid stenting procedures performed in 107 patients that were at high risk for CEA due to medical comorbidities. The 30-day incidence of ipsilateral major stroke and death was only 1.6%. At 6 months, however, there was a 4.9% incidence of asymptomatic restenosis. Lal et al.[16] reported their results from 122 carotid stent procedures performed in 118 patients. Similarly, there was a low 30-day stroke and death rate of 3.3%. This analysis applied Kaplan-Meier curves and predicted cumulative in-stent restenosis, defined as a recurrent stenosis of greater than 80%, in 6.4% of the patients at 5 years. None was associated with onset of symptoms.

The largest collection of patients undergoing carotid artery stenting comes from a review of the Global Carotid Artery Stent Registry.[17] This report, from 53 participating centers in Europe, South and North America, and Asia, is based on a survey questioning the performance and complications of carotid artery stenting. The registry began in 1997 and since then has accrued 12,392 procedures in 11,243 patients. The technical success rate was 98.9%, with technical success defined as less than 30% residual stenosis. Thirty-day complication rates were 3.07% for TIA, 2.14% for minor strokes, 1.2% for major strokes, and 0.64% for deaths. Thirty-day combined stroke and procedure-related death rate was 3.98%. In support of the use of cerebral protection devices, 4,221 patients underwent carotid artery stenting with cerebral protection, which resulted in a stroke and procedure-related death rate of 2.23%, compared with 6,753 patients who underwent a procedure without cerebral protection and had a rate of 5.29%. This difference was consistent even when patients were stratified into those who were treated for symptomatic disease and those who were asymptomatic. Restenosis rates of 5.6% were reported at 48 months, although because of the registry format Kaplan-Meier curves were not possible. A 48-month neurologic event rate was reported at 4.5%.

There are several other registries, including ARCHER (Acculink for Revascularization of the Carotids in High Risk Patients), CABERNET (Carotid Artery Revascularization using the Boston Scientific EPI Filter Wire EX/EZ and the EndoTex Nex Stent), BEACH (Boston Scientific EPI-A Carotid Stenting Trial for High Risk Surgical Patients), SHELTER (Stenting of High Risk Patients Extracranial Lesions with Emboli Removal), and MAVERIC (Evaluation of the Medtronic AVE Self-Expanding Carotid Stent with Distal Protection in the Treatment of Carotid Stenosis), that are based on high-risk entry criteria. More recent trials under way include EMPiRE (Embolic Protection with Flow Reversal) Clinical Trial, evaluating the reversal of flow device, and the ViVA (ViVEXX Carotid Revascularization) trial, employing the Bard ViVEXX carotid stent platform with the Emboshield filter device.

To better evaluate the outcomes of carotid artery stenting, in particular compared with CEA, several randomized trials have been organized and are currently under way. The first large trial of carotid angioplasty was the Carotid and Vertebral Artery Transluminal Angioplasty Study (CAVATAS).[18] This study enrolled a total of 504 patients with 251 in the endovascular arm and 253 in the carotid endarterectomy arm. Within the endovascular cohort, only 55 patients underwent stent placement with the remaining (158) being treated with balloon angioplasty alone. Distal embolic protection was not available at the time of the trial and thus not utilized for the percutaneous procedures. There were no major differences in 30-day outcomes and no difference in ipsilateral stroke in 3 years between the groups. The trial has been criticized for the lack of embolic protection, high incidence of restenosis in the balloon angioplasty arm, and higher stroke rate overall for both CEA and carotid interventions.

The Stenting and Angioplasty with Protection in Patients at High Risk for Endarterectomy (SAPPHIRE) was the first prospective randomized trial reported for carotid artery stenting.[19] The goal of this trial was to compare the safety and effectiveness of carotid artery stenting with embolic protection to CEA in high-risk patients. Patients were eligible if they had a greater than 50% stenosis and were symptomatic or had a greater than 80% stenosis and were asymptomatic. High risk was defined as patients with at least one of the following criteria: contralateral carotid artery occlusion, radiation therapy to the neck, previous CEA with recurrent stenosis, contralateral laryngeal nerve injury, difficult surgical access, heart failure, open heart surgery within the previous 6 weeks, myocardial infarction within the preceding 4 weeks, unstable angina, severe pulmonary disease, tandem lesions, or age older than 80 years. The primary outcome evaluated were rates of death, stroke, or myocardial infarction at 30 days. At 30 days, the CEA group ($n = 151$) had a composite endpoint rate of 12.6%, whereas the carotid stent group ($n = 156$) (performed with cerebral protection) had a rate of 5.8% ($p = 0.047$). At 1 year, carotid artery stenting was not statistically superior to CEA but it also wasn't inferior in the 1-year endpoints of stroke, myocardial infarction, and death. The 1-year major adverse event rate was 12.1% for carotid artery stenting and 20% for CEA. However, when the incidence of non–Q-wave myocardial infarction was removed, the difference in adverse events was not statistically different. The inclusion of myocardial infarction as a composite endpoint was controversial for several reasons. The two groups differed in types of anesthesia (general for CEA and local for carotid artery stenting) administered, as well as antiplatelet regimen (Plavix in the carotid artery stenting group and none in the CEA group). These differences may have accounted for the reduced incidence of myocardial infarction in the carotid artery stenting group. Another major criticism of the trial has been the larger number of patients assigned to the registry group (406) rather than stenting (344) due to the rationale that patients who were unfit for surgery should be directly assigned to the stent registry. The trial was halted due to the lack of enrollment and, notably, less than 50% of patients actually underwent randomization.

As was stated earlier, in order for carotid artery stenting to gain full acceptance, it must provide clinical outcomes that rival CEA. Randomized trials comparing the outcomes in patients considered to be of conventional risk, either symptomatic or asymptomatic, are under way. The Carotid Revascularization Endarterectomy versus Stent Trial (CREST) is a prospective randomized trial of symptomatic patients with carotid stenosis of greater than 50% by angiography or greater than 80% by duplex ultrasound (US). It was expanded to also include an asymptomatic arm for stenoses greater than 60% by angiography and 70% by duplex US. The enrollment goal is listed as 1,500 patients. In 2004, the CREST investigators published the interim results from the lead-in phase of CREST.[20] It showed that the periprocedural risk of stroke and death after carotid artery stenting increased with age. In this group of 749 patients, a 12.1% incidence of stoke and death was reported in patients aged 80 and older.

Recently, two European trials have been published evaluating CEA and carotid artery stenting. The Stent-Protected Percutaneous Angioplasty of the Carotid versus Endarterectomy (SPACE) trial was a European study comparing carotid artery stenting with CEA in symptomatic patients.[21] Thirty-five multinational sites participated with randomization of 1,200 patients and 1,183 patients analyzed. With stroke and death as endpoints, this study failed to demonstrate the noninferiority of carotid artery stenting. The study was terminated due to lack of funding and poor results of carotid artery stenting. Interestingly, despite a large stent group of 567 patients, only 27% were treated with embolic protection devices and the majority of patients underwent stenting without protection. Critics of the study blame the poor outcome of carotid artery stenting on the inconsistent and infrequent use of embolic protection. Similarly, the Endarterectomy Versus Angioplasty in Patients with Symptomatic Severe Carotid Stenosis (EVA-3S) study reported data comparing carotid artery stenting with CEA in high-grade symptomatic patients.[22] Thirty-five sites in France enrolled 259 patients for CEA and 261 patients for carotid artery stenting. The decision to employ cerebral protection and dual-antiplatelet therapy in the carotid artery stenting group was left to the discretion of the individual investigators. The 30-day incidence of stroke or death was 9.6% in the carotid artery stenting group and 3.9% in the CEA group, and the study failed to prove noninferiority of carotid artery stenting. It was halted prematurely due to the significantly higher stroke and death rates in the carotid artery stenting group. The study was widely criticized for the level of investigator experience and variability of carotid artery stenting technique. Proponents of carotid artery stenting felt that the operators were not appropriately skilled in the devices and procedures, which resulted in poorer outcomes for carotid artery stenting than in other studies where investigators were more experienced.

While CREST was to complete enrollment by 2008, other prospective randomized trials, such as the Transatlantic Asymptomatic Carotid Intervention Trial (TACIT), the Asymptomatic Carotid Trial (ACT-1), and the Asymptomatic Carotid Surgery Trial (ACT-2), are under way to evaluate optimal therapy with respect to asymptomatic stenosis.

MESENTERIC ARTERY INTERVENTIONS

Chronic and acute mesenteric ischemia are well-described conditions resulting from occlusive disease of the splanchnic vessels. The prevalence of mesenteric occlusive disease among the elderly has been reported at 17.5%.[23] Symptomatic disease is usually a result of occlusion or stenosis of two of the three mesenteric vessels. A delay in diagnosis and treatment of this

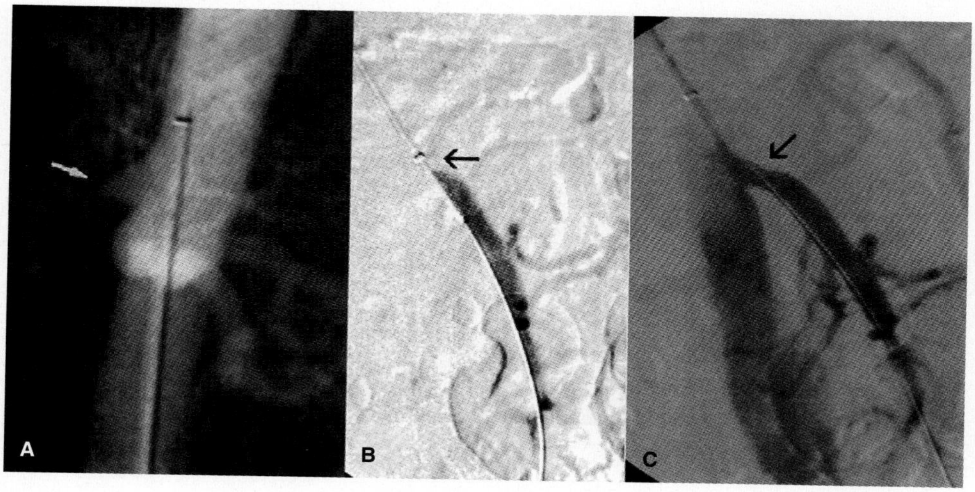

FIGURE 87.4. **A:** Lateral aortogram demonstrating occlusion of the superior mesenteric artery (SMA, *arrow*) in a patient with postprandial abdominal pain and weight loss. **B:** The occlusion was crossed with a guide wire (*arrow*) and subsequently balloon angioplastied and stented. **C:** Completion angiography reveals resolution of the occlusion with antegrade flow in the SMA. The patient's symptoms resolved.

clinical syndrome can result in bowel infarction and death. Surgical therapy with revascularization and bowel resection has been the traditional mode of treatment.

Percutaneous therapy for mesenteric occlusive disease was first described in 1980 by Furer et al. and Uflacker et al. in two separate reports.[24,25] Furer et al. reported the first balloon angioplasty of a superior mesenteric lesion with success. The early experience with percutaneous treatment favored balloon angioplasty, and several small series reported excellent initial results.[26–28] They were limited, however, by early restenosis ranging from 17% to 25% with a mean follow-up of 25 to 39 months. Failures were attributed to extrinsic compression, elastic recoil, and refractory disease. This led to the application of primary stenting, particularly in the setting of ostial disease.

Early series evaluating the efficacy of mesenteric stenting were limited by the small numbers of patients and short follow-up.[29–31] Later series have emerged with larger numbers of patients and interventions. The Cleveland Clinic experience reported by Kasirajian et al.[32] compared outcomes in 28 patients treated with endovascular therapy with those in 85 patients treated with open surgical therapy. Both groups were matched in comorbid risk factors, number of occlusive vessels involved, and duration of symptoms. They differed, however, in the age of onset and presentation. The median age for the endovascular group was 72, whereas in the open surgery group it was 65. Although both groups had similar postprocedure complication rates and 3-year restenosis rates, the percutaneous group had a higher incidence of recurrent symptoms. This may have been related to the number of lesions treated in the percutaneous group, which was one, compared to the surgical group, who had more than one vessel revascularized. Rose et al.[33] found similar results in 1995 in their retrospective review of surgical and percutaneous revascularization modes in patients. The mortality and complication rates were similar and the open surgical group underwent multivessel revascularization in the Kasirajian review.[32] Long-term pain relief was 67% at 9 months in the endovascular group and 82.7% at 34.5 months in the surgical group. The authors suggested that the differences in symptomatic relief stemmed from the number of vessels revascularized. A series by Sharafuddin et al. retrospectively evaluated 25 patients in whom 28 procedures were performed with 96% technical success and found no difference in clinical outcome or patency rates in patients who were treated for simple stenotic lesions, occlusions, or complex lesions.[33a] The patency rates and complication rates were similar to other recent studies.[34,35]

Recently, Sarac et al. investigated the results of percutaneous mesenteric revascularization and evaluated predictors of outcomes including morbidity and death.[36] Sixty-five patients underwent 87 mesenteric interventions with cumulative 1-year patency rates that included primary patency of 65%, primary assisted patency of 97%, and secondary patency of 99%. Symptomatic relief was immediate in 85% of patients and 75% experienced relief beyond 1 year. Diminished patency rates were associated with hypertension, chronic obstructive pulmonary disease (COPD), and bowel dysfunction. Patency, complications, and survival were no different despite number of vessels treated or types of stents used. Decreased survival was noted in patients with COPD, and no patient who underwent bowel resection after intervention survived. This series supports the endovascular treatment of occluded mesenteric vessels with similar patency and survival as stenotic visceral vessels.

4 With the advent of lower-profile sheaths, wires, and stents, percutaneous interventions have become more feasible and often the first-line treatment in the setting of mesenteric occlusive disease (Fig. 87.4). As with renal disease, the lesions are often ostial and respond best to stent placement. In the setting of multiocclusive lesions, solitary treatment of the superior mesenteric lesion will often suffice. The role of stent grafts and biodegradeable stents in the visceral vessels have yet to be evaluated.

RENAL ARTERY INTERVENTIONS

Renovascular hypertension is the most common cause of secondary hypertension, and obstructive renal lesions account for 5% of such cases.[37,38] Without treatment, such lesions can result in progressive renal dysfunction with ischemic nephropathy, congestive heart failure, and renal atrophy.[39] Renal revascularization options include both surgical and percutaneous interventions. Although both therapies offer similar technical results, the morbidity and mortality of surgical revascularization ranges from 17% to 31% and 2% to 7%, respectively.[40–43] Transcatheter therapy offers similar patency, with fewer complications and shorter hospital stay.

5 Percutaneous transluminal angioplasty is the treatment of choice for nonorificial atherosclerotic lesions and fibromuscular dysplasia. The first percutaneous transluminal angioplasty of the renal artery was reported by Gruntzig et al. in 1978.[44] Technical success for percutaneous transluminal angioplasty in this setting has been reported at 90% in several series.[45–47] The incidence of restenosis in the setting of angioplasty, however, is high. Reports from Martin et al. and Weibull et al. in separate series have reported a 30% incidence of restenosis.[40,45] Elastic recoil and extensive atherosclerotic aortic and orificial plaque limit the application of balloon angioplasty in patients with ostial disease and account for the high recurrence rate afterwards.

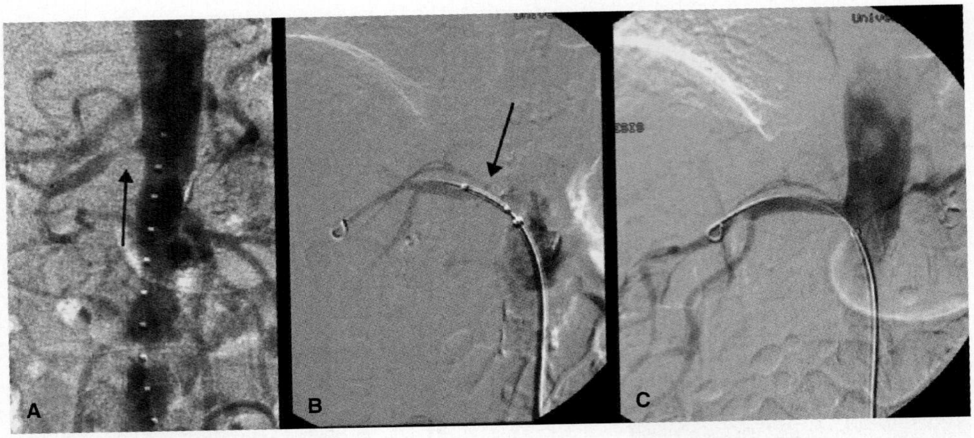

FIGURE 87.5. Angiograms from a patient undergoing angioplasty and stenting of a right renal artery stenosis. A: Flush aortogram that reveals a high-grade right renal artery stenosis (*arrow*). B: Wire access is obtained across the lesion, and a sheath is advanced up to the origin of the renal artery. A balloon-expandable stent (*arrow*, prior to deployment) is placed at the level of the stenosis (*arrow*). C: After deployment of the stent, there is no residual stenosis.

Selective placement of stents in the renal arteries (Fig. 87.5) evolved following the first report by Palmaz et al.[48] in animal models. Although first used in the setting of elastic recoil or dissection after balloon angioplasty, the use of stenting has become a primary modality for renal artery stenosis, particularly in the setting of ostial disease.[49,50] Several studies have evaluated the efficacy of stenting for ostial disease. The Erasme study prospectively assessed the safety and results of Palmaz stenting of the renal artery in 10 centers with 106 patients. The investigators demonstrated technical success in 95% of arteries and a 16.9% restenosis rate at 8 months, of which 10 out of 15 lesions were successfully redilated.[51] Rees et al.[52] reported similar success in the United States with a multicenter trial evaluating the Palmaz stent in ostial renal stenosis. Single-center reports have also verified the high technical success rate of primary stenting with restenosis rates of 15% to 20%.[53,54]

Despite the high procedural success rate and lower restenosis rate than balloon angioplasty, the effects of renal artery stenting on hypertension and renal function have varying results. Improvements in hypertension control after renal artery stenting have been demonstrated in several series and vary from 49% to 80%, whereas azotemic benefit is more variable, with most centers reporting stabilization of renal function rather than improvement.[50,53,55–57] A multicenter registry report by Dorros et al.[56] evaluated the 4-year follow-up in 1,058 patients and found significant improvement in blood pressure control, a decrease in the number of antihypertensive medications from 2.4 to 1.9, and stabilization of serum creatinine levels.

6 Results from surgical revascularization and renal interventions are comparable. Higher complication rates are reported with concurrent repair of aneurysmal disease or other visceral stenosis.[53,58] Cambria et al.[59] reviewed 285 renal revascularizations and reported an operative mortality of 5.6% and an 8.1% mortality in procedures that involved an aortic anastomosis. Hallett et al.[42] documented an operative mortality of 7.1% in a series of 652 renal operations. In contrast, complications related to renal interventions are most commonly groin hematoma and puncture site trauma, although atheroembolic phenomena and contrast nephropathy also occur.[51,60] Lower-profile systems, embolic protection devices, meticulous technique, increased experience, and nonnephrotoxic radiographic agents have been used to reduce the incidence of emboli and renal failure.[61–63]

Recently, Kashyap et al.[64] evaluated PTA and stenting in patients with renal artery stenosis and declining renal function. This study evaluated 125 patients, and 67% experienced improvement or stabilization of their glomerular filtration rate (GFR). The fate of the incidental renal artery stenosis with percutaneous treatment was evaluated in a retrospective series by Suliman et al.[65] This study evaluated 128 patients, of which 78 underwent intervention for high-grade renal artery stenosis. The authors concluded that isolated renal artery stenting resulted in the lowering of systolic and diastolic pressures in patients who had an increase in the number of antihypertensive medications. Other parameters, however, such as GFR and serum creatinine, were not affected. The management of isolated renal artery stenosis with percutaneous intervention is not clear and is not supported. Renal artery interventions have been shown to have excellent technical results and patency comparable to open surgical revascularization. The modest recurrent stenosis rate can be treated adequately with repeat intervention and balloon angioplasty. However, its long-term effect on preservation of renal function remains to be proven. Long-term outcomes with both surgery and percutaneous therapy are better in patients with normal renal function, and success with either intervention is limited in the setting of parenchymal loss and elevated serum creatinines.[66–68]

AORTIC INTERVENTIONS

Endografting for Aortic Aneurysms

Abdominal aortic aneurysm (AAA) repair has had favorable results, but a less invasive procedure with fewer physiologic stresses has evolved over time. Parodi et al.[69] reported the first clinical use of endovascular AAA repair. Since that time, the application of aortic endografting for the treatment of AAA has significantly progressed and continues to do so. The current indications for endovascular repair of AAA remain the same as for conventional operative repair. It provides many potential benefits over conventional repair, however. It requires small groin incisions instead of a large abdominal one, which may decrease the incidence of postoperative pulmonary complications. There is decreased retroperitoneal dissection and thus a lower risk of perioperative bleeding. There is no or minimal aortic occlusion, which reduces the intraoperative hemodynamic stresses compared with open aneurysm repair.[70] These benefits may broaden the scope of aneurysm repair to patients who previously were deemed untreatable due to comorbidities.

Endograft Construction. The design of an aortic endograft can greatly affect the ability to place the device in a patient. One design component that is important for effective endograft placement is the delivery system. This is the equipment that houses the endograft in a compact fashion allowing it to be delivered to the proper anatomic location. Most endografts are placed through the common femoral artery and iliac artery system. The size of the delivery system must be smaller than the lumen through which it must pass. Inadequate vessel diameter or the presence of extensive calcifications can inhibit endograft placement. The majority of available endografts easily traverse an iliofemoral segment of 7 to 8 mm in diameter. Another feature of the endograft delivery system is its flexibility, which allows it to traverse a tortuous iliac artery. Some tortuosity can be corrected or "straightened" with the use of a stiff guide wire; however, this is not always possible or desirable. Delivery systems composed of long, flexible, tapered tips pass more easily than those with short, stiff, blunt tips.[71]

Two general classifications of endograft construction exist: unibody and modular. A unibody device is a single-piece graft. This single piece includes the main body and both limbs. This composition decreases the risk of endoleaks as there are fewer sites of component apposition. However, a larger delivery system is often required, and there is less flexibility in obtaining the correct length of the graft. The modular system includes endografts that are composed of two to three pieces. Generally there is a main body that may have one attached limb and one or two docking limbs. These types of devices can be introduced through smaller delivery systems and offer a greater degree of flexibility with regard to placement. With multiple sites of graft–graft apposition, however, there is increased risk of endoleak.

Graft composition further varies by the material that is used to construct the graft and the metal "skeleton" that is used to support it. Graft material ranges from thin-walled polytetrafluoroethylene to polyester. The graft material is supported by a metal framework (stent) that is composed of stainless steel, Elgiloy, or nitinol. The graft support can be placed inside the graft material, an endoskeleton, or outside the graft material, an exoskeleton. Grafts can be fully supported, having stent material throughout, or only partially supported, with portions of the graft having only material and no metallic support. The graft skeleton provides several key elements to endograft construction. The metal skeleton provides some degree of radial force that helps to provide a seal to prevent blood flow around the graft and a point of fixation. Some devices have hooks or barbs in the proximal aspect of the skeleton that help to anchor the graft onto the aortic wall and prevent migration. Other grafts have a bare stent that extends above the level of the fabric that helps to anchor the graft in the pararenal and suprarenal portion of the aorta, at a point where less disease may be present. The other function of the metal skeleton is to provide columnar strength to the graft, which helps to prevent migration. The skeleton may play an important role in prevention of graft kinking as it crosses tortuous anatomy, but the lack of a skeleton may be important in allowing a graft to adapt more readily to morphologic changes that occur after aneurysmal exclusion, without dislodgment of attachment sites.

Anatomic Requirements for Graft Placement. There are several anatomic requirements for the successful placement of an aortic endograft. Exact requirements vary with specific device design, but the key aspects remain the same. These include an appropriate aortic neck, a distal sealing zone, and a suitable path for the endograft to be placed through. The aortic neck is defined as the area of the aorta cephalad to the aneurysm, below the level of the renal arteries, in which the aortic endograft will be placed. This area is important for two reasons: (a) it is the site of proximal fixation that will prevent the device from migrating distally and (b) a circumferential seal must be obtained in this region to prevent blood leakage around the graft and into the aneurysm sac. In general, a 15-mm length of aortic neck is required below the level of the most caudal renal artery and above the level of the aneurysm to meet these needs. Several devices employ the use of a suprarenal, uncovered stent to provide additional protection against graft migration. Other aortic neck characteristics are important in determining whether a patient is an ideal endograft candidate. These include neck angulation, the shape of the neck, and the quality of the neck. Acute angulation of the neck can greatly affect the ability to obtain a proximal seal. Aortic neck angulation greater than 60 degrees compared with the centerline is often considered prohibitive for endovascular aneurysm repair. The shape of the aortic neck will also affect the ability to obtain a seal and fixation. A conical-shaped neck, defined as an increase in diameter over the course of 15 mm by more than 10%, is felt to be a contraindication to routine aortic endografting. In addition, the presence of circumferential thrombus or severe aortic wall calcification can negatively affect the ability to obtain a seal and fixation.

The iliofemoral arterial system is important for endograft placement because it provides the route for graft placement, as well as the site for obtaining a distal seal. Many of the features important in an aortic neck for obtaining a seal and fixation are also important in the iliac arteries. The presence of thrombus, calcification, and tortuosity can significantly hinder the iliac limb seal. Most available endograft systems require at least a 15-mm segment of iliac artery to be of adequate caliber and free of significant disease to obtain a distal seal.

7 **Endograft Placement.** The most important aspect of aortic endograft placement takes place prior to graft placement in determining whether a patient is indeed a suitable candidate for endograft placement, choosing an appropriate endograft device, and properly determining the size graft to be placed. These determinations are best made based on thin-cut helical computed tomography scans and in some cases with the addition of diagnostic angiography. The majority of endografts are placed through the femoral arteries that have been operatively exposed. The aorta is cannulated with a guide wire and catheter. Small boluses of contrast agent are delivered to identify the renal arteries to avoid covering them. Due to the often angulated nature of an aneurysmal aorta, it can be necessary to focus the image intensifier at an oblique cranial-caudal view to obtain the best view of the renal arteries. The device is generally placed over a stiff guide wire and positioned to allow the most extensive coverage within the aortic neck without intruding on the ostia of the renal arteries. Every device has its own unique deployment instructions and discussion of them is beyond the scope of this chapter. Depending on the construction of the endograft, following deployment of the main body (which may include an attached ipsilateral limb), the ipsilateral limb and contralateral limbs are placed.

8 Postoperative surveillance is extremely important in patients undergoing endovascular AAA repair. Complications may be asymptomatic at first and not present clinically for several years.[72–74] Protocols for graft surveillance vary from institution to institution, but most entail four-view abdominal plain film radiographic evaluation and intravenous contrast, thin-cut computed tomography (CT) scanning. Major imaging generally occurs at 1, 6, and 12 months and then yearly thereafter. From these images, assessment can be made to evaluate for migration, changes in aneurysm size, and the presence of endoleaks. An alternative method used to track aneurysms following endograft repair is via calculation of aneurysm volume. Aneurysm volume is determined from three-dimensional reconstructions of spiral CT scans. Aneurysm morphology can change after endograft exclusion, and thus a measurement of the volume may be a more accurate assessment of changes in aneurysm size.[75,76] Duplex US would provide a less invasive and less costly means of following aortic aneurysms following endovascular exclusion, but it does not yet provide the sensitivity and specificity obtained by CT scans.[77] The addition of US contrast agents may improve its efficacy; however, its use currently is not routine.[78]

Complications Associated with Aortic Endograft Placement. A number of problems can arise during the placement of an aortic endograft, and there are several that can arise in the follow-up period. The following paragraphs outline some of the more common problems encountered.

Iliac Artery Disease. As the primary route of insertion for most endografts is via the iliofemoral arterial system, the presence of atherosclerotic disease, aneurysmal disease, and tortuosity in the iliac arteries can greatly affect the ease with which these grafts are placed. In cases of iliac artery lumen narrowing secondary to atherosclerotic disease and severe vessel tortuosity, advancement of the device despite the presence of resistance can result in vessel rupture. Iliac rupture occurs in 1% to 2% of cases of endograft placement.[79,80] Occasionally, iliac artery narrowing can be dealt with by predilation of an occlusive lesion with balloon angioplasty. Preprocedural iliac stent placement, however, can be prohibitive to endograft placement and is discouraged. An alternative is to use an iliac conduit. An iliac conduit involves suturing a prosthetic graft to the iliac artery (and occasionally the aorta), even if it is aneurysmal. The device is placed through the conduit and into the aorta. The ipsilateral limb is then "landed" in the conduit and the end of the conduit is anastomosed to the common femoral artery. The distal end of the common iliac artery can be oversewn at a level to allow continued perfusion of the hypogastric artery in a retrograde fashion. Alternatively, the hypogastric artery can be anastomosed to the iliac conduit.

Iliac artery ectasia and aneurysmal disease can cause a problem obtaining a distal seal. Enlarged common iliac arteries are present in up to 30% of patients presenting for endovascular aneurysm repair.[81–83] Some endografts allow for the placement of larger iliac limbs, or flared limbs, that can obtain seals in ecstatic iliac arteries. In those that do not, however, the distal seal may need to be obtained in the external iliac artery. This generally requires sacrifice of the hypogastric artery by coil embolization prior to the procedure. The presence of a hypogastric artery aneurysm requires the same approach. Rarely is bilateral hypogastric artery exclusion required, but, when it is, it is performed in a staged fashion. Hypogastric embolization is associated with side effects in up to 50% of patients. Buttock claudication is the predominant complaint, occurring in 12% to 50% of patients, but it generally resolves within several months.[81–83] Patients requiring embolization of the more distal branches of the hypogastric artery are at an increased risk for developing symptoms, although bilateral hypogastric embolization has not been reported.[83,84] Coil embolization of the hypogastric artery is not necessary in the presence of a common iliac artery aneurysm provided that there is a 5-mm neck of iliac artery proximal to the hypogastric origin as well as a 15-mm neck in the external iliac artery.[85] This anatomic arrangement allows for an adequate seal and can be successful in up to two thirds of patients requiring coverage of the hypogastric artery.

TABLE 87.1

ENDOLEAK CLASSIFICATION COMPLICATIONS

■ TYPE OF ENDOLEAK	■ DEFINITION
I	Arise secondary to inadequate sealing at either proximal aortic or distal aortic/iliac attachment sites
II	Arise secondary to patent branch vessels off of the aortic sac (i.e., inferior mesenteric artery or lumbar artery)
III	Arise secondary to defects in the fabric of the graft or at the junction zone between modular components
IV	Arise secondary to diffuse "leaking" of blood between the interstices of the fabric, or from suture holes at the sites where the graft is attached to the stent
V	Applied to the scenario in which the aneurysm sac remains pressurized in the absence of a discernible endoleak—termed *endotension*

Endoleaks. An endoleak is the persistence of blood flow outside of the endograft within the aneurysm sac. Endoleaks are classified according to their etiology, and currently five different types have been described (Table 87.1).[86–88] Type I endoleaks arise from inadequate sealing at either proximal aortic (allowing antegrade flow) or distal iliac (allowing retrograde flow) attachment sites. Type II endoleaks arise from patent branch vessels off of the aortic sac that allow for retrograde flow into the aneurysm. Such branches include patent lumbar arteries and a patent inferior mesenteric artery (Fig. 87.6). Type III endoleaks develop from defects in the fabric of the graft or at the junction zone between modular components. Type IV endoleaks develop secondary to diffuse "leaking" of blood between the interstices of the fabric or where the graft is sutured to a stent. Type V endoleaks are applied to the scenario in which the aneurysm sac remains pressurized resulting in subsequent aneurysmal enlargement, despite no demonstrable evidence of blood flow into the aneurysm sac. The pressure applied to the aneurysm sac causing it to continue to expand, in this situation, has been termed *endotension*.[89]

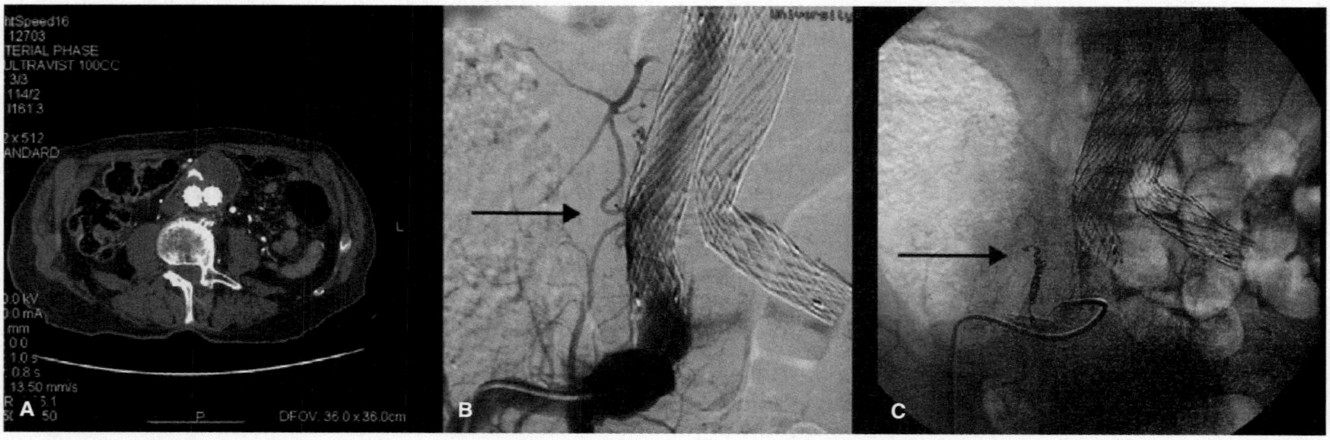

FIGURE 87.6. Radiologic images from a patient who underwent an endograft repair of an abdominal aortic aneurysm (AAA). The patient had a known type II endoleak, but subsequently developed an increase in the size of the aneurysm. **A:** Computed tomography scan revealing a type II endoleak. **B:** Angiogram revealing the branch off the hypogastric artery that was contributing to the endoleak (*arrow*). **C:** Subsequent coil embolization of this vessel (*arrow*) led to resolution of the endoleak.

Controversy with regard to this concept exists. Some argue that this merely represents a type I, II, III, or IV endoleak in which the defect is large enough to allow blood flow into the aneurysm sac, but it either occurs intermittently or is too small to be visualized by conventional means.[71]

Types I and III endoleaks are associated with an increased risk of aneurysm expansion and possible rupture, and thus should be treated.[90,91] Treatment of these lesions can be accomplished with the placement of an extension cuff over the site of the leak. Alternatively, for type I endoleaks, placement of a large balloon-expandable stent at the level of the leak may increase the radial force at that level and seal the leak. Failure to resolve a type I or III endoleak in an endovascular fashion should result in the conversion to an open procedure with standard repair of the aneurysm and removal of the endovascular device. Type II endoleaks are rarely associated with aneurysm rupture.[92] At least 10% to 15% of patients will be identified with a type II endoleak during follow-up.[93–96] Type II endoleaks are generally observed unless they are associated with an increase in aneurysm size or are associated with aortic pulsatility on physical examination. Arteriography is the next step in the evaluation of a patient with a type II endoleak associated with these findings. Superselective arterial canalization can be performed with embolization of feeding vessels. An alternative approach is via direct aneurysm sac puncture, during which sac pressures can be measured as well as the injection of contrast to identify the feeding vessels precisely.[97] Sac pressure measurements may be an indicator of the presence of an endoleak, even if it is not detected by routine imaging. The use of implantable intrasac pressure transducers to monitor patients following endovascular repair is currently under investigation.[98]

Limb Thrombosis. Thrombosis of an iliac limb of an aortic endograft occurs in up to 11% of patients.[99–102] There are a number of factors that have been suggested to place patients at increased risk for developing graft limb thrombosis. The lack of stent support within an iliac limb has been shown to increase the risk of thrombosis by nearly eightfold compared with intrinsically supported limbs.[101] Intuitively, the presence of atherosclerotic disease and luminal narrowing within the iliac artery increases the risk of limb thrombosis.[100] Oversizing of the iliac limb causes the graft material to have a significant amount of infolding, thus narrowing the intraluminal diameter and placing the limb at increased risk for thrombosis.[102] Extension of the limb into the external iliac artery can contribute to the risk of limb thrombosis due to the change in vessel diameter, as well as due to kinking caused by the acute angulation the artery takes as it exits the pelvis.[100] Most patients present with limb thrombosis within the first 6 months following endograft repair. Management of patients with acute limb thrombosis is dictated by the presenting symptoms. As many as one third of patients remain asymptomatic and require no intervention.[100] Most patients, however, are symptomatic and are managed with a femoral-femoral artery bypass. Few patients are successfully treated with thrombolysis or graft thrombectomy followed by endovascular repair of the underlying problem.

Migration. Stent graft migration complicates abdominal aortic endografting in 9% to 45% of cases.[96,103–105] Migration is a known risk factor for the delayed development of a type I endoleak and subsequent delayed aneurysm rupture or late conversion.[105] Blood flow is the main displacing force that causes graft migration. This force is counteracted by the frictional forces of the graft against the aortic wall, particularly at the aneurysm neck. These frictional forces can be affected by the length of the neck or the presence of thrombus and calcifications. Albertini et al.[104] evaluated patients that developed migration or a delayed type I endoleak. Neck angulation and neck diameter were the two factors associated with their development. Morphologic changes in the aortic aneurysm and aneurysm neck have been suggested to contribute to graft migration. Aneurysm neck dilation occurs mostly in the first 2 years after graft placement and has been shown to be independently associated with device migration.[105,106] This finding, however, has not been supported by all series.[107]

Outcomes. Endograft repair of AAA has a low mortality rate (less than 3%) and subsequent rates of aneurysm rupture are reduced to 1% per year.[91,96,108,109] The need for a secondary intervention, however, is not insignificant.[110] In the EUROSTAR registry, reporting on 1,023 patients with follow-up of 12 months or longer, 186 (18%) of patients required a secondary intervention. The majority of these (76%) were accomplished through a transfemoral approach, and the rest required an intra-abdominal or extra-anatomic procedure. The rates of freedom from intervention at 1, 3, and 4 years were 89%, 67%, and 62%, respectively. Mortality was higher in those patients requiring a secondary procedure and was more frequently associated with those requiring an intra-abdominal intervention. Similar results have been reported from single-institution series. Montefiore Medical Center reported secondary procedure rates of 10%, whereas the Cleveland Clinic Foundation had a secondary intervention rate of 15%.[108,111] Univariate analysis revealed that secondary procedures were more common in patients with large major and minor sac axes, in patients who received a large aortic stent because of a proximal endoleak present at the initial repair, and in patients who received treatment later in the course of the review. This latter finding is thought to be secondary to the increased complexity of cases.

There have been several studies comparing the results of aortic endograft repair of AAA with conventional surgery. Early studies that compared outcomes of endografting with historic controls or concomitant surgical arms suggested that endovascular repair is associated with a shorter initial hospital stay compared with open surgery. This difference, however, is negated if the total number of hospital days, including subsequent ones for secondary procedures, is taken into consideration.[112] Schermerhorn et al.[113] evaluated quality-adjusted life expectancy after endovascular AAA repair compared with open surgical repair using a Markov decision-analysis model. Endovascular data were derived from the EUROSTAR registry, whereas the open aneurysm repair data came from the 1995 Medicare claims for elective repair of nonruptured AAA. A case-based analysis of 70-year-old men revealed the life expectancy after endovascular AAA repair was 7.09 quality-adjusted life years compared with open AAA repair of 7.03 quality-adjusted life years. This represents a difference of approximately 3 weeks. Sensitivity analysis, however, revealed that for individuals younger than 64 years, open surgical repair results in a significantly greater quality-adjusted life expectancy.

There have been two direct comparisons of abdominal aortic endografting to conventional surgery.[114,115] The Dutch Randomised Endovascular Aneurysm Management (DREAM) trial group reported on the outcomes of a randomized prospective trial comparing open repair with endovascular repair in 345 patients with AAA.[114] This study demonstrated clinical equipoise between conventional surgery and endovascular aneurysm repair. Operative mortality was 4.6% in the open surgical arm and 1.2% in the endovascular arm ($p = 0.10$). The rate of moderate and severe systemic complications, however, was significantly lower in the endovascular arm (11.7%) compared to the open surgical arm (26.4%, $p < 0.001$). Endovascular Aneurysm Repair (EVAR) trial 1 evaluated a randomized controlled trial of 1,082 patients deemed anatomically suitable for endovascular repair and fit for open surgery.[115] While all-cause mortality did not differ between the two arms, there were significantly lower aneurysm-related death rates in the EVAR group (4%) compared to the surgical arm (7%, $p = 0.04$) at 4 years. This is directly related to lower operative mortality rates. There were, however, higher rates of long-term complications requiring reintervention in the EVAR group. This improvement in aneurysm-related mortality, however, does not necessarily lead to improved outcomes in those patients deemed too high risk for conventional surgery.[116]

Thoracic Aortic Endografting. Aortic endografting is no longer limited to the abdominal aorta. To date, in the United States, three thoracic aortic endografts have been approved for commercial use, and several more are undergoing clinical investigation. The construction and delivery of these devices is very similar to that of abdominal aortic endografts, and the general principles of endografting as outlined previously apply. Some differences, however, do exist. These devices are often larger in diameter than their abdominal counterparts, and thus require a larger sheath for delivery. This increased delivery system diameter can lead to more difficulty in traversing the iliac arteries and a higher rate of conversion to an iliac conduit. In addition to the size and tortuosity of the iliac arteries, the thoracic aorta can often provide an additional site of tortuosity and angulation, making it more difficult to maneuver the device into position. There can often be a significant size differential between the proximal and distal landing zones, thus requiring multiple tubular pieces in order to cross a lesion. Despite these increased difficulties, thoracic aortic endografting has been very successful. Five-year results of the Gore TAG device have been published.[117] In this trial, 140 thoracic aortic endografts were compared to standard open surgical controls ($n = 94$). At 5 years, aneurysm-related mortality was lower for the endograft arm (2.8%) compared to the surgical arm (11.7%, $p = 0.008$). In addition, major adverse events were lower in the endograft arm (57.9% vs. 78.7%, $p = 0.001$). As more data on the outcomes of thoracic aortic endografting are collected, we will be better able to assess its usefulness and long-term clinical limitations.

Thoracoabdominal Aortic Aneurysms. The current commercially available endograft systems are limited in their application to patients with suitable anatomy. This predominantly means that they are limited to patients who have sufficient normal aorta on either side of the aneurysm that will allow for the apposition of the endograft to the aortic wall, without covering any significant side branches. The future of aortic endografting, however, revolves around the development of grafts that will allow exclusion of an aneurysm but preservation of blood flow to critical branch vessels, thus allowing treatment of such complex anatomy as thoracoabdominal aortic aneurysms. Advanced endovascular technologies that allow treatment of more complex aneurysms that involve or abut the visceral segment use devices termed *fenestrated* or *branched* aortic endografts. These endovascular devices overcome problems with inadequate sealing zones by extending the sealing and fixation regions of the stent graft proximally or distally without sacrificing branch vessels. These devices require a detailed understanding of imaging studies, adjunctive endovascular devices, interventional techniques, and high-level operative/interventional facilities.

Fenestrated endografts are grafts that have a hole, or fenestration, that accommodate a single or multiple side branches. These devices are ideal for increasing the landing zone of an aortic endograft that has some neck, just not enough. The typical type of aneurysm treated with these devices would be a juxtarenal aneurysm. The wall of the endograft is in apposition to the aortic wall at the level of the vessel ostia. As this distance increases, such as when the critical vessel arises from the aneurysm itself, a branched endograft is necessary. A branched endograft allows for a cuff of fabric to bridge the gap between the endograft and the branch vessel (Fig. 87.7). The cuff or branch creates an overlap zone between the stent graft and the branch artery. The branch is often mated with the target vessel using an additional covered stent (Fig. 87.7). These types of systems have only been employed, in the United States, in clinical trials. The largest series was presented by the Cleveland Clinic.[118] This series describes the use of branched endografts in 73 patients treated for thoracoabdominal aortic aneurysms. Technical success was achieved in 93% of the patients, and there were no conversions to open repair. Five technical failures occurred: one was secondary to a death within 24 hours, and the others were related to the inability to gain access to one of the target vessels. Major complications occurred in 14% of patients and included paraplegia (2.7%), new-onset dialysis (1.4%), myocardial infarction (5.5%), and stroke (1.4%). Although this aspect of aortic endografting is still in its infancy, it is clear that the refinement of this technique will break down almost all current anatomic barriers of aortic endografting and allow for the treatment of the aorta from its origin through its bifurcation.

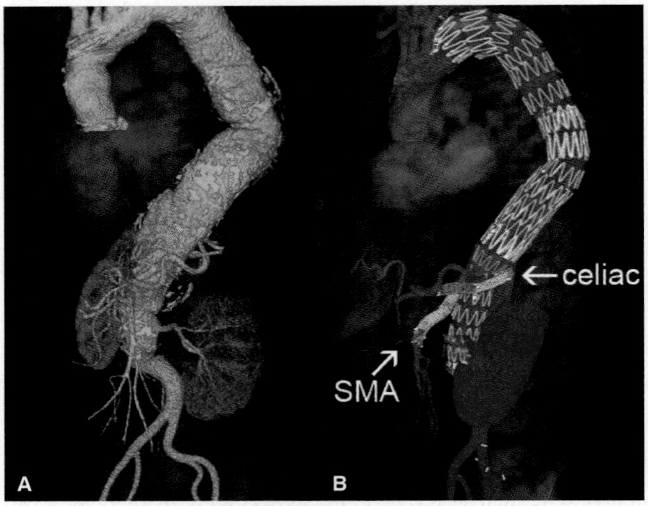

FIGURE 87.7. Three-dimensional reconstructions of an aorta from a patient with a thoracoabdominal aortic aneurysm (**A**) prior to repair and (**B**) after endovascular repair with a branched aortic endograft. The arrows demonstrate the branches arising from the endograft that supply the superior mesenteric artery and the celiac artery. SMA, superior mesenteric artery.

Aortoiliac Angioplasty and Stenting

9 Endovascular treatment of aortoiliac occlusive disease has become increasingly prominent over the past several years and has assumed a dominant role in the treatment of this disease. Factors including decreased morbidity compared with conventional surgery, shorter hospital stays, and equivalent patency rates have contributed to this change.

The specific indications for treatment of aortoiliac occlusive disease are independent of the approach to treatment, either endovascular or conventional surgery. An intervention is generally indicated if disabling claudication or limb-threatening ischemia is present. Clinically, pain starts in the thighs and buttocks and is often present in combination with lower extremity discomfort. Erectile dysfunction may be present in men. Weakened femoral pulses and decreased segmental blood pressures are indications of proximal disease. Indications for PTA, as opposed to PTA with primary stenting, are changing. Historically, PTA was the first approach and the application of a stent was reserved for suboptimal results of primary PTA, defined as a persistent reduction of the lumen diameter of 30% or more. A resting mean blood pressure gradient of 5 mm Hg or greater or a systolic blood pressure gradient exceeding 10 mm Hg is also considered significant. Provocative testing performed by the intra-arterial injection of a vasodilatory agent (25 mg papaverine or 100 to 200 μg nitroglycerine) may unmask a lesion and reveal a significant blood pressure gradient. Other indications for stent placement include eccentric stenosing plaque, arterial dissection, and when recanalization of an occluded segment is performed. With the ease with which stent placement can be performed, a more liberal approach to stenting is occurring.

Balloon dilation of iliac arteries is a relatively simple procedure. A retrograde transfemoral approach is the most widely

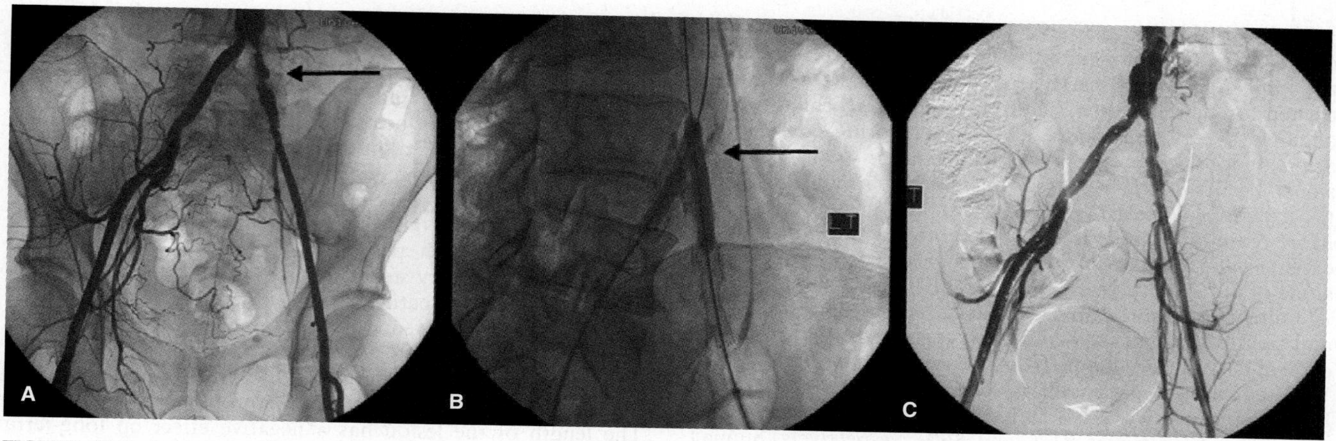

FIGURE 87.8. Angiograms from a patient who presented with disabling claudication of his left lower extremity. **A:** Aortogram revealed an area of stenosis in the proximal common iliac artery on the left (*arrow*). A pressure gradient was measured across this lesion and was found to be 30 mm Hg. **B:** The patient underwent placement of a balloon-expandable left iliac artery stent. To preserve the lumen of the right common iliac artery, a "kissing" balloon technique was performed in which a balloon was expanded in the right common iliac artery as the balloon-expandable stent was placed in the left common iliac artery (*arrow*). **C:** Angiographic resolution of the stenosis. There was also resolution of the pressure gradient.

used approach, although crossover procedures from the contralateral side can be performed. Following the use of angiography to identify the site of the lesion, a guide wire is advanced across the lesion. Once this is performed, the dilation balloon, sized to match or slightly exceed the normal vessel diameter, is inflated. The inflation device allows for the measurement of pressure within the PTA balloon, and often dilations to a pressure of 6 to 8 atmospheres of pressure are performed. Balloon dilation causes a fracture in the arterial plaque creating a local dissection, stretching the media and adventitia. Completion arteriography with or without pressure measurements is generally performed. The exact mechanism of stent deployment varies depending on the type of stent placed (balloon expandable or self-expanding) and the manufacturer. Stents are advanced across a lesion in a "protected" fashion. This entails the advancement of a sheath across the lesion, the advancement of the stent within the sheath to the level of the lesion, and then the retraction of the sheath. This protects the stent from being dislodged as it crosses a tight stenosis. If primary stent placement is considered, predeployment balloon angioplasty may be necessary to allow for advancement of the sheath and the stent.

Percutaneous treatment of chronic iliac artery occlusions is technically feasible. This is approached in a similar fashion as in a stenotic, nonocclusive lesion. Access to the artery is obtained in either a retrograde or antegrade fashion. The rate-limiting step in this scenario is obtaining wire access across the lesion. This is often accomplished with a combination of a catheter and a hydrophilic wire. Long areas of occlusion, as well as densely calcified lesions, can hinder the technical feasibility. Once wire access across the lesion is obtained, the stenosis can undergo balloon angioplasty to obtain a flow channel. This is best supported with the use of a stent after predilation.

Aortic bifurcation lesions present a unique situation as balloon angioplasty or stent placement in the origin of a common iliac artery may cause occlusion of the contralateral artery orifice. To overcome this problem, a technique termed *kissing balloon* or *kissing stent* placement is used (Fig. 87.8). This is the simultaneous placement of PTA balloons or stents that traverse the ostia of both common iliac arteries. If stents are used, it is mandatory that the proximal ends of both stents are parallel so that the flow into one stent is not hindered by the other. In most cases, the use of noncompressible, balloon-expandable stents are most beneficial in this procedure. Below the level of the aortic bifurcation, however, self-expanding stents are perfectly acceptable.

Iliac artery stent placement is technically successful in up to 97% of patients.[119] Technical complications occur in less than 6% of interventions and include subintimal dilation, dissection, arterial rupture, inability to cross the lesion with a wire, and distal embolization. Belli et al.[120] reported in their series that only 2.8% of patients developed complications requiring surgery, and only 0.9% required reconstructive bypass. Clinically significant distal embolization occurs in up to 1% of patients undergoing iliac artery PTA and stent placement. Silent peripheral embolization has been detected by Doppler ultrasound in 90% of patients immediately following iliac artery PTA, but this decreases with time.[121] Symptomatic embolization can be treated by a variety of endovascular methods, including suction thrombectomy and thrombolytic therapy. If these methods are unsuccessful, surgical thromboembolectomy is necessary.

Iliac artery dissection during PTA is reported in less than 1% of patients.[122] Half of the patients develop significant lumen compromise. Dissections are treated with prolonged balloon inflation to "tack down" the flap, or with placement of an intra-arterial stent. If endovascular therapy is unsuccessful, operative treatment includes iliac endarterectomy, iliofemoral artery bypass, femoral-femoral artery bypass, and aortobifemoral artery bypass grafting. Arterial dissection has been reported in 10% of patients undergoing iliac artery stent placement.[123] Nearly two thirds of the dissections caused a flow-limiting lesion that required the placement of an additional stent. Vessel injury is related to balloon oversizing and the degree of arterial calcification. Iliac artery rupture during balloon dilation and stent placement has been reported in up to 0.9% of cases.[124,125] Vessel disruption can present with uncontained hemorrhage, contained hemorrhage, or pseudoaneurysm formation. The key to initial management is to maintain guide wire access across the site of disruption. Control of the hemorrhage can be obtained with the insertion of an angioplasty balloon to tamponade the site of injury. If prolonged balloon tamponade does not achieve hemostasis, the placement of a covered stent is warranted. Uncontrolled hemorrhage demands operative intervention, but balloon occlusion proximal to the site of injury can afford time to prepare for surgery. Risk factors for rupture are similar to those for dissection and include the presence of a high-grade stenosis with heavy calcifications. Other risk factors include the use of oversized balloons and manual inflation without manometric control.

Results of iliac artery balloon angioplasty have been well documented. Johnston et al.[126] prospectively analyzed the results of 984 patients who underwent PTA, 684 of whom had aortoiliac angioplasty. Outcomes were assessed by Kaplan-Meier analysis. Twelve percent of the patients were treated for iliac artery occlusions, and the rest had nonocclusive stenoses. Initial success, defined as a combination of clinical factors and ankle-brachial index, was achieved in 88.6% of patients. This dropped to 48.2% at 60 months. Predictors of success included the indication for operation (with better results in patients treated for claudication vs. limb-threatening ischemia), site of angioplasty (common iliac artery lesions favoring external iliac artery lesions), and lesion severity (stenoses favoring occlusions). Becker et al.[127] reported a meta-analysis involving 2,679 procedures. Five-year patency rates for this group were 72%. More recently, Tegtmeyer et al.[119] reported a single-institution experience in 200 patients with a technical success rate of PTA alone of 88% and a 5-year patency of 85%.

Outcomes from treatment of iliac artery stenosis with PTA and stent placement have also been evaluated with long-term clinical data. The outcome from the use of the self-expanding Wallstent in 140 patients was evaluated by Martin et al.[128] Primary patency was 81% at 1 year and 71% at 2 years, and secondary patency was 91% and 86%, respectively. Similar results were obtained by Vorwerk et al.[129] They followed 118 patients with primary patency rates of 95% at 1 year, 88% at 2 years, and 82% at 4 years, and secondary patency rates were 96%, 93%, and 91%, respectively. Palmaz et al.[124] evaluated the outcomes of the use of the balloon-expandable Palmaz stent in 486 patients enrolled in a multicenter trial. Technical success occurred in 99% of patients with clinical follow-up patency of 90% at 1 year and 84% after 2 years. A meta-analysis evaluating outcomes of iliac artery PTA and stent placement in 1,300 patients, with a variety of types of stents, was performed by Bosch and Hunink.[130] Four-year primary patency rates were 77% for stenotic lesions treated with iliac stenting and 61% for occlusive lesions in patients with claudication, and 67% and 53%, respectively, in patients with limb-threatening ischemia. The risk of long-term failure was reduced by 39% after stent placement compared with PTA alone. Iliac artery stent patency rates are significantly lower in women and in patients with renal insufficiency and critical limb ischemia.[131] Kashyap et al. compared aortoiliac angioplasty and stenting to surgical reconstruction, in a retrospective fashion.[132] In this evaluation, technical success for PTA/stenting was 96%. Long-term outcomes for secondary patency, limb salvage, and survival were the same in those treated percutaneously compared to those treated operatively. These outcomes hold true even for patients with complex lesions and long-segment occlusions.[133]

LOWER EXTREMITY ARTERIAL INTERVENTIONS

Lower extremity atherosclerotic disease affects a substantial portion of the population. For a more in-depth discussion on the pathophysiology and clinical presentation of the disease, please refer to Chapter 95. Patients presenting with disabling claudication and who have failed nonoperative therapy, or those patients presenting with limb-threatening ischemia, are considered for more invasive intervention. Treatment has traditionally been bypass grafting for femoral artery, popliteal artery, and tibial artery disease. With the development of improved angioplasty and stent technology, more and more endovascular procedures are being applied to infrainguinal arterial disease.

Femoropopliteal Angioplasty and Stenting

The approach to femoropopliteal artery interventions can proceed via one of three routes. The antegrade approach via an antegrade puncture of the ipsilateral common femoral artery is perhaps one of the most utilized approaches. Alternatively, a retrograde approach through the contralateral common femoral artery can be used, with the catheters and wires traversing the aortic bifurcation. A less frequently used approach is via puncture of the ipsilateral popliteal artery. This approach is often used in patients who have had a failed attempt at an antegrade approach or in those who have severe stenotic or occlusive changes in the proximal part of the superficial femoral artery. Once arterial access is obtained, principles of wire access, balloon dilation, and stent placement (when necessary) are similar to those described for aortoiliac artery PTA and stent placement.

10 There have been mixed results reported for outcomes of patients treated with percutaneous balloon angioplasty of femoropopliteal artery stenosis. Initial technical success occurs in 88% to 93% of patients.[134–138] Primary patency rates for femoropopliteal interventions have been reported as 43% to 58% at 1 year, 41% to 46% at 2 years, 38% to 41% at 3 years, and 26% to 38% at 5 years.[134–139] Several factors have been shown to affect outcome of femoropopliteal angioplasty. The length of the lesion has a negative effect on long-term patency. Lofberg et al.[138] evaluated outcomes of 92 patients who underwent 121 PTA procedures. They reported a primary patency at 5 years of only 12% in those with occlusions longer than 5 cm and 32% in those with occlusions shorter than 5 cm. Similar results were found by Matsi et al.,[134] but they had some success with PTA of lesions up to 10 cm in length. Others have shown that treatment of patients with stenoses fared better than those with occlusions, and those with claudication fared better than those with limb-threatening ischemia.[136] The quality of outflow also affects outcome.[139] Due to the poor outcomes of femoropopliteal PTA, some argue that it should not be recommended as a first-line treatment in patients with infrainguinal occlusive disease but reserved for those who would not tolerate surgery or have no surgical options. Others, however, argue that it does not preclude surgery and may be a viable first option, reserving surgery for those who eventually fail PTA. Given the poor outcomes of PTA, few studies have attempted to evaluate whether the placement of a stent, either primarily or after failed PTA, would improve outcomes of endovascular procedures in the femoropopliteal arteries. Outcomes from many of these studies have not been shown to significantly improve patency rates. Primary patency rates for femoropopliteal artery stenting have been reported as 54% to 86% at 1 year and 29.9% to 48% at 3 years.[140–143] Secondary patency rates at 3 years increase to 68.3%.[143] Complications during PTA and stenting of the femoropopliteal arteries include arterial disruption, thrombosis, distal embolization, and arterial dissection. Complications occur more frequently in this branch of the arterial tree as compared with the aortoiliac system, and half of these complications require operative intervention.

Another technique to revascularize the lower extremity in a percutaneous fashion is the use of percutaneous intentional extraluminal (or subintimal) angioplasty and recanalization. This method overcomes some of the problems associated with conventional PTA in that the subintimal plane that is developed has a smooth neolumen, which may be less prone to thrombosis. The technique was originally described in 1990 by Bolia et al.[144] This procedure is accomplished by using a wire to enter the subintimal space of a native artery proximal to an area of hemodynamic significant stenosis or occlusion. The wire is advanced in this plane past an area of severe disease and then reenters the true lumen. The channel is then enlarged by balloon angioplasty. In the femoropopliteal region it has been specifically applied to long lesions, greater than 10 cm in length. Initial technical success rate of the procedure has varied from 82% to 90%.[145–148] Initial failure of the procedure is primarily due to inability to gain reaccess to the true lumen. Primary patency rates have been reported to be 27% to 62% at 1 year. Long-term patency rates are not known, and the application of this technique is controversial. It generally carries a low morbidity and may represent a mode of revascularization in patients with limb-threatening ischemia who do not have a surgical option.

Many failures of PTA and stenting are due to the development of neointimal hyperplasia leading to recurrent in-stent stenosis. In an attempt to address this problem, stents covered with graft material have been placed. Saxon et al.[149] reported the largest experience as part of a U.S. multicenter prospective randomized trial of PTA versus PTA and expanded polytetrafluoroethylene–covered stents. The total number of patients treated was only 28, with 13 patients receiving PTA alone and 15 patients randomized to PTA and covered stent placement. At 2-year follow-up, primary patency in the covered stent group was 87%, whereas in the PTA-alone group it was only 25% ($p = 0.002$). Further investigation is certainly warranted into the application of this technology. In addition, drug-eluting stents are being investigated for the treatment of femoropopliteal disease. One such study evaluated the use of sirolimus-eluting stents.[150] Sirolimus acts as an anti-inflammatory and cytostatic antiproliferative agent that diminishes smooth muscle cell proliferation, which may prevent the development of neointimal hyperplasia. Duda et al.[150] reported on the outcome of 36 patients recruited for the participation in a randomized, double-blind, prospective trial evaluating drug-eluting stents versus uncoated stents in the treatment of femoropopliteal occlusive disease. The in-stent mean lumen diameter was significantly larger in the sirolimus-eluting stent group compared with the uncoated stent at 6 months. Long-term patency rates are not yet known, and further investigation with this stent, as well as others, is under way.

Alternatives to PTA and stenting have been developed for percutaneous intervention of the lower extremity arterial tree, specifically utilizing debulking technologies. These entail two main technologies: directional mechanical atherectomy and laser atherectomy. Mechanical atherectomy was originally used in the coronary circulation, but has recently found new applications to the lower extremity arterial tree. These devices use either a rotational blade or a "plane"-like device that shaves the atherosclerotic debris from the arterial wall (Fig. 87.9). Most of the results for these devices are presented in small retrospective series or registry data, with the primary endpoint evaluated often being freedom from target vessel revascularization. Zeller et al.[151] reported a 76% technical success rate with these devices (defined as obtaining <30% residual stenosis). Over half of these lesions, however, required adjunctive balloon angioplasty or stent placement. The majority of data, however, come from the self-reported multicenter Treating Peripherals with Silver Hawk: Outcomes Collection (TALON) registry.[152] Similar to other series, there was a 74% technical success rate, but one quarter of patients required an adjunctive procedure. Freedom from target vessel revascularization was 80% at 12 months. Multiple lesions and increasing Rutherford stage were predictors of less favorable outcomes.

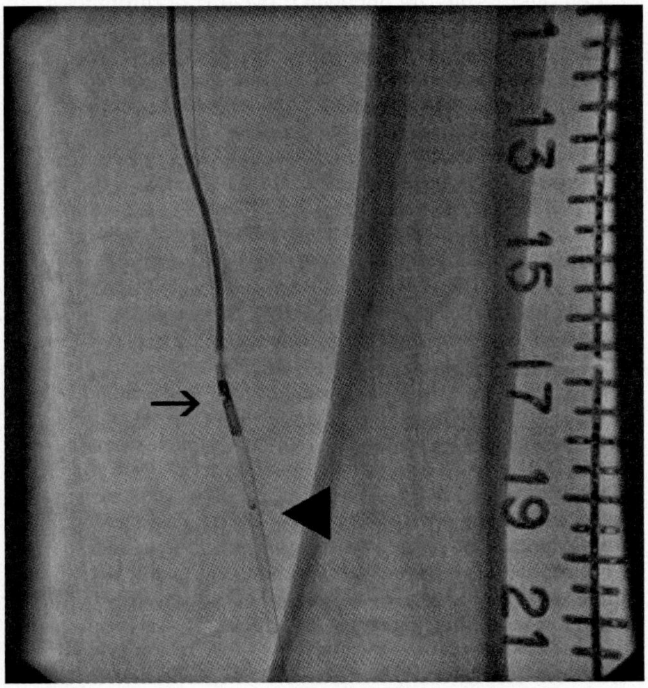

FIGURE 87.9. Radiographic picture of an atherectomy catheter within the superficial femoral artery. The "blade" (*arrow*) shaves portions of the atheroma, thus opening up the flow channel. The shaved atheroma is collected in the chamber of the catheter (*solid triangular arrow*). Multiple passes of the catheter are made to allow for a large enough flow channel and to remove the stenosis.

Lasers have also been used to treat peripheral atherosclerotic disease. Excimer laser technology uses photochemical energy, which is absorbed over a very short distance and potentially eliminates any heat generation. It is ideally suited for treating long, concentric, chronic occlusions that cannot be traversed by other means. Often, however, the bore size of the laser is small (2.5 mm) and thus almost always requires the use of adjunctive procedures once the lesion is traversed. Laser atherectomy has demonstrated usefulness in specific situations. Scheinert et al.[153] reported outcomes of its use in 318 patients with 411 chronic superficial femoral artery occlusions. Initial technical success was 83%, and all of these required an adjunctive PTA or stent. Primary patency at 1 year, however, was only 34%, but improved to a 76% secondary patency. While long-term data demonstrate its usefulness in maintaining patency, its use in crossing difficult, long, chronic occlusions appears to be beneficial.

Crural Artery Angioplasty and Stenting

Treatment of critical limb ischemia resulting from tibial vessel occlusion remains a challenge. In most situations, patients are elderly or have multiple comorbidities, which place them at high risk for surgery. Early application of angioplasty and stenting techniques to tibial vessel lesions was limited. With increased experience, however, the lack of emergent surgery to "rescue" tibial interventions has led to wider application. The technical aspects of the procedure do not differ too significantly from angioplasty in other arterial locations. Guide wire access is obtained across the lesion. Typically, a smaller guide wire is required such as one that is of 0.018 or 0.014 inches in diameter. Angioplasty is performed primarily, with stents rarely being placed as the risk of thrombosis is too great. Immediate technical success occurs in 87% to 92% of patients.[154,155] Complications related to tibial PTA that subsequently require emergent surgical intervention only occur in 0.7% of patients.

The two largest series reported on the outcomes of tibial PTA were reported by Faglia et al.[155] in 2002 and by Dorros et al.[154] in 2001. Faglia reported on the outcomes of 191 tibial PTA procedures performed in patients with critical limb ischemia (rest pain or tissue loss). Clinical recurrence occurred in 7.3% of patients at a mean time to recurrence of 4.6 months. The majority of these recurrences were successfully treated with repeat angioplasty. Major amputation was required in only 5.2% of patients. Dorros reported on the outcome of 270 PTA procedures in patients with critical limb ischemia. Over a 5-year follow-up, only 8% required a subsequent surgical revascularization and only 9% required a major amputation. Survival, however, was only 56% at 5 years. In some centers, tibial PTA for isolated tibial lesions is being considered as the primary intervention prior to tibial artery bypass, particularly in patients with multiple comorbidities.

More recently, Giles et al.[156] reported the results of infrapopliteal angioplasty in 176 limbs from 163 patients. In this series, technical success was achieved in 93% of the cases. At 1 and 2 years primary patency was 53% and 51%, respectively, while freedom from secondary restenosis and reintervention was 63% and 61%, respectively. Patients with less severe and less

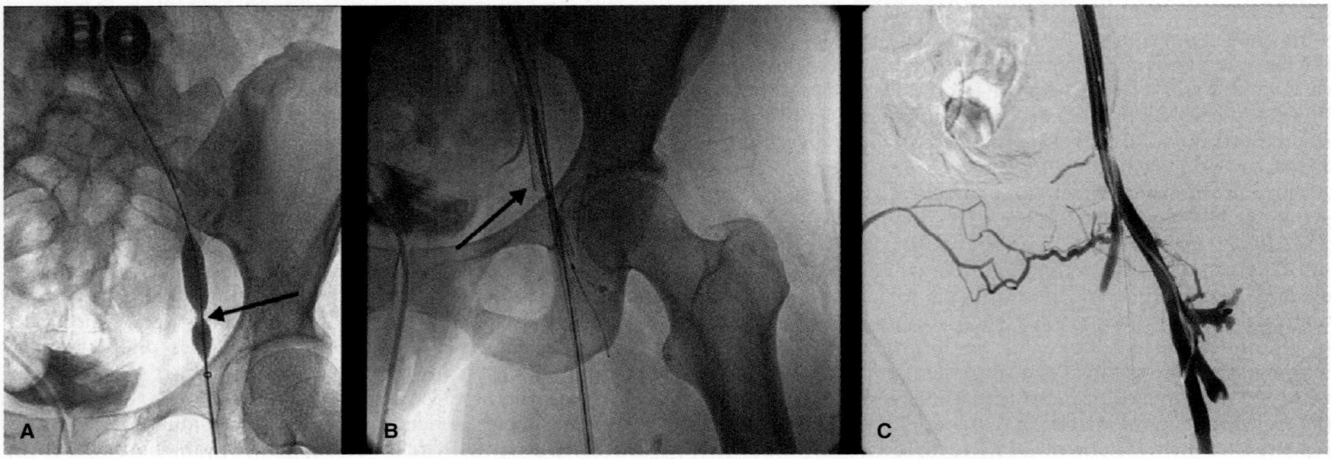

FIGURE 87.10. Venograms from a patient who presented with left common iliac vein thrombosis. After thrombolysis, areas of residual stenosis were placed in the left common iliac and external iliac veins. **A:** Balloon angioplasty of a stricture noted in the left external iliac vein. Note the "waist" depicting the stenosis that is being treated during the balloon angioplasty (*arrow*). **B:** Self-expanding stents were placed in the left common iliac and external iliac veins. Depicted is the deployment of the most distal self-expanding stent (*arrow*). **C:** Completion venogram shows resolution of the stenosis and excellent flow within the venous system.

extensive disease fared better than those with more extensive disease. As more experience is gained with this procedure, a better understanding of its outcomes and its potential applications will be attained.

VENOUS INTERVENTIONS

The pathophysiology of chronic venous disease is complex and generally results from a combination of contributing factors, such as reflux, as well as outflow obstruction. The application of angioplasty and stenting to the venous circulation is gaining increased popularity. In particular, it is being applied to the treatment of iliac venous outflow obstruction. The etiology of outflow obstruction may be secondary to previous iliac vein thrombosis or due to a primary cause of obstruction, such as May-Thurner syndrome. A more thorough discussion of venous disease is presented in Chapter 102. The technique of venous angioplasty and stenting is similar to that applied to the arterial system. Guide wire access is obtained across the area of stenosis and PTA performed to eliminate the obstruction. Placement of a stent is often necessary, and intravascular ultrasound can play an instrumental role in accurate placement (Fig. 87.10).[157]

Raju et al.[158] reviewed the results of balloon dilation and stent placement for the relief of iliac vein stenosis in 304 patients with symptomatic iliac vein stenosis. Of these patients, 57% had symptoms that were also associated with symptoms attributable to reflux disease. Approximately half of the patients had stenoses due to nonthrombotic causes (i.e., May-Thurner syndrome), whereas the other half were postthrombotic in nature. Forty-four limbs required a reintervention because of restenosis of the treated segment. Primary and secondary patency rates at 24 months were 71% and 97%, respectively. Sixty-two percent of patients with venous ulceration had healing by 2 years, and after stent placement limbs that were free from swelling increased from 12% to 47%, and limbs that were free from pain increased from 17% to 71%. Treatment of patients with occluded iliac veins is technically feasible. In general, however, these procedures require the stenting of longer segments (mean length 22 cm) and multiple in-line stents (mean stents equal to three).[159]

THROMBOLYSIS

Thrombolytic therapy is generally used to treat acute arterial or venous occlusions. There are a variety of agents that have been used for thrombolytic therapy, including streptokinase compounds, urokinase compounds (UKs), and tissue plasminogen activator and its recombinant forms (rt-PA). These agents are all plasminogen activators, which do not directly degrade fibrinogen, but rather are trypsinlike serine proteases that have high specific activity directed at the cleavage of a single peptide bond in the plasminogen zymogen, converting it to plasmin. Plasmin is the molecule that then cleaves fibrin polymer, resulting in the dissolution of thrombus. In the majority of cases of peripheral vascular disease in which thrombolytic agents are used, it is delivered in a catheter-directed fashion. Access to the blood vessel is obtained either on the contralateral side or in an "upstream" location. Best results are obtained if the area of thrombosis can be crossed with an infusion wire or catheter and the thrombolytic agent delivered directly into the thrombus burden. Specialized catheters and wires, with multiple small side holes, have been developed to allow for this. Other techniques of thrombolysis include the delivery of low-dose continuous infusion, the delivery of high-dose graded infusion, or pulse spray infusion in which periodic forceful injection of the drug into the clot is performed. Progress is assessed angiographically on a regular basis until thrombolysis is complete or no further progress is attained. In cases of acute limb ischemia, thrombolysis can generally be applied safely only to patients with category I and IIa limb ischemia, as it takes several hours to attain lysis. Patients with more severe ischemia may not tolerate the delay in recanalization and thus may require more urgent surgical intervention.

There have been two major randomized trials evaluating the use of thrombolytic therapy for lower extremity ischemia: Surgery versus Thrombolysis for Ischemia of the Lower Extremity (STILE) and Thrombolysis or Peripheral Artery Surgery (TOPAS).[160,161] In the STILE trial thrombolytic therapy was successful at restoring patency in 81% of bypass grafts and 69% of native arteries. One of the successes of thrombolytic therapy was that it reduced the extent of the planned surgical procedure in 55.8% of the patients. At 6-month follow-up, only 5.7% of patients undergoing thrombolysis required an amputation, whereas 17.9% of those randomized directly to surgery required one. In the TOPAS trial, complete lysis was obtained in 67.9% of patients. Of those treated with thrombolysis, approximately one third had underlying lesions treated percutaneously and avoided a conventional operation. Treatment was most effective in patients whose thrombosis was less than 14 days in duration.

The main risks associated with the use of thrombolytic therapy are an increased risk of bleeding. In the STILE and TOPAS trials, complications occurred at an incidence of 22% to 41% of patients and included hemorrhage, distal embolization, and catheter-related problems. Life-threatening hemorrhage occurred in 6.2% of patients undergoing thrombolytic therapy in the STILE trial and in 12.5% of patients treated with thrombolytics in the TOPAS trial. The TOPAS trial did reveal that when aspirin and therapeutic heparin were withheld during thrombolytic therapy, the rate of intracranial hemorrhage was decreased from 5% to 0.5%. In addition, aggressive control of hypertension is also beneficial at decreasing the risk of intracranial hemorrhage.[162] An analysis of data collected in a prospective, single-institution registry at the Cleveland Clinic Foundation revealed an overall complication rate of 55.9% in patients undergoing thrombolytic therapy for both arterial and venous disease. Complications rates were also analyzed according to the type of thrombolytic agent used (either UK or rt-PA). In patients receiving thrombolytic therapy for arterial disease, the complications reported were the development of a hematoma or pseudoaneurysm (30.6% UK vs. 57.7% rt-PA), any bleeding requiring a transfusion (11.9% UK vs. 18.7% rt-PA), and intracranial bleeding (0.8% UK vs. 1.6% rt-PA). Mortality rates were 2.9% for UK and 1.6% for rt-PA. For patients treated with venous thrombolysis, the complications reported were hematoma formation (18.4% UK vs. 28.6% rt-PA) and any bleeding requiring a transfusion (14.3% UK vs. 42.9% rt-PA). There were no cases of intracranial bleeding in patients undergoing venous thrombolysis.

To minimize the risks of thrombolytic therapy, several criteria have been universally accepted as contraindications to its use. Absolute contraindications include stroke or transient ischemic attack within the past 2 months, gastrointestinal bleeding within the past 10 days, and neurosurgery or intracranial trauma within the past 3 months. Relatively major contraindications include cardiopulmonary resuscitation within the past 10 days, major nonvascular surgery or trauma within the past 10 days, uncontrolled hypertension, intracranial tumor, and recent eye surgery. From a technical standpoint, the use of micropuncture needles and small catheters may decrease the risk of bleeding complications. Monitoring of laboratory values, such as fibrinogen levels, has been of no value in predicting which patients are at increased risk of bleeding.[163] In the presence of hemorrhage, heparin and thrombolytic agents should be discontinued. If necessary, thrombolytic agents can be reversed with cryoprecipitate, fresh frozen plasma, tranexamic acid, aminocaproic acid, or aprotinin. These interventions are rarely necessary as most thrombolytic agents have short half-lives, in the range of minutes.

SUMMARY

Endovascular therapy is an exciting field that offers an alternate modality of treatment to patients with a variety of peripheral vascular disorders. In most cases, the indications for the procedure are the same whether an open or endovascular option is being considered. The field of endovascular therapy continues to grow at a rapid pace and will continue to do so with the development of improving technologies. These improvements may, in the future, allow many procedures to attain clinical equipoise with open surgical procedures and in such instances may replace them. In cases in which this is not true, the endovascular interventions may remain the procedure of choice in high-risk patients.

References

1. Dotter C, Judkins M. Transluminal treatment of arteriosclerotic obstruction: description of a new technique and preliminary report of its application. *Circulation* 1969;30:645–670.
2. Leung D, Spinosa D, Hagspiel K, et al. Selection of stents for treating iliac arterial occlusive disease. *J Vasc Interv Radiol* 2003;14:137–152.
3. American Heart Association. Heart disease and stroke statistics – 2004 update. *Am Heart Assoc* 2003:1–52.
4. Executive Committee for the Asymptomatic Carotid Atherosclerosis Study. Endarterectomy for asymptomatic carotid artery stenosis. *JAMA* 1995;273:1421–1428.
5. North American Symptomatic Carotid Endarterectomy Trial Collaborators. Beneficial effect of carotid endarterectomy in symptomatic patients with high-grade carotid stenosis. *N Engl J Med* 1991;325:445–453.
6. MRC Asymptomatic Carotid Surgery Trial (ACST) Collaborative Group. Prevention of disabling and fatal strokes by successful carotid endarterectomy in patients without recent neurological symptoms: randomised controlled trial. *Lancet* 2004;363:1491–1502.
7. Kerber C, Hornwell L, Lowden O. Catheter dilation of proximal carotid stenosis during distal bifurcation endarterectomy. *Am J Neuroradiol* 1980;1:348–349.
8. Wholey M, Wholey M, Tan W, et al. A comparison of balloon-mounted and self-expanding stents in the carotid arteries: immediate and long-term results of more than 500 patients. *J Endovasc Ther* 2003;10:171–181.
9. Castriota F, Cremonesi A, Manetti R, et al. Impact of cerebral protection devices on early outcome of carotid stenting. *J Endovasc Ther* 2002;9:786–792.
10. Wilentz J, Chati Z, Krafft V, et al. Retinal embolization during carotid angioplasty and stenting: mechanisms and role of cerebral protection systems. *Catheter Cardiovasc Interv* 2002;56:320–327.
11. Macdonald S, McKevitt F, Venables G, et al. Neurological outcomes after carotid stenting protected with the Neuroshield filter compared to unprotected stenting. *J Endovasc Ther* 2002;9:777–785.
12. Martin J, Pache J, Treggiari-Venzi M, et al. Role of the distal balloon protection technique in the prevention of cerebral embolic events during carotid stent placement. *Stroke* 2001;32:479–484.
13. Wholey M, Jarmolowski C, Wholey M, et al. Carotid artery stent placement – ready for prime time? *J Vasc Interv Radiol* 2003;14:1–10.
14. Wholey M, Wholey M, Tan W, et al. Management of the neurologic complications of carotid artery stenting. *J Endovasc Ther* 2001;8:341–353.
15. Yadav J, Roubin G, Iyer S, et al. Elective stenting of the extracranial carotid arteries. *Circulation* 2004;95:376–381.
16. Lal B, Hobson R, Goldstein J, et al. In-stent recurrent stenosis after carotid artery stenting: life table analysis and clinical relevance. *J Vasc Surg* 2003;38:1162.
17. Wholey M, Al-Mubarek N, Wholey M. Updated review of the global carotid artery stent registry. *Catheter Cardiovasc Interv* 2003;60:259–266.
18. CAVATAS Investigators. Endovascular versus surgical treatment in patients with carotid stenosis in the Carotid and Vertebral Artery Transluminal Angioplasty Study (CAVATAS): a randomised trial. *Lancet* 2001;357:1729–1737.
19. Yadav J, Wholey M, Kuntz R, et al. Protected carotid-artery stenting versus endarterectomy in high-risk patients. *N Engl J Med* 2004;351(15):1493–1501.
20. Hobson R, Howard V, Roubin G, et al. Carotid artery stenting is associated with increased complications in octogenarians. 30-day stroke and death rates in the CREST lead-in phase. *J Vasc Surg* 2004;40:1106–1111.
21. The SPACE Collaborative Group. 30-day results from the SPACE trial of stent-protected angioplasty versus carotid endarterectomy in symptomatic patients: a randomized non-inferiority trial. *Lancet* 2006;368:1239–1247.
22. Mas J, Chatellier G, Beyssen B, et al. Endarterectomy versus stenting in patients with symptomatic severe carotid stenosis. *N Engl J Med* 2006;355:1660–1671.
23. Furer J, Gruntzig A, Kugelmeier J, et al. Mesenteric arterial disease in the elderly. *J Vasc Surg* 2004;40:45.
24. Furer J, Gruntzig A, Kugelmeier J, et al. Treatment of abdominal angina with percutaneous dilation for an arteria mesenterica superior stenosis. *Cardiovasc Intervent Radiol* 1980;3:43.
25. Uflacker R, Goldany M, Constant S. Resolution of mesenteric angina with percutaneous transluminal angioplasty of a superior mesenteric artery stenosis using a balloon catheter. *Gastrointest Radiol* 1980;5:367.
26. Allen R, Martin G, Rees C, et al. Mesenteric angioplasty in the treatment of chronic mesenteric ischemia. *J Vasc Surg* 1996;24:415.
27. Hallisey M, Deschaine J, Illescas F, et al. Angioplasty for the treatment of visceral ischemia. *J Vasc Interv Radiol* 1995;6:785.
28. Matsumoto A, Tegtmeyer C, Fitzcharles E. Percutaneous transluminal angioplasty of visceral artery stenosis: results and long term clinical follow-up. *J Vasc Interv Radiol* 1995;6:165.
29. Sheeran S, Murphy T, Khwaja A, et al. Stent placement for treatment of mesenteric ischemia: report of five cases. *J Vasc Interv Radiol* 1999;10:861.
30. Nyman U, Ivancev K, Lindh M, et al. Endovascular treatment of chronic mesenteric ischemia: report of five cases. *Cardiovasc Intervent Radiol* 1998;21: 305.
31. Kandarpa K, Becker G, Huniak M, et al. Transcatheter interventions for the treatment of peripheral atherosclerotic lesions: part I. *J Vasc Interv Radiol* 2001;12:695.
32. Kasirajian K, O'Hara P, Gray B, et al. Chronic mesenteric ischemia: open surgery versus percutaneous angioplasty and stenting. *J Vasc Surg* 2001;33:63.
33. Rose S, Quigley T, Raker E. Revascularization for chronic mesenteric ischemia: comparison of operative arterial bypass grafting and percutaneous transluminal angioplasty. *J Vasc Interv Radiol* 1995;6:339.

33a. Sharafuddin MJ, Olson CH, Sun S, et al. Endovascular treatment of celiac and mesenteric arteries stenoses: application and results. *J Vasc Surg* 2003;38:692–698.

34. Steinmetz E, Tatou E, Favier-Biavoux C, et al. Endovascular treatment as first choice in chronic intestinal ischemia. *Ann Vasc Surg* 2002;16:693.
35. Matsumoto A, Angle J, Spinosa D, et al. Percutaneous transluminal angioplasty and stenting in the treatment of chronic mesenteric ischemia: results and longterm follow up. *J Am Coll Surg* 2002;194:S22.
36. Sarac T, Altinel O, Kashyap V, et al. Endovascular treatment of stenotic and occluded visceral arteries for chronic mesenteric ischemia. *J Vasc Surg* 2008;47:485–491.

37. Dean R, Tribble R, Hansen K, et al. Evolution of renal artery insufficiency in ischemic nephropathy. *Ann Surg* 1991;213:446.
38. Sos T, Trost D. Renal vascular disease as a cause of hypertension. *Curr Opin Nephrol Hyperten* 1995;4:76.
39. Dean R, Tribble R, Hansen K, et al Prevalence of ischemic nephropathy in the atherosclerotic population. *Am J Kidney Dis* 1994;24:615.
40. Weibull H, Bergqvist D, Bergentz S, et al. Percutaneous transluminal renal angioplasty versus surgical reconstruction of atherosclerotic renal artery stenosis: a prospective randomized study. *J Vasc Surg* 1993;18:841.
41. Hansen K, Starr S, Sands E, et al. Contemporary surgical management of renovascular disease. *J Vasc Surg* 1992;16:319.
42. Hallett J, Fowl R, O'Brien P. Renovascular operations in patients with chronic renal insufficiency: do the benefits justify the risks? *J Vasc Surg* 1987;5:633.
43. Novick A, Ziegelbaum M, Vidt D, et al. Trends in surgical revascularization for renal artery disease: ten years' experience. *JAMA* 1987;257:498.
44. Gruntzig A, Kuhlmann U, Vetter W. Treatment of renovascular hypertension with percutaneous transluminal dilation of a renal artery stenosis. *Lancet* 1978;1:801.
45. Martin L, Cork R, Kaufman S. Long term results of angioplasty in 110 patients with renal artery stenosis. *J Vasc Interv Radiol* 1992;3:619.
46. Losinno F, Zuccala A, Busato F, et al. Renal artery angioplasty for renovascular hypertension and preservation of renal function: long term angiographic and clinical follow-up. *Am J Roentgen* 1994;162:853.
47. Klow N, Palusen D, Vatne K, et al. Percutaneous renal artery angioplasty using the coaxial technique: ten years of from 591 procedures in 419 patients. *Acta Radiol* 1998;39:594.
48. Palmaz J, Kopp D, Hayashi H. Normal and stenotic renal arteries: experience with balloon expandable intraluminal stenting. *Radiology* 1987; 164:705.
49. Blum U, Krimme B, Flugel P, et al. Treatment of ostial renal artery stenoses with vascular endoprostheses after successful balloon angioplasty. *N Engl J Med* 1997;336:459.
50. White C, Ramee S, Collins T, et al. Renal artery stent placement: utility in lesions difficult to treat with balloon angioplasty. *J Am Coll Cardiol* 1997; 30:1445.
51. Bakker J, Goffette P, Henry P, et al. The ERASME study: a multicenter study on the safety and technical results of the Palmaz stent used for the treatment of atherosclerotic ostial renal artery stenosis. *Cardiovasc Intervent Radiol* 1999;22:468.
52. Rees C, Palmaz J, Becker G, et al. Palmaz stent in the atherosclerotic stenoses involving the ostia of the renal arteries: preliminary report of a multi-center study. *Radiology* 1991;181:721.
53. Bush R, Najibi S, MacDonald M, et al. Endovascular revascularization of renal artery stenosis: technical and clinical results. *J Vasc Surg* 2001;33:2041.
54. Ivanovic V, McKusick M, Johnson C, et al. Renal artery stent placement: complications at a single tertiary care center. *J Vasc Interv Radiol* 2003;14: 217–225.
55. Yutan E, Glickerman D, Caps M, et al. Percutaneous transluminal revascularization for renal artery stenosis: Veterans Affair Puget Sound health care system experience. *J Vasc Surg* 2001;34:685.
56. Dorros G, Jaff M, Mathiak L, et al. Multicenter Palmaz stent renal artery stenosis revascularization registry report: four year follow up of 1,058 successful patients. *Catheter Cardiovasc Interv* 2002;55:182.
57. Henry M, Amor M, Henry I. Stents in the treatment of renal artery stenosis: long term follow up. *J Endovasc Ther* 1999;6:42.
58. Xue F, Bettmann M, Langdon D, et al. Outcome and cost comparison of percutaneous transluminal renal angioplasty, renal arterial stent placement and renal artery bypass grafting. *Radiology* 1999;212:378.
59. Cambria R, Brewster D, L'Italien G, et al. The durability of different reconstructive techniques for atherosclerotic renal artery disease. *J Vasc Surg* 1994;20:76.
60. Beek F, Kaate R, Beutler J, et al. Complications during renal artery stent placement for atherosclerotic ostial stenosis. *Cardiovasc Intervent Radiol* 1997;20:184.
61. Spinosa D, Matsumoto A, Angle J, et al. Safety of CO2 and gadodiamide enhanced angiography for the evaluation and percutaneous treatment of renal artery stenosis in patients with chronic renal insufficiency. *Am J Roentgen* 2001; 176:1305.
62. Feldman R, Wargovich T, Bitti J, et al. No touch technique for reducing aortic wall trauma during renal artery stenting. *Catheter Cardiovasc Interv* 1999;46:245.
63. Henry M, Henry I, Klonaris C, et al. Renal angioplasty and stenting under protection: the way of the future? *Catheter Cardiovasc Interv* 2003;60:299.
64. Kashyap V, Sepulveda R, Bena J, et al. The management of renal artery atherosclerosis for renal salvage: does stenting help? *J Vasc Surg* 2007;45: 101–108.
65. Suliman A, Imhoff L, Greenberg J, et al. Renal stenting for incidentally discovered renal artery stenosis: is there any outcome benefit? *Ann Vasc Surg* 2008;22:525–233.
66. Cambria R, Brewster D, L'Italien G, et al. Renal artery reconstruction for the preservation of renal function. *J Vasc Surg* 1996;24:371.
67. Sivamurthy N, Surowiec S, Culakova E, et al. Divergent outcomes after percutaneous therapy for symptomatic renal artery stenosis. *J Vasc Surg* 2004;39:365.
68. Steinbach F, Novick A, Campbell S, et al. Long term survival after surgical revascularization for atherosclerotic renal artery disease. *J Urol* 1997;158: 36.
69. Parodi J, Palmaz J, Barone H. Transfemoral intraluminal graft implantation for abdominal aortic aneurysms. *Ann Vasc Surg* 1991;5:491–499.
70. Baxendale B, Baker D, Hutchinson A, et al. Haemodynamic and metabolic response to endovascular repair of infra-renal aortic aneurysms. *Br J Anaesth* 1996;77:581–585.
71. Ouriel K, Greenberg R, Clair D. Endovascular treatment of aortic aneurysms. *Curr Prob Surg* 2002;39:242–345.
72. White R, Donayre C, Walot I, et al. Abdominal aortic aneurysm rupture following endoluminal graft deployment: report of a predictable event. *J Endovasc Ther* 2000;7:257–262.
73. Harris P, Vallavhaneni S, Desgranges P, et al. Incidence and risk factors of late rupture, conversion, and death after endovascular repair of infrarenal aortic aneurysms: the EUROSTAR experience. *J Vasc Surg* 2000;32:739–749.
74. Whitaker S. Imaging of abdominal aortic aneurysm before and after endoluminal stent-graft repair. *Eur J Radiol* 2001;39:3–15.
75. Harris P, Brennan J, Martin J, et al. Longitudinal aneurysm shrinkage following endovascular aortic aneurysm repair: a source of intermediate and late complications. *J Endovasc Surg* 1999;6:11–16.
76. Wolf Y, Tillich M, Lee W, et al. Changes in aneurysm volume after endovascular repair of abdominal aortic aneurysm. *J Vasc Surg* 2002;36:305–309.
77. Golzarian J, Murgo S, Dussaussois L, et al. Evaluation of abdominal aortic aneurysm after endoluminal treatment: comparison of color Doppler sonography with biphasic helical CT. *Am J Roentgen* 2002;178:623–628.
78. Bendick P, Bove P, Long G, et al. Efficacy of ultrasound scan contrast agents in the noninvasive follow-up of aortic stent grafts. *J Vasc Surg* 2003; 37:381–385.
79. Zarins C, White R, Schwarten D, et al. AneuRx stent graft versus open surgical repair of abdominal aortic aneurysm: multicenter prospective clinical trial. *J Vasc Surg* 1999;29:292–305.
80. May J, White G, Waugh R, et al. Improved survival after endoluminal repair with second-generation prostheses compared with open repair in the treatment of abdominal aortic aneurysms: a 5-year concurrent comparison using life table method. *J Vasc Surg* 2001;33:S21–S26.
81. Lee W, O'Dorisio J, Wolf Y, et al. Outcome after unilateral hypogastric artery occlusion during endovascular aneurysm repair. *J Vasc Surg* 2001;33:921.
82. Schoder M, Zaunbauer L, Holzenbein T, et al. Internal iliac artery embolization before endovascular repair of abdominal aortic aneurysms: frequency, efficacy, and clinical results. *Am J Radiol* 2001;177:599–605.
83. Mehta M, Veith F, Ohki T, et al. Unilateral and bilateral hypogastric artery interruption during aortoiliac aneurysm repair in 154 patients: a relatively innocuous procedure. *J Vasc Surg* 2001;33:S27–S32.
84. Kritpracha B, Pigott J, Price C, et al. Distal internal iliac artery embolization: a procedure to avoid. *J Vasc Surg* 2003;37:943–948.
85. Wyers M, Shermerhorn M, Fillinger M, et al. Internal iliac artery occlusion without coil embolization during endovascular abdominal aortic aneurysm repair. *J Vasc Surg* 2002;36:1138–1145.
86. White G, Yu W, May J. Endoleak: a proposed new terminology to describe incomplete aneurysm exclusion by an endoluminal graft. *J Endovasc Surg* 1996;3:124–125.
87. White G, May J, Waugh R, et al. Type I and type II endoleaks: a more useful classification for reporting results of endoluminal AAA repair. *J Endovasc Surg* 1998;5:189–191.
88. White G, May J, Waugh R, et al. Type III and type IV endoleaks: toward a complete definition of blood flow in the sac after endoluminal AAA repair. *J Endovasc Surg* 1998;5:305–309.
89. Gilling-Smith G, Brennan J, Harris P, et al. Endotension after endovascular aneurysm repair: definition, classification, and strategies for surveillance and interventions. *J Endovasc Surg* 1999;6:305–307.
90. Zarins C, White R, Hodgson K, et al. Endoleak as a predictor of outcome after endovascular aneurysm repair. *J Vasc Surg* 2000;32:90–107.
91. Holzenbein T, Kretschmer G, Thurnher S, et al. Midterm durability of abdominal aortic aneurysm endograft repair: a word of caution. *J Vasc Surg* 2001;33:S46–S54.
92. Buth J, Harris P, van Marrewijk C, et al. The significance and management of different types of endoleaks. *Semin Vasc Surg* 2003;16:95–102.
93. Chuter T, Faruqi R, Sawhney R, et al. Endoleak after endovascular repair of abdominal aortic aneurysms. *J Vasc Surg* 2001;34:98–105.
94. Buth J, Laheji R. Early complications and endoleaks after endovascular abdominal aortic aneurysm repair: report of a multicenter study. *J Vasc Surg* 2000;31:134–146.
95. Dattilo J, Brewster D, Fan C-M, et al. Clinical failures of endovascular abdominal aortic aneurysm repair: incidence, causes, and management. *J Vasc Surg* 2002;35:1137–1144.
96. Zarins C. The US AneuRx clinical trial: 6-year clinical update 2002. *J Vasc Surg* 2003;37:904–908.
97. Baum R, Cope C, Fairman R, et al. Translumbar embolization of type 2 endoleaks after endovascular repair of abdominal aortic aneurysms. *J Vasc Interv Radiol* 2001;12:111–116.
98. Ellozy S, Carroccio A, Lookistein R, et al. First experience in human beings with a permanently implantable intrasac pressure transducer for monitoring endovascular repair of abdominal aortic aneurysms. *J Vasc Surg* 2004;40:405–412.
99. Fairman R, Baum R, Carpenter J, et al. Limb intervention in patients undergoing treatment with an unsupported bifurcated aortic endograft system: a review of the phase II EVT trial. *J Vasc Surg* 2002;36:118–126.
100. Carroccio A, Faries P, Morrissey N, et al. Predicting iliac limb occlusion after bifurcated aortic stent grafting: anatomic and device-related causes. *J Vasc Surg* 2002; 36:679–684.
101. Baum R, Shetty S, Carpenter J, et al. Limb kinking in supported and unsupported abdominal aortic stent-grafts. *J Vasc Interv Radiol* 2000;11: 1165–1171.

102. Amesur N, Zajko A, Orons P, et al. Endovascular treatment of iliac limb stenosis or occlusion in 31 patients treated with the Ancure endograft. *J Vasc Interv Radiol* 2000;11:421–428.
103. Resch T, Ivancev K, Brunkwall J, et al. Distal migration of stent-grafts after endovascular repair of abdominal aortic aneurysms. *J Vasc Interv Radiol* 1997;10:257–264.
104. Albertini N, Kalliafas S, Travis S, et al. Anatomical risk factors for proximal perigraft endoleak and graft migration following endovascular repair of abdominal aortic aneurysms. *Eur J Endovasc Surg* 2000;19:308–312.
105. Cao P, Verzini F, Zannetti S, et al. Device migration after endoluminal abdominal aortic aneurysm repair: analysis of 113 cases with a minimum follow-up period of 2 years. *J Vasc Surg* 2002;35:229–235.
106. Badran M, Gould D, Raza I, et al. Aneurysm neck diameter after endovascular repair of abdominal aortic aneurysms. *J Vasc Interv Radiol* 2002;13: 887–892.
107. Lee J, Lee J, Aziz I, et al. Stent-graft migration following endovascular repair of aneurysms with large proximal necks: anatomical risk factors and long-term sequalae. *J Endovasc Ther* 2002;9:652–664.
108. Sampram E, Karafa M, Mascha E, et al. Nature, frequency, and predictors of secondary procedures after endovascular repair of abdominal aortic aneurysm. *J Vasc Surg* 2003;37:930–937.
109. Becker G, Kovacs M, Mathison M, et al. Risk stratification and outcomes of transluminal endografting for abdominal aortic aneurysm: 7-year experience and long-term follow-up. *J Vasc Interv Radiol* 2003;12:1033–1046.
110. Laheji R, Buth J, Harris P, et al. Need for secondary interventions after endovascular repair of abdominal aortic aneurysms. Intermediate-term follow-up results of a European collaborative registry (EUROSTAR). *Br J Surg* 2000; 87:1666.
111. Ohki T, Veith F, Shaw P, et al. Increasing incidence of midterm and long-term complications after endovascular graft repair of abdominal aortic aneurysms: a note of caution based on a 9-year experience. *Ann Surg* 2001;234:323–334.
112. Carpenter J, Baum R, Barker C, et al. Durability of benefits of endovascular versus conventional abdominal aortic aneurysm repair. *J Vasc Surg* 2002;35:222–228.
113. Schermerhorn M, Finlayson S, Fillinger M, et al. Life expectancy after endovascular versus open abdominal aortic aneurysm repair: results of a decision analysis model on the basis of data from EUROSTAR. *J Vasc Surg* 2002;36:1112–1120.
114. Prinssen M, Verhoeven E, Buth J, et al. A randomized trial comparing conventional and endovascular repair of abdominal aortic aneurysms. *N Engl J Med* 2004;351:1607–1618.
115. EVAR Trial Participants. Endovascular aneurysm repair versus open repair in patients with abdominal aortic aneurysm (EVAR trial 1): randomised controlled trial. *Lancet* 2005;365:2179.
116. EVAR Trial Participants. Endovascular aneurysm repair and outcome in patients unfit for open repair of abdominal aneurysm (EVAR trial 2): randomised controlled trial. *Lancet* 2005;365:2187.
117. Makaroun M, Dillavou E, Wheatley G, et al. Five-year results of endovascular treatment with the Gore TAG device compared with open repair of thoracic aortic aneurysms. *J Vasc Surg* 2008;47:912–918.
118. Roselli E, Greenberg R, Pfaff K, et al. Endovascular treatment of thoracoabdominal aortic aneurysms. *J Thor Cardiovasc Surg* 2007;133:1474–1482.
119. Tegtmeyer C, Hartwell G, Selby J, et al. Results and complications of angioplasty in aortoiliac disease. *Circulation* 1991;83:I53–I60.
120. Belli A, Cumberland D, Knox A, et al. The complication rate of percutaneous peripheral balloon angioplasty. *Clin Radiol* 1990;41:380–383.
121. Al-Hamali S, Baskerville P, Fraser S, et al. Detection of distal emboli in patients with peripheral arterial stenosis before and after iliac angioplasty: a prospective study. *J Vasc Surg* 1999;29:345–351.
122. Gardiner GJr, Meyerovitz M, Stokes K, et al. Complications of transluminal angioplasty. *Radiology* 1986;159:201–208.
123. Ballard J, Sparks S, Taylor F, et al. Complications of iliac artery stent deployment. *J Vasc Surg* 1996;24:545–555.
124. Palmaz J, Laborde J, Rivera F, et al. Stenting of iliac arteries with the Palmaz stent: experience from a multicenter trial. *Cardiovasc Intervent Radiol* 1992;15: 291–297.
125. Allaire E, Melliere D, Poussier B, et al. Iliac artery rupture during balloon dilation: what treatment? *Ann Vasc Surg* 2003;17:306–314.
126. Johnston K, Roe M, Hogg-Johnston S, et al. 5-Year results of a prospective study of percutaneous transluminal angioplasty. *Ann Surg* 1987; 206:403.
127. Becker G, Katzen B, Dake M. Non-coronary angioplasty. *Radiology* 1989;170:921–940.
128. Martin E, Katzen B, Benenati J, et al. Multicenter trial of the Wallstent in the iliac and femoral arteries. *J Vasc Interv Radiol* 1995;6:843–849.
129. Vorwerk D, Gunther R, Schurmann K, et al. Aortic and iliac stenoses: follow-up results of stent placement after insufficient balloon angioplasty in 118 cases. *Radiology* 1996;198:45–48.
130. Bosch J, Hunink M. Meta-analysis of the results of percutaneous transluminal angioplasty and stent placement for aortoiliac occlusive disease. *Radiology* 1997;204:87–96.
131. Timaran C, Stevens S, Freeman M, et al. Predictors for adverse outcome after iliac angioplasty and stenting for limb-threatening ischemia. *J Vasc Surg* 2002;36:507–513.
132. Kashyap V, Pavkov M, Bena J, et al. The management of severe aortoiliac occlusive disease: endovascular therapy rivals open reconstruction. *J Vasc Surg* 2008;48:1451–1457.
133. Laville C, Kashyap V, Clair D, et al. Endovascular management of iliac artery occlusions: extending treatment to TransAtlantic Inter-Society Consensus class C and D patients. *J Vasc Surg* 2006;43:32–39.
134. Matsi P, Manninen H, Soder H, et al. Percutaneous transluminal angioplasty in femoral artery occlusions: primary and long-term results in 107 claudicant patients using femoral and popliteal catheterization techniques. *Clin Radiol* 1995;50:237–244.
135. Stanley B, Teague B, Raptis S, et al. Efficacy of balloon angioplasty of the superficial femoral artery and popliteal artery in the relief of leg ischemia. *J Vasc Surg* 1996;23(4):679–685.
136. Matsi P, Manninen H, Vanninen R, et al. Femoropopliteal angioplasty in patients with claudication: primary and secondary patency in 140 limbs with 1–3 year follow up. *Radiology* 1994;191:727–733.
137. Golledge J, Ferguson K, Ellis M, et al. Outcome of femoropopliteal angioplasty. *Ann Surg* 1999;229(1):146–153.
138. Lofberg A, Karacagil S, Ljungman C, et al. Percutaneous transluminal angioplasty of the femoropopliteal arteries in limbs with chronic lower limb ischemia. *J Vasc Surg* 2001;34:114–121.
139. Johnston K. Femoral and popliteal arteries: reanalysis of results of balloon angioplasty. *Radiology* 1992;183:767–771.
140. Jahnke T, Voshage G, Muller-Hulsbeck S, et al. Endovascular placement of self-expanding nitinol coil stents for the treatment of femoropopliteal obstructive disease. *J Vasc Interv Radiol* 2002;13(3):257–266.
141. Cheng S, Ting A, Wong J. Endovascular stenting of superficial femoral artery stenosis and occlusions: results and risk factor analysis. *Cardiovasc Surg* 2001;9(2):133–140.
142. Strecker E, Boos I, Gottmann D. Femoropopliteal artery stent placement: evaluation of long-term success. *Radiology* 1997;205:375–383.
143. Gordon I, Conroy R, Arefi M, et al. Three-year outcome of endovascular treatment of superficial femoral artery occlusion. *Arch Surg* 2001;136: 221–228.
144. Bolia A, Miles K, Brennan J, et al. Percutaneous transluminal angioplasty of occlusions of the femoral and popliteal arteries by subintimal dissection. *Cardiovasc Intervent Radiol* 1990;13:357–363.
145. Harthun N, Cage D, Spinosa D. Subintimal recanalization is safe and effective in treating chronic critical limb ischemia in selected patients. *Am Surg* 2004;70:479–483.
146. Desgranges P, Boufi M, Lapeyre M, et al. Subintimal angioplasty: feasible and durable. *Eur J Vasc Endovasc Surg* 2004;28:138–141.
147. Laxdal E, Jenssenn G, Pedersen G, et al. Subintimal angioplasty as a treatment of femoropopliteal artery occlusion. *Eur J Vasc Endovasc Surg* 2003;25:578–582.
148. Tisi P, Mirnezami A, Baker S, et al. Role of subintimal angioplasty in the treatment of chronic lower limb ischemia. *Eur J Endovasc Surg* 2002;24: 417–422.
149. Saxon R, Coffman J, Gooding J, et al. Long term results of ePTFE stent-graft versus angioplasty in the femoropopliteal artery: single center experience from a prospective, randomized trial. *J Vasc Interv Radiol* 2003;14:303–311.
150. Duda S, Bosiers M, Pusich B, et al. Endovascular treatment of peripheral artery diseases with expanded PTFE-covered nitinol stents: interim analysis from a prospective controlled study. *Cardiovasc Intervent Radiol* 2002;25:413–418.
151. Zeller T, Rastan A, Schwarzwalder U, et al. Percutaneous peripheral atherectomy of femoropopliteal stenoses using a new-generation device: six-month results from a single-center experience. *J Endovasc Ther* 2004;11:676–668.
152. Ramaiah V, Gammon R, Kiesz S, et al. Midterm outcomes from the TALON registry: treating peripherals with Silverhawk: outcomes collection. *J Endovasc Ther* 2006;13:592–602.
153. Scheinert D, Laird J, Schroder M, et al. Excimer laser-assisted recanalization of long, chronic superficial femoral artery occlusions. *J Endovasc Ther* 2001;8: 156–166.
154. Dorros G, Jaff M, Dorros A, et al. Tibioperoneal (outflow lesion) angioplasty can be used as primary treatment in 235 patients with critical limb ischemia: five year follow up. *Circulation* 2001;104:2057–2062.
155. Faglia E, Mantero M, Caminiti M, et al. Extensive use of peripheral angioplasty, particularly infrapopliteal, in the treatment of ischaemic diabetic foot ulcers: clinical results of a multicentric study of 221 consecutive diabetic subjects. *J Int Med* 2002;252:225–232.
156. Giles K, Pomposelli F, Hamdan A, et al. Infrapopliteal angioplasty for critical limb ischemia: Relation of TransAtlantic InterSociety Consensus class to outcome in 176 limbs. *J Vasc Surg* 2008;48:128–136.
157. Hurst D, Forauer A, Bloom J, et al. Diagnosis and endovascular treatment of iliocaval compression syndrome. *J Vasc Surg* 2001;34:106–113.
158. Raju S, Owen S, Neglen P. The clinical impact of iliac venous stents in the management of chronic venous insufficiency. *J Vasc Surg* 2002;35:8–15.
159. Raju S, McAllister S, Neglen P. Recanalization of totally occluded iliac and adjacent venous segments. *J Vasc Surg* 2002;36:903–911.
160. The STILE Investigators. Results of a prospective randomized trial evaluating surgery versus thrombolysis for ischemia of the lower extremity. *Ann Surg* 1994;220:251–268.
161. Ouriel K, Veith F, Sasahara A, et al. A comparison of recombinant urokinase with vascular surgery as initial treatment for acute arterial occlusion of the legs. *N Engl J Med* 1998;338:1105–1111.
162. McNamara T, Goodwin S, Kandarpa K. Complications of thrombolysis. *Semin Intervent Radiol* 1994;11:134–144.
163. Ouriel K, Gray B, Clair D, et al. Complications associated with the use of urokinase and recombinant tissue plasminogen activator for catheter-directed peripheral arterial and venous thrombolysis. *J Vasc Interv Radiol* 2000;11:295–298.

CHAPTER 88 ■ VASCULAR INFECTIONS

G. PATRICK CLAGETT

KEY POINTS

1. Vascular infections are among the most challenging and difficult problems encountered by surgeons.
2. The overall incidence of clinically overt prosthetic infections varies according to anatomic site.
3. The majority of vascular prosthetic infections are initiated at the time of operation.
4. The principal organism responsible for infections of all implanted medical devices, including vascular prostheses, is *Staphylococcus epidermidis*.
5. The clinical presentations of vascular prosthetic infections can be protean and subtle, so that the diagnosis is difficult.
6. Imaging tests are important because the consequences of a missed diagnosis may be lethal.
7. The primary goals of treatment are to save life and limb, and this is best accomplished by eradicating infection by excision of all infected prosthetic material and vascular tissues combined with appropriate arterial reconstruction.

1 Vascular infections are among the most challenging and difficult problems encountered by vascular surgeons. Patients are often elderly, frail, desperately ill with multiple medical comorbid conditions, and unable to tolerate the extensive, complex operations usually required to treat the problem. Medical treatment based on specific antibiotic therapy is rarely successful when used alone, and complete resection and excision of all infected vascular structures are usually necessary to eradicate infection. Immediate restoration of blood flow to critical vascular beds by alternate anatomic routes or with replacement vascular conduits that minimize the risk for recurrent infection present additional challenges that tax the skill and ingenuity of vascular surgeons. Despite a great deal of progress in the treatment of vascular infections, morbidity and mortality remain among the highest of all vascular conditions.[1–3]

VASCULAR PROSTHETIC INFECTIONS

Pathogenesis

Vascular prostheses are foreign bodies that can be primarily infected by contamination at the time of placement or secondarily infected after implantation by hematogenous, lymphatic,
2 or contiguous spread of microorganisms. The overall incidence of clinically overt prosthetic infection varies according to anatomic site. Aortic prostheses confined to the abdominal or thoracic cavity rarely become infected; the incidence ranges from 0.5% to 2%.[2] The incidence is higher, from 2% to 6%, in proximal or distal anastomotic sites at the femoral level (e.g., aortofemoral or femoral-popliteal bypasses).[4]

Several features of the femoral area predispose to infectious complications. The groin is a relatively dirty area that is difficult to clean, and incisions placed in the groin are prone to infection and healing problems. Vertical groin incisions cut obliquely across the inguinal crease, tend to gape, and in obese patients lie buried in moist folds of skin. Furthermore, superficial inguinal lymph nodes are usually transected during exposure of the common femoral artery and, if not ligated, will bathe a vascular prosthesis in lymph fluid that may contain bacteria. Potential sources of prosthetic contamination in this circumstance include open, infected ischemic ulcers of a lower extremity; gangrenous toes; and wounds in any other area drained by the inguinal lymphatics, such as the perineum and perianal area. Another factor implicating the groin wound in the etiology of vascular prosthetic infections is transient local ischemia during placement of an aortic cross-clamp, which may render the wound more susceptible to infection.

3 Most authorities agree that the majority of vascular prosthetic infections are initiated at the time of operation.[2,3,5] Although direct proof of this tenet is difficult to obtain, the prevalence of *Staphylococcus epidermidis* among offending organisms suggests that skin contamination with the patient's own flora is an important mechanism.[6,7] Mucosal colonization of nasal, oropharyngeal, and gastrointestinal sites are also potential sources of *S. epidermidis* and other coagulase-negative staphylococci bacteremia and contamination.[8]

The presence of *Staphylococcus aureus* and other nosocomially acquired bacteria is also common and points to environmental sources of contamination. Other intraoperative sources of contamination include intestinal flora when the gastrointestinal tract is entered or when operations, such as cholecystectomy, are performed concomitantly. Laminated thrombus lining the wall of aneurysms has been implicated as a source of contamination and, when cultured, yields bacteria in about 10% of specimens. *S. epidermidis* is the most common isolate.[9,10]

Postoperative sources of vascular prosthetic infection include wound complications, urinary tract infections, and invasive line sepsis. Early and late hematogenous seeding of prostheses can occur during transient bacteremia associated with remote, noncontiguous infections or dental procedures.

Although bacteria are most often cultured from infected arterial prostheses, other, less common microorganisms, such as fungi, *Mycoplasma*, and *Mycobacterium*, have been encountered. *S. epidermidis* is the most common pathogen reported in modern series and outnumbers *S. aureus* infections two to one. Gram-negative and polymicrobial infections are increasingly encountered, but remain less prevalent than gram-positive infections. In many cases, negative cultures are reported despite convincing local evidence of infection, including a nonincorporated prosthesis surrounded by grossly purulent fluid.[11] These cases are most likely due to *S. epidermidis* or other low-virulence organisms that are exposed to perioperative antibiotics at the time of sampling and require fastidious microbiologic techniques for growth. Sonication of infected prosthetic material, growth in tryptic soy broth, and prolonged incubation for several days have been reported to increase the yield of cultures positive for *S. epidermidis.*[12]

The presence of a foreign body, such as an implanted device, increases the risk for infection. Early investigations documented that it takes only 10^2 *S. aureus* organisms to cause an abscess at the site of a subcutaneous silk suture, but 10^6 organisms to cause an infection in normal skin with no foreign body present. The explanations of why foreign materials are prone to infection involve physicochemical properties of the material, impairment of host defenses, and special properties of bacteria that facilitate their growth in the presence of a biomaterial.[13]

The biologic reaction to an implanted vascular prosthesis consists of an acute inflammatory response in the early stages and progresses to formation of a fibrous capsule or tissue growth into porous materials. Neutrophils rapidly become associated with any implanted biomaterial in vivo, become prematurely activated by contact with the material, and rapidly lose the capacity to become activated in response to subsequent stimuli, such as the presence of bacteria. Neutrophils in contact with biomaterials rapidly lose their ability to produce superoxide and other reactive oxygen species and become relatively impotent in their microbicidal activity.[14,15] In a sense, the biomaterial becomes a massive "decoy" that averts and diverts the ability of neutrophils to respond normally to bacteria in the microenvironment. In addition, neutrophil products released in these circumstances may promote dysfunction of new neutrophils entering the microenvironment.[16]

Vascular prosthetic biomaterials may vary in their susceptibility to infection by different microorganisms. Highly textured or rough-surfaced biomaterials, such as textiles manufactured from Dacron (woven or knitted), are more prone to bacterial adherence than smooth-surfaced biomaterials, such as expanded polytetrafluoroethylene (ePTFE) or polyurethane.[17] In vivo, adherence of platelets, plasma proteins, and other blood constituents and varying conditions of shear may dramatically alter the responses of different biomaterials to microorganisms, and all biomaterials remain susceptible to infection.[18,19]

4 The principal organism responsible for infections of all implanted medical devices, including vascular prostheses, is *S. epidermidis.* It is one species of coagulase-negative staphylococci that is a major cause of nosocomial infections and of nosocomial bacteremias in particular.[20] The organism is a ubiquitous skin commensural of relatively slow growth and low virulence. It causes chronic infections with local manifestations, but little or no systemic toxicity. Pivotal in the pathogenesis of *S. epidermidis* infection is the production of multilayered biofilms composed of exopolysaccharides, usually referred to as "slime."

The elaboration of biofilms takes place following the adherence of *S. epidermidis* to biomaterials and usually occurs when organisms adhere to one another in microcolonies.[21] Both adherence of organisms to polymer surfaces and to each other (cell–cell adhesion) is mediated by capsular polysaccharide adhesins.[21,22] Mutant bacteria that do not produce adhesins lack cell–cell adhesion and do not produce biofilms.[23] Once elaborated, biofilms form a protective shield that allows continued bacterial growth in relatively hostile environments. Bacterial nutrients and metabolic wastes freely traverse the polysaccharide biofilm, but antibiotics do not. Biofilms also alter inflammatory changes, impair host defenses, and promote tenacious adherence of microbial colonies to the biomaterial.[24] *S. epidermidis* infections tend to be persistent and refractory to antibiotics, and the implant must be removed to clear the infection.

The phenotypic transformation of *S. epidermidis* to an indolent, low-virulence organism that produces a protective biofilm is due to a phenomenon known as quorum sensing.[25] Quorum sensing is the regulation of gene expression in response to fluctuations in cell density. *S. epidermidis* and other quorum-sensing bacteria release autoinducers or pheromones that vary in concentration proportional to cell density. Oligopeptide autoinducers attach to cell surface receptors and induce transcriptional changes, resulting in dramatic changes in gene expression. In the case of *S. epidermidis,* organisms circulating alone (planktonic state) produce a low level of autoinducer in the microenvironment. Planktonic *S. epidermidis* organisms have aerobic metabolism and secrete multiple virulence and proinflammatory factors that produce signs and symptoms of sepsis. However, when these organisms attach to and aggregate in close proximity on polymer surfaces, quorum sensing results in the activation of multiple genes that result in a low-virulence organism that has anaerobic metabolism and produces abundant biofilm.[26] In addition, genes that are involved in the production of virulence factors are suppressed. In essence, the *S. epidermidis* microorganism goes into a kind of "hibernation."

Once established, bacterial infection spreads throughout a vascular prosthesis and eventually involves anastomotic sites. The eventual destruction of vascular tissue leads to the formation of an anastomotic false aneurysm. The first manifestation of a vascular prosthetic infection is often an anastomotic false aneurysm or its most frequent complication, prosthetic limb thrombosis in the case of an aortobifemoral bypass. When the false aneurysm involves the aortic anastomosis, rupture into the duodenum may occur and produce an aortoduodenal fistula with catastrophic hemorrhage.

Although all microorganisms producing vascular prosthetic infections are associated with false aneurysms, they vary in their propensity to destroy vascular tissue. Gram-negative organisms, such as *Pseudomonas aeruginosa, Proteus* species, and *Escherichia coli* are particularly notorious for their ability to digest vascular tissue.[27] These organisms elaborate elastase and alkaline protease, which break down elastin, collagen, fibronectin, and fibrin. *S. epidermidis* and other coagulase-negative staphylococci also secrete proteolytic proteins that can degrade vascular tissue. The mechanisms underlying protease elaboration and activation are highly regulated and complex.[28] In addition to causing vascular disruption and the formation of false aneurysms, many bacteria produce substances that are highly thrombogenic and may induce thrombosis that is the first manifestation of a vascular prosthetic infection.

Clinical Presentation

5 The clinical presentations of vascular prosthetic infections can be protean and subtle, so that the diagnosis is difficult. The tempo and severity of the clinical manifestations often depend on the microorganism. A patient whose infection is caused by a virulent organism, such as *S. aureus, P. aeruginosa,* or *E. coli,* presents with systemic signs of sepsis. As an example, a patient with a vascular prosthesis who has persistent fever, chills, and an elevated white blood cell count with a left shift should be suspected of having a vascular prosthetic infection. Virulent microorganisms also tend to cause earlier manifestations of infection, with the interval between implantation of the prosthesis and diagnosis of infection often being months. Very early prosthetic infections, diagnosed within weeks of implantation, are most often associated with wound infections that involve the vascular prostheses by contiguous spread.

In contrast, patients with infection caused by a low-virulence organism, such as *S. epidermidis*, present later, often years after placement.[7] Systemic signs and symptoms are usually mild or absent. These patients most often present with local manifestations, such as a chronic groin sinus that discharges small amounts of pus, a chronic wound infection exposing the prosthesis, femoral anastomotic false aneurysm, or aortofemoral bypass limb thrombosis. They may have low-grade fever and mild constitutional symptoms, but overt systemic signs of sepsis are absent. The white blood cell count is usually normal or only mildly elevated, but the erythrocyte sedimentation rate is often abnormal. A patient presenting with a femoral

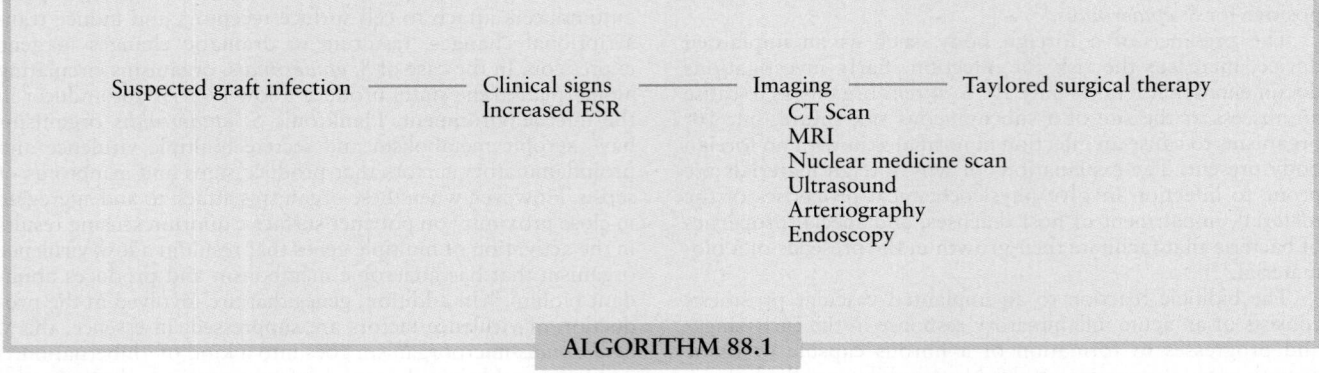

Suspected graft infection — Clinical signs / Increased ESR — Imaging — Taylored surgical therapy

Imaging:
- CT Scan
- MRI
- Nuclear medicine scan
- Ultrasound
- Arteriography
- Endoscopy

ALGORITHM 88.1

ALGORITHM 88.1. Diagnosis and treatment of prosthetic infection.

anastomotic false aneurysm or limb thrombosis who has an elevated erythrocyte sedimentation rate should be suspected of having a vascular prosthetic infection.

Patients presenting with massive gastrointestinal hemorrhage from aortoduodenal or aortoenteric fistula frequently have had lesser episodes of bleeding hours to days before the major episode. These are often referred to as "herald" or "sentinel" episodes of bleeding and offer a window of opportunity for diagnosis and management that may avert exsanguinating hemorrhage. Any patient with an intra-abdominal vascular prosthesis who has an episode of upper or lower gastrointestinal bleeding should be suspected of having an underlying aortoenteric fistula, and an expeditious workup is important.

Chronic gastrointestinal bleeding can also occur in patients with an aortoenteric fistula, but is more often associated with an enteric erosion. This condition, often referred to as "graft-enteric erosion," differs from aortoenteric fistula in that the body or limb of the vascular prosthesis erodes into bowel and the aortic suture line is not involved. This produces chronic bleeding from the eroded bowel mucosa, analogous to bleeding from an ulcer, and patients may present with chronic anemia. The diagnosis should be suspected in a patient with an intra-abdominal vascular prosthesis who has anemia, stool positive for occult blood on guaiac testing, and fever.

Another manifestation of aortofemoral and aortoiliac prosthetic infections is hydroureteronephrosis. This can develop if the ureter becomes obstructed as a result of periprosthetic inflammation and may be bilateral or unilateral, depending on the extent of infection. It is unusual for hydroureteronephrosis to be the initial manifestation of vascular prosthetic infection because the urologic condition is usually asymptomatic. This complication most often is noted during the workup of a patient with an infected vascular prosthesis who presents with other symptoms, such as a groin sinus or gastrointestinal bleeding.

Diagnosis

6 Because the manifestations of vascular prosthetic infections are so varied and subtle and because the consequences of a missed diagnosis may be lethal, imaging tests are important (Algorithm 88.1).[29] The types of imaging and other diagnostic tests used are based on the clinical presentation. Computed tomography (CT) scanning has long been the mainstay of diagnostic imaging for suspected vascular prosthetic infection. CT findings suggestive of infection include ectopic gas, periprosthetic fluid, loss of tissue planes, periprosthetic inflammatory changes, thickening of adjacent bowel, hydroureteronephrosis, and anastomotic false aneurysm (Fig. 88.1).[30] These findings are most specific and useful for late infections. During the immediate period following implantation, periprosthetic fluid, air, and inflammatory changes may be present for 2 to 3 months. After 3 months, postoperative hematoma and gas should resolve and tissue planes return to normal.[31]

Magnetic resonance imaging (MRI) has provided an alternative to CT scanning for cross-sectional imaging. In addition to demonstrating the same features seen on CT (periprosthetic air, fluid and structural abnormalities), MRI is particularly helpful in assessing periprosthetic inflammatory changes. These are seen as high-intensity signals on T2-weighted images in the tissues surrounding the prosthesis and accurately portray tissue edema (Fig. 88.2).[32] Such images can be particularly helpful in assessing the extent of infection, which may determine the operative approach. For example, in a patient with an infection localized to a single, distal limb of an aortobifemoral bypass, removal of the entire prosthesis may not be required for adequate treatment of the infection.

Radionuclide scanning has also been used in the diagnosis of vascular prosthetic infections. Scintigraphy with the use of autologous white blood cells labeled with indium oxine ^{111}In is the most common technique currently used, although the use of white cells labeled with ^{67}gallium, technetium, and other isotopes have been reported.[33,34] In addition, scintigraphy based on labeled human immunoglobulin G has been used and may be more sensitive than scintigraphy with white blood cells.[35] Most recently, positron emission tomography (PET) imaging has been found to be useful in imaging graft infection.

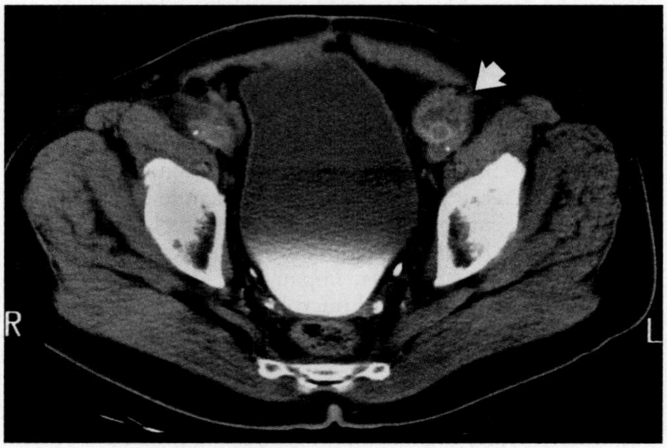

FIGURE 88.1. Computed tomography (CT) scan of lower pelvis demonstrating fluid and an enhancing ring around the left limb of an aortobifemoral bypass (*arrow*).

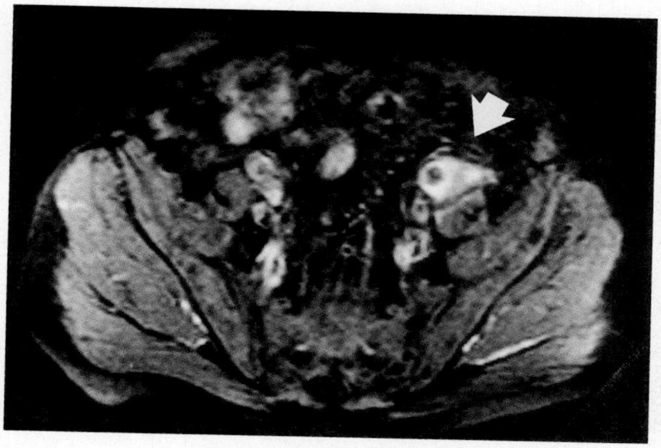

FIGURE 88.2. Magnetic resonance imaging (MRI) of the lower pelvis of the patient in Figure 88.1. The arrow points to high-intensity signals on T2-weighted images characteristic of inflammation and tissue edema.

Increased levels of fluorodeoxyglucose (FDG) tagged with isotope may be seen in areas of activated granulocytes. FDG-PET appears to have greater sensitivity and specificity in the diagnosis of graft infections in comparison to other imaging modalities.[36]

A problem with all scintigraphic methods in diagnosing vascular prosthetic infections is a lack of specificity caused by uptake in other organs or tissues that may be contiguous. In addition, faint or no uptake in the presence of limited or low-virulence infection can result in false-negative results. Scintigraphy is most helpful when occult prosthetic infection is suspected. An example would be a patient with a vascular prosthesis presenting with a fever of unknown origin or a complex of other nonspecific symptoms in whom white blood cell scintigraphy "lights up" the prosthesis.

Ultrasonography can be useful and is noninvasive and inexpensive. The finding of an echo-lucent rim or "halo" sign surrounding a vascular prosthesis is highly suggestive of a vascular prosthetic infection[37] (Fig. 88.3). In addition, duplex ultrasonography may uncover other findings such as anastomotic false aneurysms that are frequently associated with vascular prosthetic infections.

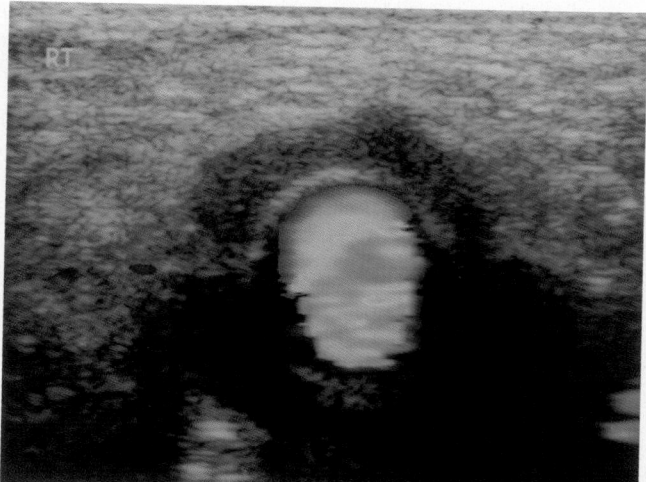

FIGURE 88.3. Duplex, color-flow scan demonstrating echo lucent rim or "halo" sign surrounding the limb of an aortofemoral bypass graft.

Arteriography is of limited usefulness in the diagnosis of vascular prosthetic infection, but it may, on occasion, demonstrate an aortic false aneurysm or even active leakage of contrast into the bowel lumen, which is pathognomonic for aortoenteric fistula. Arteriography is helpful in planning reconstruction after removal of the prosthesis and is most useful in late infection, when the vascular anatomy may have been altered by progressive occlusive disease.

In patients presenting with gastrointestinal bleeding and suspected aortoenteric fistula, complete upper gastrointestinal endoscopy with visualization of the third and fourth portions of the duodenum, the most common site of fistula, is necessary. Even if this study is incomplete, with inability to visualize the distal duodenum or the finding of gastrointestinal lesions (e.g., chronic peptic ulcer) that are not actively bleeding, an aortoenteric fistula may still be present. Continued, unexplained bleeding mandates operative exploration to rule out aortoenteric fistula. At the time of operation, the duodenum, proximal jejunum, and any other bowel in contact with a vascular prosthesis must be dissected free to make or exclude this diagnosis.

Treatment

7 The primary goals of treatment are to save life and limb, and this is best accomplished by eradicating infection and maintaining adequate circulation to portions of the body perfused by the infected prosthesis. Secondary goals include minimizing morbidity, restoring normal function, and maintaining long-term function without the need for repeated intervention and risk of amputation.

These goals are best achieved by excision of all infected prosthetic material and vascular tissues combined with appropriate arterial reconstruction. The currently favored methods of arterial reconstruction for aortic prosthetic infection include extra-anatomic bypass[38–54] and in situ replacement with the use of autogenous femoral-popliteal veins,[52,55–63] arterial allografts,[64–76] and vascular prostheses that are often treated or soaked in antibiotic solutions.[52,77–82] A recent meta-analysis of pooled data demonstrated several advantages of in situ graft replacement over extra-anatomic bypass.[83] In situ graft replacement is becoming increasingly popular because it is expedient, avoids an aortic stump with potential for lethal blowout, and is associated with a low amputation rate.

Pooled outcome data from contemporary series reported since 1985 are presented in Table 88.1. Direct comparisons of these data to judge the relative success of the various approaches are difficult because of the heterogeneity of patients with different degrees of illness and different comorbid conditions in the reported series. All of these approaches are valid and useful depending on patient-specific characteristics and circumstances. It is a mistake to think that a single surgical approach is applicable to all patients with this condition. These complicated and multifaceted patients with varying degrees of illness require individualized attention. The pros and cons of each approach are also outlined in Table 88.1.

Extra-anatomic bypass, usually involving an axillofemoral bypass, is an excellent choice for infected aortoiliac reconstructions in which femoral sites are free of sepsis and arterial runoff is good (Fig. 88.4). It is also possibly less of a physiologic insult than other procedures, particularly when the operations can be staged so that extra-anatomic bypass precedes removal of the infected aortic prosthesis by a period of days.[39] This approach has the advantage of preserving lower extremity blood flow during removal of the aortic prosthesis, so that ischemic time is minimized.

Unfortunately, the durability of an extra-anatomic bypass is limited in patients with multilevel occlusive disease and poor runoff. Most patients with infected aortic prostheses have an aortobifemoral bypass, and extra-anatomic bypass in such patients usually requires bilateral axillofemoral procedures

TABLE 88.1

TREATMENT OF AORTIC PROSTHETIC INFECTIONS[a]

	REFERENCES	NO. PATIENTS	MORTALITY (RANGE) %	MAJOR AMPUTATION (RANGE) %	REINFECTION/ ANASTOMOTIC OR VASCULAR DISRUPTION %	FIVE-YEAR PRIMARY PATENCY %	FIVE-YEAR ASSISTED/ SECONDARY PATENCY %	ADVANTAGES	DISADVANTAGES
Extra-anatomic bypass	38–54	590	21.2 (5.0–40.6)	10.7 (0–15.6)	16.0	30–73	65–90	Procedure can be staged. Less physiologic stress.	Poor patency, high long-term amputation rate. Thrombectomy, revision often required. Potential for reinfection of bypass and aortic stump blowout.
In situ femoral-popliteal vein replacement	52, 55–63	334	11.0 (6.7–20.0)	5.4 (4.9–6.7)	5.0	84	98–100	Autogenous reconstruction, resists infection. Excellent patency, low long-term amputation rate.	Complex procedure. Long ischemia time. Fasciotomy may be required in up to 20%.
In situ allograft replacement	64–76	684	22.0 (8.3–36.4)	2.0 (0–3.0)	9.7	?	?	Expeditious procedure. No aortic stump.	Reinfection. Allograft deterioration and disruption. Unavailability of allografts.
In situ prosthetic replacement	52, 77–82	169	13.0 (8.0–21.7)	0	10.3	?	?	Expeditious procedure. No aortic stump.	Reinfection rate high and unpredictable. Indefinite antibiotic therapy.

[a]Pooled data from major series reported since 1985.

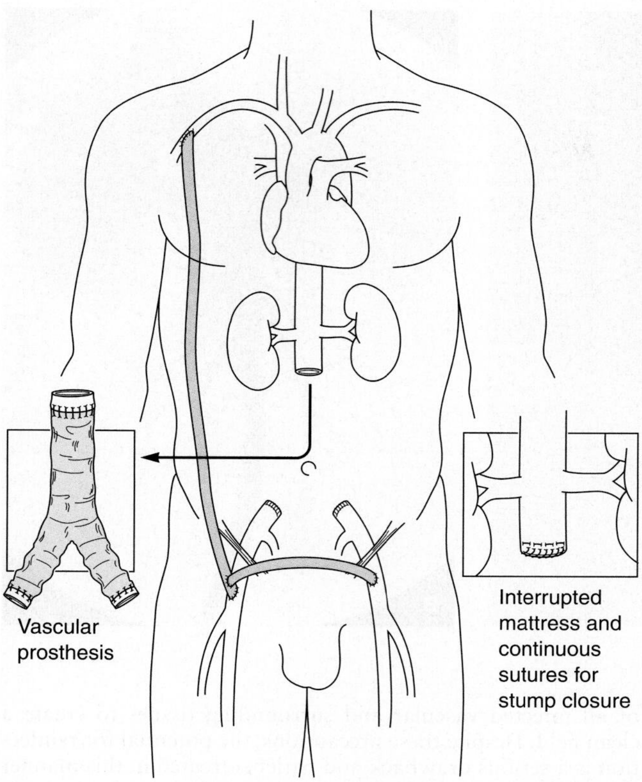

FIGURE 88.4. Standard treatment for an infected aortic vascular prosthesis. An axillobifemoral bypass is performed first. This is followed a few days later by removal of the infected aortic prosthesis and careful oversewing of the aortic stump as illustrated. This operation has its greatest usefulness in patients with infected aortoiliac prostheses and who have femoral areas free of infection and good runoff.

with distal anastomoses to diseased and, often, small profunda femoral or popliteal arteries. These are disadvantaged reconstructions with poor long-term patency despite the administration of antithrombotic agents (Table 88.1). They are prone to sudden thrombotic occlusion without warning, and amputation rates are high, even after thrombectomy and multiple revisions. In one large series, one third of patients required major amputation during long-term follow-up.[40] In addition, reinfection of the extra-anatomic bypass prostheses occurs in 10% to 20% of patients, and this condition is often lethal. A final problem with extra-anatomic bypass is continuing infection at the site of aortic closure, or aortic "stump." Although an infrequent occurrence (<10% of cases), aortic stump blowout is almost always fatal.

Dissatisfaction with the long-term patency of extra-anatomic bypass led to the development of in situ autogenous venous reconstruction.[52,55–63] Early experiences were with greater saphenous veins, but the use of femoral-popliteal veins rapidly evolved because of their large caliber and superior patency (Figs. 88.5 and 88.6).[55] This reconstruction is most applicable in patients with extensive occlusive disease and poor runoff, a circumstance in which the patency of an autogenous venous reconstruction would theoretically be better than the patency of a prosthetic bypass. The situation is analogous to the use of vein grafts for femoral-popliteal and distal bypasses because of their superior patency in comparison with prosthetic conduits. This advantage has been realized, with excellent 5-year cumulative rates of 85% to 90% for primary patency and 100% for secondary/assisted patency in superficial femoropopliteal vein aortofemoral reconstructions.[57,58,63] Long-term amputation rates have been reported to be correspondingly low.

The principal disadvantage of using femoral-popliteal veins for aortofemoral reconstruction is that the procedure is technically demanding and long. The lower extremity ischemic time is longer than with other approaches, but can be minimized by carefully sequencing the procedure to shorten aortic cross-clamp time. To minimize open body cavity exposure and lower extremity ischemia, the operation is carried out in the following order: (a) dissect femoral-popliteal veins and leave in situ until needed, (b) isolate and control femoral vessels, (c) enter abdomen and obtain aortic control, (d) remove infected prosthesis, and (e) perform reconstruction with femoral-popliteal veins.[84]

Acute venous hypertension can result in the need for leg fasciotomy in up to 20% of limbs following harvest of the femoral-popliteal vein.[85] Special risk factors that predict the need for fasciotomy include preexisting, advanced limb ischemia (preoperative ankle-brachial index <0.40) and concomitant ipsilateral harvest of the greater saphenous vein. Acute muscle swelling from venous hypertension coupled with ischemia-reperfusion injury is a major pathogenetic factor.[85]

Long-term lower extremity venous morbidity is also a potential drawback to harvesting the femoral-popliteal veins. However, venous morbidity has been surprisingly infrequent and mild.[57,63] The benign course following removal of the femoral-popliteal veins is a consequence of several compensating mechanisms.[86] First, the junction of the profunda femoral

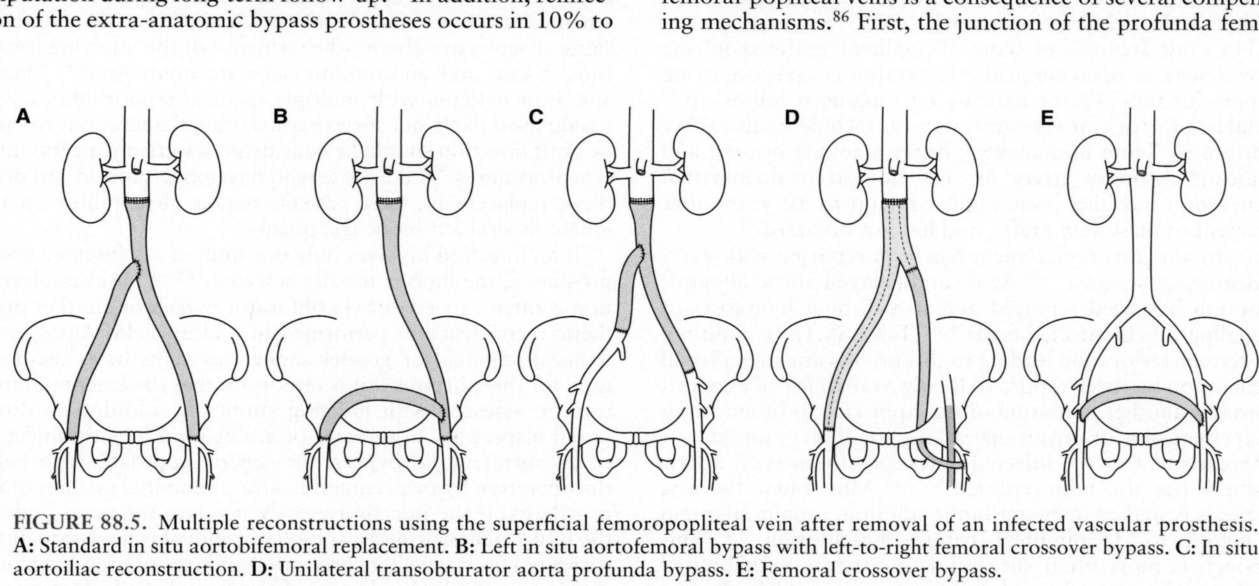

FIGURE 88.5. Multiple reconstructions using the superficial femoropopliteal vein after removal of an infected vascular prosthesis. **A:** Standard in situ aortobifemoral replacement. **B:** Left in situ aortofemoral bypass with left-to-right femoral crossover bypass. **C:** In situ aortoiliac reconstruction. **D:** Unilateral transobturator aorta profunda bypass. **E:** Femoral crossover bypass.

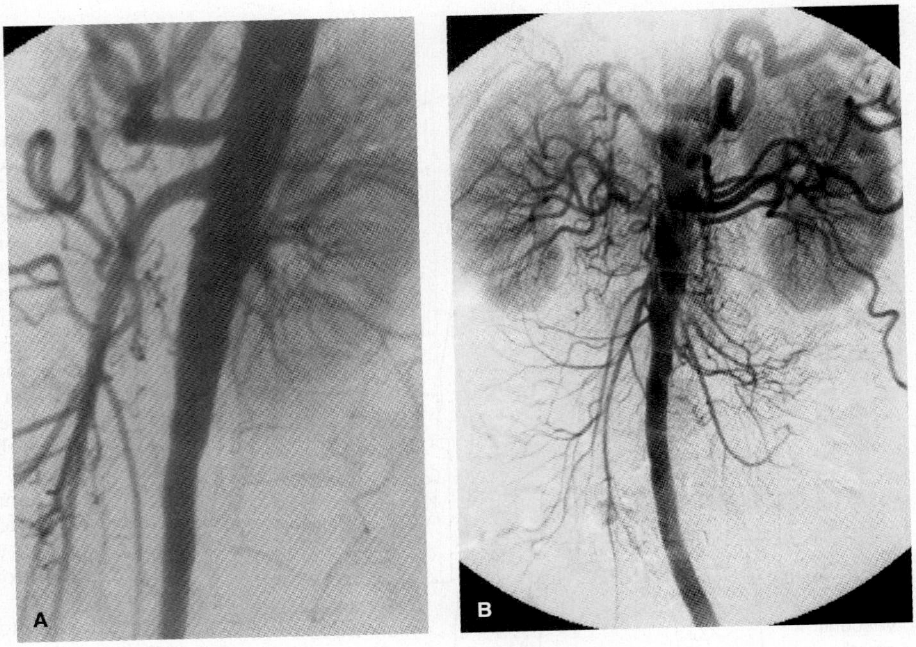

FIGURE 88.6. Lateral (A) and anteroposterior (B) arteriogram of a superficial femoropopliteal vein in situ replacement after removal of an infected aortobifemoral bypass. The left-to-right femoral crossover bypass with superficial femoropopliteal vein is not shown. The figure illustrates the excellent size match between the large-caliber superficial femoropopliteal vein and the infrarenal aorta.

and common femoral veins is carefully preserved after disconnection of the proximal femoral vein to allow unimpeded drainage via the profunda system. Second, several anatomic collateral connections are found between the remaining distal popliteal vein and the profunda system, and many of these collaterals enlarge to accommodate the increase in volume flow following removal of the femoral-popliteal vein. Finally, the valves in the tibial veins and collateral circuits remain functional, so that distal venous reflux does not occur.[87]

A final concern is that placing femoral-popliteal veins in an infected field may lead to reinfection and disruption. Experience with this approach has documented that these vein grafts resist gram-positive, gram-negative, and fungal infections, and disruption of anastomoses has been rare. In a recent large series of in situ graft replacement for infected aortic prostheses, the overall incidence of graft disruption was 5%.[58] Most were in reconstructions for aortoenteric erosion or fistula where there was breakdown of the duodenal repair. Previous experience has documented that femoral-popliteal vein graft disruption usually occurs in settings where there is ongoing contamination of the graft, severe malnutrition, immunosuppression, and a debilitated patient.[88]

Vein graft stenosis of femoral-popliteal grafts requiring endovascular or open surgical intervention is rare, occurring in approximately 5% of patients on long-term follow-up.[89] Special risk factors for vein graft stenosis include small-caliber graft (<6 to 7 mm in diameter), heavy smoking history, and significant coronary artery disease. Long-term aneurysmal degeneration has also been studied for up to 10 years after placement of these vein grafts, and has not occurred.[57]

In situ allograft replacement has been reported with varying degrees of success.[64–76] Acute and delayed aortic allograft disruption has been reported and is a distinct limitation of using allografts in infected fields[66,90] (Table 88.1). In addition, long-term deterioration leading to thrombosis and aneurysmal degeneration has been reported. Ready availability of allograft material is another limitation of this approach in situations in which emergency or urgent operations are often required.

Replacement of the infected aortic prosthesis with a new prosthesis has also been reported.[52,77–82] Most often, the new prosthesis is soaked in an antibiotic solution, usually rifampin (60 mg/mL for 15 minutes), before implantation.[79,80] This approach is most often successful in patients with limited infections of low virulence following aggressive débridement of all infected vascular and surrounding tissues to create a clean field. Despite these precautions, the potential for reinfection is a serious drawback and patients treated in this manner require close and vigilant follow-up with frequent imaging studies such as CT or MRI. They also are usually treated with lifelong oral antibiotics.

In situ prosthetic and allograft reconstructions may be most useful in very ill and unstable patients and in those with actively bleeding aortoenteric fistulas. Expeditious in situ replacement in these circumstances can be lifesaving and may be used as a "bridge" procedure, with definitive reconstruction (extra-anatomic or femoral-popliteal vein) carried out at a later date when the patient has been rendered fit for such a reconstruction.

Conservative approaches that do not involve removal of the infected prostheses have also been reported.[91–96] These are based on aggressive drainage and débridement of infected tissues; intensive, culture-specific antibiotic therapy; meticulous wound care to achieve coverage of exposed prosthetic material; and coverage of exposed prosthetic material with muscle flaps. Conservative approaches are most appropriately used when infection is extracavitary and limited in extent, systemic signs of sepsis are absent, the virulence of the infecting organisms is low, and anastomotic sites are uninvolved.[94] Elderly and frail patients with multiple medical comorbidities who would most likely not survive conventional operations for aortic graft infection should be considered selectively for less invasive procedures.[95] Like those who have undergone in situ prosthetic replacement, these patients require close follow-up and indefinite oral antibiotic treatment.

If an infection involves only one limb of a bifurcated aortic prosthesis, the limb is usually resected.[12,97–100] Revascularization is often carried out via obturator bypass or another prosthetic reconstruction performed in a clean field. Autogenous femoral-popliteal or greater saphenous veins have also been used for this purpose.[99] It is important that the extent of infection be assessed with imaging studies in addition to direct visual inspection. In the case of a unilateral femoral infection of an aortofemoral bypass, the general approach is to begin the operation by inspecting the intra-abdominal portion of the prosthesis. If the infection grossly involves the main body of the bifurcated prosthesis, complete removal is necessary. If the suspected limb is well incorporated and free of gross infection, division of the limb, closure of the tunnel, and obturator or other extra-anatomic bypass are performed. The final portion of this operation is removal of the infected limb from below, with care taken to prevent cross-contamination of other, freshly placed incisions that have been closed.

Infection of Femoropopliteal/Distal Prosthetic Bypasses

In general, the management principles for infected infrainguinal prosthetic bypasses are similar to those for infected aortic prostheses. Excision of all infected prosthetic material and creation of a new bypass through clean tissue planes are optimal.[101] Venous autografts are preferable to vascular prostheses because of the low risk of reinfection. Unfortunately, many of these patients have limited sources of adequate vein for a new vein graft bypass. Additionally, because of the limited anatomic area, cross-contamination and infection of a new prosthetic conduit are probable. In selected patients, it may be possible to couple removal of the infected lower extremity bypass graft with an endovascular intervention to revascularize and maintain viability of the limb. Endovascular treatment under these circumstances should probably avoid stenting procedures because of the possibility of infecting stents.

The overall mortality of patients undergoing operations for infected prosthetic infrainguinal bypasses approaches 20% and may be higher in patients undergoing limb salvage procedures.[101,102] These considerations have led some experts to recommend excision of the infected prosthesis and amputation in circumstances in which the limb remains in jeopardy after removal of the infected prosthesis. The rate of major amputation is approximately 40%.[101,102] If assessment with Doppler ultrasonography indicates that the limb remains viable (audible arterial signals present at the ankle level), removal of the infected prosthesis with vein patch closure of anastomotic sites is preferred. If only a limited portion of the prosthesis is involved, nonresectional, conservative measures have been successfully used.[91,103] Results with this approach are best when virulence of the infection is low, sepsis is absent, and anastomoses are free of infection.

Prevention of Vascular Prosthetic Infections

The benefit of short-term antibiotic prophylaxis in preventing wound infections after vascular surgery has been demonstrated in randomized trials.[104–106] Most often, a first-generation cephalosporin is administered intravenously shortly before operation, during operation if blood loss is extensive or the operation is prolonged, and 2 hours after operation. Evidence suggests that a more prolonged course, for up to 4 to 5 days after operation or until all invasive lines have been removed, may provide additional protection.[107] When patients have infected ischemic lesions of a lower extremity, culture-specific antibiotics should be administered perioperatively. Also, the use of more specific prophylactic antibiotic therapy should be considered in hospitals where certain organisms are prevalent, especially when exposure is increased by prolonged preoperative hospitalization.

Attention to intraoperative factors is also important in preventing vascular prosthetic infections. Patients undergoing repeated and emergency operations are especially prone to wound infections and present additional risks. Meticulous attention to hemostasis and avoidance of wound hematomas and seromas that can become secondarily infected are important surgical tenets that are often difficult to achieve in patients given anticoagulants during the operation and who are also taking antithrombotic agents, such as aspirin or clopidogrel. If possible, these agents should be discontinued 1 week before the operation. Ligation and control of the femoral lymphatics are also probably important technical features in preventing vascular prosthetic infections. Electrocautery of lymphatic tissue leads to coagulation necrosis of lymphatic vessels, but does not prevent extravasation of lymph fluid.

Patients undergoing aortic operations are prone to intraoperative hypothermia, and this condition has been shown to impair neutrophil function and increase the incidence of postoperative wound infection.[108] Maintenance of normal body temperature should be the goal during major vascular operations. Additional procedures on the gastrointestinal or biliary tract that may result in intraoperative contamination of a vascular prosthesis should be avoided unless the additional procedure is deemed necessary to avoid life-threatening postoperative complications. Hematogenous seeding of a vascular prosthesis is a continuing risk for as long as the prosthesis is in place. Dental work, procedures on the gastrointestinal and genitourinary tracts, and angiographic procedures should be carried out with the patient protected by prophylactic antibiotics (Fig. 88.7).

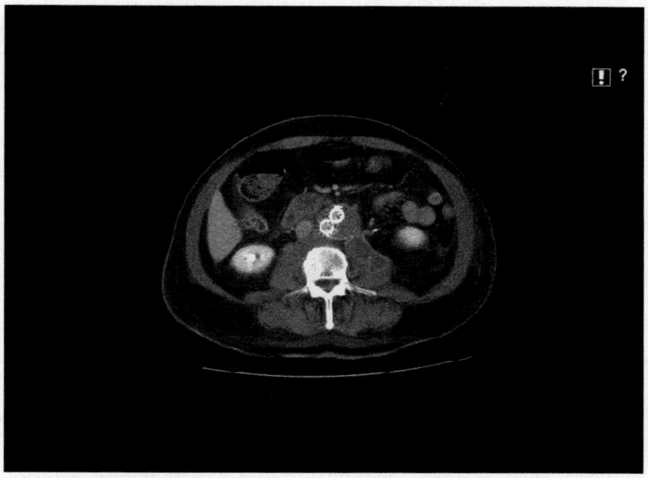

FIGURE 88.7. Patient had an uneventful endovascular aortic aneurysm repair 1 year prior to teeth cleaning. Two weeks after teeth cleaning, he presented with high fevers, chills, back pain, and an elevated white cell count. Computed tomography scan with intravascular contrast demonstrates an infected aortic stent graft with retroperitoneal extension and psoas abscesses. On explant, the aortic stent graft grew *Streptococcus viridans*, the most common microorganism found in the oral cavity.

INFECTED (MYCOTIC) ANEURYSMS

Pathogenesis

In the late 19th century, Osler first used the term *mycotic* to describe the peripheral, infected aneurysms occurring in patients with bacterial endocarditis.[109] The beaded gross appearance of the multiple aneurysms in these patients resembled a fungus growth, hence the term *mycotic*. However, he delineated the pathogenesis to be destruction of the arterial wall subsequent to embolization of bacteria-laden material from the heart. In the era before antibiotics, the presence of such lesions indicated a malignant form of endocarditis because death was inevitable.

Mycotic aneurysms, as described by Osler, are now rare, and a more comprehensive term is *infected aneurysm* or *microbial arteritis*.[110] Infected aneurysms encompass preexisting aneurysms that are secondarily infected by hematogenous or contiguous spread and infections of the arterial wall that subsequently cause aneurysmal degeneration.[111] When the arterial wall is completely disrupted and a contained rupture is present, the aneurysm may be termed an *infected false aneurysm* or *pseudoaneurysm*. Currently, fewer than 10% of infected aneurysms are caused by bacterial endocarditis.[112]

It is difficult to infect the normal arterial wall during bacteremia, but such a mechanism has been postulated in severely immunocompromised patients. Special risk factors for microbial arteritis include long-term steroid use, chemotherapy for malignancy, severe alcoholism, chronic renal failure, and extensive radiation therapy.[113,114] Such infections may be initiated by hematogenous spread of bacteria through the vasa vasorum. Much more common is infection of abnormal arterial walls with irregular luminal surfaces, to which microorganisms attach during bacteremia.[110] Arterial wall defects and irregularities associated with infected aneurysms include atherosclerotic plaque, degenerative arterial aneurysms, and congenital abnormalities, such as aortic coarctation and patent ductus arteriosus. Host compromise, malnutrition, and advanced age are also seen in many of these patients.

Contiguous spread of infection is common in infected aortic aneurysms and is seen in such conditions as spinal osteomyelitis, pancreatitis, and retroperitoneal abscess associated with diverticulitis and other gastrointestinal and severe urinary infections.[110] Trauma is becoming an increasingly common mechanism by which infected aneurysms develop; bacteria are introduced at the time of intra-arterial drug injection with contaminated needles (drug abuse)[115] or the placement of arterial catheters for diagnostic and therapeutic interventions or for monitoring.[116] Almost all infected arterial aneurysms associated with trauma are false aneurysms in which arterial wall continuity is lost.

In reports of infection of preexisting aortic aneurysms, gram-positive organisms predominate over gram-negative organisms and are present in about 60% of cases.[110,117] Of these, *Staphylococcus* species are the most prevalent, with *S. aureus* being the most commonly encountered overall. Streptococci are also etiologic agents, with *Streptococcus viridans* being the most common subtype. In iatrogenic arterial infections associated with indwelling arterial catheters, methicillin-resistant *S. aureus* and other nosocomial organisms are being seen with increasing frequency.

Salmonella is the most prevalent organism associated with infection of a nonaneurysmal aorta.[110,114,117,118] The diseased, plaque-ridden aorta has a unique susceptibility to *Salmonella* infections. *Salmonella choleraesuis* and *Salmonella enteritidis*, especially the subtype *Salmonella typhimurium,* account for more than half of reported cases of *Salmonella* aortitis.[110]

Gram-negative arterial infections are much more virulent than gram-positive infections, and arteries infected with gram-negative organisms are much more prone to rupture. Gram-negative organisms, such as *P. aeruginosa*, can elaborate alkaline proteinase and a variety of elastases that cause vascular wall neurosis.[27] In addition, many bacteria, both gram positive and gram negative, produce collagenases.[119–121] Bacteria can also upregulate collagenases and metalloproteinases in inflammatory cells associated with aneurysms.[121] Recent interest has centered on neutrophil elastase in the pathogenesis of aneurysms.[122] According to this view, bacteria may play an indirect role, acting principally through the recruitment of acute inflammatory cells, which subsequently release neutrophil elastase.

Once the arterial wall is infected, rapid, focal, and progressive deterioration occurs. This process results in the characteristic saccular or multiloculated appearance of these aneurysms and often leads to locally contained rupture and the formation of a false aneurysm. In aortas without a preexisting aneurysm, infected aneurysms tend to occur in the posterior wall of the suprarenal or supraceliac aorta[110,113,114] (Fig. 88.8). When a preexisting aortic aneurysm becomes secondarily infected, the infrarenal location is the most common site.[117,123,124]

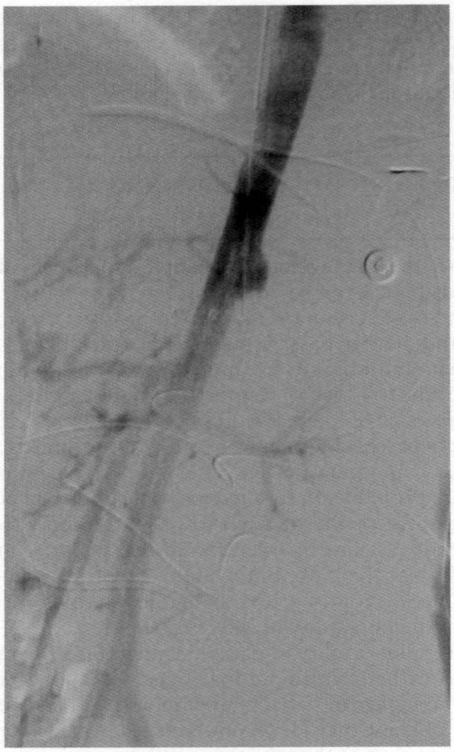

FIGURE 88.8. Infected aneurysm involving the posterior wall of the supraceliac aorta.

Clinical Presentation

The clinical presentation of an infected aneurysm depends on the virulence of the organism, the anatomic location, and the duration of infection. *Salmonella* aortic infections may appear after a febrile gastrointestinal illness. The presence of a tender abdominal aortic aneurysm in such a patient in association with continued fever and positive blood cultures strongly suggests this diagnosis. Infection of a preexisting aortic aneurysm may present as fever of unknown origin, malaise, or back and flank pain. Such patients are frequently debilitated, malnourished, and immunocompromised as the result of chronic illness, and the presence of an aortic aneurysm and positive blood cultures in this setting should arouse suspicion of an infected aneurysm. Chronic osteomyelitis or other retroperitoneal infectious processes contiguous to the aorta may also be present.

Infected aortic aneurysms are prone to rupture, even when small.[117,118] They may have been unsuspected before rupturing, and the diagnosis of infection may not be obvious at the time of emergency operation.[123] The diagnosis should be entertained in a patient presenting with a ruptured aortic aneurysm who has a fever and an elevated white blood cell count, especially when the aneurysm is small (<5 cm in diameter). At operation, additional clues include the presence of chronically inflamed retroperitoneal tissues with indistinct dissection planes and a focal aneurysm with relatively normal aorta above and below the site. Gram stains of smears from involved tissues and thrombus may be diagnostic, and cultures should be obtained even if the results of Gram stains are negative.

In contrast to aortic and other central aneurysms, peripheral infected aneurysms are usually readily apparent and the diagnosis obvious. A painful, cellulitic, warm pulsatile mass over a major artery in a febrile patient is a common clinical presentation.[115] An elevated white blood cell count and positive blood cultures are usual. The patient may have a history of drug abuse, and inadvertent or deliberate arterial injection with a contaminated needle should be suspected.[115] The common femoral artery is the most common site, and a prior history of arterial catheterization or the presence of an indwelling angiographic catheter or sheath for endovascular procedures is being increasingly seen.[116] Many of these procedures require repeated angiography and manipulation during prolonged periods, and femoral arterial sheaths or catheters are left in place for access. This increases the opportunity for arterial infection, and the risk is proportional to catheter residence time. Femoral puncture closure devices may also be sources of infection.[116]

Diagnosis

Infected aortic aneurysms can be difficult to diagnose. Leukocytosis is sensitive, but not specific, for an infected aneurysm. Blood cultures are important but may be negative in as many as 50% of patients with an infected aortic aneurysm.[110] Positive blood cultures in the presence of an abdominal aortic aneurysm should be considered evidence of an infected aneurysm until they are proven otherwise.

Radiologic studies are useful in confirming the diagnosis; CT and aortography are the most important tests.[118] MRI may also be helpful. CT and MRI will demonstrate the aneurysm and may show perivascular retroperitoneal inflammation and edema. A contained rupture may be present and suggests the diagnosis. The presence of periaortic air along with inflammatory changes is diagnostic (Fig. 88.9). Arteriography may aid in the diagnosis but is most useful in planning arterial reconstruction. A saccular aneurysm in an otherwise normal-appearing vessel or a multilobulated aneurysm strongly suggests the presence of aortic infection (Fig. 88.10).[110]

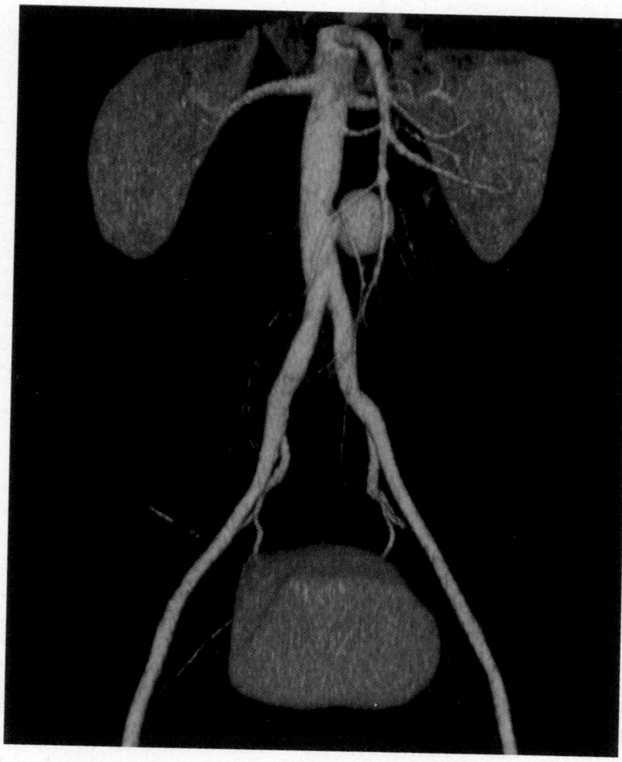

FIGURE 88.10. Computed tomography (CT) angiogram demonstrating focal, saccular infrarenal aortic aneurysm infected with *Staphylococcus aureus* in a human immunodeficiency virus–positive patient.

Treatment

Although culture-specific antibiotic therapy is important in the treatment of an infected aneurysm, surgical therapy is almost always necessary and lifesaving. Antibiotic therapy is started preoperatively and continued for at least 6 weeks after operation.[113] Surgical treatment must be expeditious because of the risk for aneurysm rupture and death. In stable patients who are dramatically improving on antibiotic therapy, withholding surgical treatment for a period to minimize, and possibly eliminate, local infection may be appropriate. However, there are reports of rupture during prolonged antibiotic therapy and the timing of operative intervention is a matter of careful judgment.[110]

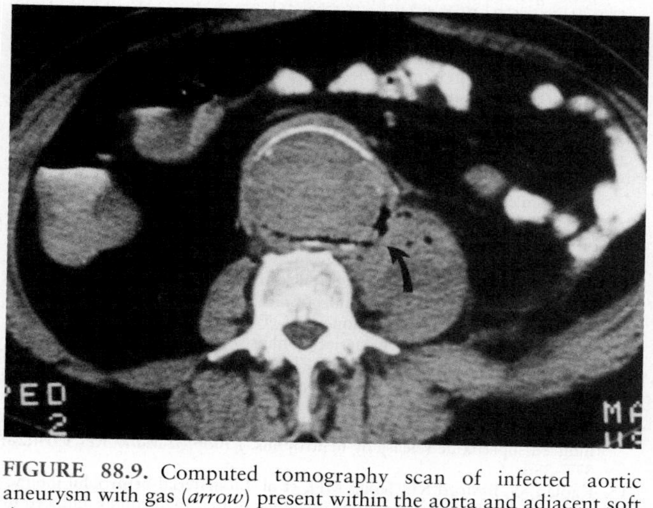

FIGURE 88.9. Computed tomography scan of infected aortic aneurysm with gas (*arrow*) present within the aorta and adjacent soft tissue.

The principles of treatment for an infected aneurysm are similar to those of surgical therapy of an infected arterial prostheses: eradication of infection by resection of the infected aneurysm and surrounding tissues and creation of a new bypass to restore circulation. Most authorities favor creating a new bypass through clean tissues. For infected aortoiliac aneurysms, axillofemoral bypass is most commonly performed.[112,114,118,123–125] For infected femoral aneurysms, an obturator bypass from the common iliac to the distal superficial femoral artery with a vascular prosthesis or vein graft routed through the obturator foramen successfully avoids the infected groin and restores distal circulation (Fig. 88.11).[115,116]

Prosthetic reconstruction in situ has been successfully used for infected aortic aneurysms when gross purulence is absent and contamination is minimal.[113,117,124,126–129] It is especially appropriate in patients with an aortic aneurysm that ruptures into the overlying duodenum, a condition usually referred to as *primary aortoduodenal fistula*. Contamination is minimal in this condition, and long-term results with prosthetic reconstruction in situ are good.[117,126–130] Patients treated in this manner require close follow-up because of the risk for recurrent infection, and most should be treated with lifelong oral antibiotics. Prosthetic reconstruction in situ is usually necessary for unstable patients with ruptured, infected aortic aneurysms.[117] Extra-anatomic bypass is not feasible in this circumstance because of the prolonged lower extremity ischemia time, especially when hypotension has been present. Overall mortality for patients with an infected aortic aneurysm is approximately 25% and is higher when rupture is present.[110]

A promising new approach involves harvesting femoral-popliteal veins to reconstruct the aortoiliac system after resection of an infected aneurysm and débridement of retroperitoneal

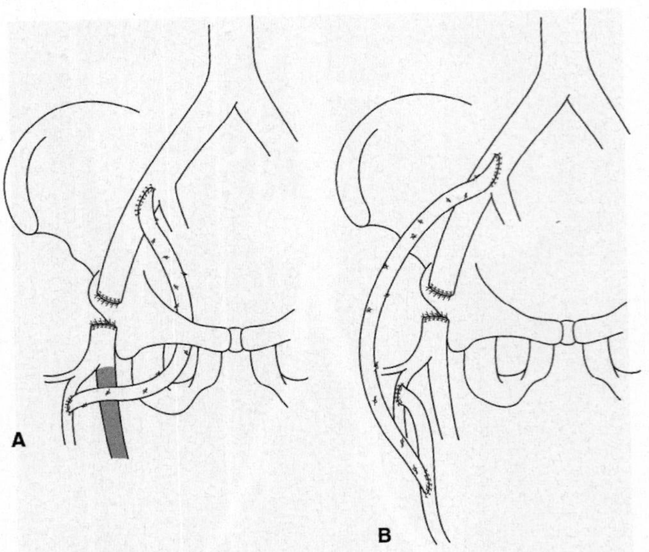

FIGURE 88.11. Extra-anatomic bypass options using superficial femoral-popliteal vein grafts for restoring lower extremity circulation for treatment of infected femoral aneurysms.

tissues.[57] These vein grafts have also been used to replace infected common femoral arterial aneurysms associated with drug abuse[115,116] (Fig. 88.11). The large vein grafts appear to be resistant to infection by most organisms, and disruption when they are placed in infected fields is rare. Because of the additional operative time for harvesting veins, reconstruction in situ with femoral-popliteal veins should be used in relatively stable patients.

There are reports of endovascular aortic stent graft placement to exclude and treat infected aneurysms. However, contamination of the stent graft with resultant graft infection is a major drawback to this approach. Stent graft treatment of patients with infected aneurysms should be reserved for only the most desperately ill patients with ruptured, infected aneurysms. Even in these individuals, stent graft treatment should be considered a "bridge" in anticipation of definitive treatment when the patient stabilizes.

SEPTIC THROMBOPHLEBITIS

Septic thrombophlebitis most commonly involves upper extremity and neck veins after the insertion of intravenous catheters and needles or intravenous drug abuse. However, venous thrombi can become secondarily infected during bacteremia or contiguity with areas of infection. Examples of contiguous infection include pelvic septic thrombophlebitis developing after obstetric infections,[131] internal jugular thrombophlebitis associated with severe pharyngitis and peritonsillar abscesses,[132] and visceral thrombophlebitis stemming from appendicitis. *S. aureus* is the most common organism cultured from patients with peripheral septic thrombophlebitis, and gram-negative and polymicrobial infections are common when a contiguous infection is the cause. Regardless of the source, infected thrombus propagates throughout the lumen of the involved vein, and septicemia with high spiking fevers and chills quickly develops. An intense perivascular inflammatory response accompanies the spread of intraluminal infection and is clinically manifested by marked edema, pain, tenderness, and erythema overlying the involved vein. *S. aureus* and other virulent organisms infecting clot can rapidly form an intravascular abscess. In this circumstance, the lumen of the vein becomes a "closed space," and excision or surgical drainage is necessary to treat the infection. Propagation of the infected clot can also give rise to septic pulmonary embolism resulting in pneumonia, metastatic pulmonary abscess, and septic pleural effusion.

The clinical diagnosis is readily apparent when peripheral veins in the extremities are involved. In addition to pain, swelling, and redness along the course of the vein, pus may be expressed at the site of catheter or needle insertion. When deep or central veins are involved, the diagnosis is more difficult. These patients may present with clinical signs of severe sepsis and occasionally with complications of septic pulmonary embolization. CT or MRI can be particularly helpful and may demonstrate enlarged, dilated veins with intravenous thrombus and perivascular inflammatory changes. These imaging modalities are most useful for septic thrombophlebitis involving ileofemoral, caval, axillary-subclavian, and pelvic veins.

The treatment of septic thrombophlebitis depends on its anatomic location. Along with antibiotic therapy, excision of a superficial vein in an extremity is curative.[133–135] One must take care to remove the entire length of involved vein to eradicate infection. When deep veins of an extremity or central veins of the chest or pelvis are involved, vein excision is difficult and associated with large losses of blood and severe morbidity. The mainstays of therapy for septic deep or central vein thrombophlebitis are intensive antibiotic therapy and heparin anticoagulation to halt the thrombotic process and prevent embolization.[136] Therapy may have to be continued for 2 to 3 weeks and is successful in most cases. If it is not successful and sepsis continues despite medical therapy, surgical intervention is indicated. Venous thrombectomy and vein excision have been reported to be successful in cases refractory to medical therapy.[131] When thrombectomy of the iliocaval system is undertaken, placement of a stainless steel caval filtration device (Greenfield filter) for protection against pulmonary embolism may be advisable.[137] Sepsis does not preclude placement of these devices. In advanced cases in which abscess forms within large veins that cannot be subjected to thrombectomy because of organization of thrombus and vein scarring, abscess drainage and débridement are indicated.

References

1. Balas P. An overview of aortofemoral graft infection. *Eur J Vasc Endovasc Surg* 1997;14(suppl A):3.
2. Kearney RA, Eisen HJ, Wolf JE. Nonvalvular infections of the cardiovascular system. *Ann Intern Med* 1994;121:219.
3. O'Brien T, Collin J. Prosthetic vascular graft infection. *Br J Surg* 1992;79:1262.
4. Lorentzen JE, Nielsen OM, Arendrup H, et al. Vascular graft infection: an analysis of sixty-two graft infections in 2411 consecutively implanted synthetic vascular grafts. *Surgery* 1985;98:81.
5. Seabrook GR. Pathobiology of graft infections. *Semin Vasc Surg* 1990;3:81.
6. Bandyk DF, Berni GA, Thiele BL, et al. Aortofemoral graft infection due to Staphylococcus epidermidis. *Arch Surg* 1984;119:102.
7. Jones L, Braithwaite BD, Davies B, et al. Mechanism of late prosthetic vascular graft infection. *Cardiovasc Surg* 1997;5:486.
8. Costa SF, Miceli MH, Anaissie EJ. Mucosa or skin as source of coagulase-negative staphylococcal bacteraemia? *Lancet Infect Dis* 2004;4:278.
9. Schwartz JA, Powell TW, Burnham SJ, et al. Culture of abdominal aortic aneurysm contents. *Arch Surg* 1987;122:777.
10. Ernst CB, Campbell HC, Daugherty ME, et al. Incidence and significance of intra-operative bacterial cultures during abdominal aortic aneurysmectomy. *Ann Surg* 1977;185:626.
11. Padberg FT Jr, Smith SM, Eng RHK. Accuracy of disincorporation for identification of vascular graft infection. *Arch Surg* 1995;130:183.
12. Bandyk DF, Bergamini TM, Kinney EV, et al. In situ replacement of vascular prostheses infected by bacterial biofilms. *J Vasc Surg* 1991;13:575.
13. Merritt K, Hitchins VM, Neale AR. Tissue colonization from implantable biomaterials with low numbers of bacteria. *J Biomed Mater Res* 1999;44:261.
14. Kaplan SS, Basford RE, Jeong MH, et al. Mechanisms of biomaterial-induced superoxide release by neutrophils. *J Biomed Mater Res* 1994;28:377–386.
15. Kaplan SS, Basford RE, Jeong MH, et al. Biomaterial-neutrophil interactions: dysregulation of oxidative functions of fresh neutrophils induced by prior neutrophil-biomaterial interaction. *B Biomed Mater Res* 1996;30:67.

16. Kaplan SS, Heine RP, Simmons RL. Defensins impair phagocytic killing by neutrophils in biomaterial-related infection. *Infect Immun* 1999;67:1640.
17. Brunstedt MR, Sapatnekar S, Rubin KR, et al. Bacterial/blood/material interactions. I. Injected and preseeded slime-forming Staphylococcus epidermidis in flowing blood with biomaterials. *J Biomed Mater Res* 1995;29: 455.
18. Wang I, Anderson JM, Jacobs MR, et al. Adhesion of Staphylococcus epidermidis to biomedical polymers: contributions of surface thermodynamics and hemodynamic shear conditions. *J Biomed Mater Res* 1995;29:485.
19. Shive MS, Hasan SM, Anderson JM. Shear stress effects on bacterial adhesion, leukocyte adhesion, and leukocyte oxidative capacity on a polyetherurethane. *J Biomed Mater Res* 1999;46:511.
20. von Eiff C, Peters G, Heilmann C. Pathogenesis of infections due to coagulase-negative staphylococci. *Lancet Infect Dis* 2002;2:677.
21. Veenstra GC, Cremers FFM, van Dijk H, et al. Ultrastructural organization and regulation of a biomaterial adhesion of Staphylococcus epidermidis. *J Bacteriol* 1996;178:537.
22. Mack D, Riedewald J, Rohde H, et al. Essential functional role of the polysaccharide intercellular adhesion of Staphylococcus epidermidis in hemagglutination. *Infect Immun* 1999;67:1004.
23. Rupp ME, Ulphani JS, Fey PD, et al. Characterization of the importance of polysaccharide intercellular adhesin/hemagglutinin of Staphylococcus epidermidis in the pathogenesis of biomaterial-based infection in a mouse foreign body infection model. *Infect Immun* 1999;67:2627.
24. Henke PK, Bergamini TM, Watson AL, et al. Bacterial products primarily mediate fibroblast inhibition in biomaterial infection. *J Surg Res* 1998; 74:17.
25. Waters CM, Bassler BL. Quorum sensing: cell-to-cell communication in bacteria. *Annu Rev Cell Dev Biol* 2005;21:319.
26. Xu L, Li H, Vuong C, et al. Role of the luxS quorum-sensing system in biofilm formation and virulence of Staphylococcus epidermidis. *Infect Immun* 2006;74:488.
27. Geary KJ, Tomkiewicz ZM, Harrison HN, et al. Differential effects of a gram-negative and a gram-positive infection on autogenous and prosthetic grafts. *J Vasc Surg* 1990;11:339.
28. Rzychon M, Sabat A, Kosowska K, et al. Staphostatins: an expanding new group of proteinase inhibitors with a unique specificity for the regulation of staphopains, Staphylococcus spp. cysteine proteinases. *Mol Microbiol* 2003;49:1051.
29. Modrall JG, Clagett GP. The role of imaging techniques in evaluating possible graft infections. *Semin Vasc Surg* 1999;12:339.
30. Low RN, Wall SD, Jeffrey RB, et al. Aortoenteric fistula and perigraft infection: evaluation with CT. *Radiology* 1990;175:157.
31. Qvafordt PG, Reilly LM, Mark AS, et al. Computerized tomographic assessment of graft incorporation after reconstruction. *Am J Surg* 1985; 150:227.
32. Auffermann W, Olofsson PA, Rabahie GN, et al. Incorporation versus infection of retroperitoneal aortic grafts: MR imaging features. *Radiology* 1989;172:359.
33. Brunner MC, Mitchell RS, Baldwin JC, et al. Prosthetic graft infection: limitations of indium white blood cell scanning. *J Vasc Surg* 1986;3:42.
34. Fiorani P, Speziale F, Rizzo L, et al. Detection of aortic graft infection with leukocytes labeled with technetium 99 m-hexametazime. *J Vasc Surg* 1993; 17:87.
35. LaMuraglia GM, Fischman AJ, Strauss HW, et al. Utility of the indium 111-labeled human immunoglobulin G scan for the detection of focal vascular graft infection. *J Vasc Surg* 1989;10:20.
36. van der Vaart MG, Meerwaldt R, Slart RH, et al. Application of PET/SPECT imaging in vascular disease. *Eur J Vasc Endovasc Surg* 2008;35: 507.
37. DeMuth RP, Kaylor C, Serrano S, et al. Hypoacoustic luminal outline (halo); an adjunct diagnostic ultrasound feature of late graft infection. *J Vasc Ultrasound* (in press).
38. O'Hara PJ, Hertzer NR, Beven EG, et al. Surgical management of infected abdominal aortic grafts: review of a 25-year experience. *J Vasc Surg* 1986; 2:725.
39. Reilly LM, Stoney RJ, Goldstone J, et al. Improved management of aortic graft infection: the influence of operation sequence and staging. *J Vasc Surg* 1987;5:421.
40. Quinones-Baldrich WJ, Hernandez JJ, Moore WS. Long-term results following surgical management of aortic graft infection. *Arch Surg* 1991;126: 507.
41. Ricotta JJ, Faggioli GL, Stella A, et al. Total excision and extra-anatomic bypass for aortic graft infection. *Am J Surg* 1991;162:145.
42. Leather RP, Darling RC 3rd, Chang BB, et al. Retroperitoneal in-line aortic bypass for treatment of infected infrarenal aortic grafts. *Surg Gynecol Obstet* 1992;175:491.
43. Olah A, Vogt M, Laske A, et al. Axillo-femoral bypass and simultaneous removal of the aorto-femoral vascular infection site: is the procedure safe? *Eur J Vasc Surg* 1992;6:252.
44. Bacourt F, Koskas F, French University Association for Research in Surgery. Axillobifemoral bypass and aortic exclusion for vascular septic lesions: a multicenter retrospective study of 98 cases. *Ann Vasc Surg* 1992; 6:119.
45. Lehnert T, Gruber HP, Maeder N, et al. Management of primary aortic graft infection by extra-anatomic bypass reconstruction. *Eur J Vasc Surg* 1993;7:301.
46. Sharp WJ, Hoballah JJ, Mohan CR, et al. The management of the infected aortic prosthesis: a current decade of experience. *J Vasc Surg* 1994;19:844.
47. Kuestner LM, Reilly LM, Jicha DL, et al. Secondary aortoenteric fistula: contemporary outcome with use of extraanatomic bypass and infected graft excision. *J Vasc Surg* 1995;21:184.
48 Hannon RJ, Wolfe JHN, Mansfield AO. Aortic prosthetic infection: 50 patients treated by radical or local surgery. *Br J Surg* 1996;83:654.
49. Schmitt DD, Seabrook GR, Bandyk DF, et al. Graft excision and extra-anatomic revascularization: the treatment of choice for the septic aortic prosthesis. *J Cardiovasc Surg* 1990;31:327.
50. Bunt TJ. Vascular graft infections: a personal experience. *Cardiovasc Surg* 1993;1:489.
51. Yeager RA, Taylor LM, Moneta GL, et al. Improved results with conventional management of infrarenal aortic infection. *J Vasc Surg* 1999;30:76.
52. Bandyk DF, Novotney ML, Back MR, et al. Expanded application of in situ replacement for prosthetic graft infection. *J Vasc Surg* 2001;34:411.
53. Seeger JM, Pretus HA, Welborn MB, et al. Long-term outcome after treatment of aortic graft infection with staged extraanatomic bypass grafting and aortic graft removal. *J Vasc Surg* 2000;32:451.
54. Dorigo W, Pulli R, Azas L, et al. Early and long-term results of conventional surgical treatment of secondary aorto-enteric fistula. *Eur J Vasc Endovasc Surg* 2003;26:512.
55. Clagett GP, Bowers BL, Lopez-Viego MA, et al. Creation of a neo-aortoiliac system from lower extremity deep and superficial veins. *Ann Surg* 1993; 218:239.
56. Nevelsteen A, Lacroix H, Suy R. Autogenous reconstruction with the lower extremity deep veins: an alternative treatment of prosthetic infection after reconstructive surgery for aortoiliac disease. *J Vasc Surg* 1995;22:129.
57. Clagett GP, Valentine RJ, Hagino RT. Autogenous aortoiliac/femoral reconstruction from superficial femoral-popliteal veins: feasibility and durability. *J Vasc Surg* 1997;25:255.
58. Ahsan AT, Modrall JG, Hocking J, et al. Treatment of aortic graft infection by in-situ replacement with femoral popliteal vein grafts in 187 patients: long-term results. *J Vasc Surg* 2009;50:30–39.
59. Franke S, Voit R. The superficial femoral vein as arterial substitute in infections of the aortoiliac region. *Ann Vasc Surg* 1997;11:406.
60. Brown Jr PM, Kim VB, Lalikos JF, et al. Autologous superficial femoral vein for aortic reconstruction in infected fields. *Ann Vasc Surg* 1999;13:32.
61. Cardozo MA, Frankini AD, Bonamigo TP. Use of superficial femoral vein in the treatment of infected aortoiliofemoral prosthetic grafts. *Cardiovasc Surg* 2002;10:304.
62. Gibbons CP, Ferguson CJ, Fligelstone LJ, et al. Experience with femoropopliteal vein as a conduit for vascular reconstruction in infected fields. *Eur J Vasc Endovasc Surg* 2003;25:424.
63. Daenens K, Fourneau I, Nevelsteen A. Ten-year experience in autogenous reconstruction with the femoral vein in the treatment of aortofemoral prosthetic infection. *Eur J Vasc Endovasc Surg* 2003;25:240.
64. Kieffer E, Bahnini A, Koskas F, et al. In situ allograft replacement of infected infrarenal aortic prosthetic grafts: results in forty-three patients. *J Vasc Surg* 1993;17:349.
65. Vogt PR, Pfammatter T, Schlumph R, et al. In situ repair of aortobronchial, aortoesophageal, and aortoenteric fistulae with cryopreserved aortic homografts. *J Vasc Surg* 1997;26:11.
66. Ruotolo C, Plissonnier D, Bahnini A, et al. In situ arterial allografts: a new treatment for aortic prosthetic infection. *Eur J Vasc Endovasc Surg* 1997; 14(suppl A):102.
67. Nevelsteen A, Feryn T, Lacroix H, et al. Experience with cryopreserved arterial allografts in the treatment of prosthetic graft infections. *Cardiovasc Surg* 1998;4:378.
68. Chiesa R, Astore S, Piccolo G, et al. Fresh and cryopreserved arterial homografts in the treatment of prosthetic graft infections: experience of the Italian Collaborative Vascular Homograft Group. *Ann Vasc Surg* 1998;12:457.
69. Leseche G, Castier Y, Petit MD, et al. Long-term results of cryopreserved arterial allograft reconstruction in infected prosthetic grafts and mycotic aneurysms of the abdominal aorta. *J Vasc Surg* 2001;34:616.
70. Verhelst R, Lacroix V, Vraux H, et al. Use of cryopreserved arterial homografts for management of infected prosthetic grafts: a multicentric study. *Ann Vasc Surg* 200;14:602.
71. Vogt PR, Brunner-LaRocca HP, Lachat M, et al. Technical details with the use of cryopreserved arterial allograft for aortic infection: influence on early and midterm mortality. *J Vasc Surg* 2002;35:80.
72. Noel AA, Gloviczki P, Cherry Jr KJ, et al. Abdominal aortic reconstruct in infected fields: early results of the United States Cryopreserved Aortic Allograft Registry. *J Vasc Surg* 2002;35:847.
73. Gabrial M, Pukacki F, Dzieciuchowicz L, et al. Cryopreserved arterial allografts in the treatment of prosthetic graft infections. *Eur J Vasc Endovasc Surg* 2004;27:590.
74. Teebken OE, Pichlmaier MA, Brand S, et al. Cryopreserved arterial allografts for in situ reconstruction of infected arterial vessels. *Eur J Vasc Endovasc Surg* 2004;27:597.
75. Lavigne JP, Postal A, Kolh P, et al. Prosthetic vascular infection complicated or not by aortoenteric fistula: comparison of treatment with and without cryopreserved allograft (homograft). *Eur J Vasc Endovasc Surg* 2003;25:416.
76. Kieffer E, Gomes D, Chiche L, et al. Allograft replacement for intrarenal aortic graft infection: early and late results in 179 patients. *J Vasc Surg* 2004;39:1009.
77. Walker WE, Cooley DA, Duncan JM, et al. The management of aortoduodenal fistula by in situ replacement of the infected abdominal aortic graft. *Ann Surg* 1987;205:727.

78. Speziale F, Rizzo L, Sbarigia E, et al. Bacterial and clinical criteria relating to the outcome of patients undergoing in situ replacement of infected abdominal aortic grafts. *Eur J Vasc Endovasc Surg* 1997;13:127.
79. Hayes PD, Nasim A, London NJM, et al. In situ replacement of infected aortic grafts with rifampicin-bonded prostheses: the Leicester experience (1992 to 1998). *J Vasc Surg* 1999;30:92.
80. Young RM, Cherry KJ Jr, Davis PM, et al. The results of in situ prosthetic replacement for infected aortic grafts. *Am J Surg* 1999;178:136.
81. Oderich GS, Bower TC, Cherry KJ, et al. Evolution from axillofemoral to in-situ prosthetic reconstruction for the treatment of aortic graft infections at a single center. *J Vasc Surg* 2006;43:1166.
82. Batt M, Magne JL, Alric P, et al. In situ revascularization with silver-coated polyester grafts to treat aortic infection: early and midterm results. *J Vasc Surg* 2003;38:983.
83. Stephen OC, Peter A, Michel B, et al. A systematic review and meta-analysis of treatments for aortic graft infection. *J Vasc Surg* 2006;44:38.
84. D'Addio VJ, Clagett GP. Surgical treatment of the infected aortic graft. In Souba WW, Harken AH, Brennan MF, eds. *ACS Surgery, Principles and Practice*. New York:WebMD Professional Publishing; 2005:1042–1047.
85. Modrall JG, Sadjadi J, Ali AT, et al. Deep vein harvest: predicting the need of fasciotomy. *J Vasc Surg* 2004;39:387.
86. Wells JK, Hagino RT, Bargmann KM, et al. Venous morbidity after superficial femoral-popliteal vein harvest. *J Vasc Surg* 1999;29:282.
87. Modrall JG, Hocking JA, Timaran CH, et al. Late incidence of chronic venous insufficiency after deep vein harvest. *J Vasc Surg* 2007;46:520.
88. Ali AT, Bell C, Modrall JG, et al. Graft-associated hemorrhage from femoral popliteal vein grafts. *J Vasc Surg* 2005;42:667.
89. Beck AW, Erin HM, Hocking JA, et al. Aortic reconstruction with femoral-popliteal vein: graft stenosis incidence, risk and reintervention. *J Vasc Surg* 2008;47:36.
90. Koskas F, Plissonnier D, Bahnini A, et al. In situ arterial allografting for aortoiliac graft infection: a 6-year experience. *Cardiovasc Surg* 1996;4:495.
91. Calligaro KD, Veith FJ, Schwartz ML, et al. Selective preservation of infected prosthetic arterial grafts. Analysis of a 20-year experience with 120 extracavitary-infected grafts. *Ann Surg* 1994;220:461.
92. Morris GE, Friend PJ, Vassallo DJ, et al. Antibiotic irrigation and conservative surgery for major aortic graft infection. *J Vasc Surg* 1994;20: 88.
93. Belair M, Soulez G, Oliva VL, et al. Aortic graft infection: the value of percutaneous drainage. *Am J Radiol* 1998;171:119.
94. Calligaro KD, Veith FJ. Graft-preserving methods for managing aortofemoral prosthetic graft infection. *Eur J Vasc Endovasc Surg* 1997; 14(suppl A):38.
95. Calligaro KD, Veith FJ, Yuan JG, et al. Intra-abdominal aortic graft infection: complete or partial graft preservation in patients at very high risk. *J Vasc Surg* 2003;38:1199.
96. Tambyraja AL, Chalmers RT. Conservative management of MRSA periaortic graft abscess. *Ann Vasc Surg* 2003;17:676.
97. Becquemin JP, Qvarfordt P, Kron J, et al. Aortic graft infection: is there a place for partial graft removal? *Eur J Vasc Endovasc Surg* 1997;14(suppl A):53.
98. Miller JH. Partial replacement of an infected arterial graft by a new prosthetic polytetrafluoroethylene segment: a new therapeutic option. *J Vasc Surg* 1993;17:546.
99. Towne JB, Seabrook GR, Bandyk D, et al. In situ replacement of arterial prosthesis infected by bacterial biofilms: long-term follow-up. *J Vasc Surg* 1994;19:226.
100. Sladen JG, Chen JC, Reid JDS. An aggressive local approach to vascular graft infection. *Am J Surg* 1998;176:222.
101. Mertens RA, O'Hara PJ, Hertzer NR, et al. Surgical management of infrainguinal arterial prosthetic graft infections: review of a thirty-five year experience. *J Vasc Surg* 1995;21:782.
102. Kikta MJ, Goodson SF, Bishara RA, et al. Mortality and limb loss with infected infrainguinal bypass grafts. *J Vasc Surg* 1987;5:566.
103. Cherry KJ, Roland CF, Pairolero PC, et al. Infected femorodistal bypass: is graft removal mandatory? *J Vasc Surg* 1992;15:295.
104. Kaiser AB, Clayson KR, Mulherin JL, et al. Antibiotic prophylaxis in vascular surgery. *Ann Surg* 1978;188:283.
105. Pitt HA, Postier RG, MacGowan WAL, et al. Prophylactic antibiotics in vascular surgery: topical, systemic, or both? *Ann Surg* 1980;192:356.
106. Hasselgren P, Ivarsson L, Risberg B, et al. Effects of prophylactic antibiotics in vascular surgery: a prospective, randomized, double-blind study. *Ann Surg* 1984;200:86.
107. Hall JC, Christiansen KJ, Goodman M, et al. Duration of antimicrobial prophylaxis in vascular surgery. *Am J Surg* 1998;175:87.
108. Kurz A, Sessler DL, Lenhardt R, et al. Perioperative normothermia to reduce the incidence of surgical-wound infection and shorten hospitalization. *N Engl J Med* 1996;334:1209.
109. Osler W. The Gulstonian lectures on malignant endocarditis. *Br Med J* 1885;1:467.
110. Reddy DJ, Ernst CB. Infected aortic aneurysms: recognition and management. *Semin Vasc Surg* 1988;1:174.
111. Patel S, Johnston KW. Classification and management of mycotic aneurysms. *Surg Gynecol Obstet* 1977;144:691.
112. Dean RH, Waterhouse G, Meacham PW, et al. Mycotic embolism and embolomycotic aneurysms. *Ann Surg* 1986;204:300.
113. Chan FY, Crawford ES, Coselli JS, et al. In situ prosthetic graft replacement for mycotic aneurysm of the aorta. *Ann Thorac Surg* 1989;47:193.
114. Oz MC, Brener BJ, Buda JA, et al. A ten-year experience with bacterial aortitis. *J Vasc Surg* 1989;10:439.
115. Benjamin ME, Cohn EJ, Purtill WA, et al. Arterial reconstruction with deep leg veins for the treatment of mycotic aneurysms. *J Vasc Surg* 1999; 30:1004.
116. Bell C, Ali A, Brawley JG, et al. Arterial reconstruction of infected femoral artery pseudoaneurysms using superficial femoral-popliteal vein. *J Am Coll Surg* 2005;200:831.
117. Fichelle JM, Tabet G, Cormier P, et al. Infected infrarenal aortic aneurysms: when is in situ reconstruction safe? *J Vasc Surg* 1993;17:635.
118. Gomes MN, Choyke PL, Wallace RB. Infected aortic aneurysms. A changing entity. *Ann Surg* 1992;215:435.
119. McGregor JA, Lawellin D, Franco-Buff A, et al. Protease production by microorganisms associated with reproductive tract infection. *Am J Obstet Gynecol* 1986;154:109.
120. Tilson MD, Newman KM. Proteolytic mechanisms in the pathogenesis of aortic aneurysms. In: Yao JST, Pearce WH, eds. *Aneurysms: New Findings and Treatments*. Norwalk, CT: Appleton & Lange; 1994:3.
121. Pierce RA, Sandefur S, Doyle GA, et al. Monocytic cell type-specific transcriptional induction of collagenase. *J Clin Invest* 1996;97:1890.
122. Buckmaster MJ, Curci JA, Murray PR, et al. Source of elastin-degrading enzymes in mycotic aortic aneurysms: bacteria or host inflammatory response? *Cardiovasc Surg* 1999;7:16.
123. Reddy DJ, Shepard AD, Evans JR, et al. Management of infected aortoiliac aneurysms. *Arch Surg* 1991;126:873.
124. Sessa C, Farah I, Voirin L, et al. Infected aneurysms of the infrarenal abdominal aorta: diagnostic criteria and therapeutic strategy. *Ann Vasc Surg* 1997;11:453.
125. Moneta GL, Taylor LM Jr, Yeager RA, et al. Surgical treatment of infected aortic aneurysm. *Am J Surg* 1998;175:396.
126. Robinson JA, Johansen K. Aortic sepsis: is there a role for in situ graft reconstruction? *J Vasc Surg* 1991;13:677.
127. Kyriakides C, Kan Y, Kerle M. et al. 11-year experience with anatomical and extraanatomical repair of mycotic aortic aneurysms. *Eur J Vasc Endovasc Surg* 2004;27:585.
128. Oderich GS, Panneton JM, Bower TC, et al. Infected aortic aneurysms: aggressive presentation, complicated early outcome, but durable results. *J Vasc Surg* 2001;34:900.
129. Hsu RB, Chen RJ, Wang SS, et al. Infected aortic aneurysms: clinical outcome and risk factor analysis. *J Vasc Surg* 2004;40:30.
130. Daugherty M, Shearer GG, Ernst CB. Primary aortoduodenal fistula: extraanatomic vascular reconstruction not required for successful management. *Surgery* 1979;86:399.
131. Kniemeyer HW, Grabitz K, Buhl R, et al. Surgical treatment of septic deep venous thrombosis. *Surgery* 1995;118:49.
132. Bach MC, Roediger JH, Rinder HM. Septic anaerobic jugular phlebitis with pulmonary embolism: problems in management. *Rev Infect Dis* 1988;10:424.
133. Leonard JD, Printen KJ. Thrombophlebitis in the elderly. *Am Surg* 1980; 46:441.
134. Munster AM. Septic thrombophlebitis: a surgical disorder. *JAMA* 1974; 230:1010.
135. Pruitt BA Jr, McManus WF, Kim SH, et al. Diagnosis and treatment of cannula-related intravenous sepsis in burn patients. *Ann Surg* 1980;191:546.
136. Ang AK, Brown OW. Septic deep vein thrombosis. *J Vasc Surg* 1986;4:563.
137. Hoffman MJ, Greenfield LJ. Central venous septic thrombosis managed by superior vena cava Greenfield filter and venous thrombectomy: a case report. *J Vasc Surg* 1986;4:606.

CHAPTER 89 ■ ATHEROSCLEROSIS AND THE PATHOGENESIS OF OCCLUSIVE DISEASE

ANTON N. SIDAWY, ROBYN R. MACSATA, MATTHEW A. GOETTSCH, NITEN SINGH, AND SUBODH ARORA

KEY POINTS

1. Susceptibility to atherosclerosis might be determined by both intrinsic (numbers of intimal masses) and extrinsic factors (hypercholesterolemia, hypertension, diabetes, cigarette smoking).
2. The initial event might be the accumulation of lipid by insudation in regions of increased susceptibility. This would lead to the production of macrophage chemotactic factors and the influx of monocytes from the blood that together with the smooth muscle cells (SMCs) would sequester lipid and become foam cells.
3. Low-density lipoprotein oxidized in the wall, as well as other extrinsic injurious agents, could produce some degree of endothelial injury and perhaps later even limited denudation. Growth factors might then be released from the endothelium, activated macrophages and other leukocytes, and the SMCs, as well as from adherent platelets.
4. Growth factors could then stimulate proliferation and migration of susceptible SMCs to form isolated smooth muscle clones and fibrous lesions.
5. Further production of matrix by the smooth muscle would permit continued accumulation of lipid.
6. Like a growing tumor, these fibrous lesions would enlarge, develop ischemic cores, and thereby induce an angiogenic response.
7. The thickened plaque with its necrotic lipid core (the atheroma) might not withstand the rigors of continued arterial pulsation and might develop hemorrhage within the lesion on account of the shearing forces on the new capillaries.
8. Breakdown of the surface and a change in the coagulation function of the endothelium would render the plaque more thrombogenic. Such changes would lead to the terminal thrombotic event, the hallmark of all ischemic complications in atherosclerotic patients.

Atherosclerosis is a disease of the intima of large arteries that causes luminal narrowing, thrombosis, and occlusion associated with ischemia of the end organ. Throughout much of its course, the disease is not detectable. Thrombosis, including vascular occlusion and embolization, produces the clinical events of importance, such as myocardial infarction, stroke, and ischemic gangrene of the extremities. The widespread prevalence of lesions in arteries of asymptomatic people, the chronicity of the process, the suddenness of the terminal vascular events, and the lack of a single etiologic factor make it impossible to give a simple explanation for atherogenesis and atherosclerosis progression. In fact, atherosclerosis might be a form of nonspecific adaptation on the part of large blood vessels to a variety of harmful stimuli and the clinical consequences, or what we might call the true disease process, appear when the compensatory mechanisms are overwhelmed.

NORMAL STRUCTURE OF BLOOD VESSELS

Normal arteries and veins, both large and small, are formed from endothelium, smooth muscle, and extracellular matrix synthesized by these vascular wall cells. The vascular wall is invariably organized into layers (Fig. 89.1). The intima, defined as the part of the wall between the blood and the internal elastic lamina, is composed of a monolayer of endothelium at the luminal surface and may overlie one or more layers of smooth muscle. The media, lying beneath the intima, constitutes the bulk of the vessel and contains smooth muscle cells arranged in layers and dispersed in a matrix made of elastin, collagen, and proteoglycan. The adventitia lies outside the external elastic lamina and forms the outer coat. It is composed of loose connective tissue, fibroblasts, capillaries, neural fibers, and occasional leukocytes. In very large arteries with greater than 28 elastic layers, a microvasculature (vasa vasorum) penetrates the media from the adventitial side and provides an alternative nutrient supply to the flux from the luminal surface.[1] Atherosclerotic lesion formation is associated with the proliferation of vaso vasorum at the site of lesion formation.[2] In thickened, atherosclerotic vessels the vasa vasora are extensive and penetrate into the diseased intima.[3,4]

EMBRYOLOGY

In the fetus, the vessel wall is derived from mesoderm. A brief review of this process is of interest because many aspects of wound healing and atherogenesis in adult vessels represent a recapitulation of the fetal program of vasculogenesis and angiogenesis. The earliest vascular primordia in the embryo are isolated "hemangioblasts" that display endothelial and hematopoietic immunologic markers.[5,6] The hemangioblasts cluster and form cords and, later, tubes that become the major vascular conduits. Some of the clusters become blood islands, the precursors for hematopoietic tissues. These structures sprout, grow, and remodel to form the primitive vascular system.[7]

Endothelial cells probably play a central role in the organization and building of vascular structures. They are derived from the hemangioblasts, organize at sites of later vessel development, and are followed by local mesenchymal cells that form the outer layers of the emerging blood vessels. These mesenchymal cells are the precursors of smooth muscle cells (SMCs) and fibroblasts. Once associated with the vessel wall,

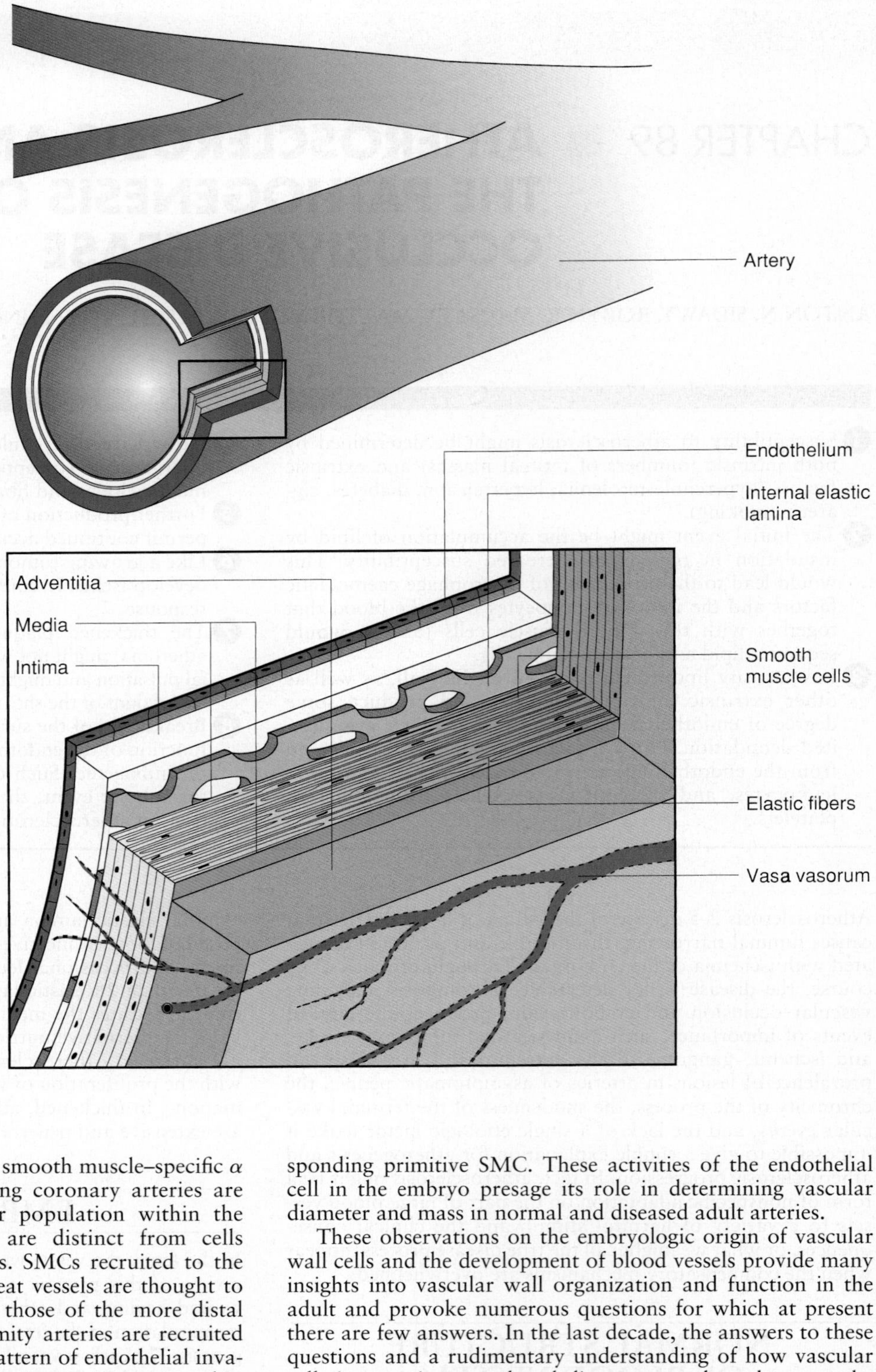

FIGURE 89.1. The artery wall is made of multiple layers (intima, media, and adventitia) that vary in composition depending on the artery.

many of these cells begin to express smooth muscle–specific α actin. SMCs recruited to developing coronary arteries are derived from a unique progenitor population within the proepicardial organ. These cells are distinct from cells recruited to coat peripheral arteries. SMCs recruited to the wall of the developing arch and great vessels are thought to derive from neural crest cells, and those of the more distal aorta and visceral and lower extremity arteries are recruited from adjacent mesenchyme.[8] This pattern of endothelial invasion followed by smooth muscle recruitment is reactivated in later life during angiogenesis in the presence of tumors and in wounds undergoing repair.

The adult form of blood vessels appears to be established by birth. In large vessels, the number of elastic and smooth muscle layers remains constant, although wall mass increases due to smooth muscle proliferation and matrix synthesis.[9,10] The vascular architecture is probably genetically determined because alterations in animal size by hormonal manipulations (e.g., excess growth hormone) are associated with increased wall mass but no change in the number of cell layers.[11] It is likely that the primitive endothelial cell regulates wall architecture because it is involved in the recruitment of the corresponding primitive SMC. These activities of the endothelial cell in the embryo presage its role in determining vascular diameter and mass in normal and diseased adult arteries.

These observations on the embryologic origin of vascular wall cells and the development of blood vessels provide many insights into vascular wall organization and function in the adult and provoke numerous questions for which at present there are few answers. In the last decade, the answers to these questions and a rudimentary understanding of how vascular cells interact in normal and disease states have begun to be realized. In the next section, recent evidence that vascular wall function and structure depend absolutely on cell–cell interactions is reviewed.

REGULATION OF LUMINAL AREA

This description of the usual arterial wall anatomy gives no clue to how a vessel adjusts its mass and dimensions in response to external stimuli (hypertension, increased blood flow, vascular injury) or to how it maintains a nonthrombogenic state at the luminal surface. For this, the array of possible

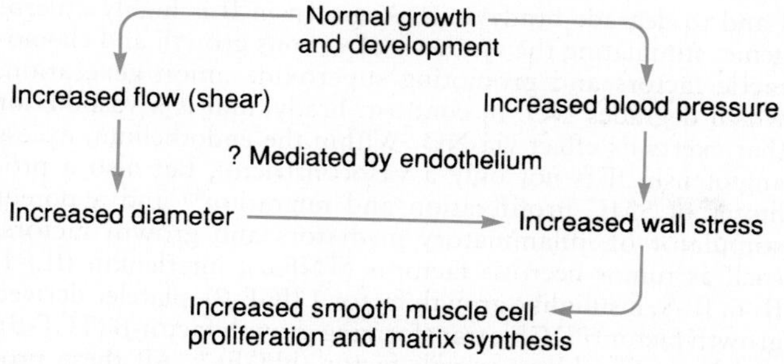

FIGURE 89.2. Changes in blood flow and pressure can have profound effects on arterial wall structure. In part, the response to hemodynamic changes might be mediated by the endothelium. (Adapted from Clowes AW. Theories of atherosclerosis. In: White RA, ed. *Atherosclerosis and Arteriosclerosis: Human Pathology and Experimental Animal Methods and Models*. Boca Raton, FL: CRC Press; 1989:3.)

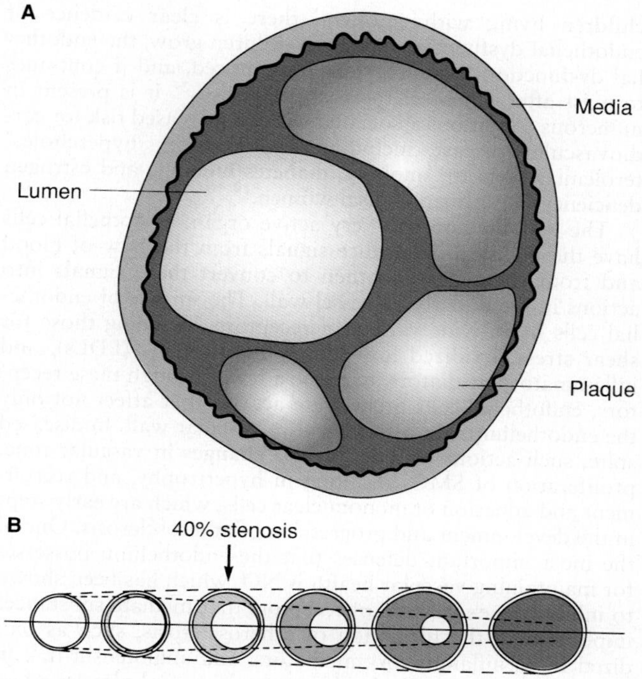

FIGURE 89.3. A: Coronary arteries dilate as atherosclerotic plaques form and maintain normal luminal dimensions. Luminal narrowing begins only after the plaque occupies more than 40% of the cross-sectional area within the internal elastic lamina and bulges outward at sites of medial atrophy. B: The course of lesion formation and luminal narrowing. (Adapted from Glagov S, Weisenberg E, Zarins CK, et al. Compensatory enlargement of human atherosclerotic coronary arteries. *N Engl J Med* 1987;316:1371.)

physiologic functions of the wall and its cellular components under normal and abnormal conditions must be considered.

Blood vessels, both large and small, become larger during growth and development and as a compensatory mechanism to increased blood flow or, more appropriately, increased blood velocity (Fig. 89.2). A particularly striking example of this is found in an artery proximal to an arteriovenous fistula; if the fistula is not treated, the artery can become frankly aneurysmal.[12] Similarly, a vessel undergoing stenosis experiences an increase in blood velocity at the point of luminal narrowing. When the stenosis is attributable to intimal thickening or to an atherosclerotic plaque, the vessel dilates at the site of the lesion. For example, a diseased coronary vessel dilates and can maintain the correct luminal dimensions despite changes in wall structure as long as the intimal lesion does not occupy more than 40% of the area inside the internal elastic lamina (Fig. 89.3).[13] At this point, pathologic narrowing begins to take place. Why vessels should dilate in each of these instances when the velocity of flow increases has not been determined. One possibility is that the cells in the wall, particularly the endothelium, are somehow capable of sensing changes in blood velocity and shear and can translate this biomechanical information into biochemical signals that then regulate the contractile state of the artery.[14–17] The effect of shear stress on the regulation of arterial vasomotility is described in more detail later in this section. Endothelial cell secretory products play a critical role in SMC function.[18] Endothelial cells secrete vasodilating (prostaglandin I_2 and E_2, adenosine, and nitric oxide) and vasoconstricting substances (endothelin). Where endothelium is damaged or absent, adherent platelets release the vasoconstrictor thromboxane A_2.

Nitric oxide (NO), previously called endothelium-dependent relaxing factor, is an important regulator in normal and diseased vessels.[19] It is a short-acting substance that is derived from the metabolic breakdown of arginine.[20–22] It is synthesized by nitric oxide synthase (NOS) by the oxidation of L-arginine. NO regulates vascular tone, downregulates endothelin, increases SMC apoptosis, and decreases SMC proliferation.[23] A number of factors stimulate endothelial cells to secrete NO, including thrombin, acetylcholine, bradykinin, serotonin, and products of platelet release. More recently it has been shown that shear stress, cyclic strain, and repetitive deformation consistently induce NO directly or increase NOS levels from vascular cells.[24] Hence, when the endothelium is present and functional, neighboring thrombotic events are likely to cause vasodilation, whereas when the endothelium is absent or dysfunctional, these same factors cause vasoconstriction. In addition, endotoxin lipopolysaccharides are a potent NOS inducer, resulting in pathologic NO production. Moreover, when the endothelium is missing, the vessel does not respond normally to changes in blood flow, either in the short term or the long term.[25] Changes in blood flow affect wall mass.[26–28] In this regard, it is interesting to note that various factors that affect smooth muscle contraction or relaxation also modulate growth (NO, endothelin, thrombin, and prostaglandins).[29–33] These observations may be the first preliminary evidence that transient signals affecting the diameter of vessels might have, in the long term, more permanent effects on wall structure. Certain pathologic conditions in which endothelium either is missing or is abnormal are associated with acute and chronic vasospasm; it is quite possible that the acute problems of atypical angina (coronary vasospasm) and cerebrovasospasm after cerebral hemorrhage are manifestations of abnormal endothelial function and decreased NO.[34] There is a relationship among shear stress exerted on the arterial lumen, the production of NO, and the development of atherosclerosis. Normal shear stress in arteries (usually >15 dynes/cm^2) is protective, whereas low shear stress (<4 dynes/cm^2) induces the formation of atherosclerotic lesions.[35] In addition, Malek et al.[36] have found that increasing shear stress led to an increase in the expression of endothelial NO synthase (eNOS) mRNA, leading to an increase in NO production, resulting in vasodilatation. Areas of low shear stress in the arterial tree, such as the carotid bifurcation, are foci for the formation of atherosclerotic lesions.[35]

Endothelial dysfunction underlies and is the earliest change in the development and progression of atherosclerosis. This role of endothelial dysfunction has been emphasized recently. It probably begins in childhood and extends through clinical events later in life. Most studies have shown that impaired endothelial function exists very early in the development of atherosclerosis, before the appearance of visible lesions. In children of parents with genetic defects of lipid transport or in children living with smokers, there is clear evidence of endothelial dysfunction. As these children grow, the endothelial dysfunction becomes more pronounced, and it continues to exist after atherosclerosis is established.[37] It is present in numerous conditions associated with an increased risk for cardiovascular disease including hypertension, hypercholesterolemia, cigarette smoking, diabetes mellitus, and estrogen deficiency in postmenopausal women.[38]

The endothelium is a very active organ. Endothelial cells have the ability to transduce signals from the flow of blood and from chemicals and then to convert these signals into actions in the underlying vessel wall. The surface of endothelial cells has a wide variety of receptors, including those for shear stress, oxidized low-density lipoproteins (LDLs), and inflammatory mediators, to name a few. Through these receptors, endothelial cells orchestrate actions that affect not only the endothelium, but also the entire vascular wall. In diseased state, such actions include adverse changes in vascular tone, proliferation of SMCs resulting in hypertrophy, and recruitment and adhesion of mononuclear cells, which are early steps in the development and progression of atherosclerosis. One of the most important defenses that the endothelium possesses for maintaining vascular health is NO, which has been shown to inhibit the expression of receptors that mediate substances implicated in the formation of atherosclerosis, such as oxidized LDL, inflammatory mediators, and angiotensin II.[39] In addition, NO prevents platelet aggregation and platelet adhesion and leukocyte chemotaxis.[23]

The chief role of NO in reversing pathologic changes appears to be its ability to counteract oxidative stress, a common pathogenic pathway for most major risk factors for atherosclerosis. Reduced eNOS may be the result of reactive oxygen species (ROS) that form peroxynitrite, which leads to oxidation of LDL and DNA injury. Peroxynitrite is known to cause accelerated SMC apoptosis and to play a significant role in vascular remodeling. Peroxynitrite and subsequent DNA injury activate poly(adenosine diphosphate [ADP]-ribose) polymerase (PARP), a nuclear enzyme that is involved in DNA damage repair and cell death via the necrotic route. PARP also regulates the release of the mitochondrial cell death factor, apoptosis-inducing factor (AIF), in cardiac myocytes during oxidative stress. AIF appears to be an important factor involved in the regulation of caspase-independent cell death in neurons and cardiac myocytes in vitro during oxidative stress. Excess PARP activation depletes nicotinamide adenine dinucleotide$^+$ (NAD$^+$) and adenosine triphosphate stores, blocks apoptosis, and results in necrosis.[40] In addition, peroxynitrite leads to degradation of tetrahydrobiopterin (BH_4), an essential cofactor of eNOS.[41,42] The classical atherosclerotic risk factors, such as hypertension, smoking, and hyperlipidemia, all act at the endothelial level by increasing oxidative stress, which inactivates NO and upsets the balance between endogenous vasodilators and vasoconstrictors, growth promoters and growth inhibitors, anti-inflammatory and proinflammatory mediators, and other factors important to endothelial function and vascular health.[43]

The normal endothelium functions in an inhibitory mode, maintaining relaxed vascular tone and inhibiting SMC growth, platelet and leukocyte adhesion and aggregation, and thrombosis. In hypertensive, hypercholesterolemic, and diabetic patients, endothelial dysfunction has been associated with decreased production or decreased activity of NO.[44] In studies of apolipoprotein E knockout mice, eNOS was ablated and accelerated atherosclerosis was noted.[45] Endothelial dysfunction is associated with most of the known risk factors for atherosclerosis and cardiovascular disease and may constitute a contributing cause for such disease. This concept has important clinical implications, especially in terms of preventive strategies.

Angiotensin-converting enzyme (ACE) acts both to produce angiotensin II, a potent vasoconstrictor, from angiotensin I and to degrade bradykinin. Angiotensin II is highly atherogenic, stimulating the synthesis of various growth and chemotactic factors and promoting superoxide anion generation, which degrades NO. In contrast, bradykinin is a vasodilator that exerts its effect via NO. Within the endothelium, excess angiotensin II is not only a vasoconstrictor, but also a promoter of SMC proliferation and migration[46] and a potent stimulator of inflammatory mediators and growth factors, such as tumor necrosis factor-α (TNF-α), interleukin (IL)-1, IL-6, IL-8, insulinlike growth factor 1 (IGF-β), platelet-derived growth factor (PDGF), transforming growth factor-β (TGF-β), and basic fibroblast growth factor (bFGF).[46] All these processes can be inhibited or reversed by ACE inhibition therapy because it decreases the level of angiotensin II and inhibits the degradation of bradykinin. ACE inhibitors prevent not only the adverse effects of hypertension, but also the effects of oxidative stress from other mechanisms. Clinical trials have shown that 6 months of ACE inhibition therapy, using quinapril, is associated with a significant improvement in endothelial function in normotensive patients with coronary artery disease.[47] ACE inhibition at the tissue level appears to be critical to prevent oxidative stress within the endothelium. This is the reason why tissue-avid ACE inhibitors, like quinapril, may have advantages over other drugs in their class. Restoring endothelial function through ACE inhibitors has become an attractive therapeutic target.

REGULATION OF MEDIAL AND INTIMAL THICKENING

Earlier it was observed that, for embryonic vessels to form, primitive endothelial cells must migrate and become aligned and then recruit smooth muscle precursors from the surrounding mesenchyme. Because endothelial cells grow as a monolayer, they can proliferate only when the vascular structure is enlarging in circumference, during vascular elongation (angiogenesis), or when injured endothelium is being replaced. Massive denudation and endothelial loss is not a normal event and probably occurs only during pathologic degeneration of the intima or during surgical instrumentation of the vessel. In any event, endothelial proliferation does not contribute significantly to an increase in wall mass; however, SMC proliferation does.

1 Under several circumstances, vessels of adult animals
2 respond by becoming thicker. In hypertensive animals and humans, arteries exhibit medial thickening, whereas after endothelial denudation or in the presence of hypercholesterolemia, they develop a thick intima.[48,49] Exactly how these responses are regulated is not clear, although it is certain that in each instance proliferation of SMCs and accumulation of extracellular matrix are important components. In addition, in hypercholesterolemic subjects, the accumulation of lipid and lipid-filled macrophages contributes to the intimal lesion.[50]

Vessel wall mass is largely determined by the accumulation of SMCs and matrix synthesized by SMCs. Hence, how smooth muscle number is regulated needs to be considered.[51] Under normal circumstances, SMCs proliferate in the vessels of young animals and enter a quiescent state at maturity. For example, SMCs in adult rat carotid artery do not increase in number and turn over at a rate of 0.06% per day.[52] In animal models of disease, these cells can readily be stimulated to enter the growth cycle by induction of hypertension or direct vascular injury. Observations made in these models provide us with insights into possible mechanisms for initiation and progression of vascular disease in humans.

Although hypertension has its greatest impact on the small "resistance vessels," in fact large arteries are equally affected. In response to increased pressure the wall thickens.[48,53] Morphometric studies have shown that this increase is largely a medial process and involves all components of the vessel wall, including the mass of SMCs and matrix. In some forms of hypertension, there is an increase in smooth muscle number, whereas in others there is an increase in the DNA content per cell. Tetraploid and octaploid cells have been detected. In venous grafts transposed from a relatively hypotensive venous environment into the normotensive arterial circulation, there is an increase in wall thickness and a corresponding increase in smooth muscle number.[51] In each instance, the change in pressure affects the mass of cells and associated matrix.

3 How a change in pressure might induce SMCs to proliferate, to change their ploidy, or to synthesize matrix is not known. In some circumstances (e.g., severe hypertension, vein grafting), there is a detectable but small amount of endothelial loss.[54] However, this is not a usual feature in more moderate or chronic forms of hypertension. Leung et al. have suggested that increased tension and stretch have a direct effect on matrix protein synthesis, but not on cell proliferation.[55] Alternatively, increased wall tension might affect the endothelium, and the endothelium might in turn secrete factors regulating smooth muscle mass.

Of the models of smooth muscle growth in vivo, perhaps the best studied is the balloon injury model first developed by Baumgartner.[52,56,57] In this model, smooth muscle proliferation is stimulated by the passage of an inflated balloon catheter along an artery. The artery is at once stretched and denuded of its endothelium. Immediately thereafter, platelets begin to adhere to the wall wherever endothelium is missing; they then spread and degranulate. In most situations, endothelial denudation and platelet adherence are followed 1 to 2 days later by the onset of medial smooth muscle proliferation. In the ballooned rat carotid (Fig. 89.4), this can be a most dramatic response with a 3-log increase in the thymidine labeling index (a measure of proliferation). This early proliferation in the media does not lead to an increase in wall thickness; the wall thickens only after SMCs migrate from the media and proliferate in the intima. In normal animals, this process continues for a period of time and subsides spontaneously whether or not endothelium reappears at the luminal surface. The intimal mass is further increased by the accumulation of extracellular matrix synthesized by the SMCs.[58]

A link between smooth muscle proliferation and earlier platelet granule release has been proposed. Among the proteins released are several growth factors including PDGF, TGF-β, and an epidermal growth factor–like protein.[59] Where these granule proteins go after being released from the platelets is not known. One hypothesis suggests that these factors accumulate in the artery wall and stimulate subsequent smooth muscle growth.[49] This hypothesis (the reaction to injury hypothesis) was first proposed many decades ago as a general mechanism for atherogenesis and has been refined in view of recent information. Although attractive in theory, it is based on rather slim evidence mainly derived from experiments in thrombocytopenic animals.[59] Injured arteries in these animals show very little intimal thickening.

The hypothesis that the decrease in intimal thickening in injured arteries of thrombocytopenic animals is attributable to decreased proliferation of SMCs has proven to be incorrect.[60] In the ballooned rat carotid model, even though intimal thickening is diminished in thrombocytopenic animals, smooth muscle proliferation and early cell cycle gene expression are the same as in controls. The interpretation of these findings is that platelet products play a role in the movement of SMCs from one vascular compartment to the next (media to intima) but do not affect the initiation of proliferation. Whether platelet factors can influence the growth of intimal smooth muscle has yet to be determined.

Although little is known of what starts or stops the intimal thickening process, there are several observations that are interesting and are perhaps important when we consider the current theories of atherosclerosis. The first is that the surface of the injured artery accumulates a single layer of platelets. Fibrin and microthrombi are seen only at the luminal surface when the artery is reinjured after an intimal thickening has formed or in small craters in association with adherent macrophages in hypercholesterolemic animals.[61–64] Active, fulminant thrombosis is not a usual feature of injured vessels; when it occurs, it must represent a major aberration of vessel function. Second, in models demonstrating early reendothelialization or partial deendothelialization without medial injury, intimal thickening does not develop, although one or two rounds of medial smooth muscle proliferation can occur.[65]

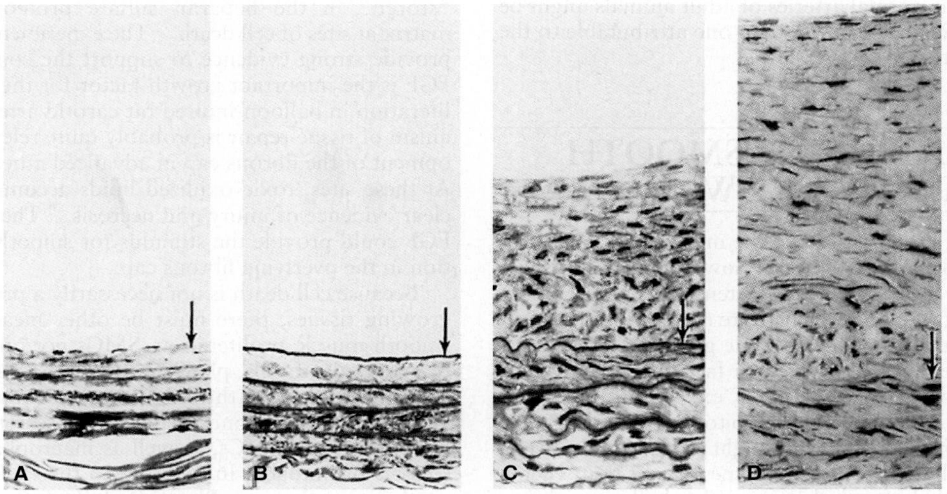

FIGURE 89.4. Elastic arteries injured by the passage of a balloon embolectomy catheter develop substantial intimal thickenings. In this series of histologic cross sections of rat carotid artery before (**A**) and after ballooning (**B–D**), the endothelium is stripped away and the inner layer of medial smooth muscle cells is damaged (**B**). **C:** By 2 weeks, the intima is thickened by the migration and proliferation of smooth muscle cells derived from the media. The mass of cells does not change significantly after this time; nevertheless, the intima is thicker at 3 months (**D**) because of matrix synthesis and accumulation. (From Clowes AW, Reidy MA, Clowes MM. Kinetics of cellular proliferation after arterial injury. I. Smooth muscle growth in the absence of endothelium. *Lab Invest* 1983:49:327, with permission.)

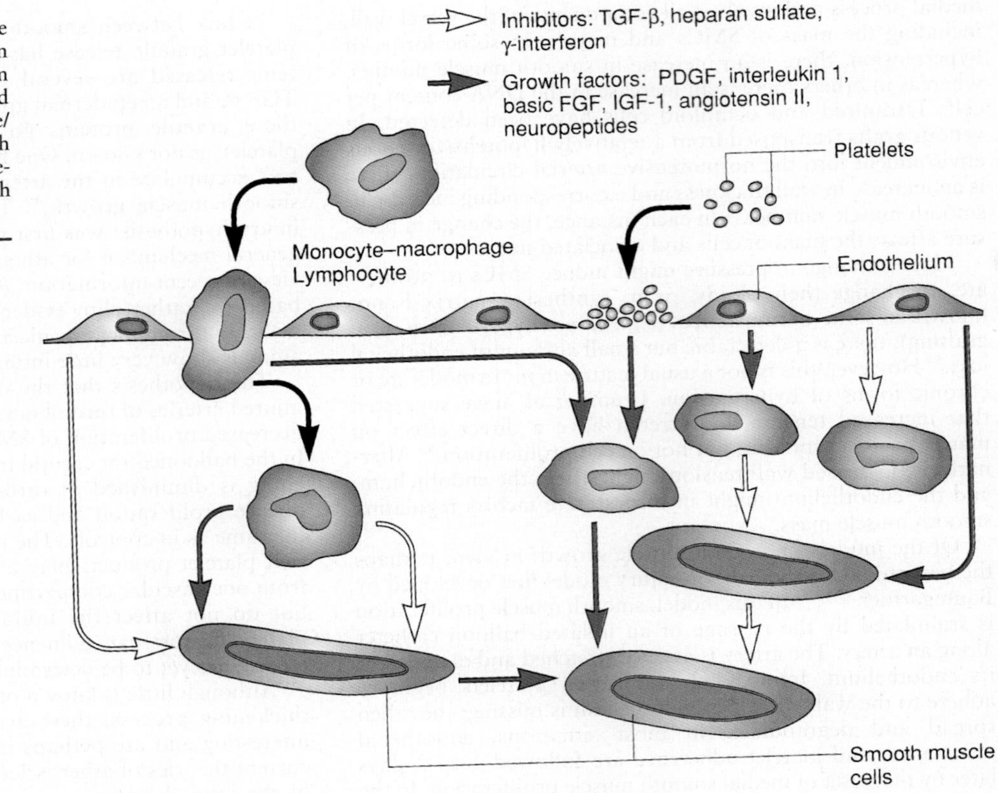

FIGURE 89.5. Diagram depicts the complexity of the interactions between vascular wall cells (endothelium and smooth muscle), platelets, and blood-borne leukocytes (monocyte/macrophage and lymphocyte). Each cell is capable of synthesizing and releasing several smooth muscle growth factors and inhibitors.

This result suggests that endothelium might play a role in suppressing smooth muscle growth and migration from the media to the intima. It is known that smooth muscle growth inhibitors can be extracted from the vessel wall, that endothelium can synthesize a heparinlike molecule that inhibits SMC growth in vitro, and that heparin itself can suppress both proliferation and migration of SMC in vitro and in vivo.[66] Taken together, these findings suggest that the endothelium can inhibit smooth muscle proliferation and that the quiescent state of SMCs in the normal arteries of adult animals might be an actively maintained one rather than one attributable to the lack of growth factors (Fig. 89.5).

REGULATION OF SMOOTH MUSCLE GROWTH

4 Platelets have long been considered the major source of mitogen for proliferating smooth muscle. However, SMCs are able to proliferate in injured and hypertensive arteries when platelets are absent. If platelet factors are not important, what, then, is the stimulus for smooth muscle growth? Three alternatives present themselves: (a) growth factors from vascular wall cells or resident leukocytes; (b) exogenous, neuroendocrine factors; or (c) loss of local inhibitors of smooth muscle proliferation. All three mechanisms might be important. Let us consider the first alternative. It is of some interest that when a rat carotid is denuded of endothelium with a balloon catheter, a substantial fraction of the medial SMCs proliferate (around 20% to 30%), but when denudation is accomplished with a fine nylon wire, there is very little proliferation (around 2% to 4%).[67] These procedures differ only in regard to the degree to which the media is damaged. Ballooning destroys 20% of the medial smooth muscle, as well as the endothelium, whereas passage of the nylon wire destroys only the endothelium. The observations become more interesting if we note that cultured cells, when damaged, release growth-promoting activity.[68,69] The predominant growth-promoting activity is due to fibroblast growth factors (FGFs).[70,71] These factors have been found in a wide variety of tissues and cell types and are synthesized by endothelium and SMCs. They are distinguished from other polypeptide mitogens by their ability to bind strongly to heparin. Furthermore, both acidic and basic FGFs are potent smooth muscle mitogens in vitro. Finally, FGFs can bind to heparinlike molecules so that released FGFs might readily be "stored" in the heparan sulfate proteoglycan–containing matrix at sites of cell death.[72] The experiments of Lindner et al. provide strong evidence to support the conclusion that basic FGF is the important growth factor for the first wave of proliferation in balloon-injured rat carotid artery.[73,74] This mechanism of tissue repair is probably quite relevant for the development of the fibrous cap in advanced atherosclerotic lesions. At these sites, toxic oxidized lipids accumulate, and there is clear evidence of injury and necrosis.[50] The release of cellular FGF could provide the stimulus for smooth muscle proliferation in the overlying fibrous cap.

Because cell death is not necessarily a prominent feature of growing tissues, there must be other means for controlling smooth muscle proliferation. SMCs not only respond to factors from dead cells, platelets (PDGF, TGF-*β*, EGF-like molecules), and plasma (thrombin, lipoproteins, IGF-1), but also synthesize and respond to their own secreted factors.[51] Both endothelial and SMCs, as well as macrophages, are potential sources of mitogen. In addition to the FGFs, these cell types synthesize and secrete PDGF, IL-1, TGF-*β*, and IGF-1.

PDGF in particular has been studied in detail.[75] The original studies on PDGF stemmed from the observation that serum prepared from whole blood contains substantially more growth-promoting activity than serum prepared from plasma. These findings led to the discovery of PDGF, a basic dimeric protein with a molecular weight of approximately 30,000. It is transported in the blood in the α granule of the platelet and is released along with other α-granule proteins. PDGF is by itself extremely potent and is active as a smooth muscle mitogen in trace amounts (nanogram per milliliter). It also exhibits a range of other activities on smooth muscle and other types of cells (stimulates smooth muscle migration, contraction, and matrix synthesis), although it is not a mitogen for endothelium. When placed in a wound chamber in vivo, it induces a granulation tissue response.[76]

An important development in the field of growth factor research in the last decade was the demonstration that the structure of the gene for PDGF is nearly identical to that of the oncogene v-sis, a gene associated with cellular transformation by the simian sarcoma virus.[77,78] This discovery, coupled with the finding that a variety of cells including normal cells synthesize and secrete active PDGF, raises the possibility that normal wound healing and malignant, unscheduled growth of tumor cells might have striking similarities with subtle differences in gene regulation. It also led to a search for growth factors in vascular wall cells. We now have solid evidence that endothelium, SMCs, and leukocytes, including macrophages, can express the PDGF gene (c-sis or PDGF B chain) in vitro and in vivo.[75] PDGF research is complicated by the observation that PDGF is not a single molecule, but is either a heterodimer or homodimer of two isoforms, PDGF A and PDGF B. The cellular receptors are also dimers of two isoforms, α and β, such that PDGF B binds to both α and β, but PDGF A binds only to the α form of the receptor. The implications of this complexity of growth factor and receptor expression have yet to be understood. At present, we know that human platelets transport mainly PDGF AB, whereas cultured SMC from human plaques, baboon graft intima, and injury-induced rat intimal thickening express mainly PDGF A-chain mRNA. This observation is probably not an artifact of cell culture because the primary lesions from which the cells are derived contain relatively large amounts of A-chain mRNA. Macrophages in atherosclerotic lesions express PDGF B protein. What role PDGF plays in wall function remains to be determined. It is not clear how the expression of the protein is regulated, nor is it clear whether regulation also occurs at the level of receptor expression. These findings suggest the intriguing possibility that the vascular wall cells, as well as the platelets, are a source of growth factors in the artery wall, and through the endogenous production of growth factors thus might be able to regulate their own growth (autocrine control) or their neighbor's growth (paracrine control). Alternatively, PDGF might control some other function than proliferation. At least after injury and in atherosclerotic mouse arteries, PDGF may act as a chemoattractant and regulate the movement of SMCs from the media into the intima or from the wall into the overlying thrombus.[79,80] In SMC migration, PDGF uses a different signaling pathway than that used for proliferation.[81]

Another alternative for regulation, in addition to factors from the blood and the cells themselves, is neuroendocrine control of smooth muscle growth.[82,83] Several neurotransmitters affect smooth muscle hypertrophy and proliferation (serotonin, neurokinin A, substance K, substance P). Furthermore, sympathectomy or inhibitors of sympathetic nerve function inhibit the increase in DNA in the media of developing arteries and arteries subjected to hypertension.[84,85] In injury models, prazosin (an α_1 antagonist) and cilazapril (an ACE inhibitor) both inhibit intimal thickening.[86,87] These recent observations provide some support for the possibility that neuroendocrine factors also influence intimal smooth muscle proliferation.

Although smooth muscle mass may be determined in large measure by the presence or absence of growth factors (i.e., positive effectors of growth), smooth muscle mass might also be influenced by endogenous inhibitors. Growth might be viewed as release from quiescence. Earlier, it was pointed out that endothelial regeneration in injured arteries is associated with cessation of underlying intimal smooth muscle growth. On the other hand, in healing vascular grafts, intimal SMCs proliferate only underneath the newly formed endothelial surface.[88] These observations are in parallel with studies of endothelial and SMCs in culture demonstrating that vascular wall cells can synthesize and secrete both inhibitors and promoters of smooth muscle growth.[15] The growth-promoting factors have already been described. Both cell types synthesize heparan sulfate, which, when released from the larger proteoglycan, can inhibit the growth of cultured SMCs.[89,90] Both cell types synthesize and secrete a TGF-β precursor,[90] and TGF-β can be found in the arterial wall after injury.[91] The precursor molecule can then be activated. In general, TGF-β acts as an inhibitor, although at times it can promote smooth muscle growth. Antibody to TGF-β administered to rats suppresses injury-induced intimal thickening.[92] There are other growth inhibitors in vivo that might be released by leukocytes present in the vascular wall. Although this mechanism is not important for the regulation of mass in normal artery, it is probably very important in diseased vessels. In atherosclerotic plaques there are large numbers of macrophages and lymphocytes. Hansson et al.[93] have shown that resident T cells secrete interferon-γ and induce the expression of class II major histocompatibility antigens. Interferon-γ also inhibits smooth muscle growth in culture, and in the injured rat carotid, there is a significant population of I_a-positive, growth-inhibited intimal SMCs.[94] Although SMCs make up the bulk of the intimal thickening, 1% or less of the intimal cells are T cells. Because I_a expression is absolutely dependent on the presence of interferon-γ, these observations strongly support the view that interferon-γ is an endogenous regulator of intimal smooth muscle growth. A recent study of the effects of interferon-γ refutes this conclusion and suggests that it may at times promote SMC growth.[95] Finally, growth of vascular wall cells might be regulated not only by secreted soluble factors, but also by direct cell–cell contact. This inhibitory mechanism is very important for endothelium and perhaps less so for SMCs.

These growth factors exert their effects via specific receptors located in the cell membrane. The majority of growth factor receptors belong to a family of peptide receptors called receptor tyrosine kinases (RTKs). A growth factor's function can be endocrine, paracrine, or autocrine in nature. A growth factor's function is said to be endocrine when it is released in the circulation and exerts its function after attaching to receptors located on cells in a distant organ. A growth factor acts in a paracrine manner when it affects cells located in the vicinity of the cell that secreted it. A growth factor can also cause its effect on the same cell that secretes it in an autocrine manner. In each of these situations, the growth factor interacts with its own specific receptors located on distant cells, on adjacent cells, or on the same cells that secreted it. The paracrine and autocrine functions are important in case of arterial injury. When endothelial cells and SMCs are injured, they secrete growth factors, such as PDGF, that bind to receptors on the same or adjacent cells, causing SMC proliferation and migration to form intimal hyperplasia.[49]

Once the growth factor binds to the extracellular domain of its receptor, the kinase function becomes activated and phosphorylates specific cytoplasmic substrates to activate pathways required for the function of the growth factor. Various growth factor receptors use different specific substrates for their actions and the same growth factor may use a different substrate depending on the ultimate action required, whether it is cell division, motion, or differentiation. Therefore, the most important events in signal transduction take place in the cytoplasm of the cell.[96] Triggered by growth factor attachment, the intracellular domains interact on a molecular level. Then, intracellular protein molecules belonging to various protein families bind to specific sites along the intracellular cytoplasmic domain of the phosphorylated receptor. These proteins carry specific recognition sites that allow a certain family of proteins to bind to a specific area of the intracellular domain. By doing so, various cellular signaling pathways are activated. Each pathway controls a specific function of the growth factor. The recognition sites found on the cellular proteins are called src homology-2 (SH-2) or src homology-3 (SH-3) domains. In addition, the SH-2 and SH-3 phosphorylated sites of the protein serve to bind them to other cellular proteins that belong to the signaling cascade. Proteins that are involved in these pathways include guanosine triphosphatase–activating protein (GAP), phospholipase C (PLC), and phosphatidylinositol-3-kinase (PI-3-K)–binding protein. These cascades of phosphorylation and specific protein binding eventually lead to a specific function of the growth factor; the function may be one of differentiation, proliferation, cell shape changes, or motility.[97]

The signaling pathways or cascades rely on the proteins' phosphorylation for the signal to be transmitted to the nucleus and cause gene activation. One of these pathways is called the Ras pathway. Once the growth factor attaches to its receptor, the receptor phosphorylates itself. Ras, a protein that attaches to the cytoplasmic aspect of the cellular membrane, undergoes phosphorylation and activates Raf-1 protein, which indirectly phosphorylates mitogen-activated protein kinase (MAPK). MAPK phosphorylates transcription factors inside the nucleus (e.g., Myc, jun) that stimulate gene activity.[97] The Jak-STAT pathway is another important signaling pathway that was recently described.[98,99] Signal transducers and activators of transcription (STATs) are families of proteins that have been found to be phosphorylated by Jaks, kinase enzymes activated in response to growth factor interaction with its receptor. The two pathways, Ras and Jak-STAT, may intersect on the way to the nucleus to cause gene activation. It is believed that MAPK from the Ras pathway enhances STAT activity by causing additional phosphorylation.[100]

Direct cell-to-cell communication and the presence of gap junctions have been demonstrated in monolayers of endothelium[101] and in mixed cell populations between endothelium and SMCs.[102] The significance of these direct links has not been defined, although a recent study has demonstrated that cultured pericytes or SMCs can inhibit endothelial growth when the cells are in contact with one another. In vivo capillary endothelial cells appear to grow when pericytes are absent and to stop growing when pericytes reappear. Endothelial cells can also regulate the growth of one another. Plasma membrane preparations from confluent large-vessel endothelium actively inhibit growing endothelial cells.[103] The intercellular links might help to regulate endothelial proliferation and endothelial-mediated vascular relaxation in collateral vessels by propagating signals from one cell to the next upstream from a large vessel occlusion. Direct cell–cell communication would also provide a mechanism for a local response in a vessel without the need for the release and wide dissemination of potent vasoactive or growth regulatory substances.

In summary, the size of a vessel wall is dependent on the mass of cells and matrix. Because SMCs and associated matrix proteins make up the bulk of the tissue, an understanding of the regulation of smooth muscle growth during development and in diseased states is extremely important. Smooth muscle number and distribution are affected by growth factors from the blood (particularly from platelets and leukocytes), growth factors and inhibitors from the vascular wall cells themselves, and neuroendocrine factors particularly from sympathetic innervation of the vessel wall. Smooth muscle quiescence in the normal adult artery might be maintained by heparinlike inhibitors synthesized by vascular wall cells or the absence of growth factor. Growth initiation might be due to a shift in the balance of these negative and positive stimuli (Fig. 89.5). For example, any condition causing injury of vascular wall cells or inducing the influx of macrophages would be expected to set up a favorable environment for smooth muscle growth. Hypercholesterolemia, a significant risk factor for atherosclerosis, is associated with macrophage migration and the accumulation of toxic oxidized LDL in susceptible large arteries. Release of endogenous FGF from dying foam cells as well as release of other growth factors (possibly PDGF) from stimulated endothelium, smooth muscle, and macrophages would increase the local concentration of growth-promoting activity. SMCs would be expected to respond by proliferating and migrating into the intima; if collections of these cells were already present in the intima as a consequence of fetal development, they might be even more responsive. These factors might also regulate the traffic of other leukocytes (macrophages, T cells) in and out of the wall, and these activated cells would in turn amplify or retard the initial smooth muscle response by the production of growth factors or inhibitors. The extent and complexity of these interactions between the cells of the wall and the blood have yet to be unraveled.

REGULATION OF THE ANTICOAGULATED STATE

Blood does not clot in normal arteries even when flow is stopped for prolonged periods. On the other hand, endothelial injury or loss provokes a dramatic thrombotic response. These observations define the importance of the endothelial layer in the maintenance of the anticoagulated state.[104,105] Studies performed primarily on cultured cells have demonstrated that endothelial cells possess an array of anticoagulant and antithrombotic functions, and it is certain that many of these are of importance in vivo. Endothelial cells also have several procoagulant functions, and the balance between procoagulant and anticoagulant functions is regulated by signals from the blood, as well as from neighboring cells.

On the anticoagulant side of the balance, the endothelium synthesizes a membrane-associated heparan sulfate that, like heparin, increases the affinity of antithrombin III for thrombin.[106] Because this interaction requires the binding of heparan sulfate to antithrombin III, the complex must be active at the level of the endothelial surface. Heparin–antithrombin III then rapidly inactivates circulating thrombin and other activated serine proteases in the clotting cascade, including factors VII, IX, and X. Thus, endothelial-derived heparin sulfate can act to impede two aspects of the injury response: the activation of the clotting cascade and the stimulation of smooth muscle proliferation, which we referred to earlier. In addition, endothelial cells can inhibit clotting by means of the protein C pathway.[100] Endothelium synthesizes and secretes a protein called thrombomodulin, which in turn is bound to a surface receptor. The receptor–thrombomodulin complex binds thrombin and in so doing inactivates the proteolytic activity for fibrinogen. The thrombomodulin–thrombin complex activates protein C, and the activated protein C binds to protein S on the endothelial surface. The protein C–protein S complex then can inactivate factor Va, thereby inhibiting the clotting cascade. That this pathway is important is amply demonstrated in homozygous protein C–deficient patients who develop spontaneous thrombosis. Finally, endothelial cells can inhibit platelet adhesion and aggregation through the synthesis of prostaglandin I_2 (PGI_2) and can degrade formed fibrin by activating plasminogen to plasmin.

On the procoagulant side, endothelial cells synthesize and secrete tissue factor, platelet-activating factor, a plasminogen activator inhibitor, and von Willebrand factor, and they express a number of receptors for factors of the clotting cascade.[104] When the cells are exposed to a variety of inflammatory mediators derived from the blood or from resident macrophages (e.g., endotoxin, IL-1, TNF), endothelial cells respond by changing the balance of anticoagulant–procoagulant activities to favor coagulation. As well, the cells synthesize and express IL-1, which potentially could affect the underlying SMCs.[107] At present, these conclusions are largely based on in vitro experiments; although they have relevance mainly for the microvasculature, they also may prove to be important for large vessels in view of the recent evidence that not only macrophages but also different populations of lymphocytes are present in the atherosclerotic plaque. Furthermore, the ability of the vascular wall cells to maintain the anticoagulant state at the luminal surface must have a direct bearing on the thrombotic complications associated with end-stage atherosclerosis.

LESIONS OF ATHEROSCLEROSIS

Atherosclerosis is a disease of the intima characterized by the accumulation of SMCs and lipid.[107,108] The earliest lesion appears to be a local accumulation of lipid in the vessel wall located either in the extracellular matrix or inside "foam cells" (lipid-filled SMCs or macrophages). The relationship between the so-called fatty streak (Fig. 89.6) made up of foam cells and the pathologic process of atherosclerosis, the fibrous plaque, and the complicated lesion has been the subject of some debate.[109] Fatty streaks are found even in young children. Although atherosclerosis has a predilection for certain countries, the extent of fatty streaks of the aorta and coronary arteries in young people is about the same in countries that have low mortality rates from heart attack as in countries with high rates. The lipid streaks have been found to be just as common in females as in males, although atherosclerosis is more prevalent in males. Finally, even though the lipid streaks are distributed throughout the aorta, end-stage disease is mostly confined to the abdominal segment. Hence, if the fatty streak is the precursor of the more advanced lesion, then there must either be a selection process or the whole concept must be wrong. The issue remains unresolved.

An alternative precursor for the atherosclerotic plaque is the intimal cell mass.[110,111] These focal accumulations of SMCs are frequently found in the vessels of children in locations that later develop fibrous plaques. In fat-fed swine, the intimal cell masses enlarge and become atherosclerotic.[112] Although the concept of the intimal cell masses as the initial lesion is attractive, there are several problems with it. First, this initial lesion is present in people throughout the world regardless of eventual risk for atherosclerosis. Second, as a general rule there is a gradual thickening of the intima throughout the arterial tree as part of the aging process; this has little to do with atherosclerosis. Finally, it has been difficult to find animal models of atherosclerotic change in intimal masses, whereas the formation of fibrofatty lesions from fatty streaks has been rather easily modeled by cholesterol feeding in a number of species. For these reasons, support for the intimal cell mass as the initial lesion has not achieved wide acceptance.

5 Whatever the initial lesion might be in atherosclerosis, it is widely agreed that the lesions characteristic of late atherosclerosis are the fibrous and the complicated plaques. The fibrous plaque is characterized by a thick fibrous luminal cap containing SMCs and leukocytes overlying a central core of necrotic debris and lipid (the "atheroma"). Animal studies have suggested that there might be either denudation or nondenuding injury of the endothelium at the surface.[63] The functional state of the endothelial cells and SMCs and leukocytes in these lesions is not known. Macrophages, by becoming foamy, clearly play a role in the metabolism of lipid, and activated macrophages also secrete a range of factors that modulate the metabolic and growth state of the vascular wall cells. Macrophages also proliferate locally in the lesions.[113,114] In addition, other leukocytes, particularly T lymphocytes, are present; because some adjacent SMCs express the class II antigen human leukocyte antigen (HLA)-DR, they must be exposed to interferon-γ presumably derived from the neighboring T cells.[115] In addition to inducing the expression of HLA-DR, interferon-γ inhibits smooth muscle proliferation. Hence, in the advanced atherosclerotic lesion these leukocytes might play a critical role in regulating smooth muscle proliferation and
6 accumulation.[116,117]

7 The complicated lesion of atherosclerosis is a fibrous
8 plaque with the additional features of ulceration, luminal thrombosis, calcification, and wall hemorrhage (Fig. 89.6). It is the source of the thromboembolic activities associated with symptomatic disease. Why a fibrous lesion evolves into a complicated plaque is not understood. This process might be accelerated by such risk factors as hypertension, whereas atherogenesis might be affected more by hypercholesterolemia and cigarette smoking. More importantly, the advent of the inflammatory cells and the release of potent mediators of inflammation must play a role in the development of the complicated lesion. Earlier it was pointed out that growth factors for smooth muscle not only were liberated from platelets, but also were synthesized and secreted by macrophages and the vascular wall cells themselves. In addition, potent cytokines, such as IL-1, TNF, and interferon-γ, alter the growth state and metabolism of the vascular wall cells. In particular, the balance of anticoagulation–coagulation at the surface of the endothelium might be shifted away from anticoagulation and toward coagulation. In the plaque, large amounts of tissue factor and plasminogen activator-1 (PAI-1) are present.[118–120] These changes, in addition to frank endothelial desquamation in response to injurious agents, including oxidized LDL, homocystinemia, and tobacco products, could promote thrombosis in the vessel, an event that is decidedly unusual. Small accretions of thrombus with subsequent fibrotic remodeling together with hemorrhage from new blood vessels in the ischemic central region of the plaque could account for the relatively rapid increase in

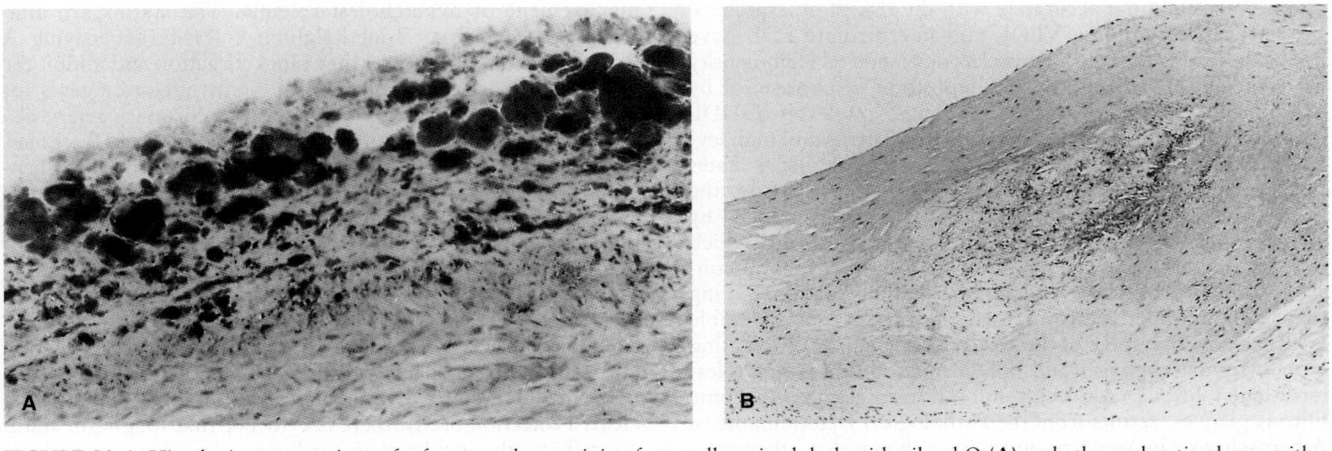

FIGURE 89.6. Histologic cross sections of a fatty streak containing foam cells stained dark with oil red O (**A**) and atherosclerotic plaque with a fibrous cap (**B**). (Courtesy of David Gordon, MD, Department of Pathology, University of Washington School of Medicine, Seattle, WA.)

plaque size and luminal narrowing that has been observed in some arterial beds.

THEORIES OF ATHEROSCLEROSIS

Some of the information on vascular wall structure and function might be relevant to general theories of atherosclerosis. From the foregoing, it should be evident that an artery is not just an inert nonthrombogenic conduit for blood; rather, it is an organ whose structure and function are very carefully modulated by interactions between vascular wall cells themselves and between vascular wall cells and the blood. Bearing this in mind, we can reexamine the prevailing theories of atherosclerosis.

Over the last century, a number of theories have been advanced to explain how atherosclerosis evolves. In reality, these theories attempt to account for one or more aspects of the disease and are therefore not mutually exclusive. Much of the controversy over these theories has to do with individual opinion concerning which of the aspects of atherosclerosis is most important.

Lipid Insudation Hypothesis

Perhaps the oldest hypothesis, termed the "lipid insudation" hypothesis, states that the lipid in the atherosclerotic lesion is derived from lipoproteins in the blood[50,121]; it thereby links the risk factor hypercholesterolemia directly to the development of the plaque foam cell, the atheroma, and eventually the complicated lesion. There is good evidence now that the lipid in the plaque comes from the blood; there is also substantial evidence correlating the severity of hypercholesterolemia (particularly elevated LDL cholesterol) with the severity of atherosclerosis both in human and in animal models. When animals are made hyperlipidemic, the initial change is a migration of macrophages through the endothelium into the subintima and media. These cells then engorge the lipids carried into the wall by lipoproteins to form foam cells. These foam cells presumably secrete chemoattractants, growth factors, and cytokines, which trigger off complex events that lead to the formation of an atherosclerotic plaque.[122] The most important study to demonstrate that blood cholesterol level is a risk factor for coronary artery disease and hence atherosclerosis is the Framingham study. A large group of healthy men and women were studied and it was found that the risk for developing clinically evident coronary artery disease was related to cholesterol levels.[123] Although a high level of LDL cholesterol is an important risk factor for atherosclerosis, epidemiologic studies have shown that levels of apolipoprotein B, the primary protein constituent of LDL, very low-density lipoprotein (VLDL), and chylomicrons, correlate more accurately with the risk of atherosclerosis. Particles resembling VLDL and intermediate LDL have been identified within the atherosclerotic plaque.[124] High-density lipoproteins (HDLs) oppose the deposition of cholesterol by transporting cholesterol to the liver. Thus, low levels of HDL correlate with an increased risk of atherosclerosis and high levels of HDL are protective. The lipid insudation theory states that the lipid in the atherosclerotic lesion is derived from the lipoproteins in the blood.[50,125] The earliest lesions induced by elevated plasma cholesterol levels are the fatty streaks, which have an impressive accumulation of lipids in them. For a considerable period of time it was thought that the lipid-containing foam cells were derived from SMCs, but there is considerable evidence now that most of these cells originate from circulating monocytes/macrophages and only a fraction represent cholesterol-laden SMCs. Although not all fatty streaks become fibrous plaques, results from the Pathological Determinants of Atherosclerosis in Youth program have shown that atherosclerosis commences as a fatty streak, which progresses to the complicated lesion, namely, the fibrous plaque.[126]

It is still unclear as to how the monocytes penetrate the endothelium to reach the subendothelial space. The endothelial injury hypothesis postulates that there is endothelial denudation that allows this penetration, but a number of experimental studies have failed to show any damage to the endothelium over the fatty streaks. Once in the subendothelial space of the intima, the monocytes take up lipoprotein cholesterol to become foam cells. Denudation of endothelial cells probably occurs later in the development of the lesion, exposing the underlying foam cells. Brown et al.,[127] however, showed that even the highest concentration of LDL could not induce the accumulation of cholesterol in monocytes/ macrophages or in SMCs, the precursors of arterial foam cells. Thus, it is not the circulating LDL that causes lipid accumulation in the monocytes/macrophages, but the oxidized LDL that is taken up avidly by the macrophages. Oxidized LDL is more atherogenic than native LDL, and in animal models antioxidant compounds can slow the rate of atherosclerotic lesion progression by 50% or more.[128] In addition, two antioxidant enzymes are associated with HDL, paraoxonase and platelet-activating factor acetylhydrolase. These factors are believed to degrade deleterious oxidized phospholipids associated with LDL.[129] There is a good deal of epidemiologic evidence correlating high intake of antioxidant vitamins with decreased risk of coronary artery disease in humans.[130] However, the results of randomized clinical trials have not demonstrated a decrease in progression of atherosclerosis. These trials have failed to demonstrate a consistent significant effect of single or multivitamin regimens on the incidence of death from coronary vascular disease.[131,132]

Regarding the role of genetic background in the development and progression of atherosclerosis, Dansky et al.[133] have demonstrated that expression of the human apo A-I transgene on the apo E–deficient background increases HDL cholesterol and greatly diminishes fatty streak lesion formation. They also demonstrated that increases in apo A-I and HDL cholesterol inhibit foam cell formation in apo E–deficient/human apo A-I transgenic mice at a stage following lipid deposition, endothelial activation, and monocyte adherence, without increases in HDL-associated paraoxonase.

The role of "statins" in delaying the progression of the atherosclerotic lesion has been investigated. Several studies, such as the Coronary Primary Prevention trial and the Helsinki Heart Study, have shown a relation between reduction in the lipoprotein profile and a reduction in the cardiac events. In the first study, a 20% reduction in LDL cholesterol yielded a more than 30% reduction in coronary events, and in the second study, gemfibrozil reduced LDL cholesterol by 8% and triglycerides by more than 35%, while causing a 15% increase in HDL and reduced coronary events by 34%.[134,135]

The discovery of the statin (e.g., simvastatin, lovastatin) group of drugs was a major advance in the pharmacologic management of hypercholesterolemia. The statins are analogues of 3-hydroxy-3-methylglutaryl (HMG)-coenzyme A (CoA) reductase; therefore, they block its action and inhibit the synthesis of cholesterol. Statins are highly effective agents for the primary and secondary prevention of coronary artery disease. Although lowering of cholesterol, especially LDL cholesterol, appears to be the most important mechanism for the beneficial effects of statins, other effects including improvement in endothelial function may also play an important role. The inhibition of cholesterol synthesis increases hepatic expression of the LDL receptor, leading to increased clearance of circulating LDL. Several studies have shown that lipid-lowering statin therapy leads to a reduction in cardiovascular events and mortality from cardiac events.[129] These studies also showed a reduction in the incidence of stroke, which has a relatively weak association with cholesterol levels. In the preliminary results of the Heart Protection Study, there is evidence that long-term statin use reduces the incidence in cardiovascular events in patients with coronary artery disease, carotid artery disease, peripheral vascular disease, or diabetes regardless of baseline LDL cholesterol level.[136,137] Simvastatin and lovastatin have been shown to reduce vascular injury from experimental stroke in a rodent model, independent of lipid changes.[138] Decreasing inflammation by lowering LDL cholesterol, and thus oxidized LDL cholesterol, is one theory on the mechanism of action of statins. Studies using C-reactive protein (CRP) as a marker of inflammation have shown a decrease in CRP along with a decrease in LDL in patients on statin therapy. However, other studies have not shown the same correlation and this has fostered a lipid-independent theory. Further studies are being conducted to elucidate the mechanism of the statins' effect.[139]

The Encrustation Hypothesis

Like the lipid insudation hypothesis, the encrustation hypothesis focuses on one aspect of the disease.[140] This hypothesis proposes that plaque initiation and progression are the consequence of repeated cycles of thrombosis and remodeling. However, autopsy studies of vessels of children and experiments with cholesterol-fed animals have shown that thrombosis is not the initial event in atherogenesis; in fact, thrombosis appears to be a feature of advanced disease. Hence, this hypothesis is applicable only to the problem of plaque progression. Furthermore, it does not explain how lipid and SMCs accumulate in the lesion.

The Reaction to Injury Hypothesis

This hypothesis attempts to explain how smooth muscle growth is regulated in atherogenesis.[49] As originally proposed, it stated that the initial event is some form of injury to the endothelium. In regions denuded of endothelium, platelets adhere and release growth factors; these growth factors accumulate in the wall and stimulate medial smooth muscle proliferation and migration into the intima. As discussed previously, this theory is based on the observation that platelets carry potent smooth muscle mitogens in their granules and that the injury-induced arterial lesion closely resembles the fibrous cap found in the atherosclerotic plaque. A modified version of this theory suggests that injuries to the endothelium, which do not produce denudation, might also cause smooth muscle growth by stimulating damaged endothelium to synthesize and release growth factors. Alternatively, monocytes might be attracted to the zone of injury; the monocyte/macrophage might then be activated and start to elaborate growth-promoting activity. The reaction to injury hypothesis suggests a possible mechanism for the accumulation of connective tissue cells and matrix; it fails to provide an explanation for the lipid accumulation or the monoclonal nature of the advanced atherosclerotic plaque.

The Monoclonal Hypothesis

This hypothesis focuses attention on smooth muscle accumulation in the lesion.[141] It states that the cells of any particular plaque are likely to arise as a clone from a single progenitor SMC. This hypothesis is based on the observation that individual plaques of human females heterozygote for the X-linked marker glucose-6-phosphate dehydrogenase (G-6-PD) frequently exhibit one, but not both, of the G-6-PD isotypes. At a certain moment in time, single cells might be stimulated to enter the growth cycle and undergo several rounds of division leading to the formation of a monoclonal lesion. The mechanism of cell activation leading to such lesions is not evident as yet; the only other known monoclonal cell masses in humans are neoplasias (e.g., leiomyomas). This would tend to suggest carcinogens or possibly viruses as possible etiologic agents and thereby might explain the link between cigarette smoking and atherosclerosis. An alternative to carcinogenesis as an explanation for monoclonality is the possibility of activation of a susceptible population of stem cells.[142,143] SMCs might have limited replicative capacity, and there might be only a small population of stem cells in the wall capable of responding to growth factors. Whatever the mechanism of activation might be, any theory attempting to provide a mechanism for the accumulation of SMCs in atherosclerotic plaques must take into account this observation of monoclonality.

The Intimal Cell Mass Hypothesis

This hypothesis was mentioned earlier and states that the accumulations of intimal SMCs are one of the two possible initial lesions in atherosclerosis.[110,111] These small accumulations of SMCs are found in children at sites where atherosclerosis later develops. How they happen to get there is unclear, nor is it evident what makes them susceptible to atherogenic stimuli. It could be that these cells are primordial rests and really are a form of stem cell capable of responding to external mitogenic stimuli. Because the intimal cell masses are found in the vessels of children throughout the world regardless of the prevalence of atherosclerosis, it is likely that the atherosclerotic change is largely determined by extrinsic risk factors, such as hypercholesterolemia.

The Infection Hypothesis

Although the role of infection in the development of atherosclerosis has been debated for many years, only recently this role has been emphasized due to a panel convened by the National Heart, Lung, and Blood Institute (NHLBI).[144] The expert panel examined the evidence linking infections to the development of the atherosclerotic process, in particular the role of cytomegalovirus (CMV) and *Chlamydia pneumoniae*. The panel reported on the seroepidemiologic evidence and the reports localizing those infectious agents to the human plaque. In addition, they examined animal studies aiming to show cause and effect among CMV, *C. pneumoniae*, and the development of atherosclerotic lesions in animal models.

CMV belongs to the herpesvirus family, which also includes the Epstein-Barr virus. Approximately 15% of adolescents, 50% of adults by age 35, and 70% of patients older than 75 years have evidence of past infection with this virus.[145] Melnick et al.[146] found significantly higher titers of CMV antibodies in patients undergoing coronary artery bypass surgery (70%) compared to matched controls (43%). Cardiac transplant recipients with CMV exposure, as evidenced by increased serum CMV immunoglobulin G (IgG) antibodies, are more likely to develop posttransplantation atherosclerosis than patients without exposure to CMV.[147] CMV infection has been associated with restenosis following coronary angioplasty.[141] In addition, CMV has been implicated in the development of carotid atherosclerosis. CMV antigens have been isolated from carotid plaque, and increased levels of CMV antibody titers are associated with carotid intimal-medial thickening.[148] Although it has been difficult to culture viral particles from atherosclerotic lesions, this by itself does not constitute strong evidence against the role of CMV infection in atherosclerosis because it is possible that the virus triggers the infection without persisting in the tissue.[145,146,148] Because of the ubiquitous nature of CMV, it is difficult to ascertain whether it is a pathogen in atherosclerosis.[149]

Three species of *Chlamydia*, *Chlamydia trachomatis*, *Chlamydia psittaci*, and *C. pneumoniae*, which are gram-negative bacteria, are known to cause human disease. *C. pneumoniae* cause upper respiratory infections and 10% of all cases of pneumonia. The prevalence of antibodies to *C. pneumoniae* is around 50% in adults.[149] *C. pneumoniae* organisms have been isolated from atherosclerotic plaque from both carotid and coronary arteries.[150,151] In a rabbit model, infection with *C. pneumoniae* has been shown to accelerate the formation of the atherosclerotic lesion. In addition, treatment with azithromycin prevented the formation of the lesion.[152] To gain insight into the mechanism by which *C. pneumoniae* infection affects the process of atherogenesis, Kol's group studied atherosclerotic plaques for the presence of chlamydial heat shock protein 60 (HSP60).[153,154] Studying plaques from human carotid atherosclerotic arteries, these investigators found that chlamydial and human HSP60 colocalize within macrophages located in the atherosclerotic lesions. They have also shown that both chlamydial and human HSP60 induced the production of TNF-α and matrix metalloproteinase (MMP) by macrophages. They concluded that, by inducing the production of such factors by macrophages, chlamydial HSP60 may represent the mechanism by which infection with *C. pneumoniae* promotes atherosclerosis.[153] In addition, the same investigators have shown that chlamydial and human HSP60 activate human endothelial cells, SMCs, and macrophages to secrete factors (e.g., E-selectin, intercellular adhesion molecule-1 [ICAM-1], and vascular cell adhesion molecule-1 [VCAM-1]) important to the pathophysiology of atherosclerosis.[154]

In addition to CMV and *Chlamydia*, *Helicobacter pylori* and herpes simplex virus are also being investigated as possible agents in atherosclerosis.[155] More work needs to be done to definitively establish the relationship between these and other agents and atherosclerosis. Establishing the role of infectious agents in the development of atherosclerosis is very important because it suggests that anti-infectious agents, such as known antibiotics, may play a role in preventing or slowing the atherosclerotic process.

Inflammatory and Immune Hypothesis

Mediators of inflammation, such as cytokines and growth factors, have been found in the atherosclerotic plaques. These mediators are involved in the synthesis and degradation of collagen by vascular SMCs. Such mediators include TGF-α and interferon-γ.[156] IL-2 receptors are markers suggesting the activation of T lymphocytes, and interferon-γ is produced and secreted by activated T lymphocytes.[157]

The involvement of macrophages and T lymphocytes in atherogenesis also suggests both an immune and an inflammatory response. The lymphocytes found in atherosclerotic lesions are polyclonal, indicating that these cells do not develop in response to a single antigen. Several different subclasses of T lymphocytes have been identified in atherosclerotic plaque, including both CD4 (helper-inducer cells) and CD8 (cytotoxic T cells).[158] In addition, accelerated coronary artery atherosclerosis is a unique variant of atherosclerosis that develops and progresses rapidly in transplanted hearts, suggesting an immunologic etiology. The lesions seen in transplanted hearts involve the entire coronary tree, and these lesions contain all the cellular elements characteristic of atherosclerosis; in addition, they have increased numbers of T lymphocytes and macrophages compared to the typical atherosclerotic lesion.[159] Mouse transplant models, using heterotopic heart transplants and arterial interposition grafts, produced arterial lesions that resembled transplant arteriosclerosis.[160,161]

Activation of the complement system is an important step in the immune process causing immune complexes to deposit in the arterial wall or precipitating the binding of specific antibodies to antigens found in vascular tissues. Cholesterol particles are potent activators of the complement system.[162] This activation of the complement system results in the production of proinflammatory molecules and the terminal membrane attack complex (MAC), which has been known to stimulate the production of cytokines, such as TNF-β and IL-8, and growth factors, such as basic FGF and PDGF by vascular smooth muscle cells (VSMCs) and endothelial cells.[162] MAC has been identified in atherosclerotic lesions, particularly fibrous plaque.[163]

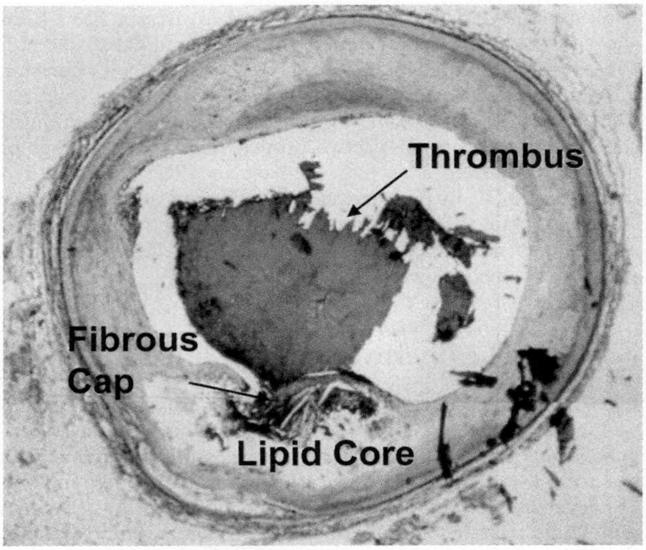

FIGURE 89.7. Plaque cap rupture exposing the lipid core of the atheroma and leading to thrombus formation. (Courtesy of Dr. Maria de Lourdes Higuchi, Department of Pathology, University of São Paulo, Brazil.)

Most complications related to atherosclerotic lesions may be due to plaque disruption or rupture. Plaque disruption exposes the circulating blood to its lipid core with subsequent formation of thrombus (Fig. 89.7), leading to acute arterial occlusion.[164,165] Plaque stability is very important in preventing plaque rupture. This stability is provided by the integrity of the extracellular matrix within the plaque. Plaque instability is related to the degree of inflammation because inflammatory cells produce cytokines that decrease the production of collagen or increase its degradation.[166] Therefore, the balance between the production of MMPs, which degrade collagen, and that of tissue inhibitors of metalloproteinases (TIMPs) regulates plaque stability.[167] The expression of both MMPs and TIMPs can be demonstrated in atheromas. TIMPs have been found in macrophages present within plaques.[167] Inflammatory cytokines, such as IL-1 and TNF, can induce the expression of MMPs by macrophages.[168] In addition, interferon-γ produced by T lymphocytes decreases collagen production, again leading to weakening of plaque extracellular matrix and rupture.[169] The foam cells express tissue factor on their surface and activate factor VII, which leads to thrombin formation and platelet aggregation, with subsequent conversion of fibrinogen to fibrin leading to thrombosis.[170] Interestingly, lipid-lowering strategies led to a decrease in plaque content of macrophages and a decrease in expression of MMP1, increasing collagen production and retention, which improve plaque stability.[168,171]

Arterial endothelial cells possess a single cilium able to detect the mechanical forces of blood flow that distinguish disturbed from laminar flow. The type of flow then dictates endothelial cell phenotype. Cells at plaque-susceptible sites have a proinflammatory phenotype. This phenotype is both permissive and causative of plaque development. The proinflammatory endothelial phenotype is permissive in that it allows the expression of proinflammatory receptors, such as Toll-like receptors (TLRs). The phenotype is also causative in that it permits the expression of cell surface adhesion molecules, like VCAM-1, which foster leukocyte accumulation in the intima. No specific disease risk has been identified that would promote a proinflammatory phenotype at only arterial bifurcations and the lesser curve of the aortic arch; however, TLRs expressed by the endothelial cells at these locations may provide an insight.[172]

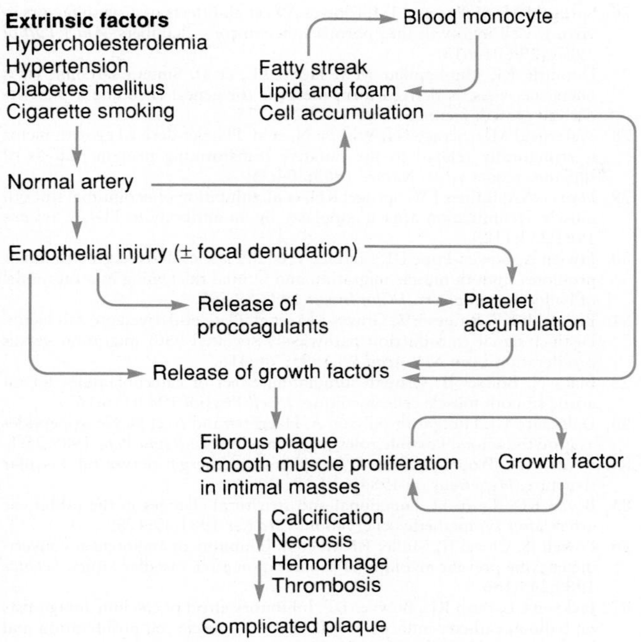

FIGURE 89.8. Atherogenesis and progression of atherosclerosis are probably the consequence of multiple factors acting on the arterial wall. (Adapted from Clowes AW. Theories of atherosclerosis. In: White RA, ed. *Atherosclerosis and Arteriosclerosis: Human Pathology and Experimental Animal Methods and Models*. Boca Raton, FL: CRC Press; 1989:3.)

Toll-like receptors are members of a larger superfamily of interleukin-1 receptors that share homology in their cytoplasmic region. There are 10 members of the TLR family identified, each with different ligands. Each member can activate distinct as well as overlapping signaling pathways, giving rise to different biologic effects. The individual ligands, as well as the location of the individual TLRs, are an active area of current research. It appears at this time that activation of TLRs is involved in the activation of the inflammatory cascade and possible initiator of plaque formation.[173]

Inflammation appears to be a common factor in all theories of atherosclerosis, and more research is being performed in this area and isolating inflammatory mediators that may be involved.[174] Each of these hypotheses attempts to explain one or more aspects of atherogenesis. It is reasonable to conclude that each might be applicable at a different time during the development of the lesion (Fig. 89.8).

References

1. Wolinsky H, Glagov S. Nature of species differences in the medial distribution of aortic vasa vasorum in mammals. *Circ Res* 1967;20:409.
2. Galili O, Hermann J, Woodrum J, et al. Adventitial vasa vasorum heterogeneity among different vascular beds. *J Vasc Surg* 2004;40:529–535.
3. Heistad DD, Armstrong ML. Blood flow through vasa vasorum of coronary arteries in atherosclerotic monkeys. *Arteriosclerosis* 1986;6:326.
4. Barger AC, Beeuwkes R III, Lainey LL, et al. Hypothesis: vasa vasorum and neovascularization of human coronary arteries. *N Engl J Med* 1984; 310:175.
5. Coffin JD, Poole TJ. Embryonic vascular development: immunohistochemical identification of the origin and subsequent morphogenesis of the major vessel primordia in quail embryos. *Development* 1988;102:735.
6. Pardanaud L, Altmann C, Kitos P, et al. Vasculogenesis in the early quail blastodisc as studied with a monoclonal antibody recognizing endothelial cells. *Development* 1987;100:339.
7. Le Douarin NM. Cell migrations in embryos. *Cell* 1984;38:353.
8. Li J, Lawrence DA, Wang X, et al. Regulator of G protein signaling 5 marks peripheral arterial smooth muscle cells and is down regulated in atherosclerotic plaque. *J Vasc Surg* 2004;40:519–528.
9. Wolinsky H, Glagov S. A lamellar unit of aortic medial structure and function in mammals. *Circ Res* 1967;20:99.
10. Wolinsky H, Glagov S. Structural basis for the static mechanical properties of the aortic media. *Circ Res* 1964;14:400.
11. Dilley RJ, Schwartz SM. Vascular remodeling in the growth hormone transgenic mouse. *Circ Res* 1989;65:1233.
12. Zarins CK, Zatina MA, Giddens DP, et al. Shear stress regulation of artery lumen diameter in experimental atherogenesis. *J Vasc Surg* 1987;5:413.
13. Glagov S, Weisenberg E, Zarins CK, et al. Compensatory enlargement of human atherosclerotic coronary arteries. *N Engl J Med* 1987;316:1371.
14. Frangos JA, Eskin SG, McIntire LV, et al. Flow effect on prostacyclin production by cultured human endothelial cells. *Science* 1985;227:1477.
15. Gibbons GH, Dzau VJ. The emerging concept of vascular remodeling. *N Engl J Med* 1994;330:1431.
16. Davies PF, Tripathi SC. Mechanical stress mechanisms and the cell. An endothelial paradigm. *Circ Res* 1993;72:239.
17. Resnick N, Collins T, Atkinson W, et al. Platelet-derived growth factor B chain promoter contains a cis-acting fluid shear-stress-responsive element. *Proc Natl Acad Sci U S A* 1993;90:4591.
18. Vanhoutte PM. The endothelium: modulator of vascular smooth-muscle tone. *N Engl J Med* 1988;319:512.
19. Furchgott RF. Role of endothelium in responses of vascular smooth muscle. *Circ Res* 1983;53:557.
20. Ignarro LJ, Buga GM, Wood KS, et al. Endothelium-derived relaxing factor produced and released from artery and vein is nitric oxide. *Proc Natl Acad Sci U S A* 1987;84:9265.
21. Palmer RMJ, Ferrige AG, Moncada S. Nitric oxide release accounts for the biological activity of endothelium-derived relaxing factor. *Nature* 1987; 327:524.
22. Ignarro LJ. Biological actions and properties of endothelium-derived nitric oxide formed and released from artery and vein. *Circ Res* 1989;65:1.
23. Ahanchi SS, Tsihlis ND, Kibbe MR. The role of nitric oxide in the pathophysiology of intimal hyperplasia. *J Vasc Surg* 2007;45:64a–73a.
24. Vouyouka AG, Jiang Y, Rostagi R, et al. Ambient pressure upregulates nitric oxide synthase in a phosphorylated-extracellular regulated kinase- and protein kinase C-dependent manner. *J Vasc Surg* 2006;44:1076–1084.
25. Langille BL, O'Donnell F. Reductions in arterial diameter produced by chronic decreases in blood flow are endothelium-dependent. *Science* 1986; 231:405.
26. Kohler TR, Jawien A. Flow affects development of intimal hyperplasia after arterial injury in rats. *Arterioscler Thromb* 1992;12:963.
27. Kohler TR, Kirkman TR, Kraiss LW, et al. Increased blood flow inhibits neointimal hyperplasia in endothelialized vascular grafts. *Circ Res* 1991; 69:1557.
28. Geary RL, Kohler TR, Vergel S, et al. Time course of flow-induced smooth muscle cell proliferation and intimal thickening in endothelialized baboon vascular grafts. *Circ Res* 1994;74:14–23.
29. Shultz PJ, Knauss TC, Mené P, et al. Mitogenic signals for thrombin in mesangial cells: regulation of phospholipase C and PDGF genes. *Am J Physiol* 1989;257:F366.
30. Bobik A, Grooms A, Millar JA, et al. Growth factor activity of endothelin on vascular smooth muscle. *Am J Physiol Cell Physiol* 1990;258:C408.
31. Libby P, Warner SJC, Friedman GB. Interleukin 1: a mitogen for human vascular smooth muscle cells that induces the release of growth-inhibitory prostanoids. *J Clin Invest* 1988;81:487.
32. Nakaki T, Nakayama M, Yamamoto S, et al. Endothelin-mediated stimulation of DNA synthesis in vascular smooth muscle cells. *Biochem Biophys Res Commun* 1989;158:880.
33. Garg UC, Hassid A. Nitric oxide-generating vasodilators and 8-bromocyclic guanosine monophosphate inhibit mitogenesis and proliferation of cultured rat vascular smooth muscle cells. *J Clin Invest* 1989;83:1774.
34. Freiman PC, Mitchell GG, Heistad DD, et al. Atherosclerosis impairs endothelium-dependent vascular relaxation to acetylcholine and thrombin in primates. *Circ Res* 1986;58:783.
35. Malek AM, Alper SL, Izumo S. Hemodynamic shear stress and its role in atherosclerosis. *JAMA* 1999;282:2035.
36. Malek AM, Izumo S, Alper SL. Modulation by pathophysiological stimuli of the shear stress-induced up-regulation of endothelial nitric oxide synthase expression in endothelial cells. *Neurosurgery* 1999;45:334.
37. Stary HC, Chandler AB, Dinsmore RE, et al. A definition of advanced types of atherosclerotic lesions and a histological classification of atherosclerosis—a report from the Committee on Vascular Lesions of the Council on Arteriosclerosis, American Heart Association. *Circulation* 1995;92:1355.
38. Celermajer DS, Sorensen KE, Gooch VM, et al. Non-invasive detection of endothelial dysfunction in children and adults at risk of atherosclerosis. *Lancet* 1992;340:1111.
39. Zeiher AM, Fisslthaler B, Schray-Utz B, et al. Nitric oxide modulates the expression of monocyte chemoattractant protein 1 in cultured human endothelial cells. *Circ Res* 1995;76:980.
40. Huang J, Lin SC, Nachershain A, et al. Role of redox signaling and poly (adenosine diphosphate-ribose) polymerase activation in vascular smooth muscle cell growth inhibition by nitric oxide and peroxynitrite. *J Vasc Surg* 2008;47:599–607.
41. Griendling KK, Fitgerald GA. Oxidative stress and cardiovascular injury. Part I: basic mechanism and in vivo monitoring of ROS. *Circulation* 2003;108:1912.
42. Milstien S, Katusic Z. Oxidation of tetrahydrobiopterin by peroxynitrite: implication for vascular endothelial function. *Biochem Biophys Res Commun* 1999;263:681.

43. Griendling KK, Alexander RW. Oxidative stress and cardiovascular disease [editorial; comment]. *Circulation* 1997;96:3264.
44. Vane JR, Anggard EE, Botting RM. Regulatory functions of the vascular endothelium. *N Engl J Med* 1990;323:27.
45. Knowles JW, Reddick RL, Jennette JC, et al. Enhanced atherosclerosis and kidney dysfunction in eNOS (−/−)ApoE (−/−) mice are ameliorated by enalapril treatment. *J Clin Invest* 2000;105:451.
46. Chuna V, Martin-McNulty B, Vinceletta J, et al. Angiotensin II induces histomorphologic features of unstable plaque in a murine model of accelerated atherosclerosis. *J Vasc Surg* 2006;44:364–371.
47. Mancini GB, Henry GC, Macaya C, et al. Angiotensin-converting enzyme inhibition with quinapril improves endothelial vasomotor dysfunction in patients with coronary artery disease. The TREND (Trial on Reversing ENdothelial Dysfunction) Study [see comments] [published erratum appears in *Circulation* 1996;94:1490]. *Circulation* 1996;94:258.
48. Wolinsky H. Long-term effects of hypertension on the rat aortic wall and their relation to concurrent aging changes: morphological and chemical studies. *Circ Res* 1972;30:301.
49. Ross R. Pathogenesis of atherosclerosis—an update. *N Engl J Med* 1986; 314:488.
50. Steinberg D, Parthasarathy S, Carew TE, et al. Modifications of low-density lipoprotein that increase its atherogenicity. *N Engl J Med* 1989;320:915.
51. Schwartz SM, Campbell GR, Campbell JH. Replication of smooth muscle cells in vascular disease. *Circ Res* 1986;58:427.
52. Clowes AW, Reidy MA, Clowes MM. Kinetics of cellular proliferation after arterial injury. I. Smooth muscle growth in the absence of endothelium. *Lab Invest* 1983;49:327.
53. Owens GK. Control of hypertrophic versus hyperplastic growth of vascular smooth muscle cells. *Am J Physiol* 1989;257:H1755.
54. Zwolak RM, Adams MC, Clowes AW. Kinetics of vein graft hyperplasia: association with tangential stress. *J Vasc Surg* 1987;5:126.
55. Leung DY, Glagov S, Mathews MB. Cyclic stretching stimulates synthesis of matrix components by arterial smooth muscle cells in vitro. *Science* 1976;191:475.
56. Baumgartner HR, Studer A. Consequences of vessel catheterization in normal and hypercholesterolemic rabbits. *Pathol Microbiol* 1966;29:393.
57. Kumagai H, Suzuki H, Matsukawa S, et al. Captopril therapy following percutaneous transluminal angioplasty for bilateral renal artery stenosis. *Arch Intern Med* 1989;149:1973.
58. Bowen-Pope DF, Ross R, Seifert RA. Locally acting growth factors for vascular smooth muscle cells: endogenous synthesis and release from platelets. *Circulation* 1985;72:735.
59. Friedman RJ, Stemerman MB, Wenz B, et al. The effect of thrombocytopenia on experimental atherosclerotic lesion formation in rabbits. Smooth muscle cell proliferation and re-endothelialization. *J Clin Invest* 1977;60:1191.
60. Fingerle J, Johnson R, Clowes AW, et al. Role of platelets in smooth muscle cell proliferation and migration after vascular injury in rat carotid artery. *Proc Natl Acad Sci U S A* 1989;86:8412.
61. Groves HM, Kinlough-Rathbone RL, Richardson M, et al. Thrombin generation and fibrin formation following injury to rabbit neointima. Studies of vessel wall reactivity and platelet survival. *Lab Invest* 1982;46:605.
62. Hatton MWC, Moar SL, Richardson M. Deendothelialization in vivo initiates a thrombogenic reaction at the rabbit aorta surface. Correlation of uptake of fibrinogen and antithrombin III with thrombin generation by the exposed subendothelium. *Am J Pathol* 1989;135:499.
63. Faggiotto A, Ross R. Studies of hypercholesterolemia in the nonhuman primate. II. Fatty streak conversion to fibrous plaque. *Arteriosclerosis* 1984;4:341.
64. Faggiotto A, Ross R, Harker L. Studies of hypercholesterolemia in nonhuman primate. I. Changes that lead to fatty streak formation. *Arteriosclerosis* 1984;4:323.
65. Reidy MA. A reassessment of endothelial injury and arterial lesion formation. *Lab Invest* 1985;53:513.
66. Clowes AW, Clowes MM. Regulation of smooth muscle proliferation by heparin in vitro and in vivo. *Int Angiol* 1987;6:45.
67. Clowes AW, Clowes MM, Fingerle J, et al. Regulation of smooth muscle cell growth in injured artery. *J Cardiovasc Pharmacol* 1989;14(suppl 6): S12.
68. Gajdusek CM, Schwartz SM. Comparison of intracellular and extracellular mitogen activity. *J Cell Physiol* 1984;121:316.
69. Gajdusek CM, Carbon S. Injury-induced release of basic fibroblast growth factor from bovine aortic endothelium. *J Cell Physiol* 1989;139:570.
70. Burgess WH, Maciag T. The heparin binding (fibroblast) growth factor family of proteins. *Annu Rev Biochem* 1989;58:575.
71. Gospodarowicz D, Neufeld G, Schwiegerer L. Fibroblast growth factor: structural and biological properties. *J Cell Physiol* 1987;(suppl 5):15.
72. Vlodavsky I, Folkman J, Sullivan R, et al. Endothelial cell-derived basic fibroblast growth factor: synthesis and deposition into subendothelial extracellular matrix. *Proc Natl Acad Sci U S A* 1987;84:2292.
73. Lindner V, Lappi DA, Baird A, et al. Role of basic fibroblast growth factor in vascular lesion formation. *Circ Res* 1991;68:106–113.
74. Lindner V, Reidy MA. Proliferation of smooth muscle cells after vascular injury is inhibited by an antibody against basic fibroblast growth factor. *Proc Natl Acad Sci U S A* 1991;88:3739.
75. Raines EW, Bowen-Pope DF, Ross R. Platelet-derived growth factor. In: Sporn MB, Roberts AB, eds. *Handbook of Experimental Pharmacology: Peptide Growth Factors and Their Receptors*. Heidelberg, Germany: Springer-Verlag; 1989:xx.
76. Sprugel KH, McPherson JM, Clowes AW, et al. Effects of growth factors in vivo. I. Cell ingrowth into porous subcutaneous chambers. *Am J Pathol* 1987;129:601–613.
77. Doolittle RF, Hunkapillar MW, Hood LE, et al. Simian sarcoma virus oncogene, v-sis, is derived form the gene (or genes) encoding a platelet-derived growth factor. *Science* 1983;221:275.
78. Waterfield MD, Scrace GT, Whittle N, et al. Platelet-derived growth factor is structurally related to the putative transforming protein p28-sis of simian sarcoma virus. *Nature* 1983;304:35.
79. Ferns GAA, Raines EW, Sprugel KH, et al. Inhibition of neointimal smooth muscle accumulation after angioplasty by an antibody to PDGF. *Science* 1991;253:1129.
80. Jawien A, Bowen-Pope DF, Lindner V, et al. Platelet-derived growth factor promotes smooth muscle migration and intimal thickening in a rat model of balloon angioplasty. *J Clin Invest* 1992;89:507.
81. Bornfeldt KE, Raines EW, Graves LM, et al. Platelet-derived growth factor. Distinct signal transduction pathways associated with migration versus proliferation. *Ann N Y Acad Sci* 1995;766:416.
82. Blaes N, Boissel JP. Growth-stimulating effect of catecholamines on rat aortic smooth muscle cells in culture. *J Cell Physiol* 1983;116:167.
83. Dalsgaard CJ, Hultgardh-Nilsson A, Haegerstrand A, et al. Neuropeptides as growth factors. Possible roles in human disease. *Regul Pept* 1989;25:1.
84. Bevan RD. Trophic effects of peripheral adrenergic nerves on vascular structure. *Hypertension* 1984;6:III-19.
85. Bevan RD, Tsuru H. Functional and structural changes in the rabbit ear artery after sympathetic denervation. *Circ Res* 1981;49:478.
86. Powell JS, Clozel JP, Muller RKM, et al. Inhibitors of angiotensin-converting enzyme prevent myointimal proliferation after vascular injury. *Science* 1989;245:186.
87. Jackson CL, Bush RC, Bowyer DE. Inhibitory effect of calcium antagonists on balloon catheter-induced arterial smooth muscle cell proliferation and lesion size. *Atherosclerosis* 1988;69:115.
88. Clowes AW, Reidy MA. Mechanisms of graft failure. The role of cellular proliferation. *Ann N Y Acad Sci* 1987;516:673.
89. Fritze LMS, Reilly CF, Rosenberg RD. An antiproliferative heparan sulfate species produced by postconfluent smooth muscle cells. *J Cell Biol* 1985; 100:1041.
90. Castellot JJ Jr, Addonizio ML, Rosenberg R, et al. Cultured endothelial cells produce a heparin-like inhibitor of smooth muscle cell growth. *J Cell Biol* 1981;90:372.
91. Majesky MW, Lindner V, Twardzik DR, et al. Production of transforming growth factor β_1 during repair of arterial injury. *J Clin Invest* 1991;88:904.
92. Wolf YG, Rasmussen LM, Ruoslahti E. Antibodies against transforming growth factor-β_1 suppress intimal hyperplasia in a rat model. *J Clin Invest* 1994;93:1172.
93. Hansson GK, Jonasson L, Seifert PS, et al. Immune mechanisms in atherosclerosis. *Arteriosclerosis* 1989;9:567.
94. Hansson GK, Jonasson L, Holm J, et al. Gamma interferon regulates vascular smooth muscle proliferation and Ia expression in vitro and in vivo. *Circ Res* 1988;63:712.
95. Tellides G, Tereb DA, Kirkiles-Smith NC, et al. Interferon-gamma elicits arteriosclerosis in the absence of leukocytes. *Nature* 2000;403:207.
96. Aaronson SA. Growth factors and cancer. *Science* 1991;254:1146.
97. Brugge JS. New intracellular targets for therapeutic drug design. *Science* 1993;260:918–919.
98. Schindler C, Shuai K, Prezioso VR, et al. Interferon-dependent tyrosine phosphorylation of a latent cytoplasmic transcription factor. *Science* 1992; 257:809.
99. Zhong Z, Wen Z, Darnell JE. Stat3: a stat family member activated by tyrosine phosphorylation in response to epidermal growth factor and interleukin. *Science* 1994;264:95.
100. Baringa M. Two major signaling pathways meet at MAP-kinase. *Science* 1995;269:1673.
101. Larson DM, Haudenschild CC, Beyer EC. Gap junction messenger RNA expression by vascular wall cells. *Circ Res* 1990;66:1074.
102. Orlidge A, D'Amore PA. Inhibition of capillary endothelial cell growth by pericytes and smooth muscle cells. *J Cell Biol* 1987;105:1455.
103. Heimark RL, Schwartz SM. The role of membrane-membrane interactions in the regulation of endothelial cell growth. *J Cell Biol* 1985;100:1934.
104. Hawiger JJ. Hemostasis, bleeding, and thromboembolic complications of trauma and infection. In: Clowes GHA Jr, ed. *Trauma, Sepsis and Shock: The Physiological Basis of Therapy.* New York: Marcel Dekker; 1988: 123–159.
105. Rodgers GM. Hemostatic properties of normal and perturbed vascular cells. *FASEB J* 1990;2:116.
106. Marcum J, McKenney J, Rosenberg R. The acceleration of thrombin-antithrombin III complex formation in rat hind quarters via heparin-like molecules bound to endothelium. *J Clin Invest* 1984;74:341.
107. Cotran RS, Kumar V, Robbins SL. *Robbins' Pathologic Basis of Disease.* Philadelphia, PA: WB Saunders; 1989:553–595.
108. Benditt EP, Gown AM. Atheroma: the artery wall and the environment. *Int Rev Exp Pathol* 1980;21:55.
109. McGill HC Jr. Persistent problems in the pathogenesis of atherosclerosis. *Arteriosclerosis* 1984;4:443.
110. Velican C, Velican D. Intimal thickening in developing coronary arteries and its relevance to atherosclerotic involvement. *Atherosclerosis* 1976;23: 345.
111. Velican C, Velican D. The precursors of coronary atherosclerotic plaques in subjects up to 40 years old. *Atherosclerosis* 1980;37:33.

112. Thomas WA, Kim DN. Atherosclerosis as a hyperplastic and/or neoplastic process. *Lab Invest* 1983;48:245.
113. Gordon D, Reidy MA, Benditt EP, et al. Cell proliferation in human coronary arteries. *Proc Natl Acad Sci U S A* 1990;87:4600.
114. O'Brien ER, Alpers CE, Stewart DK, et al. Proliferation in primary and restenotic coronary atherectomy tissue: implications for antiproliferative therapy. *Circ Res* 1993;73:223.
115. Jonasson L, Holm J, Skalli O, et al. Expression of class II transplantation antigens on vascular smooth muscle cells in human atherosclerosis. *J Clin Invest* 1985;76:125.
116. Stemme S, Rymo L, Hansson GK. Polyclonal origin of T lymphocytes in human atherosclerotic plaques. *Lab Invest* 1991;65:654.
117. Sharrett AR, Patsch W, Sorlie PD, et al. Associations of lipoprotein cholesterols, apolipoproteins A-I and B, and triglycerides with carotid atherosclerosis and coronary heart disease: the atherosclerosis risk in communities (ARIC) study. *Arterioscler Thromb* 1994;14:1098.
118. Wilcox JN, Smith KM, Schwartz SM, et al. Localization of tissue factor in the normal vessel wall and in the atherosclerotic plaque. *Proc Natl Acad Sci U S A* 1989;86:2839.
119. Schneiderman J, Sawdey MS, Keeton MR, et al. Increased type 1 plasminogen activator inhibitor gene expression in atherosclerotic human arteries. *Proc Natl Acad Sci U S A* 1992;89:6998.
120. Lupu F, Bergonzelli GE, Heim DA, et al. Localization and production of plasminogen activator inhibitor-1 in human healthy and atherosclerotic arteries. *Arterioscler Thromb* 1993;13:1090.
121. Page JH. Atherosclerosis. An introduction. *Circulation* 1954;10:1.
122. Masuda J, Ross R. Atherogenesis during low level hypercholesterolemia in the nonhuman primate. I. Fatty streak formation. *Arteriosclerosis* 1990; 10:164.
123. Castelli WP. Epidemiology of coronary heart disease: the Framingham study. *Am J Med* 1984;76:4.
124. Rapp JH, Harris HW, Hamilton RL, et al. Particle size distribution of lipoproteins from human atherosclerotic plaque: a preliminary report. *J Vasc Surg* 1989;9:81.
125. Breslow JL. Insights into lipoprotein metabolism from studies in transgenic mice. *Annu Rev Physiol* 1994;56:797.
126. Strong JP, Malcom GT, Oalmann MC, et al. The PDAY Study: natural history, risk factors, and pathobiology. Pathobiological Determinants of Atherosclerosis in Youth. *Ann N Y Acad Sci* 1997;811:226; discussion 235–237.
127. Brown MS, Basu SK, Falck JR, et al. The scavenger cell pathway for lipoprotein degradation: specificity of the binding site that mediates the uptake of negatively-charged LDL by macrophages. *J Supramol Struct* 1980;13:67.
128. Steinberg D. A critical look at the evidence for the oxidation of LDL in atherogenesis. *Atherosclerosis* 1997;131(suppl):S5.
129. Libby P. Managing the risk of atherosclerosis: the role of high-density lipoprotein. *Am J Cardiol* 2001;88:3N.
130. Rimm EB, Stampfer MJ. The role of antioxidants in preventive cardiology. *Curr Opin Cardiol* 1997;12:188.
131. Steinberg D, Witzum JL. Is the oxidative modification hypothesis relevant to human atherosclerosis? Do antioxidant trials conducted to date refute the hypothesis? *Circulation* 2002;105:2107.
132. Salonen RM, Nyyssonen K, Kaikonen J, et al. Six year effect of combined vitamin C and E supplementation on atherosclerosis progression. The Antioxidant Supplementation in Atherosclerosis Prevention (ASAP) Study. *Circulation* 2003;107:947.
133. Dansky HM, Charlton SA, Barlow CB, et al. Apo A-I inhibits foam cell formation in Apo E-deficient mice after monocyte adherence to endothelium. *J Clin Invest* 1999;104:31.
134. Lipid research clinics program [Letter]. *JAMA* 1984;252:2545.
135. Frick MH, Elo O, Haapa K, et al. Helsinki Heart Study: primary-prevention trial with gemfibrozil in middle-aged men with dyslipidemia. Safety of treatment, changes in risk factors, and incidence of coronary heart disease. *N Engl J Med* 1987;317:1237.
136. Collins R, Peto R, Armitage J. The MRC/BHF Heart Protection Study preliminary results. *Int J Clin Pract* 2002;56:53.
137. Fonarow GC, Watson KE. Effective strategies for long-term statin use. *Am J Cardiol* 2003;92:27i.
138. Endres M, Laufs U, Huang Z, et al. Stroke protection by 3-hydroxy-3-methylglutaryl (HMG)-CoA reductase inhibitors mediated by endothelial nitric oxide synthase. *Proc Natl Acad Sci U S A* 1998;95:8880.
139. Kinlay S, Selwyn AP. Effects of statins on inflammation in patients with acute and chronic coronary syndromes. *Am J Cardiol* 2003;91:9B.
140. Duguid JB. Thrombosis as a factor in the pathogenesis of aortic atherosclerosis. *J Pathol Bacteriol* 1948;60:57.
141. Benezra M, Vlodavsky I, Ishai-Michaeli R, et al. Thrombin-induced release of active basic fibroblast growth factor-heparan sulfate complexes from subendothelial extracellular matrix. *Blood* 1993;81:3324.
142. Schwartz SM, Reidy MA, Clowes AW. Kinetics of atherosclerosis, a stem cell model. *Ann N Y Acad Sci* 1985;454:292.
143. Murray CE, Gipaya CT, Bartosek T, et al. Monoclonality of smooth muscle cells in human atherosclerosis. *Am J Pathol* 1997;151:697.
144. Libby P, Egan D, Skarlatos S. Roles of infectious agents in atherosclerosis and restenosis: an assessment of the evidence and need for future research. *Circulation* 1997;96:4095.
145. Melnick JL, Adam E, DeBakey ME, et al. Possible role of cytomegalovirus atherogenesis. *JAMA* 1990;263:2204.
146. Melnick JL, Adam E, DeBakey ME. Cytomegalovirus and atherosclerosis. *Eur Heart J* 1993;14(suppl K):30.
147. Grattan MT, Moreno-Cabral CE, Starnes VA, et al. Cytomegalovirus infection is associated with cardiac allograft rejection and atherosclerosis. *JAMA* 1989;261:3561.
148. Nieto FJ, Adam E, Sorlie P, et al. Cohort study of cytomegalovirus infection as a risk factor for carotid intimal-medial thickening, a measure of subclinical atherosclerosis [see comments]. *Circulation* 1996;94:922.
149. Kuvin JT, Kimmelstiel CD. Infectious causes of atherosclerosis. *Am Heart J* 1999;137:216.
150. Grayston JT, Kuo CC, Coulson AS, et al. Chlamydia pneumoniae (TWAR) in atherosclerosis of the carotid artery [see comments]. *Circulation* 1995; 92:3397.
151. Kuo CC, Shor A, Campbell LA, et al. Demonstration of Chlamydia pneumoniae in atherosclerotic lesions of coronary arteries. *J Infect Dis* 1993; 167:841.
152. Muhlestein JB, Anderson JL, Hammond EH, et al. Infection with Chlamydia pneumoniae accelerates the development of atherosclerosis and treatment with azithromycin prevents it in a rabbit model. *Circulation* 1998; 97:633.
153. Kol A, Bourcier T, Lichtman AH, et al. Chlamydial and human heat shock protein 60s activate human vascular endothelium, smooth muscle cells, and macrophages. *J Clin Invest* 1999;103:571.
154. Kol A, Sukhova GK, Lichtman AH, et al. Chlamydial heat shock protein 60 localizes in human atheroma and regulates macrophage tumor necrosis factor-alpha and matrix metalloproteinase expression. *Circulation* 1998;98:300.
155. Danesh J, Collins R, Peto R. Chronic infections and coronary heart disease: is there a link? *Lancet* 1997;350:430.
156. Amento EP, Ehsani N, Palmer H, et al. Cytokines and growth factors positively and negatively regulate interstitial collagen gene expression in human vascular smooth muscle cells. *Arterioscler Thromb* 1991;11:1223.
157. Hansson GK, Holm J, Jonasson L. Detection of activated T lymphocytes in the human atherosclerotic plaque. *Am J Pathol* 1989;135:169.
158. Libby P, Hansson GK. Involvement of the immune system in human atherogenesis: current knowledge and unanswered questions. *Lab Invest* 1991;64:5.
159. Salomon RN, Hughes CC, Schoen FJ, et al. Human coronary transplantation-associated arteriosclerosis. Evidence for a chronic immune reaction to activated graft endothelial cells. *Am J Pathol* 1991;138:791.
160. Russell PS, Chase CM, Winn HJ, et al. Coronary atherosclerosis in transplanted mouse hearts. I. Time course and immunogenetic and immunopathological considerations. *Am J Pathol* 1994;144:260.
161. Shi C, Russell ME, Bianchi C, et al. Murine model of accelerated transplant arteriosclerosis. *Circ Res* 1994;75:199.
162. Torzewski J, Bowyer DE, Waltenberger J, et al. Processes in atherogenesis: complement activation. *Atherosclerosis* 1997;132:131.
163. Rus HG, Niculescu F, Constantinescu E, et al. Immunoelectron-microscopic localization of the terminal C5b-9 complement complex in human atherosclerotic fibrous plaque. *Atherosclerosis* 1986;61:35.
164. Richardson PD, Davies MJ, Born GV. Influence of plaque configuration and stress distribution on fissuring of coronary atherosclerotic plaques. *Lancet* 1989;2:941.
165. Cheng GC, Loree HM, Kamm RD, et al. Distribution of circumferential stress in ruptured and stable atherosclerotic lesions: a structural analysis with histopathological correlation. *Circulation* 1993;87:1179.
166. Kinlay S, Selwyn AP, Libby P, et al. Inflammation, the endothelium, and the acute coronary syndromes. *J Cardiovasc Pharmacol* 1998;32(suppl 3):S62.
167. Fabunmi RP, Sukhova GK, Sugiyama S, et al. Expression of tissue inhibitor of metalloproteinases-3 in human atheroma and regulation in lesion-associated cells: a potential protective mechanism in plaque stability. *Circ Res* 1998;83:270.
168. Libby P, Aikawa M. New insights into plaque stabilisation by lipid lowering. *Drugs* 1998;56(suppl 1):9.
169. Libby P, Schoenbeck U, Mach F, et al. Current concepts in cardiovascular pathology: the role of LDL cholesterol in plaque rupture and stabilization. *Am J Med* 1998;104:14S.
170. Dandona P, Aljada A. A rational approach to pathogenesis and treatment of type 2 diabetes mellitus, insulin resistance, inflammation, and atherosclerosis. *Am J Cardiol* 2001;90:27G.
171. Aikawa M, Rabkin E, Okada Y, et al. Lipid lowering by diet reduces matrix metalloproteinase activity and increases collagen content of rabbit atheroma: a potential mechanism of lesion stabilization. *Circulation* 1998;97:2433.
172. Akira S. Toll-like receptor signaling. *J Biol Chem* 2003;40:38105–38108.
173. Curtiss LK, Tobias PS. Emerging role of Toll-like receptors in atherosclerosis. *J Lip Res* 2009;50(suppl):S340–345.
174. Libby P. Vascular biology of atherosclerosis overview and state of the art. *Am J Cardiol* 2003;91:3A.

CHAPTER 90 ■ CEREBROVASCULAR OCCLUSIVE DISEASE

PETER H. LIN AND TAM T. HUYNH

KEY POINTS

1. Stroke remains the third most common cause of death in the United States, and atherosclerotic occlusive disease of the extracranial portion of the carotid artery is the most common cause of stroke.
2. Atherosclerosis is the pathologic process most often responsible for symptoms of cerebrovascular insufficiency.
3. Clinical risk factors for the development of carotid artery atherosclerotic lesions are the same as those for coronary artery disease: increased age, hypertension, diabetes mellitus, hyperlipidemia, hypercoagulable states, positive family history, and tobacco use.
4. Duplex ultrasound of the carotid artery is the preferred initial diagnostic study of choice to evaluate carotid occlusive disease.
5. The most common clinical presentations of extracranial cerebrovascular occlusive disease are transient ischemic attack (TIA) and hemispheric stroke.
6. The majority of asymptomatic and symptomatic carotid artery occlusive disease is caused by atherosclerosis. It is therefore important to modify risk factors to prevent progression of atherosclerotic disease.
7. Currently, carotid artery stenting should be limited to high-risk patients. The application of carotid artery stenting to patients at suitable risk to undergo endarterectomy should be limited to ongoing randomized clinical trials.

1 Carotid artery occlusive disease remains the most common cause of cerebrovascular accident, which represents the third most common cause of death in the United States.[1] The morbidity caused by a cerebrovascular accident is more disabling than that encountered with other ischemic conditions, including myocardial infarction or lower extremity ischemia. Neurologic sequelae related to cerebrovascular accident can include aphasia, paralysis, blindness, and weakness. These neurologic sequelae uniformly diminish the patient's ability to perform routine daily activities and invariably create an enormous burden with regard to health care costs. Consequently, prevention of a cerebrovascular accident, particularly the treatment of extracranial carotid occlusive disease, remains a paramount priority for all health care providers.

Atherosclerotic occlusive plaque at the origin of the internal carotid artery remains the most common cause of cerebrovascular accident. It is estimated that 40% to 60% of all ischemic strokes are related to atherosclerotic carotid bifurcation occlusive disease. Since the first reported case of carotid endarterectomy in 1954,[2] operative treatment of carotid occlusive disease has become one of the most commonly performed vascular operations in the United States. Various large, prospective, randomized clinical studies, which compared the efficacy of carotid endarterectomy plus optimal medical treatment with optimal medical treatment alone, have convincingly demonstrated the efficacy of carotid endarterectomy in reducing stroke and improving survival. The widely adopted endovascular therapy in the last decade has prompted interventional enthusiasts to establish a less invasive treatment alternative for cerebrovascular disease in selected patients. This chapter provides a comprehensive review of the epidemiology, pathophysiology, diagnosis, treatment, and relevant controversies in the management of cerebrovascular occlusive disease involving the carotid artery.

EPIDEMIOLOGY

Focal cerebral ischemic disease, or stroke, is responsible for 4.5 million deaths worldwide, with the majority occurring in nonindustrialized countries. Within the United States, it is estimated that more than 700,000 patients suffer a new or recurrent stroke annually.[1] Among them, approximately 200,000 die due to a consequence of stroke. Of the remaining survivors who suffer a stroke, two thirds are disabled and are never able to return to the workforce, while one third require prolonged hospitalization due to permanent disability. The cumulative economic burden of health care costs for these disabled patients with strokes is massive, exceeding $16 trillion annually in the United States.[1]

The term *cerebrovascular accident* (CVA) is often used interchangeably to refer to an ischemic stroke. A transient ischemic attack (TIA) is defined as a temporary focal cerebral or retinal hypoperfusion state that resolves spontaneously within 24 hours after its onset. However, the majority of TIAs resolve within minutes, and longer-lasting neurologic deficits more likely represent a stroke. The incidence of stroke is 0.2% per year in the general population but rises significantly with concurrent risk factors, age, sex, and ethnic background. Overall, the 20-year risk for a 45-year-old male is 3%, but this increases to 25% for a 40-year risk.[3] The annual incidence of stroke doubles for each decade in patients older than 55 years of age. The largest incidence of stroke is observed in patients older than 80 years of age when the prevalence is 2%. In contrast, TIA occurs far more often in the younger population. In the United States, the prevalence of TIAs in males aged between 65 and 69 years is 2.7%, which increases markedly to 3.6% for males aged between 75 and 79 years.[3]

PATHOGENESIS OF STROKE

Approximately 85% of all strokes are caused by ischemic etiologies, while the remaining are caused by hemorrhagic disease. Hemorrhagic strokes can be caused by head trauma or spontaneous disruption of intracerebral blood vessels. Ischemic strokes are due to hypoperfusion from arterial occlusion or, less commonly, decreased flow resulting from proximal arterial stenosis and a poor collateral network. Patients with ischemic neurologic deficits can be further classified into having anterior or hemispheric symptoms and posterior or vertebrobasilar symptoms. The predominant causes of hemisphere symptoms arise from the occlusive lesion of the extracranial carotid artery, which may cause internal carotid artery thrombosis, flow-related ischemic events, and/or cerebral embolization. The
3 risk factors for the development of carotid artery bifurcation disease are similar to those causing atherosclerotic occlusive disease in other vascular beds. Increasing age, male gender, hypertension, tobacco smoking, diabetes mellitus, homocysteinemia, and hyperlipidemia are well-known predisposing factors for the development of atherosclerotic occlusive disease.[4,5] Etiologic factors that can contribute to the development of cerebral ischemia or infarction are listed in Table 90.1.

Stroke due to carotid bifurcation occlusive disease is usually related to atheroembolization (Fig. 90.1). The carotid bifurcation is an area of low flow velocity and low shear stress. As the blood circulates through the carotid bifurcation, there is separation of flow into the low-resistance internal carotid artery and the high-resistance external carotid artery. Atherosclerotic plaque characteristically forms in the outer wall opposite to the flow divider (Fig. 90.2). Atherosclerotic plaque formation is complex, beginning with intimal injury, platelet deposition, smooth muscle cell proliferation, and fibroplasia, leading to subsequent luminal narrowing. With increasing degrees of stenosis in the internal carotid artery, flow becomes more turbulent, and the risk of atheroembolization escalates.

The tendency for atherosclerotic plaque to occur at the carotid bifurcation is also related to various factors, including vessel geometry, velocity profile, and shear stress. It has been demonstrated that plaque formation in the carotid artery bifurcation is increased within areas of low flow velocity and low shear stress and decreased in areas of high flow velocity and elevated shear stress. Postmortem specimens showed that atherosclerosis was particularly pronounced along the outer or lateral aspect of the proximal internal carotid artery and carotid bulb.[6] This zone corresponds to areas of low velocity and low shear stress. Conversely, the medial or inner aspect of the cadaveric carotid bulb, which was associated with high blood flow velocity and high shear stress in the flow model, was relatively free of plaque formation.

The smooth muscle cell has an important role in the initial stages of plaque development. Smooth muscle cells migrate through the intima, proliferate within the media, and promote

TABLE 90.1

ETIOLOGIC FACTORS OF CEREBRAL ISCHEMIA AND INFARCTION

■ ISCHEMIC ETIOLOGIC FACTOR	■ HEMORRHAGIC ETIOLOGIC FACTOR
1. **Atherothromboembolic**	1. **Intraparenchymal hemorrhage**
High-grade stenoses and occlusions	Hypertensive encephalopathy
Emboli	Amyloid angiopathy
Plaque	Arteriovenous malformations
Platelet–fibrin debris	Trauma
Intraplaque hemorrhage	2. **Subarachnoid hemorrhage**
2. **Cardioembolic**	Berry aneurysms
Arrhythmias	Arteriovenous malformations
Myocardial infarction with mural thrombus	Trauma
Mitral valve prolapse, calcified annulus	3. **Extracranial**
Rheumatic heart disease	Atherosclerosis
Prosthetic heart valves	Great vessels
3. **Systemic**	Carotid artery
Cardiac arrest and resuscitation	Fibromuscular dysplasia
Profound shock	Trauma
Cardiopulmonary bypass	Aortic aneurysms
4. **Venous thromboses**	Dissecting
Dural venous sinuses	Atherosclerotic
Bilateral jugular vein occlusions	Traumatic
5. **Miscellaneous causes**	Takayasu panarteritis
Lacunar infarcts	Temporal arteritis
Lipohyalinosis	Carotid dissections
Fibrinoid necrosis	Spontaneous
Charcot-Bouchard aneurysms	Trauma
Diabetes	Carotid aneurysms
Moyamoya disease	
Kawasaki syndrome	
Fibromuscular disease	
Giant cell arteritis	
Spontaneous dissections	
Trauma (extracranial cerebral vessels)	
Hypercoagulable states	
Binswanger encephalopathy	
Substance abuse	

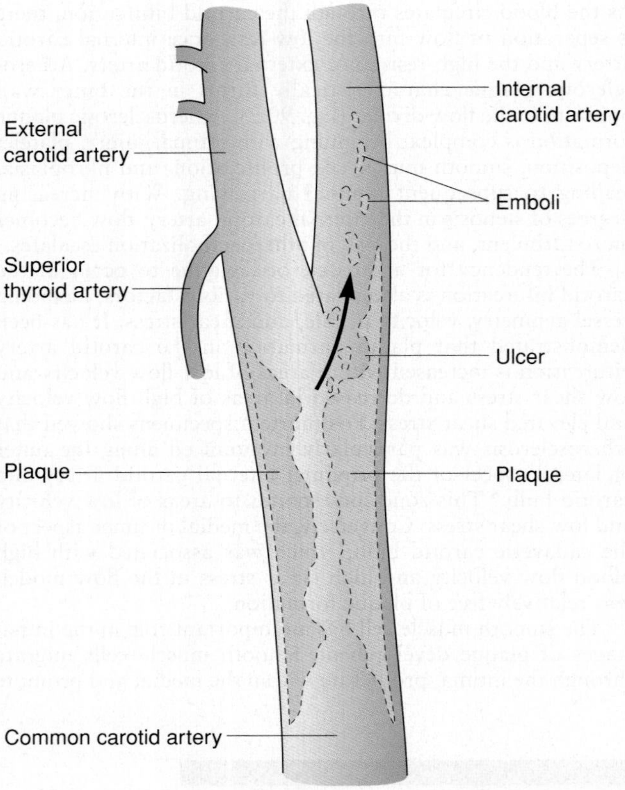

FIGURE 90.1. Stroke due to carotid bifurcation occlusive disease is usually caused by atheroemboli arising from the internal carotid artery, which provides the majority of blood flow to the cerebral hemisphere. With increasing degrees of stenosis in the carotid artery, flow becomes more turbulent, and the risk of atheroembolization escalates.

accumulation of cholesterol and other lipid molecules within the evolving lesion. Thereafter, the macrophage becomes a source of growth factor production that stimulates further smooth muscle cell proliferation and extracellular matrix production. Smooth muscle cells and macrophages initiate a secondary inflammatory cell reaction and are capable of ingesting lipid and of being transformed into vacuolated foam cells that are characteristic of atherosclerotic lesions.

In addition to these cellular components, the majority of carotid plaques have a necrotic core consisting of loose cellular debris and cholesterol crystals. The necrotic core is separated from the carotid lumen by a fibrous cap, which is composed of a rim of variable thickness comprising cellular components and extracellular matrix. The structural integrity of the fibrous cap is crucial to the final stage of plaque disruption and its clinical and pathologic sequelae. It is now generally accepted that acute changes within the plaque with exposure of the deeper lipid contents predispose toward thromboembolization. Another feature characteristic of advanced atherosclerotic plaques is intraplaque hemorrhage, which can occur in the absence of a disrupted fibrous cap. Symptomatic carotid disease is associated with increased neovascularization within the atherosclerotic plaque and fibrous cap. These vessels are larger and more irregular and may contribute to plaque instability and the onset of thromboembolic events.

CLINICAL MANIFESTATIONS OF CEREBRAL ISCHEMIA

A TIA is a focal loss of neurologic function, lasting for less than 24 hours. Crescendo TIAs refer to a syndrome consisting of repeated TIAs within a short period of time that is characterized by complete neurologic recovery in between. At a minimum, the term should probably be reserved for those with

FIGURE 90.2. **A:** The carotid bifurcation is an area of low flow velocity and low shear stress. As the blood circulates through the carotid bifurcation, there is separation of flow into the low-resistance internal carotid artery and the high-resistance external carotid artery. **B:** The carotid atherosclerotic plaque typically forms in the outer wall opposite to the flow divider due in part to the effect of the low shear stress region, which also creates a transient reversal of flow during the cardiac cycle.

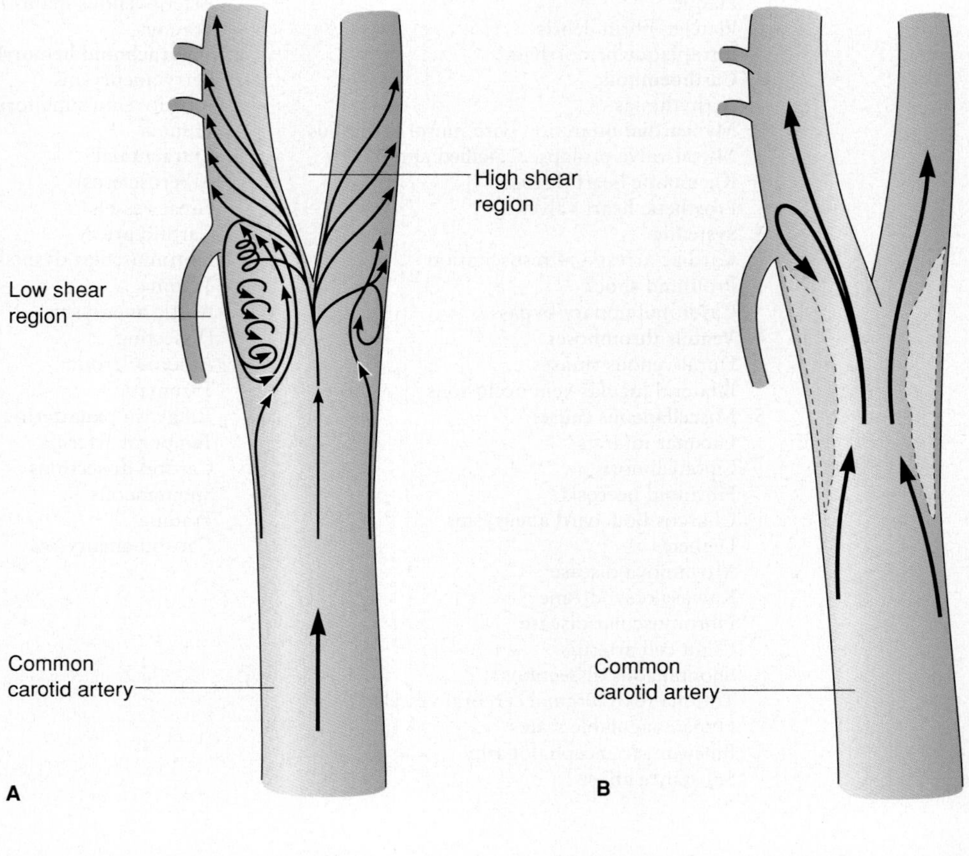

either daily events or multiple resolving attacks within 24 hours. Hemodynamic TIAs represent focal cerebral events that are aggravated by exercise or hemodynamic stress and typically occur after short bursts of physical activity, postprandially, or after getting out of a hot bath. It is implied that these are due to severe extracranial disease and poor intracranial collateral recruitment. Stroke in evolution refers to progressive worsening of the neurologic deficit, either linearly over a 24-hour period or interspersed with transient periods of stabilization and/or partial clinical improvement.[7]

The patients who suffer cerebrovascular accidents typically present with three categories of symptoms: ocular symptoms, sensory/motor deficit, and/or higher cortical dysfunction. The common ocular symptoms associated with extracranial carotid artery occlusive disease include amaurosis fugax and the presence of Hollenhorst plaques. Amaurosis fugax, commonly referred to as transient monocular blindness, is a temporary loss of vision in one eye, which patients typically describe as a window shutter coming down or gray shedding of the vision. This partial blindness usually lasts for a few minutes and then resolves. Most of these phenomena (>90%) are due to embolic occlusion of the main artery or the upper or lower divisions. Monocular blindness progressing over a 20-minute period suggests a migrainous etiology. Occasionally, the patient will recall no visual symptoms while the optician notes a yellowish plaque within the retinal vessels, which is also known as the Hollenhorst plaque. These are frequently derived from cholesterol embolization from the carotid bifurcation and warrant further investigation. Additionally, several ocular symptoms may be caused by microembolization from the extracranial carotid diseases including monocular visual loss due to retinal artery or optic nerve ischemia, the ocular ischemia syndrome, and visual field deficits secondary to cortical infarction and ischemia of the optic tracts. Typical motor and/or sensory symptoms associated with cerebrovascular accidents are lateralized or focal neurologic deficits. Ischemic events tend to have an abrupt onset, with the severity of the insult being apparent from the onset and not usually associated with seizures or paraesthesia. In contrast, they represent loss or diminution of neurologic function. Furthermore, motor or sensory deficits can be unilateral or bilateral, with the upper and lower limbs being variably affected depending on the site of the cerebral lesion. The combination of a motor and sensory deficit in the same body territory is suggestive of a cortical thromboembolic event, as opposed to lacunar lesions secondary to small-vessel disease of the penetrating arterioles. However, a small proportion of the latter may present with a sensorimotor stroke secondary to small-vessel occlusion within the posterior limb of the internal capsule. Pure sensory and motor strokes and those strokes where the weakness affects one limb only or does not involve the face are more typically seen with lacunar as opposed to cortical infarction. A number of higher cortical functions, including speech and language disturbances, can be affected by thromboembolic phenomena from the carotid artery; the most important clinical example for the dominant hemisphere is dysphasia or aphasia, while visuospatial neglect is an example of nondominant hemisphere injury.

DIAGNOSTIC EVALUATION

4 Duplex ultrasonography is the most widely used screening tool to evaluate for atherosclerotic plaque and stenosis of the extracranial carotid artery. It is also commonly used to monitor patients serially for progression of disease or after intervention (carotid endarterectomy or angioplasty). Duplex ultrasound of the carotid artery combines B-mode gray-scale imaging and Doppler waveform analysis. Characterization of the carotid plaque on gray-scale imaging provides useful information about its composition. However, there are currently no universal recommendations that can be made based solely on the sonographic appearance of the plaque. On the other hand, criteria have been developed and well refined for grading the degree of carotid stenosis based primarily on Doppler-derived velocity waveforms.

The external carotid artery has a high-resistance flow pattern with a sharp systolic peak and a small amount of flow in diastole. In contrast, a normal internal carotid artery will have a low-resistance flow pattern with a broad systolic peak and a large amount of flow during diastole. The flow pattern in the common carotid artery resembles that in the internal carotid artery, as 80% of the flow is directed to the internal carotid artery, with waveforms that have broad systolic peaks and moderate amount of flow during diastole. Conventionally, velocity measurements are recorded in the common carotid artery, external carotid artery, carotid bulb, and the proximal, mid-, and distal portions of the internal carotid artery. Characteristically, the peak systolic velocity is increased at the site of the vessel stenosis. The end-diastolic velocity is increased with greater degrees of stenosis. In addition, stenosis of the internal carotid artery can lead to color shifts, with color mosaics indicating a poststenotic turbulence. Dampening of the Doppler velocity waveforms is typically seen in areas distal to severe carotid stenosis where blood flow is reduced. It is well known that occlusion of the ipsilateral internal carotid artery can lead to a "falsely" elevated velocity on the contralateral side due to an increase in compensatory blood flow. In the presence of a high-grade stenosis or occlusion of the internal carotid artery, the ipsilateral common carotid artery displays high-flow-resistance waveforms, similar to that seen in the external carotid artery. If there is a significant stenosis in the proximal common carotid artery, its waveforms may be dampened with low velocities.

The Doppler grading systems of carotid stenosis were initially established by comparison to angiographic findings of disease. Studies have shown variability in the measurements of the duplex properties by different laboratories, as well as heterogeneity in the patient population, study design, and techniques. One of the most commonly used classifications was established at the University of Washington School of Medicine in Seattle. Diameter reduction of 50% to 79% is defined by peak systolic velocity greater than 125 cm/s with extensive spectral broadening. For stenosis in the range of 80% to 99%, the peak systolic velocity is greater than 125 cm/s and peak diastolic velocity is greater than 140 cm/s.[8] The ratio of internal carotid artery to common carotid artery (ICA/CCA) peak systolic velocity has also been part of various ultrasound diagnostic classifications. A ratio greater than 4 is a great predictor of angiographic stenosis of 70% to 99%. A multispecialty consensus panel has developed a set of criteria for grading carotid stenosis by duplex examination (Table 90.2).[8]

Magnetic resonance angiography (MRA) is increasingly being used to evaluate for atherosclerotic carotid occlusive disease and intracranial circulation. MRA is noninvasive and does not require iodinated contrast agents. MRA utilizes phase contrast or time-of-flight, with either two-dimensional or three-dimensional data sets for greater accuracy. Three-dimensional contrast-enhanced MRA allows data to be obtained in coronal and sagittal planes with improved image quality due to shorter study time. In addition, the new MRA techniques allow for better reformation of images in various planes to allow better grading of stenosis. There have been numerous studies comparing the sensitivity and specificity of MRA for carotid disease to duplex and selective contrast angiography.[9] Magnetic resonance imaging (MRI) of the brain is essential in the assessment of acute stroke patients. MRI with diffusion-weighted imaging (DWI) can differentiate areas of acute ischemia, areas still at risk for ischemia (penumbra), and chronic cerebral ischemic changes. However, computed tomography (CT) imaging remains the most expeditious test in the evaluation of acute stroke patients to rule out intracerebral hemorrhage. Recently, multidetector computed tomography angiography (CTA) has gained

TABLE 90.2

CAROTID DUPLEX ULTRASOUND CRITERIA FOR GRADING INTERNAL CAROTID ARTERY STENOSIS

DEGREE OF STENOSIS (%)	ICA PSV (cm/s)	ICA/CCA PSV RATIO	ICA EDV (cm/s)	PLAQUE ESTIMATE (%)[a]
Normal	<125	<2.0	<40	None
<50	<125	<2.0	<40	<50
50–69	125–230	2.0–4.0	40–100	≥50
≥70 to less than near occlusion	>230	>4.0	>100	≥50
Near occlusion	High, low, or not detected	Variable	Variable	Visible
Total occlusion	Not detected	Not applicable	Not detected	Visible, no lumen

[a]Plaque estimate (diameter reduction) with gray-scale and color Doppler ultrasound.
CCA, common carotid artery; EDV, end-diastolic velocity; ICA, internal carotid artery; PSV, peak systolic velocity.

increasing popularity in the evaluation of carotid disease.[10] This imaging modality can provide volume rendering, which allows rotation of the object with accurate anatomic structures from all angles (Fig. 90.3). The advantages of CTA over MRA include faster data acquisition time and better spatial resolution. However, at the time of this writing, grading of carotid stenosis by CTA requires further validation before it can be widely applied.

Historically, digital substraction angiography (DSA) has been the "gold standard" test to evaluate the extra- and intracranial circulation (Fig. 90.4). This is an invasive procedure, typically performed via a transfemoral puncture, and involves selective imaging of the carotid and vertebral arteries using iodinated contrast. The risk of stroke during cerebral angiography is generally reported at approximately 1% and is typically due to atheroembolization related to wire and catheter manipulation in the aortic arch or proximal branch vessels. Over the past decades, however, the incidence of neurologic complications following angiography has been reduced due to the use of improved guide wires and catheters, better-resolution digital imaging, and increased experience. Local access complications of angiography are infrequent and include development of hematoma, pseudoaneurysm, distal embolization, or acute vessel thrombosis. Currently, selective angiography is particularly used for patients with suspected intracranial disease and for patients in whom percutaneous revascularization is considered. The techniques of carotid angioplasty and stenting for carotid bifurcation occlusive disease are described in detail later in this chapter. We generally use CTA or MRA to gather information about the aortic arch anatomy and presence of concomitant intracranial disease and collateral pathway in planning our strategy for carotid stenting or endarterectomy.

TREATMENT OF CAROTID OCCLUSIVE DISEASE

Conventionally, patients with carotid bifurcation occlusive disease are divided into two broad categories: patients without

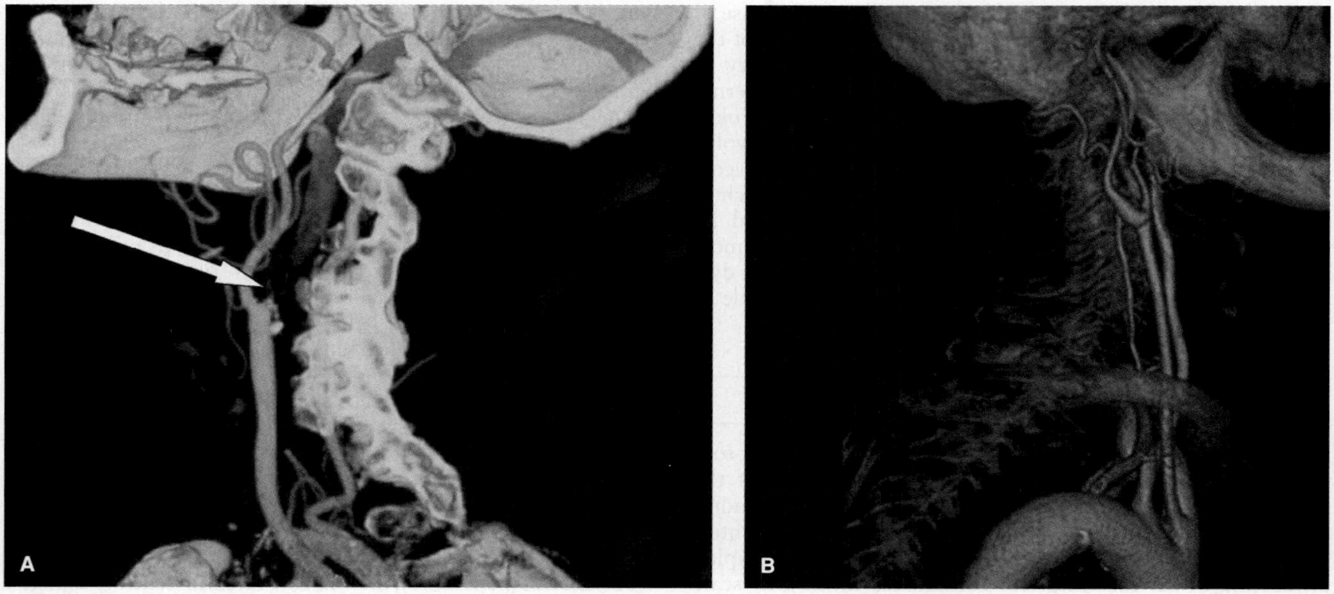

FIGURE 90.3. **A:** Carotid computed tomography angiography is a valuable imaging modality that can provide a three-dimensional image reconstruction with high image resolution. A carotid artery occlusion is noted in the internal carotid artery (*arrow*). **B:** The entire segment of extracranial carotid artery is visualized from the thoracic compartment to the base of the skull.

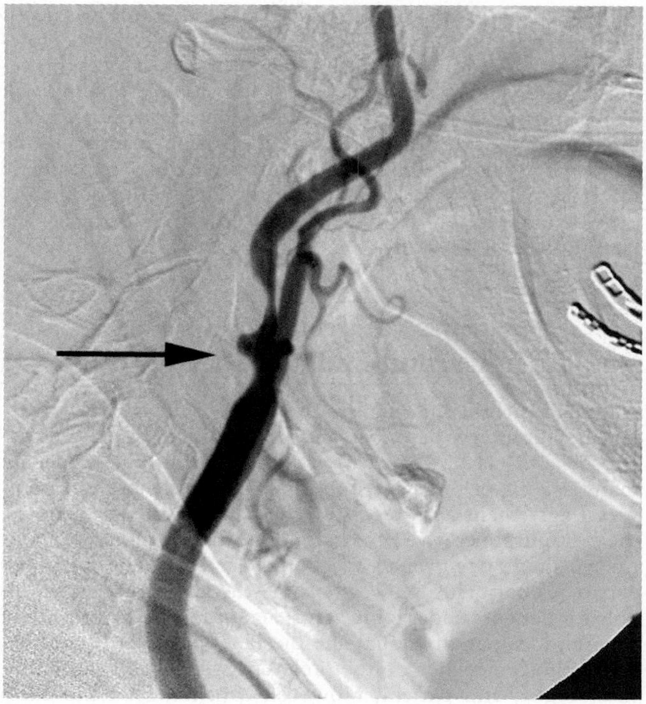

FIGURE 90.4. A carotid angiogram with digital subtraction angiography reveals an ulcerated carotid plaque (*arrow*) in the proximal internal carotid artery, which also resulted in a high-grade internal carotid artery stenosis.

prior history of ipsilateral stroke or TIA (asymptomatic) and those with prior or current ipsilateral neurologic symptoms (symptomatic). It is estimated that 15% of all strokes are preceded by a TIA. The 90-day risk of a stroke in a patient presenting with a TIA is 3% to 17%.[1] According to the Cardiovascular Health Study, a longitudinal population-based study of coronary artery disease and stroke in men and women, the prevalence of TIA in men was 2.7% between the ages of 65 and 69 and 3.6% for ages 75 to 79; the prevalence in women was 1.4% and 4.1%, respectively.[11] There have been several studies reporting on the effectiveness of stroke prevention with medical treatment and carotid endarterectomy for symptomatic patients with moderate to severe carotid stenosis. Early and chronic aspirin therapy has been shown to reduce stroke recurrence rate in several large clinical trials.[12]

Symptomatic Carotid Stenosis

Currently, most neurologists prescribe both aspirin and clopidogrel for secondary stroke prevention in patients who have experienced a TIA or stroke.[1] In patients with symptomatic carotid stenosis, the degree of stenosis appears to be the most important predictor in determining risk for an ipsilateral stroke. The risk of a recurrent ipsilateral stroke in patients with severe carotid stenosis approaches 40%. Two large, multicenter, randomized clinical trials, the European Carotid Surgery Trial (ECST) and the North American Symptomatic Carotid Endarterectomy Trial (NASCET), have both shown a significant risk reduction in stroke for patients with symptomatic high-grade stenosis (70% to 99%) undergoing carotid endarterectomy when compared to medical therapy alone.[13,14] There has been much discussion regarding the different methodology used in the measurement of carotid stenosis and calculation of the life-table data between the two studies leading to similar results.[15] Findings of these two landmark trials have also been reanalyzed in many subsequent publications. The main conclusions of the trials remain validated and widely acknowledged. Briefly, the NASCET study showed that for high-grade carotid stenosis, the cumulative risk of ipsilateral stroke was 26% in the medically treated group and 9% in the surgically treated group at 2 years. For patients with moderate carotid artery stenosis (50% to 69%), the benefit of carotid endarterectomy is less but still favorable when compared to medical treatment alone; the 5-year fatal or nonfatal ipsilateral stroke rate was 16% in the surgically treated group versus 22% in the medically treated group.[16] The risk of stroke was similar for the remaining group of symptomatic patients with less than 50% carotid stenosis, whether they had endarterectomy or medical treatment alone. The ECST reported similar stroke risk reduction for patients with severe symptomatic carotid stenosis and no benefit in patients with mild stenosis when carotid endarterectomy was performed versus medical therapy.[14]

The optimal timing of carotid intervention after acute stroke, however, remains debatable. Earlier studies showed an increased rate of postoperative stroke exacerbation and conversion of a bland to hemorrhagic infarction when carotid endarterectomy was carried out within 5 to 6 weeks after acute stroke. The dismal outcome reported in the early experience was likely related to poor patient selection. The rate of stroke recurrence is not insignificant during the interval period and may be reduced with early intervention for symptomatic carotid stenosis. Contemporary series have demonstrated acceptable low rates of perioperative complications in patients undergoing carotid endarterectomy within 4 weeks after acute stroke.[16] In a recent retrospective series, carotid artery stenting when performed early (<2 weeks) after acute stroke was associated with higher mortality than when delayed (>2 weeks).[17]

Asymptomatic Carotid Stenosis

Whereas there is universal agreement that carotid revascularization (endarterectomy or stenting) is effective in secondary stroke prevention for patients with symptomatic moderate and severe carotid stenosis, the management of asymptomatic patients remains an important controversy. Generally, the detection of carotid stenosis in asymptomatic patients is related to the presence of a cervical bruit or based on screening duplex ultrasound findings. In one of the earlier observational studies, the authors showed that the annual occurrence rate of neurologic symptoms was 4% in a cohort of 167 patients with asymptomatic cervical bruits followed prospectively by serial carotid duplex scan.[18] The mean annual rate of carotid stenosis progression to a greater than 50% stenosis was 8%. The presence of or progression to a greater than 80% stenosis correlated highly with the development of either a total occlusion of the internal carotid artery or new symptoms. The major risk factors associated with disease progression were cigarette smoking, diabetes mellitus, and age. This study supported the contention that it is prudent to follow a conservative course in the management of asymptomatic patients presenting with a cervical bruit.

One of the first randomized clinical trials on the treatment of asymptomatic carotid artery stenosis was the Asymptomatic Carotid Atherosclerosis Study (ACAS), which evaluated the benefits of medical management with antiplatelet therapy versus carotid endarterectomy.[19] Over a 5-year period, the risk of ipsilateral stroke in individuals with a carotid artery stenosis greater than 60% was 5.1% in the surgical arm. On the other hand, the risk of ipsilateral stroke in patients treated with medical management was 11%. Carotid endarterectomy produced a relative risk reduction of 53% over medical management alone. The results of a larger randomized trial from Europe, the Asymptomatic Carotid Surgery Trial (ACST), recently confirmed similar beneficial stroke risk reduction for patients with asymptomatic greater than 70% carotid stenosis undergoing endarterectomy compared to medical therapy.[20] An important point derived from this latter trial was that even with improved medical therapy, including the addition of statin drugs and clopidogrel, medical therapy was still inferior to endarterectomy in primary stroke prevention for patients with high-grade carotid artery stenosis. It is generally agreed that asymptomatic patients with severe carotid stenosis (80% to 99%) are at significantly increased risk for stroke and stand to benefit from either surgical or endovascular revascularization. However, revascularization for asymptomatic patients with a less severe degree of stenosis (60% to 79%) remains controversial.

CAROTID ENDARTERECTOMY VERSUS ANGIOPLASTY AND STENTING

Currently, medical therapy alone is inferior to surgical endarterectomy in stroke prevention for severe carotid stenosis. Now, the debate revolves around whether carotid angioplasty and stenting produces the same benefit that has been demon-
7 strated by carotid endarterectomy. Since carotid artery stenting was approved by the Food and Drug Administration for clinical application in 2004, this percutaneous procedure has become a treatment alternative in patients who are deemed "high risk" for endarterectomy (Table 90.3). In contrast to many endovascular peripheral arterial interventions, percutaneous carotid stenting represents a much more challenging procedure, because it requires complex catheter-based skills utilizing a "0.014" guide wire system and distal embolic protection device. Moreover, current carotid stent devices predominantly utilize the monorail guide wire system, which requires more technical agility, in contrast to the over-the-wire catheter system that is routinely used in peripheral interventions. This percutaneous intervention often requires balloon angioplasty and stent placement through a long carotid guiding sheath via a groin approach. Poor technical skills can result in devastating treatment complications, such as stroke, which can occur due in part to plaque embolization during the balloon angioplasty and stenting of the carotid artery. Because of these various procedural components that require high technical proficiency, many early clinical investigations of carotid artery stenting, which included physicians with little or no carotid stenting experience, resulted in alarmingly poor clinical outcomes. A recent Cochrane review noted that, before 2006, a total of 1,269 patients had been studied in five randomized controlled trials comparing percutaneous carotid intervention and surgical carotid reconstruction.[21] Taken together, these trials revealed that carotid artery stenting had a greater procedural risk of stroke and death when compared to carotid endarterectomy (odds ratio 1.33; 95% confidence interval [CI] 0.86–2.04). Additionally, a greater incidence of carotid restenosis was noted in the stenting group than the endarterectomy cohorts. However, the constant improvement of endovascular devices, procedural techniques, and adjunctive pharmacologic therapy will likely improve the treatment success of percutaneous carotid intervention. Critical appraisals of these trials comparing the efficacy of carotid stenting versus endarterectomy are available for review.[22] Several ongoing clinical trials will undoubtedly provide more insight on the efficacy of carotid stenting in the near future.

Surgical Techniques of Carotid Endarterectomy

Although carotid endarterectomy is one of the earliest vascular operations ever described and its techniques have been perfected in the last two decades, surgeons continue to debate many aspects of this procedure. For instance, there is no universal agreement with regard to the best anesthetic of choice, the best intraoperative cerebral monitoring, whether to "routinely" shunt, open versus eversion endarterectomy, and patch versus primary closure. Various anesthetic options are available for patients undergoing carotid endarterectomy, including general, local, and regional anesthesia. Typically, the anesthesia of choice depends on the preference of the surgeon, anesthesiologist, and patient. However, depending on the anesthetic given, the surgeon must decide whether intraoperative cerebral monitoring is necessary or intra-arterial carotid shunting will be used. In general, if the patient is awake, then his or her ability to respond to commands during the carotid clamp period determines the adequacy of collateral flow to the ipsilateral hemisphere. On the other hand, intraoperative electroencephalogram (EEG) or transcranial power Doppler (TCD) has been used to monitor for adequacy of cerebral perfusion during the clamp period for patients undergoing surgery under general anesthesia. Focal ipsilateral decreases in amplitudes and slowing of EEG waves are indicative of cerebral ischemia. Similarly, a decrease to less than 50% of baseline velocity in the ipsilateral middle cerebral artery is a sign of cerebral ischemia. For patients with poor collateral flow exhibiting signs of cerebral ischemia, intra-arterial carotid shunting with removal of the clamp will restore cerebral flow for the remaining part of the surgery. Stump pressures have also been used to determine the need for intra-arterial carotid shunting. Some surgeons prefer to shunt all patients on a routine basis and do not use intraoperative cerebral monitoring.

To perform a carotid endarterectomy, the patient's neck is slightly hyperextended and turned to the contralateral side, with a roll placed between the shoulder blades. An oblique incision is made along the anterior border of the sternocleidomastoid

TABLE 90.3

CONDITIONS QUALIFYING PATIENTS AS "HIGH SURGICAL RISK" FOR CAROTID ENDARTERECTOMY

■ ANATOMIC FACTORS	■ PHYSIOLOGIC FACTORS
■ High carotid bifurcation (above C2 vertebral body)	■ Age ≥80 y
■ Low common carotid artery (below clavicle)	■ Left ventricular ejection fraction ≤30%
■ Contralateral carotid occlusion	■ New York Heart Association class III/IV congestive heart failure
■ Restenosis of ipsilateral prior carotid endarterectomy	■ Unstable angina: Canadian Cardiovascular Society class III/IV angina pectoris
■ Previous neck irradiation	■ Recent myocardial infarction
■ Prior radical neck dissection	■ Clinically significant cardiac disease (congestive heart failure, abnormal stress test, or need for coronary revascularization)
■ Contralateral laryngeal nerve palsy	■ Severe chronic obstructive pulmonary disease
■ Presence of tracheostomy	■ End-stage renal disease on dialysis

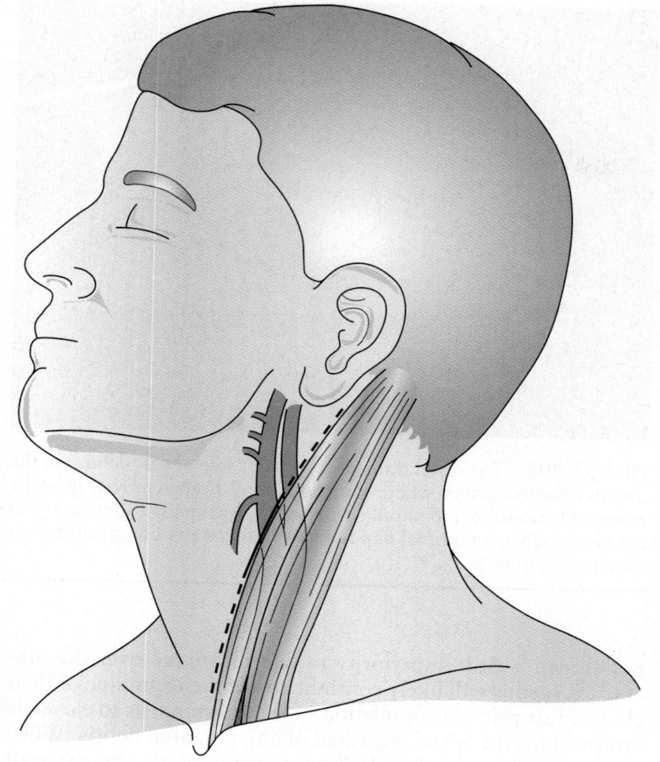

FIGURE 90.5. To perform carotid endarterectomy, the patient's neck is slightly hyperextended and turned to the contralateral side. An oblique incision is made along the anterior border of the sternocleidomastoid muscle centered on top of the carotid bifurcation.

muscle centered on top of the carotid bifurcation (Fig. 90.5). The platysma is divided completely. Typically, tributaries of the anterior jugular vein are ligated and divided. The dissection is carried medial to the sternocleidomastoid. The superior belly of the omohyoid muscle is usually encountered just anterior to the common carotid artery. This muscle can be divided. The carotid fascia is incised and the common carotid artery is exposed. The common carotid artery is mobilized cephalad toward the bifurcation. The dissection of the carotid bifurcation can cause reactive bradycardia related to stimulation of the carotid body. This reflex can be blunted with injection of 1% lidocaine into the carotid body or reversed with administration of intravenous atropine. A useful landmark in the dissection of the carotid bifurcation is the common facial vein. This vein can be ligated and divided. Frequently the 12th cranial nerve (hypoglossal nerve) traverses the carotid bifurcation just behind the common facial vein. The external carotid artery is mobilized just enough to get a clamp across. Often, a branch of the external carotid artery crossing to the sternocleidomastoid can be divided to allow further cephalad mobilization of the internal carotid artery. For high carotid bifurcations, division of the posterior belly of the digastric muscle is helpful in establishing distal exposure of the internal carotid artery.

Intravenous heparin sulfate (1 mg/kg) is routinely administered just prior to carotid clamping. The internal carotid artery is clamped first using a soft noncrushing vascular clamp to prevent distal embolization. The external and common carotid arteries are clamped subsequently. A longitudinal arteriotomy is made in the distal common carotid artery and extended into the bulb and past the occlusive plaque into the normal part of the internal carotid artery. Endarterectomy is carried out to remove the occlusive plaque (Fig. 90.6). If necessary, a temporary shunt can be inserted from the common carotid artery to

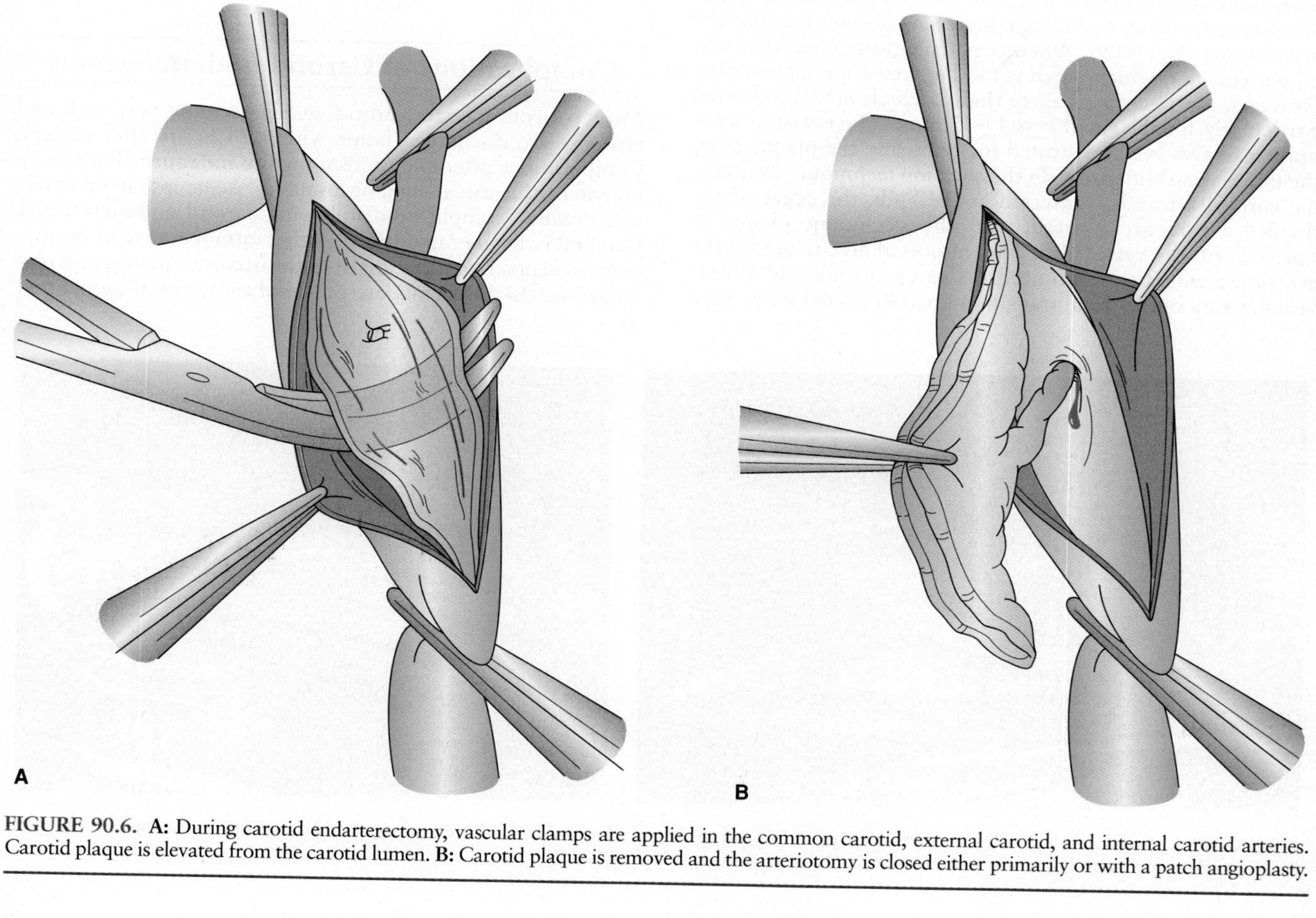

FIGURE 90.6. **A:** During carotid endarterectomy, vascular clamps are applied in the common carotid, external carotid, and internal carotid arteries. Carotid plaque is elevated from the carotid lumen. **B:** Carotid plaque is removed and the arteriotomy is closed either primarily or with a patch angioplasty.

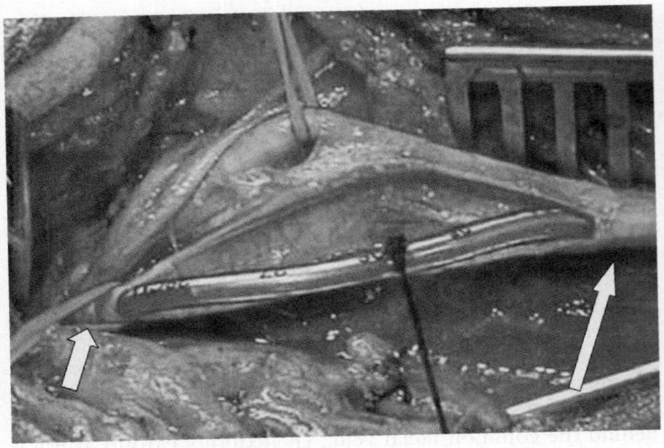

FIGURE 90.7. A temporary carotid shunt is inserted from the common carotid artery (*long arrow*) to the internal carotid artery (*short arrow*) during carotid endarterectomy to provide continuous antegrade cerebral blood flow.

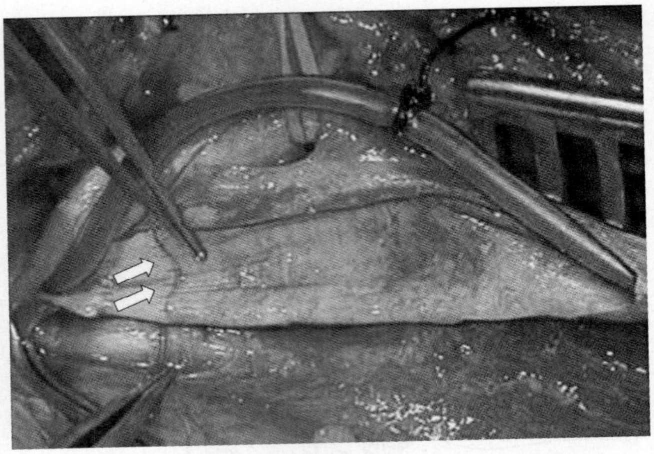

FIGURE 90.8. The distal transition line (*left side of the picture*) in the internal carotid artery where the plaque had been removed must be examined carefully and should be smooth. Tacking sutures (*arrows*) are placed when an intimal flap remains in this transition to ensure no obstruction to flow.

the internal carotid artery to maintain continuous antegrade cerebral blood flow (Fig. 90.7). Typically, a plane is teased out from the vessel wall and the entire plaque is elevated and removed. The distal transition line in the internal carotid artery where the plaque had been removed must be examined carefully and should be smooth. Tacking sutures are often placed when an intimal flap remains in this transition to ensure no obstruction to flow (Fig. 90.8). The occlusive plaque is usually removed from the origin of the external carotid artery using the eversion technique. The endarterectomized surface is then irrigated and any debris removed. A patch (autogenous saphenous vein; synthetic material, such as polyester or polytetrafluoroethylene; or biologic material) is sewn to close the arteriotomy (Fig. 90.9). Whether patch closure is necessary in all patients and which patch is the best remain controversial. However, most surgeons agree that patch closure is indicated particularly for the small vessel (<7 mm). The eversion technique has also been advocated for removing the plaque from the internal carotid artery. In the eversion technique, the internal carotid artery is transected at the bulb, the edges of the divided vessel are everted, and the occluding plaque is "peeled" off the vessel wall. The purported advantages of the eversion technique are no need for patch closure and a clear visualization of the distal transition area. Reported series have not shown a clear superiority of one technique over the others.[23] Surgeons will likely continue to use the technique of their choice. Just prior to completion of the anastomosis to close the arteriotomy, the vessel is flushed of any potential debris. When the arteriotomy is closed, flow is restored to the external carotid artery first and to the internal carotid artery second. Intravenous protamine sulfate can be given to reverse the effect of heparin anticoagulation following carotid endarterectomy. The wound is closed in layers. After surgery, the patient's neurologic condition is asserted in the operating room prior to transfer to the recovery area.

Complications of Carotid Endarterectomy

Most patients tolerate carotid endarterectomy very well and typically are discharged home within 24 hours after surgery. Complications after endarterectomy are infrequent but can be potentially life threatening or disabling. Acute ipsilateral stroke is a dreaded complication following carotid endarterectomy. Cerebral ischemia can be due to either intraoperative or postoperative events. Embolization from the occlusive plaque and prolonged cerebral ischemia are potential causes of intraoperative

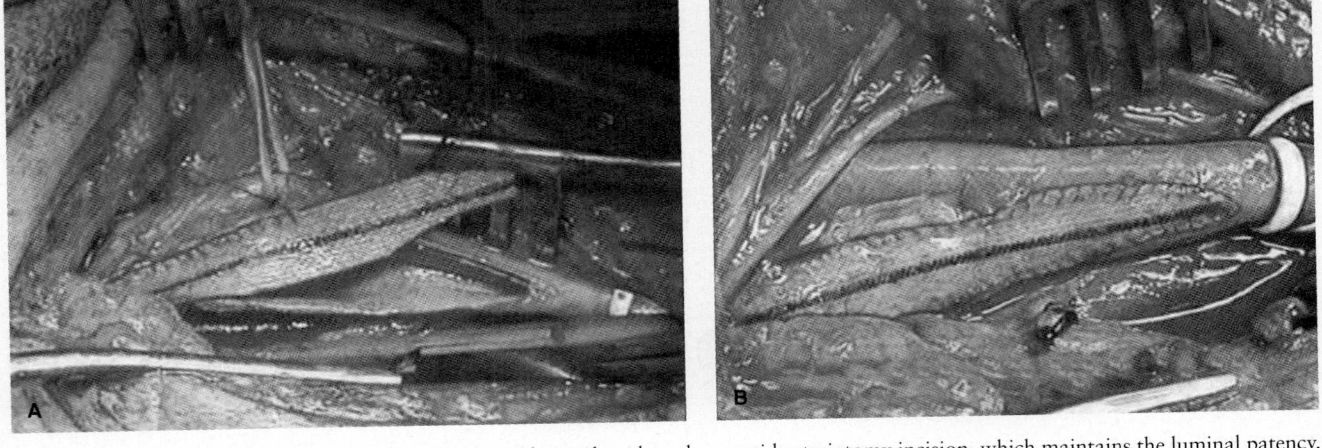

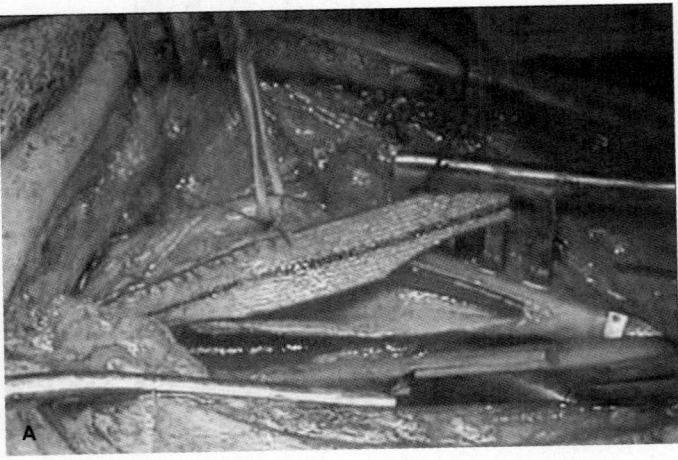

FIGURE 90.9. **A:** An autologous or synthetic patch can be used to close the carotid arteriotomy incision, which maintains the luminal patency. **B:** A completion closure of carotid endarterectomy incision using a synthetic patch.

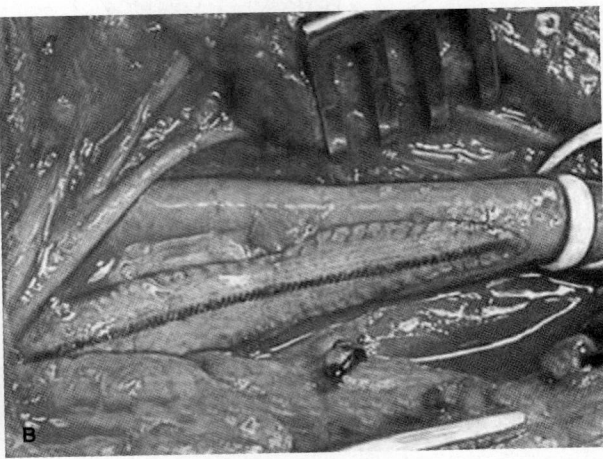

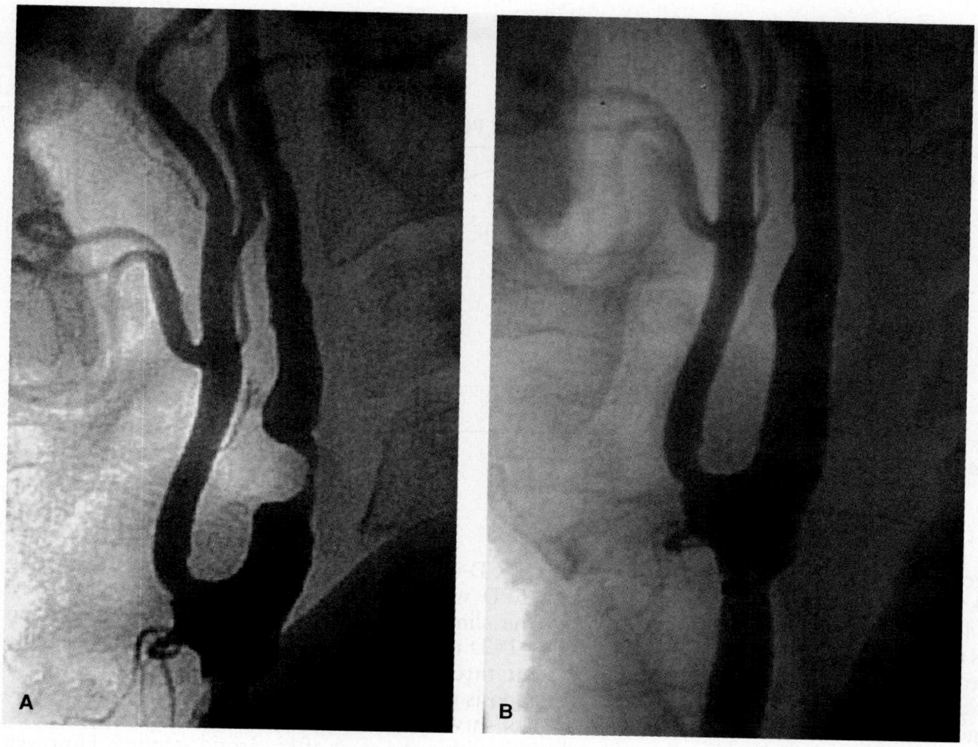

FIGURE 90.10. **A:** Carotid angiogram demonstrated a high-grade stenosis of the left internal carotid artery. **B:** Completion angiogram demonstrated a satisfactory result following a carotid stent placement.

stroke, with the most common cause of postoperative stroke being embolization. Less frequently, acute carotid artery occlusion can cause acute postoperative stroke. This is usually due to carotid artery thrombosis related to closure of the arteriotomy, an occluding intimal flap, or distal carotid dissection. When patients experience acute symptoms of neurologic ischemia after endarterectomy, immediate intervention may be indicated. Carotid duplex scan can be done expeditiously to assess patency of the extracranial internal carotid artery. Reexploration is mandated for acute carotid artery occlusion. Cerebral angiography can be useful if intracranial revascularization is considered.

Local complications related to surgery include excessive bleeding and cranial nerve palsies. Postoperative hematoma in the neck after carotid endarterectomy can lead to devastating airway compromise. Any expanding hematoma should be evacuated and active bleeding stopped. Securing an airway is critical and can be extremely difficult in patients with a large postoperative neck hematoma. The reported incidence of postoperative cranial nerve palsies after carotid endarterectomy varies from 1% to 30%.[24] Well-recognized injuries involve the marginal mandibular, vagus, hypoglossal, superior laryngeal, and recurrent laryngeal nerves. Often these are traction injuries, but they can also be due to severance of the nerve.

TABLE 90.4

UNFAVORABLE CAROTID ANGIOGRAPHIC APPEARANCE IN WHICH CAROTID STENTING SHOULD BE AVOIDED

- Extensive carotid calcification
- Polypoid or globular carotid lesions
- Severe tortuosity of the common carotid artery
- Long-segment stenoses (>2 cm in length)
- Carotid artery occlusion
- Severe intraluminal thrombus (angiographic defects)
- Extensive middle cerebral artery atherosclerosis

Techniques of Carotid Angioplasty and Stenting

Percutaneous carotid artery stenting has become an accepted alternative treatment in the management of "high-risk" patients with carotid bifurcation disease (Fig. 90.10). The perceived advantages of percutaneous carotid revascularization are related to the minimal invasiveness of the procedure compared to surgery. There are anatomic conditions based on angiographic evaluation in which carotid artery stenting should be avoided due to increased procedural-related risks (Table 90.4). In preparation for carotid stenting, the patient should be given oral clopidogrel 3 days prior to the intervention. The procedure is done in either the operating room with angiographic capabilities or in a dedicated angiography room. The patient is placed in the supine position. The patient's blood pressure and cardiac rhythm are closely monitored.

To gain access to the carotid artery, a retrograde transfemoral approach is most commonly used as the access site for carotid intervention. Using the Seldinger technique, a diagnostic 5- or 6-French sheath is inserted in the common femoral artery. A diagnostic arch aortogram is obtained. The carotid artery to be treated is then selected using a 5-French diagnostic catheter and contrast is injected to show the carotid anatomy. It is important to assess the contralateral carotid artery, vertebrobasilar circulation, and intracranial circulation if these are not known based on the preoperative noninvasive studies. Once the decision is made to proceed with carotid artery stenting, with the tip of the diagnostic catheter still in the common carotid artery, a 0.035-inch 260-cm-long stiff glide wire is placed in the ipsilateral external carotid artery. Anticoagulation with intravenous bivalirudin bolus (0.75 mg/kg) followed by an infusion rate of 2.5 mg/kg/h or heparin (1 mg/kg) for the remainder of the procedure is routinely administered. Next, the diagnostic catheter is withdrawn and a 90-cm 6-French guiding sheath is advanced into the common carotid artery over the stiff glide wire. It is critical not to advance the sheath beyond the occlusive plaque in the carotid bulb. The stiff wire is then removed and preparation is made

TABLE 90.5

COMMONLY USED EMBOLIC PROTECTION DEVICES (EPDs)

MECHANISM	NAME OF EPD	PORE SIZE (MICRONS)
Distal balloon occlusion	PercuSurge Guard Wire, Export catheter (Medtronic)	NA
Distal filter	Angioguard (Cordis)	100
	Accunet (Abbott)	150
	Emboshield (Abbott)	140
	FilterWire (Boston Scientific)	110
	SpiderRx (EV3)	<100
Flow reversal[a]	Parodi Neuro Protection (Gore)	NA

[a]Currently in clinical trial (EMPIRE) in United States.

to deploy the distal embolic protection device (EPD). Several distal EPDs are available (Table 90.5). The EPD device is carefully deployed beyond the target lesion. With regard to the carotid stent, there are several stents that have received approval from the Food and Drug Administration and are commercially available for carotid revascularization (Table 90.6). All current carotid stents use the rapid-exchange monorail 0.014-inch platform. The size selection is typically based on the size of the common carotid artery. Predilatation using a 4-mm balloon may be necessary to allow passage of the stent delivery catheter. Once the stent is deployed across the occlusive plaque, postdilatation is usually performed using a 5.5-mm or smaller balloon. It's noteworthy that balloon dilation of the carotid bulb may lead to immediate bradycardia due to stimulation of the glossopharyngeal nerve. The EPD is then retrieved and the procedure is completed with removal of the sheath from the femoral artery. The puncture site is closed using an available closure device or with manual compression. Throughout the procedure, the patient's neurologic function is closely monitored. The bivalirudin infusion is stopped or heparin is reversed with protamine, and the patient is maintained on clopidogrel (75 mg daily) for at least 1 month and on aspirin indefinitely.

Complications of Carotid Stenting

Although there have been no randomized trials comparing carotid stenting with and without EPD, the availability of embolic protection devices appears to have reduced the risk of distal embolization and stroke. The results of the various clinical trials and registries of carotid stenting have been reported and compared. It is well known that distal embolization as detected by TCD is much more frequent with carotid stenting even with EPD when compared to carotid endarterectomy. However, the clinical significance of the distal embolization detected by TCD is not clear as most are asymptomatic. Acute carotid stent thrombosis is rare. The incidence of in-stent carotid restenosis is not well known but is estimated at 10% to 30%. Duplex surveillance frequently shows elevated peak systolic velocities within the stent after carotid stenting. However, velocity criteria are being formulated to determine the severity of in-stent restenosis after carotid stenting by duplex ultrasound.[25] It appears that systolic velocities exceeding 300 to 400 cm/s would represent greater than 70% to 80% restenosis. Bradycardia and hypotension occur in up to 20% of patients undergoing carotid stenting.[26] Systemic administration of atropine is usually effective in reversing the bradycardia. Other technical complications of carotid stenting are infrequent and include carotid artery dissection and access site complications, such as groin hematoma, femoral artery pseudoaneurysm, distal embolization, and acute femoral artery thrombosis.

NONATHEROSCLEROTIC DISEASE OF THE CAROTID ARTERY

Carotid Coil and Kink

A carotid coil consists of an excessive elongation of the internal carotid artery producing tortuosity of the vessel (Fig. 90.11). Embryologically, the carotid artery is derived from the third aortic arch and dorsal aortic root, and is uncoiled as the heart and great vessels descend into the mediastinum. In children,

TABLE 90.6

CURRENTLY APPROVED CAROTID STENTS IN THE UNITED STATES

NAME OF STENT	MANUFACTURER	CELL DESIGN	TAPERED STENT	DELIVERY SYSTEM SIZE (FRENCH)
Acculink	Abbott	Open	Yes	6
Exact	Abbott	Closed	Yes	6
NexStent	Boston Scientific	Closed	Self-tapering	5
Protégé RX	EV3	Open	Yes	6
Precise RX	Cordis	Open	No	6
Exponent	Medtronic	Open	No	6

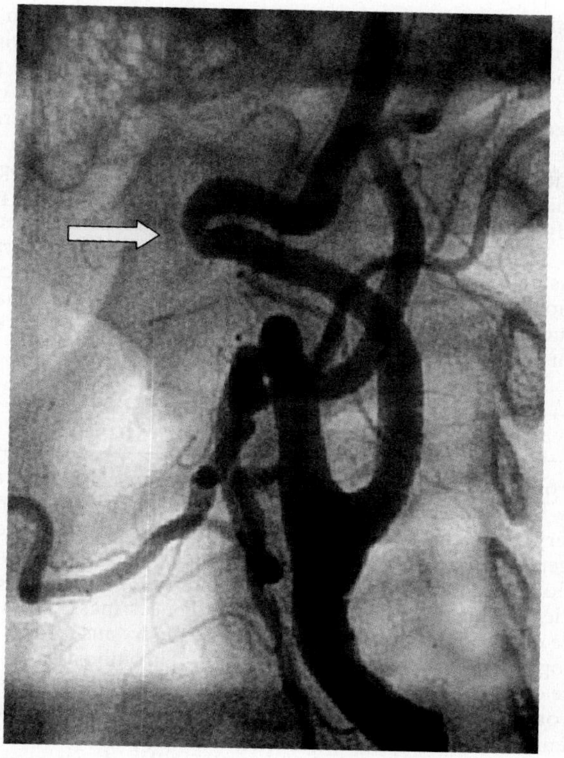

FIGURE 90.11. Excessive elongation of the carotid artery can result in carotid kinking (*arrow*), which can compromise cerebral blood flow and lead to cerebral ischemia.

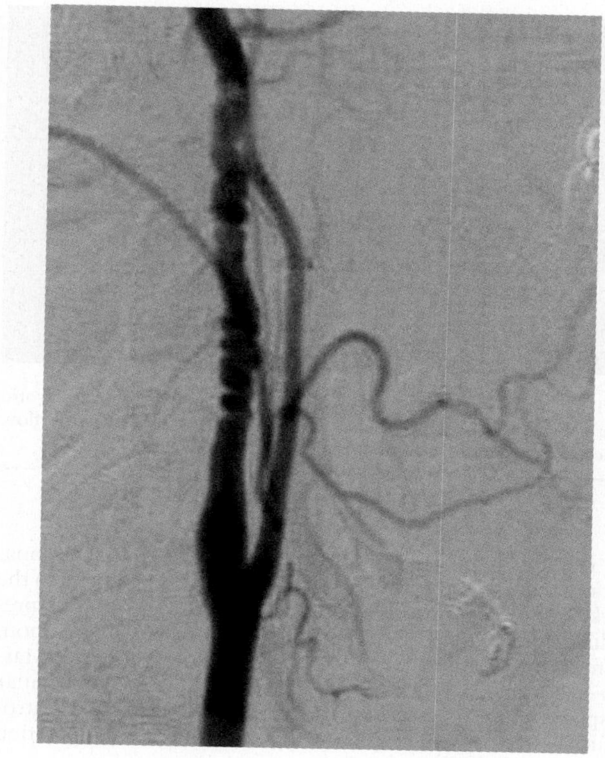

FIGURE 90.12. A carotid fibromuscular dysplasia with typical characteristics of multiple stenosis with intervening aneurysmal outpouching dilatations. The disease involves the media with the smooth muscle being replaced by fibrous connective tissue.

carotid coils appear to be congenital in origin. In contrast, elongation and kinking of the carotid artery in adults is associated with the loss of elasticity and an abrupt angulation of the vessel. Kinking is more common in women than men. Cerebral ischemic symptoms caused by kinks of the carotid artery are similar to those from atherosclerotic carotid lesions, but are more likely due to cerebral hypoperfusion than embolic episodes. Classically, sudden head rotation, flexion, or extension can accentuate the kink and provoke ischemic symptoms. Most carotid kinks and coils are found incidentally on carotid duplex scan. However, interpretation of the Doppler frequency shifts and spectral analysis in tortuous carotid arteries can be difficult because of the uncertain angle of insonation. Cerebral angiography, with multiple views taken in neck flexion, extension, and rotation, is useful in the determination of the clinical significance of kinks and coils.

Fibromuscular Dysplasia

Fibromuscular dysplasia (FMD) usually involves medium-sized arteries that are long and have few branches (Fig. 90.12). Women in the fourth or fifth decade of life are more commonly affected than men. Hormonal effects on the vessel wall are thought to play a role in the pathogenesis of FMD. FMD of the carotid artery is commonly bilateral, and in about 20% of patients, the vertebral artery is also involved.[27] An intracranial saccular aneurysm of the carotid siphon or middle cerebral artery can be identified in up to 50% of the patients with FMD. Four histologic types of FMD have been described in the literature. The most common type is medial fibroplasias, which may present as a focal stenosis or multiple lesions with intervening aneurysmal outpouchings. The disease involves the media with the smooth muscle being replaced by fibrous connective tissue. Commonly, mural dilations and microaneurysms can be seen with this type of FMD. Medial hyperplasia is a rare type of FMD with the media demonstrating excessive amounts of smooth muscle. Intimal fibroplasia accounts for 5% of all cases and occurs equally in both sexes. The media and adventitia remain normal and there is accumulation of subendothelial mesenchymal cells with a loose matrix of connective tissue causing a focal stenosis in adults. Finally, premedial dysplasia represents a type of FMD with elastic tissue accumulating between the media and adventitia. FMD can also involve the renal and external iliac arteries. It is estimated that approximately 40% of patients with FMD present with a TIA due to embolization of platelet aggregates.[27] DSA demonstrates the characteristic "string of beads" pattern, which represents alternating segments of stenosis and dilatation. The string of beads can also be shown noninvasively by CTA or MRA. FMD should be suspected when an increased velocity is detected across a stenotic segment without associated atherosclerotic changes on carotid duplex ultrasound. Antiplatelet medication is the generally accepted therapy for asymptomatic lesions. Endovascular treatment is recommended for patients with documented lateralizing symptoms. Surgical correction is rarely indicated.

Carotid Artery Dissection

Dissection of the carotid artery accounts for approximately 20% of strokes in patients younger than 45 years of age. The etiology and pathogenesis of spontaneous carotid artery dissection remains incompletely understood. Arterial dissection involves hemorrhage within the media, which can extend into the subadventitial and subintimal layers. When the dissection extends into the subadventitial space, there is an increased risk of aneurysm formation. Subintimal dissections can lead to intramural clot or thrombosis. Traumatic dissection is typically

VASCULAR

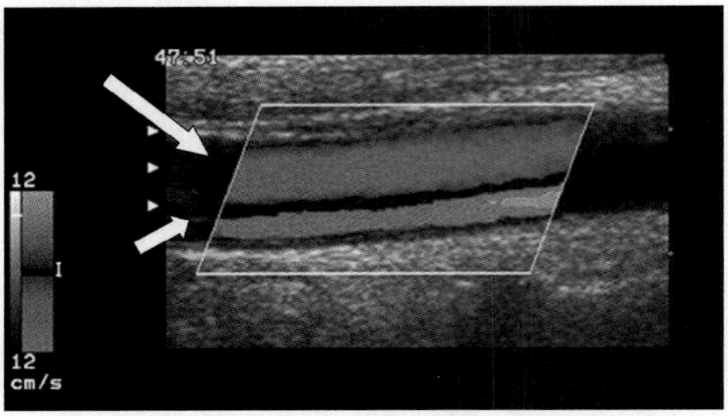

FIGURE 90.13. Carotid ultrasound reveals a patient with a carotid artery dissection in which carotid flow is separated in the true flow lumen (*long arrow*) from the false lumen (*short arrow*).

the result of hyperextension of the neck during blunt trauma, neck manipulation, strangulation, or penetrating injuries to the neck. Even in supposedly spontaneous cases, a history of preceding unrecognized minor neck trauma is not uncommon. Connective disorders, such as Ehlers-Danlos syndrome, Marfan syndrome, α_1-antitrypsin deficiency, and fibromuscular dysplasia, may predispose to carotid artery dissection. Iatrogenic dissections can also occur due to catheter manipulation or balloon angioplasty.

Typical clinical features of carotid artery dissection include unilateral neck pain, headache, and ipsilateral Horner syndrome in up to 50% of patients, followed by manifestations of cerebral or ocular ischemia and cranial nerve palsies. Neurologic deficits can result because of either hemodynamic failure (caused by luminal stenosis) or an artery-to-artery thromboembolism. The ischemia may cause TIAs or infarctions, or both. Catheter angiography has been the method of choice to diagnose arterial dissections, but with the advent of duplex ultrasonography, MRI/MRA, and CTA, most dissections can now be diagnosed using noninvasive imaging modalities (Fig. 90.13). The dissection typically starts in the internal carotid artery distal to the bulb. Uncommonly, the dissection can start in the common carotid artery or be an extension of a more proximal aortic dissection. Medical therapy has been the accepted primary treatment of symptomatic carotid artery dissection. Anticoagulation (heparin and warfarin) and antiplatelet therapy have been commonly used, although there have not been any randomized studies to evaluate their effectiveness. The prognosis depends on the severity of the neurologic deficit but is generally good in extracranial dissections. The recurrence rate is low. Therapeutic interventions have been reserved for recurrent TIAs or strokes or failure of medical treatment. Endovascular options include intra-arterial stenting, coiling of associated pseudoaneurysms, or, more recently, deployment of covered stents.

Carotid Artery Aneurysms

Carotid artery aneurysms are rare, encountered in less than 1% of all carotid operations (Fig. 90.14). The true carotid artery aneurysm is generally due to atherosclerosis or medial degeneration. The carotid bulb is involved in most carotid aneurysms, and bilaterality is present in 12% of patients. Patients typically present with a pulsatile neck mass. The available data suggest that, untreated, these aneurysms lead to neurologic symptoms from embolization. Thrombosis and rupture of the carotid aneurysm are rare. Pseudoaneurysms of the carotid artery can result from injury or infection. Mycotic aneurysms often involve a past history of syphilis but are now more commonly associated with peritonsillar abscesses caused by *Staphylococcus aureus* infection. Fibromuscular dysplasia and spontaneous dissection of the carotid artery can lead to the formation of true aneurysms or pseudoaneurysms. Whereas conventional surgery has been the primary mode of treatment in the past, carotid aneurysms are currently being treated more commonly using endovascular approaches.[28]

Carotid Body Tumor

The carotid body originates from the third branchial arch and from neuroectodermal-derived neural crest lineage. The

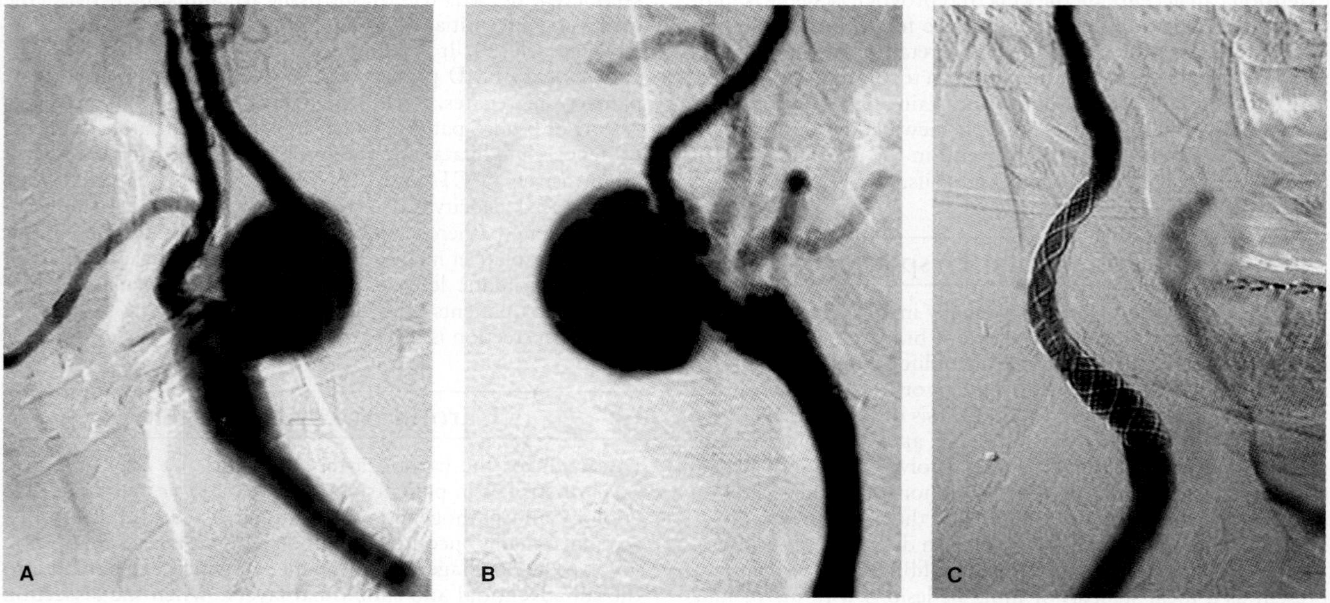

FIGURE 90.14. **A:** An anteroposterior angiogram of the neck revealing a carotid artery aneurysm. **B:** A lateral projection of the carotid artery aneurysm. **C:** Following endovascular stent graft placement, the carotid artery aneurysm is successfully excluded.

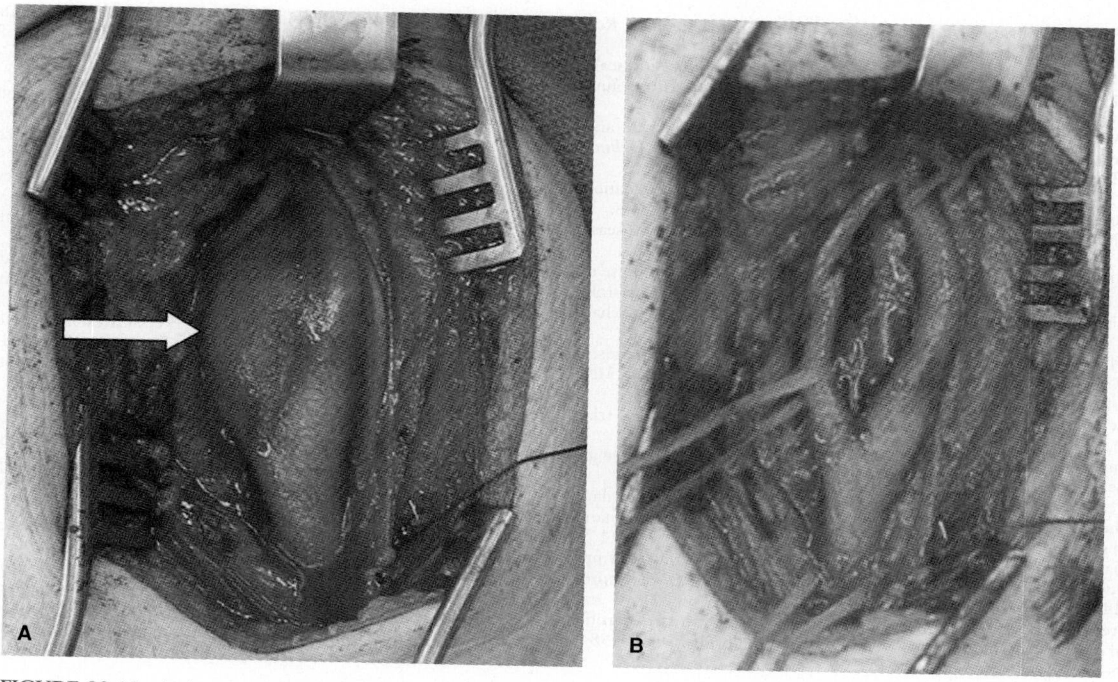

FIGURE 90.15. **A:** A carotid body tumor (*arrow*) located adjacent to the carotid bulb. **B:** Following periadventitial dissection, the carotid body tumor is removed.

normal carotid body is located in the adventitia or periadventitial tissue at the bifurcation of the common carotid artery (Fig. 90.15). The gland is innervated by the glossopharyngeal nerve. Its blood supply is derived predominantly from the external carotid artery but can also come from the vertebral artery. Carotid body tumor is a rare lesion of the neuroendocrine system. Other glands of neural crest origin are seen in the neck, parapharyngeal spaces, mediastinum, retroperitoneum, and adrenal medulla. Tumors involving these structures have been referred to as paraganglioma, glomus tumor, or chemodectoma. Approximately 5% to 7% of carotid body tumors are malignant. Although chronic hypoxemia has been invoked as a stimulus for hyperplasia of the carotid body, approximately 35% of carotid body tumors are hereditary. The risk of malignancy is greatest in young patients with familial tumors.

Symptoms related to the endocrine products of the carotid body tumor are rare. Patients usually present between the fifth and seventh decades of life with an asymptomatic lateral neck mass. The diagnosis of carotid body tumor requires confirmation on imaging studies. Carotid duplex scanning can localize the tumor to the carotid bifurcation, but CT or MRI is usually required to further delineate the relationship of the tumor to the adjacent structures. Classically, a carotid body tumor will widen the carotid bifurcation. The Shamblin classification describes the tumor extent: I, tumor is less than 5 cm and relatively free of vessel involvement; II, tumor is intimately involved but does not encase the vessel wall; and III, tumor is intramural and encases the carotid vessels and adjacent nerves.[29] With good-resolution CT and MRI, arteriography is usually not required. However, arteriography can provide an assessment of vessel invasion and intracranial circulation, and allows for preoperative embolization of feeder vessels, which has been reported to reduce intraoperative blood loss. Surgical resection is the recommended treatment for suspected carotid body tumor.

Carotid Trauma

Blunt or penetrating trauma to the neck can cause injury to the carotid artery. Notwithstanding the massive bleeding from carotid artery transection, injury to the carotid artery can result in carotid dissection, thrombosis, or pseudoaneurysm formation. Carotid duplex ultrasound can be useful to locate the site of injury in the cervical segment of the carotid artery. Spiral CTA has become the modality of choice to detect extracranial carotid artery injury. Confirmation of carotid injury by contrast cerebral angiography remains the "gold standard" diagnostic test. Injuries to the cervical segment of the common and internal carotid arteries can be repaired surgically. Acute carotid artery thrombosis is usually treated medically with anticoagulation if the patient is asymptomatic. Revascularization should be considered for patients presenting with ongoing cerebral ischemia related to carotid artery thrombosis. Traumatic carotid artery dissection can cause cerebral ischemia due to thromboembolization, decreased flow, or thrombosis. Commonly, the dissection involves the distal portion of the cervical and petrous segment of the internal carotid artery. Medical management with antiplatelet or anticoagulation therapy is usually adequate for uncomplicated traumatic carotid dissection. In patients with pseudoaneurysms of the carotid artery that are located in a segment that is out of surgical reach, the use of selective coil embolization of the pseudoaneurysm or exclusion of the pseudoaneurysm by a covered stent graft has been reported. Bare-metal stents have been used with success in the treatment of traumatic carotid artery dissection.

References

1. Donnan GA, Fisher M, Macleod M, et al. Stroke. *Lancet* 2008;371:1612–1623.
2. Debakey ME, Crawford ES, Cooley DA, et al. Cerebral arterial insufficiency: one to 11-year results following arterial reconstructive operation. *Ann Surg* 1965;161:921–945.
3. O'Rourke F, Dean N, Akhtar N, et al. Current and future concepts in stroke prevention. *CMAJ* 2004;170:1123–1133.
4. Kastrup A, Schnaudigel S, Wasser K, et al. Carotid artery disease: stenting versus endarterectomy. *Curr Atheroscler Rep* 2008;10:391–397.
5. Cucchiara B, Ross M. Transient ischemic attack: risk stratification and treatment. *Ann Emerg Med* 2008;52:S27–S39.
6. Naylor AR, Mehta Z, Rothwell PM, et al. Carotid artery disease and stroke during coronary artery bypass: a critical review of the literature. *Eur J Vasc Endovasc Surg* 2002;23:283–294.

7. Touze E. Natural history of asymptomatic carotid artery stenosis. *Rev Neurol (Paris)* 2008;164:793–800.
8. Grant EG, Benson CB, Moneta GL, et al. Carotid artery stenosis: grayscale and Doppler ultrasound diagnosis—Society of Radiologists in Ultrasound consensus conference. *Ultrasound Q* 2003;19:190–198.
9. Wardlaw JM, Chappell FM, Stevenson M, et al. Accurate, practical and cost-effective assessment of carotid stenosis in the UK. *Health Technol Assess* 2006;10:iii–iv, ix–x, 1–182.
10. Saba L, Mallarini G. MDCTA of carotid plaque degree of stenosis: evaluation of interobserver agreement. *AJR Am J Roentgenol* 2008;190:W41–W46.
11. Price TR, Psaty B, O'Leary D, et al. Assessment of cerebrovascular disease in the Cardiovascular Health Study. *Ann Epidemiol* 1993;3:504–507.
12. Chen ZM, Sandercock P, Pan HC, et al. Indications for early aspirin use in acute ischemic stroke: a combined analysis of 40 000 randomized patients from the Chinese Acute Stroke Trial and the International Stroke Trial. On behalf of the CAST and IST collaborative groups. *Stroke* 2000;31:1240–1249.
13. Kita MW. Carotid endarterectomy in symptomatic carotid stenosis: NASCET comparative results at 30 months of follow-up. *J Insur Med* 1992;24:42–46.
14. Warlow CP. Symptomatic patients: the European Carotid Surgery Trial (ECST). *J Mal Vasc* 1993;18:198–201.
15. Strandness DE, Eikelboom BC. Carotid artery stenosis—where do we go from here? *Eur J Ultrasound* 1998;7(suppl 3):S17–S26.
16. Rothwell PM, Eliasziw M, Gutnikov SA, et al. Analysis of pooled data from the randomised controlled trials of endarterectomy for symptomatic carotid stenosis. *Lancet* 2003;361:107–116.
17. Topakian R, Strasak AM, Sonnberger M, et al. Timing of stenting of symptomatic carotid stenosis is predictive of 30-day outcome. *Eur J Neurol* 2007;14:672–678.
18. Roederer GO, Langlois YE, Jager KA, et al. The natural history of carotid arterial disease in asymptomatic patients with cervical bruits. *Stroke* 1984; 15:605–613.
19. Fisher M, Martin A, Cosgrove M, et al. The NASCET-ACAS plaque project. North American Symptomatic Carotid Endarterectomy Trial. Asymptomatic Carotid Atherosclerosis Study. *Stroke* 1993;24:I24–I25; discussion I31–I32.
20. Halliday A, Mansfield A, Marro J, et al. Prevention of disabling and fatal strokes by successful carotid endarterectomy in patients without recent neurological symptoms: randomised controlled trial. *Lancet* 2004;363: 1491–1502.
21. Coward LJ, Featherstone RL, Brown MM. Safety and efficacy of endovascular treatment of carotid artery stenosis compared with carotid endarterectomy: a Cochrane systematic review of the randomized evidence. *Stroke* 2005;36:905–911.
22. Lin PH, Barshes NR, Annambhotla S, et al. Prospective randomized trials of carotid artery stenting versus carotid endarterectomy: an appraisal of the current literature. *Vasc Endovasc Surg* 2008;42:5–11.
23. Crawford RS, Chung TK, Hodgman T, et al. Restenosis after eversion vs patch closure carotid endarterectomy. *J Vasc Surg* 2007;46:41–48.
24. Organ N, Walker PJ, Jenkins J, et al. 15 year experience of carotid endarterectomy at the Royal Brisbane and Women's Hospital: outcomes and changing trends in management. *Eur J Vasc Endovasc Surg* 2008;35:273–279.
25. Zhou W, Felkai DD, Evans M, et al. Ultrasound criteria for severe in-stent restenosis following carotid artery stenting. *J Vasc Surg* 2008;47:74–80.
26. Lin PH, Zhou W, Kougias P, et al. Factors associated with hypotension and bradycardia after carotid angioplasty and stenting. *J Vasc Surg* 2007;46: 846–853; discussion 853–854.
27. Plouin PF, Perdu J, La Batide-Alanore A, et al. Fibromuscular dysplasia. *Orphanet J Rare Dis* 2007;2:28.
28. Zhou W, Lin PH, Bush RL, et al. Carotid artery aneurysm: evolution of management over two decades. *J Vasc Surg* 2006;43:493–496; discussion 497.
29. Athanasiou A, Liappis CD, Rapidis AD, et al. Carotid body tumor: review of the literature and report of a case with a rare sensorineural symptomatology. *J Oral Maxillofac Surg* 2007;65:1388–1393.

CHAPTER 91 ■ UPPER EXTREMITY ARTERIAL DISEASE

MARK D. MORASCH

KEY POINTS

1. Presenting symptoms of upper extremity occlusive disease include evidence of arterial emboli, Raynaud phenomenon, pain, and exercise-related forearm fatigue.
2. Physical examination should include the thoracic outlet and the entire upper extremity.
3. In severe bilateral hand ischemia, a systemic cause of the arterial lesions should be sought.
4. Several noninvasive tests, including plethysmography, transcutaneous Doppler examination, and duplex scan, are available for the objective evaluation of patients with upper extremity ischemia.
5. Atherosclerosis is the most common cause of upper extremity occlusive lesions.
6. Thoracic outlet syndrome is the most common condition producing upper extremity vascular complications in young adults.

In the upper extremity, a broad spectrum of arterial occlusive processes can lead to ischemic symptoms. An accurate diagnosis requires obtaining a very thorough patient history, performing careful physical examination, and applying the liberal use of ancillary testing. Appropriate endovascular or open surgical intervention depends on the location of the vascular lesion and the nature of the underlying occlusive process.

ANATOMY

The supra-aortic vessels normally develop as three separate trunks taking origin from the arch of the aorta within the superior mediastinum. The conventional definition includes the innominate artery, the subclavian arteries to involve the origins of the vertebral arteries, and the common carotid arteries proximal to their bifurcations. The left subclavian artery is the third of three trunks and it originates posterior to and to the left of the left common carotid. There may be as few as one great vessel or as many as six arising from the transverse aorta.[1] The most common variation is the bovine-type aortic arch, where the first and second branches arise from a common ostium (16%) or as a single trunk (8%). The arch configuration with an aberrant right subclavian artery that arises as the fourth of four vessels occurs in approximately 0.5% of individuals.[2,3]

The subclavian artery crosses the thoracic outlet and becomes the axillary artery. As the continuation of the subclavian, the axillary vessel commences at the outer border of the first rib and ends at the lower border of the teres major tendon. Beyond the teres major tendon, the axillary becomes the brachial artery, which runs medial to the humerus. At the bend of the elbow, the brachial artery lies midway between its two epicondyles, and below the bend of the elbow, it divides into the radial and ulnar arteries.

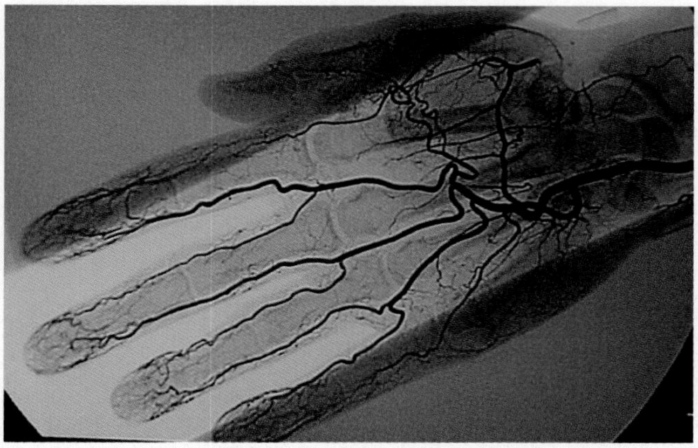

FIGURE 91.1. Incomplete palmar arch and ulnar dominant anatomy. Given radial artery occlusion, the thumb and forefinger are poorly perfused.

The anatomic variability of the upper extremity arteries, especially the palmar arches (superficial and deep), is well known,[4] and incomplete palmar arches (Fig. 91.1) play a significant role in ischemic disease. The deep palmar arch is formed by the terminal part of the radial artery and the superficial arch by the ulnar artery. In a study of 500 hand arteriograms, the deep palmar arch appeared complete in 95.2% of cases.[5] Because the ulnar artery predominates in supplying blood to the hand, the completeness of the superficial palmar arch is the determining factor in hand ischemia. In contrast to the deep arch, the superficial palmar arch exhibits many variations (Fig. 91.2). Six types of complete arch are known; a complete superficial palmar arch was seen in only 42.4% of cases in the angiographic study.[5]

MEDICAL HISTORY

Obtaining an appropriate patient history is an extremely important initial step in arriving at a diagnosis in patients with

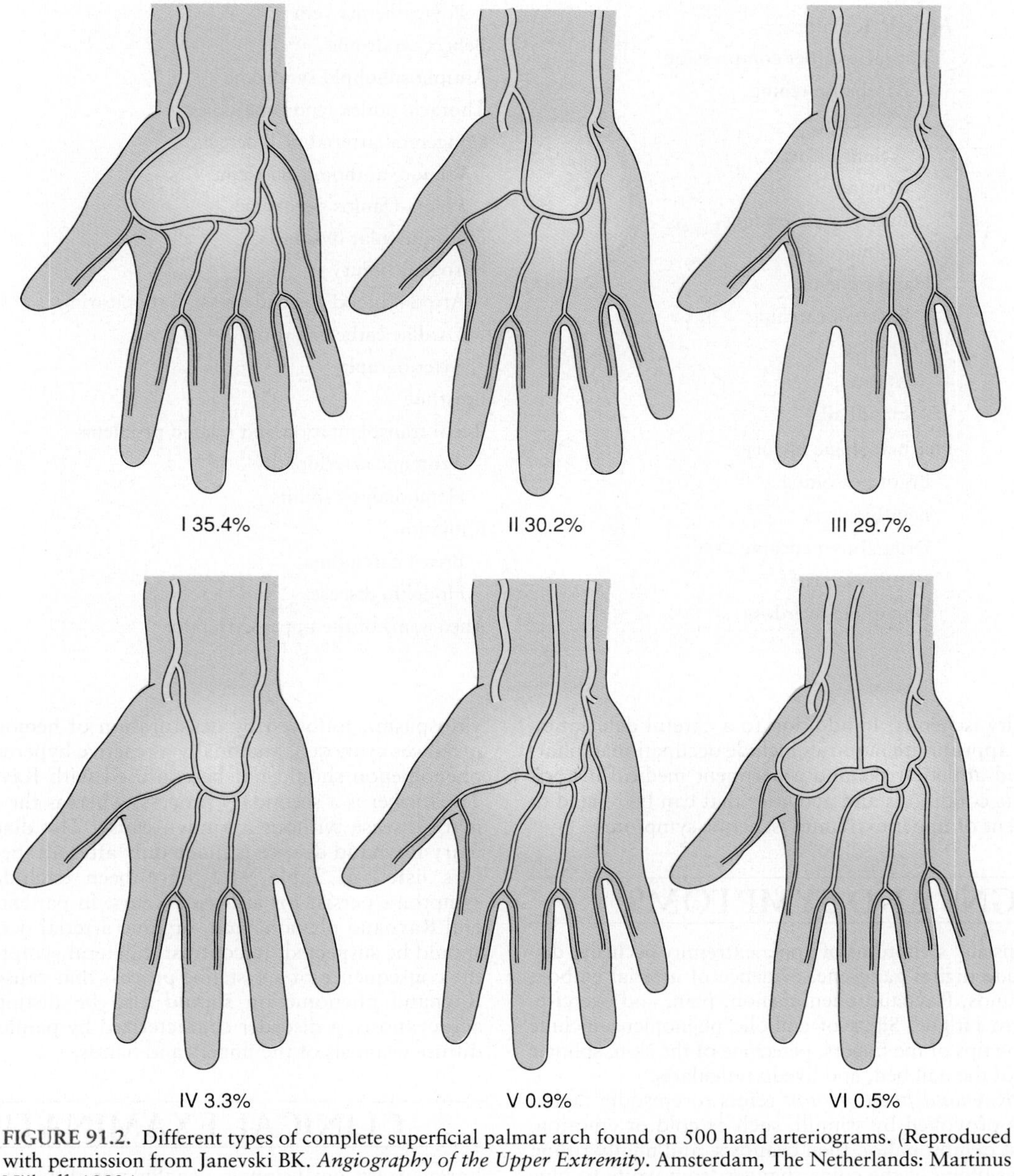

FIGURE 91.2. Different types of complete superficial palmar arch found on 500 hand arteriograms. (Reproduced with permission from Janevski BK. *Angiography of the Upper Extremity*. Amsterdam, The Netherlands: Martinus Nijhoff; 1982.)

ETIOLOGY

TABLE 91.1

CONDITIONS AND RISKS FOR UPPER EXTREMITY ISCHEMIA

Occupational injury	Medical conditions
Vibration syndrome	Atherosclerosis
Pneumatic tools	Arteritis
Chainsaws	Collagen disease
Grinders	Scleroderma
Electrical burns	Rheumatic arteritis
Hypothenar hammer syndrome	Systemic lupus erythematosus
Mechanical work or auto repair	Dermatomyositis
Lathe operation	Allergic necrotizing arteritis
Carpentry	Takayasu disease
Electrical work	Giant cell arteritis
Occupational acroosteolysis—polyvinylchloride exposure	Blood dyscrasias
Athletic activities	Cold agglutinins
Thoracic outlet compression	Cryoglobulins
Baseball pitching	Polycythemia vera
Kayaking	Behçet syndrome
Weight lifting	Antiphospholipid syndrome
Rowing	Thoracic outlet syndrome
Butterfly swimming	Congenital arterial wall defects
Golfing	Pseudoxanthoma elasticum
Hand ischemia	Ehlers-Danlos syndrome
Baseball catching	Fibromuscular dysplasia
Frisbee	Iatrogenic injury
Karate	Arterial blood gas and pressure monitoring
Handball	Cardiac catheterization
Pharmacologic history	Arteriography
Ergot poisoning	Frostbite
Beta-blockers	Renal transplantation and related problems
Drug abuse, cocaine use	Azotemic arteriopathy
Cytotoxic drugs	Hemodialysis shunts
Dopamine overdose	Radiation
	Breast carcinoma
	Hodgkin disease
	Aneurysms of the upper extremity

upper extremity ischemia. In addition to a careful delineation of symptoms, appropriate inquiries include occupational, pharmacologic, and athletic risks and a pertinent medical history. Table 91.1 lists conditions and activities that can be related to the development of upper extremity ischemic symptoms.

SIGNS AND SYMPTOMS

1 Presenting signs and symptoms of upper extremity occlusive disease can include digital gangrene, evidence of arterial emboli, persistent wounds, Raynaud phenomenon, pain, and exercise-related forearm fatigue. Signs of embolic phenomena include gangrene of the tips of the fingers, petechiae of the skin, splinter hemorrhages of the nail bed, and livedo reticularis.

The term *Raynaud phenomenon* refers to episodic digital color changes provoked by stimuli, such as cold or emotion. The digits first exhibit pallor, then cyanosis, and finally rubor. The pathophysiology of the color changes from white to blue to red is thought to be digital ischemia (resulting from vasospasm), followed by desaturation of hemoglobin (which produces cyanosis), and finally a reactive hyperemia. Raynaud phenomenon should not be confused with Raynaud disease. The former is a secondary process, whereas the latter is a primary disease without a known cause. The diagnosis of primary Raynaud disease is made only after all the etiologic factors listed in Table 91.1 have been excluded and after symptoms persist for at least 2 years. In patients with unilateral Raynaud phenomenon, organic arterial occlusive disease should be suspected. In contrast, bilateral symptoms are often the consequence of a systemic process that causes vasospasm. Raynaud phenomenon should also be distinguished from acrocyanosis, a disorder characterized by painless, persistent, diffuse cyanosis of the fingers and hands.

CLINICAL EXAMINATION

Large-artery occlusion is usually not difficult to diagnose. Careful pulse examination will usually confirm the diagnosis.

Distal arterial lesions causing hand or finger ischemia can be more difficult to delineate.

❷ Physical examination should include the thoracic outlet and the entire upper extremity. Bilateral brachial artery cuff pressure measurement and auscultation for subclavian bruits should be performed at every initial patient encounter. Palpation of the supraclavicular region may detect a subclavian artery aneurysm or a cervical rib. Auscultation with the stethoscope placed in the supraclavicular region and in the infraclavicular fossae while listening for a bruit with the patient's arm placed in both neutral and hyperabducted positions can help to establish the diagnosis of thoracic outlet compression. Pulse examination begins with the subclavian artery in the supraclavicular fossa and continues with the axillary artery under the armpit, the brachial artery at the upper arm and elbow, and the radial and ulnar arteries at the wrist level. A decreased or absent pulse in any site other than the supraclavicular fossa indicates more proximal occlusion. Conversely, a readily palpable pulse in the supraclavicular fossa may represent a subclavian artery aneurysm.

Complete examination includes an Allen test. The radial and ulnar arteries of one wrist are compressed tightly by the examiner's fingers. The patient then opens and closes the hand until the hand is devoid of blood. The fingers are extended and either the radial or the ulnar artery is released. The hand is observed for capillary return of color. The test result is judged normal if refilling of both sides of the hand is complete within a short period. If a portion of the hand does not reperfuse, continuity of the palmar vascular arch is incomplete. Examination of the hand should also include palpation of the palm for aneurysms.

LABORATORY TESTING

❸ In severe bilateral hand ischemia, a systemic cause for occlusion should be sought. Laboratory tests (Table 91.2) include serologic, immunologic, and hematologic studies to help establish the diagnosis.

The erythrocyte sedimentation rate can be a useful screening test to aid in the diagnosis of various forms of arteritis. A positive antinuclear antibody test result suggests connective tissue disease or other arteritides. When the antinuclear antibody titer is abnormal, immunofluorescent pattern analysis of antibodies can help to establish the diagnosis of various connective tissue disorders. The speckled pattern antibody is more specific for systemic lupus erythematosus. A nucleolar pattern suggests scleroderma. A positive anticardiolipin antibody is diagnostic for antiphospholipid syndrome, which is characterized by thromboembolic events in young adults.[6]

TABLE 91.2 DIAGNOSIS

LAB TESTS FOR SYSTEMIC CAUSES FOR HAND ISCHEMIA

Erythrocyte sedimentation rate
Rheumatoid factor
Antinuclear antibody
Immunoglobulin electrophoresis
Cryoglobulins
Cold agglutinins
VDRL (Venereal Disease Research Laboratory) test
Complement (C3, C4)
Anticardiolipin antibody
Blood cell counts

IMAGING

Along with laboratory testing, a combination of noninvasive vascular imaging and radiologic testing may be needed to establish the proper diagnosis. Plain radiographs can be helpful in delineating systemic disease. Soft tissue radiographs of the hand may reveal calcinosis seen in the CREST (calcinosis cutis, Raynaud phenomenon, esophageal motility disorder, sclerodactyly, and telangiectasia) syndrome or diffuse calcified arteries noted in diabetic or azotemic arteriopathy (Fig. 91.3). A chest film can detect pulmonary fibrosis consistent with systemic sclerosis or bony anomalies of the thoracic outlet, such as cervical ribs (Fig. 91.4), anomalous first ribs, or healed fractures of the first rib or clavicle.

❹ Several noninvasive tests, including plethysmography, transcutaneous Doppler examination, and duplex scan, are available for the objective evaluation of patients with upper extremity ischemia.[7] Doppler examination consists of audible signal interpretation, waveform recording with spectral analysis, and systolic pressure measurements. Bilateral examinations should be performed for comparative purposes. Systemic diseases will usually result in bilateral abnormalities, while unilateral disease indicates a more focal problem such as embolic occlusion or unilateral aneurysm.

Doppler is helpful in determining the patency of the ulnar artery, which may be difficult to palpate. In the hand, Doppler examination of the palmar arches is performed best at the midthenar and hypothenar regions. The common digital vessels should be examined at the base of the fingers, where they

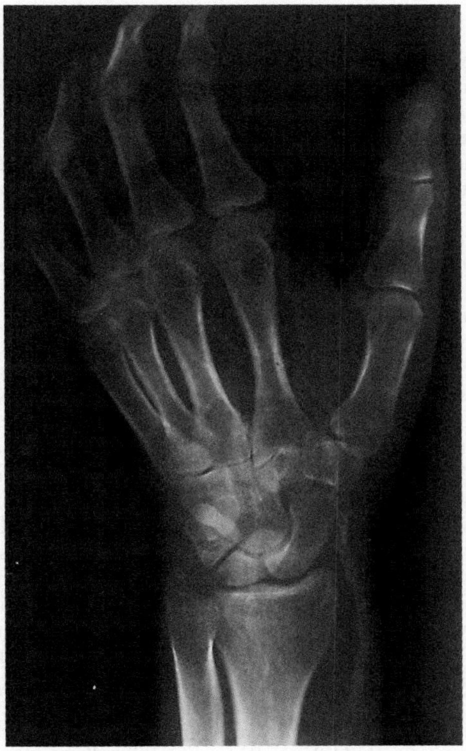

FIGURE 91.3. Typical appearance of azotemic arteriopathy (calciphylaxis) in a diabetic patient with a renal transplant. All the digital arteries are distinctly seen on plain film. The radial artery has a "lead pipe" appearance. An arteriogram shows multiple digital artery occlusions. (Reproduced with permission from Yao JST. Arterial surgery of the upper extremity. In: Haimovici H, Callow AD, DePalma RG, et al., eds. *Vascular Surgery: Principles and Techniques,* 3rd ed. Norwalk, CT: Appleton & Lange; 1989:863.)

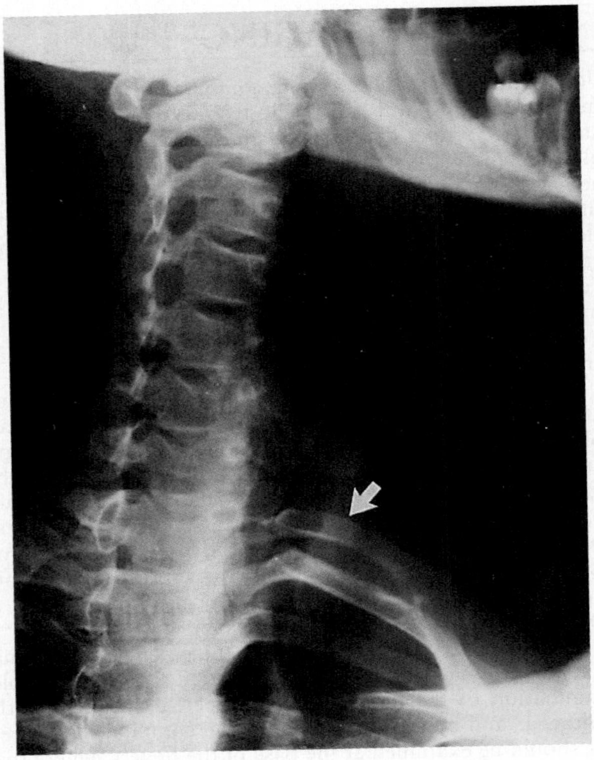

FIGURE 91.4. Cervical rib (*arrow*) in a patient with subclavian artery aneurysm caused by thoracic outlet compression.

divide into the proper digital arteries. The use of noninvasive testing to detect digital artery occlusion helps distinguish Raynaud phenomenon from disease and can pinpoint the sites of occlusive lesions.

Segmental upper extremity pressures commence with a pneumatic cuff placed on the upper arm as in routine blood pressure recording. The brachial recording reflects the pressure in all arteries proximal to the cuff. A difference of greater than 10 to 20 mm Hg compared to the other arm signifies innominate, subclavian, axillary, or brachial artery stenosis. The cuff is next applied to the forearm with the radial artery used for signal detection. A pressure drop of 20 to 30 mm Hg signifies an obstruction distal to the brachial artery. Finger pressures are measured using a 2.5-cm cuff placed at the base of the digit. Return of Doppler signals after cuff deflation is monitored at the fingertip. An arterial occlusion distal to the palmar arch is defined by a pressure gradient between the fingers of more than 15 mm Hg or a wrist-to-digit difference of 30 mm Hg. The Doppler technique is of particular value in determining palmar arch patency in a patient who is unconscious or uncooperative with an Allen test. Before arterial line placement, this simple test may help to avoid hand ischemia.

Plethysmography is used to record finger pulse contours for analysis and to differentiate between a normal state and obstructive or vasospastic disease.[7] The duplex scan is helpful in establishing the diagnosis of aneurysm.

Imaging using traditional catheter-directed contrast injection should be performed bilaterally and include all arteries from the hand. Multiplanar angiographic views of the aortic arch utilizing digital subtraction angiography are useful for planning proximal vessel revascularization. Specific emphasis should be placed on the vessel's origins with delayed views to show vascular reconstitution from steal. Arteriography is useful in defining the vascular anatomy of the hand. The use of intra-arterial vasodilators can help break spasm and lead to better delineation of the smallest hand vessels.

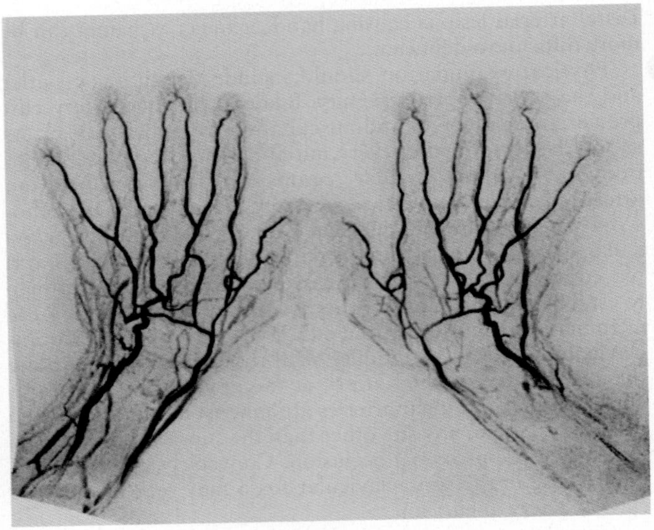

FIGURE 91.5. Focused magnetic resonance angiogram of the hand.

Magnetic resonance and computed tomography (CT) angiography provide multiplanar images of the proximal vessels that rival those of biplanar digital subtraction angiography. Gadolinium-enhanced magnetic resonance angiography and certain noncontrast magnetic resonance imaging sequences are being developed for the vessels in the hand (Fig. 91.5). CT scanning provides information regarding the extent of calcification in the aortic arch and can help delineate adjacent bony structures and their relationship to the vessels (Fig. 91.6). Transesophageal echocardiography (TEE) is used to assess myocardial function, to rule out a cardioembolic source, and, like CT, to identify significant calcific lesions or atheromata within the arch.

Proximal Arterial Lesions

5 Atherosclerosis is the most common disease affecting the supra-aortic trunk vessels. The first part of the subclavian artery is the most frequent site of involvement. The innominate artery is also a common site of disease. Lesions include total occlusion with or without associated steal phenomena, high-grade stenoses, and ulcerating plaques, which may be the source of emboli.

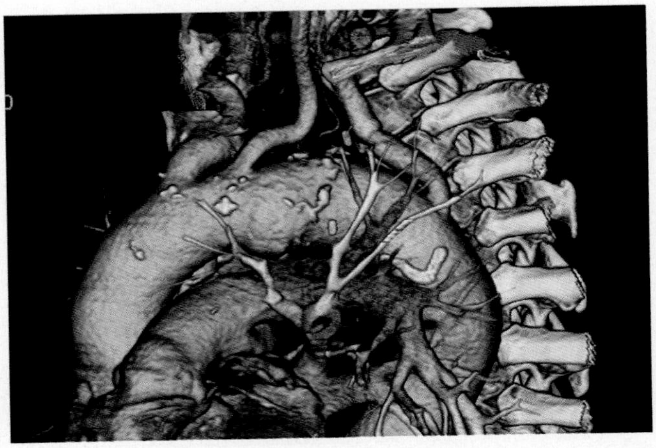

FIGURE 91.6. Thoracic outlet computed tomography scan showing bony relationship.

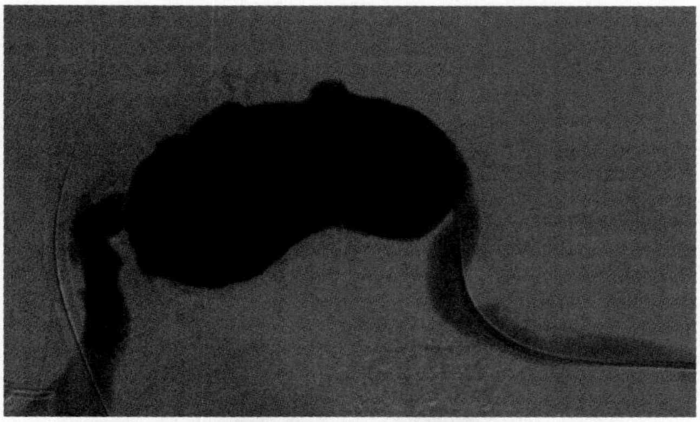

FIGURE 91.7. Large subclavian artery aneurysm.

Occlusive lesions less commonly result from congenital anomalies, arteritis, or exposure to therapeutic radiation. More distally, the subclavian arteries can be damaged from dissection, aneurysm, or the long-term effects of thoracic outlet syndrome. Symptoms from nonatherosclerotic processes account for less than 20% of the disease that requires intervention.[8–12] The more common atherosclerotic lesions tend to cause occlusive and embolic symptoms equally, while vessel obliteration from arteritis tends only to cause symptoms related to hemodynamic insufficiency.

Single-vessel atherosclerotic occlusive disease involving the great vessels is often seen in younger adults (fifth decade), while patients with extensive or multiple trunk involvement tend to be older. Cigarette smoking is certainly a significant risk factor for the development of atherosclerotic occlusive disease involving these vessels.

Subclavian artery aneurysms can develop proximally (intrathoracic aneurysms) or distally (extrathoracic aneurysms). Extrathoracic subclavian artery aneurysms usually develop distal to the vertebral artery origin and present in the form of a poststenotic dilatation or as the result of repetitive trauma to the artery in patients with arterial thoracic outlet syndrome[13] (Fig. 91.7). Causes of proximal subclavian artery aneurysm formation include atherosclerosis, infection (including those that are the result of syphilis or tuberculosis), cystic medial necrosis, Marfan syndrome, and a few other rare genetic disorders. Subclavian artery aneurysms have the potential to thrombose, embolize, and cause symptoms from local compression or rupture.

Forms of arteritis producing upper extremity ischemic symptoms include such diverse processes as Takayasu arteritis, giant cell arteritis, temporal arteritis, and polymyalgia rheumatica. Takayasu arteritis is a nonspecific inflammatory process that segmentally affects the aorta and its main branches. The process can involve the carotid, subclavian, axillary, and pulmonary arteries.[14] Takayasu arteritis frequently involves all three great vessels proximally. The true etiology of this nonspecific inflammatory disease has not been elucidated, but it is known to predominantly affect women in their second or third decades of life. The arteriographic appearance is often diagnostic. The tapered involvement of multiple arteries and a well-developed network of collaterals are characteristic. The pulmonary artery will be affected in 45% of patients. The hypertrophic occlusive lesions of Takayasu disease carry low embolic potential, and most symptoms relate to low flow as the disease progresses to multivessel occlusion (Fig. 91.8). The histopathologic appearance of the lesions depends on the phase of the disease. They appear intensely inflammatory during the acute phase and more sclerotic when the disease is "burned out." The inflammatory process is characterized by fibrosis and thickening of the arterial wall with pathologic changes usually most noticeable in the adventitial and medial layers of the involved vessels. Aneurysmal changes with embolic potential can develop during the chronic phase of the disease.

Giant cell arteritis can involve the more distal subclavian arteries and may be differentiated from Takayasu arteritis by location and by the fact that it affects an older patient population. Characteristic arteriographic findings include long segments of smooth stenosis or occlusion alternating with areas of normal or dilated artery and the absence of irregular plaques or ulceration (Fig. 91.9). The most frequently recognized clinical features of giant cell arteritis (cranial, temporal, and granulomatous arteritis) are related to involvement of the cranial arteries. The subclavian and axillary arteries are

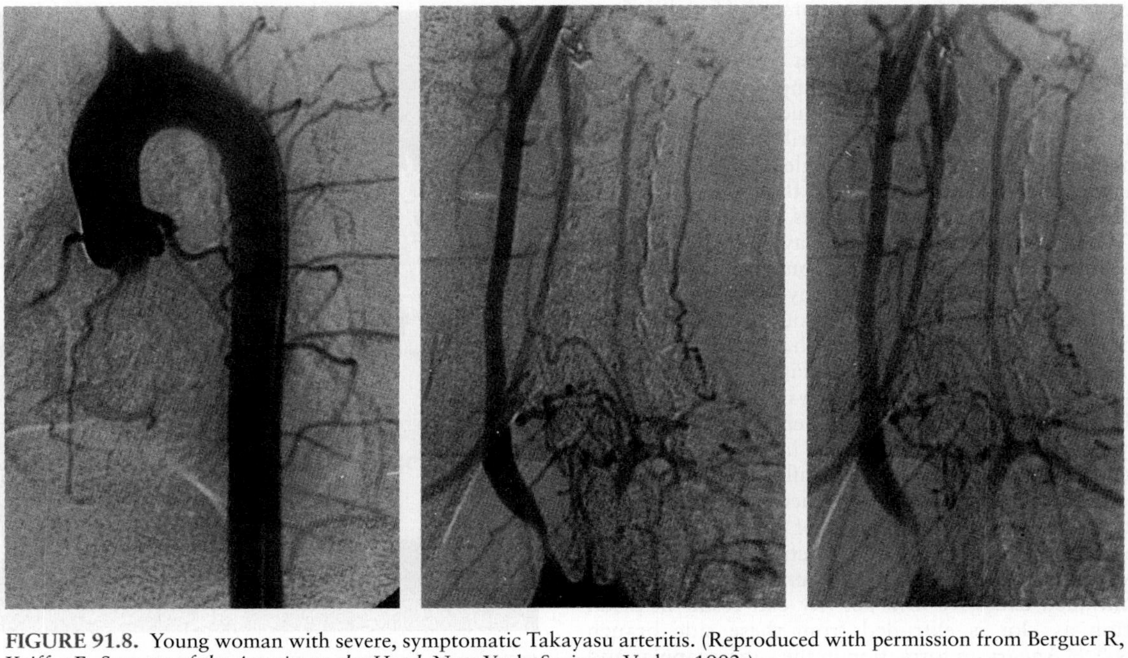

FIGURE 91.8. Young woman with severe, symptomatic Takayasu arteritis. (Reproduced with permission from Berguer R, Keiffer E. *Surgery of the Arteries to the Head*. New York: Springer-Verlag; 1992.)

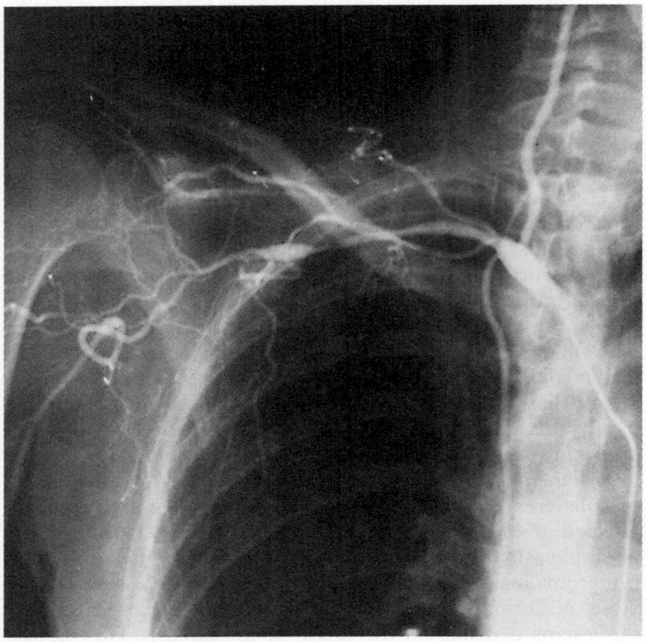

FIGURE 91.9. Characteristic long, segmental narrowing of the subclavian artery in a patient with giant cell arteritis. (Reproduced with permission from Yao JST. Arterial surgery of the upper extremity. In: Haimovici H, Callow AD, DePalma RG, et al., eds. *Vascular Surgery: Principles and Techniques,* 3rd ed. Norwalk, CT: Appleton & Lange; 1989:858.)

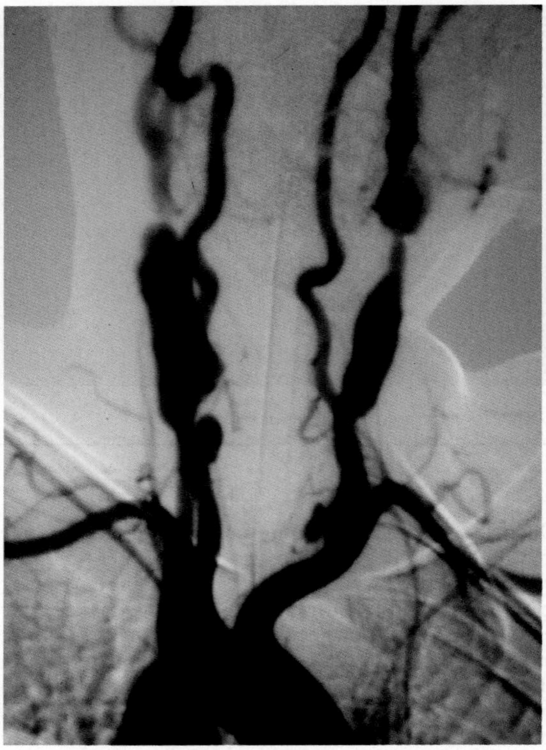

FIGURE 91.10. Severe arterial damage following high-dose cervical thoracic irradiation.

common sites of involvement.[15] In addition to upper extremity ischemic symptoms, patients with arteritis often present with fever, malaise, headache, and joint pain. The erythrocyte sedimentation rate is often elevated. The results of serologic tests may be positive, but none is sufficiently sensitive or specific to be considered diagnostic.

The subclavian artery can develop an accelerated form of atherosclerosis as a result of radiation injury (Fig. 91.10). The rate at which the process develops depends on the radiation dose and may follow radiotherapy for, among other diseases, breast cancer, intrathoracic tumors, or Hodgkin lymphoma.

6 Thoracic outlet syndrome is the most common condition producing upper extremity vascular complications in young adults. Possible sites of compression include the costoclavicular space, formed by the first thoracic rib and clavicle (Fig. 91.11); the interscalene triangle; the angle between the insertion of the pectoralis minor tendon and the coracoid process in the axilla; and the head of the humerus in extreme external rotation. Thoracic outlet compression may be caused by bony anomalies, such as a cervical rib or an abnormal first thoracic rib, or it may be secondary to hypertrophy of the anterior scalene muscle. Although a cervical rib is found in 0.5% to 1% of the population, fewer than 10% of such persons have symptoms of neurovascular compression (Fig. 91.12). Arterial complications include subclavian aneurysm formation, poststenotic dilation, thrombosis, and distal embolisms.

Aneurysmal changes can also develop in either the anterior or, more commonly, the posterior circumflex humeral arteries due to repetitive athletic activities. Tethering of the axillary artery between the chest and the loop of circumflex arteries, around the humeral neck, can lead to traction injuries. Intimal damage, subsequent thrombosis, or aneurysm formation can result. Continued excessive arm activity can result in distal embolization as clot is extruded from these side branch aneurysms.[16–19] Aneurysm formation in the suprascapular and subscapular arteries has also been reported.[17] Direct trauma from the head of the humerus can also cause compression to the axillary artery with similar sequelae.[19,20]

Distal Arterial Lesions

Several collagen vascular disorders can produce systemic signs as well as upper extremity symptoms ranging from

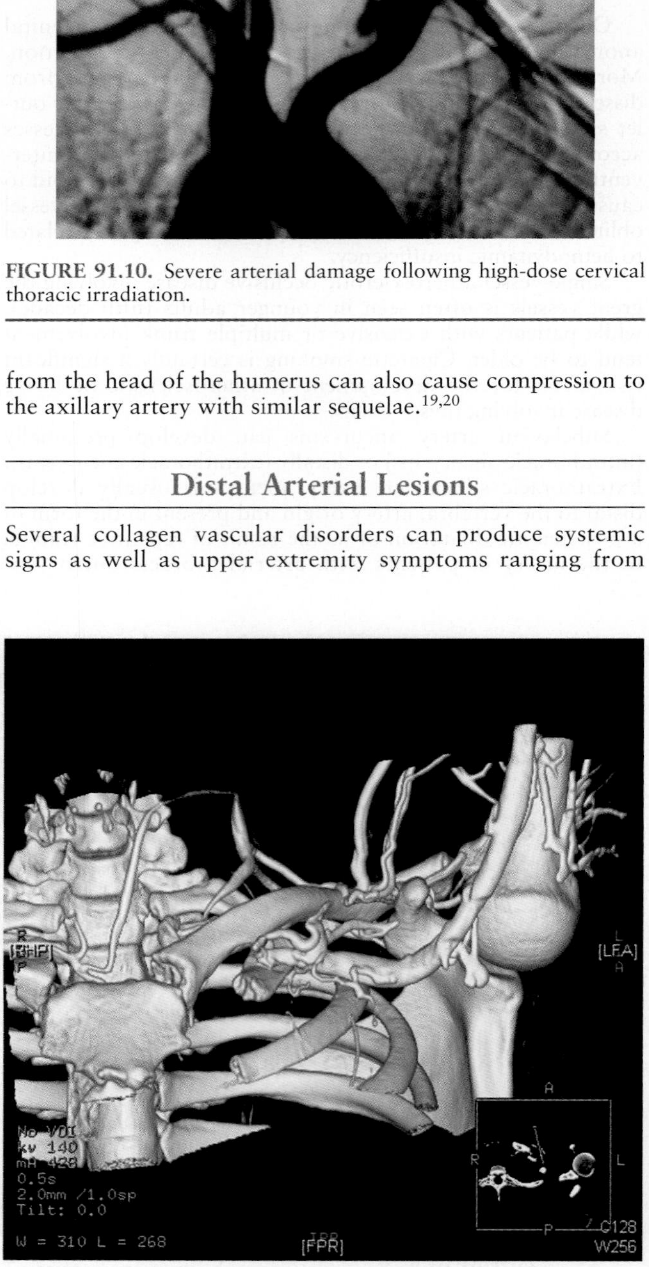

FIGURE 91.11. Thoracic outlet computed tomography scan.

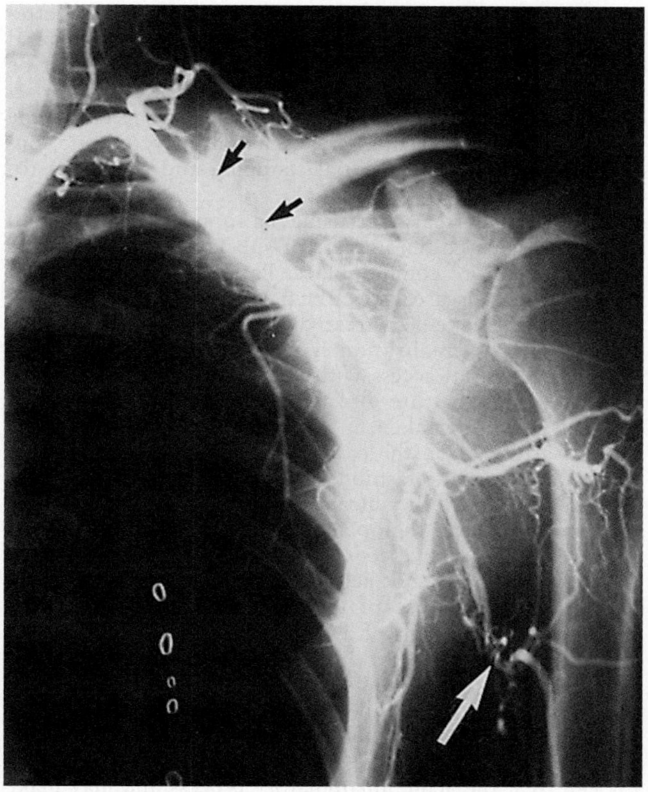

FIGURE 91.12. Arteriogram in a patient with subclavian artery aneurysm (*black arrows*) caused by a cervical rib. Multiple distal arterial occlusions have developed as a result of embolism (*white arrow*).

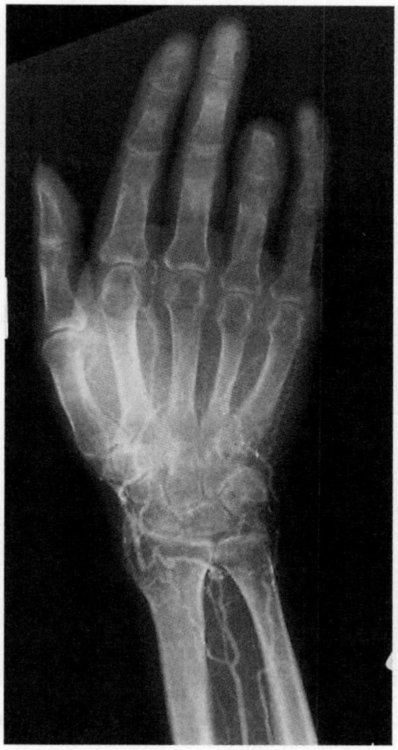

FIGURE 91.13. Arteriogram of a patient with scleroderma and digital gangrene. Extensive small-artery occlusion involves the palmar arch and digital arteries.

Raynaud phenomenon to gangrene of the digits. These disorders include scleroderma, rheumatoid arthritis, systemic lupus erythematosus, polyarteritis nodosa, and dermatomyositis. Occlusions of the palmar arches or digital arteries are common (Fig. 91.13).

Buerger disease (thromboangiitis obliterans) was initially described in male patients of Mediterranean origin who presented with digital gangrene but no occlusion of the larger arteries. Contemporary practice recognizes that men and women of many ethnic backgrounds can be affected. A persistent characteristic is a strong association with heavy smoking of a particularly addictive nature. The diagnosis of Buerger disease is based on histologic evidence of the involvement of both arteries and veins. Venous involvement can be manifested clinically as migrating phlebitis. Characteristic arteriographic findings include occlusion of the small arteries of the digits and the presence of abundant collaterals. The typical corkscrew appearance of the collaterals and lack of the large-vessel plaques characteristic of atherosclerosis are strongly suggestive. Like the symptomatic hand, the asymptomatic hand may demonstrate digital artery occlusions.

Polycythemia vera, cryoglobulinemia, and the presence of cold agglutinins are common blood dyscrasias associated with occlusion of the arteries of the hand. Occlusion of the small arteries is generally thought to be caused by local thrombosis or embolism. Specific immunologic and blood tests help to establish the diagnosis.

Iatrogenic injuries to the radial and brachial arteries have become more common because of the increasing use of diagnostic and therapeutic catheterization. These can be particularly troublesome when an incomplete palmar arch is not recognized before placement of a catheter in the radial artery. Gangrene or severe ischemia can result from the injury.

Vibration syndrome, characterized by blanching and numbness of the hands after the use of pneumatic drills, is a well-recognized clinical entity causing hand ischemia. The so-called vibratory white finger is a form of occupational trauma. Repetitive trauma to the digital arteries that initially causes spasm but ultimately causes thrombosis and permanent occlusion is believed to be the primary factor responsible for ischemic symptoms.

Hypothenar hammer syndrome is another form of occupational trauma, commonly seen in mechanics and carpenters. Injury follows repetitive use of the palm in activities that involve pounding, pushing, or twisting. The anatomic location of the ulnar artery at the area of hypothenar eminence makes it vulnerable to stress. When this area is repeatedly traumatized, ulnar artery occlusion (Fig. 91.14) or aneurysm formation can result (Fig. 91.15). Digital artery occlusion is a consequence of embolism from the injured artery.

Calciphylactic arteriopathy (heavily calcified arteries) in patients with diabetes or chronic renal failure can lead to gangrene or severe ischemia of the hand. The so-called azotemic arteriopathy (calciphylaxis) is characterized by calcification of the media of the digital arteries, which produces a "lead pipe" pattern on plain film.

TREATMENT

The type of reconstructive procedure depends on the underlying cause of ischemia, as well as the nature and location of the lesion. The results of bypass grafting in the upper extremity are similar to those of lower extremity revascularization—that is, proximal grafts fare better than distal grafts. In a recent report, the overall 5-year patency rate was 52.2% in 43 patients.[21] The patency rate for anastomosis proximal to the

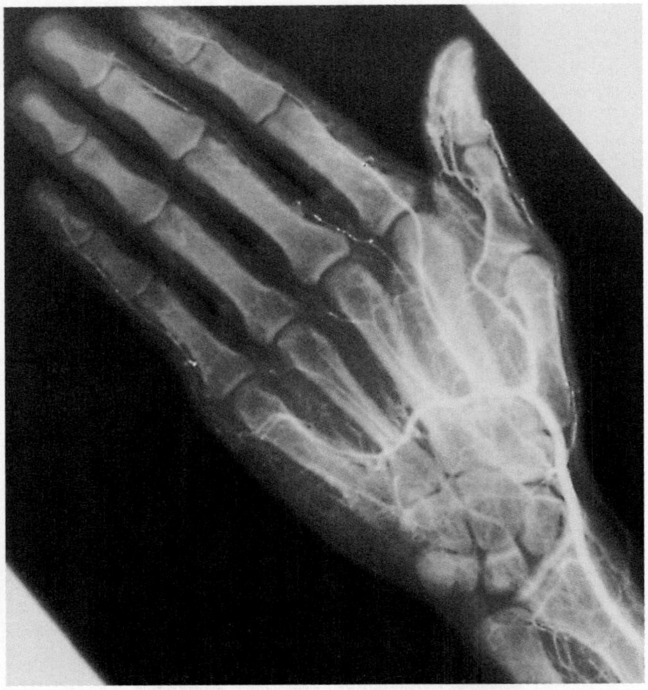

FIGURE 91.14. Occlusion of the ulnar artery over the hamate bone in a patient with hypothenar hammer syndrome.

brachial artery bifurcation was better than that for more distal placement (61.9% vs. 34.8%). Major amputation is not often required, even after graft occlusion, as it is in lower extremity surgery.

Cervical reconstruction via transposition is the surgical technique of choice for single proximal occlusive lesions involving the subclavian arteries. Multiple remote cervical bypasses or arch-based reconstruction should also be considered for patients with multiple supra-aortic trunk occlusive lesions. Arterial transpositions are completed through a short, transverse cervical incision above the clavicle. Not only is preservation of the vertebral artery critical, but also it is equally important to mobilize and preserve the valuable internal mammary artery when performing a subclavian transposition. The long-term patency rate for arterial transposition, when performed by surgeons with experience, is virtually 100%.[9,22,23]

Occasionally, it is not feasible to do a straightforward arterial transposition so the use of a bypass from the ipsilateral carotid to the subclavian becomes necessary. Care must be taken to avoid injury to the phrenic nerve during this more lateral approach. The bypass is completed to the retroscalene portion of the subclavian artery, usually using prosthetic conduit, by performing sequential clamping and serial anastomoses.[24,25]

Endoluminal treatment using balloon angioplasty and stenting of isolated innominate or subclavian artery disease is becoming more commonplace. Patients with atherosclerotic occlusive disease, as well as patients with inflammatory arteriopathies, have been treated with endovascular therapy. Endovascular recanalization is performed fluoroscopically via remote arterial access with wires, catheters, and angioplasty balloons that are directed to the target lesion. Therapy can be undertaken in antegrade fashion from the femoral artery or, in the case of innominate or subclavian lesions, a retrograde fashion, from the brachial artery. The routine use of metallic intravascular stents has become an adjuvant to balloon angioplasty in the proximal segments of these vessels and covered stent grafts may have a role as well.[26] Stents should not be placed in the postvertebral subclavian artery because of the risk of stent compression. Endoluminal treatment of arteritis results in marginal success at best.

In general, no operation should be undertaken on patients with Takayasu arteritis while in an active phase signaled by the presence of the constitutional symptoms, acute inflammation, and an elevated erythrocyte sedimentation rate. Steroid therapy can treat the acute inflammatory process and may make surgical reconstruction much safer. The indications for vascular reconstruction in patients with Takayasu disease are the same as those for treating patients with atherosclerosis.

Arterial complications of thoracic outlet obstruction often require a bypass procedure. After resection of a subclavian artery aneurysm and removal of the cervical rib, the damaged subclavian artery is reconstructed with either venous or prosthetic conduit.[27]

A bypass graft with autogenous vein (saphenous or cephalic) often relieves occlusion of the brachial artery and its major branches.[28] A short segmental occlusion of either the radial or ulnar artery may be treated by thrombectomy or endarterectomy with a vein patch. An aneurysm in the hand can be resected and continuity restored by end-to-end anastomosis or with an interposed lesser saphenous vein graft.

Distal lesions with occlusion at or distal to the palmar arch may not be amenable to direct surgical treatment. Conservative

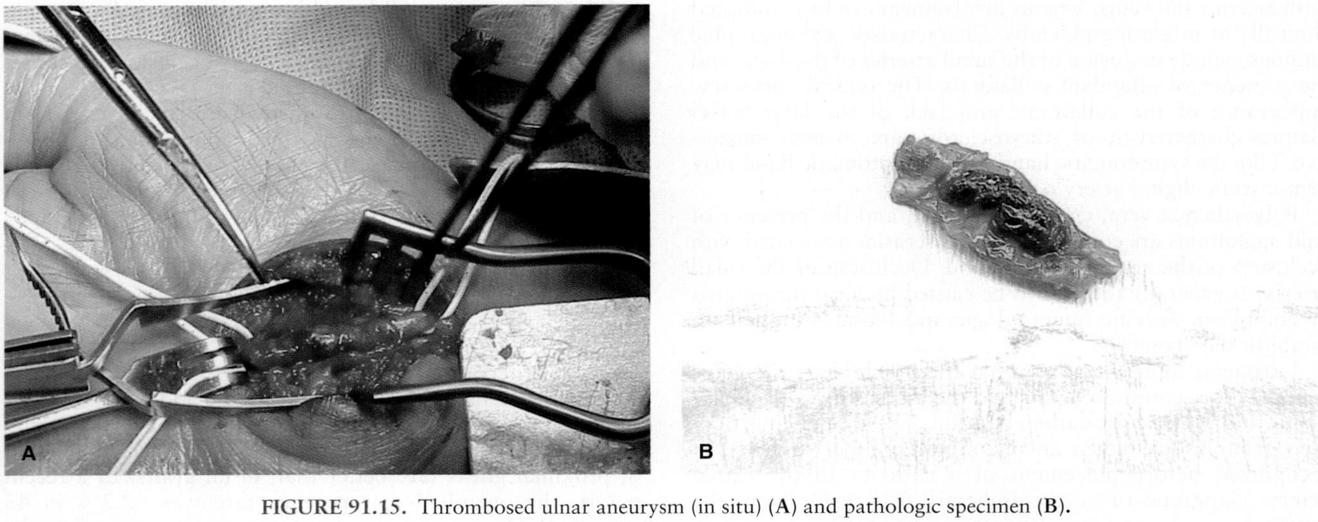

FIGURE 91.15. Thrombosed ulnar aneurysm (in situ) (A) and pathologic specimen (B).

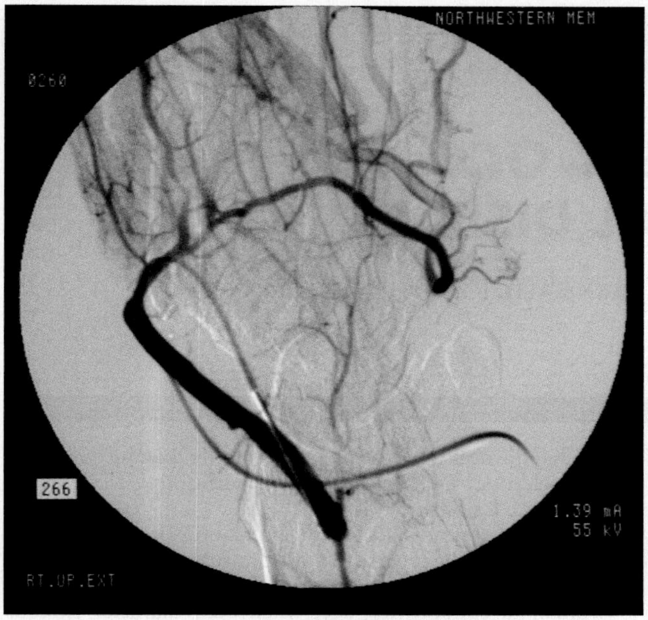

FIGURE 91.16. Bypass to the superficial palmar arch.

treatment with the use of a calcium blocker (e.g., nifedipine) may reduce the severity and frequency of attacks. A host of medications have been recommended.[29] Occasionally, a reasonable distal target for bypass is identified in the hand (Fig. 91.16). Microvascular reconstruction, with or without digital sympathectomy, may also be effective in particularly recalcitrant cases.

In all patients with upper extremity ischemia of any cause, cessation of smoking is important. Many of the constituents of tobacco smoke cause adverse vascular effects, particularly vasoconstriction, with particularly prominent effects in the upper extremity. Protective measures, such as avoiding exposure to cold temperatures and mechanical trauma, have beneficial effects when scrupulously applied.

The author would like to extend many thanks to James S.T. Yao, M.D., for his contributions to previous chapters upon which this one was based.

References

1. Bergman RA, Thompson SA, Afifi KA, et al. *Compendium of Human Anatomic Variation*. Baltimore, MD: Text, Atlas and World Literature; 1988.
2. Berguer R, Kieffer E. *Surgery of the Arteries to the Head*. New York: Springer-Verlag; 1992.
3. Molz G, Burri B. Aberrant subclavian artery (arteria lusoria): sex differences in the prevalence of various forms of the malformation. Evaluation of 1378 observations. *Virchows Arch A Pathol Anat Histol* 1978;380:303–315.
4. Coleman SS, Anson BJ. Arterial patterns in the hand based upon a study of 650 specimens. *Surg Gynecol Obstet* 1961;113:409–424.
5. Janevski BK. *Angiography of the Upper Extremity*. Amsterdam, The Netherlands: Martinus Nijhoff; 1982.
6. Levine JS, Branch DW, Rauch J. The antiphospholipid syndrome. *N Engl J Med* 2002;346:752–763.
7. Sumner DS. Noninvasive assessment of upper extremity ischemia. In: Bergan JJ, Yao JST, eds. *Evaluation and Treatment of Upper and Lower Extremity Circulatory Disorders*. Orlando, FL: Grune & Stratton; 1984:75–95.
8. Berguer R, Morasch MD, Kline RA. Transthoracic repair of innominate and common carotid artery disease: immediate and long-term outcome for 100 consecutive surgical reconstructions. *J Vasc Surg* 1998;27:34–41; discussion 42.
9. Berguer R, Morasch MD, Kline RA, et al. Cervical reconstruction of the supra-aortic trunks: a 16-year experience. *J Vasc Surg* 1999;29:239–246; discussion 246–248.
10. Kieffer E, Sabater J, Koskas F. Brachiocephalic arterial reconstruction. In: Yao JST, Pearce WH, eds. *Arterial Surgery*. Stamford, CT: Appleton and Lange; 1996:141–162.
11. Kieffer E, Sabatier J, Koskas F, et al. Atherosclerotic innominate artery occlusive disease: early and long-term results of surgical reconstruction. *J Vasc Surg* 1995;21:326–336; discussion 336–337.
12. Rhodes JM, Cherry KJ Jr, Clark RC, et al. Aortic-origin reconstruction of the great vessels: risk factors of early and late complications. *J Vasc Surg* 2000;31:260–269.
13. Bower TC, Pairolero PC, Hallett JW Jr, et al. Brachiocephalic aneurysm: the case for early recognition and repair. *Ann Vasc Surg* 1991;5:125–132.
14. Mishima Y. Leriche memorial lecture at 24th World Congress 'Takayasu's arteritis in Asia'. *Cardiovasc Surg* 2001;9:3–10.
15. Weyand CM, Goronzy JJ. Medium- and large-vessel vasculitis. *N Engl J Med* 2003;349:160–169.
16. McCarthy WJ, Yao JS, Schafer MF, et al. Upper extremity arterial injury in athletes. *J Vasc Surg* 1989;9:317–327.
17. Kee ST, Dake MD, Wolfe-Johnson B, et al. Ischemia of the throwing hand in major league baseball pitchers: embolic occlusion from aneurysms of axillary artery branches. *J Vasc Interv Radiol* 1995;6:979–982.
18. Reekers JA, den Hartog BM, Kuyper CF, et al. Traumatic aneurysm of the posterior circumflex humeral artery: a volleyball player's disease? *J Vasc Interv Radiol* 1993;4:405–408.
19. Rohrer MJ, Cardullo PA, Pappas AM, et al. Axillary artery compression and thrombosis in throwing athletes. *J Vasc Surg* 1990;11:761–768; discussion 768–769.
20. Durham JR, Yao JS, Pearce WH, et al. Arterial injuries in the thoracic outlet syndrome. *J Vasc Surg* 1995;21:57–69; discussion 70.
21. Mesh CL, Yao JST. Upper extremity bypass: five-year follow-up. In: Yao JST, Pearce WH, eds. *Long-term Results in Vascular Surgery*. Norwalk, CT: Appleton & Lange; 1993:353–365.
22. Cina CS, Safar HA, Lagana A, et al. Subclavian carotid transposition and bypass grafting: consecutive cohort study and systematic review. *J Vasc Surg* 2002;35:422–429.
23. Schardey HM, Meyer G, Rau HG, et al. Subclavian carotid transposition: an analysis of a clinical series and a review of the literature. *Eur J Vasc Endovasc Surg* 1996;12:431–436.
24. Morasch MD, Berguer R. Supra-aortic trunk revascularization. In: Yao JST, ed. *Modern Vascular Surgery*. New York: McGraw-Hill; 2000:137.
25. Ziomek S, Quinones-Baldrich WJ, Busuttil RW, et al. The superiority of synthetic arterial grafts over autologous veins in carotid-subclavian bypass. *J Vasc Surg* 1986;3:140–145.
26. Montarjeme A. Percutaneous transluminal angioplasty of supra-aortic vessels. *J Endovasc Surg* 1996;3(2):171–181.
27. Yao JST, Flinn WR, McCarthy WJ, et al. Upper extremity revascularization. In: Bergan JJ, Yao JST, eds. *Techniques in Arterial Surgery*. Philadelphia, PA: WB Saunders; 1990:328–338.
28. McCarthy WJ, Flinn WR, Yao JS, et al. Result of bypass grafting for upper limb ischemia. *J Vasc Surg* 1986;3:741–746.
29. Bowling JC, Dowd PM. Raynaud's disease. *Lancet* 2003;361:2078–2080.

CHAPTER 92 ■ RENAL ARTERY OCCLUSIVE AND ANEURYSMAL DISEASE

GILBERT R. UPCHURCH, Jr., PETER K. HENKE, JOHN E. RECTENWALD, JONATHAN L. ELIASON, AND JAMES C. STANLEY

KEY POINTS

1. Renal artery disease is recognized with increasing frequency with the advent of less invasive imaging modalities.
2. Renovascular hypertension secondary to renal artery occlusive disease is the most common form of surgically correctable hypertension, and is more common in adult patients with more severe diastolic blood pressure elevations; as many as 5% of such patients are found to have a renovascular cause of their hypertension.
3. Arteriosclerotic renal artery occlusive disease accounts for about 95% of reported cases of renovascular hypertension.
4. Medial fibroplasia is the most commonly diagnosed nonarteriosclerotic renal artery disease, accounting for 85% of dysplastic lesions.
5. Treatment of renovascular hypertension is in evolution.
6. Aneurysms of the renal artery are unusual and poorly understood vascular lesions and should generally be repaired in woman of childbearing age, when their diameter exceeds 1.5 cm, or when they are associated with hypertension.

(1) Renal artery diseases is recognized with increasing frequency with the advent of less invasive imaging modalities. The clinical importance of renal artery occlusive disease, be it due to arteriosclerosis, fibrodysplasia, or a developmental anomaly, warrants individual discussion. Similarly, renal artery aneurysms, be they true aneurysms or dissections, also warrant separate consideration.

The consequence of renal artery occlusive disease causing elevated blood pressure is well recognized and may be one of the most untreated vascular diseases in contemporary times. While true renal artery aneurysms and dissecting aneurysms are relatively uncommon, evidence suggests that they too may contribute to a hypertensive state in certain patients. The role of renal artery occlusive and aneurysmal disease as a cause of diminished renal function is less well defined.

RENAL ARTERY OCCLUSIVE DISEASE

(2) Renovascular hypertension secondary to renal artery occlusive disease is the most common form of surgically correctable hypertension. Systemic blood pressure elevations in these patients follow reductions in renal perfusion with activation of the renin-angiotensin system. This physiologic response tends to restore the renal artery perfusion pressures toward normal, although it does so in a pathologic manner by producing hypertension in the systemic circulation.

Pathophysiology of Renovascular Hypertension

The physiologic basis of renovascular hypertension is well defined. This form of hypertension was first recognized more than 60 years ago by Goldblatt et al.,[1] who produced sustained hypertension in a canine model after gradual reductions in renal artery blood flow using an externally controlled vascular clamp. Subsequent studies have discounted the importance of renal ischemia per se as the cause of renovascular hypertension, with other hemodynamic signals appearing essential in increasing renin release, the most obvious being a decrease in mean renal artery perfusion pressure. A stenosis causing an 80% reduction in renal artery cross-sectional area (a so-called critical stenosis) induces a pressure gradient sufficient to cause increased renin release from the kidney. Renin and its effects on angiotensin and aldosterone account for the elevated blood pressure of renovascular hypertension (Fig. 92.1).

Renin is produced by the juxtaglomerular apparatus of the kidney. This anatomic area consists of a variety of cells, including *myoepitheloid cells* or *granular cells*, located on the wall of the afferent arterioles; the *macula densa*, which is composed of specialized tubular epithelial cells in the glomerular hilus at the transition of the loop of Henle to the distal convoluted tubule; and *lacis cells*, located in the region of the efferent glomerular arteriole and the macula densa. Lacis cells are intimately associated with the glomerulus and are anatomically similar to mesangial cells. The interrelations between the macula densa, glomerular arteriole vasomotion, and renal tubular function are important in understanding renin kinetics.

Regulation of renin production and its release from the kidney at the cellular and molecular level is complex. Renal baroreceptors, acting as stretch receptors, affect the release of renin from juxtaglomerular cells. Activation of these receptors appears to involve the calcium ion, with increasing evidence that renin release and intracellular levels of calcium are inversely related. Alternatively, renin release can occur with changes in pressure at the afferent renal arteriole level, as well as with changes in renal interstitial volume and pressure.

Renin is a proteolytic enzyme, active at a neutral pH on its only known substrate, angiotensinogen. Renin is a single-chain polypeptide with a molecular weight of about 38 kD.[2] It is stored as granules within the juxtaglomerular cells and, in some instances, as granules within the arteriolar wall. Renin has a half-life of 20 to 30 minutes. Under usual circumstances of normal sodium balance, the sum of renin activity measured in both renal veins is about 48% greater than that in the infrarenal vena cava or peripheral arterial and venous circulations.[3] The renin levels in the peripheral circulation appear to

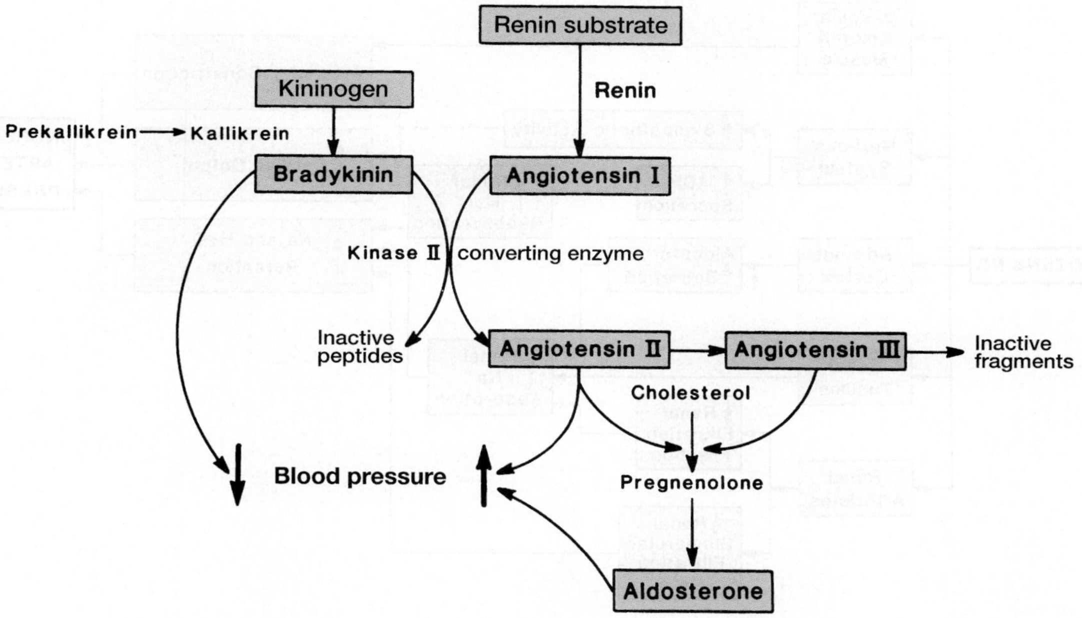

FIGURE 92.1. Renin-angiotensin system interrelation with aldosterone and bradykinin in regulation of blood pressure. (Adapted from Stanley JC, Graham LM, Whitehouse WM Jr. Renovascular hypertension. In: Miller TA, Rowland BJ, eds. *Physiologic Basis of Modern Surgical Care*. St. Louis, MO: CV Mosby; 1988:734.)

be in a steady state because of this relatively constant 48% contribution of renin from the kidneys. The liver is the primary site for removal and clearance of renin.[4] Extrarenal renin or reninlike enzymes (isorenins) exist in the submaxillary salivary gland, uterus, placenta, and brain, but there is no evidence that these substances are functionally important in elevating blood pressure.

The biochemistry of the renin-angiotensin system has been well defined (Fig. 92.2). The primary, if not sole, function of renin is the hydrolysis of renin substrate (a circulating peptide known as *angiotensinogen*) to form angiotensin I. Angiotensinogen is an α_2-globulin with a molecular weight of 60 kD. It is produced in the liver. Expression of the angiotensinogen gene is subject to a variety of physiologic and pathophysiologic stimuli, including steroid hormones, angiotensin II, salt loading, and various drugs. Angiotensinogen itself has no vasoactive properties.

Angiotensin I, a decapeptide produced by the renin–renin substrate reaction, has little vasoactivity. It does exert an effect on the adrenal medulla, the sympathetic and central nervous systems, and the renal arterioles. Angiotensin II is formed

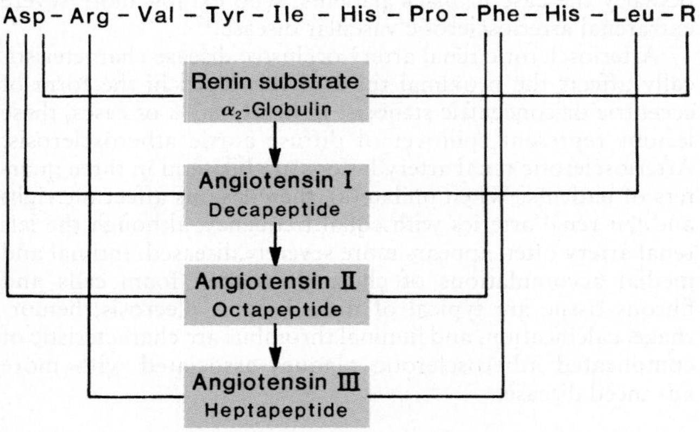

FIGURE 92.2. Biochemical composition of renin substrate and the angiotensins. (Adapted from Stanley JC, Graham LM. Renovascular hypertension. In: Miller TA, ed. *Physiologic Basis of Modern Surgical Care*, 2nd ed. St. Louis, MO: Quality Medical Publishing; 1998:918.)

when two C-terminal peptides are cleaved from angiotensin I by the carboxypeptidase angiotensin-converting enzyme (ACE). Angiotensin II, an octapeptide, represents the vasoconstrictive element of renovascular hypertension. Although angiotensin II stimulates liver production of renin substrate, in normal subjects, it provides a continuous negative feedback on renal release of renin.[5] Angiotensin II has a half-life of about 4 minutes. Angiotensin III, a heptapeptide, is produced with the aminopeptidase cleavage of angiotensin II to I-des-aspartyl-angiotensin II. Angiotensin III is known to inhibit angiotensin II, but its most relevant effect is to increase aldosterone synthesis. Nevertheless, angiotensin III has little biologic activity of physiologic importance.

Aldosterone is secreted from the zona glomerulosa of the adrenal cortex and represents the volume element of renovascular hypertension. The biosynthesis of this mineralocorticoid includes cleavage of a side chain of cholesterol to form pregnenolone. This step is facilitated by both angiotensin II and III. Aldosterone increases renal conservation of sodium and water, with a subsequent extracellular fluid volume expansion and an eventual increase in blood pressure.

ACE (dipeptidyl carboxypeptidase) is a zinc metallopeptidase responsible for producing angiotensin II from angiotensin I by removing C-terminal peptides from angiotensin I. ACE has its highest concentration in the endothelium of the pulmonary circulation. Conversion of angiotensin I to angiotensin II, at physiologic concentrations, occurs in a single passage through the lungs.[6] ACE has been found at lower levels in the blood and kidney as well as in other vascular beds. ACE is also important in the metabolism of the vasodepressor bradykinin. At least two enzymes appear to inactivate bradykinin. The first, kinase I, acts by cleaving the carboxy-terminal arginine of bradykinin. The second, kinase II, acts by cleaving the carboxy-terminal dipeptide group Phe-Arg. Kinase II and ACE appear to be similar in that they have nearly identical substrate specificities, cofactor requirements, and antigenic specificities.[7]

The actions of angiotensin on cardiac activity, vascular smooth muscle reactivity, and sodium and water metabolism contribute to increased arterial pressure (Fig. 92.3). The most important consequence of renal artery occlusive disease is the production of angiotensin II, which is one of the most potent

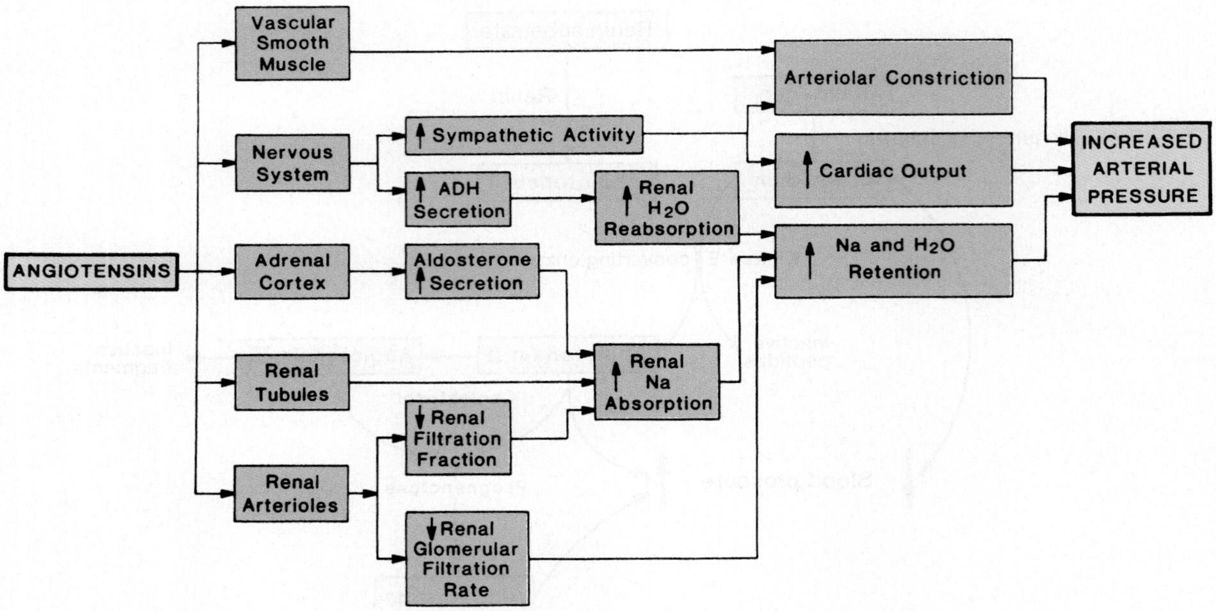

FIGURE 92.3. Effects of angiotensins contributing to increased arterial pressure. (Adapted from Stanley JC, Graham LM. Renovascular hypertension. In: Miller TA, ed. *Physiologic Basis of Modern Surgical Care,* 2nd ed. St. Louis, MO: Quality Medical Publishing; 1998:918.)

pressor substances known. Angiotensin II acts directly on arteriolar smooth muscle of nearly all vascular beds; the splanchnic, renal, and cutaneous circulations are most sensitive to its effects. There is a general acceptance of the central importance of angiotensin in the generation of renovascular hypertension.

Hemodynamic responses to an activated renin-angiotensin system depend on the rate of alterations in renal blood flow as well as on whether one or both kidneys are affected. Acute reductions in renal blood flow result in rapid increases in plasma renin and blood pressure. In the case of unilateral renovascular disease with a normal opposite kidney, the hypertension is characterized by renin hypersecretion from the affected kidney and suppression of renin production in the contralateral kidney.[8,9] Sodium retention within the affected kidney is counterbalanced by continuous sodium excretion from the normal contralateral kidney, resulting in a relative intravascular volume depletion. This vasoconstrictive form of hypertension is angiotensin II dependent and responds to ACE inhibitors.

Pathophysiologic alterations accompanying bilateral renovascular disease, or unilateral disease of a solitary kidney, relate to changes other than vasoconstriction. Angiotensin II causes sodium retention, diminutions in glomerular filtration, stimulation of aldosterone production, and stimulation of norepinephrine release from the adrenergic nervous system. In chronic bilateral or unilateral renovascular hypertension in patients with only one kidney, sodium retention accounts for late reductions in renin secretion, although it is possible that absolute renin activity is abnormally high with regard to the existing sodium balance. Blood pressure elevations do not appear as dependent on the renin-angiotensin system in sodium-replete chronic renovascular hypertension. In this setting, ACE inhibitors are more effective in reducing elevated blood pressures with sodium depletion.[10]

Pathology of Renal Artery Occlusive Disease

Different macrovascular occlusive diseases affect the renal arterial circulation.[11,12] The most common are arteriosclerosis and arterial fibrodysplasia. Developmental renal artery narrowings are a rare cause of renovascular hypertension. Although uncommon, renal artery emboli and traumatic occlusions are occasionally associated with acute renin-mediated hypertension.

3 **Arteriosclerosis.** Renal artery occlusive disease due to arteriosclerosis accounts for 95% of reported cases of renovascular hypertension (Fig. 92.4). This type of renovascular hypertension may be even more common because many earlier reported experiences were surgical series that excluded older patients who were not open operative candidates and thus not evaluated for this disease. A recent study using a large administrative database showed that the diagnosis of renovascular hypertension and renal artery atherosclerosis in the United States has increased 46% over the years 1988 to 2001.[13] Arteriosclerotic renovascular disease most commonly presents during the sixth decade of life. Men are affected twice as often as women. Although some degree of arteriosclerotic renal artery stenotic disease affects nearly half of the elderly population, it is not always associated with elevated blood pressures. Many of these patients exhibit occlusive disease of the coronary, cerebral, mesenteric, or extremity circulation.[14–16] This is particularly the case in black patients, who exhibit more severe extrarenal arteriosclerotic vascular disease.[17]

Arteriosclerotic renal artery occlusive disease characteristically affects the proximal third of the vessel in the form of eccentric or concentric stenosis. In nearly 80% of cases, these lesions represent spillover of diffuse aortic atherosclerosis. Arteriosclerotic renal artery lesions are bilateral in three quarters of patients. When unilateral, these lesions affect the right and left renal arteries with equal frequency, although the left renal artery often appears more severely diseased. Intimal and medial accumulations of cholesterol-laden foam cells and fibrous tissue are typical of these lesions. Necrosis, hemorrhage, calcification, and luminal thrombus are characteristic of complicated atherosclerotic plaques associated with more advanced disease.

Arterial Fibrodysplasia. The second most common type of renal artery disease is arteriofibrodysplasia, accounting for about 5% of reported cases of renovascular hypertension.[11,12] Dysplastic renal artery stenosis represents a heterogenous group of lesions. They are classified by the specific pathologic process and vessel wall region most affected. Included among

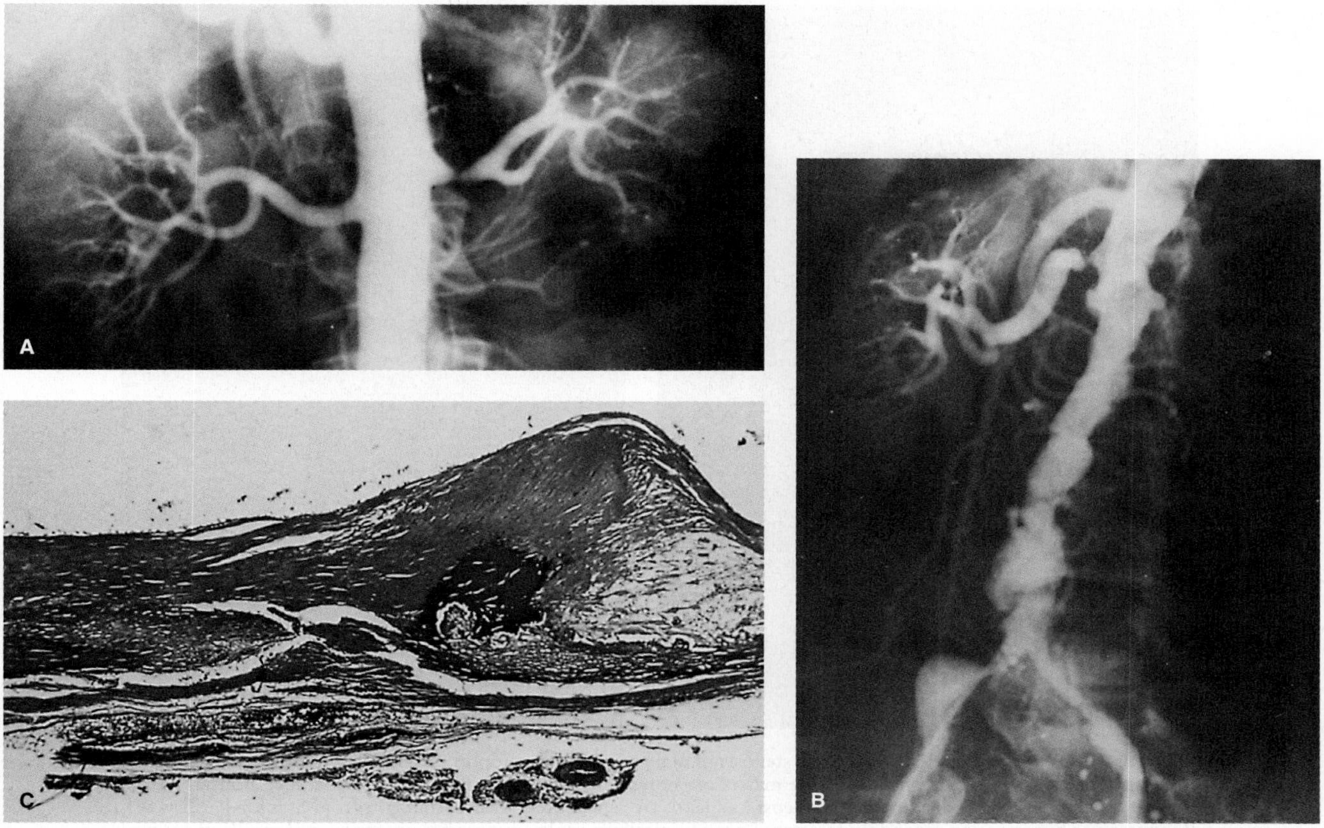

FIGURE 92.4. Renal artery arteriosclerosis. **A:** Intrinsic focal lesion of proximal renal artery. **B:** Severe aortic spillover disease affecting renal artery orifice and entire abdominal aorta. **C:** Complicated renal artery plaque exhibiting collections of cholesterol, extensive fibrosis, and calcification (hematoxin–eosin, ×60). (A and C reproduced with permission from Stanley JC. Morphologic, histopathologic and clinical characteristics of renovascular fibrodysplasia and arteriosclerosis. In: Bergan JJ, Yao JST, eds. *Surgery of the Aorta and Its Body Branches*. New York: Grune & Stratton; 1979:355; B reproduced with permission from Stanley JC, Graham LM, Whitehouse WM Jr. Renovascular hypertension. In: Miller TA, Rowland BJ, eds. *Physiologic Basis of Modern Surgical Care*. St. Louis, MO: CV Mosby; 1988:734.)

these lesions are intimal fibroplasia, medial fibroplasia, and perimedial dysplasia.[18] The last two entities appear to be a continuum of the same disease process. Each category has certain characteristic features deserving individual comment.

Intimal fibroplasia accounts for about 5% of all dysplastic renal artery stenosis (Fig. 92.5). These lesions occur in children and young adults more often than in the elderly, and they affect both genders equally. The cause of primary intimal fibroplasia is unknown but may be related to persistent embryonic myointimal cushions. Secondary intimal fibroplasia has been attributed to flow disturbances, blunt abdominal trauma, and the sequela of an earlier arteritis, such as occurs with rubella. Progression of intimal fibroplasia may cause turbulent blood flow and a rapidly accelerated fibroproliferative response that compromises the arterial lumen.

Intimal fibroplasia usually presents as a smooth, focal stenosis of the distal main renal artery. In some patients, these lesions produce long, tubular stenosis, and in rare cases, they present as webs affecting segmental arteries. Proximal ostial lesions most often represent the secondary form of this disease, associated with abdominal aortic hypoplasia and coarctation. Subendothelial accumulations of irregularly arranged mesenchymal cells surrounded by loose fibrous connective tissue are typical of all intimal fibrodysplastic lesions. The internal elastic lamina is usually intact, but partial fragmentation may occur. Medial and adventitial structures are normal in primary intimal fibrodysplasia.

4 *Medial fibroplasia* is the most commonly diagnosed dysplastic renal artery disease, accounting for 85% of these lesions (Fig. 92.6). Medial fibroplasia is invariably found in women, with cases in men being anecdotal. The clinical presentation of this disease is most common between 25 and 45 years of age. Medial fibroplasia appears to be a systemic arteriopathy, with the internal carotid arteries representing the extrarenal vessels most often affected. The cause of medial fibroplasia remains poorly understood but appears to be associated with modification of smooth muscle to myofibroblasts caused by estrogenic stimuli during the reproductive years, unusual traction forces on affected vessels, and mural ischemia from impairment of vasa vasorum blood flow.[18] The physical forces contributing to medial fibroplasia may be attributed to ptotic kidneys with stretching of the renal arteries (Fig. 92.7). The fact that renal ptosis occurs more often in women than in men may explain the almost unique involvement of the renal artery with medial fibroplasia in women.

Morphologic appearances of medial dysplasia range from a solitary stenosis to multiple constrictions with intervening mural dilations affecting the middle and distal main renal artery. The latter are responsible for this lesion's classic string-of-beads appearance. Actual macrovascular aneurysms occurring at branchings affect a little more than 10% of patients with arterial fibrodysplasia. Stenotic disease of segmental branches occurs in about 25% of cases. Bilateral disease affects nearly 60% of patients and is usually most severe on the right. Unilateral lesions affect the left and right renal arteries in 10% and 30% of cases, respectively. Progression of disease occurs in about 20% of premenopausal women.

Perimedial dysplasia accounts for nearly 10% of dysplastic renal artery stenotic disease (Fig. 92.8). These lesions invariably occur in women, usually between the ages of 30 and 50 years. Perimedial dysplasia is bilateral in 20% of patients and appears to be more progressive than medial fibrodysplasia. Perimedial dysplasia is characterized by solitary or multiple

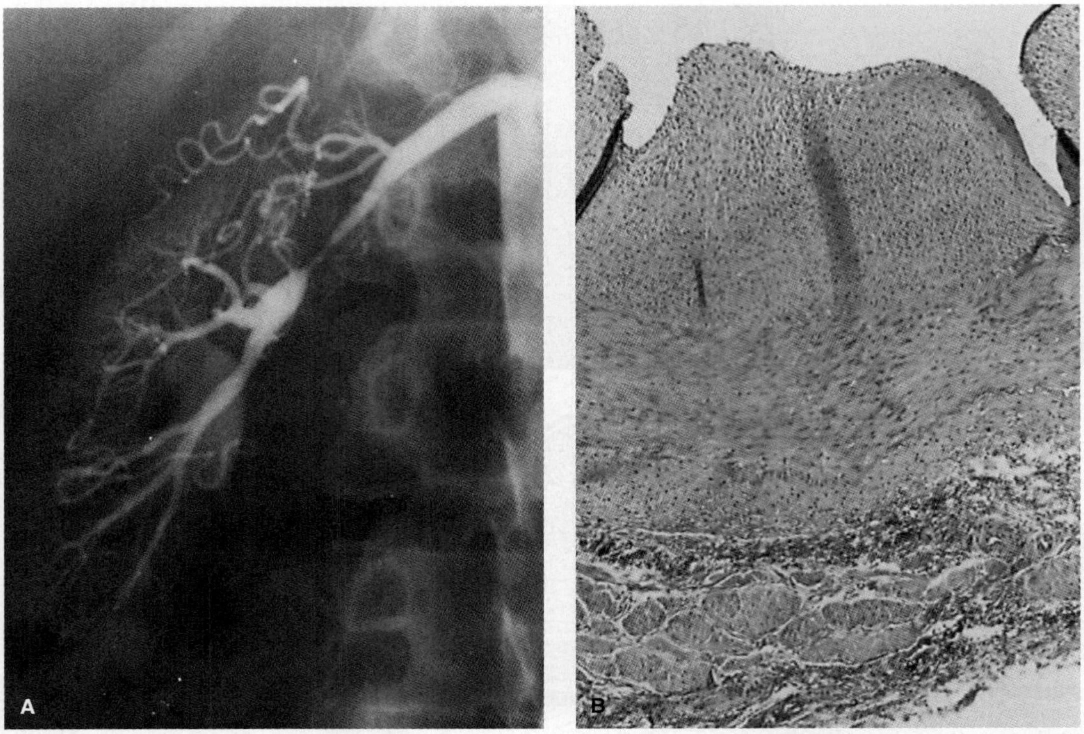

FIGURE 92.5. Intimal fibroplasia. **A:** Focal stenosis of main renal artery midportion. **B:** Subendothelial mesenchymal cells within a loose fibrous connective tissue matrix are noted above an intact internal elastic lamina, normal media, and normal adventitial tissues (hematoxin–eosin, ×120). (A reproduced with permission from Stanley JC, Fry WJ. Renovascular hypertension secondary to arterial fibrodysplasia in adults: criteria for operation and results of surgical therapy. *Arch Surg* 1975;110:922–928; B reproduced with permission from Stanley JC. Morphologic, histopathologic and clinical characteristics of renovascular fibrodysplasia and arteriosclerosis. In: Bergan JJ, Yao JST, eds. *Surgery of the Aorta and Its Body Branches*. New York: Grune & Stratton; 1979:355.)

constrictions, without intervening dilations. Most stenoses involve the distal main renal artery, without segmental branch involvement. Certain histologic features are common to both perimedial dysplasia and medial fibroplasia, and they may represent different manifestations of the same pathologic entity. Although unusual accumulations of elastic tissue in inner adventitial regions is the most prominent abnormality in perimedial dysplasia, increases in medial ground substances may also accompany this type of dysplastic disease.[18]

Developmental Renal Artery Disease. Narrowings of the renal artery occurring during fetal growth are a rare cause of renovascular hypertension. They are often associated with both abdominal aortic coarctation and splanchnic

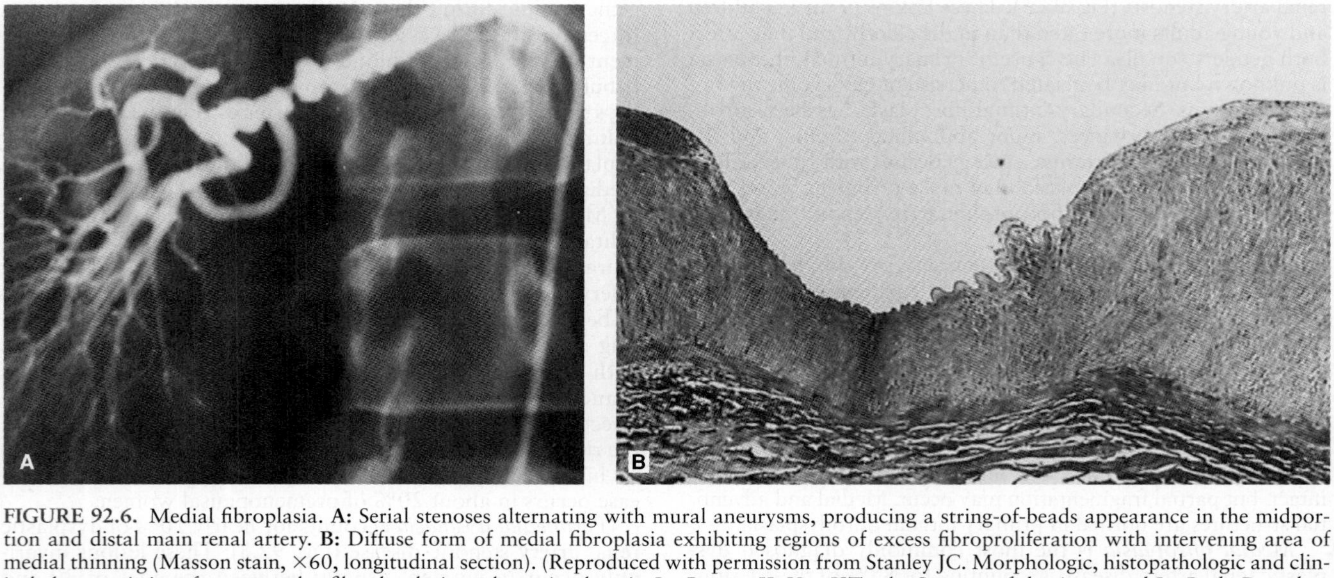

FIGURE 92.6. Medial fibroplasia. **A:** Serial stenoses alternating with mural aneurysms, producing a string-of-beads appearance in the midportion and distal main renal artery. **B:** Diffuse form of medial fibroplasia exhibiting regions of excess fibroproliferation with intervening area of medial thinning (Masson stain, ×60, longitudinal section). (Reproduced with permission from Stanley JC. Morphologic, histopathologic and clinical characteristics of renovascular fibrodysplasia and arteriosclerosis. In: Bergan JJ, Yao JST, eds. *Surgery of the Aorta and Its Body Branches*. New York: Grune & Stratton; 1979:355.)

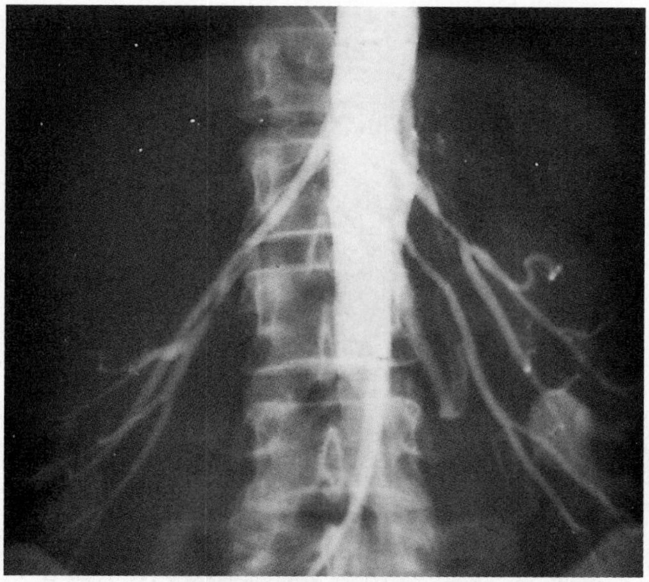

FIGURE 92.7. Medial fibrodysplasia manifested as irregular narrowings to ptotic kidneys affecting the midportion of the main renal arteries, which appear stretched during upright aortography. (Reproduced with permission from Stanley JC, Wakefield TW. Arterial fibrodysplasia. In: Rutherford RB, ed. *Vascular Surgery,* 5th ed. Philadelphia, PA: WB Saunders; 2000:387.)

arterial stenoses[19–24] (Fig. 92.9). These lesions are encountered most often in children and young adults. About 40% of children with renovascular hypertension are thought to have developmental renal artery stenosis. Similarly, nearly 20% of adults with primary intimal fibroplastic renal artery disease have stenoses that can be attributed to developmental defects. Boys slightly outnumbered girls. These stenotic lesions represent true hypoplasia of the renal artery, exhibiting an external hourglass appearance. Developmental lesions usually occur at the aortic origin of the artery. Sparse medial tissue, intimal fibroplasia, fragmentation and duplication of the internal elastic lamina, and disproportionate excesses in adventitial elastic tissue are the most common histologic abnormalities in these diminutive vessels.[20,21,23]

Developmental renal artery narrowings may be attributed to certain embryonic events occurring as the two fetal dorsal aortas fuse and all but one of their metanephric branches to the kidney regress. Abnormal transition of mesenchymal to medial smooth muscle at that time, or later impairment of its growth, can cause both aortic and renovascular anomalies. Vessels to the mesonephros within mesenchymal tissue around the two dorsal aortas are replaced during fetal growth by a more cephalic group of vessels to the metanephros. That a solitary artery to each kidney evolves from these arteries in 75% of people has been attributed to its obligate hemodynamic advantage over adjacent channels. Flow changes in the region where single central renal arteries usually arise may afford coexisting polar arteries hemodynamic advantages that ensure their persistence. Supporting such a hypothesis concerning the cause of developmental lesions is the fact that multiple stenotic renal arteries exist in more than half of those patients with central abdominal aortic coarctation or hypoplasia.

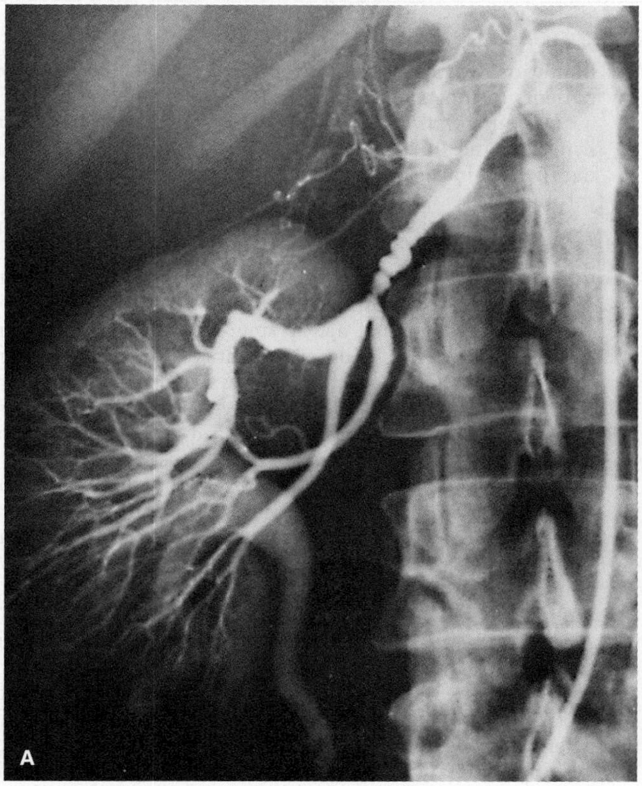

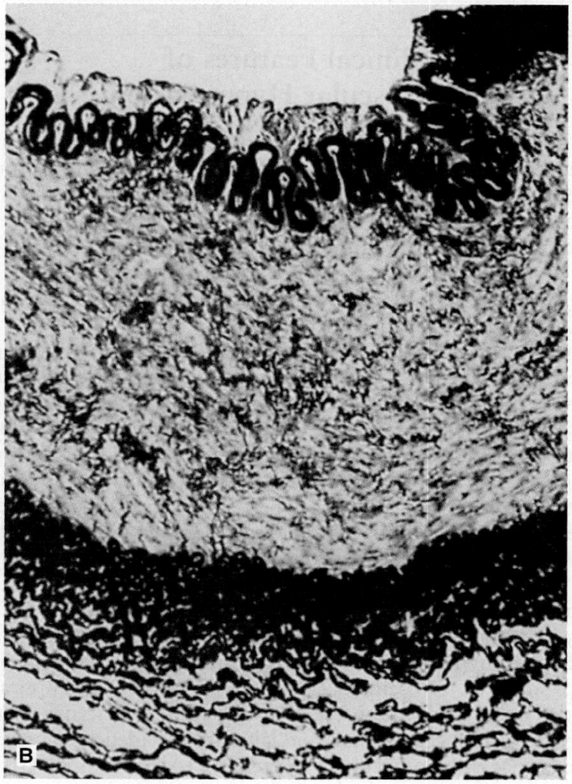

FIGURE 92.8. Perimedial dysplasia. **A:** Multiple stenoses without mural aneurysms in the midportion of the renal artery are characteristic of these lesions. **B:** These lesions are due to excessive accumulations of elastic tissue at the medial–adventitial junction (Verhoeff stain, ×120). (Reproduced with permission from Stanley JC. Morphologic, histopathologic and clinical characteristics of renovascular fibrodysplasia and arteriosclerosis. In: Bergan JJ, Yao JST, eds. *Surgery of the Aorta and Its Body Branches.* New York: Grune & Stratton; 1979:355.)

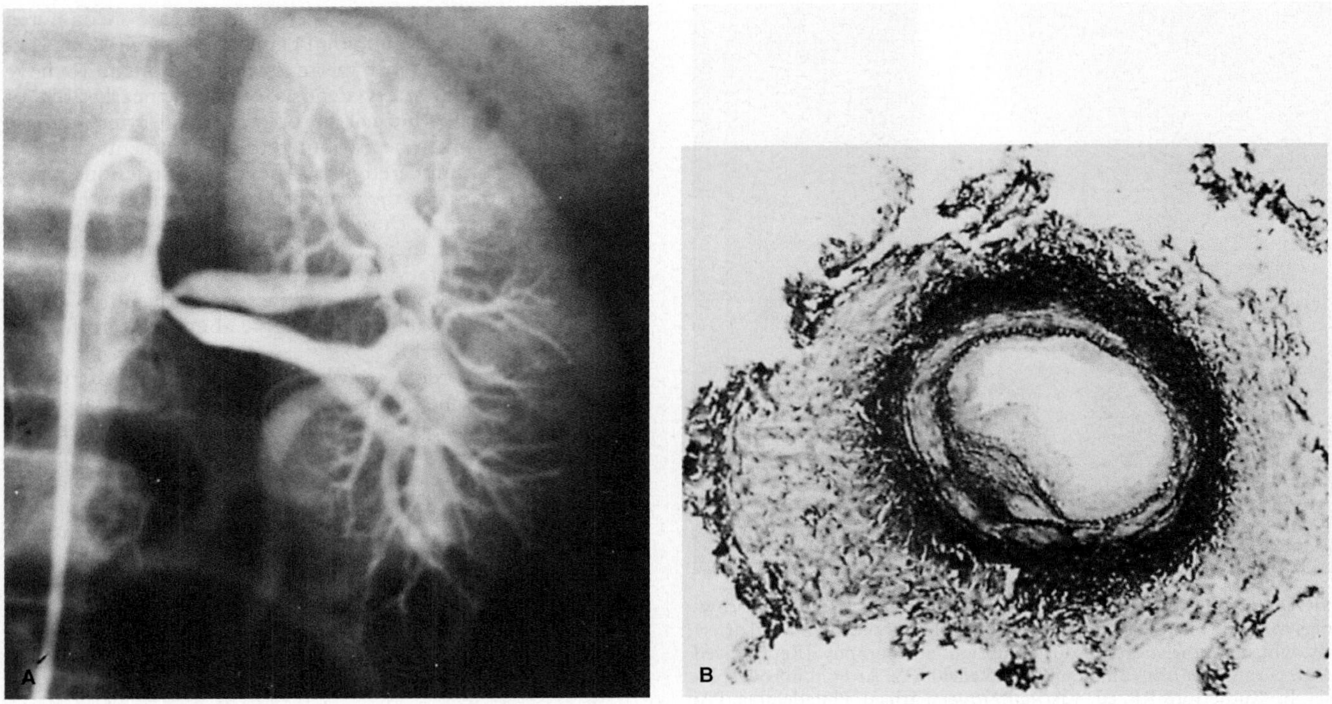

FIGURE 92.9. Developmental renal artery stenoses. **A:** Proximal vessel stenosis in a patient with neurofibromatosis and infrarenal aortic hypoplasia. **B:** Fragmentation and duplication of the internal elastic lamina and deficient medial tissues characterize these lesions. Intimal fibroplasia encroaches on the vessel lumen, which is less than 1 mm in diameter. Adventitial elastic tissues appear excessive (Movat stain, ×100). (A reproduced with permission from Stanley JC, Fry WJ. Pediatric renal artery occlusive disease and renovascular hypertension: etiology, diagnosis, and operative treatment. Developmental occlusive disease of the abdominal aorta and the splanchnic and renal arteries. *Arch Surg* 1981;116:669–676; B reproduced with permission from Stanley JC, Graham LM, Whitehouse WM Jr, et al. Developmental occlusive disease of the abdominal aorta and the splanchnic and renal arteries. *Am J Surg* 1981;142:190–196.)

Clinical Features of Renovascular Hypertension

The frequency of renovascular hypertension among adult patients who have diastolic blood pressures higher than 100 mm Hg is about 2%. It is much more common in patients with more severe diastolic blood pressure elevations; as many as 5% of such patients are found to have a renovascular cause of their hypertension. It is the second most common cause of hypertension in childhood, being outnumbered only by thoracic isthmic aortic coarctation.

Findings suggestive of renovascular hypertension include upper abdominal bruits during both systole and diastole, initial diastolic blood pressures greater than 115 mm Hg, a sudden worsening of mild to moderate essential hypertension, development of hypertension during childhood, or rapid onset of high blood pressure after the age of 50 years. Hypertension resistant to drug therapy and malignant hypertension are also more likely to be associated with this form of secondary hypertension. Similarly, patients who exhibit deterioration in renal function while receiving multiple antihypertensive drugs, especially ACE inhibitors, may have underlying renal artery stenotic disease. The costs and errors incumbent to indiscriminate evaluations for this form of hypertension that lead to unnecessary interventions are prohibitive. A useful decision algorithm in contemporary practice is based on the presenting degree of hypertension and presence or absence of clinical and laboratory evidence suggesting the existence of renovascular hypertension (Algorithm 92.1).

Diagnosis of Renal Artery Occlusive Disease and Secondary Hypertension

Most diagnostic and prognostic tests for renovascular hypertension assess either the anatomic stenosis or derangements of renal function attributed to the stenosis. The usefulness and limitations of these tests become relevant in the selection of patients for open surgical or endovascular interventions.

Deep abdominal renal artery ultrasonography may identify hemodynamically significant renal artery narrowings by imaging the renal arteries and characterizing flow velocity patterns through these vessels[25,26] (Fig. 92.10). Ultrasonography is a reasonable initial screening test. Existence of a stenosis appears established when peak systolic velocities are in the range of 180 to 200 cm/s and the ratio of these velocities to those in the aorta approaches 3.5. Unfortunately, ultrasonography does not discriminate among renal artery stenosis exceeding 60% cross-sectional narrowing. Failure to identify a main renal artery in the absence of any parenchymal flow signal suggests main renal artery occlusion. An occluded accessory or segmental renal artery, however, may not be recognized and, thus, contributes to this technology's false-negative assessments.

Computed tomographic arteriography (CTA) is another frequently used means of assessing coexistent renal artery disease (Fig. 92.11). It allows computer-generated visualization of the vessels from many different angles not possible with conventional biplanar arteriography. However, CTA carries the risk of contrast-induced nephrotoxicity.

Arteriography was central to past evaluations of patients suspected of having hypertension. Oblique aortography and multiple-plane selective renal arteriography have improved the recognition of the morphologic character and extent of renal artery stenosis in this disease entity. Collateral vessels circumventing a renal artery stenosis are evidence of the lesion's hemodynamic importance. A pressure gradient approaching 10 mm Hg is necessary for collateral vessel development, and the same degree of pressure change is associated with activation of the renin system. Thus, the functional importance of an otherwise benign-appearing stenosis is established when collateral vessels are evident (Fig. 92.12). *Intra-arterial digital subtraction angiography* allows use of smaller quantities of

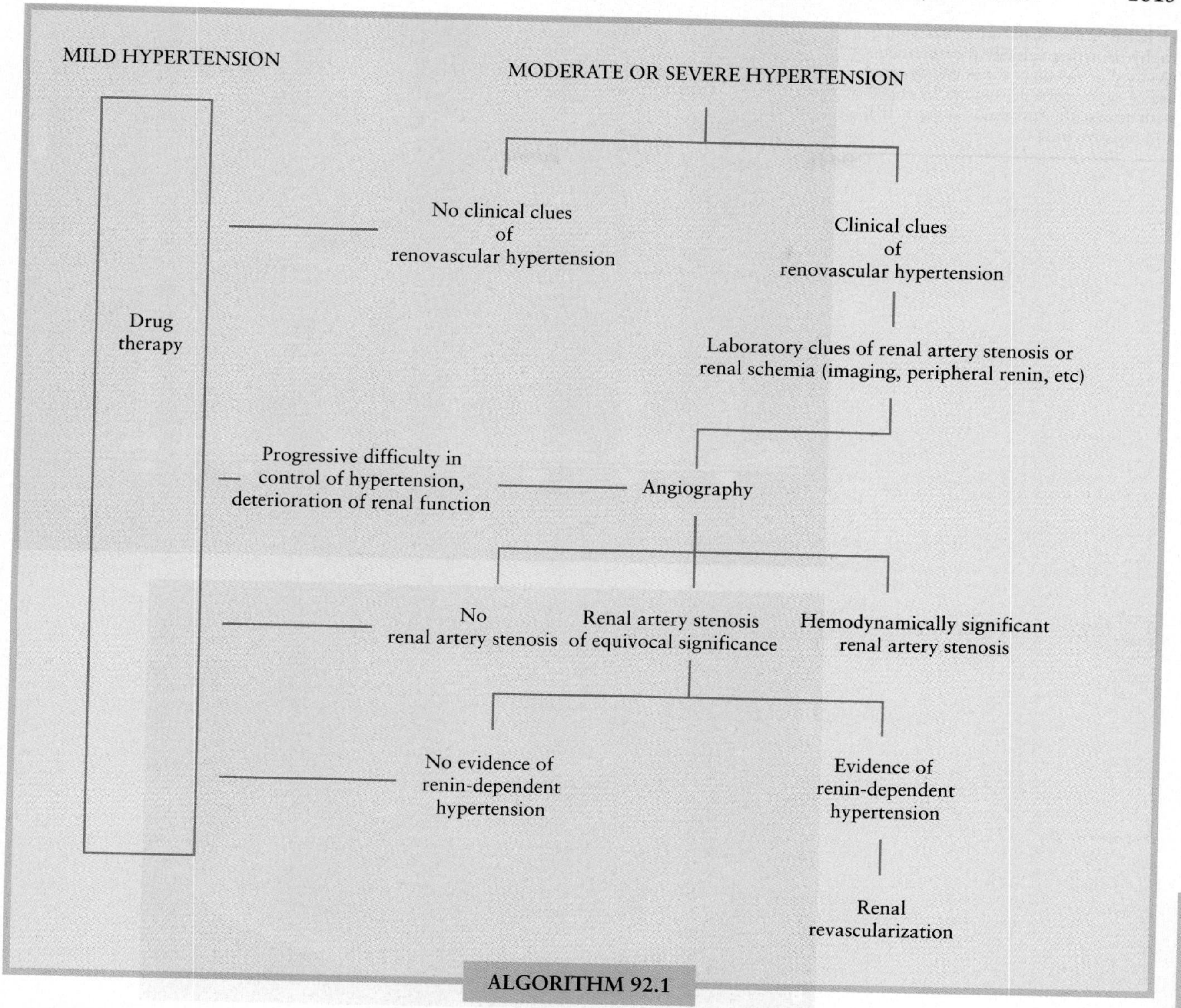

ALGORITHM 92.1. Management of renovascular hypertension. (Adapted from Stanley JC. Renal artery stenosis and hypertension. In: Brewster DC, ed. *Common Problems in Vascular Surgery*. Chicago, IL: Year Book; 1989:187.)

iodinated contrast agents compared with conventional arteriography, and it lessens the potential of contrast-induced nephrotoxicity. This is of particular relevance in patients with compromised renal function. The use of carbon dioxide in the latter circumstances is also appealing, but may not always provide sufficient anatomic detail for clinical decision making in patients with more distal segmental arterial disease.[27]

Magnetic resonance angiography (MRA), especially with breath-hold techniques and gadolinium enhancement, provides reasonable images of diseased renal arteries.[28,29] A normal study usually confirms absence of disease, but because of phase dropout with vessel tortuosity, a study may appear abnormal in a patient having a relatively minor stenotic disease. Nevertheless, MRA's noninvasiveness and lack of nephrotoxicity make it an attractive diagnostic test. The documentation of nephrogenic dermatofibrosis following the administration of gadolinium in patients with renal insufficiency has lessened the enthusiasm for the use of MRA in studying patients suspected of having renal artery stenosis.[30]

The use of physiologic tests to confirm the importance of anatomic narrowings is performed less frequently for a number of reasons, including the significant expense of the preparation required prior to these studies, as well as lack of sensitivity for certain tests.

Renin activity comparing peripheral and renal venous blood, in the past, was a recognized means of detecting functionally important renal artery disease. Today, renin assessments are undertaken in the rare patient with complex but equivocal disease, when the risk of an intervention demands a confirmed diagnosis. The *renal vein renin ratio* (RVRR) is calculated by dividing the renin activity in venous blood from the affected kidney by that from the contralateral kidney. An RVRR of greater than 1.48 is indicative of functionally important renovascular stenotic disease.[8,9] Because this test compares one kidney to another, it may not be useful in patients with bilateral disease if both kidneys exhibit elevated but equal degrees of excessive renin secretion. The *renal:systemic renin index* (RSRI) avoids this problem, and is calculated by subtracting systemic renin activity from individual renal vein renin activity and dividing the remainder by systemic renin activity.[8] It is an expression of individual kidney renin release. In nonrenovascular essential hypertensive patients, renal vein renin activity from each kidney is usually 24% higher than systemic activity.[3,9] Thus, the total of both kidneys' activity is usually

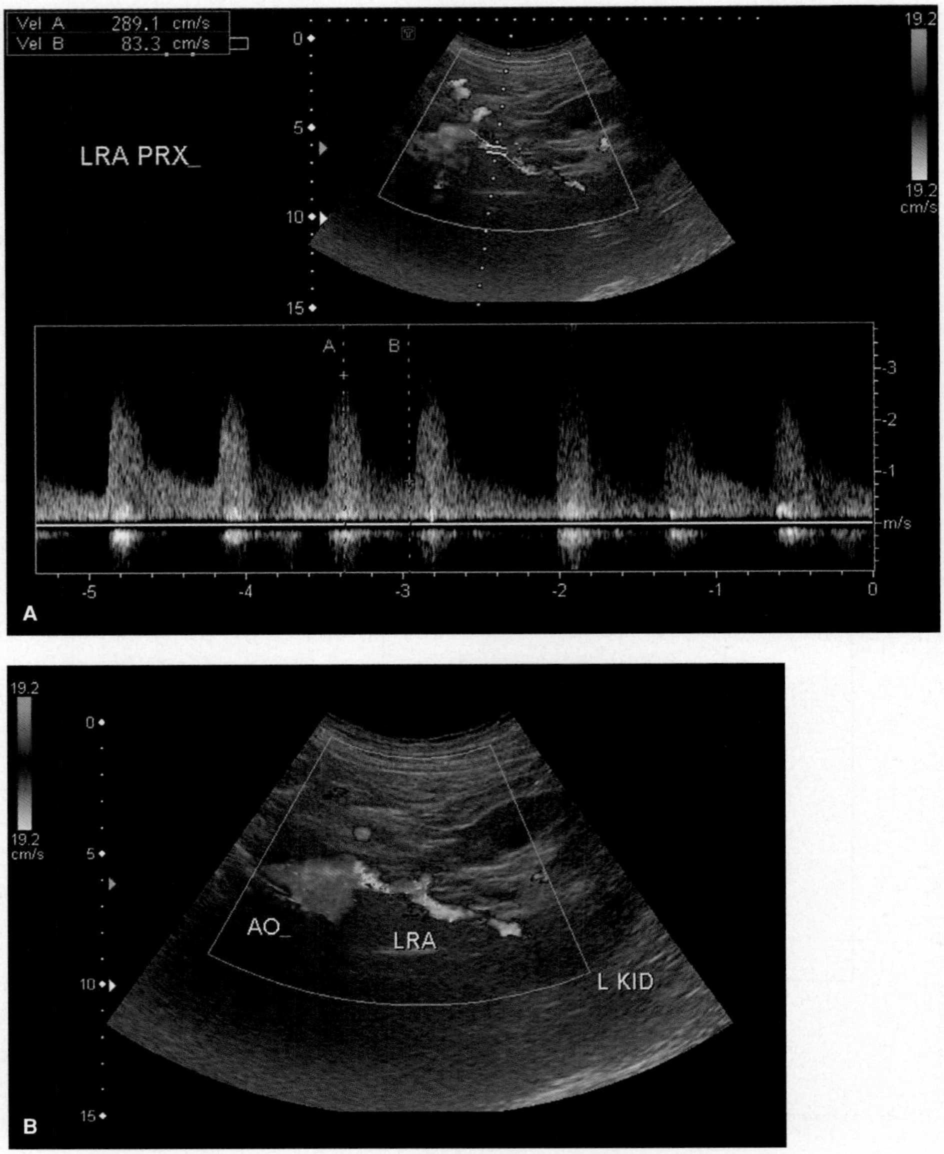

FIGURE 92.10. Renal artery ultrasonography depicting velocity measurements (**A**) used to calculate the aortic-to-renal artery ratio, percent stenosis by image with grayscale and color images (**B**), and resistive index.

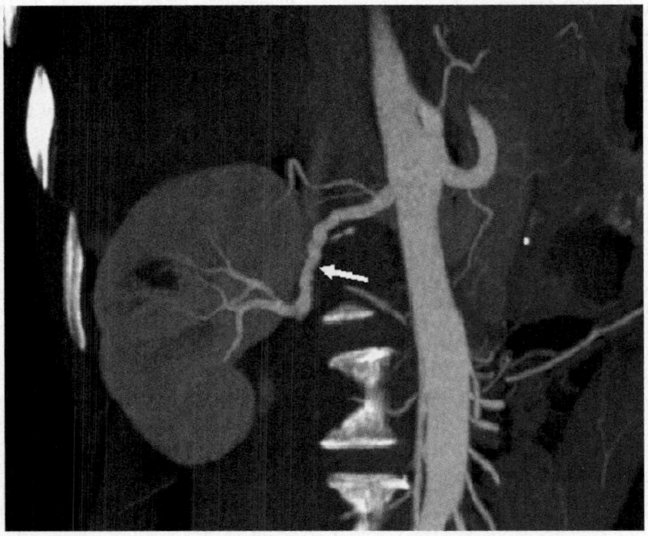

FIGURE 92.11. Computed tomographic arteriography of renal artery affected with fibromuscular dysplasia (*arrow*), exhibiting typical string-of-beads characteristic of medial fibroplasia.

48% higher than systemic activity and represents a steady state of normal renal renin release. The usefulness of ischemic kidney renin hypersecretion (RSRI more than 0.48) and contralateral kidney renin suppression (RSRI less than 0.24, approaching 0) as a means of discriminating between expected cured and improved operative outcomes has been well established.[8,31]

Hypertensive urography is not a good diagnostic test for renovascular hypertension because of its limited sensitivity.[32] Bilateral or segmental disease may interfere with the recognition of gross differences in contrast excretion between the two kidneys. In a large series of patients with proven renovascular hypertension, urograms were abnormal in only 27% of children with developmental disease, 48% of adults with arterial fibrodysplastic disease, and 72% of adults with atherosclerotic lesions.[33] Thus, use of hypertensive urography as a diagnostic or prognostic test for renovascular hypertension appears unjustified.

Isotopic renography allows both renal imaging and analysis of the washout curve of a number of radioactive tracers. A number of compounds have been used for these studies, including ^{99m}technetium-diethylenetriamine pentaacetic acid, iodine 123-orthoidohippurate or iodine 131-orthoidohippurate, ^{99m}technetium mercaptoacetyltriglycine, ^{99m}technetium-

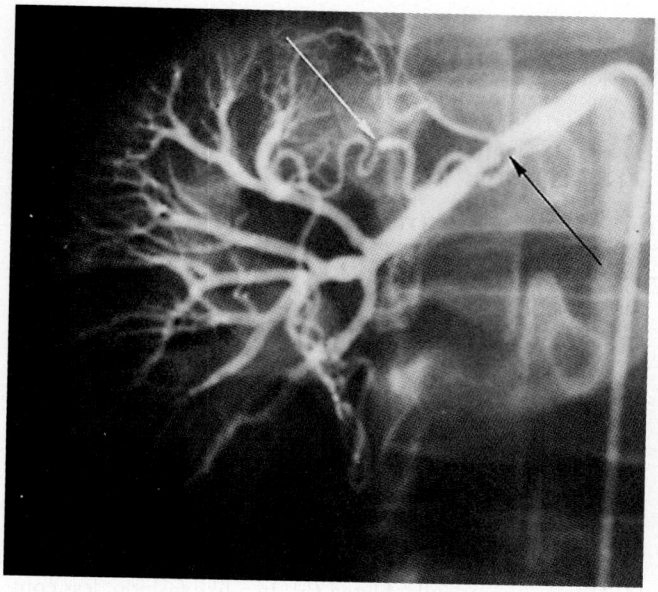

FIGURE 92.12. Arteriogram of a benign-appearing stenosis (*black arrow*) associated with a large collateral vessel (*white arrow*) circumventing the lesion, defining hemodynamic significance of the stenosis and implicating its functional importance. (Reproduced with permission from Stanley JC, Graham LM, Whitehouse WM Jr. Limitations and errors of diagnostic and prognostic investigations in renovascular hypertension. In: Bernhard VM, Towne JM, eds. *Complications in Vascular Surgery*. Orlando, FL: Grune & Stratton; 1984:213.)

dimercaptosuccinic acid, and ^{99m}glucoheptonate. These studies provide an assessment of renal blood flow as well as excretory function. Unfortunately, different states of hydration and intrarenal vascular resistance often contribute to flow abnormalities and false-positive studies in nonrenovascular hypertensives. The specificity and sensitivity of these studies are both about 75%. Administration of ACE inhibitors improves the sensitivity and specificity by blocking the compensatory change in glomerular filtration, causing it to fall in the affected kidney. The widespread use of this modified technology has not occurred, although some view ACE inhibitor–modified studies to be of greater value.[34] Renal perfusion/excretion ratios and more sophisticated computer analyses offer a potential means of increasing the predictive value of radionuclide screening for renovascular hypertension.

Treatment of Renal Artery Occlusive Disease

5 Treatment of renovascular hypertension is in evolution. Therapeutic results in the management of renovascular hypertension relate to both the proper selection of patients having clinically relevant renal artery disease as well as the execution of an appropriate intervention. Treatment options include drug therapy, percutaneous transluminal angioplasty (PTA) with or without stent placement, transcatheter renal ablation, arterial reconstructive surgery, and nephrectomy.

Drug Therapy of Renal Artery Occlusive Disease. Antihypertensive drugs are often used in the initial management of patients with renovascular hypertension. Beta-blocking agents, such as propranolol and atenolol, are commonly used as first-line therapy. Refractory hypertension, especially that caused by bilateral disease or unilateral lesions in patients with a solitary kidney or contralateral parenchymal disease, may respond to the addition of a thiazide diuretic, although with impaired renal function, the use of a loop diuretic, such as furosemide, is more effective.

ACE inhibitors, such as captopril and enalapril, have proved to be relatively effective drugs in treating renovascular hypertension. Unfortunately, ACE inhibitors may have a deleterious effect on renal function by preferentially dilating the glomerular efferent arterioles, critically decreasing the intraglomerular blood pressure, and reducing glomerular filtration. Certainly, ACE inhibitors must be used cautiously in renovascular hypertensive patients who have bilateral disease or a solitary kidney. Monitoring of renal function is mandatory after initiating treatment with ACE inhibitors. Use of angiotensin receptor blockers has not been well defined in this subgroup of hypertensive patients. Similarly, direct renin inhibitors, which have been shown to stabilize atherosclerotic plaque progression, have not been examined in the treatment of renovascular hypertension.[35]

Because stenotic disease of the renal artery often progresses with concomitant loss of renal mass and function, a definitive means of restoring normal renal blood flow may be more logical therapy than drug treatment, once a diagnosis of renovascular hypertension has been established.

Endovascular Therapy of Renal Artery Occlusive Disease. In 1978, Grüntzig was the first to report the use of PTA in the management of renovascular hypertension.[36] The less invasive nature of renal artery PTA offers certain advantages over operative intervention and this therapy is now used widely. Most renal artery stenoses can be traversed with a guide wire and subsequently dilated with or without a stent, with minimal morbidity and mortality (Fig. 92.13). To justify

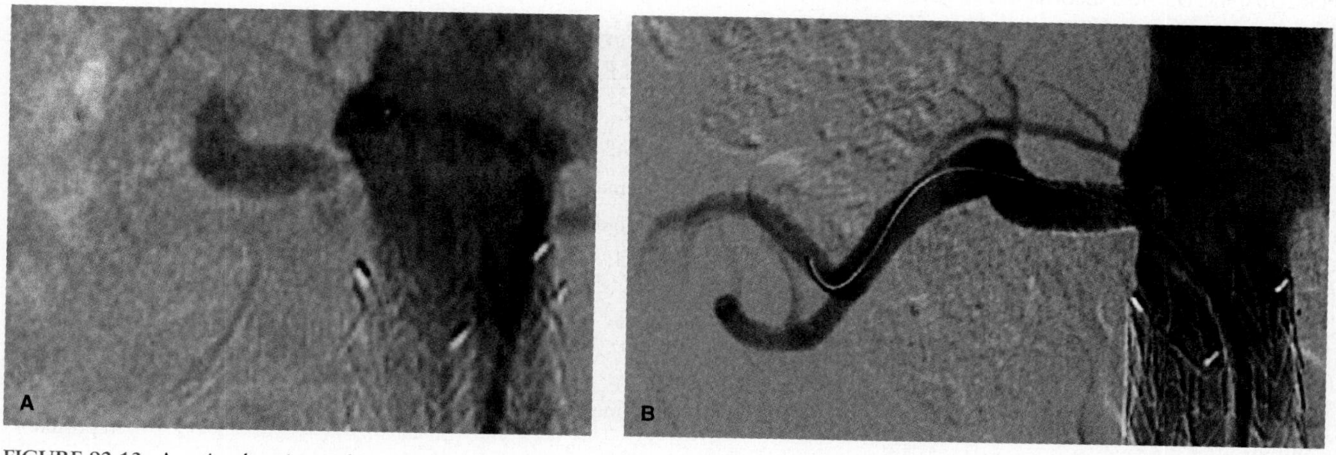

FIGURE 92.13. Arteriosclerotic renal artery stenosis (A) above an aortic endograft. Following selective cannulation of the right renal artery and stent deployment, completion angiogram documents widely patent, stented right renal artery (B).

TABLE 92.1 **RESULTS**

PERCUTANEOUS TRANSLUMINAL ANGIOPLASTY FOR FIBRODYSPLASTIC RENOVASCULAR HYPERTENSION

INSTITUTION	PATIENTS	POSTPROCEDURAL BLOOD PRESSURE RESPONSE (%)		
		CURED	IMPROVED	FAILED
Mayo Clinic	105	22	41	37
University of Virginia	66	39	59	2
University Hospital, Zurich, Switzerland	28	50	39	11
University of Florida	23	52	22	26
University Hospitals, Leuven, Belgium	22	95	—	5
Hospital Broussais, Paris	20	68	16	15

PTA, the clinical significance of the renal artery stenosis should be documented prior to initiating endovascular therapy. In addition, it is important that the patient should have adequate renal cortical reserve to recover renal function postintervention. A recent study has confirmed an explosive increase of endovascular therapy compared with open surgical therapy.[13] In many regards this therapy has been applied to what some considered functionally irrelevant renal artery narrowings, with resultant benefits being less than would occur with more carefully selected individuals for such interventions.

Arterial Fibrodysplasia. Patients with renal artery fibrodysplasia benefit the most and incur the fewest complications following renal PTA, compared to those with other types of renal artery disease. Medial dysplastic stenoses are most amenable to PTA, and this is most often the primary therapy for lesions limited to the main renal artery. Excellent early technical and clinical results usually follow renal artery PTA in these patients.[37–42] Similarly, these patients have experienced excellent long-term clinical results, with primary patency rates of around 85% (Table 92.1).[43]

Developmental Disease. In contrast, renal artery ostial stenoses in pediatric patients associated with developmental aortic anomalies represent true hypoplastic vessels that are less likely to be successfully dilated.[21,44] In a like fashion, less common causes of renovascular hypertension in children, including those associated with inflammatory arteriopathies and neurofibromatosis, do not respond to renal artery PTA.

Arteriosclerosis. The largest experience with renal artery PTA has been in treating arteriosclerotic disease.[45–60] The presence of aortic spillover arteriosclerosis versus isolated renal artery arteriosclerosis has had an important impact on long-term clinical results. Historically, PTA alone, without stent placement, has resulted in a technical success rate of only 70% to 80%. In fact, aortic spillover lesions, treated by PTA alone, have technical success rates of 30% to 50%. These latter stenoses often manifest excessive recoil and many exhibit acute dissections. As a result of high early post-PTA restenosis rates, stenting of atherosclerotic lesions is considered appropriate in these patients.

PTA with stenting for atherosclerotic renal artery disease results in outcomes that vary widely, but this therapy provides reasonable long-term technical results[61] (Table 92.2). For example, Palmaz stents placed in 64 renal arteries in 59 patients resulted in a 2-year secondary patency rate of 92%.[52] Others have documented 5-year primary and secondary patency rates of 84% and 92%, respectively.[46]

TABLE 92.2 **RESULTS**

PERCUTANEOUS TRANSLUMINAL ANGIOPLASTY WITH STENTING FOR ARTERIOSCLEROTIC RENOVASCULAR HYPERTENSION

INSTITUTION	PATIENTS	POSTPROCEDURAL RENAL FUNCTION RESPONSE (%)			POSTPROCEDURAL BLOOD PRESSURE RESPONSE (%)			
University Utrecht, Netherlands	40	17	55	28	15	—	2	14
Iowa Heart Center, Des Moines	63	36	46	18	4	35	1	14
University Freiburg, Germany	68	(No change in mean serum creatinine)			16	62	2	17
Arizona Heart Institute	82	(No change in mean serum creatinine)			13	55	2	26
Wake Forest University	99	28	65	7	1	21	8	Not reported
The Heart Institute of Spokane and Sacred Heart Medical Center, Spokane, Washington	129	16	75	9	2	46	2	14
Multicenter (G. Dorros: senior author)	163	(No change in mean serum creatinine)			1	42	7	Not reported
Duke University and University of Michigan	300	8	78	14	70	43	0	21

PTA with stenting for progressive ischemic nephropathy is not as effective at reversing renal failure. In these cases, as with open surgical interventions, benefits appear related to the degree and duration of ischemic nephropathy prior to PTA, with those having a relative rapid onset of renal insufficiency and serum creatinine of less than 3 mg/dL demonstrating the best response.[62–66] A number of prospective trials comparing PTA and medical therapy have concluded that PTA has only a modest but significant effect on blood pressure control.[67] The results of the prospective, randomized Angioplasty and Stenting for Renal Artery Lesions (ASTRAL) trial and Cardiovascular Outcomes in Renal Atherosclerotic Lesions (CORAL) trials comparing renal artery stenting versus best medical therapy may define the incremental value of PTA revascularizations.[54,68,69] Publication of their outcomes are being awaited by clinicians and health care insurers. Clearly, existing guidelines for renal PTA are controversial.[70]

Complications accompanying renal artery PTA for fibrodysplastic disease are uncommon. PTA for arteriosclerotic disease carries a 5% to 15% risk of complications, although most are not life-threatening. Intimal disruption occurs more often with proximal renal artery dilation, where the vessel elasticity is greater and medial disruption is less likely. Medial tears are more common with distal renal artery dilation where vessel elasticity is less. The exact usefulness of embolic protection devices has yet to be defined, but they may provide improved functional outcomes following renal artery stenting and PTA for arteriosclerotic disease.[48,71,72]

Surgical interventions following failed renal artery PTA are much more hazardous than primary surgical procedures, being associated with a higher incidence of emergent repair and nephrectomy. Blood pressure benefits occurred in 57% of cases after secondary operations for a failed renal artery PTA, compared to 89% following primary operations.[73]

A prospective Scandinavian, randomized controlled trial comparing endovascular treatment with open surgery was performed in 1993 for the treatment of renovascular hypertension.[74] The study documented a 2-year patency rate of 75% in the PTA group versus 96% in the surgical group, but benefits regarding hypertension were equal (90%) in each group. The former study included a large number of patients crossing over from the PTA to the surgical group, leading the authors to suggest that PTA should be first-line therapy, with repeat endovascular or open surgical intervention as necessary.

Arterial Reconstructive Surgery for Renal Artery Occlusive Disease. Despite the well-documented benefits of the open surgical treatment of renovascular occlusive disease, the number of such procedures performed in the United States is declining.[11,13,31,33,75–80] It is important that the primary revascularization procedure be successful. This point is underscored by the fact that nephrectomy accompanies nearly half of the reoperations for failed initial reconstructions. The operative mortality following primary renal artery bypass surgery in the United States has been reported to approach 10%, a figure significantly higher than that documented by most large series from individual centers.[81] Operative details vary when treating the different subgroups of renal artery disease.

Aortorenal Bypass. Aortorenal bypass in adults with arteriosclerotic and fibrodysplastic occlusive disease is most often performed using autologous reversed saphenous vein (Fig. 92.14).[11,12] Dacron or extruded Teflon conduits may also be used in reconstructing these vessels in appropriately chosen patients. Because vein grafts in children often become aneurysmal, autologous hypogastric artery grafts and direct aortic reimplantations of the renal artery are favored to reconstruct the renal arteries in pediatric-aged patients[21,23,82] (Figs. 92.15 and 92.16).

Nonanatomic Bypass Procedures. Nonanatomic bypass procedures are important in treating certain patients with renovascular hypertension.[77,83–86] The hepatic, splenic, or iliac arteries

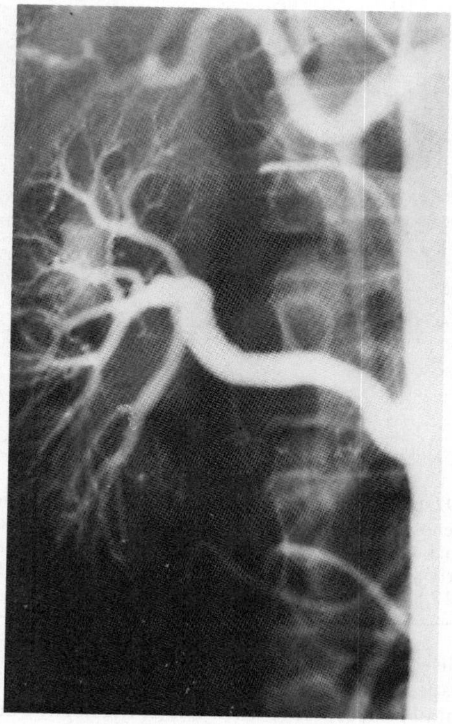

FIGURE 92.14. Autogenous saphenous vein aortorenal graft. (Reproduced with permission from Stanley JC, Graham LM. Renovascular hypertension. In: Miller DC, Roon AJ, eds. *Diagnosis and Management of Peripheral Vascular Disease*. Menlo Park, CA: Addison-Wesley; 1981.)

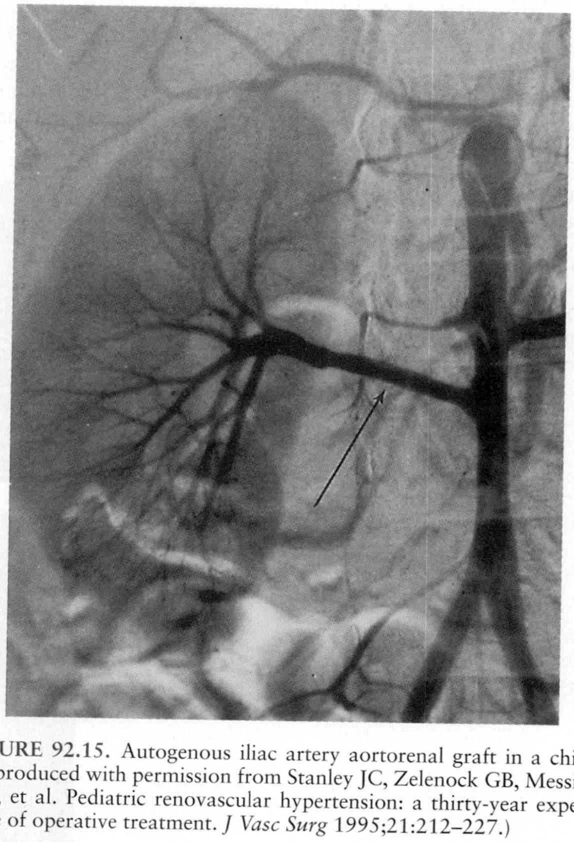

FIGURE 92.15. Autogenous iliac artery aortorenal graft in a child. (Reproduced with permission from Stanley JC, Zelenock GB, Messina LM, et al. Pediatric renovascular hypertension: a thirty-year experience of operative treatment. *J Vasc Surg* 1995;21:212–227.)

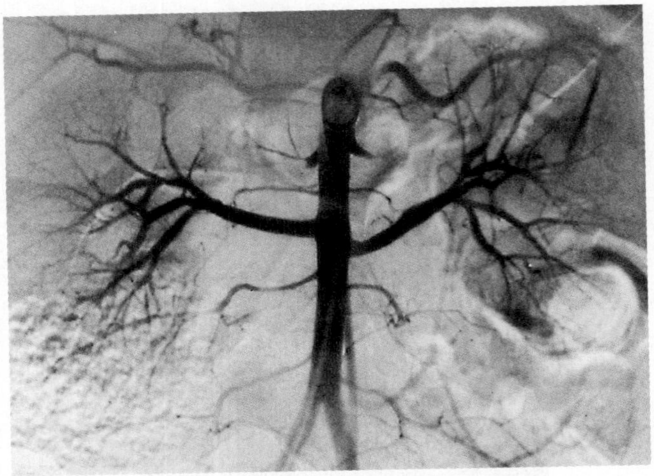

FIGURE 92.16. Aortic reimplantation of main renal arteries, beyond orificial stenoses in a child. (Reproduced with permission from Stanley JC, Zelenock GB, Messina LM, et al. Pediatric renovascular hypertension: a thirty-year experience of operative treatment. *J Vasc Surg* 1995; 21:212–227.)

may be used as sites of origin for bypass grafts to the renal artery, especially when originating a graft from the aorta would entail unacceptable risks. Use of the hepatic artery for a right-sided reconstruction or the splenic artery for a left-sided splenorenal bypass is appropriate in adults, but only after ascertaining that these vessels and the celiac trunk are free of stenotic disease. Splenorenal bypasses are not recommended in children because of potential celiac artery growth arrest that may evolve as the child becomes older, but which is not predictable at the time of the initial reconstruction.

Ex Vivo Renal Artery Reconstruction. Ex vivo renal artery reconstruction is an alternative means of treating select cases of renovascular hypertension, especially those involving revascularization of multiple distal segmental branches.[80,87,88] Disadvantages of ex vivo reconstructions include the necessity to cool the kidney, longer operating times, and perhaps most important, the disruption of preexisting collateral channels. Fortunately, most renal artery reconstructions can be successfully performed in situ.

Endarterectomy. Endarterectomy is often performed for proximal renal artery arteriosclerotic disease.[11,12,89–91] The two techniques most often used are (a) transaortic renal endarterectomy through an axial aortotomy or the transected infrarenal aorta and (b) direct renal artery endarterectomy. The extent of aortic and renal artery disease, as well as the need to perform coexistent aortic reconstructive surgery, dictates which of these procedures is most appropriate. In most cases, a linear aortotomy is begun just to the left of the superior mesenteric artery and extended in the midline to below the renal arteries. The diseased aortic arteriosclerotic tissues are elevated, and with gentle traction, the renal artery atheroma is extracted. This type of endarterectomy is particularly useful in treating bilateral disease (Fig. 92.17) or when the disease affects multiple renal arteries. Extensive plaque affecting the more distal renal artery, especially when involving bifurcations, may be better treated by a direct renal artery endarterectomy with a patch-graft closure.

Results of Operative Therapy for Renal Artery Occlusive Disease.

Renal preservation and maintenance of renal function are important in assessing clinical experiences. Nephrectomy clearly does not offer as much benefit as renal revascularization. Even when nephrectomy provides good early results, it leaves the patient at considerable risk if contralateral disease evolves later. Cumulative primary and secondary nephrectomy rates for alleged unreconstructable renal artery disease in any given practice should not exceed 5%.

Surgical treatment of renovascular hypertension affords excellent outcomes.[11,12] Differences among most individual experiences reflect variations in the prevalence of different renovascular disease categories (Table 92.3). Renovascular hypertension in childhood is most likely to exhibit a salutary outcome after restoration of normal renal blood flow (Table 92.4). Arterial fibrodysplastic renovascular hypertension (Table 92.5) is more likely to benefit from an open operation than is arteriosclerotic renovascular hypertension (Table 92.6), which is probably a reflection of coexistent essential hypertension in older patients with arteriosclerotic disease. Arteriosclerotic renovascular hypertension occurs in two subgroups of patients: (a) those with focal renal artery disease whose only clinical manifestation of

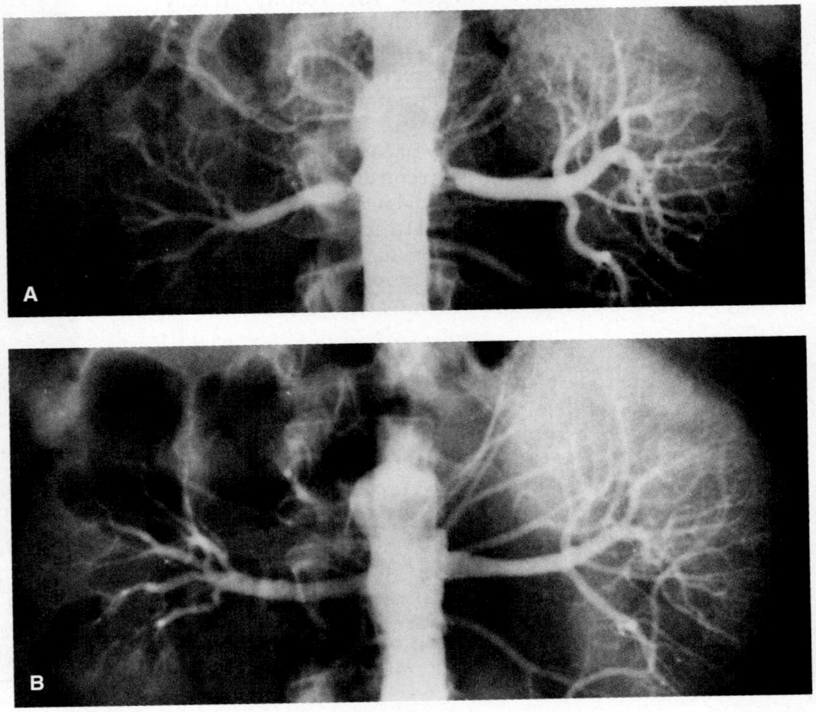

FIGURE 92.17. Transaortic bilateral renal artery endarterectomy. Preoperative (**A**) and postoperative (**B**) aortography. (Reproduced with permission from Stanley JC, Messina LM, Wakefield TW, et al. Renal artery reconstruction. In: Bergan JJ, Yao JST, eds. *Techniques in Arterial Surgery*. Philadelphia, PA: WB Saunders; 1990:247.)

TABLE 92.3

RESULTS

RESULTS OF SURGICAL TREATMENT OF RENOVASCULAR HYPERTENSION IN SPECIFIC PATIENT SUBGROUPS, THE EARLY UNIVERSITY OF MICHIGAN EXPERIENCE

SUBGROUP MORTALITY	PATIENTS	POSTOPERATIVE STATUS (%)[a]			
		CURED	IMPROVED	FAILURE	MORTALITY
Pediatric disease	34	85	12	3	0
Arterial fibrodysplasia	144	55	39	6	0
Arteriosclerosis					
Focal renal artery disease	64	33	58	9	0
Overt extrarenal disease	71	25	47	28	8.5

[a]Represents outcome of 415 operations (346 primary, 59 secondary), including initial nephrectomy in 17 patients.
Cure: Blood pressures were 150/90 mm Hg or less for a minimum of 6 months postoperatively, during which no antihypertensive medications were administered. *Improvement:* Normotensive while on drug therapy, or if diastolic blood pressures ranged between 90 and 100 mm Hg but were at least 15% lower than preoperative levels. *Failure*: Diastolic blood pressures greater than 90 mm Hg but less than 15% lower than preoperative levels or greater than 110 mm Hg. Lower pressure standards were used in evaluating children.
From Stanley JC, Whitehouse WM Jr, Graham LM, et al. Operative therapy of renovascular hypertension. *Br J Surg* 1982;63(Suppl):S63.

TABLE 92.4

RESULTS

RENOVASCULAR HYPERTENSION IN CHILDREN, OPEN SURGICAL TREATMENT

INSTITUTION	PATIENTS	OPERATIVE OUTCOME (%)			SURGICAL MORTALITY RATE (%)
		CURED	IMPROVED	FAILED	
University of Michigan	97	70	27	3	0
Cleveland Clinic	27	59	18.5	18.5	4
University of California, Los Angeles	26	84.5	7.5	4	4
Vanderbilt University	21	68	24	8	0
University of Pennsylvania	17	76.5	23.5	0	0
Argentinean Institute, Buenos Aires	15	53	13	27	7
University of California, San Francisco	14	86	7	0	7

Modified from Stanley JC. The evolution of surgery for renovascular occlusive disease. *Cardiovasc Surg* 1994;2:195–202.

TABLE 92.5

RESULTS

FIBRODYSPLASTIC RENOVASCULAR HYPERTENSION IN ADULTS, OPEN SURGICAL TREATMENT

INSTITUTION	PATIENTS	OPERATIVE OUTCOME (%)			SURGICAL MORTALITY RATE (%)
		CURED	IMPROVED	FAILED	
University of Michigan	144	55	39	6	0
Baylor College of Medicine	113	43	24	33	0
Cleveland Clinic	92	58	31	11	Unstated
University of California, San Francisco	77	66	32	1.3	0
Mayo Clinic	63	66	24	10	Unstated
University Hospital Leiden, The Netherlands	53	53	34	13	2
Vanderbilt University	44	72	24	4	2.3
Columbia University	42	76	14	10	Unstated
Bowman Gray	40	33	57	10	0
University of Lund, Malmo, Sweden	40	66	24	10	0

Modified from Stanley JC. The evolution of surgery for renovascular occlusive disease. *Cardiovasc Surg* 1994;2:195–202.

RESULTS

TABLE 92.6

ARTERIOSCLEROTIC RENOVASCULAR HYPERTENSION IN ADULTS, OPEN SURGICAL TREATMENT

INSTITUTION	PATIENTS	OPERATIVE OUTCOME (%) CURED	IMPROVED	FAILED	SURGICAL MORTALITY RATE (%)
Wake Forest University	500	12	73	15	4.6
University of Michigan	135	29	52	19	4.4
University of California, San Francisco	84	39	23	38	2.4
Cleveland Clinic	78	40	51	9	2
Columbia University	67	58	21	21	Unstated
University of Lund, Malmo, Sweden	66	49	24	27	0.9
Hospital Aiguelongue, Montpellier, France	65	45	40	15	1.1
Vanderbilt University	63	50	45	5	9

Modified from Stanley JC. The evolution of surgery for renovascular occlusive disease. *Cardiovasc Surg* 1994;2:195–202.

arteriosclerosis is secondary hypertension and (b) those with clinically overt extrarenal arteriosclerosis affecting the coronary, carotid, aorta, or extremity vessels. The severity and duration of hypertension, age, and gender in these two subgroups are similar, yet the surgical outcome regarding amelioration of hypertension is worse in patients with overt extrarenal arteriosclerotic disease. Open revascularization of a kidney with an occluded renal artery offers recovery of renal function and improvement in blood pressure control in nearly half the patients.[92,93]

RENAL ARTERY ANEURYSMAL DISEASE

Aneurysms of the renal artery are unusual, but with more frequent imaging modalities are being encountered with increasing frequency.[94–102] Complications of these aneurysms, often detected in the setting of other renal vascular disease, may have been overestimated in surgical series rather than population-based experiences. Other misperceptions regarding the importance of these aneurysms reflect unrecognized differences among their four principal types: (a) true renal artery aneurysms, (b) dissecting renal artery aneurysms, (c) aneurysmal mural dilations occurring with medial fibrodysplastic disease, and (d) arteritis-related microaneurysms. The two renal artery macroaneurysms most relevant to surgical practice are the true aneurysms and those associated with dissections (Table 92.7).

True Renal Artery Aneurysms

The precise incidence of true renal artery aneurysms in the general population is estimated to be between 0.10% and 0.7%.[101,103] Large reported series of these aneurysms are uncommon (Table 92.8). The group being studied bears greatly on the reported frequency of these lesions. For example, macroaneurysms have been identified in 0.7% of patients undergoing arteriographic studies directed at renal disease[104] and in 2.5% of those being evaluated for hypertension.[101] Women are affected with true renal artery aneurysms slightly more often than men. However, when aneurysms in patients with arterial fibrodysplasia are excluded, there appears to be no gender predilection. The predisposition of these aneurysms to affect the right renal artery may be a reflection of the greater incidence of right-sided medial fibrodysplastic disease in women.

True renal artery aneurysms are usually located at renal artery bifurcations (Fig. 92.18). Most of these aneurysms are saccular. The average diameter of true aneurysms at the time of their clinical recognition is 1.5 cm. Extraparenchymal

TREATMENT

TABLE 92.7

TRUE AND DISSECTING RENAL ARTERY ANEURYSMS

LESION	MALES/FEMALES	CONTRIBUTING FACTORS	RATE OF RUPTURE	MORTALITY WITH RUPTURE	USUAL TREATMENT
True aneurysm	1/1.2	Congenital defects Arterial fibrodysplasia Hypertension	3%	10% (during pregnancy: 55% maternal, 55% fetal)	Aneurysmectomy with renal artery reconstruction Aneurysmorrhaphy Endovascular exclusion or embolization Nephrectomy for ruptured aneurysms
Dissecting aneurysm	10/1	Blunt trauma Arterial catheterization Arterial fibrodysplasia Arteriosclerosis	Uncommon	Undefined	Renal artery reconstruction Endovascular stenting

TABLE 92.8 RESULTS

SELECTED EXPERIENCES WITH RENAL ARTERY ANEURYSMS

	PATIENTS (ANEURYSMS)	MAJOR SYMPTOMS	PRINCIPAL SURGICAL PROCEDURE				
			EXCISION AND CLOSURE	BYPASS	EX VIVO REPAIR	UNPLANNED NEPHRECTOMY	SURGICAL MORTALITY RATE (%)
University of Michigan	168 (252)	26%	63	33	0	8	0
Heinrich-Heine University	94 (136)	Unknown	37	46	4	0	0
Wake Forest University	62 (72)	11%	11	48	28	0	1.6
University of Toronto	56 (67)	51%	10	0	4	3	0
Vanderbilt University	39 (43)	15%	6	7	5	3	0
Mayo Clinic	32 (45)	34%	11	17	7	7	0

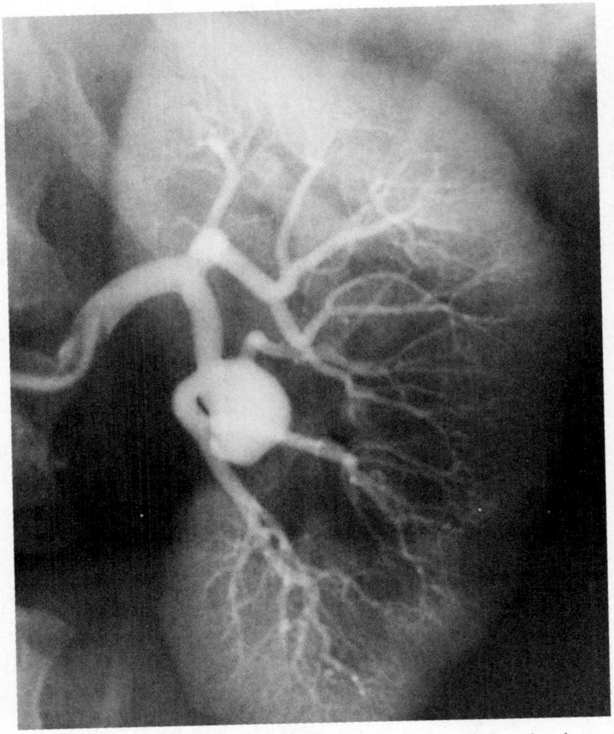

FIGURE 92.18. Renal artery aneurysm at a second-order branch. (Reproduced with permission from Stanley JC, Whitehouse WM Jr. Renal artery macroaneurysms. In: Bergan JJ, Yao JST, eds. *Aneurysms*. New York: Grune & Stratton; 1982:417.)

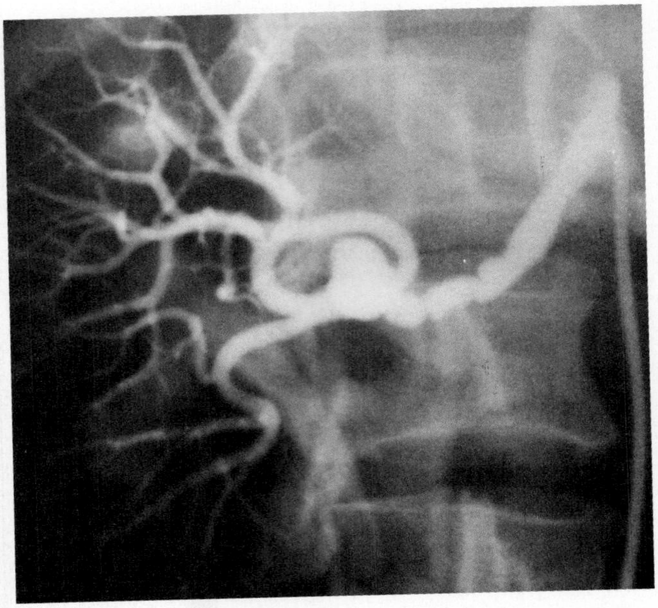

FIGURE 92.19. Saccular renal artery aneurysm occurring at the primary bifurcation of a main renal artery exhibiting medial fibroplasia. (Reproduced with permission from Stanley JC, Whitehouse WM Jr. Renal artery macroaneurysms. In: Bergan JJ, Yao JST, eds. *Aneurysms*. New York: Grune & Stratton; 1982:417.)

aneurysms are very common, accounting for more than 90% of these lesions, with more than 75% occurring at first- or second-order branchings of the main renal artery.

Two distinct histologic categories of true renal artery aneurysms exist. The first type appears to be associated with a congenital elastic tissue defect or medial degenerative process. The second type of aneurysm exhibits arteriosclerosis. Atheromatous changes often occur at irregular intervals in these aneurysms, with intervening areas composed of thin, collagenous acellular fibrous tissue. In most instances, arteriosclerosis is considered a secondary event rather than a primary etiologic event.

The high frequency of renal artery aneurysms associated with medial fibrodysplasia is well recognized (Fig. 92.19). In the latter disease state, further fragmentation and disruption of elastic tissue with loss of smooth muscle at bifurcations leaves little more than a thin layer of fibrous connective tissue to contain blood flow. The greater incidence of aneurysms among patients with hypertension secondary to dysplastic renal artery stenoses, in comparison with those with arteriosclerotic stenoses, supports the tenet that arterial fibrodysplasia is a direct contributor to aneurysmal changes.

Clinical Manifestations of the True Renal Artery Aneurysms. Most renal artery aneurysms are asymptomatic, being discovered incidentally.[85–87,91] Aneurysm expansion or renal infarction from dislodged thrombus may cause flank or abdominal pain. Hematuria and abdominal bruits have been attributed to some lesions, but are more likely due to nonaneurysmal disease. Although very uncommon, covert rupture of renal artery aneurysms into an adjacent vein may be associated with hematuria and hypertension.

Once a renal artery aneurysm is suspected, conventional catheter-based arteriography becomes the definitive diagnostic studies. However, gadolinium-enhanced magnetic resonance arteriography (MRA) and multislice three-dimensional reconstructed CT scanning (Fig. 92.20) have an increasing role in the anatomic delineation of these aneurysms.[103,105,106]

The theory that renal artery aneurysms contribute to the 80% incidence of hypertension in these patients has been a subject of continual controversy.[96,97,99,100] Embolization of aneurysmal thrombus or thrombotic occlusion of an adjacent artery may result in renal ischemia and renovascular hypertension, but this is uncommon. More often, coexisting renal artery occlusive disease in the vicinity of aneurysms may account for secondary hypertension in these patients. Indeed, renal artery stenosis may be masked by the aneurysm.[107] Because of this possibility, one should search for existence of occult stenoses in hypertensive patients with aneurysms.

Rupture is the most serious complication attending renal artery aneurysms. Exsanguinating hemorrhage from a ruptured renal artery aneurysm occurs rarely.[96,108,109] Mortality with rupture is approximately 10%, but loss of a kidney is a near-universal outcome of rupture. Overt extraparenchymal rupture occurred in 2% of patients harboring these lesions, and covert rupture causing renal arteriovenous fistulas occurred in an additional 1.5%, in one of the largest reported series from a surgical group.[96] Rupture of renal artery aneurysms during pregnancy is an exception to the generally accepted benign nature of most bland aneurysms.[110–112] Rupture of renal artery aneurysms is responsible for fetal death in nearly 85% of cases and is associated with a 55% maternal mortality rate.

An increased risk of renal artery aneurysm rupture has been attributed to large size, absence of calcification, and elevated blood pressure. However, overt rupture often has occurred in normotensive patients, as well as with calcific atherosclerotic aneurysms.[96,110] Although greater rupture rates occurring in larger aneurysms have been only inconsistently reported, a larger size remains a logical reason to assign a greater risk of rupture.

6 **Treatment of True Renal Artery Aneurysms.** Indications for surgical intervention for true renal artery aneurysms appears indicated in the following situations: (a) aneurysms with functionally important renal artery stenoses; (b) aneurysms harboring thrombus, especially with evidence of distal embolization and cortical infarcts; (c) aneurysms in women who plan to have children; (d) aneurysms with diameters greater than 1.5 cm in otherwise healthy patients; and (e) patients with flank pain attributed to their aneurysms. Size is

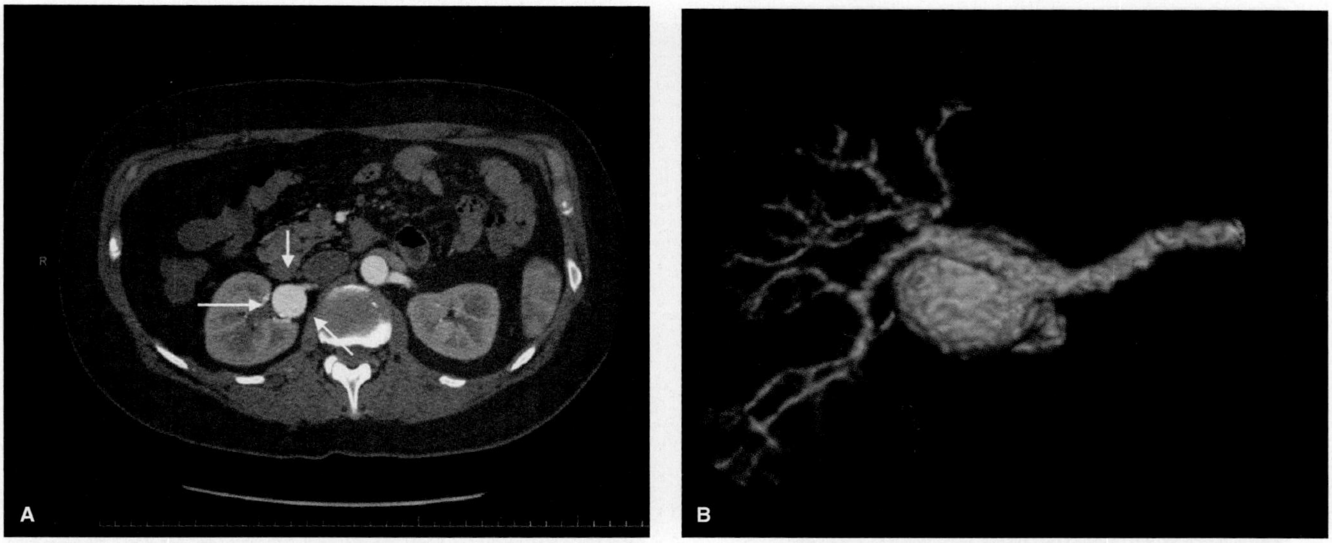

FIGURE 92.20. Computed tomography angiogram of a large renal artery aneurysm in axial cut (**A**, *arrows*) and in three-dimension (**B**).

the softest indication for surgical therapy. Cautious surgical intervention by those experienced in renovascular surgery in properly selected patients with renal artery aneurysms appears justified because of the small, but unpredictable, incidence of rupture with its attendant loss of kidney and life.

The objective of surgical therapy is to eliminate the aneurysm without losing the kidney or compromising its function.[96,113,114] Most aneurysms are best approached with a transabdominal, extraperitoneal exposure of the renal vasculature following medial displacement of the overlying colon and foregut viscera. Large aneurysms of the main renal artery can usually be excised with simple primary closure of the artery, but excision of smaller aneurysms may require arterial closure with a vein patch (Fig. 92.21). More extensive renal artery reconstructions using autogenous saphenous vein or internal iliac artery as aortorenal grafts are favored for bifurcation aneurysms, especially those associated with functionally important stenoses of the renal artery (Fig. 92.22).

Nephrectomy is the usual therapy for managing ruptured aneurysms and extensive intraparenchymal aneurysms. Long-term outcome is actually quite good following nephrectomy in carefully selected cases. No patients treated in this manner at the University of Michigan required hemodialysis during a 20-year follow-up.[96] Nevertheless, arterial reconstruction should be considered in those instances in which the kidney does not appear to have been irreparably injured from ischemia caused by the rupture.

Endovascular treatment of renal artery aneurysms has an evolving role.[115–121] Although endoluminal therapy appears to carry a higher risk of parenchymal infarction, no prospective comparison trials between endovascular and surgical treatments exist. Certainly, main renal artery aneurysms may be

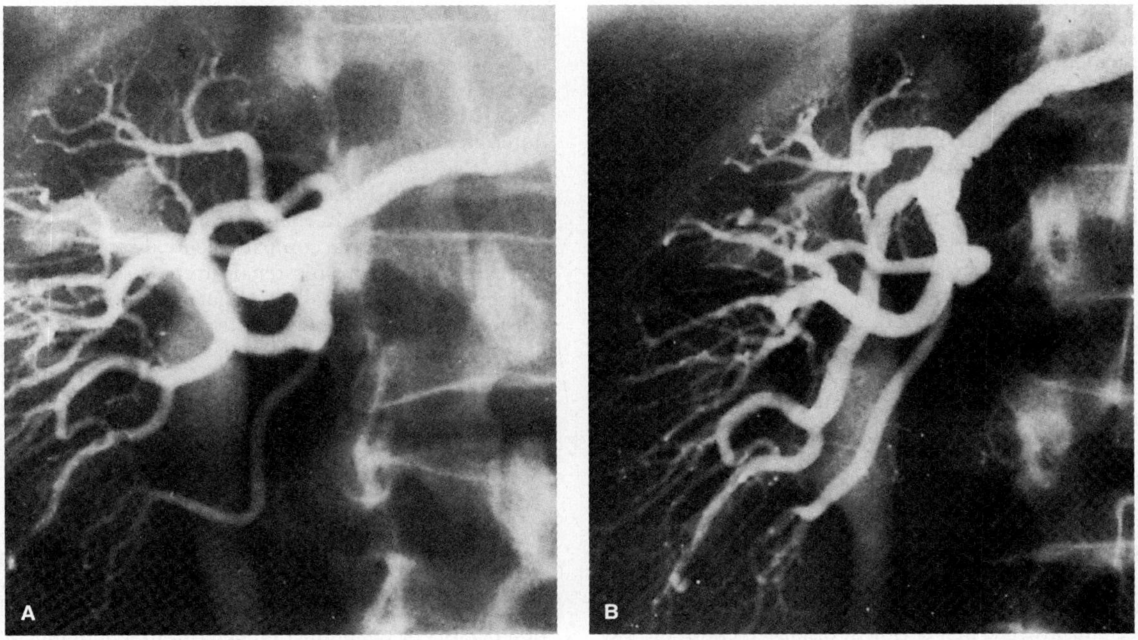

FIGURE 92.21. **A:** Renal artery aneurysm located at the bifurcation of the main renal artery. **B:** Surgical treatment included aneurysmectomy and vein patch graft closure of the artery. (Reproduced with permission from Stanley JC. Renal artery aneurysms and dissections. In: Veith FJ, ed. *Current Critical Problems in Vascular Surgery*, vol. 3. St. Louis, MO: Quality Medical Publishing; 1991:311.)

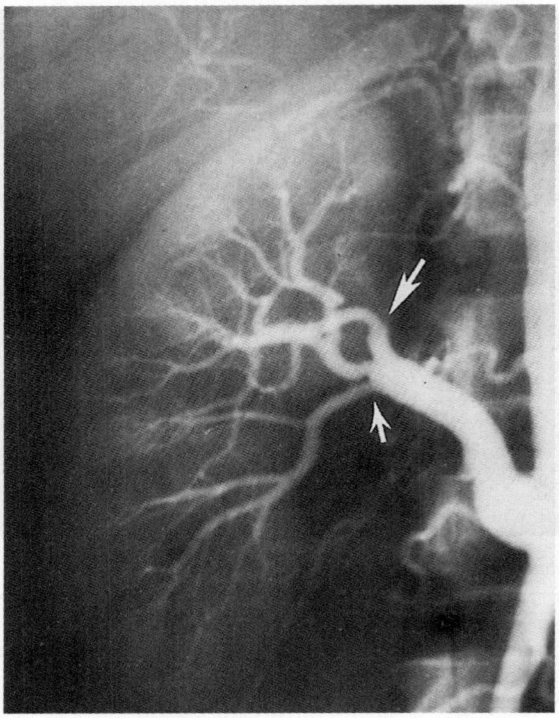

FIGURE 92.22. Aortorenal bypass with reversed autogenous saphenous vein, following excision of an aneurysm in a fibrodysplastic vessel, with end-to-end anastomosis to one first-order segmental branch (*large arrow*) and end-to-side implantation of the other first-order segmental branch (*small arrow*). (Reproduced with permission from Ernst CB, Stanley JC, Fry WJ. Multiple primary and segmental renal artery revascularization utilizing autogenous saphenous vein. *Surg Gynecol Obstet* 1973;137:1023–1026.)

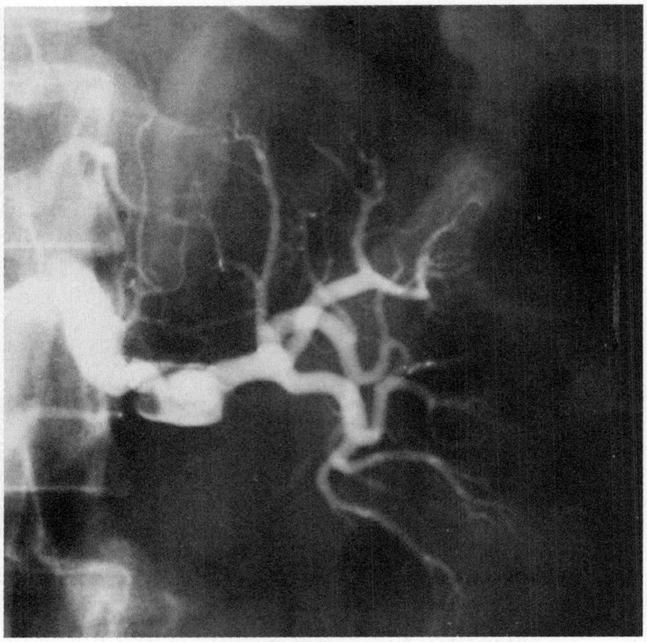

FIGURE 92.23. Saccular dissecting main renal artery aneurysm. (Reproduced with permission from Gewertz BL, Stanley JC, Fry WJ. Renal artery dissections. *Arch Surg* 1977;112:409–414.)

successfully excluded by stent graft placement, and peripheral branch aneurysms can be successfully embolized. Embolization of intraparenchymal aneurysms is an appropriate alternative to partial nephrectomy in those patients with evidence of cortical infarction. Lastly, endovascular proximal arterial occlusion may be useful in hemodynamically unstable patients having a ruptured renal artery aneurysm in whom open attempts to salvage the kidney would place the patient's life at risk.

Renal artery aneurysms not treated by operation should be subjected to long-term surveillance. Because of the relatively low incidence of complications attending most renal artery aneurysms, noninvasive studies, such as abdominal ultrasonography, CT, or MRA, performed on a regular basis are favored over repeated arteriographic studies, which may carry risks exceeding those of the aneurysmal disease itself.

Renal Artery Dissections

Isolated renal artery dissections causing aneurysms are rare.[122–126] Dissections are usually classified into two categories: (a) those due to blunt abdominal trauma or intraluminal catheter-induced injury and (b) those occurring spontaneously (Fig. 92.23). Nearly one third of renal artery dissections are bilateral. Dissections of the renal artery affect men nearly 10 times as often as women. In part, this reflects the greater likelihood of trauma-induced dissections that occur in men. Blunt abdominal trauma contributes to renal artery dissections by two specific mechanisms. The first is violent displacement of the kidney with deceleration causing marked stretching of the artery with fracture of the intima, which is the least elastic vessel wall component. This event commonly results in subintimal dissections. The second mechanism relates to traumatic compression of the renal arteries against the unyielding vertebral bodies, resulting in medial hemorrhage and false aneurysm formation.

Iatrogenic, catheter-related, renal artery injury occurring during diagnostic arteriography is another recognized cause of these aneurysms. This complication is uncommon. Iatrogenic dissections usually occur within the inner media or subintimal tissues. Dissections accompanying therapeutic catheterizations, such as balloon angioplasty, are common, although only a few cause critical narrowings or occlusion of the renal artery. In these instances, stent placement usually restores normal renal artery blood flow.

Primary or spontaneous dissections causing pseudoaneurysms affect the renal arteries more than any other peripheral artery. Most are related to coexistent arteriosclerotic or dysplastic renovascular disease. A 0.5% incidence of dissections in patients with fibrodysplastic renal arteries has been reported.[127] Spontaneous dissections usually occur within the outer media adjacent to the external elastic lamina.

Clinical Manifestations of Renal Artery Dissection.

Flank and back pain, hematuria, ileus, and elevated blood pressure frequently accompany acute dissections regardless of the cause.[123,124] Chronic renal artery dissections, when clinically relevant, are usually associated with renovascular hypertension or impaired renal function. An incorrect initial clinical diagnosis is common, occurring in more than half of patients having renal artery dissections. CT angiography can accurately define dissections and is the primary modality used most in the setting of trauma. Arteriography is used most often to diagnose and define the extent of renal artery dissections.

Treatment of Renal Artery Dissection.

Trauma-related dissections warrant emergent primary arterial reconstructions once a hemodynamic narrowing or occlusion of the main renal artery or a major segmental branch is recognized. Delayed repair is necessary for less obvious trauma-related injuries if hypertension persists or renal function deteriorates. Spontaneous dissecting aneurysms, when acute, are technically easier to treat than traumatic lesions and should be subjected to surgical therapy soon after hemodynamically significant stenoses or occlusions are recognized. Operative intervention is also pursued for chronic spontaneous dissections associated with severe renovascular hypertension or deteriorating renal function. Endovascular stent placement is an appropriate alternative therapy for short proximal renal artery dissections with a defined distal endpoint and is useful for dissections following catheter-related injuries.[128]

References

1. Goldblatt H, Lynch JP, Hazal R. Studies on experimental hypertension. I. The production of persistent elevation of systolic blood pressure by means of renal ischemia. *J Exp Med* 1934;59:347–381.
2. Pratt RE, Carleton JE, Richie JP, et al. Human renin biosynthesis and secretion in normal and ischemic kidneys. *Proc Natl Acad Sci U S A* 1987;84:7837–7840.
3. Sealey JE, Buhler FR, Laragh JH, et al. The physiology of renin secretion in essential hypertension. Estimation of renin secretion rate and renal plasma flow from peripheral and renal vein renin levels. *Am J Med* 1973; 55:391–401.
4. Schneider EG, Davis JO, Baumber JS, et al. Renin, aldosterone, and hypertension. The hepatic metabolism of renin and aldosterone. A review with new observations on the hepatic clearance of renin. *Circ Res* 1970; 27(1)(suppl 1):175–183.
5. Samuels AI, Miller ED Jr, Fray JC, et al. Renin–angiotensin antagonists and the regulation of blood pressure. *Fed Proc* 1976;35:2512–2520.
6. Oparil S, Tregear GW, Koerner T, et al. Mechanism of pulmonary conversion of angiotensin I to angiotensin II in the dog. *Circ Res* 1971;29: 682–690.
7. Oshima G, Gecse A, Erdos EG. Angiotensin I-converting enzyme of the kidney cortex. *Biochim Biophys Acta* 1974;350:26–37.
8. Stanley JC, Gewertz BL, Fry WJ. Renal: systemic renin indices and renal vein renin ratios as prognostic indicators in remedial renovascular hypertension. *J Surg Res* 1976;20:149–155.
9. Vaughan ED Jr, Buhler FR, Laragh JH, et al. Renovascular hypertension: renin measurements to indicate hypersecretion and contralateral suppression, estimate renal plasma flow, and score for surgical curability. *Am J Med* 1973;55:402–414.
10. Gavras H, Brunner HB, Vaughan ED, et al. Angiotensin-sodium interaction in blood pressure maintenance of renal hypertensive and normotensive rats. *Science* 1973;180:1369–1371.
11. Stanley JC. The evolution of surgery for renovascular occlusive disease. *Cardiovasc Surg* 1994;2:195–202.
12. Stanley JC. David M. Hume memorial lecture. Surgical treatment of renovascular hypertension. *Am J Surg* 1997;174:102–110.
13. Knipp BS, Dimick JB, Eliason JL, et al. Diffusion of new technology for the treatment of renovascular hypertension in the United States: surgical revascularization versus catheter-based therapy, 1988–2001. *J Vasc Surg* 2004; 40:717–723.
14. Louie J, Isaacson JA, Zierler RE, et al. Prevalence of carotid and lower extremity arterial disease in patients with renal artery stenosis. *Am J Hypertens* 1994;7:436–439.
15. Valentine RJ, Clagett GP, Miller GL, et al. The coronary risk of unsuspected renal artery stenosis. *J Vasc Surg* 1993;18:433–439; discussion 439–440.
16. Valentine RJ, Martin JD, Myers SI, et al. Asymptomatic celiac and superior mesenteric artery stenoses are more prevalent among patients with unsuspected renal artery stenoses. *J Vasc Surg* 1991;14:195–199.
17. Novick AC, Zaki S, Goldfarb D, et al. Epidemiologic and clinical comparison of renal artery stenosis in black patients and white patients. *J Vasc Surg* 1994;20:1–5.
18. Stanley JC, Gewertz BL, Bove EL, et al. Arterial fibrodysplasia. Histopathologic character and current etiologic concepts. *Arch Surg* 1975; 110:561–566.
19. Graham LM, Zelenock GB, Erlandson EE, et al. Abdominal aortic coarctation and segmental hypoplasia. *Surgery* 1979;86:519–529.
20. Stanley JC, Criado E, Eliason JL, et al. Abdominal aortic coarctation: surgical treatment of 53 patients with a thoracoabdominal bypass, patch aortoplasty, or interposition aortoaortic graft. *J Vasc Surg* 2008;48: 1073–1082.
21. Stanley JC, Criado E, Upchurch GR Jr, et al.; for the Michigan Pediatric Renovascular Group. Pediatric renovascular hypertension: 132 primary and 30 secondary operations in 97 children. *J Vasc Surg* 2006;44: 1219–1229.
22. Stanley JC, Graham LM, Whitehouse WM Jr, et al. Developmental occlusive disease of the abdominal aorta and the splanchnic and renal arteries. *Am J Surg* 1981;142:90–196.
23. Stanley JC, Zelenock GB, Messina LM, et al. Pediatric renovascular hypertension: a thirty-year experience of operative treatment. *J Vasc Surg* 1995; 21:212–226; discussion 226–217.
24. Upchurch GR Jr, Henke PK, Eagleton MJ, et al. Pediatric splanchnic arterial occlusive disease: clinical relevance and operative treatment. *J Vasc Surg* 2002;35:850–867.
25. Hansen KJ, Tribble RW, Reavis SW, et al. Renal duplex sonography: evaluation of clinical utility. *J Vasc Surg* 1990;12:227–236.
26. Kohler TR, Zierler RE, Martin RL, et al. Noninvasive diagnosis of renal artery stenosis by ultrasonic duplex scanning. *J Vasc Surg* 1986;4: 450–456.
27. Liss P, Eklof H, Hellberg O, et al. Renal effects of CO2 and iodinated contrast media in patients undergoing renovascular intervention: a prospective, randomized study. *J Vasc Interv Radiol* 2005;16:57–65.
28. Hertz SM, Holland GA, Baum RA, et al. Evaluation of renal artery stenosis by magnetic resonance angiography. *Am J Surg* 1994;168:140–143.
29. Prince MR, Narasimham DL, Stanley JC, et al. Breath-hold gadolinium-enhanced MR angiography of the abdominal aorta and its major branches. *Radiology* 1995;197:785–792.
30. Saxena SK, Sharma M, Patel M, et al. Nephrogenic systemic fibrosis: an emerging entity. *Int Urol Nephrol* 2008;40:715–724.
31. Stanley JC, Fry WJ. Surgical treatment of renovascular hypertension. *Arch Surg* 1977;112:1291–1297.
32. Thornbury JR, Stanley JC, Fryback DG. Hypertensive urogram: a nondiscriminatory test for renovascular hypertension. *AJR Am J Roentgenol* 1982;138:43–49.
33. Stanley JC, Whitehouse WM Jr, Graham LM, et al. Operative therapy of renovascular hypertension. *Br J Surg* 1982;69:S63–S66.
34. Meier GH, Sumpio B, Setaro JF, et al. Captopril renal scintigraphy: a new standard for predicting outcome after renal revascularization. *J Vasc Surg* 1993;17:280–285; discussion 285–287.
35. Nussberger J, Aubert JF, Bouzourene K, et al. Renin inhibition by aliskiren prevents atherosclerosis progression: comparison with irbesartan, atenolol, and amlodipine. *Hypertension* 2008;51:1306–1311.
36. Grüntzig A, Kuhlmann U, Vetter W, et al. Treatment of renovascular hypertension with percutaneous transluminal dilatation of a renal-artery stenosis. *Lancet* 1978;1:801–802.
37. Bonelli FS, McKusick MA, Textor SC, et al. Renal artery angioplasty: technical results and clinical outcome in 320 patients. *Mayo Clin Proc* 1995; 70:1041–1052.
38. Cluzel P, Raynaud A, Beyssen B, et al. Stenoses of renal branch arteries in fibromuscular dysplasia: results of percutaneous transluminal angioplasty. *Radiology* 1994;193:227–232.
39. Davidson RA, Barri Y, Wilcox CS. Predictors of cure of hypertension in fibromuscular renovascular disease. *Am J Kidney Dis* 1996;28:334–338.
40. Luscher TF, Keller HM, Imhof HG, et al. Fibromuscular hyperplasia: extension of the disease and therapeutic outcome. Results of the University Hospital Zurich Cooperative Study on Fibromuscular Hyperplasia. *Nephron* 1986;44(suppl 1):109–114.
41. Sos TA, Pickering TG, Sniderman K, et al. Percutaneous transluminal renal angioplasty in renovascular hypertension due to atheroma or fibromuscular dysplasia. *N Engl J Med* 1983;309:274–279.
42. Tegtmeyer CJ, Kellum CD, Ayers C. Percutaneous transluminal angioplasty of the renal artery. Results and long-term follow-up. *Radiology* 1984;153:77–84.
43. Tegtmeyer CJ, Hartwell GD, Selby JB, et al. Results and complications of angioplasty in aortoiliac disease. *Circulation* 1991;83(2 suppl):I53–I60.
44. Martin EC, Diamond NG, Casarella WJ. Percutaneous transluminal angioplasty in non-atherosclerotic disease. *Radiology* 1980;135:27–33.
45. Ayerdi J, Hodgson KJ. Balloon angioplasty and stenting for renovascular occlusive disease. *Perspect Vasc Surg Endovasc Ther* 2004;16:25–42.
46. Blum U, Krumme B, Flugel P, et al. Treatment of ostial renal-artery stenoses with vascular endoprostheses after unsuccessful balloon angioplasty. *N Engl J Med* 1997;336:459–465.
47. Boisclair C, Therasse E, Oliva VL, et al. Treatment of renal angioplasty failure by percutaneous renal artery stenting with Palmaz stents: midterm technical and clinical results. *AJR Am J Roentgenol* 1997;168:245–251.
48. Corriere MA, Pearce JD, Edwards MS, et al. Endovascular management of atherosclerotic renovascular disease: early results following primary intervention. *J Vasc Surg* 2008;48:580–588.
49. Dorros G, Jaff M, Jain A, et al. Follow-up of primary Palmaz-Schatz stent placement for atherosclerotic renal artery stenosis. *Am J Cardiol* 1995;75: 1051–1055.
50. Dorros G, Jaff M, Mathiak L, et al. Four-year follow-up of Palmaz-Schatz stent revascularization as treatment for atherosclerotic renal artery stenosis. *Circulation* 1998;98:642–647.
51. Harjai K, Khosla S, Shaw D, et al. Effect of gender on outcomes following renal artery stent placement for renovascular hypertension. *Cathet Cardiovasc Diagn* 1997;42:381–386.
52. Henry M, Amor M, Henry I, et al. Stent placement in the renal artery: three-year experience with the Palmaz stent. *J Vasc Interv Radiol* 1996;7: 343–350.
53. Iannone LA, Underwood PL, Nath A, et al. Effect of primary balloon expandable renal artery stents on long-term patency, renal function, and blood pressure in hypertensive and renal insufficient patients with renal artery stenosis. *Cathet Cardiovasc Diagn* 1996;37:243–250.
54. Karla PA. The ASTRAL Trial. Paper presented at: 2nd Annual Meeting of the Society for Cardiovascular Angiography and Interventions, SCA1-ACC; April 2008; Chicago, IL.
55. Lederman RJ, Mendelsohn FO, Santos R, et al. Primary renal artery stenting: characteristics and outcomes after 363 procedures. *Am Heart J* 2001; 142:314–323.
56. Leertouwer TC, Gussenhoven EJ, Bosch JL, et al. Stent placement for renal arterial stenosis: where do we stand? A meta-analysis. *Radiology* 2000; 216:78–85.
57. Rees CR, Palmaz JC, Becker GJ, et al. Palmaz stent in atherosclerotic stenoses involving the ostia of the renal arteries: preliminary report of a multicenter study. *Radiology* 1991;181:507–514.
58. Rodriguez-Lopez JA, Werner A, Ray LI, et al. Renal artery stenosis treated with stent deployment: indications, technique, and outcome for 108 patients. *J Vasc Surg* 1999;29:617–624.
59. Tuttle KR, Chouinard RF, Webber JT, et al. Treatment of atherosclerotic ostial renal artery stenosis with the intravascular stent. *Am J Kidney Dis* 1998;323:611–622.
60. van de Ven PJG, Kaatee R, Beutler JJ, et al. Arterial stenting and balloon angioplasty in ostial atherosclerotic renovascular disease: a randomised trial. *Lancet* 1999;353:282–286.

61. Costanza MJ, Strilka RJ, Edwards MS, et al. Endovascular treatment of renovascular disease. In: Rutherford RB, ed. *Vascular Surgery*, 6th ed. New York: Elsevier/Mosby; 2005:1825–1846.
62. Dean RH, Lawson JD, Hollifield JW, et al. Revascularization of the poorly functioning kidney. *Surgery* 1979;85:44–52.
63. Hansen KJ, Cherr GS, Craven TE, et al. Management of ischemic nephropathy: dialysis-free survival after surgical repair. *J Vasc Surg* 2000; 3:472–481; discussion 481–472.
64. Hansen KJ, Thomason RB, Craven TE, et al. Surgical management of dialysis-dependent ischemic nephropathy. *J Vasc Surg* 1995;21:197–209; discussion 209–211.
65. Jacobson HR. Ischemic renal disease: an overlooked clinical entity? *Kidney Int* 1988;34:729–743.
66. Jamieson GG, Clarkson AR, Woodroffe AJ, et al. Reconstructive renal vascular surgery for chronic renal failure. *Br J Surg* 1984;71:338–340.
67. Nordmann AJ, Woo K, Parkes R, et al. Balloon angioplasty or medical therapy for hypertensive patients with atherosclerotic renal artery stenosis? A meta-analysis of randomized controlled trials. *Am J Med* 2003;114: 44–50.
68. Main J, Karla PA. The ASTRAL trial. *J Renovasc Disease* 2002;1:19–23.
69. Cooper CJ, Murphy TP, Matsumoto A, et al. Stent revascularization for the prevention of cardiovascular and renal events among patients with renal artery stenosis and systolic hypertension: rationale and design of the CORAL trial. *Am Heart J* 2006;152:59–66.
70. Dear JW, Padfield PL, Webb DJ. New guidelines for drive-by renal arteriography may lead to an unjustifiable increase in percutaneous intervention. *Heart* 2007;93:1523–1532.
71. Cooper CJ, Haller ST, Colyer W, et al. Embolic protection and platelet inhibition during renal artery stenting. *Circulation* 2008;117:2752–2760.
72. Edwards MS, Craven BL, Stafford J, et al. Distal embolic protection during renal artery angioplasty and stenting. *J Vasc Surg* 2006;44:128–135.
73. Wong JM, Hansen KJ, Oskin TC, et al. Surgery after failed percutaneous renal artery angioplasty. *J Vasc Surg* 1999;30:468–482.
74. Weibull H, Bergqvist D, Bergentz SE, et al. Percutaneous transluminal renal angioplasty versus surgical reconstruction of atherosclerotic renal artery stenosis: a prospective randomized study. *J Vasc Surg* 1993;18: 841–850; discussion 850–852.
75. Anderson CA, Hansen KJ, Benjamin ME, et al. Renal artery fibromuscular dysplasia: results of current surgical therapy. *J Vasc Surg* 1995;22: 207–215; discussion 215–216.
76. Cambria RP, Brewster DC, L'Italien G, et al. Simultaneous aortic and renal artery reconstruction: evolution of an eighteen-year experience. *J Vasc Surg* 1995;21:916–924; discussion 925.
77. Cambria RP, Brewster DC, L'Italien GJ, et al. The durability of different reconstructive techniques for atherosclerotic renal artery disease. *J Vasc Surg* 1994;20:76–85; discussion 86–77.
78. Cherr GS, Hansen KJ, Craven TE, et al. Surgical management of atherosclerotic renovascular disease. *J Vasc Surg* 2002;35:236–245.
79. Hansen KJ, Starr SM, Sands RE, et al. Contemporary surgical management of renovascular disease. *J Vasc Surg* 1992;16:319–330; discussion 330–331.
80. Murray SP, Kent C, Salvatierra O, et al. Complex branch renovascular disease: management options and late results. *J Vasc Surg* 1994;20:338–345; discussion 346.
81. Modrall JG, Rosero EB, Smith ST, et al. Operative mortality for renal artery bypass in the United States: results from the National Inpatient Sample. *J Vasc Surg* 2008;48:317–322.
82. Stanley JC, Ernst CB, Fry WJ. Fate of 100 aortorenal vein grafts: characteristics of late graft expansion, aneurysmal dilatation, and stenosis. *Surgery* 1973;74:931–944.
83. Chibaro EA, Libertino JA, Novick AC. Use of the hepatic circulation for renal revascularization. *Ann Surg* 1984;199:406–411.
84. Khauli RB, Novick AC, Ziegelbaum M. Splenorenal bypass in the treatment of renal artery stenosis: experience with sixty-nine cases. *J Vasc Surg* 1985;2:547–551.
85. Novick AC, Stewart R, Hodge EE, et al. Use of the thoracic aorta for renal arterial reconstruction. *J Vasc Surg* 1994;19:605–609.
86. Moncure AC, Brewster DC, Darling RC, et al. Use of the splenic and hepatic arteries for renal revascularization. *J Vasc Surg* 1986;3:196–203.
87. Brekke IB, Sodal G, Jakobsen A, et al. Fibro-muscular renal artery disease treated by extracorporeal vascular reconstruction and renal autotransplantation: short- and long-term results. *Eur J Vasc Surg* 1992;6:471–476.
88. van Bockel JH, van den Akker PJ, Chang PC, et al. Extracorporeal renal artery reconstruction for renovascular hypertension. *J Vasc Surg* 1991;13: 101–110; discussion 110–111.
89. Dougherty MJ, Hallett JW Jr, Naessens J, et al. Renal endarterectomy vs. bypass for combined aortic and renal reconstruction: is there a difference in clinical outcome? *Ann Vasc Surg* 1995;9:87–94.
90. McNeil JW, String ST, Pfeiffer RB Jr. Concomitant renal endarterectomy and aortic reconstruction. *J Vasc Surg* 1994;20:331–336; discussion 336–337.
91. Stoney RJ, Messina LM, Goldstone J, et al. Renal endarterectomy through the transected aorta: a new technique for combined aortorenal atherosclerosis—a preliminary report. *J Vasc Surg* 1989;9:224–233.
92. Oskin TC, Hansen KJ, Deitch JS, et al. Chronic renal artery occlusion: nephrectomy versus revascularization. *J Vasc Surg* 1999;29:140–149.
93. Whitehouse WM Jr, Kazmers A, Zelenock GB, et al. Chronic total renal artery occlusion: effects of treatment on secondary hypertension and renal function. *Surgery* 1981;89:753–763.
94. Dzsinich C, Gloviczki P, McKusick MA, et al. Surgical management of renal artery aneurysm. *Cardiovasc Surg* 1993;1:243–247.
95. English WP, Pearce JD, Craven TE, et al. Surgical management of renal artery aneurysms. *J Vasc Surg* 2004;40:53–60.
96. Henke PK, Cardneau JD, Welling TH III, et al. Renal artery aneurysms: a 35-year clinical experience with 252 aneurysms in 168 patients. *Ann Surg* 2001;234:454–462; discussion 462–463.
97. Henriksson C, Bjorkerud S, Nilson AE, et al. Natural history of renal artery aneurysm elucidated by repeated angiography and pathoanatomical studies. *Eur Urol* 1985;11:244–248.
98. Henriksson C, Lukes P, Nilson AE, et al. Angiographically discovered, non-operated renal artery aneurysms. *Scand J Urol Nephrol* 1984;18:59–62.
99. Martin RS III, Meacham PW, Ditesheim JA, et al. Renal artery aneurysm: selective treatment for hypertension and prevention of rupture. *J Vasc Surg* 1989;9:26–34.
100. Pfeiffer T, Reiher L, Grabitz K, et al. Reconstruction for renal artery aneurysm: operative techniques and long-term results. *J Vasc Surg* 2003; 37:293–300.
101. Stanley JC, Rhodes EL, Gewertz BL, et al. Renal artery aneurysms. Significance of macroaneurysms exclusive of dissections and fibrodysplastic mural dilations. *Arch Surg* 1975;110:1327–1333.
102. Tham G, Ekelund L, Herrlin K, et al. Renal artery aneurysms. Natural history and prognosis. *Ann Surg* 1983;197:348–352.
103. Zhang LJ, Yang GF, Qi J, et al. Renal artery aneurysm: diagnosis and surveillance with multidetector-row computed tomography. *Acta Radiol* 2007;48:274–279.
104. Edsman G. Angionephrography and suprarenal angiography; a roentgenologic study of the normal kidney, expansive renal and suprarenal lesions and renal aneurysms. *Acta Radiol* 1957;155:1–141.
105. Sabharwal R, Vladica P, Law WP, et al. Multidetector spiral CT renal angiography in the diagnosis of giant renal artery aneurysms. *Abdom Imaging* 2007;32:17–20.
106. Browne RF, Riordan EO, Roberts JA, et al. Renal artery aneurysms: diagnosis and surveillance with 3D contrast-enhanced magnetic resonance angiography. *Eur Radiol* 2004;14:1807–1812.
107. Tanemoto M, Abe T, Satoh F, et al. Plasma renin activity revealed renal artery stenosis concealed by aneurysms. *Urology* 2005;65:592.
108. Hidai H, Kinoshita Y, Murayama T, et al. Rupture of renal artery aneurysm. *Eur Urol* 1985;11:249–253.
109. Schorn B, Falk V, Dalichau H, et al. Kidney salvage in a case of ruptured renal artery aneurysm: case report and literature review. *Cardiovasc Surg* 1997;5:134–136.
110. Cohen JR, Shamash FS. Ruptured renal artery aneurysms during pregnancy. *J Vasc Surg* 1987;6:51–59.
111. Love WK, Robinette MA, Vernon CP. Renal artery aneurysm rupture in pregnancy. *J Urol* 1981;126:809–811.
112. Rijbroek A, van Dijk HA, Roex AJ. Rupture of renal artery aneurysm during pregnancy. *Eur J Vasc Surg* 1994;8:375–376.
113. Hupp T, Allenberg JR, Post K, et al. Renal artery aneurysm: surgical indications and results. *Eur J Vasc Surg* 1992;6:477–486.
114. Mercier C, Piquet P, Piligian F, et al. Aneurysms of the renal artery and its branches. *Ann Vasc Surg* 1986;1:321–327.
115. Bui BT, Oliva VL, Leclerc G, et al. Renal artery aneurysm: treatment with percutaneous placement of a stent-graft. *Radiology* 1995;195:181–182.
116. Centenera LV, Hirsch JA, Choi IS, et al. Wide-necked saccular renal artery aneurysm: endovascular embolization with the Guglielmi detachable coil and temporary balloon occlusion of the aneurysm neck. *J Vasc Interv Radiol* 1998;9:513–516.
117. Gutta R, Lopes J, Flinn WR, et al. Endovascular embolization of a giant renal artery aneurysm with preservation of renal parenchyma. *Angiology* 2008;59:240–243.
118. Henry M, Polydorou A, Frid N, et al. Treatment of renal artery aneurysm with the multilayer stent. *J Endovasc Ther* 2008;15:231–236.
119. Ikeda O, Tamura Y, Nakasone Y, et al. Nonoperative management of unruptured visceral artery aneurysms: treatment by transcatheter coil embolization. *J Vasc Surg* 2008;47:1212–1219.
120. Manninen HI, Berg M, Vanninen RL. Stent-assisted coil embolization of wide-necked renal artery bifurcation aneurysms. *J Vasc Interv Radiol* 2008;19:487–492.
121. Tateno T, Kubota Y, Sasagawa I, et al. Successful embolization of a renal artery aneurysm with preservation of renal blood flow. *Int Urol Nephrol* 1996;28:283–287.
122. Edwards BS, Stanson AW, Holley KE, et al. Isolated renal artery dissection, presentation, evaluation, management, and pathology. *Mayo Clin Proc* 1982;57:564–571.
123. Gewertz BL, Stanley JC, Fry WJ. Renal artery dissections. *Arch Surg* 1977; 112:409–414.
124. Muller BT, Reiher L, Pfeiffer T, et al. Surgical treatment of renal artery dissection in 25 patients: indications and results. *J Vasc Surg* 2003;37: 761–768.
125. Reilly LM, Cunningham CG, Maggisano R, et al. The role of arterial reconstruction in spontaneous renal artery dissection. *J Vasc Surg* 1991; 14:468–477; discussion 477–479.
126. Smith BM, Holcomb GW III, Richie RE, et al. Renal artery dissection. *Ann Surg* 1984;200:134–146.
127. Baandrup U, Fjeldborg O, Olsen S. Spontaneous dissecting aneurysm of the renal arteries. A case and a review of the literature. *Virchows Arch A Pathol Anat Histopathol* 1983;402:73–82.
128. Mali WP, Geyskes GG, Thalman R. Dissecting renal artery aneurysm: treatment with an endovascular stent. *AJR Am J Roentgenol* 1989;153: 623–624.

CHAPTER 93 ■ SPLANCHNIC VASCULAR OCCLUSIVE AND ANEURYSMAL DISEASE

JOHN E. RECTENWALD, JONATHAN L. ELIASON, PETER K. HENKE, GILBERT R. UPCHURCH, Jr., AND JAMES C. STANLEY

KEY POINTS

1. Occlusive and aneurysmal diseases of the splanchnic vessels are relatively uncommon problems in clinical practice.
2. Approximately 50% of acute mesenteric ischemia cases are caused by an embolus, typically from a cardiac source. Atrial fibrillation and a myocardial infarction with mural thrombus formation are the most common embolic sources.
3. Acute mesenteric embolism usually results in sudden and severe epigastric or midabdominal pain, followed promptly by evacuation of the gut, with emeses or explosive diarrhea.
4. Complications of certain catheter-related procedures and operations are an increasingly common cause of acute ischemia.
5. Intestinal angina is most often a consequence of aortic spillover arteriosclerosis affecting origins of the celiac, superior mesenteric, and inferior mesenteric arteries.
6. In patients with chronic mesenteric ischemia, progression from minor symptoms to intestinal infarction is unpredictable.
7. Splanchnic artery aneurysms are uncommon, but the more frequent use of computed tomography, magnetic resonance imaging, and ultrasonography has resulted in an increase in their clinical recognition.
8. Splenic artery aneurysms are the most common splanchnic artery aneurysm, accounting for 60% of all splanchnic artery aneurysms.
9. The role of endovascular treatment of visceral artery aneurysms is becoming increasingly important, but is currently poorly defined.

1 Occlusive and aneurysmal diseases of the splanchnic vessels are relatively uncommon problems in clinical practice. However, it is important that physicians recognize the clinical presentations of these diseases and be knowledgeable regarding contemporary diagnostic studies and newer treatment options. For example, the "gold standard" diagnostic study, aortography with selective visceral arteriography, is being replaced with high-resolution computed tomographic angiography (CTA) or high-quality magnetic resonance angiography (MRA). In addition, endovascular techniques are displacing conventional open surgical treatment modalities for patients with these diseases.

SPLANCHNIC VASCULAR ANATOMY AND PHYSIOLOGY

The complex functions of the splanchnic viscera are supplied by a circulation uniquely adapted for absorbing and distributing nutrients. Persistence or regression of parts of the primitive visceral circulation results in important variations in the splanchnic arteries and their collateral circulation. Thus, a common celiacomesenteric trunk, replaced hepatic branches from the celiac artery to the superior mesenteric artery (SMA), and a persistent ventral anastomosis between the proper hepatic and a replaced right hepatic artery from the SMA denoted as an arch of Buhler are anatomic variations that are relevant in assessing occlusive diseases of the splanchnic circulation.[1]

The vascular anatomy of the splanchnic viscera follows well-described patterns[2] (Figs. 93.1 to 93.4); however, the right hepatic artery has a replaced origin from the SMA in approximately 15% to 20% of the population and the left hepatic artery is derived from the left gastric artery in about 25% of the population. In the event of occlusion or stenosis of either the celiac artery or SMA, the gastroduodenal artery becomes an important collateral vessel.

The SMA originates from the anterior surface of the aorta 1 or 2 cm below the celiac trunk. Extensive large-vessel anastomotic arcades occur among the 10 to 20 jejunal and ileal SMA branches. In addition, a well-defined anastomosis exists between the middle and left colic branches of the SMA and inferior mesenteric artery in the region of the splenic flexure. The inferior mesenteric artery arises 5 to 6 cm below the SMA, typically supplying the left half of the transverse colon and the entire descending colon through the left colic artery. The inferior mesenteric artery gives off a variable number of sigmoid branches and terminates as paired superior hemorrhoidal arteries. The marginal artery of Drummond and the arch of Riolan are discrete branch vessels capable of significant enlargement, as important collateral vessels, in the face of occlusion or stenosis of the proximal splanchnic arteries.

The venous anatomy of the gastrointestinal tract tends to parallel the arterial blood supply and drains into the portal venous system, thus perfusing the liver. The confluence of the splenic vein with the superior mesenteric vein forms the portal vein. Hepatic venous blood is drained by right, middle, and left hepatic veins, which enter the vena cava. Portal-systemic anastomoses are common and are of considerable importance in the presence of portal hypertension.

Intestinal blood flow in humans has been estimated to be between 500 and 1,200 mL/min, or about 10% to 20% of the cardiac output. Duplex ultrasound, which combines Doppler blood flow velocity determinations with B-mode grayscale images, allows precise measurement of cross-sectional areas and enables calculation of volumetric flows (Fig. 93.5). Baseline intestinal

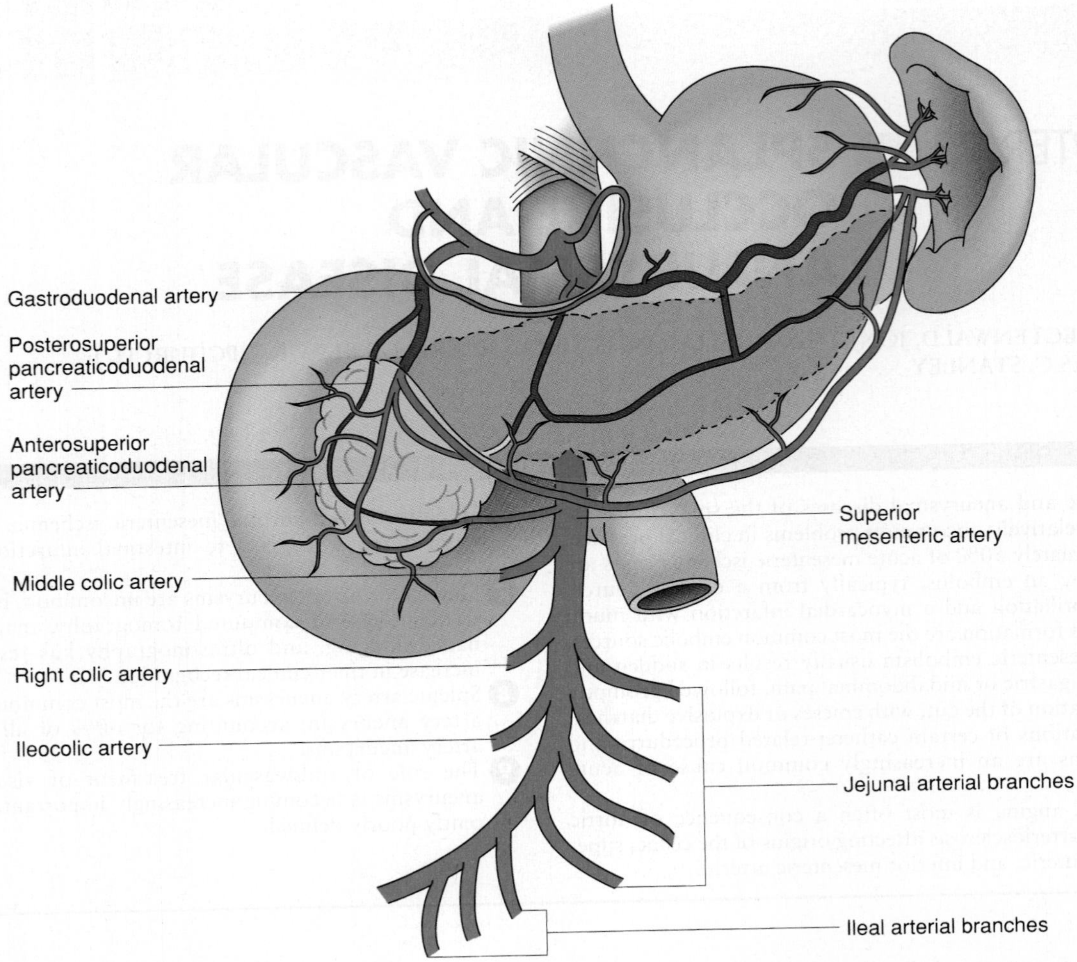

FIGURE 93.1. The celiac artery distributes blood to the stomach, duodenum, pancreas, liver, and spleen; in addition, the gastroduodenal artery and pancreaticoduodenal arcades provide important collateral flow between the celiac and superior mesenteric arteries. The superior mesenteric artery is retropancreatic but crosses anteriorly to the fourth portion of the duodenum. It supplies blood to the duodenum and head of the pancreas, jejunum, ileum, ascending colon, and right half of the transverse colon (see Fig. 93.2). Large anastomotic arcades course between the jejunal and ileal branches.

blood flow and the response to standard meals have been established, with significant increases in SMA blood flow 20 to 30 minutes after the ingestion of food that persist for up to 90 minutes. Changes in celiac artery blood flow occur with all meal types; however, these changes are not significant (Table 93.1).

SPLANCHNIC ISCHEMIC SYNDROMES

The intestinal mucosa represents 50% of the mass of the intestine, but receives 75% of the resting blood flow. The muscular and serosal layers of the intestine receive the remaining 25%. Control of blood flow in the splanchnic circulation is affected by the sympathetic nervous system and also by metabolic, myogenic, and extrinsic factors. Stimulation of sympathetic nerves increases vascular tone and decreases splanchnic blood flow, whereas parasympathetic nerve stimulation appears to have little direct effect on blood flow. Numerous intrinsic hormones, such as secretin, gastrin, cholecystokinin, glucagon, and vasoactive intestinal peptide, in addition to substances such as histamine, serotonin, bradykinin, and the prostaglandins, all have physiologic roles in regulating intestinal blood flow. Other substances, such as epinephrine, norepinephrine, and angiotensin, as well as many commonly used pharmaceuticals, also have important effects on the splanchnic circulation (Table 93.2).

The potential for bacterial translocation and toxin absorption add to the complexity of ischemia and reperfusion within the gut. These adverse effects exacerbate local injury and have important systemic effects, including myocardial depression and increased capillary permeability with edema formation and organ dysfunction.[3–7] Loss of mucosal barrier function is clearly present in acute splanchnic ischemia, with three predisposing factors: (a) physical disruption of the mucosa, (b) a change in the normal intestinal microflora (usually resulting from treatment with broad-spectrum antibiotics), and (c) impairment of host immune defenses. The repair of mucosal damage and enhancement of host defenses appear to be facilitated by early enteral feeding and by specific nutrients, such as glutamine.

Splanchnic ischemic syndromes are most conveniently categorized as acute or chronic. However, the designation of chronic ischemia is perhaps a misnomer because even in this setting, the underlying pathophysiology is characterized by repetitive, near-critical ischemic events. Acute splanchnic syndromes include mesenteric arterial embolism, mesenteric

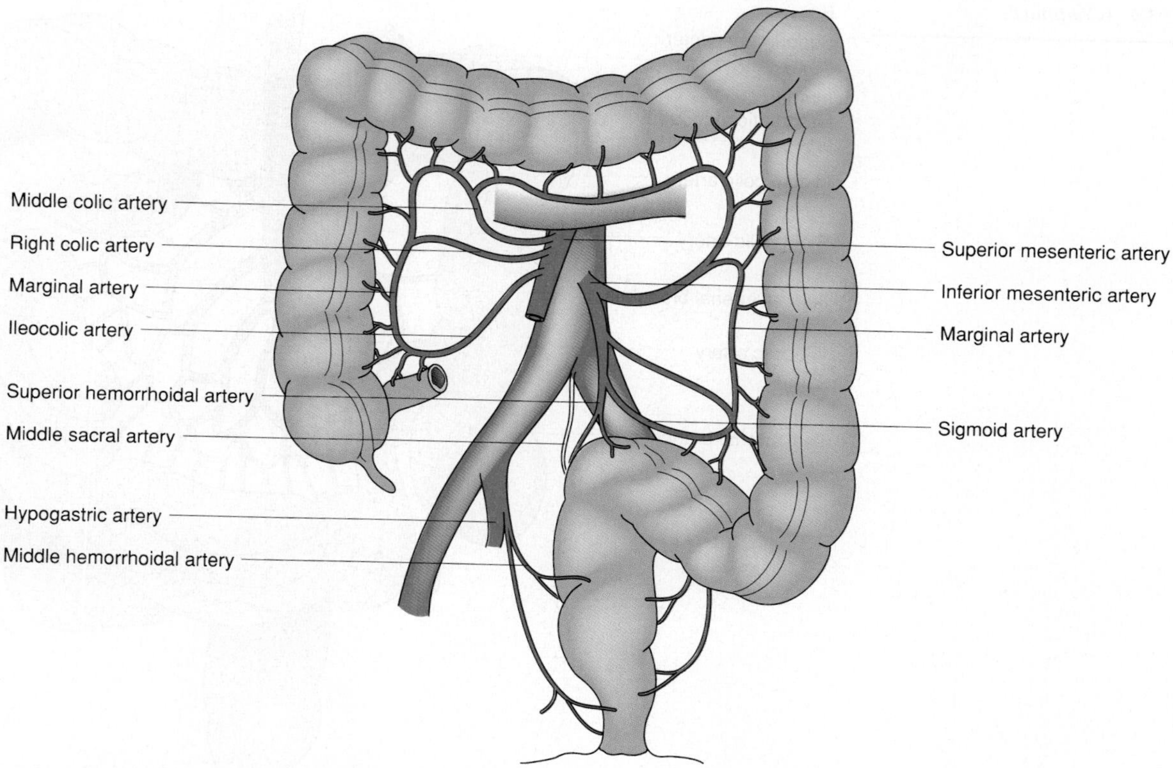

FIGURE 93.2. The inferior mesenteric artery (IMA) supplies blood to the left half of the transverse colon and the entire descending colon, including the sigmoid colon and rectum (via sigmoid and superior hemorrhoidal branches). The left branch of the middle colic artery, from the superior mesenteric artery, and the ascending portion of the left colic artery, from the IMA, form a collateral network in the region of the splenic flexure. The IMA serves as an important source of collateral blood supply when the proximal two visceral vessels are occluded.

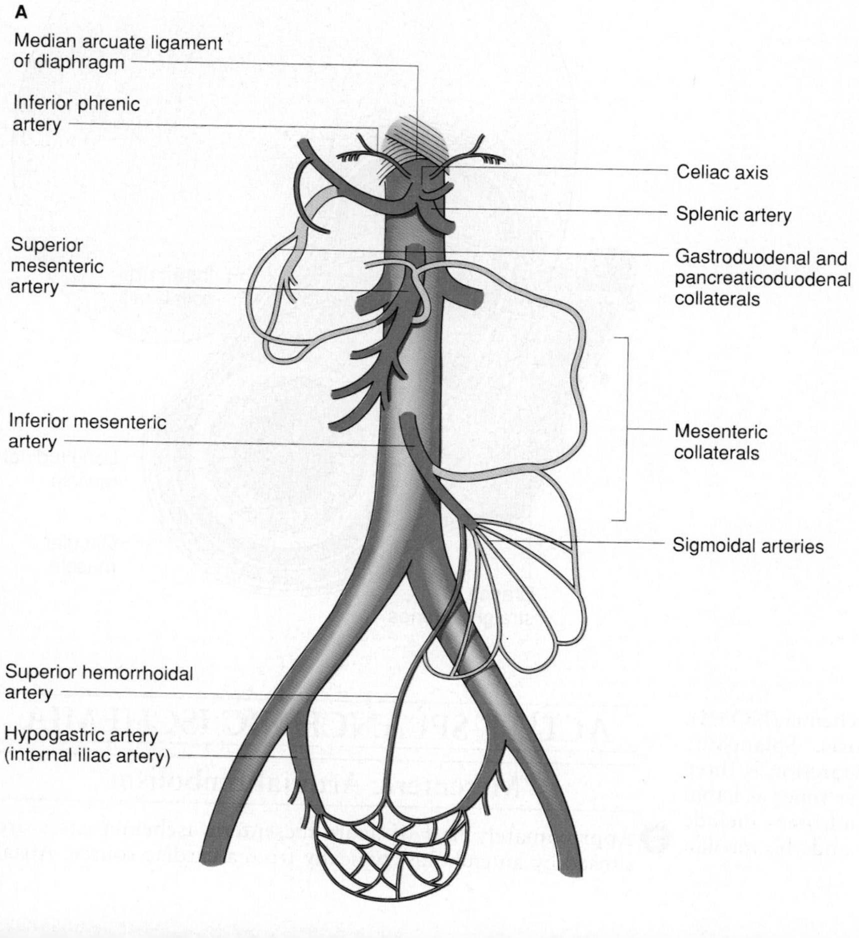

FIGURE 93.3. **A:** The collateral circulation to the intestine occurs at several levels. Well-recognized visceral-visceral and visceral-parietal collateral branches and anastomoses are important. The unnamed intestinal arcades (**B**) and the intramural anastomoses (**C**) are effective short-segment collaterals.

VASCULAR

FIGURE 93.3. (*Continued*)

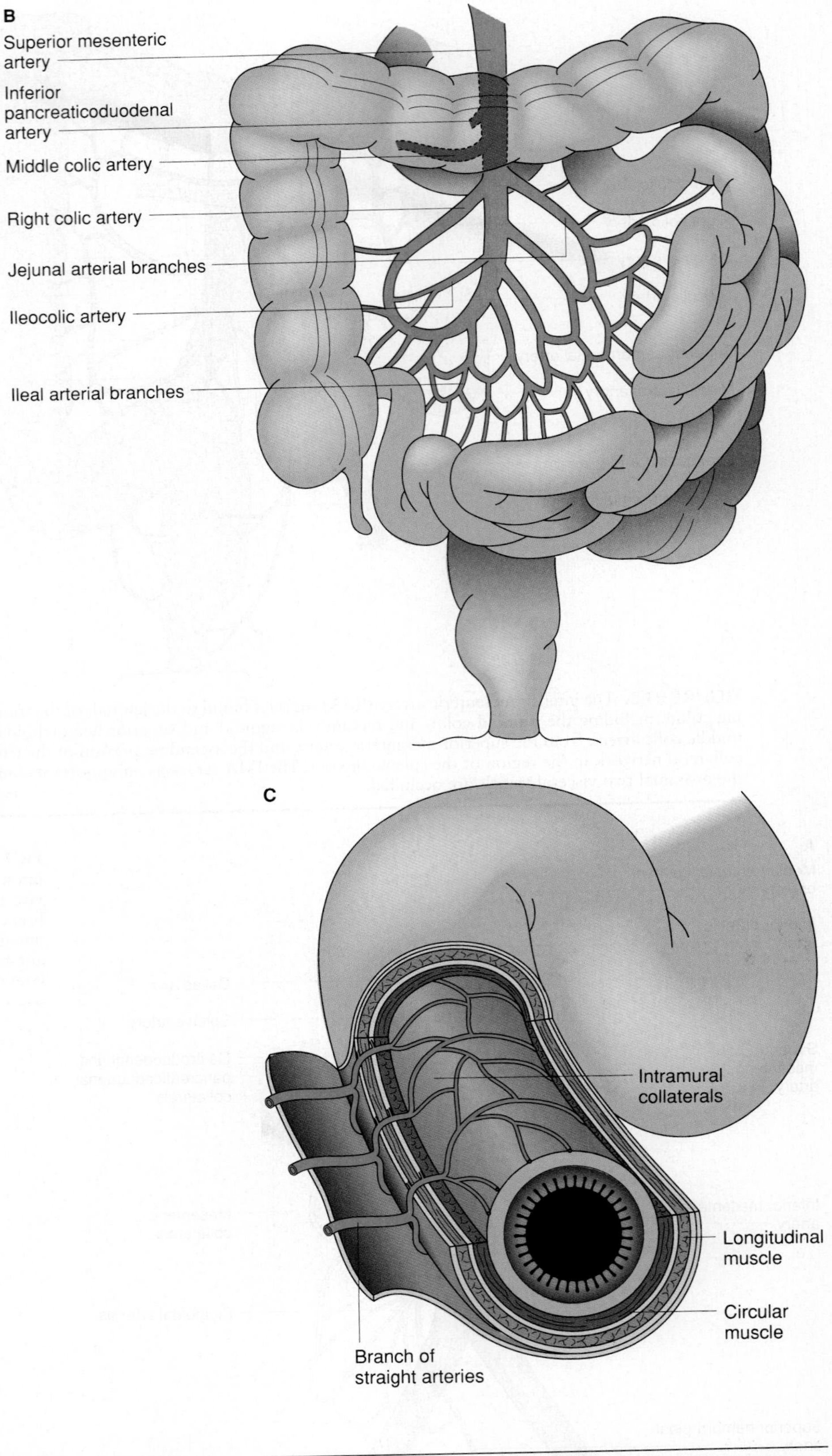

arterial thrombosis, nonocclusive mesenteric ischemia (NOMI), iatrogenic ischemia, and venous thrombosis. Splanchnic ischemia severe enough to cause intestinal infarction is three times as lethal as myocardial infarction and five times as lethal as a stroke. Chronic splanchnic ischemic syndromes include arteriosclerotic mesenteric occlusive disease and the median arcuate ligament syndrome.

ACUTE SPLANCHNIC ISCHEMIA

Mesenteric Arterial Embolism

2 Approximately half of acute mesenteric ischemia cases are caused by an embolus, typically from a cardiac source. Atrial

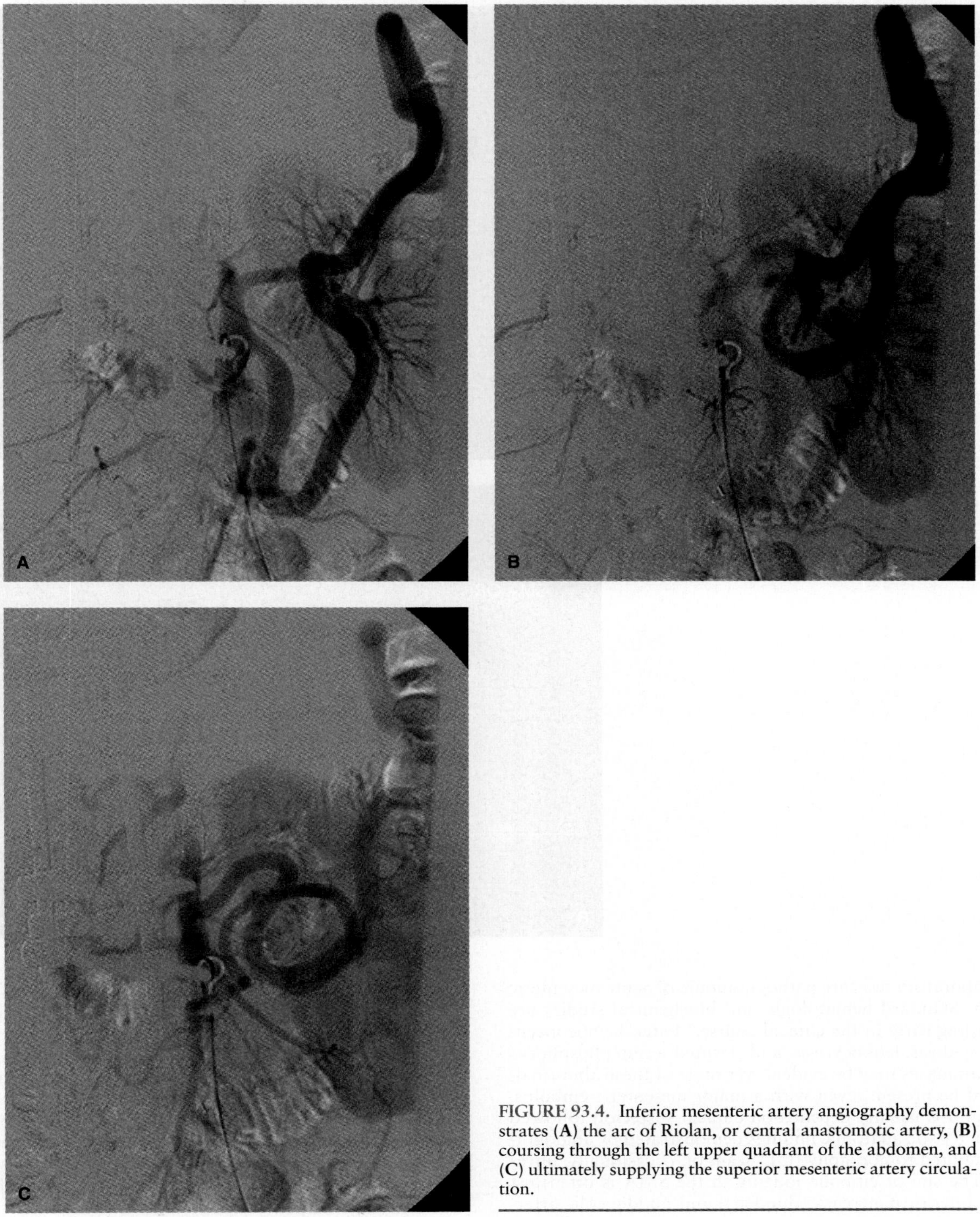

FIGURE 93.4. Inferior mesenteric artery angiography demonstrates (A) the arc of Riolan, or central anastomotic artery, (B) coursing through the left upper quadrant of the abdomen, and (C) ultimately supplying the superior mesenteric artery circulation.

fibrillation and myocardial infarction with mural thrombus formation are the most common embolic sources; however, any arrhythmia or anatomic cardiac defect may result in a mesenteric embolus. Embolism of an intracardiac tumor, such as an atrial myxoma, and a paradoxic embolus resulting from venous thromboembolism and a right-to-left cardiac communication are rare causes of mesenteric ischemia.

3 Acute mesenteric embolism usually results in sudden and severe epigastric or midabdominal pain, followed promptly by evacuation of the gut, with emeses or explosive diarrhea. The patient can often precisely pinpoint the onset of pain, and fully 25% of patients have had previous embolic events. A cardiac source of the embolus may be clinically evident if the patient has irregular heart rhythm, indicating atrial fibrillation, the classic murmur of mitral stenosis, or an enlarged heart. The abdominal examination may be normal initially, with signs of an acute abdomen evolving later. Slight to moderate abdominal distention is common. Bowel sounds are highly variable and not useful as a diagnostic finding. The classic presentation of acute mesenteric ischemia is severe abdominal pain that is out of proportion to minimal or absent physical findings. The presence of peritoneal signs and blood in the stool are late and ominous signs, implying intestinal infarction.

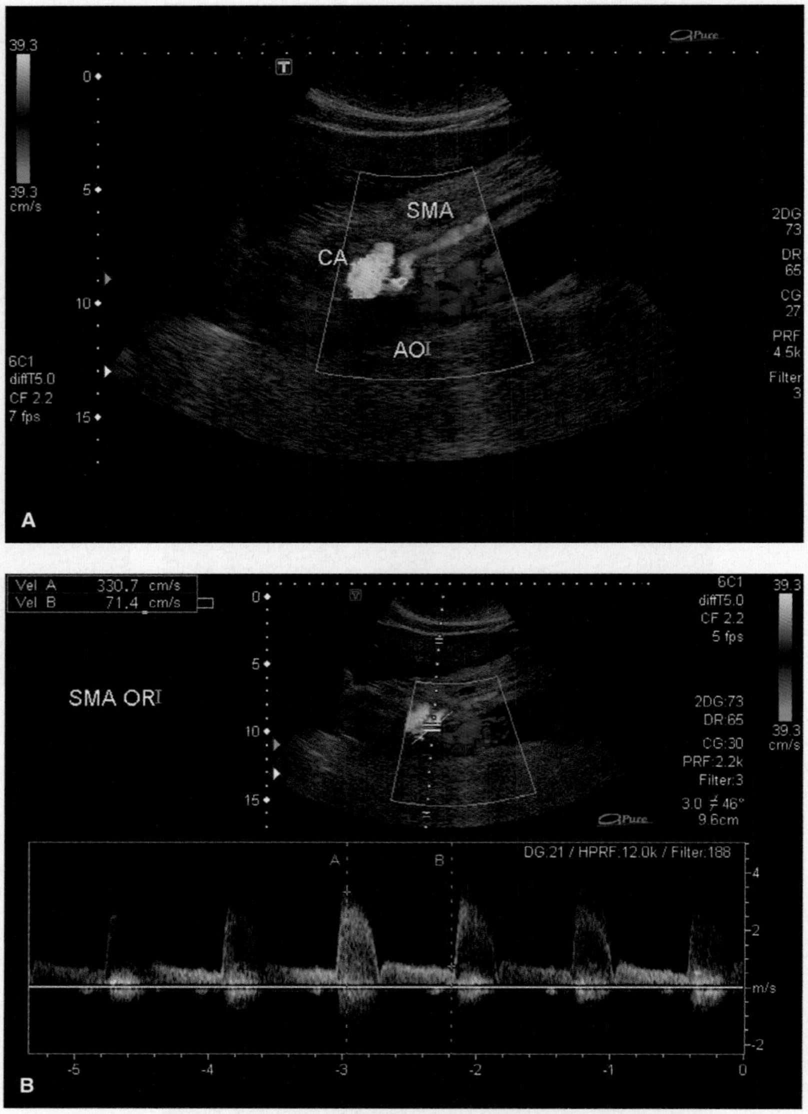

FIGURE 93.5. A: Duplex scan of the aorta and celiac and superior mesenteric arteries. Vessel diameter, flow velocity, calculated volumetric blood flow, spectral analysis, and the response to physiologic stimuli allow a precise assessment of the visceral circulation. B: Color flow Doppler scanning allows rapid identification of flow disturbances. (Courtesy of Dr. Phillip Bendick, William Beaumont Hospital, Royal Oak, MI.)

No laboratory tests are pathognomonic of acute mesenteric ischemia. Standard hematologic and biochemical studies are unrewarding early in the clinical course.[8] Later, hemoconcentration, acidosis, leukocytosis, and elevated serum phosphorus or transaminases may be evident, yet none of these abnormalities need be present, even with a major mesenteric embolus. The diagnosis usually depends on clinical suspicion followed by characteristic anatomic findings demonstrated by angiography, computed tomography (CT) scan, or, occasionally, ultrasound. The site of embolic lodging in the SMA is often just past the inferior pancreaticoduodenal and middle colic arteries, thus isolating the small bowel from its major collateral circulation (Fig. 93.6).

In the case of a suspected diagnosis, the patient should be anticoagulated with heparin, volume resuscitated, and taken to the operating room for an emergent embolectomy. Prophylactic antibiotics and full hemodynamic monitoring are mandatory. The SMA is exposed beneath the transverse mesocolon followed by achievement of proximal and distal control of the vessel. A Fogarty catheter embolectomy is then performed through either a transverse or longitudinal arteriotomy. Primary closure with interrupted sutures can typically be performed if a transverse arteriotomy is used. Patch closure of the SMA is used if the artery is small or a longitudinal incision has been made. Intestinal viability is assessed after restoration of blood flow.

Acute Mesenteric Arterial Thrombosis

A less common cause of acute splanchnic ischemia follows thrombosis of an underlying diseased SMA. The presentation is usually less abrupt than what is typically seen with an SMA embolus, with eventual development of severe midabdominal pain. These symptoms may occur de novo, as the majority of patients with chronic mesenteric artery occlusive disease are asymptomatic, or be superimposed on a background of chronic intestinal angina. A history of motility disturbances causing nausea, diarrhea, or constipation are common but of little diagnostic value.

Urgent angiography with an anteroposterior and lateral aortogram is appropriate to establish a diagnosis of mesenteric thrombosis (Fig. 93.7). The occlusive process is usually more extensive than what is readily apparent on angiography. CTA is also being used more frequently to recognize mesenteric ischemia, and in addition to excellent vascular anatomic detail for both arterial and venous phase imaging, offers additional relevant information such as changes in the bowel wall or the presence or absence of ascites.[9]

Reperfusion of the splanchnic circulation is the major priority in these acutely ill patients. Chronic weight loss with its attendant nutritional, wound-healing, and immunologic compromise makes any operative procedure hazardous. In some

TABLE 93.1

DUPLEX MEASUREMENT OF INTESTINAL BLOOD FLOW

VESSEL	AVERAGE DIAMETER (RANGE)	CHARACTERISTICS ON DUPLEX SCAN	CALCULATED FASTING VOLUME FLOW (mL/min)	CALCULATED VOLUME FLOW CHANGE FROM FASTING BY TYPE OF MEAL[a] (%)					
				MIXED	CHOLESTEROL	FAT	PROTEIN	MANNITOL	WATER
Celiac artery	0.66 cm (0.4–0.8 cm)	Continuous forward flow; no reverse flow: end-diastolic velocity about one-third peak systolic velocity	1,083 ± 75	18 ± 4	1 ± 4	10 ± 8	21 ± 6	37 ± 19	14 ± 5
		No significant changes with meals							
Superior mesenteric artery	0.59 cm (0.44–0.68 cm)	Early diastolic flow reversal; forward diastolic flow; end-diastolic velocity about zero	538 ± 37	164 ± 30	118 ± 23	117 ± 25	78 ± 15	48 ± 11	24 ± 8
		After eating, loss of reverse flow and increased peak systolic and end-diastolic velocities noted							

[a]Calculated volume flow changes that occurred after meals were not significantly increased in the celiac artery but were significantly increased with all meals except water in the superior mesenteric artery.
From Moneta GL, Taylor DC, Heiton WS, et al. Duplex ultrasound measurement of postprandial intestinal blood flow: effect of meal composition. *Gastroenterology* 1988;95:1294.

TABLE 93.2

EFFECTS OF VARIOUS SUBSTANCES ON MESENTERIC CIRCULATION AND MOTOR ACTIVITY

SUBSTANCE	INTESTINAL BLOOD FLOW	INTESTINAL O_2 UPTAKE	INTESTINAL MOTILITY
Acetylcholine	Increase	Increase	Increase
Adenosine	Increase	Variable	—
Angiotensin II	Decrease	—	Increase
Bradykinin	Variable	—	Increase
Ca^{2+}, high levels	Decrease	—	Increase
Ca^{2+} antagonists	Increase	—	Decrease
Dopamine	Variable	Decrease	—
Epinephrine	Variable	Variable	—
Gastrin	Increase	Increase	Increase
Glucagon	Increase	Increase	Decrease
Histamine	Increase	Increase	Increase
Isoproterenol	Increase	Variable	—
K^+, high levels	Decrease	—	Increase
Mg^{2+}	Increase	—	—
Nitroprusside	Increase	—	—
Norepinephrine	Decrease	Decrease	—
Papaverine	Increase	No change	—
PGE_1	Increase	Increase	—
PGF_{2a}	Decrease	Variable	Increase
PGI_2	Increase	—	—
Secretin	Variable	No change	—
Serotonin	Variable	Variable	Variable
Somatostatin	Decrease	—	Decrease
Vasopressin	Decrease	Decrease	Variable
Vasoactive intestinal	Increase	Increase	—

PG, prostaglandin.
From Wakefield TW, Stanley JC. The intestine. In: Zelenock GB, D'Alecy LG, Schlafer M, et al., eds. *Clinical Ischemic Syndromes: Mechanisms and Consequences of Tissue Injury*. St. Louis, MO: Mosby; 1990.

cases reperfusion can be quickly accomplished by angioplasty with or without stenting.[10–12] These endovascular interventions may have potential benefit, even if an open revascularization were required at a later time. Nevertheless, this approach is not appropriate when peritoneal signs suggest frankly necrotic bowel requiring resection.

Operations for an acute SMA thrombosis must be individualized. Options include (a) antegrade bypasses originating from the supraceliac aorta, (b) retrograde bypasses with inflow from the iliac arteries, (c) single versus multivessel revascularization, and (d) the use of either prosthetic or autogenous venous conduit. In the presence of frankly necrotic bowel requiring resection, autogenous vein is the preferred conduit for revascularization.

Low-flow Nonocclusive Mesenteric Ischemia

Nonocclusive mesenteric ischemia remains a problem in contemporary practice.[13,14] Vasoconstriction of the mesenteric blood vessels is common, occurring in response to diminished cardiac output, shock, hypovolemia, dehydration, or the use of vasoactive medications (Table 93.2). This form of intestinal ischemia occurs most often in critically ill patients who are hemodynamically unstable secondary to shock or congestive heart failure. Gastrointestinal mucosal sloughing and bleeding may be present. A diagnosis in these instances may be established with angiography (Fig. 93.8). Typical findings include diffuse vasoconstriction and nonopacification of branch artery vessels. The focus of intervention is the treatment of the underlying cause of shock or cardiac dysfunction. Pharmacologic support of the circulation may also aid in relieving splanchnic vasoconstriction. Patients should receive optimization of their hemodynamic and volume status, correction of contributing medical conditions, and, when possible, elimination of adverse pharmacologic agents. Selective intra-arterial infusion of vasodilators such as intra-arterial papaverine (30 to 60 mg/h)[15] or intravenous infusion of glucagon (2 to 4 mg/h) or prostaglandin E_1, which selectively increases splanchnic blood flow, has been advocated in treating this form of intestinal ischemia.[16,17]

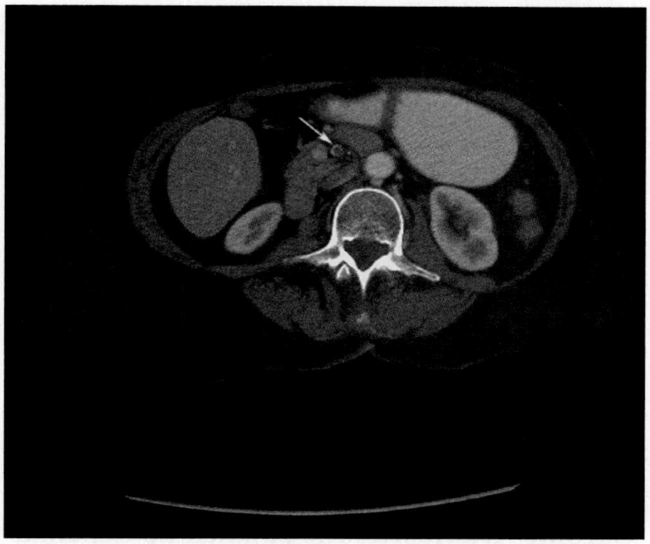

FIGURE 93.6. Axial section from thin slice contrasted CT demonstrates an obvious filling defect (*white arrow*) within the superior mesenteric artery due to an SMA embolus.

Iatrogenic Acute Splanchnic Ischemia

5 Splanchnic ischemia may also result from iatrogenic injury. Increased utilization of endovascular techniques for the treatment of occlusive and aneurysmal pathologies of the aorta and its branches may result in arterial dissections or thromboembolic events. These events are not limited to selective catheterization of the splanchnic vessels. Indeed, an atheroembolic shower from wire and/or catheter manipulation may result in multifocal ischemic necrosis of the intestine and is a highly morbid event.

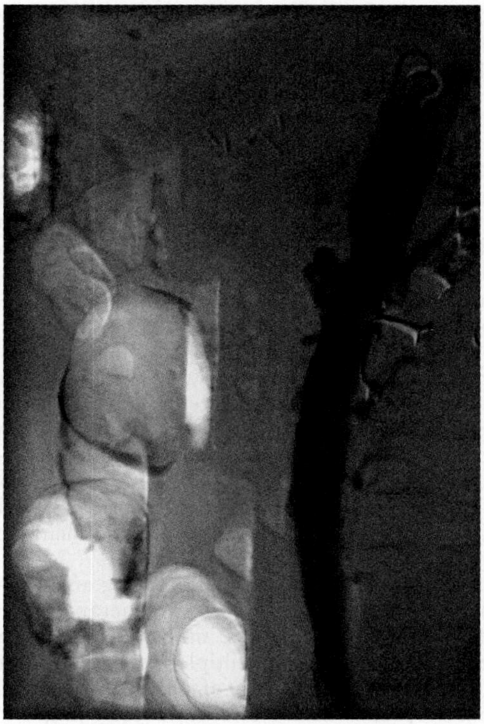

FIGURE 93.7. Lateral aortogram demonstrating acute celiac and superior mesenteric artery thrombosis, which results in widespread necrosis of the abdominal viscera.

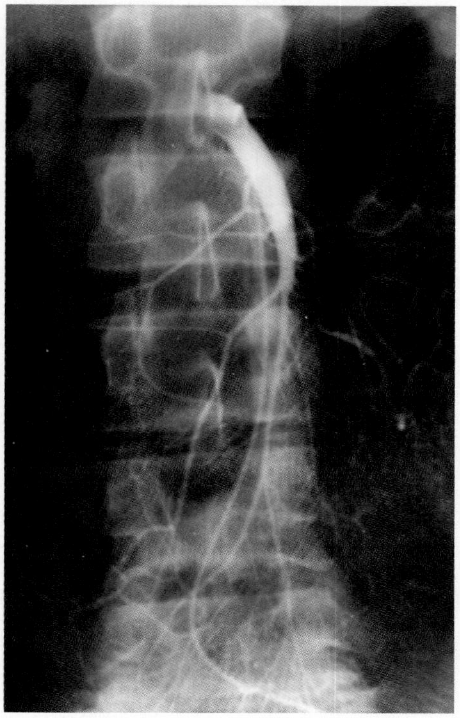

FIGURE 93.8. Low-flow nonocclusive ischemia causes profound vasoconstriction within the mesenteric arcades, which may be sufficient to cause mucosal necrosis or transmural infarction if not relieved.

Open abdominal aortic aneurysm repair is the prototypical surgical procedure associated with iatrogenic intestinal ischemia.[18] Intraoperative ligation of the inferior mesenteric artery (IMA) prior to aortic graft implantation is a typical step in this operation. The majority of patients tolerate IMA ligation without significant sequelae. However, colonic ischemia may be clinically apparent in 1% to 2% of cases and has been detected endoscopically in 6% to 8% of cases. These patients present with postoperative diarrhea and the stool is usually grossly bloody or guaiac positive. When such an event occurs, immediate colonoscopy is indicated. If the ischemia is confined to the mucosa and submucosa and subsequently heals, a stricture may form (Fig. 93.9). If the ischemia is more profound and transmural infarction occurs requiring resection, there is a 16-fold increase in mortality.[19] Intestinal ischemia is also more common with ruptured aneurysms, when occlusive and aneurysmal disease coexist, and when important collateral vessels are compromised by the aortic procedure itself.

Other Types of Acute Splanchnic Ischemia

Ischemia of the intestines may also accompany aortic dissections, traumatic injuries, or the inflammatory arteritides. The clinical presentation and diagnosis depends on the underlying cause, with superimposed symptoms of abdominal distention, an acute abdomen, or gastrointestinal bleeding.[20] Treatment must be highly individualized. In the setting of acute aortic dissection, branch revascularization or fenestration is essential. Traumatic injuries also require urgent surgical intervention. Inflammatory arteritides require treatment of the underlying medical condition, with operation reserved only for resection of clearly nonviable bowel. Intraoperative recognition of intestinal viability, the appropriate limits to resection, and

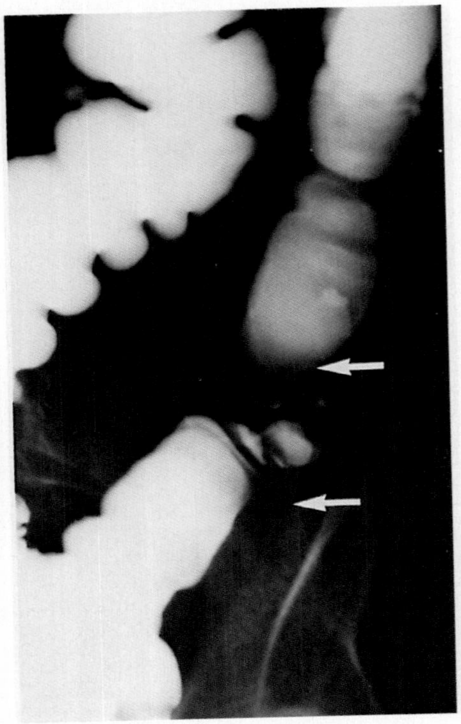

FIGURE 93.9. Stricture formation resulting from sigmoid colon ischemia after repair of a ruptured aortic aneurysm. A loss of haustrations is seen through the descending colon and the fixed narrowing in the midportion of the sigmoid colon (*arrows*).

consideration of a "second-look" procedure are critical.[21–23] Clinical parameters of color, spontaneous peristalsis, and palpable pulses are not sensitive or specific enough to provide a basis for precise and confident clinical decisions. The most common adjunctive technique to determine the extent of necessary bowel resection is Doppler ultrasonography. Fluorescein dye and Wood lamp analyses are also frequently used to assess bowel viability.

If large segments of ischemic small bowel are resected, the potential exists for the development of short-gut syndrome, in which insufficient intestine remains for adequate nutrient absorption. Contemporary clinical practice is to not resect marginally viable intestine and resect only unequivocally necrotic tissue at the initial operation. A planned "second-look" surgical procedure 24 to 48 hours later is undertaken to evaluate the status of the remaining intestine.

Mesenteric Venous Thrombosis

Thrombosis of mesenteric veins is most often subacute in its presentation. A vague prodrome of crampy abdominal pain, abdominal distention, nausea, and malaise may occur for a few days to several weeks before the disease is recognized. However, in the presence of widespread and major venous occlusions, the presentation can be acute and catastrophic. Mesenteric venous thrombosis may be secondary to an associated condition, including an intra-abdominal inflammatory process, peritonitis, portal hypertension, a hypercoagulable state, and the use of oral contraceptives. Plain films often reveal bowel wall edema. The venous phase of a selective mesenteric arteriogram may reveal the thrombus, and CT studies often demonstrate thrombus within the portal and superior mesenteric veins. In many instances, the diagnosis is made intraoperatively, with the presence of bloody ascites and dusky-appearing intestine that is thick and rubbery. The small mesenteric veins are often cordlike and exude clot when cut. Surgical therapy consists of resection of nonviable intestine, occasional large vessel venous thrombectomy, and administration of anticoagulants. Correction of any predisposing hypercoagulable state is mandatory, such as deficiency of antithrombin III and proteins C and S, as well as the presence of factor V Leiden and anticardiolipin antibodies (the lupus anticoagulant). In cases of primary mesenteric venous thrombosis, postoperative anticoagulant therapy is continued indefinitely, because if untreated, venous thrombosis recurs in 30% to 40% of patients. Anticoagulation reduces the incidence of recurrence to 3% to 5%. In cases secondary to a treatable cause, such as peritonitis, relatively short-term anticoagulation is recommended, similar to that used when treating venous thrombosis.

CHRONIC SPLANCHNIC ISCHEMIA

Chronic Arteriosclerotic Splanchnic Ischemia

Intestinal angina is most often a consequence of aortic spillover arteriosclerosis affecting the origins of the celiac, superior mesenteric, and inferior mesenteric arteries. The responsible anatomic lesions invariably involve at least two of these three arteries (Fig. 93.10). The occlusive process may also be widespread throughout the mesenteric arcades, especially in diabetics. The patient is either typically affected with generalized clinical overt arteriosclerosis or is a relatively young woman with an extensive cigarette-smoking habit.

These patients develop "food fear" and modify their pattern of eating so that they only consume small quantities of food at any one time. Intestinal angina may manifest as periumbilical discomfort, developing 15 to 30 minutes after eating and often lasting 1 to 4 hours. Patients with chronic splanchnic ischemia almost always have a profound weight loss, which raises the specter of an intra-abdominal malignancy. Many times, gastrointestinal contrast studies, endoscopy, various scans, and nonproductive exploratory laparotomies have been undertaken before a diagnosis of intestinal ischemia is considered.

6 The progression from minor symptoms to intestinal infarction is unpredictable. Frequently, patients with intestinal infarction are discovered, in retrospect, to have had preexisting symptoms of intestinal angina. Although delayed recognition is commonplace, therapeutic interventions must proceed expeditiously, because if intestinal angina progresses to transmural infarction, it is attended by an 80% mortality rate.

Duplex scanning, MRA, and CT scans support the diagnosis of this form of intestinal vascular disease. Aortography, including both anteroposterior and lateral views, however, has most commonly been used to assess this disease (Fig. 93.11). In some clinical series, 85% of the celiac, superior mesenteric, and inferior mesenteric arteries were totally occluded or severely stenotic.[24] Although often diseased, the inferior mesenteric artery frequently serves as the major remaining source of blood flow to the gut, with an occluded celiac artery and SMA. At the very least, duplex scanning of the aorta and visceral vessels should be undertaken in suspected cases. MRA, CTA, or conventional angiography can then be pursued when appropriate.[25–27]

Elective intestinal revascularization using an endovascular or open surgical approach is standard therapy in the treatment of arteriosclerotic chronic mesenteric ischemia.[20,28–37] For open revascularization, multiple-vessel revascularization with short, antegrade conduits of either autogenous saphenous vein or prosthetic material is favored (Fig. 93.12). A variety of other bypass techniques have also resulted in long-term relief of symptoms (Fig. 93.13). Endarterectomy through a "trapdoor" aortotomy with a thoracoabdominal exposure (Figs. 93.14 and 93.15) is particularly effective

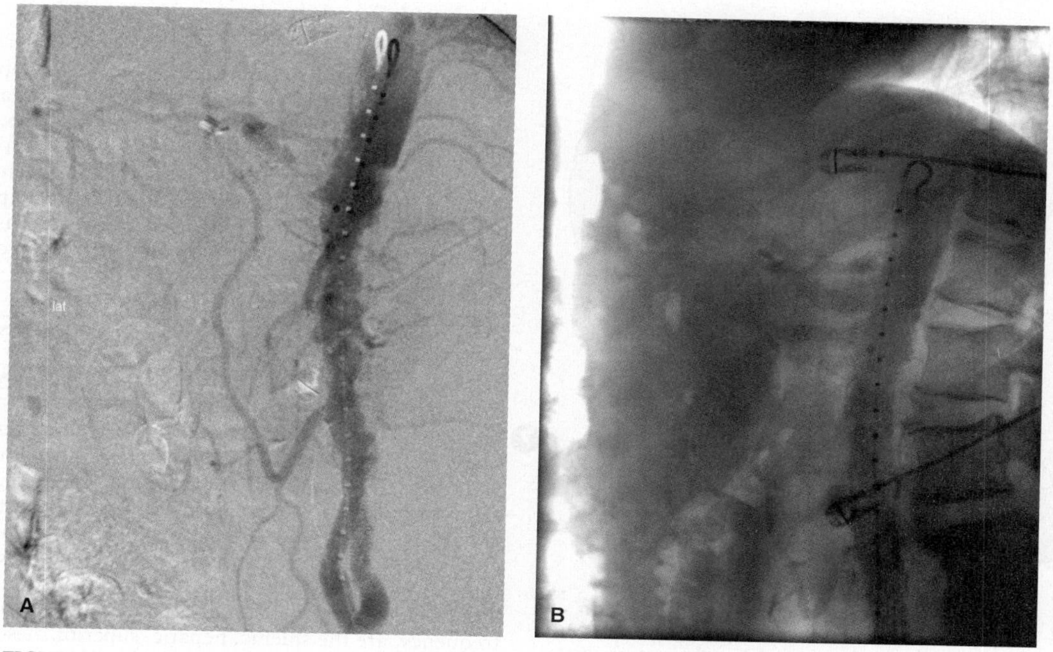

FIGURE 93.10. (A) Celiac artery stenosis and superior mesenteric artery occlusion are apparent in this lateral aortogram. (B) Lateral aortogram following primary stenting of the celiac artery, and recanalization and stenting of the superior mesenteric artery.

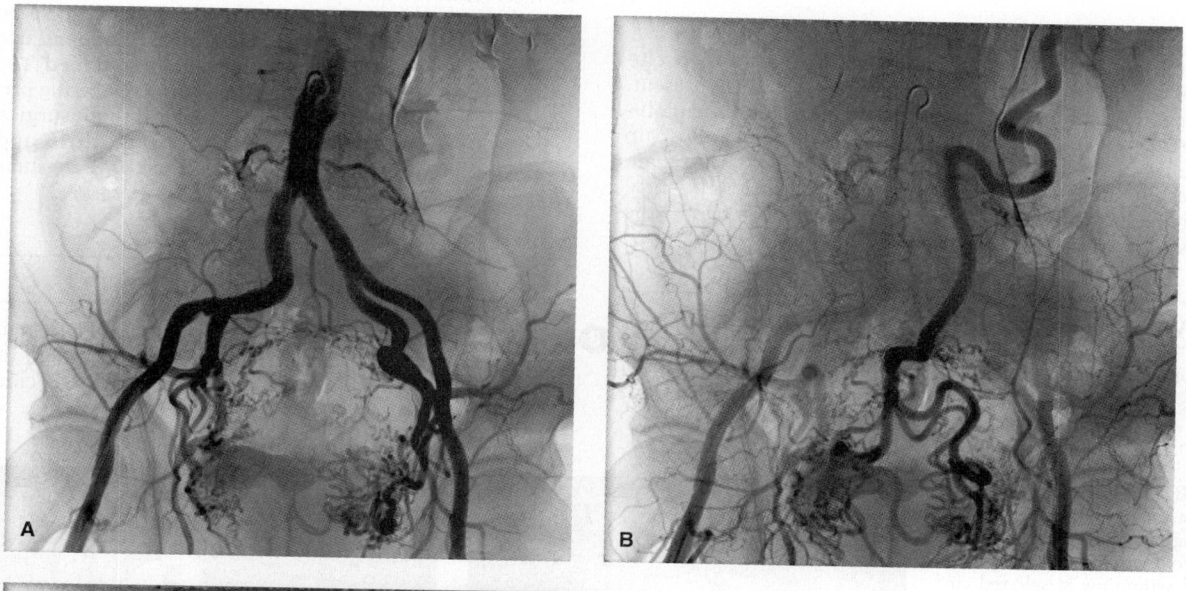

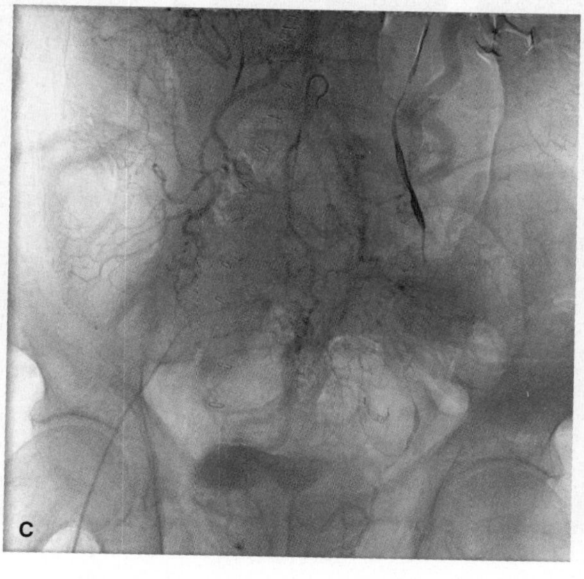

FIGURE 93.11. Chronic visceral ischemia produces visceral angina when multiple occlusions of major splanchnic blood vessels are present. Lack of apparent intestinal blood flow (A) and an unusually prominent inferior mesenteric artery (B) are angiographic signs of chronic visceral ischemia. Selective celiac injection (C) also fills the superior mesenteric artery distribution secondary to occlusions of the proximal superior and inferior mesenteric arteries.

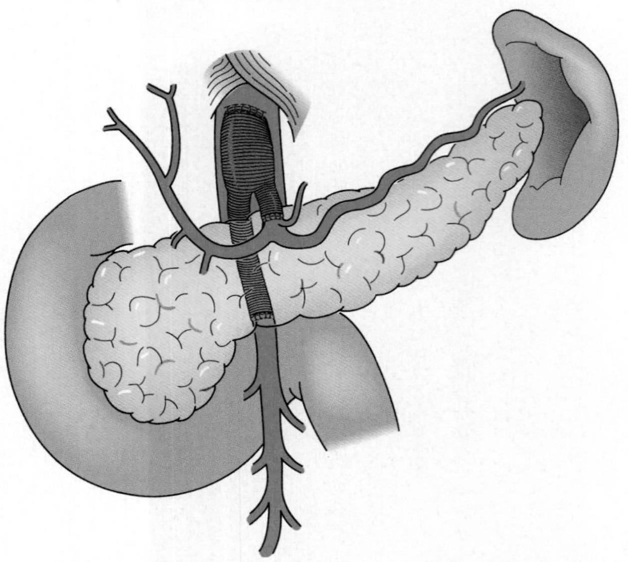

FIGURE 93.12. Bypass grafts to the visceral vessels may originate from the supraceliac aorta. Short antegrade conduits and multiple-vessel revascularization are favored.

when multiple proximal intestinal arterial stenoses or occlusions, as well as concomitant renal artery lesions, are present. Percutaneous angioplastic procedures with or without endoluminal stenting are often used. Although long-term follow-up data are lacking when compared to follow-up for open repair, initial results suggest a favorable morbidity and mortality profile with perhaps higher rates of symptom recurrence in the endovascular group.[34,38–50]

Median Arcuate Ligament Syndrome

Symptomatic entrapment of the celiac artery by the median arcuate ligament is controversial. Symptoms include postprandial periumbilical abdominal pain, but this symptom may or may not represent intestinal ischemia. Arteriography in these patients reveals a significant compression of the celiac artery by the median arcuate ligament of the diaphragm (Fig. 93.16). Lysis of the overlying median arcuate ligament and surrounding neural tissue affords relief of symptoms in approximately half of these patients, with celiac axis revascularization required, either surgical or endovascular, in an occasional case.

SPLANCHNIC ARTERY ANEURYSMAL DISEASE

7 True splanchnic artery aneurysms are uncommon, but the more frequent use of CT, magnetic resonance imaging (MRI), and ultrasonography has resulted in an increase in their clinical recognition (Table 93.3). Prompt recognition of these aneurysms is clearly clinically important considering that nearly 22% present as surgical emergencies, including 8.5% that result in the patient's death. The splanchnic vessels involved with these macroaneurysms, in decreasing order of frequency, are the splenic, hepatic, superior mesenteric, celiac, gastric–gastroepiploic, jejunal–ileal–colic, pancreaticoduodenal–pancreatic, and gastroduodenal arteries (Table 93.3). The general clinical manifestations and management of these aneurysms, including the more widespread use of endovascular interventions, have been addressed in a number of recent reviews.[51–60] Although surgical management of splanchnic artery aneurysms remains the mainstay of treatment, endovascular techniques are being increasingly applied to these aneurysms in the setting of rupture[60] and may be the preferred treatment in those patients who are deemed high surgical risk, or for aneurysms in locations that are difficult to approach surgically.[61] However, the specifics of each of these splanchnic artery aneurysms deserve individual consideration.

Splenic Artery Aneurysm

8 Splenic artery aneurysms account for 60% of all splanchnic artery aneurysms. The occurrence of these lesions in the general population is probably similar to the 0.78% incidence in

FIGURE 93.13. Retrograde conduits are an alternative bypass, and even single-vessel revascularization may provide effective long-term relief of symptoms in selected circumstances. **A:** Retrograde right external iliac artery to superior mesenteric artery (SMA) vein graft. Filling is excellent throughout the distribution of the SMA and in the branches of the celiac artery as a result of collateral flow through the gastroduodenal artery. **B:** A left common iliac artery–SMA bypass.

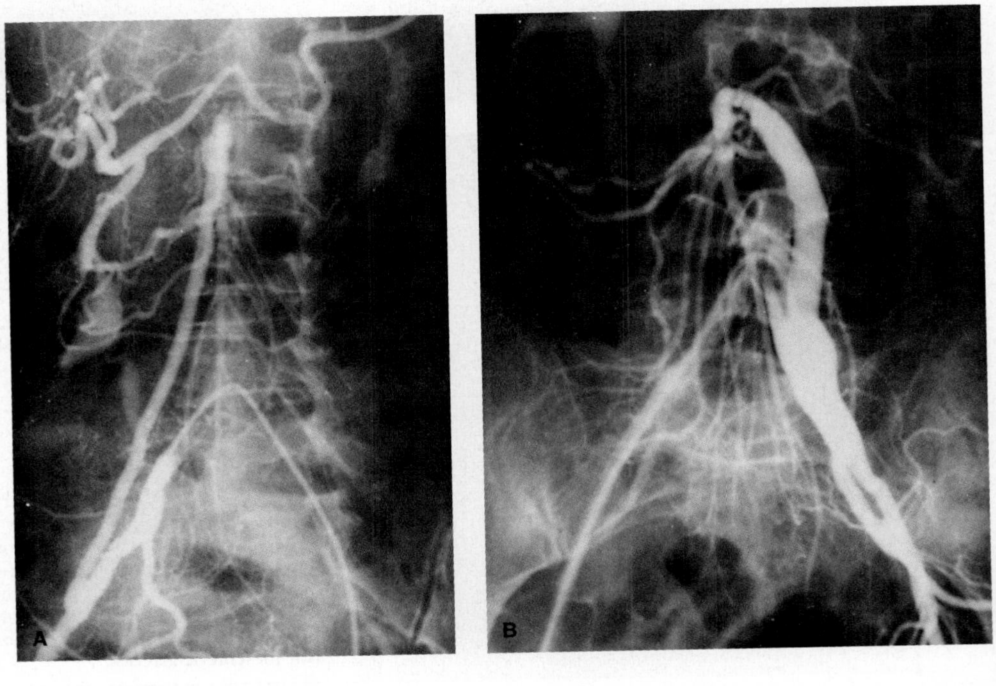

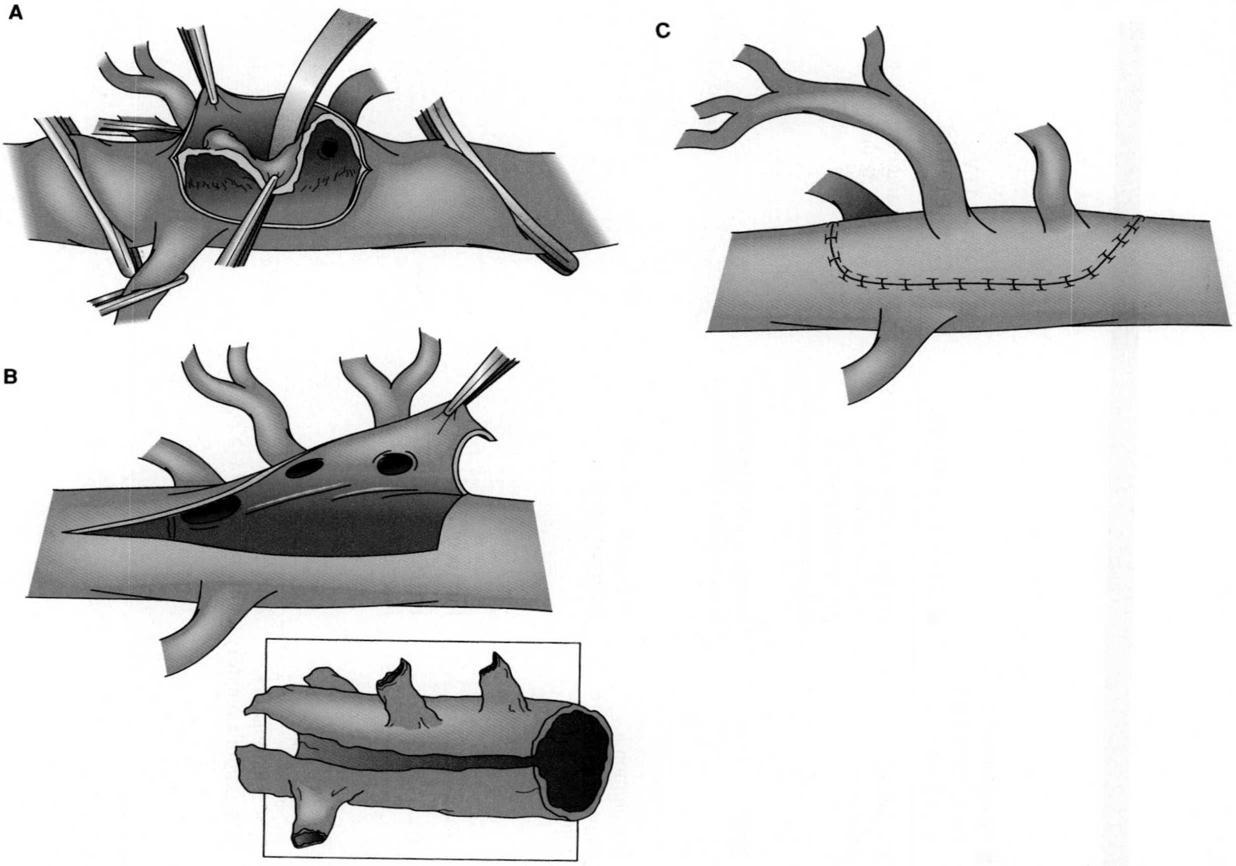

FIGURE 93.14. Endarterectomy of the celiac and superior mesenteric arteries is performed through a longitudinal trapdoor aortotomy. (Adapted from Wylie EJ. *Manual of Vascular Surgery*, vol 1. New York: Springer-Verlag; 1980:216–217.)

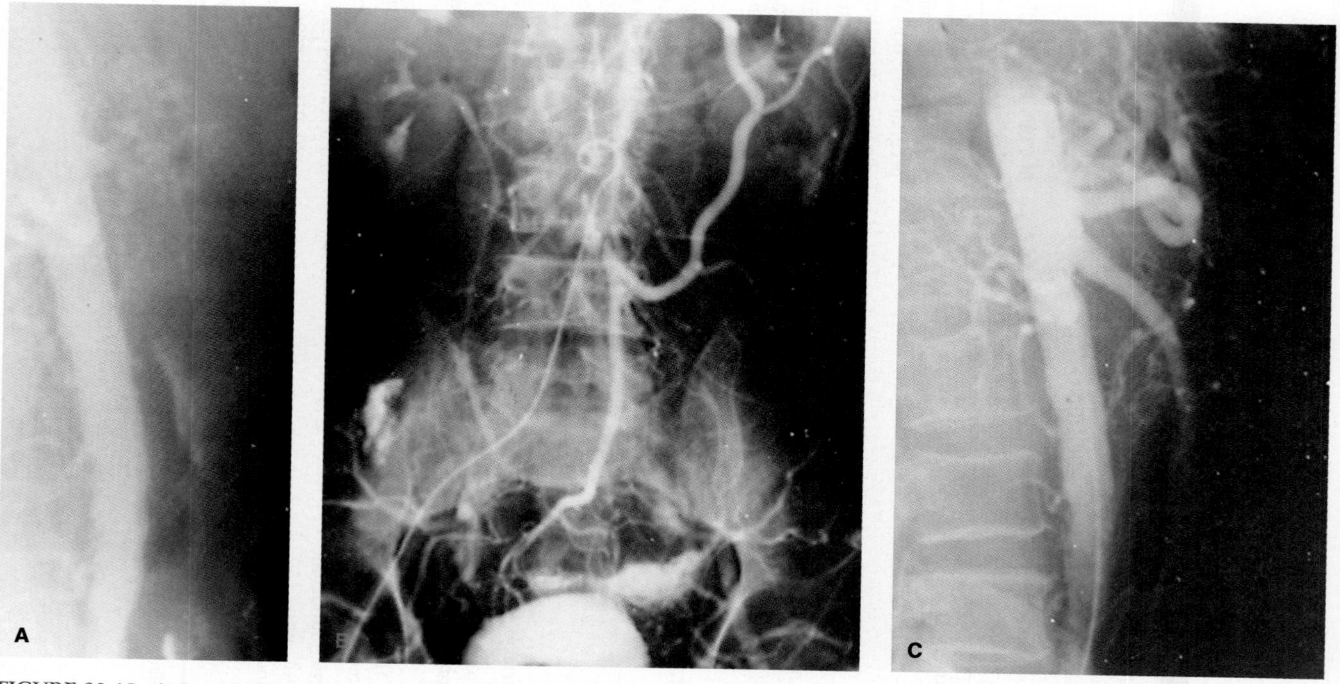

FIGURE 93.15. **A:** Preoperative lateral aortogram demonstrates total occlusion of the celiac and superior mesenteric arteries. **B:** Anteroposterior view with selective injection demonstrates large inferior-to-superior mesenteric artery collateral flow. **C:** Postoperative angiography demonstrates widely patent celiac and superior mesenteric arteries after transaortic endarterectomy.

TABLE 93.3

SPLANCHNIC ARTERY MACROANEURYSMS

ANEURYSM LOCATION	FREQUENCY WITHIN SPLANCHNIC CIRCULATION	M:F RATIO	CONTRIBUTING FACTORS	FREQUENCY OF REPORTED RUPTURE (%)	SITE OF RUPTURE	MORTALITY WITH RUPTURE
Splenic artery	60%	1:4	Medial degeneration; arterial fibrodysplasia; multiple pregnancies; portal hypertension; chronic pancreatitis with arterial erosion by pseudocysts	2% (bland aneurysms)	Intraperitoneal within lesser sac; intragastric with pancreatitis-related inflammatory aneurysms	25% bland and unassociated with pregnancy; during pregnancy 70% maternal, 75% fetal
Hepatic artery	20%	2:1	Medial degeneration; blunt and penetrating liver trauma; infection related to intravenous substance abuse	20%	Intraperitoneal and biliary tract with equal frequency	35%
Superior mesenteric artery	5.5%	1:1	Infection related to bacterial endocarditis, often associated with nonhemolytic streptococci and more recently with intravenous substance abuse; medial degeneration	Uncommon (thrombosis more common)	Intraperitoneal and retroperitoneal	50%
Celiac artery	4%	1:1	Medial degeneration	13%	Intraperitoneal	50%
Gastric and gastroepiploic arteries	4%	3:1	Periarterial inflammation; medial degeneration	90%	Intraperitoneal (30%), intestinal tract (70%)	70%
Jejunal, ileal, and colic arteries	3%	1:1	Medial degeneration; connective tissue diseases	30%		
Pancreaticoduodenal, pancreatic, and gastroduodenal arteries	2%	4:1	Pancreatitis-related arterial necrosis and arterial erosion by pseudocysts (60% of gastroduodenal, 30% of pancreaticoduodenal artery aneurysms); medial degeneration	75% inflammatory, 50% noninflammatory	Intestinal tract (85%); intraperitoneal (15%)	50%

M:F, male to female.

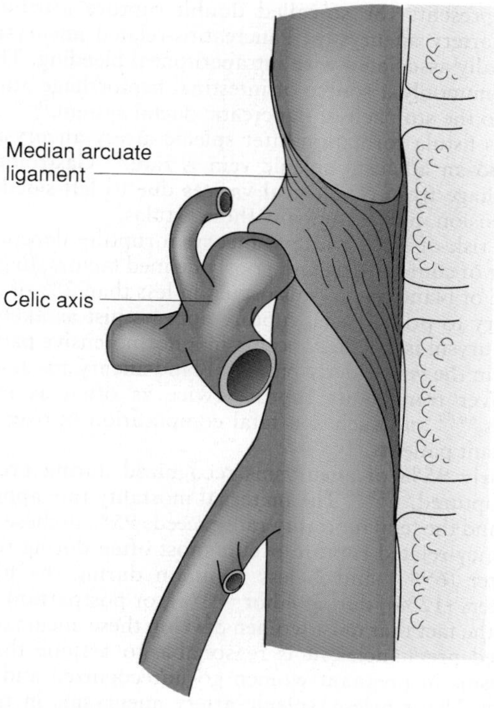

FIGURE 93.16. The median arcuate ligament syndrome is controversial. The anatomic fibrous tissue within the crura of the diaphragm is extraordinarily strong and may significantly narrow the celiac axis.

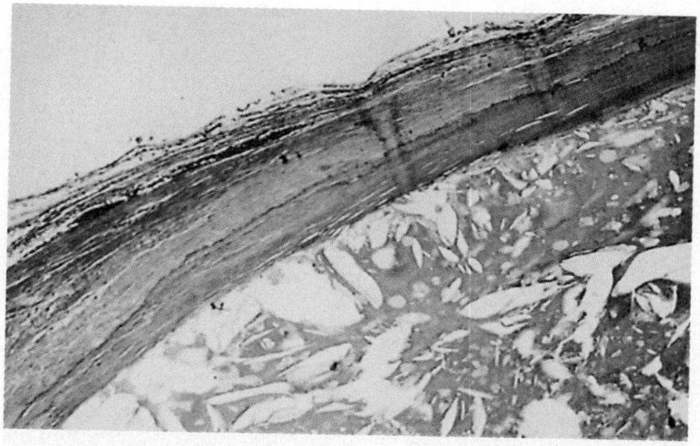

FIGURE 93.17. Splenic artery aneurysm exhibiting marked fibrosis cholesterol clefts and with calcific arteriosclerosis (hematoxylin–eosin, decalcified, ×32).

nearly 3,600 consecutive patients undergoing abdominal arteriographic studies for reasons other than suspected aneurysmal disease.[62] Women are four times more likely than men to develop splenic artery aneurysms.

The predilection for these aneurysms to affect the splenic artery reflects a peculiar group of associated disorders having an effect on the vasculature. Three distinct factors may contribute to the development of splenic artery aneurysms, including two that account for their unusual female predilection. The first factor is medial fibrodysplasia, which usually occurs in women and is most often manifested by renal artery stenosis and secondary hypertension. Approximately 2% of patients with renal artery fibrodysplasia have splenic artery aneurysms, and all of these patients have been women.[62] Systemic hypertension may contribute to aneurysm expansion in these patients. The second factor relates to the vascular consequences of pregnancy, with its known increase in splenic blood flow and reproductive hormone–related changes in elastic tissue. This factor becomes a particular problem with repeated pregnancies. Approximately 40% of women harboring these lesions have completed six or more pregnancies.[62,63] The third factor is evident in the nearly 10% of patients with portal hypertension and splenomegaly who develop splenic artery aneurysms.[62,64,65] In these cases, the vessel wall integrity may be compromised by increased splenic blood flow[66,67] and excessive estrogen activity occurring as a consequence of the underlying cirrhosis. Although splenic artery aneurysms have been described with regularity among patients after orthotopic liver transplantation,[68–71] it is speculative as to whether these represent preexisting aneurysms associated with portal hypertension or have arisen as a consequence of the transplant and attendant drug therapy, such as steroids.[68] Aneurysms in the latter patients are more likely to affect women and appear directly related to the severity of the preexisting portal hypertension.[70] Rare splenic artery aneurysms appear associated with developmental anomalies of the foregut arterial circulation.[72,73]

Certain splenic artery aneurysms exhibit extensive arteriosclerosis (Fig. 93.17). The fact that calcific arteriosclerotic changes appear limited to the aneurysm and not the intervening artery suggests that this is more likely a secondary event, rather than a primary etiologic process. Arterial disruptions caused by periarterial inflammatory disease, such as chronic pancreatitis, or penetrating trauma are less common causes of these aneurysms. Microaneurysms of smaller intraparenchymal splenic arteries are usually caused by a systemic vasculitis, such as polyarteritis nodosa, and appear to be of less clinical importance as a vascular disease than extraparenchymal aneurysms attributed to other causes.

Most aneurysms involving the distal splenic artery are saccular and occur at branchings. At such sites, discontinuities exist in the internal elastic lamina of normal vessels, and any subsequent degenerative events involving elastic tissue, as might occur with arterial fibrodysplasia or pregnancy, are likely to produce aneurysmal changes (Fig. 93.18). Such aneurysms are multiple 20% of the time, in contrast to those in patients undergoing liver transplantation for cirrhosis-related portal hypertension where multiple aneurysms occur in 90% of patients. Proximal aneurysms of the main splenic artery are usually solitary and are frequently associated with arterial erosions by pancreatitis-related pseudocysts (Fig. 93.19).

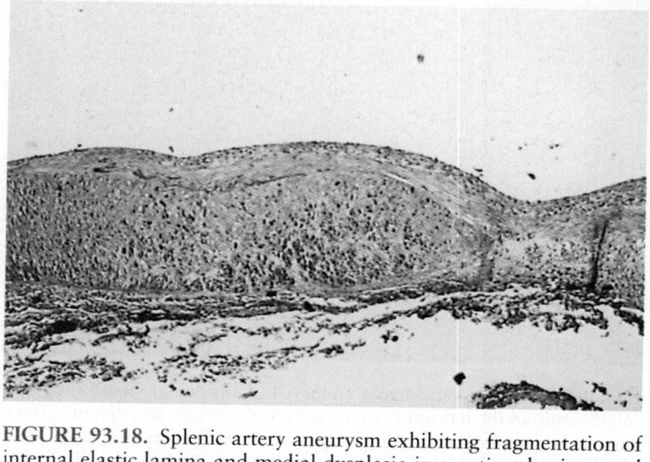

FIGURE 93.18. Splenic artery aneurysm exhibiting fragmentation of internal elastic lamina and medial dysplasia in a patient having renal arterial fibrodysplasia (Masson stain, ×32).

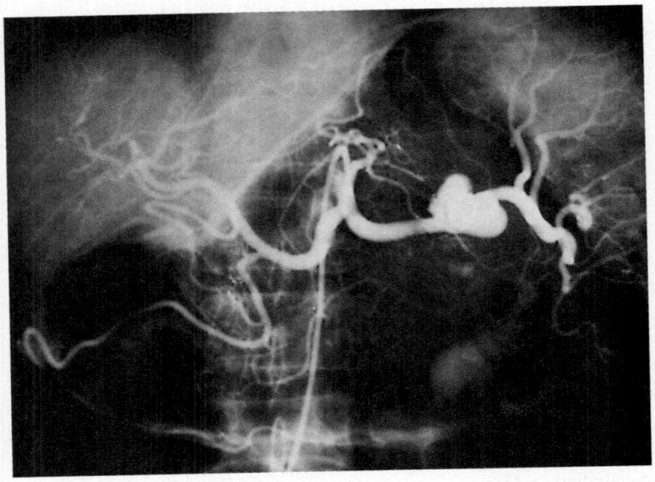

FIGURE 93.19. Splenic artery aneurysm. Arteriogram documents a pancreatitis-related aneurysm affecting the mid-splenic artery. (Stanley JC, Frey CF, Miller TA, et al. Major arterial hemorrhage: a complication of pancreatic pseudocysts and chronic pancreatitis. *Arch Surg*. 1976;111:435–440, with permission.)

Vascular calcifications on plain abdominal radiographs may be the first clinical evidence of a splenic artery aneurysm. The most characteristic of these findings are signet-ring calcifications (Fig. 93.20). However, contemporary diagnoses of splenic artery aneurysms usually follow their arteriographic demonstration during studies for nonvascular diseases. Color flow Doppler ultrasonography, CT, and MRI often establish the presence of these lesions and are often useful in identifying bleeding aneurysms.[74,75] These studies are also useful in following asymptomatic splenic artery aneurysms.

Left upper quadrant or epigastric pain may occur in patients with an intact splenic artery aneurysm. In a recent review, nearly half the patients with these aneurysms complained of abdominal pain.[58] However, the literature tends to include more spectacular cases and most bland aneurysms are likely to be asymptomatic.

In cases of splenic artery aneurysm rupture, bleeding is usually initially contained within the lesser sac, with later hemorrhage into the peritoneal cavity, and causes vascular collapse.

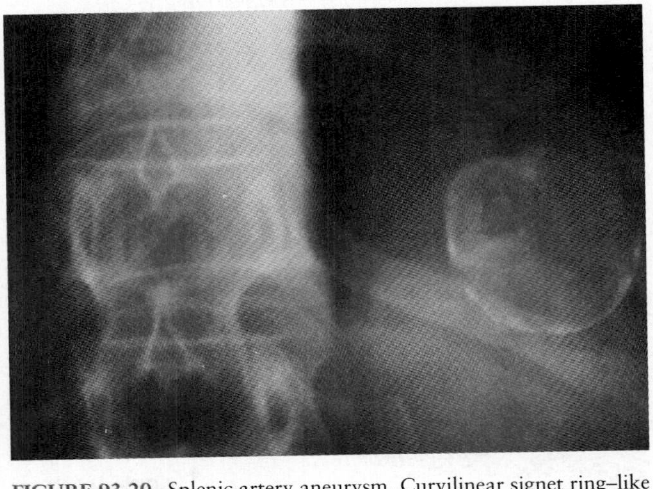

FIGURE 93.20. Splenic artery aneurysm. Curvilinear signet ring–like calcification in the left upper quadrant characteristic of a splenic artery aneurysm. (Reproduced with permission from Stanley JC, Thompson NW, Fry WJ. Splanchnic artery aneurysms. *Arch Surg* 1970;101: 689–697.)

This represents the so-called double-rupture attributed to splenic artery aneurysms. Pancreatitis-related aneurysms are not usually associated with intraperitoneal bleeding. They are more commonly a source of intestinal hemorrhage after rupture into the stomach or pancreatic ductal system.[76–80] Arteriovenous fistula formation after splenic artery aneurysm rupture into an adjacent splenic vein is rare.[81] Gastrointestinal hemorrhage from esophageal varices due to left-sided portal hypertension may accompany these fistulas.

The risk of splenic artery aneurysm rupture depends on a number of confounding and poorly defined factors. In general, rupture of bland aneurysms occurs in less than 2% of cases.[62] Contrary to prior tenets, rupture appears just as likely when the aneurysm is calcified, occurs in a normotensive patient, or occurs in the very elderly patient. Bland aneurysms associated with liver transplants rupture twice as often as in other patients,[68,69] and such is a fatal complication in over half of transplant patients.[82]

Nearly 95% of aneurysms recognized during pregnancy have ruptured.[62,83–86] The maternal mortality rate approaches 75%, and the fetal mortality rate exceeds 95% in these cases.[87] Pregnancy-related rupture occurs most often during the third trimester (69%) and is less common during the first two trimesters (12%), during labor (13%), or postpartum (6%).[85] Given the fact that most women develop these aneurysms with repeated pregnancies, it is reasonable to assume that most aneurysms in pregnant women go unrecognized and do not rupture. Nevertheless, splenic artery aneurysms in pregnant patients must be considered a threat to the life of the mother and fetus.

The reported mortality rate accompanying an open operation for rupture of a bland splenic artery aneurysm unassociated with pregnancy is 25%.[63] Thus, it would seem ill advised to undertake elective operative intervention for an asymptomatic splenic artery aneurysm if the surgical mortality rate exceeds 0.5%. This latter figure represents the product of the predicted 2% rupture rate of bland aneurysms and the known 25% risk of operative death when treating a patient following aneurysmal rupture. If intervention becomes necessary in higher-risk patients, then percutaneous transcatheter embolization of the aneurysm may represent a more appropriate therapy.

Splenectomy has been the most common form of open surgical therapy for splenic artery aneurysms in the past. However, because of the immunologic importance of the spleen even in the aged, simple ligature obliteration or excision of these aneurysms appears preferable to splenectomy.[88] Laparoscopic ligation of these aneurysms in certain instances may prove quite feasible.[89,90] Treatment of splenic artery aneurysms embedded in pancreatic tissue, especially those associated with pancreatitis, may require distal pancreatectomy.[91] In some of these cases, especially false aneurysms caused by pseudocyst erosion into the artery, treatment may entail incising the aneurysmal sac and ligating entering and exiting vessels from within. Pancreatic resection or cyst drainage in these latter cases must be individualized and depends on the extent and chronicity of the associated pancreatic inflammatory disease.

Percutaneous transcatheter embolization of splenic artery aneurysms (Fig. 93.21) often is preferred over an open operative intervention.[92–95] However, careful follow-up of endovascular-treated patients is mandatory. Splenic infarction, splenic abscess formation, and late rupture are legitimate concerns after splenic artery coil embolization. Further concerns center around issues such as transient obliteration of the aneurysm or coil migration and erosion into the adjacent viscera.[96,97] For example, coil migration into the stomach after splenic artery aneurysm treatment has been decribed.[96] Patients with multiple splenic artery aneurysms, especially near the hilum of the spleen, appear to be at particular risk for major complications.[98] Stent graft exclusion of an aneurysm with maintenance of splenic artery flow has been used in select cases,[99–101] but

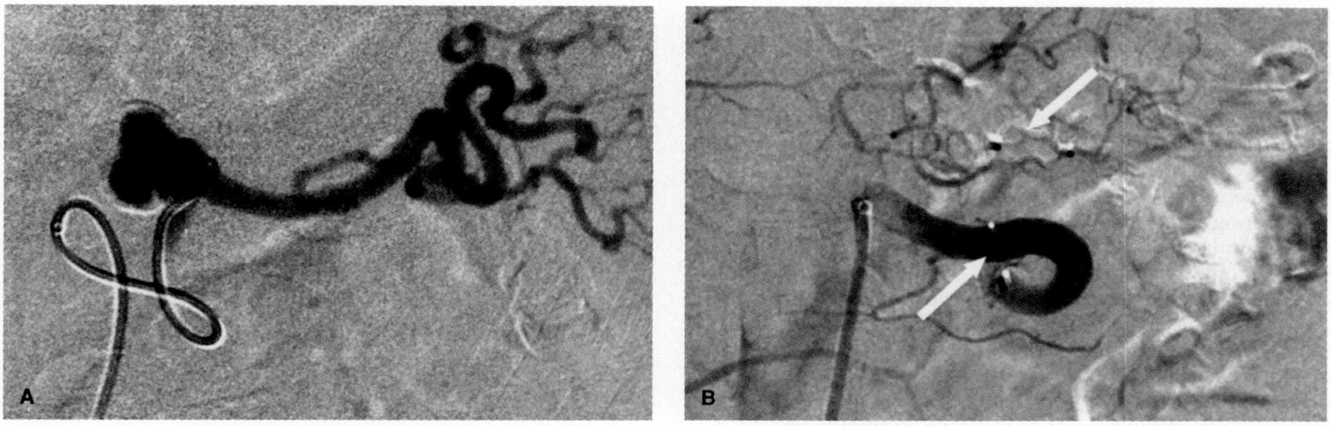

FIGURE 93.21. **A:** A 3.5 cm saccular splenic artery aneurysm on selective mesenteric angiogram. **B:** Completion splenic artery angiogram after embolization of the splenic artery. Vascular plugs (*white arrows*) in the splenic artery proximal and distal to the aneurysm.

can be particularly challenging and can result in dissection or thrombosis of the splenic artery from placement of the large-diameter catheters currently required for stent graft delivery into the tortuous artery or from apposition of the posterior wall of the artery to the relatively stiff stent lumen occluding the lumen of the stent graft ("T-bar" phenomenon).

Hepatic Artery Aneurysm

Hepatic artery aneurysms account for 20% of all previously reported splanchnic artery aneurysms (Fig. 93.22). These aneurysms are being encountered more frequently in contemporary times, and in some series outnumber splenic artery aneurysms.[58,102] Men have been twice as likely to be affected as women in the past, although gender differences are not as apparent in recent experiences.[58,103] Hepatic artery macroaneurysms are usually solitary. Large aneurysms tend to be saccular, and aneurysms less than 2 cm are usually fusiform. These aneurysms are extrahepatic in nearly 80% of cases and intrahepatic in 20%. More than one third of patients with hepatic artery aneurysms have other splanchnic aneurysms.[104]

Most noninfectious and nontraumatic hepatic artery aneurysms are usually recognized after the sixth decade of life.

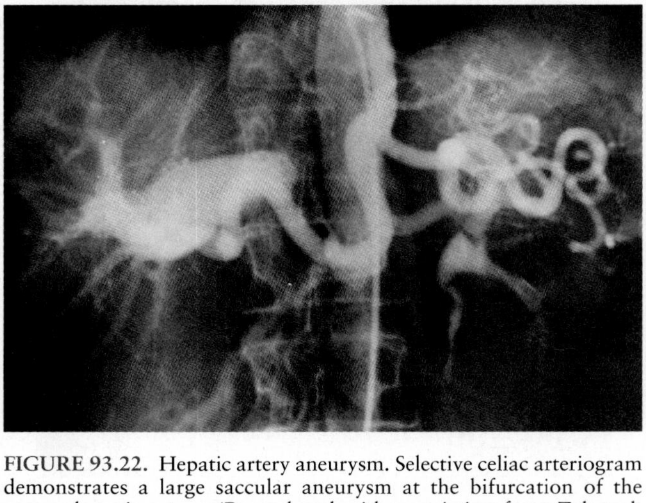

FIGURE 93.22. Hepatic artery aneurysm. Selective celiac arteriogram demonstrates a large saccular aneurysm at the bifurcation of the proper hepatic artery. (Reproduced with permission from Zelenock GB, Stanley JC. Splanchnic artery aneurysms. In: Rutherford RB, ed. *Vascular Surgery*. Philadelphia, PA: WB Saunders; 2000:1369.)

The cause of many hepatic artery aneurysms is poorly defined. Two facts regarding the cause of these aneurysms are noteworthy. First, arteriosclerosis most likely represents a secondary event rather than a primary cause of these aneurysms. Most of these lesions probably occur as a result of medial degeneration. Second, with increasing societal violence and intravenous substance abuse, the number of reported traumatic and infection-related aneurysms has markedly increased[58] (Fig. 93.23). Another common cause of intrahepatic pseudoaneurysms is arterial injury accompanying invasive percutaneous diagnostic and therapeutic procedures involving penetration of the liver.[105,106] Nearly 17% of these aneurysms encountered more recently have occurred in orthotopic liver

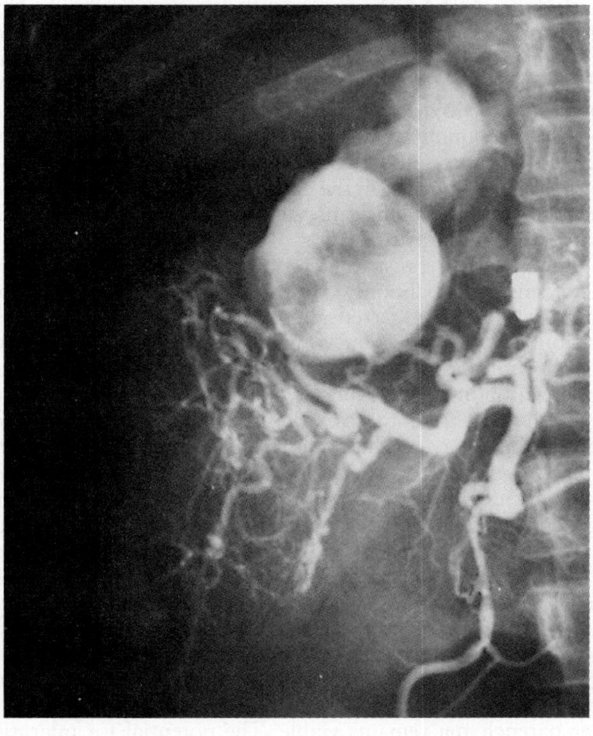

FIGURE 93.23. Traumatic hepatic artery aneurysm. Blunt abdominal injury and gunshot wounds cause most traumatic lesions. (Reproduced with permission from Whitehouse WM Jr, Graham LM, Stanley JC. Aneurysms of the celiac, hepatic, and splenic arteries. In: Bergan JJ, Yao JST, eds. *Aneurysms: Diagnosis and Treatment*. New York: Grune & Stratton; 1981:405.)

transplant patients.[58] Systemic arteriopathies, such as periarteritis nodosa, have been incriminated as a cause of occasional macroaneurysms, but are more often associated with intraparenchymal microaneurysms.[107]

Hepatic artery aneurysms may be suspected because of displacement of or indentations on intestinal structures noted on barium contrast studies. Most contemporary diagnoses of these aneurysms result from their incidental recognition during arteriography, CT, or ultrasonography for nonvascular disease. Few hepatic artery aneurysms are symptomatic. When they become symptomatic, most present with right upper quadrant or epigastric pain. Rapid expansion of these aneurysms may cause severe discomfort similar to that of acute pancreatitis. Large aneurysms have been reported to cause obstructive jaundice, although most hepatic artery aneurysms are too small to compress the major bile ducts. These lesions rarely present as pulsatile abdominal masses.

The reported incidence of hepatic artery aneurysm rupture approaches 20%, but the contemporary rate may be less. It is certainly less than the often-quoted rupture rate of 44% in cases reported a few decades ago.[63] Aneurysm rupture is associated with a 35% mortality rate, although in recent times the mortality appears less.[58] Bleeding from a ruptured hepatic artery aneurysm occurs with equal frequency into the biliary tract and peritoneal cavity. Hemobilia accompanies the former, being manifest by biliary colic, hematemesis, and jaundice.[108] Chronic, relatively asymptomatic hemorrhage is an uncommon sequela of aneurysm rupture into the biliary tract. Intraperitoneal bleeding is usually caused by rupture of inflammatory-related false aneurysms.

Common hepatic artery aneurysms are often treated by aneurysmectomy or aneurysm exclusion, without arterial reconstruction. The extensive hepatic arterial collateral circulation and parallel portal venous circulation often ensure adequate blood flow to the liver with interruption of the proximal common hepatic artery. Liver necrosis is more likely to follow ligation of arteries in the more distal hepatic circulation. Nevertheless, even in the latter vessels, complex arterial reconstructions should be avoided and simple ligation undertaken if temporary intraoperative occlusion of the involved artery does not result in obvious hepatic ischemia. If liver blood flow appears inadequate with such a maneuver, then hepatic artery reconstruction should be undertaken using either prosthetic or autologous vein grafts. In the case of rapidly bleeding ruptured intraparenchymal aneurysms, hepatic territory resection may be necessary therapy.

Percutaneous transcatheter obliteration of hepatic artery aneurysms with balloons, coils, or thrombogenic particulate matter is often a preferred alternative to open surgical intervention.[58,92,106,109,110] One must realize that transcatheter embolization may be only transiently successful, and repeated embolization or surgical therapy may subsequently be required to adequately treat these patients.[94,109] Hepatic artery coil embolization may be the preferred treatment for small intrahepatic pseudoaneurysms, especially in those patients with malignancies.[111] The reported 42% recanalization rate following hepatic artery embolic occlusion is noteworthy and mandates thoughtful postembolization follow-up. Stent graft repair of hepatic artery aneurysms has been described in the literature.[111,112] In the author's limited experience, stent grafts placed in the hepatic artery for treatment of aneurysm cause slowly progressive stenosis of the hepatic artery and the artery eventually occludes. In a small number of cases sufficient hepatic collaterals to the liver develop by the time of occlusion and the liver parenchyma remains viable. The potential for migration of embolic material or stent graft occlusion with central lobular necrosis and abscess formation is also a recognized complication of transcatheter treatment of these aneurysms. Percutaneous thrombin injection of a hepatic artery pseudoaneurysm has been reported in a liver transplant patient following repair of a perforated duodenum in the setting of bile peritonitis.[113] Transcatheter thrombin injection, coil embolization, and endograft exclusion of select aneurysms may prove useful in carefully chosen patients.[113–115]

Superior Mesenteric Artery Aneurysm

Aneurysms of the proximal SMA account for 5.5% of all splanchnic artery aneurysms. These lesions affect men twice as often as women. Infection from a cardiac source has been a common cause of these aneurysms in the past,[63,115] but are less common in recent times.[116] Nonhemolytic streptococci, as well as many common pathogens accompanying parenteral substance abuse, cause bacterial endocarditis and are the underlying source of infection in most cases. Many of these aneurysms are associated with intramural dissections (Fig. 93.24).[117] SMA aneurysms may also be caused by medial degeneration, periarterial inflammation, and trauma. Arteriosclerosis, as in the case of other splanchnic aneurysms, is usually a secondary process. SMA aneurysms are often recognized during arteriographic studies for nonvascular disease (Fig. 93.25).[59,116]

Although many patients with SMA aneurysms are asymptomatic, the majority of patients have abdominal discomfort, often suggestive of intestinal angina. SMA aneurysm rupture is not common, and in the past was considered rare.[116,117] The mortality rate with rupture approaches 50%.[118] Gastrointestinal hemorrhage associated with these aneurysms often accompanies their acute occlusion with bleeding into areas of intestinal infarction. Location of most aneurysms near the origins of the inferior pancreaticoduodenal and middle colic arteries isolates the distal mesenteric circulation when dissections or occlusions occur. In these circumstances, intestinal ischemia develops because the usual collateral network from the adjacent celiac and inferior mesenteric arterial circulations is obstructed.

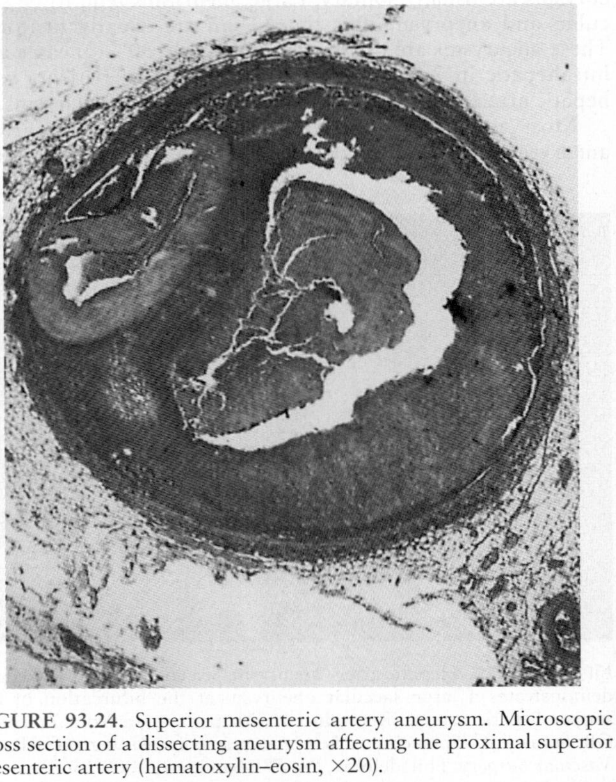

FIGURE 93.24. Superior mesenteric artery aneurysm. Microscopic cross section of a dissecting aneurysm affecting the proximal superior mesenteric artery (hematoxylin–eosin, ×20).

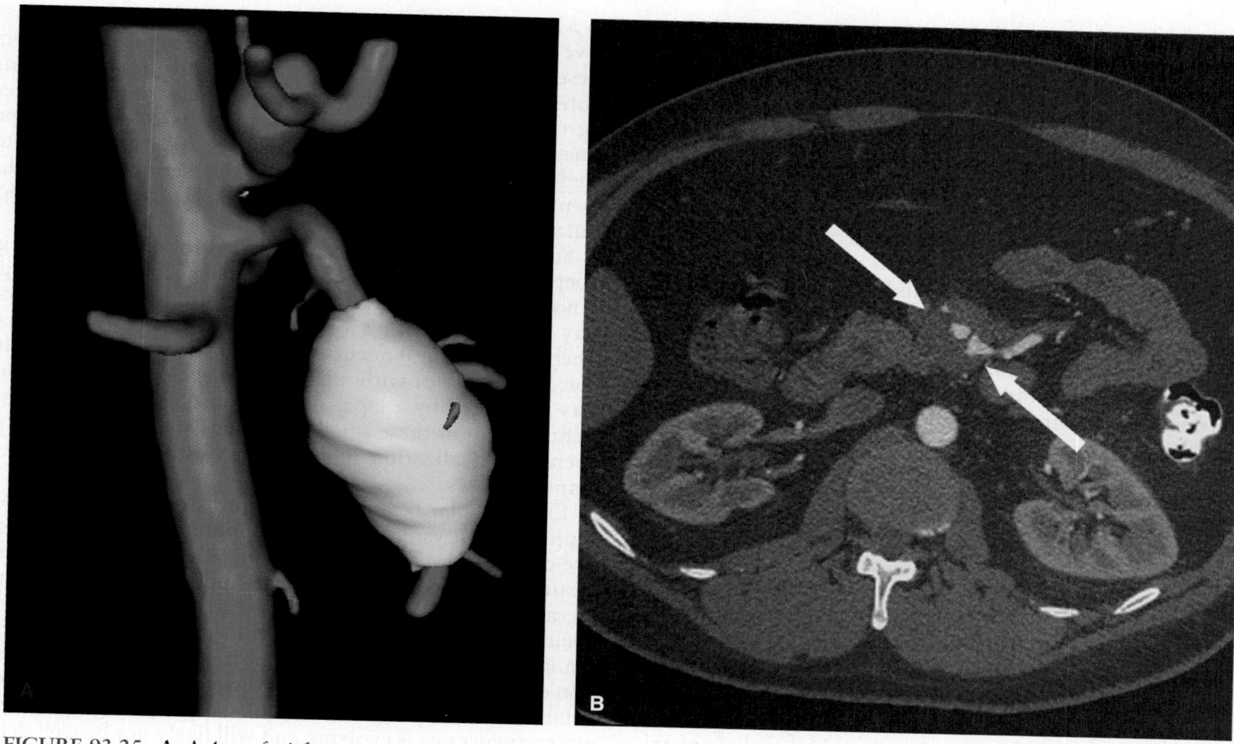

FIGURE 93.25. **A:** A 4-cm fusiform aneurysm of the superior mesenteric artery on three-dimensional computed tomographic angiographic imaging. There is an incidental finding of a 1.5 cm celiac artery aneurysm as well. **B:** Cross-sectional imaging of the same superior mesenteric aneurysm (between white *arrows*).

Operative management of SMA aneurysms is best accomplished by aneurysmectomy or aneurysm exclusion, followed by intestinal revascularization if needed with an aortomesenteric graft. Because of potential infection when bowel ischemia is present, autologous vein or artery is favored over prosthetic conduits for these reconstructions. SMA aneurysm ligation without arterial reconstruction may be successful in patients who have developed an adequate collateral circulation to their midgut. In fact, ligation and aneurysmorrhaphy have been the most commonly reported means of managing these aneurysms.[114,119–121] Temporary intraoperative occlusion of the SMA with Doppler documentation of adequate intestinal blood flow should be undertaken before proceeding with SMA ligation.

Endovascular stent graft placement for select SMA aneurysms has appeal,[122,123] although infection and thrombosis may compromise this type of treatment. Obliteration of these aneurysms by coils or direct thrombin injection may be preferred in high-risk patients having discrete aneurysm necks and adequate collateral circulation to the distal SMA.[116,124]

Celiac Artery Aneurysm

Celiac artery aneurysms account for 4% of all splanchnic artery aneurysms. Men and women appear equally affected. Those aneurysms encountered before 1950 were usually infectious in etiology, but in contemporary times have been associated with medial degeneration.[125,126] Arteriosclerosis is a common histologic finding that is considered a secondary event rather than an etiologic process. Other splanchnic artery aneurysms affect nearly 40% of these patients. Celiac artery aneurysms are usually saccular, and most are located in the distal vessel (Fig. 93.26).

Most celiac artery aneurysms are asymptomatic or appear to be associated with vague abdominal discomfort.[58,59] These aneurysms are usually recognized during ultrasonography, angiography, or other imaging studies for nonvascular diseases. In more recent times, rupture has affected 13% of these aneurysms and carried a mortality rate of 50%.[125] In contrast, rupture rates published before 1950 were often higher than 80%. Rupture usually causes exsanguinating intraperitoneal hemorrhage. Although rare, gastrointestinal bleeding may follow rupture of the aneurysm into the stomach or pancreatic ductal system.

Aneurysmectomy with celiac artery reconstruction is the preferred treatment for these lesions, although aneurysm exclusion with ligation of its branches has been performed successfully in select patients.[125–128] When simple ligature is

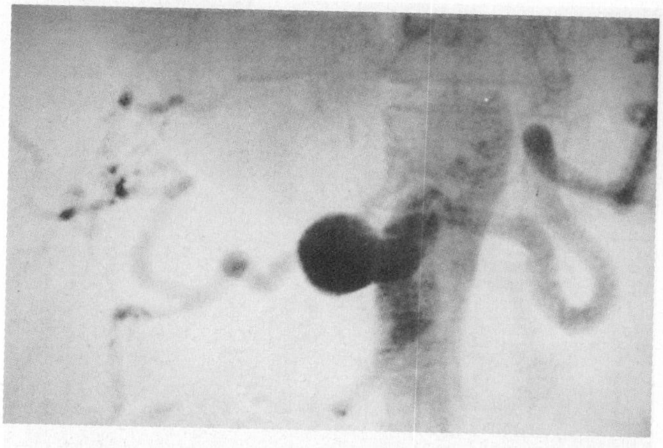

FIGURE 93.26. Celiac artery aneurysm. Aortogram reveals saccular aneurysm that exhibited medial degenerative changes and secondary arteriosclerosis. (Reproduced with permission from Stanley JC, Whitehouse WM Jr. Aneurysms of the splanchnic and renal arteries. In: Bergan JJ, Yao JST, eds. *Surgery of the Aorta and Its Body Branches*. Orlando, FL: Grune & Stratton; 1979:497.)

undertaken, the adequacy of the liver's collateral circulation must be documented. If liver ischemia is apparent after temporary intraoperative celiac artery occlusion, then hepatic revascularization becomes mandatory. An aortoceliac or aortohepatic artery bypass in these circumstances is best performed with either an autologous vein or prosthetic graft. Surgical therapy of celiac artery aneurysmal disease has been successful in more than 90% of cases.

Endovascular obliteration of a celiac artery aneurysm is not often considered because of the need to occlude the hepatic, splenic, and left gastric arteries, and perhaps the inferior phrenic arteries, in order to isolate the aneurysms. Nevertheless, in select cases catheter-based therapy may be successful.[129] Embolic occlusion of the celiac trunk with glue and treatment with coil embolization and stent graft placement have been described in the literature as viable techniques for endovascular management of celiac artery aneurysms.[111,129–131] One report describes celiac artery occlusion in a variety of aneurysms including thoracoabdominal aortic aneurysms and dissections, as well as celiac artery aneurysms. The authors report treatment of three true aneurysms of the celiac artery with coil embolization of the celiac branch vessels in two cases and of the celiac artery alone in one. There were no treatment-related complications in any case, but care was taken to ensure that collateralization to the proper hepatic artery remained intact after celiac artery or branch embolization. Normal liver function was considered a prerequisite for embolic treatment of these aneurysms.[130] Successful treatment of a large (10-cm) saccular celiac artery pseudoaneurysm in a high-risk surgical patient by exclusion of the celiac artery with an aortic stent graft has also been described.[131]

Gastric and Gastroepiploic Artery Aneurysms

Gastric and gastroepiploic artery aneurysms account for 4% of all splanchnic artery aneurysms (Fig. 93.27). Gastric artery aneurysms occur 10 times more often than gastroepiploic artery aneurysms. Men are three times more likely than women to develop these aneurysms. Most of these perigastric lesions have been encountered in patients older than 50 years of age. These aneurysms usually are solitary, occurring as a result of periarterial inflammation or medial degeneration. In many cases, there is an antecedent history of peptic ulcer disease. Arteriosclerosis, when present, is considered a secondary event, not a cause of these lesions.

Most reported gastric or gastroepiploic artery aneurysms have been symptomatic when initially recognized, frequently presenting as emergencies.[132–134] Rupture has accompanied more than 90% of reported cases, with gastrointestinal bleeding occurring slightly more than twice as often as intraperitoneal hemorrhage. Rupture carries a 70% mortality rate.[63] These figures may overestimate the seriousness of these aneurysms, with reported cases often spectacular and unrepresentative of the usual case.

Surgical treatment is recommended for all gastric and gastroepiploic artery aneurysms.[8] Vascular reconstructive surgery is not required in these cases. Intramural gastric aneurysms may be excised with a small segment of involved stomach, whereas extramural aneurysms can be treated by arterial ligation alone, with or without aneurysm excision. Certain lesions may be treated by a laparoscopic approach.[135] Intraoperative identification of these small aneurysms is often tedious if preoperative localization has not been established by arteriographic studies.

Endovascular occlusion of life-threatening bleeding from a ruptured aneurysm may be appropriate as a prelude to definitive open surgical aneurysmectomy or as potentially definitive treatment in select cases. There are multiple case reports in the literature describing catheter-based treatment of gastric artery aneurysms including treatment with embolization,[53,136] thrombin injection,[137] and even stent graft placement with preservation of arterial flow through the vessel.[138] The role of endovascular techniques in treatment of gastric and gastroepiploic artery aneurysms is evolving and will likely not be well defined in the near future due to the infrequent occurrence of these aneurysms.

Jejunal, Ileal, and Colic Artery Aneurysms

Aneurysms of the jejunal, ileal, and colic arteries account for 3% of all splanchnic artery aneurysms (Fig. 93.28). They usually occur in patients older than 60 years of age. Men and women are affected equally. Multiple aneurysms have been encountered in 10% of cases. Acquired medial defects cause most of these lesions. Although arteriosclerosis is present with 20% of these aneurysms, it is considered to represent a secondary event, not an etiologic process. An increasing number of mycotic aneurysms affect these vessels, developing as the

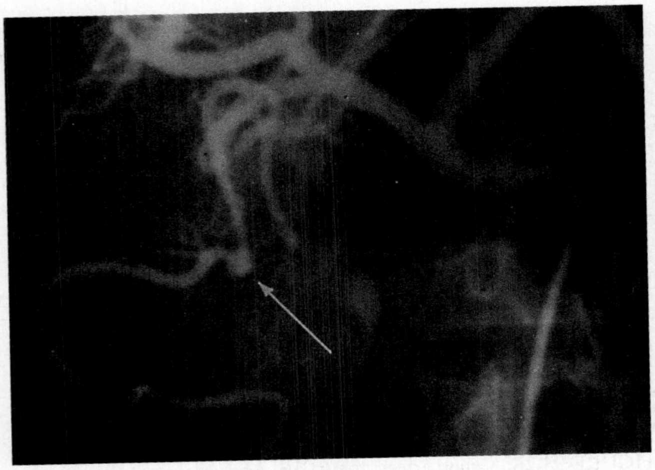

FIGURE 93.27. Gastroepiploic artery aneurysm. Selective celiac arteriogram revealing small aneurysm responsible for massive gastrointestinal hemorrhage. (Reproduced with permission from Stanley JC, Thompson NW, Fry WJ. Splanchnic artery aneurysms. *Arch Surg* 1970;101:689–697.)

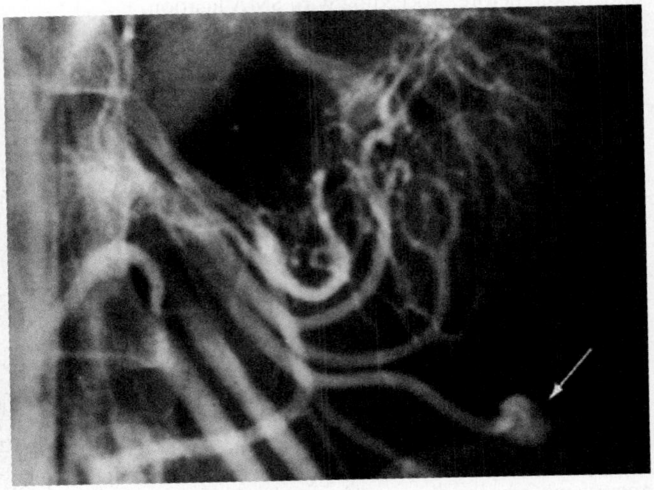

FIGURE 93.28. Ileal artery aneurysm. Mesenteric arteriogram documenting saccular aneurysm of distal ileal artery. (Reproduced with permission from Zelenock GB, Stanley JC. Splanchnic artery aneurysms. In: Rutherford RB, ed. *Vascular Surgery*. Philadelphia, PA: WB Saunders; 2000;1369.)

sequela of infected emboli originating from subacute bacterial endocarditis.[139] Periarteritis nodosa is also a common underlying cause of multiple aneurysms affecting these intestinal branch arteries.[140] Most aneurysms of these vessels have been reported to cause abdominal pain, yet many are first recognized as incidental findings during arteriography for gastrointestinal bleeding.[63,141] Jejunal, ileal, and colic artery aneurysms are reported to have ruptured in 30% of cases, but actual rupture rates are probably a third of that figure. Rupture is associated with a mortality rate of 20%. Aneurysmal rupture usually occurs into the gastrointestinal tract. Rupture into the mesentery or peritoneal cavity is uncommon.

Operation for intestinal branch aneurysms is recommended in all instances, except for bland aneurysms associated with connective tissue diseases. Expeditious surgical therapy requires careful preoperative localization with arteriographic studies. Arterial ligation, with or without aneurysmectomy, is recommended in treating extraintestinal lesions, whereas intramural aneurysms and those associated with bowel infarction require resection of the involved intestine. In select patients transcatheter embolization may be undertaken, although intestinal necrosis with perforation or late stricture formation is a recognized complication of such therapy.[142] Inferior mesenteric artery aneurysms represent a unique subset of these mesenteric aneurysms.[143,144] They are quite rare and their etiology so varied that the clinical importance of them has not been clearly established.

Endovascular treatment of this subset of visceral artery aneurysms is present but poorly described in the literature.[145,146] However, embolization of jejunal, ileal, and colic arterial vessels is certainly a well-described and accepted method of treatment in the setting of gastrointestinal bleeding and treatment of endoleaks after endovascular abdominal aortic aneurysm repair. Furthermore, given the difficulties associated with open surgical approaches in locating and surgically repairing these aneurysms, endovascular treatment of these aneurysms remains an attractive and increasingly utilized method of treatment.

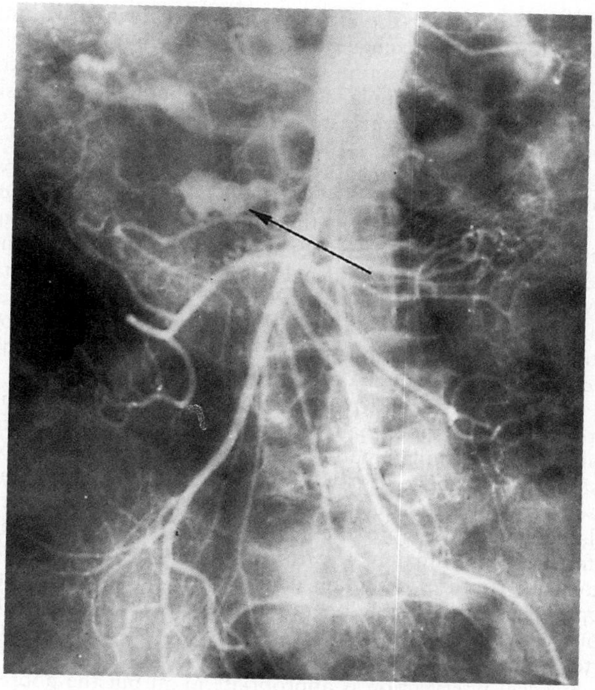

FIGURE 93.29. Inferior pancreaticoduodenal artery aneurysm. Selective superior mesenteric arteriogram revealing false aneurysm secondary to pseudocyst erosion of artery. (Reproduced with permission from Stanley JC, Frey CF, Miller TA, et al. Major arterial hemorrhage: a complication of pancreatic pseudocysts and chronic pancreatitis. *Arch Surg* 1976;111:435–440.)

Pancreaticoduodenal, Pancreatic, and Gastroduodenal Artery Aneurysms

Pancreatic and pancreaticoduodenal artery aneurysms (Fig. 93.29) account for 2% of all splanchnic artery aneurysms, and gastroduodenal artery aneurysms (Fig. 93.30) represent an additional 1.5% of these aneurysms. Men are four times more likely than women to develop these lesions. Most patients with these aneurysms are older than age 50 years. Most of these lesions are associated with pancreatitis-related vascular necrosis or vessel erosion by an adjacent pancreatic pseudocyst. Medial degeneration and trauma are less common causes of these aneurysms. Arteriosclerosis is invariably a secondary, not a causative, process. Many recently reported aneurysms have been associated with celiac artery stenoses or occlusions,

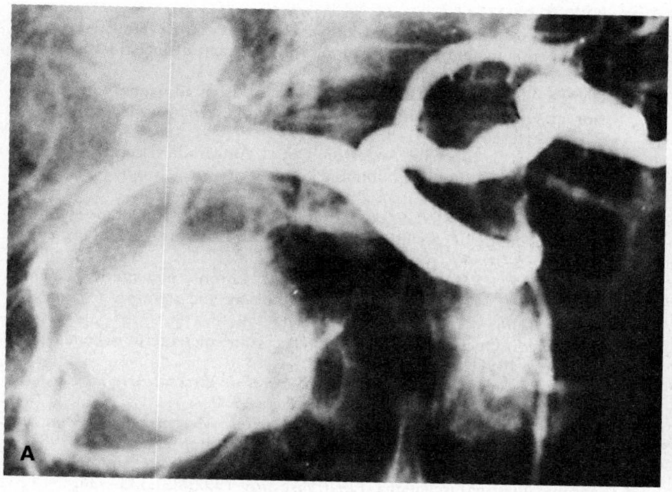

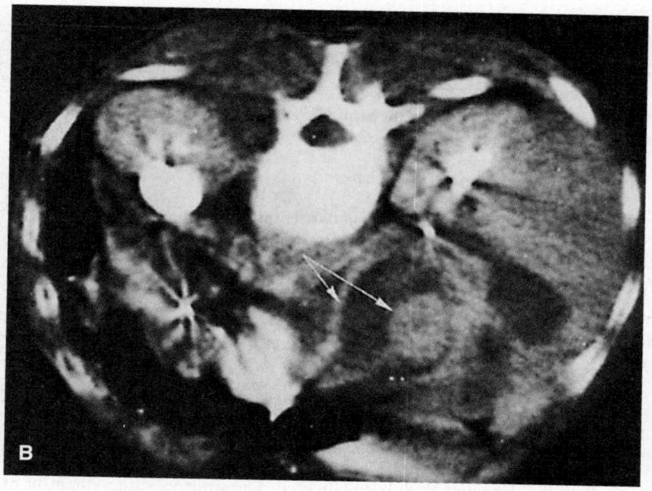

FIGURE 93.30. Gastroduodenal artery aneurysm. **A:** Selective celiac arteriogram. **B:** Computed tomography scan of a pancreatic pseudocyst (*short arrow*) containing the aneurysm (*long arrow*). (Reproduced with permission from Eckhauser FE, Stanley JC, Zelenock GB, et al. Gastroduodenal and pancreaticoduodenal artery aneurysms: a complication of pancreatitis causing spontaneous gastrointestinal hemorrhage. *Surgery* 1980;88:335–344.)

and likely represent the effect of inordinately high-volume blood flow on branchings of the collateral circulation,[147,148] where preexisting discontinuities of elastin are known to exist in normal arteries. A similar scenario contributing to aneurysm formation may exist in instances of an SMA occlusion or severe stenosis.[149]

Pancreatitis-related aneurysms are often difficult to diagnose and treat. Most are associated with epigastric pain and discomfort, which may be caused by the underlying pancreatic inflammatory disease that accompanies about 60% of gastroduodenal and 30% of pancreaticoduodenal artery aneurysms. Arteriography usually establishes the presence of these aneurysms, but CT scanning and MRI are of increasing importance in their recognition. These latter noninvasive studies are especially important in detecting rupture or associated pancreatic pathology.

Gastroduodenal and pancreaticoduodenal aneurysm rupture has affected more than 50% of the reported cases, occurring in 75% of inflammatory and 50% of noninflammatory lesions. Hemorrhage usually occurs into the stomach, biliary tract, or pancreatic ductal system. Bleeding of pancreatitis-related aneurysms into the peritoneal cavity is less likely, affecting approximately 15% of cases. The overall mortality rate with rupture, including pancreatitis-related aneurysms, approaches 25% despite operative intervention, but is nearly double that figure in the case of true pancreaticoduodenal artery aneurysms.

Surgical intervention is appropriate in all but the poorest-risk patients with gastroduodenal, pancreaticoduodenal, or pancreatic arterial aneurysms.[63,150–154] Pancreatitis-related false aneurysms are usually treated by arterial ligation from within the aneurysmal sac, rather than extra-aneurysmal arterial ligation. Extensive dissection of the pancreas affected by dense inflammatory adhesions in such circumstances is hazardous. In situations in which a pancreatic pseudocyst or abscess has eroded the artery, a drainage procedure should be undertaken. Distal pancreatectomy, or even pancreaticoduodenectomy, may be the safest mode of treatment in select cases.

9 Transcatheter embolization with coils[155] and glue[156] and electrocoagulation have an important role in treating very high-risk patients.[157–161] Thrombin injection may serve as another means of occluding small aneurysms.[162–165] Nevertheless, rebleeding and late aneurysmal rupture with these therapies can occur and restrict their universal use.[150,163,165] In select patients, however, endovascular occlusion of the bleeding aneurysm may be an appropriate lifesaving measure, followed by a later definitive open resection.

References

1. Ibukuro K, Tsukiyama T, Mori K, et al. The congenital anastomoses between hepatic arteries: angiographic appearance. *Surg Radiol Anat* 2000;22(1):41–45.
2. Reuter SR, Redman HC. *Gastrointestinal Angiography,* 2nd ed. Philadelphia, PA: WB Saunders; 1971.
3. Deitch EA. The role of intestinal barrier failure and bacterial translocation in the development of systemic infection and multiple organ failure. *Arch Surg* 1990;125(3):403–404.
4. Harward TR, Brooks DL, Flynn TC, et al. Multiple organ dysfunction after mesenteric artery revascularization. *J Vasc Surg* 1993;18(3):459–467; discussion 467–469.
5. Jamieson WG, DeRose G, Harris KA, et al. Myocardial and circulatory performance during the ischemic phase of superior mesenteric artery occlusion. *Can J Surg* 1993;36(5):435–439.
6. Paragger H, Staender S, Studer W, et al. Occlusive mesenteric ischemia and its effects on jejunal intramucosal pH, mesenteric oxygen consumption and oxygen tensions from surfaces of the jejunum in anesthetized pigs. *Intensive Care Med* 1997;23(1):91–99.
7. Park PO, Haglund U, Bulkley GB, et al. The sequence of development of intestinal tissue injury after strangulation ischemia and reperfusion. *Surgery* 1990;107(5):574–580.
8. Thompson JS, Bragg LE, West WW. Serum enzyme levels during intestinal ischemia. *Ann Surg* 1990;211(3):369–373.
9. Horton KM, Fishman EK. Multidetector CT angiography in the diagnosis of mesenteric ischemia. *Radiol Clin North Am* 2007;45(2):275–288.
10. Lim RP, Dowling RJ, Thomson KR. Angioplasty and stenting of the superior mesenteric artery in acute mesenteric ischaemia. *Australas Radiol* 2004;48(3):426–429.
11. VanDeinse WH, Zawacki JK, Phillips D. Treatment of acute mesenteric ischemia by percutaneous transluminal angioplasty. *Gastroenterology* 1986;91(2):475–478.
12. Gartenschlaeger S, Bender S, Maeurer J, et al. Successful percutaneous transluminal angioplasty and stenting in acute mesenteric ischemia. *Cardiovasc Intervent Radiol* 2008;31(2):398–400.
13. Landreneau RJ, Fry WJ. The right colon as a target organ of nonocclusive mesenteric ischemia. Case report and review of the literature. *Arch Surg* 1990;125(5):591–594.
14. Levy PJ, Krausz MM, Manny J. Acute mesenteric ischemia: improved results—a retrospective analysis of ninety-two patients. *Surgery* 1990; 107(4):372–380.
15. Mesh CL, Gewertz BL. The effect of hemodilution on blood flow regulation in normal and postischemic intestine. *J Surg Res* 1990;48(3):183–189.
16. Oshima A, Kitajima M, Sakai N, et al. Does glucagon improve the viability of ischemic intestine? *J Surg Res* 1990;49(6):524–533.
17. Kamimura K, Oosaki A, Sugahara S, et al. Survival of three nonocclusive mesenteric ischemia patients following early diagnosis by multidetector row computed tomography and prostaglandin E1 treatment. *Intern Med* 2008;47(22):2001–2006.
18. Zelenock GB, Strodel WE, Knol JA, et al. A prospective study of clinically and endoscopically documented colonic ischemia in 100 patients undergoing aortic reconstructive surgery with aggressive colonic and direct pelvic revascularization, compared with historic controls. *Surgery* 1989;106(4): 771–779; discussion 779–780.
19. Eliason JL, Wainess RM, Dimick JB, et al. The effect of secondary operations on mortality following abdominal aortic aneurysm repair in the United States: 1988–2001. *Vasc Endovascular Surg* 2005;39(6):465–472.
20. Rutherford RB, Taylor LM. Mesenteric Ischemia. *Semin Vasc Surg* 1990;3: 141.
21. Ballard JL, Stone WM, Hallett JW, et al. A critical analysis of adjuvant techniques used to assess bowel viability in acute mesenteric ischemia. *Am Surg* 1993;59(5):309–311.
22. Brolin RE, Semmlow JL, Sehonanda A, et al. Comparison of five methods of assessment of intestinal viability. *Surg Gynecol Obstet* 1989;168(1): 6–12.
23. Levy PJ, Krausz MM, Manny J. The role of second-look procedure in improving survival time for patients with mesenteric venous thrombosis. *Surg Gynecol Obstet* 1990;170(4):287–291.
24. Zelenock GB, Graham LM, Whitehouse WM Jr, et al. Splanchnic arteriosclerotic disease and intestinal angina. *Arch Surg* 1980;115(4): 497–501.
25. Burkart DJ, Johnson CD, Reading CC, et al. MR measurements of mesenteric venous flow: prospective evaluation in healthy volunteers and patients with suspected chronic mesenteric ischemia. *Radiology* 1995; 194(3):801–806.
26. Moneta GL, Lee RW, Yeager RA, et al. Mesenteric duplex scanning: a blinded prospective study. *J Vasc Surg* 1993;17(1):79–84; discussion 85–86.
27. Moneta GL, Taylor DC, Helton WS, et al. Duplex ultrasound measurement of postprandial intestinal blood flow: effect of meal composition. *Gastroenterology* 1988;95(5):1294–1301.
28. Beebe HG, MacFarlane S, Raker EJ. Supraceliac aortomesenteric bypass for intestinal ischemia. *J Vasc Surg* 1987;5(5):749–754.
29. Bjorck M, Acosta S, Lindberg F, et al. Revascularization of the superior mesenteric artery after acute thromboembolic occlusion. *Br J Surg* 2002; 89(7):923–927.
30. Foley MI, Moneta GL, Abou-Zamzam AM Jr, et al. Revascularization of the superior mesenteric artery alone for treatment of intestinal ischemia. *J Vasc Surg* 2000;32(1):37–47.
31. Gentile AT, Moneta GL, Taylor LM Jr, et al. Isolated bypass to the superior mesenteric artery for intestinal ischemia. *Arch Surg* 1994;129(9): 926–931; discussion 931–932.
32. Geroulakos G, Tober JC, Anderson L, et al. Antegrade visceral revascularisation via a thoracoabdominal approach for chronic mesenteric ischaemia. *Eur J Vasc Endovasc Surg* 1999;17(1):56–59.
33. Jimenez JG, Huber TS, Ozaki CK, et al. Durability of antegrade synthetic aortomesenteric bypass for chronic mesenteric ischemia. *J Vasc Surg* 2002; 35(6):1078–1084.
34. Kasirajan K, O'Hara PJ, Gray BH, et al. Chronic mesenteric ischemia: open surgery versus percutaneous angioplasty and stenting. *J Vasc Surg* 2001;33(1):63–71.
35. Kazmers A. Operative management of chronic mesenteric ischemia. *Ann Vasc Surg* 1998;12(3):299–308.
36. Stoney RJ, Schneider PA. *Technical Aspects of Visceral Arterial Revascularization.* Philadelphia, PA: WB Saunders; 1990.
37. Stoney RJ, Reilly LM, Ehrenfeld E. *Chronic Mesenteric Ischemia and Surgery for Chronic Visceral Ischemia.* New York: McGraw-Hill; 1987.
38. McShane MD, Proctor A, Spencer P, et al. Mesenteric angioplasty for chronic intestinal ischaemia. *Eur J Vasc Surg* 1992;6(3):333–336.
39. AbuRahma AF, Stone PA, Bates MC, et al. Angioplasty/stenting of the superior mesenteric artery and celiac trunk: early and late outcomes. *J Endovasc Ther* 2003;10(6):1046–1053.
40. Atkins MD, Kwolek CJ, LaMuraglia GM, et al. Surgical revascularization versus endovascular therapy for chronic mesenteric ischemia: a comparative experience. *J Vasc Surg* 2007;45(6):1162–1171.

41. Brown DJ, Schermerhorn ML, Powell RJ, et al. Mesenteric stenting for chronic mesenteric ischemia. *J Vasc Surg* 2005;42(2):268–274.
42. Landis MS, Rajan DK, Simons ME, et al. Percutaneous management of chronic mesenteric ischemia: outcomes after intervention. *J Vasc Interv Radiol* 2005;16(10):1319–1325.
43. Lee RW, Bakken AM, Palchik E, et al. Long-term outcomes of endoluminal therapy for chronic atherosclerotic occlusive mesenteric disease. *Ann Vasc Surg* 2008;22(4):541–546.
44. Matsumoto AH, Angle JF, Spinosa DJ, et al. Percutaneous transluminal angioplasty and stenting in the treatment of chronic mesenteric ischemia: results and longterm followup. *J Am Coll Surg* 2002;194(1 suppl): S22–S31.
45. Maspes F, Mazzetti di Pietralata G, Gandini R, et al. Percutaneous transluminal angioplasty in the treatment of chronic mesenteric ischemia: results and 3 years of follow-up in 23 patients. *Abdom Imaging* 1998; 23(4):358–363.
46. Rose SC, Quigley TM, Raker EJ. Revascularization for chronic mesenteric ischemia: comparison of operative arterial bypass grafting and percutaneous transluminal angioplasty. *J Vasc Interv Radiol* 1995;6(3):339–349.
47. Sharafuddin MJ, Olson CH, Sun S, et al. Endovascular treatment of celiac and mesenteric arteries stenoses: applications and results. *J Vasc Surg* 2003;38(4):692–698.
48. Sarac TP, Altinel O, Kashyap V, et al. Endovascular treatment of stenotic and occluded visceral arteries for chronic mesenteric ischemia. *J Vasc Surg* 2008;47(3):485–491.
49. Sivamurthy N, Rhodes JM, Lee D, et al. Endovascular versus open mesenteric revascularization: immediate benefits do not equate with short-term functional outcomes. *J Am Coll Surg* 2006;202(6):859–867.
50. Silva JA, White CJ, Collins TJ, et al. Endovascular therapy for chronic mesenteric ischemia. *J Am Coll Cardiol* 2006;47(5):944–950.
51. Carmeci C, McClenathan J. Visceral artery aneurysms as seen in a community hospital. *Am J Surg* 2000;179(6):486–489.
52. Carr SC, Pearce WH, Vogelzang RL, et al. Current management of visceral artery aneurysms. *Surgery* 1996;120(4):627–633; discussion 633–634.
53. Gabelmann A, Gorich J, Merkle EM. Endovascular treatment of visceral artery aneurysms. *J Endovasc Ther* 2002;9(1):38–47.
54. Jorgensen BA. Visceral artery aneurysms. A review. *Dan Med Bull* 1985; 32(4):237–242.
55. Panayiotopoulos YP, Assadourian R, Taylor PR. Aneurysms of the visceral and renal arteries. *Ann R Coll Surg Engl* 1996;78(5):412–419.
56. Pilleul F, Dugougeat F. Transcatheter embolization of splanchnic aneurysms/pseudoaneurysms: early imaging allows detection of incomplete procedure. *J Comput Assist Tomogr* 2002;26(1):107–112.
57. Rokke O, Sondenaa K, Amundsen SR, et al. Successful management of eleven splanchnic artery aneurysms. *Eur J Surg* 1997;163(6):411–417.
58. Shanley CJ, Shah NL, Messina LM. Common splanchnic artery aneurysms: splenic, hepatic, and celiac. *Ann Vasc Surg* 1996;10(3): 315–322.
59. Shanley CJ, Shah NL, Messina LM. Uncommon splanchnic artery aneurysms: pancreaticoduodenal, gastroduodenal, superior mesenteric, inferior mesenteric, and colic. *Ann Vasc Surg* 1996;10(5):506–515.
60. Wagner WH, Allins AD, Treiman RL, et al. Ruptured visceral artery aneurysms. *Ann Vasc Surg* 1997;11(4):342–347.
61. Pasha SF, Gloviczki P, Stanson AW, et al. Splanchnic artery aneurysms. *Mayo Clin Proc* 2007;82(4):472–479.
62. Stanley JC, Fry WJ. Pathogenesis and clinical significance of splenic artery aneurysms. *Surgery* 1974;76(6):898–909.
63. Stanley JC, Thompson NW, Fry WJ. Splanchnic artery aneurysms. *Arch Surg* 1970;101(6):689–697.
64. Lee PC, Rhee RY, Gordon RY, et al. Management of splenic artery aneurysms: the significance of portal and essential hypertension. *J Am Coll Surg* 1999;189(5):483–490.
65. Puttini M, Aseni P, Brambilla G, et al. Splenic artery aneurysms in portal hypertension. *J Cardiovasc Surg (Torino)* 1982;23(6):490–493.
66. Nishida O, Moriyasu F, Nakamura T, et al. Hemodynamics of splenic artery aneurysm. *Gastroenterology* 1986;90(4):1042–1046.
67. Ohta M, Hashizume M, Ueno K, et al. Hemodynamic study of splenic artery aneurysm in portal hypertension. *Hepatogastroenterology* 1994; 41(2):181–184.
68. Ayalon A, Wiesner RH, Perkins JD, et al. Splenic artery aneurysms in liver transplant patients. *Transplantation* 1988;45(2):386–389.
69. Bronsther O, Merhav H, Van Thiel D, et al. Splenic artery aneurysms occurring in liver transplant recipients. *Transplantation* 1991;52(4): 723–724.
70. Kobori L, van der Kolk MJ, de Jong KP, et al. Splenic artery aneurysms in liver transplant patients. Liver Transplant Group. *J Hepatol* 1997;27(5): 890–893.
71. Robertson AJ, Rela M, Karani J, et al. Splenic artery aneurysm and orthotopic liver transplantation. *Transpl Int* 1999;12(1):68–70.
72. Ailawadi G, Cowles RA, Stanley JC, et al. Common celiacomesenteric trunk: aneurysmal and occlusive disease. *J Vasc Surg* 2004;40(5): 1040–1043.
73. Settembrini PG, Jausseran JM, Roveri S, et al. Aneurysms of anomalous splenomesenteric trunk: clinical features and surgical management in two cases. *J Vasc Surg* 1996;24(4):687–692.
74. Ishida H, Konno K, Hamashima Y, et al. Splenic artery aneurysm: value of color Doppler and the limitation of gray-scale ultrasonography. *Abdom Imaging* 1998;23(6):627–632.
75. Martin KW, Morian JP Jr, Lee JK, et al. Demonstration of a splenic artery pseudoaneurysm by MR imaging. *J Comput Assist Tomogr* 1985;9(1): 190–192.
76. de Vries JE, Schattenkerk ME, Malt RA. Complications of splenic artery aneurysm other than intraperitoneal rupture. *Surgery* 1982;91(2): 200–204.
77. Harper PC, Gamelli RL, Kaye MD. Recurrent hemorrhage into the pancreatic duct from a splenic artery aneurysm. *Gastroenterology* 1984;87(2): 417–420.
78. Stabile BE, Wilson SE, Debas HT. Reduced mortality from bleeding pseudocysts and pseudoaneurysms caused by pancreatitis. *Arch Surg* 1983;118(1):45–51.
79. Stanley JC, Frey CF, Miller TA, et al. Major arterial hemorrhage: a complication of pancreatic pseudocysts and chronic pancreatitis. *Arch Surg* 1976;111(4):435–440.
80. Wagner WH, Cossman DV, Treiman RL, et al. Hemosuccus pancreaticus from intraductal rupture of a primary splenic artery aneurysm. *J Vasc Surg* 1994;19(1):158–164.
81. Brothers TE, Stanley JC, Zelenock GB. Splenic arteriovenous fistula. *Int Surg* 1995;80(2):189–194.
82. Gaglio PJ, Regenstein F, Slakey D, et al. Alpha-1 antitrypsin deficiency and splenic artery aneurysm rupture: an association? *Am J Gastroenterol* 2000;95(6):1531–1534.
83. Angelakis EJ, Bair WE, Barone JE, et al. Splenic artery aneurysm rupture during pregnancy. *Obstet Gynecol Surv* 1993;48(3):145–148.
84. Lowry SM, O'Dea TP, Gallagher DI, et al. Splenic artery aneurysm rupture: the seventh instance of maternal and fetal survival. *Obstet Gynecol* 1986;67(2):291–292.
85. Macfarlane JR, Thorbjarnarson B. Rupture of splenic artery aneurysm during pregnancy. *Am J Obstet Gynecol* 1966;95(7):1025–1037.
86. O'Grady JP, Day EJ, Toole AL, et al. Splenic artery aneurysm rupture in pregnancy. A review and case report. *Obstet Gynecol* 1977;50(5): 627–630.
87. Caillouette JC, Merchant EB. Ruptured splenic artery aneurysm in pregnancy. Twelfth reported case with maternal and fetal survival. *Am J Obstet Gynecol* 1993;168(6 Pt 1):1810–1811; discussion 1811–1813.
88. Taylor JL, Woodward DA. Splenic conservation and the management of splenic artery aneurysm. *Ann R Coll Surg Engl* 1987;69(4):179–180.
89. Arca MJ, Gagner M, Heniford BT, et al. Splenic artery aneurysms: methods of laparoscopic repair. *J Vasc Surg* 1999;30(1):184–188.
90. Hashizume M, Ohta M, Ueno K, et al. Laparoscopic ligation of splenic artery aneurysm. *Surgery* 1993;113(3):352–354.
91. de Perrot M, Buhler L, Schneider PA, et al. Do aneurysms and pseudoaneurysms of the splenic artery require different surgical strategy? *Hepatogastroenterology* 1999;46(27):2028–2032.
92. Baker KS, Tisnado J, Cho SR, et al. Splanchnic artery aneurysms and pseudoaneurysms: transcatheter embolization. *Radiology* 1987;163(1): 135–139.
93. McDermott VG, Shlansky-Goldberg R, Cope C. Endovascular management of splenic artery aneurysms and pseudoaneurysms. *Cardiovasc Intervent Radiol* 1994;17(4):179–184.
94. Salam TA, Lumsden AB, Martin LG, et al. Nonoperative management of visceral aneurysms and pseudoaneurysms. *Am J Surg* 1992;164(3): 215–219.
95. Waltman AC, Luers PR, Athanasoulis CA, et al. Massive arterial hemorrhage in patients with pancreatitis. Complementary roles of surgery and transcatheter occlusive techniques. *Arch Surg* 1986;121(4):439–443.
96. Takahashi T, Shimada K, Kobayashi N, et al. Migration of steel-wire coils into the stomach after transcatheter arterial embolization for a bleeding splenic artery pseudoaneurysm: report of a case. *Surg Today* 2001;31(5): 458–462.
97. Wholey MH, Chamorro HA, Rao G, et al. Splenic infarction and spontaneous rupture of the spleen after therapeutic embolization. *Cardiovasc Radiol* 1978;1(4):249–253.
98. Saltzberg SS, Maldonado TS, Lamparello PJ, et al. Is endovascular therapy the preferred treatment for all visceral artery aneurysms? *Ann Vasc Surg* 2005;19(4):507–515.
99. Arepally A, Dagli M, Hofmann LV, et al. Treatment of splenic artery aneurysm with use of a stent-graft. *J Vasc Interv Radiol* 2002;13(6): 631–633.
100. Brountzos EN, Vagenas K, Apostolopoulou SC, et al. Pancreatitis-associated splenic artery pseudoaneurysm: endovascular treatment with self-expandable stent-grafts. *Cardiovasc Intervent Radiol* 2003;26(1):88–91.
101. Yoon HK, Lindh M, Uher P, et al. Stent-graft repair of a splenic artery aneurysm. *Cardiovasc Intervent Radiol* 2001;24(3):200–203.
102. Guida PM, Moore SW. Aneurysm of the hepatic artery. Report of five cases with a brief review of the previously reported cases. *Surgery* 1966;60(2): 299–310.
103. Lumsden AB, Mattar SG, Allen RC, et al. Hepatic artery aneurysms: the management of 22 patients. *J Surg Res* 1996;60(2):345–350.
104. Abbas MA, Fowl RJ, Stone WM, et al. Hepatic artery aneurysm: factors that predict complications. *J Vasc Surg* 2003;38(1):41–45.
105. Czerniak A, Thompson JN, Hemingway AP, et al. Hemobilia. A disease in evolution. *Arch Surg* 1988;123(6):718–721.
106. Okazaki M, Higashihara H, Ono H, et al. Percutaneous embolization of ruptured splanchnic artery pseudoaneurysms. *Acta Radiol* 1991;32(5): 349–354.
107. Parangi S, Oz MC, Blume RS, et al. Hepatobiliary complications of polyarteritis nodosa. *Arch Surg* 1991;126(7):909–912.

108. Stauffer JT, Weinman MD, Bynum TE. Hemobilia in a patient with multiple hepatic artery aneurysms: a case report and review of the literature. *Am J Gastroenterol* 1989;84(1):59–62.
109. Kadir S, Athanasoulis CA, Ring EJ, et al. Transcatheter embolization of intrahepatic arterial aneurysms. *Radiology* 1980;134(2):335–339.
110. Thibodeaux LC, Deshmukh RM, Hearn AT, et al. Management options for hepatic artery aneurysms. *Ann Vasc Surg* 1995;9(3):285–288.
111. Sachdev U, Baril DT, Ellozy SH, et al. Management of aneurysms involving branches of the celiac and superior mesenteric arteries: a comparison of surgical and endovascular therapy. *J Vasc Surg* 2006;44(4): 718–724.
112. Larson RA, Solomon J, Carpenter JP. Stent graft repair of visceral artery aneurysms. *J Vasc Surg* 2002;36(6):1260–1263.
113. Patel JV, Weston MJ, Kessel DO, et al. Hepatic artery pseudoaneurysm after liver transplantation: treatment with percutaneous thrombin injection. *Transplantation* 2003;75(10):1755–1757.
114. De Bakey ME, Cooley DA. Successful resection of mycotic aneurysm of superior mesenteric artery; case report and review of literature. *Am Surg* 1953;19(2):202–212.
115. Friedman SG, Pogo GJ, Moccio CG. Mycotic aneurysm of the superior mesenteric artery. *J Vasc Surg* 1987;6(1):87–90.
116. Stone WM, Abbas M, Cherry KJ, et al. Superior mesenteric artery aneurysms: is presence an indication for intervention? *J Vasc Surg* 2002; 36(2):234–237; discussion 237.
117. Cormier F, Ferry J, Artru B, et al. Dissecting aneurysms of the main trunk of the superior mesenteric artery. *J Vasc Surg* 1992;15(2):424–430.
118. Blumenberg RM, David D, Slovak J. Abdominal apoplexy due to rupture of a superior mesenteric artery aneurysm: clip aneurysmorrhaphy with survival. *Arch Surg* 1974;108(2):223–226.
119. Olcott C, Ehrenfeld WK. Endoaneurysmorrhaphy for visceral artery aneurysms. *Am J Surg* 1977;133(5):636–639.
120. Geelkerken RH, van Bockel JH, de Roos WK, et al. Surgical treatment of intestinal artery aneurysms. *Eur J Vasc Surg* 1990;4(6):563–567.
121. Kopatsis A, D'Anna JA, Sithian N, et al. Superior mesenteric artery aneurysm: 45 years later. *Am Surg* 1998;64(3):263–266.
122. Appel N, Duncan JR, Schuerer DJ. Percutaneous stent-graft treatment of superior mesenteric and internal iliac artery pseudoaneurysms. *J Vasc Interv Radiol* 2003;14(7):917–922.
123. Cowan S, Kahn MB, Bonn J, et al. Superior mesenteric artery pseudoaneurysm successfully treated with polytetrafluoroethylene covered stent. *J Vasc Surg* 2002;35(4):805–807.
124. Hama Y, Iwasaki Y, Kaji T, et al. Coil compaction after embolization of the superior mesenteric artery pseudoaneurysm. *Eur Radiol* 2002;12(suppl 3): S189–S191.
125. Graham LM, Stanley JC, Whitehouse WM Jr, et al. Celiac artery aneurysms: historic (1745–1949) versus contemporary (1950–1984) differences in etiology and clinical importance. *J Vasc Surg* 1985;2(5): 757–764.
126. Stone WM, Abbas MA, Gloviczki P, et al. Celiac arterial aneurysms: a critical reappraisal of a rare entity. *Arch Surg* 2002;137(6):670–674.
127. Hertzer NR, Mullally PH. Celiac artery aneurysmectomy with hepatic artery ligation. *Arch Surg* 1972;104(3):337–339.
128. Parfitt J, Chalmers RT, Wolfe JH. Visceral aneurysms in Ehlers-Danlos syndrome: case report and review of the literature. *J Vasc Surg* 2000;31(6): 1248–1251.
129. Schoder M, Cejna M, Langle F, et al. Glue embolization of a ruptured celiac trunk pseudoaneurysm via the gastroduodenal artery. *Eur Radiol* 2000;10(8):1335–1337.
130. Waldenberger P, Bendix N, Petersen J, et al. Clinical outcome of endovascular therapeutic occlusion of the celiac artery. *J Vasc Surg* 2007;46(4): 655–661.
131. Atkins BZ, Ryan JM, Gray JL. Treatment of a celiac artery aneurysm with endovascular stent grafting—a case report. *Vasc Endovascular Surg* 2003; 37(5):367–373.
132. Funahashi S, Yukizane T, Yano K, et al. An aneurysm of the right gastroepiploic artery. *J Cardiovasc Surg (Torino)* 1997;38(4):385–388.
133. Jacobs PP, Croiset van Ughelen FA, Bruyninckx CM, et al. Haemoperitoneum caused by a dissecting aneurysm of the gastroepiploic artery. *Eur J Vasc Surg* 1994;8(2):236–237.
134. Witte JT, Hasson JE, Harms BA, et al. Fatal gastric artery dissection and rupture occurring as a paraesophageal mass: a case report and literature review. *Surgery* 1990;107(5):590–594.
135. Uchikoshi F, Sakamoto T, Imabunn S, et al. Aneurysm of the right gastroepiploic artery: a case report of laparoscopic resection. *Cardiovasc Surg* 1993;1(5):550–551.
136. Lagoudianakis EE, Filis KA, Tsekouras DK, et al. Endovascular obliteration of a ruptured right gastric artery aneurysm. *Minerva Gastroenterol Dietol* 2006;52(3):333–337.
137. Schellhammer F, Steinhaus D, Cohnen M, et al. Minimally invasive therapy of pseudoaneurysms of the trunk: application of thrombin. *Cardiovasc Intervent Radiol* 2008;31(3):535–541.
138. Lagana D, Carrafiello G, Mangini M, et al. Emergency endovascular treatment with stent graft of a gastric artery aneurysms (GAA). *Emerg Radiol* 2008;15(2):141–144.
139. Trevisani MF, Ricci MA, Michaels RM, et al. Multiple mesenteric aneurysms complicating subacute bacterial endocarditis. *Arch Surg* 1987; 122(7):823–824.
140. Sellke FW, Williams GB, Donovan DL, et al. Management of intra-abdominal aneurysms associated with periarteritis nodosa. *J Vasc Surg* 1986;4(3): 294–298.
141. Sarcina A, Bellosta R, Magnaldi S, et al. Aneurysm of the middle colic artery—case report and literature review. *Eur J Vasc Endovasc Surg* 2000; 20(2):198–200.
142. Naito A, Toyota N, Ito K. Embolization of a ruptured middle colic artery aneurysm. *Cardiovasc Intervent Radiol* 1995;18(1):56–58.
143. Graham LM, Hay MR, Cho KJ, et al. Inferior mesenteric artery aneurysms. *Surgery* 1985;97(2):158–163.
144. Raso AM, Rispoli P, Maggio D, et al. Post stenotic aneurysm of the inferior mesenteric artery: case report and discussion. *J Cardiovasc Surg (Torino)* 1996;37(4):359–362.
145. Turkbey B, Peynircioglu B, Akpinar E, et al. Isolated aneurysm of the distal branch of the jejunal artery: MDCT angiographic diagnosis and endovascular management. *Cardiovasc Intervent Radiol* 2008;31(Suppl 2):S34–S37.
146. Goffi L, Chan R, Boccoli G, et al. Aneurysm of a jejunal branch of the superior mesenteric artery in a patient with Marfan's syndrome. *J Cardiovasc Surg (Torino)* 2000;41(2):321–323.
147. Coll DP, Ierardi R, Kerstein MD, et al. Aneurysms of the pancreaticoduodenal arteries: a change in management. *Ann Vasc Surg* 1998;12(3): 286–291.
148. Suzuki K, Kashimura H, Sato M, et al. Pancreaticoduodenal artery aneurysms associated with celiac axis stenosis due to compression by median arcuate ligament and celiac plexus. *J Gastroenterol* 1998;33(3): 434–438.
149. Gouny P, Fukui S, Aymard A, et al. Aneurysm of the gastroduodenal artery associated with stenosis of the superior mesenteric artery. *Ann Vasc Surg* 1994;8(3):281–284.
150. de Perrot M, Berney T, Deleaval J, et al. Management of true aneurysms of the pancreaticoduodenal arteries. *Ann Surg* 1999;229(3):416–420.
151. Eckhauser FE, Stanley JC, Zelenock GB, et al. Gastroduodenal and pancreaticoduodenal artery aneurysms: a complication of pancreatitis causing spontaneous gastrointestinal hemorrhage. *Surgery* 1980;88(3):335–344.
152. Chiou AC, Josephs LG, Menzoian JO. Inferior pancreaticoduodenal artery aneurysm: report of a case and review of the literature. *J Vasc Surg* 1993; 17(4):784–789.
153. Gadacz TR, Trunkey D, Kieffer RF Jr. Visceral vessel erosion associated with pancreatitis. Case reports and a review of the literature. *Arch Surg* 1978;113(12):1438–1440.
154. Iyomasa S, Matsuzaki Y, Hiei K, et al. Pancreaticoduodenal artery aneurysm: a case report and review of the literature. *J Vasc Surg* 1995; 22(2):161–166.
155. Ikeda O, Tamura Y, Nakasone Y, et al. Coil embolization of pancreaticoduodenal artery aneurysms associated with celiac artery stenosis: report of three cases. *Cardiovasc Intervent Radiol* 2007;30(3):504–507.
156. Tulsyan N, Kashyap VS, Greenberg RK, et al. The endovascular management of visceral artery aneurysms and pseudoaneurysms. *J Vasc Surg* 2007;45(2):276–283; discussion 283.
157. Carr JA, Cho JS, Shepard AD, et al. Visceral pseudoaneurysms due to pancreatic pseudocysts: rare but lethal complications of pancreatitis. *J Vasc Surg* 2000;32(4):722–730.
158. Mandel SR, Jaques PF, Sanofsky S, et al. Nonoperative management of peripancreatic arterial aneurysms. A 10-year experience. *Ann Surg* 1987; 205(2):126–128.
159. Nyman U, Svendsen P, Jivegard L, et al. Multiple pancreaticoduodenal aneurysms: treatment with superior mesenteric artery stent-graft placement and distal embolization. *J Vasc Interv Radiol* 2000;11(9):1201–1205.
160. Thakker RV, Gajjar B, Wilkins RA, et al. Embolisation of gastroduodenal artery aneurysm caused by chronic pancreatitis. *Gut* 1983;24(11): 1094–1098.
161. Vujic I, Anderson MC, Meredith HC, et al. Successful embolization of the dorsal pancreatic artery to control massive upper gastrointestinal hemorrhage. *Am Surg* 1980;46(3):184–186.
162. Manazer JR, Monzon JR, Dietz PA, et al. Treatment of pancreatic pseudoaneurysm with percutaneous transabdominal thrombin injection. *J Vasc Surg* 2003;38(3):600–602.
163. McIntyre TP, Simone ST, Stahlfeld KR. Intraoperative thrombin occlusion of a visceral artery aneurysm. *J Vasc Surg* 2002;36(2):393–395.
164. Suzuki K, Tachi Y, Ito S, et al. Endovascular management of ruptured pancreaticoduodenal artery aneurysms associated with celiac axis stenosis. *Cardiovasc Intervent Radiol* 2008;31(6):1082–1087.
165. Chan RP, David E. Reperfusion of splanchnic artery aneurysm following transcatheter embolization: treatment with percutaneous thrombin injection. *Cardiovasc Intervent Radiol* 2004;27(3):264–267.

CHAPTER 94 ■ AORTOILIAC DISEASE

DANIEL J. REDDY, MITCHELL R. WEAVER, AND ALEXANDER D. SHEPARD

KEY POINTS

1. Atherosclerotic occlusive disease of the aorta and iliac arteries is one of the most common problems encountered by surgeons.
2. The aortic bifurcation is the location where the earliest atherosclerotic changes are first noted in young adults.
3. Risk factors for aortoiliac occlusive disease are those for atherosclerosis in general: smoking, hypertension, lipid abnormalities, diabetes mellitus, male sex, older age, and genetic predisposition.
4. Smoking appears to be a particularly important risk factor for the development of lower extremity atherosclerotic occlusive disease.
5. Claudication is the most common presenting symptom of patients with significant aortoiliac disease.
6. Physical examination typically reveals diminished or absent femoral pulses in patients with aortoiliac occlusive disease.
7. In the majority of cases, a diagnosis of significant aortoiliac occlusive disease can be made on the basis of the history and physical examination alone.
8. Since the very first transarterial dilation procedures, percutaneous transluminal angioplasty has become a commonly performed and, in some cases, the preferred therapy for iliac artery occlusive disease.
9. A combined open operation with endovascular surgery appears to have promising results in the treatment of aortoiliac occlusive disease.
10. Aortofemoral bypass is the most durable and reliable of all treatment options, for which reason it is the reference standard for the reconstruction of advanced aortoiliac occlusive disease.

(1) Atherosclerotic occlusive disease of the aorta and iliac arteries is one of the most common problems encountered by vascular surgeons. Alone or in combination with femoropopliteal or tibial occlusive disease, it is the most frequent cause of chronic lower extremity arterial insufficiency. Because a greater number of muscle groups are affected by aortoiliac atherosclerosis than by infrainguinal disease, the resulting symptoms may be particularly disabling. The treatment of symptomatic aortoiliac disease also represents one of the major success stories of modern vascular surgery. Since the first reconstructive procedures on the abdominal aorta were performed nearly five decades ago, treatment has undergone significant progress. Advances in noninvasive vascular diagnosis, arteriography, preoperative assessment, anesthesia, and critical care, in addition to those in surgical technique, have contributed to improved outcomes. The wide availability of magnetic resonance angiography (MRA) and multidetector computed tomography angiography (MDCTA) have facilitated even greater and earlier interventions for a variety of clinical presentations of occlusive aortoiliac arterial conditions. Endovascular and reconstructive procedures for aortoiliac disease have become routine, with low perioperative morbidity and mortality and excellent early and long-term outcomes. The excellent durability of such reconstructions is undoubtedly in large part related to the large caliber and high flow rates of the vessels involved. In recent years, endovascular methods have been added with both increasing frequency and success. This fact has broadened the scope of lesions treated and the patients' ability to undergo treatment with minimal morbidity and time lost from work and family life.

Depending on the pattern of the occlusive process and patient risk, a variety of revascularization techniques are currently available. Selection of a patient-specific treatment strategy from an increasing array of alternatives, although challenging, frequently will alleviate symptoms, avoid an amputation, and prevent or reverse organ dysfunction.

ANATOMY

The arteries supplying blood to the lower extremities are frequently divided into abdominal, or "inflow," arteries (the aorta and iliac arteries) and infrainguinal, or "outflow," arteries (the femoropopliteal and tibial arteries). The aorta enters the abdomen from the chest through the aortic hiatus, located between the 12th thoracic and first lumbar vertebrae, and ends at the level of the fourth lumbar vertebra, where it bifurcates into the right and left common iliac arteries. This terminal bifurcation roughly corresponds to the level of the umbilicus. Each common iliac artery curves posteriorly into the sacral hollow and divides into an internal and an external iliac branch. The external iliac artery then curves anteriorly and continues along the psoas muscle under the inguinal ligament to become the common femoral artery, which in turn bifurcates into the superficial and deep (profunda) femoral arteries. The internal iliac (hypogastric) artery follows the curve of the pelvic side wall and branches repeatedly to supply the pelvic viscera and gluteal musculature (Fig. 94.1).

The branches of the abdominal aorta can be divided into three groups:

1. Three unpaired arteries to the gut arise from its anterior wall; the celiac trunk supplies the foregut, the superior mesenteric artery supplies the midgut, and the inferior mesenteric artery perfuses the hindgut.
2. Arteries to the three paired genitourinary glands arise close together from the lateral wall of the aorta—the adrenal, renal, and gonadal branches.
3. Branches to the "roof" and walls of the abdominal cavity include the phrenic, lumbar, and median sacral arteries. These branches assume varying degrees of importance in the formation of collateral perfusion channels around occlusive lesions in the aorta and iliac arteries.

Because the abdominal aorta and its iliac branches are retroperitoneal structures coursing through the deepest portions

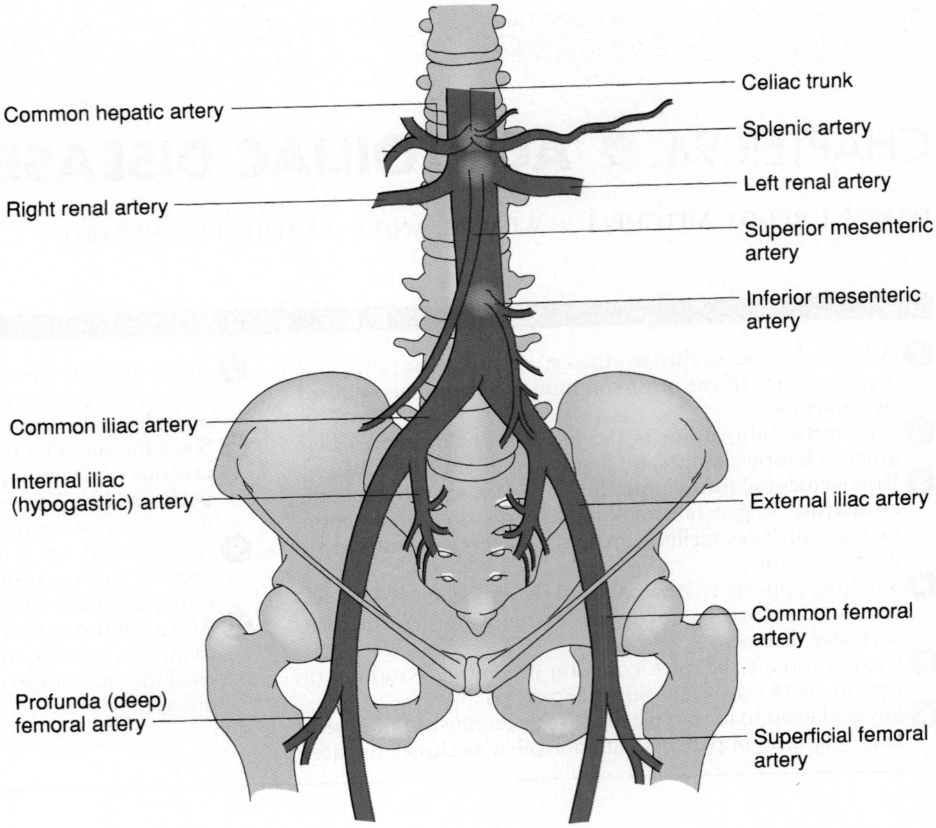

FIGURE 94.1. Anatomy of the abdominal aorta and iliac arteries.

of the abdominal cavity, a sophisticated operative technique is required to directly expose them. The proximal (suprarenal) abdominal aorta is rendered particularly inaccessible by the overlying stomach, pancreas, and colon. Occlusive lesions of this portion of the aorta are relatively uncommon, however, in comparison with those of the distal (infrarenal) aorta. The crossing left renal vein serves as a useful surgical landmark defining the usual boundary between these two segments of the abdominal aorta. Although transabdominal exposure of the infrarenal aorta is fairly routine, it requires reflection of the transverse colon superiorly and of the small bowel and its mesentery and distal duodenum to the right. The iliac bifurcations can also be difficult to expose because of their location deep in the pelvis; in addition, the bifurcation of the left iliac artery lies directly behind the sigmoid colon. When appropriate, indirect exposure with images derived from angiography or ultrasound alone may be sufficient to accomplish reconstruction percutaneously or through a remotely placed minimal incision.

PATHOPHYSIOLOGY

Although atherosclerosis is a generalized disease, the earliest and most severe lesions tend to occur at arterial bifurcations and in areas of relative fixation, where the disruption of nor-
2 mal laminar flow is greatest. The aortic bifurcation is in fact the location where the earliest atherosclerotic changes are first noted in young adults. In persons predisposed to the development of more advanced disease, plaque gradually extends proximally into the infrarenal aorta and distally into the common iliac arteries, usually along the posterior wall first. With progressive worsening of the occlusive process, hemodynamic alterations lead to the enlargement of a network of auxiliary or collateral channels around the involved segments. Important collateral arterial pathways around the aortic bifurcation and common iliac segments are the intercostal and lumbar arteries to circumflex iliac and iliolumbar arteries, the superior to inferior epigastric arteries, and the superior and inferior mesenteric arteries to rectal and internal pudendal arteries. Collateral pathways around occlusive lesions of the external iliac arteries include the hypogastric to circumflex femoral channels (Figs. 94.2 and 94.3).

With slowly developing occlusive lesions, this collateral network is usually sufficient to provide enough blood flow to meet the resting metabolic needs of the lower extremities. These channels, however, do not have the capacity to increase blood flow to the levels necessary to meet the exercise demands of the leg musculature. *Claudication* (from the Latin verb *claudicare*, "to limp") is the term used to denote the characteristic exercise-induced, cramping pain in the muscles of the lower extremity that results. With acute arterial occlusions and multiple-level disease (occlusive disease in both the aortoiliac and infrainguinal segments), collateral pathways may be inadequate to meet even the basal metabolic needs of nonexercising tissue. The outcome is critical limb ischemia associated with pain at rest, tissue loss (gangrene, nonhealing ulceration), and threatened limb viability.

PRESENTATION

3 Risk factors for aortoiliac occlusive disease are those for atherosclerosis in general—smoking, hypertension, lipid abnormalities, diabetes mellitus, male sex, older age, and genetic
4 predisposition. Smoking appears to be a particularly important risk factor for the development of lower extremity atherosclerotic occlusive disease.[1] Patients with symptoms of aortoiliac occlusive disease usually present in their 50s and 60s, whereas patients with symptoms of infrainguinal disease are generally in their 70s.[2] Patients with critical limb ischemia secondary to multiple-level disease are also generally in this older

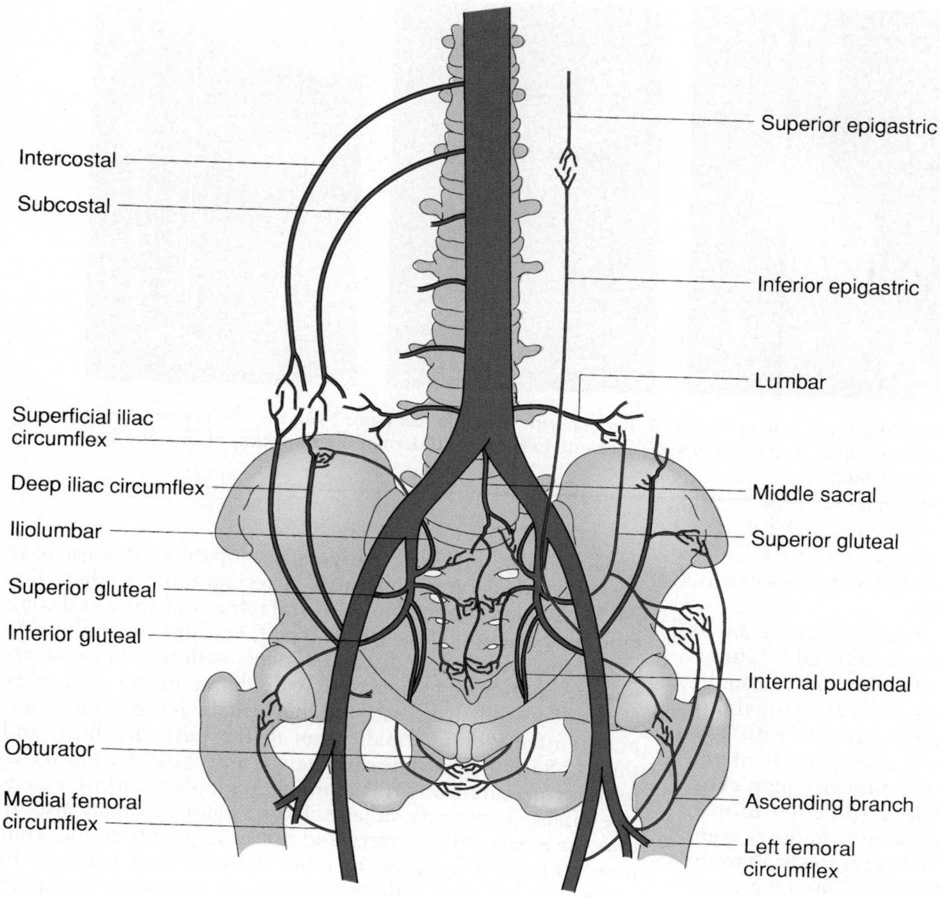

FIGURE 94.2. Major pathways of parietal–visceral collateral circulation in aortoiliac occlusive disease.

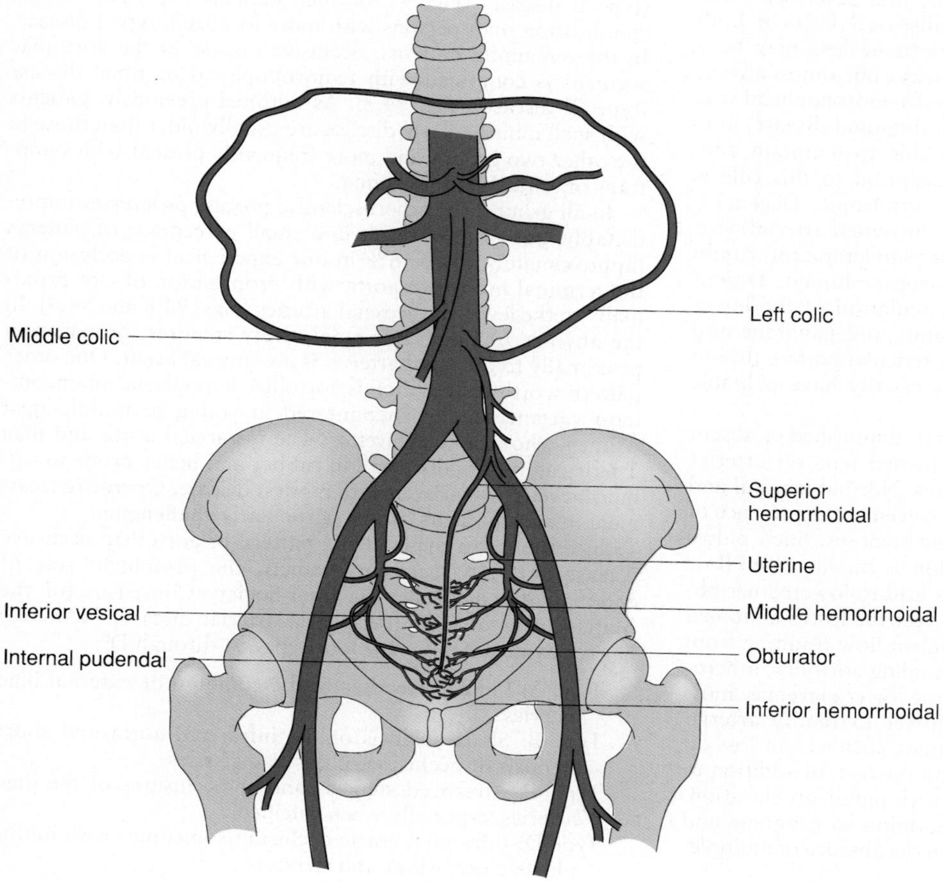

FIGURE 94.3. Major visceral collateral network available to compensate for occlusive aortoiliac disease.

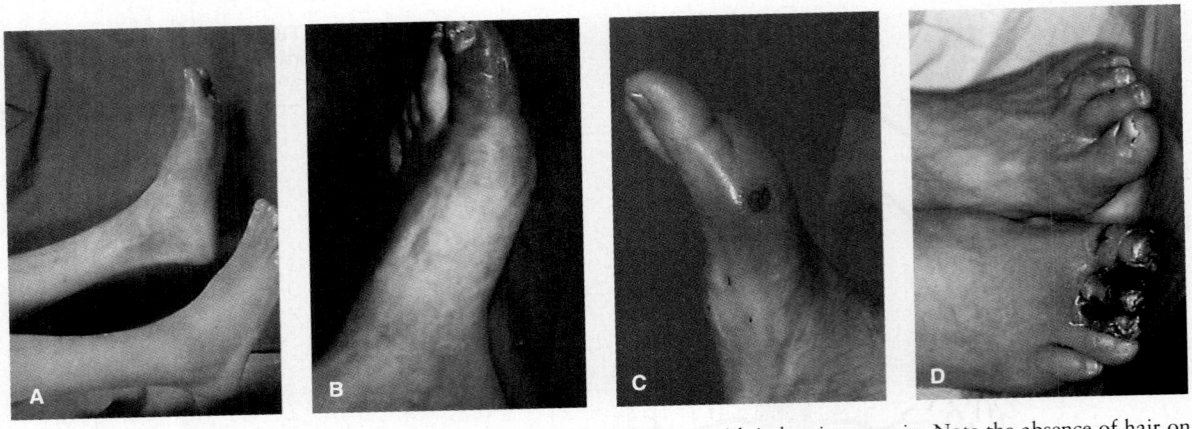

FIGURE 94.4. Clinical manifestations of critical limb ischemia. **A:** Patient with ischemic rest pain. Note the absence of hair on the atrophic shiny skin of the feet and the rubor at dependency. **B:** First-toe ischemia and dermal discoloration of blue-toe syndrome. **C:** Ischemic ulceration. **D:** Digital gangrene.

age group. The differential diagnosis includes spinal stenosis, hip arthritis, and nerve root compression.

5 Claudication is the most common presenting symptom of patients with significant aortoiliac disease. Induced by ambulation and quickly relieved by rest, claudication is usually described as a cramping pain, tiredness, or easy fatigability of the involved muscle groups. Although patients with aortoiliac disease classically present with claudication of the thighs, hips, and buttocks, a significant minority may complain of only calf claudication. Erectile dysfunction in men secondary to reduced hypogastric perfusion is another common complaint. The combination of bilateral lower extremity claudication, atrophy of the leg muscles, impotence, and diminished or absent femoral pulses is known as *Leriche syndrome,* after the French physician who first described these classic manifestations of aortoiliac disease.[3] Critical limb ischemia associated with rest pain or tissue loss may be a manifestation of aortoiliac occlusive disease, but almost always occurs in combination with more distal femoropopliteal disease (Fig. 94.4). In the absence of infrainguinal disease, aortoiliac collaterals are almost always able to maintain adequate resting tissue perfusion. An exception to this rule is atheroembolic disease, or "blue toe" syndrome. Degenerative plaque(s) in the aortoiliac (or any proximal arterial) segment can ulcerate or rupture to release platelet microthrombi and atheromatous debris into the arterial lumen. Downstream embolization into the microcirculation of the lower extremities can produce digital ischemia and gangrene and dermal discoloration in a characteristic reticular pattern (livedo reticularis) (Fig. 94.4). Such patients usually have palpable pedal pulses.

6 Physical examination typically reveals diminished or absent femoral pulses. Severely diseased, calcified femoral arteries may be palpable as firm, tubular masses. Normal femoral and distal pulses may be palpable, however, even in the presence of hemodynamically significant aortoiliac stenoses. Such pulses rapidly disappear following ambulation as the increased flow demands of the exercising leg muscles lead to lowered peripheral vascular resistance. Bruits heard over the lower abdomen or groins suggest the presence of turbulent flow resulting from occlusive plaque. Patients with longstanding aortoiliac atherosclerosis may have disuse atrophy of the lower extremity musculature. Other common signs of lower extremity arterial occlusive disease include trophic changes, such as hair loss on the legs or toes and thin, shiny skin on the feet, in addition to rubor on limb dependency coupled with pallor on elevation. Such chronic advanced changes in addition to gangrene and nonhealing ulceration(s) are unusual in the absence of multiple-level disease.

Classically, different patterns of aortoiliac disease have been identified on preoperative arteriographic studies (Fig. 94.5).[4] Disease confined to the distal infrarenal aorta and common iliac arteries, classified as type I, accounts for only 10% of patients with inflow disease. Patients with type I disease are younger and more frequently female than patients with other forms of aortoiliac disease, and they usually present with complaints of disabling claudication in the buttocks, hips, and thighs.[5] Such localized disease may be amenable to endarterectomy or percutaneous transluminal angioplasty. More extensive disease is the rule; atherosclerotic plaque extends distally into the external iliac artery and not infrequently to the common femoral bifurcation in more than 80% of patients. In somewhat less than half this group, no significant occlusive disease is present in the femoropopliteal and tibial segments (type II disease) (Fig. 94.6). Such patients experience worse claudication than persons with more localized, type I disease. In the remaining patients, occlusive disease in the aortoiliac segment is combined with femoropopliteal or tibial disease (type III disease) (Fig. 94.7). As outlined previously, patients with such multiple-level disease are usually older than those in the other two groups and more frequently present with symptoms of critical limb ischemia.

In all groups, the atherosclerotic process progresses unpredictably, but the end result in a small percentage of patients (approximately 5% to 6% in our experience) is occlusion of the terminal infrarenal aorta with propagation of clot proximally to the levels of the renal arteries (Figs. 94.8 and 94.9). In the absence of significant renal artery stenoses, propagation proximally to the renal arteries is an unusual event. One other pattern worthy of mention is aortoiliac hypoplasia, an uncommon variant usually encountered in young to middle-aged women who smoke cigarettes. The infrarenal aorta and iliac arteries are unusually small in caliber and hence prone to significant narrowing, even with modest disease. Operative treatment in such patients can be particularly challenging.

In response to the evolving pattern of aortoiliac occlusive disease (AIOD) treatment, namely, the prominent role of endovascular methods, the Inter-Society Consensus for the Management of PAD (peripheral arterial disease) (TASC II) has reclassified AIOD into four types, A through D[6]:

- Type A: Limited stenoses of the common or external iliac arteries
- Type B: Short stenosis of the infrarenal aorta and short stenosis or occlusion of the iliac arteries
- Type C: Advanced stenosis and/or occlusions of the iliac arteries, especially when calcified
- Type D: Infrarenal aortic occlusion sometimes with multiple iliac occlusions and stenoses

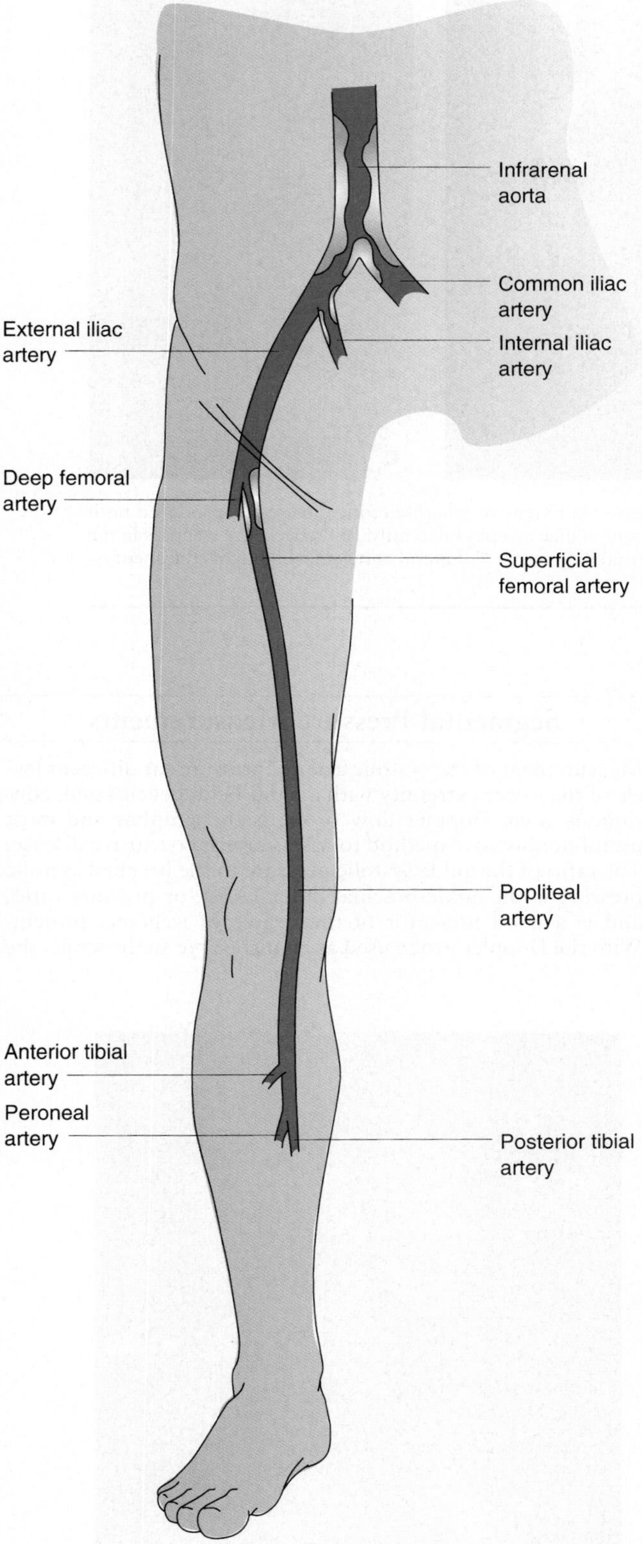

FIGURE 94.5. Common sites of arteriosclerotic lesions in aortoiliofemoral occlusive disease. Although often a generalized process, partially segmental distribution of major disease, most prominent at arterial bifurcations, usually allows surgical revascularization.

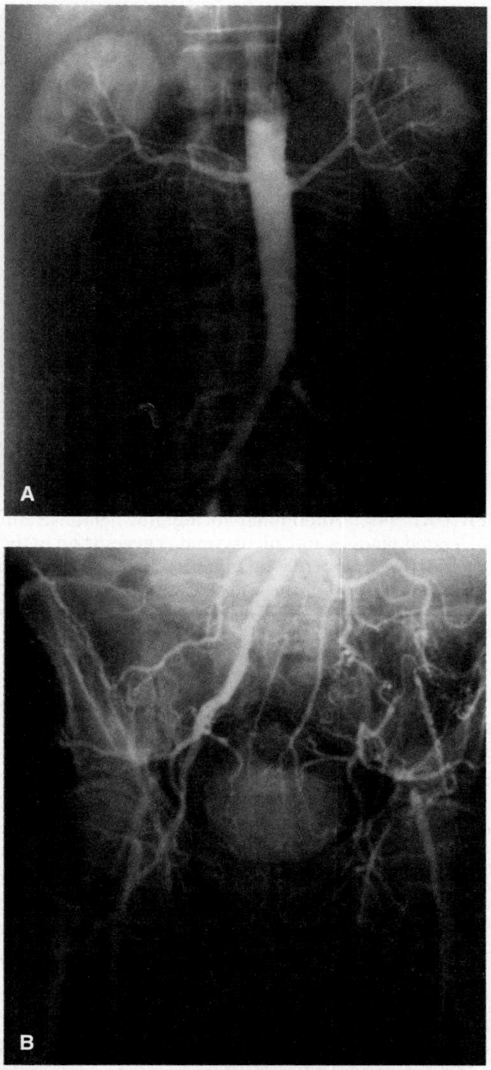

FIGURE 94.6. Abdominal aortograms demonstrating type II disease. **A:** Left common and external iliac occlusion can be seen, with reconstitution of the ipsilateral internal iliac and common femoral arteries through visceral and lumbar collaterals. **B:** The right external iliac artery is also occluded, and the right common femoral artery is reconstituted through right hypogastric-to-circumflex femoral channels.

7 The value of this and other classifications derives from its power as a template for reporting standards. Stratification of the severity and pattern of the AIOD treated measured by the matching outcomes serves to identify appropriate treatment modalities in individual patients. To simplify, the surgeon could apply endovascular treatment methods for types A and B patients and lean toward open treatment for types C and D. Nonetheless, the velocity of change in endovascular devices and their successful application has weakened the value of any classification owing to the fact that confounding variables cannot, then, be anticipated or controlled. Therefore, the vascular specialist must be conversant and expert with all methods and offer a recommendation based on evaluation, risk assessment, and preference of the individual informed patient.

EVALUATION

In the majority of cases, a diagnosis of significant aortoiliac occlusive disease can be made on the basis of the history and physical examination alone. A clinical diagnosis can and

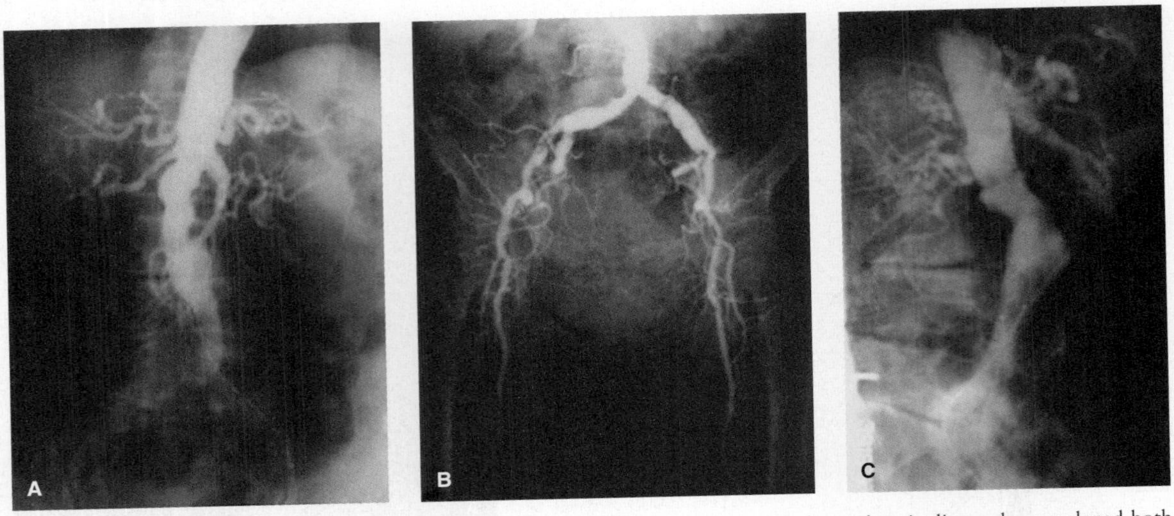

FIGURE 94.7. Abdominal aortograms demonstrating type III disease. A: Extensive atherosclerotic disease has produced both ulcerated plaques and aneurysmal degeneration in the aorta and common iliac arteries bilaterally. B: Preocclusive stenoses in the proximal right external and internal iliac arteries and in the left internal iliac artery. C: Lateral aortagram highlights the aneurysmal degeneration of the aorta.

should be supplemented by noninvasive vascular testing. Such testing provides valuable information to the treating clinician by confirming the presence of disease and objectively documenting the degree of ischemia and the arterial segment(s) involved. A baseline is established according to which the patient can be followed and interventions planned. Treatment results can be assessed by repeated testing. Such information is particularly useful in a patient with an equivocal history or pulse examination. Arteriography, MRA, and CTA may then be reserved for those patients considered suitable candidates for operative or endovascular (catheter-based) intervention.

Segmental Pressure Measurements

Measurement of the systolic arterial pressures at different levels of the lower extremity with a hand-held, pencil-sized, continuous wave Doppler flow probe is the simplest and most useful noninvasive method to assess arterial occlusive disease. The ratio of the ankle systolic pressure to the brachial systolic pressure is the ankle-brachial index (ABI), or pressure ratio, and is a good indicator of the degree of ischemia present. With the Doppler probe used as an ultrasonic stethoscope, the

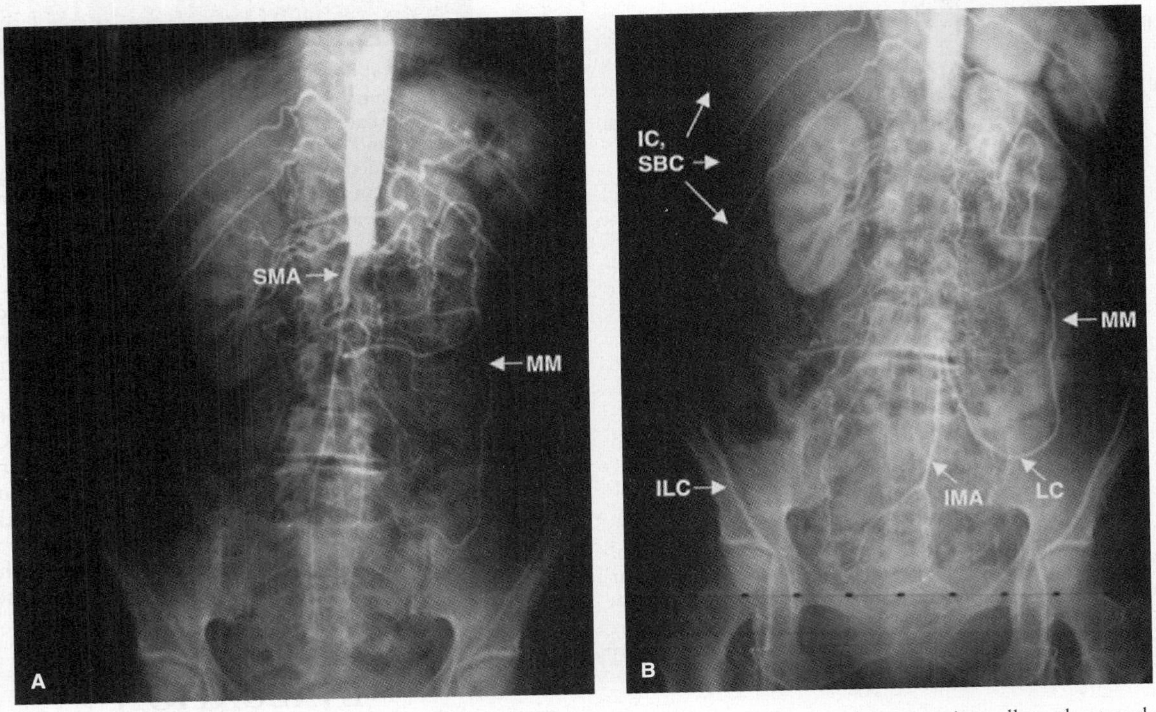

FIGURE 94.8. A, B: Abdominal aortograms demonstrating juxtarenal aortic occlusion and an extensive collateral network reconstituting the femoral arterial segments. IC, intercostal; ILC, iliac circumflex; IMA, inferior mesenteric artery; LC, left colic; MM, meandering mesenteric; SBC, subcostal; SMA, superior mesenteric artery.

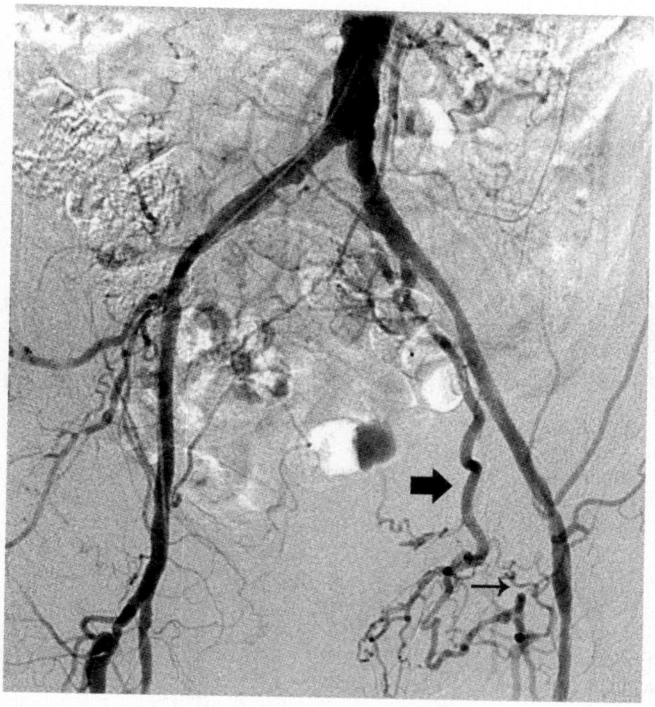

FIGURE 94.9. Pelvic aortogram showing a large collateral from the left hypogastric artery to left profunda artery.

systolic pressures in the dorsalis pedis and posterior tibial artery are measured at the ankle, and each of these values is then the numerator of a simple fraction in which the higher of the two brachial pressures is the denominator. Normal ABIs are generally equal to or slightly greater than 1. Patients with claudication usually have ABIs ranging from 0.5 to 0.9, whereas patients with rest pain and tissue loss have ABIs of less than 0.5.

Determination of limb systolic pressures at different locations (with the "four-cuff" technique, pressures are measured at the upper thigh, lower thigh, calf, and ankle) provides information about which arterial segments are involved with occlusive disease (Figs. 94.10 and 94.11). A pressure drop of more than 20 mm Hg between consecutive levels is indicative of significant disease within the intervening arterial segment. A reduced upper thigh pressure signifies occlusive disease in the aortoiliac or common femoral segments.

In patients with extensive calcification in the walls of the tibial arteries (as is frequently seen in diabetes mellitus or end-stage renal disease), the ankle pressures may not be interpretable because the vessels are too "stiff" to be compressed by the externally applied cuff. In this situation, the pressure in the digital arteries of the great toe can be measured because these small vessels are generally spared calcification. A toe pressure of less than 30 mm Hg indicates severe ischemia. Inspection of the Doppler-derived arterial waveforms can provide additional information when tibial vessels are incompressible.

Patients with claudication occasionally have a normal or nearly normal ABI. As described previously, in such cases the arterial stenosis is not severe enough to cause a pressure drop while the limb is at rest, but does produce a hemodynamic effect under conditions of higher rates of flow, as during exercise. Higher rates of flow through a moderately stenotic segment increase the energy lost at the site, so that a significant distal pressure drop results. Exercise stress testing can be used to evaluate patients suspected of having such disease. ABIs are measured before and after a treadmill exercise protocol; a drop of 15% or more in the ABI following exercise is indicative of hemodynamically significant occlusive disease.

Duplex Scanning

Duplex scanning of the aorta and iliac arteries has been advocated by some as a more precise noninvasive diagnostic tool.[7] Some authorities have even suggested that duplex scanning can be used to plan therapeutic interventions without the need

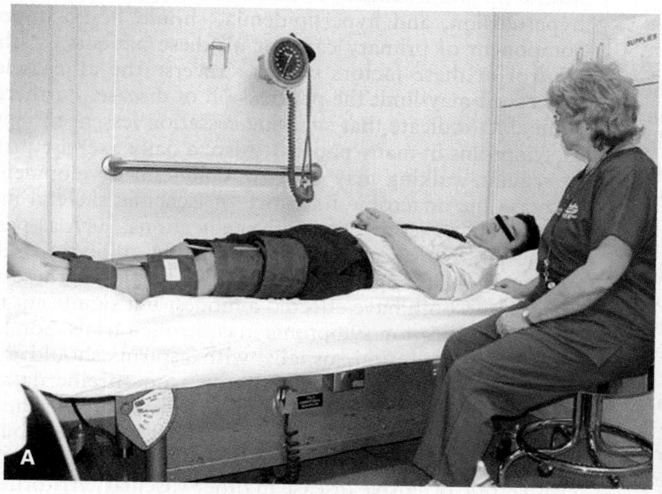

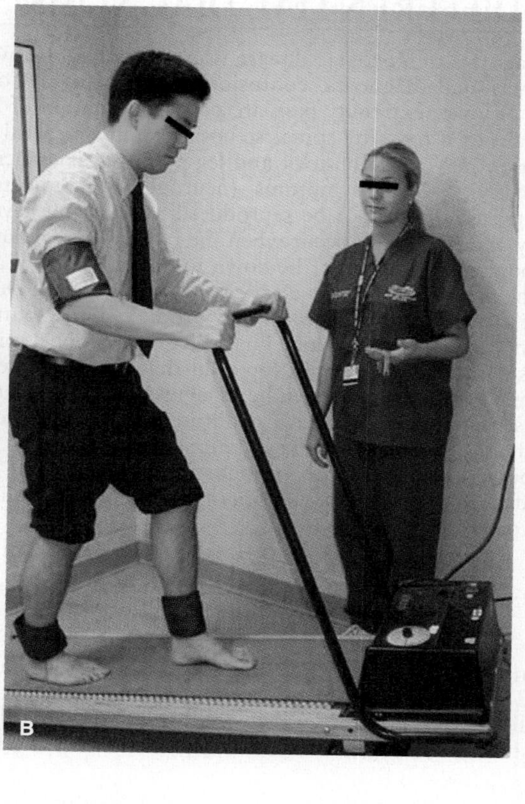

FIGURE 94.10. Noninvasive testing to evaluate lower extremity ischemia. **A:** Segmental pressure measurements with cuffs placed at the upper thigh, lower thigh, calf, and ankle. **B:** Stress testing with treadmill ergometry.

FIGURE 94.11. Segmental pressure measurements typical of normal results (A) and aortoiliac occlusive disease (B).

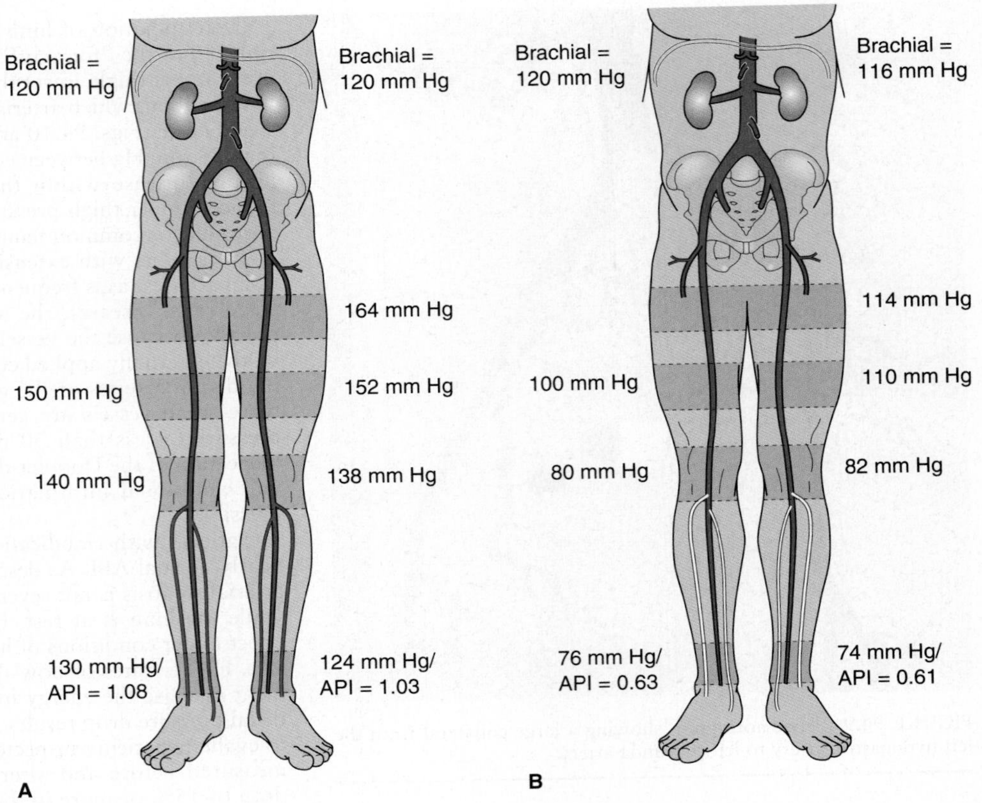

for arteriography. Imaging of the abdominal arteries, however, is difficult because of their deep retroperitoneal and pelvic locations. Many patients are not candidates for such studies because of body habitus and overlying bowel gas; even in experienced hands, this procedure is time consuming. These problems have limited the widespread use of this modality.

DIFFERENTIAL DIAGNOSIS

The diagnosis of aortoiliac disease is usually straightforward, but occasional diagnostic confusion may arise when other causes of lower extremity pain are present. Irritation of lumbosacral nerve roots by spinal stenosis or intervertebral disc herniation may cause buttock and leg pain that is associated with activity. Such symptoms (neurogenic claudication), however, usually cannot be reproduced at the same level of activity and frequently occur when the patient is standing, so that the patient must sit or lie down to obtain relief. In addition, the pain is usually in a classic sciatic distribution. Degenerative arthritis of the hip joints may produce similar buttock, hip, and referred thigh pain. Physical examination typically reveals pain directly over the hip joint that is exacerbated by movement of the joint. Peripheral neuropathy, particularly that associated with diabetes mellitus, may masquerade as ischemic rest pain. In all these situations, segmental limb pressure measurements, with or without stress testing, can be helpful in determining the contribution of arterial occlusive disease to the patient's symptoms.

TREATMENT

The aims of therapy in aortoiliac occlusive disease are to relieve symptoms and, in cases of critical limb ischemia, prevent limb loss (Algorithm 94.1). Medical therapy should be instituted in all patients with symptomatic disease, but is insufficient as sole therapy in patients with limb-threatening ischemia.

Medical Therapy

Risk factor modification, including smoking cessation and the follow-up and treatment of diabetes mellitus, systemic arterial hypertension, and hyperlipidemia, should be an important component of primary care for all these patients.[8] Although control of these factors will not reverse the atherosclerotic process, it may limit the progression of disease. Furthermore, some data indicate that smoking cessation lessens the severity of symptoms in many patients. Also, a daily exercise program of regular walking may improve collateral development and increase the anaerobic tolerance of ischemic skeletal muscle. Finally, pharmacotherapy with medications, such as pentoxifylline and cilostazol, can be a valuable adjunct in selected patients.[9,10] Although the mechanisms of action of these agents are unclear, both have effected a modest but significant reduction in claudication symptoms in controlled trials. Some form of platelet inhibition, usually with aspirin, should also be considered for all patients. Although no specific data have demonstrated that antiplatelet therapy is helpful in the treatment of lower extremity arterial occlusive disease, abundant evidence has shown it to be beneficial in the treatment of atherosclerotic occlusive disease in other vascular territories (e.g., coronary and cerebral vessels).

Revascularization

Indications. Revascularization is clearly indicated in patients with critical limb ischemia; without intervention, the vast majority progress to limb loss in a fairly short period of time. Patients with significant or repetitive atheroembolism from an aortoiliac source represent another group who clearly

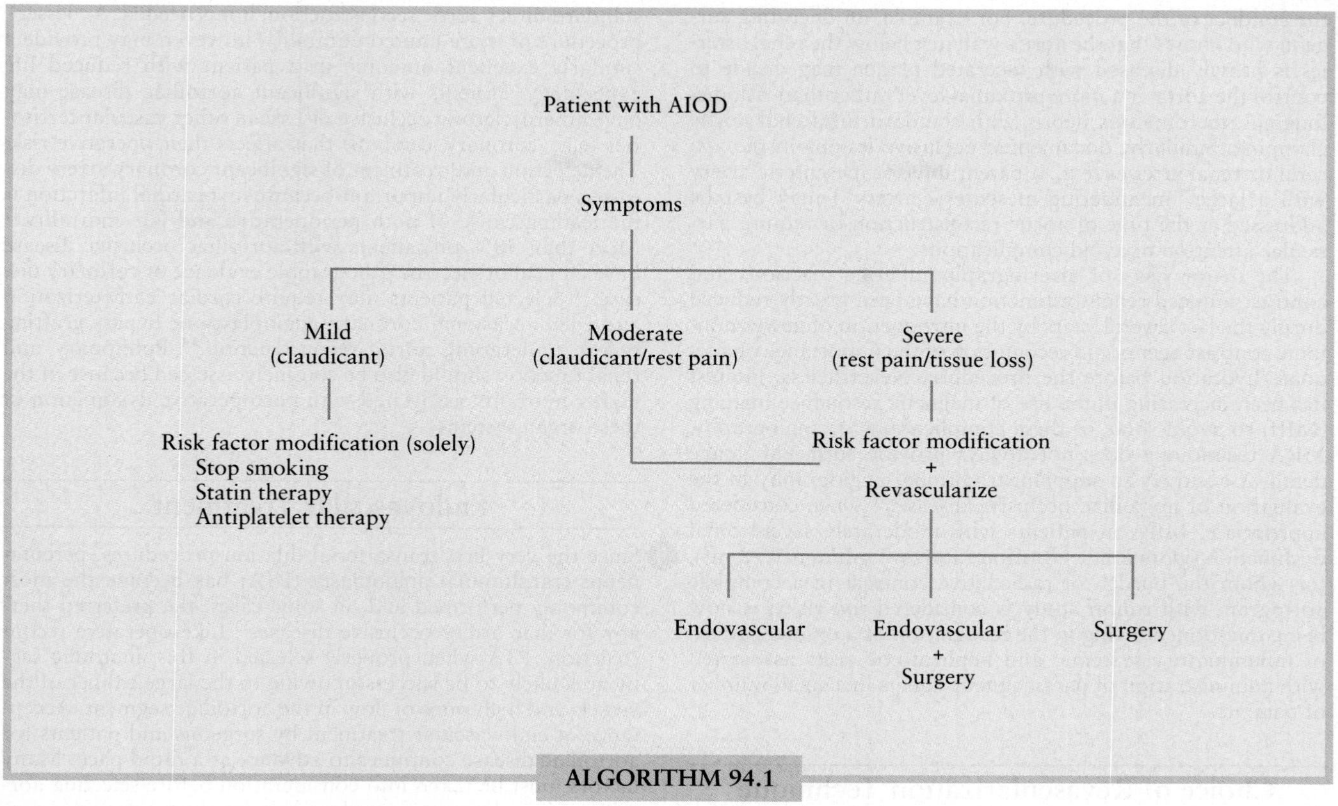

ALGORITHM 94.1. Management of aortoiliac disease.

benefit from operative therapy. Removal or bypass of the culprit lesion(s) eliminates the risk for further macroembolism and microembolism. The treatment for patients with claudication secondary to aortoiliac occlusive disease remains somewhat controversial and must be individualized. Patients with mild to moderate symptoms can be treated medically with satisfactory results. Patients with severe, disabling, lifestyle-limiting symptoms of claudication can benefit from revascularization therapy. The current safety and long-term durability of direct aortic reconstruction make this approach acceptable even for older, higher-risk patients with significant symptoms. For patients who cannot tolerate such procedures, a variety of other methods of revascularization are available that have had good long-term success rates.

Arteriography and Computed Tomography Angiography

Once a decision has been made to proceed with revascularization therapy, contrast digital subtraction arteriography is used for a detailed anatomic evaluation of the arterial circulation of the lower extremities. Such information is necessary to choose the most appropriate method of revascularization (operative or endovascular) and plan the procedure. Biplane abdominal aortography with demonstration of the arterial tree below the inguinal ligament ("runoff") is required. This procedure is most commonly performed from the femoral artery with the best pulse by means of a retrograde Seldinger technique. When neither femoral artery is available, a transaxillary or translumbar approach provides good access. Anteroposterior views of the aortoiliofemoral segments demonstrate the extent of the occlusive process and the pattern of collateral formation. Oblique views of the iliac and femoral arteries are frequently necessary to document posterior wall plaque and stenoses at the origins of the deep femoral arteries. Lateral aortography provides information about the origins of the visceral arteries, whereas anteroposterior views demonstrate the renal arteries. Views of the runoff to at least the midcalf level are required to assess the degree of associated occlusive disease; in cases of critical limb ischemia, visualization of the pedal circulation is usually necessary. CTA with reformatting also requires the administration of contrast. However, it may be administered intervenously. Access to and familiarity with sophisticated computer-based protocols is required for both image acquisition and postprocessing reformatting when CTA is the chosen imaging method. One of the added values of CTA is the ability to survey and retrieve a practically limitless array of images, allowing endovascular treatment planning and follow-up.

Occasionally, the hemodynamic effect of a stenosis or series of stenoses along an iliac arterial segment may be difficult to determine, even with oblique views. When the significance of a stenosis remains in question, pressures proximal and distal to the lesion(s) can be measured. A systolic drop of more than 5 to 10 mm Hg across the stenosis is indicative of a hemodynamically significant lesion. For borderline cases, distal pressure measurements can be obtained before and after interarterial injection of a vasodilator to simulate the hyperemic hemodynamics of exercise. A pressure drop of 20 mm Hg or more during hyperdynamic flow is considered to indicate hemodynamic significance.

The information supplied by arteriography is crucial to the success of a revascularization procedure. In addition to providing a detailed "road map" of the exact arterial segments involved and the pathology present, arteriography identifies associated anatomic variations (e.g., accessory renal arteries) and aortic wall characteristics (e.g., extensive calcification, ulcerated plaque), which may alter the operative approach and the conduct of the procedure. For example, an operating surgeon who knows that the aortic wall just below the renal arteries is heavily diseased with ulcerated plaque may decide to control the aorta at a more proximal level rather than risk dislodging atheromatous debris with standard infrarenal aortic clamping. Similarly, documented occlusive lesions in the visceral or renal arteries (e.g., a patent inferior mesenteric artery with a large "meandering mesenteric artery") may best be addressed at the time of aortic reconstruction or require particular attention to avoid complications.

The major risks of arteriography, allergic reactions and contrast-induced renal dysfunction have been greatly reduced during the last several years by the introduction of newer nonionic contrast agents and recognition of the importance of adequate hydration before the procedure. Nevertheless, interest has been increasing in the use of magnetic resonance imaging (MRI) to avoid some of these complications of angiography. MRA technology does not always provide sufficient image detail or accuracy to supplant traditional angiography in the evaluation of aortoiliac occlusive disease.[11] Once considered appropriate, MRA in patients with moderately severe renal dysfunction (glomerular filtration rate <60 mL/min/1.72 m^2), for whom the burden of radioactive contrast in a complete aortogram with runoff study is considered too risky, is now being questioned owing to the recognition of a unique pattern of inflammatory systemic and nephrotoxic risks associated with administration of paramagnetic agents in a small number of patients.

Choice of Revascularization Technique

A variety of surgical procedures, both endovascular and open, are available for revascularization of the patient with aortoiliac occlusive disease. Selection depends on a number of factors, including the pattern of the occlusive process, patient risk, and surgeon experience. Commonly used techniques include (a) catheter-based balloon dilation, with or without luminal stenting; (b) aortoiliac endarterectomy; (c) arterial reconstruction with an anatomically placed bypass prosthesis (aortofemoral or iliofemoral); and (d) arterial reconstruction with a remote or extra-anatomically placed bypass prosthesis (axillofemoral or bifemoral, femorofemoral, thoracofemoral). Catheter-based techniques are best suited for focal lesions of the common iliac arteries. Endarterectomy is limited to good-risk patients with focal occlusive disease at the aortic bifurcation and common iliac arteries. Prosthetic aortobifemoral bypass is the procedure of choice for most patients with advanced, extensive aortoiliac involvement and is considered the "gold standard" technique for aortoiliac revascularization. Axillofemoral or bifemoral bypass is reserved for the small subpopulation of patients in whom standard direct aortic reconstruction is considered too risky, either for medical reasons (usually severe pulmonary or cardiac disease) or technical reasons (aortic reoperations, multiple prior abdominal procedures with dense adhesions, prior abdominal irradiation, prosthetic graft infections). The descending thoracic aorta can be considered as an alternative arterial source for the construction of a thoracofemoral bypass in good-risk patients with a "hostile" abdomen.[12] Femorofemoral or iliofemoral bypass can be used in poor-risk patients with diffuse unilateral iliac disease or bilateral iliac involvement when the stenosis in one of the iliac arteries can be appropriately treated by balloon angioplasty, with or without intraluminal stenting.

Preoperative Evaluation

The evaluation of patients for whom aortoiliac reconstruction is being considered should include a careful assessment of overall operative risk. Age per se is not a contraindication to a standard direct aortic reconstruction, if it is needed. A "lesser" procedure of more limited durability, however, may provide a similarly excellent outcome in a patient with reduced life expectancy. Patients with significant aortoiliac disease may have atherosclerotic occlusive disease in other vascular territories (e.g., coronary, cerebral) that affects their operative risk. The detection and treatment of significant coronary artery disease is particularly important because myocardial infarction is the leading cause of both perioperative and late mortality.[13] More than 50% of patients with aortoiliac occlusive disease have clinical or electrocardiographic evidence of coronary disease.[13] Selected patients may require cardiac catheterization and even occasional coronary angioplasty or bypass grafting before undergoing aortic reconstruction.[14] Pulmonary and renal function should also be routinely assessed because of the higher mortality associated with postoperative dysfunction of these organ systems.

Endovascular Treatment

8 Since the very first transarterial dilation procedures, percutaneous transluminal angioplasty (PTA) has become the most commonly performed and, in some cases, the preferred therapy for iliac artery occlusive disease.[20] Like operative reconstruction, PTA when properly selected in this anatomic segment is likely to be successful owing to the large caliber of the vessels and high rates of flow in the aortoiliac segment. Acceptance of endovascular treatment by surgeons and patients for aortoiliac disease continues to advance at a rapid pace. Many factors must be taken into consideration before selecting aortoiliac angioplasty or stent placement for the treatment of aortoiliac occlusive disease. The continuum from claudication to limb-threatened ischemia, and patient comorbidities are primary considerations. Usually patients with mild to moderate aortoiliac disease are easily amenable to angioplasty or stent. The best results are obtained with short, focal, nonocclusive lesions in the common iliac arteries.[15] Patients with severe atherosclerotic lesions, long (>10 cm) and complex aortoiliac stenosis, or occlusions would benefit from revascularization, although many anecdotes illustrate short-term success with endovascular approaches (Fig. 94.12). Complications (thrombosis, dissection, perforation, and distal embolism) in experienced hands are uncommon and can frequently be remedied with intraluminal stenting or thrombolytic therapy. Stents have made it possible to apply angioplasty in a larger number of lesions (e.g., longer occlusions) and may improve long-term patency rates by reducing rates of restenosis.[16] This technique is particularly useful in high-risk patients, those with critical ischemia secondary to multiple-level disease, and patients in whom iliac PTA can be combined with an infrainguinal bypass for limb salvage. Even in good-risk patients with focal iliac disease, however, PTA may be the preferred initial approach, with surgical intervention reserved for the more difficult circumstances following endovascular failures. If the presence of an appropriate lesion is suspected, PTA may be considered at the same time that the diagnostic arteriogram is performed. Open surgery involves an up-front risk in the initial stages, with anesthesia and longer hospital stays. The endovascular model involves the continued surveillance and initial lower up-front risk. These patients will require follow-up angiography and repeat interventions as the disease continues to progress and, ultimately, more investment in time and resources. Complications are usually local. Long-term results depend on the initial extent of aortoiliac disease, but usually will not be as good as open surgery. Results from angioplasty of iliac arteries range from 70% to 90% over a 3-year span. This continues to decrease to as low as 50% patency at 5 years. Iliac artery occlusion with resultant endovascular recanalization shows patency of 70% at 1 year and 60% at 3 years. Nonetheless, the results of endovascular treatment are improving and the

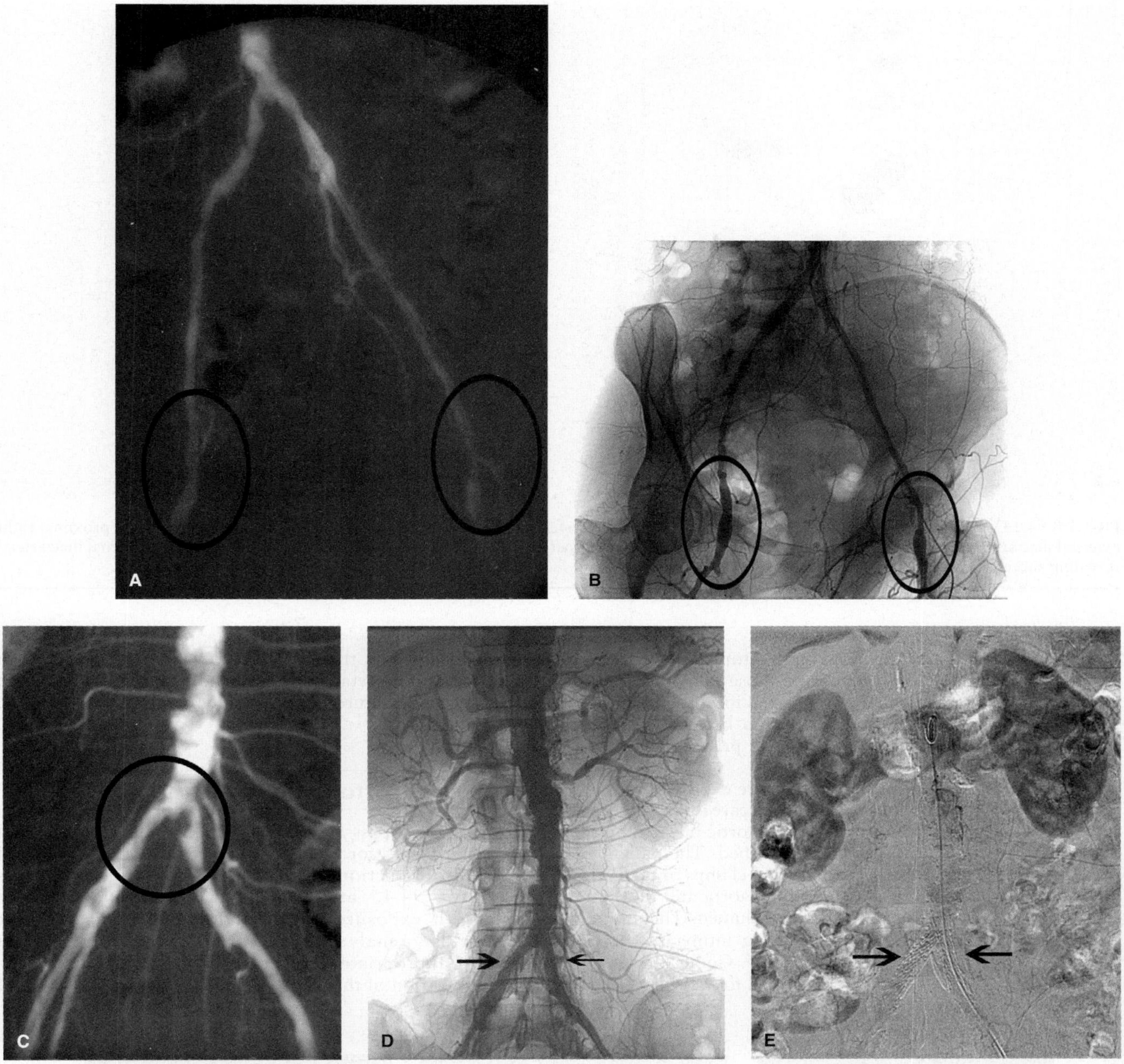

FIGURE 94.12. **A:** Abdominal aortogram demonstrating bilateral iliac and femoral artery stenosis. **B:** Bilateral iliac and femoral artery endarterectomies. **C:** Bilateral common iliac artery stenosis. **D:** Placement of bilateral common iliac artery stents. **E:** Digital subtraction view of bilateral common iliac artery stents.

proportion of patients being treated by endovascular methods has increased in recent years. Many vascular specialists now prefer endovascular treatment over open treatment. Open surgery involving an aortobifemoral bypass has been a durable operation for decades. Patency is usually greater than 85% at 5 years. Of course, the prudent vascular specialist is thoroughly conversant with both open and endovascular treatment modes and, ordinarily, will be capable of providing whichever alone or in combination is best for the patient. Clinical follow-up of the patient by the treating vascular specialist is ordinarily routine as well.

9 A combined open operation with endovascular surgery appears to have promising results and demonstrates that ideal patient care outcomes remain in the hands of the vascular surgeon (Fig. 94.13). Preliminary results show that infrainguinal bypass with concomitant aortoiliac angioplasty or stenting, or both, have a slightly higher patency of the distal bypass.[17] With the continued advancement of stents, smaller delivery devices, fluoroscopy equipment, and operator skills, endovascular intervention will continue to be a major component of care of the patient with aortoiliac occlusive disease.

Endarterectomy

Endarterectomy was more commonly performed in the era before prosthetic graft conduits were developed. Currently, direct arterial repair is reserved for the management of focal atheroocclusive disease (type I) limited to the distal aorta and common iliac arteries (Fig. 94.14). When performed for this

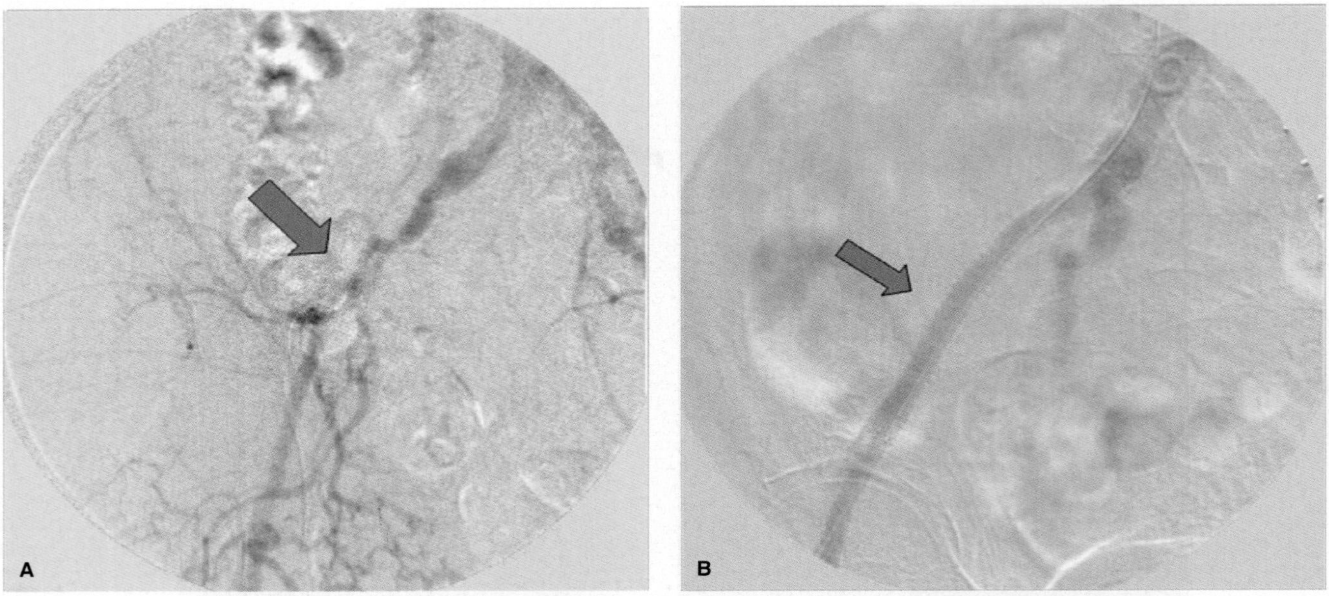

FIGURE 94.13. **A:** Initial angiogram revealing significant right iliac system occlusive disease with a chronic total occlusion of the proximal right external iliac artery. **B:** Follow-up digital subtraction arteriogram after percutaneous balloon angioplasty and stenting of right external iliac artery, revealing successful recannulization with a widely patent lumen.

specific indication, aortoiliac endarterectomy can produce excellent long-term results, similar to those of aortofemoral grafting. Endarterectomy is less well suited for disease extending in the external iliac arteries and is to be avoided when aneurysmal degeneration complicates the primary atheroocclusive aortoiliac process.

The aorta and common iliac arteries are exposed and vascular control is secured. During dissection, care is taken to preserve the autonomic nerves overlying the aortic bifurcation so that normal sexual function is not disturbed. The patient is then heparinized and atraumatic occlusion clamps or tapes are applied. Arteriotomies are made over the aorta and the common iliac arteries to expose the diseased lumen. The atherosclerotic plaque, along with the overlying intima and inner portion of the involved media, is removed. Good "breakoff" points for the removed plaques are needed to prevent postoperative thrombosis that results from the formation of an occluding flap of retained atheroma. The arteriotomies are closed by direct suture or with patch angioplasty, depending on vessel caliber.

Aortofemoral Prosthesis

10 Aortofemoral bypass is the most durable and reliable of all treatment options, for which reason it is the reference standard for the reconstruction of advanced aortoiliac occlusive disease (Figs. 94.15 and 94.16). The operative sequence starts with exposure of the abdominal aortic segment between the renal and inferior mesenteric arteries by means of appropriate retroperitoneal dissection and cephalad mobilization of the fourth portion of the duodenum and

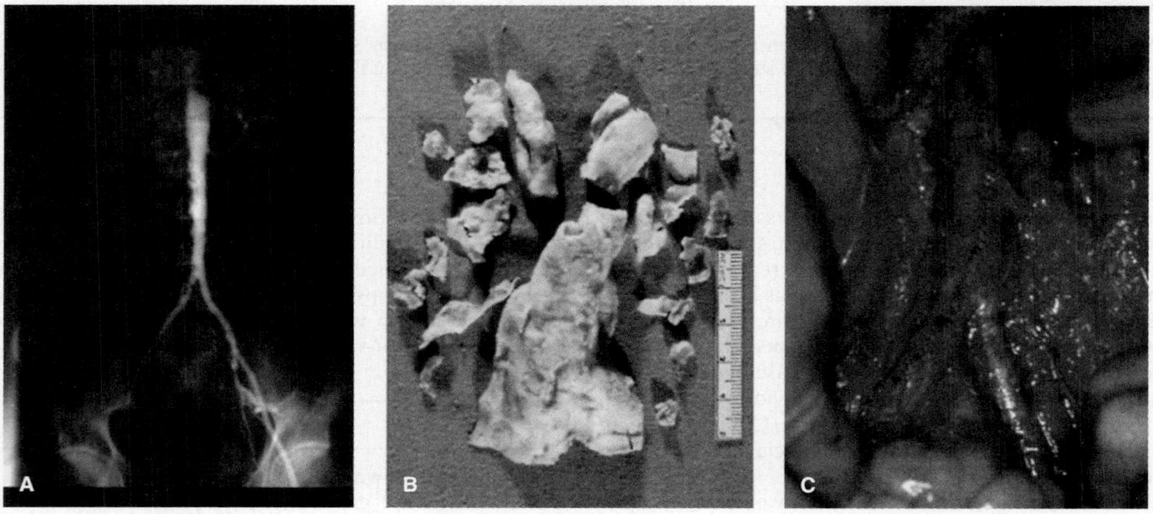

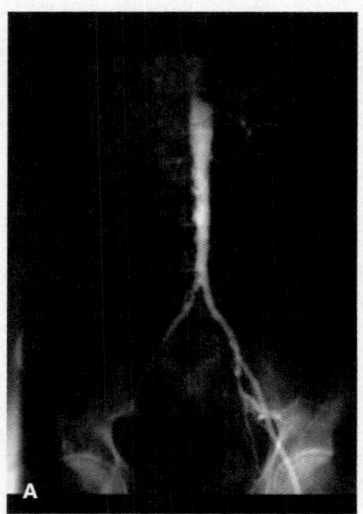

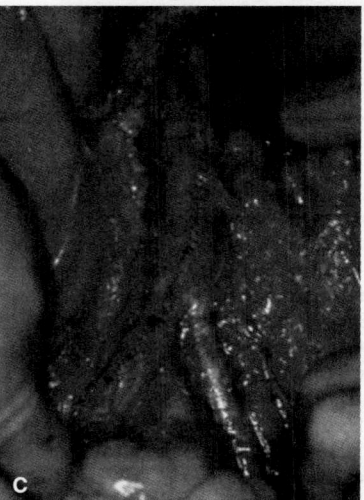

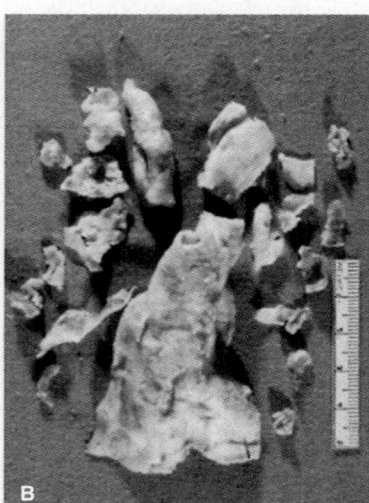

FIGURE 94.14. **A:** Preoperative aortogram demonstrating severe artherosclerosis. **B:** Large amount of plaque removal. **C:** Completion operating room photo of closed, repaired aorta and iliacs.

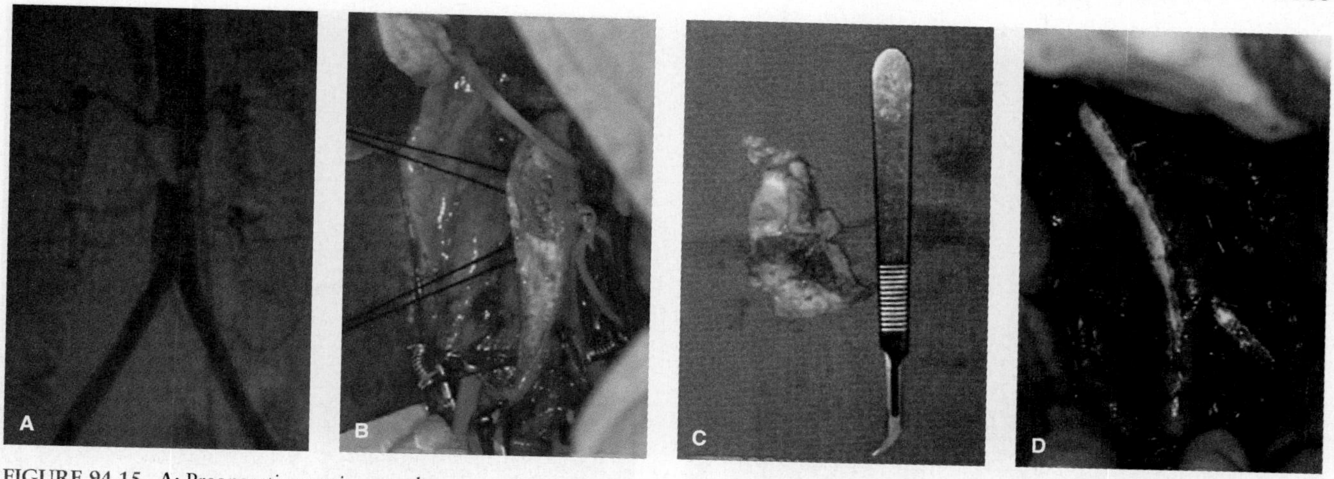

FIGURE 94.15. **A:** Preoperative angiogram demonstrates severe stenosis of the infrarenal aorta with mild stenosis bilaterally at the origin of the common iliac arteries (type I disease). **B:** Long arteriotomy over the infrarenal aorta and proximal right common iliac artery reveals advanced ulcerated luminal disease. A second, separate arteriotomy over the left common iliac artery was also created to approach plaque in that vessel. **C:** Aortic component of the atherosclerotic plaque. **D:** The two arteriotomies are closed, and polytetrafluoroethylene patches are used for angioplasty.

the left renal vein. Care is taken during dissection to avoid injury to the lumbar veins. Moreover, gentle handling of the dissected segment may lessen the risk for atheroembolism during the operation. The common, superficial, and deep femoral arteries are secured through separate groin incisions. Retroperitoneal tunnels are then developed between the exposed infrarenal aorta and the groins by means of blunt dissection. Care is taken to avoid injury to the bowel, particularly the rectosigmoid on the left. The tunnels are directed posterior to the ureter to avoid postoperative obstructive uropathy from graft limb compression of the ureter. A prosthesis of the appropriate size (polytetrafluoroethylene or Dacron) is selected, and the patient is heparinized. With an occluding clamp below the renal arteries and another just above the inferior mesenteric artery, the proximal anastomosis is performed as either an end-to-end or end-to-side graft to the aorta. The end-to-side technique has been found to be just as good, depending on the pattern of occlusive lesions and opportunity to perfuse the internal iliac arteries. The proximal anastomosis is placed as close to the renal arteries as practical to prevent future compromise of the bypass resulting from progression of atherosclerosis in the remaining infrarenal cuff. The limbs of the prosthesis are then delivered through the retroperitoneal tunnels into the groins. The distal anastomoses are performed to the common femoral arteries and may be carried into the deep femoral arteries as needed. The technique for distal femoral anastomosis is chosen to ensure adequate graft outflow, particularly if superficial femoral artery disease is present. In the patient with tissue loss secondary to type III or multiple-level aortoiliac disease associated with occluded superficial femoral arteries and compromised deep collaterals, concomitant distal reconstruction should rarely be required (Fig. 94.17).

Aortofemoral bypass has excellent 5- and 10-year graft patency rates of approximately 85% and 75%, respectively.

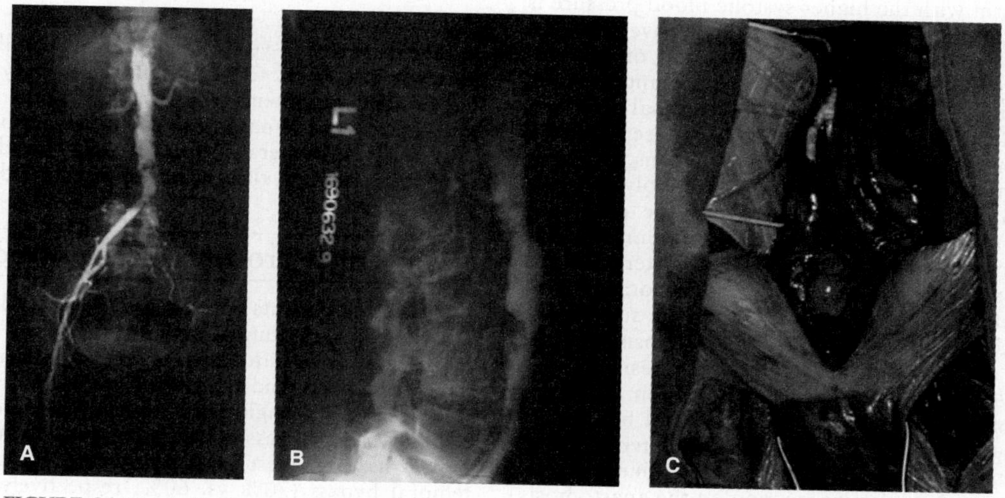

FIGURE 94.16. **A, B:** Preoperative biplane aortograms demonstrate advanced preocclusive disease of the infrarenal aorta and its bifurcation with occlusion of the left common and external iliac arteries (type II disease). **C:** The patient was treated with placement of an aortobifemoral prosthesis. The short shaft and limbs of the prosthesis are in a retroperitoneal location and are partially covered with a layer of posterior parietal peritoneum. The two groin incisions are kept open to display the anastomoses of the two limbs to the common femoral arteries.

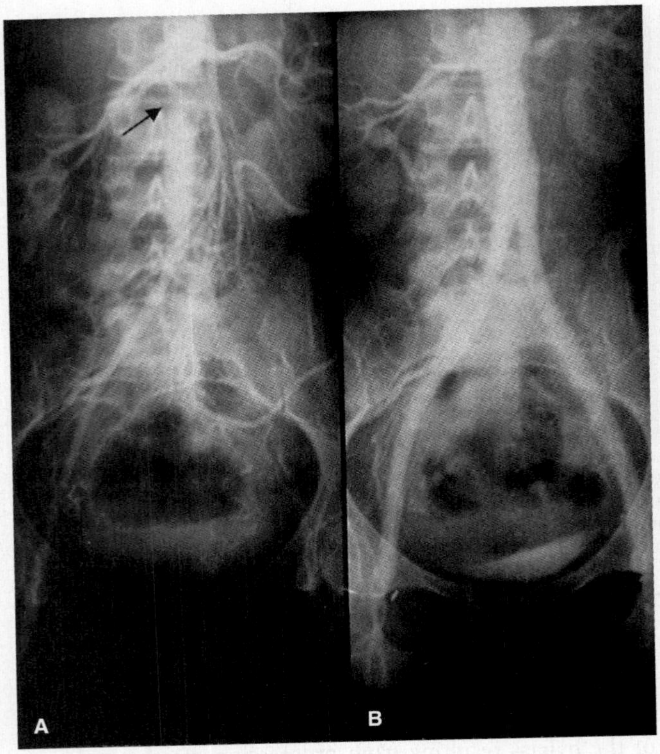

FIGURE 94.17. **A:** Preoperative aortogram demonstrates advanced preocclusive disease of the infrarenal aorta and its bifurcation with occlusion of the left common and external iliac arteries (type II disease). **B:** Aortogram after placement of an aortobifemoral prosthesis.

Perioperative morbidity and mortality are reported to be below 10% and 5%, respectively, in many centers.[13,18]

Axillofemoral Prosthesis

Axillofemoral extra-anatomic reconstruction has been used for revascularization in poor-risk patients and in those with a hostile abdomen and has been reported to be an acceptable alternative to aortofemoral prosthesis. The axillary artery supplying the arm with the higher systolic blood pressure is usually chosen as the inflow vessel. The operative sequence starts with exposure of the most proximal part of the axillary artery through an infraclavicular incision and splitting of the pectoralis major muscle between its sternal and clavicular heads. The common, superficial, and deep femoral arteries are then dissected through groin incisions. The axillary or long limb of an externally supported polytetrafluoroethylene graft is then advanced behind the pectoralis major muscle and through a subcutaneous tunnel in the anterior axillary line connecting the axillary artery and the ipsilateral groin. Next, a cross-femoral–to–femoral limb of the graft is delivered through a subcutaneous suprapubic tunnel connecting the two groins. An anastomosis between the proximal axillary artery and the prosthesis is constructed in an end-graft–to–side-of-artery fashion. The graft is positioned parallel to the axillary artery and behind the pectoral muscles for the first 10 cm, before it enters the subcutaneous channel along the anterior axillary line. Following this plan seems to minimize traction on the anastomosis during arm movement and reduces the incidence of anastomotic disruption. The distal anastomoses are performed to the common femoral arteries and may be carried over or onto the deep femoral arteries to ensure adequate graft outflow (Fig. 94.18).

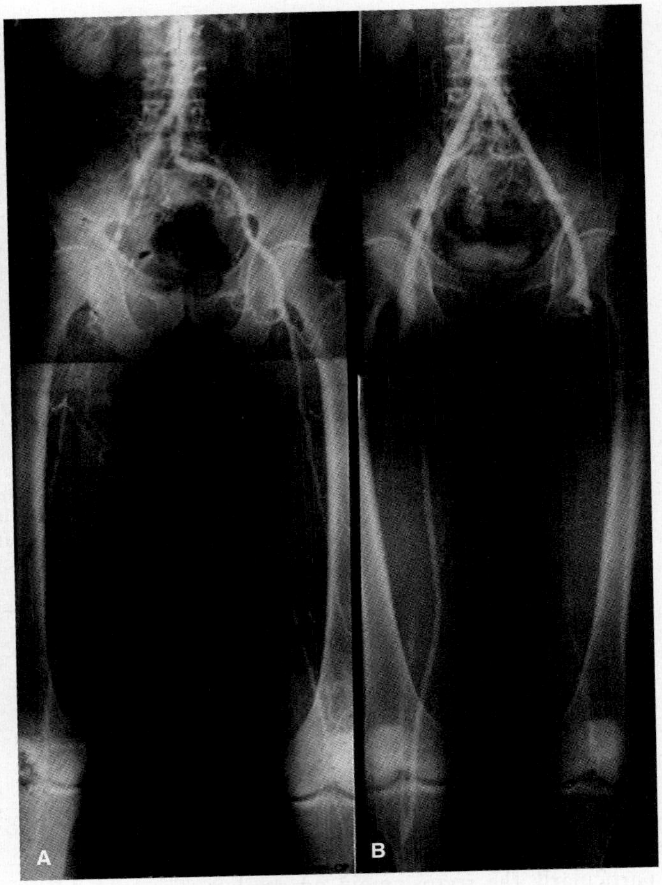

FIGURE 94.18. This diabetic patient presented with gangrene of the right first and second toes. **A:** The preoperative angiogram revealed aortic bifurcation disease, right external iliac and superficial femoral arterial occlusion, and reconstitution of a heavily diseased right deep femoral artery. On the left, occlusion of the superficial femoral artery is seen, with a patent left deep femoral artery supplying the left leg (multiple-level type III disease). **B:** The patient underwent an aortobifemoral bypass with a concomitant right femoral–to–below-knee popliteal bypass to bring pulsatile flow to the diseased forefoot.

The reported 5-year patency of the axillofemoral graft varies widely (30% to 80%), but is generally accepted to be lower than the patency of an aortofemoral prosthesis. The axillobifemoral bypass should therefore be reserved for patients with bilateral advanced aortoiliac disease who are either poor surgical risks or have a hostile abdomen.[19]

Other Prosthetic Reconstructions

For high-risk patients with diffuse advanced disease limited to one iliac artery, unilateral femorofemoral or iliofemoral bypass may be used to revascularize the ischemic extremity. If the contralateral iliac artery is normal or bears a lesion that is well treated by angioplasty or stenting, cross-femoral–to–femoral artery bypass is worthy of consideration. Iliofemoral bypass has a modest graft patency advantage over femorofemoral bypass (70% vs. 60%, respectively), but the main advantage is avoidance of a second groin incision and its associated complications. Femorofemoral bypasses are reserved for patients with occluded or heavily diseased common iliac arteries, in whom iliofemoral bypass is not advisable (Fig. 94.19).

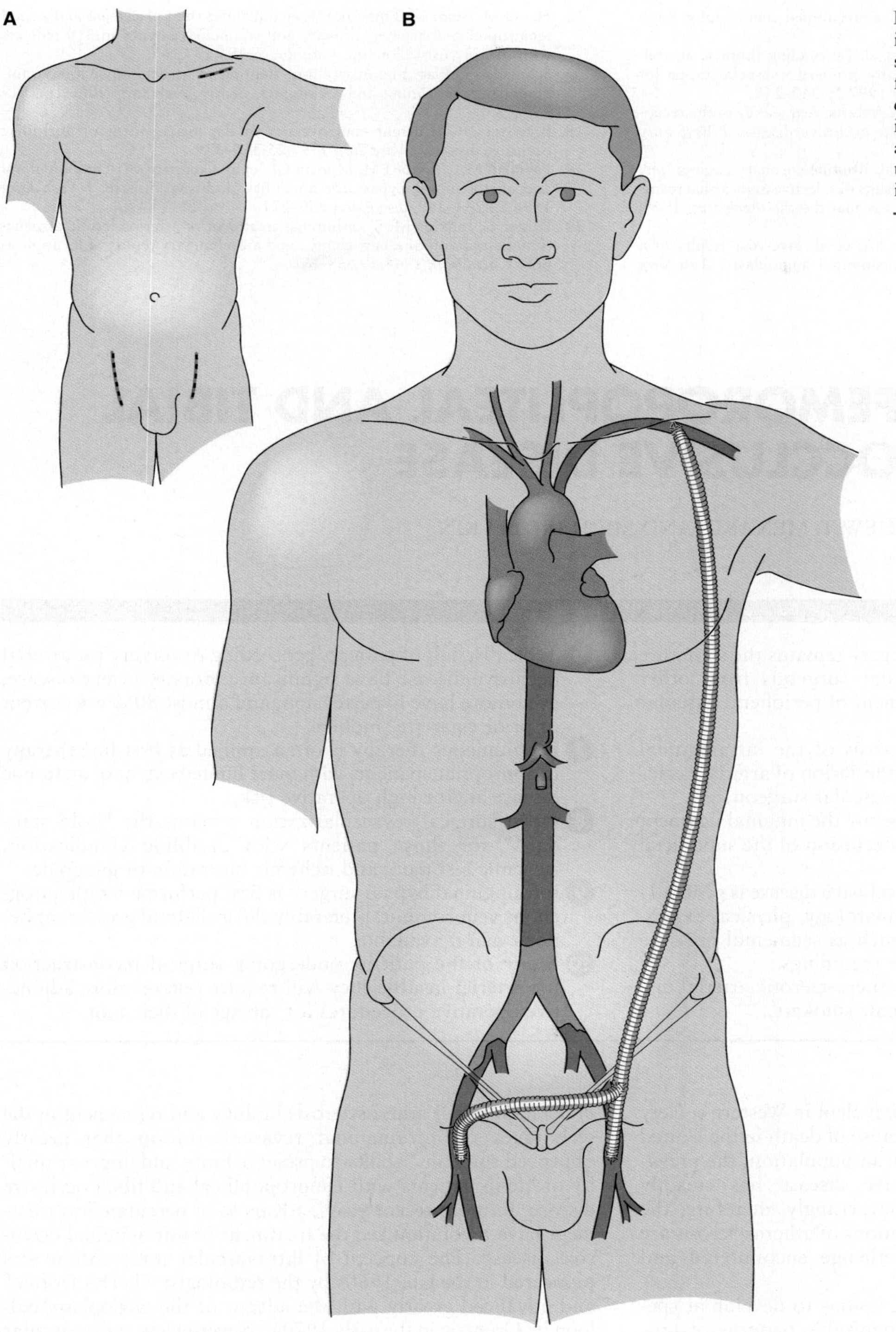

FIGURE 94.19. A unilateral axillary to ipsilateral femoral artery bypass graft is supplemented with a cross-femoral–to–femoral artery bypass graft limb. This extra-anatomic graft is frequently implanted on the right (although the artist's depiction shows the left) to allow unimpeded access to the thoracoabdominal aorta when necessary.

References

1. Kannel WB, Shurtleff D. The Framingham study: cigarettes and the development of intermittent claudication. *Geriatrics* 1973;28:61–68.
2. Hughson WG, Mann JI, Garrod A. Intermittent claudication: prevalence and risk factors. *Br Med J* 1978;1:1379–1381.
3. Leriche R, Morel A. The syndrome of thrombotic obliteration of the aortic bifurcation. *Ann Surg* 1948;127:193–206.
4. DeBakey ME, Lawrie GM, Glaeser DH. Patterns of atherosclerosis and their surgical significance. *Ann Surg* 1985;201:115–131.
5. Brewster DC, Darling RC. Optimal methods of aortoiliac reconstruction. *Surgery* 1978;84:739.
6. Norgen L, Hiatt WR. Inter-Society Consensus for the Management of PAD. *J Vasc Surg* 2007;45:S1–S67.
7. Kohler TR, Nance DR, Cramer MM, et al. Duplex scanning for diagnosis of aortoiliac and femoropopliteal disease: a prospective study. *Circulation* 1987;76:1074–1080.
8. Girolami GB, Bernardi E, Prins MH, et al. Treatment of intermittent claudication with physical training, smoking cessation, pentoxifylline, or nafronyl: a meta-analysis. *Arch Intern Med* 1999;159:337–345.
9. Porter JM, Cutler BS, Lee BY, et al. Pentoxifylline efficacy in the treatment of intermittent claudication: multicenter controlled double-blind trial with objective assessment of chronic occlusive arterial disease patients. *Am Heart J* 1982;104:66–71.
10. Money SR, Herd JA, Isaacsohn JL, et al. Effects of cilostazol on walking distances in patients with intermittent claudication caused by peripheral vascular disease. *J Vasc Surg* 1998;27:267–275.
11. Haney TF, Debatin JF, Leung DA, et al. Evaluation of the aortoiliac and renal arteries: comparison of breath-hold, contrast-enhanced,

three-dimensional MR angiography with conventional angiography. *Radiology* 1997;204:357–362.
12. Passman MA, Farber MA, Criado E, et al. Descending thoracic aortoiliofemoral artery bypass grafting: a role for primary revascularization for aortoiliac occlusive disease? *J Vasc Surg* 1999;29:249–258.
13. Szilagyi DE, Elliott JP Jr, Smith RF, et al. A thirty-year survey of the reconstructive surgical treatment of aortoiliac occlusive disease. *J Vasc Surg* 1986;3:421–436.
14. Hertzer NR, Young JR, Kramer JR, et al. Routine coronary angiography prior to elective aortic reconstruction: results of selective myocardial revascularization in patients with peripheral vascular disease. *Arch Surg* 1979; 114:1336–1344.
15. Johnston KW, Rae M, Hogg-Johnston SA, et al. Five-year results of a prospective study of percutaneous transluminal angioplasty. *Ann Surg* 1987;206:403–413.
16. Henry M, Amor M, Ethevenot G, et al. Palmaz stent placement in iliac and femoropopliteal arteries: primary and secondary patency in 310 patients with 2- to 4-year follow-up. *Radiology* 1995;197:167.
17. Schneider P. Iliac angioplasty and stenting in association with infrainguinal bypass: timing and techniques. *Semin Vasc Surg* 2003;16:291–299.
18. Brewster DC. Current controversies in the management of aortoiliac occlusive disease. *J Vasc Surg* 1997;25:365–379.
19. Passman MA, Taylor LM, Moneta GL, et al. Comparison of axillofemoral and aortofemoral bypass for aortoiliac occlusive disease. *J Vasc Surg* 1996;23:263–269; discussion 269–271.
20. Dotter C, Judkins M. Transluminal treatment of arteriosclerotic obstruction: description of a new technic and a preliminary report of its application. *Circulation* 1964;30:654–670.

CHAPTER 95 ■ FEMOROPOPLITEAL AND TIBIAL OCCLUSIVE DISEASE

WILLIAM P. ROBINSON, MATTHEW T. MENARD, AND MICHAEL BELKIN

KEY POINTS

1. Infrainguinal arterial bypass surgery remains the signature operation distinguishing vascular surgeons from other specialists involved in the treatment of peripheral vascular disease.
2. Chronic obliterative atherosclerosis of the infrainguinal vessels is the most prevalent manifestation of arterial occlusive disease encountered by the vascular surgeon.
3. The most common lesion seen below the inguinal ligament is that of a short-segment total occlusion of the superficial femoral artery.
4. The diagnosis of infrainguinal occlusive disease is generally made based on patient symptomatology, physical examination, and noninvasive tests, such as segmental pressure measurements and pulse volume recordings.
5. A particularly virulent form of atherosclerotic arterial disease is often found in young female smokers.
6. Typically, half of patients proceeding to surgery for arterial occlusive disease have significant coronary artery disease, even more have hypertension, and almost 80% are current or prior cigarette smokers.
7. Percutaneous therapy is often applied as first-line therapy in appropriate patients with more limited extent of anatomic disease and/or high operative risk.
8. Open surgical revascularization remains the "gold standard" for those patients with disabling claudication, ischemic rest pain, and ischemic ulceration or gangrene.
9. Infrainguinal bypass surgery is best performed with autogenous vein conduit, preferably the ipsilateral greater saphenous vein if available.
10. Many of the patients undergoing surgical reconstruction for arterial insufficiency will require one or more adjunctive operative procedures for salvage of their foot.

Arterial occlusive disease is highly prevalent in Western society and constitutes the leading overall cause of death in the United States. With the aging of the American population, the prevalence of lower extremity occlusive disease has steadily increased in recent decades. Not surprisingly, therefore, the clinical manifestations and complications of atherosclerosis are the most common therapeutic challenge encountered and treated by vascular surgeons.

The tendency for atherosclerotic lesions to develop at specific anatomic sites and follow recognizable patterns of progression was first appreciated in the late 1700s by the British anatomist and surgeon John Hunter. Considered one of the forefathers of vascular surgery, his dissections of atherosclerotic aortic bifurcations are preserved at the Hunterian museum in London and presage the disease process that Leriche would give his name to 150 years later.[1] The modern era of surgical reconstruction for complex atherosclerotic occlusive disease began in earnest in 1947, when the Portuguese surgeon J. Cid dos Santos successfully endarterectomized a heavily diseased common femoral artery.[2] Four years later, building on the pioneering work of Alexis Carrel,[3] Kunlin[4] would report the first long-segment vein bypass in the lower extremity. It would be another 10 years before the initial efforts to extend vein grafting to the tibial level were described by McCaughan.[5] The last three decades have seen tremendous advances in both the understanding of atherosclerosis biology and refinement in the techniques of infrainguinal revascularization that greatly improved surgeons' ability to preserve limbs and improve quality of life in patients with femoropopliteal and tibial occlusive disease. In more recent years, advances in percutaneous treatment have revolutionized the treatment of infrainguinal occlusive disease. The concept of intravascular intervention was pioneered in the late 1960s by the radiologist Charles Dotter,[6] and advanced greatly with the advent of the angioplasty balloon by Gruntzig in the early 1970s.[7] Nevertheless, endovascular intervention for infrainguinal disease was not utilized significantly until the 1990s. The technology remains in rapid development and surrounded by ongoing controversy as to its proper role.

1 Although a diverse range of technical skill is required of the contemporary vascular and endovascular surgeon, it is worth noting that infrainguinal arterial bypass surgery remains the signature operation distinguishing vascular surgeons from other specialists involved in the treatment of peripheral vascular disease. This distinction stems primarily from the fact that the outcome of infrainguinal reconstruction is highly dependent on the judgment and technical skill of the surgeon, with the end result being either successful limb salvage or major limb amputation. This chapter reviews the surgical management of femoropopliteal and tibial arterial occlusive disease

and details standard and advanced techniques underlying successful infrainguinal operative revascularization. It also briefly discusses the emerging role of endovascular surgery in the management of infrainguinal occlusive disease, though a thorough review of these techniques is beyond the scope of the chapter.

INFRAINGUINAL ARTERIAL OCCLUSIVE DISEASE

Epidemiology and Risk Factors

The prevalence of peripheral arterial disease (PAD) is between 3% and 10% overall and 15% and 20% in those over age 70.[8,9] Symptomatic PAD in the form of claudication affects approximately 10 million Americans, including 1% to 2% of those younger than 50 years, 5% of those ages 50 to 70, and 10% of those older than 70 years.[10] Of those older than 50 years of age with PAD, 1% to 3% will have critical leg ischemia (CLI) in the form of rest pain or gangrene.[11,12] The incidence of CLI ranges from 220 to 1,000 new cases per year in a European or American population of 1 million people.[13] The classic risk factors for infrainguinal occlusive disease are the same as those for the development of atherosclerosis in general and include age, male gender, hypertension, diabetes mellitus (DM), smoking, dyslipidemia, family history, and homocysteinemia. The propensity for heavy smokers to develop superficial femoral artery disease and for diabetics to develop tibial disease should be noted. More recent evidence indicates that nonwhite ethnicity, inflammatory markers such as C-reactive protein, and perhaps chronic renal insufficiency (CRI) are also associated with an increased risk of PAD.[14–16]

Presentation and Natural History

2 Chronic obliterative atherosclerosis of the infrainguinal vessels is the most prevalent manifestation of arterial occlusive disease encountered by the vascular surgeon. Patients are classified into two broad categories depending on their symptomatology: claudicants and those with CLI. Claudication, the reproducible ischemic muscle pain resulting from inadequate oxygen delivery during exercise, is the cardinal presenting symptom. Natural history studies indicate patients with claudication have increased rates of cardiovascular mortality, but an overall low risk of limb loss.[17,18] Seventy to 80% of patients with claudication demonstrate a stable pattern of disease throughout their lifetime or have improvement in their symptoms as a result of risk factor modification, whereas 20% to 30% undergo operation within 5 years as a result of disease progression. Claudication will progress to critical limb ischemia in only 5% to 10% of patients over their lifetime. However, claudication is a marker for increased cardiovascular morbidity and mortality, with 20% of patients experiencing a nonfatal myocardial infarction or stroke and 10% to 15% dying of cardiovascular-related mortality at 5 years.[12] The annual rates of mortality and limb loss in patients with claudication are approximately 2% to 5% and 1%, respectively.[12,19]

3 The most common atherosclerotic disease pattern encountered distal to the inguinal ligament is that of a short-segment total occlusion of the superficial femoral artery. Isolated disease of this nature typically presents as calf muscle claudication. It is not uncommon, however, for patients with significant single-level lesions, even those with long-segment arterial occlusions, in the superficial femoral artery or more distal arterial beds to be only minimally symptomatic or even asymptomatic. While this can sometimes be the result of exercise limitations imposed by concomitant coronary arterial disease or other physiologic impairments such as lung disease or arthritis, it is more often a result of compensatory collateral flow. Collateral perfusion from the profunda femoral artery around a heavily diseased or occluded superficial femoral artery frequently reconstitutes the distal superficial femoral artery or popliteal artery with enough well-perfused arterial blood to ensure sufficient resting tissue perfusion. Similarly, the rich network of geniculate collaterals can sometimes compensate for a diseased popliteal arterial segment to a sufficient degree to prevent rest pain or overt tissue loss, but will usually prove insufficient to meet the increased metabolic demands of ambulation and forestall claudication.

Critical limb ischemia, which must be differentiated from acute limb ischemia, refers to the presence of either rest pain or tissue loss in the lower limb. Rest pain occurs when blood flow is inadequate to meet resting metabolic requirements. In the lower extremity, ischemic rest pain is localized to the foot, frequently in the instep, and should be easily distinguishable from benign muscle cramps in the calf commonly seen in older patients. Patients with rest pain are often awakened by severe discomfort in the forefoot and hang the affected extremity over the edge of the bed for temporary symptomatic relief. Trophic changes, such as muscle wasting, thinning of skin, thickening of nails, and hair loss are frequently also seen in the distal affected limb. Rest pain is an ominous symptom and usually requires revascularization given the tendency for progression to tissue loss. Ischemia ulcerations usually begin as small, dry ulcers of the toes or heel area and progress to frankly gangrenous changes of the forefoot or heel with greater degrees of arterial insufficiency (Fig. 95.1). Patients with diabetes or renal failure are more susceptible to the development of ischemic pedal ulcers. Disease progression can be very rapid, as up to 50% of patients with CLI are asymptomatic 6 months before onset of pain or ulceration.[10] Such progressive disease, affecting multiple levels of the peripheral vasculature tree, is more frequently encountered in the elderly.

The natural history of CLI is dismal as these patients are generally of advanced age and possess significant comorbidities contributing to their advanced limb ischemia. Overall, approximately 25% of patients with CLI will die at 1 year, 30% will undergo major amputation, and 45% will be alive with two limbs.[12] The rate of amputation is 10 times higher in diabetics than nondiabetics and 5- and 10-year mortality in patients with CLI have been reported to be 60% and 85%, respectively.[10] CLI mandates revascularization for limb salvage when feasible as limb salvage with medical therapy and wound care is virtually futile; success rates for rest pain and tissue loss have been reported to be as low as 27% and 5%, respectively.[10]

Patients with rest pain or ischemic tissue loss typically manifest more extensive involvement of the femoral, popliteal, or tibial arteries than patients with claudication. Those with tissue loss also more commonly have multilevel disease involving the femoropopliteal system in combination with occlusive disease of the aortoiliac vessels or the infrageniculate runoff.[20]

Several identifiable patterns of infrainguinal occlusive disease are well recognized. Patients with an extensive history of cigarette smoking typically have lesions limited to the superficial femoral artery and corresponding symptoms of calf claudication (Fig. 95.2). Diabetes, in contrast, most often targets the tibial vessels, and patients may present with frank tissue necrosis in the presence of a palpable popliteal pulse and no prior history of claudication. Alternatively, the so-called "blue toe syndrome" is a situation in which atherosclerotic debris breaks free from a more proximal source, for example, an aortoiliac or femoropopliteal plaque or a thrombus-lined aneurysm, and embolizes to the distal vessels.[21,22] Wire manipulation during coronary or peripheral angiographic procedures and cross-clamping across a calcific aortic plaque during cardiac surgery are common sources of such emboli. The terminal target of the microembolic particles, whether cholesterol crystals, calcified plaque, thrombus, or platelet aggregates, is typically the small vessels of the toes and heel.

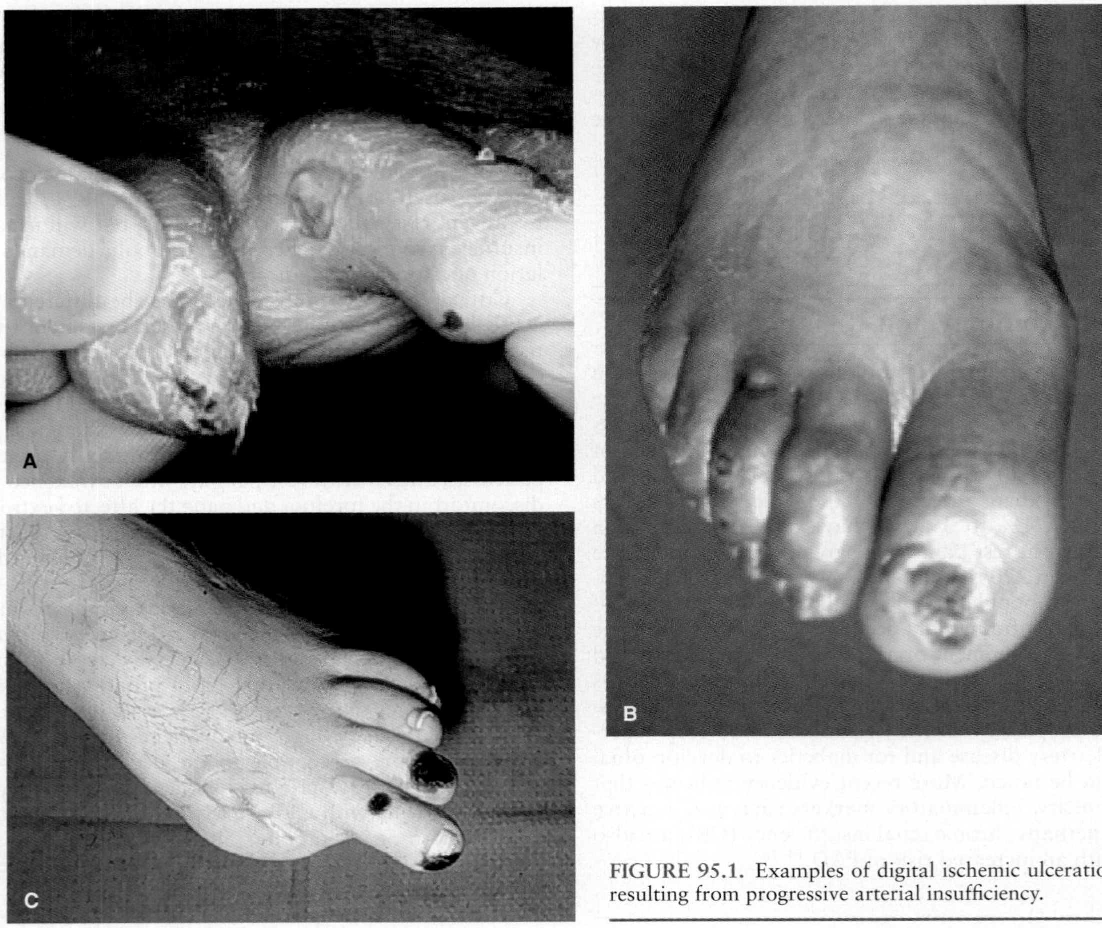

FIGURE 95.1. Examples of digital ischemic ulcerations resulting from progressive arterial insufficiency.

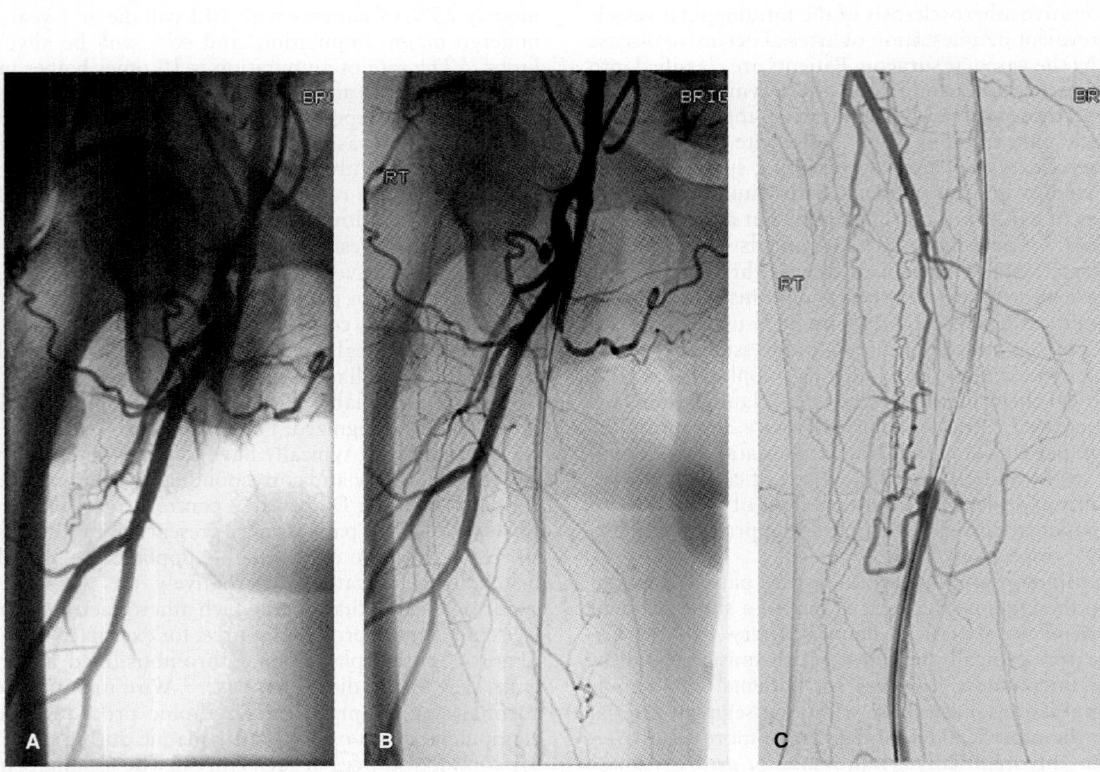

FIGURE 95.2. Long-segment total occlusion of superficial femoral artery in a patient with a long history of cigarette smoking and severe claudication.

5 A particularly virulent form of atherosclerotic arterial disease is often found in young female smokers.[23,24] Radiographic imaging in this subset of patients typically reveals atretic, narrowed vasculature with diffusely calcific atherosclerotic changes. Such patients invariably have an extensive smoking history, with or without other typical risk factors for atherosclerosis. Given the diminutive size of the inflow and outflow vessels, the durability of endovascular intervention is generally inferior in these patients, particularly in the face of continued cigarette use.

6 Typically, half of patients proceeding to surgery for arterial occlusive disease have significant coronary artery disease, even more have hypertension, and almost 80% are current or prior cigarette smokers.[25,26] The low mortality and morbidity associated with operative intervention in recent years is in large part a result of advances in the management of concomitant coronary disease. Specifically, the importance and benefit of better preoperative identification of patients in need of initial coronary revascularization, awareness of the benefit of waiting an interval period following coronary stenting prior to proceeding with major noncoronary vascular surgery, improved perioperative pharmacologic management of patients with impaired myocardium, and more focused efforts to tailor operative and postoperative fluid administration to the individual patient's myocardial reserve are all well recognized.[27,28] Appropriate beta blockade and the use of statins have been shown to reduce cardiovascular events and improve survival in patients undergoing vascular surgery, including infrainguinal bypass.[29,30] General advances in postoperative management, including pulmonary care, infection control, and blood product utilization, have further contributed to the progress seen.

Diagnosis

4 The diagnosis of infrainguinal occlusive disease is generally based on patient symptomatology, physical examination, and noninvasive tests, such as segmental pressure measurements and pulse volume recordings. Accurate history taking and physical examination are crucial to clarifying the diagnosis and guiding a treatment management aimed at maximizing symptom relief and limb preservation. Intermittent claudication (IC) indicative of infrainguinal occlusive disease is typically a cramping, aching discomfort consistently reproducible at a given distance and relieved soon after cessation of ambulation. This must be differentiated from lower extremity pain secondary to nerve root compression or spinal stenosis, which, in contradistinction to vasculogenic pain, often develops when patients maintain a stationary standing posture. Vasculogenic claudication must also be distinguished from venous claudication, hip and ankle arthritis, symptomatic Baker cyst, and chronic compartment syndrome. IC patients with isolated infrainguinal disease will likely have palpable femoral pulses but diminished popliteal and/or pedal pulses.

As is true with claudication, ischemic rest pain must be carefully distinguished from other sources of pain in the elderly population, most commonly arthralgia and neuropathy. Although tissue necrosis and gangrene are usually self-evident when caused by critical ischemia, similar lesions associated with venous stasis, severe anemia, decubitus ulcers, and diabetic neuropathy must be excluded.

Measurement of the ankle-brachial index (ABI) is frequently a useful diagnostic adjunct. A properly performed ABI in a claudicant without significant evidence for vascular calcification would be expected to be between 0.5 and 0.9. Segmental pressure measurements at the level of the upper thigh, lower thigh, upper calf, ankle, and metatarsal level also aid in localizing the level of hemodynamically significant disease. In patients with diabetes mellitus or CRI leading to extensive vascular calcification, the ABI will often be erroneously elevated due to noncompressibility of the vessels. In such circumstances, pulse volume recordings should remain a reliable indicator of perfusion to the various levels of the lower extremity. Measurement of toe pressures also effectively quantitates distal perfusion.

Only after the diagnosis of significant infrainguinal disease and the decision to pursue intervention have been made is further imaging warranted. Duplex ultrasonography, magnetic resonance angiography (MRA), and computed tomographic angiography (CTA) are increasingly being utilized as first-line modalities in planning the optimal revascularization approach, and have supplanted contrast angiography as the initial imaging study of choice in many centers. Nevertheless, due to inherent limitations with each of these techniques, digital subtraction angiography remains the "gold standard" technique for imaging of the vascular tree prior to intervention.

Although a growing literature supports the use of duplex scanning as a standalone preoperative mapping modality,[31] this use requires a highly dedicated vascular laboratory and to date has not gained wide acceptance. CTA is increasingly being utilized as a preoperative road mapping technique in institutions able to provide high-quality three-dimensional reconstructions. MRA is also particularly useful as a noninvasive screening test to determine the suitability for percutaneous therapy, as advances have solved many of the technical limitations of earlier studies (Fig. 95.3). Should a lesion amenable to percutaneous therapy be identified, angiography is then pursued. Alternatively, in some instances of femoropopliteal reconstruction, operative planning may be based solely on MRA scanning if high-quality time-of-flight and gadolinium-enhanced images are obtained.[32–34] In many cases, however, surgeons are reluctant to proceed to surgery without the confirmation afforded by standard contrast angiography. This reluctance is particularly true if the distal target is at the tibial or pedal level, where anatomic detail provided by CTA and MRA remains more limited.

When digital subtraction angiography is undertaken for preoperative planning, a retrograde femoral approach is typically utilized from the contralateral limb. In patients in whom noninvasive imaging indicates a widely patent common femoral and proximal superficial femoral artery and body habitus is not prohibitive, an antegrade approach can serve as a useful alternative. In ambiguous lesions, pull-back pressure measurements, both before and after the administration of a systemic vasodilator such as papaverine or nitroglycerine or the application of a tourniquet to induce reactive hyperemia, can be useful in documenting the hemodynamic significance of a particular stenotic zone.[35] The utilization of gadolinium[36] or carbon dioxide[37] as contrast agents in patients with compromised renal function, although perhaps less effective in the periphery than in the aortoiliac vasculature, can minimize or eliminate the nephrotoxic effects associated with standard iodinated contrast medium.

Medical Treatment

Risk factor modification remains a cornerstone of the management of lower extremity occlusive disease. Smoking cessation has been shown to reduce the risk of disease progression, amputation, and cardiovascular mortality, and may lead to symptom relief in some patients. Smoking cessation has been best achieved with repeated physician assistance, group counseling, nicotine replacement or nicotinic receptor agonists, and antidepressant drug therapy in some patients. Weight and blood pressure reduction and aggressive efforts at lipid control should be addressed with every patient with atherosclerotic disease. Lipid-lowering therapy involves dietary modifications first and utilization of hydroxymethylglutaryl-coenzyme A reductase inhibitors to lower low-density lipoprotein (LDL) cholesterol and fibrates or niacin to raise high-density lipoprotein (HDL) cholesterol. Patients with lower extremity occlusive disease should have a

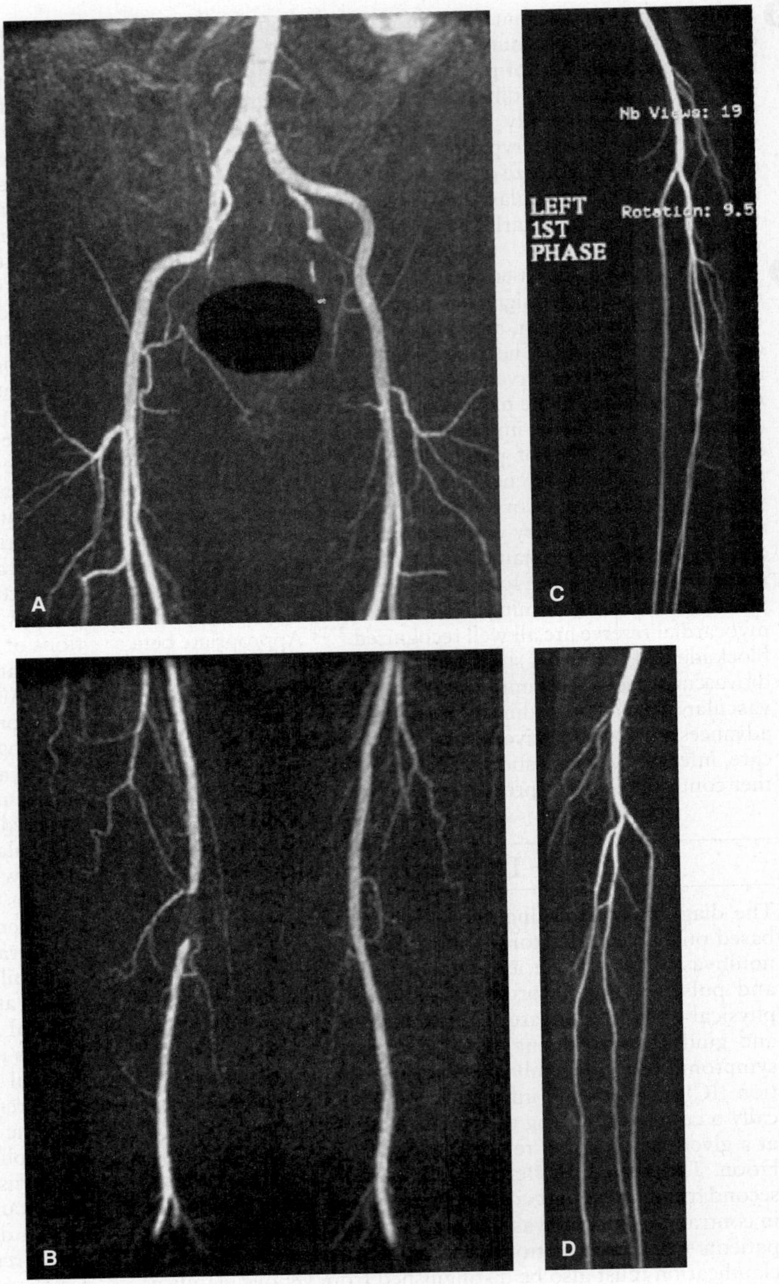

FIGURE 95.3. Magnetic resonance angiogram identifying short-segment occlusion of right superficial femoral artery, a lesion amenable to attempt at percutaneous therapy.

goal LDL cholesterol of less than 70 mg/dL.[38] Patients with diabetes should have aggressive control of blood glucose toward a goal hemoglobin A1C of less than 7%. Antiplatelet therapy in the form of either aspirin or clopidogrel is a critically important element of the treatment of established occlusive disease,[39] given its documented ability to prevent thrombosis and embolization and possibly even to arrest the progression of atherosclerosis. Aspirin and clopidogrel have both been shown to reduce cardiovascular morbidity and mortality in patients with PAD.[40,41]

Strong evidence exists supporting the benefit of a supervised structured walking program[42] in increasing the walking distance of patients with claudication. The benefit of walking outside of a structured regimen with close follow-up is more debatable.[43] Nevertheless, patients should be encouraged to "walk through" the onset of lower extremity pain, resting intermittently as required. Overall, pharmacotherapy has not had a significant impact on relieving symptoms of infrainguinal occlusive disease. There is some evidence to suggest cilostazol, a phosphodiesterase inhibitor, improves walking distance and quality of life.[44,45] While early studies showed that pentoxifylline, a rheologic agent, had beneficial effects on walking distance, later studies have questioned its clinical benefit.[46–47] Similarly, although older studies suggested that prostanoids improved healing of ischemic ulcers, the current evidence does not support the utility of any systemic drug for the relief of ischemic rest pain or the treatment of ischemic ulcerations.[48–50]

Indications for Revascularization

The two major indications for intervention of infrainguinal arterial occlusive disease are lifestyle-limiting claudication and limb-threatening critical ischemia. Less common indications for infrainguinal arterial reconstruction include trauma-related vessel disruption, popliteal artery entrapment syndrome, and femoropopliteal arterial aneurysm with thromboembolism. Infrainguinal revascularization for the treatment of peripheral vascular occlusive disease has been increasingly successful for both long-term palliation of intermittent claudication and for the salvage of limbs threatened by critical ischemia.

Critical ischemia is associated with inevitable amputation for most patients unless revascularization is undertaken. Although there are certainly cases in which primary amputation represents the safest and most advisable solution in the face of irreversible ischemia, particularly for cases in which extensive infection or tissue necrosis is present, an attempt at revascularization is almost always indicated when a limb is threatened by severe ischemia. Improvements in endovascular technology and techniques as well as perioperative management and surgical technique have allowed progressively more distal revascularizations to be successfully completed in an older, sicker, and challenging patient population. In general, high rates of relief for claudication and up to an 80% to 90% limb salvage rate may be anticipated for patients with critical ischemia at institutions devoted to peripheral bypass surgery.[51,52] Though the long-term durability of various endovascular revascularization approaches is not clear, similar rates of limb salvage in the short term to midterm have been demonstrated.

Claudication is a relative indication for intervention given the natural history of the disease, and it remains a subjective assessment on the part of both patient and surgeon as to the relative degree of disability a particular level of claudication pain represents. For example, two-block claudication in a younger patient whose livelihood depends on walking tolerance constitutes a more significant disability than the same degree of claudication in an older, retired individual able to attend to his or her daily affairs without significant consequence. Thus, proximal above-knee surgical reconstruction in a patient with disabling claudication and a patent popliteal artery with intact runoff may be justified in view of its minimal operative mortality, excellent long-term palliation, and absence of added risk of limb loss beyond that expected from the natural history of the disease process. Classically, it has been thought that the benign natural history of claudication does not warrant aggressive femorotibial reconstruction in patients with diffuse superficial femoropopliteal and tibioperoneal disease, though reconstruction will often provide symptomatic benefit and can be considered in a good-risk patient.

In recent years, the low morbidity of endovascular revascularization in combination with patient desire for intervention seems to have lowered the threshold for offering catheter-based revascularization for claudication. Patients once considered appropriate only for risk factor modification, exercise therapy, and medical treatment are now increasingly being offered percutaneous revascularization. Similarly, occlusive disease of the tibial vessels, once thought to be the exclusive domain of operative bypass, is increasingly being treated percutaneously.[53] Nevertheless, endoluminal revascularization is not without risk and is at present of limited durability. It is therefore prudent to follow the classical surgical axiom that because most patients with claudication remain stable for years, it is important to allow sufficient time for collaterals to develop; some patients may improve to such an extent that intervention proves unnecessary.[11]

Approach to Revascularization

The last two decades have seen increasing utilization of endovascular revascularization of infrainguinal occlusive disease. In this light, it cannot be overemphasized that symptom status and not anatomic findings should serve as the basis for revascularization. Once the decision to intervene has been made, a variety of factors should be considered in choosing whether to proceed with an endovascular, surgical, or combined (hybrid) approach. The goals and outcomes of revascularization should be considered in the context of the individual patient's comorbidities, operative risk and overall life expectancy, the extent of the occlusive disease present, and the expected durability of the procedure.

Anatomic variables appear to be the key determinant of the success and durability of endovascular therapy. With the promulgation of endovascular therapy has arisen the need to classify the anatomic severity of disease in order to guide potential therapy and compare outcomes between various modes of revascularization. The Trans-Atlantic Intersociety Consensus Document on Management of Peripheral Arterial Disease (TASC) was published as the result of a multidisciplinary collaboration between key medical and surgical vascular societies in 2000 and an abbreviated update was published in 2007.[13,54] This document classified infrainguinal occlusive lesions into classes A, B, C, and D based on the location of the lesion and the number, length, and severity of the stenoses and/or occlusions present. Their recommendations, which reflect current practice to a variable extent, include initial endovascular treatment for TASC A lesions, primary surgical treatment for TASC D lesions, and individualized tailoring of treatment for TASC B and C lesions depending on endovascular suitability and surgical risk. While a complete description of this classification schema and specific outcomes of endoluminal revascularization according to lesion severity are beyond the scope of this chapter, a few general principles are worth noting. The patency of endoluminal revascularization in general decreases the more distal the disease is and is less in patients with stenoses that are multiple, longer, and more severe.

Role of Endoluminal Therapy

A marked increase in the number and versatility of available balloons and stents has helped to fuel the increasing application of percutaneous technology. While a complete description of endoluminal treatment options and outcomes is beyond the scope of this chapter, a brief introduction is necessary. Percutaneous transluminal angioplasty is generally performed under local anesthesia with minimal intravenous sedation and as either a day surgical procedure or involving an overnight admission. Associated morbidity and mortality has significantly declined in recent years and overall complication rates are low. It is currently unclear whether technical failure changes the available surgical options. Contrast-induced acute renal failure remains the most common complication. With the development of hypo-osmolar and iso-osmolor contrast agents, the overall incidence has fallen to less than 6%,[55] although higher rates are found in patients with preexisting renal failure and diabetes.[56,57]

Access site complications, predominately pseudoaneurysms and arteriovenous malformations (AVMs), occur in 1% of patients.[58] Most of them can be managed conservatively, with close observation, serial hematocrit checks, and fluid and blood product replacement. Surgery is reserved for those patients with ongoing bleeding effecting hemodynamic instability or distal ischemia, or pseudoaneurysms or arteriovenous fistulas that fail to resolve on serial ultrasound imaging with several weeks of careful observation. Stable pseudoaneurysms in patients without coagulopathy can also be managed with ultrasound-guided compression therapy; more recently, ultrasound-guided thrombin injection into the sac has been used with good success.[59] Infection related to the placement of newer percutaneous closure devices utilized for puncture site control typically present several weeks to months after the percutaneous procedure. Rarely, maldeployment of these devices can lead to embolic or thrombotic sequelae causing compromise of distal flow.[60]

Percutaneous transluminal angioplasty (PTA) for femoropopliteal lesions has generally yielded 1-year patency of approximately 77% and 65% for stenoses and occlusions, respectively. Three-year patency after PTA has been reported at 55% to 68% and 40% to 55% for stenoses and occlusions, respectively. Five-year patency data are more limited but have been generally reported to be about 55% and 42% after PTA for femoropopliteal stenoses and occlusions, respectively.[13] Infrapopliteal PTA is generally even less durable, with primary patency of approximately 50% at 1 year.[53] Review of the literature does not provide compelling evidence that stent placement improves the results of femoropopliteal PTA.[61] Many practitioners thus utilize stents selectively for failure of PTA of superficial femoral artery lesions, though there is some evidence that primary stent placement yields higher short-term patency than PTA alone for femoropopliteal lesions.[62]

There is a scarcity of high-level data comparing PTA and bypass surgery. There have been only four randomized trials, and these have included a heterogeneous group of patients, measured different outcomes, and generally included limited anatomic detail.[63–66] Pooled analysis of these trials demonstrates that surgical bypass generally had superior patency to PTA at 1 year, but there were no differences in progression to amputation. Surgery was associated with increased postprocedure
7 complications in patients with CLI.[67] For patients with favorable anatomy and significant operative risk, and for the treatment of claudication in general, percutaneous therapy has
8 assumed a primary initial role. When medical therapy or percutaneous treatment has proven inadequate, open surgical revascularization remains the "gold standard" for those patients with disabling claudication. Furthermore, until the efficacy and durability of infrainguinal percutaneous intervention is better defined, surgical revascularization remains the "gold standard" for any patient with critical limb ischemia, especially those with extensive tissue loss. The relative roles of surgical and percutaneous intervention are actively being refined. It nevertheless appears that the rising popularity and success of femoral and tibial wire-based interventions may be reducing the volume, or ultimately just delay the timing, of subsequent infrainguinal reconstructive surgery. Furthermore, many patients are best treated with a combination of percutaneous and open surgical therapy, often in a single procedure (hybrid procedure). In many instances, endoluminal and open surgical revascularization are thus complementary modes of therapy.

Operative Management

Successful infrainguinal bypass grafting requires adequate arterial inflow. While aortobifemoral, femorofemoral, and axillofemoral bypass grafting remain routinely performed inflow procedures, aortoiliac angioplasty and stenting are increasingly becoming the preliminary procedures performed to attain sufficient inflow prior to construction of a more distal bypass graft. At times, the necessity of improving the inflow to support an infrainguinal graft is determined intraoperatively, either by direct visual assessment of the arterial flow at the desired donor site or by comparison of a transduced pressure tracing from the donor site with that of a systemic pressure tracing, typically obtained from a radial arterial line. Of equal importance to the outcome of any infrainguinal graft is target vessel selection. In general, the target vessel should be the least diseased artery that is the dominant supply to the foot. If tissue necrosis is present, restoration of pulsatile flow to the foot is often required to obtain full and sustained wound healing.

Infrainguinal surgical bypass can be performed under general anesthesia or, in the appropriate patient, regional spinal or epidural anesthesia. In cases involving multiple sites of dissection, such as those necessitating more tedious arm vein or lesser saphenous vein harvesting, the procedures are particularly amenable to a two-team approach, with the time saved having direct benefit in minimizing the total anesthetic load and physiologic insult. The patient is sterilely prepped and draped from the midabdomen down to the foot. It is our practice to work from proximal to distal, first exploring the inflow artery and exposing the venous conduit. We then explore the site proposed for the distal anastomosis, as high-quality preoperative imaging has already defined a suitable target vessel.

For patients with superficial femoral artery disease, the initial dissection is most commonly at the level of the common femoral artery. This vessel is exposed through a longitudinal or

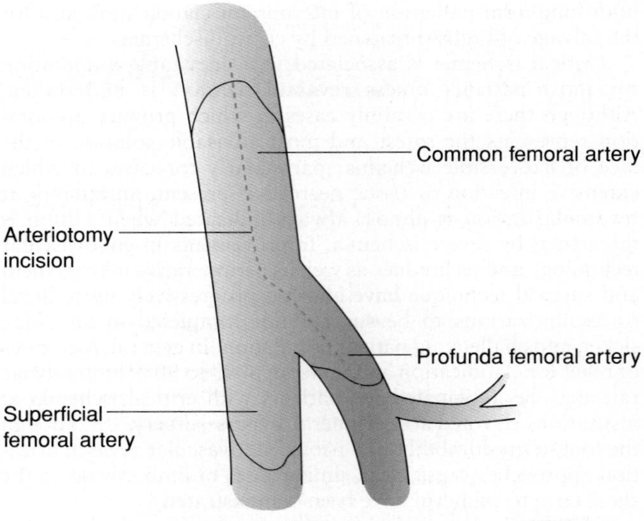

FIGURE 95.4. In the setting of orificial profunda femoral artery disease, extending the common femoral arteriotomy into the origin of the profunda and performing a profundaplasty will maximize profunda flow in the event of graft thrombosis.

oblique incision centered directly over the femoral pulse. Lymphatic tissue overlying the femoral vessels is best ligated and divided to prevent the postoperative development of lymph fistulas or lymphoceles. The severity of any concomitant common femoral and profunda femoral disease and the level of reconstruction planned dictate the extent of exposure of the femoral vessels. In most instances, the dissection extends from the inguinal ligament to the common femoral artery bifurcation, where the origins of the superficial and profunda femoral arteries are individually isolated.

If a profundaplasty is required, the dissection is extended distally along a sufficient length of the profunda femoral artery to attain an endpoint suitable for clamping and sewing (Fig. 95.4). Similarly, the inguinal ligament can be partially divided to facilitate access to the distal external iliac artery in cases in which a more extensive proximal endarterectomy is necessary. In these circumstances, it is customary to close the endarterectomized bed with a vein, bovine pericardial, or Dacron patch, onto which the proximal anastomosis can subsequently be attached.[68] In patients with a hostile groin crease from prior surgery or radiation therapy or in obese, diabetic patients with an intertriginous rash at the inguinal crease, meticulous skin preparation, close attention to draping, careful surgical technique, and judicious use of a short course of intravenous antibiotic therapy help minimize the chances of a postoperative wound or graft infection.

If all or part of the superficial femoral artery is spared of significant atherosclerotic involvement, the proximal anastomosis can be moved distally as dictated by the particular anatomic pattern of disease, and a so-called "distal origin graft" can be fashioned[69] (Fig. 95.5). This situation is particularly applicable to the diabetic population, in whom infrapopliteal disease is the rule and sparing of the superficial femoral and popliteal arteries is not uncommon. It is also utilized in situations in which conduit is sparse and a moderately diseased proximal vessel is accepted as an inflow source for a more distal origin bypass graft in the interests of performing a fully autologous vein graft rather than utilizing prosthetic material. An increasingly popular approach when only limited conduit is available is to combine, either concurrently in the operating room or as a staged preoperative procedure, catheter-based treatment of the superficial femoral or popliteal artery inflow with more distal bypass.[70]

The above-knee popliteal vessel is easily exposed through a medial thigh incision, with subsequent posterolateral retraction of the Sartorius muscle. The popliteal artery with its accompanying vein and nerve is found just posterior to the femur. The

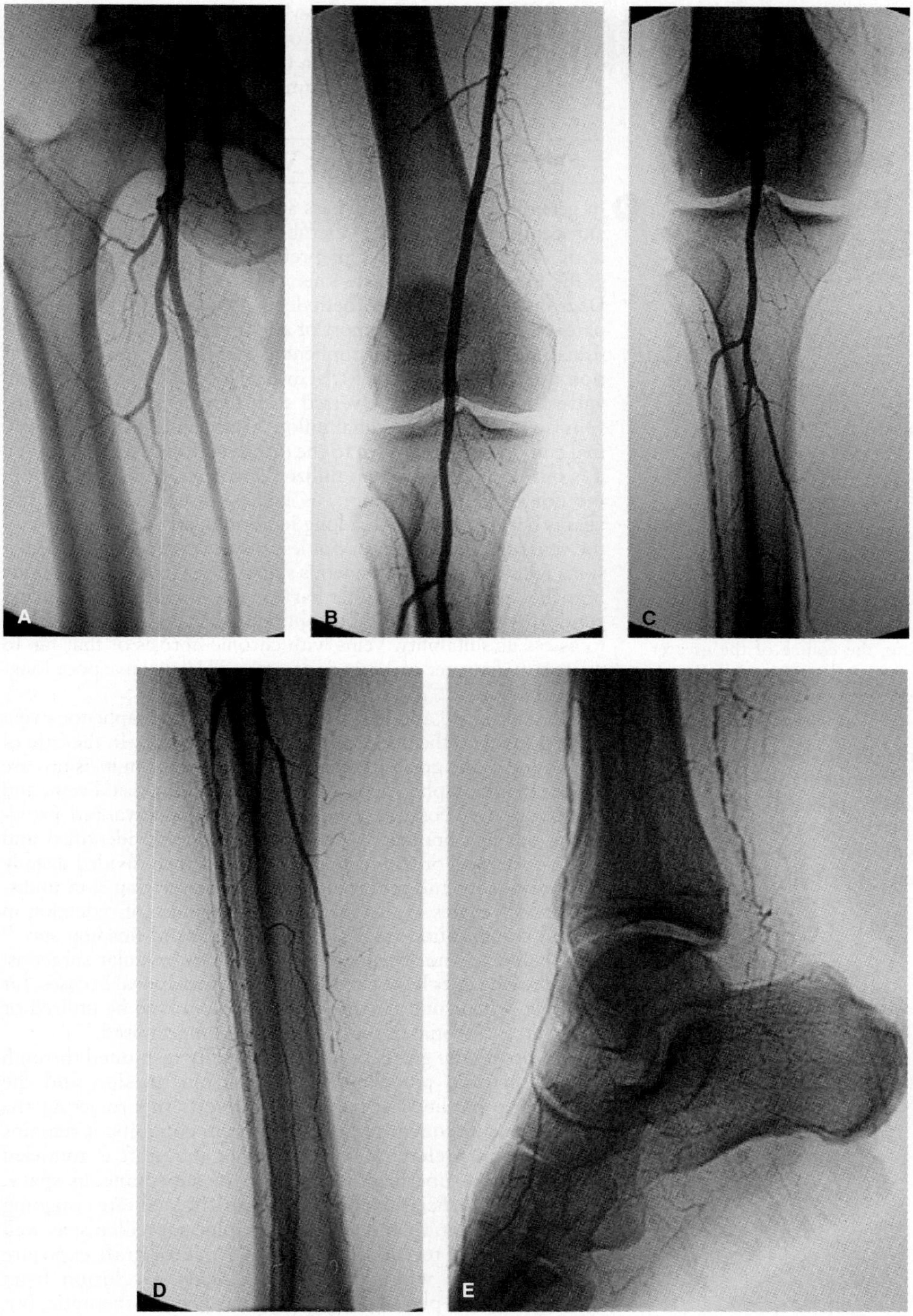

FIGURE 95.5. Arteriogram indicating preservation of the superficial femoral artery and popliteal arteries with midcalf occlusions of all three infrageniculate vessels. This anatomic pattern of disease is amenable to "distal origin" vein grafting from the below-knee popliteal or proximal posterior tibial artery to the dorsalis pedis artery.

vessel is palpated to determine the presence of atherosclerotic plaque, which will guide the extent of dissection and the optimal bypass target site. The below-knee popliteal artery is also exposed through a medial incision in the proximal calf (Fig. 95.6). If the saphenous vein is to be harvested, the incision is made directly over the vein to minimize the creation of devascularized skin flaps. With the exposed vein carefully protected, the incision is carried through the deep muscular fascia and the medial head of the gastrocnemius is reflected posterolaterally to expose the below-knee popliteal fossa. The distal popliteal artery is then dissected free from the adjacent tibial nerve posteriorly and popliteal vein medially. If the distal target is the tibioperoneal trunk, the dissection is continued along the anteromedial surface of the distal popliteal artery after dividing the origin of the soleus muscle from the tibia (Fig. 95.7). In instances in which the below-knee popliteal artery has previously been exposed or where sepsis is involved, a lateral approach with excision of a segment of proximal fibula is a useful alternative approach to the below-knee popliteal artery.

Although exposure of the proximal posterior tibial and peroneal vessels can be gained by extending the tibioperoneal trunk dissection distally, more distal exposure of these vessels is best gained through targeted medial incisions. The posterior tibial artery is found beneath the divided musculotendinous origin of the soleus muscle, and the peroneal artery is deeper and more lateral. The posterior tibial artery at the level of the ankle is a relatively easier target given the proximity of the vessel to the skin surface. The initial incision is made just posterior to the medial malleolus, and the artery exposed by division of the overlying retinaculum. Further distal dissection allows access to the bifurcation and medial and lateral plantar branches.[71] The more distal peroneal artery may be approached

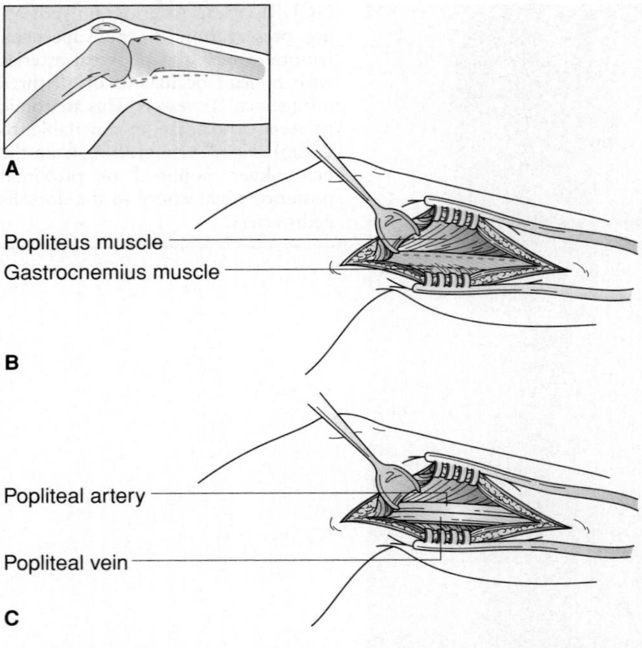

FIGURE 95.6. Exposure of the popliteal artery below the knee. The medial incision is made directly overlying the course of the greater saphenous vein.

laterally via an incision placed over the distal fibula. Excision of a short segment of fibula will expose the underlying artery.

The anterior tibial artery is typically approached from the anterolateral aspect of the calf (Fig. 95.7) and is found deep within the anterior compartment with the adjacent deep peroneal nerve and anterior tibial veins. It is best identified by developing the intermuscular plane between the tibialis anterior muscle belly medially and the extensor digitorum longus

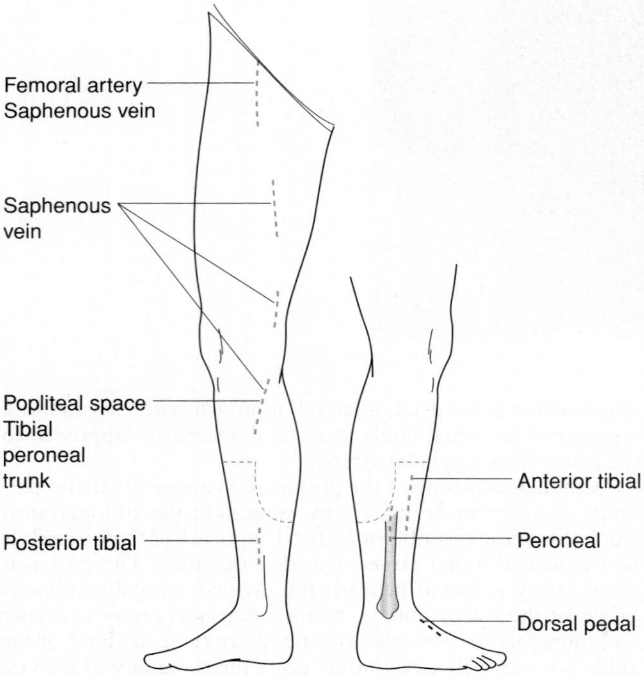

FIGURE 95.7. Placement of incisions for femoropopliteal and femorotibial bypass and for greater saphenous vein harvest. These should avoid the incision lines for a below-knee amputation.

laterally. The dorsalis pedis artery is easily exposed through an axial incision on the dorsum of the foot just lateral to the extensor hallucis longus tendon (Fig. 95.7). The artery lies just deep to the extensor retinaculum.

Autogenous Vein Bypass

9 In general, infrainguinal bypass surgery is best performed with autogenous vein conduit, preferably the ipsilateral greater saphenous vein if available.[72] This preference is particularly true for grafts extending below the knee, where prosthetic conduits of Dacron or polytetrafluoroethylene have significantly poorer patency rates. The first report of a femoropopliteal bypass graft using autogenous greater saphenous vein in a reversed orientation was by Kunlin in 1951.[4] Given the orientation of the vein valves, the vein can be reversed such that the distal end of the vein is sewn to the proximal inflow artery and the larger proximal end of the vein is sewn to the distal outflow artery. However, it is our general practice to utilize the greater saphenous vein in the nonreversed orientation, as will be discussed shortly. The vein is harvested through a long incision overlying the course of the vein or by more tedious but less invasive sequential skip incisions with intervening cutaneous skin bridges (Fig. 95.7). All side branches are ligated and after harvest, the vein is cannulated and gently dilated with a solution containing heparin and papaverine to assess its suitability. Veins with chronic fibrosis or that fail to dilate to a diameter of 3 mm or greater will likely have poor long-term function.

An alternative and less invasive approach to saphenous vein harvest involves the use of endoscopic technology. In the case of harvesting of the greater saphenous vein, small skin incisions are made over the saphenofemoral junction and the distal vein, and guided by a videoscope inserted distally and advanced proximally, the side branches of the vein are serially identified and either cauterized or clip-ligated. The vein is then divided distally and proximally and removed, leaving the overlying skin undisturbed. Advocates of this method cite a significant reduction in wound complication rates and reduced rates of hospital stay.[73] Although it has not been widely adopted by vascular surgeons, the technique does have particular theoretical appeal in cases, for example, when contralateral saphenous vein is to be utilized or the healing potential of the donor leg is compromised.

For prosthetic grafts, a tunnel is usually fashioned through the subsartorial plane between the groin incision and the above-knee popliteal space in the interests of protecting the graft from subsequent infection. For vein conduits, it remains the surgeon's preference as to whether the graft is tunneled deeply or in a superficial location in the subcutaneous space. The more superficial configuration greatly facilitates ongoing clinical examination and ultrasonographic surveillance as well as later surgical revision, but carries a risk of graft exposure should there be wound healing problems. Occlusion from trauma to grafts placed superficially has been of theoretic, but not practical, concern.

It is our practice to perform the proximal anastomosis prior to the distal anastomosis. First, this allows confirmation of adequate inflow before the bypass is performed. Second, performance of the proximal anastomosis first allows the graft to be tunneled and tailored to appropriate length under arterial pressure. This is of critical importance to prevent kinking along the length of the graft. Some surgeons also prefer to mark the distended graft to ensure against mechanical twisting of the graft during the tunneling process. An additional benefit of performing the proximal anastomosis first is that adequacy of flow through the graft can be assessed, both before and after tunneling, with brief release of the clamp.

Prior to occluding the target vessel, the patient is systemically anticoagulated with 5,000 to 10,000 units of heparin. Additional heparin is given throughout the procedure to maintain the activated clotting time near the target range of 250 to 300 seconds.

After allowing sufficient time for the heparin to circulate, atraumatic vascular clamps are placed proximally and distally and the artery is incised. The vein is then spatulated and a beveled anastomosis carried out. Typically, a 5–0 monofilament suture of polypropylene is used for the femoral anastomosis, a 6–0 used at the popliteal level, and a very fine 7–0 suture used at the tibial or pedal level. If the target tibial vessel is deep within the calf and visibility is challenging, a technique of "parachuting" the heel of the distal anastomosis is often employed. After completing the proximal anastomosis, the graft is carefully tunneled under arterial pressure. Occasionally, such extensive calcification of the target vessel is encountered that the risk of a significant injury from clamping, even with the minimally traumatic clamps in use today, is prohibitively high. In such cases, proximal inflow and distal artery backbleeding can be controlled by occlusion balloons placed intraluminally. For distal anastomoses at the knee or more distal level, another alternative technique is the use of a proximally placed sterile pneumatic tourniquet. This technique is particularly advantageous when sewing to diminutive distal tibial or pedal targets, where the impact of a crush injury or plaque dislodgment on graft function could be considerable. Removing the need for clamps by using the tourniquet has two further advantages. First, it improves the operative visibility. Second, and more importantly, given that less longitudinal and circumferential dissection is needed, the degree of vessel spasm and venous bleeding that frequently accompanies vessel exposure at this level is kept to a minimum.

Flow through the graft and the outflow arteries is assessed following completion of the bypass with a continuous wave Doppler. Ideally, a contrast angiogram is also performed after directly cannulating the proximal graft (Fig. 95.8); this allows for immediate repair of any technical defects that are identified,

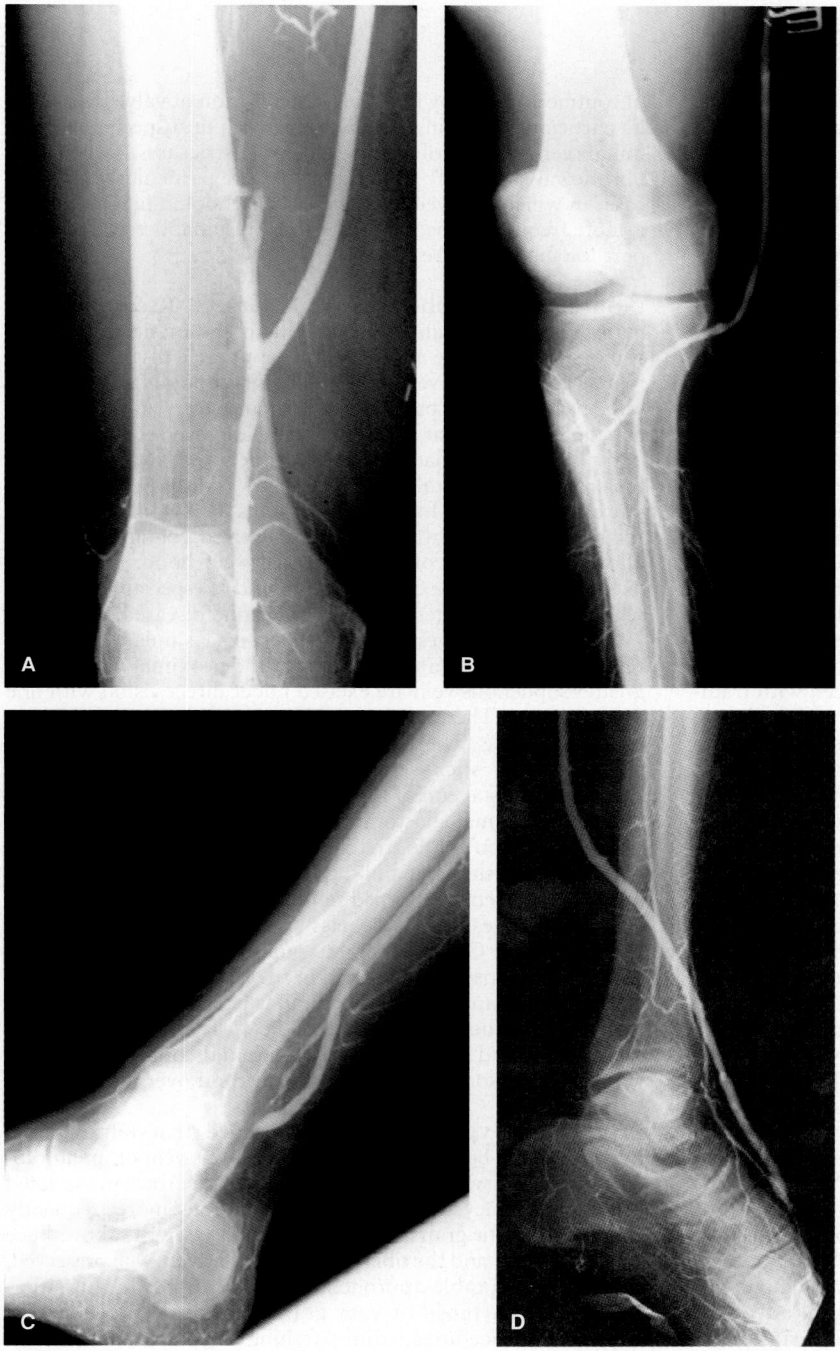

FIGURE 95.8. Intraoperative completion arteriograms of distal anastomoses to the above-knee popliteal (A), below-knee popliteal (B), distal posterior tibial (C), and dorsalis pedis (D) arteries.

TABLE 95.1 RESULTS

FIVE-YEAR PATENCY AND LIMB SALVAGE RESULTS OF INFRAINGUINAL BYPASS GRAFTING

STUDY	PATIENTS, n	CONDUIT	PRIMARY PATENCY	SECONDARY PATENCY	LIMB SALVAGE
Conte et al., 2001[79]	1,642	Autogenous vein	63	73	85
Belkin et al., 1996[51]	568	In situ vein	72	82	90
	189	Nonreversed vein	65	65	82
Shah et al., 1995[52]	2,058	In situ vein	72	81	95
Taylor et al., 1990[77]	564	Reversed vein	75	81	90
Veith et al., 1986[72]	338	PTFE to popliteal	38		70
	254	PTFE to tibial	12[a]		61[a]

PTFE, polytetrafluoroethylene.
[a]Four-year data.

such as intraluminal thrombus, twisting or kinking of the graft, or retained valve cusps.[74] Intraoperative completion duplex ultrasonography is an additional sensitive screen for hemodynamically significant abnormalities within the graft,[75,76] and its use further serves to prevent early graft loss caused by correctable technical problems.

Current reports of the 5-year results of reversed saphenous vein graft using modern techniques have been excellent, with primary and secondary patency rates of up to 75% and 80%, respectively, and limb salvage rates as high as 90%[77–79] (Table 95.1).

In Situ Grafting. There has been ongoing enthusiasm in some circles for in situ vein bypass grafting, whereby except for its proximal and distal extent, the greater saphenous vein is left undisturbed in its native bed. This technique was first described in 1962,[80] but was later popularized by Leather et al. in the late 1970s.[81] Recent reports of in situ saphenous vein grafting have indicated 5-year graft patency rates of up to 80% and limb salvage rates of 84% to 95%[51,52,78,82–84] (Table 95.1).

The in situ approach minimizes trauma to the vein during excision and handling and in theory enhances preservation of the vasa vasorum and endothelium. It further lowers the considerable risk of wound healing complications seen with traditional vein harvesting, increases vein utilization, and facilitates the creation of more technically precise anastomoses because the proximal and distal vein diameters are more closely matched to those of the inflow and outflow target vessels (Fig. 95.9). The extent of the proximal vein mobilization is dictated by the location of the saphenofemoral junction relative to the proposed site of the proximal anastomosis. It may at times be necessary to perform an endarterectomy of the superficial femoral artery if the length of proximal vein is insufficient. Lysis of the valve cusps is obligatory given the nonreversed configuration and is facilitated by newer, less traumatic valvulotomes that function safely through the blinded segments of undissected graft. Critics of this technique argue that the advantages listed previously have not translated into improved graft function or patency. They further argue that the time required and dissection involved in finding and ligating substantial side branches that can develop into physiologically important arteriovenous fistulas that "steal" distal flow obviates the stated benefits of this approach. Newer techniques using angioscopy and endoluminal coiling[85] of larger side branches may help to minimize these concerns.

Angioscopic assisted valve lysis has been employed for over a decade, but has not gained widespread favor. Although there is a significant learning curve with this technology and operative times, at least initially, are significantly prolonged, advocates cite fewer wound complications, shorter hospital stays, and decreased recuperative periods as potential benefits. Proponents of routine angioscopy for direct visualization of valve lysis stress its particular utility in demonstrating such unsuspected endoluminal venous pathology as phlebitic strictures, webs, and fibrotic valve cusps.[86] This adjunct may be particularly useful in cases in which arm vein is used because endoluminal pathology is more frequently encountered and is presumably responsible in part for suboptimal results.[87]

Nonreversed Saphenous Vein Grafts. Recognizing the many practical advantages inherent to the in situ technique, some surgeons have modified the approach to infrainguinal bypass grafting with venous conduit to incorporate several of the same principles.[51] In particular, if the harvested vein is tapered to any significant extent, it is used in a nonreversed fashion. By optimizing the size matching between the artery and vein at both the proximal and distal anastomosis sites as discussed previously, one can often accept for use smaller veins than would be suitable for reversed vein grafting. The nonreversed configuration also allows preservation of the saphenous vein hood, which both extends the available conduit length and is especially beneficial when the femoral artery is thick walled and diseased.

The vein is harvested and dilated in a similar fashion to reversed vein grafts and the cusps of the proximal valve of the greater saphenous vein are excised under direct vision with fine Potts scissors. There are currently two main types of valvulotomes available. The modified Mills valvulotome is a short, metal, hockey stick–shaped cutter that can be introduced through the distal end of the vein or through the side branches. After the proximal anastomosis is performed, and with the perfused conduit on gentle stretch, the valves are carefully lysed in a sequential fashion by pulling the valvulotome inferiorly. An alternative, recently designed self-centering valvulotome allows lysis of all valves in a single pass and is thought by some to be less traumatic. Once acceptable pulsatile flow is ensured, the distal anastomosis is performed in the standard fashion.

It is important to note that similar patency rates have consistently been demonstrated regardless of which technique is applied,[83,84] and so surgeon preference and comfort level is an acceptable reason for choosing one method over another.

Prosthetic Bypass. It is recommended that infrainguinal bypass surgery be performed with saphenous vein or an autologous substitute whenever feasible given the clearly demonstrated enhanced patency rates.[51,88] Some institutions more frequently rely on prosthetic grafts. When the distal target is the above-knee popliteal artery and the tibial outflow is relatively well preserved, this is an acceptable approach, as patency rates in this situation approach those of vein grafts.[89] A variety of surgical adjunctive procedures, from patching the distal anastomotic target vessel to the creation of a distal arteriovenous fistula or

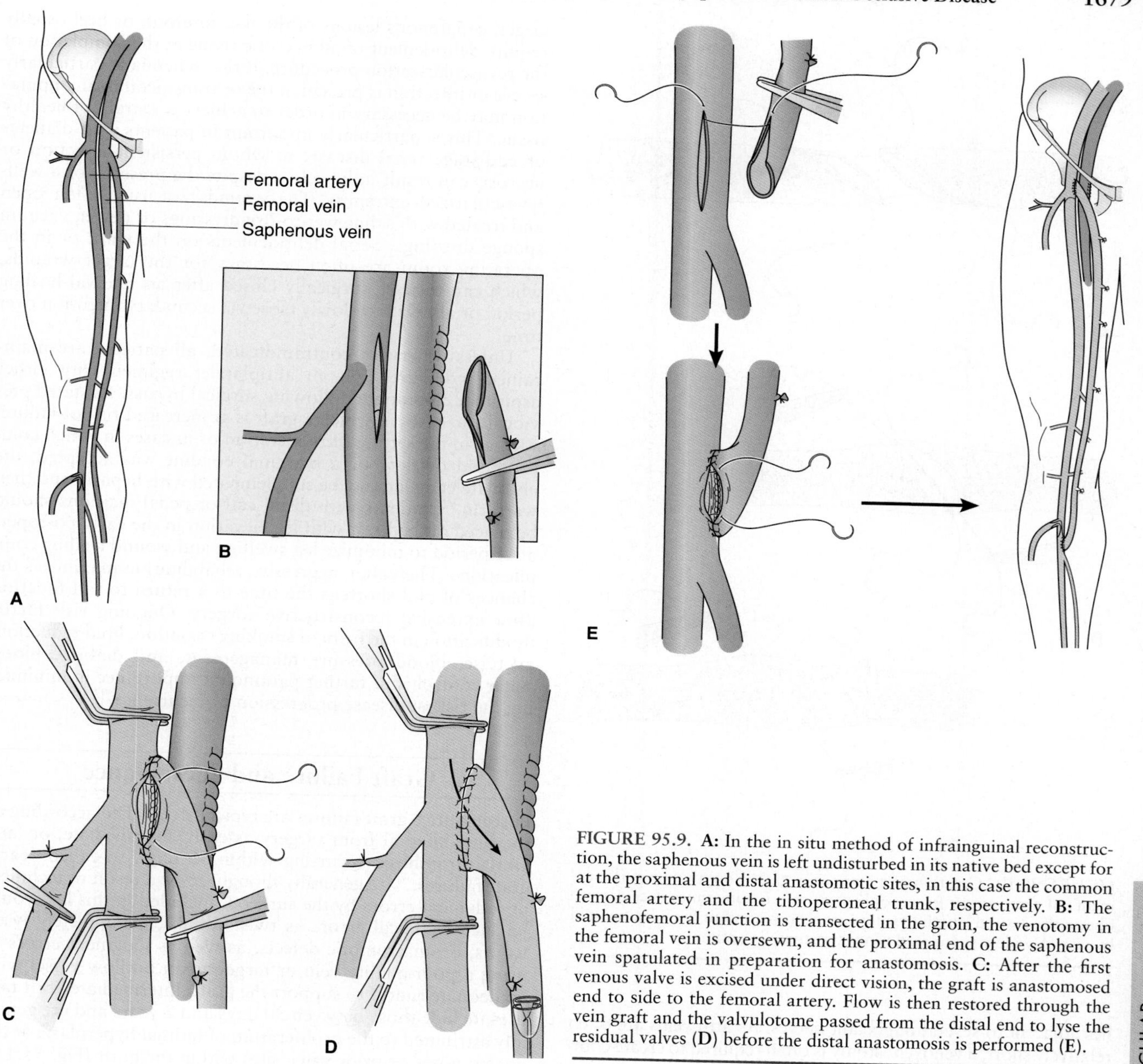

FIGURE 95.9. **A:** In the in situ method of infrainguinal reconstruction, the saphenous vein is left undisturbed in its native bed except for at the proximal and distal anastomotic sites, in this case the common femoral artery and the tibioperoneal trunk, respectively. **B:** The saphenofemoral junction is transected in the groin, the venotomy in the femoral vein is oversewn, and the proximal end of the saphenous vein spatulated in preparation for anastomosis. **C:** After the first venous valve is excised under direct vision, the graft is anastomosed end to side to the femoral artery. Flow is then restored through the vein graft and the valvulotome passed from the distal end to lyse the residual valves (**D**) before the distal anastomosis is performed (**E**).

various autogenous vein cuffs interposed between the distal prosthetic and the target artery, have all been attempted as a means of improving the patency rates of grafts extending below the knee.[90] More recently, flared grafts designed to minimize turbulence and shear stress between the prosthetic and native vessel have gained some popularity. Polyester (Dacron) and polytetrafluoroethylene (Teflon) grafts are the two main types of prosthetic available and, as in other anatomic positions, available data show generally equal results with either choice. The entire procedure is carried out through two small proximal and distal incisions between which the graft is tunneled anatomically. The selection of a 6- or 8-mm graft is dictated by the size of the native vessels.

Reoperative Bypass Surgery. As the patient population treated by vascular surgeons has increased in age, and more and more challenging cases are accepted for primary treatment, there has been a corresponding increase in the incidence of reoperative bypass surgery performed for infrainguinal arterial occlusive disease. Such reoperative procedures are particularly challenging, both because of the scarring present at the inflow and outflow target sites and because there is typically a lack of ipsilateral greater saphenous vein. Whenever possible, the first problem is addressed by choosing anastomotic sites just above or below the previous touchdown points, thereby avoiding dissection through often densely scarred tissue planes. When ipsilateral greater saphenous vein is absent because of prior infrainguinal or coronary artery bypass surgery or prior saphenous vein stripping, there are a number of alternative conduit sites available. Investigators examining the consequence of using the contralateral greater saphenous vein in these situations found it to be the optimal conduit; despite the presumably high incidence of contralateral lower extremity as well as coronary occlusive disease in this population, the short- and long-term impact was found to be minimal.[91]

In the absence of any greater saphenous vein, preoperative venous duplex ultrasonography is employed to evaluate the cephalic and basilic veins of the arms and the lesser saphenous veins of the legs in an effort to determine the best conduit available. Often the veins distal to the antecubital crease are scarred and of small caliber, but their more proximal counterparts are often of excellent size and quality. The use of arm veins in general can be extremely technically challenging and for that reason has not been universally adopted. The dissection of the basilic vein can be particularly tedious as it has multiple side branches and

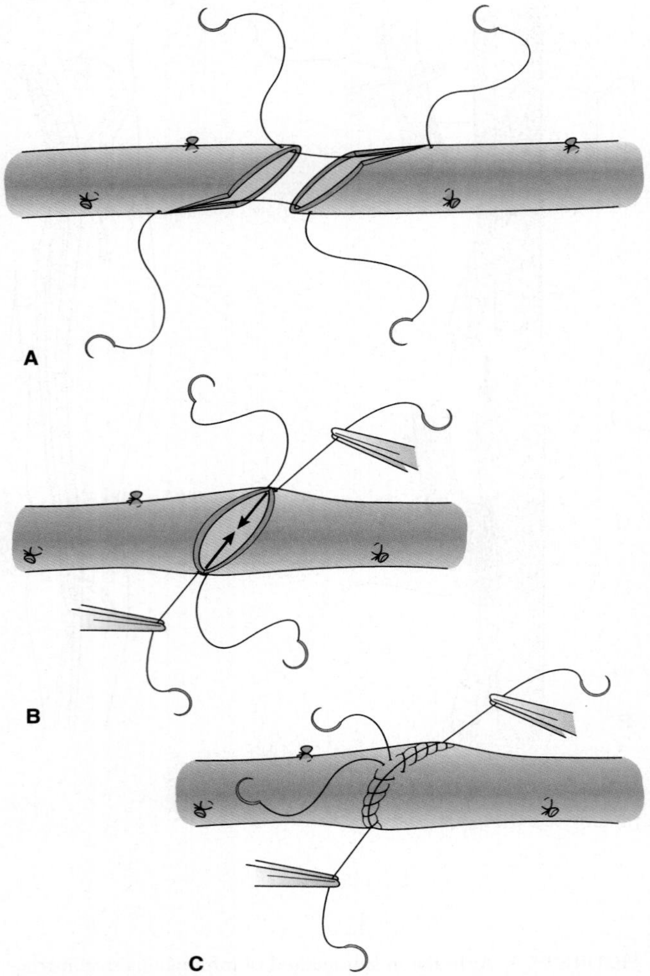

FIGURE 95.10. Creation of a composite graft from two or more segments of arm vein or lesser saphenous vein is sometimes necessary to obtain the desired length of fully autogenous conduit for infrainguinal bypass. A widely spatulated venovenostomy is optimal.

lies adjacent to several important nerves. As arm veins are often relatively short, a venovenostomy is often required to create composite grafts long enough to complete the arterial reconstruction (Fig. 95.10). This is performed with generous spatulation of each vein hood to create a widely patent vein-to-vein anastomosis. Given their thin-walled nature, arm vein grafts are also quite prone to twisting and kinking, and special care must be taken during the tunneling process to avoid these problems. The more proximal arm veins can be relatively large, and it is often advantageous to use one or more of the segments in a nonreversed fashion to better match the graft to the inflow vessel size.

Not surprisingly, the results of reoperative infrainguinal bypass surgery do not match those of primary reconstruction. With autogenous vein, 5-year patency rates of 60% and limb salvage rates of 70% to 80% have been reported.[26,91] Coumadin is often used postoperatively in patients with compromised outflow or in whom the conduit was of marginal quality and has been associated with improved long-term patency.[92]

Postreconstruction Management

10 Many patients undergoing surgical reconstruction for arterial insufficiency require one or more adjunctive operative procedures of their foot. Small, uninfected ulcerations of the toe or foot often can be safely managed conservatively. However, larger, gangrenous lesions of the toe, forefoot, or heel usually require débridement of all necrotic tissue at the completion of the revascularization procedure. If the ischemia is particularly severe or infection is present, a toe or transmetatarsal amputation may be necessary in order to achieve a margin of healthy tissue. This is particularly important in patients with diabetes or end-stage renal disease, in whom persistent infection or necrosis can result in limb loss despite the presence of a well-revascularized extremity. The wounds are usually left open and treated with saline wet-to-dry dressings or newer, vacuum sponge dressings. Serial débridements on the ward or in the operating room are often necessary for the larger wounds, which can then be surgically closed after an interval healing period or allowed to slowly close via secondary intention over time.

Unless otherwise contraindicated, all patients are maintained indefinitely on an antiplatelet regimen with either aspirin or clopidogrel following surgical bypass. As stated previously, in cases in which a graft is at increased risk of failure, such as in the setting of reoperation or in cases in which compromised outflow or a marginal conduit was accepted, the antiplatelet agent may be supplemented with heparin and then warfarin.[92] Patients with distal calf or pedal incisions should be placed on bed rest with leg elevation in the early postoperative period to minimize leg swelling and wound healing complications. Thereafter, aggressive rehabilitation maximizes the chances of and shortens the time to a return to full function after extensive reconstructive surgery. Ongoing risk factor modification in the form of smoking cessation, lipid reduction, exercise, blood pressure management, and diabetic blood sugar control is of further paramount importance in minimizing the risk of disease progression or recurrence.[93]

Graft Failure and Surveillance

Postoperative graft failures are typically classified according to the time interval from surgery as early, intermediate, or late. Graft thrombosis occurring within 30 days, so-called "early graft failures," are generally thought to be a result of technical or judgment errors by the surgeon. Included in this list would be such technical errors as twists, kinks, incompletely lysed valves, or anastomotic defects, as well as judgment errors in using a poor-quality vein or targeting an outflow vessel with inadequate runoff to support the graft. Intermediate graft failures include those between 30 days and 2 years and are generally attributed to the proliferation of intimal hyperplasia at the anastomoses or prior valve sites within the graft (Fig. 95.11). Late graft failures occurring beyond 2 years are typically a result of the progression of atherosclerotic occlusive disease within the inflow or outflow arteries.

Given the known incidence of graft failure and the potentially dire consequence in terms of limb salvage or preservation of limb function in a patient with limited options for secondary or tertiary bypass, the ability to maintain graft patency through early identification and prompt correction of graft stenoses is of paramount importance.[94] Serial postoperative surveillance scanning with a duplex ultrasound has proven an excellent means of accurately identifying hemodynamically significant stenoses within the vein graft that threaten the graft patency.[95] Velocity criteria have been developed for high-grade lesions that may warrant either more intensive surveillance or prophylactic intervention. Absolute velocities less than 40 cm/s or greater than 300 cm/s or a threefold increase in velocity in one segment compared with that of an adjacent segment are all indicative of impending graft failure. Confirmation by angiography and expeditious treatment by percutaneous cutting balloon angioplasty, surgical patch angioplasty, or interposition grafting of such significant lesions minimizes the risk of graft thrombosis and ensures optimal long-term graft patency.

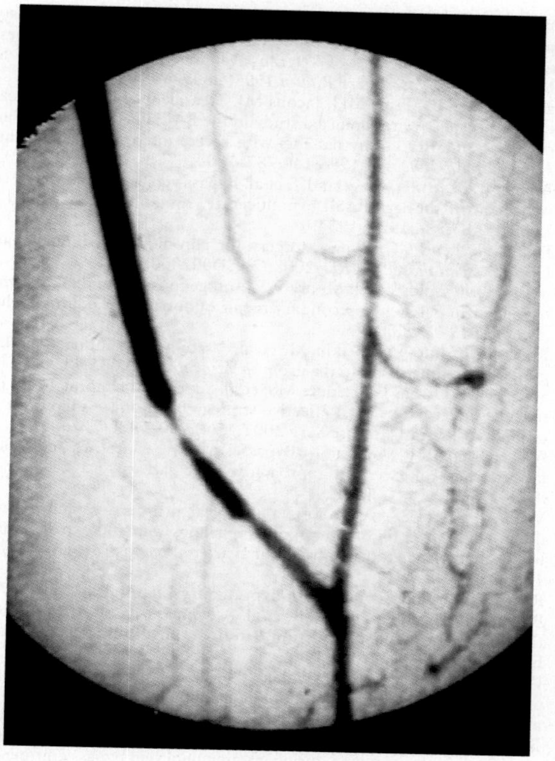

FIGURE 95.11. Arteriogram demonstrating severe stenosis of distal graft from intimal hyperplasia, likely at the prior valve site.

Complications

The most commonly seen major complications of infrainguinal bypass surgery are cardiac in nature and include myocardial infarction, congestive heart failure, and arrhythmias. In a recent review spanning 20 years and involving more than 1,600 procedures, the perioperative myocardial infarction rate was 3%, and the rate of cerebrovascular accident was 1%.[79] Patients with diabetes mellitus or preoperative renal insufficiency are at particular risk for developing postoperative renal failure (defined as an elevation of serum creatinine >3 mg/dL, doubling of the serum creatinine, or the need for hemodialysis), which is seen in up to 2% of patients overall. Patients undergoing lower extremity revascularization are also prone to wound complications, given the length of incisions and the prolonged operating times often required. Wound infection, including cellulitis, abscess formation, wound dehiscence, and skin flap necrosis, are most commonly seen and can best be avoided by gentle handling of the tissue, the use of skin bridges, and careful avoidance of skin flaps during vein harvesting. Postoperative hematomas, usually caused by slow capillary or venous oozing, or seromas are seen in 5% of patients, and less commonly encountered hemorrhage, typically a result of either a slipped vein branch ligature or anastomotic disruption, is seen in less than 1% of cases.

References

1. Gray EA. *Portrait of a Surgeon. A Biography of John Hunter.* London: Robert Hale; 1952.
2. dos Santos JC. Sur la desobstion des thromboses arterielles anciennes. *Mem Acad Chir (Paris)* 1947;73:409.
3. Carrel A. The surgery of blood vessels, etc. *John Hopkins Hosp Bull* 1907; 190:18.
4. Kunlin J. Le traitement de l'ischemie arteritique par la greffe veineuse longue. *Rev Chir* 1951;70:206.
5. McCaughan JJ Jr. Surgical exposure of the distal popliteal artery. *Surgery* 1958;44:536.
6. Dotter CT, Judkins MP. Transluminal treatment of arteriosclerotic obstruction. Description of a new technic and a preliminary report of its application. *Circulation* 1964;30:654–670.
7. Gruntzig A, Hopff H. Percutaneous recanalization after chronic arterial occlusion with a new dilator-catheter (modification of the Dotter technique) (author's transl). *Dtsch Med Wochenschr* 1974;99:2502–2510,2511.
8. Criqui MH, Fronek A, Barrett-Connor E, et al. The prevalence of peripheral arterial disease in a defined population. *Circulation* 1985;71: 510–515.
9. Selvin E, Erlinger TP. Prevalence of and risk factors for peripheral arterial disease in the United States: results from the National Health and Nutrition Examination Survey, 1999–2000. *Circulation* 2004;110:738–743.
10. Wolfe JH, Wyatt MG. Critical and subcritical ischaemia. *Eur J Vasc Endovasc Surg* 1997;13:578–582.
11. Halperin JL. Evaluation of patients with peripheral vascular disease. *Thromb Res* 2002;106:V303–V311.
12. Hirsch AT, Haskal ZJ, Hertzer NR, et al. ACC/AHA 2005 guidelines for the management of patients with peripheral arterial disease (lower extremity, renal, mesenteric, and abdominal aortic): executive summary: a collaborative report from the American Association for Vascular Surgery/Society for Vascular Surgery, Society for Cardiovascular Angiography and Interventions, Society for Vascular Medicine and Biology, Society of Interventional Radiology, and the ACC/AHA Task Force on Practice Guidelines (Writing Committee to Develop Guidelines for the Management of Patients With Peripheral Arterial Disease) endorsed by the American Association of Cardiovascular and Pulmonary Rehabilitation; National Heart, Lung, and Blood Institute; Society for Vascular Nursing; TransAtlantic Inter-Society Consensus; and Vascular Disease Foundation. *J Am Coll Cardiol* 2006;47:1239–1312.
13. Norgren L, Hiatt WR, Dormandy JA, et al. Inter-Society Consensus for the Management of Peripheral Arterial Disease (TASC II). *J Vasc Surg* 2007; 45(suppl S):S5–S67.
14. Criqui MH, Vargas V, Denenberg JO, et al. Ethnicity and peripheral arterial disease: the San Diego Population Study. *Circulation* 2005;112: 2703–2707.
15. O'Hare AM, Vittinghoff E, Hsia J, et al. Renal insufficiency and the risk of lower extremity peripheral arterial disease: results from the Heart and Estrogen/Progestin Replacement Study (HERS). *J Am Soc Nephrol* 2004; 15:1046–1051.
16. Ridker PM, Stampfer MJ, Rifai N. Novel risk factors for systemic atherosclerosis: a comparison of C-reactive protein, fibrinogen, homocysteine, lipoprotein(a), and standard cholesterol screening as predictors of peripheral arterial disease. *JAMA* 2001;285:2481–2485.
17. Imparato AM, Kim GE, Davidson T, et al. Intermittent claudication: its natural course. *Surgery* 1975;78:795.
18. McAllister FF. The fate of patients with intermittent claudication managed conservatively. *Am J Surg* 1976;132:593.
19. Walsh DB, Gilbertson JJ, Zwolak RM, et al. The natural history of superficial femoral artery stenoses. *J Vasc Surg* 1991;14:299.
20. Brewster DC, Perler BA, Robison JG, et al. Aortofemoral graft for multilevel occlusive disease: predictors of success and need for distal bypass. *Arch Surg* 1982;117:1593.
21. Wingo JP, Nix ML, Greenfield LJ, et al. The blue toe syndrome: hemodynamic and therapeutic correlates of outcome. *J Vasc Surg* 1986;3:475.
22. Karmody AM, Powers SR, Monaco VJ, et al. "Blue toe" syndrome. *Arch Surg* 1976;111:1263.
23. Cronenwett JL, Davis JT, Gooch JB, et al. Aortoiliac occlusive disease in women. *Surgery* 1980;88:775.
24. Caes F, Cham B, Van den Brande P, et al. Small artery syndrome in women. *Surg Gynecol Obstet* 1985;161:165.
25. Hertzer NR, Beven EG, Young JR, et al. Coronary artery disease in peripheral vascular patients: a classification of 1000 coronary angiograms and results of surgical management. *Ann Surg* 1984;199:223.
26. Belkin M, Conte MS, Donaldson MC, et al. Preferred strategies for secondary infrainguinal bypass: lessons learned from 300 consecutive reoperations. *J Vasc Surg* 1995;21:282.
27. Whittemore AD, Clowes AW, Hechtman HB, et al. Aortic aneurysm repair: reduced operative mortality associated with maintenance of optimal cardiac performance. *Ann Surg* 1980;192:414–421.
28. Kaluza GL, Joseph J, Lee JR, et al. Catastrophic outcomes of noncardiac surgery soon after coronary stenting. *J Am Coll Cardiol* 2000;35:1288.
29. Poldermans D, Boersma E, Bax JJ, et al. The effect of bisoprolol on perioperative mortality and myocardial infarction in high-risk patients undergoing vascular surgery. Dutch Echocardiographic Cardiac Risk Evaluation Applying Stress Echocardiography Study Group. *N Engl J Med* 1999; 341(24):1789–1794.
30. Schanzer A, Havelone N, Owens CD, et al. Statins are independently associated with reduced mortality in patients undergoing infrainguinal bypass graft surgery for critical limb ischemia. *J Vasc Surg* 2008;47(4):774–781.
31. Grassbaugh JA, Nelson PR, Rzucidlo EM, et al. Blinded comparison of preoperative duplex ultrasound scanning and contrast arteriography for planning revascularization at the level of the tibia. *J Vasc Surg* 2003;37: 1186.
32. Carpenter JP, Owen RS, Holland GA, et al. Magnetic resonance angiography of the aorta, iliac and femoral arteries. *Surgery* 1994;116:17.
33. Baum RA, Rutter CM, Sunshine JH, et al. Multicenter trial to evaluate vascular magnetic resonance angiography of the lower extremity. *JAMA* 1995;274:875.

34. Koelemay MJ, Lijmer JG, Stoker J, et al. Magnetic resonance angiography for the evaluation of lower extremity arterial disease: a meta-analysis. *JAMA* 2001;285:1338.
35. Udoff EJ, Barth KH, Harrington DP, et al. Hemodynamic significance of iliac artery stenosis: pressure measurements during angiography. *Radiology* 1979;132:289.
36. Spinosa DJ, Kaufmann JA, Hartwell GD. Gadolinium chelates in angiography and interventional radiology: a useful alternative to iodinated contrast media for angiography. *Radiology* 2002;223:319.
37. Back MR, Caridi JG, Hawkins IF, et al. Angiography with carbon dioxide (CO_2). *Surg Clin North Am* 1998;78:575.
38. Hirsch AT, Haskal ZJ, Hartzer NR, et al. ACC/AHA 2005 practice guidelines for the management of patients with peripheral arterial disease (lower extremity, renal, mesenteric, and abdominal aortic): a collaborative report from the American Association for Vascular Surgery/Society for Vascular Surgery, Society for Cardiovascular Angiography and Interventions, Society for Vascular Medicine and Biology, Society of Interventional Radiology, and the ACC/AHA Task Force on Practice Guidelines (Writing Committee to Develop Guidelines for the Management of Patients With Peripheral Arterial Disease). *Circulation* 2006;113;e463–e465.
39. Antiplatelet Trialists' Collaboration. Collaborative overview of randomised trials of antiplatelet therapy—II. Maintenance of vascular graft or arterial patency by antiplatelet therapy. *BMJ* 1994;308:159–168.
40. Clagett GP, Sobel M, Jackson MR, et al. Antithrombotic therapy in peripheral arterial occlusive disease: the Seventh ACCP Conference on Antithrombotic and Thrombolytic Therapy. *Chest* 2004;126:609S–626S.
41. A randomised, blinded, trial of clopidogrel versus aspirin in patients at risk of ischaemic events (CAPRIE). CAPRIE Steering Committee. *Lancet* 1996; 348:1329–1339.
42. Nehler MR, Hiatt WR. Exercise therapy for claudication. *Ann Vasc Surg* 1999;13:109.
43. Regensteiner JG, Meyer TJ, Krupski WC. Hospital versus home-based exercise rehabilitation for patients with peripheral arterial occlusive disease. *Angiology* 1997;48:291.
44. Dawson DL, Cutler BS, Hiatt WR, et al. A comparison of cilostazol and pentoxifylline for treating intermittent claudication. *Am J Med* 2000;109:523.
45. Moher D, Pham B, Ausejo M, et al. Pharmacological management of intermittent claudication: a meta-analysis of randomised trials. *Drugs* 2000;59: 1057–1070.
46. Hood SC, Moher D, Barber GG. Management of intermittent claudication with pentoxifylline: meta-analysis of randomized controlled trials. *CMAJ* 1996;155:1053–1059.
47. Girolami B, Bernardi E, Prins MH, et al. Treatment of intermittent claudication with physical training, smoking cessation, pentoxifylline, or nafronyl: a meta-analysis. *Arch Intern Med* 1999;159:337–345.
48. Guilmot JL, Diot E. The role of drug therapy in the treatment of critical ischemia of the lower limbs. *Presse Med* 1999;28:647–650.
49. Diehm C, Abri O, Baitsch G, et al. Iloprost, a stable prostacyclin derivative, in stage 4 arterial occlusive disease. A placebo-controlled multicenter study. *Dtsch Med Wochenschr* 1989;114:783–788.
50. Brass EP, Anthony R, Dormandy J, et al. Parenteral therapy with lipo-ecraprost, a lipid-based formulation of a PGE1 analog, does not alter six-month outcomes in patients with critical leg ischemia. *J Vasc Surg* 2006; 43:752–759.
51. Belkin M, Knox J, Donaldson MC, et al. Infrainguinal arterial reconstruction with nonreversed greater saphenous vein. *J Vasc Surg* 1996;24:957.
52. Shah DM, Darling RC, Chang BB, et al. Long-term results of in situ saphenous vein bypass: analysis of 2058 cases. *Ann Surg* 1995;222:438.
53. Giles KA, Pomposelli FB, Hamdan AD, et al. Infrapopliteal angioplasty for critical limb ischemia: relation of TransAtlantic InterSociety Consensus class to outcome in 176 limbs. *J Vasc Surg* 2008;48:128–136.
54. Dormandy JA, Rutherford RB. Management of peripheral arterial disease (PAD). TASC Working Group. TransAtlantic Inter-Society Consensus (TASC). *J Vasc Surg* 2000;31:S1–S296.
55. Berkseth RO, Kjellstrand CM. Radiologic contrast-induced nephropathy. *Med Clin North Am* 1984;68:351.
56. Kandzari DE, Rebeiz AG, Wang A, et al. Contrast nephropathy: an evidence-based approach to prevention. *Am J Cardiovasc Drugs* 2003;3:395.
57. MacNeill BD, Harding SA, Bazari H, et al. Prophylaxis of contrast-induced nephropathy in patients undergoing coronary angiography. *Catheter Cardiovasc Interv* 2003;60:458.
58. Knight CG, Healy DA, Thomas RL. Femoral artery pseudoaneurysms: risk factors, prevalence, and treatment options. *Ann Vasc Surg* 2003;17:503.
59. Lonn L, Olmarker A, Geterud K, et al. Prospective randomized study comparing ultrasound-guided thrombin injection to compression in the treatment of femoral pseudoaneurysms. *J Endovasc Ther* 2004;11:570.
60. Quinn SF, Kim J. Percutaneous femoral closure following stent-graft placement: use of the Perclose device. *Cardiovasc Intervent Radiol* 2004;27:231.
61. Twinel CP, Coulston J, Shandall A, et al. Angioplasty versus stenting for superficial femoral artery lesions. *Cochrane Database Syst Rev* 2009;(2): CD006767.
62. Schillinger M, Sabeti S, Loewe C, et al. Balloon angioplasty versus implantation of nitinol stents in the superficial femoral artery. *N Engl J Med* 2006; 354:1879–1888.
63. Holm J, Arfvidsson B, Jivegard L, et al. Chronic lower limb ischaemia. A prospective randomised controlled study comparing the 1-year results of vascular surgery and percutaneous transluminal angioplasty (PTA). *Eur J Vasc Surg* 1991;5:517–522.
64. Wolf GL, Wilson SE, Cross AP, et al. Surgery or balloon angioplasty for peripheral vascular disease: a randomized clinical trial. Principal investigators and their Associates of Veterans Administration Cooperative Study Number 199. *J Vasc Interv Radiol* 1993;4:639–648.
65. van der Zaag ES, Prins MH, Jacobs MJ. Treatment of intermittent claudication; prospective randomized study in the BAESIC-Trial (bypass, angioplasty or endarterectomy patients with severe intermittent claudication). *Ned Tijdschr Geneeskd* 1996;140:787–788.
66. Adam DJ, Beard JD, Cleveland T, et al. Bypass versus angioplasty in severe ischaemia of the leg (BASIL): multicentre, randomised controlled trial. *Lancet* 2005;366:1925–1934.
67. Fowkes F, Leng GC. Bypass surgery for chronic lower limb ischaemia. *Cochrane Database Syst Rev* 2008;(2):CD002000.
68. Malone JM, Goldstone J, Moore WS. Autogenous profundaplasty: the key to long-term patency in secondary repair of aortofemoral graft occlusion. *Ann Surg* 1978;188:817.
69. Reed AB, Conte MS, Belkin M, et al. Usefulness of autogenous bypass grafts originating distal to the groin. *J Vasc Surg* 2002;35:48.
70. Schanzer A, Owens CD, Conte MS, et al. Superficial femoral artery percutaneous intervention is an effective strategy to optimize inflow for distal origin bypass grafts. *J Vasc Surg* 2007;45(4):740–743.
71. Ascher E, Veith FJ, Gupta SK. Bypasses to plantar arteries and other tibial branches: an extended approach to limb salvage. *J Vasc Surg* 1988; 8:434.
72. Veith FJ, Gupta SK, Ascer E, et al. Six-year prospective multicenter randomized comparison of autologous saphenous vein and expanded polytetrafluoroethylene graft in infrainguinal arterial reconstruction. *J Vasc Surg* 1986;3:104.
73. Rosenthal D. Endoscopic in situ bypass. *Surg Clin N Am* 1995;75:703.
74. Baxter BT, Rizzo RJ, Flinn WR, et al. A comparative study of intraoperative angioscopy and completion arteriography following femorodistal bypass. *Arch Surg* 1990;125:997.
75. Gilbertson JJ, Walsh DB, Zwolak RM, et al. A blinded comparison of angiography, angioscopy, and duplex scanning in the intraoperative evaluation of in situ saphenous vein bypass grafts. *J Vasc Surg* 1992;15:121.
76. Bandyk D, Johnson B, Gupta A, et al. Nature and management of duplex abnormalities encountered during infrainguinal vein bypass grafting. *J Vasc Surg* 1996;24:430.
77. Taylor LM, Edwards JM, Porter JM. Present status of reversed vein bypass grafting: five-year results of a modern series. *J Vasc Surg* 1990;11:193.
78. Fogle MA, Whittemore AD, Couch NP, et al. A comparison of in situ and reversed saphenous vein grafts for infrainguinal reconstruction. *J Vasc Surg* 1987;5:46.
79. Conte MS, Belkin M, Upchurch GR, et al. Impact of increasing comorbidity on infrainguinal reconstruction: a 20-year perspective. *Ann Surg* 2001; 233:445.
80. Hall KV. The great saphenous vein used "in situ" as an arterial shunt after extirpation of vein valves. A preliminary report. *Surgery* 1962;51:492.
81. Leather RP, Powers SR, Karmody AM. A reappraisal of the in situ saphenous vein arterial bypass: Its use in limb salvage. *Surgery* 1979;86:453.
82. Donaldson MC, Mannick JA, Whittemore AD. Femoral-distal bypass with in situ greater saphenous vein: long term results using Mills valvulotome. *Ann Surg* 1991;213:457.
83. Moody AP, Edwards PR, Harris PL. In situ versus reversed femoropopliteal vein grafts: long-term follow-up of a prospective, randomized trial. *Br J Surg* 1992;79:750.
84. Wengerter KR, Veith FJ, Gupta SK, et al. Prospective randomized multicenter comparison of in situ and reversed vein infrapopliteal bypasses. *J Vasc Surg* 1991;13:189.
85. Rosenthal D, Dickson C, Rodriquez FJ, et al. Infrainguinal endovascular in situ saphenous vein bypass: ongoing results. *J Vasc Surg* 1994;20:389.
86. Panetta TF, Marin ML, Veith FJ, et al. Unsuspected pre-existing saphenous vein pathology: an unrecognized cause of vein bypass failure. *J Vasc Surg* 1992;15:102.
87. Marcaccio EJ, Miller A, Tannenbaum GA, et al. Angioscopically directed interventions improve arm vein bypass grafts. *J Vasc Surg* 1993;17:994.
88. Whittemore AD, Kent KC, Donaldson MC, et al. What is the proper role of polytetrafluoroethylene grafts in infrainguinal reconstruction? *J Vasc Surg* 1989;10:299.
89. Quinones-Baldrich WJ, Prego AA, Ucelay-Gomez R, et al. Long-term results of infrainguinal revascularization with polytetrafluoroethylene: a ten-year experience. *J Vasc Surg* 1992;16:209.
90. Miller JH, Foreman RK, Ferguson L, et al. Interposition vein cuff for anastomosis of prosthesis to small artery. *Aust N Z J Surg* 1984;54:283.
91. Chew DK, Owens CD, Belkin M, et al. Bypass in the absence of ipsilateral greater saphenous vein: safe superiority of the contralateral greater saphenous vein. *J Vasc Surg* 2002;35:1085.
92. Sarac TP, Huber TS, Back MR, et al. Warfarin improves the outcome of infrainguinal vein bypass grafting at high risk for failure. *J Vasc Surg* 1998; 28:446.
93. Creager MA. Medical management of peripheral arterial disease. *Cardiol Rev* 2001;9:238.
94. Veith FJ, Weiser RK, Gupta SK, et al. Diagnosis and management of failing lower extremity arterial reconstructions prior to graft occlusion. *J Cardiovasc Surg* 1984;25:381.
95. Bandyk DF, Schmitt DD, Seabrook GR, et al. Monitoring functional patency of in situ saphenous vein bypasses: the impact of a surveillance protocol and elective revision. *J Vasc Surg* 1989;9:286.

CHAPTER 96 ■ LOWER EXTREMITY AMPUTATION

MATTHEW J. SIDEMAN, KEVIN E. TAUBMAN, AND BRADLEY D. BEASLEY

KEY POINTS

1. More than 105,000 lower extremity amputations are performed in the United States annually.
2. The vast majority of lower extremity amputations are performed for complications of diabetes or arterial insufficiency.
3. Emergent amputation is indicated in the face of uncontrolled or ascending infection.
4. Primary amputation is occasionally indicated in cases of treatment for lower extremity trauma.
5. Revascularization is often performed in conjunction with a minor amputation, either simultaneously or as a staged procedure.
6. The choice of amputation level depends on the indication for the procedure, the condition of the patient, and the rehabilitation potential of the patient.
7. The energy required to ambulate following a lower extremity amputation increases with ascending level of amputation.

Surgeons are often involved in treating patients requiring lower extremity amputation. An increasing incidence of diabetes, peripheral arterial disease, and the aging population has put more patients at risk for amputation. Advances in the treatment of vascular disease, both surgical and endovascular, have worked to counteract these trends and keep the number of amputations performed relatively stable. Feinglass et al. demonstrated a decrease in major amputation rates in the 1980s after widespread adoption of distal bypass surgery.[1] It is believed that the substantial increase in percutaneous interventions may further contribute to improved limb salvage rates.
1 Despite these advances, recent estimates show that more than 105,000 lower extremity amputations are performed in the United States annually.[2] Clinical judgment is critical to a successful outcome. Factors to consider are primary versus staged amputation, initial versus redo revascularization, and timing and level of amputation. The surgeon must remember that the goal is to maintain maximal function of the patient, not necessarily maximal length of the limb. Consequently, experience of the surgeon has been shown to be key to a successful outcome.[3]

INDICATIONS

2 Most lower extremity amputations are performed for complications of diabetes or arterial insufficiency (Table 96.1). Chronic infection and trauma account for less than 10% of the total number of amputations. Other indications include neuroma, frostbite, malignancy, chronic pain, arterial embolization, venous insufficiency, and cryoglobulinemia.[4]

Elective lower extremity amputation in diabetic and vascular patients is indicated for gangrene (dry gangrene), gangrene with infection (wet gangrene), unremitting and nonreconstructable rest pain, and nonhealing ulcers. The goal of the operation is to remove all nonviable tissue, relieve ischemic rest pain, ensure primary wound healing, and facilitate rehabilitation. Elective amputation should only be performed following an evaluation for revascularization procedure by a surgeon capable of performing such procedures. Veith et al.[5] reported that 96% of patients who underwent lower extremity arteriography for limb-threatening infrainguinal arteriosclerosis were candidates for arterial reconstruction. Advances in percutaneous management have expanded treatment options to patients who were not otherwise operative candidates. Not all patients are candidates for arteriography, including those with chronic renal insufficiency, organic brain syndrome, nonfunctional limbs, fixed joint contractures, insensate feet, and extensive gangrene.

Spinal cord stimulation (SCS) may offer a chance for limb salvage for patients with chronic ischemia in whom reconstruction is not an option. Based on Melzack and Wall's theory for treatment of chronic pain,[6] the mechanism of pain relief and increased blood flow in end-stage peripheral vascular disease is unclear. Despite this, there is peripheral vasodilatation on the microvascular level, which leads to pain relief,[7] increased claudication distance,[8] ulcer healing,[9] and possible limb salvage.[7,10,11] The 1-year foot salvage rate is 60% to 70% on average, according to a review of the literature.[12] SCS is only appropriate when surgery for revascularization is no longer possible. Furthermore, SCS only dilates microvasculature and does nothing for the underlying, progressive peripheral vascular disease that is causing the ischemia. SCS, therefore, is only a temporizing measure, but can potentially give an extended functional period with a procedure that is well tolerated and relatively simple to perform.[12] Recently, Gersbach et al. have shown that the benefits of SCS persist longer than initially thought.[13]

3 Emergent amputation is indicated in the face of uncontrolled or ascending infection. In the case of uncontrolled sepsis, it may be a lifesaving maneuver. Similarly, a diabetic patient with a foot abscess constitutes a surgical emergency. Frequently, incision and drainage with or without a toe or a combined toe and metatarsal resection is sufficient to control the acute problem. The wounds should be left open in the setting of acute infection. If the process extends beyond the foot, a staged amputation should be performed proximal enough to control the infection. This can include an ankle disarticulation, a guillotine below-knee amputation (BKA), a knee disarticulation, or a guillotine above-knee amputation (AKA). Disarticulations have the advantage of preserving limb length and avoiding an open bone in the incision. After the infection is controlled, the appropriate amputation can be completed. A one-stage primary above-knee amputation can be considered in patients who are nonambulatory, have infection involving the entire lower leg, have a fixed knee contracture, or have a nonfunctional limb. Patients who are too unstable for surgery can be temporized with a cryoamputation.[14]

4 Primary amputation is occasionally indicated as treatment for severe lower extremity trauma. Both penetrating and blunt

VASCULAR

TABLE 96.1 INDICATIONS/CONTRAINDICATIONS

INDICATIONS FOR LOWER EXTREMITY AMPUTATION

■ INDICATION	■ PERCENTAGE
Complications of diabetes mellitus	60–80
Nondiabetic infection with ischemia	15–25
Ischemia without infection	5–10
Chronic osteomyelitis	3–5
Trauma	2–5
Miscellaneous (neuroma, frostbite, tumor, pain, nonhealing wound)	5–10

From Malone JM. Lower extremity amputation. In: Moore WS, ed. *Vascular Surgery: A Comprehensive Review*. Philadelphia, PA: WB Saunders; 1993:810.

injuries of the lower extremities are frequently associated with vascular, nerve, bone, and extensive soft tissue injuries. Several treatment guidelines have been developed for lower extremity trauma. Lange[15] recommended primary amputation for open tibial fractures with associated vascular injuries if the posterior tibial nerve was disrupted in an adult or if the duration of warm ischemia was greater than 6 hours in a crush injury. In addition, he suggested that primary amputation was relatively indicated in patients with polytrauma, severe ipsilateral foot injuries, and an expected protracted postoperative course. These suggestions are supported in work by Bosse et al.[16] demonstrating that, in the case of high-energy lower extremity trauma, amputation and reconstruction have equal functional outcomes at 2 years. Additional guidelines have been provided by Johansen et al.,[17] who devised a Mangled Extremity Severity Score (MESS) to predict the need for amputation based on the extent of skeletal or soft tissue damage, limb ischemia, shock, and age. Unfortunately, none of these guidelines are predictive of functional recovery in patients who undergo limb salvage.[18] Therefore, treatment with primary amputation is an extremely difficult decision and requires extensive clinical judgment, as well as multidisciplinary input. Contributing factors include the severity of the injury, the overall clinical status, and the ultimate rehabilitation potential of the patient.

EVALUATION FOR REVASCULARIZATION

Modern vascular surgery techniques allow successful limb salvage in situations not previously possible. All patients who present for possible lower extremity amputation, including minor amputations, should have their peripheral vascular circulation evaluated preoperatively. Any patient with absent pedal pulses or abnormal ankle-brachial indices should be evaluated by a vascular surgeon skilled in both open and endovascular revascularization techniques. The evaluation may require only a thorough history and physical examination if there is an obvious contraindication to revascularization (e.g., nonfunctional limb, severe organic brain syndrome). Noninvasive vascular laboratory examinations are a mandatory minimum for patients with abnormal vascular examinations. Additional imaging with either multidetector, helical computed tomography angiography (CTA), magnetic resonance angiography (MRA), or contrast angiography can be done based on the patient's initial evaluation and vascular laboratory results. The information obtained from these tests is heavily dependent on the quality of the machinery, the skill of the technologist, and the knowledge of the interpreting physician. All of these factors must be taken into account when deciding which test to order. Contrast arteriography should not be considered a *diagnostic* examination. It may, however, be necessary to fully define the patient's anatomy and determine suitability for reconstruction. It is preferred to perform this invasive procedure for preoperative planning or for planned percutaneous intervention.

Exponential advances in endovascular techniques have occurred over the past 10 years. These have found their way into the peripheral circulation and have applicability in limb salvage. Percutaneous techniques include conventional balloon angioplasty, stenting (including balloon-expandable, self-expanding nitinol, and covered stents), CryoPlasty, and percutaneous atherectomy (including laser, directional, and rotational). The Bypass versus Angioplasty in Severe Ischaemia of the Leg (BASIL) trial showed no significant difference in amputation-free survival among patients with critical limb ischemia when randomized to open or percutaneous revascularization.[19]

In terms of surgical reconstruction, upper extremity[20] and cryopreserved cadaver vein[21] have increased the options for conduit in limb salvage situations. Prosthetic grafts with vein cuffs[22,23] provide other alternatives when appropriate autogenous conduit is not available. More recently, a heparin-bonded prosthetic graft has been introduced and early studies show promising results.[24] An operation for limb salvage should never be denied *only* for lack of conduit.

5 Revascularization is often performed in conjunction with a minor amputation, either simultaneously or as a staged procedure. This allows management of the acute problem of sepsis and the underlying chronic ischemia. Caution must be taken if there is active infection and the only available conduit is prosthetic for fear of infecting the graft. Amputation with control of infection followed by revascularization is the more prudent course. In extreme cases, a limited amputation can be combined with revascularization and a tissue transfer (free or rotational flap) to achieve limb salvage.[25,26]

SELECTION OF AMPUTATION LEVEL

General

6 The choice of amputation level depends on the indication for the procedure, the condition of the patient, and the rehabilitation potential of the patient. The most common amputation levels are illustrated in Figure 96.1. Because most amputations are performed for complications of diabetes or arterial insufficiency, the selected level must remove all nonviable, painful tissue; allow primary healing; and maximize rehabilitation potential. Selection of the amputation level for malignant disease is dependent on the biologic characteristics of the neoplasm and is beyond the scope of this chapter.

The general medical condition and the rehabilitation potential of the patient are important factors in deciding to proceed with amputation and in selecting the appropriate level. If a patient is ambulatory and independent preoperatively, the level with the greatest likelihood of maintaining function should be selected. If the patient is not ambulatory or has significant comorbid conditions, the primary wound-healing rate should be the determining factor.

Specific Situations

Aggressive attempts to salvage a distal amputation level are not indicated for patients who are unlikely to ambulate with a prosthesis.[27] For example, patients with fixed joint contractures greater than 15 degrees at the knee or 10 degrees at the hip are unlikely to ambulate with a prosthesis. Below-knee amputations are relatively contraindicated in patients with

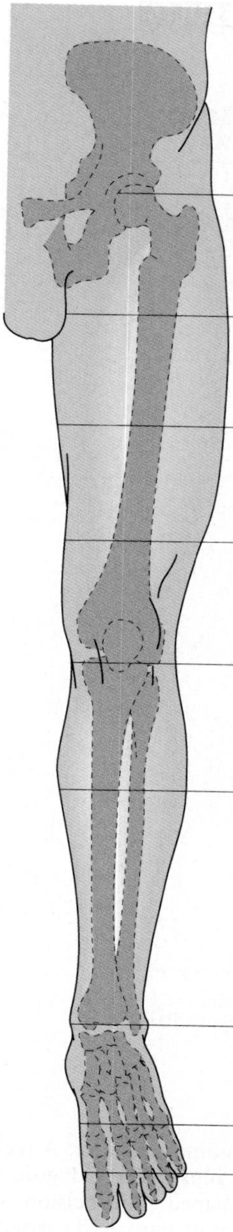

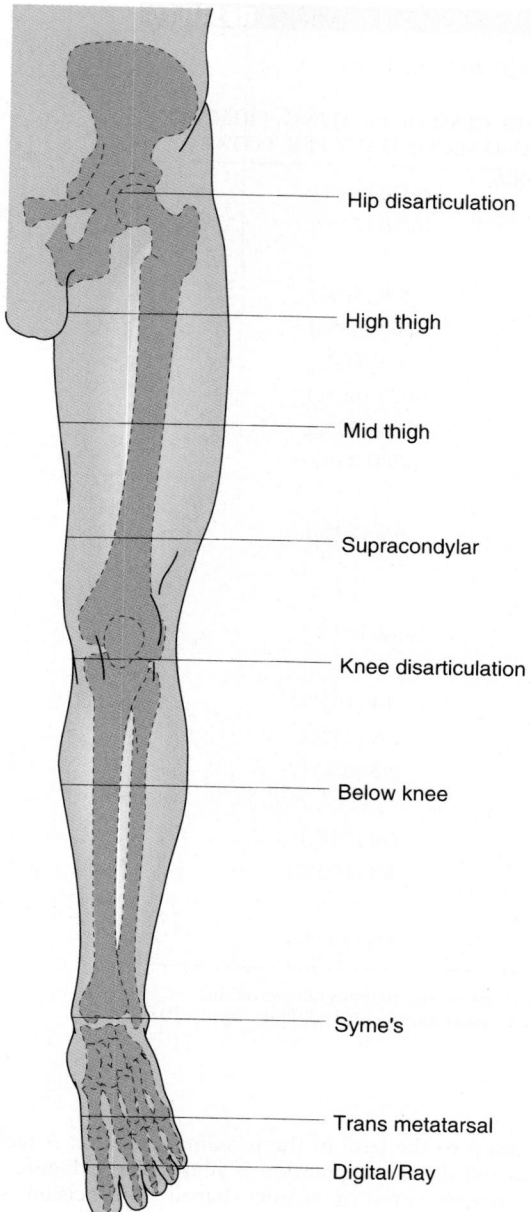

FIGURE 96.1. Common amputation levels for the lower extremity.

paraplegia because flexion contractures at the knee can lead to stump ulceration.

Energy Requirement

7 The energy required to ambulate following a lower extremity amputation increases with ascending level of amputation. The more proximal the amputation, the less likely a patient will be able to ambulate postoperatively. Table 96.2 illustrates the increased energy cost of the common lower extremity amputations. In clinical practice, the most significant increase is between below- and above-knee amputations. Ambulation on an above-knee prosthesis requires the use of muscle groups poorly suited for that purpose. These increased energy costs are minor issues for young trauma or cancer patients; however, they may represent a considerable obstacle for the older diabetic or vascular patient.

TABLE 96.2 RESULTS

REHABILITATION ENERGY COST OF AMPUTATION AT VARIOUS LEVELS

AMPUTATION LEVEL	ENERGY COST
Digital or ray	Minimal (except first ray)
Transmetatarsal	Minimal during normal walking
Below knee	30%–60% increase in energy required for ambulation
Above knee	60%–100% increase in energy required for ambulation
Hip disarticulation	100%–110% increase in energy required for ambulation

Clinical Assessment

The primary preoperative consideration for wound healing is the status of the skin and muscle blood flow. Operative technique, the patient's nutritional status, and the presence of infection also affect wound healing. Clinical judgment by an experienced surgeon accurately predicts healing of a BKA in approximately 80% of cases.[28] A palpable pulse at the level immediately proximal to the proposed amputation essentially ensures healing[29]; however, the converse is not true. Noninvasive arterial testing is the most common adjunctive test used to predict healing of a specific amputation level. Its usefulness is limited when medial sclerosis prevents vessel compression, a condition common in diabetic patients. Because the digital vessels are often spared from this process, digital pressure readings may be helpful in this setting. Transcutaneous oxygen measurement has been shown to predict primary healing, although it is less able to predict failure to heal.[30,31] It has become more widely available and has supplanted previous less reliable tests that were more limited in availability. Tables 96.3 to 96.6 summarize the results of various preoperative tests to predict wound healing for toe, foot and forefoot, below-knee, and above-knee amputations, respectively.

TABLE 96.3 RESULTS

PREOPERATIVE LEVEL SELECTION: TOE AMPUTATION

SELECTION CRITERIA	SUCCESSFUL HEALING, PRIMARY AND SECONDARY PER TOTAL
Empiric	86/115 (75%)
Presence of pedal pulses	357/365 (98%)
Doppler toe pressure >30 mm[a]	47/60 (78%)
Doppler ankle pressure >35 mm[a]	44/46 (96%)
Photoplethysmographic digit or TMA pressure >20 mm[a]	20/20 (100%)

[a]Systolic pressure (mm Hg).
TMA, transmetatarsal.
Modified from Durham JR. Lower extremity amputation levels: indications, methods of determining appropriate level, technique, prognosis. In: Rutherford RB, ed. *Vascular Surgery,* 3rd ed. Philadelphia, PA: WB Saunders; 1989:1693.

TABLE 96.4 RESULTS

PREOPERATIVE LEVEL SELECTION: FOOT AND FOREFOOT AMPUTATION

■ SELECTION CRITERIA	■ SUCCESSFUL HEALING, PRIMARY AND SECONDARY PER TOTAL
Empiric	11/24 (46%) 36/50 (72%)
Doppler ankle systolic pressure	
<40 mm Hg	5/9 (56%)
>40 mm Hg	20/60 (33%)
40–60 mm Hg	4/5 (80%)
>50 mm Hg	14/21 (66%)
>60 mm Hg	68/91 (75%)
>70 mm Hg	70/93 (75%)
Doppler toe systolic pressure	
>30 mm Hg	4/5 (80%)
Doppler ankle-brachial pressure index	
>0.45 (nondiabetic) >0.50 (diabetic)	58/60 (97%)
Photoplethysmographic toe systolic pressure	
>55 mm Hg	14/14 (100%)
>45 and <55 mm Hg	2/8 (25%)
<45 mm Hg	0/8 (0%)
Transcutaneous PO_2	
>10 mm (or a >10-mm increase on FiO_2 >1.0)	6/8 (75%)
>28 mm Hg	3/3 (100%)
Transcutaneous PCO_2	
<40 mm Hg	3/3 (100%)

Modified from Durham JR. Lower extremity amputation levels: indications, methods of determining appropriate level, technique, prognosis. In: Rutherford RB, ed. *Vascular Surgery,* 3rd ed. Philadelphia, PA: WB Saunders; 1989:1695.

OPERATIVE TECHNIQUE

General Considerations

Diabetic patients who present septic require adequate fluid resuscitation, broad-spectrum antibiotics (including anaerobic coverage), and an emergent operation. Whereas maintenance of limb length and function is admirable, control of sepsis and wide débridement of all nonviable tissue is essential and potentially lifesaving. All patients require atraumatic tissue handling. Avoid forceps on the skin edge. Excessive skin flaps and dead space are also not desired. Amputations done in the face of active infection are kept open and treated with dressing changes. Consider delayed primary closure in cases where perfusion is intact.

Postoperatively, the limb is elevated to minimize tissue edema and promote healing. Weight bearing on the amputation is delayed until healing is ensured. This patient population requires effective prophylaxis against deep venous thrombosis and venous thromboembolism.

Digital and Ray Amputations

Digital amputations are indicated for some severe and irreducible deformities as well as gangrene or osteomyelitis localized distal to the base of the proximal phalanx. A technique for partial digital amputation is illustrated in Figure 96.2A. The circumferential or racquet-shaped skin incision is made over the distal end of the proximal phalanx and carried down to bone. Nerves and tendons are transected under tension and allowed to retract. The proximal phalanx is divided with bone shears or a power saw and the transected end smoothed with a rongeur. Soft tissue coverage can be performed with either medial/lateral flaps or dorsal/plantar flaps depending on skin tension and viability. The wound is closed only with simple interrupted skin sutures. Judicious use of subcutaneous sutures is advised due to danger of vascular compromise to the small remaining flaps. Non–weight-bearing restrictions or protected weight bearing on the heel only in a rigid soled postoperative shoe or walking boot until the wound heals is recommended.

A ray amputation is indicated when the disease process extends to the metatarsal phalangeal joint. The technique is similar to a digital amputation and is illustrated in Figure 96.2B. A circumferential incision is made at the base of the involved toe and extended proximally on the dorsum of the foot over the metatarsal. The incision is extended to bone. The periosteum is cleared circumferentially and the bone is transected using a power saw at a level that will allow tension-free closure of the wound. In the case of the first or fifth toe, the incision is extended on the medial or lateral aspect of the foot, respectively. Care should be taken to bevel the distal

TABLE 96.5 RESULTS

PREOPERATIVE LEVEL SELECTION: BELOW-KNEE AMPUTATION

■ SELECTION CRITERIA	■ SUCCESSFUL HEALING, PRIMARY AND SECONDARY PER TOTAL
Empiric	794/974 (82%)
Doppler ankle systolic pressure	
>30 mm Hg	66/70 (94%)
Doppler calf systolic pressure	
>50 mm Hg	36/36 (100%)
>68 mm Hg	96/97 (99%)
Doppler thigh systolic pressure	
>100 mm Hg	31/31 (100%)
>80 mm Hg	104/113 (92%)
Transcutaneous $PO_2 = 0$	0/3 (0%)
>10 mm Hg	76/80 (95%)
(or >10-min increase on $FiO_2 = 1.0$)	
>10 and <40 mm Hg	5/7 (71%)
>20 mm Hg	25/26 (96%)
>35 mm Hg	51/51 (100%)
Transcutaneous PO_2 index >0.59	17/17 (100%)
Transcutaneous PCO_2 <40 mm Hg	7/8(88%)

Modified from Durham JR. Lower extremity amputation levels: indications, methods of determining appropriate level, technique, prognosis. In: Rutherford RB, ed. *Vascular Surgery*. 3rd ed. Philadelphia, PA: WB Saunders; 1989:1700.

metatarsal stump to minimize any prominence that may lead to skin breakdown with weight bearing or shoe gear wear. Typically, the first metatarsal is beveled from proximal medial to distal lateral and proximal plantar to distal dorsal. Metatarsals 2, 3, and 4 should be beveled from proximal plantar to distal dorsal. The fifth metatarsal is beveled from proximal lateral to distal medial and proximal plantar to distal dorsal.

In selected cases of neuropathic ulcers, the metatarsal head can be resected leaving the toe intact. A dorsal longitudinal incision is made over the metatarsal bone and the metatarsal head is resected with a power saw. Pulsed lavage and careful soft tissue inspection will help guide appropriate care for the plantar wound (i.e., packing, negative-pressure therapy, or ellipse of wound with closure). The dorsal wound is typically closed unless severe infection is encountered.

TABLE 96.6 RESULTS

PREOPERATIVE LEVEL SELECTION: ABOVE-KNEE AMPUTATION

■ SELECTION CRITERIA	■ SUCCESSFUL HEALING, PRIMARY AND SECONDARY PER TOTAL
Empiric	390/430 (91%)
Transcutaneous PO_2	
>10 mm Hg (or 10-mm increase on $FiO_2 = 1.0$)	15/23 (65%)
>20 mm Hg	12/12 (100%)
>23 mm Hg	2/2 (100%)
>35 mm Hg	21/24 (100%)
Transcutaneous PCO_2	
<38 mm Hg	5/5 (100%)

Modified from Durham JR. Lower extremity amputation levels: indications, methods of determining appropriate level, technique, prognosis. In: Rutherford RB, ed. *Vascular Surgery*, 3rd ed. Philadelphia, PA: WB Saunders; 1989:1707.

Transmetatarsal Amputation

Transmetatarsal amputation (TMA) is a useful procedure that maintains a patient's ability to ambulate without the aid of a prosthesis. It is indicated when the gangrenous or infectious process involves multiple digits or a portion of the forefoot. Care must be taken to plan for the appropriate soft tissue coverage if primary closure is desired. Maximizing the plantar flap is most common, but coverage can also be gained from medial or laterally based flaps and even filleted toe flaps. If adequate soft tissue coverage is not available and a more proximal foot amputation (i.e., Chopart joint amputation) is not desired, then an open amputation through the metatarsal bones can be performed. The wound is allowed to close secondarily or covered with a skin graft. Skin grafts in this position, however, are susceptible to breakdown secondary to the pressure related to ambulation.

The TMA technique is demonstrated in Figure 96.3. A skin incision is made on the dorsum of the foot immediately proximal to the metatarsal heads and extended medially and laterally to a point midway between the plantar and dorsal surfaces. The plantar incision is made along the digital crease and

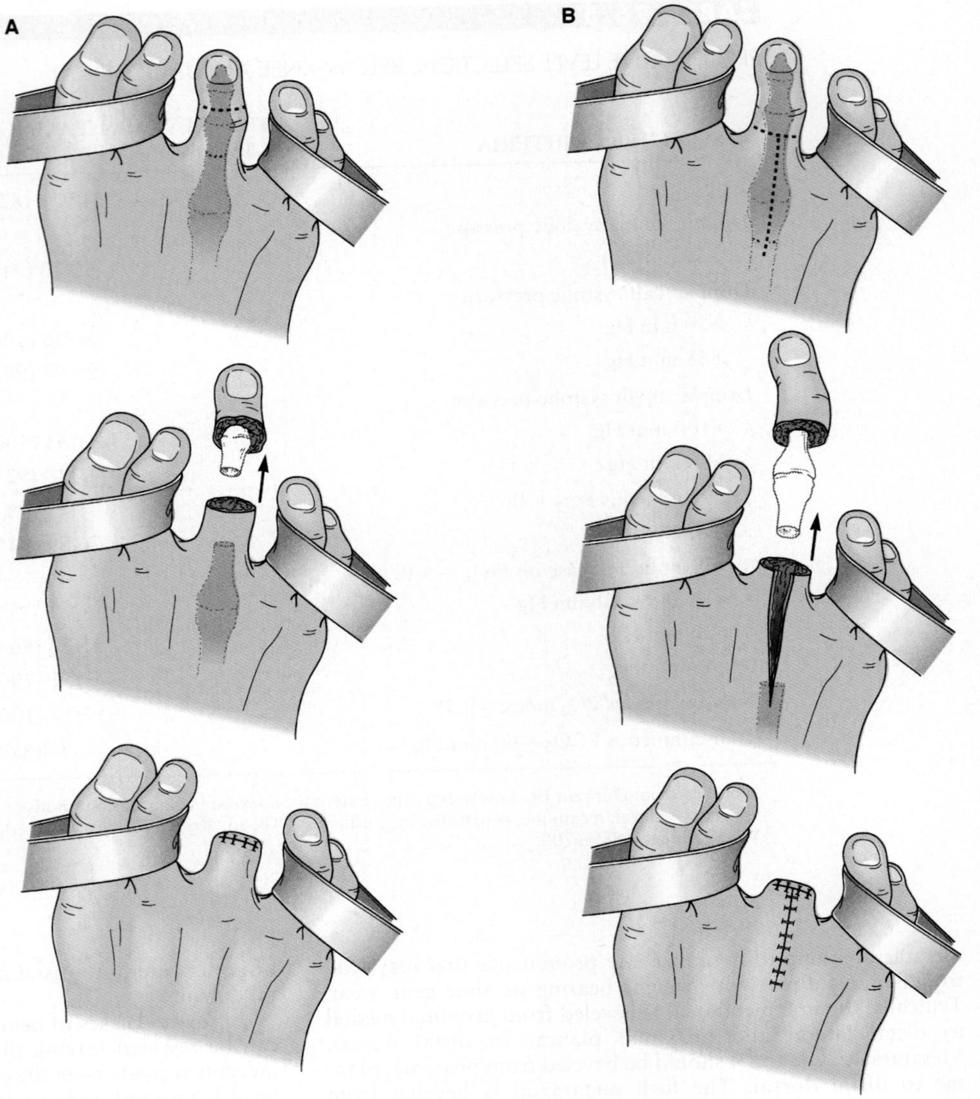

FIGURE 96.2. **A:** Digital amputation. A circumferential skin incision is made proximal to the gangrenous process. The proximal phalanx is transected and the soft tissue approximated. **B:** Metatarsal head resection (ray amputation). A racquet-shaped skin incision is made with the circular component extending circumferentially around the digit and the longitudinal component extending proximal to the metatarsal head. The metatarsal is transected proximal to the head and the soft tissue approximated.

extended diagonally medially and laterally to connect to the dorsal incision. The dorsal incision is deepened to the periosteum, which is cleared with a small periosteal elevator. The metatarsal bones are transected 0.5 to 1.0 cm proximal to the dorsal skin incision. The plantar flap is fashioned by continuing the dissection just superficial to the metatarsal heads. Care is taken to maintain plantar flap thickness. The nerves and tendons are transected sharply under tension and allowed to retract. The plantar flap is rotated anteriorly and assessed for length. Excess tissue is excised sharply and the deep tissue is approximated with absorbable suture. The skin is closed without tension using monofilament suture or skin staples.

Weight bearing is delayed for 1 month to allow adherence of the plantar flap. Either a soft dressing or a short leg cast can be used for a postoperative dressing.

Staging a tendo-Achilles lengthening (TAL) is important to consider following (or at the same time if no infection is present) a partial foot amputation. Ulcer formation at the TMA stump site is often related to equinus formation due to the ensuing flexion/extension imbalance that occurs after resection of the forefoot. A simple triple hemisection percutaneous TAL can effectively lengthen the Achilles and reduce future pressures at the stump site.[32] Other tendon-balancing procedures may be needed to control varus and valgus contraction deformities that can develop.

Syme Amputation

The Syme amputation is a foot amputation that preserves limb length and the epiphyseal growth plates and allows occasional ambulation without a prosthesis. It is indicated in cases of extensive foot trauma or other nonviable tissue conditions distal to the hindfoot. The Syme amputation is contraindicated if a supple intact heel pad and a well-vascularized hindfoot tissue flap are not available.

The procedure can be performed in one or two stages, as illustrated in Figure 96.4. The initial steps for both procedures are identical, except that the skin incision for the two-stage procedure is located 1.5 cm more distally. The skin incision for the one-stage procedure extends from the medial to the lateral malleolus in the horizontal and vertical planes. The dorsal incision is extended to the bone, and the tendons are transected under tension. The anterior tibial artery is identified, divided, and suture ligated. The dissection is carried into the tibiotalar joint space as the foot is forcibly plantar flexed. The ligaments are transected and the talus is dislocated. The plantar aspect of the incision is deepened to the calcaneus, and the calcaneus is sharply dissected from the plantar fascia. The plantar fascia is densely adherent and care must be taken to prevent damage to the heel pad, especially at the level of the Achilles tendon. The posterior tibial artery must be preserved,

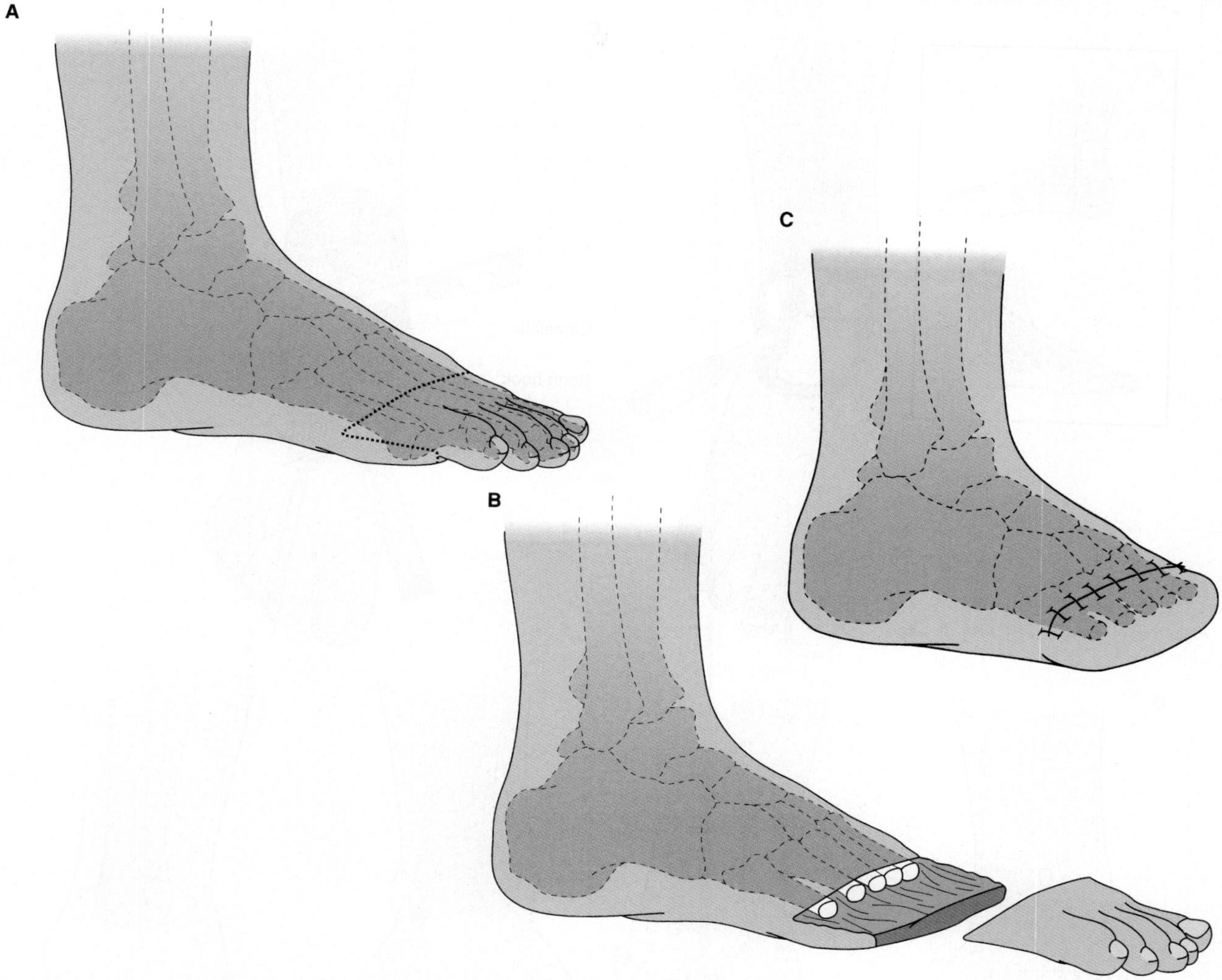

FIGURE 96.3. A: Skin incision for the transmetatarsal amputation is made on the dorsum of the foot immediately proximal to the metatarsal heads and on the plantar surface within the digital crease. B: Metatarsal heads are transected proximal to the skin incision and separated from the plantar soft tissue flap along a plane adjacent to the bone. C: Plantar soft tissue flap is rotated anteriorly and approximated.

because it perfuses the heel pad. The foot is then removed. The two procedures differ from this point forward.

In the one-stage procedure, the medial and lateral malleoli are transected flush with the tibiotalar joint space, and the heel pad is rotated over the ends of the tibia and fibula. The deep fascial layers are approximated with absorbable suture and the skin is closed with monofilament suture or skin staples. Securing the distal end of the remaining plantar fascia to a small drill hole in the distal anterior tibia will help anchor the plantar flap and reduce posterior migration. In the two-stage procedure, the heel pad is similarly positioned and the wound is closed without further bone transection. In 6 weeks, elliptical incisions are made over the medial and lateral malleoli and the distal ends of the tibia and fibula are transected flush with the ankle joint. In addition, the distal flares of the tibia and fibula are transected, creating the rectangular stump of the two-stage procedure. The wound is closed in a similar fashion. For both procedures, weight bearing is delayed for at least 4 weeks to allow heel pad fixation. A soft dressing or a short leg cast can be used.

Below-knee Amputation

The complications of diabetes and arterial insufficiency constitute most of the indications for below-knee amputations. Tables 96.5 and 96.6 outline the criteria used to decide between a BKA and an AKA in this setting.

The most common technique, using a long posterior flap, is illustrated in Figure 96.5. When gangrene, wounds, or incisions preclude the use of a posterior flap, equal anteroposterior or sagittal flaps can be used; however, the posterior flap is associated with the highest incidence of primary healing and is thus preferred whenever possible. This higher rate of healing reflects the fact that the posteriorly located gastrocnemius and soleus muscles are supplied by the sural arteries that originate proximal to the knee.

The proposed skin incision is drawn on the leg with a marker. The tibia should be transected 10 cm distal to the tibial tuberosity and the anterior aspect of the skin incision should be 1 cm distal to the site selected for the tibial transection. The anterior incision is extended medially and laterally. The length of the anterior incision should equal two thirds of the circumference of the leg at the proposed level of the tibial transection. The incision is then extended longitudinally along the medial and lateral aspects of the leg. The length of the longitudinal incisions should equal one third of circumference of the leg at the level of the tibial transection. It is prudent to err on the side of making the posterior flap too long and trim excess length at the time of closure. The medial and lateral incisions are connected posteriorly. Curving the transitions of

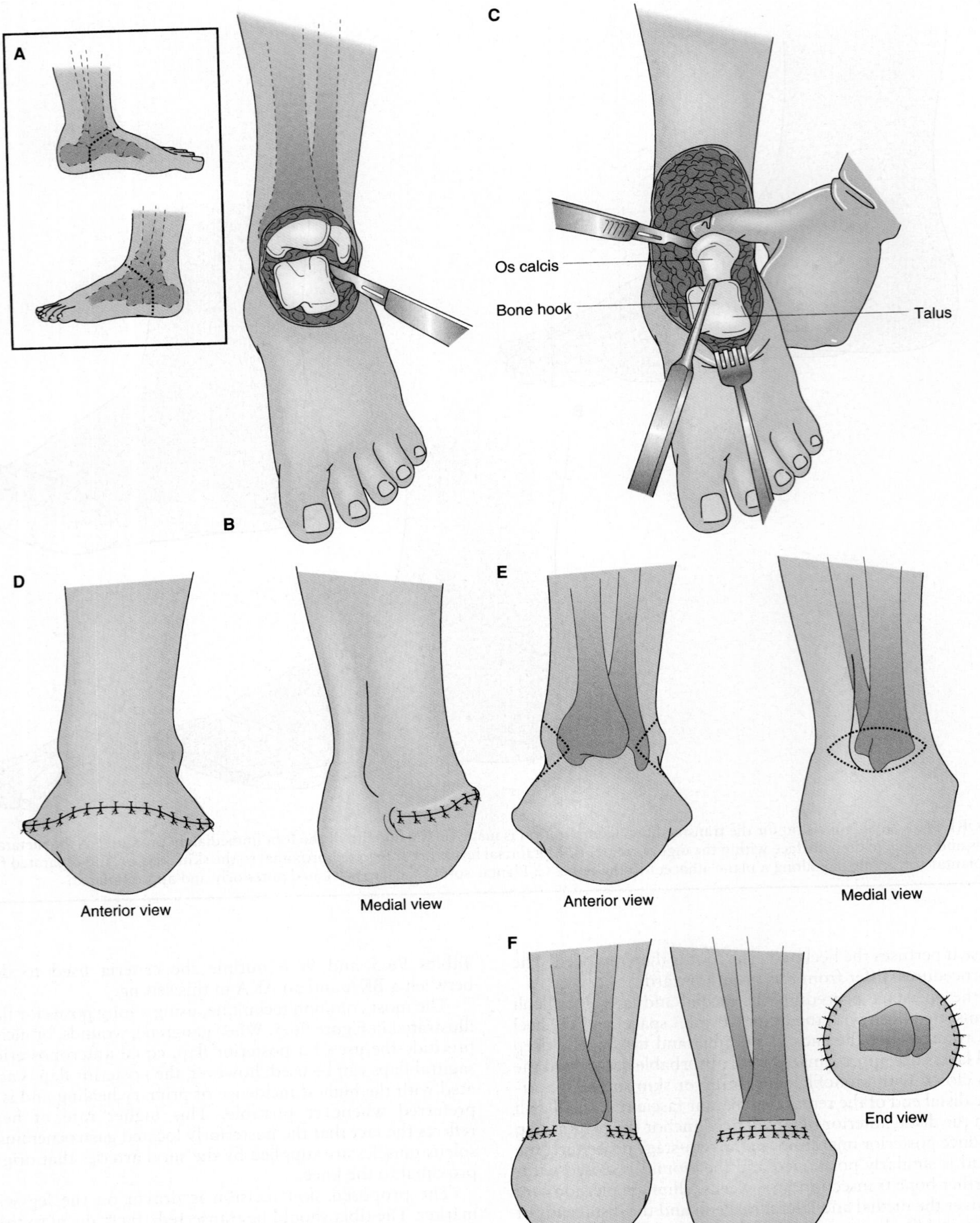

FIGURE 96.4. **A:** Skin incision for the one-stage Syme amputation connects the medial and lateral malleoli in both the horizontal and vertical planes. The skin incision for the two-stage procedure is located approximately 1.5 cm further distally. **B:** Incision is extended into the tibial–talar joint space, and the foot is placed in forced plantar flexion. **C:** Calcaneus is sharply dissected from the adherent plantar fascia along a plane adjacent to the bone. **D:** Heel pad is rotated anteriorly and approximated after the calcaneal dissection in the two-stage procedure and after the additional transection of the medial and lateral malleoli in the one-stage procedure. **E:** Elliptic incisions are made over the medial and lateral malleoli during a second operation for the staged procedure. The medial and lateral malleoli are transected flush with the ankle joint, and the distal flares of the tibia and fibula are removed. **F:** Two-stage procedure results in a less bulbous, more cosmetically acceptable residual limb.

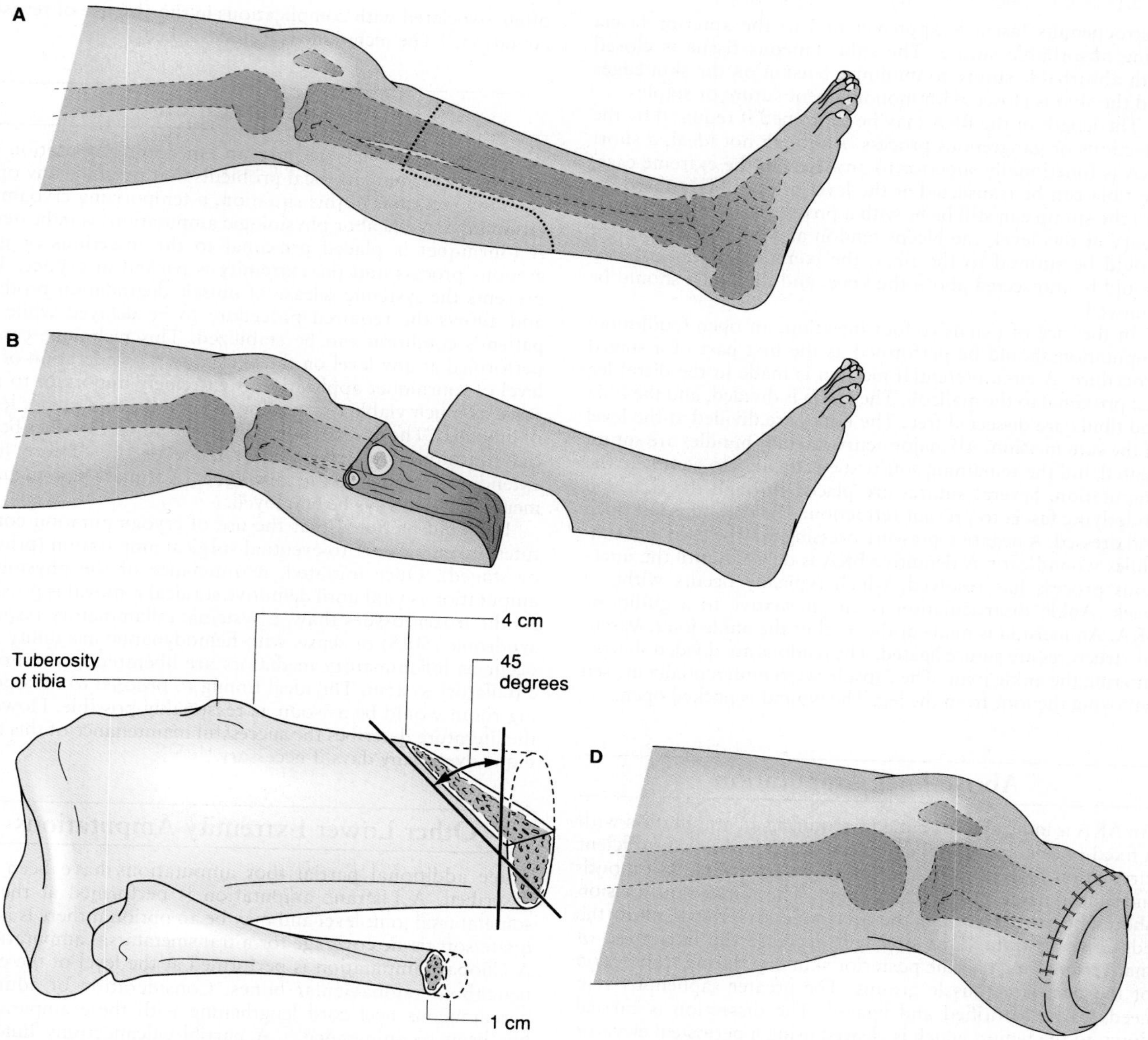

FIGURE 96.5. A: Skin incision for a below-knee amputation based on a posterior flap is made 11 cm distal to the tibial tuberosity and extended medially and laterally to the midpoint of the calf. The length of the posterior flap is about 2 cm longer than the diameter of the calf at the point of the proximal incision. B: Tibia is transected 1 cm proximal to the skin incision. The fibula is transected an additional 1 cm proximal to the level of the tibial transection, and the posterior calf muscles are incised along the plane of the skin incision. C: Anterior aspect of the tibia is beveled at an angle of about 45 degrees, and the bone edges are filed. D: Posterior flap is rotated anteriorly and approximated.

the incision prevents the accumulation of redundant tissue at the medial and lateral aspects of the completed amputation. The skin incisions should be down to the fascia to allow separation of the skin edges. This step decreases the chance of inadvertent injury to the posterior flap later in the procedure; however, the greater and lesser saphenous veins need to be ligated and transected.

The anterior aspect of the incision is deepened through the periosteum of the tibia. The muscles of the anterior compartment are divided at the level of the skin incision and the anterior tibial neurovascular bundle is identified and suture ligated. The proximal tibia is circumferentially cleared of periosteum, and transected 1 cm proximal to the skin incision. The anterior aspect of the tibia is cut on a 45-degree angle. The fibula is cleared and transected 1 cm proximal to the transected tibia. The bones are divided with either a power-driven reciprocating saw or a manual saw. Regardless, care must be taken to avoid trauma to the anterior skin flap.

The posterior tibial and peroneal neurovascular bundles are identified and suture ligated. The tibia is retracted anteriorly and the posterior musculature is divided along the plane of the longitudinal skin incisions using an amputation knife. Extreme caution must be taken to avoid injury to the skin edges of the posterior flap during this step. Often a scalpel is needed to complete the division of the gastrocnemius tendon distally. The specimen is removed; manual compression achieves temporary hemostasis while the remaining vascular structures are identified and ligated. The posterior tibial nerve is retracted distally, ligated, transected sharply, and allowed to retract. The posterior flap is rotated anteriorly to assess thickness and length. Frequently, the musculature needs to be debulked to allow a tension-free closure. Rough edges of the bones are filed smooth and the wound is irrigated. Bone wax is not used. A closed-system drain may be placed to prevent a hematoma. The end of the tibia is covered and stabilized with the deep posterior musculature using absorbable sutures. The gastrocnemius fascia is approximated to the anterior fascia using absorbable suture. The subcutaneous tissue is closed with absorbable suture to minimize tension on the skin edges and the skin is closed with monofilament suture or staples.

The length of the BKA may be shortened if required by the infectious or gangrenous process. Although not ideal, a short BKA is functionally superior to an AKA. In the extreme case, the tibia can be transected at the level of the tibial tuberosity and the stump can still be fit with a prosthesis. If a BKA is necessary at this level, the biceps tendon and collateral ligament should be sutured to the tibia, the common peroneal nerve should be transected above the knee, and the fibula should be removed.

In the face of extensive foot infection, an open (guillotine) amputation should be performed as the first part of a staged procedure. A circumferential incision is made in the distal leg just proximal to the malleoli. The fascia is divided, and the tibia and fibula are dissected free. The bones are divided at the level of the skin incision. All major neurovascular bundles are suture ligated and the remaining soft tissue is divided to complete the amputation. Several sutures are placed through the skin and underlying fascia to prevent retraction. The wound is left open and dressed. A negative-pressure dressing may be used and simplifies wound care. A definitive BKA is delayed until the infectious process has resolved, which typically occurs within a week. Ankle disarticulation is an alternative to a guillotine BKA. An incision is made at the level of the ankle joint. Vascular structures are suture ligated. The tendons are divided sharply entering the ankle joint. The capsule is circumferentially incised removing the foot from the leg. The wound is packed open.

Above-knee Amputation

An AKA is indicated for patients requiring an amputation with a fixed-knee contracture, a nonfunctional limb, or insufficient circulation to heal a BKA. Typically, a transverse fish-mouth incision is made in the lower thigh. The initial skin incision should be carried through the subcutaneous tissue to allow the edges to separate. This step will decrease the likelihood of inadvertent injury to the posterior skin flap during transection of the posterior muscle groups. The greater saphenous vein needs to be identified and ligated. The dissection is carried down to the femur, which is cleared using a periosteal elevator to a level 2 to 3 cm proximal to the skin incision. The superficial femoral artery is dissected free and suture ligated. The bone is transected with a reciprocating or manual saw, and the posterior muscle flap is divided with an amputation knife. Manual compression with a laparotomy pad on the newly divided stump will easily control hemorrhage while vessels are identified and ligated or electrocoagulated. The sciatic nerve is identified and placed on gentle traction. It is then highly ligated, sharply divided, and allowed to retract into the wound. The flaps should be power irrigated and hemostasis ensured. The fascia is then closed with absorbable suture. The subcutaneous tissue is closed with absorbable suture to minimize tension on the skin edges and the skin is closed with monofilament suture or staples. Alternative incisions can be made to accommodate surgical wounds. Most AKA wounds will heal even when the femoral pulse is nonpalpable. More proximal thigh amputations are performed when arterial perfusion is in question.

Hip Disarticulation

Lower extremity amputation at the level of the hip is an uncommon operation. The indications include malignancy, trauma, infection, and, rarely, complications of arterial insufficiency. Hip disarticulation performed for an ischemic AKA is often associated with complications in the absence of revascularization.[33] The technique is well described.

Cryoamputation

Rarely, a patient may require an emergent amputation yet have overwhelming medical problems that preclude any operative intervention. In this situation, a temporizing cryoamputation (aka, medical or physiologic amputation) is indicated.[14] A tourniquet is placed proximal to the infectious or gangrenous process and the extremity is packed in dry ice. This prevents the systemic release of muscle degradation products and allows the required procedure to be delayed while the patient's condition can be stabilized. This technique can be performed at any level on the extremity. Consideration of the level of tourniquet application is extremely important to preserve as much viable tissue as possible and avoid higher levels of limb loss. The dry ice should be placed about 3 inches below the tourniquet to reduce the chance of the "freeze line" extending proximal to the tourniquet. Adequate pain management should always be employed.

It should be noted that the use of cryoamputation constitutes a commitment to eventual surgical amputation (primary or staged). Once initiated, maintenance of the physiologic amputation is vital until definitive surgical removal is possible. As the frozen tissues thaw, a systemic inflammatory response syndrome (SIRS) or sepsis with hemodynamic instability may occur as inflammatory mediators are liberated back into the circulatory system. The ideal timing to proceed to the operating room would be as soon as reasonably possible. However, the literature describes the successful maintenance of this technique over many days if necessary.[14,34,35]

Other Lower Extremity Amputations

Three additional partial foot amputations have been well described. A Lisfranc amputation is performed at the tarsometatarsal joint level and may be an option if there is inadequate soft tissue coverage for a transmetatarsal amputation.[36] A Chopart amputation is performed at the level of the calcaneocuboid–talonavicular bones. Consideration of adding a percutaneous heel cord lengthening with these amputations has been recommended.[37] A partial calcanectomy hindfoot amputation has shown good utility for chronic posterior heel wounds and calcaneal osteomyelitis.[38,39] This amputation involves removal of the posterior body of the calcaneus behind the posterior facet of the subtalar joint. Primary closure is typically possible and patients can ambulate following this procedure using a custom orthotic with a heel filler. Knee disarticulation is a useful amputation for patients with immature growth plates. It is superior to an AKA and allows end weight bearing, improved proprioception, and improved prosthetic control. The required prosthesis is bulky and less cosmetically appealing than that used for a BKA. The technique is well described.[40] Rotationplasty is an uncommon procedure performed primarily for treatment of osteogenic sarcoma of the thigh.[41] It involves nerve-sparing resection of the femur and knee, 180-degree rotation of the leg, and reattachment of the leg. This results in a functional, sensate foot that can easily be fit with a prosthesis.

Wound Dressings

An important consideration after amputation is the type of wound dressings applied to the stump. Two important factors in the success of an amputation are time to rehabilitation and complete wound healing, both of which are influenced by postoperative wound care.[42] With transtibial amputations, there are a number of options, such as soft gauze dressings with elastic wrap, rigid plaster dressings without immediate prosthesis, rigid plaster with immediate postoperative prosthesis, and prefabricated pneumatic postoperative prosthesis. Several studies have compared two or more of these options. End points are not standardized, however, and most studies are not randomized and prospective, making comparisons and meta-analysis difficult.[42]

Benefits and drawbacks are found for each postoperative option.[42] Gauze dressings with elastic wrap are simple and low cost and provide good accessibility to evaluate wound healing. On the other hand, they may lead to higher rates of joint contraction and increased time to ambulation, and risk pressure ischemia from poorly placed elastic wrap. Despite these drawbacks, no convincing data show that soft gauze dressings are inferior to other options.[42,43] A removable knee immobilizer may be used in conjunction with gauze dressings to minimize the risk of joint contracture.

Rigid plaster helps with joint contracture and helps protect the wound from trauma. With addition of a temporary prosthesis, the rigid plaster also promotes early ambulation. The plaster, however, does not provide easy access to evaluate and care for the wound and if not fitted properly will result in sheer stress and thereby break down the wound. Consequently, a level of skill in plaster placement is required of the surgical team to make appropriate and often frequent plaster changes.[42]

Finally, a prefabricated pneumatic postoperative prosthesis allows early ambulation and weight bearing, easy wound access for examination, prevention of joint contracture, and wound protection. The prosthesis, however, is bulky and up front is more expensive than the simple gauze. Prospective studies have demonstrated statistically fewer postoperative complications with the pneumatic prosthesis and statistically fewer limbs requiring higher revisions.[44]

Complications and Outcome

Morbidity and Mortality. Operative mortality depends on the indication and the level. Mortality rates for major lower extremity amputations in vascular and diabetic patients have been reported to be up to 35%.[45] Combined mortality rates from multiple series are shown in Table 96.7.[46] Cardiovascular causes account for two thirds of these deaths, with myocardial infarction responsible for one third.[46] This data is further supported by recent studies by Sandnes et al.[47]and Aulivola et al.[48] Table 96.8 lists known complications after lower extremity amputation.

Long-term survival following major amputation in the vascular population is shown in Table 96.9. The 5-year survival rate is only 37% compared with 85% for age-matched controls.[49]

TABLE 96.7 RESULTS

AMPUTATION MORTALITY

CATEGORY	PERCENTAGE	NUMBER
Below knee	2	25/1,200
Above knee	9	54/609
Diabetic vs. nondiabetic	No difference	
After amputation revision	5.5	12/218

From Frang RD, Tayor LM, Porter JM. Amputations. In: Porter JM, Taylor LM, eds. *Basic Data Underlying Clinical Decision Making in Vascular Surgery*. St. Louis, MO: Quality Medical; 1994:154.

TABLE 96.8 COMPLICATIONS

COMPLICATIONS OF LOWER EXTREMITY AMPUTATIONS

SYSTEM	COMPLICATION
Cardiac	Arrhythmia, congestive heart failure, myocardial infarction
Pulmonary	Pneumonia, pulmonary embolism
Renal	Renal failure, urinary tract infection
Cerebrovascular	Stroke
Hematologic	Deep venous thrombosis, pulmonary embolism
Wound	Hemorrhage, hematoma, infection, failure to heal

Deep Venous Thrombosis and Pulmonary Embolism

The incidence of deep venous thrombosis following lower extremity amputation ranges from 4% to 38%.[50–52] Prophylactic measures including subcutaneous heparin, low-molecular-weight heparins, early mobilization, and pneumatic compression devices should be used as indicated.

Stump Complications

Stump complications include nonhealing, infection, hematoma, contractures, ulceration, phantom pain, and trauma. Although most amputations heal primarily, a small percentage do not. Amputation at a more proximal level usually is successful. Postoperative infections complicate 12% to 28% of all amputations, with the percentage higher in cases performed for infection.[53] Local wound care with drainage, débridement and dressing changes, and systemic antibiotics should be instituted. Wound hematomas are best treated with prevention. Meticulous hemostasis and avoidance of subcutaneous cavities decrease their incidence. Hematomas should be treated in the operating room with evacuation, irrigation, and closure of the wound.

Joint contractures complicate 1% to 3% of all amputations.[45,49] These contractures can occur rapidly postoperatively and are best treated by prevention. Rehabilitation specialists and physical therapists should evaluate patients preoperatively. Active and passive range of motion should be

TABLE 96.9 RESULTS

SURVIVAL AFTER AMPUTATION FOR ISCHEMIA

TIME (y)	SURVIVAL RATE (%)
1	75
2	60
3	50
4	45
5	37

From Frang RD, Taylor LM, Porter JM. Amputations. In: Porter JM, Taylor LM, eds. *Basic Data Underlying Clinical Decision Making in Vascular Surgery*. St. Louis, MO: Quality Medical; 1994:115, with permission.

initiated immediately postoperatively. Adequate pain medication, ideally with patient-controlled or epidural anesthesia,[54,55] is crucial. Pillows and bed positions that result in hip or knee flexion are to be strictly avoided.

Ulcers tend to develop over bony prominences. Poorly fitting prostheses or shoes are the most common causes. Diabetic patients with peripheral neuropathy are especially susceptible to the development of ulcers following toe and limited foot amputations. They can also form on the anterior aspect of AKAs secondary to the disproportional contraction of the hip flexors relative to the hip extensors. Local wound care and bed rest usually lead to healing if the ulcer is superficial. Deep skin ulcers with involvement of the soft tissue and the underlying bone are more complicated. They often suggest borderline perfusion of the stump and require formal revision to a higher level to treat definitively.

Another option in complicated wound closure is negative-pressure wound dressing, which has been used for a wide range of difficult-to-heal lesions. Studies indicate that this dressing technique decreases wound volume, whereas traditional moist gauze dressings do not.[56] The dressings result in granulation tissue and healing in otherwise difficult tissue beds, such as diabetic foot ulcers[57] and decubitus pressure ulcers.[58] In addition to helping contract the size of the wound, negative-pressure dressings also decrease the number and frequency of dressing changes drastically when compared with wet-to-dry dressings. They can also be used following open amputations to help prepare the wound bed for delayed primary closure, skin graft application, or other wound closure techniques.

Neuromas are regenerative nerve tissue that forms in response to transection. They can lead to pain if trapped in the fibrous scar or if irritated by a prosthesis. Proximal nerve division under tension during the original operation decreases the incidence of this complication. Symptomatic neuromas should be treated with proximal resection of the nerve because local excision of the neuroma is rarely adequate.

Some element of phantom extremity pain occurs in nearly all amputations,[59] although these complaints are not always directed to the treating surgeon. It is necessary to describe these common symptoms to the patient and specifically inquire about their presence. The pain is disabling in 5% to 30%[60] of patients surveyed. Currently, pain is felt to be a component of a central pain syndrome and unrelated to either a neuroma or the perception of an intact extremity. Although there is no universally effective treatment, Malone[45] has reported a low incidence with an aggressive rehabilitation program, including immediate prosthetic fitting.

Trauma to a limb following an amputation can convert a healed amputation to a nonhealing wound requiring a more proximal amputation. Perioperatively, patients with a BKA have to be observed closely to prevent attempted ambulation. Diabetic patients with retinopathy should not walk barefoot following toe and foot amputations secondary to the risk that minor trauma may lead to a major wound healing problem.

Additional Amputation

The incidence of future amputation in vascular patients is not insignificant. Snyder et al. evaluated outcomes after forefoot amputations and found that 26% underwent a subsequent forefoot amputation and 37% had a more proximal amputation over 2 years.[61] Cruz et al. demonstrated 17% contralateral amputation in their series.[62] These dismal figures reflect the systemic nature of the underlying diseases and emphasize the importance of appropriate foot care, patient education, close follow-up, and early intervention.[63] A concerted multidisciplinary approach can dramatically decrease the incidence of initial and subsequent lower extremity amputation.[64]

Special Situations

In selected cases, hyperbaric oxygen (HBO) therapy can provide benefit in treating nonhealing amputation sites. Patients require thorough evaluation of their cardiopulmonary status before initiating such treatment. In addition, the treating surgeon has to determine that revascularization is completed or is not indicated. Patients may benefit from treatment if there is a substantial increase in transcutaneous oxygen pressure ($TcPO_2$) near the wound with administration of 100% oxygen. Daily treatments are typically continued for 30 days. Platelet-derived growth factor (becaplermin, Regranex) is approved for use in the United States and has been effective in the management of diabetic foot ulcers and following open foot amputations or débridements. The wound must be clear of all necrotic tissue before initiating therapy.

REHABILITATION AND PROSTHETIC MANAGEMENT

General Considerations

Rehabilitation must be individualized. For some patients, successful rehabilitation means ambulation on a prosthesis and resumption of an independent lifestyle. For others, success may mean being able to pivot on the contralateral limb to be able to assist with transfer. Ambulating with a prosthesis depends on the physiologic status of the patient. Table 96.2 illustrates the dramatic increase in energy requirement with increasing level of the amputation. As expected, the chance of ambulating on a prosthesis decreases with ascending amputation level. The percentages of diabetic and vascular patients who can ambulate with amputations at various levels are shown in Table 96.10. The likelihood of ambulating postoperatively is inversely related to the patient's age and the length of the rehabilitation process.[65] Consideration should be given to inpatient rehab immediately after the acute care of the amputation is complete. Not only does this allow strengthening of the upper extremities and improved transfers, but it has also been shown to reduce 1-year mortality in amputees.[66]

Specific Considerations

Digital and Ray Amputations. All patients who were ambulatory preoperatively should be able to achieve their

TABLE 96.10 RESULTS

AMBULATION AFTER LOWER EXTREMITY AMPUTATION FOR DIABETES OR OCCLUSIVE DISEASE

■ AMPUTATION LEVEL	■ POSTOPERATIVE AMBULATION (%)
Digit or ray	100
Transmetatarsal	100
Syme amputation	90–100
Below knee	75
Above knee	39
Hip disarticulation	<100

From Frang RD, Taylor LM, Porter JM. Amputations. In: Porter JM, Taylor LM, eds. *Basic Data Underlying Clinical Decision Making in Vascular Surgery.* St. Louis, MO: Quality Medical; 1994:155, with permission.

preoperative functional status following a digital or ray amputation. The first digit and metatarsal head are important for weight bearing and for power. A shoe orthosis should effectively compensate for these functions when the patient has some training.

The most important component of postoperative rehabilitation for patients following a digital or ray amputation is education. The rate of repeat amputation (other toe, more proximal level, contralateral limb) is extremely high. Several studies have indicated that the rate of repeat amputation is diminished with a coordinated education program.[67,68]

Transmetatarsal Amputation. A transmetatarsal amputation minimally increases the energy requirement of ambulation; therefore, postoperative ambulation is expected following successful healing. The absence of the toes and metatarsal heads results in the loss of some forward thrust during the push-off phase of ambulation. This deficit can be overcome with either a steel shank or a rigid, roller-soled shoe. The void in the distal shoe is filled with an insert.

Syme Amputation. The prognosis for return to bipedal ambulation following a Syme amputation is excellent. The required energy expenditure is only 10% more than baseline.[69] A significant advantage of this amputation is the ability to ambulate on the stump with only a cup slipper. Even though this activity is permitted on only a limited basis in the home, it is much more convenient for the patient, especially when arising at night. For routine activity the patient uses a prosthesis composed of a nonmotion foot attached to a leg shaft. The shaft has a cutout on the medial aspect to allow passage of the flared distal end of the stump. The configuration of the distal end of the stump results in a bulbous ankle, which is less aesthetically pleasing than the typical below-knee prosthesis.

Below-knee Amputation. The rehabilitation potential following a BKA is very good. Even when the indication for amputation is arterial insufficiency, approximately 75% of patients are able to ambulate with a prosthesis.[46] Multiple design options are available; however, the patellar tendon and the medial and lateral tibial flares are the weight-bearing surfaces for most prostheses. A variety of foot designs are possible to permit extension, flexion, rotation, and energy storage.

Above-knee Amputation. Ambulation on an above-knee prosthesis is achieved by less than 40% of patients with arterial insufficiency.[46] In this patient population, the rate of ambulation on bilateral above-knee prostheses is less than 10%.[70] Most above-knee prostheses use the ischial tuberosity as the primary weight-bearing surface and are secured either by a belt or a suction socket. For younger patients, a suction socket works well. Patients with groin scars from previous revascularization attempts may benefit from a belt mechanism. The knee design depends on the patient's general condition and thigh strength. A knee that engages during the stance phase of gait is more stable and is frequently used in older patients.

References

1. Feinglass J, Brown JL, LoSasso A, et al. Rates of lower-extremity amputation and arterial reconstruction in the United States, 1979–1996. *Am J Public Health* 1999;89(8):122–127.
2. Dillingham TR, Pezzin LE, MacKenzie EJ. Limb amputation and limb deficiency: epidemiology and recent trends in the United States. *South Med J* 2002;95(8):875–883.
3. Falstie-Jensen N, Christensen K. A model for prediction of failure in amputation of the lower limb. *Dan Med Bull* 1990;37:283.
4. Sanmugarajah J, Hussain S, Schwartz J, et al. Monoclonal cryoglobulinemia with extensive gangrene of all four extremities—a case report. *Angiology* 2000;51:431–434.
5. Veith F, Gupta S, Samson R. Progress in limb salvage by reconstructive arterial surgery combined with new or improved adjunctive procedures. *Ann Surg* 1981;194:386.
6. Melzack R, Wall P. Pain mechanisms: a new theory. *Science* 1965;150: 971–979.
7. Augustinsson LE, Carlsson CA, Holm J, et al. Epidural electrical stimulation in severe limb ischemia. Pain relief, increased blood flow, and a possible limb-saving effect. *Ann Surg* 1985;202:104–110.
8. Tallis RC, Illis LS, Sedgwick EM, et al. Spinal cord stimulation in peripheral vascular disease. *J Neurol Neurosurg Psychiatry* 1983;46: 478–484.
9. Meglio M, Cioni B, Dal Lago A, et al. Pain control and improvement of peripheral blood flow following epidural spinal cord stimulation: case report. *J Neurosurg* 1981;54:821–823.
10. Horsch S, Claeys L. Epidural spinal in the treatment of severe peripheral arterial occlusive disease. *Ann Vasc Surg* 1994;5:468–474.
11. Ubbink DT, Spincemaille GH, Prins MH, et al. Microcirculatory investigations to determine the effect of spinal cord stimulation for critical leg ischemia: the Dutch multicenter randomized controlled trial. *J Vasc Surg* 1999;30:236–244.
12. Huber SJ, Vaglienti RM, Huber JS. Spinal cord stimulation in severe, inoperable peripheral vascular disease. *Neuromodulation* 2000;3:131–143.
13. Gersbach PA, Argitis V, Gardza JP, et al. Late outcome of spinal cord stimulation for unreconstructable and limb-threatening lower limb ischemia. *Eur J Vasc Endovasc Surg* 2007;33(6):717–724.
14. Winburn GB, Wood MC, Hawkins ML, et al. Current role of cryoamputation. *Am J Surg* 1991;162:647–650.
15. Lange R. Limb reconstruction versus amputation decision making in massive lower extremity trauma. *Clin Orthop* 1989;(Jun):92–109.
16. Bosse MJ, McKenzie EJ, Kellam JF, et al. An analysis of outcomes of reconstruction or amputation of leg-threatening injuries. *N Engl J Med* 2002; 347:1924–1931.
17. Johansen K, Daines M, Howey T, et al. Objective criteria accurately predict amputation following lower extremity trauma. *J Trauma* 1990;30: 568–572; discussion 572–573.
18. Ly TV, Travison TG, Castillo RC, et al. Ability of lower-extremity injury severity scores to predict functional outcome after limb salvage. *J Bone Joint Surg Am* 2008;90(8):1738–1743.
19. Adam DJ, Beard JD, Cleveland T, et al. Bypass versus Angioplasty in Severe Ischaemia of the Leg (BASIL): multicentre, randomized controlled trial. *Lancet* 2005;366(9501):1925–1934.
20. Harwood T, Coe E, Flynn T, et al. The use of arm vein conduits during infrageniculate arterial bypass. *J Vasc Surg* 1992;16:420–423.
21. Leseche G, Penna C, Bouttier S, et al. Femorodistal bypass using cryopreserved venous allografts for limb salvage. *Ann Vasc Surg* 1997;11(3): 230–236.
22. Raptis S, Miller J. Influence of vein cuff on polytetrafluoroethylene grafts for primary femoropopliteal bypass. *Br J Surg* 1995;82:478–491.
23. Stonebridge P, Prescott R, Ruckley C. Randomized trial comparing infrainguinal polytetrafluoroethylene bypass grafting with and without vein interposition cuff at the distal anastomosis. The Joint Vascular Research Group. *J Vasc Surg* 1997;26(Oct):543–550.
24. Bosiers M, Deloose K, Verbist J, et al. Heparin-bonded expanded polytetrafluoroethylene vascular graft for femoropopliteal and femorocrural bypass grafting: 1-year results. *J Vasc Surg* 2006;43(2):313–318.
25. Lepantalo M, Tukiainen E. Combined vascular reconstruction and microvascular muscle flap transfer for salvage of ischaemic legs with major tissue loss and wound complications. *Eur J Vasc Endovasc Surg* 1996;12: 65–69.
26. Briggs S, Banis JJ, Kaebnick H, et al. Distal revascularization and microvascular free tissue transfer: an alternative to amputation in ischemic lesions of the lower extremity. *J Vasc Surg* 1985;2:806–811.
27. Biancari F, Kantonen I, Alback A, et al. Limits of infrapopliteal bypass surgery for critical leg ischemia: when not to reconstruct. *World J Surg* 2000;24:727–733.
28. Keagy B, Schwartz J, Kotb M, et al. Lower extremity amputation: the control series. *J Vasc Surg* 1986;4:321–326.
29. Dwars B, Van Den Broek T, Ravwerda J, et al. Criteria for reliable selection of the lowest level of amputation in peripheral vascular disease. *J Vasc Surg* 1992;15:536.
30. Malone J, Anderson G, Halka S, et al. Prospective comparison of noninvasive techniques for amputation level selection. *Am J Surg* 1987;154:179.
31. Misuri A, Lucertini G, Nanni A, et al. Predictive value of transcutaneous oximetry for selection of the amputation level. *J Cardiovasc Surg* 2000;41: 83–87.
32. Nishimoto GS, Attinger CE, Cooper PS. Lengthening the Achilles tendon for the treatment of diabetic plantar forefoot ulceration. *Surg Clin North Am* 2003;83(3):707–726.
33. Endean ED, Schwarcz TH, Barker DE, et al. Hip disarticulation: factors affecting outcome. *J Vasc Surg* 1991;14(3):398–404.
34. Still JM, Wray CH, Moretz WH. Selective physiologic amputation: a valuable adjunct in preparation for surgical operation. *Ann Surg* 1970;171(1): 143–151.
35. Winburn GB, Hawkins ML, Wood MC. Physiologic amputation prevents myoglobinuria from lower extremity myonecrosis. *South Med J* 1993; 86(10):1101–1105.

36. Roach J, Deutsch A, McFarlane D. Resurrection of the amputations of Lisfranc and Chopart for diabetic gangrene. *Arch Surg* 1987;122: 931–934.
37. Leiberman J, Jacobs R, Goldstock L, et al. Chopart amputation with percutaneous heel cord lengthening. *Clin Orthop* 1993;292:245–249.
38. Randall DB, Phillips J, Ianiro G. Partial calcanectomy for the treatment of recalcitrant heel ulcerations. *J Am Podiatr Med Assoc* 2005;95(4): 335–341.
39. Lehmann S, Murphy RD, Hodor L. Partial calcanectomy in the treatment of chronic heel ulceration. *J Am Podiatr Med Assoc* 2001;91(7):369–372.
40. Burgess E. Disarticulation of the knee: a modified technique. *Arch Surg* 1977;112:1250.
41. Merkel K, Gebhardt M, Springfield D. Rotationplasty as a reconstructive operation after tumor resection. *Clin Orthop* 1991;270:231–236.
42. Smith DG, McFarland LV, Sangeorzan BJ, et al. Postoperative dressing and management strategies for transtibial amputations: a critical review. *J Rehabil Res Dev* 2003(May–June);40(3):213–224.
43. Kane TJ, Pollack EW. The rigid versus soft postoperative dressing controversy: a controlled study in vascular below-knee amputees. *Am Surg* 1980; 46:244–247.
44. Schon LC, Short KW, Soupiou O, et al. Benefits of early prosthetic management of transtibial amputees: a prospective clinical study of a prefabricated prosthesis. *Foot Ankle Int* 2002;23:509–514.
45. Malone J. Lower extremity amputation. In: Moore W, ed. *Vascular Surgery: A Comprehensive Review*. Philadelphia, PA: WB Saunders; 1993: 809.
46. Frang R, Taylor L, Porter J. Amputations. In: Porter J, Taylor L, eds. *Basic Data Underlying Clinical Decision Making in Vascular Surgery*. St. Louis, MO: Quality Medical Publishing; 1994:153.
47. Sandnes DK, Sobel M, Flum DR. Survival after lower extremity amputation. *J Am Coll Surg* 2004;199:394–402.
48. Aulivola B, Hile CN, Hamdan AD, et al. Major lower extremity amputation. *Arch Surg* 2004;139: 395–399.
49. Roon A, Moore W. Below-knee amputations: a modern approach. *Am J Surg* 1977;134:153.
50. Williams J, Britt L, Eades T, et al. Pulmonary embolism after amputation of the lower extremity. *Surg Gynecol Obstet* 1975;140:246–248.
51. Yeager R, Moneta G, Edwards J, et al. Deep vein thrombosis associated with lower extremity amputation. *J Vasc Surg* 1995;22:612–615.
52. Burke B, Kumar R, Vickers V, et al. Deep vein thrombosis after lower limb amputation. *Am J Phys Med Rehab* 2000;79:145–149.
53. Fisher DJ, Clagett G, Fry R, et al. One-stage versus two-stage amputation for wet gangrene of the lower extremity: a randomized study. *J Vasc Surg* 1988;8(Oct):428–433.
54. Enneking F, Morey T. Continuous postoperative infusion of a regional anesthetic after an amputation of the lower extremity. A randomized clinical trial [letter; comment]. *J Bone Joint Surg* 1997;79(Nov):1752–1753.
55. Pinzur M, Garla P, Pluth T, et al. Continuous postoperative infusion of a regional anesthetic after an amputation of the lower extremity. A randomized clinical trial [see comments]. *J Bone Joint Surg* 1996;78:1501–1505.
56. Eginton MT, Brown KR, Seabrook GR, et al. A prospective randomized evaluation of negative-pressure wound dressings for diabetic foot wounds. *Ann Vasc Surg* 2003;17(6):645–649.
57. Armstrong DG, Lavery LA; Diabetic Foot Study Consortium. Negative pressure wound therapy after partial diabetic foot amputation: a multicentre randomised controlled trial. *Lancet* 2005;366(9498):1704–1710.
58. Ford CN, Reinhard ER, Yeh D, et al. Interim analysis of a prospective, randomized trial of vacuum-assisted closure versus the healthpoint system in the management of pressure ulcers. *Ann Plast Surg* 2002;49(1): 55–61.
59. Iacono R, Linford J, Sandyk R. Pain management after lower extremity amputation. *Neurosurgery* 1987;20:496–500.
60. Sherman R, Sherman C, Parker L. Chronic phantom and stump pain among American veterans: results of a survey. *Pain* 1984;18:83.
61. Snyder DC, Salameh JR, Clericuzio CP. Retrospective review of forefoot amputations at a Veterans Affairs hospital and evaluation of post-amputation follow-up. *Am J Surg* 2006;192(5):e51–e54.
62. Cruz CP, Eidt JF, Capps C, et al. Major lower extremity amputations at a Veterans Affairs hospital. *Am J Surg* 2003;186(5):449–454.
63. Powell T, Burnham S, Johnson, GJ. Second leg ischemia. Lower extremity bypass versus amputation in patients with contralateral lower extremity amputation. *Am Surg* 1984;50:577–580.
64. Van Gils C, Wheeler L, Mellstrom M, et al. Amputation prevention by vascular surgery and podiatry collaboration in high-risk diabetic and nondiabetic patients. The Operation Desert Foot experience. *Diabetes Care* 1999; 22:678–683.
65. Harris W. Lower-extremity amputation in elderly patients. *Can J Surg* 1987;30:315.
66. Stineman MG, Kwong PL, Kurichi JE, et al. The effectiveness of inpatient rehabilitation in the acute postoperative phase of care after transtibial or transfemoral amputation: study of an integrated health care delivery system. *Arch Phys Med Rehabil* 2008;89(10):1863–1872.
67. Bild D, Selby J, Sinnock P, et al. Lower-extremity amputation in people with diabetes. Epidemiology and prevention. *Diabetes Care* 1989;12: 24–31.
68. Del Aguila M, Reiber G, Koepsell T. How does provider and patient awareness of high-risk status for lower-extremity amputation influence foot-care practice? *Diabetes Care* 1994;17:1050–1054.
69. Waters R, Perry J, Antonelli D, et al. Energy cost of walking amputees: the influence of level of amputation. *J Bone Joint Surg* 1976;58A:42.
70. Malone J. Above the knee amputation and hip disarticulation. In: Ernst C, Stanley C, eds. *Current Therapy in Vascular Surgery*. Philadelphia, PA: BC Decker; 1991:699.

CHAPTER 97 ■ PATHOGENESIS OF ANEURYSMS

B. TIMOTHY BAXTER AND G. MATTHEW LONGO

KEY POINTS

1. The principle risk factors for abdominal aortic aneurysm (AAA) are smoking, increasing age, male gender, and family history of AAA.
2. Population studies reveal a strong genetic predisposition to AAA formation, the mechanism of which is currently unknown.
3. Chronic inflammation, macrophages in particular, play a key role in the degenerative process.
4. AAAs are the result of aortic wall degeneration and defective aortic wall remodeling.
5. Digestion of elastin and collagen by proteolytic enzymes, such as the matrix metalloproteinases, is crucial to aneurysm formation.
6. Structural and hemodynamic factors unique to the infrarenal abdominal aorta most likely play a role in aneurysm pathogenesis.

An aneurysm is a permanent, localized dilation encompassing all three layers of a blood vessel wall. The Committee on Reporting Standards of the major North American vascular societies more precisely defines an aneurysm as a 50% increase in the diameter of a vessel in comparison with its expected normal diameter.[1] Aneurysms are usually classified based on their etiology and anatomic location. The most common etiology of an aneurysm is vessel wall degeneration. Other less common causes include infection, poststenotic dilation, trauma, arteritis, and various connective tissue defects (e.g., the high incidence of thoracic aneurysms in Marfan syndrome). Despite the occurrence of aneurysms throughout the arterial tree, the predominant extracranial location for aneurysms is the infrarenal aorta. Intracranial aneurysms, although common, appear to be etiologically distinct from extracranial aneurysms. This chapter focuses on the pathogenesis of the degenerative, infrarenal, abdominal aortic aneurysm (AAA).

CLINICAL RISK FACTORS

Large-scale studies have shown that patients with AAA possess many of the same risk factors as those who develop ather-
1 osclerosis. Increasing age, male gender, and smoking are the three chief risk factors for AAA recently identified within the Aneurysm Detection and Management (ADAM) cohort.[2] Of all the risk factors implicated in this cohort, the strongest modifiable risk factor appeared to be smoking. Although not all studies of AAA concur, other clinical features associated with aneurysms include hypertension, the presence of coronary artery disease, hyperlipidemia, and chronic obstructive pulmonary disease.[3–9]

Abdominal Aortic Aneurysm and Atherosclerosis

Until recently, degenerative AAAs were usually referred to as *atherosclerotic* because of the strong clinical and histopathologic associations between the two disease processes. AAA and atherosclerosis share some of the same clinical risk factors, and atherosclerotic plaque is almost always present in resected aneurysm wall.[10] Some arteries are also known to undergo compensatory remodeling in response to atherosclerotic luminal narrowing.[11] Furthermore, in human autopsy studies, increasing amounts of atherosclerotic plaque in the infrarenal aorta were associated with localized aortic dilation and thinning of the aortic media.[12,13]

Animal experiments lend support to the hypothesis that AAA may be caused by atherosclerosis. In monkeys, Zarins et al.[14] demonstrated that withdrawal of an atherogenic diet resulted in aortic atherosclerotic plaque regression and an associated development of AAAs. In another model primarily used to study atherosclerosis, transgenic mice with apolipoprotein E deficiency were found to spontaneously develop aortic aneurysms.[15] This characteristic can be augmented by giving prolonged subcutaneous infusions of angiotensin II, which has many effects including increases in blood pressure.[16] In addition, recent work has identified a sequence on 9p21 that is associated with a clinical phenotype of AAA and myocardial infarction providing evidence of a common etiologic factor in some individuals with AAA.

Although atherosclerosis may appear to be directly linked with AAA, other evidence suggests that AAA may be its own distinct pathologic process. In 1980, Tilson and Stansel[17] pointed out four important clinical differences seen in groups of AAA and aortic occlusive disease patients. They observed that AAA patients (a) exhibit a higher ratio of men to women, (b) are 10 years older on average, (c) rarely manifest symptoms of lower extremity vascular insufficiency, and (d) rarely experience problems with late graft patency compared with the aortic occlusive disease patients. In addition to these observations, multiple studies have also failed to show a consistent, positive association linking AAA with diabetes mellitus, one of the principle modifiable risk factors for atherosclerosis.[2–4] In fact, the aforementioned ADAM cohort trial found a negative relationship between AAA and diabetes mellitus.

Examination of pathologic specimens reveals histologic differences as well. A transmural process is seen with AAA; however, atherosclerosis is mainly confined with erosion into the 2
media in advanced cases. Some researchers have proposed that atherosclerosis may even be an incidental finding in AAA, citing specimens obtained from poststenotic and syphilitic aneurysms that can show atherosclerotic changes as well.[18]

In summary, it appears that the development of AAA is not simply the end result of the atherosclerotic process. Most likely, other factors of equal or greater importance are influencing aneurysm formation. Although the potential role of atherosclerosis in initiating a local inflammatory process that could lead to AAA in susceptible individuals should not be dismissed, other avenues of research aimed at sorting out the inflammatory response that leads to this susceptibility may prove to be more fruitful in understanding the pathogenesis of AAA. Identification of the protein(s) encoded by the sequence variant in 9p21 may provide critical new insight into the relationship between AAA and atherosclerosis.

CLINICAL AND BASIC SCIENCE RESEARCH IN ABDOMINAL AORTIC ANEURYSM PATHOGENESIS

Abdominal Aortic Aneurysm as a Distinct Pathologic Entity

Recognizing AAA as a distinct pathologic entity with significant morbidity, mortality, and health care costs, the National Heart, Lung, and Blood Institute has sponsored efforts to further understand its pathogenesis. These efforts are focused on four areas: (a) molecular genetics, (b) inflammation and immune responses, (c) proteolytic degradation of the aortic wall connective tissue, and (d) biomechanical wall stress.[19] The remainder of this chapter highlights past and current research in each of these four areas.

Challenges in Aneurysm Research

Before a discussion of AAA research can be fully understood and appreciated, there are two important problems that must be considered. The first is that almost all of the human AAA tissue available for study is sampled late in the course of the disease. The early changes in the human aorta during AAA pathogenesis are essentially unknown and can only be approximated through the use of animal models. The second problem is the lack of a single, well-accepted animal model that reproduces the entire spectrum of pathology found in human AAA. Currently, there are a variety of animal models, each of which develops an aneurysm through a different inciting mechanism. Although many of the models and even late-stage human AAA disease seem to ultimately converge to similar end-stage processes, the events leading to the end-stage disease may in fact be very different. Consequently, all AAA research should be evaluated within the context of these two problems and the limitations of this research should be recognized.

MOLECULAR GENETICS

The study of the genetics of AAA serves two purposes. The first is that by locating and characterizing genes suspected in AAA pathogenesis, investigators may uncover additional pathways for more detailed study. These pathways may also provide potential new targets for pharmacologic intervention. The second, and perhaps most important, purpose is to develop a means for genetic testing to help identify patients at risk for developing AAA early in the course of the disease.

Although clinicians treating large numbers of patients with AAA were undoubtedly aware of clusters of aneurysms within families, Clifton[20] was the first to describe three affected siblings in 1977. Data supporting this observation did not appear until 7 years later, when Tilson and Seashore[21] described 50 families with more than one affected member. In 1986, Johansen and Koepsell[22] reported the incidence of AAA at 19% among first-degree relatives of matched controls. A more recent study examining first-degree relatives using ultrasonography corroborated these findings, with 18% of affected siblings older than age 60 years harboring AAAs.[23]

Although these studies demonstrated a familial tendency to develop AAA, they did not use genetic models to determine the specific inheritance pattern of AAA. Two of the more conclusive studies to date have used segregation analyses of large pedigrees and both have concluded that the genetic transmission of AAA is best explained by a single gene rather than by multiple factors. However, these studies do not agree on whether the gene inheritance is recessive[24] or dominant.[25] In contrast, Kuivaniemi et al.[26] published their pedigree analysis of 233 families with at least two affected members in 2003. They concluded that AAA is a multifactorial disorder without a single inheritance mode.

In addition to traditional pedigree analysis, new techniques in molecular biology and computer technology have become available to help investigators study the genetic aspects of AAA formation. Two studies using complementary DNA microarrays analyzed the gene expression profiles of human AAA tissue compared to normal and atherosclerotic aortas. AAA tissue demonstrated a pattern showing chronic inflammation, smooth muscle cell depletion, atherosclerosis, and extracellular matrix degradation that was significantly different from the normal aortas.[27,28] Another study using whole genome scanning and linkage analysis of 36 AAA families found possible susceptibility loci on chromosomes 4 and 19, recommending further study of nearby candidate genes.[29]

In searching for a gene that might explain AAA, considerable work has focused on the genes regulating matrix protein metabolism, inflammation, and immune function. With the exception of rare cases of collagen mutations,[30] no known mutations in matrix proteins can account for the majority of AAAs.[19] Helgadottir et al.[30a] have recently identified a sequence variant on 9p21 associated with a complex of myocardial infarction, intracranial aneurysm, and AAA. Research has implicated a multitude of polymorphisms in protease, cytokine, and other immunoregulatory genes thought to be associated with AAA (Table 97.1). However, most of these studies are small and lack the statistical power to provide definitive information, so the contribution of each factor to AAA pathogenesis remains to be clarified. Given the multifactorial nature of AAA, it is possible and even likely that a combination of polymorphisms may be interacting to bring about the AAA phenotype. If so, new analytical approaches will be required to identify these combinations.

Gender differences in AAA offer perhaps the most obvious clinical risk factor associated an increased incidence of AAAs. Lederle et al. as part of the ADAM trial documented that female gender was considered a negative risk factor for developing a small AAA (odds ratio [OR] 0.47 [confidence interval (CI) 0.32–0.69] for aortic diameter (AD) 3.0–3.9 cm, OR 0.18 [CI 0.07–0.48] for AD >4.0 cm).[1] In contrast, the prevalence of AAAs among males older than 50 years is four to five times greater than age-matched females.[2] After analyzing population-based screening studies, Bengtsson et al. demonstrated that AAAs also develop 10 to 15 years later in women.[8] Speculation as to why this occurs may be due to decreased circulating levels of estrogen in postmenopausal women, as has been suggested by studies in rodents.

INFLAMMATION AND IMMUNE RESPONSES

Importance of Inflammation

3 Histologic examination of human AAA tissue demonstrates an inflammatory cell infiltrate consisting of T cells, B cells, dendritic cells, plasma cells, natural killer cells, and macrophages.[31–33] These cells are typically located throughout the intima, media, and adventitia, and in extreme cases produce what is termed *inflammatory AAA*. In contrast to the panmural inflammation of AAA, the microscopic appearance of an atherosclerotic aorta shows an infiltrate of T cells and macrophages located within the intima and media.[33] In comparing larger versus smaller AAAs, Freestone et al.[34] found that as aneurysm size increased, so did the intensity of the inflammatory cell infiltrate.

Animal models of AAA confirm the importance of inflammation in the aorta during aneurysm formation. In the elastase infusion model, transient infusion of the infrarenal rat aorta with porcine pancreatic elastase immediately renders the aorta slightly larger than its preperfusion diameter through the mechanical disruption of the elastic lamellae. The aorta then remains stable in size for nearly 3 days. When examined after 3 days, however, a 300% increase in size is seen with a concurrent inflammatory cell infiltrate.[35] This model has been adapted to mice, with the inflammation and secondary enlargement occurring closer to 2 weeks following elastase infusion.[36] A second commonly used mouse model employing the periaortic application of calcium chloride also shows an intense inflammatory cell infiltrate preceding aortic enlargement.[37] Further evidence that invading inflammatory cells play a key role in AAA progression comes again from the elastase infusion model. In these experiments, rats treated with either cyclosporine or methylprednisolone failed to develop aortic inflammation and subsequently did not develop AAAs in comparison to placebo-treated control rats.[38]

Recruitment of the Inflammatory Cell Infiltrate

The stimulus for the recruitment of the inflammatory cells into the aorta is currently unknown and is an area of ongoing research. The elastin degradation product hypothesis suggests that as the elastin in the aortic wall breaks down, specific epitopes are exposed generating an immune response with subsequent inflammatory cell invasion. Supporting experimental evidence comes from Hance et al.,[39] who studied soluble elastin degradation fragments from human AAA tissue. They found that these peptides are able to attract mononuclear phagocytes in vitro through a specific interaction with a 67-kD elastin-binding protein receptor on the phagocytes. Elastin degradation products have also been found to induce angiogenesis in the adventitia of rat aortas.[40] What remains to be explained is the inciting event leading to elastin breakdown and whether these peptides initiate or help amplify the immune response in AAAs.

Studies of human AAA tissue reveal characteristics consistent with an autoimmune process, namely large amounts of immunoglobin G[41] and the presence of plasma cells.[31] Additionally, a proposed autoantigen has been identified and characterized by Gregory et al.[42] It is a 40-kD protein similar to an extracellular matrix component that specifically binds to antibodies isolated from human AAA. However, two more recent studies have cast doubt on this autoimmune hypothesis, characterizing the immune response in AAA tissue as relatively nonspecific.[43,44]

Infection with *Chlamydia pneumoniae* has been suggested as a possible contributor in the formation of AAA. In one early study, investigators found that chlamydial antigens were present in a majority of human AAA tissue samples compared with healthy control aortas.[45] Subsequent studies have confirmed that chlamydia, or chlamydial antigens, are frequently present in AAA tissue.[46,47] In another study by Tambiah and Powell[48] using a rabbit model of AAA, topical treatment of the aorta with chlamydial antigens enhanced aneurysm formation through a process that could be attenuated by treatment with azithromycin. In this instance, the mere presence of the

TABLE 97.1

POLYMORPHISMS ASSOCIATED WITH AAA

REFERENCE	POLYMORPHISM	PATIENTS WITH AAA	PATIENTS WITHOUT AAA
Schillinger et al.[114]	Heme oxygenase-1 promotor gene	Homozygous or heterozygous for less than 25 GT repeats, 41%	Homozygous or heterozygous for less than 25 GT repeats, 59%
Pola et al.[115]	Angiotensin-converting enzyme gene	Normotension: DD genotype frequency, 70%; II genotype frequency, 5% Hypertension: DD genotype frequency, 32%; II genotype frequency, 21%	Normotensive controls DD genotype frequency, 25% II genotype frequency, 32%
Gerdes et al.[116]	Apolipoprotein E gene	E3E3 genotype: expansion rate, 2.1 mm/y E3E4 genotype: expansion rate, 1.3 mm/y E2E3 genotype: expansion rate, 3.1 mm/y E2E4 genotype: expansion rate, 4.2 mm/y	
Rossaak et al.[117]	Plasminogen activator inhibitor-1 gene promoter	Familial AAA 4G4G genotype frequency, 20% 5G5G genotype frequency, 26% Nonfamilial AAA 4G4G genotype frequency, 38% 5G5G genotype frequency, 14%	Healthy control subjects 4G4G genotype frequency, 35% 5G5G genotype frequency, 13%
Wang et al.[118]	TIMP-1 and TIMP-2 genes	Female TIMP-1 nt 434 C allele frequency, 62% T allele frequency, 38% Male TIMP-2 nt 573 G allele frequency, 91% A allele frequency, 9%	Female TIMP-1 nt 434 C allele frequency, 27% T allele frequency, 73% Male TIMP-2 nt 573 G allele frequency, 79% A allele frequency, 21%
Kotani et al.[119]	Endothelial nitric oxide synthase gene	Patients with AAA requiring operation 5 repeat intron 4 allele frequency, 79% 4 repeat intron 4 allele frequency, 21% Patients with AAA under observation 5 repeat intron 4 allele frequency, 96% 4 repeat intron 4 allele frequency, 4%	Healthy control subjects 5 repeat intron 4 allele frequency, 90% 4 repeat intron 4 allele frequency, 10%
Rasmussen et al.[120]	HLA-DR B1 gene	Patients with inflammatory AAAs HLA-DR B1*15 allele frequency, 47% HLA-DR B1*0404 allele frequency, 14%	Healthy control subjects HLA-DR B1a allele frequency, 27% HLA-DR B0404 allele frequency, 3%
Jones et al.[121]	MMP9 gene	MMP-9 nt 1562 CC genotype frequency, 62% CT genotype frequency, 35% TT genotype frequency, 2.9%	MMP-9 nt 1562 CC genotype frequency, 72% CT genotype frequency, 28% TT genotype frequency, 0.5%
Brown et al.[122]	IL-10 gene	IL-10 nt 1082 G allele frequency, 41% A allele frequency, 59%	IL-10 nt 1082 G allele frequency, 53% A allele frequency, 47%
Strauss et al.[123]	MTHFR gene	MTHFR nt 677 C allele frequency, 63% T allele frequency, 37%	MTHFR nt 677 C allele frequency, 79% T allele frequency, 21%

AAA, abdominal aortic aneurysm; GT, genotype; HLA, human leukocyte antigen; IL, interleukin; MTHFR, methylenetetrahydrofolate reductase; TIMP, tissue inhibitors of metalloproteinases.
Adapted from Ailawadi G, Eliason JL, Upchurch GR Jr. Current concepts in the pathogenesis of abdominal aortic aneurysm. *J Vasc Surg* 2003;38: 584–588.

chlamydial antigens was sufficient to enhance aneurysm development without active infection, leading the investigators to suggest that azithromycin most likely worked through an anti-inflammatory mechanism. Altogether, however, considering the high prevalence of chlamydial infection in the general population,[49] strong evidence of specificity for AAA is currently lacking.

Another possible recruitment mechanism involves the action of chemokines, a related family of low-molecular-weight cytokines that control leukocyte trafficking. Compared with controls, human AAA tissue contains greater amounts of the chemokines interleukin-8 (IL-8) and monocyte chemoattractant protein-1.[50] In mice, work using the elastase infusion model has demonstrated an increased production of the chemokine monocyte chemoattractant protein-1 and chemokines regulated on activation (normal T-cell expressed and secreted) in aneurysmal tissue. Notably, the expression of these chemokines by the aortic smooth muscle cells preceded the influx of inflammatory cells during the experimental AAA development.[51] Mactaggart et al.[51a] have investigated the role of three different chemokine receptors using a murine AAA model and mice with targeted deletions of these receptors. CCR2, but not CCR5 or CXCR3, was found to be the critical chemokine receptor for aneurysm formation.

Cytokines and Abdominal Aortic Aneurysm

Once inflammatory cells are present in the aorta, they can produce a multitude of effects. One of the most critical functions is that of coordination and direction of the ongoing immune response. This effect is achieved through the action of cytokines, which can be produced both by invading inflammatory cells and by resident mesenchymal cells. The cytokine profile of human AAA tissue has been extensively examined. Studies of homogenized AAA tissue, as well as AAA tissue culture explants, have found overexpression of proinflammatory cytokines, such as tumor necrosis factor-α, IL-6, and IL-1β.[52,53] The Th1 cytokine interferon-γ (IFN-γ) in conjunction with other Th1 cytokines, IL-2, IL-12, and IL-18,[4] has also been implicated in human AAA,[52] and elevated circulating levels of IFN-γ appear to correlate with more rapid aneurysm expansion.[54] Furthermore, a recent study using the calcium chloride AAA model in mice demonstrated that transgenic mice deficient in IFN-γ were unable to produce aneurysms. The ability to generate aneurysms was regained with the transplantation of splenocytes capable of producing IFN-γ.[55]

These findings contrast with recent work implicating the Th2 cytokine response. Schonbeck et al.[56] examined the cytokine profile of human AAA tissue and found no evidence for Th1 or IFN-γ pathway activation, but rather an abundance of IL-4, IL-5, and IL-10, all Th2 cytokines.[56] Extending these observations into an animal model, researchers transplanted wild-type mouse aortas into mice deficient in IFN-γ receptors. Despite the absence of IFN-γ receptors in all cells save for the transplanted aorta, these chimeric mice were able to form large aneurysms. Upon treatment with anti–IL-4 antibody, however, these transplanted mice were unable to form aneurysms, a finding confirmed in IL-4 knockout mice.[57] These findings had suggested that invading inflammatory cells depend on Th2 signaling pathways for aneurysm development. Recent studies have discovered the presence of natural killer (NK) and natural killer T (NKT) cells present within the media and adventitia of abdominal aortic aneurysms. These cells display a Th0 cytokine profile, and thus can produce both Th1 and Th2 cytokines. Based on this finding, it is possible that NK and NKT cells may play a role in the pathogenesis of aortic aneurysms rather than a Th2-specific cytokine response.[56,57]

Smooth Muscle Cell Depletion

The presence of inflammatory cells and the cytokine environments they produce are thought to be responsible for another unique feature found in AAA—decreased medial smooth muscle cell density. Histologic examination of AAA specimens reveal a paucity of medial smooth muscle cells as well as fragmentation of the remaining vascular smooth muscle cells compared with normal and atherosclerotic aortas.[58,59] In addition, many of the smooth muscle cells present show features consistent with apoptosis.[58] The significance of these findings is clear, as smooth muscle cells are primarily responsible for the deposition and maintenance of the aorta's normal extracellular matrix. This concept was recently illustrated using an aortic xenograft rat model, where seeding of the graft with vascular smooth muscle cells resulted in protection of the graft from inflammation, proteolysis, and aneurysm formation.[60]

Role of Prostaglandins

Several studies have examined the role of prostaglandin E_2 (PGE_2) in aneurysm formation. In these studies, researchers have found an increased expression of cyclooxygenase-2 (COX-2) localizing primarily to infiltrating macrophages. COX-2 is thought to be responsible for the increased PGE_2 levels found in both human aneurysm tissue and conditioned media from aortic tissue culture.[61,62] PGE_2 may be important in aneurysm pathogenesis by virtue of its ability to alter matrix metalloproteinase (MMP) activity, cytokine expression, and smooth muscle cell viability. Indomethacin, a nonspecific cyclooxygenase inhibitor, decreases PGE_2 in aortic tissue culture and also has been shown to decrease the size of experimental aneurysms in the rat elastase infusion model.[63]

Oxidative Stress

Inflammatory cells can also be a significant source of reactive oxygen species. These toxic substances, which may also be produced by mesenchymal cells and endothelial cells, are capable of inducing apoptosis of smooth muscle cells and activating proteases.[64,65] Miller et al.[66] have shown that reactive oxygen species and evidence of oxidative damage are increased in human AAA tissue. In rats, using the elastase infusion model, investigators have shown that genes associated with oxidative stress, such as those coding inducible nitric oxide synthase and heme oxygenase, are upregulated during aneurysm development.[67] In addition, using the same rat model, inhibition of inducible nitric oxide synthase, one of many enzymes capable of producing nitric oxide, attenuated aneurysm development.[68] Researchers studying mice using the elastase infusion model have confirmed that elevated inducible nitric oxide synthase expression and nitric oxide–mediated tissue damage are seen during aneurysm formation. However, this same study also found that mice lacking the gene for inducible nitric oxide synthase were able to form aneurysms in a similar manner to controls, casting doubt on the importance of this enzyme in AAA pathogenesis.[69] Xiong et al.[69a] recently demonstrated that inducible nitric oxide synthase–null mice were resistant to aneurysm formation using the calcium chloride aneurysm model. Among the pathways that generate reactive oxygen species, the nicotinamide adenine dinucleotide phosphate oxidase pathway was found to be the critical pathway.

Protease Production

Finally, and possibly most importantly, invading inflammatory cells are capable of producing proteases, or inducing surrounding mesenchymal cells to produce proteases, that have the ability to destroy the extracellular matrix structures necessary for maintaining aortic wall integrity. This concept has been extensively studied and is another one of the main categories of AAA pathogenesis research.

PROTEOLYTIC DEGRADATION OF AORTIC WALL CONNECTIVE TISSUE

The two principle functions of the aorta, blood transport and
4 transmission of pulsatile energy, demand both tensile
5 strength and elasticity in its structure. These properties are provided mainly by collagen and elastin, two connective tissue proteins synthesized and maintained primarily by resident mesenchymal cells in the aortic wall. Because the normal structure and function of the aorta are so dependent upon these two proteins, the study of elastin, collagen, and their metabolism has provided valuable insight into the pathogenesis of AAA.

Collagen

Collagen is present both in the aortic media and the adventitia, and is chiefly responsible for imparting tensile strength to the aorta.[70] The predominant forms of collagen in the aorta are types I and III.[71] When comparing human AAA tissue with normal control aortas and aortas with occlusive disease, it is clear that the expression of both type I and type III collagens are increased in aneurysmal tissue.[72,73] Moreover, the mass of collagen has been shown to increase progressively with increasing aneurysm size.[74] This increased expression, which appears to be regulated by a soluble tissue factor,[74] localizes to adventitial fibroblasts, medial smooth muscle cells adjacent to inflammatory infiltrates, and transformed myofibroblasts within atherosclerotic plaque.[75] Further evidence of increased collagen metabolism in AAA was demonstrated by finding elevated plasma levels of the aminoterminal propeptides of type III procollagen, a marker of type III collagen turnover, in AAA patients compared to controls.[76] Mutations in type III collagen have been identified and linked to AAA[30]; however, these mutations are rarely the cause of degenerative AAA.[19]

Elastin

Elastin, which comprises approximately 50% of the dry weight of the normal aorta,[77] is the other major aortic connective tissue protein and is responsible for the aorta's viscous and elastic properties.[78] It is synthesized and secreted as a soluble monomer, tropoelastin, which is organized and cross-linked into insoluble fibers on a preformed scaffold of microfibrillar proteins forming the medial lamellae.[79] The unique structure of elastin fibers confers resistance to proteolytic degradation and the half-life of elastin in human tissues is measured in decades.[80] Most elastin is thought to be produced by the early postnatal period, although elastin production does continue at very low levels into adulthood.[73] Recently, Krettek et al.[81] identified macrophages within human AAA tissue as a source of additional tropoelastin synthesis. This elastogenesis appeared ineffective, however, as markers of mature, organized elastin were greatly diminished.

In examining histologic sections of human AAA tissue, one of the most striking features is the fragmentation of the medial lamellae and the decreased concentration of elastin.[82,83] Paradoxically, biochemical studies looking at the absolute mass of elastin in aneurysmal aortas compared with normal aortas have shown larger amounts of elastin in the diseased tissue.[84,85] This finding is most likely explained by poor uptake of stain by the newly synthesized and unorganized elastin and also by the redistribution of the elastin over a larger aortic diameter. Nevertheless, despite an overall increase in elastin content, the increase does not keep pace with aortic expansion and its concentration is markedly decreased relative to that of collagen.[82,85] This effect results in increased stiffness in the aneurysmal aortic wall.

Proteolytic Enzymes

Because disruption of collagen and elastin is necessary for and well documented in AAA pathogenesis, investigators have focused intensely on studying the enzymes capable of degrading them. In the early 1980s, researchers began studying the proteolytic activity within human AAA tissue.[86–88] Since then, numerous studies have demonstrated the importance of the enzymatic degradation of the aortic wall in the development of AAA (Table 97.2).[124] Although there are many enzymes capable of degrading these proteins in vivo, particular emphasis has been placed on the study of metalloproteinases.

Matrix Metalloproteinases. Matrix metalloproteinases (MMPs) are a family of structurally related enzymes that are capable of digesting the various components of the extracellular matrix. They are produced by most of the cell types native to the aorta, such as endothelial cells, smooth muscle cells, and adventitial fibroblasts, and are also produced by invading inflammatory cells, such as macrophages. The normal physiologic function of these enzymes is thought to be primarily extracellular matrix remodeling, although participation in other functions, such as cell motility and cell signaling, are also known.[89] Most MMPs are secreted from cells in a proenzyme form and require some form of processing to become fully activated. Other MMPs are anchored to cell surfaces to help concentrate their activities close to the cell. Regulation of MMP synthesis and activity occurs through a number of mechanisms. MMP synthesis is primarily regulated at the level of transcription. Activity level may be regulated by the processing of the proenzyme form to its active form. Endogenous inhibitors (tissue inhibitors of metalloproteinases) and interaction with specific extracellular matrix components can also affect activity.[90] Dysregulation of MMP activity has been linked with not only vascular disease but also malignancy, rheumatoid arthritis, and a host of other pathologic conditions.

Matrix Metalloproteinase 9. MMP-9, also known as *gelatinase B*, is one of the most extensively studied MMPs within AAA research. MMP-9 has the capacity to degrade both elastin and partially hydrolyzed collagen. Using zymography and immunohistochemistry, studies of human AAA tissue have demonstrated increased amounts of MMP-9 compared with control tissue.[91] Furthermore, this MMP-9 localizes to areas surrounding infiltrating macrophages in the aortic wall. Using the elastase infusion model in mice, Pyo et al.[36] showed that mice lacking the gene for MMP-9 were resistant to AAA formation. In addition, they were able to show that the key source of MMP-9 was in fact the infiltrating macrophage, as infusion of bone marrow cells from mice with the MMP-9 gene into the MMP-9 knockout mice permitted aneurysm formation.

Matrix Metalloproteinase 2. MMP-2, also known as *gelatinase A*, is another MMP found to be important in AAA pathogenesis. MMP-2 has the capacity to degrade elastin, but unlike MMP-9, MMP-2 can degrade intact fibrillar collagen.[92] MMP-2

TABLE 97.2

ENZYMES ALTERED IN AAA

REFERENCE	ENZYME	PRIMARY SUBSTRATE	ALTERATION IN AAA	CELLS OF ORIGIN
MATRIX METALLOPROTEINASES				
Irizarry et al.[125]	MMP-1	Collagen I, III	Increased protein localized to adventitia	Epithelial, inflammatory, mesenchymal cells
Davis et al.[94]	MMP-2 (gelatinase A)	Collagen I, IV, elastin	Increased mRNA and protein localized to mesenchymal cells	SMCs, fibroblasts
Carrell et al.[126]	MMP-3	Collagen	Increased mRNA	Macrophages
Thompson et al.[91]	MMP-9 (gelatinase B)	Collagen, elastin	Increased protein localized to aortic macrophages	Macrophages, SMCs
Curci et al.[95]	MMP-12	Elastin	Increased mRNA and protein localized to aortic macrophages	Macrophages
Mao et al.[127]	MMP-13	Collagen I, II, III, IV	Increased mRNA and protein localized to mesenchymal cells	SMCs
Nollendorfs et al.[128]	MT-MMP-1 (MMP-14)	Activates pro-MMP-2	Increased mRNA and protein localized to macrophages and SMCs	Macrophages, SMCs
Tamarina et al.[129]	TIMP-1	Inhibitor of MMPs	Increased mRNA levels	SMCs
Tamarina et al.[129]	TIMP-2	Inhibitor of MMP-2	Increased mRNA levels	SMCs
Carrell et al.[126]	TIMP-3	Inhibitor of MMPs	Increased mRNA levels	Macrophages
CYSTEINE PROTEASES				
Shi et al.[96]	Cathepsin S	Elastin	Increased protein	Macrophages, SMCs
Shi et al.[96]	Cathepsin K	Elastin	Increased protein	Macrophages, SMCs
Gacko et al.[130]	Cathepsin D	Not elastin or collagen	Increased activity in AAA tissue	Inflammatory cells?
Gacko et al.[130]	Cathepsin L	Not elastin or collagen	Increased activity in AAA tissue	Inflammatory cells?
Shi et al.[96]	Cystatin C	Inhibitor of cysteine proteases	Decreased protein	SMCs, fibroblasts
SERINE PROTEASES				
Jean-Claude et al.[131]	Plasmin	Activates MMPs	Increased protein	Macrophages
Reilly et al.[132]	Tissue-plasminogen activator	Activates MMPs, plasminogen	Increased protein	Macrophages
Schneiderman et al.[133]	Urokinase-plasminogen activator	Activates MMPs, plasminogen	Increased mRNA	Macrophages

AAA, abdominal aortic aneurysm; MMP, matrix metalloproteinase; SMC, smooth muscle cell; TIMP, tissue inhibitors of metalloproteinases. Adapted from Ailawadi G, Eliason JL, Upchurch GR Jr. Current concepts in the pathogenesis of abdominal aortic aneurysm. *J Vasc Surg* 2003;38: 584–588.[124]

also differs from MMP-9 in that processing of MMP-2 to its activated form requires the presence of other membrane-bound MMPs.[89] Like MMP-9, MMP-2 levels and activity have been found to be greater in human AAA tissue compared with controls[93,94]; however, whereas MMP-9 is typically not present in disease-free aortas,[91] MMP-2 is constitutively produced by resident mesenchymal cells even in histologically normal aortas.[93] Confirmation of the importance of MMP-2 to AAA development has come from the calcium chloride mouse model of AAA. In this study, Longo et al.[37] were able to show that the targeted deletion of the MMP-2 gene inhibited AAA formation and that the key source of MMP-2 production was not invading inflammatory cells but resident mesenchymal cells. The stimulus for the increased production and activation of MMP-2 in aneurysmal aortas remains unknown.

Other Matrix Metalloproteinases. MMP-12, also referred to as *macrophage elastase*, is also elevated in human AAA tissue compared with controls. Importantly, immunohistochemical analysis has localized the enzyme to areas of elastin destruction.[95] In contrast to MMP-9 and MMP-2, however, MMP-12 has not been shown to be absolutely required for aneurysm generation in knockout mice.[36] Levels of other MMPs are altered in AAA as well, but current studies have not documented a definitive role for these enzymes in AAA development.

Other Proteases. In addition to MMPs, other proteases and their endogenous inhibitors have been suggested as potential contributors to AAA pathogenesis. Cystatin C, an endogenous inhibitor of cysteine proteases, appears to be reduced in human AAA tissue.[96] Serine proteases, particularly neutrophil elastase, have been hypothesized to play a role in AAA formation because of their potent elastase activities. However, there is currently no supporting experimental evidence. Other serine proteases, such as those from the plasminogen activator family, have been shown to play a role in AAA formation,

TABLE 97.3

POTENTIAL MEDICAL THERAPIES FOR TREATING SMALL AAA

INTERVENTION	REFERENCE	EFFECT ON AAA GROWTH	LEVEL OF EVIDENCE	CLASS OF RECOMMENDATION
Propranolol	12, 13	No inhibition	A	III
Macrolides	14	Inhibition	B	IIa
Tetracycline[a]	15	Inhibition	B	IIa
Statins	16, 134	Inhibition	B	IIb
ACE inhibitors	27, 39, 52, 53	No inhibition	B and C	IIb
AR blockers	48, 50	Animal data	C	IIb

ACE, angiotensin-converting enzyme; AR, angiotensin receptor.
[a]Inhibition at 6 and 12 months following 3 months of treatment.

although the main pathogenic mechanism involving these enzymes appears to be activation of MMPs.[97]

Potential Medical Therapy. In addition to adding to the basic knowledge of AAA pathogenesis, the study of MMPs has also led to the realization that inhibition of their activity may prevent or slow aneurysm growth. Tetracycline and its derivatives are potent inhibitors of MMPs in vitro[98] and in animal studies have inhibited aneurysm expansion.[99,100] Small trials in human AAA patients have been performed[101,102]; however, definitive evidence for their efficacy awaits large-scale randomized trials. Thus, medical therapy for the treatment of AAA, especially smaller aneurysms, may very well be an alternative to surgical therapy in the future.

Overall, four major classes of drugs have been studied as therapies for decreasing aneurysm growth rates: beta-blockers, antihypertensives (diuretics, angiotensin-converting enzyme inhibitors, calcium channel blockers), antibiotics with inhibitory function on MMPs, and anti-inflammatory agents (statins, nonsteroidal anti-inflammatory drugs) (Table 97.3). A meta-analysis of the available cohort studies suggests that beta-blockers and statins may reduce AAA growth rates. However, the results of three randomized control trials for beta-blockers do not support the conclusion that beta-blockers have an inhibitory effect on AAA growth rates.[6] To date, there are no randomized control trials investigating statins and AAA growth.[7] The human trials investigating the results of antibiotics inhibiting MMPs exhibit promise; however, they were not powered adequately to demonstrate statistical significance. Interestingly, recent data do indicate that statins also possess an inhibitory effect on MMPs, in addition to anti-inflammatory properties.[8]

BIOMECHANICAL WALL STRESS

Unique Conditions in the Infrarenal Aorta

6 The infrarenal aorta is subjected to unique hemodynamic flow patterns and also possesses specific structural characteristics that are thought to predispose it toward aneurysm formation. Reflected pressure waves from the aortic bifurcation and the presence of large renal and splanchnic artery takeoffs result in disturbed flow patterns.[103] The elastin-to-collagen ratio decreases distally, translating into increased stiffness in this section of the aorta.[104] In addition, the absence of vasa vasorum in the normal abdominal aortic media[105] and the presence of a thick intraluminal thrombus are thought to impair oxygen and nutrient delivery to the aneurysmal aorta.[106] All of these observations are plausible reasons for the development and progression of disease in the infrarenal aorta.

Aortic Wall Stress

Stress on the aortic wall is one of the key factors involved in the rupture of AAAs. Peak wall stress has been demonstrated as superior to maximal diameter for predicting the risks of AAA rupture.[9] The law of Laplace is often used to explain the propensity for larger aneurysms to rupture because it predicts wall tension to be directly proportional to the product of the radius of a tubular, thin-walled structure (AAA diameter) and its intraluminal pressure (patient blood pressure). This explanation may be an oversimplification, however, because AAAs are often asymmetric and thick walled with major and minor wall curvatures,[10] and become more spherical in shape as their size increases.[107] Because of these factors, researchers are developing improved methods to help determine patterns of stress on the aneurysmal aortic wall, as well as the effect of stress on the pathogenesis of AAA.

Raghavan et al.[108] have recently used a method termed *finite element analysis* to noninvasively determine AAA wall stress distribution and AAA rupture risk. Application of this method comparing calculated stress values obtained from patients near the time of AAA rupture with patients who have size-matched electively repaired AAA showed significantly elevated stress values in the ruptured AAA group.[109] Although still investigational, these methods could have an important impact on determining the indications for operative repair of AAAs in the future.

More recent studies have moved beyond looking at wall stress alone and have also focused on aortic wall strength. These two elements in combination provide a more accurate predictor of rupture, primarily due to the fact that as aortic size increases, wall stress increases with a concomitant decrease in wall strength.[11] Another element that remains poorly understood is the role of intraluminal thrombus. Models still need to be constructed that incorporate intraluminal thrombus to better understand its role in the rupture risk of AAA.

Hemodynamics

In addition to influencing rupture, hemodynamic factors may play an important role in aneurysm initiation and growth. Using the elastase infusion model in rats, research has established that increases in flow through the injured aorta decrease macrophage infiltration into the aortic media[110] and increase macrophage antioxidative gene expression.[111] AAAs in these high-flow groups also demonstrated a significant reduction in diameter compared with the low- and normal-flow groups. Expression of MMPs[112] and reactive oxygen species[113] is also influenced by hemodynamic factors in experimental aneurysm formation.

CONCLUSION

Significant progress has been made over the past 20 years in delineating the pathogenesis of AAA. Both clinicians and basic scientists will continue to play important roles in studying this disease process. It is hoped that by enhancing our knowledge of the underlying pathology of AAA, new and improved methods of diagnosis and treatment will follow.

References

1. Johnston KW, Rutherford RB, Tilson MD, et al. Suggested standards for reporting on arterial aneurysms. Subcommittee on Reporting Standards for Arterial Aneurysms, Ad Hoc Committee on Reporting Standards, Society for Vascular Surgery and North American Chapter, International Society for Cardiovascular Surgery. *J Vasc Surg* 1991;13:452–458.
2. Lederle FA, Johnson GR, Wilson SE, et al. The aneurysm detection and management study screening program: validation cohort and final results. Aneurysm Detection and Management Veterans Affairs Cooperative Study Investigators. *Arch Intern Med* 2000;160:1425–1430.
3. Pleumeekers HJ, Hoes AW, van der Does E, et al. Aneurysms of the abdominal aorta in older adults. The Rotterdam Study. *Am J Epidemiol* 1995;142:1291–1299.
4. Goldberg RJ, Burchfiel CM, Benfante R, et al. Lifestyle and biologic factors associated with atherosclerotic disease in middle-aged men. 20-year findings from the Honolulu Heart Program. *Arch Intern Med* 1995;155:686–694.
5. Alcorn HG, Wolfson SK Jr, Sutton-Tyrrell K, et al. Risk factors for abdominal aortic aneurysms in older adults enrolled in the Cardiovascular Health Study. *Arterioscler Thromb Vasc Biol* 1996;16:963–970.
6. Rodin MB, Daviglus ML, Wong GC, et al. Middle age cardiovascular risk factors and abdominal aortic aneurysm in older age. *Hypertension* 2003;42:61–68.
7. Vardulaki KA, Walker M, Day NE, et al. Quantifying the risks of hypertension, age, sex and smoking in patients with abdominal aortic aneurysm. *Br J Surg* 2000;87:195–200.
8. Bengtsson H, Bergqvist D, Ekberg O, et al. A population based screening of abdominal aortic aneurysms (AAA). *Eur J Vasc Surg* 1991;5:53–57.
9. Smith FC, Grimshaw GM, Paterson IS, et al. Ultrasonographic screening for abdominal aortic aneurysm in an urban community. *Br J Surg* 1993;80:1406–1409.
10. Zarins CK, Glagov S. Artery wall pathology in atherosclerosis. In: Rutherford RB, ed. *Vascular Surgery*, 5th ed. Philadelphia, PA: WB Saunders; 2000:313–330.
11. Zarins CK, Weisenberg E, Kolettis G, et al. Differential enlargement of artery segments in response to enlarging atherosclerotic plaques. *J Vasc Surg* 1988;7:386–394.
12. Xu C, Zarins CK, Glagov S. Aneurysmal and occlusive atherosclerosis of the human abdominal aorta. *J Vasc Surg* 2001;33:91–96.
13. Zarins CK, Xu C, Glagov S. Atherosclerotic enlargement of the human abdominal aorta. *Atherosclerosis* 2001;155:157–164.
14. Zarins CK, Xu C, Glagov S. Aneurysmal enlargement of the aorta during regression of experimental atherosclerosis. *J Vasc Surg* 1992;15:90–98.
15. Tangirala RK, Rubin EM, Palinski W. Quantitation of atherosclerosis in murine models: correlation between lesions in the aortic origin and in the entire aorta, and differences in the extent of lesions between sexes in LDL receptor-deficient and apolipoprotein E-deficient mice. *J Lipid Res* 1995;36:2320–2328.
16. Daugherty A, Manning MW, Cassis LA. Angiotensin II promotes atherosclerotic lesions and aneurysms in apolipoprotein E-deficient mice. *J Clin Invest* 2000;105:1605–1612.
17. Tilson MD, Stansel HC. Differences in results for aneurysm vs occlusive disease after bifurcation grafts: results of 100 elective grafts. *Arch Surg* 1980;115:1173–1175.
18. Tilson MD. Aortic aneurysms and atherosclerosis. *Circulation* 1992;85:378–379.
19. Tromp G, Wu Y, Prockop DJ, et al. Sequencing of cDNA from 50 unrelated patients reveals that mutations in the triple-helical domain of type III procollagen are an infrequent cause of aortic aneurysms. *J Clin Invest* 1993;91:2539–2545.
20. Clifton MA. Familial abdominal aortic aneurysms. *Br J Surg* 1977;64:765–766.
21. Tilson MD, Seashore MR. Fifty families with abdominal aortic aneurysms in two or more first-order relatives. *Am J Surg* 1984;147:551–553.
22. Johansen K, Koepsell T. Familial tendency for abdominal aortic aneurysms. *JAMA* 1986;256:1934–1936.
23. Baird PA, Sadovnick AD, Yee IM, et al. Sibling risks of abdominal aortic aneurysm. *Lancet* 1995;346:601–604.
24. Majumder PP, St Jean PL, Ferrell RE, et al. On the inheritance of abdominal aortic aneurysm. *Am J Hum Genet* 1991;48:164–170.
25. Verloes A, Sakalihasan N, Koulischer L, et al. Aneurysms of the abdominal aorta: familial and genetic aspects in three hundred thirteen pedigrees. *J Vasc Surg* 1995;21:646–655.
26. Kuivaniemi H, Shibamura H, Arthur C, et al. Familial abdominal aortic aneurysms: collection of 233 multiplex families. *J Vasc Surg* 2003;37:340–345.
27. Armstrong PJ, Johanning JM, Calton WC Jr, et al. Differential gene expression in human abdominal aorta: aneurysmal versus occlusive disease. *J Vasc Surg* 2002;35:346–355.
28. Tung WS, Lee JK, Thompson RW. Simultaneous analysis of 1176 gene products in normal human aorta and abdominal aortic aneurysms using a membrane-based complementary DNA expression array. *J Vasc Surg* 2001;34:143–150.
29. Shibamura H, Olson JM, van Vlijmen-Van Keulen C, et al. Genome scan for familial abdominal aortic aneurysm using sex and family history as covariates suggests genetic heterogeneity and identifies linkage to chromosome 19q13. *Circulation* 2004;109:2103–2108.
30. Kontusaari S, Tromp G, Kuivaniemi H, et al. A mutation in the gene for type III procollagen (COL3A1) in a family with aortic aneurysms. *J Clin Invest* 1990;86:1465–1473.

30a. Helgadottir A, Thorliefsson G, Mugnusson KP, et al. The same sequence variant on 9p21 associates with myocardial infarction, abdominal aortic aneurysm, and intracranial aneurysm. *Nat Genet* 2008;40:217–224.

31. Beckman EN. Plasma cell infiltrates in atherosclerotic abdominal aortic aneurysms. *Am J Clin Pathol* 1986;85:21–24.
32. Bobryshev YV, Lord RS, Parsson H. Immunophenotypic analysis of the aortic aneurysm wall suggests that vascular dendritic cells are involved in immune responses. *Cardiovasc Surg* 1998;6:240–249.
33. Koch AE, Haines GK, Rizzo RJ, et al. Human abdominal aortic aneurysms. Immunophenotypic analysis suggesting an immune-mediated response. *Am J Pathol* 1990;137:1199–1213.
34. Freestone T, Turner RJ, Coady A, et al. Inflammation and matrix metalloproteinases in the enlarging abdominal aortic aneurysm. *Arterioscler Thromb Vasc Biol* 1995;15:1145–1151.
35. Anidjar S, Dobrin PB, Eichorst M, et al. Correlation of inflammatory infiltrate with the enlargement of experimental aortic aneurysms. *J Vasc Surg* 1992;16:139–147.
36. Pyo R, Lee JK, Shipley JM, et al. Targeted gene disruption of matrix metalloproteinase-9 (gelatinase B) suppresses development of experimental abdominal aortic aneurysms. *J Clin Invest* 2000;105:1641–1649.
37. Longo GM, Xiong W, Greiner TC, et al. Matrix metalloproteinases 2 and 9 work in concert to produce aortic aneurysms. *J Clin Invest* 2002;110:625–632.
38. Dobrin PB, Baumgartner N, Anidjar S, et al. Inflammatory aspects of experimental aneurysms. Effect of methylprednisolone and cyclosporine. *Ann N Y Acad Sci* 1996;800:74–88.
39. Hance KA, Tataria M, Ziporin SJ, et al. Monocyte chemotactic activity in human abdominal aortic aneurysms: role of elastin degradation peptides and the 67-kD cell surface elastin receptor. *J Vasc Surg* 2002;35:254–261.
40. Nackman GB, Karkowski FJ, Halpern VJ, et al. Elastin degradation products induce adventitial angiogenesis in the Anidjar/Dobrin rat aneurysm model. *Surgery* 1997;122:39–44.
41. Brophy CM, Reilly JM, Smith GJ, et al. The role of inflammation in nonspecific abdominal aortic aneurysm disease. *Ann Vasc Surg* 1991;5:229–233.
42. Gregory AK, Yin NX, Capella J, et al. Features of autoimmunity in the abdominal aortic aneurysm. *Arch Surg* 1996;131:85–88.
43. Yen HC, Lee FY, Chau LY. Analysis of the T cell receptor V beta repertoire in human aortic aneurysms. *Atherosclerosis* 1997;135:29–36.
44. Walton LJ, Powell JT, Parums DV. Unrestricted usage of immunoglobulin heavy chain genes in B cells infiltrating the wall of atherosclerotic abdominal aortic aneurysms. *Atherosclerosis* 1997;135:65–71.
45. Juvonen J, Juvonen T, Laurila A, et al. Demonstration of Chlamydia pneumoniae in the walls of abdominal aortic aneurysms. *J Vasc Surg* 1997;25:499–505.
46. Halme S, Juvonen T, Laurila A, et al. Chlamydia pneumoniae reactive T lymphocytes in the walls of abdominal aortic aneurysms. *Eur J Clin Invest* 1999;29:546–552.
47. Meijer A, van Der Vliet JA, Roholl PJ, et al. Chlamydia pneumoniae in abdominal aortic aneurysms: abundance of membrane components in the absence of heat shock protein 60 and DNA. *Arterioscler Thromb Vasc Biol* 1999;19:2680–2686.
48. Tambiah J, Powell JT. Chlamydia pneumoniae antigens facilitate experimental aortic dilatation: prevention with azithromycin. *J Vasc Surg* 2002;36:1011–1017.
49. Kalayoglu MV, Libby P, Byrne GI. Chlamydia pneumoniae as an emerging risk factor in cardiovascular disease. *JAMA* 2002;288:2724–2731.
50. Koch AE, Kunkel SL, Pearce WH, et al. Enhanced production of the chemotactic cytokines interleukin-8 and monocyte chemoattractant protein-1 in human abdominal aortic aneurysms. *Am J Pathol* 1993;142:1423–1431.
51. Colonnello JS, Hance KA, Shames ML, et al. Transient exposure to elastase induces mouse aortic wall smooth muscle cell production of MCP-1 and RANTES during development of experimental aortic aneurysm. *J Vasc Surg* 2003;38:138–146.

51a. Mac Taggert, Xiong W, Knispell R, et al. Deletion of CCR2 but not CCR5 or CXCR3 inhibits aortic aneurysm formation. *Surgery* 2007;142:284–288.

52. Szekanecz Z, Shah MR, Pearce WH, et al. Human atherosclerotic abdominal aortic aneurysms produce interleukin (IL)-6 and interferon-gamma but not IL-2 and IL-4: the possible role for IL-6 and interferon-gamma in vascular inflammation. *Agents Actions* 1994;42:159–162.
53. Newman KM, Jean-Claude J, Li H, et al. Cytokines that activate proteolysis are increased in abdominal aortic aneurysms. *Circulation* 1994;90: II224–227.
54. Juvonen J, Surcel HM, Satta J, et al. Elevated circulating levels of inflammatory cytokines in patients with abdominal aortic aneurysm. *Arterioscler Thromb Vasc Biol* 1997;17:2843–2847.
55. Xiong W, Zhao Y, Prall A, et al. Key roles of CD4+ T cells and IFN-gamma in the development of abdominal aortic aneurysms in a murine model. *J Immunol* 2004;172:2607–2612.
56. Schonbeck U, Sukhova GK, Gerdes N, et al. T(H)2 predominant immune responses prevail in human abdominal aortic aneurysm. *Am J Pathol* 2002;161:499–506.
57. Shimizu K, Shichiri M, Libby P, et al. Th2-predominant inflammation and blockade of IFN-gamma signaling induce aneurysms in allografted aortas. *J Clin Invest* 2004;114:300–308.
58. Henderson EL, Geng YJ, Sukhova GK, et al. Death of smooth muscle cells and expression of mediators of apoptosis by T lymphocytes in human abdominal aortic aneurysms. *Circulation* 1999;99:96–104.
59. Lopez-Candales A, Holmes DR, Liao S, et al. Decreased vascular smooth muscle cell density in medial degeneration of human abdominal aortic aneurysms. *Am J Pathol* 1997;150:993–1007.
60. Allaire E, Muscatelli-Groux B, Mandet C, et al. Paracrine effect of vascular smooth muscle cells in the prevention of aortic aneurysm formation. *J Vasc Surg* 2002;36:1018–1026.
61. Holmes DR, Wester W, Thompson RW, et al. Prostaglandin E2 synthesis and cyclooxygenase expression in abdominal aortic aneurysms. *J Vasc Surg* 1997;25:810–815.
62. Walton LJ, Franklin IJ, Bayston T, et al. Inhibition of prostaglandin E2 synthesis in abdominal aortic aneurysms: implications for smooth muscle cell viability, inflammatory processes, and the expansion of abdominal aortic aneurysms. *Circulation* 1999;100:48–54.
63. Miralles M, Wester W, Sicard GA, et al. Indomethacin inhibits expansion of experimental aortic aneurysms via inhibition of the cox2 isoform of cyclooxygenase. *J Vasc Surg* 1999;29:884–883.
64. Li PF, Dietz R, von Harsdorf R. Reactive oxygen species induce apoptosis of vascular smooth muscle cell. *FEBS Lett* 1997;404:249–252.
65. Rajagopalan S, Meng XP, Ramasamy S, et al. Reactive oxygen species produced by macrophage-derived foam cells regulate the activity of vascular matrix metalloproteinases in vitro. Implications for atherosclerotic plaque stability. *J Clin Invest* 1996;98:2572–2579.
66. Miller FJ Jr, Sharp WJ, Fang X, et al. Oxidative stress in human abdominal aortic aneurysms: a potential mediator of aneurysmal remodeling. *Arterioscler Thromb Vasc Biol* 2002;22:560–565.
67. Yajima N, Masuda M, Miyazaki M, et al. Oxidative stress is involved in the development of experimental abdominal aortic aneurysm: a study of the transcription profile with complementary DNA microarray. *J Vasc Surg* 2002;36:379–385.
68. Johanning JM, Franklin DP, Han DC, et al. Inhibition of inducible nitric oxide synthase limits nitric oxide production and experimental aneurysm expansion. *J Vasc Surg* 2001;33:579–586.
69. Lee JK, Borhani M, Ennis TL, et al. Experimental abdominal aortic aneurysms in mice lacking expression of inducible nitric oxide synthase. *Arterioscler Thromb Vasc Biol* 2001;21:1393–1401.
70. Dobrin PB, Baker WH, Gley WC. Elastolytic and collagenolytic studies of arteries. Implications for the mechanical properties of aneurysms. *Arch Surg* 1984;119:405–409.
71. Barnes MJ. Collagens in atherosclerosis. *Coll Relat Res* 1985;5:65–97.
72. McGee GS, Baxter BT, Shively VP, et al. Aneurysm or occlusive disease—factors determining the clinical course of atherosclerosis of the infrarenal aorta. *Surgery* 1991;110:370–376.
73. Mesh CL, Baxter BT, Pearce WH, et al. Collagen and elastin gene expression in aortic aneurysms. *Surgery* 1992;112:256–262.
74. Minion DJ, Wang Y, Lynch TG, et al. Soluble factors modulate changes in collagen gene expression in abdominal aortic aneurysms. *Surgery* 1993; 114:252–257.
75. Hunter GC, Smyth SH, Aguirre ML, et al. Incidence and histologic characteristics of blebs in patients with abdominal aortic aneurysms. *J Vasc Surg* 1996;24:93–101.
76. Satta J, Juvonen T, Haukipuro K, et al. Increased turnover of collagen in abdominal aortic aneurysms, demonstrated by measuring the concentration of the aminoterminal propeptide of type III procollagen in peripheral and aortal blood samples. *J Vasc Surg* 1995;22:155–160.
77. Parks WC, Pierce RA, Lee KA, et al. Elastin. *Adv Mol Cell Biol* 1993;6: 133–182.
78. Boucek R. *Contributions of Elastin and Collagen Organization to Passive Mechanical Properties of Arterial Tissue*. Boca Raton, FL: CRC Press; 1988.
79. Mecham R, Broekelmann T, Davis E, et al. Elastic fibre assembly: macromolecular interactions. *Ciba Found Symp* 1995;192:172–184.
80. Shapiro SD, Endicott SK, Province MA, et al. Marked longevity of human lung parenchymal elastic fibers deduced from prevalence of D-aspartate and nuclear weapons-related radiocarbon. *J Clin Invest* 1991;87:1828–1834.
81. Krettek A, Sukhova GK, Libby P. Elastogenesis in human arterial disease: a role for macrophages in disordered elastin synthesis. *Arterioscler Thromb Vasc Biol* 2003;23:582–587.
82. Rizzo RJ, McCarthy WJ, Dixit SN, et al. Collagen types and matrix protein content in human abdominal aortic aneurysms. *J Vasc Surg* 1989;10: 365–373.
83. Baxter BT, McGee GS, Shively VP, et al. Elastin content, cross-links, and mRNA in normal and aneurysmal human aorta. *J Vasc Surg* 1992;16: 192–200.
84. Sumner DS, Hokanson DE, Strandness DE Jr. Stress-strain characteristics and collagen-elastin content of abdominal aortic aneurysms. *Surg Gynecol Obstet* 1970;130:459–466.
85. Minion DJ, Davis VA, Nejezchleb PA, et al. Elastin is increased in abdominal aortic aneurysms. *J Surg Res* 1994;57:443–446.
86. Busuttil RW, Abou-Zamzam AM, Machleder HI. Collagenase activity of the human aorta. A comparison of patients with and without abdominal aortic aneurysms. *Arch Surg* 1980;115:1373–1378.
87. Busuttil RW, Rinderbriecht H, Flesher A, et al. Elastase activity: the role of elastase in aortic aneurysm formation. *J Surg Res* 1982;32:214–217.
88. Cannon DJ, Read RC. Blood elastolytic activity in patients with aortic aneurysm. *Ann Thorac Surg* 1982;34:10–15.
89. Visse R, Nagase H. Matrix metalloproteinases and tissue inhibitors of metalloproteinases: structure, function, and biochemistry. *Circ Res* 2003;92: 827–839.
90. Nagase H, Woessner JF Jr. Matrix metalloproteinases. *J Biol Chem* 1999; 274:21491–21494.
91. Thompson RW, Holmes DR, Mertens RA, et al. Production and localization of 92-kilodalton gelatinase in abdominal aortic aneurysms. An elastolytic metalloproteinase expressed by aneurysm-infiltrating macrophages. *J Clin Invest* 1995;96:318–326.
92. Aimes RT, Quigley JP. Matrix metalloproteinase-2 is an interstitial collagenase. Inhibitor-free enzyme catalyzes the cleavage of collagen fibrils and soluble native type I collagen generating the specific 3/4- and 1/4-length fragments. *J Biol Chem* 1995;270:5872–5876.
93. McMillan WD, Patterson BK, Keen RR, et al. In situ localization and quantification of seventy-two-kilodalton type IV collagenase in aneurysmal, occlusive, and normal aorta. *J Vasc Surg* 1995;22:295–305.
94. Davis V, Persidskaia R, Baca-Regen L, et al. Matrix metalloproteinase-2 production and its binding to the matrix are increased in abdominal aortic aneurysms. *Arterioscler Thromb Vasc Biol* 1998;18:1625–1633.
95. Curci JA, Liao S, Huffman MD, et al. Expression and localization of macrophage elastase (matrix metalloproteinase-12) in abdominal aortic aneurysms. *J Clin Invest* 1998;102:1900–1910.
96. Shi GP, Sukhova GK, Grubb A, et al. Cystatin C deficiency in human atherosclerosis and aortic aneurysms. *J Clin Invest* 1999;104:1191–1197.
97. Carmeliet P, Moons L, Lijnen R, et al. Urokinase-generated plasmin activates matrix metalloproteinases during aneurysm formation. *Nat Genet* 1997;17:439–444.
98. Liu J, Xiong W, Baca-Regen L, et al. Mechanism of inhibition of matrix metalloproteinase-2 expression by doxycycline in human aortic smooth muscle cells. *J Vasc Surg* 2003;38:1376–1383.
99. Prall AK, Longo GM, Mayhan WG, et al. Doxycycline in patients with abdominal aortic aneurysms and in mice: comparison of serum levels and effect on aneurysm growth in mice. *J Vasc Surg* 2002;35:923–929.
100. Petrinec D, Liao S, Holmes DR, et al. Doxycycline inhibition of aneurysmal degeneration in an elastase-induced rat model of abdominal aortic aneurysm: preservation of aortic elastin associated with suppressed production of 92 kD gelatinase. *J Vasc Surg* 1996;23:336–346.
101. Mosorin M, Juvonen J, Biancari F, et al. Use of doxycycline to decrease the growth rate of abdominal aortic aneurysms: a randomized, double-blind, placebo-controlled pilot study. *J Vasc Surg* 2001;34:606–610.
102. Baxter BT, Pearce WH, Waltke EA, et al. Prolonged administration of doxycycline in patients with small asymptomatic abdominal aortic aneurysms: report of a prospective (Phase II) multicenter study. *J Vasc Surg* 2002;36:1–12.
103. Moore JE, Jr, Ku DN, Zarins CK, et al. Pulsatile flow visualization in the abdominal aorta under differing physiologic conditions: implications for increased susceptibility to atherosclerosis. *J Biomech Eng* 1992;114: 391–397.
104. Peterson L, Jensen RE, Parnell J. Mechanical properties of arteries in vivo. *Circ Res* 1960;8:622–633.
105. Wolinsky H, Glagov S. Comparison of abdominal and thoracic aortic medial structure in mammals. Deviation of man from the usual pattern. *Circ Res* 1969;25:677–686.
106. Vorp DA, Lee PC, Wang DH, et al. Association of intraluminal thrombus in abdominal aortic aneurysm with local hypoxia and wall weakening. *J Vasc Surg* 2001;34:291–299.
107. Vorp DA, Raghavan ML, Webster MW. Mechanical wall stress in abdominal aortic aneurysm: influence of diameter and asymmetry. *J Vasc Surg* 1998;27:632–639.
108. Raghavan ML, Vorp DA, Federle MP, et al. Wall stress distribution on three-dimensionally reconstructed models of human abdominal aortic aneurysm. *J Vasc Surg* 2000;31:760–769.
109. Fillinger MF, Raghavan ML, Marra SP, et al. In vivo analysis of mechanical wall stress and abdominal aortic aneurysm rupture risk. *J Vasc Surg* 2002;36:589–597.
110. Sho E, Sho M, Hoshina K, et al. Hemodynamic forces regulate mural macrophage infiltration in experimental aortic aneurysms. *Exp Mol Pathol* 2004;76:108–116.
111. Nakahashi TK, Hoshina K, Tsao PS, et al. Flow loading induces macrophage antioxidative gene expression in experimental aneurysms. *Arterioscler Thromb Vasc Biol* 2002;22:2017–2022.

112. Grote K, Flach I, Luchtefeld M, et al. Mechanical stretch enhances mRNA expression and proenzyme release of matrix metalloproteinase-2 (MMP-2) via NAD(P)H oxidase-derived reactive oxygen species. *Circ Res* 2003;92: e80–e86.
113. Howard AB, Alexander RW, Nerem RM, et al. Cyclic strain induces an oxidative stress in endothelial cells. *Am J Physiol* 1997;272:C421– C427.
114. Schillinger M, Exner M, Mlekusch W, et al. Heme oxygenase-1 gene promoter polymorphism is associated with abdominal aortic aneurysm. *Thromb Res* 2002;106:131–136.
115. Pola R, Gaetani E, Santoliquido A, et al. Abdominal aortic aneurysm in normotensive patients: association with angiotensin-converting enzyme gene polymorphism. *Eur J Vasc Endovasc Surg* 2001;21:445–449.
116. Gerdes LU, Lindholt JS, Vammen S, et al. Apolipoprotein E genotype is associated with differential expansion rates of small abdominal aortic aneurysms. *Br J Surg* 2000;87:760–765.
117. Rossaak JI, Van Rij AM, Jones GT, et al. Association of the 4G/5G polymorphism in the promoter region of plasminogen activator inhibitor-1 with abdominal aortic aneurysms. *J Vasc Surg* 2000;31: 1026–1032.
118. Wang X, Tromp G, Cole CW, et al. Analysis of coding sequences for tissue inhibitor of metalloproteinases 1 (TIMP1) and 2 (TIMP2) in patients with aneurysms. *Matrix Biol* 1999;18:121–124.
119. Kotani K, Shimomura T, Murakami F, et al. Allele frequency of human endothelial nitric oxide synthase gene polymorphism in abdominal aortic aneurysm. *Intern Med* 2000;39:537–539.
120. Rasmussen TE, Hallett JW Jr, Schulte S, et al. Genetic similarity in inflammatory and degenerative abdominal aortic aneurysms: a study of human leukocyte antigen class II disease risk genes. *J Vasc Surg* 2001;34: 84–89.
121. Jones GT, Phillips VL, Harris EL, et al. Functional matrix metalloproteinase-9 polymorphism (C-1562T) associated with abdominal aortic aneurysm. *J Vasc Surg* 2003;38:1363–1367.
122. Bown MJ, Burton PR, Horsburgh T, et al. The role of cytokine gene polymorphisms in the pathogenesis of abdominal aortic aneurysms: a case-control study. *J Vasc Surg* 2003;37:999–1005.
123. Strauss E, Waliszewski K, Gabriel M, et al. Increased risk of the abdominal aortic aneurysm in carriers of the MTHFR 677T allele. *J Appl Genet* 2003; 44:85–93.
124. Ailawadi G, Eliason JL, Upchurch GR Jr. Current concepts in the pathogenesis of abdominal aortic aneurysm. *J Vasc Surg* 2003;38:584–588.
125. Irizarry E, Newman KM, Gandhi RH, et al. Demonstration of interstitial collagenase in abdominal aortic aneurysm disease. *J Surg Res* 1993;54: 571–574.
126. Carrell TW, Burnand KG, Wells GM, et al. Stromelysin-1 (matrix metalloproteinase-3) and tissue inhibitor of metalloproteinase-3 are overexpressed in the wall of abdominal aortic aneurysms. *Circulation* 2002;105: 477–482.
127. Mao D, Lee JK, VanVickle SJ, et al. Expression of collagenase-3 (MMP-13) in human abdominal aortic aneurysms and vascular smooth muscle cells in culture. *Biochem Biophys Res Commun* 1999;261:904–910.
128. Nollendorfs A, Greiner TC, Nagase H, et al. The expression and localization of membrane type-1 matrix metalloproteinase in human abdominal aortic aneurysms. *J Vasc Surg* 2001;34:316–322.
129. Tamarina NA, McMillan WD, Shively VP, et al. Expression of matrix metalloproteinases and their inhibitors in aneurysms and normal aorta. *Surgery* 1997;122:264–272.
130. Gacko M, Glowinski S. Cathepsin D and cathepsin L activities in aortic aneurysm wall and parietal thrombus. *Clin Chem Lab Med* 1998;36: 449–452.
131. Jean-Claude J, Newman KM, Li H, et al. Possible key role for plasmin in the pathogenesis of abdominal aortic aneurysms. *Surgery* 1994;116: 472–478.
132. Reilly JM, Sicard GA, Lucore C. Abnormal expression of plasminogen activators in aortic aneurysmal and occlusive disease. *J Vasc Surg* 1994;19: 865–872.
133. Schneiderman J, Bordin GM, Engelberg I, et al. Expression of fibrinolytic genes in atherosclerotic abdominal aortic aneurysm wall. A possible mechanism for aneurysm expansion. *J Clin Invest* 1995;96:639–645.
134. Schouten O, van Laanen JH, Boersma E, et al. Statins are associated with a reduced infrarenal abdominal aortic aneurysm growth. *Eur J Vasc Endovasc Surg* 2006;32:21–26.

CHAPTER 98 THORACIC AORTIC ANEURYSMS

GORAV AILAWADI

KEY POINTS

1. The risk of thoracic aneurysm disease increases with age. Thoracic aortic aneurysms in young patients are most likely due to genetic predisposition or familial syndromes.
2. Careful planning by experienced centers is paramount to provide optimal treatment in patients with thoracic aortic aneurysms as the morbidity and mortality for surgical intervention is significant.
3. Open surgical repair remains the mainstay for aortic root, ascending aortic, and aortic arch aneurysms with very acceptable outcomes and low morbidity when performed in centers with experienced staff.
4. Endovascular techniques for the descending thoracic aorta have become the preferred treatment approach not only for aneurysms but for dissections and traumatic aortic injuries as they often can be performed with less morbidity than that associated with open surgical treatment.
5. Endovascular repair still carries the risk of endoleak. In addition, spinal cord complications are similar with endovascular compared to open approaches.

Aortic diseases constitute the 13th leading cause of death in the developed world. Aneurysms can affect the ascending, arch, descending, or abdominal aorta. Aneurysms of the thoracic aorta, including the ascending, arch, and descending aorta, in particular, are associated with high morbidity and mortality (Fig. 98.1). An aortic aneurysm is defined as a dilation of the diameter of at least 50% greater than baseline. *True aortic aneurysms* affect all the layers of the aortic wall—intima, media, and adventitia—and should be distinguished from *false aneurysms*, which occur after trauma or other injury and consist of the media and adventitia. *Aortic dissections* are intimal tears resulting in blood propagating within the medial layer. *Intramural hematoma* is the presence of blood within the wall of the aorta without a definite intimal tear.

Although understanding of the pathogenesis of aortic aneurysms is rapidly evolving, degradation of the aortic extracellular matrix proteins, collagen and elastin, and loss of smooth muscle cells are hallmark pathologic findings. In contradistinction to abdominal aortic aneurysms, ascending aneurysms less commonly display manifestations of atherosclerosis or an inflammatory infiltrate. Thoracic aortic disease is associated with high morbidity and mortality. Treatment decisions concerning operative intervention in terms of both timing and extent of resection are often complex and involve multidisciplinary management.

HISTORY

The first known description of an arterial aneurysm was by Galen, a Greek physician (A.D. 126–216), who described false aneurysms in injured gladiators.[1] It was not until 1895 that an etiology for aneurysms was hypothesized, when Dohle identified syphilitic aortitis.[2] Aneurysms were originally treated with external or internal ligation via opening the aneurysm. In the later 19th century, Rudolph Matas developed an alternate technique of obtaining proximal and distal control, aneurysm resection, and primary reconstruction. These techniques were successful in only a limited number of patients.

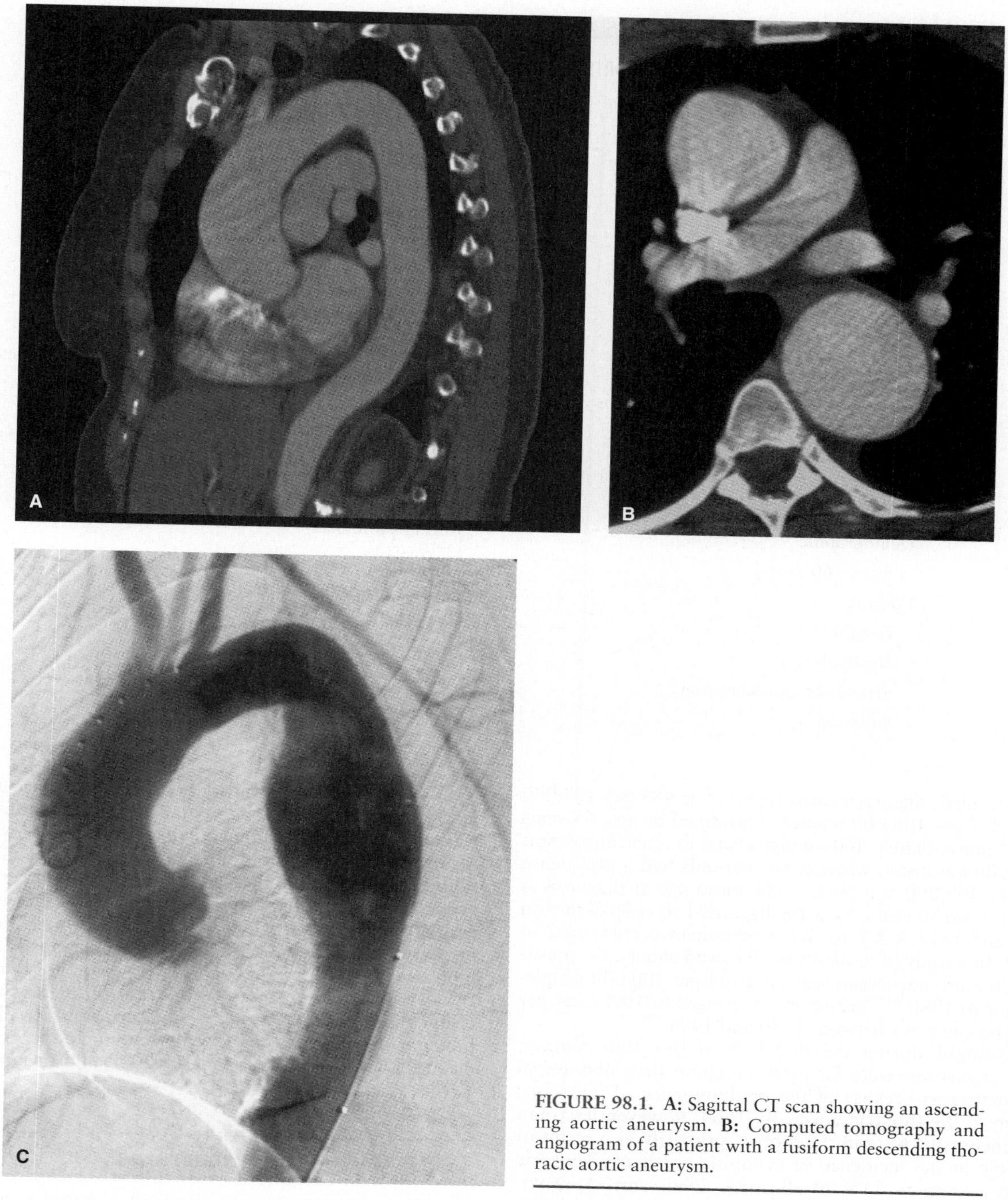

FIGURE 98.1. **A:** Sagittal CT scan showing an ascending aortic aneurysm. **B:** Computed tomography and angiogram of a patient with a fusiform descending thoracic aortic aneurysm.

The modern surgical treatment of aortic disease began in the 1950s, and the ensuing 20 to 30 years saw the development and failures of many novel techniques. In the early 1950s, the first resection of a descending thoracic aneurysm and replacement with homograft was reported.[3,4] The first excision of a saccular ascending aortic aneurysm without cardiopulmonary bypass was performed by Michael DeBakey and Denton Cooley in Houston in 1952.[5] In 1953, Dubost et al. in Paris and DeBakey and Cooley in Houston reported successful resection and reconstruction of the abdominal aorta with human aortic allograft.[6,7] The same duo performed a repair of an acute traumatic aortic transection in 1954 through a left thoracotomy with the patient's core temperature reduced to 28°C using surface cooling. They subsequently reported the first successful resection of an ascending aneurysm with cardiopulmonary bypass in 1956 and the first successful arch aneurysm repair in 1957.[8,9]

Dacron grafts, introduced by DeBakey,[2] largely replaced human allografts, avoiding the need for maintaining large tissue banks and allowing more facilities the ability to treat these patients. In addition, the development and refinement of the cardiopulmonary bypass machine, in large part by John Gibbon at Thomas Jefferson, revolutionized the open surgical repair of thoracic aortic disease. The importance of hypothermia for cerebral protection and specifically the use of hypothermic circulatory arrest was established by Randy Griepp et al. at Yale University.[10] With these techniques in place, modern surgical practice to treat aortic disease was established.

PREVALENCE

The true incidence and prevalence of thoracic aortic aneurysms is likely underreported. In a Swedish autopsy study, the prevalence

TABLE 98.1

RISK FACTORS FOR THORACIC AORTIC ANEURYSMS

Anatomic	Vascular disease
Annulo aortic ectasia	Uncontrolled hypertension
Aortic wall abnormalities	Inflammation
Bicuspid aortic valve	Aortic aneurysm
Chromosomal/genetic	Aortic arteritis
Marfan syndrome	Arthrosclerosis
Ehlers-Danlos syndrome (type IV)	Behçet disease
Noonan syndrome	Giant cell arteritis
Polycystic kidney disease	Ormond disease
Turner syndrome	Syphilis
Congenital	Takayasu arteritis
Aortic arch hypoplasia	Iatrogenic/idiopathic
Aortic coarctation	Aortic cannulation/cross-clamping
Congenital aortic stenosis	Endoluminal transcatheter therapy
Demographic	Graft anastomosis
Age (>60 years)	Instrumentation
Lifestyle	Sheehan syndrome
Cocaine	Valvular surgery
Dyslipidemia	
Pregnancy (preeclampsia)	
Smoking	

of thoracic aortic aneurysms was reported as 489 per 100,000 men and 437 per 100,000 women.[11] Stratified by age, 65-year-olds had approximately 400 asymptomatic thoracic aneurysms per 100,000 autopsies, whereas 80-year-olds had a prevalence of 670 per 100,000 autopsies.[11] The mean age at diagnosis is between 60 and 70 years. Men are diagnosed 10 years earlier on average and have a 2:1 to 3:1 predominance compared to women.[12] In a study of residents in Olmstead county, the prevalence of thoracic aneurysms was 5.9 cases per 100,000 people-years prior to 1980.[13] This number increased to 10.4 cases per 100,000 people-years between 1980 and 1994.[14]

Interestingly, during the first half of the 20th century, thoracic aneurysms were far more common than abdominal aortic aneurysms because of the predominance of infectious aneurysm in the thoracic aorta. By 1964, however, less than half of aneurysms were in the thorax, primarily as a result of the decline in the incidence of syphilitic aortitis.[15] Thoracic aneurysms compose 25% of all aortic aneurysms. Approximately 50% of thoracic aortic aneurysms involve the ascending aorta, 10% the aortic arch, and 45% the descending aorta.[13] True thoracoabdominal aneurysms constitute less than 5% of thoracic aortic aneurysms.[11]

ETIOLOGY AND RISK FACTORS

Although there has been a long-standing belief that aortic aneurysms represent a late degenerative stage of atherosclerosis,[12] this concept has been seriously challenged, and aneurysms are now viewed in terms of genetic and molecular mechanisms. Atherosclerotic disease is now thought to be associated with, rather than causative of, aneurysmal disease. Aneurysms associated with atherosclerosis of the aorta most commonly involve the descending or thoracoabdominal segments, whereas atherosclerosis is rarely associated with ascending aortic aneurysms.

Abnormal proteolysis, the presence of elastolytic serum enzymes and deficiencies of collagen and elastin have been implicated as factors contributing to the development of these aneurysms.[15] Atherosclerotic lesions of the thoracic aorta may ulcerate and penetrate the internal elastic lamina of the aortic wall, which can result in hemorrhage within the layers of the media leading to intramural hematoma, an entity on the continuum of aortic dissection. Once aneurysmal dilatation of the aorta has begun, it tends to progress. Whether this is due to a gradual but constant increase in size or episodic incremental increases is unknown. Associated chronic obstructive pulmonary disease, smoking, and hypertension are known to be risk factors and can increase the rate of aneurysm growth. Other disorders with genetic predisposition are also highly linked with thoracic aneurysms and include Marfan syndrome, Loeys-Dietz syndrome, Ehlers-Danlos syndrome, and Turner syndrome (Table 98.1).

Degenerative

The most common etiology for thoracic aortic aneurysm formation is cystic medial degeneration. Although the underlying mechanisms for this process are unknown, pathologic features include elastic fiber fragmentation, smooth muscle cell apoptosis, and local production of matrix-degrading enzymes, specifically matrix metalloproteinases (MMPs). The degree of atherosclerosis present in the aorta is dependent on the anatomy of the aneurysm. Ascending aortic aneurysms are degenerative often without extensive atherosclerosis, although atherosclerosis is often a feature associated with degenerative descending aneurysms. The pathogenesis of aortic aneurysms appears to be linked to a reduction in functional extracellular matrix proteins, elastin and collagen, either through enzymatic degradation or deficiencies in these structural proteins. Moreover, in some diseases with genetic predisposition, there is a shift in the expression of MMPs as well as the tissue inhibitors of MMPs (TIMPs) resulting in degradation of these proteins. For example, patients with bicuspid aortic valves are known to have altered expression of MMPs and TIMPs. As such, these patients have degenerative ascending aortic aneurysms often

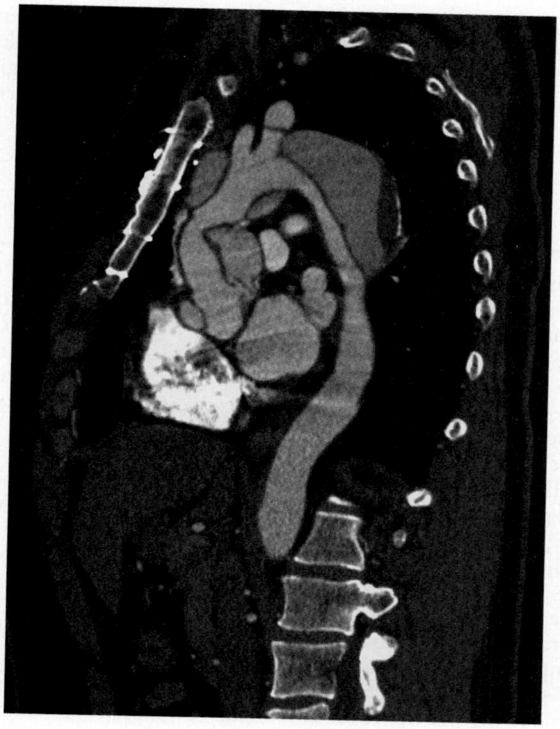

FIGURE 98.2. A CT reconstruction demonstrating a chronic Stanford type A dissection (DeBakey type I) that has undergone late aneurysmal degeneration of the proximal descending thoracic aorta.

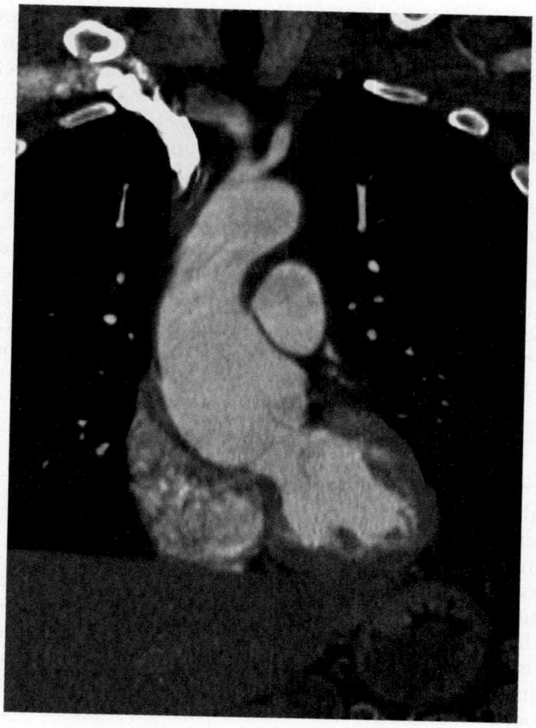

FIGURE 98.3. Reconstruction of a CT scan of an aortic root aneurysm in a patient with Marfan syndrome. Commonly the sinuses of Valsalva are involved with sparing of the aortic valve.

independent of any associated functional valve disease or atherosclerosis.

Chronic Aortic Dissection

A dissection occurs when blood enters the vessel wall through an intimal tear allowing propagation of blood between the medial and adventitial layers. Although ascending aortic aneurysms (Stanford A, or DeBakey types I and II) are treated emergently with open surgery, most descending thoracic aneurysms (Stanford B or DeBakey type III) do not rupture or result in malperfusion and are treated with medical management of hypertension and pain control. These aortas are prone to aneurysmal degeneration as the dissected aortic wall is inherently weak (Fig. 98.2). It is important to note that nearly all chronic ascending aortic dissections become aneurysmal, and roughly one third of descending thoracic aortic dissections become aneurysmal over time. Although the etiology is different with mechanical disruption of the medial and adventitial wall, the process of chronic aortic wall remodeling including production of MMPs may be similar.

Genetically Triggered

1 Although the risk of thoracic aortic aneurysm disease increases with age, thoracic aneurysms in young patients are most likely due to genetic predisposition or familial syndromes. Recently, several genetic etiologies linked to thoracic aneurysms have been elucidated. In particular, insights have been gained from a registry for the genetically triggered thoracic aortic aneurysms (TAA) and cardiovascular conditions (GenTAC) which has genetic information on more than 1,000 patients with thoracic aneurysms secondary to hereditary or genetic predisposition.[16] The most common and notorious disease is Marfan syndrome, which is an autosomal dominant defect of the fibrillin gene located on chromosome 15. Mutation of fibrillin leads to instability of the elastic fibers in the aortic media. The prevalence of aortic dilatation in Marfan syndrome is 70% to 80% and most commonly involves the aortic root and sinuses of Valsalva, rendering the aorta prone to rupture or dissection (Fig. 98.3). Marfan syndrome presents at an early age and tends to be more common in men than women. The cardinal features of the disorder include tall stature, ectopia lentis, mitral valve prolapse, aortic root dilatation, and aortic dissection. About three quarters of patients have an affected parent, while new mutations account for the remainder of cases.

Recently, mutations of transforming growth factor receptors I and II (TGFBR I, TGFBR II) termed Loeys-Dietz syndrome have been linked with thoracic aneurysms. These patients have a classic bifid uvula. Ehlers-Danlos syndrome encompasses a group of more than 10 disorders characterized by defects of collagen synthesis. The disease can range from hypermobility of the joints to extremely fragile skin and extreme muscle weakness. The common vascular Ehlers-Danlos (type 4) is caused by an autosomal dominant disorder of type III collagen. These patients are characterized by fragility of their blood vessels. Familial thoracic aortic aneurysms and dissections (FTAAD) is caused by mutations of the α actin II or myosin heavy chain (MYH11).[17] Turner syndrome is defined by the loss of an X chromosome (XO). Patients with Turner are prone to aneurysmal degeneration of their ascending aorta.

Inflammatory

A host of rare inflammatory diseases of the aorta and great vessels including Takayasu arteritis, Behçet disease, Kawasaki disease, and giant cell arteritis can result in thoracic aortic aneurysms and can require surgical treatment. Detailed descriptions of these diseases are beyond the scope of this chapter.

Infections

In current practice, primary infections of the aorta are rare but do lead to aneurysms. Mycotic aneurysms can be caused by bacterial, fungal, spirochetal, or viral agents. Prior to the antibiotic era, syphilis accounted for approximately 75% of all aneurysms. Mycotic aneurysms occur due to localized infections in the aortic or arterial walls, usually as the result of bacteremia. Infection of atherosclerotic plaques themselves can also result in mycotic aneurysms. As a result of trauma or due to infected lymph nodes, infection may also spread to blood vessel walls contiguously. Preexisting aortic aneurysms may also become infected, usually from bloodstream seeding. Although any pathogen may infect aneurysms, *Salmonella* species show a special proclivity for vascular tissues. Other organisms associated with mycotic aneurysms are *Staphylococcus* species, *Streptococcus* species, *Pasteurella multocida*, *Legionella anisa*, and *Escherichia coli*. Treatment consists of long-term antibiotics prior to and after surgical aneurysm resection.

Traumatic Pseudoaneurysm

Pseudoaneurysms are associated with trauma or previous operations on the aorta. Classically, rapid decelerating blunt trauma leads to aortic transection. In more than 50% of cases, the location of the aortic injury is just distal to the fixed ligamentum arteriosum, the remnant of the ductus arteriosus.[18,19] For the 20% of patients who survive this acute event, the rupture is partially contained by the aortic adventitia and pleura. Of survivors, aneurysmal formation around the site of injury can occur and often dilates faster because it is an unsuspected injury, and utmost care with regard to their antihypertensive therapy has to be taken to avoid rupture. Given multisystem injuries often present in these high-speed injuries, many consider endovascular aortic repair the preferred approach for most of these patients.[20] Iatrogenic pseudoaneurysms occur following aortic surgery and can form at anastomotic sites or areas where an aortic cross-clamp was placed.

DIAGNOSIS

Most thoracic aneurysms are asymptomatic and are found incidentally. Symptomatic aneurysms are often diagnosed based on their anatomic sequelae. Patients with aneurysms of the ascending aorta may also present with fullness in the chest or signs and symptoms of aortic valve insufficiency. Acute chest pain may be caused by either expansion of the aneurysm or dissection of the aortic wall. Arch and descending thoracic aneurysms can present with hoarseness secondary to stretching of the left recurrent laryngeal nerve, stridor from tracheal compression, or dysphagia from esophageal compression.

There are multiple imaging modalities to diagnose thoracic aortic aneurysms. Plain chest radiograph can be suggestive whereas computed tomography (CT), magnetic resonance imaging (MRI), and transesophageal echocardiography (TEE) are definitive studies.[21] CT is widely available and provides detailed information about the size, location, and extent of aortic disease as well as anatomic detail of surrounding mediastinal and thoracic structures. In particular, CT angiography is useful to plan endovascular approaches to repair. This is the most common means of evaluating and following the thoracic aorta although it requires exposure to radiation and nephrotoxic contrast material.

MRI offers detailed anatomy as CT does but does not require radiation. Gadolinium as a contrast agent has also recently been documented to be nephrotoxic. MRI requires lengthy image acquisition and processing times and is not as readily available as is CT. Moreover, MRI cannot be performed in patients with significant metallic implants such as pacemakers and defibrillators.

TEE avoids the use of these agents and offers good visualization of the ascending and descending thoracic aorta as well as cardiac structures. Because of the tracheal shadowing, imaging of the aortic arch is limited. In addition, the technical expertise to perform and interpret TEE is not always readily available.

The once-preferred diagnostic test, catheter-based angiography, images only the lumen and does not provide information regarding the aortic wall.

MANAGEMENT AND NATURAL HISTORY

In three large thoracic aortic aneurysm studies, rupture was the most common cause of death (42%–70% of deaths) among those patients who did not undergo operation at the time of diagnosis.[15,22,23] In all three series, the rate of rupture for aneurysms complicated by dissection substantially exceeded the rate for nondissected aneurysm.[24] Collectively, these studies indicate that an aggressive strategy to treat thoracic aneurysms is needed.

The management strategy is dictated by the aneurysm size and rate of growth. Aortic aneurysms that are large or that are rapidly enlarging are at risk of dissection or rupture. The risk of dissection or rupture increases in a nonlinear fashion as the size increases. Data from the Yale Center for Thoracic Aortic Disease, which has followed more than 3,000 patients with thoracic aortic aneurysms, has suggested that the risk of aortic complications in the ascending aorta increases significantly as the size approaches 6.0 cm, and in the descending thoracic aorta as the size approaches 7.0 cm.[25] Similarly, the Olmstead County registry (Minnesota) reported that a rupture rate of 16% at 3 years for 6-cm aneurysms compared to 31% for 7-cm aneurysms.[14] The Yale group has reported the annual risk of death or aortic-related complication exceeds 15% in patients with aneurysms of 6.0 cm or greater compared to 5% in patients with aneurysms smaller than 5.0 cm. Other studies have supported this pattern, reporting a mean rate of rupture or dissection of 2% per year for small aneurysms, 3% for aneurysms 5.0 to 5.9 cm, and 6.9% for aneurysms 6.0 cm or greater in diameter.[26,27] These data have formed the basis for size criteria to intervene prior to the attainment of the previously mentioned dimensions in an asymptomatic patient.

Recent studies have evaluated the risk of aortic complications based on aortic size individualized to body surface area (Table 98.2). In patients with a symptomatic aneurysm, however, surgical treatment should be performed irrespective of the size.

As for other aneurysms, the growth of thoracic aortic aneurysms is indolent. The typical rate of growth for ascending aortic aneurysms is 0.1 cm/year and for descending aneurysms is 0.3 cm/year.[25] The annual growth rates for patients suffering from chronic dissections are significantly higher, ranging from 0.24 cm/year for small aneurysms to 0.48 cm/year from large aneurysms.[26] Growth rates exceeding 5 to 7 mm/year for aneurysms or greater than 5 mm per 6 months for aortic dissections are considered harbingers of aortic complications, and earlier intervention should be considered.

MANAGEMENT

Since thoracic aneurysms increase in size until they rupture,[12,26] the decision to intervene is critical. Preemptive surgical therapy should be applied at a size of 5.5 cm for ascending and arch aneurysms and 6.0 cm to 6.5 cm for descending aortic aneurysms in suitable surgical candidates to avoid aortic complications or death.[26–28] These surgical threshold criteria should be modified for patients with Marfan syndrome or connective tissue disease in which preemptive surgery is appropriate at 4.5 cm for root and ascending aneurysms and 5.5 cm for descending aneurysms.[29] Some have further suggested that patients with Turner syndrome be treated surgically if the aortic diameter exceeds 4.0 cm due to the aggressive nature of aortic disease in these patients. Furthermore, any patient with

TABLE 98.2

RISK OF COMPLICATIONS BY AORTIC DIAMETER AND BODY SURFACE AREA (BSA) WITH AORTIC SIZE INDEX

	AORTIC SIZE (cm)									
BSA	3.5	4.0	4.5	5.0	5.5	6.0	6.5	7.0	7.5	8.0
1.30	2.69	3.08	3.46	3.85	4.23	4.62	5.00	5.38	5.77	6.15
1.40	2.50	2.86	3.21	3.57	3.93	4.29	4.64	5.00	5.36	5.71
1.50	2.33	2.67	3.00	3.33	3.67	4.00	4.33	4.67	5.00	5.33
1.60	2.19	2.50	2.80	3.13	3.44	3.75	4.06	4.38	4.69	5.00
1.70	2.05	2.35	2.65	2.94	3.24	3.53	3.82	4.12	4.41	4.71
1.80	1.94	2.22	2.50	2.78	3.06	3.33	3.61	3.89	4.17	4.44
1.90	1.84	2.11	2.37	2.63	2.89	3.16	3.42	3.68	3.95	4.22
2.00	1.75	2.00	2.25	2.50	2.75	3.00	3.25	3.50	3.75	4.00
2.10	1.67	1.90	2.14	2.38	2.62	2.86	3.10	3.33	3.57	3.80
2.20	1.59	1.82	2.05	2.27	2.50	2.72	2.95	3.18	3.41	3.64
2.30	1.52	1.74	1.96	2.17	2.39	2.61	2.83	3.04	3.26	3.48
2.40	1.46	1.67	1.88	2.08	2.29	2.50	2.71	2.92	3.13	3.33
2.50	1.40	1.60	1.80	2.00	2.20	2.40	2.60	2.80	3.00	3.20

Full-size table (<1K) = low risk (~4% per yr); Full-size table (<1K) = moderate risk (~8% per yr); Full-size table (<1K) = severe risk (~20% per yr).
Reproduced with permission from Davies RR, Gallo A, Coady MA, et al., Novel measurement of relative aortic size predicts rupture of thoracic aortic aneurysms. *Ann Thorac Surg* 2006;81:169–177. Article | PDF (189 K) | View Record in Scopus | Cited By in Scopus (43)

symptoms or rapid growth as seen on sequential CT scans should have surgical intervention in a timely manner.

Once the need for intervention has been determined, a full cardiac evaluation should be completed including stress testing and angiographic evaluation of coronary arteries as indicated. The basic premise of open surgical repair for aneurysms, regardless of the situation, is replacement with an interposition graft with or without cardiopulmonary bypass. Intraoperative management is essential with central venous pressure and arterial monitoring as well as large-volume intravenous infusion lines. Intraoperative transesophageal echocardiography is useful to monitor fluid status and cardiac function during the operation.

Medical Management

Medical management by aggressive antihypertensive therapy can be used in asymptomatic patients with thoracic aneurysms in whom size criteria for surgical intervention has not been reached. While β-blockers and angiotensin-converting enzyme inhibitors/angiotensin receptor blockers are common treatments, studies are currently underway to indicate their efficacy in patients with aortic aneurysms. In mouse models of Marfan syndrome, ACE inhibitors prevented aneurysms.[30] Smoking cessation may be helpful in patients who have not developed chronic obstructive pulmonary disease (COPD). The diagnosis of COPD is a significant risk factor for aortic complications. It is unclear if risk factor modification of COPD once diagnosed can influence the likelihood of aortic rupture. Frequent imaging of these patients to assess changes in size should be performed to determine if surgery should be recommended.

Open Surgical Management of TAA

2 Careful planning by experienced medical personnel is paramount to providing optimal treatment in patients with thoracic aortic aneurysms as the morbidity and mortality for surgical intervention is significant. Over the years there have been substantial improvements in the intraoperative and postoperative management in patients with TAA. The approach and techniques of repair vary widely based on the location of the thoracic aneurysm.

3 **Aortic Root and Ascending Aortic Aneurysms.** Open surgical repair remains the mainstay for aortic root, ascending aortic, and aortic arch aneurysms with very acceptable outcomes and low morbidity when performed in centers with experienced personnel. Operations to replace aortic root and ascending aorta are approached via a median sternotomy. All pathologic segments of the aorta are evaluated and replaced if abnormal, including the aortic valve, sinuses of Valsalva, the tubular portion of the ascending aorta, and the aortic arch. Cardiopulmonary bypass is established through right atrial (venous) cannulation and either aortic, femoral arterial cannulation or axillary artery cannulation. The heart is vented via the pulmonary artery or left atrium. The use of the axillary artery for cannulation allows for selective antegrade cerebral perfusion if circulatory arrest is needed during the replacement of the aorta[31] (Fig. 98.4). The axillary artery is exposed via a 4-cm transverse incision 2 cm below and parallel to the clavicle. Once through the pectoral muscles, the axillary vein is isolated and retracted superiorly isolating the axillary artery. After systemic heparinization, an 8- or 10-mm Dacron graft is anastomosed in an end-to-side fashion onto the artery. The arterial cannula is then secured to the Dacron graft. Myocardial protection is achieved by infusion of antegrade blood cardioplegia into the coronary ostia and retrograde cardioplegia into the coronary sinus accompanied by a topical hypothermia.

If the aneurysm is contained to the root or ascending aorta and does not involve the aortic arch or head vessels, the heart can be arrested with the cross-clamp proximal to the innominate artery, and mild hypothermia can be used for systemic protection while the patient is maintained on cardiopulmonary bypass. A tube graft is then anastomosed distally then proximally using running monofilament suture. The aortic valve is also assessed with the aorta open and the valve repaired or replaced as necessary (Fig. 98.5). If the dilation of the aorta extends into the arch, deep hypothermic circulatory arrest (HCA) allows for complete resection and reconstruction of the diseased aorta and an open distal anastomosis in a bloodless field. Cerebral protection can be augmented by maintaining antegrade cerebral perfusion via the right axillary

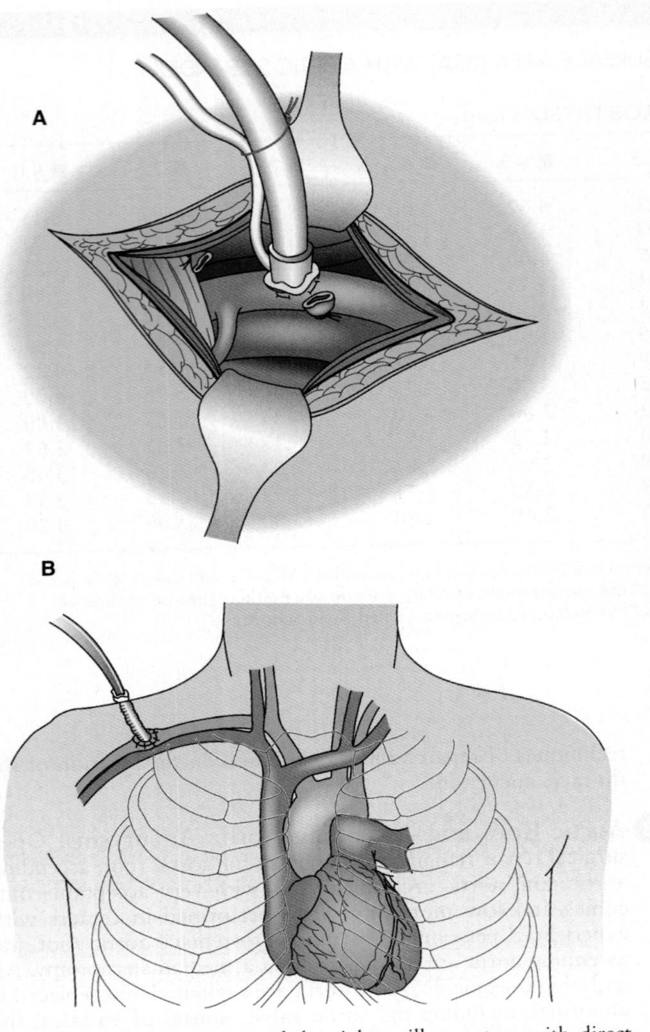

FIGURE 98.4. Cannulation of the right axillary artery with direct arterial cannulation (**A**) or with the use of a side graft (**B**). Once established, axillary artery cannulation can allow for antegrade cerebral perfusion throughout the aortic replacement procedure. (Adapted from Sabik JF, Nemeh H, Lytle BW, et al. Cannulation of the axillary artery with a side graft reduces morbidity. *Ann Thorac Surg* 2004; 77:1315–1320.)

cannula and clamping the proximal innominate artery. The distal anastomosis is then performed in a timely manner. The cross-clamp is then reapplied to the graft, and full cardiopulmonary bypass can then resume. The proximal anastomosis is then completed encompassing all diseased portions of the ascending aorta and the aortic root.

Aneurysms involving the aortic root require isolation of the right and left coronary ostia and reimplantation into the Dacron tube graft. Care must be taken to ensure the coronary arteries are not kinked. In this setting the native aortic valve can be spared (valve-sparing root replacement) if the leaflets are normal or can be replaced with a valved conduit (Bentall procedure).

Aortic Arch Aneurysms. Operations involving replacement of the thoracic aortic arch are approached from a median sternotomy or bilateral anterior thoracotomies (clamshell incision) and use hypothermic circulatory arrest (HCA). HCA allows for a bloodless field while maintaining cerebral and visceral protection. In this setting, the patient is cooled to 16° to 20°C and the cardiopulmonary bypass circuit is turned off for up to 45 to 60 minutes. The use of selective antegrade cerebral perfusion (cannulation and perfusion of the right axillary artery with a clamp on the proximal innominate artery) allows perfusion of the right carotid artery during operations of the aortic arch, maintains some perfusion to the brain, and reduces the risk of embolism and associated morbidity.[32] Individual arterial cannulation of nondiseased arch vessels can be used as well to help ensure good cerebral perfusion. Replacement of the arch is often best performed with the use of a multibranched (trifurcated) aortic graft to allow individual anastomoses to each of the three great vessels (Fig. 98.6).[32,33] This approach, rather than reimplanting an island of aortic tissue with all the great vessels, has been suggested to reduce the risk of embolization and minimizes the risk of late aneurysmal degeneration of the aortic patch.[33]

Descending Aortic Aneurysms. Open surgical repair of the descending thoracic aneurysm is performed through a left posterolateral thoracotomy. Prior to positioning, a double-lumen endotracheal tube is placed for single-lung ventilation. In addition, a lumbar drain is often placed for cerebral spinal fluid (CSF) pressure monitoring and drainage to reduce the incidence of paraparesis and paraplegia caused by spinal cord ischemia, which can accompany resection of the aorta in the distal thoracic area.[34] The use of left heart bypass has been shown to decrease the risk of visceral and spinal cord ischemia. Pharmacologic agents, including barbiturates, naloxone, and steroids, may also help reduce neurologic injury when administered during the procedure. There are two options to perform this procedure: sequential clamping versus hypothermic circulatory arrest. If the arch is relatively spared and enough normal aorta can be identified distal to the left common carotid artery, a proximal clamp can be placed, which allows for left heart bypass. In using left heart bypass, the left atrium via the left inferior pulmonary vein and the femoral artery are cannulated. A centrifugal pump, heparin-bonded tubing, and minimal heparinization can be used, which can result in less bleeding than in traditional cardiopulmonary bypass. With this technique, moderate hypothermia is used with sequential aortic clamping, reimplantation of critical intercostal arteries, and the distal anastomosis constructed with peripheral perfusion via the femoral artery (Fig. 98.7).[35–38] Conversely, for patients in whom the transverse arch cannot be safely clamped, profound hypothermic circulatory arrest is used for both cardiac protection and central and peripheral nervous system protection. With this technique, full cardiopulmonary bypass with cannulation of the femoral artery and femoral vein allows for cooling of the patient and deep hypothermic circulatory arrest and the proximal anastomoses can be performed in a bloodless field (Fig. 98.8). Other modalities used to help reduce paraparesis and paraplegia include monitoring of sensory evoked potentials and motor evoked potentials.[34] Epidural catheters are extremely beneficial for pain control and can improve early mobilization and pulmonary function. There is still great debate regarding the use of partial versus full cardiopulmonary bypass with these extensive aortic replacement surgeries.[39,40]

After clamping the aorta (or initiating HCA), the aneurysm is opened and the proximal cuff is fashioned. An interposition graft is sutured to the proximal aorta in an end-to-end fashion. Once completed, cardiopulmonary bypass can be reinstituted and the graft clamped to perform the distal anastomoses when using HCA. The distal aorta and graft are then fashioned and an anastomosis created. Significant lumbar artery identified via preoperative computed tomographic aortography or intraoperative assessment can be reimplanted into the interposition graft. There is continued controversy regarding the necessity to perform this as this process can often take more than 30 minutes during which the aorta may be clamped. Once the affected portion of aorta has been successfully replaced, the patient can be appropriately warmed and hemostasis ensured. The patient is removed from cardiac support and thoracotomy closed in the usual manner. If the diaphragm was taken down, it should be reapproximated with interrupted nonabsorbable suture.

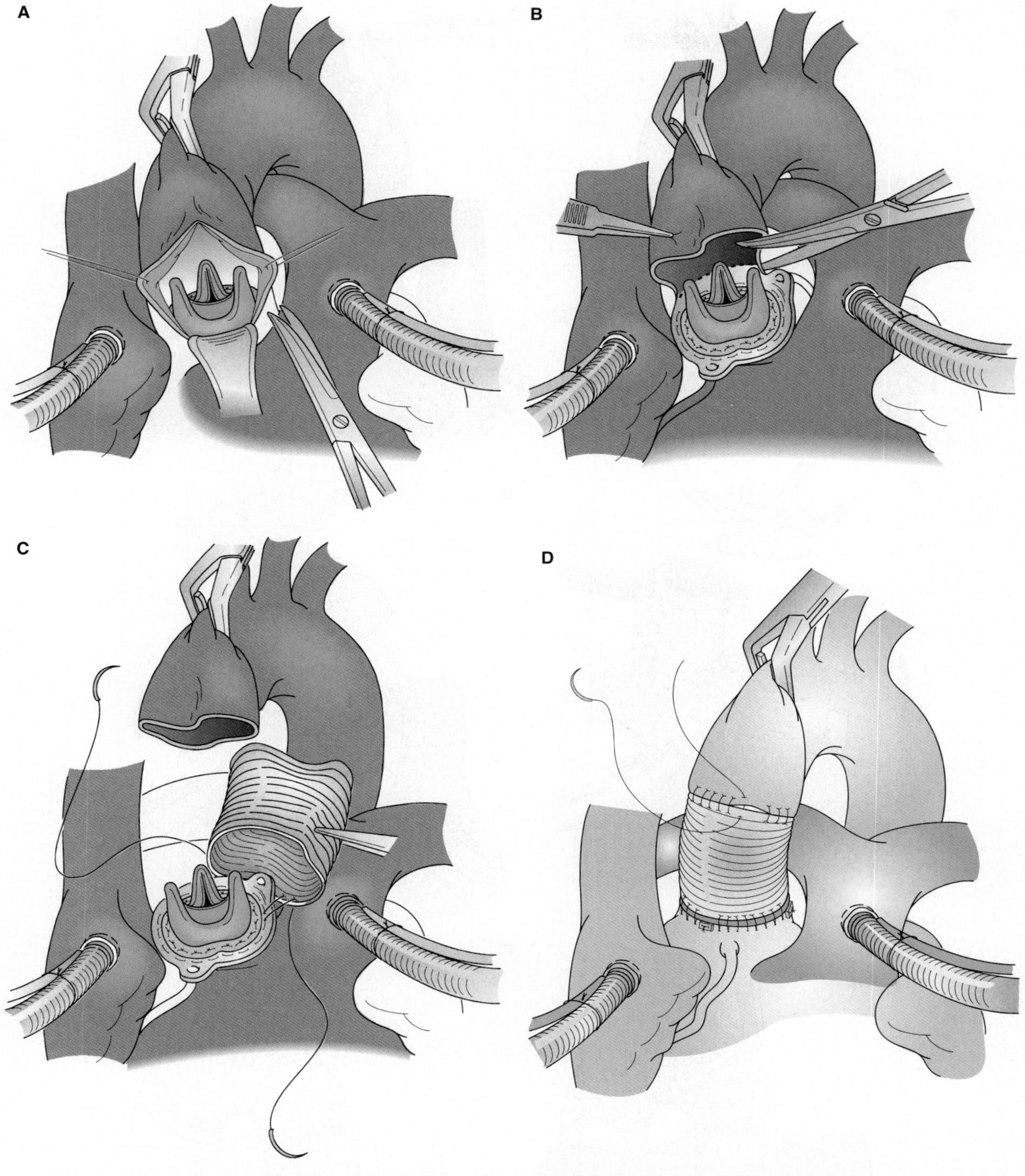

FIGURE 98.5. Operative repair of an ascending aortic aneurysm with distal clamping of the aorta. **A:** Valve replacement, when indicated, is performed after cardioplegic arrest. **B:** A full-thickness cuff of proximal aorta is developed and the aorta is transected just distal of the coronary ostia. **C:** The posterior suture line begins to the left of the left main coronary ostium and proceeds rightward, over the ostium. **D:** Completion of the distal suture line is performed prior to release of the cross-clamp. Careful measurement of the graft length ensures a tension-free distal anastomosis. (Adapted from Frist WH, Miller DC. Repair of ascending aortic aneurysms and dissections. *J Cardiac Surg* 1986;1:33–52.)

Endovascular Therapy

Open surgical procedures on the thoracic aorta, and particularly on the descending thoracic aorta, have significant mortality and morbidity. Endovascular techniques for the descending thoracic aorta have become the preferred treatment approach not only for aneurysms but for dissections and traumatic aortic injuries as they often can be performed with less morbidity than that associated with open surgical treatment. Endovascular stent graft repair was first introduced by Parodi to treat the abdominal aorta.[41] In 2005, the first commercially available device was approved by the FDA to treat descending thoracic aortic aneurysms. To date, there are three such approved devices—Gore (WL Gore Inc., Flagstaff, AZ); Medtronic (Medtronic, Minneapolis, MN); and Cook (Cook Medical, Bloomington, IN). Current grafts are as large as 45 mm and

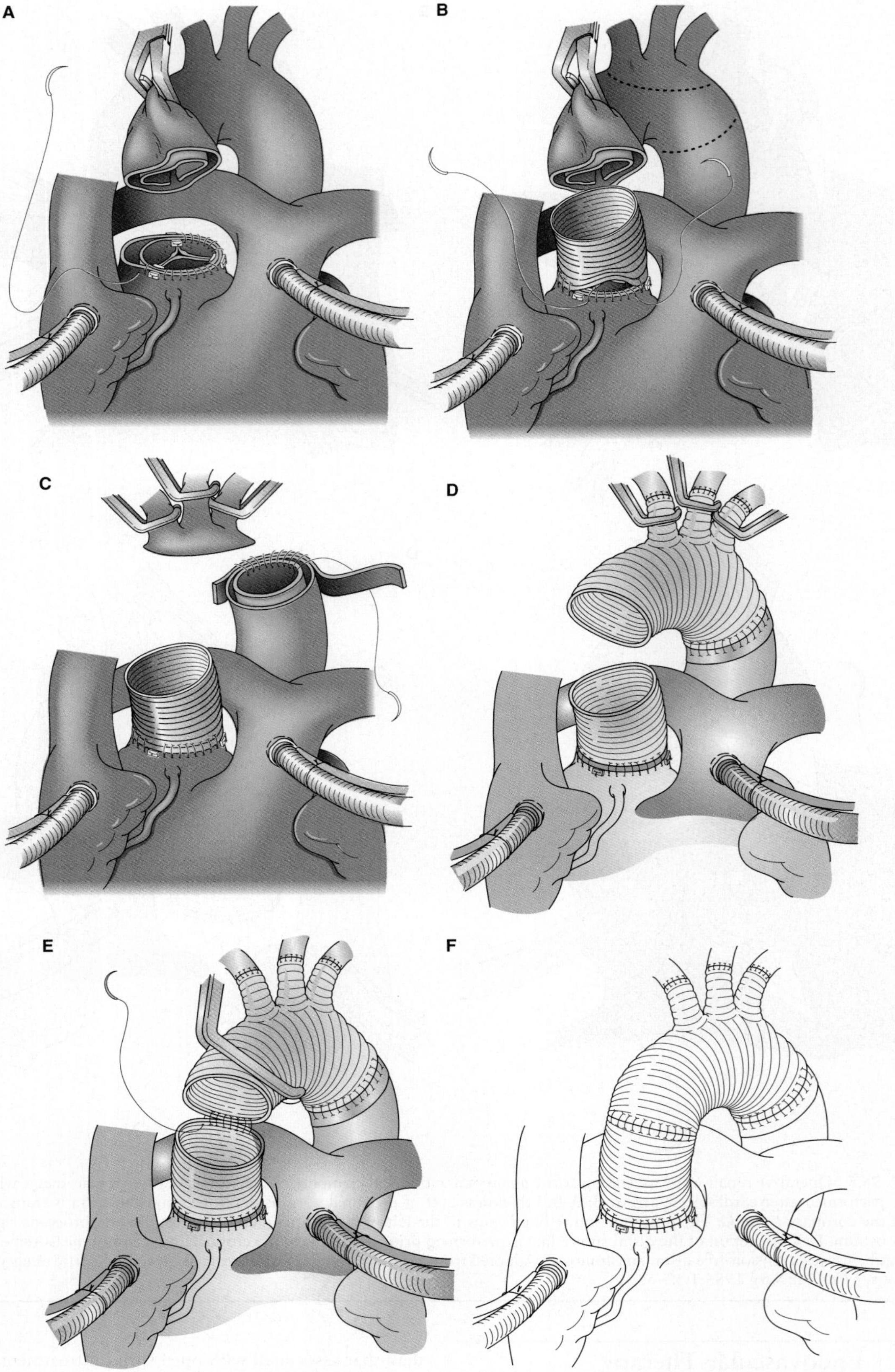

FIGURE 98.6. Repair of ascending and arch aneurysm with dissection. **A:** The ascending aorta is repaired first with the cross-clamp in place. **B:** While the ascending graft is placed proximally, the patient is cooled. **C:** During a period of hypothermic circulatory arrest (18°C), the distal aortic suture line is completed. **D:** The great vessels are reanastomosed separately using a trifurcated graft, or alternatively, an island of aorta containing the cerebral vessels can be fashioned. **E:** The cross-clamp is placed proximally, rewarming of the patient is instituted, and the proximal and distal grafts are joined. **F:** The repair as seen prior to decannulation. (Adapted from Griepp RB, Stinson EB, Hollingsworth JF, et al. Prosthetic replacement of the aortic arch. *J Thorac Cardiovasc Surg* 1975;70:1051–1063.)

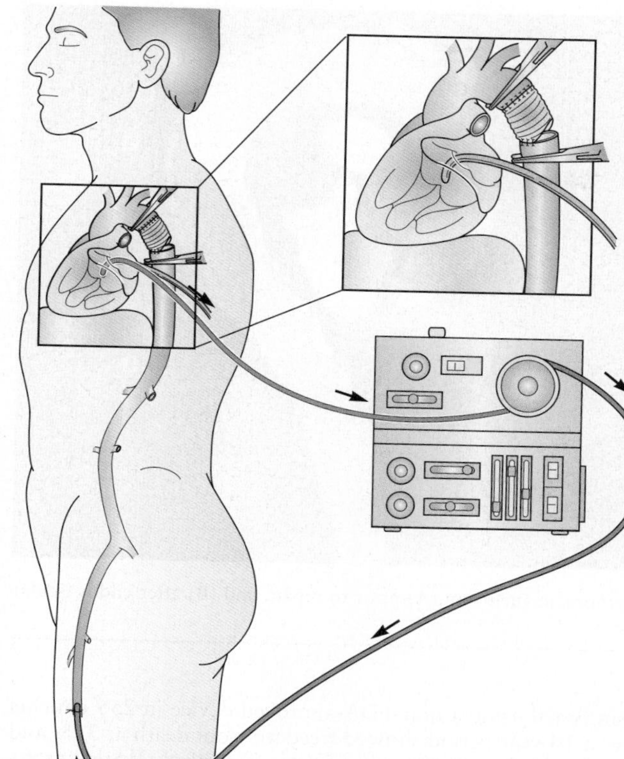

FIGURE 98.7. Schematic of left heart bypass whereby partial bypass is used to maintain perfusion to the viscera and lower extremities. The inflow to the Bio-Medicus pump is the left inferior pulmonary vein, and the outflow is the left femoral artery. This technique avoids the need for an oxygenator.

thus can treat up to 40 to 42 mm diameter aorta. Grafts are made of polytetrafluoroethylene (PTFE) or woven polyester with steel or nitinol stents to maintain their shape. Preoperative CT with arterial phase contrast of the chest, abdomen, and pelvis is essential for operative planning. Critical elements to be gained from the CT include the following:

1. Aneurysm size and extent
2. Proximal and distal landing zones (a minimum of 2 cm of "normal" aorta is required)
3. Need for coverage of the left subclavian and assessment of preoperative carotid subclavian bypass (performed in setting of dominant left vertebral artery or patent left internal mammary artery bypass to the heart)
4. Angulation of the aortic arch and descending aorta
5. Size of femoral and iliac vessels and assessment of need for iliac conduit
6. Presence of thrombus along the aortic wall.

Stent grafts are oversized by approximately 10% to 15% from the CT cross-sectional diameter to obtain sufficient seal between the aorta and the graft. With this approach, the stent graft needs to be advanced into the thoracic aorta. This requires the size of the femoral and iliac arteries to be large enough to allow safe passage of the delivery sheaths. In general, 8-mm vessels are required to pass a 24-Fr sheath, which is the current sheath size for most of the available grafts. Once in place, an aortogram is performed to ensure proper positioning. A completion angiogram is performed to ensure no positioning, presence of kinks or endoleaks, or continued filling of the aneurysm sac. Finally, the decision is made regarding the need for additional stent grafts (Fig. 98.9).

The mortality with this approach has rapidly improved. In the first 100 patients treated at Stanford University (Stanford, CA), 60% of whom were nonoperative candidates, operative mortality was 10%.[42] Homemade devices used in that study have evolved greatly. Recently, a study from the University of Virginia reported a 2% operative mortality in the first 50 patients in the FDA-approved era (2005–2006) where the treatment was

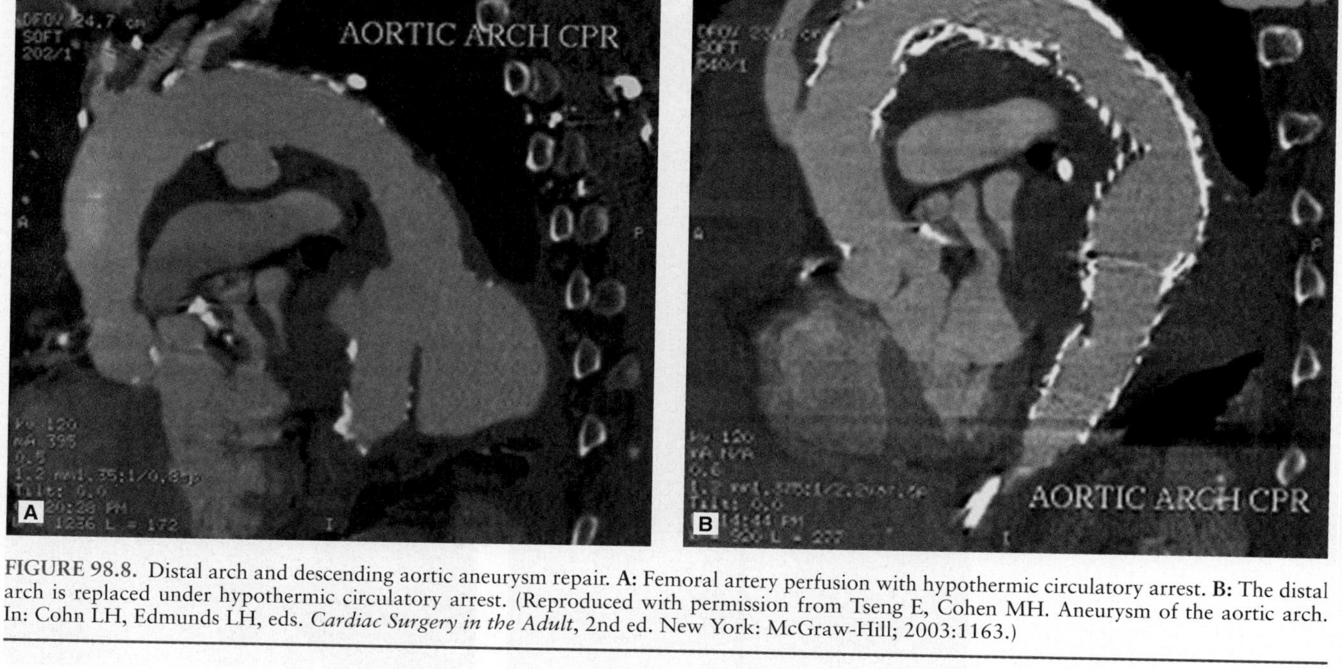

FIGURE 98.8. Distal arch and descending aortic aneurysm repair. **A:** Femoral artery perfusion with hypothermic circulatory arrest. **B:** The distal arch is replaced under hypothermic circulatory arrest. (Reproduced with permission from Tseng E, Cohen MH. Aneurysm of the aortic arch. In: Cohn LH, Edmunds LH, eds. *Cardiac Surgery in the Adult*, 2nd ed. New York: McGraw-Hill; 2003:1163.)

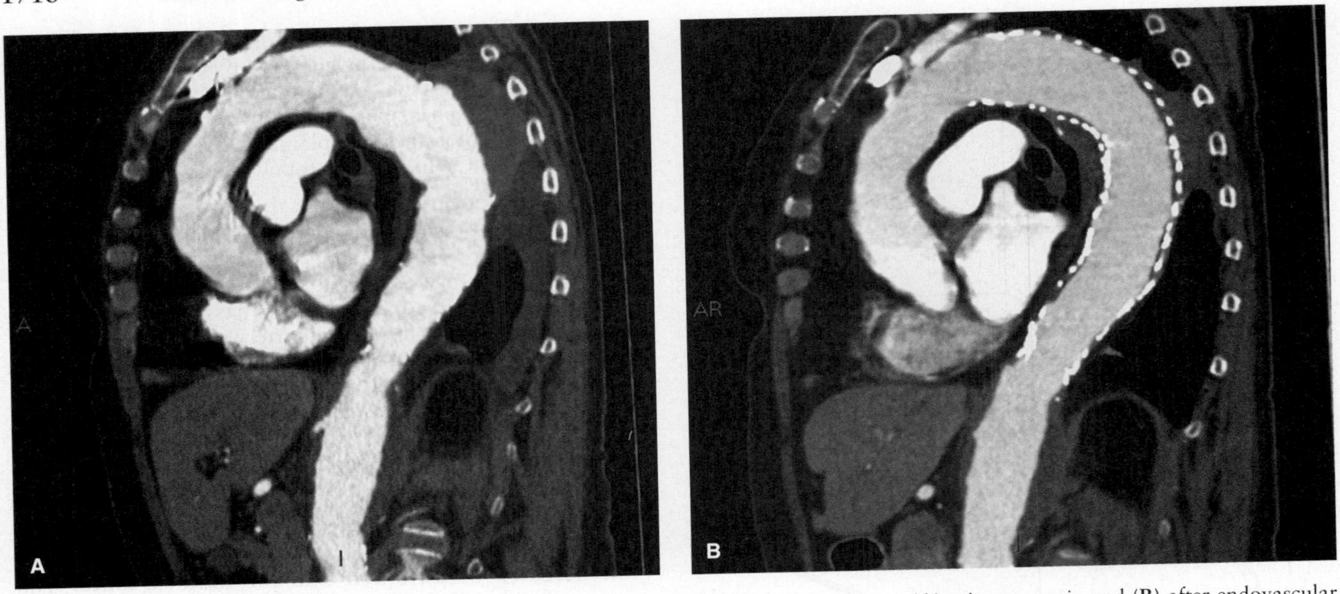

FIGURE 98.9. A reconstruction of a CT scan in a patient with a descending thoracic aneurysm (**A**) prior to repair, and (**B**) after endovascular stent graft repair showing successful exclusion of the aneurysm sac.

applied to a challenging group of patients.[30] Importantly, spinal cord ischemia occurred in 3%, stroke in 4%, and late endoleaks in 7%. Moreover, the 1-year survival was 92%.[30] Another recent study performed at the University of Pittsburgh demonstrated that the permanent paraplegia rate of 1.6% following endovascular repair was significantly better than that for open operation (5.1%, $p < 0.004$).[47] Multiple studies have supported these findings reporting lower mortality, early incidence of paraplegia, and renal failure following endovascular therapy versus open surgery for the descending thoracic aorta.[43–45]

These encouraging short-term and midterm data have led to endovascular therapy becoming the preferred technique for treatment of descending thoracic aneurysms. It is important to note that long-term data are still limited regarding device failure and migration. In one of the few long-term studies, a report from Brazil using a non–FDA-approved device in 255 patients over a 10-year period showed freedom from death at 3, 5, and 9 years of 96%, 89.1%, and 85.1%, respectively.[53] Stent grafts have been applied in other regions of the aorta. In particular, there are several reports of stent grafts placed in the ascending aorta in patients unable to undergo open operation (Fig. 98.10).

The most recent data from the Gore TAG multicenter trial show favorable implant characteristics, with decreased blood loss, intensive care unit stay, and total hospital stay compared to a nonrandomized cohort of open surgical patients.[46] Late follow-up to 2 years shows a low rate of migration (3%), low appearance of late endoleaks (9%) with most managed with new endografts, and a 17% incidence of increase in size of the aneurysm sac. There has been one open conversion, and no late ruptures, prompting the conclusion that for anatomically suitable patients,

FIGURE 98.10. Off-label stent graft repair of an ascending aortic pseudoaneurysm in an inoperable patient demonstrating good positioning of the stent graft and exclusion of the pseudoaneurysm.

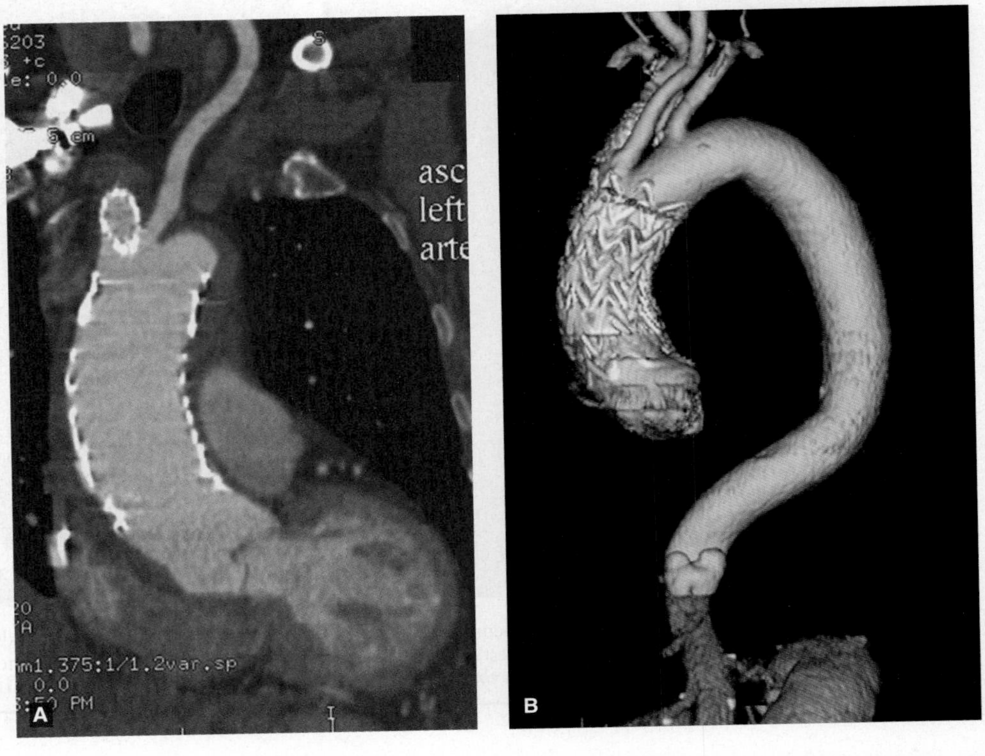

stent graft repair produced similar long-term event-free survival and was associated with less perioperative morbidity.

Hybrid Procedures

As endovascular approaches have evolved, so too have the options for hybrid procedures combining open and endovascular surgery. Patients with combined arch and descending thoracic aneurysms are often ideal candidates for hybrid procedures. The traditional approach has been a two-stage open procedure (elephant trunk). In the first operation, the arch aneurysm is repaired under HCA via a median sternotomy. The distal end of the Dacron graft replacing the arch is sewn to the proximal descending aorta with a long cuff to allow for future repair of the descending aortic aneurysm in the second stage. In the second stage, the traditional procedure has been an open descending aneurysm repair using the long cuff left at the initial operation as the proximal new aorta. Stent graft therapy has allowed for the second stage to be performed less invasively with an endovascular approach. An alternative approach to these patients is revascularization of the arch vessels via sternotomy using a trifurcated graft off the ascending aorta to the great vessels. This can be performed without the use of cardiopulmonary bypass using a side-biting clamp on the ascending aorta. This is followed by endovascular repair of the arch and descending aorta covering the native take-off of the great vessels. Other patients who benefit from hybrid procedures include those with thoracoabdominal aneurysms who require debranching of visceral vessels prior to stent graft repair. The inflow for these debranching bypasses is traditionally from the iliac vessels but can include the proximal abdominal or descending thoracic aorta.

OUTCOMES AND COMPLICATIONS

Despite continued improvement in surgical technique and postoperative care, operative morbidity and mortality remain high for patients with thoracic aortic aneurysms. These patients, in addition to aneurysmal disease, often have associated comorbidities including renal dysfunction, chronic obstructive lung disease, and ischemic heart disease. Preoperative assessment and management are paramount to facilitating good operative outcomes. Multiple studies have demonstrated the adverse effect on survival of emergent versus elective operation. Hospital mortality rates for emergency thoracic aneurysm repair can be as high as 30%, whereas elective mortality rates are less than 5%.[48] To predict risk after elective repair of ascending and aortic arch aneurysms, the Mount Sinai group analyzed multiple variables.[49] They found that the presence of diabetes and manifestations of atherosclerosis emerge as extremely important risk factors for adverse outcome after ascending and arch surgery, displacing age.

Ascending aorta replacement has relatively low mortality and morbidity. The need for circulatory arrest does increase the morbidity slightly with incrementally higher risks of stroke. Procedures on the aortic root, performed by experienced surgeons, carry mortality rates of less than 2%.[50]

Studies focusing on descending thoracic aortic replacement outcomes have shown that the use of left heart bypass or complete cardiopulmonary bypass had favorable results compared with the "clamp-and-sew" techniques without cardiopulmonary bypass. Renal failure appears to be decreased with the use of bypass. However, the rates of paraplegia and paraparesis remain dependent on the extent of repair and clamp time.[48,49] Nonetheless, use of combined adjuncts including CSF drainage, reimplantation of intercostal arteries, and distal aortic perfusion have reduced the overall early neurologic deficits rate from 7% to as low as 0.9%.[49,51]

Endovascular therapy appears to have clear advantages with less operative mortality and morbidity, although it cannot be performed in all patients due to anatomic limitations. However, stent grafts still lead to a significant number of late
5 complications to deal with postsurgery. The risk of spinal cord ischemia is not abrogated with endovascular therapy. Risk factors for spinal cord ischemia include coverage of the left subclavian artery, prior abdominal surgery, coverage of T8 to T12, and previous abdominal aortic surgery.

Moreover, endoleaks can occur late and need to be followed carefully. In our experience, early endoleaks occur in

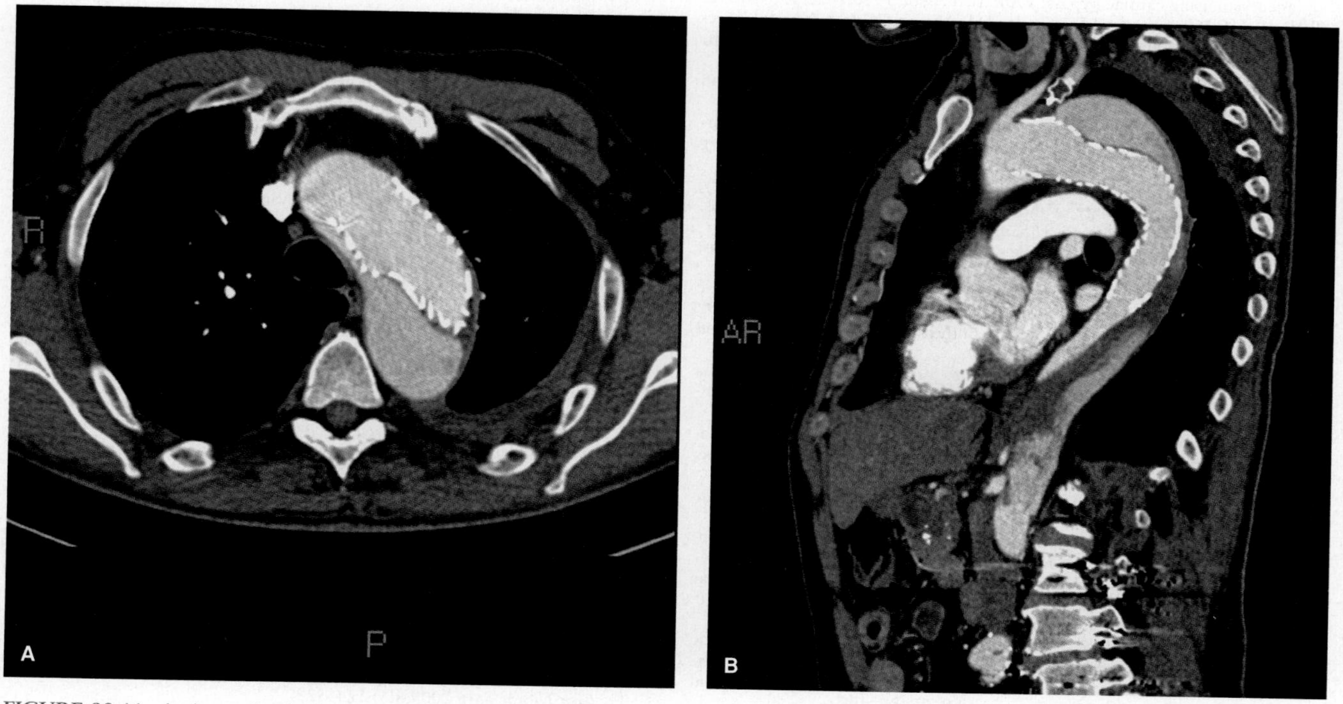

FIGURE 98.11. **A:** A proximal type I endoleak in a different patient following endovascular repair of a type B dissection. **B:** CT reconstruction demonstrates proximal type I endoleak and distal filling of the false lumen via fenestrations below the stent graft.

more than 25% whereas 7% have late endoleaks necessitating repeat procedures (Fig. 98.11). The less common complications include component separation, migration, and endograft infection.[52] Studies are still going on as to the comparative durability of the various types of endografts being used for the endovascular repair of the TAA.

CONCLUSIONS

Aneurysmal disease of the thoracic aorta has a high morbidity and mortality. Treatment of these patients requires careful preoperative planning, meticulous protection of the viscera and spinal cord, and rigorous follow-up. Endovascular therapy has become the preferred technique for descending thoracic aortic disease and offers patients less morbidity than that associated with open surgical treatment. Hybrid procedures allow the use of endovascular therapies beyond their usual anatomic limitations. The best outcomes for all patients who suffer from aneurysmal disease of the thoracic aorta are provided by a multidisciplinary approach with a firm understanding of the pathogenesis and natural history of this disease.

References

1. Kampmeier RH. Saccular aneurysms of the thoracic aorta: a clinical study of 635 cases. *Ann Intern Med* 1938;12:624.
2. Westaby S, Cecil B. Surgery of the thoracic aorta. In: Westaby S. *Landmarks in Cardiac Surgery*. Oxford, UK: Isis Medical Media; 1997: 223.
3. Swan H, Maaske C, Johnson M, Grover R. Arterial homografts: II. Resection of thoracic aortic aneurysm using a stored human arterial transplant. *AMA Arch Surg* 1950;61:732–737.
4. Lam CR, Aram HH. Resection of the descending thoracic aorta for aneurysm; a report of the use of a homograft in a case and an experimental study. *Ann Surg* 1951;134:743–752.
5. Cooley DA, De Bakey ME. Surgical considerations of intrathoracic aneurysms of the aorta and great vessels. *Ann Surg* 1952;135:660–680.
6. Dubost C, Allary M, Oeconomos N. Resection of an aneurysm of the abdominal aorta: reestablishment of the continuity by a preserved human arterial graft, with result after five months. *AMA Arch Surg* 1952;64:405–408.
7. HeldenN RA, Kirklin JW, Gifford RW Jr. The treatment of abdominal aortic aneurysms by excision and grafting. *Proc Staff Meet Mayo Clin* 1953; 28:707–713.
8. Cooley DA, De Bakey ME. Resection of entire ascending aorta in fusiform aneurysm using cardiac bypass. *J Am Med Assoc* 1956;162:1158–1159.
9. De Bakey ME, Crawford ES, Cooley DA, Morris GC Jr. Successful resection of fusiform aneurysm of aortic arch with replacement by homograft. *Surg Gynecol Obstet* 1957;105:657–664.
10. Deterling RA Jr, Bhonslay SB. An evaluation of synthetic materials and fabrics suitable for blood vessel replacement. *Surgery* 1955;38:71–91.
11. Svensjo S, Bengtsson H, Bergqvist D. Thoracic and thoracoabdominal aortic aneurysm and dissection: an investigation based on autopsy. *Br J Surg* 1996;83:68–71.
12. Coady MA, Rizzo JA, Goldstein LJ, Elefteriades JA. Natural history, pathogenesis, and etiology of thoracic aortic aneurysms and dissections. *Cardiol Clin* 1999;17(4):615–635, vii.
13. Bickerstaff LK, Pairolero PC, Hollier LH, et al. Thoracic aortic aneurysms: a population-based study. *Surgery* 1982;92:1103–1108.
14. Clouse WD, Hallett JW Jr, Schaff HV, et al. Improved prognosis of thoracic aortic aneurysms: a population-based study. *JAMA* 1998;280:1926–1929.
15. Kouchoukos NT, Dougenis D. Surgery of the thoracic aorta. *N Engl J Med* 1997;336:1876–1888.
16. Song HK, Bavaria JE, Kindem MW, et al. Surgical treatment of patients enrolled in the national registry of genetically triggered thoracic aortic conditions. *Ann Thorac Surg* 2009;88:781–787.
17. Guo DC, Papke CL, Tran-fadulu V, et al. Mutations in smooth muscle alpha-actin (ACTA2) cause coronary artery disease, stroke, and Moyamoya disease, along with thoracic aortic disease. *Am J Hum Genet* 2009;84:617–627.
18. Williams JS, Graff JA, et al. Aortic injury in vehicular trauma. *Ann Thorac Surg* 1994;57:726–730.
19. Razzouk AJ, Gundry SR, Wang N, et al. Repair of traumatic aortic rupture: a 25-year experience. *Arch Surg* 2000;135:913–918.
20. Ehrlich MP, Rousseau H, Heijman R, et al. Early outcome of endovascular treatment of acute traumatic aortic injuries: the talent thoracic retrospective registry. *Ann Thorac Surg* 2009;88:1258–1263.
21. Nguyen BT. Computed tomography diagnosis of thoracic aortic aneurysms. *Semin Roentgenol* 2001;36:309–324.
22. Pressler V, McNamara JJ. Thoracic aortic aneurysm: natural history and treatment. *J Thorac Cardiovasc Surg* 1980;79:489–498.
23. Perko MJ, Norgaard M, et al. Unoperated aortic aneurysm: a survey of 170 patients. *Ann Thorac Surg* 1995;59:1204–1209.
24. Griepp RB, Ergin MA, Galla JD, et al. Natural history of descending thoracic and thoracoabdominal aneurysms. *Ann Thorac Surg* 1999;67:1927–1930.
25. Elefteriades JA, Botta DM Jr. Indications for the treatment of thoracic aortic aneurysms. *Surg Clin North Am* 2009;89:845–67, ix.
26. Coady MA, Rizzo JA, Elefteriades JA. Developing surgical intervention criteria for thoracic aortic aneurysms. *Cardiol Clin* 1999;17:827–839.
27. Davies RR, Goldstein LJ, Coady MA, et al. Yearly rupture or dissection rates for thoracic aortic aneurysms: simple prediction based on size. *Ann Thorac Surg* 2002;73:17–27.
28. Coady MA, Rizzo JA, Hammond GL, et al. What is the appropriate size criterion for resection of thoracic aortic aneurysms? *J Thorac Cardiovasc Surg* 1997;113:476–491.
29. Di Eusanio M, Schepens MA, Morshuis WJ, et al. Brain protection using antegrade selective cerebral perfusion: a multicenter study. *Ann Thorac Surg* 2003;76:1181–1188.
30. Adams JD, Angle JF, Matsumoto AH, et al. Endovascular repair of the thoracic aorta in the post-FDA approval era. *J Thorac Cardiovasc Surg* 2009;137:117–123.
31. Strauch JT, Spielvogel D, Lauten A, et al. Technical advances in total aortic arch replacement. *Ann Thorac Surg* 2004;77:581–589.
32. Spielvogel D, Mathur MN, Lansman SL, Griepp RB. Aortic arch reconstruction using a trifurcated graft. *Ann Thorac Surg* 2003;75:1034–1036.
33. Gharagozloo F, Neville RF Jr, Cox JL. Spinal cord protection during surgical procedures on the descending thoracic and thoracoabdominal aorta: a critical overview. *Semin Thorac Cardiovasc Surg* 1998;10:73–86.
34. Rokkas CK, Kouchoukos NT. Profound hypothermia for spinal cord protection in operations on the descending thoracic and thoracoabdominal aorta. *Semin Thorac Cardiovasc Surg* 1998;10:57–60.
35. Kouchoukos NT, Daily BB, Rokkas CK, et al. Hypothermic bypass and circulatory arrest for operations on the descending thoracic and thoracoabdominal aorta. *Ann Thorac Surg* 1995;60:67–76.
36. Kouchoukos NT, Rokkas CK. Hypothermic cardiopulmonary bypass for spinal cord protection: rationale and clinical results. *Ann Thorac Surg* 1999;67:1940–1942.
37. Kouchoukos NT, Masetti P, Rokkas CK, Murphy SF. Hypothermic cardiopulmonary bypass and circulatory arrest for operations on the descending thoracic and thoracoabdominal aorta. *Ann Thorac Surg* 2002;74: S1885–S1887.
38. Coselli JS, LeMaire SA, Conklin LD, Adams GJ. Left heart bypass during descending thoracic aortic aneurysm repair does not reduce the incidence of paraplegia. *Ann Thorac Surg* 2004;77:1298–1303.
39. Coady MA, Mitchell RS. Femoro-femoral partial bypass in the treatment of thoracoabdominal aneurysms. *Semin Thorac Cardiovasc Surg* 2003;15: 340–344.
40. Kawachi Y, Nakashima A, Kosuga T, et al. Comparative study of the natural history and operative outcome in patients 75 years and older with thoracic aortic aneurysm. *Circ J* 2003;67:592–596.
41. Dake MD, Miller DC, Semba CP, et al. Transluminal placement of endovascular stent-grafts for the treatment of descending thoracic aortic aneurysms. *N Engl J Med* 1994;331:1729–1734.
42. Mitchell RS, Miller DC, Dake MD, et al. Thoracic aortic aneurysm repair with an endovascular stent graft: the "first generation." *Ann Thorac Surg* 1999;67:1971–1974.
43. Veith FJ, Lachat M, Mayer D, et al. Collected world and single center experience with endovascular treatment of ruptured abdominal aortic aneurysms. *Ann Surg* 2009;250:818–824.
44. Ehrlich M, Grabenwoeger M, Cartes-Zumelzu F, et al. Endovascular stent graft repair for aneurysms on the descending thoracic aorta. *Ann Thorac Surg* 1998;66:19–24.
45. Dillavou ED, Makaroun MS. Predictors of morbidity and mortality with endovascular and open thoracic aneurysm repair. *J Vasc Surg* 2008;48: 1114–1119.
46. Makaroun MS, Dillavou ED, Wheatley GH, et al. Five-year results of endovascular treatment with the Gore TAG device compared with open repair of thoracic aortic aneurysms. *J Vasc Surg* 2008;47:912–918.
47. Chaer RA, Makaroun MS. Late failure after endovascular repair of descending thoracic aneurysms. *Semin Vasc Surg* 2009;22:81–86.
48. Hagl C, Galla JD, Spielvogel D, et al. Diabetes and evidence of atherosclerosis are major risk factors for adverse outcome after elective thoracic aortic surgery. *J Thorac Cardiovasc Surg* 2003;126:1005–1012.
49. Svensson LG, Crawford ES, Hess KR, et al. Variables predictive of outcome in 832 patients undergoing repairs of the descending thoracic aorta. *Chest* 1993;104:1248–1253.
50. Cameron DE, Alejo DE, Patel ND, et al. Aortic root replacement in 372 Marfan patients: evolution of operative repair over 30 years. *Ann Thorac Surg* 2009;87:1344–1349.
51. Estrera AL, Rubenstein FS, Miller CC 3rd, et al. Descending thoracic aortic aneurysm: surgical approach and treatment using the adjuncts cerebrospinal fluid drainage and distal aortic perfusion. *Ann Thorac Surg* 2001;72:481–486.
52. Eagleton MJ, Greenberg RK. Late complications after endovascular thoracoabdominal aneurysm repair. *Semin Vasc Surg* 2009;22:87–92.
53. Almeida RM, Leal JC, et al.Thoracic endovascular aortic repair-a Brazilian experience in 255 patients over a period of 112 months. *Interact Cardiovasc Thorac Surg* 2009;8(5):524–528.

CHAPTER 99 ■ THORACOABDOMINAL AORTIC ANEURYSMS

HAZIM J. SAFI, ANTHONY L. ESTRERA, CHARLES C. MILLER III, ALI AZIZZADEH, AND DIANNA MILEWICZ

KEY POINTS

1. Remarkable progress has been made in the surgical treatment of thoracoabdominal aortic aneurysms.
2. The decline in mortality and complication rates can be attributed to improvements in perioperative care and in surgical technique, particularly the adoption of adjunct distal aortic perfusion and cerebrospinal fluid drainage.
3. Neurologic deficit is no longer a major threat to patients, because the use of adjuncts has lowered the incidence for all thoracoabdominal aortic aneurysms to less than 2.5%.
4. Research needs to be continued that focuses on improving organ preservation, particularly for the most troublesome extent II thoracoabdominal aortic aneurysm.

Etheredge reported the first successful repair of a thoracoabdominal aortic aneurysm (TAAA) using a homograft tube in 1955.[1] A year later, DeBakey used a Dacron tube graft to replace the descending thoracic aorta and infrarenal abdominal aorta.[2] Subsequently, Crawford introduced what became known as the *clamp-and-go technique,* encompassing three basic principles of aortic surgery: the inclusion technique, use of a Dacron tube graft conduit, and reimplantation of visceral and renal arteries.[3] Initially, the operation to repair TAAA had to be performed with haste, to avoid extended periods of
1 organ ischemia. TAAA surgery has since been transformed with the use of adjuncts that provide better organ protection and result in improved outcome; however, sudden fatal rupture of a TAAA remains a looming and unpredictable threat. Although emergency repair of ruptured TAAA can save lives, the associated morbidity and mortality remain extremely high. Elective surgical repair of TAAA is the only effective treatment for eradicating the risk of aneurysm rupture and improving patient survival (Fig. 99.1). This chapter provides a comprehensive approach to the diagnosis and management of TAAA, as well as insight into the recent surgical results and advances in organ protection.

EPIDEMIOLOGY

Abdominal aortic aneurysm remains a major cause of death in the United States. Improved imaging techniques, increasing mean age of the population, and overall heightened awareness all contribute to an apparent increase in the prevalence of aortic aneurysms. However, the incidence of TAAA from population studies of thoracic or abdominal aortic aneurysms can only be inferred. Infrarenal abdominal aortic aneurysms occur three to seven times more frequently than thoracic aortic aneurysms, as fewer than 1,000 TAAAs are repaired annually, compared with approximately 50,000 infrarenal abdominal aortic aneurysms. The estimated prevalence of abdominal aortic aneurysms varies between 2.3% and 10.7% depending on the population studied and the size used to define an aneurysm.[4–6] The incidence of TAAAs is estimated to be 10.4 cases per 100,000 person-years.[7] The mean age of patients with a TAAA is between 59 and 69 years, with a male-to-female predominance of between 2 and 4 to 1.[8]

Fewer than 40% of patients with untreated large TAAAs survive beyond 5 years, with most deaths caused by rupture.[3,8–10] TAAA studies have shown that rupture is more likely to occur when aneurysms exceed 5 cm in diameter and that the rate of rupture rises with increasing aneurysm size.[9,11–14] The median size at which TAAAs rupture is around 7 cm.[15,16] Aneurysms equal to or greater than 8 cm have an 80% risk of rupture within 1 year of diagnosis.[17] The lifetime probability of rupture for any untreated aortic aneurysm is 75% to 80%, but the size at which the aneurysm will rupture and how long it will take to reach that point cannot be easily calculated. However, the average overall rate of growth for TAAAs is 0.10 to 0.42 cm per year with an exponential growth rate for aneurysms exceeding 5 cm in diameter.[11,16,18–20]

PATHOGENESIS

An aortic aneurysm is defined as a localized or diffuse dilatation that exceeds 50% of normal aortic diameter. Most TAAAs are degenerative, with an underlying pathology similar to the more frequently encountered infrarenal abdominal aortic aneurysm. Arteriosclerosis has long been implicated in the development of aortic aneurysm; however, arteriosclerosis primarily affects the intima and typically causes occlusive disease, whereas aneurysm disease usually involves the media and adventitia. Although the pathogenesis of arteriosclerotic occlusive disease and that of aneurysm disease have been shown to be distinct, the two conditions commonly occur together. Histologically, degenerative aortic aneurysms are characterized by thinning of the media with destruction of smooth muscle cells and elastin, infiltration of inflammatory cells, and neovascularization.[21–23] A chronic inflammatory infiltrate, composed of macrophages as well as T and B lymphocytes, is consistently observed in the outer layer of the aneurysm wall. The degree of vessel wall inflammation varies and the stimulus for cell migration remains unclear. These inflammatory cells, particularly macrophages, secrete proteases and elastases that can degrade the aortic wall; in turn, elastin degradation products may act as chemotactic agents for the influx of inflammatory cells.[21] The role of matrix metalloproteinases (MMPs), the most prominent type of elastases, in the development of aortic aneurysms has emerged from both clinical and experimental studies. Increased elastases MMP-2, MMP-9, and MMP-12 have been found in aneurysmal aortic tissue.[21,24–26]

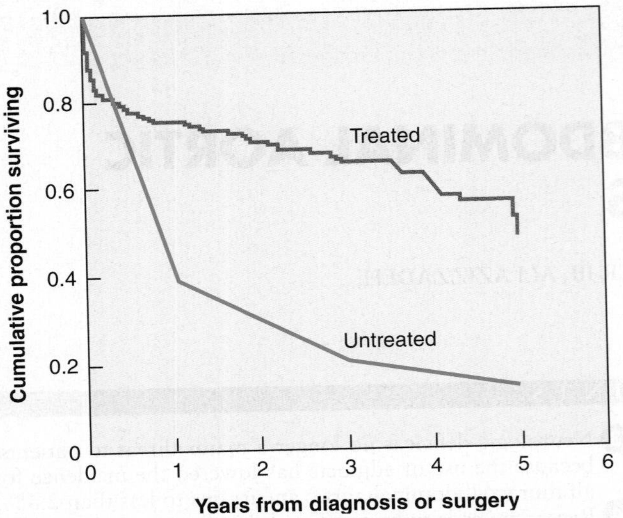

FIGURE 99.1. Thoracoabdominal aortic aneurysm: comparison of survival rates in untreated patients versus surgically treated patients.

Many TAAAs result from chronic ascending and descending aortic dissections. Familial clustering of aortic dissections is evident because up to 20% of patients with ascending thoracic aortic aneurysms that predispose to aortic dissections have one or more first-degree relatives with the same affliction.[27–29] Marfan syndrome, characterized by skeletal, ocular, and cardiovascular abnormalities, is the most common inherited connective tissue disorder related to aortic aneurysm and dissection. Marfan syndrome occurs at a frequency of 1 in 5,000 to 10,000 worldwide. Aortic dilatation observed in Marfan patients has been linked to mutations in fibrillin-1 protein, encoded by the *FBN1* gene. Other known genetic syndromes that predispose individuals to TAAA and dissection include Loeys-Dietz syndrome, Ehlers-Danlos syndrome, Turner syndrome, and polycystic kidney disease.[30–33] In addition, families with multiple members who have thoracic aortic aneurysms and dissections have been reported in the literature.[34] In most of these families, the phenotype for TAAA and dissection is inherited in an autosomal dominant manner with marked variability in the age at onset of aortic disease and decreased penetrance.[34] Four genes have been identified for familial thoracic aortic aneurysms and dissections that account for 20% of this family condition. Mutations in the smooth muscle isoform of α-actin, encoded by *ACTA2*, are responsible for 15% of familial aortic disease. Other genes responsible for less than 2% include *MYH11*, *TGFBR2*, and *TGFBR1*.[35–38]

A small percentage of TAAAs are the result of infection (mycotic aneurysms) or trauma (pseudoaneurysms). An infected aneurysm frequently results from bacterial or septic emboli that seed an atherosclerotic aorta. Another mechanism is contiguous spread from empyema or adjacent infected lymph nodes. Although any organism can infect the aortic wall, *Salmonella*, *Haemophilus influenza*, *Staphylococcus*, *Mycobacterium tuberculosis*, and *Treponema pallidum spirochetes* species are the most common.[39,40] Infected aortic aneurysms are usually saccular and thought to be at greater risk for rupture. Chronic traumatic pseudoaneurysm of the aorta related to previously unrecognized traumatic transection is also prone to rupture, and surgical repair is warranted at the time of diagnosis.

Approximately 25% of TAAAs are associated with chronic aortic dissection. An estimated 20% to 40% of patients will develop aneurysms in the thoracoabdominal aorta within 2 to 5 years following acute aortic dissection.[41–43] Persistent patency of the false aortic lumen is reported to be a significant predictor of aneurysm formation.[42,44] However, the presence of chronic aortic dissection or patent false lumen has not been linked to a higher risk of aortic rupture.[45] Aneurysmal disease occurs in more than one part of the aorta in approximately 20% of cases. The so-called "mega" aorta is an "extensive" aortic aneurysm involving the ascending, transverse arch, and entire thoracoabdominal aorta. Although associated factors include Marfan syndrome and chronic aortic dissection, the cause of extensive aortic aneurysm remains unknown.

CLINICAL MANIFESTATIONS

Aortic aneurysms can cause compressive symptoms, although most do not until they reach a large size. The most frequent complaint is ill-defined chronic back pain, although pain can also occur in the chest, flank or epigastrium. Acute changes in the characteristics and severity of pain can indicate sudden expansion or impending aortic rupture. Hoarseness, resulting from vocal cord paralysis caused by compression of the left recurrent laryngeal or vagus nerves, is frequently seen in patients with large aneurysms of the proximal descending thoracic aorta. Patients may also experience dyspnea related to compression of the tracheobronchial tree. A large aneurysm can exert pressure on the adjacent esophagus or duodenum, causing dysphagia or weight loss related to obstruction or early satiety. Direct erosion of the aneurysm into the adjacent tracheobronchial tree, esophagus, or both can cause exsanguination, presenting as massive hemoptysis or hematemesis, respectively. Less frequently, direct erosion can cause slow intermittent blood loss. Rarely, paraplegia or paraparesis can occur in patients with TAAA as a result of acute occlusion of the intercostal or spinal arteries. These findings are usually associated with acute aortic dissection, but can also result from thromboembolization. Although most aneurysms have a varying amount of mural thrombus, distal embolization causing acute mesenteric, renal, or lower extremity ischemia is infrequent.

Rupture is thought to be the first clinical manifestation of a TAAA in as many as 10% to 20% of patients. Figure 99.2 shows a CT scan of a ruptured TAAA. Note stranding in the retroperitoneum, denoting extravasation of blood. The acute onset of severe chest, abdominal, or back pain associated with

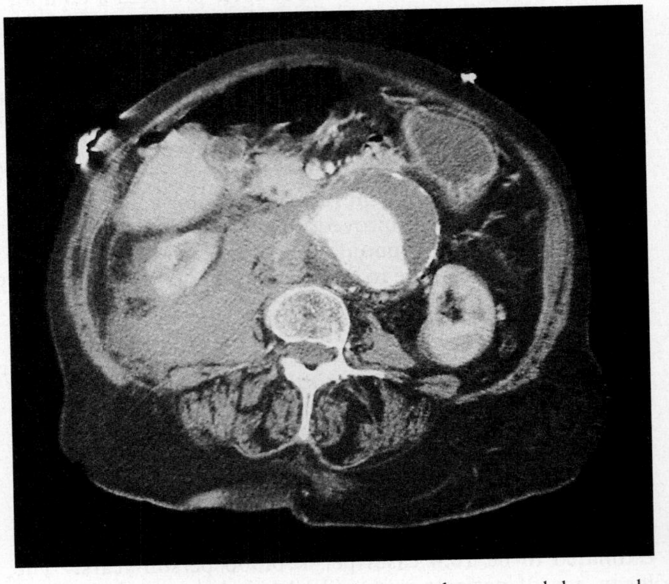

FIGURE 99.2. Computed tomography scan of a ruptured thoracoabdominal aortic aneurysm. Note stranding in the retroperitoneum denoting extravasation of blood.

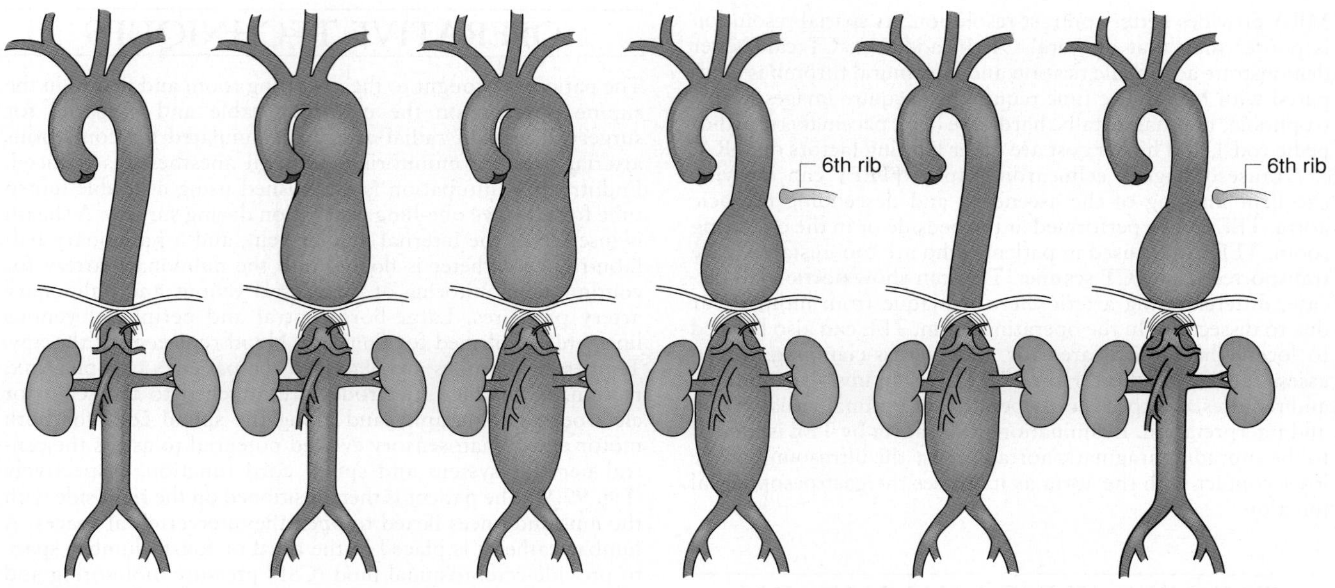

FIGURE 99.3. Thoracoabdominal aortic aneurysm classification. Extent I, distal to the left subclavian artery to above the renal arteries. Extent II, distal to the left subclavian artery to below the renal arteries. Extent III, from the sixth intercostal space to below the renal arteries. Extent IV, from the 12th intercostal space to the iliac bifurcation (total abdominal aortic aneurysm). Extent V, below the sixth intercostal space to just above the renal arteries.

hypotension must raise the suspicion of a ruptured aneurysm. A pulsatile mass may be palpable in the abdomen; however, if the larger part of the TAAA is positioned deep within the thoracic cage, the aneurysm may not be apparent on physical examination. Although most ruptured aneurysms are fatal unless treated emergently, the ruptured arterial wall may temporarily seal for several hours or days before free rupture. In patients who are brought to the hospital alive, rupture is usually contained within the pleura or retroperitoneum. Free rupture is accompanied by severe hypotension and patients are more likely to die before reaching the hospital.

DIAGNOSTIC IMAGING

The diagnosis of TAAA can be confirmed by various imaging modalities. Currently, computed tomography angiography (CTA) is the imaging modality of choice in defining the extent of TAAA per the modified Crawford classification (Fig. 99.3) and for planning operative strategy. The diameter of the entire aorta, from the ascending segment to the bifurcation, can be accurately measured at various levels on axial images. The distinction between the false and true lumens in aortic dissection can be shown on CTA images. CTA can also detect thrombus or inflammatory changes in the aortic wall. Furthermore, the presence of free (or contained) fluid or blood can indicate free (or contained) rupture. Thin-slice CTA image acquisition can also identify patent intercostal arteries. Coronal reformatting or three-dimensional reconstruction of axial CT images provides additional views of TAAA (Fig. 99.4). Intravenous iodinated contrast can be omitted in patients with impaired renal function because it is not required for simple sizing of TAAA.

Magnetic resonance angiography (MRA) has become widely available and is frequently used as a screening test to detect diseases of the aorta and its branches. The principal advantage of MRA over CTA is that MRA does not require intravenous iodinated contrast and thus can be performed safely in patients with impaired renal function. In addition, MRA avoids the radiation exposure required for CT, especially when serial follow-up examinations are required. Although

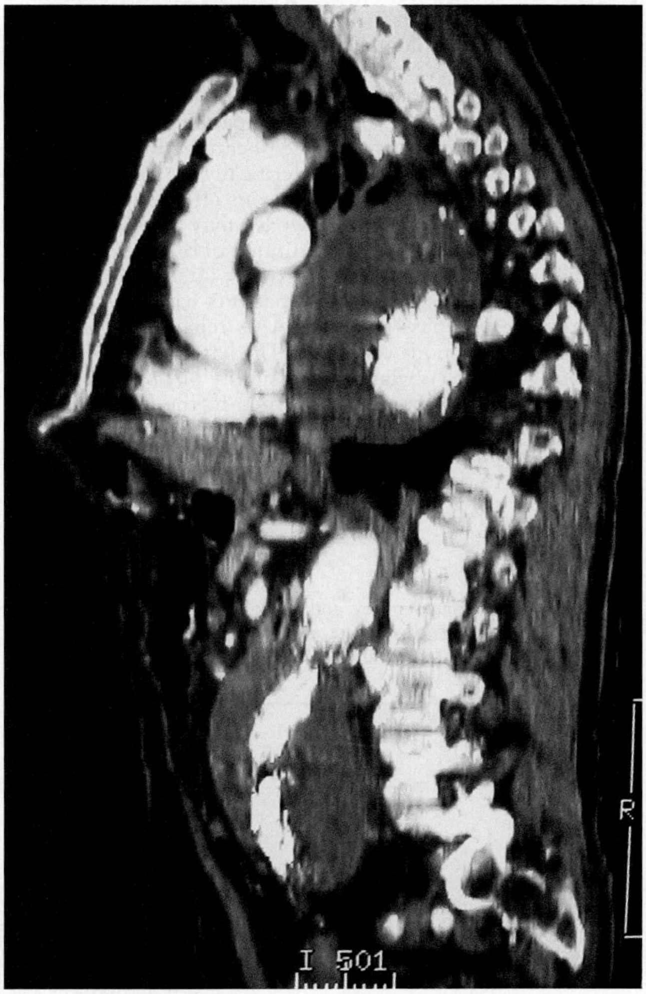

FIGURE 99.4. Sagittal computed tomography image of an extent II thoracoabdominal aortic aneurysm.

MRA provides better contrast resolution, its spatial resolution is poorer than that of spiral CT. In addition, CT can better demonstrate aortic calcification and intramural thrombus compared with MRA. The time required to acquire images, claustrophobia, internal metallic hardware (e.g., pacemakers, orthopedic rods), and higher cost are other limiting factors of MRA.

Transesophageal echocardiography (TEE) can provide excellent imaging of the ascending and descending thoracic aorta. TEE can be performed at the bedside or in the operating room. TEE can be used in patients who are too unstable to be transported to the CT scanner. TEE can show aortic wall disease, differentiating arteriosclerotic plaque from intimal tear due to dissection. In the operating room, TEE can also be used to locate the optimal area for aortic cross-clamping and to assess cardiac function. However, TEE is an invasive modality and requires an experienced operator for optimal visualization and interpretation. Examination of the aorta by TEE is limited to the supradiaphragmatic aorta because the ultrasound probe loses contact with the aorta as it crosses the gastroesophageal junction.

PREOPERATIVE EVALUATION

The initial consultation with the TAAA patient focuses on a thorough history and physical examination, primarily to detect comorbidities because there are generally few symptoms or physical signs related to the aneurysm itself. The extent of the TAAA is determined from imaging studies. Further evaluation of associated risk factors is performed, and consultation with a cardiologist, pulmonologist, or nephrologist is often necessary to aid in the stratification of risks.

Ischemic heart disease is prevalent in this population and is the most common cause of death in patients with a TAAA. TEE provides an excellent estimate of cardiac function. Coronary artery revascularization for critically stenosed coronary artery disease, using either percutaneous intervention (balloon angioplasty or stent) or surgical bypass, may be indicated prior to TAAA surgery, but the risk of rupture of the aneurysm must be weighed against the risk of coronary intervention and the delay caused by intervention. For patients who must undergo coronary artery bypass prior to TAAA repair, the conduit of choice is the saphenous vein graft. The left internal mammary artery is avoided to obviate the possibility of cardiac ischemia should aortic cross-clamping proximal to the left subclavian artery be required during the TAAA repair. Moreover, the internal mammary artery may be an important collateral blood supply to the spinal cord and chest wall.

OPERATIVE TECHNIQUES

The patient is brought to the operating room and placed in the supine position on the operating table and prepared for surgery. The right radial artery is cannulated for continuous arterial pressure monitoring. General anesthesia is induced. Endotracheal intubation is established using a double-lumen tube for selective one-lung ventilation during surgery. A sheath is inserted in the internal jugular vein, and a pulmonary balloon-tipped catheter is floated into the pulmonary artery for continuous monitoring of the central venous and pulmonary artery pressures. Large-bore central and peripheral venous lines are established for fluid and blood replacement therapy. Temperature probes are placed in the patient's nasopharynx, rectum, or bladder. Electrodes are attached to the scalp for electroencephalography and along the spinal cord for both motor and somatosensory evoked potential to assess the central nervous system and spinal cord function, respectively (Fig. 99.5). The patient is then positioned on the right side with the hips and knees flexed to open the intervertebral spaces. A lumbar catheter is placed in the third or fourth lumbar space to provide cerebrospinal fluid (CSF) pressure monitoring and drainage (Fig. 99.6). The CSF pressure is kept at 10 mm Hg or less by gravity drainage of CSF fluid throughout the procedure. The patient is then repositioned in the right lateral decubitus position with the hips slightly turned to allow access to both groins. The operative field is scrubbed using standard aseptic solution and draped.

The incision is tailored to complement the extent of the aneurysm (Fig. 99.7). The full thoracoabdominal incision begins posteriorly between the tip of the scapula and the spinous process, curving along the sixth intercostal space to the costal cartilage, then obliquely to the umbilicus, and finally in the midline to above the symphysis pubis. The latissimus dorsi muscle is divided and the insertion of the serratus anterior muscle is mobilized. The left lung is deflated and the left thoracic cavity is entered. Resection of the sixth rib facilitates exposure and is routinely performed for all TAAAs, except extent IV. Usually, a full thoracoabdominal exploration is necessary for extent II, III, and IV TAAAs. A modified thoracoabdominal incision begins similar to the full thoracoabdominal incision, but ends at the costal cartilage or above the umbilicus. The modified thoracoabdominal incision provides excellent exposure for surgery involving the descending thoracic aorta, extent I TAAA, and extent V TAAA when the aneurysm ends above the superior mesenteric artery. The thoracoabdominal incision is extended to the level of the umbilicus for extent I and V TAAAs that involve the superior mesenteric artery. A self-retaining retractor is

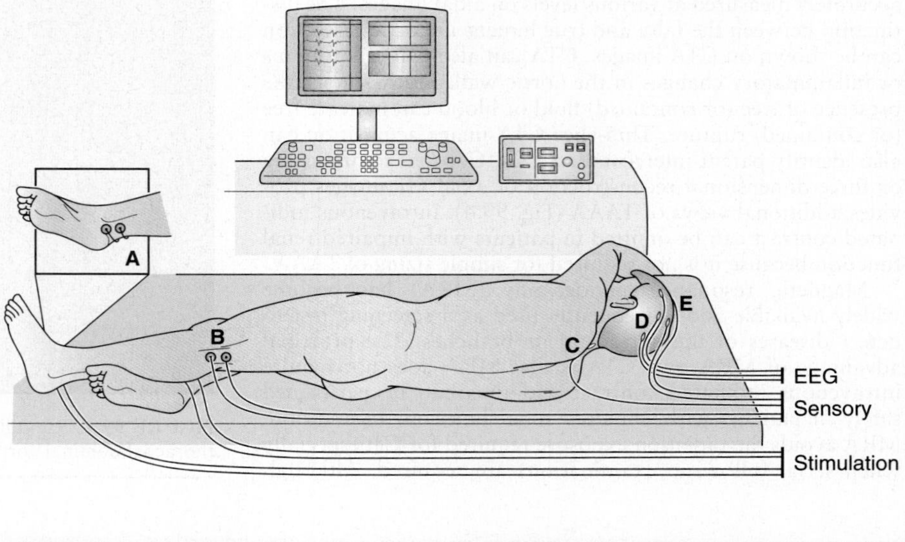

FIGURE 99.5. Somatosensory and motor evoked potentials are recorded at three sites: the popliteal fossa (**A, B**), C5 (**C**), and the vertex (**D**).

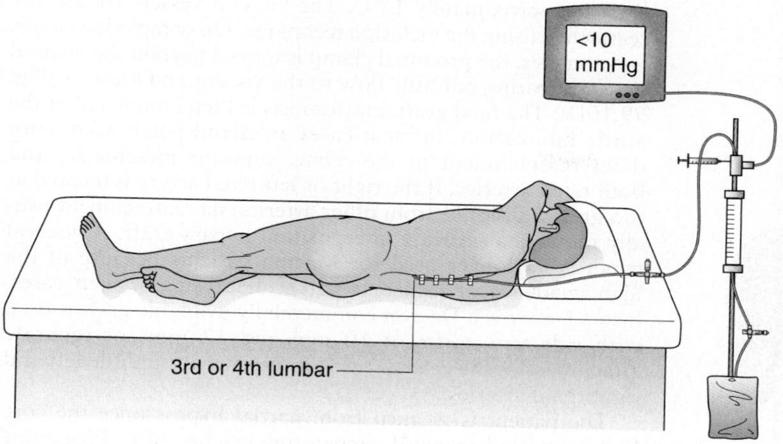

FIGURE 99.6. Placement of the lumbar catheter in the third or fourth lumbar space to provide cerebrospinal fluid drainage and pressure monitoring.

placed firmly on the edges of the incision to maintain full thoracic and abdominal exposure during the procedure.

The dissection begins at the level of the hilum of the lung cephalad to the proximal descending thoracic aorta. The ligamentum arteriosum is identified and transected, taking care to avoid injury to the left recurrent laryngeal nerve. The extent of the distal abdominal aneurysm is assessed. Only the muscular portion of the diaphragm is divided and the left phrenic nerve preserved (Fig. 99.8A, B). A retroperitoneal plane is then developed, mobilizing the spleen, bowel loops, and left kidney to the right side of the abdominal aorta (medial visceral rotation). To prepare for distal aortic perfusion, the patient is anticoagulated using intravenous heparin (1 mg/kg body weight). The pericardium is opened posterior to the left phrenic nerve to allow direct visualization of the pulmonary veins and left atrium. The left atrium is cannulated through the left inferior pulmonary vein or atrial appendage. A centrifugal pump with an in-line heat exchanger is attached to the left atrial cannula and the arterial inflow is established through the left common femoral artery, or the descending thoracic aorta, if the femoral artery is not accessible. Distal aortic perfusion is begun (Fig. 99.9).

Padded clamps are applied onto the proximal descending thoracic aorta just distal to the left subclavian artery and the midthoracic aorta. When the proximal extent of the aneurysm is too close to the left subclavian artery, the aorta between the left common and left subclavian arteries is clamped. The left subclavian artery is clamped separately. Because of the danger of graft–esophageal fistula, the inclusion technique for the proximal anastomosis is no longer used. Instead, the aorta is transected to separate it from the underlying esophagus (Fig. 99.10A). A woven Dacron graft impregnated with collagen or gelatin for replacement is preferred. The graft is sutured in an end-to-end fashion to the descending thoracic aorta, using a running 3–0 or 2–0 monofilament polypropylene suture. The anastomosis is checked for bleeding. Pledgeted polypropylene sutures for reinforcement are placed, if necessary. Sequential clamping is used for all TAAAs. After completion of the proximal anastomosis, the middescending aortic clamp is moved distally onto the abdominal aorta at the celiac axis to accommodate intercostal reattachment. Reattachment of patent, lower intercostal arteries (T8 to T12) is performed routinely, except in cases of occluded arteries, heavily calcified aorta, or acute aortic dissection. After completion of intercostal reattachment, the proximal clamp is released from the aorta and reapplied on the aortic graft beyond the intercostal patch, restoring pulsatile flow to the reattached intercostal arteries (Fig. 99.10B). The distal clamp is moved onto the infrarenal aorta, the abdominal aorta is opened, and the graft is passed through the aortic hiatus. The celiac, superior mesenteric, and renal arteries are identified and perfused using 9- or 12-French balloon-tipped catheters, depending on the size of the ostia (Fig. 99.10C). The delivery of cold perfusate (4°C) to the viscera depends on the proximal aortic pressure, which is maintained between 300 and 600 mL/min. Renal temperature is directly monitored and

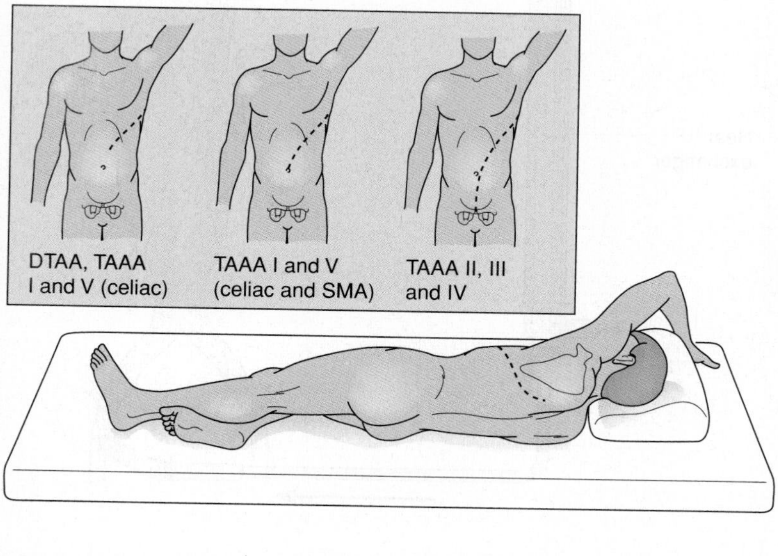

FIGURE 99.7. Tailoring of thoracoabdominal incisions for aneurysm extent. DTAA, descending thoracic aortic aneurysm; SMA, superior mesenteric artery; TAAA, thoracoabdominal aortic aneurysm.

kept at approximately 15°C. The visceral vessels are usually reattached using the inclusion technique. On completion of this anastomosis, the proximal clamp is moved beyond the visceral patch, restoring pulsatile flow to the viscera and kidneys (Fig. 99.10D). The final graft anastomosis is then completed at the aortic bifurcation. In most cases an island patch accommodates reattachment of the celiac, superior mesenteric, and both renal arteries. If the right or left renal artery is located at too great a distance from other arteries, its reattachment usually requires a separate interposition bypass graft. A visceral patch is no longer used for Marfan patients because of the high incidence of recurrent patch aneurysms in such cases. Instead, a woven Dacron commercially available graft is used with side-arm grafts of 10 mm and 12 mm for separate attachment of the celiac, superior mesenteric, and the left and right renal arteries.

The patient is weaned from partial bypass once the core body or nasopharyngeal temperature reaches 36°C. Protamine is administered (1 mg/1 mg heparin), and the atrial and femoral cannulae are removed. Once hemostasis is achieved, two or sometimes three 36-French chest tubes are placed in the pleural cavity for drainage. The diaphragm is reapproximated using running 1–0 polypropylene suture. The left lung is reinflated. Closure of the incision is done in a standard fashion. The patient is placed in the supine position, and a single-lumen endotracheal tube is exchanged for the double-lumen tube. If the vocal cords are swollen, the double-lumen tube is kept in

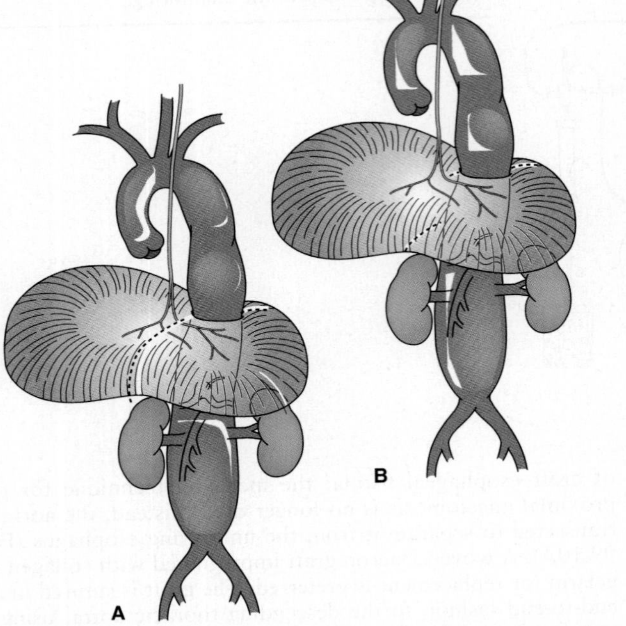

FIGURE 99.8. In previous surgical practice, the diaphragm was divided (A); currently, only the muscular portion of the diaphragm is cut (B).

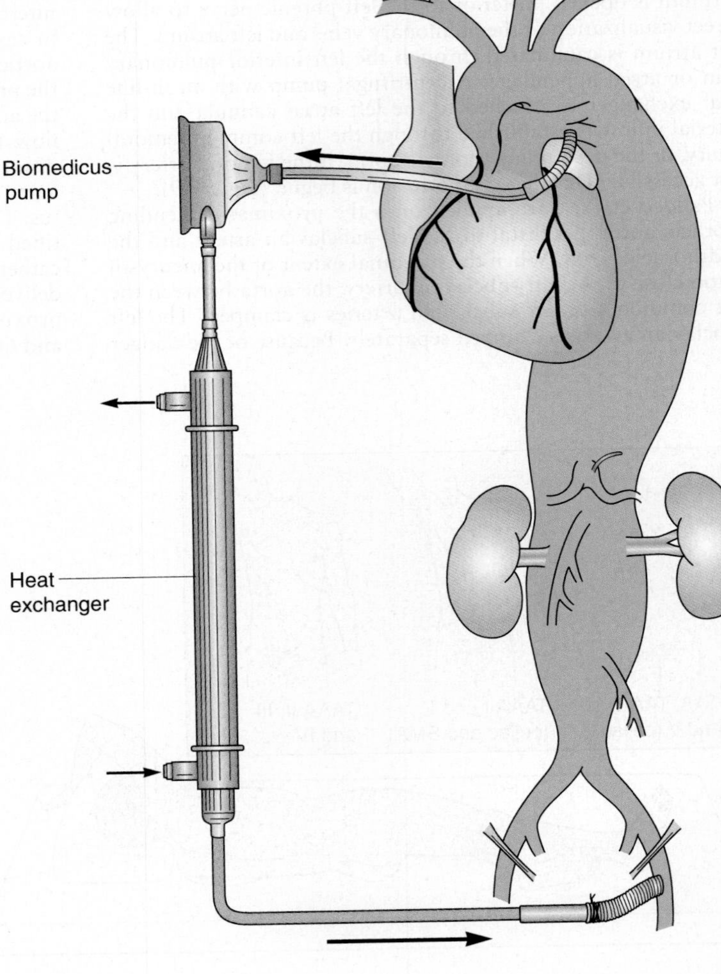

FIGURE 99.9. Distal aortic perfusion from the left inferior pulmonary vein to the left common femoral artery.

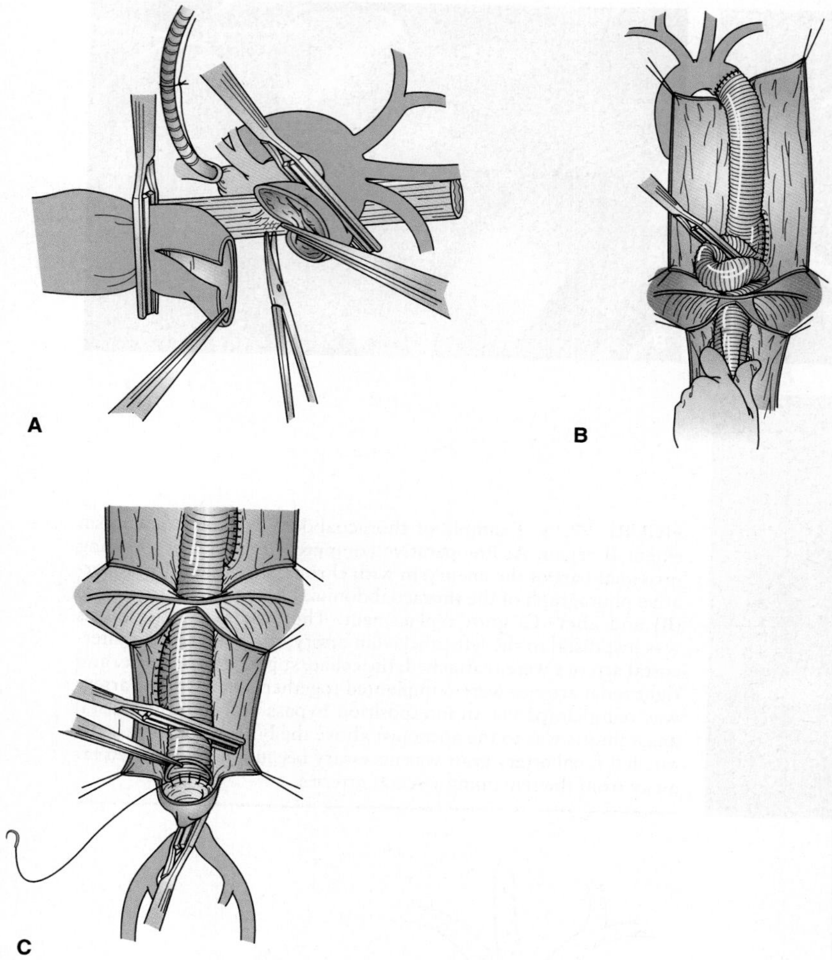

FIGURE 99.10. Sequential clamping and graft replacement. Padded clamps are placed on the proximal and middistal descending thoracic aorta. **A:** The proximal part of the aneurysm is opened. The aortic neck is completely transected and separated from the esophagus. The proximal anastomosis is fashioned. Subsequently, the patent lower intercostal arteries are reattached via an elliptical hole in the graft. **B:** The proximal clamp is then moved onto the graft to restore pulsatile flow to the intercostal arteries, and the graft is pulled through the hiatus into the abdomen. The distal clamp is reapplied onto the infrarenal aorta. The remainder of the aneurysm is opened. Balloon-tipped catheters are inserted into the celiac, superior mesenteric, and renal arteries to permit perfusion. **C:** An elliptical hole is made in the graft for reimplantation of the visceral and renal arteries.

place until the swelling resolves. The patient is then transferred to the intensive care unit (ICU). Figure 99.11 shows an extent II TAAA before and after surgery.

Elephant Trunk Technique for Extensive Aortic Aneurysms

Single-stage repair of extensive aneurysms involving the ascending, arch, and thoracoabdominal aorta greatly increases operative risks. The patient undergoes a lengthy procedure that requires multiple incisions, a daunting array of protective surgical adjuncts, protracted clamp times, and considerable blood loss. Staged repair is a practical solution. Prior to the introduction of the elephant trunk technique by Borst[46] in 1983, staged repair was fraught with complications, particularly excessive bleeding from the pulmonary artery and thoracic aorta in the second-stage repair of the thoracic or thoracoabdominal aorta. The elephant trunk technique resolves this problem because it allows the surgeon to avoid surgical manipulation and cross-clamping the proximal native descending thoracic aorta in the second stage.

The first stage of the elephant trunk technique is performed, in a similar fashion to standard surgery of the ascending aorta and transverse arch, with the exception that either an inverted distal graft or a commercially available collared graft is inserted distally (Fig. 99.12A). The folded edge of the inverted graft or the collared portion of the elephant trunk graft is sutured to the descending thoracic aorta just distal to the left subclavian artery. When the distal anastomosis is completed, the inner portion of the inverted graft is retrieved. A side hole is made in the graft, and the aortic island containing the great vessels is reimplanted. The proximal anastomosis to the ascending aorta is completed, and the distal portion of the graft, or "elephant trunk," is left dangling in the proximal descending aorta. In the first stage, cardiopulmonary bypass, profound hypothermia, circulatory arrest, and retrograde cerebral perfusion provide protection to the brain and guard against stroke.

The second stage of the elephant trunk technique is much like standard TAAA repair, using the adjuncts distal aortic perfusion and CSF drainage. After initiation of the pump, the distal clamp is applied at the middescending thoracic aorta. The proximal third of the descending thoracic aorta is opened without a proximal clamp. The elephant trunk portion of the graft, inserted in the descending thoracic aorta during stage 1, is grasped quickly and clamped (Fig. 99.12B, C). The new graft is sutured to the "elephant trunk" to replace the remaining aneurysm.

POSTOPERATIVE MANAGEMENT

In the ICU, the patient's hemodynamic status is monitored very closely. The patient is awakened as quickly as possible to check neurologic status. However, most patients are kept on mechanical ventilation the first postoperative night. Blood loss is liberally replaced using banked blood products. The patient's mean arterial pressure is maintained between 80 and 90 mm Hg to ensure adequate organ perfusion, particularly to the spinal cord. CSF

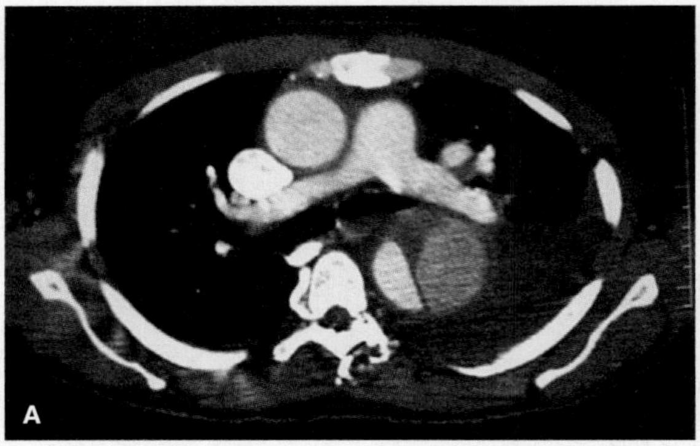

A

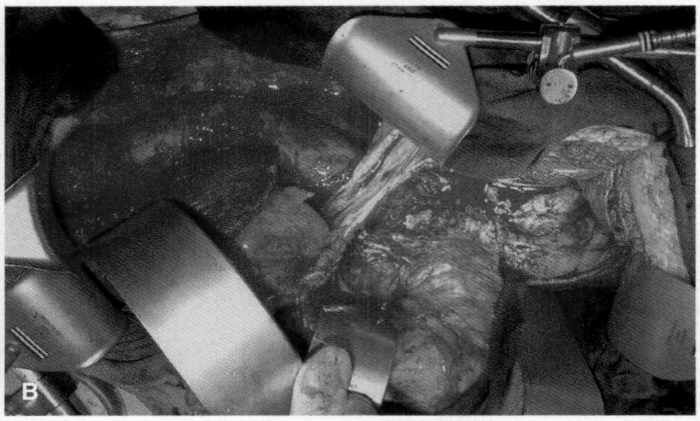

B

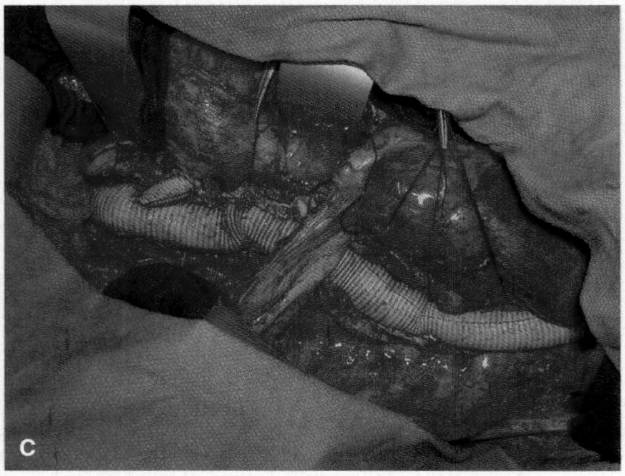

C

FIGURE 99.11. Example of thoracoabdominal aortic aneurysm extent II repair. **A:** Preoperative computed tomography showing proximal part of the aneurysm with chronic dissection. Intraoperative photograph of the thoracoabdominal aortic aneurysm before (**B**) and after (**C**) graft replacement. The proximal anastomosis was just distal to the left subclavian artery; the patent lower intercostal arteries were reattached; the celiac, superior mesenteric, and right renal arteries were reimplanted together; the left renal artery was reimplanted via an interposition bypass graft; and the distal anastomosis was to the aorta just above the bifurcation. The separate left renal artery graft was necessary because it was located far away from the remaining visceral arteries.

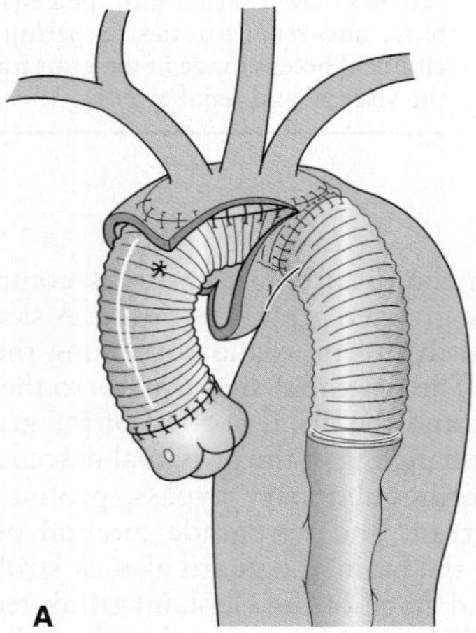

A

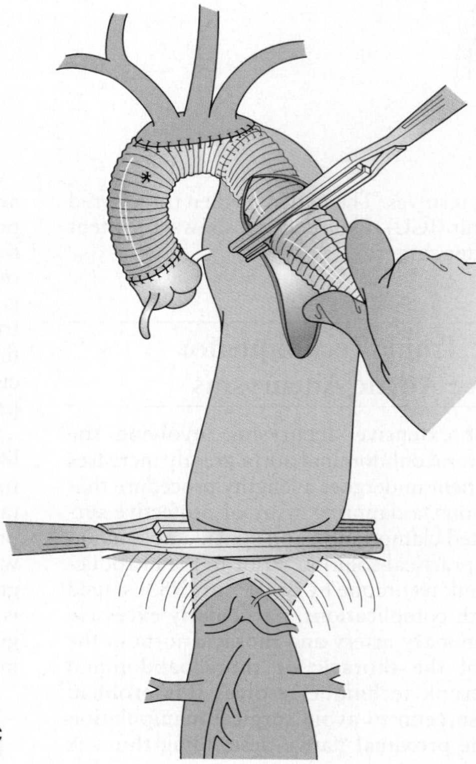

C

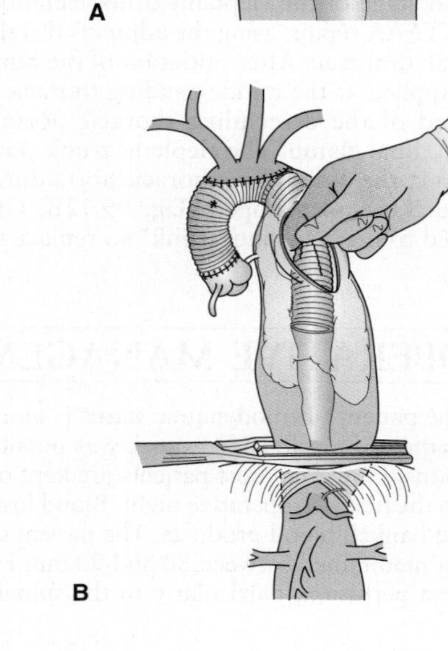

B

FIGURE 99.12. Elephant trunk technique. Illustration of completed stage 1 elephant trunk (**A**). In stage 2, the proximal aneurysm is opened and the existing graft is quickly grasped (**B**) and clamped (**C**). The remainder of the surgery follows the standard technique for thoracoabdominal aortic aneurysm.

pressure is continuously monitored. Approximately 10 to 15 mL of CSF is drained hourly to keep CSF pressure at 10 mm Hg or less. Ideally, the patient is weaned off the ventilator on the first postoperative day. Oral diet is resumed when the patient is extubated and has bowel sounds. If the patient requires longer mechanical ventilation, then a nasoduodenal feeding tube is placed and enteral feeding begins on the second or third postoperative day, when bowel activity returns. Some patients may develop postoperative ileus and require total parenteral nutrition. After the patient recovers from anesthesia and is moving all extremities, potential delayed neurologic deficit is monitored. Warning signs for delayed neurologic deficit are unstable arterial blood pressure, hypoxemia, low hemoglobin (<10 g/dL), or increased CSF pressure (>15 mm Hg). CSF drainage is discontinued on the third postoperative day. The length of stay in the ICU is about 3 or 4 days, depending on the neurologic and pulmonary status of the patient. The patient is subsequently transferred to the telemetry floor. Physical therapy is initiated in the ICU and continued throughout the patient's hospital stay. The median length of stay for patients following TAAA is 15 days.[47] Annual CT scan follow-up is recommended to screen for the development of new aneurysm or graft-related pseudoaneurysm formation. The frequency of follow-up visits or CT scans varies based on TAAA etiology. For example, patients with remaining unoperated aortic dissection, connective tissue disorders (Marfan syndrome), a family history of aortic aneurysm, or concurrent aneurysms may need closer surveillance.

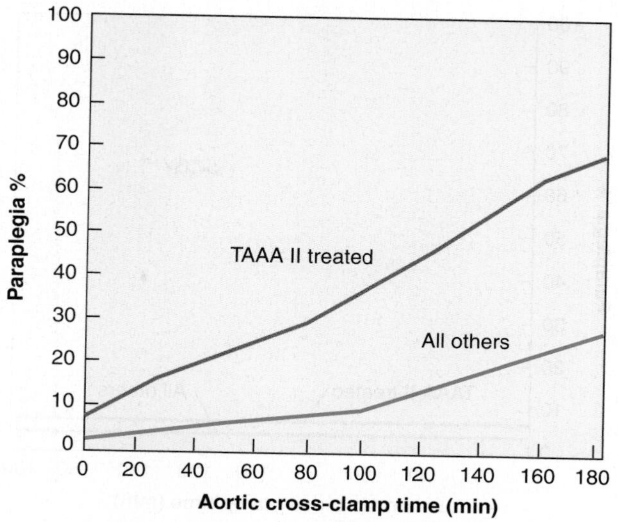

FIGURE 99.13. In extent II aneurysms, the probability of developing neurologic deficits increases with increasing clamp time, but the use of adjunct distal aortic perfusion and cerebrospinal fluid drainage reduces the chances of neurologic deficit by prolonging ischemic tolerance.

SURGICAL OUTCOMES

Mortality rates for patients undergoing TAAA and descending thoracic aortic aneurysm repair range between 4% and 21%.[12,48–50] The variable success rates are partly related to the heterogeneity of the patient population and to the expertise of the treating team. In the cumulative experience of the authors of this chapter (from January 1991 to July 2007), 1,353 patients underwent TAAA and descending thoracic aortic aneurysm repair.[51] Of these patients, 63% were men with a median age of 65 years (range, 8 to 89 years). Approximately 7% of patients had emergency surgery for free or contained rupture of TAAA or descending thoracic aortic aneurysm. Currently, the 30-day mortality rate is approximately 14%, but for patients with normal renal function (i.e., with a calculated glomerular filtration rate >90 mL/min/1.73 m^2), the early mortality was 5%. Using multivariable analysis, advanced age, renal failure, and paraplegia have been identified as important risk factors for mortality.[52] Overall, 70% of patients recover from TAAA without significant postoperative complications.[53] The 5-year survival for patients after TAAA is between 60% and 70%. Recently, negative predictors for long-term survival were found to include advanced age, extent II TAAA, renal failure, emergency surgery, cerebrovascular disease, and active tobacco smoking.[52]

Neurologic Outcome

Postoperative neurologic deficit remains the most devastating complication following TAAA repair. When the descending thoracic aorta is cross-clamped, the spinal cord is quickly rendered ischemic because of the immediate interruption of perfusion to the spinal cord and consequent increased CSF pressure. Therefore, in the "cross-clamp–and–go" era the single most important predictor of neurologic deficit was the length of clamp time. The rationale for the present method of protection is to increase the spinal cord perfusion pressure directly with distal aortic perfusion and indirectly by reducing CSF pressure to 10 mm Hg or less. Animal and human studies have confirmed that CSF drainage reduces CSF pressure and can improve spinal cord perfusion during aortic cross-clamping.[54–56]

From January 1991 to July 2007, we performed repair of the descending thoracic and thoracoabdominal aorta in 1,353 patients.[51] Nine hundred sixty-nine (71%) were male. The adjuncts distal aortic perfusion and CSF drainage with moderate hypothermia were used in 1,025 of 1,353 (76%) patients.

2 In our cumulative experience, the use of combined adjunct distal aortic perfusion and CSF drainage has been associated with a 58% reduction in the risk of neurologic deficit across all aneurysm extents. That is, the overall incidence of neurologic deficit for all patients without the use of adjunct was 5.2%, while it was 2.2% for those with adjunct. While aortic cross-clamp time remains a major predictor of paraplegia when plotted on a continuum, the curve has shifted to the right, with longer ischemic tolerance provided by the adjuncts. In high-risk extent II aneurysms, adjuncts reduced neurologic deficit from 30% to 9% at the average aortic cross-clamp time of 75
3 minutes (Fig. 99.13). When all aneurysm extents are modeled together with nonadjunct cases excluded, use of adjuncts has pushed the rates down to the range of 1% to 5% and vastly increased clamp time tolerance. This combination of results has made the current statistical models insensitive to cross-clamp time, so that although the intercept for extent II aneurysms is greater, the estimates for all extents are flat across clamp time (Fig. 99.14). Clearly, the adoption of adjunct has impacted the overall incidence of neurologic deficit, and this has led us to recategorize "low" versus "high" risk as "extent non-II" versus "extent II."[57]

Since 1991, distal aortic perfusion and CSF drainage have been utilized as adjuncts for all patients undergoing elective repair of TAAA. Overall, in a total of 1,004 patients, immediate postoperative neurologic deficit (paraplegia or paraparesis that occurs as the patient awakens from anesthesia) occurred in 2.4% of patients operated with adjuncts and in 6.8% of patients without adjuncts.[52] This combination of adjuncts has reduced the cumulative rate of neurologic deficits to 0.9% for descending thoracic aortic repair and to 3.3% for thoracoabdominal aortic repair.[52] Repair of the most extensive TAAAs (extent II) has long been known to result in the highest incidence of neurologic deficits. In the cross-clamp–and–go era, this incidence was as high as 30% to 40%.[50] With the use of adjuncts, the rate of immediate neurologic deficits for extent II TAAA has been reduced to 6.6%[52] (Fig. 99.15). In addition to the extent of the aneurysm, other perioperative risk factors for immediate neurologic deficits include age, emergency presentation, renal dysfunction, active smoking, and cerebrovascular

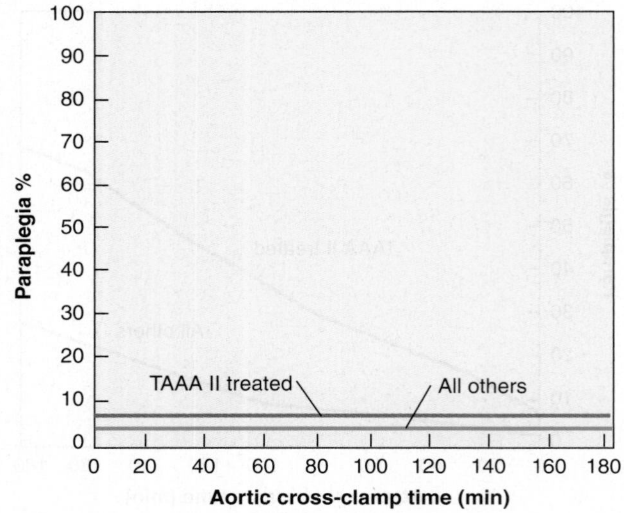

FIGURE 99.14. For thoracoabdominal aortic aneurysms and all other aneurysms, use of adjuncts has made the probability of neurologic deficits low and unrelated to cross-clamp time.

disease. The use of intraoperative distal aortic perfusion and perioperative CSF drainage, in combination, prevents one neurologic deficit in 20 cases for all patients, and one in five for extent II TAAA.[52]

Also important in spinal cord protection is the reimplantation of intercostal arteries. During the era of cross-clamp and go, reimplantation of intercostal arteries was found to be a risk factor for postoperative neurologic deficit.[58] This link was explained by the longer cross-clamp time required to reattach the intercostal arteries. The level at which the anterior radicular artery, known as the *artery of Adamkiewicz* or *arteria radicularis magna,* originates is known to be variable. Most commonly this artery branches from one of the lower intercostal arteries with or without additional collateral branches from nearby intercostal arteries. The anterior radicular artery is believed to be the major blood supply to the anterior spinal artery of the spinal cord. The relationship of neurologic deficit to ligation, reimplantation, and preexisting occlusion of intercostal arteries in patients undergoing TAAA repair using adjuncts has been studied. It was found that ligation of patent lower intercostal arteries (T9 to T12) increased the risk of paraplegia.[58] Therefore, all patent lower intercostal arteries from T9 to T12 are reattached, either together as a patch to a side hole made in the Dacron graft or, when the intercostal arteries are too far apart, separately as buttons or using interposition bypass grafts. However, if the lower intercostal arteries are occluded, the patent upper intercostal arteries will be reimplanted, because these are thought to assume a more important role in the collateral system to the anterior spinal artery in this situation.

Adequate spinal cord perfusion pressure should be maintained with avoidance of hypotension during and after surgery. Intravenous nitroprusside, in particular, can precipitate systemic hypotension, and has been shown to cause a paradoxical increase of CSF pressure.[59] Therefore, it is no longer used. A detailed account of the essential anesthetic care during TAAA
4 repair is beyond the scope of this chapter. However, the importance of adequate maintenance of systemic arterial pressure with judicious blood transfusion cannot be overemphasized, as organ perfusion greatly depends on the systemic circulation. Clearly, the era of cross-clamp and go is over, and the spinal cord must be provided with some form of protection.

Cord function can be assessed using intraoperative neurophysiologic monitoring with motor evoked potentials (MEPs) and somatosensory evoked potentials (SSEPs) as performed routinely in aortic surgery.[60,61] For SSEPs, probes are placed at the malleolus bilaterally, stimulating the posterior tibial nerve. Recordings are performed at three sites (Fig. 99.5), including the popliteal fossa, C5, and the vertex, with a positive finding defined as a drop in amplitude by 50% and/or a change in latency by 10%. For MEPs, precentral gyrus is stimulated and recording is measured at three sites including the abductor digit minimi, tibialis anterior, and abductor hallucis muscle. Compound muscle action potential is monitored, with a positive finding defined as an all-or-none potential. If there are signal changes as defined earlier, intraoperative corrective measures are performed, which include increasing the mean central pressure to over 80 mm Hg, increasing distal aortic perfusion pressure to over 60 mm Hg, lowering the CSF pressure, increasing the hemoglobin level, and attaching additional intercostal arteries.

With the current use of adjunct therapy and intraoperative SSEP and MEP monitoring, the current rate of immediate neurologic deficit remains at 3.1%.[62]

Delayed Neurologic Deficits. Delayed neurologic deficit refers to the onset of paraplegia or paraparesis after a period of observed normal neurologic function. Delayed-onset neurologic deficit after TAAA repair was first reported in 1988, at which time the condition was considered irreversible and beyond the surgeon's control.[63] Since then numerous reports have described improvements in patients' neurologic function by using CSF drainage for delayed-onset neurologic deficits.[64–66] Delayed neurologic deficit has been observed as early as 2 hours and as late as 2 weeks following surgery (median, 3 days) in 2.7% of patients.[67] No single risk factor is responsible for delayed neurologic deficit. However, using multivariable analysis, acute dissection, extent II TAAA, and renal insufficiency were identified as significant preoperative predictors for delayed-onset neurologic deficit.[67] In a subsequent case-control study, postoperative mean arterial pressure of less than 60 mm Hg and CSF drain complications were found to be predictors in the development of delayed-onset neurologic deficit, independent of preoperative predictors[68] (Fig. 99.16).

As improved spinal cord protection during TAAA surgery has reduced the incidence of neurologic complications, delayed-onset neurologic deficit has emerged as an important clinical entity. The exact mechanisms involved in the development of delayed neurologic deficit remain unknown. It is speculated that delayed neurologic deficit after TAAA repair may result from a "second hit" phenomenon. Adjuncts can protect

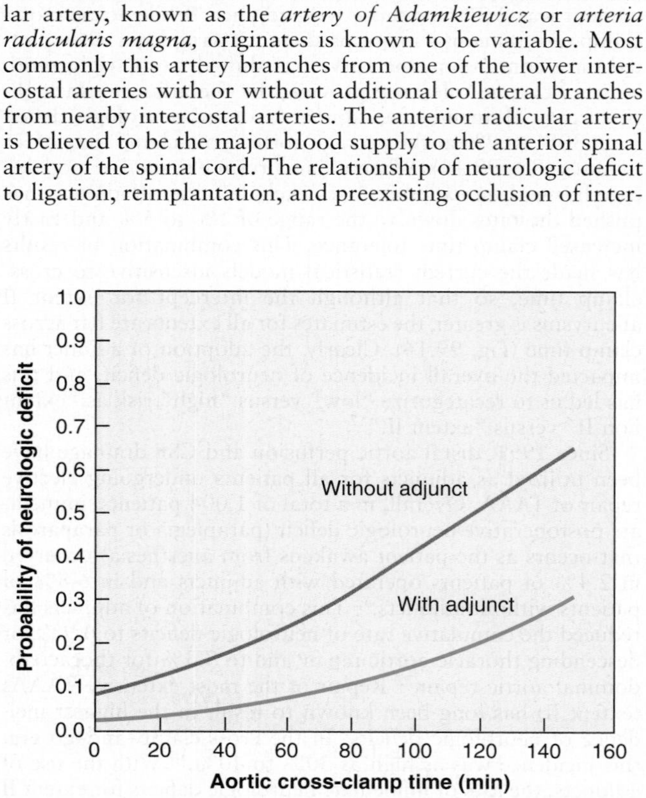

FIGURE 99.15. The probability of neurologic deficit increases with clamp time and is markedly higher in patients undergoing thoracoabdominal aortic aneurysm surgery without adjuncts.

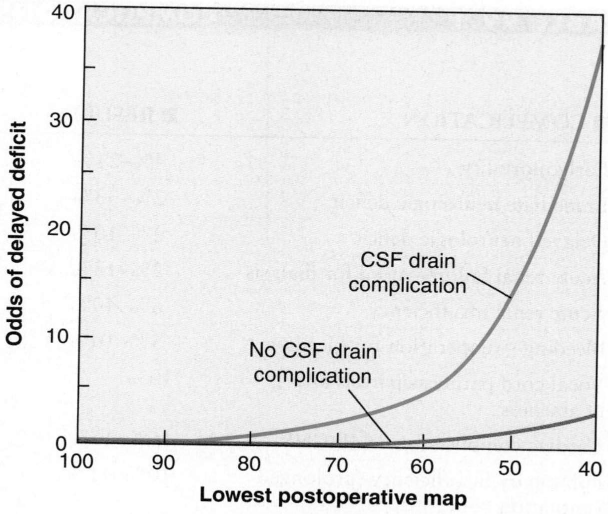

FIGURE 99.16. Odds of delayed neurologic deficit by lowest postoperative mean arterial blood pressure, with or without cerebrospinal fluid drain complication. Odds are referenced to one. For example, a patient with a mean arterial blood pressure of 40 mm Hg and a cerebrospinal fluid (CSF) drain complication would have 40:1 odds of delayed neurologic deficit.

the spinal cord intraoperatively and reduce the incidence of immediate neurologic deficit, but the spinal cord remains vulnerable during the early postoperative period. Additional ischemic insults caused by hemodynamic instability, malfunction of the CSF drainage catheter, or both may constitute a "second hit," causing delayed neurologic deficit. Furthermore, in the rigid, unyielding spinal column, any rise in CSF pressure could lead to an increase in compartment pressure, with consequent decreased spinal cord perfusion. Hence, CSF is drained freely when delayed neurologic deficit develops to relieve the compartment pressure.

To optimize postoperative spinal cord perfusion and oxygen delivery, mean arterial pressure is kept above 90 to 100 mm Hg, hemoglobin above 10 mg/dL, and cardiac index greater than 2.0 L/min. If delayed neurologic deficit occurs, measures to increase spinal cord perfusion are instituted immediately. The patient is placed flat in the supine position. The patency and function of the drain are ascertained at once. If the drain has been removed, the CSF drainage catheter is reinserted immediately and CSF is drained freely until the CSF pressure drops below 10 mm Hg. The systemic arterial pressure is raised, blood transfusion is liberally infused, and oxygen saturation is increased, as indicated earlier. CSF drainage is continued for at least 72 hours for all patients with delayed-onset neurologic deficit. Using this multifaceted approach to treating delayed-onset neurologic deficit, an improvement in neurologic function is seen in 57% of patients.[67] When the CSF drain was still in place at the onset of delayed neurologic deficit, 75% of patients recovered function; 43% recovered neurologic function if the CSF drain had to be reinserted at the time of the delayed neurologic deficit. Patients who developed delayed neurologic deficit but did not have CSF drainage failed to recover function.

Renal Failure. Acute postoperative renal failure is defined as an increase in serum creatinine of 1 mg/dL per day for 2 consecutive days or by the need for hemodialysis. The reported rate of acute renal failure from large series of patients undergoing TAAA repair falls within the range of 5% to 40% and is associated with mortality rates as high as 70%. Patients who develop acute renal failure more frequently sustain nonrenal complications, such as respiratory failure, central nervous system dysfunction, sepsis, and gastrointestinal hemorrhage. For patients who develop postoperative renal failure, early continuous venovenous hemodialysis or daily intermittent hemodialysis is initiated. In the experience of the authors of this chapter, approximately one third of patients who develop acute renal failure remain on hemodialysis, and predictably these patients have a prolonged length of hospital stay. Long-term survival for patients on hemodialysis is dismal. Preoperative chronic renal insufficiency and ruptured aneurysms are known predictors of acute postoperative renal failure. Although the authors of this chapter have theorized that patients with the most extensive extent II TAAA are at highest risk for the development of postoperative renal failure, extent of TAAA has not been shown to be a significant predictor.

The goals of perioperative renal protection are to maintain adequate renal oxygen delivery, reduce renal oxygen utilization, and reduce direct renal tubular injury. However, good strategies to protect renal function during surgical TAAA repair remain elusive. The benefit of cold temperatures for metabolic suppression in organ protection is well known. Local hypothermia has been shown to protect against renal ischemia and reperfusion injury in laboratory animals, and there is some evidence that patients with cold visceral perfusion have superior survival and recovery rates. However, this strategy has not decreased the incidence of acute renal failure. The incidence of postoperative renal failure remains troublesome and the pursuit of an optimal method of renal protection continues to be a top priority.

Glomerular Filtration Rate

Clinically apparent renal insufficiency is a known predictor of 30-day mortality. The overall 30-day mortality was 225 of 1,353 (16%), and the 5-year survival rate was 54%. We are finding increasingly that mortality cannot properly be interpreted without knowledge of preoperative glomerular filtration rate. With normal GFR (>90 mL/min/1.73 m^2), 30-day mortality was 6%, while 5-year survival was 77%. With a decline in GFR to the 65 to 90 range, 30-day mortality was 10.6%. Below a GFR of 65, 30-day mortality increases to 26%. Long-term survival stratified by quartile of GFR is shown in Figure 99.17. The effect of GFR on both short-term mortality and long-term survival was highly statistically significant ($p < 0.0001$ for both measures).

Recently, in patients undergoing TAAA repair without apparent renal disease, we have found that calculated glomerular filtration rate is a much stronger predictor for mortality than serum creatinine.[69] We have used and appraised many different forms of renal protection including distal aortic perfusion, warm blood visceral perfusion, antegrade cold blood visceral perfusion, retrograde cold blood perfusion, and the perioperative use of a renal protective pharmacologic agent, fenoldopam. None of these yielded overly promising results. Using multivariable analyses, we found that preoperative renal failure (creatinine >2.8 g/dL), left renal artery reattachment, visceral perfusion, and the clamp-and-sew technique are predictors of acute renal failure.[57]

In the past, we had used visceral perfusion without cooling or systemic heparin, and this was likely the reason for the negative effect of visceral perfusion on renal protection. We recently reviewed the impact of various adjuncts on renal function. Distal aortic perfusion has emerged as protective but only for aortic repair that does not directly involve the renal arteries. There is evidence, however, that patients treated with cold blood visceral perfusion have superior survival and recovery rates, which may be related to improved liver protection. None of the adjuncts thus far evaluated has clearly prevented acute renal failure. The major predictors of postoperative renal dysfunction remain preoperative renal function, cross-clamp time, and repair extending to the renal arteries.

Excluding patients who had clinically apparent preoperative renal failure, we found that acute renal failure occurred in

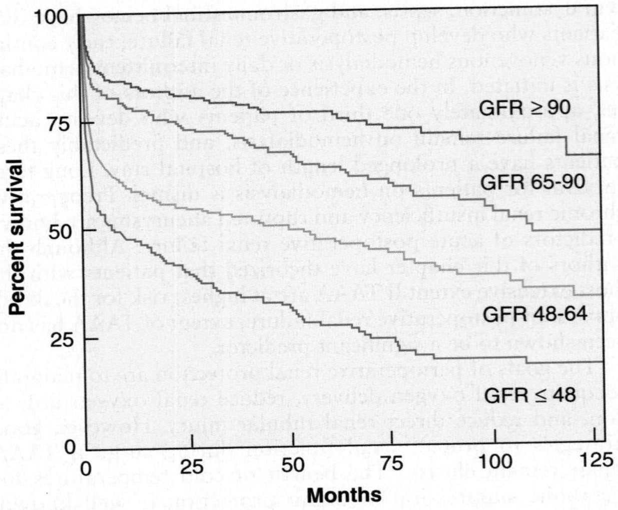

FIGURE 99.17. Long-term survival stratified by quartile of glomerular filtration rate.

344 of 1,261 (27.2%) of our patients overall. For patients with preoperative GFR above 90, renal failure was 62 of 367 (17%). When GFR was between 65 and 90, postoperative renal failure was 70 of 310 (23%). At GFRs below 65, renal failure was 212 of 584 (36%). Thirty-day mortality among patients with acute renal failure was 34% compared to 10% mortality for all other patients. Aneurysms involving the visceral vessels (extents II, III, and IV) were much more likely to produce renal failure postoperatively (39 vs. 17%, $p < 0.0001$). Approximately one third of our patients who developed acute renal failure remained on hemodialysis, and long-term survival for patients on hemodialysis has been dismal.

COMPLICATIONS

A summary of complications is shown in Table 99.1. These figures are compiled from a collection of sources.[70–80]

TABLE 99.1 COMPLICATIONS

■ COMPLICATION	■ RESULTS
Early mortality	4%–21%
Immediate neurologic deficit	2%–33%
Delayed neurologic deficit	2%–10%
Acute renal failure—need for dialysis	2%–13%
Acute renal insufficiency	6%–40%
Bleeding—reoperation for bleeding	5%–10%
Vocal cord paralysis/paresis and hoarseness	10%
Cardiac complication—MI, CHF	5%–15%
Pulmonary insufficiency (prolonged ventilation >48 h)	10%–41%
Stroke or transient ischemic attack (reversible)	2%–6%
Gastrointestinal complications (pancreatitis, ischemic colitis, small bowel, cholecystitis, hepatic insufficiency)	7%–10%
Chylothorax	<1%
Hospital length of stay	10–22 days
Survival	1 y = 60%–80% 5 y = 65%–80% 10 y = 40%

CHF, chronic heart failure; MI, myocardial infarction.

Elephant Trunk Technique

The authors of this chapter have performed the two-staged elephant trunk procedure in nearly 200 patients with extensive aortic aneurysms.[81] Mortality rates range from 5% to 9% after stage one and 6% to 7% for stage two. During the interval between the two stages (approximately 31 days to 6 weeks), mortality has averaged around 6.5%. When a 5-year follow-up of patients who failed to return for second-stage repair was performed, 32% had died. Although we were unable to determine the exact cause of death for many of these patients, it is likely that a significant number of deaths were a result of aneurysm rupture. Major complications for both stages have been relatively low, with stroke rates of 2% in the first stage and no neurologic deficits in the second. Determining the optimum length of recovery time between stages has been difficult. Because these patients are vulnerable to rupture, it is currently recommended that the second-stage repair be performed after a 4- to 6-week period of recovery.

Impact of Aortic Dissection

Aortic dissection has long been considered a risk factor for neurologic deficit in patients undergoing repair of descending thoracic and TAAAs, particularly during the clamp-and-go era.[82–85] However, in a series of 729 patients operated on for descending thoracic aneurysms and TAAAs, no differences were reported in neurologic outcome between patients with and those without chronic dissection; the rate of paraplegia was 3.6% with dissection versus 4.7% without dissection.[86] Several factors are likely responsible for the good neurologic outcome of patients with chronic dissection; they include better surgical techniques and anesthetic care, moderate hypothermia, and reimplantation of intercostal arteries. The key element in the improved spinal cord protection, however, has been the use of the adjuncts distal aortic perfusion and CSF drainage.

In acute aortic dissection, the risk of paraplegia following graft replacement of the descending thoracic or thoracoabdominal aorta remains substantial, with a neurologic deficit rate of 32%.[87] Nevertheless, acute dissection aneurysm patients are usually critically ill, undergoing surgery emergently with little time for preparation. The method of spinal cord protection employed during surgery for acute dissection is often not optimal. In particular, reimplantation of intercostal arteries is ill advised because of the risk of catastrophic bleeding from the friable dissected tissues, and the use of the adjuncts distal aortic perfusion and CSF drainage may not be possible in the presence of hemodynamic instability.

Endovascular Repair

Since the first successful reported thoracic stent graft repair in 1994,[88] endovascular management of thoracic aortic pathology has evolved at a rapid pace. Thus far, three thoracic aortic devices have received Food and Drug Administration (FDA) approval in the United States. These devices, in the order of approval, are the TAG (WL Gore, Flagstaff, AZ), the Talent Thoracic (Medtronic, Santa Rosa, CA), and the TX2 (Cook,

Bloomington, IN). The results of thoracic endovascular aortic repair (TEVAR) performed in the prospective multicenter trials that led to the FDA approval of these three devices compare favorably to open surgical controls.[89–91] Although these devices are approved for the treatment of thoracic aortic aneurysms, their off-label use for other thoracic aortic pathology is common. The use of thoracic devices for treatment of a variety of aortic conditions, including acute and chronic type B aortic dissections, traumatic aortic injury, and pseudoaneurysms, has been reported.[92–94] Although the short-term benefits of endovascular therapy are clear, with less morbidity and mortality compared with conventional surgery, the long-term durability of this treatment strategy remains to be determined.

Endovascular treatment of a TAAA would require revascularization of visceral vessels using branched and/or fenestrated devices. There are currently no FDA-approved branched and/or fenestrated devices for TAAA repair available in the United States. The feasibility of a custom-designed investigational device for endovascular TAAA repair has been reported.[95–97] Although the early results are encouraging, the technology is rapidly evolving and the widespread adoption of a custom-designed device is challenging. Moreover, a recent study showed no significant difference in mortality or spinal cord ischemia between endovascular and open repair.[98]

In addition to complete endovascular TAAA repair, "hybrid" procedures have evolved. These have combined open debranching procedures with subsequent relining of the aorta with stent grafts. The debranching procedures entail an open retroperitoneal or transperitoneal approach for extra-anatomic bypassing of the visceral and renal arteries from either iliac artery. This is subsequently followed by exclusion of the thoracoabdominal aorta with stent grafts. Although this approach is technically feasible, the risk of mortality remains discouragingly high.[99–102] Indications for this approach will likely be limited to patients with TAAA who are unfit for open repair and those who are not candidates for endovascular repair (i.e., those with tortuous vessels, inaccessible vessels, or insufficient time to order a customized stent graft). Although much progress has been made in the endovascular repair of TAAAs, the technology is still in its infancy. The next generation of endografts holds a promising future for patients with TAAAs.

Acknowledgments

The authors of this chapter are grateful to G. Ken Goodrick, editor, and to Chris Akers for assistance with the illustrations. The authors would also like to thank Kourosh Keyhani for his contributions to the chapter.

References

1. Etheredge S, Yee J, Smith J, et al. Successful resection of a large aneurysm of the upper abdominal aorta and replacement with homograft. *Surgery* 1955;38:1071–1081.
2. DeBakey ME, Cooley DA, Crawford ES, et al. Clinical application of a new flexible knitted Dacron arterial substitute. *Arch Surg* 1957;74:713–724.
3. Crawford ES, Crawford JL, Safi HJ, et al. Thoracoabdominal aortic aneurysms: preoperative and intraoperative factors determining immediate and long-term results of operations in 605 patients. *J Vasc Surg* 1986;3:389–404.
4. Bickerstaff LK, Hollier LH, Van Peenen HJ, et al. Abdominal aortic aneurysms: the changing natural history. *J Vasc Surg* 1984;1:6–12.
5. Wanhainen A, Bjorck M, Boman K, et al. Influence of diagnostic criteria on the prevalence of abdominal aortic aneurysm. *J Vasc Surg* 2001;34: 229–235.
6. Wilmink AB, Quick CR. Epidemiology and potential for prevention of abdominal aortic aneurysm. *Br J Surg* 1998;85:155–162.
7. Clouse WD, Hallett JW Jr, Schaff HV, et al. Improved prognosis of thoracic aortic aneurysms: a population-based study. *JAMA* 1998;280:1926–1929.
8. Bickerstaff LK, Pairolero PC, Hollier LH, et al. Thoracic aortic aneurysms: a population-based study. *Surgery* 1982;92:1103–1108.
9. Perko MJ, Norgaard M, Herzog TM, et al. Unoperated aortic aneurysm: a survey of 170 patients. *Ann Thorac Surg* 1995;59:1204–1209.
10. Pressler V, McNamara JJ. Thoracic aortic aneurysm: natural history and treatment. *J Thorac Cardiovasc Surg* 1980;79:489–498.
11. Cambria RA, Gloviczki P, Stanson AW, et al. Outcome and expansion rate of 57 thoracoabdominal aortic aneurysms managed nonoperatively. *Am J Surg* 1995;170:213–217.
12. Elefteriades JA, Hartleroad J, Gusberg RJ, et al. Long-term experience with descending aortic dissection: the complication-specific approach. *Ann Thorac Surg* 1992;53:11–20.
13. Juvonen T, Ergin MA, Galla JD, et al. Prospective study of the natural history of thoracic aortic aneurysms. *Ann Thorac Surg* 1997;63:1533–1545.
14. Lobato AC, Puech-Leao P. Predictive factors for rupture of thoracoabdominal aortic aneurysm. *J Vasc Surg* 1998;27:446–453.
15. Coady MA, Rizzo JA, Hammond GL, et al. Surgical intervention criteria for thoracic aortic aneurysms: a study of growth rates and complications. *Ann Thorac Surg* 1999;67:1922–1926.
16. Davies RR, Goldstein LJ, Coady MA, et al. Yearly rupture or dissection rates for thoracic aortic aneurysms: simple prediction based on size. *Ann Thorac Surg* 2002;73:17–27.
17. Dapunt OE, Galla JD, Sadeghi AM, et al. The natural history of thoracic aortic aneurysms. *J Thorac Cardiovasc Surg* 1994;107:1323–1332.
18. Coady MA, Rizzo JA, Hammond GL, et al. What is the appropriate size criterion for resection of thoracic aortic aneurysms? *J Thorac Cardiovasc Surg* 1997;113:476–491.
19. Masuda Y, Takanashi K, Takasu J, et al. Expansion rate of thoracic aortic aneurysms and influencing factors. *Chest* 1992;102:461–466.
20. Rizzo JA, Coady MA, Elefteriades JA. Procedures for estimating growth rates in thoracic aortic aneurysms. *J Clin Epidemiol* 1998;51:747–754.
21. Ailawadi G, Eliason JL, Upchurch GR Jr. Current concepts in the pathogenesis of abdominal aortic aneurysm. *J Vasc Surg* 2003;38:584–588.
22. Lopez-Candales A, Holmes DR, Liao S, et al. Decreased vascular smooth muscle cell density in medial degeneration of human abdominal aortic aneurysms. *Am J Pathol* 1997;150:993–1007.
23. Pan JH, Lindholt JS, Sukhova GK, et al. Macrophage migration inhibitory factor is associated with aneurysmal expansion. *J Vasc Surg* 2003;37:628–635.
24. Annabi B, Shedid D, Ghosn P, et al. Differential regulation of matrix metalloproteinase activities in abdominal aortic aneurysms. *J Vasc Surg* 2002; 35:539–546.
25. Longo GM, Xiong W, Greiner TC, et al. Matrix metalloproteinases 2 and 9 work in concert to produce aortic aneurysms. *J Clin Invest* 2002;110: 625–632.
26. McMillan WD, Pearce WH. Increased plasma levels of metalloproteinase-9 are associated with abdominal aortic aneurysms. *J Vasc Surg* 1999;29: 122–127.
27. Biddinger A, Rocklin M, Coselli J, et al. Familial thoracic aortic dilatations and dissections: a case control study. *J Vasc Surg* 1997;25:506–511.
28. Coady MA, Davies RR, Roberts M, et al. Familial patterns of thoracic aortic aneurysms. *Arch Surg* 1999;134:361–367.
29. Hasham SN, Willing MC, Guo DC, et al. Mapping a locus for familial thoracic aortic aneurysms and dissections (TAAD2) to 3p24–25. *Circulation* 2003;107:3184–3190.
30. Elsheikh M, Casadei B, Conway GS, et al. Hypertension is a major risk factor for aortic root dilatation in women with Turner's syndrome. *Clin Endocrinol* 2001;54:69–73.
31. Hossack KF, Leddy CL, Johnson AM, et al. Echocardiographic findings in autosomal dominant polycystic kidney disease. *N Engl J Med* 1988;319: 907–912.
32. Pepin M, Schwarze U, Superti-Furga A, et al. Clinical and genetic features of Ehlers-Danlos syndrome type IV, the vascular type. *N Engl J Med* 2000; 342:673–680.
33. Wenstrup RJ, Meyer RA, Lyle JS, et al. Prevalence of aortic root dilation in the Ehlers-Danlos syndrome. *Genet Med* 2002;4:112–117.
34. Milewicz DM, Chen H, Park ES, et al. Reduced penetrance and variable expressivity of familial thoracic aortic aneurysms/dissections. *Am J Cardiol* 1998;82:474–479.
35. Guo DC, Pannu H, Tran-Fadulu V, et al. Mutations in smooth muscle alpha-actin (ACTA2) lead to thoracic aortic aneurysms and dissections. *Nat Genet* 2007;39:1488–1493.
36. Zhu L, Vranckx R, Khau Van Kien P, et al. Mutations in myosin heavy chain 11 cause a syndrome associating thoracic aortic aneurysm/aortic dissection and patent ductus arteriosus. *Nat Genet* 2006;38:343–349.
37. Pannu H, Tran-Fadulu V, Papke C, et al. MYH11 mutations result in a distinct vascular pathology driven by insulin-like growth factor 1 and angiotensin II. *Hum Mol Genet* 2007;16:3453–3462.
38. Pannu H, Fadulu VT, Chang J, et al. Mutations in transforming growth factor-beta receptor type II cause familial thoracic aortic aneurysms and dissections. *Circulation* 2005;112:513–520.
39. Jarrett F, Darling RC, Mundth ED, et al. Experience with infected aneurysms of the abdominal aorta. *Arch Surg* 1975;110:1281–1286.
40. Bakker-de Wekker P, Alfieri O, Vermeulen F, et al. Surgical treatment of infected pseudoaneurysms after replacement of the ascending aorta. *J Thorac Cardiovasc Surg* 1984;88:447–451.
41. Bachet JE, Termignon JL, Dreyfus G, et al. Aortic dissection. Prevalence, cause, and results of late reoperations. *J Thorac Cardiovasc Surg* 1994; 108:199–205.
42. Bernard Y, Zimmermann H, Chocron S, et al. False lumen patency as a predictor of late outcome in aortic dissection. *Am J Cardiol* 2001;87:1378–1382.
43. Elefteriades JA, Lovoulos CJ, Coady MA, et al. Management of descending aortic dissection. *Ann Thorac Surg* 1999;67:2002–2005.
44. Marui A, Mochizuki T, Mitsui N, et al. Toward the best treatment for uncomplicated patients with type B acute aortic dissection: a consideration for sound surgical indication. *Circulation* 1999;100:II275–II280.

45. Juvonen T, Ergin MA, Galla JD, et al. Risk factors for rupture of chronic type B dissections. *J Thorac Cardiovasc Surg* 1999;117:776–786.
46. Borst HG, Walterbusch G, Schaps D. Extensive aortic replacement using "elephant trunk" prosthesis. *Thorac Cardiovasc Surg* 1983;31: 37–40.
47. Huynh TT, Miller CC III, Estrera AL, et al. Determinants of hospital length of stay after thoracoabdominal aortic aneurysm repair. *J Vasc Surg* 2002;35:648–653.
48. Cambria RP, Clouse WD, Davison JK, et al. Thoracoabdominal aneurysm repair: results with 337 operations performed over a 15-year interval. *Ann Surg* 2002;236:471–479.
49. Kouchoukos NT, Daily BB, Rokkas CK, et al. Hypothermic bypass and circulatory arrest for operations on the descending thoracic and thoracoabdominal aorta. *Ann Thorac Surg* 1995;60:67–76.
50. Svensson LG, Crawford ES, Hess KR, et al. Experience with 1509 patients undergoing thoracoabdominal aortic operations. *J Vasc Surg* 1993;17: 357–368.
51. Shah PJ, Estrera AL, Safi HJ. Thoracoabdominal aortic aneurysm: current surgical trends. In: Safi HJ, McPherson D, eds. *Houston Aortic Symposium*. 2008.
52. Safi HJ, Miller CC III, Huynh TT, et al. Distal aortic perfusion and cerebrospinal fluid drainage for thoracoabdominal and descending thoracic aortic repair: ten years of organ protection. *Ann Surg* 2003;238:372–380.
53. Miller CC III, Porat EE, Estrera AL, et al. Analysis of short-term multivariate competing risks data following thoracic and thoracoabdominal aortic repair. *Eur J Cardiothorac Surg* 2003;23:1023–1027.
54. Coselli JS, Lemaire SA, Koksoy C, et al. Cerebrospinal fluid drainage reduces paraplegia after thoracoabdominal aortic aneurysm repair: results of a randomized clinical trial. *J Vasc Surg* 2002;35:631–639.
55. Hollier LH, Money SR, Naslund TC, et al. Risk of spinal cord dysfunction in patients undergoing thoracoabdominal aortic replacement. *Am J Surg* 1992;164:210–213.
56. Jacobs MJ, de Mol BA, Elenbaas T, et al. Spinal cord blood supply in patients with thoracoabdominal aortic aneurysms. *J Vasc Surg* 2002;35:30–37.
57. Safi HJ, Harlin SA, Miller CC, et al. Predictive factors for acute renal failure in thoracic and thoracoabdominal aortic aneurysm surgery. *J Vasc Surg* 1996;24:338–344.
58. Safi HJ, Miller CC III, Carr C, et al. Importance of intercostal artery reattachment during thoracoabdominal aortic aneurysm repair. *J Vasc Surg* 1998;27:58–66.
59. Huynh TT, Miller CC III, Safi HJ. Delayed onset of neurologic deficit: significance and management. *Semin Vasc Surg* 2000;13:340–344.
60. Jacobs MJ, Mess W, Mochtar B, et al. The value of motor evoked potentials in reducing paraplegia during thoracoabdominal aneurysm repair. *J Vasc Surg* 2006;43:239–246.
61. Kawanishi Y, Munakata H, Matsumori M, et al. Usefulness of transcranial motor evoked potentials during thoracoabdominal aortic surgery. *Ann Thorac Surg* 2007;83:456–461.
62. Keyhani K, Miller CC III, Estrera AL, et al. Analysis of motor and somatosensory evoked potentials during thoracic and thoracoabdominal aortic aneurysm repair. *J Vasc Surg* 2009;49:36–41.
63. Crawford ES, Mizrahi EM, Hess KR, et al. The impact of distal aortic perfusion and somatosensory evoked potential monitoring on prevention of paraplegia after aortic aneurysm operation. *J Thorac Cardiovasc Surg* 1988;95:357–367.
64. Azizzadeh A, Huynh TT, Miller CC III, et al. Reversal of twice-delayed neurologic deficits with cerebrospinal fluid drainage after thoracoabdominal aneurysm repair: a case report and plea for a national database collection. *J Vasc Surg* 2000;31:592–598.
65. Safi HJ, Miller CC III, Azizzadeh A, et al. Observations on delayed neurologic deficit after thoracoabdominal aortic aneurysm repair. *J Vasc Surg* 1997;26:616–622.
66. Widmann MD, DeLucia A, Sharp J, et al. Reversal of renal failure and paraplegia after thoracoabdominal aneurysm repair. *Ann Thorac Surg* 1998;65:1153–1155.
67. Estrera AL, Miller CC III, Huynh TT, et al. Preoperative and operative predictors of delayed neurologic deficit following repair of thoracoabdominal aortic aneurysm. *J Thorac Cardiovasc Surg* 2003;126:1288–1294.
68. Azizzadeh A, Huynh TT, Miller CC III, et al. Postoperative risk factors for delayed neurologic deficit after thoracic and thoracoabdominal aortic aneurysm repair: a case-control study. *J Vasc Surg* 2003;37:750–754.
69. Huynh TT, van Eps RG, Miller CC III, et al. Glomerular filtration rate is superior to serum creatinine for prediction of mortality after thoracoabdominal aortic surgery. *J Vasc Surg* 2005;42:206–212.
70. Kouchoukos NT, Masetti P, Mauney MC, et al. One-stage repair of extensive chronic aortic dissection using the arch-first technique and bilateral anterior thoracotomy. *Ann Thorac Surg* 2008;86:1502–1509.
71. Kouchoukos NT, Masetti P, Murphy SF. Hypothermic cardiopulmonary bypass and circulatory arrest in the management of extensive thoracic and thoracoabdominal aortic aneurysms. *Semin Thorac Cardiovasc Surg* 2003; 15:333–339.
72. Tabayashi K, Motoyoshi N, Saiki Y, et al. Efficacy of perfusion cooling of the epidural space and cerebrospinal fluid drainage during repair of extent I and II thoracoabdominal aneurysm. *J Cardiovasc Surg* 2008;49: 749–755.
73. Coselli JS, Bozinovski J, LeMaire SA. Open surgical repair of 2286 thoracoabdominal aortic aneurysms. *Ann Thorac Surg* 2007;83:S862–S864.
74. Lemaire SA, Jones MM, Conklin LD, et al. Cold blood and cold crystalloid renal perfusion afford similar protection against acute renal injury during thoracoabdominal aortic aneurysm repair: results of a randomized trial. *J Vasc Surg* in press.
75. Conrad MF, Crawford RS, Davison JK, et al. Thoracoabdominal aneurysm repair: a 20-year perspective. *Ann Thorac Surg* 2007;83:S856–S861.
76. Rigberg DA, McGory ML, Zingmond DS, et al. Thirty-day mortality statistics underestimate the risk of repair of thoracoabdominal aortic aneurysms: a statewide experience. *J Vasc Surg* 2006;43:217–222.
77. Quinones-Baldrich WJ. Descending thoracic and thoracoabdominal aortic aneurysm repair: 15-year results using a uniform approach. *Ann Vasc Surg* 2004;18:335–342.
78. Fehrenbacher JW, Hart DW, Huddleston E, et al. Optimal end-organ protection for thoracic and thoracoabdominal aortic aneurysm repair using deep hypothermic circulatory arrest. *Ann Thorac Surg* 2007;83:1041–1046.
79. Etz CD, Halstead JC, Spielvogel D, et al. Thoracic and thoracoabdominal aneurysm repair: is reimplantation of spinal cord arteries a waste of time? *Ann Thorac Surg* 2006;82:1670–1677.
80. Etz CD, Di Luozzo G, Bello R, et al. Pulmonary complications after descending thoracic and thoracoabdominal aortic aneurysm repair: predictors, prevention, and treatment. *Ann Thorac Surg* 2007;83:S870–S876.
81. Safi HJ, Miller CC III, Estrera AL, et al. Staged repair of extensive aortic aneurysms: morbidity and mortality in the elephant trunk technique. *Circulation* 2001;104:2938–2942.
82. Svensson LG, Crawford ES, Hess KR, et al. Variables predictive of outcome in 832 patients undergoing repairs of the descending thoracic aorta. *Chest* 1993;104:1248–1253.
83. Okita Y, Tagusari O, Minatoya K, et al. Is distal anastomosis only to the true channel in chronic type B aortic dissection justified? *Ann Thorac Surg* 1999;68:1586–1591.
84. Gilling-Smith GL, Worswick L, Knight PF, et al. Surgical repair of thoracoabdominal aortic aneurysm: 10 years' experience. *Br J Surg* 1995;82:624–629.
85. Dudra J, Shiiya N, Matsui Y, et al. Operative results of thoracoabdominal repair for chronic type B aortic dissection. *J Cardiovasc Surg* 1997;38: 147–151.
86. Safi HJ, Miller CC III, Estrera AL, et al. Chronic aortic dissection not a risk factor for neurologic deficit in thoracoabdominal aortic aneurysm repair. *Eur J Vasc Endovasc Surg* 2002;23:244–250.
87. Safi HJ, Miller CC III, Reardon MJ, et al. Operation for acute and chronic aortic dissection: recent outcome with regard to neurologic deficit and early death. *Ann Thorac Surg* 1998;66:402–411.
88. Dake MD, Miller DC, Semba CP, et al. Transluminal placement of endovascular stent-grafts for the treatment of descending thoracic aortic aneurysms. *N Engl J Med* 1994;331:1729–1734.
89. Makaroun MS, Dillavou ED, Wheatley GH, et al. Five-year results of endovascular treatment with the Gore TAG device compared with open repair of thoracic aortic aneurysms. *J Vasc Surg* 2008;47:912–918.
90. Fairman RM, Criado F, Farber M, et al. Pivotal results of the Medtronic vascular talent thoracic stent graft system: the VALOR trial. *J Vasc Surg* 2008;48:546–554.
91. Matsumura JS, Cambria RP, Dake MD, et al. International controlled clinical trial of thoracic endovascular aneurysm repair with the Zenith TX2 endovascular graft: 1-year results. *J Vasc Surg* 2008;47:247–257.
92. Eggebrecht H, Nienaber CA, Neuhauser M, et al. Endovascular stent-graft placement in aortic dissection: a meta-analysis. *Eur Heart J* 2006;27: 489–498.
93. Xenos ES, Abedi NN, Davenport DL, et al. Meta-analysis of endovascular vs open repair for traumatic descending thoracic aortic rupture. *J Vasc Surg* 2008;48:1343–1351.
94. Buth J, Harris PL, Hobo R, et al. Neurologic complications associated with endovascular repair of thoracic aortic pathology: incidence and risk factors. A study from the European collaborators on stent/graft techniques for aortic aneurysm repair (EUROSTAR) registry. *J Vasc Surg* 2007;46: 1103–1110.
95. Roselli EE, Greenberg RK, Pfaff K, et al. Endovascular treatment of thoracoabdominal aortic aneurysms. *J Thorac Cardiovasc Surg* 2007;133: 1474–1482.
96. Greenberg RK, Lytle B. Endovascular repair of thoracoabdominal aneurysms. *Circulation* 2008;117:2288–2296.
97. Muhs BE, Verhoeven EL, Zeebregts CJ, et al. Mid-term results of endovascular aneurysm repair with branched and fenestrated endografts. *J Vasc Surg* 2006;44:9–15.
98. Greenberg RK, Lu Q, Roselli EE, et al. Contemporary analysis of descending thoracic and thoracoabdominal aneurysm repair: a comparison of endovascular and open techniques. *Circulation* 2008;118:808– 817.
99. Black SA, Wolfe JH, Clark M, et al. Complex thoracoabdominal aortic aneurysms: endovascular exclusion with visceral revascularization. *J Vasc Surg* 2006;43:1081–1089.
100. Resch TA, Greenberg RK, Lyden SP, et al. Combined staged procedures for the treatment of thoracoabdominal aneurysms. *J Endovasc Ther* 2006;13: 481–489.
101. Zhou W, Reardon M, Peden EK, et al. Hybrid approach to complex thoracic aortic aneurysms in high-risk patients: surgical challenges and clinical outcomes. *J Vasc Surg* 2006;44:688–693.
102. Chiesa R, Tshomba Y, Melissano G, et al. Hybrid approach to thoracoabdominal aortic aneurysms in patients with prior aortic surgery. *J Vasc Surg* 2007;45:1128–1135.

CHAPTER 100 ■ ABDOMINAL AORTIC ANEURYSMS

THOMAS S. HUBER AND W. ANTHONY LEE

KEY POINTS

1. An aneurysm is defined as a permanent, focal dilation of an artery that exceeds 1.5 times the normal, expected diameter.
2. The risk factors for abdominal aortic aneurysm include age, male gender, smoking, family history, hypertension, and the presence of other aortoiliac or peripheral aneurysms.
3. The diameter of an aneurysm is the greatest predictor of rupture as predicted by the tangential stress of the vessel wall.
4. The natural history of abdominal aortic aneurysms is to increase in size with a mean growth rate of 0.4 cm/y.
5. Computed tomography arteriography is both the diagnostic study of choice and the sole imaging study required for operative planning.
6. The treatment of abdominal aortic aneurysm represents a balance between the risk of rupture and the operative mortality rate.
7. Infrarenal abdominal aortic aneurysms should be repaired in men when the diameter reaches 5.5 cm and in women when the diameter reaches 5.0 cm provided they are a reasonable operative risk.
8. Endovascular aneurysm repair mandates long-term follow-up with serial imaging to confirm the integrity of the device and repair.
9. Randomized trials have not demonstrated an advantage for the endovascular approach, but it appears to be the preferred choice by both patients and providers in the United States.

Abdominal aortic aneurysms are a common problem in developed countries and represent a significant public health concern. Operative repair is the only means to reduce the risk of rupture and the associated mortality. The treatment algorithm represents a balance between the risk of operation and the future risk of rupture. The open technique has been the traditional approach since its description by Dubost et al.[1] in the early 1950s. The endovascular approach has emerged as the preferred treatment since its commercial release at the turn of the century and has truly revolutionized the care of patients with abdominal aortic aneurysms.

DEFINITIONS AND CLASSIFICATIONS

1 An aneurysm is defined as a permanent, focal dilation of an artery that exceeds 1.5 times the normal, expected diameter.[2] The diameter of a normal abdominal aorta in an adult male is approximately 2 cm (range, 1.4 to 3.0 cm), and, therefore, a 3-cm aorta would be considered aneurysmal.[3] The abdominal aorta is consistently larger in men than in women and increases slightly with age in both sexes.[4] Abdominal aortic aneurysms should be differentiated from other conditions in which the size of the aorta is increased, including ectasia and arteriomegaly. In aortic *ectasia,* the diameter is increased by less than 50% of the normal expected diameter. The term *arteriomegaly* refers to a diffuse (nonfocal) enlargement of several arterial segments with increases in diameter greater than 50% of the normal expected diameter. Arterial segments in patients with arteriomegaly may be considered aneurysmal if the diameter of a segment is increased by more than 50% of the diameter of an adjacent segment. The term *aneurysmosis* denotes the presence of multiple aneurysmal segments separated by either normal, occluded, or arteriomegalic segments.

Abdominal aortic aneurysms are classified primarily according to how far they extend cephalad (Fig. 100.1). More than 95% of all abdominal aortic aneurysms are classified as infrarenal.[5] These aneurysms start below the orifices of the renal arteries and usually have a 1.5- to 2-cm proximal segment of normal (i.e., nonaneurysmal) aorta. Approximately 10% to 20% of all abdominal aortic aneurysms are associated with aneurysms of the iliac arteries.[6,7] Aneurysmal involvement of the iliac vessels is usually confined to the common or internal iliac arteries; aneurysmal involvement of the external iliac arteries is extremely rare. The management of abdominal aortic aneurysms associated with common iliac artery aneurysms is similar to the management of abdominal aortic aneurysms alone, and these two patterns should be considered basically the same disease process. The only significant difference in the decision algorithm is the configuration of the graft for open repair (i.e., tube vs. bifurcated) and the site of the distal anastomoses. Aneurysms classified as juxtarenal extend to the level of the renal arteries, and those classified as suprarenal extend to the level of the superior mesenteric or celiac arteries. Aneurysms involving the thoracic and abdominal aorta are designated as thoracoabdominal aortic aneurysms and are classified (extent 1 through 4) according to how far they extend both cephalad and caudal. Aneurysms that extend above the renal arteries are more complicated to repair and associated with greater morbidity as might be predicted from the obligatory periods of renal and mesenteric ischemia.

MAGNITUDE OF THE PROBLEM

Abdominal aortic aneurysms and their sequelae are common problems in developed countries. The incidence of abdominal aortic aneurysms in the United States ranges from 1.5% in autopsy series to 3.2% among unselected adult patients screened with ultrasonography.[5] Predictably, the incidence increases among subsets of patients with defined risk factors for abdominal aortic aneurysms and approximates 50% among patients with either femoral or popliteal artery aneurysms.[5] It should be emphasized that these rates have been determined with the broad definition of an aneurysm (i.e., 1.5 times the normal vessel diameter) and do not necessarily reflect aneurysms that are of

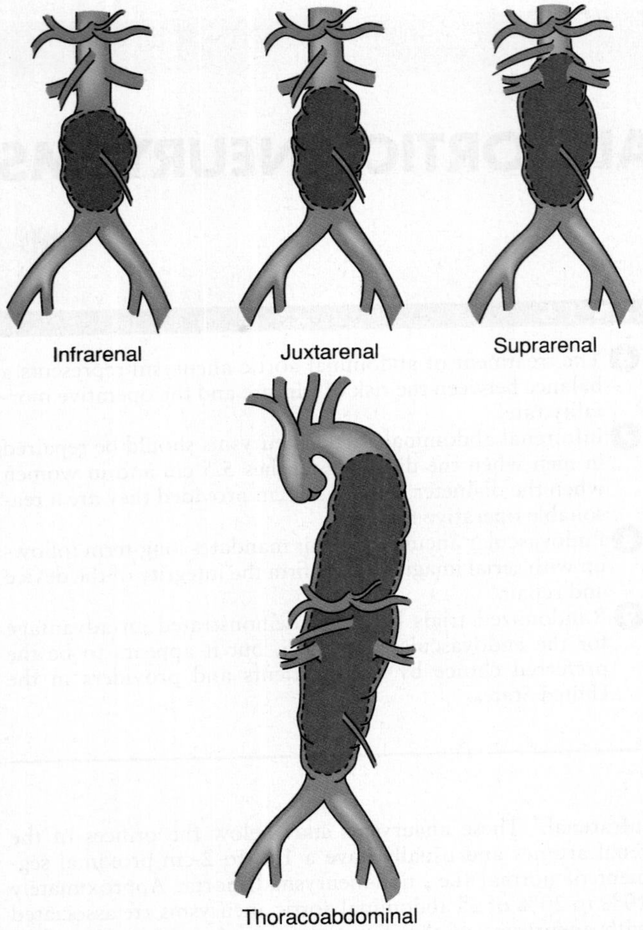

FIGURE 100.1. Classification of abdominal aortic aneurysms. More than 95% of all abdominal aortic aneurysms are infrarenal. Juxtarenal aneurysms extend cephalad to the level of the renal arteries, and suprarenal aneurysms to the level of the superior mesenteric and/or celiac arteries. Aneurysms involving the thoracic and abdominal portions of the aorta are designated as thoracoabdominal aortic aneurysms and are classified (extent 1 through 4) according to how far they extend cephalad and caudal.

sufficient size to merit repair. Furthermore, the incidence of abdominal aortic aneurysms appears to be increasing and this likely reflects an increase in the "true" incidence rather than simply an increase in detection, diagnosis, or the aging population.[8] A total of 14,751 deaths were caused by abdominal aortic aneurysms and/or dissections during 2003 and this corresponded to death rate of 5.1 per 100,000 as reported by the Centers for Disease Control and Prevention.[9] Notably, these numbers may be underestimates because a significant number of sudden deaths in elderly patients may be secondary to undiagnosed ruptured aneurysms.

PATHOGENESIS AND RISK FACTORS

The pathogenesis of abdominal aortic aneurysms remains unresolved, although it is an intense area of both experimental and clinical investigation. Multiple potential etiologic factors have been implicated including atherosclerosis,[10] hemodynamics,[11] collagen,[12] collagenase,[13] elastin,[14] elastase,[15] metalloproteinases,[16] protease inhibitors,[17] programmed cell death (apoptosis),[18] neutrophils,[19] and inflammatory mediators.[20] The etiology is likely multifactorial with interaction between both environmental and genetic factors. Unfortunately, investigation into the potential mechanisms has not resulted in any effective therapies. Elucidation of the pathogenesis has been complicated by the older age of patients at presentation and the absence of suitable animal models.

2 Multiple risk factors have been identified for the development of abdominal aortic aneurysms and include age, sex, smoking, hypertension, hyperlipidemia, peripheral vascular disease, myocardial infarction, and family history.[21–24] Identification of these risk factors is important to facilitate screening high-risk patient populations. Abdominal aortic aneurysms are a disease process of the elderly and are rare among persons younger than 50 years of age. Indeed, the mean age among patients undergoing repair across the country was 72 ± 7 years (± standard deviation [SD]) in a recent series comprising a 20% national sample.[25] A meta-analysis of the population-based screening studies for abdominal aortic aneurysms reported that male sex had the strongest association (odds ratio, 5.69).[21] The incidence of death resulting from abdominal aortic aneurysms for men 60 to 64 years of age is 11-fold higher than that for women of the same age, but it is only threefold higher for men between 85 and 90 years of age. Furthermore, men account for approximately 80% of all abdominal aortic aneurysm repairs performed nationally.[25] The Aneurysm Detection and Management Veterans Affairs Cooperative Study Group (ADAM) reported that smoking was the strongest modifiable risk factor associated with abdominal aortic aneurysms greater than 4 cm (odds ratio, 5.57) among the 73,451 veterans screened.[26] Similarly, Wilmink et al.[26,27] reported that abdominal aneurysms were 7.6 times more likely to develop in current smokers than in nonsmokers and that the duration of smoking rather than level of exposure appeared to correlate with their development. Darling et al.[28] prospectively analyzed patients undergoing repair of abdominal aortic aneurysms and reported that 15.1% had a first-degree relative with an aneurysm, in contrast to only 1.8% in the control group. Interestingly, the presence of a female family member with an aneurysm correlated with an increased risk for rupture. Larsson et al.[29] reported from a population-based control study in Sweden that the relative risk of an abdominal aortic aneurysm in first-degree relatives was 1.9 (95% confidence interval [CI], 1.6–2.2). However, the risk of an aneurysm was not affected by the gender of the index individual or relative.

The presence of an aneurysm in the aortic, iliac, femoral, or popliteal arteries dramatically increases the risk for a new or additional abdominal aortic aneurysm. In patients undergoing abdominal aortic or iliac artery aneurysm repair, there is a 5% to 15% chance that an additional aneurysm will develop that merits another repair.[30,31] This second aneurysm may develop anywhere in the remaining native aorta, commonly within the residual infrarenal aortic cuff. The incidence of aortoiliac aneurysms in patients with popliteal or femoral artery aneurysms is approximately 50%.[5] Importantly, all patients found to have one of these peripheral artery aneurysms should undergo a computed tomography scan (CT) of the entire aorta and iliac vessels to exclude a synchronous aneurysm in addition to being screened for other peripheral aneurysms. Interestingly, the reverse scenario is not true; patients with aortic or iliac artery aneurysms have a less than 5% chance of having a peripheral artery aneurysm, and evaluation beyond physical examination is likely not justified.[32]

The incidence of abdominal aortic aneurysm is increased among patients with an aortic dissection and among patients with heart transplants. Late or repeated operations are required in approximately 20% of patients by 10 years after an acute aortic dissection.[33] The aneurysms may develop in either the thoracic or abdominal aorta, although the former site is more common. The term *dissecting aneurysm* is frequently used to describe bland aneurysms, although it is a misnomer; dissection and aneurysmal degeneration are separate processes.

Simply, a dissection is a tear within the aortic wall itself that extends for a variable length resulting in "true" and "false" lumen. The prevalence of abdominal aortic aneurysms and the rate of expansion are both increased among heart transplant patients.[34–36] The responsible mechanisms remain unclear, but the obligatory chronic immunosuppression may contribute. Interestingly, several transplant centers have initiated screening programs as part of their pretransplant evaluation.

It is notable that the risk factors for abdominal aortic aneurysm are similar to those associated with the development of atherosclerosis with the noted exception of diabetes mellitus.[22,23] Furthermore, atherosclerotic changes are found almost universally within the abdominal aorta at the time of repair. However, the processes of atherosclerosis and aneurysmal degeneration are likely separate and distinct. Simplistically, atherosclerosis is a process that leads to a narrowing of the vessel lumen, whereas aneurysmal degeneration leads to dilation. Aneurysms have historically been referred to as *atherosclerotic aneurysms,* although this is also a misnomer that has been appropriately replaced by the term *nonspecific aneurysms.*

PRINCIPLES OF MANAGEMENT

The treatment goals for patients with abdominal aortic aneurysms are to prolong life, relieve symptoms, and prevent rupture. Because surgical treatment is the only effective means to achieve these goals, the crucial question that must be answered is whether the patient merits operative repair. The decision algorithm is straightforward for patients with ruptured or symptomatic aneurysms, but more difficult for patients with asymptomatic, intact aneurysms. The decision to recommend operative intervention in the elective setting is contingent on the balance between the risk of operation and the risk of expectant or nonoperative management within the context of the patient's desires or wishes. Appropriate assessment of these risks requires an understanding of the size-associated risk for rupture, the growth rate, and the mortality associated with repair. However, it should be emphasized that repair of an asymptomatic, intact aneurysm is a prophylactic operation.

Understanding the natural history of untreated abdominal aortic aneurysms requires knowledge of the physics associated with the vessel wall. The tangential stress (t) of a fluid-filled cylindric tube is determined by the following equation:

$$t = Pr/d$$

where P is the pressure exerted by the blood (dyne/cm^2), r is the internal radius (cm), and d is the thickness (cm) of the arterial wall.[37] The tangential stress of a cylinder 0.2 cm thick with an internal radius of 0.8 cm and a fluid pressure of 150 mm Hg is 8×10^5 dyne/cm^2 (Fig. 100.2). An increase in the internal radius (diameter) of the cylinder to 2.94 cm and a concomitant decrease in the wall thickness, as might occur with an aneurysm, would increase the tangential stress to 98×10^5 dyne/cm^2. Thus, a threefold increase in diameter would result in a 12-fold increase in the tangential stress. Aneurysms rupture when the tangential stress exceeds the tensile strength of the vessel wall. It should be emphasized that the tangential stress varies directly with the radius of the cylinder (vessel) but is independent of its length.

3 The diameter of an abdominal aortic aneurysm is the greatest predictor of rupture as would be predicted by the tangential stress of the vessel wall. The diameter of an aneurysm is determined by measuring its greatest diameter from outer wall to outer wall in any orientation (i.e., anterior to posterior, transverse) throughout the extent of the aneurysm. These measurements may be confounded by the tortuosity of the vessel, so every attempt should be made to obtain a cross-sectional measurement perpendicular to the long axis. The collective annual rupture risks per aneurysm diameter are shown in Table 100.1.[38] Although there is some variability in the data, it

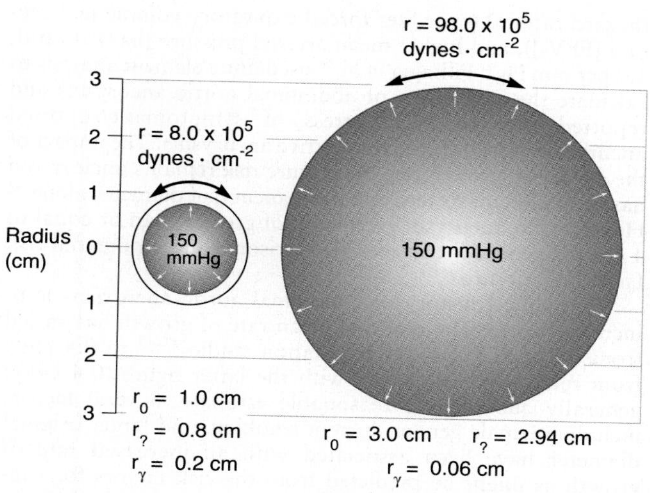

FIGURE 100.2. Cross-sectional view of a 2-cm-diameter cylinder that expands to a diameter of 6 cm while the wall cross-sectional area remains constant. Expansion of a 1-cm-diameter cylinder to a diameter of 3 cm with no change in wall cross-sectional area increases wall tensile stress 12-fold. t, wall stress; d, wall thickness; r_i, inside radius; r_o, outside radius.

is generally appreciated that the rupture risk for aneurysms less than 5 cm in diameter is small, but increases considerably for those greater than 5.5 cm. These data may be simplified by using the rule of thumb that the annual rupture risk is 5% or less for a 5-cm aneurysm, 10% for a 6-cm aneurysm, and 20% for a 7-cm aneurysm. These numbers correspond to an estimated 5-year rupture risk of 50% for 6-cm aneurysms and 100% for those 7 cm. Notably, both the ADAM[26] and UK Small Aneurysm Trial,[39] which randomized patients with small aneurysms (4.0 to 5.5 cm) to open repair or surveillance, reported that the rupture risk for surveillance was 1% or less per year.

A variety of other factors have also been reported to increase the risk of aneurysm rupture including female gender,[40–42] chronic obstructive pulmonary disease (COPD),[40,43] smoking,[40] hypertension,[40,43] family history,[44] and wall stress.[45] Notably, the UK Small Aneurysm Trial reported that the rupture risk was increased for female gender (hazard ratio, 3.0), current smoking (hazard ratio, 1.5), severe COPD

TABLE 100.1 **MANAGEMENT**

ESTIMATED ANNUAL RUPTURE RISK

■ AAA DIAMETER (cm)	■ RUPTURE RISK (%/y)
<4	0
4–5	0.5–5
5–6	3–15
6–7	10–20
7–8	20–40
>8	30–50

AAA, abdominal aortic aneurysm.
From Brewster DC, Cronenwett JL, Hallett JW Jr., et al. Guidelines for the treatment of abdominal aortic aneurysms. Report of a subcommittee of the Joint Council of the American Association for Vascular Surgery and Society for Vascular Surgery. *J Vasc Surg* 2003; 37:1106–1117.

(hazard ratio, 0.6 per liter forced expiratory volume in 1 second [FEV_1]), and higher mean arterial pressure (hazard ratio, 1.2 per mm Hg). Fillinger et al.[46] used finite element analysis to calculate the wall stress of abdominal aortic aneurysms and reported that the wall stress of symptomatic/ruptured aneurysms exceeds those for elective aneurysms. The impact of the aneurysm growth rate on rupture risk remains unclear and has been difficult to separate from aneurysm diameter alone.[42] However, an aneurysm expansion of greater than or equal to 1 cm/y is generally considered worrisome and a potential risk factor for rupture.

4 The natural history of abdominal aortic aneurysms is to increase in size. The reported mean rate of growth has varied from 0.2 to 0.3 cm/y in population studies[47–49] to 0.4 cm/y from referral practices,[50–52] with the latter figure (0.4 cm/y) generally quoted as a reasonable estimate. Several factors including female gender, current smoking, and larger original diameter have been associated with an increased rate of growth as might be predicted from the risk factors for rupture.[47,49,53] Interestingly, doxycycline and coenzyme A (CoA) reductase inhibitors (i.e., statins) may inhibit aneurysm growth.[53,54] It should be emphasized that these growth rates are mean values and that all aneurysms do not grow in a linear fashion as might be predicted. The growth curve may be somewhat erratic or "staccato," with no growth detected during consecutive 6-month intervals followed by a growth of 0.6 cm during the next one.[55] Furthermore, it should be emphasized that the past rate of growth does not predict future events; patients should not be lulled into a false sense of security if their aneurysm is relatively stable over time.

The mortality rate associated with repair of an abdominal aortic aneurysm depends on the status of the aneurysm (intact/asymptomatic, intact/symptomatic, ruptured) and the method of repair (open vs. endovascular). A recent population study from the Nationwide Inpatient Sample reported that the operative mortality rate for *open repair of intact* aneurysms in the United States was 4.2%.[25] Predictably, the operative mortality rate increased with age, ranging from 2.2% among persons 50 to 59 years of age to 9.2% among those older than age 80. Interestingly, the operative mortality rate was significantly higher among women (6.1% vs. 3.7%). Similar reports from other regional and national databases have consistently reported mortality rates less than 5% for the open repair of intact aneurysms.[56–58] The mortality rate for open repair in the randomized trials comparing operative repair with surveillance for small aneurysms (UK Small Aneurysm Trial, 5.8%; ADAM, 2.7%) and open repair with endovascular repair (Dutch Randomized Endovascular Aneurysm Management [DREAM] Trial, 4.6%; Endovascular Aneurysm Repair [EVAR] Trial, 4.6%)[59,60] are within the range of these nationwide series. Furthermore, a literature review examining the mortality rate of open abdominal aortic aneurysm repair encompassing 64 individual studies reported a collective rate of 5.5%.[61]

The reported operative mortality rate for *endovascular repair of intact* abdominal aortic aneurysms has been consistently less than those for the open approach.[56–58,62–65] Lee et al.[66] reported from the Nationwide Inpatient Sample that the operative mortality rate for endovascular repair was 1.3% in 2001. Similarly, Schermerhorn et al.[58] reported that the operative mortality after endovascular aneurysm repair was 1.2% among Medicare beneficiaries during 2001–2004. Early results from the DREAM Trial[52] and the EVAR Trial[59] comparing open and endovascular repair have reported that the perioperative mortality rate is lower for endovascular repair and within the same range (DREAM, 1.2% vs. 4.6%; EVAR, 1.7% vs. 4.7%).

The operative mortality rate for *open repair of intact/symptomatic* aneurysms among patients undergoing emergent repair exceeds that for elective repair and has ranged from 9% to 19%.[5,67,68] Various explanations have been proposed for this increased mortality rate relative to that for intact/asymptomatic aneurysms including failure to maximize preoperative medical conditions, increased incidence of inadvertent venous injuries, and less experienced operative teams, although the true explanation remains unclear. It is notable that the increased rate has been fairly consistent in the literature, in contrast to the mortality rate for intact/asymptomatic aneurysms, which has gradually decreased. Comparable data are not available for the *endovascular repair of intact/symptomatic* aneurysms, although the mortality rates are likely similar to those considered asymptomatic.

The actual mortality rate for ruptured abdominal aortic aneurysms is somewhat difficult to determine because a significant number of sudden deaths in elderly patients are likely secondary to ruptured aneurysms. It has been estimated that 50% of all patients with ruptured abdominal aortic aneurysms die outside the hospital, and that approximately 50% of those who actually undergo open repair do not survive.[5] Indeed, a recent meta-analysis spanning 50 years and 77 studies reported that the operative mortality rate for the *open repair of ruptured* aneurysms was 48%.[69] These figures correspond to an overall mortality rate of approximately 80%, although this may be an underestimate. It is remarkable that the optimization of prehospital and emergency room care, including a reduction in the mean transfer time from the emergency department to the operating room to 12 minutes, has not resulted in a decrease in the mortality rate of ruptured aneurysms.[70] Notably, the operative mortality rate for ruptured aneurysms treated with the open approach has improved slightly over the past few decades, with Bown et al.[69] reporting a 3.5% reduction per decade.

The mortality rate for the *endovascular repair of ruptured* abdominal aortic aneurysms appears to be lower than that associated with the open approach.[71–76] Rayt et al.[74] reported a collective mortality rate of 24% for the endovascular approach from 31 studies encompassing 982 patients, while other meta-analyses or systematic reviews have reported comparable rates.[72,75] The potential to treat ruptured abdominal aortic aneurysms with the endovascular approach may represent the greatest contribution or benefit of the technology. However, further validation is necessary since the reports cited previously likely reflect both patient selection and publication bias. Notably, Giles et al.[77] reported that the annual number of deaths across the country from both intact and ruptured aneurysms has decreased significantly since the introduction of the endovascular approach.

CLINICAL PRESENTATION AND DIAGNOSIS

The overwhelming majority of abdominal aortic aneurysms are asymptomatic at the time of discovery. Most aneurysms are detected by abdominal or pelvic imaging studies, such as ultrasonography and CT, performed for other indications (e.g., chronic back pain, renal cysts) rather than on physical examination. Indeed, it is often difficult to feel an abdominal aortic aneurysm on physical examination because of its anatomic location in the posterior abdomen, and these difficulties are exacerbated in the presence of truncal obesity. A recent literature review examining the accuracy of physical examination reported that the sensitivity ranged from 33% to 100%, the specificity ranged from 75% to 100%, and the positive predictive value ranged from 14% to 100%.[78] Given these fairly broad ranges, the authors concluded that physical examination could not be relied upon to exclude an abdominal aortic aneurysm. Predictably, the accuracy of primary care physicians for detecting abdominal aortic aneurysms in patients with known aneurysms is only fair because of the limitations noted earlier and the failure to actually palpate the aorta during the physical examination. Intact abdominal aortic and iliac artery aneurysms may present with symptoms that lead to further investigation and the correct diagnosis, although this is the exception rather than the rule. Enlargement of the aneurysm may cause vertebral erosion and chronic back pain. Additionally, thrombosis of an abdominal aortic aneurysm may cause acute ischemia in the lower torso, and aneurysms may be a source of arterial macroemboli or microemboli leading to acute ischemia of a lower extremity or digit, respectively.

Patients with intact/symptomatic or ruptured aneurysms present with abdominal or back pain related to the aneurysm itself. The etiology of the pain is unclear, but may be secondary to local nerve compression. The character of the pain is variable and ranges from dull to sharp. The pain is usually acute in onset and persistent. It may be superimposed on more chronic abdominal or back pain, but the presentation is usually not subtle, and the pain can be differentiated from more chronic complaints. Additionally, the pain may radiate from the abdomen to the back, flank, inguinal region, or genitalia. Approximately 10% of patients with ruptured abdominal aortic aneurysms present with signs and symptoms similar to those of ureteral colic or other acute urologic problems.[79] Indeed, the diagnosis of a ruptured aneurysm must be ruled out in a timely fashion in patients presenting with testicular pain who have a normal urinalysis and testicular examination.

Patients with a ruptured abdominal aortic aneurysm may present anywhere along the spectrum from hemodynamically stable to profound shock. Their status depends on the ability of the tissues adjacent to the aorta to tamponade the bleeding and their physiologic status. If the adjacent tissues effectively tamponade the bleeding, the patient may present in a hemodynamically stable state with essentially normal vital signs. However, it should be emphasized that this is usually a temporary situation, and health care providers should not be lulled into a false sense of security. A ruptured abdominal aortic aneurysm is a true medical emergency that requires immediate operative repair regardless of the patient's hemodynamic status. Furthermore, the vital signs may be misleading because patients can lose up to 15% of their blood volume (class 1 shock) without any appreciable change in their pulse rate or blood pressure. If the aneurysm ruptures freely into the peritoneal space, patients usually exsanguinate before they can seek medical attention.

Patients with a ruptured abdominal aortic aneurysm may also present with either an aortoenteric or an aortocaval fistula, although both are relatively rare. Patients with an aortoenteric fistula may present with massive intestinal bleeding. The aorta may rupture through any portion of the bowel, although the duodenum and proximal small bowel are the most common sites. The overwhelming majority of aortoenteric fistulas result from the erosion of a prosthetic graft into the adjacent bowel (secondary aortoenteric fistula) rather than from unrepaired aneurysm (primary aortoenteric fistula). However, the diagnosis of an aortoenteric fistula must be ruled out in all patients with gastrointestinal bleeding and either an abdominal aortic aneurysm or a previous infrarenal aortic reconstruction. Patients with an aortocaval fistula present with high-output congestive heart failure, a continuous abdominal bruit, and edema of the lower extremities. The severity of the heart failure symptoms depends on the size of the fistula and the magnitude of the systemic shunt.

Several imaging studies are available to establish or confirm the diagnosis of an abdominal aortic aneurysm. Indeed, the introduction of endovascular techniques for aneurysm repair has resulted in an evolution of these modalities. The generic imaging goals for patients with an abdominal aortic aneurysm are to establish the diagnosis, determine the presence of rupture, determine the cephalad/caudal extent of the aneurysm, determine the feasibility of endovascular repair, appropriately size the aneurysm and access vessels for endovascular repair, screen for other visceral pathology, and screen for the presence of anatomic variants that would complicate operative repair,
5 such as a left-sided vena cava or a horseshoe kidney. Although no imaging study satisfies every objective, ultrasound has emerged as the ideal *screening* study, with CT arteriography being the definitive *diagnostic* test and the preferred modality for operative planning.

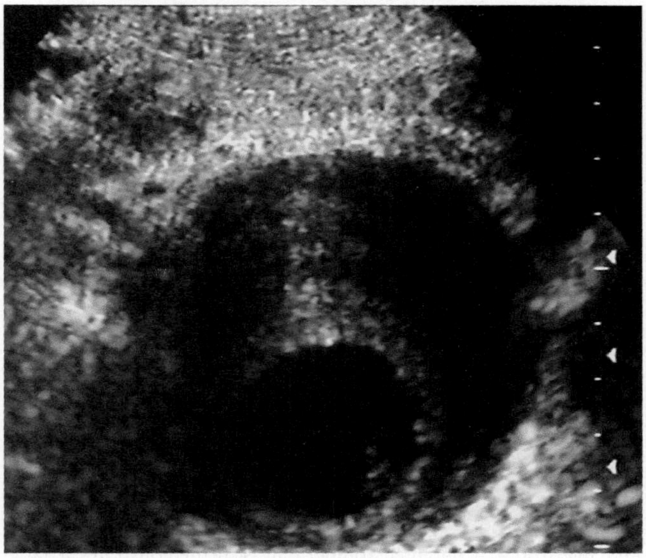

FIGURE 100.3. B-mode ultrasonogram showing a transverse view of an infrarenal abdominal aortic aneurysm. Note the vessel wall and the large quantity of intraluminal clot surrounding the smaller, blood-filled center (*dark circle*).

Abdominal ultrasound is a safe, simple, and inexpensive means of detecting abdominal aortic aneurysms (Fig. 100.3). It is relatively inexpensive and does not require the use of ionizing radiation, intravenous contrast, or arterial cannulation. Furthermore, the ultrasound units are portable and almost universally available in the hospital setting, including the emergency room.[80] The sensitivity of ultrasound for detecting abdominal aortic aneurysms is good, and the technique is reproducible within 0.3 cm.[81] However, the technique is somewhat operator dependent and potentially confounded by the presence of bowel gas. Ultrasound can accurately image the infrarenal aorta to its bifurcation but is less reliable for imaging the portions of the aorta proximal to the renal arteries and distal to the iliac vessels. Furthermore, it is not as reliable as CT for differentiating a ruptured from an intact aneurysm. It is an excellent tool for screening patients at high risk for an abdominal aortic aneurysm and for confirming the presence of an aneurysm suspected by physical examination or clinical presentation. Furthermore, it is a useful technique to follow patients with small aneurysms (<4 cm) when the exact measurement is not crucial. It should not be used to confirm the diagnosis of a ruptured aneurysm, nor should it be used as the sole imaging study before elective repair because it does not provide a complete image of the aorta and iliac arteries.

CT arteriography overcomes many of the limitations of ultrasound and represents the current "gold standard" for imaging patients with abdominal aortic aneurysms (Fig. 100.4). The technique is more expensive than ultrasound, not universally available, and potentially harmful because of the ionizing radiation and intravenous contrast. Indeed, the evolution of endovascular aneurysm repair and the requisite follow-up imaging studies have focused increased attention on the magnitude of the radiation injury. It is worth noting that the radiation dose associated with an abdominal CT scan is 10 millisieverts, while that for a routine chest radiograph is only 0.1 millisieverts. The incidence of allergic reactions to the contrast may be reduced by a steroid preparation, while the potential nephrotoxicity can be reduced by acetylcysteine or sodium

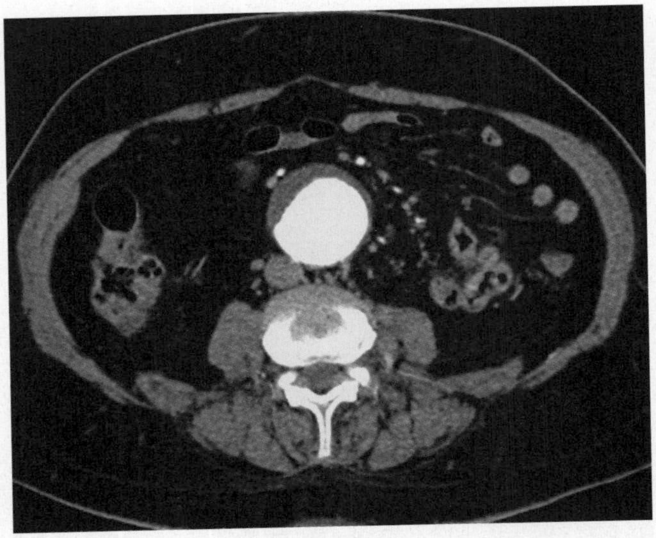

FIGURE 100.4. Computed tomography scan demonstrates a large abdominal aortic aneurysm. Note that the majority of the lumen is filled with contrast.

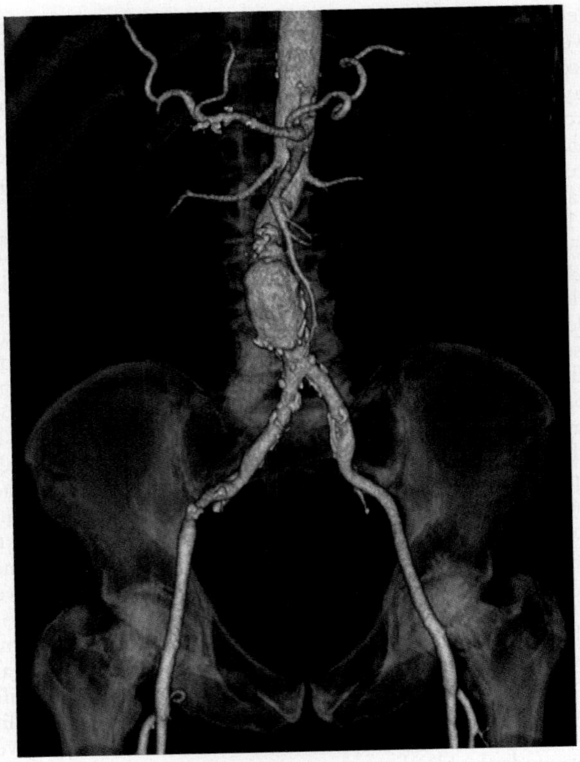

FIGURE 100.5. Three-dimensional computed tomography scan of the aorta and the iliac, femoral, and visceral arteries is shown. Note the infrarenal abdominal aortic aneurysm that extends to the aortic bifurcation.

bicarbonate.[82,83] These potential risks can be avoided altogether by not using contrast. However, the quality of the noncontrast images is less than optimal. CT is very sensitive for detecting both intact and ruptured aneurysms, and the images are reproducible within 0.2 cm.[81] The quality of the CT images has continued to improve with each new generation of scanners, and the image acquisition times have decreased. Currently, it is possible to image the aorta and iliac vessels from the ascending arch to the femoral vessels during a routine aneurysm scan with an image acquisition time of less than 45 seconds. CT arteriograms have essentially replaced traditional catheter-based diagnostic arteriograms. It is possible to reconstruct the axial CT images into three-dimensional (3D) images using special software and obtain images perpendicular to the centerline blood flow (Fig. 100.5). These 3D CT images have dramatically improved the accuracy and consistency of sizing for endovascular repair.[84] CT is also helpful for detecting other intra-abdominal pathology or anatomic variants that may impact the operative approach. Specific concerns include the location of the left renal vein and other associated venous anomalies, the location and size of the kidneys, and the characteristics of the aneurysm wall. CT is currently the sole diagnostic test performed before open surgical repair in the majority of cases and the imaging study of choice to confirm or refute the diagnosis of a ruptured abdominal aortic aneurysm. Additionally, CT is the serial imaging study of choice when aneurysms exceed 4 cm and approach the threshold for operative intervention.

Both magnetic resonance imaging (MRI) and catheter-based arteriography have been used as diagnostic imaging studies for patients with abdominal aortic aneurysms. The image quality and overall sensitivity of MRI is comparable to CT, but the technology is not as widely available and most surgeons are less familiar with interpreting the images. Furthermore, the technique is relatively contraindicated for patients with ferromagnetic devices (e.g., pacemakers, joints), and imaging critically ill patients is cumbersome, if not prohibitive. Aneurysms are frequently diagnosed during catheter-based arteriography, although this should not be viewed as a diagnostic test. An arteriogram only delineates the lumen of the vessels (i.e., aortic, iliac, and femoral arteries). Abdominal aortic aneurysms are frequently filled with laminated thrombus and have a fairly normal-appearing lumen. Importantly, the "lumenogram" produced by the contrast reflects the patent lumen rather than the "true" lumen of the vessel (and the actual size of the aneurysm). Preoperative catheter-based arteriography was formerly performed before endovascular repair to help select the appropriate-size device. Furthermore, it was considered helpful in the subset of patients undergoing open repair who had aortoiliac occlusive disease, poorly controlled hypertension/renal insufficiency, chronic mesenteric ischemia, and/or renal anomalies, including horseshoe kidneys. These concerns and indications are still relevant, but CT arteriography has largely supplanted any role for the catheter-based approach and avoids the additional inherent risks and cost.

The diagnostic approach and initial treatment for patients with a potential ruptured aneurysm merit further comment. Because of the high attendant mortality rate, prompt diagnosis and emergent repair are necessary. In a study from the Cleveland Clinic Vascular Registry, the operative mortality rate associated with ruptured abdominal aortic aneurysms increased from 35% when the initial diagnosis was correct to 75% when incorrect.[85] Admittedly, the clinical presentation may be confusing, and delays in diagnosis are not uncommon. The classic triad of hypotension, abdominal pain, and a pulsatile abdominal mass was present in only 50% of patients with ruptured aneurysms in a single institutional series.[86]

Elderly patients who present to the emergency room in a hemodynamically *unstable* state with abdominal or back pain require emergent exploratory laparotomy in most cases. The potential causes of shock (i.e., hypovolemic, cardiogenic, septic, neurogenic) can usually be quickly differentiated by a brief history and physical examination. However, this clinical scenario is most suggestive of hypovolemic or hemorrhagic shock resulting from an intra-abdominal catastrophe. The differential diagnosis is extensive and includes pancreatitis, mesenteric infarction, acute Addisonian crisis, and rupture of a visceral artery aneurysm in addition to rupture of an abdominal aortic

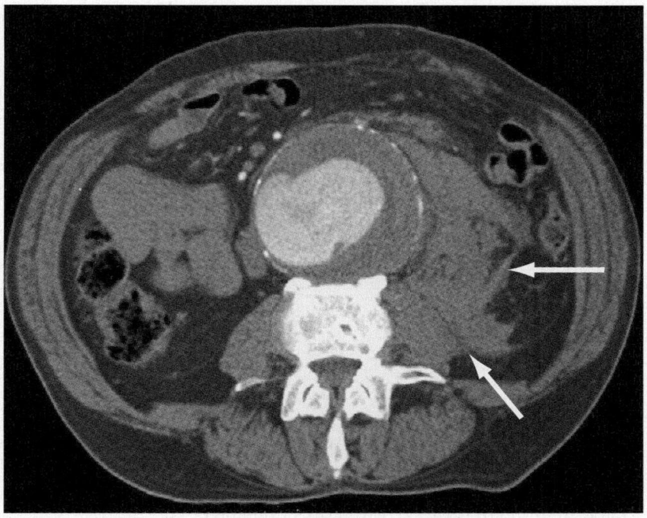

FIGURE 100.6. Contrast computed tomography scan demonstrates a ruptured abdominal aortic aneurysm. Note the large retroperitoneal hematoma and the loss of the normal fat plane anterior and lateral to the left psoas muscle.

aneurysm. A myocardial infarction can mimic a ruptured aneurysm in this patient population and potentially confounds the diagnosis, although it can usually be confirmed by the findings on electrocardiogram. Additional diagnostic imaging has not traditionally been considered necessary in this setting and, indeed, has been considered potentially harmful due to the obligatory delay in getting patients to the operating room. Due to the dramatic reduction in CT acquisition times and the potential feasibility of endovascular repair, abdominal/pelvic CT scans are likely indicated in this scenario to confirm the diagnosis and plan the operative procedure, provided it can be performed expeditiously. This approach has the added advantage of reducing the number of negative laparotomies in critically ill patients. A recent natural history study of patients with ruptured abdominal aortic aneurysms not offered operative repair reported that fewer than 15% of the patients died within 2 hours of hospital admission.[87] Based on these findings, the authors concluded that most patients with ruptured aneurysms are sufficiently stable to undergo a CT scan, and this opinion has been echoed by a recent systemic review examining the role of endovascular aneurysm repair for ruptured aneurysms.[75] Several findings on CT are suggestive of a ruptured abdominal aortic aneurysm including disruption of the calcium ring within the aortic wall, disruption of the aortic margins, retroperitoneal hematomas, mass lesions in the psoas region, displacement of the kidneys, abnormal soft tissues posterior to the aorta, effacement of the normal fat planes between the aorta and adjacent viscera, and abnormal retroperitoneal fluid collections (Fig. 100.6). Patients undergoing an emergent CT arteriogram to rule out a ruptured abdominal aortic aneurysm should not receive oral contrast because of the obligatory delay associated with administration and its confounding effects on the arteriogram or the imaging of the vessels.

The diagnosis of a ruptured abdominal aortic aneurysm should be considered in elderly patients who present to the emergency room hemodynamically *stable* with abdominal or back pain. Admittedly, the differential diagnosis for abdominal or back pain in this patient population is extensive, and the incidence of a ruptured abdominal aortic aneurysm is small. An expeditious history and physical examination can usually determine the cause of the pain. A pulsatile abdominal aortic mass, an unexplained low hematocrit, or hemodynamic instability before presentation is particularly worrisome and increases the level of suspicion. The diagnosis of an abdominal aortic aneurysm may be confirmed with a portable abdominal ultrasound in the emergency room.[80] Indeed, the current trauma algorithms include abdominal ultrasound as a diagnostic technique for blunt trauma, and many centers have ultrasound units assigned to the emergency room. If ultrasound confirms the diagnosis of an aneurysm, further evaluation with CT should be obtained to rule out rupture. Alternatively, a CT may be obtained as the sole imaging study. Any findings consistent with a ruptured aneurysm on CT mandate direct transfer to the operating room and immediate repair. Aggressive fluid resuscitation should be avoided and mild hypotension (i.e., systolic pressure >80 mm Hg) tolerated in conscious patients due to the theoretical potential to cause the aneurysm to rupture into the peritoneal cavity and/or release the tamponade effect of the retroperitoneal tissue. If an intact aneurysm is found on CT without any suggestion of rupture, the next logical question is whether the aneurysm is the source of the pain. Symptomatic aneurysms are likely associated with an increased risk of rupture, although the natural history remains poorly defined. Patients with symptomatic/intact aneurysms greater than or equal to 5 cm in diameter should be admitted to a monitored setting and scheduled for urgent operative repair, usually the following day, provided no additional causes for the pain are identified. Additional sources of the abdominal pain should be sought in patients with aneurysms smaller than 4 cm in light of the small rupture risk. The appropriate treatment for patients with aneurysms 4 to 5 cm is less clear. These aneurysms have the potential to rupture, although the risk is small. It is recommended that these patients be admitted and the source of their pain further investigated. However, urgent operative repair is recommended if no additional causes are identified.

The role of screening for abdominal aortic aneurysms in asymptomatic patients has been partially clarified. The U.S. Preventative Task Force has issued a position statement advocating a single screening ultrasound in males 65 to 75 years of age who have a smoking history.[88] These recommendations were based on the results of a best-evidence systematic review that identified four population-based, randomized, controlled trials demonstrating that screening resulted in a reduction of aneurysm-related mortality.[89] Notably, the Preventative Task Force stated that the literature did not substantiate screening for women even among those with a family history and stated that the harms of screening outweighed the risks. Screening for abdominal aortic aneurysms in this subset of elderly men has been shown to be both cost effective[90] and comparable to other screening programs in adult patients.[91] Despite the Preventative Task Force's recommendations, screening should likely be extended to other high-risk patient populations including patients with a first-degree relative with an abdominal aortic aneurysm, those with evidence of a peripheral artery aneurysm, and those undergoing evaluation for heart transplantation. Medicare currently pays for a single screening ultrasound as part of the Welcome to Medicare physical examination for men who have smoked sometime during their life and for both men and women with a family history of abdominal aortic aneurysms. Interestingly, Kim et al.[92] predicted that the introduction of a national screening program would reduce the number of emergent aneurysm repairs while increasing the number of elective repairs. They estimated that this would translate into two additional elective repairs per month for a typical district, general hospital, while saving 11 abdominal aortic aneurysm–related deaths per year.

OPERATIVE INDICATIONS

All patients with symptomatic or ruptured abdominal aortic aneurysms should undergo operative repair unless they have an underlying medical condition, such as metastatic cancer, that precludes long-term survival or their quality of life is not sufficient to justify the intervention. The latter situation entails a difficult decision, but not offering operative repair should be considered in certain cases (e.g., a debilitated, demented patient in a nursing home) after the family has been consulted.

The operative decision-making process for intact/asymptomatic abdominal aortic aneurysms is a complex one that needs to be tailored to the individual patient. Indeed, there is no single parameter that merits repair. The operative indications are contingent on the size of the aneurysm, life expectancy, comorbidities, preference, and anatomic configuration. It is important to remember that the repair of an intact/asymptomatic abdominal aortic aneurysm is a prophylactic operation that represents a balance between the operative risk and the future risk of rupture with the ultimate treatment goals to prolong life, relieve symptoms, and prevent rupture.

6

The diameter of the abdominal aortic aneurysm is the best predictor of rupture as stated earlier and has been used as the most common indication for repair. There has been a change in the diameter-based operative criteria within the past few decades, although this has been clarified more recently with level 1 evidence. It is interesting to note that the diameter threshold for good-risk patients has decreased from 6 cm to as low as 4 cm with latter recommendation from the guidelines of the national vascular surgical societies.[81] Both the UK Small Aneurysm Trial[39] and the ADAM Trial[26] concluded that it was safe to follow patients with 4.0- to 5.5-cm aneurysms and that early operation did not confer any long-term survival benefit. As noted earlier, the rupture risk for patients in the surveillance group was less than 1% per year. It is important to note that more than 60% of the patients in both studies ultimately underwent operative repair despite their initial randomization. A longer-term follow-up study from the UK Small Aneurysm Trial extending to 12 years did not demonstrate a survival benefit for the patients assigned to early surgery.[93] However, it is important to note that almost all of the patients who survived ultimately required repair since their aneurysms continued to grow and exceed the 5.5-cm threshold. Indeed, the relevant question may not be whether patients with small aneurysm need to be repaired, but rather when they need to be repaired. In a separate publication from the UK Small Aneurysm Trial, Brown et al.[40] reported that the rupture risk for women was over fourfold higher, as noted earlier, suggesting that the 5.5-cm-diameter threshold for repair may be too high for women. The proponents of smaller-diameter-based thresholds for repair (i.e., <5.5 cm) have justified their approach stating that even small aneurysms rupture, aneurysms continue to increase in diameter and will likely need to be repaired, the patients' medical conditions will likely deteriorate with age, and the operative mortality/morbidity rate for small aneurysms may be less. Although the level 1 evidence does not support this lower threshold, it is important to note that the size discrepancy between a 5.2-cm and 5.5-cm aneurysm is very small and likely within the resolution of the imaging study.

The presence of medical comorbidities predictably impacts the perioperative mortality rate and threshold for repair. Steyerberg et al.[94] identified several independent risk factors for operative mortality during open repair (Table 100.2), and these have remained consistent throughout the literature. Similarly, Beck et al.[56] developed a predictive model for both open and endovascular repair using a prospective registry from several northeastern states. They reported that chronic obstructive pulmonary disease, suprarenal aortic clamp, renal insufficiency, and advanced age (≥70) were predictive of mortality at 1 year after open repair, with the mortality ranging from 1% to 67% depending on the number of risk factors. Congestive heart failure and larger aneurysm diameter (≥6.5 cm) were the only predictive factors after endovascular repair, with the mortality ranging from 4% to 23%. The consistent, dramatic impact of renal insufficiency was further emphasized by a national series that reported a ninefold increase in mortality.

TABLE 100.2 **TREATMENT**

INDEPENDENT RISK FACTORS FOR OPERATIVE MORTALITY AFTER ELECTIVE ABDOMINAL AORTIC ANEURYSM REPAIR

RISK FACTOR	ODDS RATIO	95% CI
Creatinine >1.8 mg/dL	3.3	1.5–7.5
Congestive heart failure	2.3	1.1–5.2
ECG ischemia	2.2	1.0–5.1
Pulmonary dysfunction	1.9	1.0–3.8
Older age (per decade)	1.5	1.2–1.8
Female gender	1.5	0.7–3.0

CI, confidence interval; ECG, electrocardiogram.
From Steyerberg EW, Kievit J, de Mol Van Otterloo JC, et al. Perioperative mortality of elective abdominal aortic aneurysm surgery. A clinical prediction rule based on literature and individual patient data. *Arch Intern Med* 1995;155(18):1998–2004.

Notably, the estimated glomerular filtration rate may be a better index of renal function than serum creatinine and, therefore, likely a better predictor of adverse outcome. Life expectancy is inseparable from comorbidities, but it should be emphasized that the average life expectancy for a 60-year-old and 85-year-old man in the United States is 18 and 5 years, respectively.[95]

Patient preference should be factored into the operative decision-making process. Although the level 1 evidence suggests that it is safe to follow abdominal aortic aneurysms until they reach the 5.5-cm threshold, patients may not be willing to accept this small, finite risk and desire to have their aneurysm repaired at a lower threshold. Indeed, patients often echo the justification for early repair proposed by surgeons.

The anatomic configuration of the aneurysm and/or the associated structures should factor into the operative decision-making process. Any technical factors that complicate the repair likely increase the perioperative mortality/morbidity including the need for suprarenal clamp application due to the obligatory renal/visceral ischemia, venous anomalies (e.g., left-sided vena cava), renal anomalies (e.g., horseshoe kidney), and inflammatory aneurysms. Admittedly, many of these technical concerns are relevant only to the open approach and can be overcome/avoided by endovascular repair provided that it is an option from an anatomic standpoint.

The introduction of the endovascular approach has challenged the operative indications for intact/asymptomatic aneurysms. Indeed, the significant decrease in the perioperative mortality rate reported in both the DREAM[52] and EVAR Trials[59] appear to justify lowering the threshold. However, it is important to note that the rupture rate for aneurysms less than 5.5 cm in the UK Small Aneurysm[39] and ADAM[26] Trials was less than 1% per year, which is still lower than the perioperative mortality rate for endovascular repair reported from DREAM,[52] EVAR,[59] and most of the national databases.[57,58,66] Similarly, Finlayson et al.[96] used a decision analysis model to determine the optimal diameter for open and endovascular aneurysm repair and concluded that the endovascular approach lowers the operative threshold only for older patients in poor health.

The Joint Council of the American Association for Vascular Surgery and the Society for Vascular Surgery have released updated guidelines for the treatment of patients with abdominal aortic aneurysms that address the concerns highlighted earlier.[38] They recommend that a diameter of 5.5 cm is an appropriate threshold for repair in the "average patient" with an intact infrarenal aneurysm, but emphasize the importance of individualizing each case. They state that rapid aneurysm

expansion (>1 cm/y), symptoms related to the aneurysm, and female gender merit repair at a smaller diameter, while consideration should be given to earlier repair in young patients provided that the operative mortality rate is acceptable. Furthermore, they recommend that a larger-diameter threshold is appropriate in higher-risk patients and emphasize that there does not appear to be any justification to alter the operative
7 threshold for the endovascular approach. A reasonable approach, and one that we have adopted in our own practice, is to use 5.5 cm as a threshold for repair in men and 5.0 cm for women.

Patients who do not meet the threshold for operative repair should be followed closely. It is important to educate the patients about their underlying disease process and emphasize the importance of long-term follow-up. Notably, Valentine et al.[97] reported that 32% of patients with small aneurysms managed by "watchful waiting" were noncompliant with their follow-up plan. Furthermore, it is important to counsel patients about the presence of symptoms associated with rupture and the importance of seeking urgent medical attention. Recent guidelines have suggested that patients with aneurysms less than 3 cm in diameter should be reimaged at 5 years, while those with aneurysms between 3.0 and 3.4 cm should be reimaged at 3 years and those with aneurysms between 3.5 and 3.9 cm should be reimaged at 1 year.[98] Aneurysms greater than 4.0 cm should likely be reimaged every 6 months. As noted previously, abdominal ultrasound is likely the most appropriate imaging study for aneurysms less than 4.0 cm, with CT more appropriate above that threshold. It is important to note that up to 50% of the patients deemed a prohibitive operative risk and not offered elective repair will ultimately die from a ruptured aneurysm.[99–103] These patients who are not candidates for elective repair should not be offered emergent repair in the event that their aneurysm ruptures or becomes symptomatic.

CHOICE OF OPEN OR ENDOVASCULAR REPAIR

After the decision to recommend operative repair has been made, the technique for the repair needs to be determined. Admittedly, these decisions are somewhat interrelated since the decision to recommend operative repair in certain subsets of patients is oftentimes contingent upon whether they are candidates for the endovascular approach. The past two decades have witnessed a rapid evolution of the endovascular technique, and, indeed, this evolution has helped define our discipline. It has been clearly demonstrated that the technical success rates for endovascular graft repair are excellent and the need for intraoperative conversion to open repair negligible. The perioperative events and midterm outcomes have been defined by level 1 evidence. Many of the technical limitations inherent to the earlier endovascular devices and anatomic limitations have been overcome. Despite the lack of definitive long-term outcome data, the endovascular approach for treatment of abdominal aortic aneurysms has been widely applied. Indeed, 56% of all aneurysm repairs in the United States during 2005 were performed using the endovascular approach.[77] The choice of open or endovascular repair is complicated and contingent upon several factors including feasibility, outcome, comorbidities, compliance, cost, and preference. It is imperative that these issues, including their respective advantages/disadvantages or strengths/weaknesses, be addressed with the patients during the decision process to ensure proper informed consent.

The initial determinant of the approach is the anatomic configuration of the aorta, the aneurysm, and the access vessels. The commercially available endovascular devices come in a finite range of sizes and, thus, are suitable only if specific anatomic conditions are satisfied. Although the number of available devices and their specific characteristics are constantly evolving, the "generic" endograft consists of a fabric graft (i.e., polyester or expanded polytetrafluoroethylene) and a metallic endo/exoskeleton (i.e., stainless steel or nitinol) that facilitates proximal/distal fixation by the radial force of the stent (Fig. 100.7). In some devices, the proximal fixation is augmented by the presence of suprarenal hooks. The "generic" devices are modular and consist of either two (main body and contralateral iliac limb) or three (main body, contralateral iliac limb, and ipsilateral iliac limb) components with a variety of additional ancillary pieces that allow proximal or distal extensions at the aortic and iliac ends, respectively. The initial experiences with aortoaortic or "tube graft" configurations were unsuccessful due to problems with the distal landing site at the aortic bifurcation and have been abandoned. Indeed, the current strategy is to seat the proximal component of the bifurcated system as close to the lowest renal artery as possible and the distal components as close to the iliac bifurcation as possible. Although there is some variability among the commercially available devices in terms of their specific sizes and anatomic constraints, the general anatomic requirements are similar. The infrarenal abdominal aorta must have a suitable, nonaneurysmal landing zone for the endograft, while the diameter of the aorta at that location should be greater than or equal to 15 mm in length and greater than or equal to 17 to 19 mm, but less than or equal to 26 to 32 mm in diameter (ranges reflect differences between the commercial devices). Furthermore, the proximal neck angle should be less than or equal to 45 degrees as measured by the intersection of the centerline of the infrarenal aorta at the landing zone site and the centerline of the aneurysm through the aortic bifurcation. The infrarenal neck should be relatively free of thrombus and calcification to facilitate a seal at the implantation site. It is notable that neck length requirements have increased from greater than or equal to 1 cm to greater than or equal to 1.5 cm since release of the original devices at the turn of the century. Indeed, the longer the infrarenal neck length and, therefore, the longer the device seal zone, the better. The iliac artery should have a suitable landing zone greater than or equal to 20 mm with an associated diameter between 7 and 20 mm to facilitate both anchoring the graft and passing the main device into the aorta. The distal landing zone for the iliac limbs is usually in the common iliac artery, although the anatomic constraints with regard to the size of the access vessels and the introduction of the devices are relevant for both the common and external iliac vessels.

The percentage of patients who are anatomically suitable for an endograft remains unresolved and is likely contingent upon the nature of the individual surgeon/institution practice and the available devices. This percentage of suitable patients has been highly variable with reports of 30% in a nationwide series,[104] 55% in a regional series,[105] and 14% to 66% in institutional series.[106–108] Notably, the reasons cited for exclusion include a short infrarenal neck (54%), inadequate iliac vessels (47%), and a wide infrarenal neck (40%).[106]

A variety of techniques have been described to overcome the anatomic limitations of the endovascular approach, thereby extending its feasibility. Indeed, some modification has been described to overcome almost every anatomic contraindication. Stenoses within the access vessels can be overcome by dilation (i.e., balloon angioplasty, serial dilators) or by the use of a prosthetic conduit.[109] The prosthetic conduit is usually anastomosed to the bifurcation of the common iliac artery and then tunneled through the retroperitoneal space below the inguinal ligament. Alternatively, an aortouniiliac endograft can be configured and a femorofemoral bypass performed. Notably, the patency rates of the femorofemoral bypass graft in this setting have been reported to be excellent.[110,111] Aneurysmal degeneration of the common iliac artery can be overcome by a variety of techniques including simply using larger-diameter graft limbs, using an aortic extension as a cuff (i.e., "bell bottom" technique), occluding/embolizing the internal iliac artery and seating the iliac limb in the external iliac

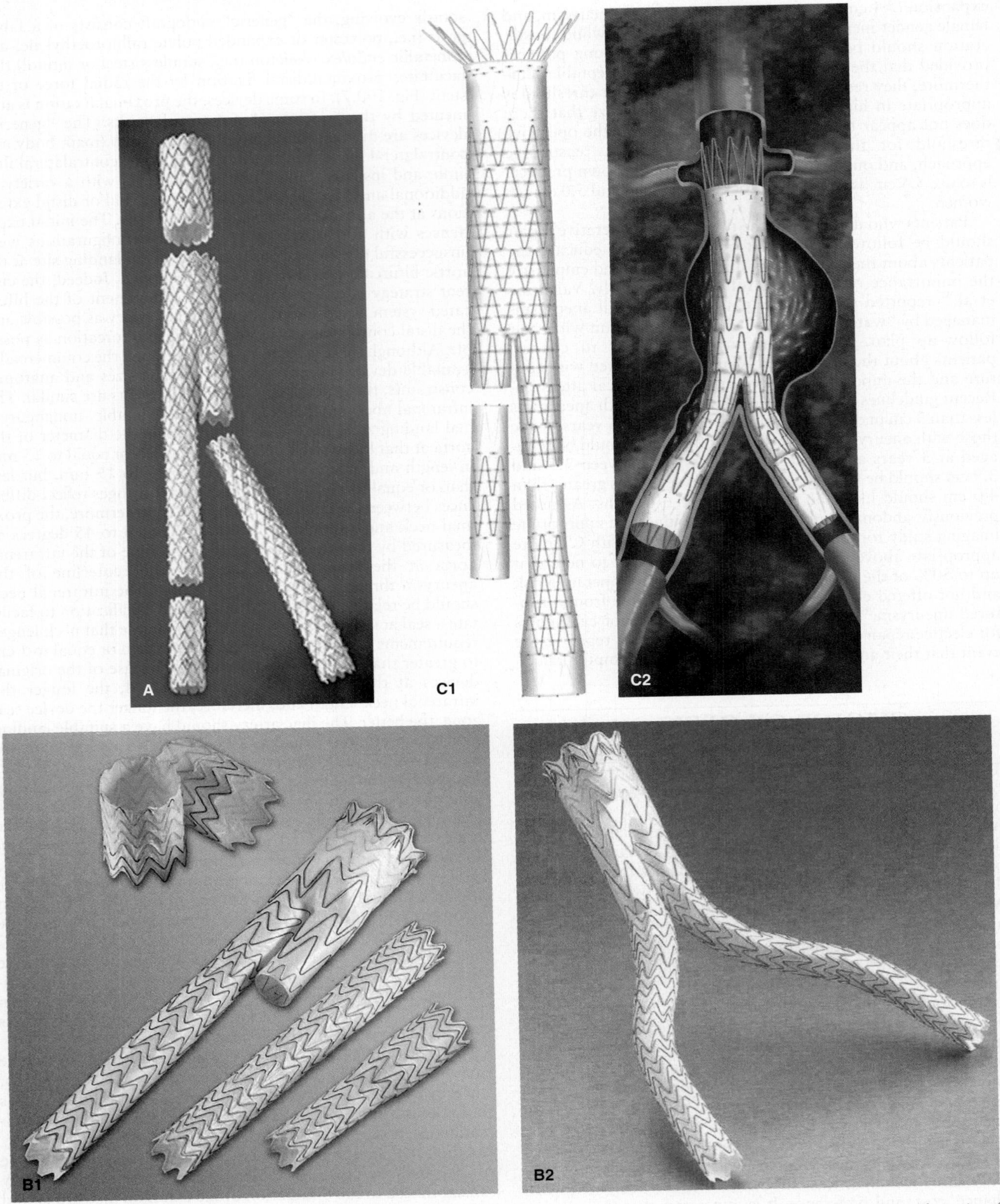

FIGURE 100.7. The commercially available endografts are shown: (A) AneuRx; (B) Excluder; (C) Zenith. All three are similar and consist of a fabric graft (polyester or expanded polytetrafluoroethylene) and a metallic exoskeleton (stainless steel or nitinol) that facilitate proximal/distal fixation by radial force with or without hooks. They are modular devices consisting of either two (main body and contralateral iliac limb) or three (main body, contralateral iliac limb, and ipsilateral iliac limb) components with a variety of additional ones that allow proximal or distal extensions at the aortic and iliac ends, respectively.

artery, or bypassing the internal iliac artery and seating the iliac limb in the external iliac artery. Although relatively simple to perform, internal iliac artery embolization has been associated with a moderate incidence of complications including buttock/thigh claudication (30% to 40%), sexual dysfunction, neurologic deficit/paraplegia, pelvic ischemia, and gluteal compartment syndrome.[112,113] The claudication improves with time in the majority of patients but can be quite debilitating, particularly in patients who did not claudicate preoperatively. Many of the other complications, although somewhat rare, are irreversible and can be catastrophic. Because of these concerns, bilateral internal iliac artery occlusion/embolization should likely be avoided. Bypass of the internal iliac artery overcomes many of these limitations and has been associated with excellent results in terms of long-term graft patency, although the procedure is somewhat challenging and adds significantly to the overall magnitude of the "less invasive" procedure.[109] Unfortunately, extending the indications for endovascular repair beyond those recommended by the manufacturers (i.e., instructions for use [IFU]) has been associated with an increase in the incidence of adverse events including decreased survival and a higher need for reintervention.[114]

Consideration of the perioperative and long-term outcomes after endovascular aneurysm repair requires introduction of the concepts of endoleak and endotension. Simply, endoleak is the perfusion of the aneurysm sac outside the lumen of the endograft, while endotension is the persistent pressurization within the excluded aneurysm sac. Endoleaks have been classified as types 1 through 4 based on the mechanism of the leak (Fig. 100.8). Type 1 leaks originate at either the proximal or

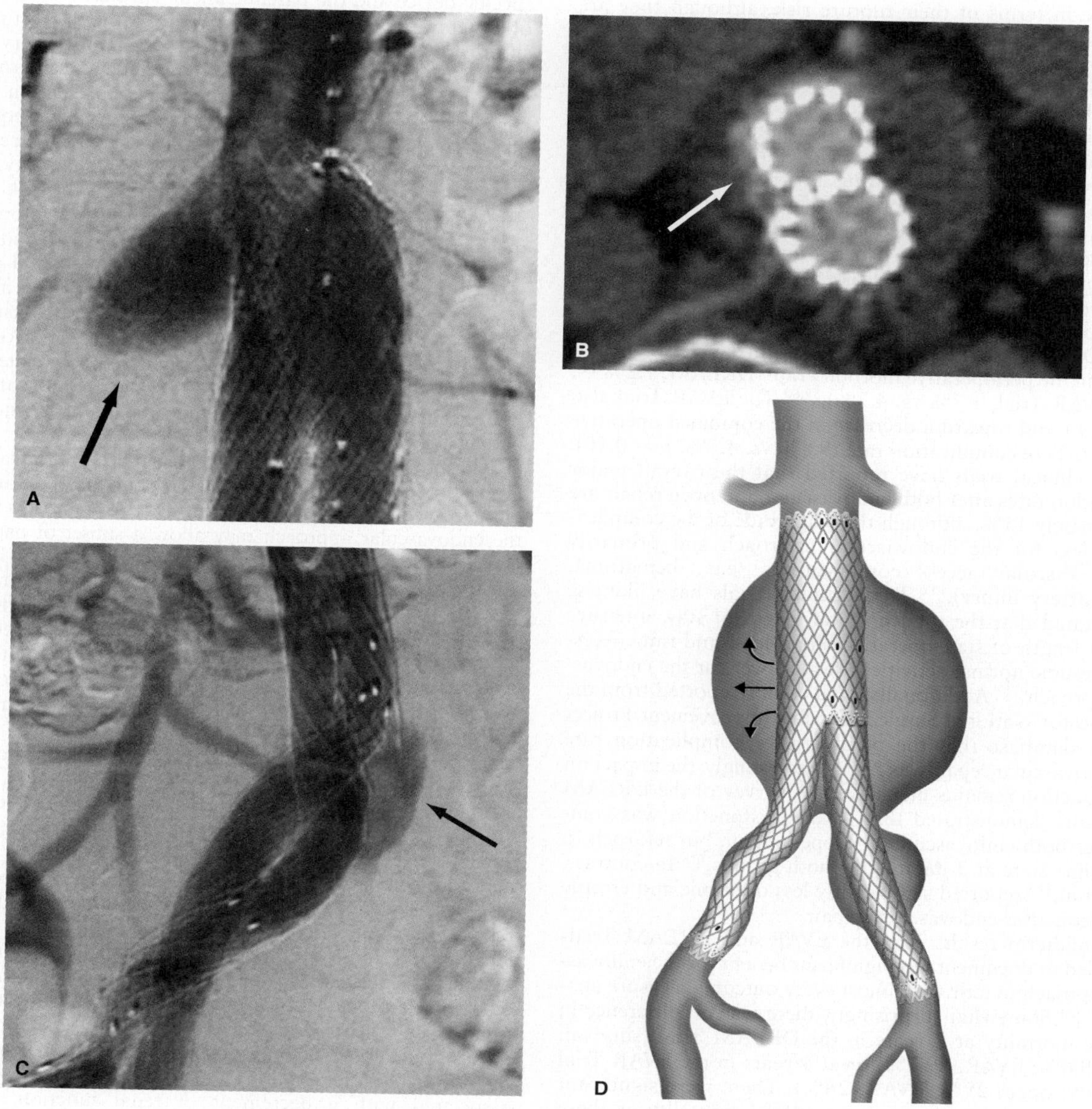

FIGURE 100.8. The various endoleaks are demonstrated. A: Type 1 leaks originate at either the proximal or distal attachment sites. Note the large blush of contrast outside of the graft lumen at the proximal fixation site. B: Type 2 leaks are from the collateral circulation originating in the lumbar or inferior mesenteric arteries. Note the contrast-filled limbs of the graft and the rim of contrast outside the limbs of the graft, but within the lumen of the aorta. The other computed tomography images demonstrated that the leak originated from the inferior mesenteric artery. C: Type 3 leaks are caused by fabric tears or problems at the graft interfaces of the modular devices. Note the contrast blush outside of the lumen of the graft at the modular interface. D: Type 4 leaks are usually transient (<24 hours) trans-graft extravasations and can result from the porosity of the graft and needle holes.

distal attachment sites. Type 2 leaks come from branch vessels such as the lumbar or inferior mesenteric arteries. Type 3 leaks are caused by fabric tears or problems at the graft interfaces of the modular devices, whereas type 4 leaks are usually transient (<24 hours) trans-graft extravasations that result from the porosity of the graft and needle holes. It should be emphasized that the entire concept of an endoleak is predicated on the ability to detect contrast or blood flow outside the lumen of the endograft and is, therefore, contingent on the sensitivity and specificity of the various imaging techniques. The major concern about both endoleaks and endotension is that the pressure transmitted to the aneurysm wall may cause the aneurysm to expand and/or rupture. The clinical significance of the various endoleak types is different. Both type 1 and 3 endoleaks are considered major adverse outcomes associated with an increased risk of rupture, and they merit urgent/emergent treatment.[115] Type 2 endoleaks are generally considered less worrisome in terms of their rupture risk, although they are associated with an increased risk for reintervention.[115] They can generally be followed with serial imaging studies, but merit evaluation/intervention if the aneurysm sac continues to enlarge. Type 4 endoleaks are self-limited and benign. The clinical significance of endotension is likewise unresolved. Indeed, the concept itself is somewhat ambiguous given the limitations of actually measuring the pressure within the aneurysm sac. It should be noted that freedom from endoleak does not necessarily mean freedom from endotension given the observation that aneurysms can continue to enlarge in the absence of an identifiable endoleak.[116]

The *perioperative* complication rates appear to be lower after endovascular repair. As noted earlier, the randomized controlled DREAM and EVAR Trials reported a significant decrease in the perioperative mortality rate (DREAM, 1.2% vs. 4.6%; EVAR Trial, 1.7% vs. 4.7%).[59,60] The EVAR Trial also reported a trend toward a decrease in the combined operative mortality/*severe* complication rate (9.8% vs. 4.7%, $p = 0.10$). Multiple clinical trials have reported that the overall major complication rates after both endovascular and open repair are approximately 15%, although the magnitude of the complications is less for the endovascular approach and primarily includes vascular access complications (e.g., hematoma, femoral artery injury).[117] These clinical trials have likewise demonstrated that the total hospital length of stay, intensive care unit length of stay, operative blood loss, and time necessary to resume normal activities are all lower for the endovascular approach.[117] Additionally, Hua et al.[57] reported from the private-sector National Surgical Quality Improvement Project (NSQIP) database that the perioperative complication rate after endovascular repair was 24%. Interestingly, the impact on sexual function remains unresolved. A survey of the DREAM participants demonstrated that sexual dysfunction was common after both endovascular and open repair, but returned to the baseline state at 3 months for both groups.[118] In contrast, Xenos et al.[119] reported significantly less orgasmic and erectile dysfunction after endovascular repair.

The midterm results after the EVAR and DREAM Trials have failed to document any significant benefit for the endovascular approach in terms of almost every outcome measure analyzed.[120,121] Somewhat surprisingly, there was no difference in all-cause mortality at 2 years in the DREAM Trial (survival: open, 89.6%; EVAR, 89.7%) or at 4 years in the EVAR Trial (mortality: open, 29%; EVAR, 26%). There were significant differences in terms of aneurysm-related mortality at these time points, although the differences were fairly minimal and their relevance suspect. Both the complication rates (EVAR, 41%; open, 9%) and costs (EVAR, £13,257; open, £9,926) were significantly greater for the endovascular approach, while there were negligible differences in the quality of life assessments.[120,122,123]

The midterm results from the DREAM and EVAR Trials have been somewhat sobering, and longer-term outcomes are necessary to further define the role of the endovascular approach. It is clear that the endovascular approach is not as secure a repair as the traditional, open alternative. The endovascular repair is associated with ongoing rupture risk that likely approaches 1% per year.[117,124] Notably, Schermerhorn et al.[58] reported a 1.8% rupture risk among Medicare patients undergoing endovascular repair between 2001 and 2004. The rupture risk has been associated with poor patient selection, operator error, unrecognized/untreated endoleaks, large aneurysms, and device migration.[117,125] Interestingly, the mortality rate associated with rupture after endovascular repair may be less than for de novo ruptures.[126] Approximately 10% to 20% of patients develop an endoleak during the first year after endovascular repair.[127–129] Admittedly, not all of these require remediation. The excluded aneurysms can continue to grow and, thereby, represent a risk for rupture. This has been correlated not only with the presence of endoleak as noted earlier but also with the specific device and the baseline aneurysm size.[130,131] Some type of structural failure including fabric tears, hook fractures, and suture breakage has been reported for almost every device. Design modifications have been implemented to overcome many of these deficiencies, although they represent an ongoing concern that may not be manifest for years. As a consequence of all these potential limitations, reintervention is necessary in about 15% of the patients per year.[58,128] The majority of these remedial procedures are catheter based with the risk of open conversion approximately 1% to 2% per year.[124] Unfortunately, the perioperative complication rate for conversion likely exceeds that for open repair as might be predicted given its complexity. It is important to emphasize that open aneurysm repair is associated with a small incidence of graft-related complications and need for remedial procedures. Approximately 2% of patients undergoing open repair require reintervention within the first 5 years,[38] while graft-related complications and graft-related deaths have been reported in 15% and 2% of patients, respectively, at 15 years.[58,132]

The presence of significant comorbidities and advanced age favors the endovascular approach. Although the operative threshold in regard to the aneurysm diameter measurement is the same, the endovascular approach may allow a subset of patients not considered suitable candidates for an open operation to have their aneurysms repaired. Indeed, endovascular aneurysm repair has been shown to be feasible in patients with hepatic insufficiency[133] and consistently safe in octogenarians.[134,135] However, a modicum of clinical judgment is necessary. It is important to reemphasize that abdominal aortic aneurysm repairs are prophylactic operations and that not every patient merits treatment. The EVAR Trial 2 randomized patients not fit for open repair to expectant management or endovascular repair and demonstrated no difference in aneurysm-related mortality, all-cause mortality, or quality of life.[122] Notably, the patients were truly "high risk," with a perioperative mortality rate of 9% and a 4-year mortality rate of almost 40%. Despite the potential nephrotoxicity associated with iodinated contrast, chronic renal insufficiency is not an absolute contraindication to endovascular repair. Strategies to reduce the associated risk can be employed including the administration of acetylcysteine and sodium bicarbonate.[82,83] Alternatively, the procedure can be performed without contrast altogether by using intravascular ultrasound. Unfortunately, chronic renal insufficiency is a significant risk factor for adverse outcome after both open and endovascular repair. Furthermore, multiple studies have shown that both approaches are associated with a decrement of renal function.[136–139] The endovascular approach may be associated with a greater decrement of function postoperatively, but the findings are somewhat equivocal; suprarenal fixation of the endovascular device does not seem to be associated with a greater decrement.[139]

8 The known device-related complications and the uncertainty about the long-term outcome after endovascular repair mandate indefinite surveillance. It is imperative that patients comply with the prescribed protocol, and their ability or desire

to fulfill these expectations should be factored into the specific choice of procedure. It is important to note that although the incidence of complications declines with the number of negative postoperative CT scans, new endoleaks have been discovered out as far as 7 years. Similarly, it is imperative that all surgeons who offer endovascular aneurysm repair provide conscientious, long-term follow-up.

The cost comparisons between the open and endovascular approach have been somewhat inconclusive, although the endovascular approach is likely more expensive. Clearly, the EVAR-1, and EVAR-2 Trials have demonstrated that the endovascular approach was more expensive.[120,122] The shorter hospital length of stay and lower incidence of major complications associated with the endovascular approach have predictably resulted in a reduction in some of the hospital costs. However, these have been offset by increases in other hospital-related costs, with the cost of the device itself representing the single largest item. Notably, Sternbergh and Money[140] reported that the cost of the device accounted for 52% of the total cost of the endovascular repair and estimated that the costs of open and endovascular repair were $12,546 and $19,985, respectively, in the AneuRx Phase II clinical trial. Analysis of the hospital costs and reimbursement associated with endovascular repair among seven medical centers (university hospital, three; community hospital, four) demonstrated a net loss of $2,162.[140,141] However, others have reported that the contribution to the hospital margin on a daily basis may be superior for endovascular repair given the associated shorter duration of stay that permits higher throughput, fuller overhead amortization, and better use of inpatient beds.[142] It is important to note that most of the analyses have focused on the hospital- and device-related costs, but have failed to include the associated professional fees and the costs associated with long-term follow-up that may be quite substantial. Kim et al.[143] reported that reimbursement for the endovascular repair is not sufficient for the long-term surveillance and secondary procedures. Indeed, it has been reported that the overall cost of endovascular repair may be twice that of the open approach.[117]

9 Despite the various advantages and disadvantages of the approaches outlined previously, patients and providers seem to prefer the endovascular approach, and these preferences appear to be one of the driving forces for the widespread application of the technique. Indeed, it is uncommon for patients who are candidates for either approach to elect open repair. Notably, Williamson et al.[144] reported that 18% of all patients undergoing open repair would not undergo the procedure again. The potential to perform the endovascular repair completely percutaneously (i.e., no femoral artery exposure) clearly adds to the appeal of the approach.[145,146] It is interesting to note that these patient preferences may not be sustained. A follow-up study from the DREAM Trial reported that patients undergoing endovascular repair had a better quality of life initially, but those undergoing open repair had a better quality at 6 months and beyond.[118]

The proverbial "bottom line" for the open versus endovascular debate remains unresolved. The Joint Council of the American Association for Vascular Surgery and the Society for Vascular Surgery have recommended that endovascular repair is most appropriate for patients at increased risk for open repair because of its uncertain long-term durability and need for surveillance.[38] The subset of patients at increased risk includes older, sicker patients and those with other mitigating anatomic concerns such as the proverbial "hostile abdomen." The recommendations further emphasize that extending the limits of the endovascular approach to patients who are poor anatomic candidates increases the incidence of adverse outcome. Similarly, the Agency for Healthcare Research Quality conducted an evidence-based review and concluded that endovascular repair for aneurysms greater than 5.5 cm did not improve patient survival or health status relative to open repair despite the fact that the perioperative outcomes were improved.[147] Furthermore, they reported that the endovascular approach was associated with increased cost, complications, need for surveillance, and need for remedial procedures. Lastly, they concluded that it did not provide a benefit for patients unfit for open repair.

OPERATIVE REPAIR

Preoperative Evaluation

The preoperative evaluation of patients undergoing elective abdominal aortic aneurysm repair is similar to that of patients undergoing any major general or vascular surgical procedure. Patients undergoing endovascular repair should likely undergo the same preoperative workup despite the perception that associated perioperative stresses are less. All patients should receive a complete history and a physical examination, an electrocardiogram, and a chest radiograph. Routine laboratory studies, including a complete blood cell count with platelets, serum electrolytes/creatinine, and coagulation studies, should be obtained. A specimen should be sent to the blood bank and the appropriate quantity of blood products cross matched. This number can be determined from the historic operative transfusion requirements obtained from the blood bank, but usually 2 to 4 units of packed red blood cells are sufficient. A thorough peripheral pulse examination should be included in the physical examination and validated with formal ankle-brachial indices. The anesthesiologist should see the patients preoperatively, and a bowel preparation with mechanical lavage should be performed the day before surgery. Additionally, patients should be started on a beta-blocker, an aspirin, and a statin (3-hydroxy-3-methylglutaryl [HMG]-CoA reductase inhibitors) agent if they are not already on them. The American College of Cardiology (ACC)/American Heart Association (AHA) Guidelines on Perioperative Cardiovascular Evaluation and Care for Noncardiac Surgery recommend that the beta-blockers should be given to vascular surgery patients who are at high cardiac risk and probably should be given to those undergoing vascular surgery with more than one clinical risk factor (risk factors: coronary artery disease, congestive heart failure, cerebral vascular occlusive disease (CVOD), diabetes mellitus, chronic renal insufficiency).[148] Furthermore, the ACC/AHA Guidelines recommend that patients undergoing vascular surgery should be on a statin. Notably, a recent study demonstrated that statins were associated with a decreased incidence of perioperative mortality and nonfatal myocardial infarction after aneurysm repair.[149] Indeed, all patients with atherosclerotic cardiovascular disease should likely be on aspirin, beta-blockers, a lipid-lowering agent, and an angiotensin-converting enzyme (ACE) inhibitor long term as part of the AHA/ACC Guidelines for Preventing Heart Attack and Death in Patients with Atherosclerotic Cardiovascular Disease.[150]

All active medical problems, including abnormalities identified during the preoperative evaluation, should be controlled as well as possible before elective aneurysm repair. However, extensive diagnostic testing is probably unnecessary. Routine pulmonary function tests and measurement of arterial blood gases are not indicated, although they may be beneficial in selected patients with advanced chronic obstructive pulmonary disease.[151] The presence of chronic obstructive pulmonary disease often complicates postoperative ventilator management, but it is unusual for a patient's pulmonary disease to be sufficiently severe to preclude operation.[152] Similarly, timed urine collections for creatinine clearance and other assessments of renal function have not proved beneficial despite the dramatic impact of preoperative renal insufficiency on perioperative outcome, although it may be beneficial to calculate the estimated glomerular filtration rate.

The appropriate cardiac workup before abdominal aortic aneurysm repair is evolving and is somewhat institution dependent. This controversy has been further complicated by the publication of the Coronary Artery Revascularization Prophylaxis (CARP) Trial that examined the role of coronary artery revascularization before major vascular surgery among patients with significant coronary artery disease.[153] Notably, the study reported that preoperative coronary artery revascularization did not reduce the incidence of either perioperative myocardial infarction or long-term mortality. It is important to emphasize that the overall objective of the preoperative cardiac workup is to optimize the cardiovascular system and thereby reduce both the perioperative and long-term risk of myocardial infarction and death. Admittedly, the prevalence of coronary artery disease among patients undergoing abdominal aortic aneurysm repair is quite high. Hertzer et al.,[154] in a landmark publication, reported that 25% of 1,000 patients undergoing evaluation for peripheral vascular surgery (cerebral vascular occlusive disease, lower extremity arterial occlusive disease, abdominal aortic aneurysm) had severe, surgically correctable lesions detected during cardiac catheterization; 6% had severe, uncorrectable disease; and only 8% had no evidence of disease. Interestingly, the incidence of surgically correctable disease was highest among patients undergoing evaluation for abdominal aortic aneurysm. The most recent edition of the ACC/AHA Guidelines have simplified the preoperative evaluation before elective vascular procedures.[148] Briefly, patients with active cardiac conditions (unstable coronary syndromes, decompensated congestive heart failure, significant arrhythmias, and significant valvular disease) should be seen in consultation by a cardiologist. Patients with good functional capacity as defined by the ability to generate at least 4 metabolic equivalents (METS, 4 METS = ability to walk up a flight of stairs) can undergo major vascular procedures without additional testing. Those patients that cannot generate 4 METS and have at least three clinical risk factors (see earlier) should be considered for further cardiac testing if the results will change the clinical management. Notably, there is insufficient evidence to support a reduced cardiac workup for patients undergoing endovascular repair.[155] It is important to emphasize that although the cardiac risk of endovascular repair may be less, the subset of patients undergoing the procedure are often older and sicker.

All patients should undergo some type of imaging modality as part of their preoperative evaluation to confirm the diagnosis and plan the procedure. Indeed, determining whether a patient is an endovascular candidate and appropriately sizing the device depend on the anatomic measurements obtained at the time of imaging. A CT arteriogram of the chest, abdomen, and pelvis is the optimal imaging study to visualize the aneurysm and is the only one required in most cases. Abdominal ultrasonography is insufficient as the sole imaging study before aneurysm repair in light of its inability to accurately define the cephalad extent of the aneurysm and the involvement of the iliac vessels.

Open Repair of Intact Abdominal Aortic Aneurysms

Technique. A significant amount of preparation is required in the operating room before making the incision, and this preparation needs to be coordinated among the surgical and anesthetic teams for both the open and endovascular approach. Although the decision about the choice of anesthesia is deferred to the anesthesiologists, inhalation agents and an endotracheal tube are used most frequently. Adjunctive epidural anesthesia may improve postoperative pain control[156] and may be beneficial in patients with severe pulmonary disease.[157] Adequate intravenous access should be established to facilitate resuscitation. Central venous access is usually obtained although not necessary. Electrocardiographic leads, an arterial catheter, and a Foley catheter should be placed for continuous monitoring of the electrocardiogram, arterial pressure, and urine output, respectively. Additionally, a nasogastric tube should be inserted. A Swan-Ganz pulmonary artery catheter or a transesophageal echocardiogram probe should be inserted in patients with significant cardiac disease. However, routine use of pulmonary artery catheters in patients undergoing aortic surgery is not recommended and may be associated with a higher rate of intraoperative complications.[158,159] Peripheral arterial pulses should be interrogated with either palpation or continuous wave Doppler ultrasound and marked to facilitate confirmation after restoration of lower extremity perfusion. Strategies to maintain core body temperature should be initiated.[158,160] Specifically, the room temperature should be increased, warming devices should be attached to all intravenous infusion lines, and either a recirculating alcohol blanket or forced-air blanket should be applied. Bush et al.[161] reported that hypothermia (<34.5°C) during abdominal aortic aneurysm repair was associated with multiple physiologic derangements and adverse outcomes. Use of an intraoperative autologous transfusion device should be considered. However, a recent meta-analysis of five randomized controlled trials reported that there is insufficient evidence to recommend its use during vascular surgery, including aortic surgery.[162] These devices should likely be used when a significant amount of blood loss is anticipated such as during suprarenal or thoracoabdominal aortic aneurysm repairs. Furthermore, they can be helpful in patients who object to blood transfusions on religious principles. An extensive operative field from "nipples to toes" should be prepared with the use of topical antimicrobial agents. A first-generation cephalosporin or vancomycin should be administered prior to the incision.

Abdominal aortic aneurysms may be repaired through several different incisions or approaches including midline, retroperitoneal, or transverse (supraumbilical straight, infraumbilical straight, infraumbilical curvilinear, bilateral subcostal). The incisions or approaches must be viewed as complementary since neither is perfect for every clinical scenario. Indeed, surgeons should be familiar with the various approaches and select the optimal one for the clinical setting. The determinants of the incision include the cephalad/caudal extent of the aneurysm, body habitus, presence of prior abdominal incisions, presence of abdominal wall stomas, comorbidities, additional intraoperative pathology, inflammatory aneurysms, renal anomalies, requirements for concomitant procedures, urgency of aortic control, and surgeon preference. The midline approach is preferable for patients with ruptured abdominal aortic aneurysms because aortic control at the level of the diaphragm can be obtained rapidly. The bilateral subcostal approach provides the best exposure and is the incision of choice for obese patients, those with extensive iliac artery aneurysms, those requiring concomitant renal artery revascularization, and those with juxtarenal aneurysms that require suprarenal aortic control. The retroperitoneal approach is optimal for patients with multiple previous abdominal incisions ("hostile abdomen"), abdominal wall stomas, suprarenal aneurysms, inflammatory aneurysms, and horseshoe kidneys. However, the retroperitoneal approach is limited by the inability to assess the intraperitoneal structures and the limited access to the right renal artery and right iliac vessels. It was previously contended that the retroperitoneal approach posed less of a physiologic insult than the transperitoneal approach and, therefore, was ideal for patients with advanced pulmonary or cardiac disease. However, this has not been supported by a prospective randomized trial.[163] A detailed description of the retroperitoneal approach is beyond the context of this chapter but is available in most standard vascular surgical texts.

The sequence of steps used to repair an intact, infrarenal abdominal aortic aneurysm after a bilateral subcostal incision can be summarized (Fig. 100.9). The abdomen is explored after the peritoneal cavity is entered, and both the gallbladder and colon are carefully examined. The lower abdominal wall

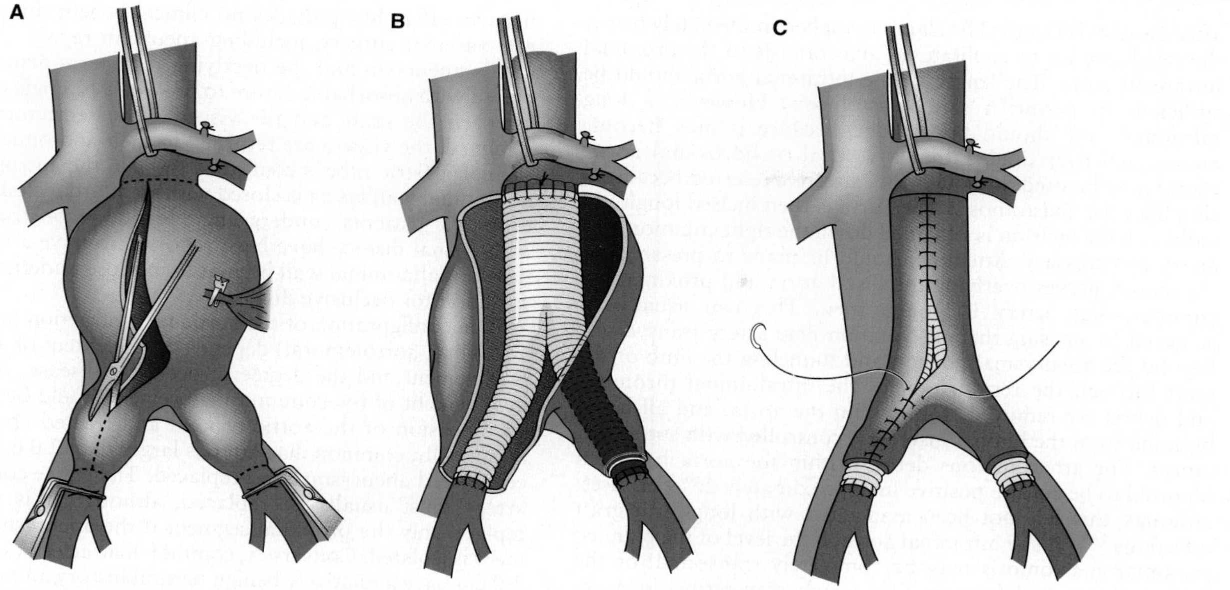

FIGURE 100.9. Steps involved in the standard repair of an infrarenal abdominal aortic aneurysm extending into the proximal common iliac arteries. **A:** The proximal duodenum is mobilized and the retroperitoneum overlying the aorta incised. The infrarenal aorta immediately below the renal vein is dissected. The iliac bifurcations are exposed, and vascular clamps are applied to the infrarenal aorta and distal common iliac arteries after adequate heparinization. A longitudinal arteriotomy is extended from the infrarenal aorta onto the right common iliac artery. **B:** Back-bleeding from the lumbar arteries is controlled with figure-of-eight sutures. The proximal anastomosis is performed in an end-to-end configuration below the renal arteries. The distal anastomoses are performed at the common iliac bifurcation beyond the aneurysmal segments. The left limb of the graft is tunneled through the intact left common iliac aneurysm shell. **C:** The residual aneurysm shell is closed over the prosthetic graft, and the retroperitoneum is reapproximated to prevent erosion of the graft into the overlying bowel.

flap is immobilized to either the drapes or the pubic towel with the use of penetrating towel clips. The small bowel is manually retracted laterally to the right, and the duodenum is mobilized by incising the ligament of Treitz. The inferior mesenteric vein may be suture-ligated at this juncture to facilitate exposure. The tissue adjacent to the inferior mesenteric vein should be palpated to rule out a large, meandering mesenteric artery. This artery is an important visceral collateral and should be preserved. The retroperitoneum over the aorta is incised with electrocautery, and the left renal vein is exposed. Self-retaining Buckwalter retractors are then placed to facilitate further exposure. The small bowel is placed in a bowel bag, eviscerated, and retracted laterally to the right with the aid of malleable retractors for the Buckwalter. The transverse colon and superior abdominal wall flap are retracted cephalad while the lower abdominal wall is further retracted caudal. The aorta immediately inferior to the renal arteries is exposed and both renal arteries visualized. The infrarenal aorta at this location is dissected circumferentially to facilitate placement of a transverse aortic clamp. However, this step may be omitted if a vertical clamp is used. It is important to identify the course of the renal vein and any venous anomalies on the preoperative CT scan to prevent inadvertently injuring these structures at this stage of the procedure. In the presence of a retroaortic renal vein or circumaortic collar, the aortic neck should not be dissected circumferentially and vascular control should be obtained with a vertical clamp. The retroperitoneum over the aorta is then incised further caudally and the incision extended along the course of the right common iliac artery. The extent of the caudal dissection depends on the anatomic configuration of the aneurysm. If the aneurysm extends to the aortic bifurcation, it is sufficient to dissect only the common iliac arteries provided a suitable site for clamp application is identified. If the aneurysm extends to the distal common iliac arteries, both the internal and external iliac vessels should be dissected free. This may be facilitated on the left side by mobilizing the sigmoid colon along its peritoneal reflection and reflecting it medially. The inferior mesenteric artery is then dissected free and vascular control obtained with a vessel loop. Patients are administered 100 units of intravenous heparin per kilogram, and the activated clotting time is confirmed to be twice the baseline value. Supplemental doses of heparin are administered throughout the procedure as dictated by the activated clotting time. Interestingly, a recent randomized controlled trial reported that heparin does not reduce thrombotic events or increase bleeding during aneurysm repair but is associated with a significant reduction in myocardial events.[164]

During the time required for adequate mixing of the heparin, the availability of the necessary equipment is reviewed and confirmed with the operating room personnel. The appropriately sized prosthetic graft is selected. The graft diameter is sized according to the infrarenal aortic neck by visual inspection or with the calibrated graft rulers (i.e. "sizers"). The general "rule of thumb" is that the smaller graft should be selected when the aorta is between two graft sizes because the aorta always appears smaller after it is transected and redundant graft material at the proximal anastomosis is more difficult to correct than the opposite problem. A variety of vascular prostheses are available. Despite the contentions of the various manufacturers, there is no clear advantage for an individual graft and the choice should be determined by surgeon preference as dictated by ease of handling, cost, availability, and requirements for preclotting. The distal vascular clamps are applied to the external, internal, or common iliac vessels depending on the extent of the aneurysm and the character of the vessels. Occasionally, the iliac vessels are so calcified that they cannot be safely occluded with a clamp. Vascular control may be obtained intraluminally in this setting with the use of a balloon thromboembolectomy catheter after the aneurysm has been incised. The proximal aortic clamp is applied in sequence after the distal clamps. The clamp is applied immediately below the renal arteries to facilitate an anastomosis to the proximal infrarenal aorta. The length of the infrarenal aorta should be sufficient to permit a safe anastomosis. However, a long infrarenal cuff should be avoided because it may become aneurysmal over time. Either a vertical or horizontal aortic clamp may be used, although the latter is preferred because it simplifies the anastomosis. The aorta is then incised longitudinally, and the incision is extended down the right common iliac artery as necessary. Attempts should be made to preserve the autonomic nerves overlying the distal aorta and proximal left common iliac artery in potent men. This can usually be achieved by incising the left common iliac artery transversely beyond the aneurysmal portion and tunneling the limb of the graft through the residual shell. The intraluminal thrombus and debris are removed from within the aorta, and all backbleeding from the lumbar arteries is controlled with suture ligatures. The atheromatous debris within the aorta has been reported to be culture positive in approximately 25% of cases, although this has not been associated with long-term graft infections.[165,166] The infrarenal aorta at the level of the planned proximal anastomosis may be completely transected, or the back wall may be left intact. Completely transecting the aorta makes the proximal anastomoses slightly easier, although leaving the back wall intact reinforces the anastomosis and provides the equivalent of an autogenous pledget. The proximal anastomosis is performed in an end-to-end configuration with a running 3–0 cardiovascular suture. All leaks in the suture line are repaired with similar 5–0 sutures and felt pledgets as necessary. The distal anastomosis or anastomoses are performed to the aortic bifurcation, common iliac arteries, or iliac bifurcation as dictated by the anatomy of the aneurysm. A 3–0 cardiovascular suture is used for anastomoses at the aortic bifurcation, and a similar 4–0 suture is used for the common iliac arteries. All anastomoses are flushed to remove any intraluminal debris before flow is restored. Blood flow is restored to the pelvis and lower extremities in sequence. Attempts should be made to flush initially into the internal iliac circulation to prevent embolization to the lower extremities. This can be facilitated by manually compressing the common femoral arteries for tube graft configurations. The lower torso should be reperfused gradually (i.e., one vessel at a time and one extremity at a time) to prevent hypotension and other acute sequelae associated with the reperfusion of the ischemic tissues. This process requires significant communication and coordination between the surgical and anesthetic teams. It is imperative that the patient is resuscitated prior to reperfusion and it is frequently necessary to delay this process to allow the anesthesiologists to achieve this objective. Reperfusion of the ischemic tissue causes the release of acid, potassium, and a variety of inflammatory mediators into the systemic circulation, all of which are potentially detrimental.

The inferior mesenteric artery may be reimplanted into either the body of the graft or the left limb if it is patent. Seeger et al.[167] reported that routine reimplantation of the inferior mesenteric artery resulted in decreased rates of colonic infarction and death after aortic reconstruction. However, a more recent randomized controlled trial demonstrated no benefit in terms of morbidity or mortality, although the authors suggested it may be beneficial for older patients and those with increased blood loss.[168] The colon and lower extremities should be interrogated with the Doppler ultrasound after reperfusion, and the heparin reversed with intravenous protamine sulfate after confirmation of adequate signals. The protamine dose is estimated based on the effectiveness of protamine (1 mg of protamine per 100 units of heparin), the initial dose of heparin, the current activated clotting time, and the elapsed time from the administration of heparin. The protamine should be administered slowly to prevent any untoward hemodynamic events.[169] Notably, a recent randomized controlled trial reported that protamine effectively reverses the heparin effect but provides no clinical benefit during peripheral vascular surgery, including aneurysm repair.[170] The shell of the aneurysm and the overlying retroperitoneum are both closed with absorbable suture to provide a biologic tissue layer between the graft and the viscera. The retractors are then removed, the viscera are returned to their anatomic positions, the nasogastric tube is confirmed to be in the antrum, and the abdominal wall fascia is closed with standard technique. Interestingly, patients undergoing aortic reconstruction for aneurysmal disease have been reported to have a higher incidence of abdominal wall hernias than those undergoing reconstruction for occlusive disease.[171–173]

The configuration of the aortic reconstruction (aortoaortic, aortoiliac, aortofemoral) depends on the extent of aneurysmal involvement and the degree of occlusive disease. Aneurysmal involvement of the common iliac vessels should be considered an extension of the aortic process and treated appropriately. Specifically, common iliac arteries larger than 2.0 cm should be considered aneurysmal and replaced. The entire common iliac artery must usually be replaced, although it is possible to replace only the proximal segment if the aneurysmal involvement is isolated. Conversely, common iliac arteries smaller than 2.0 cm have a relatively benign natural history and do not need to be replaced since only a small percentage become aneurysmal and require treatment.[30,31] Despite the fact that a patient may be a candidate for an aortic tube graft, it is often easier to perform an aortobiiliac graft because the terminal aorta is often very calcified. Aortobifemoral bypass grafts should be reserved for the small subset of patients who truly have concomitant aneurysms and severe occlusive disease since the risks of wound complications and graft infections are significantly greater. Indeed, the risk for graft infections is less than 0.5% for aortobiiliac grafts but approximately 2% for aortobifemoral grafts.[30,31,174] It is important to remember the original indication for the procedure and choose the appropriate aortic reconstruction (aortobiiliac bypass for aortoiliac aneurysm, aortobifemoral bypass for aortoiliac occlusive disease). Admittedly, there is a role for aortobifemoral reconstructions in patients with aneurysmal disease, and it is futile to attempt an aortobiiliac reconstruction in patients with severe external iliac artery disease.

The postoperative care after open repair is fairly routine and predictable for the majority of patients. Patients are transferred directly from the operating room to the intensive care unit, although selective use of the intensive care unit may be appropriate.[175] Most of the patients are extubated in the operating room or shortly after arrival in the intensive care unit. The intensive care unit length of stay is usually 1 to 2 days, and the median total length of stay is 8 days.[25] Patients are encouraged to get out of bed and begin ambulating in the early postoperative period (i.e., 24 to 48 hours). Preoperative prophylactic antibiotics are continued for a total of 24 hours. Nasogastric decompression is continued until bowel function returns. Oral feedings are initiated after removal of the nasogastric tube and advanced quickly to solids. Patients are discharged when they are ambulatory, can tolerate a regular diet, have normal bowel function, and are sufficiently able to care for themselves. A subset of people require transfer to a rehabilitation or an extended care facility. Patients are usually seen in the clinic 2 weeks after discharge and then at 6 months thereafter. Additional clinic appointments may be necessary as dictated by any ongoing medical problems. Patients are not allowed to drive until their incisional pain has resolved and they have stopped taking pain medications. Furthermore, patients are discouraged from lifting objects heavier than 10 lbs for the first 6 months to reduce the incidence of incisional hernias.

Complications and Outcome. Open repair of intact abdominal aortic aneurysms is associated with significant mortality and morbidity.[25,176,177] The attendant mortality rates have been discussed extensively in the preceding sections entitled

Principles of Management and Choice of Open or Endovascular Repair. Briefly, the contemporary mortality rate across the country has consistently been less than 5%.[56–58] The overall morbidity rate remains less clear, although the specific complications have been well defined. Huber et al.[25] reported that 33% of all patients undergoing repair of intact abdominal aortic aneurysms across the United States develop some type of complication as defined by the *International Classification of Diseases*, ninth revision (ICD-9) postoperative complication codes. Similarly, Hua et al.[57] reported from the National Surgical Quality Improvement Program Private Sector that the overall incidence of morbidity after open repair was 35%.

Intraoperative complications can result from injury to the intra-abdominal structures during dissection, although these technical complications are not specific to the aneurysm repair. The small bowel, colon, ureter, and major venous structures (inferior vena cava, iliac veins, left renal vein) are particularly susceptible. Iatrogenic bowel injury at the time of abdominal aortic aneurysm repair is particularly problematic due to the potential to infect the prosthetic graft. If the colon is injured before the aneurysm repair, the defect in the colon should be fixed and the aneurysm repair should be aborted. If the small bowel is injured before the aneurysm repair, the same course should likely be followed, although this decision requires a modicum of clinical judgment. The infectious concerns must be balanced by the fact that the small bowel contents are sterile, patients usually receive a preoperative bowel preparation, a second procedure will be required to repair the aneurysm, and there is a small risk of aneurysm rupture during the intervening delay. Injury to the bowel during or after implantation of the aortic graft should be treated with repair of the defect, extensive irrigation, and prolonged antibiotics. Admittedly, these approaches are very conservative and it is noteworthy that multiple clinical series have attested to the safety of simultaneous aortic and gastrointestinal/urologic procedures.[178–181] The ureter is susceptible to injury at the point where it crosses over the iliac bifurcation. Injury can be avoided by a heightened awareness of this anatomic location and dissection in the tissue plane immediately on top of the common iliac vessels. Inadvertent venous injury can be associated with significant bleeding. This can usually be controlled by direct pressure using sponge sticks and suture repair. The left renal vein may be transected if necessary. It should be transected near its juncture with the vena cava, and the gonadal, adrenal, and lumbar branches should be preserved to maintain venous outflow from the kidney. Although somewhat inelegant, division of the left renal vein does not appear to affect renal function after abdominal aortic aneurysm repair.[182] Transecting the common iliac artery or infrarenal aorta may facilitate exposure of the common iliac or retroaortic renal veins, respectively.

Excessive intraoperative bleeding may be encountered occasionally. Routine elective aneurysm repairs are usually associated with moderate intraoperative blood loss with a mean transfusion requirement of 1 to 2 units of packed red blood cells. Excessive bleeding may be caused by either the surgical trauma or coagulopathy. Reversal of the heparin with protamine may help correct the coagulopathic bleeding. Patients with significant bleeding and platelet counts below 50,000/mL should receive a platelet transfusion, and it should be considered for coagulopathic bleeding and counts below 100,000/mL. Transfusions of fresh frozen plasma are indicated for both patients with significant bleeding in conjunction with prolonged coagulation studies (>1.5 times control value) and those with coagulopathic bleeding. Massive bleeding, defined as more than 100% of the blood volume, may induce a dilutional coagulopathy with prolongation of the coagulation studies. Additional blood products should be set up in the blood bank in the event of significant bleeding. This may require an additional blood bank specimen. Intraoperative autologous transfusion devices should also be considered if not already in use.

Ischemia of the lower extremities has been reported to occur approximately 3% of the time after open repair.[177] The causes are multiple and include distal embolization, thrombosis, clamp injury, and technical errors. The lumen of the aneurysm is frequently filled with both thrombus and atheromatous debris that may serve as a source for both macro- and microembolization. The macroemboli usually lodge at the bifurcations of the major vessels; the microemboli usually lodge in the digital vessels and, unfortunately, are not amenable to mechanical extraction. Thrombosis may result from inadequate heparinization, hypercoagulable conditions, or poor arterial runoff. The technical conduct of the operation outlined previously is designed to minimize the ischemic complications. The specific maneuvers include anticoagulation, selection of a suitable site for distal clamp application and anastomosis, intraluminal control of severely calcified vessels, flushing of the vessels before clamp removal, and sequential removal of the vascular clamps. Further intervention is mandatory if the lower extremities are found to be ischemic. Anastomotic defects should be corrected. This may simply require dissembling and redoing the anastomosis, but often requires relocating it further distal on the outflow artery. If no problems are identified at the distal anastomosis, the femoral vessels should be explored and an intraluminal thrombus removed with a balloon embolectomy catheter. A transverse arteriotomy may be created in the common femoral artery if it is anticipated that only a thrombectomy will be required; a longitudinal incision should be created if a bypass (inflow or outflow) procedure is anticipated. The transverse arteriotomy can simply be closed with interrupted sutures without narrowing the lumen in the event that an additional bypass procedure is not necessary, whereas the longitudinal arteriotomy requires a patch closure. A bypass from the aortic graft to the femoral vessels is required if adequate inflow cannot be restored with thrombectomy alone. The popliteal artery below the knee should be explored and a thrombectomy performed if the extremity is still ischemic. This may be facilitated by creating a longitudinal arteriotomy on the below-knee popliteal artery that extends to the tibioperoneal trunk. This allows the passage of the balloon embolectomy catheter into all three tibial vessels under direct vision. A below-knee popliteal or tibial artery bypass is required if adequate perfusion to the distal extremity is not restored after patch closure of the popliteal arteriotomy. Predictably, a complex lower extremity revascularization in conjunction with an aortic reconstruction is associated with a significant degree of morbidity and dramatically increases the mortality rate.[183] The decision to proceed with an infrainguinal bypass depends on the status of the extremity and requires some clinical judgment. Aborting the procedure and allowing for a period of observation and rewarming is appropriate when popliteal Doppler signals are detected and the foot is cool yet not severely ischemic. Reoperation and definitive treatment may be necessary in the early postoperative period unless marked improvement is noted.

Many of the systemic complications that follow open aneurysm repair are not surprising, given the magnitude of the operation and the age/comorbidities of the patients. Cardiac complications (ischemia, infarction, arrhythmias, congestive heart failure) occur in up to 25%[176,177,184] and are the leading cause of death after open aneurysm repair in many series. Pulmonary complications (pneumonia, ventilator dependence greater than 48 hours, acute respiratory distress syndrome) are also quite common and approximately 10% of the patients require prolonged ventilation.[176,177] Deterioration of renal function, defined by an increase in serum creatinine or blood urea nitrogen, occurs in approximately 5% of cases, although acute renal failure requiring dialysis is rare (i.e. <1%).[177] The potential causes of renal insufficiency in the perioperative period are numerous and include contrast nephrotoxicity, hypovolemia, atheroembolization, and the inflammatory response from the lower torso ischemia/reperfusion injury.

Postoperative bleeding requiring reexploration, intra-abdominal abscess, and abdominal wound complications are all relatively infrequent complications and are associated with all major intra-abdominal procedures.

Ischemic colitis has been reported to occur in approximately 2% to 13% of cases after open aneurysm repair.[185,186] The reported incidence depends on the diagnostic algorithm and modality (routine sigmoidoscopy vs. selective sigmoidoscopy) and is dramatically increased after ruptured aneurysm repair. Indeed, the incidence of colonic ischemia after ruptured aneurysm repair in patients undergoing routine colonoscopy is approximately 25% to 40%.[185,187] Multivariate analysis of patients undergoing both open and endovascular repair demonstrated that the duration of the procedure and preoperative renal insufficiency were also predictors of colon ischemia.[186] The sigmoid colon is affected most frequently, although all the sections of the colon may be involved. The ischemia may result from inadequate resuscitation, disruption of collaterals, and/or failure to revascularize a hemodynamically significant inferior mesenteric artery. Patients usually present with bloody diarrhea in the early postoperative period. However, the diagnosis should be considered in the absence of bloody diarrhea in patients with thrombocytopenia, multiple organ dysfunction, increasing abdominal pain/peritonitis, and generalized "failure to thrive." The diagnosis may be confirmed by endoscopy. Although sigmoidoscopy is used most frequently, a complete colonoscopy is likely optimal due to the potential involvement of the other colon segments. Treatment depends on the endoscopic findings and clinical setting. The endoscopic findings range from mucosal ischemia to transmural necrosis. Unfortunately, it is often difficult to differentiate diffuse mucosal ischemia from transmural necrosis. Patients with mucosal ischemia alone should be treated with bowel rest, broad-spectrum antibiotics, total parenteral nutrition, and serial endoscopic examinations. Many of these lesions resolve spontaneously without long-term sequelae, although colonic strictures may develop in a subset of patients. Patients with transmural colonic necrosis should undergo laparotomy with resection of the involved segment, a proximal diverting colostomy, and a distal Hartmann pouch. After laparotomy, they should be maintained on broad-spectrum antibiotics and parenteral nutrition. The reported mortality rate in patients with transmural necrosis may range up to 85%.[185,186] Maintaining antegrade flow through the internal iliac vessels, routinely implanting the inferior mesenteric artery, and avoiding disruption of the colonic collateral circulation may reduce the incidence of this adverse outcome.

Several other gastrointestinal complications are common after standard infrarenal abdominal aortic aneurysm repair.[188] A postoperative ileus develops in essentially all patients, with bowel function usually returning within 3 to 5 days. An ileus may persist beyond this time period in a subset of patients, although no additional therapy is usually required. Nasogastric decompression should be continued, narcotics minimized, electrolytes normalized, and ambulation encouraged. Either calculous or acalculous cholecystitis may develop after aneurysm repair. The mortality rates reported historically for postoperative cholecystitis were significant[189] and served as the catalyst for simultaneous cholecystectomy and aneurysm repair. Although this approach has been found to be safe and not associated with an increased risk for graft infections, it is usually reserved for patients with small stones or evidence of chronic cholecystitis. Pancreatitis may develop after abdominal aortic aneurysm repair, although the incidence is surprisingly low in light of the obligatory manipulation of the pancreas during repair. The treatment of pancreatitis in this setting is conservative and includes bowel rest, parenteral nutrition, and serial imaging.

Sexual dysfunction is quite common after both open and endovascular aneurysm repair as noted earlier. Erectile and/or orgasmic dysfunction have been reported to occur in 5% to 18% of men undergoing aortoiliac reconstruction.[190] The responsible mechanisms include interruption of the pelvic perfusion and injury to the autonomic nerves that overlie the distal aorta/proximal common iliac arteries. Injury to these autonomic nerves disrupts the internal sphincter mechanism of the bladder and results in retrograde ejaculation. Care should be exercised during aneurysm repair to maintain pelvic perfusion and avoid nerve injury to prevent these untoward complications. It is imperative that these potential complications be discussed with patients preoperatively.

Paraplegia after open infrarenal abdominal aortic aneurysm repair occurs with an incidence of 0.25%.[191] The potential mechanisms for this devastating complication include embolization, thrombosis of the spinal artery, and disruption of the spinal blood supply. Paraplegia after aneurysm repair is an irreversible injury. Maintaining adequate prograde pelvic perfusion through the internal iliac arteries may minimize this complication.

The long-term outcome after open repair is generally favorable. Long-term survival is improved after aneurysm repair, although it falls short of the age-matched controls with survival rates of approximately 90%, 65%, and 40% at 1, 5, and 10 years, respectively.[2,5,192] Cardiovascular causes account for the leading cause of death.[193] This underscores the importance of long-term medical follow-up and the AHA/ACC Guidelines for preventing myocardial infarction and death.[150,193] Prosthetic aortic grafts are associated with long-term complications with a reported incidence of approximately 10% to 15% at 15 years.[117,194,195] Notably, bifurcated grafts are associated with a higher incidence of complications (13%) than tube grafts (5%).[30] The long-term graft-related complications include infection, aortoenteric fistula, thrombosis, and pseudoaneurysm formation. Additional aneurysms of a sufficient size to merit intervention develop in approximately 5% to 15% of patients in either the iliac vessels or the aorta above the prosthetic graft.[30,31] It is recommended that patients undergo CT of the complete aorta and iliac vessels 3 to 5 years postoperatively to screen for graft complications and additional aneurysms.[196] Furthermore, patients with prosthetic aortic grafts should receive prophylactic antibiotics before undergoing invasive procedures, including colonoscopy and dental extractions.

Endovascular Repair of Intact Abdominal Aortic Aneurysms

Technique. The preoperative evaluation and preparation before endovascular abdominal aortic aneurysm repair are significantly more complicated than for the open approach. The various imaging studies must be reviewed before it can be determined whether the endovascular approach is even feasible. Appropriate measurements must be taken and the necessary devices/components selected. An operative plan must be generated including specific modifications of the standard approach to overcome the patient's anatomic limitations and, thereby, extend the feasibility of the technique. Indeed, "preoperative planning, preoperative planning, and preoperative planning" have facetiously been identified as the three most important components of a successful repair.

A variety of imaging techniques (i.e., CT, catheter-based arteriography) have been employed to determine the feasibility of an aneurysm for endovascular repair and select the appropriate devices/components. However, CT arteriography with 3D reconstructions has emerged as the optimal approach. It is important to emphasize that no imaging technique is perfect and, consequently, a certain degree of flexibility is necessary for the operative plan. Measurements obtained from the 3D CT tend to overestimate the actual renal artery–internal iliac artery length assumed by the graft when deployed in vivo. Similar sizing limitations are associated with the catheter-based arteriography techniques, and these have been attributed to the course of the catheter, the presence of intraluminal thrombus, and the conformational changes in the aorta that result from the stiff guide wires and/or the device itself.

The various devices/components should be selected using the underlying principles that the main body of the device should sit as close to the orifices of the renal arteries as possible, while the iliac limbs should extend to the orifices of the internal iliac arteries. Furthermore, the manufacturers' recommendations for sizing and device selection should be followed. Grafts seated well below the orifices of the renal arteries have been associated with proximal migration,[197] while oversizing the graft diameter beyond that recommended has been associated with both graft migration and aneurysm reexpansion.[198] The endograft is sized according to the anatomic configuration of the aneurysm and adjacent arteries, and this must be performed in advance of the procedure to ensure that the appropriate devices are available. The diameter and length of the infrarenal cuff, aneurysm, and iliac vessels must be measured precisely. In addition, the distance from the lowest renal artery to the aortic bifurcation and both renal bifurcations needs to be determined. The diameter of the proximal graft is chosen to oversize the aortic cuff and iliac arteries by approximately 10% to 20%. Additional devices should be ordered for each case including two iliac limbs and an aortic extension cuff to allow for any discrepancy between the preoperative plan and the actual course of the graft in vivo. Each endograft procedure and device configuration is "custom fit" for an individual patient. Worksheets are available from the manufacturers to confirm the suitability of an aneurysm for endovascular repair and to aid in the selection of an appropriate device. Technical assistance is available from the various manufacturers to facilitate every step of the process from initial assessment to component selection to deployment. Furthermore, physicians are required to complete a training course consisting of sizing exercises and monitored deployments.

The choice of the specific endovascular device is contingent upon the anatomic constraints of the aneurysm, device-associated outcome, and surgeon preference. There are specific differences between the various grafts that lend themselves to different clinical scenarios. The specific considerations include neck diameter, neck length/angulation, renal–internal iliac artery distance, common iliac artery diameter, and access vessel diameter. For example, a graft with suprarenal fixation may be more suitable for a shorter neck, while a lower-profile system (i.e., smaller outer diameter of the delivery sheath) may be most appropriate for patients with smaller access vessels (i.e., common femoral and external iliac arteries). Despite the initial concerns about compromising renal function, suprarenal fixation has been consistently shown to be safe.[139,199] Deployment of the various endografts is reasonably involved from a technical standpoint; thus, it is not particularly surprising that most surgeons elect to concentrate on one or two devices. The ease of deployment and the precision of the deployment with regard to the location of the renal artery orifices also contribute to surgeon preference.

The need for adjunctive procedures to facilitate the endovascular repair is usually determined by the preoperative imaging and should be factored into the overall plan. The major concerns include stenotic access vessels and the absence of a suitable common iliac artery landing zone due to aneurysmal enlargement. The remedial procedures for small access vessels or significant occlusive disease include serial dilation or a retroperitoneal prosthetic iliac conduit. Repeated attempts to pass the device's sheaths through a diseased native vessel should be avoided and can result in vessel rupture at the common iliac bifurcation. Aneurysmal degeneration of the common iliac artery can be overcome by seating the iliac limb in the external iliac artery. This necessitates either embolizing or bypassing the ipsilateral internal iliac artery. Alternatively, the iliac limb of the endograft can simply occlude the internal iliac artery flush provided the iliac bifurcation is sufficiently tapered.[200] Several reports have documented that accessory renal arteries may be covered at the time of the endograft with little clinical sequelae.

The intraoperative preparation for endovascular repair is similar to that for the open approach, although there are several significant differences. The appropriate imaging equipment is mandatory. Ideally, this would entail a complete endovascular suite with a fixed fluoroscopic unit, although a portable unit with the appropriate vascular software and an imaging table is adequate. General endotracheal anesthesia is likely the standard, although a variety of techniques have been employed including both regional and local anesthesia. Indeed, the endovascular approach is well suited for these less invasive alternatives, particularly considering the feasibility of a completely percutaneous approach. Intraoperative autologous transfusion devices and a nasogastric tube are unnecessary. It is currently quite rare to convert to an open repair at the time of the initial implantation despite the early experience that reported a rate of up to 5%.[62,63,65,201] However, it should be emphasized that endovascular aneurysm repair is a surgical procedure and should be performed in an operating room with strict aseptic technique.

Although the technique for implanting the various endografts is somewhat specific to the individual device, the basic steps for deploying a "generic" modular bifurcated device using an open femoral artery exposure is illustrated (Fig. 100.10). Briefly, the common femoral arteries are exposed and an umbilical tape is wrapped circumferentially around the vessels at the level of the inguinal ligament to facilitate vascular control. A variety of femoral incisions are possible, although a 2- to 3-cm transverse incision along the caudal border of the inguinal ligament is ideal and has been associated with a low incidence of postoperative wound complications. Approximately 2 cm of the common femoral artery is dissected free. It is not usually necessary to dissect the superficial and profunda femoral branches. While the dissection is being performed, the various device components are prepared on the back table by the surgical technologist. A pursestring suture using a 5–0 cardiovascular suture can be placed on the anterior aspect of the common femoral artery and left untied until the completion of the procedure. The various catheters/sheaths may be introduced through the center of the pursestring, thereby facilitating a rapid/simple closure of the artery at the completion of the procedure. The common femoral artery on the side chosen to introduce the main body of the device (ipsilateral groin) is punctured using an angiographic needle, and a 0.035-inch standard working wire (e.g., Bentsen) is passed into the abdominal aorta using fluoroscopic guidance. A 5-French introducer sheath is advanced over the guide wire using a Seldinger technique and vessel entry is confirmed by manual contrast injection. The working wire is further advanced into the thoracic aorta and exchanged for a longer 0.035-inch stiffened guide wire (e.g., Meier) using a catheter. Attention is then directed to the contralateral groin and in a similar manner a guide wire is advanced into the aorta and an appropriate-sized introducer sheath is inserted over the guide wire into the body of the aneurysm at approximately the L3 vertebral space. An angiographic catheter is advanced to the L1 vertebral body through the contralateral sheath and the catheter connected to the power injector. The patient is then anticoagulated with heparin using a standard protocol (100 units/kg) and therapeutic anticoagulation (activated clotting time twice baseline) is maintained throughout the procedure. The main body delivery catheter is introduced over the stiff wire through the ipsilateral groin and the upper limit of the main body positioned between the L1-2 vertebral bodies. Devices that do not have an integral sheath as part of their delivery system require an 18- to 22-French sheath to be inserted prior to introduction of the actual delivery catheter. Radiopaque markers on the graft facilitate the positioning and orientation of the main body.

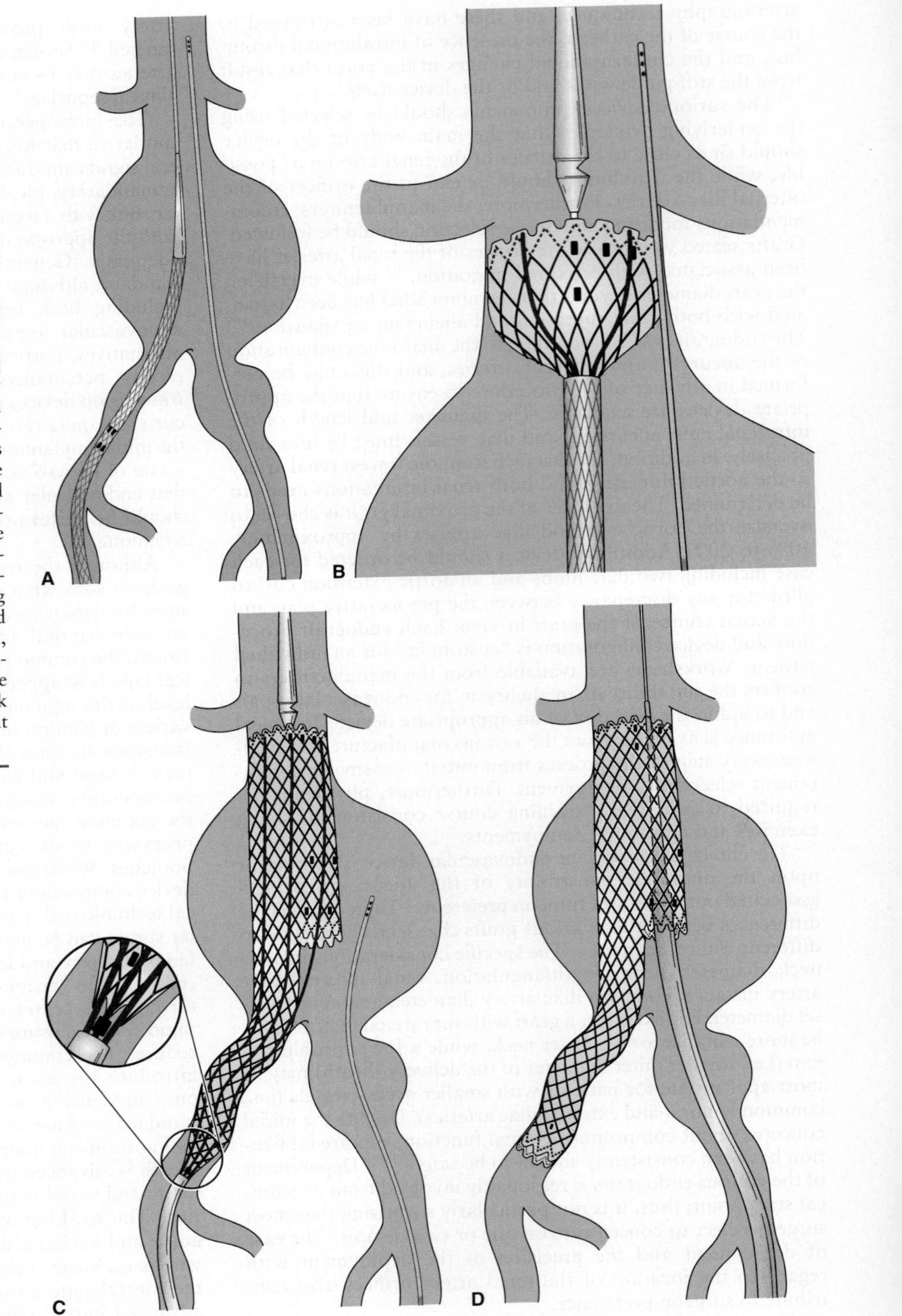

FIGURE 100.10. General steps involved in the endovascular repair of an abdominal aortic aneurysm. The common femoral arteries are exposed bilaterally and stiff wires are introduced into the thoracic aorta under fluoroscopic guidance. An appropriate-sized large-diameter introducer sheath is inserted over the stiff wire into the body of the aneurysm at approximately the L3 vertebral space on the side contralateral to the one chosen for the main device. **A:** The main body delivery catheter is introduced over the stiff wire through the ipsilateral groin and the upper limit of the main body positioned between the L1-2 vertebral bodies. An aortogram is obtained and the location of the renal arteries identified. The location of the renal arteries is marked on the imaging screen and the position of the main body finely adjusted. **B, C:** The main body is deployed exposing the opening of the contralateral docking limb. The contralateral docking limb is cannulated and a stiff wire advanced into the thoracic aorta. Deployment of the contralateral limb is started by obtaining a retrograde arteriogram through the contralateral sheath in the opposite oblique projection to identify the orifice of the internal iliac artery. **D–F:** The location of the orifice is marked on the imaging screen; the contralateral limb is then introduced over the stiff wire, appropriately positioned, and deployed. A compliant aortic occlusion balloon is advanced over the ipsilateral stiff wire and inflated in the region of the infrarenal neck to mold the proximal and distal attachment sites. *(continued)*

An aortogram is obtained and the location of the renal arteries identified. The fluoroscope should be adjusted to optimize visualization of the infrarenal neck. A 5- to 10-degree craniocaudal angulation is usually sufficient to account for the anterior angulation of the infrarenal neck caused by the natural lumbar lordosis of the spine and the posterior bulging of the aneurysm sac. However, the optimal angulation or orientation may be estimated based on the preoperative CT images. The location of the renal arteries is marked on the imaging screen and the position of the main body adjusted. The main body is now deployed exposing the opening of the contralateral docking limb. Using a combination of a hydrophilic wire and a curved catheter, the contralateral docking limb is cannulated. This can be challenging at times and requires a modest degree of catheter skills. Various maneuvers including different fluoroscopic projections, different shaped catheters, and proper orientation of the contralateral docking limb prior to deployment of the main body device can facilitate this step. It is imperative to confirm that the cannulating guide wire is actually within the body of the main endograft. This can be rapidly performed by visualizing the guide wire in two orthogonal projections and confirming that the stents of the endograft can be seen on either side of the cannulating guide wire. Alternatively, an arteriogram can be performed using a catheter within the main body. The contralateral wire is advanced into the ascending thoracic aorta under fluoroscopic guidance and exchanged for a stiff wire using a catheter.

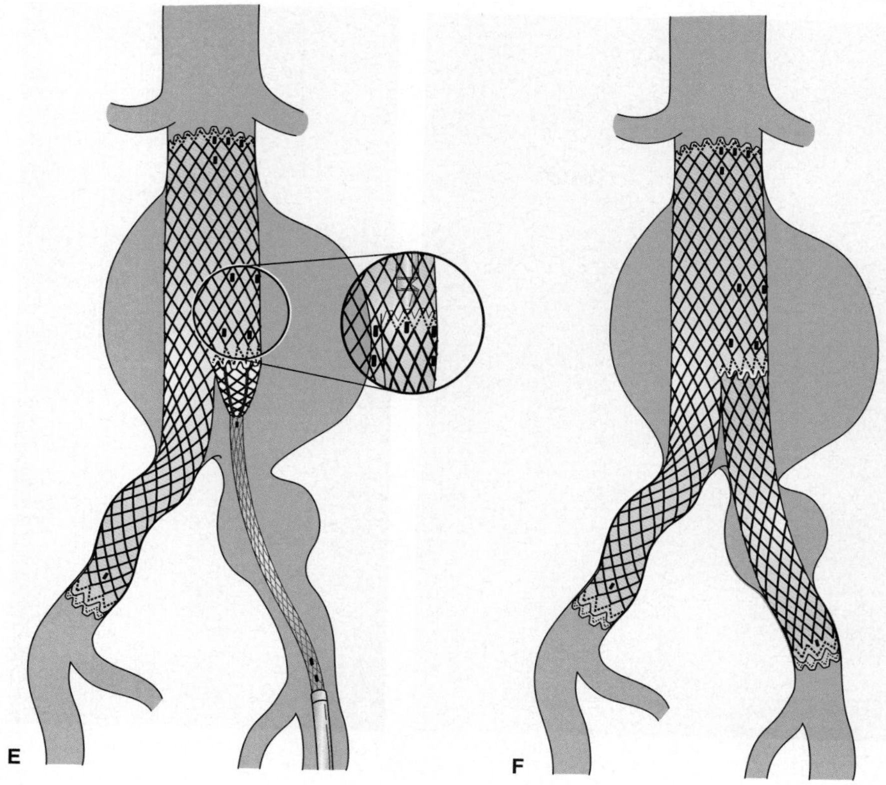

FIGURE 100.10. (*Continued*)

Deployment of the contralateral limb is started by obtaining a retrograde arteriogram through the contralateral sheath in the opposite oblique projection (e.g., right anterior oblique projection for left limb) to identify the orifice of the internal iliac artery. The location of the orifice is marked on the imaging screen and a marker catheter is used to measure the distance from the contralateral docking limb to confirm the preoperative measurements and device selection. The contralateral limb is then introduced over the stiff wire, appropriately positioned relative to the docking limb and the orifice of the internal iliac artery, and then deployed.

After deployment of all the devices, a compliant aortic occlusion balloon is advanced over the ipsilateral stiff wire and inflated in the region of the infrarenal neck to mold the proximal attachment sites. The aortic balloon is then withdrawn and gently expanded at the main body/iliac limb overlap zone and both distal iliac artery fixation sites. A completion arteriogram is then obtained using an angiographic catheter placed through one of the introducer sheaths (Fig. 100.11). The arteriogram should adequately evaluate the proximal–distal fixation sites, the graft–graft overlap zones, and the orifices of the renal–internal iliac arteries. Additionally, it should include a delayed phase to help identify any endoleaks. Problems identified on the completion study should be corrected if possible. The potential remedial procedures include balloon dilation or aortic/iliac extension cuffs.

All sheaths, catheters, and wires are removed after the completion of the arteriogram. The common femoral arteriotomy is closed using the pursestring suture, although additional interrupted sutures are frequently necessary. The heparin is reversed with protamine (1 unit protamine/100 units heparin) after adequate signals are detected at the feet by Doppler ultrasound. The groin wounds are closed in layers with a continuous suture and the final skin later is closed with a subcuticular technique.

The immediate postoperative course is fairly uneventful. Patients are transferred to the general care ward after recovery in the postanesthesia care unit. Patients are started on an appropriate diet the evening of the procedure and encouraged to get out of bed. Plain radiographs of the abdomen (four views, optimized for metal) are obtained on the first postoperative day, and patients are discharged thereafter. Patients are seen in the outpatient clinic at 1 month with an abdominal/pelvic CT scan. It is important to note that mild fever and the

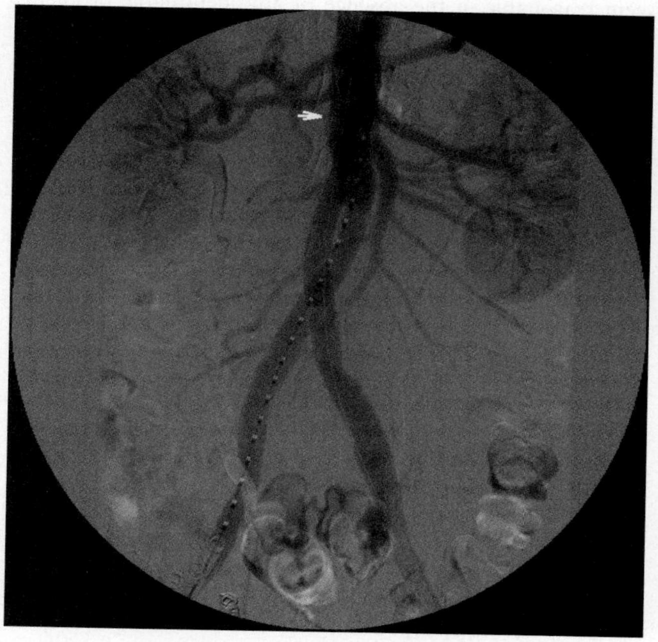

FIGURE 100.11. Completion arteriogram after an endovascular aneurysm repair is shown. The arrow marks the caudal extent of the stent graft. Note that the iliac limbs have been intentionally crossed to facilitate the cannulation of the contralateral gate.

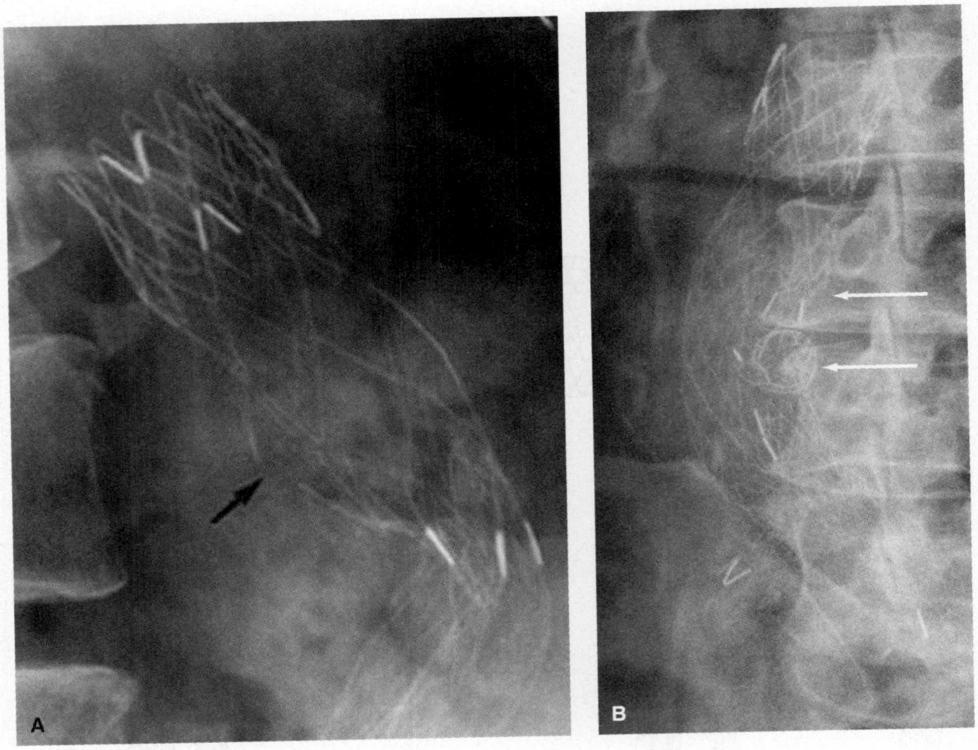

FIGURE 100.12. Plain radiographs of an endovascular graft demonstrating (A) strut fracture and (B) modular disruption. (Reproduced with permission from Magennis R, Joekes E, Martin J, et al. Complications following endovascular abdominal aortic aneurysm repair. *BJR* 2002;75:700–707.)

finding of air around the graft on CT are common occurrences immediately after endograft repair and have not been associated with graft infection.[202]

It is imperative that patients are followed long term given the uncertainty associated with the endovascular repair and the need for remedial procedures. As noted previously, new endoleaks have been identified as late as 7 years postoperatively.[203] A variety of protocols and imaging techniques have been described, although an abdominal/pelvic CT scan with contrast at 12 months and then yearly noncontrast studies seem reasonable in the absence of any identifiable problems and an aneurysm sac that is not increasing in size. Indeed, Sternbergh et al.[204] reported from a multicenter trial that the absence of an endoleak at 1 and 12 months predicted favorable long-term outcome. More frequent imaging may be indicated if the aneurysm continues to grow or there is evidence of an endoleak. The surveillance CT scans should include noncontrast and biphasic contrast views with delayed images to help identify any late endoleaks.[205] Although not part of all surveillance protocols, early plain radiographs are very helpful to identify structural changes/problems with the grafts (Fig. 100.12). Duplex ultrasound has been employed as a surveillance study, but its accuracy is dependent on the local expertise of the vascular laboratory.[206–208]

Complications and Outcome. The overall mortality and complication rates after endovascular repair have been reviewed in the sections entitled Principles of Management and Choice of Open or Endovascular Repair. Briefly, the mortality rate in the recent randomized trials and national series is approximately less than 2%,[58–60,66,66] the perioperative complication rate is less than 25%,[57,117] the rupture risk is approximately 1% per year,[117,124] and the incidence of remedial procedures is approximately 10% per year.[128] Many of the same complications that can occur after open repair can occur after endovascular repair. However, the relative incidence of the various complications is significantly different, and several complications inherent to the endovascular repair have been identified.

A variety of potential complications may arise during insertion of the delivery catheter or introducer sheath. Indeed, access problems secondary to iliac stenoses and/or tortuosity are the most common procedure-related complication. The outer diameters of the delivery sheaths are device dependent, but can range up to 24 French. These correspond to an outer diameter of approximately 7 mm (1 French corresponds to the circular cross-sectional diameter of $1/\pi$ millimeter, e.g., 24 French = 24/3.14 mm or 7.6 mm). A variety of techniques are available to correct or overcome the access vessel stenoses, and these should be factored into the preoperative plan. Excessive force during insertion of these large sheaths or delivery catheters can result in serious injury and perforation of the vessels. Predictably, this can lead to significant hemorrhage and hemodynamic changes. The diagnosis can be confirmed by arteriography and the bleeding controlled intraluminally using the device sheath or a balloon catheter. A variety of endovascular salvage techniques are possible in this setting, including deployment of either the main device or a covered stent over the disrupted artery. Indeed, nearly all major arterial disruptions, with the possible exception of the proximal aorta, may be treated using endovascular techniques and do not necessitate emergent laparotomy. Safe conduct of an endovascular aneurysm repair is predicated by sufficient knowledge of the various salvage techniques, the necessary catheter and guide wire skills to execute them, and a complement of ancillary equipment. However, the adage that "prevention is better than the cure" holds true and endovascular surgeons should maintain a low threshold for constructing a retroperitoneal iliac conduit. Dissection within the arterial wall of the iliac vessels or aorta may also result from misdirection or excessive force during cannulation of the vessels. It can usually be corrected by cannulating the "true" lumen and reestablishing its integrity by deploying a peripheral (uncovered) stent.

Graft deployment can be associated with mechanical problems related to the delivery system or inappropriate positioning. A host of mechanical problems have been described, and the list will likely expand with widespread application of the devices and the introduction of newer systems. Many of the mechanical problems are device specific and related to the actual sequence of events and manipulations required. Troubleshooting guidelines and specific recommendations are available from the manufacturers. Deployment of the endovascular graft below the proximal target site on the infrarenal aorta may be corrected using an aortic extension cuff. Attempting to reposition the graft further proximally after deployment has not been successful and is not recommended. Deployment of the endovascular graft across the orifices of the renal arteries can potentially be corrected by displacing the graft caudally. A guide wire can be passed over the flow divider and out the contralateral groin. The entire graft can then be retracted caudally by pulling on the wires. Alternatively, a large balloon can be inflated above the flow divider and retracted. Extreme care must be exercised during these maneuvers to prevent complete dislodgement of the proximal main body from the neck. Deployment of the graft across part of the renal orifice can be corrected by placing a stent within the lumen of the renal artery and thereby displacing part of the main body caudally. Deployment of the endograft across the lumen of one internal iliac artery is usually tolerated provided the contralateral vessel is patent and relatively free of occlusive disease. Indeed, it is relatively common to embolize a single internal iliac artery in patients with common iliac artery aneurysms to facilitate fixation of the graft limb in the external iliac artery. Occlusion of both internal iliac arteries or occlusion of one vessel in the presence of contralateral disease may render the pelvis ischemic. Occasionally, one of the iliac limbs can be pushed cephalad using a sheath and its dilator. It should be emphasized that many of these remedial procedures are not manufacturer approved and should only be attempted by experienced endovascular surgeons. Due to the advanced age of many of these patients and their attendant comorbidities, open surgical conversion should be contemplated only as a last resort after the endovascular options have been exhausted, again emphasizing the need for advanced endovascular skills.

It is relatively common to see an endoleak on the completion arteriogram. Treatment is contingent upon the specific type of leak and its associated natural history, although the majority of these early endoleaks ultimately resolve.[209] The type 1 (attachment site) and type 3 (fabric tear or module interface) endoleaks are particularly concerning and every reasonable attempt to correct these defects should be made. The aneurysm sac is presumably still exposed to systemic pressure in the presence of a type 1 or type 3 endoleak, and, therefore, the rupture risk likely approaches that associated with the untreated aneurysm. Both the type 1 and 3 endoleaks can potentially be corrected by repeat balloon angioplasty at the proximal/distal attachment sites or at the modular interface. If these measures are not successful, additional extension devices can be deployed. With the exception of large proximal type 1 endoleaks, it is reasonable to manage most perioperative endoleaks expectantly since many seal spontaneously after reversal of the anticoagulation or within the first 6 months. Furthermore, it should be kept in mind that the inability to obtain a satisfactory exclusion of the aneurysm at the time of endograft implantation does not mandate a surgical conversion at the same setting. Consideration should be given to completing the procedure, allowing for a brief recovery, and discussing potential options in an elective, outpatient setting with the patient and his or her family. The potential options at this point include referral to another center with more expertise, open surgical repair with removal of any or all implanted devices, or no further treatment if the patient is a poor surgical risk. Type 2 endoleaks (retrograde branch vessel related) have a relatively benign natural history and do not merit aggressive intervention unless the aneurysm continues to increase in size over time. Type 4 (trans-graft) endoleaks are self-limiting and do not merit treatment at all. They are identified as a diffuse contrast "blush" at the time of the completion arteriography. They represent a diagnosis of exclusion and mandate that the more worrisome type 1 endoleak be excluded.

The spectrum of immediate postoperative complications after endovascular aneurysm repair is comparable to that outlined for after open repair and will not be repeated. However, the incidence of major, systemic complications after endovascular aneurysm repair is quite small. It is noteworthy that the incidence of both paraplegia and bowel ischemia are comparable after endovascular and open repair, although the mechanisms are different and likely due to atheroembolism.[186,210,211] Indeed, diffuse embolization to the small bowel has been reported after endovascular repair and is almost uniformly fatal.[210]

The long-term complications after endovascular repair include endoleak, structural failure, need for remedial procedures, need for open conversion, and rupture. These ongoing risks further emphasize the importance of conscientious lifelong surveillance. All type 1 and 3 endoleaks identified during surveillance merit further evaluation and correction given their ongoing rupture risk. Device migration has been reported to cause type 1 endoleaks and has been associated with neck length, site of deployment below the renal arteries, and surgeon/center experience.[197] The treatment of these late-occurring type 1 and 3 leaks is identical to that for those occurring earlier and includes identification of the specific site and remediation with either balloon angioplasty or an additional endovascular device, although the latter is most common. Type 2 endoleaks merit intervention and treatment if the aneurysm continues to increase in diameter. Identification of the type 2 endoleak can be challenging and may require selective catheterization of the superior mesenteric or internal iliac arteries.[212] A variety of approaches have been described to treat the type 2 endoleaks including coil embolization, laparoscopic ligation of the feeder vessels, and direct translumbar injection of the aneurysm sac with glue or other thrombotic agents.

Aneurysms that continue to increase in size after endovascular repair merit further intervention and may require open conversion due to their ongoing rupture risk. Continued aneurysm growth has been associated with the type of prosthesis and baseline size in addition to the presence of endoleak.[130] It should be emphasized that the goal of aneurysm repair is to prevent rupture/death from rupture and that endoleak and even sac enlargement are surrogate markers of potential late failure of the therapy. Indeed, even the clinical significance of an enlarging sac in the absence of a visible endoleak is controversial as long as a secure proximal and distal fixation of the endograft has been demonstrated. To confound the issue further, rupture of aneurysms without an endoleak or a change in sac diameter has also been reported, leading some to describe the phenomenon teleologically as endotension. A presumed endoleak that is not detected on a properly performed contrast CT scan is typically not identified on a catheter-based arteriogram. The proper diagnostic investigation of an endoleak should include interrogation of all the fixation sites and modular interfaces and selective injections of mesenteric and hypogastric arteries with sufficient contrast dose and proper acquisition techniques. It should be emphasized that open conversion and explant of the endovascular graft is technically more challenging than a de novo open repair and usually requires suprarenal or supraceliac aortic control. It is not always possible (or necessary) to remove the whole endovascular graft, particularly when the device has suprarenal fixation. It is possible to transect the endovascular graft near the usual site of the infrarenal aortic anastomosis and incorporate the fabric/stents of the graft into the anastomosis. Temporary distal vascular control can be achieved by clamping the limbs of the endovascular graft. The limbs of a bifurcated surgical graft may be anastomosed directly to the endograft limbs if they are securely attached to the iliac artery.

A variety of device-specific complications, including strut fracture, fabric tears, and buckling of the graft, have been identified, and the list will likely increase with the introduction of newer systems. These may present at any time throughout the postoperative period. An extensive discussion of all the potential device-related complications and their treatment is beyond the scope of this chapter. Disturbingly, regression of the aneurysm has been associated with significant conformational changes in the endografts and has resulted in limb thrombosis and disruption of the distal attachment sites.[213] These adverse outcomes in the presence of decrease in the aneurysm size have been termed the "paradox of success."

Repair of Ruptured Abdominal Aortic Aneurysms

Open Repair. The approach to the patient with a ruptured abdominal aortic aneurysm is similar to the elective one, although several points merit further comment. It is important to realize that operative repair is the only acceptable treatment and the only effective means to prevent further hemorrhage. The diagnosis should be made in an expeditious fashion and the appropriate treatment initiated. The endovascular approach appears to be associated with a lower mortality rate, but this remains to be further documented given the inherent bias in terms of patient selection and publication.[71,72,74–76]

The patient should be taken emergently to the operating room once the diagnosis of a ruptured aneurysm has been made. Unnecessary delays to complete the preoperative evaluation should be avoided. Unfortunately, the diagnosis is not always made in a setting where an operating room is immediately available. Given this scenario, the patient should be transferred to a setting in which an operating room is available or the necessary resources should be mobilized. The decision to transfer or treat locally should be dictated by the ultimate time necessary to get the patient to the operating room and the institutional resources. The operating room and anesthesia personnel should be notified immediately upon diagnosis and instructed that the patient is en route. The necessary instrument trays should be opened, the room temperature in the operating room increased, adjunctive measures to maintain body temperature obtained, and the intraoperative autologous salvage device prepared. Notably, hypothermia has been shown to be a strong, independent predictor of mortality after ruptured aneurysm repair.[214] The blood bank should be notified and instructed to send 6 units of blood to the operating room. This should be type O negative or type specific if cross matched units are not available. Furthermore, the blood bank should be instructed to expedite the cross match of additional red blood cells, fresh frozen plasma, and platelets. The patient should be prepared and draped before intubation and the induction of anesthesia. Simultaneously, the surgeon and assistants should be prepared to make the incision at the time of induction. Patients with ruptured aneurysms frequently become hypotensive after the induction of anesthesia because of its vasodilator effect.

A midline incision should be made and supraceliac aortic control obtained. This is facilitated by bluntly dissecting the gastrohepatic ligament, the crus of the diaphragm, and the connective tissue enveloping the aorta. The latter may be somewhat tenacious and requires a moderate amount of force. Vascular control can be achieved manually by either occluding the aorta between the fingers and thumb or compressing it against the vertebral bodies. Definitive control should be obtained with an aortic clamp, which can be guided along the arm, hand, and digits. Care should be utilized during these maneuvers to prevent injury to the esophagus or the aorta itself. Inexperienced surgeons may mistake the esophagus for the aorta in hypotensive patients. The presence of a nasogastric tube or pulse may aid in differentiating the aorta from the esophagus. Aortic control can also be achieved through a variety of other means: thoracotomy with occlusion of the descending thoracic aorta, intraluminal control of the infrarenal aorta with a Foley balloon, supraceliac control via a retroperitoneal approach, and intraluminal control with an aortic balloon catheter inserted through the femoral arteries. The aortic surgeon should be familiar with these various techniques because they can be helpful in certain clinical settings, but the midline approach with supraceliac control is recommended for most ruptured infrarenal aneurysms. After supraceliac aortic control has been obtained, the infrarenal aorta is dissected and vascular control is achieved below the level of the renal arteries. The hematoma from the ruptured aneurysm often facilitates the dissection by displacing the normal tissue planes. However, the normal tissues may be obscured, and care should be taken not to injure the venous structures, particularly the left renal vein. The supraceliac aortic clamp can be released after infrarenal control has been obtained, and flow can be restored to the visceral vessels. It is imperative that these various steps are coordinated with the anesthesia team, and it is recommended that the supraceliac clamp be left in position to facilitate reapplication if necessary. Distal vascular control can be achieved with either vascular clamps or intraluminal balloons, depending on the character of the iliac vessels.

Patients can be heparinized after proximal and distal vascular control has been obtained, provided that the patient is doing well and the case is proceeding expeditiously.[215] However, the decision to anticoagulate the patient is contingent on a variety of factors, including the quantity of blood lost, presence of coagulopathic bleeding, body temperature, and hemodynamic status. Anticoagulation potentially reduces thrombotic complications, but it exacerbates coagulopathic bleeding. Before completion of the distal anastomoses, thromboembolectomy catheters should be passed distally through the iliac vessels to remove any thrombus or debris. It is recommended that the inferior mesenteric artery be implanted (if patent) to reduce the risk of postoperative colonic ischemia. The heparin effect can be reversed with protamine after confirmation of distal lower extremity arterial signals. The administration of fresh frozen plasma, platelets, or both should be considered at this point if any evidence of coagulopathic bleeding is noted.

The postoperative course after repair of a ruptured aneurysm is predictably more complicated and protracted than the course after elective repair.[216–220] Both the intensive care unit and total hospital length of stay are significantly increased. The mortality and complication rates are likewise significantly increased. As noted earlier, the mortality rate for patients with ruptured abdominal aortic aneurysms who make it to the operating room is approximately 50%.[5] The spectrum of postoperative complications after repair of a ruptured aneurysm is essentially the same as after elective repair, although the incidences are increased. The incidence of bowel ischemia may be as high as 40% and routine colonoscopy may be indicated.[187] Abdominal compartment syndrome[221] and adrenal insufficiency[222] have been reported after ruptured aneurysm repair and merit consideration in patients who are not doing well. Notably, adrenal insufficiency was identified in almost 70% of patients with unexplained postoperative hypotension after ruptured aneurysm repair.[222] Predictably, long-term survival is decreased relative to patients undergoing elective repair,[200] although the overall quality of life is comparable.[223]

Endovascular Repair. The endovascular approach has the potential to impact the operative mortality rate for ruptured abdominal aortic aneurysms. Although the worldwide experience is relatively small, the early outcomes are impressive, particularly given the significant mortality/morbidity associated with the open repair, which has remained relatively constant over the past few decades.[69] Despite the appeal of the endovascular approach, its application requires a defined protocol/approach consisting of an experienced endovascular surgeon, a committed team, an available operating room with the necessary imaging equipment, and an inventory of suitable devices. Furthermore, the patient must be an acceptable anatomic candidate. Several recent studies have estimated that approximately 20% to 50% of patients with ruptured aneurysms are anatomically suitable for endovascular repair using conventional devices, although this number may increase with the introduction of newer devices and/or the extension beyond the manufacturers' instructions for use.[199,224–226]

The endovascular approach for the treatment of ruptured abdominal aortic aneurysms can be briefly summarized and has recently been described by Lee et al.[227] Patients with a presumed diagnosis of a ruptured abdominal aortic aneurysm who are hemodynamically stable, as defined by a systolic blood pressure greater than 80 mm Hg and normal mentation, should undergo a rapid CT arteriogram to determine their suitability. Notably, aggressive fluid resuscitation should be avoided during this period to avoid the theoretical risk of releasing the retroperitoneal tamponade. The anatomic criteria for endovascular repair include an acceptable neck anatomy (length ≥10 mm, diameter ≤32 mm) and adequate access vessels (≥7 mm diameter). The operative plan is generated and the appropriate devices selected based on the CT findings, and patients are taken directly to the operating room from the scanner. Oversizing of the aortic neck greater than or equal to 20% and encroachment on the orifices of the renal arteries with adjunctive stenting are both tolerated in an attempt to limit the necessary inventory and increase the proximal fixation zone, respectively. Access to the common femoral arteries is obtained using a percutaneous approach with direct exposure and repair delayed until the completion of the procedure. The remaining conduct of the procedures is essentially the same as described in the elective setting. It is not usually necessary to occlude the aorta with an intraluminal balloon, although one should be readily available in the event that the patients become hemodynamically unstable.[228,229] It should be noted that the criteria for an acceptable result are somewhat less in this setting and persistent attempts to achieve a perfect radiographic result should be avoided. The ultimate goal is to prevent further hemorrhage and to allow the patient to be resuscitated. Further interventions including conversion to open repair may be necessary at a later date, but these can usually be performed in an elective fashion.

ADDITIONAL CONSIDERATIONS

Isolated Iliac Artery Aneurysms

Isolated iliac artery aneurysms are rare and have been reported to occur with an incidence ranging from 0.03% in autopsy series[6] to 2.2% in single-institution series.[230] The common iliac artery is involved in approximately 70% of the cases, and the internal iliac artery in the remainder.[231] Aneurysmal involvement of the external iliac artery, either in combination with the common iliac artery or alone, is distinctly rare. These isolated iliac artery aneurysms should be differentiated from the common iliac artery aneurysms that occur concomitantly with abdominal aortic aneurysms. Simultaneous aneurysmal involvement of the aorta and common iliac arteries occurs in about 10% to 20% of all abdominal aortic aneurysms[6,7]; this pattern should be considered as one disease process and treated accordingly.

The natural history of isolated iliac artery aneurysms is poorly defined because of their low incidence. The clinical risk factors appear to be similar to those for abdominal aortic aneurysms with the highest incidence seen among elderly men. Unlike patients with abdominal aortic aneurysms, a significant proportion of patients with isolated iliac artery aneurysms present with symptoms.[231] These symptoms may result from either rupture or compression of adjacent structures including the bowel, ureters, iliac veins, and nerves. The clinical presentation of patients with a ruptured iliac artery aneurysm is similar to that of ruptured abdominal aortic aneurysms, and the diagnosis should be included in the differential for patients with genitourinary symptoms and normal findings on urinalysis and testicular examination. CT arteriography is optimal for confirming the diagnosis of an isolated iliac artery aneurysm. The utility of ultrasonography is limited by the posterior course of the iliac vessels and the overlying bowel. Large iliac artery aneurysms may occasionally be palpated during rectal or gynecologic examination, and ruptured iliac artery aneurysms may present with ecchymosis of the perineum.

The principles of treatment for asymptomatic, isolated iliac artery aneurysms are similar to those for abdominal aortic aneurysms, and operative repair is justified when the risk for rupture offsets the risk of repair. Unfortunately, the natural history of isolated iliac artery aneurysms and the appropriate threshold for repair remain unresolved. The reported growth rate for iliac artery aneurysms less than 3 cm is 0.11 cm/y, while that for aneurysms 3 to 5 cm is 0.26 cm/y.[232] Although rupture has been reported for aneurysms smaller than 2 cm, it is rare for aneurysms smaller than 3 cm to rupture.[230,233] Operative repair is generally recommended for good-risk patients with isolated iliac artery aneurysms greater than or equal to 3.5 cm. The frequency of surveillance imaging studies should be dictated by the size of the aneurysm, with yearly studies appropriate for aneurysms less than 3 cm and 6-month intervals appropriate for aneurysms between 3 and 3.5 cm.[230]

The treatment or repair of isolated iliac artery aneurysms depends on the specific vessel involved and the extent of the aneurysm. Theoretically, common iliac artery aneurysms can be repaired with an interposition graft or a covered stent provided that there is a sufficient proximal and/or distal neck to sew the anastomosis or seat the graft. However, this is rarely an option because the aneurysmal involvement of the vessel usually extends over its whole length. Therefore, repair necessitates replacing the whole common iliac artery with a bifurcated graft similar to the approach for patients with combined aortic and iliac artery aneurysms. Both open and endovascular approaches are available and the concerns about the individual choice (i.e., open vs. endovascular) are likely similar to that outlined for abdominal aortic aneurysms. Additionally, the principles of treatment for both the open and endovascular approach of isolated iliac artery aneurysms are similar to abdominal aortic aneurysms. In the case of open repair, the proximal anastomosis should be performed immediately below the renal arteries to prevent subsequent aneurysmal degeneration of the infrarenal cuff, while the distal anastomosis should be performed at the common iliac bifurcation on the involved side. The distal anastomosis on the uninvolved common iliac artery can be performed to a nonaneurysmal segment. For the endovascular repair, the graft should be seated immediately below the renal arteries and at the takeoff of the internal iliac artery on the side opposite the aneurysm. The iliac limb on the side of the aneurysm is seated in the external iliac artery and necessitates embolization or bypass of the ipsilateral internal iliac artery.

The treatment of internal iliac artery aneurysms is exclusion. This can be performed using either an endovascular or open approach, although the former is likely preferred due to its simplicity. Bypass of an internal iliac artery aneurysm is not usually possible because there is rarely a proximal or distal neck. Indeed, the aneurysmal involvement usually extends to the common iliac bifurcation and the distal aspect usually arborizes into multiple smaller vessels. The principles of the endovascular treatment include obliterating both the arterial inflow and the outflow of the aneurysm. The outflow is usually thrombosed using selective coil embolization, although a variety of other agents have been described. Placing a covered stent across its orifice extending from the common to the external iliac vessels eliminates the inflow. The open approach requires vascular control of the distal common iliac and proximal external iliac arteries. The internal iliac artery is then opened by incising the aneurysm, and the branches are oversewn from within. The proximal internal iliac artery can be either oversewn at its takeoff or the resultant defect at the common iliac bifurcation can be repaired with patch angioplasty. The appropriate treatment for patients with bilateral internal iliac arteries remains unclear. Exclusion of both vessels has the potential to cause severe pelvic ischemia that may not be remediable. A conservative approach is likely justified in this setting with a higher threshold for intervention appropriate for the second vessel. Treatment options include excluding only the larger vessel, attempted revascularization, and staged exclusion after sufficient time has elapsed to facilitate potential collateral development. Regardless of the treatment option, it is important to assess the status of the pelvic circulation including the profunda femoral artery.

Inflammatory Abdominal Aortic Aneurysms

Approximately 5% of all abdominal aortic aneurysms are described or considered inflammatory.[234] These are characterized by a dense inflammatory response encasing the anterior and lateral walls of the infrarenal aorta with sparing of the posterior aspect. The inflammatory response consists of a dense cellular infiltrate that has a white, glistening appearance on inspection. The inflammation results in an increase in wall thickness with the difference between the inner and outer diameters of the aorta ranging from 1 to 5 cm. The cause of this inflammatory process remains unresolved, but it is likely an autoimmune phenomenon. Indeed, some type of autoimmune disorder has been identified in up to 20% of patients with inflammatory aneurysms.[235]

Patients with an inflammatory abdominal aneurysm are predominantly male and frequently present with symptoms of back or abdominal pain. The triad of a pulsatile abdominal aortic mass, abdominal pain, and an elevated sedimentation rate has been described. Abdominal ultrasonography or CT may confirm the diagnosis. The anterior and lateral aspects of the aortic wall are thickened and hypoechoic on the sonogram. The CT findings are characteristic and include a thick, contrast-enhancing wall in the distribution described. An inexperienced observer may confuse the CT findings with those of a ruptured abdominal aortic aneurysm. Hydronephrosis with medial displacement of the ureters is frequently seen in contradistinction to the lateral displacement seen with noninflammatory aneurysms. Indeed, this entity may share some pathogenetic pathways with retroperitoneal fibrosis.

The treatment of inflammatory abdominal aortic aneurysms is essentially the same as that for the more common, noninflammatory variety. Nonoperative treatment with corticosteroids has been advocated in the past, although this approach is likely ineffective and has largely been abandoned.[236] It has been suggested that the rupture risk of inflammatory aneurysms is less than that for the noninflammatory variety because the wall thickness is increased. However, this is not true, and patients should not be lulled into a false sense of security. It should be emphasized that most aneurysms rupture through their posterior or posterolateral aspect, which is not involved in the inflammatory process. The open repair of an inflammatory abdominal aortic aneurysm is complicated by the fact that the adjacent structures, including the duodenum, colon, and ureters, may be involved in the process and densely adherent to the aortic wall. The operative blood loss and procedure time associated with the open repair of inflammatory abdominal aortic aneurysms may be greater than the more common, uninvolved type. These potential technical difficulties should be factored into the operative indications and size-related threshold for the open approach.

The endovascular approach may be the optimal treatment for patients with inflammatory abdominal aortic aneurysms due to the concerns about the inflammatory process and adherent structures outlined previously.[237–240] Notably, Puchner et al.[240] performed a meta-analysis of patients undergoing endovascular repair for inflammatory aneurysms and reported that the inflammatory process resolved in approximately 50% of the cases. The technical difficulties associated with the open repair can be reduced by using the retroperitoneal approach. Inflammatory aneurysms can be repaired through a transperitoneal approach, and this scenario occasionally arises when the diagnosis is not suspected preoperatively. Regardless of the open approach, no attempt should be made to mobilize the adherent structures, specifically the duodenum, because of the potential for accidental injury. Proximal aortic control can be achieved either immediately above the renal arteries or above the visceral vessels. Alternatively, intraluminal aortic control can be achieved with a balloon catheter, although this approach is less appealing. Distal control can usually be achieved at the common iliac arteries or at the level of their bifurcation. The duodenum and other adherent structures should be mobilized by incising the wall of the aneurysm and then reflecting them laterally. The proximal anastomosis can usually be performed to the infrarenal aorta after the aneurysm wall has been incised. The preoperative placement of ureteral catheters may facilitate their identification intraoperatively and can be helpful in patients with hydronephrosis. An increased incidence of anastomotic pseudoaneurysms has been demonstrated in patients with inflammatory aneurysms after open repair and likely justifies long-term surveillance.[241,242]

Juxtarenal and Suprarenal Abdominal Aortic Aneurysms

The management of aneurysms extending to the level of the renal arteries or more cephalad is complicated, and, predictably, the morbidity and mortality rates associated with open repair are increased.[243–245] Interestingly, several recent reports from centers of excellence have documented mortality rates comparable to those reported for infrarenal repairs, although it is unlikely that these findings are applicable nationwide.[246–248] Repair of these complex aneurysms is complicated by the obligatory period of renal and visceral ischemia associated with aortic occlusion during the proximal anastomosis. Indeed, the renal complication rates range from 15% to 20% even from these select centers of excellence.[246–248] These increased morbidity and mortality rates should be factored into the decision algorithm and threshold for operative repair. Elective operative repair is usually recommended for patients with aneurysms 6 cm or larger in diameter in this setting, although the 5.5-cm criterion may be appropriate for very good-risk patients and those with juxtarenal aneurysms who will require only a short period of suprarenal aortic occlusion.

Abdominal aortic aneurysms extending to the renal arteries or more cephalad may be repaired via either a retroperitoneal or a transperitoneal approach, although the former is optimal. The *retroperitoneal* approach, with elevation of the left kidney, obviates the concerns about the left renal vein and simplifies exposure of the abdominal aorta. Furthermore, the distal descending thoracic aorta may be exposed by incising the diaphragm and its crus. Admittedly, it is more difficult to expose the right renal and common iliac arteries. The proximal anastomosis may be fashioned as a large hood incorporating the orifices of the renal and visceral arteries. Separate revascularization of the left renal artery is occasionally necessary if the orifices of the renal arteries are splayed too far apart by the aneurysm. The *transperitoneal* repair requires exposing the suprarenal aorta for clamp application. This is facilitated by retracting the left renal vein inferiorly after ligating its adrenal, gonadal, and lumbar branches. As noted earlier, the left renal vein may be ligated near its confluence with the cava without adverse sequelae.[182] However, the named collaterals of the left renal vein (e.g., adrenal) should be preserved with this approach. The anterior surface of the aorta at the level of the visceral vessels is encased by dense neural tissue that can be incised. Incising the crus of the diaphragm that envelops the lateral aspect of the aorta further facilitates clamp application. The configuration of the proximal anastomosis in the setting of the transperitoneal approach depends on the extent of the aneurysm and the vessels involved. Juxtarenal aneurysms can be repaired by obtaining suprarenal control and sewing the proximal anastomosis at the level of the renal orifices. The proximal anastomosis for suprarenal aneurysms can be performed by fashioning an anastomotic hood that incorporates most of the visceral vessels, although this frequently requires separate revascularization of one renal artery.

Endovascular aneurysm repair has been reported to be feasible for juxtarenal and suprarenal abdominal aortic aneurysms.[249–252] The approach is based on constructing a suitable landing zone for the more traditional endograft in patients with an inadequate or short infernal neck. This is accomplished using an individually designed fenestrated endograft that contains orifices that correspond to the renal and visceral vessel. These fenestrations permit the introduction of individual covered stents. Although the worldwide experience is somewhat limited and the devices are not commercially available in the United States, the technique has been shown to be feasible and safe and to prevent aneurysm rupture in the short term.[249–252] The technique likely represents the proverbial "next frontier" for endovascular aneurysm and may dramatically impact the care of another group of complex patients not amenable to open repair.

Combined endovascular and open (i.e., "hybrid") approaches have also been used to treat the juxtarenal and more complex proximal aneurysms. These techniques, somewhat similar to the fenestrated graft approach, are based on constructing a suitable aortic neck to land a traditional endograft by "debranching" the renal or visceral vessels. For example, a suitable landing zone below the superior mesenteric artery could be created for a juxtarenal aneurysm by performing bilateral iliorenal bypasses. Although theoretically appealing, early reports have demonstrated that the mortality rates for the hybrid approach for complex aneurysms have been comparable to open repair.[253,254] Indeed, the magnitude of the revascularization procedure appears to be comparable to that of the more traditional open repair and, accordingly, the approach does not appear to extend the indications for aneurysm repair to older, sicker patients.

Infected Abdominal Aortic Aneurysms

Infected abdominal aortic aneurysms comprise a small subset of all abdominal aortic aneurysms, accounting for less than 1% of all repairs.[255] The term *mycotic aneurysm* has traditionally been used to refer to infected aneurysms, although it is a misnomer that has led to a significant amount of confusion. A newer classification system, proposed to clarify the situation, consists of four groups based on the underlying mechanism: (a) mycotic aneurysm, in which a septic embolus from the heart infects an artery; (b) microbial arteritis, in which bacteria infects an atherosclerotic but nonaneurysmal artery and cause aneurysmal degeneration; (c) existing aneurysms that become infected; (d) traumatic pseudoaneurysm with concomitant bacterial inoculation.[256] Microbial arteritis resulting from hematogenous bacterial spread currently accounts for approximately 80% of all cases of infected aortic aneurysms.[257,258] *Salmonella* causes approximately 40% of all aneurysmal infections in contemporary series with the remainder caused by *Streptococcus, Staphylococcus, Bacteroides, Arizona hinshawii, Escherichia coli,* and *Pseudomonas aeruginosa*.[256]

The diagnosis of infected aortic aneurysm is often difficult and the clinical presentation insidious. Patients may present with fever, back/abdominal pain, or both. The physical examination is often remarkable for a palpable abdominal mass and the presence of peripheral emboli. Laboratory studies are notable for an elevated leukocyte count and positive blood cultures, although the latter are present only 50% of the time[258,259] and negative blood cultures do not exclude the diagnosis. CT is the most useful diagnostic study, and the features suggestive of an infected aneurysm include a periaortic mass, an aneurysm in an atypical location, periaortic fluid or gas, retroperitoneal inflammation, and frank rupture. The angiographic finding of a saccular or eccentric aneurysm in an atypical location is also suggestive of an infected aneurysm.

The treatment of an infected aneurysm requires control of hemorrhage in the presence of rupture, removal of all infected tissues, and restoration of perfusion to the viscera and lower torso. Indeed, these treatment concerns and the management options are identical to those for patients with infected aortic grafts, a far more common problem. Patients should be started on broad-spectrum antibiotics when the diagnosis is suspected, although antibiotic therapy alone is not sufficient and the operative intervention should not be delayed in an attempt to sterilize the retroperitoneum. Patients with suspected rupture should undergo emergent exploration through either a transperitoneal or retroperitoneal approach. After vascular control has been obtained, the retroperitoneum should be explored, and intraoperative cultures with an immediate Gram stain should be obtained. Several options for arterial reconstruction are available, including in situ replacement with a prosthetic or cadaveric graft, ligation of the infrarenal aorta with extra-anatomic bypass (axillofemoral, femorofemoral configuration), or in situ replacement with staged extra-anatomic bypass and subsequent removal of the in situ graft. The choice is contingent on the character of the aorta, degree of inflammation in the retroperitoneum, suspected organism, and hemodynamic status. In situ replacement of the infected aneurysm with a prosthetic or cadaveric graft is a reasonable option if retroperitoneal inflammation is minimal and the Gram stain is negative. Ligation of the infrarenal aorta with extra-anatomic bypass at the same session is the recommended approach in most settings, although this is a major undertaking. The three-stage approach of in situ replacement followed by extra-anatomic bypass and graft explant is reserved for patients who cannot tolerate the simultaneous procedure because of underlying comorbidities or hemodynamic instability. The integrity of the aortic stump at the time of ligation and the potential for dehiscence or breakdown of the suture line are major concerns. The aorta should be débrided back to grossly uninvolved tissue and sutured in two layers with a running horizontal mattress and a simple continuous technique using nonabsorbable monofilament suture. A pedicle of omentum can be mobilized and approximated next to the aortic stump to help control the retroperitoneal inflammation and minimize the risk for stump dehiscence. When the diagnosis is suspected preoperatively and no evidence of rupture is found, the staged approach with extra-anatomic bypass followed by graft removal is recommended. The procedures are usually performed 2 to 3 days apart to allow the patients a period of recovery. Patients should be anticoagulated between procedures to prevent thrombosis of the extra-anatomic bypass resulting from competitive flow. Fortunately, the risk of graft thrombosis and graft infection during the intervening period is small. Endovascular repair of infected aortic aneurysm has been reported and should be considered an additional alternative.[260] Although the long-term safety of the endovascular approach remains unclear in this setting, it may serve as a temporizing approach that converts an urgent problem to an elective one. A recent meta-analysis by Kan et al.[261] reported that the endovascular approach was reasonable, but the incidence of subsequent endograft infection was significant in patients with ruptured aneurysms and those with fevers. They concluded that endovascular repair could be used as a bridge in this setting (i.e., ruptured aneurysm, febrile) prior to definitive open repair. Mycotic aneurysms involving the suprarenal aorta pose a particularly challenging problem, but fortunately they are uncommon. In situ replacement with a prosthetic or cadaveric graft is frequently the only available option. Extra-anatomic bypass (hepatorenal and splenorenal) of the renal arteries with ligation of the suprarenal aorta is an option but represents a significant undertaking and should be reserved for select cases.

Patients with infected aneurysms, regardless of the arterial reconstruction, require long-term antibiotics and follow-up. Patients should receive intravenous antibiotics for 6 weeks, with the specific choice depending on the culture results. After completing the intravenous antibiotics, patients should be started on oral antibiotics, although the duration of treatment remains unresolved. Patients should be treated with at least 6 months of oral antibiotics and suppressive, lifelong therapy may be appropriate. Additionally, patients should undergo serial CT scans to assess the retroperitoneum and the status of the in situ graft when applicable. A CT scan is usually performed at 2 weeks, 3 months, and 6 months, and then at 6-month intervals thereafter. This is not necessary for patients with extra-anatomic revascularization in the absence of retroperitoneal inflammation. Predictably, the morbidity and mortality rates associated with infected abdominal aortic aneurysms are significant, with a 40% mortality rate reported in a recent publication.[262]

Aortoenteric Fistulas

An aortoenteric fistula is a communication between the aorta and the bowel. The duodenum is involved most commonly at the site where it crosses over the aorta, but the communication can develop between almost any portion of the intestine. Primary aortic fistulas result when nonspecific abdominal aortic aneurysms erode into the bowel and are distinctly rare, with a reported incidence of 0.04% to 0.07% in autopsy series.[263] Debonnaire et al.[264] identified 18 primary aortoenteric fistulas through a survey of 196 Belgian surgeons and reported a mortality rate of 30%. Secondary aortic fistulas result from the erosion of a prosthetic aortic graft into the bowel; they are significantly more common, with a reported incidence of 0.1% to 2.0% after aortic reconstruction.[265] Notably, they can occur after endovascular aneurysm repair.[266] The management of both primary and secondary aortic fistulas is the same.

The diagnosis of an aortoenteric fistula is often difficult and mandates a high index of suspicion. Patients usually present with gastrointestinal bleeding manifested as either hematemesis or melena. The initial episode of gastrointestinal bleeding is often self-limited and has been described as a "herald" bleed. The diagnosis of aortoenteric fistula should be foremost among the differential when a patient with a known aneurysm or prior aortic reconstruction presents with intestinal bleeding. Patients should undergo endoscopic evaluation of the upper and lower intestinal tract to determine the source of bleeding. It is imperative that the clinical suspicion of an aortoenteric fistula be communicated to the endoscopist to ensure that the third and fourth portions of the duodenum are adequately examined. This occasionally requires the use of a pediatric colonoscope. The endoscopic findings of erosion, thrombus, active bleeding, or visible prosthetic graft in the third or fourth portion of the duodenum are diagnostic of an aortoenteric fistula and mandate emergent laparotomy. Mild duodenitis and gastritis are frequently seen at the time of endoscopy and do not exclude the diagnosis of an aortoenteric fistula. Notably, the findings during upper endoscopy are normal in up to 30% of patients with a documented aortoenteric fistula.[267] A CT should be performed if the results of endoscopy are inconclusive. The findings on CT that suggest an aortoenteric fistula include inflammation within the retroperitoneum, an anastomotic pseudoaneurysm, close approximation of the bowel and the prosthetic aortic graft or aneurysm, and loss of the normal tissue planes between the third portion of the duodenum and the aorta or prosthetic graft. Occasionally, both endoscopy and CT are nondiagnostic despite the clinical suspicion of an aortoenteric fistula. Exploratory laparotomy is recommended in this setting for both diagnosis and treatment. Adherence of the bowel to the aorta at the time of the initial exploration suggests an aortoenteric fistula and mandates obtaining suitable proximal and distal control of the aorta, iliac vessels, or prosthetic graft before further dissection. The diagnosis cannot be excluded until the bowel is entirely separated from the retroperitoneum.

The treatment of an aortoenteric fistula requires repair of the defect in the gastrointestinal tract in addition to repair of the aneurysm or treatment of the infected prosthetic graft. Treatment of the gastrointestinal defect is usually straightforward and is based on standard surgical principles.[268] After the fistula is disassembled, the edges of the bowel can be débrided and a primary closure performed with either a stapler or sutures. A limited bowel resection or diversion of the enteral tract may be necessary. The intraoperative and longer-term management of the aortic aneurysm or prosthetic graft is the same as that outlined earlier for infected aortic aneurysms. Indeed, aortoenteric fistulas represent a variant of infected aortic aneurysms. In situ replacement of the prosthetic graft or infrarenal aorta, ligation of the infrarenal aorta with excision of the prosthetic graft and extra-anatomic bypass, and in situ replacement with staged extra-anatomic bypass and subsequent graft excision are all reasonable options. The clinical scenario usually dictates the choice. Ligation of the infrarenal aorta with excision of the graft and extra-anatomic bypass is recommended in most cases. However, in situ repair is appropriate for patients who are older or sicker, those with minimal retroperitoneal inflammation or evidence of hemodynamic instability, and those in whom ligation of the infrarenal aorta would compromise the renal arteries. Additionally, patients should be maintained on long-term antibiotics and undergo serial imaging studies, as outlined for infected aneurysms.

Venous Anomalies

Anomalies of the vena cava and renal veins are occasionally encountered at the time of aortic reconstruction. The common anomalies are related to the embryologic development of the iliac veins and vena cava. The four most clinically relevant anomalies include duplication of the inferior vena cava (0.2% to 3.0%), left-sided vena cava (0.2% to 0.5%), circumaortic left renal vein (1.5% to 8.7%), and retroaortic renal vein (1.2% to 2.4%).[269] Patients with a duplicated inferior vena cava have large veins that run parallel to the infrarenal aorta and join together either anterior or posterior to the aorta at the level of the renal vein. In the case of a left-sided inferior vena cava, a large vein runs parallel to the left side of the aorta, and the traditional right-sided vena cava is absent. The left-sided vena cava crosses the aorta at the level of the renal vein to become the suprarenal inferior vena cava. The gonadal and adrenal veins on the right drain directly into the renal vein in a mirror image of the normal anatomy. The circumaortic left renal vein forms a collar of veins that surrounds the aorta at the normal level. In the case of a retroaortic left renal vein, a single vein runs posterior to the aorta at a slightly more caudal location. Notably, both duplication of the inferior vena cava and left-sided vena cava can be associated with other venous anomalies, including a circumaortic or retroaortic renal vein.

The diagnosis of the various venous anomalies can usually be made preoperatively on CT. Identification of the vena cava and left renal vein should be part of the mental checklist used when the preoperative CT scans are reviewed. The various anomalies may not become evident immediately in the operating room if missed on the preoperative imaging studies. A very prominent left renal vein at the usual location or slightly inferior is suggestive of a left-sided vena cava, whereas the absence of a left renal vein despite dissection along the anterior aspect of the aorta at the level of the superior mesenteric artery is suggestive of a retroaortic renal vein.

The open repair of an infrarenal abdominal aortic aneurysm in a patient with a venous anomaly is essentially the same as the standard approach, although additional care should be exercised to prevent inadvertent injury. Exposure of the infrarenal neck is more difficult in the presence of a duplicated or left-sided vena cava. However, sufficient exposure can usually be obtained by gentle dissection and mobilization of the venous structures. The presence of a duplicated or left-sided vena cava is a relative contraindication to the left retroperitoneal approach. A circumaortic left renal collar or retroaortic left renal vein presents a potential hazard when the proximal aortic clamp is applied. A vertical aortic clamp is recommended and obviates the dissection on the posterior aspect of the aorta. Transecting the aorta may facilitate exposure of a retroaortic renal vein when significant bleeding is encountered.

Renal Anomalies

Congenital variations in the renal anatomy may complicate the repair of an abdominal aortic aneurysm. Specifically, their presence may complicate the dissection during open repair because they are frequently associated with multiple renal arteries, aberrant venous return, and abnormally positioned ureters. The various congenital anomalies of the upper urinary system have been classified in an attempt to standardize the approach for vascular surgeons.[270] The anomalies have been broken down into abnormalities of position, including simple ectopia, and abnormalities of both form and fusion, including horseshoe kidney, crossed renal ectopia without fusion, and crossed renal ectopia with fusion. An ectopic kidney may be positioned anywhere from the pelvis to the thorax. Common forms of ectopic kidney include the pelvic kidney, located opposite the sacrum and below the aortic bifurcation; the lumbar kidney, located opposite the sacral promontory in the iliac fossa and anterior to the iliac vessels; the abdominal kidney, located above the iliac crest adjacent to the second lumbar vertebra; and the thoracic kidney, which can be located above the diaphragm in the posterior mediastinum. In a horseshoe kidney, two distinct renal masses are fused together by either a bridge of renal parenchyma or fibrous tissue; in the overwhelming majority, the lower poles are fused. In crossed renal ectopia, the kidney mass is located on the side opposite to its insertion in the bladder. Multiple configurations of crossed ectopia with and without fusion have been described.

The preoperative objective for the various renal anomalies is to image the renal mass adequately, delineate the course of the ureter, and establish the arterial and venous supply. The approach is simplified by the fact that most patients undergo abdominal/pelvic CT as part of the preoperative evaluation. The location and position of both the kidneys and ureters, like the position of the left renal vein, should be established as part of the review of every CT scan for patients with aneurysms. Formerly, it was recommended that patients with renal anomalies undergo preoperative arteriography to confirm the location and number of renal arteries. However, this information can now be obtained from the CT arteriogram, which is now part of the routine preoperative evaluation.

Patients with renal anomalies can safely undergo repair of an abdominal aortic aneurysm using either an open or endovascular approach.[271–273] However, the anomalies must be factored into the operative plan. The specific operative approach depends on the location of the renal mass, blood supply, course of the ureters, and presence of fusion. A left-sided retroperitoneal or transperitoneal approach with medial visceral rotation is the most helpful for open repair, particularly in patients with a horseshoe kidney. A standard transperitoneal approach with transection of the fused parenchyma can be used in patients with a horseshoe kidney, although this may be associated with both significant bleeding and a urine leak and, therefore, is discouraged. The frequently encountered multiple renal arteries can be handled most expeditiously by using a Carrel patch technique, in which a cuff of aorta including the renal artery orifices is reimplanted into the aortic graft after completion of the proximal anastomosis. Endovascular repair is possible in many cases, with the feasibility dictated by the location of the renal arteries in addition to the other standard anatomic considerations. Use of the endovascular approach may require covering at least one of the renal vessels and has been associated with loss of some renal parenchyma.[271]

Coexistent Renal or Visceral Artery Occlusive Disease

Coexistent renal or visceral artery occlusive disease is frequently found in patients undergoing abdominal aortic aneurysm repair. The optimal management of patients with coexistent lesions remains unresolved. The options include repair of the aneurysm alone, simultaneous repair of the aneurysm and revascularization of the renal or visceral vessels, and staged repair, with either aneurysm repair or revascularization performed first. Furthermore, the specific treatment options include both open and endovascular alternatives for the aneurysm repair and visceral/ renal revascularization (i.e., angioplasty/stent). The rapid expansion of the endovascular technologies has afforded effective, safe approaches that have widely replaced open surgical revascularization for both renal and visceral artery lesions. Regardless, the optimal approach represents a balance between the indications for the procedure and the associated added risk.

Renal/visceral revascularization is mandatory at the time of open aneurysm repair if the affected vessels are involved in the aneurysm, as in a suprarenal aneurysm or a horseshoe kidney. More commonly, a lower pole or accessory renal artery may come off the aneurysm. The decision to perform a concomitant revascularization with either reimplantation or a bypass graft in this setting depends on the size of the vessel and the quantity of kidney parenchyma perfused. Revascularization is recommended for larger vessels (>2 mm) that supply a significant portion of the renal mass. The presence of any accessory renal arteries should factor into the operative plan and the general feasibility for endovascular repair. Covering small, accessory renal arteries has been reported to be safe, although it must be appreciated that this approach sacrifices some renal parenchyma.[274]

Combined aneurysm repair with renal or visceral artery revascularization may be justified if the indications for renal or visceral artery revascularization are satisfied. The traditional indications for renal revascularization included poorly controlled hypertension in a patient with a significant renal artery stenosis and rapidly progressive renal insufficiency in a patient with adequate renal mass and bilateral renal artery stenoses. However, the antihypertensive agents have improved so much that renal revascularization is currently reserved for patients with poor blood pressure control despite optimal medical therapy encompassing three or more, separate medications.[275] The indication for renal revascularization in patients with atherosclerotic renal artery disease and progressive renal insufficiency is even less compelling although the focus of several ongoing randomized trials. Endovascular treatment of the renal artery stenoses (when indicated) can be performed prior to open aneurysm repair or simultaneous with the endovascular approach. Although feasible, simultaneous open aneurysm repair and renal artery bypass is associated with a significant increase in the operative mortality rate relative to the aneurysm repair alone.[276,277]

The traditional indications for mesenteric revascularization include symptoms of chronic mesenteric ischemia and critical stenosis of either the superior mesenteric artery alone or two of the three visceral vessels. Patients with chronic mesenteric ischemia and abdominal aortic aneurysms should have their visceral occlusive disease corrected prior to aneurysm repair. Repairing the aneurysm first potentially increases the risk of developing acute mesenteric ischemia, while the simultaneous open approach is likely prohibitive given the significant morbidity/mortality associated with open mesenteric revascularization alone.[278–280] Endovascular treatment with balloon angioplasty and stenting is probably the optimal treatment for the visceral lesions in this setting because of its simplicity despite the concerns about its longer-term durability.[281,282]

The optimal treatment for patients with aneurysms and *asymptomatic* renal or visceral artery lesions remains even less clear. Natural history studies with the use of both arteriography[283] and duplex scanning[284] have suggested that significant renal artery stenoses are preocclusive lesions that may merit intervention. However, analysis of patients with asymptomatic renal artery stenosis who underwent aortic reconstruction found that the natural history of the renal artery lesions is fairly benign when untreated and is associated only with an increase in the antihypertensive requirements.[285] Little is known about the natural history of asymptomatic mesenteric occlusive lesions. However, a recent small report suggested that patients with asymptomatic severe mesenteric occlusive disease involving all three visceral vessels have a high incidence of bowel infarction.[286] Consideration should be given for mesenteric revascularization prior to aneurysm repair in patients with severe visceral artery occlusive disease due to the potential risk of mesenteric infarction at the time of aneurysm repair as noted earlier.

Additional Concurrent Intra-abdominal Disease

The finding of an abdominal aortic aneurysm and an additional intra-abdominal process that may require operative repair is a frequent event. A second surgical problem may be identified as part of the preoperative evaluation or discovered at the time of the exploratory laparotomy during open aneurysm repair. Alternatively, an abdominal aortic aneurysm may be identified during the surgical treatment of another problem. No algorithms have been defined for the management of such concurrent problems, and the overall approach requires a modicum of clinical judgment. Options include simultaneous repair or staged repair with repair of the abdominal aortic aneurysm as either the first or second procedure. The approach depends on the risk for aneurysm rupture, natural history of the second surgical problem, and potential for infection of the prosthetic graft during simultaneous repair. Notably, both the laparoscopic and endovascular approaches have impacted the approach to patients with combined problems due to their reduced morbidity and mortality that facilitates a more rapid, definitive treatment.

The generic recommendation for patients with an abdominal aortic aneurysm and an additional intra-abdominal surgical problem is that the most life-threatening or imminent problem be addressed first. The natural history of untreated abdominal aortic aneurysm has been defined reasonably well and has been outlined extensively earlier in this chapter. It has been suggested that the risk for aneurysm rupture is increased after major intra-abdominal surgery and that it is potentially related to an increase in collagenase activity.[287] However, this reported increased rupture risk is speculative and should not necessarily be factored into the decision algorithm. The management of concurrent colon cancer and abdominal aortic aneurysm is a frequent treatment dilemma that provides an excellent illustration of the approach to these problems. Indeed, the reported incidence of colon cancer and an abdominal aortic aneurysm occurring simultaneously ranges from 0.5% to 2.1%.[181] The treatment principles promulgated by Szilagyi et al.[288] include the following: (a) aneurysm repair first in the presence of rupture; (b) colon resection first in the presence of hemorrhage, perforation, or obstruction; (c) aneurysm repair first in the presence of a large aneurysm and a small colon cancer; (d) colon resection first in the presence of a large colon cancer and a small aneurysm.

Simultaneous abdominal aortic aneurysm repair and cholecystectomy is probably safe for patients with cholelithiasis or evidence of chronic cholecystitis. The safety of these simultaneous procedures has been documented in several series, and the concerns about an increased incidence of aortic graft infection have not been substantiated.[289] Advocates of the simultaneous approach justify the cholecystectomy by the potential requirement for a cholecystectomy in the future and the morbidity and mortality associated with cholecystitis after aneurysm repair.[289] Although a consensus is not found in the literature, simultaneous abdominal aortic aneurysm repair and cholecystectomy are recommended only if evidence of chronic cholecystitis or multiple small stones is present. Regardless, the cholecystectomy and other simultaneous procedures should not be performed until after the aneurysm repair is completed and the retroperitoneum closed in an attempt to reduce the hypothetical risk for graft infection.

The safety and utility of other simultaneous procedures remain poorly defined, although a wide range of procedures have been combined with open aneurysm repair.[178–181] The repair of ventral hernias is often mandatory to achieve a tension-free abdominal closure and should be viewed more as an extension of the aneurysm repair than as a simultaneous procedure. Inguinal hernias may be repaired at the time of aneurysm repair, but it is uncertain whether the small risk associated with a subsequent procedure at a later date offsets the obligatory additional time for the simultaneous repair. Appendectomy[290] and small-bowel excision for Meckel diverticulum[289] have been reported to be safe when performed concomitantly with aneurysmectomy, although the natural history of the associated underlying problems in the usual age group of patients undergoing abdominal aortic aneurysm repair is relatively benign.

References

1. Dubost C, Allary M, Oeconomos N. Resection of an aneurysm of the abdominal aorta: reestablishment of the continuity by a preserved human arterial graft, with result after five months. *AMA Arch Surg* 1952;64(3): 405–408.
2. Ernst CB. Abdominal aortic aneurysm. *N Engl J Med* 1993;328(16): 1167–1172.
3. Collin J, Araujo L, Walton J, et al. Oxford screening programme for abdominal aortic aneurysm in men aged 65 to 74 years. *Lancet* 1988; 2(8611):613–615.
4. Ouriel K, Green RM, Donayre C, et al. An evaluation of new methods of expressing aortic aneurysm size: relationship to rupture. *J Vasc Surg* 1992; 15(1):12–18.
5. Taylor LM, Porter JM. Abdominal aortic aneurysms. In: Porter JM, Taylor LM, eds. *Basic Data Underlying Clinical Decision Making in Vascular Surgery*. St. Louis, MO: Quality Medical; 1994:98–100.
6. Brunkwall J, Hauksson H, Bengtsson H, et al. Solitary aneurysms of the iliac arterial system: an estimate of their frequency of occurrence. *J Vasc Surg* 1989;10(4):381–384.
7. Lowry SF, Kraft RO. Isolated aneurysms of the iliac artery. *Arch Surg* 1978;113(11):1289–1293.
8. Best VA, Price JF, Fowkes FG. Persistent increase in the incidence of abdominal aortic aneurysm in Scotland, 1981–2000. *Br J Surg* 2003; 90(12):1510–1515.
9. Hoyert DL, Kung H, Smith BL. Deaths: preliminary data for 2003. *Natl Vital Stat Rep* 2005;53(15):1–48.

10. Zarins CK, Glagov S. Aneurysms and obstructive placques: differing local responses to atherosclerosis. In: Bergan JJ, Yao J, eds. *Aneurysms: Diagnosis and Treatment*. New York: Grune and Stratton; 1982:61.
11. Sho E, Sho M, Hoshina K, et al. Hemodynamic forces regulate mural macrophage infiltration in experimental aortic aneurysms. *Exp Mol Pathol* 2004;76(2):108–116.
12. Tilson MD, Elefteriades J, Brophy CM. Tensile strength and collagen in abdominal aortic aneurysm disease. In: Greenhalgh RM, Mannick JA, Powell JT, eds. *The Cause and Management of Aneurysms*. Philadelphia: W.B. Saunders; 1990:97.
13. Busuttil RW, Abou-Zamzam AM, Machleder HI. Collagenase activity of the human aorta. A comparison of patients with and without abdominal aortic aneurysms. *Arch Surg* 1980;115(11):1373–1378.
14. Baxter BT, McGee GS, Shively VP, et al. Elastin content, cross-links, and mRNA in normal and aneurysmal human aorta. *J Vasc Surg* 1992;16(2): 192–200.
15. Lindholt JS, Jorgensen B, Klitgaard NA, et al. Systemic levels of cotinine and elastase, but not pulmonary function, are associated with the progression of small abdominal aortic aneurysms. *Eur J Vasc Endovasc Surg* 2003;26(4):418–422.
16. Newman KM, Ogata Y, Malon AM, et al. Identification of matrix metalloproteinases 3 (stromelysin-1) and 9 (gelatinase B) in abdominal aortic aneurysm. *Arterioscler Thromb* 1994;14(8):1315–1320.
17. Brophy CM, Marks WH, Reilly JM, et al. Decreased tissue inhibitor of metalloproteinases (TIMP) in abdominal aortic tissue: a preliminary report. *J Surg Res* 1991;50:653.
18. Rowe VL, Stevens SL, Reddick TT, et al. Vascular smooth muscle cell apoptosis in aneurysmal, occlusive, and normal human aortas. *J Vasc Surg* 2000;31(3):567–576.
19. Eliason JL, Ailawadi G, Sinha I. Neutrophil depletion inhibits experimental aortic aneurysm formation unrelated to MMP-2 and MMP-9. Vascular Annual Meeting 2003, June 2003, Chicago, IL.
20. Newman KM, Jean-Claude J, Li H, et al. Cytokines that activate proteolysis are increased in abdominal aortic aneurysms. *Circulation* 1994;90(5 Pt 2): II224–II227.
21. Cornuz J, Sidoti PC, Tevaearai H, et al. Risk factors for asymptomatic abdominal aortic aneurysm: systematic review and meta-analysis of population-based screening studies. *Eur J Public Health* 2004;14(4):343–349.
22. Baumgartner I, Hirsch AT, Abola MT, et al. Cardiovascular risk profile and outcome of patients with abdominal aortic aneurysm in out-patients with atherothrombosis: data from the Reduction of Atherothrombosis for Continued Health (REACH) Registry. *J Vasc Surg* 2008;48(4):808–814.
23. Lederle FA, Larson JC, Margolis KL, et al. Abdominal aortic aneurysm events in the women's health initiative: cohort study. *BMJ* 2008;337: a1724.
24. Lederle FA, Johnson GR, Wilson SE, et al. Prevalence and associations of abdominal aortic aneurysm detected through screening. Aneurysm Detection and Management (ADAM) Veterans Affairs Cooperative Study Group. *Ann Intern Med* 1997;126(6):441–449.
25. Huber TS, Wang JG, Derrow AE, et al. Experience in the United States with intact abdominal aortic aneurysm repair. *J Vasc Surg* 2001;33(2): 304–310.
26. Lederle FA, Wilson SE, Johnson GR, et al. Immediate repair compared with surveillance of small abdominal aortic aneurysms. *N Engl J Med* 2002;346(19):1437–1444.
27. Wilmink TB, Quick CR, Day NE. The association between cigarette smoking and abdominal aortic aneurysms. *J Vasc Surg* 1999;30(6):1099–1105.
28. Darling RC III, Brewster DC, Darling RC, et al. Are familial aortic aneurysms different? *J Vasc Surg* 1989;10:39–43.
29. Larsson E, Granath F, Swedenborg J, et al. A population-based case-control study of the familial risk of abdominal aortic aneurysm. *J Vasc Surg* 2009;49(1):47–50.
30. Calcagno D, Hallett JW Jr, Ballard DJ, et al. Late iliac artery aneurysms and occlusive disease after aortic tube grafts for abdominal aortic aneurysm repair. A 35-year experience. *Ann Surg* 1991;214(6): 733–736.
31. Kalman PG, Rappaport DC, Merchant N, et al. The value of late computed tomographic scanning in identification of vascular abnormalities after abdominal aortic aneurysm repair. *J Vasc Surg* 1999;29:442–450.
32. Cutler BS. Arteriosclerotic femoral artery aneurysms. In: Ernst CB, Stanley JC, eds. *Current Therapy in Vascular Surgery*, 3rd ed. St. Louis, MO: Mosby; 1995:315.
33. Haverich A, Miller DC, Scott WC, et al. Acute and chronic aortic dissections–determinants of long-term outcome for operative survivors. *Circulation* 1985;72(3 Pt 2):II22–II34.
34. Ammori BJ, Madan M, Bodenham AR. A review of the management of abdominal aortic aneurysms in patients following cardiac transplantation. *Eur J Vasc Endovasc Surg* 1997;14(3):185–190.
35. Muluk SC, Steed DL, Makaroun MS, et al. Aortic aneurysm in heart transplant recipients. *J Vasc Surg* 1995;22(6):689–694.
36. Vantrimpont PJ, van Dalen BM, van Riemsdijk-van Overbeeke IC, et al. Abdominal aortic aneurysms after heart transplantation. *J Heart Lung Transplant* 2004;23(2):171–177.
37. Zierler RE, Strandness DE Jr. Hemodynamics for the vascular surgeon. In: Moore WS, ed. *Vascular Surgery: A Comprehensive Review*, 4th ed. Philadelphia: W.B. Saunders; 2005:179–204.
38. Brewster DC, Cronenwett JL, Hallett JW Jr., et al. Guidelines for the treatment of abdominal aortic aneurysms. Report of a subcommittee of the Joint Council of the American Association for Vascular Surgery and Society for Vascular Surgery. *J Vasc Surg* 2003;37(5):1106–1117.
39. Mortality results for randomised controlled trial of early elective surgery or ultrasonographic surveillance for small abdominal aortic aneurysms. The UK Small Aneurysm Trial Participants. *Lancet* 1998;352(9141): 1649–1655.
40. Brown LC, Powell JT. Risk factors for aneurysm rupture in patients kept under ultrasound surveillance. UK Small Aneurysm Trial Participants. *Ann Surg* 1999;230(3):289–296.
41. Mofidi R, Suttie SA, Howd A, et al. Outcome from abdominal aortic aneurysms in Scotland, 1991–2006. *Br J Surg* 2008;95(12):1475–1479.
42. Brown PM, Zelt DT, Sobolev B. The risk of rupture in untreated aneurysms: the impact of size, gender, and expansion rate. *J Vasc Surg* 2003;37(2):280–284.
43. Cronenwett JL, Murphy TF, Zelenock GB, et al. Actuarial analysis of variables associated with rupture of small abdominal aortic aneurysms. *Surgery* 1985;98(3):472–483.
44. Verloes A, Sakalihasan N, Koulischer L, et al. Aneurysms of the abdominal aorta: familial and genetic aspects in three hundred thirteen pedigrees. *J Vasc Surg* 1995;21(4):646–655.
45. Fillinger MF, Marra SP, Raghavan ML, et al. Prediction of rupture risk in abdominal aortic aneurysm during observation: wall stress versus diameter. *J Vasc Surg* 2003;37(4):724–732.
46. Fillinger MF, Raghavan ML, Marra SP, et al. In vivo analysis of mechanical wall stress and abdominal aortic aneurysm rupture risk. *J Vasc Surg* 2002;36(3):589–597.
47. Brady AR, Thompson SG, Fowkes FG, et al. Abdominal aortic aneurysm expansion: risk factors and time intervals for surveillance. *Circulation* 2004;110(1):16–21.
48. Nevitt MP, Ballard DJ, Hallett JW Jr. Prognosis of abdominal aortic aneurysms. A population-based study. *N Engl J Med* 1989;321(15): 1009–1014.
49. Solberg S, Singh K, Wilsgaard T, et al. Increased growth rate of abdominal aortic aneurysms in women. The Tromso study. *Eur J Vasc Endovasc Surg* 2005;29(2):145–149.
50. Bernstein EF, Chan EL. Abdominal aortic aneurysm in high-risk patients. Outcome of selective management based on size and expansion rate. *Ann Surg* 1984;200(3):255–263.
51. Delin A, Ohlsen H, Swedenborg J. Growth rate of abdominal aortic aneurysms as measured by computed tomography. *Br J Surg* 1985;72(7): 530–532.
52. Guirguis EM, Barber GG. The natural history of abdominal aortic aneurysms. *Am J Surg* 1991;162(5):481–483.
53. Baxter BT, Terrin MC, Dalman RL. Medical management of small abdominal aortic aneurysms. *Circulation* 2008;117(14):1883–1889.
54. Mosorin M, Juvonen J, Biancari F, et al. Use of doxycycline to decrease the growth rate of abdominal aortic aneurysms: a randomized, double-blind, placebo-controlled pilot study. *J Vasc Surg* 2001;34(4):606–610.
55. Kurvers H, Veith FJ, Lipsitz EC, et al. Discontinuous, staccato growth of abdominal aortic aneurysms. *J Am Coll Surg* 2004;199(5):709–715.
56. Beck AW, Goodney PP, Nolan BW, et al. Predicting 1-year mortality after elective abdominal aortic aneurysm repair. *J Vasc Surg* 2009;49(4): 838–843.
57. Hua HT, Cambria RP, Chuang SK, et al. Early outcomes of endovascular versus open abdominal aortic aneurysm repair in the National Surgical Quality Improvement Program-Private Sector (NSQIP-PS). *J Vasc Surg* 2005;41(3):382–389.
58. Schermerhorn ML, O'Malley AJ, Jhaveri A, et al. Endovascular vs. open repair of abdominal aortic aneurysms in the Medicare population. *N Engl J Med* 2008;358(5):464–474.
59. Greenhalgh RM, Brown LC, Kwong GP, et al. Comparison of endovascular aneurysm repair with open repair in patients with abdominal aortic aneurysm (EVAR trial 1), 30-day operative mortality results: randomised controlled trial. *Lancet* 2004;364(9437):843–848.
60. Prinssen M, Verhoeven EL, Buth J, et al. A randomized trial comparing conventional and endovascular repair of abdominal aortic aneurysms. *N Engl J Med* 2004;351(16):1607–1618.
61. Hallin A, Bergqvist D, Holmberg L. Literature review of surgical management of abdominal aortic aneurysm. *Eur J Vasc Endovasc Surg* 2001; 22(3):197–204.
62. Blum U, Voshage G, Lammer J, et al. Endoluminal stent-grafts for infrarenal abdominal aortic aneurysms. *N Engl J Med* 1997;336(1): 13–20.
63. May J, White GH, Yu W, et al. Concurrent comparison of endoluminal versus open repair in the treatment of abdominal aortic aneurysms: analysis of 303 patients by life table method. *J Vasc Surg* 1998;27(2): 213–220.
64. Moore WS, Rutherford RB. Transfemoral endovascular repair of abdominal aortic aneurysm: results of the North American EVT phase 1 trial. EVT Investigators. *J Vasc Surg* 1996;23(4):543–553.
65. Zarins CK, White RA, Schwarten D, et al. AneuRx stent graft versus open surgical repair of abdominal aortic aneurysms: multicenter prospective clinical trial. *J Vasc Surg* 1999;29(2):292–305.
66. Lee WA, Carter JW, Upchurch G, et al. Perioperative outcomes after open and endovascular repair of intact abdominal aortic aneurysms in the United States during 2001. *J Vasc Surg* 2004;39(3):491–496.
67. Haug ES, Romundstad P, Aadahl P, et al. Emergency non-ruptured abdominal aortic aneurysm. *Eur J Vasc Endovasc Surg* 2004;28(6):612–618.

68. Soisalon-Soininen S, Salo JA, Perhoniemi V, et al. Emergency surgery of non-ruptured abdominal aortic aneurysm. *Ann Chir Gynaecol* 1999;88: 38–43.
69. Bown MJ, Sutton AJ, Bell PR, et al. A meta-analysis of 50 years of ruptured abdominal aortic aneurysm repair. *Br J Surg* 2002;89(6):714–730.
70. Johansen K, Kohler TR, Nicholls SC, et al. Ruptured abdominal aortic aneurysm: the Harborview experience. *J Vasc Surg* 1991;13(2):240–245.
71. Egorova N, Giacovelli J, Greco G, et al. National outcomes for the treatment of ruptured abdominal aortic aneurysm: comparison of open versus endovascular repairs. *J Vasc Surg* 2008;48(5):1092–1100, 1100.e1–e2.
72. Mastracci TM, Garrido-Olivares L, Cina CS, et al. Endovascular repair of ruptured abdominal aortic aneurysms: a systematic review and meta-analysis. *J Vasc Surg* 2008;47(1):214–221.
73. Mureebe L, Egorova N, Giacovelli JK, et al. National trends in the repair of ruptured abdominal aortic aneurysms. *J Vasc Surg* 2008;48(5): 1101–1107.
74. Rayt HS, Sutton AJ, London NJ, et al. A systematic review and meta-analysis of endovascular repair (EVAR) for ruptured abdominal aortic aneurysm. *Eur J Vasc Endovasc Surg* 2008;36(5):536–544.
75. Sadat U, Boyle JR, Walsh SR, et al. Endovascular vs open repair of acute abdominal aortic aneurysms–a systematic review and meta-analysis. *J Vasc Surg* 2008;48(1):227–236.
76. Verhoeven EL, Kapma MR, Groen H, et al. Mortality of ruptured abdominal aortic aneurysm treated with open or endovascular repair. *J Vasc Surg* 2008;48:1396–1400.
77. Giles KA, Pomposelli F, Hamdan A, et al. Decrease in total aneurysm-related deaths in the era of endovascular aneurysm repair. *J Vasc Surg* 2009;49(3):543–550.
78. Lynch RM. Accuracy of abdominal examination in the diagnosis of non-ruptured abdominal aortic aneurysm. *Accid Emerg Nurs* 2004;12(2): 99–107.
79. Moursi MM, Stanley JC. Surgical treatment of ruptured infrarenal aortic aneurysms. In: Ernst CB, Stanley JC, eds. *Current Therapy in Vascular Surgery*, 3rd ed. St. Louis, MO: Mosby; 1995:224–226.
80. Moore CL, Holliday RS, Hwang JQ, et al. Screening for abdominal aortic aneurysm in asymptomatic at-risk patients using emergency ultrasound. *Am J Emerg Med* 2008;26(8):883–887.
81. Hollier LH, Taylor LM, Ochsner J. Recommended indications for operative treatment of abdominal aortic aneurysms. Report of a subcommittee of the Joint Council of the Society for Vascular Surgery and the North American Chapter of the International Society for Cardiovascular Surgery. *J Vasc Surg* 1992;15(6):1046–1056.
82. Liu R, Nair D, Ix J, et al. N-acetylcysteine for the prevention of contrast-induced nephropathy. A systematic review and meta-analysis. *J Gen Intern Med* 2005;20(2):193–200.
83. Merten GJ, Burgess WP, Gray LV, et al. Prevention of contrast-induced nephropathy with sodium bicarbonate: a randomized controlled trial. *JAMA* 2004;291(19):2328–2334.
84. Sprouse LR, Meier GH III, Parent FN, et al. Is three-dimensional computed tomography reconstruction justified before endovascular aortic aneurysm repair? *J Vasc Surg* 2004;40(3):443–447.
85. Hoffman M, Avellone JC, Plecha FR, et al. Operation for ruptured abdominal aortic aneurysms: a community-wide experience. *Surgery* 1982;91(5): 597–602.
86. Wakefield TW, Whitehouse WM Jr, Wu SC, et al. Abdominal aortic aneurysm rupture: statistical analysis of factors affecting outcome of surgical treatment. *Surgery* 1982;91(5):586–596.
87. Lloyd GM, Bown MJ, Norwood MG, et al. Feasibility of preoperative computer tomography in patients with ruptured abdominal aortic aneurysm: a time-to-death study in patients without operation. *J Vasc Surg* 2004;39(4):788–791.
88. U.S. Preventive Services Task Force. Screening for abdominal aortic aneurysm: recommendation statement. *Ann Intern Med* 2005;142(3): 198–202.
89. Fleming C, Whitlock EP, Beil TL, et al. Screening for abdominal aortic aneurysm: a best-evidence systematic review for the U. S. Preventive Services Task Force. *Ann Intern Med* 2005;142(3):203–211.
90. Lindholt JS, Juul S, Fasting H, et al. Hospital costs and benefits of screening for abdominal aortic aneurysms. Results from a randomised population screening trial. *Eur J Vasc Endovasc Surg* 2002;23(1):55–60.
91. Wilmink AB, Quick CR, Hubbard CS, et al. Effectiveness and cost of screening for abdominal aortic aneurysm: results of a population screening program. *J Vasc Surg* 2003;38(1):72–77.
92. Kim LG, Scott RA, Thompson SG, et al. Implications of screening for abdominal aortic aneurysms on surgical workload. *Br J Surg* 2005;92(2): 171–176.
93. Powell JT, Brown LC, Forbes JF, et al. Final 12-year follow-up of surgery versus surveillance in the UK Small Aneurysm Trial. *Br J Surg* 2007;94(6): 702–708.
94. Steyerberg EW, Kievit J, de Mol Van Otterloo JC, et al. Perioperative mortality of elective abdominal aortic aneurysm surgery. A clinical prediction rule based on literature and individual patient data. *Arch Intern Med* 1995;155(18):1998–2004.
95. Cronenwett JL. Factors influencing the long-term results of aortic aneurysm surgery. In: Yao J, Pearce WH, eds. *Vascular Surgery: Long Term Results*. East Norwalk: Appleton and Lange; 1993:171–179.
96. Finlayson SR, Birkmeyer JD, Fillinger MF, et al. Should endovascular repair lower the threshold for repair of abdominal aortic aneurysms? *J Vasc Surg* 1999;29:973–985.
97. Valentine RJ, Decaprio JD, Castillo JM, et al. Watchful waiting in cases of small abdominal aortic aneurysms – appropriate for all patients? *J Vasc Surg* 2000;32:441–448.
98. McCarthy RJ, Shaw E, Whyman MR, et al. Recommendations for screening intervals for small aortic aneurysms. *Br J Surg* 2003;90(7): 821–826.
99. Conway KP, Byrne J, Townsend M, et al. Prognosis of patients turned down for conventional abdominal aortic aneurysm repair in the endovascular and sonographic era: Szilagyi revisited? *J Vasc Surg* 2001;33(4): 752–757.
100. Englund R, Perera D, Hanel KC. Outcome for patients with abdominal aortic aneurysms that are treated non-surgically. *Aust N Z J Surg* 1997; 67(5):260–263.
101. Jones A, Cahill D, Gardham R. Outcome in patients with a large abdominal aortic aneurysm considered unfit for surgery. *Br J Surg* 1998;85(10): 1382–1384.
102. Tambyraja AL, Stuart WP, Sala TA, et al. Non-operative management of high-risk patients with abdominal aortic aneurysm. *Eur J Vasc Endovasc Surg* 2003;26(4):401–404.
103. Walker EM, Hopkinson BR, Makin GS. Unoperated abdominal aortic aneurysm: presentation and natural history. *Ann R Coll Surg Engl* 1983; 65(5):311–313.
104. Woodburn KR, Chant H, Davies JN, et al. Suitability for endovascular aneurysm repair in an unselected population. *Br J Surg* 2001;88(1):77–81.
105. Arko FR, Filis KA, Seidel SA, et al. How many patients with infrarenal aneurysms are candidates for endovascular repair? The Northern California experience. *J Endovasc Ther* 2004;11(1):33–40.
106. Carpenter JP, Baum RA, Barker CF, et al. Impact of exclusion criteria on patient selection for endovascular abdominal aortic aneurysm repair. *J Vasc Surg* 2001;34(6):1050–1054.
107. Elkouri S, Martelli E, Gloviczki P, et al. Most patients with abdominal aortic aneurysm are not suitable for endovascular repair using currently approved bifurcated stent-grafts. *Vasc Endovascular Surg* 2004;38(5): 401–412.
108. Wolf YG, Fogarty TJ, Olcott C IV, et al. Endovascular repair of abdominal aortic aneurysms: eligibility rate and impact on the rate of open repair. *J Vasc Surg* 2000;32(3):519–523.
109. Lee WA, Berceli SA, Huber TS, et al. Morbidity with retroperitoneal procedures during endovascular abdominal aortic aneurysm repair. *J Vasc Surg* 2003;38(3):459–463.
110. Clouse WD, Brewster DC, Marone LK, et al. Durability of aortouniiliac endografting with femorofemoral crossover: 4-year experience in the Evt/Guidant trials. *J Vasc Surg* 2003;37(6):1142–1149.
111. Hinchliffe RJ, Alric P, Wenham PW, et al. Durability of femorofemoral bypass grafting after aortouniiliac endovascular aneurysm repair. *J Vasc Surg* 2003;38(3):498–503.
112. Lee WA, O'Dorisio J, Wolf YG, et al. Outcome after unilateral hypogastric artery occlusion during endovascular aneurysm repair. *J Vasc Surg* 2001; 33(5):921–926.
113. Lyden SP, Sternbach Y, Waldman DL, et al. Clinical implications of internal iliac artery embolization in endovascular repair of aortoiliac aneurysms. *Ann Vasc Surg* 2001;15(5):539–543.
114. Greenberg RK, Clair D, Srivastava S, et al. Should patients with challenging anatomy be offered endovascular aneurysm repair? *J Vasc Surg* 2003; 38(5):990–996.
115. Buth J, Harris PL, van Marrewijk C, et al. The significance and management of different types of endoleaks. *Semin Vasc Surg* 2003;16(2):95–102.
116. Gilling-Smith GL, Martin J, Sudhindran S, et al. Freedom from endoleak after endovascular aneurysm repair does not equal treatment success. *Eur J Vasc Endovasc Surg* 2000;19(4):421–425.
117. Rutherford RB, Krupski WC. Current status of open versus endovascular stent-graft repair of abdominal aortic aneurysm. *J Vasc Surg* 2004;39(5): 1129–1139.
118. Prinssen M, Buskens E, Nolthenius RP, et al. Sexual dysfunction after conventional and endovascular AAA repair: results of the DREAM trial. *J Endovasc Ther* 2004;11(6):613–620.
119. Xenos ES, Stevens SL, Freeman MB, et al. Erectile function after open or endovascular abdominal aortic aneurysm repair. *Ann Vasc Surg* 2003; 17(5):530–538.
120. EVAR Trial Participants. Endovascular aneurysm repair versus open repair in patients with abdominal aortic aneurysm (EVAR trial 1): randomised controlled trial. *Lancet* 2005;365(9478):2179–2186.
121. Blankensteijn JD, de Jong SE, Prinssen M, et al. Two-year outcomes after conventional or endovascular repair of abdominal aortic aneurysms. *N Engl J Med* 2005;352(23):2398–2405.
122. EVAR Trial Participants. Endovascular aneurysm repair and outcome in patients unfit for open repair of abdominal aortic aneurysm (EVAR trial 2): randomised controlled trial. *Lancet* 2005;365(9478):2187–2192.
123. Prinssen M, Buskens E, Blankensteijn JD. Quality of life endovascular and open AAA repair. Results of a randomised trial. *Eur J Vasc Endovasc Surg* 2004;27(2):121–127.
124. Harris PL, Vallabhaneni SR, Desgranges P, et al. Incidence and risk factors of late rupture, conversion, and death after endovascular repair of infrarenal aortic aneurysms: the EUROSTAR experience. European Collaborators on Stent/graft techniques for aortic aneurysm repair. *J Vasc Surg* 2000;32(4): 739–749.
125. van Marrewijk CJ, Fransen G, Laheij RJ, et al. Is a type II endoleak after EVAR a harbinger of risk? Causes and outcome of open conversion and

aneurysm rupture during follow-up. *Eur J Vasc Endovasc Surg* 2004; 27(2):128–137.
126. May J, White GH, Stephen MS, et al. Rupture of abdominal aortic aneurysm: concurrent comparison of outcome of those occurring after endovascular repair versus those occurring without previous treatment in an 11-year single-center experience. *J Vasc Surg* 2004;40(5): 860–866.
127. Lifeline Registry of Endovascular Aneurysm Repair Steering Committee. Lifeline Registry of Endovascular Aneurysm Repair: Registry data report. *J Vasc Surg* 2002;35(3):616–620.
128. Laheij RJ, Buth J, Harris PL, et al. Need for secondary interventions after endovascular repair of abdominal aortic aneurysms. Intermediate-term follow-up results of a European collaborative registry (EUROSTAR). *Br J Surg* 2000;87(12):1666–1673.
129. Schurink GW, Aarts NJ, van Bockel JH. Endoleak after stent-graft treatment of abdominal aortic aneurysm: a meta-analysis of clinical studies. *Br J Surg* 1999;86(5):581–587.
130. Bertges DJ, Chow K, Wyers MC, et al. Abdominal aortic aneurysm size regression after endovascular repair is endograft dependent. *J Vasc Surg* 2003;37(4):716–723.
131. Greenberg RK, Deaton D, Sullivan T, et al. Variable sac behavior after endovascular repair of abdominal aortic aneurysm: analysis of core laboratory data. *J Vasc Surg* 2004;39(1):95–101.
132. Biancari F, Leo E, Ylonen K, et al. Value of the Glasgow Aneurysm Score in predicting the immediate and long-term outcome after elective open repair of infrarenal abdominal aortic aneurysm. *Br J Surg* 2003;90(7):838–844.
133. Hall J, Singh G, Hood D, et al. Management of an abdominal aortic aneurysm in a patient with end-stage liver disease. *Am J Transplant* 2004; 4(4):666–668.
134. Biebl M, Lau LL, Hakaim AG, et al. Midterm outcome of endovascular abdominal aortic aneurysm repair in octogenarians: a single institution's experience. *J Vasc Surg* 2004;40(3):435–442.
135. Henebiens M, Vahl A, Koelemay MJ. Elective surgery of abdominal aortic aneurysms in octogenarians: a systematic review. *J Vasc Surg* 2008;47(3): 676–681.
136. Garcia JM, Monzon EO, Martinez AP, et al. Comparative analysis of renal function after treatment of infrarenal abdominal aortic aneurysms with a suprarenal fixation device as opposed to open surgery. *Ann Vasc Surg* 2008;22(4):513–519.
137. Gawenda M, Brunkwall J. Renal response to open and endovascular repair of abdominal aortic aneurysm: a prospective study. *Ann Vasc Surg* 2008; 22(1):1–4.
138. Mills JL Sr, Duong ST, Leon LR Jr, et al. Comparison of the effects of open and endovascular aortic aneurysm repair on long-term renal function using chronic kidney disease staging based on glomerular filtration rate. *J Vasc Surg* 2008;47(6):1141–1149.
139. Walsh SR, Boyle JR, Lynch AG, et al. Suprarenal endograft fixation and medium-term renal function: systematic review and meta-analysis. *J Vasc Surg* 2008;47(6):1364–1370.
140. Sternbergh WC III, Money SR. Hospital cost of endovascular versus open repair of abdominal aortic aneurysms: a multicenter study. *J Vasc Surg* 2000;31(2):237–244.
141. Bertges DJ, Zwolak RM, Deaton DH, et al. Current hospital costs and Medicare reimbursement for endovascular abdominal aortic aneurysm repair. *J Vasc Surg* 2003;37(2):272–279.
142. Rosenberg BL, Comstock MC, Butz DA, et al. Endovascular abdominal aortic aneurysm repair is more profitable than open repair based on contribution margin per day. *Surgery* 2005;137(3):285–292.
143. Kim JK, Tonnessen BH, Noll RE Jr, et al. Reimbursement of long-term postplacement costs after endovascular abdominal aortic aneurysm repair. *J Vasc Surg* 2008;48:1390–1395.
144. Williamson WK, Nicoloff AD, Taylor LM Jr, et al. Functional outcome after open repair of abdominal aortic aneurysm. *J Vasc Surg* 2001;33(5): 913–920.
145. Lee WA, Brown MP, Nelson PR, et al. Total percutaneous access for endovascular aortic aneurysm repair ("Preclose" technique). *J Vasc Surg* 2007;45(6):1095–1101.
146. Lee WA, Brown MP, Nelson PR, et al. Midterm outcomes of femoral arteries after percutaneous endovascular aortic repair using the Preclose technique. *J Vasc Surg* 2008;47(5):919–923.
147. Wilt TJ, Lederle FA, MacDonald R, et al. *Comparison of Endovascular and Open Surgical Repairs for Abdominal Aortic Aneurysm.* Evidence Report/Technology Assessment No. 144. Rockville, MD: Agency for Heathcare Research and Quality; 2006. AHRQ Publication No. 06-E017.
148. Fleisher LA, Beckman JA, Brown KA, et al. ACC/AHA 2007 Guidelines on Perioperative Cardiovascular Evaluation and Care for Noncardiac Surgery: executive summary: a report of the American College of Cardiology/American Heart Association Task Force on Practice Guidelines (writing committee to revise the 2002 Guidelines on Perioperative Cardiovascular Evaluation for Noncardiac Surgery): developed in collaboration with the American Society of Echocardiography, American Society of Nuclear Cardiology, Heart Rhythm Society, Society of Cardiovascular Anesthesiologists, Society for Cardiovascular Angiography and Interventions, Society for Vascular Medicine and Biology, and Society for Vascular Surgery. *Circulation* 2007;116(17):1971–1996.
149. Kertai MD, Boersma E, Westerhout CM, et al. A combination of statins and beta-blockers is independently associated with a reduction in the incidence of perioperative mortality and nonfatal myocardial infarction in patients undergoing abdominal aortic aneurysm surgery. *Eur J Vasc Endovasc Surg* 2004;28(4):343–352.
150. Smith SC Jr, Blair SN, Bonow RO, et al. AHA/ACC Guidelines for Preventing Heart Attack and Death in Patients With Atherosclerotic Cardiovascular Disease: 2001 update. A statement for healthcare professionals from the American Heart Association and the American College of Cardiology. *J Am Coll Cardiol* 2001;38(5):1581–1583.
151. Jayr C, Matthay MA, Goldstone J, et al. Preoperative and intraoperative factors associated with prolonged mechanical ventilation. A study in patients following major abdominal vascular surgery. *Chest* 1993;103(4): 1231–1236.
152. Upchurch GR Jr, Proctor MC, Henke PK, et al. Predictors of severe morbidity and death after elective abdominal aortic aneurysmectomy in patients with chronic obstructive pulmonary disease. *J Vasc Surg* 2003; 37(3):594–599.
153. McFalls EO, Ward HB, Moritz TE, et al. Coronary-artery revascularization before elective major vascular surgery. *N Engl J Med* 2004;351(27): 2795–2804.
154. Hertzer NR, Beven EG, Young JR, et al. Coronary artery disease in peripheral vascular patients. A classification of 1000 coronary angiograms and results of surgical management. *Ann Surg* 1984;199(2):223–233.
155. Cuypers PW, Buth J. Does endovascular aortic aneurysm repair justify a reduced cardiology work-up? *J Cardiovasc Surg (Torino)* 2003;44(3): 437–442.
156. Boylan JF, Katz J, Kavanagh BP, et al. Epidural bupivacaine-morphine analgesia versus patient-controlled analgesia following abdominal aortic surgery: analgesic, respiratory, and myocardial effects. *Anesthesiology* 1998;89(3):585–593.
157. Major CP Jr, Greer MS, Russell WL, et al. Postoperative pulmonary complications and morbidity after abdominal aneurysmectomy: a comparison of postoperative epidural versus parenteral opioid analgesia. *Am Surg* 1996;62(1):45–51.
158. Eagle KA, Berger PB, Calkins H, et al. ACC/AHA Guideline Update for Perioperative Cardiovascular Evaluation for Noncardiac Surgery–executive summary. A report of the American College of Cardiology/American Heart Association Task Force on Practice Guidelines (committee to update the 1996 Guidelines on Perioperative Cardiovascular Evaluation for Noncardiac Surgery). *Anesth Analg* 2002;94(5):1052–1064.
159. Valentine RJ, Duke ML, Inman MH, et al. Effectiveness of pulmonary artery catheters in aortic surgery: a randomized trial. *J Vasc Surg* 1998; 27(2):203–211.
160. Elmore JR, Franklin DP, Youkey JR, et al. Normothermia is protective during infrarenal aortic surgery. *J Vasc Surg* 1998;28:984–992.
161. Bush HL Jr, Hydo LJ, Fischer E, et al. Hypothermia during elective abdominal aortic aneurysm repair: the high price of avoidable morbidity. *J Vasc Surg* 1995;21(3):392–400.
162. Alvarez GG, Fergusson DA, Neilipovitz DT, et al. Cell salvage does not minimize perioperative allogeneic blood transfusion in abdominal vascular surgery: a systematic review. *Can J Anaesth* 2004;51(5):425–431.
163. Sicard GA, Reilly JM, Rubin BG, et al. Transabdominal versus retroperitoneal incision for abdominal aortic surgery: report of a prospective randomized trial. *J Vasc Surg* 1995;21(2):174–181.
164. Thompson JF, Mullee MA, Bell PR, et al. Intraoperative heparinisation, bloodloss and myocardial infarction during aortic aneurysm surgery: a joint vascular research group study. *Eur J Vasc Endovasc Surg* 1996;12:86–90.
165. Marques dS, Lingaas PS, Geiran O, et al. Multiple bacteria in aortic aneurysms. *J Vasc Surg* 2003;38(6):1384–1389.
166. van der Vliet JA, Kouwenberg PP, Muytjens HL, et al. Relevance of bacterial cultures of abdominal aortic aneurysm contents. *Surgery* 1996;119:129–132.
167. Seeger JM, Coe DA, Kaelin LD, et al. Routine reimplantation of patent inferior mesenteric arteries limits colon infarction after aortic reconstruction. *J Vasc Surg* 1992;15(4):635–641.
168. Senekowitsch C, Assadian A, Assadian O, et al. Replanting the inferior mesentery artery during infrarenal aortic aneurysm repair: influence on postoperative colon ischemia. *J Vasc Surg* 2006;43(4):689–694.
169. Wakefield TW, Hantler CB, Wrobleski SK, et al. Effects of differing rates of protamine reversal of heparin anticoagulation. *Surgery* 1996;119(2): 123–128.
170. Dorman BH, Elliott BM, Spinale FG, et al. Protamine use during peripheral vascular surgery: a prospective randomized trial. *J Vasc Surg* 1995;22(3): 248–255.
171. Hall KA, Peters B, Smyth SH, et al. Abdominal wall hernias in patients with abdominal aortic aneurysmal versus aortoiliac occlusive disease. *Am J Surg* 1995;170(6):572–575.
172. Liapis CD, Dimitroulis DA, Kakisis JD, et al. Incidence of incisional hernias in patients operated on for aneurysm or occlusive disease. *Am Surg* 2004;70(6):550–552.
173. Raffetto JD, Cheung Y, Fisher JB, et al. Incision and abdominal wall hernias in patients with aneurysm or occlusive aortic disease. *J Vasc Surg* 2003;37(6):1150–1154.
174. Yeager RA, Porter JM. Arterial and prosthetic graft infection. In: Porter JM, Taylor LM, eds. *Basic Data Underlying Clinical Decision Making in Vascular Surgery.* St. Louis, MO: Quality Medical; 2005:90–97.
175. Bastounis E, Filis K, Georgopoulos S, et al. Selective use of the intensive care unit after elective infrarenal abdominal aortic aneurysm repair. *Int Angiol* 2003;22(3):308–316.
176. Akkersdijk GJ, Van der GY, Moll FL, et al. Complications of standard elective abdominal aortic aneurysm repair. *Eur J Vasc Endovasc Surg* 1998; 15(6):505–510.

177. Johnston KW. Multicenter prospective study of nonruptured abdominal aortic aneurysm. Part II. Variables predicting morbidity and mortality. *J Vasc Surg* 1989;9(3):437–447.
178. Georgopoulos S, Pikoulis E, Bacoyiannis C, et al. Combined abdominal aortic aneurysmectomy and other abdominal operations. *Scand J Surg* 2004;93(1):61–63.
179. Grego F, Lepidi S, Bassi P, et al. Simultaneous surgical treatment of abdominal aortic aneurysm and carcinoma of the bladder. *J Vasc Surg* 2003; 37(3):607–614.
180. Illuminati G, Calio' FG, D'Urso A, et al. Simultaneous repair of abdominal aortic aneurysm and resection of unexpected, associated abdominal malignancies. *J Surg Oncol* 2004;88(4):234–239.
181. Kiskinis D, Spanos C, Melas N, et al. Priority of resection in concomitant abdominal aortic aneurysm (AAA) and colorectal cancer (CRC): review of the literature and experience of our clinic. *Tech Coloproctol* 2004;8(suppl 1): s19–s21.
182. Komori K, Furuyama T, Maehara Y. Renal artery clamping and left renal vein division during abdominal aortic aneurysm repair. *Eur J Vasc Endovasc Surg* 2004;27(1):80–83.
183. Harward TR, Ingegno MD, Carlton L, et al. Limb-threatening ischemia due to multilevel arterial occlusive disease. Simultaneous or staged inflow/ outflow revascularization. *Ann Surg* 1995;221(5):498–503.
184. Blankensteijn JD. Influence of study design on reported mortality and morbidity rates after abdominal aortic aneurysm repair. *Br J Surg* 1998;85(12): 1624–1630.
185. Tollefson DF, Ernst CB. Colon ischemia following aortic reconstruction. In: Porter JM, Taylor LM Jr, eds. *Basic Data Underlying Clinical Decision Making Vascular Surgery*. St. Louis, MO: Quality Medical; 1994: 111–115.
186. Becquemin JP, Majewski M, Fermani N, et al. Colon ischemia following abdominal aortic aneurysm repair in the era of endovascular abdominal aortic repair. *J Vasc Surg* 2008;47(2):258–263.
187. Champagne BJ, Darling RC III, Daneshmand M, et al. Outcome of aggressive surveillance colonoscopy in ruptured abdominal aortic aneurysm. *J Vasc Surg* 2004;39(4):792–796.
188. Valentine RJ, Hagino RT, Jackson MR, et al. Gastrointestinal complications after aortic surgery. *J Vasc Surg* 1998;28(3):404–411.
189. Ottinger LW. Acute cholecystitis as a postoperative complication. *Ann Surg* 1976;184(2):162–165.
190. Yao J. Vasculogenic impotence. In: Ernst CB, Stanley JC, eds. *Current Therapy in Vascular Surgery*, 3rd ed. St. Louis, MO: Mosby; 1995: 397–400.
191. Szilagyi DE. A second look at the etiology of spinal cord damage in surgery of the abdominal aorta. *J Vasc Surg* 1993;17(6):1111–1113.
192. Feinglass J, Cowper D, Dunlop D, et al. Late survival risk factors for abdominal aortic aneurysm repair: experience from fourteen Department of Veterans Affairs hospitals. *Surgery* 1995;118(1):16–24.
193. McFalls EO, Ward HB, Santilli S, et al. The influence of perioperative myocardial infarction on long-term prognosis following elective vascular surgery. *Chest* 1998;113(3):681–686.
194. Biancari F, Ylonen K, Anttila V, et al. Durability of open repair of infrarenal abdominal aortic aneurysm: a 15-year follow-up study. *J Vasc Surg* 2002;35(1):87–93.
195. Hallett JW Jr, Marshall DM, Petterson TM, et al. Graft-related complications after abdominal aortic aneurysm repair: reassurance from a 36-year population-based experience. *J Vasc Surg* 1997;25(2):277–284.
196. Conrad MF, Crawford RS, Pedraza JD, et al. Long-term durability of open abdominal aortic aneurysm repair. *J Vasc Surg* 2007;46(4):669–675.
197. Zarins CK, Bloch DA, Crabtree T, et al. Stent graft migration after endovascular aneurysm repair: importance of proximal fixation. *J Vasc Surg* 2003;38(6):1264–1272.
198. Sternbergh WC III, Money SR, Greenberg RK, et al. Influence of endograft oversizing on device migration, endoleak, aneurysm shrinkage, and aortic neck dilation: results from the Zenith Multicenter Trial. *J Vasc Surg* 2004; 39(1):20–26.
199. Ricotta JJ. What's new in vascular surgery. *J Am Coll Surg* 2004;198(4): 600–625.
200. Wyers MC, Fillinger MF, Schermerhorn ML, et al. Endovascular repair of abdominal aortic aneurysm without preoperative arteriography. *J Vasc Surg* 2003;38(4):730–738.
201. Becquemin JP, Lapie V, Favre JP, et al. Mid-term results of a second generation bifurcated endovascular graft for abdominal aortic aneurysm repair: the French Vanguard trial. *J Vasc Surg* 1999;30(2):209–218.
202. Velazquez OC, Carpenter JP, Baum RA, et al. Perigraft air, fever, and leukocytosis after endovascular repair of abdominal aortic aneurysms. *Am J Surg* 1999;178(3):185–189.
203. Corriere MA, Feurer ID, Becker SY, et al. Endoleak following endovascular abdominal aortic aneurysm repair: implications for duration of screening. *Ann Surg* 2004;239(6):800–805.
204. Sternbergh WC III, Greenberg RK, Chuter TA, et al. Redefining postoperative surveillance after endovascular aneurysm repair: recommendations based on 5-year follow-up in the US Zenith multicenter trial. *J Vasc Surg* 2008;48(2):278–284.
205. Rozenblit AM, Patlas M, Rosenbaum AT, et al. Detection of endoleaks after endovascular repair of abdominal aortic aneurysm: value of unenhanced and delayed helical CT acquisitions. *Radiology* 2003;227(2): 426–433.
206. Elkouri S, Panneton JM, Andrews JC, et al. Computed tomography and ultrasound in follow-up of patients after endovascular repair of abdominal aortic aneurysm. *Ann Vasc Surg* 2004;18(3):271–279.
207. Raman KG, Missig-Carroll N, Richardson T, et al. Color-flow duplex ultrasound scan versus computed tomographic scan in the surveillance of endovascular aneurysm repair. *J Vasc Surg* 2003;38(4):645–651.
208. Wolf YG, Johnson BL, Hill BB, et al. Duplex ultrasound scanning versus computed tomographic angiography for postoperative evaluation of endovascular abdominal aortic aneurysm repair. *J Vasc Surg* 2000;32(6): 1142–1148.
209. Matsumura JS, Moore WS. Clinical consequences of periprosthetic leak after endovascular repair of abdominal aortic aneurysm. Endovascular Technologies Investigators. *J Vasc Surg* 1998;27(4):606–613.
210. Rockman CB, Riles TS, Landis R. Lower extremity paraparesis or paraplegia subsequent to endovascular management of abdominal aortic aneurysms. *J Vasc Surg* 2001;33(1):178–180.
211. Zhang WW, Kulaylat MN, Anain PM, et al. Embolization as cause of bowel ischemia after endovascular abdominal aortic aneurysm repair. *J Vasc Surg* 2004;40(5):867–872.
212. Kasirajan K, Matteson B, Marek JM, et al. Technique and results of transfemoral superselective coil embolization of type II lumbar endoleak. *J Vasc Surg* 2003;38(1):61–66.
213. Harris P, Brennan J, Martin J, et al. Longitudinal aneurysm shrinkage following endovascular aortic aneurysm repair: a source of intermediate and late complications. *J Endovasc Surg* 1999;6(1):11–16.
214. Janczyk RJ, Howells GA, Bair HA, et al. Hypothermia is an independent predictor of mortality in ruptured abdominal aortic aneurysms. *Vasc Endovascular Surg* 2004;38(1):37–42.
215. Chinien G, Waltham M, Abisi S, et al. Systemic administration of heparin intraoperatively in patients undergoing open repair of leaking abdominal aortic aneurysm may be beneficial and does not cause problems. *Vascular* 2008;16(4):189–193.
216. Bradbury AW, Makhdoomi KR, Adam DJ, et al. Twelve-year experience of the management of ruptured abdominal aortic aneurysm. *Br J Surg* 1997; 84(12):1705–1707.
217. Halpern VJ, Kline RG, D'Angelo AJ, et al. Factors that affect the survival rate of patients with ruptured abdominal aortic aneurysms. *J Vasc Surg* 1997;26(6):939–945.
218. Maziak DE, Lindsay TF, Marshall JC, et al. The impact of multiple organ dysfunction on mortality following ruptured abdominal aortic aneurysm repair. *Ann Vasc Surg* 1998;12(2):93–100.
219. van Dongen HP, Leusink JA, Moll FL, et al. Ruptured abdominal aortic aneurysms: factors influencing postoperative mortality and long-term survival. *Eur J Vasc Endovasc Surg* 1998;15(1):62–66.
220. Johnston KW. Ruptured abdominal aortic aneurysm: six-year follow-up results of a multicenter prospective study. Canadian Society for Vascular Surgery Aneurysm Study Group. *J Vasc Surg* 1994;19(5):888–900.
221. Papavassiliou V, Anderton M, Loftus IM, et al. The physiological effects of elevated intra-abdominal pressure following aneurysm repair. *Eur J Vasc Endovasc Surg* 2003;26(3):293–298.
222. Parikshak M, Shepard AD, Reddy DJ, et al. Adrenal insufficiency in patients with ruptured abdominal aortic aneurysms. *J Vasc Surg* 2004; 39(5):944–950.
223. Hennessy A, Barry MC, McGee H, et al. Quality of life following repair of ruptured and elective abdominal aortic aneurysms. *Eur J Surg* 1998; 164(9):673–677.
224. Reichart M, Geelkerken RH, Huisman AB, et al. Ruptured abdominal aortic aneurysm: endovascular repair is feasible in 40% of patients. *Eur J Vasc Endovasc Surg* 2003;26(5):479–486.
225. Rose DF, Davidson IR, Hinchliffe RJ, et al. Anatomical suitability of ruptured abdominal aortic aneurysms for endovascular repair. *J Endovasc Ther* 2003;10(3):453–457.
226. Slater BJ, Harris EJ, Lee JT. Anatomic suitability of ruptured abdominal aortic aneurysms for endovascular repair. *Ann Vasc Surg* 2008;22(6): 716–722.
227. Lee WA, Hirneise CM, Tayyarah M, et al. Impact of endovascular repair on early outcomes of ruptured abdominal aortic aneurysms. *J Vasc Surg* 2004;40(2):211–215.
228. Malina M, Veith F, Ivancev K, et al. Balloon occlusion of the aorta during endovascular repair of ruptured abdominal aortic aneurysm. *J Endovasc Ther* 2005;12(5):556–559.
229. O'Donnell ME, Badger SA, Makar RR, et al. Techniques in occluding the aorta during endovascular repair of ruptured abdominal aortic aneurysms. *J Vasc Surg* 2006;44(1):211–215.
230. Richardson JW, Greenfield LJ. Natural history and management of iliac aneurysms. *J Vasc Surg* 1988;8(2):165–171.
231. Krupski WC, Bass A, Rosenberg GD, et al. The elusive isolated hypogastric artery aneurysm: novel presentations. *J Vasc Surg* 1989;10(5): 557–562.
232. Santilli SM, Wernsing SE, Lee ES. Expansion rates and outcomes for iliac artery aneurysms. *J Vasc Surg* 2000;31(1 Pt 1):114–121.
233. Huang Y, Gloviczki P, Duncan AA, et al. Common iliac artery aneurysm: expansion rate and results of open surgical and endovascular repair. *J Vasc Surg* 2008;47(6):1203–1210.
234. Money SR, Hollier LH. Surgical treatment of inflammatory abdominal aortic aneurysms. In: Ernst CB, Stanley JC, eds. *Current Therapy in Vascular Surgery*, 3rd ed. St. Louis, MO: Mosby; 1995:229–231.

235. Haug ES, Skomsvoll JF, Jacobsen G, et al. Inflammatory aortic aneurysm is associated with increased incidence of autoimmune disease. *J Vasc Surg* 2003;38(3):492–497.
236. Baskerville PA, Browse NL. Peri-aortic fibrosis: progression and regression. *J Cardiovasc Surg (Torino)* 1987;28(1):30–31.
237. Chuter T, Ivancev K, Malina M, et al. Inflammatory aneurysm treated by means of transfemoral endovascular graft insertion. *J Vasc Interv Radiol* 1997;8(1 Pt 1):39–41.
238. Nevelsteen A, Lacroix H, Stockx L, et al. Inflammatory abdominal aortic aneurysm and bilateral complete ureteral obstruction: treatment by endovascular graft and bilateral ureteric stenting. *Ann Vasc Surg* 1999; 13(2):222–224.
239. Ruppert V, Verrel F, Kellner W, et al. Endovascular repair of inflammatory abdominal aortic aneurysms: a valuable alternative?–Case report and review of literature. *Ann Vasc Surg* 2004;18(3):357–360.
240. Puchner S, Bucek RA, Loewe C, et al. Endovascular repair of inflammatory aortic aneurysms: long-term results. *AJR Am J Roentgenol* 2006;186(4): 1144–1147.
241. Bonati L, Rubini P, Japichino GG, et al. Long-term outcome after inflammatory abdominal aortic aneurysm repair: case-matched study. *World J Surg* 2003;27(5):539–544.
242. Dalainas I, Nano G, Ranucci M, et al. Inflammatory abdominal aortic aneurysms. A 20-year experience. *J Cardiovasc Surg (Torino)* 2007;48(3): 305–308.
243. Crawford ES, Beckett WC, Greer MS. Juxtarenal infrarenal abdominal aortic aneurysm. Special diagnostic and therapeutic considerations. *Ann Surg* 1986;203(6):661–670.
244. Jean-Claude JM, Reilly LM, Stoney RJ, et al. Pararenal aortic aneurysms: the future of open aortic aneurysm repair. *J Vasc Surg* 1999;29(5):902–912.
245. Martin GH, O'Hara PJ, Hertzer NR, et al. Surgical repair of aneurysms involving the suprarenal, visceral, and lower thoracic aortic segments: early results and late outcome. *J Vasc Surg* 2000;31(5):851–862.
246. Chong T, Nguyen L, Owens CD, et al. Suprarenal aortic cross-clamp position: a reappraisal of its effects on outcomes for open abdominal aortic aneurysm repair. *J Vasc Surg* 2009;49(4):873–880.
247. Knott AW, Kalra M, Duncan AA, et al. Open repair of juxtarenal aortic aneurysms (JAA) remains a safe option in the era of fenestrated endografts. *J Vasc Surg* 2008;47(4):695–701.
248. Pearce JD, Edwards MS, Stafford JM, et al. Open repair of aortic aneurysms involving the renal vessels. *Ann Vasc Surg* 2007;21(6):676–686.
249. Greenberg RK, Haulon S, O'Neill S, et al. Primary endovascular repair of juxtarenal aneurysms with fenestrated endovascular grafting. *Eur J Vasc Endovasc Surg* 2004;27(5):484–491.
250. Bicknell CD, Cheshire NJ, Riga CV, et al. Treatment of complex aneurysmal disease with fenestrated and branched stent grafts. *Eur J Vasc Endovasc Surg* 2009;37(2):175–181.
251. Greenberg RK, West K, Pfaff K, et al. Beyond the aortic bifurcation: branched endovascular grafts for thoracoabdominal and aortoiliac aneurysms. *J Vasc Surg* 2006;43(5):879–886.
252. Scurr JR, Brennan JA, Gilling-Smith GL, et al. Fenestrated endovascular repair for juxtarenal aortic aneurysm. *Br J Surg* 2008;95(3):326–332.
253. Black SA, Wolfe JH, Clark M, et al. Complex thoracoabdominal aortic aneurysms: endovascular exclusion with visceral revascularization. *J Vasc Surg* 2006;43:1081–1089.
254. Lee WA, Brown MP, Martin TD, et al. Early results after staged hybrid repair of thoracoabdominal aortic aneurysms. *J Am Coll Surg* 2007;205(3): 420–431.
255. Reddy DJ, Shepard AD, Evans JR, et al. Management of infected aortoiliac aneurysms. *Arch Surg* 1991;126(7):873–878.
256. Ellenby MI, Ernst CB. Surgical treatment of infected abdominal aortic aneurysms. In: Ernst CB, Stanley JC, eds. *Current Therapy in Vascular Surgery*, 3rd ed. St. Louis, MO: Mosby; 1995:232–235.
257. Brown SL, Busuttil RW, Baker JD, et al. Bacteriologic and surgical determinants of survival in patients with mycotic aneurysms. *J Vasc Surg* 1984; 1(4):541–547.
258. Oz MC, Brener BJ, Buda JA, et al. A ten-year experience with bacterial aortitis. *J Vasc Surg* 1989;10(4):439–449.
259. Ewart JM, Burke ML, Bunt TJ. Spontaneous abdominal aortic infections. Essentials of diagnosis and management. *Am Surg* 1983;49(1):37–50.
260. Koeppel TA, Gahlen J, Diehl S, et al. Mycotic aneurysm of the abdominal aorta with retroperitoneal abscess: successful endovascular repair. *J Vasc Surg* 2004;40(1):164–166.
261. Kan CD, Lee HL, Yang YJ. Outcome after endovascular stent graft treatment for mycotic aortic aneurysm: a systematic review. *J Vasc Surg* 2007; 46(5):906–912.
262. Fillmore AJ, Valentine RJ. Surgical mortality in patients with infected aortic aneurysms. *J Am Coll Surg* 2003;196(3):435–441.
263. Taheri SA, Kulaylat MN, Grippi J, et al. Surgical treatment of primary aortoduodenal fistula. *Ann Vasc Surg* 1991;5(3):265–270.
264. Debonnaire P, Van RO, Arts J, et al. Primary aorto enteric fistula: report of 18 Belgian cases and literature review. *Acta Gastroenterol Belg* 2008; 71(2):250–258.
265. Pitrowski JJBVM. Management of vascular graft infection. In: Bernhard VM, Towne JB, eds. *Complications in Vascular Surgery*. St. Louis, MO: Quality Medical Publishing; 1991:235.
266. French JR, Simring DV, Merrett N, et al. Aorto-enteric fistula following endoluminal abdominal aortic aneurysm repair. *ANZ J Surg* 2004;74(5): 397–399.
267. Berman SS, Bernhard VM. Management of primary aortoenteric fistula. In: Ernst CB, Stanley JC, eds. *Current Therapy in Vascular Surgery*. St. Louis, MO: Mosby; 1995:262–264.
268. Cendan JC, Thomas JB, Seeger JM. Twenty-one cases of aortoenteric fistula: lessons for the general surgeon. *Am Surg* 2004;70(7):583–587.
269. Giordano JM. Venous anomalies encountered during aortic reconstruction. In: Ernst CB, Stanley JC, eds. *Current Therapy in Vascular Surgery*. St. Louis, MO: Mosby; 1995:252–255.
270. Gaspar MR, Waters HJ, Averbook AW. Renal ectopia and renal fusion in patients requiring abdominal operations. In: Ernst CB, Stanley JC, eds. *Current Therapy in Vascular Surgery*. St. Louis, MO: Mosby; 1995: 246–250.
271. Davidovic LB, Kostic DM, Jakovljevic NS, et al. Abdominal aortic surgery and horseshoe kidney. *Ann Vasc Surg* 2004;18(6):725–728.
272. Jackson RW, Fay DM, Wyatt MG, et al. The renal impact of aortic stent-grafting in patients with a horseshoe kidney. *Cardiovasc Intervent Radiol* 2004;27(6):632–636.
273. Kaplan DB, Kwon CC, Marin ML, et al. Endovascular repair of abdominal aortic aneurysms in patients with congenital renal vascular anomalies. *J Vasc Surg* 1999;30(3):407–415.
274. Kim B, Donayre CE, Hansen CJ, et al. Endovascular abdominal aortic aneurysm repair using the AneuRx stent graft: impact of excluding accessory renal arteries. *Ann Vasc Surg* 2004;18(1):32–37.
275. Nordmann AJ, Logan AG. Balloon angioplasty versus medical therapy for hypertensive patients with renal artery obstruction. *Cochrane Database Syst Rev* 2003;(3):CD002944.
276. Benjamin ME, Hansen KJ, Craven TE, et al. Combined aortic and renal artery surgery. A contemporary experience. *Ann Surg* 1996;223(5): 555–565.
277. Huber TS, Harward TR, Flynn TC, et al. Operative mortality rates after elective infrarenal aortic reconstructions. *J Vasc Surg* 1995;22(3):287–293.
278. Gentile AT, Moneta GL, Taylor LM Jr, et al. Isolated bypass to the superior mesenteric artery for intestinal ischemia. *Arch Surg* 1994;129(9):926–931.
279. Mateo RB, O'Hara PJ, Hertzer NR, et al. Elective surgical treatment of symptomatic chronic mesenteric occlusive disease: early results and late outcomes. *J Vasc Surg* 1999;29(5):821–831.
280. Derrow AE, Seeger JM, Dame DA, et al. The outcome in the United States after thoracoabdominal aortic aneurysm repair, renal artery bypass, and mesenteric revascularization. *J Vasc Surg* 2001;34(1):54–61.
281. Sarac TP, Altinel O, Kashyap V, et al. Endovascular treatment of stenotic and occluded visceral arteries for chronic mesenteric ischemia. *J Vasc Surg* 2008;47(3):485–491.
282. Silva JA, White CJ, Collins TJ, et al. Endovascular therapy for chronic mesenteric ischemia. *J Am Coll Cardiol* 2006;47(5):944–950.
283. Tollefson DF, Ernst CB. Natural history of atherosclerotic renal artery stenosis associated with aortic disease. *J Vasc Surg* 1991;14(3):327–331.
284. Zierler RE, Bergelin RO, Isaacson JA, et al. Natural history of atherosclerotic renal artery stenosis: a prospective study with duplex ultrasonography. *J Vasc Surg* 1994;19(2):250–257.
285. Williamson WK, Abou-Zamzam AM Jr, Moneta GL, et al. Prophylactic repair of renal artery stenosis is not justified in patients who require infrarenal aortic reconstruction. *J Vasc Surg* 1998;28(1):14–20.
286. Thomas JH, Blake K, Pierce GE, et al. The clinical course of asymptomatic mesenteric arterial stenosis. *J Vasc Surg* 1998;27(5):840–844.
287. Swanson RJ, Littooy FN, Hunt TK, et al. Laparotomy as a precipitating factor in the rupture of intra-abdominal aneurysms. *Arch Surg* 1980; 115(3):299–304.
288. Szilagyi DE, Elliott JP, Berguer R. Coincidental malignancy and abdominal aortic aneurysm. Problems of management. *Arch Surg* 1967;95(3): 402–412.
289. String ST. Management of concurrent intra-abdominal disease and abdominal aortic aneurysms. In: Ernst CB, Stanley JC, eds. *Current Therapy in Vascular Surgery*. St. Louis, MO: Mosby; 1995:235–237.
290. Oshner JL, Cooley DA, DeBakey ME. Associated intra-abdominal lesions encountered during resection of aortic aneurysms. *Dis Colon Rectum* 1960; 3:485–490.

CHAPTER 101 ■ LOWER EXTREMITY ANEURYSMS

AMY B. REED

KEY POINTS

1. Femoral and popliteal aneurysms may be asymptomatic, being an incidental finding on routine physical examination, but they are potentially limb threatening and are frequently associated with life-threatening abdominal aortic aneurysms.
2. Femoral artery aneurysms are the most common peripheral aneurysm if both true and false aneurysms are considered together.
3. Anastomotic aneurysms result from a disrupted suture line between a graft and the host artery.
4. Catheter-induced pseudoaneurysms result from failed hemostasis.
5. Popliteal artery aneurysms often develop limb-threatening complications if not treated, and results of surgical therapy are much better if treatment is undertaken prior to the development of complications.
6. Thrombolytic therapy is a useful adjuvant in patients presenting with acute limb ischemia secondary to occlusion of a popliteal artery aneurysm and the outflow arteries.

PERIPHERAL ANEURYSMS

1 Popliteal artery aneurysms are the most frequently encountered peripheral aneurysm. Their significance comes from their potential for limb-threatening complications, rather than rupture, and their association with life-threatening abdominal aortic aneurysms. True femoral artery aneurysms are rare, with iatrogenic and anastomotic pseudoaneurysms being more common.

Incidence

While the exact incidence of femoral and popliteal aneurysms is difficult to determine, the number being recognized is increasing. An aging population, increased arterial trauma, more common use of invasive therapies for vascular disease, and increased use of imaging modalities all contribute to the rise in number of peripheral aneurysms being diagnosed. In a screening study of men between the ages of 65 and 74 years, abdominal aortic aneurysms were identified in 4.9% of patients.[1] In patients with abdominal aortic aneurysms, 6.8% had femoral artery aneurysms and 9.6% had popliteal artery aneurysms.[2] Screening of men between the ages of 65 and 80 years identified popliteal artery aneurysms in 1%.[3]

An increasing number of false aneurysms—"pseudoaneurysms"—are occurring coincident with the increased use of catheter-based diagnostic and therapeutic interventions in addition to lower extremity bypass surgery. Pseudoaneurysms can be iatrogenic, infectious, or traumatic in nature and are identified by their lack of involvement of all three vessel wall layers, as is typically seen in true aneurysms. The incidence of pseudoaneurysm after diagnostic procedures is approximately 0.3% and slightly higher at 1.5% after therapeutic procedures, in general due to use of larger sheaths.[4] False aneurysms can also arise from trauma during surgery, such as orthopedic procedures. Femoral pseudoaneurysms develop after 0.08% of total hip arthroplasties, and popliteal aneurysms arise following 0.17% of total knee arthroplasties.[5]

Degenerative (often called atherosclerotic) femoral and popliteal artery aneurysms are encountered far more frequently in men than women. The male-to-female ratio in patients with femoral and popliteal aneurysms is about 30:1.[6,7] This predilection for men is markedly different from aortic aneurysms where the male-to-female patient ratio is approximately 4:1.[2]

Pathogenesis

The cause of femoral and popliteal artery aneurysms has changed significantly since they were first recognized centuries ago. Once primarily mycotic or syphilitic in origin, most true aneurysms in the 21st century have a degenerative cause commonly called *atherosclerotic aneurysms*, whereas false aneurysms usually follow surgery or trauma. True tibial artery aneurysms are rare.

The cause of degenerative aneurysms of the femoral and popliteal vessels is not clear. One factor believed to contribute to aneurysm formation is turbulent flow beyond a relative stenosis resulting in poststenotic dilatation beyond the inguinal ligament at the groin or beyond the tendinous hiatus of the adductor magnus or the arcuate popliteal ligament and the heads of the gastrocnemius muscle at the popliteal level. Arterial wall fatigue resulting from vibration and turbulence proximal to a major branching or caused by stress during hip and knee flexion may also contribute to aneurysm formation.

The frequent occurrence of multiple peripheral aneurysms in the same patient suggests a systemic abnormality in the arterial wall, which promotes aneurysmal degeneration at locations where hemodynamic or mechanical factors put unusual stress on the arterial wall. The multiple factors that contribute to aneurysmal degeneration are reviewed in Chapter 100 and are felt to contribute to degenerative femoral and popliteal aneurysms, as well as aortic aneurysms. The presence of an inflammatory infiltrate has been noted in the wall of femoral and popliteal aneurysms, similar to aortic aneurysms.[8] The exact role of this inflammatory process, with potential release of reactive oxygen species and matrix metalloproteinases, is unknown. Apoptosis of smooth muscle cells may also play a role in the formation of aneurysms by limiting the ability of the arterial wall to respond to the degenerative process.[9] These factors, however, do not explain the male predilection for femoral and popliteal aneurysm formation. X-linked genetic abnormalities for aneurysm formation have not been noted in humans.

Clinical Manifestations

Femoral and popliteal aneurysms are often asymptomatic, being detected on routine physical examination by a bounding, expansile pulse. Both femoral and popliteal artery aneurysms, however, may be accompanied by symptoms of local fullness, pain caused by pressure on the adjacent nerve, limb edema, and venous distention or thrombosis caused by compression of the adjacent vein. Patients may also present with lower extremity ischemia with intermittent claudication, rest pain, or gangrene secondary to complications of a femoral or popliteal aneurysm, including thrombosis or distal embolization. Because the natural history and complication rate in femoral and popliteal aneurysms differ, they are considered separately here.

FEMORAL ARTERY ANEURYSMS

2 Femoral artery aneurysms are the most common peripheral aneurysm if both true and false aneurysms are considered together, with the vast majority being false aneurysms. Their clinical importance rests in the fact that they are limb-threatening lesions and can jeopardize the viability of the leg if thrombosis, embolization, or rupture occurs. The vast majority of true aneurysms are degenerative lesions commonly called *atherosclerotic aneurysms*, whereas false aneurysms include anastomotic, traumatic, and mycotic lesions. Rarely, femoral aneurysms develop secondary to connective tissue disorders. The femoral region is the most common site for both anastomotic aneurysms and mycotic aneurysms associated with trauma; so the presentation and surgical repair of these lesions are discussed.

Degenerative (Atherosclerotic) Aneurysms

Incidence. The exact incidence of degenerative (atherosclerotic) common femoral artery aneurysms in the general population remains undefined. They are found in 6.8% of all patients with abdominal aortic aneurysms, and 85% of patients with femoral artery aneurysms have abdominal aortic aneurysms.[2,6]

Pattern of Disease. Femoral aneurysms most frequently affect the common femoral artery. They may be classified as *type I*, those limited to the common femoral artery, or *type II*, those involving the orifice of the profunda femoris artery.[10] Type I and type II aneurysms occur with nearly equal frequency. This classification becomes important in reference to vascular reconstructive procedures, with type II aneurysms requiring more complex reconstructions to ensure continued patency of both the superficial and profunda femoris arteries. Isolated lesions of the profunda femoris artery are rare (2% of femoral artery aneurysms) and are prone to rupture because they are difficult to diagnose at the asymptomatic stage. Isolated superficial femoral artery aneurysms are also uncommon, but one third of patients present with rupture and one quarter with thrombosis.[11]

Femoral artery aneurysms can be limb-threatening lesions and are frequently associated with limb-threatening popliteal aneurysms and life-threatening abdominal aortic aneurysms. Multiple aneurysms are common in patients with femoral artery aneurysms. In a series of 100 patients with degenerative femoral artery aneurysms seen at a single institution, 72% of patients had bilateral femoral artery aneurysms.[6] In addition, aortoiliac aneurysms were detected in 85% of patients, thoracic aortic aneurysms in 6%, and popliteal aneurysms in 44%, of which 55% were bilateral.

Clinical Manifestations. The typical patient with a degenerative femoral artery aneurysm is a male in his 60s or 70s with the usual risk factors for atherosclerosis. Of these patients, 86% are cigarette smokers, 36% have hypertension, and 14% have diabetes mellitus.[6] Associated cardiovascular disease is common, with clinical manifestations of coronary artery disease and cerebrovascular disease present in 34% and 7%, respectively.

The clinical manifestations of femoral artery aneurysms cover the spectrum from asymptomatic to severe ischemia of the lower extremity. Although 40% of patients are asymptomatic at the time of diagnosis, the majority present with local symptoms or complaints of lower extremity ischemia.[6] Local pain or observation of a groin mass is the only complaint in 18% of patients. Lower extremity venous disease is present in 8%, being attributable to venous obstruction by the femoral artery aneurysm in 4%; but venous obstruction is rarely the sole sign of an aneurysm. Lower extremity ischemic symptoms of claudication, rest pain, or gangrene are present in 42% of patients and often lead to the diagnosis of the femoral artery aneurysm.

As with aneurysms in other locations, femoral artery aneurysms may be complicated by embolization, thrombosis, or, rarely, rupture. Peripheral embolization may be identified incidentally on angiography or produce signs as mild as spotty discoloration of the toes to as severe as peripheral gangrene. Although embolization is reported in about 10% of aneurysms, the femoral artery aneurysm is not necessarily the source of these emboli because many patients have a concomitant popliteal aneurysm.[6] In larger clinical series, 1% to 16% of patients with degenerative femoral artery aneurysms present with an acute thrombosis, whereas 1% to 16% have a chronically thrombosed lesion.[6,10] Rupture is reported in 1% to 14% of aneurysms.[6,10]

Natural History. The natural history of degenerative femoral artery aneurysms is poorly defined. Most publications have reviewed aneurysms that were treated surgically. A small asymptomatic femoral artery aneurysm does not appear to pose the same threat to the limb as does a popliteal artery aneurysm. In a series of 100 patients with atherosclerotic femoral artery aneurysms, serious limb-threatening complications were documented in only 2.9% of the 105 aneurysms followed nonoperatively.[6]

Diagnosis. In most cases the diagnosis of femoral artery aneurysm is suspected by the finding of a pulsatile groin mass on routine physical examination or during evaluation for vascular disease. If the femoral artery aneurysm is small or thrombosed, detection on physical examination may be difficult. Although a radiograph of the region may occasionally demonstrate the calcified rim of the aneurysm, only ultrasonography, computed tomography (CT), or magnetic resonance imaging (MRI) can reliably establish the diagnosis of the femoral aneurysm. In addition, these modalities are useful in accurately defining the size of the lesion and evaluating associated aneurysmal disease in the distal aorta and popliteal regions. These findings are particularly important because life-threatening abdominal aortic aneurysms are missed on physical examination in 50% of patients with multiple aneurysms.[12] The diagnostic accuracy of arteriography is limited because it demonstrates only the residual lumen and an aneurysm filled with smooth mural thrombus may be missed, but the definition of the vascular anatomy of the lower extremity provided by angiography is helpful in planning the appropriate operative procedure (Fig. 101.1).

Treatment. Management of femoral artery aneurysms can be found in Algorithm 101.1. Operative treatment is indicated for aneurysms causing local symptoms and presenting with limb-threatening complications. Asymptomatic aneurysms greater than 2.5 cm in diameter should also be repaired unless the patient is a prohibitive risk for operative intervention. In patients with small, asymptomatic aneurysms, observation may be appropriate, particularly in the patient with multiple medical problems who would be high risk for surgery. When nonoperative management is selected, the size of the aneurysm should be documented by ultrasonography. The patient should be followed at regular intervals with ultrasound scans and

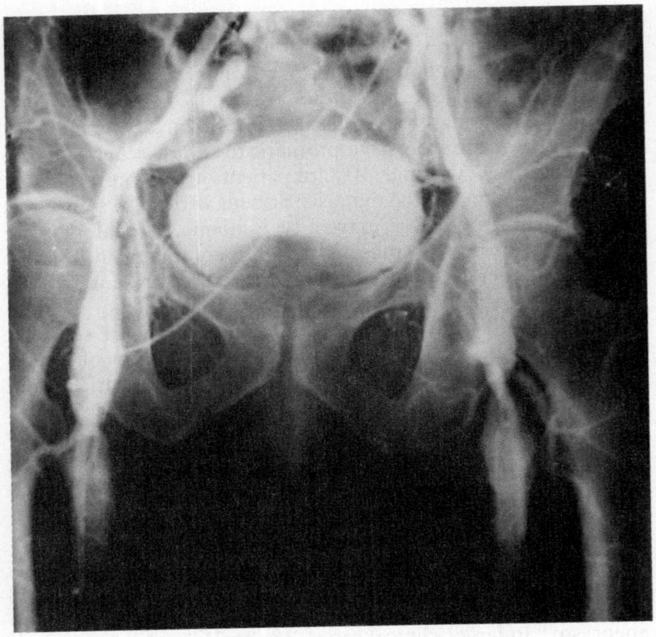

FIGURE 101.1. Arteriogram demonstrating bilateral femoral artery aneurysms that extend into the superficial femoral arteries. Unlike many patients with femoral artery aneurysms, this patient did not have an associated aortic aneurysm or popliteal aneurysms.

careful examination for occult complications. Operative treatment should be undertaken without undue delay if the femoral aneurysm enlarges, produces symptoms, or is complicated by embolization, thrombosis, or rupture.

Surgical Strategy. The operative approach is individualized based on associated aneurysmal disease. In patients with multiple asymptomatic aneurysms, treatment is staged. The life-threatening aortic lesions are treated before limb-threatening femoropopliteal lesions. Femoral artery aneurysms are addressed after popliteal lesions unless the femoral aneurysm is repaired in combination with treatment of the aortic or popliteal aneurysm. If an aortofemoral bypass is necessary, the femoral aneurysm should be treated at the same time, to avoid later anastomotic aneurysm formation. The graft limb can be anastomosed into an interposition graft that has replaced the femoral aneurysm. Similarly, if a stent graft is placed for treatment of an abdominal aortic aneurysm in a patient with femoral artery aneurysms, the aneurysm should be repaired with an interposition graft. In patients with severe lower extremity ischemia, the femoral aneurysm is treated with an interposition graft, from which the proximal anastomosis of the required femoropopliteal or femorotibial bypass is based.

Technique. The operative procedure for treatment of an isolated femoral artery aneurysm is determined by aneurysmal involvement of the superficial and deep femoral arteries as well as by the existence of lower extremity occlusive disease. The femoral artery aneurysm is usually approached through a longitudinal groin incision. When addressing an unusually large aneurysm or a ruptured aneurysm, however, initial proximal control of the external iliac artery through a retroperitoneal approach is advisable. After proximal and distal arterial control is obtained, the aneurysm sac is opened and the atheromatous debris removed. Small aneurysms may be excised, but routine excision of large aneurysms is not recommended as these lesions can often be adherent to the adjacent vein and nerve. For type I aneurysms, the preferred treatment is reconstruction with an interposition graft of Dacron or expanded polytetrafluoroethylene with the proximal anastomosis at the distal external iliac artery or proximal common femoral artery and the distal anastomosis at the femoral bifurcation.

For type II aneurysms with patent superficial and profunda femoris arteries, an interposition graft to the profunda femoris artery with reimplantation of the superficial femoral artery is one

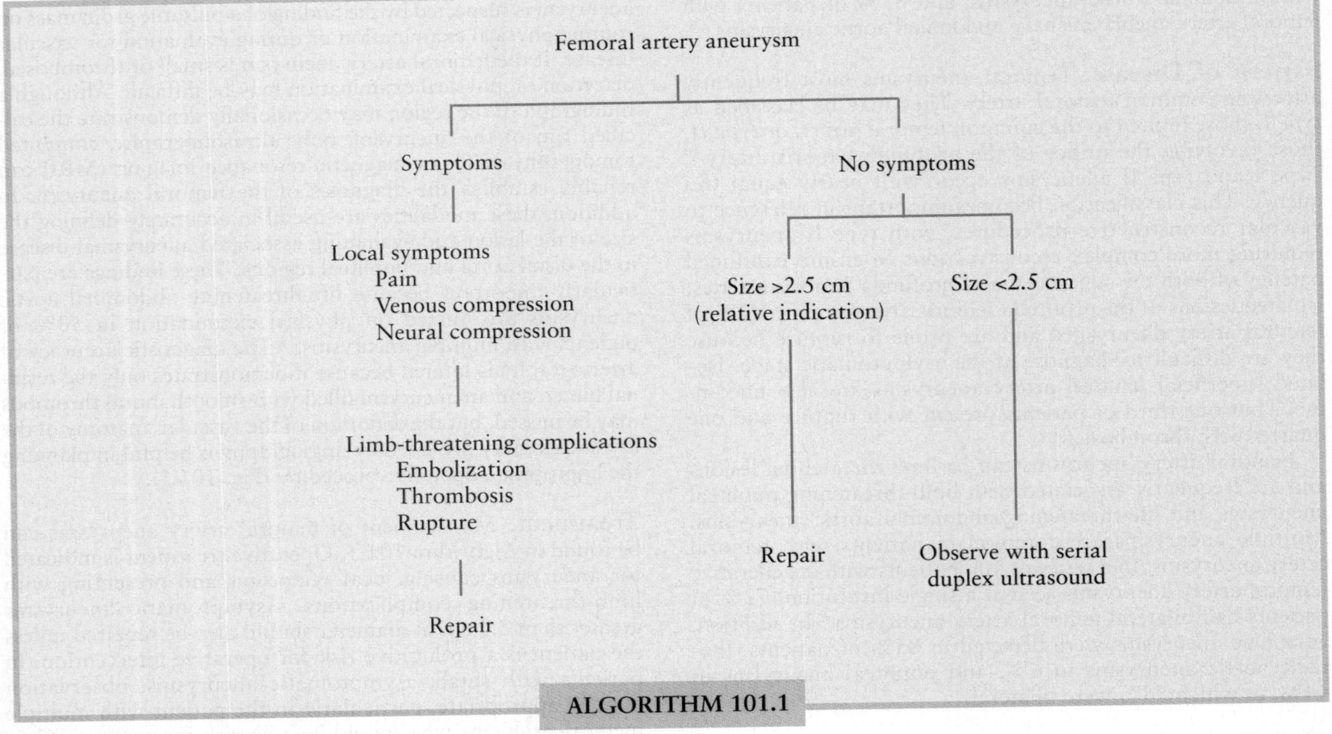

ALGORITHM 101.1. Management of femoral artery aneurysm.

standard configuration. If the superficial femoral artery is chronically occluded and the patient has minimal symptoms, an interposition graft to the profunda femoris artery alone is sufficient. If the patient has severe lower extremity ischemia, this is typically followed by a standard distal reconstruction. If recent emboli or in situ thrombosis have occluded the outflow tract, percutaneous mechanical thromboembolectomy or catheter-directed thrombolytic therapy is useful before open arterial reconstruction is undertaken.

Results. Results of surgical therapy depend on the patency of the distal vasculature. More than 80% of asymptomatic patients have excellent long-term results, whereas 68% of those presenting with lower extremity ischemia achieve satisfactory long-term outcomes.[6]

Anastomotic Pseudoaneurysms

3 **Incidence.** Anastomotic pseudoaneurysms result from a disrupted suture line between a graft and the host artery. The incidence varies with the location of the anastomosis and the type of graft that is used. Involvement of the femoral artery accounts for nearly 80% of these lesions, and 3% of all femoral anastomoses or 6% of femoral anastomoses after aortofemoral bypass develop this complication compared with 0.2% of aortic anastomoses.[14,15] Patient factors that are associated with increased likelihood of developing a femoral anastomotic aneurysm after aortofemoral bypass include chronic obstructive pulmonary disease, current smoking, and postoperative groin wound infection.[16] After infrainguinal bypass procedures, the incidence is higher with prosthetic grafts than with autogenous vein grafts, with 6% of femoral anastomoses developing aneurysms when Dacron is used compared with 0.9% when a vein graft is placed.[14] Anastomotic pseudoaneurysms are a late complication of bypass procedures; the mean interval from primary procedure to recognition is more than 6 years.[17,18]

Pathogenesis. Several factors contributing to anastomotic pseudoaneurysm formation have been identified, including weakness of the arterial wall, the type of graft material and suture utilized, the presence of infection, the method of construction of the anastomosis, and the stress on the suture line from hypertension, leg motion, or excess tension on the graft limb.[14,17,18] Progressive degeneration of the recipient artery accounts for most anastomotic pseudoaneurysms, and an increased incidence has been noted following endarterectomy of the artery at the anastomosis. False aneurysms occur less frequently with saphenous vein grafts than synthetic vascular grafts, a reflection of more complete healing of autogenous tissue. With the use of monofilament synthetic suture, anastomotic pseudoaneurysms rarely result from a loss of suture integrity, although occasionally a broken suture is a factor in pseudoaneurysm formation. Although most anastomotic aneurysms are not accompanied by overt graft infection, occult infections with coagulase-negative *Staphylococcus* species may be an important factor in the development of anastomotic aneurysms.[18] A higher incidence is noted in patients with wound healing complications, and the use of anticoagulants may increase such complications.

Clinical Manifestations. Femoral anastomotic pseudoaneurysms usually present as a pulsatile groin mass, which may or may not be accompanied by pain, redness, or symptoms of venous obstruction. Acute complications include hemorrhage, embolization, and occlusion. The latter may cause lower extremity ischemia with claudication, rest pain, or gangrene.

Diagnosis. The diagnosis of a false aneurysm is usually made on physical examination by the presence of a pulsatile groin mass in a patient who has undergone a femoral arterial reconstructive procedure. The differential diagnosis includes nonpulsatile groin masses, such as hernia, lymphocele, or abscess, through which pulsation is transmitted from an underlying normal femoral artery. Diagnosis of an anastomotic disruption in one region should raise suspicion of other anastomotic pseudoaneurysms because multiple lesions are found in at least 30% of patients,[17] and their presence suggests infection. Evaluation of an anastomotic aneurysm includes ultrasonography or CT of all anastomoses of the graft. Angiography done prior to repair of the anastomotic aneurysm is helpful in defining the proximal and distal arterial anatomy (Fig. 101.2).

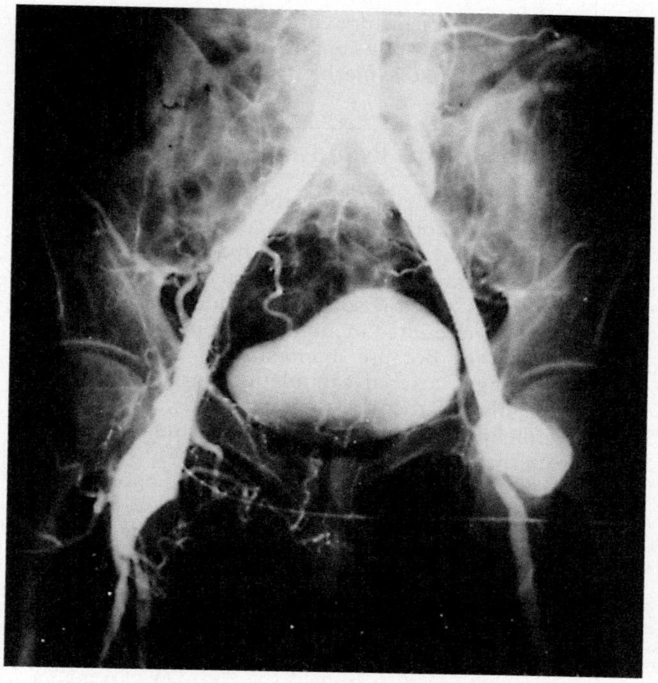

FIGURE 101.2. Arteriogram demonstrating bilateral femoral anastomotic aneurysms after an aortofemoral bypass and a left femoropopliteal bypass.

Treatment. Because of the progressive nature of anastomotic pseudoaneurysms, surgical treatment is undertaken for all lesions except those which are small (<2 cm) in high-risk patients. Principles of surgical therapy are those of primary aneurysms: obtain proximal and distal control and replace the aneurysmal segment. Securing proximal control often requires dividing the inguinal ligament to isolate the graft limb. Distal control is most easily obtained using intraluminal balloon catheters. If intrinsic arterial disease requires extension of the graft distally on the profunda femoris or superficial femoral artery, these arteries can be identified by dissection through unscarred tissue distal to the previous exposure. After débridement of the degenerated artery, an interposition graft is placed between the prosthetic graft limb and the healthy native artery. Cultures of the graft and vessel wall are essential to exclude infection as an etiologic factor in the development of the anastomotic aneurysm. If infection is obvious at the time of surgery, the approach is the same as that of any infected graft with removal of infected prosthetic material and reestablishment of blood flow, if necessary, with a bypass through an uninfected tissue route, such as an obturator, lateral femoral, or axillofemoral bypass.

Results. Results of elective operations on uncomplicated anastomotic aneurysms are excellent with 2% operative mortality, 97.5% graft patency at 2 years, and 2% amputation within 2 years of surgery.[17] Recurrence is reported in less than

16% of cases.[14,15] Patients presenting with aneurysms complicated by hemorrhage, occlusion, or embolization have significantly increased operative morbidity and mortality.

Femoral Pseudoaneurysms

Incidence. The femoral artery is the preferred site for percutaneous access for both diagnostic and therapeutic angiography, including endovascular grafts. In recent years, diagnostic studies for coronary and peripheral artery occlusive disease have increased as have the subsequent endovascular interventions, which have resulted in an increased number of femoral pseudoaneurysms. Because interventional techniques often require prolonged arterial cannulation, large-bore sheaths, and anticoagulation, they are accompanied by a higher rate of arterial complications than are diagnostic studies. Review of recent experience shows that pseudoaneurysms form after about 0.3% of diagnostic catheterizations and about 1.5% of catheter-based therapeutic procedures.[4] The use of percutaneous closure devices decreases the risk of developing a pseudoaneurysm at the arterial access site for an interventional procedure by a factor of 10 to an incidence of about 0.1%.[19,20]

Pathogenesis. Pseudoaneurysms from iatrogenic catheter trauma are classically defined as collections of blood in continuity with the arterial system that is not enclosed by all three lay-
4 ers of the arterial wall. These lesions form because of failed hemostasis at the arterial wall defect created by sheath insertion. Normally, hemostasis, aided by direct focal application of pressure or hemostatic devices, seals the defect promptly, and the arterial wall repairs itself. When hemostasis is not successfully obtained, blood under arterial pressure leaks from the artery, dissects surrounding tissue planes, and forms what is perceived on physical examination to be a pulsatile mass. The gross findings at surgery are a blood-filled cavity surrounded by a capsule. Like all pseudoaneurysms, these lesions can cause symptoms by rupture or compression of surrounding structures.

Diagnosis. The diagnosis of femoral pseudoaneurysm is suspected when a pulsatile groin mass is noted after arterial catheterization. The differential diagnosis includes hematoma, lymphadenopathy, and abscess. Arterial duplex scanning or CT is typically used to establish the diagnosis, differentiate pseudoaneurysm from hematoma, and aid in defining the communication between the mass and the arterial lumen. Color-flow duplex scanning is the diagnostic test of choice, providing accurate diagnosis, localization, and sizing of the false aneurysms.

Natural History. Color-flow duplex scanning has been used to define the incidence and natural history of pseudoaneurysms after percutaneous transluminal coronary angioplasty.[21] Many pseudoaneurysms will thrombose spontaneously within 4 weeks; however, this is less likely to occur in anticoagulated patients and those with pseudoaneurysms more than 2.0 cm in diameter. About 30% of patients with pseudoaneurysms will require intervention.[22]

Treatment. Therapy of femoral pseudoaneurysms is influenced by aneurysm size and symptoms, and whether the patient requires continuous anticoagulation (Algorithm 101.2). Surgical therapy is mandatory for all pseudoaneurysms that are acutely expanding, compressing adjacent nerves, or compromising the overlying skin. Proximal and distal arterial control is obtained, and the arterial defect is repaired directly, rarely requiring placement of more than one to two sutures.

An excellent alternative to a surgical approach, when urgent evacuation of the hematoma and arterial repair are not required, is the use of ultrasound-directed compression therapy or thrombin injection into the false aneurysm. The pseudoaneurysm is identified with a color-flow ultrasound probe and then compressed with the scan head. Real-time observation of flow in the underlying artery allows compression of the pseudoaneurysm while maintaining flow in the native vessel to prevent arterial occlusion.[23] Pseudoaneurysm thrombosis is documented by absence of flow signals on release of scan-head pressure in the case of compression therapy. While effective, this can often be quite uncomfortable for the patient and take upwards of 30 minutes of compression by the vascular technologist.

Another nonoperative treatment option of femoral pseudoaneurysms is percutaneous ultrasound-guided injection of 0.5 to 1.0 mL thrombin (1,000 U/mL) into the pseudoaneurysm away from the neck of the aneurysm.[23–25] Thrombin injection avoids the discomfort of prolonged compression and is effective in anticoagulated patients. Continuous ultrasonographic imaging is used to monitor thrombosis of the pseudoaneurysm.

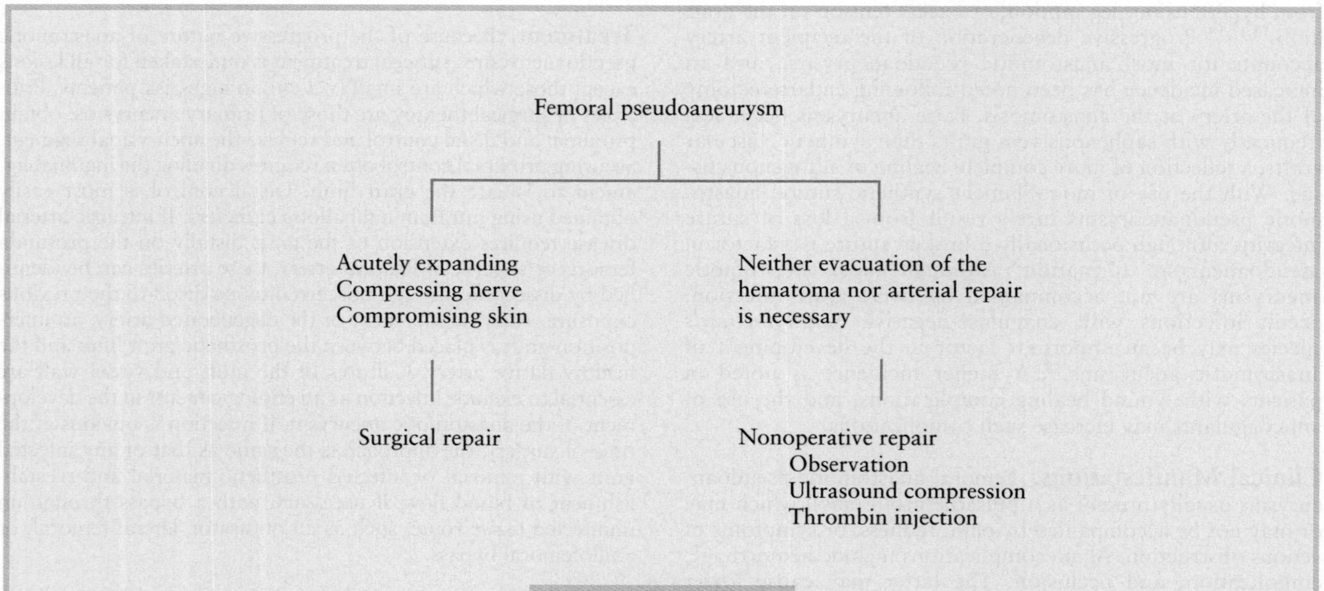

ALGORITHM 101.2

ALGORITHM 101.2. Management of femoral pseudoaneurysm.

Results. Ultrasound-guided compression therapy for femoral pseudoaneurysms results in thrombosis in 80% to 90% of cases. The initial success rate is similar in patients who are anticoagulated and in those who are not, although long-term success appears to be better in patients not receiving anticoagulant therapy. In one of the largest series of pseudoaneurysms treated with ultrasound-guided compression, thrombosis was achieved in 86% of anticoagulated patients and in 98% of those not anticoagulated, with a 20% recurrence rate in less than 24 hours in anticoagulated patients.[26] Success using this therapeutic modality requires a knowledgeable ultrasonographer and meticulous postcompression follow-up.

Thrombin injection to induce thrombosis of pseudoaneurysms is successful in 94% to 98% of patients, with thrombosis occurring in less than 1 minute.[23–25] This technique can be complicated by arterial thrombosis if an excessive volume of thrombin is used and may not be appropriate for pseudoaneurysms with large necks. Remote thromboembolic events are rare and probably are not a result of a systemic effect of the thrombin. Allergic reactions to bovine thrombin occasionally occur. Large pseudoaneurysms, greater than 8 cm in diameter, and an associated arteriovenous fistula (AVF) are predictors of failure with thrombin injection.[27]

Mycotic Aneurysms

The term *mycotic aneurysm* is currently used to refer to any infected aneurysm. Mycotic aneurysms today are often a complication of parental drug abuse, but can follow arterial trauma of any form, including invasive diagnostic and therapeutic procedures. In the past, septic emboli from bacterial endocarditis were a major cause of mycotic aneurysmal degeneration, but this is less common today. With the advent of antibiotics, aneurysms secondary to syphilis or tuberculosis are rare. With the change in cause, the location of mycotic aneurysms has shifted from central to peripheral arteries, with the femoral artery being the most common site.[29,30] The importance of mycotic aneurysms comes from their propensity to rupture.

Pathogenesis. The pathogenesis of mycotic aneurysms can be divided into four major categories, although other less common causes also exist.[29] First, septic emboli from bacterial endocarditis may lodge in normal arteries, causing infection that weakens the arterial wall, resulting in aneurysm formation. These lesions are often multiple. Second, during an episode of bacteremia, microorganisms may lodge in a preexisting atherosclerotic plaque or aneurysm and begin to multiply with the same result. A third cause of mycotic aneurysms is the contiguous spread of bacteria from a local abscess. The inflammatory process destroys the arterial wall, causing pseudoaneurysm formation. Finally, trauma to the artery with concomitant contamination may result in formation of an infected pseudoaneurysm. This mechanism of mycotic aneurysm formation is being seen more frequently, coincident with the increased use of catheter-based procedures. Bacteria may be introduced concomitantly with needle puncture or by migration during prolonged arterial catheterization. Mycotic aneurysms accompanying drug abuse may be secondary to direct contamination of the arterial wall, or they may result from destruction of the vessel wall by a local abscess.

The bacteriology of arterial infections depends on the cause of the lesion. Aneurysms secondary to bacterial endocarditis grew *Pneumococcus*, *Streptococcus*, and *Enterococcus* species most frequently in the past, but recently *Staphylococcus*, *Salmonella*, *Escherichia coli*, and *Proteus* organisms also have been cultured.[30] *Staphylococcus aureus* is the most common pathogen in mycotic femoral artery aneurysms secondary to trauma and drug abuse, occurring in more than 65% of cases.[31] In this population, at least 50% of the *S. aureus* organisms are resistant to methicillin.

Clinical Manifestations. The typical patient with a mycotic femoral aneurysm presents with a history of chills and fever and a tender, enlarging, pulsatile groin mass. The patient may have a history of intravenous drug use, recent arterial catheterization, penetrating trauma, or bacterial endocarditis. Local signs of infection, including tenderness, erythema, and warmth, are noted on physical examination. Lower extremity edema may occur secondary to venous or lymphatic obstruction. Petechial skin lesions, splinter hemorrhages, cutaneous abscesses, and septic arthritis may occur as a result of emboli originating from a mycotic aneurysm. A "sentinel bleed" may occur and signals impending rupture and life-threatening hemorrhage. Emergency surgery is indicated.

Diagnosis. The diagnosis of a mycotic aneurysm is usually straightforward, but distinguishing an abscess adjacent to the femoral artery from a femoral mycotic aneurysm may be difficult. In the patient with a pulsatile groin mass, laboratory findings including a leukocytosis, elevated erythrocyte sedimentation rate, and positive blood cultures are suggestive, but not specific, for a mycotic aneurysm. Multiple blood cultures or downstream arterial blood cultures may be necessary to yield positive results. Ultrasonography and CT angiography are helpful in establishing the diagnosis of an aneurysm (Fig. 101.3), but lack precision in distinguishing infected from bland aneurysms. The diagnosis of a mycotic aneurysm is confirmed at operation by demonstration of organisms on Gram stain or by positive cultures of the aneurysm wall.

Treatment. Mycotic aneurysms represent a serious life- and limb-threatening disease because their natural history is one of expansion and rupture. Therefore, mycotic aneurysms should be addressed surgically. The goal of treatment is eradication of the infection by excision of the aneurysm and débridement of adjacent infected tissue as well as by long-term antibiotic therapy. Secondly, adequate distal circulation must be restored. Before operative intervention is performed, the patient is started on antibiotics that are modified based on sensitivity testing of intraoperative cultures. Stent grafts have been used in selected cases of mycotic aneurysms when other approaches were not feasible; however, concern about latent infection of the stent graft oftentimes renders this more of a bridging technique than a long-term solution.

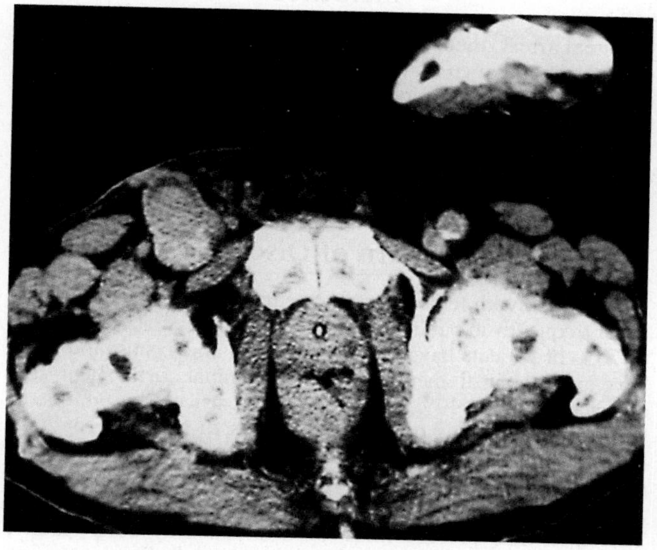

FIGURE 101.3. Computed tomography scan of an infected femoral anastomotic aneurysm that was diagnosed 5 years after aortofemoral graft placement.

The complexity of the operative procedure varies with the location and extent of the mycotic aneurysm. Although a direct approach to the femoral artery may be taken, a retroperitoneal exposure of the distal external iliac artery for proximal control is sometimes preferred for large or proximal femoral lesions to avoid excessive hemorrhage. When an infected femoral artery aneurysm is confined to only one arterial segment (common, superficial, or deep femoral artery), the aneurysm is excised and the proximal and distal arteries are ligated in emergent situations. In these cases in which an isolated arterial segment is ligated, severe ischemia resulting in amputation is unusual. In more than 50% of cases, however, the mycotic aneurysm involves the femoral artery bifurcation, and treatment requires resection of the femoral bifurcation and débridement to healthy arterial wall. The distal external iliac or proximal common femoral artery as well as the superficial and deep femoral arteries are oversewn with nonabsorbable monofilament suture. This results in significant ischemia in most patients, but with the patient heparinized, symptoms gradually improve as collateral circulation increases. The majority of patients will not need revascularization for limb salvage,[32] but up to one third of patients will have limb-threatening ischemia.[31] In patients in whom sepsis can be adequately controlled at the initial procedure, aggressive débridement may be followed by immediate revascularization using autogenous saphenous vein graft as the conduit and covering the graft with a sartorius muscle flap.[31] Another option is to observe patients for 24 hours after arterial ligation and selectively revascularize only those patients in whom limb-threatening ischemia persists. Use of prosthetic material is avoided because of the high incidence of early and late septic complications, although it can occasionally be necessary through uninfected tissue planes such as the obturator or lateral femoral route. Antibiotics are begun preoperatively and continued for at least 6 weeks postoperatively.

POPLITEAL ARTERY ANEURYSMS

5 Popliteal aneurysms are limb-threatening lesions, the vast majority of which are degenerative in etiology. Occasionally, anastomotic or traumatic popliteal aneurysms, and rarely mycotic aneurysms, are encountered in contemporary clinical practice. The remainder of this section addresses only popliteal aneurysms that are degenerative in etiology.

Incidence

Popliteal artery aneurysms are the most common degenerative true peripheral aneurysm. They occur slightly more frequently than femoral artery lesions; however, popliteal aneurysms are relatively unusual compared to abdominal aortic aneurysms. Aortic aneurysms are diagnosed with about 10 times the frequency of popliteal aneurysms.[33,34]

Pattern of Disease

Like patients with femoral artery aneurysms, multiple aneurysms occur frequently in patients with popliteal aneurysms. About 60% to 70% of patients have bilateral popliteal aneurysms, and 55% have extrapopliteal aneurysms.[35,36] Abdominal aortic aneurysms are encountered in 40% to 50%, and are particularly common in patients with bilateral popliteal aneurysms, of whom about 70% have aortic aneurysms.[35–37] Femoral artery aneurysms occur in nearly 40% of patients.[36,37] The importance of this multiplicity of aneurysms is that they may be missed on physical examination. Therefore, their presence must be determined by other studies, such as ultrasonography or CT, so that potentially life-threatening abdominal aortic aneurysms and other limb-threatening lesions are identified and managed appropriately. Even when popliteal aneurysms are initially asymptomatic, patients will develop symptoms at a mean rate of 14% per year, and one third will develop complications requiring emergent intervention within 5 years, resulting in poorer outcomes for both life and limb.[38,39]

Clinical Manifestations

The typical patient with a popliteal aneurysm is a male in his 60s or 70s with the usual risk factors for atherosclerosis. Of patients with popliteal aneurysms, 50% to 75% are smokers, 40% to 60% have hypertension, and about 15% have diabetes mellitus.[35–37,40] Other manifestations of cardiovascular disease are also common, with 10% of patients having manifestations of cerebrovascular disease and more than 40% having evidence of significant cardiac disease.[37]

The clinical manifestations of popliteal artery aneurysms range from an asymptomatic pulsatile mass to severe lower extremity ischemia. About 40% of patients are asymptomatic at diagnosis.[7] More than 50% of patients present with symptoms of limb ischemia, usually claudication, but the ischemia may be more advanced and manifested as rest pain or gangrene. Local symptoms, including sensation of a mass, local pain, and leg swelling or phlebitis secondary to compression of the adjacent vein, account for the remainder of symptoms. A popliteal artery aneurysm may be complicated by thrombosis, embolization, or, rarely, rupture. Thrombosis is reported in approximately 40% of patients,[36] and embolization occurs in about 25% of cases.[36] Some patients present with classic "blue toe syndrome," but more commonly, repeated episodes of embolization occlude the outflow vessels and result in thrombosis of the aneurysm. Rupture occurs in fewer than 5% of popliteal aneurysms[35,36]; in these cases, the hemorrhage is usually confined to the popliteal space, thus permitting surgical intervention and arterial reconstruction in a timely fashion.

Natural History

The natural history of popliteal aneurysms is not well defined because most series are composed primarily of aneurysms that have been treated surgically. In a review of 29 reports in the English literature published between 1980 and 1994, subgroups of patients were identified whose aneurysms had been observed.[7] A mean of 35% of patients with conservative follow-up developed ischemic complications, and 25% of these required amputation even with modern therapy. Thus, a significant percentage of popliteal aneurysms will develop a complication if left untreated, and although this is not synonymous with limb loss, the amputation rate is high.

Diagnosis

The diagnosis of popliteal aneurysm is usually first suspected on physical examination. Palpation of the popliteal space with the knee flexed reveals a pulsatile mass in approximately two thirds of patients. Small aneurysms may not be palpable on physical examination, and if thrombosis has occurred the mass may be nonpulsatile. Radiographs of the knee demonstrating a calcified arterial wall occasionally suggest the diagnosis of a popliteal artery aneurysm, but it must be confirmed by duplex ultrasonography, CT (Fig. 101.4), or MRI. These diagnostic modalities can establish diagnosis of popliteal artery aneurysms and exclude other entities that could be responsible for a nonpulsatile popliteal fossa mass (tumor or Baker cyst). Ultrasonography, CT, or MRI is also useful in the detection of associated aneurysms, particularly abdominal aortic and femoral artery aneurysms. Angiography can be misleading in the diagnosis of aneurysms because intraluminal thrombus may obscure the true size of the vessel (Fig. 101.5); however, it is essential for visualization of the inflow and outflow vessels necessary for revascularization. CT angiography can be a noninvasive way to provide this information (Fig. 101.6).

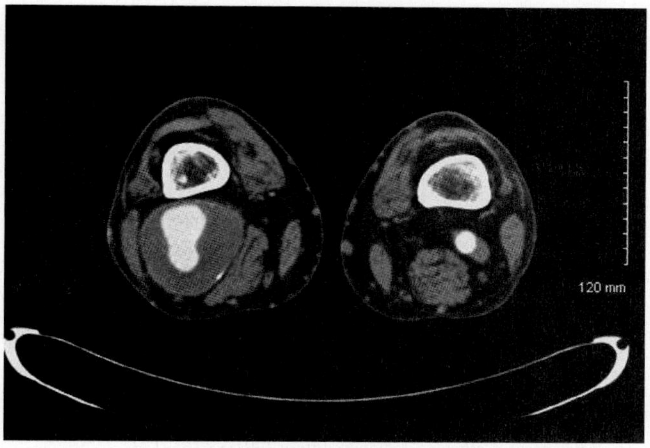

FIGURE 101.4. Computed tomography of large right popliteal aneurysm with significant laminar thrombus present.

Treatment

Indications. Surgical treatment is indicated for all symptomatic and many asymptomatic aneurysms. Controversy exists regarding the optimal management of small asymptomatic popliteal aneurysms because the natural history is not well defined. The incidence of complications with popliteal artery aneurysms is high, and the occurrence of complications does not correlate with the size of the aneurysm because the most common complications are embolization and thrombosis, which are not size related. In fact, in some reports the average diameter of symptomatic aneurysms is smaller than asymptomatic lesions.[41,42] These considerations, and the significantly higher limb loss rate after complications develop even when intervention is undertaken, have resulted in the recommendation for operative treatment when a popliteal aneurysm is diagnosed.

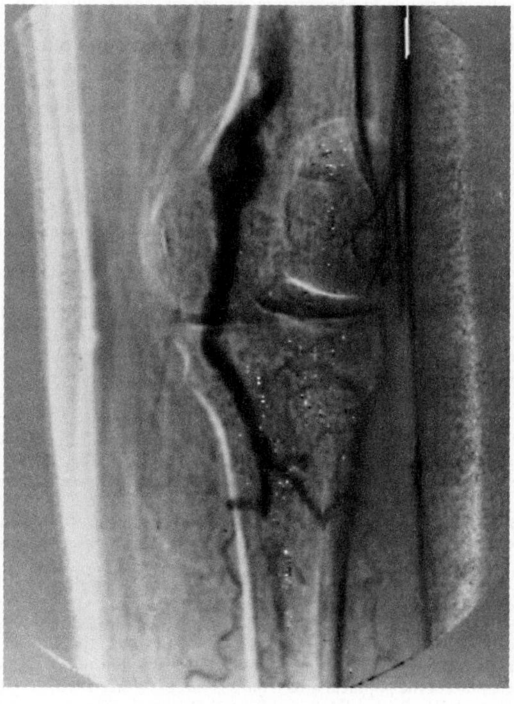

FIGURE 101.5. Arteriogram demonstrating a popliteal aneurysm associated with occlusion of the outflow tract presumably from repeated episodes of embolization. A bypass to the distal posterior tibial artery was successful.

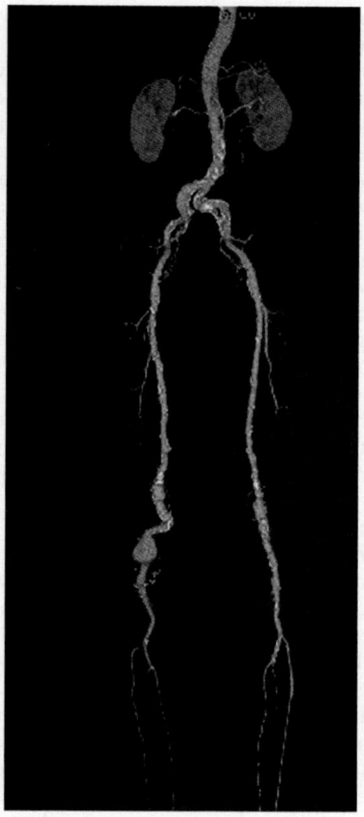

FIGURE 101.6. Computed tomography arteriogram demonstrating right popliteal artery aneurysm and associated inflow and outflow.

The goals of surgical treatment are to eliminate the potential for complications and to preserve or restore adequate blood flow to the limb. In patients with multiple aneurysms, the operative approach must be individualized. Generally, the life-threatening aortic aneurysm is treated first, followed by repair of the popliteal aneurysm. On the other hand, if a limb-threatening complication has occurred, treatment of the popliteal aneurysm usually takes precedence, followed by expeditious aortic aneurysm repair.

Surgical Technique. Most popliteal aneurysms are easily approached through standard medial thigh and calf incisions for exposure of the distal superficial femoral artery and the distal popliteal artery, respectively. The proximal anastomosis will need to originate from the common femoral artery if the entire superficial femoral artery is aneurysmal. Occasionally, the posterior approach is preferred for lesions confined to the popliteal fossa, especially when accompanied by symptoms due to compression of adjacent structures. Most aneurysms are left in situ, bypassed using a segment of saphenous vein, and ligated proximally and distally. The conduit of choice for bypass is autologous saphenous vein, which is harvested from the thigh, reversed, and tunneled along the course of the popliteal artery. The proximal and distal anastomosis may be either end to end or end to side in configuration, with the aneurysm excluded from the circulation by proximal and distal ligatures. Ligation should be adjacent to the aneurysm to minimize the number of patent collaterals that are in continuity with the aneurysm.[41,43] Late expansion and rupture of a bypassed and ligated popliteal aneurysm can occur when patent geniculate arteries continue to perfuse and pressurize the aneurysm. When the distal popliteal and proximal tibial vessels are occluded with recent emboli, they can sometimes be cleared using a balloon catheter or intraoperative thrombolytic therapy. Frequently, bypass grafts must be carried to the distal tibial arteries. Extensive femoral and popliteal aneurysms may require a femoral-popliteal or femoral-tibial bypass using in situ saphenous vein that originates from a prosthetic graft replacing a common femoral artery aneurysm.

Popliteal aneurysms have been treated by an endovascular approach. Small series show a primary patency rate of about 50% at 14 to 18 months[13,44] and a cumulative patency of 74%,[45] suggesting that this approach should be reserved for the more high-risk patient who requires intervention.

The patient who presents with an acutely ischemic extremity secondary to popliteal aneurysm thrombosis is a management challenge. Popliteal aneurysms often thrombose because of repeated episodes of emboli to the outflow vessels, which results in their occlusion. An expeditious arteriogram may identify a 6 suitable outflow vessel for the bypass graft. If no target vessel is identified, intra-arterial thrombolytic therapy should be initiated with the goal of lysing thrombus in the tibial arteries to identify a suitable outflow vessel for vascular reconstruction. Although the embolic process may be chronic, results with thrombolytic therapy followed by bypass of the aneurysm have been much better than surgical therapy alone for the patient with an acutely occluded aneurysm and severe leg ischemia.

Results. Excellent results are obtained in asymptomatic aneurysms with intact distal vasculature. Patients with thrombosed aneurysms or those in whom multiple episodes of embolization have occluded the tibial arteries have less optimal results. Operative mortality is in the 0% to 2% range, with asymptomatic patients faring better than those presenting with acutely symptomatic lesions.[46,47] In patients undergoing revascularization before ischemic complications occur, 5- and 10-year graft patency rates are greater than 80% and limb salvage is 93% to 98%.[35,48] Graft patency rates in patients undergoing surgery after developing complications of their aneurysms are 60% and 48% at 5 and 10 years, respectively, and limb salvage rates are 60% to 80%.[35,48,49] Thrombolytic therapy, when successful, improves primary graft patency in patients presenting with acute limb ischemia.[50]

References

1. Ashton HA, Buxton MJ, Day NE, et al. The Multicentre Aneurysm Screening Study (MASS) into the effect of abdominal aortic aneurysm screening on mortality in men: a randomised controlled trial. *Lancet* 2002; 360:1531–1539.
2. Diwan A, Sarkar R, Stanley JC, et al. Incidence of femoral and popliteal artery aneurysms in patients with abdominal aortic aneurysms. *J Vasc Surg* 2000;31:863–869.
3. Trickett JP, Scott RA, Tilney HS. Screening and management of asymptomatic popliteal aneurysms. *J Med Screen* 2002;9:92–93.
4. Lange P, Houe T, Helgstrand UJV. The efficacy of ultrasound-guided compression of iatrogenic femoral pseudo-aneurysms. *Eur J Vasc Endovasc Surg* 2001;21:248–250.
5. Calligaro KD, Dougherty MJ, Ryan S, et al. Acute arterial complications associated with total hip and knee arthroplasty. *J Vasc Surg* 2003;38: 1170–1177.
6. Graham LM, Zelenock GB, Whitehouse WM Jr, et al. Clinical significance of arteriosclerotic femoral artery aneurysms. *Arch Surg* 1980;115:502–507.
7. Dawson I, Sie RB, Van Bockel JH. Atherosclerotic popliteal aneurysm. *Br J Surg* 1997;84:293–299.
8. Faggioli GL, Gargiulo M, Bertoni F, et al. Parietal inflammatory infiltrate in peripheral aneurysms of atherosclerotic origin. *J Cardiovasc Surg* 1992; 33:331–336.
9. Thompson RW, Liao SX, Curci JA. Vascular smooth muscle cell apoptosis in abdominal aortic aneurysms. *Coronary Artery Dis* 1997;8:623–631.
10. Cutler BS, Darling RC. Surgical management of arteriosclerotic femoral aneurysms. *Surgery* 1973;74:764–773.
11. Jarrett F, Makaroun MS, Rhee RY, et al. Superficial femoral artery aneurysms: an unusual entity? *J Vasc Surg* 2002;36:571–574.
12. Dent TL, Lindenauer SM, Ernst CB, et al. Multiple arteriosclerotic artery aneurysms. *Arch Surg* 1972;105:338–344.
13. Henry M, Amor M, Henry I, et al. Percutaneous endovascular treatment of peripheral aneurysms. *J Cardiovasc Surg* 2000;41:871–883.
14. Szilagyi DE, Smith RF, Elliott JP, et al. Anastomotic aneurysms after vascular reconstruction: problems of incidence, etiology, and treatment. *Surgery* 1975;78:800–816.
15. Szilagyi DE, Elliott JP Jr, Smith RF, et al. A thirty-year survey of the reconstructive surgical treatment of aortoiliac occlusive disease. *J Vasc Surg* 1986;3:421–436.
16. Ylönen K, Biancari F, Leo E, et al. Predictors of development of anastomotic femoral pseudoaneurysms after aortofemoral reconstruction for abdominal aortic aneurysm. *Am J Surg* 2004;187:83–87.
17. Dennis JW, Littooy FN, Greisler HP, et al. Anastomotic pseudoaneurysms. A continuing late complication of vascular reconstructive procedures. *Arch Surg* 1986;121:314–317.
18. Seabrook GR, Schmitt DD, Bandyk DF, et al. Anastomotic femoral pseudoaneurysm: an investigation of occult infection as an etiologic factor. *J Vasc Surg* 1990;11:629–634.
19. Knight CG, Healy DA, Thomas RL. Femoral artery pseudoaneurysms: risk factors, prevalence, and treatment options. *Ann Vasc Surg* 2003;17: 503–508.
20. La Perna L, Olin JW, Goines D, et al. Ultrasound-guided thrombin injection for the treatment of postcatheterization pseudoaneurysms. *Circulation* 2000;102:2391–2395.
21. Kresowik TF, Khoury MD, Miller BV, et al. A prospective study of the incidence and natural history of femoral vascular complications after percutaneous transluminal coronary angioplasty. *J Vasc Surg* 1991;13:328–335.
22. Kent KC, McArdle CR, Kennedy B, et al. A prospective study of the clinical outcome of femoral pseudoaneurysms and arteriovenous fistulas induced by arterial puncture. *J Vasc Surg* 1993;17:125–133.
23. Hertz SM, Brener BJ. Ultrasound-guided pseudoaneurysm compression: efficacy after coronary stenting and angioplasty. *J Vasc Surg* 1997;26: 913–916.
24. Fram DB, Giri S, Jamil G, et al. Suture closure of the femoral arteriotomy following invasive cardiac procedures: a detailed analysis of efficacy, complications, and the impact of early ambulation in 1,200 consecutive, unselected cases. *Catheter Cardiovasc Interv* 2001;53:163–173.
25. Mohler ER III, Mitchell ME, Carpenter JP, et al. Therapeutic thrombin injection of pseudoaneurysms: a multicenter experience. *Vasc Med* 2001;6: 241–244.
26. Maleux G, Hendrickx S, Vaninbroukx J, et al. Percutaneous injection of human thrombin to treat iatrogenic femoral pseudoaneurysms: short- and midterm ultrasound follow-up. *Eur Radiol* 2003;13:209–212.
27. Cox GS, Young JR, Gray BR, et al. Ultrasound-guided compression repair of postcatheterization pseudoaneurysms: results of treatment in one hundred cases. *J Vasc Surg* 1994;19:683–686.
28. Kumins NH, Landau DS, Montalvo J, et al. Expanded indications for the treatment of postcatheterization femoral pseudoaneurysms with ultrasound-guided compression. *Am J Surg* 1998;176:131–136.
29. Anderson CB, Butcher HR Jr, Ballinger WF. Mycotic aneurysms. *Arch Surg* 1974;109:712–717.
30. Brown SL, Busuttil RW, Baker JD, et al. Bacteriologic and surgical determinants of survival in patients with mycotic aneurysms. *J Vasc Surg* 1984; 1:541–547.
31. Reddy DJ, Smith RF, Elliott JP, et al. Infected femoral artery false aneurysms in drug addicts: evolution of selective vascular reconstruction. *J Vasc Surg* 1986;3:718–724.
32. Gan JP, Leiberman DP, Pollock JG. Outcome after ligation of infected false femoral aneurysms in intravenous drug abusers. *Eur J Vasc Endovasc Surg* 2000;19:158–161.
33. Szilagyi DE, Schwartz RL, Reddy DJ. Popliteal arterial aneurysms. Their natural history and management. *Arch Surg* 1981;116:723–728.
34. Ramesh S, Michaels JA, Galland RB. Popliteal aneurysm: morphology and management. *Br J Surg* 1993;80:1531–1533.
35. Anton GE, Hertzer NR, Beven EG, et al. Surgical management of popliteal aneurysms: trends in presentation, treatment, and results from 1952 to 1984. *J Vasc Surg* 1986;3:125–134.
36. Vermilion BD, Kimmins SA, Pace WG, et al. A review of one hundred forty-seven popliteal aneurysms with long-term follow-up. *Surgery* 1981; 90:1009–1014.
37. Whitehouse WM Jr, Wakefield TW, Graham LM, et al. Limb-threatening potential of arteriosclerotic popliteal artery aneurysms. *Surgery* 1983;93: 694–699.
38. Michaels JA, Galland RB. Management of asymptomatic popliteal aneurysms: the use of a Markov decision tree to determine the criteria for a conservative approach. *Eur J Vasc Surg* 1993;7:136–143.
39. Bowyer RC, Cawthorn SJ, Walker WJ, et al. Conservative management of asymptomatic popliteal aneurysm. *Br J Surg* 1990;77:1132–1135.
40. Lowell RC, Gloviczki P, Hallett JW Jr, et al. Popliteal artery aneurysms: the risk of nonoperative management. *Ann Vasc Surg* 1994;8:14–23.
41. Ascher E, Markevich N, Schutzer RW, et al. Small popliteal artery aneurysms: are they clinically significant? *J Vasc Surg* 2003;37:755–760.
42. Michaels JA, Galland RB. Management of asymptomatic popliteal aneurysms: the use of a Markov decision tree to determine the criteria for a conservative approach. *Eur J Vasc Surg* 1993;7:136–143.
43. Jones WT III, Hagino RT, Chiou AC, et al. Graft patency is not the only clinical predictor of success after exclusion and bypass of popliteal artery aneurysms. *J Vasc Surg* 2003;37:392–398.
44. Gerasimidis T, Sfyroeras G, Papazoglou K, et al. Endovascular treatment of popliteal artery aneurysms. *Eur J Endovasc Surg* 2003;26:506–511.
45. Tielliu IFJ, Verhoeven ELG, Prins TR, et al. Treatment of popliteal artery aneurysms with the Hemobahn stent-graft. *J Endovasc Ther* 2003;10: 111–116.
46. Varga ZA, Locke-Edmunds JC, Baird RN, et al. A multicenter study of popliteal aneurysms. *J Vasc Surg* 1994;20:171–177.
47. Reilly MK, Abbott WM, Darling RC. Aggressive surgical management of popliteal artery aneurysms. *Am J Surg* 1983;145:498–502.
48. Roggo A, Brunner U, Ottinger LW, et al. The continuing challenge of aneurysms of the popliteal artery. *Surg Gynecol Obstet* 1993;177:565–572.
49. Dawson I, Van Bockel JH, Brand R, et al. Popliteal artery aneurysms: long-term follow-up of aneurysmal disease and results of surgical treatment. *J Vasc Surg* 1991;13:398–407.
50. Dorigo W, Pulli R, Turini F, et al. Acute leg ischaemia from thrombosed popliteal artery aneurysms: role of preoperative thrombolysis. *Eur J Vasc Endovasc Surg* 2002;23:251–254.

CHAPTER 102 ■ VENOUS DISEASE

THOMAS W. WAKEFIELD AND MICHAEL C. DALSING

KEY POINTS

1. The diagnosis and treatment of acute and chronic venous disease has made significant advances in the last few years.
2. New drug therapies exist or are on the verge of impacting the treatment of acute DVT.
3. Chronic venous disease has experienced a resurgence of interest in the United States with new endoluminal and surgical interventions being investigated and used clinically.
4. Characterization of the disease is being scrutinized to allow for a better understanding of how treatment impacts patient outcomes.
5. The care of patients with venous disease is an active and maturing discipline within the realm of the surgical disciplines.

ACUTE VENOUS THROMBOEMBOLIC DISEASE

Incidence, Risk Factors, and Categories

Venous thromboembolism (VTE), including deep venous thrombosis (DVT) and pulmonary embolism (PE), is a national healthcare concern. DVT affects more than 250,000 patients annually, whereas PE affects more than 200,000 patients per year. The incidence has remained constant since 1980 and increases with age.[1] The cost of treatment for both DVT and PE (termed VTE) is in the billions of dollars per year. Although the Virchow triad of stasis, vessel wall injury, and hypercoagulability has defined the events that predispose to DVT formation for the past 150 years, today the understanding of events that occur at the level of the vein wall, including the influence of the inflammatory response, on thrombogenesis is increasingly becoming recognized.

Acquired risk factors for VTE include increasing age, malignancy, immobilization, surgery and trauma, oral contraceptive use, hormone replacement therapy, pregnancy and the puerperium, neurologic disease, cardiac disease, obesity, and antiphospholipid antibodies.[2] Genetic risk factors include deficiencies of antithrombin, protein C and protein S, factor V Leiden, prothrombin 20210 A, blood group non-O, dysfibrinogenemia, dysplasminogenemia, hyperhomocystinemia, reduced heparin cofactor II activity, elevated levels of clotting factors (e.g., factors XI, IX, VII, VIII, X, and II), and elevations in plasminogen activator inhibitor-1 (PAI-1).[3] When a patient presents with an idiopathic VTE, there is family history of VTE, there is recurrent thrombosis, or there is thrombosis in unusual locations, workup for a hypercoagulable state may be indicated (Table 102.1).[2,3] Hematologic diseases associated with VTE include heparin-induced thrombocytopenia and thrombosis syndrome (HITTS), disseminated intravascular coagulation (DIC), antiphospholipid antibody syndrome, thrombotic thrombocytopenic purpura (TTP), hemolytic uremic syndrome (HUS), and myeloproliferative disorders.

Most DVT affect the iliac, femoral, or popliteal lower limb veins. Presenting symptoms include unilateral leg pain and swelling, but some DVTs are silent, with the first manifestation a PE. A recent study of 5,451 patients with ultrasound-confirmed DVT revealed the most common comorbidities to be hypertension, surgery within 3 months, immobility within 30 days, cancer, and obesity.[4]

Venous Thromboembolism Diagnosis

1 **Deep Venous Thrombosis.** The diagnosis of DVT must be made with confirmatory laboratory testing, as patients will be asymptomatic at presentation in up to half the time. Patients complain of a dull ache or pain in the calf or leg. The most common physical finding is edema, although Wells et al.[5] have classified patients into a scoring system that emphasizes physical presentation. Characteristics that score points include the presence of active cancer, paralysis or paresis, recent plaster immobilization of the lower extremity, being recently bedridden for 3 days or more, localized tenderness along the distribution of the deep venous system, the entire leg being swollen, calf swelling that is at least 3 cm larger on the involved side as compared to the noninvolved side, pitting edema in the symptomatic leg, and a history of previous DVT. With extensive proximal iliofemoral DVT there may be significant swelling, cyanosis, and dilated superficial collateral veins.

Massive iliofemoral DVT may result in the development of phlegmasia alba dolens (white swollen leg) or phlegmasia cerulea dolens (blue swollen leg). Venous gangrene may occur if the phlegmasia is not aggressively treated. This occurs when the arterial inflow becomes obstructed due to the effects of the venous hypertension. Alternatively, arterial emboli or spasm may occur and contribute to the pathology. Skin blisters and toes on the limb may turn black. Venous gangrene is often associated with an underlying malignancy and is always preceded by phlegmasia cerulea dolens. Amputation rates of 20% to 50%, PE rates of 12% to 40%, and mortality rates of 20% to 40% are associated with venous gangrene.[6]

Tests of historical interest for making the diagnosis of DVT include indirect flow examinations. Presently, duplex ultrasound imaging has replaced these indirect tests due to its high sensitivity, specificity, and reproducibility. Duplex has also replaced the invasive test contrast phlebography. Duplex ultrasound imaging includes both a B-mode image and Doppler flow pattern. Duplex imaging demonstrates sensitivity and specificity rates greater than 95%.[7] According to the grade criteria for the strength of medical evidence, duplex ultrasound is given a 2 C level of evidence.[7–9] Other tests include magnetic resonance imaging (especially good for assessing central pelvic vein and inferior vena cava [IVC] thrombosis), and spiral CT scanning (especially with chest imaging during examination for PE).[10] Even at the level of the calf, a level in which duplex imaging is less accurate, it has become an acceptable technique in symptomatic patients. Duplex imaging is painless, requires no

VASCULAR

TABLE 102.1 **DIAGNOSIS**

HYPERCOAGULABLE TESTING

Standard coagulation tests
APC resistance test
Factor V Leiden genetic analysis
Prothrombin 20210A genetic analysis
Homocysteine level
Protein C antigen/activity
Protein S antigen
Antithrombin antigen/activity
Antiphospholipid/anticardiolipin antibody
Platelet count/platelet aggregation testing
Factor VIII, XI, IX, VII, X, II levels
Functional plasminogen
Heparin antibodies (if indicated)
Mixing studies (if aPTT is elevated)

APC, activated protein C; aPTT, activated thromboplastin time.

contrast, can be repeated, and is safe during pregnancy. It is important that it also identifies other causes of a patient's symptoms other than DVT.[8]

A single complete technically adequate negative duplex scan is accurate enough to justify withholding anticoagulation with liminal long-term adverse thromboembolic complications.[11] This requires that all venous segments of the leg have been imaged and evaluated. If the duplex scan is indeterminate, treatment may be based on other factors, such as biomarkers, with the duplex scan repeated in 24 to 72 hours. Combining clinical characteristics with a D-dimer assay may decrease the number of negative duplex scans performed.[5] Also, repeat imaging should be performed if the patient's symptoms change or worsen. Although clinical characteristics and D-dimer levels are useful to rule out thrombosis, the converse is not true. A positive D-dimer and a positive risk assessment is associated with DVT in only approximately 70% of cases.[12] Ongoing efforts to establish a panel of biomarkers that may be used to make a positive diagnosis of DVT based on the inflammatory response to DVT are under investigation.[13]

Other conditions that may be confused with DVT include lymphedema, muscle strains, and muscle contusion. Iliac vein obstruction may lead to unilateral leg edema (May-Thurner Syndrome), whereas the presence of a cyst behind the knee may produce unilateral lower leg pain and edema. Other causes of leg swelling include systemic problems such as cardiac, renal, or hepatic abnormalities. However, these systemic problems usually lead to bilateral edema.

Pulmonary Embolism. In the past, the diagnosis of PE was made with ventilation-perfusion (V/Q) scanning and pulmonary angiography. However, newer techniques include spiral computed tomographic scanning and magnetic resonance imaging. The sensitivity of V/Q scanning was defined in PIOPED I at 98%, but specificity was low at 10%.[14] By combining clinical factors with V/Q scan, levels of sensitivity and specificity greater than 95% were achieved. With a high-probability V/Q scan, two risk factors positive for PE, the sensitivity was 97%; with one risk factor, 84%; and with no risk factors, 82%. Similarly, with a normal V/Q scan, the chance of PE was essentially 0, irrespective of the risk factor status.[15] Thus, a normal V/Q scan or a high-probability scan provided good diagnostic information on which treatment could be based. However, only a small portion of V/Q scans are in one of these two categories, leaving many patients needing further testing. Due to its invasive nature, pulmonary angiography is used less often today. Pulmonary arteriography is indicated with acute massive PE, IVC interruption, and when planning interventional therapy, such as thrombolysis or pulmonary embolectomy.

Spiral computed tomographic scanning has demonstrated excellent specificity and sensitivity as the technology has improved. Now emboli at the subsegmental level can be identified.[16] The sensitivity for isolated chest CT imaging is increased greater than 90% when clinical analysis is added. Additionally, sensitivity improved when a lower extremity imaging study was added to the chest scan.[10] Results from PIOPED II demonstrate that if the clinical presentation and spiral CT scan results are concordant, therapies can be safely recommended. However, if results are discordant between clinical presentation and spiral CT, then other confirmatory tests are necessary. For the diagnosis of PE, spiral CT imaging is given a 1 A level of evidence. Magnetic resonance imaging is currently being investigated in PIOPED III.

Axillary/Subclavian Vein Thrombosis. Thrombosis of the axillary/subclavian vein accounts for less than 5% of all cases of acute DVT. However, it may be associated with PE in up to 10% to 15% of cases and additionally can also be the source of significant disability.[17] Primary axillary/subclavian vein thrombosis results from obstruction of the axillary vein in the thoracic outlet, the so-called Paget-von Schrötter syndrome, noted especially in healthy muscular athletic individuals. Such thrombosis may also occur in patients with hypercoagulable states. Secondary axillary/subclavian vein thrombosis results include mediastinal tumors, congestive heart failure, and nephrotic syndrome. Patients with axillary-subclavian venous thrombosis often present with arm pain, edema, and cyanosis. Superficial venous distention may be apparent over the arm, forearm, shoulder, and even the anterior chest wall.

Upper extremity venous duplex ultrasound is used to make the diagnosis of suspected axillary-subclavian vein thrombosis. Thrombolysis and phlebography are often considered next. If phlebography is performed, it is important that the patient undergo positional phlebography with arm abduction to 120 degrees to confirm extrinsic subclavian vein compression at the thoracic outlet. Venous compromise is further evidenced by prominent collateral veins. Since a cervical rib may be the cause of such obstruction, chest x-ray views should be obtained to exclude its presence.

STANDARD THERAPY FOR VTE

The primary treatment of VTE is systemic anticoagulation (Algorithm 102.1). This reduces the risk of PE, extension of thrombosis, and thrombus recurrence. Since it has been shown that the recurrence rate for VTE is higher if anticoagulation is not therapeutic in the first 24 hours, immediate anticoagulation should be undertaken.[18] However, recurrent DVT may still occur in up to one third of patients over an 8-year period, even with appropriate anticoagulant therapy.[19]

Unfractionated heparin or low-molecular-weight heparin (LMWH) is undertaken for 5 days during which time oral anticoagulation with vitamin K antagonists (usually warfarin) is started. It is recommended that international normalized ratios (INRs) be therapeutic for two consecutive days before stopping heparin or LMWH.[20] LMWHs, derived from the lower-molecular-weight range of standard heparin, have become the standard for treatment. They can be given by subcutaneous route, require no monitoring except in certain circumstances (morbid obesity, pregnancy, or renal insufficiency), and are associated with a lower bleeding potential.[21] Additionally, they

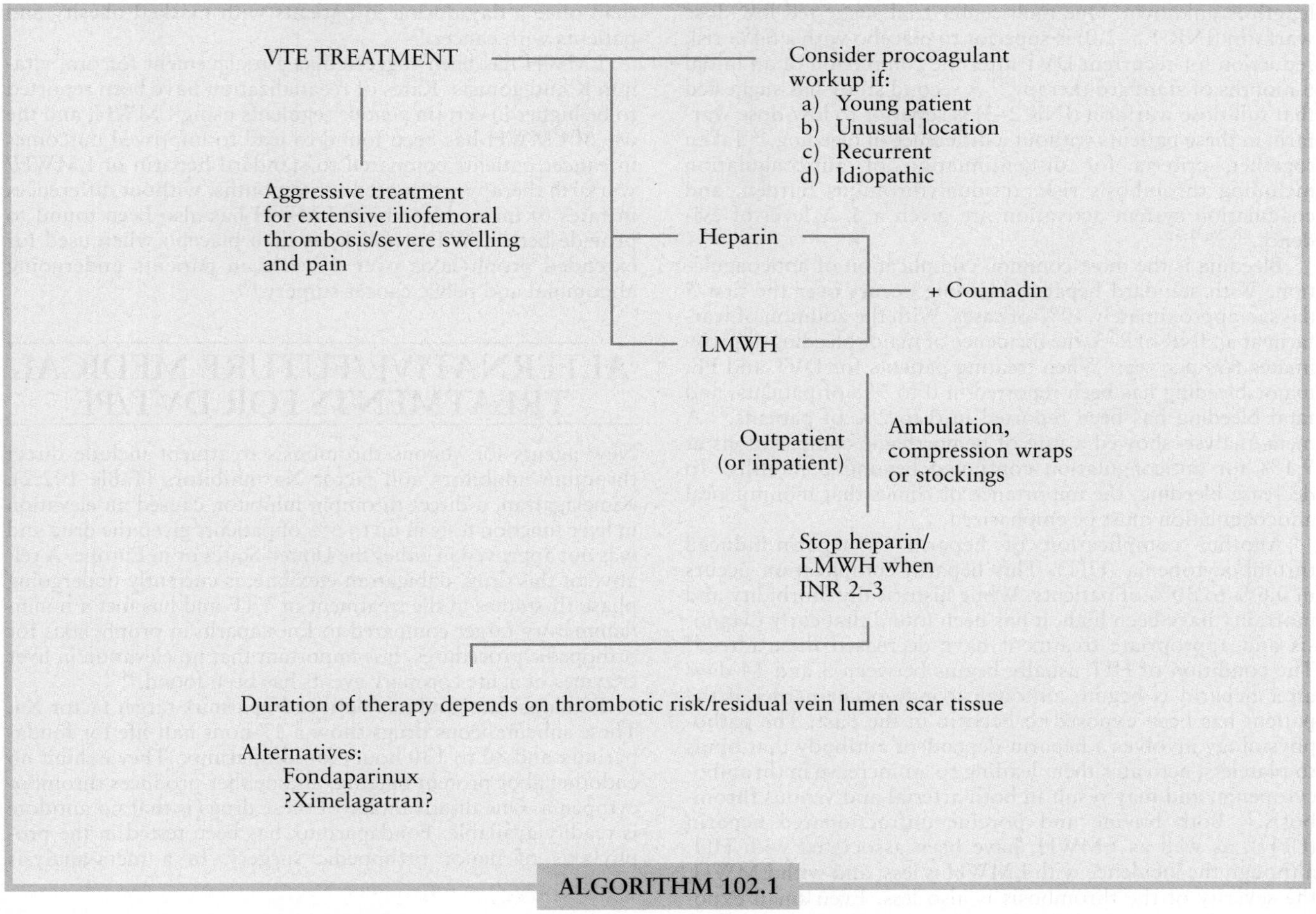

ALGORITHM 102.1. Treatment of venous thromboembolism.

demonstrate less direct thrombin inhibition and more factor Xa inhibition. Compared to standard unfractionated heparin, LMWHs have significant improvement in bioavailability, less endothelial cell binding and protein binding as compared to standard unfractionated heparin, and due to this an improved pharmacokinetic profile.[22] Additionally, other potential advantages of LMWHs compared to standard unfractionated heparin include less bleeding, less antiplatelet activity, less frequent heparin-induced thrombocytopenia, less interference with protein C and complement activation, and less osteoporosis. LMWHs are administered in a weight-based fashion subcutaneously. However, the use in outpatient settings usually requires a coordinated effort of multiple healthcare providers. LMWH may also decrease the incidence of postthrombotic syndrome.[23] Based on all of the available evidence, LMWH is now preferred over standard unfractionated heparin for the initial treatment of VTE with a 1 A level of evidence.[24]

Warfarin should be started after heparinization is therapeutic to prevent warfarin-induced skin necrosis. For standard unfractionated heparin, this would mean after a therapeutic aPTT was obtained, whereas for LMWH, this would mean after an appropriate weight-based dose was administered and had been allowed to circulate. Warfarin causes inhibition of protein C and S before factors II, IX, and X. Thus, patients can be transiently hypercoagulable on the initiation of warfarin therapy. The goal for warfarin dosing is an INR between 2.0 and 3.0. The duration of anticoagulation depends on several factors, including the presence of continuing thrombogenic risk factors, the type of thrombosis (idiopathic, for example), the number of times thrombosis has occurred, the status of the veins when stopping anticoagulation, and the level of D-dimer noted 1 month after warfarin therapy stops. The recommended duration of anticoagulation after a first episode of VTE is 3 to 6 months.[25] Calf thrombi may be treated with a shorter course of warfarin, usually 6 weeks to 3 months. After a second episode of VTE, the usual recommendation is prolonged warfarin unless the patient is very young at the time of presentation or there are other mitigating factors. In aggregate, criteria for discontinuation of warfarin are given a 1 A level of evidence.[26]

VTE recurrence is increased with homozygous factor V Leiden and prothrombin 20210 A mutation, protein C/S deficiency, antithrombin deficiency, antiphospholipid antibodies, and cancer until resolved. In these conditions, long-term warfarin is usually recommended. However, heterozygous factor V Leiden and prothrombin 20210 A genetic abnormalities do not carry the same risk as their homozygous counterparts, and the length of oral anticoagulation is shortened correspondingly.

Although the amount of scar tissue inside the venous circulation leading to stasis has recently been suggested to be an important factor, a better validated factor involves D-dimer testing obtained one month after warfarin is complete. If D-dimer is elevated above normal, warfarin should be continued, as this result suggests that the patient is still prothrombotic.[27–29] One study demonstrated a statistically significant advantage to resuming Coumadin if the D-dimer assay is elevated over an average 1.4 year follow-up (odds ratio [OR] 4.26, $p = 0.02$).[30]

Regarding idiopathic DVT, most believe this diagnosis requires more than 6 months of anticoagulation, but the actual length is unknown. One multicenter trial suggested low-dose warfarin (INR 1.5–2.0) is superior to placebo with a 64% risk reduction for recurrent DVT after the completion of an initial 6 months of standard therapy.[31] A second study has suggested that full-dose warfarin (INR 2–3) is superior to low-dose warfarin in these patients without a difference in bleeding.[32] Taken together, criteria for discontinuation of anticoagulation including thrombosis risk, residual thrombus burden, and coagulation system activation are given a 1 A level of evidence.[26–29,31,32]

Bleeding is the most common complication of anticoagulation. With standard heparin, bleeding occurs over the first 5 days in approximately 10% of cases. With the addition of warfarin at an INR of 2–3, the incidence of major bleeding approximates 6% per year. When treating patients for DVT and PE, major bleeding has been reported in 0 to 7% of patients, and fatal bleeding has been reported in 0 to 2% of patients.[33] A meta-analysis showed a rate of hemorrhagic complications at 9.1% for anticoagulation continued beyond 3 months. To decrease bleeding, the importance of clinics that monitor oral anticoagulation must be emphasized.

Another complication of heparin is heparin-induced thrombocytopenia (HIT). This heparin complication occurs in 0.6% to 30% of patients. While historically morbidity and mortality have been high, it has been found that early diagnosis and appropriate treatment have decreased these rates.[34] The condition of HIT usually begins between 3 and 14 days after heparin is begun, although it may occur earlier if the patient has been exposed to heparin in the past. The pathophysiology involves a heparin-dependent antibody that binds to platelets, activates them leading to an increase in thrombocytopenia, and may result in both arterial and venous thrombosis.[35] Both bovine and porcine unfractionated heparin (UFH), as well as LMWH, have been associated with HIT, although the incidence with LMWH is less, and with LMWH, the severity of the thrombosis is also less. Even small exposures to heparin, such as heparin coating on indwelling catheters, has caused the syndrome. The diagnosis should be suspected with a 50% or greater drop in platelet count, when the platelet count falls below 100,000/μL during heparin therapy, or when thrombosis occurs during heparin or LMWH therapy.[36] Although there are many tests for this diagnosis, the most useful is an enzyme-linked immunosorbent assay (ELISA) that detects the antiheparin antibody in
2 plasma. This test is highly sensitive but poorly specific. The serotonin release assay is another test that can be used. This test is more specific but less sensitive than the ELISA test.[37] When the diagnosis is made, cessation of heparin is most important. Warfarin should not be given until an adequate alternative anticoagulant has been established to prevent paradoxical thrombosis as warfarin-induced thrombosis has been reported with this condition. As LMWHs demonstrate high cross-reactivity with standard heparin antibodies, they cannot be substituted for standard heparin in patients with HIT. Agents that have been FDA approved as alternatives for HIT include the direct thrombin inhibitors hirudin (lepirudin/Refludan) and argatroban. Other agents have also been found to be effective, such as fondaparinux, but they are not FDA approved for this indication.[38,39] The use of these alternative agents is given either a 2 C or 1 C level of evidence.[26,36,38,39]

Low-Molecular-Weight Heparin Special Features

When considering once a day to twice a day LMWH dosing, a meta-analysis of more than 1,500 patients with VTE demonstrated a nonsignificant difference in the incidence of recurrent thromboembolism, thrombosis size, hemorrhagic events, and mortality.[40] Twice a day dosing may still be more appropriate than once a day dosing in patients with marked obesity and patients with cancer.[41]

LMWH has been suggested as a replacement for oral vitamin K antagonists. Rates of recanalization have been reported to be higher in certain venous segments using LMWH, and the use of LMWH has been found to lead to improved outcomes in cancer patients compared to standard heparin or LMWH/warfarin therapy when used for 6 months, without differences in rates of major bleeding.[42] LMWH has also been found to provide better DVT prophylaxis than placebo when used for extended prophylaxis over 4 weeks in patients undergoing abdominal and pelvic cancer surgery.[43]

ALTERNATIVE/FUTURE MEDICAL TREATMENTS FOR DVT/PE

New agents for venous thrombosis treatment include direct thrombin inhibitors and factor Xa inhibitors (Table 102.2). Ximelagatran, a direct thrombin inhibitor, caused an elevation in liver function tests in up to 6% of patients given the drug and was not approved in either the United States or in Europe. A relative of this drug, dabigatran etexilate, is currently undergoing phase III studies in the treatment of VTE and has met a noninflammatory target compared to Enoxaparin in prophylaxis for orthopedic procedures. It is important that no elevation in liver enzymes or acute coronary events has been found.[44]

Fondaparinux and its relative idraparinux target factor Xa. These subcutaneous drugs show a 17-hour half-life for fondaparinux and 80 to 130 hours for idraparinux. They exhibit no endothelial or protein binding, and neither produces thrombocytopenia. One disadvantage of these drugs is that no antidote is readily available. Fondaparinux has been tested in the prophylaxis of major orthopedic surgery. In a meta-analysis

TABLE 102.2

ALTERNATIVE ANTICOAGULANTS

■ DRUGS	■ MECHANISM OF ACTION
Dabigatran etexilate	Direct thrombin (FIIa) inhibitor
Lepirudin	Direct thrombin (FIIa) inhibitor
Bivalirudin	Direct thrombin (FIIa) inhibitor
Argatroban	Direct thrombin (FIIa) inhibitor
Fondaparinux	Indirect FXa inhibitor
Idraparinux	Indirect FXa inhibitor
Rivaroxaban	Direct FXa inhibitor
Apixaban	Direct FXa inhibitor
Oral heparins/LMWH	Same as heparin/LMWH with passage through GI tract
Ancrod	Defibrinating agent
P-selectin inhibitors	Anti-inflammatory preventing thrombus amplification
Factor VIIa inhibitors	Competes with FVIIa for binding to TF
Tissue factor pathway inhibitor	FVIIa/TF complex inhibitor
Activated protein C	Inactivates FVa, FVIIIa, inhibitor to tPA

FIIa, factor IIa; FXa, factor Xa; FVIIa, factor VIIa; FVIIIa, factor VIIIa; FVa; factor Va; TF, tissue factor; tPA, tissue plasminogen activator.

involving more than 7,000 patients, there was a greater than 50% risk reduction for VTE using fondaparinux begun 6 hours after surgery compared to LMWH begun 12 to 24 hours after surgery.[45] Critical bleeding was not different, although major bleeding was increased. Fondaparinux has also been effective in prophylaxis of general medical patients, abdominal surgery patients, and for extended prophylaxis after hip fracture.[46–48] For DVT treatment, fondaparinux was found equal to LMWH whereas for PE, it was found equal to standard heparin.[49,50] Dosage is based on body weight—5 mg per body weight less than 50 kg; 7.5 mg per body weight 50 to 100 kg; and 10 mg per body weight greater than 100 kg. Treatment for at least 5 days with concurrent administration of oral anticoagulation is recommended, until the INR is therapeutic at a level of 2 to 3. Fondaparinux has been approved for the treatment of DVT/PE and for thrombosis prophylaxis in total hip, total knee, and hip fracture patients; in the extended prophylaxis of hip fracture patients; and in abdominal surgery patients. Idraparinux with the longer half-life in an open label, noninferiority trial of 2,904 DVT patients and 2,215 PE patients was found to meet the noninferiority requirement of DVT, but not of PE.[51] This may have been due to a dose problem. Additionally, in a study of long-term treatment, major bleeding was found with three intracranial bleeding episodes noted.[51] Thus, idraparinux development has been halted. However, biotinylated idraparinux is being tested; this drug, called SSR 126517, can be reversed with avidin. Phase III trials are currently underway with this drug.[52]

New oral anti–factor Xa agents are being developed. Rivaroxaban and apixaban are the two agents furthest along in development. Rivaroxaban has 66% renal excretion, whereas apixaban has only 25% renal excretion.[44,53] Other antithrombotic agents being evaluated include oral heparins, other direct thrombin inhibitors, such as lepirudin, bivalirudin, and argatroban; defibrinating agents such as ancrod; anti-inflammatory agents, such as P-selectin inhibitors; factor VIIa inhibitors; tissue factor pathway inhibitor; and activated protein C.[54,55] Lepirudin and argatroban have been approved for patients with HIT. The use of P-selectin inhibitors, an area of ongoing research, uses an anti-inflammatory approach to limit thrombus amplification without causing anticoagulation.

NONPHARMACOLOGIC TREATMENTS

Pain and swelling after an above the knee DVT can be decreased by approximately 50% by the use of strong compression stockings.[56] Additionally, walking with good compression does not increase the risk of PE, while significantly decreasing the incidence and severity of pain and swelling after DVT.[57,58] Once patients are on therapeutic anticoagulants, they should ambulate while wearing compression stockings. The use of strong compression and early ambulation after DVT treatment can significantly reduce the pain and swelling resulting from the DVT and carries a 1 A level of evidence.[26,56,57]

IVC Filters

The traditional indications for the use of IVC filters include a complication of anticoagulation, a contraindication to anticoagulation, and failure of anticoagulation. Protection from PE has been greater than 95% using cone-shaped wire-based permanent IVC filters.[59] The success achieved with filters has expanded the indications including free-floating thrombus longer than 5 cm, when bleeding risk with anticoagulation is excessive, when the risk of PE is felt to be very high, and to allow for the use of perioperative epidural anesthesia.[60–62] Filters can be permanent or optional (retrievable). If a retrievable filter is left in to become a permanent filter, the long-term fate of that filter has not yet been defined.

Filters are usually placed in an infrarenal location. However, they may also be placed in the suprarenal location or in the superior vena cava. Indications for suprarenal placement include high-lying clot, pregnancy, women of childbearing potential, or a previous device that has failed or become filled with clot. Sepsis is not a contraindication to the use of wire-based filters since the trapped material can be sterilized with antibiotics. Although filters have been placed under x-ray guidance, percutaneous techniques for filter insertion using bedside external ultrasound or intravascular ultrasound are now being recommended. Transabdominal external ultrasound is difficult in the setting of morbid obesity, overlying bowel gas, or open abdominal wounds. In these instances, intravascular ultrasound has been found to be more successful.[63] Other than one randomized prospective study on the use of filters as treatment of DVT (which is not how filters are traditionally used), evidence for the use of filters is given a 2 C level of evidence.[26,64]

Thrombolytic and Surgical Procedures for Deep VTE

The incidence of chronic venous insufficiency after appropriate anticoagulant treatment for DVT has been reported to be as high as 23% after 2 years, 28% after 5 years, and 29% after 8 years.[19] Thus the use of thrombolytic agents more rapidly to clear venous thrombosis has been suggested (Algorithm 102.1). By duplex ultrasound, spontaneous lysis time is 2.3- to 7.3-fold longer in segments with reflux than in segments without reflux.[65] Systemic thrombosis in two small series revealed a decrease in the incidence of chronic venous insufficiency with streptokinase, as opposed to systemic UFH. However, results depend on complete thrombolysis. Because of this inability to predict complete lysis, combined with its bleeding potential, thrombolysis is recommended infrequently. However, urokinase administered directly into venous thrombi has led to an increase in enthusiasm and the publication of a national thrombolysis registry.[66,67] In 473 patients, 287 of whom underwent follow-up, 312 urokinase infusions in 303 limbs were reported. Venous thrombi occurred in the iliofemoral segment in 71% of cases alone, without IVC involvement in 79%, and including the IVC in 21% of cases. Patients had acute disease in approximately two thirds of cases, 16% had chronic disease, and 19% had combined acute and chronic disease. Approximately 30% had prior DVT. Complete thrombolysis was achieved in 31% and partial lysis in 52% of cases. The mean amount of urokinase used was 7.8 million units, and the mean time of infusion was 53.4 hours. Successful lysis was predicated by acute DVT and no history of prior DVT. Complications included major bleeding necessitating blood products in 11% and minor bleeding in 16%. The mortality rate was 0.4%, the intracranial hemorrhage rate was 0.2%, and the subdural hemorrhage rate was 0.2%. Total lysis was noted in only 31% of the entire series; however, in patients with acute iliofemoral DVT, no previous symptoms, and the use of the popliteal vein access site, total lysis was more frequent. At 12 months, patency was 79% if lysis was complete, 58% with greater than 50% lysis, and 32% with less than 50% lysis. Absence of valvular reflux was found in 72% of cases with complete lysis, whereas overall valvular reflux was seen in 58% of cases.

It is important that aggressive therapies have been found to improve quality of life. A small randomized study demonstrated that thrombolysis is superior to anticoagulation in patients with iliofemoral DVT.[68] The use of lytic agents for DVT is now given a 2 B level of evidence.[26]

Thrombolytic therapy for PE remains controversial. Although agents lysed thrombus effectively, recurrence rates and patient mortality were not improved. However, the original studies were not powered to address this outcome. Results are best if patients are young, the embolus is less than 48 hours old, and the embolus is large. Streptokinase, urokinase, and tissue plasminogen activator have all been used.[69] All agents rapidly dissolve clot, but by 7 days, the advantages for all three agents decrease. The benefit of thrombolytic agents for PE thus appears to be greatest in patients who would die as a result of massive PE in the first hour after the PE occurs, which can occur in up to 10% of cases. However, more recent data suggest that thrombolysis may be useful in patients with right ventricular dysfunction without hemodynamic instability, and it has been suggested that thrombolysis will improve outcomes if patients have evidence of right heart changes.[70–75] Additionally, thrombolysis therapy has been recommended in patients without pulmonary hypertension who are judged to have a low risk of bleeding.[26]

Venous Thrombectomy. Iliofemoral venous thrombectomy has been advocated to prevent impending venous gangrene. This technique results in mechanical clearing of the venous circulation and may be combined with a temporary arteriovenous fistula. Thrombectomy uses a Fogarty balloon catheter passed from the femoral vein during Valsalva maneuvers. An arteriovenous fistula is constructed so that it can be taken down by nonsurgical techniques. Complete venography in the operating room is recommended, as back-bleeding is unreliable for the assessment of complete thrombus clearance. Thrombosis recurrence rates less than 20% have been reported. The incidence of PE during the first week after thrombectomy is equivalent to the incidence with anticoagulation only. The frequency of clinical success has been reported to be between 42% and 93%.[76] The largest series of 77 legs with a follow-up period of between 5 and 13 years revealed maintenance of patency but a steady decline in valvular competence over time.[77]

In the only comparative study of iliofemoral venous thrombosis treatment comparing thrombectomy with anticoagulation (31 patients) versus anticoagulation alone (32 patients), iliofemoral vein patency was improved (76% vs. 35%), femoropopliteal patency was improved (52% vs. 26%), and the clinical outcome was better at 6 months (40% asymptomatic vs. 7%).[77] At 10 years, the number of patients available for follow-up had decreased to 13 in the thrombectomy group and 17 in the anticoagulation-alone group. Patency remained improved in the thrombectomy group (83% vs. 41%), and absence of popliteal reflux was found in 78% of the thrombectomy-plus-anticoagulation group compared to 43% of the anticoagulation-alone group.

Pulmonary Embolectomy. Surgical approaches for PE are indicated for patients with massive PE with hypotension who require large doses of vasopressors. These are often patients in whom thrombolytic agents have been unsuccessful. Open pulmonary embolectomy is associated with high rates of morbidity and mortality. Today, open pulmonary embolectomy is limited to those who require manual cardiac massage for hypotension or those in whom catheter pulmonary embolectomy fails. However, there may be a more expanded role for pulmonary embolectomy in the future.[78]

Superficial Thrombophlebitis

Superficial vein thrombophlebitis (SVT) is a well-recognized clinical entity characterized by a painful erythematous and palpable cordlike structure, usually compromising the lower extremities but capable of affecting any superficial vein in the body. Thrombophlebitis is believed to have a multifactorial etiology, in which the Virchow triad of altered blood flow, changes in the vessel wall, and abnormal coagulation are recognized to play a significant role. SVT has been considered a benign disease requiring only conservative management with compression, nonsteroidal anti-inflammatory medications, and lower extremity elevation. Recently SVT, especially above the knee superficial thrombophlebitis, has been reported to coexist with DVT, to propagate to popliteal or femoral level, and even to cause PE.[79–83] A medical approach using anticoagulant therapy appears as the treatment of choice when there is above knee SVT with deep venous system involvement.

The incidence of SVT occurs in approximately 125,000 people in the United States per year.[84] However, the actual incidence is likely far greater as these statistics may be outdated and many cases go unreported. Approximately 54% to 65% of the reported cases affect females with an average age of 58 years old.[79,85] The most frequent predisposing risk factor for SVT is varicose veins, occurring in 62% of patients. Other risk factors include the following: immobilization, trauma, postoperative states, age older than 60 years, obesity, tobacco use, history of DVT or SVT, pregnancy, puerperium, autoimmune disease, use of oral contraceptives or hormonal replacement therapy, and hypercoagulable state.[79,85,86] Hypercoagulable screening should be considered in patients with ascending or worsening thrombophlebitis despite initial treatment.[87,88] Malignancy has been reported as a risk factor for developing SVT, affecting 13% to 18% of patients.[82,89]

The overall recurrence of SVT was described as 18% over 15 months, equally frequent in varicose and nonvaricose phlebitis. Deep venous reflux increases the recurrence rate to 33%, whereas hypercoagulable states increase the recurrence rate to 42% over the same period of time.[90]

The clinical symptoms and signs for SVT are overt. Duplex ultrasound imaging of the affected extremity should be performed to rule out extension of the process into the deep venous system or concomitant DVT.[87,91] Duplex ultrasound shows the extent of the SVT, its relation to the veins connecting with the deep vein system, and the presence of concomitant DVT. Additionally, duplex ultrasound allows checking the competence of the valves in the superficial and deep veins.[91]

Complete thrombophilia workup is not routinely recommended. However, it may be indicated in selected patients with recurrent primary thrombophlebitis or aggressive thrombophlebitis.[91] Screening for underlying diseases, including malignancy or vasculitis, is performed if signs or symptoms suggest the presence of such problem.[91]

Treatment. Several therapeutic approaches have been proposed for patients with SVT. These include ligation or vein stripping of the affecting vein, elastic stockings, nonsteroidal anti-inflammatory drugs to reduce pain and inflammation, and variable doses of unfractionated heparin or LMWH followed by oral anticoagulant therapy. There is no consensus on the optimal treatment of SVT in clinical practice.

It seems clear that the course of treatment for SVT should be tailored accordingly to its location, concomitant DVT and if there is any associated infectious process. Thrombus locations in trunks of either the great or small saphenous vein may have the highest risk of extension into the deep vein system and thus require more aggressive treatment than other locations. The treatment for primary SVT localized in the distal great saphenous vein and tributary veins consists of ambulation, warm soaks, compression, and nonsteroidal anti-inflammatory (NSAID) agents.[92,93] If the patient presents risk factors for DVT, pharmacologic prophylaxis should be considered seriously.[91]

Titon et al.[94] were among the first to compare different approaches in the medical treatment of SVT. In a multicenter study, 117 patients were randomized into three groups: fixed dose LMWH calcium nadroparin (n = 38), adjusted-dose LMWH calcium nadroparin (n = 39), and the NSAID naproxen (n = 40) for 6 days. At day 7, heat and redness were significantly less ($p < 0.001$) in both groups treated with LMWH compared to those given the NSAID. Additionally at 8 weeks, persistence of symptoms and signs was less frequent in the LMWH treated groups ($p = 0.007$). Efficacy did not differ between the fixed and weight-adjusted dose of LMWH.

The management of SVT was further addressed in a randomized double-blind study describing 427 patients with documented acute symptomatic SVT of the legs.[95] Patients were randomly assigned to receive 40 mg enoxaparin sodium subcutaneously; 1.5 mg/kg enoxaparin sodium subcutaneously; oral tenoxicam 20 mg; or placebo, all once daily for 8 to 12 days. LMWH was associated with a lower incidence of SVT extension and/or recurrence, compared with placebo (OR 0.32; 95% confidence interval [CI], 0.16–0.65, and OR 0.33; 95% CI, 0.16–0.68, respectively), without major bleeding or HIT. There was no statistical difference with respect to 12-day outcomes between the active treatment groups. However, there was a trend in favor of LMWH.

The Vesalio Investigator Group compared two regimens of LMWH with each other.[96] A total of 164 patients were enrolled and randomized into two groups: prophylaxis group ($n = 81$) and treatment group ($n = 83$). After completion of 3 months, the cumulative rate of SVT progression and venous thromboembolism complications did not differ between the prophylactic (8.6%; 95% CI, 3.5–17.0) and therapeutic (7.2%; 95% CI, 2.8–15.1) groups. No patient in either group developed major bleeding, although one patient in each group developed clinically asymptomatic HIT. Clinical symptoms improved to a similar extent in both groups, and similar rates of minor extension or recurrent thrombophlebitis were observed during the follow-up period.

Prophylactic-dose intravenous (IV) UFH was compared in two studies.[97] Relative to elastic stocking alone, prophylactic IV UFH plus elastic stockings was associated with an 86% reduction in SVT extension and/or recurrence (OR 0.14; 95% CI, 0.03–0.67). Marchiori et al.[98] compared high- versus low-dose IV UFH. A nonsignificant 86% reduction in VTE (OR 0.14; 95% CI 0.02–1.23) and a 37% (OR 0.63; 95% CI, 0.21–1.88) lower rate of SVT extension and/or recurrence were observed in those patients treated with high-dose UFH. There were no episodes of major bleeding or HIT.

Low-molecular-weight heparin was compared with saphenofemoral disconnection for the treatment of proximal great saphenous vein thrombophlebitis in a prospective, randomized clinical study.[99] In this study, 84 consecutive patients diagnosed as presenting SVT alone, were divided into two groups treated with either saphenofemoral disconnection under local anesthesia with a short hospital stay ($n = 45$) or enoxaparin on an outpatient basis for 4 weeks ($n = 39$). In all, 30 patients per group completed the study requirements. In the surgical group, two patients (6.7%) presented complications of the surgical wound, one (3.3%) had SVT recurrence, and two (6.7%) had nonfatal pulmonary embolism. In the enoxaparin group, there was no progression of the thrombosis to the deep venous system or PE; there were two cases (6.7%) of minor bleeding and three (10%) recurrences of SVT. Even when the study found no statistically significant difference between the two groups in the treatment of SVT, the LMWH group demonstrated a significant socioeconomic advantage and confirmed the efficacy of LMWH treatment in resolving symptoms and signs and preventing DVT and PE.

Prophylactic-dose LMWH has the advantage over other equally efficacious techniques in resolving symptoms and signs and preventing DVT and PE in cases without concomitant DVT. Patients treated with LMWH do not require hospitalization, present less adverse effects, do not require laboratory monitoring in most situations, have a low risk of bleeding, and treatment is less expensive if hospitalization is not required. It is generally felt that medical management with anticoagulants versus surgical treatment is somewhat superior for minimizing complications and preventing subsequent DVT and PE development. On the other hand, surgical treatment with ligation at the saphenofemoral junction combined with stripping (with or without perforator interruption) appears to minimize superficial venous thrombus extension, which ultimately provides improved pain relief.[100]

Septic thrombophlebitis requires treatment with broad-spectrum intravenous antibiotics. If rapid resolution of the cellulitis occurs, no treatment beyond a short course of antibiotics and standard treatment for the superficial thrombophlebitis are required. However, if the patient becomes septic, excision of the infected vein is required. With positive blood cultures, an extended course of antibiotics specific for the identified organism is indicated additionally.

Most episodes of uncomplicated superficial thrombophlebitis respond to conservative management. However, the recurrence rate for superficial thrombophlebitis has been estimated as between 15% and 20%.[101–103]

CHRONIC VENOUS DISEASE

Normal Venous Anatomy

The lower extremity venous system is composed of deep, perforating, and superficial veins (Fig. 102.1).[104] The common femoral, femoral, deep (profunda) femoral veins in addition to the popliteal and tibial/peroneal veins make up the deep system. There is a concerted effort to replace the once named "superficial" femoral vein with simply "femoral vein" to alleviate the confusion the term "superficial" implies when treating what is actually a deep vein. The deep veins lie beneath the investing fascia of the muscles of the leg and thigh (the deep compartment). The saphenous veins have similarly undergone a change in name to the great saphenous (GSV) and small saphenous vein (SSV) to standardize the abbreviations that are otherwise extremely confusing. It has also become clear that the GSV and SSV lie within the superficial compartment and also within a saphenous compartment. The saphenous nerve lies within the GSV compartment, which places the nerve at risk of injury during surgery, but if the associated sensory loss occurs, it appears to have little impact on the patient's quality of life.[105] The sural nerve lies in close proximity to the SSV within its compartment. The superficial veins outside the saphenous compartment are called accessory saphenous veins and lie parallel to the GSV or SSV. The term *communicating*

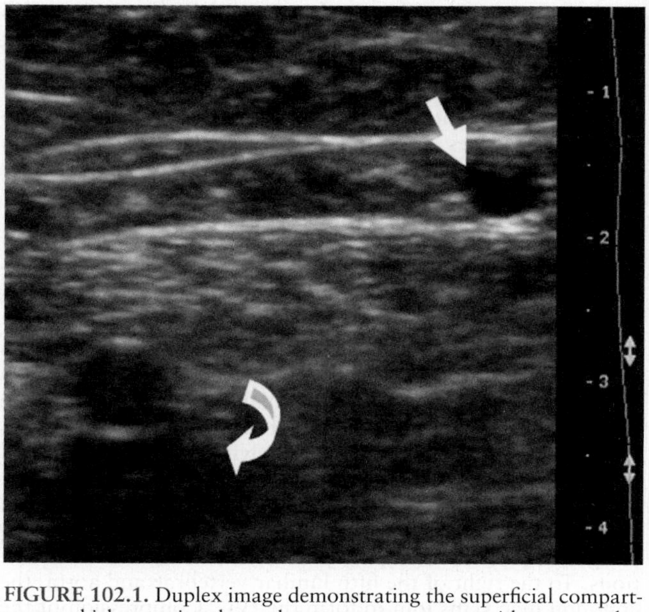

FIGURE 102.1. Duplex image demonstrating the superficial compartment, which contains the saphenous compartment with great saphenous vein (GSV) (*straight arrow*) lying within and the deep compartment with femoral vessels (*curved arrow*) lying within.

vein is now reserved for those veins that interconnect with other veins of the same system, and the term *perforating vein* is reserved for those that penetrate the muscular fascia to connect superficial to deep.[104] In the past, perforating veins with rather constant anatomic location have been named for their discoverer (e.g., Crockett, Boyd perforators), but more descriptive terms designating location are now preferred.[104]

The variability of the lower extremity venous system is well known, but only certain anatomic variations are of importance for current surgical practice. The popliteal and femoral veins have variable anatomy and are often duplicated much like the tibial veins. The deep femoral vein often connects directly or though tributaries to the popliteal vein. Although duplication of the GSV has been estimated to be present in up to 50% of patients in some studies, it is becoming evident that duplications of the true GSV lying within the saphenous compartment may be less common.[106,107] The saphenofemoral junction often has at least four branches in addition to the GSV, but the arrangement and precise location of the branches is quite variable. The most cephalic branch is generally the superficial epigastric vein and is of some importance in new techniques for managing GSV reflux. The SSV is rarely duplicated (4%).[108] Although the SSV appears to pierce the deep fascia in the upper third of the calf, in reality the membranous layer forming the roof of the SSV compartment is thickened, while the muscular fascia disappears, which positions the SSV between the gastrocnemius muscle bellies.[108] In only 62% of limbs does the SSV actually end in the popliteal fossa.[108] The anatomy of the perforating veins becomes extremely important when considering surgery aimed at preventing reflux in the lower leg. Certainly, removing the GSV may not prevent the impact of perforator reflux if one ignores the fact that the posterior tibial vein perforators connect the posterior accessory GSV with the posterior tibial veins, rather than forming a direct connection with the GSV proper. Similarly, not recognizing the presence of paratibial perforators can result in an unsuccessful operation aimed at preventing calf perforator reflux.[109]

With the exception of foot veins, the valves promote blood flow from superficial to deep and from caudal to cephalad in direction. The valves are made of a fine connective tissue skeleton covered by endothelium and are generally bicuspid, delicate, and extremely strong. The tibial and peroneal veins contain about 7 to 19 valves each. The popliteal vein contains one or two valves, and the femoral vein generally has three. About 70% of common femoral veins have a valve located within 1 cm of the inguinal ligament. Twenty-five percent of external iliac and 10% of the internal iliac veins have a valve.[110] The common iliac vein generally has no valves. Within like lengths of the superficial venous system when compared to the deep veins, fewer valves are found (approximately seven to nine in the GSV and SSV). Perforating veins and even larger venules have venous valves.[110]

Variable numbers of venous lakes (1 to 18 sinuses) are found in the soleus muscle. These sinuses are valveless, floppy channels linked to small-valved venous channels that prevent reflux to the superficial system. The sinuses empty into the posterior tibial vein in the proximal calf. Within the gastrocnemius muscle, there are interlacing valved venous networks that coalesce to form a pair of venous channels that empty into the popliteal vein. These intramuscular venous chambers store venous blood and are crucial to calf muscle pump function.

The veins of the abdomen and pelvis begin at the inguinal ligament as the external iliac vein, which is joined medially by the internal iliac to form the common iliac vein. The internal iliac veins drain the pelvis via connections, such as the obturator, gluteal, and internal pudendal veins and their interconnections. To the right of the fifth lumbar vertebrae and aorta, the common iliac veins join to form the IVC. Compression of the left iliac vein by the right common iliac artery can lead to a venous obstructive condition, the May-Thurner syndrome. The IVC typically ascends to the right of the aorta and vertebral column terminating in the right atrium. Its direct tributaries are the lumbar veins, the right gonadal vein, the renal veins, the right suprarenal vein, the right inferior phrenic vein, and the hepatic veins. Other named veins generally join one of these tributaries to empty into the IVC. Because of the embryonic evolutions that lead to the "normal" IVC and its branches, variations are common. Duplication of the IVC occurs in 0.2% to 0.3% of cases, transposition or a left-sided IVC can occur in 0.2% to 0.5% of cases, and a retroaortic left renal (1.2%–2.4%) and circumaortic left renal vein (1.5%–8.7%) have also been reported.[111] In the face of IVC occlusion, veins of the chest and abdominal wall, the azygos and hemiazygos systems, and vertebral plexuses may play a prominent role in venous decompression.

Normal Venous Physiology

Under conditions of low volume or external pressure, many veins lying within muscle are demonstrated by duplex scanning to collapse in an elliptical configuration consistent with a thin vein wall and the lack of in situ external support.[112] With muscular relaxation, veins within these compartments change from an elliptical to a circular configuration to accept venous blood being emptied from the superficial system and delivered to the lower extremity by arterial inflow. Compliance is very high; in fact, increasing the venous volume by over two and one half times results in only a 0- to 15-mm Hg increment rise in pressure.[113] This allows a significant amount of blood (at least 500 mL in the standing position) to become sequestered in the lower limb without a significant buildup of intraluminal pressure. However, once a vein reaches its full circular shape, further increases in venous volume result in a proportional increase in intraluminal pressure. The capacitance of the venous system has been met, and sustained venous hypertension results in decompensation noted as edema. Normally, modest exercise of the muscles will expel the blood volume and reset the capacitance of the venous system.

In contrast to intramuscular veins, duplex scanning demonstrates that large axial veins (e.g., femoral, popliteal) collapse in a circular manner. Supported/tethered on all sides by connective tissue, these veins are subject to equal external pressures along the vein wall and expand or collapse in a direct response to changes in volume.[114] Their compliance mimics that of an artery in that pressure changes are more reflective of volume changes. They are conduit rather than compliance vessels.

The calf muscle and possibly the thigh muscles act as a pump, the "peripheral heart," which can generate pressures of up to 300 mm Hg during exercise.[110] Muscle contraction propels the blood toward the heart and lungs via the cephalad conduit veins. The valves in the proximal superficial and deep veins open to allow blood to move forward. The perforating vein valves close to prevent venous blood reflux from deep to superficial veins, thereby preventing high pressures generated in the deep system from affecting superficial structures (i.e., skin, soft tissues). In addition, blood moves centrally during exercise by compression of the superficial veins between the deep fascia and skin, but the pressure generated is only 100 to 150 mm Hg.[110] As the calf muscle relaxes, the flow/pressure gradient falls and proximal vein valve closure prevents reflux. Arterial blood then slowly fills the venous system; valves in the foot veins and perforating veins open to allow the deep veins to fill from the superficial system replenishing the calf muscle pump venous sinuses.

The vein valve functions in a four-phase cycle: opening, equilibrium, closing, and closed phase. During equilibrium, flow separation occurs at the valve edge, the flow splits into two streams with one of the streams directed into the valve sinus possibly aiding in a self-cleaning step (preventing stasis). When maximally open, the two cusps create about a 35% narrowing of the outflow lumen, which may aid in outflow.[115] It is interesting that most of the cycle has the valve in the open position. Valve closure normally occurs within 0.5 to 1.0 second in response to retrograde blood flow and the loss of a pressure/flow gradient.[116,117] Closure time is somewhat dependent on the stimulus to closure, and a flow velocity of at least 30 cm per second is required.[118]

An intravenous catheter placed into a foot vein can measure changes in venous pressure over time and with movement. These measurements reflect normal venous hemodynamics in the distal superficial venous system.[110] When lying flat, a person's normal lower extremity intravenous pressure is about 15 mm Hg, but with standing the pressure rises to reflect the hydrostatic pressure of a column of blood from the heart to the foot catheter most reflective of the patient's height (generally ±90 mm Hg). A hemodynamic study of venous function involves pressure measurements obtained during controlled exercise. The venous filling time (VFT) is the time required to arrive at a steady-state pressure after standing. Ten steps (one per second) causes a drop in pressure, and the lowest pressure, called the ambulatory venous pressure (AVP), is generally less than 45 mm Hg. The venous refilling time (VRT) is the time required, following exercise, to reach the baseline erect pressure. It is normally greater than 20 seconds. This rather simplistic measurement reflects a complex interaction of the venous conduits, the property of the veins, and the action of the peripheral pump.[119] If one measures the venous pressure in deeper veins and in more central locations, the measurements would be considerably different, but such measurements are not commonly obtained in clinical practice.

Prevalence and Impact

Chronic venous disease (CVD) is a common, costly malady in Western countries. If one considers the entire spectrum of the disease, it affects more than 30 million Americans (more than half women).[120,121] Varicose veins are observed in 15% to 25% of the adult population.[122,123] Chronic venous insufficiency (CVI) is defined as venous pathology that results in advanced clinical symptoms (edema to venous ulceration). Skin changes suggestive of venous disease are noted in 6 to 7 million U.S. citizens, and venous ulcers occur in up to 2% of those with CVI (approximately 500,000 patients).[120,124] Population studies confirm these earlier clinical observations.[125] The most recent population-based study supported by duplex imaging and using a modified CEAP classification (see later) demonstrated that 5.8% of those studied presented with edema, whereas 6.2% had skin changes and/or prior or active venous ulcers.[123] Furthermore, the annual cost to treat venous ulcers is estimated at greater than $1 billion.[126] It is interesting that similar findings are noted throughout Europe.[127–131] Relevant risk factors for varicose veins are advanced age, a positive family history, female gender, multiparity, and obesity based on epidemiologic studies.[120,123,127,128,130–132] Risk factors for CVI are advanced age, positive family history, and obesity.[123,127,131]

Pathophysiology and Etiology

Three pathophysiologic states exist: obstruction, valvular insufficiency, and calf muscle pump malfunction. These conditions reflect a failure of one or more of the components of the normal venous system and are not mutually exclusive.

Venous obstruction causes an increased resistance to blood exiting the lower extremity. It was once thought that venous obstruction was rarely the major underlying hemodynamic problem in patients with CVD. However, there are currently data to suggest that venous occlusive disease in combination with venous insufficiency is found in 55% of patients with CVI, especially those with the most severe symptoms.[133] Certainly, evidence exists that past estimates of venous occlusive disease in the pathophysiology of CVI were underestimates of its importance and prevalence.[133–135] The result is elevated intravenous pressure noted clinically as pain especially after exercise.[133] If the deep system is primarily involved, the increased pressure generated with each calf compression may impact the perforating veins resulting in valvular malfunction and leading to venous hypertension in the superficial system and its capillary network. Asymptomatic primary iliac venous compression is quite common with intraluminal (27 ± 5%) and varying degrees of external compression (66%–88%) observed in the general population.[136–141] Left common iliac vein compression by the right common iliac artery, as well as external iliac vein compression from the internal iliac artery on either side, have been described.[140,142] It has been suggested that the nonthrombotic iliac occlusive lesion is a "permissive lesion" not clinically significant until other components of the lower extremity venous circulation fail, often presenting as valvular insufficiency.[143] The good results of iliac vein stenting in patients with CVI even in the presence of untreated reflux might be explained by eliminating this permissive lesion. In one of the largest experiences treating ileofemoral venous occlusive disease involving nearly 1,000 patients, compression of the common iliac vein was seen in 36%, external iliac vein in 18%, and both sites in 46% of limbs.[143] Of these patients, 53% of limbs had nonthrombotic compressive lesions (absent history of DVT, no venographic or ultrasound findings indicating previous DVT); 40% had postthrombotic obstruction; and 7% had a combined etiology. Furthermore, 20% of the patients were men, and 25% of the symptomatic lower limbs were on the right side. Intraluminal webs from repetitive trauma have been reported in 14% to 30% of symptomatic cases of the May-Thurner syndrome.[142] Extrinsic compression of the iliac and pelvic veins may also be caused by tumor, fibrosis, or infection. Contents of a femoral hernia can crush the femoral vein, as can soft tissue tumors of the thigh. Arterial aneurysms can impinge on the femoral vein. The popliteal vein can be obstructed by a popliteal aneurysm or Baker cyst.[144] Aplasia of the vein or tumors of the vein wall have been described.[144,145] Deep venous thrombosis is associated with inflammation and thrombus resolution resulting in external vein wall scarring with stiffening and thickening, as well as intraluminal recannulation with webs and bands. The venous valves are generally incorporated in the scarring process, leading to even more occlusive debris within the lumen. It is a common cause of venous occlusive disease due to its overall prevalence and association with chronic venous disease and clearly can involve any part of the venous system.

Valvular insufficiency may occur in any part of the lower extremity venous systems. It accounts for 85% of symptomatic CVD cases with a 70% incidence of primarily superficial and 30% primarily deep venous insufficiency (DVI) as determined by clinical experiences.[134,135] Duplex imaging studies suggest that patients with minimal disease (varicose veins or less) have superficial reflux while those with edema, skin changes, and past or present ulcers have increasing presence of perforator and deep disease. In those with more advanced venous disease, reflux alone is observed in 80%, reflux and obstruction in 17%, and only 29% had obstructive disease alone.[146,147] The presence of obstructive and reflux disease had the worse prognosis for the development of skin changes.[148] No matter the clinical stage, the superficial system is most commonly affected (90%) with GSV involvement in 70% to 80%, SSV in 15% to 20%, and nonsaphenous veins in approximately 10%. The deep veins are involved in about 30% and perforator veins in about 20%.[146,147] Those with the most severe sequelae of venous disease have superficial reflux in 74% to 93% with 17% to 54% having only superficial disease.[149–153] Fifty percent of patients have superficial with or without perforator disease, and less than 10% have isolated deep venous reflux.[152–155] In those patients with venous ulcers, two vein systems were involved in 50% to 70% of patients, and all three systems were involved in 16% to 50% of patients. Since these duplex imaging studies mainly involve imaging of the lower extremity veins, the influence of proximal venous occlusive disease may well be underestimated. Reflux allows the transmission of high venous pressures to the lower leg, while standing, that cannot be relieved by exercise. Primary valvular insufficiency may rarely be a consequence of congenital absence of valves.[156] More commonly, venous valve prolapse (elongated, floppy valves) or defects in the vein wall that cause the valve ring to dilate can result in malfunctioning valve cusps with retained valve architecture.[157,158] The muscle cell dilating effect of estrogens may explain the genesis of varicose veins noted in the first trimester. Prolonged exposure to high venous pressures can cause vein dilation as occurs from an arteriovenous fistula or occupations requiring prolonged periods of standing. Roughly 50% of deep vein valvular dysfunction occurs secondary to DVT, whereas the remainder appears to be of a primary etiology with a 10% to 20% variance depending on the clinical experience being reported.[134,159–161] Inflammation and thrombosis associated with DVT tends to cause valve scarring, whether or not recanalization is complete, leaving damaged valve architecture in contradistinction to primary valvular insufficiency. This classic differentiation between primary and secondary (or postthrombotic) pathology does not clearly exist when subjected to direct observation of the veins and valves at surgery. In fact, the two conditions can be present in the same patient as noted some 20 years ago.[162] In these cases, the vein wall is thickened/fibrotic at the valve station or there is thickening of the valve cusps and/or intima. Pathologic study of eleven such veins demonstrated clear postthrombotic changes in six, but phlebosclerosis of a nonthrombotic origin in the remaining five.[163] Clearly, preservation of a rather normal valve architecture can be explained if primary reflux and sustained high pressure on the wall is the cause of the changes noted. Another theory is that rapid resolution of acute thrombi, an event known to occur, may have allowed these valves to escape damage or the valve itself may not have been directly involved in the thrombotic process.[164] The fibrotic process involves only the vein wall, and the valve cusps become floppy by virtue of a decrease in wall diameter resulting from a thickened, noncompliant vein wall.[163] The valve remains architecturally intact and can be repaired surgically, a situation once thought impossible in the postthrombosis patient.

There can be failure of calf muscle pump function. The pump becomes unable to generate the force needed to eject blood from the leg while standing, resulting in sustained venous hypertension. Patients with muscle disuse (e.g., paraplegia, traumatic injury, elderly or bedridden patients) may not have sufficient muscle for effective exercise. Pathologic conditions that result in muscle fibrosis (e.g., muscular dystrophy, multiple sclerosis) can destroy the calf muscle pump. Thrombus and scarring in the gastrocnemius and soleal veins can prevent blood from entering the pump resulting in a deficient ejection volume with contraction. Calf pump function and ankle range of motion are progressively diminished with increasing severity of CVI.[165–168] Physical conditioning to improve calf pump function as a therapeutic maneuver has been studied in a small, randomized controlled trial and demonstrated improvement in both pump function and muscle strength.[169] With the exception of muscle rehabilitation, very little can be offered patients with some of these disorders.

Regardless of the etiology, the sequelae of venous hypertension/stasis are changes observed in the lower leg skin and subcutaneous tissues. Originally, ischemia from various causes was considered the etiology of the damage noted in the skin and soft tissue of the lower leg, especially ulceration.[170] More recent observations suggest that far from being simply an ischemic event, the end-organ response to venous hypertension is highly dynamic. The final answer is likely to involve a complex interaction of multiple factors that favor either continued destruction or the ultimate healing of the ulcer. Leukocytes, extracellular matrix, fibroblasts, and a host of other factors are recruited to heal the early endothelial injury and the more delayed soft tissue injury.[170] The soft tissue injury may result in a chronic ulcer that requires growth factors to force the process to healing.[171] Research remains active in this component of venous pathophysiology.

Clinical Signs and Symptoms

Venous disease presents in many ways. A telangiectasia, spider vein, is a confluence of dilated intradermal venules less than 1 mm in caliber. A reticular vein is a dilated bluish subdermal vein, usually 1 mm to less than 3 mm in diameter and usually tortuous. These venous abnormalities may or may not be accompanied by a larger, more deeply located, pathologic vein.

Hereditary varicose veins usually appear during the second decade of life. If a secondary etiology is involved (e.g., thrombosis, trauma), varicosities often present several years after the inciting event. These veins appear alone or in clusters as dilated, often bluish, serpentine, and palpable protrusions of branches of the GSV, SSV, or collateral veins lying beneath the skin within the subcutaneous tissues. Symptoms may be those associated with any type of CVD.

CVD can result in pain, edema, hyperpigmentation, stasis dermatitis or eczema, and/or venous ulcers. These changes often occur in the "gaiter" area just above the medial malleolus. Important perforating veins lie in this area. The observed hyperpigmentation is thought to result from extruded red blood cells that are degraded by macrophages leaving hemosiderin deposits.

Venous claudication is a pain syndrome experienced when walking and is associated with cyanosis, a sensation of increased swelling, and increased prominence of the superficial veins, which is relieved with rest in combination with elevation of the extremity.[133,172,173] It may be so severe in rare cases that amputation is requested.[174] The most severe form is observed when venous incompetence is associated with obstruction and when the obstructive process is in a more proximal locale.[175]

Critical to patient management and treatment evaluation is an accurate classification of the disease at any given time. Each patient should be stratified according to the *c*linical picture, the *e*tiology, the *a*natomic distribution, and the *p*athophysiology (CEAP) classification system.[176] This classification system helps the physician to define the venous disease so that a focused and appropriate management strategy can be formulated. An extension of the clinical classification system is available to quantify the extent of venous disease and, therefore, to evaluate the patient's clinical response to treatment.[177,178] The anatomic and pathophysiologic improvement following a treatment of venous disease can be scored using the Venous Segmental Disease Score,[178] whereas the Venous Disability Score provides some information of what a person can do while afflicted with venous disease.[178] Quality of life (QOL) surveys have been developed specifically for patients with venous disease to help determine the impact of the disease on the patient's life and the effect therapy has on the patient's overall well-being.[179–182] Consistent application of these surveys to the postsurgical outcome of patients has yet to be achieved, but is imperative to improve our ability to precisely determine the effect and benefit of a given intervention.

Diagnostic Evaluation

The diagnosis of CVD begins with a thorough history and physical examination. The history is important to provide hints to familial coagulation disorders or events in the patient's history that may impact the care of the chronic disorder. Use of the CEAP clinical classification (Table 102.3) will provide a snapshot of the patient being examined, whereas use of the more detailed venous clinical severity score (Table 102.4) will allow some impression of how any therapy is performing on the patient's behalf.

TABLE 102.3 CLASSIFICATION

CLINICAL CLASSIFICATION OF CHRONIC VENOUS DISEASE

■ CLASS	■ DESCRIPTION
0	No visible or palpable signs of venous disease
1	Telangiectases and/or reticular veins
2	Varicose veins
3	Edema
4a	Skin changes (pigmentation and/or eczema)
4b	Skin changes (lipodermatosclerosis and/or atrophie blanche)
5	Healed venous ulcer
6	Active venous ulcer
S (in addition to the class)	Symptoms including ache, pain, tightness, skin irritation, heaviness, muscle cramps as well as other complaints attributable to venous dysfunction
A (in addition to the class)	Asymptomatic

Venous duplex ultrasonography provides a B-mode image of the vein as well as spectral analysis of the blood flow within it. It is essential to clarify the etiology (*E* of CEAP; congenital, primary, or secondary), better define the anatomic location (*A* of CEAP; specific veins can be imaged with spectral analysis to determine reflux), and aid in determining the pathophysiology (*P* of CEAP; reflux, obstruction, or both) of the venous problem. Once considered unnecessary in the evaluation of patients with simple varicose veins, it has become common practice prior to intervention for superficial reflux due to anatomic variability, variability in veins affected, and the need for precise targeting of veins during endoluminal intervention.[106,183–185] Venous duplex imaging clearly visualizes deep and perforator veins and valves as well.

Valvular insufficiency is defined as prolonged reflux time through a valve following a provocative test. A reflux time of more than 0.5 second is considered abnormal with a rapidly deflating distal cuff during the provocative test, whereas longer than 1.0 second is considered the cutoff following manual compression.[116,117] A recent study suggests that these values may be appropriate for the deep calf veins, but that 1.0 second should be the cutoff for larger femoropopliteal veins even when using the rapidly deflating distal cuff method.[186] The latter has yet to be confirmed by other investigators. The examination is performed in the upright position in these

TABLE 102.4 DIAGNOSIS

VENOUS CLINICAL SEVERITY SCORE

■ ATTRIBUTE	■ ABSENT 0	■ MILD 1	■ MODERATE 2	■ SEVERE 3
Pain	None	Occasional, not restricting activity or requiring analgesics	Daily, moderate activity limitation, occasional analgesics	Daily, severely limiting activities, regular use of analgesics
Varicose veins[a]	None	Few, scattered: branch VVs with competent GS/SS	Multiple: single-segment GS/SS reflux	Extensive: multisegment GS/SS reflux
Venous edema[b]	None	Evening ankle edema only	Afternoon edema, above ankle	Morning edema above ankle and requiring activity change, elevation
Skin pigmentation[c]	None or focal, low intensity (tan)	Diffuse, but limited in area and old (brown)	Diffuse over gaiter distribution (lower 1/3) *or* recent pigmentation (purple)	Wider distribution (above lower 1/3) *and* recent pigmentation
Inflammation	None	Mild cellulitis, limited to marginal area around ulcer	Moderate cellulitis, involves most of gaiter area	Severe cellulitis (lower 1/3 and above) or venous eczema
Induration	None	Focal, circummalleolar (<5 cm)	Medial or lateral, less than lower third	Entire lower third of leg or more
No. of active ulcers	0	1	2–4	>4
Active ulceration, duration	None	≤3 mo	>3 mo and ≤1 y	Not healed >1 y
Active ulcer, size[d]	None	<2 cm diameter	2–4 cm diameter	>4 cm diameter
Compressive therapy[e]	Not used or not compliant	Intermittent use of stockings	Wears elastic stockings most days	Full compliance: stockings + elevation

GS, greater saphenous; SS, small saphenous; VV, varicose vein.

[a]Varicose veins must be >4 mm diameter to qualify so that differentiation is ensured between C1 and C2 venous pathology. Occasional or mild edema and focal pigmentation over varicose veins does not qualify for C3 or C4.

[b]Presumes venous origin by characteristics (e.g., brawny [not pitting or spongy] edema), with significant effect of standing/limb elevation and/or other clinical evidence of venous etiology (i.e., varicose veins, history of DVT). Edema must be regular finding (e.g., daily occurrence). Occasional or mild edema does not qualify.

[c]Focal pigmentation over varicose veins does not qualify.

[d]Largest dimension/diameter of largest ulcer.

[e]Sliding scale to adjust for background differences in use of compressive therapy.

Reproduced with permission from Rutherford RB, Padberg FT Jr, Comerota AJ, et al. Venous severity scoring: an adjunct to venous outcome assessment. *J Vasc Surg* 2000;31:1307.

reports. Many other provocative maneuvers to generate venous reflux exist (Valsalva, standardized Valsalva, etc.) in addition to performing the test in different positions (e.g., 15% Trendelenburg, sitting).[187] Each may be acceptable if standardized for an individual laboratory and supported by the literature. Venous obstruction is seen as thickened, scarred, and constricted veins with poor flow and diminished augmentation following distal and/or proximal compression. Respiratory variation is lost as a result of local disease or proximal occlusion. Similar imaging and spectral analysis can be performed to determine obstruction or insufficiency in the superficial and perforator veins. Reflux in the superficial system is considered abnormal with parameters similar to the deep calf veins and is determined by provocative compression.[187] Disease within the SSV should not be ignored because it can have a significant clinical impact as an isolated event.[188] Incompetent perforating veins are generally larger in diameter, thereby allowing a larger volume of blood flow during reflux, and are considered to demonstrate reflux with a reflux time longer than 0.5 second.[185] There is some thought that this cutoff should be decreased to 0.35 second, but currently the 0.5-second cutoff remains used in most laboratories.[186] By imaging the entire lower leg venous system, the surgeon is provided a detailed roadmap of all veins with confirmation of obstruction or reflux if present within segments commonly separated by valves. Of course, isolated venous valvular insufficiency or obstruction may have little clinical impact on the patient, and therefore clinicians have attempted to quantify the pathology by adding up segmental disease, determining mean duration of reflux, determining peak reverse flow velocity, and so forth.[117,174] Although average scores correlate with disease severity, individual results have little predictive value, and therefore, these methods have not been widely adapted. The issue of common standards for the performance and interpretation of venous duplex studies still plagues efforts to define venous disease, but many find it the most versatile and reproducible imaging device currently available.[187,189] This is often the only diagnostic evaluation needed for the evaluation of superficial and even perforator disease requiring treatment as a first stage in patient management.

A difficult area of investigation from a noninvasive perspective is the pelvic, abdominal, and chest veins. CT and MRI can provide details of anatomy and the effect of surrounding structures in areas not visualized by duplex evaluation.[190–192] However, as with all vascular laboratory studies, clinical correlation is mandatory because anatomic presence does not necessarily translate into a clinical problem. For example, iliac vein compression is commonly seen in an asymptomatic population.[136–141] These studies can be particularly useful in evaluating for pelvic congestion syndrome.[193]

Plethysmography assesses the overall hemodynamics of the lower extremity venous system. Air plethysmography (APG) can measure several venous hemodynamic parameters and is the study currently most used. A plastic cylinder filled with air is fitted over the calf and foot. Changes in leg volume with positional change or exercise are detected by pressure changes in the cylinder. The venous filling index is 90% of resting standing venous volume (VV) divided by the time it takes to reach 90% of VV as the patient shifts from the supine to standing position (mL/s). A venous filling index of 2 mL/s or less is indicative of a competent venous system, and higher values suggest venous insufficiency.[194,195] The use of tourniquets to separate superficial from deep or perforator disease has not been reliable, but it can be useful in specific cases.[196] After an erect baseline reading, patients exercise by dorsiflexion or heel raises to empty the calf veins. The ejection fraction is the amount of blood propelled cephalad with a single muscle contraction divided by VV. After a series of 10 ankle flexions, the volume remaining in the leg is referred to as the residual volume and when divided by the VV is called the residual volume fraction. An ejection fraction of greater than 60% and residual volume fraction of less than 35% suggests that the calf pump is working well.[167,197] The residual volume fraction is relatively equivalent to the AVP.[126,196] Significant outflow obstruction is determined by occluding venous outflow until a stable plateau is reached. The thigh cuff causing the venous occlusion is rapidly deflated, and the difference between maximal volume and that volume present 1 second later divided by the total calf volume is called the outflow fraction (OF). Normally, 38% or more of venous blood is expelled from the leg in 1 second.[195] Several other plethysmographic methods (e.g., impedance, photo) and even light reflex rheography have evaluated similar venous parameters. The ability of these techniques to reliably eliminate the presence of significant venous occlusion in patients with CVD is questioned.[178,198] Although these plethysmographic methods can differentiate patients with severe CVI (class 3 or greater) from those without disease, stratification by symptom severity is not possible, and therefore, its use in the treatment of patients with minor symptoms, such as varicose veins or telangiectases, is also questionable.[187] Because these studies do not provide an anatomic image of the venous system or evaluation of individual venous valve function, many physicians combine one of these studies as an estimate of global hemodynamics, in patients with advanced disease (clinical grade 3 or higher), with ultrasonography to complete the venous evaluation.

As in acute venous disease, venography has no significant role in the initial evaluation of patients with CVD. Ascending venography can suggest venous occlusion when duplex imaging clearly demonstrates an open system.[189] Even the presence of significant collaterals on transfemoral venography may underestimate the degree of venous occlusion documented by intravascular ultrasound.[133,199] The use of ascending venography is selectively used in specific cases to complement noninvasive studies when considering intervention in the deep venous system.

The technique of descending venography has been well described.[200] Descending venography is used to determine valve leaflet integrity and anatomic location, and to demonstrate the extent of reflux.[200] Assessment of the competence of the profunda femoris venous system in addition to the femoral system is imperative. If it is a competent system, it may be a source for a valve transposition or may predict success with an isolated proximal femoral vein repair.[201–203] Certainly, descending venography is not infallible in determining the presence or absence of a normal valve.[163] Raju et al. report that descending venography misrepresented the presence of a valve in 11% of cases (a valve considered present was not at operation) and missed an intact valve in 25% of cases (a valve thought absent was actually present).[163] However, when combined with a careful venous duplex examination, it is currently the best method available to determine preoperatively if an in situ reconstruction will be possible.

Intravenous pressure measurements can aid in the diagnosis of venous disease, but is invasive and generally used only when invasive surgery of the deep system is being considered. This study can help to determine the overall magnitude of reflux.[126] AVP has been shown to correlate with the presence of venous ulceration, with each 10-torr increase above 30 torr corresponding to a 10% to 15% increase in the incidence of venous ulceration.[204] Direct lower limb intravenous pressure measurements obtained prior to and after thigh cuff compression and compared to arm intravenous pressure have been suggested as a method to determine the presence or absence of venous obstruction and to determine if obstruction is compensated or not.[163,205] The inventors of this intravenous measurement now question the reliability of this or any other hemodynamic studies to accurately rule out significant iliac obstruction and recommend intravenous ultrasonography to clarify the issue.[198] Although intravenous pressure measurements and venography were once the gold standard for evaluating venous disease, duplex scanning with the addition of plethysmographic or intravascular ultrasonographic techniques, in specific cases, are the anatomic and functional tests of choice in current medical practice.[194]

Treatment Options and Results

Medical Therapy. Compression has been the mainstay of the medical treatment for all stages of CVI for centuries. The goals are to manage clinical symptoms and to control venous hypertension. Roughly speaking there are two types of compression: elastic (e.g., support stockings or long stretch bandages) and inelastic (e.g., Unna paste boot, short stretch bandages, multilayer (four-layer) bandage or Velcro band devices). The degree to which any particular bandaging is one or the other will depend on the care provider who applies the compression along with other factors. The mechanical effect is dependent on the level and type of compression as well as the underlying venous pathology. Initial narrowing of deep and superficial calf veins on standing as determined by duplex imaging is observed at 20 mm Hg.[206] There is a trend to decreasing residual venous volume and venous filling index, which translates into decreased edema and improved quality of life (QOL) data in those with early mild disease.[207–210] Consistent narrowing of superficial and calf veins occurs at a median of 30 to 40 mm Hg pressure on standing, whereas complete occlusion occurs at a median pressure of 70 mm Hg. Complete occlusion is not the goal. At 30 mm Hg and standing, inelastic bandages significantly decrease the venous filling index and venous volume in patients with venous ulcers and deep venous reflux.[207] It took 40 mm Hg to decrease the venous filling index when using elastic stockings. The higher the pressure exerted up to 60 mm Hg, the more impressive the changes in residual venous volume and decrease in venous filling index.[207] Therapeutic calf compression improves calf muscle pump function expressed as a reduction in residual volume fraction during walking as well.[211] Thigh compression was helpful in reducing great saphenous and femoral vein diameter (by duplex imaging) at a constant pressure of ≥40 mm Hg and reduced venous reflux (by APG) at 60 mm Hg.[212] Overall, these effects on the underlying veins help to improve the venous pump and decrease the venous volume in the lower extremity. It is interesting that elastic stockings maintain a rather constant pressure during exercise and at rest. Alternatively, inelastic wraps demonstrate a more dramatic increase in pressure during exercise since they do not stretch but have decreasing pressure with recumbence as the edema exits the leg and the bandage maintains its shape.[213] This may explain why inelastic wraps are much better tolerated when left on day and night. It also explains why such compression should be changed more frequently early in treatment and less frequently later as the degree of edema requiring control lessens.

There are data to suggest that extended use of elastic compression may impede the microcirculation and thereby jeopardize tissue viability.[214] However, it is also apparent that compression has a positive influence on the local skin and soft tissues in the face of edema. A compression stocking at 30 mm Hg of compression will significantly improve the capillary filtration rate in patients with C_{4-6} disease, and stiffer stockings do better.[215] By decreasing the subcutaneous pressure in the perimalleolar area, medium and strong compression can promote extracellular fluid reabsorption and improve sodium subcutaneous tissue clearance.[216,217] There are data to indicate that skin transcutaneous oxygen tension is diminished and the skin capillary density depressed as a result of venous insufficiency, but this can be improved with compression (edema reduction).[218,219] Compression can increase microcirculatory flow velocity and may ameliorate the inflammatory injury and fibrosis associated with chronic venous insufficiency.[213,218,220,221] Cytokines, such as vascular endothelial growth factor and tumor necrosis factor, decrease with compression therapy and correlate with ulcer healing.[222] Furthermore and in contradistinction to the first statement in this paragraph, standard compression can actually increase arterial blood flow in some circumstances.[213,223] The lymphatic system is involved in this derangement, which can also be improved with compression.[219] In those with significant arterial occlusive disease (especially with ABI <0.50 and even 0.80 in some cases), compression is contraindicated since an external pressure could decrease the distal perfusion to critical levels.[213,224–226] This may especially be true for elastic compression garments since constant pressure is applied. However, inelastic bandages applied with a resting pressure of less than 20 mm Hg and used with active exercise reduce edema and increase arterial flow similar to the use of intermittent pneumatic compression.[227]

Evidence-based medicine confirms our clinical impression and has been applied to the use of compression garments for the treatment of CVI. Two areas have substantial evidence to demonstrate that compression is statistically beneficial. First, elastic compression stockings (30–40 mm Hg) significantly reduce the incidence of the postthrombotic syndrome after an episode of DVT.[228,229] Second, compression increases ulcer healing rates when compared to no compression. Multilayered systems are more effective than single-layered systems, and high compression (25–35 mm Hg at ankle) is more effective than low compression, but there is no clear difference in the effectiveness of different types of high-compression dressings (three layer, four layer, short stretch, Unna boot) (recommendation grade A).[228,229] High-compression (30–40 mm Hg) stockings can be used to heal ulcers with an expected 90+% rate of healing within 6 months.[230,231] The compliant patient can expect healing rates in the 90% range, whereas those noncompliant may have healing in only 50% of cases.[230,231] The evidence for the use of compression for other clinical stages of CVI is less clear and best studied by an initiative of the International Union of Phlebology with grade B recommendations defined as those based on only one large or several smaller randomized controlled trials (RCTs) and grade C recommendations based on observational studies or consensus meetings. Certainly, compression aids in preventing the recurrence of venous ulcers, but the optimal pressure and type of compression is not clearly defined (recommendation grade B).[213,229,232] In one study, recurrence of the ulcer was nearly ensured if the patient was noncompliant in the use of maintenance compression, whereas only 29% of those compliant experienced a recurrence.[230] The prophylactic use of compression in patients with a prior venous ulcer appears cost-effective.[233] There is Grade B evidence for the use of compression stockings in $C_{0S,1S,3}$ afflicted patients (10–21 mm Hg in the first two and 23–32 mm Hg in the latter) to relieve symptoms.[213,229] Patients with varicose veins both asymptomatic (23–32 mm Hg) and symptomatic (34–46 mm Hg) may be helped with compression stockings (recommendation grade C).[213,229]

In the final analysis, inelastic wraps or multilayer wraps are preferred for the *therapy phase* of venous disease (ulcer healing), but compression stockings of sufficient strength are also effective. When the ulcers are healed and the extremity is relatively free from edema, elastic wraps such as compression stockings are used to maintain a stable clinical condition (*maintenance phase*). In addition, elevating the legs when possible during the day, avoiding prolonged periods of standing or sitting, and elevating the foot of the bed 4 to 6 inches above the heart while sleeping are adjuvant components of conservative therapy.[234,235]

Intermittent pneumatic compression (IPC) provides pulsatile emptying of the venous system and can have a positive impact on the inflammatory injury and fibrosis associated with CVI.[213,220] A Cochrane review with last update in 2008 found conflicting results when IPC was used alone or as an adjuvant to compression therapy to heal venous ulcers.[236] Certainly, one

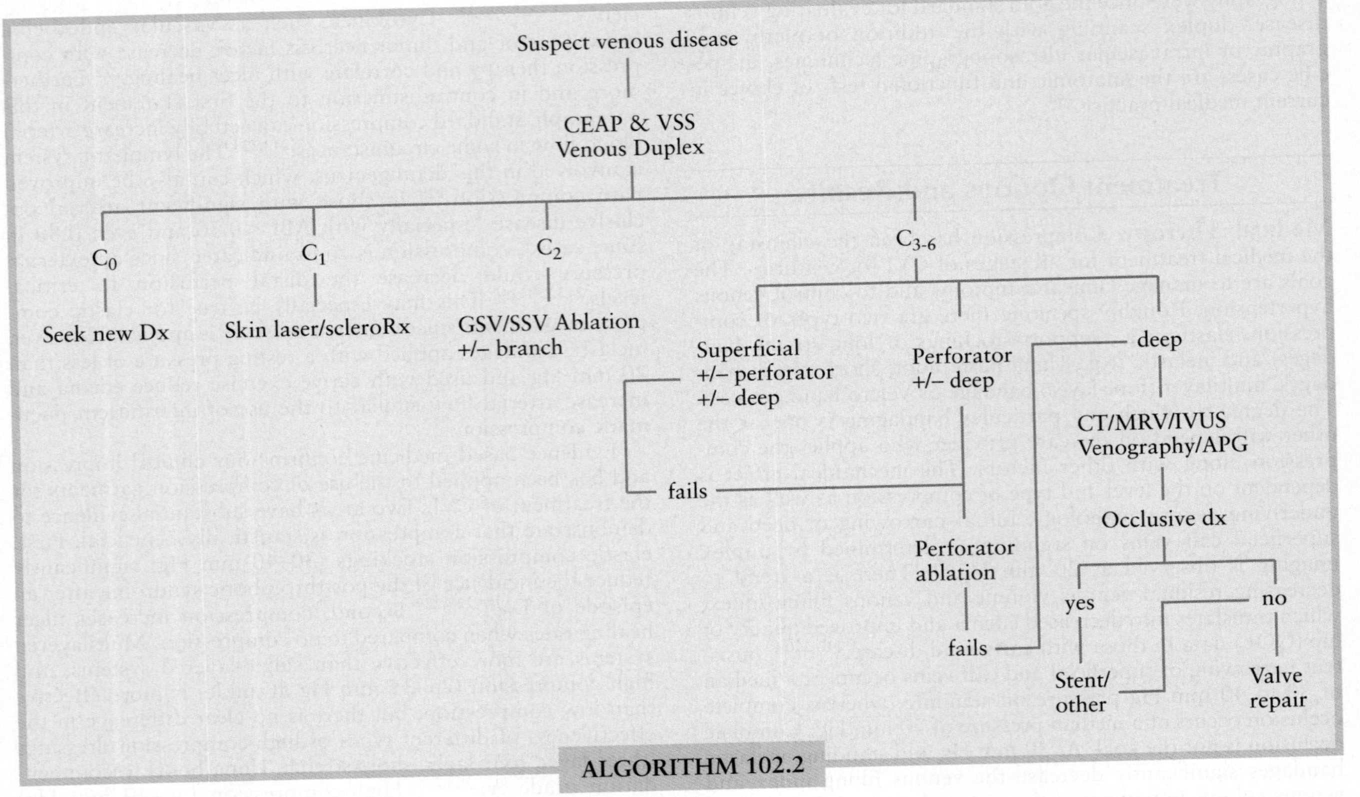

ALGORITHM 102.2. Treatment of chronic venous insufficiency.

RCT of 45 patients has demonstrated its use in patients with long-standing ulcers (at least 3 months' duration) comparing standard ambulatory compression with or without the addition of IPC. At 3 months, 10 of 21 ulcers healed with the addition of IPC, whereas only 1 of 24 healed with standard care.[237] It does appear to aid in healing very recalcitrant ulcers with sufficient raw data to allow Centers for Medicare & Medicaid Services (CMS) to permit payment after all other compression therapies have been unsuccessful.

Structured exercise can improve dynamic muscle strength and calf muscle pump function in patients with essentially all levels of CVI from varicose veins to venous ulceration.[169,238,239] It is unclear whether such exercise improves ulcer healing rates per se.

In Europe, various oral agents (e.g., diosmin, rutoside) have been touted to improve the feeling of heaviness, fatigue, and even edema of CVD, but these agents are not available in the United States. Drugs potentially useful in treating patients with venous ulcers are available in the United States. Pentoxifylline provides a small incremental benefit in ulcer healing and works best as an adjunct to compressive therapy.[240] The trade-off appears to be a greater percentage of gastrointestinal adverse effects. Prophylactic use of systemic antibiotics in the treatment of venous ulcers is not recommended and may select only resistant organisms. One randomized clinical trial in 47 patients compared elastic support bandages only versus those also treated with systemic antibiotics. There was no statistical difference in healing rates of ulcers or in changes of the microbiologic flora.[241] Certainly, an established infection (cellulitis or deeper) must be treated as it would be at any site.

Topical pharmaceuticals have been evaluated as a means of improving venous ulcer wound healing. Topical antibiotics have found little use in this capacity and may retard wound healing and cause allergic reactions.[242] Growth factors and cytokines, in addition to compression, when provided as isolated topically applied agents, have not demonstrated efficacy when compared to placebo. Reviews of the literature demonstrate inconsistent results or studies with insufficient data to determine with any certainty the efficacy of such adjuvants.[243,244] Several topical dressings applied on the ulcer bed and beneath the compression dressing have been investigated to determine if ulcer healing could be improved. Hydrocolloids (e.g., DuoDERM), foams (e.g., Allevyn), alginates (e.g., Sorbsan), hydrogels (e.g., Intra-Site gel or Debrisan) and others (e.g., OpSite) have been studied. Insufficient data are available to make firm conclusions, but it is clear that the nature and amount of the exudates present may provide a rationale for the benefit of one or the other of these dressings in a given patient.[245–247] The failure of medical measures or patient dissatisfaction with the results being obtained initiates a more invasive approach.

Surgical Therapy. The use of surgical intervention in the realm of venous disease as in all areas of vascular surgery is driven by the documented presence of disease, the risk of the intervention planned, and the expected outcome (Algorithm 102.2).

Telangectasia, Reticular Veins, Branch Varicose Veins. Percutaneous laser energy can be used to treat telangiectasias up to 0.7 mm in diameter with reasonable success. For matting and telangiectasias less than 0.5 mm diameter, the flashlamp pumped dye laser (595-nm wavelength) is well studied.[248] The potassium titanylphosphate (KTP) laser of wavelength 532 nm is applicable to those 0.7 mm or less.[249] Since melanin is the prime competing light absorber to hemoglobin in the body, the increased epidermal melanin in the tanned skin risks long-lasting hyperpigmentation, and therefore, percutaneous laser therapy should not be preformed in those with a suntan.

Sclerotherapy (needle injection of caustic solutions directly into superficial veins) has long been advocated for treating varicosities remaining after saphenous ablation, small isolated varicosities, telangiectasias, and reticular veins.[250–252] Sclerotherapy alone appears an effective treatment for branch varicosities in patients without major saphenous reflux and appears effective when combined with GSV ablation to control branch varicosities.[253–255] The most common sclerosing agents are sodium tetradecyl sulfate, sodium morrhuate and hypertonic saline (23.4%) with some use of combination of 25% dextrose with 10% saline. Polidocanol used extensively in Europe is not yet commercially available in the United States. Most agents are not specifically approved by the FDA for sclerosing veins but have been used for decades in many cases and in some were available before FDA approval was required (e.g., sodium morrhuate).[256] All act to damage the vein endothelium, inducing inflammation and scarring with ultimate lumen collapse.[250,256] Foam sclerotherapy is the addition of air to liquid sclerosing agents, particularly detergent sclerosants, to allow a more protracted contact of sclerosing agent to the vein wall. The technique is the current technique of choice for many phlebologists, especially for larger veins.[253,257] Modification of the sclerosing agents, by producing a foam, adds a component to the agent that converts its use to off-label. The exact concentration of sclerosant, liquid or foam, used for sclerotherapy is dependent on vein size and agent used.[250,256] These interventions are generally outpatient procedures.

Common complaints including burning, stinging, itching, and muscle spasm are observed with sclerotherapy injections.[258,259] Extravasation of the agent can cause fat or skin necrosis, ulcerations, and/or hyperpigmentation of the surrounding skin.[258] Posttreatment veins are often brown as opposed to the blue-red pretreatment color. Microthrombectomy appears to reduce postsclerotherapy pigmentation, especially in veins 1 mm or less in diameter.[260] Other potential complications of sclerotherapy include allergic reactions and toxicity if too much agent is used at one sitting.[250,258] Therefore, a limited amount of sclerosing agent is typically injected during a single setting. Rarely, ocular events or even cerebrovascular events have been observed following foam sclerotherapy and, therefore, must be discussed with the patient prior to its use.[259,261]

Phlebectomy (ambulatory phlebectomy, stab avulsion, stab phlebectomy, microphlebectomy, and microextraction are synonymous terms) is a technique in which varicose veins are removed through small stab incisions with hooks or small mosquito clamps used to pull the vein from its bed. Several phlebectomy instruments are available.[262] It can be performed in an ambulatory setting with local anesthesia or in conjunction with a more invasive procedure and more extensive anesthesia. One small randomized controlled study suggests that this approach may have improved results over sclerotherapy.[263] Which approach is best remains a point of contention in the literature. In some cases, the need for reintervention may be tolerable based on the minimally invasive nature of the procedures. Complications are generally minor and of low risk (<2%) including development of telangiectasia, blistering, hyperpigmentation, and missed varix.[264] Tumescent anesthesia has allowed for extensive interventions with little pain on an ambulatory basis.[265] Such field anesthesia allows for another method of phlebectomy, powered phlebectomy, involving a modified arthroscopic shaver with transillumination, which allows venous clusters to be illuminated, morcellized, and aspirated. When compared to ambulatory phlebectomy, there is no benefit in patient cosmetic scores or satisfaction, and the recurrence rate at one year is 15% higher.[266] The added cost and lack of patient preference will likely prevent this technique from becoming widely adopted.

Saphenous Vein Stripping/Ablation. Duplex imaging of patients prior to invasive saphenous treatment has proven that not all saphenous veins per se are incompetent when varicosities exist. In such cases, saphenous preservation leads to good results.[267] If saphenous insufficiency is present, some method of controlling reflux is required for best results. Removing the refluxing vein from the venous system is the current best solution. The vein can be stripped from its bed and discarded. The procedure is called saphenous vein high ligation and stripping. Lower leg deep venous occlusive disease is not an absolute contraindication to removal of the saphenous system and may actually be indicated in patients with mixed obstruction/reflux disease and is often the first step in cases of combined deep and superficial insufficiency.[268,269] Preoperatively, with the patient standing to fully dilate the veins, the varicosities are marked with a permanent marker for later operative visualization. The operation includes ligation and disconnection of the GSV at the saphenofemoral junction followed by complete removal of the vein to the knee. If the below knee greater saphenous vein is incompetent based on preoperative diagnostic studies, it may also be excised. The method of vein removal may involve the introduction of long metal or plastic stripping wires with removable heads of varying size (i.e., Codman), the perforate invagination (PIN) stripper, or various other devices aimed at pulling the vein from the leg.[270,271] Both GSV and SSV can be treated by these methods, taking into account required patient positioning and anatomic variability especially of concern in the case of the SSV.[270] Among properly selected patients undergoing GSV high ligation and stripping, recurrent saphenous varicosities will be noted in less than 25% of cases at 2 years, but increases to 41% at 5 years and 62% at 11 years depending on the rigor of patient evaluation.[271–273] These results serve to highlight the chronicity of varicose vein disease and places in perspective the expectations for other forms of saphenous ablation.

Another method of removing the GSV from the venous circulation is to thermally heat the inside with radiofrequency-generated heat.[274,275] Placed percutaneously or rarely by venous cutdown, the probe is sequentially heated throughout the length of the GSV. Tumescent anesthesia is administered within the saphenous compartment providing anesthesia, a heat sink, and some venous compression during the procedure. The cumulative vein occlusion rate reported from a venous registry is 87.2% at 5 years.[276] Nearly 6% of patients had SSV and accessory saphenous vein interventions in this registry. Direct comparison to standard GSV vein stripping demonstrated comparable results in terms of recurrent varicose veins (14.3% vs. 20.9%) with an improved quality of life score even 2 years after surgery.[277] The newest rendition of this procedure involves using a 7-cm-long heating probe placed at the end of the catheter, which is heated to 120°C for 20-second intervals sequentially down the length of the vein. The time for ablation is significantly decreased, and early work would suggest that at 6 months all veins were effectively removed from the venous circulation (99.6%).[278] Long-term results are not available for this latest technical modification.

Alternatively, laser energy of various wavelengths (810–1,320 nm) delivered via a 600-μm bare-tipped fiber will cause a localized thermal injury to the vein wall.[279–281] Early success is excellent with 90% to 100% freedom from recurrent varicosities. Elimination of reflux at a rate of 80% has been documented in 3-year follow-up.[282] Some have found utility of this newer method for the SSV.[280] High-volume tumescent anesthesia provides a heat sink and, therefore, protection from collateral heat damage. When delivering endoluminal therapy aimed at obliterating the vein lumen, energy is delivered beginning about 1 to 2 cm below the superficial epigastric vein to preserve lower abdominal wall venous drainage and to prevent thrombosis of the deep system, and this is true for any technique using thermal energy for these procedures.

Hamel-Desnos et al.[257] found GSV ultrasonography-directed foam sclerotherapy to be 84% effective in eliminating reflux for 1 year. Midterm results with ultrasonographic-directed foam sclerotherapy in 175 patients reports a 2-year primary success rate of 55% with a 77% secondary success rate in preventing recurrent reflux.[283] The long-term results of the VEDICO trial would suggest that substantially more veins are present at 10 years when foam is used as a single modality than when surgery or surgery and foam are used.[253] If recurrence without reintervention is the goal, sclerotherapy appears to be at a disadvantage. A meta-analysis suggests that over time sclerotherapy loses any advantage over older methods of vein ablation, which is also confirmed by individual case series.[250,254,257,284,285] Newer techniques of sclerotherapy lack long-term evaluation.

Complications of GSV surgery are rare but include wound infection, DVT, nerve damage, and hematoma formation to mention the more prominent.[272,286,287] Saphenous nerve injury can result in an area of numbness around the knee or foot but is often clinically irrelevant.[105,122] Complications from SSV stripping are also typically rare but include bleeding, hematoma formation, sural nerve damage, DVT, and wound infection.[288] These same complications are reported for radiofrequency and laser ablations, possibly at a slightly lower incidence for some such as nerve paresthesia. DVT risk is about 1% for all procedures.[272,275,281,282,286,287] A complication unique to radiofrequency and laser procedures is thermal damage to adjacent structures, such as nerve or skin that appear to be mitigated by tumescent anesthesia.[274] Complications as well as short-term and midterm freedom from recurrence for both radiofrequency and laser saphenous vein ablation compare favorably with standard stripping, and both may provide some early patient benefit.[275,281,282]

Perforator Vein Ablation. Ligation of perforating veins can be an effective treatment for patients with isolated perforator vein incompetence. This procedure can be performed in conjunction with saphenous vein removal. Perforating vein ligation can be performed via an open or minimally invasive endoscopic technique. A Linton-type procedure uses an incision along the medial or posterior lower leg and creation of subfascial flaps.[289] The perforating veins are directly ligated. If a skin ulcer is present, this can be débrided. If a large amount of soft tissue and/or fascia is involved, a skin graft can be placed to aid healing once the diseased tissues are removed.[289] Alternatively, an endoscopic technique (subfascial endoscopic perforator surgery [SEPS]) can be used.[290] Subfascial dissection is performed using sharp and blunt balloon dissection to allow direct video-enhanced ligation and division of perforating veins with or without CO_2 subfascial insufflation to increase visualization and decrease the risk of air embolization. The SEPS procedure has demonstrated decreased symptoms and a near 90% ulcer healing rate at 2 years.[291] Wound complications are less common after SEPS (0–10%) compared to the open method (12%–53%) with comparable outcomes.[292]

Both of the aforementioned procedures are more invasive than several percutaneous methods of perforator ablation, which can be accomplished under local anesthesia and with minimal skin disruption. No matter the ablating energy delivered (radiofrequency, laser, or chemical), ultrasonographic access, operative monitoring and confirmation of results is routine. Prevention of energy delivery to the deep system prevents unwanted thrombosis. Various sclerosing agents have been used with minimal risk of DVT or skin infection, and with an immediate success of 90% to 98% and a 2-year maintenance of occlusion of nearly 80%.[293–295] Radiofrequency ablation demonstrates a greater than 90% early ablation rate with more than 90% free of reflux at 1 year.[296,297] Laser energy of various wavelengths have been used for this procedure with reports of about 100% occlusions immediately and 85% to 90% occlusion rate at 6 months.[297,298] Whether perforator ligation is required in addition to saphenous surgery for advanced CVD when both systems demonstrate insufficiency remains debatable.[292]

Iliac Stenting and Venous Bypass. Endovascular stenting of iliac vein stenosis/obstruction has improved the symptoms of venous occlusive disease including decreased edema and pain symptoms, and improved quality of life parameters.[111,133,173,299–301] It will often result in healing of venous ulcers, many of which have associated untreated lower leg venous insufficiency, at an initial rate of 68% with only 8 of 101 healed ulcers recurring within 5 years whether performed for primary or postthrombotic occlusion.[301] Parameters of venous reflux are not worsened following resolution of the occlusive iliac vein occlusive disease.[301] The primary and assisted primary stent patency rates at 3 years are 75% and 92%, respectively, and at 6 years 69% and 89%, respectively (Fig. 102.2).[301,302] Intervention was performed in the presence of significant clinical symptoms (C_3 or C_2 with pain) and greater than 50% morphologic stenosis found on transfemoral venography or intravascular ultrasonography.[133,301,302] Potential complications include DVT, access site complications, retroperitoneal hematoma, and other catheter- and balloon-related problems with essentially no mortality associated with the procedure.[198,301–303] When technically feasible, endovascular intervention has replaced more invasive approaches.

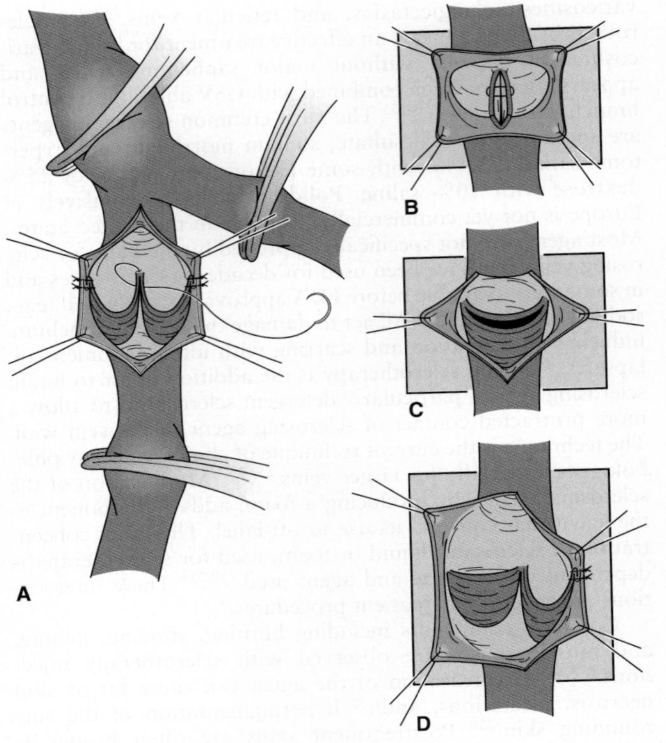

FIGURE 102.2. Open valvuloplasty to repair an insufficient valve can be accomplished by various venotomy incisions. **A:** The method of Kistner. **B:** The method of Raju. **C:** The method of Sottiurai. **D:** The method of Tripathi and his colleagues.

The open surgical procedures use native saphenous vein or polytetrafluoroethylene (PTFE) graft material as the conduit to bypass from a nondiseased distal vein to a disease-free proximal vein. Vena cava reconstructions often use PTFE grafts to allow a proper size match.[304] Preoperative venous pressure studies are often obtained to document venous hypertension.[305] Iliac vein decompression has been used in the instance of extrinsic compression by an overlying right iliac artery (e.g., May-Thurner syndrome). If the iliac vein is severely stenosed or occluded, cross-femoral venous bypass or direct repair of the iliac vein can be performed.[191,306] Patient survival should be considered prior to aggressive intervention if iliac vein compression is due to a cancerous encroachment. The cross-femoral venous bypass (Palma procedure) is performed by passing a vein graft or graft material via a suprapubic subcutaneous tunnel to the contralateral femoral vein. The saphenous vein or prosthetic graft is then connected to the unaffected femoral vein by an end-to-side technique. The key to success of this surgery may be graft diameter. If the native vein is less than 4.5 mm in diameter, better success may be achieved with a 10-mm diameter PTFE graft, although others would question whether PTFE is superior to vein in this location.[304,305] An arteriovenous fistula is generally used to increase flow through the graft in the immediate postoperative period. This fistula can then be ligated in 1 to 3 months or left open long-term if no unwanted sequelae are noted. In one series, venous reconstruction for iliofemoral and IVC obstruction reported a 62% 3-year patency with the Palma procedure demonstrating the overall patency of 83% at 4 years.[304] Mortality was minimal and wound complications rare. In current practice, these procedures are generally used only when a percutaneous approach has failed.

Indications for a saphenopopliteal bypass are symptomatic patients with isolated femoral or popliteal vein occlusion, a patent common femoral and iliocaval system, a nonvaricose saphenous vein, and femoral phlebitis inactive for at least 1 year. In addition, conservative therapy must have failed and venous hypertension must be documented. These distal to proximal venous bypasses use autogenous vein as the conduit of choice, and bypasses extend from distal to proximal nondiseased segments.[305] This operation is rarely performed.

Although not yet proven as a method of treating occlusive venous disease due to prior thrombosis, some data suggest that endophlebectomy (operative removal of synechiae and septa) of iliac, femoral, popliteal, and even tibial veins is possible and can result in a 77% primary patency rate at 8 months.[307]

Venous Valve Repair or Replacement. During the conduct of these operations, several observations influence what the surgeon does for a given patient. If operative handling of the suspect valve results in vasoconstriction and secondary competence (often determined by a standard strip test), an external valvuloplasty or a prosthetic sleeve technique may be viable options.[308] For a valve station requiring in situ repair, careful adventitial dissection of the valve attachment lines facilitates proper venotomy when required and helps to verify the feasibility of valve repair.[160] A lack of valve attachment lines may signify the destruction of the valve as a postthrombotic sequela, prompting other than an in situ repair.[160] Valvuloplasty of any sort is most commonly performed in the femoral or popliteal location due to size and hemodynamic considerations.

An internal valvuloplasty or an open direct valve repair has been the mainstay for the repair of primary venous valvular reflux for decades. This technique involves venotomy and suturing of the elongated valve leaflets under direct visualization with fine polypropylene suture (7 or 6-0) to tighten the valve cusps. Kistner[309] reported success with a longitudinal venotomy extending through the valve commissure in 1968 (Fig. 102.3). Raju championed a supracommissural approach involving a transverse venotomy at least 2.5 cm above the valve.[310] Sottiurai devised a hybrid approach (a T-shaped venotomy), using a supravalvular transverse venotomy with distal extension into the valve sinus.[311] A "trapdoor" approach involving two transverse incisions (supravalvular and infravalvular) connected by a single vertical incision through the commissure has been described (Fig. 102.3).[312] Plication of approximately 20% of the valve leaflet length tends to restore valve competency in most cases.[313]

The technique of external valvuloplasty offers the advantage of valve repair without venotomy.[314] It is performed by placing sutures transmurally through the valve attachment lines, and when tied, reduces the commissural angle and vein diameter resulting in a competent valve. The valve leaflets are generally not captured or reefed by this method. Reported results suggest that it may be less durable than the more precise open valvuloplasty, but patient selection plays a key role.[314] A modification (limited anterior plication) involves only anterior vein dissection and then reefing of the cusps using a running mattress suture from a point 3 to 4 mm proximal to the angle of the valve cusp insertion lines up to the angle of valve cusp insertion.[315] About 3 mm of the vein wall is incorporated into the stitch to approximate the cusps. This technique was developed with the aim of decreasing vein dissection and resultant external scarring. It has been described in conjunction with saphenous vein stripping and limited to the femoral vein valve. Results after 10-year follow-up demonstrated improved VRT and decreased AVP in patients with moderate deep venous valvular incompetence.[315] Thus, it shows promise as a mode of therapy for highly selected patients. Another modification of this technique features the use of an angioscope.[316] A side branch of the GSV allows introduction of an angioscope, which is advanced into the femoral vein to a position above the incompetent valve, and external sutures are then placed under direct vision.[316] Following a learning curve while using the angioscope, Raju et al. demonstrated good clinical and competency data with the transcommissural technique without the use of the angioscope with 30 months of follow-up.[317] In these last two methods, the venous valve cusps are actually engaged with the suture, and

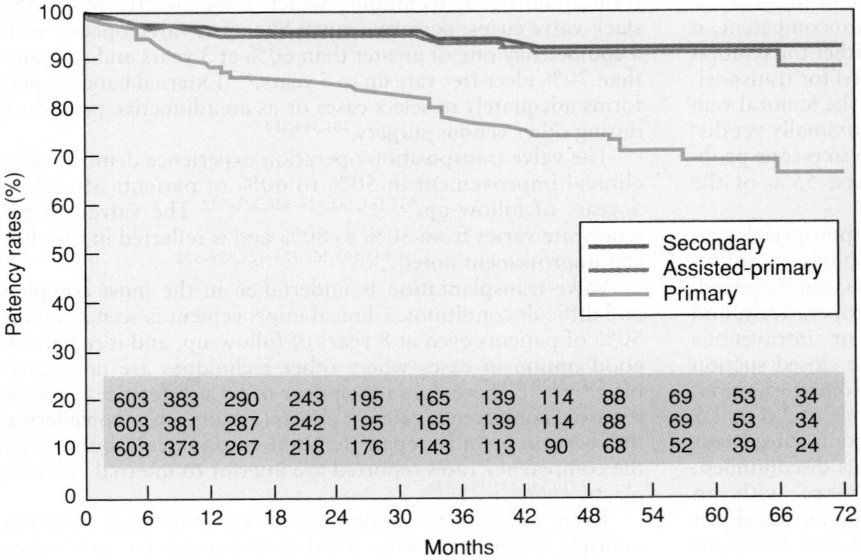

FIGURE 102.3. Cumulative primary, assisted-primary, and secondary patency rates of 603 limbs after iliofemoral stenting. The lower numbers represent limbs at risk for each time interval (all standard error of the mean <10%). (Adapted from Neglén P, Hollis KC, Olivier J, et al. Stenting of the venous outflow in chronic venous disease: long-term stent-related outcome, clinical and hemodynamic results. *J Vasc Surg* 2007;46:979–990.)

therefore, the cusps are tightened directly much as in the open method of repair.

External banding has been used when dissection vasospasm renders a valve spontaneously competent. The technique uses an external sleeve made of synthetic material wrapped circumferentially around the vein at the site of the valve and tightened to diminish the size of the vein lumen until the valve is competent. The sleeve is then anchored in place to the adventitia by sutures to avoid slippage. It has achieved good results when used in select patients.[201,318,319] One group of investigators have been more aggressive with this approach, using the technique in patients with more severe valvular reflux and often placing multiple external cuffs.[318]

Venous valve transplantation is an option when the valve is absent or destroyed. This procedure was first reported clinically by Taheri et al. in 1982.[320] A 2- to 3-cm segment of upper extremity vein containing a competent valve (or a reparable one) is first removed. The incompetent femoral vein is opened below the takeoff of the profunda femoris vein, and the axillary vein segment is sutured into place following the removal of an appropriate length of femoral vein. The popliteal location may be more appropriate if the femoral location does not control all axial reflux into the leg, for example, if the profunda femoral vein system is also incompetent. The proximal anastomosis may be accomplished first to confirm the competence of the newly transplanted valve and to allow distention and lengthening of the vein/valve to facilitate the distal anastomosis. For vein transplantation in trabeculated postthrombotic veins, investigators have excised intraluminal synechiae to create one acceptable lumen for transplantation.[321] Interrupted sutures are preferred to avoid suture line stenosis.[313] Valve competence is determined by the intraoperative strip test. An external sleeve can then be placed to prevent late dilatation of the repaired segment, and because approximately 40% of axillary vein valves are incompetent at explant, a bench repair may be required to restore competency.[160,313] Should a bench repair be necessary, the transcommissural external valvuloplasty technique appears to have better results than the standard external valvuloplasty,[160] and success has been achieved with internal open valvuloplasty.[322]

A less common option for the postthrombotic syndrome is valve transposition. If a venous valve is competent in one of the major thigh venous systems, then a transposition procedure can be performed placing the incompetent venous system below the competent valve. Most commonly, the femoral system is incompetent and the profunda femoris valve remains competent. Here, the incompetent femoral vein can be transected and reimplanted distal to the competent valve in the profunda femoris vein. Alternatively, the incompetent femoral system can be placed below a competent valve in the GSV, or when the profunda femoris venous system is incompetent, it may be placed distal to a competent valve in either the femoral vein or the GSV. A technique has been described for transposition of the ipsilateral valve-competent GSV to the femoral vein and subsequent ligation of the femoral vein proximally yet distal to the takeoff of the profunda femoris vein to escape problems with diameter mismatch.[323] At 10 years, 55% of the patients were reported to be ulcer free.

Aggressive venous valve surgery requires appropriate consideration of perioperative adjunctive care: prophylactic antibiotics, intraoperative heparin use especially if the vein is opened, the use of pneumatic compression devices postoperatively, and the use of low-molecular-weight heparin or intravenous heparin in the postoperative period. Some use closed suction drainage of wounds to avoid hematoma and seroma formation. Warfarin should have an initial target INR range of 2.0 to 2.5 for the first 6 weeks and some would advocate a subsequent decrease to 1.7 to 2.0 until 4 months when it is discontinued. Adjustments are made to accommodate those with an increased risk of thrombosis. One suggested long-term regimen is minidose warfarin, which uses daily doses of 1 to 2.5 mg to

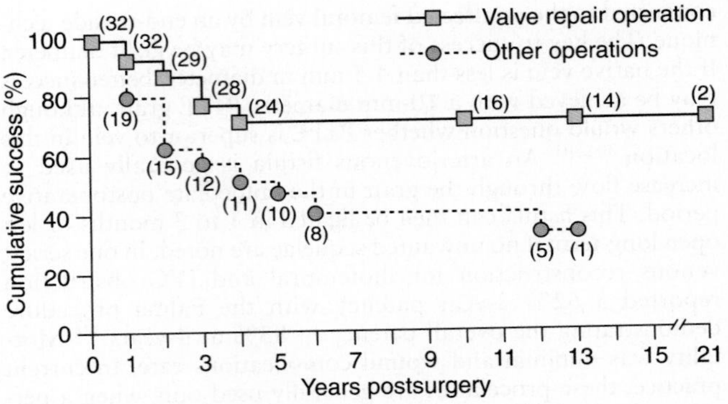

FIGURE 102.4. Life-table demonstrates cumulative clinical success rate based on type of valve reconstruction procedure. The valve repair operation is valvuloplasty as performed by Kistner and associates via the Kistner technique. "Other operations" refer to valve transpositions (n = 14), superficial femoral vein valve transplantations (n = 2), and combined valve repair and transposition procedures (n = 3). Numbers in parentheses indicate the number of valve repairs remaining in the study at that time point. Significant difference exists between valve repair versus other operations. (Adapted from Masuda EM, Kistner RL. Long-term results of venous valve reconstruction: a four to twenty-one year follow-up. *J Vasc Surg* 1994;19:391.)

prevent thrombosis.[160,324] Although many surgeons encourage the use of compressive support, patients often do not comply but still have an acceptable clinical result.[162,163]

Valve repair procedures are well tolerated by most patients and have a low morbidity, as well as essentially zero mortality in most series.[135] Hematoma and seroma formation are noted in less than 15% of cases depending on the level of anticoagulation used.[162,313,325–327] DVT occurs in less than 10% of cases in most series and even if higher is not associated with clinical sequelae, while the PE risk is well less than 1%.[160–162,313,325–327] Wound infections have been seen in 2% to 7% of cases.[160,162,313,327]

The Kistner et al.[328] long-term follow-up of internal valvuloplasty spans decades and is reported in life-table format (Fig. 102.4). Valve competency is 60% to 70% at 5 years in most series.[161–163,201,310,312,327–333] In general, a patent and competent valve translates into clinical improvement and a healed ulcer, whereas the reverse is true with recurrent reflux. This is true for all types of single-station venous valvular reconstructions. External valvuloplasty without direct cusp repair (isolated wall diameter reduction) appears to perform less well in all aspects than open valvuloplasty.[201,327] However, the transcommissural technique, which does directly repair the slack valve cusps, performs much like open valvuloplasty with a competency rate of greater than 60% at 3 years and a greater than 70% ulcer-free rate up to 5 years.[317] External banding performs adequately in select cases or as an adjunctive procedure during other venous surgery.[201,318,319]

The valve transposition operation experience demonstrates clinical improvement in 50% to 60% of patients after 3 to 5 years of follow-up.[135,161,162,323–326,328–332] The valve competency rate varies from 30% to 80% and is reflected in the clinical improvement noted.[135,161,162,323–326,328–332]

Valve transplantation is undertaken in the most complex and difficult conditions. Clinical improvement is seen in about 50% of patients even at 8 years of follow-up, and it remains a good option in cases where other techniques are not possible.[134,135,313] There does not appear to be a difference between reported competency rates or clinical results when considering the location of valve repair (femoral vs. popliteal), but overall the competency rates reported are inferior to internal valvuloplasty.[310,320,332,334–339]

There are data to support the observation that repairing multiple valves in the same axial system translates into longer clinical benefit, but this approach does, of course, add risks at the initial operative intervention.[317,318,327,340]

In general, patients with postthrombotic reflux tend to have more problems maintaining healed ulcers than those with a primary etiology of reflux, as noted from the results of internal valvuloplasty (generally a primary etiology) versus those requiring transplantation or a transposition operative approach.[162]

Valve Substitutes. For those patients with chronic DVI and no autogenous valve available, a valve substitute is the only alternative. Many experimental attempts using allografts and synthetics have been unsuccessful.[341] Three substitute valves—a cryopreserved venous valve containing allograft, a cadaveric cryopreserved pulmonary monocusp patch, and a small intestinal submucosa bicuspid stent mounted valve—have had isolated, but often unsustained success when reaching the clinical arena.[342–344] The stent design and percutaneous route of the last-mentioned device is quite innovative; however, substrate fibrosis has lead the investigators to study the use of an autogenous valve with good preliminary animal results.[345]

Autogenous tissue appears to be the only material which currently can act as a substitute valve with some hope of success in the clinical arena. Using donor vein, after trimming adventitia and part of the media, to fashion semilunar cusps within the deficient recipient vein, Raju and Hardy[160] have reported acceptable clinical results. Another approach invaginates a stump of the long saphenous vein into the femoral vein to fashion a bicuspid valve; 19 of 20 reconstructions were patent and competent at a mean of 10 months with one valve demonstrating reflux.[346] No other series have reproduced these findings to date. The newest innovation has been to use an ophthalmic knife or other fine tool to dissect the intima/media wall of the thickened postthrombotic vein wall into one or two sheets and thereby fashion the valve cusp(s).[347] This technique has been reproduced by another investigator.[348] A recent improvement has been to place two sutures on the cusp(s) to hold the valve in the semiopen position and thereby to prevent valve collapse and improve neovalve competence. The results with this modification include 21 operations (mean follow-up 11 months) with all valves competent, a 95% ulcer-healing rate, and two recurrences (9.5%).[349]

Surgical Wound Care

Débridement to healthy tissue when required benefits the rate of ulcer healing and does not lead to a higher risk of systemic infection.[242,350,351] It is especially beneficial when evaluated as adjuvant care to the standard methods of venous ulcer wound care.[246,352]

For resistant venous ulcers, skin grafting is an option. These ulcers can be extensive, and skin grafting allows for coverage of raw surfaces to speed the healing process. Once the ulcer has a clean base of granulation tissue, a split-thickness skin graft can be applied. There are reports on improved healing with skin grafting for chronic venous ulceration.[353] Skin grafting is generally considered only when ulcer healing has not occurred following diligent conservative management. An alternative or precursor to an autologous skin graft may be one of several skin substitutes. Various skin substitutes have been used to aid in venous ulcer healing (e.g., fresh allografts, porcine dermis, etc.), but for most there are insufficient data available to determine whether venous ulcer healing is improved.[354] However, the biologically active bilayered human skin equivalent with an allogenic epidermal and dermal layer has demonstrated more promise.[246,354] Falanga et al.[355,356] randomized 309 patients into one of two groups but only 275 were fully analyzed: Group 1 received human skin equivalent and compression, while group 2 received dressing (made to look the same as the intervention) and compression. At 6 months, 92 of 146 (63%) in group 1 and 63 of 129 (48%) in group 2 healed ($p < 0.05$), and time to complete healing averaged 61 days in group 1 and 181 days in group 2.[355,356] Porcine small intestine submucosa (SIS) is primarily a collagen-based extracellular matrix with retained biologically active components. Sixty-two patients received SIS plus a nonadherent dressing covered by a four-layer compression bandage, whereas 58 patients received the same treatment without SIS application. With SIS, 63% healed in 12 weeks, while only 40% did so in the same period without the addition of SIS ($p = 0.02$), and when adjusted for ulcer size SIS was three times as likely to heal as treatment for the control group ($p = 0.007$).[352] Of those that healed, none recurred in 6 months in the SIS group, whereas 30% of the control group experienced a recurrent ulcer. This manuscript was included in a recent review of the literature as a RCT demonstrating significance when used to heal venous ulcers.[246]

The Pelvic Congestion Syndrome

This distressing clinical condition can result from gonadal vein and/or hypogastric vein reflux. Pelvic pain is a constant complaint. Gonadal vein reflux may be best managed with gonadal vein excision due to its many areas of potential reflux, but an endovascular approach using coils, sclerosants, or a combination can also be successful and is gaining in popularity.[357] Hypogastric vein reflux may be best managed by percutaneous embolization.[358] When the elimination of proximal reflux does not resolve superficial varicosities, the management involves techniques used for saphenous vein branch varicosities.

References

1. Heit JA. The epidemiology of venous thromboembolism in the community. *Arterioscler Thromb Vasc Biol* 2008;28(3):370–372.
2. Bauer KA, Rosendaal FR, Heit JA. Hypercoagulability: too many tests, too much conflicting data. *Hematology Am Soc Hematol Educ Program* 2002: 353–368.
3. Henke PK, Schmaier A, Wakefield TW. *Thrombosis Due to Hypercoagulable States*, 6th ed. Vol 1. Philadelphia: Elsevier Saunders; 2005: Chapter 34.
4. Goldhaber SZ, Tapson VF. A prospective registry of 5,451 patients with ultrasound-confirmed deep vein thrombosis. *Am J Cardiol* 2004;93: 259–262.
5. Wells PS, Anderson DR, Rodger M, et al. Evaluation of d-dimer in the diagnosis of suspected deep-vein thrombosis. *N Engl J Med* 2003;349(13): 1227–1235.
6. Perkins JM, Magee TR, Galland RB. Phlegmasia caerulea dolens and venous gangrene. *Br J Surg* 1996;83(1):19–23.
7. Fowl RJ, Strothman GB, Blebea J, et al. Inappropriate use of venous duplex scans: an analysis of indications and results. *J Vasc Surg* 1996; 23(5):881–885; discussion 885–886.
8. Douglas MG, Sumner DS. Duplex scanning for deep vein thrombosis: has it replaced both phlebography and noninvasive testing? *Semin Vasc Surg* 1996;9(1):3–12.
9. Guyatt G, Shünemann HJ, Cook D, et al. Applying the grades of recommendation for antithrombotic and thrombolytic therapy: the seventh ACCP Conference on Antithrombiotic and Thrombolytic Therapy. *Chest* 2004;126:179S–187S.
10. Stein PD, Fowler SE, Goodman LR, et al. Multidetector computed tomography for acute pulmonary embolism. *N Engl J Med* 2006;354(22): 2317–2327.
11. Schellong SM, Schwarz T, Halbritter K, et al. Complete compression ultrasonography of the leg veins as a single test for the diagnosis of deep vein thrombosis. *Thromb Haemost* 2003;89(2):228–234.
12. Cornuz J, Ghali WA, Hayoz D, et al. Clinical prediction of deep venous thrombosis using two risk assessment methods in combination with rapid quantitative D-dimer testing. *Am J Med* 2002;112(3):198–203.
13. Rectenwald JE, Myers DD Jr, Hawley AE, et al. D-dimer, P-selectin, and microparticles: novel markers to predict deep venous thrombosis. A pilot study. *Thromb Haemost* 2005;94(6):1312–1317.
14. Value of the ventilation/perfusion scan in acute pulmonary embolism. Results of the prospective investigation of pulmonary embolism diagnosis (PIOPED). The PIOPED Investigators. *JAMA* 1990;263(20):2753–2759.
15. Worsley DF, Alavi A. Comprehensive analysis of the results of the PIOPED Study. Prospective Investigation of Pulmonary Embolism Diagnosis Study. *J Nucl Med* 1995;36(12):2380–2387.
16. Remy-Jardin M, Remy J. Spiral CT angiography of the pulmonary circulation. *Radiology* 1999;212(3):615–636.

17. Prandoni P, Bernardi E. Upper extremity deep vein thrombosis. *Curr Opin Pulm Med* 1999;5(4):222–226.
18. Hull RD, Raskob GE, Brant RF, et al. Relation between the time to achieve the lower limit of the APTT therapeutic range and recurrent venous thromboembolism during heparin treatment for deep vein thrombosis. *Arch Intern Med* 1997;157(22):2562–2568.
19. Prandoni P, Lensing AW, Cogo A, et al. The long-term clinical course of acute deep venous thrombosis. *Ann Intern Med* 1996;125(1):1–7.
20. Bates SM, Ginsberg JS. Clinical practice. Treatment of deep-vein thrombosis. *N Engl J Med* 2004;351(3):268–277.
21. Ageno W, Turpie AG. Low-molecular-weight heparin in the treatment of pulmonary embolism. *Semin Vasc Surg* 2000;13(3):189–193.
22. van Dongen CJ, Carlo J, van den Belt AG, et al. Fixed-dose subcutaneous low molecular weight heperin versus adjusted dose unfractionated heperin for venous thromboembolism. *Cochrane Database Syst Rev* 2009;1.
23. Hull RD, Pineo GF, Mah AF, et al. A randomized trial evaluating long-term low-molecular-weight heparin therapy out-of-hospital versus warfarin sodium comparing the post-phlebitic outcomes at three months. 2001; 98:447A.
24. van Dongen CJ, van den Belt AG, Prins MH, et al. Fixed dose subcutaneous low molecular weight heparins versus adjusted dose unfractionated heparin for venous thromboembolism. *Cochrane Database Syst Rev* 2004; (4):CD001100.
25. Hyers TM, Agnelli G, Hull RD, et al. Antithrombotic therapy for venous thromboembolic disease. *Chest* 2001;119(1 suppl):176S–193S.
26. Kearon C, Kahn SR, Agnelli G, et al.; American College of Chest Physicians. Antithrombotic therapy for venous thromboembolic disease: ACCP Evidence-Based Clinical Practice Guidelines (8th Edition). *Chest* 2008; 133(6):454S–545S. (Erratum in *Chest* 2008;134(4):892.)
27. Prandoni P, Lensing AW, Prins MH, et al. Residual venous thrombosis as a predictive factor of recurrent venous thromboembolism. *Ann Intern Med* 2002;137(12):955–960.
28. Hull RD, Marder VJ, Mah AF, et al. Quantitative assessment of thrombus burden predicts the outcome of treatment for venous thrombosis: a systematic review. *Am J Med* 2005;118(5):456–464.
29. Cosmi B, Legnani C, Cini M, et al. D-dimer levels in combination with residual venous obstruction and the risk of recurrence after anticoagulation withdrawal for a first idiopathic deep vein thrombosis. *Thromb Haemost* 2005;94(5):969–974.
30. Palareti G, Cosmi B, Legnani C, et al. D-dimer testing to determine the duration of anticoagulation therapy. *N Engl J Med* 2006;355(17): 1780–1789.
31. Ridker PM, Goldhaber SZ, Danielson E, et al. Long-term, low-intensity warfarin therapy for the prevention of recurrent venous thromboembolism. *N Engl J Med* 2003;348(15):1425–1434.
32. Kearon C, Ginsberg JS, Kovacs MJ, et al. Comparison of low-intensity warfarin therapy with conventional-intensity warfarin therapy for long-term prevention of recurrent venous thromboembolism. *N Engl J Med* 2003;349(7):631–639.
33. Linkins LA, Choi PT, Douketis JD. Clinical impact of bleeding in patients taking oral anticoagulant therapy for venous thromboembolism: a meta-analysis. *Ann Intern Med* 2003;139(11):893–900.
34. Almeida JI, Coats R, Liem TK, et al. Reduced morbidity and mortality rates of the heparin-induced thrombocytopenia syndrome. *J Vasc Surg* 1998;27(2):309–314; discussion 315–306.
35. Greinacher A, Michels I, Mueller-Eckhardt C. Heparin-associated thrombocytopenia: the antibody is not heparin specific. *Thromb Haemost* 1992; 67(5):545–549.
36. Alving BM. How I treat heparin-induced thrombocytopenia and thrombosis. *Blood* 2003;101(1):31–37.
37. Baldwin ZK, Spitzer AL, Ng VL, et al. Contemporary standards for the diagnosis and treatment of heparin-induced thrombocytopenia (HIT). *Surgery* 2008;143(3):305–312.
38. Greinacher A, Volpel H, Janssens U, et al. Recombinant hirudin (lepirudin) provides safe and effective anticoagulation in patients with heparin-induced thrombocytopenia: a prospective study. *Circulation* 1999;99(1): 73–80.
39. Kovacs MJ. Successful treatment of heparin induced thrombocytopenia (HIT) with fondaparinux. *Thromb Haemost* 2005;93(5):999–1000.
40. van Dongen CJ, Mac Gillary MR, Prins MH. Once versus twice daily LMWH for theititial treatment of venous thromboembolism. *Cochrane Database Syst Rev* 2005;3:CO003074.
41. Merli G, Spiro TE, Olsson CG, et al. Subcutaneous enoxaparin once or twice daily compared with intravenous unfractionated heparin for treatment of venous thromboembolic disease. *Ann Intern Med* 2001;134(3): 191–202.
42. Lee AY, Levine MN, Baker RI, et al. Low-molecular-weight heparin versus a coumarin for the prevention of recurrent venous thromboembolism in patients with cancer. *N Engl J Med* 2003;349(2):146–153.
43. Bergqvist D, Agnelli G, Cohen AT, et al. Duration of prophylaxis against venous thromboembolism with enoxaparin after surgery for cancer. *N Engl J Med* 2002;346(13):975–980.
44. Gross PL, Weitz JI. New anticoagulants for treatment of venous thromboembolism. *Arterioscler Thromb Vasc Biol* 2008;28(3):380–386.
45. Turpie AG, Bauer KA, Eriksson BI, et al. Fondaparinux vs enoxaparin for the prevention of venous thromboembolism in major orthopedic surgery: a meta-analysis of 4 randomized double-blind studies. *Arch Intern Med* 2002;162(16):1833–1840.
46. Wolozinsky M, Yavin YY, Cohen AT. Pharmacological prevention of venous thromboembolism in medical patients at risk. *Am J Cardiovasc Drugs* 2005;5(6):409–415.
47. Agnelli G, Bergqvist D, Cohen AT, et al. Randomized clinical trial of post-operative fondaparinux versus perioperative dalteparin for prevention of venous thromboembolism in high-risk abdominal surgery. *Br J Surg* 2005; 92(10):1212–1220.
48. Eriksson BI, Lassen MR. Duration of prophylaxis against venous thromboembolism with fondaparinux after hip fracture surgery: a multicenter, randomized, placebo-controlled, double-blind study. *Arch Intern Med* 2003;163(11):1337–1342.
49. Buller HR, Davidson BL, Decousus H, et al. Fondaparinux or enoxaparin for the initial treatment of symptomatic deep venous thrombosis: a randomized trial. *Ann Intern Med* 2004;140(11):867–873.
50. Buller HR, Davidson BL, Decousus H, et al. Subcutaneous fondaparinux versus intravenous unfractionated heparin in the initial treatment of pulmonary embolism. *N Engl J Med* 2003;349(18):1695–1702.
51. Buller HR, Cohen AT, Davidson B, et al. Idraparinux versus standard therapy for venous thromboembolic disease. *N Engl J Med* 2007;357(11): 1094–1104.
52. Spyropoulos AC. Investigational treatments of venous thromboembolism. *Expert opin investig drugs* 2007;16(4):431–440.
53. Agnelli G, Gallus A, Goldhaber SZ, et al. Treatment of proximal deep-vein thrombosis with the oral direct factor Xa inhibitor rivaroxaban (BAY 59-7939): the ODIXa-DVT (Oral Direct Factor Xa Inhibitor BAY 59-7939 in Patients With Acute Symptomatic Deep-Vein Thrombosis) study. *Circulation* 2007;116(2):180–187.
54. Weitz JI, Hirsh J, Samama MM. New anticoagulant drugs: the seventh ACCP Conference on Antithrombotic and Thrombolytic Therapy. *Chest* 2004;126(3 suppl):265S–286S.
55. Saiah E, Soares C. Small molecule coagulation cascade inhibitors in the clinic. *Curr Top Med Chem* 2005;5(16):1677–1695.
56. Prandoni P, Lensing AW, Prins MH, et al. Below-knee elastic compression stockings to prevent the post-thrombotic syndrome: a randomized, controlled trial. *Ann Intern Med* 2004;141(4):249–256.
57. Aschwanden M, Labs KH, Engel H, et al. Acute deep vein thrombosis: early mobilization does not increase the frequency of pulmonary embolism. *Thromb Haemost* 2001;85(1):42–46.
58. Partsch H. Ambulation and compression after deep vein thrombosis: dispelling myths. *Semin Vasc Surg* 2005;18(3):148–152.
59. Greenfield LJ, Proctor MC. Twenty-year clinical experience with the Greenfield filter. *Cardiovasc Surg* 1995;3(2):199–205.
60. Berry RE, George JE, Shaver WA. Free-floating deep venous thrombosis. A retrospective analysis. *Ann Surg* 1990;211(6):719–722; discussion 722–713.
61. Langan EM III, Miller RS, Casey WJ III, et al. Prophylactic inferior vena cava filters in trauma patients at high risk: follow-up examination and risk/benefit assessment. *J Vasc Surg* 1999;30(3):484–488.
62. Sugerman HJ, Sugerman EL, Wolfe L, et al. Risks and benefits of gastric bypass in morbidly obese patients with severe venous stasis disease. *Ann Surg* 2001;234(1):41–46.
63. Chiou AC. Bedside placement of IVC filters. *Endovascular Today* 2005;4: 60–63.
64. Decousus H, Leizorovicz A, Parent F, et al. A clinical trial of vena caval filters in the prevention of pulmonary embolism in patients with proximal deep-vein thrombosis. Prevention du Risque d'Embolie Pulmonaire par Interruption Cave Study Group. *N Engl J Med* 1998;338(7):409–415.
65. Meissner MH, Manzo RA, Bergelin RO, et al. Deep venous insufficiency: the relationship between lysis and subsequent reflux. *J Vasc Surg* 1993; 18(4):596–605; discussion 606–608.
66. Semba CP, Dake MD. Iliofemoral deep venous thrombosis: aggressive therapy with catheter-directed thrombolysis. *Radiology* 1994;191(2): 487–494.
67. Mewissen MW, Seabrook GR, Meissner MH, et al. Catheter-directed thrombolysis for lower extremity deep venous thrombosis: report of a national multicenter registry. *Radiology* 1999;211(1):39–49.
68. Elsharawy M, Elzayat E. Early results of thrombolysis vs anticoagulation in iliofemoral venous thrombosis. A randomised clinical trial. *Eur J Vasc Endovasc Surg* 2002;24(3):209–214.
69. Turpie AG. Thrombolytic agents in venous thrombosis. *J Vasc Surg* 1990; 12:196–197.
70. Goldhaber SZ. Pulmonary embolism. *Lancet* 2004;363(9417): 1295–1305.
71. Sharma GV, Folland ED, McIntyre KM, et al. Long-term benefit of thrombolytic therapy in patients with pulmonary embolism. *Vasc Med* 2000; 5(2):91–95.
72. Goldhaber SZ, Haire WD, Feldstein ML, et al. Alteplase versus heparin in acute pulmonary embolism: randomised trial assessing right-ventricular function and pulmonary perfusion. *Lancet* 1993;341(8844):507–511.
73. Jerjes-Sanchez C, Ramirez-Rivera A, Arriaga-Nava R, et al. High dose and short-term streptokinase infusion in patients with pulmonary embolism: prospective with seven-year follow-up trial. *J Thromb Thrombolysis* 2001; 12(3):237–247.
74. Konstantinides S, Geibel A, Olschewski M, et al. Association between thrombolytic treatment and the prognosis of hemodynamically stable patients with major pulmonary embolism: results of a multicenter registry. *Circulation* 1997;96(3):882–888.
75. Eid-Lidt G, Gaspar J, Sandoval J, et al. Combined clot fragmentation and aspiration in patients with acute pulmonary embolism. *Chest* 2008;134(1): 54–60.

76. Eklof B, Kistner RL. Is there a role for thrombectomy in iliofemoral venous thrombosis? *Semin Vasc Surg* 1996;9(1):34–45.
77. Juhan CM, Alimi YS, Barthelemy PJ, et al. Late results of iliofemoral venous thrombectomy. *J Vasc Surg* 1997;25(3):417–422.
78. Meneveau N, Seronde MF, Blonde MC, et al. Management of unsuccessful thrombolysis in acute massive pulmonary embolism. *Chest* 2006;129(4): 1043–1050.
79. Lutter KS, Kerr TM, Roedersheimer LR, et al. Superficial thrombophlebitis diagnosed by duplex scanning. *Surgery* 1991;110(1):42–46.
80. Bjorgell O, Nilsson PE, Jarenros H. Isolated nonfilling of contrast in deep leg vein segments seen on phlebography, and a comparison with color Doppler ultrasound, to assess the incidence of deep leg vein thrombosis. *Angiology* 2000;51(6):451–461.
81. Talbot S. Use of real-time imaging in identifying deep venous obstruction: a preliminary report. *Bruit* 1982;7:41–42.
82. Barrellier MT. Superficial venous thromboses of the legs. *Phlebologie* 1993;46(4):633–639.
83. Blumenberg RM, Barton E, Gelfand ML, et al. Occult deep venous thrombosis complicating superficial thrombophlebitis. *J Vasc Surg* 1998;27(2): 338–343.
84. De Wees M. Non-operative treatment of acute superficial thrombophlebitis and deep femoral thrombosis. In: Ernst CB, Stanley JC, eds. *Current Therapy in Vascular Surgery.* Phildelphia: BC Decker; 1991:952–960.
85. Martinelli I, Cattaneo M, Taioli E, et al. Genetic risk factors for superficial vein thrombosis. *Thromb Haemost* 1999;82(4):1215–1217.
86. Hanson JN, Ascher E, DePippo P, et al. Saphenous vein thrombophlebitis (SVT): a deceptively benign disease. *J Vasc Surg* 1998;27(4):677–680.
87. Meissner MH, Wakefield TW, Ascher E, et al. Acute venous disease: venous thrombosis and venous trauma. *J Vasc Surg* 2007;46(suppl S): 25S–53S.
88. Sullivan V, Wakefield TW. Superficial venous thrombosis. In: Pearce WH, Yao JST, eds. *Trends in Vascular Surgery.* Chicago: Precept Press; 2002: 463–472.
89. Krause U, Kock HJ, Kroger K, et al. Prevention of deep venous thrombosis associated with superficial thrombophlebitis of the leg by early saphenous vein ligation. *Vasa* 1998;27(1):34–38.
90. Gillet JL, Perrin M, Cayman R. Thromboembolic recurrence after superficial thrombophlebitis of the lower limbs. *J Phlebol* 2002;2:103–110.
91. Blattler W, Schwarzenbach B, Largiader J. Superficial vein thrombophlebitis–serious concern or much ado about little? *Vasa* 2008;37(1): 31–38.
92. Verlato F, Zucchetta P, Prandoni P, et al. An unexpectedly high rate of pulmonary embolism in patients with superficial thrombophlebitis of the thigh. *J Vasc Surg* 1999;30(6):1113–1115.
93. Samlaska CP, James WD. Superficial thrombophlebitis: I. Primary hypercoagulable states. *J Am Acad Dermatol* 1990;22(6 pt 1):975–989.
94. Titon JP, Auger D, Grange P, et al. Therapeutic management of superficial venous thrombosis with calcium nadroparin. Dosage testing and comparison with a non-steroidal anti-inflammatory agent. *Ann Cardiol Angeiol (Paris)* 1994;43(3):160–166.
95. [No authors listed.] The Superficial Thrombophlebitis Treatment by Enoxaparin Study Group. A pilot randomized double-blind comparison of a low-molecular-weight heparin, a nonsteroidal anti-inflammatory agent, and placebo in the treatment of superficial vein thrombosis. *Ann Cardiol Angeiol Paris* 2003;43(3):160–166.
96. Group TVI. High vs. low doses of low-molecular-weight heparin for the treatment of superficial vein thrombosis of the legs: a double-blind, randomized trial. *J Thromb Haemost* 2005;3:1152–1157.
97. Belcaro G, Nicolaides AN, Errichi BM, et al. Superficial thrombophlebitis of the legs: a randomized, controlled, follow-up study. *Angiology* 1999; 50(7):523–529.
98. Marchiori A, Verlato F, Sabbion P, et al. High versus low doses of unfractionated heparin for the treatment of superficial thrombophlebitis of the leg. A prospective, controlled, randomized study. *Haematologica* 2002; 87(5):523–527.
99. Lozano FS, Almazan A. Low-molecular-weight heparin versus saphenofemoral disconnection for the treatment of above-knee greater saphenous thrombophlebitis: a prospective study. *Vasc Endovascular Surg* 2003; 37(6):415–420.
100. Sullivan V, Denk PM, Sonnad SS, et al. Ligation versus anticoagulation: treatment of above-knee superficial thrombophlebitis not involving the deep venous system. *J Am Coll Surg* 2001;193(5):556–562.
101. Hafner CD, Cranley JJ, Krause RJ, et al. A Method of managing superficial thrombophlebitis. *Surgery* 1964;55:201–206.
102. Ascer E, Lorensen E, Pollina RM, et al. Preliminary results of a nonoperative approach to saphenofemoral junction thrombophlebitis. *J Vasc Surg* 1995;22(5):616–621.
103. Husni EA, Williams WA. Superficial thrombophlebitis of lower limbs. *Surgery* 1982;91(1):70–74.
104. Caggiati A, Bergan JJ, Gloviczki P, et al. Nomenclature of the veins of the lower limbs: an international interdisciplinary consensus statement. *J Vasc Surg* 2002;36(2):416–422.
105. Morrison C, Dalsing MC. Signs and symptoms of saphenous nerve injury after greater saphenous vein stripping: prevalence, severity, and relevance for modern practice. *J Vasc Surg* 2003;38(5):886–890.
106. Corrales NE, Irvine A, McGuinness CL, et al. Incidence and pattern of long saphenous vein duplication and its possible implications for recurrence after varicose vein surgery. *Br J Surg* 2002;89(3):323–326.
107. Caggiati A, Bergan JJ. The saphenous vein: derivation of its name and its relevant anatomy. *J Vasc Surg* 2002;35(1):172–175.
108. Caggiati A. Fascial relationships of the short saphenous vein. *J Vasc Surg* 2001;34(2):241–246.
109. Mozes G, Gloviczki P, Menawat SS, et al. Surgical anatomy for endoscopic subfascial division of perforating veins. *J Vasc Surg* 1996;24(5):800–808.
110. Browse NL, Burnand KG, Thomas ML. Disease of the veins: pathology, diagnosis, and treatment. London: Edward Arnold; 1988:53–69.
111. Giordano JM, Trout HH III. Anomalies of the inferior vena cava. *J Vasc Surg* 1986;3(6):924–928.
112. Nehler M, Moneta GL. The lower extermity venous disease: I. Anatomy and physiology. *Perspect Vasc Surg* 1991;4:104.
113. Moreno AH, Katz AI, Gold LD, et al. Mechanics of distension of dog veins and other very thin-walled tubular structures. *Circ Res* 1970;27(6): 1069–1080.
114. Moneta GL, Bedford G, Beach K, et al. Duplex ultrasound assessment of venous diameters, peak velocities, and flow patterns. *J Vasc Surg* 1988; 8(3):286–91.
115. Lurie F, Kistner RL, Eklof B, et al. Mechanism of venous valve closure and role of the valve in circulation: a new concept. *J Vasc Surg* 2003;38(5): 955–961.
116. van Bemmelen PS, Bedford G, Beach K, et al. Quantitative segmental evaluation of venous valvular reflux with duplex ultrasound scanning. *J Vasc Surg* 1989;10(4):425–431.
117. Mattos MA, Summer D. Direct noninvasive tests (duplex scan) for the evaluation of chronic venous obstruction and valvular incompetence. In: Gloviczki P, Yao JST, eds. *Handbook of Venous Disorders.* London: Arnold; 2001:120–131.
118. van Bemmelen PS, Beach K, Bedford G, et al. The mechanism of venous valve closure. Its relationship to the velocity of reverse flow. *Arch Surg* 1990;125(5):617–619.
119. Raju S, Fredericks R, Lishman P, et al. Observations on the calf venous pump mechanism: determinants of postexercise pressure. *J Vasc Surg* 1993;17(3):459–469.
120. Brand FN, Dannenberg AL, Abbott RD, et al. The epidemiology of varicose veins: the Framingham Study. *Am J Prev Med* 1988;4(2):96–101.
121. Coon WW, Willis PW III, Keller JB. Venous thromboembolism and other venous disease in the Tecumseh community health study. *Circulation* 1973;48(4):839–846.
122. Dale WL, Cranley JJ, DeWeese JA, et al. Symposium: management of varicose veins. *Contemp Surg* 1975;6:86.
123. Criqui MH, Jamosmos M, Fronek A, et al. Chronic venous disease in an ethnically diverse population: the San Diego Population Study. *Am J Epidemiol* 2003;158(5):448–456.
124. Baker SR, Stacey MC, Jopp-McKay AG, et al. Epidemiology of chronic venous ulcers. *Br J Surg* 1988;78(7):864–867.
125. Heit JA, Rooke TW, Silverstein MD, et al. Trends in the incidence of venous stasis syndrome and venous ulcer: a 25-year population-based study. *J Vasc Surg* 2001;33(5):1022–1027.
126. Nicolaides AN. Investigation of chronic venous insufficiency: a consensus statement (France, March 5–9, 1997). *Circulation* 2000;102(20):E126–E163.
127. Rabe EP-FF, Pannier-Fischer F, Bromen K, et al. Bonner Venestudie der Deutschen Gesellschaft fur Phlebologie-epidemiologische Untersuchung zur Frage der Haufigkeit und Auspragung von chronischen Venekrankheiten in der stadtischen und landlichen Wohnbevolkerung. *Phlebologie* 2003;32:1–14.
128. Carpentier PH, Maricq HR, Biro C, et al. Prevalence, risk factors, and clinical patterns of chronic venous disorders of lower limbs: a population-based study in France. *J Vasc Surg* 2004;40(4):650–659.
129. Chiesa R, Marone EM, Limoni C, et al. Demographic factors and their relationship with the presence of CVI signs in Italy: the 24-cities cohort study. *Eur J Vasc Endovasc Surg* 2005;30(6):674–680.
130. Chiesa R, Marone EM, Limoni C, et al. Chronic venous insufficiency in Italy: the 24-cities cohort study. *Eur J Vasc Endovasc Surg* 2005;30(4): 422–429.
131. Jawien A, Grzela T, Ochwat A. Prevalence of chronic venous insufficiency in men and women in Poland: multicenter cross-sectional study in 40095 patients. *Phlebology* 2003;18:110–121.
132. Jukkola TM, Makivaara LA, Luukkaala T, et al. The effects of parity, oral contraceptive use and hormone replacement therapy on the incidence of varicose veins. *J Obstet Gynaecol* 2006;26(5):448–451.
133. Neglen P, Thrasher TL, Raju S. Venous outflow obstruction: an underestimated contributor to chronic venous disease. *J Vasc Surg* 2003;38(5): 879–885.
134. O'Donnell TF Jr. Chronic venous insufficiency: an overview of epidemiology, classification, and anatomic considerations. *Semin Vasc Surg* 1988;1:60.
135. Eklof BG, Kistner RL, Masuda EM. Venous bypass and valve reconstruction: long-term efficacy. *Vasc Med* 1998;3(2):157–164.
136. May R, Thurner J. The cause of the predominately sinistral occurence of thrombosis of the pelvic veins. *Angiology* 1957;8:419–427.
137. Ehrich WE, Krumbhaar EB. A frequent obstructive anmaly of the mouth of the left common iliac vein. *Am Heart J* 1943;26:737–750.
138. McMurrich J. The occurrence of congential adhesions in the common iliac veins, and their relation to thrombosis of the femoral and iliac veins. *Am J Med Sci* 1943;135:342–346.
139. Cockett FB, Thomas ML, Negus D. Iliac vein compression. Its relation to iliofemoral thrombosis and the post-thrombotic syndrome. *Br Med J* 1967;2(5543):14–19.

140. Cockett FB, Thomas ML. The iliac compression syndrome. *Br J Surg* 1965;52(10):816–821.
141. Kibbe MR, Ujiki M, Goodwin AL, et al. Iliac vein compression in an asymptomatic patient population. *J Vasc Surg* 2004;39:937–943.
142. Lalka SG. Management of chronic obstructive venous disease of the lower extermity. In: Rutherford RB, ed. *Vascular Surgery*, 4th ed. Phildelphia: WB Saunders; 1995:1862–1882.
143. Raju S, Neglen P. High prevalence of nonthrombotic iliac vein lesions in chronic venous disease: a permissive role in pathogenicity. *J Vasc Surg* 2006;44:136–144.
144. Browse NL, Burnand KG, Thomas ML. Disease of the veins: pathology, diagnosis, and treatment. London: Edward Arnold; 1988:271–287.
145. Martin-Pedrosa JM, Del Blanco I, Carrera S, et al. Intravascular lipoma of the external iliac vein and common femoral vein. *Eur J Vasc Endovasc Surg* 2002;23(5):470–472.
146. Kistner RL, Eklof B, Masuda EM. Diagnosis of chronic venous disease of the lower extremities: the "CEAP" classification. *Mayo Clin Proc* 1996; 71(4):338–345.
147. Labropoulos N. CEAP in clinical practice. *Vasc Surg* 1997;31:224–225.
148. Johnson BF, Manzo RA, Bergelin RO, et al. Relationship between changes in the deep venous system and the development of the postthrombotic syndrome after an acute episode of lower limb deep vein thrombosis: a one- to six-year follow-up. *J Vasc Surg* 1995;21(February):307–313.
149. Labropoulos N, Delis K, Nicolaides AN, et al. The role of the distribution and anatomic extent of reflux in the development of signs and symptoms in chronic venous insufficiency. *J Vasc Surg* 1996;23(3):504–510.
150. Labropoulos N, Giannoukas AD, Nicolaides AN, et al. The role of venous reflux and calf muscle pump function in nonthrombotic chronic venous insufficiency. Correlation with severity of signs and symptoms. *Arch Surg* 1996;131(4):403–406.
151. Labropoulos N, Leon M, Geroulakos G, et al. Venous hemodynamic abnormalities in patients with leg ulceration. *Am J Surg* 1995;169(6): 572–574.
152. Labropoulos N, Giannoukas AD, Nicolaides AN, et al. New insights into the pathophysiologic condition of venous ulceration with color-flow duplex imaging: implications for treatment? *J Vasc Surg* 1995;22(1): 45–50.
153. Hanrahan LM, Araki CT, Rodriguez AA, et al. Distribution of valvular incompetence in patients with venous stasis ulceration. *J Vasc Surg* 1991;13(6):805–811; discussion 811–802.
154. Barwell JR, Davies CE, Deacon J, et al. Comparison of surgery and compression with compression alone in chronic venous ulceration (ESCHAR study): randomised controlled trial. *Lancet* 2004;363(9424):1854–1859.
155. Yamaki T, Nozaki M, Sasaki K. Color duplex ultrasound in the assessment of primary venous leg ulceration. *Dermatol Surg* 1998;24(10):1124–1128.
156. Plate G, Brudin L, Eklof B, et al. Physiologic and therapeutic aspects in congenital vein valve aplasia of the lower limb. *Ann Surg* 1983;198(2): 229–233.
157. Rose SS, Ahmed A. Some thoughts on the aetiology of varicose veins. *J Cardiovasc Surg (Torino)* 1986;27(5):534–543.
158. Clarke H, Smith SR, Vasdekis SN, et al. Role of venous elasticity in the development of varicose veins. *Br J Surg* 1989;76(6):577–580.
159. Kistner RL, Eklof B, Masuda EM. Deep venous valve reconstruction. *Cardiovasc Surg* 1995;3(2):129–140.
160. Raju S, Hardy JD. Technical options in venous valve reconstruction. *Am J Surg* 1997;173(4):301–307.
161. Perrin M. Reconstructive surgery for deep venous reflux: a report on 144 cases. *Cardiovasc Surg* 2000;8(4):246–255.
162. Masuda EM, Kistner RL. Long-term results of venous valve reconstruction: a four- to twenty-one-year follow-up. *J Vasc Surg* 1994;19(3):391–403.
163. Raju S, Fredericks RK, Hudson CA, et al. Venous valve station changes in "primary" and postthrombotic reflux: an analysis of 149 cases. *Ann Vasc Surg* 2000;14(3):193–199.
164. Killewich LA, Bedford GR, Beach KW, et al. Spontaneous lysis of deep venous thrombi: rate and outcome. *J Vasc Surg* 1989;9(1):89–97.
165. Meissner MH, Moneta G, Burnand K, et al. The hemodynamics and diagnosis of venous disease. *J Vasc Surg* 2007;46(suppl S):4S–24S.
166. Kugler C, Strunk M, Rudofsky G. Venous pressure dynamics of the healthy human leg. Role of muscle activity, joint mobility and anthropometric factors. *J Vasc Res* 2001;38(1):20–29.
167. Araki CT, Back TL, Padberg FT, et al. The significance of calf muscle pump function in venous ulceration. *J Vasc Surg* 1994;20(6):872–877; discussion 878–879.
168. Back TL, Padberg FT Jr, Araki CT, et al. Limited range of motion is a significant factor in venous ulceration. *J Vasc Surg* 1995;22(5):519–523.
169. Padberg FT Jr, Johnston MV, Sisto SA. Structured exercise improves calf muscle pump function in chronic venous insufficiency: a randomized trial. *J Vasc Surg* 2004;39(1):79–87.
170. Pappas PJ, Duran WN, Hobson RW. Pathology and cellular physiology of chronic venous insufficiency. In: Gloviczki P, Yao JST, eds. *Handbook of Venous Disorders*. New York, NY: Arnold; 2001:58–67.
171. Stanley AC, Park HY, Phillips TJ, et al. Reduced growth of dermal fibroblasts from chronic venous ulcers can be stimulated with growth factors. *J Vasc Surg* 1997;26(6):994–999; discussion 999–1001.
172. Killewich LA, Martin R, Cramer M, et al. Pathophysiology of venous claudication. *J Vasc Surg* 1984;1(4):507–511.
173. Raju S, Owen S Jr, Neglen P. The clinical impact of iliac venous stents in the management of chronic venous insufficiency. *J Vasc Surg* 2002;35(1): 8–15.
174. Danielsson G, Eklof B, Grandinetti A, et al. Deep axial reflux, an important contributor to skin changes or ulcer in chronic venous disease. *J Vasc Surg* 2003;38(6):1336–1341.
175. Labropoulos N, Volteas N, Leon M, et al. The role of venous outflow obstruction in patients with chronic venous dysfunction. *Arch Surg* 1997; 132(1):46–51.
176. Eklof B, Rutherford RB, Bergan JJ, et al. Revision of the CEAP classification for chronic venous disorders: consensus statement. *J Vasc Surg* 2004; 40(6):1248–1252.
177. Porter JM, Moneta GL. Reporting standards in venous disease: an update. International Consensus Committee on Chronic Venous Disease. *J Vasc Surg* 1995;21(4):635–645.
178. Rutherford RB, Padberg FT Jr, Comerota AJ, et al. Venous severity scoring: an adjunct to venous outcome assessment. *J Vasc Surg* 2000;31(6): 1307–1312.
179. Lamping DL, Schroter S, Kurz X, et al. Evaluation of outcomes in chronic venous disorders of the leg: development of a scientifically rigorous, patient-reported measure of symptoms and quality of life. *J Vasc Surg* 2003;37(2):410–419.
180. Launois R, Reboul-Marty J, Henry B. Construction and validation of a quality of life questionnaire in chronic lower limb venous insufficiency (CIVIQ). *Qual Life Res* 1996;5(6):539–554.
181. Garratt AM, Macdonald LM, Ruta DA, et al. Towards measurement of outcome for patients with varicose veins. *Qual Health Care* 1993;2(1): 5–10.
182. Smith JJ, Guest MG, Greenhalgh RM, et al. Measuring the quality of life in patients with venous ulcers. *J Vasc Surg* 2000;31(4):642–649.
183. Wong JK, Duncan JL, Nichols DM. Whole-leg duplex mapping for varicose veins: observations on patterns of reflux in recurrent and primary legs, with clinical correlation. *Eur J Vasc Endovasc Surg* 2003;25(3): 267–275.
184. Mercer KG, Scott DJ, Berridge DC. Preoperative duplex imaging is required before all operations for primary varicose veins. *Br J Surg* 1998; 85(11):1495–1497.
185. Labropoulos N, Mansour MA, Kang SS, et al. New insights into perforator vein incompetence. *Eur J Vasc Endovasc Surg* 1999;18(3):228–234.
186. Labropoulos N, Tiongson J, Pryor L, et al. Definition of venous reflux in lower-extremity veins. *J Vasc Surg* 2003;38(4):793–798.
187. Lynch TG, Dalsing MC, Ouriel K, et al. Developments in diagnosis and classification of venous disorders: non-invasive diagnosis. *Cardiovasc Surg* 1999;7(2):160–178.
188. Labropoulos N, Giannoukas AD, Delis K, et al. The impact of isolated lesser saphenous vein system incompetence on clinical signs and symptoms of chronic venous disease. *J Vasc Surg* 2000;32(5):954–960.
189. Mantoni M, Larsen L, Lund JO, et al. Evaluation of chronic venous disease in the lower limbs: comparison of five diagnostic methods. *Br J Radiol* 2002;75(895):578–583.
190. Stanson AW, Breen JF. Computed tomography and magnetic resonance imaging in venous disorders. In: Gloviczki P, Yao JST, eds. *Handbook of Venous Disorders*. London: Arnold; 2001:153–176.
191. Wolpert L. Magnetic resonance venography in the diagnosis and management of May-Thurner syndrome. *Vasc Endovascular Surg* 2002;36:51–57.
192. Butty S, Hagspiel KD, Leung DA, et al. Body MR venography. *Radiol Clin North Am* 2002;40(4):899–919.
193. Coakley FV, Varghese SL, Hricak H. CT and MRI of pelvic varices in women. *J Comput Assist Tomogr* 1999;23(3):429–434.
194. Bays RA, Healy DA, Atnip RG, et al. Validation of air plethysmography, photoplethysmography, and duplex ultrasonography in the evaluation of severe venous stasis. *J Vasc Surg* 1994;20(5):721–727.
195. Nicolaides AN, Christopoulos D. Quantification of venous reflux and outflow obstruction with air-plethysmography. In: Berstein EF, ed. *Vasculas Diagnosis*. St. Louis, MO: Mosby; 1993:915–921.
196. Criado E, Farber MA, Marston WA, et al. The role of air plethysmography in the diagnosis of chronic venous insufficiency. *J Vasc Surg* 1998;27(4): 660–670.
197. Cordts PR, Hartono C, LaMorte WW, et al. Physiologic similarities between extremities with varicose veins and with chronic venous insufficiency utilizing air plethysmography. *Am J Surg* 1992;164(3):260–264.
198. Neglen P, Raju S. Proximal lower extremity chronic venous outflow obstruction: recognition and treatment. *Semin Vasc Surg* 2002;15(1):57–64.
199. Neglen P, Raju S. Intravascular ultrasound scan evaluation of the obstructed vein. *J Vasc Surg* 2002;35(4):694–700.
200. Kistner RL, Ferris EB, Randhawa G, et al. A method of performing descending venography. *J Vasc Surg* 1986;4(5):464–468.
201. Raju S, Fredericks RK, Neglen PN, et al. Durability of venous valve reconstruction techniques for "primary" and postthrombotic reflux. *J Vasc Surg* 1996;23(2):357–366; discussion 366–357.
202. Cheatle TR, Perrin M. Venous valve repair: early results in fifty-two cases. *J Vasc Surg* 1994;19(3):404–413.
203. Kistner RL, Sparkuhl MD. Surgery in acute and chronic venous disease. *Surgery* 1979;85(1):31–43.
204. Nicolaides AN, Hussein MK, Szendro G, et al. The relation of venous ulceration with ambulatory venous pressure measurements. *J Vasc Surg* 1993;17(2):414–419.
205. Raju S. New approaches to the diagnosis and treatment of venous obstruction. *J Vasc Surg* 1986;4(1):42–54.
206. Partsch B, Partsch H. Calf compression pressure required to achieve venous closure from supine to standing positions. *J Vasc Surg* 2005;42(4): 734–738.

207. Partsch H, Menzinger G, Mostbeck A. Inelastic leg compression is more effective to reduce deep venous refluxes than elastic bandages. *Dermatol Surg* 1999;25(9):695–700.
208. Benigni JP, Sadoun S, Allaert FA, et al. Efficacy of Class 1 elastic compression stockings in the early stages of chronic venous disease. A comparative study. *Int Angiol* 2003;22(4):383–392.
209. Partsch H, Winiger J, Lun B. Compression stockings reduce occupational leg swelling. *Dermatol Surg* 2004;30(5):737–743; discussion 743.
210. Labropoulos N, Leon M, Volteas N, et al. Acute and long-term effect of elastic stockings in patients with varicose veins. *Int Angiol* 1994;13(2):119–123.
211. Ibegbuna V, Delis KT, Nicolaides AN, et al. Effect of elastic compression stockings on venous hemodynamics during walking. *J Vasc Surg* 2003;37(2):420–425.
212. Partsch H, Menzinger G, Borst-Krafek B, et al. Does thigh compression improve venous hemodynamics in chronic venous insufficiency? *J Vasc Surg* 2002;36(5):948–952.
213. Partsch H. Mechanism and effects of compression therapy. In: Bergan JJ, ed. *The Vein Book*. Burlington, MA: Elsevier; 2007:103–109.
214. Murthy G, Ballard RE, Breit GA, et al. Intramuscular pressures beneath elastic and inelastic leggings. *Ann Vasc Surg* 1994;8(6):543–548.
215. van Geest AJ, Veraart JC, Nelemans P, et al. The effect of medical elastic compression stockings with different slope values on edema. Measurements underneath three different types of stockings. *Dermatol Surg* 2000;26(3):244–247.
216. Nehler MR, Moneta GL, Woodard DM, et al. Perimalleolar subcutaneous tissue pressure effects of elastic compression stockings. *J Vasc Surg* 1993;18(5):783–788.
217. Jones NA, Webb PJ, Rees RI, et al. A physiological study of elastic compression stockings in venous disorders of the leg. *Br J Surg* 1980;67(8):569–572.
218. Junger M, Steins A, Hahn M, et al. Microcirculatory dysfunction in chronic venous insufficiency (CVI). *Microcirculation* 2000;7(6 pt 2):S3–S12.
219. Franzeck UK, Haselbach P, Speiser D, et al. Microangiopathy of cutaneous blood and lymphatic capillaries in chronic venous insufficiency (CVI). *Yale J Biol Med* 1993;66(1):37–46.
220. Dai G, Tsukurov O, Orkin RW, et al. An in vitro cell culture system to study the influence of external pneumatic compression on endothelial function. *J Vasc Surg* 2000;32(5):977–987.
221. Abu-Own A, Shami SK, Chittenden SJ, et al. Microangiopathy of the skin and the effect of leg compression in patients with chronic venous insufficiency. *J Vasc Surg* 1994;19(6):1074–1083.
222. Murphy MA, Joyce WP, Condron C, et al. A reduction in serum cytokine levels parallels healing of venous ulcers in patients undergoing compression therapy. *Eur J Vasc Endovasc Surg* 2002;23(4):349–352.
223. Mayrovitz HN. Compression-induced pulsatile blood flow changes in human legs. *Clin Physiol* 1998;18(2):117–124.
224. Kakkos SK, Perrin M, Cutting KF, et al. Conservative treatments: medical therapies: medical/drug therapies. In: Labropoulos N, Stansky G, eds. *Venous and Lymphatic Diseases*. New York, NY: Taylor and Francis Group; 2006:257–276.
225. Chauveau MVF, Houot B. Lack of tourniquet effect of below-knee stockings. *Phlebology* 2000;15(2):60–63.
226. Griswold ME, Monetta GL. Nonoperative treatment of chronic venous insufficiency. In: Rutherford RB, ed. *Vascular Surgery*, 6th ed. Philadelphia: Elsevier; 2005:2241–2250.
227. Mayrovitz HN, Sims N. Effects of ankle-to-knee external pressures on skin blood perfusion under and distal to compression. *Adv Skin Wound Care* 2003;16(4):198–202.
228. Kolbach DN, Sandbrink MWC, Hamulyak HAM, et al. Non-pharmaceutical measures for prevention of post-thrombotic syndrome [Review]. In: *The Cochrane Collaboration*. John Wiley and Sons. The Cochrane Library; 2007(3):11–14.
229. Partsch H, Flour M, Coleridge-Smith P, et al. Evidence based compression-therapy. An initiative of the International Union of Phlebology (IUP). *VASA* 2004;34(suppl 63):3–39.
230. Mayberry JC, Moneta GL, Taylor LM Jr, et al. Fifteen-year results of ambulatory compression therapy for chronic venous ulcers. *Surgery* 1991;109(5):575–581.
231. Motykie GD, Caprini JA, Arcelus JI, et al. Evaluation of therapeutic compression stockings in the treatment of chronic venous insufficiency. *Dermatol Surg* 1999;25(2):116–120.
232. Nelson EA, Bell-Syer SEM, Cullum NA. Compression for preventing recurrence of venous ulcers. *Cochrane Database Syst Rev* 2000;(4):CD002303.
233. Korn P, Patel ST, Heller JA, et al. Why insurers should reimburse for compression stockings in patients with chronic venous stasis. *J Vasc Surg* 2002;35(5):950–957.
234. Erickson CA, Lanza DJ, Karp DL, et al. Healing of venous ulcers in an ambulatory care program: the roles of chronic venous insufficiency and patient compliance. *J Vasc Surg* 1995;22(5):629–636.
235. Nicoloff AD, Moneta, GL, Porter JM. Compression treatment of chronic venous insufficiency. In Gloviczki P, Yao JST, eds. *Handbook of Venous Disorders*, 2nd ed. London: Arnold; 2001:303–308.
236. Mani R,Vowden K, Nelson EA. Intermittent pneumatic compression for treating venous leg ulcers [Review]. *Cochrane Database Syst Rev* 2008;(2):CD001899.
237. Coleridge-Smith PSS, Hasty J, Scurr JH. Sequential gradient pneumatic compression enhances venous ulcer healing. A randomized trial. *Surg* 1990;108:871–875.
238. Kan YM, Delis KT. Hemodynamic effects of supervised calf muscle exercise in patients with venous leg ulceration: a prospective controlled study. *Arch Surg* 2001;136(12):1364–1369.
239. Pittler MH, Ernst E. Horse-chestnut seed extract for chronic venous insufficiency. A criteria-based systematic review. *Arch Dermatol* 1998;134(11):1356–1360.
240. Jull A, Arroll B, Parag V, et al. Pentoxifylline for treating venous leg ulcers. *Cochrane Database Syst Rev* 2007;(3):CD00173.
241. Alinovi A, Bassissi P, Pini M. Systemic administration of antibiotics in the management of venous ulcers. A randomized clinical trial. *J Am Acad Dermatol* 1986;15(2 pt 1):186–191.
242. Chukwuemeka NE, Phillips TJ. Venous ulcers. *Clin Dermatol* 2007;25(1):121–130.
243. Stacey MC, Mata SD, Trengove NJ, et al. Randomised double-blind placebo controlled trial of topical autologous platelet lysate in venous ulcer healing. *Eur J Vasc Endovasc Surg* 2000;20(3):296–301.
244. Khan MN, Davies CG. Advances in the management of leg ulcers–the potential role of growth factors. *Int Wound J* 2006;3(2):113–120.
245. Palfreyman SJ, Nelson EA, Lochiel R, et al. Dressings for healing venous leg ulcers. *Cochrane Database Syst Rev* 2006;3:CD001103.
246. Lau J, Tatsioni E, O'Donnell TF. Usual care in management of chronic wounds: a review of the recent literature. Quality AfHRa. 2005;:513–516.
247. Limova M, Troyer-Caudle J. Controlled, randomized clinical trial of 2 hydrocolloid dressings in the management of venous insufficiency ulcers. *J Vasc Nurs* 2002;20(1):22–32; quiz 33–34.
248. Hohenleutner U, Walther T, Wenig M, et al. Leg telangiectasia treatment with a 1.5 ms pulsed dye laser, ice cube cooling of the skin and 595 vs 600 nm: preliminary results. *Lasers Surg Med* 1998;23(2):72–78.
249. Bernstein EF, Kornbluth S, Brown DB, et al. Treatment of spider veins using a 10 millisecond pulse-duration frequency-doubled neodymium YAG laser. *Dermatol Surg* 1999;25(4):316–320.
250. Villavicencio JL. Sclerotherapy guidelines. In: Gloviczki P, Yao JST, eds. *Handbook of Venous Disorders*, 2nd ed. New York: Arnold; 2001:253–266.
251. Kern P, Ramelet AA, Wutschert R, et al. Single-blind, randomized study comparing chromated glycerin, polidocanol solution, and polidocanol foam for treatment of telangiectatic leg veins. *Dermatol Surg* 2004;30(3):367–372; discussion 372.
252. Alos J, Carreno P, Lopez JA, et al. Efficacy and safety of sclerotherapy using polidocanol foam: a controlled clinical trial. *Eur J Vasc Endovasc Surg* 2006;31(1):101–107.
253. Belcaro G, Cesarone MR, Di Renzo A, et al. Foam-sclerotherapy, surgery, sclerotherapy, and combined treatment for varicose veins: a 10-year, prospective, randomized, controlled, trial (VEDICO trial). *Angiology* 2003;54(3):307–315.
254. Miyazaki K, Nishibe T, Sata F, et al. Stripping operation with sclerotherapy for primary varicose veins due to greater saphenous vein reflux: three-year results. *World J Surg* 2003;27(5):551–553.
255. Iwamoto S, Ikeda M, Kawasaki T, et al. Treatment of varicose veins: an assessment of intraoperative and postoperative compression sclerotherapy. *Ann Vasc Surg* 2003;17(3):290–295.
256. Field C. Sclerosing solutions. In: Bergan JJ, ed. *The Vein Book*. Boston, MA: Elsevier Academic Press; 2007:125–131.
257. Hamel-Desnos C, Desnos P, Wollmann JC, et al. Evaluation of the efficacy of polidocanol in the form of foam compared with liquid form in sclerotherapy of the greater saphenous vein: initial results. *Dermatol Surg* 2003;29(12):1170–1175; discussion 1175.
258. Goldman M. Complications and adverse sequelae of sclerotherpy. In: Bergan JJ, ed. *The Vein Book*. Burlington, MA: Elsevier Academic Press; 2007:139–155.
259. Guex JJ, Allaert FA, Gillet JL, et al. Immediate and midterm complications of sclerotherapy: report of a prospective multicenter registry of 12,173 sclerotherapy sessions. *Dermatol Surg* 2005;31(2):123–128; discussion 128.
260. Scultetus AH, Villavicencio JL, Kao TC, et al. Microthrombectomy reduces postsclerotherapy pigmentation: multicenter randomized trial. *J Vasc Surg* 2003;38(5):896–903.
261. Morrison N, Neuhardt DL, Rogers CR, et al. Comparisons of side effects using air and carbon dioxide foam for endovenous chemical ablation. *J Vasc Surg* 2008;47(4):830–836.
262. Bergan JJ. Varicose veins: hooks, clamps, and suction. Application of new techniques to enhance varicose vein surgery. *Semin Vasc Surg* 2002;15(1):21–26.
263. de Roos KP, Nieman FH, Neumann HA. Ambulatory phlebectomy versus compression sclerotherapy: results of a randomized controlled trial. *Dermatol Surg* 2003;29(3):221–226.
264. Ramelet AA. Complications of ambulatory phlebectomy. *Dermatol Surg* 1997;23(10):947–954.
265. Smith SR, Goldman MP. Tumescent anesthesia in ambulatory phlebectomy. *Dermatol Surg* 1998;24(4):453–456.
266. Aremu MA, Mahendran B, Butcher W, et al. Prospective randomized controlled trial: conventional versus powered phlebectomy. *J Vasc Surg* 2004;39(1):88–94.
267. Criado E, Lujan S, Izquierdo L, et al. Conservative hemodynamic surgery for varicose veins. *Semin Vasc Surg* 2002;15(1):27–33.

268. Raju S, Easterwood L, Fountain T, et al. Saphenectomy in the presence of chronic venous obstruction. *Surgery* 1998;123(6):637–644.
269. Padberg FT, Pappas PJ, Araki CT. Hemodynamic and clinical improvement after superficial vein ablation in primary combined venous insufficiency with ulceration. *J Vasc Surg* 1997;26:169.
270. Dalsing MC. Lower extremity varicose vein disease. In: Cameron JL, ed. *Current Surgical Therapy*, 7th ed. St. Louis: Mosby; 2001:992–998.
271. Dwerryhouse S, Davies B, Harradine K, et al. Stripping the long saphenous vein reduces the rate of reoperation for recurrent varicose veins: five-year results of a randomized trial. *J Vasc Surg* 1999;29(4):589–592.
272. Larson RH, Lofgren EP, Myers TT, et al. Long-term results after vein surgery. Study of 1,000 cases after 10 years. *Mayo Clin Proc* 1974;49(2): 114–117.
273. Winterborn RJ, Foy C, Earnshaw JJ. Causes of varicose vein recurrence: late results of a randomized controlled trial of stripping the long saphenous vein. *J Vasc Surg* 2004;40(4):634–639.
274. Chandler JG, Pichot O, Sessa C, et al. Treatment of primary venous insufficiency by endovenous saphenous vein obliteration. *J Vasc Surg* 2000;34: 201.
275. Lurie F, Creton D, Eklof B, et al. Prospective randomized study of endovenous radiofrequency obliteration (closure procedure) versus ligation and stripping in a selected patient population (EVOLVeS Study). *J Vasc Surg* 2003;38(2):207–214.
276. Merchant RF, Pichot O. Long-term outcomes of endovenous radiofrequency obliteration of saphenous reflux as a treatment for superficial venous insufficiency. *J Vasc Surg* 2005;42(3):502–509; discussion 509.
277. Lurie F, Creton D, Eklof B, et al. Prospective randomised study of endovenous radiofrequency obliteration (closure) versus ligation and vein stripping (EVOLVeS): two-year follow-up. *Eur J Vasc Endovasc Surg* 2005; 29(1):67–73.
278. Proebstle TM, Vago B, Alm J, et al. Treatment of the incompetent great saphenous vein by endovenous radiofrequency powered segmental thermal ablation: first clinical experience. *J Vasc Surg* 2008;47(1):151–156.
279. Navarro L, Min RJ, Bone C. Endovenous laser: a new minimally invasive method of treatment for varicose veins–preliminary observations using an 810 nm diode laser. *Dermatol Surg* 2001;27(2):117–122.
280. Proebstle TM, Gul D, Kargl A, et al. Endovenous laser treatment of the lesser saphenous vein with a 940-nm diode laser: early results. *Dermatol Surg* 2003;29(4):357–361.
281. Min RJ, Khilnani N, Zimmet SE. Endovenous laser treatment of saphenous vein reflux: long-term results. *J Vasc Interv Radiol* 2003;14(8): 991–996.
282. Myers K, Fris R, Jolley D. Treatment of varicose veins by endovenous laser therapy: assessment of results by ultrasound surveillance. *Med J Aust* 2006;185(4):199–202.
283. Myers K, Cluugh A. Treatment of small saphenous vein reflux. In: Bergan JJ, ed. *The Vein Book*. Burlington, MA: Elsevier Academic Press; 2007: 139–155.
284. Neglen P, Einarsson E, Eklof B. The functional long-term value of different types of treatment for saphenous vein incompetence. *J Cardiovasc Surg (Torino)* 1993;34(4):295–301.
285. Rigby KA, Palfreyman SJ, Beverley C, et al. Surgery versus sclerotherapy for the treatment of varicose veins. *Cochrane Database Syst Rev* 2004;(4): CD004980.
286. Keith LM Jr, Smead WL. Saphenous vein stripping and its complications. *Surg Clin North Am* 1983;63(6):1303–1312.
287. Ramsheyi A, Soury P, Saliou C, et al. Inadvertent arterial injury during saphenous vein stripping: three cases and therapeutic strategies. *Arch Surg* 1998;133(10):1120–1123.
288. Seror P. Sural nerve neuropathy (external saphenous) linked to a disease of the small saphenous vein. Apropos of 5 cases [in French]. *J Mal Vasc* 2000; 25(2):128–131.
289. Depalma R. Management of incompetent perforators: conventional techniques. In: Gloviczki P, ed. *Handbook of Venous Disorders,* 2nd ed. London: Arnold; 2001:384–390.
290. Gloviczki P, Bergan JJ, Menawat SS, et al. Safety, feasibility, and early efficacy of subfascial endoscopic perforator surgery: a preliminary report from the North American registry. *J Vasc Surg* 1997;25(1):94–105.
291. Gloviczki P, Bergan JJ, Rhodes JM, et al. Mid-term results of endoscopic perforator vein interruption for chronic venous insufficiency: lessons learned from the North American subfascial endoscopic perforator surgery registry. The North American Study Group. *J Vasc Surg* 1999;29(3): 489–502.
292. Kalra M, Gloviczki P. Subfascial endoscopic perforator vein surgery: who benefits? *Semin Vasc Surg* 2002;15(1):39–49.
293. Masuda EM, Kessler DM, Lurie F, et al. The effect of ultrasound-guided sclerotherapy of incompetent perforator veins on venous clinical severity and disability scores. *J Vasc Surg* 2006;43(3):551–556; discussion 556–557.
294. Thibault PK, Lewis WA. Recurrent varicose veins: 2. Injection of incompetent perforating veins using ultrasound guidance. *J Dermatol Surg Oncol* 1992;18(10):895–900.
295. Guex JJ. Ultrasound guided sclerotherapy (USGS) for perforating veins (PV). *Hawaii Med J* 2000;59(6):261–262.
296. Peden E, Lumsden A. Radiofrequency ablation of incompetent perforator veins. *Perspect Vasc Surg Endovasc Ther* 2007;19(1):73–77.
297. Elias S, Peden E. Ultrasound-guided percutaneous ablation for the treatment of perforating vein incompetence. *Vascular* 2007;15(5):281–289.
298. Proebstle TM, Herdemann S. Early results and feasibility of incompetent perforator vein ablation by endovenous laser treatment. *Dermatol Surg* 2007;33(2):162–168.
299. Raju S, Owen S Jr, Neglen P. Reversal of abnormal lymphoscintigraphy after placement of venous stents for correction of associated venous obstruction. *J Vasc Surg* 2001;34(5):779–784.
300. Raju S, McAllister S, Neglen P. Recanalization of totally occluded iliac and adjacent venous segments. *J Vasc Surg* 2002;36(5):903–911.
301. Neglen P, Hollis KC, Olivier J, et al. Stenting of the venous outflow in chronic venous disease: long-term stent-related outcome, clinical, and hemodynamic result. *J Vasc Surg* 2007;46(5):979–990.
302. Neglen P. In-stent recurrent stenosis in stents placed in the lower extremity venous outflow tract. *J Vasc Surg* 2004;39:181–188.
303. Hartung O, Otero A, Boufi M, et al. Mid-term results of endovascular treatment for symptomatic chronic nonmalignant iliocaval venous occlusive disease. *J Vasc Surg* 2005;42(6):1138–1144; discussion 1144.
304. Jost CJ, Gloviczki P, Cherry KJ Jr, et al. Surgical reconstruction of iliofemoral veins and the inferior vena cava for nonmalignant occlusive disease. *J Vasc Surg* 2001;33(2):320–327; discussion 327–328.
305. Lalka S. Autogenous venous bypass grafts for chronic iliac or infrainguinal venous occlusive disease. In: Gloviczki P, ed. *Handbook of Venous Disorders,* 2nd ed. London: Arnold; 2001:362–373.
306. Akers DL Jr, Creado B, Hewitt RL. Iliac vein compression syndrome: case report and review of the literature. *J Vasc Surg* 1996;24(3):477–481.
307. Puggioni A, Kistner RL, Eklof B, et al. Surgical disobliteration of postthrombotic deep veins—endophlebectomy—is feasible. *J Vasc Surg* 2004; 39(5):1048–1052; discussion 1052.
308. Camilli S, Guarnera G. External banding valvuloplasty of the superficial femoral vein in the treatment of primary deep valvular incompetence. *Int Angiol* 1994;13(3):218–222.
309. Kistner RL. Surgical repair of a venous valve. *Straub Clin Proc* 1968;24: 41.
310. Raju S. Venous insufficiency of the lower limb and stasis ulceration. Changing concepts and management. *Ann Surg* 1983;197(6):688–697.
311. Sottiurai VS. Technique in direct venous valvuloplasty. *J Vasc Surg* 1988; 8(5):646–648.
312. Tripathi R, Ktenidis KD. Trapdoor internal valvuloplasty—a new technique for primary deep vein valvular incompetence. *Eur J Vasc Endovasc Surg* 2001;22(1):86–89.
313. Raju S, Fredericks R. Valve reconstruction procedures for nonobstructive venous insufficiency: rationale, techniques, and results in 107 procedures with two- to eight-year follow-up. *J Vasc Surg* 1988;7(2):301–310.
314. Kistner RL. Surgical technique of external venous valve repair. *Straub Found Proc* 1990;55:15.
315. Belcaro G, Nicolaides AN, Ricci A, et al. External femoral vein valvuloplasty with limited anterior plication (LAP): a 10-year randomized, follow-up study. *Angiology* 1999;50(7):531–536.
316. Gloviczki P, Merrell SW, Bower TC. Femoral vein valve repair under direct vision without venotomy: a modified technique with use of angioscopy. *J Vasc Surg* 1991;14(5):645–648.
317. Raju S, Berry MA, Neglen P. Transcommissural valvuloplasty: technique and results. *J Vasc Surg* 2000;32(5):969–976.
318. Lane RJ, Cuzzilla ML, McMahon CG. Intermediate to long-term results of repairing incompetent multiple deep venous valves using external valvular stenting. *ANZ J Surg* 2003;73:267–274.
319. Guarnera G, Furgiuele S, Mascellari L, et al. External banding valvuloplasty of the superficial femoral vein in the treatment of recurrent varicose veins. *Int Angiol* 1998;17(4):268–271.
320. Taheri SA, Lazar L, Elias SM, et al. Vein valve transplant. *Surgery* 1982; 91(1):28–33.
321. Raju S, Neglen P, Doolittle J, et al. Axillary vein transfer in trabeculated postthrombotic veins. *J Vasc Surg* 1999;29(6):1050–1062; discussion 1062–1054.
322. Sottiurai V. Supravalvular incision for valve repair in primary valvular insufficiency. In: Bergan JJ, Kistner RL, eds. *Atlas of Venous Surgery.* Phildelphia: WB Saunders; 1992:137–138.
323. Cardon JM, Cardon A, Joyeux A, et al. Use of ipsilateral greater saphenous vein as a valved transplant in management of post-thrombotic deep venous insufficiency: long-term results. *Ann Vasc Surg* 1999;13(3):284–289.
324. Poller L, McKernan A, Thomson JM, et al. Fixed minidose warfarin: a new approach to prophylaxis against venous thrombosis after major surgery. *Br Med J (Clin Res Ed)* 1987;295(6609):1309–1312.
325. Welch HJ, McLaughlin RL, O'Donnell TF Jr. Femoral vein valvuloplasty: intraoperative angioscopic evaluation and hemodynamic improvement. *J Vasc Surg* 1992;16(5):694–700.
326. Jamieson WG, Chinnick B. Clinical results of deep venous valvular repair for chronic venous insufficiency. *Can J Surg* 1997;40(4):294–299.
327. Tripathi R, Sieunarine K, Abbas M, et al. Deep venous valve reconstruction for non-healing leg ulcers: techniques and results. *ANZ J Surg* 2004; 74(1–2):34–39.
328. Kistner RL. Surgical repair of the incompetent femoral vein valve. *Arch Surg* 1975;110(11):1336–1342.
329. Ferris EB, Kistner RL. Femoral vein reconstruction in the management of chronic venous insufficiency. A 14-year experience. *Arch Surg* 1982; 117(12):1571–1579.
330. Eriksson I, Almgren B. Influence of the profunda femoris vein on venous hemodynamics of the limb. Experience from thirty-one deep vein valve reconstructions. *J Vasc Surg* 1986;4(4):390–395.

331. Lurie F, Makarova NP, Hmelniker SM. Results of deep-vein reconstruction. *Vasc Surg* 1997;31:275.
332. Perrin M. Results of deep-vein reconstruction. *Vasc Surg* 1997;31:273.
333. Perrin M, Hiltbrand B, Bayon JM. Results of valvuloplasty in patients presenting deep venous insufficiency and recurring ulceration. *Ann Vasc Surg* 1999;13(5):524–532.
334. Taheri SA, Elias SM, Yacobucci GN, et al. Indications and results of vein valve transplant. *J Cardiovasc Surg (Torino)* 1986;27(2):163–168.
335. O'Donnell TF Jr, Mackey WC, Shepard AD, et al. Clinical, hemodynamic, and anatomic follow-up of direct venous reconstruction. *Arch Surg* 1987; 122(4):474–482.
336. Nash T. Long term results of vein valve transplants placed in the popliteal vein for intractable post-phlebitic venous ulcers and pre-ulcer skin changes. *J Cardiovasc Surg (Torino)* 1988;29(6):712–716.
337. Rai DB, Lerner R. Chronic venous insufficiency disease. Its etiology. A new technique for vein valve transplantation. *Int Surg* 1991;76(3):174–178.
338. Bry JD, Muto PA, O'Donnell TF, et al. The clinical and hemodynamic results after axillary-to-popliteal vein valve transplantation. *J Vasc Surg* 1995;21(1):110–119.
339. Sottiurai V. Results of deep-vein reconstruction. *Vasc Surg* 1997;31:276.
340. Rosales A, Slagsvold CE, Kroese AJ, et al. External venous valve plasty (EVVP) in patients with primary chronic venous insufficiency (PCVI). *Eur J Vasc Endovasc Surg* 2006;32(5):570–576.
341. Dalsing MC, Ricotta JJ, Wakefield T, et al. Animal models for the study of lower extremity chronic venous disease: lessons learned and future needs. *Ann Vasc Surg* 1998;12(5):487–494.
342. Garcia-Rinaldi R, Soltero E, Gaviria J, et al. Implantation of cryopreserved allograft pulmonary monocusp patch to treat nonthrombotic femoral vein incompetence. *Tex Heart Inst J* 2002;29(2):92–99.
343. Pavcnik D. Update on venous valve replacement: long-term clinical results. *Vascular* 2006;14(suppl 1):S106.
344. Neglen P, Raju S. Venous reflux repair with cryopreserved vein valves. *J Vasc Surg* 2003;37(3):552–557.
345. Pavcnik D, Yin Q, Uchida B, et al. Percutaneous autologous venous valve transplantation: short-term feasibility study in an ovine model. *J Vasc Surg* 2007;46(2):338–345.
346. Plagnol P, Ciostek P, Grimaud JP, et al. Autogenous valve reconstruction technique for post-thrombotic reflux. *Ann Vasc Surg* 1999;13(3):339–342.
347. Maleti O, Lugli M. Neovalve construction in postthrombotic syndrome. *J Vasc Surg* 2006;43(4):794–799.
348. Corcos L, Peruzzi G, Procacci T, et al. A new autologous venous valve by intimal flap. One case report. *Minerva Cardioangiol* 2003;51(4):395–404.
349. Lugli M, Guerzoni S, Maleti O. Neovalve construction in deep venous incomptence: comparison between two subsequent case series and related technical details. Paper presented at: 20th Annual Meeting of the American Venous Forum; February 20–23, 2008; Charleston, SC.
350. Williams D, Enoch S, Miller D, et al. Effect of sharp débridement using curette on recalcitrant nonhealing venous leg ulcers: a concurrently controlled, prospective cohort study. *Wound Repair Regen* 2005;13(2): 131–137.
351. Brem H, Sheehan P, Boulton AJ. Protocol for treatment of diabetic foot ulcers. *Am J Surg* 2004;187(5 A):1S–10S.
352. Mostow EN, Haraway GD, Dalsing M, et al. Effectiveness of an extracellular matrix graft (OASIS Wound Matrix) in the treatment of chronic leg ulcers: a randomized clinical trial. *J Vasc Surg* 2005;41(5):837–843.
353. Schmeller W, Gaber Y. Surgical removal of ulcer and lipodermatosclerosis followed by split-skin grafting (shave therapy) yields good long-term results in "non-healing" venous leg ulcers. *Acta Derm Venereol* 2000; 80(4):267–271.
354. Jones JE, Nelson EA. Skin grafting for venous leg ulcers. *Cochrane Database Syst Rev* 2007;(2):CD001737.
355. Falanga V, Sabolinski M. A bilayered living skin construct (APLIGRAF) accelerates complete closure of hard-to-heal venous ulcers. *Wound Repair Regen* 1999;7(4):201–207.
356. Falanga V, Margolis D, Alvarez O, et al. Rapid healing of venous ulcers and lack of clinical rejection with an allogeneic cultured human skin equivalent. Human Skin Equivalent Investigators Group. *Arch Dermatol* 1998; 134(3):293–300.
357. Richardson G, Driver B. Ovarian vein ablation: coils or surgery? *Phlebology* 2006;21:16–23.
358. Scultetus AH, Villavicencio JL, Gillespie DL, et al. The pelvic venous syndromes: analysis of our experience with 57 patients. *J Vasc Surg* 2002; 36(5):881–888.

CHAPTER 103 ■ SURGICAL PHYSIOLOGY OF INFANTS AND CHILDREN

FEDERICO G. SEIFARTH AND DAVID K. MAGNUSON

KEY POINTS

1. During the 8-week embryonic period, developmental events transform a fertilized egg into a "preorganism" that is composed of all the specialized tissues and organ systems required for future independent life; the subsequent 32-week fetal period involves accelerated growth and continuous organ maturation.
2. The fetus utilizes glucose as its primary energy substrate.
3. Maternal and placental mechanisms maintain an optimal temperature for fetal development; the net heat produced by fetal metabolic activity must be transferred away from the fetal environment to avoid a rise in temperature.
4. Neonates and children have significantly higher energy requirements than adults.
5. Breast milk is a complex mixture of macromolecules that changes as the growing infant's needs change; the usable energy content of milk is divided almost equally between carbohydrates and lipids.
6. At 12 weeks' gestation, water constitutes 95% of fetal mass; this declines to about 80% by 32 weeks' gestation and to 75% at term.
7. The determinants of gas exchange are total alveolar ventilation, ventilation/perfusion matching, diffusion, and extrapulmonary shunt; the mechanical properties of the lung affect gas exchange primarily by determining the amount and distribution of ventilation. Regulation of pulmonary blood flow determines ventilation/perfusion matching and the efficiency of gas exchange.
8. Respiratory distress syndrome, or hyaline membrane disease, is the most common cause of respiratory distress in neonates and one of the primary causes of neonatal mortality in developed countries.
9. The variations of extracorporeal membrane oxygenation share underlying principles: the partial diversion of blood from the patient to an external membrane oxygenator, ex vivo exchange of oxygen and carbon dioxide, and return of blood to the circulatory system.
10. At birth, circulatory patterns, hemodynamics, and gas exchange transition are characterized by the cessation of placental blood flow and gas exchange and the simultaneous increase in blood flow and gas exchange in the lungs.
11. Most mechanisms of physiologic control in the gastrointestinal tract are present at birth, although continued postnatal maturation results in ongoing adjustments over time.

This chapter introduces a variety of physiologic issues relevant to the care of infants and children with surgical disease. Reviewed are some of the basic physiologic concepts that govern clinical management, delineating some of the differences between pediatric and adult patients. These differences may be merely quantitative when comparing adults with adolescents and older children. The distinction between neonates and older patients, however, is frequently of a more dramatic and qualitative nature. These differences are the consequences of two unique conditions: the functional immaturity of organ systems during the transition from fetal to neonatal life and the demands placed on the physiologic machinery of the neonate by the overriding priority of growth. Whereas homeostasis is a valid concept on a small scale, in a larger sense the concept of a "steady state" is paradoxical in the newborn infant. Virtually every physiologic function in the infant is influenced in some way by the exponential growth that occurs during the first year of life. That growth, and the metabolic activity it demands, is perhaps the single most important property that differentiates the neonatal patient from the adult.

GROWTH AND METABOLISM

Growth, Development, and Prematurity

The 40-week gestational period is divided by convention into an
1 8-week embryonic period and a 32-week fetal period. During the embryonic period, developmental events occur that transform a fertilized egg into a "preorganism" that is composed of all the specialized tissues and organ systems required for future independent life. The subsequent fetal period is characterized by accelerated growth and continuous organ maturation, both of which are required to translate embryonic potential into biologic reality. Many of the congenital defects encountered in the practice of pediatric surgery have their beginnings in some developmental miscue during the embryonic period that prevents normal growth and maturation during the fetal period. At birth, the consequences of these antecedent events often are manifested by serious physiologic derangements.

Fetal maldevelopment is complicated frequently by prematurity, that is, entry into the extrauterine world before fetal growth and maturation have been completed. Most fetal growth and organ maturation occur in the third trimester, and so premature birth interrupts development at a time when the rate of biologic change is most rapid. In many cases, prematurity is the direct consequence of intrauterine developmental abnormalities, such as those that produce polyhydramnios (excess amniotic fluid that results in increased uterine size and early labor). In others, prematurity occurs in an otherwise normal fetus and is the result of maternal factors. In both cases, prematurity causes significant morbidity by forcing the neonate to contend with extrauterine challenges using physiologic systems that are not yet prepared to do so and also forces the neonate to complete simultaneously a schedule of preprogrammed fetal tasks.

Although the "normal" gestational period is generally agreed to be 40 weeks, infants are considered to be full term at 37 weeks. Neonates born before 37 weeks are referred to as premature or preterm. A normal-term birthweight is defined as 2,500 g or more. Infants born at less than 2,500 g are considered to be low birthweight, regardless of gestational age. More precise classifications include moderately low birthweight (1,500 to 2,500 g), very low birthweight (1,000 to 1,500 g), and extremely low birthweight (<1,000 g).

Mortality rates are directly related to both gestational age and birthweight. The current thresholds for survival appear to be approximately 22 weeks' gestation and 350 g birthweight. Above this threshold, survival rates increase rapidly, achieving 50% survival at approximately 24 to 25 weeks' gestation and 700 g.[1] Three additional independent variables predict increased survival in premature infants: female gender, exposure to corticosteroids in utero, and singleton gestation.[2] Continued gains in survival have come at an increasingly high cost of long-term morbidity. The most common types of serious long-term morbidity resulting from prematurity are neurodevelopmental conditions (e.g., cerebral palsy, mental retardation, seizure disorders), retinopathy, and chronic lung disease.

Although virtually all premature infants are born at low birthweights, a distinction is drawn between those whose weights are appropriate for their gestational age and those who are small for gestational age (SGA). SGA infants are defined as those in the 10th percentile or less with respect to age-adjusted birthweight. Normal intrauterine growth is a sensitive indicator of fetal well-being. Infants who qualify as SGA, whether term or preterm, are presumed to have experienced some intrauterine event that has compromised development. This phenomenon, referred to as intrauterine growth retardation (IUGR), can be caused by a plethora of factors that either reduce oxygen and nutrient delivery to the fetus or result in their decreased utilization. These abnormalities include maternal factors (tobacco, alcohol, and drug use; malnutrition; systemic disease), fetal factors (congenital defects, genetic or chromosomal anomalies), and placental factors (vascular anomalies, placental infarction, placental separation).

Both prematurity and IUGR may have detrimental consequences for the newborn. Both groups are challenged by insufficient energy reserves, poor thermal insulation, and increased heat and water loss. The premature infant must confront the extrauterine world with physiologically immature organ systems but may have a good eventual outcome if properly supported. Prenatal development may have been otherwise normal but prematurely terminated by maternal factors. On the other hand, the full-term SGA infant may have functionally mature organ systems and not require extensive physiologic support. When IUGR is the result of maternal or placental factors, premature birth separates the fetus from those factors and often results in compensatory growth and a good prognosis. When IUGR results from fetal or genetic factors, however, a poor prognosis may be anticipated. In general, an SGA infant has a better prognosis than a premature infant of the same birthweight because physiologic immaturity is less pronounced in the former.[3]

The rapid somatic growth and maturation occurring during the last trimester continues into the postnatal period and accounts for many of the unique metabolic events and nutritional requirements of the newborn surgical patient. This explosive growth phase is regulated largely by growth hormone (GH) and its peptide intermediates insulinlike growth factor-1 (IGF-1) and -2 (IGF-2), IGF-binding proteins (IGFBPs), and glucocorticoids, and is also influenced by insulin and thyroid hormone.[4,5] Recently defined mediators of growth and metabolic activity such as leptin and ghrelin have also been implicated in fetal and neonatal growth. Ghrelin, a 28-amino-acid peptide produced by the stomach, placenta, and intestinal tract, stimulates the release of GH.[6,7] In neonates, ghrelin has a potent orexigenic (appetite-stimulating) effect, and has been shown to be active in fetuses. It may play a role in prenatal programming and behavioral activities such as sucking and swallowing in preparation for postnatal feeding.[8] Ghrelin levels peak in late infancy and decline to puberty, coinciding with the rapid growth rate that characterizes early childhood.[8] Leptin, a hormone produced by adipocytes, also appears to regulate the metabolic rate and substrate utilization in fetuses and neonates. Leptin is detected in the fetal circulation and, like ghrelin, stimulates the secretion of GH. The widespread abundance of leptin receptors in fetal tissues, especially in developing cartilage and bone, has led to the suggestion that leptin is involved in the control of growth in accordance with nutrient availability in utero.[9,10] In adults, leptin plays an important role in the control of appetite and energy expenditure.

The normal-term baby will nearly double its birthweight by 4 months of age and will triple it by 1 year. The near-exponential rate of growth declines gradually thereafter until late adolescence. This pattern of growth is so constant in normal infants that significant departures from it are commonly the earliest indication of previously unrecognized disease. Any metabolic stress contributed by an acute disease or injury event will therefore be superimposed on the existing stringent demands for energy substrates.

As the neonate transitions to later infancy, childhood, and adolescence, its metabolic processes and responses gradually approximate those of the adult. As this transition represents a continuum, no clear delineation between these stages can be made. It is reasonable, however, to consider the metabolic responses of the neonate to starvation and stress as being qualitatively different from those of the adult, whereas those of older infants and children should be considered as only quantitatively different.

Basic Patterns of Energy Metabolism

In general, two basic patterns of energy metabolism are recognized: anabolic and catabolic. Anabolic processes characterize growth and involve the consolidation of nutrient substrates into structural and storage molecules. Catabolic processes involve the breakdown and redistribution of preexisting reserves to meet the short-term needs of specific tissues for specific substrates. Although persistent catabolism is pathologic and ultimately fatal, short-term catabolism is a necessary adaptive response to both starvation and stress.

The endocrine and cytokine environments that promote these two states are likewise distinct. Anabolic metabolism is mediated principally by insulin, IGF-1, and growth hormone. These mediators promote conversion of circulating glucose into glycogen (glycogenesis), storage of excess carbohydrate as fat (lipogenesis), and synthesis of new structural proteins from amino acids. The presence of available substrate and the absence of physiologic stress elicit a neuroendocrine environment conducive to these processes.

Catabolic metabolism is mediated by "counterregulatory" cytokines and hormones that have effects that are diametrically opposed to the anabolic mediators. These agents include tumor necrosis factor, interleukins, glucagon, cortisol, and catecholamines. These mediators promote an increase in glucose availability through hepatic glycogenolysis and gluconeogenesis and by inhibition of the peripheral effects of insulin on target organs. The objective of short-term catabolism is to generate adequate substrate for critical glucose-obligate tissues such as the brain, red and white blood cells, and renal medulla. The fetal and newborn heart depends on carbohydrates as a primary energy source and contains high concentrations of stored glycogen, allowing anaerobic glycolysis.[11] In contrast, oxidation of free fatty acids provides the main substrate for the myocardial metabolism in the adult heart.

Gluconeogenesis requires a supply of three-carbon fragments that reenter the glycolytic pathway under conditions that favor the reverse flow of intermediates and the synthesis of glucose. These three-carbon fragments are supplied by amino acids from protein breakdown (especially alanine and glutamine) and by glycerol from the hydrolysis of triglycerides. An additional source of gluconeogenic substrate is the Cori

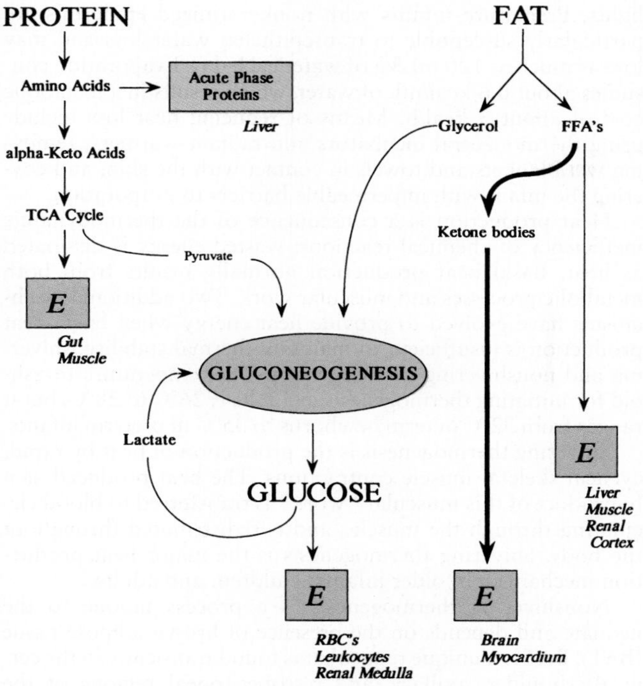

FIGURE 103.1. Energy production (E) during simple starvation. Ketoadaptation by brain and other glucose-obligate tissues allows free fatty acids (FFAs) to be used for energy production and limits the requirement for protein catabolism to generate gluconeogenic precursors via the tricarboxylic acid (TCA) cycle. (Adapted from Magnuson DK, Maier RV. In: Eichelberger MR, ed. *Pediatric Trauma: Prevention, Acute Care, Rehabilitation*. St. Louis, MO: Mosby; 1993.)

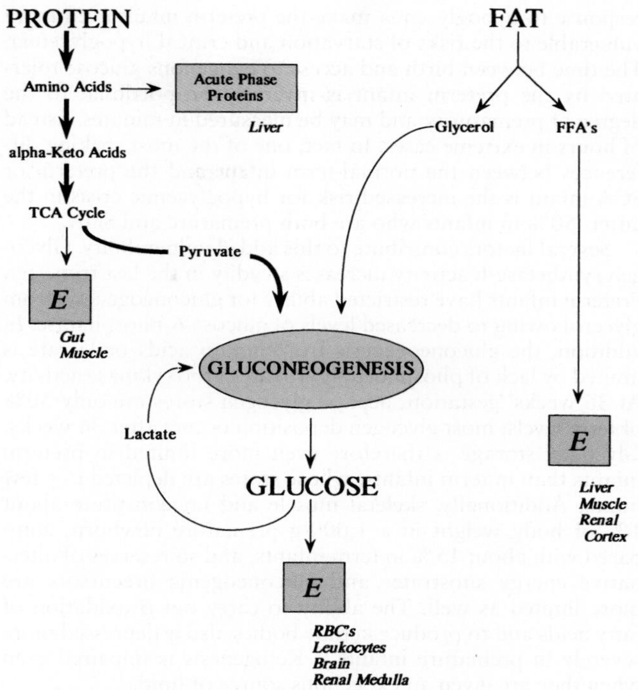

FIGURE 103.2. Energy production (E) during stress catabolism. Inhibition of ketoadaptation results in persistent protein catabolism to produce gluconeogenic precursors for glucose-obligate tissues. (Adapted from Magnuson DK, Maier RV. In: Eichelberger MR, ed. *Pediatric Trauma: Prevention, Acute Care, Rehabilitation*. St. Louis, MO: Mosby; 1993.)

cycle, in which lactate from anaerobic metabolism in compromised tissues (e.g., surgical or traumatic wounds) is transported to the liver and converted to pyruvate, a substrate for gluconeogenesis.

Catabolic metabolism can be separated into two distinct patterns: simple starvation and the stress response. In simple starvation, the brain (which accounts for the greatest demand for glucose) undergoes a gradual process called ketoadaptation, in which receptors and enzymes are expressed that allow for the utilization of ketone bodies as fuel (Fig. 103.1). Fatty acid metabolism then is altered to allow for the diversion of some fatty acids away from oxidative energy production and into the production of ketone bodies. The increased production of ketone bodies (ketogenesis), and their utilization by brain and myocardium, gradually reduces the demand for glucose and the degradation of visceral protein to gluconeogenic precursors.

In stress metabolism, however, the transition to the chronic starvation response of ketoadaptation is inhibited, and an ongoing requirement for glucose drives the continued breakdown of proteins to amino acids. Most of the amino acids produced by proteolysis during stress catabolism are rechanneled into gluconeogenesis (Fig. 103.2). The remainder is used in the synthesis of acute-phase proteins, in the synthesis of structural proteins for tissue repair, and for direct energy production by conversion to α-keto acids and entry into the tricarboxylic acid cycle. The mechanism of this inhibition is not well defined but most likely involves the persistence of stress-related neuroendocrine and cytokine mediators.

Metabolic Patterns in Neonates

2 The fetus utilizes glucose as its primary energy substrate. Transplacental movement of glucose by facilitated diffusion maintains fetal glucose levels at about 75% of maternal levels. At birth, the neonate experiences an abrupt withdrawal of placental support and plasma glucose levels fall. In response to hypoglycemia, secretion of catecholamines, cortisol, and glucagon mediates a shift to acute stress metabolism, relying initially on glycogenolysis because the capacity for gluconeogenesis is markedly decreased in newborns. During the third trimester of pregnancy, glucose is stored as glycogen in the fetal liver and in small quantities in the skeletal muscle, kidneys, and intestine. The hepatic glycogen stores are limited in the neonate, and available glycogen reserves are depleted within 2 to 3 hours. Thereafter, gluconeogenesis is the sole supply of endogenous glucose until feeding provides new substrate. Protein and triglyceride breakdown provide direct energy substrates and gluconeogenic precursors, but fetal adipose and muscle mass are relatively modest, and this endogenous supply of fuel is also soon depleted. At this point, plasma glucose levels of 40 to 50 mg/dL are expected. As the infant begins to feed, absorption of exogenous substrates reverses the catabolic pattern, and an anabolic phase mediated by insulin begins. Plasma glucose levels usually rebound to 70 to 80 mg/dL by 3 days of age.

Neonatal demand for exogenous glucose is therefore immediate, and the provision of enteral or parenteral glucose soon after birth is critical. Not only does the neonate have a higher relative energy demand than older children and adults, but also a much greater proportion of the total caloric demand is generated by glucose-obligate tissues, and the availability of endogenous glucose from glycogen and gluconeogenesis is limited. Furthermore, fat stores and lipolytic pathways are both poorly developed at birth, requiring more metabolically versatile tissues to utilize glucose as well.

The metabolic priorities of the premature or SGA infant are identical to those of the full-term neonate, but relative deficiencies in substrate stores and immaturity of the counterregulatory response to hypoglycemia make the preterm infant even more vulnerable to the risks of starvation and critical hypoglycemia. The time between birth and access to exogenous glucose tolerated by the preterm infant is inversely proportional to the degree of prematurity and may be measured in minutes instead of hours in extreme cases. In fact, one of the most striking differences between the normal-term infant and the preterm or SGA infant is the increased risk for hypoglycemic crisis in the latter: 50% in infants who are both premature and SGA.

Several factors contribute to this added vulnerability. Glycogen synthetase-b activity increases steadily in the last trimester. Preterm infants have restricted ability for gluconeogenesis from glycerol owing to decreased levels of glucose-6-phosphatase. In addition, the gluconeogenesis from amino acids or lactate is limited by lack of phosphoenolpyruvate carboxykinase activity. At 36 weeks' gestation, hepatic glycogen stores are only 30% of term levels; most glycogen deposition occurs after 36 weeks. Glycogen storage is therefore even more limited in preterm infants than in term infants, whose stores are depleted in a few hours. Additionally, skeletal muscle and fat constitute about 1% of body weight in a 1,000-g premature newborn, compared with about 15% in term infants, and so reserves of alternative energy substrates and gluconeogenic precursors are more limited as well. The ability to carry out β-oxidation of fatty acids and to produce ketone bodies also is depressed more severely in premature infants.[12] Ketogenesis is impaired even when they are given an exogenous source of lipid.

Thermoregulation

Temperature governs the kinetics of complex biochemical processes that have evolved to be maximally efficient within a narrow temperature range. Regulation of core body temperature has a high priority in the metabolic activities of the neonate and is a significant contributor to energy consumption. 3 The fetal environment is one of thermal constancy: maternal and placental mechanisms maintain an optimal temperature for fetal development and obviate the need for fetal energy expenditure to regulate temperature. In fact, the net heat produced by fetal metabolic activity must be transferred away from the fetal environment to avoid a rise in temperature.

Thermal equilibrium is a balance between heat production and heat loss. Newborns, particularly premature newborns, are characterized both by diminished capacity for heat production and by increased vulnerability to heat loss compared with older children and adults. The surface area–to–volume ratio of the neonate is greater than that of older patients, and so the area across which heat can be lost is disproportionately large compared with the mass of metabolically active tissue-generating energy. The body surface area–to–mass ratio averages approximately 250 cm^2/kg in the adult and may be as high as 1,400 cm^2/kg in the premature infant.[13] The paucity of insulating fat and the lower muscular activity level contribute to the problem.

Heat loss in the neonate occurs chiefly through four mechanisms. Conduction refers to the transfer of heat by direct contact with another static heat acceptor. The rate and direction of heat flow depend on the heat gradient and the heat capacities of the two objects. Convection refers to the transfer of heat from the skin surface to a fluid, such as air, which carries heat energy away from the body. Radiation is the loss of heat as electromagnetic energy in the infrared spectrum. Evaporation of water at the skin surface consumes heat energy by transforming water from its liquid into gas state.

The physical environment surrounding the sick neonate provides limitless opportunities for heat loss. Contact with cold surfaces, particularly wet sheets and blankets, is a principal cause of heat loss. The flow of cold air over exposed skin surfaces transfers heat by both convection and evaporation. Evaporation is exacerbated by radiant warmers and phototherapy lights. Premature infants with nonkeratinized epidermis are particularly susceptible to transepithelial water loss and may lose as much as 120 mL/kg of water each day. Evaporation consumes about 0.6 kcal/mL of water, which results in a metabolic cost of about 3 kcal/h. Means of reducing heat loss include using thermoneutral incubators and radiant warmers, removing wet blankets and towels in contact with the skin, and covering the infant with impermeable barriers to evaporation.

Heat production is a consequence of the thermodynamic inefficiency of chemical reactions; wasted energy is dissipated as heat. Basal heat production normally results from both metabolic processes and muscular work. Two additional mechanisms have evolved to provide heat energy when basal heat production is insufficient to maintain thermal stability: shivering and nonshivering thermogenesis. The temperature threshold for initiating thermogenesis in adults is 26°C to 28°C, but it ranges from 32°C in term newborns to 35°C in preterm infants.

Shivering thermogenesis is the production of heat by rapid, cyclical skeletal muscle contractions. The heat produced as a byproduct of this muscular "work" is transferred to blood circulating through the muscles and is redistributed throughout the body. Shivering thermogenesis is the major heat production mechanism in older infants, children, and adults.

Nonshivering thermogenesis is a process unique to the neonate and depends on the presence of brown adipose tissue (BAT). BAT is a unique tissue that is found transiently in the cervical, shoulder, axillary, and retroperitoneal regions of the neonate, and it is distinguished by its ability to generate metabolic heat by the inefficient metabolism of fatty acids. BAT is well established by 22 weeks' gestation. Sympathetic activation by cold stress causes norepinephrine to be released in BAT, bind to β-adrenergic receptors on adipocyte membranes, and initiate the hydrolysis of fatty acids. This process is facilitated by the presence of thyroid hormone. The fatty acids are shuttled into mitochondria where β-oxidation takes place. Normally, fatty acid oxidation is coupled to the phosphorylation of adenosine diphosphate (ADP) to adenosine triphosphate (ATP), preserving potential energy in the high-energy phosphate bond. In brown adipocytes, however, a unique peptide called uncoupling protein 1 (UCP1) "uncouples" the oxidative phosphorylation of ADP, allowing energy liberated by oxidation to be released as heat. The high density of mitochondria present in brown adipocytes attests to its role in heat production. Leptin also modulates UCP1, suggesting that BAT may play a role in overall energy balance regulation in infants.[14]

Nonshivering thermogenesis is the principal means of heat production in neonates, but it has severe limitations. It is a costly means of producing heat from a metabolic standpoint and rapidly depletes precious energy stores in term infants. Premature and SGA infants, with relatively reduced fat composition, are poorly equipped to use this strategy effectively. In term neonates, BAT constitutes about 10% of body fat and is gradually replaced by white adipose tissue in later infancy. Neonates who undergo surgery under general anesthesia run a high risk of hypothermia due not only to environmental exposure, but also to the inhibitory effects of general anesthetic agents on neonatal nonshivering thermoregulation.[15,16]

NUTRITIONAL SUPPORT

Energy Requirements

4 Neonates and children have significantly higher energy requirements than adults. These requirements diminish gradually throughout childhood, but they do not reach adult levels until physical maturity is attained. The two principal reasons for this discrepancy are a higher basal metabolic rate (BMR) and an additional energy requirement for growth. The total energy expenditure (TEE) consists of the BMR, the energy

TABLE 103.1

AGE-SPECIFIC ENERGY REQUIREMENTS

■ AGE (y)	■ ENERGY REQUIREMENT (kcal/kg/d)
0–1	120–90
1–7	90–75
7–12	75–60
12–18	60–30
>18	30

required to process substrates, energy for activity, energy for thermoregulation, and the energy cost of growth. The resting energy expenditure (REE), which may be substituted for BMR, is estimated to be 45 to 50 kcal/kg per day in term neonates and 50 to 60 kcal/kg daily in premature infants.[17,18] This compares with an REE of 20 to 25 kcal/kg daily in adolescents and adults.

Neonates and infants expend a much higher percentage of their total energy production on somatic growth than do older children. Growth consumes 35% to 40% of an infant's caloric intake during the first 6 months of life, a value that declines to about 5% at 2 years of age.[19] The energy cost of growth, which includes the energy used in new tissue synthesis plus the energy content of the synthesized tissue, approximates 40 to 50 kcal/kg daily in the neonate and progressively less in the older child. Add to these the energy requirements for nutrient processing, cold stress, and activity, and the baseline energy requirements for a term neonate are about 100 to 110 kcal/kg daily. The preterm neonate may require 120 kcal/kg per day or more to sustain growth. Caloric requirements for intravenous nutrition are perhaps 10% less because of the absence of obligate energy loss in fecal output.

The energy requirements of older infants and children gradually approach adult levels of 30 to 35 kcal/kg daily as BMR, cold stress, and rate of growth all decline with age (Table 103.1). This downward trend is moderated somewhat by an increase in energy expended in physical activity. Although many methods of estimating caloric requirements exist, the most straightforward estimation simply uses a weight-based calculation of caloric needs (Table 103.2).

It is important to recognize that these guidelines represent estimates for unstressed children. Energy requirements are altered in a variety of clinical settings commonly encountered in pediatric surgical patients. Both congenital heart disease and pulmonary disease can be associated with reduced pulmonary compliance and increased work of breathing, which can substantially increase energy expenditure. The healing of wounds related to major surgical procedures, trauma, and burns also increases caloric requirements. Sepsis, pancreatitis, and other conditions associated with generalized inflammatory activation may increase energy requirements dramatically.

TABLE 103.2

WEIGHT-SPECIFIC ENERGY REQUIREMENTS

■ WEIGHT (kg)	■ ENERGY REQUIREMENT (kcal/d)
0–10	100/kg
10–20	1,000 + 50/kg over 10
>20	1,500 + 20/kg over 20

It is equally important to appreciate that, in certain circumstances, caloric requirements in stressed children may be decreased because of changes in REE and the energy consumption related to growth. As opposed to older children and adults, infants actually may experience a decrease in REE during periods of postsurgical stress.[20,21] As previously discussed, the metabolic pattern that characterizes acute stress states is one of catabolism and growth postponement. This temporary growth inhibition is a consequence of, among other things, a cytokine and neuroendocrine environment that opposes the anabolic actions of insulin. Because 30% to 40% of a healthy neonate's caloric requirement represents energy required for growth, administration of the same caloric load to the stressed infant or child may result in significant overfeeding. The complications of overfeeding are not commonly recognized but include fluid overload, hepatic steatosis, and increased lipogenesis. Lipogenesis is associated with increased CO_2 production and is reflected in an increased respiratory quotient. Increased CO_2 production requires an increase in minute ventilation that may not be tolerated by critically ill neonates and children with respiratory disease and limited ventilatory reserve.

In the stressed infant or child, therefore, it may be prudent to reduce caloric administration transiently by as much as 25% to 30% during the acute stress phase, when growth is inhibited and the metabolic rate depressed. Determining when the metabolic environment has reverted back to one more permissive for growth and caloric utilization can be difficult. Direct calculation of the respiratory quotient by indirect calorimetry and measurement of nitrogen balance may be helpful in detecting a capacity to utilize more energy substrate. More frequently, however, a clinical judgment must be based on resolution of the hyperdynamic response to adrenergic stimulation or infection and the restoration of normal hemodynamics and fluid requirements.

Substrate Requirements

Carbohydrates. Carbohydrates constitute the major source of energy substrate for infants and older children, although they have a lower caloric density (3.4 kcal/g of intravenous hydrated dextrose, 4 kcal/g of enteral glucose) than either proteins (4 kcal/g) or fats (9 kcal/g). As discussed, glucose is the preferred fuel in a variety of tissues, including brain and blood cells. The obligate glucose consumption rate in neonates is about 4 to 6 mg/kg per minute. This compares with a glucose utilization rate of about 1 mg/kg per minute in adults. The discrepancy is explained in part by the fact that the neonatal brain accounts for 10% of body weight in the newborn and only 2% of body weight in adults. This contrast is even more striking in SGA infants whose brain growth is preserved in the face of generalized IUGR. In these infants, brain size and glucose consumption are even more disproportionately large. Most of the demand for glucose in newborns is for brain energy production, with relatively little remaining available for other tissues. Consequently, prolonged hypoglycemia may cause profound neurologic impairment.

The addition of small amounts of glucose to intravenous fluids prevents protein catabolism by providing a fuel source for glucose-obligate tissues and obviating gluconeogenesis. In adults, this protein-sparing glucose requirement is about 1 mg/kg per minute and is conveniently provided by administering 5% dextrose in water (D_5W) intravenously at maintenance fluid rates. In neonates, who require 4 to 6 mg/kg per minute of glucose to avoid protein catabolism, it is usually necessary to administer maintenance intravenous fluids as 10% dextrose in water ($D_{10}W$). The relatively higher fluid administration rate and dextrose concentration provide the increased glucose supply necessary to avert protein catabolism in the short term.

Normal plasma glucose values are variable and depend on gestational age, weight, and postnatal age. The definition of hypoglycemia is therefore somewhat fluid, but it is generally agreed that plasma glucose levels less than 35 mg/dL in term infants and less than 25 mg/dL in preterm infants constitute metabolic emergencies and require immediate intervention. Healthy full-term infants of appropriate birthweight rarely develop hypoglycemia. Infants at risk for hypoglycemia include those who are premature, SGA infants, multiple gestations, infants of diabetic mothers, infants of toxemic mothers, and infants who are critically ill for some other reason. Neurologic injury resulting from an inadequate supply of substrate to brain cells depends on both the degree and duration of hypoglycemia. Signs of hypoglycemia are late and nonspecific and include poor feeding, respiratory irregularity, apnea, bradycardia, hypothermia, cyanosis, irritability, tremors, seizures, lethargy, hypotonia, and coma.

Mild, asymptomatic hypoglycemia usually can be managed simply by initiating early oral feedings with breast milk or $D_{10}W$. Severe or symptomatic hypoglycemia requires intravenous dextrose administration. Dextrose concentrations of 10% to 12.5% are the maximum that can be tolerated by peripheral veins; higher concentrations of dextrose require a central (e.g., umbilical) venous catheter. Treatment consists of administering glucose at a rate of 6 to 8 mg/kg per minute (3.6 to 4.8 mL/kg per hour of $D_{10}W$). Profoundly hypoglycemic infants may require an initial dextrose "minibolus" of 200 mg/kg (2 mL/kg $D_{10}W$) over 1 to 2 minutes. The dextrose infusion rate then is increased by 2 mg/kg per minute every 3 to 4 hours until stable plasma glucose levels of 40 to 50 mg/dL are achieved.

Most neonatal hypoglycemia is transient, allowing dextrose administration to be weaned down as feeding or intravenous nutritional support is begun. Persistent hypoglycemia, particularly in infants requiring more than 12 to 15 mg/kg per minute of dextrose, may indicate a pathologic cause for hypoglycemia. Causes of pathologic hypoglycemia in neonates include hyperinsulinism (Beckwith-Wiedemann syndrome, nesidioblastosis or islet cell dysmaturation syndrome), congenital adrenal insufficiency, and other inborn errors of metabolism. In these circumstances, treatment options include corticosteroids, glucagon, epinephrine, somatostatin analogues, diazoxide, calcium channel blockade, intramuscular growth hormone, and near-total pancreatectomy.[22]

Fats. Lipids are the other main source of energy substrate. Nutrient lipids consist primarily of triglycerides—a glycerol backbone to which three fatty acids are esterified. During energy metabolism, the fatty acids are cleaved off the glycerol moiety and transported into mitochondria, where they undergo β-oxidation to produce energy stored in ATP. In addition to providing an energy source of high caloric density (9 kcal/g), lipids are essential for cell membrane structure, steroid hormones, the synthesis of inflammatory mediators such as prostaglandins and leukotrienes, and thermal insulation.

Most dietary triglycerides contain long-chain fatty acids 16 to 18 carbons long. Most fatty acids derived from animal sources have no double bonds within the carbon chain (saturated), whereas those derived from fish and vegetables have one or more double bonds (unsaturated). Because most fatty acids can be synthesized from carbohydrate precursors, there is no absolute dietary requirement for most fats as long as adequate calories are being provided from sugars. The fatty acids linoleic and α-linolenic acids are considered to be "essential" from a dietary standpoint because they cannot be synthesized de novo. α-Linolenic acid is a "triene" characterized by three double bonds in its carbon chain. Linolenic acid deficiency has been associated with neurologic dysfunction, which suggests a role in brain development. Linoleic acid has two double carbon bonds, but is converted into arachidonic acid, which contains four double bonds and is therefore a "tetraiene." Linoleic acid deficiency is marked by dryness and thickening of the skin, hair loss, and delayed wound healing. An increased triene-to-tetraiene ratio indicates essential fatty acid deficiency.

Proteins. Although amino acids can be converted to their keto acid counterparts, enter the tricarboxylic acid cycle, and yield usable energy (4 kcal/g), they are ideally reserved for the synthesis of new structural and functional proteins. The need for protein precursors is particularly acute in the neonate who is undergoing accelerated somatic growth. As the infant ages and the rate of growth declines, the requirements for dietary protein diminish somewhat. Recommendations for protein requirements in infants and children are variable. Premature infants may require 3 to 4 g/kg each day, whereas term newborns require 2 to 3 g/kg each day, older infants 1.5 to 2 g/kg per day, and children and adolescents 1 to 1.5 g/kg daily. These recommendations are somewhat controversial given that healthy newborn infants on a breast milk diet maintain normal growth with an average protein intake of 1.5 to 2 g/kg daily.

Eight of the 20 amino acids are unable to be produced by enzymatic conversion of other existing amino acids and therefore must be obtained from dietary sources. These essential amino acids are threonine, leucine, isoleucine, valine, lysine, methionine, phenylalanine, and tryptophan. Several other amino acids may be considered essential in the neonate because the specific enzyme systems for their conversion are consistently slow to mature in the postnatal period. These include histidine, tyrosine, cysteine, taurine, and possibly proline. Although clinical consequences of deficiencies in these amino acids have not been clearly defined, amino acid formulations designed for administration to adults may not contain them (especially cysteine and taurine), and specialized pediatric formulations supplemented with these amino acids are available.

Although not usually considered an essential amino acid, glutamine is of critical importance to many tissues and has been the subject of intense investigation.[23] Glutamine is produced from glutamate by the enzyme glutamine synthetase and has many physiologic functions. It participates in nitrogen transport in both the ammonia and urea cycles. It serves as a precursor for nucleic acid synthesis and an energy source in tissues with rapid cell proliferation. Intestinal epithelium is the primary consumer of glutamine, extracting a significant fraction from the circulation as well as the intestinal lumen. Within the continuously dividing enterocytes, glutamine is a necessary precursor to nucleic acid synthesis as well as the principal energy substrate. Maintenance of mucosal health and barrier function is directly dependent on the availability of glutamine for enterocyte metabolism.

Because glutamine synthetase is present in both infants and adults, and because glutamine is unstable in solution, this amino acid is not included in commercial amino acid formulations. During episodes of physiologic and metabolic stress, glutamine levels may fall despite the intravenous administration of other amino acids, suggesting a stress-induced alteration in glutamine synthesis. Intestinal mucosal atrophy and loss of barrier function may occur during prolonged periods of intestinal rest when only parenteral nutrition is administered. The addition of glutamine modified to increase stability in standard intravenous amino acid formulations and enteral administration of glutamine-containing formulas are being investigated as strategies for improving mucosal function and promoting intestinal growth in infants and children with severe gut injury.

Types of Nutritional Support

Enteral Support. The provision of all fluids, electrolytes, and substrates through the gastrointestinal tract is the ultimate goal of nutritional therapy. Using the gastrointestinal tract, even if only for a fraction of the patient's needs, provides trophic substances and enteroendocrine stimulation for intestinal growth and development, maintains the integrity of intestinal barrier function, and mitigates against the cholestatic liver complications of prolonged gut rest. Enteral feeding is associated with significantly fewer complications than parenteral nutrition and can be administered at a much lower cost. Equally important, early oral feeding is crucial for the maintenance of an intact suck and swallow reflex and the prevention of behavioral feeding aversion.

5 Breast milk is the optimal nutritional vehicle. Human milk is a complex mixture of macromolecules that evolves over time as the growing infant's needs change. The usable energy content of milk is divided almost equally between carbohydrates and lipids. The carbohydrate fraction is predominately lactose, but it includes more than 100 other oligosaccharides that have putative immunologic functions. A variety of lipids constitute the fat component, including both linoleic and linolenic acids. The protein content of human milk is relatively low compared with cow's milk and commercial formulas. As opposed to cow's milk, human milk has more whey than casein. The whey fraction includes many proteins, some with antibacterial functions, including the lactalbumins, albumin, lactoferrin, lysozyme, secretory immunoglobulin A (IgA), enzymes, growth factors, and hormones. In addition to these macromolecules, human milk contains a variety of cellular elements, including B and T lymphocytes, macrophages, and neutrophils.

When human breast milk is not available, a wide variety of commercial formulations are available from which to choose (Table 103.3). The nutritional compositions of these formulas are modeled on breast milk, but they differ with respect to the specific carbohydrate, protein, and fat content. Commercial formulas contain slightly more protein and less fat as a percentage of total calories than breast milk. Considerable variation in the specific nutritional components provides multiple options for optimizing nutrition in neonates with gastrointestinal derangements.

Most of the available formulas have a caloric density equal to that of human milk: 20 kcal/oz (0.67 kcal/mL). Formulas with higher caloric densities are available for infants with restrictions on fluid intake, or may be provided by fortifying standard formulas with polymeric glucose or other additives. Children between 6 months and 1 year of age may be transitioned to pediatric formulas with a higher caloric density of 30 kcal/oz.

The amount of formula required to supply adequate energy substrate to the growing infant can be estimated easily. Assuming an energy requirement of 110 kcal/kg daily, a feeding regimen of eight feedings per day, and a caloric density of 20 kcal/30 mL, the calculation of the required feeding volume can be reduced to a single "nutritional coefficient" of 22:

$$\text{Wt (kg)} \times 22 = \text{Volume of breast milk or formula required every 3 h}$$

This coefficient reduces to 7.3 for 24-hour continuous drip feedings.

A number of specialized formulas are available for infants with specific abnormalities of substrate absorption. The most important carbohydrate source for infants is lactose, the predominant disaccharide in human milk, which is hydrolyzed by intestinal lactase to glucose and galactose. Lactase and other disaccharidases are sensitive to changes in the villous environment and exhibit reduced activity in the setting of mucosal disease. Lactase is the most labile of brush-border enzymes, being among the first to exhibit decreased activity in disease and the last to increase during recovery. Inflammatory disorders that cause increased epithelial turnover result in a population of immature enterocytes with reduced lactase activity. Prolonged gut rest also results in reduced disaccharidase activity as a result of villous atrophy and mucosal loss.

Premature infants have reduced intestinal brush-border enzyme activity as a result of epithelial immaturity, especially with respect to lactase, but they also have deficiencies in fat and protein absorption for the same reason. Premature-specific formulas provide carbohydrates largely as glucose polymers (corn syrup) with or without lactose. They also provide a fat mixture of long-chain and medium-chain triglycerides to improve fat absorption. In the extremely premature or stressed infant, formulations providing hydrolyzed proteins (oligopeptides) have advantages over those that contain complex, intact proteins. Formulas for premature infants also provide increased concentrations of various other components, such as calcium and phosphorous, to meet the needs of accelerated bone mineralization (a fetal task under normal circumstances).

Hypersensitivity to bovine protein antigens may cause inflammation of the gastrointestinal tract and malabsorption in some infants. Soy-based formulas are usually the initial option for infants with cow's milk protein allergy because the protein content derives exclusively from soy proteins. As many as 30% of these infants will develop hypersensitivity to soy proteins as well and may require the use of a formula containing only protein hydrosylates, which are less allergenic than intact proteins.

Synthetic medium-chain triglycerides (MCTs) containing fatty acid moieties 8 to 10 carbons long are commercially available and have some advantages over long-chain triglycerides in certain clinical settings. MCTs are efficiently metabolized in the gut lumen to their constituent parts, are readily absorbed, and produce a nearly identical caloric yield. More importantly, they appear to have the capability of being transported directly into the enterocyte without prior degradation to glycerol and fatty acid. Hence, they offer the advantage of improved absorption in prematurity and other conditions that impair lipid digestion. These states include biliary obstruction (e.g., biliary atresia), bile salt insufficiency (e.g., ileal resection), pancreatic insufficiency (e.g., cystic fibrosis), and decreased absorptive surface area (e.g., short-gut syndrome). Because they bypass lymphatic absorption, they also may be useful in reducing lymphatic flow in treating chylous ascites and chylothorax. Because MCTs do not contain the essential fatty acids, periodic supplementation is necessary to avoid deficiency states.

Total Parenteral Nutrition. Few developments in clinical medicine have had a more profound impact on the survival of premature and critically ill neonates than the capability of administering hypertonic solutions of nutritional substrates by central venous catheter. The management of total parenteral nutrition (TPN) is complicated and covered more thoroughly elsewhere. Several issues related specifically to the management of TPN in infants and children are discussed here.

Indications for TPN depend on age, size, and clinical condition. In general, the younger the patient, the more intolerant he or she is of the effects of prolonged fasting. Although a healthy child may tolerate a week of inadequate nutrition or longer, infants and neonates are not so resilient. It is reasonable to consider initiating TPN in any neonate expected to fast for at least 2 to 3 days. Extremely premature neonates with multiple medical problems are commonly started on TPN within the first 2 days of life. Substrate concentrations are initially low and are gradually weaned up to calculated maintenance values over several days to avoid hyperglycemia and acidosis.

Estimations of caloric needs are made using the same assumptions discussed in the previous section. It is reasonable to divide total caloric requirements between carbohydrates and fats. The energy content of proteins should not be calculated to contribute to caloric requirements because the exogenous amino acids are expected to be used primarily for new protein synthesis. The appropriate distribution of calories between carbohydrates and fats may differ between individual patients, but in general fats should account for 40% to 50% of nonprotein calories, and carbohydrates usually account for 50% to 60%. Carbohydrates are administered as dextrose, and standard lipid emulsions containing essential fatty acids also are used. Although essential fatty acids can be supplied in adequate quantities with once-weekly lipid infusions, the high caloric density and low respiratory quotient characteristic of

TABLE 103.3

COMPOSITION OF SPECIALIZED INFANT FORMULAS (PER 100 mL)

FORMULA	CARBO	GRAMS	% kcal	PROTEIN	GRAMS	% kcal	FAT	GRAMS	% kcal	Osm	USES
Human milk	Lactose	7.2	42	Casein 20% Whey 80%	1.1	6	Human	3.9	52	290	Infants
Cow's milk	Lactose	4.8	30	Casein 80%	3.4	21	Butterfat	3.4	49	260	Older children
COW'S MILK BASED											
Enfamil 20	Lactose	7.3	43	Nonfat cow's milk	1.5	9	Coconut, soy oils	3.6	48	300	Healthy infants
Similac 20 SMA											
SOY BASED											
Isomil	Corn syrup	6.9	41	Soy isolate	1.7	10	Coconut, soy	3.7	49	240	Lactose intolerance, milk protein allergy
Prosobee		6.7	40		2.0	12		3.5	48	200	
PREMATURE											
Enfamil premature	Corn syrup + lactose	7.4	44	Nonfat cow's milk	2.0	12	MCT 40% +coconut, soy	3.4	44	260	Premature infants
Similac special care	Cornstarch + lactose	7.2	42				MCT 50% +coconut, soy	3.7	47	250	
PROTEIN HYDROSYLATES											
Pregestamil	Corn syrup, cornstarch + dextrose	6.9	41	Hydrolyzed casein +cysteine, tyrosine, tryptophan	1.9	11	MCT 60% + corn, safflower	3.8	48	320	Malabsorption
Nutramigen	Corn syrup, cornstarch	7.4	44	Hydrolyzed casein + amino acid mix	1.9	11	Corn oil	3.4	45	320	
Alimentum	Tapioca starch + sucrose	6.9	41	Hydrolyzed casein	1.9	11	MCT 50% + corn, safflower	3.8	48	370	
ELEMENTAL DIET											
Neocate	Corn syrup	7.9	47	L-amino acids	2.1	12	Safflower, vegetable oils	3.1	41	342	Malabsorption
Elecare	Corn syrup	10.7	43	L-amino acids	3.1	15	Safflower, MCT, soy oils	4.8	42	350	Malabsorption
HIGH MCT											
Portagen	Corn syrup + sucrose, lactose	7.7	46	Sodium caseinate	2.3	14	MCT 85% + corn oil	3.1	40	220	Lymphatic leak

MCT, medium-chain triglycerides.

intravenous lipids make them attractive as a primary energy source for most neonates who may have difficulty handling large fluid and CO_2 loads.

Protein requirements in parenteral nutrition are age dependent because of the changing requirements for somatic growth. As discussed previously, premature infants typically require 3 to 4 g/kg daily, whereas term newborns require 2 to 3 g/kg daily, and older infants 1.5 to 2 g/kg daily. To promote efficient utilization of amino acids for protein synthetic purposes, the nonprotein calorie-to-nitrogen ratio should be 150:1 to 200:1. Special formulations, including amino acids thought to be essential specifically in neonates, are widely available. Pediatric requirements for electrolytes, fat- and water-soluble vitamins, and trace elements must be provided as well.

The administration of both enteral and parenteral nutrition involves many assumptions and estimations. One of the most important aspects of nutritional management, then, is monitoring the response to therapy. In the older child and adolescent, maintenance of weight is an important goal. In the rapidly growing neonate, measurable nonedema weight gain is the objective. A daily weight gain of about 0.5% to 1% is a reasonable goal (15 to 30 g daily in the average term neonate). Measurements of white blood count, serum albumin, prealbumin and its binding proteins, and transferrin are helpful in assessing protein synthetic status in the neonate, just as they are in the adult. Routine surveillance of serum electrolytes, plasma and urine glucose, and liver function studies are mandatory to recognize metabolic complications of TPN administration.

FLUID, ELECTROLYTE, AND RENAL PHYSIOLOGY

Fluid Compartments

Like the adult, but to a greater degree, the infant and child are composed primarily of water. This simple fact influences many clinical phenomena, ranging from fluid balance to the volume of distribution for electrolytes and drugs. The percentage of body weight that is water, as well as its distribution within physiologic compartments, is in a state of rapid flux during the fetal and neonatal period. Body fluid distribution approaches a steady state by approximately 1 year of age and remains reasonably constant thereafter.

The greatest changes in total body water (TBW) occur dur-
6 ing fetal development. At 12 weeks' gestation, water constitutes 95% of fetal mass. This percentage declines to about 80% by 32 weeks' gestation and to 75% at term. Prematurity results in the birth of a fetus at a stage of rapid change in water content, a fact that needs to be appreciated when caring for the preterm surgical patient. A further decline in TBW occurs in a roughly linear fashion over the first year of life and reaches a plateau of about 65% by 1 year of age (Fig. 103.3).

Within the body, water is distributed between two main compartments: intracellular and extracellular. Although the extracellular compartment predominates early in fetal life, continued cellular proliferation and growth cause the intracellular and extracellular compartments to approach equivalence (about 40% each) at term. Postnatal diuresis of extracellular fluid causes the extracellular compartment to be reduced further within the first few weeks. Continued growth and fat deposition cause extracellular fluid to decline to about 25% at 1 year of age, whereas at the same time the intracellular compartment rises to a plateau of 40% to 45%.

The extracellular compartment is divided further into the interstitial and intravascular compartments. Generally, intravascular water accounts for only 25% of extracellular water, but this value is highly variable and depends on changeable factors, such as hematocrit and oncotic pressure. Blood volume itself is relatively high in the fetus because it includes blood circulating in the umbilical-placental vessels. At term, the normal fetal blood volume after cord occlusion is about 90 mL/kg (higher in premature infants). Blood volume declines gradually to 80 mL/kg in toddlers, 75 mL/kg in school-aged children, and 65 mL/kg in adolescents.

Fetal stress is often accompanied by the generalized accumulation of extracellular fluid, a condition referred to as hydrops fetalis. Fluid accumulates both as soft tissue edema and as effusions in the peritoneal, pleural, and pericardial spaces. This condition is readily diagnosed by prenatal ultrasound, which can detect cavitary fluid accumulations and quantify soft tissue edema by measuring the increased thickness of cervical soft tissues between the spine and the skin (nuchal thickening).

The mechanism of fluid accumulation is ill defined but most likely involves hydrostatic forces related to in utero congestive heart failure and venous hypertension. A principal cause of hydrops fetalis is autoimmune hemolytic anemia secondary to maternal–fetal Rh antigen incompatibility (erythroblastosis fetalis). The high fetal oxygen demand continues in the face of ongoing red cell destruction, resulting in a compensatory increase in cardiac output and the eventual development of high-output cardiac failure. Other causes of hydrops fetalis

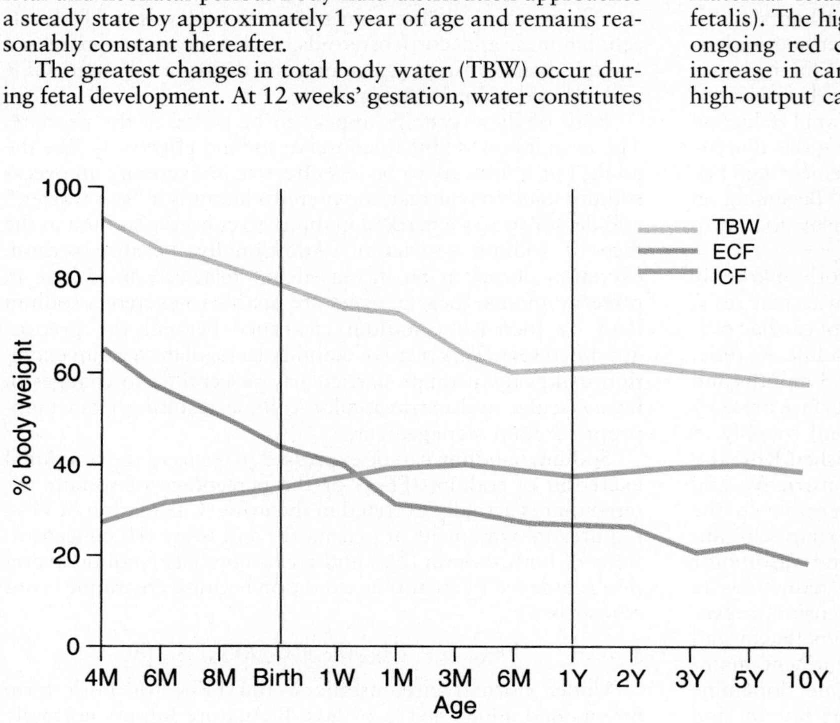

FIGURE 103.3. Changes in total body water distribution during prenatal and postnatal growth and development. (Adapted from Friis-Hansen B. Changes in body water compartments during growth. *Acta Pediatr* 1957;46[suppl 110]:1.)

also involve congestive heart failure: fetal arrhythmias, structural heart defects, mediastinal shift resulting from diaphragmatic hernia or developmental lung anomalies, and arterial "steal" syndromes caused by fetal tumors such as giant sacrococcygeal teratomas and hemangiomas. Additional causes are generalized infections, conditions of reduced oncotic pressure due to liver disease or nephropathies, maternal substance abuse, or chromosomal abnormalities.

These causes of fetal extracellular fluid accumulation are referred to as nonimmune hydrops and carry a poor prognosis. About 80% of fetuses identified with this condition die in utero, and only half of those that are liveborn survive beyond the neonatal period.

Renal Physiology

Maintenance of water and electrolyte balance within the body's fluid compartments is the responsibility of the kidneys. Renal function in infants and children relies on the same physiologic principles as adults, but it differs in the relative capacities to excrete and conserve water and solutes. These differences mainly affect infants and small children; by the age of 2 years, a child's renal function approaches that of the adult.

Renal function depends on two interrelated processes: the glomerular ultrafiltration of plasma and the tubular modification of the ultrafiltrate by selective reabsorption of water and solutes. Glomerular filtration is a passive event in which water and low–molecular-weight solutes percolate through the glomerular capillary membrane into the glomerular lumen. About 20% of renal plasma flow is filtered through the glomeruli in this fashion. The glomerular filtration rate (GFR) is dependent on renal blood flow, which is autoregulated by a tubuloglomerular feedback mechanism between specialized renal tubular cells (macula densa) and proximal arterioles. Modification of the ultrafiltrate occurs in the tubular system and collecting ducts through active transport of some solutes and passive diffusion of water and other solutes. A detailed description of these physiologic events is beyond the scope of this chapter, but certain generalizations can be made regarding age-related differences in renal function.

Urine output in the immediate postnatal period is characterized by three distinct phases: prediuretic, diuretic, and postdiuretic. The prediuretic phase occupies the first 24 hours and is marked by a fixed, low urine output of 1 mL/kg per hour or less. Urine output during the second and third day of life increases dramatically, to 5 to 10 mL/kg per hour, and is largely insensitive to exogenous fluid administration. Much of the rapid reduction in TBW seen in the postnatal period occurs during this diuretic phase. The unloading of excess water has an extremely high priority and is observed even in premature infants.[24] Beginning on the fourth day of life, urine output begins to display an appropriate responsiveness to fluid balance.

Renal blood flow (RBF) and GFR are both markedly reduced in the neonate because of elevated renovascular resistance. In the newborn, RBF represents only 6% of cardiac output, compared with 25% in the older child and adult. As resistance falls, RBF increases by fourfold in the first 3 months and doubles again to adult levels (indexed to body surface area) by 1 or 2 years of age. Changes in GFR correspond roughly to those in RBF. Because of this preexisting diminished RBF and GFR and the delicate balance between vasoconstrictive and vasodilatory forces, neonates are highly susceptible to the development of renal insufficiency under certain circumstances. Both acute tubular necrosis (ATN) and vasomotor nephropathy (VMNP) can occur secondary to reductions in renal perfusion because of hypovolemia, hypotension, sepsis, neonatal asphyxia, and administration of indomethacin and angiotensin-converting enzyme inhibitors. Treatment mainstays include optimization of intravascular volume, dopamine administration for infants with congestive heart failure, and furosemide administration in infants with indomethacin-induced ATN.[25]

Tubular function also varies according to age. The ability to concentrate urine is dependent on mechanisms that cause reabsorption of free water in renal collecting ducts to regulate serum osmolarity. Free water absorption is governed by the actions of antidiuretic hormone (ADH), which is secreted by the posterior pituitary in response to increased serum osmolarity and decreased blood pressure, and which acts on tubular epithelium in the collecting ducts to increase permeability to water. Water diffuses out of the ductal lumen and into the interstitium and capillary network, as directed by the concentration gradient.

Although the capacity to produce ADH is fully developed both in preterm and term infants, the sensitivity of tubular epithelium to ADH appears to be diminished in all neonates. The mechanism for reduced sensitivity appears to be related to the diminished production and increased degradation of prostaglandin E_2. On stimulation by ADH, renal collecting duct cells increase the expression of aquaporin-2 transmembrane water channels, increasing the translocation of water from the collecting duct lumen to the interstitium. The expression of aquaporin-2 in neonates is diminished as well.[26] These differences account for the fact that infants have a reduced capability to excrete concentrated urine relative to adults. The neonatal kidney can concentrate urine to a maximum of 500 to 600 mOsm/L. By 1 year of age, maximum concentrating capacity reaches about 1,000 mOsm/L, and by 2 years of age, the concentrating capacity attains adult levels of 1,200 to 1,400 mOsm/L. In contrast, the ability of the neonate to excrete free water and to produce dilute urine appears to exceed that of the adult. Maximal urine dilution capacity in the preterm and term neonate is about 30 to 50 mOsm/L, compared with 70 to 100 mOsm/L in the adult.

The other primary tubular function is the regulation of sodium balance, which in turn determines TBW and affects intravascular volume. Sodium regulation is governed largely by two counterregulatory hormones: aldosterone and atrial natriuretic peptide (ANP). Aldosterone is secreted by the adrenal cortex in response to activation of the renin-angiotensin system, and it acts on renal tubular epithelium to increase active sodium resorption and passive water resorption. Active sodium resorption is tightly coupled to potassium excretion. ANP is secreted in response to atrial distention and increased levels of ADH, catecholamines, and corticosteroids, and it promotes increased sodium excretion and water diuresis through enhanced GFR and reduced sodium resorption.

Both of these systems appear to be active in the neonate. The term infant is able to conserve sodium effectively, like the adult, but it appears to be less effective in excreting an excess sodium load. In contrast, the preterm infant is a "salt waster," and demonstrates a marked inability to conserve sodium in the face of sodium restriction. Additionally, because sodium excretion occurs at an increased but relatively fixed rate in preterm infants, these patients are unable to excrete a sodium load by increasing sodium clearance beyond the preprogrammed rate. This relative inability to regulate sodium excretion makes the neonate particularly susceptible to changes in intravascular and extravascular volume resulting from inappropriate fluid management.

Sodium handling can be expressed in terms of the fractional excretion of sodium (FE_{Na}) or the percentage of sodium filtered that is actually excreted in the urine. Calculation of FE_{Na} requires measurement of plasma (P) and urine (U) concentrations of both sodium (Na) and creatinine (Cr) (sodium excretion is indexed to creatinine excretion because creatinine is not reabsorbed):

$$FE_{Na}\ \% = (U_{Na})(P_{Cr})/(U_{Cr})(P_{Na}) \times 100$$

Under normal circumstances, the FE_{Na} for both term infants and adults is 1% or less. Premature infants normally have elevated FE_{Na} values of 3% to 9%. Calculation of the FE_{Na} can be helpful in assessing the cause of oliguria by determining whether renal tubular function indicates increased sodium resorption. Recent diuretic use invalidates the FE_{Na} as an indicator of tubular function. Oliguria associated with an appropriately low FE_{Na} implies renal hypoperfusion. Oliguria associated with an abnormally high FE_{Na} (>1 in term infants, >3 in preterm infants) indicates inappropriate sodium excretion and suggests a renal parenchymal cause for the oliguria (e.g., ischemic acute tubular necrosis).

Fluid and Electrolyte Management

Neonates and young children are exquisitely sensitive to small changes in body chemistry and do not have mature homeostatic mechanisms to compensate for rapid changes in fluid and electrolyte flux and to maintain internal balance. Additionally, the requirements for chemical homeostasis in the neonate are superimposed on a background of ongoing change. Iatrogenic alterations of body chemistry in the child are therefore quickly and easily produced by inattention to the details of fluid and electrolyte administration, causing impairments of cardiovascular, pulmonary, neurologic, and gastrointestinal function.

The systematic approach to fluid and electrolyte management requires an estimate of maintenance requirements, which then are adjusted to take into account both preexisting imbalances and ongoing losses. Once therapy is initiated, frequent reassessment and readjustment are necessary to ensure that the patient is responding as initially predicted. This involves documenting reversal of the symptoms and signs of dehydration, correction of any electrolyte or acid–base abnormalities, and normalization of urine output.

When normal renal function is present, the most reliable and easily measured indicator of adequate hydration is urine output. In the adult, the production of urinary output at a rate of 0.5 mL/kg per hour (30 to 40 mL/h) is adequate to excrete a normal renal solute load, given the concentrating capacity of the adult kidney. Because the immature kidney has diminished concentrating capacity compared with that of the adult, and because the pediatric solute load requiring excretion is relatively higher owing to the increased requirements for energy metabolism and growth, normal urinary outputs in children are higher. A desirable urine output in preterm infants is 3 to 4 mL/kg per hour, dropping to 2 mL/kg per hour in neonates and infants, and 1 mL/kg per hour in toddlers and school-age children.

Maintenance Requirements

Maintenance fluid and electrolyte requirements are those required to replenish normal, anticipated losses. Obligate fluid losses can be estimated by considering water lost in the excretion of solutes in the urine, excretion of stool, transepithelial water and sweat lost by evaporation, water lost through respiration, water utilized in anabolic metabolism for growth, and water gained through oxidation of nutrient substrates. Obviously, the actual "maintenance" fluid requirements in individual patients will vary widely according to the variables listed, but certain generalizations can be helpful in estimating requirements and initiating therapy.

Maintenance fluid requirements are related primarily to patient size and can be estimated by the Holliday-Segar method (Table 103.4). Many neonates, however, will require much higher maintenance fluid volumes (100 to 150 mL/kg daily) as a result of increased obligatory losses from a variety of causes. Increased transepithelial losses occur with fever, with the use of radiant warmers, with exposure to phototherapy for hyperbilirubinemia, and in premature infants with thin, nonkeratinized skin. Neonates with tachypnea or those undergoing mechanical ventilation may have increased lung water loss despite inspired gas humidification. It is common practice to reduce the fluid volumes for the first 2 to 3 days of life to about 70% of maintenance to accommodate the obligatory diuresis of extracellular fluid.

TABLE 103.4

HOLLIDAY-SEGAR METHOD FOR ESTIMATING FLUID REQUIREMENTS

■ WEIGHT (kg)	■ FLUID REQUIREMENT (mL/d)
0–10	100/kg
10–20	1,000 + 50/kg over 10
>20	1,500 + 20/kg over 20

Maintenance requirements of sodium are about 2 to 3 mEq/kg daily in term infants and children. This value may be somewhat higher in premature infants who cannot conserve sodium as effectively. Potassium requirements are also approximately 2 mEq/kg daily. Requirements for exogenous calcium are low in older infants and children with adequate skeletal stores, but calcium supplementation may be necessary in the premature infant with little skeletal ossification, particularly in those with cardiac disease, and in all children receiving prolonged TPN. As discussed in the preceding section, glucose is administered along with maintenance fluids to provide sufficient caloric support to meet the needs of glucose-obligate tissues and to prevent protein catabolism for gluconeogenesis.

Taking these requirements into consideration, maintenance fluids composed of one-fourth normal saline in 10% dextrose (D_{10}1/4NaCl) should be appropriate for most healthy neonates. Half-normal saline in 10% dextrose may be required in the premature infant. After the infant transitions into the postnatal diuretic phase on the second or third day of life, 10 to 20 mEq/L of KCl may be added to replenish obligate potassium losses and avoid hypokalemia. Depending on prior nutritional status and ongoing illness, it may be appropriate to reduce glucose intake to 5% dextrose after 1 to 2 weeks.

Preexisting Imbalances

Frequently, maintenance fluid administration must be superimposed on a significant preexisting deficit or excess. A complete history and physical examination are invaluable in detecting evidence of fluid imbalance and understanding its cause. Protracted vomiting or diarrhea, copious enterostomal output, chronic diuretic therapy, mechanical ventilation, phototherapy, and the like are all clues to extraordinary fluid losses. Physical examination is paramount in assessing current fluid status in all children. Because of the absence of comorbidity in most cases, physical signs of volume status are frequently more reliable in children than in adults.

Signs of both intravascular and extravascular fluid imbalance should be sought. Signs of extravascular fluid deficit, which are apparent with mild to moderate dehydration (<10%), include poor skin turgor, recessed eyes, sunken or soft fontanel, dry mucous membranes, absence of tears, and orthostatic hypotension and tachycardia. Signs of intravascular fluid deficit, which usually indicate more severe dehydration (>10%), include resting tachycardia and hypotension, oliguria, delayed capillary refill, reduced extremity temperature, diminished peripheral pulses, and altered mental status.

Signs of intravascular volume depletion usually indicate a need for intravenous resuscitation, which is usually initiated before proceeding with maintenance therapy. Isotonic crystalloid resuscitation with serial boluses of lactated Ringer solution (10 to 20 mL/kg) is usually appropriate and followed by careful assessment of the response to therapy. For dehydration associated with hyponatremia and hypochloremia, normal saline boluses may be preferable. In most conditions, however, repeated boluses of saline may be associated with iatrogenic hypernatremia and a normal anion gap metabolic acidosis resulting from hyperchloremia with a compensatory decrease in serum bicarbonate anion.

Preexisting fluid excesses are encountered less frequently in children, but it is important to recognize them to avoid exacerbating the underlying condition by instituting ill-advised maintenance therapy. Fluid excesses occur most frequently as a result of iatrogenic mismanagement, but they also may be seen in acute renal failure and congestive heart failure. Signs may include peripheral and pulmonary edema, hypertension, and increased heart size on chest radiography. Obviously, maintenance therapy may need to be postponed until euvolemia is achieved through diuresis.

Ongoing Losses: Body Secretion Compositions

Before a final strategy can be established, it is important to anticipate and account for the presence of extraordinary ongoing fluid losses. These losses usually result from increased gastrointestinal losses caused by nasogastric suction, enterostomal output, diarrhea, pancreatic or biliary drainage, or drainage of chylous ascites or chylothorax. Another common, although "occult" cause of ongoing fluid loss is the unavoidable sequestration of extracellular fluid in regions of surgical, inflammatory, or traumatic injury, often referred to as third spacing.

Because gastrointestinal secretions from various levels of the gastrointestinal tract have differing electrolyte profiles, they are most safely replaced on an equal volume (mL per mL) basis with fluid of similar composition. This can be accomplished by periodically measuring the electrolyte composition of the lost fluid or by estimating the composition according to known values (Table 103.5). In practice, upper gastrointestinal secretions in the setting of paralytic ileus or mechanical obstruction frequently approach isotonicity and may be safely replaced with lactated Ringer solution as long as careful monitoring of serum electrolytes is maintained. Pancreatic, biliary, and some ileostomy-related fluids are safely replaced with 0.45% NaCl supplemented with sodium bicarbonate at a concentration of 25 to 50 mEq/L. Chylous drainage may require the addition of albumin to avoid a progressive decrease in serum oncotic pressure over time. Third-space losses are best replaced with lactated Ringer solution administered by intermittent bolus (10 to 20 mL/kg), because the exact rate of fluid loss is not measurable and adequacy of resuscitation can be judged best by physiologic response.

Specific Examples

Abnormalities of Sodium Concentration. Changes in serum sodium concentration reflect changes in free water balance. Mild hyponatremia (serum sodium of 125 to 135 mEq/L) is a common electrolyte abnormality in children and is seen frequently in postoperative patients with excessive ADH secretion in response to perceived intravascular volume depletion. It is also seen in patients with chronic conditions associated with fluid retention, such as cirrhosis, nephrotic syndrome, and congestive heart failure. Severe, acute hyponatremia (serum sodium <120 mEq/L) usually is associated with volume contraction from hypertonic fluid loss, as can occur with vomiting, diarrhea, excessive stomal output, or inappropriate ADH secretion (SIADH).

Acute hyponatremia can cause severe neurologic symptoms, including headache, nausea, vomiting, lethargy, seizure activity, and coma. These symptoms are referred to as water intoxication and result from diffusion of water into relatively hypertonic brain cells, causing cerebral edema and intracranial hypertension. Treatment of severe or symptomatic hyponatremia involves correction of the underlying cause and administration of hypertonic saline (3% NaCl) over 30 to 60 minutes to correct serum sodium to about 125 mEq/L, followed by a more gradual elevation of serum sodium levels to normal over the ensuing 24 to 48 hours. The sodium deficit can be calculated by using a volume of distribution for sodium of 0.6:

$$\text{Sodium deficit} = [\text{Na}^+_{\text{target}} - \text{Na}^+_{\text{measured}}] \times \text{weight (kg)} \times 0.6$$

Hyponatremia of a more chronic, gradual nature should be corrected more slowly, particularly if asymptomatic. When hyponatremia develops gradually, compensatory loss of osmotic agents from brain cells prevents water intoxication. Rapid normalization of serum sodium levels may therefore cause a rapid fluid shift out of compensated brain cells, occasionally causing permanent neurologic injury. This is referred to as *osmotic demyelination* or *central pontine myelinolysis*, although demyelination often is diffuse and not necessarily involving the

TABLE 103.5

COMPOSITION OF BODY FLUIDS

SOURCE	Na* (mEq/L)	K* (mEq/L)	Cl⁻ (mEq/L)	HCO⁻ (mEq/L)	PROTEIN (g/dL)	SUGGESTED REPLACEMENT
Gastric	20–80	5–20	100–150	—	—	0.45% NaCl + 10 mEq/L Cl
Pancreatic	120–140	5–15	40–80	115	—	LR or 0.45% NaCl + 50 mEq/L $NaHCO_3$
Bile	120–140	5–15	80–120	100–115	—	LR or 0.45% NaCl + 50 mEq/L $NaHCO_3$
Ileostomy	45–135	3–15	20–115	30–50	—	LR or 0.45% NaCl + 25 mEq/L $NaHCO_3$
Diarrhea	10–90	10–80	10–110	30–50	—	LR or 0.45% NaCl + 25 mEq/L $NaHCO_3$
Pleural or peritoneal	140	5	100	25	6–8	LR 5% albumin or Plasmanate

LR, lactated Ringer solution.

pons. Osmotic demyelination can manifest as quadriparesis or pseudobulbar palsy. Mild, chronic hyponatremia in conditions associated with fluid retention usually can be corrected with free water restriction alone.

Hypernatremia is an uncommon electrolyte abnormality in children. Neurologic symptoms are related to brain-cell dehydration and shrinkage, causing disruption of bridging veins and intracranial hemorrhage. Recommendations for correction include calculation of the free water deficit and slow correction with D_5W over 24 to 48 hours. As a result of the production of cytoplasmic osmotic substances (ideogenic osmoles) by brain cells to offset increased extracellular sodium concentration, chronic hypernatremia is usually well tolerated and should be corrected gradually to avoid precipitating acute cerebral edema.

Abnormalities of Acid–Base Status. Metabolic acidosis can be categorized as having an increased anion gap or normal anion gap. The causes of an increased anion gap metabolic acidosis in children are the same as in adults: lactic acidosis or ketoacidosis accounts for most cases. Their implications and management in children do not differ from that in the adult. Normal anion gap metabolic acidosis, however, is much more common in infants than in older children and adults. The immature kidney is less efficient both at bicarbonate reclamation in the proximal tubule and at hydrogen ion excretion in the distal tubule. These functional deficits are considered a transient form of renal tubular acidosis type II (proximal), which is one of a heterogeneous group of disorders characterized by abnormal hydrogen ion and bicarbonate handling in the nephron. The vast majority of neonates outgrow this condition in the first year of life.

One of the most commonly encountered acid–base abnormalities in infants is metabolic alkalosis associated with hypochloremia, hypokalemia, and volume contraction. This pattern is typical of that seen in infants with protracted vomiting resulting from hypertrophic pyloric stenosis. Persistent vomiting of acidic gastric secretions causes the progressive depletion of both hydrogen and chloride ions. The loss of hydrogen ions results in alkalosis. Hypochloremia is associated with an increase in serum bicarbonate ion to maintain electroneutrality and with a decrease in renal hydrogen ion excretion. Renal tubular sodium resorption increases to reverse extracellular volume contraction. Sodium resorption is coupled with excretion of potassium. This potassium loss is facilitated by systemic alkalosis, which drives hydrogen ions out of renal tubular cells in exchange for potassium, raising renal tubular availability of potassium. As potassium becomes progressively depleted, a shift to hydrogen excretion occurs, resulting in the creation of urine with an inappropriately low pH: paradoxical aciduria. Treatment is directed at restoring extracellular fluid volume and chloride and potassium ions, and correcting the underlying pathology.

RESPIRATORY PHYSIOLOGY AND SUPPORT

Pulmonary Development

Abnormal or incomplete pulmonary development accounts for much of the clinical pathophysiology observed in infants with respiratory distress syndrome, bronchopulmonary dysplasia, and pulmonary hypoplasia related to congenital diaphragmatic hernia or cystic adenomatoid malformation. All these conditions manifest physiologic disturbances related to immature or altered development of the tracheobronchial tree, pulmonary vasculature, or alveolar parenchyma. A general knowledge of normal lung development is therefore necessary to understand these pathologic entities and their management.

Normal lung development can be described as occurring in roughly five phases. The embryonic phase begins in the third week of gestation, when a ventral diverticulum appears in the proximal foregut. This lung bud grows caudally, undergoing a series of binary branchings to form first the carina and then the lobar and segmental bronchi. The developing lung buds are composed of entodermal cells destined to become both bronchial epithelium and alveolar parenchyma. As the primitive lung bud branches, it grows into mesoderm destined to differentiate into cartilage, smooth muscle, and vascular structures. This phase is largely complete by 6 weeks.

The pseudoglandular phase extends from week 7 to week 16 and is characterized by continued dichotomous branching of the primitive airways. Under normal conditions, the developing airway branches about 23 times and acquires a glandular appearance as the epithelial tubes are surrounded by amorphous mesenchymal tissue. Entodermal differentiation into bronchial and alveolar epithelium occurs, as does mesenchymal differentiation into muscle, blood vessels, and connective tissue. Physical contact between the entodermal and mesodermal components is necessary for reciprocal induction of differentiation. By the end of this phase, all tracheobronchial branching is complete.

The canalicular phase extends from week 17 to 24 and is characterized by development of the gas-exchange architecture of the lung parenchyma. Primitive epithelial channels evolve into more complex groupings, interstitial tissue diminishes, and capillary ingrowth occurs. Alveolar epithelial cells differentiate into type I and II pneumocytes. Type I pneumocytes make up the alveolar wall and have a flattened morphology with scant cytoplasm, which is appropriate for the diffusion interface between the alveolar lumen and the capillary blood. Type II pneumocytes contain cytoplasmic lamellar bodies that identify these cells as future surfactant producers. A considerable body of evidence suggests that type I pneumocytes differentiate from existing type II pneumocytes. The earliest time at which functional gas exchange is possible is at the end of the canalicular phase.

The terminal saccular phase follows the canalicular phase at 24 weeks and lasts until the end of gestation. Two principal events occur during this time: (a) further morphologic change in the gas-exchange units with thinning of the interstitium and increased exposure of capillaries to the epithelial interface and (b) production of surfactant in preparation for extrauterine life. At this stage, each capillary is exposed to only one respiratory surface.

At birth, each lung contains approximately 20 million immature gas-exchange units, referred to as terminal sacs. In the postnatal alveolar phase, these structures proliferate and mature, reaching 300 million mature alveoli by the time the child is 8 years old. The terminal sacs multiply in number and mature morphologically. During this final phase, the respiratory membrane thins out further and presents more surface area to the capillary network. In the mature alveolus, each capillary is exposed simultaneously to at least two alveolar surfaces. After the end of this phase, when the child is 8 years of age, further lung growth occurs only by increasing individual alveolar size.

Apoptosis, the process of programmed cell death without inflammation, plays an important role in both prenatal and postnatal lung development. As the airway epithelium proliferates into the mesenchyme, apoptosis is involved in the formation of branch points. As the airways develop further, mesenchymal apoptosis is necessary for the thinning out of the interstitial connective tissue and the creation of the blood–alveolar interface. Apoptosis is also involved in the consolidation of the microvascular network into a single capillary layer between alveoli. Apoptosis in the developing lung appears to be upregulated by transforming growth factor-β and insulinlike growth factor and downregulated by nitric oxide.[27] Apoptosis combined with selective local morphogenesis forms the developing lung. Local expression of fibroblast growth factor-10 (FGF-10) seems to induce the latter.[28]

Lung growth during prenatal development appears to be linked to the secretion of fetal lung liquid. Fetal breathing movements provide for amniotic fluid flow into and out of the

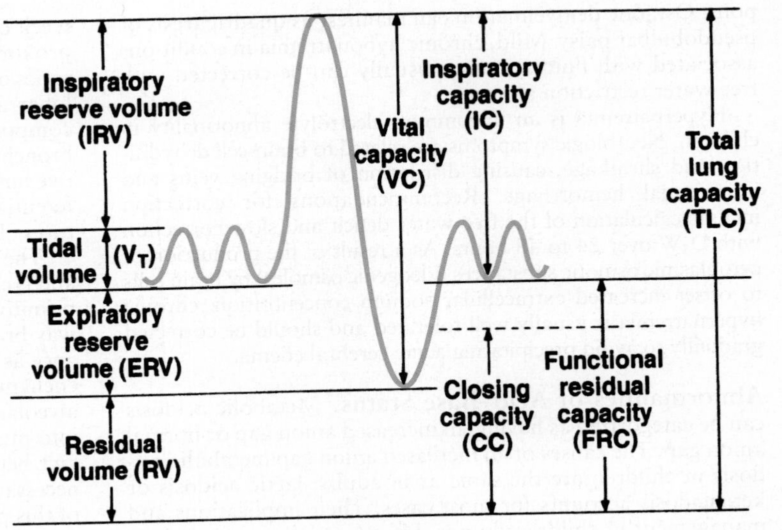

FIGURE 103.4. Lung volumes and capacities. (Adapted from Wilson JM, DiFiore JW. In: O'Neill JA, Rowe MI, Grosfeld JL, et al., eds. *Pediatric Surgery*, 5th ed. St. Louis, MO: Mosby; 1998.)

developing lungs. Net fluid flow appears to be outward, however, implying that lung fluid is secreted into the airway and flows out during the fetal respiratory cycle. Lung liquid production seems to stimulate lung growth, perhaps by providing a positive distending pressure in the fluid-filled fetal lung. The mechanism by which physical distention leads to cell proliferation or apoptosis is referred to as mechanotransduction. This process appears to depend on cell deformation and changes in cell–cell and cell–matrix adhesion, which are transduced into cytoskeletal changes and activation of intracellular kinases.

Pulmonary Physiology in the Neonate

Lung Volumes. Total lung capacity is composed of four distinct lung volumes: tidal volume, inspiratory and expiratory reserve volumes, and residual volume (Fig. 103.4). Residual volume is the volume of gas left in the lung after complete, forced expiration. The sum of the three lung volumes above residual volume (expiratory reserve, tidal, and inspiratory reserve) is the vital capacity, or the maximal volume of gas that can be voluntarily inspired or expired. Two functional parameters with great relevance to the physiologic management of lung pathophysiology are the functional residual capacity (FRC), which is the total volume of gas remaining in the lung after passive expiration during tidal breathing when alveolar pressure has equilibrated to atmospheric pressure, and the closing capacity (CC), which is the volume below which small conducting airways and alveoli begin to collapse.

Alterations in FRC occur in many pathologic states and significantly impact the efficiency of gas exchange. Normally, FRC exceeds CC, and alveoli in most regions of the lung remain open for gas exchange during tidal breathing. In disease states in which FRC is reduced, usually because of diminished compliance, FRC may drop below CC, causing regional atelectasis and impaired gas exchange. Common conditions associated with reduced FRC include respiratory distress syndrome (RDS), adult respiratory distress syndrome (ARDS), cardiogenic pulmonary edema, pneumonia, and postoperative hypoventilation caused by pain and splinting. Management focuses on recruiting collapsed alveoli by restoring and maintaining a higher FRC. This usually entails applying positive intra-alveolar distending pressure in the form of positive end-expiratory pressure (PEEP) or continuous positive airway pressure (CPAP).

Mechanical Properties and Their Effects on Ventilation. The bulk flow of gas can be described by the simple equation:

$$\Delta P = VR$$

where ΔP is the pressure gradient, V is volume flow per unit time, and R is resistance. The mechanical properties that govern clinically important aspects of lung ventilation include compliance, elastic recoil, and airway resistance. Compliance describes the distensibility of lung tissue and reflects the energy required to effect a volume change. Compliance is defined as the change in lung volume per unit change in pressure: $\Delta V/\Delta P$, with higher values signifying greater distensibility. Dynamic compliance (C_{dyn}) uses peak inspiratory pressure (PIP) in the calculation, whereas static compliance (C_{st}) uses plateau inspiratory pressure; hence, C_{dyn} is always lower than C_{st}. From a clinical standpoint, compliance is a critical determinant of lung volume, which in turn determines the efficiency of ventilation/perfusion matching and gas exchange. Conditions that reduce compliance make it more difficult to maintain volumes above closing capacity and therefore promote atelectasis. Low compliance states are caused by increased structural wall tension (edema or fibrosis), increased alveolar surface tension (surfactant deficiency), or decreased alveolar radius (reduced FRC).

Compliance is the inverse of elastic recoil, defined as the tendency for stretched tissue to return to its prestretched state. Whereas elastic recoil depends in part on intrinsic properties of lung and chest-wall tissue structure, the elastic recoil of lung parenchyma is closely related to alveolar wall tension. Wall tension tends to cause collapse of the alveolus unless opposed by some internal "splinting" pressure within the alveolus. The interaction between wall tension, alveolar radius, and pressure is defined by the Laplace relationship:

$$P = 2T/R$$

where P equals the splinting pressure, T the wall tension, and R the alveolar radius. This relationship states that the internal distending pressure required to counteract alveolar collapse is directly proportional to wall tension and inversely proportional to alveolar radius. At low alveolar radii (volumes), higher splinting pressures are required to counteract wall tension and oppose alveolar collapse. This explains both the tendency for low lung volumes to promote regional atelectasis and the high energy investment required to reopen collapsed alveoli. The most important component of total wall tension in the neonate is surface tension, which is the tension created by the physiochemical properties of the gas–liquid interface. In the mature lung, surface tension is dramatically reduced by surfactant, a phospholipoprotein that coats the alveolar surface and stabilizes it against collapse. Therefore, alveolar collapse is facilitated both by small lung volumes and by surfactant insufficiency.

The relationship between pressure and lung volume, referred to as the static compliance curve, is not linear (Fig. 103.5). At

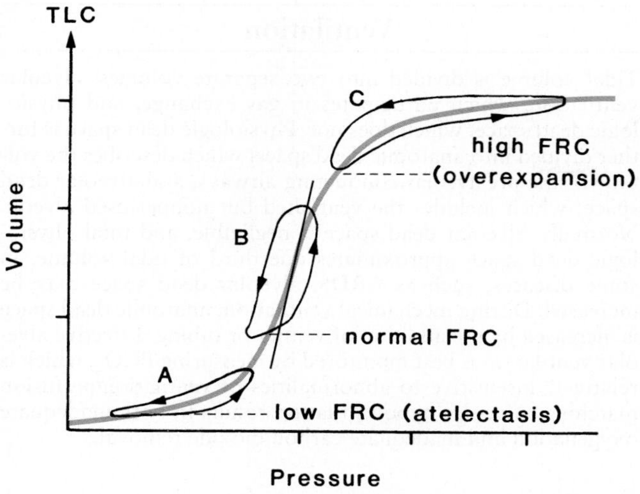

FIGURE 103.5. Static compliance curve. Nonlinear relationship between inflation pressure and volume change illustrated at low, normal, and high functional residual capacities (FRCs). Volume represented as fraction of total lung capacity (TLC). (Adapted from Harris TR, Wood BR. In: Goldsmith JP, Karotkin EH, eds. *Assisted Ventilation of the Neonate*, 3rd ed. Philadelphia, PA: WB Saunders; 1996.)

low lung volumes, atelectatic alveoli initially require a large energy input to reopen. As more alveoli are recruited, further increases in pressure bring about much larger increases in lung volume. At high lung volumes, alveoli are overdistended and less compliant. Pulmonary management aims at maintaining FRC in the steep portion of the static compliance curve, where lung compliance is optimal.

Extrinsic compliance refers to the component of lung compliance related to extrapulmonary structures, primarily chest wall, diaphragm, and abdomen. Under normal circumstances, chest wall compliance in the infant is high and contributes little to total compliance, which then is determined mostly by intrinsic lung compliance. In some instances, such as increased chest-wall edema caused by sepsis, hydrops fetalis, persistent fetal circulation, or superior vena caval thrombosis, reduced extrinsic compliance can have a significant impact on total compliance and ventilation. Chest-wall compliance also can decrease with the use of intravenous fentanyl, which affects muscle tone. Extrinsic compliance also decreases when intra-abdominal pressures are increased (e.g., ileus, closure of abdominal wall defects), in the presence of pleural fluid collections, and after diaphragmatic plication or diaphragmatic hernia repair.[29]

Ventilation is inversely related to resistance, which has both viscous and airway components. Viscous resistance is the friction generated by contiguous tissues moving against each other. It accounts for up to 40% of total resistance in neonates and is increased with conditions of high tissue density caused by edema (e.g., RDS, bronchopulmonary dysplasia, and anatomic left-to-right shunts). Airway resistance, on the other hand, reflects friction caused by gas molecules interacting with each other and with the airway walls.

Airway resistance is related to length, radius, turbulence, and density. According to Poiseuille's law, resistance is directly related to the length of the conducting tube and inversely related to the fourth power of radius:

$$\Delta P = V8hL/pr^4$$

where h is viscosity, L is tube length, and r is radius. Radius is a powerful determinant of resistance in simple tubes, but in the branching bronchial tree, the impact of progressively smaller radii is offset by the large total cross-sectional area of the distal airways. This is particularly true for older children and adults, in whom occult small-airway disease may exist without affecting total resistance. The small airways in infants contribute a much larger percentage of total airway resistance, however, so conditions affecting these airways, such as bronchospasm and bronchiolitis, have a more significant effect on airflow. Although tube length has few important clinical ramifications, it is interesting to note that infants with pulmonary hypoplasia resulting from congenital diaphragmatic hernia have truncated development of the bronchial tree and lower airway resistance than normal infants.[30]

Turbulence refers to the random swirling of gas molecules during bulk flow, in contrast to laminar flow, which is characterized by organized streaming of gas molecules along the same axis. Turbulence is induced as flow rates increase, and it makes ventilation less efficient because it consumes energy. Gas density is directly and linearly related to resistance. Although this has little clinical relevance in most settings, the use of low-density gas mixtures improves ventilation with anatomic abnormalities that produce high resistance, such as tracheal stenosis and bronchopulmonary dysplasia. Heliox, a mixture of 80% helium and 20% oxygen, has a density one-third that of room air and therefore generates one-third the resistance.[31]

The calculated product of resistance and compliance is a useful parameter that integrates two of the primary determinants of airflow and is referred to as the time constant (TC):

$$TC = RC_{dyn}$$

where R is resistance and C_{dyn} is dynamic compliance. The time constant reflects the time required for pressure equilibration to occur as air flows down a pressure gradient. During one time constant, 63% of an inspiratory or expiratory tidal volume can occur, whereas about four time constants are required for completion of flow. Conditions that increase either resistance or compliance will increase the time constant. During mechanical ventilation, consideration of this effect is required to allow adequate expiratory time before initiation of the next ventilatory cycle. Inadequate expiratory time results in "breath stacking" and overdistention of alveoli. Additionally, most focal lung diseases result in considerable heterogeneity in regional time constants. Inspiratory times need to be adjusted to allow for the longest time constants to ensure even distribution of ventilation. Conditions associated with low compliance result in short time constants. Therefore, an increase in minute ventilation is accomplished more efficiently by increasing ventilatory rate, which is permitted by the short time constant, than by increasing tidal volume, which requires high pressures in low-compliance lungs.

Pulmonary Blood Flow. Although the pathophysiology of pulmonary hypertension is covered more thoroughly in the subsequent section, the basic principles governing the regulation of pulmonary vascular resistance and flow are introduced here because they determine the matching of ventilation and perfusion, and hence the efficiency of gas exchange. Blood flow in the lung is influenced by a variety of mechanical and vasoreactive phenomena, which combine to determine local vascular resistances and, therefore, the regional distribution of blood flow.

As discussed, resistance is inversely related to the fourth power of vessel radius, making vessel caliber the most important determinant of resistance and flow. Pulmonary vascular caliber is determined both by mechanical factors acting on vessel walls and by muscular contraction within vessel walls. The mechanical factors that influence vessel caliber include radial traction on larger vessels produced by parenchymal expansion and compressive pressure imparted on microvessels within the alveolar walls by air pressure within the alveolus.

These mechanical forces come into play primarily at the extremes of lung volume. At low lung volumes, the lack of radial traction reduces caliber and increases resistance within the larger parenchymal vessels. At high volumes, excessive intra-alveolar pressures are imparted to the alveolar arterioles, capillaries, and venules as they transit through the alveolar unit. If this intra-alveolar pressure exceeds downstream pulmonary venous pressure (or pulmonary capillary wedge pressure), it becomes a determinant of the pressure gradient driving flow across the alveolar capillary. Normally, the pressure gradient is determined by the difference between mean pulmonary arterial pressure (P_{PA}) and pulmonary venous pressure (P_{PV}) ($\Delta P = P_{PA} - P_{PV}$). When alveolar pressure exceeds P_{PV}, it acts as the downstream pressure ($\Delta P = P_{PA} - P_{Alv}$). The anatomic arrangement of vessels "suspended" within the alveolar unit and influenced by external alveolar pressures is referred to as a Starling resistor. The phenomenon of the Starling resistor allows the lung to be viewed as a continuum of zones in which capillary blood flow depends on the relationship between hydrostatic venous pressure and intra-alveolar pressure.

In addition to mechanical forces, the distribution of blood flow within the pulmonary circulation is affected by a variety of vasoconstrictive stimuli. Extensive autoregulation of pulmonary blood flow ensures that perfusion is directed toward capillaries adjoining well-ventilated alveoli and away from collapsed or fluid-filled alveoli. This autoregulation is accomplished by increasing pulmonary vascular tone in vessels leading to poorly ventilated alveoli with low partial pressures of oxygen, a process referred to as hypoxic pulmonary vasoconstriction (HPV).

Factors that influence HPV include (a) the partial pressure of oxygen within the alveolus (PAO_2), (b) the partial pressure of oxygen within arteriolar blood (PaO_2), (c) the partial pressure of carbon dioxide in arteriolar blood ($PaCO_2$), and (d) the pH of arteriolar blood. Pulmonary vascular tone is inversely related to the partial pressure of oxygen in both the alveolus and the capillary blood, but PAO_2 appears to be a more important factor. In fact, alveolar hypoxia is the single most powerful stimulus to pulmonary vasoconstriction. The pH of capillary blood also affects blood flow; local acidosis is an important stimulus to pulmonary vasoconstriction. Increased $PaCO_2$ increases vascular tone both by lowering pH and by acidosis-independent mechanisms.

Physiologic mediators of vascular smooth muscle contraction common to these stimuli have not yet been fully identified. The caliber of pulmonary vessels at any given time is dependent on the balance of mediators causing vascular smooth muscle contraction and relaxation. Mediators of vasodilatation include bradykinin, prostaglandins E_1 and A_1 (PGE_1, PGA_1), prostacyclin (PGI_2), and nitric oxide. Mediators of vasoconstriction include the leukotrienes, endothelin-1 (ET-1), prostaglandin D_2 (PGD_2), and histamine. Histamine, ET-1, and PGD_2 appear to have biphasic effects mediated by different receptor populations, causing vasodilatation in the fetal and early neonatal periods and vasoconstriction after the first few days of life.[32–34] Most of these mediators originate from local sources, such as pulmonary endothelial cells and mast cells.

Gas-Exchange Determinants. The ultimate goal of respiratory function is gas exchange, which is the transfer of oxygen from inspired air to capillary blood and the reciprocal transfer
7 of carbon dioxide from blood to alveolar gas. The principal determinants of gas exchange are total alveolar ventilation, ventilation/perfusion matching, diffusion, and extrapulmonary shunt. The mechanical properties discussed previously affect gas exchange primarily by determining the amount and distribution of ventilation. Regulation of pulmonary blood flow determines ventilation/perfusion matching and the efficiency of gas exchange. Extrapulmonary shunt occurs primarily through cardiac septal defects and the ductus arteriosus and is discussed in the section on cardiac physiology. Diffusion abnormalities are uncommon causes of gas-exchange problems in children. Total ventilation and ventilation/perfusion matching are the most important causes of impaired gas exchange and merit further discussion.

Ventilation

Tidal volume is divided into two separate volumes: alveolar ventilation, which participates in gas exchange, and physiologic dead space, which does not. Physiologic dead space is further divided into anatomic dead space, which describes the volume of the prealveolar conducting airways, and alveolar dead space, which includes the ventilated but nonperfused alveoli. Normally, alveolar dead space is negligible, and total physiologic dead space approximates one third of tidal volume. In some diseases, such as ARDS, alveolar dead space may be increased. During mechanical ventilation, anatomic dead space is increased by the addition of ventilator tubing. Effective alveolar ventilation is best monitored by measuring PCO_2, which is relatively insensitive to abnormalities of ventilation/perfusion matching. Alveolar hypoventilation results in both inadequate oxygenation and inadequate carbon dioxide removal.

Ventilation/Perfusion Matching

The appropriate matching of ventilation and perfusion is the single most important determinant of gas exchange in the normal lung. Most disease states that cause abnormal gas exchange do so by promoting an imbalance between ventilation and perfusion. Perfusion is matched to regional ventilation by the mechanisms governing pulmonary blood flow discussed previously. When the normal mechanisms of pulmonary vascular autoregulation are impaired, ventilation/perfusion ratio ($\dot{V}/\dot{Q}$) mismatch ensues.

Normal alveoli with matched ventilation and perfusion are considered to have a $\dot{V}/\dot{Q}$ ratio of 1. Those with relatively less ventilation have a $\dot{V}/\dot{Q}$ less than 1, and those with relatively less perfusion have a $\dot{V}/\dot{Q}$ greater than 1. Those with ventilation but no perfusion define alveolar dead space, whereas those with perfusion but no ventilation contribute to intrapulmonary shunt, which is microcirculatory bypass of alveolar exchange. Between these two extremes lies a spectrum of $\dot{V}/\dot{Q}$ relationships that may contribute to abnormal gas exchange. $\dot{V}/\dot{Q}$ mismatch generally results in hypoxemia with normocarbia. Because carbon dioxide diffuses through the capillary–alveolar interface much more readily than does oxygen, $\dot{V}/\dot{Q}$ mismatch has relatively little effect on PCO_2 levels.

Mismatching of ventilation and perfusion is responsible for the hypoxemia encountered in most clinical settings. These include the disease states in which lung compliance is reduced, FRC drops below closing volume, and regional alveolar collapse occurs: pneumonitis, aspiration, RDS, ARDS, cardiogenic pulmonary edema, postoperative splinting, and others. Simply increasing forced inspiratory oxygen (FiO_2) does little to rectify the situation because the venous admixture of blood passing through low $\dot{V}/\dot{Q}$ units remains low in oxygen saturation, and blood passing through normal $\dot{V}/\dot{Q}$ units cannot further increase oxygen content to compensate. Therapeutic efforts must be directed at reopening closed alveoli and restoring homogenous alveolar ventilation.

Although diuresis, antibiotic therapy, and chest physiotherapy may have important roles in restoring FRC and matched ventilation and perfusion, perhaps the most effective therapeutic intervention is the use of continuous positive intra-alveolar distending pressure: CPAP or PEEP, which recruit and maintain previously closed or underventilated alveoli and improve $\dot{V}/\dot{Q}$ matching and oxygenation. They also shift ventilation up on the static compliance curve, producing a higher tidal volume with less pressure trauma.

The use of positive-pressure mechanical ventilation and PEEP must be managed judiciously because they can have both beneficial and deleterious effects on $\dot{V}/\dot{Q}$ matching. It is important to remember that positive airway pressure is transmitted to the alveolar capillaries that carry blood flow through the alveolar network. The alveolar pressure surrounding these capillaries acts as a Starling resistor and can impede capillary blood flow if it exceeds downstream venous pressure. The use of high peak ventilatory pressures without the use of PEEP, or the excessive use of PEEP itself, can cause overdistention of alveoli, reduced compliance, increased alveolar capillary resistance, and diminished alveolar capillary perfusion. The result is redirection of blood flow to underventilated alveoli, which actually worsens $\dot{V}/\dot{Q}$ mismatch. Similarly, the use of PEEP in focal lung disease may be counterproductive because its effects are preferentially directed to the normal, more compliant alveoli. This causes overdistention of normal $\dot{V}/\dot{Q}$ units and redistribution of blood flow to diseased alveoli, canceling the benefits of hypoxic pulmonary vasoconstriction.

Surfactant and Respiratory Distress Syndromes

8 Respiratory distress syndrome, or hyaline membrane disease (HMD), is the most common cause of respiratory distress in neonates and one of the primary causes of neonatal mortality in developed countries. RDS occurs as a direct result of pulmonary immaturity and surfactant deficiency. Because surfactant is not produced and secreted by type II alveolar epithelial cells until the third trimester, prematurity causes newborns to rely on lungs of variable maturity to support extrauterine respiration. Preterm infants born during the terminal saccular phase of lung development face the challenge of supporting gas exchange with lungs characterized by relatively thicker epithelial barriers, suboptimal capillary architecture, and a tendency toward alveolar collapse. This last feature is the most important cause of respiratory failure in premature infants and is directly related to the lack of surfactant, which lowers surface tension at the alveolar liquid–gas interface.

Surfactant is a complex substance composed of phospholipids (80%), proteins (10%), and cholesterol (10%). The phospholipid profile changes during lung maturation, but phosphatidylcholine predominates and is the principal substance responsible for the surface tension–lowering properties of surfactant. Phosphatidylinositol is present in immature surfactant, but it is largely replaced by phosphatidylglycerol in mature lungs, a useful fact when assessing fetal lung maturity. Surfactant also contains at least four specific proteins: surfactant protein-A (SP-A), SP-B, SP-C, and SP-D. SP-A and SP-D are important in host lung defense, facilitating the uptake of bacterial and viral pathogens by local immune cells. SP-C participates in phospholipid layer formation in the alveolus. SP-B is critical for processing, storage, and secretion of surfactant from the type II pneumocytes. Genetic mutations that result in the absence of functional SP-B are lethal in the perinatal period.

The physiologic role of surfactant is to stabilize alveolar units against collapse and thereby to facilitate homogeneous lung ventilation and $\dot{V}/\dot{Q}$ matching. LaPlace's law states that the pressure required to overcome the retracting force of surface tension in a sphere is inversely related to radius. In clinical terms, this means that smaller alveoli actually require greater distending pressure to maintain stability. This is analogous to the phenomenon one experiences when trying to inflate a balloon: the initial pressure required to begin inflation is high and becomes progressively less as the balloon radius increases. Because the lung is a collection of alveoli of varying sizes, and all alveoli are exposed to the same atmospheric pressure through a shared network of airways, the natural tendency is for the smaller alveoli to collapse and transfer their volume of air to larger neighboring alveoli, which become overdistended. In both cases, the effect on compliance is deleterious: FRC declines, the work of breathing increases, $\dot{V}/\dot{Q}$ matching is compromised, and respiratory failure ensues. Surfactant not only reduces absolute surface tension, but it also does so in a graded fashion. In small-radius alveoli, the phospholipid layer is condensed and its effect on surface tension is great. As the alveolus expands, the phospholipid molecules spread out and impart a gradually decreasing effect on surface tension. This differential efficiency of surfactant function allows alveoli of different sizes to coexist in a stable fashion.

Surfactant composition is an important determinant and predictor of fetal lung maturity. By the 20th week of gestation, collections of surfactant appear in type II cells within cytoplasmic granules called lamellar bodies. Thereafter, surfactant begins to appear in the developing terminal sacs. Infants born at 25 weeks occasionally survive without respiratory support; at 30 weeks' gestation, the risk of respiratory distress approaches 50%, and by 35 weeks' gestation, nearly all fetuses are capable of unassisted extrauterine respiration. There is considerable variability with respect to the timing of lung maturity, however, and clinical indices that assess lung maturity are useful in planning early delivery. The most common index of lung maturity is the amniotic fluid ratio of lecithin (phosphatidylcholine) to sphingomyelin, that is, the L/S ratio. Because amniotic phosphatidylcholine is derived solely from surfactant and sphingomyelin derives from all cell membranes, this provides a convenient self-indexed measurement of surfactant production that is independent of changes in amniotic fluid volume. An L/S ratio of 2.0 is achieved in the normal fetus by 35 weeks' gestation and is associated with an extremely low risk of RDS. Values of 1.5 to 2.0 are considered "immature" but of low risk. Values below 1.5 are associated with increased risk, and those below 1.0 are considered high risk. A more detailed test, the Lung Profile, utilizes the L/S ratio as well as percentages of phosphatidylglycerol and phosphatidylinositol to predict more accurately the risk of RDS. More recently developed tests of fetal lung maturity include the direct measurement of amniotic fluid surfactant concentration by fluorescence polarization and the quantitation of amniotic fluid lamellar bodies.

The fact that some infants born before 35 weeks' gestation do not manifest RDS led to the idea of stress-induced lung maturation. Fetal stress that promotes preterm labor also appears to promote accelerated lung maturation. This observation prompted the use of exogenous maternal corticosteroid administration to promote early lung maturation in fetuses expected to deliver early because of preterm labor or induced delivery. Exogenous corticosteroids appear to accelerate the maturation of surfactant phospholipids as well as increasing the synthesis of surfactant proteins.[35]

Postnatal administration of exogenous surfactant has become a mainstay of treatment not only for prematurity-associated RDS but also for a wide variety of neonatal lung diseases associated with reduced compliance. Surfactant replacement therapy has been proved to decrease the incidence and severity of RDS, especially when used in conjunction with antenatal maternal corticosteroids, and it appears to be efficacious in both prophylactic and rescue strategies. Natural surfactant preparations derived from animal lungs contain SP-B and SP-C, and have demonstrated superiority over synthetic surfactants that do not contain these proteins. Synthetic surfactants (which are safer and less immunogenic) containing SP-B/C protein analogues are under development. These preparations are aerosolized into the airway through an endotracheal tube with positive-pressure ventilation. Although initially designed for treatment of RDS, they appear to reduce ventilatory requirements and complications in a variety of diseases characterized by reduced compliance, including congenital diaphragmatic hernia, meconium aspiration, persistent pulmonary hypertension of the newborn (PPHN), and ARDS in older patients.[36]

Pulmonary Hypoplasia

Pulmonary hypoplasia refers to a condition in which pulmonary parenchymal tissue is abnormally reduced relative to body size. It is defined pathologically by reduced lung dry weight or DNA content relative to body mass and reduced alveolar number per unit volume. Although pulmonary hypoplasia may occur rarely as a primary disease, it is usually a stereotypical consequence of mechanical compression during lung development. Clinically, secondary pulmonary hypoplasia is associated most commonly with congenital diaphragmatic hernia, giant omphaloceles, and oligohydramnios caused by fetal renal dysfunction or urinary obstruction. Whether the true cause of pulmonary hypoplasia is mechanical compression, some alteration in fetal lung fluid dynamics, or a combination of both has not yet been elucidated.

Whatever the cause, pulmonary hypoplasia results from arrested development of the tracheobronchial tree and pulmonary vasculature. Depending on the severity of compression, the sequential binary branching of the developing airway may be arrested well before the usual 22 or 23 divisions, resulting in fewer respiratory units and a reduced pulmonary capillary network. The pulmonary arterial tree is not just quantitatively diminished, but it is histologically and functionally abnormal as well. The pulmonary arterioles in affected lungs are characterized by thickening of the muscular media, abnormal extension of the muscular media into terminal arterioles, and hyperreactivity of the vascular smooth muscle cells to vasoconstrictive stimuli. Endothelin is a potent vasoconstrictor that also acts as a smooth muscle mitogen, and may have a role in the development of fetal pulmonary vascular hyperplasia.[37] The pathophysiologic effects of pulmonary hypoplasia, therefore, include both inadequate gas exchange and persistent pulmonary hypertension.

In most cases of pulmonary hypoplasia, the life-threatening consequences of hypoplasia are related to persistent pulmonary hypertension, not to inadequate gas exchange. Most patients with congenital diaphragmatic hernia, for instance, have one or more blood gas measurements that document the potential for adequate gas exchange. Subsequent physiologic deterioration and death result from progressive, refractory pulmonary hypertension; extrapulmonary right-to-left shunting; and global hypoxemia. These subjects are covered more thoroughly in the discussion of persistent fetal circulation.

Ventilatory Support

Ventilatory management of pediatric patients has become increasingly complex as technologic innovation has expanded the number of available options. These advances have been motivated by a need to improve gas distribution in diseased lungs, to avoid complications associated with barotrauma, and to provide better synchronized and tolerated ventilation. Although conventional positive-pressure ventilation remains the mainstay of management for most infants and children requiring ventilatory support, a number of nonconventional technologies have gained increasing acceptance in certain situations where conventional techniques have proved inadequate.

Conventional Mechanical Ventilation

Conventional positive-pressure ventilators deliver a bulk flow of oxygen-enriched gas to the lungs through an endotracheal tube. In general, they are classified according to the method used to initiate and terminate a single ventilatory cycle. Volume-cycled ventilators deliver a predetermined tidal volume of gas. Respiratory rate (cycles/min), flow rate (L/min), inspiratory-to-expiratory ratio, and inspired oxygen concentration are manipulated to achieve certain respiratory goals, but the actual termination of the positive-pressure breath occurs when the preset tidal volume has been delivered. Volume-cycled ventilation has the advantage of providing precise control of minute ventilation regardless of lung compliance, and it is used routinely in adults and older children.

Infants and small children historically have not been managed with volume-cycled ventilators. Although control of minute ventilation is equally important in this group, the risks of barotrauma are high, particularly in neonates with pulmonary immaturity. A reduction in compliance will result in a reciprocal increase in pressure during volume-cycled ventilation, leading to overdistention of ventilated alveoli, $\dot{V}/\dot{Q}$ mismatching, alveolar rupture and pneumothorax, and the chronic lung changes observed with barotrauma. For this reason, precise control of inspiratory pressure is preferable to volume control.

Most neonatal and pediatric ventilators are technically not pressure cycled, but instead are time cycled and pressure limited. Instead of ventilatory flow ceasing when a preset pressure is reached, flow continues at a plateau pressure until the inspiratory time is reached. This improves tidal volume consistency and distribution. Constant monitoring of respiratory function (e.g., continuous transcutaneous oximetry) is imperative to prevent hypoventilation in the event of a sudden decrease in compliance and tidal volume.

The usual options for ventilatory modes in pediatric ventilator management are essentially identical to those used in adults: control, assist control, intermittent mandatory ventilation (IMV), synchronized IMV, and pressure support. The function and utility of these modes in children are similar to their use in adults. Pressure support, in which each spontaneous breath is assisted by supplemental positive pressure, is becoming the preferred mode in many settings where the patient is conscious and breathing spontaneously. It is particularly effective in the weaning of mechanical ventilation and restoring respiratory muscle strength.

For most modes, parameters are selected that determine gas exchange: FiO_2, respiratory rate, PIP, and PEEP. Inspiratory flow rates may need to be adjusted to provide an appropriate inspiratory/expiratory ratio within the constraints of the preset respiratory rate. PEEP is adjusted to optimize compliance and FRC; PIP is adjusted to provide an adequate tidal volume. Flow rates are adjusted to match the time constant requirements of particular disease processes. The FiO_2 is minimized to avoid pulmonary oxygen toxicity and retinopathy. The mean airway pressure (MAP), which is measured and represents the area under the time–pressure curve, is probably the single best parameter to follow for monitoring changes in the level of ventilatory support required as well as the risk of barotrauma.

Complications of Mechanical Ventilation in Infants and Children. Conventional breathing and mechanical ventilation both involve the bulk transport of air through conducting airways to gas-exchange chambers (alveoli), where diffusion occurs across the alveolar–capillary membrane. In many disease states associated with reduced lung compliance, the high pressures necessary to produce this bulk flow of gas during mechanical ventilation result in considerable iatrogenic lung injury. Ventilator-associated lung injury (VALI) is manifested both by parenchymal changes and edema, which further reduce compliance and diffusion, and mechanical disruption of small bronchi and alveoli resulting in pulmonary interstitial emphysema (PIE), mediastinal emphysema, and pneumothorax. Excessively high inspiratory pressures also impair venous return to the right atrium, thereby reducing preload, lung perfusion, gas exchange, and global cardiac output.

Whether VALI is caused by pressure itself or by physical overdistention of the more compliant alveoli is a subject of considerable debate. Current evidence seems to favor the structural overdistention of alveoli as the principal cause of iatrogenic lung injury, leading some to prefer the term *volutrauma* to the more accepted term *barotrauma*.[38–40] Volutrauma consists of two distinct entities: alveolar overdistention and cyclical atelectasis, in which the repetitive collapse of some alveoli creates shear forces that damage the walls of adjacent alveoli. The consequences of alveolar overdistention include disrupted endothelial and epithelial barrier function, increased permeability, interstitial edema, protein deposition, and fibrosis.

Although alveolar volume and overdistention may be the most important cause of VALI, the use of high ventilatory pressures in volutrauma-injured lungs increases the risk of interstitial emphysema and pneumothorax. Since small changes in alveolar volume are difficult to accurately measure in the ventilated patient, inspiratory pressures are still more commonly used to monitor and predict lung injury. Peak inspiratory pressures in settings of low compliance and high respiratory rate are often exaggerated, and inspiratory plateau pressures are now thought to correlate better with the eventual development of VALI.

Innovations in Pediatric Conventional Ventilation. Numerous developments in ventilation management have occurred in recent years that aim to make ventilation more effective, more physiologic, and less damaging.[41–43] Trends in both neonatal and pediatric respiratory support have favored the widespread adoption of less invasive and more natural techniques. The simplest of these techniques is the application of CPAP by mask—essentially, the application of PEEP in a nonintubated patient. Like PEEP, CPAP recruits and maintains FRC and improves $\dot{V}/\dot{Q}$ matching and compliance. A more recent development is bilevel CPAP, or BiPAP, in which positive airway pressure is incrementally increased during the inspiratory phase, more precisely reproducing the advantages of PEEP. These noninvasive ventilatory support techniques have been useful in reducing the need for, and duration of, invasive mechanical ventilation in infants and children with respiratory compromise.

In patients requiring mechanical ventilation where high pressures would traditionally have been employed, newer strategies using small tidal volumes have been devised to reduce VALI. In "open lung ventilation," higher-than-usual levels of PEEP are applied to recruit and maintain alveoli against cyclic atelectasis, and very small tidal volumes are delivered in volume-control mode to avoid alveolar overdistention. In this strategy, the use of "permissive hypercapnia" allows for a reduced minute ventilation that keeps ventilator rates acceptably low.

With advances in ventilator technology, volume-controlled ventilation has again become safe for use in neonatal and pediatric patients, and may have some distinct advantages over pressure-limited ventilation in certain circumstances. In "volume guarantee" mode, ventilators provide pressure-regulated volume control (PRVC) ventilation in which tidal and minute volumes are preset, and which the ventilator delivers in a pressure-limited fashion. The ventilator calculates compliance changes continuously and adjusts flow rates to minimize inspiratory pressure with each breath. The resulting ventilation mode is a hybrid of volume- and pressure-regulated techniques and may be helpful in infants with bronchopulmonary dysplasia and rapidly changing compliance who are at risk for alveolar injury.[44]

Although not currently employed in neonatal ventilation, airway pressure release ventilation (APRV) is gaining attention in pediatric ventilatory management. In APRV, continuous positive pressure is maintained at a high level during spontaneous ventilation by the use of a CPAP valve. These longer periods of high CPAP are punctuated by rapid, brief drops in airway pressure that are controlled by a "release" valve. During airway decompression, the lungs deflate and CO_2 is expelled. During rapid inflation, the lungs expand again and FRC is preserved. APRV has the advantage of allowing spontaneous ventilation to be superimposed on a high-PEEP/high-compliance system with decreased work of breathing while avoiding overinflation due to breath-stacking. Studies in adults have not demonstrated a survival advantage over conventional ventilation, but other parameters such as total time on ventilatory support and incidence of VALI may be decreased.[45]

Currently, the area of most rapid change in ventilatory management in infants and children relates to the synchronization of patient-initiated respiratory efforts and ventilator-delivered respiratory support. While pressure support ventilation (PSV) represented a significant advance in patient participation during ventilatory support, patients on PSV still experienced significant complications related to asynchrony with the ventilator. The inaccurate matching of respiratory triggering and demand with ventilator support results in several major problems for the ventilated patient. Breath-stacking, or auto-PEEP, occurs when asynchrony results in the accumulation of inspired volumes before complete exhalation, resulting in excessive FRC and alveolar overdistention. At high levels this causes VALI, but even at modest levels this results in the creation of steady-state lung volumes associated with reduced compliance, impaired gas flow, and diminished venous return. Another important consequence of ventilatory asynchrony is patient discomfort and anxiety, which leads to the overuse of sedative medications that suppress spontaneous ventilation.

Two novel ventilator technologies that address this important limitation in conventional ventilation are proportional assist ventilation (PAV) and neurally adjusted ventilatory assist (NAVA).[46,47] In PAV, fine adjustments in ventilator pressures and flows are continuously made based on calculated parameters, resulting in a more precise and variable delivery of breath-to-breath ventilator support targeted to predicted patient demand. In practice, the reliance on complicated formulas using difficult-to-measure physiologic parameters has limited the usefulness of PAV in pediatric settings. The recent development of NAVA has eliminated many of the shortcomings of PAV while still maintaining many of its touted advantages. In NAVA, intrinsic diaphragm activity is monitored by an array of bipolar electrodes in the distal esophagus that measure diaphragmatic action potentials, or electrical activity of the diaphragm (EADi). The timing and strength of EADi potentials correspond precisely with the initiation of a central nervous system trigger event and with the predicted demand for tidal volume. This allows ventilatory assistance to be matched and timed much more closely to patient activity, improving comfort and reducing inspiratory pressures and auto-PEEP.[48,49]

Unconventional Mechanical Ventilation. Several novel ventilatory techniques have emerged recently that attempt to mitigate barotrauma and hemodynamic compromise by providing effective ventilation without excessive pressures. These techniques employ extremely high ventilatory rates and tidal volumes less than or equal to anatomic dead space. Although numerous variations exist, the most popular modes are high-frequency jet ventilation (HFJV) and high-frequency oscillatory ventilation (HFOV). In HFJV, a small cannula is advanced through the endotracheal tube and used to deliver rapid, low-volume bursts of inspired gas. Ventilation does not require bulk flow, but it relies on several poorly defined physical processes, the most important of which is probably coaxial flow. In coaxial flow, the jet stream induces continuous rotational flow of inspired gas down the center of the airway and reverse rotational flow of expired gas along the perimeter of the airway (Fig. 103.6). In HFOV, ventilation is driven by the oscillations of a diaphragm within a closed noncompliant system. The cyclical compression and expansion of gas within the system generate high-velocity, streaming flow patterns that are similar to the coaxial flow seen in HFJV. The major difference between the two is that the expiratory phase is active in HFOV, as opposed to the passive expiration seen in both HFJV and conventional ventilation. This difference may make HFOV more effective in reducing air leaks from bronchopleural fistulas and less likely to cause air trapping and overdistention in lungs with longer and more heterogeneous time constants.

Unconventional ventilator management is often unpredictable and counterintuitive. For instance, in HFOV the FiO_2, MAP, frequency (cycles per second, or Hz), and amplitude (volume displacement caused by oscillation of the diaphragm) are preset. The amplitude is not an accurate reflection of the

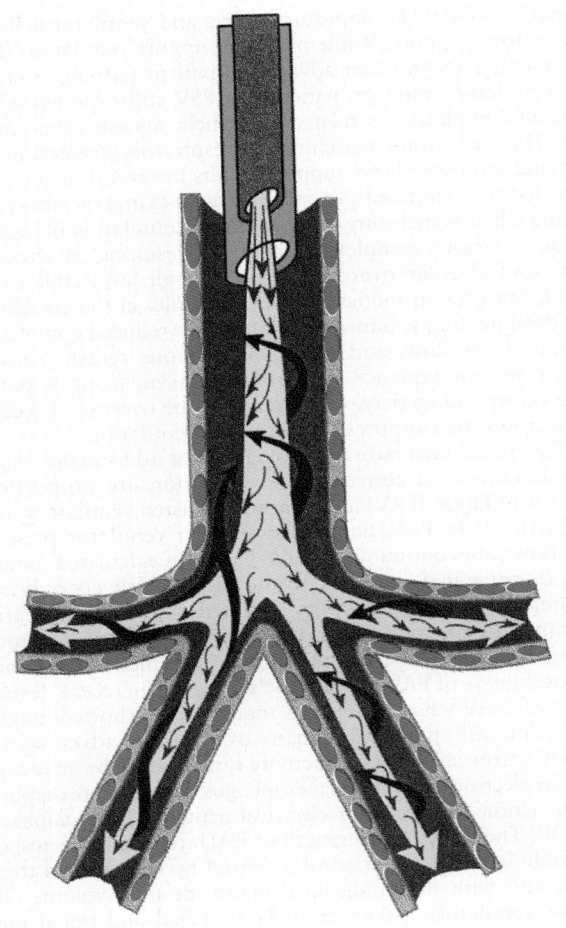

FIGURE 103.6. Proposed coaxial flow pattern during high-frequency jet and oscillatory ventilation. Gas inflow is confined to the center of the airway lumen, and outflow is confined to the periphery. (Adapted from Harris TR, Wood BR. In: Goldsmith JP, Karotkin EH, eds. *Assisted Ventilation of the Neonate*, 3rd ed. Philadelphia, PA: WB Saunders; 1996.)

tiny tidal volume produced at the end of the endotracheal tube and is therefore useful as a relative, "unitless" measurement only. In practice, the adequacy of the amplitude can be judged subjectively by observing chest-wall vibration. Increasing PaO_2 usually requires increasing the FiO_2 or the MAP, which recruits alveoli and increases FRC similar to the use of PEEP. In some conditions, the MAP required actually may be higher than that required in conventional ventilation, but the PIP is far less. Reducing $PaCO_2$ actually may require reducing the oscillatory rate to allow more time for gas displacement and more effective gas streaming.

In general, high-frequency ventilatory techniques are effective at promoting improved CO_2 elimination at lower pressures than conventional ventilation. Improved oxygenation is less reliable. HFJV and HFOV are both helpful in providing respiratory support in infants with preexisting barotrauma and air leaks. The ability of HFOV to actively promote enhanced CO_2 removal and generate a respiratory alkalosis at lower pressures has made it useful in managing infants with persistent pulmonary hypertension, particularly those with congenital diaphragmatic hernia.

HFOV has largely supplanted jet ventilation as the preferred modality in unconventional ventilation, and has been widely adopted by neonatologists as the most reliable and efficacious form of advanced ventilatory support. Despite this widespread clinical endorsement, a metastudy of recent reports of the safety and efficacy of HFOV in neonates with respiratory distress secondary to prematurity did not show any benefit for HFOV over conventional ventilation. The role of HFOV in neonates with other causes of respiratory failure (congenital diaphragmatic hernia, developmental lung anomalies, bronchopleural fistula) has not been delineated.

Liquid ventilation is a novel, experimental approach to respiratory support that currently is undergoing clinical trials in a variety of settings. In this approach, a liquid perfluorocarbon solution is instilled into the lungs instead of a gas mixture. Because many forms of respiratory failure are associated with surfactant insufficiency and reduced compliance, the substitution of liquid for gas in the alveolus eliminates the liquid–gas interface, reduces surface tension, and improves compliance. The improvement of mechanical properties in the perfluorocarbon-filled lung allows ventilation to occur at lower pressures and less barotrauma. The solubility of oxygen and carbon dioxide in perfluorocarbon solutions is extremely high, allowing respiratory gases to diffuse easily across the alveolar–capillary membrane.

Although total liquid ventilation requires a closed circuit and is clinically impractical, a partial liquid ventilation technique has been developed that is logistically feasible and promises to provide ventilatory benefits to some patients with reduced lung compliance.[50] In partial liquid ventilation, perfluorocarbon is instilled at a volume equal to FRC, and conventional ventilation then is superimposed on the liquid-phase FRC. In essence, this is analogous to providing "liquid PEEP," and improves pulmonary mechanics with little increase in alveolar distending pressure. The optimal role for partial or total liquid ventilation remains a subject for further investigation.

Extracorporeal Support

In certain situations, both conventional and unconventional ventilatory techniques are inadequate to provide gas exchange in the face of overwhelming pulmonary dysfunction. Under these circumstances, the use of extracorporeal membrane oxygenation (ECMO) may succeed in sustaining oxygen delivery and carbon dioxide removal until the underlying cause of respiratory failure is reversed and physiologic improvement occurs. It is important to recognize that, like conventional ventilation, ECMO is a supportive rather than therapeutic technique and has a limited window of utility imposed by the adverse effects of the technology itself.

9 Several variations of ECMO technology exist, but all share the same underlying principles: the partial diversion of blood from the patient to an external oxygenator (membrane or hollow fiber), the ex vivo exchange of oxygen and carbon dioxide, and return of blood to the circulatory system. The circuit is driven by either a roller or centrifugal pump similar to that used for routine cardiopulmonary bypass. Systemic anticoagulation is necessary to prevent thrombosis from occurring in the extracorporeal circuit.

Two basic methods of providing ECMO support are currently available: venoarterial (VA) and venovenous (VV). In VA ECMO, the right common carotid artery (RCCA) and jugular vein are cannulated in infants. In adolescents and young adults, the femoral artery is preferred. Venous inflow to the system results from passive drainage of the right atrium; arterial flow back to the patient occurs in the aortic arch (Fig. 103.7). As return flow is into the aorta, partial cardiac bypass occurs, which may provide significant benefit when respiratory failure is accompanied by compromised cardiac performance. The pump flow rate is advanced to 100 to 120 mL/kg per minute, which approximates 60% to 80% of cardiac output. Although VA ECMO directly augments cardiac output, the return of oxygenated blood to the descending aorta and the flow of desaturated blood through the pulmonary circuit and left heart results in both pulmonary vasoconstriction and reduced delivery of oxygen to the coronary arteries.

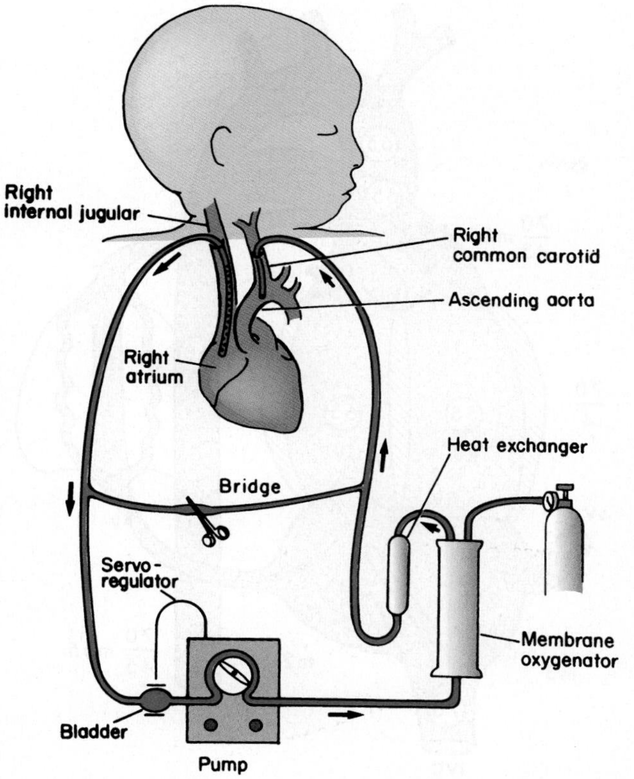

FIGURE 103.7. Components of a standard venoarterial extracorporeal membrane oxygenation (ECMO) circuit. (Adapted from O'Rourke PP. In: Holbrook PR, ed. *Textbook of Pediatric Critical Care*. Philadelphia, PA: WB Saunders; 1993.)

The consequences of RCCA cannulation in infants are undefined, and the long-term effects of carotid occlusion are the subject of increasing clinical investigation.[51–53] Although infants subjected to ECMO have a slightly increased incidence of neurologic injury, radiologic evidence for cerebral hypoxia does not seem to be lateralized to the right side. Carotid artery reconstruction (as opposed to ligation) at the time of decannulation has been studied extensively, with conflicting reports of long-term patency. Even (or especially) when patency is established, the theoretical risks of platelet embolism or plaque disruption later in life at a stenotic anastomosis are undefined. Longer-term neurodevelopmental studies are necessary to assess the potential benefits of this practice.

In VV ECMO, the circuit is interposed into the venous side of the circulation, with blood returning to the right atrium. This mode of extracorporeal support is less efficient than VA ECMO, resulting in a lower maximal SaO_2 because of the phenomenon of recirculation. Because both cannulas are positioned on the venous side, some of the oxygenated perfusate will be siphoned back into the venous return instead of flowing forward to perfuse end organs. The degree of recirculation is monitored by comparing oxygen saturations of the venous drainage and the arterial blood: the venous drainage saturation should be less than the arterial saturation. Although it provides no direct support of cardiac output, this method obviates the ligation and sacrifice of a carotid artery, avoids some of the risk of arterial embolization, and provides well-oxygenated blood for pulmonary and coronary circulation. Even in patients with decreased cardiac contractility, the improvement in oxygen delivery to the myocardium afforded by VV ECMO results in significant enhancement of cardiac output and may obviate VA ECMO. For most infants and children with adequate cardiac function, VV ECMO may become the modality of choice for extracorporeal support.[54]

Indications for ECMO vary among institutions. Because of the high cost and potential for complications, ECMO is justifiable only when all other available therapies for respiratory failure have proved inadequate and when quantifiable parameters predict a mortality rate of 80% or greater with conventional management. Several methods of providing a quantitative estimate of respiratory failure have been used to predict mortality with conventional ventilation and guide the use of ECMO. Perhaps the most widely used index is the oxygenation index (OI), which compares ventilatory support parameters (MAP and FiO_2) with gas-exchange results (postductal PaO_2):

$$OI = (MAP)(FiO_2)/P_aO_2 \times 100$$

An OI greater than 40 predicts a mortality rate of 80% and is a commonly cited threshold indicator for the use of ECMO. Another useful, although more burdensome, parameter for quantifying respiratory failure and predicting mortality is the alveolar–arterial oxygen gradient ($PAO_2 - PaO_2$), which when greater than 600 predicts a mortality rate of 80%. Other inclusion criteria for ECMO include the absence of a major intrinsic cardiac defect, chromosomal abnormality, or significant intraventricular hemorrhage; a gestational age greater than 33 weeks; weight greater than 2 kg; and an underlying respiratory pathology that is judged to be reversible.

The use of exogenous surfactant, oscillatory ventilation, and inhaled nitric oxide has had two major effects on ECMO utilization: many infants have avoided ECMO support altogether, while others have become candidates for less-invasive VV support. Consequently, the reduced number of patients requiring VA ECMO support is a more varied, complicated, and physiologically challenged group.[55,56] Results for extracorporeal support are age and diagnosis dependent. Infants with respiratory failure (meconium aspiration syndrome, RDS, sepsis) appear to benefit most from extracorporeal support. This is most likely because neonatal respiratory failure often is associated with reversible pulmonary hypertension, and ECMO allows for the normalization of PO_2, PCO_2, pH, and pulmonary vascular resistance without the aggressive ventilatory support that frequently causes iatrogenic lung injury and chronic lung disease. Neonates with reversible, idiopathic PPHN benefit from ECMO for the same reasons.

Neonates with respiratory failure and pulmonary hypertension attributable to congenital diaphragmatic hernia and pulmonary hypoplasia appear to benefit from ECMO, but the improvement in survival over conventional management is not as significant. This may reflect the irreversible problems related to inadequacy of alveolar number and microvascular development associated with pulmonary hypoplasia. The results of ECMO in children and adolescents with respiratory failure resulting from ARDS, trauma, bronchopleural fistula, viral pneumonia, or aspiration are less convincing, and the role of ECMO in these diseases is not yet well defined.[57]

CARDIOVASCULAR PHYSIOLOGY AND SUPPORT

Fetal Circulation

Fetal circulation has evolved to utilize an external organ of gas exchange, the placenta, while maintaining the anatomic relationships that will later be necessary in extrauterine life when responsibility for gas exchange transitions abruptly to the lungs. The fetal circulatory system is characterized by asymmetric ventricles that function in parallel, an arrangement made possible by two anatomic shunts—the *foramen ovale* and *ductus arteriosus*. These shunts make possible the nonrandom

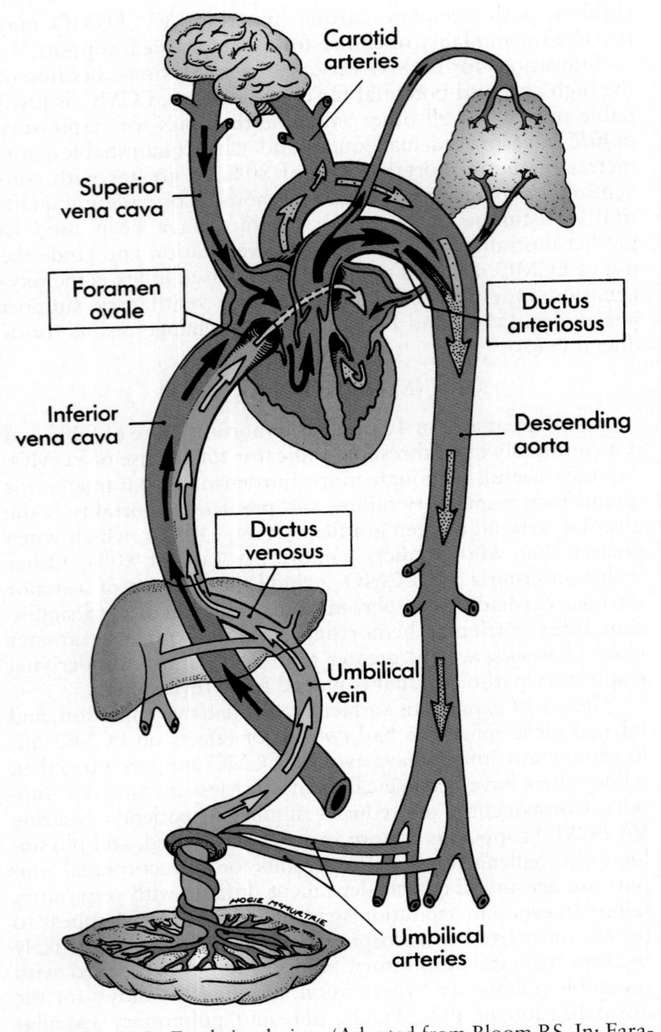

FIGURE 103.8. Fetal circulation. (Adapted from Bloom RS. In: Fanaroff AA, Martin RJ, eds. *Neonatal–Perinatal Medicine: Diseases of the Fetus and Infant*, 6th ed. St. Louis, MO: Mosby; 1997.)

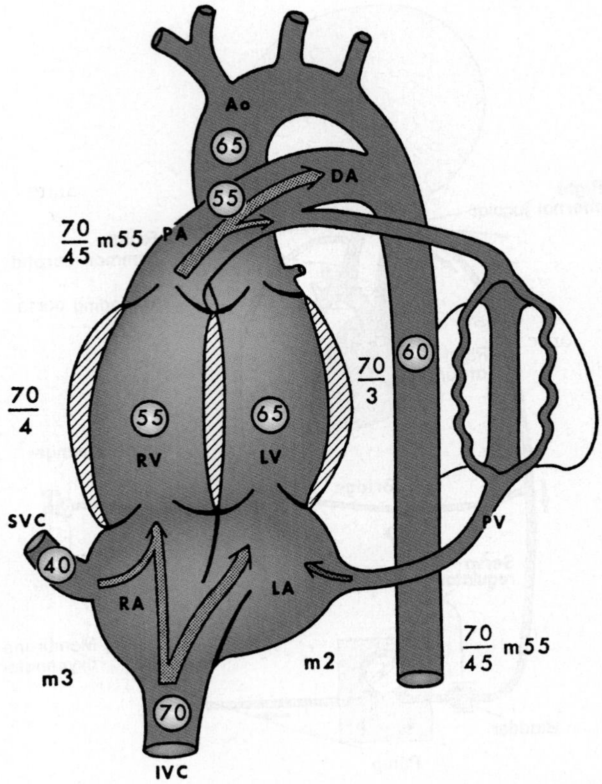

FIGURE 103.9. Oxyhemoglobin saturations in the fetal circulation. Preferential flow of saturated blood from the inferior vena cava (IVC) into the left atrium (LA) and desaturated blood from the superior vena cava (SVC) into the right atrium (RA) results in the distribution of blood with higher oxygen content to the aortic arch (Ao) and developing brain. (Adapted from Rudolph AM. Changes in the circulation after birth. In: Rudolph AM, ed. *Congenital Diseases of the Heart*. Chicago, IL: Year Book Medical; 1974.)

distribution of blood of varying oxygen contents and the delivery of adequate amounts of oxygen and substrate to developing organs (Fig. 103.8).

Well-oxygenated blood returning from the placenta and umbilical cord passes through the hepatic *ductus venosus*, into the inferior vena cava (IVC) and immediately into the right atrium. Ductus venosus blood mixes little with the less oxygenated blood in the infrahepatic IVC and flows relatively undisturbed (in a laminar fashion referred to as streaming) along the medial wall of the IVC, through the right atrium, across the foramen ovale, and into the left atrium. This oxygen-rich blood then is pumped by the left ventricle into the aortic arch, where it is distributed to the developing heart, brain, and upper body (Fig. 103.9). The less oxygenated blood in the IVC and superior vena cava (SVC) flows preferentially through the right atrium to the right ventricle and is pumped into the pulmonary artery, where most of it is shunted through the ductus arteriosus into the descending aorta. A small amount of pulmonary artery flow provides substrate to the lungs. Descending aortic flow is distributed to the developing organs of the lower body, with most of the flow being diverted back to the placenta through the two umbilical arteries. Flow through the placental circulation approximates 40% of cardiac output.

The fetal pattern of blood flow is made possible by high pulmonary vascular resistance, which directs the flow of oxygen-poor blood from the pulmonary artery into the descending aorta. Only 5% to 10% of pulmonary artery flow actually traverses the pulmonary capillary bed. This minimizes the return of less-oxygenated blood through the pulmonary veins and prevents mixing with the oxygen-rich blood in the left ventricle destined for the heart and brain. The relatively low afterload presented to the right ventricle by the low-resistance shunt across the ductus arteriosus accounts for the fact that fetal right ventricular output exceeds left ventricular output, in some estimates by 40% to 100%.[58,59] Mechanisms of increased pulmonary resistance in the fetus include mechanical compression of pulmonary vessels in the fluid-filled lung and vasoconstriction secondary to hypoxemia, leukotrienes, and the peptide mediator endothelin-1.[60]

Transitional Circulation

10 At birth, profound changes in circulatory patterns, hemodynamics, and gas exchange occur as a result of the abrupt withdrawal of placental support. Transitional physiology is characterized by the cessation of placental blood flow and gas exchange and the simultaneous increase in blood flow and gas exchange in the lungs. As amniotic fluid is expelled from the lungs by compression during birth and the lungs expand with the infant's first breath, alveolar expansion causes an immediate reduction in pulmonary vascular resistance secondary to increased traction on larger parenchymal vessels and decreased intra-alveolar pressure transmitted to alveolar microvessels.

These purely mechanical changes account for a fourfold reduction in pulmonary vascular resistance (PVR), contributing significantly to the 15-fold overall reduction in PVR that occurs at birth. Pulmonary artery pressures fall more slowly over the first weeks of life and may approximate systemic pressures for the first several days of life.

Increased local oxygen concentrations reduce hypoxic pulmonary vasoconstriction through mechanisms mediated by endothelial-derived intermediates, such as nitric oxide (NO) and prostacyclin.[61,62] The enzymes responsible for the production of NO and prostacyclin in the pulmonary circulation, NO synthase and cyclooxygenase, undergo developmental maturation late in gestation, and their activity increases rapidly in response to birth-related stimuli, ventilation, and oxygenation. NO and prostacyclin act on pulmonary vascular smooth muscle cells to increase intracellular concentrations of cyclic guanosine monophosphate (GMP) and cyclic adenosine monophosphate (cAMP), respectively, which results in relaxation and vasodilation. ATP, released directly from oxygenated red blood cells in the pulmonary circulation, is also a potent mediator of vasodilation. These vasodilatory mediators are countered by vasoconstrictor substances such as endothelin, thromboxane, and cytochrome P450 pathway products.

The sudden decrease in pulmonary vascular resistance causes a dramatic increase in pulmonary blood flow and left atrial return. Left ventricular preload increases, resulting in increased left ventricular stroke volume and output. Right atrial return is reduced as placental flow ceases. Elevated left atrial pressure and reduced right atrial pressure cause closure of the flaplike foramen ovale, eliminating one of the fetal extrapulmonary shunts.

The other shunt, the ductus arteriosus, begins to close by vasoconstriction immediately. This process is mediated by both a withdrawal of placental-derived prostaglandins and an increase in oxygen tension, a potent vasoconstrictive stimulus for ductal tissue. Physiologic duct closure usually occurs by 24 hours but may take up to 3 days. Anatomic duct obliteration resulting from thrombosis and fibrosis may take several weeks or months. When spontaneous closure of the ductus arteriosus does not occur, as often happens in the premature infant whose immature ductal tissue is unresponsive to vasoconstrictive mediators, significant physiologic problems may occur. If pulmonary artery pressures remain abnormally high, an anatomic right-to-left shunt may occur that diverts desaturated blood around the pulmonary system, drastically lowering systemic oxygen delivery. If pulmonary artery pressure falls normally, a left-to-right shunt will occur, increasing pulmonary blood flow above cardiac output. Pulmonary overcirculation causes pulmonary edema and congestive heart failure in the short term and irreversible pulmonary hypertension in the long term, if uncorrected. Indomethacin administration, which inhibits prostaglandin synthetase, is effective in promoting ductal closure in most premature infants if given within the first 2 weeks of life. Failure of medical therapy indicates the need for surgical duct ligation.

Another event in the transition to extrauterine circulation involves vasoconstrictive or mechanical occlusion of the cord vessels. The abolishment of this "shunt" increases left ventricular afterload and systemic blood pressure and, along with increased left ventricular preload, accounts for an immediate increase in blood flow to target organs. Ductus venosus closure occurs by stasis and thrombosis as return flow through the umbilical vein ceases.

Postnatal Circulation and Cardiac Performance

Following the transition from fetal to neonatal life, the circulatory system is characterized by two separate cardiovascular circuits operating in a "series" configuration. By definition, right and left heart cardiac outputs are identical and can be considered symmetric despite discrepancies in system pressures and contractile properties. The series configuration has great significance in that it imposes a degree of interdependence on the two circuits that does not exist in utero. Pathologic changes in one circuit necessarily impact the other circuit by virtue of alterations in the other circuit's preload or afterload. Failure of complete separation of the two circuits results in the deleterious shunting of blood from the pulmonary to systemic circuit or vice versa.

Cardiac output is determined by the same parameters in the neonate as in the adult: heart rate and stroke volume. Stroke volume, in turn, is dependent on three factors: preload, contractility, and afterload. Although a detailed discussion of these four determinants of cardiac performance is beyond the scope of this chapter, it is instructive to consider some of the differences between pediatric and adult cardiac function relative to these four variables. These differences account for the fact that, in general, neonatal and pediatric patients have less cardiovascular reserve than do adolescents and young adults.

Heart rate, an important determinant of cardiac output in infants, becomes less important in childhood and adolescence. In fact, neonates are commonly referred to as rate dependent. The normal range for heart rate in neonates is higher than that in adults and decreases gradually throughout childhood to adult levels (Table 103.6). In adults, changes in heart rate result in little change in cardiac output because of compensatory

TABLE 103.6

NORMAL RANGE OF VITAL SIGNS

■ AGE	■ HEART RATE (BEATS/MIN)	■ SYSTOLIC BLOOD PRESSURE (mm Hg)	■ DIASTOLIC BLOOD PRESSURE (mm Hg)	■ RESPIRATORY RATE (BREATHS/MIN)
Premature infant				
1 kg	120–140	36–58	18–38	40
3 kg	120–140	50–72	26–46	40
Term infant	120	65–80	30–50	40
0–12 mo[a]	100–120	105	65	40
1–6 y	100	105–110	70	30
6–12 y	80	110–125	70–80	20

[a]90th percentile.
Adapted from Horan MU. Report of the second task force on blood pressure control in children—1987. *Pediatrics* 1987;79:1.

changes in other parameters. When heart rate decreases, ventricular filling and stroke volume increase, and cardiac output is minimally altered. Reciprocal changes occur when heart rate increases. In neonates and, to a lesser extent, in children, these compensatory changes are less effective and changes in heart rate produce corresponding changes in cardiac output. The explanation for this observation lies in the fact that increased ventricular filling times and pressures fail to generate increased end-diastolic and stroke volumes because of decreased myocardial compliance and a blunted Frank-Starling mechanism, as discussed later.

The sympathetic innervation of the heart is relatively underdeveloped in the neonate, resulting in an autonomic imbalance with respect to cardiac function. Neonates respond to physiologic challenges in a predominantly vagal, or parasympathetic, fashion. Sinus bradycardia is therefore a common stereotypical response in the critically ill neonate to many stimuli, including hypoxemia, acidosis, hypoglycemia, intracranial hypertension, abdominal distention, and pulmonary aspiration. Because bradycardia is also more likely to result in an uncompensated decrease in cardiac output, prompt recognition and treatment of bradycardia are more urgent in these patients.

Preload refers to the myocardial fiber stretch at end diastole. Fiber stretch is related to end-diastolic volume, which in turn is related to end-diastolic pressure. The Frank-Starling mechanism describes this relationship: an increase in end-diastolic volume and fiber length produces an increase in stroke volume (Fig. 103.10). This phenomenon most likely is explained by changes in contractile fiber geometry that result from increased stretch. The Frank-Starling mechanism is not synonymous with an increase in contractility, which would produce an increased stroke volume at the same preload. This mechanism is less effective in neonates than in adults in producing an increase in myocardial performance. The immature heart is less compliant than the adult heart, so increases in end-diastolic pressure therefore do not produce similar increases in end-diastolic volume and fiber length. Furthermore, neonatal and infant hearts operate at a higher baseline end-diastolic volume (nearer the maximal fiber length) under normal circumstances, leaving less reserve for further effective increases in preload. These observations explain why the neonatal cardiovascular response to preload enhancement is less pronounced than in adults and why the neonate is generally more susceptible to congestive failure when challenged with a volume load.

Contractility refers to the magnitude and velocity of tension development by the cardiac myocytes in response to contractile stimuli. The contractile, or inotropic, state of the heart is influenced by many factors, including the availability of oxygen, calcium, and catecholamines. An increase in contractility does not result in a shift upward along the Frank-Starling curve, but rather it results in a shift of the entire curve to reflect a greater stroke volume generated at every preload. The neonatal heart is immature in several respects compared with the adult heart. Most importantly, the neonatal heart has a lower concentration of contractile fibers, generating less tension during contraction.[63] This is reflected in the lower mean arterial pressures observed throughout childhood. About 60% of the adult cardiac myocyte mass consists of contractile myofibrils, compared with 30% in fetal myocytes. Additional causes of reduced contractility include an underdeveloped sarcoplasmic reticulum and T-tubule system for releasing calcium, a lower concentration of myocyte cell surface β-adrenergic receptors, and decreased sympathetic innervation.[64] The structural and functional immaturity of the infant heart account for the relatively greater sensitivity to negative inotropic stimuli, the greater requirement for calcium to maintain the inotropic state, and the requirement for higher concentrations of inotropic agents to achieve measurable hemodynamic effects. In contrast, the neonatal heart is more resistant to the negative inotropic effects of hypoxemia and acidosis than the adult heart, possibly conferring some advantage with respect to the success of cardiopulmonary resuscitation.[65]

Afterload refers to the resistance (or impedance) to ventricular output and is directly related to mean arterial pressure. During the transitional phase of circulation, afterload drops abruptly in the right ventricle as pulmonary vascular resistance drops. Left ventricular afterload increases immediately as the placental shunt is abolished but then falls as its output distributes to both the upper and lower body and a larger vascular bed. After the transitional phase, left ventricular afterload slowly increases throughout infancy and childhood, stimulating asymmetric growth of the left ventricle compared with that of the right. This growth is caused primarily by hyperplasia until 2 to 3 months of age, when hypertrophy becomes more important. Before adaptive left ventricular growth occurs, the neonatal heart is exquisitely sensitive and decompensates rapidly when exposed to increases in afterload, such as those that occur in aortic stenosis and aortic coarctation.

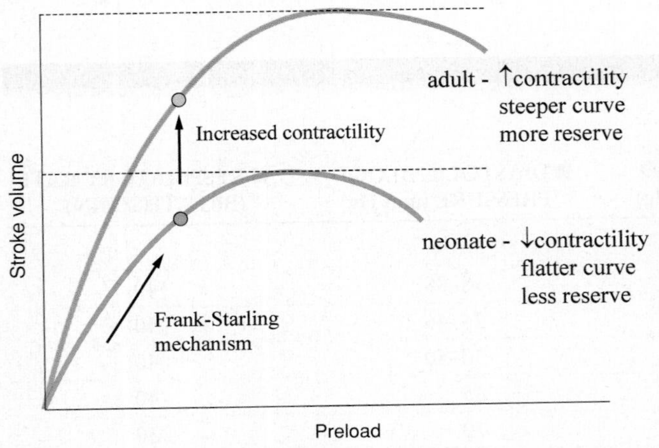

FIGURE 103.10. Conceptual differences in cardiac performance between neonates and adults. The neonatal heart displays reduced contractility, a reduced response to augmented preload, and less reserve compared with the adult heart.

Oxygen Content and Delivery

Oxygen delivery is the product of cardiac output and oxygen content. Arterial oxygen content (CaO_2) is determined by the same set of variables in children as in adults:

$$CaO_2 = (Hb)(1.34 \text{ mL } O_2/\text{g Hb})(\%\text{Hb saturation}) + \text{Dissolved } O_2$$

where Hb = hemoglobin.

Under most circumstances, dissolved oxygen is negligible. The main difference in the oxygen-carrying capacity of blood between neonates and older patients is the presence of fetal hemoglobin (HbF). The fetal red blood cell contains primarily HbF, a hemoglobin isomer with a higher affinity for oxygen than hemoglobin A (HbA), which predominates in adults. This gives HbF a lower P_{50} (the partial pressure of oxygen at which hemoglobin saturation is 50%), which is reflected in a leftward shift of the oxyhemoglobin dissociation curve relative to HbA (Fig. 103.11). This difference in affinities promotes the transfer of oxygen from maternal to fetal hemoglobin in the placenta. Following birth, neonatal red blood cells gradually accumulate HbA at the expense of HgF, which disappears by 4 months of age.

The presence of HbF in the neonate has several clinical consequences. Adequate hemoglobin saturation may occur at lower PaO_2 levels, but the benefits of this in the ex utero environment are deceiving. Greater oxygen affinity makes the unloading

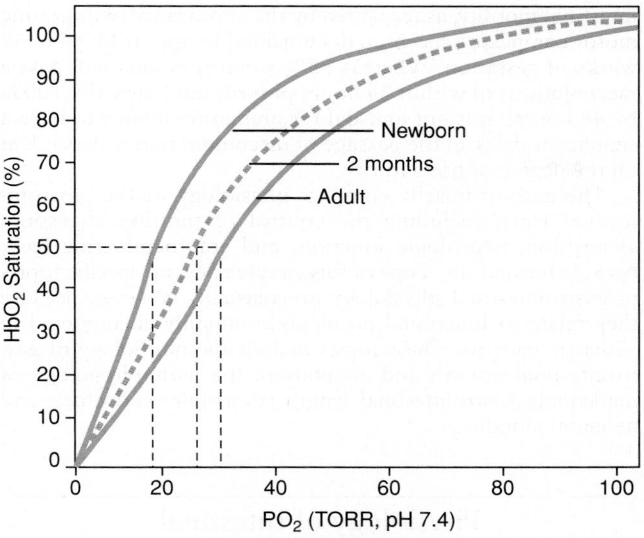

FIGURE 103.11. Representative oxyhemoglobin (HbO_2) saturation curves for newborn, infant, and adult. (Adapted from Hodson WA, Truog WE. In: Avery GB, Fletcher MA, MacDonald MG, eds. *Neonatology: Pathophysiology and Management of the Newborn.* 5th ed. Philadelphia, PA: Lippincott Williams & Wilkins; 1999.)

of oxygen in peripheral tissues more difficult. Increasing oxygen extraction during periods when oxygen demand temporarily exceeds supply is therefore less efficient. Increased difficulty in extracting oxygen from hemoglobin in peripheral tissues makes the neonate less tolerant than the older child of decreased oxygen delivery resulting from reduced hemoglobin concentration, hemoglobin saturation, or cardiac output. Constant attention to adequate oxygen content and cardiac output is therefore of paramount importance in the stressed neonate.

Pulmonary Hypertension and Persistent Fetal Circulation

In the older infant and child, PVR is normally low, which allows right ventricular output to equal that of the left ventricle at considerably lower pressure and contractile work. The instability of PVR in the neonate during the transitional period, along with the presence of anatomic connections between the pulmonary and systemic circuits, accounts for severe derangements in respiratory and hemodynamic performance in a wide variety of clinical disorders. These include acquired conditions (e.g., sepsis and meconium aspiration syndrome), congenital conditions (e.g., pulmonary hypoplasia associated with congenital diaphragmatic hernia [CDH]), idiopathic abnormalities in pulmonary vascular function (e.g., PPHN), and chronic microangiopathy, alveolar–capillary dysplasia, and fibrosis ("fixed" pulmonary hypertension secondary to uncorrected anatomic left-to-right shunting and pulmonary overcirculation).

The common denominator in these conditions is an abnormally high PVR, related both to vascular tone and to vascular anatomy. Pulmonary vascular tone is governed by the balance between molecular factors produced by vascular endothelium, including endothelin-1, nitric oxide, and prostacyclin. Endothelin-1 stimulates vascular smooth muscle contraction and proliferation, while both nitric oxide and prostacyclin cause vascular smooth muscle relaxation and inhibit proliferation. These mediators are important in prenatal, transitional, and postnatal regulation of pulmonary blood flow.

It is useful to categorize the etiologies of elevated PVR as related to vascular underdevelopment, maldevelopment, and maladaptation. Pulmonary vascular underdevelopment occurs in pulmonary hypoplasia when the normal number of airway and vascular branchings is abbreviated due to extrinsic compression during lung development (e.g., CDH, congenital cystic adenomatoid malformation [CCAM]) and causes a reduced total capillary cross-sectional area. This condition may be moderated over time with compensatory alveolar and capillary growth, but it represents a fixed limitation to pulmonary blood flow during the initial postnatal period. Pulmonary hypoplasia also results in vascular maldevelopment characterized by medial smooth muscle hypertrophy and hyperplasia, resulting in exaggerated responses to vasoconstrictive stimuli. Maladaptation refers to the deleterious responses of a normal pulmonary vascular bed to pathologic stimuli, as occurs in bacteremia (e.g., β-streptococcal sepsis).

Not uncommonly, increased PVR results from a combination of these factors. For example, pulmonary hypoplasia not only causes a decreased cross-sectional area but also results in hyperreactive arterioles prone to vasospasm. In "fixed" pulmonary hypertension, both fibrosis and decreased vessel numbers have been demonstrated. In perinatal aspiration of meconium or blood, ventilation is delayed and pulmonary hypertension ensues. Fetal exposure to maternally ingested nonsteroidal anti-inflammatory drugs causes spasm of the ductus arteriosus, increased fetal pulmonary flows and pressures, diminished NO synthase activity, and harmful pulmonary vascular remodeling.

Whatever the cause, increased PVR has several deleterious consequences. Increased right ventricular afterload results in decreased output, diminished pulmonary perfusion, and reduced left ventricular preload. Hypoxemia, hypercarbia, and globally decreased cardiac output result, which in turn cause metabolic acidosis. Increased PVR also promotes anatomic right-to-left shunting at the levels of the patent ductus arteriosus (PDA) and foramen ovale, a phenomenon referred to as persistent fetal circulation (PFC). This profoundly exacerbates the hypoxemia, hypercarbia, and acidosis already present. Because hypoxemia, hypercarbia, and acidosis are all potent mediators of pulmonary vasoconstriction, PVR is further increased. For this reason, pulmonary hypertension and PFC in the neonate frequently deteriorate into a vicious cycle that culminates in circulatory and metabolic collapse.

Therapy for pulmonary hypertension and PFC is directed at treating the underlying cause, removing the physiologic stimuli for pulmonary vasoconstriction, and introducing pharmacologic mediators of pulmonary vasodilatation. Analgesia, sedation, and neuromuscular blockade are commonly used to decrease endogenous stimulation of pulmonary vasoconstriction by catecholamines. The historical mainstays of management included aggressive ventilatory support to maximize PaO_2 and minimize $PaCO_2$, and systemic alkalinization (pH 7.50 to 7.60) with sodium bicarbonate or tris-hydroxymethylaminomethane (THAM) if an adequate respiratory alkalosis could not be induced. Because aggressive ventilatory strategies result in lung injury, current management targets a normal pH and $PaCO_2$ while maintaining adequate oxygenation, often with HFOV. Pharmacologic agents with the ability to promote direct pulmonary vasodilatation would obviously be desirable.

Selective pulmonary vasodilation is presently unrealistic from a clinical standpoint. No pharmacologic substance has yet been identified that has vasodilatory effects specifically limited to the pulmonary circulation. Intravenous administration of nitroprusside, nitroglycerine, and PGE_1 all produce systemic vasodilatation as well, negating the reduction of resistance and pressure in the pulmonary circuit, and resulting in an unaltered right-to-left shunt. Tolazoline hydrochloride was commonly used in the past as a pulmonary vasodilator in neonates with pulmonary hypertension. Its vasodilatory effects can be ascribed both to α-adrenergic blockade and to stimulation of pulmonary vascular histamine receptors.[66] Unfortunately, responses to tolazoline are unpredictable and nonselective, and no consistent clinical benefit has been convincingly demonstrated.

Perhaps the most promising pharmacologic approach to pulmonary vasodilation is the administration of inhaled nitric oxide (iNO). NO is a ubiquitous, potent vasodilator that serves as the final common pathway for vascular smooth muscle relaxation induced by a wide variety of other agents with known vasodilatory properties.[67,68] Endogenous NO is generated from L-arginine by the action of NO synthase in endothelial cells (eNOS) and diffuses to adjacent smooth muscle cells, where it promotes muscular relaxation via a cyclic guanosine monophosphate (GMP)-dependent mechanism.[69] Although smooth muscle relaxation induced by NO is not specific for the pulmonary circulation, vasodilatation is limited to the pulmonary circulation because iNO is immediately scavenged and inactivated in the pulmonary bloodstream by binding to hemoglobin and forming methemoglobin. Thus, iNO is able to bind to pulmonary vascular smooth muscle cell receptors and induce relaxation before it diffuses into the capillary lumen and becomes inactivated. The fact the iNO diffuses directly to the smooth muscle cells makes this therapy ideal in the presence of endothelial cell injury, which is commonly seen in PPHN.

iNO is administered by mixing minute quantities of NO (5 to 20 ppm) into the gas mixture during mechanical ventilation. Although toxicity from methemoglobin has been suggested as a potential adverse effect, clinically significant methemoglobinemia has not been observed when NO is delivered at such low concentrations. A more significant difficulty with inhaled NO therapy is the development of tachyphylaxis, which frequently occurs after as little as 2 to 3 days of treatment.[70] Despite this potential obstacle, this novel strategy of selective delivery of a potent, nonspecific vasodilator to the pulmonary circulation represents a major new development in the treatment of pulmonary hypertension in infants.

A better understanding of the mechanisms of pulmonary vasoreactivity has suggested alternate approaches to iNO therapy for PPHN.[71] Direct infusion of L-arginine provides both increased substrate for endogenous NO generation and stimulation of increased eNOS activity. Phosphodiesterase inhibitors such as sildenafil delay the degradation of both cyclic AMP and cyclic GMP, resulting in higher intracellular concentrations of these vasodilatory compounds. Sildenafil use may be limited by systemic hypotension, and studies are currently ongoing to establish the safety and efficacy of this drug in PPHN. Adenosine and ATP may also produce selective pulmonary vasodilation when infused intravenously, though their use in neonates with PPHN has not been studied.

Failure to promote pulmonary vasodilatation through physiologic or pharmacologic manipulation may indicate a need to use extracorporeal techniques to reverse hypoxemia, hypercarbia, hypoperfusion, and acidosis. As discussed, ECMO has become a widely accepted therapy for refractory pulmonary hypertension associated with a variety of causes. It is important to recognize that extracorporeal support for pulmonary hypertension (or respiratory failure) is indicated only when the underlying cause is thought to be reversible.

GASTROINTESTINAL AND HEPATIC PHYSIOLOGY

11 Most mechanisms of physiologic control in the gastrointestinal tract are present at birth, although continued postnatal maturation results in ongoing adjustments over time. Prematurity, however, is associated with a delay in gastrointestinal function, just as it is in the cardiovascular and pulmonary systems. For example, immaturity of gastrointestinal motility and digestive enzyme activity in the preterm infant frequently results in early feeding intolerance. The functional immaturity of small-intestinal "brush-border" enzymes in premature infants has already been mentioned with respect to the particular nutritional requirements of preterm infants. Normal intestinal motility, as measured by the appearance of migrating motor complexes, has been documented to appear by 36 to 38 weeks of gestation. Whereas 95% of term infants will pass a meconium stool within 24 hours of birth (and virtually 100% by 48 hours), it is not unusual for premature infants to have a significant delay in the passage of meconium that is dependent on the degree of prematurity.

The extraordinarily complex physiology of the gastrointestinal tract, including the control of motility, digestion, absorption, neurologic function, and enteroendocrine feedback, is beyond the scope of this chapter. Several specific topics in gastrointestinal physiology are relevant, however, because they relate to functional problems commonly encountered in pediatric patients. These topics include the physiology of gastrointestinal growth and adaptation, the pathophysiology of inadequate gastrointestinal length (short-gut syndrome), and neonatal jaundice.

Physiology of Intestinal Growth and Adaptation

To meet the needs of the growing child for energy and structural substrates, the absorptive surface area of the intestinal tract must increase along with somatic growth. At 28 weeks of gestation the small bowel measures about 100 cm and grows to 120 cm at 34 weeks to reach a mean length of 160 cm at full term.[72] Postnatally, the small intestine increases from a length of about 150 to 200 cm and a diameter of about 1.5 cm at birth to a length of 600 to 800 cm and a diameter of 4 cm at maturity. Further growth and maturation of the villous architecture and the development of *plicae circulares* increase the total absorptive surface area from approximately 900 cm^2 to 7,500 cm^2 over the same period.[73]

After growing to full length in childhood, the small intestine enters a state of dormancy and remains quiescent unless some major change occurs. Following massive intestinal resection, various adaptive responses occur in the small intestine; these responses are designed to enhance the absorptive function of the remaining bowel. These adaptive changes include an increase in diameter, an increase in the number and size of the plicae circulares, and epithelial hyperplasia manifested as increased villous height and crypt depth. These changes augment the absorptive surface area significantly, but they do not constitute a physiologically equivalent substitute for intestine of normal length and caliber. The markedly dilated, adapted intestine displays abnormal motility as a result of muscular hypertrophy and an inability to sustain normal peristalsis by coaptation. These dyskinetic contractions do not provide consistent, unidirectional flow and, therefore, allow stasis and bacterial colonization of the proximal intestine.

Although the factors governing stimulation of intestinal growth and adaptation are poorly understood, it is becoming increasingly clear that trophic stimulation from both enteroendocrine mediators and intraluminal substances is necessary. The gastrointestinal mucosa is richly populated with a variety of peptide-secreting enteroendocrine cells that produce local signaling and mediator molecules in response to specific stimuli (Fig. 103.12). Some of these enteroendocrine peptides are expressed only during fetal development. Virtually every known postnatal enteroendocrine cell is present and functionally mature at term.[74] The levels of many of these peptides rise sharply in the first days of life in fed infants, but not in fasting infants.[75] The observation that intestinal growth and maturation are inhibited by withholding enteral feeds suggests that enteroendocrine stimulation is one of the processes responsible for normal postnatal intestinal growth. Glucagon, glucagon-like peptides 1 and 2, and gastrin are present in the fetal and neonatal gut, and appear to be leading candidates for the principal enteroendocrine mediators of epithelial proliferation and

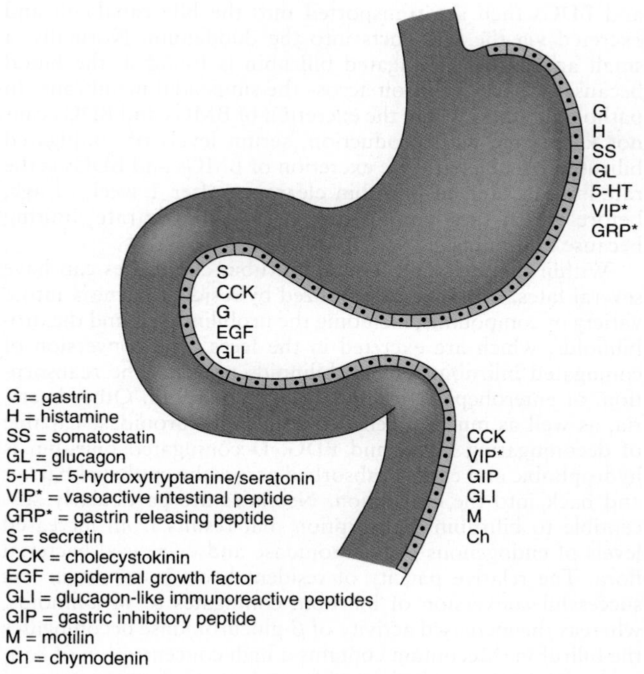

FIGURE 103.12. Distribution of selected enteroendocrine and neuroendocrine (*asterisks*) cells and their products in the proximal gastrointestinal tract. (Adapted from Magnuson DK, Schwartz MZ. In: Oldham KT, Colombani PM, Foglia RP, eds. *Surgery of Infants and Children*. Philadelphia, PA: Lippincott–Raven; 1997.)

overall gut growth, both by direct stimulation and through generation of other mediators such as insulin.[76–78] Recent studies reveal members of the PACAP (pituitary adenylate cyclase–activating peptide)/glucagon family to be involved in gastrointestinal signaling and growth regulation. This group of related neuropeptides is found throughout the intestine. Like vasoactive intestinal peptide (VIP), PACAP is a potent vasodilator. To date, there is no evidence that VIP or PACAP administration is directly trophic for small bowel after resection or injury.[79]

Direct stimulation of mucosal growth by luminal nutrients plays a major role in intestinal adaptation. The fact that villous height and absorptive capacity are greatest in the proximal jejunum and gradually decrease through the remaining jejunum and ileum suggests that progressive depletion of luminal nutrients results in relatively diminished growth of the distal intestine. Reciprocal transposition of ileal and jejunal segments results in hypertrophy of the proximally transposed ileal segment and atrophy of the distally transposed jejunal segment. The "underdevelopment" of the distal small bowel may be viewed, to a certain extent, as built-in reserve potential.

In various experimental models, adaptive growth will not occur after resection unless some level of luminal nutrition is provided. Studies in animal models have shown that complex nutrients that require enzymatic degradation (e.g., long-chain fatty acids, disaccharides, and complex proteins) are more potent stimulators of growth than are more elemental nutrients.[80–82] This effect may result from the trophic properties of pancreaticobiliary secretions, which are stimulated by complex nutritional substrates. The amino acid glutamine is the preferred energy substrate for enterocytes and a necessary constituent of growth-promoting enteral nutrition formulas. It is not clear whether glutamine acts in a permissive fashion only by providing energy substrate for growth or whether it also has trophic properties separate from its energy content. Intravenous glutamine administration can preserve intestinal mucosal health in the absence of enteral glutamine, but whether it can promote long-term gut adaptation and growth also is not known. Epidermal growth factor (EGF), present in duodenal and biliary secretions, and growth hormone are both potent growth stimuli. The administration of enteral glutamine and EGF (or growth hormone or both) may have a therapeutic benefit in stimulating intestinal growth after bowel resection.

Clinical Aspects of Short-gut Syndrome

Although intestinal growth is commonly taken for granted in health, its importance is brought into sharp focus by conditions in which inadequate intestinal length causes malabsorption and malnutrition: the short-gut syndrome. This syndrome usually occurs after massive intestinal resection for a variety of diseases. The most common causes in the neonatal period are necrotizing enterocolitis and midgut volvulus, although gastroschisis also may be associated with decreased intestinal length in the absence of resection.[83,84] In older children, volvulus and inflammatory bowel disease predominate.[85] The extent of resection likely to result in short-gut syndrome is difficult to quantify and is influenced by patient age, site of intestinal loss, and status of the ileocecal valve (ICV). It is commonly held that a term newborn who retains at least 25 cm of small intestine with an intact ICV, or 40 cm without an ICV, has a reasonable potential for resuming full enteral feedings at some point. In older patients, loss of 75% to 80% of intestinal length may be tolerated as long as the ICV is preserved.

The loss of intestinal surface area diminishes absorptive capacity, brush-border digestive enzyme activity, and enteroendocrine mediator production. These deficiencies all lead to malnutrition and weight loss. Unabsorbed sugars pass through to the colon and produce an osmotic diarrhea. Presentation of undigested carbohydrates to the colon also provides fuel for bacterial proliferation. The bacteria metabolize the undigested sugars to lactate and short-chain fatty acids, which stimulate colonic secretion of water and electrolytes. Thus, a secretory diarrhea exacerbates the osmotic one. After ileal resections, bile salt recirculation is impaired and bile salts reach the colon, providing more bacterial fuel and further stimulating the secretory diarrhea. Bile salt wasting eventually depletes the hepatic bile salt pool, resulting in fat malabsorption and steatorrhea, and leading to lithogenic bile and gallstones. Extensive ileal resections also result in impaired absorption of vitamin B_{12} and the fat-soluble vitamins A, D, E, and K.

Bacterial overgrowth in the residual small intestine occurs in most patients with short-gut syndrome. It is related primarily to the loss of the ICV and reflux of colonic bacteria into the small intestine. Overgrowth also is promoted by stasis and hypomotility, which occur in adapted, dilated, dyskinetic intestine. Bacterial overgrowth in the proximal intestine leads to further increases in carbohydrate, protein, and fluid and electrolyte loss caused by diarrhea.

Gastric hypersecretion of fluid and acid is well documented in short-gut syndrome. Acid hypersecretion has been linked to hypergastrinemia, possibly because of the loss of somatostatin and gastrin-inhibiting peptide production. Gastric hypersecretion results in peptic complications, reduced enzymatic digestion caused by low intraluminal pH, and further exacerbation of diarrhea.

Management of short-gut syndrome is complex and may include any combination of the following: parenteral nutrition, limited enteral feeding with easily absorbed substrates (glucose polymers, medium-chain triglycerides, protein hydrosylates), judicious enteral exposure to trophic substrates (complex carbohydrates, intact protein, long-chain triglycerides, and glutamine), antibiotic suppression of bacterial overgrowth, supplementation of vitamins and minerals, and control of diarrhea with antimotility agents. Clinical trials have not demonstrated any benefit with respect to enhanced intestinal adaptation from the intravenous administration of glutamine or growth hormone.[86] Surgical treatment of short-gut syndrome by intestinal lengthening procedures and transplantation has been disappointing. In contrast, recent advances in small-bowel transplantation have resulted in improved 5-year patient survivals of 60% to 70% at centers of excellence.[87,88]

Long-term parenteral nutrition, as it is applied in many patients with short-gut syndrome, is associated with numerous complications. Among these are catheter-related sepsis, growth failure, metabolic disorders, bone disease, and, most importantly, parenteral nutrition–associated liver disease (PNALD). PNALD is characterized by steatosis, cholestasis, hepatic fibrosis, and ultimate progression to biliary cirrhosis, portal hypertension, and end-stage liver disease. The reported incidence of PNALD varies greatly and is reported to be up to 30% in children on long-term parenteral nutrition and almost 90% in infants with similar risk exposure. The incidence of PNALD in neonates receiving parenteral nutrition ranges from 14% after 2 to 4 weeks and reaches 72% for those receiving parenteral nutrition for more than 100 days. The risk for PNALD seems to correlate inversely with birthweight.[89]

Currently, parenteral lipid emulsions contain safflower and soybean oils. The administration of those plant oils may play a role in the onset of liver injury. Studies indicate that fish oil–based lipid emulsions provide a promising alternative, leading to dramatic reduction of PNALD in children receiving long-term parenteral nutrition. Due to the high concentrations of omega-3 poly-unsaturated fatty acids, administration of fish oil modulates the inflammatory response by reducing levels of proinflammatory cytokines.[90–92]

Neonatal Jaundice

Hepatic function in the older child is essentially the same as in the adult. In the neonatal period, however, liver function may be altered in a number of ways by hepatocyte immaturity. Although fetal hepatocytes begin to manifest synthetic capabilities early in gestation, the quantitative capacity to produce, modify, and detoxify various substances develops gradually and is often incompletely developed at birth, particularly in premature infants. This functional immaturity affects a range of processes, including glycogen metabolism and the biotransformation of many drugs, but most notably it affects the excretion of bilirubin.

Bilirubin Metabolism. Bilirubin is produced by the degradation of heme-containing compounds, primarily hemoglobin from senescent red blood cells, but also myoglobin, cytochromes, catalases, and other molecules. Because infants have a relatively greater red cell mass than adults, as well as a shorter red cell life span and higher turnover, bilirubin production is proportionately greatest in the first weeks of life. The conversion of heme to bilirubin occurs in reticuloendothelial cells in the liver, spleen, and elsewhere. In the first step, the ring structure of heme is opened by the oxidative removal of a carbon atom through heme oxygenase, which also releases a reduced iron atom. The resulting product, biliverdin, is a linear molecule that is further reduced by biliverdin reductase to bilirubin. Bilirubin is held in a tightly folded configuration by extensive hydrogen bonding, resulting in a highly hydrophobic and insoluble molecule. As such, transport of bilirubin from sites of production to the liver for excretion requires binding to albumin as a carrier molecule.

Bilirubin is extracted from hepatic sinusoidal blood and transported by a specific membrane carrier protein into the hepatocyte, where it is attached to the cytoplasmic carrier protein ligandin (glutathione S-transferase). Within the cytoplasm, bilirubin is conjugated with glucuronic acid by bilirubin glucuronosyltransferase (BGT) to form bilirubin monoglucuronides (BMGs) and diglucuronides (BDGs). Both BMGs and BDGs then are transported into the bile canaliculi and excreted via the bile ducts into the duodenum. Normally, a small amount of conjugated bilirubin is found in the blood because of back-diffusion across the sinusoidal membrane. In pathologic states where the excretion of BMGs and BDGs cannot keep pace with production, serum levels of conjugated bilirubin rise. Hepatocyte excretion of BMGs and BDGs is the rate-limiting step in bilirubin clearance after 1 week of age, before which time conjugation of bilirubin is rate limiting because of diminished activity of BGT.

Within the intestinal lumen, bilirubin conjugates can have several fates. Most are metabolized by resident bacteria into a variety of compounds, including the urobilinogens and the urobilinoids, which are excreted in the feces. The conversion of conjugated bilirubin into urobilinoids prevents the reabsorption, or enterohepatic recirculation, of bilirubin. Other bacteria, as well as mucosal cells, contain β-glucuronidase capable of deconjugating BMG and BDG. Deconjugated bilirubin is hydrophobic and easily reabsorbed across the epithelial barrier and back into the circulation. Neonates are particularly susceptible to bilirubin reabsorption that results from increased levels of endogenous β-glucuronidase and decreased bacterial flora. The relative paucity of resident bacteria results in less successful conversion of bilirubin conjugates to urobilinoids, whereas the increased activity of β-glucuronidase deconjugates the bilirubin. Meconium contains a high concentration of conjugated bilirubin, which readily undergoes deconjugation if impaired motility delays its excretion.

Neonatal Hyperbilirubinemia. Transient, unconjugated hyperbilirubinemia is a ubiquitous finding in neonates and represents a normal stage in early postnatal life. For this reason, it is often referred to as physiologic jaundice. The exact cause of physiologic jaundice is unclear, but it appears to involve a combination of increased enterohepatic circulation of bilirubin and decreased BGT activity.[93] Both the duration and magnitude of the hyperbilirubinemia are variable but, in general, plasma levels of unconjugated bilirubin peak at about 5 to 6 mg/dL at 3 days of life and resolve by 7 to 10 days in healthy term infants.

In addition to physiologic jaundice, numerous conditions are associated with more severe unconjugated hyperbilirubinemia in the early postnatal period. These include breast-milk jaundice, hemolytic diseases (ABO or Rh incompatibility, hemoglobinopathies), reabsorption of extravascular blood, neonatal hepatitis, inborn errors of metabolism, and sepsis. Unconjugated hyperbilirubinemia can cause both a reversible encephalopathy and an irreversible neurologic injury termed *kernicterus*. The predilection of unconjugated bilirubin for neural tissue is related to its nonpolar structure, which makes it highly hydrophobic and lipophilic. Deposition of bilirubin in the basal ganglia and cranial nerve nuclei is the most common pathologic feature, although clinical manifestations include a wide variety of cognitive, developmental, motor, and sensory dysfunction. The risks of neurologic injury are related to peak sustained bilirubin levels; kernicterus is likely when sustained plasma levels exceed 30 mg/dL and is virtually unknown when levels do not exceed 20 mg/dL. Between 20 and 30 mg/dL, the incidence of reversible encephalopathy is greatest, but increasing risk of kernicterus is a concern.

Indications for intervention include early onset or prolonged duration of jaundice and exaggerated absolute levels of unconjugated bilirubin. The precise level at which therapeutic intervention is considered depends on postnatal and gestational age, weight, and presence of comorbidity, and is the subject of considerable debate. First-line therapies include stimulation of intestinal motility by oral feeding and rectal stimulation to promote the passage of meconium and reduce enterohepatic circulation. When levels become high or sustained enough to elicit genuine concern, the treatment of choice is phototherapy. Light in the blue spectrum with wavelengths of 420 to 480 nm is absorbed by unconjugated bilirubin. The absorbed energy alters the double-bond structure of bilirubin in a process termed *photoisomerization*. The new isomers are less capable of forming internal hydrogen bonds and, therefore, become unfolded and more polar. This configurational change makes them more soluble, promotes their mobilization from central nervous system tissues, and allows their excretion in the bile without further conjugation. When extremely high levels of bilirubin are encountered and phototherapy is deemed insufficiently rapid, exchange transfusion provides the most reliable method of rapidly reducing serum bilirubin levels into a nontoxic range.

In contrast to unconjugated hyperbilirubinemia, elevation of serum conjugated bilirubin is always pathologic and mandates expeditious evaluation. The presence of isolated conjugated hyperbilirubinemia in the first weeks of life usually suggests the presence of a condition associated with reduced bile excretion. These include extrahepatic biliary atresia, Alagille syndrome (arteriohepatic dysplasia or intrahepatic biliary hypoplasia), nonsyndromic intrahepatic bile duct paucity, Byler syndrome (progressive familial intrahepatic cholestasis), choledochal cyst, and TPN-related cholestasis. Not all episodes of conjugated hyperbilirubinemia result from biliary obstruction, however. Because hepatocyte excretion of BMGs and BDGs is rate limiting after the first week of life, increased bilirubin loads generated by hemolysis or reabsorption may result in the production of bilirubin conjugates at a rate exceeding the hepatocyte's ability to excrete them into the canaliculi. Intracellular buildup results in back-diffusion of conjugated bilirubin into the sinusoidal and systemic circulation.

References

1. Bottoms SF, Paul RH, Mercer BM, et al. Obstetric determinants of neonatal survival: antenatal predictors of neonatal survival and morbidity in extremely low birth weight infants. *Am J Obstet Gynecol* 1999;180(Pt 1):665–669.
2. Tyson JE, Parikh NA, Langer J, et al. Intensive care for extreme prematurity—moving beyond gestational age. *N Engl J Med* 2008;358(16):1672–1681.
3. Horbar JD, Onstad L, Wright E. Predicting mortality risk for infants weighing 501 to 1500 grams at birth. *Crit Care Med* 1993;21:12–18.
4. Fowden AL, Forhead AJ. Endocrine regulation of feto-placental growth. *Horm Res* 2009;72(5):257–265.
5. Fuglsang J, Sandager P, Moller N, et al. Peripartum maternal and foetal ghrelin, growth hormones, IGFs and insulin interrelations. *Clin Endocrinol (Oxf)* 2006;64(5):502–509.
6. Takaya K, Ariyasu T, Kanamoto N, et al. Ghrelin strongly stimulates growth hormone release in humans. *J Clin Endocrinol Metab* 2000;85(12):4908–4911.
7. Gualillo O, Caminos J, Blanco M. Ghrelin, a novel placental-derived hormone. *Endocrinology* 2001;142(2):788–794.
8. Soriano-Guillen L, Barrios V, Chowen JA, et al. Ghrelin levels from fetal life through early adulthood: relationship with endocrine and metabolic and anthropometric measures. *J Pediatr* 2004;144(1):30–35.
9. Forhead AJ, Fowden AL. The hungry fetus? Role of leptin as a nutritional signal before birth. *J Physiol* 2009;587(Pt 6):1145–1152.
10. Forhead AJ, Lamb CA, Franko KL. Role of leptin in the regulation of growth and carbohydrate metabolism in the ovine fetus during late gestation. *J Physiol* 2008;586(9):2393–2403.
11. Onay-Besikci A. Regulation of cardiac energy metabolism in newborn. *Mol Cell Biochem* 2006;287(1–2):1–11.
12. Hawdon JM, Ward Platt MP. Metabolic adaptation in small for gestational age infants. *Arch Dis Child* 1993;68:262–268.
13. Lee H, Jain L. Physiology of infants with very low birth weight. *Semin Pediatr Surg* 1990;9:50–55.
14. Sell H, Deshaies Y, Richard D. The brown adipocyte: update on its metabolic role. *Int J Biochem Cell Biol* 2004;36:2098–2104.
15. Albanese CT, Nour BM, Rowe MI. Anesthesia blocks nonshivering thermogenesis in the neonatal rabbit. *J Pediatr Surg* 1994;29(8):983–986.
16. Ohlson KB, Lindahl SG, Cannon B, et al. Thermogenesis inhibition in brown adipocytes is a specific property of volatile anesthetics. *Anesthesiology* 2003;98(2):437–448.
17. Whyte RK, Campbell D, Stanhope R, et al. Energy balance in low birth weight infants fed formula of high or low medium chain triglyceride content. *J Pediatr* 1986;108:964–971.
18. Sauer PJ, Dane HF, Visser HK. Longitudinal studies on metabolic rate, heat loss, and energy cost of growth in low birth weight infants. *Pediatr Res* 1984;18:254–259.
19. Holliday MA. Body composition and energy needs during growth. In: Faulkner F, Tanner JM, eds. *Human Growth: A Comprehensive Treatise,* 2nd ed. New York: Plenum Press; 1986:101–117.
20. Groner JI, Brown MF, Stallings VA, et al. Resting energy expenditure in children following major operative procedures. *J Pediatr Surg* 1989;24:825–827.
21. Mitchell IM, Davies PS, Day JM, et al. Energy expenditure in children with congenital heart disease, before and after cardiac surgery. *J Thorac Cardiovasc Surg* 1994;107:374–380.
22. Dekelbab BH, Sperling MA. Hyperinsulinemic hypoglycemia of infancy: the challenge continues. *Diabetes Metab Res Rev* 2004;20:189–195.
23. Souba WW, Herskowitz K, Austgen TR, et al. Glutamine nutrition: theoretical considerations and therapeutic impact. *JPEN J Parenter Enteral Nutr* 1990;14(5 suppl):237S–243S.
24. Lorenz JM, Kleinman LI, Ahmed G, et al. Phases of fluid and electrolyte homeostasis in the extremely low birth weight infant. *Pediatrics* 1995;96(3Pt 1):484–489.
25. Patzer L. Nephrotoxicity as a cause of acute kidney injury in children. *Pediatr Nephrol* 2008;23(12):2159–2173.
26. Bonilla-Felix M. Development of water transport. *Am J Physiol Renal Physiol* 2004;287:F1093–F1101.
27. Del Riccio V, Van Tuyl M, Post M. Apoptosis in lung development and neonatal lung injury. *Pediatr Res* 2004;55:183–189.
28. Galambos C, Demello DE. Regulation of alveologenesis: clinical implications of impaired growth. *Pathology* 2008;40(2):124–140.
29. Nakayama DK, Motoyama EK, Tagge EM. Effect of preoperative stabilization on respiratory system compliance and outcome in newborn infants with congenital diaphragmatic hernia. *J Pediatr* 1991;118:793–799.
30. Helms P, Stocks J. Lung function in infants with congenital pulmonary hypoplasia. *J Pediatr* 1982;101:918–922.
31. Wolfson MR, Bhutani VK, Shaffer TH, et al. Mechanics and energetics of breathing helium in infants with bronchopulmonary dysplasia. *J Pediatr* 1984;104:752–757.
32. Cassin S, Tod M, Philips J, et al. Effects of prostaglandin D2 in the perinatal circulation. *Am J Physiol* 1981;240:H755–H760.
33. Chatfield BA, McMurtry IF, Hall SL, et al. Hemodynamic effects of endothelin-1 on the ovine fetal pulmonary circulation. *Am J Physiol* 1991;261:R182–R187.
34. Ivy DD, Kinsella JP, Abman SH. Physiologic characterization of endothelin A and B receptor activity in the ovine fetal pulmonary circulation. *J Clin Invest* 1994;93:2141–2148.
35. Bunt JE, Carnielli VP, Darcos Wattimena JL, et al. The effect in premature infants of prenatal corticosteroids on endogenous surfactant synthesis as measured with stable isotopes. *Am J Respir Crit Care Med* 2000;162:844–849.
36. Gregory TJ, Steinberg KP, Spragg R, et al. Bovine surfactant therapy for patients with acute respiratory distress syndrome. *Am J Respir Crit Care Med* 1997;155:1309–1315.
37. Galie N, Manes A, Branzi A. The endothelin system in pulmonary arterial hypertension. *Cardiovasc Res* 2004;61:227–237.
38. Dreyfuss D, Soler P, Basset G, et al. High inflation pulmonary edema. *Am Rev Respir Dis* 1988;137:1159–1164.
39. Hernandez LA, Peevy KJ, Moise AA, et al. Chest wall restriction limits high airway pressure-induced lung injury in young rabbits. *J Appl Physiol* 1989;66:2364–2368.
40. Dreyfuss D, Saumon G. Role of tidal volume, FRC, and end-inspiratory volume in the development of pulmonary edema following mechanical ventilation. *Am Rev Respir Dis* 1993;148:1194–1203.
41. McCallion N, Davis PG, Morley CJ. Volume-targeted versus pressure-limited ventilation in the neonate. *Cochrane Database Syst Rev* 2005;(3):CD003666.
42. Greenough A, Dimitriou G, Prendergast M, et al. Synchronized mechanical ventilation for respiratory support in newborn infants. *Cochrane Database Syst Rev* 2008;(1):CD000456.
43. Ramanathan R, Sardesai S. Lung protective ventilatory strategies in very low birthweight infants. *J Perinatol* 2008;28(suppl):S41–S46.
44. Marraro GA. Innovative practices of ventilatory support with pediatric patients. *Pediatr Crit Care Med* 2003;4:1–26.
45. Putensen C, Zech S, Wrigg H, et al. Long-term effects of spontaneous breathing during ventilatory support in patient with acute lung injury. *Am J Respir Crit Care Med* 2001;164(1):43–49.
46. Sinderby C, Beck J. Proportional assist ventilation and neurally adjusted ventilatory assist – better approaches to patient ventilator synchrony? *Clin Chest Med* 2008;29(2):329–342.
47. Navalesi P, Costa R. New modes of mechanical ventilation: proportional assist ventilation, neurally adjusted ventilatory assist, and fractal ventilation. *Curr Opin Crit Care* 2003;9(1):51–58.
48. Breatnach C, Conlon NP, Stack M, et al. A prospective crossover comparison of neurally adjusted ventilatory assist and pressure support ventilation in a pediatric and neonatal intensive care population. *Pediatr Crit Care Med* 2010;11:7–10.
49. Hummler H, Schultze A. New and alternative modes of mechanical ventilation in neonates. *Semin Fetal Neonatal Med* 2009;14(1):42–48.
50. Leach CL, Fuhrman BP, Morin FC III, et al. Perfluorocarbon-associated gas exchange (partial liquid ventilation) in respiratory distress syndrome: a prospective, randomized, controlled study. *Crit Care Med* 1993;21:1270–1278.
51. Levy MS, Share JC, Fauza DO, et al. Fate of the reconstructed carotid artery after extracorporeal membrane oxygenation. *J Pediatr Surg* 1995;30(7):1046–1049.
52. Desai SA, Stanley C, Gringlas M, et al. Five-year follow-up of neonates with reconstructed right common carotid arteries after extracorporeal membrane oxygenation. *J Pediatr* 1999;134(4):428–433.

53. Buesing KA, Kilian AK, Schaible T, et al. Extracorporeal membrane oxygenation in infants with congenital diaphragmatic hernia: follow-up MRI evaluating carotid artery reconstruction and neurologic outcome. *AJR Am J Roentgenol* 2007;188(6):1636–1642.
54. Hansell DR. Extracorporeal membrane oxygenation for perinatal and pediatric patients. *Respir Care* 2003;48:352–362.
55. Lequier L. Extracorporeal life support in pediatric and neonatal critical care: a review. *J Intensive Care Med* 2004;19:243–249.
56. Kugelman A, Gangitano E, Taschuk R, et al. Extracorporeal membrane oxygenation in infants with meconium aspiration syndrome: a decade of experience with venovenous ECMO. *J Pediatr Surg* 2005;40(7):1082–1089.
57. Moler FW, Custer JR, Bartlett RH, et al. Extracorporeal life support for severe pediatric respiratory failure: an updated experience 1991–1993. *J Pediatr* 1994;124:875–880.
58. St. John Sutton MG, Raichlen JS, Reichek N, et al. Quantitative assessment of right and left ventricular growth in the human fetal heart: a pathoanatomic study. *Circulation* 1984;70:935–941.
59. Rudolph AM, Heymann MA. Circulatory changes during growth in the fetal lamb. *Circ Res* 1970;26:289–299.
60. Fineman JR, Soifer SJ, Heymann MA. Regulation of pulmonary vascular tone in the perinatal period. *Annu Rev Physiol* 1995;57:115–134.
61. Shaul PW, Farrar MA, Magness RR. Oxygen modulation of pulmonary arterial prostacyclin synthesis is developmentally regulated. *Am J Physiol* 1993;265(2pt 2):H621–H628.
62. Shaul PW, Farrar MA, Zellers TM. Oxygen modulates endothelium-derived relaxing factor production in fetal pulmonary arteries. *Am J Physiol* 1992;262(2 Pt 2):H355–H364.
63. Anderson P. Physiology of the fetal, neonatal, and adult heart. In: Polin RA, Fox WW, eds. *Fetal and Neonatal Physiology*. Philadelphia, PA: WB Saunders; 1992:722–758.
64. Artman M, Graham TP Jr, Boucek RJ Jr. Effects of postnatal maturation on myocardial contractile responses to calcium antagonists and changes in contraction frequency. *J Cardiovasc Physiol* 1985;7:850–855.
65. Talner NS, Lister G, Fahey JT. Effects of asphyxia on the myocardium of the fetus and newborn. In: Polin RA, Fox WW, eds. *Fetal and Neonatal Physiology*. Philadelphia, PA: WB Saunders; 1992:759–769.
66. Goetzman BG, Milstein JM. Pulmonary vasodilator action of tolazoline. *Pediatr Res* 1979;13:942–944.
67. Palmer RMJ, Ferrige AG, Moncada S. Nitric oxide release accounts for the biological activity of endothelium-derived relaxing factor. *Nature* 1987; 327:524–526.
68. Ignarro LJ, Byrns RE, Buga GM, et al. Endothelium-dependent relaxing factor from pulmonary artery and vein possesses pharmacologic and chemical properties identical to those of nitric oxide radical. *Circ Res* 1987;61: 866–879.
69. Moncada S, Palmer RMJ, Higgs EA. Nitric oxide: physiology, pathophysiology, and pharmacology. *Pharmacol Rev* 1991;43:109–142.
70. Kinsella JP, Nelsh SR, Ivy DD, et al. Clinical responses to prolonged treatment of persistent pulmonary hypertension of the newborn with low doses of inhaled nitric oxide. *J Pediatr* 1993;123:103–108.
71. Konduri GG. New approaches for persistent pulmonary hypertension of newborn. *Clin Perinatol* 2004;31:591–611.
72. Struijs MC, Diamond IR, de Silva N, et al. Establishing norms for intestinal length in children. *J Pediatr Surg* 2009;44(5):933–938.
73. Klish WJ, Putnam TC. The short gut. *Am J Dis Child* 1981;135:1056–1061.
74. Bryant MG, Buchan AM, Gregor M, et al. Development of intestinal regulatory peptides in the human fetus. *Gastroenterology* 1982;83(1 Pt 1):47–54.
75. Lucas A, Bloom SR, Aynsley-Green A. Metabolic and endocrine consequences of depriving preterm infants of enteral nutrition. *Acta Paediatr Scand* 1983;72:245–249.
76. Bloom SR. Gut hormones in adaptation. *Gut* 1987;28(suppl 1):31–35.
77. Fuller PJ, Beveridge DJ, Taylor RG. Ileal proglucagon gene expression in the rat: characterization in intestinal adaptation using in situ hybridization. *Gastroenterology* 1993;104:459–466.
78. Drucker DJ, Ehrlich P, Asa SL, et al. Induction of intestinal epithelial proliferation by glucagon-like peptide 2. *Proc Natl Acad Sci U S A* 1996;93: 7911–7916.
79. Martin GR, Beck PL, Sigalet DL. Gut hormones and short bowel syndrome: the enigmatic role of glucagon-like peptide-2 in the regulation of intestinal adaptationn. *World J Gastroenterol* 2006;12(26):4117–4129.
80. Lentze MJ. Intestinal adaptation in short-bowel syndrome. *Eur J Pediatr* 1989;148:294–299.
81. Weser E, Babbitt J, Hoban M. Intestinal adaptation: different growth responses to disaccharides compared with monosaccharides in rat small bowel. *Gastroenterology* 1986;91:1521–1527.
82. Vanderhoof JA, Grandjean CJ, Burkley KT, et al. Effect of casein versus casein hydrosylate on mucosal adaptation following massive small bowel resection in infant rats. *J Pediatr Gastroenterol Nutr* 1984;3:262–267.
83. Grosfeld JL, Rescorla FJ, West JW. Short bowel syndrome in infancy and childhood. *Am J Surg* 1986;151:41–46.
84. Grosfeld JL, Rescorla FJ, West JW, et al. Gastrointestinal injuries in childhood: analysis of 53 patients. *J Pediatr Surg* 1989;24:580–583.
85. Ricour C, Duhamel JF, Arnaud-Battendier F, et al. Enteral and parenteral nutrition in the short-bowel syndrome in children. *World J Surg* 1985;9: 310–315.
86. Li L, Irving M. The effectiveness if growth hormone, glutamine, and a low-fat diet containing high-carbohydrate on the enhancement of the function of remnant intestine among patients with short bowel syndrome: a review of published trials. *Clin Nutr* 2001;20(3):199–204.
87. Mazariegos GV, Squires RH, Sindhi RK. Current perspectives on pediatric intestinal transplantation. *Curr Gastroenterol Rep* 2009;11(3):226–233.
88. Vianna RM, Mangus RS. Present prospects and future perspectives of intestinal and multivisceral transplantation. *Curr Opin Clin Nutr Metab Care* 2009;12(3):281–286.
89. Christensen RD, Henry E, Wiedmeier SE, et al. Identifying patients on the first day of life at high-risk of developing parenteral nutrition-associated liver disease. *J Perinatol* 2007;27(5):284–290.
90. Puder M, Valim C, Meisel JA, et al. Parenteral fish oil improves outcomes in patients with parenteral nutrition-associated liver injury. *Ann Surg* 2009;250(3):395–402.
91. Wessel JJ, Kocoshis SA. Nutritional management of infants with short bowel syndrome. *Semin Perinatol* 2007;31(2):104–111.
92. de Meijer VE, Gura KM, Le HD, et al. Fish oil based lipid emulsions prevent and reverse parental nutrition-associated liver disease: the Boston experience. *JPEN* 2009;33(5):541–547.
93. Kawade N, Onishi S. The prenatal and postnatal development of UDP-glucuronyltransferase activity towards bilirubin and the effect of premature birth on this activity in the human liver. *Biochem J* 1981;196:257–260.

CHAPTER 104 ■ FETAL INTERVENTION

GEORGE B. MYCHALISKA AND DARRELL L. CASS

KEY POINTS

1. Four fetal conditions clearly benefit from fetal intervention: congenital cystic adenomatoid malformation, fetal sacrococcygeal teratoma, a fetus with airway obstruction from a giant neck mass or laryngeal atresia, and twin-to-twin transfusion syndrome.
2. Any fetal therapy requires (a) accurate diagnosis of the condition and any associated anomalies that may have an impact on outcome, (b) reliable prediction of which individual fetuses will die or suffer serious long-term morbidity without fetal intervention, and (c) that the procedure improves the outcome of the fetus with little to no maternal risk.
3. Preterm labor is the single biggest concern during the operation and in the postoperative period.
4. For a fetus with a lung mass, the only indication for fetal intervention is the presence of hydrops.
5. For a fetus with sacrococcygeal teratoma, increased aortic velocity, increased combined cardiac output, increased cardiac-to-thoracic ratio, a dilated inferior vena cava, or reversed end-diastolic umbilical blood flow are sensitive early predictors of impending hydrops and fetal demise; before 28 weeks' gestation, open fetal surgery and resection is the treatment of choice.
6. Fetal intervention may play a role in the management of a small cohort of fetuses with the most severe form of congenital diaphragmatic hernia.
7. An ex utero intrapartum treatment procedure is the treatment of choice for fetuses with a giant neck mass or congenital high airway obstruction syndrome.

Fetal surgery has emerged as an independent subspecialty at the intersection of pediatric surgery and maternal–fetal medicine. It is a field that has arisen from clinical necessity. Pediatric surgeons, maternal–fetal medicine specialists, and neonatologists became frustrated with the management of a number of congenital structural anomalies in which the baby died or suffered severe lifelong disability despite all efforts at postnatal treatment. With the advent of prenatal ultrasound in the 1970s, many conditions were diagnosed before birth. Fetuses were followed, and the prenatal natural history was elucidated. It became clear that a component of organ failure was acquired because of ongoing alterations in fetal development caused by the anomaly. Thus, it made sense that fetal interventions may be of benefit to correct the pathophysiology and restore normal fetal development in the hope of improving survival and decreasing morbidity.

The first successful fetal intervention was reported by Sir A.W. Liley, who successfully transfused a hydropic fetus for Rh disease.[1] Although a few attempts were made at exchange transfusion by an open technique in the 1960s, modern fetal surgery was envisioned and developed by Dr. Michael Harrison at the University of California, San Francisco (UCSF) in the late 1970s.[2] It was at UCSF that the concept of a fetal treatment program was developed, permitting a true multidisciplinary approach to fetal diagnosis and treatment. The first open fetal operation was performed in 1982, at which bilateral ureterostomies were performed in a 21-week-gestation fetus with obstructive uropathy.[3] In the intervening years, tremendous progress has been made in the development of fetal surgery techniques, including advances in maternal–fetal anesthesia, tocolysis (prevention of preterm labor), and the development of less invasive surgical techniques. During this same period there have been significant advances in neonatal surgical critical care that has improved the outcome of fetuses with congenital anomalies. Thus, fetal surgery indications must be continually reassessed in the context of emerging pre-
❶ natal and postnatal therapies. At the present time there are only three fetal conditions that show clear benefit from fetal surgery during pregnancy: congenital cystic adenomatoid malformation, fetal sacrococcygeal teratoma, and twin-to-twin transfusion syndrome. Open fetal surgery at the end of pregnancy, the ex utero intrapartum treatment (EXIT) procedure, has proven effective for treatment of giant neck masses and laryngeal atresia. The EXIT procedure has been expanded to treat conditions that result in impending respiratory failure at birth using the EXIT-ECMO (extracorporeal membrane oxygenation) strategy, but the efficacy of this technique is still unproven. Fetal interventions, including open, fetoscopic, and percutaneous, have been used to treat a number of other fetal disorders, such as congenital diaphragmatic hernia, myelomeningocele, urologic obstruction, chylothorax, and, most recently, congenital heart malformations. Many of these procedures are promising, but questions remain regarding the natural history of these disorders, selection criteria, and efficacy.

FETAL IMAGING AND PRENATAL DIAGNOSIS

Fetal imaging is a critical component of the decision-making
❷ process in fetal surgery. Criteria that must be met to consider fetal surgery include (a) accurate diagnosis of the condition and any associated anomalies that may have an impact on outcome, (b) reliable prediction of which individual fetuses will die or suffer serious long-term morbidity without fetal intervention, and (c) demonstration of improved fetal outcome with minimal maternal risk.

Most congenital defects can now be detected before birth with the use of high-resolution ultrasound, color Doppler, and fetal magnetic resonance imaging (MRI). Frequently diagnosed anomalies include diaphragmatic hernia (Fig. 104.1), congenital lung lesions (Fig. 104.2), obstructive uropathy, neural tube defects, neck masses (Fig. 104.3), congenital heart defects, and sacrococcygeal teratoma. Other surgical disorders include abdominal wall defects (gastroschisis and omphalocele), intestinal atresias, and cystic and solid abdominal masses. Although ultrasound is the predominant prenatal screening and diagnostic modality, fetal MRI has proven particularly helpful in the further evaluation of central nervous system, chest, and neck anomalies.[4–6] Fetal echocardiography is essential in the evaluation of congenital heart disease and is also useful in evaluating abnormal cardiac function associated with other birth defects.[7–9]

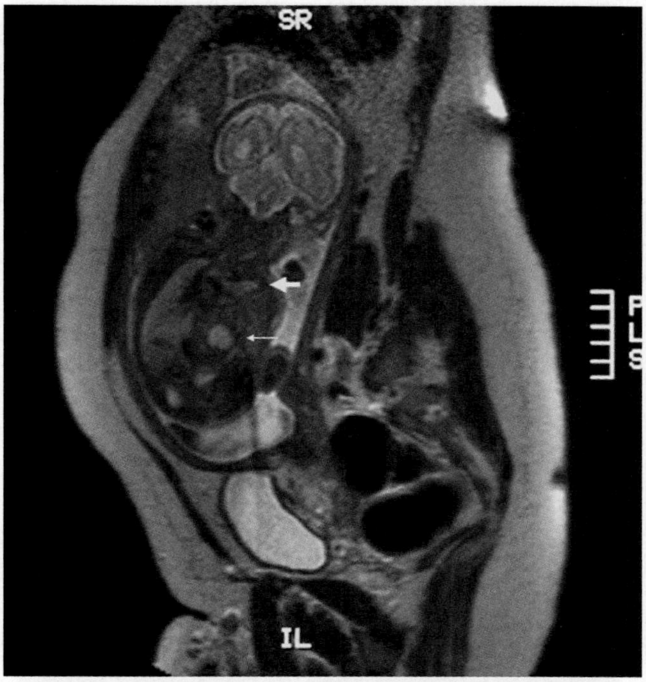

FIGURE 104.1. Coronal section of fetal magnetic resonance image (MRI) of a 30-week fetus with left congenital diaphragmatic hernia (CDH). The stomach (*small arrow*) and intestines are herniated into the left chest. The left lung is severely hypoplastic (*large arrow*).

Prenatal detection and serial ultrasonographic evaluation of these disorders has enhanced our understanding of their natural history, and has significantly improved perinatal management. Pediatric surgeons familiar with the management of congenital malformations before and after birth, along with obstetricians, neonatologists, geneticists, and other specialists, participate in family counseling and together contribute to optimal maternal–fetal management. Such multidisciplinary teams may recommend that the timing, mode (cesarean vs. vaginal delivery), or location of delivery be altered. Furthermore, in rare circumstances prenatal diagnosis permits in utero treatment of the developing fetus to prevent, reverse, or minimize fetal organ injury or death. In one study, prenatal consultation led to a change in pregnancy management in 67% of 221 pregnancies, of which 11 patients (5% of total) benefited from fetal intervention.[10]

Although most congenital anomalies are best managed with the use of appropriate medical and surgical therapy after delivery at term, rare fetal anomalies may benefit from surgery before birth. The innovations required for fetal surgery include the development of new surgical, anesthetic, and tocolytic techniques, as well as the resolution of such ethical issues as maternal safety and future maternal reproductive potential.[11–13]

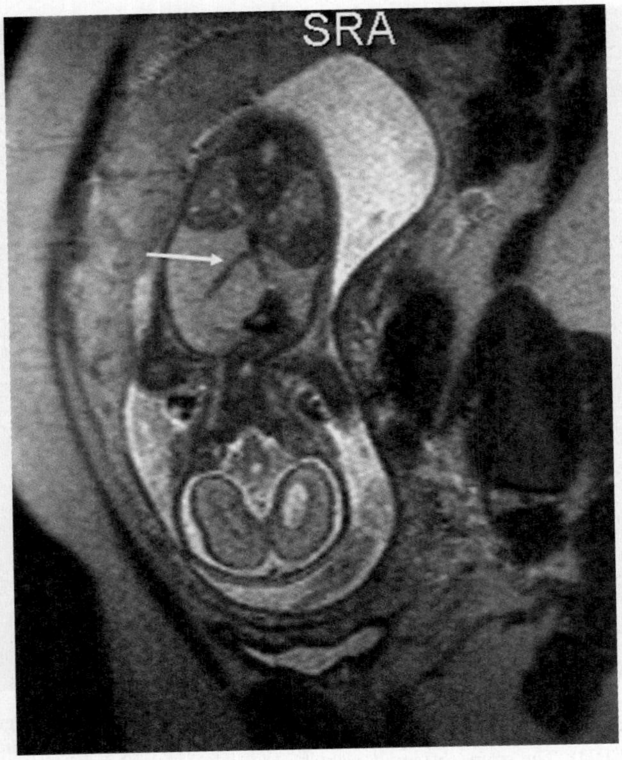

FIGURE 104.2. Coronal section of a fetal magnetic resonance image (MRI) of a 24-week fetus with a large left lung mass (bronchopulmonary sequestration). The left diaphragm is flattened and there is moderate dextroposition of the heart. A large vessel is seen coming from the low thoracic aorta (*arrow*). The congenital cystic adenomatoid malformation volume ratio (CVR) was 1.96; however, hydrops did not develop and the baby "grew around" the mass.

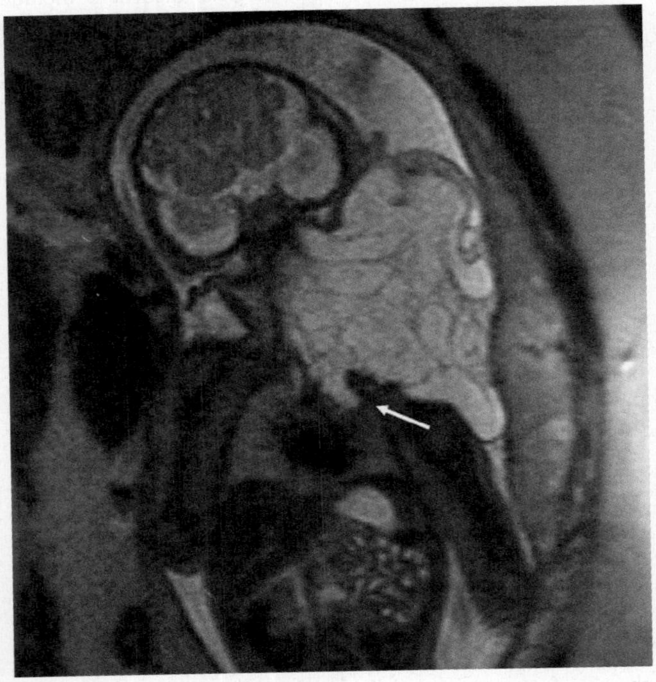

FIGURE 104.3. Coronal section of a fetal magnetic resonance image (MRI) of a 31-week fetus with a large left neck lymphatic malformation. The mass extends to the apex of the left chest (*arrow*). There is moderate left-to-right tracheal deviation. This fetus was delivered with an ex utero intrapartum treatment (EXIT) procedure.

MATERNAL–FETAL RISKS

Fetal surgery is unlike all other surgical specialties in that it involves two patients; the surgeon must operate on a healthy maternal patient to fix a disease in the affected fetus. This paradigm presents challenging moral and ethical conflicts that must be considered and balanced in each circumstance. Chervenak and McCullough[14] and others have helped to provide an ethical framework within which fetal surgery should exist. The keys to this framework are that (a) the fetal operation has significant chance of being lifesaving or of preventing serious or irreversible disease in the fetus; (b) the procedure involves low mortality and morbidity risk to the fetus; and (c) the operation has very low mortality and morbidity risk to the pregnant woman, including risks to future pregnancies. In light of these considerations, a number of contraindications to fetal intervention exist, including chromosomal abnormalities, the presence of other major anomalies, and significant maternal comorbidities.

There are significant maternal and fetal risks associated with fetal surgery that must be weighed for each patient. For the fetus, there is risk of preterm delivery, fetal death, or survival with poor outcome. Most indications for fetal surgery, however, are ones in which the fetus would die without it, and therefore the risk-to-benefit ratio is very favorable. For those interventions aimed at improving the outcome of fetuses with nonlethal conditions, the risk-benefit ratio is much more difficult to assess. For example, the efficacy of fetal surgery for spina bifida is being evaluated with a prospective randomized trial.[15]

The risks and benefits to the mother depend on the invasiveness of the fetal surgical operation. In any intervention, benefits to the mother include the psychological reward from doing everything possible to improve the condition of the unborn baby. In select cases, there is physiologic benefit in preventing the possibility of "mirror syndrome," a preeclampsialike condition in which the mother's condition "mirrors" that of a sick or dying fetus.[16] In the presence of this syndrome, fetal surgery is contraindicated and urgent fetal delivery is important to ensure maternal health. For the mother, fetal surgery adds the discomfort of one or two operations that would not have been required otherwise. For mothers who have hysterotomy other than low transverse, and for all mothers having open fetal surgery, there are theoretical risks to subsequent pregnancies and future fertility. When maternal fertility following fetal surgery was studied, however, it was found that 32 of 35 mothers were able to achieve successful subsequent pregnancies and 31 live births resulted.[11] Furthermore, if a classic cesarean section is performed during open fetal surgery, subsequent deliveries must be performed by cesarean section. Specific complications resulting from a classic cesarean section in subsequent pregnancies include uterine dehiscence and uterine rupture.[17] Postoperatively, nonhydrostatic pulmonary edema may occur in the mother. This problem was more prevalent in the early experience of open fetal surgery, but it still persists. In a recent trial reported by Harrison et al.,[18] 3 of 11 mothers developed pulmonary edema and required oxygen after fetal surgery. In each of these patients the symptoms were mild and resolved within 48 hours. The cause of this phenomenon remains unclear, but is likely related to uterine manipulation and the release of prostaglandins or thromboplastins that alter maternal lung vascular permeability.[19] As with all obstetric surgery, blood loss may be significant and mothers undergoing fetal surgery occasionally require blood transfusion.[20] Chorioamniotic membrane separation and preterm labor remain the Achilles' heel of fetal interventions.[21,22] Surgical approaches that involve a smaller hysterotomy and more minimally invasive techniques appear to lower these risks.[23] Specifically, fetoscopic and percutaneous approaches lessen the maternal and fetal risks.[24] These techniques allow vaginal delivery after fetal surgery and appear to decrease the incidence of preterm delivery.[25] Thus far, no maternal deaths have occurred at the major fetal surgery centers in the United States and Europe.

SURGICAL TECHNIQUES: OPEN, FETOSCOPIC, AND PERCUTANEOUS APPROACHES

Numerous technical aspects of fetal surgical procedures have evolved over 30 years of experimental and clinical work and have been reviewed in detail elsewhere.[26–29] The comprehensive care of the fetal surgery patient is labor intensive and requires multidisciplinary cooperation between all team members. In the operating room, the leader of the fetal surgery team is either a pediatric surgeon or maternal–fetal medicine specialist with specific training in fetal surgical techniques. The leader should be chosen depending on the procedure and specific expertise.[30] Responsibility for the patient's anesthesia is shared between an obstetric anesthesiologist for the mother and a pediatric anesthesiologist for the fetus. Both anesthesiologists should have special expertise in maternal–fetal anesthesia and work together as a team. A high-resolution ultrasound machine with color and enhanced Doppler is essential and used throughout the procedure to assess fetal and placental position; monitor fetal heart rate, cardiac function, and volume status; and assess amniotic fluid levels.[31] A pulse oximetry probe is placed on the fetal hand to assess fetal oxygen saturation and continuous heart rate. A peripheral intravenous catheter is often placed in the fetus for fluid, blood, and medication delivery. A surgical nursing team trained in the specific aspects of fetal surgical procedures and instrumentation is mandatory.

Open fetal surgery is performed with general and epidural anesthesia. Epidural delivery of a fentanyl/bupivacaine mixture provides optimal postoperative analgesia and minimizes uterine irritability. Intraoperatively, inhaled isoflurane titrated to an end-tidal concentration of 2% or higher is used to achieve uterine relaxation, which is critical to successful outcomes. Because of the risk of postoperative pulmonary edema, the mothers are fluid restricted during these procedures and receive as little as 500 mL of crystalloid. The patient is positioned supine with a roll under the right side to avoid compression of the inferior vena cava by the gravid uterus. The uterus is exposed through a low transverse abdominal incision. If the placenta is positioned posteriorly, subcutaneous flaps and a midline incision from the umbilicus to the pubis permit adequate uterine exposure. In cases of an anterior placenta, the fascia and rectus muscles are divided transversely so that the uterus can be tilted forward for a posterior hysterotomy. A large abdominal ring retractor is useful for abdominal wall retraction. After uterine relaxation is confirmed by palpation, the orientation of the fetus and placenta is confirmed by ultrasound. For open fetal surgery during pregnancy, a classical cesarean section incision is made. For the EXIT procedure, it is preferable to perform a low transverse hysterotomy. Two opposing traction sutures are placed with ultrasound guidance to provide hemostasis and to secure the fetal membranes to the uterine wall. The myometrium is then incised, and a hemostatic uterine stapler is used to open the uterine wall in both directions. A rubber catheter connected to a rapid infuser is inserted

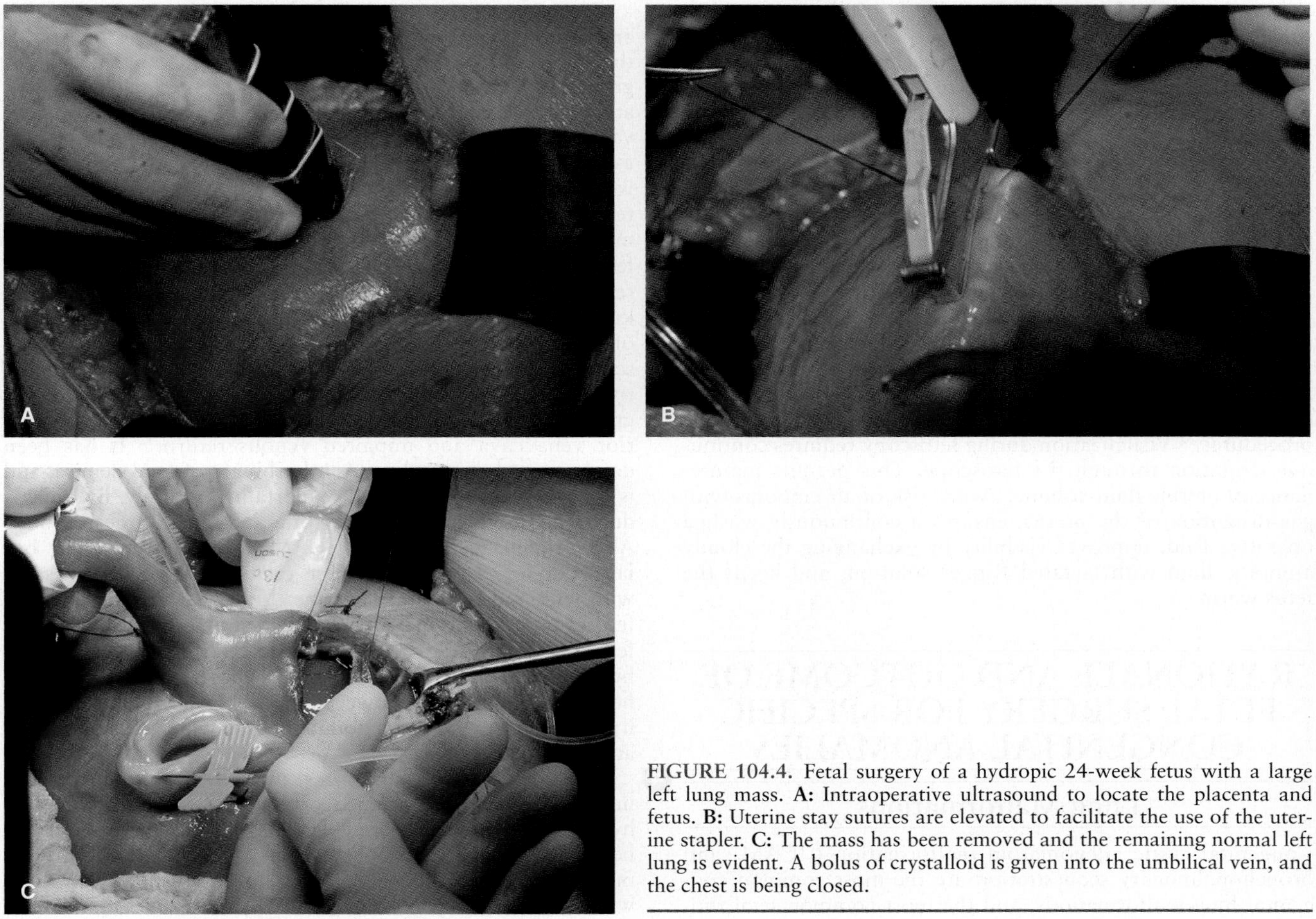

FIGURE 104.4. Fetal surgery of a hydropic 24-week fetus with a large left lung mass. **A:** Intraoperative ultrasound to locate the placenta and fetus. **B:** Uterine stay sutures are elevated to facilitate the use of the uterine stapler. **C:** The mass has been removed and the remaining normal left lung is evident. A bolus of crystalloid is given into the umbilical vein, and the chest is being closed.

into the amniotic space to replace egress of amniotic fluid with warmed Ringer lactate. Infusion of warmed fluids is critical to maintain fetal temperature and amniotic volume and to minimize the risk of uterine contractions and umbilical cord compression (Fig. 104.4).

One of the unique requirements of fetal surgery is that the surgeon must operate on the fetus and then return the fetus to the amniotic environment in such a way as to minimize disturbance to the continuing pregnancy. The uterine closure must have adequate strength to prevent rupture, must have membrane reapproximation to prevent amniotic fluid leakage, and must limit risks for preterm labor or future infertility. Currently, the uterus is closed in two layers using an outer layer of full-thickness 0 polydioxanone (PDS) retention sutures and an inner running layer of 2–0 PDS to close the myometrium and membranes. Before the closure is complete, the rapid infuser is used to restore amniotic volume and administer antibiotics. An omental pedicle is secured over the hysterotomy to seal any small leaks from the full-thickness sutures.

3 Preterm labor is the single biggest concern during the operation and in the postoperative period. The mother receives a 50-mg indomethacin suppository 4 hours before surgery, and remains on indomethacin for 48 hours postoperatively. Daily echocardiography is essential; if there is evidence of patent duct arteriosus (PDA) restriction, then the indomethacin is stopped. During the operation terbutaline or nitroglycerin infusion can be used to help control uterine irritability and enhance relaxation. During closure of the hysterotomy, the mother is given a 6-g bolus dose of magnesium sulfate followed by a continuous infusion of 2 to 4 g/h. Postoperatively the mother is observed in an intensive care unit (ICU) setting for close monitoring for pulmonary edema, fluid management, and uterine irritability. The magnesium sulfate is continued for 48 to 72 hours with close monitoring of magnesium levels and signs of toxicity. On the second to third postoperative day, usually the magnesium and indomethacin can be weaned, and the patient is converted to subcutaneous terbutaline or oral nifedipine. The patient is maintained on bedrest until the time of delivery. Postoperatively, daily ultrasound examinations help to assess the ductus arteriosus, amniotic fluid index (estimate of fetal urine output or of amniotic fluid leak), and fetal movement (marker of fetal well-being).

Fetoscopic surgery has been used most recently to permit a number of fetal surgical interventions, such as tracheal occlusion, laser ablation of communicating vessels in twin-to-twin transfusion syndrome, and fetoscopic ablation of posterior urethral valves for fetuses with obstructive uropathy. Initially, these procedures were performed by exposing the uterus through a maternal laparotomy. More recently, surgeons have placed trocars percutaneously into the uterus through the intact maternal abdominal wall. Specially designed fetoscopic instruments have been developed that have allowed for single-port procedures.[32] Visualization during fetoscopy requires continuous irrigation through the fetoscope. This permits maintenance of uterine fluid volume, avoids risk of air embolus with gas distention of the uterus, ensures a continuously washed operative field, improves visibility by exchanging the cloudy amniotic fluid with lactated Ringer solution, and keeps the fetus warm.

RATIONALE AND OUTCOME OF FETAL SURGERY FOR SPECIFIC CONGENITAL ANOMALIES

Lung Malformations

Congenital cystic adenomatoid malformation (CCAM) and bronchopulmonary sequestration are the most common congenital lung malformations, and the most common fetal thoracic lesions that may benefit from fetal intervention.[33] The incidence of these lesions has been estimated at 1 in 25,000 to 35,000 pregnancies[34]; however, current referral patterns to fetal therapy centers suggest they may occur more frequently. Grossly, a CCAM is a discrete, space-occupying intrapulmonary mass that contains variable-sized cysts. These lesions do not function in normal gas exchange; however, airspaces within these masses communicate with the tracheobronchial tree. Histologically, CCAM is distinguished from other lesions and normal lung by (a) polypoid projections of the mucosa, (b) an increase in smooth muscle and elastic tissue within cyst walls, (c) an absence of cartilage (except that found in "entrapped" normal bronchi), (d) the presence of mucus-secreting cells, and (e) the absence of inflammation. In contrast, bronchopulmonary sequestrations (BPSs) (intralobar or extralobar) are masses of nonfunctioning lung tissue that are supplied by an anomalous systemic artery and do not have connection to the native tracheobronchial tree. The pathogenesis of both lesions is unknown, but they are thought to arise during the fifth to sixth week in embryonic development, and may result from abnormalities in growth signals between the branching airway epithelium and pulmonary mesenchyme.[35,36] Congenital lung lesions are commonly diagnosed by prenatal ultrasound as an echogenic solid, or cystic and solid thoracic mass. Not infrequently, these lesions may be seen to have a systemic blood supply on Doppler ultrasound. Although CCAM and BPS have been distinguished prenatally in the past by the presence or absence of a systemic vessel, it is now recognized that these lung lesions represent a continuum of pulmonary maldevelopment and there are lesions that have clinicopathologic features of both.[37,38] Fetal MRI may enhance diagnostic accuracy in examining these lesions and distinguishing them from other thoracic abnormalities, such as congenital lobar emphysema, bronchial atresia, bronchogenic cyst, and congenital diaphragmatic hernia.[39,40]

The natural history and clinical spectrum of these anomalies are variable, but they appear to depend mostly on the size of the mass and the secondary physiologic derangement. The growth of CCAMs usually plateaus between 25 and 28 weeks, at which time the fetus appears to grow around the lesion. The vast majority of small to moderate-sized CCAMs remain asymptomatic during fetal life. Approximately 15% of CCAMs will shrink significantly before birth.[41] In contrast, large lesions represent 5% to 10% of CCAMs and may produce significant mass effect, which can lead to pulmonary hypoplasia, impaired fetal swallowing and polyhydramnios, and impaired venous return and heart failure. Congestive heart failure in the fetus, known as nonimmune fetal hydrops, is defined by the presence of skin or scalp edema, or by fluid accumulation in one or more serous cavities (ascites or pericardial or pleural effusions). The risk of hydrops appears to depend on the size and rate of growth of the mass, and results from compression of the superior vena cava and impaired venous return.[42] It has been demonstrated that hydrops is a harbinger of fetal demise, and is associated with near 100% mortality.[43] Rarely, hydrops is due to a tension hydrothorax from extralobar sequestration.[43] As a prognostic factor, the CCAM volume ratio (CVR) has been developed to correlate the relative size of these lesions with fetal and postnatal outcome.[44] In one series in which 58 fetuses with a lung mass were followed prospectively, 75% of fetuses (12 of 16) with a CVR greater than 1.6 developed hydrops, whereas only 17% (7 of 42) with a CVR of 1.6 or less had this complication. However, the CVR was not predictive of hydrops if a CCAM had a dominant cyst, which may enlarge at an unpredictable rate.

4 For a fetus with a lung mass, the only indication for fetal intervention is the presence of hydrops. Most commonly, hydrops occurs in the period of rapid growth of these lesions between 19 and 26 weeks' gestation.[33,43,44] Fetuses with a lung mass should be followed closely. It is recommended that those with a CVR less than 1.6 receive weekly ultrasound up to about

28 weeks' gestation, whereas those with a CVR greater than 1.6 should be examined as frequently as two to three times per week. If signs of hydrops appear, the treatment options include percutaneous placement of a thoracoamniotic shunt for lesions with a dominant cyst, and open fetal thoracotomy and mass resection for more solid lesions. Use of the laser or radiofrequency ablation to debulk a large CCAM cannot be recommended now because of technical limitations and inability to control energy distribution and postprocedure swelling.[45,46]

Fetal surgery for fetal lung masses requires open hysterotomy (Fig. 104.4). Intraoperative echocardiography is critical to assess fetal intravascular volume and right ventricle filling. These fetuses have tamponade physiology and generally benefit from a fluid bolus before thoracotomy. A relatively large thoracotomy is required to permit adequate exposure, and the mass is delivered slowly to prevent rapid decreased cardiac venous return. At resection, the presence of a systemic vessel must be considered.

The first successful open fetal surgery for CCAM was reported in 1990 by Harrison et al. at UCSF.[47] Since then, there have been reports of 22 open fetal resections of lung masses, with 50% survival.[33] Delays in referral and intervention, the presence of maternal "mirror" syndrome, preterm labor, chorioamnionitis, and technical difficulties associated with the procedure have limited outcomes in half of the cases. Recent evidence suggests that administration of maternal steroids may reverse the pathophysiology of hydrops, but this strategy requires further validation.[48,49]

Sacrococcygeal Teratoma

Sacrococcygeal teratoma (SCT) is the most common neonatal tumor, with an incidence of 1 in 35,000 live births.[50,51] Thought to arise from totipotent somatic cells originating in the caudal cell mass, this tumor contains multiple neoplastic tissues that lack organ specificity, are foreign to the sacrococcygeal region, and are derived from all three germ layers. The postnatal mortality of SCT is low, despite that about 10% of neonatal lesions are malignant. However, the prenatal mortality from SCT is greater than 50%. The causes of death in fetal SCT are multifactorial, but primarily involve dystocia with tumor rupture and bleeding at the time of delivery, or high-output cardiac failure and hydrops from high blood flow within the mass.[52] The evolution of high-output cardiac failure before the development of placentomegaly and hydrops in a fetus with SCT is the sole indication for fetal surgical intervention. Furthermore, SCT may lead to maternal mirror syndrome (Ballantine syndrome).[53] In this condition, the mother experiences progressive preeclampsialike symptoms, including vomiting, hypertension, peripheral edema, proteinuria, and pulmonary edema, caused by the release of placental vasoactive factors or endothelial cell toxins from the edematous placenta. This syndrome is reversed only by delivering the child and the placenta, but not by removing the SCT prenatally.

The diagnosis of SCT can be made by fetal ultrasound as early as 14 weeks' gestation.[54] The sonographic appearance may be cystic, solid, or mixed, and may demonstrate irregular echogenic patterns secondary to areas of tumor necrosis, cystic degeneration, internal hemorrhage, or calcification. Ultrasound is important to assess abdominal or pelvic extension, evidence of bowel or urinary tract obstruction, and the integrity of the fetal spine, and to document lower extremity function. Fetal MRI is helpful to delineate the anatomy and may be useful to distinguish these lesions from myelomeningocele, meconium pseudocyst, and obstructive uropathy. Fetal echocardiography and Doppler ultrasound measurements are important in the diagnostic assessment and follow-up of fetuses with these conditions. 5 Increased aortic velocity, increased combined cardiac output, increased cardiac-to-thoracic ratio, a dilated inferior vena cava, or reversed end-diastolic umbilical blood flow appear to be sensitive early predictors of impending hydrops and fetal demise.[8,55] For fetuses greater than 28 weeks' gestation, these findings are an indication for emergency cesarean delivery and postnatal resection. For fetuses less than 28 weeks, open fetal surgery and resection is the treatment of choice. Minimally invasive approaches to interrupt the tumor's blood supply with radiofrequency ablation have had limited success[56] but may be alternatives for a fetus that is a poor candidate for open fetal resection.

Adzick et al.[57] reported the first successful outcome for fetal surgery resection of a fetus with a large SCT and hydrops in 1997. More recently, investigators from that center have reported 75% survival (three of four) for fetal resection of SCT. A similar high-output heart failure physiology can occur with teratomas in other locations. A fetus with a cervical teratoma and hydrops had successful fetal resection of the lesion at 24 weeks' gestation.[58]

Congenital Diaphragmatic Hernia

At present, the role of fetal intervention in the management of fetuses with congenital diaphragmatic hernia (CDH) is not clear. A hole in the posterolateral diaphragm, left sided in 80% to 85% of cases, permits abdominal viscera to herniate into the chest during fetal development, resulting in pulmonary hypoplasia and pulmonary hypertension. In current practice, more than half of the infants with CDH are diagnosed before birth. At times it can be difficult to distinguish CDH from a cystic lung mass or other cystic lesions. Fetal MRI is useful to enhance diagnostic accuracy, confirm liver position, calculate lung volumes, and further exclude associated anomalies.[6,59]

Outcome for patients with CDH varies widely, depending on the severity of disease when the disease is diagnosed.[60] The overall survival of CDH in the United States is 68%.[61] Although the survival has improved in select centers,[62–65] the morbidity of some survivors remains high.[66] Fetuses with CDH have lower survival rates than those for live-born infants or for infants presenting to a neonatal surgical center. This paradigm has been termed the "hidden mortality" by Harrison et al.,[67] and has been confirmed by multiple investigators.[68–70] In 2000, Dillon et al.[71] reviewed the outcomes from a large series of fetuses with CDH registered in the Northern Region Congenital Abnormality Survey in the United Kingdom. Between 1985 and 1997, 201 fetuses were evaluated for diaphragmatic problems, of which 187 had congenital diaphragmatic hernia (14 had diaphragm eventration). From this cohort, 38 pregnancies were terminated, 26 of which had "multiple abnormalities," and 14 pregnancies (7%) were complicated by spontaneous miscarriage or stillbirth. The overall 1-year survival was 37%, but for live-born fetuses the survival was 50%. Furthermore, for those live-born babies with isolated CDH, the overall survival was 59%.

Ultrasound (and more recently MRI) can be used to predict fetal CDH severity. Herniation of the liver into the fetal chest and marked lung hypoplasia as estimated by a lung-to-head ratio (LHR) less than 1.0 are strong predictors of perinatal death.[72,73] Fetuses without liver herniation through the diaphragm have a reported survival rate between 75% and 93%, whereas those with "liver up" have a survival rate as low as 43%.[74] In a report that included evaluation of 174 patients with CDH, an LHR less than 0.9 was associated with only 13% survival, whereas survival was 68% for an LHR 0.9 to 1.2 and 88% for an LHR greater than 1.2.

For select infants with severe CDH, fetal surgery has been performed in an attempt to reverse the high mortality rate. Initially, complete in utero repair of the diaphragmatic defect was attempted.[75] This approach, however, led to fetal bradycardia and immediate death after attempts to reduce the liver from the fetal chest resulted in kinking of the ductus venosus.[76] Subsequently, in utero tracheal occlusion has been used to treat fetuses with severe CDH. It has been shown that temporary tracheal occlusion, performed either as an open procedure or fetoscopically, can prevent the normal egress of lung fluid and enhance growth of the fetal lungs.[77] In a review of 15 patients treated by open fetal tracheal occlusion at Children's Hospital of Philadelphia (CHOP), survival was 100% for patients with right-sided defects (two of two) and 23% for patients with left-sided defects (3 of 13), compared with 0% survival for a matched group of seven infants with left-sided lesions managed by conventional treatment alone. Endoscopic approaches to fetal tracheal occlusion, termed "fetoscopic" or "FETENDO," showed more promising outcomes.[78] Recently, however, Harrison et al.[18] from UCSF reported results from a National Institutes of Health (NIH)-sponsored, prospective randomized trial that compared fetoscopic tracheal occlusion with standard postnatal care for fetuses with left-sided CDH, "liver up," and an LHR less than 1.4. Twenty-four fetuses were randomized, but at this point the trial was stopped because of an unexpected high survival in the standard treatment group and the expectation that fetal therapy in this design would show no benefit. In this study of fetuses with liver-up CDH, the overall 90-day survival rate was 75%, a number much higher than those reported previously. Whereas 8 of 11 (73%) fetuses survived following fetoscopic tracheal occlusion, 10 of 13 (77%) survived with postnatal treatment alone, thus showing no benefit to fetal therapy in this study. As expected, a striking difference in the gestational ages was noted between the two groups. Whereas the standard treatment group delivered at a mean gestation of 37 weeks, the tracheal occlusion group delivered at a mean of 30.8 (range of 28 to 34) weeks' gestational age. Although fetoscopic tracheal occlusion likely had an effect on lung growth, this response may have been limited by preterm labor, early delivery, and associated lung immaturity. As has been demonstrated in the treatment of other conditions, chorioamniotic membrane separation and preterm labor limit outcomes from fetal surgery.[21,22] The lack of benefit from fetal therapy may also result from the excellent outcomes that were achieved in the control group. These results certainly suggest that a standardized protocol involving prenatal steroids and expert pre- and postnatal care may improve outcome for fetuses with severe CDH.

Deprest et al. from Europe[23] have reported initial results from the fetoscopic tracheal occlusion (FETO) task group, an ongoing prospective multicenter study of patients with severe CDH treated by fetoscopic approaches. This study involves patients with isolated CDH, liver up, and an LHR of less than 1.0. Using epidural anesthesia, a single 10-French cannula is placed through the intact maternal abdominal wall and uterus. A specially designed fetoscope is placed, the fetus is endotracheally intubated, and a detachable balloon is deployed in the midtrachea of these patients. Initially, fetuses were delivered by an EXIT procedure; however, more recently investigators have performed a second fetoscopic procedure later in gestation to remove the balloon and permit vaginal delivery. Results from the first 21 patients treated between April 2002 and October 2003 showed 47% overall survival in the treatment group, with a mean gestation of 34 weeks. In comparison, a matched cohort of fetuses with severe CDH had only 8% survival (1 of 12). More recently, Deprest reported results from the use of FETO in 210 patients. The procedure was performed at a median gestational age of 27 weeks. Although spontaneous preterm prelabor rupture of membranes occurred in 47% of patients, the median gestational age at delivery was 35.3 weeks. The authors estimated that in fetuses with left CDH treated with FETO, the survival rate increased from 24% to 49%.[25] The results from this trial are promising but still limited due to a lack of a randomized design and lack of standardized, centralized postnatal care in the control group of fetuses.

6 It is likely that fetal intervention may play a role in the management of a small cohort of fetuses with the most severe form of CDH. Current work is directed at accurate identification of this cohort and optimizing minimally invasive treatment approaches.

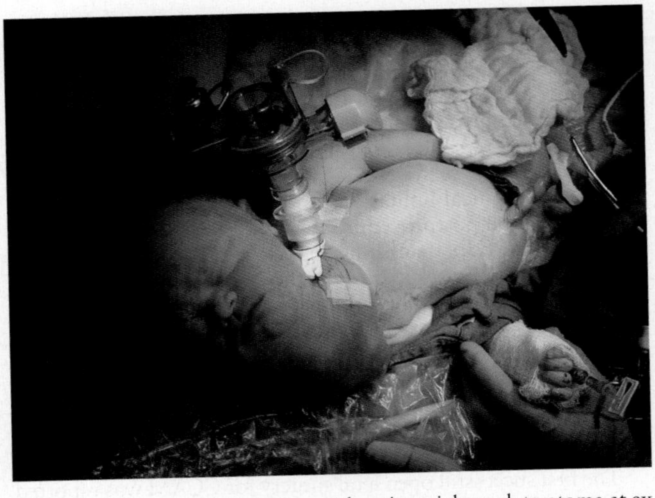

FIGURE 104.5. A 36-week fetus with a giant right neck teratoma at ex utero intrapartum treatment (EXIT) procedure. Due to significant tracheal deviation, a tracheostomy was performed on placental support.

Fetal Surgery at the End of Pregnancy

Ex Utero Intrapartum Treatment Procedure. As an outgrowth of the fetal intervention efforts, the EXIT procedure was devised to treat fetal airway obstruction caused by large neck masses or intrinsic airway problems.[79] This approach involves a planned hysterotomy and delivery with preservation of the maternal–fetal placental circulation for oxygenation of the fetus. While on "placental bypass," up to 2 hours is available for direct laryngoscopy, bronchoscopy, endotracheal intubation, tumor resection, or tracheostomy to secure the airway (Fig. 104.5). The umbilical cord is then divided, and the fetus delivered. Indications for an EXIT procedure include the presence of a large cervical mass with evidence of airway deviation or compression. Polyhydramnios, caused by esophagus compression, is one marker for fetal tracheal compression. Recently, the tracheoesophageal displacement index (TEDI) has been described to assess the degree of tracheal deviation
7 on fetal MRI.[80] Multiple centers have used the EXIT procedure to stabilize the airway in fetuses with large cervical tumors (e.g., teratomas or lymphatic malformations) with excellent fetal outcomes and very little additional maternal risk[81–83] (Fig. 104.5).

An EXIT procedure is the treatment of choice for fetuses with congenital high airway obstruction syndrome (CHAOS). This syndrome is usually caused by laryngeal or tracheal atresia, tracheal stenosis, or a mucosal web. A fetus with this condition develops overdistended, echogenic lungs, which may compress the mediastinum, flatten or evert the diaphragm, and cause hydrops because of compromise of venous return. Fetuses with CHAOS should be delivered with an EXIT procedure to permit tracheostomy and airway control while maintaining the maternal–fetal placental circulation. For fetuses with CHAOS who develop hydrops, early delivery or prenatal tracheostomy are treatment options, depending on gestational age.[84–86]

EX UTERO INTRAPARTUM TREATMENT–EXTRACORPOREAL MEMBRANE OXYGENATION

The EXIT-ECMO procedure has been developed to treat anticipated respiratory failure at birth. The rationale for this procedure is to transition from a stable intrauterine environment to ECMO while avoiding hypoxemia, barotrauma, hemodynamic

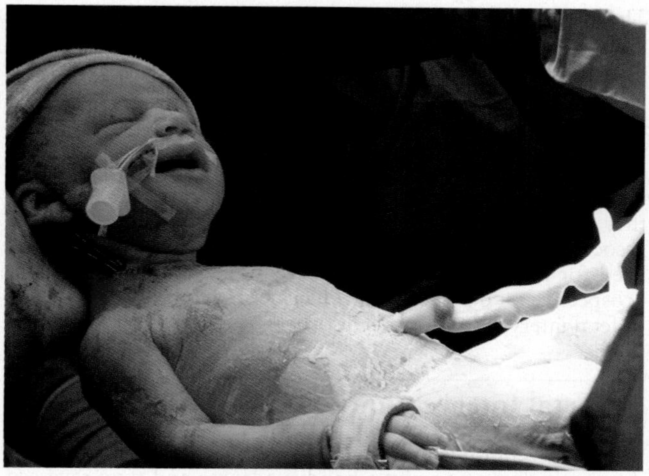

FIGURE 104.6. A 37-week fetus with severe congenital diaphragmatic hernia (CDH) delivered using the ex utero intrapartum treatment (EXIT)-extracorporeal membrane oxygenation (ECMO) procedure. The airway was secured and ECMO cannulas were placed on placental support.

instability, and acidosis. This strategy has been applied to severe CDH. Kunisaki et al. reported the largest series of 14 patients who had EXIT-ECMO for treatment of severe CDH.[87] Inclusion criteria included liver herniation, an LHR less than 1.4, percentage of predicted lung volume by fetal MRI less than 15, and/or congenital heart disease. Overall survival was 64% for this severe subset of CDH patients. Although this therapy is promising, at this time its efficacy is unproven. Variations of this procedure include EXIT-resection for lung lesions,[88] EXIT-ECMO for fetal thoracic masses,[89] and EXIT-resection-ECMO for giant chest masses[90] (Fig. 104.6).

Myelomeningocele

Myelomeningocele (MMC) was the first nonlethal anomaly to be treated by fetal surgery.[91–93] MMC, or spina bifida, is a midline defect of the spine and spinal cord that leads to exposure of the contents of the neural canal. It is relatively common, and occurs in 1 of every 2,000 live births. The natural history of fetuses with this condition is variable, but generally mortality is low. Instead, affected newborns suffer lifelong disabilities, which include a combination of paraplegia, abnormalities in bowel or bladder control, sexual dysfunction, skeletal deformations, hydrocephalus, and mental impairment. More than 80% of fetuses with MMC can be identified before birth by maternal serum α-fetoprotein screening. Fetal ultrasound may detect the characteristic spine abnormalities as early as 16 weeks' gestation.

The rationale for fetal intervention for MMC is based on compelling evidence that associated neurologic deficits do not simply result from incomplete neurulation but rather from chronic mechanical and chemical trauma caused by exposure of the neural tissue to the amniotic environment. Support for this conclusion includes the observation that fetal leg movements decrease with advancing gestational age. Furthermore, in animal models of MMC, in utero repair leads to improved neurologic function and reversal of hindbrain herniation.[94]

Human fetal interventions for MMC were initially designed to reduce intrauterine exposure of neural elements. Both fetoscopic and open techniques were attempted; however, open methods are considered the current standard. The first successful outcome of fetal surgery repair of MMC was reported by Adzick et al. in 1998.[91] Since that time multiple centers have reported positive outcomes that suggest that surgical repair of MMC before 25 weeks' gestation can preserve neurologic function, reverse the hindbrain herniation, decrease the incidence of clubfoot, and obviate the need for postnatal placement of a ventriculoperitoneal shunt compared with historical controls.[92,93,95] No consistent improvement was seen in neurologic or bladder function, however, and these interventions did come at the cost of fetal prematurity (preterm labor) and increased maternal risk. Furthermore, lack of accurate prenatal indicators of neurologic function and absence of matched controls and long-term follow-up hamper evaluation of this approach. To better assess the merit of fetal surgery for this condition, an NIH-sponsored multicenter, prospective, randomized trial is currently under way.

Urinary Obstruction

Obstructive uropathy, one of the most common fetal structural anomalies, occurs in about 1 of 1,000 live births. Of all fetuses with urinary tract dilatation, as many as 90% do not require fetal intervention, such as those with low-pressure dilation, continued good urine output, adequate amniotic fluid volume, unilateral urinary obstruction, or advanced irreversible renal dysplasia.[96,97] Fetuses with urethral obstruction, severe bilateral hydronephrosis, and preserved renal function may be candidates for fetal intervention. Urethral obstruction, usually caused by posterior urethral valves in a male fetus, leads to decreased fetal urine output, oligohydramnios, and eventually pulmonary hypoplasia, which is often the most important factor affecting postnatal outcome. Fetuses with oligohydramnios present in the early second trimester have mortality rates in excess of 90%.[98,99]

Prenatal ultrasound is very accurate in the detection of fetal hydronephrosis and in determining the level of urinary obstruction. Because most of the amniotic fluid in middle and late pregnancy is the product of fetal urination, the presence of a normal amniotic fluid index implies the excretion of urine from at least one kidney. Decreasing amniotic fluid volume on serial ultrasound usually indicates deteriorating renal function. Furthermore, renal function can be assessed by the sonographic appearance of the renal parenchyma and by the laboratory analysis of fetal urine via percutaneous bladder aspiration. The presence of cortical cysts or increased echogenicity is highly predictive of renal dysplasia, but the absence of these findings does not exclude it.[100] Normal fetal urine chemistry includes a urinary sodium less than 100 mEq/dL, chloride less than 90 mEq/dL, osmolarity less than 200 mOsm/L, and β_2-microglobulin less than 4 mg/dL. Values greater than these suggest that the fetal kidney is unable to reabsorb these molecules and predict poor postnatal renal function.

The greatest challenge is selecting fetuses that have severe urinary obstruction yet reversible or salvageable renal function. Presently, selection criteria for fetal intervention are a male fetus less than 30 weeks' gestation with evolving oligohydramnios, normal renal function, and no associated anomalies. Fetuses older than this are best treated by postnatal approaches. If there is evidence of lung maturation, then early delivery is recommended. The goal of fetal therapy is to adequately drain the urinary obstruction and to restore normal amniotic fluid volume. Methods of urinary tract decompression include percutaneous vesicoamniotic shunt placement, fetoscopic or open vesicostomy, and fetoscopic fulguration of posterior urethral valves.[101,102] Open fetal surgery, including vesicostomy or ureterostomy, has resulted in 50% survival, with two of eight children in one series having normal renal function.[103] Today, the most widely used and accepted means of treating bladder outlet obstruction is percutaneous insertion of a double-J vesicoamniotic shunt. Placement of a vesicoamniotic shunt is associated with 50% survival, but shunt complication rates as high as 45% may result. Direct fetoscopic ablation of posterior urethral valves holds promise for the future, though currently limited data are available to assess selection criteria and outcomes for fetuses treated by this approach.

Twin-to-twin Transfusion Syndrome

Twin-to-twin transfusion syndrome (TTTS), present in 5% to 35% of monochorionic twin pregnancies, occurs when there is unequal sharing of the monochorionic placenta. Generally, this finding can be made on prenatal ultrasound, and often the communicating placental vessels can be characterized by Doppler. Arteriovenous anastomoses lead to a net shunting of blood from the donor to recipient. The donor twin often suffers intrauterine growth retardation, cardiac failure, and oligohydramnios, whereas the recipient twin may suffer polyhydramnios, cardiomyopathy, and fetal hydrops. The smaller twin's placental cord insertion is often marginal or velamentous, whereas the larger twin's cord inserts into the placenta centrally.[104] Quintero et al.[105] have described a staging system for this condition. In stage 1, polyhydramnios and oligohydramnios occur, but the donor bladder is still visible. In stage 2, the bladder is no longer visible, and in stage 3 abnormal Doppler signals are detected in the respective umbilical arteries or veins. Stage 4 is characterized by findings of hydrops, and stage 5 is fetal death. In addition to the Quintero staging, recent studies suggest that comprehensive cardiac assessment by echocardiography may improve patient risk stratification.[9] Overall, TTTS before 26 weeks' gestation is associated with a high rate of fetal loss and perinatal death and a high incidence of brain damage in survivors.[106,107] In severe forms of TTTS, perinatal mortality rates of up to 90% have been reported.[108]

Treatment options include aminoreduction of the recipient sac, amniotic membrane septostomy, and fetoscopic ablation of communicating vessels.[109–111] Recently, endoscopic laser coagulation has become the treatment of choice for severe TTTS diagnosed before 26 weeks' gestation. In a multicenter European trial, twins with severe TTTS of all Quintero stages were randomized to undergo fetoscopic laser ablation or standard amnioreduction therapy. The trial was stopped after 142 women were randomized, because of the clear benefit of the laser approach. Endoscopic laser ablation led to improved outcomes in all variables examined, including increased fetal survival and decreased incidence of neurologic complications.[106]

Congenital Heart Defects

Fetal intervention may play a role in the management of some fetuses with rare congenital heart defects, including those with severe aortic or pulmonary stenosis, and hypoplastic left heart syndrome with intact or highly restrictive atrial septum.[112–114] There is evidence that fetuses with aortic or mitral valve stenosis may progress to hypoplastic left heart syndrome, presumably as a result of decreased ventricular filling. Furthermore, critical pulmonary stenosis or atresia with intact ventricular septum may progress to the so-called "hypoplastic right heart syndrome." Staged palliative surgery is the only therapeutic option for newborns with these conditions, and mortality remains significant. The goals of fetal intervention for these anomalies are to relieve the obstruction, restore normal cardiac physiology, and reverse the progression toward ventricular hypoplasia. In an initial report from investigators at Children's Hospital, Boston, in which 20 fetuses underwent balloon dilation of a stenotic aortic valve at 21 to 29 weeks' gestation, five fetuses died following the procedure.[114] Of 14 who were thought to have a technically successful procedure, three had evidence of a two-ventricle heart postnatally, thus supporting the experimental rationale. More recently, Tworetzky reported the predictors of technical success and postnatal biventricular outcome after in utero aortic valvuloplasty in 70 fetuses. The technical success rate was 74%, and 17 had biventricular circulation postnatally. The authors developed a multivariable threshold scoring system allowing highly sensitive and moderately specific identification of fetuses able to survive postnatally with a biventricular circulation.[115] Tworetzky also reported the outcomes of in utero atrial septoplasty in fetuses with hypoplastic left heart syndrome. Of 21 procedures attempted, 19 were technically successful. Although the authors could not conclude that this particular procedure improved survival given the small patient size, they did find that creation of a defect greater than 3 mm was associated with better postnatal oxygenation and less frequent need for emergent postnatal intervention.[112] It is likely that a prospective randomized trial will be needed to prove the efficacy of fetal intervention for this disorder.

Fetal Intervention for Other Anomalies

Fetal intervention is indicated for a number of other fetal conditions, including amniotic band syndrome and twin reversed arterial perfusion (TRAP) sequence. Fetoscopic lysis of constricting amniotic bands may lead to limb salvage and improved outcome.[116–118] Similarly, in the TRAP sequence, fetoscopic ligation or ablation of the acardiac twin's umbilical cord is the treatment of choice.[119]

FUTURE OF FETAL INTERVENTION

There will always be a role for fetal intervention in the treatment of certain specific congenital structural abnormalities. The exact nature of this role, however, is under constant reevaluation and change. The primary goal of fetal therapy is to improve the outcome of the affected fetus while minimizing maternal risks. If fetal outcomes can be improved by alternative means, such as lung liquid ventilation or other postnatal therapies that pose no risks to the mother, then indications for fetal therapy will decrease. On the other hand, as the risks and complications of fetal surgery continue to decrease, such as those related to preterm labor and chorioamniotic membrane separation, then the role for fetal interventions may increase. Increased miniaturization of fetoscopic equipment and optics, advances in robotics, newer approaches to closure of the uterus and fetal membranes, and advances in our understanding and treatment of preterm labor will enhance our ability to change the outlook for an increased number of fetuses with congenital malformations.

References

1. Liley AW. Intrauterine transfusion of foetus in haemolytic disease. *Br Med J* 1963;5365:1107–1109.
2. Bruner JP. In their footsteps: a brief history of maternal-fetal surgery. *Clin Perinatol* 2003;30:439–447.
3. Harrison MR, Golbus MS, Filly RA, et al. Fetal surgery for congenital hydronephrosis. *N Engl J Med* 1982;306:591–593.
4. Chung R, Kasprian G, Bruffer PC, et al. The current state and future of fetal imaging. *Clin Perinatol* 2009;36:685–699.
5. Estroff JA. The growing role of MR imaging in the fetus. *Pediatr Radiol* 2009;39:209–210.
6. Hubbard AM, Crombleholme TM, Adzick NS, et al. Prenatal MRI evaluation of congenital diaphragmatic hernia. *Am J Perinatol* 1999;16:407–413.
7. Bakiler AR, Ozer EA, Kanik A, et al. Accuracy of prenatal diagnosis of congenital heart disease with fetal echocardiography. *Fetal Diagn Ther* 2007;22:241–244.
8. Hedrick HL, Flake AW, Crombleholme TM, et al. Sacrococcygeal teratoma: prenatal assessment, fetal intervention, and outcome. *J Pediatr Surg* 2004; 39:430–438; discussion 430–438.
9. Shah AD, Border WL, Crombleholme TM, et al. Initial fetal cardiovascular profile score predicts recipient twin outcome in twin-twin transfusion syndrome. *J Am Soc Echocardiogr* 2008;21:1105–1108.
10. Crombleholme TM, D'Alton M, Cendron M, et al. Prenatal diagnosis and the pediatric surgeon: the impact of prenatal consultation on perinatal management. *J Pediatr Surg* 1996;31:156–162; discussion 162–163.
11. Farrell JA, Albanese CT, Jennings RW, et al. Maternal fertility is not affected by fetal surgery. *Fetal Diagn Ther* 1999;14:190–192.

12. Howell LJ, Adzick NS. Establishing a fetal therapy center: lessons learned. *Semin Pediatr Surg* 2003;12:209–217.
13. Myers LB, Cohen D, Galinkin J, et al. Anaesthesia for fetal surgery. *Paediatr Anaesth* 2002;12:569–578.
14. Chervenak FA, McCullough LB. A comprehensive ethical framework for fetal research and its application to fetal surgery for spina bifida. *Am J Obstet Gynecol* 2002;187:10–14.
15. Fichter MA, Dornseifer U, Henke J, et al. Fetal spina bifida repair–current trends and prospects of intrauterine neurosurgery. *Fetal Diagn Ther* 2008; 23:271–286.
16. Longaker MT, Golbus MS, Filly RA, et al. Maternal outcome after open fetal surgery. A review of the first 17 human cases. *JAMA* 1991;265: 737–741.
17. Wilson RD, Johnson MP, Flake AW, et al. Reproductive outcomes after pregnancy complicated by maternal-fetal surgery. *Am J Obstet Gynecol* 2004;191:1430–1436.
18. Harrison MR, Keller RL, Hawgood SB, et al. A randomized trial of fetal endoscopic tracheal occlusion for severe fetal congenital diaphragmatic hernia. *N Engl J Med* 2003;349:1916–1924.
19. DiFederico EM, Burlingame JM, Kilpatrick SJ, et al. Pulmonary edema in obstetric patients is rapidly resolved except in the presence of infection or of nitroglycerin tocolysis after open fetal surgery. *Am J Obstet Gynecol* 1998;179:925–933.
20. Harrison MR. Fetal surgery. *Am J Obstet Gynecol* 1996;174:1255–1264.
21. Sydorak RM, Hirose S, Sandberg PL, et al. Chorioamniotic membrane separation following fetal surgery. *J Perinatol* 2002;22:407–410.
22. Wilson RD, Johnson MP, Crombleholme TM, et al. Chorioamniotic membrane separation following open fetal surgery: pregnancy outcome. *Fetal Diagn Ther* 2003;18:314–320.
23. Deprest J, Gratacos E, Nicolaides KH. Fetoscopic tracheal occlusion (FETO) for severe congenital diaphragmatic hernia: evolution of a technique and preliminary results. *Ultrasound Obstet Gynecol* 2004;24:121–126.
24. Fowler SF, Sydorak RM, Albanese CT, et al. Fetal endoscopic surgery: lessons learned and trends reviewed. *J Pediatr Surg* 2002;37:1700–1702.
25. Jani JC, Nicolaides KH, Gratacos E, et al. Severe diaphragmatic hernia treated by fetal endoscopic tracheal occlusion. *Ultrasound Obstet Gynecol* 2009;34:304–310.
26. Adzick NS, Harrison MR, Glick PL, et al. Fetal surgery in the primate. III. Maternal outcome after fetal surgery. *J Pediatr Surg* 1986;21:477–480.
27. Bianchi DW, Crombleholme TM, D'Alton ME. *Fetology: Diagnosis and Management of the Fetal Patient*. New York: McGraw-Hill; 2000.
28. Harrison MR, Adzick NS. Fetal surgical techniques. *Semin Pediatr Surg* 1993;2:136–142.
29. Harrison MR, Evans MI, Adzick NS, et al. *The Unborn Patient: The Art and Science of Fetal Therapy*. Philadelphia, PA: W.B. Saunders; 2001.
30. Harrison M. Fetal surgery: trials, tribulations, and turf. *J Pediatr Surg* 2003;38:275–282.
31. Keswani SG, Crombleholme TM, Rychik J, et al. Impact of continuous intraoperative monitoring on outcomes in open fetal surgery. *Fetal Diagn Ther* 2005;20:316–320.
32. Klaritsch P, Albert K, Van Mieghem T, et al. Instrumental requirements for minimal invasive fetal surgery. *BJOG* 2009;116:188–197.
33. Adzick NS. Management of fetal lung lesions. *Clin Perinatol* 2003;30: 481–492.
34. Laberge J, Flageole H, Pugash D. Outcome of the prenatally diagnosed congenital cystic adenomatoid lung malformation. *Fetal Diagn Ther* 2001; 16:179–186.
35. Cass DL, Quinn TM, Yang EY, et al. Increased cell proliferation and decreased apoptosis characterize congenital cystic adenomatoid malformation of the lung. *J Pediatr Surg* 1998;33:1043–1046; discussion 1047.
36. Liechty KW, Crombleholme TM, Quinn TM, et al. Elevated platelet-derived growth factor-B in congenital cystic adenomatoid malformations requiring fetal resection. *J Pediatr Surg* 1999;34:805–809; discussion 809–810.
37. Cass DL, Crombleholme TM, Howell LJ, et al. Cystic lung lesions with systemic arterial blood supply: a hybrid of congenital cystic adenomatoid malformation and bronchopulmonary sequestration. *J Pediatr Surg* 1997; 32:986–990.
38. Langston C. New concepts in the pathology of congenital lung malformations. *Semin Pediatr Surg* 2003;12:17–37.
39. Hubbard AM, Adzick NS, Crombleholme TM, et al. Congenital chest lesions: diagnosis and characterization with prenatal MR imaging. *Radiology* 1999;212:43–48.
40. Olutoye OO, Coleman BG, Hubbard AM, et al. Prenatal diagnosis and management of congenital lobar emphysema. *J Pediatr Surg* 2000;35: 792–795.
41. Adzick NS. Management of fetal lung lesions. *Clin Perinatol* 2009;36: 363–376, x.
42. Rice HE, Estes JM, Hedrick MH, et al. Congenital cystic adenomatoid malformation: a sheep model of fetal hydrops. *J Pediatr Surg* 1994;29: 692–696.
43. Adzick NS, Harrison MR, Crombleholme TM, et al. Fetal lung lesions: management and outcome. *Am J Obstet Gynecol* 1998;179:884–889.
44. Crombleholme TM, Coleman B, Hedrick H, et al. Cystic adenomatoid malformation volume ratio predicts outcome in prenatally diagnosed cystic adenomatoid malformation of the lung. *J Pediatr Surg* 2002;37:331–338.
45. Bruner JP, Jarnagin BK, Reinisch L. Percutaneous laser ablation of fetal congenital cystic adenomatoid malformation: too little, too late? *Fetal Diagn Ther* 2000;15:359–363.
46. Milner R, Kitano Y, Olutoye O, et al. Radiofrequency thermal ablation: a potential treatment for hydropic fetuses with a large chest mass. *J Pediatr Surg* 2000;35:386–389.
47. Harrison MR, Adzick NS, Jennings RW, et al. Antenatal intervention for congenital cystic adenomatoid malformation. *Lancet* 1990;336:965–967.
48. Peranteau W, Wilson R, Liechty K, et al. Effect of maternal betamethasone administration on prenatal congenital cystic adenomatoid malformation growth and fetal survival. *Fetal Diagn Ther* 2007;22:365–371.
49. Tsao K, Hawgood S, Vu L, et al. Resolution of hydrops fetalis in congenital cystic adenomatoid malformation after prenatal steroid therapy. *J Pediatr Surg* 2003;38:508–510.
50. Berry CL, Keeling J, Hilton C. Teratomata in infancy and childhood: a review of 91 cases. *J Pathol* 1969;98:241–252.
51. Grosfeld JL, Ballantine TV, Lowe D, et al. Benign and malignant teratomas in children: analysis of 85 patients. *Surgery* 1976;80:297–305.
52. Langer JC, Harrison MR, Schmidt KG, et al. Fetal hydrops and death from sacrococcygeal teratoma: rationale for fetal surgery. *Am J Obstet Gynecol* 1989;160:1145–1150.
53. Kuhlmann RS, Warsof SL, Levy DL, et al. Fetal sacrococcygeal teratoma. *Fetal Ther* 1987;2:95–100.
54. Holzgreve W, Mahony BS, Glick PL, et al. Sonographic demonstration of fetal sacrococcygeal teratoma. *Prenat Diagn* 1985;5:245–257.
55. Olutoye OO, Johnson MP, Coleman BG, et al. Abnormal umbilical cord Doppler sonograms may predict impending demise in fetuses with sacrococcygeal teratoma. A report of two cases. *Fetal Diagn Ther* 2004;19:35–39.
56. Paek BW, Jennings RW, Harrison MR, et al. Radiofrequency ablation of human fetal sacrococcygeal teratoma. *Am J Obstet Gynecol* 2001;184: 503–507.
57. Adzick NS, Crombleholme TM, Morgan MA, et al. A rapidly growing fetal teratoma. *Lancet* 1997;349:538.
58. Hirose S, Sydorak RM, Tsao K, et al. Spectrum of intrapartum management strategies for giant fetal cervical teratoma. *J Pediatr Surg* 2003;38: 446–450; discussion 446–450.
59. Walsh DS, Hubbard AM, Olutoye OO, et al. Assessment of fetal lung volumes and liver herniation with magnetic resonance imaging in congenital diaphragmatic hernia. *Am J Obstet Gynecol* 2000;183:1067–1069.
60. Doyle NM, Lally KP. The CDH Study Group and advances in the clinical care of the patient with congenital diaphragmatic hernia. *Semin Perinatol* 2004;28:174–184.
61. The Congenital Diaphragmatic Hernia Study Group. *Report from the Congenital Diaphragmatic Hernia Study Group*. http://cdhsg.net. Accessed September, 2008.
62. Boloker J, Bateman DA, Wung JT, et al. Congenital diaphragmatic hernia in 120 infants treated consecutively with permissive hypercapnea/spontaneous respiration/elective repair. *J Pediatr Surg* 2002;37:357–366.
63. Downard CD, Jaksic T, Garza JJ, et al. Analysis of an improved survival rate for congenital diaphragmatic hernia. *J Pediatr Surg* 2003;38:729–732.
64. Javid PJ, Jaksic T, Skarsgard ED, et al. Survival rate in congenital diaphragmatic hernia: the experience of the Canadian Neonatal Network. *J Pediatr Surg* 2004;39:657–660.
65. Kays DW, Langham MR Jr, Ledbetter DJ, et al. Detrimental effects of standard medical therapy in congenital diaphragmatic hernia. *Ann Surg* 1999; 230:340–348; discussion 348–351.
66. Cortes RA, Keller RL, Townsend T, et al. Survival of severe congenital diaphragmatic hernia has morbid consequences. *J Pediatr Surg* 2005;40: 36–45; discussion 45–46.
67. Harrison MR, Bjordal RI, Langmark F, et al. Congenital diaphragmatic hernia: the hidden mortality. *J Pediatr Surg* 1978;13:227–230.
68. Betremieux P, Lionnais S, Beuchee A, et al. Perinatal management and outcome of prenatally diagnosed congenital diaphragmatic hernia: a 1995–2000 series in Rennes University Hospital. *Prenat Diagn* 2002;22:988–994.
69. Skari H, Bjornland K, Haugen G, et al. Congenital diaphragmatic hernia: a meta-analysis of mortality factors. *J Pediatr Surg* 2000;35:1187–1197.
70. Stege G, Fenton A, Jaffray B. Nihilism in the 1990s: the true mortality of congenital diaphragmatic hernia. *Pediatrics* 2003;112:532–535.
71. Dillon E, Renwick M, Wright C. Congenital diaphragmatic herniation: antenatal detection and outcome. *Br J Radiol* 2000;73:360–365.
72. Lipshutz GS, Albanese CT, Feldstein VA, et al. Prospective analysis of lung-to-head ratio predicts survival for patients with prenatally diagnosed congenital diaphragmatic hernia. *J Pediatr Surg* 1997;32:1634–1636.
73. Metkus AP, Filly RA, Stringer MD, et al. Sonographic predictors of survival in fetal diaphragmatic hernia. *J Pediatr Surg* 1996;31:148–151; discussion 151–152.
74. Albanese CT, Lopoo J, Goldstein RB, et al. Fetal liver position and perinatal outcome for congenital diaphragmatic hernia. *Prenat Diagn* 1998;18: 1138–1142.
75. Harrison MR, Adzick NS, Longaker MT, et al. Successful repair in utero of a fetal diaphragmatic hernia after removal of herniated viscera from the left thorax. *N Engl J Med* 1990;322:1582–1584.
76. Harrison MR, Adzick NS, Flake AW, et al. Correction of congenital diaphragmatic hernia in utero: VI. Hard-earned lessons. *J Pediatr Surg* 1993;28:1411–1417; discussion 1417–1418.
77. Hedrick MH, Estes JM, Sullivan KM, et al. Plug the lung until it grows (PLUG): a new method to treat congenital diaphragmatic hernia in utero. *J Pediatr Surg* 1994;29:612–617.
78. Harrison MR, Albanese CT, Hawgood SB, et al. Fetoscopic temporary tracheal occlusion by means of detachable balloon for congenital diaphragmatic hernia. *Am J Obstet Gynecol* 2001;185:730–733.

79. Mychaliska GB, Bealer JF, Graf JL, et al. Operating on placental support: the ex utero intrapartum treatment procedure. *J Pediatr Surg* 1997;32:227–230; discussion 230–231.
80. Cass DL, Cassady CI, O'Day MP, et al. *Predictors of Airway Obstruction and Outcome of Fetuses with Giant Neck Masses.* San Francisco, CA: Surgical Section, American Academy of Pediatrics; 2004.
81. Hedrick HL. Ex utero intrapartum therapy. *Semin Pediatr Surg* 2003;12:190–195.
82. Hirose S, Farmer DL, Lee H, et al. The ex utero intrapartum treatment procedure: looking back at the EXIT. *J Pediatr Surg* 2004;39:375–380; discussion 375–380.
83. Noah MM, Norton ME, Sandberg P, et al. Short-term maternal outcomes that are associated with the EXIT procedure, as compared with cesarean delivery. *Am J Obstet Gynecol* 2002;186:773–777.
84. Crombleholme TM, Sylvester K, Flake AW, et al. Salvage of a fetus with congenital high airway obstruction syndrome by ex utero intrapartum treatment (EXIT) procedure. *Fetal Diagn Ther* 2000;15:280–282.
85. DeCou JM, Jones DC, Jacobs HD, et al. Successful ex utero intrapartum treatment (EXIT) procedure for congenital high airway obstruction syndrome (CHAOS) owing to laryngeal atresia. *J Pediatr Surg* 1998;33:1563–1565.
86. Paek BW, Callen PW, Kitterman J, et al. Successful fetal intervention for congenital high airway obstruction syndrome. *Fetal Diagn Ther* 2002;17:272–276.
87. Kunisaki SM, Barnewolt CE, Estroff JA, et al. Ex utero intrapartum treatment with extracorporeal membrane oxygenation for severe congenital diaphragmatic hernia. *J Pediatr Surg* 2007;42:98–104; discussion 104–106.
88. Hedrick HL, Flake AW, Crombleholme TM, et al. The ex utero intrapartum therapy procedure for high-risk fetal lung lesions. *J Pediatr Surg* 2005;40:1038–1043; discussion 1044.
89. Kunisaki SM, Fauza DO, Barnewolt CE, et al. Ex utero intrapartum treatment with placement on extracorporeal membrane oxygenation for fetal thoracic masses. *J Pediatr Surg* 2007;42:420–425.
90. Mychaliska GB, Bryner BS, Nugent C, et al. Giant pulmonary sequestration: the rare case requiring the EXIT procedure with resection and ECMO. *Fetal Diagn Ther* 2009;25:163–166.
91. Adzick NS, Sutton LN, Crombleholme TM, et al. Successful fetal surgery for spina bifida. *Lancet* 1998;352:1675–1676.
92. Bruner JP, Tulipan N, Paschall RL, et al. Fetal surgery for myelomeningocele and the incidence of shunt-dependent hydrocephalus. *JAMA* 1999;282:1819–1825.
93. Sutton LN, Adzick NS, Bilaniuk LT, et al. Improvement in hindbrain herniation demonstrated by serial fetal magnetic resonance imaging following fetal surgery for myelomeningocele. *JAMA* 1999;282:1826–1831.
94. Meuli M, Meuli-Simmen C, Hutchins GM, et al. In utero surgery rescues neurological function at birth in sheep with spina bifida. *Nat Med* 1995;1:342–347.
95. Farmer DL, von Koch CS, Peacock WJ, et al. In utero repair of myelomeningocele: experimental pathophysiology, initial clinical experience, and outcomes. *Arch Surg* 2003;138:872–878.
96. Glick PL, Harrison MR, Golbus MS, et al. Management of the fetus with congenital hydronephrosis II: prognostic criteria and selection for treatment. *J Pediatr Surg* 1985;20:376–387.
97. Harrison MR, Golbus MS, Filly RA, et al. Management of the fetus with congenital hydronephrosis. *J Pediatr Surg* 1982;17:728–742.
98. Crombleholme TM, Harrison MR, Golbus MS, et al. Fetal intervention in obstructive uropathy: prognostic indicators and efficacy of intervention. *Am J Obstet Gynecol* 1990;162:1239–1244.
99. Mandelbrot L, Dumez Y, Muller F, et al. Prenatal prediction of renal function in fetal obstructive uropathies. *J Perinat Med* 1991;19(suppl 1):283–287.
100. Mahony BS, Filly RA, Callen PW, et al. Fetal renal dysplasia: sonographic evaluation. *Radiology* 1984;152:143–146.
101. Quintero RA, Johnson MP, Romero R, et al. In-utero percutaneous cystoscopy in the management of fetal lower obstructive uropathy. *Lancet* 1995;346:537–540.
102. Quintero RA, Shukla AR, Homsy YL, et al. Successful in utero endoscopic ablation of posterior urethral valves: a new dimension in fetal urology. *Urology* 2000;55:774.
103. Cortes RA, Farmer DL. Recent advances in fetal surgery. *Semin Perinatol* 2004;28:199–211.
104. Fries MH, Goldstein RB, Kilpatrick SJ, et al. The role of velamentous cord insertion in the etiology of twin-twin transfusion syndrome. *Obstet Gynecol* 1993;81:569–574.
105. Quintero RA, Morales WJ, Allen MH, et al. Staging of twin-twin transfusion syndrome. *J Perinatol* 1999;19:550–555.
106. Senat MV, Deprest J, Boulvain M, et al. Endoscopic laser surgery versus serial amnioreduction for severe twin-to-twin transfusion syndrome. *N Engl J Med* 2004;351:136–144.
107. Ville Y, Hyett J, Hecher K, et al. Preliminary experience with endoscopic laser surgery for severe twin-twin transfusion syndrome. *N Engl J Med* 1995;332:224–227.
108. De Lia JE. Surgery of the placenta and umbilical cord. *Clin Obstet Gynecol* 1996;39:607–625.
109. De Lia JE, Kuhlmann RS, Harstad TW, et al. Fetoscopic laser ablation of placental vessels in severe previable twin-twin transfusion syndrome. *Am J Obstet Gynecol* 1995;172:1202–1208; discussion 1208–1211.
110. Feldstein VA, Machin GA, Albanese CT, et al. Twin-twin transfusion syndrome: the 'Select' procedure. *Fetal Diagn Ther* 2000;15:257–261.
111. Hecher K, Diehl W, Zikulnig L, et al. Endoscopic laser coagulation of placental anastomoses in 200 pregnancies with severe mid-trimester twin-to-twin transfusion syndrome. *Eur J Obstet Gynecol Reprod Biol* 2000;92:135–139.
112. Marshall AC, van der Velde ME, Tworetzky W, et al. Creation of an atrial septal defect in utero for fetuses with hypoplastic left heart syndrome and intact or highly restrictive atrial septum. *Circulation* 2004;110:253–258.
113. Tworetzky W, Marshall AC. Fetal interventions for cardiac defects. *Pediatr Clin North Am* 2004;51:1503–1513, vii.
114. Tworetzky W, Wilkins-Haug L, Jennings RW, et al. Balloon dilation of severe aortic stenosis in the fetus: potential for prevention of hypoplastic left heart syndrome: candidate selection, technique, and results of successful intervention. *Circulation* 2004;110:2125–2131.
115. McElhinney DB, Marshall AC, Wilkins-Haug LE, et al. Predictors of technical success and postnatal biventricular outcome after in utero aortic valvuloplasty for aortic stenosis with evolving hypoplastic left heart syndrome. *Circulation* 2009;120:1482–1490.
116. Crombleholme TM, Dirkes K, Whitney TM, et al. Amniotic band syndrome in fetal lambs. I: fetoscopic release and morphometric outcome. *J Pediatr Surg* 1995;30:974–978.
117. Keswani SG, Johnson MP, Adzick NS, et al. In utero limb salvage: fetoscopic release of amniotic bands for threatened limb amputation. *J Pediatr Surg* 2003;38:848–851.
118. Quintero RA, Morales WJ, Phillips J, et al. In utero lysis of amniotic bands. *Ultrasound Obstet Gynecol* 1997;10:316–320.
119. Farmer DL, Hirose S. Fetal intervention for complications of monochorionic twinning. *World J Surg* 2003;27:103–107.

CHAPTER 105 ■ PEDIATRIC HEAD AND NECK

KEITH T. OLDHAM AND JOHN J. AIKEN

KEY POINTS

1. Airway obstruction is the most serious complication of neck masses in children, and in infants presents with restlessness, followed by tachypnea, dyspnea, chest-wall retractions, and respiratory arrest.
2. Infants are obligate nasal breathers; thus, congenital lesions that obstruct the nasal passages or nasopharynx (choanal atresia, encephalocele, teratoma) typically cause early respiratory distress.
3. Acute epiglottitis presents as a rapidly progressive illness with severe stridor, airway obstruction, drooling, and difficulty swallowing and with signs of systemic toxicity, including an elevated temperature and white blood cell count, tachypnea, and tachycardia.
4. Branchial cleft sinuses present as cutaneous openings and are most often noted in infancy or at an early age, whereas cysts typically appear later in childhood when they accumulate secretions; treatment is complete surgical removal.
5. Thyroglossal duct cysts or remnants arise when embryonic elements persist along the tract of descent of the thyroid gland; treatment requires complete removal of the cyst, its entire tract, and the central portion of the hyoid bone.

6 Benign cervical lymphadenopathy is the most common neck mass in childhood.

7 Lymphangiomas are masses of disorganized, dilated lymph channels that arise when communications with the internal jugular system fail to develop in portions of the lymphatic channels; the larger lesions with macrocystic dilated lymphatic channels are often referred to as *cystic hygromas*.

Surgical lesions of the head and neck are common in infants and children and include a broad spectrum of congenital and acquired disorders. Most lesions of the head and neck in children are benign (80% to 90%) and the etiology is congenital or inflammatory, but occasionally neoplastic lesions are encountered. Congenital lesions include vascular malformations, hemangiomas, branchial cleft anomalies, thyroglossal duct cysts, dermoid and epidermoid cysts, and others. The most common inflammatory neck masses are lymph nodes, but it is not uncommon for congenital lesions to be unnoticed until they become infected and present as a neck abscess. Neck masses in children may present clinically as asymptomatic masses or as life-threatening emergencies due to airway obstruction.

Malignant lesions of the head and neck in children are rare and may be primary tumors or represent metastatic disease to neck lymph nodes. Malignant lymphoma is the most common primary malignancy of the head and neck region in children. Other malignant neck masses occasionally encountered include rhabdomyosarcoma, thyroid carcinoma, and neuroblastoma.

An understanding of the relevant embryology and developmental anatomy of head and neck structures is important to enable efficient assessment, workup, and management of these lesions. Early biopsy is essential if there is any question of malignancy. This chapter focuses on the general principles and management of airway obstruction in infants and children and the most common head and neck lesions seen in pediatric surgical practice.

IMAGING STUDIES

In most head and neck masses in infants and children, an understanding of the pertinent developmental anatomy and embryology allows for a diagnosis on physical examination and diagnostic imaging is not required. In atypical cases or if the diagnosis is in question, an ultrasound, computed tomography (CT) scan, magnetic resonance imaging (MRI) scan, or fine-needle aspiration (FNA) may be helpful.

With the advent of cross-sectional imaging, the traditional cervical triangle method of organizing the anatomy of the neck has been largely replaced by a system that defines neck spaces according to the cervical fascial planes. The cervical spaces of the suprahyoid and infrahyoid neck include the sublingual space, submandibular space, buccal space, parotid space, parapharyngeal space, carotid space, masticator space, pharyngeal mucosal space, visceral space, retropharyngeal space, posterior cervical space, and perivertebral space.

Ultrasound is particularly helpful in distinguishing cystic from solid masses and identifying the presence of fluid within a lesion, as within a maturing deep cervical abscess. In addition, Doppler ultrasound can evaluate the vascularity of the lesion. Ultrasound should be considered as the first-line investigation because it has advantages of being noninvasive, does not involve ionizing radiation, and does not require sedation.

CT scan and MRI are used selectively to provide more detailed anatomic information and delineate extensions of head and neck lesions into the thorax, axilla, or intracranial space. While both CT scan and MRI can provide detailed multiplanar images of anatomic landmarks and tumor extension, CT is better able to demonstrate invasiveness and bony destruction. MRI provides three-dimensional soft tissue detail and is particularly useful for spinal cord involvement or intracranial extension of neck masses, but has higher costs and frequently requires sedation of younger patients. T2-weighted imaging identifies areas of increased vascularity, and T1-weighted images enhanced with gadolinium allow precise localization of central nervous system tumors. T1 can also delineate the position of the facial nerve with respect to a parotid tumor.

Gallium-67 scanning is useful in the initial staging and monitoring of disease response and recurrence in high-grade lymphomas. Positron emission tomography (PET) scanning is a functional imaging technique that maps the location and concentration of the intravenously injected radioactive glucose analogue 2-fluoro-2-deoxy-D-glucose (FDG) in metabolically active tumors. In contrast to CT and MRI, which are modalities primarily depicting anatomic details, PET provides information about metabolism. Neoplastic cells incorporate more of the glucose analogue and thus produce more-intense images than surrounding normal tissue.

Additional radiographic studies that may be needed to evaluate a neck mass include chest radiograph, bone scan, and CT scans of the abdomen, pelvis, chest, and brain as part of a metastatic workup if a malignant tumor is suspected or diagnosed. A chest radiograph can demonstrate pulmonary involvement in tuberculosis or a potentially systemic fungal disease.

AIRWAY OBSTRUCTION

Many lesions, both congenital and acquired, can produce airway obstruction in infants and children. They may be intrinsic or extrinsic to the airway and vary from clinically insignificant to universally fatal.[1]

1 Airway obstruction is the most serious complication of neck masses in children. Often the first significant sign of respiratory distress in an infant is restlessness, followed by tachypnea, dyspnea, chest-wall retractions, and respiratory arrest if the obstruction is not relieved. It is crucial to establish an adequate airway and to administer respiratory support while proceeding with the diagnostic evaluation. Supportive interventions may include simple measures such as repositioning the infant, clearing or suctioning the nose and mouth, and administering supplemental oxygen, or more-extreme measures, such as endotracheal intubation or tracheostomy. Evaluation includes a careful history and physical examination, chest radiography, and arterial blood gas analysis. A nasogastric tube should be passed into the stomach, as gastric distention limits excursion of the diaphragm and can significantly contribute to respiratory compromise. Laryngoscopy and bronchoscopy are employed as needed.

2 Because infants are obligate nasal breathers, congenital lesions that obstruct the nasal passages or nasopharynx (choanal atresia, encephalocele, teratoma) typically cause early respiratory distress. These disorders are readily identified by physical examination and emergent management is usually placement of an oropharyngeal airway. Airway obstruction at the level of the oral cavity in newborn infants is often a consequence of macroglossia or structural abnormalities such as micrognathia. Macroglossia may be a consequence of muscular hyperplasia and hypertrophy, as in Beckwith-Wiedemann syndrome and congenital hypothyroidism, or of diffuse involvement of the tongue with tumor (hemangiopericytoma, lymphangioma, neurofibromatosis).[2] Structural abnormalities, such as Pierre-Robin syndrome (hypoplastic mandible with cleft palate), cause respiratory distress as the tongue falls posterior and obstructs the airway. Cysts or tumors of the pharynx or a mass arising at the base of the tongue, such as a lingual thyroid, may also obstruct the

airway.[3] Clinically, upper airway obstruction, above the glottis or larynx, is characterized by dyspnea, tachypnea, and suprasternal, intercostal, and costal margin retractions, but the child has no significant difficulty exhaling, and the voice and cry are normal. Emergency management consists of placing an oropharyngeal airway. Placing the infant in a prone position allows the tongue to fall forward and often provides significant relief. The infant may be fed through an orogastric feeding tube pending definitive correction of the obstruction. In extreme cases, a tracheostomy may be necessary.

Laryngeal obstruction can result from congenital or acquired vocal cord paralysis or tumors or cysts originating in the neck. Hemangiomas, lymphatic malformations (cystic hygromas), and teratomas are the most common cervical tumors in infants and young children. Laryngoscopy may be required to differentiate these lesions. Emergency management of such malformations frequently requires placement of an endotracheal tube or tracheostomy. Endotracheal intubation can be difficult in the setting of a large neck mass, possibly causing displacement of the larynx, and bronchoscopy may be necessary with passage of the tube over a flexible bronchoscope. After the airway is stabilized, further diagnostic evaluation may include neck and chest radiography, CT, MRI, and laryngobronchoscopy. Tracheostomy may be necessary at the time of definitive surgical excision, and placement of a gastrostomy tube may also be indicated if feeding problems are anticipated. Hemangiomas are the most common tumors involving the larynx; they often respond to intralesional or systemic steroids, or may regress spontaneously.[4]

Acquired Obstruction

Foreign body aspiration and acute epiglottitis are common causes of acquired airway obstruction in children. Acute epiglottitis most commonly occurs in children 2 to 4 years of age, and *Haemophilus influenza* type B can be isolated in greater than 90% of cases. Since the introduction of *H. influenzae* vaccine in 1991, the incidence of this illness has been reduced in children.[5] Pneumococci and β-hemolytic streptococci are also causative
3 organisms in epiglottitis. Acute epiglottitis typically presents as a rapidly progressive illness with symptoms of severe stridor, airway obstruction, drooling, and difficulty swallowing and with signs of systemic toxicity, including an elevated temperature and white blood cell count, tachypnea, and tachycardia. Prolonged inspiratory stridor that worsens in the supine position is characteristic. In advanced cases, the child usually sits erect and leans forward, is anxious, drools, and becomes increasingly exhausted with air hunger. Attempts to examine or visualize the larynx may result in sudden airway occlusion with aspiration and respiratory arrest and therefore should be performed only in the operating room with personnel prepared to perform endotracheal intubation or tracheostomy. If the child's condition permits, lateral neck radiographs with soft tissue techniques are obtained and should confirm the diagnosis by demonstrating edema of the epiglottis and ballooning of the hypopharynx.

The most important aspect of management is establishing a definitive diagnosis without delay. Once the diagnosis is established, maintaining an adequate airway is vital. Because of the high risk for progressive airway obstruction, standard therapy often involves short-term endotracheal intubation performed in the operating room under general anesthesia. The surgeon should be prepared to perform a tracheostomy in the event that the airway cannot be secured with an endotracheal tube or flexible bronchoscope. The inflammatory process typically resolves rapidly with administration of intravenous antibiotics, and intubation is seldom required beyond 3 days. Ampicillin is no longer recommended because of the high incidence of resistant *Haemophilus*. The drug of choice is usually a third-generation cephalosporin, such as cefoxitin or cefuroxime. The timing of extubation should be determined by resolution of clinical signs and symptoms and direct visualization of the supraglottic area by fiberoptic nasopharyngoscopy. In the past, tracheostomy was the standard therapy, but comparative reviews demonstrate that short-term endotracheal intubation is associated with less morbidity and fewer complications.[6]

BRANCHIAL CLEFT REMNANTS

Remnants of the embryonic branchial apparatus (cysts, sinuses, fistulas, and cartilaginous rests) are common in children. Although congenital by definition, they are often unrecognized or misdiagnosed until symptoms or complications initiate an evaluation. Sinuses, fistulas, and cartilaginous remnants are usually apparent at birth and noticed early in life, whereas cysts are more likely to present later in childhood as a neck mass when they fill with secretions. All of these lesions have a risk of infection and can present as an abscess or with drainage and surrounding erythema. Rarely, these remnants may harbor malignancy.[7]

Anatomy and Embryology

During the fourth to eighth week after fertilization, four pairs of well-developed ridges (branchial arches) and associated clefts are prominent in the lateral cervicofacial region of the human embryo. Each consists of a cartilaginous center (mesoderm), an intervening cleft (ectoderm), an internal pouch (endoderm), and a parent nerve. The mature structures of the head and neck are derivatives of these paired branchial arches, clefts, and pouches in the embryo.[8] The contributions of the branchial arches and clefts to the structures of the neck and jaw are summarized in Figure 105.1. Incomplete closure or resorption of these primordial elements, particularly clefts, may result in development of cysts, sinuses, fistulas, and masses.

The first branchial arch forms the mandible and the maxillary process of the upper jaw. The dorsal portion of the first branchial cleft remains open as the external auditory canal; the other external clefts are obliterated. The closing plate between the first pouch and cleft becomes the tympanic membrane. The first pouch becomes the eustachian tube, the middle-ear cavity,

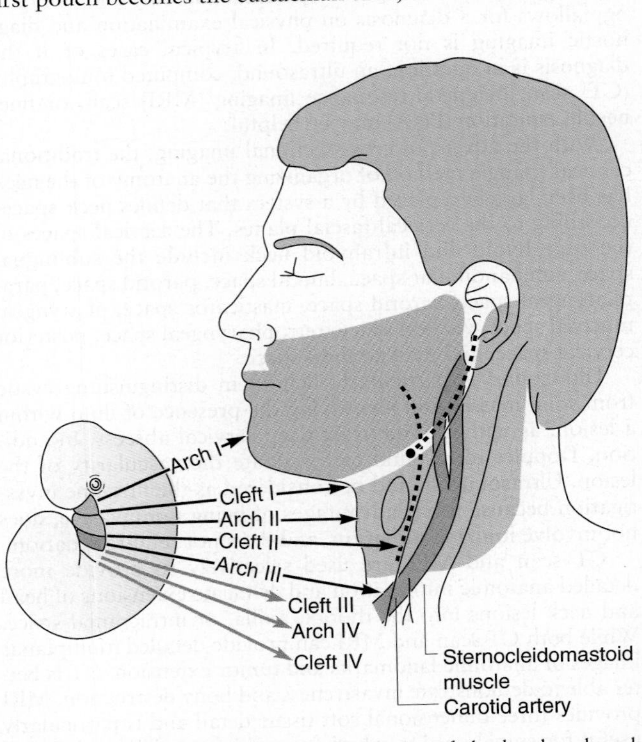

FIGURE 105.1. Derivation of various areas of the head and neck from the branchial arches and clefts of the embryo.

and the mastoid air cells. Abnormal development of the first branchial arch results in a host of facial deformities including cleft lip and palate, abnormal shape and contour of the external ear, and malformation of the internal ossicles. The second branchial arch and its internal pouch form the hyoid bone and the cleft of the tonsillar fossa. The palatine tonsil and the supratonsillar fossa are also remnants of the second branchial pouch.

Remnants of the first branchial cleft are found along the base of an imaginary fold extending from the auditory canal behind and below the angle of the mandible to just below the midpoint of the mandible. The critical anatomic relationship for first branchial cleft remnants is their intimate association to the facial nerve and its proximal branches.

Second branchial cleft remnants are found along any part of a line extending from the tonsillar fossa inferiorly to a point on the lower third of the anterior border of the sternocleidomastoid muscle. The third cleft migrates low in the neck to form the inferior parathyroid glands and the thymus. The fourth cleft also migrates but stops higher up in the neck and forms the superior parathyroid glands and C cells of the thyroid gland.

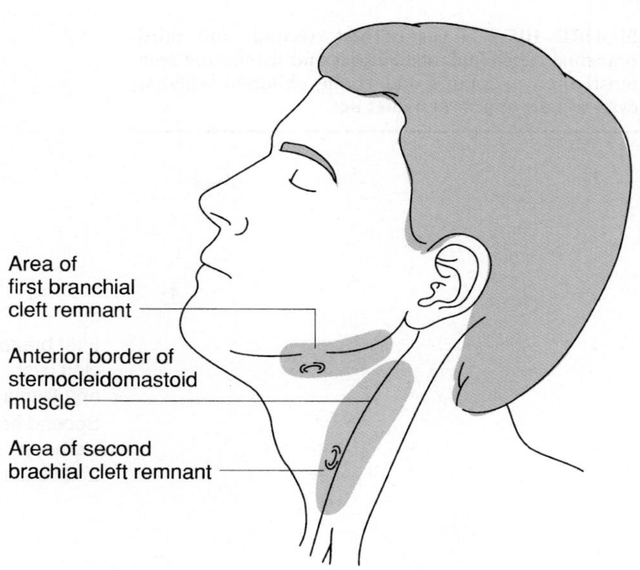

FIGURE 105.2. Areas of the neck in which cysts and sinuses originating from the first and second branchial clefts are usually found.

Clinical Aspects

4 All abnormal branchial remnants are congenital abnormalities and therefore are present at birth. Branchial cleft sinuses present as cutaneous openings and are most often noted in infancy or at an early age, whereas cysts typically appear later in childhood when they accumulate secretions. Branchial cleft sinuses and fistulas frequently produce mucoid drainage from the skin opening, and the cutaneous openings are occasionally marked by skin tags or subcutaneous cartilaginous remnants. The tract is often palpable.

First branchial cleft remnants present as a sinus opening near the angle of the mandible in the region of the submandibular triangle or preauricular region. These sinus tracts extend from their submandibular opening superficial to the mandible up to the external auditory canal. The tract is intimately associated with the superficial lobe of the parotid gland and facial nerve.[9] First branchial anomalies are less common than those of the second cleft and are often misdiagnosed. A history of recurrent infection, often leading to incision and drainage, is generally present. A key to the diagnosis is a history of nonpurulent drainage before infection.

Second branchial anomalies are six times more common than first branchial anomalies and present as an opening along the anterior border of the sternocleidomastoid muscle in its lower third and may be bilateral (10% of cases) (Figs. 105.2 and 105.3). The sinus tract of a second branchial anomaly passes through the subcutaneous tissues beneath the platysma muscle, over the bifurcation of the carotid artery, and between the external and internal carotid arteries, and enters the lateral wall of the pharynx at the tonsillar fossa. The tract may be complete (fistula) or incomplete (sinus).

Cysts or infections arising from the third and fourth branchial arch and cleft are rare and much more challenging to diagnose and treat than first and second branchial remnants.[10–12] For both third and fourth remnants, the internal opening is located in the piriform sinus (Fig. 105.4). Radiographic imaging is typically not necessary for first and second branchial anomalies, but barium studies and CT may be useful in demonstrating a piriform sinus fistula. The third branchial cleft sinus presents as a mass lower in the neck than the second branchial sinus. Its course is superior and posterior to the carotid sheath, most commonly on the left side (90%). Third and fourth branchial anomalies generally present before age 10 years, often as a left thyroid abscess. Contrast esophagram may demonstrate the fistula between the piriform sinus and the neck.[13,14] Because of the risk of the development of infection in any of the branchial cleft anomalies, excision is recommended at diagnosis of a noninfected lesion. Surgery in infants may be delayed until age 3 to 6 months.

Treatment and Outcome

The goal of treatment of any branchial cleft remnant is complete surgical excision. The operation is usually performed once the diagnosis is secure, provided no active inflammation or infection is present. If infection is found, antibiotics are administered initially, and the operation is delayed several weeks to allow the inflammation to resolve. This approach provides the best opportunity for complete excision of the tract. Abscesses are managed initially with limited incision and drainage to control infection. Formal excision of branchial cleft lesions in the presence of active inflammation or infection is associated with a higher recurrence rate secondary to incomplete excision[15] and an increased likelihood of injury to nerves (facial, hypoglossal) and other vital structures. Important principles for neck dissection for excision of branchial cleft remnants include avoidance of muscle relaxants, selective use of a nerve stimulator, and cautious use of retractors and electrocautery.

The operation is performed under general anesthesia. The patient is positioned with the head and neck slightly extended. A small elliptical incision along the Langer lines incorporates

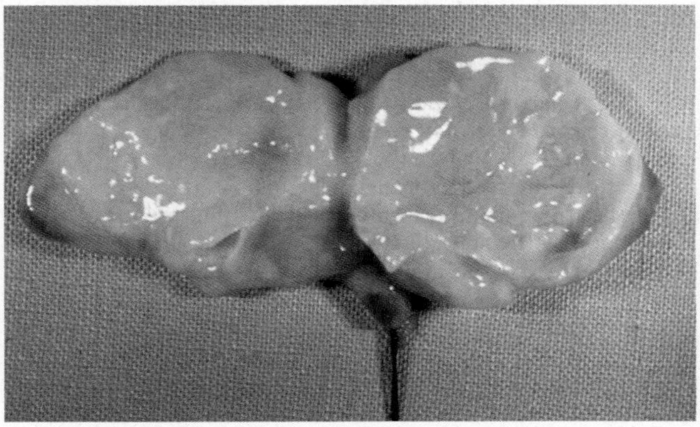

FIGURE 105.3. Branchial cyst. Most of these cysts arise from the second branchial cleft and occur laterally in the neck. The cysts have a thin wall, contain turbid fluid, and are lined by stratified squamous or respiratory-type epithelium. (From Rubin E, Farber JL. *Pathology,* 3rd ed. Philadelphia, PA: Lippincott Williams & Wilkins; 1999, with permission.)

PEDIATRICS

FIGURE 105.4. Types of first, second, and third branchial cleft remnants. Sinuses and fistulas are seen most often in infants and young children, whereas cysts usually appear at a later age.

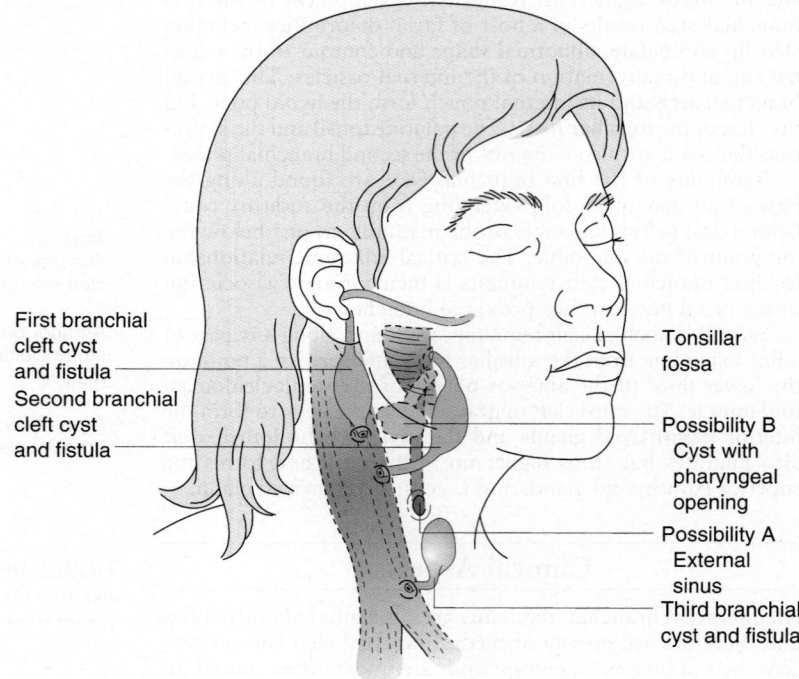

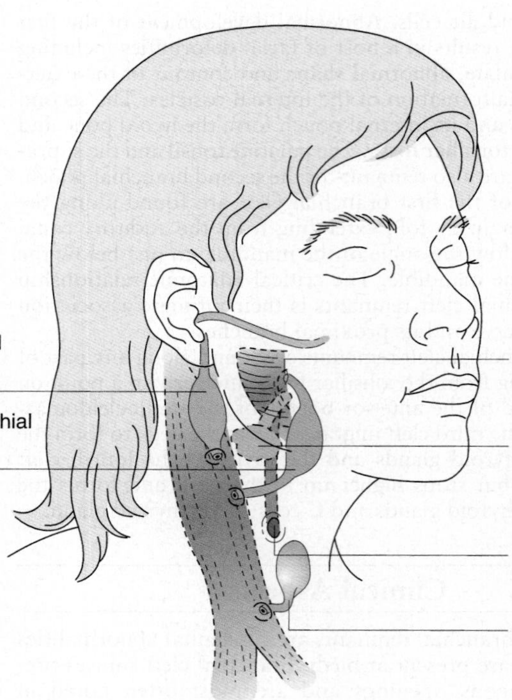

the sinus opening, excising the ellipse of skin without dividing the attachment to the sinus tract. The tract is identified and dissection continues cephalad immediately along the tract to avoid injury to contiguous structures. The dissection for a second branchial remnant penetrates the platysma muscle and cervical fascia, ascends along the carotid sheath to the level of the hyoid bone, turns medially between the branches of the carotid artery, and courses behind the posterior belly of the digastric muscle and stylohyoid muscle and in front of the hypoglossal nerve before ending in the pharynx, most often in the tonsillar fossa. A finger in the mouth pressing downward gently in the tonsillar fossa helps identify the endpoint of the dissection, where the tract is suture ligated with absorbable suture and divided (Fig. 105.5). Occasionally, in older patients with a long tract, a second, "stepladder" incision may be required to complete the dissection.

The tract for a first branchial cleft remnant typically courses from its sinus opening along the angle of the mandible cephalad in proximity to the parotid gland and facial nerve and ends at the external auditory canal (Fig. 105.6).[16] Draping should allow visualization of the lateral aspect of the eye and corner of the mouth. A nerve stimulator for electrophysiologic localization may be helpful to avoid injury to the main trunk of the facial nerve or its proximal branches. The superficial lobe of the parotid gland may need to be reflected upward to expose the tract or may require excision in cases of chronic infection.

For third and fourth branchial remnants, the dissection follows the tract to its termination in the piriform sinus. Endoscopy at the start of the operation may enable cannulation of the tract from above with a Fogarty catheter or small feeding tube, which greatly facilitates localization of the tract during excision.[14] Third or fourth branchial remnants almost all occur on the left side (90%). The thyroid gland is exposed through a standard collar incision, and the appropriate lobe is mobilized. The recurrent and superior laryngeal nerves and parathyroid glands should be identified and protected. If no discrete cyst or tract is found, the fistula may be located at the laryngeal level near the cricothyroid membrane. This is an anatomic area where the recurrent laryngeal nerve is particularly at risk for injury. The fibers of the inferior constrictor muscle are bluntly spread to expose the piriform recess. Extreme caution should be exercised in this region to preserve the external branch of the superior laryngeal nerve. The tract typically passes inferior and external to the recurrent laryngeal nerve along the trachea to the superior pole of the thyroid gland. It may end blindly near the gland or penetrate the capsule to terminate in the parenchyma of the left thyroid lobe. Thyroid lobectomy or resection of the superior pole is carried out as indicated by the extent of the cyst (Fig. 105.7).[17] Once surgical extirpation is complete, the wound is closed in layers with absorbable suture. Drainage is only used if infection is encountered during the dissection. Recurrence is rare (<5%) and implies that the entire epithelium-lined tract was not excised.

When remnants of the branchial apparatus persist as cartilaginous rests, these masses are generally small and present subcutaneously along the anterior border of the sternocleidomastoid muscle. The lesion is typically visible and palpable on physical examination and may be bilateral (10% of cases). An accompanying sinus or cyst is uncommon and infection is rare. Excision is for cosmetic reasons.

Preauricular cysts and sinuses are also common in infants and children. They are believed to arise as a result of anomalies in the formation of the external ear and represent vestiges of the first two branchial arches. These pits are lined with squamous epithelium and may contain hair and other skin appendages. They differ from first branchial cleft cysts in that they are more common, often bilateral, often inherited, and only rarely are complicated by infection, involvement of the facial nerve, or entrance into the external auditory canal.[18] They extend from the skin surface down through the subcutaneous tissue in close proximity to the superficial temporal artery and typically terminate in the cartilage of the external auditory canal. Operative excision is recommended to avoid infection. Draining sinuses and infected cysts require antibiotic treatment, incision and drainage for failure to resolve, and delayed excision to prevent recurrence. Complete surgical excision of the sinus tract and cyst to the level of the temporalis fascia is the treatment of choice in the uninfected draining sinus. The cyst or sinus may have multiple branches, making complete resection difficult, and some clinicians have advocated an extended incision and

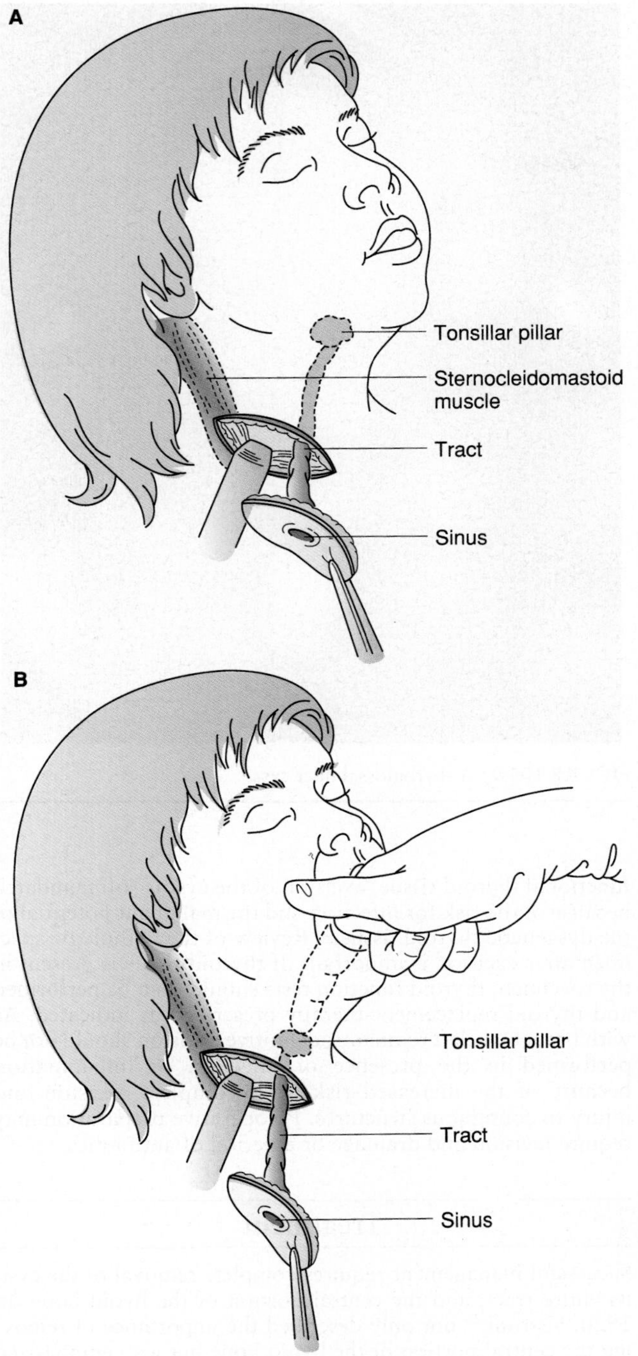

FIGURE 105.5. **A:** Single incision in the lower part of the neck with the sinus tract developed to usual length. **B:** The anesthesiologist's finger depresses the tonsillar fossa to facilitate complete dissection of the sinus tract through the single incision.

removal of a small portion of adjacent cartilage to reduce the risk of missing one of these branching tracts.[19,20]

THYROGLOSSAL DUCT CYST

Thyroglossal duct cysts are the most common neck mass in children. Most thyroglossal duct cysts are diagnosed in early childhood. The gender incidence is approximately equal, in contrast to thyroid disorders, in which girls are predominantly affected. Rare cases of familial inheritance with an autosomal dominant distribution have been described.

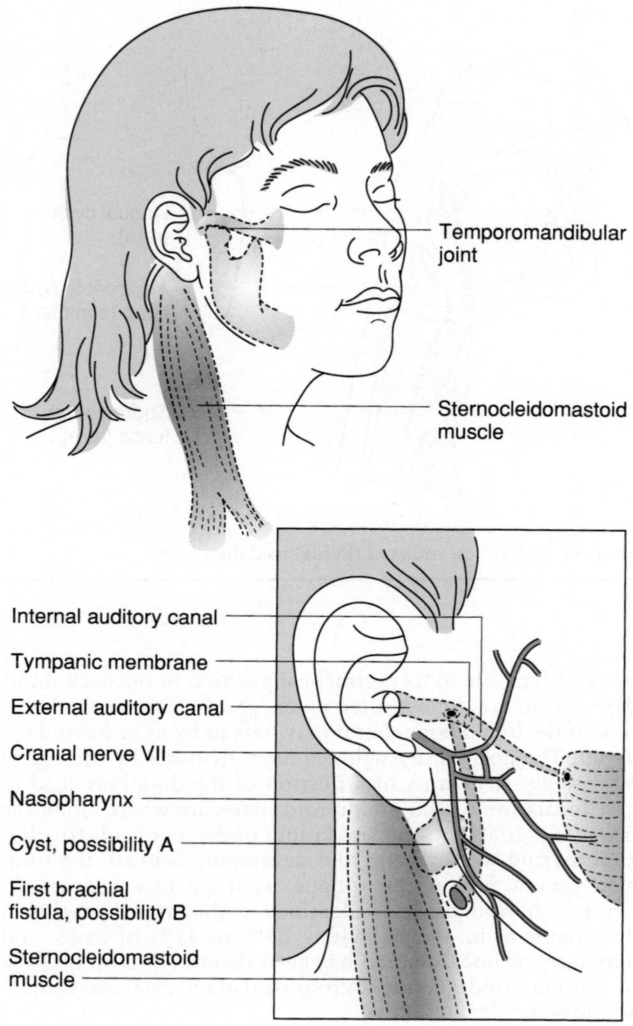

FIGURE 105.6. Relations of cyst or sinus of the first branchial cleft. Note especially the proximity to the facial nerve and external auditory canal.

Anatomy and Embryology

5 Thyroglossal duct cysts arise when embryonic elements persist along the tract of descent of the developing thyroid gland. The thyroid gland starts as a diverticulum at the foramen cecum at the base of the tongue and descends in the sixth

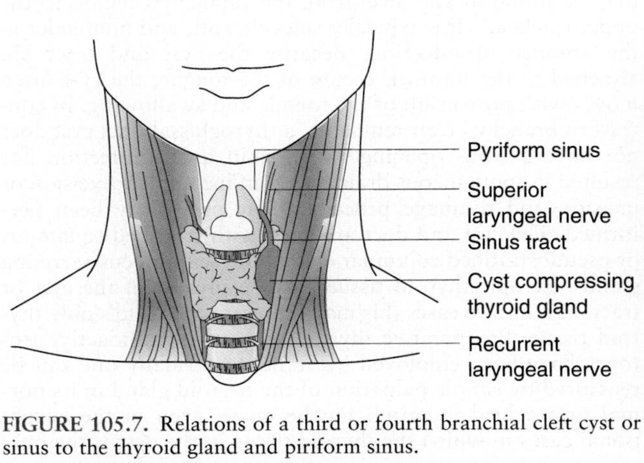

FIGURE 105.7. Relations of a third or fourth branchial cleft cyst or sinus to the thyroid gland and piriform sinus.

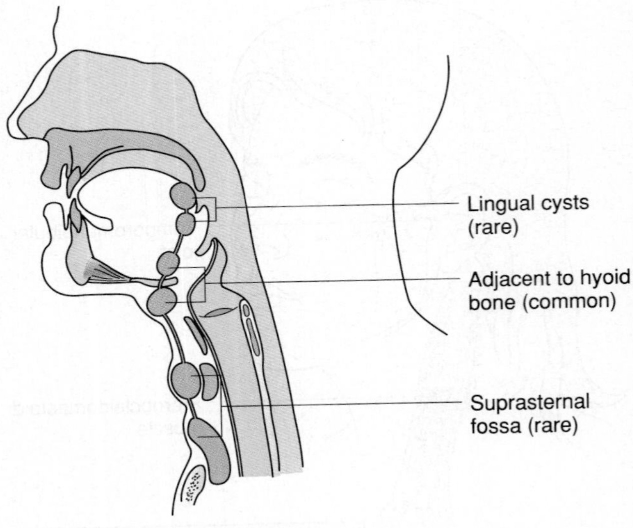

FIGURE 105.8. Locations of thyroglossal duct cysts.

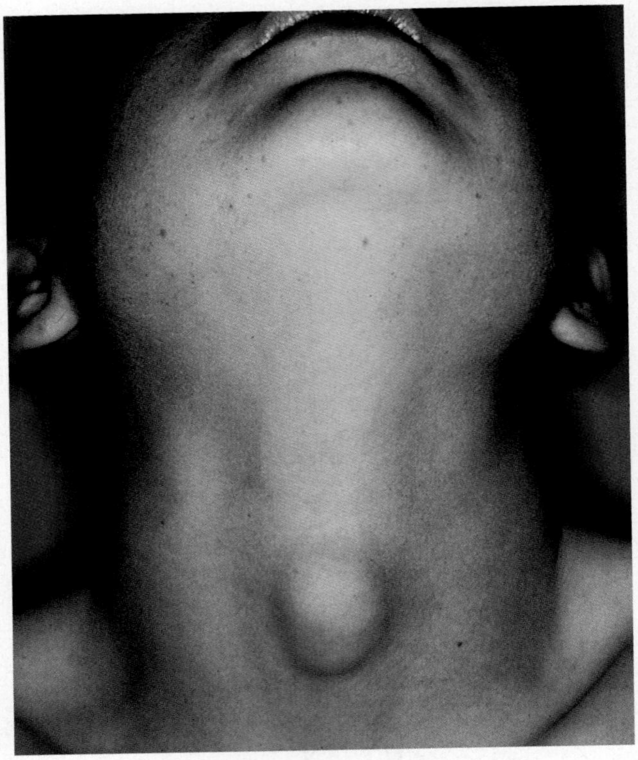

FIGURE 105.9. A thyroglossal duct cyst.

week of fetal life to its pretracheal position in the neck. In its descent, the tract most often passes through the central portion of the hyoid bone, but it may pass in front or behind the hyoid. The normal thyroglossal duct involutes by the eighth fetal week. Remnants of a portion of the duct may lead to cyst formation or ectopic thyroid tissue anywhere along the tract (Fig. 105.8). Complete failure of descent leads to a lingual thyroid, with the thyroid developing beneath the foramen cecum within the tongue itself or just beneath it. Ectopic thyroid tissue is identified within the thyroglossal duct remnant in approximately 25% to 35% of cases, and papillary adenocarcinoma has been described in up to 10% of patients undergoing thyroglossal duct cyst excision in adulthood.[11,21,22]

Clinical Aspects

Thyroglossal duct cysts are present at birth but rarely present clinically in infancy. The most common presentation is a midline cystic neck mass (Fig. 105.9) or draining sinus in early childhood, most by age 5 years.[23,24] Infection and abscess formation frequently arise because of communication with the mouth and contamination by oral flora. If it is not infected, the cyst is usually apparent by palpation. The cyst is at or near the midline, most commonly overlying the hyoid bone, but may be found at any level from the submental region to the upper trachea.[15] It is typically smooth, soft, and nontender in the absence of infection. Because the cyst and tract are attached to the foramen cecum of the tongue, the cyst often moves with protrusion of the tongue and swallowing. In contrast to branchial cleft remnants, a thyroglossal duct cyst does not have a sinus opening to the skin unless infection has resulted in spontaneous drainage or an incomplete excision or incision and drainage procedure has previously been performed. The cyst and duct are lined with stratified squamous or pseudostratified columnar epithelium with mucus-secreting glands. Ectopic thyroid tissue may be present in the cyst or tract, and in rare cases this may represent the child's only thyroid tissue. Preoperative thyroid scans with radioactive isotopes have been employed by some, but usually one can be reassured by simple palpation of the thyroid gland in its normal pretracheal location. Furthermore, even in the exceptional cases in which the thyroid tissue in the cyst is the only functional thyroid tissue, excision of the cyst is still mandated because of the risk for infection and the malignant potential of the dysgenetic thyroid tissue.[25] Review of the pathologic specimen after excision is important. If thyroid tissue is present in the specimen, thyroid function tests should then be performed and thyroid replacement therapy prescribed as indicated. As with branchial cleft remnants, definitive excision should not be performed in the presence of infection or inflammation because of the increased risk for incomplete excision and injury to contiguous structures. Preoperative preparation may require incision and drainage or a period of antibiotics.

Treatment

Successful management requires complete removal of the cyst, its entire tract, and the central portion of the hyoid bone. In 1920, Sistrunk[26] not only described the importance of removing the central portion of the hyoid bone but also emphasized the possible existence of multiple tracts and therefore the importance of an en bloc dissection and removal of a core of tissue to the base of the tongue. Before these operative principles were elucidated, most series reported a recurrence rate of 20% or higher. The operation is performed under general endotracheal anesthesia. The patient's neck is extended, and often a roll is placed beneath the shoulders. A transverse skin incision is made directly over the cyst, usually in the infrahyoid region. If a sinus opening exists to the skin from prior infection or surgery, an elliptical incision to include the sinus is used. The cyst is easily identified beneath the platysma muscle. Dissection adjacent to the cyst wall mobilizes the cyst, and the tract is identified. Dissection is continued cephalad up to the hyoid bone. The muscular attachments to the superior and inferior portions of the body of the hyoid bone are divided, and the central portion of the hyoid bone is removed in continuity with the cyst and tract. Beyond the hyoid bone, a core of tissue 5 to 10 mm in diameter is excised through the muscles of the base of the tongue to the foramen cecum, where the tract is suture ligated with absorbable suture.[27,28] Identification of the endpoint of the dissection at the foramen cecum may be facilitated by having the anesthesiologist place downward pressure on the base of the tongue with a gloved finger. The ends of the hyoid bone are not reapproximated. The wound is copiously irrigated and closed in layers. A drain may be used, particularly if the patient has a history of infection, but most often it is not required. Complete excision of a thyroglossal duct cyst is generally curative. Contemporary recurrence rates generally are less than 10% and usually related to prior infection or incomplete surgical excision. Thyroid neoplasia (<1%) has been described in ectopic thyroid tissue, both associated and unassociated with thyroglossal duct cysts.[11,21,22]

Other midline neck masses that occur in children include dermoid and epidermoid inclusion cysts, pathologic lymph nodes, cervical thymic cysts, and bronchogenic cysts. Dermoid and epidermoid cysts consist of ectodermal elements that were sequestered beneath the skin or failed to separate from the neural tube.[29,30] Dermoids are distinguished histologically from epidermoids by the accessory glandular structures they possess, including sebaceous glands, hair follicles, connective tissues, and papillae. The most common location of dermoids in infants and children is the lateral orbital ridge. They are usually soft, mobile, and nontender, and typically demonstrate slow growth along with the child's linear growth, becoming clinically apparent in early childhood.

Midline dermoid cysts probably represent entrapment of epithelium of branchial arch origin at the time of embryologic midline fusion.[31,32] Differentiation from thyroglossal duct cysts can usually be accomplished on physical examination, with dermoid cysts typically smaller and more superficial and that do not move with protrusion of the tongue. Midline dermoid cysts overlying the nasal bridge occasionally penetrate the bone, forming a dumbbell-shaped mass with dermoid elements on either side of the bone. CT imaging and occasionally MRI should be performed for midline facial dermoid cysts or fixed or atypical lesions in other locations to exclude intracranial extension. Complete surgical excision is the treatment of choice for all dermoid and epidermoid cysts to confirm the diagnosis, to prevent rupture or infection, and for cosmetic reasons. This is generally performed as an open operation, although increasing experience is accruing using endoscopic minimally invasive techniques.[33] Although exceedingly rare, malignant degeneration has been reported.

LYMPHADENOPATHY

6 Benign cervical lymphadenopathy is the most common neck mass in childhood.[34] Cervical nodes up to 1 cm in diameter are normal in children younger than 12 years of age, and many children in all age groups have palpable lymph nodes that are not associated with infection or systemic illness. The anterior cervical, occipital, retroauricular, and submandibular nodal groups are the ones most often enlarged. Bacterial and viral infections, particularly upper respiratory tract infections, otitis media, and pharyngitis, are the most common cause, with bacterial infections most likely to progress to acute suppurative lymphadenitis. Unilateral nodal enlargement is usually the result of pyogenic infection originating in the tonsils and oropharynx, while bilateral disease is frequently observed in viral upper respiratory tract infections.

Fungal infections are an uncommon cause of lymphadenopathy in children with the exception of immunocompromised patients. Other important inflammatory causes of cervical lymphadenopathy include cat scratch disease, mononucleosis, atypical mycobacteria (AMB) infections, and tuberculosis. Enlarged cervical or supraclavicular lymph nodes may also be the presenting manifestation of certain malignancies, both primary and metastatic, particularly lymphoma.[35] Rare noninfectious causes of cervical lymphadenopathy include Kawasaki disease, sarcoidosis, sinus histiocytosis (Rosai-Dorfman syndrome), and histiocytosis X.

Acute suppurative cervical lymphadenitis most frequently occurs in young children, between 6 months and 3 years of age. Typically, enlargement of the lymph node is preceded by an episode of pharyngitis or an upper respiratory tract infection. The most common causative organisms are penicillin-resistant *Staphylococcus aureus* and group A β-hemolytic streptococci.[36] Bacterial lymphadenitis is often characterized by rapid nodal enlargement. The enlarged node initially becomes erythematous and tender, with surrounding cellulitis. Systemic signs of infection are usually present—fever, tachycardia, and elevated white blood cell count with a leftward shift. Fluctuance develops as the abscess forms. Management includes systemic antibiotics to cover *Streptococcus* and *Staphylococcus* organisms. Occasionally, aspiration of the purulent and necrotic material with a large-bore needle provides fluid for culture, and in combination with antibiotics, may effect resolution without formal incision and drainage. More frequently, fluctuant nodes require incision and drainage, with the use of either conscious sedation and local anesthesia, or general anesthesia in the operating room. The most important consideration when performing incision and drainage of a fluctuant neck mass is control of the airway. A skin-line incision is made over the area of maximal fluctuance and the abscess cavity is drained, with care to disrupt any loculations. The incision should be designed with concern for complete drainage; avoidance of vital structures, particularly the branches of the facial nerve; and cosmesis. Incisions high or low in the neck should be made in parallel with the angle of the mandible or clavicle and at least 1 cm away from these structures to avoid hypertrophic scar formation. The wound is loosely packed open and covered with a dry gauze dressing. Drains may be used in cases of deep or complex neck abscesses, but are not generally necessary in uncomplicated cases. Recurrence is rare and should prompt evaluation for an underlying immunodeficiency or congenital anomaly. Viral infections are also associated with the development of acute cervical lymphadenitis, which is typically bilateral, rarely suppurative, and generally self-limited with spontaneous resolution.

Lymphadenitis is chronic or subacute when enlargement of lymph nodes persists long after any evidence of infection has disappeared or the patient has no history or evidence of a precipitating infectious illness. The child may have a history of frequent upper respiratory infections, otitis media, tonsillitis, sinusitis, or allergic rhinitis or eczema. Systemic signs of infection are not present. The nodes are usually solitary, nontender, mobile, and soft. Enlarged nodes that are asymptomatic, less than 1 cm in diameter, and soft and that have been present for less than 8 weeks do not require treatment. Excisional biopsy should be performed for any lymph node that is larger than 2 cm in diameter, persists beyond 8 weeks, or demonstrates worrisome characteristics such as firmness, immobility, or rapid growth. Communication between the surgeon and pathologist is important to ensure that complete culture data is obtained, including cultures for tuberculosis, atypical mycobacterial infection, and cat scratch disease, as well as histopathologic and flow cytometry studies for possible malignancy. Most of the lymph nodes that come to biopsy are benign and the histologic examination reveals "reactive hyperplasia."

Mycobacterial lymphadenitis and cat scratch disease also commonly cause lymphadenopathy in children.[37] Mycobacterial lymphadenitis is usually caused by atypical mycobacteria of the *Mycobacterium avium-intracellulare-scrofulaceum* (MAIS) complex.[38–40] Pathogens typically enter the body through breaks in the mucus membranes of the oropharynx during the eruption of teeth. Unlike *Mycobacterium tuberculosis*, person-to-person transmission of MAIS has not been demonstrated.

Infection with *M. tuberculosis* is uncommon in children in the United States, and when present, it is usually accompanied by positive findings on chest radiographs because the lung is the site of entry for this organism.

Atypical mycobacterial lymphadenitis occurs predominantly in children 1 to 5 years of age and is rare after the age of 12. The lymphadenopathy observed with AMB infection is typically asymptomatic with enlarged but nontender nodes and no associated fever or leukocytosis. The nodes are initially rubbery and firm, and submandibular or preauricular areas are most common. They later become matted together to form a confluent mass. If no treatment is given, drainage and sinus formation may occur spontaneously.

The child with tuberculosis scrofula is typically symptomatic with pulmonary tuberculosis. The results of chest radiography and skin testing with purified protein derivative standard are usually positive. For *M. tuberculosis* infection, a trial of antituberculosis chemotherapy is recommended. Current treatment regimens consist of multiple-agent chemotherapy with isoniazid and rifampin for 9 to 12 months and a third drug (pyrazinamide, streptomycin, or ethambutol) for the first 2 months.[41]

Atypical mycobacterial infections generally respond poorly to chemotherapy. When a lymph node biopsy is planned, if tuberculosis or atypical mycobacterial infection is suspected, complete excision is required. Incision and drainage or incomplete nodal excision in cases of atypical mycobacterial infection invariably leads to recurrence or cutaneous draining sinuses. Complete excision is generally curative, although there may be a role for adjunctive antimicrobial therapy with clarithromycin and rifabutin.[42]

Cat scratch disease is a common cause of lymphadenitis in children in Western countries.[43] In most cases, the history reveals direct contact with a cat with the development of tender regional lymphadenopathy within 2 weeks of inoculation. Other animals, such as dogs and monkeys, have also been implicated in transmission. The site of inoculation is most commonly an extremity, resulting in inguinal, epitrochlear, or axillary adenopathy; however, cervical nodes are involved in as many as 25% of cases.[44,45] The disease is believed to be caused by a gram-negative bacillus, *Bartonella henselae*, and typically begins as a superficial infection at the inoculation site on a limb. The diagnosis can be confirmed by several methods, including skin test antigen, *B. henselae*–based serologic indirect fluorescent antibody test, and enzyme immunoassays. The clinical presentation usually is lymphadenopathy with only mild tenderness and without systemic symptoms; however, severe complications including encephalitis, follicular conjunctivitis, and neuroenteritis can occur. No treatment is necessary if the diagnosis is secure (positive skin test result) because the illness is generally self-limited and lymphadenopathy resolves in most cases in 6 to 8 weeks without specific treatment. Antibiotics are not generally effective despite in vitro sensitivities. If the diagnosis is in doubt, complete excision is recommended and curative.

Although most lymphadenopathy in children is benign, malignant conditions such as Hodgkin disease and non-Hodgkin lymphoma are also common in children and frequently present as primary neck lymphadenopathy. Any case of a neck mass that has concerning examination characteristics, or that persists despite appropriate antibiotic therapy, requires FNA for cytology and likely excisional biopsy for definitive diagnosis.

VASCULAR MALFORMATIONS

Hemangioma

Hemangiomas are endothelial tumors characterized by an increased proliferation and turnover of endothelial cells, and this differentiates them from other vascular malformations. Hemangiomas display a unique biologic behavior—they grow rapidly, regress slowly, and never recur. Hemangiomas can occur anywhere in the body and the craniofacial region is common with frequent involvement of the tongue, subglottic area, and parotid glands. Single lesions predominate, but there also can be multiple lesions in up to 20% of infants, with the head, neck, and trunk being the areas most often affected. A superficial hemangioma is a well-demarcated, elevated, bright red mass or plaque that blanches incompletely with pressure. Sometimes a hemangioma can have a deep component that is a soft, flesh-colored, rubbery, ill-defined subcutaneous mass with a bluish hue. Risk factors for the development of infantile hemangiomas include female sex, Caucasian race, preterm birth, and low birth weight. Most hemangiomas are not clinically evident at birth but become apparent in the first few months of life, and 90% are evident by age 6 months.

Hemangiomas can be extensive and typically have a red or blue coloration and a spongy or rubbery texture on palpation. The presenting symptom for subglottic hemangioma is often stridor that is not present at birth but presents at age 1 to 3 months. Parotid hemangioma typically presents as an enlarging soft tissue mass in the parotid gland in the first 1 to 3 months of infancy. Cutaneous capillary hemangiomas may be present on the face, neck, or chest. Evaluation by ultrasonography with Doppler flow studies is usually diagnostic.[46] The natural history of these lesions is for significant growth (proliferative phase) in the first 6 to 12 months of life, followed by a period of minimal growth, after which involution and spontaneous resolution occurs by thrombosis and epithelialization.[47] If involution takes place, it is complete by age 5 years in 80% of patients. Biopsy of these lesions was recommended in the past but is no longer routinely performed in most centers. CT with intravenous contrast and magnetic resonance angiographic imaging are very useful in selected cases for evaluating the extent of tissue involvement. Angiography is invasive and rarely necessary for diagnostic purposes, but may be useful for treatment of large lesions by embolization. Biopsy remains important when the diagnosis is in question, particularly to rule out kaposiform hemangioendothelioma (KHE), a vascular tumor associated with profound thrombocytopenia.

Although most hemangiomas spontaneously resolve, up to 24% of infants will have complications, such as hemorrhage, ulceration, infection, and necrosis. Rarely (3% to 5%), hemangiomas may become quite large, involve vital organs, or produce life-threatening complications including hemorrhage, thrombocytopenia, and coagulopathy owing to platelet trapping, airway obstruction, or congestive heart failure. Periorbital hemangiomas should be recognized as particularly problematic with potential to lead to the development of astigmatism, ptosis, strabismus, amblyopia, and blindness.

Treatment of hemangiomas is challenging given the wide spectrum of disease, unpredictable biologic behavior, and natural tendency for involution. Most hemangiomas will follow the natural history of rapid growth followed by gradual spontaneous involution, and observation is appropriate. Aggressive treatment is necessary for infants at highest risk of complications. Lesions that, because of their location or growth, are obstructing the airway, involving the eye, or causing tissue destruction are generally treated with oral corticosteroids due to their antiproliferative effect (Fig. 105.10). The response is typically excellent. Other treatment options include topical and intralesional corticosteroids, pulsed-dye laser therapy, and surgical excision.

LYMPHATIC MALFORMATIONS

Anatomy and Embryology

At about the sixth week of gestation, a system of clefts develops in the cervical mesenchyme that subsequently forms lymph channels. These channels give rise to jugular lymph sacs that become the cervical lymph nodes and lymphatics, ultimately

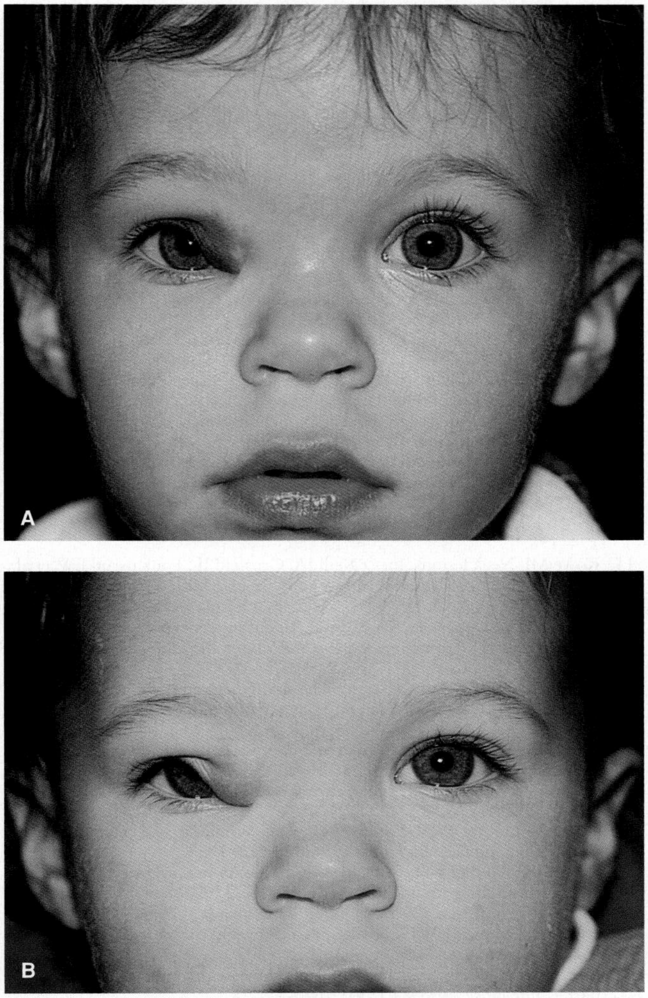

FIGURE 105.10. Capillary hemangioma. **A:** The lesion of the upper lid is large enough to partially occlude the visual axis and induced a significant astigmatic error and strong visual preference for the left eye, requiring occlusion therapy. Because it is located in the deeper tissue layers, this hemangioma appears more bluish than more superficially located lesions. **B:** Three days after intralesional steroid injection, the hemangioma has shrunk out of the visual axis. (From Tasman W, Jaeger E. *The Wills Eye Hospital Atlas of Clinical Ophthalmology*, 2nd ed. Philadelphia: Lippincott Williams & Wilkins; 2001, with permission.)

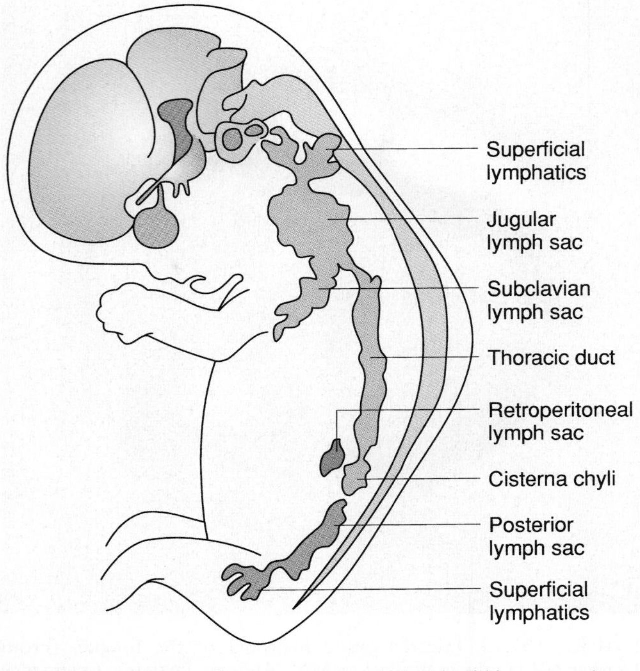

FIGURE 105.11. Lymphatic system in an 8-week-old human embryo. Development of the major and minor lymphatic sacs is well under way. The jugular lymphatic sac in the neck is prominent. Sequestration of tissue from any of the developing lymphatic structures leads to formation of a lymphangioma or cystic hygroma.

draining into the internal jugular venous system (Fig. 105.11). 7 Lymphatic malformations are benign masses of disorganized dilated lymph channels that arise when portions of these primitive embryonic lymph sacs fail to develop communications with the internal jugular venous system. Although sequestered from the normal lymphatic channels, these sequestered lymph channels are lined by endothelial cells and continue to produce lymph fluid. In contrast to hemangiomas, the proliferative rate of the lining endothelial cells is normal. Lymphatic malformations can vary in size from a few centimeters in diameter to massive tumorlike lesions extending into the mediastinum. Radiologically and histologically, they are characterized as microcystic, macrocystic, or combined.

Lymphatic malformations tend to develop in close proximity to large veins and lymphatic ducts. Large macrocystic lesions are commonly found in the lateral cervical and submandibular region and are often termed *cystic hygromas*. Lesions that involve the tongue or extend into the mediastinum may result in stridor, cyanosis, apnea, or dysphagia with failure to thrive. Other locations for lymphatic malformations are the axilla/chest, extremities, retroperitoneum, and perineum. Most lymphatic malformations are evident early in life, with 65% present at birth, 80% evident within the first year of life, and 90% diagnosed by the age of 2 years.[48] They are more common (2:1) on the left side of the neck, presumably because the thoracic duct enters the subclavian vein on the left side. The physical examination characteristics of a soft, discrete, cystic, multiloculated mass are often sufficient for a definitive diagnosis. Spontaneous resolution is rare. Hemorrhage can occur within the lesion and is often the reason for the rapid enlargement sometimes noted clinically. When this occurs there is sudden swelling and ecchymosis. Intralesional bleeding is a predisposing factor for infection, and antibiotics should be initiated (Fig. 105.12).

Cellulitis is common in lymphatic malformations, particularly those in the head, neck, and perineum. This also commonly results in rapid expansion of the lesion with erythema, fever, and tenderness. In the newborn, large neck lesions may cause significant airway compromise or esophageal and pharyngeal obstruction. Symptoms such as pain or discomfort are rare unless the lesion has hemorrhaged or become infected. Approximately 10% of cervical lymphatic malformations extend into the chest.

Lymphatic malformations can be detected by prenatal ultrasonography, most often as septated or nonseptated lesions in the nuchal region. When associated with fetal hydrops, chromosomal abnormalities, or structural anomalies, early fetal death frequently is noted by 22 weeks' gestation. Lymphatic malformations demonstrated after parturition generally have a favorable prognosis. The physical examination findings of a soft, cystic, multiloculated mass are often sufficient for a definitive diagnosis. Ultrasonography, particularly with Doppler flow studies, is often useful to confirm the diagnosis. CT with intravenous contrast or magnetic resonance angiography is used selectively to evaluate extension of the lesion from one body space to another and delineate associated vital structures when planning for resection.

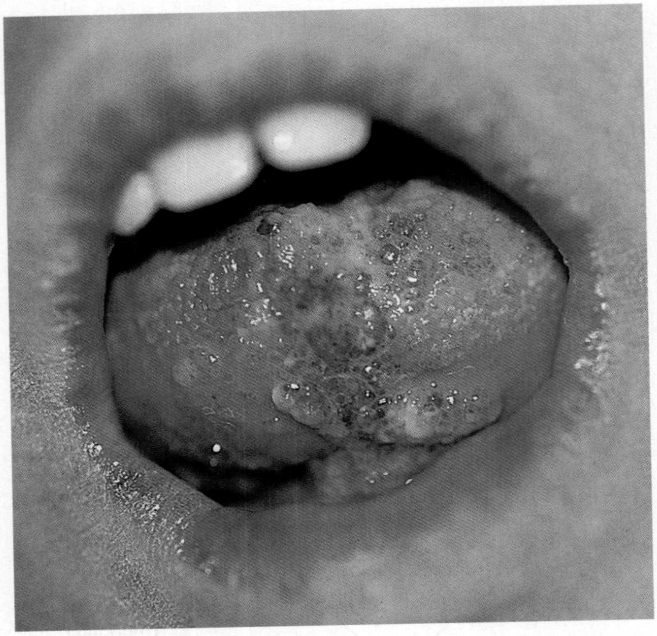

FIGURE 105.12. Infected cystic hygroma of the tongue. (From Fleisher GR, Ludwig W, Baskin MN. *Atlas of Pediatric Emergency Medicine*. Philadelphia, PA: Lippincott Williams & Wilkins; 2004, with permission.)

Treatment

Complete surgical excision is the optimal treatment for lymphatic malformations, but the tendency for these benign malformations to insinuate in and around vital structures can make complete resection difficult. With incomplete excision, disease recurrence is high (10% to 15%). Radical extirpative resections resulting in loss of function or severe deformity are not indicated. Spontaneous regression of these lesions is unusual but may occur after acute inflammation. Only two thirds of lymphatic malformations will be amenable to complete excision and one third will require partial excision or in the case of extensive or complex lesions staged excision due to involvement of vital structures within the lesion. Percutaneous aspiration usually is followed by prompt recurrence and may result in hemorrhage or infection and is not recommended except to emergently decompress a cyst and relieve airway obstruction. Radiation treatment has not been of benefit in the treatment of lymphatic malformations and has significant morbidity in the growing child. Injection of sclerosing agents, most commonly bleomycin, has been used but has significant potential complications of infection, gastrointestinal problems, and pulmonary fibrosis.[49] More recently, large cystic lesions in locations difficult to manage surgically have been treated by injection of OK-432, a monoclonal antibody produced by incubation and interaction of *Streptococcus pyogenes* with penicillin.[50] At present this treatment remains experimental but has demonstrated success in some difficult cases.

References

1. DeLorimer AA. Congenital malformations and neonatal problems of the respiratory tract. In: Welch KJ, Randolph JG, Ravitch MM, et al., eds. *Pediatric Surgery,* 4th ed. Chicago, IL: Year Book; 1986:631.
2. Alpers CE, Rosenau W, Finkbeiner WE, et al. Congenital (infantile) hemangiopericytoma of the tongue and sublingual region. *Am J Clin Pathol* 1984;81:377–382.
3. Weider DJ, Parker W. Lingual thyroid: review, case reports, and therapeutic guidelines. *Ann Otol Rhinol Laryngol* 1977:86:841–848.
4. Fonkalsrud EW. Malformations of the lymphatic system and hemangiomas. In: Holder TM, Ashcraft KW, eds. *Pediatric Surgery*. Philadelphia, PA: WB Saunders; 1980:1042.
5. Adams WG, Deaver KA, Cochi SL, et al. Decline of Haemophilus influenzae type B (HIB) disease in the HIB vaccine era. *JAMA* 1993;269:221–226.
6. Kinnefors A, Olofsson J. Acute epiglottitis in children: experience with tracheostomy and intubation. *Clin Otolaryngol Allied Sci* 1983;8:25–30.
7. Soper RT, Pringle KC. Cysts and sinuses of the neck. In: Welch KJ, Randolph JG, Ravitch MM, et al., eds. *Pediatric Surgery,* 4th ed. Chicago, IL: Year Book; 1986:539.
8. Gray SW, Skandalakis JE. *Embryology for Surgeons: The Embryological Basis for the Treatment of Congenital Defects*, 2nd ed. Baltimore: Williams and Wilkins; 1994:17–64.
9. Triglia JM, Nicollas R, Dueroz V, et al. First branchial cleft anomalies. A study of 39 cases and a review of the literature. *Arch Otolaryngol Head Neck Surg* 1998;124:291–295.
10. Lin JN, Wang KL. Persistent third branchial apparatus. *J Pediatr Surg* 1991;26:663–665.
11. Brown RL, Azizkhan RG. Pediatric head and neck lesions. *Pediatr Clin North Am* 1998;45:889–905.
12. Rosenfeld RM, Biller HF. Fourth branchial pouch sinus: diagnosis and treatment. *Otolaryngol Head Neck Surg* 1991;105:44–50.
13. Roback SA, Telander RL. Thyroglossal duct cysts and branchial cleft anomalies. *Semin Pediatr Surg* 1994;3:142–146.
14. Godin MS, Kearns DB, Pransky SM, et al. Fourth branchial pouch sinus: principles of diagnosis and management. *Laryngoscope* 1990;100: 174–178.
15. Rowe MI. Neck lesions. In: O'Neill JA, Grosfeld JL, Fonkalsrud EW, et al., eds. *Essentials of Pediatric Surgery*. St. Louis, MO: Mosby–Year Book; 1998:765.
16. D'Souza AR, Uppal HS, De R, et al. Updating concepts of first branchial cleft defects: a literature review. *Int J Pediatr Otorhinolaryngol* 2002;62: 103–109.
17. Miller D, Hill JL, Sun CC, et al. The diagnosis and management of pyriform sinus fistulae in infants and young children. *J Pediatr Surg* 1983;18: 377–381.
18. Burge D, Middleton A. Persistent pharyngeal pouch derivatives in the neonate. *J Pediatr Surg* 1983;18:230–234.
19. Singer R. A new technique for extirpation of preauricular cysts. *Am J Surg* 1966;111:291–295.
20. Currie AR, King WW, Vlantis AC, et al. Pitfalls in the management of preauricular sinuses. *Br J Surg* 1996;83:1722–1724.
21. LiVolsi VA, Perzin KH, Safetsky L. Carcinoma arising in ectopic thyroid tissue (including thyroglossal duct tissue). *Cancer* 1974;34:1303–1131.
22. Page CP, Kemmerer WT, Hatt RC, et al. Thyroid carcinoma arising in thyroglossal ducts. *Ann Surg* 1974;180:799–803.
23. Guarisco JL. Congenital head and neck masses in infants and children: part 1. *Ear Nose Throat J* 1991;70:40–47.
24. Guarisco JL. Congenital head and neck masses in infants and children: part I. *Ear Nose Throat J* 1991;70:75–82.
25. Radkowski D, Arnold J, Healy GB, et al. Thyroglossal duct remnants: preoperative evaluation and management. *Arch Otolaryngol Head Neck Surg* 1991;117:1378–1381.
26. Sistrunk WE. The surgical management of cysts of the thyroglossal tract. *Ann Surg* 1920;71:121–122.
27. Hoffman MA, Schuster SR. Thyroglossal duct remnants in infants and children: reevaluation of histopathology and methods for resection. *Ann Otol Rhinol Laryngol* 1988;97:483–486.
28. Ein SH, Shandling B, Stephens CA, et al. Management of recurrent thyroglossal duct remnants. *J Pediatr Surg* 1984;19:437–439.
29. Gold BC, Skeinkopf DE, Levy B. Dermoid, epidermoid, and teratomatous cysts of the tongue and floor of the mouth. *J Oral Surg* 1974;32:107–111.
30. Smirniotopoulos JG, Chiechi MV. Teratomas, dermoids, and epidermoids of the head and neck. *Radiographics* 1995;15:1437–1455.
31. McAvoy JM, Zuckerbraun L. Dermoid cysts of the head and neck in children. *Arch Otolaryngol* 1976;102:529–531.
32. Waldhausen JA, Tapper D. Head and neck sinuses and masses. *Pediatr Clin North Am* 1998;45:889–905.
33. Huang MG, Cohen SR, Burstein FD, et al. Endoscopic pediatric plastic surgery. *Ann Plast Surg* 1997;38:1–8.
34. Telander RL, Filston HC. Review of head and neck lesions in infancy and childhood. *Surg Clin North Am* 1992;72:1429–1447.
35. LaQuaglia MP. Non-Hodgkin lymphoma of the head and neck in childhood. *Semin Pediatr Surg* 1994;3:207–215.
36. Bodenstein L, Altman RP. Cervical lymphadenitis in infants and children. *Semin Pediatr Surg* 1994;3:134–141.
37. Zitelli BJ. Neck masses in children: adenopathy and malignant disease. *Pediatr Clin North Am* 1981;28:813–821.
38. Altman RP, Margileth AW. Cervical lymphadenopathy from atypical mycobacteria: diagnosis and surgical management. *J Pediatr Surg* 1975; 10:419–422.
39. Taha AM, Davidson PT, Bailey WC. Surgical treatment of atypical mycobacterial lymphadenitis in children. *Pediatr Inf Dis J* 1985;4:664–667.
40. Sigalet D, Lees G, Fanning A. Atypical tuberculosis in the pediatric patient: implications for the pediatric surgeon. *J Pediatr Surg* 1992;27:1381–1384.
41. Speck WT. Tuberculosis. In: Behrman RE, Kliegman R, Jensen HB, eds. *Nelson Textbook of Pediatrics,* 17th ed. Philadelphia, PA: Saunders; 2004:967–975.

42. Starke JR. Management of nontuberculous mycobacterial cervical adenitis. *Pediatr Infect Dis J* 2000;19:674–676.
43. Jackson LA, Perkins BA, Wenger JD. Cat-scratch disease in the United States: an analysis of three national databases. *Am J Public Health* 1993; 83:1707–1711.
44. Carithers HA. Cat-scratch disease: an overview based on the study of 1,200 patients. *Am J Dis Child* 1985;139:1124–1133.
45. Committee on Infectious Diseases. Summaries of infectious diseases. In: Dickering CK, Baker CJ, Overturf GD, et al., eds. *Red Book*, 26th ed. Elk Grove Village, IL: American Academy of Pediatrics; 2003:232–234.
46. Welch KJ. The salivary glands. In: Welch KJ, Randolph JG, Ravitch MM, et al., eds. *Pediatric Surgery*, 4th ed. Chicago, IL: Year Book; 1986.
47. Mulliken JB, Young AE. *Vascular Birthmarks: Hemangiomas and Malformations.* Philadelphia, PA: WB Saunders; 1988:1511–1518.
48. Bill AH, Sumner DS. A unified concept of lymphangioma and cystic hygroma. *Surg Gynecol Obstet* 1965;120:79–86.
49. Tanaka K, Inomata Y, Utsunomiya H, et al. Sclerosing therapy with bleomycin emulsion for lymphangioma in children. *Pediatr Surg Int* 1990;5:270.
50. Ogita S, Tsuto T, Deguchi E, et al. OK-432 therapy for unresectable lymphangiomas in children. *J Pediatr Surg* 1991;26:263–270.

CHAPTER 106 ■ THE PEDIATRIC CHEST

TONY CAPIZZANI, RONALD B. HIRSCHL, AND ROBERT E. CILLEY

KEY POINTS

1. Pectus excavatum results from abnormal regulation of the growth of the costal cartilages with a corresponding posterior curve in the body of the sternum beginning at the manubrium and extending to the xiphoid; the deformity is rarely precisely symmetric, with one side (usually the right) slightly more curved in than the other.
2. Pectus excavatum repair should occur in late childhood or adolescence and is now most frequently performed with a rigid transversely oriented bar (Lorenz bar) that pushes the deformity back into place.
3. Pectus carinatum occurs less frequently than pectus excavatum and does not cause physiologic impairment; for operative repair, osteotomies and sternal fracture are performed in such a way as to depress the sternum.
4. Pulmonary sequestrations (PS) are abnormal lung tissue with anomalous systemic blood supply that can be either intralobar or extralobar lesions based on their relationship with the investing visceral pleura and adjacent normal lung tissue. They do not communicate normally with the trachea or a bronchus.
5. Congenital cystic adenomatoid malformations (CCAMs) have a normal vascular supply and communicate with the normal tracheobronchial tree. They result from excessive proliferation of bronchial structures without the development of the corresponding alveoli.
6. Benign cysts of the mediastinum are relatively common and include thymic cysts, enterogenous cysts, dermoid cysts, lymphatic malformations (cystic hygromas), and pericardial cysts. Resection is usually recommended because of the possibility of progressive enlargement with compression, hemorrhage, or infection.
7. Primary lung tumors in children include bronchial adenoma, rarely bronchogenic carcinoma, pulmonary blastoma, inflammatory pseudotumor (composed of inflammatory cells), and hamartoma. Resection is generally appropriate initial therapy.
8. Mediastinal tumors include neurogenic tumors (usually from the sympathetic chain), lymphoma (Hodgkin or non-Hodgkin), teratoma, neurilemmoma, sarcoma, and thymic tumors.
9. Tracheoesophageal fistula can occur as esophageal atresia with proximal pouch and distal tracheoesophageal fistula (most common, at 85% to 95%), esophageal atresia without fistula (5% to 7%), tracheoesophageal fistula without esophageal atresia H type (2% to 6%), and rarer forms of this anomaly including esophageal atresia with proximal tracheoesophageal fistula and esophageal atresia with both proximal and distal tracheoesophageal fistula.
10. Vascular rings result from faulty embryogenesis of the aortic arch and great vessels resulting in vascular structures and dense connective tissue that surround the esophagus and trachea and can result in symptoms of airway or esophageal obstruction.
11. Approximately 200 children die from foreign body aspiration or ingestion each year. Bronchoscopic evaluation and foreign body removal are performed in the operating room under general anesthesia, where the rigid bronchoscope with optical forceps can be used to remove most aspirated foreign bodies safely.
12. Left-sided congenital diaphragmatic hernia (CDH) is a 2- to 4-cm posterolateral defect in the diaphragm through which the abdominal viscera have translocated into the ipsilateral thoracic cavity. Through a right-sided defect, the large right lobe of the liver can occupy most of the hemithorax.
13. CDH is a physiologic emergency and not a surgical emergency. The newborn with CDH should be stabilized by nonsurgical means and delayed, well-planned surgical repair undertaken subsequently.

CHEST WALL DEFORMITIES

Deformities of the chest wall may be obvious at birth but often become more noticeable at the time of preadolescent and adolescent growth. The physical appearance may vary from barely detectable to grotesquely deforming. Although there may be some physiologic benefit from surgical correction of these deformities, restoration of a more normal appearance is equally important in the decision to operate. The impact of these deformities on normal psychosocial development, as well as the less certain evidence of cardiorespiratory impairment, constitutes adequate justification in the affected child.

Embryology, Development, and Etiology of Chest Wall Deformities

In the embryo, the ribs are derived from individual somites as mesoderm differentiates into cartilage and advances ventrally toward the developing sternum. The rib cartilage eventually approaches the sternum. The sternum itself is derived independently from two parallel bands of mesoderm that develop away from the midline. The two sternal bands fuse in a cranial to caudal direction and become progressively chondrified. Transverse divisions of the cartilaginous sternum differentiate into segments opposite each end of the rib pairs. At birth, small ossification centers are present in the sternum and the ribs have largely ossified. Final ossification is usually complete by mid adolescence. The process is sufficiently predictable that sternal ossification is a reliable method of determining bone age. There is a sharp demarcation in each rib between the ossified portion and the cartilaginous portion, with the latter becoming ossified only much later in life. The etiology of chest wall deformities is poorly understood.[1] Explanations include abnormal intrauterine pressure applied to the chest, abnormalities of diaphragmatic development, connective tissue abnormalities, and genetic predisposition. Abnormal, excessive, or asymmetric growth of the costal cartilages associated with the 3rd to 10th ribs is most implicated. Sternal clefts are understood as a failure of fusion of some portion of the sternal bands.

Pectus Excavatum

Pectus excavatum, from the Latin phrase "hollowed chest," is
1 the most common deformity of the anterior chest wall. Pectus excavatum results from abnormal regulation of the growth of the costal cartilages. There is a corresponding posterior curve in the body of the sternum beginning at the manubrium and extending to the xiphoid. The deformity is rarely precisely symmetric, with one side (usually the right) slightly more curved in than the other. Asymmetry may be pronounced with the sternum rotated nearly to the sagittal plane. The deformity may be apparent at birth but may become more apparent during growth and development, particularly during adolescence. Pectus excavatum occurs more frequently in males than females. Another affected relative, most often a father or uncle, is found in one third of cases. Scoliosis is present at increased incidence in this population although rarely requires surgical correction. Patients often have an asthenic build and stoop-shouldered posture. Marfan syndrome predisposes to pectus excavatum. The diagnosis of Marfan syndrome should be considered when patients are referred for evaluation of a chest wall deformity.

At the time of surgical consultation, concerns about the cardiopulmonary implications of the chest wall deformity are often paramount in the mind of the referring physician as well as the family. Many patients will have complaints of chest pain and/or shortness of breath. Most patients are disturbed by the appearance of the deformity, and some may be profoundly depressed and dysfunctional. The physiologic consequences of the deformity are less certain. Invasive and echocardiographic assessment of cardiovascular performance have demonstrated improvement in cardiac function and resolution of mitral valve prolapse in some patients following surgical correction of pectus excavatum.[2–6] There is no consensus on the exact nature of the cardiopulmonary impairment or on the pulmonary benefit of surgical correction. Although more difficult to measure, the psychological benefit of correcting this severe chest wall anatomic defect has demonstrated excellent results and patient satisfaction.

Clinically, pectus excavatum patients typically complain of chest discomfort and shortness of breath. Dynamic testing can be used to further explore a patient's complaints, but this methodology is not always routinely utilized. Clinical assessment of the severity of the deformity has included chest radiographs, computerized tomography (CT), caliper measurements, and contrast volume measurements of the cavity. The "pectus index" is defined as the ratio of the maximum internal transverse diameter of the thorax to the minimum sternovertebral distance.[7] If cardiac disease is suspected on the basis of the history and physical examination, an echocardiogram may be indicated. Pulmonary function testing is rarely helpful.

Surgical Correction of the Pectus Excavatum. The ossification of key components of the anterior chest wall is not completed until the teenage years. The further understanding of this physiology has led to a more uniform timing of surgical correction for pectus excavatum in the past decade. Infants and young children should not undergo surgical correction
2 because of the risk of acquired thoracic dystrophy.[8,9] Most pediatric surgeons agree that the optimal timing is in late childhood and adolescence.

Traditional Operations. Traditional surgical correction[3,10] is performed through a transverse incision centered on the defect in the line of the inframammary crease (Fig. 106.1). The necessary incision is quite small and may be kept well within the nipple lines. An alternative that may be useful, especially in older females, uses a small incision in each inframammary crease. The operation requires exposure of the costal cartilages by incision into or elevation of the pectoral muscles from the chest wall. Subperiochondrial excision is made to the involved costal cartilages. The 3rd through 7th cartilages are excised

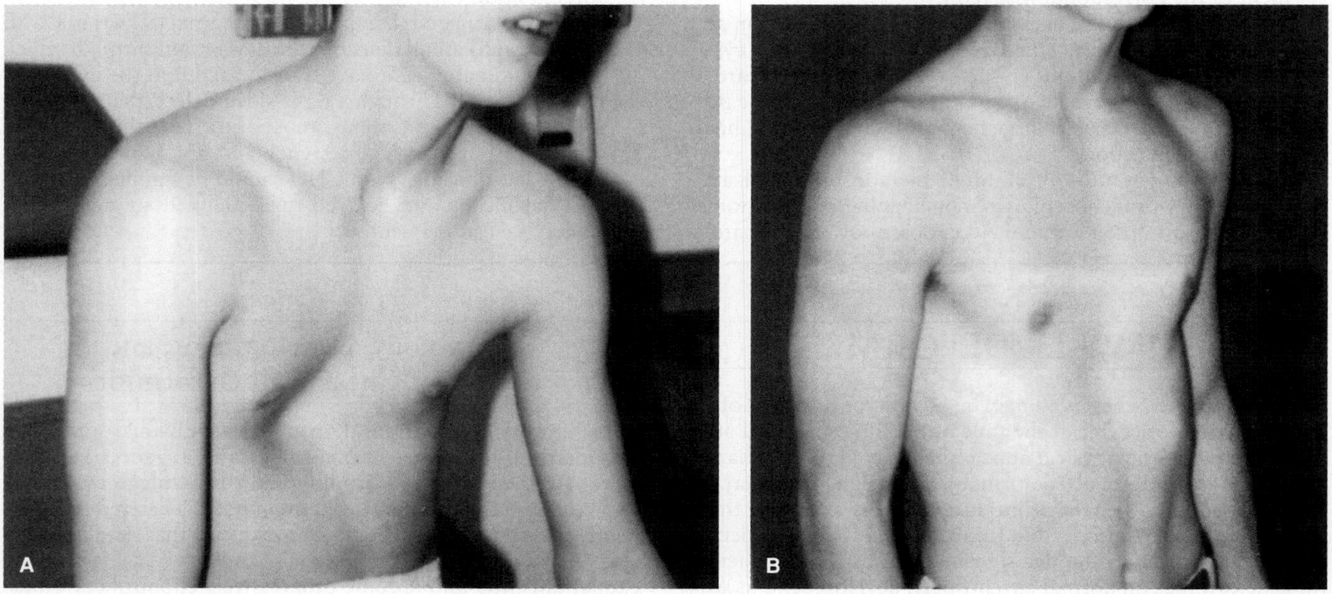

FIGURE 106.1. Pectus excavatum. **A:** Appearance of an adolescent male with a typical depression deformity. Note "stoop-shouldered" posture. **B:** Postoperative appearance at 6 months. Erect posture and subpectoral incision give a good cosmetic result.

along with portions of the 8th, 9th, or 10th cartilages if there is particularly prominent flaring of the costal margin. The xiphoid is detached from the sternum, and the rectus muscles are detached inferiorly. The undersurface of the sternum is dissected free from the pericardium and pleura. An anterior osteotomy is created in the sternum at the point where the sternum deflects posteriorly and the posterior cortex is fractured. Closure of the osteotomy elevates the lower sternum. Asymmetric deformities may require insinuation of the osteotome into the sternotomy site on the right and left, which allows rotation of the inferior aspect of the sternum. Some degree of overcorrection is usually performed to help maintain the correction over time. A strut is usually placed beneath or through the sternum to maintain the corrected sternal position. The choice of material and configuration for the strut is variable. Struts may be left in permanently but are usually removed after an interval of 2 to 12 months. The pectoral and rectus muscles are reapproximated. Closed suction drains are used to drain the substernal, submuscular, and/or subcutaneous spaces. Patients are discharged when they are able to tolerate a diet and their pain is controlled by oral analgesics. Drains are removed either as an inpatient or an outpatient. In current practice, patients are often discharged on the second postoperative day. Multimodal pain management including regional anesthesia, postoperative epidural analgesia, nonsteroidal anti-inflammatory agents, and narcotics are used. Complications are generally limited to wound infections and pneumothorax that rarely requires tube drainage. Recurrence rates in large series with long-term follow-up range from 5% to 15%.[3] The incidence of reactive pectus carinatum after excavatum repair is 1%.[11] Migration of implanted struts and bars has caused the most serious problems, including cardiac injury.

The Lorenz Bar/Nuss Procedure. The Lorenz bar/Nuss procedure has gained widespread popularity. A rigid U-shaped bar inserted transversely across the chest pushes the deformity back into place[12] (Fig. 106.2). The procedure is best performed in late childhood and early adolescence, when there is more pliability of the costal cartilages. Long-term follow-up data is encouraging.[13] Complications have been reported as the procedure has become more widely practiced, including pneumothorax, cardiac injury, bar displacement, chronic pain, pericarditis, and extraosseous bone formation.[14] The bar is left in for up to 3 years during a period of development when most children are active and may engage in contact sports. Activity restrictions that are necessary while the bar is in place are not well defined. This technique is an important addition to the surgical treatment of chest wall deformities. Recent techniques utilizing thorascopic windows have been developed to hopefully reduce more life-threatening complications such as cardiac injury.[15] Other modifications include dual bar placement, bending the bar in a skewed fashion to correct an angled sternum, and bar placement to correct recurrent pectus excavatum development after an open surgical approach.[16]

Other Techniques. Implantation of submuscular silastic molds to alter the chest contour may result in a very acceptable appearance.[17,18] This technique does not address any of the potential physiologic problems associated with pectus excavatum and has not been used widely.

Externally applied suction may also be used to treat depression deformities of the chest wall.[19] Finally, implanted devices that use magnetic forces to pull the sternum forward show promise in correcting the defect in patients with pectus excavatum.[20]

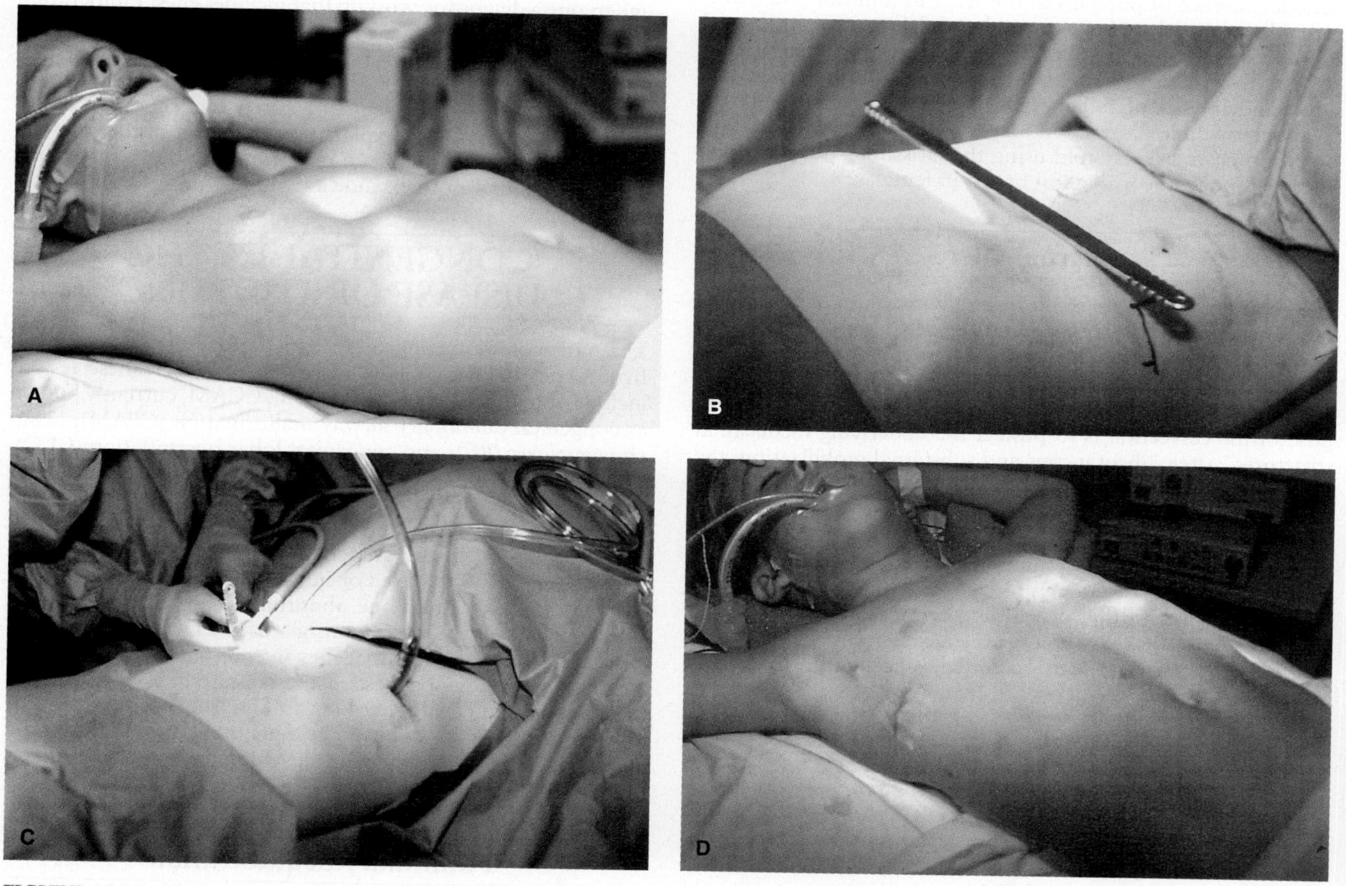

FIGURE 106.2. Thoracoscopically assisted Lorenz Bar insertion (Nuss procedure). **A:** Preoperative appearance with symmetrical depression deformity. **B:** Lorenz bar. **C:** Lorenz bar inserted with thoracoscopic guidance. **D:** Immediate postoperative appearance. (Digital images provided by William Hardin, M.D., University of Alabama, used with permission.)

Pectus Carinatum

Pectus carinatum, from the Latin phrase for "keel," is a chest wall defect where there is a protrusion of the sternum and ribs.
3 This type of defect occurs less commonly than pectus excavatum and presents in approximately 1 in 1,000 teenagers. Physiologic impairment is absent; however, the concern for appearance may be even greater than with depression deformities of the chest wall. Protrusion deformities may be very difficult to hide even when fully clothed. Rapid growth of the costal cartilages occurring during puberty makes the deformity more pronounced at that time. The operative correction of a pectus carinatum deformity is similar to that described for pectus excavatum. An osteotomy and sternal fracture are often not required, but when necessary they are performed in such a way as to depress the sternum. A strut is usually not required to maintain sternal position. The postoperative course and results are similar to pectus excavatum. In the immediate postoperative period, cardiac pulsation may be particularly visible; however, with healing this finding disappears. External compression devices have shown some efficacy in larger trials with a minimal complication rate.[21] Success depends on prolonged application of the compression device. The Nuss bar has also been applied to force the sternum in a corrective posterior direction.[22]

Poland Syndrome

Named after the English surgeon Sir Alfred Poland, this rare congenital syndrome occurs in from 1 in 10,000 to 1 in 100,000 births and includes a range of skeletal and muscle defects. These features include absence of the sternal portions of the pectoralis major muscle; absence of the pectoralis minor muscle; absence of portions of the serratus anterior and external oblique muscles; forearm and hand deformities; ipsilateral hypoplasia of the nipple, breast, and chest wall subcutaneous tissues; absence or deformity of the second to fifth costal cartilages; and absence of axillary hair on the affected side. Surgical treatment includes correction of any deformed ribs, formation of the anterior axillary fold using the latissimus dorsi muscle, and creation of the ipsilateral breast in females.[23]

Sternal Clefts

Congenital sternal clefts result from failure of midline fusion of the paired sternal bands. The cleft is usually in the superior portion of the sternum and may extend to but not include the xiphoid. The defects are rare and are usually repaired in the neonatal period when the chest is more pliable.[24] The purpose of the correction is to protect the underlying mediastinal structures. After subcutaneous and substernal mobilization, the fibrocartilaginous sternal bars are approximated in the midline. Typically, the cleft is incomplete and a V-shaped excision of the sternum at the most inferior aspect of the cleft may be required to avoid buckling of the sternum in that region.[24] Cantrell pentology refers to a distal sternal cleft, omphalocele, diaphragmatic defect, pericardial defect, and intracardiac defect. Thoracic ectopia cordis (exstrophy of the heart) may occur as a part of this abnormality and until recently has been uniformly fatal.

Jeune Asphyxiating Thoracic Dystrophy

Jeune asphyxiating thoracic dystrophy is a rare developmental abnormality that results in the failure of chest wall growth. Surgical correction involves the expansion of the thoracic cavity by rib resection and frame shifting of the ribs. Most recently, the use of a vertical expandable prosthetic titanium rib (VEPTR) device allows division of the most posterior aspect of approximately the third to ninth ribs and division at the costochondral junction of the same ribs. The rib plate is then elevated to the curved VEPTR strut by wires, thus expanding the chest. This is done for both chests, and the device is serially expanded every 4 to 6 months to promote chest enlargement.[25]

The "Slipping Rib" Syndrome

The slipping rib syndrome is an unusual abnormality that has been ascribed to abnormal development of the costal cartilages along the costal margin such that the 9th or 10th rib is free floating. Positive findings on examination include a click with anterior displacement of the rib by either gently pulling on the inferior costal margin or by pushing on the suspected rib in a lateral direction at the midaxillary line. Patients typically complain of either sharp thoracic or abdominal pain and typically have had a thorough imaging workup that is nonrevealing. Surgical therapy involves excising the involved rib and cartilage, thereby relieving pressure on the involved intercostal nerve.

"Flaring" of the Costal Margin

Patients are sometimes referred for surgical opinions regarding unusual prominence of the costal margin. The "flaring" is most pronounced when the patient is supine. This finding represents a variation of the normal development of the chest wall. Surgical correction should be avoided.

Costochondral "Tumor"

Prominence of a single costal cartilage may present as a concern of a tumor of cartilage or bone. This abnormality is usually found in preadolescents and adolescents. Patients may have undergone a diagnostic workup that includes chest radiographs, ultrasound, CT, or magnetic resonance imaging (MRI) prior to surgical consultation. This abnormality most likely represents a minor variation of a chest wall deformity, such as a pectus carinatum. The area of enlargement is rarely tender so that costochondritis is an unlikely explanation. Excision of the involved cartilage is rarely helpful. Plain radiographs or thoracic imaging are usually sufficient to exclude a tumor.

CONGENITAL CYSTIC DISEASE OF THE LUNG

The most common congenital cystic lesions of the lung result from abnormalities of lung embryogenesis.[26,27] These lesions include pulmonary sequestration (PS); CCAM, currently known as congenital pulmonary airway malformation (CPAM); bronchogenic cyst (BC); and congenital lobar overinflation (CLO). The first three (PS, CPAM, and BC) are part of the spectrum of bronchopulmonary foregut malformations. The abnormality may be primarily characterized by aberrant blood supply (PS), hamartomatous lung parenchyma (CPAM), or an isolated epithelial cyst (BC). Mixed or intermediate forms that contain elements of more than one abnormality are common.[28] The coexistence of these malformations with CDH and congenital heart defects emphasizes that they may be part of a generalized problem with organogenesis. CLO is more likely a secondary response of the developing lung to abnormal compression or obstruction of a bronchus. The retention of fetal lung fluid during critical phases of lung development adversely affects the development of the lung.

Pulmonary Sequestration

4 PS are divided into intralobar or extralobar lesions based on their relationship with the investing visceral pleura and adjacent normal lung tissue. Structurally, sequestrations represent

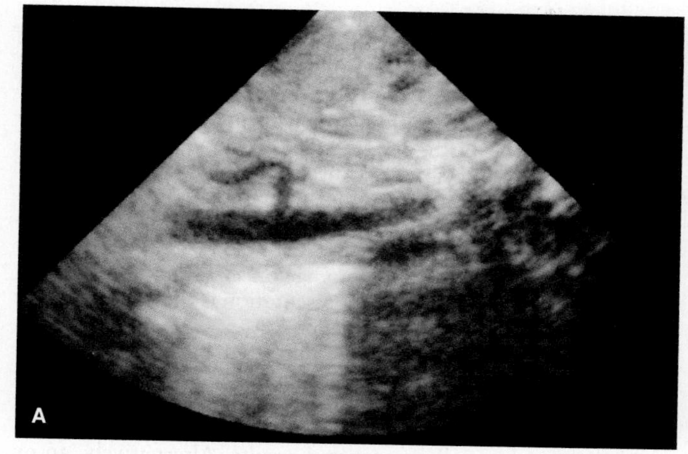

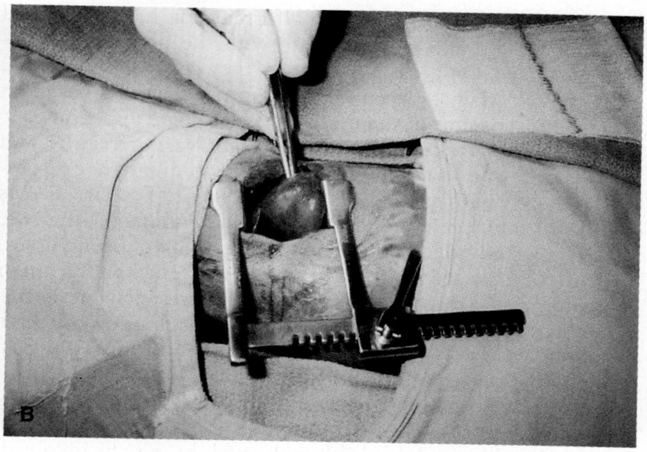

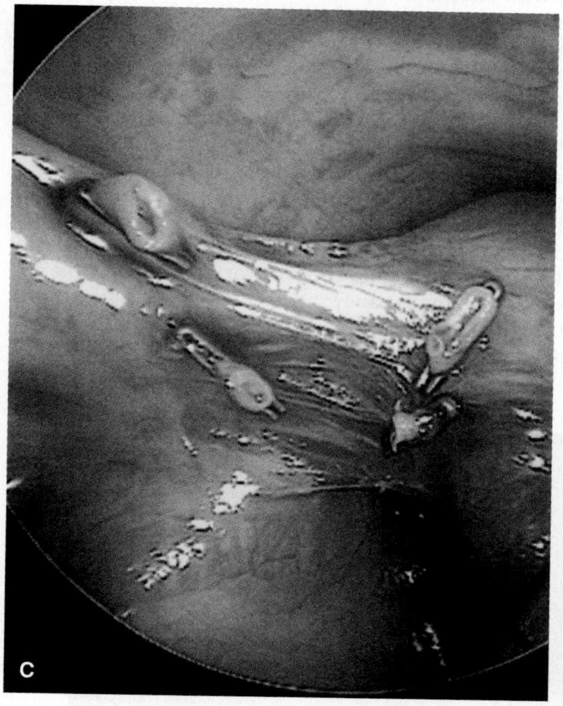

FIGURE 106.3. Pulmonary sequestration (PS). **A:** Sagittal ultrasound view of the aortic branch supplying an extralobar PS. **B:** Left-sided extralobar PS excised via a muscle-sparing thoracotomy. **C:** Intraoperative view of extralobar sequestration removed thoracoscopically. Note the main blood supply with clips.

abnormal lung tissue with anomalous systemic blood supply. They do not communicate normally with the trachea or a bronchus. They are found most commonly in the lower lobes, predominantly on the left.

Intralobar sequestrations lie within a lobe of the lung and are invested by its visceral pleura. They are most common in the posterior segment of the left lower lobe but can occur elsewhere. The anomalous arterial blood supply comes from either the thoracic or abdominal aorta and may traverse the diaphragm to supply the sequestration. Venous drainage from this aberrant tissue may be either pulmonary or systemic but is usually into the pulmonary vein. Aberrant air space connections with adjacent normal lung tissue may permit air trapping within the sequestration, causing it be to aerated on radiographs. Although most often asymptomatic at birth, intralobar PS may present during childhood as recurrent localized pneumonia due to these aberrant air space connections.

Extralobar sequestrations occur outside the pleura of the normal lung. They are most common in the lower left side of the chest but have been reported in various locations, including in the retroperitoneum below the diaphragm.[29] In this location, they may be difficult to distinguish from an intra-abdominal tumor such as neuroblastoma. Rarely, extralobar sequestration is associated with CDH. In extralobar sequestration, both the arterial and venous blood supplies are usually systemic, and the arterial blood supply frequently arises from the aorta below the diaphragm. The lesion itself is usually a spongy consolidated mass with no aeration, which can resemble a congenital pulmonary hemangioma.[30] Although infection is rarely present, these lesions can be associated with hemorrhage, arteriovenous shunting, or mediastinal compression. Occasionally, the amount of blood shunted through the lesion is sufficient to result in symptomatic congestive heart failure. Pulmonary malignancies have occurred within these lesions. CPAMs may occur in sequestrations; in fact, sequestrations and CPAMs may be mixed.[28]

Radiographic evaluation of these lesions involves plain films of the chest and CT scans with care taken to identify a systemic arterial blood supply. Intralobar sequestrations are usually treated with thoracotomy and lobectomy (Fig. 106.3A,B). Sequestrations may be removed with minimally invasive surgical techniques[31] (Fig. 106.3C). In dealing with both lesions, particular attention must be paid to safe ligation of the vascular supply.

Congenital Pulmonary Airway Malformations

5 CCAMs or CPAMs result from excessive proliferation of bronchial structures without the development of the

corresponding alveoli. These malformations have a normal vascular supply and communicate with the normal tracheobronchial tree. On gross appearance, they can be solid, cystic, or both. CPAMs have been classified into three types based on size, shape, spacing of the cysts, and histologic appearance.[32] Type I CPAMs are composed of cysts with large irregular and widely dispersed spaces larger than 2 cm in diameter or a single large cyst with small cysts surrounding it. Type II CPAMs consist of multiple cysts less than 1 cm in diameter that are closely packed together and resemble dilated bronchioles. Type III CPAMs are made up of small cysts less than 0.5 cm in diameter, and the parenchymal tissue represents late gestational age fetal lung. Cartilage is usually lacking in all three types of CPAMs. Type I cysts account for almost 50% of cases, while type II cysts make up an additional 40%. CPAMs usually affect only one lobe, but multilobar and bilateral involvement also occurs. The most common lobes affected are the left-sided and lower lobes, although any lobe may be involved. On a molecular level, there have been evidence of at least three genes involved in the development of CCAMs: HOXB5, Fgf7, and platelet-derived growth factor-B (PDGF-B).[33]

Prenatal diagnosis is common. In fact, with the advent of prenatal diagnosis, the number of CPAM resections has tripled and the number of asymptomatic CPAMs increased 20% based on the National Inpatient Sample Database (O. S. Soldes, pers. comm.). If the CPAM has sufficient pathophysiologic effects, the fetus may develop life-threatening hydrops. Open fetal surgical resection and thoracoamniotic shunting has resulted in survival of some of these severely affected fetuses.[34] As a result of serial prenatal ultrasounds, spontaneous in utero resolution has been observed to occur in as many as one third of these infants.[35] Even cystic lesions that are large enough to cause mass effect on nearby structures may spontaneously regress and not require fetal lobectomy or thoracoamniotic shunting.[36]

The incidence of CPAM is thought to occur in 1 in 25,000 to 1 in 35,000 live births, and approximately 14% of all CPAM patients are stillborn. Although newborns with CPAM can be asymptomatic at birth, nearly 80% of CPAM patients present with some type of respiratory distress in the neonatal period.[33] The usual radiologic appearance after birth is that of a solid mass because of retained fetal lung fluid (Fig. 106.4A). As ventilation occurs and fluid is reabsorbed, the mass appears larger and cystic and may begin to impinge on surrounding structures (Fig. 106.4B). A less common presentation is the appearance of recurrent pneumonia later in life.

Infants with symptomatic lesions after birth require resection of the involved lobe. Those with severe physiologic affects may require extracorporeal support with resection of the involved lung on extracorporeal membrane oxygenation (ECMO) with excellent expected results. Alternatively, an ex utero intrapartum treatment (EXIT)-to-ECMO approach may be used when gas exchange is predicted to be compromised.[37] Asymptomatic lesions can be followed closely to allow for growth and development. In cases where there is no CPAM evident on plain radiograph, a CT scan of the chest should be obtained after birth to document residual parenchymal abnormalities and to look for systemic arterial blood supply.

Operation is clearly recommended if symptoms occur. Although recommendations among pediatric surgeons differ, most recommend elective resection in the setting of asymptomatic CPAM because of the concern for future infection and the possibility of malignancy[38,39] (see below). Studies have demonstrated that CPAMs evident in the postnatal period rarely spontaneously resolve.[40] A CT scan prior to operation

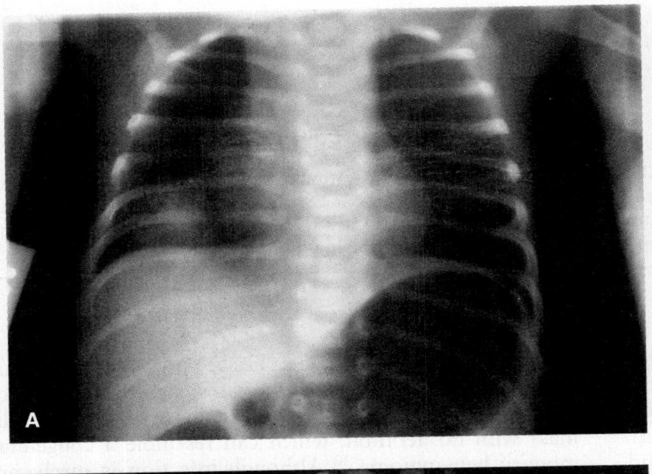

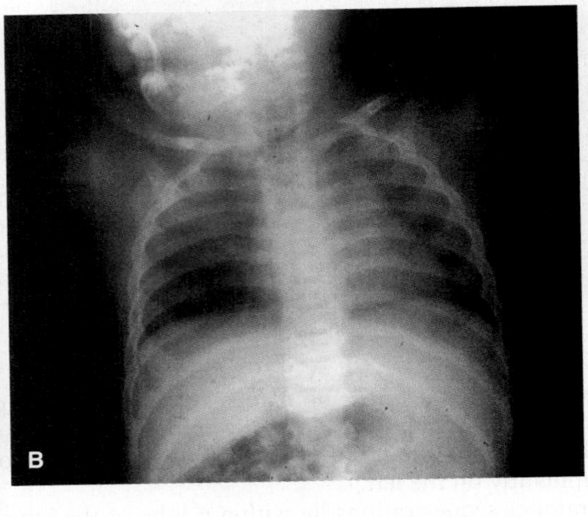

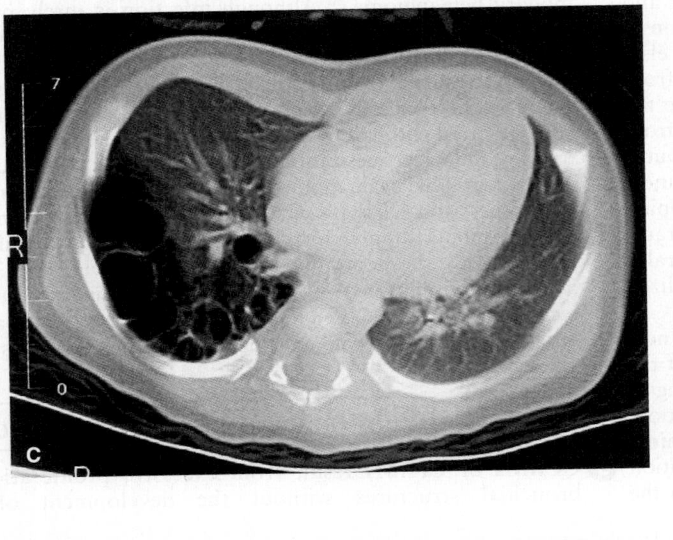

FIGURE 106.4. Congenital cystic adenomatoid malformation (CCAM). **A:** Newborn chest x-ray of a patient with prenatal diagnosis of CCAM. Note that immediately after birth, the mass is fluid-filled and appears as a density in the right hemithorax. **B:** Chest x-ray of the same child at 5 months of age prior to surgical excision. Note the air-filled cystic appearance of CCAM. **C:** Transverse thoracic computerized tomographic view of CCAM.

confirms the diagnosis and assists in surgical planning in infants with asymptomatic lesions (Fig. 106.4C). Elective resection is then performed at 2 to 12 months of age and can usually be accomplished by a minimally invasive approach. Proponents of early intervention point to data demonstrating inflammation in most CPAM specimens, which makes resection more difficult.[41] When bilateral and/or multilobar involvement is found, CT scans may assist in planning lung-conserving resections and in follow-up of residual disease. Lung-preserving resections should be used for CPAMs that involve multiple lung lobes.[42]

Bronchogenic Cysts

BCs represent groups of epithelial cells from the developing trachea and lung that have become separated from the tracheobronchial tree. These cysts exist as discrete masses, usually in the paratracheal region, and do not incorporate pulmonary mesenchyme on which further lung development is dependent. If cells separate from the bronchopulmonary foregut structures early in development, these cysts tend to originate from the esophageal portion of the foregut. Separation that occurs later in development is from the ventral or tracheal portion of the foregut, resulting in BCs. BCs are usually extrapulmonary masses that do not communicate with the normal tracheobronchial tree. They do not have a unique blood supply. Resection of these lesions with either a thoracotomy or video-assisted thoracoscopy is recommended because of the risk of bleeding, infection, or enlargement with compression of adjacent mediastinal structures[43,44] (Fig. 106.5).

Congenital Lobar Overinflation

CLO (previously referred to as congenital lobar emphysema) is caused by abnormal development or compression of a lobar bronchus, resulting in retention of fluid during fetal lung development and subsequent air trapping and overinflation after birth. The lung tissue is intrinsically normal but has been secondarily altered due to the trapping of fluid and gas. The

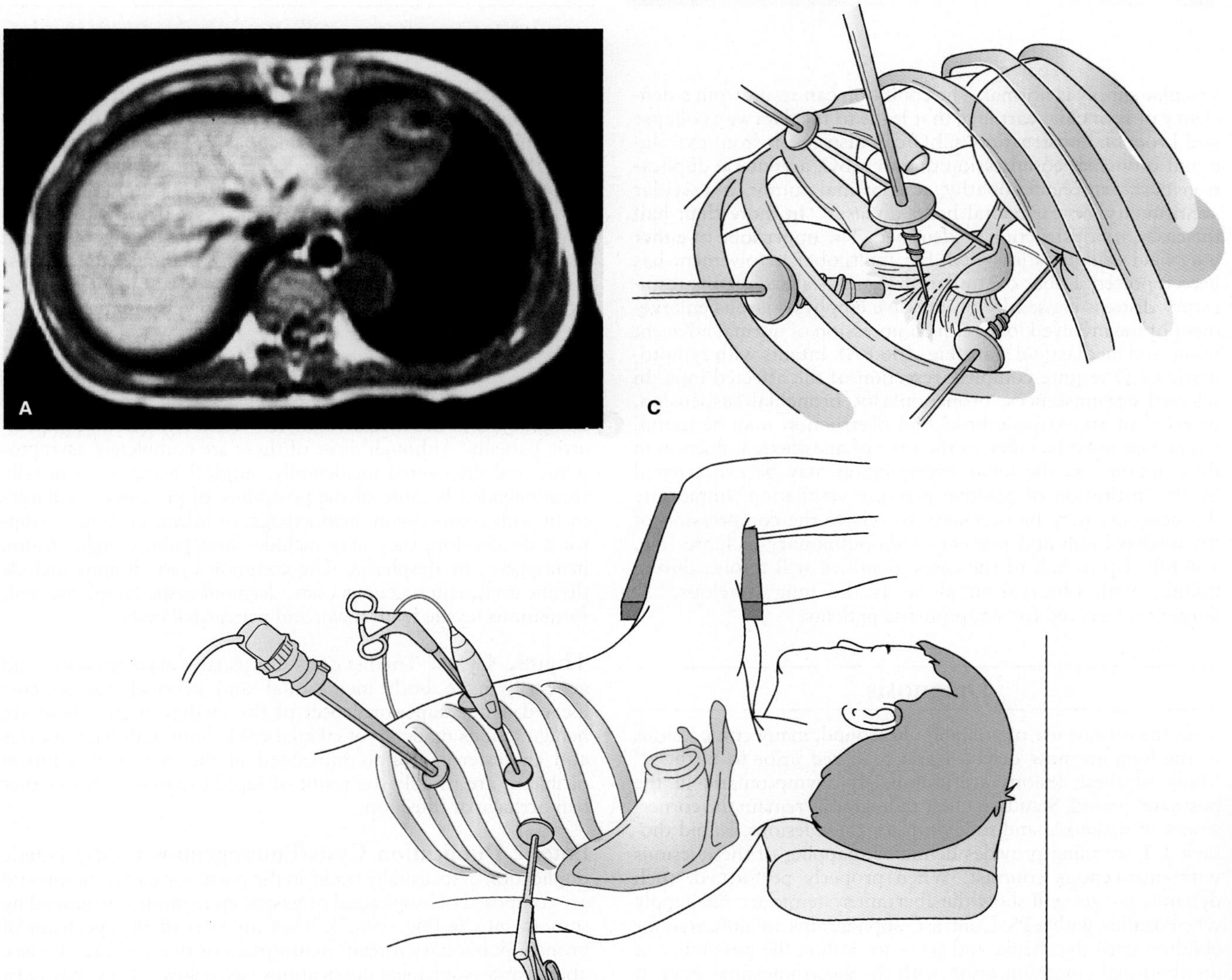

FIGURE 106.5. Bronchogenic cyst (BC). **A:** Transverse thoracic computerized tomographic view of a BC located in the inferior pulmonary ligament. **B:** Illustrative representation of thoracoscopic instrumentation for excision of a BC. **C:** Operative detail. (Adapted from Dillon PW, Cilley RE, Krummel TM. Video-assisted thoracoscopic excision of intrathoracic masses in children: report of two cases. *Surg Laparosc Endosc* 1993;3:433–436.)

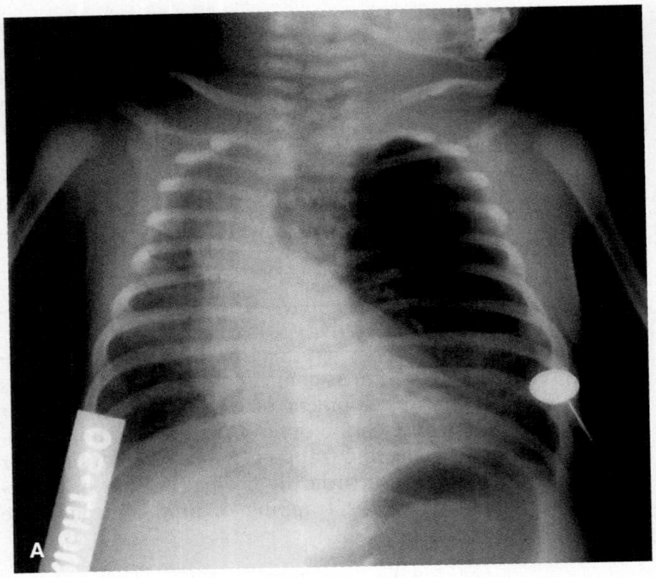

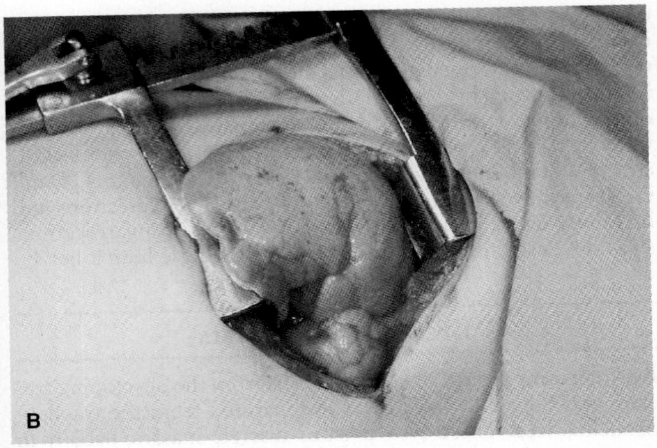

FIGURE 106.6. Congenital lobar overinflation. **A:** Chest radiograph demonstrating overinflation of the left upper lobe in an infant. Note the mediastinal shift. **B:** Operative photograph demonstrating an overexpanded left upper lobe decompressing through the incision.

vascular supply is normal. The condition can result from a deficiency of bronchial cartilage that leads to focal airway collapse and bronchial obstruction. CLO can also result from extraluminal bronchial compression due to a BC, an enteric duplication cyst, lymphadenopathy, mediastinal tumor, a vascular abnormality, or congenital heart disease.[45] In more than half the cases, no obstruction is identified. The upper lobe of either lung field usually is involved, but multilobar involvement has been reported. Lobar overinflation presents as worsening respiratory distress caused by progressive emphysematous enlargement of the involved lobe with compression of normal adjacent tissue and mediastinal shift (Fig. 106.6A). Infants with symptomatic CLO require complete resection of the affected lobe. In selected circumstances, bronchoplasty, bronchial suspension, or relief of an extrinsic bronchial obstruction may be useful. Great care must be taken at the time of anesthetic induction in these infants, as the lobar overinflation may be exacerbated by the institution of positive pressure ventilation. Immediate thoracotomy may be necessary to relieve the compression of the mediastinum and prevent cardiopulmonary collapse (Fig. 106.6B). Up to half of the cases identified will resolve during infancy with observation alone as the lung develops.[46–48] Surgery is reserved for symptomatic patients.

Diagnosis

With the routine use of prenatal ultrasound, many cystic lesions of the lung are now detected and followed prior to birth.[35,49] Many of these lesions are completely asymptomatic in the postnatal period. Standard chest radiographs remain the cornerstones of diagnosis and follow-up for these lesions. Rapid thoracic CT scanning provides definitive mapping of these lesions with intravenous contrast. When properly performed, such dynamic images will show the aberrant systemic arterial supply when dealing with a PS. Contrast esophagrams are indicated for children with dysphagia and serve to outline the possibility of an abnormal communication with the gastrointestinal tract. If aberrant vascular supply is suspected but not demonstrated on a CT scan, then MRI angiography of the chest can be obtained.

Treatment

Asymptomatic pulmonary cysts should be removed because of the possibility of infection as well as the rare association of malignant pulmonary neoplasms in these congenital cysts, including myxosarcoma, embryonal rhabdomyosarcoma, pleuropulmonary blastoma, and bronchoalveolar carcinoma.[33] Any cyst that is enlarging on serial chest radiographs should be resected because of the respiratory compromise that may ensue and the possibility of infection either in the cyst or in the surrounding lung tissue. The only reason for following a lesion in the long term would be if serial CT scans demonstrate progressive resolution, indicating the possibility of an acquired infectious pulmonary cyst, most of which resolve spontaneously.

Cysts of the Mediastinum

6 Benign cysts of the mediastinum are relatively common in pediatric patients. Although most of these are completely asymptomatic and discovered incidentally, surgical resection is usually recommended because of the possibility of progressive enlargement with compression, hemorrhage, or infection. When symptoms do develop, they may include chest pain, cough, stridor, hemoptysis, or dysphasia. The common cystic lesions include thymic cysts, enterogenous cysts, dermoid cysts, lymphatic malformations (cystic hygromas), and pericardial cysts.

Thymic Cysts. Thymic cysts are usually asymptomatic and generally have both mediastinal and cervical components located in the superior aspect of the mediastinum. These are benign lesions made up of ciliated epithelium with lymphocytes and cholesterol crystals imbedded in the cyst wall. Clinical problems are usually the result of rapid expansion from either hemorrhage or infection.

Enteric Duplication Cysts/Enterogenous Cysts. Enteric duplication cysts usually occur in the posterior mediastinum and are composed of esophageal or gastric epithelium surrounded by smooth muscle (Fig. 106.7). They are part of the spectrum of bronchopulmonary foregut malformations that include BCs (see above) and esophageal duplications (see below). They may exist completely separate from the structure of origin or may communicate with the gastrointestinal tract above or below the diaphragm. In rare instances, they may attach to or communicate with the spinal canal. A number of large thoracoabdominal enteric cysts have been reported. These cysts may penetrate the diaphragm and end blindly in the peritoneal cavity or communicate with the gastrointestinal tract. If gastric mucosa is present within the cyst, peptic ulceration with erosion and bleeding has

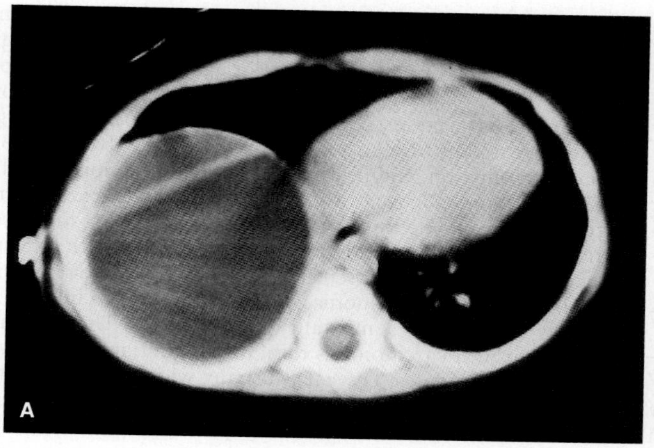

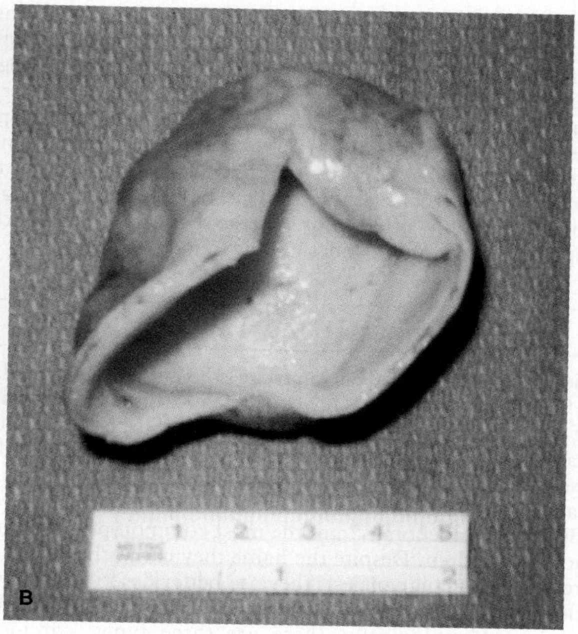

FIGURE 106.7. Enterogenous cyst. This represents another abnormality in the spectrum of bronchopulmonary foregut malformations. **A:** Computerized tomography demonstrating a large mass occupying the right hemithorax. **B:** Surgical specimen.

been reported. Therefore, removal of these cysts is recommended to avoid these possible complications.

Lymphatic Malformations. Lymphatic malformations in the head, neck, and mediastinal region have been classically referred to as cystic hygromas. They are multilocular, thin-walled cysts derived from primitive, aberrant lymphatic sacs. Their mediastinal involvement can be quite extensive, as they insinuate around the great vessels and nervous structures of the superior mediastinum. As with other cystic structures, these lesions are usually asymptomatic. However, with enlargement (most frequently due to hemorrhage) or infection, symptoms may develop with life-threatening potential. Surgical resection of these lesions is usually recommended without sacrificing important anatomic structures within the mediastinum. Most of the intrathoracic components can be resected via a cervical approach. Recurrence develops in approximately one third of cases. Recently, clinical series of successful sclerotherapy of cystic hygromas with large cysts have been reported and may be an effective approach to such lesions.[50]

Pericardial Cysts. Pericardial cysts are almost always asymptomatic lesions discovered as incidental findings on chest radiographs. They appear in the cardiophrenic sulcus as small discrete masses. They are thin-walled cysts containing clear fluid and lined by mesothelium. Resection can be performed with either an open thoracotomy or video-assisted thoracoscopy.

THORACIC TUMORS IN CHILDREN

Thoracic tumors in children are rare. Neoplasms originate from the chest wall, the mediastinum, and the lung. Lung metastases from extrathoracic cancers are more common than primary neoplasms. Surgical treatment may involve removal of the primary tumor, resection of adjacent structures, chest wall reconstruction, lung resection (including wedge resection, lobectomy, pneumonectomy), and tracheobronchial resection and reconstruction. The role of minimally invasive surgery/thoracoscopic surgery is increasing in both the diagnosis and treatment of thoracic tumors in children.[51]

Metastatic Lung Tumors

In order for surgical excision of metastatic lung tumors to be beneficial, the primary tumor must be eradicated and the patient should be free of other metastatic disease. Osteogenic sarcoma, other soft tissue sarcomas, and Wilms tumor are the tumors with lung metastases that are most often considered for surgical treatment.[52,53]

Osteogenic Sarcoma. Although the reported experience in the treatment of metastatic osteogenic sarcoma to the lung is based on retrospective review, there is good evidence that resection of lung metastases is beneficial. The success of surgical removal of metastatic lung disease depends upon effective chemotherapy to eliminate other micrometastatic disease. The metastases are calcified and palpable, which facilitates their surgical removal. Fewer than four nodules, complete resection of all disease, and lack of penetration through the parietal pleura favor survival. Treatment failures and late recurrence are common, mandating careful follow-up. Available data support aggressive attempts at surgical resection, including the removal of many metastatic nodules and multiple resections. A thoracoscopic approach has been felt to be inappropriate by some because of the inability to palpate small lesions.[54] Prophylactic exploration of both lungs via thoracotomy has also been suggested in order to eradicate small lesions that may not be appreciated on CT.

Soft Tissue Sarcoma. Chemotherapy and radiation-resistant tumors (liposarcoma, leiomyosarcoma, synovial sarcoma, fibrosarcoma, neurogenic sarcoma, epithelioid sarcoma, alveolar soft parts sarcoma) may benefit from resection when the primary tumor has been controlled.[53] Rhabdomyosarcoma and Ewing sarcoma are chemo- and radiation sensitive. Lung excision for metastatic disease is generally not helpful, although chest wall resection for a Ewing sarcoma chest wall primary is critical to disease cure. For sarcomas in general, surgery for lung metastases may aid in diagnosis and may be beneficial in removing a large focus of residual disease.

Wilms Tumor. There is little advantage to excision of lung metastases in Wilms tumor. Chemotherapy is required for treatment, and surgical removal offers no added benefit. The role of whole lung radiation (previously used for lung metastases) will be evaluated in the next phase of the National Wilms Tumor Study under the auspices of the Children's Oncology Group. There are special cases that may benefit from surgery, including very young patients (in whom radiation therapy causes the most lung injury) with few or solitary lesions. Surgery may also be necessary for diagnostic purposes and to determine the effects of therapy. This tissue histiopathologic diagnosis arguably offers more therapy direction than radiographic evidence of indistinct lesions found on CT scans.[55]

Primary Lung Tumors

Reviews by Hartman and Shochat[56] in 1983 and Hancock et al.[57] in 1993 have catalogued fewer than 500 reported primary
7 lung neoplasms in children (Table 106.1). Surgical resection remains the mainstay therapy for these primary lesions, and a consensus is developing that surgery may also play a role in metastatic lesions.[58]

Bronchial "adenomas" are the most common primary lung tumors in children. Despite the name they carry, these tumors represent true malignancies. They are better described as low-grade adenocarcinomas of the lung. The incidence of metastasis is low. Histologically, there are three types: carcinoid (85%), mucoepidermoid (10%), and adenoid cystic carcinoma (5%). Bronchial adenomas most commonly arise in primary and secondary brochi. Presenting symptoms include cough, hemoptysis, airway obstruction, pneumonia, atelectasis, and reactive airway disease. The chest radiographs may show air trapping or pneumonia and atelectasis. The clinical presentation may be most suspicious for an airway foreign body. CT may demonstrate the lesion. Bronchoscopy is required for diagnosis. Biopsy must be done with great care and with some peril since life-threatening bleeding may result from biopsy attempts. Surgical resection with clean intraoperative margins is the treatment of choice. Resection may involve lobectomy, bi-lobectomy, pneumonectomy, or sleeve resection as well as regional lymphadenectomy with intraoperative frozen section to assure complete tumor resection while limiting lung resection. Bronchial carcinoids are rarely associated with carcinoid syndrome and are radiosensitive if residual disease remains.

Bronchogenic carcinomas are uncommon in children and highly lethal with a mortality rate of 90%. Unlike adults, squamous cell carcinoma is rare; undifferentiated adenocarcinoma predominates. Disease is usually widespread at the time of diagnosis, compromising survival. Rarely, with early discovery and localized disease, cure is possible. Bronchioalveolar carcinoma is a rare lung tumor in children that carries a good prognosis with surgical resection.[59] This tumor is particularly observed in CPAM lung lesions.[60]

Pulmonary blastoma is a malignant lung tumor occurring most often in children under 4 years of age. It is composed of cells that histologically resemble fetal lung. This tumor usually is located peripherally in the lung and presents with cough, chest pain, and hemoptysis. Pulmonary blastoma is treated by lobectomy, with half of the patients being long-term survivors.

TABLE 106.1

PRIMARY PULMONARY NEOPLASMS IN CHILDREN

TYPE OF TUMOR	NUMBER (%)[a]
Benign (*n* = 92)	
Inflammatory	48 (52.2)
Hamartoma	22 (23.9)
Neurogenic tumor	9 (9.8)
Leiomyoma	6 (6.5)
Mucous gland adenoma	3 (3.3)
Myoblastoma	3 (3.3)
Benign teratoma	1 (1.1)
Malignant (*n* = 291)	
Bronchial "adenoma"	118 (40.5)
Bronchogenic	49 (16.8)
Pulmonary blastoma	45 (15.5)
Fibrosarcoma	28 (9.6)
Rhabdomyosarcoma	17 (5.8)
Leiomyosarcoma	11 (3.8)
Sarcoma	6 (2.1)
Hemangiopericytoma	4 (1.4)
Plasmacytoma	4 (1.4)
Lymphoma	3 (1.0)
Teratoma	3 (1.0)
Mesenchymoma	2 (0.7)
Myxosarcoma	1 (0.3)

[a]"(%)" is percent of benign or percent of malignant tumors.
Modified from Hancock.

Other Malignant Tumors

Sarcomas, including fibrosarcoma, rhabdomyosarcoma, and leiomyosarcoma, are the next most common primary malignant lung neoplasms found in children. They arise endobronchially as well as peripherally. It is also of note that 9% of all reported malignant lung neoplasms in children were associated with previously documented cystic lung disease.[57]

Inflammatory pseudotumor is the most common "benign" lung tumor in children. Variable nomenclature relates to the description of the inflammatory cells involved. The terms *plasma cell granuloma*, *histiocytoma*, *xanthofibroma*, *fibroxanthoma*, and *inflammatory myofibroblastic tumor* have been used to describe these tumors. They may present as peripheral lesions or as obstructing endobronchial masses, often following a previous pulmonary infection. Symptoms include cough, chest pain, hemoptysis, fever, and airway obstruction (Fig. 106.8). Although there may be some tendency for spontaneous resolution, aggressive local invasion is often seen. As such, it may be more accurate to describe these lesions as low-grade malignancies.[61] Unresectable tumors may respond to nonsteroidal anti-inflammatory agents.[62] Complete resection, even if extensive in nature, should be undertaken since no adjuvant therapies have proven effective.

Hamartoma. Hamartomatous lung nodules are usually discovered in adults but may be large enough or calcified to be discovered on chest radiographs in children.[63] These tumors may be endobronchial and result in airway obstruction or, more commonly, peripheral and asymptomatic unless very large. Conservative pulmonary resection is the best treatment, but large lesions may require lobectomy or even pneumonectomy.

8 **Mediastinal Tumors.** Mediastinal tumors in children may be benign or malignant. Certain tumors have a predilection for arising from the anterior, middle, or posterior mediastinum.[64]

Neurogenic tumors are the most common thoracic tumors in the pediatric population (Fig. 106.9). The tumors originate in the posterior mediastinum, often from elements of the sympathetic chain. They may grow very large before detection and may be found incidentally. Symptoms of Horner syndrome or tracheal displacement may be apparent. Occasionally,

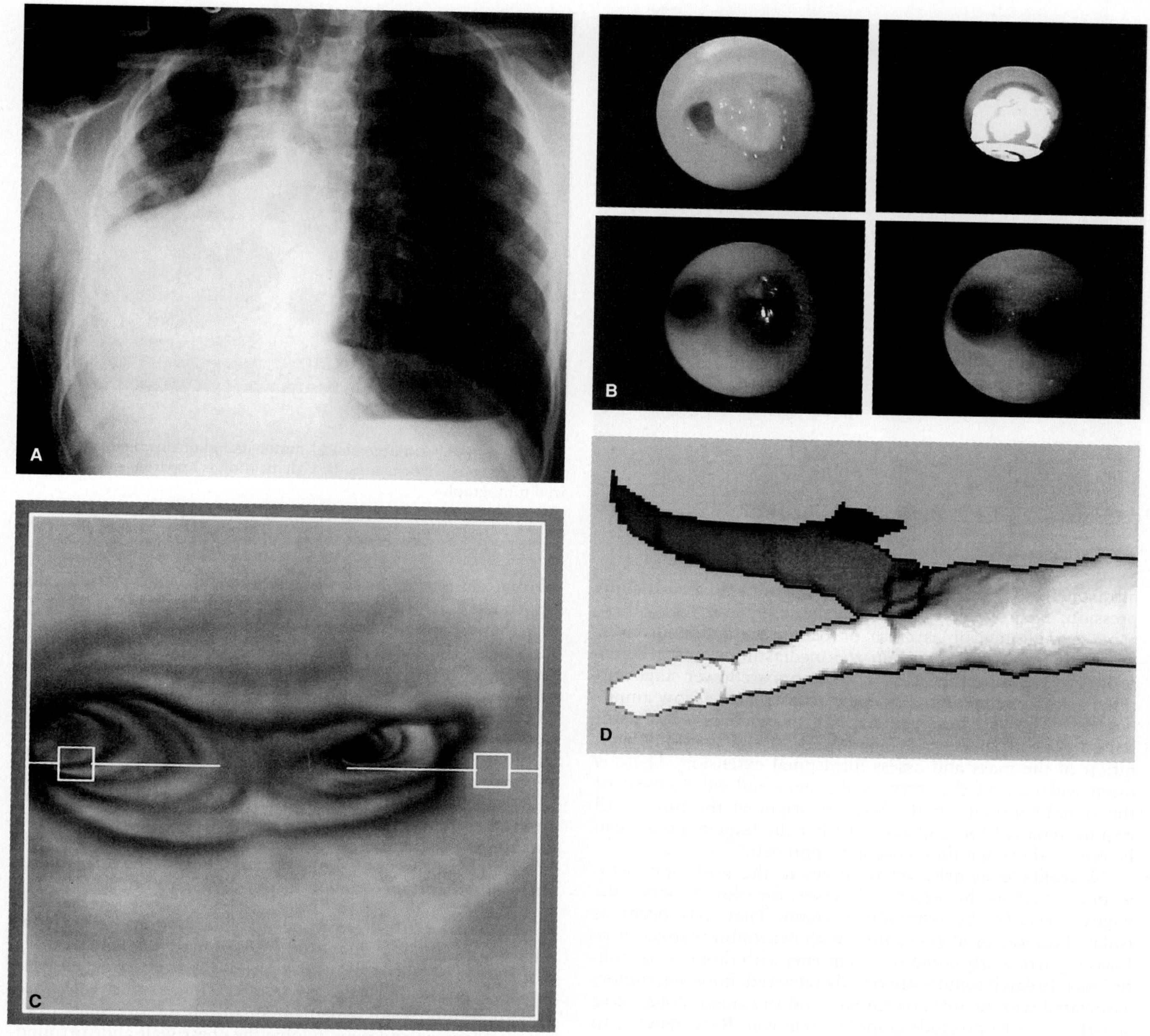

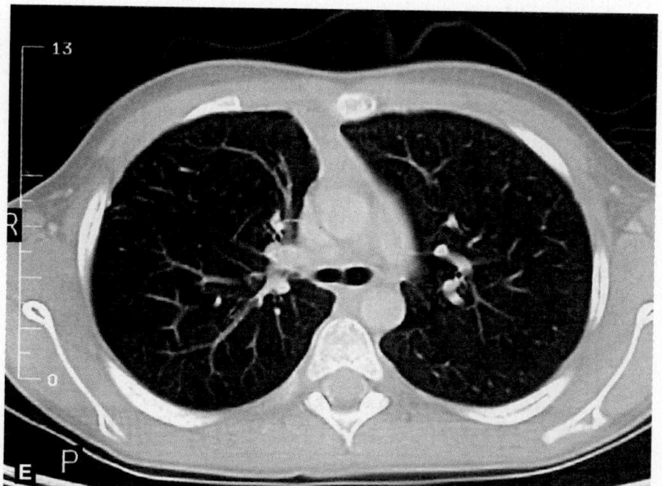

FIGURE 106.8. Lung neoplasm in an 8-year-old child: inflammatory pseudotumor. **A:** Presenting chest radiograph with right lung collapse. **B:** Biopsy of an obstructing endobronchial mass demonstrates inflammatory pseudotumor (inflammatory myofibroblastic tumor). **C:** Computerized tomographic "virtual bronchoscopy" image after initial biopsy demonstrates deformation of the right main stem bronchus and carina due to tumor infiltration. **D:** Computerized tomography reconstruction of the external appearance of airways demonstrating the deformation of the carina and right main stem bronchus. The child underwent excision of the right main stem bronchus and carina and tracheobronchial reconstruction. **E:** Postoperative transverse thoracic computerized tomography at the level of the reconstruction of the carina.

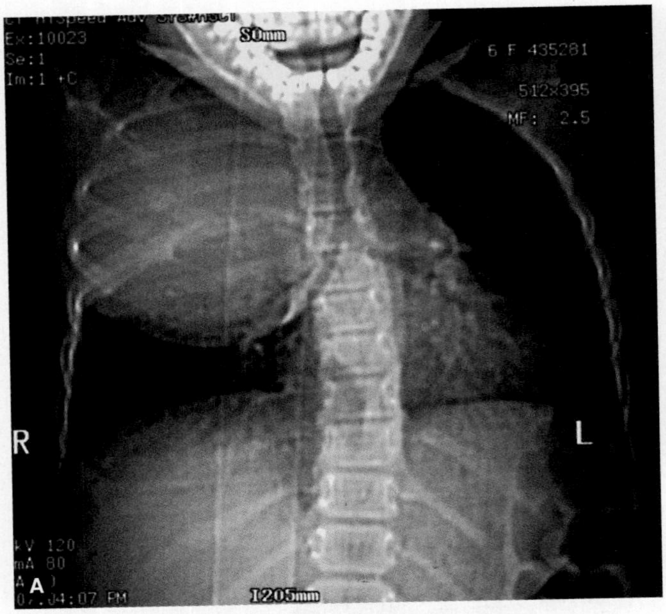

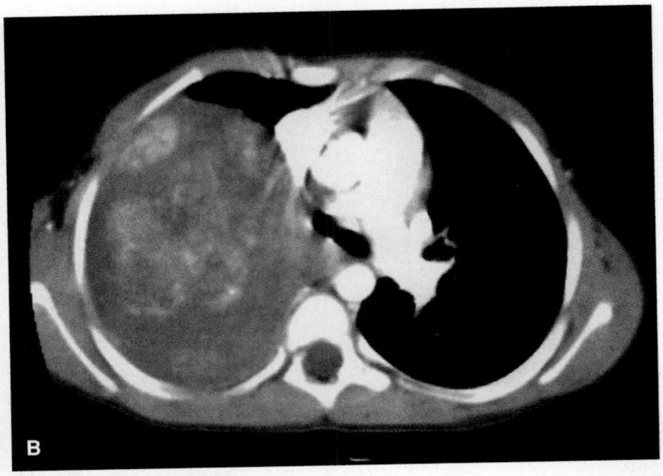

FIGURE 106.9. **A:** Large neural tumor (ganglioneuroma arising from the right sympathetic chain). **B:** Calcification is apparent on computerized tomography.

intraspinal extension results in symptoms of spinal cord compression. Neurogenic tumors may be malignant (neuroblastoma, ganglioneuroblastoma) or benign (ganglioneuroma). Neuroblastoma originating in the mediastinum has a better prognosis than in other sites. The tumors are lower stage and often have more favorable biologic activity such as low amplification of N-myc; however, stage IV mediastinal tumors still have a poor prognosis.[65] CT and MRI provide anatomic definition of the mass and assess intraspinal extension. There is often widening of the intercostal spaces and enlargement of the spinal foramina at the level of origin of the tumor. All require removal for diagnosis. All but the largest tumors can be removed using a thoracoscopic approach.[66]

Neurofibromas arise from nerves in the posterior mediastinum, such as the intercostal nerves, the phrenic nerve, the vagus nerve, or the sympathetic chain. They may occur as isolated tumors or in association with neurofibromatosis. Scoliosis is particularly common in patients with thoracic neurofibromas. Isolated tumors are readily removed; however, tumors associated with neurofibromatosis tend to extend along nerve sheaths so as to preclude complete removal. Recurrence is to be expected in neurofibromatosis, and malignant degeneration to neurofibrosarcoma can occur in large tumors, mandating periodic monitoring. Neuroblastoma is also increased in patients with neurofibromatosis.[67]

Hodgkin and non-Hodgkin lymphoma may present as an anterior or middle mediastinal mass. Surgical removal is not required, but the pediatric surgeon often participates in the diagnostic workup.[68] Tissue sampling from cervical lymph nodes, thoracoscopy, or open biopsy may be needed for diagnosis. Special anesthetic risks, including difficulty with ventilation and compromise of cardiac output, exist in the case of bulky anterior mediastinal tumors that compress the large airways. Specifically, patients with greater than 50% reduction in tracheal cross-sectional area or with dyspnea or orthopnea are at special risk.[69] Under these circumstances, biopsy of a supraclavicular lymph node under local anesthesia or mass biopsy under general anesthesia without paralyzing agents and with ECMO standby should be considered.[70]

Teratomas arise in the anterior mediastinum and may contain elements of all three embryonic germ layers. The lesions are either solid or cystic well-rounded masses that frequently contain calcification on imaging. The most common form of a cystic teratoma consists of mature ectodermal elements known as a dermoid cyst. This lesion is characterized by a thick-walled fibrous sac with squamous epithelium in which various skin appendages including hair and teeth can be found. Occasionally, they are found within the pericardium. The tumors may be large (Fig. 106.10). Patients typically present with cough, dyspnea, or chest pain, although many will be asymptomatic. Surgical removal of these cysts is indicated because of the risk of infection, erosion into the pleura or pericardium, and local compression. The rare occurrence of malignant components within the tumor mandates assessment of preoperative serum α-fetoprotein and β-HCG and tumor removal.

Other neoplasms of the mediastinum are very rare in children but often require surgical biopsy or extirpation. These include neurolemmoma, pheochromocytoma, primitive neuroectodermal tumors, germ cell tumors, mesenchymal tumors including rhabdomyosarcoma, and thymic tumors.

Chest Wall Tumors. Ewing sarcoma, chondrosarcoma, and liposarcoma are malignant tumors that may originate from the chest wall. Local control of disease may require extensive chest wall excision and prosthetic reconstruction. Primitive neuroectodermal tumors are malignant small-cell tumors that carry a poor prognosis and may involve the chest wall and surrounding tissues. Multimodal therapy with surgery, chemotherapy, and radiation may be of benefit.[71,72]

Respiratory Papillomatosis. Recurrent respiratory papillomatosis is a viral-induced disorder caused by the same human papilloma viruses that cause genital condylomata.[73] It is likely transmitted at birth, and there may be some protective prophylactic benefit from cesarean section in selected high-risk expectant mothers. Airway-obstructing papillomas develop in the first several years of life and are treated with laser ablation. Often, many sessions are required to clear the airways. Children who develop symptoms before age 3 years are more likely to have severe disease.[74]

ESOPHAGEAL ATRESIA/ TRACHEOESOPHAGEAL FISTULA

Esophageal atresia and tracheoesophageal fistula were first described by Thomas Gibson in 1697. A London-based physician, Gibson visited a baby who was unable to swallow without constant regurgitation of food. At autopsy, Gibson discovered two blind ends of esophagus that did not interconnect.

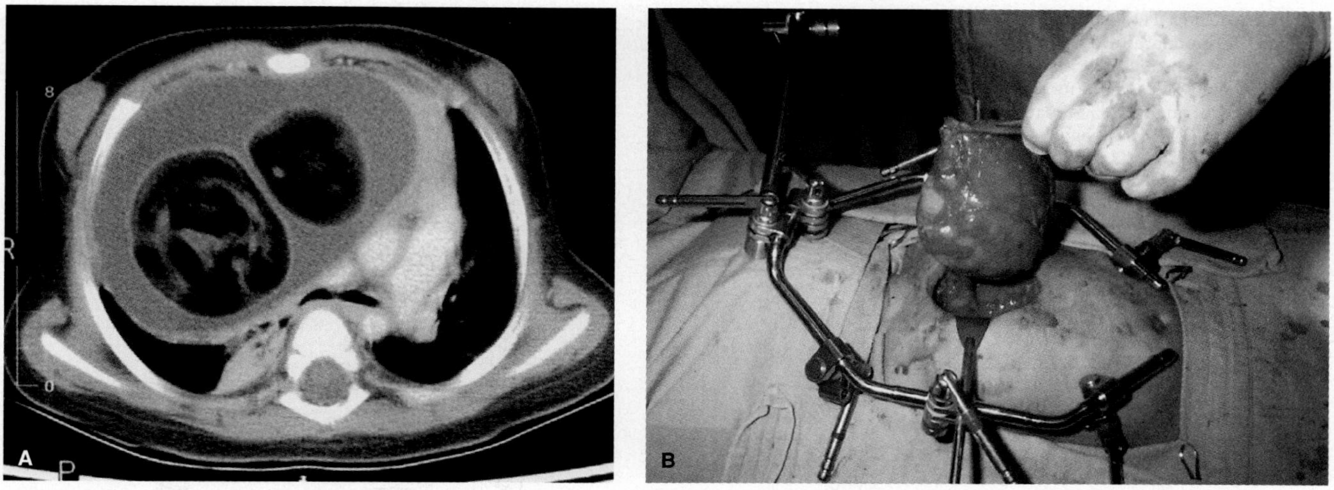

FIGURE 106.10. Mediastinal teratoma. **A:** Transverse thoracic computerized tomography of a large anterior mediastinal teratoma presenting with airway compression symptoms in a 9-month-old female. **B:** Tumor removal via a median sternotomy.

As the subjects of anatomy and physiology exploded with new information, the understanding of esophageal atresia and fistula drastically improved. Initial attempts at both corrective and palliative surgery in the early part of the 20th century were unsuccessful. On March 15, 1941, Dr. Cameron Haight performed the first successful primary repair of esophageal atresia at the University of Michigan.[75] Refinements in surgical technique and postoperative critical care have resulted in a steady improvement in survival for such patients over the ensuing five decades.[76] In the modern era, survival is determined almost exclusively by severe prematurity and the presence of associated anomalies, in particular cardiac disease, and not by the esophageal abnormality itself.[77]

Embryology

Development of the human respiratory tract begins as primitive epithelial cells branch off of the ventral foregut of the embryo into the surrounding mesenchyme at the beginning of the fourth week of gestation. There are ongoing processes that involve both elongation and separation of the foregut (esophagus) and the airway (trachea). By the end of the fourth week of gestation, the esophagus and trachea have completely separated to the level of the larynx. This developmental program is under the control of master regulatory genes that are turned on and off in an orderly fashion. Interruption of this developmental process during the fourth week of gestation probably results in the various forms of esophageal atresia with or without tracheoesophageal fistula. By the end of the sixth week of gestation, the circular muscular coat of the esophagus develops, followed by vagal innervation. The segmental blood supply from the aorta appears by the seventh week, and the muscular coat has differentiated into two layers by the ninth week. The malformation can be recapitulated in an animal model by the administration of Adriamycin at specific times and doses to pregnant rats during organogenesis.[78,79]

Classification

9 Descriptive terminology is used to indicate the anatomic configuration of a patient with esophageal atresia (Fig. 106.11). Esophageal atresia with proximal pouch and distal tracheoesophageal fistula is by far the most common type encountered by the pediatric surgeon, accounting for 85% to 95% of all cases. Esophageal atresia without fistula (pure atresia) occurs in 5% to 7% of patients. Tracheoesophageal fistula without esophageal atresia (so-called "H-type" or "N-type" fistula) occurs in 2% to 6% of patients. The more rare forms of this anomaly include esophageal atresia with proximal tracheoesophageal fistula and esophageal atresia with both proximal and distal tracheoesophageal fistula. The frequency of these rare forms is less than 1% in most reports. Alphabetical and numeric classification schemes, devised by Haight,[80] Gross,[81] and Kluth[82] are of historical interest. The most common variety (proximal pouch, distal fistula) is still commonly referred to as "Gross type C."

Incidence and Epidemiology

The incidence of esophageal atresia varies among populations and races in the range of 1 in 2,500 to 1 in 20,000 births. The overall incidence is about 1 in 5,000. There is a slight male preponderance of 1.26:1. First pregnancy, advanced maternal age, hormonal exposure in pregnancy, and an affected parent and affected siblings are risk factors. Chromosomal abnormalities, twinning, and associated anomalies are more common than expected.

Clinical Findings, Diagnosis, and Pathophysiology

The diagnosis of esophageal atresia may be suspected by the finding of maternal polyhydramnios. Specific ultrasonic identification of the blind-ending upper pouch may be diagnostic. However, many patients go undiagnosed until after birth. Most infants are asymptomatic in the first hours of life. Excessive drooling may be noted. Choking, coughing, and regurgitation may be present and worsened by attempts at feeding. Respiratory distress and cyanosis due to aspiration may occur. Occasionally, in the breast-fed infant, the diagnosis may be unrecognized for more than a day as the volume of feeding associated with colostrum ingestion prior to milk flow may be very low. The inability to pass a nasogastric or orogastric tube is confirmatory of the diagnosis. Radiographs confirm the position of the tube in the proximal blind-ending pouch. Injection of air during the radiograph outlines the pouch. The child with esophageal atresia and a tracheoesophageal fistula will have a full abdomen and gas visible throughout the bowel on the abdominal radiograph. A scaphoid abdomen and gasless

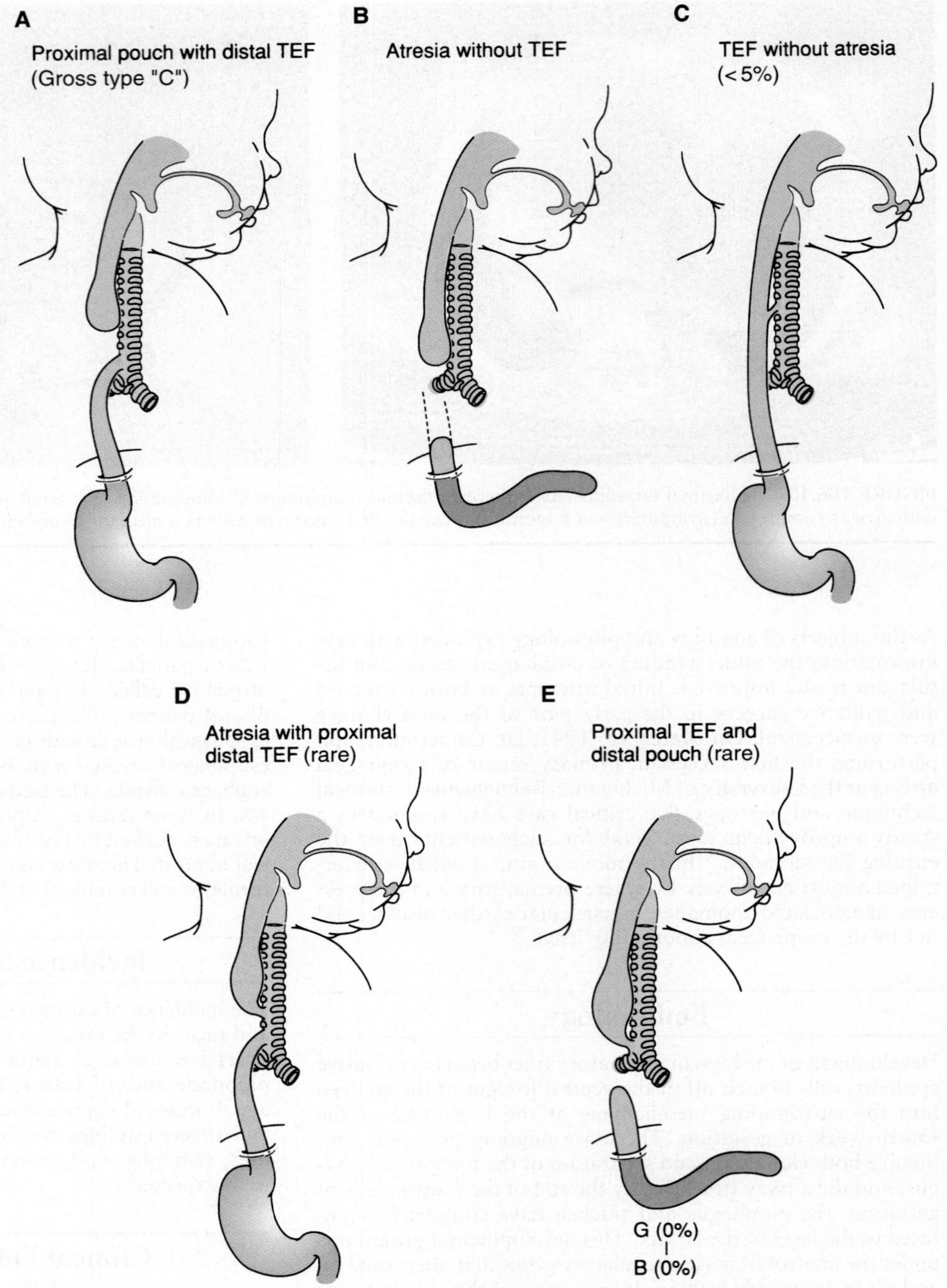

FIGURE 106.11. The anatomy of the variants of esophageal atresia and tracheoesophageal fistula (TEF). **A:** Proximal pouch with distal TEF (most common type occurring in 85% of patients; Gross type "C"). **B:** Esophageal atresia without TEF (5%). **C:** TEF without esophageal atresia (<5%). **D:** Esophageal atresia with proximal and distal TEF (rare). **E:** Proximal TEF and distal pouch (rare). (After Manning PB, Morgan RA, Coran AG, et al. Fifty years' experience with esophageal atresia and tracheoesophageal fistula. *Ann Surg* 1988;204:446.)

radiograph indicate pure esophageal atresia with no fistula. Isolated tracheoesophageal fistula without esophageal atresia does not result in esophageal obstruction and therefore is diagnosed later in infancy or childhood as a result of respiratory symptoms such as aspiration pneumonia, choking with feeds, and gastric distention with crying. Exact delineation of the anatomy may require endoscopic evaluation at the time of surgical correction (Fig. 106.12). If a distal fistula is present, gastroesophageal reflux into the respiratory tract will result in chemical pneumonitis. This may be made worse by air distention of the stomach through the fistula. This is less of a problem if the respiratory tract is mature and the infant can breathe normally. If significant respiratory failure is present, lung compliance is decreased, and positive pressure mechanical ventilation is required, ventilating gases may flow preferentially through the fistula into the gastrointestinal tract. Progressive abdominal distention may preclude adequate ventilation requiring emergency decompression of the stomach and control of the fistula.

Associated Anomalies

Associated anomalies are present in about half of newborns with esophageal atresia, indicating that other systems are affected by the early organogenic insult that disturbs the development of the trachea and esophagus. The most common associated anomalies are cardiovascular defects. Genitourinary, gastrointestinal, skeletal, neurologic, and craniofacial defects are found with increased frequency in patients with esophageal atresia as well. The particular occurrence of vertebral anomalies, anorectal malformations, and cardiac, tracheoesophageal, renal and (radial) limb defects is known as the VACTERL association. Two or more of these defects need to be

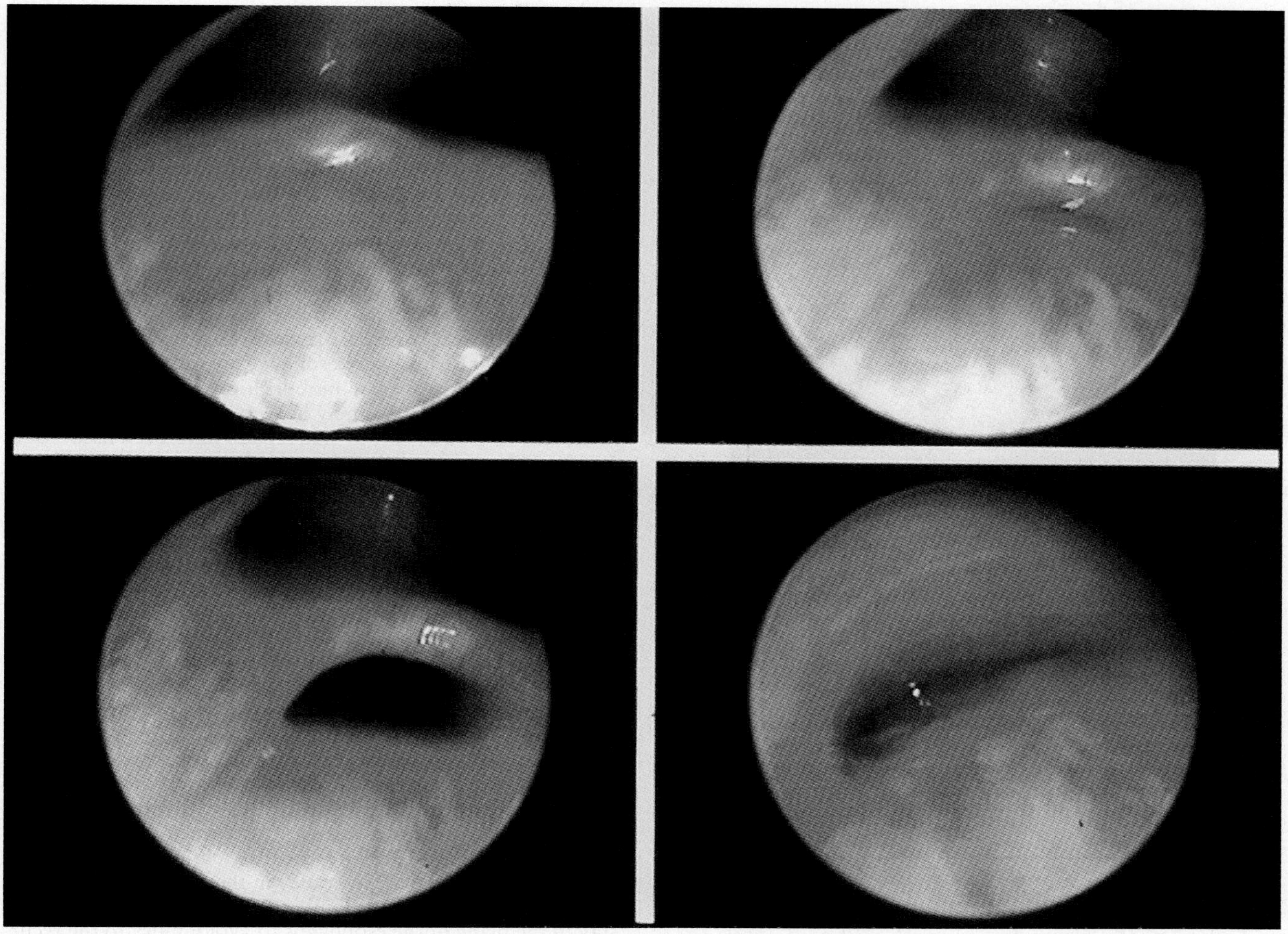

FIGURE 106.12. Bronchoscopic view of the trachea in a patient with common esophageal atresia and tracheoesophageal fistula (TEF). Note that during the inspiratory phase of positive pressure ventilation the fistula opens widely, demonstrating the "face" of TEF (**lower left**). The more proximal view in the trachea demonstrates tracheomalacia with coaptation of the anterior trachea and posterior membranous trachea (**lower right**).

present to assign the association to a given patient. Nearly half of tracheoesophageal atresia patients will exhibit one of the VACTERL malformations.[83]

Preoperative Treatment

Preoperatively, attempts at feeding are stopped and intravenous fluids are started. Further aspiration is minimized by placement of a sump catheter in the upper esophageal pouch. To avoid further lung injury, antacids and antibiotics should be considered. Additionally, standard precautions such as head-up positioning should be universally accepted. Endotracheal intubation is avoided unless necessary since positive pressure ventilation may result in preferential flow of ventilatory gases through the fistula. Ventilation strategies such as high-frequency oscillatory ventilation (HFOV) should be employed if respiratory failure is associated with decreased lung compliance and to potentially avoid filling the stomach with gas. Early use of surfactant to improve lung compliance should be considered in premature infants with respiratory failure. Bedside decompressive gastrostomy may be needed if gastric distention compromises ventilation or a prolonged interval is planned prior to surgery. One of the more difficult issues in pediatric surgery is the decision making around ligating the fistula in a newborn with esophageal atresia and distal tracheoesophageal fistula prior to onset of severe respiratory insufficiency. The lung retraction required to ligate the fistula is prohibitive once respiratory insufficiency has progressed. Thus, the surgeon must be prepared at the first signs of respiratory compromise to control the fistula by emergency operative ligation. An alternative is to place an occluding distal esophageal balloon via a gastrostomy under fluoroscopic guidance or bronchoscopic guidance if ventilation cannot be maintained.[84]

The goal of modern operative treatment is to correct the anomaly completely with a single operation, avoiding a gastrostomy if possible. Immediate surgery is rarely required, and a day or two may be utilized to complete the assessment of the infant, including the echocardiographic evaluation to determine the position of the aortic arch and the presence of structural heart disease. This time period will also allow a complete transition from fetal circulation. Respiratory hygiene, positioning, and antibiotics may improve the infant's overall condition.

High-risk infants who cannot safely undergo surgical correction of their esophageal abnormality may be treated with delayed repair. A decompressive gastrostomy, proximal pouch suctioning, and parenteral nutrition are used until the infant is ready for operation. Severe respiratory failure (usually from prematurity) and structural heart disease are the most common reasons to delay esophageal surgery. A staged repair that employs gastrostomy, surgical division of the tracheoesophageal fistula, followed by esophageal anastomosis as a second thoracic operation is rarely used except as a lifesaving approach.

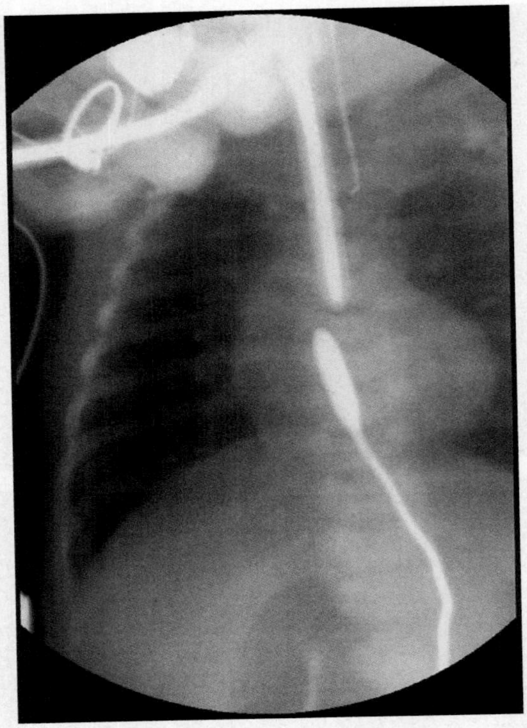

FIGURE 106.13. Patient with pure esophageal atresia treated initially with feeding gastrostomy, and proximal pouch stretching. This "gap-o-gram" demonstrates close approximation of a dilator in the proximal pouch and a probe placed in the distal esophagus via the gastrostomy. The child subsequently underwent primary repair of the esophagus.

In the case of pure esophageal atresia without fistula, a prolonged period of delay prior to repair may be used to improve the likelihood of completing a primary repair of the esophagus. A feeding gastrostomy is performed initially. This may be technically challenging since microgastria is present with pure atresia. Intragastric feeding and somatic growth result in shortening of the interval between the upper pouch and lower esophageal segment over the course of several weeks. The upper pouch may be stretched by daily or twice-daily passage of a blunt flexible bougie. Radiographic determination of the distance between the two esophageal ends guides the timing of operation (Fig. 106.13).

The Waterston classification stratified infants into good, moderate, and high-risk groups based on birth weight, pneumonia, and associated anomalies.[85] The risk group was used to help determine the timing and staging of surgical correction and to compare the results at different centers. Low birth weight/prematurity has less of an impact on survival than in the past. Currently, the presence of major cardiac disease and chromosomal abnormalities are the most important predictors of survival.[86–89]

Surgical Technique

In most patients, it is not necessary to perform a gastrostomy at the time of repair. With typical anatomy (left aortic arch), the repair is performed via a right thoracotomy (Fig. 106.14). Although the approach may be either transplural or extraplural, the extrapleural approach is preferred by most pediatric surgeons. A standard posterolateral right thoracotomy may be employed. There is no need to divide the latissimus or serratus muscles, and a muscle-sparing approach may have long-term benefits.[90] A more posterior approach through the auscultatory triangle affords excellent exposure with a very small skin incision. The extrapleural plane is established at the fourth intercostal space and developed sufficiently to allow control of the fistula and adequate mobilization of the proximal pouch. The distal tracheoesophageal fistula is divided and closed. The proximal pouch is identified and mobilized to whatever extent is needed to bring the ends together for anastomosis. If a proximal fistula is present, it is closed.

Various lengthening techniques may be used when the gap is long between the esophageal ends. These techniques include circular myotomies, spiral myotomies, flap tubularization of the proximal pouch, and extensive mobilization of the proximal pouch through a supplementary cervical incision. Contrary to earlier teaching, the distal esophagus may be mobilized as well when there is a long distance between the upper pouch and lower esophagus, or in the case of pure esophageal atresia. Distal mobilization may extend to the stomach. An anastomosis may heal, even under tension. One-layer, two-layer, and end-to-side repairs have been used. Most surgeons use a single layer end-to-end anastomosis.

A staged repair has been described that has been successfully employed in pure and long gap esophageal atresia. Traction sutures are initially placed in the upper pouch and lower segment. Daily tensioning results in lengthening of the esophagus that allows anastomosis within a few weeks[91] (Fig. 106.15).

In the worst cases of long gap atresia, pure atresia, or failed initial operative repairs, esophageal replacement may be performed at a later date using stomach, gastric tube, or colon.[92–94] Such conditions may be temporized with a cervical esophagostomy ("spit fistula") and gastrostomy with initiation of sham feeds.

Tracheoesophageal fistula without esophageal atresia is referred to as H-type atresia. The orientation of the fistula is such that the opening into the trachea is always proximal to the esophageal entry site. Repair is performed through a cervical approach after bronchoscopically stenting the fistula with a small catheter. The catheter aids in the precise identification of the fistula during dissection in the neck. Care must taken to stay in the plane of the esophagus to avoid injury to the recurrent laryngeal nerves.

Minimally invasive techniques using modifications of thoracoscopy may be used to treat esophageal atresia.[95,96] In fact, the thoracoscopic approach is now used by many surgeons with equivalent outcomes except, perhaps, an increased rate of stricture formation.[97]

Results, Complications, and Outcomes. Technical mishaps during the procedure occur when the anatomy is misidentified or dissection is carried out improperly. Unplanned injury to the vagus nerves, recurrent laryngeal nerves, posterior trachea, and adjacent vessels must be avoided.

Anastomotic leak is said to occur in 10% to 20% of patients. The vast majority of such leaks will heal spontaneously. The presence of a leak prolongs hospitalization and increases the likelihood of stricture formation at the anastomotic site. When a leak is detected, the retropleural chest tube is left in place, the infant is not fed by mouth, and antibiotics may be administered. Repeat contrast documents healing prior to the initiation of feeds.

Esophageal stricture at the site of the repair is found in as many as 40% of patients after repair. Many strictures will respond to a few sessions of dilation. Dilations are performed in the operating room with endoscopic and fluoroscopic assistance, as necessary, to assure the safe traverse of the narrowing by guide wires and dilators. More recalcitrant strictures may require many dilation sessions, steroid injection, and medical or surgical control of gastroesophageal reflux for resolution. Occasionally reoperation, with resection of the stricture and reanastomosis of the esophagus, may be required.

Recurrent tracheoesophageal fistula is reported to occur in up to 10% of patients. Recurrent fistulas may respond to endoscopic ablation, a combined Tisseel/Gelfoam construct

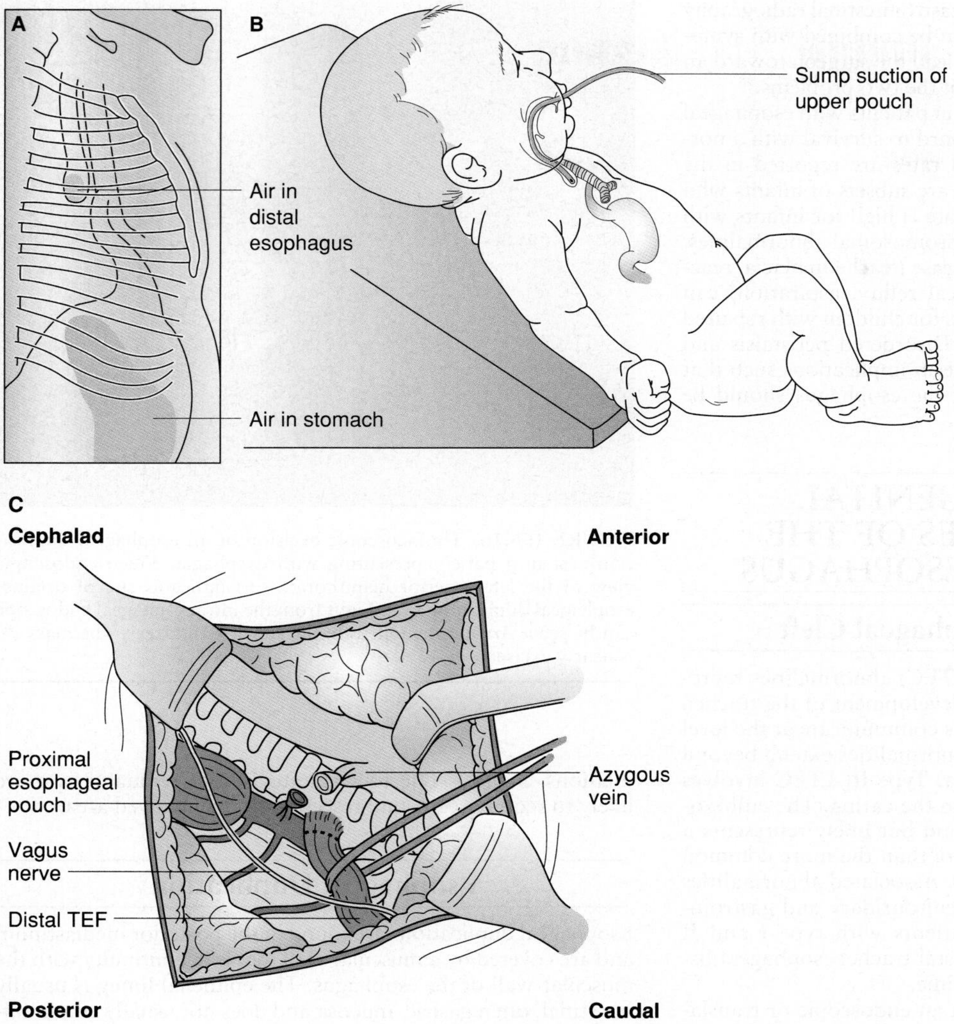

FIGURE 106.14. **A:** Schematic illustration of esophageal atresia with distal tracheoesophageal fistula. **B:** The initial management of this anomaly includes upright or prone posture, sump suction of the blind esophageal pouch. **C:** The right extrapleural operative approach. After division and closure of the fistula, primary esophagoesophagostomy is performed. (After Coran AG. Congenital abnormalities of the esophagus. In: Zuidema GD, Orringer MD, eds. *Shackelford's Surgery of the Alimentary Tract*. 2nd ed. Philadelphia, PA: WB Saunders; 1990.)

placed into the fistula, or require operative division with interposition of pleura, muscle, or pericardium.

Gastroesophageal reflux is present in nearly all infants with esophageal atresia. It is symptomatic in many and may contribute to respiratory symptoms and stricture formation.

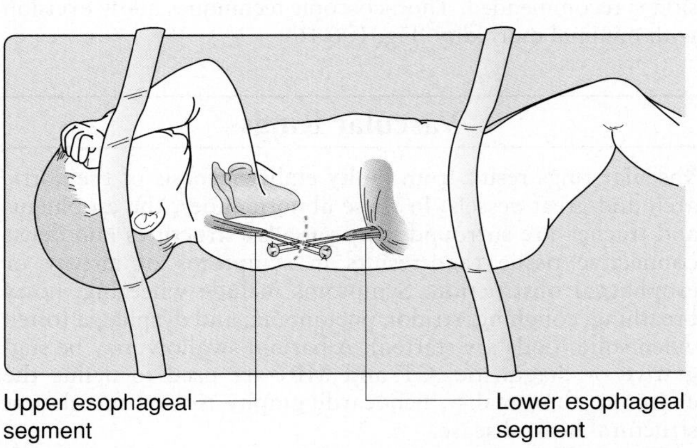

FIGURE 106.15. In patients with ultra-long-gap esophageal atresia, traction sutures are placed on the upper pouch and lower segment. Tension is increased daily until the segments lengthen, allowing primary repair. (Adapted from Foker JE, Kendall TC, Catton K, et al. A flexible approach to achieve a true primary repair for all infants with esophageal atresia. *Semin Pediatr Surg* 2005;14:8–15.)

Medical treatment consists of thickened feedings, upright positioning after feeds, frequent burping, small frequent feeds, acid reduction, and prokinetic agents. In many infants, medical treatments will be inadequate to control symptoms and surgical control of reflux will be required.

Esophageal dysmotility is present to some degree in all patients with esophageal atresia. Dysmotility contributes to gastroesophageal reflux and may be responsible for dysphagia and recurrent respiratory problems.

Tracheomalacia may result in symptoms after the correction of esophageal atresia. Bronchoscopically, the trachea appears oval in shape rather than round. The anterior and posterior walls coapt during the respiratory cycle (Fig. 106.12). Fluoroscopic examination of the trachea demonstrates narrowing or "fish-mouthing" in the anteroposterior dimensions during spontaneous expiration. Tracheomalacia "fits" occur as the infant becomes agitated and develops worsening chest retractions with inspiration. The condition may deteriorate to complete inspiratory block and unconsciousness. When spontaneous respiration resumes in a quiet fashion, the "spell" is over. Intubation and resuscitation may be required. The symptoms are completely relieved by endotracheal intubation. Infants with less severe symptoms may improve over time as the trachea grows. Severe symptoms require either tracheostomy or tracheal suspension with an aortopexy under bronchoscopic guidance to ensure effectiveness of the aortopexy. There can be difficulty in determining whether cyanotic spells or an acute life-threatening event are due to tracheomalacia or gastroesophageal reflux. Data from bronchoscopy to evaluate the degree of tracheomalacia and upper gastrointestinal radiography and pH probe to assess for reflux can be combined with symptoms noted prior to the event to help lead the surgeon toward an operation to resolve the most likely of the two problems.[98]

Long-term results have improved in patients with esophageal atresia. Most children can look forward to survival with a normal existence.[99–103] Overall survival rates are reported in the 85% to 95% range. However, there are subsets of infants who do not fare as well. The mortality rate is high for infants with severe congenital heart defects and chromosomal abnormalities. Late deaths related to respiratory disease (tracheomalacia, reactive airway disease, gastroesophageal reflux, aspiration) can occur.[88] The very long term outcomes for children with repaired esophageal atresia are not known. Disordered peristalsis and chronic esophagitis may have long-term implications such that periodic endoscopic surveillance of the esophagus should be performed in select patients.[104]

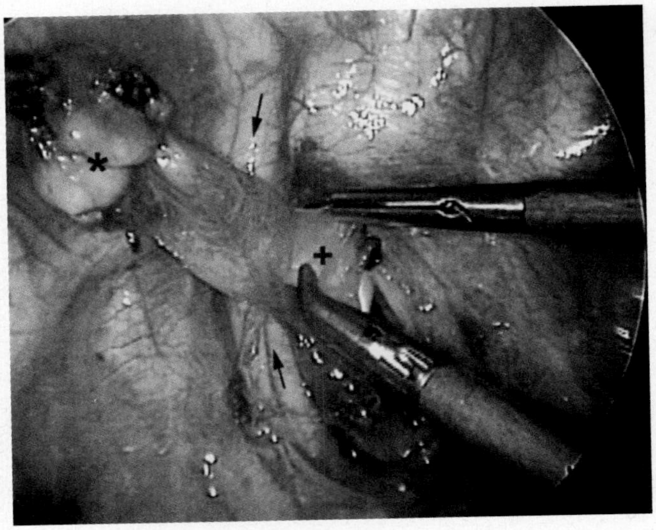

FIGURE 106.16. Thoracoscopic excision of an esophageal duplication cyst in a patient presenting with dysphagia. Video endoscopic view of the left superior hemithorax. (+) indicates site of original esophageal duplication cyst. Light from the intraesophageal endoscope can be seen. *Arrows* demonstrate the subclavian artery. The mass (*) is nearly excised.

OTHER CONGENITAL ABNORMALITIES OF THE TRACHEA AND ESOPHAGUS

Laryngotracheoesophageal Cleft

Laryngeotracheoesophageal cleft (LTEC) abnormalities represent the most severe anomalies of development of the trachea and esophagus. Type I abnormalities communicate at the level of the larynx and cricoid. Type II abnormalities extend beyond the cricoid into the cervical trachea. Type III LTEC involves the entire trachea from the larynx to the carina. The embryogenesis of LTEC is poorly understood but likely represents a disruption similar to but more severe than the more common esophageal atresia/TEF abnormality. Associated abnormalities of the cardiovascular system and genitourinary and gastrointestinal tracts are common. In patients with type I and II defects, esophageal atresia and a distal tracheoesophageal fistula is present about a third of the time.

Type I clefts may be repaired via an endoscopic or translaryngeal approach. Type II clefts require cervical exposure, either laterally or by dividing the larynx and trachea in the midline. This anterior midline approach provides excellent exposure and avoids injury to the recurrent laryngeal nerves. Type III clefts extending to the carina, or beyond, require direct exposure through a right extrapleural thoracotomy as well as cervical exposure. The trachea and esophagus are separated longitudinally in such a way as to leave a remnant of the esophagus with the trachea to be used in reconstructing the posterior membranous portion of the trachea. The esophagus is then tubularized. A multilayered repair of the larynx is completed through the cervical exposure. Breakdown of the repair and prolonged need for tracheostomy are common. Oromotor dysfunction and chronic aspiration are long-term problems. Most children will require a gastrostomy for feedings. Gastroesophageal reflux is common and may require surgical control.

Congenital Esophageal Stenosis

Acquired peptic strictures of the esophagus are relatively common and may occur early in life. True congenital stenosis is very uncommon. The stenotic areas may be (a) a membranous, weblike diaphragm; (b) fibromuscular thickening characterized by submucosal proliferation of smooth muscle cells and connective tissue; or (c) due to sequestration of respiratory tract remnants in the form of respiratory epithelium and cartilage. The cartilage remnants may form a complete nondistensible ring in the esophagus. Dysphagia may be present from infancy or become apparent when solid foods are introduced. The diagnosis is confirmed by esophagoscopy. Stenoses are initially treated with dilations. Stenosis due to respiratory tract remnants is more likely to require segmental resection of the involved area.

Esophageal Duplication

Esophageal duplications are found in the posterior mediastinum and are covered by a muscular wall that is in continuity with the muscular wall of the esophagus. The epithelial lining is usually intestinal, often gastric, mucosa and does not usually communicate with the esophagus. These cysts may also have a respiratory epithelium lining underscoring the relatedness of the various bronchopulmonary foregut malformations. Neurenteric cysts will communicate with the spinal canal. Masses are discovered incidentally or as a result of compression on adjacent organs. Acid-peptic ulceration from gastric mucosa within the cyst may result in symptoms such as pain, bleeding, or erosion into adjacent structures (lung parenchyma, bronchus, esophagus). Excision is recommended. Thoracoscopic techniques allow excision with minimal morbidity (Fig. 106.16).

Vascular Rings

10 Vascular rings result from faulty embryogenesis of the aortic arch and great vessels. In these abnormalities, the esophagus and trachea are surrounded by vascular structures and dense connective tissue that results in symptoms of airway or esophageal obstruction. Symptoms include wheezing, noisy breathing, coughing, stridor, pneumonia, and dysphagia (often when solid foods are started). A barium swallow may be suggestive or diagnostic. CT and MRI are used to define the anatomic abnormality. Echocardiography is used to rule out structural heart disease.

The most common abnormality encountered is a double aortic arch, resulting from the persistence of both the left and the right embryologic aortic arches. The ascending aorta bifurcates, surrounding the trachea and esophagus, then rejoins as the descending aorta. Other developmental abnormalities may result in complete or incomplete rings that compress the trachea and/or the esophagus. When the vascular ring is symptomatic, the patient should be treated surgically by appropriate division of the ring and the lysis of the fibrous bands that surround the trachea and esophagus.

Congenital Tracheal Stenosis

Failure of tracheal growth and development results in a wide variety of abnormalities. Short segments of the trachea may be narrowed, or the entire trachea may be hypoplastic. Often, complete tracheal cartilaginous rings are present. Short stenotic areas may occasionally respond to balloon dilation, which splits the complete tracheal rings. Segmental stenoses may be amenable to resection and anastomosis. Longer stenoses may be corrected with placement of a graft to widen the lumen of the trachea. Most recently, the slide tracheoplasty technique has been used to reconstruct narrowed regions of the trachea.[105,106]

FOREIGN BODIES OF THE TRACHEOBRONCHIAL TREE

Foreign body ingestion and aspiration occur commonly in the pediatric population. Endoscopic removal of foreign bodies that lodge in the esophagus is covered in Chapter 45. Any foreign body that could obstruct the airway represents a poten-
11 tially life-threatening problem. The National Safety Council estimates that 200 deaths (most in children under 5 years of age) occur each year in persons under the age of 15 years as a result of suffocation by an ingested object.[107] The Hopkins rod lens optical system with fiberoptic illumination, developed in the 1970s, combined with rigid pediatric bronchoscopes and specialized grasping devices has resulted in a safe and reliable method for airway foreign body extraction.

Pathophysiology

Complete obstruction of the airway and asphyxiation can occur at the level of the laryngeal inlet, the subglottis, or the trachea. Back blows (recommended in infants), abdominal thrust, or the Heimlich maneuver may dislodge the obstruction and save a life. An inhaled foreign body that lodges at the bronchial level can create a ball-valve phenomenon in the affected bronchus, allowing bi-directional but unequal flow of air. Air trapping and hyperinflation in the affected lobe or lung leads to mediastinal shift to the opposite side. Complete blockage of the bronchus by the foreign body results in loss of volume in the affected lobe or lung. In this case, the resulting volume loss from atelectasis will shift the mediastinum to the ipsilateral side.

Clinical Presentation

Most affected children are under 4 years of age, with a peak incidence between 1 and 2 years. Twenty percent of foreign body aspirations occur after the age of 4 years. Foreign bodies are more likely to lodge in the right side of the tracheobronchial tree. Most will be found in the main stem bronchus.[108] Peanuts are commonly aspirated and particularly troublesome. They become soft, fracture readily, and may require piecemeal removal. Other types of food, such as carrots and popcorn, or inorganic material, such as pins, wood, paper, and metallic and plastic parts, may be aspirated.

The aspiration event may have been witnessed or suggested by a history of a coughing or choking spell. The most common symptoms include cough, wheezing, dyspnea, and fever, while the most common signs are unilateral decreased breath sounds, unilateral wheezing, and rhonchi. Inspiratory and expiratory chest radiographs (or bilateral decubitus views in the case of children too young to cooperate) may demonstrate hyperinflation on the affected side due to air trapping. Although physical signs, symptoms, and radiographic findings are often present, a suggestive history alone is an adequate indication to proceed with bronchoscopy.[109]

Management

Bronchoscopic evaluation and foreign body removal is performed in the operating room under general anesthesia (Fig. 106.17). The rigid bronchoscope with optical forceps can be used to remove most aspirated foreign bodies safely. The flexible grasper, Fogarty balloon catheters, and baskets can be useful, especially when the foreign body has migrated distally or has

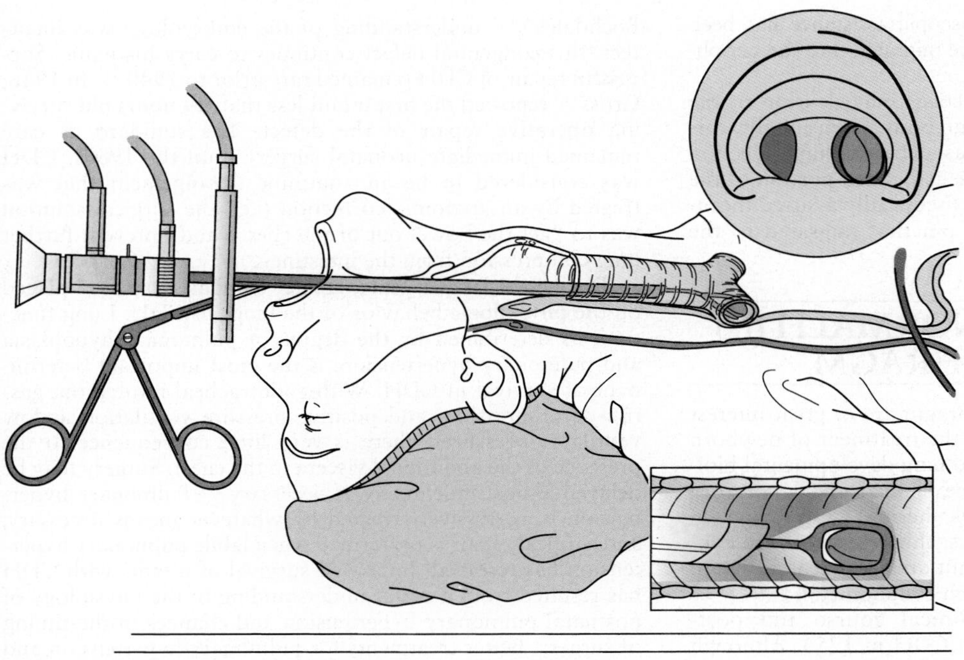

FIGURE 106.17. Schematic illustration of a peanut foreign body being extracted from the right main stem bronchus under direct vision.

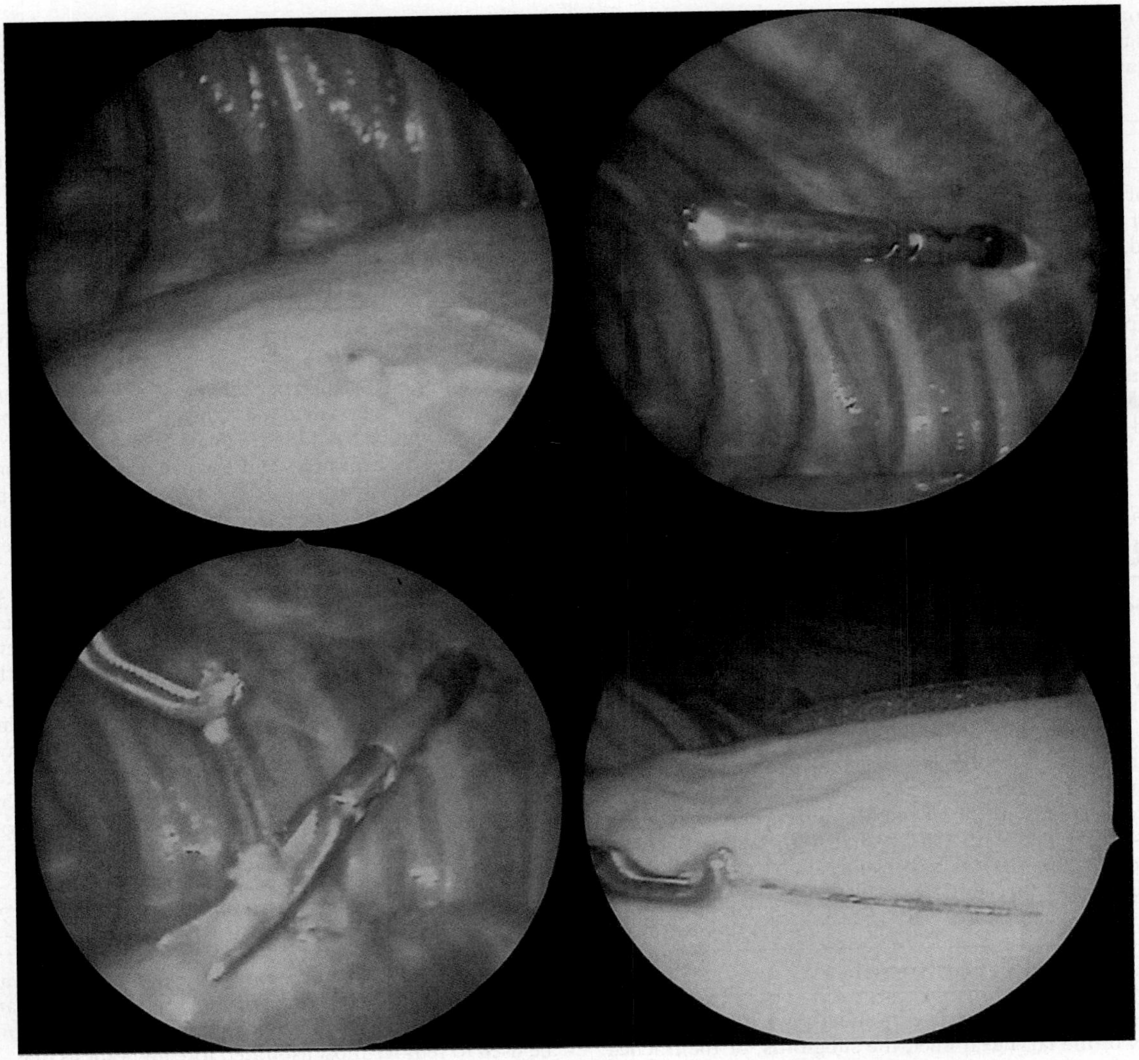

FIGURE 106.18. Four-panel operative photograph of the removal of a pin from lung periphery. The tip of the pin is seen on the lung surface. Thoracoscopic instrumentation. Grasping pin. Pin removed.

a smooth or round surface. Fluoroscopic assistance has been used for radiopaque objects that have migrated into the peripheral airways.

Over time, pneumonia or atelectasis may develop in the lobe or lung associated with a foreign body. Occasionally, foreign body aspiration that presents as a chronic lung infection will require surgical resection of the associated portion of the lung. Figure 106.18 shows the fluoroscopically assisted thoracoscopic removal of an aspirated pin that migrated to the peripheral lung surface.

CONGENITAL ABNORMALITIES OF THE DIAPHRAGM

Developmental defects of the diaphragm are of great interest to pediatric surgeons. Advances in the treatment of newborn respiratory failure, fetal surgery, and lung developmental biology have grown directly out of the clinical and laboratory investigation of CDH (Bochdalek hernia). Occurring in approximately 1 in 3,000 newborns, this relatively rare congenital disease represents a significant area of research within the clinical and basic science research community.

McCauley[110] described the clinical course and postmortem anatomy of an infant with CDH in 1754. Although Bochdalek's[111] understanding of the embryology was incorrect, this congenital defect continues to carry his name. Successful repair of CDH remained rare prior to 1940.[112] In 1946, Gross[113] reported the first infant less than 24 hours old surviving operative repair of the defect. The standard of care remained immediate neonatal surgery until the 1980s. CDH was considered to be an anatomic derangement that was treated by an anatomic correction (i.e., the surgical solution was to "get the bowel out of the chest" and "prevent further lung compression from the intestines").

During the last 25 years, greater emphasis has been placed on the physiologic behavior of the lungs in CDH. Lung function, as determined by the degree of pulmonary hypoplasia and pulmonary hypertension, is the most important determinant of survival in CDH. With endotracheal intubation, gastric decompression, and positive pressure ventilation at low ventilator pressures, there is very little consequence to the presence of the abdominal viscera in the chest. Surgery may be delayed almost indefinitely, if necessary.[114] Pulmonary hypertension is aggressively treated by whatever means necessary, and surgical repair is performed when labile pulmonary hypertension has resolved. Improved survival of infants with CDH has resulted from a better understanding of the physiology of postnatal pulmonary hypertension and changes in the timing of surgery. Better treatments for pulmonary hypertension and therapies aimed at augmenting the development of hypoplastic lungs will no doubt result in further improvements in the survival and long-term morbidity of CDH infants.[115]

Embryology of the Lung and Diaphragm

Mammalian lung development occurs in vivo as a coordinated developmental process that includes (a) airway and acinar development, (b) cellular differentiation, (c) biochemical maturation, (d) interstitial development including vasculature and extracellular matrix, and (e) physical growth or enlargement. These parallel developmental processes occur in such a fashion that at any one time during development, there are characteristic relationships among each component that define the so-called stages of lung development.[116–118] Pulmonary development is marked by a series of programmed events regulated by master genes such as the homeobox genes, nuclear transcription factors, hormones, and growth factors. These processes involve genes regulating epithelial and endothelial interactions as well as temporal and spatial interactions of several hormones and growth factors.[119,120] Hormones such as the glucocorticoids, thyroid hormone, and retinoic acid have been shown to regulate several of the crucial cellular interactions required for proper pulmonary organogenesis and differentiation. In the human embryo, respiratory tract development begins in the fourth week of gestation as a ventral out pouching of the foregut that soon has bifurcated and begun branching into the surrounding mesenchyme. The primitive, pluripotent epithelial cells differentiate into both bronchial and alveolar cell lines, under the control of the surrounding mesenchyme. By a process of asymmetric branching, the divisions are complete by the 16th week of gestation. Lung at this phase has columnar epithelium with thick mesenchyme giving rise to the descriptive term *pseudoglandular phase of development* because of its histologic appearance. The canalicular phase that follows and continues up to about the 24th gestational week is characterized by flattening of the epithelium of the distal airways, thinning of the mesenchyme, and the growth of the capillary network that surrounds the terminal airways. Gas exchange becomes functionally possible at the end of this phase. The terminal sac period that follows refers to the appearance of a thin respiratory epithelium in apposition to a capillary network capable of supporting gas exchange. True alveolar formation in humans begins shortly before or around the time of birth. Alveolar maturation and multiplication takes place after birth and may continue up to 8 years of age.

The precursors of the mesoderm-derived diaphragm begin to form during the fourth week of gestation with the appearance of the peritoneal folds from lateral mesenchymal tissue. At the same time, the septum transversum forms from the inferior portion of the pericardial cavity and serves to delineate the thoracic from the abdominal cavities. Eventually, the septum transversum leads to the formation of the central tendinous area of the fully developed diaphragm. The pleuroperitoneal folds extend from the lateral body wall and grow medially and ventrally until they fuse with the septum transversum and dorsal mesentery of the esophagus during the sixth gestational week. Complete closure of the canal takes place during the eighth week of gestation, with the right side closing before the left.[121] Muscularization of the diaphragm appears to develop from the innermost layer of thoracic mesoderm, although other mechanisms have been proposed.[122] A cell-based computer model system supports a pleuroperitoneal fold–dominated diaphragm morphogenesis theory in the rodent model, which creates a posteromedial diaphragm defect, whereas the posterolateral defect seen in humans would be supported by an alternate cellular development.[123] A contribution from cervically derived myoblasts is also present, as evidenced by the innervation of the diaphragm by the phrenic nerve originating from the third, fourth, and fifth cervical nerve roots. Posterolaterally, at the junction of the lumbar and costal muscle groups, the fibrous lumbocostal trigone remains as a small remnant of the pleuroperitoneal membrane and relies for its strength on the fusion of the two muscle groups in the final stages of development. It is in this area that the defect of CDH occurs (Fig. 106.19).

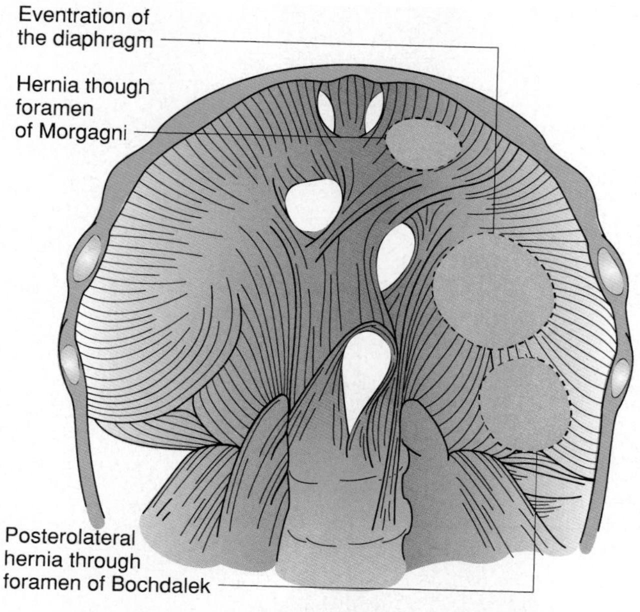

FIGURE 106.19. Anatomy of the diaphragm showing the location of congenital diaphragmatic defects.

Congenital Diaphragmatic Hernia Pathology and Pathophysiology

The reported incidence of CDH is estimated to be between 1 in 2,000 and 1 in 5,000 births, making it one of the most common congenital abnormalities.[124] Approximately one third of infants with CDH are stillborn, but these deaths are usually due to associated fatal anomalies such as neural tube defects (anencephaly, myelomeningocele, hydrocephalus, and encephaloceles) and cardiac defects. Defects are more common on the left side (80% left, 20% right) based on the CDH registry.[114] CDH is thought to represent a sporadic developmental anomaly, although a number of familial cases have been reported. The expected recurrence risk in a first-degree relative has been estimated to be 1 in 45.[124] One third of affected infants have associated major defects. The combination of CDH and an abnormal karyotype is associated with a poor outcome.[125] Associated significant heart disease is also a predictor of poor outcome.[126]

The cause of CDH is unknown, but it is presumed that some combination of intrinsic predisposition (genetic factors) and environmental insult (teratogen or deficiency) results in abnormal diaphragm and lung development. Exposure to a number of pharmacologic agents has been implicated in its development, including certain drugs and insecticides such as phenmetrazine, thalidomide, quinine, and nitrofen.[124] Vitamin A deficiency in CDH infants and the effects of vitamin A administration in nitrofen-induced pulmonary hypoplasia have strengthened the evolving hypothesis that alterations in retinoid-regulated target genes may be responsible for CDH development.[127] Diaphragmatic hernia and pulmonary hypoplasia can be created in animal models, both surgically and pharmacologically.[128–131] Genetically, there is currently no established inheritance pattern in patients afflicted with CDH.

During the early development of the diaphragm, the midgut is largely extracoelomic. If closure of the pleuroperitoneal canal has not occurred by the time the midgut returns to the

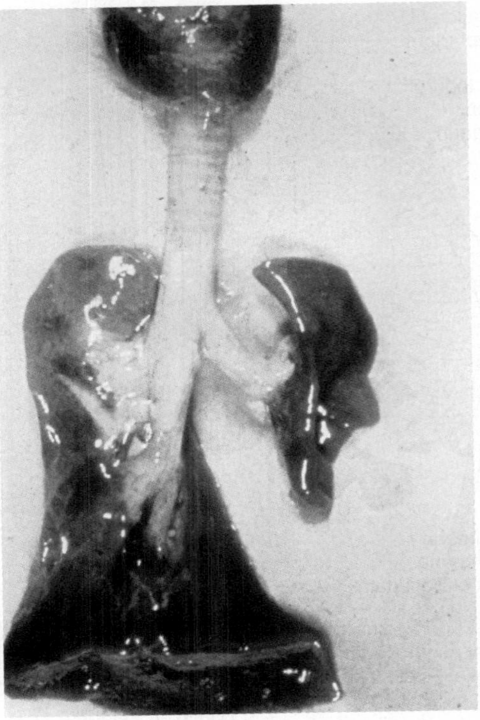

FIGURE 106.20. Autopsy specimen of an infant with severe pulmonary hypoplasia secondary to congenital diaphragmatic hernia. Pulmonary hypoplasia is bilateral, but the left lung is most severely affected.

abdomen during the 9th and 10th weeks of gestation, the abdominal viscera herniate through the lumbocostal trigone into the ipsilateral thoracic cavity. The resulting abnormal position of the bowel prevents its normal counterclockwise rotation and fixation. No hernia sac is present if the event occurs before complete closure of the pleuroperitoneal canal, but a nonmuscularized membrane forms a hernia sac in 10% to 15% of CDH patients. In addition to the small bowel, other intra-abdominal organs such as the spleen, stomach, colon, and liver may also herniate through the diaphragmatic defect.

12 Left-sided CDH is characterized by a 2- to 4-cm posterolateral defect in the diaphragm through which the abdominal viscera have translocated into the ipsilateral thoracic cavity. On a right-sided defect, the large right lobe of the liver can occupy most of the hemithorax. The hepatic veins may drain ectopically into the right atrium, and the liver and lung may be fused.[132]

The pathophysiology of CDH has been attributed to pulmonary parenchymal compression by the herniated organs and its effect on growth and maturation of the lung. An emerging school of thought attributes the pulmonary hypoplasia to an early mesenchymal developmental insult to the lung and diaphragm.[119,120,133] Unilateral diaphragmatic hernia is associated with both ipsilateral and contralateral abnormal pulmonary development, although hypoplasia is more severe on the ipsilateral side. The lung on the side of the hernia is much smaller than its contralateral counterpart, and both are strikingly smaller than normal lungs (Fig. 106.20). The pulmonary vascular bed is abnormal in lungs from patients with CDH. There is a reduction in the total number of arterial branches in both the ipsilateral and contralateral pulmonary parenchyma. The small preacinar and intra-acinar arterioles feature inappropriate and significant medial muscular hyperplasia (Fig. 106.21). The physiologic consequence of this abnormal arteriolar muscularization may be an increased susceptibility to development of pulmonary hypertension.

Pulmonary blood flow accounts for only 7% of cardiac output during normal fetal development. Pulmonary vascular resistance is high. The fetus preferentially shunts oxygenated blood from the placenta through the foramen ovale and ductus arteriosus in a right to left direction into the systemic circulation. With the institution of breathing at birth, oxygen levels rise causing pulmonary vascular resistance to fall, which in turn allows an increase in pulmonary blood flow. Increased arterial oxygen tension then also induces spontaneous closure of the ductus arteriosus. Persistent fetal circulation may develop if this process is interrupted. Elevated pulmonary vascular resistance results in right to left shunting of blood at either the atrial or ductal levels with the delivery of unsaturated blood into the systemic circulation. As shunting increases, the oxygen saturation in the systemic circulation falls. The resulting hypoxia further increases pulmonary vascular resistance and compromises pulmonary blood flow while increasing the right to left shunt flow. Factors that contribute to the persistence of high pulmonary vascular resistance in CDH lungs are thought to be the structural changes of decreased total arteriolar cross-sectional area in the involved lungs and the increased muscularization of the arterial structures that are present. Additional exacerbations of pulmonary vascular resistance may be induced by the known stimulators of pulmonary hypertension, which include hypoxia, acidosis, hypothermia, and

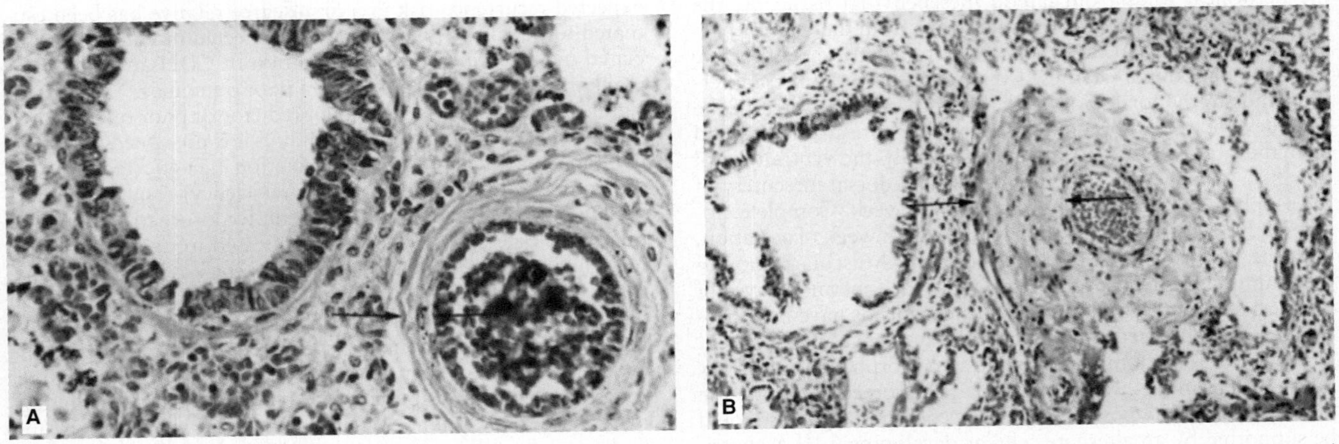

FIGURE 106.21. Histology of pulmonary arteries. Pulmonary artery branches of similar size and location are shown in a normal infant (A) and in an infant with Bochdalek diaphragmatic hernia (B). There is increased muscle mass associated with the arterial wall in (B) (*arrows*). This vascular smooth muscle is exquisitely sensitive to chemical, hormonal, and paracrine mediators in the neonatal period. Pulmonary arterial vasospasm is an important cause of persistent fetal circulation and respiratory failure. Treatment of pulmonary hypertension is the primary objective in the immediate care of the newborn with congenital diaphragmatic hernia.

stress. Alternations in the levels of prostaglandins, leukotrienes, catecholamines, and the renin angiotensin system had been implicated as mediators of this complex process. The combination of hypoplastic lungs and lungs prone toward increased vascular resistance often proves to be deadly: A vicious cycle may ensue in which hypoplastic lungs and associated hypoxia leads to pulmonary hypertension in a lung vasculature already prone toward reactive vasospasm. The increase in pulmonary pressures results in a greater shunt, which in turn further reduces oxygen levels.

Diagnosis

The diagnosis of CDH is often made on a prenatal ultrasound examination, although studies have shown that up to 60% of routine ultrasounds may fail to demonstrate a diaphragmatic hernia.[134] Polyhydramnios is common. Prenatal MRI evaluation is being now used routinely when obstetric sonography has detected a complex fetal anomaly and is ideally suited for fetuses with CDH.[135,136] After birth, the spectrum of respiratory symptoms in an infant with CDH is determined by the degree of pulmonary hypoplasia and reactive pulmonary hypertension. Severely affected infants develop respiratory distress at birth, and most demonstrate respiratory symptoms within the first 24 hours of life. On physical examination, these infants have a scaphoid abdomen. A plain chest radiograph that demonstrates loops of intestines in the chest confirms the diagnosis of a CDH (Fig. 106.22). The location of the stomach is confirmed by placement of a nasogastric tube and may be predictive of survival.[125] The chest radiograph shows

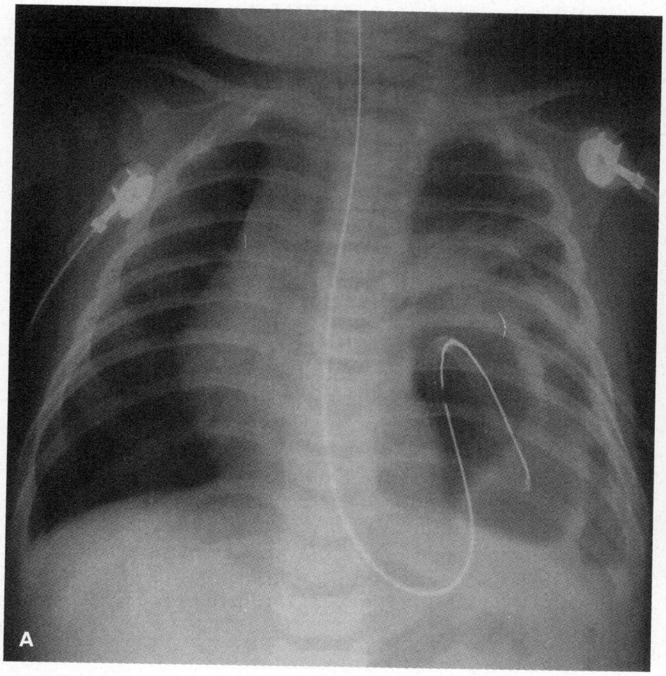

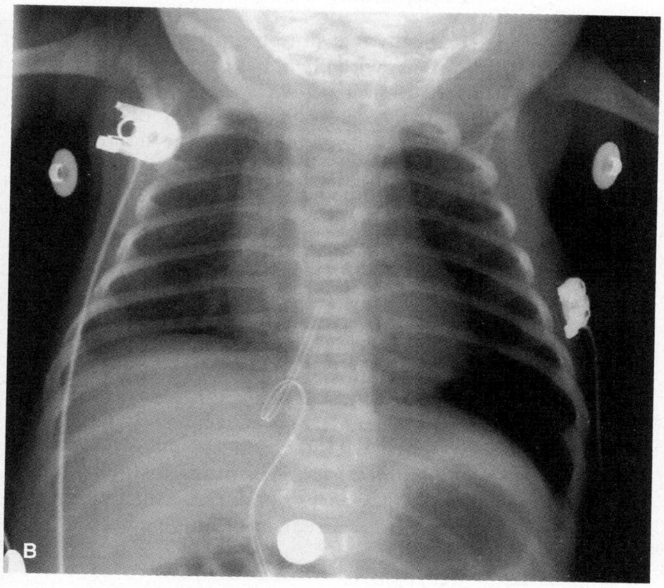

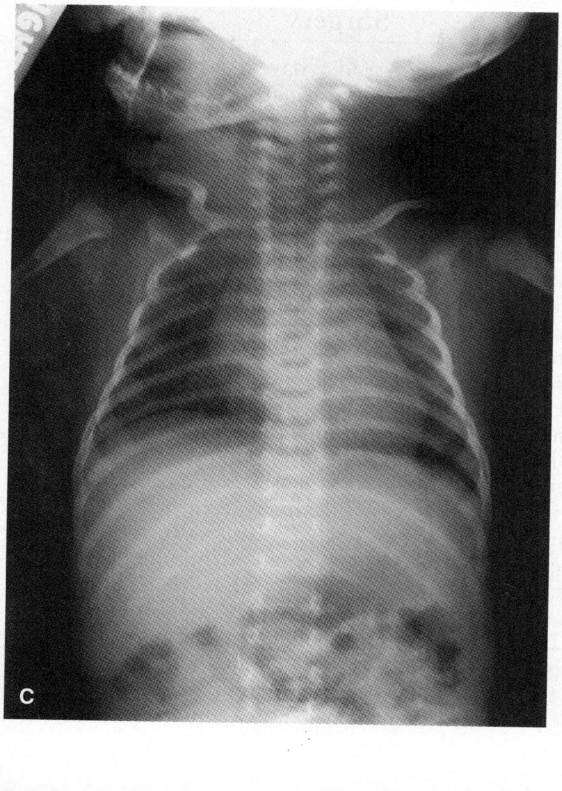

FIGURE 106.22. A: Chest radiograph of a newborn with a left congenital diaphragmatic hernia. Mediastinal structures are shifted to the right. Abdominal viscera occupy the left hemithorax. The nasogastric tube locates the stomach. The child underwent repair of the congenital diaphragmatic hernia after treatment and resolution of pulmonary hypertension. **B:** Immediate postoperative photograph demonstrates return of mediastinal structures to a more normal position. The hypoplastic left lung is apparent. **C:** Chest x-ray 1 month later is unremarkable.

angulation of the mediastinum and a shifting of the cardiac silhouette into the contralateral thorax. Chest radiographs are unreliable for estimating the degree of pulmonary hypoplasia. Once the diagnosis of a CDH is confirmed, additional radiographic and ultrasonographic examination should be carried out to search for associated anomalies. Echocardiography should also be obtained. Diagnosis is made in 10% to 20% of infants after the first day of life. The diagnosis of a CDH can be confused with a number of other congenital thoracic conditions, including eventration of the diaphragm, anterior diaphragmatic hernia of Morgagni, congenital cystic disease of the pulmonary parenchyma, unilateral pulmonary effusion, and primary agenesis of the lung.[137]

Prognostic Factors

Attempts to define clinically relevant prognostic factors to predict the outcome of infants with CDH have largely been unsuccessful. A prenatal anatomic parameter that appears to have predictive correlation is the determination of the lung to head ratio. The ratio is determined by multiplying the simultaneous sonographic measurements of size of the contralateral lung in an anteroposterior and lateromedial direction and dividing that multiple by the head circumference. Ratios less than 1.0 have been associated with poor outcomes.[138–141] Anatomic factors such as the position of the stomach either above or below the diaphragmatic rim and the size of the diaphragmatic defect itself are also predictive of outcome. In fact, the CDH Registry suggests that the most powerful predictors of outcome are the presence of cardiac defects and the need for reconstruction of the diaphragm with a patch that serves as a surrogate for defect size.[142] Physiologic parameters have been difficult to define and are limited to variations of arterial blood gas analyses, such as whether blood was obtained before or after treatment intervention and whether the blood was obtained preductal or postductal. MRI has allowed measurement of lung volume, which may be predictive of outcome.[143]

Treatment

The fetus and mother should be referred to an appropriate tertiary perinatal center where the full array of respiratory care strategies including inhaled nitric oxide (iNO), oscillating ventilators, and ECMO are immediately available. Anything less may potentially compromise the best possible outcome. A spontaneous vaginal delivery is preferred unless obstetric issues
13 supervene. CDH is a physiologic emergency and not a surgical emergency. The respiratory distress associated with a CDH in newborn infants results from a combination of uncorrectable pulmonary hypoplasia and potentially reversible pulmonary hypertension. The balance between these two factors determines the response to therapy and ultimately the outcome.

Resuscitation should begin with standard Neonatal Resuscitation Program guidelines and then proceed with endotracheal intubation and nasogastric tube insertion. Bag-mask ventilation is discouraged to avoid distention of the stomach and intestines that may be in the thoracic cavity. Meticulous attention must be paid to maintaining proper temperature regulation, glucose homeostasis, and volume status in the neonate. Systemic hypotension and inadequate tissue perfusion may be reversed with intravenous fluid administration including crystalloid, blood products, and colloid. Inotropic drugs such as dopamine or dobutamine may be required. Most infants can be successfully managed with a simple pressure-cycled ventilator with the goal of ventilatory support being a preductal p_aO_2 greater than 60 (S_aO_2 90% to 100%) with a corresponding p_aCO_2 of less than 60.[144,145] The extremes of hyperventilation, particularly with high rates and high ventilatory pressures, should be avoided to prevent ventilator-induced lung injury. If conventional mechanical ventilatory techniques cannot reverse the hypoxemia or hypercarbia, then high-frequency techniques using either the jet ventilator or the oscillating ventilator may be tried, although there are little data to suggest that these approaches are effective.

A broad spectrum of drugs and antihypertensive agents have been used in attempts to modify the pulmonary vascular resistance in infants with CDH and respiratory failure. Agents such as tolazoline (α-receptor blocker) have had marginal benefit in CDH infants. Other drugs, such as nitroprusside, isoproterenol, nitroglycerin, and captopril, have not been effective. The administration of various prostaglandin derivatives, including prostaglandin D_2 (PGD_2), prostaglandin 1 (PGE_1), and prostacyclin as well as the cyclo-oxygenase inhibitor indomethacin has also been disappointingly unsuccessful. Clinical and experimental studies have demonstrated surfactant deficiencies in infants with CDH. A multicenter review of surfactant administration in CDH patients showed no overall benefit to its use and demonstrated a lower survival rate in preterm infants compared to full-term infants.[146] At this time, there is no clinical data to support the administration of surfactant in the management of CDH infants. The combined administration of thyrotropin-releasing hormone and glucocorticoid therapy has been demonstrated to have positive effects on lung maturity.[147] However, a multicenter trial of prenatal steroid administration in fetuses with CDH failed to demonstrate enhanced lung function or survival.[148] Nitric oxide (NO) is a potent mediator of vasodilatation and particularly suited for administration to the pulmonary vasculature using inhalation techniques. It has been shown to be effective in improving oxygen saturation levels in neonates with respiratory failure due to prematurity and persistent pulmonary hypertension of the newborn. Unfortunately, its effects in CDH infants with respiratory failure have been disappointing. In fact, a multicenter trial of iNO in newborns with CDH suggested that the need for ECMO was increased in the iNO when compared to controls.[149] As a result, iNO should only be used as a temporizing measure in the deteriorating newborn with CDH.[150] Patients who do not respond to conventional treatments, HFOV, and NO are considered for ECMO treatment (see below).

Surgery

Multiple single-institution studies have reported improved survival rates with delayed surgery as part of their treatment protocols, while others have found no changes in overall outcome. No study has shown a decrease in survival rates with this technique.[151] Although delayed surgical repair is now widely practiced, there is no statistical evidence that supports this approach over immediate repair.[152] What the data does suggest, however, is that immediate repair does not show benefit over delayed repair.

The diaphragm defect is usually approached through a subcostal incision, although the repair can be performed through a thoracotomy incision (Fig. 106.23). Both thoracoscopic and laparoscopic techniques have been used to repair these defects, although the majority of surgeons tend to use a thoracoscopic approach because of the domain in the chest created by reducing the viscera into the abdomen.[153] Minimally invasive techniques may have a higher incidence of physiologic consequences in the newborn, specifically hypercarbia.[154] However, recent studies have demonstrated advances in the ability to close the larger defects that prevented minimally invasive repair of the diaphragm.[155] Once the abdominal contents are reduced, the defect in the diaphragm in the posterolateral position can be examined. In some patients, a hernia sac formed by parietal pleura and peritoneum is present and must be excised. Usually, there is an anterior rim of diaphragm of varying size, while the posterior rim must be exposed in the retroperitoneal

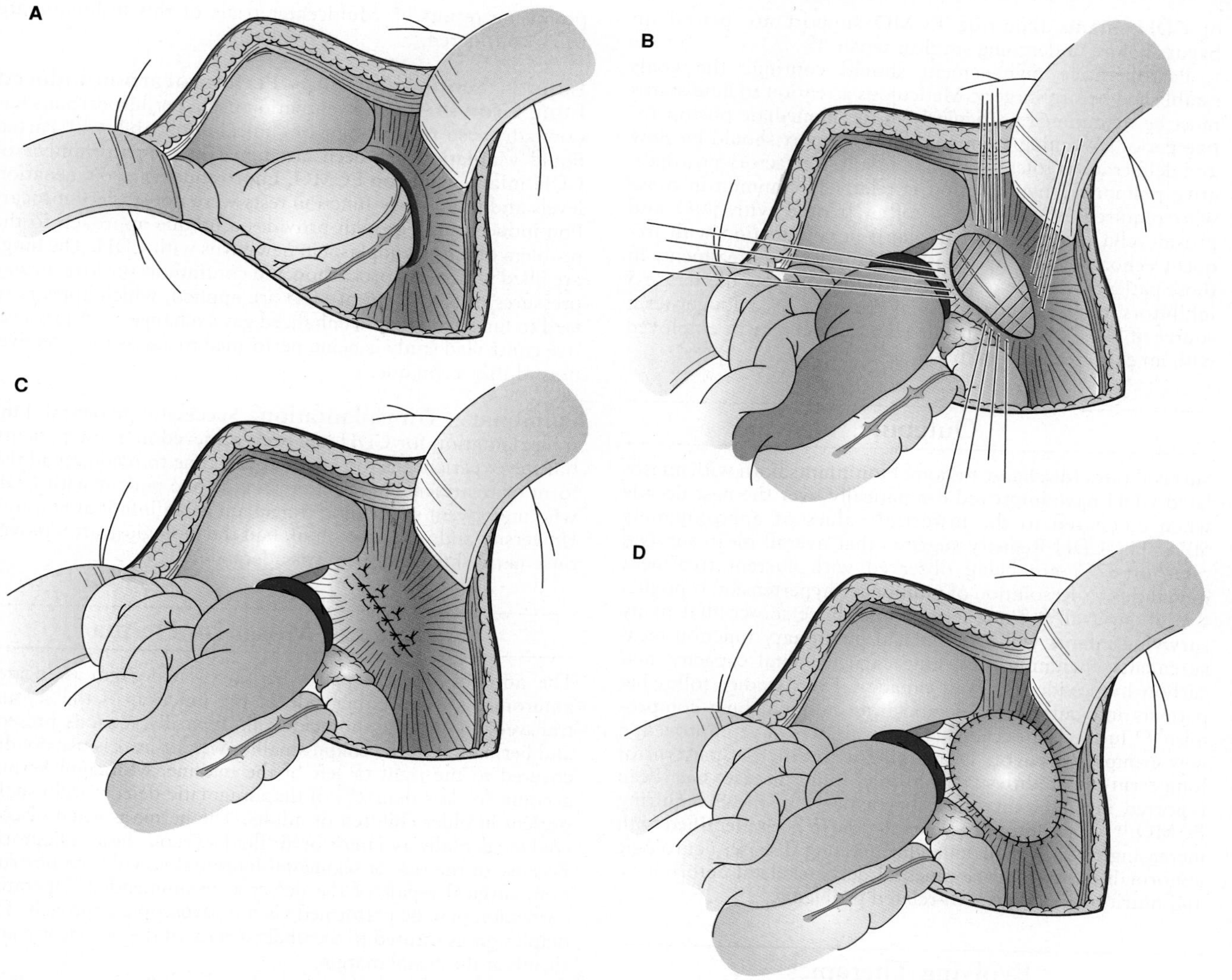

FIGURE 106.23. Repair of a congenital diaphragmatic hernia (CDH). A: Operative appearance of CDH. B: Placement of sutures for repair of a typical left posterolateral diaphragmatic defect. C: Completed repair. D: Prosthetic material may be used for large defects to avoid tension. (Adapted from Stollar CJH. Congenital diaphragmatic hernia. In: Spitz L, Coran AG, eds. *Rob and Smith's Operative Surgery: Pediatric Surgery.* 5th ed. London: Chapman and Hall; 1995.)

tissue. When diaphragmatic tissue is adequate, a primary repair with nonabsorbable suture material can be performed. If the defect is too large to be closed in a primary fashion, a number of reconstructive techniques have been described using rib structures and abdominal wall muscle flaps. The use of prosthetic material, such as Goretex, to complete the diaphragmatic closure has gained widespread acceptance. A floppy, tensionfree diaphragmatic repair can be accomplished that may lessen the degree of intra-abdominal pressure when closing the abdominal wall. The major drawback to using a prosthetic patch closure is the risk of infection as well as the risk of reherniation, which occurs in nearly 25% of patients with a patch repair. It has been suggested that the innervated latissimus dorsi muscle can be used to reconstruct the diaphragm in the setting of recurrence.[153] Tissue engineering may offer new materials for repair.[156]

With the loss of intra-abdominal domain, abdominal wall closure may not be possible. In this situation, simple closure of the skin can be accomplished with prosthetic patch repair of the ventral wall. If increased abdominal pressures inhibit respiratory mechanics, a silo abdominal apparatus has been used effectively.[157] A tube thoracostomy may be placed, although many surgeons find this unnecessary. The tube thoracostomy is of advantage in the nearly 30% of patients who develop chylothorax following diaphragmatic repair. The cause of frequent chylothorax is unclear and may require maintaining the patient as NPO (nothing by mouth), performance of pleurectomy, or ligation of the thoracic duct.[158]

ECMO is a form of partial cardiopulmonary bypass with the goal of maintaining oxygen delivery to the body for an extended period of time when ventilator therapy has failed. It has become the cornerstone for managing infants who have life-threatening respiratory failure with CDH.[159] ECMO allows respiratory support without the risks of barotrauma and oxygen toxicity associated with conventional ventilation. Initially, infants were placed on ECMO after developing respiratory failure following the immediate repair of the diaphragmatic defect. With the evolution of delayed surgical repair, ECMO is now considered a part of the preoperative stabilization process. Failure to improve in the setting of severe pulmonary hypertension and progressive hypoxemia despite maximum medical intervention remains a valid qualifying criterion for ECMO support. As a result of the acceptance of delayed surgical repair as a treatment strategy, more than 90%

of CDH infants requiring ECMO support are placed on bypass before undergoing surgical repair.[160]

Postoperative management should continue the goals established before surgery. Meticulous attention to fluid status must be maintained particularly in the immediate postoperative period. Weaning from ventilator support should be slow and deliberate as tolerated by the infant. Refractory postoperative pulmonary hypertension is relatively common in those who required ECMO and is often treated with iNO and prostacyclin (epoprostenol [Flolan]) in conjunction with frequent echocardiography to assess the effect of treatment. In those patients who are responsive to iNO, phosphodiesterase-5 inhibitors such as sildanefil may be used as a longer-term source of NO.[161] A second course on ECMO may be employed with an expected survival of 47%.[162]

Outcome

Survival rates (discharge to home) for infants born with an isolated CDH have improved dramatically over the past decade when compared to the historical values of approximately 50%. The CDH Registry suggests that overall mean survival rates of 67% are being observed with current treatment modalities.[163] Resolution of pulmonary hypertension is predictive of survival.[164] Long-term studies have shown that many surviving infants will have normal pulmonary function measurements, including total lung capacity, vital capacity, and carbon monoxide diffusing capacity. Even studies following patients into adulthood demonstrate minimal lung compromise.[165] In the last decade, as survival rates have improved, a new group of survivors is emerging with different patterns of long-term morbidities.[166] Chronic lung disease has been reported in CDH survivors, particularly in those requiring ECMO.[167] Long-term problems that have been identified with increasing frequency include chronic lung disease, neurologic abnormalities with developmental delay, skeletal deformities, and nutritional and growth-related problems.

Evolving Therapies

Even with the increasing success of current treatment strategies such as permissive hypercapnea, delayed surgery, antihypertensive pharmacology, and advanced ventilatory techniques, a cohort of infants refractory to these interventions continue to be candidates for novel treatments.

In Utero Repair of Diaphragmatic Hernia. The concept of fetal surgical intervention evolved from the experimental observation in lambs that reduction of compressive forces on the lung resulted in continued pulmonary growth and development.[168] Although technically and theoretically exciting, the clinical results have been disappointing.[169,170] A direct advancement of these initial attempts at in utero repair was the observation that fetal tracheal ligation accelerated fetal lung growth and reversed pulmonary hypoplasia.[171,172] Tracheal occlusion or PLUG therapy (plug the lung until it grows) resulted in improved oxygenation and ventilation after birth when compared to untreated control animals.[173] A randomized clinical trial comparing fetal endoscopic tracheal occlusion to current standard postnatal care for severe CDH showed no benefit in survival.[174] Early-onset labor was a major problem for both trials studying in utero CDH repair and in utero tracheal ligation. In fact, the early delivery of fetuses in the treatment arm may have masked evidence of benefit for either approach. European centers have been applying transuterine fetal bronchoscopy at 26 weeks gestation with balloon tracheal ligation followed by removal of the balloon at 34 weeks. This minimally invasive approach has decreased the incidence of early delivery and has been used extensively with promising results.[175] Multicenter trials of this technique are being considered.

Liquid Ventilation and Perfluorocarbon-induced Lung Growth. Liquid ventilation using perflurocarbons has now advanced to the point of clinical applicability.[176] Partial liquid ventilation has been attempted in a small number of CDH infants while on ECMO. Improvements in oxygenation levels and pulmonary function tests were noted. Perfluorocarbon-induced lung growth provides a unique approach to the problem of lung hypoplasia in newborns with CDH. The lungs are filled with perfluorocarbon and continuous positive airway pressures of 5 to 8 cm of H_2O are applied, which appears to lead to lung growth and enhanced gas exchange.[177] A prospective controlled study is being performed to assess the effectiveness of this technique.

Pulmonary Transplantation. Successful neonatal lung transplantation for CDH has been achieved in a few patients, but the experience is too small at this time to recommend this form of treatment. Most interesting is one patient with CDH who underwent single lung transplant as an infant at Stanford University and who, as a child, had the biologic graft removed once native lung function was adequate.[178]

Foramen of Morgagni Hernia

The anterior diaphragmatic hernia of Morgagni is located anteromedially on either side of the junction of the septum transversum and the thoracic wall. Typically, a sac is present, and herniation of the colon, small bowel, or liver is usually discovered to the right or left of the midline. Morgagni hernias account for less than 2% of diaphragmatic defects and usually present in older children or adults. The hernia is often discovered incidentally as a mass or air fluid level on chest radiograph. Because of the risk of segmental intestinal volvulus or obstruction, surgical repair of the defect is recommended. Operative correction may be performed via a laparoscopic approach. The diaphragm is sutured to the undersurface of the posterior rectus sheath at the costal margin.

Eventration of the Diaphragm

Eventration of the diaphragm may be either congenital or acquired. The congenital form may be indistinguishable from a diaphragmatic hernia with a sac, and symptoms are similar, although the presentation is typically clinically less severe. The acquired form is due to paralysis of the phrenic nerve. The phrenic nerve is vulnerable to surgical trauma from a wide variety of cervical, thoracic, and diaphragmatic procedures. Phrenic nerve injuries and a variety of neuromuscular disorders including primary myopathies and degenerative diseases may produce diaphragmatic paralysis and require operative plication of the diaphragm in infants and young children. The most common cause of phrenic nerve injury in children is associated with thoracic and mediastinal surgery. Cervical stretching at birth may result in phrenic nerve injury. The diaphragmatic muscle is usually present in its normal distribution but is attenuated and nonfunctional. When an acquired nerve palsy is present, initial treatment may be expectant.

An eventration may be completely asymptomatic and noted only on chest x-ray. Clinical findings may range from mild respiratory compromise with wheezing, frequent respiratory infections, and exercise intolerance to extreme respiratory distress. Diagnosis is usually made by fluoroscopic examination of the chest with examination of diaphragmatic motion. In such cases, the diaphragm moves paradoxically with respiration. A small or asymptomatic eventration may be left untreated and observed. It has been postulated that an eventration that involves a large area of the diaphragm may adversely affect pulmonary function and lung growth and should be repaired. However, there are no long-term data assessing the effect of an asymptomatic, high-riding diaphragm on future lung function. Under most circumstances where the respiratory status of the infant remains compromised, surgical intervention should be considered. Repair may be either through the abdomen or the chest, but in most cases a thoracoscopic approach is preferred.[179] The diaphragm is plicated with nonabsorbable sutures placed in an anteroposterior orientation. The redundant diaphragmatic tissue is reefed up until it is taut.

Diaphragm Pacing

Ventilator-dependent children with spinal cord injury or central hypoventilation syndromes may benefit from diaphragm pacing.[180] The application of repetitive stimulus patterns to the phrenic nerves causes rhythmic contractions of the diaphragm. Phrenic nerve pacing wires are implanted at the cervical or intrathoracic level. Receivers are implanted in subcutaneous pockets, while an external microprocessor-controlled transmitter/antenna assembly activates the receiver. Patients with injured phrenic nerves (high spinal cord injury) may benefit from diaphragm pacing after intercostal to phrenic nerve transfer.[181]

PLEURAL DISEASES

Empyema

Empyema is an accumulation of purulent material within the pleural space. In children, empyema occurs most often as a sequelae of bacterial pneumonia. Empyema develops when a parapneumonic effusion becomes infected or necrotizing pneumonia erodes through the lung into the pleural space. Empyema may also develop after penetrating thoracic trauma, intrathoracic or cervical esophageal perforation, or surgery on the chest. Empyema is divided into three stages:

- *Exudative:* Thin free-flowing fluid with a low cell count
- *Fibrinopurulent:* Thick purulent material resulting in multiple loculations and encasement of the lung parenchyma
- *Organizing:* Fibroblasts that have grown into the exudate and have produced a fibrotic peel

Haemophilus influenzae, *Streptococcus pneumoniae*, and *Staphylococcus aureus* are the most common pathogens in pediatric pneumonia, with anaerobes, gram-negative bacteria, and atypical organisms also being occasionally found. The signs and symptoms of an empyema in a child are usually those of worsening pneumonia with fever, tachypnea, shortness of breath, and sometimes cyanosis. Abdominal pain with distention and ileus may intensify the respiratory difficulty.

Diagnosis is confirmed by the presence of pleural fluid and loculation on conventional chest radiographs (Fig. 106.24A). CT scan of the chest cavity is the best method of determining the extent of loculated effusion and underlying parenchymal involvement (Fig. 106.24B).

When a small parapneumonic effusion develops, it may resolve with antibiotics alone. Larger effusions will require adequate pleural space drainage with a tube thoracostomy in addition to antibiotic therapy. It is reasonable to place the thoracostomy tube in the operating room and, at the same time, perform thoracoscopic decortication/pneumolysis and pleural debridement along with evacuation of loculated pleural fluid. This video-assisted thoracoscopic surgery (VATS) approach has proven to be very effective in the treatment of pediatric empyema, shortening hospitalization and resulting in more rapid recovery[182,183] (Fig. 106.24C,D).

Instillation of intrapleural streptokinase or urokinase also has been utilized for loculated effusions. In fact, a randomized controlled study of VATS versus tissue plasminogen activator therapy with thoracostomy tube drainage demonstrated a reduction in cost with tissue plasminogen activator treatment with equivalent efficacy.[184]

Pneumothorax

Spontaneous pneumothorax is seen in previously healthy older children and teenagers who are usually tall and thin. They often have apical blebs seen on chest radiographs. CT scanning is more sensitive to detect bleb disease, but is not necessary prior to operation. Pneumothorax may also complicate advanced pulmonary disease due to cystic fibrosis. Other causes include both blunt and penetrating thoracic trauma, severe asthmatic attack, or pulmonary infection. The classic presentation of a spontaneous pneumothorax is the sudden onset of chest pain and shortness of breath.

Diagnosis is best confirmed by chest radiograph. In patients with significant symptoms, tube thoracostomy should be immediately performed and the chest tube placed to water seal suction drainage.

Recurrent pneumothoraces can be treated nonoperatively with the intrapleural instillation of various sclerosing agents such as talc or tetracycline through the chest tube. Patients with recurrent pneumothorax and apical blebs are treated with bleb removal and pleurodesis. The blebs will be found at the apex of the upper lobe or at the apex of the superior segment of the lower lobe. Excision of the blebs and pleurodesis may be performed through a VATS approach.[185]

Chylothorax

In the newborn, chylothorax may occur in association with manipulation during a difficult delivery as a result of congenial diaphragmatic hernia repair, from a malformation of the thoracic duct, or spontaneously without an obvious cause. In older infants and children, cardiothoracic procedures can be complicated by postoperative chylothorax in 0.5% of the cases. The thoracic duct has also been known to rupture during violent bouts of coughing or with hyperextension of the spine. Obstruction or erosion of the duct may occur as a result of malignant disease within the mediastinum such as lymphoma. Other causes include inflammatory processes, subclavian vein or superior vena caval thrombosis, and misplaced central venous devices.

A defect in the lower portion of the duct frequently results in an effusion into the right pleural space, while an effusion on the left results from a defect in the upper region of the duct. Clinically, the patient presents with a large pleural effusion resulting in pulmonary compression, mediastinal displacement, and the progressive development of respiratory distress. Radiographs will generally show a massive effusion on the evolved side. The diagnosis should be suspected at the initial thoracentesis with the retrieval of milky, lipid-laden fluid. Laboratory values will confirm a chylothorax if a pleural fluid cell count differential is greater than 90% lymphocytes, which is the primary means of diagnosis in patients who are not being fed.

Initial treatment consists of tube thoracostomy for evacuation of the chylous fluid and expansion of the collapsed lung. Minimizing the flow of lymph within the thoracic duct by placing the patient on complete bowel rest using parenteral nutrition has been shown to permit healing of the thoracic duct lymph fistula over time. With newborns, spontaneous chylothorax usually ceases spontaneously with adequate drainage. If the chylothorax persists, fluid and protein losses may complicate the management of the newborn with chylothorax and predispose the patient to sepsis. As such, if no

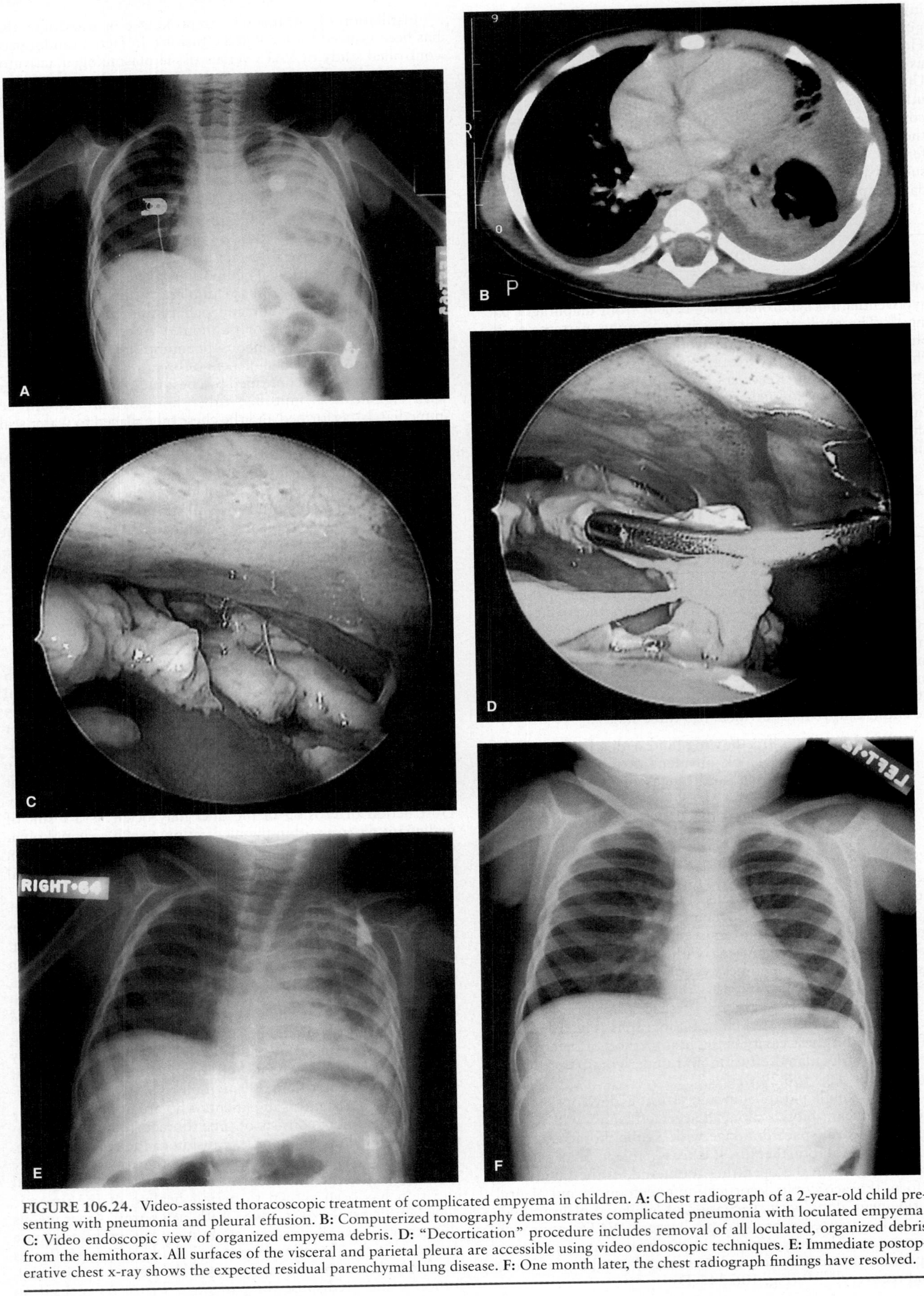

FIGURE 106.24. Video-assisted thoracoscopic treatment of complicated empyema in children. **A:** Chest radiograph of a 2-year-old child presenting with pneumonia and pleural effusion. **B:** Computerized tomography demonstrates complicated pneumonia with loculated empyema. **C:** Video endoscopic view of organized empyema debris. **D:** "Decortication" procedure includes removal of all loculated, organized debris from the hemithorax. All surfaces of the visceral and parietal pleura are accessible using video endoscopic techniques. **E:** Immediate postoperative chest x-ray shows the expected residual parenchymal lung disease. **F:** One month later, the chest radiograph findings have resolved.

improvement is noted after a brief period of conservative therapy, then surgical intervention should be considered. Through either an open thoracotomy or with video-assisted thoracoscopy, the surgical therapy involves ligation of the thoracic duct just above the diaphragm within the right chest. This goal can be accomplished with surgical ligation, direct clipping, the use of fibrin glue, and pleurodesis. Administration of cream via a nasogastric tube in the hours prior to operation may make identification of the thoracic duct and an associated leak more obvious. For intractable conditions, unilateral or bilateral pleurectomy may be effective. Pleural peritoneal shunting can also be considered. Octreotide is of questionable value in the treatment of postoperative chylothorax.[186]

References

1. Sadler TW. Embryology of the sternum. *Chest Surg Clin N Am* 2000; 10(2):237–244.
2. Kowalewski J, Brocki M, Dryjanski T, et al. Pectus excavatum: increase of right ventricular systolic, diastolic, and stroke volumes after surgical repair. *J Thorac Cardiovasc Surg* 1999;118(1):87–93.
3. Shamberger RC. Congenital chest wall deformities. In: O'Neill JA Jr, Rowe MI, Grosfeld JL, et al, eds. *Pediatric Surgery*. 5th ed. St. Louis, MO: Mosby; 1998.
4. Sigalet DL, Montgomery M, Harder J. Cardiopulmonary effects of closed repair of pectus excavatum. *J Pediatr Surg* 2003;38(3):380–385.
5. Shamberger RC. Cardiopulmonary effects of anterior chest wall deformities. *Chest Surg Clin N Am* 2000;10(2):245–252.
6. Malek MH, Fonkalsrud EW, Cooper CB. Ventilatory and cardiovascular responses to exercise in patients with pectus excavatum. *Chest* 2003;124(3):870–882.
7. Haller JA Jr, Scherer LR, Turner CS, et al. Evolving management of pectus excavatum based on a single institutional experience of 664 patients. *Ann Surg* 1989;209:578–582.
8. Haller JA Jr, Colombani PM, Humphries CT, et al. Chest wall constriction after too extensive and too early operations for pectus excavatum. *Ann Thorac Surg* 1996;61(6):1618–1625.
9. Robicsek F, Rokin AA. How not to do it; restrictive thoracic dystrophy after pectus excavatum repair. *Interact Cardiovasc Thorac Surg* 2004;3(4): 566–568.
10. Ravitch MM. The chest wall. In: Welch KJ, Randolph JG, Ravitch MM, et al, eds. *Pediatric Surgery*. 4th ed. Chicago: Year Book.
11. Swanson JW, Colombani PM. Reactive pectus carinatum in patients treated for pectus excavatum. *J Pediatr Surg* 2008;43(8):1468–1473.
12. Nuss D, Kelly RE Jr, Croitoru DP, et al. A 10-year review of a minimally invasive technique for the correction of pectus excavatum. *J Pediatr Surg* 1998;33(4):545–552.
13. Croitoru DP, Kelly RE Jr, Goretsky MJ, et al. Experience and modification update for the minimally invasive Nuss technique for pectus excavatum repair in 303 patients. *J Pediatr Surg* 2002;37(3):437–445.
14. Moss RL, Albanese CT, Reynolds M. Major complications after minimally invasive repair of pectus excavatum: case reports. *J Pediatr Surg* 2001; 36(1):155–158.
15. Hendrickson RJ, Bensard DD, Janik JS, et al. Efficacy of left thoracoscopy and blunt mediastinal dissection during Nuss procedure for pectus excavatum. *J Pediatr Surg* 2005;40(8):1312–1314.
16. De Ugarte DA, Choi E, Fonkalsrud EW. Repair of recurrent pectus deformities. *Am Surg* 2002;68(12):1075–1079.
17. Horch RE, Springer O. Minimally-invasive endoscopic correction of funnel chest deformity via an umbilical incision. *Aesthetic Plast Surg* 2002; 26(4):295–298.
18. Marks MW, Iacobucci J. Reconstruction of congenital chest wall deformities using solid silicone onlay prostheses. *Chest Surg Clin N Am* 2000; 10(2):341–355.
19. Schier F, Bahr M, Klobe E. The vacuum chest wall lifter: an innovative, nonsurgical addition to the management of pectus excavatum. *J Pediatr Surg* 2005;40(3):496–500.
20. Harrison MR, Estefan-Ventura D, Fechter R, et al. Magnetic mini-mover procedure for pectus excavatum: I. Development, design, and simulations for feasibility and safety. *J Pediatr Surg* 2007;42(1):81–85; discussion 85–86.
21. Martinez-Ferro M, Fraine C, Benard S. Dynamic compression system for correction of pectus carinatum. *Semin Pediatr Surg* 2008;17(3):194–200.
22. Abramson H, D'Agostino J, Wuscovi S. A five-year experience with a minimally invasive technique for pectus carinatum repair. *J Pediatr Surg* 2009;44(1):118–123; discussion 123–124.
23. Borshcel GH, Costantino DA, Cederna PS. Individualized implant-based reconstruction of Poland syndrome breast and soft tissue deformities. *Ann Plast Surg* 2007;59(5):507–514.
24. Mogilner J, Siplovich L, Bar-Ziv J, et al. Surgical management of the cleft sternum. *J Pediatr Surg* 1998;23(10):889–891.
25. Hell AK, Campbell RM, Hefti F. The vertical expandable prosthetic titanium rib implant for the treatment of thoracic insufficiency syndrome associated with congenital and neuromuscular scoliosis in young children. *J Pediatr Orthop B* 2005;14(4):287–293.
26. Luck SR, Reynolds M, Raffensperger JG. *Current Problems in Surgery*. Chicago, IL: Year Book Medical Publishers, Inc.; 1986.
27. Coran AG, Drongowski R. Congenital cystic disease of the tracheobronchial tree in infants and children. *Arch Surg* 1994;129:521–527.
28. Conran RM, Stocker JT. Extralobar sequestration with frequently associated congenital cystic adenomatoid malformation, type 2: report of 50 cases. *Pediatr Dev Pathol* 1999;2(5):454–463.
29. Gross E, Chen MK, Lobe TE, et al. Infradiaphragmatic extralobar pulmonary sequestration masquerading as an intra-abdominal, suprarenal mass. *Pediatr Surg Int* 1997;12(7):529–531.
30. Capizzani TR, Hirenkumar P, Hines MH, et al. A unique case of a giant congenital pulmonary hemangioma in a newborn. *J Pediatr Surg* 2008; 43(3):574–578.
31. Jesch NK, Leonhardt J, Sumpelmann R, et al. Thoracoscopic resection of intra- and extralobar pulmonary sequestration in the first 3 months of life. *J Pediatr Surg* 2005;40(9):1404–1406.
32. Stocker JT, Madewell JE, Drake RM. Congenital cystic adenomatoid malformation of the lung: classification and morphologic spectrum. *Hum Pathol* 1977;8:155–171.
33. Azizkhan RG, Crombleholme TM. Congenital cystic lung disease: contemporary antenatal and postnatal management. *Pediatr Surg Int* 2008; 24:643–657.
34. Adzick NS, Flake AW, Crombleholme TM. Management of congenital lung lesions. *Semin Pediatr Surg* 2003;12(1):10–16.
35. Adzick NS, Harrison MR, Crombleholme TM, et al. Fetal lung lesions: management and outcome. *Am J Obstet Gynecol* 1998;179(4):884–889.
36. Kunisaki SM, Barnewolt CE, Estroff JA, et al. Large fetal congenital cystic adenomatoid malformations: growth trends and patient survival. *J Pediatr Surg* 2007;42(2):404–410.
37. Marwan A, Crombleholme TM. The EXIT procedure: principles, pitfalls, and progress. *Semin Pediatr Surg* 2006;15(2):107–115.
38. Van Leeuwen K, Teitelbaum DH, Hirschl RB, et al. Prenatal diagnosis of congenital cystic adenomatoid malformation and its postnatal presentation, surgical indications, and natural history. *J Pediatr Surg* 1999;34(5): 794–798.
39. Aspirot A, Puligandla PS, Bouchard S, et al. A contemporary evaluation of surgical outcome in neonates and infants undergoing lung resection. *J Pediatr Surg* 2008;43:508–512.
40. Yan-Sin A, Jones S. Lack of consensus among Canadian pediatric surgeons regarding the management of congenital cystic adenomatoid malformation of the lung. 2008;43(5):797–799.
41. Vu LT, Farmer DL, Nobuhara KK, et al. Thoracoscopic versus open resection for congenital cystic adenomatoid malformations of the lung. 2008; 43(1)35–39.
42. Mentzer SJ, Filler RM, Phillips J. Limited pulmonary resections for congenital cystic adenomatoid malformation of the lung. *J Pediatr Surg* 1992; 27(11):1410–1413.
43. Merry C, Spurbeck W, Lobe TE. Resection of foregut-derived duplications by minimal-access surgery. *Pediatr Surg Int* 1999;15(3–4):224–226.
44. Dillon PW, Cilley RE, Krummel TM. Video-assisted thoracoscopic excision of intrathoracic masses in children: report of two cases. *Surg Laparosc Endosc* 1993;3:433–436.
45. Scully RE, Mark EJ, McNeely WF, et al. Case records of the Massachusetts General Hospital—Case 30–1997. *N Engl J Med* 1997;337(13):916–924.
46. Nuchtern JG, Harberg FJ. Congenital lung cysts. *Semin Pediatr Surg* 1994; 3(4):233–243.
47. Stigers KB, Woodring JH, Kanga JF. The clinical and imaging spectrum of findings in patients with congenital lobar emphysema. *Pediatr Pulmonol* 1992;14(3):160–170.
48. Karnak I, Senocak ME, Ciftci AO, et al. Congenital lobar emphpysema: diagnostic and therapeutic considerations. *J Pediatr Surg* 1999;34(9): 1347–1351.
49. Davenport M, Warne SA, Cacciaguerra S, et al. Current outcome of antenally diagnosed cystic lung disease. *J Pediatr Surg* 2004;39(4):549–556.
50. Okazaki T, Iwatani S, Yanai T, et al. Treatment of lymphangioma in children: our experience of 128 cases. *J Pediatr Surg* 2007;42(2):386–389.
51. Rothenberg SS. Thoracoscopy in infants and children. *Semin Pediatr Surg* 1998;7(4):194–201.
52. Black CT. Current recommendations for the resection of pulmonary metastases of pediatric malignancies. *Pediatr Pulmonol Suppl* 1997; 16:181.
53. Quaglia LA. The surgical management of metastases in pediatric cancer. *Semin Pediatr Surg* 1993;2:75–82.
54. Su WT, Chewning J, Abramson S, et al. Surgical management and outcome of osteosarcoma patients with unilateral pulmonary metastases. *J Pediatr Surg* 2004;39(3):418–423; discussion 418–423.
55. Ehrlich PF, Hamilton TE, Grundy P, et al. The value of surgery in directing therapy for patients with Wilms' tumor with pulmonary disease. A report from the National Wilms' Tumor Study Group (National Wilms' Tumor Study 5). *J Pediatr Surg* 2006;(41):162–167.
56. Hartman GE, Shochat SJ. Primary pulmonary neoplasms of childhood: a review. *Ann Thorac Surg* 1983;36(1):108–119.
57. Hancock BJ, DiLorenzo M, Youssef S, et al. Childhood primary pulmonary neoplasms. *J Pediatr Surg* 1993;28(9):1133–1136.
58. Weldon CB, Shamberger RC. Pediatric pulmonary tumors: primary and metastatic. *Semin Pediatr Surg* 2008;17:17–29.

59. Ohye RG, Cohen DM, Caldwell S, et al. Pediatric bronchioloalveolar carcinoma: a favorable pediatric malignancy? *J Pediatr Surg* 1998;33(5):730–732.
60. Granata C, Gambini C, Balducci T, et al. Bronchioloalveolar carcinoma arising in congenital cystic adenomatoid malformation in a child: a case report and review on malignancies originating in congenital cystic adenomatoid malformation. *Pediatr Pulmonol* 1998;25(1):62–66.
61. Mentzel T, Fletcher CDM. Recent advances in soft tissue tumor diagnosis. *Am J Clin Pathol* 1998;110:660–670.
62. Su W, Ko A, O'Connell TX, et al. Treatment of pseudotumors with nonsteroidal antiinflammatory drugs. *J Pediatr Surg* 2000;35(11):1635–1637.
63. Eggli KD, Newman B. Nodules, masses and pseudomasses in the pediatric lung. *Radiol Clin North Am* 1993;31:651.
64. Grosfeld JL, Skinner MA, Rescorla FJ, et al. Mediastinal tumors in children: experience with 196 cases. *Ann Surg Oncol* 1994;1:121–127.
65. Suita S, Tajiri T, Sera Y, et al. The characteristics of mediastinal neuroblastoma. *Eur J Pediatr Surg* 2000;10(6):353–359.
66. Petty JK, Bensard DD, Partrick DA, et al. Resection of neurogenic in children: is thoracoscopy superior to thoracotomy? *J Am Coll Surg* 2006;203(5):699–703.
67. Tonini GP, Lo Cunsolo C, Cusano R, et al. Loss of heterozygosity for chromosome 1P in familial neuroblastoma. *Eur J Cancer* 1997;33(12):1953–1956.
68. Glick RD, LaQuaglia MP. Lymphomas of the anterior mediastinum. *Semin Pediatr Surg* 1999;8(2):69–77.
69. Shamberger RC. Preanesthetic evaluation of children with anterior mediastinal masses. *Semin Pediatr Surg* 1999;8(2):61–68.
70. Takeda S, Miyoshi S, Omori K, et al. Surgical rescue for life-threatening hypoxemia caused by a mediastinal tumor. *Ann Thorac Surg* 1999;68(6):2324–2326.
71. Taneli C, Genc A, Erikci V, et al. Askin tumors in children: a report of four cases. *Eur J Pediatr Surg* 1998;8(5):312–314.
72. Sawin RS, Conrad EU III, Park JR, et al. Preresection chemotherapy improves survival for children with Askin tumors. *Arch Surg* 1996;131(8):877–880.
73. Kashima HK, Mounts P, Shah K. Recurrent respiratory papillomatosis. *Obstet Gynecol Clin North Am* 1996;131(8):877–880.
74. Armstrong LR, Derkay CS, Reeves WC. Initial results from the national registry for juvenile-onset recurrent respiratory papillomatosis. RRP Task Force. *Arch Otolaryngol Head Neck Surg* 1999;125(7):743–748.
75. Haight C, Towsley HA. Congenital atresia of the esophagus with tracheoesophageal fistula: extrapleural ligation of fistula and end-to-end anastomosis of esophageal segments. *Surg Gynecol Obstet* 1943;76:672–688.
76. Manning PB, Morgan RA, Coran AG, et al. Fifty years' experience with esophageal atresia and tracheoesophageal fistula. Beginning with Cameron Haight's first operation in 1935. *Ann Surg* 1986;204:446–451.
77. Lopez PJ, Keys C, Pierro A, et al. Oesophageal atresia: improved outcome in high risk group? *J Pediatr Surg* 2006;41(2):331–334.
78. Oi BQ, Beasley SW. Pathohistological study of adriamycin-induced tracheal agenesis in the fetal rat. *Pediatr Surg Int* 1999;15(1):17–20.
79. Possogel AK, Diez-Pardo JA, Morales C, et al. Embryology of esophageal atresia in the adriamycin rat model. *J Pediatr Surg* 1998;33(4):606–612.
80. Haight C. Congenital esophageal atresia and trachesophageal fistula. In: Mustard WT, Ravitch MM, Snyder WH Jr, et al, eds. *Pediatric Surgery*. Chicago, IL: Year Book Medical Publishers; 1969.
81. Gross RE. The surgery of infancy and childhood. Philadelphia, PA: WB Saunders; 1953.
82. Kluth D. Atlas of esophageal atresia. *J Pediatr Surg* 1976;11:901–919.
83. McMullen KP, Karnes PS, Moir CR, et al. Familial recurrence of tracheoesophageal fistula and associated malformations. *Am J Med Genet* 1996;63(4):525–528.
84. Filston HC, Chitwood WR Jr, Schkolne B, et al. The Fogarty balloon catheter as an aid to management of the infant with esophageal atresia and tracheoesophageal fistula complicated by severe RDS or pneumonia. *J Pediatr Surg* 1982;17(2):149–151.
85. Waterston DJ, Carter RE, Aberdeen E. Esophageal atresia: tracheo-oesophageal fistula. A study of survival in 218 infants. *Lancet* 1962;1:819–822.
86. Randolph JG, Newman KD, Anderson KD. Current results in repair of esophageal atresia with tracheoesophageal fistula using physiologic status as a guide to therapy. *Ann Surg* 1989;209:526–530.
87. Choudhury SR, Ashcraft KW, Sharp RJ, et al. Survival of patients with esophageal atresia: influence of birth weight, cardiac anomaly, and late respiratory complications. *J Pediatr Surg* 1999;34(1):70–74.
88. Dunn JC, Fonkalsrud EW, Atkinson JB. Simplifying the Waterston's stratification of infants with tracheoesophageal fistula. *Am Surg* 1999;65(10):908–910.
89. Deurloo JA, de Vos R, Ekkelkamp S, et al. Prognostic factors for mortality of oesophageal atresia patients: Waterston revived. *Eur J Pediatr* 2004;163:624–625.
90. Cilley RE, Dillon PW. Pulmonary resection and thoracotomy. In: Stringer MD, Oldham KT, Mouriquand PDE, eds. *Pediatric Surgery and Urology: Long-Term Outcomes*. London: WB Saunders Company Limited; 1998.
91. Foker JE, Kendall TC, Catton K, et al. A flexible approach to achieve a true primary repair for all infants with esophageal atresia. *Semin Pediatr Surg* 2005;14:8–15.
92. Spitz L, Kiely E, Pierro A. Gastric transposition in children—a 21-year experience. *J Pediatr Surg* 2004;39(3):276–281.
93. Puri P, Khurana S. Delayed primary esophageal anastomosis for pure esophageal atresia. *Semin Pediatr Surg* 1998;7(2):126–129.
94. Othersen HB Jr, Hebra A, Tagge EP. Esophageal replacement for atresia without fistula. *Semin Pediatr Surg* 1998;7(2):134–136.
95. Lobe TE, Rothenberg S, Waldschmidt J, et al. Thoracoscopic repair of esophageal atresia in an infant: a surgical first. *Pediatr Endosurg Innov Tech* 1999;3(3):141–148.
96. Rothenberg SS. Thoracoscopic repair of tracheoesophageal fistula in newborns. *J Pediatr Surg* 2002;37(6):869–872.
97. Holcomb GW III, Rothenberg SS, Bax KM, et al. Thoracoscopic repair of esophageal aresia and tracheoesophageal fistula: a multi-institutional analysis. *Ann Surg* 2005;242(3):422–428; discussion 428–430.
98. Delius RE, Wheatley MJ, Coran AG. Etiology and management of respiratory complications after repair of esophageal atresia with tracheoesophageal fistula. *Surgery* 1992;112(3):527–532.
99. Spitz L. Esophageal atresia: past, present, and future. *J Pediatr Surg* 1996;31(1):19–25.
100. Bouman NH, Koot HM, Hazebroek FW. Long-term physical, psychological, and social functioning of children with esophageal atresia. *J Pediatr Surg* 1999;34(3):399–404.
101. Tonz M, Kohli S, Kaiser G. Oesophageal atresia: what has changed in the last 3 decades? *Pediatr Surg Int* 2004;20(10):768–772.
102. Orford J, Cass DT, Glasson MJ. Advances in the treatment of oesophageal atresia over three decades: the 1970s and the 1990s. *Pediatr Surg Int* 2004;20(6):402–407.
103. Little DC, Rescorla FJ, Grosfeld JL, et al. Long-term analysis of children with esophageal atresia and tracheoesophageal fistula. *J Pediatr Surg* 2003;38(6):852–856.
104. Beasley SW. Esophageal atresia: surgical aspects. In: Stringer MD, Oldham KT, Mouriquand PDE, eds. *Pediatric Surgery and Urology: Long-Term Outcomes*. London: WB Saunders Company Limited; 1998.
105. Rutter MJ, Cotton RT, Azizkhan RG, et al. Slide tracheoplasty for the management of complete tracheal rings. *J Pediatr Surg* 2003;38(6):928–934.
106. Backer CL, Mavroudis C, Holinger LD. Repair of congenital tracheal stenosis. *Semin Thorac Cardiovasc Surg Pediatr Card Surg Annu* 2002;5:173–186.
107. National Safety Council Accident Facts. http://www.nsc.org. February, 2000.
108. Manning PB, Wesley JR, Polley TZ, et al. Esophageal and tracheobronchial foreign bodies in infants and children. *Pediatr Surg Int* 1987;2:346.
109. Ciftci AO, Binqöl-Koloqlu M, Senocak ME, et al. Bronchoscopy for evaluation of foreign body aspiration in children. 2003;38(8):1170–1176.
110. McCauley G. An account of viscera herniation. *Phil Trans R Coll Phys* 1754;6:25.
111. Bochdalek VA. Einige Betrachtungen uber die Enstehung des angeborenen Zwerfekkbruches. Als Bietrag Zur pathologischen Anatomie der Hernien. *Vjscher Prakt Heilk* 1848;18:89.
112. Ladd WE, Gross RE. Congenital diaphragmatic hernia. *N Engl J Med* 1940;223:917.
113. Gross RE. Congenital hernia of the diaphragm. *Am J Dis Child* 1946;71:579.
114. Doyle NM, Lally KP. The CDH Study Group and advances in the clinical care of the patient with congenital diaphragmatic hernia. *Semin Perinatol* 2004;28(3):174–184.
115. Cilley RE. Invited commentary. Weber TR, Kountzman B, Dillon PA, et al. Improved survival in congenital diaphragmatic hernia with evolving therapeutic strategies. *Arch Surg* 1998;133:503.
116. Cilley RE. Respiratory physiology and extracorporeal life support. In: Oldham KT, Foglia RP, Colombani PM, eds. *Surgery of Infants and Children: Scientific Principles and Practice*. Philadelphia, PA: Lippincott–Raven Publishers; 1997:183–222.
117. DiFiore JW, Wilson JM. Lung development. *Semin Pediatr Surg* 1994;3:221–232.
118. Davies GM, Reid L. Growth of the alveoli and pulmonary arteries in childhood. *Thorax* 1970;25:669–681.
119. Chinoy MR. Lung growth and development. *Front Biosci* 2003;8:d392.
120. Chinoy MR. Pulmonary hypoplasia and congenital diaphragmatic hernia: advances in the pathogenetics and regulation of lung development. *J Surg Res* 2002;106(1):209.
121. Moore KL. *The Developing Human*. 3rd ed. Philadelphia, PA: WB Saunders;1982.
122. Iritani I. Experimental study on embryogenesis of congenital diaphragmatic hernia. *Anat Embryol* 1984;169:133–139.
123. Fisher JC, Bodenstein L. Computer simulation analysis of normal and abnormal development of the mammalian diaphragm. *Theor Biol Med Model* 2006;3:9.
124. Stolar CJH, Dillon PW. Congenital diaphragmatic hernia and eventration. In: O'Neill JA, Rowe MI, Grosfeld JL, et al, eds. *Pediatric Surgery*. 5th ed. St. Louis, MO: Mosby–Year Book, Inc; 1998.
125. Dott MM, Wong LY, Rasmussen SA. Population-based study of congenital diaphragmatic hernia: risk factors and survival in metropolitan Atlanta, 1968–1999. *Birth Defects Res A Clin Mol Teratol* 2003;67(4):261.
126. Graziano JN; Congenital Diaphragmatic Hernia Study Group. Cardiac anomalies in patients with congenital diaphragmatic hernia and their

prognosis: a report from the Congenital Diaphragmatic Hernia Study Group. *J Pediatr Surg* 2005;40(6):1045–1049; discussion 1049–1050.
127. Greer JJ, Babiuk RP, Thebaud B. Etiology of congenital diaphragmatic hernia: the retinoid hypothesis. *Pediatr Res* 2003;53(5):726.
128. DeLorimier AA, Tierney DF, Parker HR. Hypoplastic lungs in fetal lambs with surgically produced congenital diaphragmatic hernia. *Surgery* 1967; 62:12–17.
129. Harrison MR, Jester JA, Ross NA. Correction of congenital diaphragmatic hernia in utero. I. The model: intrathoracic balloon produces fatal pulmonary hypoplasia. *Surgery* 1980;88:174–182.
130. Brandsma AE. *Lung Development in Congenital Diaphragmatic Hernia*. Rotterdam: Offsetdrukkerij Ridderprint B.V.; 1995.
131. Cilley RE, Zgleszewski SE, Krummel TM, et al. Nitrofen dose-dependent gestational day-specific murine lung hypoplasia and left-sided diaphragmatic hernia. *Am J Physiol* 1997;272(2 Pt 1):L362–L371.
132. Keller RL, Aaroz PA, Hawgood S, et al. MR imaging of hepatic pulmonary fusion in neonates. *AJR Am J Roentgenol* 2003;180(2):438.
133. Tibboel D, Hazebroek F, Mooi W, eds. *Pathogenetic and Experimental Aspects of Congenital Diaphragmatic Hernia*. Netherlands Symposium: Erasmus University Rotterdam; 1999.
134. Lewis DA, Reickert C, Bowerman R, et al. Prenatal ultrasonography frequently fails to diagnose congenital diaphragmatic hernia. *J Pediatr Surg* 1997;32(2):352–356.
135. Hubbard AM, Crombleholme TM, Adzick NS, et al. Prenatal MRI evaluation of congenital diaphragmatic hernia. *Am J Perinatol* 1999;16(8): 407.
136. Leung JW, Coakley FV, Hricak H, et al. Prenatal MR imaging of congenital diaphragmatic hernia. *AJR Am J Roentgenol* 2000;174(6):1607.
137. Kasales CJ, Coulson CC, Meilstrup JW, et al. Diagnosis and differentiation of congenital diaphragmatic hernia from other noncardiac thoracic fetal masses. *Am J Perinatol* 1998;15(11):623–628.
138. Keller RL, Glidden DV, Paek BW, et al. The lung-to-head ratio and fetoscopic temporary tracheal occlusion: prediction of survival in severe left congenital diaphragmatic hernia. *Ultasound Obstet Gynecol* 2003;21(3): 244.
139. Laudy JA, Van Gucht M, Van Dooren MF, et al. Congenital diaphragmatic hernia: evaluation of the prognostic value of the lung-to-head ratio and other prenatal parameters. *Prenat Diagn* 2003;23(8):634.
140. Lipshutz GS, Albanese CT, Feldstein VA, et al. Prospective analysis of lung-to-head ratio predicts survival for patients with prenatally diagnosed congenital diaphragmatic hernia. *J Pediatr Surg* 1997;32(11):1634.
141. Harrison MR, Mychaliska GB, Albanese CT, et al. Correction of congenital diaphragmatic hernia in utero X: fetuses with poor prognosis (liver herniation and low lung-to-head ratio) can be saved by fetoscopic temporary tracheal occlusion. *J Pediatr Surg* 1998;33(7):1017–1023.
142. Congenital Diaphragmatic Hernia Study Group. Treatment evolution in high-risk congenital diaphragmatic hernia: ten years' experience with diaphragmatic agenesis. *Ann Surg* 2006;244(4):505–513.
143. Jani J, Cannie M, Sonigo P, et al. Value of prenatal magnetic resonance imaging in the prediction of postnatal outcome in fetuses with diaphragmatic hernia. *Ultrasound Obstet Gynecol* 2008;32(6):793–799.
144. Wung JT, Sahni R, Moffitt ST, et al. Congenital diaphragmatic hernia: survival treated with very delayed surgery, spontaneous respiration, and no chest tube. *J Pediatr Surg* 1995;30:406–409.
145. Boloker J, Bateman DA, Wung JT, et al. Congenital diaphragmatic hernia in 120 infants treated consecutively with permissive hypercapnea/spontaneous respiration/elective repair. *J Pediatr Surg* 2002;37(3):357.
146. Lally KP, Lally PA, Langham MR, et al; Congenital Diaphragmatic Hernia Study Group. Surfactant does not improve survival rate in preterm infants with congenital diaphragmatic hernia. *J Pediatr Surg* 2004;39(6):829.
147. Suen HC, Losty P, Donahoe PK, et al. Combined antenatal thyrotropin-releasing hormone and low-dose glucocorticoid therapy improves the pulmonary biochemical immaturity in congenital diaphragmatic hernia. *J Pediatr Surg* 1994;29:359–363.
148. Lally KP, Bagolan P, Hosie S, et al; Congenital Diaphragmatic Hernia Study Group. Corticosteroids for fetuses with congenital diaphragmatic hernia: can we really show benefit? *J Pediatr Surg* 2006;41(4):668–674; discussion 668–674.
149. The Neonatal Inhaled Nitric Oxide Study Group (NINOS). Inhaled nitric oxide and hypoxic respiratory failure in infants with congenital diaphragmatic hernia. *Pediatrics* 1997;99(6):838–845.
150. Finer NN, Barrington KJ. Nitric oxide for respiratory failure in infants born at or near term. *Cochrane Database Syst Rev* 2001;(4):CD000399.
151. Nio M, Haase G, Kennaugh J, et al. A prospective randomized trial of delayed versus immediate repair of congenital diaphragmatic hernia. *J Pediatr Surg* 1994;29(5):618–621.
152. Rozmiarek AJ, Qureshi FG, Cassidy L, et al. Factors influencing survival in newborns with congenital diaphragmatic hernia: the relative role of timing of surgery. *J Pediatr Surg* 2004;39(6):821–824; discussion 821–824.
153. St Peter SD, Valusek PA, Tsao K, et al. Abdominal complications related to type of repair for congenital diaphragmatic hernia. *J Surg Res* 2007; 140(2):234–236.
154. Arca MJ, Barnhart DC, Lelli JL Jr, et al. Early experience with minimally invasive repair of congenital diaphragmatic hernias: results and lessons learned. *J Pediatr Surg* 2003;38(11):1563.
155. Yang EY, Allmendinger N, Johnson SM, et al. Neonatal thoracoscopic repair of congenital diaphragmatic hernia: selection criteria for successful outcome. *J Pediatr Surg* 2005;40(9):1369–1375.
156. Fuchs JR, Kaviani A, Oh JT, et al. Diaphragmatic reconstruction with autologous tendon engineered from mesenchymal amniocytes. *J Pediatr Surg* 2004;39(6):834–838.
157. Rana AR, Khouri JS, Teitelbaum DH, et al. Salvaging the severe congenital diaphragmatic hernia patient: is a silo the solution? *J Pediatr Surg* 2008;43(5):788–791.
158. Teitelbaum DH, Teich S, Hirschl RB. Successful management of a chylothorax in infancy using a pleurectomy. *Pediatr Surg Int* 1996;11: 166–168.
159. Cilley RE, Bartlett RH. Extracorporeal life support for respiratory failure. In: Gravlee GP, ed. *Principles and Practice of Cardiopulmonary Bypass*. Baltimore, MD: Williams & Wilkins; 1993.
160. Lally KP; The CDH Study Group. The use of ECMO for stabilization of infants with congenital diaphragmatic hernia—a report of the CDH Study Group. Presented at the 20th annual meeting of the surgical section of the American Academy of Pediatrics; October 2002; Boston, MA.
161. Rashid A, Ivy D. Severe paediatric pulmonary hypertension: new management strategies. *Arch Dis Child* 2005;90(1):92.
162. Lally KP, Breaux CW Jr. A second course of extracorporeal membrane oxygenation in the neonate—is there a benefit? *Surgery* 1995;117(2): 175–178.
163. Tsao K, Lally KP. The Congenital Diaphragmatic Hernia Study Group: a voluntary international registry. *Semin Pediatr Surg* 2008;17(2):90–97.
164. Dillon PW, Cilley RE, Mauger D, et al. The relationship of pulmonary artery pressure and survival in congenital diaphragmatic hernia. *J Pediatr Surg* 2004;39(3):307.
165. Peetsold MG, Vonk-Noordegraaf A, Heij HH, et al. Pulmonary function and exercise testing in adult survivors of congenital diaphragmatic hernia. *Pediatr Pulmonol* 2007;(4):325–331.
166. Iocono JA, Cilley RE, Mauger DT, et al. Postnatal pulmonary hypertension after repair of congenital diaphragmatic hernia: predicting risk and outcome. *J Pediatr Surg* 1999;34:349–353.
167. Muratore CS, Kharasch V, Lund DP, et al. Pulmonary morbidity in 100 survivors of congenital diaphragmatic hernia monitored in a multidisciplinary clinic. *J Pediatr Surg* 2001;36(1):133.
168. Kitano Y, Flake AW, Crombleholme TM, et al. Open fetal surgery for life-threatening fetal malformations. *Semin Perinatol* 1999;23(6):448–461.
169. Harrison MR, Adzick NS, Flake AW, et al. Correction of congenital diaphragmatic hernia in utero. VI. Hard earned lessons. *J Pediatr Surg* 1993;28:1411–1418.
170. Harrison MR, Adzick NS, Bullard KM, et al. Correction of congenital diaphragmatic hernia in utero VII: a prospective trial. *J Pediatr Surg* 1997; 32(11):1637–1642.
171. DiFiore JW, Fauza DO, Slavin R, et al. Experimental fetal tracheal ligation reverses the structural and physiological effects of pulmonary hypoplasia in congenital diaphragmatic hernia. *J Pediatr Surg* 1994;29:248–257.
172. DiFiore JW, Fauza DO, Slavin R, et al. Experimental fetal tracheal ligation and congenital diaphragmatic hernia: a pulmonary vascular morophometric analysis. *J Pediatr Surg* 1995;30:917–924.
173. Hedrick MH, Estes JM, Sullivan KM, et al. Plug the lung until it grows (PLUG): a new method to treat congenital diaphragmatic hernia in utero. *J Pediatr Surg* 1994;29:612–617.
174. Harrison MR, Keller RL, Hawgood SB, et al. A randomized trial of fetal endoscopic tracheal occlusion for severe fetal congenital diaphragmatic hernia. *N Engl J Med* 2003;349(20):1916.
175. Deprest J, Gratacos E, Nicolaides KH, et al; FETO Task Group. Fetoscopic tracheal occlusion (FETO) for severe congenital diaphragmatic hernia: evolution of a technique and preliminary results. *Ultrasound Obstet Gynecol* 2004;24(2):121.
176. Hirschl RB. Respiratory failure: current status of experimental therapies. *Semin Pediatr Surg* 1999;8:155–170.
177. Hirschl RB, Philip WF, Glick L, et al. A prospective randomized pilot trial of perfluorocarbon-induced lung growth in newborns with congenital diaphragmatic hernia. *J Pediatr Surg* 2003;38(3):283–289; discussion 283–289.
178. DeAnda A Jr, Cahill JL, Bernstein D, et al. Elective transplant pneumonectomy. *J Pediatr Surg* 1998;33(4):655–656.
179. Hines MH. Video-assisted diaphragm plication in children. *Ann Thorac Surg* 2003;76(1):234–236.
180. Ali A, Flageole H. Diaphragmatic pacing for the treatment of congenital central aveolar hypoventilation syndrome. *J Pediatr Surg* 2008; 43(5):792–796.
181. Krieger LM, Krieger AJ. The intercostal to phrenic nerve transfer: an effective means of reanimating the diaphragm in patients with high cervical spine injury. *Plast Reconstr Surg* 2000;105:1255–1261.
182. Kalfa N, Allal H, Montes-Tapia F, et al. Ideal timing of thoracoscopic decortication and drainage for empyema in children. *Surg Endosc* 2004; 18(3):472–477.
183. Gates RL, Caniano DA, Hayes JR, et al. Does VATS provide optimal treatment of empyema in children? A systematic review. *J Pediatr Surg* 2004; 39(3):381–386.
184. St Peter SD, Tsao K, Harrison C, et al. Thoracoscopic decortication vs. tube thorascostomy with fibrinolysis for empyema in children: a prospective, randomized trial. *J Pediatr Surg* 2009;44(1):106–111; discussion 111.
185. Tsao K, St Peter SD, Sharp SW, et al. Current application of thoracopy in children. *J Laparoendosc Adv Surg Tech A* 2008;18(1):131–135.
186. Chan SY, Lau W, Wong WH, et al. Chylothorax in children after congenital heart surgery. *Ann Thorac Surg* 2006;82(5):1650–1656.

CHAPTER 107 ■ PEDIATRIC ABDOMEN

THOMAS T. SATO AND KEITH T. OLDHAM

KEY POINTS

1. Gastroschisis occurs with an incidence rate of 1 in 3,000 to 8,000 live births and is characterized by exposed intestine herniating through a defect to the right of the umbilicus. In contrast, omphalocele is an abdominal wall defect of varying size characterized by herniated visceral contents contained in a sac, and has a high incidence rate of associated congenital anomalies.
2. A congenital, indirect inguinal hernia is an abnormal, patent continuation of the peritoneum through the internal inguinal ring; inguinal hernia repair is the most common elective procedure in pediatric surgery.
3. Neonatal bilious emesis should be considered the result of an acute mechanical intestinal obstruction until proven otherwise; emergent surgical evaluation is warranted to determine if intestinal malrotation with midgut volvulus is present.
4. Necrotizing enterocolitis (NEC) is a progressive, inflammatory intestinal condition of the surviving premature neonate. Perforated NEC is the most common neonatal surgical emergency.
5. Hirschsprung disease is caused by aganglionosis of the myenteric nervous system in the rectum, and it will involve the contiguous bowel for varying lengths proximally, most commonly to the rectosigmoid colon. Both propulsion and reflexive relaxation is disordered or absent in the rectum, leading to functional bowel obstruction in the neonate and chronic constipation in the older child or adolescent. Enterocolitis associated with Hirschsprung disease is a potentially life-threatening condition.
6. Intussusception is the invagination or telescoping of a proximal segment of intestine into an adjacent distal segment and is the most common cause of intestinal obstruction in infants and children 3 months to 3 years of age.
7. The incidence of biliary atresia is 1 in 8,000 to 12,000 live births and is the most common cause of chronic cholestasis in infants and children as well as the most frequent indication for pediatric liver transplantation. Early diagnosis and management is necessary for optimal outcome.

ABDOMINAL WALL DEFECTS

Gastroschisis

1 Gastroschisis occurs with an incidence rate of 1 in 3,000 to 8,000 live births, and for unknown reasons, the incidence rate is increasing. Infants with gastroschisis tend to be born prematurely, have lower birth weights, and have younger mothers.[1,2] Familial cases of gastroschisis have been reported and are distinctly rare.[3] Associated congenital anomalies are uncommon and occur in about 10% of cases, most commonly intestinal atresia or stenosis. These anomalies are thought to reflect mechanical or vascular compromise to the herniated bowel. Rarely, infants with gastroschisis have complete loss of small bowel secondary to in utero volvulus.

The pathophysiology of gastroschisis remains unknown. In normal fetal development, there are two paired umbilical veins. As the intestine returns to the abdominal cavity through the umbilicus, the right umbilical vein undergoes resorption, leaving the left umbilical vein intact. Weakness of the umbilical membrane at the site of umbilical vein resorption may allow for evisceration of the intestine through the defect. This explanation is consistent with the clinical observation that the gastroschisis defect is almost always located to the right of the umbilicus. Routine antenatal ultrasonography has documented the sequential development of gastroschisis as a consequence of a ruptured hernia of the umbilical cord in utero.[4] Therefore, gastroschisis should be considered an isolated mechanical defect of the developing umbilical cord rather than a global defect in embryogenesis.

The amount of bowel eviscerated in gastroschisis can be extensive because the bowel has not undergone complete mesenteric rotation and fixation. Typically, the bowel is thickened and the mesentery may be foreshortened secondary to the inflammatory response induced by direct exposure to amniotic fluid. Given the typical small size of the abdominal wall defect, herniation of the liver in gastroschisis is distinctly unusual (Fig. 107.1).

Omphalocele

Anatomy, Embryology, and Pathophysiology. The incidence rate of omphalocele is approximately 1 in 6,000 to 10,000 live births and has been stable over the past several decades. *Omphalocele* is an abdominal wall defect of varying size characterized by the presence of herniated visceral contents into a translucent sac. The sac is composed of amniotic membrane, mesenchymal tissue known as *Wharton jelly,* and peritoneum. The umbilical cord attaches to the sac and may be eccentric in origin (Fig. 107.2). The sac may be inadvertently ruptured before or during delivery, but it is always present. As in gastroschisis, intestinal malrotation is usually present. Unlike in gastroschisis, the bowel is normal in appearance because it has not been directly exposed to the amniotic fluid. Small omphaloceles are abdominal wall defects 2 to 5 cm in diameter and may have only a small amount of herniated bowel within the sac. Giant omphaloceles greater than 8 cm in diameter can lead to extensive herniation of the stomach, bowel, liver, and spleen with subsequent underdevelopment of the abdominal cavity (Fig. 107.3).

Omphalocele results from incomplete closure of the anterior abdominal wall at the umbilicus during embryogenesis. During week 4 of gestation, the midgut undergoes progressive elongation in the yolk sac outside the embryonic coelomic cavity. The midgut returns to the abdominal cavity during week 10, where it undergoes normal rotation and fixation of the mesentery to the posterior abdominal wall. Normal closure of

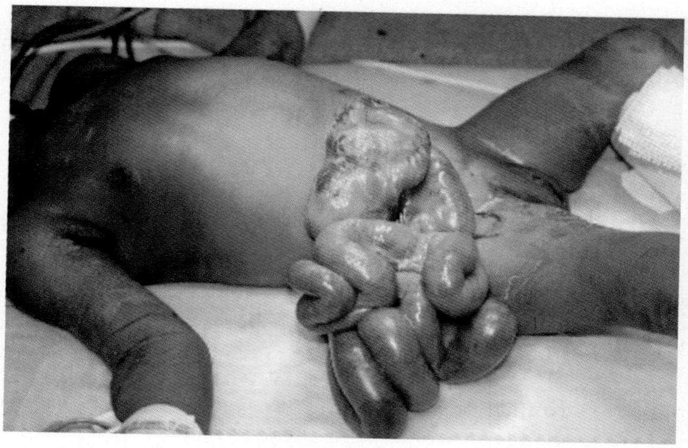

FIGURE 107.1. Gastroschisis. The defect is to the right of the normal umbilicus, and the bowel is thickened and inflamed.

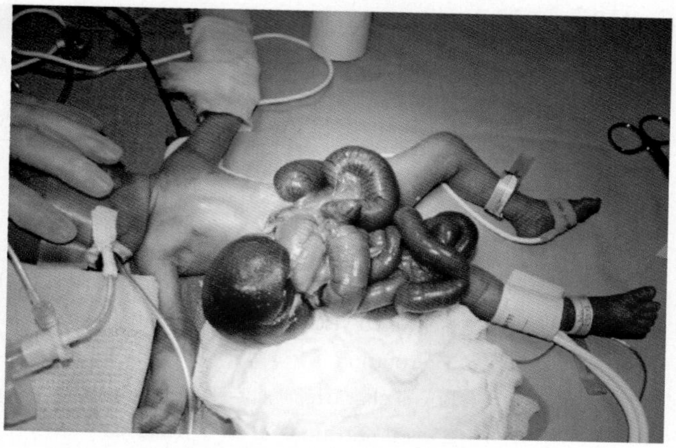

FIGURE 107.3. Ruptured omphalocele. Although the bowel is relatively normal in appearance, the abdominal cavity is extremely underdeveloped.

the anterior abdominal wall requires return of the midgut to the abdominal cavity, along with growth and fusion of the anterior body folds (cephalic, caudal, and two lateral) at the base of the umbilicus. Failure of growth, migration, or fusion of the lateral body folds leads to omphalocele. Failure of growth and fusion of the cephalic folds may lead to either a supraumbilical omphalocele associated with a midline sternal defect (Fig. 107.4) and a herniated heart, termed *ectopia cordis*, or a constellation of defects known as the *pentalogy of Cantrell*.[5] This sequence includes a sternal cleft, an absence of the septum transversum of the diaphragm, a pericardial defect, a cardiac defect, and an epigastric omphalocele. Infants born with either ectopia cordis or pentalogy of Cantrell have significant morbidity, and often these conditions are lethal.

Associated anomalies are more common in infants with omphalocele than with gastroschisis, reflecting the more global abnormality of embryogenesis in omphalocele. About 50% to 60% of infants with omphalocele have at least one associated congenital anomaly.[6,7] These infants are at moderate to high risk for anomalies of the skeleton, gastrointestinal tract, nervous system, genitourinary system, and cardiopulmonary system. In addition, infants with omphalocele have a higher incidence of chromosomal abnormalities and other conditions such as Beckwith-Wiedemann syndrome. A comparison of gastroschisis and omphalocele is summarized in Table 107.1.

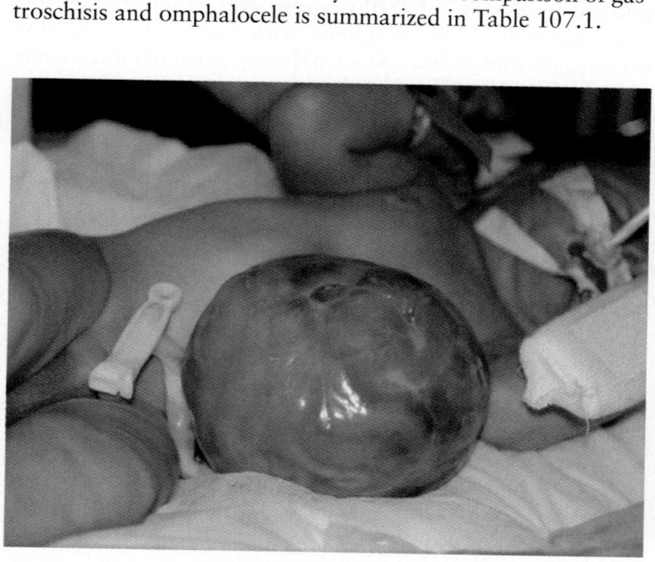

FIGURE 107.2. Omphalocele. The herniated intestines and liver are visible inside the sac. The umbilical cord attaches to the sac.

Perioperative Management for Gastroschisis and Omphalocele. In the absence of fetal distress, whether elective cesarean section improves neonatal outcome in infants with gastroschisis or omphalocele remains controversial.[8–10] Some investigators advocate elective delivery of infants with gastroschisis following the establishment of lung maturity. A prospective study that alternated vaginal delivery with elective cesarean section for infants with gastroschisis demonstrated no significant differences in outcome.[11] To prevent birth-related hepatic injury, cesarean section is preferable for prenatally diagnosed infants with giant omphaloceles.

After delivery, infants with either gastroschisis or omphalocele have similar initial management priorities. Attention must be given to the establishment of an adequate airway with effective ventilation and oxygenation. The infant should be maintained under either an external warmer or a humidified incubator. An orogastric sump tube should be inserted early and placed on suction to prevent further intestinal distention. The herniated viscera should be covered with warm, saline-soaked gauze and covered with plastic wrap to prevent further contamination; this maneuver also helps to prevent hypothermia and volume depletion. Alternatively, the infant's entire lower torso can be placed inside a plastic bowel bag. Regardless of the method, the initial therapeutic goal is to provide rapid, effective temporary coverage of the viscera. Adequate support of the herniated viscera must be provided to prevent intestinal

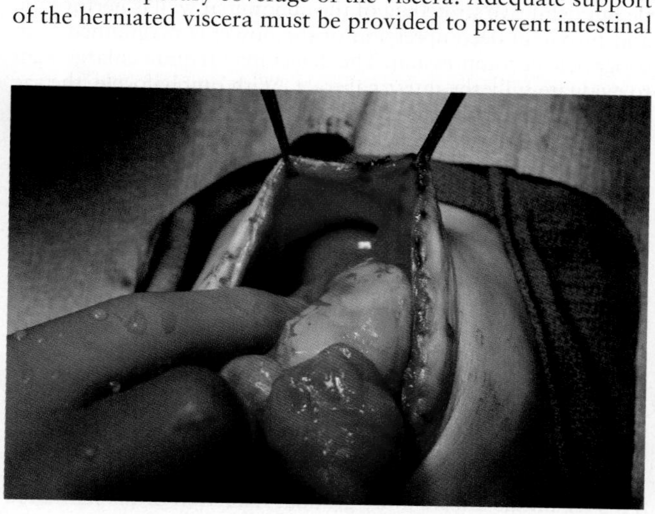

FIGURE 107.4. Operative exploration of giant omphalocele with abdominal wall defect, absence of the septum transversum of the diaphragm, and pericardial defect, cardiac defect.

PEDIATRICS

TABLE 107.1 DIAGNOSIS

COMPARISON OF GASTROSCHISIS AND OMPHALOCELE

CHARACTERISTIC	GASTROSCHISIS	OMPHALOCELE
Defect size (diameter)	2–3 cm	2–15 cm
Sac	Never	Always, may be ruptured
Gestational age	Prematurity	Term
Umbilical cord	Adjacent (left side) of defect	Attached to sac
Herniated viscera	Small bowel, stomach, colon	Small bowel, stomach, colon, liver
Malrotation	Yes	Yes
Bowel character	Inflammatory, edematous	Normal
Enteral nutrition	Delayed	Normal
Associated anomalies	Uncommon (10% atresia)	Common (50%)

ischemia. With large omphaloceles, the position of the infant's liver and viscera may impair venous return from the inferior vena cava when the infant is supine, and these infants may preferentially require a left-side-down position to maintain normal hemodynamic status. Intravenous dextrose and broad-spectrum antibiotics are administered. Given the inflammatory nature of the intestine, infants with gastroschisis will have higher intravenous fluid requirements to maintain euvolemia. If the infant is not delivered at a center where definitive surgical care can be provided, urgent transport should be arranged.

Given the high incidence of associated anomalies, infants with an intact omphalocele should undergo preoperative diagnostic investigation, guided by the clinical presentation and physical examination of the infant. These studies include a chest film, echocardiogram, and renal ultrasound, in addition to baseline blood work. Until the decision is made with respect to the timing and method of repair, the omphalocele should remain covered and protected with a dressing. If the omphalocele is ruptured or torn, immediate closure or coverage is necessary.

Once the infant has been stabilized and assessment for other anomalies is complete, the infant is taken to the operating room for correction of the abdominal wall defect. Reduction of the herniated viscera with primary fascial closure of the abdominal wall is an achievable goal in approximately 60% to 70% of infants with either gastroschisis or omphalocele. Gentle but definitive stretching of the abdominal wall is performed, and proximal decompression of the bowel is maintained with orogastric decompression. The defect may require enlargement to evaluate fully the intestinal tract. With omphalocele, the sac is usually resected. The limiting factor in primary closure of a congenital abdominal wall defect is the increased intra-abdominal pressure generated by the reduction of the herniated viscera. Increased intra-abdominal pressure can lead to abdominal compartment syndrome. Features of neonatal abdominal compartment syndrome include impaired venous return caused by compression of the inferior vena cava, reduction of splanchnic blood flow leading to mesenteric ischemia, and respiratory compromise secondary to impaired diaphragmatic excursion. Intraoperative measurement of intragastric or intravesical pressure, end-tidal CO_2, central venous pressure, or regional oximetry may be helpful in determining the safety of primary abdominal wall closure.[12] If the herniated viscera cannot be reduced primarily, a silicone elastomer pouch or silo is constructed and daily partial reduction of the silo is performed. This technique allows more gradual reduction of the herniated viscera into the abdominal cavity, and complete reduction usually is obtained within 3 to 7 days. The infant is returned to the operating room for removal of the temporary silo with delayed primary closure of the abdominal wall defect (Fig. 107.5). Staged closure of gastroschisis using commercially available silicone elastomer silos has been reported to decrease the risk of long-term bowel dysfunction and need for reoperation by avoiding abdominal compartment syndrome.[13] Alternatively, a large abdominal wall defect may be effectively covered with abdominal skin flaps with delayed repair of the ventral hernia months to years later.

Infants with intact, giant omphaloceles may also be managed nonoperatively. The sac can be physically supported and left undisturbed, allowing epithelialization of the sac over several weeks to months. Antibiotic solutions or ointments are usually applied to control desiccation. Delayed repair of the ventral hernia is required. This delay is particularly useful in the infant with a giant omphalocele and a small, underdeveloped abdominal cavity that prohibits primary closure.

Infants with repaired omphalocele usually have relatively prompt return of bowel function after definitive repair. In comparison, nearly all infants with gastroschisis have delayed intestinal function following closure. The use of total parenteral nutrition (TPN) is essential in the treatment of these infants because it allows nutritional support while the bowel inflammatory process resolves. It is not unusual for these infants to require up to 4 weeks after repair to have bowel function normalize, and time taken to achieve full enteral feeding is not affected by the use of erythromycin as a prokinetic agent.[14] Approximately 15% of infants with gastroschisis develop necrotizing enterocolitis (NEC), a diffuse, often life-threatening

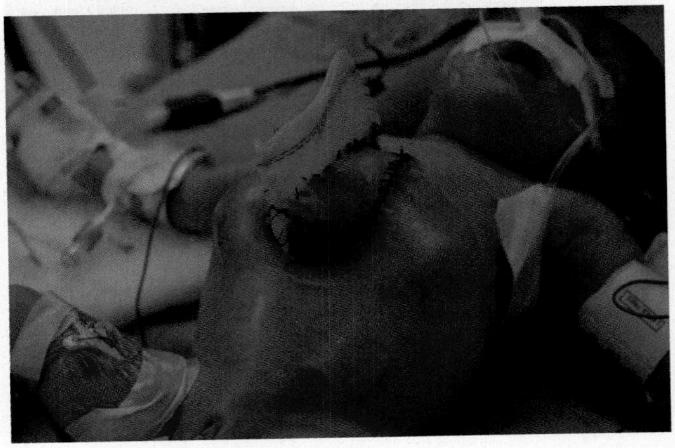

FIGURE 107.5. Silastic chimney or silo for temporary coverage and staged reduction of giant omphalocele.

inflammatory complication of the neonatal intestinal tract.[15] In addition, infants with gastroschisis are at risk for nutrient malabsorption and intestinal dysmotility with inability to tolerate full enteral feeding. In particular, infants with gastroschisis and associated intestinal atresia may have pronounced intestinal dysmotility and may require long-term, sometimes lifelong, dependence on TPN for caloric intake.[16]

Long-term outcome of infants operated on for gastroschisis or omphalocele is usually dependent on the morbidity and mortality of associated conditions rather than the abdominal wall defect itself. Surgical conditions such as undescended testicles, Meckel diverticulum, and adhesive small bowel obstruction are encountered with moderate frequency. Adhesive small bowel obstruction most commonly occurs in the first year of life and requires operative management in most.[17] Most children with repaired abdominal wall defects enjoy satisfactory health and quality of life, although they have been reported to have a lower degree of physical fitness measured by exercise time and maximal oxygen consumption.[18]

Umbilical Hernia

Anatomy and Embryology. Congenital umbilical hernia is the most common abdominal wall defect in infants and children. The umbilical ring begins to contract circumferentially after birth and normally is reinforced by the paired lateral umbilical ligaments (the obliterated umbilical arteries), the singular round ligament (the obliterated umbilical vein), the urachal remnant, and the transversalis fascia. Incomplete growth or impaired development of any one of these structures can lead to weakness at the umbilical ring and cause a congenital umbilical hernia.

Clinical Issues and Management. Congenital umbilical hernias generally do not pose significant problems during childhood. Rarely, an umbilical hernia presents with incarceration of intra-abdominal contents within the sac.[19] Infants and children may also present with infection or drainage at the umbilicus from associated urachal or vitelline duct remnants. The incidence rate of congenital umbilical hernia has been reported to be 25% to 50% in black infants and 4% to 9% in white infants in the first few months of life.[20] There is an increased incidence of umbilical hernia in premature infants, and there is a tendency for familial inheritance.

Diagnosis of umbilical hernia is usually made after separation of the umbilical cord remnant from the umbilicus and is often initially noted by parents or pediatrician. The defect size may vary from a few millimeters to several centimeters and is typically reducible and asymptomatic. Age and size of the defect are the most important factors determining spontaneous closure rates.[21] Many umbilical hernias spontaneously close within the first 2 to 3 years of life. Parents should be reassured that complications related to untreated umbilical hernia are rare. Given the high rate of spontaneous closure and the relatively asymptomatic nature of most umbilical hernias, operative repair is generally not performed during the first 2 years of life. Skin ulceration or an episode of incarceration should prompt earlier repair. Large defects with significant protrusion may necessitate surgery, and parents may desire repair if an older child appears to be self-conscious about the hernia.

Nearly all umbilical hernia repairs can be performed as outpatient surgical procedures. An incision is made along the umbilicus and the hernia sac is dissected free circumferentially. The sac is completely excised and primary fascial closure is performed. The umbilical skin is typically preserved and sutured to the fascial closure, and an acceptable cosmetic result is almost always achievable. Large umbilical hernias with redundant skin may require umbilicoplasty. The incidence of complications such as wound infection and recurrence is low.

Inguinal Hernia and Hydrocele

Anatomy, Embryology, and Pathophysiology. Inguinal hernias constitute one of the major surgical problems of infancy and childhood. Inguinal hernia repair is the most common elective general surgical procedure performed by pediatric surgeons. Three distinct anatomic types of inguinal hernias are observed in children: congenital indirect (99% of infants and children), direct (0.5%), and femoral (<0.5%). An *indirect inguinal hernia* is an abnormal, patent continuation of the peritoneum through the internal inguinal ring. The hernia sac originates lateral to the deep inferior epigastric vessels and descends along the spermatic cord within the cremasteric fascia. The sac can reside completely within the inguinal canal or descend through the external inguinal ring into the scrotum. A *direct inguinal hernia* originates medial to the deep inferior epigastric vessels and is external to the cremasteric fascia. The hernia sac protrudes directly through the posterior wall of the inguinal canal and can descend through the external inguinal ring and into the scrotum. A *femoral hernia* originates medial to the femoral vein and descends inferior to the inguinal ligament along the femoral canal. A femoral hernia never enters the scrotum or labia.

The developing testicle is initially adjacent to the mesonephros and subsequently descends to the scrotum during the third trimester of gestation. The peritoneal extension that descends alongside the chorda gubernaculum of the testicle is called the processus vaginalis. A slightly higher incidence rate of right-sided indirect inguinal hernia is thought to reflect delay of right-sided testicular descent from the developing inferior vena cava and right external iliac vein. As the testicle descends into the scrotum, the processus vaginalis forms a serous covering around the testicle known as the tunica vaginalis. Normally, the patent processus vaginalis undergoes obliteration, closing the communication between the peritoneal cavity and the inguinal canal. A patent processus vaginalis can lead to various anatomic conditions of the inguinal region (Fig. 107.6).

The incidence of patent processus vaginalis has been reported to be as high as 80% to 94% in newborn infants undergoing autopsy,[22] whereas in adulthood, the incidence is 20% to 30%. Infants with unilateral inguinal hernias have been found to have a patent contralateral processus vaginalis in 60% during the first few months of life. By the age of 2 years, 20% of these hernias were obliterated, and half of the remaining 40% became clinical hernias.[23] At least 30% of infants requiring placement of a ventriculoperitoneal shunt for hydrocephalus have been observed to have a patent processus vaginalis in the first few months of life, with a rapid decline in patency in older children.[24] These studies, along with contemporary use of laparoscopic exploration of the contralateral internal ring, demonstrate that although a patent processus vaginalis is common in infancy, there is some degree of obliteration that occurs with increasing age, and a patent processus vaginalis by itself does not constitute a clinical inguinal hernia.

Clinical Issues. Inguinal hernias occur in 1% to 3% of all children and in 3% to 5% of premature infants. There is no known inheritance pattern, but there is an increased incidence of inguinal hernia in children with connective tissue disorders such as Ehlers-Danlos syndrome and Marfan syndrome. There is a 6:1 predominance of males to females. At least 30% of children are younger than 6 months of age at the time of operative repair. Inguinal hernia more commonly presents as right-sided (56.2%) compared with left-sided (27.5%) or bilateral (16.2%).[25]

Most infants and children have a history of an intermittent inguinal mass or bulge that may descend into the scrotum or labia. The hernia may become more pronounced during times of increased intra-abdominal pressure, such as crying or having a bowel movement. Most inguinal hernias in children reduce

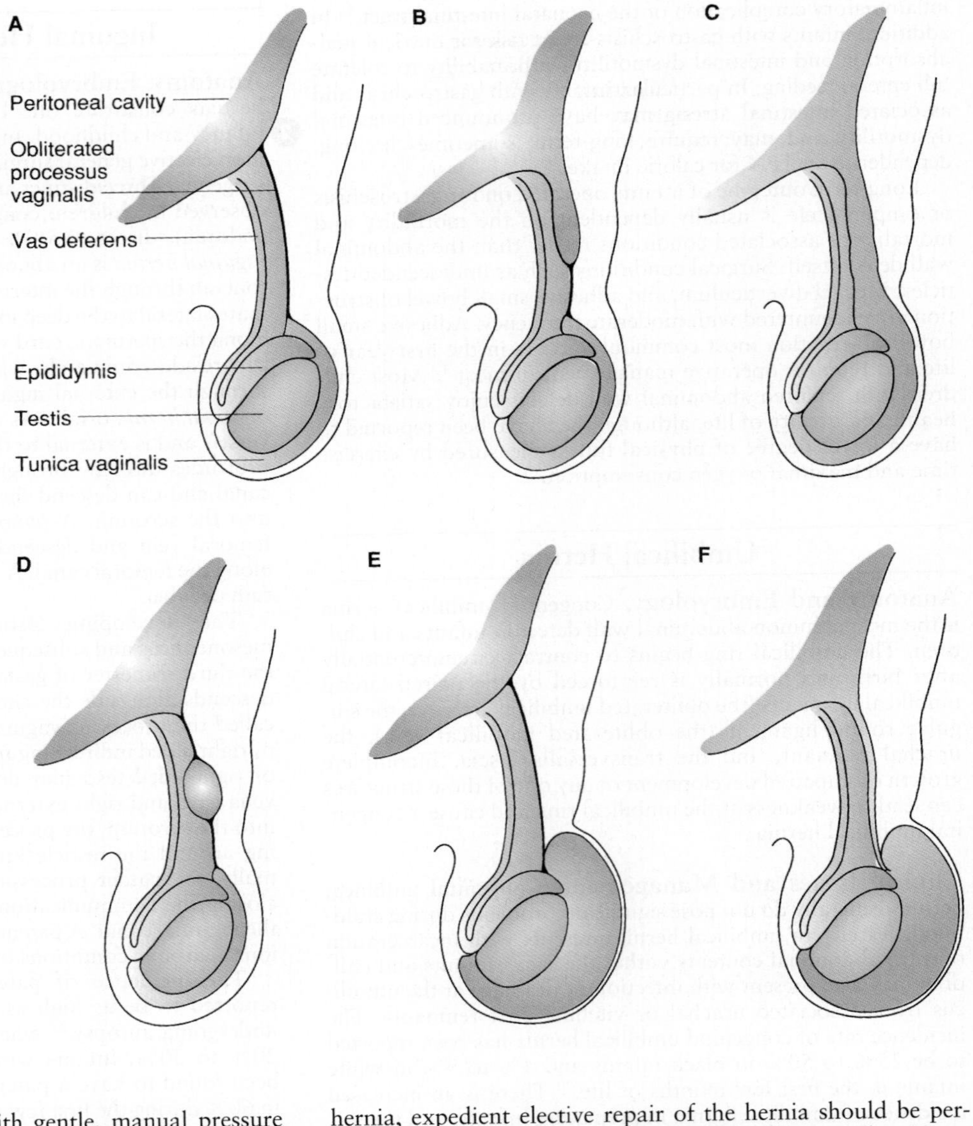

FIGURE 107.6. Anatomic variations that occur with different degrees of obliteration of the processus vaginalis. A: Normal; obliterated processus vaginalis. B: Proximal hernia sac; distal obliterated processus. C: Hernia sac extending into scrotum; no obliteration. D: Proximal and distal obliteration with hydrocele of the cord. E: Hydrocele of the scrotum, obliterated processus. F: Patent processus with communicating hydrocele.

spontaneously or are reducible with gentle, manual pressure along the inguinal canal. Female infants may have an ovary and fallopian tube in the hernia sac, identified clinically as a firm, slightly mobile, nontender mass in the labia or inguinal canal. Most parents or pediatricians give a characteristic history that is sufficient to warrant inguinal exploration, even in children in whom the hernia cannot be clinically demonstrated at the time of examination. Depending on institution and surgeon preference, infants and children with a strong history consistent with inguinal hernia and an equivocal clinical examination may be offered ultrasound or diagnostic laparoscopy to effectively confirm the diagnosis before groin exploration.[26]

Incarceration is a common consequence of untreated inguinal hernia and presents as a nonreducible mass in the inguinal canal, scrotum, or labia.[27] Clinical symptoms and signs are related to the duration of incarceration. If the incarceration has been present for several hours, the infant may be inconsolable and have feeding intolerance, pain, abdominal distention, vomiting, and lack of flatus or stool, signaling complete intestinal obstruction. The affected groin may become quite edematous, and a reactive scrotal hydrocele may evolve. Elevation of the infant's lower extremities with a pillow may help to encourage spontaneous reduction. Attempts at manually reducing an incarcerated inguinal hernia should be performed by an experienced surgeon. If necessary, sedation to calm the infant before attempting manual reduction may be cautiously used. Ice packs should be avoided in infants and children. Following successful reduction of an incarcerated hernia, expedient elective repair of the hernia should be performed after the edema has subsided. If reduction of an incarcerated hernia requires several attempts and is difficult, overnight inpatient observation is warranted to rule out reduction of strangulated bowel; fortunately, this is an uncommon occurrence in the pediatric population. Inability to reduce an incarcerated hernia is a clear indication for urgent operative exploration and repair. Incarcerated inguinal hernia must be differentiated from an acute, noncommunicating hydrocele or inguinal lymphadenitis. With acute hydrocele, it is usually possible to transilluminate the hydrocele and palpate normal cord structures above the scrotal mass. Additionally, symptoms of bowel obstruction are absent with acute hydrocele. Acute lymphadenitis typically is associated with fever, erythema, and tenderness, and there may be a history of lower-extremity infection on the ipsilateral side. If the inguinal mass is not reducible and an incarcerated hernia cannot be excluded, urgent groin exploration is required.

Operative Considerations and Outcome. The diagnosis of inguinal hernia in an infant or child is an indication for operative repair. The rationale for elective repair is to prevent the complications associated with incarceration. At least 71% of infants who require operative reduction of incarcerated inguinal hernia are younger than 11 months.[28] Therefore, an approach emphasizing timely elective repair of inguinal hernia is warranted, particularly during infancy. Delay of elective repair may be necessary in premature, extremely low birthweight (<1,500 g) infants and in children with other conditions such as congenital heart disease, pulmonary disease, infection, or metabolic disease.

Elective inguinal hernia repair in the pediatric age group is usually performed as an outpatient surgical procedure using general anesthesia, although spinal anesthesia is an effective alternative in selected high-risk infants.[29] A regional caudal block or local inguinal nerve block using local anesthetic is useful to diminish perioperative pain and increase patient comfort. These techniques, along with the use of rapid-acting general anesthetics, allow the vast majority of children to be discharged home within hours of operation. Overnight observation and monitoring are required for high-risk infants and children with disorders that increase anesthetic risk for postoperative apnea.

Repair of pediatric inguinal hernia relies on high ligation of the hernia sac at the internal inguinal ring. Sensory nerves deep to the external oblique aponeurosis should be identified and preserved. Careful identification and dissection of the hernia sac from the vas deferens and the testicular blood supply must be performed. The vas deferens must be carefully dissected free from the sac, and direct handling or pinching of the vas with forceps is avoided. The absence of a vas deferens or a blind-ending vas may be observed in children with cystic fibrosis (CF). In female infants, opening the hernia sac to visualize the ovary and fallopian tube may help to avoid inadvertent injury to these structures during suture ligation of the sac. The distal component of the hernia sac is opened widely, and any fluid in the sac is evacuated. If the internal inguinal ring is attenuated or enlarged, it can be repaired with a few sutures. Experience with laparoscopic inguinal hernia repair using purse-string suture closure of the patent internal ring without direct inguinal exploration has been described.[30] The testicle is returned to its scrotal position by gentle traction on the gubernaculum, and the spermatic cord is carefully aligned along the inguinal canal. Postoperative pain is managed with oral acetaminophen for 24 to 48 hours; older children may require postoperative narcotics.

Operative exploration of the asymptomatic contralateral groin remains controversial but is often performed in infants younger than 2 years because of the reported 60% to 70% incidence of a patent processus vaginalis on the opposite side.[31] In a survey of the surgical section of the American Academy of Pediatrics, 65% of the respondents perform contralateral exploration in male patients younger than 2 years, and 84% perform exploration for female infants up to age 4 years.[32] Direct visualization of the contralateral groin can be performed using a laparoscope inserted either through the umbilicus or through a side-viewing laparoscope inserted through the hernia sac. Experience with diagnostic laparoscopy demonstrates that approximately one third to one half of children have a patent processus vaginalis on the contralateral, asymptomatic groin, with higher rates in infants younger than 1 year.[33,34] This approach avoids unnecessary contralateral groin exploration in about half of all children who undergo surgery for unilateral inguinal hernia. However, the presence of a patent processus alone does not necessarily translate into a clinically significant hernia, and via systematic review, the reported risk of developing a metachronous contralateral inguinal hernia following open unilateral hernia repair in children is 7.2%.[35]

The major risk of inguinal hernia repair in infants and children is related to general anesthesia. Complications in pediatric inguinal hernia repair include wound infection, injury to the vas deferens or testicular vessels, injury or displacement of the testicle, and recurrence. Fortunately, all these complications are infrequent. The overall complication rate is higher for children requiring emergent operation for incarcerated or strangulated hernia. Recurrent inguinal hernia following elective repair is unusual and may be an indication of an underlying connective tissue disorder such as Ehlers-Danlos syndrome.

Hydrocele

A *hydrocele* is a fluid collection that resides in the tunica vaginalis in the scrotum or the processus vaginalis in the inguinal canal. A hydrocele may be present at birth, or it may occur acutely as a result of an incarcerated hernia or torsion of the appendix testis. On examination, a hydrocele transilluminates with a bright handheld light. A hydrocele is described as either *communicating* or *noncommunicating* depending on whether there is direct patency between the hydrocele and the peritoneal cavity. A history of intermittent fluctuation in the size of the hydrocele is generally diagnostic for communicating hydrocele. A communicating hydrocele is synonymous with a patent processus vaginalis, and therefore, a communicating hydrocele is treated operatively in the same fashion. In male patients, a hydrocele of the cord is a collection of fluid in the processus vaginalis separate from the tunica vaginalis. In female patients, fluid trapped in the processus vaginalis is considered a hydrocele of the canal of Nuck. In noncommunicating hydrocele, the isolated fluid collection is typically asymptomatic and tends to spontaneously resolve before age 12 months. Operative management of noncommunicating hydrocele is usually reserved for lesions that persist after this age, acute enlargement of the hydrocele, or if there is any question of communication.

GASTROINTESTINAL DISORDERS

Neonatal Intestinal Obstruction

Various congenital anatomic defects, inherited metabolic diseases, and acquired physiologic disorders may present as intestinal obstruction in a newborn. **3** Neonatal intestinal obstruction is characterized clinically by bilious emesis and is often associated with abdominal distention. Bilious emesis in a neonate must be considered to be acute mechanical intestinal obstruction until proven otherwise. Emergent surgical evaluation is warranted for any newborn with bilious emesis. Table 107.2 provides differential diagnoses for neonatal intestinal obstruction along with salient features of the history, physical examination, and diagnostic studies.

The clinical presentation of neonatal intestinal obstruction depends, in part, on the site of obstruction and the age of the infant. Clinical examination of the infant typically provides the surgeon with a preliminary diagnosis and helps guide further diagnostic studies. Abdominal distention is a characteristic physical finding with distal bowel obstruction, whereas the abdomen may be flat in proximal obstruction. The presence of bile in the gastric contents or stool provides clinical evidence of the location of an obstruction relative to the ampulla of Vater. Bilious emesis in an infant or child should be considered an anatomic obstruction requiring emergent surgical evaluation. An infant with bilious emesis who has already passed meconium and has tolerated feeding is unlikely to have intestinal atresia and more likely to have intestinal malrotation with midgut volvulus. If volvulus is suspected, emergent evaluation must be performed to diagnose and prevent catastrophic bowel injury or death.

Definitive diagnosis of neonatal intestinal obstruction may often be made by physical examination and readily available radiologic studies. Incarcerated inguinal hernia is an important cause of neonatal bowel obstruction, and examination leads to a straightforward diagnosis. Some congenital conditions have clearly recognizable features and may be associated with anatomic intestinal obstruction. For example, infants with trisomy 21 have a higher probability of having duodenal atresia or Hirschsprung disease than the general population. An approach to imaging the neonate suspected of having an intestinal obstruction is to obtain a plain abdominal radiograph, followed by either a contrast enema or an upper gastrointestinal series. Plain films of the newborn abdomen can be

TABLE 107.2 **DIAGNOSIS**

NEONATAL INTESTINAL OBSTRUCTION

■ DIAGNOSIS	■ HISTORY	■ PHYSICAL EXAMINATION	■ DIAGNOSTIC STUDIES
Intestinal atresia or stenosis	Bilious emesis	Abdominal distention	Plain abdominal film
	Failure to pass meconium	Abdominal distention	Contrast enema
Duodenal atresia or stenosis	Bilious or nonbilious emesis	Gastric distention	Plain abdominal film
	Feeding intolerance	Trisomy 21	Upper GI contrast study
Imperforate anus	Failure to pass meconium	Absent anus or visible fistula	Plain chest, abdominal film
	Bilious emesis (late)	Abdominal distention	Ultrasound kidneys, sacrum, rectum
		VACTERL association	Echocardiogram
Necrotizing enterocolitis	High-risk, premature infant	Abdominal distention	Plain abdominal film
		Abdominal wall erythema	
	Bilious emesis	Hematochezia, guaiac-positive stool	
Meconium ileus	Cystic fibrosis (10%)	Acholic meconium	Plain abdominal film
	Bilious emesis	Abdominal distention	Contrast enema
Malrotation	Bilious emesis	No abdominal distention	Plain abdominal film
	Term, healthy infant		Upper GI contrast study
Hirschsprung disease	Delayed passage of meconium	Abdominal distention	Plain abdominal film
	Bilious emesis	Trisomy 21	Contrast enema
Uncommon causes of obstruction (intussusception, Meckel diverticulum, duplication)		Abdominal mass, incarcerated hernia	Variable
Medical conditions associated with ileus	Bilious emesis	Sepsis, hypothyroidism, etc.	Plain abdominal film

GI, gastrointestinal; VACTERL, vertebral, anal, cardiac, tracheal, esophageal, renal, and limb anomalies.

extremely useful because swallowed gas acts as a contrast agent. For example, duodenal atresia gives rise to a dilated, gas-filled stomach and duodenum proximal to the obstruction; the remainder of the bowel remains gasless, giving rise to the "double-bubble" appearance on plain films. Other causes of proximal intestinal obstruction may lead to a microcolon on contrast enema, which is a small, unused but otherwise normal colon. If a retrograde contrast enema does not pass into the dilated segment of bowel, an upper gastrointestinal series may be useful to identify a more proximal obstruction. Upper gastrointestinal series is also the most useful diagnostic test for intestinal malrotation.

Several medical conditions of the newborn appear clinically similar to mechanical intestinal obstruction (Table 107.2). In particular, bilious emesis from ileus secondary to neonatal sepsis is not uncommon. Congenital hypothyroidism is an infrequent and medically treatable condition that can produce delayed intestinal motility that mimics mechanical intestinal obstruction.

Intestinal Atresia or Stenosis

Embryology and Anatomy. The embryonic intestine undergoes segmental development during the third week of gestation. The septum transversum demarcates the developing foregut from the midgut. The midgut can be considered a tubular structure that progressively undergoes several predictable, developmental stages: (a) elongation; (b) herniation from and reduction into the coelomic cavity; (c) rotation; and (d) fixation of the mesentery to the posterior body wall.

Several different types of intestinal atresia are clinically observed (Fig. 107.7). *Type I* atresia is an intraluminal web or diaphragm that can either be complete or fenestrated with intact seromuscular layers of bowel. *Types II* and *IIIa* atresia are believed to be a result of in utero mesenteric vascular accidents. Experimental interruption of the fetal mesenteric blood supply in utero leads to this type of atresia.[36,37] *Type IIIb* atresia, also known as the *apple-peel* or *Christmas tree deformity,* has complete mesenteric discontinuity, with the distal bowel concentrically surrounding a singular mesenteric blood supply. *Type IV* atresia has multiple segmental areas of discontinuous bowel. Types IIIb and IV atresia are thought to be consequences of major and multiple fetal mesenteric vascular interruption.

At least 90% of infants with congenital intestinal obstruction of the small bowel have complete atresia, whereas the remaining children have either stenoses or fenestrated intraluminal webs. The most common location is the distal ileum, and multiple areas of atresia are discovered in 3.6% to 20% of these infants.[38] Infants with fenestrated intraluminal webs may have a small, often eccentric opening only millimeters in diameter. These infants may not have obstructive symptoms until the introduction of solid food at 6 to 12 months of age and present with feeding intolerance, failure to thrive, or abdominal pain.

Congenital colonic atresia is a distinctly unusual condition. In a contemporary series of 277 infants treated with intestinal atresia, only 21 children had colonic atresia.[38] Similar to small bowel atresia, colonic atresia is believed to reflect fetal mesenteric vascular injury. Given the distal nature of colonic atresia, initial feeding may be well tolerated and definitive diagnosis may be delayed for several days. The diagnostic evaluation

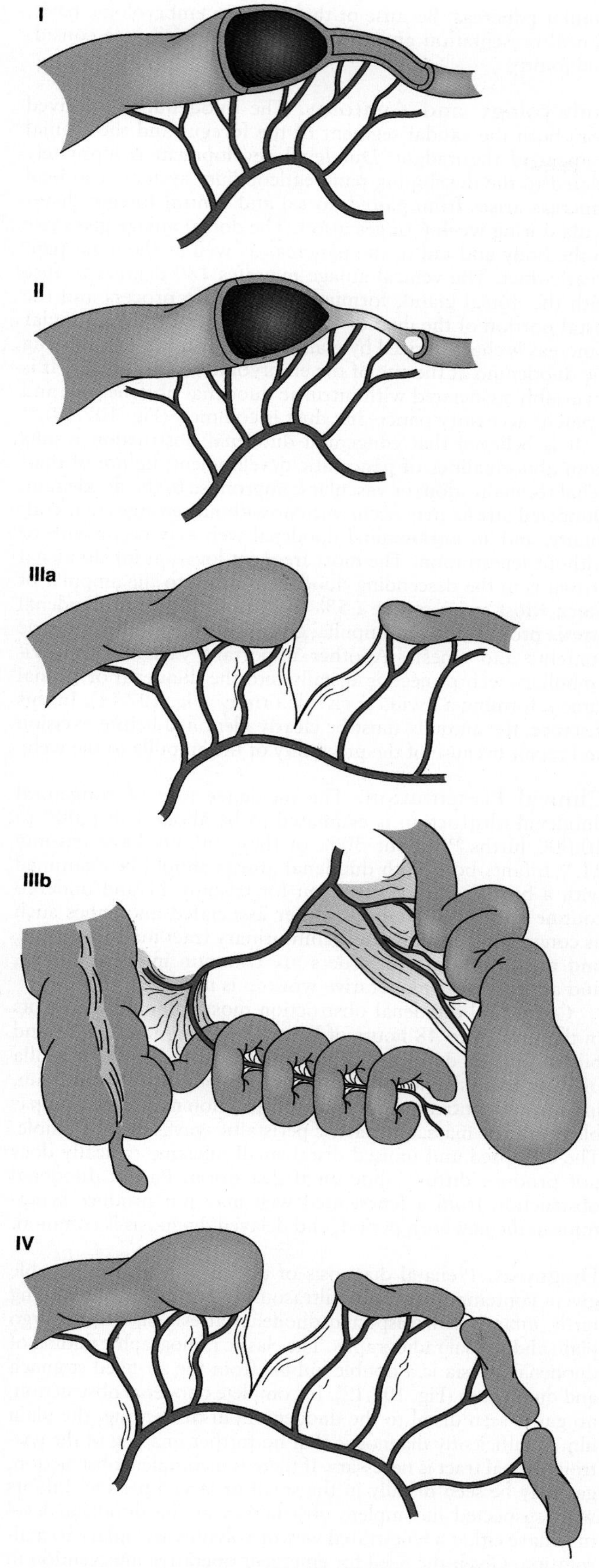

FIGURE 107.7. Classification of intestinal atresia. Type I, muscular continuity with a complete web. Type II, mesentery intact, fibrous cord. Type IIIa, muscular and mesenteric discontinuous. Type IIIb, apple-peel deformity. Type IV, multiple atresias. (Adapted from Grosfeld JL. Jejunoileal atresia and stenosis. In: O'Neill JA Jr, Rowe MI, Grosfeld JL, et al. eds. *Pediatric Surgery,* 5th ed. St. Louis, MO: Mosby; 1998:1145–1158.)

and surgical treatment of colonic atresia is identical to the approach used for small bowel atresia. Colonic atresia may be associated with abdominal wall defects, skeletal or cardiac defects, or coexisting small intestinal atresia.

Clinical Presentation. The actual incidence rate of congenital intestinal atresia is unknown. Reported estimates in the United States are 3.5 to 3.75 cases per 10,000 total births.[39] Infants with jejunal or ileal atresia have a low incidence rate of significant associated anomalies. Approximately10% of infants with gastroschisis have intestinal atresia or stenosis secondary to mechanical interruption of the mesenteric vascular supply.

Detection of maternal polyhydramnios on routine prenatal ultrasound screening can be an indication of proximal bowel obstruction caused by the interruption of normal amniotic fluid absorption in the fetal gut.[40] Following delivery, the classic clinical presentation of intestinal atresia is bilious emesis, abdominal distention, and failure to pass meconium. The degree of abdominal distention depends on the site of obstruction, the infant's age, and the efficacy of proximal decompression. Abdominal distention may be absent with proximal intestinal atresia. Distal intestinal atresia may lead to abdominal distention with visible or palpable intestinal loops on examination. Rectal examination and evaluation of stool character remains important when intestinal obstruction is suspected.

Diagnosis. Following history and physical examination, plain radiographic abdominal films should be obtained. Plain films in jejunal or ileal atresia demonstrate marked gaseous distention of the proximal intestine with gasless distal small bowel and colon. Haustral markings are normally not apparent in the neonatal colon, and therefore discrimination between small bowel and colon in the newborn is difficult without intraluminal contrast. A contrast enema is generally obtained to confirm the diagnosis of jejunoileal atresia. A diminutive, unused but otherwise normal microcolon is typical of proximal intestinal obstruction. The inability to reflux contrast into the proximal, dilated small bowel segment is diagnostic for congenital intestinal obstruction. This radiographic finding, in conjunction with the clinical setting, warrants operative exploration. An upper gastrointestinal series is unnecessary and may increase the risk of further emesis and aspiration in the newborn with obstruction. Incomplete obstruction from a fenestrated intraluminal web may require more sophisticated imaging techniques such as catheter-directed enteroclysis.

Treatment. Anatomic lesions causing neonatal intestinal obstruction require operative treatment. Whereas malrotation with midgut volvulus requires emergent diagnostic workup and operative intervention, obstruction resulting from intestinal atresia is generally not associated with life-threatening physiologic disturbances. Therefore, initial treatment is aimed at treating any other associated problems, confirming diagnosis, and preparing the infant for an operation. During this period, the infant always should have an orogastric or nasogastric tube in place to provide proximal decompression of the obstructed bowel.

The operative strategy in treating intestinal atresia is to restore gastrointestinal tract continuity while preserving as much intestinal length as possible. The operation is straightforward, and an end-to-end or end-to-oblique (end-to-back) anastomosis is typically performed (Fig. 107.8). Short segmental bowel resection and excision of an intraluminal web or diaphragm are used when necessary. Visual inspection and instillation of intraluminal saline or air to exclude distal atresia or web prior to anastomosis is important to evaluate patency of the downstream bowel. The size discrepancy between the proximal and distal bowel is usually considerable, and delayed postoperative bowel motility is common. Some surgeons advocate the use of technical procedures to improve emptying of the proximal bowel by reducing overall bowel diameter. These procedures include resection, plication, and tapering enteroplasty.

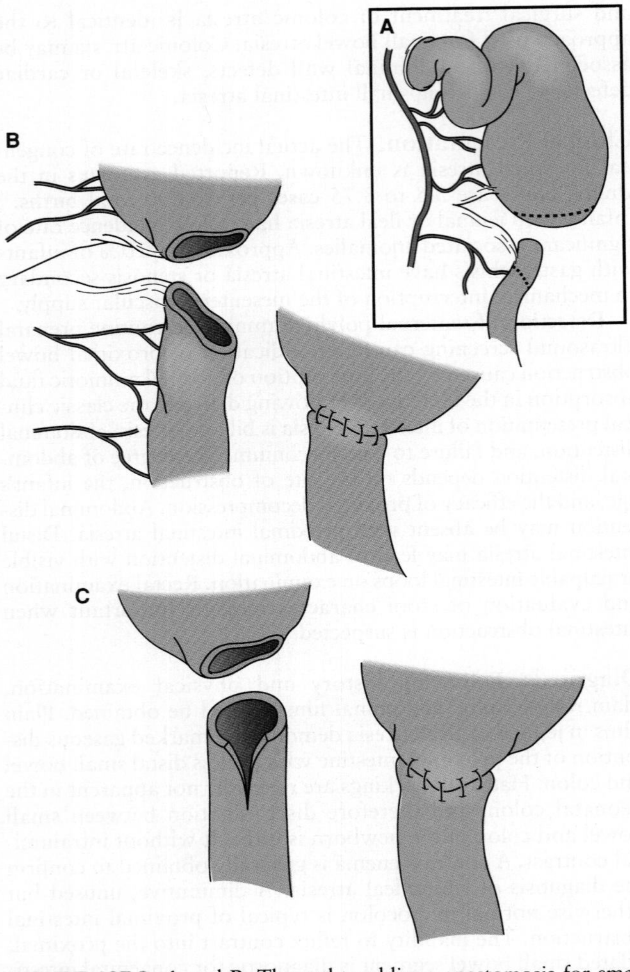

FIGURE 107.8. A and B: The end-to-oblique anastomosis for small bowel atresia. C: An extension of the distal enterostomy along the antimesenteric border may be used to create proximal and distal lumens of equal size for anastomosis.

Complex atresia associated with apple-peel deformity or multiple segmental atresias may require multiple serial anastomoses to preserve as much bowel length as possible. The ileocecal valve is preserved whenever possible, allowing improved tolerance of enteral nutrition in infants with limited small bowel length. It is estimated that approximately 40 cm of small bowel without an ileocecal valve, compared with 15 to 20 cm with an ileocecal valve, is sufficient for long-term enteral feeding tolerance in the neonate.[41] Contemporary management of colonic atresia includes primary anastomosis when technically possible.

Results and Outcome. Currently, the overall survival rate for infants treated for intestinal atresia or stenosis (including duodenal atresia) exceeds 93% in most large series.[38,42] Mortality in these infants is generally related to cardiac anomalies, birthweight less than 2 kg, and associated congenital anomalies.[43] Infants with a limited amount of intestinal length for nutritional absorption (short bowel syndrome with less than 40 cm) usually require long-term TPN and are at moderate to high risk for sepsis and liver injury. Infants with normal gastrointestinal length may still have prolonged intestinal dysfunction and dysmotility for several weeks.

Congenital Duodenal Obstruction

Causes of duodenal obstruction in the newborn include duodenal atresia or stenosis, duodenal intraluminal web, and annular pancreas. Because of the common embryologic basis, clinical presentation and treatment, these entities are considered jointly.

Embryology and Anatomy. The duodenum is derived from both the caudal segment of the foregut and the cranial segment of the midgut. Duodenal development is intimately related to the developing pancreaticobiliary system. The fetal pancreas arises from paired dorsal and ventral foregut diverticula during week 6 of gestation. The dorsal anlage gives rise to the body and tail of the pancreas as well as the main pancreatic duct. The ventral anlage migrates 180 degrees to fuse with the dorsal gland, forming the uncinate process and the distal portion of the duct of Wirsung (Fig. 107.9). An annular pancreas is characterized by glandular persistence surrounding the duodenum at the site of the embryonic ventral anlage. It is invariably associated with intrinsic duodenal obstruction, and a patent accessory pancreatic duct is common (Fig. 107.10).[44]

It is believed that congenital duodenal obstruction results from abnormalities of pancreatic development, failure of duodenal recanalization, or vascular compromise to the duodenum. Duodenal atresia may occur with or without seromuscular continuity, and an intraluminal duodenal web may occur with or without fenestration. The most frequent location for duodenal atresia is in the descending duodenum distal to the ampulla of Vater. Most series report a 5% to 10% incidence of duodenal atresia proximal to the ampulla, giving rise to nonbilious gastric contents and emesis. Another important variant is a periampullary web projecting distally into the duodenal or jejunal lumen, forming a "wind sock" deformity (Fig. 107.11). In this instance, the ampulla must be clearly identified before excision and repair because of the proximity of the ampulla to the web.

Clinical Presentation. The incidence rate of congenital duodenal obstruction is estimated to be about 1 in 6,000 to 10,000 births.[45] About 30% of these infants have trisomy 21.[46] Infants born with duodenal atresia should be examined with a high degree of suspicion for trisomy 21 and undergo routine karyotype analysis. Other associated anomalies such as congenital heart disease, genitourinary tract malformations, and musculoskeletal disorders are common in these infants, and appropriate preoperative workup is necessary.

Congenital duodenal obstruction most commonly presents in the first 24 to 48 hours of life with feeding intolerance and bilious emesis; duodenal obstruction proximal to the ampulla of Vater results in nonbilious emesis. On physical examination, infants with untreated duodenal obstruction may have a palpable epigastric mass, and gastric peristaltic waves may be visible. The collapsed and unused distal small intestine typically does not produce diffuse abdominal distention. Partial duodenal obstruction from a fenestrated web may not produce symptoms in the newborn period, and delayed diagnosis is common.

Diagnosis. Prenatal diagnosis of duodenal atresia is possible given contemporary fetal ultrasound techniques. Following birth, infants with suspected duodenal atresia should undergo plain abdominal radiographs. The classic radiographic finding of duodenal atresia is a double bubble from the air-filled stomach and duodenum (Fig. 107.12). In complete duodenal obstruction, no gas is seen distal to the duodenum; in this setting, the plain film is sufficiently diagnostic that no further imaging of the gastrointestinal tract is necessary. If there is incomplete obstruction, gas may be seen distally in the small or large intestine. Infants with suspected incomplete obstruction at the duodenal level may have either a fenestrated web or volvulus secondary to malrotation. Given the need for emergent operative intervention in malrotation with acute volvulus, an urgent upper gastrointestinal series with contrast should be strongly considered to exclude a neonatal surgical emergency. It is important that all anatomic lesions causing neonatal duodenal obstruction require operative repair using a similar approach.

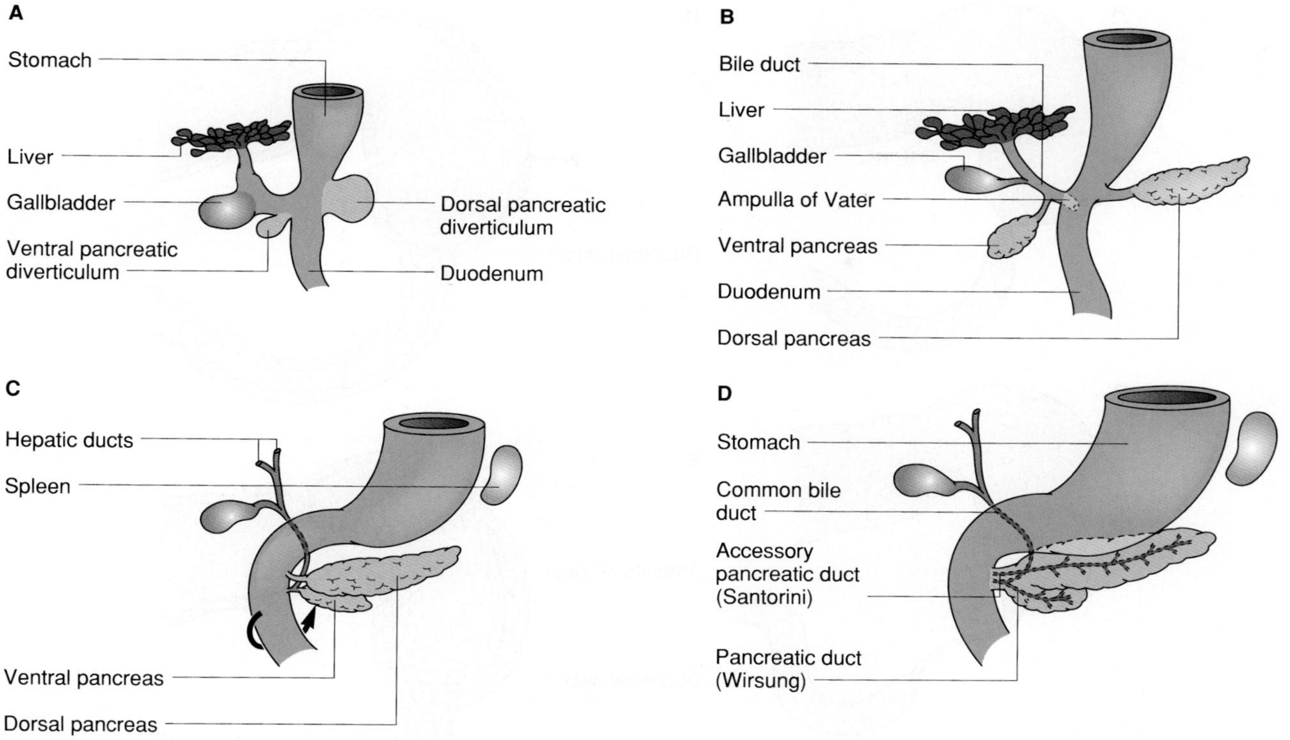

FIGURE 107.9. Normal embryologic development of the duodenum, pancreas, and bile ducts. **A:** Fifth gestational week. **B:** Sixth week. **C:** Seventh week. **D:** Eighth week.

Treatment. Following expedient treatment of any associated life-threatening medical conditions and preoperative evaluation, the operative goals are to restore gastrointestinal continuity without sacrificing intestinal length or absorptive surface area. Because most lesions causing congenital duodenal obstruction are near the ampulla of Vater, great care must be exercised in treatment to avoid inadvertent injury to the ampulla or pancreas.

Congenital duodenal atresia is treated by duodenoduodenostomy. Duodenal obstruction secondary to annular pancreas is also treated by duodenoduodenostomy. Direct division of annular pancreas is not performed because this does not address the underlying intraluminal duodenal obstruction, and there is significant risk of injury to the accessory pancreatic duct (Fig. 107.10).

Duodenoduodenostomy is performed by making a transverse incision in the dilated, proximal duodenum and a longitudinal incision in the unused, downstream duodenum. The lumens are sutured together to form a diamond-shaped anastomosis (Fig. 107.13).[47] Downstream duodenal patency should

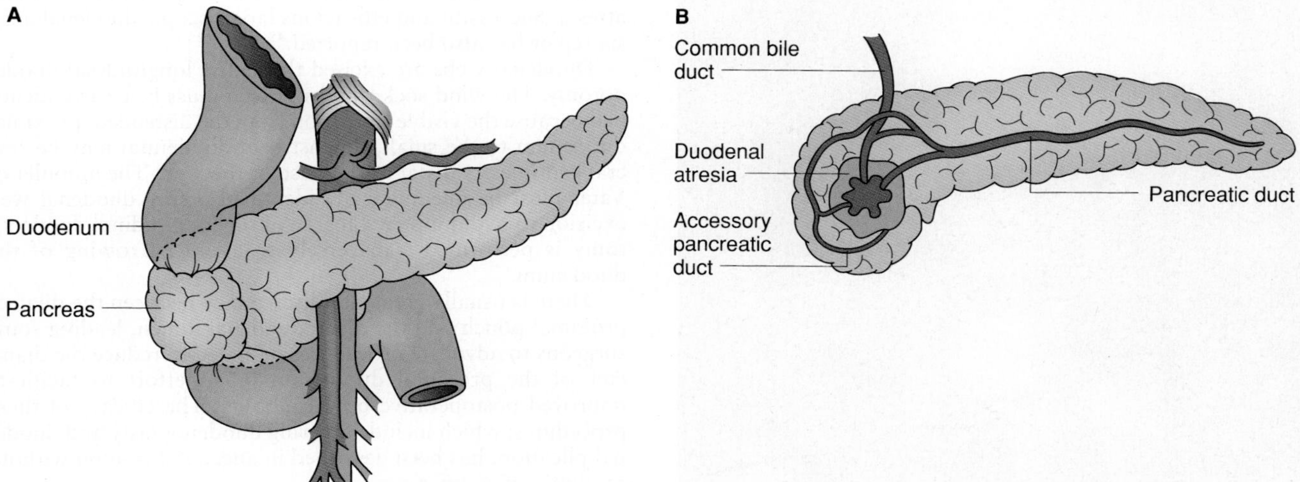

FIGURE 107.10. Annular pancreas. **A:** The associated duodenal atresia is shown. **B:** The relationships of the annular pancreas to the common bile duct and main and accessory pancreatic ducts are shown in cross section.

PEDIATRICS

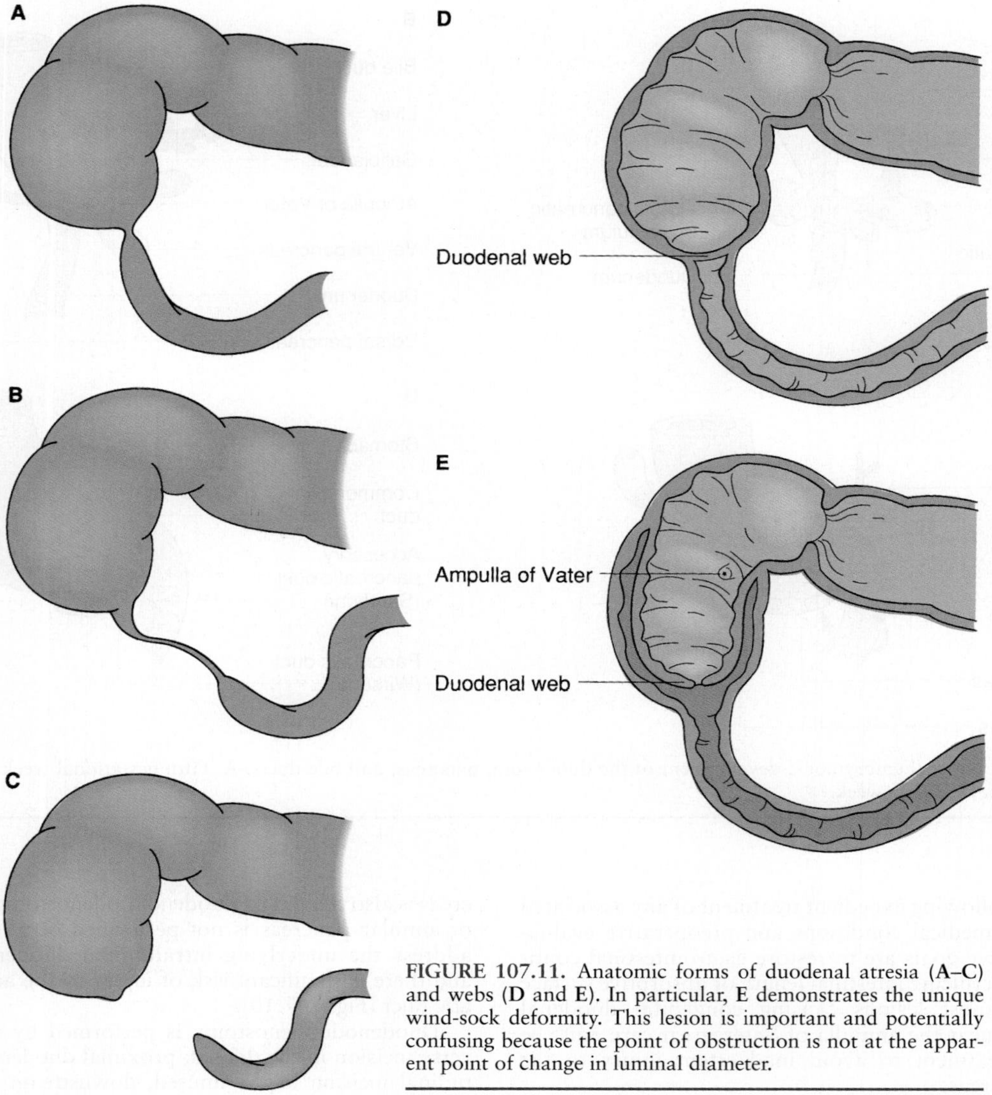

FIGURE 107.11. Anatomic forms of duodenal atresia (A–C) and webs (D and E). In particular, E demonstrates the unique wind-sock deformity. This lesion is important and potentially confusing because the point of obstruction is not at the apparent point of change in luminal diameter.

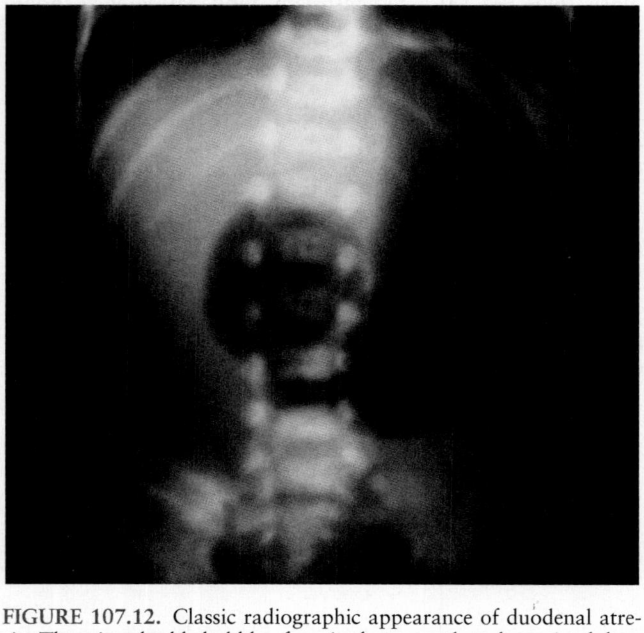

FIGURE 107.12. Classic radiographic appearance of duodenal atresia. There is a double bubble of gas in the stomach and proximal duodenum, with no gas in the distal intestinal tract.

be demonstrated by passing a catheter or infusing saline or air distally to avoid overlooking synchronous distal intestinal atresia. Successful and efficacious laparoscopic duodenal atresia repair has also been reported.[48]

Duodenal webs are excised through a longitudinal duodenotomy. The wind sock duodenal web must be clearly identified because the visible transition from the distended, proximal duodenum to the small, downstream duodenum may be several centimeters distal to the base of the web. The ampulla of Vater must be unequivocally identified before duodenal web excision to avoid injury. Closure of the longitudinal duodenotomy is performed transversely to avoid narrowing of the duodenum.

There is usually great size discrepancy between the dilated, proximal pouch and the distal duodenal lumen, leading some surgeons to advocate procedures designed to reduce the diameter of the proximal duodenum in an effort to facilitate improved postoperative bowel motility. The efficacy of these procedures, which include tapering duodenoplasty and duodenal plication, has been described in anecdotal fashion without randomized comparison.

Results and Outcome. After successful operative repair of duodenal atresia or stenosis, delayed gastric emptying is common and typically manifests as enteral feeding intolerance.

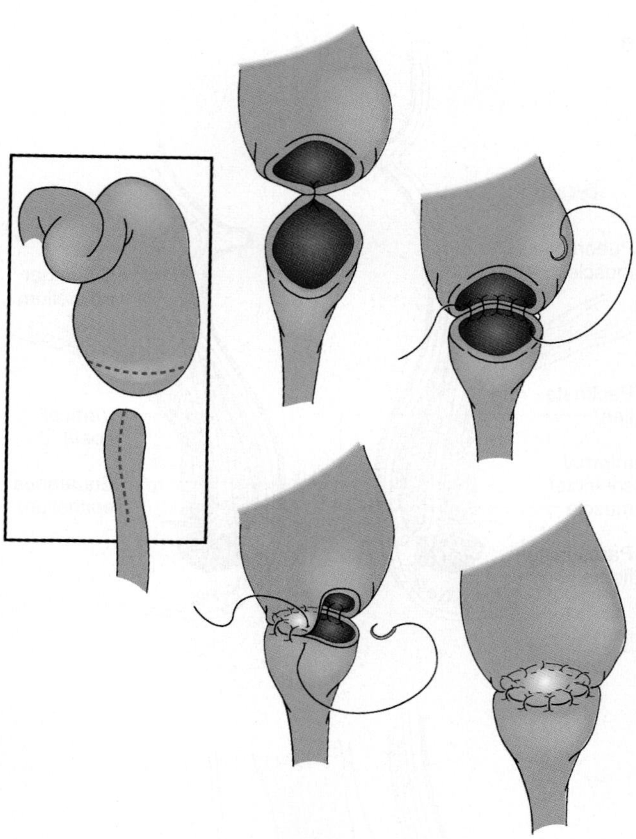

FIGURE 107.13. Diamond-shaped duodenoduodenostomy for repair of duodenal atresia.

Patience and persistence are essential during the postoperative period. Surgical outcomes after repair of congenital duodenal obstruction are excellent,[46–49] with perioperative survival exceeding 95%. Perioperative mortality is generally related to other congenital anomalies, and in particular, congenital heart disease in infants with trisomy 21. Other late problems may be encountered that reflect gastroduodenal motility issues such as poor gastric emptying, gastroesophageal reflux, and duodenal dilatation. These symptoms may appear several months to years following repair, and therefore, long-term surgical follow-up remains important.

Anorectal Malformations (Imperforate Anus)

Embryology. By week 5 of gestation, the fetal cloaca is identifiable with the adjacent hindgut, allantois, and vestigial tailgut (Fig. 107.14). The mesoderm of the urorectal septum extends caudally to fuse with the cloacal closing plate. Fusion of the lateral cloacal ridges completes division of the cloaca into the rectum and the urogenital sinus. The caudal aspect of the urorectal septum forms the perineal body. The anal membrane normally ruptures during week 8 of gestation, completing the patency of the distal rectum to the skin. Further development of the urogenital sinus leads to the formation of the urethra and bladder. In female infants, the uterus and proximal vagina develop from the müllerian ducts. The diverse anatomic variation observed with anorectal malformations is thought to reflect anomalous or interrupted development of these structures during normal embryogenesis.

Anatomy and Classification. The normal anatomy of the anus and rectum is reviewed in previous chapters. Normally, the rectum descends to the perineum and ultimately, to the anal orifice through a striated muscle complex in the pelvis resembling a funnel. The striated muscle complex is under voluntary control and is responsible for providing fecal continence (Fig. 107.15). Contiguous portions of the *levator ani,* the *external sphincter,* and the *puborectalis* muscles compose the *striated muscle complex*. These anatomically indistinct components of the muscle complex act together to provide control of defecation. The concept of the striated muscle complex and anatomic relationships leading to normal fecal continence with respect to anorectal malformations has evolved from both clinical and anatomic data as described by Peña.[50]

Because of the variety of anorectal malformations observed, different classification systems have been proposed in an attempt to characterize the defects. A summary of the Wingspread classification is provided in Table 107.3. This anatomically descriptive classification scheme is useful in planning the operative management of anorectal malformations.

In male subjects, the two most common anorectal malformations observed are low imperforate anus with a perineal fistula (Fig. 107.16) and high anorectal agenesis with a rectoprostatic

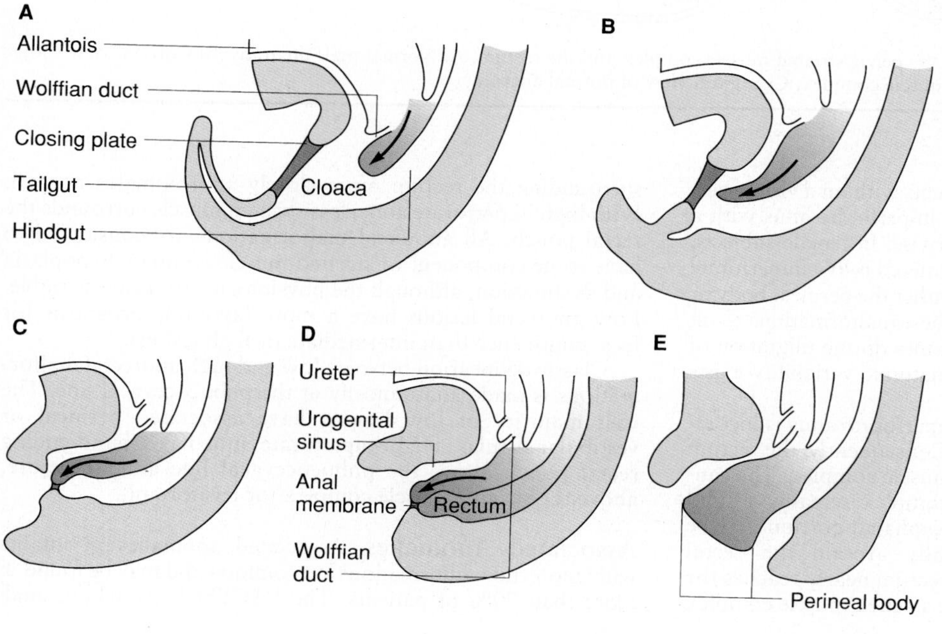

FIGURE 107.14. Normal embryologic division of the cloaca by the urorectal septum into the ventral urinary tract and the dorsal rectum. This process is normally completed by the ninth or tenth week of gestation.

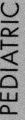

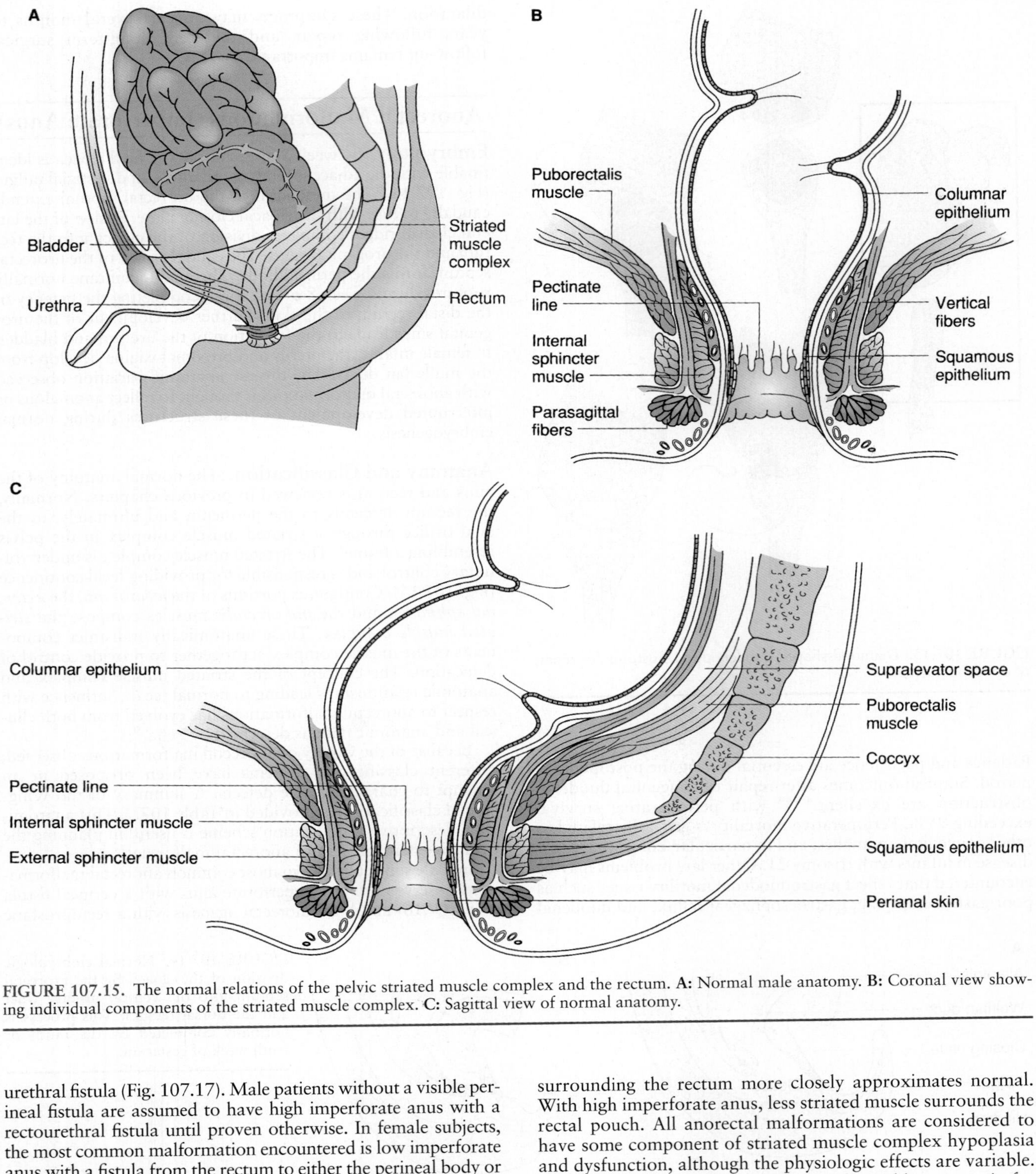

FIGURE 107.15. The normal relations of the pelvic striated muscle complex and the rectum. **A:** Normal male anatomy. **B:** Coronal view showing individual components of the striated muscle complex. **C:** Sagittal view of normal anatomy.

urethral fistula (Fig. 107.17). Male patients without a visible perineal fistula are assumed to have high imperforate anus with a rectourethral fistula until proven otherwise. In female subjects, the most common malformation encountered is low imperforate anus with a fistula from the rectum to either the perineal body or the vaginal vestibule (Fig. 107.18). As these malformations result from developmental arrest at various times during migration of the urogenital septum, considerable anatomic variability exists in both male and female subjects.

A common anatomic feature of imperforate anus is incomplete rectal descent to the perineum. Consequently, the rectum is not completely within the striated muscle complex. The caudal portion of the striated muscle complex remains a solid mass of striated muscle, whereas the cephalad portion may be normally positioned circumferentially around the rectal pouch. In low imperforate anus, the rectum nearly reaches the perineum and the configuration of the striated muscle complex surrounding the rectum more closely approximates normal. With high imperforate anus, less striated muscle surrounds the rectal pouch. All anorectal malformations are considered to have some component of striated muscle complex hypoplasia and dysfunction, although the physiologic effects are variable. Low anorectal lesions have a more favorable prognosis for fecal continence than intermediate or high lesions.

Classic delineation between low and high anorectal malformations is made anatomically at the pubococcygeal line. The vast majority of low lesions have associated perineal or vestibular fistulas. High imperforate anus has a blind-ending rectal pouch above the pubococcygeal line and, therefore, above the striated muscle complex (or levator ani).

Associated Anomalies. Associated anomalies in infants with anorectal malformations are common and may be found in more than 70% of patients. The VACTERL (vertebral, anal,

TABLE 107.3 CLASSIFICATION

ANATOMIC CLASSIFICATION OF ANORECTAL MALFORMATIONS

■ FEMALE	■ MALE
HIGH	
Anorectal agenesis with rectovaginal fistula with or without fistula	Anorectal agenesis with rectoprostatic urethral fistula* with or without fistula
Rectal atresia	Rectal atresia
INTERMEDIATE	
Rectovestibular fistula	Rectobulbar urethral fistula
Rectovaginal fistula	Anal agenesis without fistula
Anal agenesis without fistula	
LOW	
Anovestibular fistula[a]	Anocutaneous fistula[a]
Anocutaneous fistula[a,b]	Anal stenosis[a,c]
Anal stenosis[c]	Rare malformations
RARE MALFORMATIONS	
Cloacal malformations[d]	

[a]Relatively common lesion.
[b]Includes fistulas occurring at the posterior junction of the labia minora, often called *fourchette fistulas* or *vulvar fistulas.*
[c]Previously called *covered anus.*
[d]Previously called *rectocloacal fistulas.* Entry of the rectal fistula into the cloaca may be high or intermediate, depending on the length of the cloacal canal.

cardiac, tracheal, esophageal, renal and limb) association is important and requires consideration in any infant with imperforate anus. *Vertebral anomalies* are common and include sacral dysplasia and agenesis. Infants with sacral anomalies commonly have high imperforate anus and sacral nerve dysfunction that can lead to poor long-term fecal continence and neurogenic bladder. Various spinal cord malformations also can be

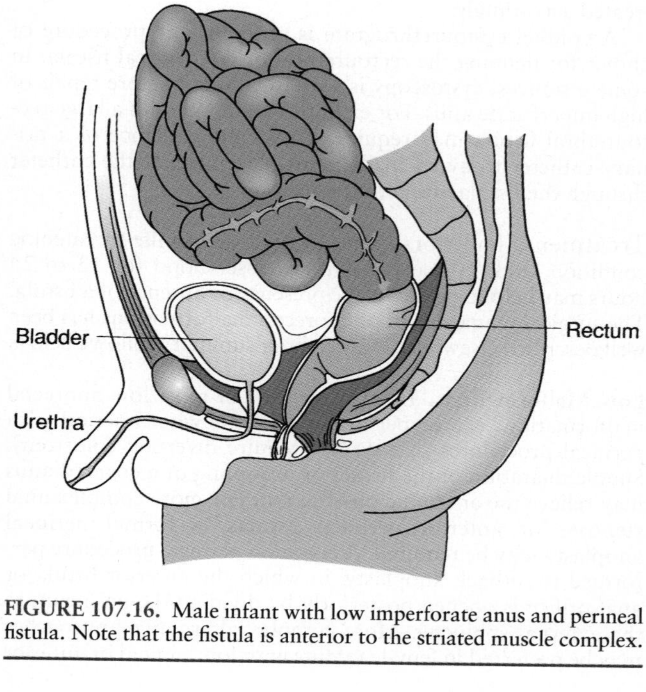

FIGURE 107.16. Male infant with low imperforate anus and perineal fistula. Note that the fistula is anterior to the striated muscle complex.

observed in these infants, including tethered spinal cord syndromes and some myelodysplastic syndromes. During the neonatal period, these spinal lesions may be detected by using ultrasound or magnetic resonance imaging (MRI), and surgical treatment may be necessary within the first 8 to 18 months of life. *Tracheoesophageal* fistula with or without esophageal atresia is estimated to occur in about 10% of infants with anorectal malformations. *Renal anomalies* are the most common associated abnormalities with anorectal malformations and include both upper and lower tract conditions. Genitourinary screening in the form of a renal ultrasound and voiding cystourethrogram is routinely performed. *Cardiac* anomalies are common, and screening echocardiography is clinically indicated. *Limb abnormalities,* in particular, involvement of the radius, complete the associated anomalies defined by the acronym.

Clinical Presentation. The incidence rate of anorectal malformations is estimated at 1 in 2,524 to 5,000 live births,[51] with a slightly higher rate in males. Careful examination of the neonatal perineum reveals the diagnosis. If unrecognized and left untreated, high imperforate anus eventually leads to signs and symptoms of complete bowel obstruction characterized by abdominal distention, feeding intolerance, and bilious emesis. Because of the nearly uniform rectourethral or rectovesicular fistula in males with high lesions, some of these infants will pass meconium or gas through the urethra during urination. In contrast, infants with low malformations typically pass meconium through a perineal or vestibular fistula within the first 24 hours of life. Occasionally, infants with large perineal fistulas are not diagnosed with an anorectal malformation until progressive constipation is noted weeks to months after birth.

In male infants, more than 95% of low malformations are associated with either a thin anal membrane or a fistula to the perineum or scrotal raphe. The presence of a "bucket handle" skin deformity at the presumptive anal dimple is also diagnostic of a low lesion. Infants with high malformations typically lack anal skin dimpling, have a flat gluteal contour, and may have little or absent contraction of the external sphincter with cutaneous stimulation. In female infants, 90% to 95% of low malformations have a perineal or vestibular fistula. In both male and female infants, a perineal fistula may not become apparent in the first 12 to 24 hours of life until meconium progresses distally through the rectum into the fistula.

Diagnosis. Because surgical treatment of a high or intermediate anorectal malformation is different from that for low lesion, a primary diagnostic goal is to determine whether an infant with imperforate anus has a high or low malformation. A secondary diagnostic goal is to determine the specific anorectal malformation as it relates to the rectourethral or rectovesicular fistula.

Clinical examination of an infant with low imperforate anus almost always reveals an external fistula to the perineum or vestibule. The classic radiographic study of newborns with imperforate anus is the Wangensteen-Rice invertogram, with a lateral view of the pelvis obtained 12 to 24 hours after birth with the infant in a head-down position. This technique has been largely replaced by ultrasound-directed imaging.[52] Real-time ultrasound is currently well accepted as an accurate method of determining the distal extent of the rectal pouch. Computed tomography (CT) imaging and MRI can be useful in evaluating the pelvic striated muscle complex in difficult cases, and in particular, cloacal malformations. MRI is also useful in evaluation of the distal spinal cord in these infants.

If there is a suspected perineal fistula or covered anus, diagnostic needle aspiration under anesthesia may be useful. Aspiration of meconium not only localizes the rectum or fistula, but it also can provide an estimation of the distance between the perineum and the rectum or the fistula. In general, low lesions are within 1 cm of the perineum. An infant not clearly found to have a low lesion by physical examination, radiographic studies, or examination under anesthesia should

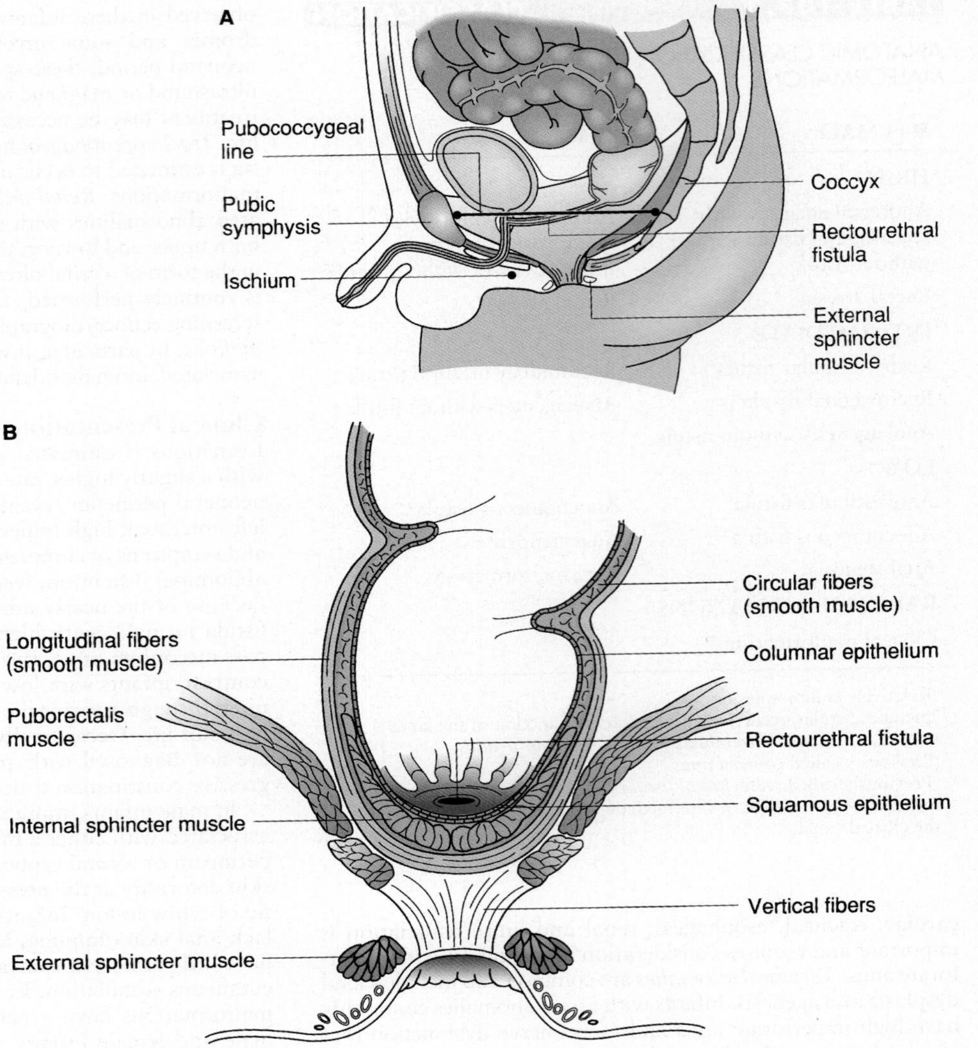

FIGURE 107.17. Male infant with high imperforate anus, showing the pubococcygeal line, ischium, and striated muscle complex. **A:** The rectal pouch ends cephalad to the pubococcygeal line. This location of the rectourethral fistula is typical. **B:** Coronal view showing incomplete development of the rectal pouch within the striated muscle complex. The rectourethral fistula is shown.

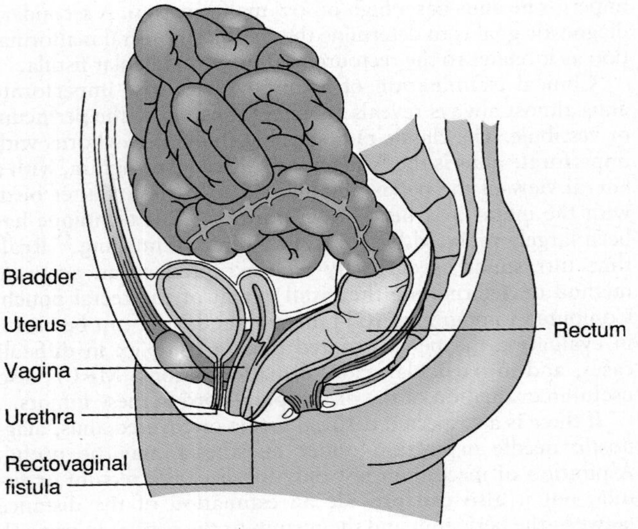

FIGURE 107.18. Female infant with low imperforate anus and vestibular fistula.

be considered to have a high anorectal malformation and treated accordingly.

A voiding cystourethrogram is generally the procedure of choice for defining the rectourethral or rectovesical fistula. In some instances, cystoscopy is a useful adjunct before repair of high imperforate anus. For example, an infant with a large rectourethral fistula may require cystoscopic guidance of a urinary catheter to avoid inadvertent placement of the catheter through the fistula and into the rectum.

Treatment. Imperforate anus by itself is not a life-threatening condition, and, in many instances, observation for 12 to 24 hours may help to delineate the presence or absence of a fistula. The surgical management of anorectal malformations has been well described elsewhere,[50] and a brief summary follows below.

Low Malformations. Definitive repair of most low anorectal malformations can be performed in the newborn period with perineal procedures that do not require diverting colostomy. Simple dilatation of the fistula or unroofing of a covered anus may relieve the anatomic obstruction. For more complex anal stenoses or anterior perineal fistulas, a formal perineal anoplasty may be required. A common perineal procedure performed is cutback anoplasty, in which the anterior fistula or anal orifice is opened posteriorly by dividing the perineum to the external sphincter. More complex alternative approaches may be preferred in female infants with low vaginal or anterior perineal fistulas. These lesions generally require circumferential mobilization of the anterior fistula with transposition to the center of the external sphincter. Anterior reconstruction of the perineal body is then performed. Transposition anoplasty is designed to position the neoanus within the center of the external sphincter and separate the neoanus from the vaginal introitus.

Intermediate and High Malformations. Infants determined to have an intermediate, high, or indeterminate anorectal malformation generally require diverting divided colostomy as initial surgical management. Care must be taken to ensure that the proximal diverting colostomy provides adequate length and mobility of the distal colon in anticipation of eventual anorectoplasty. A divided colostomy is preferred over a loop colostomy by many surgeons to provide maximal fecal diversion from the downstream rectourinary fistula. Following diverting colostomy, a distal contrast study into the rectal pouch can also define the fistula and delineate the position of the rectum relative to the perineum.

Anorectoplasty is generally performed when the infant is approximately 8 to 12 months of age. Many different approaches have been described, and considerable personal and institutional variation is common. No single approach has superior results, and all have technical merits and difficulties. The common surgical objectives in the treatment of anorectal malformations include the following: (a) relieve the rectal obstruction; (b) create a new anus; (c) position the rectum as normally as possible within the striated muscle complex; and (d) divide the rectourinary fistula. In addition, preservation of the surrounding structures (prostate, urethra, seminal vesicles, vaginal wall) is essential.

For repair of high and intermediate anorectal malformations, the most widely used procedure in the United States is the posterior sagittal anorectoplasty described in detail by Peña.[50] The infant is placed prone, and a posterior sagittal incision following the gluteal crease is used. The external sphincter and the striated muscle complex are divided posteriorly along the midline to expose the rectal pouch. A muscle stimulator is used to define and map the striated muscle complex and to confirm symmetric dissection along the midline. Typically, the rectal pouch can be adequately dissected by this approach to allow enough length to reach the perineum. Infrequently, a combined abdominoperineal approach is required. The mobilized rectal pouch is opened and the rectourinary fistula identified and closed directly. The rectal pouch is placed centrally within the striated muscle complex, which is reconstructed circumferentially around the rectum. The neoanus is centered within the external sphincter, and the mucosa is sutured to the perineum.

Other accepted and practiced surgical approaches to imperforate anus include a sacroperineal approach as proposed by Stephens,[53] and an approach that uses components of endorectal dissection as attributed to Rehbein.[54] Both these surgical procedures are characterized by blind pull-through of the distal rectum to the perineum without direct visualization of the striated muscle complex. Experience with laparoscopic dissection and division of the rectourinary fistula with perineal pull-through reconstruction has been reported.[55] It appears that personal preference, experience, and familiarity rather than differences in outcome dictate the selection of procedure. In general, diverting colostomy in all of these procedures is maintained until the anorectoplasty has completely healed, after which the colostomy is closed electively.

Results, Complications, and Outcome. Mortality following anorectoplasty is related to the presence of associated congenital anomalies other than imperforate anus. A careful review of 284 infants undergoing repair of anorectal malformations observed an 18.7% mortality,[56] suggesting that this group is at moderate to high risk for complications and death secondary to coexisting congenital anomalies.

Complications are similar to other gastrointestinal surgical procedures and include infection, leak, recurrent fistula, or anastomotic stricture. Leak or stricture formation is observed in 5% to 10% of infants undergoing tapering rectoplasty during posterior sagittal anorectoplasty. Anorectal strictures are treated by gradual postoperative anal dilatation for weeks to months. Recurrent rectourethral fistula or urethral stricture is uncommon.

Long-term functional outcome in infants with low malformations is generally good given the relatively normal descent of the distal rectum within the striated muscle complex. Infants with higher lesions have a less predictable prognosis and are much more likely to have difficulty with fecal continence. Currently, the outcomes appear to be independent of the type of surgical reconstruction performed and more related to anatomic patient factors, including degree of rectal descent, integrity of the striated muscle complex, and sacral innervation. Few or perhaps none of these children have completely normal bowel habits after operation. About half of the infants have acceptable to good results with episodic fecal soilage that can be improved with bowel management programs, enemas, and cathartics.[57–59] A comprehensive bowel management program is essential in preventing fecal impaction and subsequent motility dysfunction in the rectum. The remaining children require major adjustments in lifestyle secondary to fecal incontinence, chronic constipation, or fecal smearing and odor. In some instances, socially acceptable continence can be assisted by the use of daily antegrade enemas via a cecostomy or appendicostomy. In other situations, a permanent diverting colostomy may be desirable.

Necrotizing Enterocolitis

4 **Pathophysiology.** NEC is a neonatal disease characterized by an initial intestinal mucosal injury that may ultimately progress to transmural bowel necrosis. NEC is the most frequently encountered neonatal surgical emergency and a major cause of morbidity and mortality in the premature infant. Despite its frequency and extensive study, the pathogenesis remains obscure, and surgical treatment is directed largely at controlling the complications of intestinal necrosis. The development of NEC occurs in association with various associated conditions, including perinatal stress, sepsis, respiratory failure, hypoxemia, hypotension, and congenital cardiac defects. In general, NEC is observed in the premature infant with multiple risk factors and potential etiologic events and conditions. Current clinical and experimental data support the concept that the pathophysiology of NEC remains enigmatic and multifactorial.

The intestinal mucosal injury observed in NEC is likely to be the end result of an ischemic insult in a susceptible host. Normally, the neonatal pulmonary and systemic vascular smooth muscle undergoes rapid structural and physiologic changes shortly after birth. The premature infant appears to be particularly vulnerable to vasoconstriction. With regard to NEC, it is hypothesized that hypoperfusion and ischemia of the premature neonatal intestinal tract may be the result of uncontrolled splanchnic vasoconstriction. This situation may be worsened in critically ill premature infants with low cardiac output states impairing oxygen delivery to the intestines.

A common characteristic of NEC is the host inflammatory response to the initiating mucosal injury. Experimental data are consistent with an important role for inflammatory mediators in the propagation of intestinal injury in NEC.[60] More than 90% of cases of NEC occur after the initiation of enteral feeding, and several studies document that the osmolarity or rate of initial feeding may be important. Although controversy exists, most neonatal centers now avoid rapid advancement of hyperosmolar enteral feedings and attempt to prevent excessive fluid volume in premature infants.[61,62] A multicenter, randomized controlled clinical trial using *Bifidobacterium* and

Lactobacillus as a probiotic given with initial feeding demonstrated significant reduction in death from NEC in very low birthweight premature infants.[63]

The most common site of involvement of NEC is the terminal ileum and right colon. NEC may be localized, segmental, or it may involve the entire gastrointestinal tract. Histopathologic examination of intestinal tissue from infants with NEC demonstrates submucosal edema, hemorrhage, and microvascular thrombosis leading to transmural necrosis. The histopathology of NEC resembles that of experimental intestinal ischemia, with areas of reversible mucosal injury adjacent to areas of transmural necrosis. Dissection of intraluminal gas through the injured mucosa leads to gas within the bowel wall, known as *pneumatosis intestinalis*. The finding of pneumatosis intestinalis is a classic radiographic and pathologic feature of NEC. Initially, the gas may be localized in the submucosa or lymphatic vessels, but it may dissect into the muscularis, the portal venous tract, or into the subserosa. Intestinal perforation, inflammatory phlegmon, and diffuse peritonitis are common with advanced NEC.

Clinical Presentation. Over the past three decades, advancements in technology, prenatal care, and neonatology have improved overall outcome in premature infants who were previously unable to survive. In the United States alone, low birthweight infants (less than 2,500 g) account for more than 250,000 births a year. At least half of all infants with NEC are extremely low birthweight infants weighing less than 1,500 g. In a study of 302 infants with NEC treated over two decades, the average birth weight fell from 1,645 to 1,505 g, and in similar fashion, the mean gestational age fell from 32.4 weeks to 30.4 weeks.[64] NEC is estimated to occur in 1 to 3 of 1,000 live births and 30 per 1,000 low birthweight births.[65] NEC may also occur in term infants, and in this group, it has a tendency to involve the colon and may present without classic signs.[66] The actual incidence of NEC remains difficult to determine because the diagnosis is subjective; classic signs on physical examination and diagnostic imaging are not always uniformly present. The classic clinical signs of NEC include abdominal distention, feeding intolerance, bilious emesis, and either occult or gross blood in the stool. Gastrointestinal mucosal bleeding is present in the vast majority of cases (80%–90%) but is rarely significant from a hemodynamic standpoint. On physical examination, abdominal tenderness with distention is common, and individual loops of thickened or fixed bowel may be palpable. Edema, erythema, crepitus, or discoloration of the abdominal wall suggests intestinal necrosis, perforation, or intra-abdominal abscess (Fig. 107.19). Hematochezia or guaiac-positive stool is typical. Systemic signs of inflammation and sepsis such as temperature instability, apnea, bradycardia, hypoxemia, acidosis, and thrombocytopenia are also common. The primary diagnostic goal during initial clinical evaluation is to determine whether irreversible, transmural intestinal necrosis is present. There is no single physical finding or laboratory test that makes this distinction.

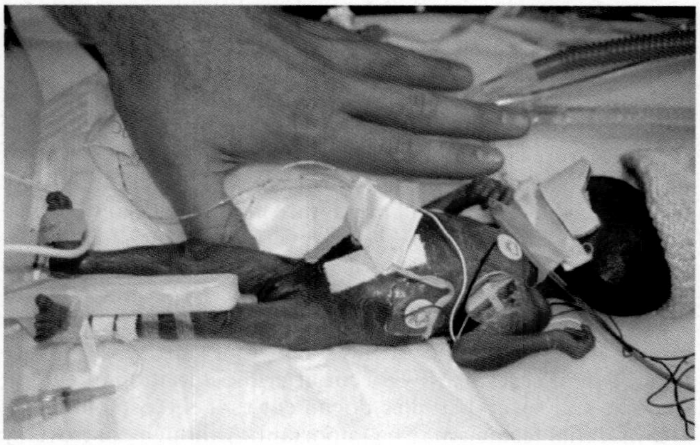

FIGURE 107.19. Clinical presentation of diffuse staining of abdominal wall in an extremely low birthweight infant with perforated necrotizing enterocolitis.

Diagnosis. The diagnosis of NEC relies on clinical evaluation and judgment based on symptoms and signs in the appropriate setting. Table 107.4 summarizes diagnostic criteria and a staging system for NEC most commonly used in the United States.[67] Radiographic confirmation of NEC requires only plain abdominal films. During the acute inflammatory phase, contrast studies may be hazardous and are contraindicated. The classic radiographic finding of pneumatosis intestinalis (Fig. 107.20) confirms the diagnosis in the appropriate clinical setting but is variably present. Other radiographic findings consistent with NEC include thickened bowel loops, ascites, and portal venous gas. Serial abdominal films, including a left

TABLE 107.4 **STAGING**

NECROTIZING ENTEROCOLITIS

STAGE I NEC (SUSPECTED)
Any one or more historical factors producing perinatal stress
Systemic manifestations
Temperature instability
Lethargy
Apnea
Bradycardia
Gastrointestinal manifestations
Poor feeding
Increasing pregavage residuals
Emesis
Mild abdominal distention
Occult blood in stool
Abdominal radiographs showing distention with mild ileus
STAGE II NEC (DEFINITE)
Any one or more historical factors
Above signs and symptoms, plus:
Persistent occult or gross gastrointestinal bleeding
Marked abdominal distention
Abdominal radiographs showing significant intestinal distention with:
Ileus
Small bowel edema
Pneumatosis intestinalis
Portal venous gas
STAGE III NEC (ADVANCED)
Any one or more historical factors
Above signs and symptoms, plus: Deterioration of vital signs
Evidence of septic shock
Marked gastrointestinal hemorrhage
Abdominal radiographs showing pneumoperitoneum in addition to findings listed for stage II

Reproduced from Bell MJ, Kosloske AM, Benton C, et al. Neonatal necrotizing enterocolitis: prevention of perforation. *J Pediatr Surg* 1973; 8:601–605, with permission.

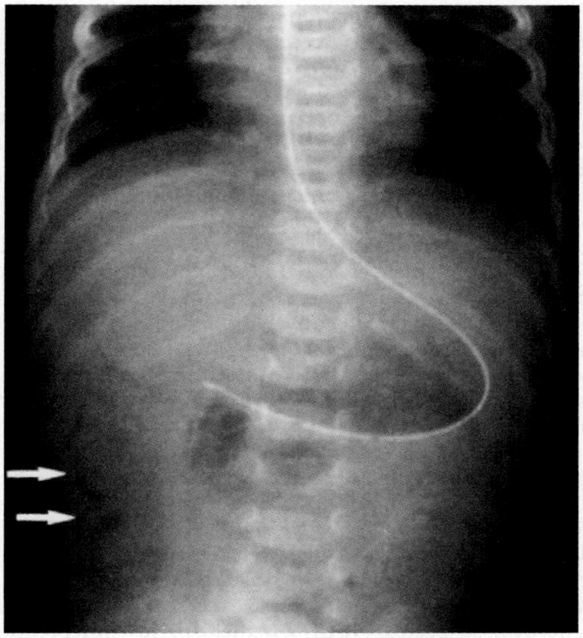

FIGURE 107.20. Plain abdominal film demonstrating pneumatosis intestinalis (*arrows*) in an infant with necrotizing enterocolitis.

lateral decubitus or upright film, should be obtained every 6 to 8 hours during the early course of the disease. These sequential studies help to document the progression or resolution of the inflammatory process and, importantly, evaluate for the presence of intestinal perforation presenting as free intraperitoneal gas or pneumoperitoneum. The presence of pneumoperitoneum mandates operative intervention; however, up to half of infants with perforated NEC do not have discernible pneumoperitoneum on plain films.

Treatment

Nonoperative. The vast majority of infants with NEC can be managed medically. Initial management of NEC includes proximal decompression with a nasogastric or orogastric tube, bowel rest, and broad-spectrum intravenous antibiotics. Prompt correction of hypotension, hypoxemia, and inadequate ventilation must be undertaken. Intravenous fluid management, with particular attention to electrolytes and acid–base status, is essential. Central venous access is secured and TPN is initiated. Oxygen delivery and cardiac performance must be maintained, which in a premature neonate may require operative closure of a patent ductus arteriosus; this approach is preferable over the use of indomethacin in the setting of NEC.[68] Serial physical examinations and blood work are useful in monitoring disease progress.

Most infants with NEC improve with medical management. Typically, reversal of the systemic inflammatory response occurs rapidly, and the abdominal distention and ileus resolve over a period of days. Nasogastric tube decompression and intravenous antibiotics are usually continued for 7 to 14 days. Enteral feeding usually is resumed once antibiotics have been discontinued and there has been return of gastrointestinal function. The usual course of medically treated NEC is rapid clinical response and stabilization in the first 24 to 36 hours. Infants with significant intestinal necrosis typically have signs of either pneumoperitoneum or clinical deterioration during the initial 24 to 72 hours of treatment.

Indications to abandon medical management and escalate surgical therapy include evidence of intestinal perforation or clinical deterioration with persistent or progressive systemic illness despite maximal medical therapy. Evidence of persistent or progressive systemic sepsis includes temperature instability, refractory hypotension, acidosis, hypoglycemia, neutropenia, and thrombocytopenia. Local findings such as portal venous gas, abdominal wall cellulitis, or crepitus also may signal intestinal necrosis and the need for operative intervention. A palpable, fixed abdominal mass consistent with intestinal perforation with an inflammatory phlegmon or abscess also may be a relative indication for operation. Because there is not complete agreement on what constitutes clinical deterioration, some controversy exists regarding operative indications for NEC in the absence of pneumoperitoneum. Because the interpretation of clinical deterioration criteria remains subjective, the decision to operate remains a multifactorial clinical judgment. In equivocal situations, abdominal paracentesis of ascitic fluid may be helpful in diagnosing intestinal necrosis with perforation in the absence of pneumoperitoneum if the aspirate contains bacteria or stool.[69]

Operative. Operative indications in NEC include the presence of intestinal necrosis with or without frank intestinal perforation. Conventional operative intervention is aimed at treating the complications of NEC (i.e., intestinal necrosis). In general, resection of intestine involved with NEC does not prevent further extension of disease in other involved areas of the bowel. For isolated segmental disease, the traditional surgical treatment of NEC is resection of necrotic bowel with proximal enterostomy and distal mucous fistula placement. In infants with diffuse NEC, multiple resections with several enterostomies may be required. The primary operative goal is an expedient operation with preservation of as much intestinal length as possible, including the ileocecal valve. Because the risk of developing short-gut syndrome is substantial in infants with diffuse disease, preservation of marginal areas of involved intestine with a planned second-look operation to reevaluate intestinal viability may be useful. Accurate measurement of the remaining bowel length is important from a diagnostic and prognostic standpoint, with the length of bowel resected determined by the extent of transmural intestinal necrosis. Resection with primary anastomosis in selected infants with NEC has been reported,[70] with a recent study observing recurrent NEC in 22% and strictures in 17% of 18 treated infants following primary anastomosis.[71] Complete intestinal necrosis of the small intestine and colon is uncommon and is not compatible with long-term survival without the sequelae of short-gut syndrome and the potential need for intestinal transplantation (Fig. 107.21).

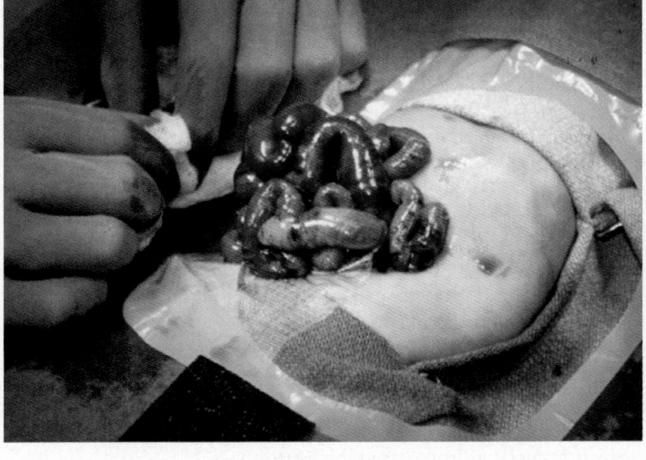

FIGURE 107.21. Fulminant necrotizing enterocolitis involving the entire gastrointestinal tract in a premature infant. Note the presence of pneumatosis intestinalis.

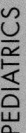

Infants with NEC are typically fragile and premature, and complications in this population are not well tolerated. Survival in this situation may be more dependent on disease severity and coexisting medical problems than the operative approach. For the high-risk, low birthweight infant, initial management with primary bedside peritoneal drainage rather than laparotomy and bowel resection may be useful as either a temporizing measure or, in some instances, a definitive procedure.[72] A multicenter, randomized, controlled surgical trial comparing laparotomy with primary peritoneal drainage in premature infants with perforated NEC found that overall survival, dependence on TPN, and length of stay were independent of the type of operation performed.[73]

Complications, Results, and Outcome. Most infants with NEC are treated successfully without operative intervention. Morbidity and mortality for this group are related primarily to problems associated with prematurity. Given the delay of bowel function and the need for TPN, cholestatic jaundice commonly occurs but is generally reversible. Infants placed on broad-spectrum antibiotics for an extended period are at risk for developing fungal sepsis. For infants with intestinal necrosis from NEC, infectious complications including wound sepsis, central venous catheter infections, and pneumonia with respiratory failure may occur.

The overall surgical complication rate in infants with NEC is at least 20% to 40%. Virtually every infant with NEC has a significant complication, an associated medical problem, or both. Immediate technical complications in treating NEC include intestinal leak, fistula formation, stoma necrosis, bleeding, and liver injury during exploration (Table 107.5). These complications are obviously magnified in the extremely low birthweight infant with preexisting intestinal injury. Fluid and electrolyte losses from proximal diverting enterostomies can be significant and even life threatening in extremely low birthweight infants whose circulating blood volume is less than 50 to 100 mL. A review of 68 infants treated surgically for NEC observed a 26% mortality rate and a 68% complication rate related to the stoma or its closure in the perioperative survivors.[74] Complications included intestinal stricture, incisional or parastomal hernia, stoma prolapse, intussusception, wound dehiscence or infection, small bowel obstruction, and anastomotic failure. The complications associated with diverting enterostomy in this unique population provide a compelling rationale for early enterostomy closure once the inflammation from peritonitis has resolved. A prospective, randomized trial comparing resection and enterostomy with resection and primary anastomosis in the treatment of NEC has not been reported.

TABLE 107.5 COMPLICATIONS

OPERATIONS FOR NECROTIZING ENTEROCOLITIS

Infection (wound, intra-abdominal, central venous catheter, pneumonia)
Bleeding
Stoma-related complications (stenosis, retraction, prolapse)
Electrolyte or nutritional disturbances from enterostomy output
Enterocutaneous fistula
Anastomotic leak, stenosis, failure
Adhesive small bowel obstruction
TPN-associated cholestasis
Short bowel syndrome, malabsorption
Sepsis, cardiopulmonary failure
Intraventricular hemorrhage

Intestinal stricture formation following NEC, whether managed operatively or nonoperatively, is common. This consequence usually results from a normal host inflammatory response to transmural intestinal injury. The degree of fibrosis and subsequent stricture formation are clearly related to the severity and extent of disease. Less frequently, mesenteric vascular compromise secondary to an intra-abdominal adhesion may lead to stricture formation. Although stricture can develop anywhere in the gastrointestinal tract involved with NEC, a higher rate of demonstrable stricture is observed in the left colon, occurring in as many as 36% of medically treated infants.[75] Routine contrast enema 4 to 6 weeks after clinical resolution of NEC treated operatively or nonoperatively has been advocated in some institutions. Symptomatic strictures generally require segmental resection with anastomosis, although fluoroscopically guided balloon catheter dilatation has been reported.

Overall survival rates for infants with NEC have improved significantly over the past three decades and are currently about 60% to 80% for both operative and nonoperative groups.[76] The observed improvement in survival is thought to reflect improved neonatal intensive care, the use of TPN, and early, aggressive treatment for suspected NEC. Most neonatal intensive care units initiate aggressive medical treatment in any infant with suspected NEC. Whether surgical interventions such as resection with primary anastomosis or limited primary peritoneal drainage can improve morbidity and mortality in these critically ill infants remains to be fully determined. Long-term outcome for NEC survivors generally reflects associated problems of prematurity. In particular, many of these infants have persisting neurodevelopmental, ophthalmologic, and pulmonary disease, but morbidity from the gastrointestinal system generally is limited to infants with short-gut syndrome following extensive bowel resection. These infants present complex ethical and management issues beyond the scope of this review. Most NEC survivors (75%) enjoy a good to excellent quality of life, suggesting that the treatment cost relative to the potential benefit for these infants is worthwhile.[77]

Meconium Ileus

Meconium ileus is a descriptive term for small bowel obstruction in a newborn infant with cystic fibrosis (CF). About 10% to 20% of infants with CF initially present with meconium ileus. A review of CF is useful to understand the pathophysiology and treatment of meconium ileus.

CF is the most common fatal hereditary disease in Europe and North America. It is an autosomal recessive disorder found with a heterozygous carrier incidence rate of 1 in 20 to 25 in white populations. The estimated incidence rate of homozygous gene expression and phenotypic manifestation of CF is about 1 in 2,000 to 2,500 in this population.[78] The CF gene has been cloned and the single most common mutation characterized.[79,80] The most common point mutation is a three-base-pair deletion found in 70% to 75% of the carrier population. This mutation leads to deletion of a phenylalanine residue in amino acid position 508 of the CF transmembrane conductance regulator (*CFTR*) gene. In addition, there are about 200 more infrequent mutations of the *CFTR* gene that lead to clinical CF. The molecular heterogeneity of *CFTR* gene mutations produces practical implications in the development and use of carrier screening tests in the general population. Currently, widespread use of molecular genetic screening tests in the general population to identify asymptomatic carriers and at-risk couples without a family history of CF is not recommended; there are significant technical, ethical, and social issues that must be prospectively addressed.[81] Screening of at-risk couples with a family history of CF is recommended, however, and in this setting, carrier discovery approaches 100% so that appropriate genetic counseling can be provided.

Molecular genetic screening also should be offered to parents and infants with clinically suspected CF as well as asymptomatic infants born to at-risk couples. This approach allows rapid identification and confirmation of virtually all infants homozygous for CF.

Pathophysiology. The clinical manifestations of CF are caused by an epithelial electrolyte transport defect that results in impermeability to the chloride (Cl^-) ion.[82] The epithelial defect occurs in apocrine sweat glands and the tracheobronchial tree as well as the pancreas, gastrointestinal tract, and liver. In sweat glands, failure of normal Cl^- ion reabsorption following beta-adrenergic stimulation leads to an obligate sodium chloride loss despite a normal adenosine triphosphate (ATP)-dependent sodium-potassium pump. This mechanism is the basis for the traditional diagnostic *sweat chloride test.*

Reduction of Cl^- permeability in the tracheobronchial tree leads to diminished secretion volume as well as increased absorption of sodium chloride. As a result, airway secretions in CF patients are low in volume and particularly viscous. Because of the tenacious nature of the airway secretions, airway clearance is impaired, which leads to chronic, recurrent infection with bronchitis and pneumonia. As the disease advances, bronchiectasis and progressive pulmonary parenchymal destruction ensues. Recurrent pulmonary bacterial infection is common, and airway colonization by *P. aeruginosa* is predictable. Chronic pulmonary disease accounts for more than 90% of the deaths in advanced CF, with a mean life expectancy approaching 30 years.

Pancreatic exocrine function is also affected by impaired Cl^- permeability. Pancreatic duct obstruction resulting from inspissated viscous secretion is followed by glandular autolysis, acinar atrophy, and pancreatic fibrosis. Pancreatic exocrine insufficiency is a classic early clinical feature of CF and is thought to account for some of the gastrointestinal manifestations of the disease. In particular, the deficiency of pancreatic proteinases, impaired chloride permeability, and abnormal epithelial mucous secretion lead to meconium ileus in the newborn, characterized by abnormally thick and viscid, protein-laden meconium that causes mechanical gastrointestinal obstruction. The obstruction is usually observed in the terminal ileum just proximal to the ileocecal valve (Fig. 107.22). Infants with meconium ileus have small pellets, or concretions, of pale, nonbilious meconium in the terminal ileum with a distal microcolon. Proximal to the obstruction, the meconium is variably mixed with gas and often is thick and tarry in consistency. The bowel containing the thick meconium is often grossly distended and thickened. Microscopically, the muscularis is hypertrophied; distended mucous glands with prominent goblet cells may be present. The most proximal jejunum is typically normal.

In utero events such as proximal volvulus of the dilated segment of ileum, perforation from distention, or atresia occur in approximately one third to one half of fetuses with meconium ileus. These clinical entities are characterized together as *complicated meconium ileus*. A classic clinical presentation of complicated meconium ileus is in utero intestinal perforation with sterile meconium peritonitis and formation of a calcified pseudocyst (Fig. 107.23). Gastrointestinal conditions presenting later in life occur in 10% of children with CF and include acute appendicitis, recurrent rectal prolapse, and intussusception. These conditions reflect abnormal transit of thick, inspissated stool causing proximal distention or obstruction of the bowel lumen. Small bowel obstruction in CF outside the neonatal period was historically called *meconium ileus equivalent,* and is now termed *distal intestinal obstruction syndrome (DIOS)*. Treatment of DIOS is similar to initial nonoperative management of uncomplicated meconium ileus in the newborn discussed later. Prevention of DIOS relies on conscientious pancreatic enzyme replacement. Finally, children with CF are at risk of cholestasis secondary to obstruction of small intrahepatic bile ducts. Chronic hepatic inflammation can occur with subsequent fibrosis and cirrhosis, causing hepatic failure and portal hypertension in approximately 5% of CF patients.

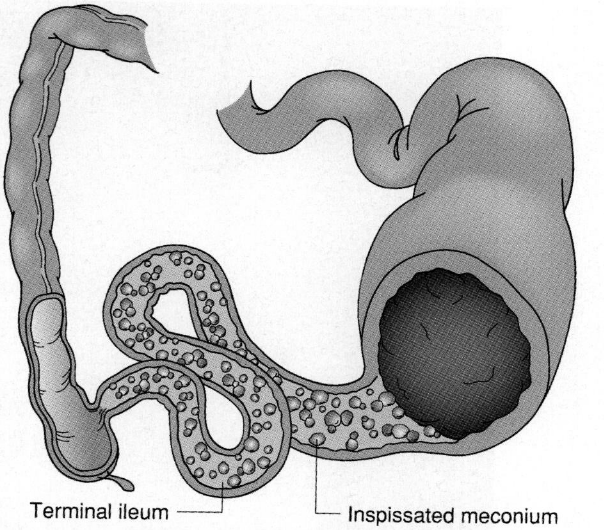

FIGURE 107.22. Meconium ileus causing obstruction of the terminal ileum from abnormally thick, inspissated meconium.

Diagnostic Evaluation. In nearly all newborns with CF, the diagnosis is clinically apparent by the presence of meconium ileus, a family history of CF in a sibling, or a positive newborn screening test. Laboratory confirmation of *CFTR* gene dysfunction is performed in several ways. The historical standard for detection of CF has been analysis of the sodium chloride content of the sweat. The most commonly used and reliable technique uses pilocarpine iontophoresis, with positive sweat test results showing sodium and chloride concentrations exceeding 60 mEq/L.[83] This test is less useful during the first 4 to 6 weeks of age because normal neonates do not reliably conserve sodium chloride in sweat. Generally, abnormal *CFTR* gene is documented by two elevated sweat chloride tests obtained on separate days. With the emergence of genetic technology capable of providing accurate assessment of *CFTR* gene mutations, the sweat test is now largely used to provide clinical confirmation of *CFTR* gene dysfunction along with molecular diagnosis of CF.

Clinical Presentation. With routine prenatal ultrasound practices along with selected fetal DNA screening, the prenatal diagnosis of CF or meconium ileus is feasible, potentially allowing for improved management of anticipated clinical problems following delivery.[84] Initial signs of meconium ileus include neonatal bowel obstruction with abdominal distention, bilious emesis, and failure to pass meconium. On examination, the neonate may have palpable loops of meconium-filled intestine with a texture on palpation described as "doughy." Similar to other causes of proximal neonatal intestinal obstruction, rectal examination and evaluation of the meconium typically reveals clear white mucus or thick gray meconium. In utero intestinal perforation with pseudocyst formation in complicated meconium ileus may cause a palpable abdominal mass that is not particularly tender. On plain films or ultrasound, calcification is visible in the pseudocyst wall. In contrast, volvulus or intestinal perforation secondary to meconium ileus following birth generally results in diffuse peritonitis and sepsis. Intestinal atresia may also be seen as a consequence of complicated meconium ileus.

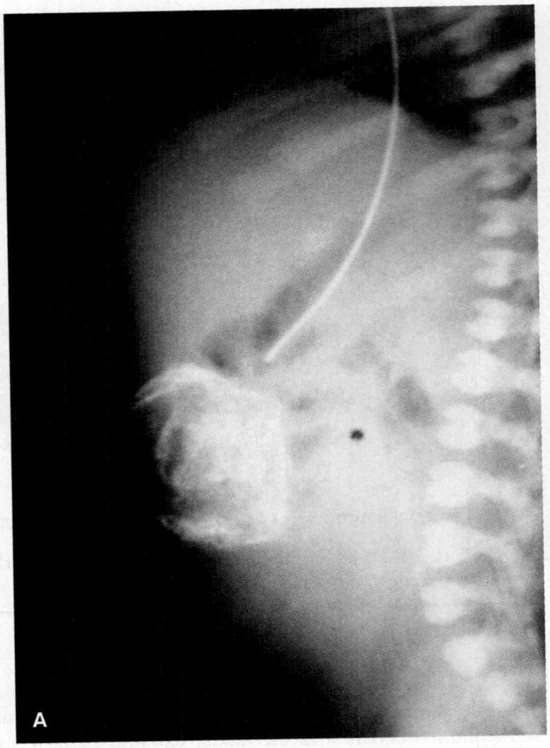

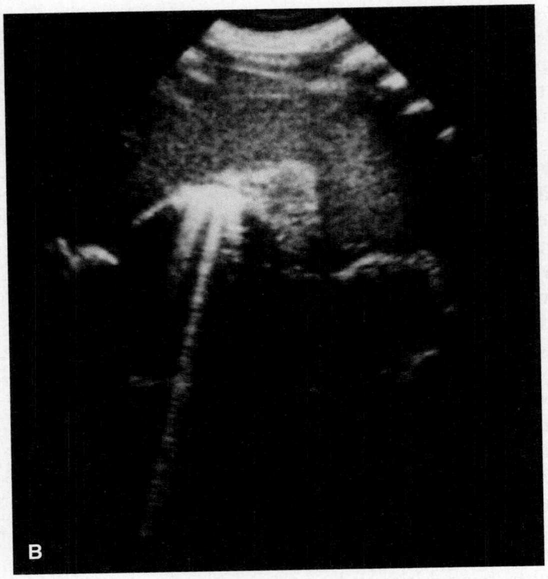

FIGURE 107.23. **A:** Plain-film radiograph of calcified pseudocyst in complicated meconium ileus. **B:** In utero ultrasound demonstrating calcified pseudocyst.

Diagnosis. Abdominal plain films may be diagnostic in meconium ileus, demonstrating multiple, distended loops of bowel (Fig. 107.24A). Fluid- or meconium-filled loops of bowel mixed with gas give a characteristic "soap bubble" or "ground glass" appearance. Classic air–fluid levels seen in other causes of intestinal obstruction are not expected because of the tenacious, sticky intraluminal meconium. The presence of intraperitoneal calcifications or a calcified cyst is consistent with prenatal intestinal perforation of sterile meconium.

A contrast enema is useful in the evaluation and treatment of simple meconium ileus. This study usually demonstrates an unused but functionally normal microcolon (Fig. 107.24B). Reflux of contrast into the terminal ileum may confirm the presence of inspissated meconium pellets. In conjunction with a family history and plain films, this finding is sufficient evidence to confirm the diagnosis of neonatal meconium ileus. Upper gastrointestinal contrast studies are generally unnecessary and may complicate further therapeutic efforts.

Treatment

Nonoperative. Nonoperative management of simple meconium ileus is achieved in about 60% to 70% of newborns. Once the diagnosis of meconium ileus is confirmed, the initial

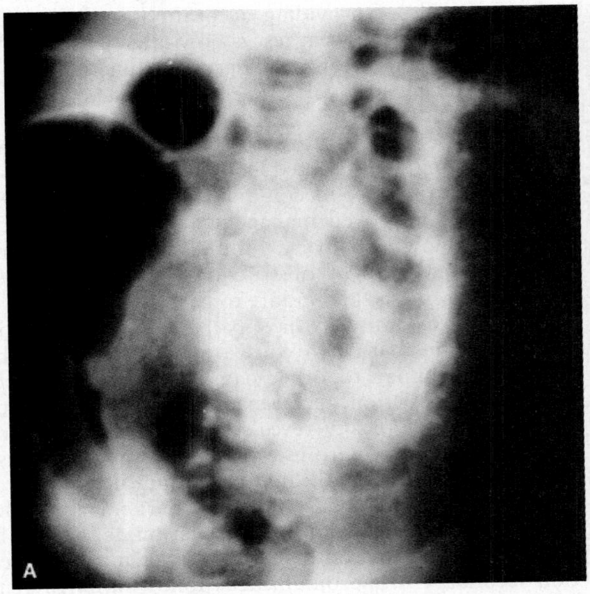

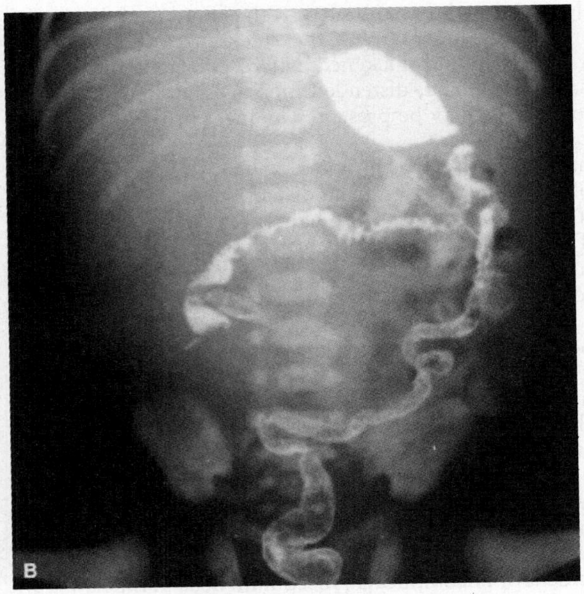

FIGURE 107.24. **A:** Plain radiograph of neonate with meconium ileus. **B:** Contrast enema in an infant with meconium ileus demonstrating an unused but intrinsically normal microcolon.

treatment of choice is to perform retrograde irrigation of the terminal ileum with one of several solutions designed to dissipate the obstructing meconium. In the United States, several different enema techniques and various contrast media have been described, including normal saline, hyperosmolar contrast agents, and dilute N-acetylcysteine. Initially, it was believed that using hyperosmolar contrast material was necessary to create an osmolar gradient. The resultant influx of fluid into the intestinal lumen was thought to solubilize the inspissated meconium. Recent data suggest that successful meconium clearance is not necessarily related to the osmolality of the contrast agent; however, a significantly higher overall success rate is reported with the use of water-soluble x-ray contrast (sodium and meglumine amidotrizoate) and the use of other solubilizing agents such as Tween-80 and N-acetylcysteine.[85] As long as clinical progress is being made, sequential enemas may be required to disimpact the inspissated meconium from the terminal ileum. In similar fashion, children and older patients presenting with DIOS are treated with retrograde enemas until the obstruction resolves. The distinct advantage of this treatment approach is the avoidance of general anesthesia and exploratory laparotomy. Reported complications with this approach include rare intestinal perforation, intestinal mucosal injury, and persistent obstruction resulting from meconium concretions.

Operative. The major indications for operative intervention are either failure to clear the obstruction by retrograde enema or complicated meconium ileus with cyst formation, volvulus, atresia, or perforation. For simple meconium ileus with persistent obstruction despite contrast enemas, the operative goals are meconium disimpaction from the ileum and evacuation of the remaining stool from the small intestine. These steps can be accomplished by either milking the meconium downstream into the colon or solubilizing the meconium by transmural needle instillation of irrigant. However, enterotomy or enterostomy and direct irrigation of the bowel lumen are usually required to completely clear the inspissated meconium. Simple closure of the enterotomy is preferred, but segmental resection may be required if marginal or compromised intestine is found. End-to-end anastomosis is the appropriate reconstruction technique following segmental bowel resection. A temporary enterostomy may be required, and several historical techniques have been described. Another surgical option is the placement of a T-tube into the ileum for continued irrigation with dilute N-acetylcysteine. Following clearance of meconium from the intestine and the return of bowel function, the T-tube can be safely and simply removed.[86]

Complicated meconium ileus occurs in about one third of patients. The surgical management of this entity is individualized. Intestinal atresia is not uncommon in meconium ileus, and the entire length of the intestine must be inspected for patency. When possible, resection of nonviable, stenotic, or perforated intestine is performed with immediate reconstruction via primary anastomosis. Patency of the downstream bowel must be confirmed to prevent anastomotic leak resulting from distal obstruction. If the infant is critically ill or has diffuse peritonitis, a safe primary anastomosis may not be possible and a diverting enterostomy is required. Stoma closure may be performed promptly after resolution of peritonitis and inflammation.

Postoperative Care and Results. If the meconium has been successfully cleared without opening the intestine, dilute N-acetylcysteine may be given through the nasogastric tube or by enema. Alternatively, if a T-tube has been placed, dilute N-acetylcysteine or other irrigant can be used directly into the ileum. These efforts are aimed at keeping the meconium soluble and preventing recurrent ileal obstruction. Following return of bowel function, enteral feeding using breast milk or an elemental formula is started along with oral pancreatic enzyme replacement. Vigilant pulmonary therapy is routine and includes mucolytics and antibiotics when indicated. Nutritional assessment and support are essential in long-term management.

Successful nonoperative management of simple meconium ileus historically was associated with a more favorable outcome; however, the operative mortality rates of infants with meconium ileus have improved dramatically over the past several decades, and current short-term operative survival rates of 70% to 100% are reported.[87,88] Long-term survival following meconium ileus is generally determined by the course of the underlying pulmonary disease. Contemporary management of CF has produced a mean survival age that approaches 30 years in most centers. With the exception of the development of portal hypertension in about 5% of patients, intestinal manifestations of the CF are treatable. Future medical and surgical efforts to improve the long-term outcome in these patients include direct replacement of the diseased pulmonary system by lung transplantation, manipulation of the epithelial chloride transport defect with pharmacologic agents, and gene therapy directed at *CFTR* gene transfer into respiratory epithelial cells.

Meconium Plug Syndrome

Meconium plug syndrome is characterized by functional obstruction of the colon or rectum by a meconium plug. It affects both normal and premature infants with immature gastrointestinal motility and must be differentiated from other causes of neonatal intestinal obstruction. Unlike meconium ileus, in meconium plug syndrome the colon is of normal caliber and the meconium is not inspissated. The infant's symptoms within the first few days of life are abdominal distention and bilious emesis. Spontaneous passage of meconium is often absent. On examination, the infant is normal with a patent anus and a distended abdomen. Digital rectal examination may deliver the meconium plug. Plain films of the abdomen demonstrate dilated loops of bowel consistent with distal bowel obstruction. The diagnosis is confirmed by contrast enema, which is also therapeutic in helping the meconium plug pass. The meconium plug is followed by bile-stained meconium of normal consistency. It is important that, although the vast majority of these infants are normal, a few have Hirschsprung disease or CF. Therefore, infants presenting with meconium plug syndrome should undergo routine rectal suction biopsy and have CF screening tests performed.

Malrotation

Embryology. Normal midgut fixation requires sequential growth, elongation, and rotation of the intestine beginning as early as week 5 of gestation as illustrated in Figure 107.25. Three distinct events occur during normal midgut fixation. The first stage involves herniation of the primary midgut loop into the base of the umbilical cord, where it remains until week 10 of gestation. The axis of the midgut loop is the superior mesenteric artery (SMA), with the omphalomesenteric duct at the apex of the midgut loop. The midgut loop rotates 180 degrees counterclockwise so that the proximal half passes posterior to the SMA. The proximal portion gives rise to the proximal duodenum, which lies to the right of midline. A portion of this segment becomes the third and fourth portions of the duodenum. The distal duodenum is normally fixed to the left of the aorta at the ligament of Treitz, having rotated 270 degrees counterclockwise from its original position. The jejunoileal segment undergoes dramatic elongation, forming about six primary intestinal loops. The distal midgut loop gives rise to the cecum and the right colon, which also undergoes growth and elongation with concomitant rotation 270 degrees counterclockwise. Therefore, the cecum is initially positioned to the left, then anterior, and finally to the right of the SMA before reaching its final location.[89]

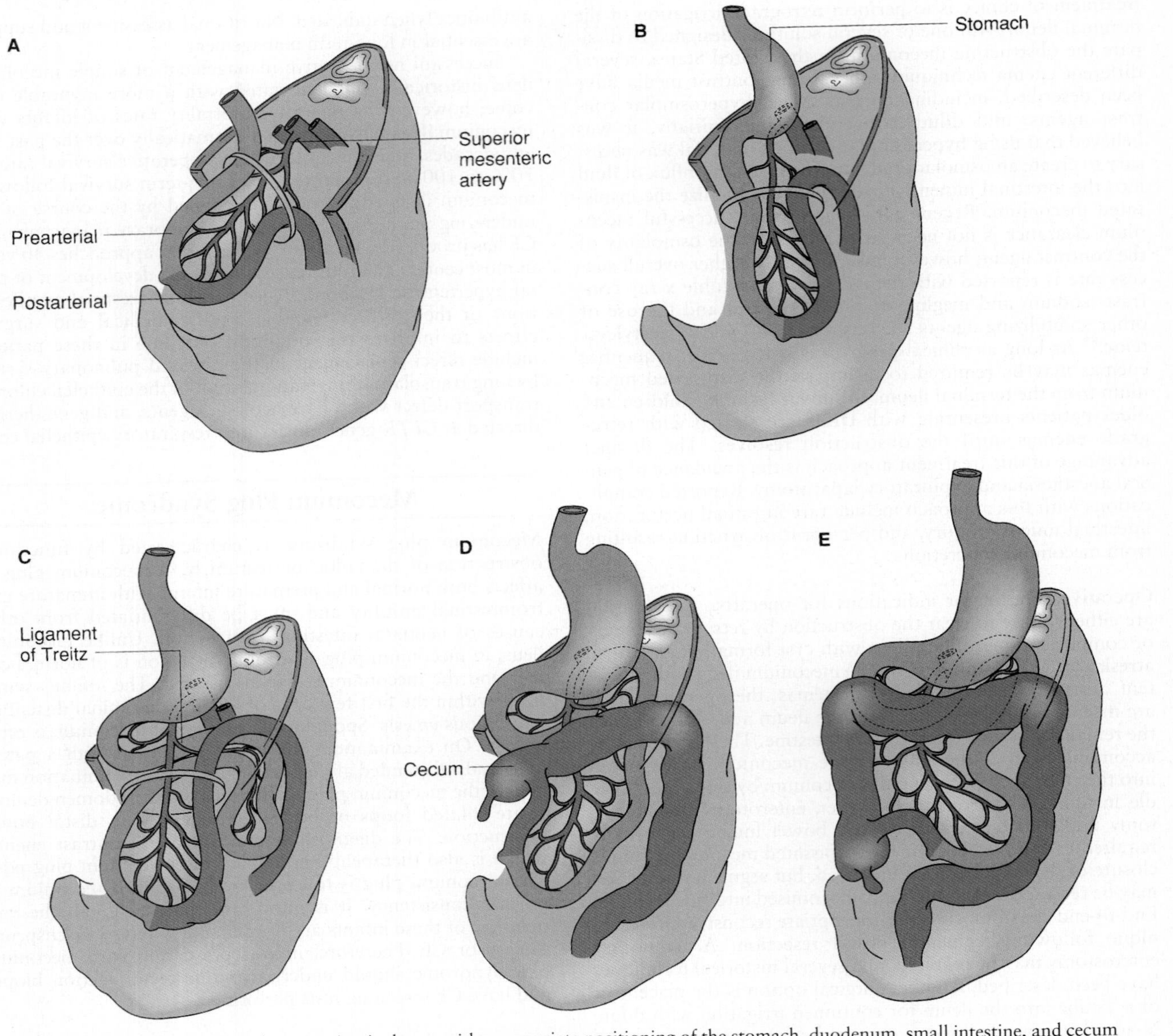

FIGURE 107.25. Normal midgut rotation is shown with appropriate positioning of the stomach, duodenum, small intestine, and cecum from the fifth gestational week (**A**) through completion by the 12th week (**E**).

Reduction of the extracoelomic gut is the second stage of midgut development and fixation, occurring between weeks 10 and 12 of gestation. By this time, the duodenojejunal junction has passed posterior to the SMA and the midgut has rotated 180 degrees counterclockwise; however, the small intestine initially remains to the right side of midline, and the cecum and ascending colon are anterior to the SMA after return of the gut into the abdomen. Many common abnormalities of intestinal fixation occur as a result of arrested development during this 2-week period.

The final stage of midgut development is fixation of the intestine to the posterior body wall, occurring after week 12 of gestation. Cecal descent occurs at this time. Normal points of fixation include the cecum in the right iliac fossa and the duodenojejunal junction at the ligament of Treitz just to the left of the aorta and anterior to the left renal vein (Fig. 107.26). Therefore, the normal intestinal mesentery is fixed with a broad base extending from the ligament of Treitz to the cecum. This broad-based mesenteric attachment prevents volvulus from occurring. In contrast, in disorders of intestinal rotation, the base of the mesentery is neither fixed nor broad, placing the entire midgut at risk for volvulus.

Anatomy. The normal sequence required for intestinal positioning and fixation can be interrupted at any developmental stage, producing a diverse spectrum of rotational abnormalities. Some neonatal surgical conditions are nearly always associated with abnormal intestinal rotation or fixation resulting from displacement of the midgut from the abdominal cavity during embryologic development. These anomalies include omphalocele, gastroschisis, and congenital diaphragmatic hernia. The term *malrotation* has been applied generically to describe disorders of intestinal rotation and fixation, although specific definitions of the more commonly encountered lesions are provided in the following sections.

Nonrotation. This common anomaly is characterized by inadequate counterclockwise rotation of the midgut around the SMA. Instead of the normal 270-degree arc, rotation is either absent or arrested before exceeding 90 degrees (Fig. 107.27). The small

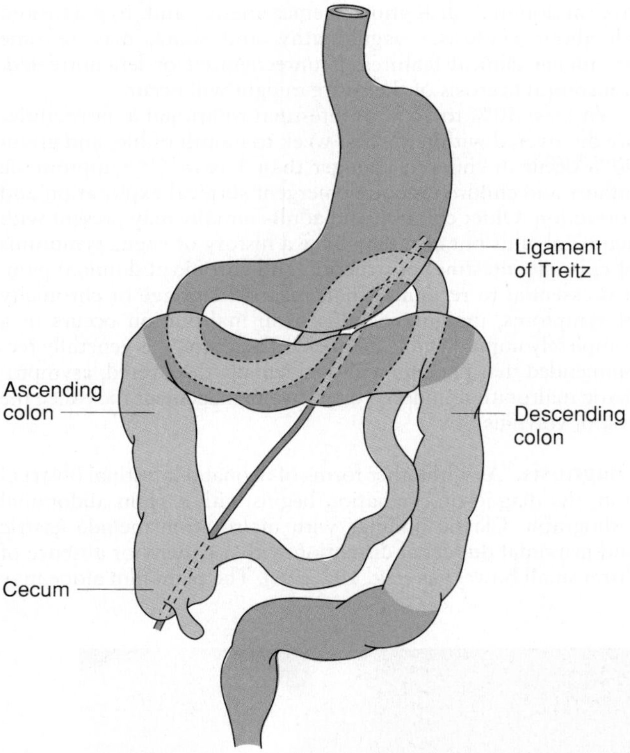

FIGURE 107.26. Normal oblique fixation of the midgut mesentery at the ligament of Treitz and in the right lower quadrant. The blue portions of the colon are extraperitoneal.

intestine resides on the right side of midline, the colon resides on the left, and the cecum is anterior and near the midline. The duodenojejunal junction is to the right of midline and more caudal and anterior in position. Nonrotation carries a significant clinical risk of midgut volvulus because the mesenteric vascular pedicle is narrow. Duodenal obstruction also may occur as a result of

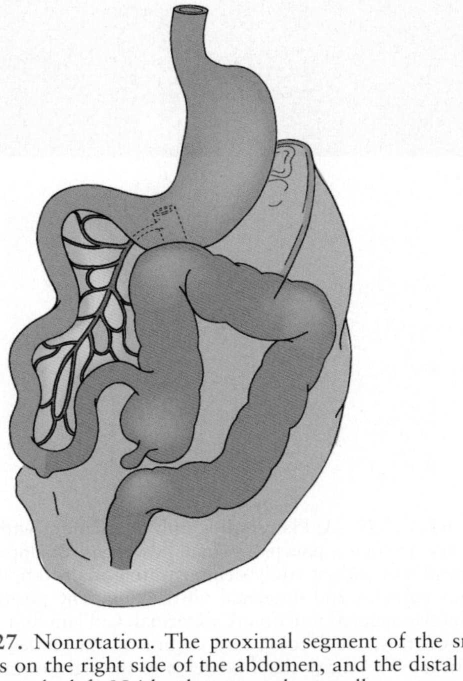

FIGURE 107.27. Nonrotation. The proximal segment of the small intestine resides on the right side of the abdomen, and the distal segment (colon) is on the left. Neither has rotated normally.

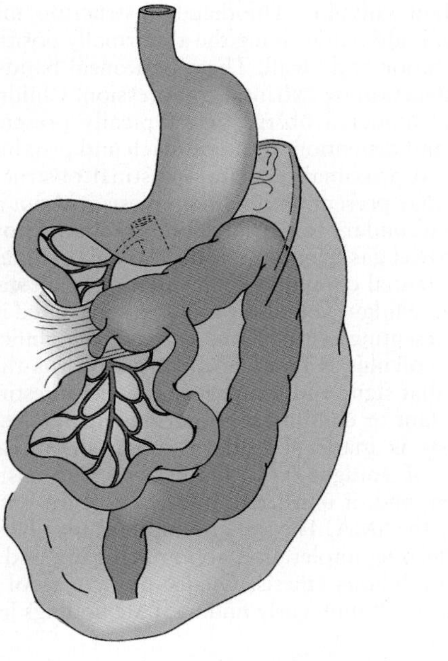

FIGURE 107.28. Incomplete rotation. The proximal segment has failed to rotate and is on the right. The distal segment has rotated to reside anterior to the duodenum so that cecal bands to the posterior abdominal wall may compress and obstruct the duodenum.

peritoneal attachments known as *Ladd bands*. These peritoneal bands fix the cecum to the posterior body wall by passing anterior and lateral to the distal duodenum.

Mixed or Incomplete Rotation. This rotational abnormality is characterized by arrest of the normal rotation at or near 180 degrees rather than the normal 270 degrees (Fig. 107.28). Instead of rotating posterior and to the left of the SMA, incomplete or arrested rotation of the prearterial segment leaves the duodenojejunal junction to the right of midline. The cecum also does not complete its counterclockwise passage anterior to the SMA; it usually resides in the upper abdomen just to the left of the SMA. Similar to nonrotation, fixation of the cecum to the posterior body wall by Ladd bands places the duodenum at risk for compression or obstruction. Additionally, the SMA pedicle is narrow and places the midgut at risk for volvulus.

Mesocolic Hernias. Mesocolic hernias are rare but important anomalies characterized by failure of fixation of either the right or left mesocolon to the posterior body wall. Small bowel can become entrapped in the resulting potential cavities on either side of the abdomen. A right-sided mesocolic defect (paraduodenal hernia) is associated with nonrotation of the proximal midgut segment. Small bowel entrapment posterior to the right colon and cecum may occur. Similar entrapment of small bowel may occur from an incompletely fixed left mesocolon but is associated with normal colonic and cecal position. Entrapped small bowel in a left mesocolic hernia usually is contained within a hernia sac with the neck composed of the inferior mesenteric vein and peritoneal bands extending to the posterior body wall. Both left and right mesocolic hernias carry the potential risks of obstruction, incarceration, and strangulation of bowel.

Clinical Presentation. Abnormalities of intestinal rotation are estimated to be present in about 1% of the population. Most persons with intestinal rotational anomalies are clinically asymptomatic; therefore, some children are found to have malrotation incidentally by upper gastrointestinal contrast studies conducted for other reasons. Symptomatic malrotation usually is encountered clinically in the setting of duodenal obstruction or midgut volvulus. Duodenal obstruction may occur as a result of Ladd bands fixing the abnormally positioned cecum to the posterior body wall. These peritoneal bands cause duodenal obstruction by extrinsic compression. Children with symptomatic duodenal obstruction typically present with bilious emesis and distention of the stomach and proximal duodenum. Similar to proximal neonatal intestinal obstruction, newborn infants may present with bilious emesis without abdominal distention secondary to partial duodenal obstruction. A paucity of small bowel gas may be seen on plain abdominal films.

A potential consequence of intestinal malrotation is midgut volvulus. Midgut volvulus should be considered in any infant or child presenting with bilious emesis. The clinical outcome of midgut volvulus is time dependent, which is the fundamental reason that signs and symptoms of acute intestinal obstruction in an infant or child must be pursued aggressively until a clear diagnosis is made. The devastating, life-threatening consequence of midgut volvulus is vascular insufficiency, gut ischemia, and, if untreated, infarction of the entire bowel supplied by the SMA. The initial symptoms may be subtle and limited to feeding intolerance, abdominal pain, and irritability followed by bilious emesis. Guaiac-positive stool from mucosal injury is a common early finding. Late findings include progressive abdominal distention, hematemesis, and hypotension. Metabolic acidosis, coagulopathy, and shock may become prominent clinical features. If unrecognized or left untreated, transmural necrosis of the entire midgut will occur.

At least 50% to 75% of intestinal rotational abnormalities are discovered within the first week to month of life, and about 90% occur in children younger than 1 year.[90,91] Symptomatic infants and children require emergent surgical exploration and correction. Older children and adults initially may present with acute volvulus but also may have a history of vague symptoms of episodic intestinal obstruction and chronic abdominal pain. It is essential to recognize that, regardless of age or chronicity of symptoms, midgut volvulus from malrotation occurs in a completely unpredictable manner.[92] Therefore, it is generally recommended that patients with incidentally discovered, asymptomatic malrotation undergo operative management to reduce the risk of volvulus.

Diagnosis. As with other forms of neonatal intestinal obstruction, the diagnostic evaluation begins with a plain abdominal radiograph. Classic findings with malrotation include gastric and proximal duodenal distention with a paucity or absence of distal small bowel gas (Fig. 107.29A). The plain film alone may

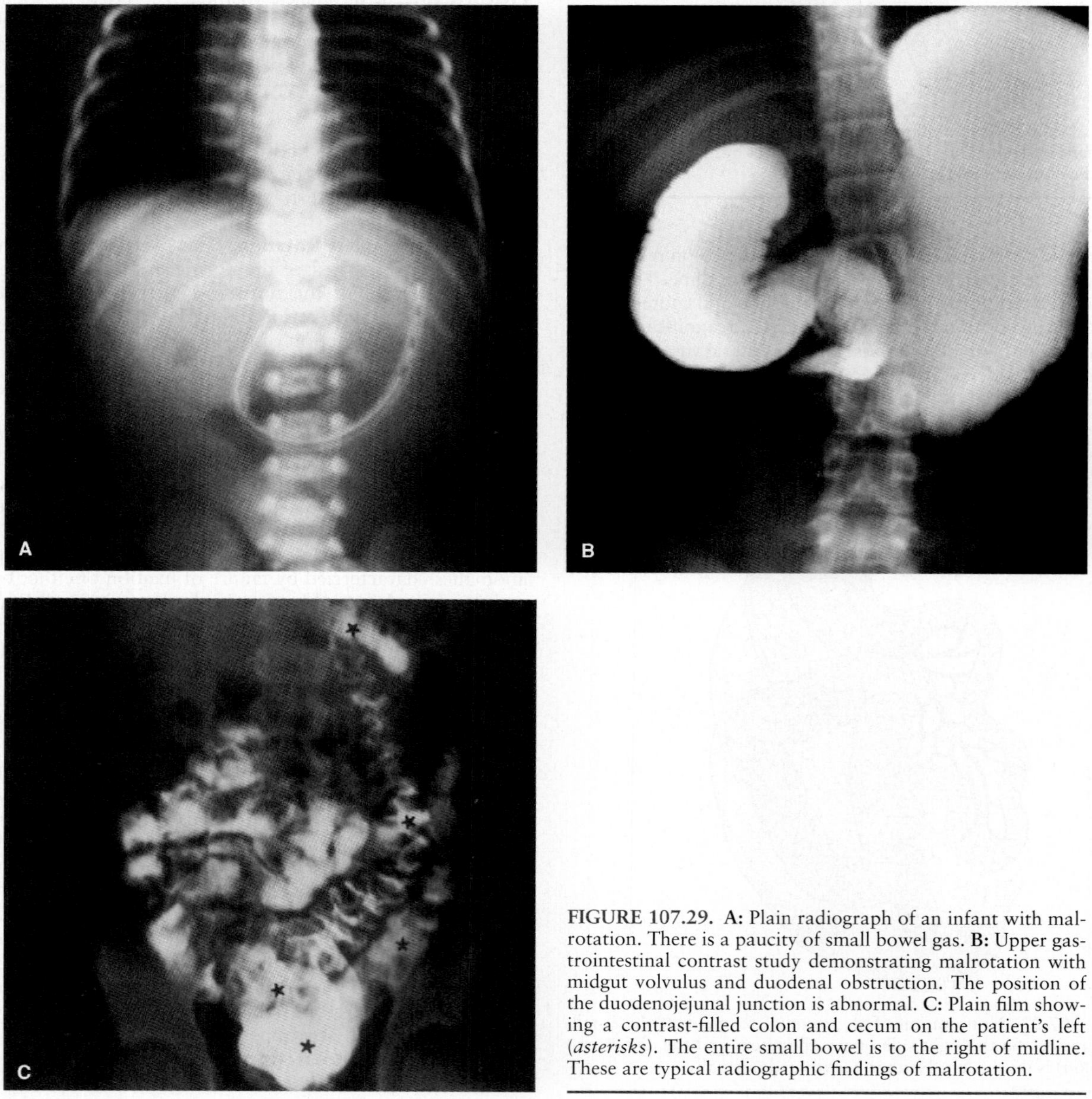

FIGURE 107.29. **A:** Plain radiograph of an infant with malrotation. There is a paucity of small bowel gas. **B:** Upper gastrointestinal contrast study demonstrating malrotation with midgut volvulus and duodenal obstruction. The position of the duodenojejunal junction is abnormal. **C:** Plain film showing a contrast-filled colon and cecum on the patient's left (*asterisks*). The entire small bowel is to the right of midline. These are typical radiographic findings of malrotation.

not differentiate malrotation from duodenal atresia or stenosis. In most cases of suspected duodenal obstruction with concern of malrotation, an upper gastrointestinal series is a conclusive imaging study (Fig. 107.29B). Malrotation with volvulus typically produces incomplete duodenal obstruction with a corkscrew or coiled appearance in the distal duodenum. Extrinsic compression of the duodenum by Ladd bands may be visible on contrast study. Duodenal atresia and stenosis may occur anywhere within the duodenum but tend to be more proximal. Complete absence of small bowel gas is typical of duodenal atresia, whereas diminished but discernable distal gas is characteristic of duodenal stenosis or malrotation with volvulus.

Other radiographic findings in malrotation include incorrect position of the duodenojejunal junction, particularly to the right of midline. Failure to achieve normal cephalad and posterior fixation is typical in malrotation and may be best appreciated on lateral views. The small bowel resides in the right side of the abdomen, the colon and cecum on the left (Fig. 107.29C). In a symptomatic infant or child, radiographic evidence of malrotation alone is enough to warrant emergent exploration. A contrast enema is helpful in the evaluation of neonatal intestinal obstruction, although it may not be the initial study of choice if malrotation is suspected. The classic finding on contrast enema for malrotation is cecal malposition, usually in the left abdomen or near the midline. Finally, the relative position of the SMA to the superior mesenteric vein may be assessed by ultrasound. Normally, the superior mesenteric vein is to the right of the SMA on transverse sonograms. Abnormal position of the superior mesenteric vein either ventral or to the left of the SMA is associated with malrotation.[93]

Treatment. The management of bowel obstruction from malrotation or an internal hernia is operative. Initial assessment, resuscitation, and preoperative preparation in a symptomatic newborn should be conducted simultaneously so that confirmation of malrotation can be followed immediately by laparotomy. Urgent laparotomy is required to reduce the ischemic injury to the intestine. Shock, if present, must be treated aggressively by ensuring adequate gas exchange and establishing restoration of intravascular volume prior to the induction of general anesthesia. Volvulus with complete infarction of the midgut, if not immediately lethal, is survivable only with enterectomy followed by permanent or long-term TPN support. In older, asymptomatic children with incidentally discovered malrotation, operative repair remains controversial. Given the devastating consequences of midgut volvulus, however, elective surgical correction appears warranted in most asymptomatic individuals as well.

Operative repair of malrotation is performed by the Ladd procedure.[94] The first objective is to relieve the midgut volvulus, if present. This is accomplished by delivery and detorsion of the affected midgut, usually in a counterclockwise direction. Recurrent volvulus is prevented by broadening the base of the mesenteric vascular pedicle by dividing the peritoneal bands that tether the cecum, small bowel mesentery, mesocolon, and duodenum around the base of the SMA (Fig. 107.30). Once completed, the mesentery and mesocolon open widely and the mesenteric pedicle is at low risk for recurrent volvulus.

The second objective of the Ladd procedure is to divide the abnormal peritoneal attachments between the cecum and the abdominal wall. A modified Kocher maneuver involving meticulous and complete mobilization of the entire duodenum with division of all anterior, lateral, and posterior attachments is performed. Duodenal and distal small bowel patency should be demonstrated using intraluminal air or saline because synchronous intestinal webs and atresia have been reported. An appendectomy is performed to eliminate potential confusion from acute appendicitis developing in an abnormally positioned appendix. Performance of a laparoscopic Ladd procedure has been demonstrated to be feasible and may help to reduce time to enteral feeding and hospital length of stay; however, the long-term efficacy of this approach has been debated.[95] Fixation of the mesentery by cecal or duodenal plication to the body wall has been abandoned for lack of data supporting efficacy. Postoperative small bowel obstruction secondary to adhesions is reported in about 10% of patients.

Volvulus with intestinal necrosis is treated by preserving as much bowel length as possible. If bowel viability is unclear during initial exploration, a second-look procedure may be helpful to delineate reversible from irreversible injury. The management of nonviable bowel from volvulus is not different from other situations in which intestinal necrosis is encountered, and clinical decisions regarding resection and anastomosis are individualized. In situations where the entire small intestine is lost and long-term survival doubtful, treatment decisions must be made with the family.

Surgical management of right mesocolic hernia is directed at dividing the lateral peritoneal attachments of the cecum and right colon to eliminate the hernia. In addition, given the associated nonrotation of the proximal bowel, the vascular pedicle should be broadened as much as possible. Left mesocolic hernia is treated by mobilization of the inferior mesenteric vein, reduction of the small bowel from the hernia sac, and closure of the neck of the hernia sac to eliminate the potential space.

Results and Complications. Results following surgical correction of intestinal rotational abnormalities should be excellent, and life expectancy should be normal in the absence of intestinal necrosis. Recurrent volvulus and recurrent duodenal obstruction are distinctly unusual if the initial procedure is technically complete. Adhesive small bowel obstruction following the Ladd procedure is reported in 1% to 10% of patients. Long-term outcome is obviously less favorable in patients with intestinal necrosis at the time of exploration.

Congenital Aganglionosis (Hirschsprung Disease)

5 **Embryology.** Congenital aganglionosis of the intestine (Hirschsprung disease) is characterized by the absence of intestinal ganglion cells. The pathogenesis of aganglionosis remains unknown. In normal development, neuroblasts derived from neural crest precursors become evident by week 5 of gestation. The neuroblasts begin maturation and caudal migration along with vagal nerve fibers. The initial caudal migration in an intermuscular plane is followed by intramural dispersal into both superficial and deep submucosal nerve plexuses. Ultimately, the neuroblasts give rise to the ganglion cells of the myenteric nervous system, with functional maturation continuing well into infancy. The orderly migration pathway of myenteric innervation has been documented in human embryos; normally, ganglion cells can be identified in the esophagus at week 6 of gestation, in the transverse colon at week 8 of gestation, and in the rectum by week 12 of gestation.[96]

Anatomy. Hirschsprung disease is characterized by a lack of ganglion cells in the distal intestine. The length of aganglionosis is variable but most commonly involves the distal rectosigmoid colon in 75% to 80% of affected infants. In about 5% of cases, the transition zone between the normal, proximal bowel and the distal, aganglionic segment occurs in the small intestine.[97] Discontinuous aganglionosis has been reported but should be considered distinctly unusual. Therefore, in virtually all cases, the aganglionic intestinal segment is continuous with the distal rectum to the anal verge and also includes the internal sphincter. Because of this distribution, the pathogenesis of congenital aganglionosis is often attributed to failure of neuroblast migration. The characteristic lesion in the distal bowel is the aganglionosis in the intermuscular and submucosal

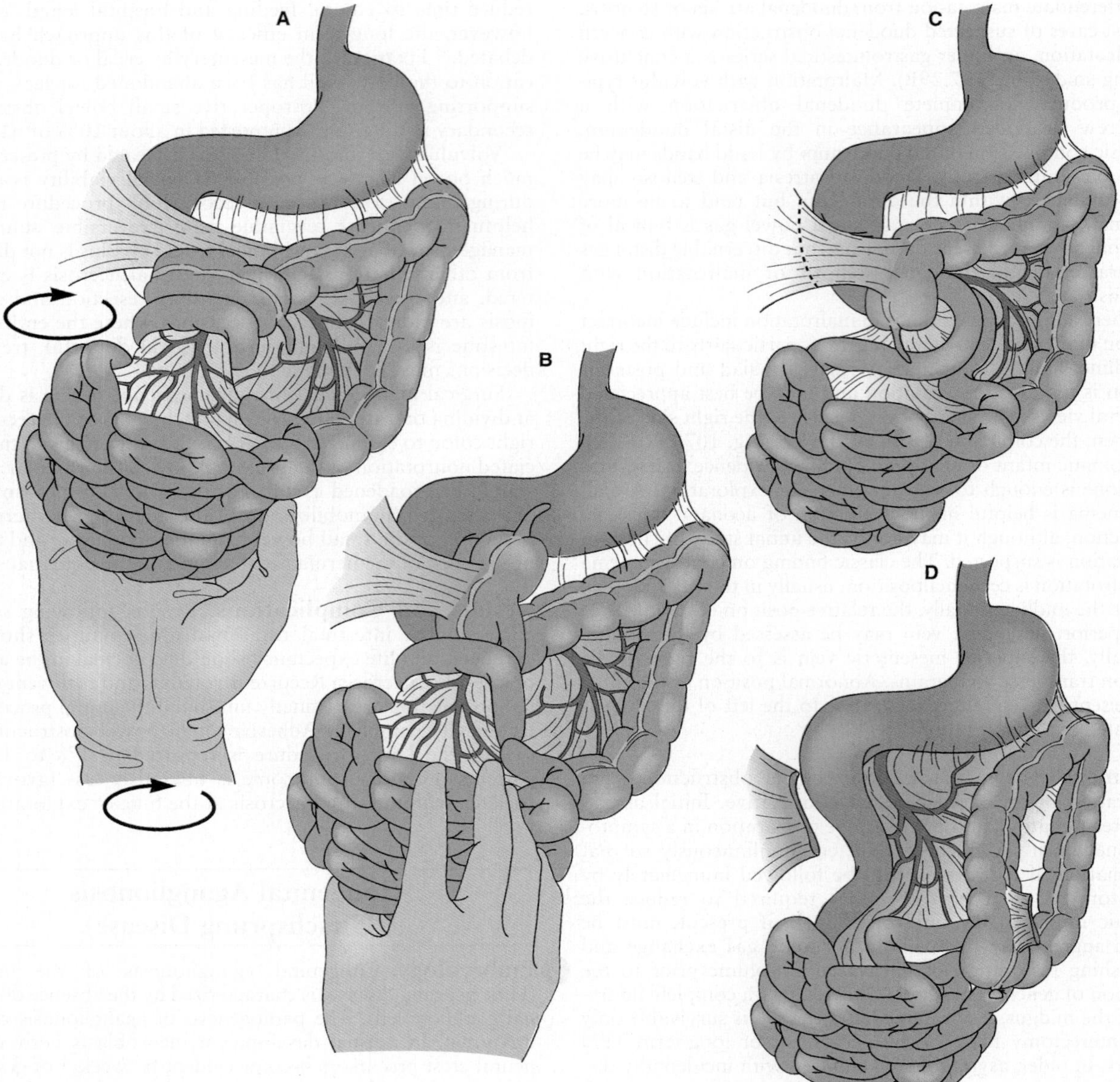

FIGURE 107.30. Correction of malrotation with volvulus. A and B: Detorsion of midgut. C and D: Division of peritoneal attachments (Ladd bands) of cecum to abdominal cavity.

plexuses. Large, hypertrophied, nonmyelinated nerve fibers are present within the muscularis mucosa, lamina propria, submucosa, and Auerbach intermuscular plexus. Both adrenergic and cholinergic fibers are prominent in the aganglionic segment, and acetylcholinesterase staining is useful diagnostically. Abnormalities in the peptidergic nervous system, including vasoactive intestinal peptide, substance P, and neurotensin immunoreactive fibers, also are described in the aganglionic bowel segment.[98] Deficient neuronal nitric oxide synthase mRNA and subsequent decreased local nitric oxide synthase activity in the aganglionic bowel have also been described.[99] These experimental data are consistent with the concept that a defect in nitric oxide–mediated smooth-muscle relaxation may account for some of the characteristic clinical features of Hirschsprung disease.

The transition zone between the normal proximal bowel and the aganglionic distal bowel is distinguished grossly by distention of the proximal bowel with histologic evidence of muscular hypertrophy. The transition zone often becomes evident to direct inspection or on contrast enema during the first few weeks of life as functional obstruction leads to progressive proximal dilatation. On gross inspection, the transition zone may appear as a short funnel or cone-shaped colonic segment. The discrepancy in bowel lumen diameter is somewhat age dependent and may be subtle in a newborn or in a child with total colonic aganglionosis. Therefore, it may be difficult for the surgeon or radiologist to define the exact transition zone site based on gross inspection or contrast enema. Gross examination alone is not sufficient for surgical decision making, and histologic confirmation of the level of ganglion cell transition is required. Given the continuous nature of aganglionosis, a rectal biopsy performed 1 to 1.5 cm above the dentate line demonstrating ganglion cells effectively excludes Hirschsprung disease.

Neuronal intestinal dysplasia is a clinically described entity similar to or associated with Hirschsprung disease.[100,101] Despite the presence of ganglion cells, dysplastic changes in the myenteric nervous system affect bowel motility in similar fashion to aganglionosis. Clinical presentation and treatment are similar to those of classic Hirschsprung disease. There is considerable controversy regarding neuronal intestinal dysplasia, but it is reasonable to suggest that this represents an entity within the spectrum of abnormalities found in the intestinal myenteric nervous system.

Pathophysiology. Normal intestinal motility depends on coordinated propagation of segmental contraction waves immediately preceded by relaxation of the enteric smooth muscle. Patients with Hirschsprung disease lack a functional myenteric nervous system in the aganglionic segment; therefore, both propulsion and reflexive relaxation are disordered or absent in the distal bowel. Loss of neuronal nitric oxide synthase activity appears to play an important role. The internal sphincter is aganglionic and lacks the normal reflexive relaxation following rectal distention. In fact, patients with Hirschsprung disease may exhibit a paradoxical increase in sphincter tone in response to rectal distention. The functional result is tonic contraction of the aganglionic segment of bowel with ineffective peristalsis. Clinically, this presents as incomplete distal intestinal obstruction in the newborn or as chronic constipation in the older child or adult.

Hirschsprung disease has been associated with mutations in at least three specific genes: the *RET* protooncogene, the endothelin B receptor (*EDNRB*) gene,[102] and the endothelin 3 (*EDN3*) gene. Additionally, several other candidate genes are under investigation. In mice, natural and in vitro induced mutations affecting the *RET, EDNRB,* and *EDN3* genes generate intestinal aganglionosis identical to Hirschsprung disease.[103,104] Although widely accepted, it is still unknown whether the primary event in aganglionosis is failure of neuroblast migration to the distal bowel. Alternatively, ineffective microenvironmental support of neuroblasts that have already migrated may fail to promote normal neuroblast development and survival.[105]

Clinical Features

Incidence and Associations. The incidence rate of Hirschsprung disease is estimated at 1 per 5,000 live births with a marked male-to-female (4:1) preponderance. Most cases are sporadic, but long-segment, total colonic aganglionosis and female gender are strongly associated with familial inheritance. Genetic chromosomal analysis suggests that multiple loci may be involved, including chromosomes 13q22, 21q22, and 10q, among others.[106] Familial Hirschsprung disease has been clearly associated with *RET* protooncogene mutations. From a clinical standpoint, mutations of the *RET* protooncogene are associated with disorders of neural crest development, namely, multiple endocrine neoplasia (MEN) types IIA and IIB as well as familial medullary thyroid carcinoma, and patients with familial Hirschsprung disease associated with RET mutation are at risk for the development of medullary thyroid carcinoma.[107] Congenital cardiac defects are present in 2% to 5% of patients with Hirschsprung disease. Other rare congenital anomalies have been reported, but a consistent and important association is a 5% to 15% incidence of trisomy 21.[108] Infants presenting with meconium plug syndrome should undergo rectal suction biopsy to exclude aganglionosis.

Presentation. Most infants with Hirschsprung disease fail to pass meconium within the first 24 to 48 hours of life. Nonspecific signs of neonatal intestinal obstruction (feeding intolerance, abdominal distention, and bilious emesis) may develop. About half of patients with Hirschsprung disease are diagnosed as neonates. Infrequently, older children or adults are diagnosed with aganglionosis during evaluation for chronic constipation. In this setting, symptoms may be minimal to disabling, and parents or patients often develop elaborate strategies to deal with chronic constipation. Abdominal distention is characteristic, and sometimes failure to thrive and malnutrition may occur. Digital rectal examination may demonstrate spasm, and, in the presence of enterocolitis, forceful expulsion of foul-smelling, liquid stool may occur.

Enterocolitis occurs in about 10% to 30% of infants and children with Hirschsprung disease and may be the presenting clinical manifestation. Enterocolitis associated with Hirschsprung disease has an unknown pathophysiology, but obstructive stasis and bacterial overgrowth are thought to be important factors. *C. difficile* and rotavirus have been implicated as important pathogenic organisms; diagnostic and treatment plans should consider these possibilities. The early presenting symptoms and signs of enterocolitis include fever, abdominal distention, and diarrhea, which may be explosive, foul-smelling, and bloody. Systemic sepsis, transmural intestinal necrosis, and perforation are all possible later findings. The clinical progression can be rapid, with death occurring in as few as 12 to 24 hours if treatment is not initiated. Infants are particularly vulnerable to this complication, and enterocolitis accounts for virtually all mortality directly related to Hirschsprung disease in modern pediatric surgical practice. Infants with known Hirschsprung disease and suspected enterocolitis should be treated aggressively. Initial treatment includes resuscitation, broad-spectrum antibiotics, cessation of feeding, and rectal irrigation. If the enterocolitis does not respond promptly, emergent intestinal decompression with an enterostomy proximal to the transition zone is indicated.

Diagnosis. A high index of suspicion for Hirschsprung disease should be maintained for any newborn infant with abdominal distention failing to pass meconium in 24 to 48 hours. The signs of neonatal intestinal obstruction should lead to a stereotypical workup. In the presence of characteristic findings on history, examination, or radiographic studies, any infant suspected of having Hirschsprung disease should undergo rectal biopsy.

Plain Abdominal Radiographs. Plain-film radiographs of the neonate with Hirschsprung disease are nonspecific and typically demonstrate distended, air-filled loops of bowel throughout the abdomen. It is often difficult to discriminate between small and large intestine on plain films at this age, but the pattern is consistent with distal intestinal obstruction. Older children or adults may have a stool-filled megacolon on plain radiographs. In the presence of enterocolitis, thickened, dilated intestinal loops and pneumatosis intestinalis may be present.

Contrast Enema. When distal neonatal intestinal obstruction is suspected on plain abdominal films, a contrast enema should be performed. With an experienced pediatric radiologist, findings consistent with Hirschsprung disease can be accurately detected in most instances. The classic radiographic finding in Hirschsprung disease is a transition zone (Fig. 107.31A). A definitive transition zone may not be apparent in a neonate because proximal dilatation takes some time to develop. Additionally, infants with short-segment disease or total colonic aganglionosis may not have obvious transition zones on contrast enema. In these instances, a lateral view of the rectum may show abnormal spasm (Fig. 107.31B). Contrast remaining in the rectum more than 24 hours following a study is suggestive of Hirschsprung disease.

Rectal Biopsy. The diagnostic standard for aganglionosis is the rectal biopsy. Several commercially available instruments capable of performing rectal suction biopsies are in widespread use. The rectal suction biopsy can be performed at bedside or in clinic without anesthesia in all newborns and most children up to several months of age. The desire for early diagnosis and the technical simplicity of the procedure allow liberal use of this technique. When applied liberally, the vast majority (85%–90%) of infants undergoing this procedure have normal ganglion cells on biopsy, effectively excluding Hirschsprung

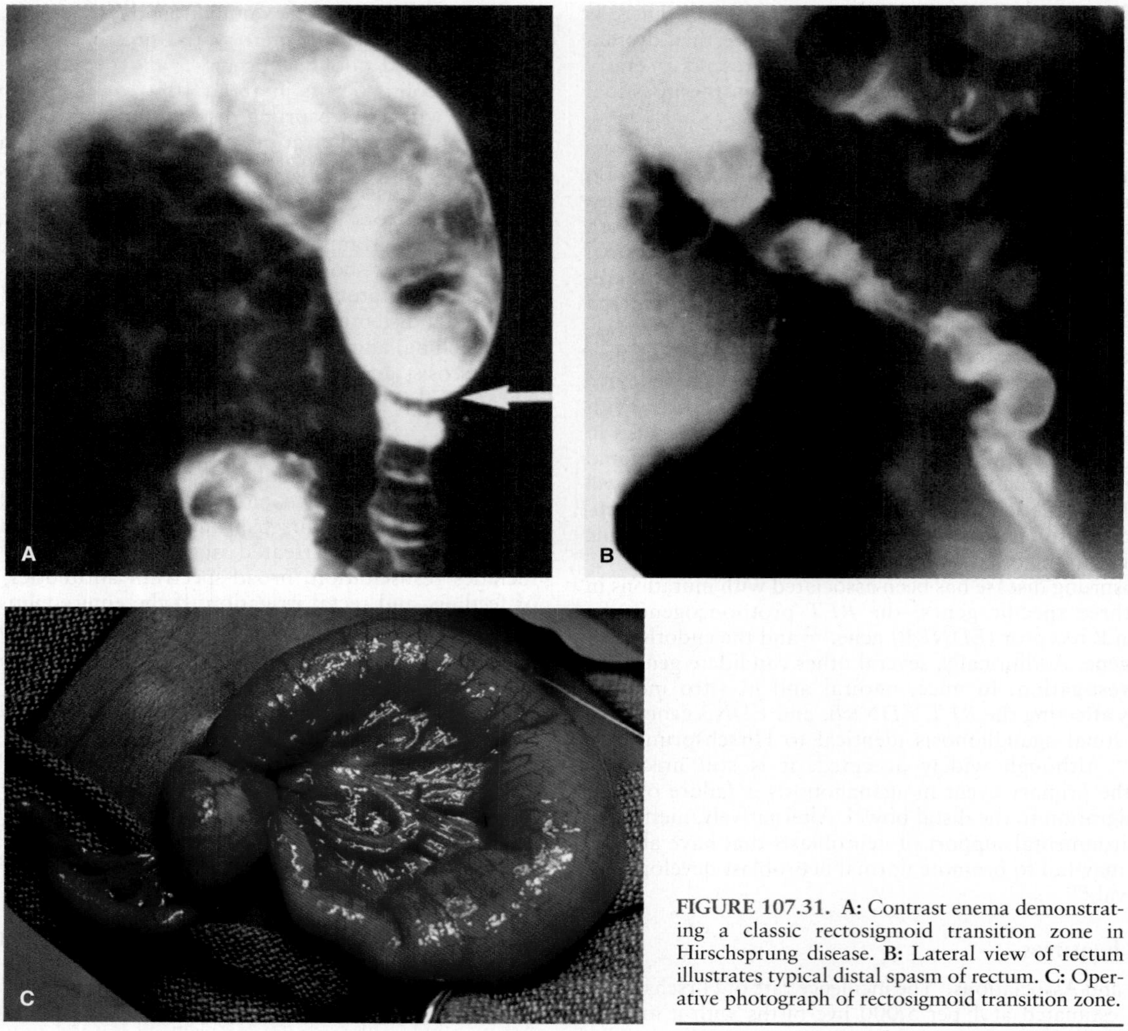

FIGURE 107.31. **A:** Contrast enema demonstrating a classic rectosigmoid transition zone in Hirschsprung disease. **B:** Lateral view of rectum illustrates typical distal spasm of rectum. **C:** Operative photograph of rectosigmoid transition zone.

disease. Using the rectal suction biopsy technique, a biopsy of the mucosa and submucosa is obtained. This is sufficient to establish the diagnosis because ganglion cells are absent from all intramural plexuses in Hirschsprung disease. The biopsy must be taken 1 to 1.5 cm proximal to the dentate line. Complications of infection, perforation, and bleeding with rectal suction biopsy are infrequent. Full-thickness rectal biopsy under general anesthesia is reserved for older children and in infants in whom suction biopsy is inadequate. An experienced pediatric pathologist must read the biopsies for maximal diagnostic accuracy. Evaluation for ganglion cells and the axons of the myenteric neurons is performed (Fig. 107.32), which may be accomplished using conventional hematoxylin-eosin staining or histochemical staining for acetylcholinesterase. Similar histochemical staining for nitric oxide synthase can be performed. These adjunctive techniques are used routinely in some centers and can help to provide additional evidence of Hirschsprung disease rather than simply demonstrating aganglionosis in the biopsy specimen. Diagnostic accuracy for Hirschsprung disease is excellent with a correctly obtained rectal suction biopsy and an experienced pediatric pathologist.[109]

Anorectal Manometry. The absence of sphincter relaxation in response to rectal dilatation is consistent with Hirschsprung disease. Because of the relative ease and accuracy of rectal suction biopsy, anorectal manometry is not widely used in the United States for the primary diagnosis of Hirschsprung disease in infancy; however, this is used in some centers around the world, and when applied carefully with an appropriate transduction probe, accurate manometric diagnosis is achievable in 85% to 90% of cases.

Treatment. Diverting colostomy should be considered for a newborn infant with Hirschsprung disease who has enterocolitis or multiple associated medical problems or anomalies. In the presence of enterocolitis, rectal irrigation and decompression can be an effective temporizing measure while resuscitation and broad-spectrum antibiotics are being instituted. Prompt proximal diversion will be required once the patient has stabilized. In the neonate, one approach following diagnosis is to perform proximal diversion by means of a colostomy (or enterostomy) placed in normal, ganglionated intestine. The diverting colostomy must be proximal to the histologic transition zone, and a series of biopsies examined by frozen section may be necessary to find the correct level for diversion. For classic rectosigmoid disease, a leveling colostomy is placed just proximal to the transition zone. This approach is generally done in two stages, with takedown of the stoma and definitive pull-through operation performed together weeks to months later, typically when the infant reaches 9 to 12 months of age. In older children, definitive pull-through is deferred until the colon has decompressed to relatively normal caliber.

For many infants and children without enterocolitis, a single-stage approach that eliminates the diverting colostomy has been advocated.[110,111] Despite several different operative techniques in performing a single-stage pull-through, results and outcomes

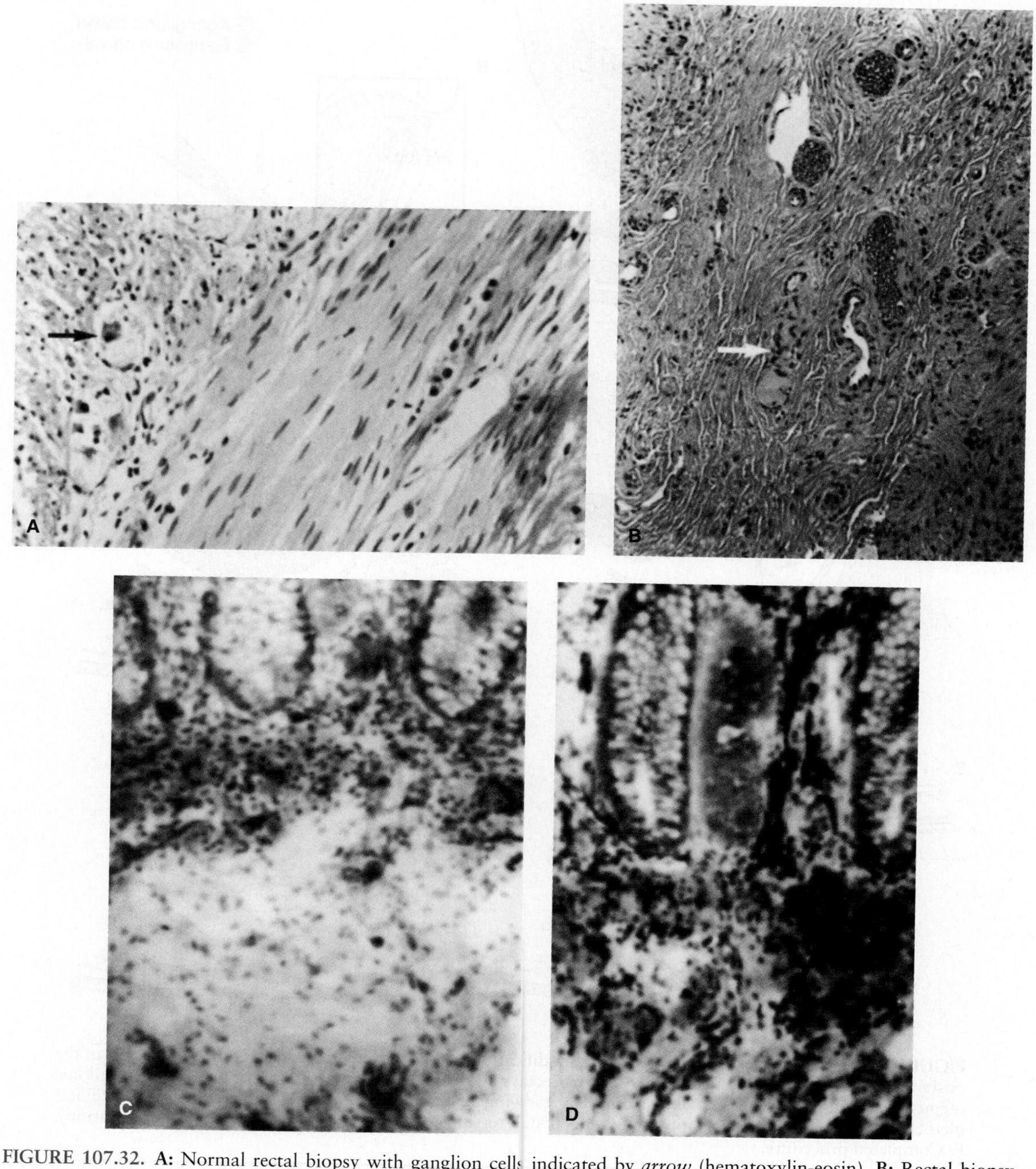

FIGURE 107.32. **A:** Normal rectal biopsy with ganglion cells indicated by *arrow* (hematoxylin-eosin). **B:** Rectal biopsy specimen with aganglionosis (hematoxylin-eosin). Note the characteristic thickened nerve fiber (*arrow*). **C:** Normal rectal biopsy using acetylcholinesterase histochemical staining. **D:** Similarly stained specimen from a patient with Hirschsprung disease. Many thickened submucosal nerve fibers stain densely black.

appear nearly equivalent. Definitive repair of Hirschsprung disease with a single operation is desirable from technical and economical standpoints and essentially eliminates the complications associated with neonatal stomas. As with most aspects of pediatric surgery, an increasing experience with laparoscopically assisted, single-stage pull-through operations has been reported.[112] The contemporary, laparoscopic single-stage approach in the management of Hirschsprung disease has gained wide acceptance in the pediatric surgical community and is considered by many surgeons as the current standard of care for most infants and children.

Definitive Operations for Hirschsprung Disease. The major goal of operative therapy in the treatment of Hirschsprung disease is to provide resection or bypass of the distal aganglionic rectum with the performance of a low rectal anastomosis with normally innervated proximal intestine. Numerous definitive procedures have been designed to treat Hirschsprung disease, and a brief description of the principal procedures in use follows. In general, the selection of a procedure depends on a surgeon's individual training and preference rather than compelling differences in outcome.[113,114]

Duhamel Procedure (Martin Modification). The key elements of the Duhamel procedure are illustrated in Figure 107.33. After minimal pelvic dissection, resection of the aganglionic colon is performed. The aganglionic rectum is left in situ. Normal proximal colon is brought caudad into the retrorectal

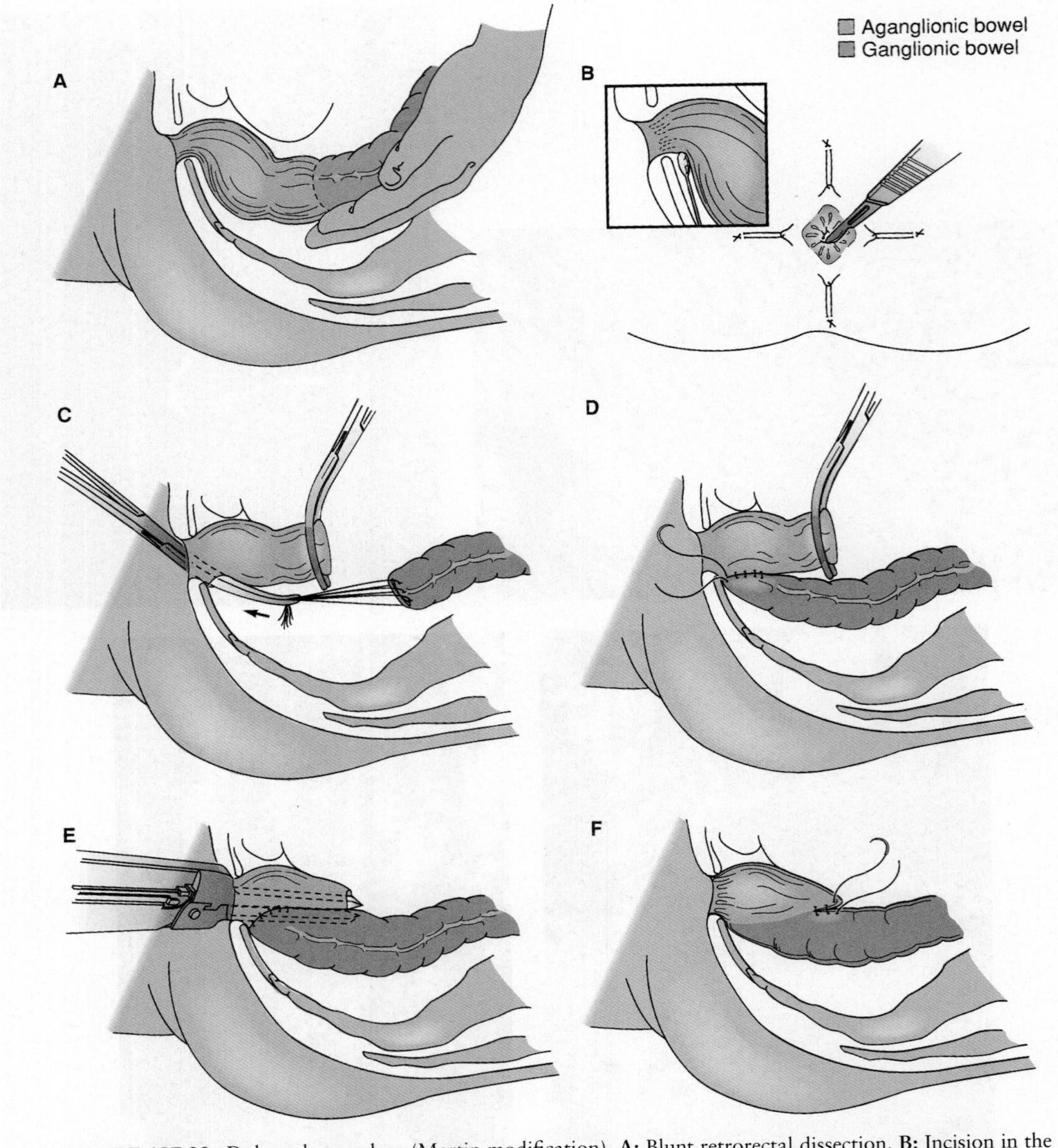

FIGURE 107.33. Duhamel procedure (Martin modification). **A:** Blunt retrorectal dissection. **B:** Incision in the posterior wall of the aganglionic rectum. **C:** Retrorectal pull-through after resection of the proximal aganglionic segment. **D:** End-to-side colorectal anastomosis preserving aganglionic rectum (as originally described). **E:** Stapled conversion of anastomosis into an extended side-to-side colorectal anastomosis (Martin modification). **F:** Completed procedure.

space, and a colorectal anastomosis is performed 1 cm above the dentate line. The original operation left the defunctionalized rectal pouch as shown, which proved problematic. The procedure has been modified by Martin to include a longer side-to-side colorectal anastomosis. Advantages of this procedure include its relative technical ease and limited pelvic dissection. Adoption of the stapled anastomosis has simplified this procedure significantly.

Soave Procedure. The Soave procedure is illustrated in Figure 107.34. Following resection of aganglionic colon, an endorectal dissection in the submucosal plane is performed from proximal rectum to anus. The endorectal dissection is started in the extraperitoneal rectum. This dissection is typically much easier than similar dissection for ulcerative colitis given the lack of mucosal inflammation. The dissected rectal mucosal tube is everted through the anus, excised, and normal proximal bowel is pulled through the rectal muscular cuff. The original operation did not suture the pull-through segment of proximal bowel to the rectum. A formal sutured colorectal anastomosis is now universally performed. Care must be taken to ensure that the pull-through segment is not obstructed by the muscular cuff.

Swenson Procedure. The Swenson procedure is the original definitive procedure for the treatment of Hirschsprung disease. It is somewhat more demanding from a technical standpoint, and, as such, it has been reported to have a slightly higher incidence of postoperative complications. However, long-term outcome in children who undergo a properly performed Swenson procedure is equivalent to other procedures. The basic strategy is outlined in Figure 107.35. The aganglionic segment of colon is resected and a careful, nearly complete extramural dissection of the distal rectum is performed. Care must be taken to avoid inadvertent injury to the seminal vesicles, vas deferens, ureters, and pelvic splanchnic nerves. The dissected rectum is everted through the anus onto the perineum and

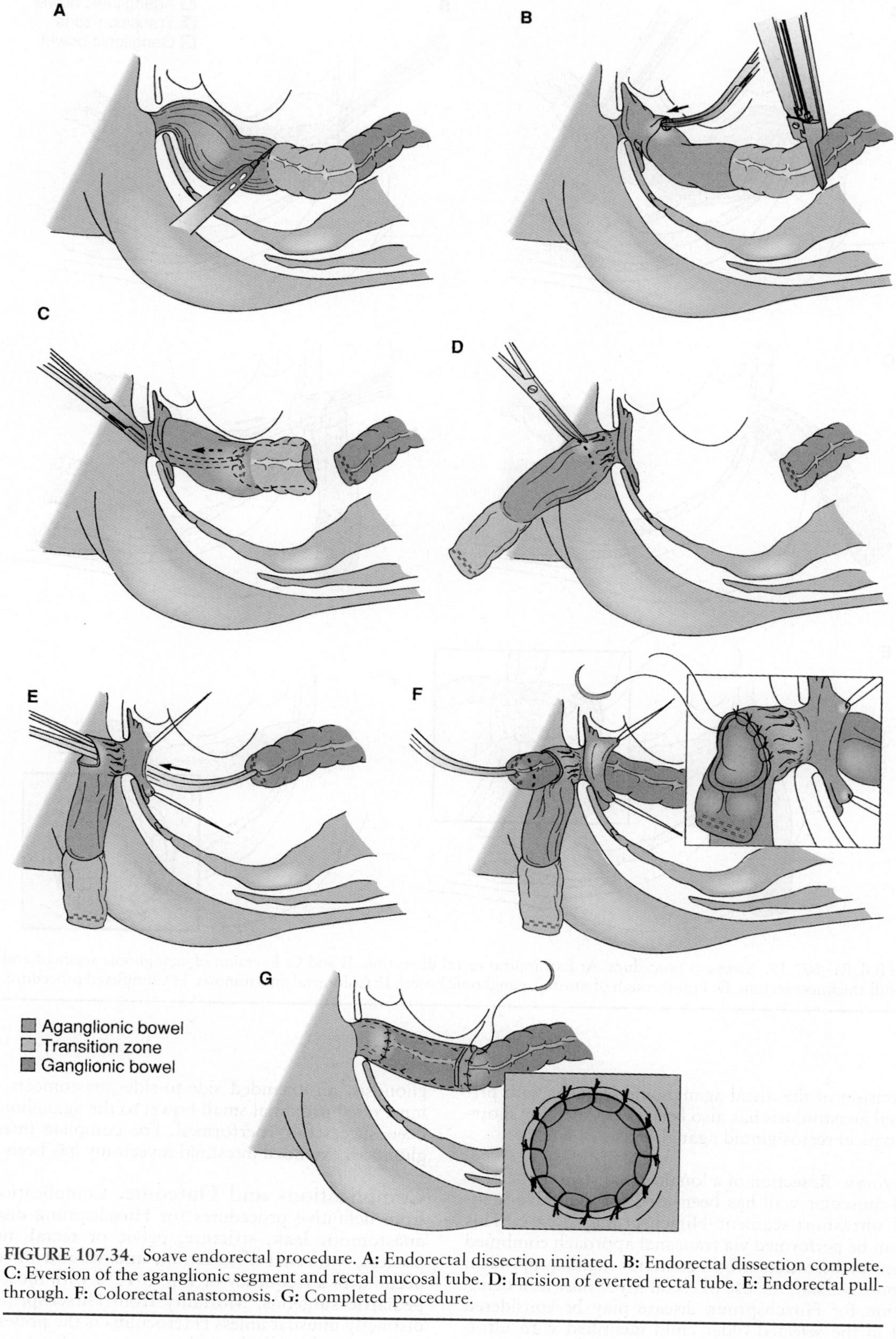

FIGURE 107.34. Soave endorectal procedure. **A:** Endorectal dissection initiated. **B:** Endorectal dissection complete. **C:** Eversion of the aganglionic segment and rectal mucosal tube. **D:** Incision of everted rectal tube. **E:** Endorectal pull-through. **F:** Colorectal anastomosis. **G:** Completed procedure.

excised. Normal proximal bowel is pulled through and a colorectal anastomosis is performed.

Laparoscopically Assisted Endorectal Pull-through. A multi-institutional clinical experience with a laparoscopically assisted endorectal pull-through technique for the treatment of Hirschsprung disease has been reported.[112] Potential advantages of this approach include excellent visibility of the distal rectum during dissection, early return of postoperative bowel function, and decreased length of hospital stay. The early results report outcomes similar to the other established procedures. The procedure is reviewed in Figure 107.36. Complete

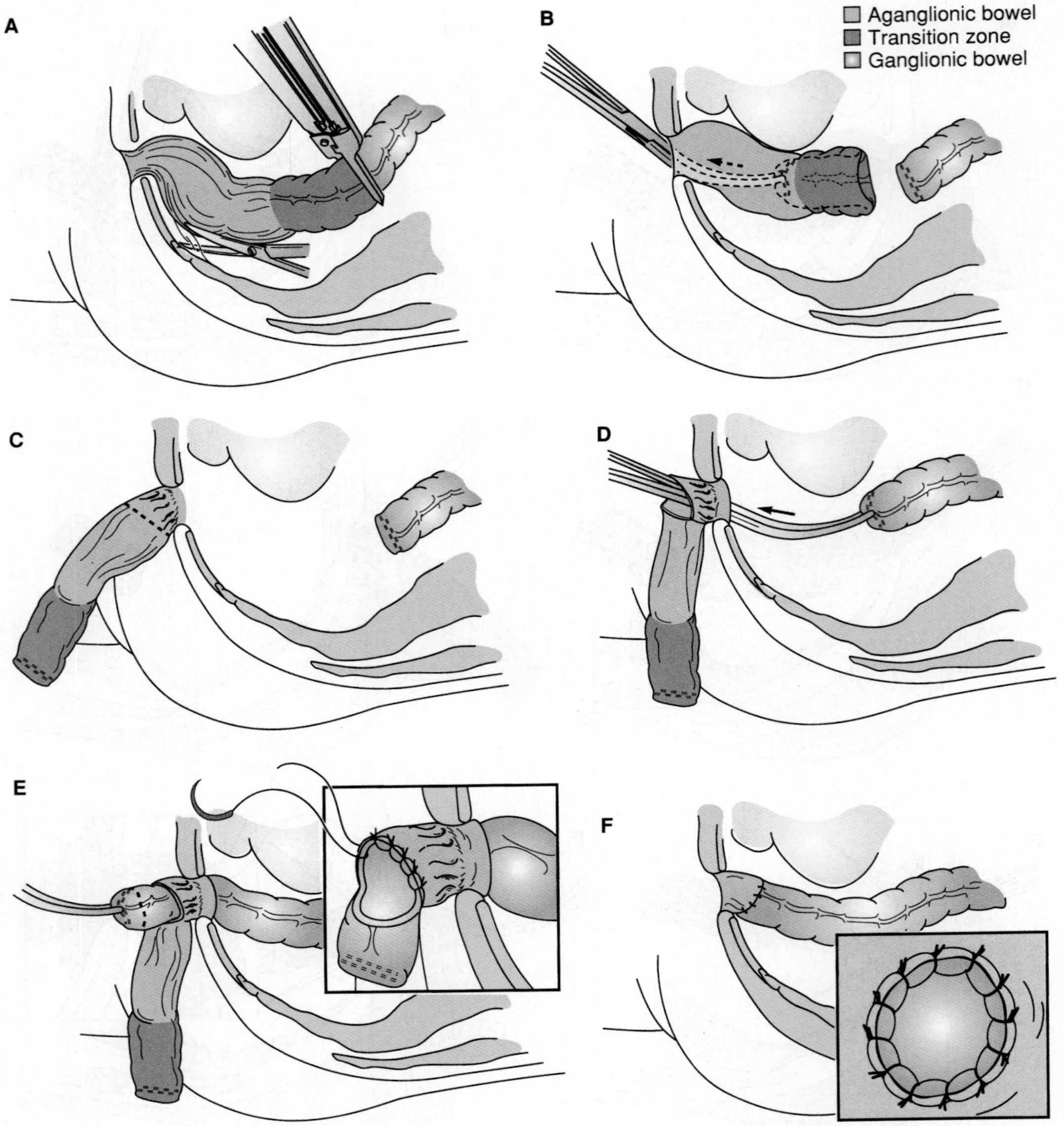

FIGURE 107.35. Swenson procedure. **A:** Extramural rectal dissection. **B** and **C:** Eversion of aganglionic segment and full-thickness rectum. **D:** Pull-through of normal, ganglionic bowel. **E:** Colorectal anastomosis. **F:** Completed procedure.

transanal excision of the distal aganglionic segment with primary coloanal anastomosis has also been performed for short-segment or typical rectosigmoid aganglionosis as well.

Rectal Myectomy. Resection of a longitudinal strip of the posterior rectal muscular wall has been used for definitive management of ultrashort-segment Hirschsprung disease. This procedure can be performed via transanal approach combined with submucosal dissection or by a posterior sagittal approach. Although controversial, the use of rectal myectomy as a definitive operation for Hirschsprung disease may be considered most useful in the selected older child identified with ultrashort-segment disease.[115]

Total Colonic Aganglionosis. Total colonic aganglionosis is complex and, fortunately, relatively rare. Several different operative procedures have been described, and treatment must be individualized. The endorectal pull-through with ileoanal anastomosis has been used with good success when most or all of the small bowel is normal. For extensive small bowel aganglionosis, an extended side-to-side anastomosis of normally innervated proximal small bowel to the aganglionic colon has been successfully performed. For complete intestinal aganglionosis, extended intestinal myectomy has been described.

Complications and Outcome. Complications resulting from definitive procedures for Hirschsprung disease include anastomotic leak, stricture, pelvic or rectal muscular cuff abscess, intestinal obstruction, and wound infection. These occur with a frequency of 1% to 10% with most experienced pediatric surgeons. Mortality from Hirschsprung disease is distinctly unusual unless enterocolitis is the presenting feature or associated medical problems or anomalies are present.

A unique complication following definitive repair of Hirschsprung disease is postoperative enterocolitis. The clinical presentation and pathogenesis have been discussed, and it remains an important and significant cause of morbidity. The incidence of postoperative enterocolitis ranges from 10% to 30% in most large series. Although rare, Hirschsprung enterocolitis can occur even in the presence of a diverting colostomy.

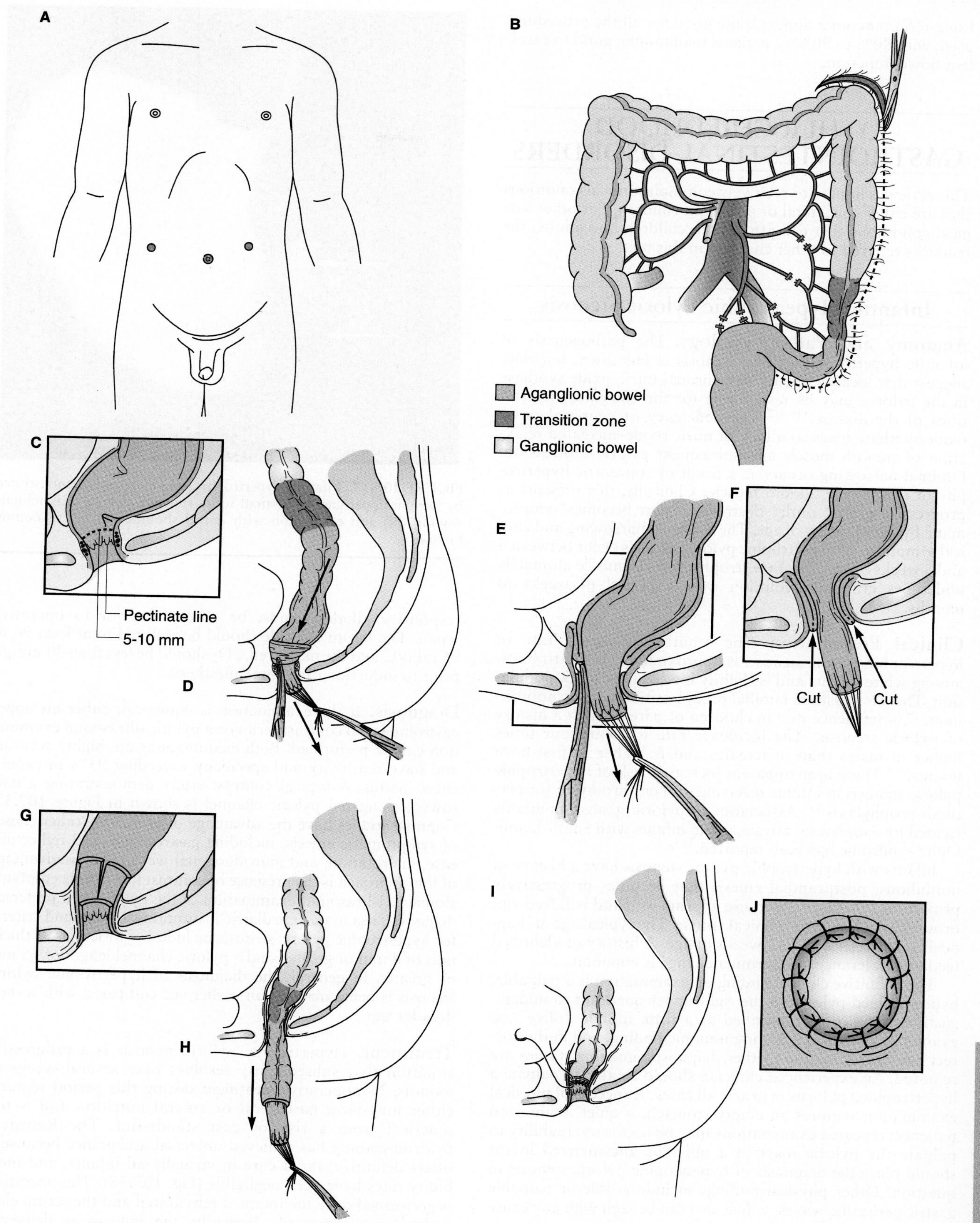

FIGURE 107.36. Laparoscopically assisted pull-through for Hirschsprung disease. **A:** Sites for operative trocar placement. **B:** Division of colon and rectal mesentery with mobilization of proximal colon. **C:** Circumferential incision in rectal mucosa 5 to 10 mm cephalad to the pectinate line. **D:** Mucosal traction sutures to facilitate further dissection from rectal muscular cuff. **E:** Transanal submucosal dissection is continued cephalad to meet the caudal extent of the transperitoneal rectal dissection. **F:** Circumferential incision of rectal muscular cuff. **G:** Rectal muscular cuff is split posteriorly to accommodate the pull-through segment (the pull-through segment is not shown here to clarify this maneuver). **H:** Rectum and sigmoid colon are pulled through the rectal muscular cuff to the anastomotic site. **I:** Colon is transected at appropriate site with confirmation of ganglion cells by frozen section. **J:** Transanal, end-to-end single layer colorectal anastomosis.

Long-term outcomes appear quite good for all the procedures used, with 80% to 90% of patients maintaining good to excellent bowel function.

OTHER CHILDHOOD GASTROINTESTINAL DISORDERS

This review is limited to relatively common surgical conditions that are either congenital or unique in children. For other surgical conditions that can affect both children and adults, the reader is referred to other chapters in this text.

Infantile Hypertrophic Pyloric Stenosis

Anatomy and Pathophysiology. The pathogenesis of infantile hypertrophic pyloric stenosis is unknown, but data suggest that local deficiency of neuronal nitric oxide synthase in the pylorus may be responsible for the clinical manifestations of the disease.[116,117] The deficiency of neuronal nitric oxide synthase leads to a lack of nitric oxide–mediated relaxation of smooth muscle and subsequent pyloric obstruction. Luminal narrowing occurs as a result of concentric hypertrophy of the pyloric smooth muscle. Clinically, this presents as progressive gastric outlet obstruction that becomes symptomatic by 2 to 4 weeks of age. The maximal narrowing and clinical symptoms of hypertrophic pyloric stenosis occur between 4 and 8 weeks of age. The hypertrophic pyloric muscle ultimately undergoes gradual involution over a period of weeks to months.

Clinical Presentation. The reported incidence rate of hypertrophic pyloric stenosis is approximately 0.1% to 0.4% among white infants and is slightly lower in the black population. There is a distinct familial predisposition with an approximate 7% incidence rate in children of parents with a history of pyloric stenosis. The incidence rate is about four times higher in males than in females and is higher in first-born infants.[118] There is an apparent increased risk of hypertrophic pyloric stenosis in infants receiving oral erythromycin for pertussis prophylaxis.[119] Association of pyloric stenosis in infants treated for esophageal atresia and in infants with Smith-Lemli-Opitz syndrome has been reported.[120]

Infants with hypertrophic pyloric stenosis have a history of nonbilious, postprandial emesis that becomes progressively projectile. The infant otherwise appears well and will feed vigorously until late in the clinical course. The typical age at diagnosis is between 2 and 12 weeks of age. A history of identified feeding intolerance and formula change is common.

The definitive clinical finding on examination is a palpable, hypertrophied pylorus in the right upper quadrant to midepigastric region, often described as a firm, mobile "olive" on examination. This is a pathognomonic finding, and in the correct clinical setting, no further diagnostic imaging studies are required. An experienced clinician should be able to palpate a hypertrophied pylorus in nearly all cases. A successful physical examination requires an empty stomach, a quiet infant, and patience; repeated examinations may be necessary. Inability to palpate the pyloric mass in a quiet or anesthetized infant should place the diagnosis of hypertrophic pyloric stenosis in question. Other physical findings include visible or palpable gastric peristaltic waves, which also can be seen with any cause of gastric or duodenal obstruction.

Late findings with advanced symptoms include dehydration and a hypochloremic, hypokalemic metabolic alkalosis from gastric fluid losses. Profound metabolic alkalosis is less common in current practice but occasionally can be encountered in an extremely dehydrated infant with a long-standing history of emesis. The intravascular volume depletion and chloride-responsive alkalosis must be corrected prior to operative repair. The serum chloride should be restored to at least 90 to 95 mEq/L, and the measured CO_2 should be less than 30 mEq/L prior to induction of general anesthesia.

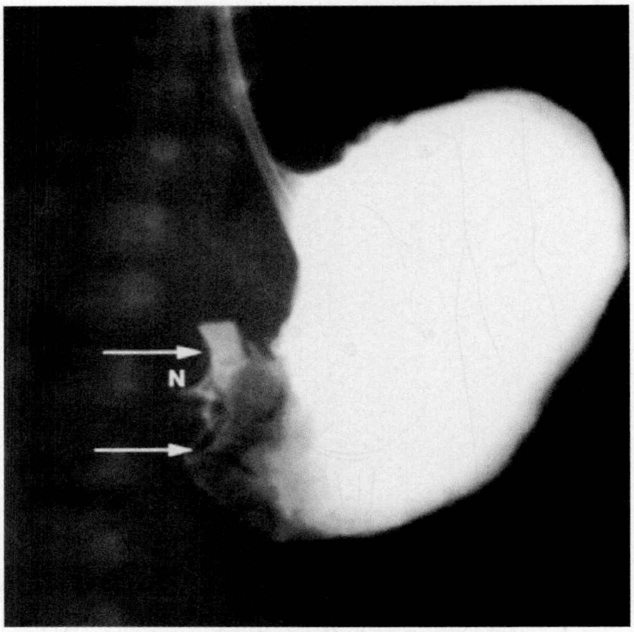

FIGURE 107.37. Infantile hypertrophic pyloric stenosis demonstrated by barium upper gastrointestinal series showing pyloric channel narrowing (*N*) and elongation with antral shouldering or cushioning (*arrows*).

Diagnosis. If the examination is equivocal, either an upper gastrointestinal contrast series or a pyloric ultrasound examination can be performed. Both examinations are highly accurate and have sensitivity and specificity exceeding 95% in experienced hands. A typical contrast study demonstrating a narrowed, elongated pyloric channel is shown in Figure 107.37. Contrast studies have the advantage of evaluating other causes of symptomatic emesis, including gastroesophageal reflux disease, malrotation, and antroduodenal webs. The disadvantage of this approach is the presence of contrast in a poorly emptying stomach. Ultrasound examination of the pylorus is a preferred diagnostic test in most pediatric institutions. Ultrasound criteria for hypertrophic pyloric stenosis include a pyloric muscle thickness of 4 mm or greater, and a pyloric channel length of 15 mm or greater. In general, the diagnosis of hypertrophic pyloric stenosis is being made at an earlier age compared with several decades ago.

Treatment. Hypertrophic pyloric stenosis is a progressive situation that subsequently resolves over several weeks to months. Nonoperative treatment during this period requires either long-term parenteral or enteral nutrition and is not practical from a risk or cost standpoint. The Ramstedt pyloromyotomy has achieved universal acceptance because it offers definitive, rapid cure in virtually all infants, and morbidity rates have been negligible (Fig. 107.38). The operation is performed once the infant is rehydrated and the serum electrolytes are corrected. Typically, the pylorus is delivered through a transverse right upper quadrant incision. A single longitudinal incision is made in the hypertrophied pyloric muscle. The hypertrophied circular pyloric muscle must be meticulously divided from the stomach to the junction of the proximal duodenum. An adequate pyloromyotomy is achieved when the submucosa bulges into the myotomy site and both

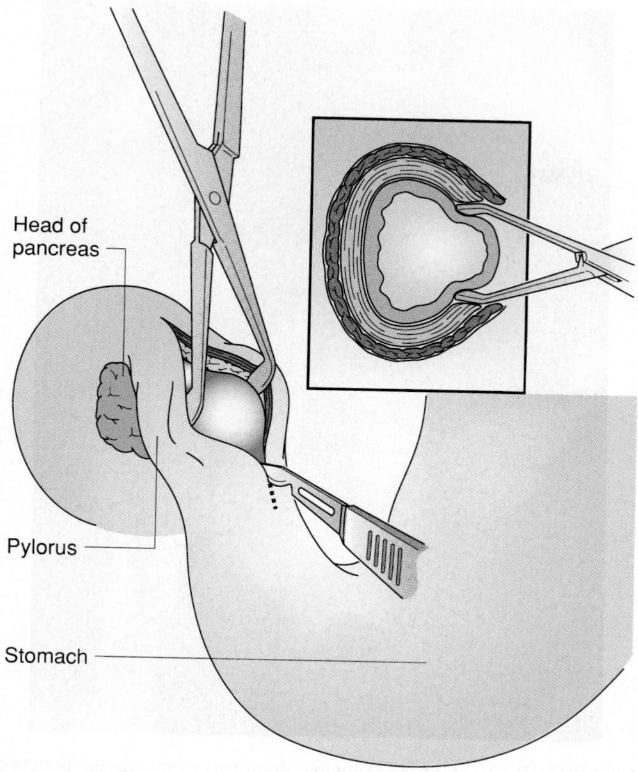

FIGURE 107.38. Ramstedt pyloromyotomy for infantile hypertrophic pyloric stenosis. The cross-sectional view shows herniation of the submucosa into the myotomy site, indicative of an adequate myotomy.

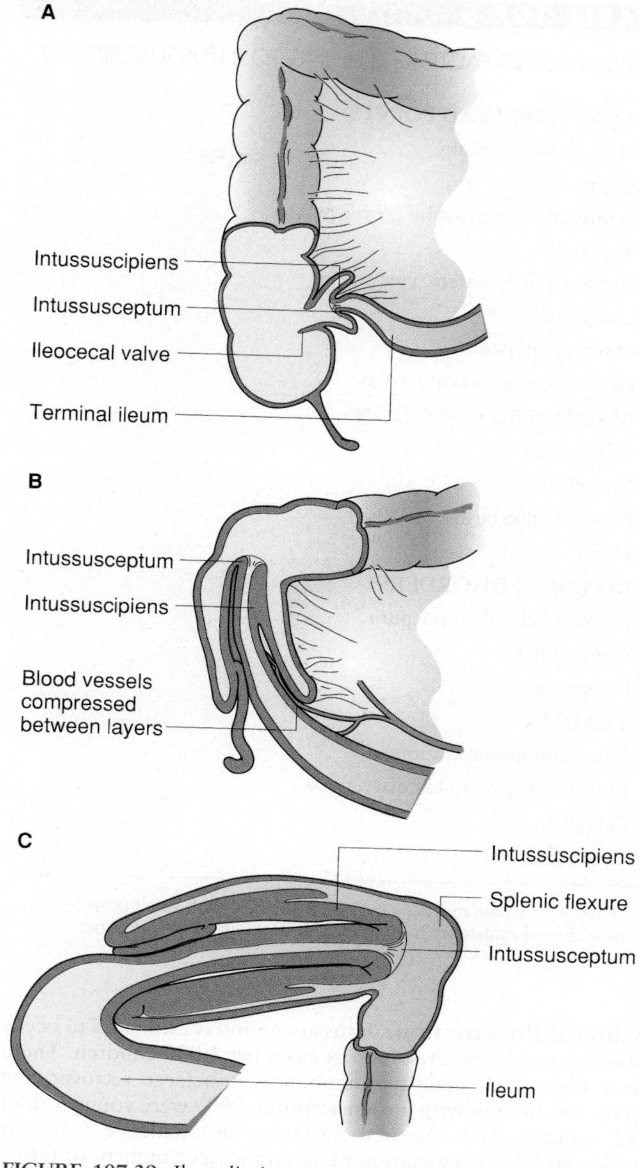

FIGURE 107.39. Ileocolic intussusception with the intussusceptum and intussuscipiens indicated.

edges of the divided pyloric muscle are freely mobile. Laparoscopic pyloromyotomy has been demonstrated to be efficacious and safe with similar operative times and outcome to the open repair; laparoscopic pyloromyotomy has become a standard approach at most children's hospitals.[121,122]

Postoperative feeding typically is started within 6 to 8 hours after recovery from anesthesia. Most infants are tolerant of enteral feeding and can be discharged home safely within 24 hours of operation. The surgical treatment of pyloric stenosis is straightforward, and the recovery is typically uncomplicated. A population-based study reviewing 1,777 infants with pyloric stenosis demonstrated a shorter length of stay and a lower overall complication rate in infants operated on by specialty-trained pediatric surgeons compared to general surgeons.[123] Mortality following pyloromyotomy is distinctly unusual in the absence of concomitant medical problems. Complications are rare and usually represent either wound infection, technical failures related to an inadequate pyloromyotomy, or inadvertent entry into the duodenum or stomach. Rarely, infants with inadequate pyloromyotomy may require reexploration and a second myotomy on the posterior pyloric wall. Inadvertent duodenotomy or gastrotomy must be recognized and repaired.

Intussusception

6 **Anatomy and Physiology.** *Intussusception* is defined as the invagination or telescoping of a proximal segment of intestine into an adjacent distal segment and is the most common cause of intestinal obstruction in infants and children age 3 months to 3 years (Fig. 107.39). The invaginated proximal bowel is referred to as the *intussusceptum*, and the recipient distal bowel is called the *intussuscipiens*. This process most commonly originates in the small intestine either at or near the ileocecal valve, with the terminal ileum passing into the cecum and colon (ileocolic intussusception). In the pediatric population, the vast majority (95%) of cases are considered idiopathic because of a lack of an identifiable anatomic lesion causing the intussusception. Older children are more likely to have a pathologic lead point causing the intussusception. In similar fashion, infants and children with repeated episodes of intussusception have a greater probability of a pathologic lead point. Table 107.6 describes several factors that have been associated with the development of intussusception.

Many cases of idiopathic intussusception in infants are probably caused by the normally prominent intramural lymph nodes (Peyer patches) in the terminal ileum acting as functional lead points. The anatomic consequence of intussusception is obstruction of the distal bowel. As bowel edema and inflammation progress, mesenteric vascular insufficiency from compression and congestion may occur. Incarceration, strangulation, and intestinal perforation ultimately may result if this condition remains unrecognized or untreated.

PEDIATRICS

TABLE 107.6

PREDISPOSING FACTORS LEADING TO INTUSSUSCEPTION

ANATOMIC LEAD POINTS
Meckel diverticulum
Polyp
Lymphatic hypertrophy (Peyer patch)
Appendix
Duplication or enteric cyst
Lymphoma
Other neoplasm
Heterotopic pancreatic tissue
ASSOCIATED INFECTIONS
Adenovirus
Rotavirus
Parasitic infestation
Other
BLEEDING DISORDERS[a]
Henoch-Schönlein purpura
Hemophilia
Leukemia
TRAUMA
Blunt abdominal trauma
Major retroperitoneal dissections
OTHER
Cystic fibrosis

[a]These factors are more likely to be associated with small bowel–to–small bowel intussusception than with ileocolic intussusception.

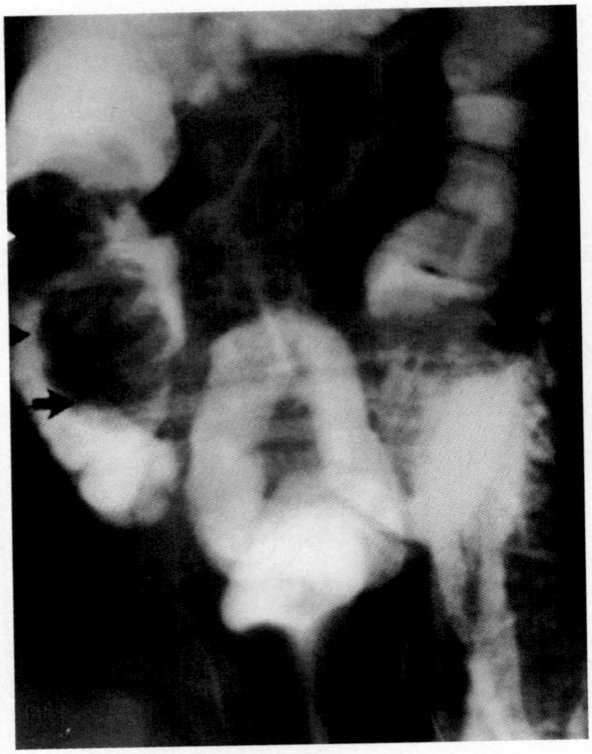

FIGURE 107.40. Contrast enema demonstrating classic ileocolic intussusception with the intussusceptum visible in the ascending colon (*arrows*).

Clinical Presentation. Intussusception is estimated to occur with an incidence rate of 1 to 4 cases per 1,000 children. There is a slight (3:2) male predominance; in a large retrospective series of children with intussusception, 79% were younger than 12 months, and seasonal variation in incidence was not observed.[124] An association between the development of intussusception and the administration of a previously available, tetravalent rhesus-based rotavirus vaccine (RotaShield, Wyeth Laboratories, Inc., Marietta, PA) was reported.[125] The currently available rotavirus vaccine does not appear to be associated with intussusception.[126]

Otherwise healthy infants who develop intussusception may have a characteristic clinical triad of abdominal pain, vomiting, and bloody stool. The typical infant develops an acute onset of severe, colicky abdominal pain. Intermittent episodes of irritability and crying may be associated with drawing the legs up to the abdomen. Between bouts of colic, the infant is often lethargic or sleepy. During periods of relative exhaustion, the abdominal examination may not be impressive; however, on careful physical examination, a palpable mass in the right abdomen may be appreciated in 80% to 90% of cases. Emesis is common and is often the presenting complaint. As intestinal obstruction progresses, intractable vomiting with abdominal distention and intravascular volume depletion may occur. Guaiac-positive stool is present in 90% to 95% of infants as a result of the ischemic mucosal injury to the intussusceptum. The passage of bloody stool mixed with mucus, classically described as *currant-jelly stool*, may be observed.

Diagnosis. Plain radiographs of the abdomen are generally nonspecific and may show a paucity of gas in the right lower quadrant with a mass effect in the ascending colon. Late findings demonstrate mechanical small bowel obstruction with proximal distention, air–fluid levels, and a decrease or absence of gas distally. Diagnostic enema techniques using either air or contrast approach 100% accuracy with typical ileocolic intussusception (Fig. 107.40). An approach using hydrostatic or pneumatic enema allows therapeutic reduction of intussusception as well. Ultrasound examination typically reveals a mass resembling a bull's-eye or target sign, corresponding to the intussusceptum within the intussuscipiens. The target sign of intussusception also may be demonstrated by CT scan imaging. Neither of these latter modalities allows for potential therapeutic reduction, and both may be more useful in diagnosing suspected cases of proximal jejunoileal or enteroenteral intussusception.

Treatment. Any infant with suspected intussusception in the absence of peritonitis should undergo diagnostic hydrostatic or pneumatic enema. A high index of clinical suspicion and liberal application of this approach should be maintained. The incidence of normal contrast enema examinations in this setting may exceed 75% in most pediatric centers, and this is justified by the considerable risk inherent in a missed diagnosis. An experienced pediatric radiologist and surgical evaluation are essential. Intravenous access and resuscitation should occur before attempts are made at diagnostic or therapeutic enemas.

Successful hydrostatic or pneumatic reduction of ileocolic intussusception is achieved in 60% to 80% of infants in most pediatric centers in the United States. Some centers prefer pneumatic enema using air as a contrast agent, and this technique appears comparable to the hydrostatic approach in both diagnosis and therapeutic reduction of intussusception. The ability to reduce intussusception using these techniques is time dependent and diminishes substantially after the duration of symptoms exceeds 24 hours. In this setting, a contrast enema is still diagnostic and potentially therapeutic if carefully performed.[127] With most experienced pediatric radiologists, the risk of perforation or reduction of a strangulated intussusceptum is low.

The technique of retrograde reduction of intussusception is straightforward. Contrast or air is introduced into the rectum by a balloon catheter, with the height of the hydrostatic column 1 m or less. Most centers use three attempts at reduction, with each attempt no longer than 3 minutes in duration. As long as progress is being made, however, attempts can be repeated until reduction is achieved. Successful reduction of ileocolic intussusception is demonstrated by observing retrograde flow of contrast or air into the terminal ileum. Inability to demonstrate retrograde flow into the ileum suggests incomplete reduction requiring surgical exploration.

Operative Management. Infants presenting with peritonitis and small bowel obstruction with a clinical diagnosis of intussusception should undergo immediate resuscitation and exploration without attempts at retrograde enema. Surgical exploration also is required after incomplete retrograde enema reduction of intussusception or in the relatively infrequent situation of bowel perforation during diagnostic or therapeutic enema. The operative strategy is dictated by the findings. Spontaneous reduction of the intussusception is reported to occur in up to 20% to 30% of infants following induction of general anesthesia. In this situation, exploration confirming the reduction and examining the bowel for a pathologic lead point is sufficient. With persistent intussusception and viable bowel, the bowel is manually reduced, generally pushing the intussusceptum out of the distal bowel. If manual reduction cannot be performed or the intussusceptum is strangulated, then segmental resection with primary anastomosis is performed. Attempts at reducing intussusception with clearly necrotic bowel should be avoided. Diverting enterostomy as a result of peritoneal contamination usually is not required. Appendectomy is routinely performed in all infants undergoing operative exploration for intussusception. As with many aspects of pediatric surgery, a successful laparoscopic approach to the diagnosis and management of intussusception has been reported in approximately two thirds of selected patients.[128–130]

Complications and Outcome.

Retrograde techniques are successful at reducing idiopathic ileocolic intussusception in 60% to 80% of cases. Following successful enema reduction, the infant is given intravenous fluids and usually observed for 24 hours. Tolerance of oral feeding is predictably rapid. Recovery from operative reduction or bowel resection is generally no different than from other similar gastrointestinal procedures. Most infants enjoy a complete recovery with minimal or no morbidity. Recurrent intussusception after either nonoperative or operative reduction occurs in about 5% of infants and usually can be treated with repeat enema. Mortality from intussusception is rare and is almost always the result of systemic sepsis and shock from unrecognized, strangulated intestine.

Meckel Diverticulum and Related Disorders

Embryology and Anatomy.

The most frequently encountered congenital anomaly of the gastrointestinal tract is the Meckel diverticulum, representing one of several malformations resulting from persistence of the yolk stalk (synonymous with *vitelline duct* and *omphalomesenteric duct*) and its components. The embryonic yolk stalk connects the yolk sac and the developing midgut (Fig. 107.41). Between weeks 5 and 7 of gestation, the yolk sac involutes and the stalk fuses with the umbilical cord. Developmental failure or arrest of yolk sac involution creates a spectrum of clinical malformations as outlined in Figure 107.42, with Meckel diverticula constituting greater than 95% of these anomalies. The Meckel diverticulum is a true diverticulum of variable size derived from the intestinal remnant of the yolk stalk. Typically, it is found on the antimesenteric border of the terminal ileum approximately 40 to 50 cm from the ileocecal valve in adults. The blood supply is derived from persistent vitelline vessels supplied from the SMA. About 25% of the diverticula have a fibrous or vascular attachment to the anterior abdominal wall at the umbilicus (Fig. 107.42C). Heterotopic gastric mucosa or pancreatic tissue is found in about half of the diverticula examined at autopsy. In about 75% of patients with symptomatic diverticula, gastric mucosa is present. When symptoms occur, bleeding or perforation is generally the result of peptic ulceration of the adjacent ileal mucosa and not from the diverticulum itself.

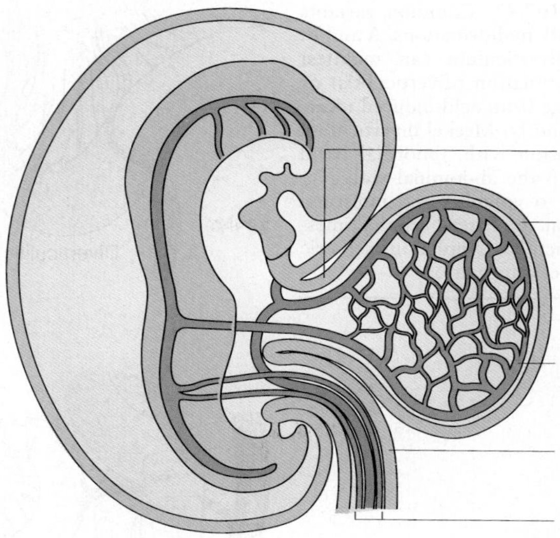

FIGURE 107.41. Normal embryonic relations of the yolk sac, yolk stalk, and developing gut.

Clinical Presentation.

Symptomatic yolk stalk anomalies are usually diagnosed by history and clinical examination. Umbilical drainage from a persistent fistula or sinus tract may be noted in a newborn following separation of the umbilical cord. Intestinal prolapse or passage of stool from the umbilicus signifies a patent omphalomesenteric duct. Small bowel obstruction in an otherwise healthy infant without a history of laparotomy may be a result of volvulus around an omphalomesenteric band or intussusception from a Meckel diverticulum acting as a lead point.

The incidence rate of Meckel diverticula in the general population is about 2%, with a 2:1 male-to-female predominance. The risk of developing symptoms from the diverticulum decreases with age, and the vast majority of subjects remain asymptomatic. About half of the persons who do become symptomatic are younger than 2 years of age. Table 107.7 outlines several of the more common clinical presentations of symptomatic Meckel diverticulum.

Hemorrhage. Gastrointestinal bleeding related to Meckel diverticulum generally results from peptic ulceration of the adjacent ileal mucosa. Clinically, it manifests as painless, episodic hemorrhage that is typically bright red to maroon; melena is not characteristically seen. Bleeding from a Meckel diverticulum is generally not hemodynamically significant or exsanguinating, but it can be persistent enough to require transfusion. The diagnostic test of choice is the ^{99m}Tc-pertechnetate radioisotope scan (Meckel scan) because of the high affinity of the isotope for gastric mucosa and the high probability of gastric mucosa within a symptomatic Meckel diverticulum. Diagnostic accuracy is reported to be as high as 90% for

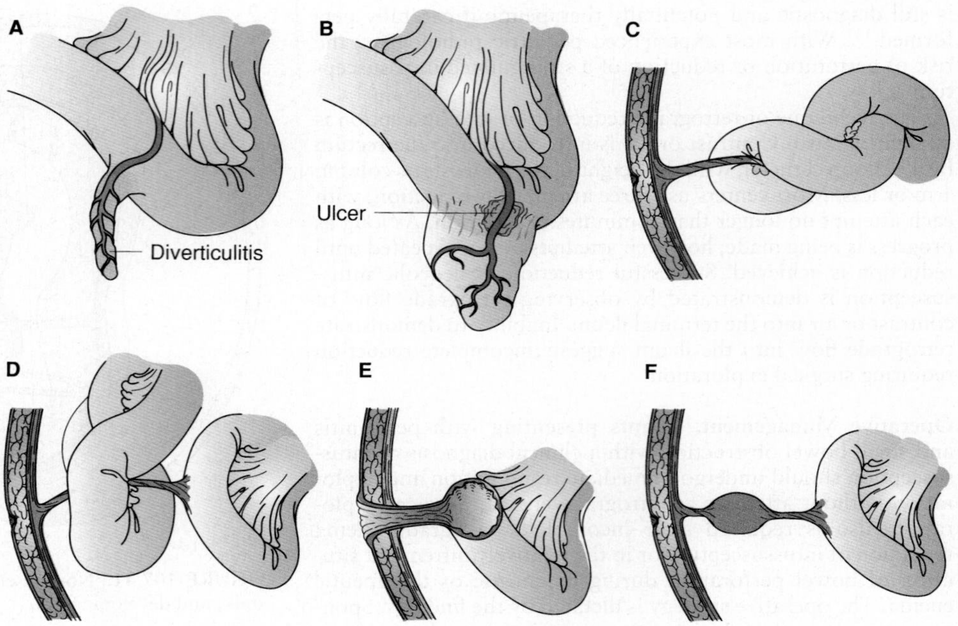

FIGURE 107.42. Common variants of yolk stalk malformations. **A** and **B**: Meckel diverticulum can manifest with inflammation (diverticulitis) or hemorrhage from acid-induced ulceration. **C** and **D**: Meckel diverticulum in association with abnormal band attached to the abdominal wall predisposing to volvulus and intestinal obstruction. **E**: Patent omphalomesenteric duct. **F**: Omphalomesenteric sinus and cyst formation.

Meckel-related bleeding. Contrast studies and endoscopy have a limited role when the problem is hemorrhage from a Meckel diverticulum.

Obstruction. Intestinal obstruction associated with omphalomesenteric duct anomalies usually results from either intussusception or volvulus around an abnormal attachment between the bowel and the abdominal wall. In about 5% to 10% of persons with symptomatic Meckel diverticula, intussusception is the initial symptom. In patients with Meckel diverticula whose initial symptom is small bowel obstruction, about half have intussusception and the remainder have volvulus, internal hernias, or other mechanical causes. Intussusception secondary to a Meckel diverticula has a decreased likelihood for successful enema reduction. Small bowel obstruction from volvulus around an omphalomesenteric band requires operative exploration and treatment.

Diverticulitis. About one third of patients with symptomatic Meckel diverticulum have acute diverticulitis. Similar to appendicitis, intraluminal obstruction at the base of a Meckel diverticulum can lead to distal inflammation, gangrene, and subsequent perforation. Peptic ulceration also can lead to local inflammation and perforation with the development of peritonitis. The signs and symptoms of Meckel diverticulitis are virtually indistinguishable from appendicitis, and exploration is both diagnostic and therapeutic.

TABLE 107.7 **DIAGNOSIS**

SIGNS AND SYMPTOMS OF MECKEL DIVERTICULUM

■ CLINICAL PRESENTATION	■ APPROXIMATE FREQUENCY (%)
Hemorrhage	30–35
Small bowel obstruction	30–35
Diverticulitis	20–25
Umbilical fistula	10
Other	Uncommon

Umbilical Anomalies. About 10% of patients with yolk stalk or persistent omphalomesenteric duct anomalies have umbilical problems. The usual clinical presentation is persistent drainage or intestinal mucosa found at the umbilicus. The diagnosis can be confirmed by contrast sonogram of the umbilical orifice or tract. Occasionally, ultrasound examination may be useful to demonstrate omphalomesenteric cysts. Ultimately, surgical exploration may be required for both diagnosis and treatment.

Meckel Diverticulum as an Incidental Finding. The management of an incidentally discovered Meckel diverticulum during abdominal exploration for other reasons is controversial. The risk of resecting an asymptomatic diverticulum must be weighed against the reasons for the operative exploration, patient age, and the potential for future symptoms from the diverticulum. Infants younger than 2 years are at greater probability of becoming symptomatic from a Meckel diverticula. Resection is clearly indicated with demonstration of heterotopic gastric mucosa in the diverticulum to prevent peptic ulceration. This finding may occasionally be determined by direct palpation because the gastric mucosa is thicker than ileal mucosa. Abnormal omphalomesenteric bands to the abdominal wall also should be excised. If clinical judgment suggests that the diverticulum is at risk for luminal obstruction, resection is warranted.

Treatment.

Infants and children with symptomatic umbilical abnormalities from yolk stalk remnants are usually well, and umbilical exploration with possible laparotomy can be undertaken electively. The yolk stalk remnant is excised, and, if present, the communication with the ileum is closed primarily with minimal morbidity and mortality. Operative exploration is required for patients with symptomatic Meckel diverticula. Typically, exploration can be accomplished through a variety of incisions. The treatment of choice is resection through either antimesenteric wedge excision or segmental bowel resection with primary closure or anastomosis. Laparoscopic diagnosis and management of a Meckel diverticulum has also been described.[131] In the absence of associated medical problems, excellent functional outcome is expected with minimal morbidity and essentially no mortality unless intestinal necrosis has occurred.

Foreign Bodies

Ingestion of foreign bodies by infants and children is common. Toddlers in the age range of 9 months to 2 years are at particular risk given newly acquired mobility and the tendency for oral exploration. The type of foreign body and the location in the gastrointestinal tract on discovery dictate overall management.

Esophagus. Typical foreign bodies found in the esophagus include coins and small toys. In normal children, these objects become impacted at predictably narrow portions of the esophagus, including the cricopharyngeus, the esophagus at the level of the left mainstem bronchus, and the gastroesophageal junction. Previous areas of esophageal repair or injury predispose to points of obstruction. In particular, infants and children with repaired esophageal atresia, gastroesophageal reflux, or caustic esophageal injury are at risk for impaction at these sites.

Esophageal foreign bodies produce clinical symptoms of drooling, feeding intolerance (particularly to solids), dysphagia, and pain. Unrecognized foreign bodies with unusual configuration or sharp points and edges may cause esophageal perforation and mediastinitis. The diagnosis is straightforward on plain radiographs if the object is metallic or radiopaque. If a radiolucent object is suspected, an upper gastrointestinal contrast study is usually required to confirm the diagnosis. Lateral plain films of the neck or chest may be useful to differentiate between small foreign bodies in the esophagus or trachea.

Foreign bodies impacted in the esophagus cause partial esophageal obstruction and can cause complications including aspiration, erosion, perforation, and late stricture formation. Therefore, all esophageal foreign bodies should be removed. Extraction of foreign objects can be accomplished by using balloon catheter retrieval under fluoroscopic guidance or direct visualization using endoscopy. Performed within 24 hours of ingestion, balloon catheter retrieval of esophageal foreign bodies is relatively straightforward. This technique is limited to smooth radiopaque objects such as coins to minimize the risk of esophageal perforation. The most significant risk with balloon catheter retrieval is potential aspiration from an unprotected airway, and this must be anticipated as the foreign body traverses the pharynx. Alternatively, for esophageal coin impaction of less than 24 hours' duration in children without a history of esophageal surgery or injury, esophageal bougienage with clearance of the coin into the stomach has been successful.[132]

Retrieval of esophageal foreign bodies under direct endoscopic vision requires general anesthesia. Either flexible or rigid endoscopy systems are widely available and used with individual and institutional preferences. Esophageal perforation, the major risk, occurs in fewer than 5% of cases in most reported series. Long-standing esophageal foreign bodies may erode into the aorta and cause life-threatening hemorrhage from aorto-esophageal fistula.[133]

Distal Gastrointestinal Tract. More than 95% of foreign bodies that pass beyond the gastroesophageal junction proceed uneventfully through the gastrointestinal tract. The transit time for an asymptomatic foreign body is highly variable and can take hours to weeks. Progress of an asymptomatic radiopaque foreign body can be followed by abdominal plain films, but this is rarely useful from a clinical standpoint unless it is a battery. The stool may also be screened to confirm passage of a known foreign body.

Operative exploration or endoscopic retrieval of distal gastrointestinal foreign bodies is generally reserved for clinical symptoms related to either obstruction or intestinal injury heralded by abdominal pain, vomiting, fever, or peritonitis. Additionally, persistence of an asymptomatic foreign body in the stomach for several weeks is a relative indication for upper endoscopic retrieval, particularly with foreign bodies with irregular shape, configuration, or sharpness. This is a clinical judgment that is best reserved for an experienced pediatric surgeon because remarkably complex and improbable objects may pass uneventfully through the gastrointestinal tract. For asymptomatic foreign bodies lodged distal to the stomach, a relative indication for operative removal is a fixed, persistent location in the intestine for longer than 1 week.

Ingested batteries, in particular alkaline disc batteries, are a potentially serious hazard to children and require a more aggressive approach. Disruption of the battery casing and spillage of the contents have been reported to cause intestinal injury and perforation, presumably because of leakage of potassium or sodium hydroxide. Esophageal impaction of a battery warrants prompt removal when recognized because the risk of acquired esophageal injury, perforation, and development of traumatic tracheoesophageal fistula is present.[134] In the distal bowel, cathartics may be helpful to expedite passage of the battery. Operative removal may be necessary if the battery fails to progress distally over a few days or if symptoms related to the battery occur. Notably, the vast majority of batteries pass through the gastrointestinal tract uneventfully. Ingestion of multiple magnets can cause problems with small bowel obstruction or enteroenteric fistula formation.

Gastrointestinal Hemorrhage

The subject of gastrointestinal hemorrhage and general principles of management are discussed elsewhere in this book. The following section reviews some of the important and age-dependent clinical causes and unique issues of gastrointestinal bleeding in the pediatric population. These causes are age dependent and are summarized in Tables 107.8 and 107.9.

Diagnostic workup of an infant or child with gastrointestinal hemorrhage requires coordinated participation between pediatricians, surgeons, gastroenterologists, and radiologists. Several general principles governing the diagnostic approach to gastrointestinal bleeding in infants and children follow:

a. A clear diagnosis can be made in most situations; given the current technology available to assist with diagnosis, an aggressive approach is warranted. Diagnostic procedures such as flexible fiberoptic endoscopy, radioisotope imaging, and angiography are widely available, safe, and applicable to any age group, including the newborn. Despite these measures, in approximately 16% of cases, the cause of guaiac-positive stools in a neonate or infant remains unknown,[135] and the bleeding is self-limited.
b. The primary diagnostic investigation of choice for upper gastrointestinal bleeding is esophagogastroduodenoscopy. This procedure is optimally performed within the first 24 hours after cessation of active hemorrhage and usually requires general anesthesia. Imaging studies for active upper gastrointestinal hemorrhage are limited in their ability to aid with diagnosis.
c. Infants and children presenting with minor lower gastrointestinal bleeding are best evaluated by a careful perineal and digital rectal examination followed by anoscopy.
d. Massive lower gastrointestinal hemorrhage in an infant or child outside the newborn period is most likely the result of a bleeding Meckel diverticulum.
e. If a definitive source for lower gastrointestinal hemorrhage is not found on colonoscopy, evaluation for an upper gastrointestinal source, including upper endoscopy and diagnostic laparoscopy, is warranted.
f. Pain is an uncommon symptom with pediatric gastrointestinal hemorrhage and implies a more complex problem such as volvulus, ischemic bowel, or inflammatory bowel disease. Painful gastrointestinal hemorrhage in a pediatric patient requires urgent evaluation and prompt diagnostic workup.
g. In contrast to that in adults, gastrointestinal bleeding in children is rarely a symptom or sign of gastrointestinal neoplasm.

TABLE 107.8 ETIOLOGY

CAUSES OF UPPER GASTROINTESTINAL HEMORRHAGE[a]

PATIENT AGE GROUP	COMMON CAUSES	LESS COMMON CAUSES
Neonatal (0 to 30 days)	Gastritis Esophagitis Ingested maternal blood Peptic ulcer	Iatrogenic trauma Primary coagulopathy Vascular malformation (hemangioma, telangiectasia, arteriovenous malformation) Nasal or pharyngeal bleeding Miscellaneous (leiomyoma, gastric polyp, duplication)
Infant (30 days to 1 year)	Gastritis Esophagitis Peptic ulcer	Same as neonate, with addition of: Drugs (steroids, nonsteroidal anti-inflammatory drugs) Foreign body, caustic ingestion Esophageal varices
Child (1 to 12 years)	Esophageal varices Esophagitis Peptic ulcer	Same as infant, with addition of: Acquired thrombocytopenia (chemotherapy)
Older child (12 years to adult)	Esophageal varices Esophagitis Peptic ulcer	Same as for child

[a]Order in appearance approximates clinical frequency.
Adapted from Oldham KT, Lobe TE. Gastrointestinal hemorrhage in children. A pragmatic update. *Pediatr Clin North Am* 1985;32:1247–1263, with permission.

Neonates (0 to 30 Days of Age). The most common cause of gastrointestinal hemorrhage in a neonate is gastritis. Endoscopic evaluation of newborns with symptomatic upper gastrointestinal hemorrhage demonstrates gastritis or esophagitis in 50% to 75% of cases. About 10% to 15% have swallowed maternal blood during birth, and 10% of newborns are found to have an underlying coagulopathy. Anatomic lesions requiring operative control are distinctly unusual in this age group. Significant and sometimes massive upper gastrointestinal hemorrhage may occur in a neonate without a definable anatomic lesion despite endoscopic evaluation. This finding is usually the result of gastritis, and treatment is directed at blood and volume replacement and correction of any underlying coagulopathy.

Significant conditions responsible for lower gastrointestinal bleeding in the newborn include NEC, malrotation with volvulus, enterocolitis, or bowel obstruction secondary to an incarcerated inguinal hernia. These clinical entities present with characteristic histories, findings on clinical examination, and surgical treatment guidelines previously discussed. Anorectal fissure is also common and easy to diagnose in neonates, and bleeding is typically self-limited.

Infants (30 Days to 1 Year). Infants with upper gastrointestinal bleeding deserve comprehensive evaluation, including endoscopy, to identify potential lesions requiring operative intervention. The most common causes of lower gastrointestinal hemorrhage in this age group include infectious diarrhea, intussusception, food allergy, and bleeding Meckel diverticulum. Most of these lesions have distinct symptoms, signs, and diagnostic findings to facilitate diagnosis. Infectious diarrhea is usually accompanied by fever, feeding intolerance, possibly emesis, and abdominal pain. Fecal leukocytes may be present on stool examination, and enteric pathogens or their toxins can be identified by stool culture.

Children (1 to 12 Years). An important surgical cause of upper gastrointestinal bleeding in this age group includes esophageal variceal bleeding from portal hypertension. Children with biliary atresia or extrahepatic portal venous obstruction account for most cases of variceal bleeding in this age group. In the acute setting, endoscopic sclerotherapy or banding is used as a temporizing measure for hemorrhage control; some investigators advocate maintenance sclerotherapy. Ultimately, for these children, orthotopic liver transplantation may offer definitive surgical treatment. The use of operative portosystemic shunts for acute variceal hemorrhage is not widely used in pediatric surgical practice in the United States.

Conditions causing lower gastrointestinal bleeding in this age group include juvenile polyps. These are benign, hamartomatous polyps and represent the single most common cause of lower gastrointestinal bleeding in children. About 20% to 30% of the polyps are palpable on digital rectal examination. A history of painless, bright red blood per rectum during a bowel movement is typical. The bleeding results from mucosal irritation, involution, and sloughing of a pedunculated polyp and is usually not associated with hemodynamically significant hemorrhage. Tissue may be passed or the pedunculated polyp may prolapse out the anus. A hypochromic, microcytic anemia may be present. Diagnostic workup generally involves a contrast enema to identify the polyp and evaluate the colon for synchronous lesions. Colonoscopy may require general anesthesia in this age group, and endoscopic snare polypectomy is the treatment of choice for appropriate-sized polyps. Infrequently, transanal excision or open resection of larger polyps is required. In the case of multiple juvenile polyps not

TABLE 107.9

CAUSES OF LOWER GASTROINTESTINAL HEMORRHAGE[a]

PATIENT AGE GROUP	COMMON CAUSES	LESS COMMON CAUSES
Neonatal (0 to 30 days)	Benign anorectal lesions (fissure) Upper gastrointestinal hemorrhage Milk allergy Necrotizing enterocolitis Midgut volvulus	Iatrogenic trauma Primary coagulopathy Vascular malformations Enterocolitis (Hirschsprung disease, other) Miscellaneous (duplication, lymphoma, lymphangiectasia)
Infant (30 days to 1 year)	Incarcerated inguinal hernia Benign anorectal lesions Idiopathic intussusception Meckel diverticulum Infectious diarrhea Upper gastrointestinal hemorrhage Milk allergy	Same as neonate, with addition of: Acquired thrombocytopenia Ingestion of colored foodstuff (pseudohematochezia)
Child (1 to 12 years)	Benign anorectal lesions Juvenile polyps Intussusception Meckel diverticulum Infectious diarrhea Upper gastrointestinal hemorrhage	Same as infant, with addition of: Juvenile polyposis coli/familial polyposis coli Hemolytic uremic syndrome Henoch-Schönlein purpura Systemic vasculitis (dermatomyositis, lupus) Acquired thrombocytopenia (as above plus idiopathic thrombocytopenic purpura)
Older child (12 years to adult)	Juvenile polyps Benign anorectal lesions Inflammatory bowel disease Upper gastrointestinal hemorrhage	Same as child, except: Henoch-Schönlein purpura and hemolytic uremic syndrome less likely Meckel diverticulum

[a]Order in appearance approximates clinical frequency.
Adapted from Oldham KT, Lobe TE. Gastrointestinal hemorrhage in children. A pragmatic update. *Pediatr Clin North Am.* 1985;32:1247–1263, with permission.

amenable to endoscopic polypectomy, management may be expectant based on the benign natural history characterized by involution during adolescence. Histologic confirmation is necessary to differentiate these lesions from adenomatous polyps seen in familial polyposis syndromes or Gardner syndrome.

Older Children and Adolescents (Older than 12 Years). Causes of both upper and lower gastrointestinal hemorrhage in this age group include most etiologic conditions found in adults. It is important that inflammatory bowel disease is significant in this age group.

Intestinal Duplication

The embryologic origin of enteric duplication formation remains controversial, but duplication likely represents abnormal development of either a diverticulum or adjacent portion of the developing gut. In some cases, duplication cysts of the upper gastrointestinal tract may be associated with thoracic spinal cord or vertebral defects; this association appears to reflect abnormal sequestration and integration of developing primitive notochord elements in addition to duplication. The resulting lesions are described as either *cystic* or *tubular* based on their gross appearance (Fig. 107.43). All types of gastrointestinal-derived epithelia are found, but the clinically relevant finding is ectopic gastric mucosa. Duplications are commonly found along the mesenteric border of the native bowel. The muscular wall is typically well developed and intimately attached to the functional bowel. Additionally, the blood supply is also shared with the functional intestine, an important surgical consideration.

Cystic Duplications. Cystic duplications may be found throughout the gastrointestinal tract. They are frequently located in the esophagus and the hindgut, particularly the rectum. Direct communication between a duplication cyst and the functional gut lumen is unusual. Typically, asymptomatic duplications are discovered as incidental mass lesions during diagnostic imaging studies, particularly when the location is the thoracic cavity or the rectum. Duplications also may present as symptomatic lesions from ectopic gastric mucosa leading to ulceration and bleeding. Other potential presenting symptoms of enteric duplication include obstruction, intussusception, perforation or traumatic rupture, torsion, infection, and occasional malignant degeneration. Useful examinations to define the extent of the lesion include ultrasound, CT scanning, MRI studies, and contrast studies. The identification of enteric duplication on routine prenatal ultrasound examination has been reported.

The treatment for all cystic duplications is operative. Even in asymptomatic infants and children, uncertainty regarding the nature of the mass and the potential for subsequent problems dictates surgical exploration. Esophageal and rectal duplication cysts are generally amenable to simple excision. In

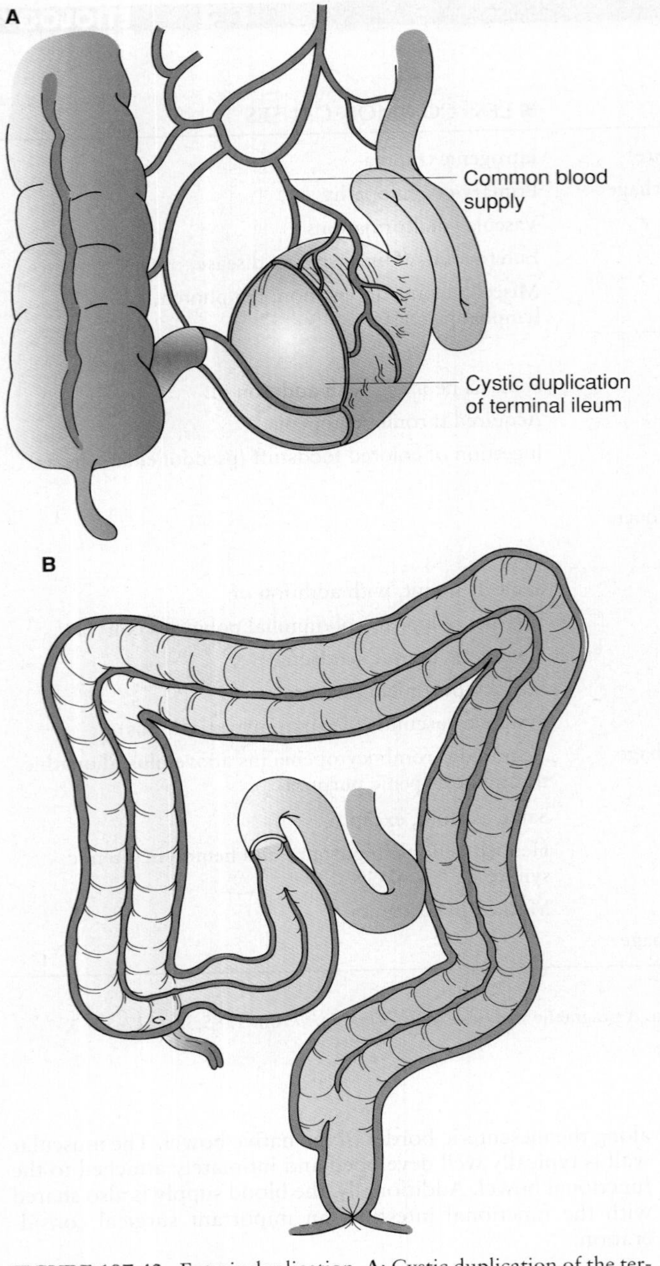

FIGURE 107.43. Enteric duplication. **A:** Cystic duplication of the terminal ileum. **B:** Tubular duplication of the terminal ileum and colon.

contrast, duplication cysts of the small intestine usually require segmental resection and primary anastomosis, given the intimate attachment and shared blood supply with the native bowel. For large cystic duplications involving longer segments of native bowel, individualized treatment strategies are required. One option is cyst marsupialization with resection of the duplication cyst wall with preservation of the common blood supply and wall between the cyst and native bowel. This technique is combined with submucosal dissection and stripping of the remaining epithelium from the cyst wall. Another approach is internal drainage of the cyst into the adjacent native intestine, for example, creation of a cystoduodenostomy for duodenal duplication not amenable to local resection and anastomosis; this would be distinctly unusual.

Tubular Duplications. Tubular duplications may be found anywhere along the length of the gastrointestinal tract. They are less frequent than cystic duplications and have a tendency to involve the ileum and the colon. It is believed that tubular duplication generally reflects abnormal, disordered recanalization of the gastrointestinal tract. Similar to cystic duplications, tubular lesions share a common wall and blood supply with the native bowel. Communication between the tubular duplication and native bowel lumen is common. Tubular duplications may be extensive and can involve the entire length of terminal ileum and colon. Malformations of the entire colon and rectum are associated with genitourinary anomalies, particularly duplications of the external genitalia or bladder.

Tubular duplications manifest clinically in similar fashion to cystic lesions. Symptomatic lesions most commonly present with gastrointestinal bleeding or obstruction. Treatment is operative, and an individualized strategy is required that is based on the location and nature of the duplication. Resection with primary anastomosis may require removal of an unacceptable length of normal bowel. Marsupialization with submucosal stripping of the duplication epithelium may be particularly helpful if ectopic gastric mucosa is suspected or found. Obstruction from a long, blind-ending parallel duplication that communicates with the functional gut lumen can be treated effectively with a reentry procedure such as a distal enteroenterostomy. This approach avoids a potentially complex resection of a significant length of bowel.

The outcomes of surgical management of enteric duplications are generally excellent in the absence of other associated anomalies or medical problems. Mortality attributable to the duplication itself is unusual. Postoperative morbidity is generally dependent on the nature and location of the duplication.

Mesenteric and Omental Cysts

Mesenteric and omental cysts are rare lesions thought to result from the sequestration of lymphatic tissue during development. Mesenteric cysts are twice as common as omental cysts. Both are characterized by thin, often incomplete walls lined with endothelial cells absent of surrounding smooth muscle. They may be filled with either serous lymphatic fluid or chyle and may be unilocular or multilocular. These cysts may become extraordinarily large before producing symptoms.

Most infants and children with mesenteric or omental cysts are diagnosed prior to adolescence. Asymptomatic children are usually diagnosed incidentally during studies for other reasons. Symptomatic children present with abdominal pain, and, on examination, a soft, mobile abdominal mass is characteristic. Bleeding, rupture, obstruction, torsion, or cyst infection may be observed. Most of these lesions can be diagnosed by ultrasound or CT scan imaging. Ascites, duplication cysts, pancreatic pseudocysts, and large ovarian cysts may have a similar appearance on diagnostic imaging. Peripheral calcification and evidence of recent hemorrhage may be seen in mesenteric or omental cysts (Fig. 107.44).

The treatment for these lesions is simple excision. Total excision of mesenteric or omental cysts is generally preferable over partial excision with marsupialization. Limited resection with primary anastomosis may be required for a mesenteric cyst located adjacent to the intestinal wall, particularly if there is concern that the cyst actually may be an enteric duplication. Morbidity and mortality are generally limited to concurrent problems associated with the intestine. In particular, volvulus of a mesenteric cyst may cause vascular compromise and infarction of the adjacent intestine.

Primary Peritonitis

Bacterial peritonitis without a specific, identifiable cause is referred to as *primary peritonitis*. Spontaneous bacterial peritonitis in children with ascites or nephrosis is generally

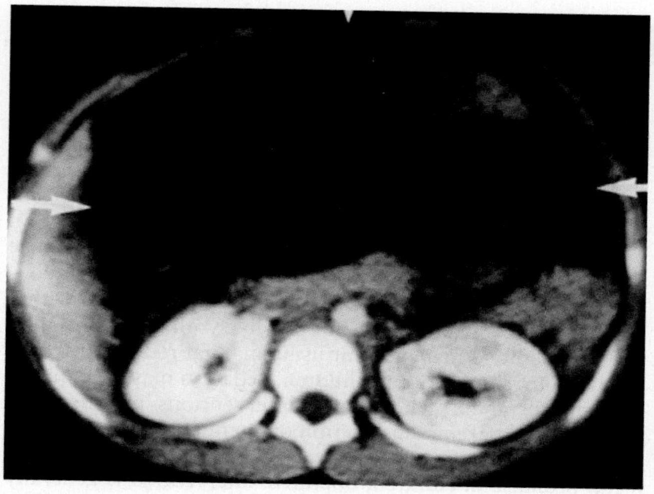

FIGURE 107.44. Computed tomography scan image from a child after abdominal trauma. Hemorrhage into large omental cyst is apparent (*arrows*).

included in this group. Hematogenous seeding of ascitic fluid is probably responsible for the development of spontaneous bacterial peritonitis. The infecting bacterial organisms were classically gram-positive with various staphylococcal, streptococcal, and other species accounting for most cases. In a series of infants and children with primary peritonitis, more than two thirds of the cases were caused by gram-negative organisms such as *Escherichia coli*.[136] This trend may reflect the use of antibiotic prophylaxis directed against gram-positive organisms.

The other etiologic mechanism for the development of primary peritonitis is believed to involve retrograde inoculation of the peritoneal cavity via the genitourinary tract. This etiology is characteristic of prepubertal girls 5 to 10 years of age, accounting for as many as half of the cases of primary peritonitis. The initial signs and symptoms in these children are virtually identical to children with perforated appendicitis: fever, emesis, abdominal pain, and tenderness on examination. Leukocytosis is characteristic, and an ileus is observed on plain abdominal films. On exploration, these children have inflammatory peritonitis without an identifiable enteric cause. Gram-negative enteric organisms are commonly cultured from the peritoneal fluid.

Infants and children with peritonitis in association with an indwelling peritoneal dialysis catheter or ventriculoperitoneal shunt may be treated successfully with intravenous broad-spectrum antibiotics. The catheter or shunt should be removed or exteriorized promptly if peritonitis does not resolve within 24 to 48 hours.[137] In association with ascites or nephrosis, diagnostic paracentesis should be performed and the peritoneal fluid examined by Gram stain and culture. If there is any diagnostic uncertainty, laparoscopic or open operative exploration may be required to exclude intestinal perforation as a cause of peritonitis. If the appendix is normal, peritoneal cultures should be obtained and a thorough, complete abdominal exploration for other causes should be performed. Appendectomy is generally performed when the diagnosis of primary peritonitis is established by a right lower-quadrant incision. Other than perforated appendicitis, distinct causes of intestinal perforation or peritonitis in this age group include perforated Meckel diverticulum, duodenal ulcer, and acute pancreatitis. About half of the peritoneal fluid cultures are positive for a single organism. Treatment with specific antibiotics is continued until the patient is afebrile with a normal white blood cell count and normal clinical examination. Following operative exploration in primary peritonitis, the morbidity is no different than that for appendectomy, and the recovery is generally uneventful.

TABLE 107.10 **ETIOLOGY**

COMMON CAUSES OF NEONATAL ASCITES

Maternal-fetal Rh incompatibility (rare)
Structural malformations
Urinary obstruction
Congenital heart disease
Malrotation, duplications, cyst (associated with intestinal volvulus)
Biliary perforation
Ovarian ascites
Pulmonary abnormalities
Chylous ascites
Hematologic disorders
α-Thalassemia
Infection
Toxoplasmosis
Cytomegalovirus
Others
α_1-Antitrypsin deficiency
Idiopathic

Ascites

The common causes of neonatal and childhood ascites are listed in Tables 107.10 and 107.11. The clinical presentation is that of abdominal distention with bulging flanks and demonstrable fluid on palpation and percussion. Ultrasound or CT scan imaging may be useful to confirm the clinical diagnosis. Paracentesis and routine examination of the fluid for Gram stain, cell count, cytology, protein, chemistries, and culture should be performed. Chylous ascites is characterized by a white milky appearance, high lymphocyte count, and high triglyceride content. Bile-stained fluid in the absence of demonstrable bowel perforation is characteristic of biliary ascites. High fluid amylase content is seen in pancreatic ascites, and a low protein count (<3 g/dL) is consistent with serous ascites. Elevated urea nitrogen or creatinine in the fluid may suggest urinary ascites, particularly in a male patient. Cytology should be performed to exclude peritoneal ascites secondary to malignancy, particularly in pubertal and adolescent females.

If the initial fluid does not provide a diagnosis in an otherwise normal-appearing child, a comprehensive diagnostic imaging evaluation is warranted. An echocardiogram should be performed and either ultrasound or CT scan imaging performed to evaluate the genitourinary system, the hepatobiliary system, and the pancreas. A voiding cystourethrogram may also be indicated.

Treatment of neonatal or childhood ascites depends on the establishment of a specific diagnosis. In the absence of anatomic lesion or injury, spontaneous resolution of chylous ascites occurs in 50% to 75% of cases with the temporary cessation of enteral feeding and administration of parenteral nutrition. Persistence of chylous ascites for longer than 4 to 6 weeks is an indication for operative attempts to ligate the cisterna chyli. Neonatal biliary ascites may result from spontaneous bile duct perforation, in which case a diagnosis of CF must be considered. Transient bile duct obstruction typically leads to perforation at the junction of the cystic duct with the common duct. Simple external drainage is the treatment of choice, and complex hepatobiliary tract reconstruction in this setting is unnecessary and potentially hazardous. Urinary ascites in a male patient requires

TABLE 107.11 **ETIOLOGY**

COMMON CAUSES OF CHILDHOOD ASCITES

SEROUS ASCITES
Cirrhosis
Budd-Chiari syndrome
Nephrosis
Right-sided heart failure
Postoperative ascites (after renal transplantation, peritoneal dialysis, ventriculoperitoneal shunt)
α_1-Antitrypsin deficiency
Other rare metabolic disorders
CHYLOUS ASCITES
Malrotation with volvulus
Small bowel obstruction
Incarcerated hernia
Lymphangioma
Trauma (includes operative trauma)
BILIARY ASCITES
Neonatal bile duct perforation
Cystic fibrosis
Biliary atresia
Hepatitis
Cytomegalovirus infection
URINARY ASCITES (7:1 MALE PREDOMINANCE)
Urinary obstruction
Posterior urethral valves
Bladder perforation
Ureterocele
Neurogenic bladder
PANCREATIC ASCITES
Acute pancreatitis (drugs, trauma, gallstones, infection)
Pancreatic pseudocysts
OVARIAN ASCITES
Cysts (torsion, rupture)
Tumors
MALIGNANT ASCITES
Intra-abdominal neoplasm
IDIOPATHIC

a workup that includes a voiding cystourethrogram to exclude posterior urethral valves. Urinary ascites resolves with treatment of obstructive uropathy. Pancreatic ascites is typically self-limited, and treatment by drainage procedures is generally not required or limited for relief of persistent symptoms.

Massive neonatal ascites may cause hypoventilation secondary to impairment of diaphragmatic excursion, and therapeutic paracentesis may be required. Childhood ascites generally responds to adequate treatment of the underlying problem and occasionally requires medical therapy. Placement of a peritoneovenous shunt in children for intractable ascites is rare.

Rectal Prolapse

Spontaneous rectal prolapse is relatively common in toddlers and children up to 5 years of age. A peak incidence occurs at or near the time of toilet training. There is an association between straining during bowel movement and rectal prolapse; it may be more commonly observed in children with CF, myelodysplasias with sacral neuropathy, congenital anorectal malformations, Hirschsprung disease, and colorectal polyps. However, most children presenting with rectal prolapse are normal.

A history of protrusion of mucosa or full-thickness rectum with or without bleeding is usually described. Other lesions of childhood that have a similar appearance are prolapse of an intussusceptum or passage of a polyp through the anus. The rectal examination is diagnostic. If the protruding intestine is an intussusceptum, a finger can be placed adjacent to it within the rectum; this maneuver is not possible with rectal prolapse.

Nonoperative management using manual reduction is successful in most infants and children. Sedation may be required in some instances. Therapeutic interventions include stool softeners and parental instruction on manual reduction. Spontaneous resolution over a few weeks is typical. For persistent rectal prolapse in children, operative intervention is generally governed by doing the least invasive procedure possible. Unlike in adults, complex operations involving bowel resection and pelvic suspension are generally unnecessary in children with rectal prolapse. The most useful and commonly used procedure is rectal submucosal injection using a sclerosant (Fig. 107.45). With the patient under general anesthesia, injection with 5% sodium morrhuate or cow's milk[138] has been performed successfully on an outpatient basis. About 90% of children can be treated successfully with a single four-quadrant sclerosant technique, but on occasion further sclerosis is necessary. Submucosal dissection or cauterization is also successful but may have a higher incidence of postoperative bleeding or stricture formation and usually requires a short period of hospitalization. The major objective in treating childhood rectal prolapse is to create a local extraperitoneal inflammatory process in the perirectal space. Morbidity is low and the long-term outcome is excellent.

PEDIATRIC LIVER

Tumors of the Liver

Primary hepatic tumors are rare in children, and at least 60% to 70% are malignant.[139,140] Table 107.12 reviews the incidence rates and types of hepatic tumors presenting during infancy and childhood. Pediatric hepatic tumors often manifest as asymptomatic abdominal masses discovered by parents or pediatricians. Symptoms related to the tumor, such as pain, hemorrhage, hypertension, and precocious puberty, are less frequent. Initial diagnostic imaging studies include plain abdominal radiographs and ultrasound to assist in early determination as to whether the mass is cystic or solid and whether calcifications are present. CT scan imaging and MRI remain definitive in the ability to discern anatomic characteristics of the mass and its relationship to adjacent structures. Most children require operative exploration for either definitive excision or for incisional biopsy in lesions deemed unresectable.

Benign Tumors. Of all primary liver tumors of childhood, 30% are benign. The most common benign tumors are hemangiomas, hemangioendotheliomas, mesenchymal hamartomas, cysts, focal nodular hyperplasia, and hepatic adenoma. In most large series, hemangiomas constitute about 50% of the benign hepatic tumors observed.[141]

Vascular Tumors. Infantile hepatic hemangiomas represent a clinically diverse spectrum of vascular endothelial anomalies. They are characterized by a phase of proliferative growth over the first year of life, with subsequent involution over several years. The International Society for the Study of Vascular Anomalies classifies vascular tumors into two categories based

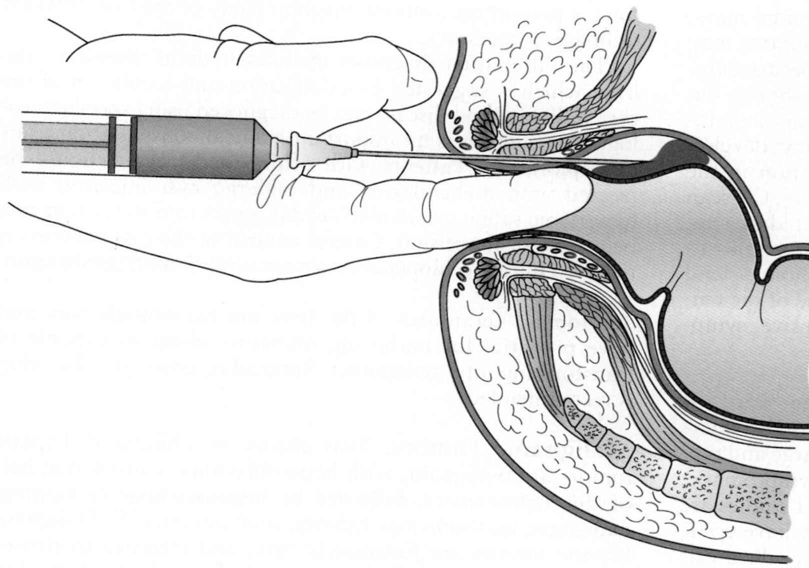

FIGURE 107.45. Four-quadrant injection of sclerosant into the rectal submucosa for the treatment of childhood rectal prolapse.

on the presence or absence of GLUT-1, an erythrocyte-type glucose transporter protein expressed in the endothelium of the placenta and hemangiomas.[142] Therefore, hemangiomas are GLUT-1 positive, and other, more heterogeneous vascular anomalies such as vascular malformations are GLUT-1 negative. Most asymptomatic infantile hepatic hemangiomas are detected as incidental findings on diagnostic imaging studies performed for unrelated reasons. A smaller proportion will create symptoms of enlarging abdominal mass, progressive hepatic failure, high-output cardiac failure due to shunting, thrombocytopenia, or hypothyroidism from excess production of type III iodothyronine deiodinase.[143]

Most benign vascular lesions of the pediatric liver do not require operative management. Operative intervention is generally reserved for bleeding secondary to traumatic rupture symptoms not controllable with medical management. Treatment strategies remain highly individualized based on whether the lesions are focal, multifocal, or diffuse.[144] In the face of multifocal or diffuse disease associated with congestive heart failure and thrombocytopenia secondary to sequestration, medical treatment with corticosteroid therapy may be useful. More invasive procedures such as irradiation, selective hepatic arterial ligation, angiographic embolization, or hepatic transplantation remain useful in selected patients with uncontrollable symptoms. Chemotherapeutic agents, including recombinant alpha-interferon, low-dose vincristine, and cyclophosphamide have been used for life-threatening vascular lesions. Hepatic resection is generally reserved for mass lesions of unknown diagnosis, ruptured vascular lesions with signs of active hemorrhage, or for symptomatic, locally resectable lesions.

Hemangioendotheliomas are important vascular anomalies encountered in infants. The lesions vary in size from 1 cm to several cm in diameter and may be multiple (Fig. 107.46).

TABLE 107.12

INCIDENCE OF LIVER TUMORS IN CHILDHOOD

■ TUMOR TYPE	■ INCIDENCE RATE (%)
BENIGN	
Vascular tumors	13
Hemangioma	9
Hemangioendothelioma	4
Mesenchymal hamartoma	6
Focal nodular hyperplasia	2
Adenoma	2
Teratoma	2
Other	3
MALIGNANT	
Hepatoblastoma	43
Hepatocellular carcinoma	23
Malignant mesenchymal tumor	4
Sarcoma	2
Embryonal cell carcinoma	2
Angiosarcoma	1

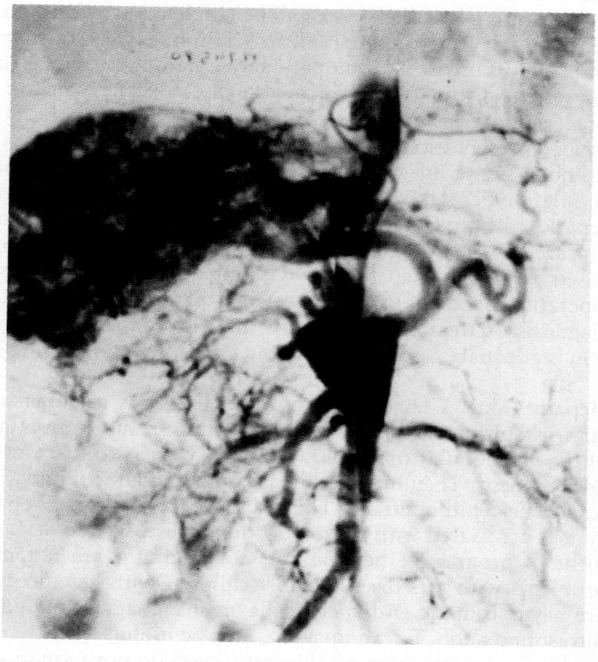

FIGURE 107.46. Selective visceral angiogram demonstrating large hepatic vascular malformation in a neonate with congestive heart failure. This finding is consistent with a bilobar hemangioendothelioma.

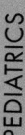

Symptomatic neonates may present with an abdominal mass, hepatomegaly, and congestive heart failure. These infants may also experience spontaneous rupture and hemoperitoneum, with tachycardia, tachypnea, and hypovolemic shock. On examination, the infant may have other cutaneous hemangiomas visible on the skin. Affected infants may develop thrombocytopenia secondary to platelet sequestration in the vascular malformation (*Kasabach-Merritt syndrome*). CT scan imaging or MRI is diagnostic. Treatment is directed at controlling symptoms using medical management principles as discussed previously; however, hemangioendotheliomas tend to be more problematic than hemangiomas because of the tendency to occur during infancy and the more extensive, symptomatic nature of the lesions.

Mesenchymal Hamartomas. Approximately one third of benign hepatic tumors in children are mesenchymal hamartomas. A mesenchymal hamartoma is often quite large and typically presents within the first year of life as an asymptomatic, solitary abdominal mass. CT scan imaging or MRI studies are usually diagnostic and show a solid mass that may have cystic components within the liver parenchyma. Definitive diagnosis may require open tissue biopsy, and the therapy of choice is complete excision, although spontaneous involution has been described. Simple enucleation may be adequate because these tumors tend to be well circumscribed. On occasion, formal hepatic resection may be required.[145] Recurrence is low after adequate resection.

Focal Nodular Hyperplasia. This tumor occurs primarily in female children and in adults and may be associated with the use of oral contraceptives or focal hepatic injury. Focal nodular hyperplasia is usually a well-defined, solitary mass that has characteristic findings on CT scan imaging. Open or percutaneous biopsy may be required to differentiate the lesion from hepatic adenoma. This lesion results from a focal inflammatory response of normal hepatic parenchyma surrounded by areas of micronodular fibrosis and cirrhosis. Operative management is generally unnecessary unless there is a question of diagnosis or active hemorrhage from the lesion.

Hepatic Adenoma. Adenomas are rare in infants and children and constitute less than 5% of all benign hepatic lesions in the pediatric age group. There is an association between the use of oral contraceptives, exogenous anabolic steroid use, and glycogen storage disease type I (von Gierke disease). These tend to be large, solitary lesions located in the right hepatic lobe. The typical presentation is an asymptomatic abdominal mass, although symptoms are seen more commonly than with focal nodular hyperplasia. About 20% to 25% of patients with hepatic adenoma present with hemoperitoneum from tumor rupture. On histologic examination, these lesions are composed of normal hepatocytes without evidence of dysplasia. Operative therapy is usually directed at either making definitive diagnosis or treating hemorrhage. Enucleation or local resection is adequate, and recurrence rates are low.

Hepatic Cysts. Congenital cysts of the liver may be either solitary or multiple. These cysts are thought to result from failure of the intralobular or interlobular biliary ducts to fuse during development. They may be lined with cuboidal, columnar, or squamous epithelium.[146] The presence of multiple hepatic cysts is associated with polycystic kidney disease, and development of progressive hepatic and renal failures are potential problems with this disease. Most children with hepatic cysts are asymptomatic. Adjunctive diagnostic imaging, including ultrasound and CT scan imaging, may be useful.

Asymptomatic congenital hepatic cysts do not require surgical therapy. Operative therapy is reserved for symptomatic cysts. Resection or drainage by marsupialization or hepaticocystoenterostomy may be required. If patency to the biliary tract is present on contrast injection study of the cyst, internal drainage is necessary.

The differential diagnosis includes hydatid disease of the liver, which is suggested by calcification and loculation of the cyst wall. Hydatid disease can be diagnosed using specific serologic tests, which is an important surgical consideration prior to exploration. Patients with echinococcal cysts should be treated with mebendazole and undergo cyst injection with hypertonic saline or other scolicidal agents into the parent cyst before surgical excision. Careful control of the cyst contents is required during echinococcal cyst excision or marsupialization.

Teratomas. Teratomas of the liver are exceedingly rare and have potential for harboring immature elements capable of transforming into malignancy. Surgical resection on discovery is recommended.

Malignant Tumors. Two thirds of childhood hepatic tumors are malignant, with hepatoblastoma constituting half of the malignancies, followed by hepatocellular carcinoma, malignant mesenchymal tumors, and sarcoma.[139] Malignant hepatic tumors are fortunately rare, and effective treatment requires a multidisciplinary approach that is best achieved in an experienced pediatric center.

Hepatoblastoma. Most hepatoblastomas are discovered in children younger than 2 years of age. There is a 2:1 male-to-female predominance. Hepatoblastomas usually are found as either an asymptomatic abdominal mass or symptoms of gastrointestinal obstruction from extrinsic compression by the mass. There is an association of hepatoblastoma in patients with Beckwith-Wiedemann syndrome and hemihypertrophy. On examination, a firm, palpable upper abdominal mass is notable. Obstructive jaundice is unusual. More than 90% of children with hepatoblastoma have elevated levels of alphafetoprotein, which is a useful serum tumor marker for postoperative surveillance. In a few instances, children have initial symptoms and signs of excess androgen secretion, including virilization and precocious puberty. Diagnostic imaging with CT scan imaging or MRI is essential to evaluate the extent of the tumor and evaluate for metastatic disease (Fig. 107.47).

Most children presenting with hepatoblastoma initially have unresectable disease. In the absence of metastatic disease, however, an aggressive surgical approach is used. Cure and long-term survival with hepatoblastoma requires complete surgical excision of the primary lesion. Therefore, localized, resectable tumors usually are excised by formal hepatic lobectomy or extended trisegmentectomy. Children with hepatoblastomas considered initially unresectable or with metastatic

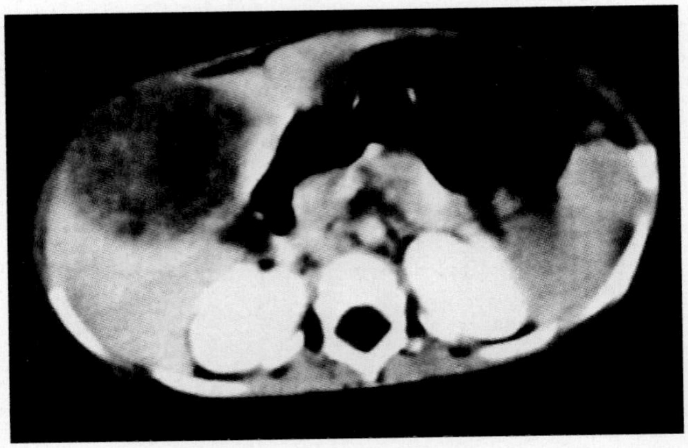

FIGURE 107.47. Computed tomography scan of the abdomen demonstrating an infant with hepatoblastoma of the right hepatic lobe.

disease should undergo percutaneous or incisional biopsy to confirm the histologic diagnosis, followed by multiagent chemotherapy to reduce the size of the primary tumor and control metastases.[147,148] Delayed resection is appropriate if enough functional, normal hepatic parenchyma remain after resection. More than half of the patients who initially have unresectable hepatoblastoma can be rendered disease-free with the combination of chemotherapy and subsequent surgery. Cure rates for hepatoblastoma range from 60% to 80% if histologically clear margins and no metastatic disease are present. All patients with hepatoblastoma, regardless of stage, receive chemotherapy after resection. Unfortunately, cure cannot be expected in children treated with chemotherapy and radiation therapy alone without complete surgical resection.

Hepatocellular Carcinoma. Hepatocellular carcinoma is significantly more common in adults but is occasionally seen in older children and adolescents. There is a male predilection (2:1), and except for the age at diagnosis, the clinical presentation is similar to that for hepatoblastoma. Children with hepatocellular carcinoma are more likely to have jaundice and abnormal liver enzymes. The high association of cirrhosis in adults (80%) is not seen in children with hepatocellular carcinoma; only 5% of children develop hepatocellular carcinoma in the background of cirrhosis. An increased risk of hepatocellular carcinoma is seen in children with Beckwith-Wiedemann syndrome, hemihypertrophy, von Gierke disease, hepatitis B, and Fanconi syndrome. Exposure to oral contraceptives, anabolic steroids, and some chemotherapeutic agents also has been associated with hepatocellular carcinoma. This malignancy carries a poor prognosis with an overall survival rate of 10% to 20% despite aggressive surgical resection and multiagent chemotherapy. A histologic variant, fibrolamellar hepatocellular carcinoma, carries a more favorable prognosis. As with hepatoblastoma, complete surgical resection with clear histologic margins is necessary for long-term survival and cure. In the absence of metastatic disease, unresectable hepatoblastoma or hepatocellular carcinoma in children has been successfully treated by orthotopic liver transplantation. A review of data from the United Network for Organ Sharing database demonstrates good long-term survival for both hepatoblastoma (66% 10-year survival) and hepatocellular carcinoma (58% 10-year survival) treated with liver transplantation.[149]

Malignant Mesenchymal Tumors. These rare hepatic malignancies occur in children 5 to 10 years of age; initial signs are fever, pain, and an abdominal mass, which is usually quite large on diagnosis and may have both solid and cystic components. Multidisciplinary treatment, including complete surgical resection, multiagent chemotherapy, and radiation therapy is required for cure. In general, the prognosis of primary malignant mesenchymal tumors of the liver remains poor.

Sarcomas. Children may rarely have a primary sarcoma of the liver. Embryonal rhabdomyosarcoma of the biliary tract is distinctly unusual. It may manifest with obstructive jaundice attributable to both extrinsic and intrinsic biliary tract obstruction. Undifferentiated, embryonal sarcoma of the liver has also been described. Angiosarcoma developing in the liver may be associated with exposure to toxins such as arsenic. Aggressive surgical resection may be required, but long-term survival is uncommon. Despite radical surgery, chemotherapy, and radiation therapy, the prognosis and long-term survival of children with these malignancies remains poor, and data regarding effective drug regimens are limited.[150,151]

Liver Resection

Operative principles and techniques for hepatic resection are discussed elsewhere in this book. Several unique issues in the safe performance of hepatic resection in children should be emphasized.[152] Contemporary management of hepatic resection for tumors in children requires adequate preoperative assessment and the liberal use of intraoperative monitoring techniques. The circulating blood volume of an infant or child is small compared to that of an adult, and children are sensitive to compression of the inferior vena cava causing decreased venous return to the right heart. Blood must be available for transfusion, and adequate intravenous access is essential. Resection can be performed through either a subcostal or a right thoracoabdominal incision; in general, the ability to perform the operation safely should not be limited by the size of the incision. In children, the right and left hepatic veins are difficult to control near the inferior vena cava because of their short lengths, and intraparenchymal control from an anterior approach may be safer (Fig. 107.48). Resection may be performed using total hepatic vascular isolation by

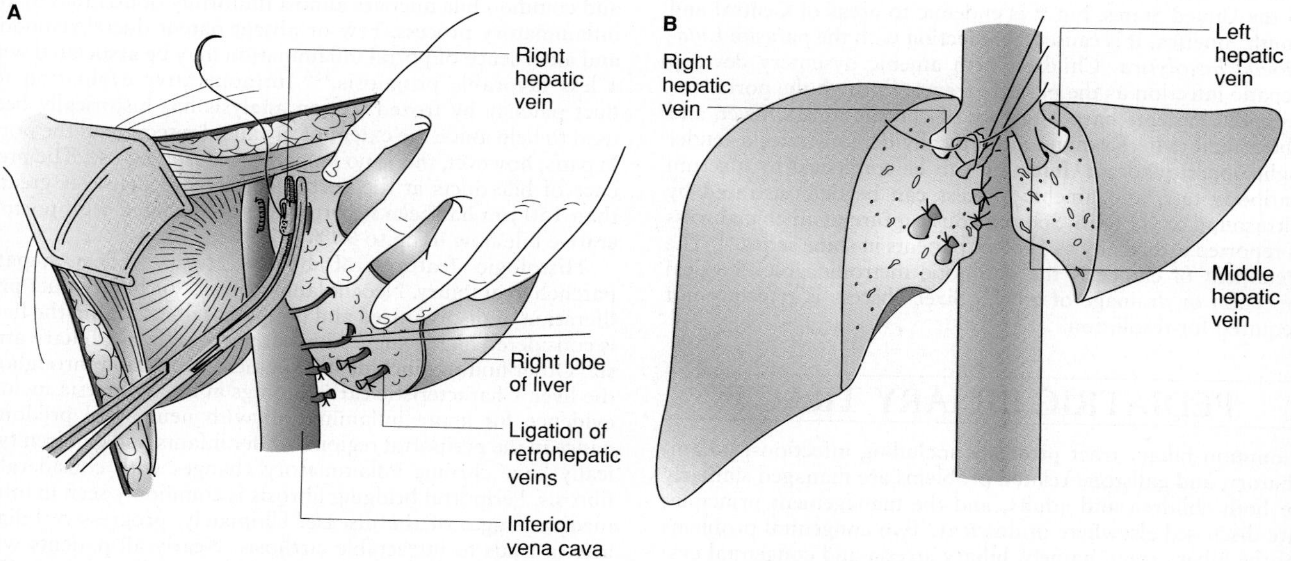

FIGURE 107.48. A: The hepatic veins in infants and children may be extremely short, making extrahepatic control impossible or dangerous. **B:** Intrahepatic control of the hepatic veins via an anterior approach may be safer in infants and children.

controlling the hepatic and portal inflow, the suprahepatic inferior vena cava, and the suprarenal inferior vena cava caudal to the liver. When extrahepatic biliary duct reconstruction is required, T-tube drainage is not routinely performed given the small diameter of the ducts in most children.

Hepatic Infections

Hepatic infections are generally rare in the pediatric population, and their management is similar to that used in adults. An important issue is the development of hepatic abscess in an immunocompromised child, and in particular, the association of chronic granulomatous disease with pyogenic hepatic abscess formation.

Pyogenic Abscess. The most common cause of pyogenic liver abscess before the advent of antibiotic therapy was perforated appendicitis. Now the most common causative factor in the development of pyogenic hepatic abscess in children with chronic granulomatous disease and other causes of immunosuppression.[153] Chronic granulomatous disease is an inherited disorder characterized by a defect in oxidative burst-mediated bacterial killing by neutrophils. These children develop skin, soft tissue, and solid organ abscesses. A significant number of children with pyogenic liver abscesses have chronic granulomatous disease or other inherited/acquired immunodeficiency states. Liver abscesses are infrequently seen as a complication of umbilical vein catheterization, omphalitis, biliary tract disease, and hepatobiliary operations.

Patients with pyogenic liver abscess present with fever, jaundice, and leukocytosis. Hepatosplenomegaly and a tender liver may be found on physical examination. Diagnostic imaging with ultrasound, CT scan imaging, or MRI is useful. Common responsible organisms include staphylococcal species, streptococcal species, and *E. coli*. Gram-negative organisms and anaerobic bacteria are becoming increasingly prevalent. Treatment involves the use of broad-spectrum antibiotics. Large abscess cavities may require image-guided percutaneous drainage to expedite resolution of sepsis. Currently, few hepatic abscesses require open operative drainage. The outcome is dependent on the underlying disease process. Recovery from the abscess is predictably good following adequate antibiotic therapy and drainage when necessary.

Amebic Abscess. Amebic abscess of the liver is uncommon in the United States, but it is endemic to areas of Central and South America. It is caused by infection with the parasite *Entamoeba histolytica*. Children with amebic dysentery develop hepatic infection as the parasite travels through the portal circulation. Patients have a history of chronic illness, fever, and abdominal pain. Examination typically demonstrates a tender right upper quadrant. Infection can be confirmed by a serum antibody test, and amebic abscess can be demonstrated by ultrasound or CT scan. Spontaneous rupture of amebic abscess is reported in as many as 10% of patients in some series.[154] The treatment of choice is the antibiotic metronidazole. Surgical resection or drainage of amebic liver abscess is typically not required for resolution.

PEDIATRIC BILIARY TRACT

Common biliary tract problems including infectious, inflammatory, and gallstone-related problems are managed similarly in both children and adults, and the management principles are discussed elsewhere in this text. Two congenital problems of the biliary tract, namely, biliary atresia and congenital cystic disease of the biliary tract (choledochal cyst), are somewhat unique to infants and children in presentation and management and are reviewed in the following discussion.

Embryology

The fetal liver and biliary tract develop between weeks 4 and 10 of gestation, representing the fusion of an endodermal foregut diverticulum with a mesodermal component from the septum transversum. The hepatocytes are derived from cords of endodermal cells in the hepatic diverticulum and ultimately give rise to the hepatic sinusoidal endothelium. The proximal hepatic diverticulum gives rise to the extrahepatic biliary tract, including the gallbladder, cystic duct, and common bile duct. As the intrahepatic and extrahepatic ductal systems develop, they unite to form a connected, arborizing system of cords composed of primitive ductular epithelial cells. These epithelial cells assume tubular configuration with ductal patency established between weeks 6 and 12 of gestation. Bile flow from the hepatocytes and into the biliary duct system is apparent by the beginning of the second fetal trimester.

This embryologic sequence appears to take place normally in infants who develop biliary atresia. In fact, the term *biliary atresia* does not reflect embryologic atresia resulting from failure of recanalization of the biliary tree. Rather, biliary atresia is caused by an uncontrollable inflammatory process that produces progressive obliteration of the normally developed extrahepatic biliary tract.

Biliary Atresia

7 **Anatomy.** The overall incidence rate of biliary atresia is about 1 in 8,000 to 12,000 live births and is the most common cause of chronic cholestasis in infants and children as well as the most frequent indication for pediatric liver transplantation.[155] Extrahepatic biliary atresia must be differentiated from biliary hypoplasia. Biliary hypoplasia describes a diminutive but patent biliary system and can result from many underlying situations such as neonatal hepatitis and alpha$_1$-antitrypsin deficiency. Biliary hypoplasia involves both intrahepatic and extrahepatic ductal systems.

Microscopic Anatomy. Biliary atresia is characterized by replacement of the extrahepatic biliary tract with dense, fibrous inflammatory tissue. In most cases, complete obliteration of the extrahepatic biliary tract, including the gallbladder, occurs. There appears to be gradual progression of the inflammatory process with advancing age. The common hepatic duct and common bile duct are almost uniformly obliterated by the inflammatory process. Few or absent patent ductal remnants and an absence of portal inflammation may be associated with a less favorable prognosis.[156] Intraoperative evaluation for duct patency by frozen section analysis has historically been used to help guide the extent of proximal resection at the porta hepatis; however, this is no longer in widespread use. The presence of bile ducts at the porta hepatis with diameter greater than 150 μm has been reported to be associated with postoperative bile flow in up to 90% to 95% of cases.[157]

Histologic features of biliary atresia reflect hepatic parenchymal injury. Neocholangiogenesis, or biliary duct proliferation of disorganized and nonpatent ducts within the liver, is considered highly suggestive but not specific for biliary atresia. Other findings include bile pigment deposition throughout the liver. Characteristic early findings in biliary atresia include evidence for acute inflammation with neutrophil predominance in the periportal regions. Older infants and children typically have chronic inflammatory changes with considerable fibrosis. Periportal bridging fibrosis is commonly seen in intermediate stages of the disease. Ultimately, progressive biliary atresia leads to intractable cirrhosis. Nearly all patients with biliary atresia have histologic evidence of liver injury. The severity and extent of liver damage may be the most important predictor of long-term outcome and survival in biliary atresia.

Pathophysiology. Despite numerous investigations, the mechanism causing biliary atresia remains unknown. The current, widely accepted concept is that the normally developed biliary tract undergoes inflammatory sclerosis and subsequent obliteration. This process appears to occur during the first few weeks to months of life. Infants who develop biliary atresia are rarely jaundiced at birth, and biliary atresia is either rare or nonexistent in fetal autopsy studies. Clinical data are consistent with the fact that biliary atresia appears to be a progressive, dynamic inflammatory response that is acquired during the perinatal period and targets the extrahepatic biliary tract. Early establishment of biliary drainage via portoenterostomy within the first 2 to 4 months of age may be associated with reversal of liver injury and subsequent long-term survival. Conversely, infants operated on after 120 days of life typically have obliterated bile ducts. Neonatal biliary atresia shares some clinical and morphologic features of sclerosing cholangitis in adults. Data supporting an infectious etiologic agent, and in particular reoviruses, rotaviruses, and hepatitis C, have been reported and may play a role in some cases. Additionally, other noninfectious stimuli may trigger an inflammatory response directed at the neonatal extrahepatic bile duct.[158] The actual mechanism may reflect a stereotypical inflammatory response initiated by various different stimuli that is ultimately directed preferentially against the neonatal bile duct.

Clinical Presentation and Diagnosis. The cardinal sign of biliary atresia is progressive neonatal jaundice during the first few weeks of life. Dark urine and acholic stools are expected findings. Progressive hyperbilirubinemia produces clinical jaundice around 2 to 4 weeks of age. The physical examination is generally unremarkable except for jaundice and possibly mild hepatomegaly. Alagille syndrome, which presents with neonatal jaundice, can usually be distinguished from biliary atresia on physical examination. Children with Alagille syndrome have biliary hypoplasia and distinctly abnormal facies, growth retardation, vertebral defects, and pulmonic stenosis.

A characteristic laboratory finding is conjugated hyperbilirubinemia consistent with obstructive jaundice. A direct fraction of bilirubin greater than 50%, or greater than 2 mg/dL in an infant, requires prompt investigation. Mild elevation of hepatic transaminases is commonly seen. The alkaline phosphatase is significantly elevated, often in the range of 500 to 1,000 IU/L. There are no specific biochemical markers for biliary atresia, as these serum profiles can be seen in other causes of neonatal cholestasis. Late findings in biliary atresia include failure to thrive, feeding intolerance, stigmata of portal hypertension, and fat-soluble vitamin deficiency.

Table 107.13 is a partial list of the causes of neonatal cholestatic syndromes. Neonatal physiologic jaundice is commonly encountered. This condition is self-limited once the glucuronyl transferase system matures, allowing the hepatocytes to conjugate bilirubin efficiently. Because of the numerous causes of neonatal jaundice and the relative infrequency of biliary atresia, a delay in diagnosis is common. Given the age-sensitive nature of biliary atresia and the improved outcome in younger infants, the diagnostic workup should be expedient.

TABLE 107.13 ETIOLOGY

CAUSES AND ASSOCIATIONS OF NEONATAL CHOLESTASIS

CONGENITAL INFECTIOUS CAUSES
Cytomegalovirus[a]
Rubella virus[a]
Herpes virus
Hepatitis virus B[a]
Echovirus 14, 19
Coxsackievirus B
Toxoplasmosis
Syphilis
GENETIC ASSOCIATIONS
Galactosemia
Tyrosinemia
Congenital fructose intolerance
$alpha_1$-Antitrypsin deficiency
Cystic fibrosis
Niemann-Pick disease
Trisomy 17, 18, 21
Turner syndrome
Menkes syndrome
Zellweger syndrome
Polysplenia syndrome[b]
MISCELLANEOUS ASSOCIATIONS
Hemolytic disease
Bacterial sepsis
Pyelonephritis
Total parenteral nutrition (prolonged)
Congestive heart failure
Hypoplastic left heart syndrome
Necrotizing enterocolitis, gastroschisis, omphalocele
Neonatal hypopituitarism
Inspissated bile syndrome (without hemolysis), neonatal shock, respiratory distress syndrome, acidosis

[a]Rarely associated with biliary atresia.
[b]Frequently associated with biliary atresia.

Radioisotope Scanning. Technetium 99m–iminodiacetic acid (^{99m}Tc-IDA) analogues are widely used for hepatobiliary imaging and provide the basis for a sensitive and specific test for biliary atresia. The sensitivity of this diagnostic examination for biliary atresia can be 100% with a specificity of 94%.[159] To improve sensitivity, infants are administered oral phenobarbital (5 mg/kg daily) to induce hepatic microsomal enzymes and increase hepatocyte processing of ^{99m}Tc-IDA. Both hepatic uptake of radionuclide and excretion into the gastrointestinal tract are evaluated over a timed interval. Infants with primary hepatocellular disorders characteristically have impaired hepatocyte uptake of radionuclide, whereas normal infants and infants with biliary atresia have prompt uptake. Normal infants excrete the isotope rapidly into the gut through the biliary tract. In biliary atresia, there is no excretion into the gut because of the obliteration of the extrahepatic bile ducts (Fig. 107.49). The hepatobiliary scan is a rapid test that can be performed simultaneously with other diagnostic examinations, for example, ultrasound. This test reliably identifies infants with choledochal cyst as well.

Other Diagnostic Tests. Several other diagnostic tests are of interest in the workup of an infant with conjugated hyperbilirubinemia in whom obstructive jaundice is suspected. MRI cholangiography is emerging as a sensitive, specific examination for identification of extrahepatic anatomy. The important management principle is that prompt operative exploration, liver biopsy, and cholangiogram should be performed in any infant in whom biliary atresia is suspected. An aggressive approach is warranted in that unnecessary delay in definitive drainage may lead to a less favorable outcome.

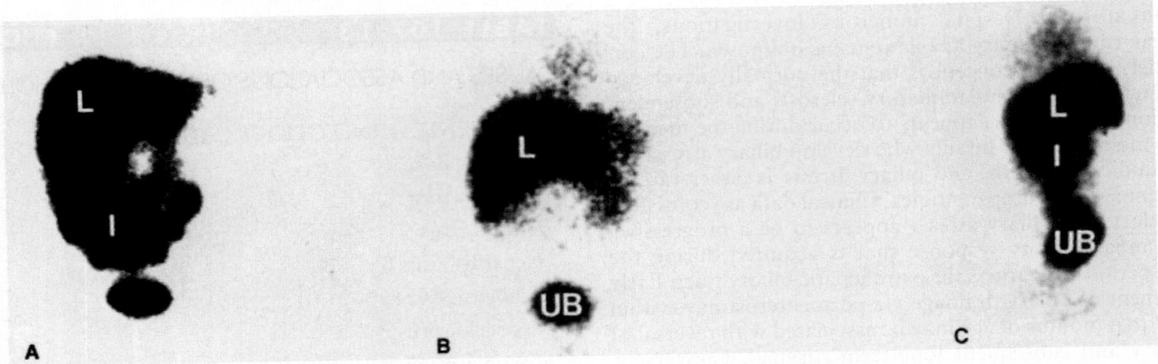

FIGURE 107.49. **A:** Normal scan using p-isopropylacetanilidoiminodiacetic acid (PIPIDA) as the hepatobiliary scanning agent. At 45 minutes, isotope is clearly visible in the liver (L) and intestine (I). **B:** Scan after phenobarbital administration in infant with biliary atresia. Even after 8 hours, isotope is apparent only in the liver and urinary bladder (UB). **C:** Patient with cholestatic jaundice. At 65 minutes, isotope is visible in the liver (L) and intestine (I). Hepatocyte uptake is variable but usually decreased or normal, whereas excretion into the gut is predictably present with cholestatic jaundice or hepatocellular disease.

Ultrasound. A standard examination of the jaundiced infant is a comprehensive abdominal ultrasound, with particular attention given to the liver and biliary tract. The most common ultrasonographic finding in biliary atresia is a diminutive or absent gallbladder without associated intrahepatic duct dilatation. Biliary tract obstruction from a choledochal cyst also can be reliably identified by ultrasound. Other rare causes of extrahepatic biliary duct obstruction are associated with proximal duct dilatation.

Liver Biopsy. Because the histologic findings in biliary atresia are not specific, about 20% to 25% of infants who undergo percutaneous liver biopsy remain undiagnosed. Liver biopsy is often performed in conjunction with the workup of conjugated hyperbilirubinemia following hepatobiliary scanning and ultrasonography, but in the setting of biliary atresia, it has limited utility. The histologic examination of a percutaneous liver biopsy is probably most helpful in diagnosing nonoperative causes of neonatal jaundice, thus avoiding anesthesia and operative exploration.

Alpha$_1$-Antitrypsin Deficiency. Alpha$_1$-antitrypsin deficiency is perhaps the single most important medical condition that may be difficult or impossible to differentiate from biliary atresia. All jaundiced infants should have plasma alpha$_1$-antitrypsin levels determined before operative exploration for suspected biliary atresia. Infants with alpha$_1$-antitrypsin deficiency do not benefit from operative exploration or portoenterostomy.

Treatment. Infants with biliary atresia require surgical therapy as the initial management intervention. Medical therapy is directed to the postoperative management of the chronic liver disease. The use of sequential surgical treatment, using portoenterostomy in infancy and orthotopic liver transplantation for children with progressive hepatic failure, provides improvement in overall survival.[160,161] Limited organ availability and a higher rate of perioperative complications limit primary liver transplantation for most infants with biliary atresia younger than 1 year. In the rare instance of unrecognized biliary atresia in an older child with established hepatic dysfunction, primary orthotopic liver transplantation may be a reasonable option.

Portoenterostomy. The recommended initial procedure for the treatment of biliary atresia is portoenterostomy. Before the development of portoenterostomy in Japan by Morio Kasai during the late 1950s, all infants with biliary atresia died of chronic liver disease and cirrhosis. Current management dictates that operative exploration and portoenterostomy be performed promptly. Early intervention by portoenterostomy to provide biliary drainage has been proposed to arrest or reverse the parenchymal liver injury, but the point at which the liver injury becomes irreversible remains unknown. From a clinical standpoint, most long-term success with portoenterostomy alone appears to be achieved in infants younger than 2 to 3 months, whereas infants older than 3 to 4 months appear to have a less favorable prognosis. Portoenterostomy for this "late" group has been reported successful in approximately one third of infants, however, and should be considered a potential alternative in the absence of available liver transplant donors.[162]

The initial approach to the infant with suspected biliary atresia is to perform an operative cholangiogram. If the diagnosis is confirmed, a portoenterostomy is constructed (Fig. 107.50). To maximize the potential for effective biliary drainage with portoenterostomy, several technical caveats are worthy of mention. An open liver biopsy is routinely performed to document the state of parenchymal injury. The cholangiogram is generally attempted through the gallbladder. In the 10% to 15% instances of a patent distal biliary tree, treatment still requires portoenterostomy. A nonpatent, fibrous cord rather than a normal common bile duct is found in the hepatoduodenal ligament. This cord is dissected free proximally to the level of the porta hepatis between the portal vein bifurcation. The fibrous remnant is sharply transected at this level to preserve any patent bile ducts. A short, 15- to 25-cm retrocolic, jejunal Roux-Y limb is constructed. There has been no clear advantage with longer or modified conduits with intussusception-type antireflux valves in the prevention of cholangitis.[163,164]

Previously, some surgeons preferred to exteriorize the biliary conduit (Fig. 107.51). With an exteriorized biliary conduit, postoperative bile flow is directly visible. The diverting stoma must be closed, however, and there is potential to develop parastomal variceal hemorrhage from progressive portal hypertension. Additionally, fluid and electrolyte losses from the biliostomy can be significant, and there are no reported survival differences between patients with exteriorized and closed biliary conduits following portoenterostomy. Because many of these infants may ultimately require liver transplantation, there is a trend toward using a simple, closed biliary conduit with portoenterostomy. Therefore, the use of a stoma to divert the bile flow in the Roux limb has been largely abandoned.

Results and Complications. Following portoenterostomy, bile flow occurs in about 66% to 75% of all infants when operated on at less than 60 days of age; however, establishment of bile flow may take weeks to months. The probability of bile flow appears related to age at the time of operation.

Cholangitis is a constant concern and an important postoperative problem after portoenterostomy. The clinical signs

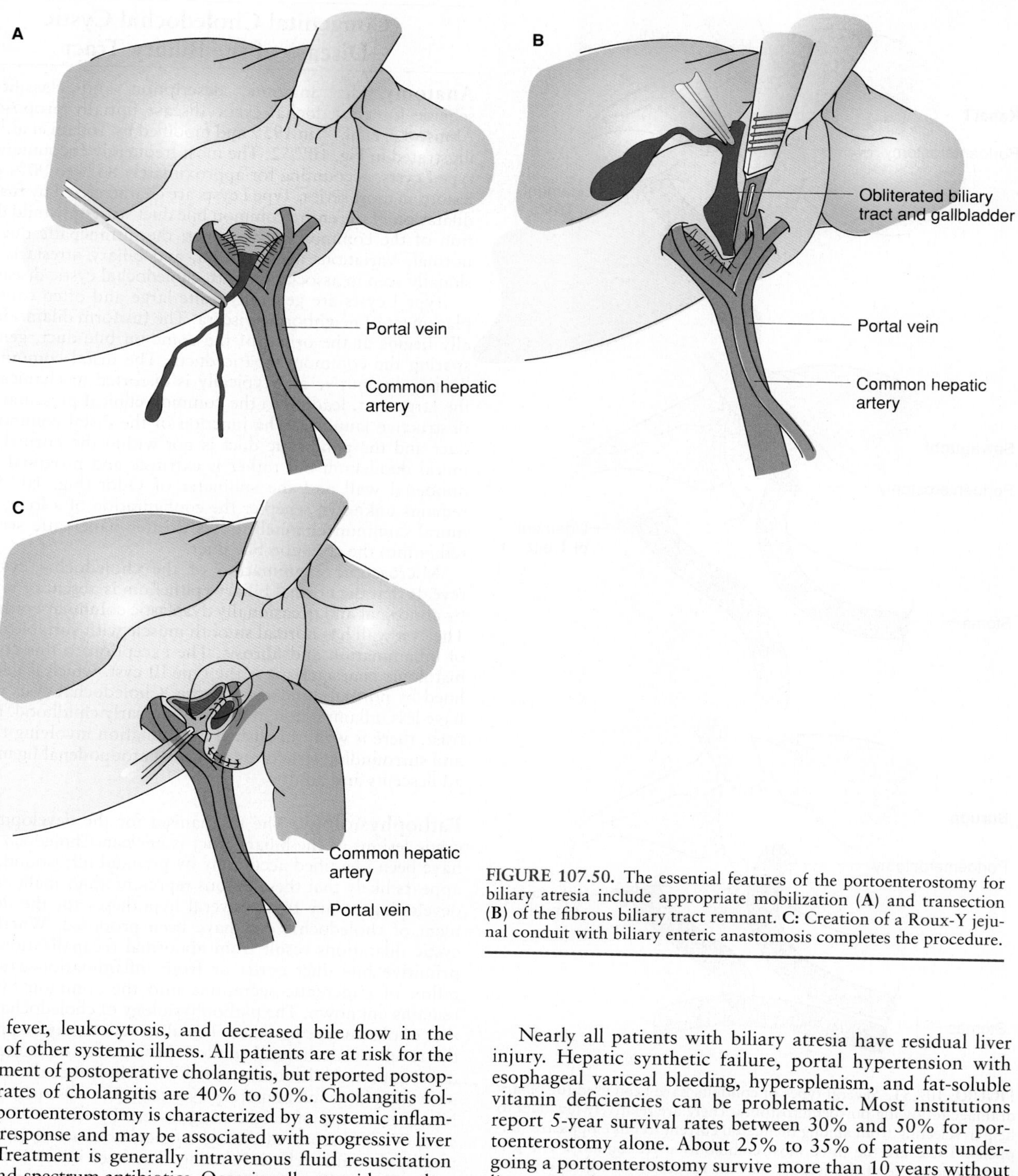

FIGURE 107.50. The essential features of the portoenterostomy for biliary atresia include appropriate mobilization (**A**) and transection (**B**) of the fibrous biliary tract remnant. **C:** Creation of a Roux-Y jejunal conduit with biliary enteric anastomosis completes the procedure.

include fever, leukocytosis, and decreased bile flow in the absence of other systemic illness. All patients are at risk for the development of postoperative cholangitis, but reported postoperative rates of cholangitis are 40% to 50%. Cholangitis following portoenterostomy is characterized by a systemic inflammatory response and may be associated with progressive liver injury. Treatment is generally intravenous fluid resuscitation and broad-spectrum antibiotics. Occasionally, steroids or other anti-inflammatory agents may be helpful, whereas reoperation or endoscopic revision of the portoenterostomy usually is not.[165] In an effort to determine the optimal treatment of infants with biliary atresia, a group of investigators have formed the Biliary Atresia Research Consortium (BARC).[166] The primary objectives of the consortium are to establish a clinical database and tissue repository. A retrospective BARC study of 104 children with biliary atresia treated in the United States demonstrated that at 2 years of age, 58 patients were alive with their native liver and 42 had undergone liver transplantation.[167] Data from the United Kingdom demonstrated improved measurable outcomes in children with biliary atresia treated with Kasai portoenterostomy by regionalization of care to three centers in the U.K. health care system.[168]

Nearly all patients with biliary atresia have residual liver injury. Hepatic synthetic failure, portal hypertension with esophageal variceal bleeding, hypersplenism, and fat-soluble vitamin deficiencies can be problematic. Most institutions report 5-year survival rates between 30% and 50% for portoenterostomy alone. About 25% to 35% of patients undergoing a portoenterostomy survive more than 10 years without liver transplantation. The remaining two thirds of children with biliary atresia ultimately require liver transplantation for survival. Although the failure rate for portoenterostomy is high, the possibility of long-term success is notable. Additionally, the limited availability of infant donor organs and the technical limitations of liver transplantation in infants younger than 1 year of age make portoenterostomy an accepted initial treatment of biliary atresia in most centers.

Hepatic Transplantation. Hepatic transplantation is discussed in detail elsewhere in this text. For biliary atresia, transplantation offers a means of long-term survival in children with failed portoenterostomies. The current 5-year survival of children with biliary atresia who undergo liver transplantation ranges from 75% to 94.4%.[169,170] Additionally, with the use

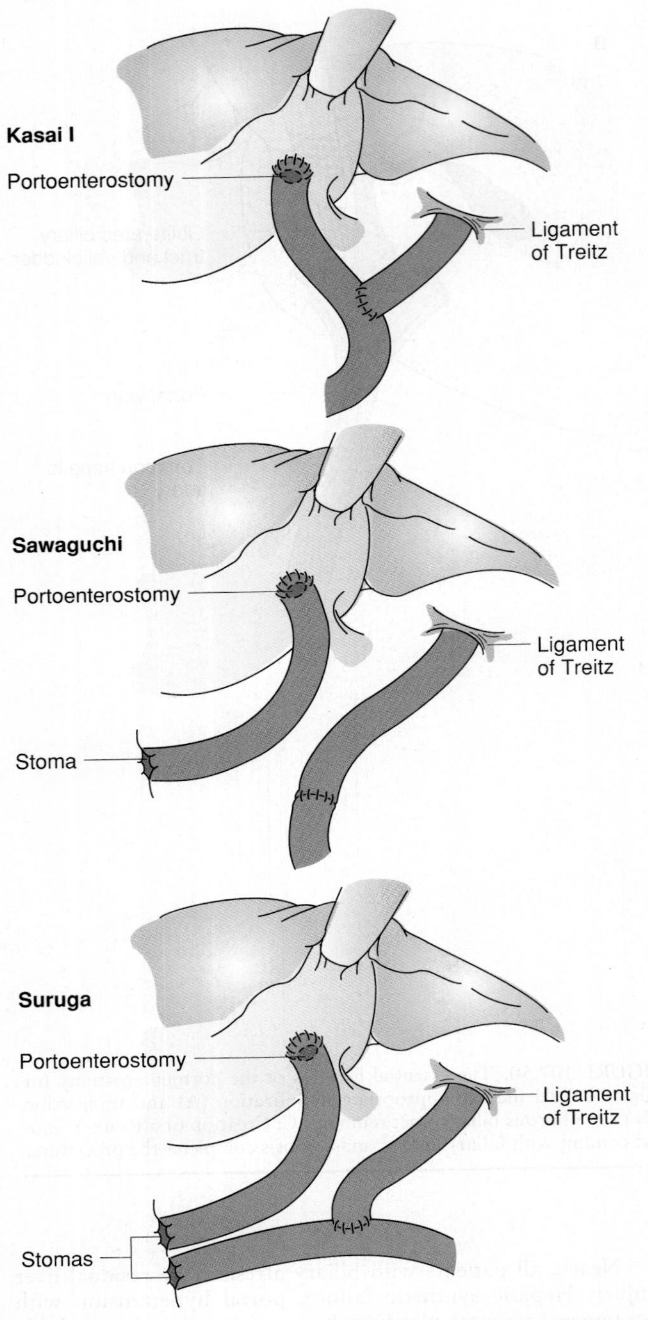

FIGURE 107.51. Several types of conduits have been used for biliary drainage following portoenterostomy. There are relatively few data to help in selecting from among them, and current trends emphasize simplicity. These are the three most commonly used conduits. The primary importance of this issue is that the reoperative surgeon must be familiar with the anatomic variations.

of reduced-size cadaveric donor livers as well as living-related donor livers, the mortality rate for infants on transplant waiting lists may be decreasing. Indications for liver transplantation in biliary atresia include progressive hepatic failure despite portoenterostomy, growth retardation, and complications of portal hypertension. It is important to consider the consequences of lifelong immunosuppression in these children, including the risks of infection and treatment-related malignancy.

Congenital Choledochal Cystic Disease of the Biliary Tract

Anatomy. The anatomic description and classification scheme for choledochal cystic disease initially proposed by Alonso-Lej et al.[171] in 1959 and modified by Todani et al.[172] are illustrated in Fig. 107.52. The most frequently encountered are type I cysts, accounting for approximately 85% to 90% of the lesions in most series. Type I cysts are characterized by fusiform dilatation of the entire common bile duct with only mild dilatation of the common hepatic duct; the intrahepatic ducts are normal. Variations are common, and biliary atresia is occasionally seen in association with choledochal cystic disease.

Type I cysts are generally quite large and often cause displacement of neighboring viscera. The fusiform dilatation usually begins at the origin of the common bile duct, generally sparing the common hepatic ducts. The distal common bile duct is diminutive and typically is distorted mechanically by the large cyst, leading to the common clinical presentation of obstructive jaundice. The junction of the distal common bile duct and the pancreatic duct is not within the normal intramural duodenum but rather is extrinsic and proximal to the duodenal wall and the sphincter of Oddi (Fig. 107.53). It remains unknown whether the configuration of a long, extramural common channel allows greater pancreatic secretion reflux into the common bile duct.

Microscopic examination of the choledochal cyst wall reveals that the normal biliary epithelium is absent or replaced by abnormal and occasionally dysplastic columnar epithelium. The cyst wall has normal smooth muscle with variable degrees of inflammation and fibrosis. The exception to this common histologic characteristic is the type III cyst, which is generally lined by normal duodenal mucosa. Choledochal cysts tend to have less inflammation in infancy and early childhood. In contrast, there is well-established inflammation involving the cyst and surrounding structures in the hepatoduodenal ligament in adolescents and adults.

Pathophysiology. The mechanism for the development of cystic lesions of the biliary tract is unclear. Choledochal cysts have been identified accurately by prenatal ultrasound, and it appears likely that these lesions represent abnormalities in the developing biliary tract. Several hypotheses for the development of choledochal cyst have been proposed. Whether the cystic dilatations result from abnormal recanalization of the primitive bile duct cords or from inflammation caused by reflux of pancreatic secretions into the common bile duct remains unknown. The pathophysiology of choledochal cyst is that of obstructive jaundice. The obstruction may be primarily the result of mechanical outflow obstruction of a diminutive distal common bile duct with a dilated choledochal cyst. Alternatively, a large inflammatory cyst can cause obstruction of the biliary tract and of neighboring viscera by extrinsic compression. When discovered during infancy, obstructive jaundice is usually the initial clinical finding. The liver injury is typically reversible, and progression to biliary cirrhosis is rare. The exception to this situation is type V disease, which is associated with a high incidence of hepatic fibrosis.

Other initial clinical situations include cholelithiasis and acute bacterial cholangitis secondary to diminished bile drainage. Children with type III cysts may have acute pancreatitis. Infrequently, extrinsic compression of the portal vein by a large choledochal cyst may produce symptoms and signs of portal hypertension. Abdominal pain and tenderness following minor injury may lead to an incidental diagnosis of choledochal cyst on imaging studies.

Carcinoma of the biliary tract occurs in about 3% to 5% of patients with choledochal cyst. The number of reported cases remains small in the literature, but the incidence for biliary tract neoplasm is about 1,000 times that of the normal

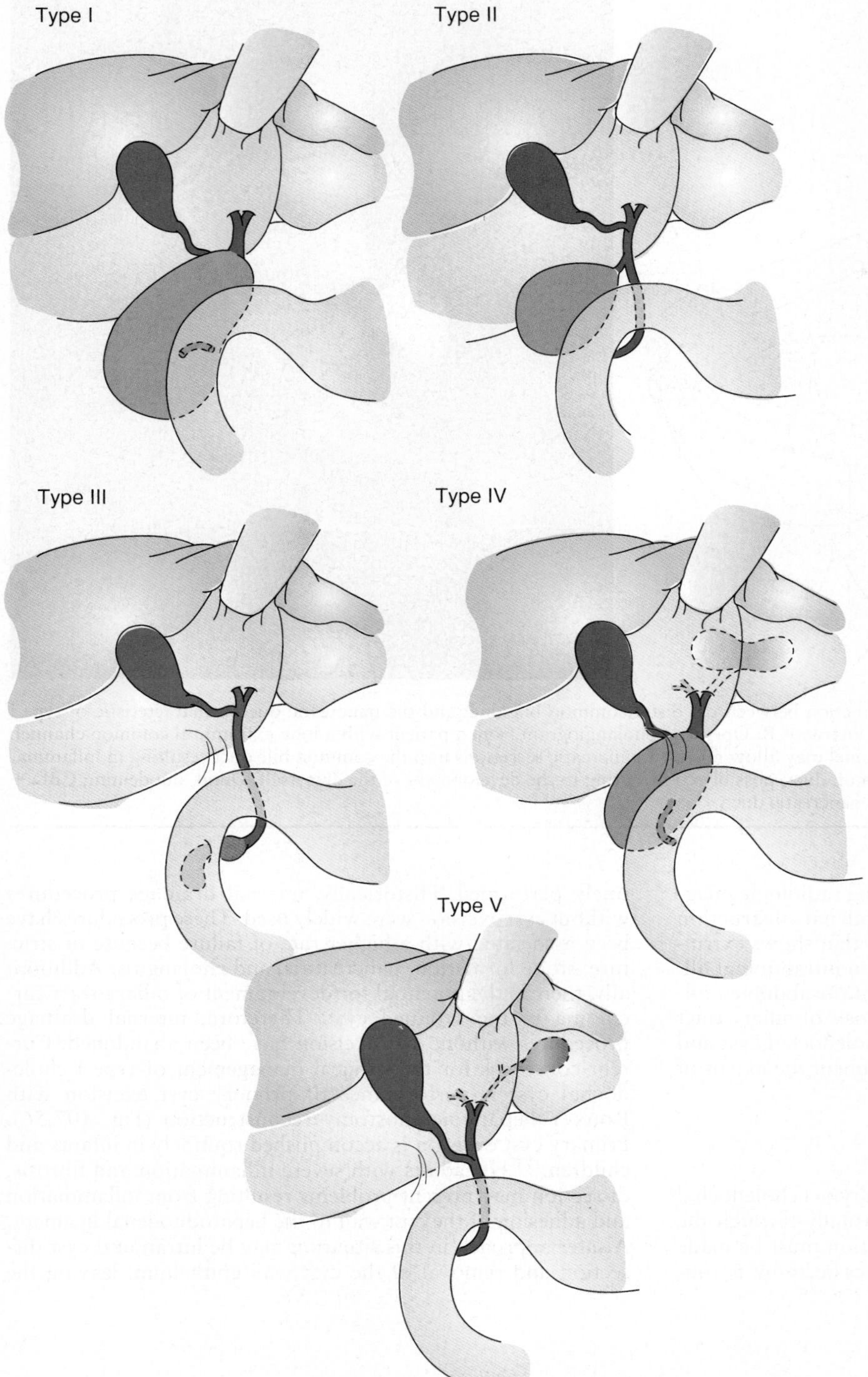

FIGURE 107.52. Classification of choledochal cyst.

population.[173] Patients with choledochal cyst are at increased risk for the development of biliary tract carcinoma in adolescence or early adulthood. The dysplastic cyst epithelium may be susceptible to malignant change from chronic inflammation. It is interesting that there appears to be an increased risk of malignancy to develop anywhere in the biliary tract, gallbladder, or pancreas, and not just in the choledochal cyst itself.[174] Therefore, current treatment emphasizes complete cyst excision of the cyst epithelium while providing adequate biliary drainage to prevent stasis and chronic inflammation. Infants and children treated for choledochal cyst should have long-term follow-up for complications and potential malignancy.

Clinical Presentation and Diagnosis. Choledochal cysts present most commonly in infancy and early childhood with symptoms of obstructive jaundice. In older children and adults, the classic clinical triad of episodic abdominal pain, a palpable right upper-quadrant mass, and jaundice occurs in fewer than 50% of patients. Adults occasionally present with hepatomegaly or evidence of portal hypertension. The diagnosis in infants and most children can be confirmed by ultrasound examination and ^{99m}Tc-IDA imaging studies (Figs. 107.54 and 107.55). In older children, both MRI cholangiography and endoscopic retrograde cholangiopancreatography (ERCP) are highly sensitive and specific in confirming diagnosis. These

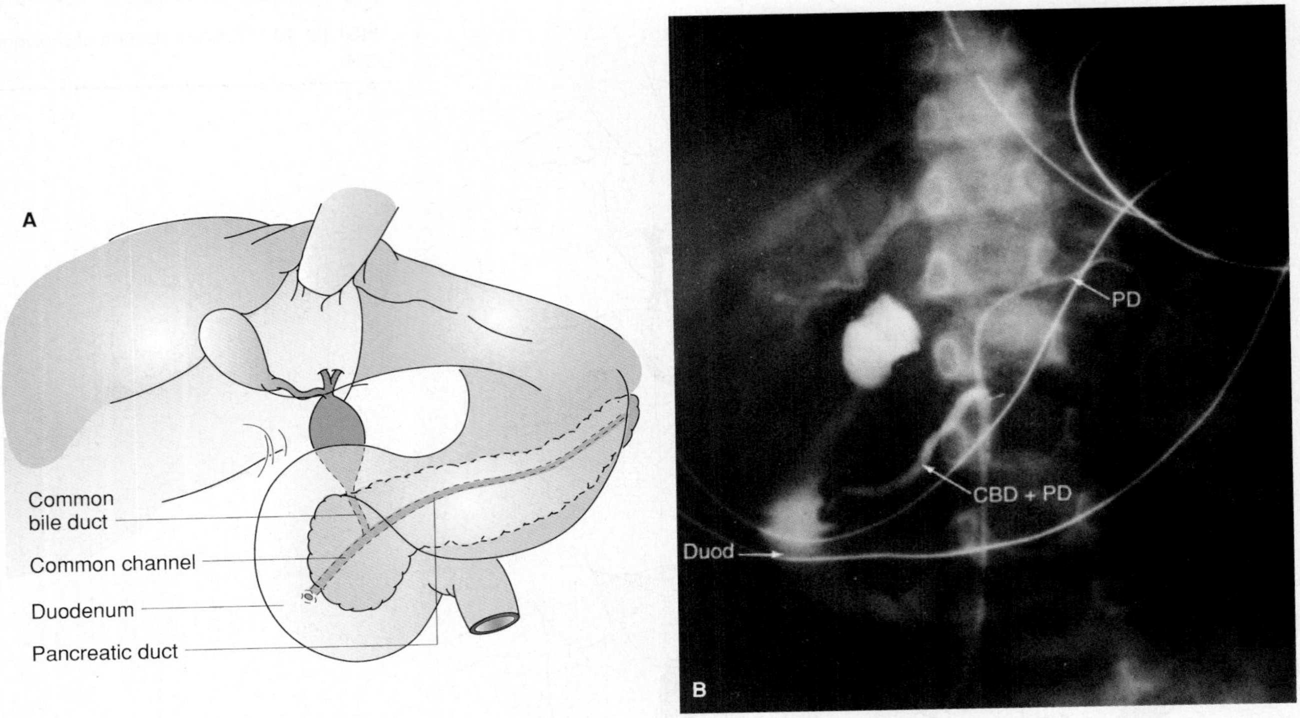

FIGURE 107.53. An anomalous, extramural junction between the distal common bile duct and the pancreatic duct is characteristic of type I choledochal cyst. **A:** Schematic depiction of this anatomy. **B:** Operative cholangiogram from a patient with a long extramural common channel. It has been suggested that the long common channel may allow reflux of pancreatic secretions into the common bile duct resulting in inflammation and proteinase-mediated injury to the common duct, possibly contributing to the development of the cyst itself. Duod, duodenum; CBD + PD, common bile duct and pancreatic duct; PD, pancreatic duct.

lesions also are diagnosed incidentally during radiologic imaging studies for other reasons. Partial duodenal obstruction may lead to an upper gastrointestinal series that shows extrinsic compression from a large type I cyst or an intraluminal filling defect from a type III cyst. CT imaging of the abdomen following blunt trauma may lead to the diagnosis of biliary tract dilatation. Liver biopsy is not specific in choledochal cyst and has little diagnostic role other than to document the extent of liver injury.

Treatment

Type I Cysts. Initial operative strategy for a type I choledochal cyst is exploration and cholangiography, usually through the gallbladder, but occasionally contrast injection must be made directly into the common bile duct. Cholecystectomy is routinely performed. Historically, internal drainage procedures without cyst excision were widely used. These procedures have been associated with a higher rate of failure because of stricture, stone formation, pancreatitis, and cholangitis. Additionally, there is the potential for development of biliary tract carcinoma in the retained cyst. Therefore, internal drainage procedures without cyst excision have been abandoned. Current consensus for the surgical management of type I choledochal cyst is performance of primary cyst excision with Roux-Y hepaticojejunostomy reconstruction (Fig. 107.56). Primary cyst excision is accomplished routinely in infants and children.[175] For adults with severe inflammation and fibrosis, dissection may present problems resulting from inflammation and adhesion of the cyst wall to the hepatoduodenal ligament. A safer approach in this situation may be intramural cyst dissection and removal of the cyst wall epithelium, leaving the

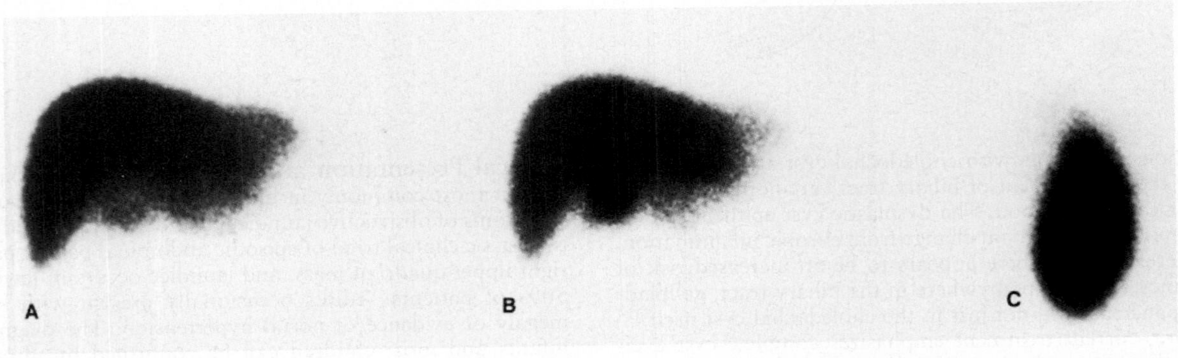

FIGURE 107.54. Typical ^{99M}Tc iminodiacetic acid (HIDA) scan from a child with a type I choledochal cyst. Images were made in 5 minutes (**A**), 30 minutes (**B**), and 3 hours (**C**) after isotope injection. The isotope is retained within the choledochal cyst more than 24 hours, and the pattern of hepatocyte uptake is normal.

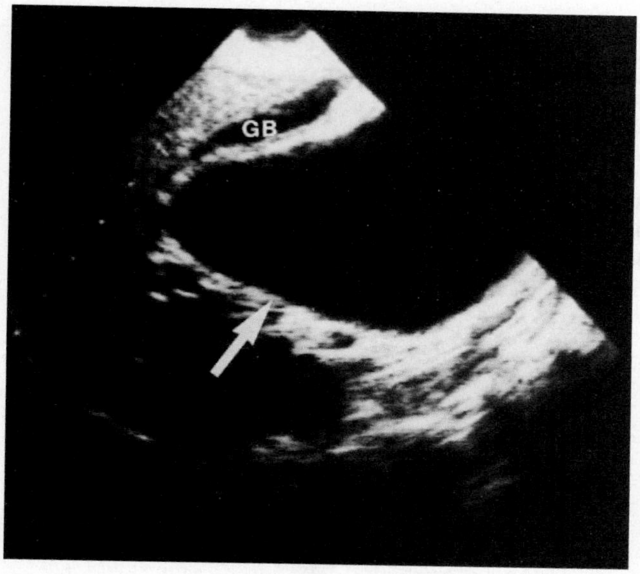

FIGURE 107.55. Ultrasound image of a type I choledochal cyst (*arrow*; longitudinal image). The gallbladder (GB) is also shown.

posteromedial outer cyst wall adjacent to the portal vein and hepatic artery intact.

Other Types of Cysts. Type II cysts are excised completely and the choledochotomy closed primarily. Type III choledochoceles require a transduodenal approach with either marsupialization or excision of the cyst. Care must be taken to identify the ampulla, and a formal sphincteroplasty may be required to ensure adequate drainage from the biliary tract and the pancreas. Types IV and V intrahepatic cystic disease must be approached on an individualized basis. In general, unilobar or focal cystic disease can be either resected or drained with Roux-Y jejunostomy reconstruction. In cases of bilobar intraparenchymal disease, particularly in the setting of hepatic fibrosis, it may be difficult, if not impossible, to obtain complete, adequate drainage.

Complications and Outcome. The major complications associated with operative repair of choledochal cyst include cholangitis, stricture formation, choledocholithiasis, and development of biliary tract malignancy. A summary of the incidence of complications, mortality, and reoperation for the different procedures in 955 cases reported in the literature demonstrated a clear advantage for primary cyst excision in terms of morbidity and need for reoperation, and no significant increase in mortality occurred using this approach.[176] Subsequent to this analysis in 1975, internal drainage procedures without cyst excision have been essentially replaced by primary cyst excision with hepaticojejunostomy reconstruction. Currently, several series have reported excellent results with little or no mortality using total transmural excision of choledochal cysts.[177] Primary transmural excision with biliary tract reconstruction continues to be a safe and desirable operative approach for cystic lesions of the biliary tract.

PEDIATRIC PANCREAS

Disorders of the pancreas are uncommon in infants and children. Pancreatic disorders in children include congenital anatomic disorders, inflammatory pancreatitis, rare neoplastic lesions, and pancreatic endocrinopathies.[178] Several significant issues are relative to the pancreatic problems in the pediatric age group, and a brief overview is presented in the following discussion.

Embryology

The fetal pancreas arises from the paired dorsal and ventral foregut diverticular buds during the sixth week of gestation.

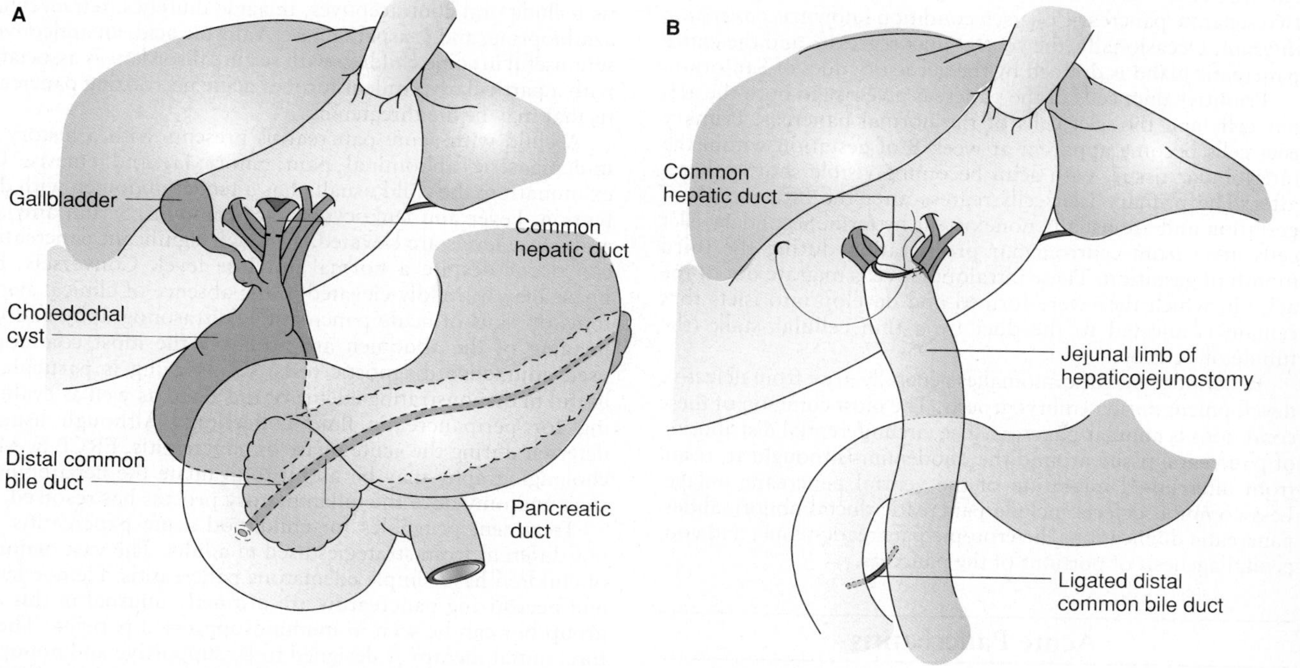

FIGURE 107.56. The preferred operative treatment of type I choledochal cyst consists of primary total transmural cyst excision with Roux-Y hepaticojejunostomy.

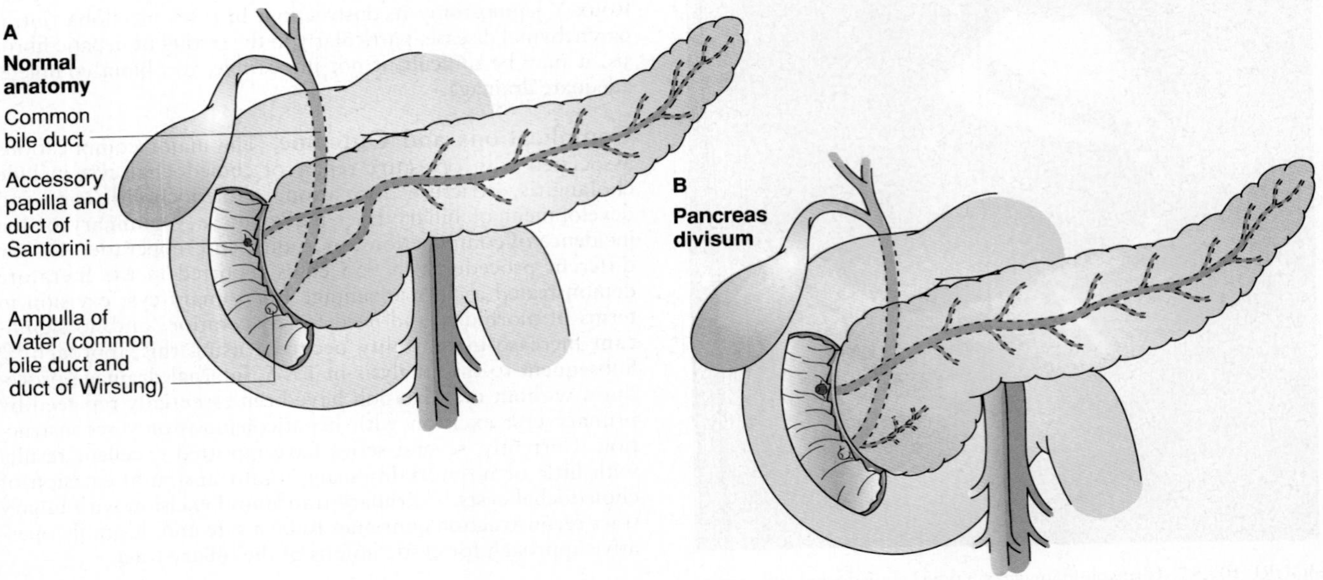

FIGURE 107.57. **A:** Normal pancreatic ductal anatomy. **B:** Pancreas divisum. There is no communication between the duct of Wirsung and the duct of Santorini. The duct of Wirsung is short or absent. Most of the pancreas is drained by the duct of Santorini through the accessory papilla. This anatomy is found in about 10% to 15% of normal individuals.

The dorsal pancreatic anlage gives rise to the body and tail of the pancreas as well as the main pancreatic duct. The ventral pancreatic anlage migrates 180 degrees to fuse with the dorsal gland, forming the uncinate process and the distal portion of the duct of Wirsung (Fig. 107.57). The independent ductal systems of the developing pancreatic anlage fuse. The dorsal (Santorini) duct opens directly into the duodenum, and this anatomy is persistent in 10% to 15% of normal subjects. The ventral (Wirsung) duct opens into the duodenum by fusion with the common bile duct. Normally, the dorsal duct fuses with the ventral duct just to the right of the mesenteric vessels. Failure of the dorsal and ventral ducts to fuse normally leads to two separate pancreatic ducts, a condition known as *pancreatic divisum*. Occasionally, the ventral duct regresses and the entire pancreatic gland is drained by the accessory duct of Santorini.

Primitive duct cells of the pancreas give rise to both the acinar cells and the islet cells of the normal pancreas. Primary islet cells become apparent at week 8 of gestation within the interlobular tissue, with acini becoming visible shortly thereafter. The primary islet cells regress after the fifth month of gestation and are usually nonexistent by term. Secondary islet cells arise from centroacinar proliferation during the third month of gestation. These intralobular cells migrate out of the acini in which they were formed and develop into islets that remain connected to the duct by a thin cellular stalk (the tubule of Bensley).

Exocrine pancreatic anomalies generally arise from defective development during embryogenesis. The most common of these conditions is annular pancreas. The circumferential distribution of pancreatic tissue around the duodenum is thought to result from interrupted migration of the ventral pancreatic anlage. Less common defects include pancreatic ductal abnormalities, pancreatic duplications, heterotopic pancreatic tissue, and congenital agenesis of portions of the pancreas.

Acute Pancreatitis

Acute pancreatitis is often overlooked as a cause of abdominal pain in children; however, it is the most common disorder of the pancreas in both infants and children. Adult pancreatitis is often caused by either alcohol ingestion or gallstones. In contrast, 50% to 80% of cases in children, particularly adolescents, are posttraumatic or idiopathic in origin. An important clinical condition seen with moderate frequency is acute pancreatitis in the setting of immunosuppression, in particular, high-dose corticosteroids. Steroid-induced acute pancreatitis typically accounts for the third most common cause of pancreatitis in most children's hospitals. Other causes of acute pancreatitis include gallstones, CF, hyperlipidemia, juvenile diabetes mellitus, mumps, coxsackievirus infection, infectious mononucleosis, collagen vascular diseases, and anatomic lesions such as choledochal cyst. Medications significantly associated with acute pancreatitis include oral contraceptives, thiazide diuretics, tetracyclines. azathioprine, and L-asparaginase. Valproic acid, an anticonvulsant useful in some children with seizure disorders, is associated with a particularly virulent form of acute necrotizing pancreatitis that may be life threatening.

A child with acute pancreatitis presents with a history of midepigastric abdominal pain, anorexia, and emesis. On examination, the child usually has a tender abdomen with distention. Fever and leukocytosis are common. Serum amylase and lipase levels are elevated, although significant pancreatitis can occur despite a normal amylase level. Conversely, the lipase may be mildly elevated in the absence of clinical symptoms or signs of acute pancreatitis. Ultrasonography and CT imaging of the abdomen are probably the most commonly used adjunctive diagnostic tests. CT imaging is particularly useful in demonstrating edema of the gland as well as evaluating for peripancreatic fluid collections. Although usually deferred during the acute phase of pancreatitis, ERCP or MRI cholangiography may be useful to evaluate the hepatobiliary tract anatomy once the inflammatory process has resolved.

Treatment principles for childhood acute pancreatitis are not different from strategies used in adults. The vast majority of children have simple edematous pancreatitis. Hemorrhagic and necrotizing pancreatitis are distinctly unusual in this age group but can be seen in immunosuppressed patients. Therefore, initial therapy is designed to be supportive and nonoperative in approach. Endotracheal intubation and mechanical ventilation may be required. Intravenous fluid resuscitation, pancreatic rest by nasogastric tube decompression, analgesia, and TPN are provided. No clinical efficacy data are available to support the widespread use of anticholinergics or somatostatin analogues for acute pancreatitis in children. Operative intervention is reserved for complications of pancreatitis such as hemorrhage, infected pancreatic necrosis, or pancreatic pseudocyst.

Recurrent pancreatitis in a child usually is associated with an anatomic abnormality or specific physiologic problem. Following recovery from the acute inflammatory event, an aggressive diagnostic workup, including consideration of ERCP or MRCP to define ductal anatomy, should be performed. In particular, the presence of pancreas divisum with stenosis of the accessory papilla should be considered. Children with pancreatitis in the setting of cholelithiasis should undergo laparoscopic cholecystectomy after resolution of the pancreatitis.

Pancreas Divisum

Pancreas divisum occurs with failure of normal fusion between the dorsal and ventral pancreatic ducts. About 10% to 15% of normal persons have two separate pancreatic ducts, and up to 10% of asymptomatic persons undergoing ERCP have two complete ductal systems. The anatomic variant of pancreas divisum is not necessarily pathologic, but if the orifice of the accessory papilla is stenotic or obstructed, pancreatitis can occur.[179] Approximately 25% of affected individuals are thought to be at risk for developing pancreatitis. Because pancreas divisum is characterized by a dominant dorsal duct system dependent on secretion through the accessory papilla, stenosis of the accessory (lesser) papilla is probably necessary to produce pancreatic symptoms. Most of the experience with surgical treatment of pancreas divisum is reported in adults. Successful surgical management of children presenting with recurrent pancreatitis secondary to accessory papilla stenosis with pancreas divisum also has been reported.[180]

To diagnose pancreas divisum, ERCP is required. Endoscopic visualization of the major and accessory papillae is essential. Radiographic findings with pancreas divisum demonstrate a short or absent duct of Wirsung that does not communicate with the duct of Santorini (Fig. 107.57). Definitive diagnosis of pancreas divisum is made by demonstrating two separate, parallel ductal systems.

Few pediatric patients with pancreatitis and pancreas divisum requiring operation have been reported. Most of these children were female patients who had a history of recurrent pancreatitis. The primary operative goal is to provide adequate drainage of the duct of Santorini by performing a sphincterotomy of the accessory duct. An open dorsal duct sphincterotomy appears to be more durable than endoscopic sphincterotomy. Some surgeons advocate sphincterotomy of the main papilla as well, but dorsal duct sphincterotomy alone appears effective in preventing acute pancreatitis associated with pancreas divisum. The reported surgical outcome in the limited number of children treated for pancreatitis associated with pancreas divisum is favorable.

Pancreatic Cysts

Pancreatic pseudocysts are uncommon in the pediatric age group and are usually the result of blunt traumatic abdominal injury or acute pancreatitis. Children typically present with abdominal pain, nausea, emesis, and weight loss. There may be a palpable midepigastric mass on examination. Diagnosis usually is made with ultrasound or CT imaging of the abdomen. The serum amylase and lipase are usually elevated.

In children, many small asymptomatic pseudocysts regress spontaneously with resolution of the pancreatic inflammation. Larger or symptomatic pseudocysts may require drainage. Symptoms and potential complications of untreated pseudocysts include hemorrhage, infection, perforation, gastrointestinal or biliary tract obstruction, or, rarely, development of pancreaticoenteric fistula. The decision to use either external or internal drainage procedures for a pseudocyst depends on the status of the pancreatic duct. In many centers, definitive external drainage of a large or symptomatic pseudocyst is performed with acceptable morbidity and mortality rates by an ultrasound- or CT-guided percutaneous approach.[181] Pseudocyst recurrence or persistent external drainage without resolution suggests significant pancreatic duct injury or complete ductal transection. Determination of whether a major pancreatic ductal injury is associated with a pseudocyst may be made by either percutaneous contrast injection of the pseudocyst or ERCP.[182] Pseudocysts associated with pancreatic duct injury may not resolve with percutaneous external drainage or endoscopic pancreatic duct stenting, so internal drainage procedures such as cystgastrostomy or cystojejunostomy with or without distal pancreatectomy may be required.[183]

Epithelial cysts of the pancreas are rare in children. Congenital cysts are lined by epithelium and acinar tissue and are seen most commonly in the body and tail of the pancreas. They may be associated with other syndromes such as von Hippel-Lindau disease, which is characterized by hereditary cerebellar cysts, retinal hemangioma, and pancreatic cysts. Congenital pancreatic cysts are typically asymptomatic unless they are large enough to cause compression or obstruction of the stomach or colon. In the absence of trauma, spontaneous rupture of a pancreatic epithelial cyst is rare. Treatment is cyst excision or internal drainage into the stomach or jejunum.

Other rare cystic lesions of the pancreas in children include retention cysts. These cysts result from chronic ductal obstruction. They are characteristically lined by epithelium unless inflammatory obliteration has occurred. Enteric duplication cysts of the stomach or duodenum can also be associated intimately with the pancreas and communicate with the pancreatic duct. Treatment of both retention cysts and enteric duplication cysts either within or associated with the pancreas includes excision, occasionally internal drainage, and, if necessary, distal pancreatectomy. Not all pancreatic cysts in children can be uniformly considered benign. Suspicious lesions should be investigated thoroughly and biopsy performed. Cystadenoma, cystadenocarcinoma, and rhabdomyosarcoma associated with a pancreatic cyst have been reported. These neoplasms are treated by anatomic pancreatic resection following histologic confirmation on biopsy.

Pancreatic Neoplasms

Childhood malignant neoplasms of the pancreas are uncommon. Typically, pancreatic malignancy in childhood is found on discovery of an asymptomatic abdominal mass. Infrequently, the lesion may be found incidentally or during a diagnostic imaging workup for abdominal trauma. Jaundice may occur with a lesion in the pancreatic head causing common bile duct obstruction. The most frequently encountered lesions include islet cell carcinoma and adenocarcinoma. The treatment of choice for localized malignant neoplasms of the pancreas is surgical resection.[184] Pancreaticoduodenectomy in children can successfully control some malignancies of the pancreatic head. To promote adequate nutrient absorption and growth, children undergoing pancreaticoduodenectomy should be considered for oral pancreatic enzyme replacement and fat-soluble vitamin supplementation.[185]

Two pancreatic neoplasms seen in childhood and adolescence deserve further discussion. The *papillary cystic neoplasm* of the pancreas occurs predominantly in younger female children, is typically slow growing with low malignant potential, and is highly curable with surgical resection.[186] This tumor is thought to be a neoplasm of the ductuloacinar primordial cells of the pancreas. The other lesion is the *pancreatoblastoma*, also referred to as *juvenile adenocarcinoma of the pancreas*. Pancreatoblastoma is somewhat more common in boys than girls and typically has slow growth with low malignant potential as well. Histologic examination demonstrates undifferentiated ductular and acinar areas with nodules of squamous epithelium, suggesting that these tumors arise from primordial pancreatic cells. Both papillary cystic neoplasm and pancreatoblastoma have more favorable prognoses than adenocarcinoma following surgical resection.

Endocrine Lesions of the Pancreas

Zollinger-Ellison Syndrome. Childhood tumors of the endocrine pancreas are exceedingly rare. The diagnosis and management of these tumors do not differ greatly from those of the adult population. The most common of these lesions include gastrinoma and insulinoma. The functional endocrine tumors of the pancreas are characterized by secreted peptide products such as glucagon, vasoactive intestinal peptide, somatostatin, and pancreatic polypeptide.

Similar to adults, children with Zollinger-Ellison syndrome clinically present with symptoms related to gastric hypersecretion. Peptic ulcer disease with or without gastrointestinal hemorrhage, abdominal pain, and diarrhea are common presenting symptoms. The diagnosis is confirmed by finding elevated serum gastrin levels. The basal acid output typically is elevated as well. A paradoxical increase in serum gastrin levels is found following intravenous administration of secretin (secretin stimulation test).

Contemporary management of Zollinger-Ellison syndrome in children relies on control of gastric acid hypersecretion with the oral administration of a proton-pump inhibitor. Diagnostic imaging studies, including helical CT scanning and MRI, are useful in localization of a primary gastrinoma and evaluating for metastatic disease before exploration. Definitive treatment relies on complete excision of the primary gastrinoma, which typically is found in the right of the superior mesenteric vessels in the head of the pancreas or the duodenum. The growth and progression of gastrinoma appear to be less aggressive in children than in adults; however, total gastrectomy occasionally is required in a child to control intractable symptoms related to persistent hypergastrinemia or metastatic disease.[187]

About 25% of gastrinomas occur in the setting of MEN syndrome, reviewed elsewhere in this book. At least 90% of patients with MEN type I have hyperparathyroidism secondary to hyperplasia. Additionally, 30% to 80% of patients have pancreatic islet cell tumors, and 15% to 50% have pituitary tumors.

Hypoglycemia. There are diverse metabolic causes for hypoglycemia in infancy and childhood. These include endocrinopathies such as panhypopituitarism, hypothyroidism, adrenal insufficiency, and congenital adrenal hyperplasia (adrenogenital syndrome). Several inborn errors of metabolism interrupt normal glucose regulatory mechanisms. Systemic disease states, perinatal stress, and sepsis can predispose an otherwise normal infant to low blood glucose levels. Infants who remain unresponsive to glucose infusion typically have inappropriately high circulating insulin levels for a given blood glucose level. Hyperinsulinemia should be suspected in any infant or child younger than 1 year of age with persistent hypoglycemia. There are heterogeneous causes for hyperinsulinemic hypoglycemia, but the most common historical cause in infancy is nesidioblastosis, which is characterized by uncontrolled development of the pancreatic endocrine tissue that functions abnormally during infancy.[188,189] Clinically, these cells secrete inappropriately high amounts of insulin, causing clinical hypoglycemia in infants. Two distinct histologic lesions appear to be responsible for congenital hyperinsulinism. Mutations in the beta cell K_{ATP} channel genes may lead to either focal, adenomatous hyperinsulinism or diffuse hyperinsulinism; both genotypes lead to phenotypic hypoglycemia if left untreated.

Infants with congenital hyperinsulinism usually become symptomatic from hypoglycemia within the first few hours or days of life. These infants commonly present with neurologic symptoms such as lethargy or generalized seizures and have corresponding fasting blood glucose levels less than 40 mg/dL. The diagnosis of hyperinsulinemia is supported by the clinical features of the Whipple triad, which includes (a) neurologic changes with fasting or activity, (b) fasting blood glucose levels less than 40 to 50 mg/dL, and (c) neurologic symptoms reversed by the administration of glucose. The diagnosis is made by demonstrating inappropriately high levels of circulating insulin for a given level of blood glucose. An insulin (IU/mL) to glucose (mg/dL) ratio that is greater than 0.5 in a fasting patient is consistent with hyperinsulinemic hypoglycemia. In infants and children, an absolute insulin level greater than 5 IU/mL in the presence of a blood glucose less than 40 mg/dL is diagnostic. Ketone body production is impaired in infants with congenital hyperinsulinism.

The initial management of a hypoglycemic infant with congenital hyperinsulinism is to provide adequate glucose concentrations to prevent permanent neurologic injury. Dextrose-containing intravenous solutions are titrated to maintain blood glucose levels greater than 40 mg/dL and may require a central venous catheter. The short-term administration of somatostatin analogues to increase blood glucose levels in hyperinsulinemic states has been demonstrated to be useful.[190] Other pharmacologic agents used to reduce insulin levels and raise blood glucose concentration include diazoxide (15 mg/kg daily). The use of streptozocin to control hyperinsulinemia most often is reserved for adults with metastatic islet cell carcinoma and is not widely used in infants because of the potential side effects.

Following initial control of blood glucose and clinical confirmation of hyperinsulinemia, operative intervention should be considered as a means of providing definitive control of hypoglycemia. Diagnostic imaging using CT scan imaging, MRI, or more recently,[18] F-FDOPA PET scanning may be useful either to identify or to exclude a focal lesion.[191] Localization of focal lesions is important in that this approach may lead to effective glucose control with selective partial pancreatectomy and allow for preservation of normal pancreatic tissue and function.[192,193]

Operatively, the abdomen is explored thoroughly, and the entire pancreas must be visualized. Preoperative localization data guided by intraoperative ultrasound and frozen section analysis may identify focal lesions amenable to partial resection. In the absence of a focal lesion, the infant is presumed to have diffuse islet cell hyperplasia. In this setting, the general operative strategy is total or near-total pancreatectomy.[194] Lesser procedures such as subtotal (80%) pancreatectomy do not effectively treat diffuse congenital hyperinsulinism, and recurrent hypoglycemia places the infant at risk for hypoglycemic encephalopathy. Near-total pancreatectomy involves resection of the distal 95% of the gland with preservation of the spleen. The entire distal pancreas, including the uncinate process, is resected, leaving a small rim of pancreatic tissue adjacent to the duodenum (Fig. 107.58). Total pancreatectomy is usually reserved for persistent or recurrent hypoglycemia following lesser procedures. Near-total pancreatectomy controls hypoglycemia in 90% of infants with diffuse congenital hyperinsulinism. The remaining infants with persistent hypoglycemia may require further pancreatic resection. With extensive pancreatic resection, the typical postoperative course is a transient period of hyperglycemia with subsequent stabilization of blood glucose levels. Pancreatic exocrine function is ablated, and oral replacement therapy is required. Despite clinical remission following resection, however, diabetes mellitus may occur as a long-term consequence in children treated either medically or surgically for diffuse congenital hyperinsulinism.[195] Therefore,

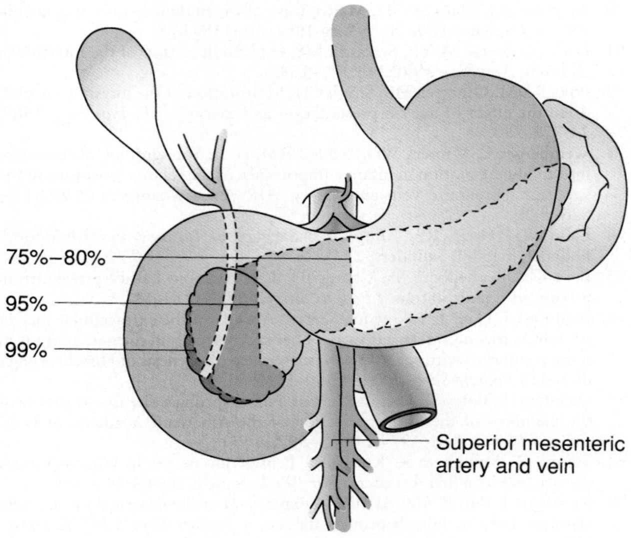

FIGURE 107.58. Illustration of the various degrees of pancreatic resection.

these infants need long-term metabolic follow-up for both pancreatic endocrine and exocrine function.

References

1. Nichols CR, Dickinson JE, Pemberton PJ. Rising incidence of gastroschisis in teenage pregnancies. *J Matern Fetal Med* 1997;6:225–229.
2. Blakelock RT, Upadhyay V, Pease PW, et al. Are babies with gastroschisis small for gestational age? *Pediatr Surg Int* 1997;12:580–582.
3. Torfs CP, Curry CJ. Familial cases of gastroschisis in a population-based registry. *Am J Med Genet* 1993;45:465–467.
4. Glick PL, Harrison MR, Adzick NS. The missing link in the pathogenesis of gastroschisis. *J Pediatr Surg* 1985;20:406–407.
5. Cantrell JR, Haller JA Jr, Ravitch MM. A syndrome of congenital defects involving the abdominal wall, sternum, diaphragm, pericardium, and heart. *Surg Gynecol Obstet* 1958;107:602–605.
6. Calzolari E, Bianchi F, Dolk H, et al. Omphalocele and gastroschisis in Europe: a survey of 3 million births 1980–1990. EUROCAT Working Group. *Am J Med Genet* 1995;58:187–194.
7. Boyd PA, Bhattacharjee A, Gould S, et al. Outcome of prenatally diagnosed anterior abdominal wall defects. *Arch Dis Child Fetal Neonatal Ed* 1998;78:F209–F213.
8. Lurie S, Sherman D, Bukovsky I. Omphalocele delivery enigma: the best mode of delivery still remains dubious. *Eur J Obstet Gynecol Reprod Biol* 1999;82:19–22.
9. Sipes SL, Weiner CP, Sipes DR, et al. Gastroschisis and omphalocele: does either antenatal diagnosis or route of delivery make a difference in perinatal outcome? *Obstet Gynecol* 1990;76:195–199.
10. Hadidi A, Subotic U, Goeppl M, et al. Early elective cesarean delivery before 36 weeks vs late spontaneous delivery in infants with gastroschisis. *J Pediatr Surg* 2008;43:1342–1346.
11. Bethel CA, Seashore JH, Touloukian RJ. Cesarean section does not improve outcome in gastroschisis. *J Pediatr Surg* 1989;24:1–4.
12. Puffinbarger NK, Taylor DV, Tuggle DW, et al. End-tidal carbon dioxide for monitoring primary closure of gastroschisis. *J Pediatr Surg* 1996;31:280–282.
13. Kidd JN Jr, Jackson RJ, Smith SD, et al. Evolution of staged versus primary closure of gastroschisis. *Ann Surg* 2003;237:759–765.
14. Curry JJ, Lander AD, Stringer MD, et al. A multicenter, randomized, double-blind, placebo-controlled trial of the prokinetic agent erythromycin in the postoperative recovery of infants with gastroschisis. *J Pediatr Surg* 2004;39:565–569.
15. Jayanthi S, Seymour P, Puntis JW, et al. Necrotizing enterocolitis after gastroschisis repair: a preventable complication? *J Pediatr Surg* 1998;33:705–707.
16. Phillips JD, Raval MV, Redden C, et al. Gastroschisis, atresia, dysmotility: surgical treatment strategies for a distinct clinical entity. *J Pediatr Surg* 2008;43:2208–2212.
17. van Eijck FC, Wijnen RMH, van Goor H. The incidence and morbidity of adhesions after treatment of neonates with gastroschisis and omphalocele: a 30-year review. *J Pediatr Surg* 2008;43:479–483.
18. Zaccara A, Iacobelli BD, Calzolari A, et al. Cardiopulmonary performances in young children and adolescents born with large abdominal wall defects. *J Pediatr Surg* 2003;38:478–481.
19. Papagrigoriadis S, Browse DJ, Howard ER. Incarceration of umbilical hernias in children: a rare but important complication. *Pediatr Surg Int* 1998;14:231–232.
20. Evans A. The comparative incidence of umbilical hernias in colored and white infants. *J Natl Med Assoc* 1941;33:158–162.
21. Snyder CL. Current management of umbilical abnormalities and related anomalies. *Semin Pediatr Surg* 2007;16:41–49.
22. Snyder WH Jr, Greaney EM Jr. Inguinal hernia. In: Benson CD, Mustard WT, Ravitch MM, et al., eds. *Pediatric Surgery*. Chicago: Year Book Medical; 1962.
23. Rowe MI, Copelson LW, Clatworthy HW. The patent processus vaginalis and the inguinal hernia. *J Pediatr Surg* 1969;4:102–107.
24. Clarnette TD, Lam SK, Hutson JM. Ventriculo-peritoneal shunts in children reveal the natural history of closure of the processus vaginalis. *J Pediatr Surg* 1998;33:413–416.
25. Sato TT, Oldham KT. Pediatric abdomen. In: Mulholland MW, Lillemoe KD, Doherty GM, et L., eds. *Greenfield's Surgery: Scientific Principles and Practice*,, 4th ed. Philadelphia: Lippincott Williams & Wilkins; 2006.
26. Chou TY, Chu CC, Diau GY, et al. Inguinal hernia in children: US versus exploratory surgery and intraoperative contralateral laparoscopy. *Radiology* 1996;201:385–388.
27. Palmer BV. Incarcerated inguinal hernia in children. *Ann R Coll Surg Engl* 1978;60:121–124.
28. Rowe MI, Clatworthy HW. Incarcerated and strangulated hernias in children: a statistical study of high-risk factors. *Arch Surg* 1970;101:136–139.
29. Somri M, Gaitini L, Vaida S, et al. Postoperative outcome in high-risk infants undergoing herniorrhaphy: comparison between spinal and general anesthesia. *Anaesthesia* 1998;53:762–766.
30. Chan KL, Chan HY, Tam PKH. Towards a near-zero recurrence rate in laparoscopic inguinal hernia repair for pediatric patients of all ages. *J Pediatr Surg* 2007;42–1993–1997.
31. Hrabovszky Z, Pinter AB. Routine bilateral exploration for inguinal hernia in infancy and childhood. *Eur J Pediatr Surg* 1995;5:152–155.
32. Wiener ES, Touloukian RJ, Rodgers BM, et al. Hernia survey of the Section on Surgery of the American Academy of Pediatrics. *J Pediatr Surg* 1996;31:1166–1169.
33. Tackett LD, Breuer CK, Luks FI, et al. Incidence of contralateral inguinal hernia: a prospective analysis. *J Pediatr Surg* 1999;34:684–687.
34. Owings EF, Georgeson, KE. A new technique for laparoscopic exploration to find contralateral patent processus vaginalis. *Surg Endosc* 2000;14:114–116.
35. Ron O, Eaton S, Pierro A. Systematic review of the risk of developing a metachronous contralateral inguinal hernia in children. *Br J Surg* 2007;94:804–811.
36. Haller JA Jr, Tepas JJ, Pickard LR, et al. Intestinal atresia: current concepts of pathogenesis, pathophysiology, and operative management. *Am Surg* 1983;49:385–391.
37. Koga Y, Hayashida Y, Ikeda K, et al. Intestinal atresia in fetal dogs produced by localized ligation of mesenteric vessels. *J Pediatr Surg* 1975;10:949–953.
38. Dalla Vecchia LK, Grosfeld JL, West KW, et al. Intestinal atresia and stenosis: a 25-year experience with 277 cases. *Arch Surg* 1998;133:490–496.
39. James LM, Erickson JD, McClean AB. *Prevalence of Birth Defects*. Atlanta: Centers for Disease Control; 1992.
40. Filkins K, Russo J, Flowers WKD. Third trimester ultrasound diagnosis of intestinal atresia following clinical evidence of polyhydramnios. *Prenat Diagn* 1985;5:215–220.
41. Wilmore DW. Factors correlating with a successful outcome following extensive intestinal resection in newborn infants. *J Pediatr* 1972;80:88–95.
42. Touloukian RJ. Intestinal atresia. *Clin Perinatol* 1978;5:3–18.
43. Piper HG, Alesbury J, Waterford SD, et al. Intestinal atresias: factors affecting clinical outcomes. *J Pediatr Surg* 2008;43:1244–1248.
44. Menardi G. Duodenal atresia, stenosis, and annular pancreas. In: Freeman NV, Burge DM, Griffiths M, et al. eds. *Surgery of the Newborn*. Edinburgh: Churchill Livingstone; 1994:107–115.
45. Stauffer UG, Schwoebel M. Duodenal atresia and stenosis–annular pancreas. In: O'Neill JA Jr, Rowe MI, Grosfeld JL, et al. eds. *Pediatric Surgery*. St. Louis, MO: Mosby; 1998:1133–1143.
46. Stauffer UG, Irving I. Duodenal atresia and stenosis—long-term results. *Prog Pediatr Surg* 1977;10:49–60.
47. Kimura K, Mukohara N, Nishijima E, et al. Diamond-shaped anastomosis for duodenal atresia: an experience with 44 patients over 15 years. *J Pediatr Surg* 1990;25:977–979.
48. Valusek PA, Spilde TL, Tsao K, et al. Laparoscopic duodenal atresia repair using surgical U-clips: a novel technique. *Surg Endosc* 2007;21:1023–1024.
49. Weber TR, Lewis JE, Mooney D, et al. Duodenal atresia: a comparison of techniques of repair. *J Pediatr Surg* 1986;21:1133–1136.
50. Peña A. *Atlas of Surgical Management of Anorectal Malformations*. New York: Springer-Verlag; 1990.
51. Spouge D, Baird PA. Imperforate anus in 700,000 consecutive liveborn infants. *Am J Med Genet* 1986;2(suppl):151–161.
52. Schuster SR, Teele RL. An analysis of ultrasound scanning as a guide in determination of "high" or "low" imperforate anus. *J Pediatr Surg* 1979;14:798–800.
53. Ong NT, Beasley SW. Long-term continence in patients with high and intermediate anorectal anomalies treated by sacroperineal (Stephens) rectoplasty. *J Pediatr Surg* 1991;26:44–48.
54. Ito Y, Yokoyama J, Hayashi A, et al. Reappraisal of endorectal pull-through procedure: I. Anorectal malformations. *J Pediatr Surg* 1981;16:476–483.

55. Georgeson KE, Inge TH, Albanese CT. Laparoscopically assisted anorectal pull-through for high imperforate anus—a new technique. *J Pediatr Surg* 2000;35:927–930.
56. Kiesewetter WB, Hoon A. Imperforate anus: an analysis of mortalities during a 25-year period. *Prog Pediatr Surg* 1979;13:211–220.
57. Kiesewetter WB, Chang JH. Imperforate anus: a five- to thirty-year follow-up perspective. *Prog Pediatr Surg* 1977;10:111–120.
58. Bliss DP Jr, Tapper D, Anderson JM, et al. Does posterior sagittal anorectoplasty in patients with high imperforate anus provide superior fecal continence? *J Pediatr Surg* 1996;31:26–30.
59. Rintala RJ, Pakarinen MP. Imperforate anus: long- and short-term outcome. *Semin Pediatr Surg* 2008;17:79–89.
60. Lin PW, Nasr TR, Stoll BJ. Necrotizing enterocolitis: recent scientific advances in pathophysiology and prevention. *Semin Perinatol* 2008;32:70–82.
61. Anderson DM, Kliegman RM. The relationship of neonatal alimentation practices to the occurrence of endemic necrotizing enterocolitis. *Am J Perinatol* 1991;8:62–67.
62. Rayyis SF, Ambalavanan N, Wright L, et al. Randomized trial of "slow" versus "fast" feed advancements on the incidence of necrotizing enterocolitis in very low birth weight infants. *J Pediatr* 1999;134:293–297.
63. Lin HC, Hsu CH, Chen HL, et al. Oral probiotics prevent necrotizing enterocolitis in very low birth weight preterm infants: a multicenter, randomized, controlled trial. *Pediatrics* 2008;122:693–700.
64. Grosfeld JL, Cheu H, Schlatter M, et al. Changing trends in necrotizing enterocolitis: experience with 302 cases in two decades. *Ann Surg* 1991;214:300–306.
65. Pokorny WJ, Garcia-Prats JA, Barry YN. Necrotizing enterocolitis: incidence, operative care, and outcome. *J Pediatr Surg* 1986;21:1149–1154.
66. Andrews DA, Sawin RS, Ledbetter DJ, et al. Necrotizing enterocolitis in term neonates. *Am J Surg* 1990;159:507–509.
67. Bell MJ, Kosloske AM, Benton C, et al. Neonatal necrotizing enterocolitis: prevention of perforation. *J Pediatr Surg* 1973;8:601–605.
68. Grosfeld JL, Chaet M, Molinari F, et al. Increased risk of necrotizing enterocolitis in premature infants with patent ductus arteriosus treated with indomethacin. *Ann Surg* 1996;224:350–355.
69. Ricketts RR. The role of paracentesis in the management of infants with necrotizing enterocolitis. *Am Surg* 1986;52:61–65.
70. Cooper A, Ross AJ, O'Neill JA Jr, et al. Resection with primary anastomosis for necrotizing enterocolitis: a contrasting view. *J Pediatr Surg* 1988;23:64–68.
71. Ade-Ajayi N, Kiely E, Drake D, et al. Resection and primary anastomosis in necrotizing enterocolitis. *J R Soc Med* 1996;89:385–388.
72. Sato TT, Oldham KT. Abdominal drain placement versus laparotomy for necrotizing enterocolitis with perforation. *Clin Perinatol* 2004;31:577–589.
73. Moss RL, Dimmitt RA, Barnhart DC, et al. Laparotomy versus peritoneal drainage for necrotizing enterocolitis and perforation. *N Engl J Med* 2006;354:2225–2234.
74. O'Connor A, Sawin RS. High morbidity of enterostomy and its closure in premature infants with necrotizing enterocolitis. *Arch Surg* 1998;133:875–880.
75. Schwartz MZ, Hayden CK, Richardson CJ, et al. A prospective evaluation of intestinal stenosis following necrotizing enterocolitis. *J Pediatr Surg* 1982;17:764–770.
76. Moss RL, Dimmitt RA, Henry MC, et al. A meta-analysis of peritoneal drainage versus laparotomy for perforated necrotizing enterocolitis. *J Pediatr Surg* 2001;36:1210–1213.
77. Patel JC, Tepas JJ III, Huffman SD, et al. Neonatal necrotizing enterocolitis: the long-term perspective. *Am Surg* 1998;64:575–579.
78. [No authors listed.] Statement from the National Institutes of Health workshop on population screening for the cystic fibrosis gene. *N Engl J Med* 1990;323:70–71.
79. Riordan JR, Rommens JM, Kerem B, et al. Identification of the cystic fibrosis gene: cloning and characterization of complementary DNA. *Science* 1989;245:1066–1073.
80. Kerem B, Rommens JM, Buchanan JA, et al. Identification of the cystic fibrosis gene: genetic analysis. *Science* 1989;245:1073–1080.
81. Rosenstein BJ, Cutting GR. The diagnosis of cystic fibrosis: a consensus statement. Cystic Fibrosis Foundation Consensus Panel. *J Pediatr* 1998;132:589–595.
82. Quinton PM. Cystic fibrosis: a disease in electrolyte transport. *FASEB J* 1990;4:2709–2717.
83. Quinton PM, Bijman J. Higher bioelectric potentials due to decreased chloride absorption in the sweat glands of patients with cystic fibrosis. *N Engl J Med* 1983;308:1185–1189.
84. Irish MS, Ragi JM, Karamanoukian H, et al. Prenatal diagnosis of the fetus with cystic fibrosis and meconium ileus. *Pediatr Surg Int* 1997;12:434–436.
85. Kao SC, Franken EA Jr. Nonoperative treatment of simple meconium ileus: a survey of the Society for Pediatric Radiology. *Pediatr Radiol* 1995;25:97–100.
86. Mak GZ, Harberg FJ, Hiatt P, et al. T-tube ileostomy for meconium ileus: four decades of experience. *J Pediatr Surg* 2000;35:349–352.
87. Del Pin CA, Czyrko C, Ziegler MM, et al. Management and survival of meconium ileus: a 30-year review. *Ann Surg* 1992;215:179–185.
88. Docherty JG, Zaki A, Coutts JA, et al. Meconium ileus: a review 1972–1990. *Br J Surg* 1992;79:571–573.
89. Sato TT. Abnormal rotation and fixation of the intestine. In: Wyllie R, Hyams JS, eds. *Pediatric Gastrointestinal and Liver Disease*. Elsevier: London; 2006.
90. Andrassy RJ, Mahour GH. Malrotation of the midgut in infants and children: a 25-year review. *Arch Surg* 1981;116:158–160.
91. Ford EG, Senac MO Jr, Srikanth MS, et al. Malrotation of the intestine in children. *Ann Surg* 1992;215:172–178.
92. Powell DM, Othersen HB, Smith CD. Malrotation of the intestines in children: the effect of age on presentation and therapy. *J Pediatr Surg* 1989;24:777–780.
93. Weinberger E, Winters WD, Liddell RM, et al. Sonographic diagnosis of intestinal malrotation in infants: importance of the relative positions of the superior mesenteric vein and artery. *AJR Am J Roentgenol* 1992;159:825–828.
94. Ladd WE, Gross RE. *Abdominal Surgery of Infancy and Childhood*. Philadelphia: WB Saunders; 1941.
95. Bass KD, Rothenberg SS, Chang JH. Laparoscopic Ladd's procedure in infants with malrotation. *J Pediatr Surg* 1998;33:279–281.
96. Fujimoto T, Hata J, Yokoyama S, et al. A study of the extracellular matrix protein as the migration pathway of neural crest cells in the gut: analysis in human embryos with special reference to the pathogenesis of Hirschsprung's disease. *J Pediatr Surg* 1989;24:550–556.
97. Kleinhaus S, Boley SJ, Sheran M, et al. Hirschsprung's disease—a survey of the members of the Surgical Section of the American Academy of Pediatrics. *J Pediatr Surg* 1979;14:588–597.
98. Tomita R, Munakata K, Kurosu Y. Peptidergic nerves in Hirschsprung's disease and its allied disorders. *Eur J Pediatr Surg* 1994;4:346–351.
99. Kusafuka T, Puri P. Altered mRNA expression of the neuronal nitric oxide synthase gene in Hirschsprung's disease. *J Pediatr Surg* 1997;32:1054–1058.
100. Puri P, Wester T. Intestinal neuronal dysplasia. *Semin Pediatr Surg* 1998;7:181–186.
101. Meier-Ruge WA, Ammann K, Bruder E, et al. Updated results on intestinal neuronal dysplasia (IND B). *Eur J Pediatr Surg* 2004;14:384–391.
102. Tanaka H, Moroi K, Iwai J, et al. Novel mutations of the endothelin B receptor gene in patients with Hirschsprung's disease and their characterization. *J Biol Chem* 1998;273:11378–11383.
103. Kusafuka T, Puri P. Genetic aspects of Hirschsprung's disease. *Semin Pediatr Surg* 1998;7:148–155.
104. Robertson K, Mason I, Hall S. Hirschsprung's disease: genetic mutations in mice and men. *Gut* 1997;41:436–441.
105. Puri P, Ohshiro K, Wester T. Hirschsprung's disease: a search for etiology. *Semin Pediatr Surg* 1998;7:140–147.
106. Puffenberger EG, Kauffman ER, Bolk S, et al. Identity-by-descent and association mapping of a recessive gene for Hirschsprung disease on human chromosome 13q22. *Hum Mol Genet* 1994;3:1217–1225.
107. Romeo G, Ronchetto P, Luo Y, et al. Point mutations affecting the tyrosine kinase domain of the RET protooncogene in Hirschsprung's disease. *Nature* 1994;367:377–378.
108. Quinn FM, Surana R, Puri P. The influence of trisomy 21 on outcome in children with Hirschsprung's disease. *J Pediatr Surg* 1994;29:781–783.
109. Qualman SJ, Jaffe R, Bove KE, et al. Diagnosis of Hirschsprung disease using the rectal biopsy: multi-institutional survey. *Pediatr Dev Pathol* 1999;2:588–596.
110. Ramesh JC, Ramanujam TM, Yik YI, et al. Management of Hirschsprung's disease with reference to one-stage pull-through without colostomy. *J Pediatr Surg* 1999;34:1691–1694.
111. Albanese CT, Jennings RW, Smith B, et al. Perineal one-stage pull-through for Hirschsprung's disease. *J Pediatr Surg* 1999;34:377–380.
112. Georgeson KE, Cohen RD, Hebra A, et al. Primary laparoscopic-assisted endorectal colon pull-through for Hirschsprung's disease: a new gold standard. *Ann Surg* 1999;229:678–682.
113. Skinner MA. Hirschsprung's disease. *Curr Probl Surg* 1996;33:389–460.
114. Saleh W, Rasheed K, Al Mohaidly M, et al. Management of Hirschsprung's disease: a comparison of Soave's and Duhamel's pull-through methods. *Pediatr Surg Int* 2004;20:590–593.
115. Sawin R, Hatch E, Schaller R, et al. Limited surgery for lower-segment Hirschsprung's disease. *Arch Surg* 1994;129:920–924.
116. Vanderwinden JM, Mailleux P, Schiffmann SN, et al. Nitric oxide synthase activity in infantile hypertrophic pyloric stenosis. *N Engl J Med* 1992;327:511–515.
117. Saur D, Vanderwinden J, Seidler B, et al. Single-nucleotide promoter polymorphism alters transcription of neuronal nitric oxide synthase exon 1c in infantile hypertrophic pyloric stenosis. *Proc Natl Acad Sci U S A* 2004;101:1662–1667.
118. Rasmussen L, Green A, Hansen LP. The epidemiology of infantile hypertrophic pyloric stenosis in a Danish population, 1950–84. *Int J Epidemiol* 1989;18:413–417.
119. Honein MA, Paulozzi LJ, Himelright IM, et al. Infantile hypertrophic pyloric stenosis after pertussis prophylaxis with erythromycin: a case review and cohort study. *Lancet* 1999;354:2101–2105.
120. Schechter R, Torfs CP, Bateson TF. The epidemiology of infantile hypertrophic pyloric stenosis. *Paediatr Perinat Epidemiol* 1997;11:407–427.
121. Hall NJ, Van Der Zee J, Tan HL, et al. Meta-analysis of laparoscopic versus open pyloromyotomy. *Ann Surg* 2004;240:774–778.
122. St Peter SD, Holcomb GW, Calkins CM, et al. Open versus laparoscopic pyloromyotomy for pyloric stenosis. *Ann Surg* 2006;244:363–370.
123. Langer JC, To T. Does pediatric surgical specialty training affect outcome after Ramstedt pyloromyotomy? A population-based study. *Pediatrics* 2004;113:1342–1347.
124. Kim YS, Rhu JH. Intussusception in infancy and childhood: analysis of 385 cases. *Int Surg* 1989;74:114–118.

125. From the Centers for Disease Control and Prevention. Withdrawal of rotavirus vaccine recommendation. *JAMA* 1999;282:2113–2114.
126. Postmarketing monitoring of intussusception after RotaTeq vaccination—United States, February 1, 2006–February 15, 2007. *MMWR Morb Mortal Wkly Rep* 2007;56:218–222.
127. Okuyama H, Nakai H, Okada A. Is barium enema reduction safe and effective in patients with a long duration of intussusception? *Pediatr Surg Int* 1999;15:105–107.
128. Poddoubnyi IV, Dronov AF, Blinnikov OI, et al. Laparoscopy in the treatment of intussusception in children. *J Pediatr Surg* 1998;33:1194–1197.
129. Cheung ST, Lee KH, Yeung TH, et al. Minimally invasive approach in the management of childhood intussusception. *ANZ J Surg* 2007;77:778–781.
130. Bonnard A, Demarche M, Dimitriu C, et al. Indications for laparoscopy in the management of intussusception: a multicenter retrospective study conducted by the French Study Group for Pediatric Laparoscopy (GECI). *J Pediatr Surg* 2008;43:1249–1253.
131. Schier F, Hoffmann K, Waldschmidt J. Laparoscopic removal of Meckel's diverticula in children. *Eur J Pediatr Surg* 1996;6:38–39.
132. Bonadio WA, Jona JZ, Glicklich M, et al. Esophageal bougienage technique for coin ingestion in children. *J Pediatr Surg* 1988;23:917–918.
133. Stuth EA, Stucke AG, Cohen RD, et al. Successful resuscitation of a child after exsanguination due to aortoesophageal fistula from undiagnosed foreign body. *Anesthesiology* 2001;95:1025–1026.
134. Maves MD, Carithers JS, Birck HG. Esophageal burns secondary to disc battery ingestion. *Ann Otol Rhinol Laryngol* 1984;93:364–369.
135. Thompson EC, Brown MF, Bowen EC, et al. Causes of gastrointestinal hemorrhage in neonates and children. *South Med J* 1996;89:370–374.
136. McDougal WS, Izant RJ Jr, Zollinger RM Jr. Primary peritonitis in infancy and childhood. *Ann Surg* 1975;181:310–313.
137. Zurowska A, Feneberg R, Warady BA, et al. Gram-negative peritonitis in children undergoing long-term peritoneal dialysis. *Am J Kidney Dis* 2008;51:455–462.
138. Zganjer M, Cizmic A, Cigit I, et al. Treatment of rectal prolapse in children with cow milk injection sclerotherapy: 30-year experience. *World J Gastroenterol* 2008;14:737–740.
139. Newman KD. Malignant liver tumors of children. *Semin Pediatr Surg* 1992;1:145–151.
140. Bowman LC, Riely CA. Management of pediatric liver tumors. *Surg Oncol Clin N Am* 1996;5:451–459.
141. Luks FI, Yazbeck S, Brandt ML, et al. Benign liver tumors in children: a 25-year experience. *J Pediatr Surg* 1991;26:1326–1330.
142. Hernandez F, Navarro M, Encinas JL, et al. The role of GLUT1 immunostaining in the diagnosis and classification of liver vascular tumors in children. *J Pediatr Surg* 2005;40:801–804.
143. Huang SA. Tu HM, Harney JW, et al. Severe hypothyroidism caused by type 3 iodothyronine deiodinase in infantile hemangioma. *N Engl J Med* 2000;343:185–187.
144. Christison-Lagay ER, Burrows PE, Alomari A, et al. Hepatic hemangiomas: subtype classification and development of a clinical practice algorithm and registry. *J Pediatr Surg* 2007;42:62–68.
145. Isaacs H Jr. Fetal and neonatal hepatic tumors. *J Pediatr Surg* 2007;42:1797–1803.
146. Ein SH, Stephens CA. Benign liver tumors and cysts in childhood. *J Pediatr Surg* 1974;9:847–851.
147. Tiao GM, Bobey N, Allen S, et al. The current management of hepatoblastoma: a combination of chemotherapy, conventional resection, and liver transplantation. *J Pediatr* 2005;146:204–211.
148. Pham TH, Iqbal CW, Grams JM, et al. Outcomes of primary liver cancer in children: an appraisal of experience. *J Pediatr Surg* 2007;42:834–839.
149. Austin MT, Leys CM, Feurer ID, et al. Liver transplantation for childhood hepatic malignancy: a review of the United Network for Organ Sharing (UNOS) database. *J Pediatr Surg* 2006;41:182–186.
150. Urban CE, Mache CJ, Schwinger W, et al. Undifferentiated (embryonal) sarcoma of the liver in childhood: successful combined-modality therapy in four patients. *Cancer* 1993;72:2511–2516.
151. Finegold MJ, Egler RA, Goss JA, et al. Liver tumors: pediatric population. *Liver Transpl* 2008;14:1545–1556.
152. Randolph JG, Altman RP, Arensman RM, et al. Liver resection in children with hepatic neoplasms. *Ann Surg* 1978;187:599–605.
153. Larsen LR, Raffensperger J. Liver abscess. *J Pediatr Surg* 1979;14:329–331.
154. Wells CD, Arguedas M. Amebic liver abscess. *South Med J* 2004;97:673–682.
155. Balistreri WF, Grand R, Hoofnagle JH, et al. Biliary atresia: current concepts and research directions. *Hepatology* 1996;23:1682–1692.
156. Tan CE, Davenport M, Driver M, et al. Does the morphology of the extrahepatic biliary remnants in biliary atresia influence survival? A review of 205 cases. *J Pediatr Surg* 1994;29:1459–1464.
157. Chandra RS, Altman RP. Ductal remnants in extrahepatic biliary atresia: a histopathologic study with clinical correlation. *J Pediatr* 1978;93:196–200.
158. Schmeling DJ, Oldham KT, Guice KS, et al. Experimental obliterative cholangitis: a model for the study of biliary atresia. *Ann Surg* 1991;213:350–355.
159. Kobayashi H, Stringer MD. Biliary atresia. *Semin Perinatol* 2003;8:383–391.
160. Ryckman FC, Alonso MH, Bucuvalas JC, et al. Biliary atresia—surgical management and treatment options as they relate to outcome. *Liver Transpl Surg* 1998;4(5 suppl 1):S24–S33.
161. Visser BC, Suh I, Hirose S, et al. The influence of portoenterostomy on transplantation for biliary atresia. *Liver Transpl* 2004;10:1279–1286.
162. Davenport M, Puricelli V, Farrant P, et al. The outcome of the older (>100 days) infant with biliary atresia. *J Pediatr Surg* 2004;4:575–581.
163. Ogasawara Y, Yamataka A, Tsukamoto K, et al. The intussusception antireflux valve is ineffective for preventing cholangitis in biliary atresia: a prospective study. *J Pediatr Surg* 2003;38:1826–1829.
164. Kasai M, Suzuki H, Ohashi E, et al. Technique and results of operative management of biliary atresia. *World J Surg* 1978;2:571–579.
165. Rothenberg SS, Schroter GP, Karrer FM, et al. Cholangitis after the Kasai operation for biliary atresia. *J Pediatr Surg* 1989;24:729–732.
166. Dolgin, SE. Answered and unanswered controversies in the surgical management of extra hepatic biliary atresia. *Pediatr Transplant* 2004;8:628–631.
167. Shneider BL, Brown MB, Haber B, et al. A multicenter study of the outcome of biliary atresia in the United States, 1997–000. *J Pediatr* 2006;148:467–474.
168. Stringer MD. Biliary atresia: service delivery and outcomes. *Semin Pediatr Surg* 2008;17:116–122.
169. Goss JA, Shackleton CR, Swenson K, et al. Orthotopic liver transplantation for congenital biliary atresia: an 11-year, single-center experience. *Ann Surg* 1996;224:276–284.
170. Cowles RA, Lobritto SJ, Ventura KA, et al. Timing of liver transplantation in biliary atresia—results in 71 children managed by a multidisciplinary team. *J Pediatr Surg* 2008;43:1605–1609.
171. Alonso-Lej F, Revor WB, Pessagno DJ. Congenital choledochal cyst, with a report of 2, and an analysis of 94 cases. *Surg Gynecol Obstet* 1959;108:1–30.
172. Todani T, Watanabe Y, Narusue M, et al. Congenital bile duct cysts: classification, operative procedures, and review of thirty-seven cases including cancer arising from choledochal cyst. *Am J Surg* 1977;134:263–269.
173. Todani T, Tabuchi K, Watanabe Y, et al. Carcinoma arising in the wall of congenital bile duct cysts. *Cancer* 1979;44:1134–1141.
174. Fieber SS, Nance FC. Choledochal cyst and neoplasm: a comprehensive review of 106 cases and presentation of two original cases. *Am Surg* 1997;63:982–987.
175. Miyano T, Yamataka A, Kato Y, et al. Hepaticoenterostomy after excision of choledochal cyst in children: a 30-year experience with 180 cases. *J Pediatr Surg* 1996;31:1417–1421.
176. Flanigan PD. Biliary cysts. *Ann Surg* 1975;182:635–643.
177. Lipsett PA, Pitt HA, Colombani PM, et al. Choledochal cyst disease: a changing pattern of presentation. *Ann Surg* 1994;220:644–652.
178. Werlin SL. Disorders of the pancreas in children. *Curr Opin Pediatr* 1998;10:507–511.
179. Warshaw AL, Richter JM, Schapiro RH. The cause and treatment of pancreatitis associated with pancreas divisum. *Ann Surg* 1983;198:443–452.
180. Adzick NS, Shamberger RC, Winter HS, et al. Surgical treatment of pancreas divisum causing pancreatitis in children. *J Pediatr Surg* 1989;24:54–58.
181. Kagan RJ, Reyes HM, Asokan S. Pseudocyst of the pancreas in childhood: current advances in diagnosis. *Arch Surg* 1981;116:1200–1203.
182. Rescorla FJ, Plumley DA, Sherman S, et al. The efficacy of early ERCP in pediatric pancreatic trauma. *J Pediatr Surg* 1995;30:336–340.
183. Cooney DR, Grosfeld JL. Operative management of pancreatic pseudocysts in infants and children: a review of 75 cases. *Ann Surg* 1975;182:590–596.
184. Grosfeld JL, Vane DW, Rescorla FJ, et al. Pancreatic tumors in childhood: analysis of 13 cases. *J Pediatr Surg* 1990;25:1057–1062.
185. Shamberger RC, Hendren WH, Leichtner AM. Long-term nutritional and metabolic consequences of pancreaticoduodenectomy in children. *Surgery* 1994;115:382–388.
186. Wang KS, Albanese C, Dada F, et al. Papillary cystic neoplasm of the pancreas: a report of three pediatric cases and literature review. *J Pediatr Surg* 1998;33:842–845.
187. Wilson SD. Zollinger-Ellison syndrome in children: a 25-year follow-up. *Surgery* 1991;110:696–702.
188. Sempoux C, Poggi F, Brunelle F, et al. Nesidioblastosis and persistent neonatal hyperinsulinism. *Diabetes Metab* 1995;21:402–407.
189. Aynsley-Green A, Polak JM, Bloom SR, et al. Nesidioblastosis of the pancreas: definition of the syndrome and the management of the severe neonatal hyperinsulinaemic hypoglycaemia. *Arch Dis Child* 1981;56:496–508.
190. Hirsch HJ, Loo S, Evans N, et al. Hypoglycemia of infancy and nesidioblastosis: studies with somatostatin. *N Engl J Med* 1977;296:1323–1326.
191. Adzick NS, Thornton PS, Stanley CA, et al. A multidisciplinary approach to the focal form of congenital hyperinsulinism leads to successful treatment by partial pancreatectomy. *J Pediatr Surg* 2004;39:270–275.
192. Becherer A, Szabo M, Karanikas G, et al. Imaging of advanced neuroendocrine tumors with 18 F-FDOPA PET. *J Nucl Med* 2003;45:1161–1167.
193. Viola KV, Sosa JA. Current advances in the diagnosis and treatment of pancreatic endocrine tumors. *Curr Opin Oncol* 2005;17:24–27.
194. Willberg B, Muller E. Surgery for nesidioblastosis—indications, treatment, and results. *Prog Pediatr Surg* 1991;26:76–83.
195. Leibowitz G, Glaser B, Higazi AA, et al. Hyperinsulinemic hypoglycemia of infancy (nesidioblastosis) in clinical remission: high incidence of diabetes mellitus and persistent beta-cell dysfunction at long-term follow-up. *J Clin Endocrinol Metab* 1995;80:386–392.
196. Grosfeld JL. Jejunoileal atresia and stenosis. In: O'Neill JA Jr, Rowe MI, Grosfeld JL, et al. eds. *Pediatric Surgery,* 5th ed. St. Louis, MO: Mosby; 1998:1145–1158.

CHAPTER 108 ■ THE PEDIATRIC GENITOURINARY SYSTEM

EUGENE MINEVICH AND CURTIS A. SHELDON

KEY POINTS

1. The nephric system develops progressively through three stages.
2. Horseshoe kidney is the most common type of renal fusion and occurs in 0.25% of the population.
3. Renal cystic disease, congenital or acquired, is one of the most common causes of the pediatric abdominal mass.
4. Multicystic dysplastic kidney is the most common type of renal cystic disease.
5. The ureteropelvic junction is the most common site of obstruction in the urinary tract and the most common cause of neonatal hydronephrosis.
6. Ureteral duplication is the most common anomaly of the urinary tract.
7. The incidence of vesicoureteral reflux in otherwise normal children is approximately 1%; the incidence is up to 40% in patients undergoing evaluation for urinary tract infection.
8. Epispadias in boys consists of a dorsally placed urethral meatus, and the degree of penile deformity is related to the extent of the meatal displacement.
9. Posterior urethral valves are the most common obstructive urethral lesions in male infants and consist of a membrane or mucosal leaflet within the prostatic urethra.
10. Descent of the testis from its original position near the kidney into the cooler scrotum is necessary for its normal development and production of fertile sperm. True undescended testes fail to reach the scrotum despite following a normal line of descent.
11. Prepubertal testis tumors account for approximately 2% of all testicular tumors, with a peak patient age of approximately 2 years.

THE NEPHRIC SYSTEM

1 The nephric system develops progressively through three stages. The initial stage, *the pronephros*, disappears completely by the fourth week of embryonic life. *The mesonephros*, the second stage, degenerates as well, although part of its system becomes associated with the reproductive system. The caudal portion of the mesonephric duct, which communicates with the cloaca, forms a ureteral bud between the fourth and sixth weeks of gestation. The cranial portion of the ureteral bud joins with the metanephric blastema, branching into the renal pelvis and the calyces and inducing nephron formation during the final stage of development, *metanephros*. The kidneys undergo ascent and rotation before assuming their final position.

ANOMALIES OF THE KIDNEY

Supernumerary Kidney

The supernumerary kidney is a very rare anomaly of the urinary system and represents a distinct extra kidney (or kidneys). Embryologically, an additional ureteral bud develops a separate metanephric mass, resulting in the formation of an extra kidney, which is usually caudal to the dominant kidney. This anomaly is usually an incidental finding on abdominal imaging for unrelated reasons, although some adults may occasionally present with abdominal pain, hypertension, or symptoms of urinary tract infections (UTIs).

Renal Agenesis

Absence of a ureteral bud or its failure to join the metanephric blastema results in renal agenesis. A bilateral anomaly occurs in approximately 1 per 4,000 births (*Potter syndrome*). This is manifested by characteristic faces, pulmonary hypoplasia, and orthopedic abnormalities.[1] These infants are stillborn or rapidly die of respiratory failure.

The incidence of unilateral renal agenesis is about 1 in 1,200 births. The ipsilateral ureter is absent in more than 50% of cases, although an adrenal gland is usually present. The most common contralateral anomalies are vesicoureteral reflux (30%), renal malrotation, or renal ectopia (15%). Genital anomalies are more often observed in girls (25% to 50%) than in boys (10% to 15%); malformations of the rectum, anus, and lower spine frequently occur in both sexes. Other associated congenital anomalies may involve the cardiovascular, gastrointestinal, or musculoskeletal systems. Unilateral renal agenesis is usually asymptomatic and found incidentally.

Renal Ectopy

Failure of the *metanephros* to ascend leads to an ectopic kidney, which occurs in about 1 in 1,100 people. An ectopic kidney may be on the ipsilateral side (*simple ectopy*) or on the contralateral side (*crossed ectopy*) with or without fusion. The adrenal gland develops separately from the kidney and is therefore found in its normal position, despite anomalies in renal position. Further classification of renal ectopia is based on the position of the kidney in the retroperitoneum: abdominal, lumbar, or pelvic kidney. Rarely, the kidney is located above the ipsilateral diaphragm (*intrathoracic kidney*) because of delayed closure of the diaphragm or accelerated kidney ascent.

Most ectopic kidneys are clinically asymptomatic and detected incidentally. Almost half of ectopic kidneys have hydronephrosis secondary to malrotation, aberrant renal vessels compressing the renal pelvis, or ureteropelvic junction (UPJ) obstruction.[2] If surgical correction of the obstructed kidney is required, the anomalous renal vasculature may be important. Ectopic kidney function should be preserved because the contralateral kidney is abnormal in up to 50% of patients, with hydronephrosis or vesicoureteral reflux (VUR) being the most common abnormality. Genital anomalies have been reported in 15% to 45% of patients with renal ectopia.

Horseshoe Kidney

2 Horseshoe kidney is the most common type of renal fusion and occurs in 0.25% of the population. Patients with Turner syndrome and trisomy 18 have a significantly higher incidence. The anomaly consists of two renal masses connected by the isthmus at the midline, usually at the lower poles. The isthmus, which consists of renal parenchyma or fibrous tissue, usually lies just below the junction of the inferior mesenteric artery and aorta and anterior to the great vessels. The pelvises and ureters of horseshoe kidney are usually anteriorly placed, crossing the isthmus ventrally.

The horseshoe kidney does not usually produce symptoms unless it is associated with other anomalies. The most commonly associated abnormality is VUR and UPJ obstruction, which can lead to UTI or urolithiasis, with corresponding symptomatology. If surgical repair of UPJ obstruction is required, a standard dismembered pyeloplasty with or without division of the renal isthmus is recommended. The retroperitoneal flank approach is usually successful, but the surgeon should be prepared for a transperitoneal approach as well. The incidence of Wilms tumor seems to be increased in patients with horseshoe kidney.[3]

Cystic Disease of the Kidney

3 Renal cystic disease, congenital or acquired, is one of the most common causes of pediatric abdominal masses. Several classifications have been proposed, based on the clinical or radiologic presentation, pathologic studies, and genetic associations.[4]

Autosomal recessive ("infantile") polycystic kidney disease results from dilated collecting ducts and has a spectrum of severity, with the severest forms appearing in infancy. This congenital disorder affects both kidneys and liver (ranging from biliary ectasia to congenital hepatic fibrosis). The affected infant usually presents with large flank masses. Renal ultrasound (RUS) demonstrates enlarged, homogeneously hyperechogenic kidneys. Most children develop progressive renal and/or hepatic failure.

4 *Multicystic dysplastic kidney (MCDK)* is the most common type of renal cystic disease. This anomaly represents a severe form of renal dysplasia with complete replacement of renal parenchyma by different-sized cysts (Fig. 108.1). RUS is usually definitive in making the correct diagnosis, although renal scintigraphy is necessary to demonstrate the absence of renal function in the involved kidney and occasionally differentiate MCDK from severe obstructed hydronephrosis. The high incidence of VUR in the solitary functioning contralateral kidney (18% to 43%) makes a voiding cystourethrogram (VCUG) an essential part of the evaluation. Involution of MCDK may occur to the point that the involved kidney disappears from subsequent sonograms. Potential long-term sequelae of retained MCDK, including hypertension, infection, and pain, are very rare. Sporadic reports of renal cell carcinoma and Wilms tumor in MCDK raise concern of the persistent potential for malignant degeneration in the dysplastic kidney. Patients with MCDK should be followed with ultrasonic surveillance, especially in early childhood.[5] Nephrectomy is reserved for the symptomatic child, the patient with equivocal radiologic appearance, or MCDK that fails to regress.

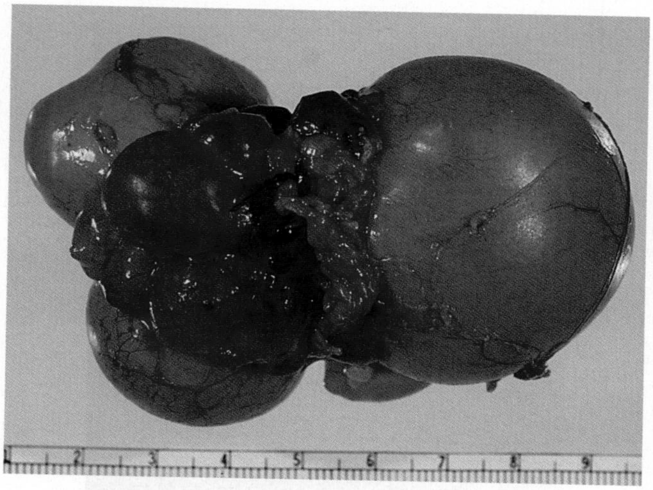

FIGURE 108.1. Multicystic dysplastic kidney.

Ureteropelvic Junction Obstruction

5 The UPJ is the most common site of obstruction in the urinary tract and the most common cause of neonatal hydronephrosis. The pathogenesis of this disorder is variable. Of the intrinsic factors, the adynamic segment is associated most often with classic UPJ obstruction. This obstruction is thought to be a congenital absence or abnormal arrangement of the muscular fiber at the transition zone of the upper ureter and renal pelvis leading to failure of peristaltic wave propagation. Extrinsic causes include fibrous bands, aberrant accessory vessels, and various organ-compressing factors. Most cases of UPJ obstruction are diagnosed in utero and such patients are initially asymptomatic. Some children present with abdominal or flank pain, hematuria, or UTI. Occasionally, previously asymptomatic UPJ obstruction may be discovered in the patient with renal injury following relatively minor abdominal trauma.

RUS is the test of choice to determine the degree of renal pelvic dilatation, parenchymal thickness, and associated abnormalities of the bladder and the ureter. Diuretic renography and occasionally Whitaker antegrade pressure perfusion studies are necessary to confirm UPJ obstruction. The VCUG and occasional excretory urogram (intravenous pyelogram [IVP]) may define anatomic details (Fig. 108.2). Retrograde pyelography is used to rule out other causes of obstruction and is usually performed just before surgery.

A dismembered pyeloplasty, with removal of an adynamic segment, remains the surgical treatment of choice because it provides dependant drainage of the renal pelvis. With utilization of optical magnification and careful attention to surgical technique, a successful outcome should be expected in over 95% of cases.[6] Laparoscopic pyeloplasty can be performed in older children.

ANOMALIES OF THE URETER

Ureteral Duplication

6 Ureteral duplication is the most common anomaly of the urinary tract. Early branching of the single ureteral bud results in *incomplete (partial) duplication* with a single ureteral orifice and bifid proximal ureters (1 in 125 individuals). An accessory ureteral bud creates *complete duplication* (1 in 500 individuals), with the upper ureter usually inserting into the bladder

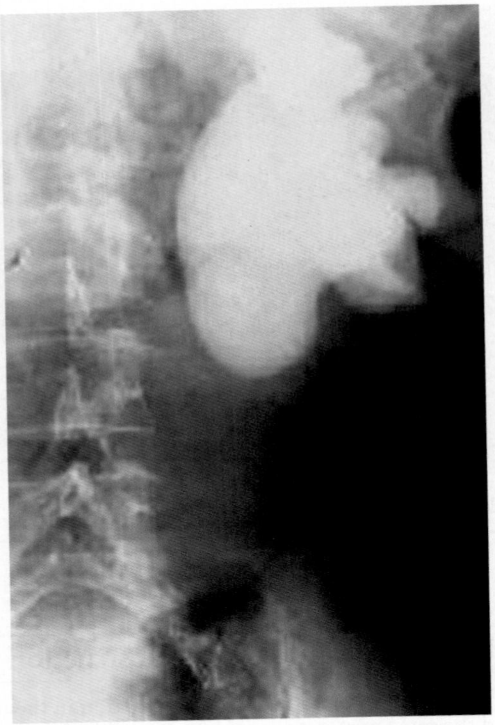

FIGURE 108.2. Intravenous pyelogram showing hydronephrosis secondary to ureteropelvic junction obstruction.

more medially and inferiorly than the lower ureter. The upper ureter is more likely to be associated with ectopic insertion, ureterocele, or obstruction, whereas the lower ureter is frequently associated with VUR. Most patients with ureteral duplication are asymptomatic, although they occasionally present with UTI.

Ureteral Ectopia and Ureterocele

The ectopic ureteral orifice lies in a position caudal to the normal insertion of the ureter on the bladder trigone. Ureteral ectopia is much more common in association with complete ureteral duplication. In the boy, ectopic ureteral orifices are most frequently found at the prostatic urethra and even along the course of the male genital ductal system. In the girl, ectopic ureters can be found draining into the bladder neck, urethra, vagina, or even the uterus. Boys with bilateral anomaly and girls with termination of an ectopic ureter below the external urinary sphincter usually present with urinary incontinence.

Ureteroceles are congenital cystic dilatations of the distal ureter. Those associated with a single ureter (simple ureterocele) are usually located in an orthotopic trigonal position. Ureteroceles found in association with duplicated ureters usually drain the upper pole kidney and are located in an ectopic position. Ectopic ureteroceles are commonly associated with obstruction and varying degrees of dysplasia of the affected renal segment. Decompression of the obstructed renal moiety from above (ureteropyelostomy) or from below (excision of ureterocele with ureteral reimplantation) is usually successful. Transurethral puncture of a ureterocele is usually reserved for infants, whereas a severely dysplastic moiety can be managed by partial nephrectomy. Large ureteroceles obstructing other renal moieties and the bladder neck will most likely require secondary procedures to restore normal urinary tract anatomy.[7]

Vesicoureteral Reflux

Vesicoureteral reflux refers to the retrograde passage of urine from the bladder into the ureter. The incidence of VUR in otherwise normal children is approximately 1%; a much higher incidence of up to 40% is reported in patients undergoing evaluation for UTI. A significant familial association has been encountered. A sufficient tunnel length of submucosal ureter is the most important component of the competent ureterovesical junction. This provides a predominantly passive valve mechanism compression of the ureter, preventing retrograde passage of urine. Marginal tunnel pressure can be made to reflux primarily or secondarily because of loss of compliance of the valve roof (during UTI), structural weakness of the detrusor floor (bladder diverticulum, ureterocele), or excessively high intravesical pressure caused by neurovesical dysfunction or bladder outlet obstruction. VUR is graded according to the International Classification System based on the proximal extent of retrograde urine flow, ureteral and pelvic dilatation, and the resultant anatomy of the calyceal fornices.

Reflux-induced renal injury is usually caused by the association of VUR with UTI and may range from clinically silent focal scar formation to generalized scarring and renal atrophy (reflux nephropathy) with hypertension and even end-stage renal failure. Children of either sex should be investigated at the time of the initial infection. The diagnosis of VUR is accomplished by cyclic VCUG, with either contrast medium or isotope (Fig. 108.3). Imaging of the upper tracts (kidneys and ureters) is extremely important and can be accomplished by ultrasonography, isotope renography, or, rarely, intravenous urography. Ultrasonography is helpful in quantifying renal growth or atrophy, whereas isotope renography is particularly sensitive in detecting focal scarring. Patients with voiding dysfunction should be considered strongly for urodynamic studies.

Because the submucosal ureter tends to lengthen with age, the ratio of tunnel length to ureteral diameter increases, and the propensity for reflux may disappear. In general, a lower reflux

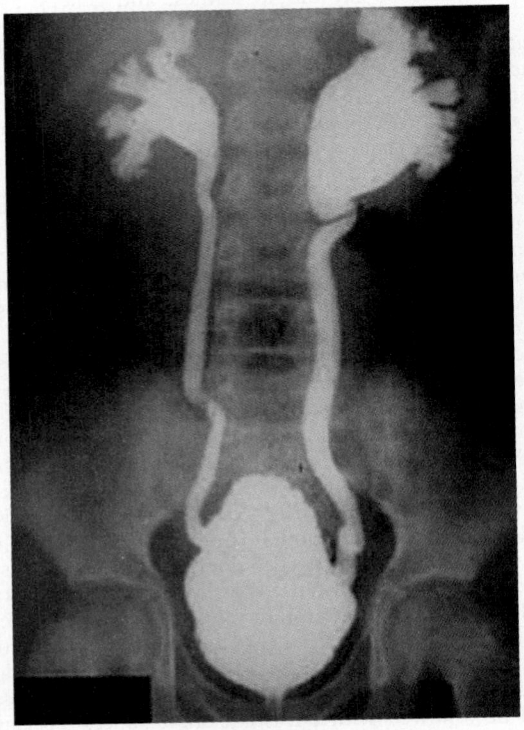

FIGURE 108.3. Voiding cystourethrogram of bilateral vesicoureteral reflux.

grade correlates with a better chance of spontaneous resolution. Nonoperative management of VUR (which is successful in most patients) requires prevention of UTI with suppression antibiotics, treatment of symptomatic voiding dysfunction, and long-term strict surveillance. Patients with breakthrough UTIs, significant renal injury, high-grade reflux, or pubertal age or those who fail to respond to 4 to 5 years of suppression therapy may require surgical correction. The principle of open ureteral reimplantation is the creation of a capacious subepithelial tunnel with the ratio of its length to ureteral diameter equal to 5:1. In general, excellent results are attained with most open intravesical or extravesical procedures. The extravesical approach, which preserves the integrity of the bladder lumen and doesn't require a ureteral anastomosis, eliminates postoperative hematuria, minimizes bladder spasms, decreases the risk of postoperative obstruction, and shortens hospital stay.[8] Since the initial report of successful endoscopic subureteral injection of polytetrafluoroethylene (Teflon) for correction of VUR, this minimally invasive technique has been widely used worldwide with different injectable materials. The only injectable substance with Food and Drug Administration approval is dextranomer/hyaluronic acid copolymer (Deflux). This substance is biodegradable, has no immunogenic properties, and seems to have no potential to cause malignant transformation.[9]

Megaureter

The term *megaureter* refers to an enlarged ureter, of which there are four categories: refluxing, obstructing, refluxing or obstructing, and nonrefluxing or nonobstructing, with an additional subdivision of each group into primary or secondary. Most patients are asymptomatic with an incidental finding of hydroureteronephrosis on screening renal ultrasound. The most common clinical presentation is UTI. The VCUG is necessary to rule out VUR, although its presence does not exclude the possibility of a coexistent obstruction. Diuretic renography is helpful to establish the presence of ureteral obstruction, which is usually at the level of the ureterovesical junction.

Megaureter secondary to severe VUR or obstruction is usually managed with ureteral reimplantation to prevent deterioration of renal function. Reduction of ureteral caliber by excision of the distal redundant ureter to achieve a satisfactory antireflux mechanism is usually necessary. Patients without reflux or obstruction may demonstrate radiographic improvement of the megaureter with preservation of renal function without surgical intervention. Therefore, initial nonoperative management with close follow-up of patients with nonobstructing or nonrefluxing megaureters is advisable.[10]

VESICOURETHRAL SYSTEM

The cloaca forms from the blind caudal end of the hindgut. The division of the cloaca by the urorectal septum into a ventral portion (the urogenital sinus [UGS]) and a dorsal portion (the rectum) is completed by the seventh week of gestation. Simultaneously, the mesodermal growth of the lower abdominal wall separates the umbilical cord from the genital tubercle. The mesonephric duct and ureteral bud have independent opening sites. The mesonephric duct (which will become the ejaculatory duct) migrates downward and medially, while the opening of the ureteral bud (which will become the ureteral orifice) migrates upward and laterally. The UGS can be divided into two segments at the point where the müllerian ducts join the dorsal wall of the UGS. The ventral portion forms the bladder, part of the prostatic urethra in the male, and the entire female urethra. The caudal portion gives rise to a portion of the prostatic and the entire membranous urethra in males and forms the lower part of the vagina and the vaginal vestibule in females.

ANOMALIES OF THE BLADDER

Urachal Abnormality

Embryologically, the urachus represents the apical attachment of the cloaca to the allantois. During fetal development it is obliterated and eventually represented by a fibrous retroperitoneal cord extending from the dome of the bladder to the umbilicus. Symptomatic urachal anomalies are rare and clinical syndromes most often arise from a patent urachus or a urachal cyst. The former condition is suggested by a persistently wet umbilicus and can occur in patients with bladder outlet obstruction. Excision of the urachus with bladder closure is usually necessary.

The urachal cyst is an inclusion cyst lined with transitional epithelium. If infected, it can present with abdominal pain and tenderness as well as fever, nausea, and leucocytosis, closely mimicking the acute abdomen. Radiologic evaluation should include abdominal US and/or computed tomography (CT). The infected urachal cyst is best managed by initial drainage of the abscess and delayed excision of the urachal remnant. Exploratory laparotomy is indicated if signs of peritonitis are present[11] (Algorithm 108.1).

Exstrophy–Epispadias Complex

The overgrowth and delayed rupture of the cloacal membrane prevents medial mesenchymal migration and proper lower abdominal wall development. Depending on the extent of the infraumbilical defect and the stage of development at which rupture occurs, bladder exstrophy, epispadias, or cloacal exstrophy results.

8 Epispadias in boys, as an isolated defect, consists of a dorsally placed urethral meatus and the degree of penile deformity is related to the extent of the meatal displacement. Most often, epispadias is associated with exstrophy of the bladder (Fig. 108.4). This defect usually involves pubic diastasis with separation of the rectus abdominis muscles, inguinal hernias, and anterior displacement of the anus. Male external genitalia have a characteristic epispadiac appearance, while females have a bifid clitoris with a stenotic and short vagina. Complete primary closure of the bladder plate with simultaneous repair of epispadias within the first 72 hours of life is the most appropriate treatment of this complicated anomaly.[12]

Cloacal exstrophy is the most severe defect that can occur in the formation of the ventral abdominal wall. Anatomically, there is exstrophy of the shortened hindgut or cecum, which displays its bulging mucosa between the two hemibladders. There is no

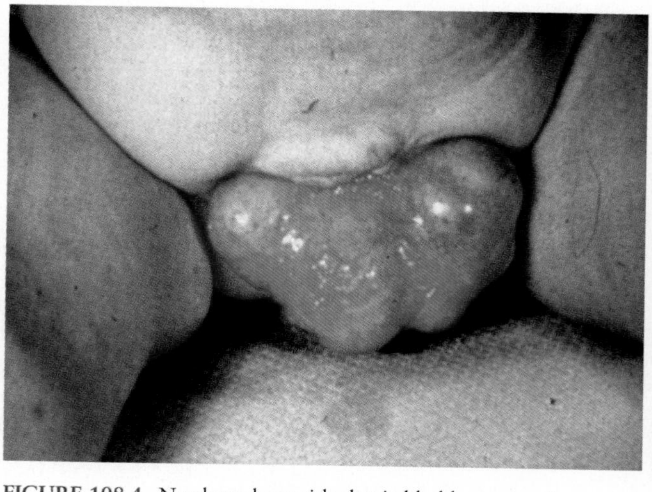

FIGURE 108.4. Newborn boy with classic bladder exstrophy.

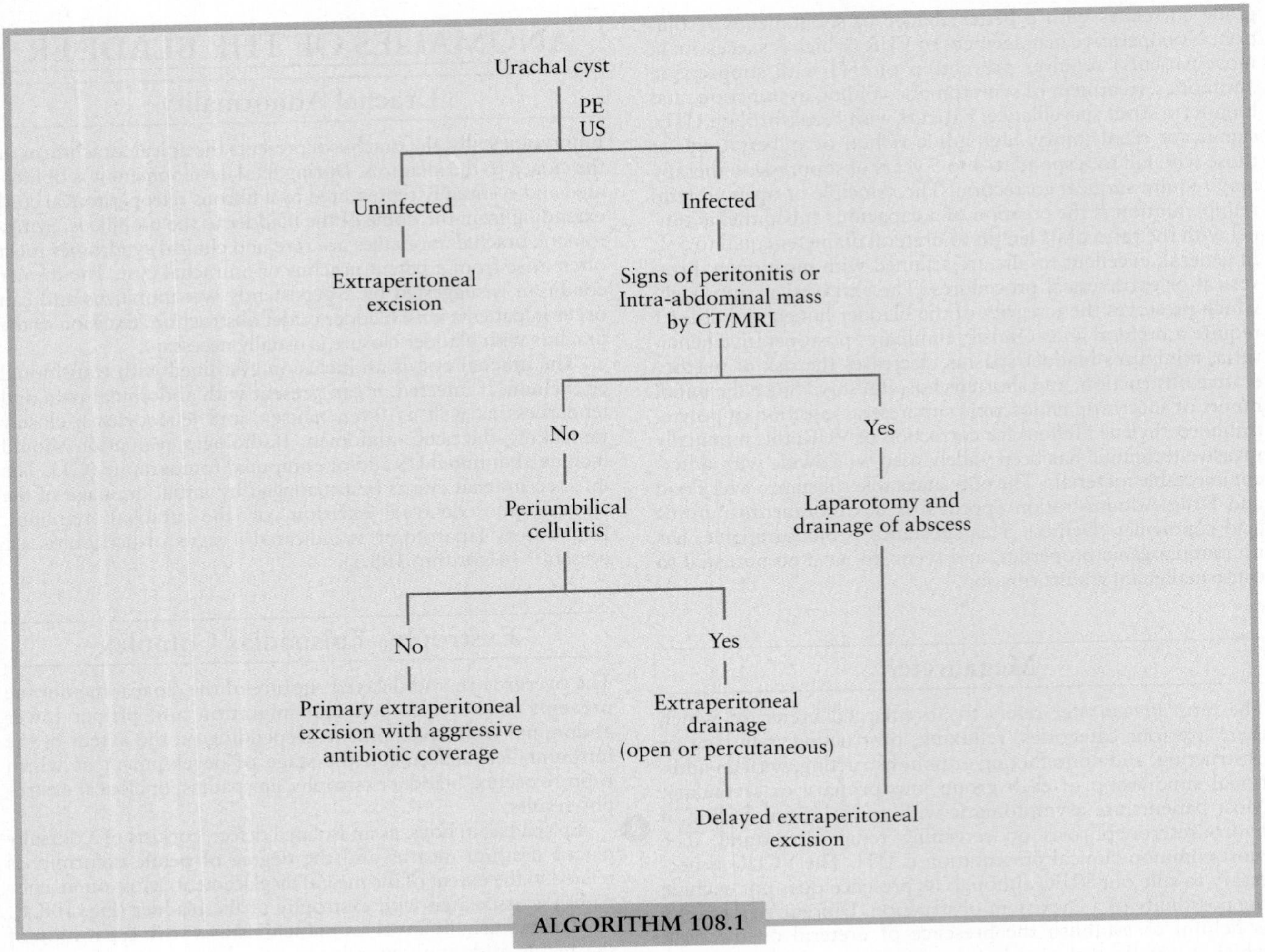

ALGORITHM 108.1. Algorithm of surgical management of urachal cyst. PE, physical examination; US, ultrasound. (Adapted from Minevich E, Wacksman J, Lewis AG, et al. The infected urachal cyst: primary excision versus a staged approach. *J Urol* 1997;157:1869.)

anus or rectum, and an omphalocele is present (Fig. 108.5). The initial surgical approach (in the neonatal period) includes closure of the omphalocele, separation of the bladder from the bowel, and closure of the bladder. Considerable reconstructive surgery remains to be done later to restore acceptable anatomic appearance and functioning urinary and intestinal tracts.

Neurogenic Bladder

An abnormal spinal column development affecting spinal cord function (myelodysplasia) is the most common cause of neurogenic bladder (NGB) in children. Myelomeningocele (MM) accounts for over 90% of open spinal dysraphic states. Bladder dysfunction usually results in urinary incontinence, although the poorly compliant bladder with leak point pressure over 40 cm H_2O may cause VUR and hydronephrosis, leading to deterioration of renal function.[13] Presumably at this point the ureterovesical junction can no longer protect the transmission of this pressure to the upper tracts. Urinary continence depends on bladder capacity and bladder outlet (bladder neck and urethral sphincter) resistance. The most important contribution affecting management of these children was the introduction of clean intermittent catheterization

FIGURE 108.5. Diagram depicting cloacal exstrophy.

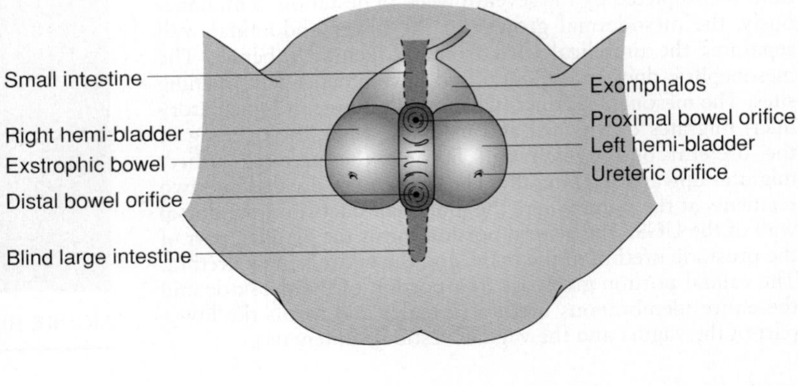

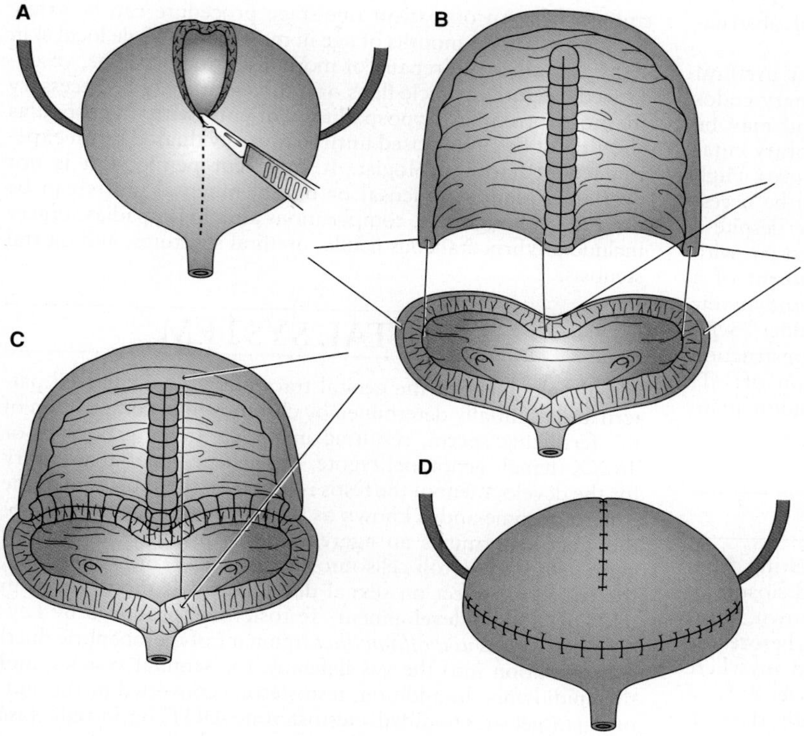

FIGURE 108.6. Bladder augmentation employing an intestinal segment. A: The bladder is opened as a "clam shell." B: The intestinal segment is detubularized by longitudinal incision along the antimesenteric border. A cup-patch is fashioned by suturing one edge of the resultant rectangle to itself. C: The cup-patch is sutured to the remnant bladder plate. D: Final appearance. (Reproduced with permission from Sheldon CA, Bukowski T. Bladder function. In: Rowe MI, O'Neal JA, Grosfeld JL, et al., eds. *Essentials of Pediatric Surgery*. St. Louis, MO: Mosby Year Book; 1995.)

(CIC) to facilitate timely bladder emptying. Evaluation of infants with urodynamic studies, RUS, and VCUG identifies those ultimately at risk for renal damage.

The primary goal in children with NGB is maintenance of safe intravesical pressure, the ultimate achievement of urinary continence, and preservation of renal function. If anticholinergic therapy with or without CIC is unsuccessful in achieving these goals, surgical reconstruction is necessary. Owing to the high incidence of upper tract deterioration with time and the significant sequelae of altered body image following cutaneous urinary diversion, incontinent diversion is no longer considered an acceptable alternative to reconstruction in the pediatric population. The goals of reconstructive surgery are to achieve a large-capacity, low-pressure reservoir; adequate bladder outlet resistance; and easy access for catheterization. A variety of donor tissue sources including bowel segments, stomach, or ureter are available for bladder augmentation (Fig. 108.6). Potential complications of enterocystoplasty include electrolyte abnormalities, spontaneous perforation of the bowel segment, and tumor formation. Bladder outlet resistance can be increased by bladder neck reconstruction, implantation of an artificial urinary sphincter, urethral or bladder neck suspension, submucosal injection of collagen, or a combination of these procedures. A Mitrofanoff neourethra (appendiceal or ileal) is usually necessary to provide bladder access for decompression and continence, and is highly successful in even the most devastating cases.[14]

Significant neurogenic bladder is frequently accompanied by refractory fecal incontinence. This may severely compromise care with respect to UTI, incontinence, and achieving independent self-care. When preoperative conventional therapy (dietary modification, timed toileting, cathartics, bulking agents, and enemas) is unsuccessful to control complete evacuation of the colon, an antegrade continence enema (ACE) procedure, performed through a continent cecostomy utilizing appendix or tapered ileum, is a viable option. The ACE procedure has been successfully utilized in the management of intractable fecal incontinence, even in the most debilitating childhood recto-urogenital anomalies.[15]

ANOMALIES OF THE URETHRA

Posterior Urethral Valves

9 Posterior urethral valves are the most common obstructive urethral lesions in male infants and consist of a membrane or mucosal leaflet within the prostatic urethra. The diagnosis is usually suspected in neonates because of abnormal findings of prenatal hydronephrosis (bilateral hydronephrosis, distended bladder) and oligohydramnios. Some of them are found to have flank masses, ascites, and urinary retention. Older children usually present with voiding symptoms, UTI, or hematuria. VCUG is diagnostic in most cases (Fig. 108.7), although cystoscopy may be necessary in an equivocal setting. Patients with significant bilateral hydronephrosis should be screened for renal insufficiency, and nuclear

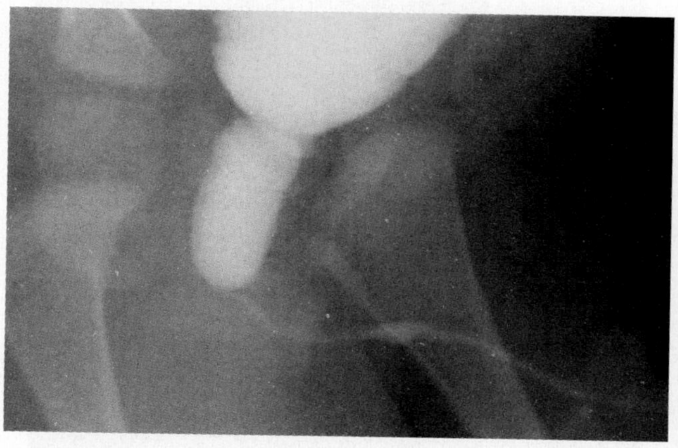

FIGURE 108.7. Voiding cystourethrogram showing dilated posterior urethra secondary to posterior urethral valves.

scintigraphy may be indicated to rule out ureteral obstruction and/or renal dysplasia.

Other than temporary urinary drainage with a urethral catheter (feeding tube), in critically ill patients primary endoscopic valve ablation is the preferred approach and may be accomplished safely in most instances. Initial temporary cutaneous vesicostomy is useful in occasional circumstances. High upper urinary tract diversion may on rare occasion be necessary in infants who demonstrate a rising creatinine despite a lower tract drainage. Long-term follow-up is necessary with special attention directed to the possible development of a poorly compliant, high-pressure bladder.[16] Careful urodynamic evaluation and timely treatment of the "valve bladder" with anticholinergics, CIC, and very selective vesical reconstruction (including enterocystoplasty) as well as prevention of UTI ensure the best chance for successful prevention and/or management of chronic renal failure.

Hypospadias

Hypospadias is a common congenital defect resulting from incomplete tubularization of the urethral plate and closure of the genital folds. The cause of this anomaly is unknown, but is probably related to inadequate androgenization before the 20th week of gestation. The meatus may be located anywhere from the perineum to the glans penis, although in over 85% of cases it is distal to the midshaft (Fig. 108.8). Typically, the ventral prepuce is deficient and ventral penile chordee occurs more frequently with proximal hypospadias.

Principles of hypospadias repair include meticulous surgical technique with sufficient optical magnification to advance the urethral meatus to a normal glanular position and to correct penile chordee if necessary. Numerous operations have been described for surgical correction of hypospadias and the surgeon treating this anomaly should be familiar with all possible approaches. An outpatient one-stage procedure can be safely performed after 6 months of age in most cases. While local skin flaps are utilized in repairs of more distal hypospadias, vascularized preputial pedicle flaps or a tube-graft may be necessary in more proximal hypospadias. Patients with hypospadias should not be circumcised until they are evaluated by an experienced pediatric urologist. If sufficient penile skin is not available, bladder mucosal or buccal mucosal grafts can be utilized. Although rare, complications after hypospadias surgery include urethrocutaneous fistula, urethral strictures, and meatal stenosis.

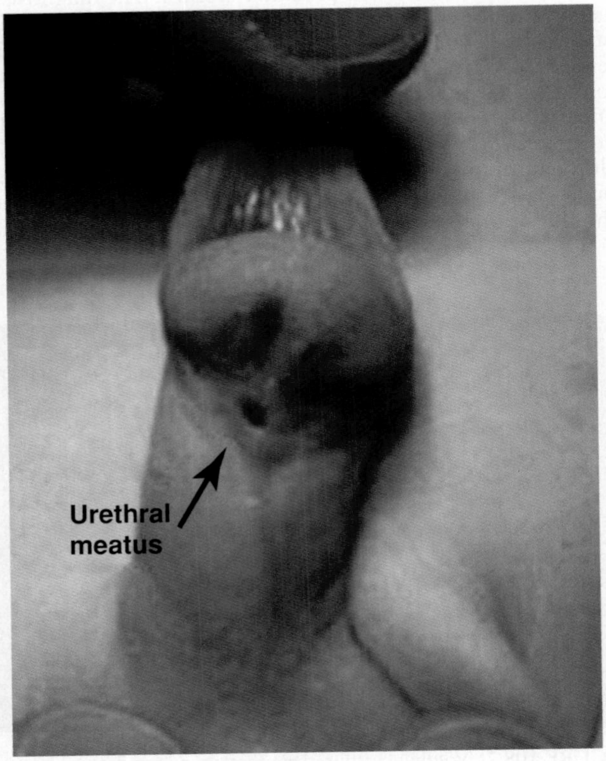

FIGURE 108.8. Coronal hypospadias.

GENITAL SYSTEM

The development of the genital tract follows a sequential pattern and is initially determined by chromosomal composition of the fertilizing sperm, resulting in 46,XY (male genotype) or 46,XX (female genotype) zygote. The genetic material necessary for the development of the testis is found on the short arm of the Y chromosome and is known as the SRY gene. The presence of this gene determines an aggregation of primitive indifferent germ cells and Sertoli cells into the testicular cord. Thereafter, the endocrine effect on sexual development is most crucial in male phenotype development. Testosterone, produced by Leydig cells, results in *wolffian duct* (remnant of mesonephric duct) differentiation into the vas deferens, the seminal vesicles, and the epididymis. In addition, testosterone converted at the end-organ target sites to dihydrotestosterone (DHT) by 5a-reductase regulates the virilization of the urogenital sinus and external genitalia at around the ninth week of gestation. Only at this point, the previously indifferent genital tubercle starts to differentiate into a penis while the genital swelling fuses to form the scrotum. At the same time, müllerian-inhibiting substance (MIS) produced by testicular Sertoli cells results in an almost complete regression of the *müllerian ducts*.

In the absence of the SRY gene, the primitive gonads differentiate into an ovary. The female development of the *müllerian (paramesonephric)* duct system into fallopian tube, uterus, and cervix; feminization of the external genitalia; and involution of the *wolffian duct*s are automatic processes in the absence of testosterone and MIS.

AMBIGUOUS GENITALIA

The term *ambiguous genitalia* refers to genitalia in the spectrum of sexual development that are not clearly male or female. This situation represents a true medical and social emergency. Rapid but careful determination of the genetic composition, gonadal sex, and genitourinary anatomy of the affected newborn is essential to enable gender assignment, acceptance of the child by the family, and ultimately surgical reconstruction.

Patients with ambiguous genitalia can be divided in four categories: female and male pseudohermaphroditism, true hermaphroditism, and gonadal dysgenesis. Complete evaluation of the infant with ambiguous genitalia should include the following:

1. Thorough physical examination (special attention to palpable gonads, phallic structure, vaginal orifice, and anus)
2. Complete family history (genital anomalies in other family members, unexplained neonatal death in previous children)
3. Evaluation of the pregnancy (especially maternal exposure to androgenic agents)
4. Blood karyotype
5. Biochemical evaluation (serum electrolytes, adrenal steroids and precursors, serum gonadotropins, and testosterone)
6. Radiologic evaluation (renal and pelvic US, genitogram)

Occasionally, diagnostic laparoscopy and gonadal biopsy are necessary to guide the gender assignment. After the chromosomal and gonadal composition is established, sex assignment is determined, based mostly on the potential for sexual function. Surgical reconstruction is aimed at matching the external genitalia to the gender assigned to the child and is usually undertaken at 6 to 12 months of age.[17]

Female Pseudohermaphroditism

Female pseudohermaphroditism is the largest diagnostic category and, within this category, the leading cause is congenital adrenal hyperplasia (CAH). CAH results from a deficiency in the enzymes responsible for the synthesis of mineralocorticosteroids and glucocorticosteroids, resulting in overproduction of adrenal androgens. A deficiency of 21-hydroxylase represents 95% of patients with CAH. All of these patients are genetic females (46,XX karyotype, ovarian gonads) with masculinization of the external genitalia ranging from an enlarged clitoris to a normal-appearing male phallus with complete labial fusion (Fig. 108.9). These patients are potentially fertile regardless of how severe the degree of virilization.

A high index of suspicion allows for early diagnosis of this condition and initiation of hormonal replacement (glucocorticosteroids and mineralocorticosteroids) to prevent adrenal insufficiency, salt-wasting syndrome, and continued virilization. Because internal müllerian structures are always present, these children are reared as females and feminizing genitoplasty is performed to correct the cosmetic and functional deformities of external genitalia. If the vagina enters the urogenital sinus distally, a cutback or flap vaginoplasty can be combined with clitoroplasty (reduction and relocation of the clitoris with preservation of glanular sensation) and labioplasty in a single procedure. If the vagina enters the urogenital sinus more proximally, a total urogenital sinus mobilization, pedicle skin flap, or segmental bowel interposition vaginoplasty is deferred to a later date.

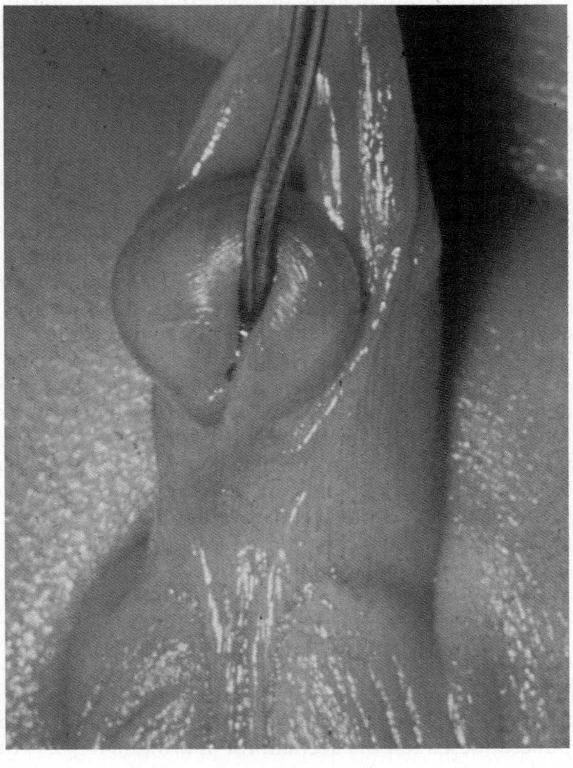

FIGURE 108.9. Severe masculinization of the external genitalia in a girl with congenital adrenal hyperplasia.

Male Pseudohermaphroditism

Male pseudohermaphrodites are genetic males (46,XY) with decreased virilization of the external genitalia. This anomaly can result from abnormal testosterone synthesis, 5a-reductase deficiency leading to decreased levels of DHT, and androgen insensitivity syndrome (defect of the androgen receptor). The phallic structure may be inadequate for the male gender role. In this setting, consideration should be given to female gender assignment.

Testicular feminization syndrome (complete androgen insensitivity) is the most common form of male pseudohermaphroditism, although affected individuals appear as normal phenotypic females with a short vagina. They are usually diagnosed at puberty with primary amenorrhea, although infrequently diagnosis is made during routine childhood herniorrhaphy, at which time testes are found. Bilateral gonadectomy is indicated because of an increased risk of gonadoblastoma development in the intra-abdominal testis. It can be delayed until puberty in selected cases. Short vagina can be managed with vaginal dilatation, but vaginal reconstruction or vaginal replacement will be necessary in some patients.

True Hermaphroditism

In this condition, patients have both ovarian and testicular tissue (ovary and testis, ovotestis, or a combination of these). True hermaphroditism is the rarest form of intersex abnormality. The internal genital structures conform with the ipsilateral gonad. The most common karyotype is 46,XX, although mosaicism and a 46,XY karyotype occur as well. The appearance of external genitalia varies widely. After gender is assigned, gonadal tissue of the opposite sex is removed and surgical reconstruction is undertaken.

Mixed Gonadal Dysgenesis

This is the second most frequent cause of genital ambiguity, and the majority of neonates exhibit a 45,XO/46,XY mosaic karyotype. They generally present with a dysgenetic testis on one side and a streak of gonads on the other. The appearance of external genitalia is variable; however, the majority are poorly virilized and consequently most infants will be raised as females. Appropriate genital reconstruction is required. Early gonadectomy is indicated because of the high risk of malignant degeneration (gonadoblastoma, seminoma, and dysgerminoma) of the dysgenetic gonad.

ANOMALIES OF MALE GENITALIA

Anomalies of the Foreskin

At birth, the prepuce is retractable in only 4% of boys. No special care of the uncircumcised penis is required. During the first years of life, spontaneous separation occurs physiologically in most boys secondary to intermittent erections and epithelialization of the inner prepuce. It is unnecessary to retract the prepuce on any routine basis to promote retractability or to hasten physiologic separation. This usually results in pain, bleeding, and, occasionally, paraphimosis.

Much confusion exists as to the indications for neonatal circumcision. The most important arguments are those of custom and tradition. In infants, circumcision may be performed using the Gomco clamp under local penile block. The most important principles of neonatal circumcision are complete lysis of penile adhesions, adequate but not excessive excision of outer and inner preputial layers, hemostasis, and protection of the glans penis.

Truly pathologic phimosis, paraphimosis, and recurrent balanitis are definitive indications for circumcision. It is estimated that as many as 18% of uncircumcised boys may develop one of the aforementioned indications by 8 years of age. Phimosis is a fibrotic contraction of the foreskin preventing its retraction over the glans. This pathologic condition should be differentiated from physiologic phimosis of infancy. Paraphimosis is the entrapment of a phimotic prepuce proximal to the coronal sulcus. The skin ring causes venous congestion initially, but as the condition progresses, arterial occlusion and necrosis of the glans penis may occur. If persistent manual compression does not reduce paraphimosis, emergency circumcision or the creation of a dorsal slit is indicated. Circumcision in infancy undoubtedly prevents cancer of the penis. If the decision is made not to circumcise a male infant, there must be a lifetime commitment to genital hygiene to minimize the risks of developing penile cancer. Circumcision should be encouraged in boys with a history of UTI, VUR, or other urinary abnormalities to decrease the chance of ascending infection. Patients with hypospadias, penile chordee, penile torsion, epispadias, buried penis, or megalourethra are not candidates for routine circumcision. To correct these conditions, a sufficient amount of foreskin must be available.

Cryptorchidism

10 Descent of the testis from its original position near the kidney into the cooler scrotum is necessary for its normal development and production of fertile sperm. Various mechanisms including gubernacular traction and intra-abdominal pressure have been proposed to be responsible for testicular descent, but endocrine factors of the hypothalamic-pituitary-testicular axis also play a major role in this process. Between the 12th and 17th weeks of gestation, the testis undergoes transabdominal migration to a location near the internal inguinal ring. It is not until the seventh month of gestation that transinguinal migration of the testis to its final position takes place.

True undescended testes fail to reach the scrotum despite following a normal line of descent. Ectopic testes follow the usual course of descent until they emerge from the external inguinal ring, but are then misdirected to an ectopic position (superficial inguinal pouch, perineal, femoral, transverse scrotal). While approximately 3.4% of full-term boys have undescended testes, 30% of premature infants have this anomaly. By 1 year of age, the incidence of cryptorchidism is about 1% and remains at this level thereafter. Actually, most cryptorchid testes descending during the first year of life do so within the first 3 months after birth. The diagnosis of cryptorchidism relies upon gentle and patient genital examination. Relaxation of the patient and warming of the examiner's hand aid in successful examination. Reexamination of the child in the cross-legged position may also reveal the gonad. A functional classification that provides a practical approach to therapy is based on whether the testis is palpable or impalpable (20%). While endocrine testing is reliable in predicting bilateral anorchidism, radiologic means including abdominal sonography, computed tomography, magnetic resonance imaging, and gonadal arteriography are inaccurate in localization of nonpalpable testes. Diagnostic laparoscopy will provide diagnosis of vanishing testis by identification of blind-ending spermatic vessels or accurate localization of the intra-abdominal testis in this situation.[18] Undescended testes must be distinguished from retractile testes that may reside above the scrotum but, with careful positioning, can be made to stay within the lower scrotum without continuous traction.

Although the correction of undescended testes eliminates any coexisting inguinal hernia (found in 95% of all cases) and prevents possible testicular injury or torsion (the risk of which is increased in these patients), the central issues in managing these patients revolve around future fertility and the risk of developing a testicular neoplasm. There is an increased risk of testicular carcinoma in undescended testes, and orchidopexy facilitates self-examination and early detection of the cancer. Because germ cell count of the infant undescended testis deteriorates after 1 year of life, correction of cryptorchidism is indicated between 6 and 12 months of age. For palpable undescended testes, routine inguinal orchidopexy is successful in most patients. For high intra-abdominal testes, testicular microsurgical autotransplantation[19] provides the highest success rate among different surgical options.[20]

Torsion of the Testis and Appendages

Torsion of the testicle is classified as a surgical emergency because it causes strangulation of gonadal blood supply with subsequent testicular necrosis and atrophy. Testicular salvage is likely if the duration of torsion is less than 6 to 8 hours.[21] Torsion presenting in the neonatal period most commonly develops prenatally in the spermatic cord proximal to the attachments of the tunica vaginalis (*extravaginal torsion*). Although possible at any age, testicular torsion is most common in adolescents, being distal to the insertion of the tunica vaginalis (*intravaginal torsion*). A bell-clapper deformity predisposes to this condition.

Prenatal torsion presents with a firm, hard scrotal mass that does not transilluminate in an otherwise asymptomatic newborn male. Salvage of the testis is extremely rare,[22] but timely surgical exploration is indicated to anchor the contralateral testis, since bilateral (synchronous or asynchronous) neonatal testicular torsion has been described. In older boys sudden onset of severe testicular pain followed by scrotal swelling is the classic presentation of testicular torsion. On physical examination, a swollen, tender testis with shortening of the cord is noticed. If testicular torsion is clinically suspected, an immediate surgical scrotal exploration is indicated. A negative exploration of the scrotum is more acceptable than the loss of a testis that might have been salvaged. In situations with a low suspicion of testicular torsion, scrotal color Doppler US or testicular nuclear scan can be helpful to differentiate torsion from acute epididymitis. At surgical exploration, the testis is untwisted and observed for viability. A frankly necrotic testis is removed, while viable gonads (return of color, return of Doppler flow, signs of arterial blood after incision of tunica albuginea) are fixed to the scrotal wall to prevent subsequent torsion. Exploration and anchoring of the contralateral testis, which can be done through the same incision, is mandatory to prevent its subsequent torsion. Manual detorsion of the torsed testis is usually difficult because of acute pain during manipulation but, if successful (and confirmed by color Doppler US in a patient with complete resolution of symptoms), definitive surgical fixation of the testes should be performed before the patient leaves the hospital as an urgent rather than emergency procedure.

The testicular appendix, a müllerian duct remnant, is the most common genital appendage susceptible to torsion. Although frequently presenting with symptoms similar to testicular torsion, this condition can usually be diagnosed by a finding of a tender focal induration or a blue dot near the upper pole of the testis. Appendix testis torsion is best managed by several days of bed rest and oral preventive antibiotics. If a reliable diagnosis cannot be made, scrotal color Doppler US or even surgical exploration is indicated to rule out testicular torsion.

Prepubertal Testicular Tumor

In boys presenting with a painless palpable scrotal mass, a testicular tumor should be included in the differential diagnosis.
11 Prepubertal testis tumors account for approximately 2% of all testicular tumors, with a peak patient age of approximately 2 years. The most common lesion is a yolk sac tumor, which is a variant of embryonal cell carcinoma. When spread occurs, it

is usually a hematogenous spread to the lungs and, less commonly, lymphatic spread to the retroperitoneal nodes. Scrotal US is usually definitive in visualizing an intratesticular mass, while abdominal and chest CT scans are necessary for metastatic evaluation. Tumor markers (α-fetoprotein and β-human chorionic gonadotropin) are helpful for initial evaluation and during follow-up. In young children, prognosis is excellent and the radical inguinal orchiectomy is the initial treatment. Retroperitoneal lymph node dissection and multidrug chemotherapy are necessary in cases of disseminating disease. In the absence of metastasis and/or elevated tumor marker levels, the applicability of these treatment modalities remains controversial.

Varicocele

Varicocele is a dilation of the veins of the spermatic cord and is reported to occur at a 15% incidence in adolescent boys, which correlates with that in the general male population. In the majority of adolescents the varicocele is grade I, while in 35% it is grade II or III. Varicocele is generally visible or palpable in the upright position. Most urologists agree that scrotal discomfort and ipsilateral testicular growth failure are reliable indications for varicocele surgery in this population. Additionally, some authors have advocated surgical repair in patients demonstrating a progressive increase in varicocele size, bilateral varicoceles, or a large varicocele associated with a change in testicular consistency. Incisional surgery with an inguinal, retroperitoneal, or modified approach is the basis of varicocelectomy in adolescents. The optical magnification allows reliable identification and preservation of the testicular artery and lymphatics during ligation of the venous channels. As a result, the postoperative development of hydrocele or recurrence of the varicocele may be prevented.[23]

VAGINAL ANOMALIES AND UROGENITAL SINUS MALFORMATIONS

The urogenital sinus is apparent by 6 weeks of gestation. After it receives the fused müllerian ducts, the distal potion of the UGS forms the lower one third of the vagina, while the fused müllerian ducts form the upper two thirds of the vagina and uterus. Although most vaginal anomalies occur in conjunction with intersex disorders, isolated vaginal anomalies or those occurring in association with a urogenital sinus are also seen (Fig. 108.10). Vaginal agenesis may occur in isolation or as a component of the Mayer-Rokitansky syndrome, which refers to normal phenotypic females with vaginal and occasional uterine dysgenesis. Because the distal vagina is normally formed in most of these patients, the diagnosis is not usually made until puberty, at which time the patient presents with amenorrhea. Approximately one third of these patients have urologic anomalies, the most common being unilateral renal agenesis. Vaginoplasty is indicated in almost all patients and depends on the anatomy present. Several techniques using tubularized skin flaps, skin grafts, and bowel segments have been described for vaginal reconstruction.[24] Careful preoperative counseling and evaluation of the patient's and parents' motivation are essential for a good result since long-term vaginal dilatation is occasionally required until the patient is old enough to participate in sexual intercourse.

UGS anomalies occur because of a failure of the urethra and the vagina to separate. These children have two perineal openings, including the anus, because the rectum is usually normal. Many of these girls have some degree of bladder dysfunction and CIC may be necessary. If CIC of the bladder is not possible, temporary vesicostomy may be indicated. To separate the urethral and vaginal orifices, urethral lengthening or vaginal pull-through procedures are required.[24–26]

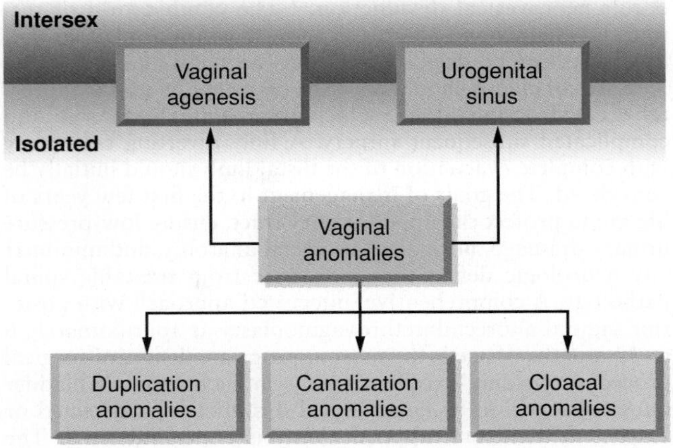

FIGURE 108.10. Classification of vaginal anomalies. (Reproduced with permission from Sheldon CA. Imperforate anus, urogenital sinus and cloaca. In: Kelalis PP, King LR, Belman AB, eds. *Clinical Pediatric Urology*. Philadelphia: WB Saunders; 2000.)

OTHER GENITOURINARY DISORDERS

Eagle-Barrett Syndrome

The Eagle-Barrett syndrome, also referred to as prune-belly syndrome (PBS), is a set of genitourinary malformations with a deficiency or absence of the abdominal wall musculature accompanied by a broad spectrum of associated organ system anomalies. It was theorized that delayed canalization of the urethral membrane resulted in a temporary total urinary obstruction causing massive dilatation of the ureters, a large bladder frequently associated with a patent urachus, and a dilated proximal urethra with a hypoplastic prostate. The wrinkled, prunelike skin of the abdominal wall in the newborn is a characteristic manifestation. Renal dysplasia occurs frequently and in severe cases is associated with pulmonary hypoplasia, resulting in stillbirth or death in the neonatal period. Bilateral cryptorchidism with intra-abdominal testes is a characteristic feature of PBS. Extraurinary problems are associated with this syndrome in 73% of patients and usually involve defects of the cardiovascular, musculoskeletal, respiratory, or central nervous systems.[27] Since the dilatation of the urinary tract is usually nonobstructive, a favorable outcome in these patients can be expected with a conservative approach of observation, prevention of UTI, and surgical drainage, with reconstruction only being performed when absolutely required.

Urologic Implications of Imperforate Anus

Anorectal malformations (ARMs) encompass a broad spectrum of abnormalities of termination of the hindgut and urogenital sinus, ranging from the simple covered anus to complex cloacal malformations involving the gastrointestinal, urinary, and genital tracts. Morbidity and mortality in these cases are largely attributed to associated structural and functional genitourinary anomalies, ranging from vesicoureteral reflux (57%) to renal dysplasia and agenesis (65%). Therefore, neonatal screening with renal US and VCUG is essential in all patients with ARMs.[28] The assessment of bladder function is also critical because of a reportedly high incidence of occult neurovesical dysfunction.[29] The combination of rectourinary fistula and neurovesical dysfunction or bladder outlet obstruction predisposes to critical neonatal illness.

Cases of cloaca should never be managed by initial anorectal reconstruction alone, which necessitates extensive and complicated subsequent surgery. A fully diverting colostomy with complete evacuation of the distal limb should initially be considered. The goals of management in the first few years of life are to protect the upper urinary tract, ensure low-pressure urinary drainage, normalize anorectal anatomy, and minimize any neurologic deficit that may arise from treatable spinal pathology. A comprehensive, integrated approach with posterior sagittal anorectalurethrovaginoplasty at approximately 6 to 12 months of age is the most appropriate definitive surgical procedure yielding excellent results in such cases. If bladder outlet obstruction or neurovesical dysfunction is detected or suspected, incidental appendectomy is contraindicated. The goals of management of the preschool and school-aged child with ARMs are to ensure social urinary and fecal continence and to promote self-esteem and self-care.[24]

References

1. Potter EL. Bilateral absence of ureters and kidneys: a report of 50 cases. *Obstet Gynecol* 1965;25:3.
2. Gleason PE, Kelalis PP, Husman DA, et al. Hydronephrosis in renal ectopia: incidence, etiology and significance. *J Urol* 1994;151:1660.
3. Mesrobian HJ, Kelalis PP, Hrabovsky E, et al. Wilms tumor in horseshoe kidneys: a report from the National Wilms Tumor Study. *J Urol* 1985;133:1002.
4. Glassberg KI, Stephens FD, Lebowitz RL, et al. Renal dysgenesis and cystic disease of the kidney: a report of the Committee on Terminology, Nomenclature and Classification. *J Urol* 1987;138:1085.
5. Minevich E, Wacksman J, Phipps L, et al. Importance of accurate diagnosis and early close follow-up in patients with suspected MCDK. *J Urol* 1997;158:1301.
6. Minevich E, Wacksman J. Pyeloplasty. In: Graham SD, ed. *Glenn's Urologic Surgery*. Philadelphia, PA: Lippincott-Raven; 1998.
7. DeFoor W, Minevich E, Tackett L, et al. Ectopic ureterocele: clinical application of classification based on renal unit jeopardy. *J Urol* 2003;169(3):1092–1094.
8. Minevich E, Sheldon CA. Urinary tract infection and vesicoureteral reflux. In: Ascraft K, Holder T, eds. *Pediatric Surgery*. Philadelphia, PA: WB Saunders; 2004.
9. Elder JS, Diaz M, Caldamone AA, et al. Endoscopic therapy for vesicoureteral reflux: a meta-analysis. I. Reflux resolution and urinary tract infection. *J Urol* 2006;175(2):716–722.
10. Keating MA, Escola J, Snyder HM, et al. Changing concepts in management of primary obstructive megaureter. *J Urol* 1989;142:636.
11. Minevich E, Wacksman J, Lewis AG, et al. The infected urachal cyst: primary excision versus a staged approach. *J Urol* 1997;157:1869.
12. Shnorhavorian M, Grady RW, Andersen A, et al. Long-term followup of complete primary repair of exstrophy: the Seattle experience. *J Urol* 2008;180(4 suppl):1615–1619; discussion 1619–1620.
13. McGuire EJ, Woodside JR, Borden TA, et al. Prognostic value of urodynamic testing in myelodysplastic patients. *J Urol* 1981;126:205.
14. Minevich E, Sheldon CA. Structural disorders of the bladder, augmentation. In: Grosfeld JL, O'Neill JA, Coran AG, et al., eds. *Pediatric Surgery*. Philadelphia: Mosby; 2006:1823.
15. Sheldon CA, Minevich E, Wacksman J, et al. Role of the antegrade continence enema in the management of the most debilitating childhood rectourogenital anomalies. *J Urol* 1997;158:1277.
16. Peters CA, Bolkier M, Bauer SB, et al. The urodynamic consequences of posterior urethral valves. *J Urol* 1990;144:122.
17. Sheldon CA. Intersex states. In: Oldham KT, Colombani PM, Foglia RT, eds. *Surgery of Infants and Children: Scientific Principles and Practice*. Philadelphia, PA: Lippincott-Raven; 1997:1608.
18. Weiss RM, Seashore JH. Clinical implications of laparoscopy in the management of a nonpalpable undescended testis. *J Urol* 1986;135:332.
19. Tackett LD, Wacksman J, Billmire D, et al. The high intra-abdominal testis: technique and long-term success of laparoscopic testicular autotransplantation. *J Endourol* 2002;16(6):359–361.
20. Docimo SG. Results of surgical therapy for cryptorchidism: literature review and analysis. *J Urol* 1995;154:1148.
21. Ransler CW, Allen TD. Torsion of the spermatic cord. *Urol Clin North Am* 1982;9:245.
22. Brandt MT, Sheldon CA, Wacksman J, et al. Prenatal testicular torsion: principles of management. *J Urol* 1992;147:670.
23. Minevich E, Wacksman J, Lewis AG, et al. Inguinal microsurgical varicocelectomy in the adolescent: technique and preliminary results. *J Urol* 1998;159:1022.
24. Sheldon CA. Imperforate anus, urogenital sinus and cloaca. In: Kelalis PP, King LR, Belman AB, eds. *Clinical Pediatric Urology*. Philadelphia, PA: WB Saunders; 2000:836.
25. Jenak R, Ludwikowski B, Gonzalez R. Total urogenital sinus mobilization: a modified perineal approach for feminizing genitoplasty and urogenital sinus repair. *J Urol* 2001;165(6 Pt 2):2347–2349.
26. Sheldon CA, Gilbert A, Lewis AG. Vaginal reconstruction: critical technical principles. *J Urol* 1994;152:190.
27. Geary DF, MacLusky IB , Chirchill BM, et al. A broader spectrum of abnormalities in the prune belly syndrome. *J Urol* 1986;135:324.
28. Sheldon CA, Gilbert A, Lewis AG, et al. Surgical implications of genitourinary tract anomalies in patients with imperforate anus. *J Urol* 1994;152:196.
29. Sheldon CA, Cormier M, Crone K, et al. Occult neurovesical dysfunction in children with imperforate anus and its variants. *J Pediatr Surg* 1991;26:49.

CHAPTER 109 ■ CHILDHOOD TUMORS

BARRIE S. RICH AND MICHAEL P. LA QUAGLIA

KEY POINTS

1. In childhood, neuroblastoma is the most common extracranial solid tumor, followed in incidence by Wilms tumor; rhabdomyosarcoma is less common than neuroblastoma and Wilms tumor but has a biphasic age distribution, with 40% of cases occurring in the age range 10 to 19 years.
2. Patients with neuroblastoma and an increased number of copies of the *MYCN* gene have a much worse prognosis.
3. High-risk neuroblastoma remains one of the central problems in pediatric oncology, with overall survival rates less than 30% despite multidisciplinary therapy and the use of multiagent chemotherapy and myeloablative regimens.
4. The standard of care for Wilms tumor in the United States is initial surgical resection, with exceptions to this rule only for extensive intracaval tumors that require cardiopulmonary bypass for extraction, obviously unresectable tumors with documented invasion of contiguous structures, and possibly bilateral tumors, especially if it is unclear which side is most heavily involved; all patients with resectable Wilms tumor receive postoperative chemotherapy.
5. Clear cell sarcoma of the kidney is a distinct histopathologic and clinical entity from Wilms tumor with an age distribution similar to that observed in Wilms tumor but a markedly worse prognosis; it has been called the *bone-metastasizing renal tumor of childhood.*
6. Modern treatment of rhabdomyosarcoma is multidisciplinary and includes multiagent chemotherapy, judicious resection, and radiation therapy; the intensity of therapy should be tailored to the risk of subsequent relapse as a function of tumor, node, or metastasis stage.

The focus of this chapter is malignant solid tumors of infancy, childhood, and adolescence. Fortunately, these conditions are rare, especially compared with major adult solid malignancies. This rarity, however, poses special problems to the cancer researcher. For the clinician studying the effectiveness of a particular drug or surgical technique, fewer patients are available for randomized trials. Similarly, basic scientists analyzing the effect of a particular genetic mutation of a tumor have limited materials at their disposal. The solution to this problem has been the establishment of The Children's Oncology Group (COG) and the Societé Internacionale Oncologique Pediatrique (SIOP) in Europe for the clinical and basic scientific study of pediatric malignancies. Despite the progress these groups have made, less than 30% of children with high-risk neuroblastomas survive more than 5 years. Of children with lymphomas and germ cell tumors, 10% to 30% relapse or become resistant to treatment. Approximately 10% of children with hepatocellular carcinomas survive more than 5 years after diagnosis, and almost no patients who have rhabdoid tumor, pediatric colon cancer, or renal cell carcinoma in childhood survive more than 5 years. This has resulted in a 70% increase in the overall survival rate for pediatric cancer over the last 50 years.[1] Overall 5-year survival rates for all stages are approximately 85% for Wilms tumor, 70% for hepatoblastoma, and 60% (83% to 31% by stage, age, and site[2]) for rhabdomyosarcoma. In comparison, the survival rate was less than 20%, and closer to zero, respectively, for these malignancies before the advent of multidisciplinary therapy.

Future progress will depend on myriad biologic analyses done on each tumor system. As in the past, the pediatric surgical oncologist, the first line of defense in tumor diagnosis and staging, will be instrumental to advances in the field.[3–5] It is crucial that biopsy specimens be adequate both in size and quality. Snap freezing of portions of a tumor biopsy should become routine. Because molecular biologic studies often require a biopsy larger than 1 cm,[3] this factor should be kept in mind when planning the operative approach.

INCIDENCE OF SOLID TUMORS IN CHILDHOOD

The percent distribution for all races and sexes of various pedi-
1 atric solid tumors are compared in Figure 109.1.[6] Neuroblastoma is the most common extracranial solid tumor, followed in incidence by Wilms tumors. Rhabdomyosarcomas account for about three-quarters of the previous two but have a biphasic age distribution, with 40% of cases occurring in the 10- to 19-year-old age range. Hepatoblastomas occur much less frequently, and hepatocellular carcinomas are, fortunately, extremely rare. Many germ cell tumors occur in adolescents or young adults.

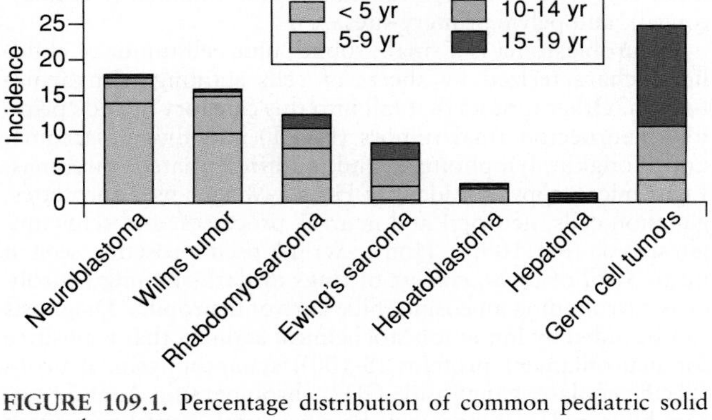

FIGURE 109.1. Percentage distribution of common pediatric solid tumors by age group.

NEUROBLASTOMA

Epidemiology and Associated Conditions

Neuroblastoma is the most common extracranial solid tumor and the most common abdominal malignancy of childhood. High-risk neuroblastoma remains one of the central problems of pediatric oncology, with long-term survival less than 40%.[7,8] Neuroblastoma represents 8% to 10% of cancers diagnosed in children and approximately 15% of cancer deaths in this population.[9,10] The age-adjusted incidence for patients younger than 15 years is 10.5 per million. The overall male-to-female incidence is 1.2:1, and there is no racial disparity.[10] Neuroblastoma is much more likely to occur in infancy, with a median age of diagnosis at 23 months.[10] Forty percent of tumors are identified in the first year of life, and 75% of tumors are seen by the fourth birthday.[11] The overall incidence of neuroblastoma has remained stable over a 21-year period.

Despite overall stable rates, neuroblastoma incidence among infants has increased somewhat during recent years. This increase may be a result of mass screening in certain areas. However, screening does not identify tumors with poor prognosis in older children and does not reduce mortality.[12–14]

Case reports associating neuroblastoma with fetal exposures, such as fetal alcohol syndrome, hydantoin exposure, or phenobarbital exposure, have not been supported by larger studies.[15,16] The occurrence of neuroblastoma has also been associated with neurofibromatosis type I (NF1), Beckwith-Wiedemann syndrome, Hirschsprung disease, musculoskeletal and cardiovascular malformations, Turner syndrome, and neurodevelopmental abnormalities.[17–19] However, data for these associations remains conflicting. Mutations in PHOX2B gene, which is often associated with congenital central hypoventilation disorder, have been recognized in those with familial neuroblastoma and in 2.3% of those with sporadic neuroblastomas.[20] Possible but unproven environmental risk factors include parental exposure to solvents or electromagnetic fields, maternal hormone use during pregnancy, and parental cigarette smoking.[21]

Recently, it was discovered that genetic mutations in the anaplastic lymphoma kinase (*ALK*) gene explain most hereditary neuroblastomas and also activating mutations can be somatically acquired.[22] This has set the scene for the development of therapeutic strategies based on *ALK* inhibition.[23]

Basic Science

Neuroblastoma was the first tumor in which molecular biologic advances in the field of oncogenes were translated into a clinically useful tool. The *MYCN* oncogene (formerly N-myc), was empirically shown to be a useful predictor of sur-
2 vival and risk. Patients with an increased number of copies of the *MYCN* gene have a much worse prognosis.[24] Most authorities consider a copy number of more than 10 to be significant. It has also been shown that when *MYCN* is amplified in the primary tumor, it is amplified in any metastatic deposits or recurrent tumors. One study demonstrated that *MYCN* amplification is an independent predictor of outcome in infants with neuroblastoma, although it remains a strongly adverse prognostic indicator in children diagnosed after 12 months of age. This finding is supported by an Italian study that showed that *MYCN* amplification was an adverse prognostic factor except in patients with stage 4s disease.[25] More recent studies, however, have shown that the poor prognostic value is present in 4s disease as well.[26,27] The *MYCN* oncogene has been identified in 25% to 35% of diagnosed neuroblastomas; amplification is present in 30% to 40% of stage III and IV neuroblastomas and only 5% of those with localized or 4s disease.[10]

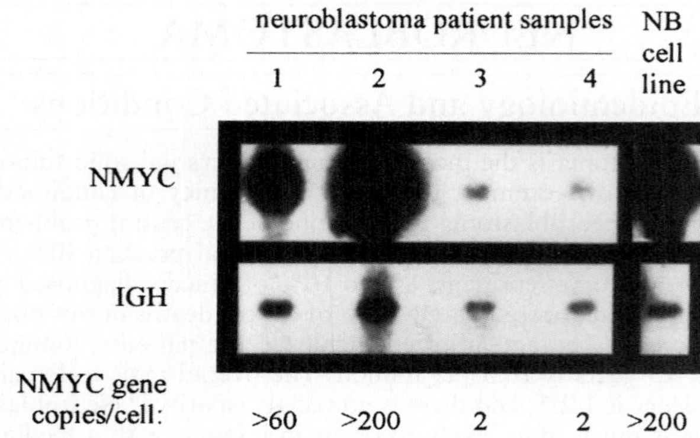

FIGURE 109.2. Example of *MYCN* amplification analysis by Southern blotting in neuroblastoma samples from four patients. The Southern blot hybridization signal obtained with the *MYCN* probe is normalized to that obtained on the same blot with a control probe for a gene not subject to amplification, such as the immunoglobulin heavy chain gene (IGH). The signals are then normalized to a negative control (placental DNA, not illustrated). A neuroblastoma cell line with *MYCN* amplification is used as a positive control. The IGH signals show that similar amounts of DNA are present in each lane, but the *MYCN* signals are grossly different from each other, indicating amplification in cases 1 and 2 and in the control cell line. Samples 1 and 2 show high-level *MYCN* amplification, exceeding 60 and 200 copies of *MYCN* per cell, respectively, which corresponds to greater than 30-fold and 100-fold amplification. Samples 3 and 4 contain two copies of *MYCN* per cell, as expected in diploid cells without amplification. (Courtesy of Marc Ladanyi, M.D., Department of Pathology, Memorial Sloan-Kettering Cancer Center.)

Rapid assessment of the *MYCN* copy number can be performed using the process of in situ fluorescent hybridization. An example of a tumor analysis from a patient is presented in Figure 109.2. The mechanism of *MYCN* amplification in neuroblastoma remains unknown. *MYCN* is a DNA-binding protein and has been shown to increase the levels of endogenous MDM2 mRNA and protein with consequent p53 inhibition. Modulation of MDM2 levels by *MYCN* may partially explain its role in neuroblastoma resistance to therapy.[28,29]

The most common cytogenetic abnormalities in neuroblastoma are 1p deletion and a gain of genetic material on 17q.[30] The presence of a 1p deletion correlates with a worse outcome in neuroblastoma and has been used as a prognostic factor.[31–33] It has been shown using cell fusion that replacement of this deleted segment is associated with a marked reduction in tumorigenicity.[34] More recently, interest has focused on the unbalanced gain of genetic material on the long arm of chromosome 17. In one multivariate analysis, a gain at 17q was a significant predictor of outcome and was associated with a worse prognosis.[35] Likely involved genes on 17q include *NM23* and the *BIRC5* (surviving gene).[10] This factor had a greater impact on outcome than either stage or 1p status. In addition, 11q loss is seen in approximately 35% to 45% of neuroblastoma patients.[36–38] Deletions of 11q have an inverse relationship with *MYCN* amplification and thus detect a high-risk population as well.[10]

Another active area of neuroblastoma research is the relation of nerve growth factor receptors to differentiation and clinical risk. The low-affinity nerve growth factor receptor gene *LNGFR* and the *TRK* proto-oncogene, which is a component of the high-affinity nerve growth factor receptor, are expressed in human neuroblastoma tissue. Several authors have shown that *LNGFR* and *TRK* (*TRK-A*) expression are inversely correlated with *MYCN* amplification and associated with lower stage at diagnosis and improved prognosis.[39–41] The absence of *TRK-A* expression was highly correlated with *MYCN* amplification in one study, in which 96% of *MYCN*-amplified tumors lacked *TRK-A* expression.[42] *TRK-C* expression is also a favorable prognostic factor in neuroblastoma, whereas *TRK-B* expression is associated with poor survival.[43] One recent study used microarray analysis to identify targets affected by TRK gene expression. In this report, TRK-A expression was associated with upregulation of proapoptotic factors and angiogenesis inhibitors. In contrast, TRK-B expression correlated with the upregulation of genes involved with invasion and therapy resistance.[44] Its activation is seen with enhanced proliferation, migration, angiogenesis, and chemotherapy resistance of neuroblastoma cells.[45]

Disturbances of conventional apoptotic pathways are also involved in neuroblastoma, both in spontaneous regression and therapy resistance. The BCL2 family, survivin, and caspase-8 have all been identified to be involved.[46–48] In neuroblastoma, Cp-G-island hypermethylation is seen to be the means for functional gene inactivation for caspase-8, TRAIL apoptosis receptors, and the caspase-8 inhibitor, among others.[47,49] Since gene hypermethylation, therefore, may lead to resistance patterns to therapies, demethylating agents, such as decitabine, are currently being investigated in preclinical studies.[10] Other features associated with resistance patterns seen in neuroblastoma include expression of MYCN, TrkB/BDNF signaling or loss of p53 expression.[45,50,51]

Molecular mechanisms have also been studied regarding involvement in local invasiveness and metastases. Metalloproteinases (mainly MMP9), activating matrix-degrading proteolytic enzymes, and molecules regulating tumor cell adhesion and migration, such as CD44 and NM23-H1, have all been identified to be involved.[52–55]

DNA index of neuroblastoma is also linked to prognosis and responsiveness of therapy. Hyperdiploid DNA content is coupled with a better prognosis and early-stage disease. Alternatively, diploid DNA content is found in approximately 66% of advanced-stage disease and frequently portends resistance to chemotherapy treatment.[56,57]

Pathology

Neuroblastoma is one of several peripheral neuroblastic tumors (pNTs). Neuroblastoma cells are derived from the primitive neural crest, as are melanocytes; Schwann cells; neuroendocrine or amine precursor uptake and decarboxylation (APUD) cells; and C cells of the thyroid gland, the autonomic nervous system, and the adrenal medulla. Neuroblastoma cells are thought to arise from primitive sympathoblasts functioning as stem cells and sometimes called *I cells*.[58] Under certain circumstances, these pluripotential cells demonstrate an ability to differentiate along a separate neural crest lineage. For instance, pure ganglioneuroma is thought to arise from complete differentiation of primitive neuroblasts into ganglion cells. Both Schwann cell and melanocytic differentiation are well-reported in these tumors. Finally, because the sympathetic nervous system extends along the entire neuraxis, neuroblastoma can arise from cervical, thoracic, abdominal (retroperitoneal), and pelvic primary sites.

Neuroblastoma is a small, round, blue cell tumor of childhood characterized by sheets of cells staining with hematoxylin. Other tumors that fall into this category include primitive neuroectodermal tumors (PNET) and Ewing sarcoma, non-Hodgkin lymphomas, and undifferentiated sarcomas. Light microscopy can identify Homer-Wright pseudorosettes, ganglion cells, neuropil and neuritic processes, and schwannian stroma (Fig. 109.3). Homer-Wright pseudorosettes, seen in up to 50% of cases, consist of rings of dark-staining neuroblasts surrounding an eosinophilic core of neuropil.[59] Diagnosis can be aided by immunohistochemical staining that is positive for neurofilament proteins (S-100), synaptophysin, neuron-specific enolase, ganglioside GD2, chromogranin A, and tyrosine hydroxylase (improved diagnosis with negative staining for markers found in other small round cell tumors).[60] PNETs

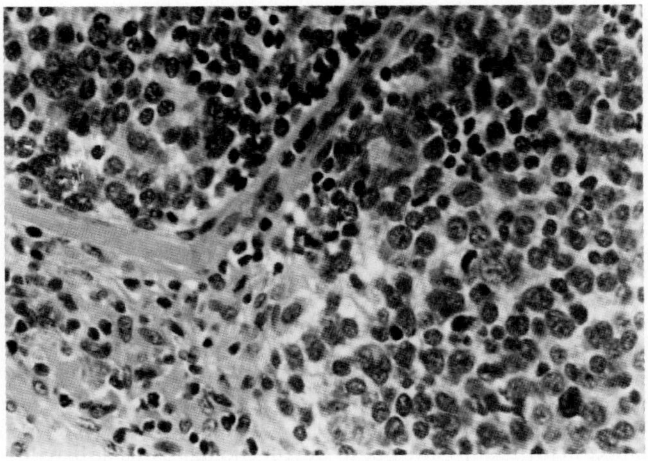

FIGURE 109.3. Typical neuroblastoma with monotonous cellular patterns. Note the mitotic figure (*center*) (×450).

may express neuron-specific enolase but not the other neural markers.[61]

At presentation, most neuroblastomas are highly cellular and have a uniform appearance. After chemotherapy, the tumor often appears to have rests of neuroblasts contained in a schwannian stroma. This histologic appearance is called *ganglioneuroblastoma,* and although it appears more differentiated, there is no impact on clinical risk, which is determined by the findings at initial diagnosis. It is also possible for tumors to contain significant amounts of stroma at diagnosis, which is associated with improved outcome. This observation is the basis of the Shimada grading system, which is summarized in Table 109.1.[62] To help predict risk, all neuroblastomas should undergo Shimada classification at diagnosis.

A new, rare yet aggressive, phenotype of neuroblastoma has been described called large cell neuroblastoma. It is a poorly differentiated schwannian stroma-poor tumor with large cells that have sharply outlined nuclear membranes and one to four prominent nucleoli. It is classified with the undifferentiated and poorly differentiated subtypes.[63]

TABLE 109.1 CLASSIFICATION

SHIMADA HISTOPATHOLOGIC CLASSIFICATION OF NEUROBLASTOMA

FAVORABLE
Stroma rich, all ages, no nodular pattern
Stroma poor, age 1.5–5 y, MKI <100
C, 1.5 y, MKI, 200
UNFAVORABLE
Stroma rich, all ages, nodular pattern
Stroma poor, age >5 y
Stroma poor, age 1.5–5 y, undifferentiated
Stroma poor, age 1.5–5 y, differentiated, MKI >100
Stroma poor, age > 1y, MKI >200
MKI, mitosis–karyorrhexis index (number of mitoses and karyorrhexis per 5,000 cells).

Reprinted from Shimada H, Ambros IM, Dehner LP, et al. The International Neuroblastoma Pathology Classification (the Shimada system). *Cancer* 1999;86(2):364–372. Permission granted for previous edition.

Neuroblastoma metastasizes to regional lymph nodes and distant sites, most frequently bone marrow and cortical bone. The liver and, rarely, lungs can also be sites of metastatic spread. Cortical bone involvement as manifested by a positive bone scan is a particularly poor prognostic indicator.[64]

Presentation, Workup, and Staging

Clinical presentation depends on site of origin, age at diagnosis, and the biologic aggressiveness of the tumor. The primary site of tumor is not located in 1% of patients.[10] Patients with metastatic or large, bulky tumors, especially if older than 1 year, may appear generally ill or anemic. The proportion of patients with cervical or pelvic tumors is higher in patients younger than 1 year than in older children. Cervical tumors present as a lateral neck mass, yet rarely cause any airway compromise. Because they arise from cervical sympathetic ganglia, cervical tumors may be associated with Horner syndrome, which is often permanent after resection and should be discussed before surgery with the parents. Regional nodal involvement is common, but distant metastases are rare and most tumors are of low risk. Primary thoracic tumors can present with respiratory distress; however, they are often detected on incidental chest radiographs.

Pelvic tumors usually are diagnosed after palpation of a mass. Bladder symptoms, bowel symptoms, and hydronephrosis can occur when pelvic tumors reach great size and compress these organs. Epidural extension to the sacrum can also be noted, and neurologic evaluation documenting somatic motor and sphincter function is mandatory.

The most common presentation among all age groups is an abdominal tumor that is often hard and fixed. The tumor arises from the midline sympathetic nerves or the adrenal gland. Often, regional nodal echelons are involved along the aorta. These involved nodes can be bulky and may extend distally to the aortic bifurcation and proximally into the mediastinum, overshadowing the primary tumor. Invasion of epidural or intradural spaces can occur, and therefore, focal neurologic deficits may be present.

Several syndromes are particularly associated with neuroblastoma: periorbital ecchymoses (raccoon eyes), opsoclonus–myoclonus syndrome, and the secretory diarrhea syndrome. Periorbital ecchymoses are caused by orbital metastases with subsequent obstruction and rupture of veins in the periorbital skin (Fig. 109.4). Vision is not usually threatened, and the ecchymoses often take months to resolve even after the orbital tumors have regressed. Opsoclonus–myoclonus, seen in 2% to 4% of patients with neuroblastoma, is a paraneoplastic syndrome thought to be caused by the development of antibodies against the tumor that cross-react with Purkinje cells in the cerebellum. It consists of rapid eye movements, ataxia, and irregular muscle movements.[65] Unfortunately, the symptoms may not resolve after tumor resection and can therefore result in devastating neurologic injury. Secretory diarrhea syndrome is caused by release of vasoactive intestinal peptide by the tumor. The watery diarrhea may require intravenous support but usually resolves with treatment and resection of the tumor.[56] This condition is an indication of tumor differentiation and is associated with low-risk lesions.

The workup is directed toward delineation of tumor extent in the primary site and identification of metastatic deposits. The primary site is usually evaluated by computed tomography (CT) or magnetic resonance imaging (MRI). CT is effective for characterizing the primary tumor site and its lymphatic extension. The lower chest should be included in scans of cervical primaries; the upper abdomen and lower neck in thoracic tumors; and the entire abdomen, pelvis, and lower chest for abdominal primaries. CT of the skull can detect widespread disease. Recently, MRI has been shown to be superior to CT for staging of neuroblastoma, as it demonstrates bone marrow and cortical

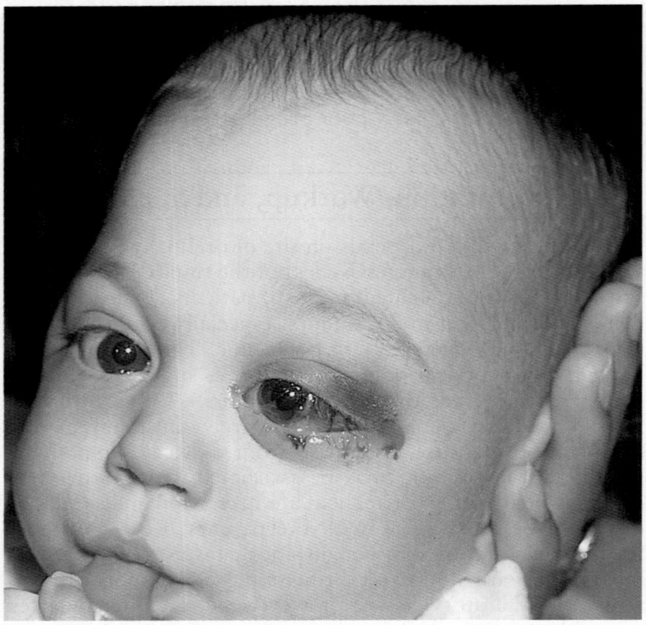

FIGURE 109.4. Periorbital neuroblastoma. (From Fleisher GR, Ludwig W, Baskin MN. *Atlas of Pediatric Emergency Medicine*. Philadelphia: Lippincott Williams & Wilkins; 2004, with permission.)

bone involvement, better characterization of intrahepatic lesions, and intraspinal extension.[66] When CT scans are used, they should be performed with both gastrointestinal and intravenous contrast. This is true even for cervical and thoracic primaries so that the position and course of the pharynx and esophagus are precisely determined. If CT or MRI scans include the liver, appropriate windows can be used to identify hepatic metastases. Ultrasound can also be used in this regard, and plain chest films are used to identify pulmonary metastases. If pulmonary metastases are present, Doppler ultrasonography can be used to identify intracaval tumor extension. It is also useful to perform a^{67} I (or^{68} I) metaiodobenzylguanidine scan to assess metastatic sites and as a baseline for evaluation of therapeutic response in the primary site.[68] I scans are more sensitive and preferable for imaging. About 10% of neuroblastomas do not take up metaiodobenzylguanidine (MIBG) and a useful surrogate is a positron emission tomography (PET) scan.[69] One study on MIBG use for diagnosis of neuroblastoma showed that using scintigraphy with CT significantly increased the detection of stage 4 disease.[70] Likewise, MIBG has been shown to locate bone marrow or cortical bone disease not otherwise found.[71] However, because of the high incidence of cortical bone involvement, especially in children older than 1 year, bone scans are performed routinely. The bone marrow is assessed by bone marrow aspiration at four iliac crest sites and bone biopsy at two sites. Finally, a 24-hour urine collection for measurement of metanephrine, dopamine, and vanillylmandelic acid may help diagnostically and as a tumor marker to assess therapeutic response. Diagnosis of neuroblastoma requires histologic confirmation either by direct tumor biopsy or by demonstration of malignant cells in bone marrow samples. Because of the wide range of molecular biologic studies that have prognostic importance, many groups attempt to obtain enough tissue at diagnosis to allow full molecular biologic and cytogenetic analysis in addition to histologic diagnosis. When possible, several grams of tumor tissue should be obtained, and a portion should be snap frozen. Biopsy can usually be achieved through a minilaparotomy or laparoscopic approach. Some groups have questioned the ethics of open biopsy when diagnosis can be obtained by examination of the bone marrow and assessment of urinary catecholamines. Some groups have tried to avoid initial minilaparotomy and base the diagnosis on elevation of urinary catecholamines and bone marrow aspirates. In this situation, biologic studies are dependent on the number of tumor cells in the aspirate with *MYCN* copy number assessed by fluorescent in situ hybridization.

The most widely used staging system for neuroblastoma is based on the international system, which is listed in Table 109.2.[72–74] This system evolved from previous systems developed by Evans et al. and the Pediatric Oncology Group (POG).[75] Tumor size and location relative to the midline remain important determinants of stage, as does the presence and degree of metastatic disease. The present system is also highly dependent on surgical resection of the primary tumor in patients with nonmetastatic disease. Recently, the International Neuroblastoma Risk Group developed a staging system based on tumor imaging and bone marrow morphology, rather than surgical resection, for pretreatment risk assessment, which is listed in Table 109.3.[76] This was developed to be used concurrently with the international system. The midline is not

TABLE 109.2 **STAGING**

INTERNATIONAL STAGING CRITERIA FOR NEUROBLASTOMA

		THREE-YEAR SURVIVAL RATE (%)	
STAGE	CRITERIA	OVERALL	RELAPSE-FREE
1	Localized tumor confined to site of origin; complete gross resection with or without microscopic margin; all identifiable regional nodes negative, including contralateral	97	88
2A	Unilateral tumor with incomplete gross excision; nodes negative	87	72
2B	Unilateral tumor with incomplete or complete gross excision with positive ipsilateral but negative contralateral nodes	86	63
3	Infiltration across the midline with or without regional nodal involvement; unilateral tumor with positive contralateral nodes; midline tumor with bilateral nodes	62	58
4	Distant metastases to lymph nodes (4 N), bone, bone marrow, liver, or other organs	<40	<40
4S	Localized primary tumor as described for stage 1 or 2 with distant metastases limited to liver, skin, and bone marrow (<10% involvement)	−75	−75

TABLE 109.3 **STAGING**

INTERNATIONAL NEUROBLASTOMA RISK GROUP STAGING SYSTEM

STAGE	DESCRIPTION
L1	Localized tumor not involving vital structures as defined by the list of image-defined risk factors and confined to one body compartment
L2	Locoregional tumor with presence of one or more image-defined risk factors
M	Distant metastatic disease (except stage MS)
MS	Metastatic disease in children younger than 18 months with metastases confined to skin, liver, and/or bone marrow

Note: Patients with multifocal primary tumors should be staged according to the greatest extent of disease as defined in the table.
Reprinted from Monclair T, Brodeur GM, Ambros PF, et al; The International Neuroblastoma Risk Group (INRG) staging system: an INRG Task Force report. *J Clin Oncol* 2009;27(2):298–303, with permission.

incorporated into this assessment.[76] Prospective analyses to validate this new system are ongoing.

Risk Groups

Neuroblastoma patients are categorized into high-, intermediate-, and low-risk groups at diagnosis. This assessment is based on age, stage, Shimada classification, and the results of specialized studies, including flow cytometry, analysis for *MYCN* amplification, cytogenetics, and *TRK* gene expression. Ancillary criteria include serum ferritin, lactate dehydrogenase, and neuron-specific enolase determinations at diagnosis and before blood transfusion. Table 109.4 lists criteria for the risk groups.[10] Risk assignment is important because it strongly determines therapy. Although 1 year was previously the cutoff age to differentiate between low and high risk, recent studies have demonstrated that diagnosis before 18 months improves prognosis. Investigations with less aggressive treatments are ongoing regarding the treatment of children ages 12 to 18 months with locoregional or metastatic disease.[10]

Treatment

Neuroblastoma treatment depends on degree of risk, as noted earlier. In general, low-risk tumors do not require chemotherapy or radiation. Resection of the primary lesion to obtain the

TABLE 109.4

CHILDREN'S ONCOLOGY GROUP NEUROBLASTOMA RISK STRATIFICATION

RISK GROUP	STAGE	AGE	*MYCN* AMPLIFICATION STATUS	PLOIDY	SHIMADA
Low	1	Any	Any	Any	Any
Low	2a/2b	Any	Not amplified	Any	Any
High	2a/2b	Any	Amplified	Any	Any
Intermediate	3	<547 d	Not amplified	Any	Any
Intermediate	3	≥547 d	Not amplified	Any	FH
High	3	Any	Amplified	Any	Any
High	3	≥547 d	Not amplified	Any	UH
High	4	<365 d	Amplified	Any	Any
Intermediate	4	<365 d	Not amplified	Any	Any
High	4	365–<547 d	Amplified	Any	Any
High	4	365–<547 d	Any	DI = 1	Any
High	4	365–<547 d	Any	Any	UH
Intermediate	4	365–<547 d	Not amplified	DI >1	FH
High	4	≥547 d	Any	Any	Any
Low	4s	<365 d	Not amplified	DI >1	FH
Intermediate	4s	<365 d	Not amplified	DI = 1	Any
Intermediate	4s	<365 d	Not amplified	Any	UH
High	4s	<365 d	Amplified	Any	Any

DI, DNA index; FH, favorable histology; UH, unfavorable histology.
Courtesy of Children's Oncology Group.

diagnosis and biologic markers is followed by observation. Serial imaging studies of the primary and possible metastatic sites in low-risk patients are performed. Urinary catecholamines should fall to normal levels and remain there. Chemotherapy is an option for those with low-risk neuroblastoma as a salvage therapy only for those who relapse after surgery.[77,78] Since those with Stage 4s without MYCN amplification often have spontaneous regression of disease, chemotherapy or low-dose radiotherapy is used only in those patients who are symptomatic from tumor burden, including substantial hepatomegaly leading to bowel obstructions or respiratory distress.[79,80]

Intermediate-risk neuroblastoma is treated with both surgical resection and moderate-dose, multiagent chemotherapy, which includes cisplatin/carboplatin, doxorubicin, etoposide, and cyclophosphamide.[10] For those whose tumor has favorable histology, survival is often greater than 95%.[81] Studies are ongoing in the hopes of minimizing treatment regimens for this group of patients.

3 High-risk neuroblastoma remains one of the central problems in pediatric oncology, with overall survival rates less than 30% despite multidisciplinary therapy and the use of multiagent chemotherapy and myeloablative regimens. Standard therapy for patients with high-risk neuroblastoma involves induction chemotherapy, local control with aggressive surgical resection and external-beam radiotherapy, consolidation therapy, and treatment of minimal disease with biologic agents. Local control is completed despite a response to induction therapy.[10]

Initial surgery should be confined to acquisition of diagnostic tissue, staging, and placement of a vascular access device. Surgical complications are higher after initial attempts at complete resection without impact on survival.[82] After a course of chemotherapy, usually four or five cycles, second-look surgery is performed (Fig. 109.5). Although perspectives on resection in high-risk patients vary, most authorities agree that complete gross resection, which is associated with excellent local control, should be the goal of second-look procedures.[83] The approach is dictated by the particular properties of the primary tumor. For upper abdominal lesions, especially those involving major midline branches of the abdominal aorta or the vena cava, thoracoabdominal exposure is helpful and well tolerated. The goal of resection is a complete vascular dissection and should encompass not only the primary but also all involved regional nodal echelons.

Chemotherapy for neuroblastoma has evolved toward higher dose intensities of multiple agents. In one meta-analysis, increased dose intensity correlated with improved overall and disease-free survival rates. In another report, primary tumor resectability correlated with increased chemotherapy intensity. There is no widely accepted regimen, and the major cooperative groups as well as larger single institutions have differing protocols. Standard induction regimens include a combination of anthracyclines, alkylators, platinum compounds, and topoisomerase II inhibitors. The COG is considering topotecan as an agent during induction. During induction therapy, stem cells are harvested and allocated for later use in the consolidation phase of treatment.[9]

Local control is achieved after induction therapy with a combination of surgery and external-beam radiotherapy. Neuroblastoma is one of the most radiosensitive solid tumors in pediatric oncology.[84] Doses of 2,160 cGy are given daily in 180 cGy fractions to the primary site of tumor. Risk of local recurrence is higher if residual tumor remains after induction therapy. Current studies are investigating higher doses of external-beam radiation for improved local control.

After induction and local control with second-look resection, patients will receive consolidation therapy with a high-dose chemotherapy and hematopoietic stem cell transplant. Chemotherapeutic agents used for consolidation include carboplatin, etoposide, and melphalan.[85] Studies looking at high-dose chemotherapy with stem cell rescue compared to maintenance chemotherapy alone have shown improved event-free survival.[7,86] Survival has been improved further with the use of purged, peripheral blood hematopoietic stem cells.[87] Early studies have shown increased event-free survival with rapid sequential tandem transplant consolidation therapy, which has spurred the ongoing phase III COG trial testing single versus tandem transplant as consolidation therapy.[87] The CCG-3891 study indicated that treatment with 13-*cis*-retinoic acid after bone marrow transplantation was associated with an improved survival rate.[7] Recently, investigators from the COG have observed, in phase III trials, improvements in overall survival and event-free survival with *cis*-retinoic acid plus a three-part immunotherapy: chimeric anti GD-2 antibody ch14.18, interleukin-2 (IL-2), and granulocyte-macrophage colony-stimulating factor (GM-CSF) for patients with high-risk neuroblastoma, after induction with dose intensive chemotherapy.[88] Chimeric anti GD-2 antibodies recognize the surface ganglioside GD2 that is usually highly expressed on the surface of human neuroblastoma cells. Further trials for this regimen are in progress.

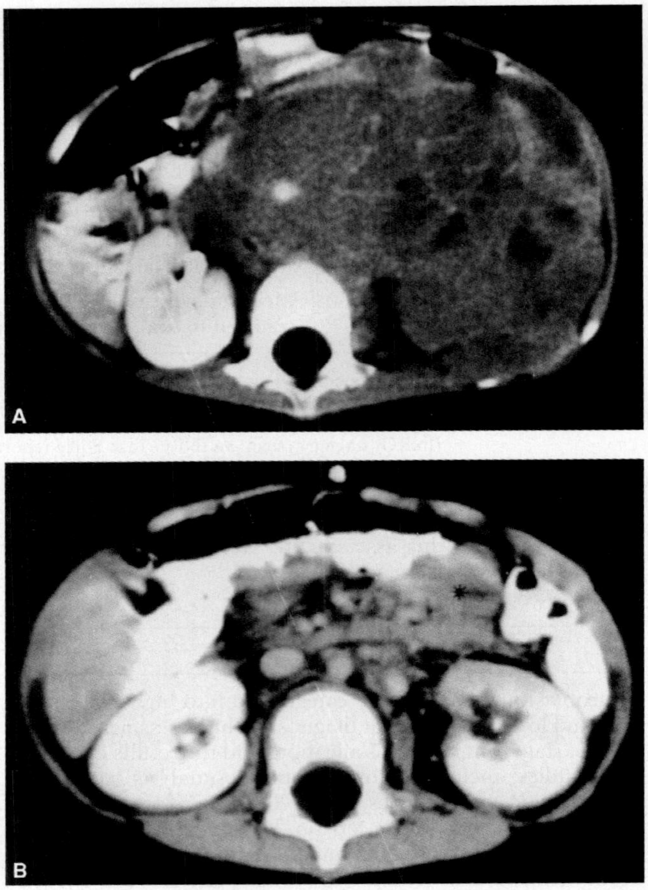

FIGURE 109.5. **A:** Initial computed tomography (CT) scan of a child with stage 4 neuroblastoma. **B:** CT scan of the same child after incisional biopsy and cytoreductive chemotherapy. Residual tumor is present despite dramatic reduction in overall tumor size.

Future Directions

Even with aggressive treatment, less than 30% of those diagnosed will survive.[89,90] Therefore, new methods for treatment continue to be studied. As neuroblastoma is typically a radiosensitive tumor,[67] IMIBG infusion signifies a way to specifically deliver radiotherapy to malignant cells. The COG is planning a pilot trial to evaluate the efficacy of MIBG with high-dose chemotherapy regimens. Bisphosphonates are under investigation as a possible agent to delay bone metastases. Nifurtimox, an antiparasitic agent, has shown some cytotoxic effects against neuroblastoma cell lines, and a phase I study is currently in progress. Rapamycin (an immunosuppressive drug also known as sirolimus) affects a pathway that is important for the cell growth and continued existence of neuroblastoma tumors through interactions with mTOR (mammalian target of rapamycin). Phase II trials including mTOR inhibitors are ongoing. Preliminary studies demonstrated a benefit to those with recurrent neuroblastoma.[91] Further studies are investigating the AKT pathway, as activation of AKT correlates with worse event-free and overall survival; however, no specific inhibitors are clinically available at this time.[92–94] Tumor vaccines and techniques of adoptive immunotherapy are being evaluated in clinical trials but so far are not curative. Biologic agents, such as histone deacetylase inhibitors, Trk tyrosine kinase inhibitors, MYCN inhibitors, and anaplastic lymphoma kinase (ALK) inhibitors, and various antiangiogenic agents have been proposed for use in minimal disease states and are undergoing clinical trials. In intermediate-risk neuroblastoma, there is a strong trend to eliminate or minimize chemotherapy.

WILMS TUMOR

Epidemiology and Associated Conditions

Malignancies of the kidney represent 6.3% of all cancer diagnoses among children younger than 15 years, with an incidence of 7.9 per million.[95] In the United States each year, approximately 550 children younger than 20 years are diagnosed with a renal cancer, 500 of which are Wilms tumors. The overall incidence of Wilms tumor or nephroblastoma is 8 per 1 million children younger than 15 years.[96] The incidence is highest among African Americans and lowest among patients of East Asian descent. The sex ratio is approximately 1:1, and the peak incidence occurs between 2 and 3 years.[97] Most Wilms tumors occur in patients younger than 5 years. Median ages reported from the National Wilms Tumor Study (NWTS) were 36 months for boys and 43 months for girls with unilateral disease, whereas boys and girls with bilateral disease presented at median ages of 23 and 30 months, respectively.[98] Rhabdoid tumors of the kidney, clear cell sarcomas, and renal cell carcinomas make up 1.0%, 1.6%, and 2.6%, respectively, of renal cancers occurring in children younger than 15 years.[95] Wilms tumors can arise from areas other than the kidney, but this is extremely rare. The most common extrarenal site is the retroperitoneum, followed by the pelvis and inguinal canal. Stage for stage, extrarenal Wilms tumors have a prognosis similar to that of renal primary tumors and therapy should be guided by principles developed by NWTS.[99–101]

Table 109.5 lists conditions associated with development of Wilms tumor along with the associated increase in relative risk. In general, the presence of any of these conditions or syndromes should initiate a workup to rule out the presence of Wilms tumor. Known risk factors include race, aniridia,

TABLE 109.5

SYNDROMES ASSOCIATED WITH INCREASED SUSCEPTIBILITY TO WILMS TUMOR[a]

■ SYNDROME	■ LOCUS/GENE	■ PHENOTYPE
WAGR (Wilms tumor, aniridia, genitourinary abnormalities, and mental retardation)	11p13/*WT1*: large deletions (also involving *PAX6*)	Absence of the iris (aniridia), genitourinary defects, and mental retardation; 30% of patients develop Wilms tumors
Denys-Drash	11p13/*WTI*: point mutations (in the zinc-finger domain)	Genitourinary defects, renal mesangial sclerosis and intersex disorder; 90% of patients develop Wilms tumors
Frasier	11p13/*WT1*: point mutations (in the KTS donor splice site)	Genitourinary defects, focal glomerular sclerosis, and intersex disorder; patients rarely develop Wilms tumor
Beckwith-Wiedemann	11p15/Several genes implicated (*IGF2*, *H19*, *p57*, and *LIT1*)	Abnormally enlarged organs (organomegaly) including the tongue (macroglossia), overgrowth of one side of the body (hemihypertrophy), hypoglycemia, umbilical hernia, and increased risk of several tumors (including Wilms tumor, hepatoblastoma, and adrenal carcinoma); 5% of patients develop Wilms tumors
Simpson-Golabi-Behmel	Xq26/*GPC3*: point mutations, microdeletions	Organomegaly, renal dysplasia, excess digits (polydactyly), diaphragmatic and heart defects; 7.5% of patients develop Wilms tumors
Sotos	5q35/*NSD1*: point mutations, microdeletions	Overgrowth, craniofacial dysmorphism, mental retardation, and increased risk of several tumors (including Wilms tumor, neuroblastoma, and acute lymphocytic leukemia); 5% of patients develop Wilms tumor
Perlman	Unknown	An abnormally large body (macrosomia), enlarged viscera (visceromegaly), undescended testes (cryptorchidism), excess amniotic fluid (polyhydramnios), characteristic facial features; 30% of patients develop Wilms tumors
Familial Wilms tumor 1 (FTW1)	17q12–21	20% of patients develop Wilms tumors
Familial Wilms tumor 2 (FWT2)	19q13.4	70% of patients develop Wilms tumors

[a]Several syndromes are associated with an increased incidence of Wilms tumor. There is a wide variation in the risk of Wilms tumor among these conditions. Other syndromes that have also been reported to have an increased incidence of Wilms tumor include neurofibromatosis type 1 and the Li-Fraumeni, hyperparathyroid-jaw tumor, and Bloom syndromes.
GPC3, glypican 3; *IGF2*, insulin-like growth factor 2; KTS, lysine, threonine, serine; *NSD1*, nuclear-receptor–binding SET-domain protein 1; *PAX6*, paired box gene 6; *WT1*, Wilms tumor protein 1.
Reprinted from Rivera MN, Haber DA. Wilms' tumour: connecting tumorigenesis and organ development in the kidney. *Nat Rev Cancer* 2005;5(9):699–712. Permission requested from publisher 11/24/2009.

genitourinary anomalies, WAGR syndrome (Wilms tumor, aniridia, genitourinary anomalies, mental retardation), Beckwith-Wiedemann syndrome, Perlman syndrome, Denys-Drash syndrome, and Simpson-Golabi-Behmel syndrome.[95]

Basic Science

For Wilms tumor, cytogenetic abnormalities have been identified on chromosomes 11p13, 1p, and 16q.[102–104] *WT1*, a gene responsible for genitourinary development, is expressed in the kidney, gonads, spleen, and mesothelium. It was cloned from 11p13 to encode four zinc finger transcriptional factors that have regulatory functions on cell growth, differentiation, and apoptosis.[105] Reduced *WT1* has been linked to stromal predominant Wilms tumor,[106] and lack of *WT1* expression has been seen in WAGR and Denys-Drash syndromes.[107,108] Only a small percentage of those with sporadic Wilms tumors are found to have mutations of *WT1*.[56] *WT2* gene, located on 11p15, has been shown to be related to insulin-like growth factor 2, and has been associated with Beckwith-Wiedemann syndrome.[105,109] In one study, *WTX*, which is located on the X chromosome, was present in 29% of patients with Wilms tumor.[110] *WTX* has been shown to be a tumor suppressor gene that controls WNT/beta-catenin signal transduction.[111] Mutations in H19, beta-catenin, and $p57^{Kip2}$ have been observed in Wilms tumor patients as well. Another study found the p53 tumor suppressor gene in 75% of patients with anaplastic histology.[112] *FWT1* (17q) and *FWT2* (19q) have been associated with several familial Wilms tumors.[113] The NWTS-5 trial reported that loss of heterozygosity at chromosomes 1p and 16q is associated with unfavorable outcomes.[114] In addition, abnormal E2F3 expression is often seen in Wilms tumors but not other renal tumors. Furthermore, miRNAs (such as miR-17–92 and oncomiR-1) have been shown to be upregulated in Wilms tumors. Since oncomiR-1 is a transcriptional target of E2F3, it has been suggested that this pathway may be involved in tumorigenesis.[115,116]

Pathology

It is hypothesized that Wilms tumor arises from primitive metanephric blastema. Individual tumors often contain primitive metanephric cells but also cartilage, skeletal muscle, and squamous epithelium. Most tumors arise unifocally within the kidney, but approximately 7% of unilateral Wilms tumors are multicentric.[97] The proportion of synchronous bilateral tumors among all patients with nephroblastoma ranges from 4.4% to 7%, whereas that of metachronous tumors is 1.0% to 1.9%.[117] Wilms tumors have equally distributed laterality and may occur with no apparent connection to the kidneys. Usually, extrarenal Wilms tumor occurs in the retroperitoneal area, but other reported sites include the pelvis, scrotum, and inguinal region.

Grossly, the tumors are globular or spherical and uniformly pale gray or tan on sectioning. Calcification is not usually apparent, unlike the stippled calcifications seen in neuroblastoma; Wilms tumors may have "eggshell" calcification in tumors that have undergone significant spontaneous hemorrhage. Cysts may be present, and in infants, polypoid extension into the pelvicalyceal system may cause confusion with botryoid rhabdomyosarcoma. Also, a pseudocapsule of compressed renal parenchyma is often found. Most tumors, unless composed of a large proportion of stromal elements, are friable and easily ruptured. This is of great significance to the operating surgeon, who must recognize preoperative rupture and avoid intraoperative spillage. The consequence of either of these events is upstaging of the lesion and the need for whole-abdomen radiation therapy with its attendant morbidity.

Microscopically, these tumors demonstrate a triphasic pattern of blastemic, stromal, and epithelial cells. Biphasic tumors with blastemic and stromal cells are common, and some specimens consist of only a single type (Fig. 109.6). The diffuse blastemal type, although often seen in patients who present with advanced-stage tumors, responds well to chemotherapy.[56] Tumors with mainly epithelial differentiation are typically less aggressive.[118]

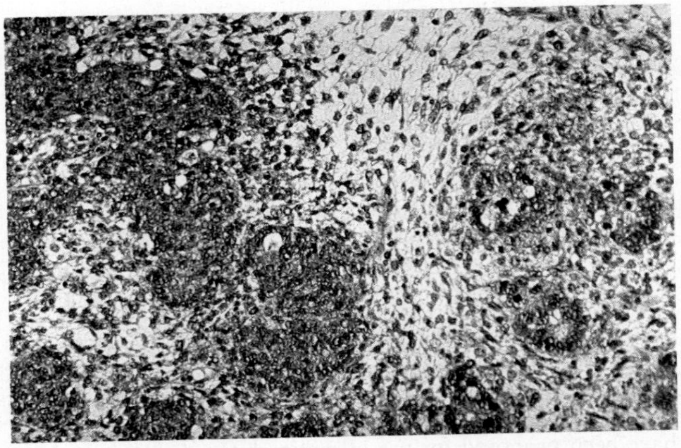

FIGURE 109.6. Wilms tumor (nephroblastoma). This photomicrograph of the tumor shows highly cellular areas composed of undifferentiated blastema, loose stroma containing undifferentiated mesenchymal cells, and immature tubules. (From Rubin E, Farber JL. *Pathology*. 3rd ed. Philadelphia: Lippincott Williams & Wilkins; 1999, with permission.)

A major parameter predictive of tumor aggressiveness and patient survival is the histologic finding of anaplasia, defined by the presence of hyperdiploid mitotic figures, threefold or greater nuclear enlargement, and hyperchromasia of enlarged nuclei. The effect of anaplasia on prognosis is so marked that tumors with these findings are designated "unfavorable histology" by the NWTS. Anaplastic tumors, which compose approximately 5% of all Wilms tumors, are rare in the first 2 years of life, but their incidence increases to 13% of patients with a Wilms diagnosis at 5 years or older. These tumors are often resistant to chemotherapy.[56]

Nephrogenic rests are persistent metanephric tissue in the kidney after 36 weeks' gestation. They have been deemed precursors of Wilms tumor, as they are seen in 30% to 40% of resected kidneys with Wilms. The NWTS-4 study documented that nephrogenic rests were present in approximately half of the unilateral and most of the bilateral tumors.[119] Rests can involute, remain quiescent, go through hyperplastic changes, or advance to focal neoplastic lesions.[56,119] Controversy remains over how to treat incidentally found nephrogenic rests.

Presentation, Workup, and Staging

Most Wilms tumors are first diagnosed after appreciation of an asymptomatic abdominal mass, which can be very large. The mass is usually discovered during routine pediatric examination or while the children are handled by a relative. Parents may need reassurance, as they are usually surprised and feel guilty that such a mass could have gone unnoticed. In a subset of patients, rapid abdominal enlargement develops, associated with pain, fever, and gross hematuria. This is attributed to intratumoral hemorrhage and may be associated with spontaneous rupture. Rarely, patients can present with symptoms of a paraneoplastic syndrome that include hypertension, hypercalcemia, erythrocytosis, and von Willebrand disease.[120,121]

The NWTS recommends the following workup for patients with suspected nephroblastoma. An excretory urogram is obtained to identify the tumor site; pelvicaliceal distortion is demonstrated, thus localizing the process to the kidney; and the function of the contralateral kidney is assessed. It is acceptable

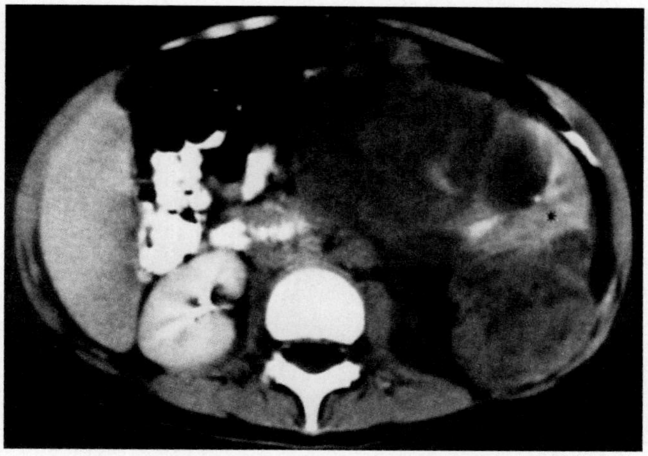

FIGURE 109.7. Initial computed tomography scan of a child with a left-sided Wilms tumor. The distortion of the calyceal system is characteristic of intrinsic renal tumor. A kidney (*asterisk*) is identifiable.

to substitute CT scanning of the abdomen with intravenous and oral contrast for excretory urography (Fig. 109.7). Indeed, almost every center performs this study routinely. Abdominal, real-time Doppler ultrasonography is performed to identify intracaval tumor extension, liver metastases, or enlarged retroperitoneal lymph nodes. Finally, good posteroanterior and oblique plain films of the chest are obtained to identify pulmonary metastases. All data in the NWTS studies concerning stage IV patients are based on a diagnosis made using plain chest radiographs. Several studies support the validity of this approach. In particular, patients with pulmonary metastases diagnosed by CT but not by plain chest films did as well as patients with nonmetastatic disease when staged and treated on the basis of their abdominal tumor alone. Some recommend that patients with pulmonary nodules identified by CT scan, but not plain chest radiographs, undergo biopsy to verify the diagnosis.[122] Because this recommendation has obvious cost-of-care and quality-of-life implications, some effort to resolve this controversy is needed, given the prevalence of CT scanning.

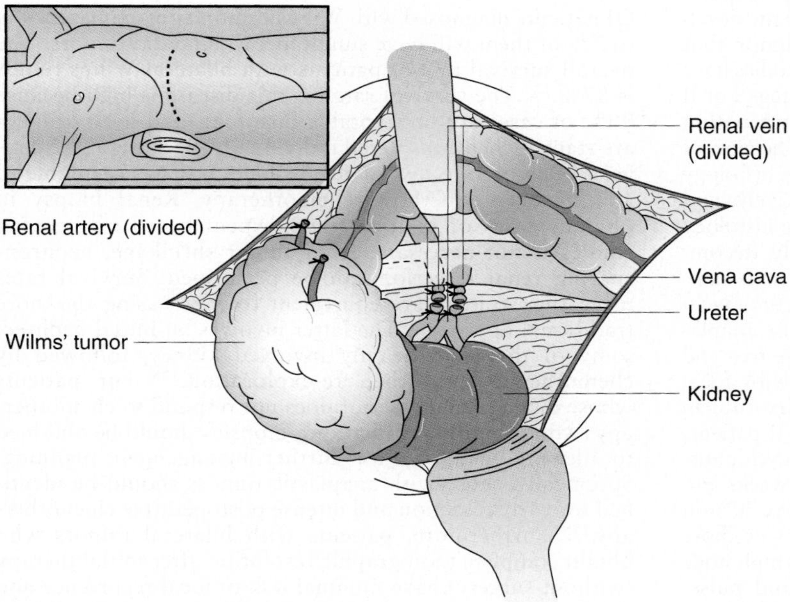

In the United States, this initial workup is followed by surgical resection of the tumor if possible (Fig. 109.8), which allows surgical and histologic parameters to be included in staging. The surgeon must pay strict attention to the local tumor extent or tumor rupture and status of the regional periaortic, interaortocaval, paracaval, and perirenal lymph nodes. Previously, direct visualization and manual palpation of the contralateral kidney was considered mandatory in all cases, even when CT scans did not indicate involvement. *Surgeons should be aware that the Renal Tumor Committee of the COG no longer recommends this approach.* Finally, the liver should be carefully palpated and the peritoneal and diaphragmatic surfaces inspected for metastases. Recently, initial treatment with chemotherapy has been recommended in cases of bilateral Wilms tumor in patients who have significant vascular invasion (discussed later in this chapter).

Once the imaging and surgical and pathologic data are acquired, a tumor stage is assigned based on the current NWTS staging schema (see Table 109.6).

Treatment

With modern treatment protocols, overall survival rates approximate 90%.[118] The focus remains on optimizing tumor response for a cure, while reducing side effects from treatment. 4 The standard of care in the United States is initial surgical resection. Exceptions to this rule include extensive intracaval tumors that require cardiopulmonary bypass for extraction, obviously unresectable tumors with documented invasion of contiguous structures, and possibly bilateral tumors, especially if it is unclear which side is most heavily involved. The European (SIOP) approach is neoadjuvant chemotherapy, and the overall survival is comparable to that found in the United States. For most patients, exploration and resection should be performed through a wide transverse incision that allows comfortable inspection and palpation of the contralateral kidney. As noted earlier, complete sampling of regional nodal echelons is mandatory, as is careful assessment of the tumor margins and possible areas of metastases. Lack of lymph nodes in the surgical specimen confers treatment as stage III disease.[118] Although most authors recommend early ligation of the renal vein, most surgeons admit to not perform this maneuver because it is often difficult or unsafe owing to the size of the tumor. The available

FIGURE 109.8. Operative approach to resection of a right renal Wilms tumor.

PEDIATRICS

STAGING

TABLE 109.6

STAGING CRITERIA FOR WILMS TUMOR

	WILMS TUMOR STAGING SYSTEM[a]	FOUR-YEAR SURVIVAL RATE (%)
Stage 1	Tumor limited to kidney and completely excised; surface intact with no evidence of rupture	97
Stage 2	Tumor extends beyond kidney but completely excised; infiltration through the renal capsule, or extension into vessels outside the kidney substance, or local open biopsy or spillage confined to the flank; no residual tumor	95
Stage 3	Residual nonhematogenous tumor	91
Stage 4	Hematogenous metastases to lung, liver, bone, brain, etc.	78
Stage 5	Bilateral renal involvement at diagnosis	Same as for highest-stage unilateral

[a]Survival based on outcome for patients with favorable histologic types in the National Wilms Tumor Study-3.
Courtesy of the National Wilms Tumor Study.

data indicate that later ligation of the renal vein after tumor mobilization does not adversely affect prognosis. After the kidney and accompanying Gerota fascia is mobilized, the renal artery is most easily identified by posterior dissection. Radical ureterectomy does not affect outcome, but the ureter should be divided well distal to the calyceal system to ensure any polypoid pelvicalyceal extensions are encompassed. It is essential to perform *en bloc* resection without tumor spillage as this produces a sixfold increase in local abdominal recurrence.[118]

Nephron-sparing surgery (NSS) is considered for patients with a solitary kidney in addition to those with bilateral Wilms tumor. NSS in those children with unilateral Wilms tumor is controversial. The size of most of the tumor contradicts this method as it would be impossible to obtain negative margins. However, tumors that may allow for the use of NSS include those that involve a single pole of the kidney, if the collecting system and vessels are not involved with the tumor, if there are clear margins between the tumor and adjacent structures, and if the tumor-bearing kidney is adequately functional.[123] Laparoscopic resection of renal tumors in children was examined; however, the risks of tumor spillage and inaccurate staging in those without chemotherapy pretreatment hinder this method.[124] Complications involved with surgical resection of Wilms include bleeding, bowel obstruction, and chylous leak.

All patients with resectable Wilms tumor receive postoperative chemotherapy. A major effort by the NWTS was the development of chemotherapy protocols for Wilms tumor that minimize toxicity while maintaining efficacy. These studies have shown survival improvements among patients with stage I or II favorable histology disease who undergo combination chemotherapy with vincristine and actinomycin D. The current 4-year relapse-free and overall survival for favorable histology stage I Wilms tumors are 94% and 98%, respectively, and relapse-free and overall 4-year survival for favorable histology stage II Wilms tumors are 85% and 96%, respectively. Recommended treatment is initial nephrectomy and lymph node sampling followed by 18 weeks of vincristine and dactinomycin chemotherapy. For stage I patients with focal or diffuse anaplasia, a similar regimen is used, and the 2-year relapse-free and overall survival is about 86%. Stage II patients with focal anaplasia receive vincristine, dactinomycin, and doxorubicin for 24 weeks as well as abdominal radiation. Stage II patients with diffuse anaplasia are treated with vincristine, cyclophosphamide, doxorubicin, etoposide, and mesna for 24 weeks and also receive abdominal radiation. Four-year survival is 70% in this group.[68,125] Favorable histology stage III tumors or those with focal anaplasia are treated with nephrectomy, lymph node sampling, 24 weeks of vincristine, doxorubicin, and pulse-intensive dactinomycin and abdominal radiation.[68] This regimen results in a 90% 4-year relapse-free survival and 95% 4-year overall survival. For stage III patients with diffuse anaplasia, nephrectomy, lymph node sampling, abdominal radiation, and 24 weeks of vincristine, doxorubicin, cyclophosphamide, and etoposide are given, resulting in a 56% 4-year survival.[126]

Patients with stage III favorable histology disease generally undergo external beam radiation therapy. The usual dose is 1,000 cGy. The entire kidney bed and areas of gross residual disease are targeted and radiation delivered to the entire vertebral column at the level of involvement to minimize the risk of scoliosis. Patients with stage IV disease should have their primary tumor staged as if metastases were not present. If the primary kidney tumor is stage I or II, no local radiation is delivered; the previously noted guidelines are followed for primary stage III tumors. Pulmonary metastases, nonresectable liver metastases, bulky nodal brain metastases, and skeletal metastases are treated with external-beam radiation therapy. The COG is currently undergoing trials regarding both radiation treatment and chemotherapy to further improve risk-stratified therapies for Wilms tumor.

Bilateral Wilms Tumor

Of patients diagnosed with Wilms tumor, approximately 4% to 7% of them will have simultaneous bilateral tumors. The overall survival rate of patients with bilateral Wilms tumor is 87%.[127] The survival rate for this disease is high because 90% of cases are of favorable histology, and most kidneys are stage I when considered individually. Because of the danger of debilitating loss of renal function, it is acceptable to administer preoperative chemotherapy. Renal biopsy in obvious cases of bilateral involvement based on imaging studies is not necessary. After tumor shrinkage, nephron-sparing renal resection can be performed. Survival rates using this strategy are equivalent to those using the more traditional approach. The latter involves an initial nephrectomy of the most heavily involved kidney, followed by chemotherapy and then re-exploration.[128] For patients whose disease progresses or does not respond to chemotherapy (with or without radiation), biopsies should be obtained to identify histology for further management planning. Specifically, those with anaplastic tumors should be identified for early resection and intense postoperative chemotherapy.[129] Furthermore, patients with bilateral tumors who obtain complete radiographic resolution after initial therapy (without surgery) have minimal risk of local recurrence and can be monitored by serial imaging.[130]

Renal Vein and Inferior Vena Cava Involvement

A study from NWTS-3 included 164 patients with gross involvement and 47 patients with microscopic involvement of the renal vein beyond the kidney (11.3%). Two-year survival rates for patients with stages I, II, and III disease were 90%, 79%, and 72%, respectively. Important predictors of outcome were histologic pattern and stage. The authors suggested that complete *en bloc* resection of the primary tumor and the renal vein extension constituted the most effective initial management.[131] In a second report from the NWTS, 165 of 2,731 Wilms tumor patients had intravascular extension (6%).[67] Vascular extension involved the inferior vena cava in 134 cases and the atrium in 31. Of these, 69 patients received preoperative neoadjuvant chemotherapy for a median of 8 weeks; 55 were treated for caval extension and 14 for atrial extension. The intravascular extension regressed in 39 of 49 patients. The overall complication rate was not statistically different in patients undergoing neoadjuvant chemotherapy compared with those treated with immediate surgery and occurred in 36.7% of patients with atrial extension compared with 17.2% of those with tumors localized to the inferior vena cava. The authors suggest that neoadjuvant chemotherapy be used in most patients with vascular extension.

Three-year relapse-free survival rates of patients with intravascular tumor extension (76.9%) do not statistically differ from the overall Wilms tumor rates (80.3%).[67] It has been suggested that a complicated operation involving cardiopulmonary bypass can be safely avoided by administration of preoperative chemotherapy. A second-look procedure should then be performed and all residual tumors resected. Second-look surgery is usually less complicated, and resection can be accomplished using conventional means. Tumor shrinkage usually is rapid when cytotoxic drugs are first administered but stabilizes after four to five cycles of therapy. At this point, no further tumor reduction can be expected and resection should be planned with appropriate preoperative consultation from other services (e.g., cardiovascular) as indicated. Nevertheless, a preoperative workup that includes Doppler ultrasonography should always be performed before operation. Contrast vena cavography has become less critical with advances in contrast-enhanced CT or MRI techniques, which now provide detailed information concerning the vascular anatomy. Nevertheless, the anatomic extent of the tumor thrombus must be determined before surgery. If tumor thrombus continues to extend to the proximal vena cava or right atrium, resection should be coordinated and performed under cardiopulmonary bypass. Without resection, intraoperative tumor embolism, which is often fatal, may be the result.

Adult and Neonatal Wilms Tumor

Wilms tumors that occur at both ends of the age spectrum are rare.[132,133] In a recent review from 1960 to 2007 including 47 fetuses and 163 infants with renal tumors, 139 had congenital mesoblastic nephromas, 41 had Wilms tumors, 23 rhabdoid tumors, and 7 clear cell sarcomas. Of those with Wilms tumor, 65.9% were stage I, none were stage IV, and 12.2% were bilateral.[134] Fetal and neonatal Wilms is treated with initial surgery, which is often curative. [134] Chemotherapy is used for those with stage IV disease or inoperable tumors.[135–137] When chemotherapy is used in children less than 1 year of age and stage greater than II, a 50% reduction in the dose of chemotherapy is recommended.[135,137] Adult Wilms tumors are associated with worse outcomes, even in patients with favorable histology. A 3-year overall survival rate reported by NWTS supports the use of aggressive therapy in all adult patients with Wilms tumor.[138–140]

Future Directions

Future work will focus on individualizing treatment to patients based on risk stratifications and minimizing side effects. As loss of heterozygosity (LOH) of 1p and 16q has worse outcomes, current COG studies are looking into more intensive treatment for this subset of patients. Other areas of investigation include the role of autologous bone marrow transplantation in patients with relapsed favorable and unfavorable histology disease, and attempts to improve outcome in the non-Wilms renal tumors in childhood. In this regard, sarcoma-like protocols, using agents such as cisplatin, ifosfamide, and etoposide, are being evaluated.

NON-WILMS RENAL TUMORS OF CHILDHOOD AND ADOLESCENCE

Clear Cell Sarcoma

5 Clear cell sarcoma of the kidney is considered a distinct histopathologic and clinical entity from Wilms tumor.[141] It has an age distribution similar to that observed in Wilms tumor but a markedly worse prognosis. Male-to-female ratio is 2:1. This tumor is characterized by a proclivity to metastasize to bones and has been called the *bone-metastasizing renal tumor of childhood* by British workers. Grossly, the tumors are soft, tan-grey, and well-demarcated. Histopathologically, the tumor consists of cords and nests of pale-stained tumor cells separated by vascular structures. Confusion with classic Wilms tumor is possible, however, and central pathologic review is recommended. Clear cell sarcoma can metastasize not only to bone but also to brain. Bony metastases are usually polyostotic, but the skull is almost invariably involved. A CT scan of the abdomen or intravenous urogram, chest radiograph, MRI of the brain, and bone scan are recommended as part of the workup. The staging system is similar to that for Wilms tumor, but high rates of tumor relapse are associated with even stage I tumors, supporting the use of aggressive systemic chemotherapy in all stages. Relapse and death occur in 75% of patients treated with actinomycin-D and vincristine alone, with more than half dying within 1 year of diagnosis. The addition of doxorubicin to the treatment regimen for these children has resulted in significant survival improvement with a 6-year relapse-free survival of 64.6%.[142] Treatment recommendations include radical resection of the primary tumor when possible as well as involved regional lymph nodes, followed by a postoperative chemotherapy regimen that includes doxorubicin, actinomycin D, and vincristine. In one randomization, a 15-month course of chemotherapy compared with 6 months improved relapse-free survival but not overall survival.[143] Preliminary results of NWTS-5 patients treated with 6 months of vincristine, doxorubicin, and actinomycin D alternating with cyclophosphamide/etoposide with radiotherapy report a 5-year event-free survival of 79% and an overall survival of 89%.[144] Postoperative radiation therapy to the tumor bed is recommended regardless of stage. Usually, 1,080 cGy of postoperative flank irradiation is administered. Patients should be followed with serial chest radiographs or CT scans and 6-monthly brain MRI scans and bone scans for at least 3 years after treatment.

Rhabdoid Tumor

Rhabdoid tumors are rare malignancies that most commonly involve the kidney in childhood; they also can occur primarily in the mediastinum or brain.[145–147] Rhabdoid tumors of the kidney occur in infancy, with a median age at presentation of 13 months (range, 2 months to 5 years). Some rhabdoid tumors may be associated with the coincident development of PNETs of the brain. Extrarenal rhabdoid tumors occur in older patients. The most common presentation is hematuria. Imaging shows a large, central, heterogeneous soft tissue mass that involves the renal hilum and has subcapsular fluid collections, tumor lobules separated by dark areas of necrosis or hemorrhage, and calcifications.[148] Metastasis, mainly found in the lungs, liver, and brain, is present in approximately 80% of those diagnosed.[149] Outcome is particularly poor, and there is no proved chemotherapy regimen. Abnormalities in the *hSNF5/INI1* tumor suppressor genes on chromosome 22 are typically found.[150] The tumor is characterized grossly as poorly circumscribed and soft with areas of hemorrhage and necrosis.[149] Histopathologically, these tumors have a rhabdomyosarcomatoid or myoblastic appearance, but the tumors do not express muscle markers and are not myoblastic in origin. The survival rate is almost zero, and even patients with stage I disease fare poorly. Therefore, patients should undergo aggressive therapy including surgical resection, local radiation therapy, and systemic chemotherapy. Because these tumors have been refractory to historical protocols, use of experimental dose-intensive chemotherapy regimens or new chemotherapeutic agents is warranted. A study of NWTS-5 looks at surgery followed by carboplatin and etoposide and alternating with cyclophosphamide for 24 weeks, and radiotherapy. Preliminary results show overall survival of 25.8%.[151,152] Current COG studies are looking at regimens for metastatic disease.

Congenital Mesoblastic Nephroma

Congenital mesoblastic nephroma was first described by Bolande[153] in 1969 and differentiated from Wilms tumor. This tumor usually occurs in infants and typically follows a benign course; however, well-documented cases have resulted in metastases and death. It usually presents as a palpable abdominal mass on physical exam and less often hematuria. However, many cases are diagnosed using prenatal ultrasound.[149] Imaging shows a large, intrarenal mass with cystic hemorrhagic or necrotic foci. Mesoblastic nephroma has been reported in adults and in patients with Beckwith-Wiedemann syndrome. A translocation, t (12;15), has been reported and is associated with an *ETV6–NTRK3* gene fusion that may link mesoblastic nephroma to congenital fibrosarcoma.[154] Histologically, the tumor consists of bundles of spindle cells, tubules of basophilic cells, and invasion into the renal parenchyma or perinephric soft tissue. The cells resemble fibroblasts or smooth muscle. Congenital mesoblastic nephroma is usually curable by radical nephrectomy alone. Wide surgical margins are essential as this tumor often infiltrates locally into perinephric tissues. Tumors with high cellularity on light microscopic examination, however, and those with evident metastases, require more aggressive treatment. In particular, older patients with densely cellular lesions or high mitotic indices should be considered for systemic chemotherapy.

Renal Cell Carcinoma

There are several reported series as well as scattered case reports of renal cell carcinoma (RCC) occurring in childhood, adolescence, and young adults. In one study,[155] the median age was 15.5 years (range, 3–21 years). Histologically, the tumor is an adenocarcinoma similar to that seen in older patients. Most reported cases are of the clear cell variant of renal adenocarcinoma. There is no predilection for the right or left side, and the tumors are equally distributed between upper and lower poles and midkidney. Bilateral disease is associated with von Hippel-Lindau syndrome. Genetic abnormalities lead to approximately 33% to 50% of pediatric renal cell carcinomas, many of which include translocations involving chromosome Xp11.2. This translocation is considered pathognomonic for pediatric RCC and results in the fusion of the *TFE3* gene.[149,150] This subtype of RCC is similar to those of clear cell RCCS; however, they contain papillary structures, eosinophilic cytoplasm, and calcifications.[149] A further genetic abnormality described is t(6.11)(p21;q12) translocation tumors, which are less aggressive than those of Xp11.2.[149] Presentation is typically with hematuria, loin pain, and a palpable mass; however, approximately 25% are found incidentally on imaging. Imaging often shows a solid, nondescript lesion with little enhancement. There may be foci of hemorrhage and necrosis.[149] Sites of metastases include lung (64%), liver (57%), bone (42%), and pleura or brain (7%). Staging is based on the adult staging system, and survival is stage dependent. Unfortunately, many of these patients present with stage IV disease. Outcome analysis shows a correlation of survival with complete resection, although resectability was also associated with adverse prognostic factors such as lymph node involvement or distant metastases. Recommended therapy is complete resection by radical nephrectomy, if feasible. Recent studies show that partial nephrectomy has outcomes similar to radical nephrectomy in patients with stage I and II disease; however, longer-term data are necessary.[156,157] In addition, immunotherapy has shown some beneficial effect on survival; however, further studies are necessary. The role of chemotherapy is undefined, but given the poor outcome associated with higher-stage disease, it is reasonable to administer postoperative chemotherapy as an experimental protocol. This should probably be performed as part of a national cooperative study.

RHABDOMYOSARCOMA

Epidemiology and Associated Conditions

In the United States, 850 to 900 children and adolescents younger than 20 years receive a diagnosis of soft tissue sarcoma each year, 350 of which are rhabdomyosarcomas.[158] Rhabdomyosarcoma is the most common soft tissue sarcoma in children younger than 14 years, accounting for almost 50% of soft tissue sarcomas in this age group. Two major histologic subtypes occur in childhood, embryonal and alveolar. Embryonal rhabdomyosarcoma constitutes approximately 75% of cases.[158] The alveolar subtype is more common in older children and extremity lesions. The incidence of rhabdomyosarcoma in the United States is 4 cases per 1 million white children younger than 15 years and approximately half that rate for black children.[159] The male-to-female ratio is 1.4:1, and 80% of patients are white, 12% are black, and 8% are of another race.

Rhabdomyosarcoma (RMS) can develop in any muscle throughout the body, and is the one tumor for which primary site affects survival.[160] Rhabdomyosarcoma has been observed in patients with neurofibromatosis and Beckwith-Wiedemann syndrome. The Li-Fraumeni cancer family syndrome involves the occurrence of sarcoma, in particular rhabdomyosarcoma, in addition to breast, bone, or brain cancer; lung and laryngeal cancer; and adrenocortical neoplasia. In this syndrome, children with rhabdomyosarcoma have first-degree relatives with the other malignancies. An autopsy study from the Intergroup Rhabdomyosarcoma Study (IRS) showed that 32% of patients with rhabdomyosarcoma had congenital anomalies that included (in order of frequency) genitourinary, central nervous system, and cardiovascular malformations.[161] Also, basal cell carcinoma has been observed in conjunction with rhabdomyosarcoma.

Basic Science

The two histologic subtypes of RMS, embryonal and alveolar, are associated with individual genetic abnormalities that are likely involved in tumorigenesis. Alveolar RMS has translocations between the long arm of chromosome 2 and the long arm of chromosome 13, t(2;13)(q35;q14), which is present in approximately 55% of cases of alveolar RMS. The translocation results in the fusion of the *PAX3* gene, which is involved with transcription during neuromuscular development, with the *FKHR* gene, also a transcription factor but in the fork-head family. Another variant is with t(1;13)(p36;q14), seen in approximately 22% of alveolar RMS, which gives rise to a *PAX7-FKHR* fusion in younger patients, mainly those with extremity lesions, and has a better prognosis. Abnormalities of the *PAX* gene cause abnormal muscle development. Currently, polymerase chain reaction (PCR) assays can confirm a diagnosis of alveolar RMS by detecting these fusion genes.[162–165] No translocations have been reported for embryonal RMS; however, it is associated with hyperdiploidy and loss of heterozygosity at chromosome 11p15 or other genes.[158,166]

Pathology

Rhabdomyosarcomas are malignant tumors that arise from the ubiquitously distributed primitive mesenchyme found in the fetus. These tumors display characteristics of striated muscle, including immunohistochemical expression of skeletal muscle myosin and actin, desmin, myoglobin, and Z-band protein. Electron microscopy may show actin–myosin bundles or Z-band material. Expression of the DNA-binding protein, MyoD1, has been shown to be a lineage marker for rhabdomyosarcoma.[167]

Based on classic pathology, rhabdomyosarcoma has been divided into four main histopathologic subtypes: embryonal, alveolar, botryoid, and pleomorphic. The most common type in children is embryonal (75%). Botryoid tumors are really of the embryonal subtype but growing into a hollow space (e.g., vagina, bladder) so that they assume a characteristic grapelike appearance. Alveolar tumors are so named because of a resemblance to the microscopic structure of the lung (Fig. 109.9). Rhabdomyosarcomas are identified as alveolar if any alveolar elements are found in the tumor. Pleomorphic tumors usually occur in older adults. For all histologic types, sites of occurrence include the following: (a) head and neck (orbit, infratemporal fossa); (b) genitourinary tract, including perineum and perianal area; (c) extremities; (d) trunk (chest wall, paraspinal area); (e) retroperitoneum; and (f) biliary tract. Histologically, RMS is composed of small round blue cells, contains muscle-specific antigens including desmin and Myo, and is composed of eosinophilic rhabdomyoblasts.[165]

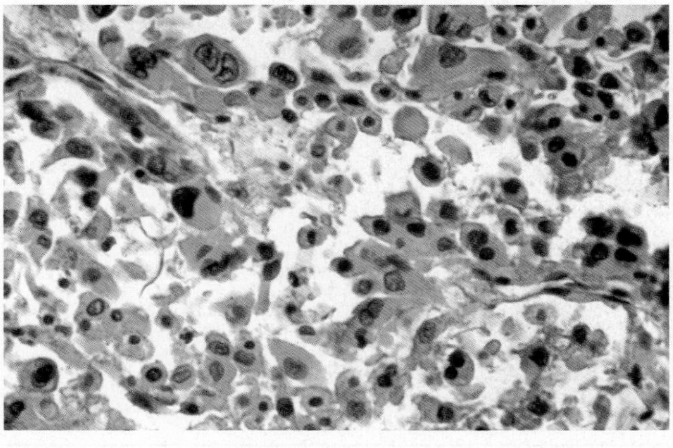

FIGURE 109.9. Photomicrograph illustrating the typical lung-like appearance of an alveolar rhabdomyosarcoma. (From Rubin E, Farber JL. *Pathology*. 3rd ed. Philadelphia: Lippincott Williams & Wilkins; 1999, with permission.)

The initial biopsy should be generous enough for cytogenetic and immunohistochemical studies. Light microscopy alone is no longer adequate to secure the diagnosis and establish histopathologic subtype as polymerase chain reaction is used to detect translocations of minimal residual disease.[168]

Presentation and Workup

The incidence of rhabdomyosarcoma is biphasic, with one peak in infancy followed by a second peak in the adolescent years. Presentation is site dependent. Head and neck lesions, found in approximately 35% of patients with rhabdomyosarcoma, can cause facial or cervical swelling and associated pain or skin discoloration. Sinusitis or middle ear infections can occur because the tumor blocks the normal drainage from these sites (i.e., sinusal ostia, eustachian tubes). Epistaxis, proptosis, or cranial nerve palsies may also be evident in head and neck lesions. Orbital sites, which occur in 75% of all head and neck tumors, have a favorable outlook in younger but not in older children. They are the least likely head/neck tumors to invade the meninges. Parameningeal involvement has a very poor outcome. Regional node sampling may be important in determination of risk status.[169]

Genitourinary tumors can present with gross or microscopic hematuria, a suprapubic mass, and urinary tract infection or obstruction. Vaginal and cervical primary tumors often prolapse through the vaginal orifice as a friable polypoid mass and may hemorrhage.

Paratesticular lesions are most often observed in adolescence as a hard mass above and separable from the testis. Extremity tumors present as a painless or painful expanding mass, and there may be an associated limp or overlying skin change. Local bony invasion may result in pathologic fractures.

Rational management depends on a thorough pretreatment workup that completely defines local tumor extent as well as evaluating regional and distant sites of metastases. Table 109.7 lists the standard workup for pediatric patients with sarcoma. An extensive history, including a family history of malignancy, and a thorough physical examination are elementary. CT scans and MRI are used for evaluation of the primary tumor and metastatic disease. However, recent retrospective studies have shown PET to be an effective addition to the current imaging modalities, with a sensitivity of 77% and specificity of 95% for defining extent of disease.[170] Prospective studies are needed. Figure 109.10 depicts a CT scan of a large pelvic rhabdomyosarcoma originating from the bladder.

Staging

An evolution in sarcoma staging has occurred since the late 1980s, with most groups adopting the tumor, node, metastasis (TNM) system defined by the International Union Against Cancer. This staging system, which is used with the older IRS grouping, is listed in Table 109.8. The grouping system is listed in Table 109.9 and has been shown to be one of the main predictors of response to treatments.[171] The TNM schema divides each stage into definable clinical components and is applied before any therapeutic interventions (although a second staging based on histologic findings of the primary tumor and regional lymph nodes after resection can also be performed). The IRS grouping schema is retained as well, although it remains operator dependent. The TNM system for rhabdomyosarcoma is unique in that it takes into account the site of disease origin, which affects prognosis.

The reported overall percentage of patients with tumors greater than 5 cm ranges from 50% to 68%, based on the TNM system. The proportions of other staging variables include invasive tumors, 37% to 71%; regional nodal involvement, 7% to 28%; and distant metastases at diagnosis, 20% to 23%.

DIAGNOSIS

TABLE 109.7

DIAGNOSTIC EVALUATION FOR SUSPECTED RHABDOMYOSARCOMA

■ EXAMINATION OR TEST	■ RATIONALE
History and physical examination	Search for lymph nodes, size of primary mass, general condition, underlying conditions.
Complete blood count	Bone marrow replacement associated with anemia or thrombocytopenia; bone marrow toxicity is the major side effect of chemotherapy.
Electrolytes, renal and hepatic function tests, creatinine clearance	Renal toxicity associated with cisplatin and other alkylators; genitourinary tumors may obstruct ureters; hepatic toxicity with dactinomycin.
Four-site bone marrow aspirations, two-site bone biopsies	Bone marrow metastases reported in up to 6% of patients at diagnosis (29% of stage 4 patients have marrow involvement); bone marrow assessment before chemotherapy.
Bone scan	Possibility of bone and bone marrow metastases
CT scan of the primary site	Evaluation of tumor size, invasiveness, enlargement of regional nodes, and complicating ureteral, biliary, bowel, or airway patency.
CT scan of possible metastatic sites	CT scanning of the lungs and liver should be done to rule out parenchymal metastases. CT scanning is superior to MRI in assessing the degree of bone destruction in paraspinal, extremity, and head and neck (base of skull) lesions.
MRI	MRI is done for the same rationale as CT scanning. It may give more detailed information regarding the extent of viable tumor (T_2-weighted imaging) and the presence of hepatic metastases. It is also the most useful tool for evaluation of the epidural space in paraspinal or base of skull primaries.
Gallium scanning	Both the primary tumor and metastatic deposits may be identified by gallium scanning.

[a]The same workup is applicable to other high-grade sarcomas.
CT, computed tomography; MRI, magnetic resonance imaging.

It is preferable to sample metastatic regional lymph nodes, but extensive nodal dissections are not indicated. In the special case of paratesticular rhabdomyosarcoma, a limited dissection of ipsilateral, periaortic nodes is used as a determinant of the need for nodal radiation. The current recommendation for paratesticular rhabdomyosarcoma is for ipsilateral, nerve-sparing lymph node dissection, especially in boys older than 10 years at diagnosis, the cohort seriously understaged by imaging studies alone. Patients 10 years or younger are staged with computed axial tomography. The use of sentinel lymph node mapping has been investigated for patients with RMS, and preliminary results are optimistic.[172,173]

Excisional biopsy should be performed on small, accessible primary lesions, with the surgeon attempting to obtain a clear microscopic margin. Patients with larger infiltrating lesions or lesions for which removal would cause debilitation or deformity

STAGING

TABLE 109.8

TNM PRETREATMENT STAGING SYSTEM

■ STAGE	■ SITES	■ T	■ TUMOR SIZE	■ N	■ M
I	Orbit Head and neck (excluding parameningeal) GU-nonbladder/nonprostate	T1 or T2	a or b	N0 or N1 or N2	M0
II	Bladder/Prostate Extremity Head and neck parameningeal Other (including trunk, retroperitoneum, etc.)	T1 or T2	a	N0 or Nx	M0
III	Bladder/Prostate Extremity Head and neck parameningeal Other (including trunk, retroperitoneum, etc.)	T1 or T2	a b	N1 N0 or N1 or Nx	M0
IV	All	T1 or T2	a or b	N0 or N1	M1

GU, genitourinary.
Reprinted from Lawrence W Jr, Anderson JR, Gehan EA, et al. Pretreatment TNM staging of childhood rhabdomyosarcoma: a report of the Intergroup Rhabdomyosarcoma Study Group. Children's Cancer Study Group. Pediatric Oncology Group. *Cancer* 1997;80(6):1165–1170. Permission requested from Wiley 11/20/2009.

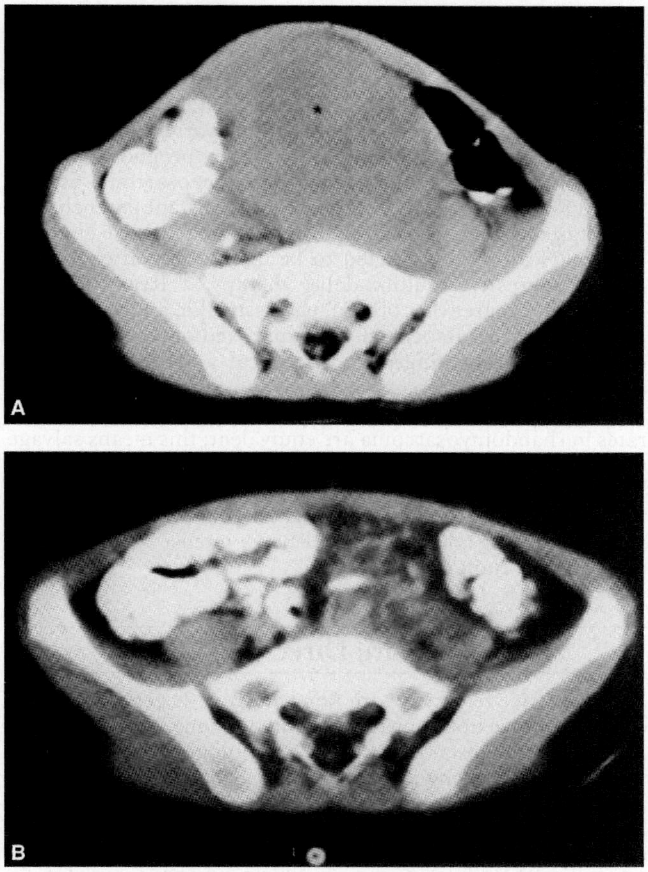

FIGURE 109.10. **A:** Initial computed tomography (CT) scan of a child with a large pelvic rhabdomyosarcoma. **B:** CT scan of the same child after biopsy and cytoreductive chemotherapy. No tumor was demonstrable by diagnostic imaging.

TABLE 109.9 **RESULTS**

SURGICAL-HISTOPATHOLOGIC CLINICAL GROUPING SYSTEM FOR THE INTERGROUP RHABDOMYOSARCOMA STUDIES I AND II

Group I	Localized disease, completely resected
	A. Confined to organ or muscle of origin
	B. Infiltration outside organ or muscle of origin; regional nodes not involved
Group II	Compromised or regional resection including
	A. Grossly resected tumors with "microscopic" residual
	B. Regional disease, completely resected, in which nodes may be involved and/or tumor extends into an adjacent organ
	C. Regional disease with involved nodes, grossly resected, but with evidence of microscopic residual
Group III	Incomplete resection or biopsy with gross residual disease
Group IV	Distant metastases, present at onset

Reprinted from Crist WM, Garnsey L, Beltangady MS, et al. Prognosis in children with rhabdomyosarcoma: a report of the Intergroup RhabdomyosarComa Studies I and II. Intergroup Rhabdomyosarcoma Committee. *J Clin Oncol* 1990;8(3):433–452, with permission. © American Society of Clinical Oncology.

(i.e., amputation or cystectomy) should undergo limited incisional or endoscopic biopsy. It is acceptable to perform transperineal needle core biopsies for bladder neck or perineal primary tumors. Enough biopsy material for light and electron microscopic analysis, immunohistochemistry, and cytogenetics should be obtained and frozen in liquid nitrogen as soon as possible after biopsy.

Risk Status

Presently the soft tissue sarcoma committee of the COG, the successor of the IRS, uses risk group assessment to determine therapy. Risk status is dependent on IRS group or stage but also age, anatomic location, and histopathology.[174–176] Favorable anatomic sites include the orbit; nonparameningeal head and neck; paratestis; vagina and non–bladder-prostate genitourinary sites; and the biliary tract.[177–179] High-risk sites include extremities, retroperitoneum, bladder-prostate, and parameningeal primaries.

Low-risk patients have embryonal rhabdomyosarcoma at favorable anatomic sites (stage 1, groups I, II, or III), or embryonal rhabdomyosarcoma at unfavorable sites but completely resected, or resected with only a positive microscopic margin (groups I or II). Intermediate-risk patients have embryonal rhabdomyosarcoma at unfavorable sites with residual gross disease (group III). The intermediate-risk group also includes patients with metastatic rhabdomyosarcoma who are younger than 10 years and patients with localized disease who have alveolar histology or undifferentiated sarcoma. High-risk patients have metastatic rhabdomyosarcoma or undifferentiated sarcoma at presentation, excepting patients younger than 10 years.

Treatment

6 The modern treatment of rhabdomyosarcoma is multidisciplinary and includes multiagent chemotherapy, judicious resection, and radiation therapy. The intensity of therapy should be tailored to the risk of subsequent relapse, which is a function of TNM stage. In general, agents are combined to limit drug resistance while attaining a synergistic antitumor effect.

A surgical procedure is typically done to confirm the diagnosis of rhabdomyosarcoma. However, often there remains gross residual tumor or positive surgical margins.[180,181] Adequate margins of 0.5 cm should be obtained surrounding the tumor, which is easier to accomplish in tumors of the extremities or trunk. Clear margins are necessary but are not achievable when this would result in removing normal tissue that cannot be resected; or serious disfigurement or disability; or when it technically cannot be completed.[180]

Surgical resection of the primary tumor was the mainstay of treatment 50 years ago but resulted in overall survival rates of only approximately 20%. The addition of chemotherapy improved the rate to 50%. Resection of primary tumors should be undertaken either before chemotherapy for small, noninvasive lesions or after documented response with more formidable primary tumors. An example of the operative approach for a lower extremity rhabdomyosarcoma involving anterior thigh muscles is depicted in Figure 109.11. In certain situations in which chemotherapy results in complete or very good tumor regression, external beam irradiation may be used as a primary means of local control. Even in these circumstances, it is important to obtain biopsy specimens to document complete tumor eradication. Debilitating or disfiguring surgery should be performed only if residual tumor is present after both chemotherapy and therapeutic irradiation. Amputation of extremity rhabdomyosarcomas does not enhance cure and should be performed only when lesions are bulky, invade bone or neurovascular structures, or are recurrent and cannot be resected by lesser procedures. Similarly, radical cystectomy is reserved for situations in which complete tumor eradication

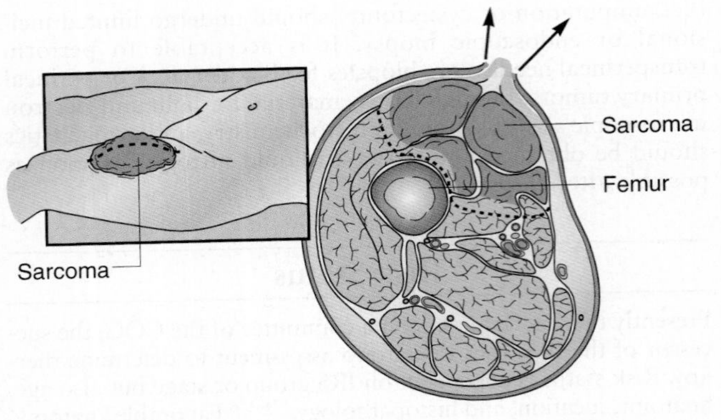

FIGURE 109.11. Technique for resection of a proximal lower-extremity rhabdomyosarcoma. Longitudinal incisions are always used. It is important to excise the tumor completely, with a surrounding 1- to 2-cm margin if feasible.

has not been accomplished by chemotherapy and external-beam irradiation.

Second-look operations are often done after a partial response or no response to chemoradiation therapy, and after relapse. The guiding principle of rhabdomyosarcoma surgery is complete tumor resection, but removal of large amounts of normal tissue (i.e., muscle group resection, amputation) alone does not affect outcome.

The trend since the early 1990s has been to minimize treatment toxicity for genitourinary rhabdomyosarcoma.[182–186] Currently, all patients with these tumors receive neoadjuvant chemotherapy after cystoscopic or transperineal biopsies confirm the diagnosis. This therapy is followed by repeat evaluations, including cystoscopic or percutaneous biopsies as well as imaging studies. A complete response after chemotherapy may obviate the need for external-beam radiation therapy in some cases, but most patients require local radiation. Surgery is reserved for recurrent or poorly responsive cases with residual gross tumor.[187] Exenterative cystectomy has decreased from more than 50% to 30% with the use of neoadjuvant chemoradiation.[188] When anatomically feasible, partial cystectomy is effective and preserves bladder function.[184] Newer techniques of urinary reconstruction involving stomas that can be catheterized may improve patients' quality of life.

Most patients with low-risk rhabdomyosarcoma are treated with vincristine and dactinomycin. Intermediate-risk patients receive cyclophosphamide in addition to these two drugs, and current studies are evaluating other agents. High-risk patients have a very poor outlook, and new therapies—including the use of irinotecan, melphalan, ifosfamide, and etoposide—are in development.

External-beam radiation therapy of the primary site or involved regional nodal echelons has contributed to locoregional control. All patients with group II to IV disease, in addition to group I alveolar tumors, receive radiotherapy.[189] Orbital and genitourinary primaries receive radiation therapy as the primary means of local control, with surgery reserved for very specific indications in patients with refractory or recurrent disease. Clinical data suggest that doses from 26 Gy to 50.4 Gy can be used in combination with chemotherapy. There is no difference in locoregional control rates between patients treated with conventional versus hyperfractionated radiotherapy.[189] Recent improvements in administration of radiation therapy include intensity-modulated radiation therapy (IMRT) and computer-modulated radiotherapy.[190,191] The COG is currently studying "up-front" radiotherapy with chemotherapy administered earlier than currently given.[160]

Outcome

The overall 5-year survival for children with rhabdomyosarcoma is approximately 64%. Table 109.10 lists the estimated 5-year failure-free survival and overall survival of patients with nonmetastatic rhabdomyosarcoma by prognostic factors based on the COG's Intergroup Rhabdomyosarcoma Studies III and IV.[192] As expected, the presence of distant parenchymal metastases at diagnosis has an overwhelming adverse effect on survival, with 25% expected to be disease free after 3 years despite aggressive multimodality therapy.[180] Regarding site, most authors agree that orbital, paratesticular, and vaginal primary tumors are associated with improved outcome, whereas extremity, parameningeal, and truncal and retroperitoneal sites carry a worse prognosis. Survival is stage dependent.

Most studies conclude that overall and disease-free survival rates in rhabdomyosarcoma are equivalent; this means salvage after initial relapse is low and may depend on initial stage and histopathologic subtype. Therefore, primary therapy is crucial for long-term survival.[193] This suggests that, after risk assessment by staging, therapy should be as intense as possible to eradicate the tumor.

Future Directions

Myeloablative regimens with bone marrow or peripheral stem cell rescue have not improved overall outcome in patients with recurrent or metastatic disease.[194–197] Biologic or immunologic therapy for rhabdomyosarcoma is not available. There is great interest in reducing the intensity of therapy for patients with low-risk tumors. Most clinical research for the worst-risk cases has focused on development of new chemotherapeutic regimens with activity against this tumor. There is also an interest in combining the use of chemotherapy and radiotherapy and in using pre-resection radiotherapy.

NONRHABDOMYOMATOUS SOFT TISSUE SARCOMAS

Epidemiology

Nonrhabdomyomatous soft tissue sarcoma (NRSTS) is a heterogeneous collection of tumors that accounts for 3% to 5% of pediatric tumors.[198] These tumors are different from rhabdomyosarcomas in histology, clinical characteristics, and prognosis. There is a bimodal age distribution, with tumors occurring most commonly in infants and adolescents, with slightly higher incidence among males. This group of tumors is composed of diverse histologic tumor types, no subtype of which represents more than 15% of all cases.[199] Since these tumors are rare, they are often analyzed as a group. The most common of the NRSTS tumors in children are dermatofibrosarcoma protuberans, malignant fibrous histiocytoma, synovial sarcoma, malignant peripheral nerve sheath tumor, and fibrosarcoma.

Pathology and Genetics

NRSTS are tumors of somatic tissue, derived from primitive mesenchyme. Table 109.11 characterizes these tumors. Each tumor type corresponds to normal cell types that develop from mesenchymal cells. The International Classification of Childhood Cancer has classified these tumors into four subgroups: fibrosarcoma category, Kaposi sarcoma category, the "other specified" soft tissue sarcomas, and the "unspecified" soft tissue sarcomas, none of which have any prognostic or therapeutic relevance.[199]

TABLE 109.10 **RESULTS**

ESTIMATED 5-YEAR FFS AND OVERALL SURVIVAL OF CHILDREN WITH NONMETASTATIC RMS BY PROGNOSTIC FACTORS (n = 1,258)

PATIENT SUBSET AND FACTOR	NO. OF PATIENTS	ESTIMATED 5-YEAR FFS RATE		ESTIMATED 5-YEAR OVERALL SURVIVAL RATE	
		%	95% CI	%	95% CI
Alveolar RMS/UDS	370	65	60–70	72	67–76
Stage 1 or 2, group I or II	119	80	72–87	86	78–91
Stage 1 or 2, group III	56	76	63–86	78	64–87
Age 1+ years	49	83	70–92	83	69–91
Age <1 year	7	29	4–61	43	10–73
Stage 3, group I or II	73	66	54–76	77	65–85
Stage 3, group III	122	45	36–54	52	43–61
N0	60	56	42–67	66	52–77
N1	51	31	19–44	34	21–47
Embryonal RMS888	82	79–84	88	86–90	
Low-risk subset A[a]	403	90	86–92	97	94–98
Age <10 years	324	92	88–94	97	94–99
Age ≥10 years	79	82	71–89	94	85–98
Low-risk subset B[b]	80	87	77–93	96	88–99
Size ≤5 cm	37	100	—	100	—
Size >5 cm	42	77	60–87	93	79–98
Intermediate	405	73	69–77	78	74–82
T1, age 1–9 years, nonextremity	73	90	80–95	90	80–95
T2, age 1–9 years, nonextremity	197	75	69–81	81	74–86
T1, age <1 or ≥10 years, nonextremity	19	73	45–88	89	62–97
T2, age <1 or ≥10 years, nonextremity	73	56	43–67	61	48–71
Extremity	18	43	20–64	46	21–68

CI, confidence interval; FFS, failure-free survival; RMS, rhabdomyosarcoma; UDS, undifferentiated sarcoma.
[a]Low-risk subset A: stage 1, group I or IIa; stage 2, group I; and group III orbit disease.
[b]Low-risk subset B: stage 1, group IIb or IIc; stage 1, group III nonorbit; stage 2, group II; and stage 3, group I or II.
Reprinted from Meza JL, Anderson J, Pappo AS, et al. Analysis of prognostic factors in patients with nonmetastatic rhabdomyosarcoma treated on. Intergroup Rhabdomyosarcoma Studies III and IV: The Children's Oncology Group. *J Clin Oncol* 2006;24(24):3844–3851, with permission.

Presentation and Diagnostic Evaluation

Patients with NRSTS typically present with a painless mass that is often slow growing. Further symptoms may be present, secondary to compression by the tumor or invasion of adjacent tissues. Tumors that occasionally develop in the head and neck, such as fibrosarcomas, can be associated with swallowing and airways problems, which may require lifesaving tracheostomy. Approximately 15% of patients present with metastatic disease, most commonly in the lungs.[201] Bone marrow invasion is uncommon.

Workup for NRSTS begins with imaging, typically MRI, to provide anatomic definition; however, CT of the chest, abdomen, and pelvis is useful for staging. Core needle biopsies, which have higher sensitivity and specificity, are often used for diagnosis.[202–204] In addition to routine histopathology, immunohistochemistry, cytogenetic and molecular studies, flow cytometry, and electron microscopy are recommended for accurate diagnosis.

Staging

There is currently no validated staging system for pediatric NRSTS. The Intergroup Rhabdomyosarcoma Study Group's surgicopathologic system for rhabdomyosarcoma is often extrapolated to NRSTS. Staging systems for adults, which take into account tumor size, tumor extent, and tumor grade, are also used. The COG is currently working on a staging/grading system for NRSTS.

Treatment

The primary treatment modality for NRSTS is surgery. These tumors are resistant to chemotherapy and radiotherapy, so gross total resections are crucial when possible. A 1-cm margin is recommended. However, wide resections may not be attainable secondary to functional or cosmetic effects. When complete resection would require mutilating surgery such as amputation or laryngectomy, simple observation may be the best treatment. Often, the tumor mass is dormant for years, allowing growth of the affected part and the possibility of a less debilitating or deforming resection later. Radiation is often used to treat residual disease and has been shown to reduce the risk of local recurrence.[205] Optimal dose and timing of radiation therapy is unclear. Although intraoperative radiation therapy (IORT) and IMRT have been used with

RESULTS

TABLE 109.11

NONRHABDOMYOSARCOMA TUMOR CHARACTERISTICS

TUMOR TYPE	INCIDENCE[a]	NORMAL COUNTERPART[a]	CYTOGENIC ABNORMALITY[a]	GENES INVOLVED[a]	COMMON PRIMARY SITES
Fibrosarcoma	0.6	Fibroblast	t(12; 15)	TEL (ETV6), NTRK3 (TRKC)	Lower extremity > upper extremity
Desmoplastic round cell tumor[b]	Approximately 200 case reports[c]	Lineage from epithelial, neural, and myogenic cells	T(11; 22)	EWS, WT1	Abdomen, paratesticular, thoracic cavity
Leiomyosarcoma	0.3	Smooth muscle	Variable	Multiple gene alterations	Gastrointestinal or genitourinary tract, superficial dermis, retroperitoneum, lungs, uterus, vascular wall
Alveolar soft parts tumor	0.1	Unknown	t(x; 17)	ASPL, TFE3	Thigh, buttocks, abdominal and chest walls
Neurofibrosarcoma	0.6	Schwann cell	Variable, abnormalities of chromosome 17	Multiple gene alterations, associated with NF1	Extremity > retroperitoneum > trunk
Liposarcoma	0.1	Adipocyte	t(12;16)	FUS, CHOP	Lower extremity > upper extremity > retroperitoneum
Tendosynovial sarcoma	0.7	Synovial cells	T(X; 18)	SYT, SSX-1, or SSX-2	Lower extremity (thigh, foot posterior knee) > upper extremity (shoulder, forearm)
Dermatofibrosarcoma protuberans	1.0	Fibroblast	t(17; 22)	COL1A1, PDGF	Trunk > proximal extremities

[a]From Gurney J, Young J Jr, Roffers S, et al. In: Ries LAG, Smith MA, Gurney JG, et al., eds. *Cancer Incidence and Survival among Children and Adolescents: United States SEER Program 1975–1995*. Bethesda, MD: National Cancer Institute, SEER Program; 1999.
[b]From Saab R, Khoury JD, Krasin M, et al. Desmoplastic small round cell tumor in childhood: the St. Jude Children's Research Hospital experience. *Pediatr Blood Cancer* 2007;49:274–279.
[c]Incidence age-adjusted per million younger than 20 years old (excluding desmoplastic round cell tumor).

encouraging results, data for the pediatric population is inadequate. NRSTS tumors are chemoresistant; however, chemotherapy may be used in patients with unresectable disease with the goal of making these patients surgical candidates. Chemotherapy is also sometimes used for residual disease after surgery. It is also often used for patients with distant spread or at high risk for distant spread, although this use is controversial. Doxorubicin and ifosfamide are typically used.[206,207] Novel therapies, including targeted therapies, are currently being studied, including antibody 8H9 in desmoplastic round cell tumors.

Outcome

Characteristics of NRSTS that affect outcomes include disease extent, histologic grade, tumor size, and degree of resection.[201,208–214] Survival in patients with high risk or metastatic disease is approximately 15%. Survival in patients deemed intermediate risk (those with unresectable disease, or high grade with >5 cm) is approximately 50%. Patients with resectable tumors, or low risk, have a survival of approximately 90%.[215]

HEPATIC TUMORS

Hepatoblastoma versus Hepatocellular Carcinoma

Epidemiology and Genetics. In Europe and North America, primary liver tumors constitute approximately 1.1% of childhood malignant neoplasms (1.4 cases per 1 million children in the United States).[216] The ratio of hepatoblastoma to hepatocellular carcinoma is variously reported from 1.3:1 to 6.5:1, accounting for approximately two thirds of all liver tumors in children[217,218]. In areas endemic for hepatitis B, the ratio may be reversed and as low as 0.2:1. No geographic clustering of cases of hepatoblastoma has been noted. A male predominance is usually reported for both tumors, the ratio ranging from 1.5:1 to 3.1:1 for hepatoblastoma and from 1.3:1 to 3.2:1 for hepatocellular carcinoma. Between 1973 and 1997, 67% of hepatic malignancies in patients younger than 20 years were hepatoblastomas and 33% hepatocellular carcinomas.[219] Among children younger than 5 years, hepatoblastoma accounted for 91%. In children 15 to 19 years, hepatocellular carcinoma accounted for 87%. Hepatoblastoma is more common in children born premature than at full-term. [220–222]

Hepatoblastoma occurs sporadically in adults, but the tumor usually presents in the first 3 years of life. Congenital presentation and antenatal diagnosis have also been reported.[218] Hepatocellular carcinoma, in contrast, is rare in infancy. The median age for diagnosis of hepatoblastoma in children is 18 months, whereas most cases of hepatocellular carcinoma are diagnosed after children are 10 years old.[223] Historical series without pathologic review may report a higher rate of infantile hepatoma because of misdiagnosis of some early hepatoblastomas.

Hepatoblastoma has been linked to various genetic syndromes and familial conditions, such as familial adenomatous polyposis and Beckwith-Wiedemann syndrome.[224,225] Erroneous imprinting at the 11–15 locus; alterations in the beta-catenin/Wnt pathway; and trisomies of chromosomes 2, 8, and 20 and rearrangements of chromosome 1 are seen in hepatoblastoma as well.[226–231]

Clinical Presentation

Children with hepatoblastoma most commonly present with abdominal mass or diffuse abdominal swelling. Not infrequently, the child is in good health, and the lesion may be discovered on routine examination. Accompanying symptoms, such as pain, irritability, minor gastrointestinal disturbances, fevers, and pallor, occur in fewer patients. Significant weight loss is unusual, although patients may fail to thrive.

In contrast, although children and adolescents with hepatocellular carcinoma frequently present with palpable abdominal masses, these are rarely incidental. Pain is frequently present and can occur in the absence of an obvious mass. Constitutional disturbances, such as anorexia, malaise, nausea and vomiting, and significant weight loss, occur with greater frequency. Jaundice is an uncommon feature of either disease.

In most series of hepatoblastoma and hepatocellular carcinoma, a few patients present acutely with tumor rupture. Hepatoblastoma can present with sexual precocity caused by androgen synthesis or beta-HCG, although this is rare.

Laboratory Studies

Mild anemia is common in both conditions, and thrombocytosis is most often seen in patients with hepatoblastoma but occasionally in patients with hepatocellular carcinoma.[232] The cause for thrombocytosis in these conditions is unknown but may be related to release of tumor-derived cytokines.

Liver function test results are usually nonspecifically deranged in both conditions. A high serum cholesterol level is present in 50% to 60% of cases, and evidence suggests that higher elevations may correlate with a poorer prognosis. Beta-HCG is commonly secreted by liver tumors, and serum assays are often elevated. The most useful tumor marker is the serum α-fetoprotein (AFP). Elevation, often extreme, occurs in approximately 84% to 91% of cases of hepatoblastoma. Fewer patients with hepatocellular carcinoma have elevated AFP levels, and the elevation tends to be less marked. Patients with fibrolamellar variant of hepatocellular carcinoma rarely have elevated AFP. Although nonspecific for epithelial liver tumors, the AFP marker is used extensively to monitor both disease reduction in patients undergoing nonoperative therapy and disease recurrence in treated patients. Some reports concluded that a rise in AFP above normal in a patient with quiescent disease is more sensitive than radiology or surgical exploration to detect recurrence. Of note, AFP is often elevated in healthy children younger than 6 months and also may be elevated during liver damage, liver regeneration, or with other tumors.

Imaging Studies

Abdominal CT scanning is the investigation of choice both for diagnostic discrimination and to assess operability. The chest should be included to identify pulmonary metastases. Hepatoblastoma typically appears as a solitary mass with lower attenuation values than a normal liver (Fig. 109.12). Dramatic contrast enhancement (as in benign vascular neoplasms), invasion of the portal vein, and lymph node involvement are unusual. Hepatocellular carcinomas have a similar appearance but are more likely to be multifocal, invade the portal vein, and metastasize to draining lymph nodes. Distinction between the two lesions cannot be definite because the pattern of disease may be atypical in either instance.

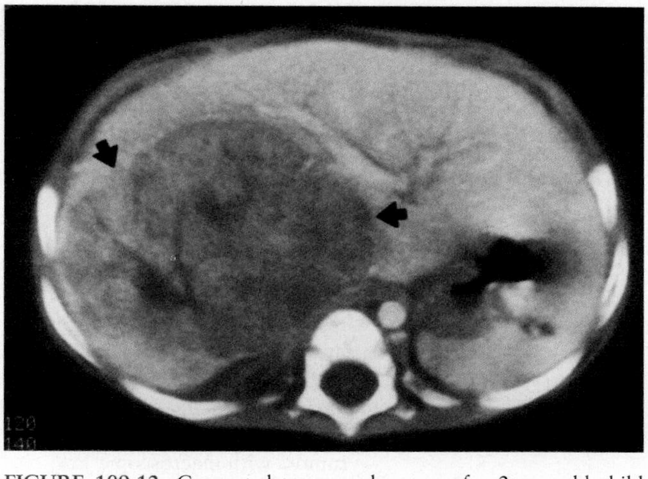

FIGURE 109.12. Computed tomography scan of a 2-year-old child with a large right lobar hepatoblastoma (*arrows*). Despite the large size, these lesions can often be completely resected before chemotherapy. Hepatocellular carcinoma, in contrast, often involves multiple hepatic segments, and there is a significant incidence of extrahepatic extension.

The diagnostic ability of MRI is similar to that of CT. The particular features of both hepatoblastoma and hepatocellular carcinoma on MRI are low signal intensity on T_1-weighted images and high intensity on T_2-weighted images. The two lesions cannot be distinguished by appearance alone.

Plain radiographs and liver-spleen scans usually indicate abnormalities but do not often contribute to diagnosis or assist in planning therapy. Angiography is indicated if embolization or infusion chemotherapy is contemplated, but this test is invasive, technically difficult in childhood, and not universally available. Similar information is available from dynamic CT scan or MRI such that these methods are considered adequate in most instances.

An abdominal ultrasound, in view of the low cost and ready accessibility, is probably the most useful screening investigation for children with large livers. This technique allows distinction between space-occupying lesions and diffuse hepatomegaly. Anatomic detail of the tumor margin is not usually sufficiently well delineated to assess resectability. Doppler ultrasound is also useful to evaluate patency of the inferior vena cava and hepatic veins, but extreme compression of these vessels may prevent useful interpretation.

The ability of imaging studies to predict resectability is questionable. Resectable lesions must usually be confined to the right lobe, right lobe plus medial left lobe, or the left lobe; in addition, the hepatic veins, inferior vena cava, and portal vein must be free of disease. On occasion, the distinction between compression versus invasion of liver adjacent to the lesion cannot be made, nor can the patency of vessels be established with certainty. In rare instances, it may be obvious that metastases in the remaining liver, portal or periaortic nodes, or other intra-abdominal organs preclude complete resection.

The available data do not establish any superiority of MRI or CT scan for evaluating the resectability of hepatic malignancies in children. In view of the possible advantage of

TABLE 109.12 **STAGING**

CHILDREN'S ONCOLOGY GROUP STAGING FOR HEPATOBLASTOMA

Stage I	Complete resection
Favorable histology	Purely fetal histology with a low mitotic index
Other histology	All other stage I tumors
Stage II	Gross total resection with microscopic residuals or total resection with preoperative or intraoperative rupture
Stage III	Unresectable tumors as determined by the attending surgeon, partially resected tumors with macroscopic residual, or any tumor with lymph node involvement
Stage IV	Measurable metastatic disease to lungs or other organs

Courtesy of the Children's Oncology Group.

TABLE 109.13

COMPARISON OF RELATIVE RISK OF DEATH FOR HISTOLOGIC SUBTYPES OF HEPATOBLASTOMA

HISTOPATHOLOGIC SUBTYPE	RELATIVE RISK FOR DEATH OF DISEASE[a]
Fetal	1.07
Embryonal	1.74
Mixed	0.53
Macrotrabecular pattern	1.20
Small cell undifferentiated	3.71

[a]Risk of death adjusted for age, sex, and stage compared with other histologic subtypes.

primary resection, a more reliable option is to judge resectability at formal laparotomy.

Early diagnosis by screening patients with genetic defects and families with hepatitis B is unlikely to have a major impact in Western nations. In Taiwan a program of early vaccination significantly reduced the incidence of hepatocellular carcinoma.[233,234]

Staging

A staging system was derived and has been modified by the COG (Table 109.12) based on surgical findings and outcome of a primary operation before systematic therapy has been administered. Alternatively, a TNM classification has been proposed by the International Union Against Cancer and the American Joint Committee on Cancer and another by the Japanese Society for Pediatric Surgery. More recently, the PRETEXT (PRE-Treatment EXTent of disease) system has been advocated by SIOPEL (International Society of Pediatric Oncology Liver Tumor Group). This is a pretreatment, radiographic staging system that emphasizes the anatomic site of involvement as well as the number of involved Couinaud hepatic segments.[235] A recent report from COG on the role of PRETEXT showed that COG stage and PRETEXT are good predictors of mortality and long-term survival.[236]

Pathology

Hepatoblastoma usually presents as a single, pseudoencapsulated lesion, often reaching large proportions before becoming clinically apparent. The tumor grows in an expansive fashion such that the umbilical fissure usually is not breached. Thus, despite a 30% to 40% incidence of bilobar disease, successful extended resection may still be possible. Multicentricity or massive diffuse disease within the liver occurs in less than 20% of patients, and cirrhosis of the surrounding liver is unusual.

In contrast, hepatocellular carcinoma usually lacks a distinct capsule. The tumor spreads diffusely through the liver in up to 70% of patients, often with satellite nodules well separated from the main tumor mass. Bilobar involvement occurs in 50% to 70% of cases, and the umbilical fissure does not constitute a barrier to spread. As a result, hepatocellular carcinoma is usually unresectable. Finally, because of the association of hepatocellular carcinoma with hepatitis B infection, cirrhosis may be present in the surrounding nonneoplastic liver. This may preclude complete tumor resection if the volume of liver to be removed is likely to compromise liver function further.

Hepatoblastoma is made up of embryonal-like cells, similar to hepatic stem cells. It contains five histologic subtypes including pure fetal, embryonal, mixed epithelial, mesenchymal/macrotubular, and small cell undifferentiated. The fetal subtype has the best outcome and small cell/undifferentiated the worst.[237–239] One analysis showed that resected patients with pure fetal histologic type have a 2-year survival rate of 92%, which is significantly better than that for patients with embryonal or anaplastic tumor components (63% and zero 2-year survival rates, respectively).[240] A comparison of the relative mortality risks for subtypes of hepatocellular carcinoma is listed in Table 109.13. In addition to the epithelial element, hepatoblastoma may contain varying amounts of immature stromal tissue, often containing osteoid.

The fibrolamellar subtype of hepatocellular carcinoma is characterized by broad fibrous septa that separate the cellular component into nodules and is most commonly seen in late childhood and adolescence. It is associated with a better prognosis and a higher resection rate. This difference, however, may not be independent of stage.

Of patients with hepatoblastoma, 10% to 20% present with distant metastases. The locations of metastases at autopsy in 46 patients in one report were the lungs in 46%, portal and periaortic nodes in 11%, brain in 7%, and peritoneum and diaphragm in 4% each.[241] The incidence of metastases is reportedly higher in patients with embryonal and anaplastic histologic types compared with fetal differentiation.

Hepatocellular carcinoma presents with metastatic disease in 30% to 50% of patients. The location of metastases at autopsy was reported by the Liver Cancer Study Group of Japan.[242] The lungs were involved in 48% of patients, lymph nodes in 37%, intraperitoneal organs in 16%, peritoneum in 15%, adrenal in 11%, bone in 10%, brain in 2%, and skin in 1%. Tumor emboli were detected in the portal vein in 59.7% and in the hepatic vein in 26.6% of patients. The higher incidence of lymphatic and intra-abdominal spread in hepatocellular carcinoma is relevant to local resectability and recurrence. Nodal disease in the porta hepatis and periaortic region is not readily resectable, and recurrence is inevitable if such disease is present.

Treatment

Hepatoblastoma. Complete surgical resection remains the major objective of therapy for hepatoblastoma (Fig. 109.12).

At presentation, approximately 60% of patients with hepatoblastoma have resectable tumors, and one review reported no survivors among children who underwent biopsy only or incomplete resection. More recently, sporadic patients who received nonoperative treatments have achieved complete response,[243,244] and chemotherapy and radiation therapy have shown good results for some patients whose tumors were incompletely resected at the primary site.

A nonanatomic resection, wedging out the tumor with a satisfactory margin, may be feasible in the uncommon instance of a small peripheral or pedunculated lesion. More often, a major anatomic resection is required, depending on tumor location and extent. As much as 85% of hepatic substance may be removed, with subsequent full and rapid regeneration despite the administration of postoperative chemotherapy.[245] The principles of safe hepatic resection are now well developed, and a considerable reduction in operative mortality rates has been possible since the 1970s. In two historical series, the mortality rate was reported to be approximately 22%, but in more recent series, it was as low as 0% to 3%.[246,247]

The surgical principles include wide exposure using a generous bilateral subcostal incision and dissection at the liver hilum with isolation of vascular and ductal structures of the segment or lobe to be resected. After hepatic arterial and portal venous inflow to the relevant area is ligated, a color demarcation acts a guide to the correct plane of division of liver substance and allows this to proceed with minimal blood loss. Technologic advances such as the Cavitron Ultrasonic Surgical Aspirator (CUSA; Cooper Lasersonics, Santa Clara, CA) and metallic clip applicators have reduced the risk of hemorrhage, although finger-fracture technique with individual vessel and duct suture–ligation remains an acceptable alternative. Hemostasis of the transected surface can be completed with use of the argon beam coagulator or electrocautery and topical agents such as thrombin and Gelfoam (Pharmacia & Upjohn, Kalamazoo, MI). A trend to eliminate use of abdominal drains in uncomplicated cases has emerged.

Approximately 40% of patients with hepatoblastoma have inoperable tumors at presentation. Bilaterality, diffuse multicentricity, and metastatic lesions may all preclude resection. Various techniques have been used to increase the resectability rates, including preoperative chemotherapy, profound hypothermia with circulatory arrest, and total hepatic vascular occlusion. These maneuvers are a useful part of the surgical armamentarium in selected instances. During the 1990s, it became evident that some of these tumors may be rendered resectable by preoperative therapy. When the tumor is large, multicentric, has portal/hepatic venous involvement, or pulmonary metastasis, curative resection may be more likely after neoadjuvant chemotherapy.[239] For truly unresectable disease, aside from transplantation, chemotherapy is the major treatment option available. If the tumor is unresectable at the time of the operation (stage III or IV), patients should receive four cycles of cisplatin, 5-fluorouracil, and vincristine, and then undergo either re-resection or transplantation. Doxorubicin is often added when the response is minimal. Furthermore, adjuvant chemotherapy is used after resection for patients with nonfetal histology stage I disease and stage II disease.

The role of radiation therapy is not clearly defined. In treating patients with bulky disease, the tolerance of normal liver is not compatible with the doses that would be required for tumor ablation, although temporary stability may be achieved. Hepatic toxicity has been described at doses to the whole liver of greater than 25 Gy. Focal radiation up to 45 Gy can be safely administered. There may be a place for radiation in a dose range of 25 to 45 Gy combined with chemotherapy in inoperable hepatoblastoma and in patients with postresection residual disease. In one report, eight patients were treated after incomplete resections (four with gross and four with microscopic residual disease) with combined irradiation and chemotherapy; six of these patients were free of disease at 4 to 83 months' follow-up.[243]

The use of liver transplantation in those with unresectable primary tumors is growing. A recent study showed up to 80% long-term disease-free survival in children receiving transplantation in large, solitary, or multifocal tumors invading all four sectors of the liver.[248] The United Network for Organ Sharing database contains 237 patients from 1987 to 2006 who underwent orthotopic liver transplantation for hepatoblastoma. The median age of these children was 2.9 years. The overall survival at 1, 5, and 10 years was 80%, 69%, and 66%, respectively, with recurrence in approximately 50% of patients.[249] Another recent multicenter study reviewed 147 patients with hepatoblastoma who had liver transplantation. Seventy-two percent of these patients underwent orthotopic liver transplantation as the first surgery, while the other 28% had an initial incomplete resection or had recurrent disease. The latter cohort had a worse outcome, with 30% overall disease-free survival versus 82% in those patients who received transplantation as their primary surgery.[250] These results were replicated in other single-center studies.[251–253] Patients, however, require long-standing immunosuppressive therapy after transplantation. In addition, the risk of hepatic artery thrombosis in transplant patients is 3 to 4 times greater in children than in the adult population.[254] Recurrence and/or metastases are the primary causes of death in children with liver transplantation for hepatoblastoma, leading to 54% of deaths.[249] Upcoming COG studies involve liver transplantation, and an international registry of all patients with childhood liver tumors has been established.

Other treatments with encouraging results are in developmental phases. Transcatheter selective arterial chemoembolization (TACE), which involves transarterial administration of chemotherapy in addition to a vascular occlusive agent, has been studied as potential neoadjuvant therapy in the hope of making unresectable disease resectable or for palliative therapy. The intra-arterial route allows the administration of agents directly to the tumor with the theoretic advantage of less systemic toxicity. One recent study looked at the feasibility and effectiveness of this technique. Cycles of cisplatin and Adriamycin mixed with lipiodol were given, followed with gelatin foam particles or stainless steel coils. TACE allowed for successive complete surgical resection in 13 of 16 patients and partial resection in the remaining three. Overall survival rates were 87.5%, 68.7%, and 50% at 1, 3, and 5 years, respectively. There was no major chemotherapeutic toxicity noted. Multicenter, randomized studies are needed.[255]

With improving management of the primary lesion, mortality is increasingly the result of metastatic relapse in the lungs. If metastases demonstrate progression or relapse on therapy, surgical resection is an option. Cure of pulmonary metastatic disease has not been demonstrated with radiation therapy. The use of pulmonary metastasectomy is not adequately studied in prospective studies; however, a recent report concludes that resection of lung metastases may be beneficial in patients with disease present at diagnosis that is not responsive to neoadjuvant treatment.[256] Another series reported the operative treatment of five cases of pulmonary metastatic disease that developed after successful management of the primary tumor.[257] All lesions developed during or soon after chemotherapy. Four patients were free of disease at 8 to 83 months' follow-up, despite having multiple lesions and requiring more than one resection in two cases. No patients with hepatoblastoma with metastases to sites other than lung or regional nodes have been reported cured.

Hepatocellular Carcinoma. Despite recent progress in the treatment of hepatoblastoma, treatment of children with hepatocellular carcinoma remains problematic and their outcome poor. Analogous to hepatoblastoma, complete surgical resection is a prerequisite for cure in hepatocellular carcinoma of childhood. Patients with incompletely resected tumors do not survive, as these tumors are very chemoresistant. In one study, the response rate to chemotherapy was less than 50%, with many patients having disease progression despite systemic chemotherapy.[258] Although patients undergoing resection survive longer than those who do not undergo resection, the gain is small owing to the high local and systemic relapse rates. The Japanese Liver Cancer Study Group reported a 40% 1-year survival rate for resectable disease and 10% for unresectable lesions.[242]

Stage for stage, the prognosis of hepatocellular carcinoma is no worse than that for hepatoblastoma. Many more patients present with advanced hepatocellular carcinoma, however, because the prevalence of bilobar and multicentric tumors and extrahepatic extension renders them unresectable. Nodal and systemic metastatic disease is more common at the outset. The liver may be cirrhotic in some instances, precluding an extensive resection short of transplantation.

Most series report the percentage of children with resectable hepatocellular carcinoma (HCC) to be approximately 10% to 20%. Patients with fibrolamellar histologic pattern may be an exception, with a resection rate of 48% to 60%, and essentially no association with cirrhosis. Relapse after resection is common. A POG and CCG intergroup study showed no impact of either cisplatin plus doxorubicin, or cisplatin, vincristine, and 5-fluorouracil on outcome in patients with hepatocellular carcinoma. The overall survival rate in the pediatric age group for hepatocellular carcinoma is rarely reported to exceed 20% and more realistically approaches zero. A role for external-beam radiation therapy has not been established. Only temporary stability of bulky disease has been demonstrated, and radiation has also failed to decrease the relapse rate in patients with minimal disease after surgical resection. Intra-arterial chemotherapy and chemoembolization have been used for patients with HCC as well, although studies do not show great responses. In addition, metronomic chemotherapy and adjuvant antiangiogenic treatments are currently under investigation and are preliminarily showing promising results.[239,259–261] Given the poor results for conventional therapy, there may be a place for liver transplantation. However, transplantation is limited to tumors that fulfill the Milan criteria (single tumor ≤5 cm in diameter or up to three tumors each 3 cm or less in diameter, absence of macroscopic portal vein invasions, and absence of extrahepatic disease). These criteria are often used for adults, and it is unclear if they should be altered for the use of transplantation in children. The United Network for Organ Sharing database from 1987 to 2006 contained 41 pediatric patients with HCC who received orthotopic liver transplantation. The overall 1-, 5-, and 10-year patient survival rates were 86%, 63%, and 58%, respectively. As with hepatoblastoma, the main cause of mortality was relapse; however, relapse occurred more frequently in those patients with HCC (compared to the 54% in hepatoblastoma).[249]

Outcome. After a successful complete surgical resection, the 5-year event-free survival is 83% versus 41% for those patients with residual tumor after surgical resection.[262] Classifying tumors by grade, the COG has shown a 3-year event-free survival of 90% for stage 1 or 2 disease, 50% for stage 3 disease, and 20% for stage 4 disease.[263] These patients have better outcomes than those with HCC, as a recent COG trial showed a 5-year overall survival of those with stage 1 tumors is 88%, stage 3 tumors is 23%, and stage 4 tumors is 10%.[264]

References

1. O'Leary M, Krailo M, Anderson J, et al. Progress in childhood cancer: 50 years of research collaboration, a report from the Children's Oncology Group. *Semin Oncol* 2008;35:484–493.
2. Punyko J, Mertens A, Baker K, et al. Long-term survival probabilities for childhood rhabdomyosarcoma. A population-based evaluation. *Cancer* 2005;103:1475–1483.
3. Bleyer W. The U. S. pediatric cancer clinical trials programmes: international implications and the way forward. *Eur J Cancer* 1997;33:1439–1447.
4. Kramer S, Meadows A, Jarrett P, et al. Incidence of childhood cancer: experience of a decade in a population-based registry. *J Natl Cancer Inst* 1983;70:49–55.
5. Miller R, Dalager N. U.S. childhood cancer deaths by cell type, 1960–68. *J Pediatr* 1974;85:664–668.
6. Ries LAG, Percy CL, Benin G. Introduction. In: Ries LAG, Smith MA, Gurney JG, et al., eds. *Cancer Incidence and Survival among Children and Adolescents: United States SEER Program 1975–1995*, National Cancer Institute, SEER Program. Bethesda, MD: National Cancer Institute, SEER Program; 1999.
7. Matthay K, Villablanca J, Seeger R, et al. Treatment of high-risk neuroblastoma with intensive chemotherapy, radiotherapy, autologous bone marrow transplantation, and 13-cis-retinoic acid. Children's Cancer Group. *N Engl J Med* 1999;341:1165–1173.
8. De Bernardi B, Nicolas B, Boni L, et al. Disseminated neuroblastoma in children older than one year at diagnosis: comparable results with three consecutive high-dose protocols adopted by the Italian Co-Operative Group for Neuroblastoma. *J Clin Oncol* 2003;21:1592–1601.
9. Maris J, Hogarty M, Bagatell R, et al. Neuroblastoma. *Lancet* 2007;369: 2106–2120.
10. Park J, Eggert A, Caron H. Neuroblastoma: biology, prognosis, and treatment. *Pediatr Clin North Am* 2008;55:97–120, x.
11. Brodeur G. Neuroblastoma: biological insights into a clinical enigma. *Nat Rev Cancer* 2003;3:203–216.
12. Schilling F, Spix C, Berthold F, et al. Neuroblastoma screening at one year of age. *N Engl J Med* 2002;346:1047–1053.
13. Woods W, Gao R, Shuster J, et al. Screening of infants and mortality due to neuroblastoma. *N Engl J Med* 2002;346:1041–1046.
14. Yamamoto K, Hayashi Y, Hanada R, et al. Mass screening and age-specific incidence of neuroblastoma in Saitama Prefecture, Japan. *J Clin Oncol* 1995;13:2033–2038.
15. Allen RJ, Ogden B, Bentley F, et al. Fetal hydantoin syndrome, neuroblastoma, and hemorrhagic disease in a neonate. *JAMA* 1980;244:1464–1465.
16. Kinney H, Faix R, Brazy J. The fetal alcohol syndrome and neuroblastoma. *Pediatrics* 1980;66:130–132.
17. Blatt J, Olshan A, Lee P, et al. Neuroblastoma and related tumors in Turner's syndrome. *J Pediatr* 1997;131:666–670.
18. Pivnick E, Furman W, Velagaleti G, et al. Simultaneous adrenocortical carcinoma and ganglioneuroblastoma in a child with Turner syndrome and germline p53 mutation. *J Med Genet* 1998;35:328–332.
19. Geraci A, de Csepel J, Shlasko E, et al. Ganglioneuroblastoma and ganglioneuroma in association with neurofibromatosis type I: report of three cases. *J Child Neurol* 1998;13:356–358.
20. van Limpt V, Schramm A, van Lakeman A, et al. The Phox2B homeobox gene is mutated in sporadic neuroblastomas. *Oncogene* 2004;23:9280–9288.
21. Goodman MT, Gurney JG, Smith MA, et al. *Sympathetic Nervous System Tumors*. Bethesda, MD: National Cancer Institute SEER Program, 1999.
22. Mosse YP, Laudenslager M, Longo L, et al. Identification of ALK as a major familial neuroblastoma predisposition gene. *Nature* 2008;455:930–935.
23. Mosse YP, Wood A, Maris JM. Inhibition of ALK signaling for cancer therapy. *Clin Cancer Res* 2009;15:5609–5614.
24. Brodeur G, Seeger R, Schwab M, et al. Amplification of N-myc in untreated human neuroblastomas correlates with advanced disease stage. *Science* 1984;224:1121–1124.
25. Tonini G, Boni L, Pession A, et al. MYCN oncogene amplification in neuroblastoma is associated with worse prognosis, except in stage 4s: the Italian experience with 295 children. *J Clin Oncol* 1997;15:85–93.
26. Maris J. The biologic basis for neuroblastoma heterogeneity and risk stratification. *Curr Opin Pediatr* 2005;17:7–13.
27. Westermann F, Schwab M. Genetic parameters of neuroblastomas. *Cancer Lett* 2002;184:127–147.
28. Tweddle D, Pearson A, Haber M, et al. The p53 pathway and its inactivation in neuroblastoma. *Cancer Lett* 2003;197:93–98.
29. Slack A, Chen Z, Tonelli R, et al. The p53 regulatory gene MDM2 is a direct transcriptional target of MYCN in neuroblastoma. *Proc Natl Acad Sci U S A* 2005;102:731–736.
30. Caron H, van Sluis P, de Kraker J, et al. Allelic loss of chromosome 1p as a predictor of unfavorable outcome in patients with neuroblastoma. *N Engl J Med* 1996;334:225–230.
31. Rubie H, Delattre O, Hartmann O, et al. Loss of chromosome 1p may have a prognostic value in localised neuroblastoma: results of the French NBL 90 Study. Neuroblastoma Study Group of the Société Française d'Oncologie Pédiatrique (SFOP). *Eur J Cancer* 1997;33:1917–1922.
32. Maris J, White P, Beltinger C, et al. Significance of chromosome 1p loss of heterozygosity in neuroblastoma. *Cancer Res* 1995;55:4664–4669.
33. Maris J, Weiss M, Guo C, et al. Loss of heterozygosity at 1p36 independently predicts for disease progression but not decreased overall survival probability in neuroblastoma patients: a Children's Cancer Group study. *J Clin Oncol* 2000;18:1888–1899.
34. Bader S, Fasching C, Brodeur G, et al. Dissociation of suppression of tumorigenicity and differentiation in vitro effected by transfer of single human chromosomes into human neuroblastoma cells. *Cell Growth Differ* 1991;2:245–255.
35. Bown N, Lastowska M, Cotterill S, et al. 17q gain in neuroblastoma predicts adverse clinical outcome. U.K. Cancer Cytogenetics Group and the U.K. Children's Cancer Study Group. *Med Pediatr Oncol* 2001;36:14–19.
36. Guo C, White P, Weiss M, et al. Allelic deletion at 11q23 is common in MYCN single copy neuroblastomas. *Oncogene* 1999;18:4948–4957.
37. Plantaz D, Vandesompele J, Van Roy N, et al. Comparative genomic hybridization (CGH) analysis of stage 4 neuroblastoma reveals high frequency of 11q deletion in tumors lacking MYCN amplification. *Int J Cancer* 2001;91:680–686.

38. Spitz R, Hero B, Ernestus K, et al. Deletions in chromosome arms 3p and 11q are new prognostic markers in localized and 4s neuroblastoma. *Clin Cancer Res* 2003;9:52–58.
39. Nakagawara A, Arima M, Azar C, et al. Inverse relationship between trk expression and N-myc amplification in human neuroblastomas. *Cancer Res* 1992;52:1364–1368.
40. Nakagawara A, Arima-Nakagawara M, Scavarda N, et al. Association between high levels of expression of the TRK gene and favorable outcome in human neuroblastoma. *N Engl J Med* 1993;328:847–854.
41. Kogner P, Barbany G, Dominici C, et al. Coexpression of messenger RNA for TRK protooncogene and low affinity nerve growth factor receptor in neuroblastoma with favorable prognosis. *Cancer Res* 1993;53:2044–2050.
42. Kramer K, Cheung N, Gerald W, et al. Correlation of MYCN amplification, Trk-A and CD44 expression with clinical stage in 250 patients with neuroblastoma. *Eur J Cancer* 1997;33:2098–2100.
43. Rydén M, Sehgal R, Dominici C, et al. Expression of mRNA for the neurotrophin receptor trkC in neuroblastomas with favourable tumour stage and good prognosis. *Br J Cancer* 1996;74:773–779.
44. Schulte J, Schramm A, Klein-Hitpass L, et al. Microarray analysis reveals differential gene expression patterns and regulation of single target genes contributing to the opposing phenotype of TrkA- and TrkB-expressing neuroblastomas. *Oncogene* 2005;24:165–177.
45. Ho R, Eggert A, Hishiki T, et al. Resistance to chemotherapy mediated by TrkB in neuroblastomas. *Cancer Res* 2002;62:6462–6466.
46. Castle V, Heidelberger K, Bromberg J, et al. Expression of the apoptosis-suppressing protein bcl-2, in neuroblastoma is associated with unfavorable histology and N-myc amplification. *Am J Pathol* 1993;143:1543–1550.
47. Eggert A, Grotzer M, Zuzak T, et al. Resistance to tumor necrosis factor-related apoptosis-inducing ligand (TRAIL)-induced apoptosis in neuroblastoma cells correlates with a loss of caspase-8 expression. *Cancer Res* 2001;61:1314–1319.
48. Hopkins-Donaldson S, Bodmer J, Bourloud K, et al. Loss of caspase-8 expression in highly malignant human neuroblastoma cells correlates with resistance to tumor necrosis factor-related apoptosis-inducing ligand-induced apoptosis. *Cancer Res* 2000;60:4315–4319.
49. van Noesel M, van Bezouw S, Salomons G, et al. Tumor-specific down-regulation of the tumor necrosis factor-related apoptosis-inducing ligand decoy receptors DcR1 and DcR2 is associated with dense promoter hypermethylation. *Cancer Res* 2002;62:2157–2161.
50. Jaboin J, Kim C, Kaplan D, et al. Brain-derived neurotrophic factor activation of TrkB protects neuroblastoma cells from chemotherapy-induced apoptosis via phosphatidylinositol 3'-kinase pathway. *Cancer Res* 2002; 62:6756–6763.
51. Scala S, Wosikowski K, Giannakakou P, et al. Brain-derived neurotrophic factor protects neuroblastoma cells from vinblastine toxicity. *Cancer Res* 1996;56:3737–3742.
52. Almgren M, Henriksson K, Fujimoto J, et al. Nucleoside diphosphate kinase A/nm23-H1 promotes metastasis of NB69-derived human neuroblastoma. *Mol Cancer Res* 2004;2:387–394.
53. Chantrain C, Shimada H, Jodele S, et al. Stromal matrix metalloproteinase-9 regulates the vascular architecture in neuroblastoma by promoting pericyte recruitment. *Cancer Res* 2004;64:1675–1686.
54. Gross N, Balmas Bourloud K, Brognara C. MYCN-related suppression of functional CD44 expression enhances tumorigenic properties of human neuroblastoma cells. *Exp Cell Res* 2000;260:396–403.
55. Jodele S, Chantrain C, Blavier L, et al. The contribution of bone marrow-derived cells to the tumor vasculature in neuroblastoma is matrix metalloproteinase-9 dependent. *Cancer Res* 2005;65:3200–3208.
56. Kim S, Chung D. Pediatric solid malignancies: neuroblastoma and Wilms' tumor. *Surg Clin North Am* 2006;86:469–487, xi.
57. Look A, Hayes F, Nitschke R, et al. Cellular DNA content as a predictor of response to chemotherapy in infants with unresectable neuroblastoma. *N Engl J Med* 1984;311:231–235.
58. Walton J, Kattan D, Thomas S, et al. Characteristics of stem cells from human neuroblastoma cell lines and in tumors. *Neoplasia* 2004;6: 838–845.
59. Comito M, Savell V, Cohen M. CD44 expression in neuroblastoma and related tumors. *J Pediatr Hematol Oncol* 1997;19(4):292–296.
60. Look A, Hayes F, Shuster J, et al. Clinical relevance of tumor cell ploidy and N-myc gene amplification in childhood neuroblastoma: a Pediatric Oncology Group study. *J Clin Oncol* 1991;9:581–591.
61. Triche TJ Askin FB, Kissane JM. Neuroblastoma, Ewing's sarcoma, and the differential diagnosis of small-, round-, blue-cell tumors. Philadelphia: WB Saunders; 1986.
62. Shimada H, Ambros I, Dehner L, et al. The International Neuroblastoma Pathology Classification (the Shimada system). *Cancer* 1999;86:364–372.
63. Tornóczky T, Kálmán E, Kajtár P, et al. Large cell neuroblastoma: a distinct phenotype of neuroblastoma with aggressive clinical behavior. *Cancer* 2004;100:390–397.
64. Katzenstein H, Cohn S, Shore R, et al. Scintigraphic response by 123I-metaiodobenzylguanidine scan correlates with event-free survival in high-risk neuroblastoma. *J Clin Oncol* 2004;22:3909–3915.
65. Matthay K, Blaes F, Hero B, et al. Opsoclonus myoclonus syndrome in neuroblastoma a report from a workshop on the dancing eyes syndrome at the advances in neuroblastoma meeting in Genoa, Italy, 2004. *Cancer Lett* 2005;228:275–282.
66. Papaioannou G, McHugh K. Neuroblastoma in childhood: review and radiological findings. *Cancer Imaging* 2005;5:116–127.
67. Shamberger R, Ritchey M, Haase G, et al. Intravascular extension of Wilms tumor. *Ann Surg* 2001;234:116–121.
68. Green D, Breslow N, Beckwith J, et al. Comparison between single-dose and divided-dose administration of dactinomycin and doxorubicin for patients with Wilms' tumor: a report from the National Wilms' Tumor Study Group. *J Clin Oncol* 1998;16:237–245.
69. Kushner B, Yeung H, Larson S, et al. Extending positron emission tomography scan utility to high-risk neuroblastoma: fluorine-18 fluorodeoxyglucose positron emission tomography as sole imaging modality in follow-up of patients. *J Clin Oncol* 2001;19:3397–3405.
70. Siegel M, Ishwaran H, Fletcher B, et al. Staging of neuroblastoma at imaging: report of the radiology diagnostic oncology group. *Radiology* 2002; 223:168–175.
71. Kushner B. Neuroblastoma: a disease requiring a multitude of imaging studies. *J Nucl Med* 2004;45:1172–1188.
72. Ikeda H, Iehara T, Tsuchida Y, et al. Experience with International Neuroblastoma Staging System and Pathology Classification. *Br J Cancer* 2002;86:1110–1116.
73. Brodeur G, Seeger R, Barrett A, et al. International criteria for diagnosis, staging, and response to treatment in patients with neuroblastoma. *J Clin Oncol* 1988;6:1874–1881.
74. Brodeur G, Pritchard J, Berthold F, et al. Revisions of the international criteria for neuroblastoma diagnosis, staging, and response to treatment. *J Clin Oncol* 1993;11:1466–1477.
75. Evans A, Albo V, D'Angio G, et al. Factors influencing survival of children with nonmetastatic neuroblastoma. *Cancer* 1976;38:661–666.
76. Monclair T, Brodeur G, Ambros P, et al. The International Neuroblastoma Risk Group (INRG) staging system: an INRG Task Force report. *J Clin Oncol* 2009;27:298–303.
77. Alvarado C, London W, Look A, et al. Natural history and biology of stage A neuroblastoma: a Pediatric Oncology Group Study. *J Pediatr Hematol Oncol* 2000;22(3):197–205.
78. Perez C, Matthay K, Atkinson J, et al. Biologic variables in the outcome of stages I and II neuroblastoma treated with surgery as primary therapy: a Children's Cancer Group study. *J Clin Oncol* 2000;18:18–26.
79. Nickerson H, Matthay K, Seeger R, et al. Favorable biology and outcome of stage IV-S neuroblastoma with supportive care or minimal therapy: a Children's Cancer Group study. *J Clin Oncol* 2000;18:477–486.
80. Katzenstein H, Bowman L, Brodeur G, et al. Prognostic significance of age, MYCN oncogene amplification, tumor cell ploidy, and histology in 110 infants with stage D(S) neuroblastoma: the Pediatric Oncology Group experience–a Pediatric Oncology Group study. *J Clin Oncol* 1998;16: 2007–2017.
81. Matthay K, Perez C, Seeger R, et al. Successful treatment of stage III neuroblastoma based on prospective biologic staging: a Children's Cancer Group study. *J Clin Oncol* 1998;16:1256–1264.
82. Shamberger R, Allarde-Segundo A, Kozakewich H, et al. Surgical management of stage III and IV neuroblastoma: resection before or after chemotherapy? *J Pediatr Surg* 1991;26:1113–1117; discussion 1117–1118.
83. La Quaglia M, Kushner B, Su W, et al. The impact of gross total resection on local control and survival in high-risk neuroblastoma. *J Pediatr Surg* 2004;39:412–417; discussion 412–417.
84. Brodeur GM Maris JM. Neuroblastoma, 4th ed. Philadelphia: Lippincott; 2002.
85. Wagner L, Danks M. New therapeutic targets for the treatment of high-risk neuroblastoma. *J Cell Biochem* 2009;107:46–57.
86. Berthold F, Boos J, Burdach S, et al. Myeloablative megatherapy with autologous stem-cell rescue versus oral maintenance chemotherapy as consolidation treatment in patients with high-risk neuroblastoma: a randomised controlled trial. *Lancet Oncol* 2005;6:649–658.
87. Fish J, Grupp S. Stem cell transplantation for neuroblastoma. *Bone Marrow Transplant* 2008;41:159–165.
88. Yu A, MF G, WB O, et al. A phase III randomized trial of the chimeric anti-GD2 antibody ch 14.19 with GM-CSF and IL2 as immunotherapy following dose intensive chemotherapy for high-rish neuroblastoma: Children's Oncology Group (COG) study ANBL0032. 2009.
89. Pearson A, Pinkerton C, Lewis I, et al. High-dose rapid and standard induction chemotherapy for patients aged over 1 year with stage 4 neuroblastoma: a randomised trial. *Lancet Oncol* 2008;9:247–256.
90. Zage P, Kletzel M, Murray K, et al. Outcomes of the POG 9340/9341/9342 trials for children with high-risk neuroblastoma: a report from the Children's Oncology Group. *Pediatr Blood Cancer* 2008;51: 747–753.
91. SL S, S G, T V, et al. Phase I safety pharmacokinetic and exploratory biomarker study of intravenous temsirolimus in children with advanced solid tumors. *Proc Am Soc Ped Hem/Onc* 2008;.
92. Opel D, Poremba C, Simon T, et al. Activation of Akt predicts poor outcome in neuroblastoma. *Cancer Res* 2007;67:735–745.
93. Radhakrishnan S, Halasi M, Bhat U, et al. Proapoptotic compound ARC targets Akt and N-myc in neuroblastoma cells. *Oncogene* 2008;27: 694–699.
94. Sartelet H, Oligny L, Vassal G. AKT pathway in neuroblastoma and its therapeutic implication. *Expert Rev Anticancer Ther* 2008;8:757– 769.
95. Bernstein L, Linet M, Smith MA, et al. Renal tumors. In: Ries LAG, Smith MA, Gurney JG, et al., eds. *Cancer Incidence and Survival among Children and Adolescents: United States SEER Program 1975–1995*. Bethesda, MD: National Cancer Institute, SEER Program; 1999:79–90.
96. Bernstein L, Linet M, Smith MA, et al. Chapter VI: Renal tumors. In: Health NIo, ed 1999.

97. Breslow N, Beckwith J, Ciol M, et al. Age distribution of Wilms' tumor: report from the National Wilms' Tumor Study. *Cancer Res* 1988;48: 1653–1657.
98. Breslow N, Beckwith J. Epidemiological features of Wilms' tumor: results of the National Wilms' Tumor Study. *J Natl Cancer Inst* 1982;68: 429–436.
99. Ward S, Dehner L. Sacrococcygeal teratoma with nephroblastoma (Wilm's tumor): a variant of extragonadal teratoma in childhood. A histologic and ultrastructural study. *Cancer* 1974;33:1355–1363.
100. Lüchtrath H, de Leon F, Giesen H, et al. Inguinal nephroblastoma. *Virchows Arch A Pathol Anat Histopathol* 1984;405:113–118.
101. Naito K, Yokoyama O, Yamaguchi K, et al. Extrarenal nephroblastoma: report of a case and review of the literature. *Hinyokika Kiyo* 1985;31: 1773–1780.
102. Maw M, Grundy P, Millow L, et al. A third Wilms' tumor locus on chromosome 16q. *Cancer Res* 1992;52:3094–3098.
103. Francke U, Holmes L, Atkins L, et al. Aniridia-Wilms' tumor association: evidence for specific deletion of 11p13. *Cytogenet Cell Genet* 1979;24: 185–192.
104. Rose E, Glaser T, Jones C, et al. Complete physical map of the WAGR region of 11p13 localizes a candidate Wilms' tumor gene. *Cell* 1990;60: 495–508.
105. Varan A. Wilms' tumor in children: an overview. *Nephron Clin Pract* 2008;108:c83–c90.
106. Lee S, Haber D. Wilms tumor and the WT1 gene. *Exp Cell Res* 2001;264: 74–99.
107. Fischbach B, Trout K, Lewis J, et al. WAGR syndrome: a clinical review of 54 cases. *Pediatrics* 2005;116:984–988.
108. Büyükpamukçu M, Kutluk T, Büyükpamukçu N, et al. Renal tumors with pseudohermaphroditism and glomerular disease. *Acta Oncol* 1992;31: 745–748.
109. Niemitz E, Feinberg A, Brandenburg S, et al. Children with idiopathic hemihypertrophy and Beckwith-Wiedemann syndrome have different constitutional epigenotypes associated with Wilms tumor. *Am J Hum Genet* 2005;77:887–891.
110. Rivera M, Kim W, Wells J, et al. An X chromosome gene, WTX, is commonly inactivated in Wilms tumor. *Science* 2007;315:642–645.
111. Major M, Camp N, Berndt J, et al. Wilms tumor suppressor WTX negatively regulates WNT/beta-catenin signaling. *Science* 2007;316:1043–1046.
112. Bardeesy N, Falkoff D, Petruzzi M, et al. Anaplastic Wilms' tumour, a subtype displaying poor prognosis, harbours p53 gene mutations. *Nat Genet* 1994;7:91–97.
113. Dome J, Coppes M. Recent advances in Wilms tumor genetics. *Curr Opin Pediatr* 2002;14:5–11.
114. Grundy P, Telzerow P, Breslow N, et al. Loss of heterozygosity for chromosomes 16q and 1p in Wilms' tumors predicts an adverse outcome. *Cancer Res* 1994;54:2331–2333.
115. Kort E, Farber L, Tretiakova M, et al. The E2F3-Oncomir-1 axis is activated in Wilms' tumor. *Cancer Res* 2008;68:4034–4038.
116. Saal S, Harvey S. MicroRNAs and the kidney: coming of age. *Curr Opin Nephrol Hypertens* 2009;18:317–323.
117. Horwitz J, Ritchey M, Moksness J, et al. Renal salvage procedures in patients with synchronous bilateral Wilms' tumors: a report from the National Wilms' Tumor Study Group. *J Pediatr Surg* 1996;31:1020–1025.
118. Ko EY, Ritchey ML. Current management of Wilms' tumor in children. *J Pediatr Urol* 2009;5:56–65.
119. Beckwith J, Kiviat N, Bonadio J. Nephrogenic rests, nephroblastomatosis, and the pathogenesis of Wilms' tumor. *Pediatr Pathol* 1990;10:1–36.
120. Voûte PJ, van der Meer J, Staugaard-Kloosterziel W. Plasma renin activity in Wilms' tumour. *Acta Endocrinol (Copenh)* 1971;67:197–202.
121. Coppes M, Ye Y, Rackley R, et al. Analysis of WT1 in granulosa cell and other sex cord-stromal tumors. *Cancer Res* 1993;53:2712–2714.
122. Ehrlich P, Hamilton T, Grundy P, et al. The value of surgery in directing therapy for patients with Wilms' tumor with pulmonary disease. A report from the National Wilms' Tumor Study Group (National Wilms' Tumor Study 5). *J Pediatr Surg* 2006;41:162–167; discussion 162–167.
123. Wilimas J, Magill L, Parham D, et al. The potential for renal salvage in nonmetastatic unilateral Wilms' tumor. *Am J Pediatr Hematol Oncol* 1991;13:342–344.
124. Duarte R, Dénes F, Cristofani L, et al. Further experience with laparoscopic nephrectomy for Wilms' tumour after chemotherapy. *BJU Int* 2006; 98:155–159.
125. Green D, Breslow N, Beckwith J, et al. Effect of duration of treatment on treatment outcome and cost of treatment for Wilms' tumor: a report from the National Wilms' Tumor Study Group. *J Clin Oncol* 1998;16:3744–3751.
126. Green D, Beckwith J, Breslow N, et al. Treatment of children with stages II to IV anaplastic Wilms' tumor: a report from the National Wilms' Tumor Study Group. *J Clin Oncol* 1994;12:2126–2131.
127. Malcolm A, Jaffe N, Folkman M, et al. Bilateral Wilm's tumor. *Int J Radiat Oncol Biol Phys* 1980;6:167–174.
128. Montgomery B, Kelalis P, Blute M, et al. Extended followup of bilateral Wilms tumor: results of the National Wilms Tumor Study. *J Urol* 1991;146:514–518.
129. Shamberger R, Haase G, Argani P, et al. Bilateral Wilms' tumors with progressive or nonresponsive disease. *J Pediatr Surg* 2006;41:652–657; discussion 652–657.
130. Hamilton T, Ritchey M, Argani P, et al. Synchronous bilateral Wilms' tumor with complete radiographic response managed without surgical resection: a report from the National Wilms' Tumor Study 4. *J Pediatr Surg* 2008;43:1982–1984.
131. Ritchey M, Othersen HJ, de Lorimier A, et al. Renal vein involvement with nephroblastoma: a report of the National Wilms' Tumor Study-3. *Eur Urol* 1990;17:139–144.
132. Wexler H, Poole C, Fojaco R. Metastatic neonatal Wilms' tumor: a case report with review of the literature. *Pediatr Radiol* 1975;3:179–181.
133. Hrabovsky E, Othersen HJ, deLorimier A, et al. Wilms' tumor in the neonate: a report from the National Wilms' Tumor Study. *J Pediatr Surg* 1986;21:385–387.
134. Isaacs HJ. Fetal and neonatal renal tumors. *J Pediatr Surg* 2008;43: 1587–1595.
135. Ritchey M, Azizkhan R, Beckwith J, et al. Neonatal Wilms tumor. *J Pediatr Surg* 1995;30:856–859.
136. Maes P, Delemarre J, de Kraker J, et al. Fetal rhabdomyomatous nephroblastoma: a tumour of good prognosis but resistant to chemotherapy. *Eur J Cancer* 1999;35:1356–1360.
137. Corn B, Goldwein J, Evans I, et al. Outcomes in low-risk babies treated with half-dose chemotherapy according to the third National Wilms' Tumor Study. *J Clin Oncol* 1992;10:1305–1309.
138. Babaian R, Skinner D, Waisman J. Wilms' tumor in the adult patient: diagnosis, management, and review of the world medical literature. *Cancer* 1980;45:1713–1719.
139. Byrd R, Evans A, D'Angio G. Adult Wilms tumor: effect of combined therapy on survival. *J Urol* 1982;127:648–651.
140. Hupperets P, Havenith M, Blijham G. Recurrent adult nephroblastoma. Long-term remission after surgery plus adjuvant high-dose chemotherapy, radiation therapy, and allogeneic bone marrow transplantation. *Cancer* 1992;69:2990–2992.
141. Argani P, Perlman E, Breslow N, et al. Clear cell sarcoma of the kidney: a review of 351 cases from the National Wilms Tumor Study Group Pathology Center. *Am J Surg Pathol* 2000;24:4–18.
142. Green D, Breslow N, Beckwith J, et al. Treatment of children with clear-cell sarcoma of the kidney: a report from the National Wilms' Tumor Study Group. *J Clin Oncol* 1994;12:2132–2137.
143. Seibel N, Li S, Breslow N, et al. Effect of duration of treatment on treatment outcome for patients with clear-cell sarcoma of the kidney: a report from the National Wilms' Tumor Study Group. *J Clin Oncol* 2004;22: 468–473.
144. NL S, S L, NE B, et al. Outcome of clear cell sarcoma of the kidney (CCSK) treated on the National Wilms Tumor Study-5 (NWTS). 2006.
145. Eftekhari F, Erly W, Jaffe N. Malignant rhabdoid tumor of the kidney: imaging features in two cases. *Pediatr Radiol* 1990;21:39–42.
146. Weeks D, Beckwith J, Mierau G, et al. Rhabdoid tumor of kidney. A report of 111 cases from the National Wilms' Tumor Study Pathology Center. *Am J Surg Pathol* 1989;13:439–458.
147. Beckwith J. Histopathology as a prognostic indicator in tumors of childhood. *Prog Clin Biol Res* 1983;132E:159–164.
148. Lowe L, Isuani B, Heller R, et al. Pediatric renal masses: Wilms tumor and beyond. *Radiographics* 2000;20(6):1585–1603.
149. Ahmed H, Arya M, Levitt G, et al. Part I: Primary malignant non-Wilms' renal tumours in children. *Lancet Oncol* 2007;8:730–737.
150. Sebire N, Vujanic G. Paediatric renal tumours: recent developments, new entities and pathological features. *Histopathology* 2009;54:516–528.
151. Kodet R, Newton WJ, Sachs N, et al. Rhabdoid tumors of soft tissues: a clinicopathologic study of 26 cases enrolled on the Intergroup Rhabdomyosarcoma Study. *Hum Pathol* 1991;22:674–684.
152. Hilden J, Watterson J, Longee D, et al. Central nervous system atypical teratoid tumor/rhabdoid tumor: response to intensive therapy and review of the literature. *J Neurooncol* 1998;40:265–275.
153. Bolande R. Congenital mesoblastic nephroma of infancy. *Perspect Pediatr Pathol* 1973;1:227–250.
154. Knezevich S, Garnett M, Pysher T, et al. ETV6-NTRK3 gene fusions and trisomy 11 establish a histogenetic link between mesoblastic nephroma and congenital fibrosarcoma. *Cancer Res* 1998;58:5046–5048.
155. Aronson D, Medary I, Finlay J, et al. Renal cell carcinoma in childhood and adolescence: a retrospective survey for prognostic factors in 22 cases. *J Pediatr Surg* 1996;31:183–186.
156. Ahmed H, Arya M, Levitt G, et al. Part II: Treatment of primary malignant non-Wilms' renal tumours in children. *Lancet Oncol* 2007;8:842–848.
157. Cook A, Lorenzo A, Salle J, et al. Pediatric renal cell carcinoma: single institution 25-year case series and initial experience with partial nephrectomy. *J Urol* 2006;175:1456–1460; discussion 1460.
158. Gurney J, Roffers S, Smith M, et al. e. Soft tissue sarcomas 1999.
159. Young JJ, Miller R. Incidence of malignant tumors in U.S. children. *J Pediatr* 1975;86:254–258.
160. Hayes-Jordan A, Andrassy R. Rhabdomyosarcoma in children. *Curr Opin Pediatr* 2009;21:373–378.
161. Ruymann F, Maddux H, Ragab A, et al. Congenital anomalies associated with rhabdomyosarcoma: an autopsy study of 115 cases. A report from the Intergroup Rhabdomyosarcoma Study Committee (representing the Children's Cancer Study Group, the Pediatric Oncology Group, the United Kingdom Children's Cancer Study Group, and the Pediatric Intergroup Statistical Center). *Med Pediatr Oncol* 1988;16:33–39.
162. McDowell H. Update on childhood rhabdomyosarcoma. *Arch Dis Child* 2003;88:354–357.
163. Seale P, Sabourin L, Girgis-Gabardo A, et al. Pax7 is required for the specification of myogenic satellite cells. *Cell* 2000;102:777–786.

164. Lam P, Sublett J, Hollenbach A, et al. The oncogenic potential of the Pax3-FKHR fusion protein requires the Pax3 homeodomain recognition helix but not the Pax3 paired-box DNA binding domain. *Mol Cell Biol* 1999; 19: 594–601.
165. Loeb D, Thornton K, Shokek O. Pediatric soft tissue sarcomas. *Surg Clin North Am* 2008;88:615–627, vii.
166. Bridge J, Liu J, Weibolt V, et al. Novel genomic imbalances in embryonal rhabdomyosarcoma revealed by comparative genomic hybridization and fluorescence in situ hybridization: an intergroup rhabdomyosarcoma study. *Genes Chromosomes Cancer* 2000;27:337–344.
167. Dias P, Parham D, Shapiro D, et al. Myogenic regulatory protein (MyoD1) expression in childhood solid tumors: diagnostic utility in rhabdomyosarcoma. *Am J Pathol* 1990;137:1283–1291.
168. Kelly K, Womer R, Barr F. Minimal disease detection in patients with alveolar rhabdomyosarcoma using a reverse transcriptase-polymerase chain reaction method. *Cancer* 1996;78:1320–1327.
169. Kraus D, Saenz N, Gollamudi S, et al. Pediatric rhabdomyosarcoma of the head and neck. *Am J Surg* 1997;174:556–560.
170. Klem M, Grewal R, Wexler L, et al. PET for staging in rhabdomyosarcoma: an evaluation of PET as an adjunct to current staging tools. *J Pediatr Hematol Oncol* 2007;29:9–14.
171. Neville H, Andrassy R, Lobe T, et al. Preoperative staging, prognostic factors, and outcome for extremity rhabdomyosarcoma: a preliminary report from the Intergroup Rhabdomyosarcoma Study IV (1991–1997). *J Pediatr Surg* 2000;35:317–321.
172. McMulkin H, Yanchar N, Fernandez C, et al. Sentinel lymph node mapping and biopsy: a potentially valuable tool in the management of childhood extremity rhabdomyosarcoma. *Pediatr Surg Int* 2003;19:453–456.
173. Neville H, Andrassy R, Lally K, et al. Lymphatic mapping with sentinel node biopsy in pediatric patients. *J Pediatr Surg* 2000;35:961–964.
174. La Quaglia M, Heller G, Ghavimi F, et al. The effect of age at diagnosis on outcome in rhabdomyosarcoma. *Cancer* 1994;73:109–117.
175. Joshi D, Anderson J, Paidas C, et al. Age is an independent prognostic factor in rhabdomyosarcoma: a report from the Soft Tissue Sarcoma Committee of the Children's Oncology Group. *Pediatr Blood Cancer* 2004;42: 64–73.
176. Raney R, Anderson J, Barr F, et al. Rhabdomyosarcoma and undifferentiated sarcoma in the first two decades of life: a selective review of Intergroup Rhabdomyosarcoma Study group experience and rationale for Intergroup Rhabdomyosarcoma Study V. *J Pediatr Hematol Oncol* 2001; 23:215–220.
177. Spunt S, Lobe T, Pappo A, et al. Aggressive surgery is unwarranted for biliary tract rhabdomyosarcoma. *J Pediatr Surg* 2000;35:309–316.
178. Crist W, Gehan E, Ragab A, et al. The third Intergroup Rhabdomyosarcoma Study. *J Clin Oncol* 1995;13:610–630.
179. Crist W, Anderson J, Meza J, et al. Intergroup Rhabdomyosarcoma Study-IV: results for patients with nonmetastatic disease. *J Clin Oncol* 2001;19: 3091–3102.
180. Leaphart C, Rodeberg D. Pediatric surgical oncology: management of rhabdomyosarcoma. *Surg Oncol* 2007;16:173–185.
181. Hays D, Lawrence WJ, Wharam M, et al. Primary reexcision for patients with 'microscopic residual' tumor following initial excision of sarcomas of trunk and extremity sites. *J Pediatr Surg* 1989;24:5–10.
182. LaQuaglia M. Genitourinary rhabdomyosarcoma in children. *Urol Clin North Am* 1991;18:575–580.
183. Corpron C, Andrassy R, Hays D, et al. Conservative management of uterine pediatric rhabdomyosarcoma: a report from the Intergroup Rhabdomyosarcoma Study III and IV pilot. *J Pediatr Surg* 1995;30:942–944.
184. Hays D, Raney R, Wharam M, et al. Children with vesical rhabdomyosarcoma (RMS) treated by partial cystectomy with neoadjuvant or adjuvant chemotherapy, with or without radiotherapy. A report from the Intergroup Rhabdomyosarcoma Study (IRS) Committee. *J Pediatr Hematol Oncol* 1995;17:46–52.
185. Andrassy R, Hays D, Raney R, et al. Conservative surgical management of vaginal and vulvar pediatric rhabdomyosarcoma: a report from the Intergroup Rhabdomyosarcoma Study III. *J Pediatr Surg* 1995;30:1034–1036; discussion 1036–1037.
186. Andrassy R, Wiener E, Raney R, et al. Progress in the surgical management of vaginal rhabdomyosarcoma: a 25-year review from the Intergroup Rhabdomyosarcoma Study Group. *J Pediatr Surg* 1999;34:731–734; discussion 734–735.
187. Lobe T, Wiener E, Andrassy R, et al. The argument for conservative, delayed surgery in the management of prostatic rhabdomyosarcoma. *J Pediatr Surg* 1996;31:1084–1087.
188. Hays DM. Bladder/prostate rhabdomyosarcoma: results of the multi-institutional trials of the Intergroup Rhabdomyosarcoma Study. *Semin Surg Oncol* 1993;9:520–523.
189. Paulino A, Okcu M. Rhabdomyosarcoma. *Curr Probl Cancer* 2008:32: 7–34.
190. Arndt C, Hawkins D, Meyer W, et al. Comparison of results of a pilot study of alternating vincristine/doxorubicin/cyclophosphamide and etoposide/ifosfamide with IRS-IV in intermediate risk rhabdomyosarcoma: a report from the Children's Oncology Group. *Pediatr Blood Cancer* 2008;50:33–36.
191. McDonald M, Esiashvili N, George B, et al. Intensity-modulated radiotherapy with use of cone-down boost for pediatric head-and-neck rhabdomyosarcoma. *Int J Radiat Oncol Biol Phys* 2008;72:884–891.
192. Meza J, Anderson J, Pappo A, et al. Analysis of prognostic factors in patients with nonmetastatic rhabdomyosarcoma treated on Intergroup Rhabdomyosarcoma Studies III and IV: the Children's Oncology Group. *J Clin Oncol* 2006;24:3844–3851.
193. Blakely M, Spurbeck W, Pappo A, et al. The impact of margin of resection on outcome in pediatric nonrhabdomyosarcoma soft tissue sarcoma. *J Pediatr Surg* 1999;34:672–675.
194. Carli M, Colombatti R, Oberlin O, et al. High-dose melphalan with autologous stem-cell rescue in metastatic rhabdomyosarcoma. *J Clin Oncol* 1999;17:2796–2803.
195. Carli M, Colombatti R, Oberlin O, et al. European intergroup studies (MMT4-89 and MMT4-91) on childhood metastatic rhabdomyosarcoma: final results and analysis of prognostic factors. *J Clin Oncol* 2004;22: 4787–4794.
196. Koscielniak E, Klingebiel T, Peters C, et al. Do patients with metastatic and recurrent rhabdomyosarcoma benefit from high-dose therapy with hematopoietic rescue? Report of the German/Austrian Pediatric Bone Marrow Transplantation Group. *Bone Marrow Transplant* 1997;19: 227–231.
197. Boulad F, Kernan N, LaQuaglia M, et al. High-dose induction chemoradiotherapy followed by autologous bone marrow transplantation as consolidation therapy in rhabdomyosarcoma, extraosseous Ewing's sarcoma, and undifferentiated sarcoma. *J Clin Oncol* 1998;16:1697–1706.
198. Grovas A, Fremgen A, Rauck A, et al. The National Cancer Data Base report on patterns of childhood cancers in the United States. *Cancer* 1997; 80:2321–2332.
199. Gurney J, Young J Jr, Roffers S, et al. *Cancer Incidence and Survival among Children and Adolescents: United States SEER Program 1975–1995.* Bethesda, MD: National Cancer Institute, SEER Program; 1999.
200. Saab R, Khoury JD, Krasin M, et al. Desmoplastic small round cell tumor in childhood: the St. Jude Children's Research Hospital experience. *Pediatr Blood Cancer* 2007;49:274–279.
201. Pappo A, Rao B, Jenkins J, et al. Metastatic nonrhabdomyosarcomatous soft-tissue sarcomas in children and adolescents: the St. Jude Children's Research Hospital experience. *Med Pediatr Oncol* 1999;33:76–82.
202. Ball A, Fisher C, Pittam M, et al. Diagnosis of soft tissue tumours by Tru-Cut biopsy. *Br J Surg* 1990;77:756–758.
203. Barth RJ, Merino M, Solomon D, et al. A prospective study of the value of core needle biopsy and fine needle aspiration in the diagnosis of soft tissue masses. *Surgery* 1992;112:536–543.
204. Heslin M, Lewis J, Woodruff J, et al. Core needle biopsy for diagnosis of extremity soft tissue sarcoma. *Ann Surg Oncol* 1997;4:425–431.
205. Yang J, Chang A, Baker A, et al. Randomized prospective study of the benefit of adjuvant radiation therapy in the treatment of soft tissue sarcomas of the extremity. *J Clin Oncol* 1998;16:197–203.
206. Edmonson J, Ryan L, Blum R, et al. Randomized comparison of doxorubicin alone versus ifosfamide plus doxorubicin or mitomycin, doxorubicin, and cisplatin against advanced soft tissue sarcomas. *J Clin Oncol* 1993;11: 1269–1275.
207. Verweij J, van Oosterom A, Somers R, et al. Chemotherapy in the multidisciplinary approach to soft tissue sarcomas. EORTC Soft Tissue and Bone Sarcoma Group studies in perspective. *Ann Oncol* 1992;3(suppl 2): S75–S80.
208. Spunt S, Pappo A. Childhood nonrhabdomyosarcoma soft tissue sarcomas are not adult-type tumors. *J Clin Oncol* 2006;24:1958–1959; author reply 1959–1960.
209. Pappo A, Devidas M, Jenkins J, et al. Phase II trial of neoadjuvant vincristine, ifosfamide, and doxorubicin with granulocyte colony-stimulating factor support in children and adolescents with advanced-stage nonrhabdomyosarcomatous soft tissue sarcomas: a Pediatric Oncology Group Study. *J Clin Oncol* 2005;23:4031–4038.
210. Pratt C, Pappo A, Gieser P, et al. Role of adjuvant chemotherapy in the treatment of surgically resected pediatric nonrhabdomyosarcomatous soft tissue sarcomas: a Pediatric Oncology Group Study. *J Clin Oncol* 1999;17: 1219.
211. Ferrari A, Casanova M, Collini P, et al. Adult-type soft tissue sarcomas in pediatric-age patients: experience at the Istituto Nazionale Tumori in Milan. *J Clin Oncol* 2005;23:4021–4030.
212. Spunt S, Hill D, Motosue A, et al. Clinical features and outcome of initially unresected nonmetastatic pediatric nonrhabdomyosarcoma soft tissue sarcoma. *J Clin Oncol* 2002;20:3225–3235.
213. Spunt S, Poquette C, Hurt Y, et al. Prognostic factors for children and adolescents with surgically resected nonrhabdomyosarcoma soft tissue sarcoma: an analysis of 121 patients treated at St Jude Children's Research Hospital. *J Clin Oncol* 1999;17:3697–3705.
214. Pratt C, Maurer H, Gieser P, et al. Treatment of unresectable or metastatic pediatric soft tissue sarcomas with surgery, irradiation, and chemotherapy: a Pediatric Oncology Group study. *Med Pediatr Oncol* 1998;30:201–209.
215. Spunt SL, Skapek SX, Coffin CM. Pediatric nonrhabdomyosarcoma soft tissue sarcomas. *Oncologist* 2008;13:668–678.
216. Ni Y, Chang M, Hsu H, et al. Hepatocellular carcinoma in childhood. Clinical manifestations and prognosis. *Cancer* 1991;68:1737–1741.
217. Multerys M, Goodman M, Smith M, et al. Hepatic tumors. In: Ries LAG, Smith MA, Gurney JG, et al., eds. *Cancer Incidence and Survival among Children and Adolescents: United States SEER Program 1975–1995.* SEER Program, NIH Pub. No. 99–4649. Bethesda, MD: National Cancer Institute; 1999.
218. Weinberg A, Finegold M. Primary hepatic tumors of childhood. *Hum Pathol* 1983;14:512–537.

219. Darbari A, Sabin K, Shapiro C, et al. Epidemiology of primary hepatic malignancies in U.S. children. *Hepatology* 2003;38:560–566.
220. Ikeda H, Matsuyama S, Tanimura M. Association between hepatoblastoma and very low birth weight: a trend or a chance? *J Pediatr* 1997;130: 557–560.
221. Reynolds P, Urayama K, Von Behren J, et al. Birth characteristics and hepatoblastoma risk in young children. *Cancer* 2004;100:1070–1076.
222. Spector L, Feusner J, Ross J. Hepatoblastoma and low birth weight. *Pediatr Blood Cancer* 2004;43:706.
223. Litten J, Tomlinson G. Liver tumors in children. *Oncologist* 2008;13: 812–820.
224. Kingston J, Herbert A, Draper G, et al. Association between hepatoblastoma and polyposis coli. *Arch Dis Child* 1983;58:959–962.
225. DeBaun M, Tucker M. Risk of cancer during the first four years of life in children from the Beckwith-Wiedemann Syndrome Registry. *J Pediatr* 1998;132:398–400.
226. Rainier S, Dobry C, Feinberg A. Loss of imprinting in hepatoblastoma. *Cancer Res* 1995;55:1836–1838.
227. Park W, Oh R, Park J, et al. Nuclear localization of beta-catenin is an important prognostic factor in hepatoblastoma. *J Pathol* 2001;193:483–490.
228. Monga S, Mars W, Pediaditakis P, et al. Hepatocyte growth factor induces Wnt-independent nuclear translocation of beta-catenin after Met-beta-catenin dissociation in hepatocytes. *Cancer Res* 2002;62:2064–2071.
229. Tomlinson G, Douglass E, Pollock B, et al. Cytogenetic evaluation of a large series of hepatoblastomas: numerical abnormalities with recurring aberrations involving 1q12-q21. *Genes Chromosomes Cancer* 2005;44: 177–184.
230. Schneider N, Cooley L, Finegold M, et al. The first recurring chromosome translocation in hepatoblastoma: der(4)t(1;4)(q12;q34). *Genes Chromosomes Cancer* 1997;19:291–294.
231. Parada L, Limon J, Iliszko M, et al. Cytogenetics of hepatoblastoma: further characterization of 1q rearrangements by fluorescence in situ hybridization: an international collaborative study. *Med Pediatr Oncol* 2000;34:165–170.
232. Nickerson H, Silberman T, McDonald T. Hepatoblastoma, thrombocytosis, and increased thrombopoietin. *Cancer* 1980;45:315–317.
233. Chang M, Shau W, Chen C, et al. Hepatitis B vaccination and hepatocellular carcinoma rates in boys and girls. *JAMA* 2000;284:3040–3042.
234. Huang K, Lin S. Nationwide vaccination: a success story in Taiwan. *Vaccine* 2000;18(suppl 1):S35–S38.
235. Aronson D, Schnater J, Staalman C, et al. Predictive value of the pretreatment extent of disease system in hepatoblastoma: results from the International Society of Pediatric Oncology Liver Tumor Study Group SIOPEL-1 study. *J Clin Oncol* 2005;23:1245–1252.
236. Meyers R, Rowland J, Krailo M, et al. Predictive power of pretreatment prognostic factors in children with hepatoblastoma: a report from the Children's Oncology Group. *Pediatr Blood Cancer* 2009;53:1016–1022.
237. Malogolowkin M, Katzenstein H, Krailo M, et al. Intensified platinum therapy is an ineffective strategy for improving outcome in pediatric patients with advanced hepatoblastoma. *J Clin Oncol* 2006;24:2879–2884.
238. Haas J, Feusner J, Finegold M. Small cell undifferentiated histology in hepatoblastoma may be unfavorable. *Cancer* 2001;92:3130–3134.
239. Meyers R. Tumors of the liver in children. *Surg Oncol* 2007;16:195–203.
240. Haas J, Muczynski K, Krailo M, et al. Histopathology and prognosis in childhood hepatoblastoma and hepatocarcinoma. *Cancer* 1989;64: 1082–1095.
241. Lack E, Neave C, Vawter G. Hepatocellular carcinoma. Review of 32 cases in childhood and adolescence. *Cancer* 1983;52:1510–1515.
242. [No authors listed.]. Primary liver cancer in Japan. Sixth Report. The Liver Cancer Study Group of Japan. *Cancer* 1987;60:1400.
243. Habrand J, Nehme D, Kalifa C, et al. Is there a place for radiation therapy in the management of hepatoblastomas and hepatocellular carcinomas in children? *Int J Radiat Oncol Biol Phys* 1992;23:525–531.
244. Weinblatt M, Siegel S, Siegel M, et al. Preoperative chemotherapy for unresectable primary hepatic malignancies in children. *Cancer* 1982;50: 1061–1064.
245. Taylor P, Filler R, Nebesar R, et al. Experience with hepatic resection in childhood. *Am J Surg* 1969;117:435–441.
246. Lee C, Sung J, Hwang L, et al. Surgical treatment of 109 patients with symptomatic and asymptomatic hepatocellular carcinoma. *Surgery* 1986; 99:481–490.
247. Exelby P, Filler R, Grosfeld J. Liver tumors in children in the particular reference to hepatoblastoma and hepatocellular carcinoma: American Academy of Pediatrics Surgical Section Survey–1974. *J Pediatr Surg* 1975;10: 329–337.
248. Otte J, de Ville de Goyet J, Reding R. Liver transplantation for hepatoblastoma: indications and contraindications in the modern era. *Pediatr Transplant* 2005;9:557–565.
249. Austin M, Leys C, Feurer I, et al. Liver transplantation for childhood hepatic malignancy: a review of the United Network for Organ Sharing (UNOS) database. *J Pediatr Surg* 2006;41:182–186.
250. Otte J, Pritchard J, Aronson D, et al. Liver transplantation for hepatoblastoma: results from the International Society of Pediatric Oncology (SIOP) study SIOPEL-1 and review of the world experience. *Pediatr Blood Cancer* 2004;42:74–83.
251. Pham T, Iqbal C, Grams J, et al. Outcomes of primary liver cancer in children: an appraisal of experience. *J Pediatr Surg* 2007;42:834–839.
252. D'Alessandro A, Knechtle S, Chin L, et al. Liver transplantation in pediatric patients: twenty years of experience at the University of Wisconsin. *Pediatr Transplant* 2007;11:661–670.
253. Reyes J, Carr B, Dvorchik I, et al. Liver transplantation and chemotherapy for hepatoblastoma and hepatocellular cancer in childhood and adolescence. *J Pediatr* 2000;136:795–804.
254. Jain A, Costa G, Marsh W, et al. Thrombotic and nonthrombotic hepatic artery complications in adults and children following primary liver transplantation with long-term follow-up in 1000 consecutive patients. *Transpl Int* 2006;19:27–37.
255. Li J, Chu J, Yang J, et al. Preoperative transcatheter selective arterial chemoembolization in treatment of unresectable hepatoblastoma in infants and children. *Cardiovasc Intervent Radiol* 2008;31:1117–1123.
256. Meyers R, Katzenstein H, Krailo M, et al. Surgical resection of pulmonary metastatic lesions in children with hepatoblastoma. *J Pediatr Surg* 2007; 42:2050–2056.
257. Black C, Luck S, Musemeche C, et al. Aggressive excision of pulmonary metastases is warranted in the management of childhood hepatic tumors. *J Pediatr Surg* 1991;26:1082–1085; discussion 1085–1086.
258. Czauderna P, Mackinlay G, Perilongo G, et al. Hepatocellular carcinoma in children: results of the first prospective study of the International Society of Pediatric Oncology group. *J Clin Oncol* 2002;20:2798–2804.
259. Gille J, Spieth K, Kaufmann R. Metronomic low-dose chemotherapy as antiangiogenic therapeutic strategy for cancer. *J Dtsch Dermatol Ges* 2005;3:26–32.
260. Pang R, Poon R. Angiogenesis and antiangiogenic therapy in hepatocellular carcinoma. *Cancer Lett* 2006;242:151–167.
261. Meng F, Henson R, Patel T. Chemotherapeutic stress selectively activates NF-kappa B-dependent AKT and VEGF expression in liver cancer-derived endothelial cells. *Am J Physiol Cell Physiol* 2007;293:C749–C760.
262. Ortega J, Douglass E, Feusner J, et al. Randomized comparison of cisplatin/vincristine/fluorouracil and cisplatin/continuous infusion doxorubicin for treatment of pediatric hepatoblastoma: a report from the Children's Cancer Group and the Pediatric Oncology Group. *J Clin Oncol* 2000;18:2665–2675.
263. Malogolowkin M, Katzenstein H, Krailo M, et al. Redefining the role of doxorubicin for the treatment of children with hepatoblastoma. *J Clin Oncol* 2008;26:2379–2383.
264. Katzenstein H, Krailo M, Malogolowkin M, et al. Hepatocellular carcinoma in children and adolescents: results from the Pediatric Oncology Group and the Children's Cancer Group intergroup study. *J Clin Oncol* 2002;20:2789–2797.

CHAPTER 110 THE PREGNANT PATIENT

COSMAS J. M. VANDEVEN, N. SCOTT ADZICK, AND ALEXANDER S. KRUPNICK

KEY POINTS

1. The general surgeon should be familiar with the physiologic changes associated with pregnancy in order to distinguish maternal physiologic changes from signs or symptoms of disease.
2. When the uterus reaches the umbilicus, precise assessment of gestational age is recommended, which may require consultation with the obstetric service. Fetal monitoring should be considered to optimize uterine physiology, starting at approximately 20 weeks of gestation.
3. Concerns regarding medicolegal repercussions should not interfere with the proper medical care of the pregnant patient. Optimal care, including imaging studies, surgery, and the use of medications, benefit the mother and therefore the unborn child.
4. Perforated appendicitis in pregnancy rapidly leads to diffuse peritonitis, premature labor, and fetal loss. The rate of preterm labor and fetal loss with perforated appendicitis ranges from 26% to 66%, compared with 0% to 5% for uncomplicated appendicitis.
5. Laparoscopic cholecystectomy is a safe and reliable modality to treat gallstone disease during pregnancy. Symptomatic cholelithiasis treatment during the first trimester includes conservative measures until elective cholecystectomy can be performed safely during the second trimester of gestation. Second trimester disease can be dealt with surgically, whereas that presenting later in gestation can probably be managed symptomatically until the postpartum period.
6. Adhesions are the most common cause of intestinal obstruction in the gravid patient, but intestinal volvulus is a much more common complication than in the population as a whole. Intussusception, hernia, and carcinoma are responsible for a minority of cases of bowel obstruction.

In the United States alone, approximately 13 million conceptions occur annually, resulting in over 4 million live births each year.[1] Despite the continuous presence of this patient population, little emphasis has been placed on educating the general surgeon in the diagnosis and treatment of surgical problems in (1) the pregnant patient. Although obstetricians routinely deal with pregnancy-related maternal disease and surgery, in many medical and surgical diseases the general surgeon is consulted. It is therefore imperative that he or she understands the normal physiologic changes occurring during pregnancy as well as the presentation of surgical disease in pregnancy. The surgeon often is the first person to evaluate a pregnant patient after trauma or for abdominal pain or learns of the pregnancy during the initial workup. The incidence of most surgical diseases remains the same in the pregnant patient, although some, like cholelithiasis, may actually increase. In addition, the surgeon must be aware of the changes in presentation as well as be conversant with the safety and utility of diagnostic imaging modalities. Pathways and algorithms for diagnosis and treatment of diseases in the nonpregnant woman must be altered to ensure the safety and well-being of the mother as well as that of the fetus. The purpose of this chapter is to review the physiologic changes that occur in pregnancy, discuss the risks and benefits of diagnostic imaging modalities and medications in pregnancy, and review the role of fetal monitoring and assessment of preterm labor. In addition, the presentation, frequency, and treatment of some common surgical diseases during pregnancy as well as their adverse effects on the pregnancy are described. Pregnancy is one of the rare situations when surgical decisions directly affect the lives of two people, and although mistakes can be twice as costly, rewards can double.

UTERINE PHYSIOLOGY AND PRETERM LABOR

Full-term delivery is delivery at 37 weeks of gestation or beyond. Twelve percent of live births are premature, at less than 37 weeks of gestation. Seventy-five percent of all perinatal morbidity and mortality is associated with premature delivery.[2]

The uterus is a smooth muscle organ responsible for reception, implantation, development, and expulsion of the fetus. In the nonpregnant woman, the uterus is an exclusively pelvic organ weighing approximately 70 g with a cavity volume of 10 mL. During pregnancy, the uterus gradually becomes an intra-abdominal organ weighing close to 1,100 g and expanding to a total volume of 5 L at term. By the 12th week of gestation, the uterus becomes too large to reside exclusively in the pelvis (2) and extends into the abdominal cavity. By the 20th week, the uterine fundus reaches the umbilicus; by the third trimester, it reaches almost to the liver (Fig. 110.1). As the uterus continues to rise, it exerts pressure on the anterior abdominal wall, displaces the intestines superiorly and laterally, and changes the relationship between the abdominal visceral organs. In the upright position, the uterus is supported by the anterior abdominal wall and usually undergoes a dextrorotation because of the presence of the rectosigmoid on the left. In the supine position, most of the uterine weight falls on the spinal column, but compression of the surrounding great vessels, especially the flaccid inferior vena cava, can occur.

Uterine activity and contractions are coupled to the electrical changes in the myometrium, which is physiologically arranged to maximize the efficiency of uterine contractions for the expulsion of the fetus at term. The resting membrane potential of the uterine myocyte ranges from −40 to −60 mV. It becomes more negative (−60 mV) early in gestation and increases to −40 mV near term. Early in pregnancy, the myometrium exhibits irregular electrical activity, termed *slow waves*. These rhythmic alterations in the membrane potential occasionally reach the threshold potential and lead to an action potential at the top of the slow wave. Entry of Ca^{2+} through voltage-sensitive Ca^{2+} channels allows for actin–myosin interaction and electromechanical coupling, leading to uterine contraction. By the second trimester, irregular contractions can be palpated through the abdominal wall and are known as Braxton Hicks contractions.[3] These irregular contractions during

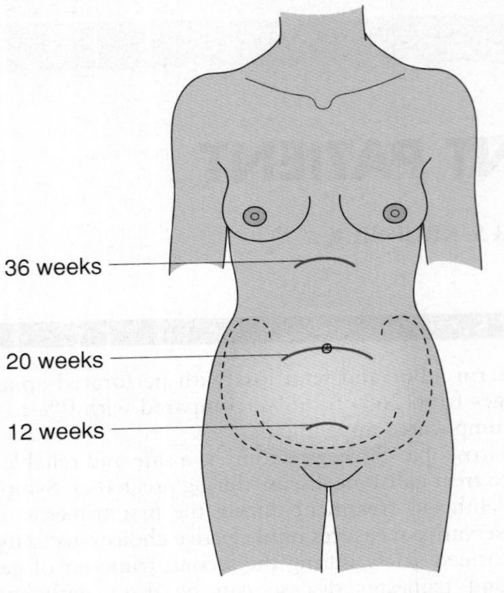

FIGURE 110.1. Enlarging uterus during gestation. At 12 weeks, the uterus rises out of the pelvis into the abdomen. At 20 weeks, the fundus is at the height of the umbilicus, and at 36 weeks the uterus reaches to the upper abdomen.

pregnancy lead to relatively small increases in uterine pressure and do not result in cervical effacement or dilatation. At term, gap junctions are formed between the uterine myocytes, which allow for electrical and metabolic communication. The increase in gap junctions results in rapid and efficient conduction of the action potential throughout the uterine smooth muscle with resulting coordinated, purposeful contractions generating pressures up to 80 mm Hg. These coordinated contractions ultimately result in effacement and dilatation of the cervix and delivery of the baby.

The mechanisms behind human parturition are still poorly understood. Numerous hormones, peptides, and local mediators act on the myometrium both to stimulate and down-regulate its activity (Table 110.1). Parturition begins when forces favoring uterine activity override those of quiescence and tip the balance toward contraction and ultimately birth. Progesterone maintains uterine relaxation during most of the pregnancy by blocking Ca^{2+} flux through cell membranes and opposing the action of estrogen. Close to term, the concentration of estrogen increases relative to that of progesterone, leading to uterine activation. Synthesis and surface expression of contraction-associated proteins, including gap junctions, ion channels, and oxytocin receptors, is initiated, and the uterus is transformed from its pliable, relaxed state to one of responsiveness and excitability. A shift in arachidonic acid metabolism from lipoxygenase products to those of cyclooxygenase, especially prostaglandin E_2 and F_{2a}, favors activation of the uterine musculature as well as the onset of uterine contractions. Prostaglandins raise local Ca^{2+} concentrations by increasing Ca^{2+} flux across the cell membrane and stimulating Ca^{2+} release from intracellular stores. Inflammatory cytokines, especially interleukin (IL)-1 and IL-6, are produced locally by placental tissues and act in concert with other stimulatory factors to propagate uterine activity.[3,4]

Oxytocin is a nonapeptide synthesized in the hypothalamus and secreted from the posterior pituitary. Its name means "quick birth," and it was the first uterotonin to be implicated in parturition. Oxytocin stimulates Ca^{2+} flux across myometrial plasma membranes and has distinct receptors located in the myometrium and other reproductive tissues. Uterine responsiveness to oxytocin is directly related to receptor concentration, which can increase 300-fold during pregnancy. The uterine smooth muscle surface expression of oxytocin receptors is increased by maternal estrogen and opposed by progesterone. Although it was originally isolated from the posterior pituitary, the placental content of oxytocin is approximately five times that of the pituitary, and the placenta is most likely the main source of oxytocin during pregnancy and parturition.[4]

TABLE 110.1

MEDIATOR OF UTERINE ACTIVITY

■ STIMULATES UTERINE ACTIVITY	■ DOWN-REGULATES UTERINE ACTIVITY
Estrogen	Progesterone
Oxytocin	
PGE_2, $PGF_{2\alpha}$	
IL-1, IL-6	

IL, interleukin; PG, prostglalndin.

Preterm Onset of Labor

Preterm onset of labor is uterine contractions producing cervical change prior to 37 weeks of gestation. Despite many attempted interventions, the rate of premature deliveries has increased in the last 40 years and is currently about 12%.[2] Prematurity is responsible for 75% of all neonatal morbidity, mortality, and cost of neonatal care.[5] Survival has increased with improvement in neonatal intensive care units, but the premature infant still experiences a wide variety of ailments with long-term sequelae in many organ systems.

The cause of preterm labor is often multifactorial, but the onset of labor during surgical manipulation or intra-abdominal inflammatory processes is of most concern to the surgeon. Increased prostaglandin production in the presence of an infective process can activate preterm labor. Bacterial infection of the amniotic tissues or peritoneum leads to a local increase in eicosanoids and the onset of labor.[6] Endotoxin acts on inflammatory cells to increase production of IL-1 and IL-6, which also amplify local prostaglandin production. All these factors can act in concert to initiate and propagate preterm labor. Uterine activation and increased expression of gap junctions as well as oxytocin receptors can be induced by uterine stretch.[7] Uterine trauma caused by surgical manipulation could affect these same mechanisms, leading to premature uterine contractions. The interrelations at various levels between the inflammatory response, uterine and maternal trauma, and the initiation of labor can represent the body's attempt to expel the fetus from a hostile intrauterine environment.

Tocolysis

Tocolytic therapy attempts to reverse or alleviate the premature onset and/or progression of labor. In most clinical presentations, the etiology of the preterm onset of uterine contractions is not known. Intervention is directed at decreasing the uterine smooth muscle activity through inhibition of the muscle contraction. Despite 40 years of research, there has been little success in the prevention or treatment of preterm labor. Tocolytic treatments may result in the delay of delivery by approximately 48 hours, which allows for the administration of steroids to promote fetal lung maturation through the release of surfactant. The use of antenatal steroids is associated with a decreased risk of respiratory distress syndrome and multiorgan failure in the preterm neonate.[8] Prostaglandin synthesis inhibitors, magnesium sulfate, β-adrenergic agonists, and calcium channel blockers are the four most common pharmacologic agents used as tocolytics.[9] The choice of tocolytic agent may vary between institutions.

Magnesium sulfate is often used as a first-line tocolytic agent when the onset of premature contractions is documented. Most data support the theory that magnesium exerts its effects by calcium antagonism. High intracellular magnesium concentrations inhibit Ca^{2+} entry into myometrial cells, interfering with actin–myosin coupling. High magnesium concentrations also increase the sensitivity of K^+ channels, favoring hyperpolarization and uterine relaxation. Maternal serum levels necessary to inhibit myometrial contractility are not well established but may range between 4 and 9 mg/dL, two to six times normal levels. These serum concentrations of magnesium needed for tocolysis are not far from levels causing ablation of deep tendon reflexes (9 to 13 mg/dL) or respiratory depression (14 mg/dL). Concern regarding magnesium toxicity requires careful monitoring of the patient, particularly in patients with compromised renal function.

Because of the importance of prostaglandins in the promotion of uterine contractions, prostaglandin synthetase inhibitors, especially nonsteroidal anti-inflammatory drugs, are used to stop premature labor. Indomethacin is the nonsteroidal drug used most frequently for tocolysis because of its quick onset of action and ease of dosing.

β_2-Adrenergic agonists used in the treatment of preterm labor include ritodrine and terbutaline. Stimulation of uterine β_2 receptors leads to activation of adenylate cyclase and an increase in intracellular cyclic adenosine monophosphate (cAMP) concentration. Activation of cAMP-dependent protein kinase A inhibits myosin light-chain phosphorylation and actin–myosin coupling. Protein kinase A activity is also associated with increased Ca^{2+} efflux, decreased Ca^{2+} influx, and increased K^+ conductance. All these actions lead to myometrial relaxation.

Calcium channel blockers inhibit entry of calcium through voltage-dependent Ca^{2+} channels. The use of oral nifedipine can abolish uterine activity and prevent delivery with minimal toxicity or side effects.

The role of tocolytic therapy remains controversial. The benefit appears to be limited to delaying premature delivery by 48 hours, allowing for administration of steroids to enhance fetal lung maturity. Maternal and fetal side effects can be serious, so close observation is necessary with all forms of tocolysis. The decision to use tocolytics must be made only after the diagnosis of premature onset of labor is confirmed and the benefits of prolonging gestation outweigh the risks of tocolysis.

When nonobstetric surgery is required in a pregnant patient, prophylactic use of prostaglandin synthesis inhibitors such as indomethacin is recommended. A preoperative dose of 50 to 100 mg of indomethacin can be administered orally. Postoperative continued prophylaxis using indomethacin 50 mg by mouth, every 6 hours for a total of 48 hours, should be considered.

For intra-abdominal surgery in the preterm pregnant patient, preoperative steroid administration should be considered. Either two doses of betamethasone 12 mg, 24 hours apart, or four doses of dexamethasone 6 mg, 12 hours apart, should be administered to the mother, ideally beginning 48 hours prior to surgery.[8]

PHYSIOLOGIC CHANGES OF PREGNANCY THAT MIMIC DISEASE

The maternal physiologic homeostasis adapts in order to promote a physiologic environment that benefits the development and growth of the fetus. These physiologic changes may mimic or mask the diagnosis of medical disorders.

Progesterone levels increase throughout the pregnancy.[3] Progesterone is a smooth muscle relaxant that plays a major role in assuring relaxation of the uterine smooth muscle in order to prevent premature delivery. In addition, vascular, gastrointestinal, and urogenital smooth muscle relaxes, resulting in common pregnancy-associated signs and symptoms. Progesterone-induced smooth muscle relaxation appears to be dose dependent and can be blocked by increasing the extracellular concentration of Ca^{2+}, at least in vitro, suggesting that progesterone may alter the effective Ca^{2+} available for actin–myosin coupling.[10]

Plasma volume increases by up to 50% and red blood cell volume by 20% to 30%. This increase in intravascular (blood) volume leads to a 50% increase in cardiac output (CO).[11] In order to allow for this increase in CO, pregnancy is associated with marked venous and arterial vasodilatation. Vasodilatation occurs to such an extent that the blood pressure actually decreases during pregnancy, with the nadir around 24 weeks and a return to baseline by term.[12] Vasodilatation is facilitated by a decrease in vasoconstrictor sensitivity and an increase in the production of nitric oxide and prostacyclin.[13] Common clinical signs and symptoms associated with this increase in CO and associated vasodilatation include decreased exercise tolerance, mild peripheral edema, spider angiomata, complaints of stuffy sinuses, an increase in lower extremity varicosities, and hemorrhoids.

In order to increase oxygen delivery to the fetus and remove the increased supply of CO_2 produced by the fetus, the mother hyperventilates throughout the pregnancy.[14] Arterial pO_2 values increase while pCO_2 levels decrease, and pH increases (mild alkalosis). Maternal oxygen metabolism increases by 20% to 30% and functional reserve capacity decreases. Therefore, a pregnant patient may desaturate much quicker compared to a nonpregnant patient. When intubation is needed, there is significantly less time to establish an airway and assure continued oxygenation of the mother and baby. Fetal CO_2 is cleared by passive diffusion. In case of mechanical ventilation, maternal pCO_2 levels should be targeted at lower levels in order to prevent acidosis of the fetus. It is common for the pregnant patient to have the sensation of shortness of breath, specifically in the second and third trimester when the uterus increases in size and displaces the diaphragm upward.

The lower esophageal sphincter tone gradually decreases, as does gastric emptying time. Nausea and vomiting of pregnancy is a common occurrence affecting between 50% and 90% of all women.[15] This correlation with pregnancy was documented as early as 2000 BC. Although a clear cause has not been established, it rarely extends beyond the first trimester. Other causes must be investigated if the nausea and vomiting persist or occur later in pregnancy.

The gallbladder empties more slowly during pregnancy and undergoes a gradual increase in residual volume, both during fasting and after meals. With these changes, combined with supersaturation of bile by cholesterol, pregnancy becomes a lithogenic state.[16] The effects of pregnancy are transient, and gallbladder motility and volumes return to normal as early as 2 weeks after pregnancy, but the gallstones, if formed, may persist.

Prolonged small bowel transit time and decreased colonic emptying work to maximize nutrient and water absorption but also contribute to the constipation reported by 38% of pregnant women.[17]

Abdominal pain may be related to a surgical pathologic process but can have many pregnancy-associated causes.[18] Round ligament pain is described as an aching, dragging pain that typically is unilateral. It is provoked by physical activity or even turning while sleeping. It is a common occurrence until the third trimester. Pain in the hypochondrium can result from uterine pressure on the lower ribs. The patient describes a very localized, sharp, nonradiating pain that more often is on the right compared to the left upper quadrant.

Hemoglobin concentrations may drop to 10 mg/dL, and hematocrit values may go as low as 30%. Pregnancy may be associated with an increase in the white blood cell (WBC)

TABLE 110.2

CHANGE IN LABORATORY VALUES DURING PREGNANCY

■ PARAMETER	■ CHANGE	■ NORMAL NONPREGNANT VALUE	■ LATE PREGNANCY VALUE
Albumin (g/dL)	↓	3.2–3.8	2.4–3.1
Alkaline phosphatase (IU/L)	↑	30–115	100–210
Total bilirubin (mg/dL)	↔	0.26–1.00	Unchanged
Aspartate aminotransferase (IU/L)	↔	0–31	Unchanged
Hemoglobin (g/dL)	↓	12.0–16.0	10.5–14
Leukocyte count ($\times 10^3$/mm^3)	↑	4.5–11.0	6.0–16.0

From Martin C, Varner MW. Physiologic changes in pregnancy surgical implications. *Clin Obstet Gynecol.* 1994;37:241–255.

count, up to levels of 13,000 WBCs per mL. Intrapartum and immediate postpartum (<24 hours) counts may be as high as 25,000 WBCs per mL. Platelet counts may slightly decrease as the pregnancy progresses. Thrombocytopenia is relatively common (up to 8%) in pregnancy. The most common cause is gestational thrombocytopenia.[19] The patient is typically asymptomatic, and platelet counts recover to normal levels within a few weeks following the delivery. Renal blood flow and glomerular filtration rates increase by over 50%. Creatinine levels decrease appropriately, resulting in normal levels of 0.5 to 0.6 mg/dL. Serum alkaline phosphatase levels gradually increase because of production of an alkaline phosphatase isozyme by the placenta. This does not reflect biliary or bone disease. Albumin levels may be lower, associated with the increase in plasma volume, and osmotic pressure may be decreased (Table 110.2).

IMAGING MODALITIES IN THE PREGNANT PATIENT

Advances in radiology have revolutionized surgical practice. By visualizing the lesion before exploration, surgical intervention can focus on the area of disease or avoid it altogether. Emergency medicine physicians, radiologists, and surgeons are frequently hesitant to use the proper diagnostic imaging modalities for pregnant patients because of the perceived danger to the developing fetus. In almost all clinical presentations, the risks of misdiagnosis by avoiding the proper imaging tests are greater compared to the risks of sequelae from ionizing 3 radiation to the fetus. The physician should not avoid proper diagnostic and therapeutic interventions because of medicolegal concerns. Although experimental data regarding the effects of ionizing radiation on the developing human fetus are impossible to obtain, animal exposure and follow-up of those inadvertently exposed to radiation have provided some information: Retrospective studies of atomic bomb survivors in Hiroshima and Nagasaki have allowed for evaluation of the effects of massive radiation exposure in utero.[20]

Ionizing Radiation

Fetal effects of ionizing radiation depend on the dose absorbed by the fetal tissue and the stage of fetal development during exposure. Exposure is defined as the amount of ionic charge created by the radiation on passing through a defined mass of air. The roentgen is a common unit of exposure, producing 0.26 millicoulomb per kilogram of air or 2 billion ion pairs per cubic centimeter of exposed air. Although exposure is useful for measuring radiation output, the absorbed dose is the radiation imparted to tissue that creates a biologic effect. One gray (Gy) is strictly defined as the deposition of 1.0 joule of energy per kilogram of tissue. One rad is 1% of 1 Gy. As a gross estimate, exposure to 1 roentgen gives an absorbed dose of 1 rad or 10 mGy.

It is a misconception to assume that the radiation absorbed by the mother is the same as that absorbed by the fetus. Dosing of radiation to the uterus and conceptus can vary several fold based on abdominal wall depth and the anteverted or retroverted position of the uterus. Radiographic evaluation of the abdomen and pelvis is most likely to expose the fetus to direct ionizing radiation, whereas examination of the extremities and chest leads to exposure from scatter radiation only[21] (Table 110.3).

Radiation-induced ionization of vital cellular structures can result in damage to the DNA. DNA damage may be repaired or may result in cell death, rapid cell growth, abnormal cell growth, or genetic mutation. Cellular destruction either leads to the death of the embryo if a significant amount of tissue is affected or has no effect if the damaged cells are replaced by healthy ones. Growth impairment of organs occurs if the population of cells cannot be replaced or damage occurs to a small population of progenitor cells at a vital stage of development. All these effects are produced at threshold doses, and exposure to radiation levels below the threshold does not have biologic consequences compared with control populations.[22] The outcome of radiation exposure depends on the absorbed dose and the stage of

TABLE 110.3

RADIATION DOSING TO THE CONCEPTUS AND UTERUS FROM SELECTED RADIOGRAPHIC EXAMINATIONS[21]

■ EXAMINATION	■ DOSE (mrad)
Routine chest radiograph	0.5–1.0
Abdominal flat plate	140
Intravenous pyelogram	78
Computed tomography, chest (uterus shielded, not exposed)	16–23
Computed tomography, abdomen (uterus shielded, not exposed)	150–190
Computed tomography, pelvis	2,000

development during exposure, with potential death early in gestation, teratogenesis during organogenesis (4 to 10 weeks of gestation), and growth retardation at later gestational stages.

Lethal Effects

The multicellular embryo, before the blastocyst stage, is most sensitive to the lethal effects of radiation but resistant to teratogenesis if it survives. The cause of this phenomenon is uncertain but could relate to the totipotent nature of the embryo at this stage and its ability indiscriminately to replace a specific volume of tissue below the lethal threshold. Because more than 50% of all human pregnancies abort, mostly without any recognition that fertilization has even occurred,[23] determining the lethal dose of radiation at this stage is difficult. Significant radiation exposure in the first 2 weeks of human development, which corresponds to gestational weeks 3 and 4, results in loss of the pregnancy. If the pregnancy is not lost, the patient can be reassured that the risk for teratogenicity is very low.

Teratogenic Effects

Teratogenic effects of radiation can occur during early organogenesis in animal studies. Exposure of rats to 100 rads at various points of development reveals a very narrow window for teratogenesis. This window corresponds to weeks 2 to 8 in human development (4 to 10 weeks of gestation), consistent with early organ formation. Despite these experimental data, it is difficult to link any specific human malformation with radiation exposure other than those of the central nervous system (CNS). Microcephaly, pigmentary changes in the retina, hydrocephalus, and optic nerve atrophy have been reported at a significantly higher rate after exposure to radiation in pregnancy.[24] All patients were exposed to a minimum estimated dose of 100 rads, and no visceral, limb, or other malformations were found unless the child also exhibited CNS abnormalities. One explanation for this discrepancy is that the developmental period of the CNS is much longer, continuing throughout gestation and into the neonatal period, whereas other organs have a very narrow period during which morphologic alterations can be produced. Exposure to high doses of radiation during this narrow window is rare, and even if an isolated congenital abnormality were to occur, it would be difficult to separate this event from the background malformation rate. Current data suggest that exposure less than 5 rads does not increase the risk for birth defects. Although there is concern about teratogenicity of exposure from 5 to 10 rads, only exposure greater than 10 rads is proven to create serious risk to the fetus.[25]

Intrauterine Growth Restriction

Intrauterine growth restriction results from radiation-induced cellular depletion. Although catch-up growth can occur if exposure happens early in gestation, permanent cell depletion and growth restriction occur with exposure during the second and third trimester.[26] Wood et al.[27,28] studied growth retardation of children exposed in utero to the Japanese atomic blasts. Those within 1,500 m from the center of the explosion were exposed to over 25 rads and, when followed through age 17 years, were 2 to 3 cm shorter, 3 kg lighter, and had a head circumference 1 cm smaller than normal. Those beyond 1,500 m from the blast received less than 25 rads and had a normal head circumference, height, and weight. Further animal and human data support the contention that exposures of less than 5 rads should not cause either anatomic malformation or growth retardation.[22]

Oncogenic Potential

The correlation between childhood cancer and in utero exposure to radiation has been reported,[29,30] although conclusions regarding the cause-and-effect relationship of this correlation could not be definitively established. In addition, the severity of the effect appears unrelated to the dose. In analyses of Japanese A-bomb survivors who were exposed in utero, no significant increase in rates of childhood or adult cancer were reported.[31] Expert consensus estimates the increased risk of lifetime cancer associated with at least 10 rad in utero exposure to increase by 1%, from 20% to 21%.[32]

Ultrasound

Ultrasonography uses high-frequency, nonionizing, acoustic radiation to create images. A surface transducer sets up vibratory motions that are transmitted through matter as acoustic waves. The boundaries between different densities of tissue reflect some of these sound waves back to be detected by a transducer. Ultrasonic images therefore detect acoustic boundaries between different biologic materials in the body. Audible sound ranges from 20 to 20,000 vibrations per second, whereas ultrasonography uses frequencies of 1 million to 10 million vibrations per second. Since its initial use in the 1950s, diagnostic ultrasonography has not been shown to produce fetal damage or harmful effects;[26,33] however, theoretic dangers do exist. Rapid compression and decompression of tissue by sound waves could cause tissue damage. Conversion of mechanical energy to thermal energy, especially at the bone–soft tissue interface, could lead to local hyperthermia, whereas the phenomenon known as cavitation could cause microscopic bubbles already present in tissues to grow in size because of absorption of surrounding diffused gases. However, there is no consistent evidence that properly used diagnostic ultrasound is detrimental to the conceptus.[33]

Magnetic Resonance Imaging

Like ultrasonography, magnetic resonance imaging (MRI) uses no ionizing radiation and instead relies on the magnetic properties of tissues to create images. Four magnetic fields interact during an MRI examination to create the image. The intrinsic magnetic field of an atomic nucleus, usually that of a hydrogen proton, is combined with a strong, uniformly applied external magnetic field and a weaker magnetic field gradient. In addition, a magnetic field is intermittently generated by pulsed radiofrequency waves. When this external radiofrequency is applied to nuclei in an existing magnetic field, the nuclei absorb some of the energy and change their orientation. When the radiofrequency ceases, the nuclei return to their previous orientation and emit the radiofrequency they absorbed. These signals are detected, stored, and processed by a computer to create an image.

Based on current data, it is unlikely that magnetic fields of the intensity used for diagnostic MRI pose any danger to the developing fetus, but biologic mechanisms do exist that could, at least theoretically, lead to damage. Charged particles and molecules moving in a strong magnetic field create an electrostatic potential difference, and normal red blood cells can alter their shape and create a charge when moving within an electric field.[34] Changing magnetic fields can induce visual light flashes because of magnetic effects on the photoreceptors in the eye,[34,35] and heat can be generated during the application of radiofrequencies. All these effects, however, occur with applications well above those used for diagnostic purposes. Based on these and other data, the International Radiation Protection Association has concluded that despite the lack of evidence that mammalian embryos are sensitive to the magnetic fields encountered during MRI examination, elective examination of pregnant women by MRI should be postponed until after the first trimester and completion of organogenesis. Ultrasonography should be the diagnostic modality of choice during pregnancy, with MRI limited to cases in which unique diagnostic information is required.[36] MRI, however, is not absolutely contraindicated even in the first trimester in situations when ultrasound cannot suffice.

Medications in Pregnancy

Many pregnant patients will require medical interventions, including the use of medications. In contrast to common belief, most medications are relatively safe in pregnancy. Medications contraindicated in pregnancy include but are not limited to coumarin derivatives, isotretinoin, methotrexate, diethylstilbestrol, thalidomide, angiotensin-converting enzyme (ACE) inhibitors and ACE antagonists, tetracycline, and quinolones. However, the risks to the fetus may be less compared to the risk to the mother when not using the proper medication. Optimizing maternal physiology and maternal well-being almost always benefits the fetus. When medications are needed to accomplish this, the benefits most commonly outweigh the risks. Particularly in clinical emergencies or trauma, immediate initiation of the proper medications may be required to save the life of the mother and therefore the life of the fetus as well. Many resources are available to the clinician to assess the risks to the fetus.[37] The widely used Food and Drug Administration (FDA) classification is of limited value since it does not incorporate data from pregnancy registries and other resources.[38] The most detailed information is available through a national database called *Reprotox*. Consultation with the obstetric service may assist in choosing the optimal medications for both the mother and the fetus.

FETAL MONITORING

Fetal heart rate (FHR) monitoring is used in obstetric practice as an indirect assessment of fetal well-being. Electronic FHR monitoring was introduced in the late 1950s,[39] has gained wide acceptance, and is now used in over 85% of all pregnancies.[40] The FHR can be monitored externally, using a Doppler device that is placed on the maternal abdomen. Uterine activity is monitored by using a tocodynometer, also applied to the maternal abdomen (Fig. 110.2). Since direct evaluation of fetal oxygenation and acid–base status is not possible except for a few rare unusual circumstances, monitoring of fetal well-being is based on indirect methods. It is believed that the FHR patterns may change in response to altered uterine–placental perfusion or decreased oxygen content in the maternal blood. In trauma or during surgery, uterine perfusion or maternal oxygenation may be altered, and monitoring the FHR may assist the surgical team in correcting placental perfusion and oxygenation in order to improve the fetal status.

Internal fetal monitoring is used intrapartum and relies on analysis of fetal cardiac patterns from electrocardiogram leads placed directly on the exposed part of the fetus. A transcervical intrauterine pressure catheter may be used concurrently to monitor the strength of the uterine contractions.[40]

Fetal Heart Rate Interpretation

A normal FHR during pregnancy ranges between 110 and 160 beats per minute (bpm). A prolonged baseline (≥10 minutes) above 160 bpm is considered fetal tachycardia, whereas that below 110 bpm is considered fetal bradycardia.[41]

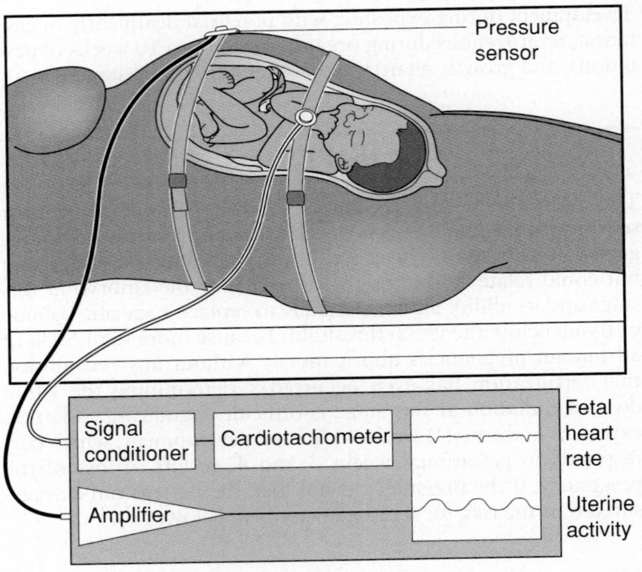

FIGURE 110.2. Intraoperative and postoperative fetal monitoring using noninvasive surface Doppler and pressure sensor to monitor uterine contractions.

Accelerations are defined as an increase in the FHR of at least 15 bpm for at least 15 seconds. The presence of accelerations is reassuring. FHR accelerations are normal findings in the second half of pregnancy and occur as a result of increased sympathetic and decreased parasympathetic stimulation with fetal movements.

Changes in blood pressure and oxygenation are detected by the chemoreceptors and baroreceptors of the aortic arch and carotid bodies, resulting in a change in the heart rate to maintain a steady state. Normal FHR tracings express continuous adjustment in the vagal tone through variability in the heart rate. The FHR demonstrates continuous variability from the baseline, with fluctuations of peaks and troughs ranging from 6 to 25 bpm. Decreased heart rate variability can be a physiologic response of the fetal sleep–wake cycle or maternal medications such as sedatives. Persistently decreased variability may be associated with altered fetal perfusion or oxygenation. Decelerations usually occur intrapartum and are related to the uterine contractions (periodic decelerations). The decelerations are classified as "early," or simultaneous with the contraction; "late," or starting when the contraction is in progress and recovering after the contraction is over; and "variable," or variable in relation to the contractions. Early decelerations are uniform, gradual drops in the FHR that mirror the uterine contractions and reflect an increased vagal tone from a transient increase in intracranial pressure. This pattern is a benign physiologic manifestation of a functioning autonomic nervous system and is not associated with adverse outcome. Variable decelerations result from umbilical cord compression by uterine contractions. Isolated variable decelerations have little clinical significance, but if persistent with inadequate recovery between contractions, intervention may be indicated. Late decelerations may indicate poor uterine perfusion or decreased oxygenation. Causes include maternal hypotension caused by inferior vena cava compression, blood loss, or regional anesthesia. Persistent late decelerations warrant investigation to correct the cause and sometimes delivery of the child.

A sinusoidal heart rate pattern is an uncommon baseline abnormality. It has the characteristics of a smooth sine wave with a frequency of 3 to 5 cycles per minute. Variability is minimal (0 to 5 bpm). This pattern has been associated with mild hypoxia in the setting of fetal anemia.[42]

Fetal Monitoring for Trauma or Surgical Patients

Utility of both FHR and uterine contraction monitoring lies in the ability to intervene based on the acquired information. The most optimal environment for a fetus is optimal maternal physiology. While providing care to the mother, fetal monitoring may assist in improving maternal perfusion and/or oxygenation, may diagnose fetal distress requiring a cesarean section, or may detect uterine contractions that may require tocolytic treatment when the fetus is premature. Depending on the availability of neonatal care, fetal survival is possible starting at around 24 weeks of gestation. The uterus rises above the umbilicus at approximately 20 weeks. Fetal and uterine monitoring is suggested when the gestational age is 20 weeks or beyond. Whenever possible, discussion with the mother or family should occur prior to operation to delineate the expectations regarding fetal survival and quality of life of an extreme premature infant. Consultation with obstetrics or neonatology/pediatrics may be helpful. Intraoperative fetal distress as indicated by an ominous heart rate tracing must be treated by correcting maternal hypotension or increasing oxygen delivery with increased fraction of inspired oxygen (FiO_2), blood transfusion, or more aggressive fluid resuscitation. The inability to improve the intrauterine milieu can necessitate an emergent cesarean section to prevent fetal demise. Even when delivery is not an option because of prematurity, fetal and uterine monitoring may still assist in the management of the mother optimizing the intrauterine environment.

Concern for premature labor may necessitate the use of tocolytic agents. In most cases, indomethacin 50 mg by mouth every 6 hours can be used. When the pregnancy is at high risk for premature delivery, steroid administration prior to operation should be considered (refer to the Preterm Onset of Labor section).

APPENDICITIS IN THE PREGNANT PATIENT

Appendicitis affects 250,000 patients every year in the United States. As a disease of the young, its peak incidence corresponds to the childbearing years. Appendicitis is the most common nonobstetric indication for operation during pregnancy, with an average incidence of 1 in 1,500 deliveries. Although some smaller studies have suggested that this condition is more common later in gestation,[42–44] larger series show an equal distribution throughout pregnancy.[45] The incidence is similar to that in nonpregnant women, but the anatomic and physiologic changes of the gravid state make the diagnosis difficult.

Classic appendicitis in the nonpregnant patient presents with a constellation of signs and symptoms suggesting the disorder. Luminal obstruction of the appendiceal orifice, whether by fecalith or lymphoid hyperplasia, leads to an increase in intraluminal pressure by blocking the normal egress of mucus. Progressive obstruction of venous outflow followed by capillary and arterial thrombosis leads to mucosal ulceration, transmural wall necrosis, and, if unabated, perforation. Because early appendiceal distention is relayed by stretch receptors to the 10th thoracic ganglion, referred pain is perceived in the distribution corresponding to the epigastric region. Once the ongoing inflammation extends to involve the parietal peritoneum, the pain localizes to the right lower quadrant. Anorexia, nausea, and vomiting, initiated by visceral mechanisms similar to those responsible for the referred pain, follow the onset of pain. Findings on physical examination arise from this pathophysiologic process. Voluntary guarding of the right lower quadrant reflects the patient's anticipation of pain with palpation in the area. Rigidity or involuntary guarding indicates reflex spasm of the abdominal musculature caused by the nearby inflammatory process, whereas psoas and obturator signs indicate respective irritation of these muscles. Tenderness on rectal examination can be elicited with a low-lying appendix, whereas fever and leukocytosis indicate systemic inflammation. Although none of these signs or symptoms is 100% diagnostic, the presence of right lower quadrant pain, rigidity, and migration of pain was found to have the highest likelihood ratio for the presence of appendicitis in a large multifactorial analysis.[46] All the aforementioned signs and symptoms are altered by pregnancy (Table 110.4).

In a classic 1932 study, Baer et al.[47] evaluated the migration of the appendix through the duration of pregnancy with barium enemas. Beginning in the third month of pregnancy, the appendix and cecum are gradually displaced by the uterus and start a craniad migration out of the pelvis into the upper abdomen. By the third trimester, the appendiceal tip can abut the gallbladder (Fig. 110.3). The vague, referred epigastric pain caused by early appendiceal obstruction is not changed by this anatomic consideration, but the location of the somatic pain is. In a large study of pregnant women with proved appendicitis, abdominal pain was present in all patients. Location of pain in the right lower quadrant, however, was common only early in gestation, and a portion of patients reported pain in the right upper quadrant. This change in symptomatology is easily understood if the anatomic changes of the appendix are taken into consideration.[45] Both guarding and rigidity are valuable findings on physical examination but are common only in the first trimester. Elevation of the abdominal wall from the more laterally placed, upward-directed appendix and the laxity of the abdominal wall musculature caused by this distention decrease the reliability of these findings. Only 42.9% of patients in the third trimester are reported to have abdominal spasm and guarding, compared with 80% during the first trimester.[48] Psoas and obturator signs are similarly obscured as the appendix is moved from its normal location.

Anorexia, nausea, and vomiting occur in 58% to 77% of pregnant patients with appendicitis.[45,49] Although nausea and

TABLE 110.4

VARIATION IN SIGNS AND SYMPTOMS OF APPENDICITIS DURING PREGNANCY

SIGNS AND SYMPTOMS	FIRST TRIMESTER (%)	SECOND TRIMESTER (%)	THIRD TRIMESTER (%)
Right lower quadrant pain	100	50	14
Right upper quadrant pain	0	17	57
Guarding (muscle spasm)	80	50	43
Nausea and vomiting	53	60	23
Tenderness on rectal examination	60	17	0
Perforation rate	20	49	70

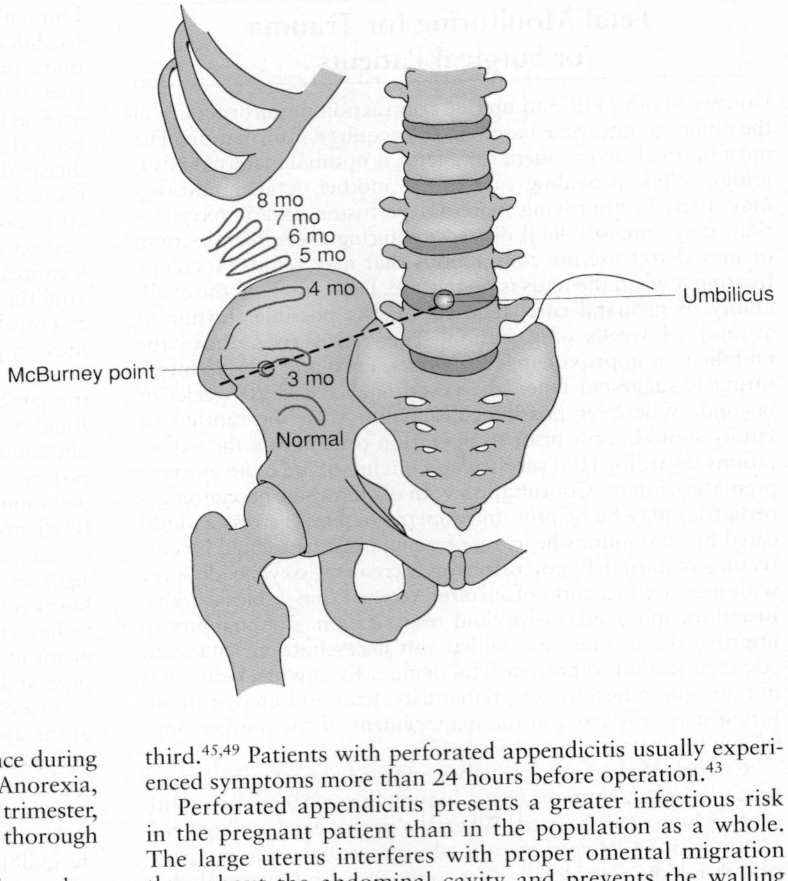

FIGURE 110.3. Changing location of the appendix throughout gestation. (From Baer JL, Reis RA, Arens RA. Appendicitis in pregnancy. *JAMA* 1932;98:1963, with permission.)

vomiting in the first trimester is common, its occurrence during the later stages of pregnancy should raise suspicion. Anorexia, nausea, and vomiting during the second and third trimester, especially if associated with abdominal pain, require a thorough investigation.

The results of laboratory examinations commonly used to assist in the diagnosis of appendicitis are also obscured by pregnancy. The physiologic leukocytosis of pregnancy, ranging from 5,000 to 12,000 WBCs per mL, overlaps that of appendicitis. In one collected series, the WBC counts of pregnant patients with proved appendicitis was not significantly elevated over these values, and only 25% of patients had a WBC count over 15,000. Most patients (50%) had WBC counts ranging between 10,000 and 15,000, and 25% had less than 10,000 WBCs per mL.[45] Urinalysis is a useful adjunct in the workup of appendicitis but again presents a dilemma in pregnancy. Urinary tract infection is common in pregnancy as the enlarging uterus compresses the right ureter. Dilatation and stagnant flow in the right collecting system can contribute to bacterial overgrowth and infection, and an inflamed and enlarging appendix can contribute to the urinary tract infection by further compressing this system. Pyuria without bacteria can also indicate involvement of the right ureter in the appendiceal inflammatory process. Pus or bacteria in the urine does not rule out appendiceal inflammation, as the two conditions often coexist. Attributing abdominal pain to pyelonephritis and choosing a course of antibiotics rather than further investigation only leads to a delay in diagnosis and missed appendicitis.[44]

These complicating factors and the physician's fear of surgically induced premature labor can contribute to delay of appendectomy in pregnancy. One series documented a correlation between a delay in the diagnosis and gestational age. In the first trimester, all the diagnoses were made promptly and timely surgical intervention undertaken. A delay in diagnosis occurred in 18% of patients presenting in the second trimester, but in the third trimester delay was the rule. Numerous patients were discharged from the emergency room with various misdiagnoses ranging from false labor to nausea and vomiting of pregnancy to gastroenteritis. All presented with vague signs and symptoms obscuring the true diagnosis.[50] Other series have documented the same delay in operation with a high rate of perforation, as high as 49% in the second trimester and 70% in the third.[45,49] Patients with perforated appendicitis usually experienced symptoms more than 24 hours before operation.[43]

Perforated appendicitis presents a greater infectious risk in the pregnant patient than in the population as a whole. The large uterus interferes with proper omental migration throughout the abdominal cavity and prevents the walling off of the inflammatory process. Braxton Hicks contractions disrupt adhesion formation, and the general increase in vascularity of the abdomen with greater lymphatic drainage allows rapid dissemination of infection. The high circulatory levels of adrenocorticoids in pregnancy have also been hypothesized to diminish the tissue inflammatory response
4 and hinder containment of infection.[51,52] Perforated appendicitis in pregnancy rapidly leads to diffuse peritonitis, premature labor, and fetal loss. The rate of preterm labor and fetal loss with perforated appendicitis ranges from 26% to 66%, compared with 0% to 5% for uncomplicated appendicitis.[45,49,53]

Although history and clinical examination for suspected appendicitis during pregnancy are not ideal, they are still the best tools for detecting the disease. A patient with appendicitis during the first trimester might present with right lower quadrant pain, guarding, and nausea and vomiting, whereas a women in the third trimester would most likely have pain in another location and a more confusing clinical picture. The adage "If you cannot rule it out, take it out" applies in pregnancy as well as the nongravid state.[45] In applying this principle, the average negative laparotomy rate is 19% to 35% in the pregnant patient, a rate similar to that in the population as a whole.[54] Negative laparotomy rates as high as 75% in the third trimester, however, have been reported.[55] Although complication rates are low for negative explorations, fetal loss does occur. Imaging studies offer the potential of increasing the accuracy of the diagnosis of appendicitis.

Imaging Modalities

Ultrasonography is safe for the developing fetus and the study of choice in the pregnant patient. Findings that suggest appendicitis include visualization of a tubular structure with a diameter greater than 6.0 mm, a wall thickness above 3.0 mm,[55] and

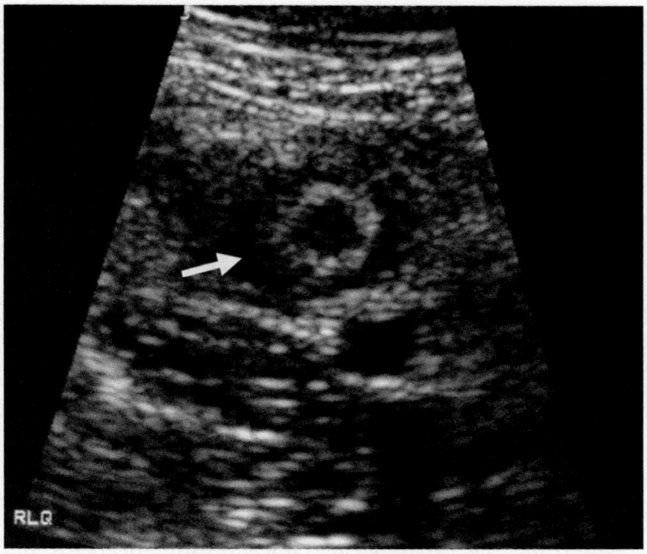

FIGURE 110.4. Ultrasonographic appearance of appendicitis. The appendix appears as a thick, noncompressible tubular structure with central hypoechogenicity. The walls are 5 mm thick, over the 3-mm limit for a normal appendix. (Courtesy of Dr. Beverly Coleman, Department of Radiology, Hospital of the University of Pennsylvania, Philadelphia, PA.)

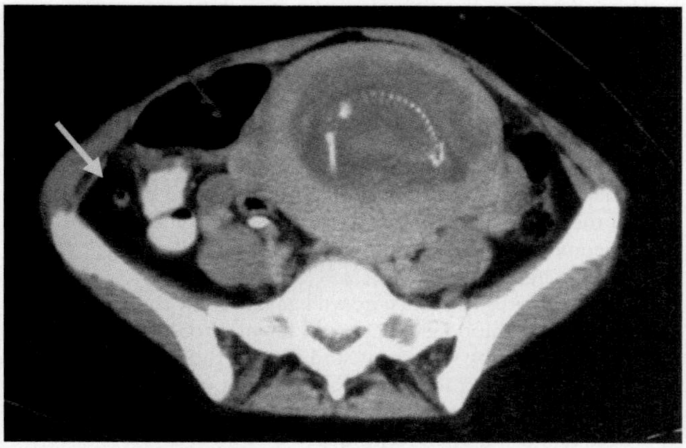

FIGURE 110.5. Computed tomography (CT) scan of a woman in the 18th week of gestation presenting with a 12-hour history of right-sided abdominal pain. Abdominal examination on presentation revealed significant tenderness; after a nondiagnostic ultrasound, a laparotomy is considered for presumed appendicitis. A CT scan is obtained instead, revealing a normal, air-filled appendix with no sign of periappendiceal inflammation (*arrow*). The laparotomy was postponed, and 12 hours later the patient aborted a septic fetus. An unnecessary laparotomy for an atypical presentation of chorioamnionitis was avoided by the judicious use of the CT scan. (Courtesy of Dr. David Weiss, Chestnut Hill Hospital, University of Pennsylvania Health System, Chestnut Hill, PA.)

lack of peristalsis (Fig. 110.4). Because a normal appendix is difficult to identify, simply seeing the appendix combined with tenderness on palpation with the ultrasound probe is suggestive of appendicitis. Ultrasonography, however, has been criticized for being operator dependent and situation specific. Sensitivity varies widely, from 68% to 89%,[48,56] and examination can be prohibitive because of abdominal guarding, pain during examination, and a thick abdominal wall. Distortion of anatomic landmarks and the displacement of the appendix by the gravid uterus complicate the diagnosis. Other structures such as an inflamed salpinx can also mimic appendicitis on ultrasound,[57] and a dilated uterine vein during pregnancy has been mistaken for an acutely inflamed appendix.[56] Despite these limitations, ultrasound is readily available in the emergency department or office and often can add diagnostic information to a confusing clinical picture. If the patient's history and physical examination do not warrant an immediate operation, abdominal ultrasonography should be the first study obtained.

Computed tomography (CT) has emerged as a highly reliable modality in the diagnosis of appendicitis. Appendiceal CT, using rectally administered contrast, can be performed within 10 to 20 minutes, does not require a waiting period for oral contrast to progress down through the cecum, and exposes the patient to only one third the radiation of a regular CT scan.[58] Results at one center[59] have indicated that CT interpretation can be 98% sensitive and 98% specific for the diagnosis of appendicitis. Routine use of this modality reduces costs, expedites the diagnosis, and reduces perforation rates from 22% to 14% while decreasing the incidence of negative laparotomy from 20% to 7%.[59,60] Although radiation risks to the developing fetus do exist, it is unlikely that fetal loss or malformations occur with the dosing needed for an abdominal CT. Because even low levels of radiation in utero can increase the incidence of childhood cancer, widespread use of this modality in the pregnant patient with abdominal pain may be detrimental. Reserving the CT scan for those cases where the clinical history, physical examination, and ultrasonography are indeterminate should decrease the rate of perforation and negative exploration, just as it has in the nonpregnant population (Fig. 110.5).

MRI uses no ionizing radiation and, like CT, has the potential to image the whole abdomen. It is generally considered safe in pregnancy, and initial experimentation has shown that the higher water content of an inflamed appendix can be detected by MRI.[61] Reported sensitivity for appendicitis approaches 100%, at least in children.[62] Routine use of MRI may be hindered by availability and limited experience for detecting appendicitis using this modality. Future studies of MRI in appendicitis are warranted.

Laparoscopy

Pregnancy is no longer a contraindication to laparoscopy. Although earlier studies reported a high rate of fetal and maternal complications, it is likely the underlying pathologic process rather than laparoscopy contributed to maternal morbidity and fetal demise.[63] Fetal acidosis with experimental maternal CO_2 pneumoperitoneum has been reported but can be minimized in the clinical setting with arterial blood gas monitoring and careful attention to maternal ventilation and acid–base balance.[64] Concerns regarding the effect of increased intra-abdominal pressure are questionable considering the high uterine pressures during delivery. Experimental pneumoperitoneum in itself does not alter hemodynamics in the fetus until pressures of 20 torr are reached.[64] Reduced insufflation pressures of 8 to 12 mm Hg should not contribute to fetal morbidity and mortality. Patients undergoing nongynecologic laparoscopic surgery begin a regular diet sooner, have lower narcotic requirements, and are discharged from the hospital earlier than patients undergoing open surgery.[65]

Laparoscopy to evaluate the appendix is a feasible diagnostic modality during pregnancy but may be difficult during later gestation. Anatomic changes alter placement of trocars above the gravid uterus[66] and require the use of the open Hasson technique of trocar placement under direct visualization rather than blind insufflation with a Veress needle. Maneuvers to enhance operative safety of laparoscopy in pregnancy have been outlined by the Society of American Gastrointestinal and Endoscopic Surgeons[67] (Table 110.5).

TABLE 110.5

GUIDELINES FOR LAPAROSCOPIC SURGERY DURING PREGNANCY

1. Defer operative intervention until the second trimester, when the fetal risk is lowest, whenever possible.
2. Pneumatic compression devices must be used because of the enhancement of lower venous stasis with pneumoperitoneum and pregnancy-induced hypercoagulable state.
3. Fetal and uterine status, as well as maternal end-tidal CO_2 and arterial blood gases, should be monitored.
4. Use fluoroscopy selectively and protect the uterus with lead shield if intraoperative cholangiography is possible.
5. Given enlarged gravid uterus, abdominal access should be obtained using open technique.
6. Dependent positioning should be used to shift the uterus off the inferior vena cava.
7. Pneumoperitoneum pressures should be minimized (to 8–12 mm Hg) and not allowed to exceed 15 mm Hg.
8. Obstetric consultation should be obtained before operation.

From SAGES Committee on Standard Practice. Guidelines for laparoscopic surgery during pregnancy. *Surg Endosc* 1998;12: 189–190.

Appendectomy

Once the diagnosis of appendicitis is made, treatment is strictly surgical. The type of incision can vary based on surgeon preference but becomes an issue during later pregnancy. Because of the migration of the appendix, an incision over the McBurney point in the late second and third trimester is inadequate. A low midline incision is favored by some to allow treatment of other conditions that mimic appendicitis but may require excessive retraction of the uterus.[50] A right-sided transverse incision over the point of maximal tenderness is usually the safest approach because the appendix typically lies beneath that point.[43,45,49] A similar incision at the level of the umbilicus allows good exposure of most of the right upper and lower abdomen. By tilting the patient 30 degrees to the left, the uterus is shifted away from the operative field and off of the inferior vena cava. A right paramedian incision usually necessitates medial retraction of the uterus for exposure and increases the risk of precipitating premature labor. The laparoscopic approach, although useful for both diagnosis and treatment, can be difficult in later gestation. While the potential benefits over the open appendectomy include less uterine manipulation and decreased incidence of preterm labor, its utility depends heavily on surgeon experience and comfort with the procedure.[65,66]

If exploration reveals a normal appendix, an appendectomy still should be performed. Although some authors question this approach because of the suggested high rate of preterm labor with a normal appendectomy,[68] most believe this to be untrue. Taking out the normal appendix adds little to morbidity while eliminating potential confusion if symptoms should recur.[45] Perforated appendicitis or pus in the abdominal cavity demands thorough peritoneal toilet along with the appendectomy. Drainage of the perforated appendectomy bed was avoided in the past because of fears that foreign material increased the risk of premature labor,[47] but these fears have not been substantiated and drainage of the appendiceal stump has been performed without complications.

BILIARY TRACT DISEASE IN PREGNANCY

Acute cholecystitis is the second most common general surgery diagnosis during pregnancy. Progesterone-induced relaxation of the gallbladder combined with estrogen-induced supersaturation of bile predispose to gallstone formation.[38,69] The risk for development of gallstones is related to the number of pregnancies, doubling after two pregnancies and nearly quadrupling after four.[69–71] Although gallstones are found in approximately 4% of all pregnant patients undergoing routine ultrasonography early during pregnancy, the rate can be as high as 12.2% immediately after delivery in high-risk populations.[70] Despite this high prevalence of gallstones, the incidence of acute cholecystitis during pregnancy is relatively low—1 to 8 in 10,000 pregnancies (0.01% to 0.08%).[72,73] Inhibition of gallbladder contraction by progesterone is most likely the reason for this discrepancy. Although gallstones and sludge can form, weaker contractions prevent cystic duct obstruction until delivery. Postpartum, the progesterone concentrations decrease and the increased force of gallbladder contraction potentiates gallstone-induced cystic duct obstruction. An increased prevalence of cholecystitis in the year after childbirth has been noted.[74–76]

Symptoms of cholecystitis or biliary colic caused by cystic duct obstruction are similar in the pregnant and nonpregnant patient. Crampy right upper quadrant or epigastric pain after a meal can last several minutes to hours. The pain may radiate to the back and accompany nausea and vomiting. Tenderness on palpation of the right upper quadrant is usually present with acute cholecystitis, but laboratory evaluation may be obscured by the normal leukocytosis and elevated alkaline phosphatase during pregnancy. Increased bilirubin or visible jaundice, however, is unlikely without common bile duct obstruction.[73]

The differential diagnosis for cholecystitis during pregnancy includes hepatitis, acute fatty liver of pregnancy, and appendicitis. The diagnosis can be strengthened by the history and physical examination and confirmed by abdominal ultrasound. Ultrasonography is more than 97% accurate in detecting cholecystitis, with typical findings of echogenic shadowing, gallbladder wall thickening, and pericholecystic fluid.[77] Pain on palpation with the ultrasound transducer, or a sonographic Murphy sign, is confirmatory of inflammation.

Historically, medical management was the definitive treatment of cholecystitis during pregnancy. The pregnant patient was given nothing orally, maintained on intravenous hydration, and treated with antibiotics for signs of infection. A low-fat diet was started once symptoms abated, antibiotics were discontinued, and the patient was discharged to home. Most women had initial relief of symptoms with this management, and surgery was reserved for those with persistent symptoms, severe toxicity, sepsis, peritonitis, or obstructive jaundice.[78] Fear of surgical complications prompted some to place pregnant patients with disabling biliary symptoms on total parenteral nutrition until delivery.[65,79] Analysis of patient outcomes throughout the course of pregnancy, however, has put strict medical management into question. Between 57% and 70% of patients treated for gallstone disease during pregnancy have recurrence at some time during gestation.[80,81] This risk is close to 92% for those who present in the first trimester, 64% for those presenting during the second trimester, and 44% for those who present during the third. Of these patients, 90% require hospitalization for management of the relapse,[80] and a significant portion of those presenting in the first trimester experience pregnancy loss as a complication of the disease.[79,82] Complications of gallstones such as choledocholithiasis and pancreatitis can also arise with future attacks and have been associated with a maternal mortality rate of 15% and a 60% chance of fetal demise.[78,83–85]

5 Laparoscopic cholecystectomy is a safe and reliable modality to treat gallstone disease during pregnancy. Numerous reports and case control studies comparing laparoscopic with open cholecystectomy have supported the laparoscopic approach. Overall, patients have a shorter postoperative stay, resume oral intake earlier, have fewer postoperative hernias, and experience less pain with lower narcotic requirements by avoiding a large open incision.[63,65,86] Because fetal loss is most likely related to the underlying maternal illness and extent of uterine manipulation during surgery,[81,87] laparoscopic cholecystectomy offers a solution to both problems. Removing the diseased gallbladder eliminates the potential for recurrence, and the minimal uterine retraction needed with laparoscopic access to the right upper quadrant should decrease the risk for preterm labor. Although no randomized studies exist, preliminary data seem to support these assumptions. The incidence of premature uterine contractions with laparoscopic cholecystectomy has been reported at 0% to 21%, but contractions are usually well controlled by tocolytics. Most series report rates of premature birth or spontaneous abortion ranging from 0% to 7% with the laparoscopic approach.[66,80,81,87] After an open cholecystectomy, the reported rate of premature labor ranges from 0% to 40%, based on trimester,[88] and a spontaneous abortion or premature birth rate of up to 22% has been reported.[7] Based on the available data, laparoscopic cholecystectomy is safe during pregnancy and is preferable to open cholecystectomy.[88] An isolated report of three laparoscopic cholecystectomies ending in abortion, however, has been published, emphasizing that this procedure is not without risk, so careful attention must be paid to the timing, indications, and maternal physiology before any procedure.[89]

Because most biliary symptoms can be controlled, at least initially, with conservative management, the management of symptomatic gallstones varies based on the stage of gestation. The second trimester is the optimal time to perform an elective cholecystectomy. Organogenesis is complete, and the gravid uterus is not yet large enough to impinge on the operating field.[85] Clinical studies of open cholecystectomy confirm that this is the safest time to perform the operation. Spontaneous abortion rates after an open cholecystectomy are 12% during the first trimester, whereas the incidence of premature labor can be as high as 40% during the third trimester. The second trimester offers the ideal compromise, with the low spontaneous abortion rate of 5.6%.[88] Laparoscopic cholecystectomy offers the potential to decrease fetal loss even further over these values. Suggested management for symptomatic cholelithiasis during the first trimester consists of conservative measures until elective cholecystectomy can be performed safely during the second trimester of gestation. Second trimester disease can be dealt with surgically, whereas those presenting later in gestation can probably be managed symptomatically until the postpartum period. If symptoms are unremitting and cannot be handled with diet alone, surgical intervention might be necessary regardless of the period of gestation.[76,81]

FHR monitoring is an essential part of laparoscopic procedures. Because pneumoperitoneum can have detrimental physiologic effects on both the mother and fetus, any evidence of fetal distress should result in immediate desufflation.[67] FHR aberrations can also be treated by increasing uterine perfusion with maternal intravascular volume and changing the mother's position on the operating room table to decrease uterine compression of the inferior vena cava. Because the transabdominal signal is lost with pneumoperitoneum, transvaginal monitoring should be used during surgery,[65] whereas an external tocodynamometer should be placed on the abdomen immediately after the completion of the operation to monitor for uterine contractions. Tocolytic agents need not be used prophylactically but can be administered if the patient demonstrates uterine irritability or contractions. The rate of successful tocolysis after laparoscopic procedures with minimal uterine manipulation is close to 100%.[63,65,76,83,87,90]

Choledocholithiasis

Indications for evaluation of the common bile duct are no different in the pregnant patient from the population as a whole, namely a bilirubin above 1.5 mg/dL, a dilated common bile duct, or gallstone pancreatitis.[66] Endoscopic retrograde cholangiopancreatography (ERCP) can be performed safely in pregnancy. With proper lead shielding, judicious use of fluoroscopy time, and avoidance of permanent roentgenographic films, ERCP has been performed with no direct exposure of the fetus to radiation. Calculated scatter radiation on the order of 4 mrads during the whole examination presents the only risk from ionizing radiation.[84] Evaluation of the biliary tree, stone retrieval, and sphincterotomy can be performed under these conditions without maternal or fetal complications.[91] Other methods avoid radiation altogether and include imaging of choledocholithiasis with endoscopic ultrasonography,[92] endoscopic papillotomy under ultrasonographic control,[93] and magnetic resonance cholangiography for choledocholithiasis.[94] Success with all these modalities has been reported but can be limited by operator experience and availability. [Au5]

SURGICAL SPECIALITIES

INTESTINAL OBSTRUCTION DURING PREGNANCY

The incidence of intestinal obstruction during pregnancy rose throughout the 20th century. In the presurgical era, cases were cited as infrequently as 1 in every 68,000 deliveries. Since the 1940s, however, the incidence has increased to 1 in 2,500 to 3,500 deliveries.[95] This change reflects the increased number of laparotomies in young women and the prevalence of post-
6 operative adhesions during pregnancy. Adhesions remain the most common cause of intestinal obstruction in the gravid patient, but intestinal volvulus is a much more common complication than in the population as a whole. Intussusception, hernia, and carcinoma are responsible for a minority of cases of bowel obstruction (Table 110.6).

TABLE 110.6

CAUSES OF INTESTINAL OBSTRUCTION COMPLICATING PREGNANCY AND THE PUERPERIUM IN 66 PATIENTS

Adhesions	39 (59%)
Volvulus	15 (23%)
Sigmoid	7
Cecal	3
Midgut	3
Volvulus around vitellointestinal band	2
Intussusception	3 (5%)
Hernia	2 (3%)
Carcinoma	1 (1%)
Appendicitis	1 (1%)
Idiopathic (ileus)	5 (8%)

From Perdue PW, Johnson HW, Stafford PW, et al. Intestinal obstruction complicating pregnancy. *Am J Surg* 1992;164:385.

Obstruction during pregnancy classically presents during three peak periods because of the change in the interrelationship between the abdominal viscera caused by the gravid uterus. The first peak occurs during the fourth to fifth months of gestation as the uterus becomes an intra-abdominal organ, stretching any previously formed adhesions. The second peak occurs during the eighth to ninth months, when the fetal head descends into the pelvis, decreasing the uterine size. The third peak occurs after delivery as the sudden decrease in uterine size drastically changes the association of adhesions to surrounding bowel. The incidence of adhesion-related obstruction is highest during the first pregnancy after an operation, when the association between the viscera and adhesions is initially tested.[89,95]

In the general population, incarceration of bowel in groin hernias is the second most common cause of small bowel obstruction, but in the pregnant patient volvulus becomes the number two cause. As the enlarging uterus displaces the bowel out of the pelvis and away from the inguinal region, symptomatic groin hernias diminish in frequency.[96] Volvulus increases in prevalence during pregnancy because of changes in colon and small bowel anatomy and causes one fourth of all bowel obstructions. Sigmoid volvulus normally occurs owing to a long and redundant sigmoid colon. In the United States, this usually occurs in debilitated, institutionalized, or chronically constipated people. In countries such as Africa, a high incidence of sigmoid volvulus has been attributed to the high-fiber vegetable diet characteristic of that population. Anatomic changes of pregnancy further exacerbate this condition by causing the redundant sigmoid colon to rise out of the pelvis and twist around its point of fixation.[97] It is the most common site of volvulus during pregnancy.[98]

Cecal volvulus occurs because of failure of lateral peritoneal fixation during development. As the uterus enlarges during pregnancy, it raises the redundant or abnormally mobile cecum out of the pelvis. If a transition point or distal obstruction should occur from uterine pressure or an adhesive band, the colonic distention raises the colon even higher, producing torsion around this fixed point.[99] Volvulus of the small bowel also results from a congenital abnormality of rotation and fixation. Because clinical presentation usually occurs in infancy or childhood, the true incidence of malrotation in adulthood is unknown. The enlarging uterus potentially predisposes to the presentation of this anomaly during pregnancy by pushing the nonfixed, mobile portions of the small bowel into the upper abdomen, initiating the volvulus.[100]

Presentation and Diagnosis

Symptoms of intestinal obstruction are similar to those in the nonpregnant patient and commonly include abdominal pain and vomiting. Proximal small bowel obstruction results in short periods between vomiting episodes with poorly localized, crampy upper abdominal pain. Colonic obstruction can present with less frequent feculent vomiting and lower abdominal pain. Findings on physical examination such as abdominal distention are often difficult to evaluate because of the gravid uterus. Obstipation, although characteristic of distal obstruction such as sigmoid volvulus, may not occur with proximal obstruction. Laboratory studies, although useful to rule out other conditions, are not reliable enough to be considered diagnostic of obstruction. Significant leukocytosis can occur with necrosis and bowel strangulation, but mild elevations are not definitive because of the physiologic leukocytosis of pregnancy. Tachycardia and hypotension are also late signs suggesting bowel compromise and shock.

The murky clinical picture combined with the tendency to treat the progressive vomiting as a normal part of pregnancy and crampy abdominal pain as early contractions lead to a delay in presentation and diagnosis. The median time from the onset of symptoms to admission in one series was 48 hours, and the median time from admission to a necessary laparotomy was also 48 hours. This delay in diagnosis and treatment contributed to excessive maternal and fetal mortality.[96] Abdominal pain and vomiting in a pregnant patient with an abdominal scar should raise the serious suspicion of small bowel obstruction.

If intestinal obstruction is suspected, upright and flat films of the abdomen are the diagnostic studies of choice. Although some authors[95] believe that radiographs are nonspecific early in obstruction, serial films obtained every 4 to 6 hours usually show progressive changes confirming the diagnosis. Small bowel obstruction gives the appearance of a progressive stepladder formation with dilatation and multiple air–fluid levels. Large bowel obstruction can produce a similar picture or reveal a grossly dilated bowel loop suggestive of volvulus. Contrast studies are also useful, and a "bird's bill" shape of contrast with gradual narrowing after a barium enema can be diagnostic of colonic volvulus, whereas dilute diatrizoate (Gastrografin) or barium by mouth can usually differentiate partial from complete obstruction. Fetal radiation risks from the plain radiographs are negligible and greatly outweighed by those from the possibility of misdiagnosis.

Treatment

The initial treatment for bowel obstruction in the pregnant patient is no different from that of a nonpregnant patient. Nasogastric tube decompression and fluid resuscitation are the cornerstones of therapy. By the time an obstruction is visible on plain film, the fluid deficit from vomiting and intraluminal losses is estimated at 1,000 to 1,500 mL. In advanced cases of dehydration presenting with tachycardia and hypotension, fluid losses may be as high as 4 to 6 L.[95] Prompt fluid resuscitation is essential in the pregnant patient because compromise of uterine blood flow leads to fetal distress and demise.

Surgical intervention plays a prominent and earlier role in the management of the pregnant patient with bowel obstruction. Although adhesion-related small bowel obstruction in the nonpregnant patient usually resolves with nasogastric decompression and fluid administration, numerous series have documented failure of conservative management of small bowel obstruction in the pregnant woman. Of all patients, 89% to 100% eventually require an operation, and 13% to 23% require resection of gangrenous bowel at the time of laparotomy.[96,101] Based on these outcomes, some have stated that once the diagnosis of small bowel obstruction is made in a pregnant patient, the only role of nasogastric decompression and fluid resuscitation is to prepare the patient for an operation.[101] Cecal volvulus is also treated surgically, and although sigmoid volvulus in the nonpregnant patient can be managed with sigmoidoscopic decompression and placement of a rectal tube, the large gravid uterus may act as a mechanical impediment to detorsion. A laparotomy is usually necessary for treatment.[96,97]

A generous midline incision allows for maximum exposure of the abdomen with minimal manipulation of the uterus. During lysis of small bowel adhesions, bowel viability must be carefully assessed. Definitive management of cecal volvulus requires resection of necrotic cecum or detorsion and cecopexy. Sigmoid volvulus should also be treated by resection if necrotic, but simple detorsion and placement of a rectal tube can be performed if the sigmoid is viable. Although resection of the redundant sigmoid is the definitive treatment for this disease, it can be delayed until the postpartum period. Aggressive surgical treatment has been credited with reducing the maternal and fetal mortality rates from 20% and 50%, respectively, in the 1930s to 6% and 26% today.[96] Increased awareness of this disease and expeditious management can reduce those rates even further.

COLORECTAL CANCER DURING PREGNANCY

Colon cancer is a rare disease during pregnancy but one with lethal consequences. The incidence of colon cancer was estimated as 1 in 50,000 pregnancies based on a 1955 report.[102] More recent reviews estimate the incidence as 1 in 13,000 deliveries,[103] with the increasing prevalence attributable to increasing maternal age with the delay in pregnancy until later in life.[104] Presenting symptoms are similar to those in nonpregnant patients and include rectal bleeding, constipation, and abdominal pain and distention as well as nausea and vomiting.[105] All of these symptoms are common during pregnancy. Even the findings of occult blood in the stool and hematochezia are often attributed to pregnancy-related hemorrhoids and ignored.

The anatomic distribution and stage of colorectal cancer in the pregnant patient differ from those in the population as a whole. A nationwide survey of the members of the American Society of Colon and Rectal Surgeons who had cared for pregnant patients with colorectal cancer revealed a predominance of rectal cancer in this patient population. Of tumors, 64% were distributed below the peritoneal reflection and 36% were in the more proximal colon. A review of more than 200 pregnancy-associated colorectal cancers reported in the literature disclosed a similar distribution with 86% of tumors located in the rectum and only 14% above the peritoneal reflection.[106] This is in contrast to the general population, where most tumors (69%) are located in the colon and only 31% in the rectum. This trend could reflect a presentation bias because of frequent rectal examinations during prenatal care or the change in pelvic anatomy and symptoms of rectal compression by the gravid uterus.

Pregnant patients present with more advanced cancers than the population as a whole. In the study mentioned previously,[106] no pregnant patient was Dukes stage A at presentation, whereas 41% were Dukes stage B, 44% were stage C, and 15% were stage D. Although increased hormonal stimulation during pregnancy could cause rapid tumor growth and progression of disease,[106–108] not all colon cancers have estrogen or progesterone receptors and respond to this stimulation.[109] The advanced stage of disease on presentation most likely results from a delay in the diagnosis and the low clinical suspicion of malignancy in this patient population. This trend is similar to that in the young population as a whole, and although only 4% to 8% of all colon cancer occurs in those younger than 40 years, these patients also have a delayed presentation with more advanced disease.[110] The average interval between the onset of symptoms and diagnosis of colon cancer in those younger than 40 years is 6.4 months, and 32% of patients wait longer than 1 year before seeking medical attention for symptoms.[111] The stage of disease on presentation in this patient population is similar to that in the pregnant patient (Table 110.7), and colonic malignancy during gestation most likely represents pregnancy superimposed on colon cancer rather than a pregnancy-related disease.

Diagnosis

Diagnosis of colorectal cancer during pregnancy demands a very high level of suspicion. Patients with rectal bleeding, occult blood–positive stools, and anemia below physiologic levels of pregnancy should be evaluated for a colonic malignancy. Sigmoidoscopy is not contraindicated during pregnancy and does not appear to induce labor or congenital malformations. Because most cancers are located below the peritoneal reflection, they can be easily accessed and sampled for biopsy through a limited sigmoidoscopic examination. Because of the 5% risk of a second, synchronous primary, a more extensive colonoscopic evaluation might be necessary, especially if findings were to change the treatment or extent of surgical resection. Colonoscopy during pregnancy is still considered experimental and may be technically difficult because of colonic compression by the gravid uterus. Maneuvers to increase safety include use of only gentle pressure when manipulating the colonoscope, maternal administration of supplemental oxygen, and FHR monitoring during the procedure.[112]

Transrectal ultrasonographic staging of rectal cancer is particularly helpful during pregnancy because of its ability to evaluate cancerous invasion of the uterus or encroachment on the cervix that could prevent vaginal delivery.[112] Serum carcinoembryonic antigen levels are not normally elevated during pregnancy, and although of limited use as a screening tool, levels can be obtained before resection for early detection of recurrence.[113] Evaluation of metastatic disease to the liver can be performed with transabdominal ultrasonography at no risk to the fetus, and a CT scan can be obtained in more difficult cases.

Treatment

Treatment of colorectal cancer during pregnancy presents as an ethical dilemma for both the patient and the physician.

TABLE 110.7

STAGE AT PRESENTATION OF COLORECTAL CANCER DURING PREGNANCY AND THOSE YOUNGER THAN 40 YEARS OF AGE

DUKES STAGE	PREGNANT PATIENTS (%)	PATIENTS <40 Y (%)
A	0	2
B	41	30
C	44	45
D	15	23

Data from Bernstein MA, Madoff RD, Caushaj PF. Colon and rectal cancer in pregnancy. *Dis Colon Rectum* 1993;36:172°178; Smith C, Butler JA. Colorectal cancer in patients younger than 40 years of age. *Dis Colon Rectum* 1989;32:843–846.)

Aside from the difficulty in dealing with a potentially lethal disease in a young person, there is an inherent conflict between the treatment of the mother and fetus. Treatment of other surgical conditions encountered during pregnancy, such as appendicitis or cholecystitis, equally benefits both the mother and the unborn child. Treatment of colon cancer puts the two at odds. Although early tumor resection can improve the prognosis for the mother, this treatment might be detrimental to the fetus. Adjuvant chemotherapy or radiation therapy can improve survival of the mother but is generally contraindicated during pregnancy, especially early in gestation. Careful attention must be paid to the wishes of the family while explaining the risks and benefits for both the mother and child.

If the cancer is discovered in the first half of gestation, a definitive resection should be performed. Waiting months until adequate fetal maturation for delivery can allow cancer dissemination and disease progression.[105,112] In most cases, a colon resection can be handled without disturbing the pregnancy, and resection of even low-lying tumors can be performed before 20 weeks of gestation.[109,113] Total abdominal hysterectomy is recommended only if tumor invasion into the uterus has occurred, a technically complete operation cannot be performed without it, or the mother's life expectancy is shorter than the time needed to reach fetal viability. If the tumor is unresectable, a colostomy is performed for palliation until fetal viability is documented.

Treatment of tumors discovered after the 20th week can be postponed until term or fetal viability. Vaginal delivery is not contraindicated unless the tumor is obstructing the birth canal or presents a risk of episiotomy entering the tumor bed. Tumor resection is undertaken several days after the birth to allow uterine involution and resolution of pelvic vascular congestion. If a cesarean section is performed for obstetric reasons or because of tumor impingement on the birth canal, resection can be performed immediately, but the operation may be technically easier if done as a separate procedure and postponed for several days. This is especially important with low rectal lesions, where decreased pelvic vasculature can facilitate a low anterior or abdominoperineal resection.[105]

Management of the ovaries is a controversial issue. The incidence of colon carcinoma metastasizing to the ovaries is estimated to be between 3% and 8%[114] in the general population but can be as high as 25% during pregnancy and in young patients.[111,115] Bilateral salpingo-oophorectomy at the time of tumor resection has been advocated by some,[114] but during pregnancy the procedure carries a high chance of spontaneous abortion, especially during the first half of gestation. Although resection should be performed if the ovaries are grossly involved with tumor or a hysterectomy is undertaken, bilateral ovarian wedge biopsies with frozen section evaluation can be safely carried out without disturbing the pregnancy. Salpingo-oophorectomy is then performed only if the ovaries are involved with tumor.[105]

Adjuvant chemotherapy conveys a survival advantage to patients with Dukes stage C colon cancer. The classic adjuvant chemotherapy includes 5-fluorouracil, an antimetabolite that inhibits DNA synthesis. The safety of this drug during pregnancy is questionable, and evidence of fetal toxicity exists in animal models. Limited data on the human fetal safety of this drug are available, and it is considered a category D drug during pregnancy by the FDA: generally unsafe during pregnancy, but the risk may be justifiable in certain circumstances. Chemotherapy during the first trimester is usually contraindicated and should be limited to those patients with Dukes stage C lesions who may choose to accept the risks of fetal teratogenesis or demise. Chemotherapy during the second and third trimesters is less teratogenic because of the completion of organogenesis but still carries some risk for the fetus.[112,116]

Adjuvant radiation therapy reduces the local recurrence of rectal cancer. Because the most effective dose to eradicate microscopic disease is on the order of 50 Gy and the fetus cannot be effectively shielded from pelvic exposure, radiation therapy cannot be safely performed during pregnancy. Therapeutic pelvic radiation also results in permanent and irreversible female sterility, so the mother considering this form of therapy must be fully aware of the risks to the current and future pregnancies.[112,117]

References

1. Hamilton B, Martin J, Ventura S. Births: preliminary data for 2007. *Natl Vit Stat Rep* 2009:57:12.
2. Martin J, Hamilton B, Sutton P, et al. Births: final data for 2005. *Natl Vit Stat Rep* 2007;56:6.
3. Norwitz E, Lye S. Biology of parturition. In: Creasy R, Resnik R, Iams J, et al., eds. *Maternal–Fetal Medicine*. 6th ed. Philadelphia, PA: WB Saunders; 2009:69–86.
4. Petraglia F, Florio P, Nappi C, et al. Peptide signaling in human placenta and membranes: autocrine, paracrine, and endocrine mechanisms. *Endocr Rev* 1996;17:156–186.
5. Copper RL, Goldenberg RL, Creasy RK, et al. A multicenter study of preterm birth weight and gestational age-specific neonatal mortality. *Am J Obstet Gynecol* 1993;168:78–84.
6. Romero R, Avila C, Brekus CA, et al. The role of systemic and intrauterine infection in preterm parturition. *Ann N Y Acad Sci* 1991;622:355–375.
7. Ou CW, Orsino A, Lye S. Expression of connexin-43 and connexin-26 in the rat myometrium during pregnancy and labor is differentially regulated by mechanical and hormonal signals. *Endocrinology* 1997;138: 5398–5407.
8. Bonanno C, Wapner R. Antenatal corticosteroid treatment: what's happened since Drs Liggins and Howie? *Am J Obstet Gynecol* 2009;200: 448–457.
9. Iams J, Romero R, Creasy R. Preterm labor and birth. In: Creasy R, Resnik R, Iams J, et al., eds. *Maternal–Fetal Medicine*. 6th ed. Philadelphia, PA: WB Saunders; 2009:545–582.
10. Katz PO, Castell DO. Gastroesophageal reflux during pregnancy. *Gastroenterol Clin North Am* 1998;27:153–167.
11. Lund C, Donovan J. Blood volume during pregnancy. *Am J Obstet Gynecol* 1967;98:393.
12. Duvekot J, Cheriex E, Pieters F, et al. Early pregnancy changes in hemodynamics and volume homeostasis are consecutive adjustments triggered by a primary fall in systemic vascular tone. *Am J Obstet Gynecol* 1993;169: 1382.
13. Duvekot J, Pieters F. Maternal cardiovascular hemodynamic adaptation to pregnancy. *Obstet Gynecol Surv* 1994;49:S1.
14. Awe R, Nicotra M, Newsome T, et al. Arterial oxygenation and alveolar-arterial gradients in term pregnancy. *Obstet Gynecol* 1979;53:182.
15. Broussard CN, Richter JE. Nausea and vomiting of pregnancy. *Gastroenterol Clin North Am* 1998;27:123–151.
16. Everson GT, McKinley C, Lawson M, et al. Gallbladder function in the human female: effect of the ovulatory cycle, pregnancy, and contraceptive steroids. *Gastroenterology* 1982;82:711–719.
17. Bonapace ES, Fisher RS. Constipation and diarrhea in pregnancy. *Gastroenterol Clin North Am* 1998;27:197–211.
18. Baker PN, Madeley RJ, Symonds EM. Abdominal pain of unknown aetiology in pregnancy. *Br J Obstet Gynaecol* 1989;96:688–691.
19. Silver R, Berkowitz R, Bussel J. Thrombocytopenia in pregnancy. *ACOG Pract Bulletin* 1999;6:1
20. Yoshimoto Y, Soda M, Schull WJ, et al. Studies of children in utero during the atomic detonations. In: Proceedings of the 203rd national meeting of the American Chemical Society; April 5, 1992; San Francisco, CA.
21. Goodsitt MM, Christodoulou EG. Imaging safety in the fetus. In: Pearlman MD, Tintinalli JE, eds. *Emergency Care of the Woman*. New York: McGraw-Hill; 1998:A2, 719.
22. Brent RL. The effects of embryonic and fetal exposure to x-ray, microwaves, and ultrasound: counseling the pregnant and non-pregnant patient about these risks. *Semin Oncol* 1989;16:347–368.
23. Boklage CE. Survival probability of human conceptions from fertilization to term. *Int J Fertil* 1990;35:75–94.
24. Brent RL. Radiation teratogenesis. *Teratology* 1980;21:281–298.
25. Schwartz HM, Reichling BA. Hazards of radiation exposure for pregnant women. *JAMA* 1978;239:1908.
26. Brent RL. The effects of embryonic and fetal exposure to x-ray, microwaves, and ultrasound. *Clin Perinatol* 1986;13:615–649.
27. Wood JW, Johnson KG, Omori Y, et al. Mental retardation in children exposed in utero to the atomic bombs in Hiroshima and Nagasaki. *Am J Public Health* 1967;57:1381–1390.
28. Wood JW, Keehan RJ, Kawamoto S, et al. The growth and development of children exposed in utero to the atomic bombs in Hiroshima and Nagasaki. *Am J Public Health* 1967;57:1374–1380.
29. Harvey EB, Boice JD, Honeyman M, et al. Prenatal x-ray exposure and childhood cancer in twins. *N Engl J Med* 1985;312:541–545.
30. Doll R, Wakeford R. Risk of childhood cancer from fetal irradiation. *Br J Radiol* 1997;70:130–139.
31. UNSCEAR 1994 United Nations Scientific Committee on the Effects of Atomic Radiation. Annex A: Epidemiological studies of radiation

carcinogenesis. In: *Sources and Effects of Ionizing Radiation*, Publication E.94.IX.11. New York: United Nations Publications; 1994.
32. NCRP Commentary No. 9. *Considerations Regarding the Unintended Radiation Exposure of the Embryo, Fetus or Nursing Child*. Bethesda, MD: National Council on Radiation Protection; 1994.
33. Reece AE, Goldstein I, Hobbins JC. *Fundamentals of Obstetric and Gynecologic Ultrasound*. Norwalk, CT: Appleton & Lange, 1994.
34. Kanal E, Shellock FG, Talagala L. Safety considerations in MR imaging. *Radiology* 1990;176:593–606.
35. Schenck JF, Dumoulin CL, Redington RW. Human exposure to 4.0-Tesla magnetic fields in a whole-body scanner. *Med Phys* 1992;19:1089–1098.
36. IRPA/INIRC. Protection of the patient undergoing a magnetic resonance examination. *Health Phys* 1991;61:923–928.
37. Briggs G, Freeman R, Yaffe S. *Drugs in Pregnancy and Lactation: A Reference Guide to Fetal and Neonatal Risk*. 8th ed. Philadelphia: Lippincott Williams & Wilkins; 2008.
38. *Fed Regist* 1980;44:37434–37467.
39. Hon EH. The fetal heart rate patterns preceding death in utero. *Am J Obstet Gynecol* 1959;78:47.
40. Chauhan S, Macones G. Intrapartum fetal heart rate monitoring. *ACOG Pract Bulletin* 2005;70:1.
41. Macones G, Hankins G, Spong C, et al. The 2008 National Institute of Child Health and Human Development Workshop Report on electronic fetal monitoring. Update on definitions, interpretation, and research guidelines. *Obstet Gynecol* 2008;112:661–666.
42. Al-Mulhim AA. Acute appendicitis in pregnancy. *Int Surg* 1996;81: 295–297.
43. Tamir IL, Bongard FS, Klein SR. Acute appendicitis in the pregnant patient. *Am J Surg* 1990;160:571–576.
44. Masters K, Levine BA, Gaskill HV, et al. Diagnosing appendicitis during pregnancy. *Am J Surg* 1984;148:768–771.
45. Babaknia A, Parsa H, Woodruff JD. Appendicitis during pregnancy. *Obstet Gynecol* 1977;50:40–44.
46. Wagner JM, McKinney WP, Carpenter JL. Does this patient have appendicitis? *JAMA* 1996;276:1589–1594.
47. Baer JL, Reis RA, Arens RA. Appendicitis in pregnancy. *JAMA* 1932;98: 1359–1364.
48. Schwerk WB, Wichtrup B, Rothmund M, et al. Ultrasonography in the diagnosis of acute appendicitis: a prospective study. *Gastroenterology* 1989;97:630–639.
49. Weingold AB. Appendicitis in pregnancy. *Clin Obstet Gynecol* 1983;26: 801–809.
50. Cunningham FG, McCubbin JH. Appendicitis complicating pregnancy. *Obstet Gynecol* 1975;45:415–420.
51. Black WP. Acute appendicitis in pregnancy. *BMJ* 1960;1:1938–1941.
52. Parker RB. Acute appendicitis in late pregnancy. *Lancet* 1954;1: 1252–1257.
53. Horowitz MD, Gomez GA, Santiesteban R, et al. Acute appendicitis during pregnancy. *Arch Surg* 1985;120:1362–1367.
54. Varner MW. Surgical diseases in pregnancy. *Clin Obstet Gynecol* 1994;37: 239–315.
55. Worrell JA, Drolshagen LF, Kelly TC, et al. Graded compression ultrasound in the diagnosis of appendicitis: a comparison of diagnostic criteria. *J Ultrasound Med* 1990;9:145–150.
56. Abu-Yousef MM, Phillips ME, Franken EA, et al. Sonography of acute appendicitis: a critical review. *Crit Rev Diagn Imaging* 1989;29:381–408.
57. Paulman AA, Huebner DM, Forrest TS. Sonography in the diagnosis of acute appendicitis. *Am Fam Physician* 1991;44:465–468.
58. Rao PM, Rhea JT, Novelline RA, et al. Helical CT combined with contrast material administered only through the colon for imaging of suspected appendicitis. *AJR Am J Roentgenol* 1997;169:1275–1280.
59. Rao PM, Rhea JT, Rattner DW, et al. Introduction of appendiceal CT impact on negative appendectomy and appendiceal perforation rates. *Ann Surg* 1999;229:344–349.
60. Rao PM, Rhea JT, Novelline RA, et al. Effects of computed tomography of the appendix on treatment of patients and use of hospital resources. *N Engl J Med* 1998;338:141–146.
61. Jacobs DO, Settle RG, Clarke JR, et al. Identification of human appendicitis by in vitro nuclear magnetic resonance. *J Surg Res* 1990;48:107–110.
62. Hormann M, Paya K, Eibenberger K, et al. MR imaging in children with nonperforated acute appendicitis: value of unenhanced MR imaging in sonographically selected cases. *AJR Am J Roentgenol* 1998;171:467–470.
63. Conron RW, Abbruzzi K, Cochrane SO, et al. Laparoscopic procedures in pregnancy. *Am Surg* 1998;65:259–263.
64. Hunter JG, Swanstrom L, Thornburg K. Carbon dioxide pneumoperitoneum induces fetal acidosis in a pregnant ewe model. *Surg Endosc* 1995; 9:272–279.
65. Curet MJ, Allen D, Josloff RK, et al. Laparoscopy during pregnancy. *Arch Surg* 1996;131:546–551.
66. Gurbuz AT, Peetz ME. The acute abdomen in the pregnant patient. *Surg Endosc* 1997;11:98–102.
67. SAGES. Guidelines for laparoscopic surgery during pregnancy. *Surg Endosc* 1998;12:189–190.
68. Saunders P, Milton PJD. Laparotomy during pregnancy: an assessment of diagnostic accuracy and fetal wastage. *BMJ* 1973;3:165–167.
69. Everson GT. Gastrointestinal motility in pregnancy. *Gastroenterol Clin North Am* 1992;21:751–776.
70. Valdivieso V, Covarrubias C, Siegel F, et al. Pregnancy and cholelithiasis: pathogenesis and natural course of gallstones diagnosed in early puerperium. *Hepatology* 1993;17:1–4.
71. Barbara L, Sama C, Morselli Labate AM, et al. A population study on the prevalence of gallstone disease: the Sirmione Study. *Hepatology* 1987;7: 913–917.
72. Basso L, McCollum PT, Darling MN, et al. A study of cholelithiasis during pregnancy and its relationship with age, parity, menarche, breast-feeding, dysmenorrhea, oral contraception, and a maternal history of cholelithiasis. *Surgery* 1992;175:41–46.
73. Mayer IE, Hussain H. Abdominal pain during pregnancy. *Gastroenterol Clin North Am* 1998;27:1–36.
74. Gerwig WH, Thistlethwaite JR. Cholecystitis and cholelithiasis in young women following pregnancy. *Surgery* 1950;28:983–996.
75. Scott LD. Gallstone disease and pancreatitis in pregnancy. *Gastroenterol Clin North Am* 1992;21:803–815.
76. Steinbrook RA, Brooks DC, Datta S. Laparoscopic cholecystectomy during pregnancy review of anesthetic management: surgical considerations. *Surg Endosc* 1996;10:511–515.
77. Epstein FB. Acute abdominal pain in pregnancy. *Emerg Med Clin North Am* 1994;12:151–165.
78. Simon JA. Biliary tract disease and related surgical disorders during pregnancy. *Clin Obstet Gynecol* 1983;26:810–821.
79. Dixon NP, Faddis DM, Silberman H. Aggressive management of cholecystitis during pregnancy. *Am J Surg* 1987;154:292–294.
80. Glasgow RE, Visser BC, Harris HW, et al. Changing management of gallstone disease during pregnancy. *Surg Endosc* 1998;12:241–246.
81. Graham G, Baxi L, Tharakan T. Laparoscopic cholecystectomy during pregnancy: a case series and review of the literature. *Obstet Gynecol Surv* 1998;53:566–574.
82. Hiatt JR, Hiatt JCG, Williams RA, et al. Biliary disease in pregnancy: strategy for surgical management. *Am J Surg* 1986;151:263–265.
83. Eichenberg BJ, Vanderlinden J, Miguel C, et al. Laparoscopic cholecystectomy in the third trimester of pregnancy. *Am Surg* 1996;62:874–877.
84. Baillie J, Cairns SR, Cotton PB. Endoscopic management of choledocholithiasis during pregnancy. *Surgery* 1990;171:1–4.
85. Printen KJ, Ott RA. Cholecystectomy during pregnancy. *Am Surg* 1978; 44:432–434.
86. Pucci RO, Seed RW. Case report of laparoscopic cholecystectomy in the third trimester of pregnancy. *Am J Obstet Gynecol* 1991;165:401–402.
87. Elerding SC. Laparoscopic cholecystectomy in pregnancy. *Am J Surg* 1993; 165:625–627.
88. McKellar DP, Anderson CT, Boynton CJ, et al. Cholecystectomy during pregnancy without fetal loss. *Surg Gynecol Obstet* 1992;174:465–468.
89. Hill LM, Symmonds RE. Small bowel obstruction in pregnancy: a report and review of four cases. *Obstet Gynecol* 1976;49:170–173.
90. Lanzafame RJ. Laparoscopic cholecystectomy during pregnancy. *Surgery* 1995;118:627–633.
91. Axelrad AM, Fleischer DE, Strack LL, et al. Performance of ERCP for symptomatic choledocholithiasis during pregnancy: techniques to increase safety and improve patient management. *Am J Gastroenterol* 1994;89: 109–112.
92. Amouyal P, Amouyal G, Levy P, et al. Diagnosis of choledocholithiasis by endoscopic ultrasonography. *Gastroenterology* 1994;106:1062–1067.
93. Parada AA, Goncalves MOL, Tafner E, et al. Endoscopic papillotomy under ultra-sonographic control. *Int Surg* 1991;76:75–76.
94. Yu-leung C, Chan ACW, Lam WWM, et al. Choledocholithiasis: comparison of MR cholangiography and endoscopic retrograde cholangiography. *Radiology* 1996;200:85–89.
95. Davis MR, Bohon CJ. Intestinal obstruction in pregnancy. *Clin Obstet Gynecol* 1983;26:832–842.
96. Perdue PW, Johnson HW, Stafford PW. Intestinal obstruction complicating pregnancy. *Am J Surg* 1992;164:384–388.
97. Lord SA, Boswell WC, Hungerpiller JC. Sigmoid volvulus in pregnancy. *Am Surg* 1996;62:380–382.
98. Kantor HM. Midgut volvulus in pregnancy: a case report. *J Reprod Med* 1990;35:577–580.
99. Pratt AT, Donaldson RC, Evertson LR, et al. Cecal volvulus in pregnancy. *Obstet Gynecol* 1981;57:37S–40S.
100. Rothstein RD, Rombeau JL. Intestinal malrotation during pregnancy. *Obstet Gynecol* 1993;81:817–819.
101. Meyerson S, Holtz T, Ehrinpreis M, et al. Small bowel obstruction in pregnancy. *Am J Gastroenterol* 1995;90:299–302.
102. McLean DW, Arminski TC, Bradley GT. Management of primary carcinoma of the rectum diagnosed during pregnancy. *Am J Surg* 1955;90: 816–825.
103. Woods JB, Martin JN Jr, Ingram FH, et al. Pregnancy complicated by carcinoma of the colon above the rectum. *Am J Perinatol* 1992;9:102–110.
104. Antonelli NM, Dotters DJ, Katz VL, et al. Cancer in pregnancy: a review of the literature, part 1. *Obstet Gynecol Surv* 1996;51:125–142.
105. Nesbitt JC, Moise KJ, Sawyers JL. Colorectal carcinoma in pregnancy. *Arch Surg* 1985;120:636–640.
106. Bernstein MA, Madoff RD, Caushaj PF. Colon and rectal cancer in pregnancy. *Dis Colon Rectum* 1993;36:172–178.
107. Francavilla A, Leo D, Polimeno L, et al. Nuclear and cytosolic estrogen receptors in human colon carcinoma and in surrounding noncancerous colonic tissue. *Gastroenterology* 1987;93:1301–1306.
108. Stedman KE, Moore GE, Morgan RT. Estrogen receptor proteins in diverse human tumors. *Arch Surg* 1980;115:244–248.

109. Wobbes T, Beex LV, Koenders AM. Estrogen and progestin receptors in colonic cancer? *Dis Colon Rectum* 1984;27:591–592.
110. Smith C, Butler JA. Colorectal cancer in patients younger than 40 years of age. *Dis Colon Rectum* 1989;32:843–846.
111. Pitluk H, Poticha SM. Carcinoma of the colon and rectum in patients less than 40 years of age. *Surg Gynecol Obstet* 1983;157:335–337.
112. Cappell MS. Colon cancer during pregnancy: the gastroenterologist's perspective. *Gastroenterol Clin North Am* 1998;7:225–256.
113. McCall JL, Black RB, Rich CA, et al. The value of serum carcinoembryonic antigen in predicting recurrent disease following curative resection of colorectal cancer. *Dis Colon Rectum* 1994;37:875–881.
114. Mason MH III, Kovalcik PJ. Ovarian metastases from colon carcinoma. *J Surg Oncol* 1981;17:33–38.
115. Walsh C, Fazio VW. Cancer of the colon, rectum, and anus during pregnancy: the surgeon's perspective. *Gastroenterol Clin North Am* 1998;27: 257–267.
116. Zemlickis D, Lishner M, Degendorfer P, et al. Fetal outcome after in utero exposure to cancer chemotherapy. *Arch Intern Med* 1992;152: 573–576.
117. Mayr NA, Wen B-C, Saw CB. Radiation therapy during pregnancy. *Obstet Gynecol Clin North Am* 1998;25:301–321.

SURGICAL SPECIALITIES

CHAPTER 111 ■ CUTANEOUS NEOPLASMS

MICHAEL S. SABEL, TIMOTHY M. JOHNSON, AND CHRISTOPHER K. BICHAKJIAN

KEY POINTS

1. Cutaneous neoplasms are the most commonly diagnosed malignant tumors in the United States, with an incidence of approximately 1.4 million new cases annually.
2. Risk factors for development of cutaneous melanoma include ultraviolet (UV) light exposure, fair complexion/inability to tan, blue or green eyes, blonde or red hair, freckling, history of actinic keratosis or nonmelanoma skin cancer (NMSC), history of blistering or peeling sunburns, immunosuppression, personal or family history of melanoma, CDKN2A/p16/MC1R mutation, xeroderma pigmentosa, atypical (dysplastic) nevus, more than 100 normal nevi, and giant congenital melanocytic nevus.
3. The ABCD rule is used to assess skin lesions for melanoma risk: A is for *a*symmetry; B is *b*order irregularity; C is *c*olor, and D is *d*iameter greater than 6 mm.
4. Melanoma prognosis is inverse correlated to tumor thickness; ulceration and increased mitotic rate are independent survival risk factors; and nodal tumor burden (uninvolved vs. microscopic vs. macroscopic disease) has an inverse correlation with survival.
5. For melanoma in situ, excision margins of 0.5 to 1.0 cm are indicated; for invasive melanoma, wide excision of the primary tumor with margins generally ranging from 1 to 2 cm is indicated for local control.
6. Clinically involved lymph nodes should be resected; patients with primary melanomas of 1 mm thickness or greater and clinically negative nodes should be considered for sentinel lymph node biopsy.
7. Basal cell and squamous cell skin carcinoma account for 96% of new NMSCs.
8. Dermatofibrosarcoma protuberans (DFSP) is a rare soft tissue sarcoma (1% of all soft tissue sarcomas) with a propensity for local recurrence rather than systemic metastasis.

1 Cutaneous neoplasms are the most commonly diagnosed malignant tumors in the United States, with an incidence of approximately 1.4 million new cases annually.[1,2] One in five Americans born today will be diagnosed with skin cancer in their lifetime. More than half of all cancers diagnosed in the United States are skin cancers. The most common skin cancer types are basal cell carcinoma (BCC) and squamous cell carcinoma (SCC). Cutaneous melanoma accounts for 4% of skin cancer diagnoses but accounts for 75% of skin cancer deaths, with 8,420 deaths due to melanoma in 2008, or about one every hour. Approximately 62,480 new cases of invasive melanoma were diagnosed in the United States in 2008 (34,950 men and 27,530 women). The incidence of melanoma has dramatically increased, with the lifetime risk of melanoma increasing from 1 in 600 in the 1960s to 1 in 41 in men and 1 in 61 in women in 2008.[1] Invasive melanoma is the sixth most common cancer in men and the seventh most common cancer in women.[1] The early diagnosis and surgical treatment of these skin cancers can be curative.

MELANOMA

Etiology and Risk Factors

Numerous environmental and genetic risk factors have been implicated in the development of cutaneous melanoma, many
2 of which center around sun exposure.[2] Risk factors include factors related to exposure to UVA and UVB, such as geography, occupation, a history of blistering or peeling sunburns, and the use of tanning beds/salons, as well as factors related to increased sensitivity to UV light, such as decreased pigmentation, a fair complexion (blue or green eyes, blonde hair, freckling), or xeroderma pigmentosa. Melanoma incidence is subject to large geographic and ethnic variations, mainly because of an inverse correlation with latitude and with degree of skin pigmentation. Populations residing closer to the equator have a higher incidence of melanoma. Many factors that increase risk for melanoma are surrogates for a history of excess sun exposure, such as actinic keratosis, a history of either melanoma or an NMSC, atypical nevi, or multiple normal nevi. Finally, there are inheritable risk factors, such as a family history of melanoma, CDKN2A/p16/MC1R mutation, or MC1R mutation.

Adults with more than 100 clinically normal-appearing nevi, children with more than 50 clinically normal-appearing nevi, and any patient with atypical or dysplastic nevi are at risk. A prior history of melanoma places a patient at increased risk, with 5% to 10% of individuals developing a second primary melanoma. This risk of developing a second primary is lifelong and can occur anywhere on the skin. Therefore, long-term surveillance with a thorough total body examination is recommended.

A genetic component has been implicated in the pathogenesis of melanoma. Of patients with melanoma, 10% to 15% report a positive family history. The most common chromosomal mutation associated with melanoma involves CDKN2A, also known as p16. However, the mutation accounts for only a small percentage of melanoma cases observed, estimated at 0.2%. A MC1R gene mutation is clearly a risk factor for cutaneous melanoma.[3] The combination of MC1R mutation and red hair is associated with a very high risk of melanoma development. In addition, MC1R R151 C modifies the effect of another cutaneous melanoma susceptibility gene, CDKN2A.[4] The genetic etiology of melanoma represents an area of future discovery.

The hereditary nature of cutaneous melanoma was also noted in the 1970s.[5] Members afflicted with the "B-K mole syndrome," named after two families, acquired large, irregular, and dysplastic nevi, often in sun-protected regions of the body such as the scalp and trunk. During this time period, Lynch et al.[6] independently reported a familial association of melanoma among individuals with atypical nevi, which he termed *familial atypical multiple mole melanoma syndrome*, or FAMMM syndrome, with an autosomal dominant inheritance pattern. The 10-year melanoma risk in the setting of atypical mole syndrome is reported to be 10.7% compared with 0.62% in control patients. Greene et al.[7] approximated a 56% cumulative risk from age 20 to 59 years, with 100% of atypical mole syndrome patients developing melanoma by age 76. An atypical nevus is not a premelanoma but represents a genetic marker for increased risk of development of melanoma, which may occur anywhere on the skin surface including sun-protected sites. In fact, more than 50% to 75% of melanomas develop on clinically normal skin de novo, not in pre-existing melanocytic lesions.

Xeroderma pigmentosa is a rare autosomal recessive disorder associated with a reduced or absent ability to repair DNA damaged by UV light. Consequently, this disorder results in the development of multiple primary cutaneous malignancies, including melanoma as well as BCC and SCC. Individuals are usually diagnosed with their first cancer before the age of 10 years. Unfortunately, the development of skin cancers is relentless.

Congenital melanocytic nevi (CMN) are present at birth or appear within the first 6 months of infancy.[8] An estimated 1% to 6% of children are born with CMN. The nevi are classified by size. Small CMN measure less than 1.5 cm in diameter and account for the majority of lesions. Medium CMN measure between 1.5 and 19.9 cm in diameter. Large CMN, also termed *giant congenital nevi*, measure 20 cm or greater. This large size can lead to significant cosmetic and psychosocial implications. The risk of melanoma development in small- and medium-sized CMN is similar to any other area of skin. Melanoma development in small and medium CMN usually occurs after childhood and arises from the dermoepidermal junction, making early detection feasible. Routine prophylactic removal of small and medium CMN is rarely indicated in the absence of signs or symptoms for malignant progression. Conversely, giant congenital nevi carry an increased risk for melanoma, with an estimated rate of 5% to 20%. Of giant congenital nevi that progress to melanoma, 70% are diagnosed prior to age 10 years. Melanoma can originate deep in the epidermis in giant congenital nevi. Consequently, diagnosis within the setting of giant congenital nevi is challenging and may develop deep in the skin with a more advanced primary lesion.

Patients with a giant congenital nevus, especially on the posterior axis, or in conjunction with many satellite lesions are also at risk for neurocutaneous melanocytosis (NCM).[9,10]

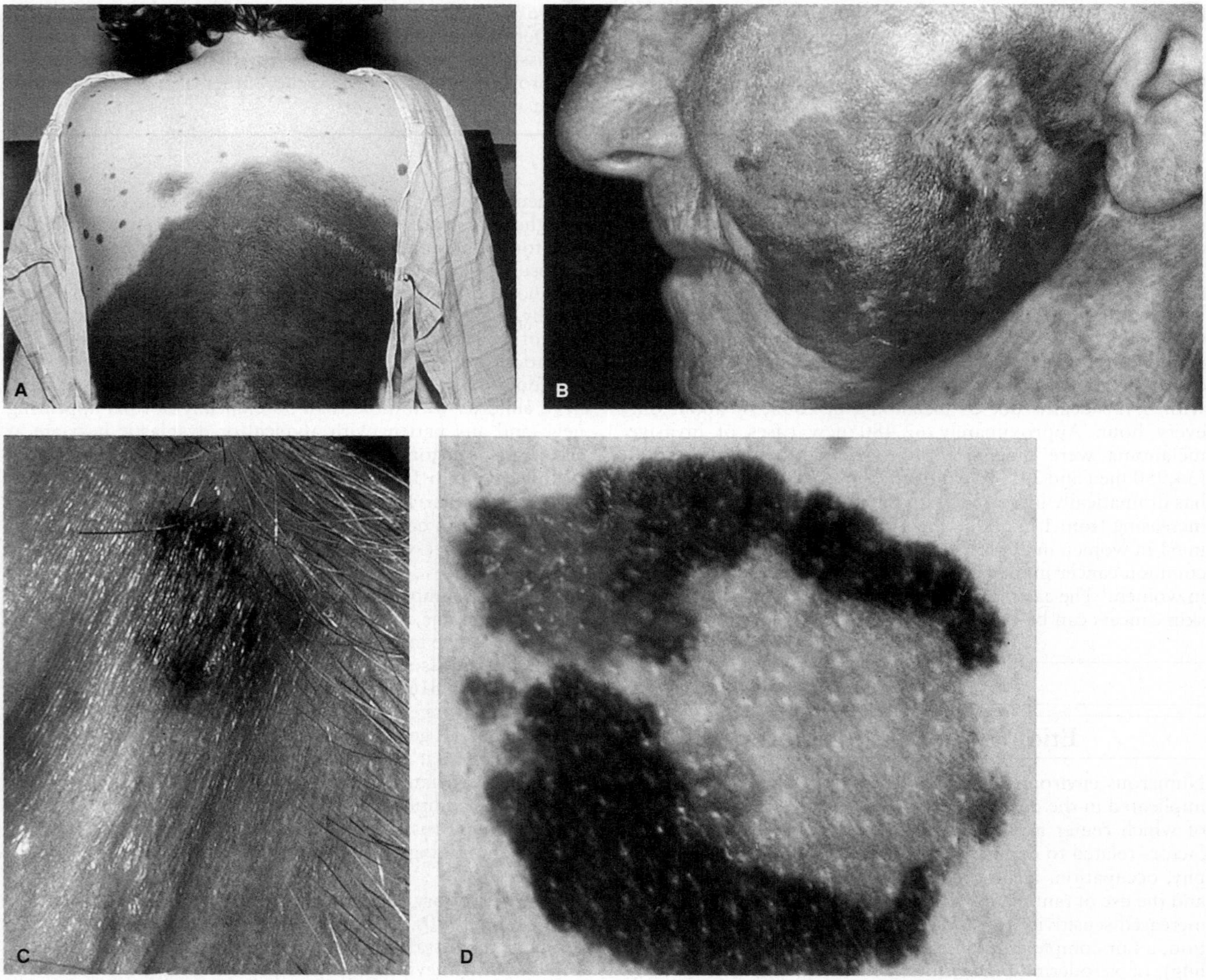

FIGURE 111.1. Examples of skin lesions. **A:** Giant congenital nevus. **B:** Lentigo maligna (Hutchinson freckle). **C:** Melanoma arising in a lentigo maligna (lentigo maligna melanoma). **D:** Superficial spreading melanoma. *(continued)*

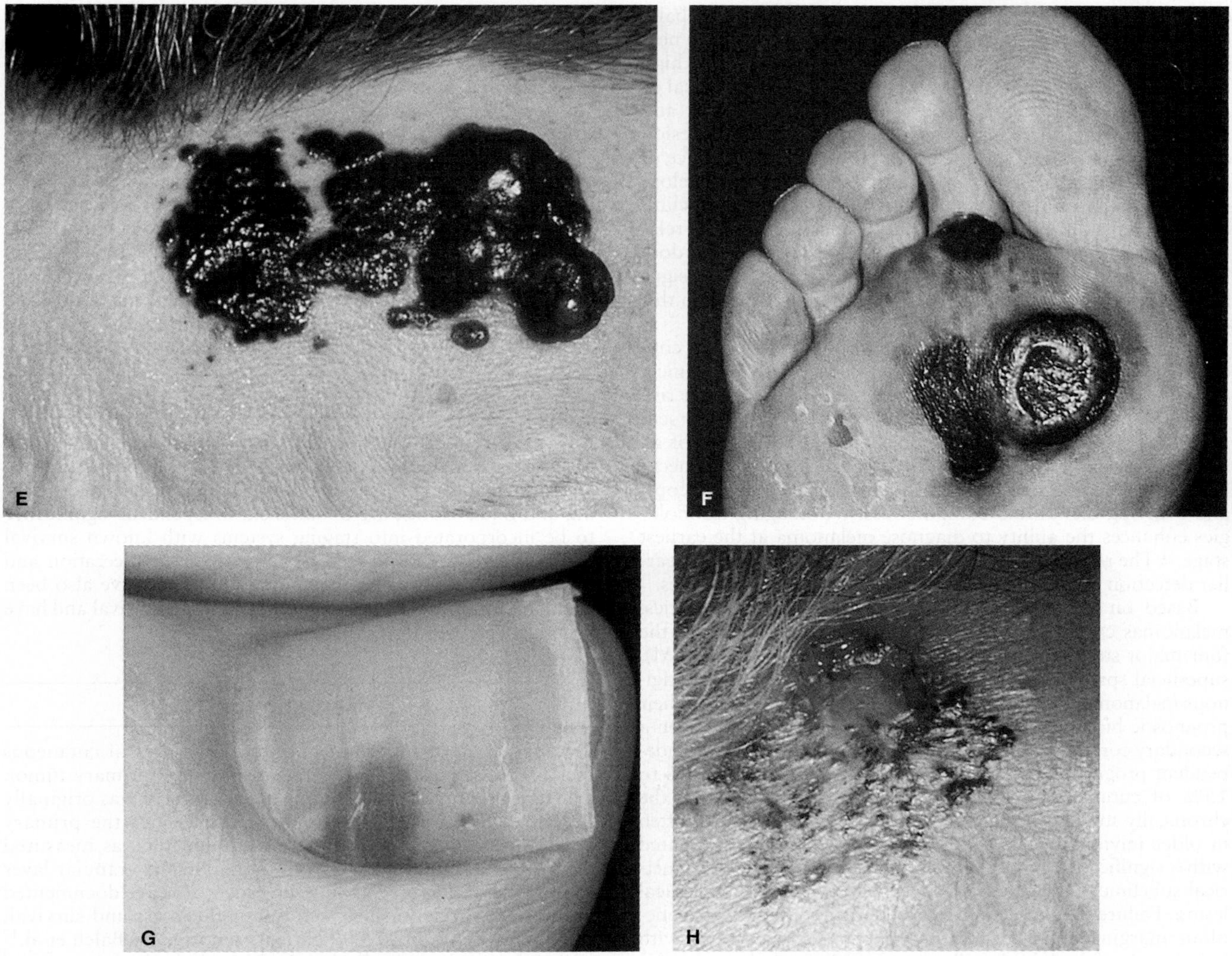

FIGURE 111.1. (*Continued*) E: Nodular melanoma. F: Acral lentiginous melanoma (ulcerated nodular plantar melanoma with satellite lesions). G: Subungual melanoma. H: Pigmented basal cell carcinoma.

NCM is characterized by the presence of benign or malignant leptomeningeal tumors. Most patients present in the first 2 years of life with neurologic manifestations of increased intracranial pressure, mass lesions, or malignant transformation to melanoma. Magnetic resonance imaging (MRI) findings of NCM may be present, even in asymptomatic children. NCM is associated with an increased risk of development of central nervous system melanoma. Symptomatic NCM is associated with a poor prognosis, even in the absence of malignancy. Chemotherapy is not effective, but shunt placement to reduce intracranial pressure may be palliative.

Clinical Diagnosis and Classification

Melanoma may have a characteristic appearance (Fig. 111.1). 3 Early detection is key. The ABCD rule, which outlines the warning signs of melanoma, was developed decades ago.[11] A stands for *a*symmetry—one half of the lesion does not match the other half when drawing an imaginary line through the center of the lesion. B is *b*order irregularity—the edges of the lesion are ragged, notched, or fuzzy. C is *c*olor—the pigmentation is not uniform throughout the lesion. Varying shades of tan, dark brown to black, or shades of red, white, and/or blue may be present with a mottled appearance. And D is *d*iameter—the width is greater than 6 mm (about the size of a pencil eraser). The seven-point checklist used in Europe incorporates several of the ABCD features with the addition of change. Another useful diagnostic aid is the "ugly duckling" sign. A pigmented lesion that is different from the others should be carefully approached with a high index of suspicion.

The goal of any diagnostic aid is early detection and the ability to differentiate between benign and malignant, with 100% sensitivity combined with high specificity. The ABCD rule, seven-point checklist, and ugly duckling sign all provide relatively highly sensitivity but none fulfills all of these criteria, especially with respect to specificity, to distinguish melanoma from benign lesions.

The ABCD criteria may fail to detect an important subset of nodular melanoma (NM), which often does not exhibit the ABCDs and is often less than 6 mm in early development. The ABCD rule is also relatively static without the important critical characteristic of change. Studies have documented early signs of a change in size, shape, or color and the early symptom of persistent itching. One of the best tools for diagnosis of early lesions that may fail to exhibit many of the standard melanoma features is the importance of *change*. Thus, the authors and others have used the D in the ABCD rule to signify "*d*ifference." A difference or change in lesions, especially with respect to size, shape, color, or persistent itching, warrants evaluation. Furthermore, the nevi on the body should globally share a common look or family resemblance. If one of the nevi seems different from the rest, it should be evaluated with a high index of suspicion. Additionally, if all of the nevi are atypical or irregular but are morphologically similar to one another and are not changing, there may be no reason for individual lesion concern (atypical or dysplastic nevi). However, the presence of atypical nevi represents a risk factor for melanoma development anywhere on the skin surface with development in clinically normal skin, normal nevi, and dysplastic nevi with relatively equal frequency. Thus, excision of all atypical nevi does little for prevention. Education of the patient for early signs and symptoms, particularly change or difference, is key in this clinical scenario.

It must be emphasized that critical diagnostic decisions concerning skin lesions should still always be based on clinical assessments and the history, with attention to melanoma risk factors. The optimum diagnostic aid that combines 100% sensitivity and specificity currently does not exist. The use of all available means including the ABCD and seven-point checklists, ugly duckling sign, difference, photography, dermoscopy, and evolving digital and computer-assisted imaging technologies enhances the ability to diagnose melanoma at the earliest stage.[11] The result of using these multiple diagnostic aids is earlier detection of melanoma with higher overall survival rates.

Based on histologic patterns and clinical characteristics, melanomas can be classified into multiple categories, with the four major subtypes being lentigo maligna melanoma (LMM), superficial spreading melanoma (SSM), NM, and acral lentiginous melanoma (ALM).[12] In general, these subtypes derive their prognostic biologic behavior and risk of metastasis based on a secondary correlation with Breslow depth and are thus not independent prognostic factors. Invasive LMM constitutes 10% to 15% of cutaneous melanomas and typically occurs on the chronically sun exposed areas of the head and neck, most often in older inividuals. Clinically, the LMM pattern is associated with a significantly higher rate of often extensive and asymmetrical subclinical growth several centimeters beyond the clinical lesion. Failure to completely excise the entire lesion with meticulous margin control results in higher recurrence rates with lethal potential. Additionally, amelanotic and desmoplastic melanoma with neurotropism is more frequent in the lentigo maligna (LM) lesion subtype. LM is not a benign disease as once thought. LM represents in situ melanoma and, with time, progresses to invasive LMM. LMM often begins as a flat brown lesion on chronically sun exposed areas with progression to black and other classic melanoma features over time.

SSM accounts for approximately 70% of cutaneous melanomas. This pattern is the most common in melanomas arising in a pre-existing nevus. SSM is typically characterized by variation in color, irregular borders, and irregular surface and often exhibits the classic melanoma clinical features.

NM occurs in approximately 15% to 30% of patients with cutaneous melanoma and is often the most aggressive of the four types of melanoma because of later detection and rapid growth. In general, NM may be more uniform in coloration than the other types, have regular borders with size less than 6 mm in early lesions, and lack the classic melanoma features initially. Lesion change and difference is important for early detection.

ALM is a distinct clinicopathologic variant of melanoma that most commonly occurs on the hands, feet, fingers, and toes as well as in subungual locations (Fig. 111.1). ALM represents only 2% to 8% of melanoma in whites but 35% to 60% in people of color. Later detection frequently occurs because of location that is not easily or routinely examined and a low index of suspicion. When corrected for Breslow depth, the overall prognosis for ALM appears similar to the other subtype categories. In subungual locations, this phase can appear as an irregular, tan-brown streak in the nail that originates from the base of the nail bed. More than three fourths of subungual melanomas involve the great toe or thumb, and they can be confused with subungual hematoma.

Other rare melanoma subtypes deserve brief mention. Mucosal, anal, and vulvovaginal melanomas are associated with a poorer prognosis, possibly related to advanced disease at presentation with late detection and high vascularity at the lesion site. Desmoplastic melanoma is associated with a higher rate of neurotropism and lower rate of lymph node metastases.[13–15] Small cell or nevoid melanoma often lacks any of the classic features, is difficult to accurately diagnose without expert dermatopathology interpretation, and thus may be initially more frequently misdiagnosed. And amelanotic melanoma, occurring in 3% to 4% of cases, is often associated with late detection due to lack of pigment and failure to diagnose early.

Staging and Prognostic Factors

4 A great deal of information is available regarding various factors that correlate with the clinical outcome of patients with melanoma. Some of these prognostic factors, such as microstaging and nodal status, are of sufficient independent significance to be incorporated into staging systems with known survival rates. Other prognostic factors, such as tumor ulceration and microscopic versus macroscopic nodal disease, have also been found to be significant variables that influence survival and have been incorporated into the staging system.

Microstaging

One of the most important prognostic features of cutaneous melanoma is the stage of development of the primary tumor. The microstaging method that is used routinely was originally described by Breslow.[16] This method classifies the primary tumor according to its thickness in millimeters, as measured with an ocular micrometer, from the top of the granular layer to the base of the tumor. Many investigators have documented an inverse correlation between tumor thickness and survival. The largest series of 17,600 patients reported by Balch et al.[17] is summarized in Table 111.1. The ulceration status and mitotic rate are also independent factors that are used to determine microstaging of the primary lesion.[17,18] Prior to the use of the Breslow microstaging method, melanomas were staged according to the level of invasion into the histologic layer of skin. This was known as the Clark level of invasion and comprised five levels (I, in situ lesions; V, subcutaneous involvement). Several studies have confirmed that Breslow thickness conveys more accurate prognostic information than does the determination of Clark level.[17,19]

The presence of regional lymph node metastases is associated with a worsening prognosis. The tumor burden (microscopic vs. macroscopic disease) of involved lymph nodes has an inverse correlation with long-term survival.[17,19] The 5-year survival rate for patients with involved lymph nodes ranges from 70% to 25%, based primarily on tumor burden and ulceration status of the primary lesion (Table 111.2). The use of sentinel lymph node biopsy (SNLB) has identified a subgroup of patients with micrometastatic nodal disease who have a favorable prognosis compared with patients with macroscopic nodal involvement. This information has been incorporated in the staging system as well.

Clinical and Pathologic Staging

The American Joint Committee on Cancer (AJCC) developed a five-stage system that divides melanomas according to tumor thickness (T), nodal status (N), and metastatic disease (M).[17,19] The current system was updated in 2009 and is summarized in Table 111.3. There are five stages based on prognosis: stage 0

TABLE 111.1 RESULTS

SURVIVAL RATES FOR MELANOMA TNM AND STAGING CATEGORIES

STAGE	TNM	THICKNESS (mm)	ULCERATION	POSITIVE NODES (No.)	NODAL SIZE	DISTANT METASTASIS	PATIENTS (No.)	SURVIVAL 1-YEAR	2-YEAR	5-YEAR	10-YEAR
IA	T1a	†1	No	0	—	—	4,510	99.7	99.0	95.3	87.9
IB	T1b	†1	Yes or level IV, V	0	—	—	1,380	99.8	98.7	90.9	83.1
	T2a	1.01–2.0	No	0	—	—	3,285	99.5	97.3	89.0	79.2
IIA	T2b	1.01–2.0	Yes	0	—	—	958	98.2	92.9	77.4	64.4
	T3a	2.01–4.0	No	0	—	—	1,717	98.7	94.3	78.7	63.8
IIB	T3b	2.01–4.0	Yes	0	—	—	1,523	95.1	84.8	63.0	50.8
	T4a	>4.0	No	0	—	—	563	94.8	88.6	67.4	53.9
IIC	T4b	>4.0	Yes	0	—	—	978	89.9	70.7	45.1	32.3
IIIA	N1a	Any	No	1	Micro	—	252	95.9	88.0	69.5	63.0
	N2a	Any	No	2–3	Micro	—	130	93.0	82.7	63.3	59.6
IIIB	N1a	Any	Yes	1	Micro	—	217	93.3	75.0	52.8	37.8
	N2a	Any	Yes	2–3	Micro	—	111	92.0	81.0	49.6	35.9
	N1b	Any	No	1	Macro	—	122	88.5	78.5	59.0	47.7
	N2b	Any	No	2–3	Macro	—	93	76.8	65.6	46.3	39.2
IIIC	N1b	Any	Yes	1	Macro	—	98	77.9	54.2	29.0	24.4
	N2b	Any	Yes	2–3	Macro	—	109	74.3	44.1	24.0	15.0
	N3	Any	Any	4	Micro/Macro	—	396	71.0	49.8	26.7	18.4
IV	M1a	Any	Any	Any	Any	Skin, SQ	179	59.3	36.7	18.8	15.7
	M1b	Any	Any	Any	Any	Lung	186	57.0	23.1	6.7	2.5
	M1c	Any	Any	Any	Any	Other	793	40.6	23.6	9.5	6.0
Total							17,600				

From Balch M, Buzaid AC, Soong SJ, et al. Final version of the American Joint Committee on Cancer Staging System for Cutaneous Melanoma. *J Clin Oncol* 2001;19:3635–3648.
Reprinted with permission from the American Society of Clinical Oncology.

TABLE 111.2 RESULTS

FIVE-YEAR SURVIVAL RATES FOR PATIENTS WITH STAGE III MELANOMA STRATIFIED BY NUMBER OF NODES WITH METASTASIS, ULCERATION, AND TUMOR BURDEN

■ POSITIVE NODES (No.)	■ NODAL BURDEN	■ ULCERATION	■ 5-YEAR SURVIVAL ± STANDARD ERROR (%)	■ PATIENTS IN STUDY GROUP (No.)
1	Microscopic	Absent	69 ± 3.7	252
1	Microscopic	Present	52 ± 4.1	217
2–3	Microscopic	Absent	63 ± 5.6	130
2–3	Microscopic	Present	50 ± 5.7	111
>3	Microscopic	Absent	27 ± 9.3	57
>3	Microscopic	Present	37 ± 8.8	46
1	Macroscopic	Absent	59 ± 4.7	122
1	Macroscopic	Present	29 ± 5.0	98
2–3	Macroscopic	Absent	46 ± 5.5	93
2–3	Macroscopic	Present	25 ± 4.4	109
>3	Macroscopic	Absent	27 ± 4.6	109
>3	Macroscopic	Present	13 ± 3.5	104

Modified from Balch M, Soong SJ, Gershenwald JE, et al. Prognostic factors analysis of 17,600 melanoma patients: validation of the American Joint Committee on Cancer Melanoma Staging System. *J Clin Oncol* 2001;19:3622–3634.

(in situ melanoma), stage I (local disease), stage II (local disease), stage III (regional nodal, in-transit, or satellite metastases), and stage IV (distant metastases; Table 111.4). In general, increasing stage is associated with decreasing survival (Table 111.1).

Other Prognostic Factors

The major prognostic factors that predict survival in melanoma patients have been accounted for in the AJCC staging system—namely, tumor microstaging, ulceration, nodal status, and distant metastases.[17,19] The presence of ulceration in a melanoma appears to be associated with a poorer prognosis. Men have a higher proportion of ulcerated lesions than women (27% vs. 19%, respectively). Although ulceration appears to correlate with thickness of the melanoma, the presence of ulceration is an independent prognostic factor and has been included in the staging system.[17,19] Additionally, a higher mitotic rate of 1.0 mm^2 or greater is an independent prognostic factor of both nodal involvement and survival.[18,20,21] The presence of angiolymphatic invasion is also a poor prognostic sign.

Treatment of Primary Melanoma

Biopsy. For localized melanoma, the tumor thickness (Breslow depth of invasion) is the single variable that most accurately determines therapy and prognosis. The ulceration status and mitotic rate also represent independent prognostic variables. A full-thickness biopsy with 1- to 2-mm margins only, to the adipose tissue, is preferred for any lesion highly suspect for melanoma.[22] If the melanoma is transected with a partial-thickness shave biopsy, the ability to obtain an accurate measurement of tumor thickness is lost. Therefore, a superficial shave biopsy is never recommended for a suspect pigmented lesion. Saucerization, which uses a curved blade to perform a deeper shave biopsy down to the subcutaneous fat, is acceptable.

Excisional biopsy with 1- to 2-mm margins is the preferred method for suspect lesions to provide the pathologist a total specimen for histologic interpretation and accurate microstaging. Performing a wide excision as the first step, especially on the trunk or head and neck, is not recommended, as several benign and malignant lesions can mimic melanoma and because doing so may result in the inability to accurately perform SLNB. Formalin-fixed, paraffin-embedded, permanent sections should be used for biopsy diagnosis of primary cutaneous melanoma to accurately determine tumor thickness and other histopathologic prognostic variables. Frozen sections have no role in the diagnosis or microstaging of primary melanoma. If the lesion is a melanoma, the excisional biopsy represents the first stage of a two-stage procedure. The second stage is re-excision with margins generally ranging from 0.5 to 2.0 cm, with or without SLNB, depending primarily on the tumor thickness. When biopsying a suspected melanoma on the extremities, it is critical that the biopsy be oriented on the long axis of the extremity, parallel to the lymphatics. Performing a biopsy oriented transversely on the extremity may not only compromise the accuracy of lymphatic mapping but also may obligate the patient to a skin graft to close the subsequent wide exision defect.

For suspicious lesions that are too large for complete excision and those that are located where the amount of skin is critical in terms of functional or cosmetic results, an incisional biopsy may be performed with an elliptical incision, deep saucerization shave to adipose or deep dermis in thick skin areas, or a punch biopsy. Incisional biopsies for melanoma do not increase the risk of local recurrence and distant metastasis or affect patient survival. They should generally be performed on the most raised or most pigmented area of the lesion to maximize the obtainable diagnostic and prognostic information. The most raised area usually corresponds to the maximal thickness of the lesion, but not always. Several incisional biopsies can be obtained from different areas for large lesions with multiple morphologic features. In the scenario of incisional biopsy with significant remaining lesion, complete excision for accurate microstaging should be considered prior to definitive treatment, unless the lesion is already 1 mm or greater in Breslow depth.

TABLE 111.3 **STAGING**

AMERICAN JOINT COMMISSION ON CANCER MELANOMA STAGING SYSTEM, TNM DEFINITIONS

PRIMARY TUMOR	
TX:	Cannot be assessed (shave biopsy, regressed lesion)
T0:	Unknown primary
Tis:	In situ melanoma
T1:	≤1-mm Breslow thickness
	a. Without ulceration and mitosis <1 mm^2
	b. With ulceration or mitosis ≥ 1 mm^2
T2:	1.01 to 2.00 mm
	a. Without ulceration
	b. With ulceration
T3:	2.01 to 4.00 mm
	a. Without ulceration
	b. With ulceration
T4:	>4 mm
	a. Without ulceration
	b. With ulceration
REGIONAL LYMPH NODE INVOLVEMENT	
NX:	Cannot be assessed (previously removed)
N0:	No regional node metastasis
N1:	Metastasis in one regional node
	a. Micrometastasis (diagnosed by SLNB or elective lymph node dissection)
	b. Macrometastasis (clinically palpable or found on imaging studies, confirmed histologically, or gross extracapsular extension)
N2:	Metastasis in two to three regional nodes
	a. Micrometastasis
	b. Macrometastasis
	c. In-transit or satellite metastasis without nodal metastasis
N3:	Metastasis in ≥4 regional nodes, matted nodes, or in-transit or satellite metastasis with positive metastatic nodes
DISTANT METASTASIS	
MX:	Cannot be assessed
M0:	No distant metastasis
M1a:	Distant skin, subcutaneous, or lymph node metastasis with normal LDH
M1b:	Lung metastasis with normal LDH
M1c:	All other visceral metastases with a normal LDH or any distant metastases with an elevated LDH

SLNB, sentinel lymph node biopsy; LDH, lactate dehydrogenase.

Metastatic Workup

In an attempt to standardize staging workup for melanoma, the National Comprehensive Cancer Network (NCCN) has published guidelines.[23] There are three basic reasons to perform a metastatic workup following the diagnosis of primary cutaneous melanoma: (a) for staging and prognosis, (b) to detect an early metastasis with potential survival benefit, and (c) to avoid morbidity of an extensive surgical procedure by detection of a distant metastasis.[24] The best test for the staging workup still starts with a history (a focused review concentrating on constitutional, respiratory, neurologic, hepatic, musculoskeletal, gastrointestinal, skin, and lymphatic systems) and physical examination (total body skin examination, palpation of lymph nodes). Routine imaging (chest x-ray, computed tomography [CT] scans, positron emission tomography [PET] scans) and blood studies (complete blood count, comprehensive metabolic profile, liver function tests, serum lactate dehydrogenase levels) in asymptomatic, clinically node-negative patients are low in both sensitivity and specificity and are not necessary.[25–28] False-positive staging tests are common and lead to more tests and patient distress. SLNB represents the best baseline staging test, with both relatively high sensitivity and specificity in patients at significant risk for metastasis. The ability to detect stage IV disease with routine studies is small if the SLNB is negative. Both ultrasound and PET scanning have been examined as methods of identifying nodal metastases prior to surgery. While they detect disease in a minority of patients, the size of most metastases to the regional nodes are below the threshold of ultrasound or PET to detect, so this is not a cost-effective strategy.[29–31] If a thorough history and physical and detailed review of systems reveals no signs or

TABLE 111.4 **STAGING**

STAGE GROUPINGS FOR CUTANEOUS MELANOMA

	CLINICAL STAGING[a]			PATHOLOGIC STAGING[b]		
	T	N	M	T	N	M
0	Tis	N0	M0	Tis	N0	M0
IA	T1a	N0	M0	T1a	N0	M0
IB	T1b	N0	M0	T1b	N0	M0
	T2a	N0	M0	T2a	N0	M0
IIA	T2b	N0	M0	T2b	N0	M0
	T3a	N0	M0	T3a	M0	M0
IIB	T3b	N0	M0	T3b	N0	M0
	T4a	N0	M0	T4a	N0	M0
IIC	T4b	N0	M0	T4b	N0	M0
		N1				
III[c]	Any T	N2	M0			
		N3				
IIIA				T1–4a	N1a	M0
				T1–4a	N2a	M0
				T1–4b	N1a	M0
				T1–4b	N2a	M0
IIIB				T1–4a	N1b	M0
				T1–4a	N2b	M0
				T1–a/b	N2c	M0
				T1–4b	N1b	M0
IIIC				T1–4b	N2b	M0
				Any T	N3	M0
IV	Any T	Any N	Any M1	Any T	Any N	Any M1

[a]Clinical staging includes microstaging of the primary melanoma and clinical/radiologic evaluation for metastasis. By convention, it should be used after complete excision of the primary melanoma with clinical assessment for regional and distant metastases.
[b]Pathologic staging includes microstaging of the primary melanoma and pathologic information about the regional lymph nodes after partial or complete lymphadenectomy. Pathologic stage 0 or stage IA patients are the exception; they do not require pathologic evaluation of their lymph nodes.
[c]There are no stage III subgroups for clinical staging.
From Balch M, Buzaid AC, Soong SJ, et al. Final version of the American Joint Committee on Cancer Staging System for Cutaneous Melanoma. *J Clin Oncol.* 2001;19:3635–3648. Reprinted with permission from the American Society of Clinical Oncology.

symptoms suspicious for regional or distant disease, then no further staging is necessary. However, a high index of suspicion should be maintained and a thorough symptom-directed workup should be initiated for any worrisome finding on the history and physical.

Approximately 5% to 10% of newly diagnosed melanoma patients present with clinically involved lymph nodes. Any clinically suspicious node should be confirmed by fine needle aspiration (FNA) biopsy, as enlarged lymph nodes may be reactive (particularly after a biopsy). Ultrasound-guided FNA biopsy can be useful in cases where the suspicious node is difficult to biopsy by hand. Patients documented to have macroscopic regional disease should undergo complete staging prior to definitive surgery, as a significant percentage may have more advanced regional or distant disease that may alter surgical therapy.[32,33] Staging should include a serum lactate dehydrogenase (LDH) level; MRI of the head and either CT of the chest, abdomen, and pelvis; PET scan; or combined CT/PET scan. For patients with involved groin nodes, CT scan is recommended to visualize the pelvic nodes, as this may help to determine the extent of inguinal node dissection. Workup for stage IV disseminated melanoma is often dictated by clinical trial protocols. Follow-up test guidelines are similar to these workup principles (Table 111.5).

Surgical Excision of Primary Melanoma

The primary purpose of a melanoma excision is to prevent local 5 recurrence due to persistent disease. For melanoma in situ, excision margins of 0.5 cm are indicated. For invasive melanoma, wide excision of the primary tumor, with margins generally ranging from 1 to 2 cm, is indicated for local control. The optimal margin width remains somewhat controversial. The historical approach of excising all primary melanomas with a 3- to 5-cm margin is extinct. At least five randomized controlled trials failed to demonstrate a difference in overall survival or local recurrence with narrow (1- to 2-cm) versus wide (3- to 5-cm)

TABLE 111.5 **TREATMENT**

FOLLOW-UP GUIDELINES: INTERVAL FREQUENCY AND TESTS

	■ NCCN	■ UMMC
In situ	Periodic skin examination for life	q6mo for 1 yr, then annually
Local disease: <1 mm or >1 mm with a negative SLNB and without ulceration	q3–12mo	q6mo for 3 yr, then annually
Local disease: 1 mm; no SLNB or negative SLNB with ulceration	q3–12mo for 3 yr, then 4–12mo for 2 yr, then annually	q6mo for 3 yr, then annually; tests based on H&P
Regional disease	q3–12mo for 3 yr, then 4–12mo for 2 yr, then annually CXR, LDH, CBC q3–12mo (optional); other imaging studies (optional)	q6mo for 3 yr, then annually; tests based on H&P
Distant disease	Medical oncology trials	Medical oncology trials

NCCN, National Comprehensive Cancer Network; UMMC, University of Michigan Multidisciplinary Melanoma Clinic; SLNB, sentinel lymph node biopsy; H&P, histology and pathology; CXR, chest x-ray; LDH, lactate dehydrogenase; CBC, complete blood count.
Shorter intervals may be considered for patients with dysplastic nevus syndrome or those who have difficulty with self-examinations. Coordination is necessary dermatologist and primary care provider/internist/or medical oncology team.

margins[34] (Table 111.6). Of note, one trial[35] demonstrated an increased risk of locoregional recurrence with 1-cm versus 3-cm margins for melanoma more than 2 mm thick. Based on these trials, current consensus guidelines recommend margins of 1 cm for melanomas 1 mm or less thick, 2 cm for melanomas greater than 2 mm thick, and 1 to 2 cm for melanomas 1 to 2 mm thick. For this last group, the size of the margins should be based on the anatomic location of the melanoma and the morbidity of excising 2 cm versus 1 cm, including the need for an advancement flap or skin graft (Table 111.7). For several locations, such as melanomas on the head and neck, the maximum margins attainable are dictated by anatomic limitations. Subungal melanomas require amputation of the digit. Perianal melanoma can often be treated by wide excision, but melanoma of the anal mucosa may require abdominoperineal resection (APR). A complete staging workup should be performed before proceeding with APR, as these patients have a very high rate of regional and distant disease.[36]

For the clinically ill-defined LMM, histologic confirmation of negative margins is important, and it should be emphasized that these margin recommendations may not apply to in situ LM and invasive LMM on the head and neck.[37,38] LM and LMM are often associated with extensive subclinical involvement to as much as several centimeters beyond the clinical component. Careful and complete margin control, including excision of the lesional trailing edge of atypical melanocytic hyperplasia, often beyond the standard margins, may be necessary for complete surgical resection of LM/LMM on the head and neck.

Treatment of Regional Metastatic Melanoma

Lymphadenectomy Results and Indications. Surgical excision of metastases to regional lymph nodes is potentially curative therapy. The 5-year survival rate for patients who undergo lymphadenectomy for clinically positive involved

TABLE 111.6 **RESULTS**

RANDOMIZED CONTROLLED TRIALS: NARROW VERSUS WIDE EXCISION MARGINS

■ TRIAL[a]	■ SUBJECTS (No.)	■ NARROW RESECTION MARGIN (cm)	■ WIDE RESECTION MARGIN (cm)	■ TUMOR THICKNESS (mm)	■ TUMOR SITE	■ MEDIAN LENGTH FOLLOW-UP (yrs)
French 2003	326	2	5	<2.1	T, E, H&N	10.0
Intergroup 1996	470	2	4	1.0–4.0	T, E	7.6
Swedish 2000	989	2	5	0.8–2.0	T, E	11.0
WHO 1991	612	1	3	<2.0	T, E	7.5
UK 2004	900	1	3	>2.0	T, E	5.0

T, trunk; E, extremity; H&N, head and neck; WHO, World Health Organization; UK, United Kingdom.
[a]There was no difference in any outcomes in the first four trials. UK 2004 showed increased locoregional recurrence but no difference in local or in-transit recurrence.

TABLE 111.7 **TREATMENT**

RECOMMENDED SURGICAL MARGINS FOR MELANOMA EXCISION

■ MELANOMA THICKNESS (mm)	■ CLINICAL EXCISION MARGIN (cm)
In situ	0.5 to 1.0
≤1.0	1.0
1.1 to 2.0	1.0 to 2.0
>2.0	2.0

Margins may need to be modified based on anatomic considerations but still require histologic confirmation of tumorfree margins. For clinically ill-defined lentigo maligna/lentigo maligna melanoma, wider margins may be required for histologic confirmation of tumorfree margins.

nodes (AJCC stage III) ranges from 25% to 70%. In addition, for those patients not cured by lymphadenectomy, resection can avoid potential pain associated with tumor enlargement, skin breakdown, and tumor necrosis (Fig. 111.2). Only 5% to 10% of patients who first present with the diagnosis of melanoma have clinical evidence of nodal metastases, approximately 85% to 90% have localized disease, and the remaining 5% have distant metastases. In less than 3% of patients, a diagnosis of melanoma is made in the absence of a definable primary lesion.[39] When patients present with isolated nodal disease from an unknown primary site, the results of lymphadenectomy are similar to those for patients with known 6 primary tumors. For patients with melanoma 1 mm thick or greater who present with clinically negative nodes, SLNB should be considered to determine whether therapeutic lymphadenectomy is indicated.[40]

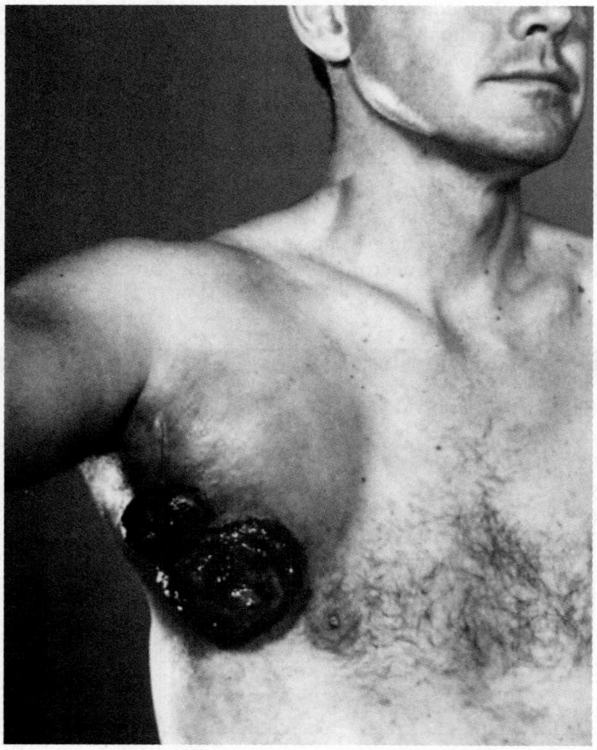

FIGURE 111.2. Patient with large melanoma axillary involvement with skin ulceration.

Sentinel Lymph Node Biopsy

Morton et al.[41] were the first to develop the concept of "sentinel lymph nodes" in the nodal basins draining cutaneous melanomas. They hypothesized that melanoma involvement of a nodal basin develops in an orderly fashion with metastasis to the sentinel lymph node as the first step in that process. With the intradermal injection of a blue dye, these investigators were able to identify sentinel lymph nodes 90% of the time. If the sentinel node was negative for melanoma, the remaining lymph nodes were also free of involvement in at least 96% of cases. These results have been confirmed by multiple other groups.[42–44]

Two tracers are typically used for identifying the sentinel lymph nodes: a blue dye—1% isosulfan blue (Lymphazurin)—and a radiolabeled colloid solution. Lymphazurin carries a risk of allergic reaction in 0.5% to 2.0% of patients, which can be life threatening.[45] Methylene blue dye can also be used, without risk of allergic reaction, although this should be diluted as it can cause skin necrosis if not completely resected. One to 4 hours before surgery, a radiolabeled colloid solution is injected intradermally. The injection site is around the primary tumor site or excision site, taking care to avoid injecting directly into any residual tumor. Lymphoscintigraphy imaging is then performed, which is critical in that it can identify sentinel nodes outside the traditional nodal basin. The blue dye is injected intradermally in the operating room a few minutes before the procedure. Using a handheld gamma detector probe, the surgeon is able to identify the sentinel lymph node location through the skin, thereby limiting the incision necessary to find the node. Blue-stained lymphatics and lymph nodes can be directly visualized (Fig. 111.3). The combined use of the blue dye plus the radiolabeled colloid enables the detection of the sentinel node in more than 95% of cases.[44] The technique of SLNB is most often performed in conjunction with the wide excision of the primary tumor. It can routinely be performed as an outpatient procedure.

Once the sentinel lymph node is removed, it is processed by the pathologist by step sectioning the entire node into multiple sections for routine hematoxylin and eosin staining. This is done to examine for micrometastases that could be missed by the standard approach to examining nodes, which involves bivalving the lymph node and performing an examination of only one section. If serial sectioning and staining are negative for metastasis, then immunohistochemical staining for melanoma markers such as S-100, Melan-A, and HMB-45 is performed.[46] These stains can identify microscopic clusters of tumor cells that are hard or impossible to identify by hematoxylin and eosin staining. The thoroughness of assessing the

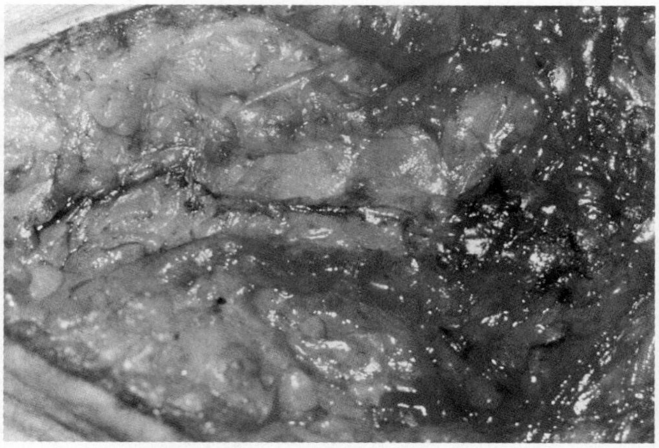

FIGURE 111.3. Blue dye tracking up a lymphatic vessel to a blue-stained lymph node.

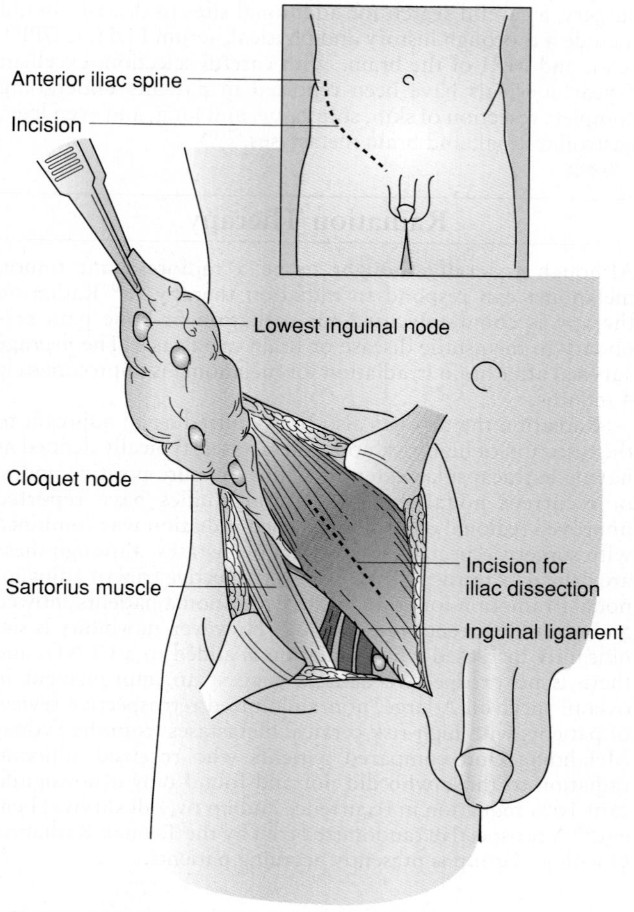

FIGURE 111.4. Technique of groin dissection.

sentinel lymph nodes for metastatic disease has resulted in much more accurate staging of patients. Micrometastases to lymph nodes has been incorporated in the current staging system as described above.

If the sentinel lymph node is positive for melanoma, then complete lymph node dissection (CLND) (Fig. 111.4) is indicated based on potential survival and clinical benefit. The interim results of the Multicenter Selective Lymphadenectomy Trial I (MSLT-I), which randomized patients to wide local excision (WLE) alone or WLE in combination with SLNB and CLND for a positive lymph node demonstrated that the survival of patients with regional metastases detected by SLNB who underwent CLND was significantly improved over those patients who underwent CLND for a regional recurrence (66.2% vs. 54.2%, $p < 0.02$).[47] An unresolved question is whether every patient with a positive sentinel lymph node requires CLND. Several attempts to retrospectively identify clinical or histologic factors that may predict the absence or presence of disease within the non–sentinel nodes have not identified any absolute way to determine who requires additional surgery, although a combination of the Breslow depth and amount of disease within the sentinel lymph node seems promising. The results of the ongoing MSLT-II trial, which randomizes patients with a positive sentinel lymph node to CLND or serial ultrasonography of the regional basin, will provide more information regarding the benefit of CLND for sentinel lymph node–positive patients. Until that time, CLND for a positive sentinel lymph node remains the standard of care in the treatment of melanoma.

Patients with primary melanomas equal to or greater than 1 mm thickness and clinically negative nodes should be considered for SLNB. For some subgroups of patients with melanoma Breslow depth of 0.75 to 1.0 mm, SLNB may be considered. These subgroups include younger patients, evidence of ulceration or angiolymphatic invasion, extensive dermal regression to 1 mm, or 1 mitosis/mm^2 or greater in the primary tumor.[20,48–50] Reasons not to perform SLNB include significant medical comorbidities or the patient does not desire SLNB after an informed discussion.

Adjuvant Therapy

Although the prognosis for patients with early-stage cutaneous melanoma is quite good, less than 50% of patients with thick primaries (i.e., >4 mm) or regional node involvement are cured by surgery alone. The development of effective adjuvant therapy capable of increasing postsurgical survival in high-risk groups of patients has been a long-standing goal of clinicians. Unfortunately, numerous randomized trials evaluating systemic chemotherapeutic agents (most notably dacarbazine), nonspecific immunotherapy (such as bacille Calmette-Guérin), and tumor-specific vaccines in the adjuvant setting have failed to demonstrate any impact on survival.[51–53]

Interferon-α2b (IFN-α) has a variety of modulatory effects on the immune system that could enhance antitumor reactivity. IFN-α has been reported to have antitumor activity in patients with metastatic disease. In 1996, Kirkwood et al.[54] reported the effectiveness of IFN-α to improve diseasefree and overall survival rates of patients with stage IIb (>4 mm) or III disease after surgery. In this multi-institutional prospective randomized trial, 287 high-risk patients with deep primary (>4-mm) tumors or positive nodes were randomly assigned after surgery to either postoperative adjuvant treatment with IFN-α2b or to observation. IFN-α2b therapy significantly increased median overall survival by 1 year and produced a 24% improvement in the 5-year overall survival rate (46% for IFN-α2b patients vs. 37% for observation patients). Based on these results, the Food and Drug Administration (FDA) approved the use of adjuvant IFN-α2b after surgical resection of stage IIb or III melanoma. Follow-up studies have raised concerns about the relative efficacy of IFN-α in this setting; however, in healthy melanoma patients at high risk of relapse, this is the only known adjuvant therapy that should be considered.[55]

Treatment of In-Transit Disease

In-transit disease and satellitosis develop in 5% to 8% of patients with melanomas thicker than 1.5 mm.[56] These are classified as stage III disease but portend not only a poor prognosis but can be a challenge to treat. Treatment involves either local excision or ablation, or regional chemotherapy. Surgical excision is the optimal management when the number of lesions is small and complete excision is possible. Prior to proceeding with surgery, a complete staging workup for metastatic disease is recommended, as these patients often harbor distant disease. When surgery is not feasible, a number of intralesional therapies (such as granulocyte-macrophage colony-stimulating factor) or ablative therapies (radiation, cryotherapy, electrodessication, laser ablation, photodynamic therapy) have been employed with limited success. When the in-transit disease is unresectable but limited to an extremity, regional administration of high-dose chemotherapy can be effective in controlling disease.

Isolated limb perfusion (ILP) uses an extracorporeal membrane oxygenator (as is used with cardiac surgery) to deliver chemotherapy doses 15 to 25 times higher than can be obtained with systemic delivery. The surgeon isolates the vessels and uses a tourniquet to prevent systemic uptake of the agent(s). Using the bypass machine, the limb is perfused with hyperthermic (38°C to 40°C) chemotherapy solutions, most commonly melphalan. After 60 to 90 minutes of treatment, the drug is flushed from the circulation and systemic circulation is restored. Response rates between 80% and 90% are reported, with complete response rates between 40% and 65%.[56–58] In some cases, these can be quite durable. Toxicities can range from mild erythema and edema to epidermolysis, functional impairment, and in extremely rare cases a need for amputation.

Because of the complexities involved in scheduling and performing ILP, it is currently available at only a few select centers. A less invasive and less toxic approach is the use of isolated limb infusion. Rather than surgical isolation of the vessels, percutaneous catheters are placed radiologically in the artery and vein and connected to an extracorporeal circuit incorporating a heating coil. A tourniquet is placed on the extremity, but because some systemic uptake is anticipated, lower doses of chemotherapeutic agents are used. Some studies have reported response rates equal to ILP, although others report slightly lower response rates.[59,60]

Treatment of Disseminated Melanoma

Evaluation for Metastatic Disease and Clinical Course. The follow-up evaluation for patients with AJCC stage I, II, or III melanoma who are rendered tumorfree by surgery should include regular histories and physical examinations. The use of extensive and frequent radiographic studies and blood work in asymptomatic, clinically diseasefree patients is rarely productive.[23,24] For AJCC stage IA (≤1 mm), the NCCN recommends that patients should undergo a history and physical examination with emphasis on skin and nodal examinations every 3 to 12 months as clinically indicated. For AJCC stage IB to III, patients should undergo a history and physical examination every 3 to 6 months for 3 years, then every 4 to 12 months for 2 years, then annually as clinically indicated (Table 111.5). The use of chest radiographs and blood work, as well as other imaging scans, when clinically indicated, is based on the history and physical examination.

Melanoma can disseminate to any organ. The most common sites of recurrence are skin, subcutaneous tissues, and distant lymph nodes, followed by visceral sites. Common visceral sites of metastasis, in order of decreasing occurrence, are the lung, liver, brain, bone, and gastrointestinal tract. Most patients who die with disseminated disease have multiple organ involvement. Frequently, the cause of death is respiratory failure or brain complications. Patients with disseminated disease have a poor prognosis, with a mean survival of approximately 6 months. Cure with any treatment is rare. Selection of treatment or a decision against treatment should be based on several factors, including the patient's medical condition, the potential for palliation, and the impact of treatment on quality of life.

Surgery

While surgery is rarely considered for patients with metastases, melanoma remains an exception, with documented long-term survival among patients who undergo resection of metastatic lesions. Surgery should be strongly considered for palliative purposes, but also should be considered in select patients with stage IV melanoma with a goal of prolonged diseasefree survival. Careful selection is key, and most patients who present with metastases are not candidates for resection. The decision to pursue surgery should be made on the age and health of the patient, the number and locations of the metastases and ability to achieve negative margins, the morbidity of the operation, and the diseasefree interval. Patients with single versus multiple lesions and longer diseasefree intervals, as well as those in good overall health, are the ideal candidates. Before surgery, a careful search for additional sites of disease should include a thorough history and physical, serum LDH, CT/PET scan, and MRI of the brain. With careful selection, excellent 5-year survivals have been reported in patients undergoing complete resection of skin, soft tissue, and lung, and even liver, gastrointestinal, and brain metastases.[61–68]

Radiation Therapy

Although generally thought to be a radioresistant tumor, melanoma can respond to radiation therapy.[69,70] Radiation therapy is commonly used for palliation of bone pain secondary to metastatic disease or brain metastasis. The average survival after brain irradiation for melanoma is approximately 4 months.

Radiation therapy has also been utilized as an adjuvant to the resection of high-risk nodal metastases, typically defined as having extracapsular extension, four or more positive nodes, or recurrent nodal disease. Several studies have reported improved regional control rates when radiation was combined with surgery, especially for cervical metastases, although these are primarily retrospective.[71–74] A prospective trial of adjuvant nodal irradiation for node-positive melanoma patients showed an in-field recurrence rate of 7%.[75] However, morbidity is significantly increased when radiation is added to a CLND, and there is no prospective data to suggest an improvement in overall survival. A large, nonrandomized retrospective review of patients with high-risk cervical metastases from the Sydney Melanoma Unit compared patients who received adjuvant radiation to those who did not and found only a nonsignificant 10% reduction in recurrence and no overall survival benefit.[76] A prospective randomized trial by the Tasman Radiation Oncology Group is presently accruing patients.

Chemotherapy

Melanoma is responsive to few chemotherapeutic drugs.[49–53] The best single agents for treatment of melanoma are dacarbazine (DTIC), the nitrosoureas, vinca alkaloids, and cisplatin, which have objective response rates in the range of 10% to 20%. Conventionally, objective responses have included complete disappearance of all known tumor sites (complete response) and reduction of more than half in all assessable tumor (partial response). Complete responses are rare and nearly always of brief duration (<6 months). Responses are more frequently observed in patients with tumor in the skin, subcutaneous tissue, lymph nodes, or lung. Combination chemotherapy with the potential of drug synergy has been used with limited success in the treatment of metastatic melanoma. No evidence indicates that combination chemotherapy offers better results than single-agent DTIC at this time.

Immunotherapy

The rapid evolution of recombinant DNA technology has resulted in the availability of cytokines, such as the interferons and interleukins, that can be administered to modulate a patient's immune response.[36–40] These biologic agents have been used in immunotherapeutic trials for metastatic melanoma and demonstrate that an antitumor immune response can be generated in select patients. A significant advance in melanoma immunotherapy has been associated with the use of interleukin-2 (IL-2). IL-2 is a cytokine secreted by antigen-activated helper T cells and was initially discovered because it was a T-cell growth factor. Subsequently, it was found to have many other immunologic effects, and it appears to have an important role in the enhancement of immune responses. Mulé et al.[77] discovered that the in vivo administration of IL-2 in preclinical animal

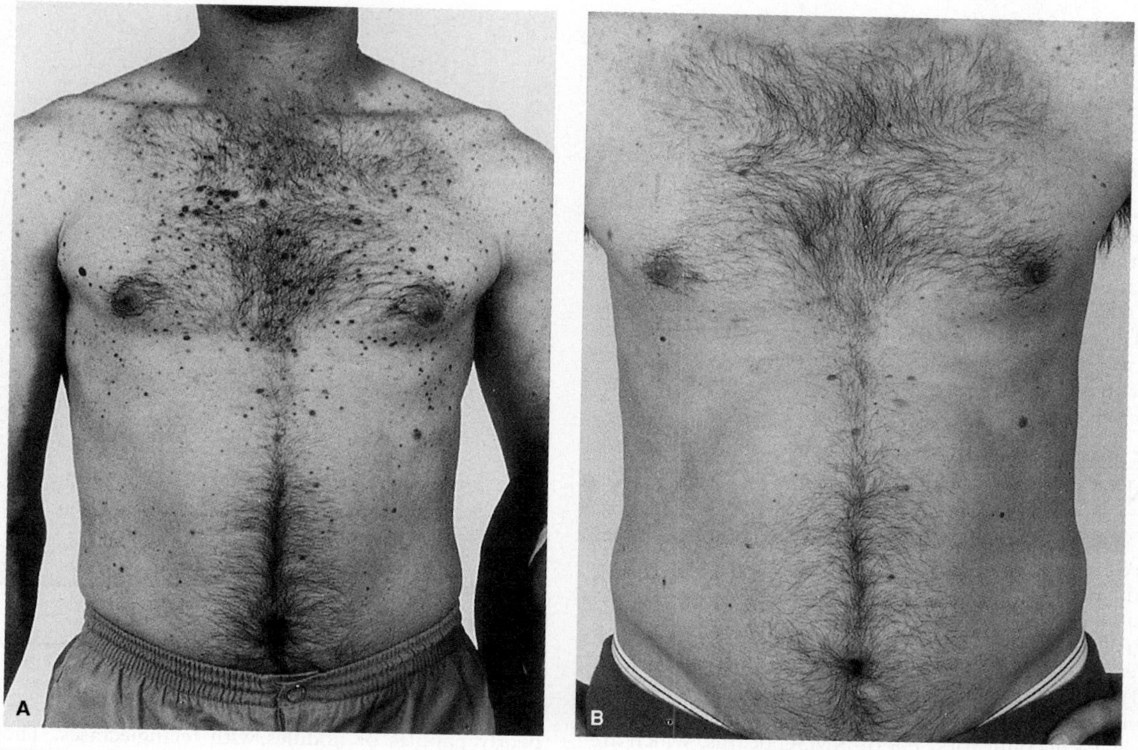

FIGURE 111.5. **A:** Patient with disseminated melanoma metastatic to multiple cutaneous sites. **B:** After several courses of therapy with lymphokine-activated killer cells and interleukin-2, the patient had a complete response. (Courtesy of Steven A. Rosenberg, M.D., Surgery Branch, National Cancer Institute, Bethesda, MD.)

models resulted in dramatic tumor regression. In clinical studies, the administration of IL-2 resulted in a 15% to 20% response rate in patients with advanced melanoma.[78] Approximately 5% of patients have a complete response that has been durable for prolonged periods (Fig. 111.5). This latter result prompted the FDA to approve IL-2 for the treatment of metastatic melanoma.

There has been significant interest in the use of vaccines as a treatment for malignant melanoma, fueled by the lack of efficacy of standard chemotherapy, evidence of the immune system's ability to recognize and eradicate melanoma, and the discovery of unique melanoma tumor–associated antigens. Unfortunately, results of using peptides, gangliosides, or allogeneic cells have been disappointing.[79,80] A more promising approach may be the use of dendritic cells (DCs). DCs are potent antigen-presenting cells of the immune system that are capable of sensitizing naive T cells to respond against tumor antigen. DCs can be "pulsed" with tumor antigen in the form of peptides, whole tumor cells, lysates of tumor cells, or genes encoding antigen. Animal studies have shown that antigen-pulsed DCs can cause the regression of established tumors by intradermal or intravenous administration. The administration of IL-2 with DC therapy has improved the antitumor response rate in animal studies.[81] In humans, antigen-pulsed DCs have resulted in complete responses in patients with stage IV melanoma.[82] Numerous studies are being conducted to evaluate DC vaccine therapy in the treatment of melanoma.

A promising area of research in melanoma is direct immune modulation through the blockade of cytotoxic T-lymphocyte–associated antigen 4 (CTLA-4), a cell surface molecule on T cells that is upregulated in activated cells and serves as an immunologic "brake." Humanized monoclonal antibodies (mAb) that block CTLA-4, thus releasing the brake on T cells, have been shown to augment the antitumor response.[83] Two such antibodies, MDX-010 and ticilimumab, have been tested in stage IV melanoma with promising results.[84,85] Several studies of anti-CTLA-4 mAb alone or in combination with other immunotherapies, in both the adjuvant and metastatic settings, are ongoing.

As opposed to active immunotherapy, where an agent is delivered with the goal of stimulating or augmenting the host's immune response (such as a vaccine), passive immunotherapy involves delivering components of the immune system that have already been sensitized to tumor antigens. One example of this in the treatment of metastatic melanoma is the use of antitumor reactive T cells, known as *adoptive immunotherapy*. One source of these T cells is from the tumor itself, known as tumor-infiltrating lymphocytes (TIL). In clinical studies, Rosenberg et al.[86,87] have reported that patients with advanced melanoma treated with the combination of TIL, IL-2, and chemotherapy can result in response rates between 35% and 50%. Lymphodepletion of patients before adoptive immunotherapy may improve these results. One drawback to the use of TIL for adoptive immunotherapy is the need to harvest adequate tumor from patients with stage IV disease, which may be difficult. Alternative approaches include delivering a vaccine to the patient and then using T cells from the vaccine-draining lymph nodes,[88–90] or retroviral gene transduction of peripheral blood mononuclear with the genes for the TCR-α and β chains against a melanoma-associated antigen.[91]

Biochemotherapy

Combinations of IL-2 and/or IFN-α with chemotherapy, known as biochemotherapy, have shown significant improved response rates compared with chemotherapy alone or cytokines alone. As might be expected, these regimens are more toxic than the component therapies by themselves. One of the biochemotherapy regimens that has demonstrated a significant response rate (i.e., 64%, including 21% complete and 43% partial) with moderate toxicity is a combination of cisplatin, vinblastine, dacarbazine, IL-2, and IFN-α.[92–95] Unfortunately, a randomized trial comparing this regimen to cisplatin, vinblastine, and dacarbazine alone demonstrated that while the addition of the cytokines produced slightly higher response rates and improved median progressionfree survival than chemotherapy alone, this was not associated with improved overall survival or durable responses.[96] In addition, a meta-analysis of trials of biochemotherapy versus chemotherapy in patients with metastatic melanoma also showed that although biochemotherapy improves response rates, this does not appear to translate into a survival benefit.[97] Clinical trials of other regimens are still ongoing, and biochemotherapy may be considered in select patients with advanced melanoma who are thought to be able to tolerate the toxicities of the therapy.

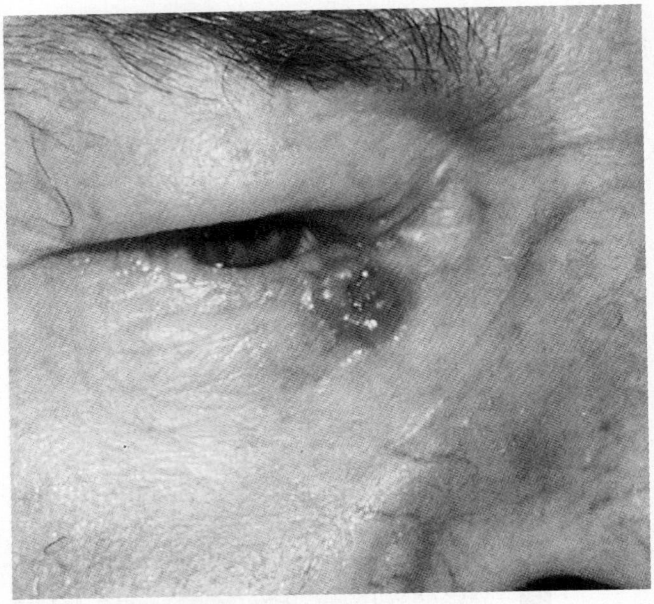

FIGURE 111.6. Basal cell carcinoma near the eye.

NONMELANOMA SKIN TUMORS

7 BCC and SCC account for 96% of new NMSCs. These tumors are derived from epithelial origin.[1–3] The ratio of BCC to SCC is approximately 4:1. The annual incidence of BCC and SCC in the United States alone exceeds 1 million cases. The public health burden on the U.S. population from NMSC, for which the incidence is rapidly rising, is highly significant. Patients with NMSC have an excellent prognosis, with 90% to 99% curable with appropriate treatment and less than 1% resulting in death. SCCs account for 75% of NMSC deaths, which are estimated at 2,000 to 2,500 per year.

Etiology

Both BCC and SCC are most commonly induced by significant exposure to UV light from the sun or tanning booths.[2] These cancers are the predominant neoplasms of the head, neck, trunk, lower legs, and extensor arms and hands where sun exposure is common. Skin cancer is a significant occupational hazard for people who work outdoors. The phenotype at increased risk is one with fair skin who sunburns and freckles easily, has blue eyes, and has red or blonde hair. Melanin pigment in the skin appears to be the protective factor.

A number of genetic syndromes are associated with an increased risk of developing NMSC, including Gorlin syndrome, xeroderma pigmentosa, and albinism. Gorlin syndrome is an autosomal dominant disorder associated with multiple BCCs, palmoplantar pits, jaw cysts, frontal bossing, and hypertelorism. Albinism is a disorder characterized by a partial or complete deficiency in melanin production and, thus, loss of protective pigment. Another factor associated with NMSC, primarily SCC, is chronic exposure to chemicals such as arsenic and hydrocarbons (found in coal tars, soot, and asphalt). Cigarette smoking has been associated with SCC of the lip and mouth. Human papillomavirus has been associated with cutaneous SCC in the genital and acral/periungual areas. Radiation has been associated with both SCC and BCC.

Basal Cell Carcinoma

BCC is the most common form of skin cancer. These epithelial-derived tumors can be divided into various subtypes according to clinical appearance, histologic pattern, and biologic behavior. Although BCCs rarely metastasize, they are characterized by slow but relentless and destructive local invasion that results in high morbidity without treatment. The subclinical local invasion may be deep, extensive, and asymmetric, with finger-like extensions several centimeters beyond the clinical borders.

The most common subtype of BCC is the well-circumscribed nodular variety. These tumors often present as pearly papules or nodules with telangiectases. They may be pruritic and bleed occasionally. With time, the center ulcerates to create peripheral "rolled" borders; such ulcerating BCCs are called *rodent ulcers* (Fig. 111.6). Occasionally, the lesions are deeply pigmented and nodular and can be confused with melanoma. This variant has been called *pigmented* BCC (Fig. 111.1H). The histologic features of these tumors demonstrate isolated areas of basaloid tumor islands arising from the epidermis with peripheral palisading of nuclei and stromal retraction. In some cases, the BCC has histologic features of squamous metaplasia with keratinization. These tumors have basosquamous differentiation and can become more aggressive and develop regional lymphatic spread.

The most locally agressive type of BCC is characterized by a diagnostic histopathologic aggressive growth pattern, known as morpheaform, sclerosing, or fibrosing BCC (Fig. 111.7). Clinically, these tumors may be more subclinical, are flat, and appear to be scarlike. They have a significant incidence of

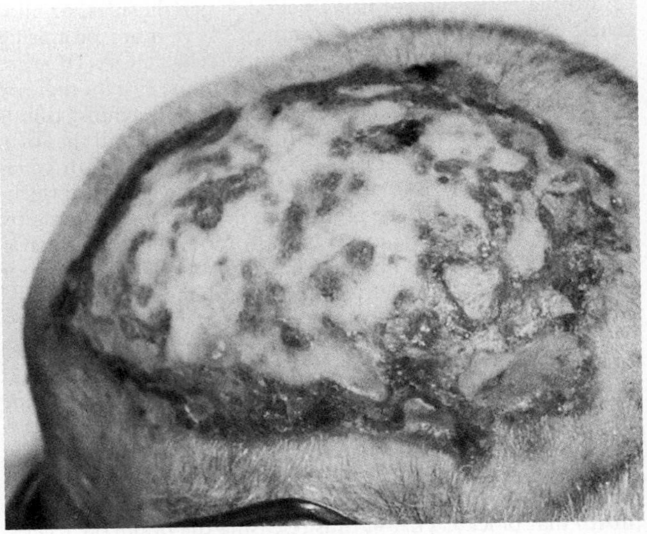

FIGURE 111.7. Morpheaform basal cell carcinoma of the scalp.

TABLE 111.8

BASAL CELL CARCINOMA: HIGHER RISK FACTORS FOR SUBCLINICAL INVASION AND RECURRENCE

- Recurrent tumor
- Anatomic location

  High risk: Central face, eyelid, eyebrow, periorbital, nose, lip, chin, mandible, temple, ear, in front or behind the ear, genitalia, hand and foot

  Medium risk: Cheeks, forehead, scalp, and neck

  Low risk: Trunk, extremity (excluding hand/foot)
- Size

  Lesions ≥6 mm on high-risk area

  Lesions ≥10 mm on medium-risk area

  Lesions ≥20 mm on low-risk area
- Histologic subtype pattern

  Aggressive growth (morpheaform, fibrosing, sclerosing, infiltrating)

  Micronodular
- Ill-defined clinical borders
- Perineural invasion
- Development in sites of prior radiation
- Immunosuppression

From Sondak VK, Sabel MS, Mulé JJ. Allogeneic and autologous melanoma vaccines: where have we been and where are we going? *Clin Cancer Res* 2006;12:2337s–2341s.

recurrence because of the isolated, fingerlike fronds of basal cell tumor cells that may deeply invade the surrounding structures well beyond the clinical margins of the lesion. These small, fingerlike islands are often missed with standard histologic margin control.

Clinically, superficial BCCs are scaly pink to red lesions. Frequently, they are confused with psoriasis or other eczematous, scaly dermatoses. Although these tumors are usually relatively superficial, extensive superficial subclinical involvement is common. Numerous risk factors are associated with possible extensive subclinical invasion and increased rates of local recurrence for BCC after standard treatment, including surgical excision (Table 111.8).

Squamous Cell Carcinoma

SCC is the second most common form of skin cancer and is derived from the epithelial keratinocyte. SCC can deeply invade surrounding structures and metastasizes most commonly to regional lymph nodes. In immunosuppressed transplant individuals, SCC is the most common skin cancer, occurring 65 to 250 times more frequently than in the general population. SCC in these individuals tends to have more aggressive behavior.

Several precursor lesions to invasive SCC exist, most commonly actinic keratoses and Bowen disease (in situ SCC). Erythroplasia of Queyrat, another precursor lesion, represents SCC in situ on the glans penis. Histologically, SCC shows malignant degeneration of epithelial cells with differentiation toward keratin formation. SCC often appears clinically as a nonhealing sore with ulceration and inflammatory pink borders or an erythematous papulonodule with overlying keratotic crust or ulceration (Figs. 111.8 and 111.9). These tumors most often arise in chronically actinically damaged skin or within an actinic keratosis, but they may also develop in burn scars or chronic inflammatory wounds. These lesions may infiltrate widely. Metastasis to regional lymph nodes accounts for approximately 80% to 90% of metastatic cases. Distant sites, such as the lung, liver, brain, bone, and skin, account for the other 10% to 20%. Metastatic SCC portends a poor prognosis with a 10-year survival rate for regional lymph node disease of less than 20% and for distant disease of 10%.[72]

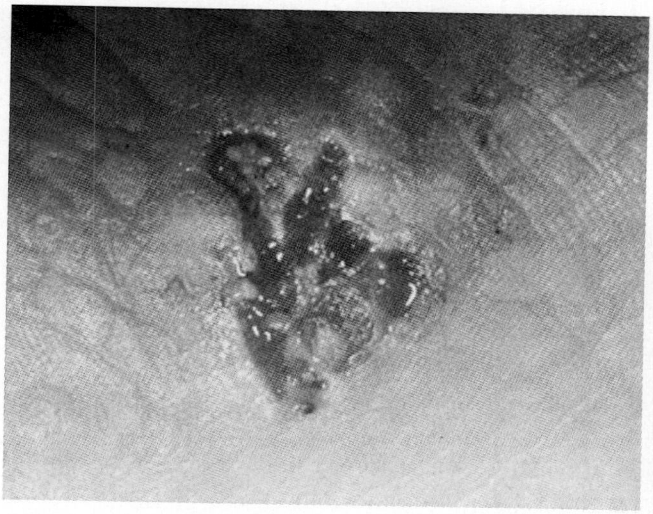

FIGURE 111.8. Squamous cell carcinoma of the hand secondary to exposure to arsenic in welding flux.

Accurate assessment of the higher-risk cutaneous SCCs is handicapped because of the lack of large prospective studies using multivariate analysis. Nine variables, however, have been identified as prognostic risk factors by retrospective analysis. Factors that may determine a higher risk for local recurrence, extensive subclinical invasion, and metastasis are noted in Table 111.9.

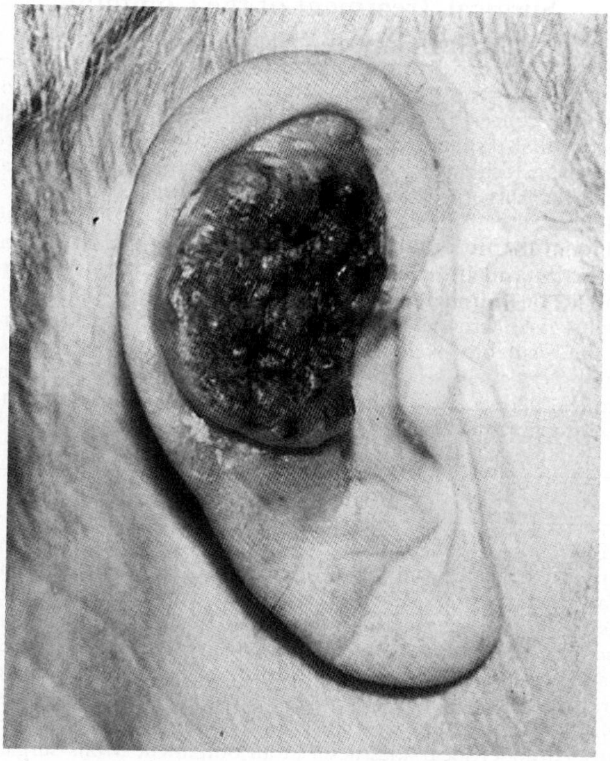

FIGURE 111.9. Ulcerative squamous cell carcinoma.

TABLE 111.9

SQUAMOUS CELL CARCINOMA: HIGHER RISK FACTORS FOR SUBCLINICAL INVASION AND RECURRENCE

- Recurrent tumor
- Anatomic location
  High risk: Central face, eyelid, eyebrow, periorbital, nose, lip, chin, mandible, temple, ear, in front or behind the ear, genitalia, hand and foot
  Medium risk: Cheeks, forehead, scalp, and neck
  Low risk: Trunk, extremity (excluding hand/foot)
- Size
  Lesions ≥6 mm on high-risk area
  Lesions ≥10 mm on medium-risk area
  Lesions ≥20 mm on low-risk area
- Histology
  Poorly differentiated
- Depth of invasion
  Clark level IV (lesion that involves the reticular dermis), V (lesion that invades into subcutaneous fat), or ≥4 mm
- Perineural invasion
- Rapid growth
- Etiology
  Scar, chronic ulcer or inflammatory process, sinus tract, sites of prior radiation therapy
- Immunosupression

From Sondak VK, Sabel MS, Mule JJ. Allogeneic and autologous melanoma vaccines: where have we been and where are we going? *Clin Cancer Res* 2006;12:2337s–2341s.

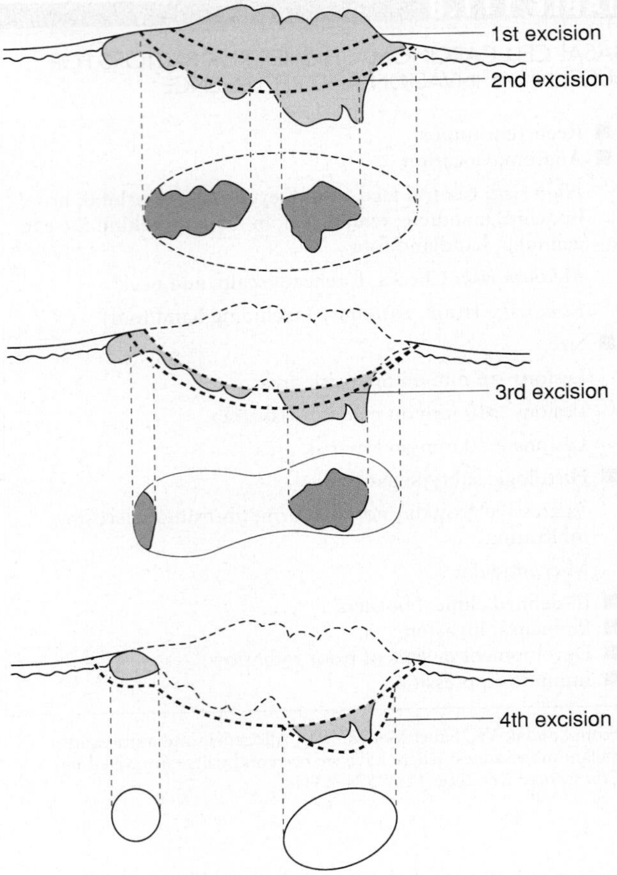

FIGURE 111.10. Mohs micrographic surgical technique.

Surgical Treatment of the Common Nonmelanoma Skin Cancers

A skin biopsy for diagnosis is important before treatment of any skin cancer. Fortunately, most NMSCs are small, low-risk lesions that respond with 90% to 95% cure rates to standard treatment techniques, including curettage and electrodesiccation, cryosurgery, radiation therapy, and surgical resection.[79] Many skin cancers can be removed with elliptical excisions. Margins for low-risk SCC range from 0.5 to 1.0 cm. Margins for low-risk BCC range from 0.3 to 0.5 cm. Mohs surgery should be considered for BCCs and SCCs that exhibit the higher-risk factors in Tables 111.8 and 111.9. If Mohs surgery is not available, excision with careful frozen section control (with permanent section confirmation) is indicated. The fundamental oncologic principle of tumor clearance first and reconstruction second should be followed.

Mohs Surgery

Mohs surgery was developed by Frederick E. Mohs, a general surgeon from the University of Wisconsin, in the 1940s. Initially, a chemical fixative paste was applied to the skin to fix the tissue in situ; hence, the now outdated term *Mohs chemosurgery*. The fresh tissue technique, which omitted the chemical paste, was developed and refined in the 1970s. Mohs micrographic surgery is most useful for the treatment of higher risk NMSC (Tables 111.8 and 111.9). Mohs surgery is usually performed under local anesthesia in an outpatient Mohs surgical unit.[80–82] After removal of all gross tumor, the surgeon excises a thin layer of tissue with 2- to 3-mm margins. The tissue is mapped, color-coded for orientation, and sent to the technician for frozen section processing. The specimen is flexible and flattened, with the beveled peripheral skin edge placed in the same horizontal plane with the deep margin. In this plane, both the deep and peripheral margins are examined in one horizontal cut by frozen section analysis with total (theoretically 100%) margin control. Good-quality frozen sections may be achieved only by a skilled and experienced Mohs histotechnician. The Mohs surgeon functions as both surgeon and pathologist. After histologic interpretation of the frozen section specimens, the precise anatomic location of any residual tumor can be identified and re-excised until all margins are tumor free (Fig. 111.10). The Mohs surgeon's ability microscopically to track subclinical tumor extensions results in the highest cure rate with maximal preservation of normal tissue. Soft tissue reconstruction can then be performed on the same day, after completion of Mohs surgical excision of the tumor (Fig. 111.11). A multidisciplinary approach involving Mohs, plastic, head and neck, and oculoplastic surgeons and radiation oncologists may be needed for extensive tumors. Mastering the Mohs technique is based on a steep learning curve that requires extensive training for optimal competence. Numerous 1- to 2-year Accreditation Council for Graduate Medical Education (ACGME) postgraduate fellowship training programs in procedural dermatology are available.

Based on a review of all studies from all disciplines since 1950, the 5-year cure rate for treatment of previously untreated primary BCC by Mohs surgery is 99%, versus 90% to 93% for all non-Mohs modalities, including standard surgical excision.[83] For previously treated recurrent BCC, the 5-year cure rates are 94% for Mohs versus 60% to 84% for non-Mohs modalities.[84] In general, Mohs surgery should be considered for NMSCs that are associated with a higher risk of recurrence after standard treatment and for tumors for which conservation of normal tissue is important. Risk factors for recurrence after standard

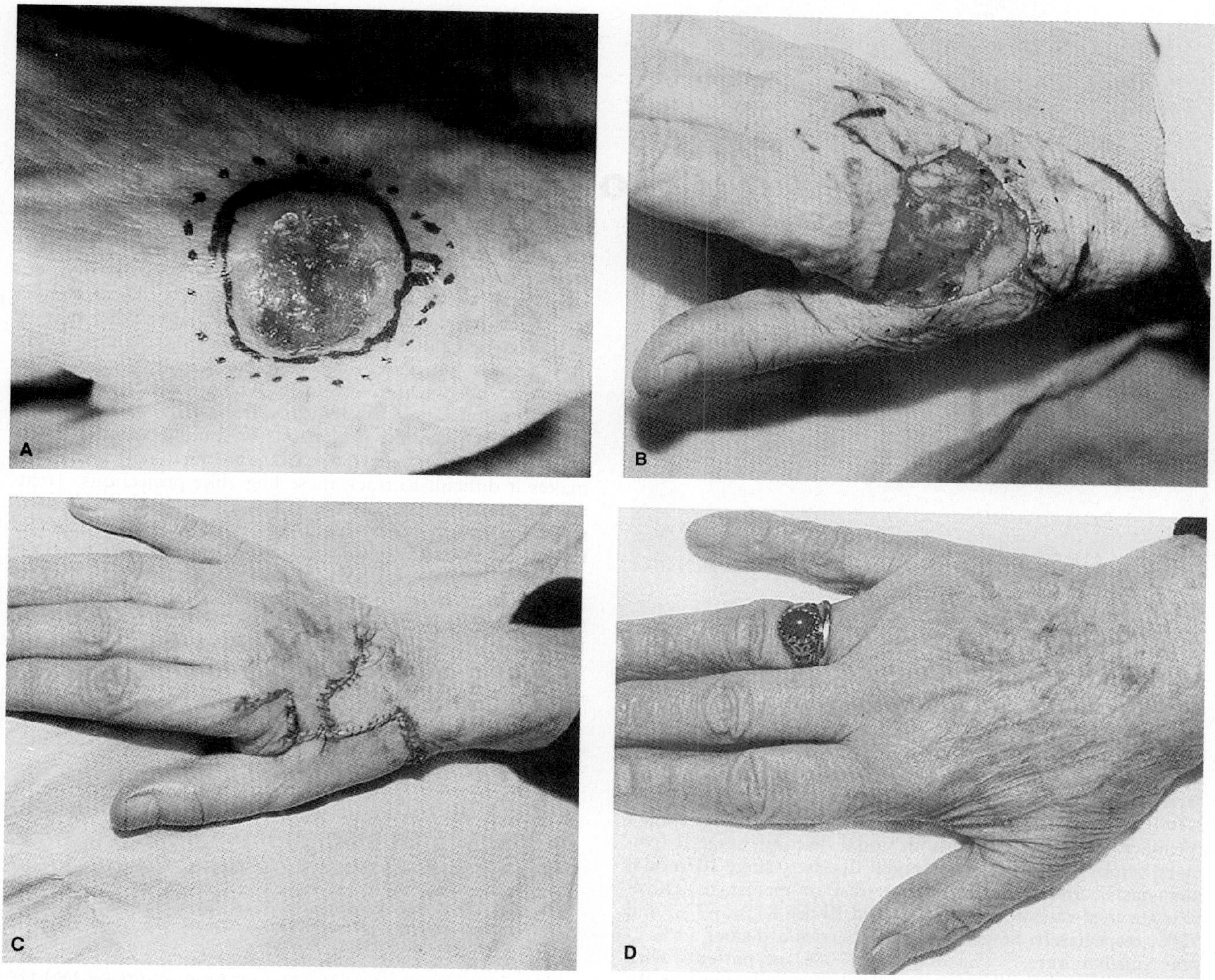

FIGURE 111.11. A: Patient with a 3 × 3 cm basal cell carcinoma on the right dorsal hand with mixed nodular and aggressive growth histologic pattern. B: Final Mohs surgery defect measuring 4.0 × 4.8 cm to the underlying tendon with preservation of tendon and nerve structures. Complete excision of the tumor required two Mohs stages (10 frozen sections). C: The defect was reconstructed immediately after achievement of clear margins under local anesthesia in the Mohs surgery unit using birhombic flap soft tissue reconstruction. D: Result 3 months after surgery.

treatment have been mentioned previously. Tumors for which maximal conservation of tissue may be important include tumors in the high-risk locations and tumors in young patients.

Adjuvant and Primary Radiation Therapy

Radiation therapy may be useful for primary treatment of low-risk NMSCs. In experienced hands, primary radiation therapy may also be useful for higher-risk tumors with high cure rates. For cutaneous SCC with many high-risk factors and for those with extensive neurotropism, adjuvant prophylactic radiation therapy to the primary site and the primary draining lymph nodes may decrease the risks of local recurrence and regional nodal metastasis. Prophylactic adjuvant radiation therapy should also be considered for highly aggressive, deeply invasive BCCs that exhibit extensive neurotropism.

Other Tumors of Interest

Hundreds of cutaneous tumors exist, and their description is beyond the scope of this chapter. Tumors that may be encountered by the surgeon for further management include Merkel cell carcinoma (MCC), sweat gland carcinoma, and DFSP.

MCC, or primary cutaneous neuroendocrine carcinoma, is an aggressive skin cancer with a higher overall mortality than melanoma (approximately 33% vs. 15%, respectively).[98] The incidence of MCC is low compared to other cutaneous malignancies (approximately 1,500 annually in the United States), but the number of cases has tripled over the last two decades.[99] While UV radiation and immunosuppression are considered important pathogenetic factors, recent findings suggest a virus (Merkel cell polyomavirus) as a contributing factor in the pathogenesis of MCC.[100] MCC most commonly occurs in older, white individuals, with only 5% diagnosed before age 50 years. The majority of tumors (90%) are located on sun-exposed skin, equally distributed between the head and neck and extremities. The remaining 10% are located on the trunk and buttocks. Primary MCC typically presents as a new-onset, growing, red or purple, dome-shaped or subcutaneous nodule, frequently mistaken for a cyst, lipoma, or BCC (Fig. 111.12). The most common location of metastasis is the draining lymph node basin, followed by distant skin, lung, central nervous system, bone, and liver.[101] MCC is a dermal small blue cell tumor with positive immunohistochemical staining for

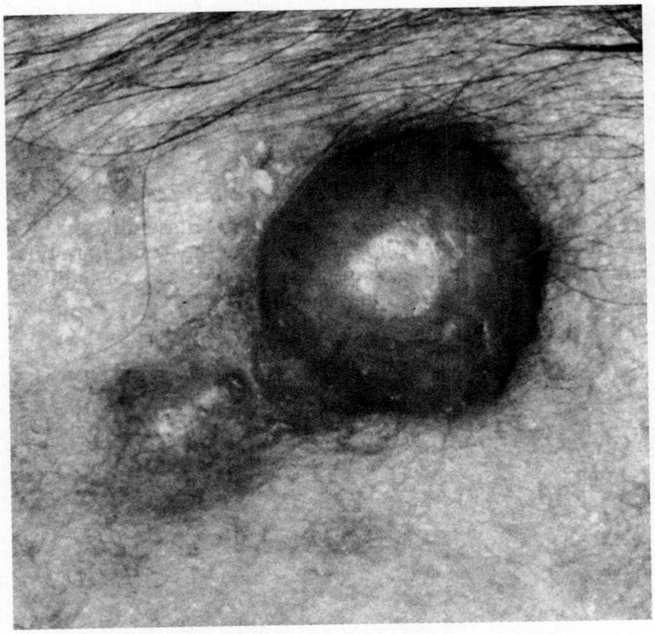

FIGURE 111.12. Merkel cell carcinoma.

cytokeratin-20 (CK-20) in a characteristic paranuclear dot-like pattern. Small cell lung cancer, another neuroendocrine carcinoma histologically indistinguishable from MCC and occasionally CK-20 positive, expresses thyroid transcription factor-1 (TTF-1), which is consistently absent in MCC.[102] Newly proposed AJCC staging for MCC distinguishes stage I (primary tumor <2 cm without nodal disease), stage II (primary tumor ≥2 cm without nodal disease), stage III (nodal metastasis), and stage IV disease (distant metastasis). Five-year survival rates for stage I, II, and III are 81%, 67%, and 52%, respectively. Stage IV disease carries a dismal 11% 2-year survival rate.[98] The majority (70%) of patients with MCC present clinically with localized disease (stage I or II), 25% have palpable lymphadenopathy (stage III), and 5% present with distant metastases (stage IV).[101] Multidisciplinary management of MCC is encouraged by the NCCN.[103,104] Treatment consists of WLE with 1- to 2-cm margins. Adjuvant radiation therapy to the primary site should be considered and is recommended for stage II disease. SLNB with immunostaining using CK-20 is highly recommended for all primary MCC to stage the nodal basin and guide regional nodal therapy.[103,105] Regional lymph node metastases can be treated by regional therapeutic lymphadenectomy and/or radiation therapy. Adjuvant radiation therapy to the regional nodal basin should be considered if SLNB is not performed or is thought to be false negative. For nonsurgical candidates, primary treatment of MCC with radiation therapy may also be considered.[106] Chemotherapy has failed to demonstrate a survival benefit in an adjuvant setting in the treatment of localized or regional MCC and should be reserved for distant metastatic (stage IV) disease.[107]

Sweat gland carcinomas represent a broad scope of neoplasms with variable risk for local, regional, or distant metastasis, most commonly of eccrine or apocrine origin.[108] These are rare tumors (0.005% of skin malignancies) that have multiple histologic subtypes, giving rise to a diverse and confusing nomenclature. The aggressive types of sweat gland carcinomas have a propensity for both local recurrence and regional or systemic metastasis. Clinically, these tumors appear as indurated plaques, papules, or nodules commonly on the head and neck or extremities and are red, blue, pink, or skin colored. Histologic subtypes that are associated with a risk of regional lymph node or systemic metastasis include aggressive digital papillary adenocarcinoma, hidradenocarcinoma, and eccrine carcinoma. Recommended treatments have included wide excision of the primary tumor with consideration of SLNB for high-risk lesions commonly based on size, mitotic rate, growth rate, or immunosuppression.[108] Postoperative radiation may also be considered as adjuvant therapy.

8 DFSP is a rare soft tissue sarcoma (1% of all soft tissue sarcomas) with a propensity for local recurrence rather than systemic metastasis. It is a spindle cell tumor that characteristically demonstrates immunoreactivity to CD34.[109,110] Adults in their third to fifth decades are most commonly affected, but DFSP may occur in children or the elderly. These tumors appear as firm flesh-colored to dull red plaques that may be mistaken for keloids or hypertrophic scars. Although DFSPs may appear discrete, they characteristically demonstrate extensive subclinical involvement, which makes this sarcoma difficult to manage. Histologically, these sarcomas are identified by their fingerlike projections of spindle cells that likely account for tumor recurrence. Standard histologic processing makes it difficult to track these fingerlike projections. Treatment commonly consists of WLE with more comprehensive margin assessment or Mohs surgery, depending on patient and tumor factors. A multidisciplinary approach utilizing the expertise from several fields (Mohs surgery, surgical subspecialties, pathology) may be needed to achieve the goals of tumor excision and reconstructive repair. Radiation may also be beneficial in surgically unresectable cases.[109,110] Imatinib mesylate has shown promsing results in the treatment of unresectable or metastatic DFSP.[111]

References

1. Jemal A, et al. Cancer statistics, 2008. *CA Cancer J Clin* 2008;58:71–96.
2. Diepgen TL, Mahler V. The epidemiology of skin cancer. *Br J Dermatol* 2002;146:1–6.
3. Raimondi S, et al. MC1R variants, melanoma and red hair color phenotype: a meta-analysis. *Int J Cancer* 2008;122:2753–2760.
4. Goldstein AM, et al. Association of MC1R variants and risk of melanoma in melanoma-prone families with CDKN2A mutations. *Cancer Epidemiol Biomarkers Prev* 2005;14:2208–2212.
5. Lynch HT, Shaw TG, Lynch JF. Inherited predisposition to cancer: a historical overview. *Am J Med Genet C Semin Med Genet* 2004;129: 5–22.
6. Lynch HT, Frichot BC, Lynch JF. Famililal atypical multiple mole-melanoma syndrome. *J Med Genet* 1978;15:352–356.
7. Greene MH, et al. High risk of malignant melanoma in melanoma-prone families with dysplastic nevi. *Ann Intern Med* 1985;102(4):458–465.
8. Marghoob AA, Borrego JP, Halpern AC. Congential melanocytic nevi: treatment modalities and management options. *Semin Cutan Med Surg* 2003;22:21–32.
9. Di Rocco F, et al. Neurocutaneous melanosis. *Childs Nerv Syst* 2004;20: 23–28.
10. Bittencourt FV, et al. Large congenital melanocytic nevi and the risk for development of malignant melanoma and neurocutaneous melanocytosis. *Pediatrics* 2000;106:736–741.
11. Abbasi NR, et al. Early diagnosis of cutaneous melanoma: revisiting the ABCD criteria. *JAMA* 2004;292:2771–2776.
12. Buettner PG, et al. Development of prognostic factors and survival in cutaneous melanoma over 25 years: an analysis of the Central Malignant Melanoma Registry of the German Dermatological Society. *Cancer* 2005; 103:616–624.
13. Arora A, et al. Wide excision without radiation for desmoplastic melanoma. *Cancer* 2005;104:1462–1467.
14. Su LD, et al. Desmoplastic and neurotropic melanoma. Analysis of 33 patients with lymphatic mapping and sentinel node biopsy. *Cancer* 2004; 100:598–604.
15. Hawkins WG, et al. Desmoplastic melanoma: a pathologically and clinically distinct form of cutaneous melanoma. *Ann Surg Oncol* 2005;12(3): 207–213.
16. Breslow A. Thickness, cross-sectional area, and depth of invasion in prognosis of cutaneous melanoma. *Ann Surg* 1970;172:902–908.
17. Balch CM, et al. Final version of 2009 American Joint Committee on Cancer staging system for cutaneous melanoma. *J Clin Oncol* 2009;27(36): 6199–6206.
18. Azzola MF, et al. Tumor mitotic rate is a more powerful prognostic indicator than ulceration in patients with primary cutaneous melanoma: an analysis of 3661 patients from a single center. *Cancer* 2003;97(6): 1488–1498.

19. Balch CM, et al. Prognostic factors analysis of 17,600 melanoma patients: validation of the American Joint Committee on Cancer melanoma staging system. *J Clin Oncol* 2001;19(16):3622–3634.
20. Sondak VK, et al. Mitotic rate and younger age are predictors of sentinel lymph node positivity: lessons learned from the generation of a probabilistic model. *Ann Surg Oncol* 2004;11:247–258.
21. Francken AB, et al. The prognostic importance of tumor mitotic rate confirmed in 1317 patients with primary cutaneous melanoma and long follow-up. *Ann Surg Oncol* 2004;11:426–433.
22. Arca MJ, et al. Biopsy techniques for skin, soft-tissue, and bone neoplasms. *Surg Oncol Clin N Am* 1995;4:157–174.
23. http://www.nccn.org/professionals/physician_gls/f_guidelines.asp. August 1, 2010.
24. Johnson TM, et al. Staging workup, sentinel node biopsy, and follow-up tests for melanoma: update of current concepts. *Arch Dermatol* 2004; 140(1):107–113.
25. Wang TS, et al. Evaluation of staging chest radiographs and serum lactate dehydrogenase for localized melanoma. *J Am Acad Dermatol* 2004;51(3): 399–405.
26. Terhune MH, Swanson N, Johnson TM. Use of chest radiography in the initial evaluation of patients with localized melanoma. *Arch Dermatol* 1998;134(5):569–572.
27. Hafner J, et al. Baseline staging in cutaneous malignant melanoma. *Br J Dermatol* 2004;150:677–686.
28. Sabel MS, Wong SL. Review of evidence-based support for pretreatment imaging in melanoma. *JCNN* 2009;7:281–289.
29. Starritt EC, et al. Ultrasound examination of sentinel nodes in the initial assessment of patients with primary cutaneous melanoma. *Ann Surg Oncol* 2005;12:18–23.
30. Crippa F, et al. Which kinds of lymph node metastases can FDG PET detect? A clinical study in melanoma. *J Nucl Med* 2000;41:1491–1494.
31. Wagner JD, et al. Inefficacy of F-18 flourodeoxy-D-glucose-positron emission tomography scans for initial evaluation in early-stage cutaneous melanoma. *Cancer* 2005;104:570–579.
32. Brady MS, et al. Utility of preoperative (18)F flourodeoxyglucose-positron emission tomography scanning in high-risk melanoma patients. *Ann Surg Oncol* 2006;13(4):525–532.
33. Tyler DS, et al. Positron emission tomography scanning in malignant melanoma. Clinical utility in patients with stage III disease. *Cancer* 2000; 89:1019–1025.
34. Blazer DG, Sondak VK, Sabel MS. Surgical therapy of cutaneous melanoma. *Semin Oncol* 2007;34:270–280.
35. Thomas JM, et al. Excision margins in high-risk malignant melanoma. *N Engl J Med* 2004;350(8):757–766.
36. Yeh JJ, et al. The role of abdominoperineal resection as surgical therapy for anorectal melanoma. *Ann Surg* 2006;244:1012–1017.
37. Anderson KW, et al. Treatment of head and neck melanoma, lentigo maligna subtype: a practical surgical technique. *Arch Facial Plast Surg* 2001;3:202–206.
38. Agarwal-Antal N, Bowen GM, Gerwels JW. Histologic evaluation of lentigo maligna with permanent sections: implications regarding current guidelines. *J Am Acad Dermatol* 2002;47:743–748.
39. Chang AE, Karnell LH, Menck HR. The National Cancer Data Base report on cutaneous and noncutaneous melanoma: a summary of 84,836 cases from the past decade. The American College of Surgeons Commission on Cancer and the American Cancer Society. *Cancer* 1998;83: 1664–1678.
40. Johnson TM, et al. The role of sentinel lymph node biopsy for melanoma: evidence assessment. *J Am Acad Dermatol* 2006;54(1):19–27.
41. Morton DL, et al. Technical details of intraoperative lymphatic mapping for early stage melanoma. *Arch Surg* 1992;127:392–399.
42. McMasters KM, et al. Sentinel lymph node biopsy for melanoma: controversy despite widespread agreement. *J Clin Oncol* 2001;19(11):2851–2855.
43. Gershenwald JE, et al. Patterns of recurrence following a negative sentinel lymph node biopsy in 243 patients with stage I or II melanoma. *J Clin Oncol* 1998;16(6):2253–2260.
44. Gershenwald JE, et al. Multi-institutional melanoma lymphatic mapping experience: the prognostic value of sentinel lymph node status in 612 stage I or II melanoma patients. *J Clin Oncol* 1999;17(3):976–983.
45. Cimmino VM, et al. Allergic reactions to isosulfan blue during sentinel node biopsy—a common event. *Surgery* 2001;130:439–442.
46. Karimipour DJ, et al. Standard immunostains for melanoma in sentinel lymph node specimens: which ones are most useful? *J Am Acad Dermotol* 2003;50(5):759–764.
47. Morton DL, et al. Sentinal-node biopsy or nodal observation in melanoma. *NEJM* 2006;355:1307–1317.
48. Puleo CA, et al. Sentinel node biopsy for thin melanomas: which patients should be considered? *Cancer Control* 2005;12(4):230–235.
49. Paek SC, et al. The impact of factors beyond Breslow depth on predicting sentinel lymph node positivity in melanoma. *Cancer* 2007;109(1): 100–108.
50. Bleicher RJ, et al. Role of sentinel lymphadenectomy in thin invasive cutaneous melanomas. *J Clin Oncol* 2003;21(7):1326–1331.
51. Sondak VK, Wolfe JA. Adjuvant therapy for melanoma. *Curr Opin Oncol* 1997;9:189–204.
52. Sosman JA, et al. Adjuvant immunotherapy of resected, intermediate-thickness, node-negative melanoma with an allogeneic tumor vaccine: impact of HLA class I antigen expression on outcome. *J Clin Oncol* 2002; 20(8):2067–2075.
53. Morton DL, et al. An international, randomized, phase II trial of bacillus Calmette-Guerin (BCG) plus allogeneic melanoma vaccine (MCV) or placebo after complete resection of melanoma metastatic to regional or distant sites [Abstract]. *J Clin Oncol* 2007;25(18S):Abstract 8508.
54. Kirkwood JM, et al. Interferon alfa-2b adjuvant therapy of high-risk resected cutaneous melanoma: the Eastern Cooperative Oncology Group Trial EST 1684. *J Clin Oncol* 1996;14(1):7–17.
55. Sabel MS, Sondak VK. Pros and cons of adjuvant interferon in the treatment of melanoma. *Oncologist* 2003;8(5):451–458.
56. Eggermont AMM, et al. The role of isolated limb perfusion for melanoma confined to the extremities. *Surg Clin North Am* 2003;83(2):371–384.
57. Lens MB, Dawes M. Isolated limb perfusion with melphalan in the treatment of malignant melanoma of the extremities: a systematic review of randomised controlled trials. *Lancet Oncol* 2003;4(6):359–364.
58. Fraker DL. Management of in-transit melanoma of the extremity with isolated limb perfusion. *Curr Treat Options Oncol* 2004;5(3):173–184.
59. Thompson JF, Kam PC. Isolated limb infusion for melanoma: a simple but effective alternative to isolated limb perfusion. *J Surg Oncol* 2004;88(1): 1–3.
60. Thompson JF, et al. Isolated limb infusion with cytotoxic agents: a simple alternative to isolated limb perfusion. *Semin Surg Oncol* 1998;14: 238–247.
61. Markowitz JS, et al. Prognosis after initial recurrence of cutaneous melanoma. *Arch Surg* 1991;126:703–707.
62. Karakousis CP, et al. Metastatectomy in malignant melanoma. *Surgery* 1995;115:295–302.
63. Meyer T, et al. Surgical therapy for distant metastases of malignant melanoma. *Cancer* 2000;89:1983–1991.
64. Wong JH, Euhus DM, Morton DL. Surgical resection for metastatic melanoma to the lung. *Arch Surg* 1988;123(9):1091–1095.
65. Tafra L, et al. Resection and adjuvant immunotherapy for melanoma metastatic to the lung and thorax. *J Thorac Cardiovasc Surg* 1995;110: 119–128.
66. Leo F, et al. Lung metastses from melanoma: when is surgical treatment warranted? *Br J Cancer* 2000;83:569–557.
67. Pawlik TM, et al. Hepatic resection for metastatic melanoma: distinct patterns of recurrence and prognosis for ocular versus cutaneous disease. *Ann Surg Oncol* 2006;13(5):712–720.
68. Ollila DW, et al. Surgical resection for melanoma metastatic to the gastrointestinal tract. *Arch Surg* 1996;131:975–979.
69. Stone A, et al. A comparison of survival rates for treatment of melanoma metastatic to the brain. *Cancer Invest* 2004;22:492–497.
70. Ang KK, et al. Postoperative radiotherapy for cutaneous melanoma of the head and neck region. *Int J Radiat Oncol Biol Phys* 1994;30:795–798.
71. Ballo MT, et al. Adjuvant irradiation for cervical lymph node metatases from melanoma. *Cancer* 2003;97(7):1789–1796.
72. Ballo MT, Ang KK. Radiation therapy for malignant melanoma. *Surg Clin N Am* 2003;83(2):323–342.
73. O'Brian CJ, et al. Adjuvant radiotherapy following neck dissection and parotidectomy for metastatic malignant melanoma. *Head Neck* 1997; 19(7):589–594.
74. Chang DT, et al. Adjuvant radiotherapy for cutaneous melanoma: comparing hypofractionation to conventional fractionation. *Int J Radiat Oncol Biol Phys* 2006;66(4):1051–1055.
75. Burmeister BH, et al. A prospective phase II study of adjuvant postoperative radiation therapy following nodal surgery in malignant melanoma: Trans Tasman Radiation Oncology Group (TROG) study 96.06. *Radiother Oncol* 2006;81(2):136–142.
76. Moncrieff MD, et al. Adjuvant postoperative radiotherapy to the cervical lymph nodes in cutaneous melanoma: is there any benefit for high-risk patients? *Ann Surg Oncol* 2008;15(11):3022–3027.
77. Mulé JJ, et al. Adoptive immunotherapy of established pulmonary metastases with LAK cells and recombinant interleukin-2. *Science* 1984;225: 1487.
78. Rosenberg SA, Lotze MT, Muul LM, et al. A progress report on the treatment of 157 patients with advanced cancer using lymphokine activated killer cells and interleukin-2 or interleukin-2 alone. *N Engl J Med* 1987; 316(15):889–897.
79. Sondak VK, Sabel MS, Mulé JJ. Allogeneic and autologous melanoma vaccines: where have we been and where are we going? *Clin Cancer Res* 2006; 12:2337s–2341s.
80. Tsai S, Sabel MS. Translational research in melanoma. *Surg Oncol Clin N Am* 2008;17:391–419.
81. Shimizu K, et al. Systemic administration of interleukin 2 enhances the therapeutic efficacy of dendritic cell-based tumor vaccines. *Proc Natl Acad Sci U S A* 1999;96:2268.
82. Nestle FO, et al. Vaccination of melanoma patients with peptide- or tumor lysate-pulsed dendritic cells. *Nat Med* 1998;4(3):328–332.
83. Sabel MS, et al. CTLA-4 blockade augments human T lymphocyte-mediated suppression of lung tumor xenografts in SCID mice. *Cancer Immunol Immunother* 2005;54:944–952.
84. Attia P, et al. Autoimmunity correlates with tumor regression in patients with metastatic melanoma treated with anti-CTLA4. *J Clin Oncol* 2005; 23:6043–6053.
85. Ribas A, et al. Antitumor activity in melanoma and anti-self responses in a phase I trial with the anti-CTLA-4 monoclonal antibody CP-675206. *J Clin Oncol* 2005;23:8968–8977.

86. Rosenberg SA, et al. Treatment of patients wtih metastatic melanoma with autologous tumor-infiltrating lymphocytes and interleukin-2. *J Natl Cancer Inst* 1994;86:1159–1166.
87. Rosenberg SA, Dudley ME. Cancer regression in patients with metastatic melanoma after the transfer of autologous antitumor lymphocytes. *Proc Natl Acad Sci U S A* 2004;101(suppl 2):14639–14645.
88. Chang AE, et al. Adoptive immunotherapy with vaccine-primed lymph node cells secondarily activated with anti-CD3 and interleukin-2. *J Clin Oncol* 1997;15:796–807.
89. Chang AE, et al. Clinical observations on adoptive immunotherapy with vaccine-primed T-lymphocytes secondarily sensitized to tumor in vitro. *Cancer Res* 1993;53:1043–1050.
90. Chang AE, Li Q, Jiang G, et al. Phase II trial of autologous tumor vaccination, anti-CD3-activated vaccine-primed lymphocytes, and interleukin-2 in stage IV renal cell cancer. *J Clin Oncol* 2003;21(5):884–890.
91. Morgan RA, et al. Cancer regression in patients after transfer of genetically engineered lymphocytes. *Science* 2006;314:126–129.
92. Buzaid AC. Management of metastatic cutaneous melanoma. *Oncology (Huntington)* 2004;18:1443–1450.
93. Legha SS, et al. Development of a biochemotherapy regimen with concurrent administration of cisplatin, vinblastine, dacarbazine, interferon alfa and interleukin-2 for patients with metastatic melanoma. *J Clin Oncol* 1998;16:1752–1759.
94. Ridolfi R, Chiarion-Sileni V, Guida M, et al; Italian Melanoma Intergroup. Cisplatin, dacarbazine with or without subcutaneous interleukin-2, and inteferon alpha-2b in advanced melanoma outpatients: results from an Italian multicenter phase III randomized clinical trial. *J Clin Oncol* 2002; 20:1600–1607.
95. Eton O, et al. Sequential biochemotherapy versus chemotherapy for metastatic melanoma: results from a phase III randomized trial. *J Clin Oncol* 2002;20:2045–2052.
96. Atkins MB, et al. Phase III trial comparing concurrent biochemotherapy with cisplatin, vinblastine, dacarbazine, interleukin-2 and interferon alfa-2b with cisplatin, vinblastine, and dacarbazine alone in patients with metastatic malignant melanoma (E3695): a trial coordinated by the Eastern Cooperative Oncology Group. *J Clin Oncol* 2008;26(35):5748–5754.
97. Ives NJ, et al. Chemotherapy compared with biochemotherapy for the treatment of metastatic melanoma: a meta-analysis of 18 trials involving 2,621 patients. *J Clin Oncol* 2007;25(34):5426–5434.
98. Allen PJ, et al. Merkel cell carcinoma: prognosis and treatment of patients from a single institution. *J Clin Oncol* 2005;23(10):2300–2309.
99. Hodgson NC. Merkel cell carcinoma: changing incidence trends. *J Surg Oncol* 2005;89(1):1–4.
100. Feng H, et al. Clonal integration of a polyomavirus in human Merkel cell carcinoma. *Science* 2008;319(5856):1096–1100.
101. Medina-Franco H, et al. Multimodality treatment of Merkel cell carcinoma: case series and literature review of 1024 cases. *Ann Surg Oncol* 2001;8:204–208.
102. Bobos M, et al. Immunohistochemical distinction between Merkel cell carcinoma and small cell carcinoma of the lung. *Am J Dermatopathol* 2006; 28:99–104.
103. Bichakjian CK, et al. Merkel cell carcinoma: critical review with guidelines for multidisciplinary management. *Cancer* 2007;110(1):1–12.
104. National Comprehensive Cancer Network. http://www.nccn.org/professionals/physician_gls/PDF/mcc.pdf. Accessed December 7, 2008.
105. Su LD, et al. Immunostaining for cytokeratin 20 improves detection of micrometastatic Merkel cell carcinoma in sentinel lymph nodes. *J Am Acad Dermatol* 2002;46(5):661–666.
106. Mortier L, Mirabel X, Fournier C, et al. Radiotherapy alone for primary Merkel cell carcinoma. *Arch Dermatol* 2003;139(12):1587–1590.
107. Poulsen MG, et al. Does chemotherapy improve survival in high-risk stage I and II Merkel cell carcinoma of the skin? *Int J Radiat Oncol Biol Phys* 2006;64(1):114–119.
108. Bogner PN, et al. Lymphatic mapping and sentinel lymph node biopsy in the detection of early metastases from sweat gland carcinoma. *Cancer* 2003;97:2285–2289.
109. Dubay D, et al. Low recurrence rate after surgery for dermatofibrosarcoma protuberans: a multidisciplinary approach from a single institution. *Cancer* 2004;100:1008–1016.
110. National Comprehensive Cancer Network. http://www.nccn.org/professionals/physician_gls/pdf/dfsp.pdf. Accessed December 7, 2008.
111. McArthur GA, et al. Molecular and clinical analysis of locally advanced dermatofibrosarcoma protuberans treated with imatinib: Imatinib Target Exploration Consortium Study B2225. *J Clin Oncol* 2005;23(4):866–873.

CHAPTER 112 ■ SARCOMAS OF SOFT TISSUE AND BONE

SANDRA L. WONG

KEY POINTS

1. Sarcomas are a rare and heterogeneous group of cancers that arise from mesoderm-derived elements such as muscle, fat, nerve/nerve sheath, cartilage, blood vessels, bone, and other connective tissue. They are distinguished from cancers of epithelial origin.
2. Clinical behavior and prognosis are largely defined by anatomic location, tumor grade, size, and completeness of surgical resection.
3. For extremity sarcomas, limb-sparing procedures are used to maximize functional outcomes. Radiotherapy is used for high-risk tumors to decrease disease relapse and improve survival.
4. Surgical resection is the cornerstone of treatment for intra-abdominal or retroperitoneal sarcomas. Complete resection may require en bloc resection of adjacent organs, most commonly of the kidney and colon.
5. The successful use of imatinib, a selective tyrosine kinase inhibitor, in the contemporary management of gastrointestinal stromal tumors is a paradigm for targeted molecular therapies.
6. Use of multimodality therapies including surgical resection, chemotherapy, and radiotherapy have dramatically improved outcomes for bone sarcomas such as osteosarcoma and Ewing sarcoma.

Sarcomas are a heterogeneous group of cancers that arise from mesenchymal cells, or mesoderm-derived elements, including muscle, fat, nerve/nerve sheath, cartilage, blood vessels, bone, and other connective tissue. Sarcomas of soft tissue and bone are considered two distinct categories. Though mesoderm-derived elements constitute nearly two thirds of the body's mass, sarcomas are relatively rare. In 2010, an estimate of just over 10,000 new cases of soft tissue sarcoma were expected to
1 be diagnosed in the United States,[1] which accounts for less than 1% of all new cancers. Sarcomas also represent an extremely heterogeneous group of cancers, but taken together, 5-year overall survival is about 50% to 60%.[2,3] Anatomic location, tumor size, grade, and histopathology are important determinants of clinical presentation, treatment, and prognosis.

The Greek word "sarkoma," meaning 'fleshy excrescence,' is the origin for the term *sarcoma*. As early as CE 130–200, these fleshy tumors were regarded as cancerous by Galen.[4] With the evolution of light microscopy and cellular pathology, there was increasing recognition of soft tissue sarcomas. Sarcomas, then called "soft cancers," were differentiated from carcinomas by neuroanatomist Charles Bell as early as 1816. Virchow refined the definition of sarcoma as "new formations of connective tissue" and developed classifications according to microscopic features that separated sarcomas from carcinomas of epithelial origin. Modern foundations for the description and histogenic descriptions of sarcoma are attributed to the work of James Ewing, who over the course of his pathology career refined the classification of sarcomas, including the importance of grade in disease outcome.[5]

Multimodality therapies, including surgery, radiation, and chemotherapy, have been combined to improve local and systemic tumor control. Over the past few decades, a multidisciplinary approach has moved treatment options from radical amputation to limb-sparing procedures. As refinements in pathologic classification continue, so does progress in the use of treatment modalities. Modern molecular diagnostics are increasingly being translated to clinical practice, and tailored treatment options are being developed as the histologic diversity of soft tissue sarcomas is continually elucidated.

Epidemiology

Soft tissue sarcomas can occur in all age groups and are equally distributed between genders. Although the median age at diagnosis varies by histopathologic subtype, sarcomas are among the most common cancers that occur in children and young adults. Though sarcomas are relatively rare in the adult population, these tumors represent approximately 15% of pediatric malignancies and often occur in children younger than 5 years of age.[6] Sarcomas can occur at any anatomic site, though most arise in the extremities and trunk (Fig. 112.1). Histopathologic subtype distribution is variable by anatomic site, and anatomic site influences treatment and outcomes (Fig. 112.2).

Although the vast majority of sarcomas arise spontaneously, there are some predisposing conditions to consider. Sarcomas are not thought to be the result of malignant degeneration of a long-standing benign lesion such as a lipoma. A traumatic incident may lead to the initial recognition of a mass, but there are no data to support the notion that antecedent trauma leads to the development of soft tissue or bony sarcomas. Clinical evaluation and subsequent workup, including biopsy if indicated, should be able to distinguish malignant growths from various benign posttraumatic lesions, such as myositis ossificans, which must be differentiated from an extraosseous osteogenic sarcoma.

Toxic exposures leading to the development of sarcoma are largely of historic interest. For example, industrial use of thorium dioxide (Thorotrast), arsenic, and vinyl chloride led to accumulation of toxins in the liver and were associated with the development of hepatic angiosarcomas. Various types of radiation have been implicated in the later development of sarcomas. For example, ingestion of luminous paint containing ^{226}radium by factory workers led to the development of osteosarcomas. With the increasing use of external beam radiation in cancer treatment, there has been a noted increase in the modern incidence of sarcoma in patients treated with radiation for various malignancies. Following median latent periods of approximately 8 years (range 6–20 years), radiation-associated sarcomas are being increasingly diagnosed in previously radiated areas. Common radiation-associated sarcoma subtypes are malignant fibrous histiocytoma, fibrosarcoma, angiosarcoma, and leiomyosarcoma, and they are commonly, but not uniformly, high grade.[7,8] Notably, with the advent of breast conservation therapy for breast cancer (lumpectomy and radiation therapy), there should be an appropriate index of suspicion for breast angiosarcomas with findings of skin changes on the breast (Fig. 112.3).

Several other predisposing conditions are known to be associated with the development of sarcoma. The classic Stewart-Treves syndrome was originally described in patients with lymphedema following radical mastectomy and radiation for breast cancer who then developed lymphangiosarcoma of the affected arm.[9] Since then, long-standing extremity edema from other causes has also been linked to the development of lymphangiosarcomas. Kaposi sarcoma was previously an

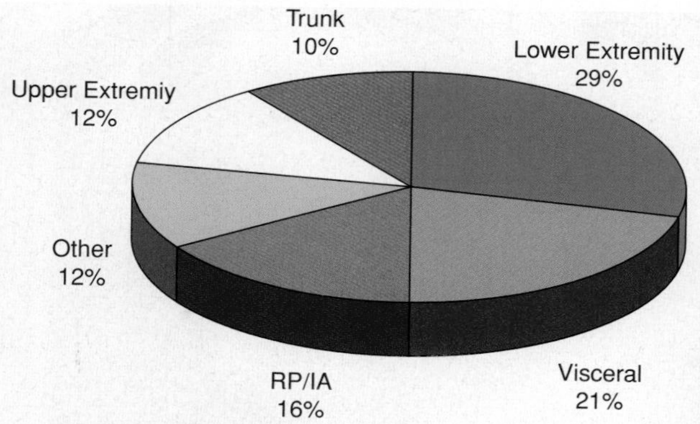

FIGURE 112.1. Classification of sarcomas by anatomic location. More than 50% of sarcomas are located in the trunk or extremities. RP/IA, retroperitoneum intra-abdominal sites. Visceral sites include gastrointestinal tract, gynecologic, and genitourinary tract tumors. From 7,527 cases at Memorial Sloan-Kettering Cancer Center, July 1982 to December 2007. (Courtesy of Murray F. Brennan, MD, Memorial Sloan-Kettering Cancer Center, New York, NY.)

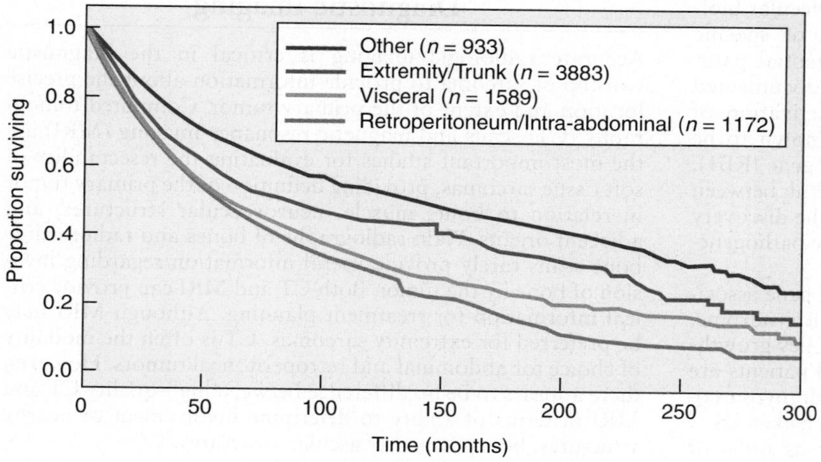

FIGURE 112.2. Classification of sarcomas by anatomic location and long-term outcomes. Overall survival is influenced by primary site of disease. Visceral category includes gastrointestinal tract, gynecologic, and genitourinary tract tumors. From 7,527 cases at Memorial Sloan-Kettering Cancer Center, July 1982 to December 2007. (Courtesy of Murray F. Brennan, MD, Memorial Sloan-Kettering Cancer Center, New York, NY.)

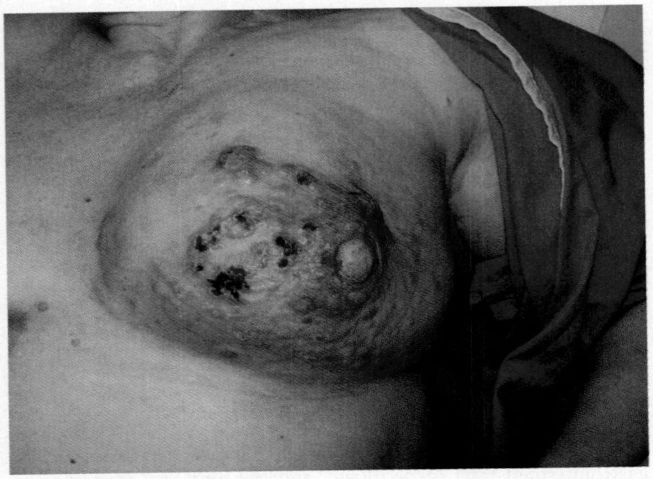

FIGURE 112.3. Radiation-associated angiosarcoma. This 79-year-old woman developed skin changes on her breast 7 years after breast conservation therapy (lumpectomy and radiation therapy) for a 2 cm invasive ductal adenocarcinoma. Salvage mastectomy was performed.

uncommon cutaneous vascular tumor thought limited to elderly men of Mediterranean origin. In the early 1980s it became one of the first described opportunistic diseases associated with HIV infection. Though the incidence of HIV-associated Kaposi sarcoma has markedly declined with effective antiretroviral therapy, it remains an important cause of morbidity among HIV-infected patients and other immunosuppressed patients such as renal allograft recipients.[10–12]

A genetic predisposition to sarcoma occurs in patients with neurofibromatosis type 1 (NF-1, or von Recklinghausen disease), and malignant peripheral nerve sheath tumors (MPNST) develop in an estimated 5% of patients over a lifetime.[13] A genetic predisposition to desmoid tumors or desmoid fibromatosis is associated with familial adenomatous polyposis (FAP), or Gardner syndrome.[14,15] Intra-abdominal and extremity desmoids are a common extracolonic manifestation of FAP and can be a source of increased morbidity in these patients following proctocolectomy for the prevention or treatment of colon cancer.[16]

MOLECULAR BIOLOGY AND DIAGNOSTICS

Although the vast majority of sarcomas are sporadic, numerous genetic alterations are associated with both bone and soft tissue sarcomas.[17] Better understanding of the molecular biology of sarcomas has revolutionized diagnosis of specific histopathologic subtypes and has elucidated potential pathways for targeted molecular therapy. One well-documented mechanism of sarcoma development is the inactivation of tumor suppressor genes. Retinoblastoma was known to be associated with a mutation in the retinoblastoma gene (RB1), a 13q chromosomal deletion. Investigation of the link between familial retinoblastoma and osteosarcoma led to the discovery that a genetic defect in RB1 also plays a role in the pathogenesis of sarcomas.[18,19]

Another inherited defect of a tumor suppressor gene associated with soft tissue sarcomas is the Li-Fraumeni syndrome, caused by an inherited mutation in the p53 gene, a key growth-regulatory gene.[20] Germline mutations in affected patients are associated with high incidences of childhood rhabdomyosarcomas, breast cancer, brain tumors, lung cancer, and leukemias.[21] p53 abnormalities may be present in as many as 60% of osteosarcomas and malignant fibrous histiocytomas, as well as approximately 33% of other sarcomas.[22] Several oncogenes that can induce malignant transformation and drive proliferation have also been associated with sarcoma development, including amplifications of N-myc, c-erbB2, and members of the *ras* family.[23]

Cytogenetic aberrations have been recognized in several soft tissue sarcomas.[17] Several histologic subtypes of sarcomas have each been found to have specific genetic alterations—usually simple karyotypes including fusion genes due to reciprocal translocations or specific point mutations (Table 112.1). These chromosomal translocations serve as powerful diagnostic markers and may be important in determining tumor biology and subsequent tumor behavior. For example, identification of the translocation of t(X;18)(p11;q11) can confirm the diagnosis of synovial sarcoma if there is any doubt of its histopathology. There are data to suggest that the SYT-SSX1 fusion transcript carries a worse prognosis than the SYT-SSX2 fusion transcript, with median survivals of 6.1 years and 13.7 years, respectively.[24,25]

SOFT TISSUE SARCOMAS

Clinical Presentation

The most common presentation of a soft tissue sarcoma is that of an asymptomatic mass. Sarcomas tend to grow in a centrifugal fashion, pushing surrounding structures away rather than directly invading them. Such compression generally does not produce pain, swelling, or obstructive symptoms until the tumors become quite large. Because of surrounding anatomic structures, tumors of the extremities tend to be detected at a relatively smaller size, whereas tumors of the retroperitoneum are infrequently smaller than 10 cm at time of presentation.[5] Even very large abdominal or retroperitoneal sarcomas present with nonspecific abdominal symptoms such as fullness, early satiety, or minor abdominal discomfort (Fig. 112.4). The differential diagnosis for a soft tissue sarcoma includes many types of benign lesions (e.g., lipomas, leiomyomas, neuromas) but also other malignant lesions (e.g., primary or metastatic carcinoma, melanoma, lymphoma).

In general, the vast majority of soft tissue masses tend to be benign, but concerning features that should prompt a higher index of suspicion for malignancy include large size (>5 cm), deep location (subfascial, intramuscular, intra-abdominal), variations in texture on examination, immobile nature or noted fixation to underlying structures, or changes to an existing lesion (increasing size or worsening compressive symptoms). No tumor markers for sarcomas exist, so serum blood work is generally not useful in the evaluation of soft tissue masses.

Diagnostic Imaging

Accurate radiologic imaging is critical in the diagnostic workup of sarcoma to provide information about the precise location and extent of the primary tumor. Computed tomography (CT) scans and magnetic resonance imaging (MRI) are the most important studies for evaluating the resectability of soft tissue sarcomas, providing definition of the primary tumor in relation to bone, muscle, neurovascular structures, and adjacent organs. Plain radiographs of bones and radionuclide bone scans rarely provide useful information regarding invasion of bone by the tumor. Both CT and MRI can provide critical information for treatment planning. Although MRI may be preferred for extremity sarcomas, CT is often the modality of choice for abdominal and retroperitoneal tumors. However, there appears to be no difference between high-quality CT and MRI in terms of ability to determine involvement of nearby structures, bone, or neurovascular structures.[26–28]

TABLE 112.1

CYTOGENETIC ABNORMALITIES IN SOFT TISSUE SARCOMA SUBTYPES

HISTOLOGIC SUBTYPE	CHROMOSOMAL TRANSLOCATION	FUSION GENE
Alveolar rhabdomyosarcoma	t(2;13)(q35;q14)	PAX3-FKHR
	t(1;13)(p36;q14)	PAX7-FKHR
Alveolar soft part sarcoma	t(X;17)(p11;q25)	ASPL-TFE3
Clear cell sarcoma	t(12;22)(q13;q12)	EWS-ATF1
Desmoplastic small round cell tumor	t(11;22)(p13;q12)	EWS-WT1
Dermatofibrosarcoma protuberans	t(17;22)(q21;q13)	COL1A1-PDGFB
Endometrial stromal sarcoma	t(7;17)(p15;q21)	JAZF1-JJAZ1
Ewing sarcoma/PNET	t(11;22)(q24;q12)	EWS-FLI1
	t(11;22)(q22;q12)	EWS-ERG
Extraskeletal myxoid chondrosarcoma	t(9;22)(p13;q12)	EWS-CHN
	t(9;17)(q22;q11)	TAF2 N-NR4A3
	t(9;15)(q22;q11)	TCF12-NR4A3
Fibrosarcoma	t(12;15)(p13;q26)	ETV6-NTRK3
Inflammatory myofibroblastic tumor	t(1;2)(q22;p23)	TPM3-ALK
	t(2;19)(p23;p13)	TPM4-ALK
	t(2;17)(p23;q23)	CLTC-ALK
	t(2;2)(p23;q13)	RANB2-ALK
Fibromyxoid sarcoma	t(7;16)(q33;p11)	FUS-CREB3L2
	t(11;16)(p11;p11)	FUS-CREB3L1
Myxoid and round cell liposarcoma	t(12;16)(q13;p11)	TLS-CHOP
	t(12;16)(q13;p12)	
Synovial sarcoma	t(X;18)(p11;q11)	SYT-SSX1
		SYT-SSX2

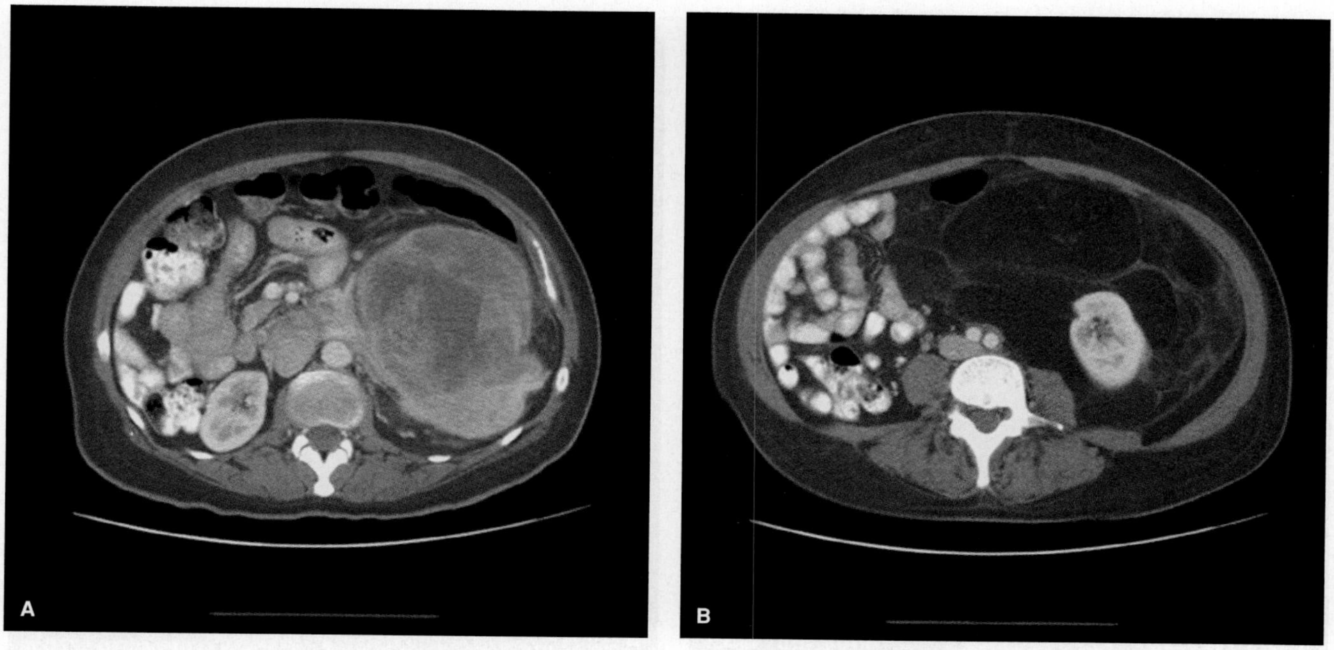

FIGURE 112.4. Dedifferentiated liposarcoma of the retroperitoneum. This 51-year-old woman presented with only vague symptoms of abdominal fullness from a very large retroperitoneal mass. The CT scan demonstrates a heterogeneous soft tissue mass in the upper abdomen (**A**), which blends into a more fatty component (**B**) that encases the left kidney and displaces abdominal contents. She underwent radical resection en bloc left nephrectomy, distal pancreatectomy, splenectomy, left colectomy, and segmental resection of inferior vena cava.

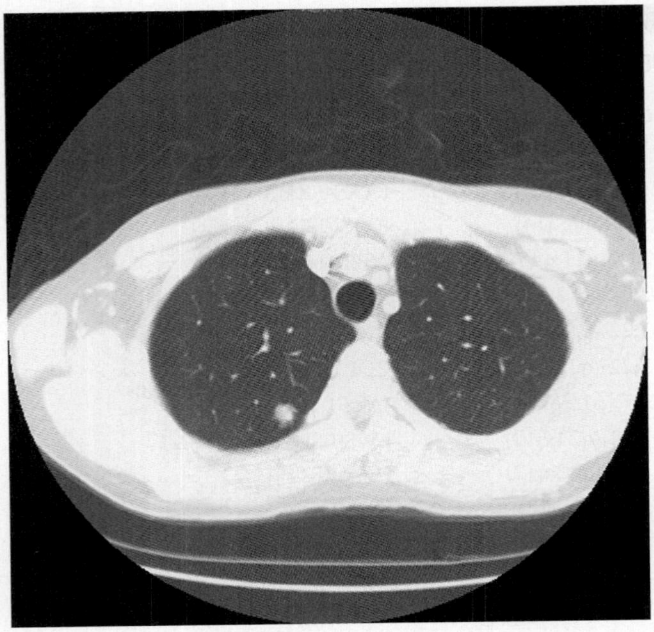

FIGURE 112.5. Pulmonary metastasis. A noncontrasted CT scan of the thorax demonstrates a 1.1-cm noncalcified nodule consistent with pulmonary metastasis in the upper lobe of the right lung.

Imaging is also important as part of the extent of disease workup. Because sarcomas are known to metastasize predominantly to the lungs, directed chest imaging should be performed at time of diagnosis. Chest radiography (CXR) may be used, but CT scans are increasingly being used as the screening examination of choice for patients with high-grade lesions or tumors larger than 5 cm.[29] Any abnormal CXR must be followed by a CT scan for more detailed evaluation of potential pulmonary metastases (Fig. 112.5). CT of the chest, abdomen, and pelvis should be considered in any patient with a myxoid liposarcoma of an extremity because this subtype often metastasizes to the abdomen or other "fat pads" such as the axilla.[30]

MRI is the most commonly used imaging modality for extremity sarcomas.[26,31] Sequencing routinely involves axial T2-weighted and precontrast/postcontrast T1-weighted images. Contrast enhancement with gadolinium is crucial for detecting and characterizing lesions with coronal, sagittal, and other reconstructions. This imaging modality can accurately delineate between muscle groups and distinguish among tumor and neurovascular structures (Fig. 112.6). Magnetic resonance angiography (MRA) can be performed if more accurate delineation of vascular structures is required for treatment planning.

Positron emission tomography (PET) scanning using fluoro-13-deoxyglucose also offers the potential for noninvasive analysis of tumor metabolism and has been shown to correlate with both tumor grade and response to treatment for many types of cancers.[32–35] PET may be helpful in distinguishing between benign and malignant lesions and may be useful for assessing response to treatment.[36] However, its accuracy and potential for false-negative results are still incompletely defined so its use is not routine.

Diagnostic Biopsy

Properly performed biopsies are critical in directing a multimodality treatment approach. Image-guided techniques are increasingly being applied so that open biopsy is not mandatory. Fine-needle aspiration (FNA) is frequently used for the evaluation of enlarged lymph nodes, thyroid nodules, or breast masses. However, FNA often does not provide sufficient material for histopathologic diagnosis. Core-needle biopsy (CNB) is considered the initial procedure of choice for diagnosis of soft tissue sarcomas.[37] CNB retrieves sufficient material for immunohistochemical staining, and when necessary, for cytogenetic analysis or flow cytometry. Image-guided CNB, using either computed tomography (CT) or ultrasound (US), allows for the biopsy of deep masses that may not be easily palpable and can help target suspicious areas for better diagnostic value. An adequate sample

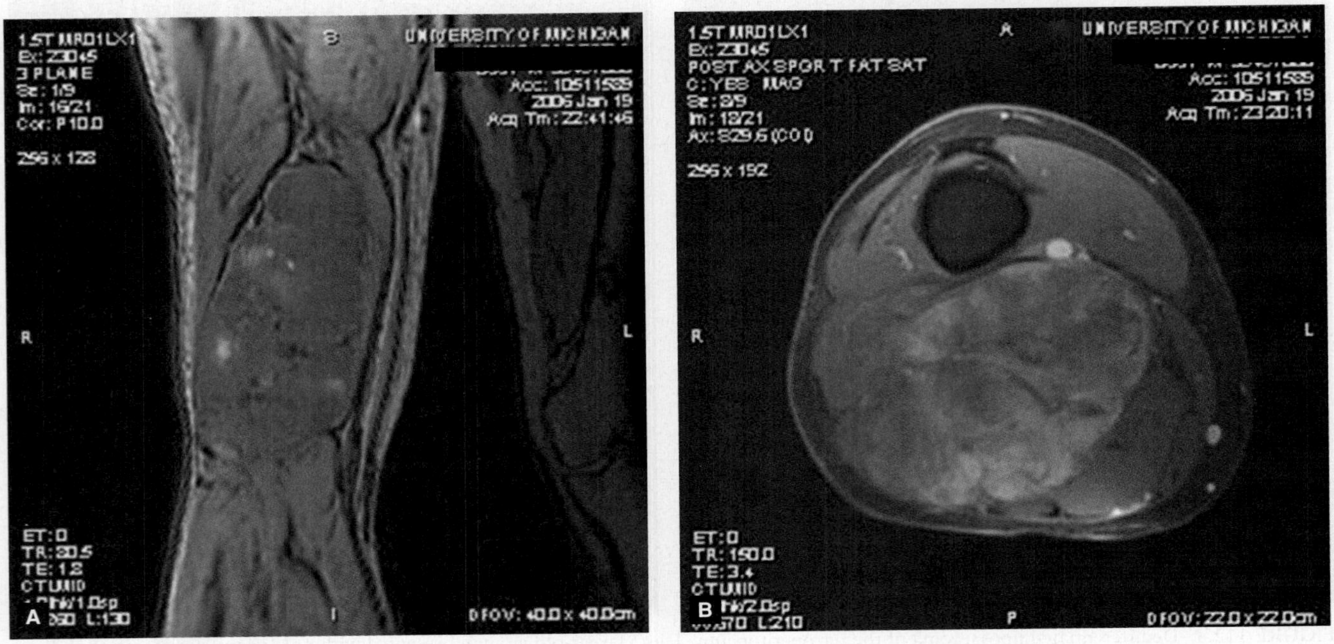

FIGURE 112.6. Extremity sarcoma. MRI demonstrates a 2-cm low-grade myxoid liposarcoma. **A:** Coronal reconstruction demonstrates location in the distal right thigh. **B:** Axial images show displacement of the popliteal vessels and vastus medialis anteriorly; the common tibioperoneal nerve and biceps femoris laterally; and the semimembranosus and semitendinosus muscles medially.

from a viable area of sarcoma is required for definitive diagnosis and accurate grading.

Open surgical biopsy, or incisional biopsy, is uncommonly needed with increasing success of CNB. However, open biopsy should be considered when core-needle specimens yield nondiagnostic findings and if preoperative diagnosis is definitely required for treatment planning. Several important technical factors must be considered when performing an incisional biopsy. Incisions must be oriented along the long axis of extremities to facilitate definitive management. A transverse incision in the extremity often commits the patient to more extensive procedures than would be otherwise necessary, potentially compromising the ability to obtain clear margins with definitive limb-sparing procedures. Attempts to enucleate the sarcoma within its pseudocapsule are discouraged though excisional biopsy can be considered as the primary approach for small, superficial lesions.[5]

Pathologic Classification

Histopathologic designations of soft tissue sarcomas reflect an extremely heterogeneous group of tumors. Sarcomas are generally classified according to the tissues they mimic rather than the type of tissue from which the tumor arises. Some sarcomas have no recognizable normal tissue counterpart and are characterized by other distinguishing histologic features.[5,38] The various types of benign and malignant soft tissue tumors are noted in Table 112.2. The development of specialized markers for identifying individual types of sarcoma has led to greater precision in their classification. Helpful immunohistochemical stains include the intermediate filaments (i.e., vimentin, keratin) and muscle markers (i.e., desmin, actin). More specific markers can be instrumental in diagnosis, such as myoglobin staining for rhabdomyosarcomas. In a small proportion of tumors (approximately 10% in most series), the tumor cells are so poorly differentiated that no specific histogenesis can be determined, and these may be designated as spindle cell sarcomas or pleomorphic sarcomas.

One of the most critical pieces of pathologic information for clinicians treating sarcoma patients is histologic grade. Histologic grade is assessed based on the degree of cellular atypia, the frequency of mitotic figures, and the presence or absence of spontaneous tumor necrosis. Although grading criteria have undergone numerous revisions over the years, in general, low-grade tumors have relatively little cellular atypia, few mitoses, and no tumor necrosis. High-grade tumors show a significant degree of necrosis in addition to atypia and frequent mitotic figures (Fig. 112.7). A consistently applied grading system discriminates between tumors with good prognosis (low grade) and those with poorer prognosis (high grade). In the past, a three-grade system has been used (low, intermediate, high), and until recently the American Joint Commission on Cancer (AJCC) used a classification system ranging from well-differentiated (G1) to undifferentiated (G4)[39–41] tumors, though in 2010, that was changed to a three-teir system. There can be disagreement about grading schemas, and expert pathology opinion can vary from center to center.[42,43] As such, it is important to take note of tumor classification when interpreting results from clinical trials or retrospective reports.[44] The metastatic potential for low-grade lesions is approximately 5% to 10% and up to 50% to 60% for high-grade tumors.[2] For lesions in which disparate areas exist, the highest grade encountered is generally used to categorize the tumor.

Staging

Because of the prognostic importance of staging, stage classification of the primary tumor is based on both clinical and
2 histologic information. The usual TNM classification used by the AJCC[41] for other solid tumors is modified to a GTNM system (Table 112.3) for soft tissue sarcomas. For the practical purposes of staging, well-differentiated and moderately differentiated tumors (grades 1 and 2) are considered together as low grade, whereas poorly differentiated and undifferentiated tumors (grades 3 and 4) are considered together as high grade.

TABLE 112.2 **CLASSIFICATION**

HISTOLOGIC CLASSIFICATION OF SOFT TISSUE TUMORS

■ CONNECTIVE TISSUE	■ BENIGN SOFT TISSUE TUMOR	■ MALIGNANT SOFT TISSUE TUMOR (SARCOMA)
Fat	Lipoma	Liposarcoma
Fibrous tissue	Fibroma	Fibrosarcoma
Skeletal muscle	Rhabdomyoma	Rhabdomyosarcoma
Smooth muscle	Leiomyoma	Leiomyosarcoma
Bone	Osteoma	Osteosarcoma
Cartilage	Chondroma	Chondrosarcoma
Synovium	Synovioma	Synovial sarcoma
Blood vessels	Hemangioma Hemangiopericytoma	Angiosarcoma
Lymphatics	Lymphangioma	Lymphangiosarcoma
Nerve	Neurofibroma	Neurofibrosarcoma
Mesothelium	Benign mesothelioma	Malignant mesothelioma
Histiocytes	Benign fibrous histiocytoma	Malignant fibrous histiocytoma
Uncertain		Ewing sarcoma Alveolar soft parts tumor Epithelioid sarcoma

SURGICAL SPECIALITIES

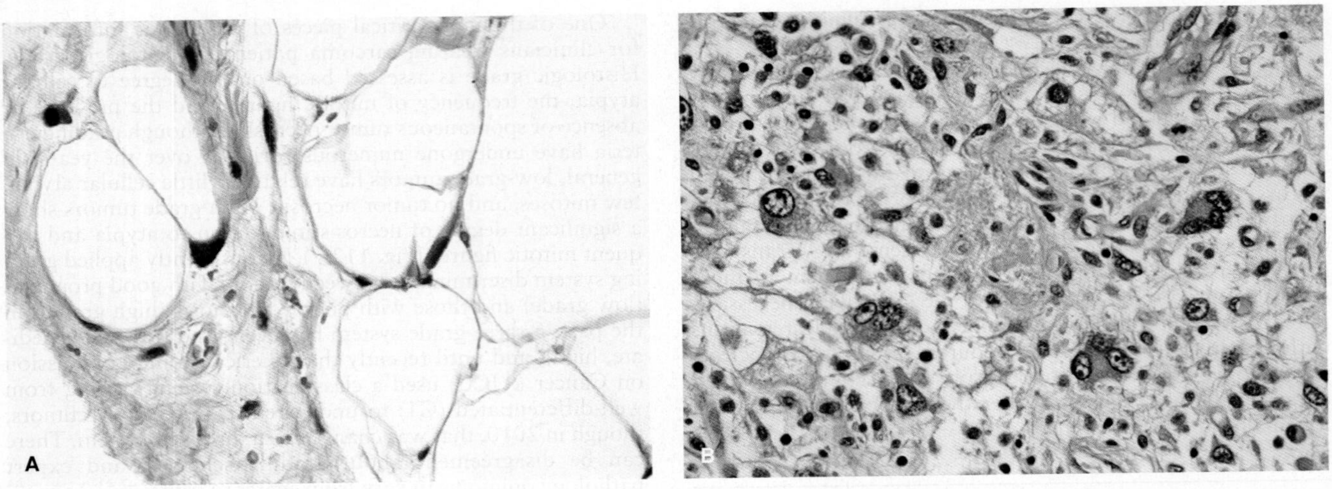

FIGURE 112.7. Histologic grading of sarcomas. Photomicrographs demonstrate the appearance of different grades within the same histologic subtype. **A:** Well-differentiated liposarcoma (lipoma-like) of the retroperitoneum with noted few atypical lipoblasts. **B:** High-grade, dedifferentiated liposarcoma of the retroperitoneum with highly atypical lipoblasts. (Courtesy of David R. Lucas, MD, University of Michigan, Ann Arbor, MI.)

The primary tumor is categorized according to size (<5 cm = T1, >5 cm = T2) and depth relative to the fascia (entirely above the fascia, or superficial = a; invading or entirely below the fascia, or deep = b). Because depth of tumor seemed to add significant prognostic information, this distinction was added to the 1998 edition of the AJCC staging system. One series of 215 patients with superficial extremity sarcomas documented a 10-year survival rate of 85% although 53% of tumors were high grade and 25% of tumors were 5 cm or larger.[45] Though the cutoff between small and large tumors is 5 cm, tumors larger than 10 cm seem to have an even worse prognosis.[46] When 316 patients with soft tissue sarcoma were grouped into four subgroups (<5 cm, 5–10 cm, 10–15 cm, and >15 cm) each subgroup had a distinct prognosis (84%, 70%, 50%, and 33%, respectively).[47]

For nonmetastatic sarcomas, the AJCC staging system is clinically useful because it assigns patients into groups with clearly different prognoses (Fig. 112.8). Nodal metastasis of soft tissue sarcomas is rare (less than 5% of cases), with the exception of a few histologic subtypes for which the incidence of nodal involvement may be between 10% and 20%. These subtypes include angiosarcoma, embryonal rhabdomyosarcoma, epithelioid sarcoma, synovial sarcoma, and clear cell sarcoma.[48] By far the most common site of metastasis is the lungs though metastases to other sites do occur. Unlike other solid organ tumors, when node involvement occurs in sarcomas, it conveys essentially the same prognosis as distant metastatic disease and therefore is classified as stage IV disease.

Treatment

Principles of Surgical Resection. Complete surgical resection remains the cornerstone of treatment for soft tissue sarcomas. Performing a wide excision of the tumor with negative margins is the goal of resection with curative intent. Compartmental excision, or enucleation, usually results in inadequate resection and should be avoided. Technical aspects of resection must take into consideration the anatomic location and extent of disease. Often, soft tissue sarcomas are surrounded by a zone of compressed reactive tissue that forms a pseudocapsule. Care should be taken to avoid entry into the tumor and pseudocapsule during the course of dissection. Enucleation commonly results in microscopically positive margins, and patients evaluated after such resections should undergo re-resection, even if they have no clinical or radiographic evidence of residual tumor, recognizing that anatomic location may preclude effective clearance of margins even with a second operation.

Metallic clips placed in the tumor bed following resection can help define the limits of resection and aid in planning of future treatment. Suction drainage catheters are routinely used to obviate postoperative seroma formation following resection of extremity or truncal sarcomas. Drains should be placed

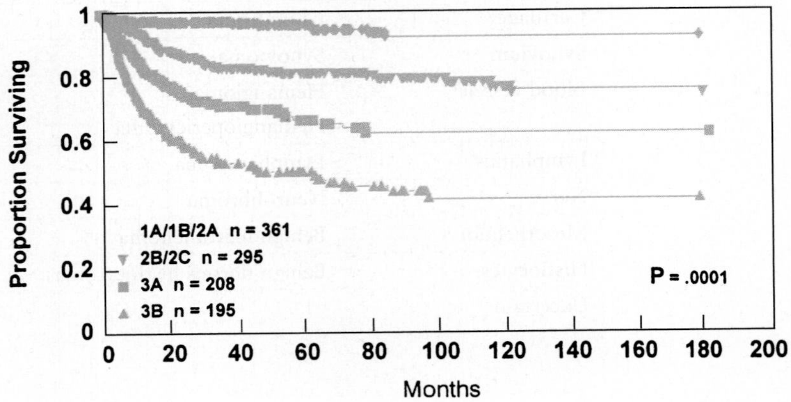

FIGURE 112.8. Survival rates according to the American Joint Committee on Cancer (AJCC) staging system. Patients with soft tissue sarcoma were categorized by tumor depth, grade, and size. 3A designates stage III tumors of 5 to 10 cm, and 3B designates stage III tumors greater than 10 cm in size. (Reproduced with permission from Brennan MF. Staging of soft tissue sarcomas. *Ann Surg Oncol.* 1999;6:8–9.)

TABLE 112.3 CLASSIFICATION

AMERICAN JOINT COMMISSION ON CANCER (AJCC): GTNM CLASSIFICATION AND STAGE GROUPING OF SOFT TISSUE SARCOMAS

■ CLASSIFICATION	■ DESCRIPTION
TUMOR GRADE	
GX	Grade cannot be assessed
G1	Well differentiated
G2	Moderately differentiated
G3	Poorly differentiated
G4	Undifferentiated
PRIMARY TUMOR	
TX	Primary tumor cannot be assessed
T0	No evidence of a primary tumor
T1	Tumor <5 cm in greatest diameter
T1a	Superficial tumor
T1b	Deep tumor
T2	Tumor <5 cm in greatest diameter
T2a	Superficial tumor
T2b	Deep tumor
LYMPH NODE INVOLVEMENT	
NX	Regional lymph nodes cannot be assessed
N0	No known metastases to lymph nodes
N1	Verified metastases to lymph nodes
DISTANT METASTASIS	
MX	Presence of distant metastasis cannot be assessed
M0	No known distant metastasis
M1	Known distant metastasis
STAGE GROUPING	
Stage I	G1–2, T1a, N0, M0
	G1–2, T1b, N0, M0
	G1–2, T2a, N0, M0
	G1–2, T2b, N0, M0
Stage II	G3–4, T1a, N0, M0
	G3–4, T1b, N0, M0
	G3–4, T2a, N0, M0
Stage III	G3–4, T2b, N0, M0
Stage IV	Any G, Any T, N1, M0
	Any G, Any T, N0, M1

Adapted from Greene F, Page D, Fleming I, et al. eds. *AJCC Cancer Staging Manual*, 6th ed. New York: Springer-Verlag; 2002.

close to the incision so that the site can be included in a postoperative radiation field and to minimize the extent of proximal involvement if amputation ever becomes necessary. A unique characteristic of sarcoma is the lack of metastasis to regional lymph nodes. If regional lymphadenopathy is discovered in conjunction with a diagnosis of sarcoma, therapeutic lymphadenectomy can be considered since clearance of disease may be associated with improved outcomes.[48,49] In selected patients with clinically negative node examination, there may be a role for sentinel lymph node biopsy to identify occult micrometastatic disease.[50]

Taken together, sarcomas of the upper and lower extremities and trunk make up most soft tissue sarcomas. Large truncal tumors may require reconstruction with a myocutaneous flap or prosthetic materials if resultant defects cannot be closed primarily (Fig. 112.9). Largely of historic interest now, radical amputations were once the mainstay of treatment for extremity sarcoma, but modern surgical approaches involve limb-sparing procedures (Fig. 112.10), which maximize functional outcomes. As recently as the 1970s, more than 50% of all soft tissue sarcomas of the extremity were treated with radical amputations. The accepted standard of care changed after a group at the National Cancer Institute, led by Rosenberg,[51] published the results of a randomized trial of limb-sparing resection plus adjuvant radiation therapy compared to amputation, finding no differences in disease-free survival rates (71% vs. 78%, respectively) and the overall survival rates (83% vs. 88%, respectively) at 5 years. This trial demonstrated that amputation was

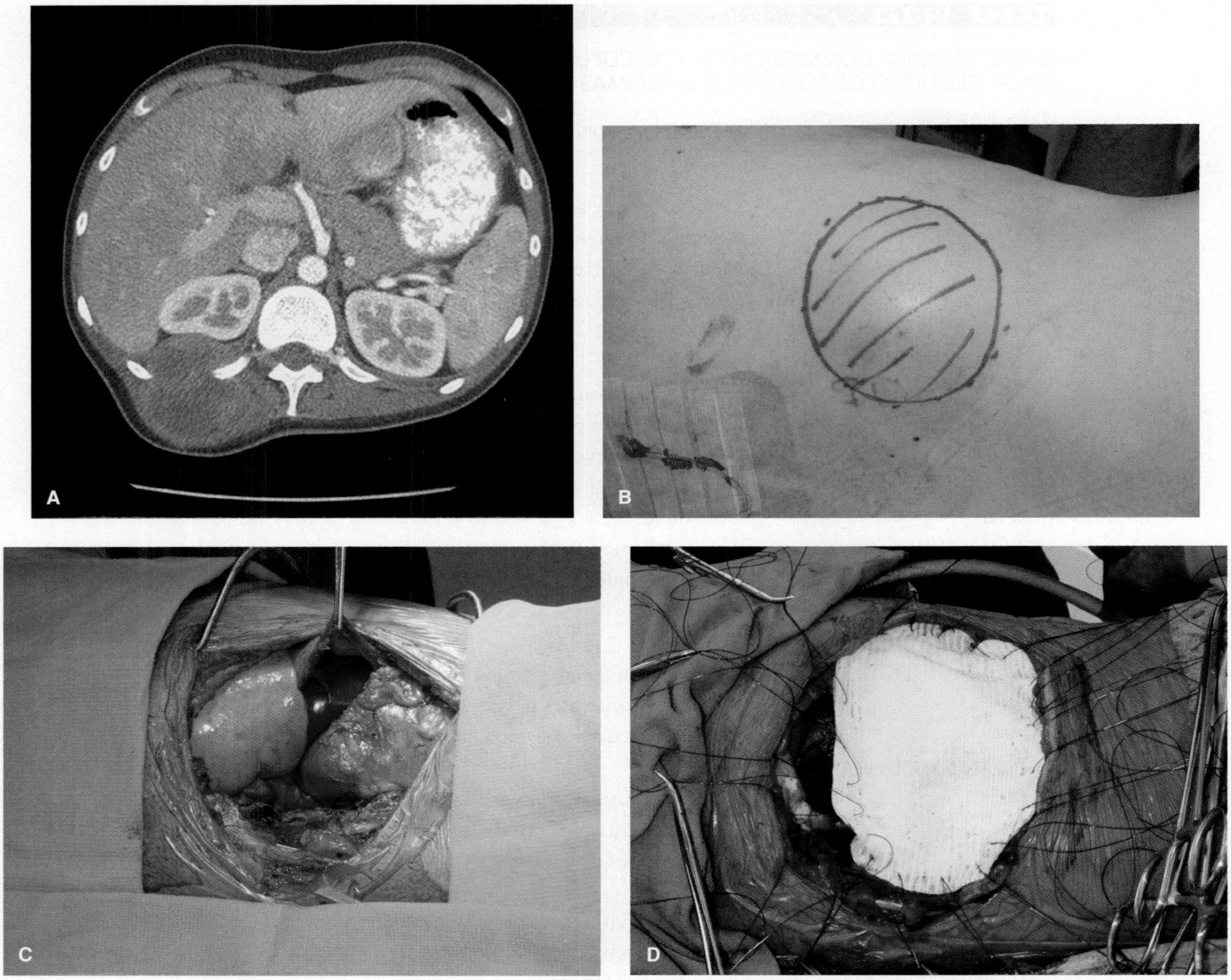

FIGURE 112.9. Chest wall sarcoma. A 20-year-old man with a 7.5-cm right posterior chest wall epithelioid sarcoma involves the 11th and 12th ribs as demonstrated on CT scan (**A**) and on physical exam (**B**). Chest wall resection was performed, including a portion of diaphragm. Resulting chest wall defect (**C**) was repaired using prosthetic mesh (**D**).

not mandatory, and in 1985, a National Institute s of Health consensus statement recommended limb-sparing procedures for most patients with high-grade extremity sarcomas.[52] Radical amputations, such as hemipelvectomy, hip disarticulation or forequarter amputation, are now reserved for patients who are not suitable candidates for limb-sparing approaches, usually because of extent of disease, bony or joint invasion, or for otherwise unsalvageable recurrence after previous limb-sparing surgery (Fig. 112.11). There is no improvement in survival with this approach under these circumstances.[53]

Acceptance of multimodality therapy has led to the ability 3 to perform wide excisions while preserving function when treating extremity or truncal soft tissue sarcomas.[5,54,55] Judicious use of radiation has allowed for the sparing of major neurovascular structures, though if necessary, arteries and/or veins can be resected en bloc with the tumor and subsequent reconstruction can be done with autologous or prosthetic graft materials. In cases of neurologic compromise, customized adjuncts from experienced physical medicine departments can help restore reasonable function. For instance, resultant foot drop from peroneal neuropathy can be managed with an ankle-foot orthotic and gait training. In some cases, resection should be planned in conjunction with a plastic surgeon to provide complex soft tissue reconstruction with microvascular free flaps if the size of defect following resection prohibits primary closure.

Adjuvant and Neoadjuvant Therapies. The role of external beam radiotherapy is best defined by a trial comparing limb-sparing surgery alone with limb-sparing surgery with adjuvant radiation, showing improved 10-year local recurrence rates with radiation. In high-grade sarcomas, the recurrence rate was 0% versus 22%, respectively, though no significant effect on overall survival was appreciated.[56] Certainly, in the setting of involved surgical margins that could not otherwise be resected, adjuvant radiation therapy is associated with improved local control.[3,57]

There is controversy regarding the optimal use of radiation in the preoperative setting compared to the postoperative setting for extremity and truncal sarcomas. Radiation in the adjuvant setting with either external beam radiation or brachytherapy has long been the standard approach.[3] Typically, the entire surgical bed and drain sites are included in the field, along with wide margins around the sarcoma. Hemoclips marking the site of resection can be placed at the time of resection to help with radiation planning. It is important that an individual approach be taken with each patient since radiation can result in severe complications when used inappropriately (Table 112.4). For

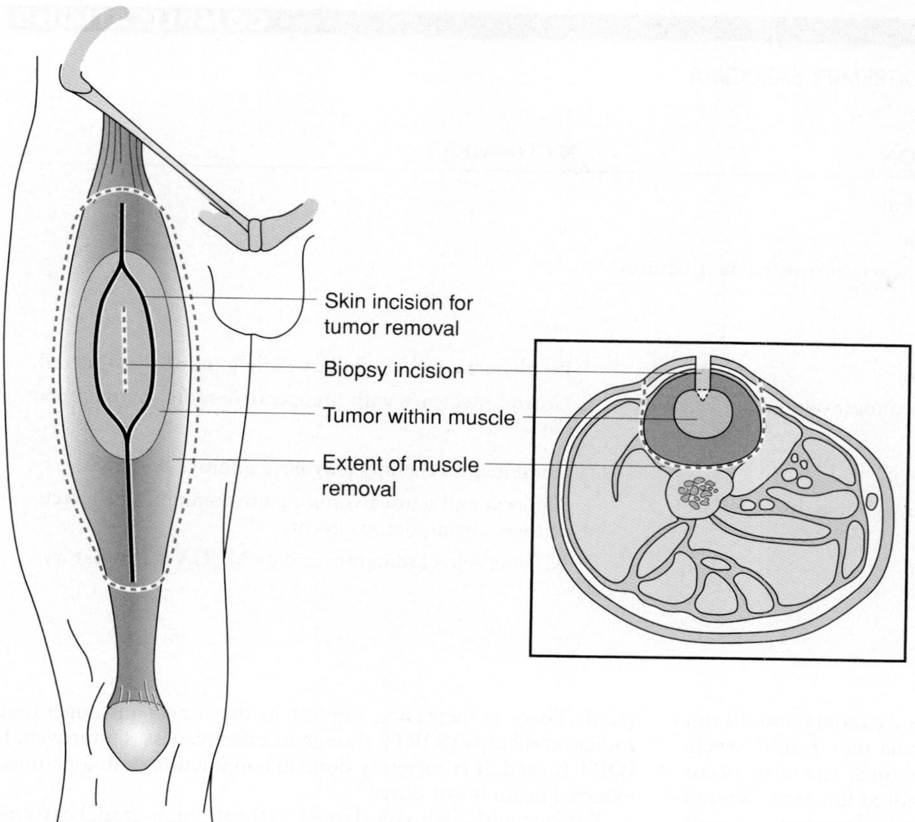

FIGURE 112.10. Wide excision involves removal of the tumor with a margin of normal tissue. If necessary, major vascular structures or nerves may be resected.

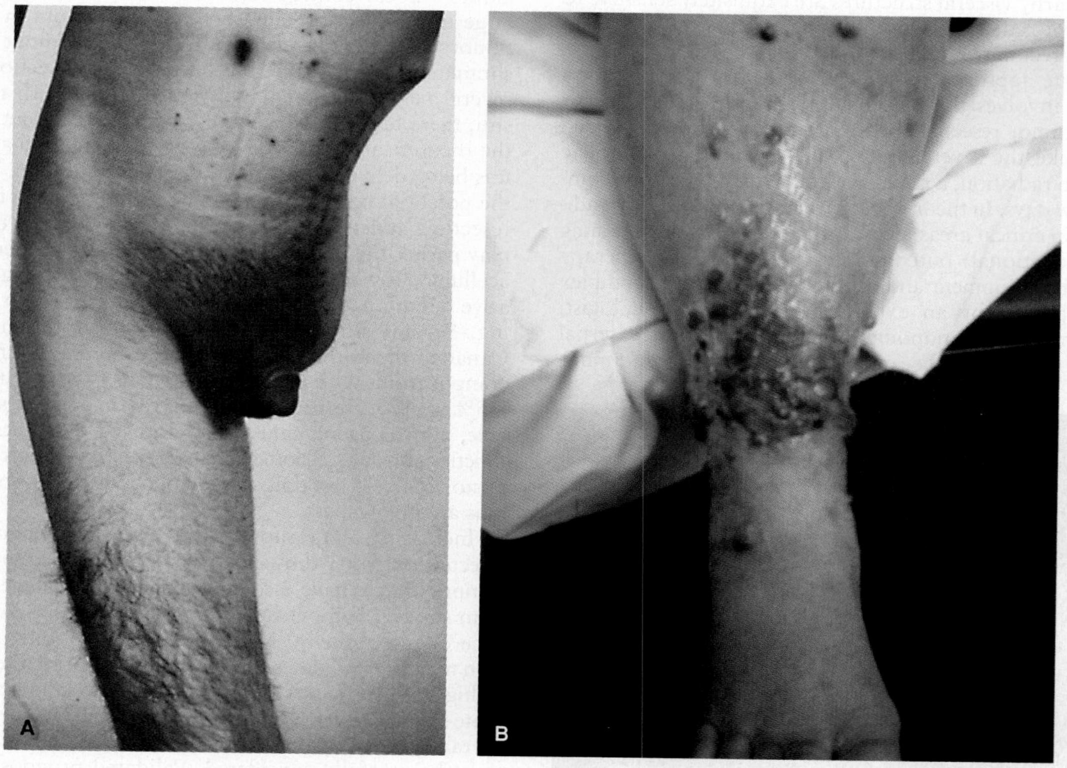

FIGURE 112.11. A: Radical amputations for extremity sarcomas include one joint above the most proximal extent of tumor. Now largely of historic interest, tumors of the proximal thigh or buttock were previously routinely treated with hemipelvectomy. **B:** Although limb-sparing procedures are now done whenever possible, amputation may be necessary for certain cases. This 60-year-old woman had high-grade angiosarcoma of the right leg with extensive satellite metastases extending above her knee. She required above-knee amputation.

TABLE 112.4 **COMPLICATIONS**

COMPLICATIONS OF TREATMENT FOR EXTREMITY SARCOMA

■ TREATMENT MODALITY	■ COMPLICATION	■ COMMENT
Surgical resection	Wound complications	
	Seroma/hematoma	
	Inadvertent damage to neurovascular structures	
Radiation	Fibrosis	
	Edema	
	Pathologic fracture	Prophylactic intramedullary nailing may be considered.
	Delayed wound healing/wound complications	Greater incidence with preoperative radiation treatment.
Chemotherapy		
Doxorubicin	Myelosuppression	Combination therapy may have additive toxicities.
	Cardiotoxicity (arrhythmia, heart failure)	Alopecia and nausea/vomiting are common side effects of these chemotherapy agents.
		Baseline echocardiogram and/or MUGA is mandatory.
Ifosfamide	Myelosuppression	
	Neurotoxicity	
	Nephrotoxicity	

example, the entire circumference of the extremity should not be irradiated because massive lymphedema may result. Severe fibrosis, necrosis, fractures, and contractures can also occur with focused treatment and result in impaired function. Wound healing may be compromised in patients undergoing adjuvant radiation, and in selected cases, use of rotational flaps for coverage can prevent or minimize chronic wound healing problems.[58] Similarly, radiation must be used judiciously in sensitive areas since nearby visceral structures are exquisitely sensitive to higher doses of radiation. Dose-limiting toxicity must be considered when recommending such therapies.

An alternate approach to adjuvant radiation is brachytherapy,[56] which involves the placement of multiple catheters or seeds in the tumor resection bed to administer iridium^{192} (Fig. 112.12). Unlike the several-week course needed to complete external beam radiation, a course of brachytherapy can be completed in a few days. In theory, brachytherapy produces less radiation scatter in critical areas, decreasing toxicity while obtaining equivalent functional outcome.[59] However, brachytherapy requires special equipment and can involve technically complex treatment planning by an experienced radiation oncologist. From a therapeutic standpoint, brachytherapy and external beam radiation appear to be equivalent when properly administered. There is increasing interest in the use of intraoperative radiation therapy (IORT), though its effectiveness is unproven. If IORT is used, it is currently done in conjunction with a planned external beam boost dose.[60]

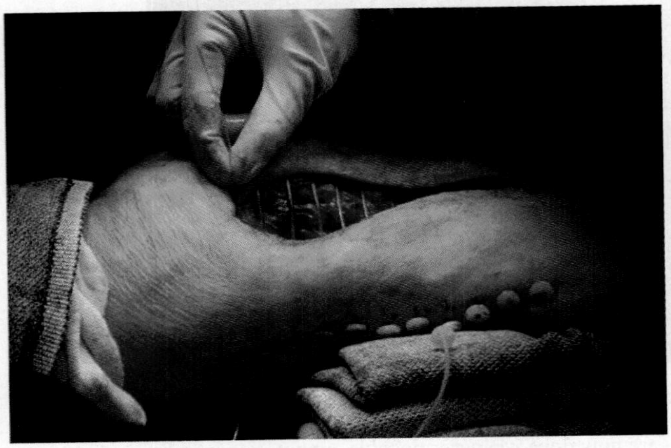

FIGURE 112.12. Adjuvant brachytherapy for extremity sarcoma. Brachytherapy catheters are shown in a resected tumor bed.

Patients with high-risk (large [>10 cm], high-grade) extremity sarcomas should be considered for preoperative treatment with chemotherapy or with chemoradiation since overall local control rates are disappointing with postoperative radiation alone.[54] Local control rates were considerably higher when large tumors were treated before surgery, and in some cases, tumors initially considered unresectable without amputation shrank sufficiently to permit limb-sparing resection. There are several benefits of preoperative radiation. With the tumor in situ, there tends to be a smaller overall treatment volume and the theoretical advantages of more effective radiation because it is being delivered to an undisturbed tumor bed. There is also the potential benefit of decreased seeding during the course of resection and improved margin status because the radiation may shrink the tumor's pseudocapsule and render it relatively acellular. However, there is one major disadvantage to preoperative radiation and that is its detrimental effect on wound healing. Several studies, including a large randomized trial in Canada,[61] demonstrated significant differences in major wound complications with preoperative versus postoperative radiation (35% vs. 17%, respectively). Longer-term outcomes seem acceptable, even boasting similar or improved outcomes in terms of functional results.[62] Some groups have used an intraoperative or postoperative boost dose of radiation to the resection bed if margins are involved.

Increasing data support the use of resection alone for selected patients; those who have small (<5 cm), low-grade tumors seem to have acceptable local control and excellent long-term survival without radiation if wide margins are obtained at time of resection.[63,64] Most patients undergoing surgical excision may be candidates for additional radiation therapy because of high risk for recurrence, though its role in lower- or intermediate-risk patients is somewhat undefined, and the so-called therapeutic ratio of risk and benefits to radiation treatment must be carefully considered. Validated prognostic tools may be helpful for individual patients weighing the benefits of available treatment options. Kattan et al.[65] developed a nomogram to help better predict individual risk for 12-year disease-specific mortality in sarcoma patients using multiple prognostic factors simultaneously.

For extremity sarcomas, the importance of pathologically negative margins must be emphasized. Although differing widths of margins have been called optimal, it is generally agreed that 1 to 2 cm are adequate, but that microscopically clear margins may be sufficient. Involved margins, along with age, recurrent presentation, and fibrosarcoma or MPNST subtypes, significantly increase the risk of local recurrence.[3,66] Patients presenting with involved margins following the index operation should be offered re-resection to obtain surgical clearance of margins. Several studies have shown no compromise in survival if complete resection is achieved with a second operation.[67] Interestingly, it is unclear if local recurrence predisposes to subsequent distant metastasis or if margin status is merely a proxy for aggressive disease.[66,68]

Since the main cause of death in patients with soft tissue sarcoma is distant metastatic disease, continued efforts have been made to develop effective systemic therapies.[5,69] Postoperative adjuvant chemotherapy has been controversial because risk of adverse toxic effects may not be outweighed by the relatively low response rates and lack of durable results. The histologic subtypes of sarcoma vary in their responsiveness to chemotherapy. For example, osteogenic sarcoma, rhabdomyosarcoma, and Ewing sarcoma (the pediatric sarcomas) have had high rates of success with multimodality treatments including adjuvant chemotherapy.[54] Unfortunately, most randomized trials are underpowered to detect modest differences in survival, and promising response rates reported in smaller nonrandomized clinical trials are not duplicated in subsequent larger randomized trials. In general, adjuvant chemotherapy is not ever indicated for patients with low-grade sarcomas and patients with small sarcomas of higher grades. Initial interest in adjuvant chemotherapy for extremity soft tissue sarcoma was piqued by a randomized trial reported by Rosenberg et al.,[70] which demonstrated an improvement in disease-free and overall survival with adjuvant doxorubicin, cyclophosphamide, and high-dose methotrexate. After a longer follow-up period (median follow-up 7.1 years), however, both disease-free and overall survival were not statistically significant.[71]

Over the years, single agents as well as combination chemotherapy regimens have been used in the adjuvant treatment of soft tissue sarcomas. Two of the more active agents include doxorubicin and ifosfamide. However, multiple randomized trials of postoperative chemotherapy have not demonstrated an improvement in disease-free or overall survival with intermediate- or long-term follow-up though there was a trend toward chemotherapy in many studies.[54,72–74] The Sarcoma Meta-analysis Collaboration evaluated the effect of adjuvant doxorubicin-based chemotherapy in 1,568 patients from 14 trials.[75] Although the time to local and distant recurrences, as well as recurrence-free survival, were significantly better in the treatment group, an overall survival advantage was not observed (HR 0.89, $p = 0.12$). Because of the rarity of disease and heterogeneity of tumor characteristics, most studies are too small to provide adequate power for testing responses in specific histologic subtypes. In general, many regimens have combined two of the most active agents, doxorubicin (or other anthracycline) and ifosfamide, and results from a randomized trial did show improved disease-free survival and overall survival; distant relapse rates were not different, however.[76] Outside of clinical trials, doxorubicin and ifosfamide combination therapy is commonly used for high-risk, primary extremity, and truncal sarcomas in the adjuvant setting. Newer regimens with promising results include the combination of gemcitabine and docetaxel, which was initially discovered to be active in heavily pretreated uterine leiomyosarcomas and is currently being considered for use in that subtype as well as in high-grade undifferentiated pleomorphic sarcomas and other high-risk subtypes.[77–79]

One potential advantage of upfront systemic chemotherapy is the ability to assess tumor response in situ. By seeing whether the tumor responds to the chemotherapy, both radiologically and pathologically, it may be possible to spare patients prolonged therapy if they have not shown a response, or to continue therapy postoperatively if there is response. However, data from a trial of preoperative doxorubicin and ifosfamide-based chemotherapy conducted by the European Organisation for Research and Treatment of Cancer (EORTC) and the National Cancer Institute of Canada did not demonstrate any survival benefit compared to surgery alone.[80] Some agents such as gemcitabine may have chemosensitizing properties,[81] making preoperative chemoradiation strategies attractive. Based on current evidence, neoadjuvant chemoradiation, either concurrent or sequential, should be offered only to selected high-risk patients on clinical protocol.[82] It is important to follow patients on neoadjuvant therapy closely since tumor progression occurs in approximately 30% of patients.[83,84]

Commonly used measures of radiologic response to treatment may not be good surrogate endpoints for treatment response.[36] The pathologic correlations of treatment-induced necrosis or histologic response to therapy with clinical outcomes have also not been well defined in soft tissue sarcoma.[85] Some patients who have a clinical or pathologic response to chemotherapy may have improved local control and decreased distant disease-free survival, but no overall survival advantage.[86] In other cases, lack of measurable response did not seem to predict significant differences in event-free endpoints.[83] These issues must be carefully considered in the design of future trials.

Alternative approaches to standard systemic therapy have been attempted with limited success. For example, preoperative radiation therapy in combination with intra-arterial doxorubicin chemotherapy initially showed good local control, but results could not be duplicated in subsequent randomized trials and treatments were associated with high morbidity.[87,88] Regional chemotherapy administered via hyperthermic isolated limb perfusion has been attempted for advanced extremity sarcomas. Extracorporeal circulation allows the delivery of drug concentrations 10 to 20 times higher than with systemic delivery, and a European study showed a limb-salvage rate of 71% for unresectable extremity sarcomas using melphalan and tumor necrosis factor-α.[89,90] However, this technique is uncommonly used in the United States and usually reserved for highly selected patient populations. Hyperthermia in combination with systemic chemotherapy is being evaluated for high-risk extremity sarcomas, but long-term data have not yet been reported.[91]

RETROPERITONEAL AND INTRA-ABDOMINAL SARCOMAS

Management of intra-abdominal (visceral) and retroperitoneal sarcomas deserves special consideration since specific anatomic location may dictate workup and subsequent management. The grouping of visceral sarcomas generally includes tumors of the gastrointestinal tract and gynecologic organs, and less commonly, genitourinary organs. Location often precludes early diagnosis, unless the mass is found incidentally. Though some patients have noted increased abdominal girth, an abdominal mass can be appreciated with focused physical examination, but it is uncommonly the presenting complaint. Typically, vague symptoms of mass effect intra-abdominally trigger a medical evaluation. Neurovascular symptoms related to compression or invasion can occur and manifest as paresthesia, dysesthesia, weakness, and swelling or varicosities in the lower extremities.

Complete history and physical examination should exclude signs and symptoms of lymphoma (e.g., B-symptoms such as fevers and night sweats) and presence of scrotal masses concerning for testes cancer. Serum laboratory testing can be helpful if lymphoma (e.g., elevated lactate dehydrogenase [LDH]), germ-cell tumors (e.g., elevated beta-human chorionic gonadotropin

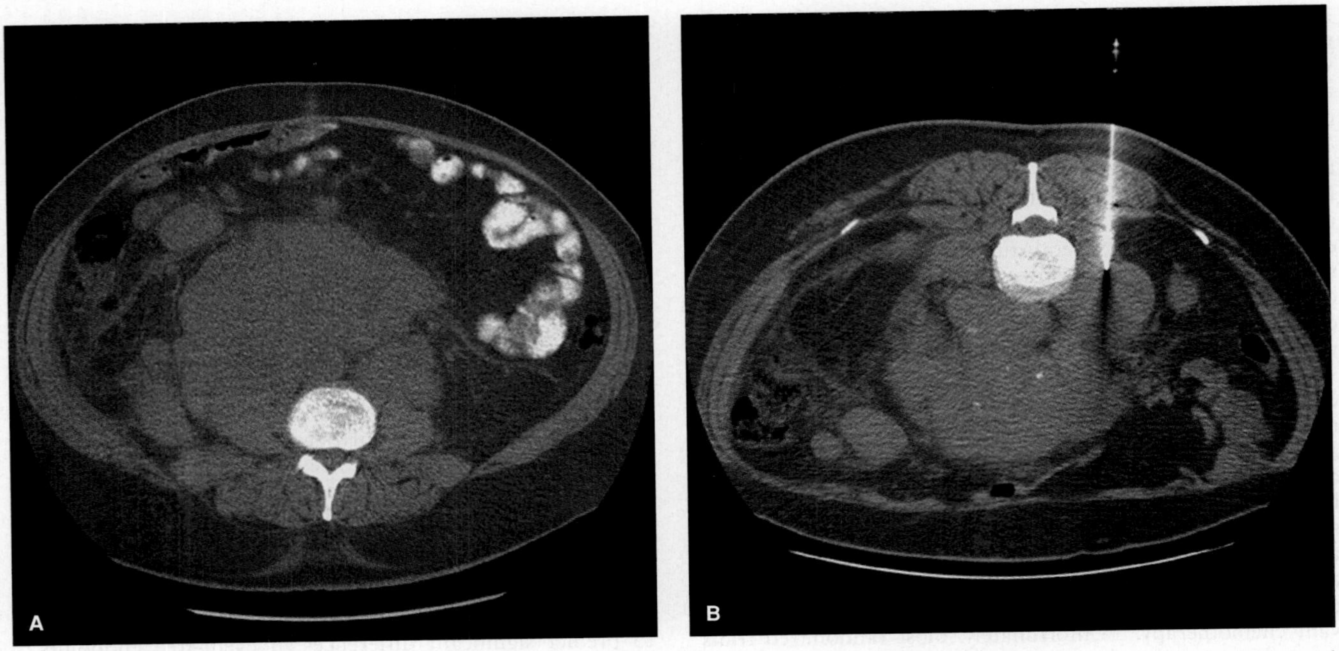

FIGURE 112.13. Biopsy can be helpful in the workup of retroperitoneal masses. **A:** CT scan shows a retroperitoneal mass encasing the IVC and aorta. **B:** Image-guided biopsy is demonstrated here. Pathology confirmed a diagnosis of large B-cell lymphoma.

[B-HCG] or alpha-fetoprotein [AFP]), or adrenal tumors (e.g., cortisol levels or adrenocorticotropic hormone [ACTH]) are in the differential diagnosis. High-quality cross-sectional imaging with CT or MRI is critical for diagnosis and treatment planning. Use of oral and intravenous contrast defines the extent of primary disease and the relationship of the tumor to nearby structures. Chest imaging should be obtained to assess for presence of pulmonary metastases. Hepatic involvement is the second most common site of distant spread in intra-abdominal and retroperitoneal sarcomas, so a CT scan that includes the proper contrast phasing for examination of the liver should be done.

For large tumors, preoperative image-guided biopsy can almost always be performed by experienced interventional radiologists (Fig. 112.13). However, preoperative biopsy is not mandatory[5,92] if management would not be altered by findings. Use of biopsy is reserved for cases in which a diagnosis of sarcoma is in question or if neoadjuvant approaches are being considered for large, high-grade lesions or lesions that are locally advanced and potentially unresectable. Complete resection is the treatment of choice for intra-abdominal (visceral) and retroperitoneal sarcomas whenever possible. Only complete resection is associated with long-term survival benefit, with retroperitoneal liposarcomas being a possible exception.[93,94] For retroperitoneal sarcomas, median survival for those with an incomplete resection is similar to those who were observed (unresectable)[95] (Fig. 112.14). In general, incomplete resection should be considered only for palliation of intractable symptoms. Although successful palliation may be achieved in carefully selected patients, aggressive tumor biology limits the ability to maintain sustained relief of symptoms.[96]

4 To attain complete removal of the sarcoma, en bloc resection of nearby structures should be considered when necessary. Resectability is more a function of location than of size, grade, or histologic subtype. Common reasons for unresectability include distant metastasis, peritoneal metastasis, extensive multifocality, and prohibitive vascular involvement. Though sarcomas do not uniformly invade other structures, involvement of vascular structures or mesentery (mesocolon) may lead to resection of solid organs or bowel that may not be directly involved. When nephrectomy may be necessary, it is important to assess bilateral renal function with preoperative contrast scanning. Concomitant nephrectomy, when necessary, is associated with comparable outcomes for retroperitoneal sarcomas overall.[97] Commonly resected organs include the following: kidney, colon, adrenal gland, pancreas, and spleen[98] (Table 112.5). For tumors located in the pelvis, it may be necessary to perform en bloc resection of the colon/rectum, bladder, and uterus. When vascular structures limit complete resection of tumor, resection with ligation or reconstruction of vessels must be considered if technically feasible (Fig. 112.15).

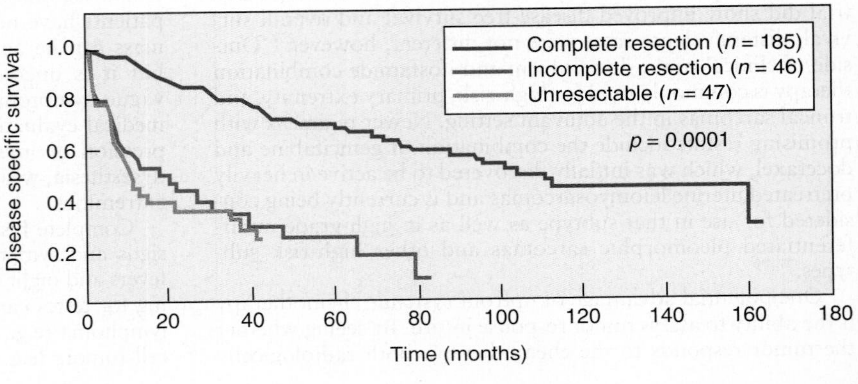

FIGURE 112.14. Kaplan-Meier plot of disease-specific survival for patients with retroperitoneal sarcomas treated at Memorial Sloan-Kettering Cancer Center. Disease-specific survival is 103 months in patients who underwent complete resection of retroperitoneal sarcomas, compared to 18 months in those who had an incomplete resection or just observation. (Reproduced with permission from Lewis JJ, Leung D, Woodruff JM, et al. Retroperitoneal soft-tissue sarcoma: analysis of 500 patients treated and followed at a single institution. *Ann Surg* 1998;228(3):355–365.)

TABLE 112.5

EN BLOC RESECTIONS FOR PRIMARY RETROPERITONEAL SARCOMAS

■ ORGAN	■ CASES IN WHICH ORGAN IS RESECTED (%)
Kidney	46
Colon	24
Pancreas	15
Spleen	10
Major vessels (vena cava, iliac artery or vein)	10

Adapted from Jaques DP, Coit DG, Hajdu SI, et al. Management of primary and recurrent soft-tissue sarcoma of the retroperitoneum. *Ann Surg* 1990;212:51–59.

Even when surgical resection is possible and complete gross resection is achieved, margin status is often compromised by constraints of visceral anatomy. A transperitoneal approach allows for excellent exposure and facilitates en bloc resection with early control of the vascular supply to the tumor. Even with aggressive surgical management, local recurrence rates range from 40% to 70% for high grade tumors.[17,99] Unlike in extremity sarcomas, local progression is associated with decreased survival. Difficulty obtaining negative margins and high recurrence rates support a possible role for multimodality treatments.

However, the benefits of radiation for extremity sarcomas have not been similarly appreciated for retroperitoneal sarcomas, and no improvement in disease-free intervals have been noted.[100] Large field sizes and the dose-limiting toxicity of abdominal viscera limit the utility of postoperative radiation, and preoperative radiation warrants consideration. The major advantage of preoperative radiation is the displacement of small bowel and other structures by the in situ tumor. Similar to preoperative radiation for extremity tumors, a possible advantage in the abdomen/retroperitoneum is that the radiation may prevent later seeding of tumor cells because radiation is administered to tumor and surrounding peritoneum. With the advent of conformal technology, or intensity-modulated radiation therapy (IMRT), further selective application of radiotherapy may be possible with minimal toxicity.[101,102] The role of chemotherapy, either in the preoperative or postoperative setting, is unproven for intra-abdominal and retroperitoneal sarcomas.[103,104] Several trials of postoperative adjuvant chemotherapy do not show any benefit for patients with retroperitoneal sarcoma, and in one series, treated patients fared worse than those not receiving chemotherapy.[105] In one trial of an aggressive multimodality approach, there was an improvement in locoregional control but no overall survival advantage and significant toxicity from

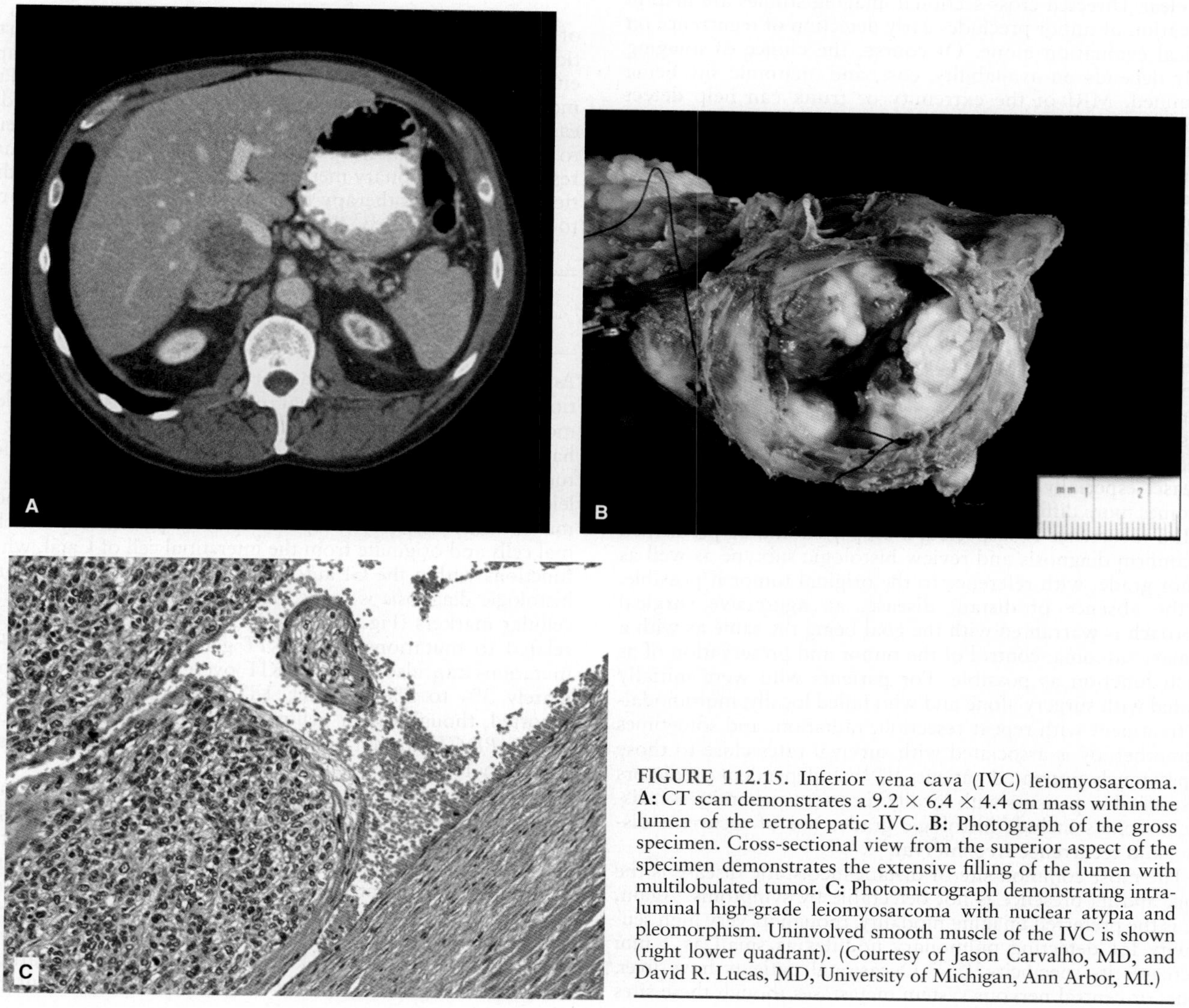

FIGURE 112.15. Inferior vena cava (IVC) leiomyosarcoma. **A:** CT scan demonstrates a 9.2 × 6.4 × 4.4 cm mass within the lumen of the retrohepatic IVC. **B:** Photograph of the gross specimen. Cross-sectional view from the superior aspect of the specimen demonstrates the extensive filling of the lumen with multilobulated tumor. **C:** Photomicrograph demonstrating intraluminal high-grade leiomyosarcoma with nuclear atypia and pleomorphism. Uninvolved smooth muscle of the IVC is shown (right lower quadrant). (Courtesy of Jason Carvalho, MD, and David R. Lucas, MD, University of Michigan, Ann Arbor, MI.)

the chemotherapy and radiation therapy.[106] Though some histologic subtypes, such as leiomyosarcoma, pleomorphic sarcoma, or myxoid/round cell liposarcoma, may be relatively more responsive to systemic treatments, a paucity of data exist to guide appropriate use of therapy.

Special consideration is also given to complete resection with functional preservation in head and neck sarcomas and genitourinary sarcomas. As is true of sarcomas in other anatomic locations, histologic grade and size adversely affect prognosis for head and neck sarcomas.[107] Resections with negative margins may not require adjuvant radiotherapy treatments. Grade, size, location, and histologic subtype predict disease-specific survival for genitourinary sarcomas.[108] Regional relapse is influenced by margin status so radical resections are necessary. Unfortunately, recurrences are not uncommon and may be difficult to control due to anatomic location.

RECURRENT OR METASTATIC DISEASE

About two thirds of soft tissue sarcoma recurrences occur in the first 2 years after diagnosis and treatment, though recurrences may occur at any time.[109] Recurrences may be classified as locoregional or distant. Though no standardized follow-up regimens exist, routine history and physical examination (clinical follow-up) and interval chest imaging are recommended for the first 2 to 3 years. Site-specific imaging guidelines are less clear. Directed cross-sectional imaging studies are helpful if location of tumor precludes early detection of recurrence on clinical evaluation alone. Of course, the choice of imaging study depends on availability, cost, and anatomic site being examined. MRI of the extremity or trunk can help detect locoregional recurrences when they are relatively small. CT scans may be useful for detection of intra-abdominal or retroperitoneal recurrences that would otherwise be undetectable. However, there is no evidence that earlier detection improves survival for retroperitoneal sarcomas,[95] so a less aggressive imaging schedule may be appropriate.

If chest radiography is used, abnormal findings should be followed with a CT scan of the chest. Low-grade lesions infrequently metastasize in the absence of local recurrence though they can recur locally up to 20 years after original resection. For high-grade lesions, surveillance should be directed toward detecting recurrence and metastatic disease. Patients with locally recurrent or even metastatic sarcomas can be considered for surgical resection if tumor biology supports potential cure or effective palliation with removal of known disease. Recurrent disease, especially within the abdomen or retroperitoneum, becomes more difficult to treat with each recurrence.[109]

If a recurrence is suspected, a biopsy should be performed to confirm diagnosis and review histologic subtype as well as tumor grade, with reference to the original tumor if possible. In the absence of distant disease, an aggressive surgical approach is warranted with the goal being the same as with a primary sarcoma: control of the tumor and preservation of as much function as possible. For patients who were initially treated with surgery alone and who failed locally, multimodality treatment with repeat resection, radiation, and sometimes chemotherapy is associated with survival rates close to those of previously untreated patients.[110–112] Independent predictors of survival in patients with locally recurrent extremity soft tissue sarcomas include histologic grade, size of recurrent disease, and recurrence-free interval.[113]

The most common site of distant metastatic disease is the lung, and its presence is not detectable by symptoms. Again, CT is the preferred imaging modality, though its very high sensitivity for detecting pulmonary nodules as small as 2 mm decreases its specificity.[114,115] Occasional patients have liver, bone, or central nervous system metastases though these sites of disease are relatively uncommon. Once diagnosed, metastatic disease is best approached with systemic chemotherapy, either as a single agent or with combination treatments. Pulmonary metastases are the most common form of distant disease, and metastasectomy in carefully selected patients seems to improve outcomes. Taking patient selection into account, resection of pulmonary metastases in combination with radiation and/or chemotherapy may improve outcomes compared to resection alone[116,117] (Fig. 112.16).

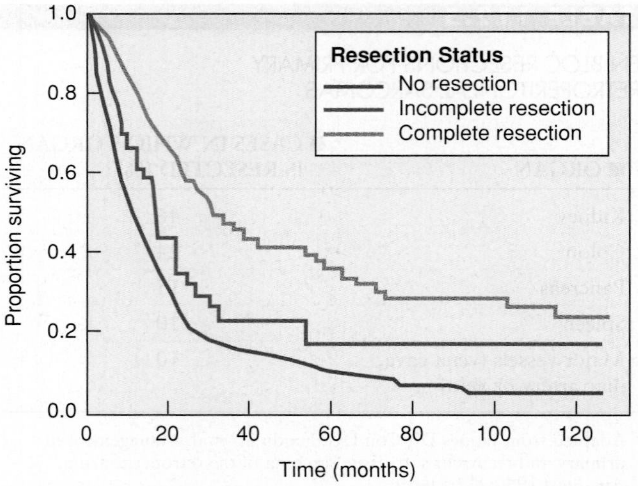

FIGURE 112.16. Kaplan-Meier plot of disease-specific survival for patients with pulmonary metastases treated at Memorial Sloan-Kettering Cancer Center. Patients treated with complete resection had a median survival of 33 months. Patients who underwent incomplete resection or who did not undergo resection had median survival of 16 months and 11 months, respectively. (Reproduced with permission from Billingsley KG, Burt ME, Jara E, et al. Pulmonary metastases from soft tissue sarcoma: analysis of patterns of diseases and post-metastasis survival. *Ann Surg* 1999;229(5):602–610.)

GASTROINTESTINAL STROMAL TUMORS (GIST)

Another subtype of sarcoma that deserves separate consideration is gastrointestinal stromal tumor (GIST). Prior to modern molecular diagnostic techniques, these tumors were likely to have been considered leiomyosarcomas based on histologic features.[17] It is now known that GIST are differentiated from GI leiomyosarcoma based on lack of well-differentiated smooth muscle cells. GIST are composed of more primitive mesenchymal cells and originate from the interstitial cell of Cajal, which functions within the GI autonomic nervous system. Immunohistologic diagnosis is made via expression of KIT (CD 117) cellular markers (Fig. 112.17). KIT overexpression is usually related to mutations in the *KIT* gene, although *PDGFR-α* mutations can also result in KIT overexpression in approximately 3% to 5% of GIST. KIT-negative GIST have been reported, though tumor genotyping should be done to either *KIT* or *PDGFR-α* mutations even with negative immunohistochemistry for KIT.[118]

The *KIT* protooncogene encodes for KIT protein, a transmembrane glycoprotein receptor with an intracellular tyrosine kinase domain. Binding of the KIT ligand induces dimerization and autophosphorylation of KIT, activating a cascade of intracellular signaling that results in cell proliferation and tumorigenesis. A gain of function mutation in KIT occurs in up to 90% of GIST[119] and results in ligand-independent (constitutive) activation of tyrosine kinase function.[120] KIT mutation is found in 90% of GIST, and the most frequent sites of mutation

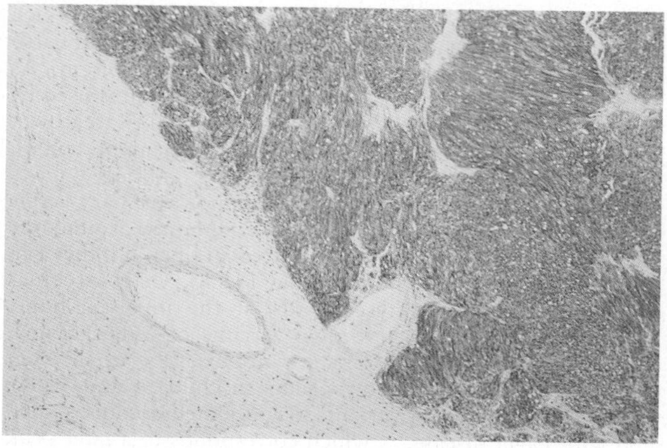

FIGURE 112.17. Strong and diffuse kit immunoreactivity is demonstrated in a gastrointestinal stromal tumor. (Reproduced with permission from Kelsen DP, Daly JM, Kern SE, et al. *Gastrointestinal Oncology: Principles and Practice.* Philadelphia: Lippincott Williams & Wilkins; 2002.)

are found in exon 11 (70%) or exon 9 (10%), whereas rare mutations are found in exon 13 or exon 17.[121] Mutation status may affect prognosis, though it is not routinely tested for.

The exact incidence of GIST has been difficult to determine because of its relatively new recognition as a distinct pathologic entity. Swedish epidemiologic data estimate 14.5 cases per million, which translates to an annual U.S. incidence of 4,000 to 5,000 cases.[122] GIST are nearly all sporadic, but they have occurred in association with hereditary syndromes such as von Recklinghausen disease and the Carney triad, and familial germline mutations have been identified. Clinical presentation can be indolent: Most patients have nonspecific symptoms such as nausea, emesis, or abdominal discomfort. Infrequently, GIST can rupture or bleed, leading to a more emergent presentation. GIST are most commonly found in the stomach (50%–60%), with 30% to 40% of tumors in the small bowel, 5% in the colon or rectum, and 5% in the esophagus. Rarely, GIST develop within the mesentery, omentum, or retroperitoneum. Most GIST are found in adults older than 40 years of age, with a median age of 60 years. Tumors found in children or young adults are considered a separate entity since pediatric GIST have a more epithelioid histology and wild-type KIT or PDGFR-α genotype.[123]

Complete surgical resection is the treatment of choice for GIST, but recurrences are common and 5-year survival following resection of a localized tumor is approximately 50%.[124] Recurrences are common and thought to occur at 18 to 24 months from the time of the index operation. Lymph node dissection is not warranted because GIST very rarely metastasize to regional nodes. Treatment of GIST has been revolutionized with the development of imatinib mesylate (Gleevec), an orally administered, molecularly targeted agent that is a selective tyrosine kinase inhibitor. The proof of concept for this treatment paradigm was demonstrated in 2000 when a patient with diffuse metastatic disease achieved a near-complete metabolic response[125] on PET and with 75% reduction in tumor size at 8 months and histologic evidence of myxoid degeneration and lack of mitotic activity. Contemporary use of imatinib in patients with metastatic GIST results in approximately 80% partial response or stable disease,
3 and imatinib is considered appropriate first-line treatment of metastatic disease (Fig. 112.18).

The use of imatinib in the neoadjuvant or adjuvant setting is still under investigation.[126] It is reasonable to consider the use of imatinib for large or borderline resectable lesions prior to surgical resection. Postoperative use of imatinib has been suggested for high-risk tumors, including tumors that are

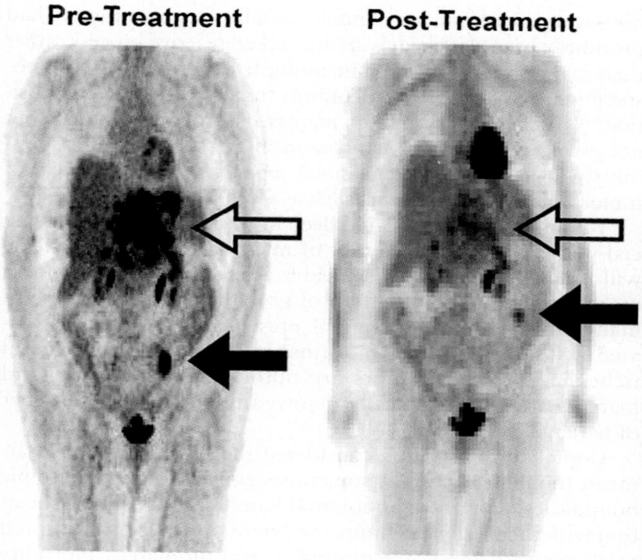

FIGURE 112.18. ^{18}FDG-PET scan showing response of metastatic GIST to imatinib mesylate. This patient presented with primary disease in the small bowel and synchronous metastatic disease in the liver. The scan at presentation (**left**) compared to the one obtained after 3 weeks of therapy (**right**) shows decrease in size of tumors and decreased ^{18}FDG uptake in both the small bowel and liver tumors consistent with a good response to imatinib. The patient eventually went on to complete surgical resection. (Reproduced with permission from Gold JS, DeMatteo RP. Combined surgery and molecular therapy: the gastrointestinal stromal tumor model. *Ann Surg* 2006;244(2): 176–184.)

greater than 5 to 10 cm in size or contain more than 5 mitoses per 50 HPFs (high-powered fields). Risk-stratification must be approached with care; other factors that need to be considered include location of tumor and mutation status. Isolated surgical resection of recurrences has limited utility, and imatinib should be considered in addition to resection.

DESMOID TUMORS/ DESMOID FIBROMATOSIS

Desmoid tumors warrant separate notation in the discussion of soft tissue tumors because of their distinct biologic behavior.[14,127] Desmoid tumors, or aggressive deep-seated fibromatosis, are part of a rare group of fibrous tissue proliferations that have no propensity for metastasis but tend to be locally aggressive. The natural history of desmoid tumors is poorly understood and not well defined. Clinical behavior and, therefore, recommended treatments are often dictated by anatomic site. Location of tumors can limit therapeutic options and result in significant morbidity with or without surgical resection.

Desmoid tumors are uncommon with an estimated incidence rate of 2 to 4 cases per million per year. The median age of diagnosis is 35 years, range 16 to 79 years. Desmoids are slightly more common in women than men. Desmoid tumors are classically described as an abdominal wall tumor that develops in young women during the postpartum period.[128] However, desmoids can occur at any site in the body, and three main anatomic sites are described: (i) trunk or extremity, (ii) abdominal wall, and (iii) intra-abdominal (bowel and mesentery). Fibromatosis is usually sporadic but can be associated with familial adenomatous polyposis.

Desmoids are characterized by a monoclonal fibroblastic proliferation arising from muscular or aponeurotic structures. On gross examination, the tumors appear firm and smooth with a surrounding pseudocapsule. However, microscopically, the tumor characteristically extends beyond this pseudocapsule with fibrous septae of tumor extending radially. Desmoid tumors had previously been classified as an unchecked reactive process rather than a neoplastic process, but uniform patterns of X-chromosome inactivation seems to confirm tumors of clonal composition.[129] There appears to be an increased estrogen receptor-β, but not estrogen receptor-α, expression in 80% of desmoid specimens.[130] These findings lend some support for the treatment of tumors with adjuvant agents such as tamoxifen.

Tumors tend to be located deep in the muscles or along fascial planes, such as at a point of muscular insertion. Patients will usually present with a greater than 5-cm, localized, firm mass with an indolent pattern of growth, which can be minimally painful. Intra-abdominal presentations can be associated with mass effect, intestinal obstruction, or mucosal ischemia. Desmoid tumors are notoriously infiltrative, and margins are microscopically involved in a significant number of patients.

Complete resection is considered the best course of treatment, though resection is sometimes constrained by anatomic boundaries. For intra-abdominal tumors, extensive association with the mesentery limits the extent of resection and could predispose to significant morbidity and ultimately, mortality due to bowel involvement. Resection of large abdominal wall tumors often requires prosthetic reconstruction of the resulting defect. Ability to accomplish complete resection at the first attempt defines likelihood of recurrence, so it is important to have a sufficient preoperative suspicion of fibromatosis and to be circumspect in surgical technique. Positive margins do not inevitably lead to recurrent disease, just as patients with a complete microscopic resection are often found to have local recurrences.[131] There are no data to support the use of radiation therapy in the adjuvant setting following a complete surgical resection. The utility of radiation in the setting of positive resection margins is thought to be quite minimal given the difficulty in predicting risk of recurrence in these patients. Several systemic treatment regimens have been used in the past and in present practice with varying results.

BONE SARCOMAS

Various primary bone tumors are well described (Table 112.6). The vast majority (>70%) of bone malignancies represent metastasis from another site or are of hematologic origin (lymphoma or myeloma). Primary bone cancers, however, are relatively rare types of cancer and account for less than 0.2% of all cancers, with only an estimated 2,380 new cases in 2008.[1] The three main types of bone sarcomas are osteosarcoma (which arises from bone), chondrosarcoma (which arises from cartilage), and Ewing sarcoma (which has an undefined origin). As with soft tissue sarcomas, a GTNM staging system is used by the AJCC[41] (Table 112.7). Modern multimodality treatment approaches have been associated with excellent outcomes, including cures for most osteosarcoma cases.

Osteosarcomas are the most common primary bone tumors. Osteosarcomas occur most commonly around the knee, either in the distal femur or proximal tibia, but they can be encountered in any bone (Table 112.8). Osteosarcomas originate in the metaphyseal ends of the involved bone. Although there are eleven known variants of osteosarcoma, classic osteosarcoma accounts for nearly 80% of incident cases. This tumor commonly occurs in children and young adults. Other important variants include osteosarcoma associated with Paget disease,[132] which corresponds to a later peak in incidence at 60 years of age. Other well-described etiologies of osteosarcoma include prior radiation or history of retinoblastoma,[133] Classic osteosarcoma is of intramedullary origin and is high grade. Osteosarcoma patients are at high risk for metastatic disease; metastases to the lung are the most common, though bony metastases are not uncommon. Low-grade variants do exist, and these less aggressive tumors are usually parosteal or periosteal in location. Elevated serum alkaline phosphatase and lactate dehydrogenase is associated with reduced disease-free survival and overall survival rates.

Chondrosarcomas are typically classified as either primary or central tumors arising from previously normal-appearing bone, or secondary or peripheral tumors that develop from preexisting benign cartilage lesions.[134,135] The secondary or peripheral lesions are usually low grade and infrequently metastasize. Chondrosarcomas usually occur in middle-aged or elderly people, though they can appear at any age. Ewing sarcomas are broadly considered a family of small round cell neoplasms and include the following subtypes: Ewing sarcoma, primitive neuroectodermal tumor (PNET), and extraosseous Ewing sarcoma. Most Ewing sarcomas occur in adolescents and young adults, but they can develop in older individuals. These tumors may arise in soft tissues as well as bone, and most commonly occur in the femur, pelvic bones, and chest wall (Askin tumor).

Clinical Presentation

A painful mass is the most common presenting complaint with an extremity osteosarcoma, though symptoms of chondrosarcoma

TABLE 112.6 **CLASSIFICATION**

HISTOLOGIC CLASSIFICATION OF BONE TUMORS

■ TISSUE CATEGORY	■ BENIGN TUMOR	■ MALIGNANT TUMOR (BONE SARCOMA)
Bone	Osteoid osteoma	Osteogenic sarcoma
	Osteoblastoma	Parosteal osteogenic sarcoma
Cartilage	Osteochondroma	Periosteal osteogenic sarcoma
	Endochondroma	Chondrosarcoma
	Chondroblastoma	Mesenchymal chondrosarcoma
Fibrous lesions	Benign fibrous histiocytoma	Malignant fibrous histiocytoma
	Giant cell tumor	Adamantinoma
	Fibrous dysplasia	Fibrosarcoma
Vascular	Aneurysmal bone cyst	Angiosarcoma
Other	Glomus tumor	Hemangiopericytoma
		Ewing sarcoma

TABLE 112.7 **CLASSIFICATION**

AMERICAN JOINT COMMISSION ON CANCER (AJCC): GTNM CLASSIFICATION AND STAGE GROUPING OF BONE SARCOMAS

■ CLASSIFICATION	■ DESCRIPTION
TUMOR GRADE	
GX	Grade cannot be assessed
G1	Well differentiated
G2	Moderately well differentiated
G3	Poorly differentiated
G4	Undifferentiated
PRIMARY TUMOR	
TX	Primary tumor cannot be assessed
T0	No evidence of primary tumor
T1	Tumor ≤8 cm in greatest dimension
T2	Tumor >8 cm in greatest dimension
T3	Discontinuous tumors in the primary bone site
LYMPH NODE INVOLVEMENT	
NX	Regional lymph nodes cannot be assessed
N0	No regional lymph node metastasis
N1	Regional lymph node metastasis
DISTANT METASTASIS	
MX	Presence of distant metastasis cannot be assessed
M0	No distant metastasis
M1	Distant metastasis
STAGE GROUPING	
Stage IA	G1–2, T1, N0, M0
Stage IB	G1–2, T2, N0, M0
Stage IIA	G3–4, T1, N0, M0
Stage IIB	G3–4, T2, N0, M0
Stage III	Any G, T3, N0, M0
Stage IVA	Any G, any T, N0, M1a
Stage IVB	Any G, any T, N1, any M
	Any G, any T, any N, M1b

Adapted from Greene F, Page D, Fleming I, et al. eds. *AJCC Cancer Staging Manual*, 6th ed. New York: Springer-Verlag; 2002.

may be quite mild. Tumor location in the axial skeleton may also be associated with a more insidious presentation. Limitation of motion is often present when the tumor arises in proximity to a joint. Patients occasionally present with a pathologic fracture of the involved bone. Plain radiographs of the affected area often suggest a diagnosis. High-grade osteosarcomas lead to rapid destruction of bone evidenced by cortical destruction and demonstrate periosteal reaction with new bone formation; an extensive, poorly defined destructive bony lesion, often with an extraosseous component is often evident (Fig. 112.19). Ewing sarcomas have a classic "onion skin" periosteal reaction, and underlying bone often appears mottled. Primary or central chondrosarcomas show cortical destruction and calcification. Further radiologic evaluation with MRI (or CT scan) provides excellent detail of the anatomic extent of tumor and aids operative planning. Chest imaging should be used to determine if there is metastatic disease. Evaluation with radionuclide bone scanning and/or PET scans may also be useful.[136]

After the radiologic evaluation establishes the extent of the bony lesion, diagnostic biopsy should be performed. Either CNB or open biopsy techniques can be used. Placement of the incision should be carefully planned to avoid jeopardizing subsequent options for a limb-sparing procedure. Consideration should also be given to stabilization techniques if there is risk of pathologic fracture during treatment.

TABLE 112.8

DISTRIBUTION OF ANATOMIC LOCATIONS OF OSTEOSARCOMA

■ ANATOMIC SITE	■ PERCENTAGE (%)
Lower extremity	83
Upper extremity	9
Other (pelvis, shoulder, vertebrae)	7

Adapted from Bieling et al. *J Clin Oncol* 1996;14:848–858.

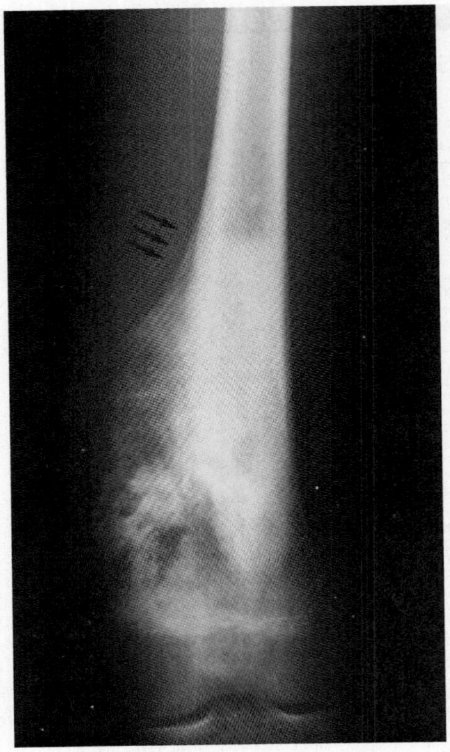

FIGURE 112.19. Plain radiograph of the femur showing a high-grade osteosarcoma. The tumor is an ill-defined destructive lesion with an extensive soft tissue involvement. The Codman triangles (*arrows*) indicate periosteal reaction, which are characteristic, but not pathognomonic, of osteosarcoma.

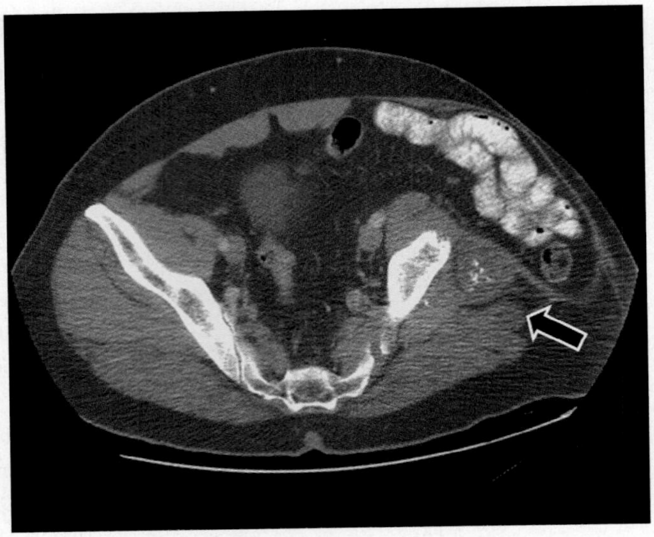

FIGURE 112.20. Chondrosarcoma recurrence. A 60-year-old man had previously undergone resection of a low-grade chondrosarcoma of the left pelvis, necessitating resection of the left iliac bone. After many local bony recurrences, he was found to have an extraskeletal site of disease. On the CT scan, adjacent to the remaining bone, there is a 4.4 × 3.6 cm soft tissue mass (*arrow*), which contains dystrophic calcifications. Recurrent disease was completely resected.

Cytogenetic analysis for evaluation of the t(11;22) translocation should be done if Ewing sarcoma is suspected.[17] Presenting features associated with poor prognosis in Ewing sarcoma include elevated serum lactate dehydrogenase levels, fever, anemia, large tumor volume, mutation in p53 or deletion of p16/p14ARF, and pelvic location. Most patients have at least micrometastatic disease at presentation, and bone marrow biopsy can be considered because it is a common site of distant disease.

Treatment

Standard treatment for Ewing sarcoma involves combination chemotherapy, followed by surgical resection. Regimens have evolved over time and currently involve some combination (or all) of the following agents: ifosfamide, cyclophosphamide, etoposide, doxorubicin, and vincristine.[137–139] Investigations continue to define the trade-offs between survival benefit and toxicity of high-dose combination chemotherapy.[140] Adjuvant radiation can be considered or used as definitive treatment in some cases. Most patients will receive additional chemotherapy in the postoperative period as well. The aggressive use of multimodality therapy has led to excellent outcomes for patients with localized disease over time. Five-year survival rates have improved from 44% in the 1970s to 68% in the 6 1990s. Even outcomes with advanced disease at presentation have improved dramatically, increasing from 16% to 39% over the same time period.[141]

Surgical resection is the definitive treatment for most chondrosarcomas (Fig. 112.20). Intracompartmental lesions can be considered for intralesional resection with wide margins. Radiation can be considered as an adjuvant therapy, but chemotherapy is generally not very effective. If lesions are unresectable, radiation may be considered as a possible definitive treatment modality.

Historically, patients with clinically localized osteosarcoma treated by surgery alone had a 5-year survival rate of approximately 20%. Adjuvant systemic chemotherapy after surgery has generally improved that figure up to 55% to 70% in most randomized trials.[142–146] Contemporary protocols that incorporate preoperative chemotherapy into the regimen have been associated with event-free survival rates of up to 70%.[147] The following agents have shown to be active, and regimens have used differing combinations of those agents: doxorubicin, cisplatin, ifosfamide, high-dose methotrexate. Progressive disease carries a poor prognosis. Disease relapse should be treated with further chemotherapy and resection if possible.

Extremity osteosarcomas are ideally treated with limb-sparing approaches when possible to maximize functional outcomes. Limb-sparing operations include complete removal of the affected bone and soft tissues. Various reconstructive techniques are available after resection of an extremity osteosarcoma. Autografts (such as vascularized or nonvascularized fibular grafts), cadaver allografts, and sophisticated endoprostheses can be used. Because the osteosarcoma population includes many children who continue to grow, modular prostheses that can periodically be expanded are increasingly being used.

References

1. Jemal A, Siegel R, Ward E, et al. Cancer statistics, 2008. *CA Cancer J Clin* 2008;58(2):71–96.
2. Coindre JM, Terrier P, Bui NB, et al. Prognostic factors in adult patients with locally controlled soft tissue sarcoma. A study of 546 patients from the French Federation of Cancer Centers Sarcoma Group. *J Clin Oncol* 1996;14(3):869–877.
3. Pisters PW, Leung DH, Woodruff J, et al. Analysis of prognostic factors in 1,041 patients with localized soft tissue sarcomas of the extremities. *J Clin Oncol* 1996;14(5):1679–1689.
4. Long ER. *History of Pathology*. Baltimore: Williams & Wilkins; 1928.
5. Brennan MF, Lewis JJ. *Diagnosis and Management of Soft Tissue Sarcoma*. London: Martin Dunitz; 2002.
6. King T. Epidemiology. In: Pollock R, ed. *Soft Tissue Sarcomas*. London: BC Decker; 2002:1–10.
7. Cha C, Antonescu CR, Quan ML, et al. Long-term results with resection of radiation-induced soft tissue sarcomas. *Ann Surg* 2004;239(6): 903–909; discussion 909–910.
8. Abbott R, Palmieri C. Angiosarcoma of the breast following surgery and radiotherapy for breast cancer. *Nat Clin Pract Oncol* 2008;5(12):727–736.

9. Stewart FW, Treves N. Lymphangiosarcoma in postmastectomy lymphedema; a report of six cases in elephantiasis chirurgica. *Cancer* 1948; 1(1):64–81.
10. Safai B, Johnson KG, Myskowski PL, et al. The natural history of Kaposi's sarcoma in the acquired immunodeficiency syndrome. *Ann Intern Med* 1985;103(5):744–750.
11. Dittmer DP, Krown SE. Targeted therapy for Kaposi's sarcoma and Kaposi's sarcoma-associated herpesvirus. *Curr Opin Oncol* 2007;19(5):452–457.
12. Clayton G, Omasta-Martin A, Bower M. The effects of HAART on AIDS-related Kaposi's sarcoma and non-Hodgkin's lymphoma. *J HIV Ther* 2006;11(3):51–53.
13. Sorensen SA, Mulvihill JJ, Nielsen A. Long-term follow-up of von Recklinghausen neurofibromatosis. Survival and malignant neoplasms. *N Engl J Med* 1986;314(16):1010–1015.
14. Posner MC, Shiu MH, Newsome JL, et al. The desmoid tumor. Not a benign disease. *Arch Surg* 1989;124(2):191–196.
15. Fraumeni JF Jr, Vogel CL, Easton JM. Sarcomas and multiple polyposis in a kindred. A genetic variety of hereditary polyposis? *Arch Intern Med* 1968;121(1):57–61.
16. Latchford AR, Phillips RK. Duodenal adenoma and cancer in FAP. *Gut* 2005;54(1):171.
17. Borden EC, Baker LH, Bell RS, et al. Soft tissue sarcomas of adults: state of the translational science. *Clin Cancer Res* 2003;9(6):1941–1956.
18. Bennicelli JL, Barr FG. Genetics and the biologic basis of sarcomas. *Curr Opin Oncol* 1999;11(4):267–274.
19. Stratton MR, Williams S, Fisher C, et al. Structural alterations of the RB1 gene in human soft tissue tumours. *Br J Cancer* 1989;60(2):202–205.
20. Li FP, Fraumeni JF Jr. Prospective study of a family cancer syndrome. *JAMA* 1982;247(19):2692–2694.
21. Malkin D, Li FP, Strong LC, et al. Germ line p53 mutations in a familial syndrome of breast cancer, sarcomas, and other neoplasms. *Science* 1990; 250(4985):1233–1238.
22. Andreassen A, Oyjord T, Hovig E, et al. p53 abnormalities in different subtypes of human sarcomas. *Cancer Res* 1993;53(3):468–471.
23. Levine EA. Prognostic factors in soft tissue sarcoma. *Semin Surg Oncol* 1999;17(1):23–32.
24. Kawai A, Woodruff J, Healey JH, et al. SYT-SSX gene fusion as a determinant of morphology and prognosis in synovial sarcoma. *N Engl J Med* 1998;338(3):153–160.
25. Ladanyi M, Antonescu CR, Leung DH, et al. Impact of SYT-SSX fusion type on the clinical behavior of synovial sarcoma: a multi-institutional retrospective study of 243 patients. *Cancer Res* 2002;62(1):135–140.
26. Demas BE, Heelan RT, Lane J, et al. Soft-tissue sarcomas of the extremities: comparison of MR and CT in determining the extent of disease. *AJR Am J Roentgenol* 1988;150(3):615–620.
27. Jelinek JS, Kransdorf MJ, Shmookler BM, et al. Liposarcoma of the extremities: MR and CT findings in the histologic subtypes. *Radiology* 1993;186(2):455–459.
28. Panicek DM, Gatsonis C, Rosenthal DI, et al. CT and MR imaging in the local staging of primary malignant musculoskeletal neoplasms: Report of the Radiology Diagnostic Oncology Group. *Radiology* 1997;202(1):237–246.
29. Arca MJ, Sondak VK, Chang AE. Diagnostic procedures and pretreatment evaluation of soft tissue sarcomas. *Semin Surg Oncol* 1994;10(5):323–331.
30. Pearlstone DB, Pisters PW, Bold RJ, et al. Patterns of recurrence in extremity liposarcoma: implications for staging and follow-up. *Cancer* 1999; 85(1):85–92.
31. Hanna SL, Fletcher BD. MR imaging of malignant soft-tissue tumors. *Magn Reson Imaging Clin N Am* 1995;3(4):629–650.
32. Jones DN, McCowage GB, Sostman HD, et al. Monitoring of neoadjuvant therapy response of soft-tissue and musculoskeletal sarcoma using fluorine-18-FDG PET. *J Nucl Med* 1996;37(9):1438–1444.
33. Benz MR, Allen-Auerbach MS, Eilber FC, et al. Combined assessment of metabolic and volumetric changes for assessment of tumor response in patients with soft-tissue sarcomas. *J Nucl Med* 2008;49(10):1579–1584.
34. Kumar R, Chauhan A, Kesav Vellimana A, et al. Role of PET/PET-CT in the management of sarcomas. *Expert Rev Anticancer Ther* 2006;6(8): 1241–1250.
35. Heron DE, Andrade RS, Beriwal S, et al. PET-CT in radiation oncology: the impact on diagnosis, treatment planning, and assessment of treatment response. *Am J Clin Oncol* 2008;31(4):352–362.
36. Schuetze SM, Baker LH, Benjamin RS, et al. Selection of response criteria for clinical trials of sarcoma treatment. *Oncologist* 2008;13(suppl 2): 32–40.
37. Heslin MJ, Lewis JJ, Woodruff JM, et al. Core needle biopsy for diagnosis of extremity soft tissue sarcoma. *Ann Surg Oncol* 1997;4(5):425–431.
38. Czerniak B, Kram A. Pathology. In: Pollock R, ed. *Soft Tissue Sarcomas.* London: BC Decker; 2002:11–42.
39. Rubin BP, Goldblum JR. Pathology of soft tissue sarcoma. *J Natl Compr Canc Netw* 2007;5(4):411–418.
40. Deyrup AT, Weiss SW. Grading of soft tissue sarcomas: the challenge of providing precise information in an imprecise world. *Histopathology* 2006;48(1):42–50.
41. Greene F, Page D, Fleming I, et al. eds. *AJCC Cancer Staging Manual*, 6th ed. New York: Springer-Verlag; 2002.
42. Coindre JM, Trojani M, Contesso G, et al. Reproducibility of a histopathologic grading system for adult soft tissue sarcoma. *Cancer* 1986; 58(2):306–309.
43. Guillou L, Coindre JM, Bonichon F, et al. Comparative study of the National Cancer Institute and French Federation of Cancer Centers Sarcoma Group grading systems in a population of 410 adult patients with soft tissue sarcoma. *J Clin Oncol* 1997;15(1):350–362.
44. Tierney JF, Mosseri V, Stewart LA, et al. Adjuvant chemotherapy for soft-tissue sarcoma: review and meta-analysis of the published results of randomised clinical trials. *Br J Cancer* 1995;72(2):469–475.
45. Brooks AD, Heslin MJ, Leung DH, et al. Superficial extremity soft tissue sarcoma: an analysis of prognostic factors. *Ann Surg Oncol* 1998;5(1):41–47.
46. Brennan MF. Staging of soft tissue sarcomas. *Ann Surg Oncol* 1999;6(1): 8–9.
47. Ramanathan RC, A'Hern R, Fisher C, et al. Modified staging system for extremity soft tissue sarcomas. *Ann Surg Oncol* 1999;6(1):57–69.
48. Fong Y, Coit DG, Woodruff JM, et al. Lymph node metastasis from soft tissue sarcoma in adults. Analysis of data from a prospective database of 1772 sarcoma patients. *Ann Surg* 1993;217(1):72–77.
49. Al-Refaie WB, Andtbacka RH, Ensor J, et al. Lymphadenectomy for isolated lymph node metastasis from extremity soft-tissue sarcomas. *Cancer* 2008;112(8):1821–1826.
50. Blazer DG III, Sabel MS, Sondak VK. Is there a role for sentinel lymph node biopsy in the management of sarcoma? *Surg Oncol* 2003;12(3): 201–206.
51. Rosenberg SA, Tepper J, Glatstein E, et al. The treatment of soft-tissue sarcomas of the extremities: prospective randomized evaluations of (1) limb-sparing surgery plus radiation therapy compared with amputation and (2) the role of adjuvant chemotherapy. *Ann Surg* 1982;196(3):305–315.
52. National Institute of Health Consensus Development Panel on Limb-sparing Treatment of Adult Soft-Tissue Sarcoma and Osteosarcomas. Proceedings of Cancer Treatment Symposium. 1985:1–5. Limb-sparing Treatment of Adult Soft-Tissue Sarcomas and Osteosarcomas. NIH Consensus Statement Online. 1984;5(6):1–7.
53. Stojadinovic A, Jaques DP, Leung DH, et al. Amputation for recurrent soft tissue sarcoma of the extremity: indications and outcome. *Ann Surg Oncol* 2001;8(6):509–518.
54. Pisters PW, O'Sullivan B, Maki RG. Evidence-based recommendations for local therapy for soft tissue sarcomas. *J Clin Oncol* 2007;25(8): 1003–1008.
55. Cormier JN, Ballo MT. Functional outcome after treatment of lower extremity soft tissue sarcoma: what should we tell our patients? *Ann Surg Oncol* 2004;11(5):453–454.
56. Yang JC, Chang AE, Baker AR, et al. Randomized prospective study of the benefit of adjuvant radiation therapy in the treatment of soft tissue sarcomas of the extremity. *J Clin Oncol* 1998;16(1):197–203.
57. Alektiar KM, Velasco J, Zelefsky MJ, et al. Adjuvant radiotherapy for margin-positive high-grade soft tissue sarcoma of the extremity. *Int J Radiat Oncol Biol Phys* 2000;48(4):1051–1058.
58. Spierer MM, Alektiar KM, Zelefsky MJ, et al. Tolerance of tissue transfers to adjuvant radiation therapy in primary soft tissue sarcoma of the extremity. *Int J Radiat Oncol Biol Phys* 2003;56(4):1112–1116.
59. Alektiar KM, Leung D, Zelefsky MJ, et al. Adjuvant brachytherapy for primary high-grade soft tissue sarcoma of the extremity. *Ann Surg Oncol* 2002;9(1):48–56.
60. Tran QN, Kim AC, Gottschalk AR, et al. Clinical outcomes of intraoperative radiation therapy for extremity sarcomas. *Sarcoma* 2006;2006(1):91671.
61. O'Sullivan B, Davis AM, Turcotte R, et al. Preoperative versus postoperative radiotherapy in soft-tissue sarcoma of the limbs: a randomised trial. *Lancet* 2002;359(9325):2235–2241.
62. Davis AM, O'Sullivan B, Bell RS, et al. Function and health status outcomes in a randomized trial comparing preoperative and postoperative radiotherapy in extremity soft tissue sarcoma. *J Clin Oncol* 2002;20(22): 4472–4477.
63. Pisters PW, Pollock RE, Lewis VO, et al. Long-term results of prospective trial of surgery alone with selective use of radiation for patients with T1 extremity and trunk soft tissue sarcomas. *Ann Surg* 2007;246(4):675–681; discussion 681–682.
64. Baldini EH, Goldberg J, Jenner C, et al. Long-term outcomes after function-sparing surgery without radiotherapy for soft tissue sarcoma of the extremities and trunk. *J Clin Oncol* 1999;17(10):3252–3259.
65. Kattan MW, Leung DH, Brennan MF. Postoperative nomogram for 12-year sarcoma-specific death. *J Clin Oncol* 2002;20(3):791–796.
66. Lewis JJ, Leung D, Heslin M, et al. Association of local recurrence with subsequent survival in extremity soft tissue sarcoma. *J Clin Oncol* 1997; 15(2):646–652.
67. Lewis JJ, Leung D, Espat J, et al. Effect of reresection in extremity soft tissue sarcoma. *Ann Surg* 2000;231(5):655–663.
68. Herbert SH, Corn BW, Solin LJ, et al. Limb-preserving treatment for soft tissue sarcomas of the extremities. The significance of surgical margins. *Cancer* 1993;72(4):1230–1238.
69. Huth JF, Eilber FR. Patterns of metastatic spread following resection of extremity soft-tissue sarcomas and strategies for treatment. *Semin Surg Oncol* 1988;4(1):20–26.
70. Rosenberg SA, Tepper J, Glatstein E, et al. Prospective randomized evaluation of adjuvant chemotherapy in adults with soft tissue sarcomas of the extremities. *Cancer* 1983;52(3):424–434.
71. Chang AE, Kinsella T, Glatstein E, et al. Adjuvant chemotherapy for patients with high-grade soft-tissue sarcomas of the extremity. *J Clin Oncol* 1988;6(9):1491–1500.
72. Antman K, Crowley J, Balcerzak SP, et al. An intergroup phase III randomized study of doxorubicin and dacarbazine with or without ifosfamide and mesna in advanced soft tissue and bone sarcomas. *J Clin Oncol* 1993; 11(7):1276–1285.

73. Bramwell V, Rouesse J, Steward W, et al. Adjuvant CYVADIC chemotherapy for adult soft tissue sarcoma—reduced local recurrence but no improvement in survival: a study of the European Organization for Research and Treatment of Cancer Soft Tissue and Bone Sarcoma Group. *J Clin Oncol* 1994;12(6):1137–1149.
74. Cormier JN, Huang X, Xing Y, et al. Cohort analysis of patients with localized, high-risk, extremity soft tissue sarcoma treated at two cancer centers: chemotherapy-associated outcomes. *J Clin Oncol* 2004;22(22): 4567–4574.
75. [No authors listed.] Adjuvant chemotherapy for localised resectable soft-tissue sarcoma of adults: meta-analysis of individual data. Sarcoma Meta-analysis Collaboration. *Lancet* 1997;350(9092):1647–1654.
76. Frustaci S, Gherlinzoni F, De Paoli A, et al. Adjuvant chemotherapy for adult soft tissue sarcomas of the extremities and girdles: results of the Italian randomized cooperative trial. *J Clin Oncol* 2001;19(5):1238–1247.
77. Hensley ML, Maki R, Venkatraman E, et al. Gemcitabine and docetaxel in patients with unresectable leiomyosarcoma: results of a phase II trial. *J Clin Oncol* 2002;20(12):2824–2831.
78. Maki RG, Wathen JK, Patel SR, et al. Randomized phase II study of gemcitabine and docetaxel compared with gemcitabine alone in patients with metastatic soft tissue sarcomas: results of sarcoma alliance for research through collaboration study 002 [corrected]. *J Clin Oncol* 2007;25(19): 2755–2763.
79. Leu KM, Ostruszka LJ, Shewach D, et al. Laboratory and clinical evidence of synergistic cytotoxicity of sequential treatment with gemcitabine followed by docetaxel in the treatment of sarcoma. *J Clin Oncol* 2004;22(9): 1706–1712.
80. Gortzak E, Azzarelli A, Buesa J, et al. A randomised phase II study on neo-adjuvant chemotherapy for 'high-risk' adult soft-tissue sarcoma. *Eur J Cancer* 2001;37(9):1096–1103.
81. Murphy JD, Lucas DR, Somnay YR, et al. Gemcitabine-mediated radiosensitization of human soft tissue sarcoma. *Transl Oncol* 2008;1(1): 50–56.
82. Grobmyer SR, Maki RG, Demetri GD, et al. Neo-adjuvant chemotherapy for primary high-grade extremity soft tissue sarcoma. *Ann Oncol* 2004; 15(11):1667–1672.
83. Pisters PW, Patel SR, Varma DG, et al. Preoperative chemotherapy for stage IIIB extremity soft tissue sarcoma: long-term results from a single institution. *J Clin Oncol* 1997;15(12):3481–3487.
84. Meric F, Hess KR, Varma DG, et al. Radiographic response to neoadjuvant chemotherapy is a predictor of local control and survival in soft tissue sarcomas. *Cancer* 2002;95(5):1120–1126.
85. Lucas DR, Kshirsagar MP, Biermann JS, et al. Histologic alterations from neoadjuvant chemotherapy in high-grade extremity soft tissue sarcoma: clinicopathological correlation. *Oncologist* 2008;13(4):451–458.
86. Eilber FC, Rosen G, Eckardt J, et al. Treatment-induced pathologic necrosis: a predictor of local recurrence and survival in patients receiving neoadjuvant therapy for high-grade extremity soft tissue sarcomas. *J Clin Oncol* 2001;19(13):3203–3209.
87. Rossi CR, Vecchiato A, Foletto M, et al. Phase II study on neoadjuvant hyperthermic-antiblastic perfusion with doxorubicin in patients with intermediate or high grade limb sarcomas. *Cancer* 1994;73(8):2140–2146.
88. Nijhuis PH, Pras E, Sleijfer DT, et al. Long-term results of preoperative intra-arterial doxorubicin combined with neoadjuvant radiotherapy, followed by extensive surgical resection for locally advanced soft tissue sarcomas of the extremities. *Radiother Oncol* 1999;51(1):15–19.
89. Eggermont AM, Schraffordt Koops H, Lienard D, et al. Isolated limb perfusion with high-dose tumor necrosis factor-alpha in combination with interferon-gamma and melphalan for nonresectable extremity soft tissue sarcomas: a multicenter trial. *J Clin Oncol* 1996;14(10):2653–2665.
90. Hoekstra HJ, van Ginkel RJ. Hyperthermic isolated limb perfusion in the management of extremity sarcoma. *Curr Opin Oncol* 2003;15(4):300–303.
91. Issels RD. High-risk soft tissue sarcoma: clinical trial and hyperthermia combined chemotherapy. *Int J Hyperthermia* 2006;22(3):235–239.
92. Wong S, Brennan MF. Therapeutic management of intra-abdominal and retroperitoneal soft tissue sarcomas. *Chirurg* 2004;75(12):1174–1181.
93. Bevilacqua RG, Rogatko A, Hajdu SI, et al. Prognostic factors in primary retroperitoneal soft-tissue sarcomas. *Arch Surg* 1991;126(3):328–334.
94. Shibata D, Lewis JJ, Leung DH, et al. Is there a role for incomplete resection in the management of retroperitoneal liposarcomas? *J Am Coll Surg* 2001;193(4):373–379.
95. Lewis JJ, Leung D, Woodruff JM, et al. Retroperitoneal soft-tissue sarcoma: analysis of 500 patients treated and followed at a single institution. *Ann Surg* 1998;228(3):355–365.
96. Yeh JJ, Singer S, Brennan MF, et al. Effectiveness of palliative procedures for intra-abdominal sarcomas. *Ann Surg Oncol* 2005;12(12):1084–1089.
97. Russo P, Kim Y, Ravindran S, et al. Nephrectomy during operative management of retroperitoneal sarcoma. *Ann Surg Oncol* 1997;4(5):421–424.
98. Jaques DP, Coit DG, Hajdu SI, et al. Management of primary and recurrent soft-tissue sarcoma of the retroperitoneum. *Ann Surg* 1990;212(1): 51–59.
99. Henricks WH, Chu YC, Goldblum JR, et al. Dedifferentiated liposarcoma: a clinicopathological analysis of 155 cases with a proposal for an expanded definition of dedifferentiation. *Am J Surg Pathol* 1997;21(3):271–281.
100. Jones JJ, Catton CN, O'Sullivan B, et al. Initial results of a trial of preoperative external-beam radiation therapy and postoperative brachytherapy for retroperitoneal sarcoma. *Ann Surg Oncol* 2002;9(4):346–354.
101. Webb S. Advances in three-dimensional conformal radiation therapy physics with intensity modulation. *Lancet Oncol* 2000;1(1):30–36.
102. Leibel SA, Fuks Z, Zelefsky MJ, et al. Intensity-modulated radiotherapy. *Cancer J* 2002;8(2):164–176.
103. Raut CP, Pisters PW. Retroperitoneal sarcomas: combined-modality treatment approaches. *J Surg Oncol* 2006;94(1):81–87.
104. Singer S, Corson JM, Demetri GD, et al. Prognostic factors predictive of survival for truncal and retroperitoneal soft-tissue sarcoma. *Ann Surg* 1995;221(2):185–195.
105. Singer S, Corson JM, Gonin R, et al. Prognostic factors predictive of survival and local recurrence for extremity soft tissue sarcoma. *Ann Surg* 1994;219(2):165–173.
106. Glenn J, Sindelar WF, Kinsella T, et al. Results of multimodality therapy of resectable soft-tissue sarcomas of the retroperitoneum. *Surgery* 1985; 97(3):316–325.
107. Bentz BG, Singh B, Woodruff J, et al. Head and neck soft tissue sarcomas: a multivariate analysis of outcomes. *Ann Surg Oncol* 2004;11(6):619–628.
108. Dotan ZA, Tal R, Golijanin D, et al. Adult genitourinary sarcoma: the 25-year Memorial Sloan-Kettering experience. *J Urol* 2006;176(5): 2033–2038; discussion 2038–2039.
109. Stojadinovic A, Leung DH, Allen P, et al. Primary adult soft tissue sarcoma: time-dependent influence of prognostic variables. *J Clin Oncol* 2002;20(21):4344–4352.
110. Midis GP, Pollock RE, Chen NP, et al. Locally recurrent soft tissue sarcoma of the extremities. *Surgery* 1998;123(6):666–671.
111. Karakousis CP, Proimakis C, Rao U, et al. Local recurrence and survival in soft-tissue sarcomas. *Ann Surg Oncol* 1996;3(3):255–260.
112. Giuliano AE, Eilber FR, Morton DL. The management of locally recurrent soft-tissue sarcoma. *Ann Surg* 1982;196(1):87–91.
113. Eilber FC, Brennan MF, Riedel E, et al. Prognostic factors for survival in patients with locally recurrent extremity soft tissue sarcomas. *Ann Surg Oncol* 2005;12(3):228–236.
114. Davis SD. CT evaluation for pulmonary metastases in patients with extrathoracic malignancy. *Radiology* 1991;180(1):1–12.
115. Pfannschmidt J, Bischoff M, Muley T, et al. Diagnosis of pulmonary metastases with helical CT: the effect of imaging techniques. *Thorac Cardiovasc Surg* 2008;56(8):471–475.
116. Billingsley KG, Burt ME, Jara E, et al. Pulmonary metastases from soft tissue sarcoma: analysis of patterns of diseases and postmetastasis survival. *Ann Surg* 1999;229(5):602–610; discussion 610–612.
117. van Geel AN, Pastorino U, Jauch KW, et al. Surgical treatment of lung metastases: the European Organization for Research and Treatment of Cancer-Soft Tissue and Bone Sarcoma Group study of 255 patients. *Cancer* 1996;77(4):675–682.
118. Medeiros F, Corless CL, Duensing A, et al. KIT-negative gastrointestinal stromal tumors: proof of concept and therapeutic implications. *Am J Surg Pathol* 2004;28(7):889–894.
119. Rubin BP, Singer S, Tsao C, et al. KIT activation is a ubiquitous feature of gastrointestinal stromal tumors. *Cancer Res* 2001;61(22):8118–8121.
120. Hirota S, Isozaki K, Moriyama Y, et al. Gain-of-function mutations of c-kit in human gastrointestinal stromal tumors. *Science* 1998;279(5350): 577–580.
121. Antonescu CR, Sommer G, Sarran L, et al. Association of KIT exon 9 mutations with nongastric primary site and aggressive behavior: KIT mutation analysis and clinical correlates of 120 gastrointestinal stromal tumors. *Clin Cancer Res* 2003;9(9):3329–3337.
122. Nilsson B, Bumming P, Meis-Kindblom JM, et al. Gastrointestinal stromal tumors: the incidence, prevalence, clinical course, and prognostication in the preimatinib mesylate era—a population-based study in western Sweden. *Cancer* 2005;103(4):821–829.
123. Prakash S, Sarran L, Socci N, et al. Gastrointestinal stromal tumors in children and young adults: a clinicopathologic, molecular, and genomic study of 15 cases and review of the literature. *J Pediatr Hematol Oncol* 2005; 27(4):179–187.
124. DeMatteo RP, Lewis JJ, Leung D, et al. Two hundred gastrointestinal stromal tumors: recurrence patterns and prognostic factors for survival. *Ann Surg* 2000;231(1):51–58.
125. Joensuu H, Roberts PJ, Sarlomo-Rikala M, et al. Effect of the tyrosine kinase inhibitor STI571 in a patient with a metastatic gastrointestinal stromal tumor. *N Engl J Med* 2001;344(14):1052–1056.
126. Katz SC, DeMatteo RP. Gastrointestinal stromal tumors and leiomyosarcomas. *J Surg Oncol* 2008;97(4):350–359.
127. Wong SL. Diagnosis and management of desmoid tumors and fibrosarcoma. *J Surg Oncol* 2008;97(6):554–558.
128. Gansar GF, Markowitz IP, Cerise EJ. Thirty years of experience with desmoid tumors at Charity Hospital. *Am Surg* 1987;53(6):318–319.
129. Li M, Cordon-Cardo C, Gerald WL, et al. Desmoid fibromatosis is a clonal process. *Hum Pathol* 1996;27(9):939–943.
130. Deyrup AT, Tretiakova M, Montag AG. Estrogen receptor-beta expression in extraabdominal fibromatoses: an analysis of 40 cases. *Cancer* 2006; 106(1):208–213.
131. Merchant NB, Lewis JJ, Woodruff JM, et al. Extremity and trunk desmoid tumors: a multifactorial analysis of outcome. *Cancer* 1999;86(10): 2045–2052.
132. Shaylor PJ, Peake D, Grimer RJ, et al. Paget's osteosarcoma—no cure in sight. *Sarcoma* 1999;3(3–4):191–192.
133. Tucker MA, D'Angio GJ, Boice JD Jr, et al. Bone sarcomas linked to radiotherapy and chemotherapy in children. *N Engl J Med* 1987;317(10): 588–593.
134. Mankin HJ, Cantley KP, Lippiello L, et al. The biology of human chondrosarcoma: I. Description of the cases, grading, and biochemical analyses. *J Bone Joint Surg Am* 1980;62(2):160–176.

135. Mankin HJ, Cantley KP, Schiller AL, et al. The biology of human chondrosarcoma: II. Variation in chemical composition among types and subtypes of benign and malignant cartilage tumors. *J Bone Joint Surg Am* 1980;62(2):176–188.
136. Brenner W, Bohuslavizki KH, Eary JF. PET imaging of osteosarcoma. *J Nucl Med* 2003;44(6):930–942.
137. Nesbit ME Jr, Gehan EA, Burgert EO Jr, et al. Multimodal therapy for the management of primary, nonmetastatic Ewing's sarcoma of bone: a long-term follow-up of the First Intergroup study. *J Clin Oncol* 1990;8(10):1664–1674.
138. Burgert EO Jr, Nesbit ME, Garnsey LA, et al. Multimodal therapy for the management of nonpelvic, localized Ewing's sarcoma of bone: intergroup study IESS-II. *J Clin Oncol* 1990;8(9):1514–1524.
139. Grier HE, Krailo MD, Tarbell NJ, et al. Addition of ifosfamide and etoposide to standard chemotherapy for Ewing's sarcoma and primitive neuroectodermal tumor of bone. *N Engl J Med* 2003;348(8):694–701.
140. Schuetze SM. Chemotherapy in the management of osteosarcoma and Ewing's sarcoma. *J Natl Compr Canc Netw* 2007;5(4):449–455.
141. Esiashvili N, Goodman M, Marcus RB Jr. Changes in incidence and survival of Ewing sarcoma patients over the past 3 decades: Surveillance Epidemiology and End Results data. *J Pediatr Hematol Oncol* 2008;30(6):425–430.
142. Meyers PA, Heller G, Healey J, et al. Chemotherapy for nonmetastatic osteogenic sarcoma: the Memorial Sloan-Kettering experience. *J Clin Oncol* 1992;10(1):5–15.
143. Eilber F, Giuliano A, Eckardt J, et al. Adjuvant chemotherapy for osteosarcoma: a randomized prospective trial. *J Clin Oncol* 1987;5(1):21–26.
144. Link MP, Goorin AM, Miser AW, et al. The effect of adjuvant chemotherapy on relapse-free survival in patients with osteosarcoma of the extremity. *N Engl J Med* 1986;314(25):1600–1606.
145. Rosen G, Caparros B, Huvos AG, et al. Preoperative chemotherapy for osteogenic sarcoma: selection of postoperative adjuvant chemotherapy based on the response of the primary tumor to preoperative chemotherapy. *Cancer* 1982;49(6):1221–1230.
146. Souhami RL, Craft AW, Van der Eijken JW, et al. Randomised trial of two regimens of chemotherapy in operable osteosarcoma: a study of the European Osteosarcoma Intergroup. *Lancet* 1997;350(9082):911–917.
147. Bacci G, Picci P, Ferrari S, et al. Primary chemotherapy and delayed surgery for nonmetastatic osteosarcoma of the extremities. Results in 164 patients preoperatively treated with high doses of methotrexate followed by cisplatin and doxorubicin. *Cancer* 1993;72(11):3227–3238.

CHAPTER 113 ■ PLASTIC AND RECONSTRUCTIVE SURGERY

DAVID L. BROWN, STEVEN R. BUCHMAN, PAUL S. CEDERNA, KEVIN C. CHUNG, EDWIN G. WILKINS, AND WILLIAM M. KUZON, Jr.

KEY POINTS

1. Because all open wounds are contaminated, the designation of a wound as "infected" should be contingent on the physical examination findings of local inflammation: erythema, pain, swelling, fluctuance, purulence, and loss of function.
2. Once a wound has been fully evaluated, the treatments should be designed to achieve specific goals. In order of greatest priority, these goals are (a) preventing complications resulting from the wound, (b) preserving or restoring critical functions, (c) achieving wound closure, and (d) restoring aesthetics.
3. Skin grafts are classified as either split thickness, where the epidermis and a portion of the dermis are harvested, or full thickness, where the epidermis and the entire dermis are harvested.
4. The rediscovery of the musculocutaneous perforator as a predominant vascular supply to the skin in many areas of the body has led to the wide use of musculocutaneous flaps. These flaps derive their inflow from a major muscular artery. Perforators emanating vertically from the muscle surface supply the skin overlying the muscle.
5. A variety of operative procedures have been described for breast reconstruction following mastectomy. These approaches can be categorized as implant based, autogenous (natural) tissue, and "hybrid" procedures.
6. A variety of autogenous (natural) tissue options have been described for postmastectomy breast reconstruction. Currently, the most commonly performed of these procedures is the transverse rectus abdominis myocutaneous flap.
7. The absolute indications for replantation (i.e., situations in which replantation should always be attempted) are (a) thumb amputation, (b) multiple finger amputations, (c) pediatric population amputations, and (d) midhand, wrist, or distal forearm amputations.
8. Rigid skeletal fixation, revascularization using vein grafts, and immediate wound coverage are crucial factors in successful limb salvage.
9. Aesthetic surgery requires meticulous attention to detail, careful patient selection, rigorous procedural planning, and precise execution of technically challenging procedures. If patients are carefully selected and their goals are realistic, then the chances for a successful outcome are good. However, if a patient is poorly selected or they have unrealistic goals, then a technically successful operation with an aesthetically pleasing outcome may be a dismal failure in the eyes of the patient.
10. Patients who smoke are at a significantly increased risk for developing postoperative complications, including skin flap necrosis, infection, or wound dehiscence, and are consequently instructed to quit prior to undergoing elective aesthetic surgery.
11. A cleft lip deformity can be bilateral or unilateral and is considered complete if it extends into the nose and incomplete if it does not. The cleft lip can extend into the gum partially or completely through the alveolus, creating a bony defect. The cleft lip deformity affects the nose as well as the lip, and therefore both of these structures must be addressed in the reconstruction of the deformity.
12. Craniosynostosis is defined as the premature fusion of one or more of the cranial sutures. The child afflicted with craniosynostosis displays abnormalities in the size and shape of the cranial vault. Virchow's law proposes that the growth of the skull will be restricted in the direction perpendicular to a synostosed suture while compensatory growth occurs in a parallel direction.

Plastic and reconstructive surgery can be defined as a discipline that addresses problem wounds using a diverse array of nonsurgical and, especially, surgical therapies. In this definition, the term *problem wounds* is taken in the broadest sense; plastic surgeons treat traumatic, congenital, developmental, and even psychological wounds. Perhaps it is this latter aspect of plastic surgery that most fully sets it apart from other surgical specialties:

TABLE 113.1 COMPLICATIONS

THE SPECTRUM OF PLASTIC SURGERY

Aesthetic surgery
Burns: acute and reconstructive surgery
Craniofacial surgery
Cutaneous and soft tissue oncology
Hand and upper extremity surgery
Head and neck oncology
Microvascular surgery
Maxillofacial and orthognathic surgery
Peripheral nerve surgery
"General" reconstructive surgery
Face (ear, lip, nose, eyelid)
Breast
Trunk
Lower extremity

We restore and make whole those parts which nature or ill fortune have taken away, not so much to delight the eye but to buoy up the spirit of the afflicted.

—Gaspare Tagliacozzi, 1597

In more concrete terms, plastic surgery is an approach to surgical problems. Plastic surgeons operate "from the top of the head to the tip of the toes," and they envision themselves as surgical innovators. Plastic surgeons have been instrumental in the development of microvascular surgery, craniofacial surgery, head and neck reconstruction, nerve grafting, and even renal transplantation.[1] Although the field of plastic surgery can be arbitrarily divided into "cosmetic" surgery (surgery to improve the appearance of a normal phenotype) and "reconstructive" surgery (repair of damaged anatomy or an abnormal phenotype), in many circumstances, both functional reconstruction and aesthetic improvement are paramount. Plastic surgery is truly "general surgery," with a broad and growing list of subspecialties (Table 113.1).

PRINCIPLES OF MANAGEMENT FOR PROBLEM WOUNDS

Regardless of the etiology or location of a wound, the principles of management are universal and can be embodied by a straightforward algorithm:

1. Evaluate and, if possible, eliminate the factors contributing to the presence of the wound.
2. Control or optimize the wound prior to closure.
3. Close the wound using the simplest method, unless specific factors mitigate a more complex approach.

Although it is the nature of surgeons to focus on the technical details of operative procedures, the first two steps in this algorithm are most critical for the successful reconstruction of problem wounds. This algorithmic approach allows plastic surgeons to treat diabetic foot ulcers, infected sternotomy wounds, major defects after composite resection of the head and neck, pressure ulcers, lower extremity wounds after open tibial fractures, venous stasis ulcers, and other difficult defects with a high degree of success. *This rational approach is the core of plastic surgery*. In plastic surgery there is no one-to-one correlation between a surgical problem and a specific operation. There is no "right" way to reconstruct a given defect, and a spectrum of options must be considered for every reconstructive problem. Selecting the best option for a given patient is the challenge.

Evaluation of Problem Wounds

The evaluation of patients with difficult wounds is best approached by considering local and systemic (or intrinsic and extrinsic) contributing factors for each phase of the workup. In the history, local factors of importance include the mechanism that resulted in the wound, symptoms such as pain or loss of function, the time course and progression of the wound, any previous nonsurgical or surgical treatments for the wound, and any history of previous injury, irradiation, malignancy, or other local factors that contributed to the presence of the wound. The history should also uncover systemic factors that impair wound healing, including immunosuppression (e.g., chemotherapy, immune deficiencies), medical conditions known to impair healing (e.g., diabetes, renal failure), medications (e.g., steroids, cyclosporin A), cigarette smoking, and general debility (e.g., nutritional deficiencies, old age).

The physical examination of patients with problem wounds should be focused on local and systemic signs that affect wound healing. For the wound itself, the location, size, depth, exposure of deep or vital structures, presence of necrotic material, presence of foreign bodies, or signs of any neoplastic processes should be carefully noted. Because all 1 open wounds are contaminated, the designation of a wound as "infected" should be contingent on the physical examination findings of local inflammation: erythema, pain, swelling, fluctuance, purulence, and loss of function. Physical examination should be the primary criterion for the diagnosis of local wound infection; surface swabs indicating the presence of pathogenic bacteria do not correlate with clinically significant infection.[2] In addition to the wound itself, surrounding tissue should be examined for signs of injury (e.g., actinic changes), previous irradiation, arterial or venous insufficiency, lymphedema, loss of sensation, and dermal thinning (e.g., aging, steroid therapy). For all wounds on an arm or leg, a careful neurovascular examination for the entire limb is mandatory. In addition to the local examination, a focused systematic physical examination is mandatory in patients with problem wounds. Systemic signs of infection (e.g., fever, hypotension) are of particular importance. Obesity is a major risk factor that impairs wound healing. The general physical examination should focus on the systemic factors that affect wound healing as noted previously. Table 113.2 lists some of the local and systemic factors that impair wound healing; history and physical examination are the principal modalities for diagnosing these problems.

Laboratory examinations can be invaluable in the management of problem wounds. However, laboratory tests are often misused in wound patients, and a rational, evidence-based approach is necessary to efficiently utilize this expensive resource. Again, the local–systemic paradigm is useful in determining which laboratory examinations are warranted.

For local evaluation, as already mentioned, wound swabs can be valuable for surveillance of the flora contaminating a wound but should not be used as a trigger to initiate therapy for wound infection. Wound biopsy and quantitative bacteriology have proved valuable in the management of burns and chronic wounds.[3,4] Bacterial loads in excess of 10^5/g tissue indicate contamination at a level that precludes skin graft take and jeopardizes wound closure of any kind. The use of quantitative cultures, however, is not justified for most acute or uncomplicated chronic wounds. In general, quantitative cultures are reserved for "high stakes" wounds, where a failure of closure on the initial attempt may leave an unreconstructable situation with grave consequences, such as amputation or death. Wound biopsies can be invaluable for diagnosing invasive burn wound infection and are preferred over quantitative

TABLE 113.2 CLASSIFICATION

LOCAL AND SYSTEMIC FACTORS THAT AFFECT WOUND MANAGEMENT

LOCAL FACTORS	SYSTEMIC FACTORS
Infection	Immune deficiencies
Local malignancy	Distant malignancy
Foreign bodies	Diabetes mellitus
Local toxins	Cigarette smoking
Radiation	Chemotherapeutic agents
Ischemia	Hereditary healing disorders
Venous insufficiency	Nutritional deficiency
Lymphatic insufficiency	Old age
Repetitive trauma	Uremia
Reduced sensation	Glucocorticoid therapy, immunosuppressive agents

culture for this purpose.[5] The presence of bacteria in the deep dermis on biopsy is highly correlated with the risk of systemic sepsis in burn patients. Bone biopsy demonstrating bacteria within the bone is the preferred test for making the diagnosis of osteomyelitis. Standard radiographs are most useful for diagnosing and delineating acute fractures and are much less useful in the setting of chronic, open wounds. Ultrasound, computed tomography (CT) scan, or magnetic resonance imaging (MRI) may be useful for delineating fluid collections, necrotic tissue, or inflammation in selected circumstances. In contrast, radionuclide bone scans have little role to play in patients with open wounds or fractures. In the face of an open wound or recent fracture, a "hot" bone scan (even a triple-phase bone scan) is not specific for osteomyelitis and has little value. Therefore, obtaining bone scans in patients with suspected sternal osteomyelitis after recent midline sternotomy, in pressure sore patients with exposed bone, or in other patients with open wounds overlying exposed bone is unwarranted. Under these circumstances, bone biopsy is preferred for making a diagnosis of osteomyelitis and for determining the responsible pathogen; MRI is preferred for delineating the extent of bony involvement. Magnetic resonance angiography (MRA) or standard angiography may be indicated if vascular insufficiency is suspected or if a free-tissue transfer is planned.

The use of systemic laboratory investigations should be limited to specific indications; "routine" blood work is not required for patients with acute or chronic wounds. White blood cell differential counts and blood cultures can confirm the diagnosis of systemic infection. Serum albumin and transferrin determinations may be valuable in determining nutritional status. A greatly elevated erythrocyte sedimentation rate can help confirm the diagnosis of osteomyelitis. Other laboratory tests to confirm the diagnosis and severity of associated medical conditions may be justified for specific indications.

Treatment of the Problem Wound

2 Once a wound has been fully evaluated, the treatments should be designed to achieve specific goals. In order of greatest priority, these goals are (a) preventing complications resulting from the wound, (b) preserving or restoring critical functions, (c) achieving wound closure, and (d) restoring aesthetics. Again, each of these goals may require specific local or systemic interventions.

Preventive Treatment. The preventive measures that should be taken for patients with open wounds depend on the setting. For an acute laceration, tetanus prophylaxis should be considered. For patients with pressure sores, a strict adherence to pressure-relief protocols and an assessment of nutritional status take priority. In wounds caused by human or animal bites, prophylactic antibiotics are warranted. In addition, any associated medical conditions that are contributing to the wound must be aggressively optimized. It is the responsibility of the surgeon to ensure that a patient with a wound does not develop a complication from that wound and that the patient does not develop more wounds from the same mechanism. This is of particular importance in bedridden, obtunded, or paralyzed patients, in whom it should be possible to completely prevent pressure sores with proper nursing care.

Preservation of Function. Preserving joint motion must always be considered for patients with open wounds of the extremities. Aggressive physiotherapy to maintain or improve joint motion can be instituted in the presence of an open wound. Splinting should be used to minimize joint contractures and any plans for wound closure should include measures to maintain joint function. In the case of facial defects, especially if facial paralysis is present, oral competence and the maintenance of eye protection should weigh heavily into any reconstructive plan. Function takes precedence over form in the reconstructive algorithm.

Nonsurgical Therapy. After careful consideration of preventive measures and the preservation of critical function, a strategy for wound closure can be formulated. The basic tenet is: "débride dirty wounds, close clean wounds." Therefore, the first step in wound closure is achieving control of the wound by eliminating necrotic debris and controlling any infection present. Nonsurgical therapies are used in conjunction with surgical therapy to achieve a clean wound. The mainstay of local, nonsurgical therapy is the use of wound dressings. It is beyond the scope of this chapter to review the wide range of options available to dress wounds. Recent articles contain a contemporary review of this topic.[6–8] However, the basic principle is to employ débriding dressings for dirty wounds and occlusive dressings for clean wounds. The most commonly employed débriding dressing is the "wet-to-dry" dressing. Gauze made damp with normal saline, weak acetic acid, weak bleach, or various other solutions is applied to the wound. Over a period of hours, evaporation dries the dressing, which becomes slightly adherent to the wound surface. When the dressing is removed, necrotic debris is pulled off with the dressing, but healthy tissue is left behind. Wet-to-dry dressings work through *mechanical débridement,* and the most important component of their use is how often they are changed. Wet-to-dry dressings must be changed a minimum of twice per day; they should not be "soaked" off to reduce patient discomfort because this technique completely defeats their purpose. Enzymatic dressings have also been used to débride wounds, but their use can be limited by patient tolerance to the pain they cause. Débriding dressings are indicated for infected wounds and wounds containing necrotic debris.

If a wound is "clean," meaning that it does not contain necrotic debris and has an acceptable bacterial load, a dressing that maintains a moist wound environment to encourage wound healing should be used.[8] For many simple wounds, allowing a scab to provide the moist healing environment or the application of a nonadherent sterile dressing is all that is required. In the case of more complex wounds, occlusive dressings that maintain a moist environment to maximize wound healing are preferred. Options include hydrocolloid dressings, alginate dressings, and various hydrogels. Again, occlusive dressings must not be used on infected or dirty wounds. For many wounds, judicious application of hydrocolloid dressings may allow closure by secondary intention in a reasonable period of time.

Under some circumstances, it is appropriate to use antibiotic dressings. Burn wounds are most commonly dressed with silver sulfadiazine or mafenide Sulfamylon (Bertek Pharmaceuticals, Inc., Research Triangle Park, North Carolina) dressings. The low toxicity and excellent antibiotic properties of elemental silver have led to the development and widespread use of wound dressings containing nanocrystalline silver. Acticoat (Smith & Nephew, London, UK) is particularly useful for the management of large burn wounds and for dressing skin grafts applied to chronic wounds.[9,10] In general, however, antibiotic dressings are not required for clean wounds, even if they are chronic.

Last, it should be noted that we are entering a new era of nonsurgical wound management. A rapid advance in our understanding of wound healing has led to the development of growth factor therapy, cellular therapy, and new physical modalities for the treatment of chronic wounds.[6] Although recombinant platelet-derived growth factor appears to be a useful adjunct to the dressing regimen for pressure sores and diabetic foot ulcers,[11,12] there is general agreement that exogenously administered growth factors currently play a limited role in the management of acute and chronic wounds.[13] Similarly, laboratory data point to the potential for the use of stem cells as a modality to treat difficult wounds, but cellular therapy for clinical wounds is still largely investigational.[6,14]

A bigger clinical impact has been realized from tissue-engineered dressings and skin substitutes.[15,16] Integra (Integra Life Sciences Corp., Plainsboro, New Jersey), a bilaminar skin substitute composed of a collagen matrix base with a silicone rubber barrier layer, has proven extremely useful in the management of complex wounds. Integra is most useful for burn wounds and wounds where a poorly vascularized base precludes immediate skin grafting. While the silicone membrane serves as a barrier and maintains a moist environment, the collagen matrix supports the ingrowth of vascularized granulation tissue. Integra is now an integral part of the management of burn wounds, with the silicone layer providing a temporary barrier function that allows excision of eschar when autograft supply is limited.[15] In poorly vascularized wounds, the ingrowth of vascularized tissue allows skin grafting at a second operation. That is, this strategy converts a complex wound, requiring a flap reconstruction, to a much simpler wound that can be managed with skin grafting. Integra has proven to be of considerable utility in the management of wounds of the scalp resulting from the excision of skin cancers where bare skull is exposed in a previously irradiated field. Integra placement supports the development of a vascularized base and has allowed many such wounds to be closed with skin grafts.[17] Likewise, the management of wounds of the hand after trauma or tumor excision with Integra and delayed grafting can often prevent the need for flap surgery or even, in the case of squamous cell carcinomas of the fingers, amputation.[18] The development of new tissue-engineered adjuncts to wound healing remains a very active area of research in plastic surgery.

Negative-pressure wound therapy has become widespread and has been demonstrated to be efficacious and cost effective when applied appropriately for complex wounds.[19,20] The commercially available VAC system (KCI, San Antonio, Texas) employs an open cell sponge that is applied to the wound and then sealed with an impermeable plastic dressing; negative pressure is applied to the sponge via tubing and pump. Extensive experimental and clinical data confirm that the VAC system promotes tissue perfusion, reduces edema, favorably alters wound fluid composition, and stimulates the formation of granulation tissue.[19] The VAC system is easy to use; its primary limitation is related to cost. Additional cost-utility studies to justify its higher daily cost compared with simple dressings are required.

Multiple other modalities, such as hyperbaric oxygen treatment, are in use and are being developed on an ongoing basis, underscoring the high prevalence, the significant cost, and the clinical challenge that are posed by complex wounds. Despite these ongoing developments, the basic algorithm for evaluation and nonsurgical management of wounds will not change.

Surgical Therapy

Wound Preparation. For problem wounds, surgical therapy is primarily aimed at wound preparation and wound reconstruction. For dirty wounds with necrotic debris, a judicious but thorough surgical débridement can convert a contaminated, chronic wound into a fresh surgical wound ready for immediate closure. Although débriding dressings can prepare wounds for closure under some circumstances, an operative débridement is preferred to a long course of débriding dressings for most problem wounds. Consequently, most complex wounds require an operative débridement prior to definitive reconstruction. In the case of chronic osteomyelitis, a formal resection of the sequestrum is required before formal wound closure. Prolonged treatment with intravenous or oral antibiotics cannot clear bacteria from a focus of dead bone; chronic osteomyelitis is a surgical disease cured with a saw, rongeur, bur, or bone curette. Therefore, the common practice of placing patients with chronic osteomyelitis on 6 weeks of antibiotic therapy is irrational unless performed in conjunction with a formal sequestrectomy.

Reconstructive Principles. As stated earlier, there is no "right" way to close any given wound. Plastic surgeons use a straightforward set of principles in delineating the optimum way to close a given wound for a given patient. The predominant principle is that the simplest method to close a wound is usually the best choice. This principle is embodied in the "reconstructive ladder," which is a hierarchy of reconstructive options progressing from simple to complex (Table 113.3). Therefore, when engaging options for wound closure, plastic surgeons "climb" the reconstructive ladder, usually stopping on the lowest rung that will achieve a closed wound. However, other principles of reconstruction sometimes override a slavish adherence to the reconstructive ladder. The choice of a technique for wound closure should take into consideration the need for subsequent procedures and other factors that might mitigate skipping over simpler options for wound closure. An example would be an avulsion injury to the palm of the hand. Although it might be possible to close this wound with a skin graft, the need to restore flexor tendon function is preeminent in the hand, so that the use of a distant flap to provide a suitable bed for tendon grafting may be the preferred choice. In addition to the reconstructive ladder, other examples of guiding reconstructive principles are as follows: function takes precedence over form, single-stage reconstructions are preferred over multistage approaches, and autologous tissue is preferred over alloplastic reconstructions. Other factors to be considered are the durability of the reconstruction over many years, the psychological impact on the patient, and data indicating that some options are sometimes preferred for specific reasons. For example, muscle flaps are known to be superior to skin flaps in their ability to resist or eradicate infection.[21] Therefore, a muscle flap may be chosen over a simpler option if the eradication of osteomyelitis or mediastinitis is the goal.

TABLE 113.3 **ETIOLOGY**

THE RECONSTRUCTIVE LADDER

1. Primary wound closure
2. Healing by secondary intention
3. Skin grafting
4. Local flaps
5. Regional flaps
6. Distant flaps

As mentioned earlier, weighing this complex array of factors to arrive at the optimal reconstruction for a given patient is the true challenge in reconstructive surgery.

Reconstructive Techniques. Regardless of the reconstructive method chosen, plastic surgeons strive for technical virtuosity in the operating room. To maximize healing and minimize scar formation, atraumatic technique includes delicate tissue handling, the use of skin hooks and sharp rakes, bipolar electrocautery, sharp dissection, and loupe magnification. When reconstructing difficult wounds, the margin for error is minimal, and small errors in technical execution can result in failure. The general surgical methods used by reconstructive surgeons are briefly considered in this chapter.

Primary Closure. If a laceration or other wound can be closed primarily, consideration is given to a meticulous, layered closure. Emphasis is placed on eversion of skin edges without strangling tissue. Nonabsorbable skin stitches that provoke minimal inflammatory response are preferred, but they must be removed promptly to minimize cross-hatching. Therefore, for most wounds, deep dermal, absorbable stitches are placed to allow early removal of skin stitches while still providing prolonged support to the repair; this may minimize the chances of a dehiscence or scar spread. It is preferable to place a closed-suction drain to eliminate dead space rather than suturing fat or other easily devascularized tissue. If a technically perfect, tension-free repair cannot be achieved with primary closure, it is preferable to use a more complex surgical option.

3 *Skin Grafting.* Skin grafting was one of the foundations on which the specialty of plastic surgery was established. Skin grafts are classified as either split thickness, where the epidermis and a portion of the dermis are harvested, or full thickness, where the epidermis and the entire dermis are harvested. Both full-thickness and split-thickness skin grafts can be used to resurface open wounds in cases in which primary closure is not possible. Skin graft take is contingent on the successful revascularization of the graft within a narrow time window (48 to 72 hours). Initially, grafts are nourished by a process of plasmatic imbibition, wherein serum from the wound bed diffuses into the adjacent graft. Revascularization occurs by the process of inosculation. Vessels from the wound bed grow into the graft, forming functional circulatory connections with the vasculature of the graft. For plasmatic imbibition and inosculation to be successful, two criteria must be met. First, the wound bed must be appropriately vascularized. Therefore, skin grafts cannot be placed on poorly vascularized wound surfaces, including bone denuded of periosteum, tendon denuded of peritenon, or cartilage. Second, a bolster dressing or splint must be used to ensure absolute immobilization of the graft on the bed to prevent shearing of the nascent vascular connections during inosculation. If either of these criteria cannot be met, a more complex reconstructive option must be considered.

Random Skin Flaps. The use of tissue (usually skin) immediately adjacent to the defect as the tissue for reconstruction is referred to as a local flap reconstruction. Skin rearrangement can range in complexity from simple undermining to complex, geometric skin flaps. Which method is appropriate is dependent on multiple factors, including the etiology of the defect, the desired direction of the scar, the fragility or mobility of underlying structures, and the need to avoid distortion to adjacent free margins such as the lip or eyelid. Significant experience is required for the optimal utilization of skin rearrangement. When plastic surgeons think of "classical" skin flaps, they are referring to random skin flaps, without an axial blood supply. These skin flaps rely on a dermal plexus of vessels for their survival, and the perfusion of the distal end of the flap is inadequate to allow tissue survival if the flap design is inappropriate. It was previously thought that survival of the distal part of random skin flaps could be ensured by adhering to length-to-width ratios established for various areas of the body. It is now recognized that these ratios have no basis in circulatory physiology, and the surviving length of a random skin flap does not depend on flap width.[22] In practice, most of the commonly employed skin flaps have been developed empirically. There are three basic types of random skin flaps: rotation, advancement, and transposition, depending on how adjacent skin is shifted into the defect. Each type of flap has specific design criteria. Many eponyms are used to describe variations on these basic three flap designs; examples are the Romberg transposition flap, the Mustarde rotation flap, and the Rintala advancement flap. Excellent reviews of the use of skin flaps in reconstructive surgery are available.[23,24]

As mentioned earlier, the concern with flap viability limits the utility of random skin flaps. Several strategies have been developed to circumvent this problem. The first of these is the concept of surgical delay. Delay is defined as the partial interruption of blood flow to a defined piece of tissue. At present, surgical delay is the only method available to augment the surviving length of random skin flaps (Fig. 113.1). Another strategy is the use of tissue expanders. Tissue expanders are implantable balloons that are inserted in a deflated state and are inflated with sterile saline via percutaneous injection into a self-sealing valve. Except for the scalp, where expanders are placed in the subgaleal plane, tissue expanders are usually placed subcutaneously. In fact, the insertion of the tissue expander into a subcutaneous pocket effects a surgical delay, and the slow expansion has been demonstrated to result in the formation of new skin. However, the most important strategy to circumvent the use of random skin flaps has been to develop axial pattern flaps that do not rely on a random blood supply.

Flaps with Axial Blood Supply. Regional flaps are defined as the transfer of tissue that is not immediately adjacent to the defect without the disruption of blood supply to the transferred tissue. For this approach to be practical, an axial blood supply to the transferred tissue must be present.

Axial Skin Flaps. The pioneering work of Bakamjian[25] and McGregor and Jackson[26] identified longitudinal blood vessels of large caliber traversing a defined region of skin. Their descriptions of the deltopectoral and groin flaps, respectively, opened a new era of reconstructive surgery. Surgeons were no longer constrained to the use of random skin flaps; any piece of tissue in the body with an axial blood supply could be transposed on a vascular pedicle with a high degree of assurance that the tissue would survive. Taylor and Palmer's[27] description of the angiosome concept solidified our ability to design flaps based on a sound knowledge of vascular anatomy. An angiosome is defined as a region of tissue supplied by an identifiable, and usually named, artery and its venae comitantes. Because of the ability of choke vessels crossing angiosome boundaries to enlarge, flaps can be designed to encompass an adjacent angiosome. However, flaps crossing two angiosome boundaries are destined to undergo partial necrosis. In practice, there are relatively few axial skin flaps, most being better classified as fasciocutaneous flaps.

Fasciocutaneous Flaps. Cormack and Lamberty[28] further expanded our understanding of the blood supply to the skin with their description of fasciocutaneous flaps. They pointed out that the dermal plexus derives its inflow from vertically oriented vessels arising at the level of the deep fascia. The vessels at the deep facial level have horizontal orientation relative to the skin's surface and form a subfacial plexus. This subfacial plexus can form the basis for the design of fasciocutaneous flaps based on several defined anatomic patterns.[28] Several fasciocutaneous flaps have enjoyed widespread use. The radial forearm flap has become a workhorse for hand reconstruction and as a free flap

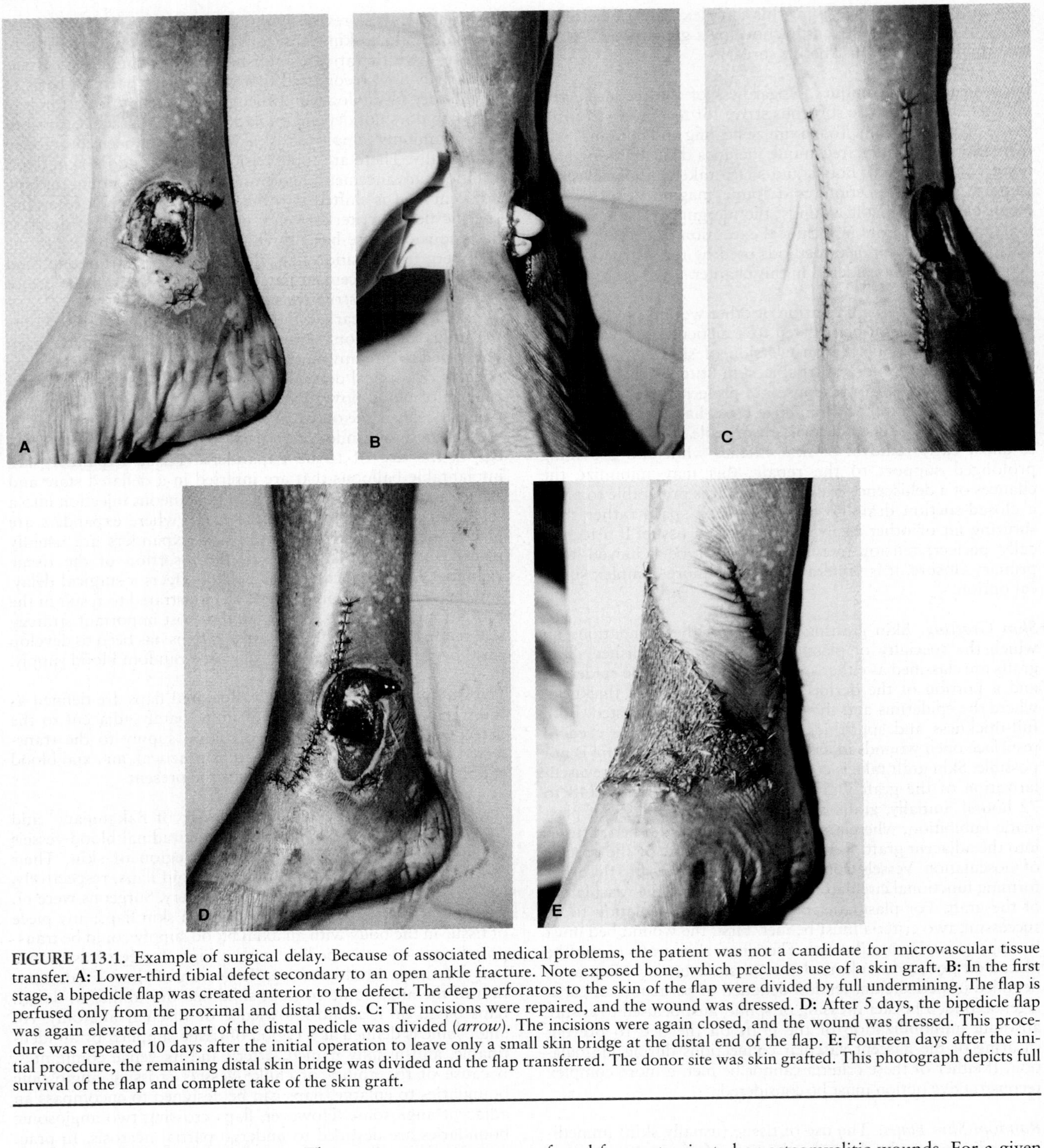

FIGURE 113.1. Example of surgical delay. Because of associated medical problems, the patient was not a candidate for microvascular tissue transfer. **A:** Lower-third tibial defect secondary to an open ankle fracture. Note exposed bone, which precludes use of a skin graft. **B:** In the first stage, a bipedicle flap was created anterior to the defect. The deep perforators to the skin of the flap were divided by full undermining. The flap is perfused only from the proximal and distal ends. **C:** The incisions were repaired, and the wound was dressed. **D:** After 5 days, the bipedicle flap was again elevated and part of the distal pedicle was divided (*arrow*). The incisions were again closed, and the wound was dressed. This procedure was repeated 10 days after the initial operation to leave only a small skin bridge at the distal end of the flap. **E:** Fourteen days after the initial procedure, the remaining distal skin bridge was divided and the flap transferred. The donor site was skin grafted. This photograph depicts full survival of the flap and complete take of the skin graft.

for head and neck reconstruction. The osteoseptocutaneous fibula free flap has been widely used for intraoral reconstruction during reconstruction of oromandibular defects.

Muscle and Myocutaneous Flaps. Based on the knowledge that tissue with an axial blood supply can be reliably transferred, muscle and myocutaneous flaps came into widespread use in the 1980s, thanks in large part to the classification system by Mathes and Nahai.[29] Whole muscles can be transferred as a pedicled or free flap if a dominant vascular pedicle is present. Segmental muscle transfers are sometimes possible on minor vascular pedicles. Muscle flaps have enjoyed wide use for a diverse array of indications. As mentioned earlier, muscle flaps have an enhanced ability to eradicate infection and are preferred for contaminated or osteomyelitic wounds. For a given defect, muscle flaps are chosen by their size and arc of rotation.

4 The rediscovery of the musculocutaneous perforator as a predominant vascular supply to the skin in many areas of the body has led to the wide use of musculocutaneous flaps. These flaps derive their inflow from a major muscular artery. Perforators emanating vertically from the muscle surface supply the skin overlying the muscle. Table 113.4 lists "workhorse" muscle and myocutaneous flaps. Of particular note is the transverse rectus abdominis myocutaneous (TRAM) flap, based on periumbilical myocutaneous perforators from the rectus abdominis muscle, which has been widely employed for breast reconstruction.[30] An extension of this concept has led to the increasing use of "perforator" flaps. Perforator flaps are based

TABLE 113.4 CLASSIFICATION

WORKHORSE MUSCLE, MYOCUTANEOUS, AND PERFORATOR FLAPS

■ FLAP	■ MYOCUTANEOUS	■ PERFORATOR	■ COMMON USES
Temporalis	No	No	Orbital and intraoral reconstruction, facial reanimation (pedicled flap)
Pectoralis major	Yes	No	Intraoral and neck reconstruction; reconstruction of sternal defects (muscle only)
Latissimus dorsi	Yes	Yes	Breast reconstruction, neck reconstruction, free flap for very large defects
Rectus abdominis	Yes, including TRAM	Yes, including DIEP	Breast reconstruction, sternal reconstruction, reconstruction of groin defects, free flap for medium-sized defects
Gluteus maximus	Yes	Yes, including SGAP	Ischial pressure sores, sacral pressure sores, SGAP used for breast reconstruction
Biceps femoris	Yes	No	Ischial pressure sores
Tensor fascia lata	Yes	No	Trochanteric pressure sores, abdominal wall reconstruction
Gracilis	Yes	Yes	Perineal reconstruction, vaginal reconstruction, facial reanimation (muscle free flap), free flap for small defects
Rectus femoris	Yes	No	Infected hip wounds, abdominal wall reconstruction
Medial gastrocnemius	Rarely	No	Knee defects, proximal third tibial defects
Soleus	No	No	Middle third tibial defects

DIEP, deep inferior epigastric perforator; SGAP, superior gluteal artery perforator; TRAM, transverse rectus abdominis myocutaneous.

on fasciocutaneous or myocutaneous perforating vessels. Dissection isolates the skin and subcutaneous tissue to be transferred on one or more perforating vessels; the underlying muscle is left intact, eliminating the functional disturbance that would result if a whole muscle was harvested. Because of their robust vascularity and ability to minimize donor deficit, perforator flaps are a "growth area" in reconstructive surgery, and a large number of perforator flaps have now been described and are used as both pedicled and free flaps.[31]

Microvascular Tissue Transfer. Historically, pedicled flaps were used to reconstruct distant defects. The distant transfer was accomplished in one of two ways. Flaps could be moved to the defect in a series of pedicled transfers (waltzing or tumbling flaps). Alternatively, flaps could be attached directly to the defect with a temporary pedicle to the donor site being maintained temporarily. At a second stage the flap was detached from the donor site, after it had developed sufficient blood supply from the recipient bed (e.g., cross-leg flaps, pedicled groin flaps). Although the distant transfer of pedicled flaps still has definitive indications (e.g., the median forehead flap for nasal reconstruction), reconstruction using distant tissue is now most commonly performed via microvascular tissue transfer, or "free" flaps. First described clinically by Daniel and Taylor,[32] free flaps have revolutionized reconstructive surgery. Any tissue with an axial blood supply with pedicle vessels 1 mm in diameter or larger can be reliably transferred microsurgically. Circulation in the transferred tissue is established via microvascular anastomoses between the axial flap vessels and vessels in the recipient site. Microvascular anastomoses are performed with 9–0 or 10–0 suture with the aid of an operating microscope; success rates for free-flap transfers exceed 90%.[33] The greatest advantage of free-flap reconstruction is that the surgeon is not restricted to the use of available, local tissues; any flap or composite block of tissue that has feeding vessels large enough for microvascular anastomoses (1 mm diameter or larger) can be transferred with this technique. By using composite tissue flaps, massive, complex tissue defects can be reconstructed replacing "like with like"[34] (Fig. 113.2). Bowel, skin, bone, muscle, fascia, and composite tissue can be transferred microsurgically. Free flaps are the primary modality for reconstruction of major head and neck defects after composite resection of squamous cell carcinoma and for the reconstruction of traumatic defects in the distal foreleg. As already mentioned, perforator flaps are increasingly used as microsurgical tissue transfers. The anterior lateral thigh (ALT) perforator flap has become a workhorse for reconstruction for a diverse array of complex defects, especially after extirpative surgery of the head and neck,[35] and the deep inferior epigastric artery perforator (DIEP) flap now rivals the TRAM as the workhorse for autologous breast reconstruction.[36]

RECONSTRUCTIVE AND AESTHETIC SURGERY OF THE BREAST

Plastic surgery of the female breast includes both reconstructive and aesthetic procedures. Breast reconstruction following mastectomy and reduction mammaplasty for macromastia (oversized breasts) are the most common examples of reconstructive breast surgery. By contrast, breast augmentation (enlargement) and mastopexy (breast lift) generally are performed for aesthetic reasons. Although some surgical approaches may be applicable to both categories of breast procedures, the relative benefits, risks, and costs of reconstructive versus aesthetic breast surgery may be quite different, particularly as viewed by patients, providers, and payers.

Before advising women on reconstructive or aesthetic breast procedures, the surgeon should carefully assess the patient's

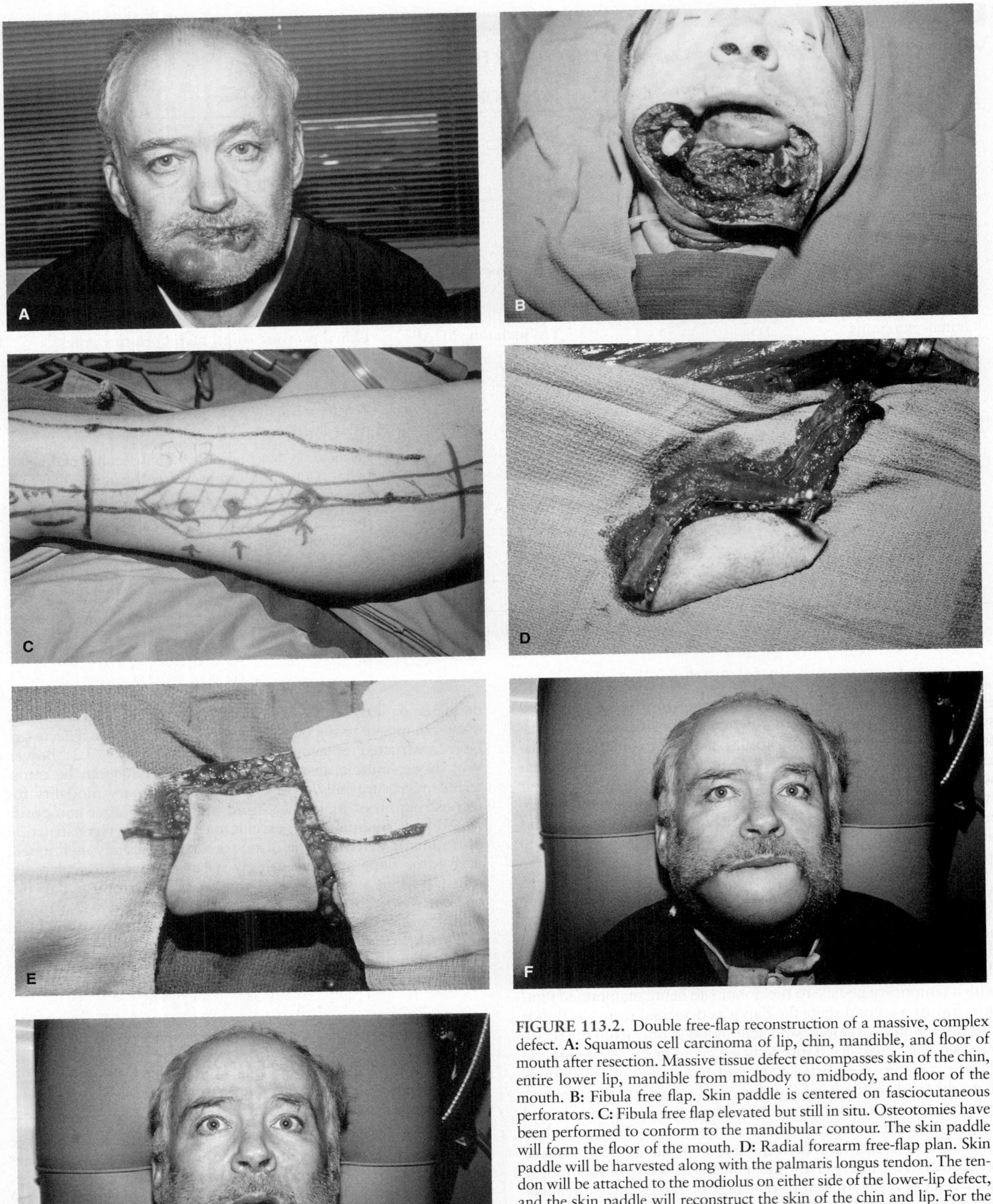

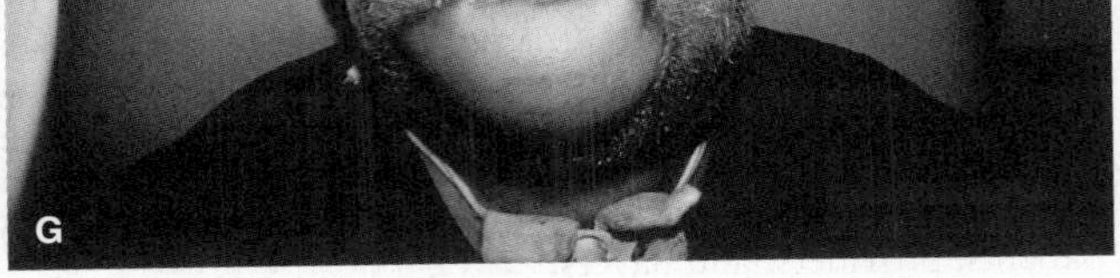

FIGURE 113.2. Double free-flap reconstruction of a massive, complex defect. **A:** Squamous cell carcinoma of lip, chin, mandible, and floor of mouth after resection. Massive tissue defect encompasses skin of the chin, entire lower lip, mandible from midbody to midbody, and floor of the mouth. **B:** Fibula free flap. Skin paddle is centered on fasciocutaneous perforators. **C:** Fibula free flap elevated but still in situ. Osteotomies have been performed to conform to the mandibular contour. The skin paddle will form the floor of the mouth. **D:** Radial forearm free-flap plan. Skin paddle will be harvested along with the palmaris longus tendon. The tendon will be attached to the modiolus on either side of the lower-lip defect, and the skin paddle will reconstruct the skin of the chin and lip. For the lip, the skin paddle will be draped over the tendon like a bed sheet on a clothesline. **E:** Radial forearm flap elevated but in situ. **F:** Postoperative result, mouth closed. **G:** Postoperative result, mouth open. (Reproduced with permission from Kuzon WM Jr, Jejurikar S, Wilkins EG, et al. Double free-flap reconstruction of massive defects involving the lip, chin, and mandible. *Microsurgery* 1998;18:372–378.)

current preferences, concerns, history, and physical findings. Initially, any history of breast disease (as well as familial history of breast pathologies) should be evaluated. On physical examination, careful linear measurements and preoperative photographs should be taken to document existing contour deformities, asymmetries, or other findings. A standard breast examination should be carried out to detect previously undiagnosed masses, nipple discharge, or lymphadenopathy. Finally, it is also advisable that women age 40 years or older undergo mammography unless this study has been performed in the previous 12 months.

Preoperative consultation should include a thorough discussion covering the relative benefits and risks of the various surgical options. The surgeon is well advised to provide comprehensive information in an understandable format. To enhance patient satisfaction with the eventual surgical result, providers should elicit patients' preferences and expectations for surgical outcomes and tailor treatment options accordingly. Because of the prevalence of breast cancer in North American women, the impact of reconstructive or aesthetic procedures on breast cancer monitoring also should be discussed.

Reconstructive Breast Surgery

5 **Postmastectomy Reconstruction.** A variety of operative procedures have been described for breast reconstruction following mastectomy. These approaches can be categorized as implant-based, autogenous (natural) tissue, and "hybrid" procedures. For purposes of this discussion, the term *hybrid* is applied to procedures combining elements of both implant and autogenous tissue techniques. This overview describes the advantages and disadvantages of the most common techniques. Ultimately, procedure selection is based on a range of patient variables, including size and shape of the desired reconstructed breast; availability of local, regional, and distant donor tissues; coexisting medical problems; and, perhaps most important, patient preferences.

Implant-based Techniques. As most commonly practiced, the implant approach usually requires two operative procedures to reconstruct the female breast. In the first stage, a temporary tissue expander is placed in a soft tissue pocket, usually located deep to the pectoralis major muscle. The tissue expander is a deflated Silastic (silicone) envelope with an integrated or remote injection port through which saline solution can be percutaneously injected. Following expander placement and meticulous closure of the overlying muscle and skin, saline is periodically injected beginning at 10 to 21 days (Fig. 113.3A). As the device enlarges, growth is induced in the overlying skin, recreating soft tissue coverage for the new breast.[37]

Following completion of expansion, most surgeons delay the second stage of reconstruction for 1 to 4 months to allow for maximal skin growth. At the conclusion of this hiatus, the second procedure is performed, consisting of removal of the expander and placement of the reconstructive implant (Fig. 113.3B). Currently available breast implants include a range of options, including variations in shape (round vs. "anatomic" or teardrop configurations), fill material (silicone gel vs. saline), and surface configuration (smooth vs. textured envelopes). The relative advantages and disadvantages of these options are discussed in the Breast Augmentation section later in this chapter. As the most common option for postmastectomy reconstruction in the United States, the expander–implant approach offers several advantages. The surgical procedures associated with this approach usually are relatively brief (often 1 hour or less) and are technically straightforward. Particularly when employed in concert with procedures on the contralateral breast (i.e., breast reduction, mastopexy, or augmentation), resulting symmetry and aesthetic outcomes are relatively good.

Patients considering implant reconstruction should also be mindful of the disadvantages of these procedures. The expander–implant approach usually requires two surgical procedures, multiple visits for expansion, and approximately 4 to 6 months to complete. For patients eager to return to a normal lifestyle following breast cancer treatment, this delay can be particularly frustrating. In addition, tissue expanders and

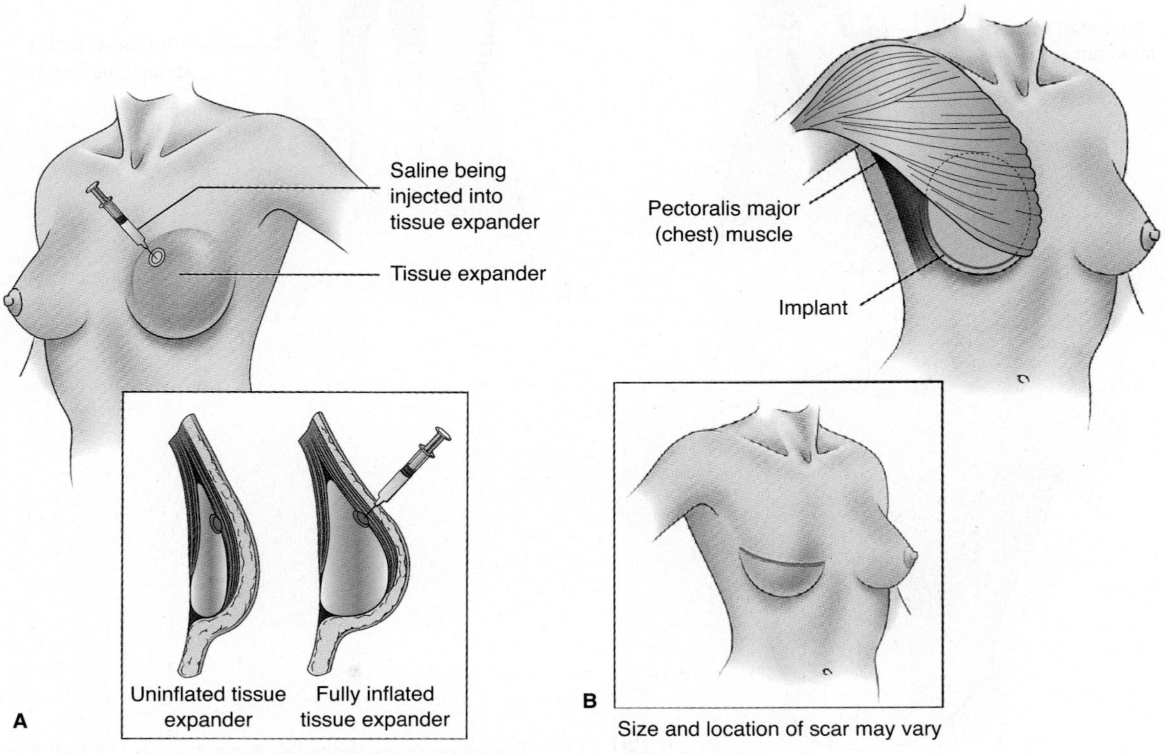

FIGURE 113.3. Expander–implant reconstruction.

reconstructive implants have been associated with a number of complications. Early in the postoperative period, these devices may be troubled by delays in wound healing, at times resulting in implant exposure and requiring explantation. Implant infections also may necessitate removal of the prosthetic device. Late complications include expander or implant leakage. Also, the development of excessive scar tissue surrounding the implant (termed a *capsular contracture*) can produce a hard, painful, or deformed breast requiring surgical revision.

6 *Autogenous Tissue Reconstruction.* A variety of autogenous (natural) tissue options have been described for postmastectomy breast reconstruction. Currently, the most commonly performed of these procedures is the TRAM flap. Originally popularized by Hartrampf et al.,[30] the TRAM flap is most commonly performed as a pedicle muscle flap; that is, the transferred rectus muscle is left partially attached to the costal margin, preserving the superior epigastric artery and vein as the flap's blood supply (Fig. 113.4A, B). In pedicle TRAM reconstruction, the rectus muscle serves as the vascular carrier for a large ellipse of lower abdominal skin and fat. These tissues are tunneled subcutaneously into the mastectomy defect, where they are sculpted into the desired breast size and shape. Meanwhile, the abdominal donor site is closed by reapproximating the anterior rectus sheath and by advancing the remaining superior skin edge of the donor site as a modified abdominoplasty (Fig. 113.4C).

Pedicle TRAM reconstruction offers several benefits. Because the TRAM flap usually provides a generous amount of lower abdominal adipose tissue for breast bulk, implants are rarely needed with this approach. The TRAM flap can be inset and sculpted in a virtually infinite number of ways, giving the reconstructive surgeon considerable latitude in the creation of breast shapes and sizes. Furthermore, in contrast to implant approaches, TRAM reconstruction is a one-stage technique, requiring only a single surgery to recreate the breast mound. An additional advantage of TRAM flaps is their tendency to gain or lose volume in association with weight changes and body mass, thereby maintaining better symmetry than implant reconstructions over time. Among reconstructive surgeons, there appears to be a growing consensus that TRAM flaps produce superior aesthetic results compared with other techniques.

Despite these advantages, TRAM flaps also are associated with several disadvantages. Compared with implant approaches, TRAM reconstruction requires longer operations, hospitalizations, and recovery times. Furthermore, TRAM procedures can produce a range of complications, including partial and total flap loss as a result of vascular compromise of the transferred tissue. Also, occurrences of postoperative abdominal hernias or (more commonly) abdominal wall laxity remain persistent issues for some patients choosing TRAM reconstruction.[38]

Although the pedicle TRAM flap is the most frequently employed option for autogenous tissue breast reconstruction, free tissue transfer has received growing attention as a potentially useful technique for recreating the breast mound. In particular, the free TRAM flap has been promoted by Kroll and Baldwin,[39] Grotting et al.,[40] and Allen and Treece[41] as

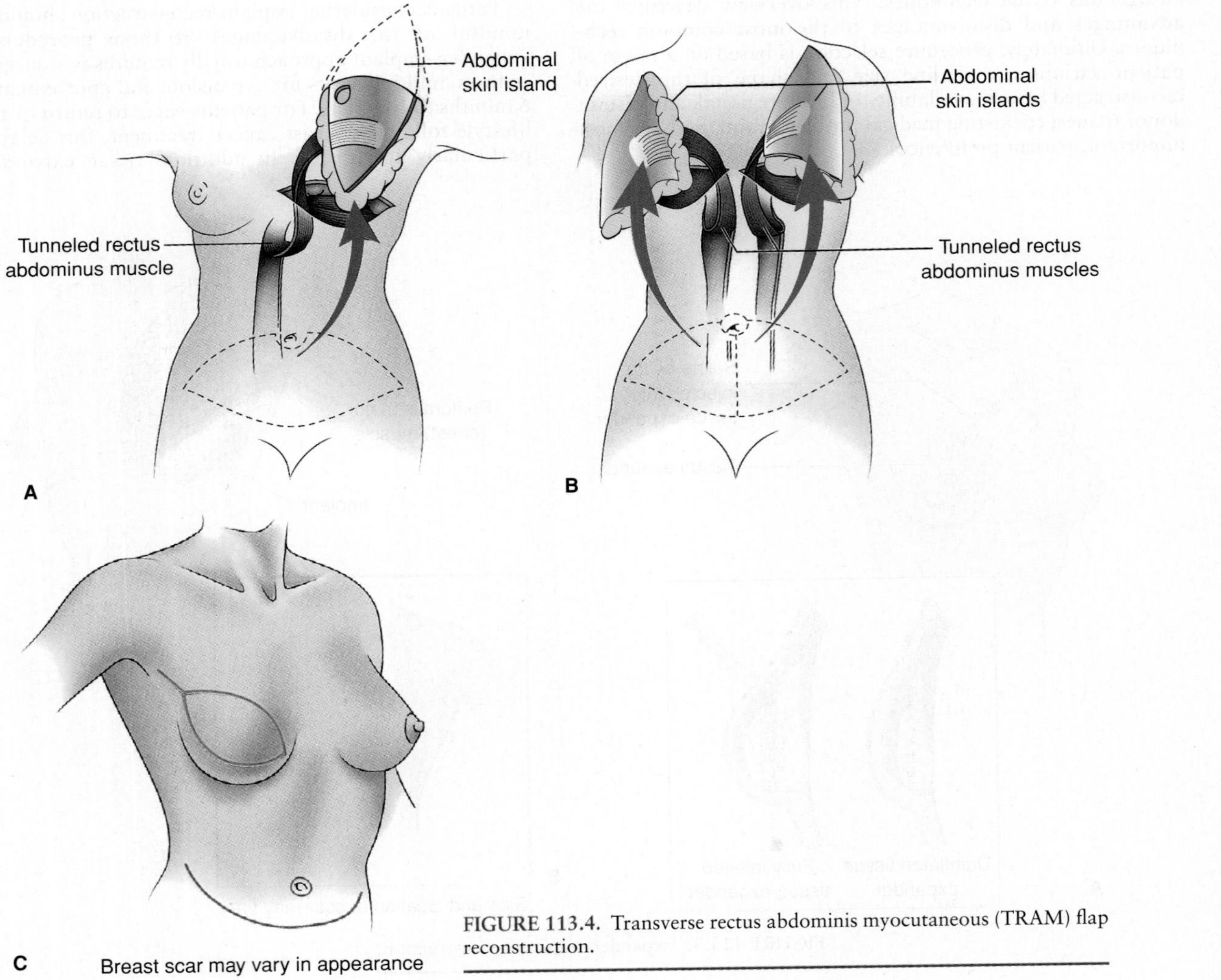

FIGURE 113.4. Transverse rectus abdominis myocutaneous (TRAM) flap reconstruction.

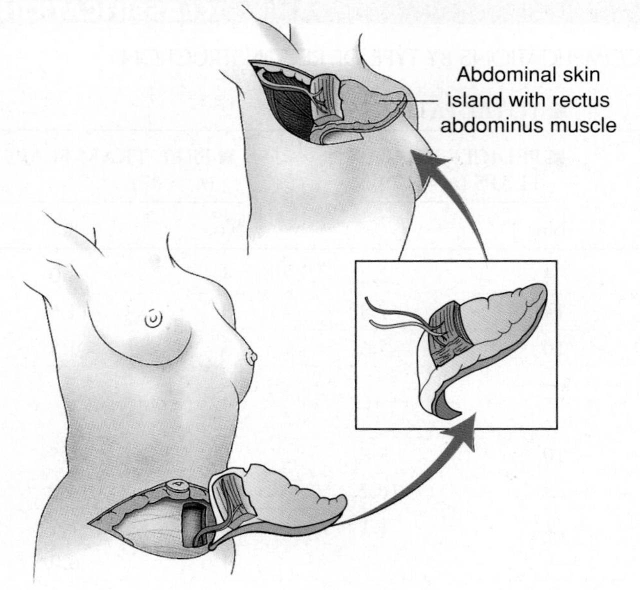

FIGURE 113.5. Free transverse rectus abdominis myocutaneous (TRAM) flap reconstruction.

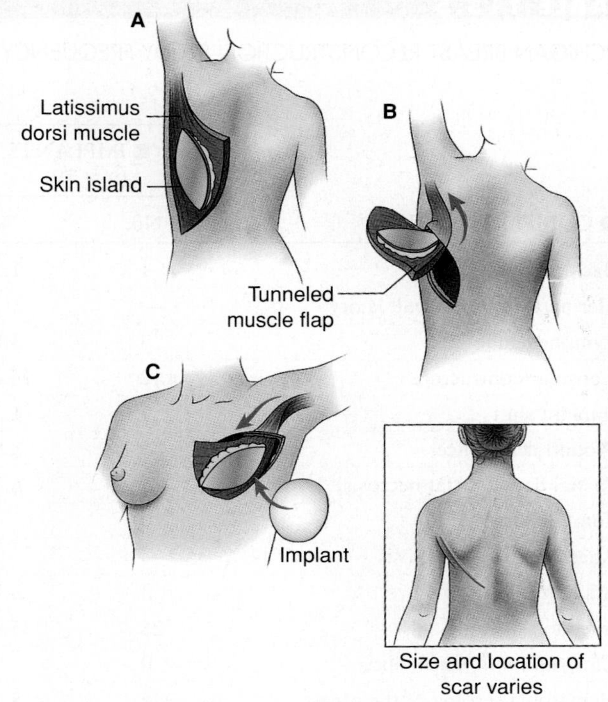

FIGURE 113.6. Latissimus dorsi flap reconstruction.

producing superior results compared with the pedicle version of the flap. With the free TRAM flap, a lower abdominal segment of skin and fat is harvested based on the deep inferior epigastric artery and vein. A small island of rectus abdominis muscle also is included with the flap, mainly to facilitate inclusion of small perforating vessels that travel from the deep inferior epigastric artery and vein into the overlying skin and fat (Fig. 113.5). Using microsurgical techniques, the flap's vascular pedicle is then anastomosed to recipient vessels (usually the thoracodorsal, subscapular, or internal mammary vessels) adjacent to the mastectomy site. In the views of Grotting et al.[40] and other investigators,[29] free TRAM flaps offer the potential advantages of greater flap reliability, superior aesthetics, and preservation of abdominal wall integrity.

Allen and Treece[41] and Allen and Tucker[42] have taken the free TRAM flap a step further with their development of the deep inferior epigastric perforator flap: by meticulously dissecting vascular perforators from the deep inferior epigastric pedicle into the overlying abdominal fat, these investigators have been able to avoid removal of any rectus abdominis muscle with free TRAM harvest, thereby minimizing disruption of abdominal wall structures.[41] The free perforator flap concept also has been applied to other donor sites for breast reconstruction, most notably the superior gluteal artery perforator flap.[42,43] Although they appear to avoid the functional deficits associated with muscle flap harvest, perforator flaps (like all free tissue transfers) entail long, technically difficult operations requiring special facilities, equipment, and expertise. Also, because the blood supply for the entire flap depends on two or three microsurgical anastomoses (each usually involving vessels no more than 2 to 3 mm in diameter), there is the potential for complete flap loss in the event of anastomotic thrombosis.

"Hybrid" Breast Reconstruction Techniques. As an additional alternative for breast reconstruction, flaps can be used in concert with saline or silicone gel implants. Most commonly, the ipsilateral latissimus dorsi and a segment of overlying skin are harvested as a musculocutaneous pedicle flap and are tunneled anteriorly into the mastectomy defect (Fig. 113.6A–C). Although the latissimus dorsi and its associated skin island constitute an extremely reliable flap when used for wound coverage, this approach usually provides insufficient bulk for breast volume. Tissue expanders or implants are often used to address this volume deficiency. The combination of a latissimus dorsi flap and tissue expansion may be particularly appropriate for cases in which the remaining mastectomy skin is of insufficient quality or quantity to tolerate tissue expansion. Following transfer and expansion of a latissimus dorsi musculocutaneous flap, an appropriately sized breast implant usually can be safely placed in a secondary operation.

From 1994 to 2000, the Michigan Breast Reconstruction Outcome Study evaluated long-term results in women undergoing expander–implant, pedicle TRAM, and free TRAM procedures in 12 centers across the United States. A variety of outcomes were assessed, including complications. Table 113.5 summarizes the complications by procedure type.[44]

Nipple–Areolar Reconstruction. Reconstruction of the nipple–areolar complex (NAC) can be accomplished at the conclusion of breast mound reconstruction or at a later date. Following recreation of the mound, many surgeons prefer to allow several months for tissue healing and settling before proceeding with nipple–areolar reconstruction. To recreate the papule, common options usually rely on local skin flaps or a segment of redundant contralateral papule. For the areola, a full-thickness skin graft or tattooing of the surrounding skin can be used.

Breast Reduction (Reduction Mammaplasty).

Because reduction mammaplasty is intended to alleviate functional problems and symptoms of macromastia, this procedure is considered a reconstructive rather than an aesthetic operation. In general, appropriate candidates for reduction mammaplasty are women with macromastia and associated back, neck, or shoulder pain; limitations in daily work or recreational activities; or difficulties obtaining proper fit in bras or other clothing. Although reduction mammaplasty usually is a covered benefit by most health care payers, patients' symptomatic and functional concerns must be carefully assessed and documented before proceeding with surgery. As noted earlier in this section, patients' preferences and expectations regarding postoperative breast size, shape, and functional results should also be carefully evaluated.

TABLE 113.5 **CLASSIFICATION**

MICHIGAN BREAST RECONSTRUCTION STUDY FREQUENCY OF COMPLICATIONS BY TYPE OF RECONSTRUCTION

	TOTAL PATIENTS: 325					
	IMPLANTS (n = 79)		PEDICLE TRAM FLAPS (n = 179)		FREE TRAM FLAPS (n = 67)	
COMPLICATION	No.	%	No.	%	No.	%
Back pain	1	1.3	4	2.2	4	6.0
Hernia/abdominal wall laxity	—		14	7.8	8	11.9
Lymphedema	3	3.8	10	5.6	3	4.5
Capsular contracture	12	15.2	—		—	
Implant shift	1	1.3	—		—	
Wound dehiscence	3	3.8	10	5.6	1	1.5
Partial flap loss (fat necrosis)	5	6.3	29	16.2	10	14.9
Total flap loss	0		2	1.1	1	1.5
Anastomotic thrombosis	—		—		4	6.0
Implant failure	3	3.8	—		—	
Infection	28	35.4	21	11.7	12	17.9
Clostridium difficile colitis	0		1	0.5	0	
Hematoma/seroma of the breast	4	5.1	7	3.9	6	9.0
Hematoma/seroma of the abdomen	—		7	3.9	3	4.5
Abdominal wall necrosis	—		3	1.7	0	
Cardiac/pulmonary complications	1	1.3	6	3.4	6	9.0

TRAM, transverse rectus abdominis myocutaneous.

Although a variety of approaches have been described for breast reduction, common surgical options share a number of characteristics. Most techniques of breast reduction resect both breast parenchyma and redundant skin. Also, reduction procedures generally reposition the NAC to a more superior point on the breast mound. To maintain nipple viability and sensation, the NAC usually is mobilized as part of a pedicle of breast parenchyma or dermis. Following dissection of the nipple pedicle and reduction of the surrounding breast skin and parenchyma, the pedicle is transferred superiorly with its vascular and neural supplies intact, while the remaining breast is reapproximated around the nipple pedicle.

In categorizing reduction mammaplasty techniques, surgical options often are described in terms of the nipple pedicle design. For example, the most common approaches rely on an inferiorly or centrally based dermal-parenchymal pedicle to maintain vascular and nerve supplies to the NAC (Figs. 113.7A–C and 113.8A–C).[45–47] In designing skin incisions, traditional methods of reduction often have incorporated a modification of a pattern originally described by Wise.[48] While allowing considerable flexibility in resection of redundant breast skin, the modified Wise pattern produces an inverted T-shaped scar, the inferior portion of which runs along the inframammary fold (IMF). In an effort to eliminate the IMF scar, Lejour[49] and Hammond[50] have described a vertical scar reduction mammaplasty.

Prospective outcome analysis of women undergoing reduction mammaplasty indicate that this surgical intervention produces considerable improvements in somatic pain and in functional status.[51,52] However, patients and providers also should

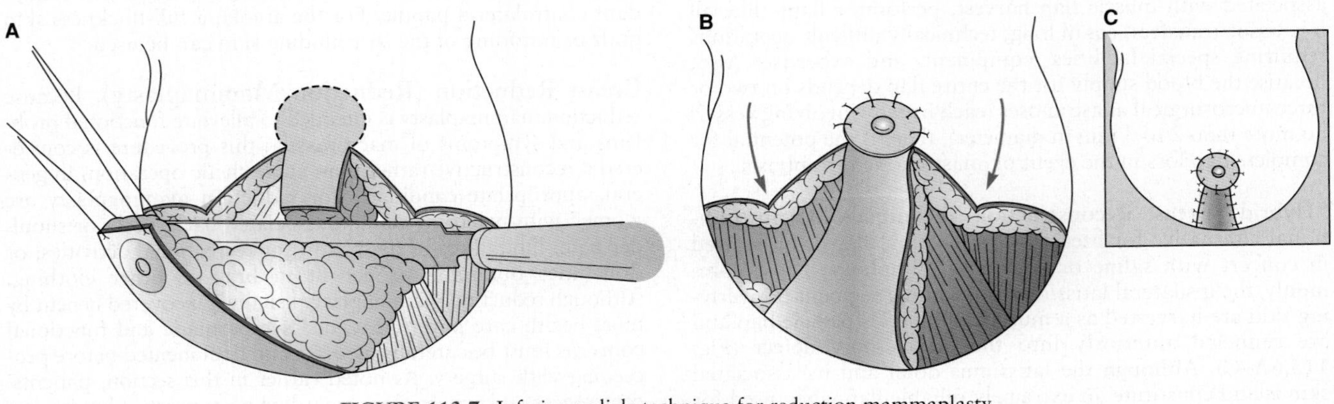

FIGURE 113.7. Inferior pedicle technique for reduction mammaplasty.

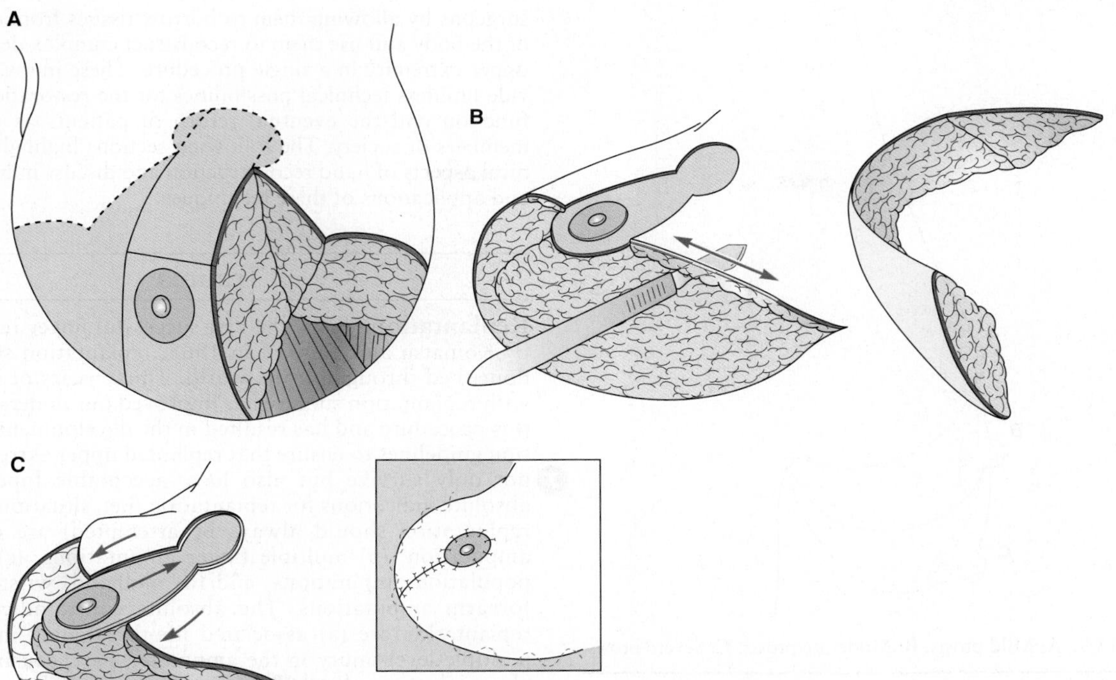

FIGURE 113.8. Central pedicle technique for reduction mammaplasty.

be aware of the potential risks associated with reduction. Complications reported with these procedures include instances of nipple or skin loss, changes in levels of nipple sensation, hypertrophic scarring or keloid formation, contour deformities, and breast asymmetry.

Aesthetic Breast Surgery

Breast Augmentation (Augmentation Mammaplasty). Augmentation or breast enlargement is one of the most commonly performed aesthetic procedures. Evaluation of patients seeking breast augmentation should follow the guidelines described earlier. Particular attention should be focused on thoroughly assessing several factors, including patient preferences for postoperative breast size and shape, history of breast disease, and physical findings. The preoperative examination should evaluate and document any possible breast masses as well as existing breast size, asymmetries, and contour deficits.

In planning augmentation mammaplasty, a variety of approaches and options are available. Decisions regarding these choices are best reached in consultation with the patient. Implants can be placed through a variety of incisions including periareolar, inframammary fold, and transaxillary approaches. With the advent of endoscopic techniques in recent years, transaxillary augmentation now can be carried out with direct visualization of the implant pocket. This latter approach commonly produces excellent aesthetic results with minimal visible skin scarring.

Location of the implant pocket is another critical decision in augmentation mammaplasty. Implants can be placed anterior to the pectoralis major muscle ("subglandular" location) or posterior to the muscle ("subpectoral" location). Subglandular placement usually results in less postoperative pain, but a submuscular implant location may produce lower rates of capsular contracture[53] and may pose fewer difficulties in obtaining subsequent mammograms.[54]

Several choices also exist in selection of implant types. Since the mid-1990s, many surgeons have relied on the use of implants with textured surfaces to reduce capsular contracture rates. Although textured surfaces appear to lessen scar tissue contracture,[55] some patients and surgeons assert that, compared with the smooth-walled envelope, the thicker, less pliable textured envelope gives the augmented breast a less natural appearance and feel. With the recent reintroduction of silicone gel–filled implants under research protocols in selected centers, patients and providers also have a choice of implant fill materials. Although gel implants may produce aesthetically superior results compared with saline implants in some patients, diagnosis and surgical treatment of implant rupture may be more challenging with gel devices.

Whatever options are chosen for breast augmentation, surgeons should clearly communicate with patients about the potential risks of these procedures. The most commonly reported complications include implant rupture, capsular contracture, implant infection, contour deformities, and breast asymmetries.[56] Despite the potential for local complications, there currently is no substantial evidence that silicone gel filler material or implant envelopes are associated with increased risk for systemic disease. At this writing, concerns voiced in the early 1990s about adverse "health effects" of silicone breast implants appear to be unfounded.[57]

Mastopexy. Mastopexy (or "breast lift") describes a category of surgical procedures designed to address redundancy or laxity of the breast's skin envelope, a condition termed *ptosis of the breast*. Breast ptosis can be classified as mild, moderate, or severe, depending on the location of the NAC relative to the inframammary fold (Fig. 113.9). Ptosis occurs when an imbalance exists between the volume of breast parenchyma and the quantity of overlying skin. Mastopexy procedures usually reduce ptosis by removing redundant breast skin and by relocating the NAC to a more superior position. These goals can be achieved through a variety of skin incisions and excisions, many of which closely resemble techniques described earlier for reduction mammaplasty. Fundamentally, mastopexy differs from breast reduction in that mastopexy removes redundant skin while leaving most or all of the breast

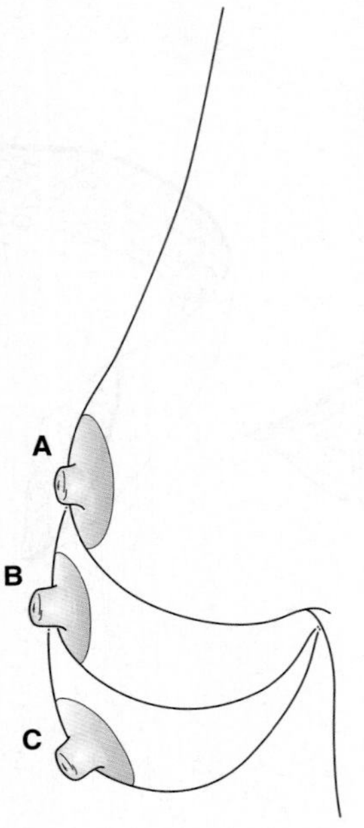

FIGURE 113.9. A: Mild ptosis. B: Moderate ptosis. C: Severe ptosis.

parenchyma. Approaches to mastopexy range from minimal periareolar techniques to more extensive skin resections using more extensive vertical incisions (Fig. 113.10A, B). As always, patients considering this procedure must weigh the potential benefits of mastopexy (most notably, diminished ptosis) with the disadvantages (scars and risks of complications) associated with the operation. Although relatively rare, the potential complications of mastopexy closely parallel those described for reduction mammaplasty.

RECONSTRUCTIVE SURGERY OF THE HAND

Advances in plastic surgery have improved our ability to reconstruct hands that have been mutilated by trauma, destroyed by arthritic diseases, or impaired by congenital conditions. Innovations in microvascular techniques, wound management, and rigid fracture fixation have expanded the capabilities of plastic surgeons by allowing them to borrow tissues from other parts of the body and use them to reconstruct complex defects in the upper extremity in a single procedure. These innovations provide limitless technical possibilities for the restoration of hand function and the eventual return of patients as productive members of society. The following sections highlight the technical aspects of hand reconstruction and discuss indications for and applications of these techniques.

Trauma

Replantation. Since the first successful finger replantation by Komatsu and Tamai[58] in 1968, replantation surgery has flourished throughout the world. Thirty years of experience with replantation surgery has improved our understanding of this procedure and has resulted in the development of indication guidelines to ensure that replanted upper extremity parts 7 not only survive but also have acceptable function. The absolute indications for replantation (i.e., situations in which replantation should always be attempted) are (a) thumb amputation, (b) multiple finger amputations, (c) pediatric population amputations, and (d) midhand, wrist, or distal forearm amputations. The absolute contraindications for replantation are (a) associated life-threatening injuries; (b) multiple-level injury in the amputated part, causing injuries along the vessels and preventing blood flow into the replanted part; and (c) severe contamination of the part, which carries a high probability of systemic infection if replanted. There are other situations in which the benefit of replantation is debatable because outcome data are not available. For example, single finger amputation at zone II (a tight fibro-osseous tunnel extending from the insertion of the superficialis tendon at the middle phalange to the first annular pulley) is generally not recommended. Tendon adhesion after zone II replantation may result in a stiff finger, which can interfere with the overall performance of the hand. On the other hand, single-finger amputation at zone I (distal to the superficialis insertion) is often recommended (Fig. 113.11). A stiff distal interphalangeal joint generally does not cause much impairment, and nerve regeneration to the replanted part is quite rapid because of the short distance to the terminal sensory organs. Furthermore, the aesthetic appearance of zone I replantation is far superior to that of an amputation stump. In the future, the use of patient-related outcome instruments and an increased body of replantation experience among centers will help to define the utility of various digit replantation procedures.

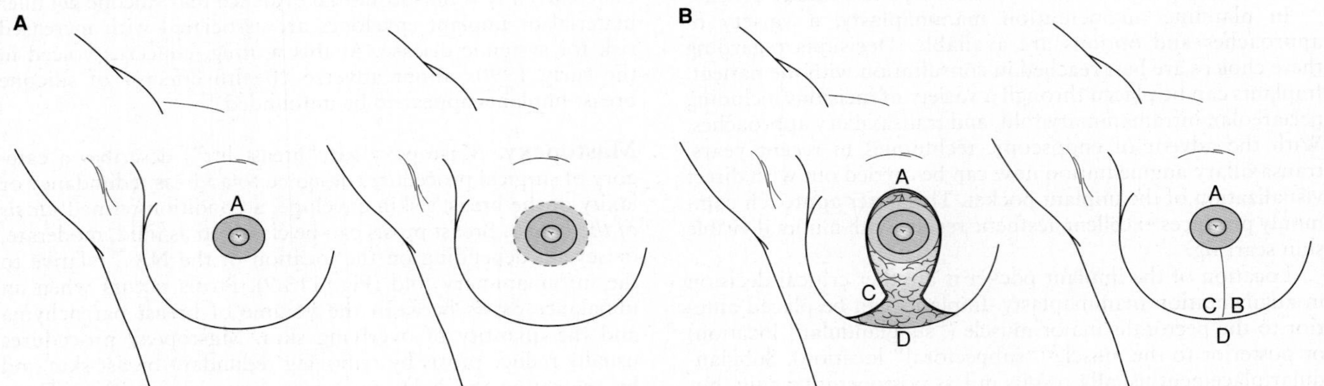

FIGURE 113.10. Mastopexy procedures. (Redrawn from Bostwick J. *Plastic and Reconstructive Breast Surgery*. St. Louis, MO: Quality Medical Publishing; 1990.)

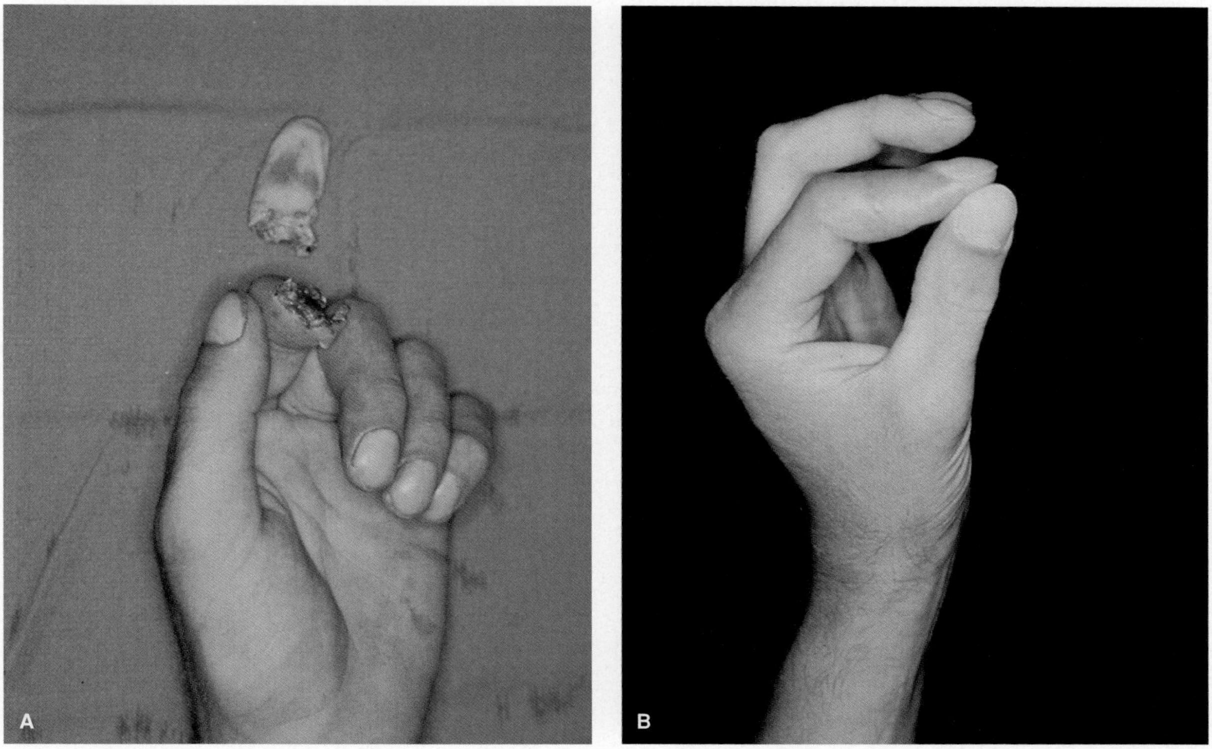

FIGURE 113.11. **A:** Amputation of the index finger at zone 1 in a mechanic. The patient requested replantation because his work requires fine manipulative tasks. **B:** Successful replantation with good aesthetic outcome and function.

Toe Transfer

When finger replantation is not possible or not successful, patients are left with significant functional loss. Disability is most severe when the thumb has been amputated at or proximal to the metacarpophalangeal joint or when all of the fingers have been amputated in machine injuries. In these cases, toe transfer to the hand is an effective procedure in restoring grasp and pinch function. Although a prosthesis is available to mimic the thumb, lack of sensation is a major drawback and often leads to disuse of the prosthesis. For a patient who has had a thumb amputation at or proximal to the metacarpophalangeal joint, big toe or second toe transfer to the thumb can create a sensate digit that will oppose to the other fingers. Big toe transfer is advantageous because it provides a broad contact surface and closely resembles the shape of the thumb, particularly when the big toe is trimmed and sculptured to match the size of the thumb. However, the disadvantage of the big toe transfer is the conspicuous donor site appearance in the foot and potential gait problems with foot push-off if the head of the first metatarsal is taken along with the big toe. For these reasons, the second toe has become the preferred method of transfer in some centers (Fig. 113.12). The disadvantage of the second toe transfer procedure is the slender appearance of the digit as compared to the original thumb, but the donor site appearance is quite acceptable. A recent outcome study, using objective physical measurements and validated outcome questionnaires, demonstrated that toe-to-thumb transfer is an effective procedure in restoring hand function.[59] In addition, patients did not complain of gait difficulty after either big toe or second toe transfer.

One of the most complex problems in hand surgery is the reconstruction of a hand without digits. To create a new hand capable of tripod pinch, plastic surgeons can transfer multiple toes from both feet to the hand (Fig. 113.13). This type of reconstruction can restore function to an otherwise useless hand and has allowed two farmers who were treated at one center to return to heavy farm labor.

Complex Hand Injuries

Although crush injuries to the hand are common, injuries associated with sufficient force to disrupt the structural integrity of the wrist and to sever the blood supply to the hand are uncommon events (Fig. 113.14). Because multiple structures are traumatized in injuries of this kind, a systematic treatment approach is important in salvaging the hand and in restoring its function. Crucial steps in the management of this injury are (a) ruling out other injuries, (b) aggressive débridement, (c) skeletal fixation, (d) decompression of fascial compartments in the hand, (e) revascularization, (f) tendon repair, (g) nerve repair, and (h) early soft tissue coverage (within 1 week of injury) (Table 113.6).

Excluding Other Injuries. In devastating trauma, attention is often focused on the obvious injury, and injuries to other organ systems may be ignored. In a review of 1,100 patients referred for emergent microsurgery over a 7-year

TABLE 113.6 COMPLICATIONS

COMPLICATIONS OF TREATMENT OF COMPLEX HAND INJURIES

Inadequate débridement of contaminated tissue
Poor fixation technique for bone injuries
Postponement of soft tissue coverage, over 1 wk after injury
Free-flap pedicle anastomosis within the zone of injury
Delay in hand therapy

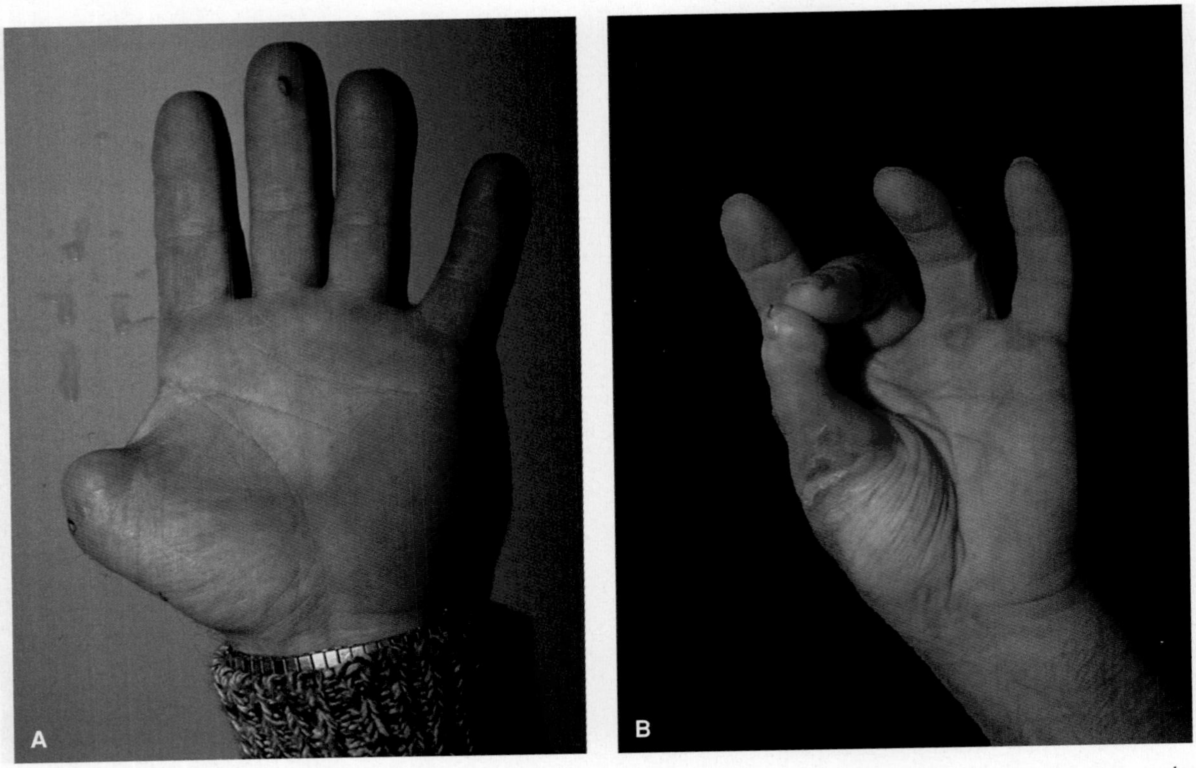

FIGURE 113.12. **A:** Second-toe transfer for thumb reconstruction in a carpenter. He sustained a thumb amputation at the metacarpophalangeal joint while using a saw at work. **B:** Good function with restoration of fine pinch. The patient returned to work as a carpenter 3 months after the toe reconstruction.

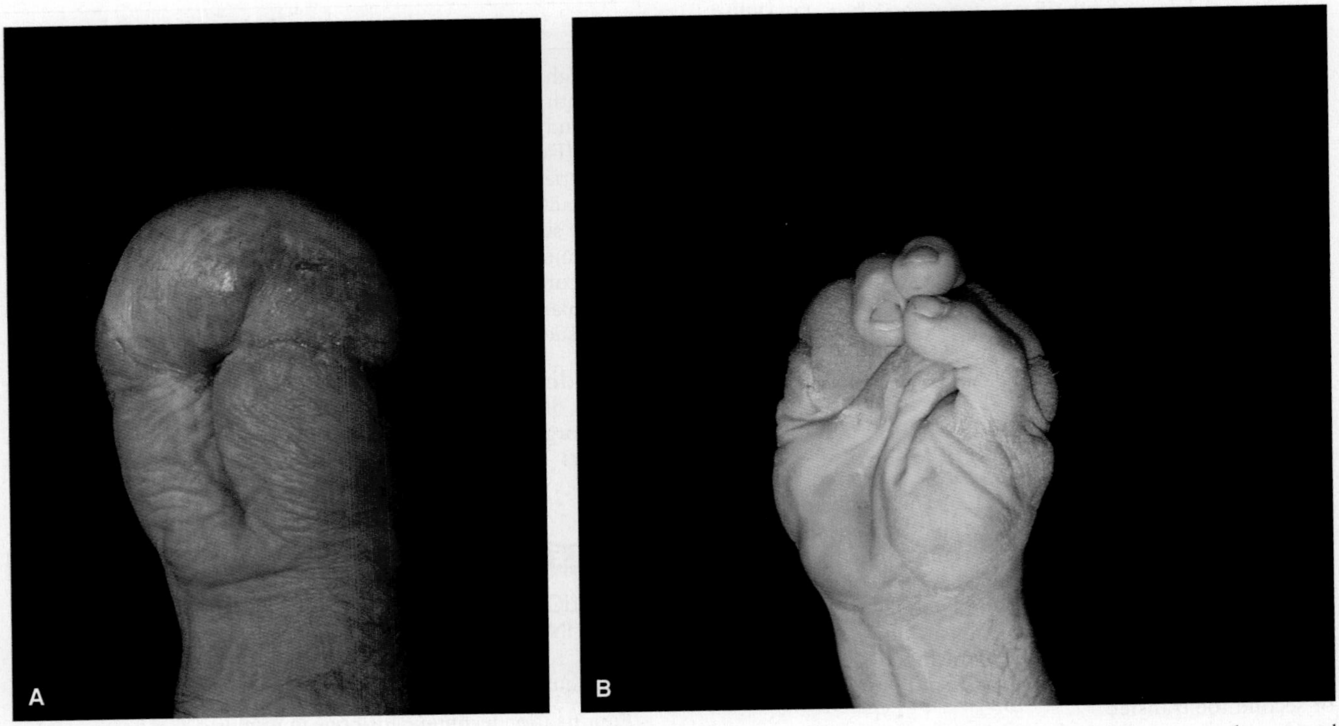

FIGURE 113.13. **A:** A farmer who lost all his fingers when he was injured by a corn picker. A groin skin flap was used to cover the exposed metacarpal heads. **B:** A second toe was removed from one foot to reconstruct the thumb, and the second and third toes were removed together from the other foot to reconstruct the fingers. Note the good opposition of the thumb and acceptable flexion of the digits. The patient returned to work on his dairy farm after the hand reconstruction.

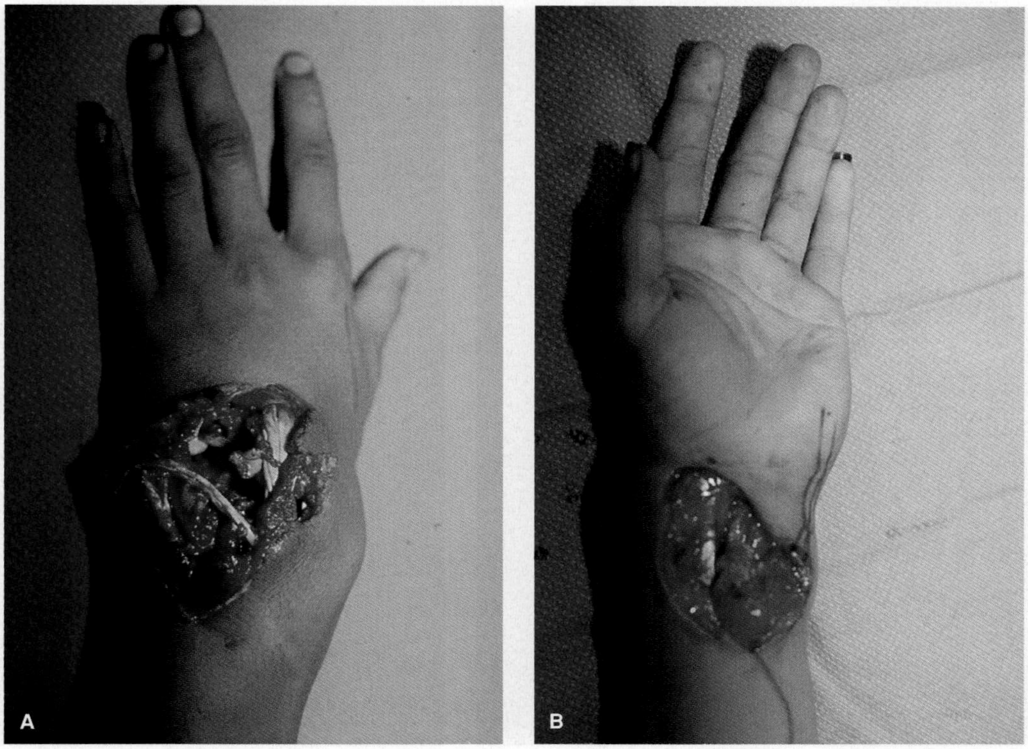

FIGURE 113.14. A: Accidental shotgun blast injury in a 16-year-old boy. Both the radial and ulnar arteries were ruptured, and the hand was ischemic. The wrist was destroyed, and multiple tendons and nerves were severed. B: Volar wrist wound. Markings show incision lines for ulnar artery exposure.

period, investigators found nine cases (0.8%) of unrecognized life-threatening injuries that required abandonment of the microsurgical procedures.[60] Therefore, systematic trauma evaluation and ruling out other associated injuries should precede treatment of the hand injury.

Débridement. Severe crush and blast injuries are associated with large zones of injury, and the wounds may be contaminated with foreign materials such as grease or paint, as in printing-press injuries. In these cases, aggressive débridement is important in preventing infection. Except for critical structures that include nerves and tendons, all devitalized soft tissues and bone fragments must be excised. The concept of radical débridement has been shown to decrease wound infection and improve the success of microvascular reconstruction.[61]

Skeletal Fixation. After débridement, the next priority is to stabilize the wrist and to rigidly fix hand fractures. A stable wrist provides a platform for repairing other injured structures. If the crush injury is associated with comminuted fractures of multiple carpal bones and rupture of the intercarpal ligaments, wrist fusion may be the best option because it is often impossible to reconstitute the normal anatomy of the distal and proximal carpal rows in the face of severe comminution of the carpal bones. To avoid possible bone graft contamination with primary wrist fusion, external fixators are placed for provisional fixation during the initial débridement. Definitive wrist fusion with bone grafting is performed after adequate débridements and during the flap coverage procedure. Two 2.7-mm fixator pins are placed through an incision along the radial index metacarpal, and two proximal 3.5-mm pins are placed into the radius using an incision along the radial border of the distal radius, between the brachioradialis and the extensor carpi radialis longus. The superficial radial nerve, which lies under the brachioradialis, is dissected free and retracted away from the pins. External fixator rods are then secured to the pins with nuts and screws. If the wound is clean during the second-look procedure at 24 or 48 hours, total wrist fusion is then undertaken (Fig. 113.15). Otherwise, the external fixator is left in place until the wound is suitable for fusion using internal plating and cancellous bone grafts. This stable skeletal fixation allows early hand therapy, usually instituted on postinjury day 7 when tissue edema is subsiding.

Revascularization. In a crush injury of the wrist, the zone of injury can be extensive. Use of vein grafts is essential in performing the arterial anastomosis away from the zone of injury. The ulnar artery is chosen for repair because it is the dominant artery in most patients and because it can be exposed readily in the hypothenar area. If the ulnar artery is contused in the palm, distal anastomosis can be performed to the superficial palmar arch. Because soft tissue bridges are often present, venous outflow is not a problem and venous anastomosis is not necessary.

Decompression of Fascial Compartments. Increased edema associated with crush injuries often raises the compartmental pressures in the intrinsic muscle compartments and in the carpal tunnel. Prior reviews have shown a high incidence of ischemia and resultant fibrosis of the intrinsic muscles following crushing trauma to the hand.[62] Consequently, surgeons perform prophylactic carpal tunnel releases and intrinsic muscle decompressions in severe crush injuries of this kind.

Soft Tissue Coverage. After aggressive débridement, a soft tissue defect is often present around the wrist. A split-thickness autograft is placed over the vein graft to prevent desiccation. Other open wounds can be covered temporarily with homografts. If wrist fusion is undertaken during the second-look procedure, primary wound closure can be achieved. For residual wound defects, split-thickness autografts are used to cover the exposed muscle bellies. However, if tendons or nerves are

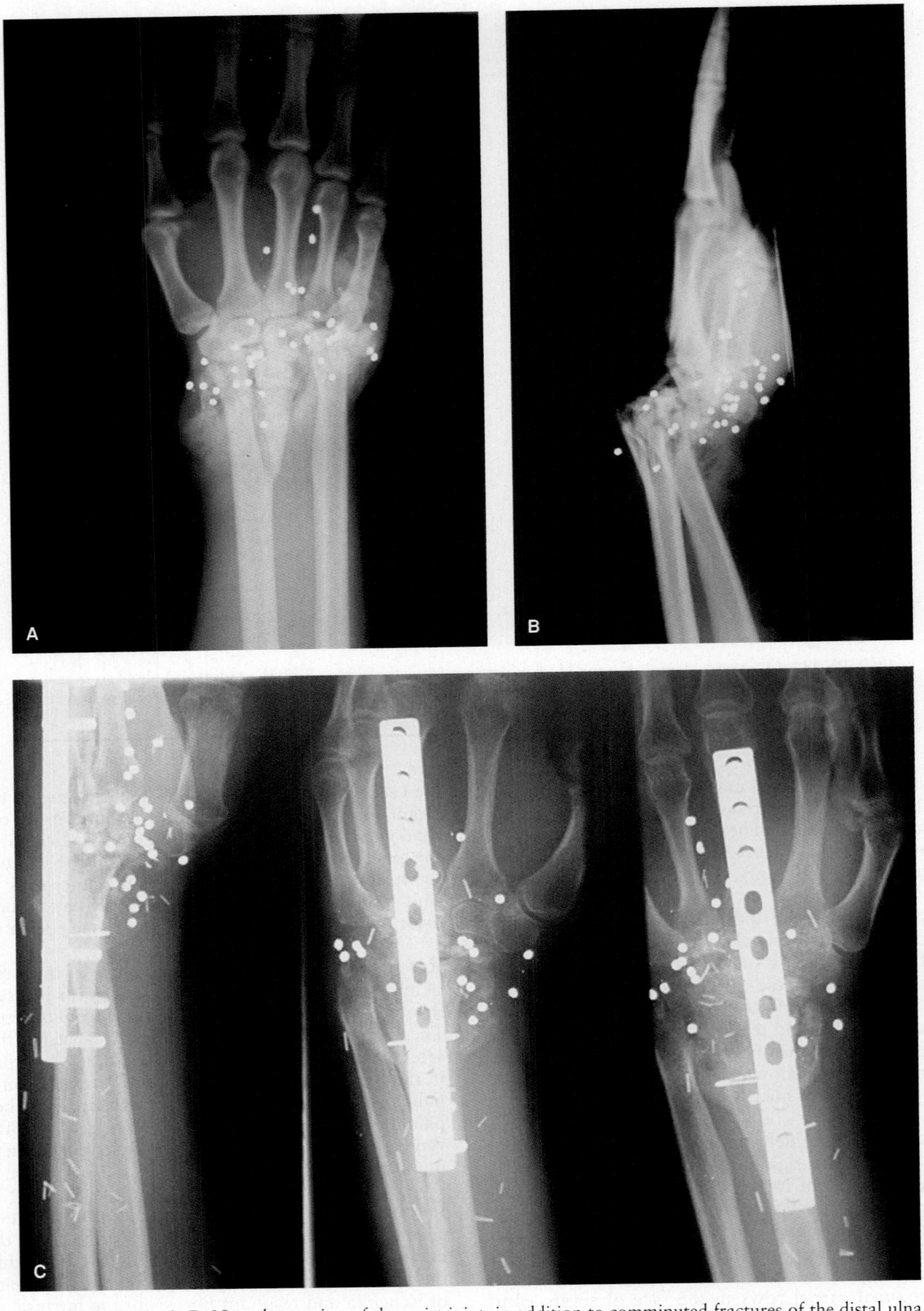

FIGURE 113.15. A, B: Note destruction of the wrist joint, in addition to comminuted fractures of the distal ulna and radius. C: Total wrist fusion was performed 48 hours after the initial injury.

exposed, coverage with either fasciocutaneous or muscle free flaps will allow earlier tendon mobilization and prevent tendon adhesions. Definitive early wound coverage is important in protecting vital structures and avoiding wound colonization with bacteria (Fig. 113.16).

Nerve Repair. When nerves are crushed, the delineation between viable and nonviable nerve fascicles is difficult to assess in the acute setting. Therefore, the traditional approach is to delay the nerve grafting procedures until 2 or 3 months after injury. To prevent retraction of the nerve ends, we suture the nerve ends to the surrounding soft tissues. However, secondary nerve grafting is often difficult because of the amount of scar in the wound. One way to deal with this situation is to primarily graft the nerve injury at the expense of more aggressive resection of the traumatized nerve ends.

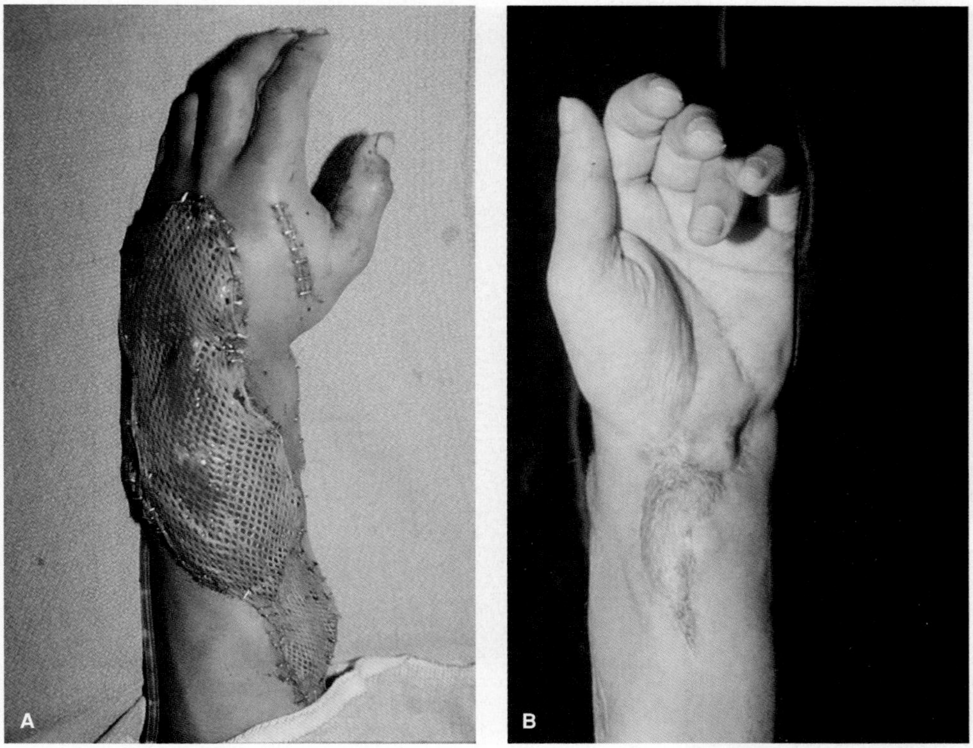

FIGURE 113.16. A: A free rectus muscle was used for immediate coverage of the reconstructed wrist and tendons. B: The hand was salvaged, and the patient has acceptable hand function after secondary nerve and tendon reconstruction.

8 In conclusion, rigid skeletal fixation, revascularization using vein grafts, and immediate wound coverage are crucial factors in successful limb salvage.

Congenital Anomalies

Syndactyly. Syndactyly is a condition in which the fingers are fused. Syndactyly can be classified as complete or incomplete. Complete syndactyly is the union of the digits extending to the distal phalanx. Incomplete syndactyly is the union of the digits proximal to the distal phalanx but distal to the normal webbing at the midproximal phalanx. Syndactyly is further categorized as simple or complex. In simple syndactyly, there is no bony union between the digits, whereas complex syndactyly includes bony union.

Typically, syndactyly can be separated when the child is 1 year of age. Surgery should be performed earlier if syndactyly affects the thumb–index finger or ring–little finger web space and causes deviation of the shorter digits during growth. Separating the fingers requires meticulous design of the skin flaps, and the dorsal skin flap is most crucial to creating a web space that is not prone to contracture (Fig. 113.17). Distally, triangular skin flaps are designed to drape the sides of the fingers. A full-thickness skin graft from the groin is often required to cover open areas in the fingers.

Thumb Duplication. Although thumb duplication does not often cause a functional problem for the child, the presence of this prominent hand malformation can have a significant impact on the child's psychosocial development. Surgery can be undertaken when the child is about 2 years old to prevent

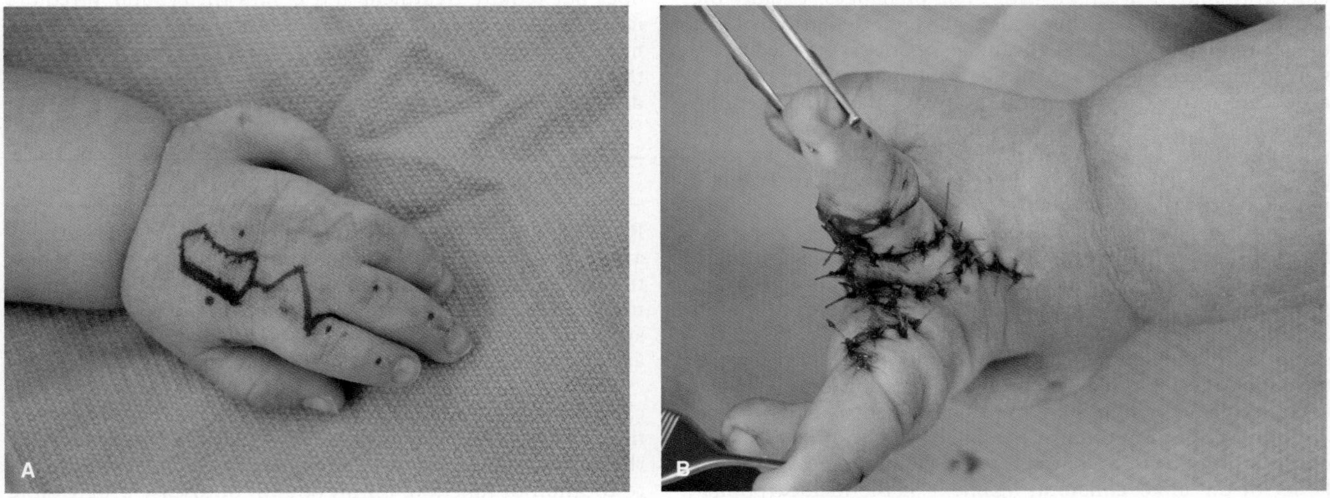

FIGURE 113.17. A: A simple, complete syndactyly in a 1-year-old child. Note the design of the dorsal skin flap to reconstruct the web space and the interdigitating distal skin flaps. B: Immediate postoperative photograph of the syndactyly release.

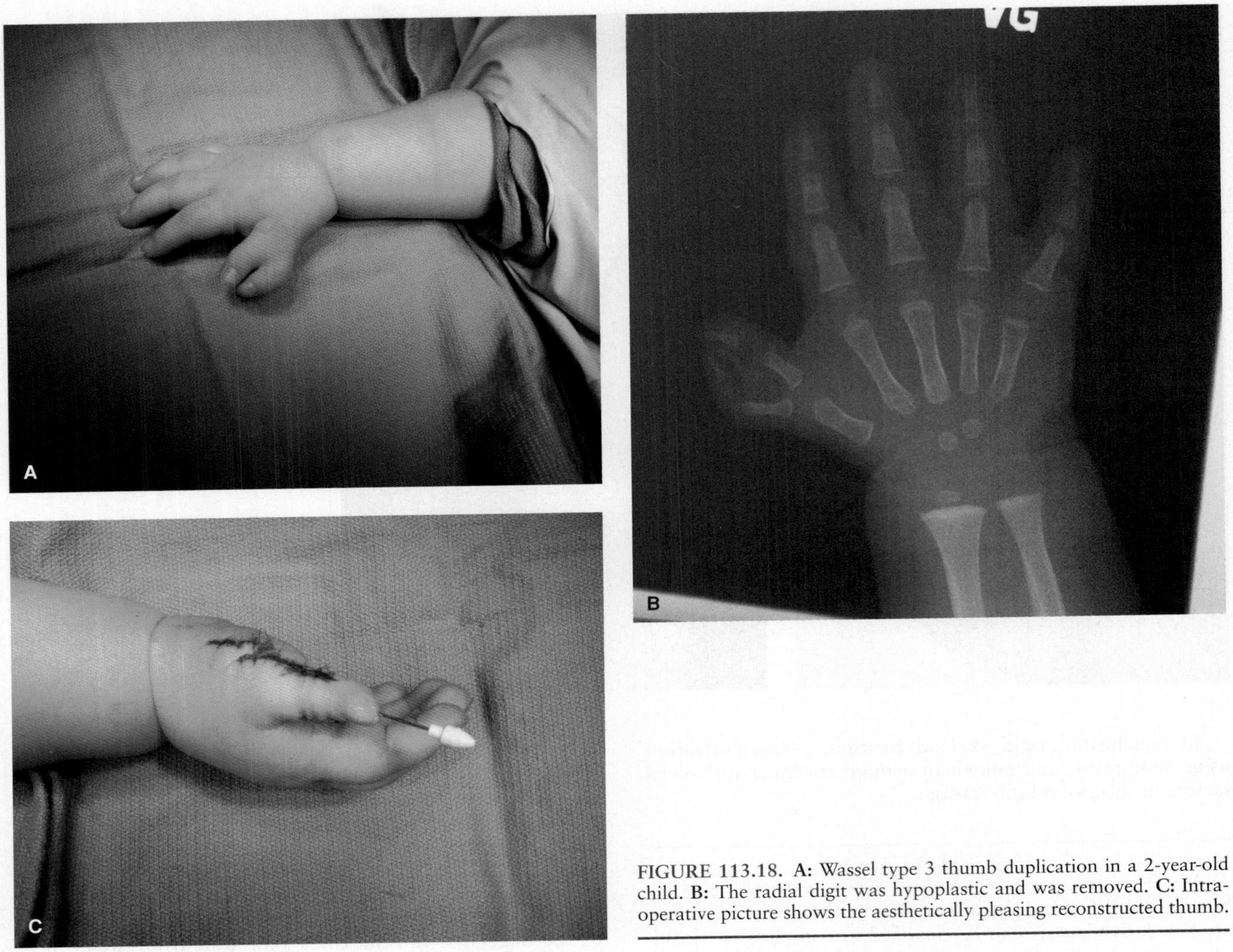

FIGURE 113.18. **A:** Wassel type 3 thumb duplication in a 2-year-old child. **B:** The radial digit was hypoplastic and was removed. **C:** Intraoperative picture shows the aesthetically pleasing reconstructed thumb.

progressive deviation of the thumb during growth. Thumb duplication can be classified into seven groups, depending on the level of the duplication. Type I consists of a bifid distal phalanx, whereas type II is a complete duplication of the distal phalanx. Types III and IV involve the proximal phalanx, and types V and VI involve the metacarpal. Type VII is a triphalangeal thumb or a thumb with three phalanges. Usually the radial, less developed thumb is removed. Retention of the ulnar thumb has the added advantage of preserving the important stabilizing ulnar collateral ligament. The surgery requires a delicate reconstruction of the bone, ligament, and tendon structures to sculpture the remaining thumb as normally as possible (Fig. 113.18). After the immediate postsurgical period, these patients are followed once a year to evaluate potential growth abnormality.

Hypoplasia and Aplasia of the Thumb. The thumb contributes about 50% of hand function and is important in pinch and grip. Reconstruction of the underdeveloped thumb is critical in improving hand function for the child. Hypoplasia of the thumb can be classified into five grades, and treatment options are often based on this classification. Grade I consists of minor hypoplasia; all components of the thumb are present, but the thumb is smaller than normal. Grade II consists of adduction contracture of the first web space and laxity of the ulnar collateral ligament at the metacarpophalangeal joint; the thenar musculature is hypoplastic but the skeletal framework of the thumb is normal. Grade III includes severe hypoplasia of the thumb with absent intrinsic muscles and underdeveloped extrinsic tendons; the skeletal framework is hypoplastic and the carpometacarpal joint is vestigial. Grade IV is characterized by a floating, nonfunctional thumb (pouce flottant), with soft tissue attachment of the thumb at the metacarpophalangeal joint of the index finger. Grade V is defined by total absence of the thumb. Grade I hypoplasia does not require treatment and grades III, IV, and V require index pollicization (reconstructing a thumb using the index finger) for optimal function (Fig. 113.19). In grade II, the thumb can be reconstructed by using a combination of tendon, joint, and soft tissue procedures.

Rheumatoid Arthritis

Rheumatoid arthritis (RA) is a crippling disease that severely affects the quality of life for millions of Americans. RA is postulated to be an autoimmune disease mediated by inflammatory cells that attack the synovial tissues in the body. Persistent synovitis in the joints causes erosion of the articular surfaces and disrupts their soft tissue supports.

Because the hand is often damaged by RA, effective surgical treatment of hand deformities can improve patient function and restore independence. The goals of surgery for the rheumatoid hand include (a) pain control, (b) improvement or restoration of function, (c) prevention of disease progression, and (d) aesthetic improvement. To accomplish these goals, the surgeon must have good rapport with both the rheumatologist and the patient as priorities of treatment are determined. By

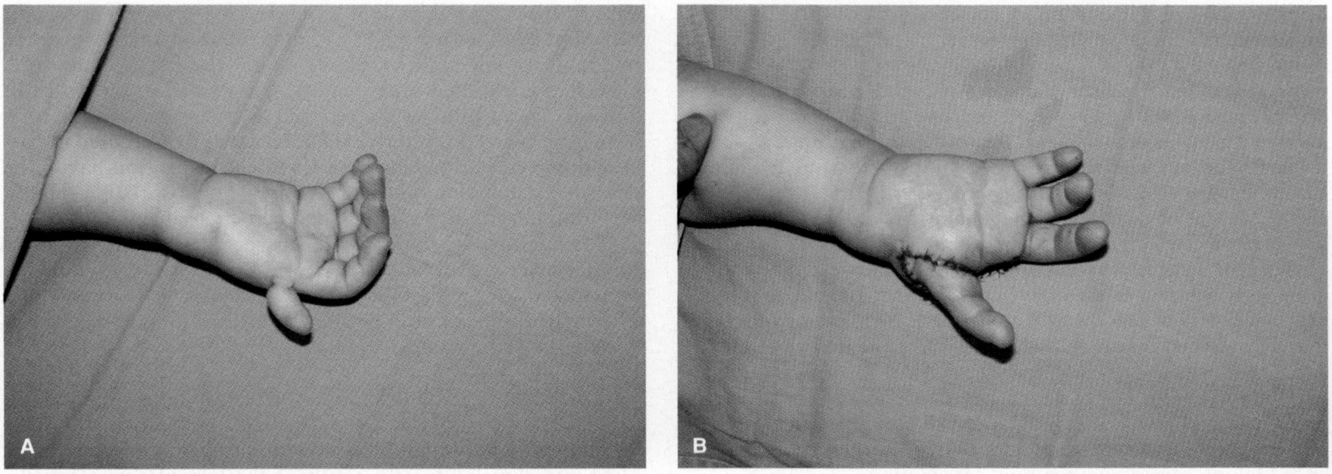

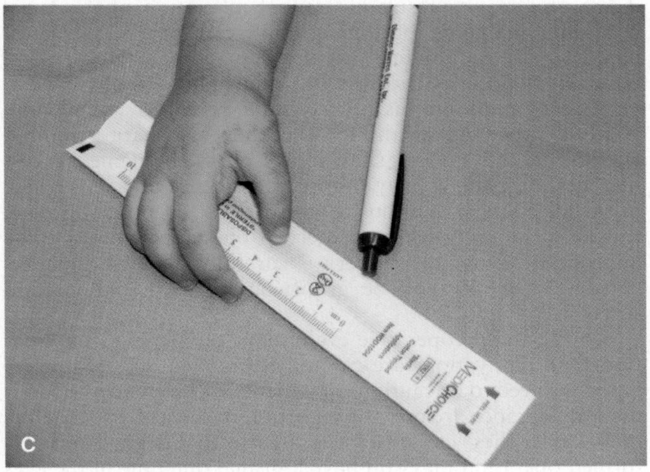

FIGURE 113.19. **A:** Absence of a thumb in a 2-year-old child. Note the floating thumb attached to the index finger. **B:** Immediate appearance in the operating room after pollicization. **C:** Three months after index pollicization, the child is able to use the new thumb for grasp and fine pinch.

listening to patients with RA describe their impairments and their goals, the surgeon can gain insight into the surgical plan that will offer the patient the most benefit.

Surgical treatment can be classified as preventive, corrective, or salvage.[63] Preventive procedures include tenosynovectomy to avoid tendon rupture and synovectomy to ameliorate ongoing joint destruction from erosive synovitis in the joints. Corrective procedures include tendon transfers for tendon ruptures and nerve decompression for carpal tunnel syndrome. Salvage procedures consist of joint arthroplasty and joint fusion.

A common hand deformity in RA consists of subluxation and ulnar deviation of the fingers at the level of the metacarpophalangeal joints (MPJs) (Fig. 113.20). Synovitis at the MPJs distends the joints and attenuates the supporting ligaments. Wrist destruction in RA contributes to the radial deviation of the metacarpals, which accentuates the ulnar deviation of the fingers. With progressive MPJ disease, patients have great difficulty opening their hands because of subluxation of the MPJs and difficulty with fine pinch because of the ulnar deviation of the fingers. In addition to pain at the MPJs secondary to their worn articular surfaces, RA patients often complain of the aesthetic appearance of their hands.

The Swanson metacarpophalangeal joint arthroplasty (SMPA) is an effective procedure that will meet all four goals of RA surgery. By replacing the arthritic joints with prosthetic spacers and realigning the soft tissue envelope around the MPJs, surgeons are able to markedly improve function and enhance the aesthetic appearance of RA hands. A recent systematic overview of the world's literature on this procedure showed that SMPA is an effective procedure in improving the health-related quality of life for RA patients.[64]

AESTHETIC SURGERY

Plastic and reconstructive surgery is a discipline that adapts broad surgical principles to a multitude of unique clinical problems by altering form and function. Plastic surgery not only restores physical function but also enhances a patient's

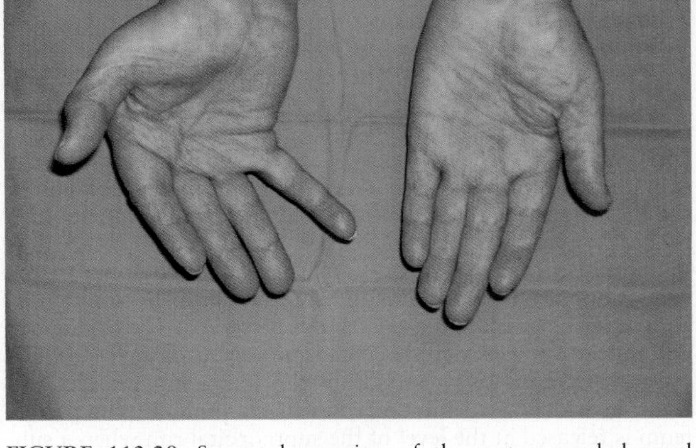

FIGURE 113.20. Severe destruction of the metacarpophalangeal joints with ulnar deviation of the fingers of the left hand. Note restoration of normal finger alignment of the right hand after Swanson metacarpophalangeal joint arthroplasty.

body image and self-esteem. In no other area of surgery is this more true than in aesthetic surgery. A blepharoplasty may not only improve the appearance of baggy, tired eyes but also may treat visual field defects caused by eyelid ptosis or blepharochalasis. A rhinoplasty can improve the outward appearance of a nose as well as nasal airflow and breathing.

9 Aesthetic surgery requires meticulous attention to detail, careful patient selection, rigorous procedural planning, and precise execution of technically challenging procedures. If patients are carefully selected and their goals are realistic, then the chances for a successful outcome are good. However, if patients are poorly selected or they have unrealistic goals, then a technically successful operation with an aesthetically pleasing outcome may be a dismal failure in the eyes of the patient. The aesthetic surgeon must not only diagnose the clinical deformity but also carefully evaluate the patient's expectations and motivations for surgery. Through the application of sound surgical principles and technical expertise, the aesthetic surgeon can experience lifelong career and personal satisfaction.

Cosmetic Procedures for the Head and Neck

Brow Lift. Brow ptosis is a natural consequence of the biologic process of aging. If left uncorrected, patients can appear angry, tired, or older than their chronologic age. If severe, brow ptosis may cause visual field obstruction on upward gaze; correction of this deformity can produce dramatic functional and aesthetic improvements. Patients frequently present with the complaint of looking tired or angry and request a blepharoplasty. In many cases, the etiology of their complaint is brow ptosis rather than upper eyelid ptosis or blepharochalasis. These patients will require a brow lift alone, or in combination with a blepharoplasty, to correct their functional and aesthetic concerns.

Correction of brow ptosis can be achieved with either an open or endoscopic approach. The traditional open approach requires a transcoronal incision with resection of excess scalp or forehead. Unfortunately, this approach results in a long scar, potential scar alopecia, and anesthesia of the scalp and forehead. In addition, an open brow lift in male patients with a receding hairline requires resection of hair-bearing scalp, which is an undesirable outcome. To reduce these complications, the endoscopic brow lift was developed and has become the primary approach for repair of brow ptosis.[54] The endoscopic brow lift requires only three to five 1-cm incisions behind the hairline to gain access to the forehead and glabellar rhytids, producing less of an aesthetic deformity and limiting the amount of scarring. There is also evidence to suggest that the endoscopic approach produces a more lasting result than the traditional approach.[55] Lastly, it has been reported that anesthesia of the forehead and scalp is significantly reduced when an endoscopic approach is utilized for correction of brow ptosis, as compared to an open, transcoronal approach.

Endoscopic and open brow lifts may be performed under local or general anesthesia. Patients are marked preoperatively in the upright position. The desired brow position is at the level of the orbital rim in male patients and 1 cm above the orbital rim in female patients. The position of the brow in relation to the supraorbital rim changes from medial to lateral; the lateral brow should be more elevated than the medial brow. During an open brow lift, a coronal incision is made and the entire forehead is mobilized in a subgaleal or subperiosteal plane down to the orbital rim. The supraorbital and supratrochlear nerves are dissected free of surrounding tissues and preserved. The corrugator and procerus muscles are resected if prominent glabellar rhytids are present. Excessive resection of the corrugator muscles will result in widening of the eyebrows in the midline. The periosteum is released at the level of the supraorbital rim when a subperiosteal plane is utilized for mobilization of the forehead; the dissection is carried down to the level of the supraorbital rim when a subgaleal plane is used for forehead mobilization. The forehead is then elevated and redraped posteriorly, the redundant scalp is resected, and the wound is closed. In an endoscopic brow lift, incisions are made within the hair-bearing scalp at the midpupillary line and over the temporal fossa. The entire forehead flap is elevated under endoscopic guidance, the procerus and corrugator muscles are resected as necessary, and the forehead is retracted posteriorly. The forehead is then secured into its new position. Various methods of forehead fixation have been described including absorbable and nonabsorbable plates, screws, multipronged anchors, and cortical tunnels.[65,66]

Postoperatively, patients are instructed to avoid vigorous physical exercise for at least 6 weeks. Bruising and swelling are anticipated for the first 2 to 3 weeks following the procedure. The final result is not expected for at least 6 to 8 weeks following the procedure.

Rhytidectomy. The deleterious effects of aging, gravity, sun exposure, and smoking are particularly evident on the face. Ultraviolet radiation and tobacco use produce fine facial wrinkling and skin laxity as a result of the loss of skin elasticity. Aging and gravity result in gradual relaxation of the facial retaining ligaments producing midfacial ptosis, deepened nasolabial folds, "jowling" along the mandibular border, and redundancy of cervical skin.[67] Old family photographs and driver license photographs are constant reminders of a more youthful appearance with high cheekbones, a sharp mandibular border, and smooth skin. However, as the aging process marches on, patients may lose self-confidence and self-esteem in social, political, and business situations, encouraging them to seek facial rejuvenation surgery. If the patients are selected appropriately and the surgery is carefully planned and executed, the results will be gratifying for both patient and surgeon.[68]

During the preoperative evaluation, the patient's expectations and motivations are carefully evaluated and addressed. Surgeons need to be cautious of patients whose concerns about their appearance are out of proportion to their physical deformity. Under these circumstances, a perfectly designed and performed operation may still have a dismal outcome in the eyes of the patient.

10 Patients who smoke are at a significantly increased risk for developing postoperative complications, including skin flap necrosis, infection, or wound dehiscence, and are consequently instructed to quit prior to undergoing elective aesthetic surgery. Many surgeons will refuse to perform a cervicofacial rhytidectomy in any patient who is actively smoking or utilizing any products containing nicotine. Urine cotinine levels can be determined to confirm whether a patient has been utilizing nicotine in any form. Older patients with coexisting medical illnesses are referred to a general practitioner for optimization of their medical condition preoperatively. If the patient is deemed a moderate or high risk for general anesthesia because of medical comorbidities, then the operation may be postponed until those medical conditions are optimized. Occasionally, if the risk of anesthesia is too high for a patient, then the operation may need to be cancelled.

Younger patients (40 to 50 years old) with good skin quality, mild midfacial ptosis, and early "jowling" may benefit from a minimally invasive facelift. This operation is typically combined with an endoscopic brow lift to provide upper and lower facial rejuvenation with minimal scarring. The operation is performed under local or general anesthesia. Bilateral temporal and superior buccal sulcus incisions are made. The temporal fossa dissection is carried down to the level of the superficial layer of the deep temporal fascia. Under endoscopic guidance, the superficial layer of the deep temporal fascia is then incised to expose the temporal fat pad. The dissection then proceeds caudally until the zygomatic arch is identified. A subperiosteal plane of dissection provides access to the midface while preserving the integrity of the frontal branch of the facial nerve. The subperiosteal plane of dissection is continued into the midface with care taken to avoid the infraorbital nerves. The masseter is mobilized from its lateral attachments.

The superior buccal sulcus incisions are made, and a midface subperiosteal dissection is performed under both direct visualization and endoscopic guidance. Once the dissection is completed, the entire midface is suspended in the desired position with sutures or specialized anchors spanning from the superficial layer of the deep temporal fascia to the midface periosteum. Symmetry of the suspension is then confirmed and the wounds are closed in layers. This technique will nicely correct mild midface ptosis, mild jowling, and early nasolabial fold prominence. However, this technique will not correct deformities from significant skin laxity. Under these circumstances, a traditional cervicofacial rhytidectomy will be required.[65,69]

In patients who require resection of excess skin, a traditional rhytidectomy can be performed under local or general anesthesia. The skin incision is made over the temporal fossa 4 to 5 cm cephalad to the root of the helix and extended caudally toward the apex of the ear. The incision is then extended anterior to the ear, behind the tragus, around the base of the earlobe into the retroauricular sulcus, across the mastoid, and caudally along the anterior hairline of the neck. The skin flap is then elevated just superficial to the superficial musculoaponeurotic system (SMAS) and platysma. This plane of dissection maintains a thin layer of subcutaneous fat on the skin flap to preserve viability while avoiding injury to the facial nerve branches, greater auricular nerve, parotid gland, and jugular vein. The flaps are elevated medially to the nasolabial fold in the face and to the midline in the neck. Occasionally a platysmal diastasis may exist, which creates platysmal banding, an obtuse cervicomental angle, and a prominent neck. Under these circumstances, a platysmal plication may be performed through a 2- to 3-cm submental incision to correct the diastasis and improve the appearance of the neck. At this point, there are many variations in how the remainder of the cervicofacial rhytidectomy is performed with the goal of repositioning all of the tissues that have migrated into dependent positions creating facial aging changes. The surgeon may simply chose to not perform any additional dissection at this point and simply reposition the skin, resect the excess skin, and close the incisions. In other circumstances, the surgeon may choose to do one of the following: SMAS plication, standard SMAS dissection, extended SMAS dissection, or deep plane dissection. These operations are all designed to improve control of facial and cervical tightening while reducing the tension on the skin closure. Once the dissection of the facial tissues is completed and all planes are mobilized optimally, the SMAS and platysma are placed under tension and secured to create the desired facial appearance. The skin flaps are then redraped posteriorly, the patient is examined for symmetry, and a skin resection is performed. Hemostasis is obtained through judicious use of bipolar electrocautery. The wounds are closed in layers and a pressure dressing is applied. Drains are typically used in the face and neck.[70–74]

Postoperatively, the patient is evaluated in the recovery room for any evidence of a hematoma or facial nerve injury. It is crucial to identify a hematoma early to avoid overlying skin necrosis. Facial nerve injuries occur in only 2% to 3% of cases. On the first postoperative day, the pressure dressings and drains are removed and the patient is examined for evidence of a late hematoma, unrecognized facial nerve injury, or compromised skin flap. Patients should expect to have significant swelling and bruising for at least 2 weeks following the procedure. The final postoperative result is not realized until approximately 6 months following the procedure (Fig. 113.21).

Blepharoplasty. Eyelid surgery may be performed to correct functional or aesthetic deformities. Excessive skin and fat of the eyelids can give the patient an angry, aged, or tired look and may cause visual field obstruction. Older patients typically present with redundant skin and fine wrinkling, whereas younger patients commonly complain of persistent bags under their eyes or fine wrinkling ("crow's feet") at the lateral canthus. Treatment of each clinical entity requires a unique approach based on the diagnosis and presentation.[75] All patients being evaluated for blepharoplasty require a complete ophthalmologic examination preoperatively to evaluate visual acuity, upper eyelid ptosis, exophthalmos, lower eyelid laxity, and symptoms of "dry" eye. Meticulous attention to detail is critical for the successful outcome of blepharoplasty surgery.[66] If there is lower lid laxity preoperatively, and a standard blepharoplasty is performed, the patient may develop a lower lid ectropion postoperatively. Symptoms of dry eye can also be significantly worsened by a blepharoplasty. As a result, it is critically important to perform a comprehensive evaluation of the health of the eye prior to performing any eyelid surgery.

Once a complete evaluation has been performed and a diagnosis has been made, an operative plan can be formulated to correct the concerns of the patient. The operation can be performed under local or general anesthesia. Older patients frequently require skin excisions and removal or repositioning of orbital fat. The blepharoplasty incisions are designed preoperatively with the patient in the upright position. Local anesthesia with epinephrine is then infiltrated for pain control and hemostasis. The upper eyelid blepharoplasty then begins with an elliptical excision of upper eyelid skin and orbicularis oculi muscle. The skin excision is designed based on the amount and location of the blepharochalasis. Very rarely will a patient require removal of fat from the upper eyelids. Excessive fat resections will produce a "hollowed-out" appearance. However, occasionally there may be a substantial amount of excess orbital fat in the upper eyelids and conservative fat resection may be helpful to achieve the desired postoperative outcome. If a fat resection is to be performed, small openings are made in the orbital septum to gain access to the two compartments of periorbital fat. A conservative fat resection is then performed to avoid a postoperative hollowed-out appearance. The skin is then redraped and the wounds are closed in a single layer. If an upper lid blepharoplasty is being performed in conjunction with a brow lift, the brow lift should be performed first, so that the amount of excess upper eyelid skin can be determined after the brow has been elevated.

The traditional lower eyelid blepharoplasty begins with a subciliary incision. A 4- to 5-mm rim of orbicularis oculi is then preserved along the lower eyelid margin. The dissection is then carried deep to the orbicularis oculi muscle until the orbital septum is identified. The orbital septum is then divided to gain access to the three compartments of periorbital fat in the lower lid. Fat may be resected in cases of prominent herniation, but overresection must be avoided. A trend in blepharoplasty surgery has emphasized periorbital fat repositioning rather than resection. Simply repositioning the herniated periorbital fat over the inferior orbital rim, rather than resecting fat, can dramatically improve the appearance of the lower eyelids.[76] The approach of repositioning the orbital septum medially has proven to be very helpful in eliminating tear trough deformities. Once the periorbital fat has been resected or repositioned, the skin/muscle flap is redraped superiorly and the redundant tissue is excised. The lower eyelid wounds are closed with interrupted sutures of 6–0 silk. Ancillary procedures may also be necessary to improve the position of the lower eyelid, including a medial canthoplasty, lateral canthoplasty, lateral canthopexy, or horizontal lid shortening. If a lower lid blepharoplasty is being performed in conjunction with a rhytidectomy, the rhytidectomy should be performed first, so that the amount of excess lower eyelid skin can be determined after the facial soft tissues have been elevated.

In younger patients, the tired appearance of the lower eyelids is commonly a result of excessive or herniated periorbital fat. A lower lid blepharoplasty through a transconjunctival approach allows removal or repositioning of the periorbital fat without an external scar. The conjunctiva is divided transversely 1 mm above the sulcus to gain access to the orbital septum. The septum is divided and the periorbital fat is removed or repositioned from all three compartments. Once again, the

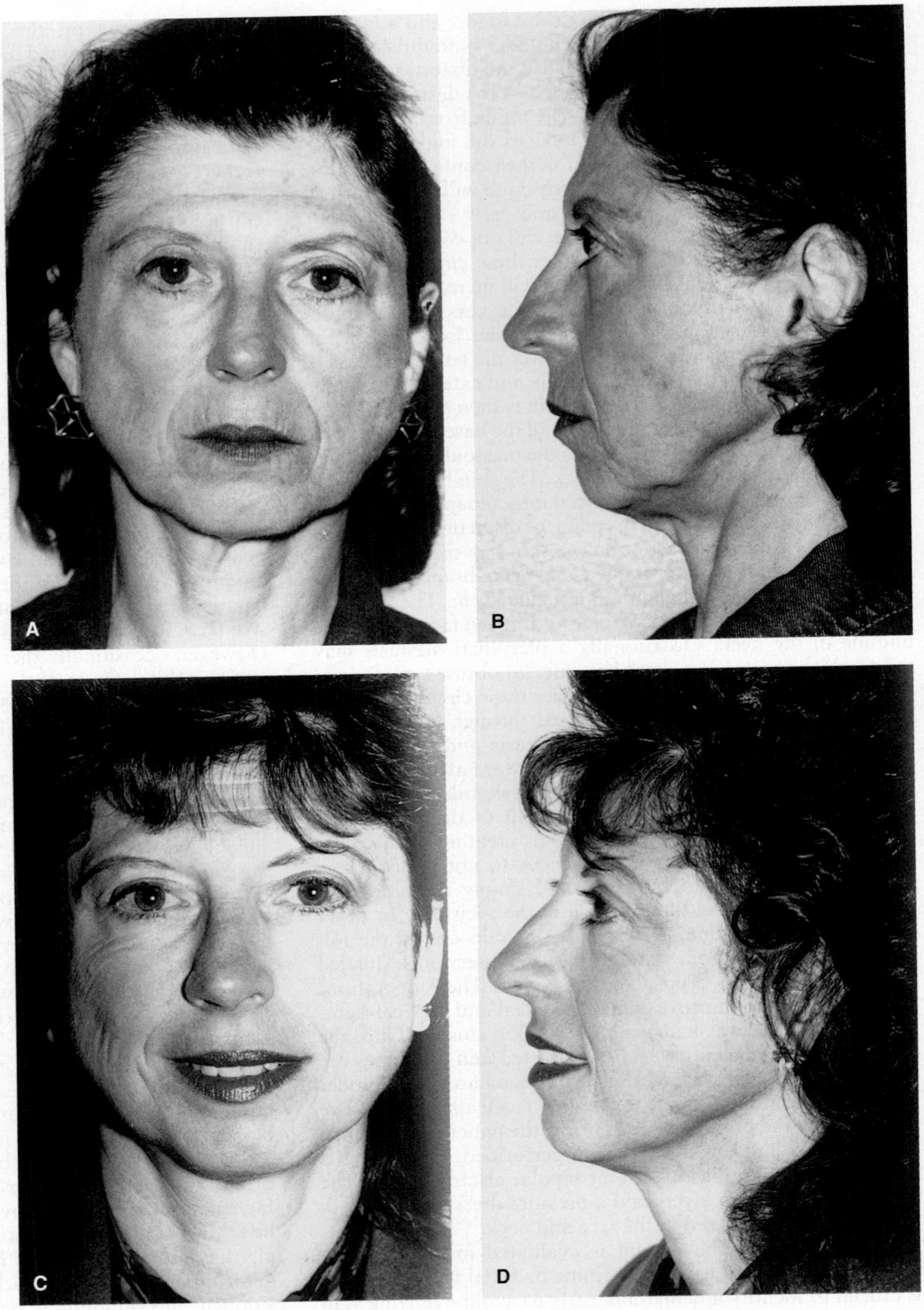

FIGURE 113.21. Cervicofacial rhytidectomy with superficial musculoaponeurotic system resection, platysma plication, submental suction-assisted lipectomy, endoscopic browlift, and bilateral subciliary lower eyelid blepharoplasty. A, B: Preoperative appearance. C, D: Postoperative appearance. Note the dramatic improvement in the appearance of her neck, flattened nasolabial folds, improved definition of the mandibular border, and improved prominence of the malar regions.

emphasis has been to preserve periorbital fat and simply reposition the orbital septum into a more optimal location obviating the need for fat resections. The transconjunctival incision is then allowed to heal by secondary intention, allowing rejuvenation of the lower lids without an external incision.

Recently, a multiplanar approach for the rejuvenation of the lower eyelids has been employed to reduce the incidence of lower eyelid ectropion postoperatively. These approaches combine both subciliary incisions for removal of excess skin and a transconjunctival incision for repositioning or resection of the periorbital fat. Clinical case series from experienced plastic surgeons have demonstrated outstanding outcomes with this approach.

Postoperatively, patients are evaluated in the recovery room for corneal abrasions, changes in visual acuity, or hematomas, which may require emergent intervention. No vigorous physical exercise is permitted during the early postoperative period. Artificial tears are used to maintain appropriate lubrication. Sutures are removed 5 to 7 days postoperatively. Patients are informed that they will be bruised and swollen for approximately 2 weeks and that it will be approximately 6 to 8 weeks before the final result will be seen.

Rhinoplasty. Rhinoplasty is an exacting operation to alter the external appearance and internal anatomy of the nose. The nose may be aesthetically unappealing or functionally impaired as a result of trauma, surgery, or a congenital deformity. Clearly, many familial and ethnic traits result in a multitude of nasal appearances. As a result, it is crucial that the patient and surgeon discuss the goals of the procedure and the likelihood of achieving

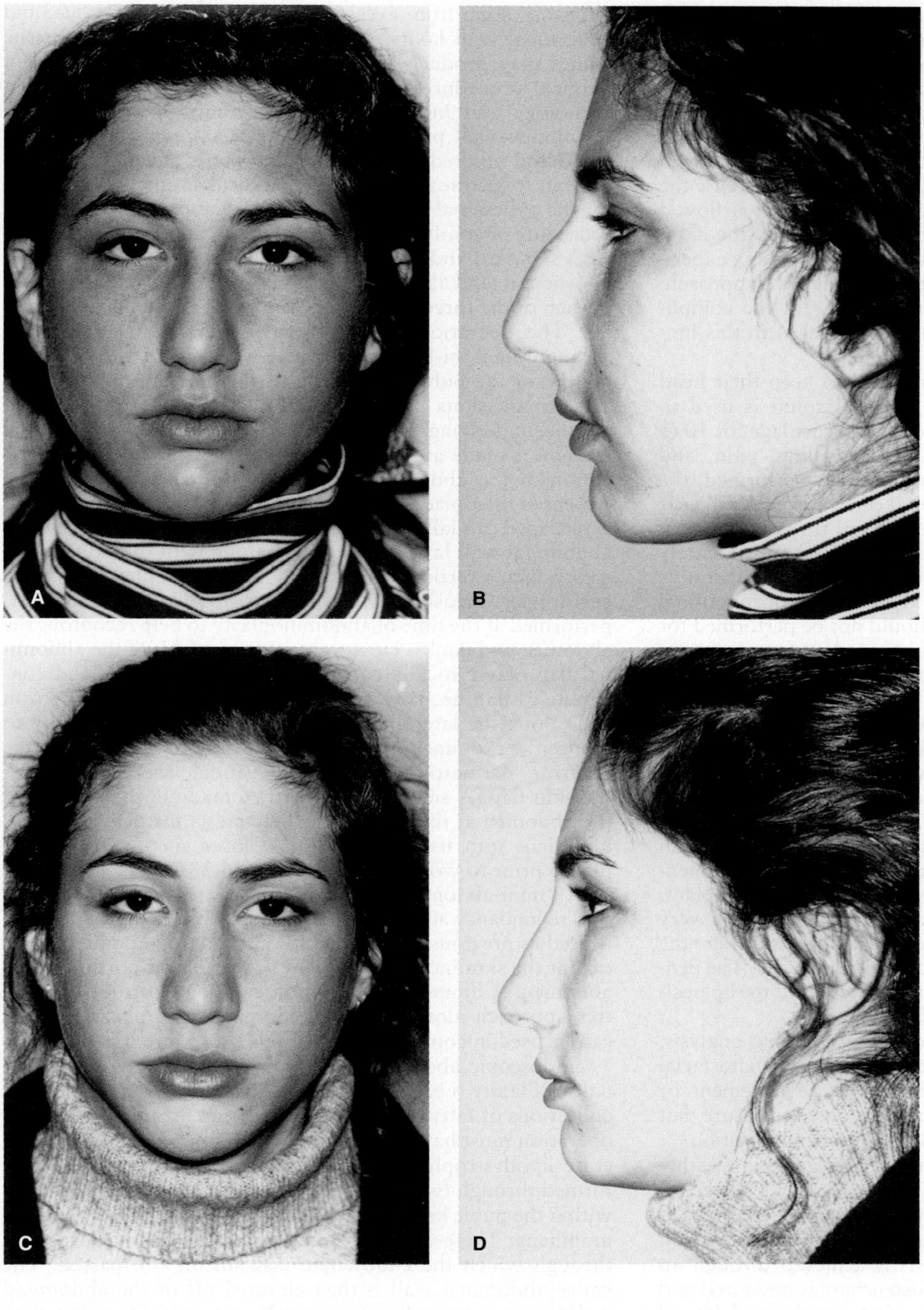

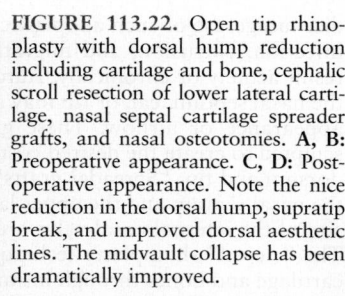

FIGURE 113.22. Open tip rhinoplasty with dorsal hump reduction including cartilage and bone, cephalic scroll resection of lower lateral cartilage, nasal septal cartilage spreader grafts, and nasal osteotomies. **A, B:** Preoperative appearance. **C, D:** Postoperative appearance. Note the nice reduction in the dorsal hump, supratip break, and improved dorsal aesthetic lines. The midvault collapse has been dramatically improved.

those goals. The patient must have realistic expectations and be prepared for the operation both physically and mentally.

To successfully achieve the goals of rhinoplasty, a complete nasal history is obtained with particular attention paid to nasal airway obstruction, allergies, trauma, and previous surgery. A photographic analysis is performed to evaluate facial and nasal dimensions. The photographs are examined with the patient, the operative plan is discussed, and the potential structural and functional outcomes are reviewed.[77]

Rhinoplasty may be performed under local or general anesthesia. The patient is prepared for surgery by intranasal injections of vasoconstrictors containing lidocaine and epinephrine. Topical vasoconstrictors are applied to the nasal lining and septum. The operation can be performed in an "open" or "closed" fashion. The open technique requires a transcolumellar incision extended intranasally to allow exposure of the cartilage and bones of the nose. Direct visualization of the structure of the nose allows greater precision in cartilaginous sculpting, grafting, and nasal bone repositioning. The paired lower lateral cartilages create the shape and provide the support for the nasal tip. Any deformity involving the nasal tip requires manipulations of this cartilage, including resections for a bulbous or overprojecting tip, suturing to reposition an asymmetric nasal tip, or cartilage grafting to increase tip projection. The paired upper lateral cartilages and nasal bones define the shape of the nasal dorsum and control nasal airflow. A prominent dorsal hump may require resections of both the upper lateral cartilages and nasal bones. Osteotomies of the nasal bones may be required to narrow nasal width by disconnecting the base of the nasal bones from the maxilla (Fig. 113.22). In contrast, "saddle nose" deformities may require cartilage or bone grafting to provide dorsal augmentation. Alloplastic materials have been described for use as dorsal grafts, tip grafts, or columellar struts to increase nasal projection. However, many surgeons discourage use of such alloplastic grafts due to problems with infection, extrusion, and migration producing a suboptimal result acutely or chronically. Autogenous cartilage grafts from the nasal septum, ear, or rib may also be used to improve nasal appearance or airflow. These grafts can be harvested and sculpted to create the desired cosmetic appearance of the nasal dorsum and tip. "Spreader grafts" can also be placed between the nasal septum and the upper lateral cartilage to increase the size of the internal nasal valve area, improving nasal airflow.[78] The "closed" rhinoplasty technique allows access to the nasal cartilage and bones through intranasal incisions. Many experienced rhinoplastic surgeons prefer this less invasive approach. Unfortunately, it is difficult to perform many of the complicated cartilage grafting and suturing techniques with this limited exposure.

Postoperatively, patients are instructed to keep their head elevated and apply ice packs. An external splint is used to maintain the position of the nasal bones and cartilage for 10 to 14 days. Patients should expect nasal swelling, pain, and bruising for 2 to 3 weeks; if osteotomies are performed, the patient may also experience periorbital ecchymosis. A full year is required for complete resolution of nasal tip swelling, particularly following an open tip rhinoplasty. Approximately 10% of primary rhinoplasty patients will require an operative revision due to dissatisfaction with the cosmetic or functional outcome; the revision rhinoplasty should not be performed for at least 1 year following the original procedure to ensure that all postoperative swelling and tissue remodeling has stabilized.

Genioplasty. Genioplasties are common plastic surgical procedures to manipulate the position of the chin and thereby improve facial appearance. Based on the design of the mandibular symphysis osteotomy, the vertical height and anterior projection of the chin can be adjusted.[79] Patients with a "weak" chin may undergo an advancement genioplasty to enhance chin projection and improve the cervicomental angle. Chin augmentation may also be accomplished with an alloplastic implant, eliminating the need for an osteotomy. Patients with a very prominent chin can undergo a reduction genioplasty where the vertical height and anterior projection can be reduced. The dental occlusion is not affected by these procedures, but the lip position and neck appearance may be altered.[80]

A complete physical examination, photographic analysis, and radiographic evaluation are performed to evaluate facial harmony and determine the extent of the advancement or reduction. Dental occlusion is carefully examined to ensure that orthognathic surgery is not required to correct chin position.

Operations are typically performed under general anesthesia, but can also be performed under local anesthesia if desired. Local anesthesia containing epinephrine is injected intraorally for hemostasis and postoperative pain control. Access to the mandibular symphysis is achieved through an inferior buccal sulcus incision. The osteotomy is measured and marked based on the preoperative photographs and lateral radiographs; the mental foramen is avoided. The bony segment is mobilized and secured in its new position with plates and screws. If an alloplastic chin augmentation is to be performed, incisions can be performed in the submental region or intraorally for placement of the implant. Postoperatively, swelling and pain persist for approximately 4 to 6 weeks. During this time, the patient should perform meticulous oral hygiene and avoid foods that may traumatize the inferior buccal sulcus incision.

Cosmetic Procedures of the Trunk and Extremities (Body Sculpting)

Abdominoplasty. Abdominoplasties encompass a wide array of surgical procedures used to correct abdominal deformities resulting from excess abdominal skin, fatty tissue, and abdominal wall laxity. Abnormalities in any of these tissue planes may produce an aesthetically unappealing abdomen. Surgical procedures are designed to correct the underlying pathology and include dermatolipectomy, liposuction, and abdominal wall plication. These procedures are often combined and tailored to fit the surgical needs and desires of the patient. It is critical to define the physical anomaly responsible for the abdominal deformity so that the appropriate operative procedure or combination of procedures can be performed.[81,82]

A standard abdominoplasty combines a dermatolipectomy, liposuction, and abdominal wall plication to correct deformity in each of the three previously mentioned abdominal wall layers. The operation is performed under general anesthesia through a bikini-line incision extending from the cephalad margin of the pubic escutcheon to the iliac crests bilaterally. The skin incisions are made and the abdominal flap is elevated off the underlying abdominal wall fascia. A circumferential incision is made around the umbilicus to allow complete elevation of the abdominal flap up to the costal margin. The patient is then placed in a flexed position, the abdominal flap is redraped caudally, and the redundant skin is resected. If any abdominal wall laxity is identified along with the skin redundancy, then a vertical, midline abdominal wall plication is also performed. Occasionally, suction-assisted lipectomy (SAL) is performed at the time of abdominoplasty to help recontour the abdomen and flanks. However, aggressive SAL of the abdominal flap may critically compromise flap vascularity and contribute to flap necrosis. Occasionally, it is helpful to perform SAL along the lateral and posterior iliac crests bilaterally to reduce the prominence that may have developed following the anterior dermatolipectomy and caudal repositioning of the skin flap. A small incision is then made in the midline of the abdomen at the level of the iliac crests for delivery of the umbilicus into its new position. Closed-suction drains are placed prior to wound closure (Fig. 113.23).

A "mini-abdominoplasty" is used to treat mild abdominal skin redundancy and abdominal wall laxity. The same approach is used as previously described for a standard abdominoplasty except the skin incision is limited to the central portion of the abdomen. A limited skin resection can be performed through this approach along with an abdominal wall plication. SAL can be used in combination with this procedure if necessary.

Endoscopic abdominoplasty can be used to treat abdominal wall laxity (i.e., postpartum rectus diastasis) and localized collections of fatty tissue. Patients who are candidates for this operation must have good skin quality and only mild to moderate lipodystrophy. The endoscopic abdominoplasty is performed through two incisions, a 3- to 5-cm transverse incision within the pubic hair and a circumferential incision around the umbilicus. These incisions function as the two access ports through which the endoscopic instruments are passed. The entire abdominal wall is then elevated off of the abdominal wall fascia under endoscopic visualization with electrocautery. The midline of the abdominal wall is plicated from pubis to xiphoid. The abdominal wall is then recontoured with SAL, which is performed through the two access ports.[65]

Liposuction. Liposuction is a surgical procedure designed to resect collections of fat from isolated anatomic regions. Liposuction is not a form of weight loss and is not indicated in obese patients. Liposuction is ideally suited to patients who are within 20% to 30% of their ideal body weight and have localized collections of fat that are refractory to dietary modifications and exercise. A complete evaluation of skin elasticity is very important in patients considering liposuction because once fat is surgically removed, the skin must be able to contract down to the contour of the remaining subcutaneous tissue. If the skin quality is poor, then wrinkling, dimpling, or skin ptosis may severely compromise the aesthetic result.[81–83]

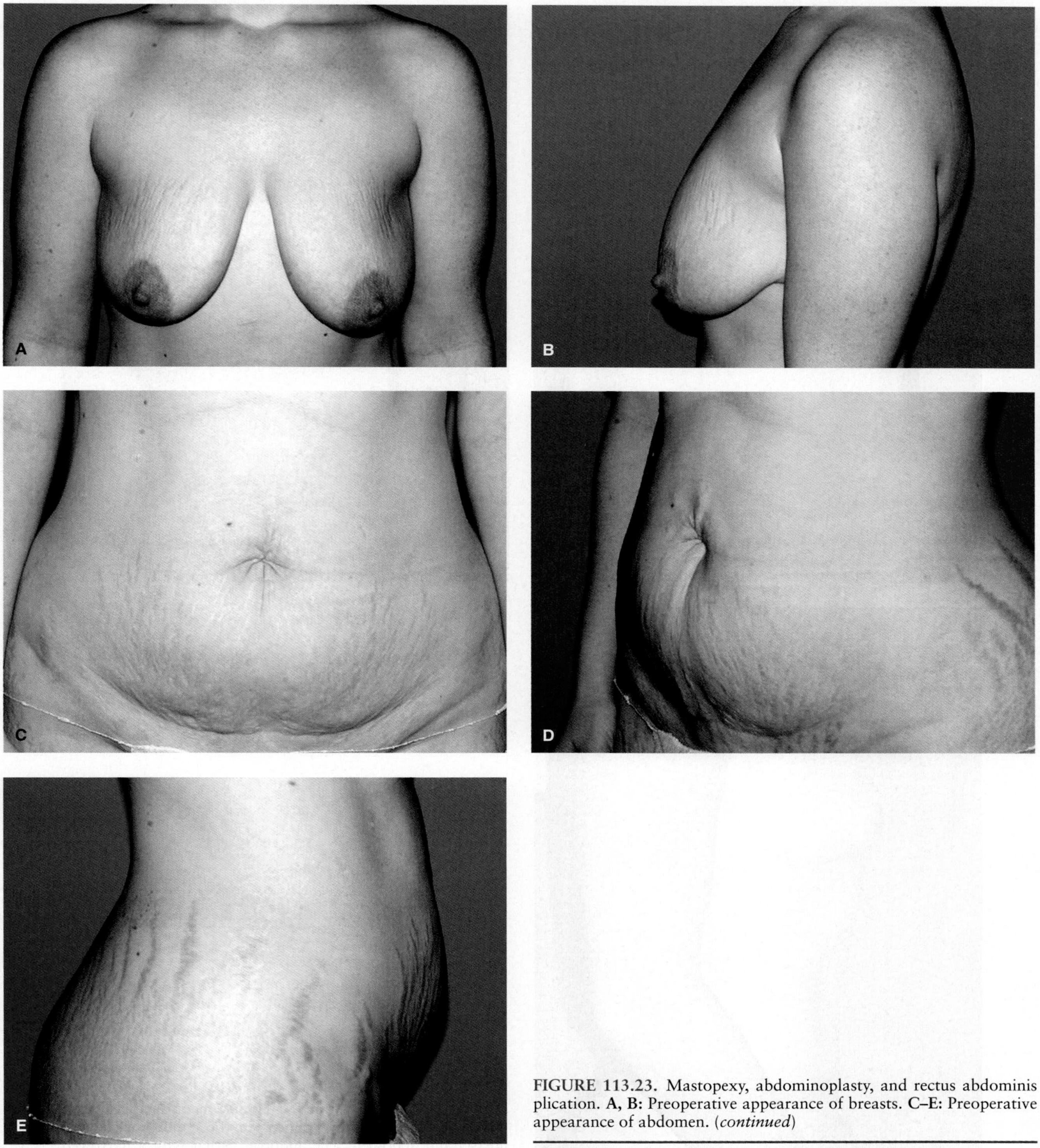

FIGURE 113.23. Mastopexy, abdominoplasty, and rectus abdominis plication. **A, B:** Preoperative appearance of breasts. **C–E:** Preoperative appearance of abdomen. (*continued*)

Two forms of liposuction are currently used: SAL and ultrasonic-assisted liposuction (UAL). SAL is used in all areas of the body but may not be as effective as UAL in more fibrous anatomic regions such as the flank, upper abdomen, or male breast. Treatment of lipodystrophy in these regions is more effective with UAL alone or UAL in combination with SAL.[84,85,87] A number of technologic advances have led to new techniques for performance of liposuction or liposculpting (i.e., Lipodissolve, Endermologie, Smart-lipo). However, none of these newer devices or techniques has proven to be efficacious in rigorous clinical trials, nor have they been shown to be as effective as standard SAL or UAL.

As with all aesthetic procedures, careful patient selection is of paramount importance. All patients must undergo a complete evaluation preoperatively to ensure that their goals can be achieved by performance of liposuction. Preoperative photographic documentation is performed on all patients. Markings are then made with the patient in the upright position. Access ports (6 to 8 mm), through which the SAL or UAL is performed, are marked in concealable areas. Patients can

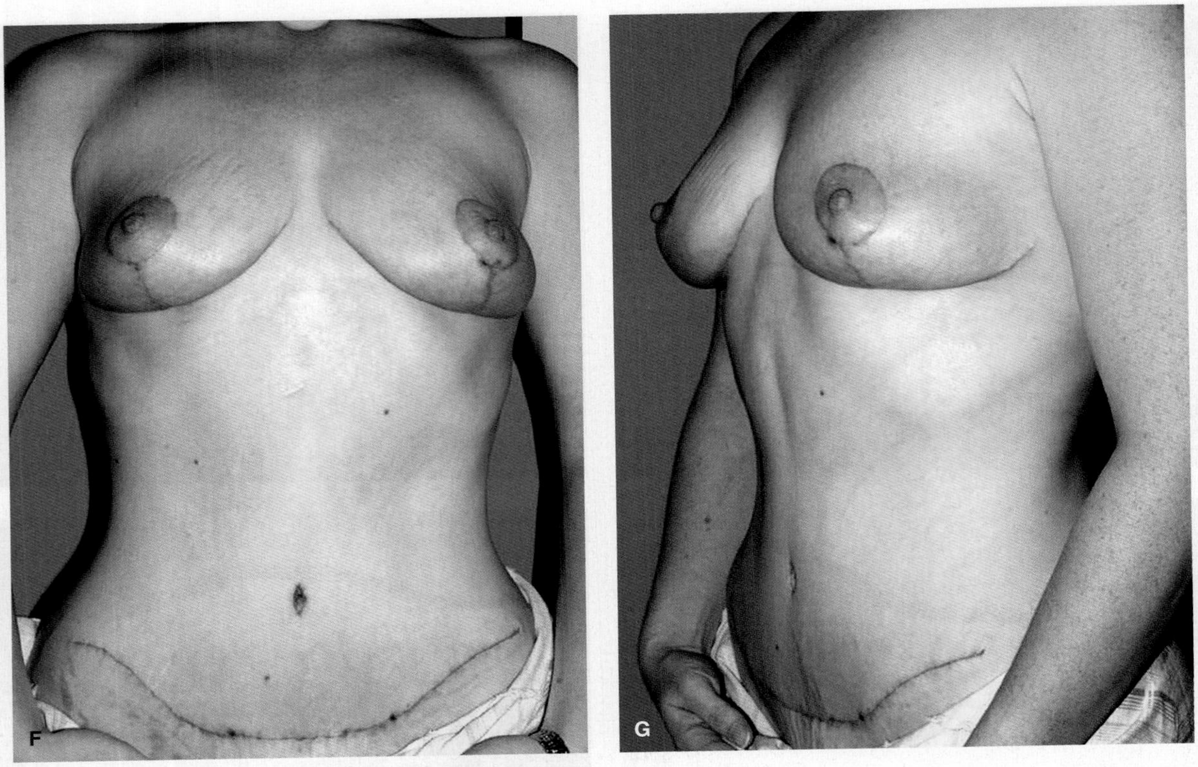

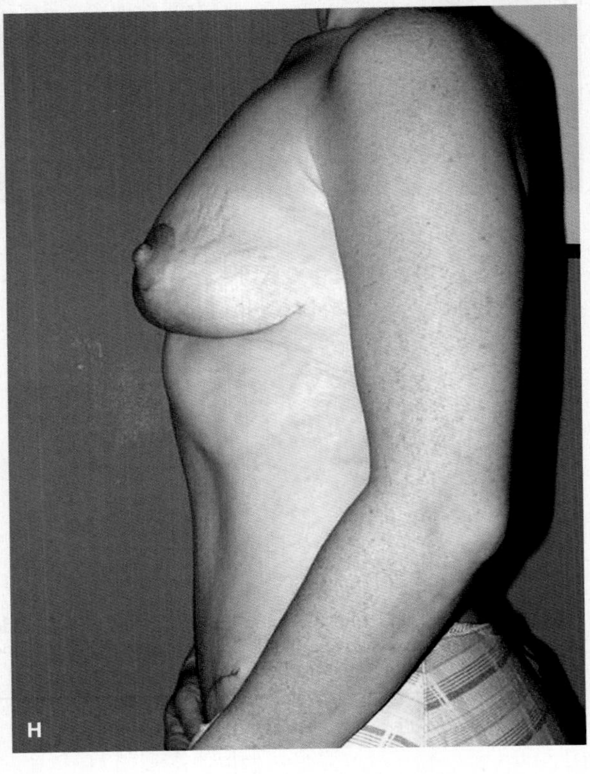

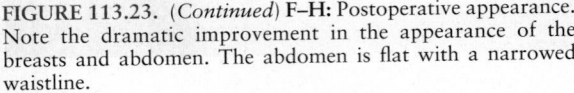

FIGURE 113.23. (*Continued*) **F–H:** Postoperative appearance. Note the dramatic improvement in the appearance of the breasts and abdomen. The abdomen is flat with a narrowed waistline.

undergo these procedures under local or general anesthesia. Tumescent fluid (1,000 mL of lactated Ringer, 50 mL of 1% lidocaine, and 1 mg of epinephrine) is then infiltrated for pain control and hemostasis.

SAL is performed with metal cannulas connected to an aspirating device that generates a negative pressure of 1 atmosphere. Various cannula configurations are used to perform the resection. Fatty tissue is aspirated into the holes of the cannula and then resected by movement of the cannula tip. The operation is performed through multiple access ports, starting with large (6- to 8-mm-diameter) cannulas and progressing to smaller (3- to 4-mm-diameter) cannulas with fewer holes to allow more precise body contouring. Overlapping patterns of resection are used to avoid contour irregularities.

UAL is a surgical technique that allows body contouring through the liquefaction and aspiration of fatty tissue. When employed alone or in combination with traditional SAL, UAL is effective for treating lipodystrophy in fibrous anatomic regions such as the flank, upper abdomen, and male breast. The UAL probe tip produces sound waves at an ultrasonic frequency of 20 to 30 kHz. The effect of these sound waves is to cavitate and liquefy to low-density lipocytes. Low-power suction is then employed to remove the resultant fluid. If UAL is used inappropriately, patients may experience severe complications, including full-thickness skin loss from thermal injury.[86]

All patients are placed in a compressive garment 24 hours per day for 6 weeks postoperatively. Early postoperative compression reduces the chances of hematoma formation. Prolonged compression reduces swelling and the potential for skin wrinkling. All patients experience some degree of ecchymosis, swelling, and decreased sensibility. The end result will not be realized for approximately 2 to 3 months following the procedure.

PEDIATRIC PLASTIC SURGERY

The specialized area of pediatric plastic surgery focuses on the reconstruction of abnormalities in children with congenital malformations and acquired deformities. Utilizing a sound knowledge of embryology as well as the changes inherent during growth and development, pediatric plastic surgeons employ a combination of innovation and technical expertise to restore both form and function to their patients. Although the manifestations of congenital malformations may be diverse, the approach to reconstruction is always based on solid fundamental surgical principles. Similarly, the management of traumatic or other acquired maladies in the pediatric population is founded on essential surgical tenets influenced by the special considerations of maturation and growth. This section concentrates on the most salient aspects of pediatric plastic surgery to give the clinician an accurate grasp of the subspecialty.

Cleft Lip and Palate

Perhaps the area of expertise that best exemplifies the specialty of pediatric plastic surgery is the management of children with cleft lip and palate deformity. The cleft lip and palate pose a variety of structural and functional deficits that must be addressed with respect to growth and development as well as psychosocial concerns of the individual patient and family. The care of these children requires exacting surgical technique in combination with the efforts of a team of allied health professionals to effect a comprehensive level of rehabilitation.

The overall incidence of cleft lip and palate deformity is approximately 1 in 750 children. This incidence is significantly higher in the Asian population, 1 in 300, and significantly lower in the black population, 1 in 2,000.[87–90] The distribution of cleft types is approximately 46% combined cleft lip and palate, 21% isolated cleft lip, and 33% isolated cleft palate.[90]

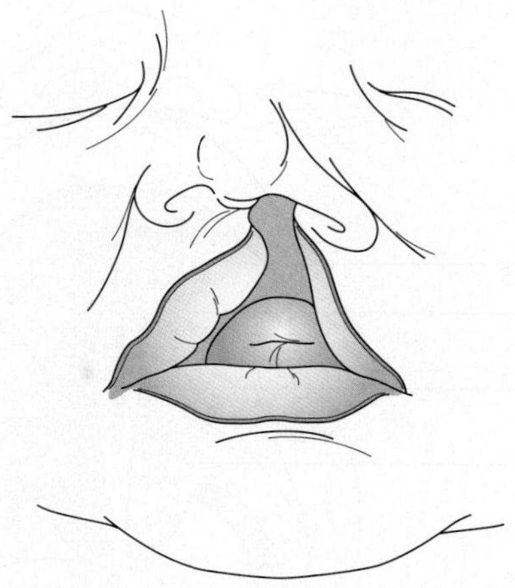

FIGURE 113.24. Left unilateral complete cleft lip. (Adapted from Jurkiewicz MJ, Krizek TJ, Mathes SJ, eds. *Plastic Surgery: Principles and Practice*, Vol 1. St. Louis, MO: Mosby; 1990:64.)

Almost 30% of children with cleft lip and palate deformity have associated birth defects that vary in scope and extent and therefore require vigilance in the physical examination.[91] The chance of having a second child with cleft lip and palate to unaffected parents is approximately 4%, as is the chance of one affected parent producing an offspring with a cleft.[91,92] Genetic counseling is usually helpful in both educating the parents and screening for other associated congenital anomalies.

11 A cleft lip deformity can be bilateral or unilateral and is considered *complete* if it extends into the nose and *incomplete* if it does not (Fig. 113.24). The cleft lip can extend into the gum partially or completely through the alveolus, creating a bony defect. The cleft lip deformity affects the nose as well as the lip, and therefore both of these structures must be addressed in the reconstruction of the deformity. Although the timing of cleft lip repair is controversial, the repair of the cleft lip is most often addressed in about the third month of life, after the child shows sufficient weight gain. This timing permits a potentially safer anesthetic administration.

There are multitudes of cleft lip repairs, but the goals of the repairs remain the same: an anatomic reconstruction with minimal scarring and normal function. In general, the skin around the cleft is cut into flaps that are brought together in a way that will give adequate length to the lip and restore the continuity of the orbicularis musculature (Fig. 113.25). Symmetry is the mainstay of reconstructive procedures to the cleft lip, allowing the normal side of a unilateral cleft to serve as a template for restoration and ensuring equal balance and proportion in a bilateral cleft repair.

The cleft palate can affect the soft palate alone or include the hard palate. A unilateral cleft of the hard palate exposes only one side of the vomer, whereas a bilateral cleft of the hard

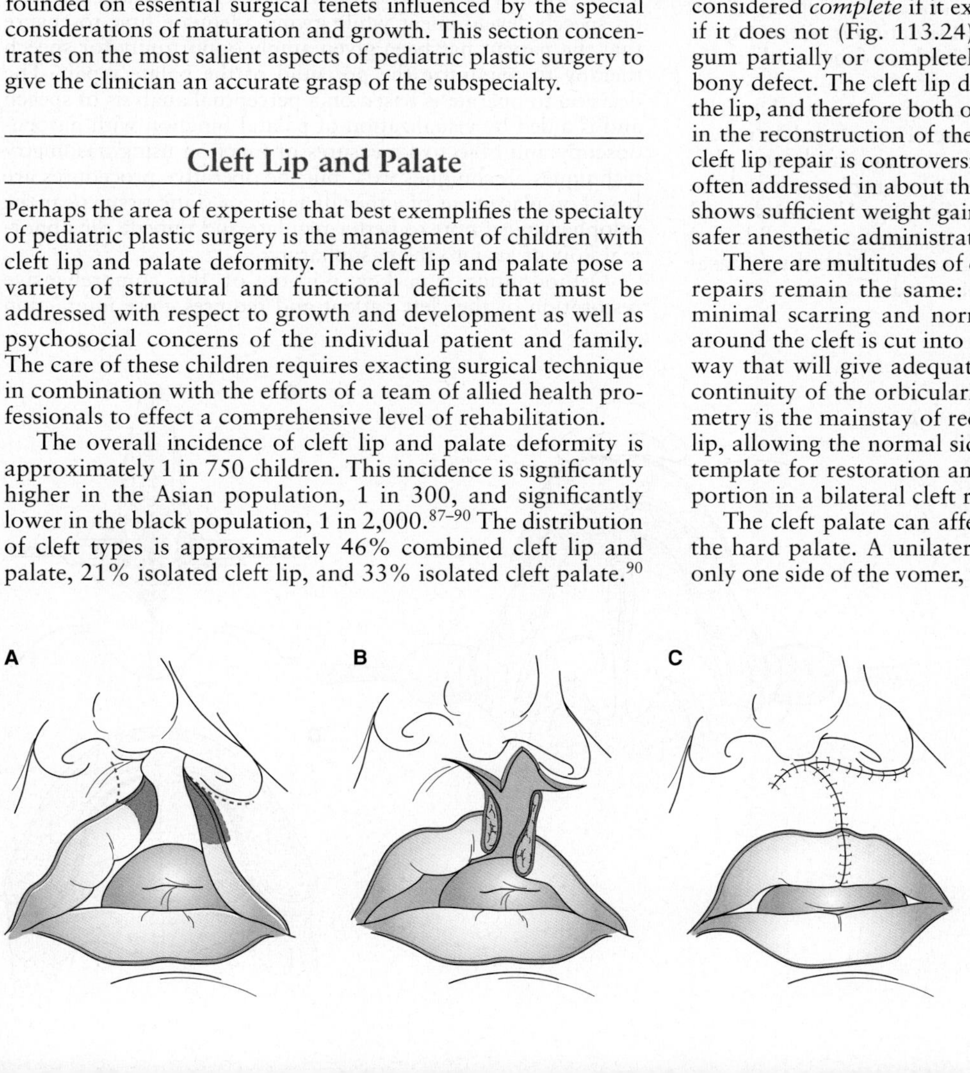

FIGURE 113.25. Millard rotation—advancement lip repair. (Adapted from Jurkiewicz MJ, Krizek TJ, Mathes SJ, et al. *Plastic Surgery: Principles and Practice,* Vol 1. St. Louis, MO: Mosby; 1990:71.)

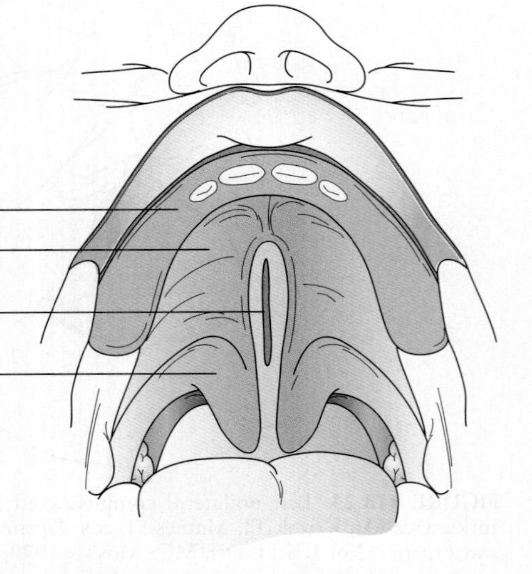

FIGURE 113.26. Cleft palate. (Adapted from Jurkiewicz MJ, Krizek TJ, Mathes SJ, et al. *Plastic Surgery: Principles and Practice*, Vol 1. St. Louis, MO: Mosby; 1990:84.)

palate exposes both sides of the vomer (Fig. 113.26). The cleft of the hard palate can be continuous with an alveolar defect from a cleft lip, resulting in an opening that runs from the most anterior portion of the lip through to the back of the uvula. In some cases, a cleft palate may have no mucosal separation at all and display only a separation or clefting of the underlying musculature. This special situation is referred to as a submucous cleft palate and may also have functional consequences for the patient.

Functionally, the hard palate acts as a structural barrier between the oropharynx and the nose. The soft palate moves superiorly and articulates with the posterior and lateral pharyngeal walls to effect a seal between the oropharynx and the nasopharynx during speech and swallowing. The coordinated activity of the soft palate prevents regurgitation of solids and liquids into the nose while eating and prevents hypernasal speech while producing strictly oral sounds.

As with cleft lip, there are a multitude of cleft palate repairs but the goals of the repairs remain the same: an anatomic reconstruction with minimal scarring and normal function. Reconstructive procedures are based on reconstituting the oral and nasal lining of the palate and reapproximating and realigning the palatal musculature. A purely soft palatal cleft may require only the separation of the layers of the palate, reapproximation of the muscles, and simple closure. The wider clefts and many of the hard palatal clefts, however, require relaxing incisions and release of the mucosa from the underlying bone. The lateral mucosa from both sides is transposed over the midline cleft and sewn closed (Fig. 113.27). Flaps derived from the vomer may be required to achieve closure without tension, a chief precept for any repair of the palate. The dissection of mucosal tissue off the bone is thought to contribute to the severe growth restriction of the midface and bony palate exhibited by many of the children with this deformity.[93,94] A delay in the procedure is thought to enhance the growth of the midface and palate, whereas early intervention is thought to improve speech. For this reason, the timing of the repair of the cleft palate is controversial; however, the cleft palate repair is most often addressed by the age of 1 year.

Speech therapy is almost always required for children with a cleft palate and is instituted as soon as the child develops the necessary language skills. "Early on" programs have arisen for preschoolers, and speech programs are often available through local school systems. Unfortunately, the palate repair alone is successful in normalizing speech in only about 80% of patients.[95] The remainder of patients will require a supplemental operation to decrease residual hypernasality and improve speech. The operations directed at salvaging speech are performed early enough to have the most beneficial effect on speech development while giving adequate time to ensure that the patient has been given ample opportunity for speech therapy to maximize the potential of the palate repair. The decision to operate is based on a perceptual analysis of speech and is aided by visualization of palatal function with nasoendoscopy and objective measures of function using nasometry techniques. Techniques vary, but the operative procedures are based on placement of either dynamic or static tissue near the velopharyngeal port to better regulate and impede the abnormal flow of air into the nasopharynx.

Orthodontics is a key portion of the comprehensive restoration of the cleft patient and requires close interaction

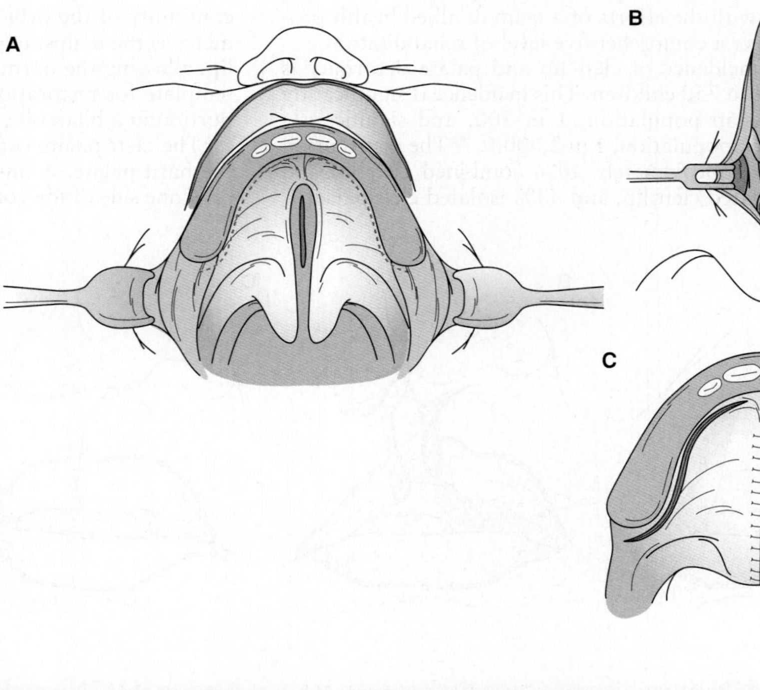

FIGURE 113.27. **A:** Von Langenbeck palatoplasty. **B:** Nasal mucosa and levator muscles approximated. **C:** Layered closure of oral mucosa and lateral relaxing incisions. (Adapted from Jurkiewicz MJ, Krizek TJ, Mathes SJ, et al. *Plastic Surgery: Principles and Practice*, Vol 1. St. Louis, MO: Mosby; 1990:91.)

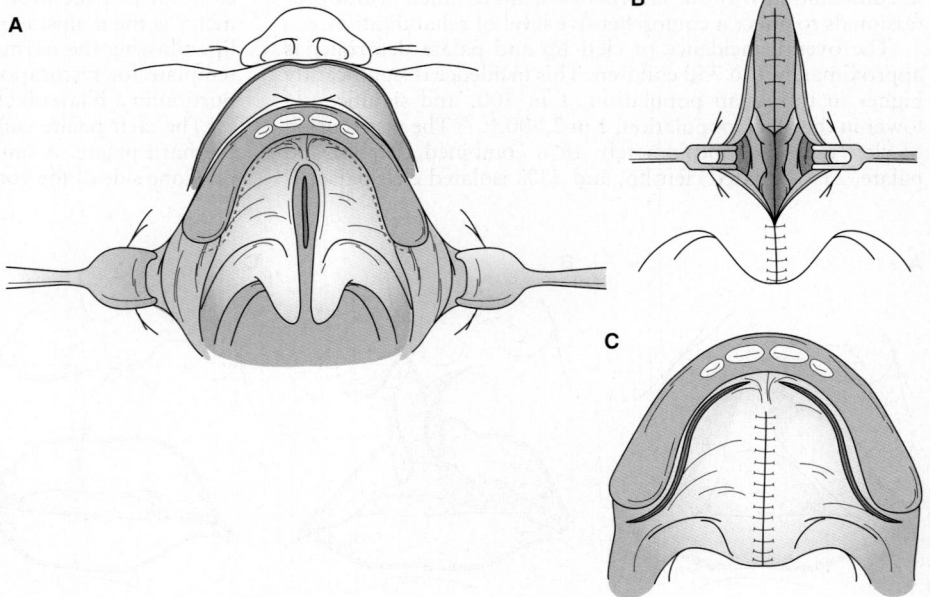

between the pediatric plastic surgeon and the orthodontist. One of the early interactions involves the repair of any residual clefting of the alveolus. Bone grafting is required for reconstruction of the alveolar cleft to restore the continuity of the upper maxillary dental arch, allow the normal emergence of the canine tooth, close the persistent oral nasal fistula, and provide structural support for the recessed nasal alar base. The orthodontist will monitor tooth eruption and may institute early-phase therapy to align the teeth in preparation for bone grafting. The timing of alveolar bone grafting is also controversial but is mandatory for normal tooth emergence. Bone grafting is often performed at about 7 to 8 years of age and entails the surgical isolation and excision of the oral nasal fistula, the reconstruction of the adjacent nasal floor and palatal roof, the placement of bone graft in the alveolar defect, and coverage anteriorly with gingival flaps. The bone grafts are most often cancellous in composition and can be taken from the iliac crest or the cranial diploe.

Many patients respond favorably to the skilled implementation of a long-term orthodontic plan, but some patients display bony hypoplasia as mentioned earlier and require orthognathic surgery of the maxilla, and possibly the mandible, to assist in establishing normal occlusion. Operations to restore a normal occlusion should await the cessation of growth so that the surgical registration of occlusion will be permanent and not require additional procedures. The most common operation to address midfacial hypoplasia and restore occlusion in the cleft patient is the Le Fort I osteotomy. The orthodontist helps the pediatric plastic surgeon to determine the best postoperative occlusion for the patient based on the orthodontic plan, and an oral surgical splint is fashioned to allow easy registration intraoperatively. The patient undergoes a horizontal osteotomy above the level of the tooth roots and across the nasomaxillary and zygomaticomaxillary buttresses below the level of the zygomatic body (Fig. 113.28). The bones of the midface are separated from the cranial base by performing a pterygomaxillary disjunction, and the floating maxilla is then repositioned into the planned occlusion by registering the teeth in the splint. The bones of the maxilla are then fixed using plates and screws. In severe malocclusion cases, the mandible may also need to be cut and reregistered into a position that results in an anatomic orthognathic bite.

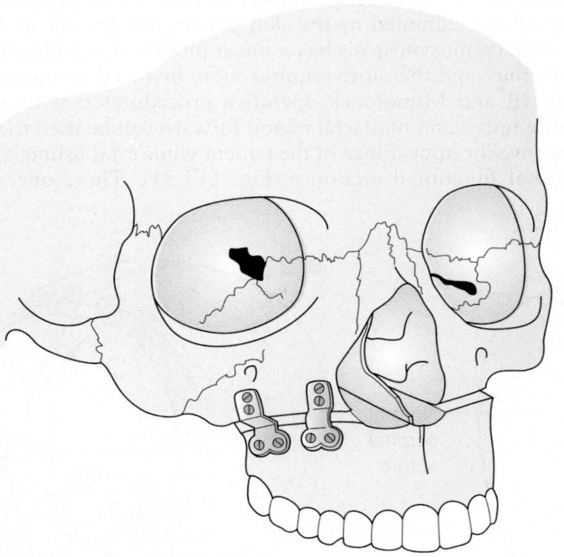

FIGURE 113.28. Le Fort I osteotomy in an advanced position. One side has been plated into position. (Adapted from Jurkiewicz MJ, Krizek TJ, Mathes SJ, et al. *Plastic Surgery: Principles and Practice*, Vol 1. St. Louis, MO: Mosby; 1990.)

The last operation to be performed on the patient with a cleft lip and nasal deformity is often the formal rhinoplasty. There is almost always a septal deviation that must be addressed in these patients and is an important part of the procedure. Each rhinoplasty is necessarily individualized, but the procedure usually entails repositioning and trimming of the nasal tip cartilages, added support to the nasal tip and slumping lower lateral cartilages to achieve projection, straightening of the septum, and finally infracturing of the widened nasal bones.

Although the care of the cleft patient requires interaction with the pediatric plastic surgeon and the cleft team throughout the patient's childhood, it should remain a small and unobtrusive part of life. The number of operations is kept to the minimum needed to attain an adequate reconstruction as deemed necessary by both the patient and the doctor. Revisional surgery is usually an important part of cleft care but should be guided by the principle that the intervention is done *for* the child and not *to* the child, with an attempt to empower the patient as often as possible.

Craniosynostosis

12 Craniosynostosis is defined as the premature fusion of one or more of the cranial sutures. The child afflicted with craniosynostosis displays abnormalities in the size and shape of the cranial vault. Virchow's law proposes that the growth of the skull will be restricted in the direction perpendicular to a synostosed suture while compensatory growth occurs in a parallel direction.[96] The ensuing skull shape of the patient provides the nomenclature of the deformity and is primarily empiric in nature (Fig. 113.29). Synostosis of the metopic suture most often results in a triangular forehead and is referred to as *trigonocephaly*. Unilateral coronal suture involvement often results in a recessed or slanted supraorbital bar and forehead and is referred to as *plagiocephaly,* whereas bilateral coronal synostosis often results in a shortened and flattened forehead referred to as *brachycephaly*. The sagittal suture is the most commonly fused suture and results in a boat- or keel-shaped head referred to as *scaphocephaly*.

The abnormal shape of a craniosynostotic skull can often be severe and progressively worsen with time as the expanding brain reinforces and emphasizes the deformity. In addition, a small percentage of patients with a single-suture synostosis, and a much larger percentage of children with multiple-suture synostoses, are at risk for the development of increased intracranial pressure.[97,98] The care of these patients, therefore, requires close interaction between a pediatric neurosurgeon and a pediatric craniofacial plastic surgeon. A thorough clinical evaluation is mandatory and an ophthalmologic evaluation to check for papilledema can be beneficial. A CT scan is also useful in these patients to confirm the diagnosis and assess the ventricular system as well as the neuroanatomy for possible associated developmental anomalies of the brain.

Once the functional aspects of craniosynostosis are evaluated and addressed, the operative strategy is then aimed at restoring normal morphology. The operation is tailored to the individual diagnosis and malformation, but the underlying surgical principles remain the same. A sinusoidal coronal incision in the scalp is used to afford access to the cranium and to hide the scar. The pediatric neurosurgeon performs a craniotomy to provide access to the cranial vault. In the case of plagiocephaly and trigonocephaly, the craniofacial pediatric plastic surgeon removes the frontal bar by performing a bilateral osteotomy at the lateral orbital rim and along the orbital roof, meeting in the midline with a cut across the region just above the glabella. The frontal bar is removed, bent and reshaped, and replaced in an advanced position as a bandeau or with interposition bone grafts placed to support the reconstruction. The bones of the forehead are similarly cut, bent and reshaped, and placed into a normal anatomic position. The bones are fixed with small

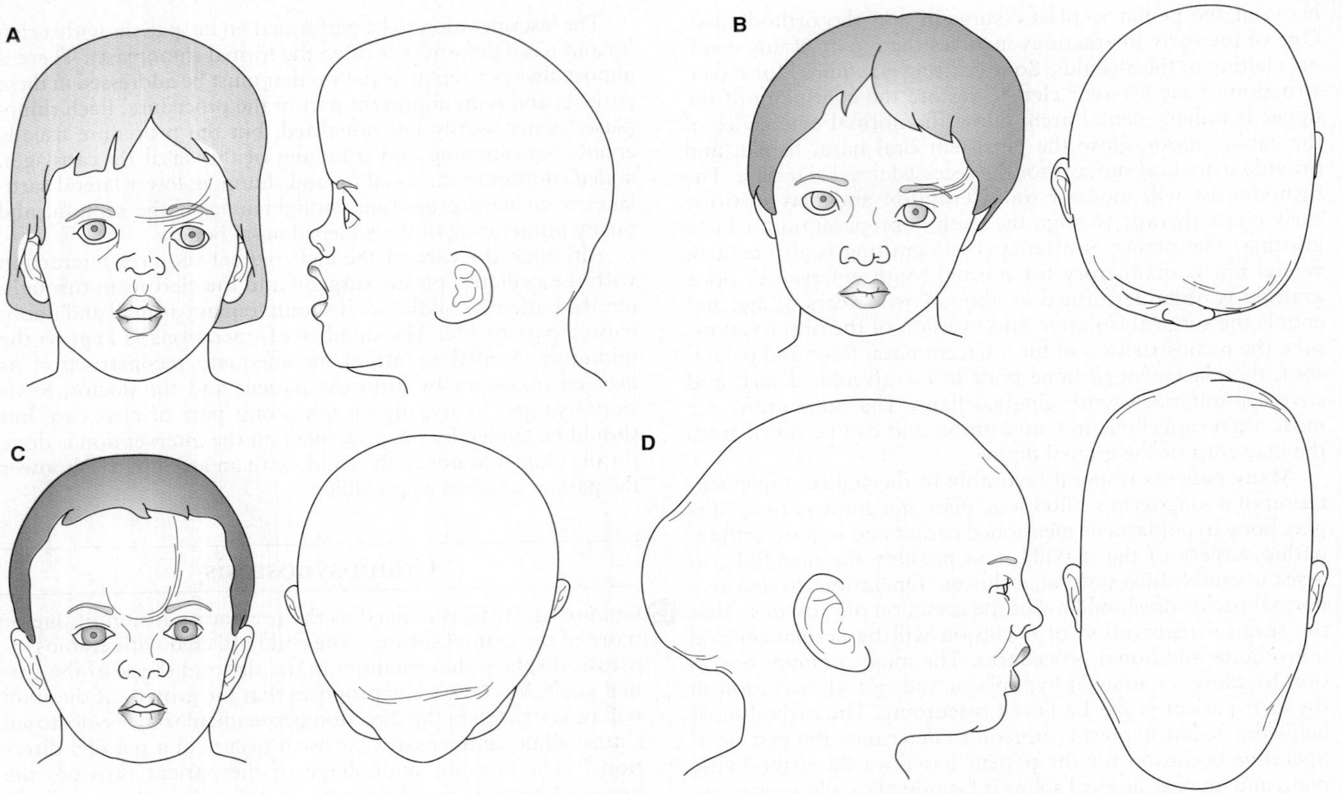

FIGURE 113.29. **A:** Turribrachycephaly (short, flat head). **B:** Plagiocephaly (slanted head). **C:** Trigonocephaly (triangular head). **D:** Scaphocephaly (keel-shaped head). (Adapted from Jurkiewicz MJ, Krizek TJ, Mathes SJ, et al. *Plastic Surgery: Principles and Practice*, Vol 1. St. Louis, MO: Mosby; 1990:119.)

metal or resorbable plates and screws (Fig. 113.30). A gap is left in the area of the coronal suture to allow growth and expansion of the brain. During infancy the dura is osteogenic and fills the gap in slowly with newly formed bone. In the case of a sagittal synostosis, the frontal bar often need not be removed; the operation entails the creation of barrel stave osteotomies in the parietal skull and outfracturing of the bone. The forehead is then back-fractured and gently posteriorly repositioned, the occipital bone is then fractured and gently anteriorly repositioned, and the bones are then fixed into position with the aid of bone grafts. During gentle repositioning the brain takes on a rounder shape filling out behind the parietal bone outfracture. This arrangement encourages subsequent growth to fill out the parietal region and secure a more anatomic shape. Other approaches to sagittal craniosynostosis include "strip craniectomy" whereby the synostosed suture and a few-centimeter margin of bone on either side are removed as a strip. Due to unpredictability of the repair, postoperative helmeting protocols are often added to coax subsequent growth and remodeling of the skull into a more normal shape.

In the case of syndromic craniosynostosis patients, such as those with Apert, Crouzon, or Pfeiffer syndrome, similar reconstructions may be required for the cranial vault. Additional operations are often needed, however, to address deformities of the orbits and midface. In contrast to the midfacial hypoplasia exhibited by the cleft patient, the patient with syndromic craniosynostosis has a much more severe and extensive deformity and therefore requires more involved operations. Le Fort III and Monoblock operative procedures that move the entire upper and midfacial region forward can be used to vastly improve the appearance of the patient while establishing a more normal functional anatomy (Fig. 113.31). These operations

FIGURE 113.30. **A:** Plagiocephalic head viewed from above. **B:** The surgeon removes the bone of the forehead and advances the forehead to allow the brain to grow and the skull to resume a normal shape. (Adapted from Sidhu SR, Zang L, Schultz KL, et al. *Craniosynostosis and Craniofacial Surgery: A Parent's Guide*. Ann Arbor, MI: University of Michigan; 1996:9.)

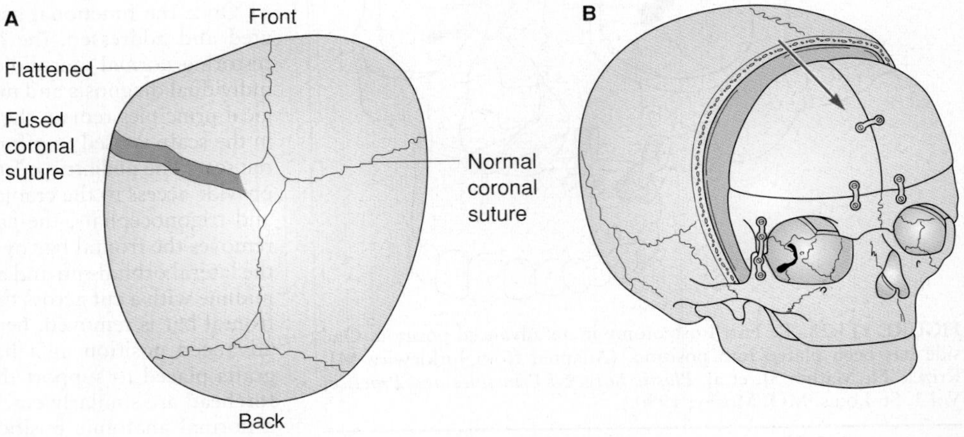

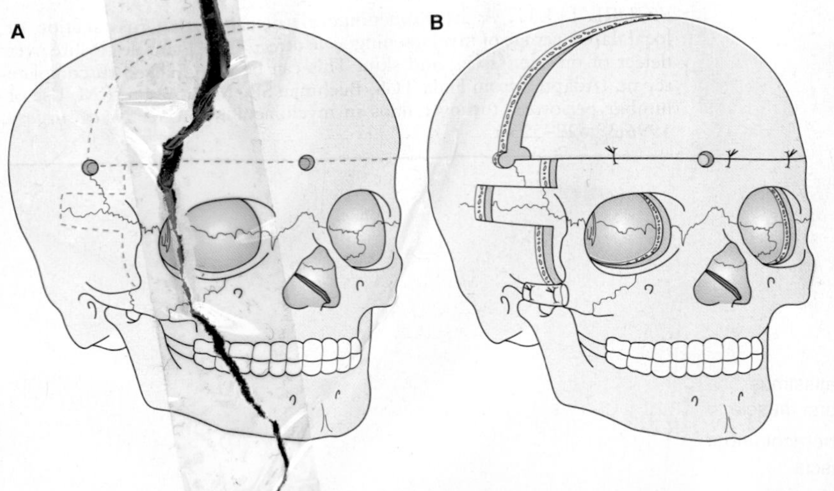

FIGURE 113.31. Monoblock frontofacial advancement. (Adapted from Jurkiewicz MJ, Krizek TJ, Mathes SJ, et al. *Plastic Surgery: Principles and Practice*, Vol 1. St. Louis, MO: Mosby; 1990:119.)

address the bulging eyes, malar hypoplasia, and recessed and diminutive nasopharyngeal airway of these patients, restoring normal eye position and opening up the breathing passages to relieve obstructions of the airway and symptoms of sleep apnea.[99]

Hemangiomas and Vascular Malformation. The pediatric plastic surgeon is often the primary caregiver for children afflicted with cutaneous hemangiomas and vascular malformations. These lesions may present at birth or in the neonatal period and require careful diagnosis and management. Hemangiomas are benign tumors that most often arise just after birth and undergo a spontaneous rapid growth phase followed by a slow involutional stage.[100,101] In general, management of hemangiomas is nonoperative; however, ulceration or interference with function may require intervention. The use of systemic or local steroids may induce an involutional regression, but operative intercession may be necessary. Surgical strategies should strive to conserve tissue and function, avoiding the creation of significant deformities that would necessitate extensive and delayed reconstruction.

Vascular malformations are usually made up of veins, lymphatic vessels, capillaries, or a combination of each. The malformations are usually present at birth and grow in proportion to the patient. There is usually neither a growth phase, as in a hemangioma, nor an involutional stage. Small capillary hemangiomas such as port-wine stains are well treated with pulse dye laser therapy, and larger, more involved lesions may be better treated with a combination of surgical intervention and laser treatment. Lymphangiomas are difficult to treat because they are diffuse and often adjacent to vital structures. Staged partial excisions can be performed if there are functional indications for intervention.

Nevi

Congenital nevi are perhaps the most common benign tumor seen by the pediatric plastic surgeon. The small- to moderate-size nevi are usually of little consequence but need to be monitored closely for any significant changes in size, shape, color, bleeding, or ulceration. The potential for malignant degeneration into a melanoma for small- to moderate-size congenital nevi is controversial. The figures reported in several studies range so widely as to make a reasonable estimation difficult.[89] Serial examination and even photographs can be helpful to document changes over time, and the "gold standard" for any doubtful skin lesion is still excisional biopsy.

Giant hairy congenital nevi are larger and rarer, but they can be quite devastating to a child and the family. These lesions can affect the entire body or vast areas, including vital structures such as the eyelids, anus, and external sexual organs. A reasoned and conservative approach to such difficult cases is mandatory. It is often helpful to enlist the aid of a dermatologist and the patient's pediatrician to assist in monitoring these lesions. Again, photographic documentation is helpful in serially assessing these lesions. Areas that show significant change warrant incisional biopsy and pathologic evaluation. The aesthetic consequences of these lesions often can be severe, and the parents often want them to be excised. The surgical approaches to benign giant hairy congenital nevi are varied and range from excision and grafting to serial excision as well as the use of tissue expansion.

The use of extensive skin grafting as a reconstructive option for the reconstruction of giant hairy congenital nevi is usually reserved for malignant or dysplastic lesions. Skin grafts are not particularly durable long term, and they are often aesthetically displeasing and require subsequent resection and reconstruction. Serial excision can be useful in limited giant hairy congenital nevi, especially in locations near tissues that stretch well. The tissues adjacent to the lesion are undermined and advanced over the nevus to determine the amount that can be resected, and then a portion of the nevus is excised and the tissues are then reapproximated and allowed to heal. After 4 to 6 months the same procedure is performed until the nevus is fully excised. Tissue expansion requires the placement of a tissue expander adjacent to the lesion with slow instillation of saline into the expander over time, allowing stretching and recruitment of new tissue near the nevus to assist in excision and closure. If the expansion is not adequate in size, it can be removed after full expansion and replaced with a larger expander to fully expand the tissue. The quality and thickness of the skin, the possibility of exposure and infection, and the cooperation of the young patient at times limit the usefulness of this technique.

Prominent Ears

Prominent ears are a deformity that is mainly in the domain of the pediatric plastic surgeon. Children with prominent ears are prone to ridicule by classmates in school, teasing by siblings, and thoughtless comments by insensitive adults. The deformity does not usually present with an enlarged ear but rather with a lack of an antihelical fold, either with or without conchal hypertrophy. The remedy is aimed specifically at the deformity. An incision is made on the posterior portion of the ear exposing the cartilage, and sutures are placed in a mattress fashion to reconstruct an antihelical fold. The stiff conchal cartilage can be shaved, and the concha is then secured to the mastoid fascia using permanent suture. A strict postoperative head-banding protocol may be used to avoid trauma to the ear and allow undisturbed healing. Successful otoplasty is one of the most rewarding procedures performed by a pediatric

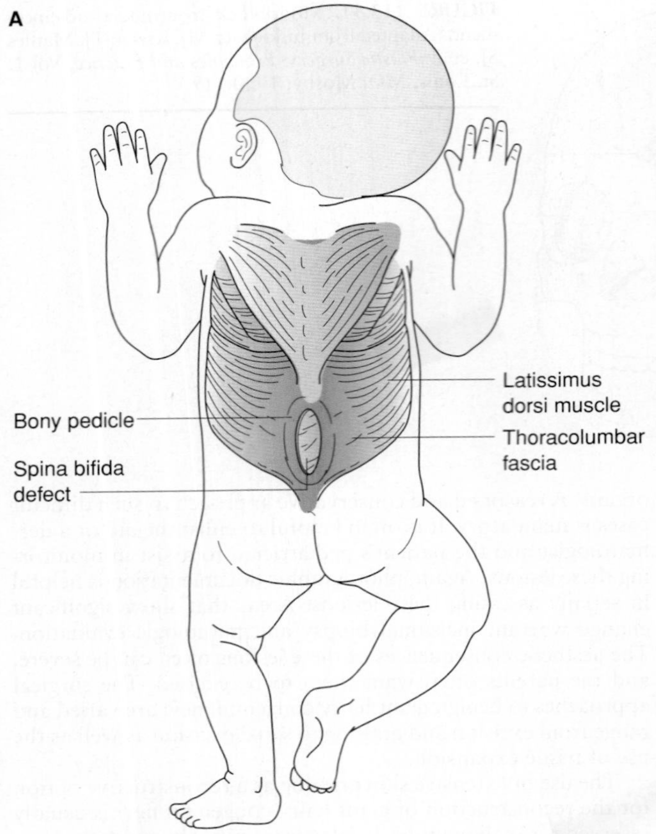

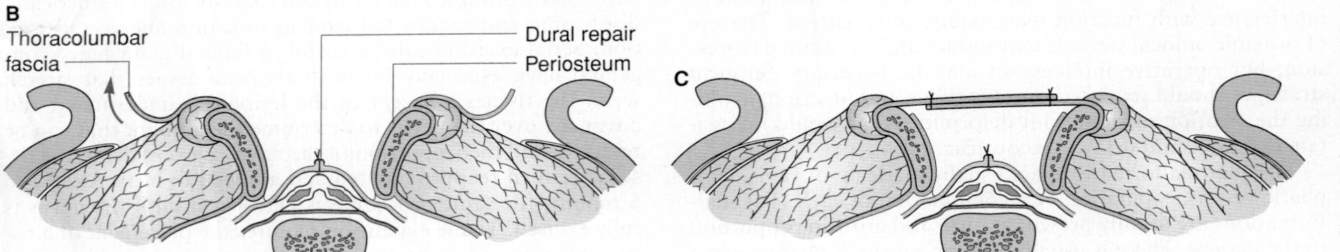

FIGURE 113.32. A: Myelomeningocele defect. B: Cross section of local flap coverage of myelomeningocele defect. C: Durable closure over defect of muscle, fascia, and skin. This can be mobilized to complete repair. (Adapted from Fiala TGS, Buchman SR, Muraszko KM. Use of lumbar periosteal turnover flaps in myelomeningocele. *Neurosurgery* 1996;39:522–525.)

plastic surgeon because the child usually wants the surgery and is rewarded with immense satisfaction.

Myelomeningocele

The interaction between the pediatric neurosurgeon and the pediatric plastic surgeon often extends beyond the realm of craniofacial surgery. A prime example of the symbiotic interaction between the two specialties is in the repair and reconstruction of the myelomeningocele, which is a form of spina bifida. The neurosurgeon is often presented with an exposed dural sac and a wide-open skin defect. The neurosurgeon may be faced with a tenuous dural closure and may need to resort to the use of a homograft to achieve an adequate dural repair. The pediatric plastic surgeon can assist by closing the defect over the dural reconstruction with stable, reliable coverage using well-vascularized tissue, protecting the neurosurgeon's repair. The soft tissue coverage may require local paraspinous muscle flaps or various fasciocutaneous flaps, but the goal of a durable reconstruction with a normal contour is paramount so as to avoid persistent long-term complications both at the level of the skin and at the level of the dural repair (Fig. 113.32).

SUMMARY

Although there are a multitude of additional procedures and topics in the specialized domain of the pediatric plastic surgeon, such as pediatric facial trauma, facial reanimation surgery, and various deformities resulting from congenital hypoplasia and hyperplasia, this chapter has focused on some of the major and more common areas of patient management. In fact, the pediatric plastic surgeon is often a chief collaborator with many of the pediatric surgical services when presented with a case of challenging wound care or any case that poses a reconstructive dilemma. Continuing innovation and technical advances combined with an appreciation for sound fundamental surgical principles allow the specialty to continue meeting that challenge.

References

1. Murray JE. Reminiscences for the "50-year retrospective" of transplantation. *Transplant Proc* 1999;34:3101–3102.
2. Brown DL, Smith DJ. Bacterial colonization/infection and the surgical management of pressure ulcers. *Ostomy Wound Manage* 1999;45:109S–118S.
3. Robson M, Heggers J. Delayed wound closure based on bacterial counts. *J Surg Oncol* 1970;2:379–384.

4. Pruitt BA Jr, McManus AT, Kim SH, et al. Burn wound infections: current status. *World J Surg* 1998;22:135–145.
5. McManus AT, Kim SH, McManus WF, et al. Comparison of quantitative microbiology and histopathology in divided burn-wound biopsy specimens. *Arch Surg* 1987;122:74–76.
6. Ladin DA. Understanding dressings. *Clin Plast Surg* 1998;25:433–441.
7. Cho CY, Lo JS. Dressing the part. *Dermatol Clin* 1998;16:25–47.
8. Lionelli GT, Lawrence WT. Wound dressings. *Surg Clin North Am* 2003; 83:617–638.
9. Fong J, Wood F, Fowler B. A silver coated dressing reduces the incidence of early burn wound cellulitis and associated costs of inpatient treatment: comparative patient care audits. *Burns* 2005;31(5):562–567.
10. Silver GM, Robertson SW, Halerz MM, et al. A silver-coated antimicrobial barrier dressing used postoperatively on meshed autografts: a dressing comparison study. *J Burn Care Res* 2007;28(5):715–719.
11. Rees RS, Robson MC, Smiell JM, et al. Becaplermin gel in the treatment of pressure ulcers: a phase II randomized, double-blind, placebo-controlled study. *Wound Repair Regen* 1999;7:141–147.
12. Piascik P. Use of Regranex gel for diabetic foot ulcers. *J Am Pharm Assoc (Wash)* 1998;38:628–630.
13. Bennett SP, Griffiths GD, Schor AM, et al. Growth factors in the treatment of diabetic foot ulcers. *Br J Surg* 2003;90(2):133–146.
14. Volk SW, Radu A, Zhang L, et al. Stromal progenitor cell therapy corrects the wound-healing defect in the ischemic rabbit ear model of chronic wound repair. *Wound Repair Regen* 2007;15(5):736–747.
15. Pham C, Greenwood J, Cleland H, et al. Bioengineered skin substitutes for the management of burns: a systematic review. *Burns* 2007;33(8): 946–957.
16. Jeng JC, Fidler PE, Sokolich JC, et al. Seven years' experience with Integra as a reconstructive tool. *J Burn Care Res* 2007;28(1):120–126.
17. Wilensky JS, Rosenthal AH, Bradford CR, et al. The use of a bovine collagen construct for reconstruction of full-thickness scalp defects in the elderly patient with cutaneous malignancy. *Ann Plast Surg* 2005;54(3): 297–301.
18. Dantzer E, Queruel P, Salinier L, et al. Dermal regeneration template for deep hand burns: clinical utility for both early grafting and reconstructive surgery. *Br J Plast Surg* 2003;56(8):764–774.
19. Hunter JE, Teot L, Horch R, et al. Evidence-based medicine: vacuum-assisted closure in wound care management. *Int Wound J* 2007;4(3): 256–269.
20. Hess CL, Howard MA, Attinger CE. A review of mechanical adjuncts in wound healing: hydrotherapy, ultrasound, negative pressure therapy, hyperbaric oxygen, and electrostimulation. *Ann Plast Surg* 2003;51: 210–218.
21. Chang N, Mathes SJ. Comparison of the effect of bacterial inoculation in musculocutaneous and random-pattern flaps. *Plast Reconstr Surg* 1982; 70:1–10.
22. Milton SH. The effects of "delay" on the survival of experimental pedicled skin flaps. *Br J Plast Surg* 1969;22:244–252.
23. Grabb WC, Myers MB, eds. *Skin Flaps*. Philadelphia, PA: Williams and Wilkins; 1975.
24. Jackson IT. *Flaps in Head and Neck Reconstruction*. St. Louis, MO: Harcourt Health Sciences Group; 1985.
25. Bakamjian VY. Total reconstruction of pharynx with medially based deltopectoral skin flap. *N Y State J Med* 1968;68:2771–2778.
26. McGregor IA, Jackson IT. The groin flap. *Br J Plast Surg* 1972;25:3–16.
27. Taylor GI, Palmer JH, The vascular territories (angiosomes) of the body: experimental study and clinical applications. *Br J Plast Surg* 1987;40: 113–141.
28. Cormack GC, Lamberty BG. A classification of fascio-cutaneous flaps according to their patterns of vascularisation. *Br J Plast Surg* 1984;37: 80–87.
29. Mathes SJ, Nahai F. Classification of the vascular anatomy of muscles: experimental and clinical correlation. *Plast Reconstr Surg* 1981;67: 177–187.
30. Hartrampf CR, Scheflan M, Black PW. Breast reconstruction with a transverse abdominal island flap. *Plast Reconstr Surg* 1982;69:216–225.
31. Blondeel P, Morris S, Hallock G, et al., eds. *Perforator Flaps: Anatomy, Technique, and Clinical Applications*. St. Louis, MO: Quality Medical Publishers; 2006.
32. Daniel RK, Taylor GI. Distant transfer of an island flap by microvascular anastomoses. A clinical technique. *Plast Reconstr Surg* 1973;52:111–117.
33. Khouri RK, Cooley BC, Kunselman AR, et al. A prospective study of microvascular free-flap surgery and outcome. *Plast Reconstr Surg* 1998; 102:711–721.
34. Kuzon WM Jr, Jejurikar S, Wilkins EG, et al. Double free-flap reconstruction of massive defects involving the lip, chin, and mandible. *Microsurgery* 1998;18:372–378.
35. Valentini V, Cassoni A, Marianetti TM, et al. Anterolateral thigh flap for the reconstruction of head and neck defects: alternative or replacement of the radial forearm flap? *J Craniofac Surg* 2008;19(4):1148–1153.
36. Granzow JW, Levine JL, Chiu ES, et al. Breast reconstruction with the deep inferior epigastric perforator flap: history and an update on current technique. *J Plast Reconstr Aesthet Surg* 2006;59(6):571–579.
37. Argenta LC. Reconstruction of the breast by tissue expansion. *Clin Plast Surg* 1984;11:257–264.
38. Wilkins EG. *Donor Site Morbidity in TRAM Breast Reconstruction*. Presented at the Annual Meeting of the American Society of Plastic Surgeons; October 1999, New Orleans.
39. Kroll SS, Baldwin B. A comparison of outcomes using three different methods of breast reconstruction. *Plast Reconstr Surg* 1992;90:455–462.
40. Grotting JC, Urist MM, Maddox WA, et al. Conventional TRAM flap versus free microsurgical TRAM flap for immediate breast reconstruction. *Plast Reconstr Surg* 1989;83:828–844.
41. Allen RJ, Treece P. Deep inferior epigastric perforator flap for breast reconstruction. *Ann Plast Surg* 1994;32:32–38.
42. Allen RJ, Tucker C. Superior gluteal artery perforator free flap for breast reconstruction. *Plast Reconstr Surg* 1995;95:1207–1212.
43. Blondeel PN. The sensate free superior gluteal perforator (S-GAP) flap: a valuable alternative in autologous breast reconstruction. *Br J Plast Surg* 1999;52:185–193.
44. Alderman AK, Wilkins EG, Kim HM, et al. Complications in postmastectomy breast reconstruction: two-year results of the Michigan Breast Reconstruction Outcome Study. *Plast Reconstr Surg* 2002;109:2265–2274.
45. Mandrekas AD, Zambacos GJ, Anastasopoulos A, et al. Reduction mammaplasty with the inferior pedicle technique: early and late complications in 371 patients. *Br J Plast Surg* 1996;49:442–446.
46. Wallace WH, Thompson WOB, Smith RA, et al. Reduction mammaplasty with the inferior pedicle technique. *Ann Plast Surg* 1998;40:235–240.
47. Hester TR Jr, Bostwick J, Miller L, et al. Breast reduction utilizing the maximally vascularized central breast pedicle. *Plast Reconstr Surg* 1985; 76:890–900.
48. Wise RJ. Preliminary report on a method of planning the mammaplasty. *Plast Reconstr Surg* 1956;17:367–375.
49. Lejour M. Vertical mammaplasty and liposuction of the breast. *Plast Reconstr Surg* 1994;94:100–114.
50. Hammond DC. Short scar periareolar inferior pedicle (SPAIR) mammaplasty. *Plast Reconstr Surg* 1999;103:890–901.
51. Mizgala CL, MacKenzie KM. Breast reduction outcome study. *Ann Plast Surg* 2000;44:125–134.
52. Behmand RA, Tang DH, Smith DJ Jr. Outcomes in breast reduction surgery. *Ann Plast Surg* 2000;45:575–580.
53. Gruber RP, Kahn RA, Lash H, et al. Breast reconstruction following mastectomy: a comparison of submuscular and subcutaneous techniques. *Plast Reconstr Surg* 1981;67:312–317.
54. Handel N, Silverstein MJ, Gamagami P, et al. Factors affecting mammographic visualization of the breast after augmentation mammaplasty. *JAMA* 1992;268:1913–1917.
55. Maxwell GP, Falcone PA. Eighty-four consecutive breast reconstructions using a textured silicone tissue expander. *Plast Reconstr Surg* 1992;89: 1022–1036.
56. Gutowski KA, Mesna GT, Cunningham BL. Saline-filled breast implants: a plastic surgery educational foundation multicenter outcome study. *Plast Reconstr Surg* 1997;100:1019–1027.
57. Janowsky EC, Kupper LL, Hulka BS. Meta-analysis of the relation between silicone breast implants and the risk of connective-tissue diseases. *N Engl J Med* 2000;342:781–790.
58. Komatsu A, Tamai S. Successful replantation of a completely cut-off thumb. Case report. *Plast Reconstr Surg* 1968;42:374–377.
59. Chung KC, Wei FC. An outcome study of thumb reconstruction using microvascular toe transfer. *J Hand Surg Am* 2000;25:651–658.
60. Partington MT, Lineaweaver WC, O'Hara M, et al. Unrecognized injuries in patients referred for emergency microsurgery. *J Trauma* 1993;34:238–241.
61. Godina M. Early microsurgical reconstruction of complex trauma of the extremities. *Plast Reconstr Surg* 1986;78:285–292.
62. Weinzweig N, Sharzer LA, Starker I. Replantation and revascularization at the transmetacarpal level: long-term functional results. *J Hand Surg Am* 1996;21:877–883.
63. Chung KC, Pushman A. Current concepts in the management of the rheumatoid hand. *J Hand Surg*; In press.
64. Chung KC, Kowalski CP, Kim HM, et al. Patient outcomes following Swanson Silastic metacarpophalangeal arthroplasty in the rheumatoid hand: systematic overview. *J Rheumatol* 2000;27:1395–1402.
65. Bostwick J, Eaves F, Nahai F, eds. *Endoscopic Plastic Surgery*. St. Louis, MO: Quality Medical Publishers; 1995.
66. Romo T III, Sclafani AP, Yung RT. Endoscopic foreheadplasty: temporary vs. permanent fixation. *Aesthetic Plast Surg* 1999;23:388–394.
67. Furnas D. Facial aesthetic surgery: art, anatomy, anthropometrics, and imaging. *Clin Plast Surg* 1987;14:579–788.
68. Antell D, Taczanowski E. How environment and lifestyle choices influence the aging process. *Ann Plast Surg* 1999;43:585–588.
69. Ramirez O, Pozner J. Subperiosteal endoscopic techniques in secondary rhytidectomy. *Aesthetic Surg* 1997;17:22.
70. Barton FE Jr. Rhytidectomy and the nasolabial fold. *Plast Reconstr Surg* 1992;90:601–607.
71. Pitanguy I. Facial cosmetic surgery: a 30 year perspective. *Plast Reconstr Surg* 2000;105:1517–1527.
72. Owsley J. Face lifting: problems, solutions, and an outcome study. *Plast Reconstr Surg* 2000;105:302–315.
73. Rees T. In search of the perfect facelift: a personal odyssey. *Aesthetic Surg* 1997;17:29.
74. Menick F, ed. Aesthetic surgery of the face. *Clin Plast Surg* 1997;24:2.
75. Smith B, ed. *Ophthalmic Plastic and Reconstructive Surgery*. St. Louis, MO: Mosby-Year-Book; 1987.
76. Goldberg R. Transconjunctival orbital fat repositioning: transposition of orbital fat pedicles into a subperiosteal pocket. *Plast Reconstr Surg* 2000; 105:743–751.

77. Constantian MB. Four common anatomic variations that predispose to unfavorable rhinoplasty results: a study based on 150 consecutive secondary rhinoplasties. *Plast Reconstr Surg* 2000;105:316–333.
78. Godley FA, Nemeroff RF, Josephson JS. Current trends in rhinoplasty and the nasal airway. *Med Clin North Am* 1993;77:643–656.
79. Zide BM, Pfeifer TM, Longaker MT. Chin surgery: I. Augmentation–the allures and the alerts. *Plast Reconstr Surg* 1999;104:1843–1862.
80. Guyuron B, Kadi JS. Problems following genioplasty: diagnosis and treatment. *Clin Plast Surg* 1997;24:507–514.
81. Pitanguy I. Evaluation of body contouring surgery today: a 30-year perspective. *Plast Reconstr Surg* 2000;105:1499–1516.
82. Matarasso A, Swift RW, Rankin M. Abdominoplasty and abdominal contour surgery: a nation plastic surgery survey. *Plast Reconstr Surg* 2006; 117(6):1797–1808.
83. Rohrich RJ, Gosman AA, Conrad MH, et al. Simplifying circumferential body contouring: the central body lift evolution. *Plast Reconstr Surg* 2006;118(2):525–535, discussion 536–538.
84. Zocchi M. Ultrasonic liposculpturing. *Aesthetic Plast Surg* 1992;16: 287–298.
85. Zocchi ML. Ultrasonic assisted lipoplasty. Technical refinements and clinical evaluations. *Clin Plast Surg* 1996;23:575–598.
86. Troilius C. Ultrasound-assisted lipoplasty: is it really safe? *Aesthetic Plast Surg* 1999;23:307–311.
87. Fogh-Andersen P. *Inheritance of Harelip and Cleft Palate*. Copenhagen, Denmark: Arnold Busck; 1942.
88. Millicovsky G, Johnston MC. Maternal hypoxia greatly reduces the incidence of phenytoin-induced cleft lip and palate in A/J mice. *Science* 1981;212:671.
89. Neel JV. A study of major congenital defects in Japanese. *Am J Hum Genet* 1958;10:398–445.
90. Sando WC, Jurkiewicz MJ. Cleft lip. In: Jurkiewicz MJ, Krizek TJ, Mathes SJ, et al., eds. *Plastic Surgery: Principles in Practice*. St. Louis, MO: Mosby-Year Book; 1990.
91. Gosman. Cleft lip and palate. Part 1: embryology, anatomy, epidemiology, and clinical outcomes. *Selected Readings Plast Surg* 2007;10:16.
92. Cohen MM Jr. Syndromes with cleft lip and cleft palate. *Cleft Palate J* 1978;15:306.
93. Gosman. Cleft lip and palate. Part 2: surgical management. *Selected Readings Plast Surg* 2007;10:16.
94. Shinbashi T, O'Hata N, Hayashi Y, et al. Changes in bone remodeling after palatal surgery. *Ann Plast Surg* 1985;14:267.
95. Morris HL. Velopharyngeal competence and primary cleft palate surgery 1960–1971: a critical review. *Cleft Palate J* 1973;10:621.
96. Virchow R. Uber den cretinismus nametlich in franken, und uber pathologische schadelforamen. *Ver Phys Med Cesselsch (Wurzburg)* 1891;2: 230.
97. Marchac D. Radical forehead remodeling for craniostenosis. *Plast Reconstr Surg* 1978;61:823–835.
98. Renier D, Sainte-Rose C, Marchac D, et al. Intracranial pressure in craniostenosis. *J Neurosurg* 1982;57:370.
99. Buchman SR, Muraszko K. Syndromic craniosynostosis. In: Thaller S, Bradley JP, Garr JI, eds. *Craniofacial Surgery*. New York: Informa Healthcare USA, Inc.; 2008:103–126.
100. Buchman SR, Smith DJ. Congenital vascular lesions in infancy and childhood. In: Ernst CB, Stanley JC, eds. *Current Therapy and Vascular Surgery*. St. Louis, MO: C.V. Mosby and Company; 1995.
101. Kaplan EN. The risk of malignancy in large congenital nevi. *Plast Reconstr Surg* 1974;53(4):421–423.

Note: Page numbers followed by *f* indicate figure; those followed by *t* indicate table.

O

P

Q

R